Feigin and Cherry's

Textbook of

Pediatric Infectious Diseases

Feigin and Cherry's *Textbook of* Pediatric Infectious Diseases

EIGHTH EDITION

JAMES D. CHERRY, MD, MSc
Distinguished Research Professor of Pediatrics
David Geffen School of Medicine at UCLA;
Attending Physician
Pediatric Infectious Diseases
Mattel Children's Hospital UCLA
Los Angeles, California

GAIL J. HARRISON, MD
Professor
Department of Pediatrics
Section of Infectious Diseases
Baylor College of Medicine;
Attending Physician
Infectious Diseases Service
Texas Children's Hospital
Houston, Texas

SHELDON L. KAPLAN, MD
Professor and Executive Vice-Chair
Head, Section of Infectious Diseases
Department of Pediatrics
Baylor College of Medicine;
Chief, Infectious Disease Service
Head, Department of Pediatric Medicine
Texas Children's Hospital
Houston, Texas

WILLIAM J. STEINBACH, MD
Professor of Pediatrics
Professor in Molecular Genetics and Microbiology
Chief, Pediatric Infectious Diseases
Director, Duke Pediatric Immunocompromised Host Program
Director, International Pediatric Fungal Network
Duke University School of Medicine
Durham, North Carolina

PETER J. HOTEZ, MD, PhD
Dean, National School of Tropical Medicine
Professor, Pediatrics and Molecular & Virology and Microbiology
Head, Section of Pediatric Tropical Medicine
Baylor College of Medicine;
Endowed Chair of Tropical Pediatrics
Center for Vaccine Development
Texas Children's Hospital;
Professor, Department of Biology
Baylor University
Waco, Texas;
Baker Institute Fellow in Disease and Poverty
Rice University
Houston, Texas;
Co-Editor-in-Chief, *PLoS Neglected Tropical Diseases*

ELSEVIER

ELSEVIER

1600 John F. Kennedy Blvd.
Ste 1800
Philadelphia, PA 19103-2899

FEIGIN AND CHERRY'S TEXTBOOK OF PEDIATRIC INFECTIOUS DISEASES, EIGHTH EDITION ISBN: 978-0-323-37692-1

Hookworm and tick images courtesy of Anna Grove Photography. Staphylococcus aureus image from CDC Public Health Image Library (provided by Frank DeLeo, National Institute of Allergy and Infectious Diseases). Mosquito scanning electron micrograph from DCD Public Health Imaging Library (provided by Dr. Paul Howell, CDC).

ISBN: 978-0-323-37692-1

Senior Acquisitions Editor: Kate Dimock
Senior Content Development Specialist: Jennifer Shreiner
Publishing Services Manager: Patricia Tannian
Senior Project Manager: Carrie Stetz
Design Direction: Maggie Reid

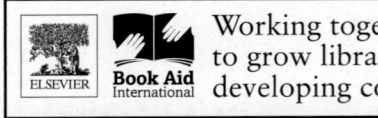

Printed in China

Last digit is the print number: 9 8 7 6 5 4 3 2 1

To my wife, Jeanne M. Cherry, who passed away on June 2, 2017
To my children, James Cherry, Jeffrey Cherry and Kass Hogan,
Susan Cherry, and Kenneth and Jennifer Cherry
To my grandchildren, Ferguson, Dennis, and Siena Rose Cherry
James Cherry

To my husband, Neil Harrison
To my children and sons-in-law, Emily Wolfe and Josh Wolfe,
Kelly Green and Daniel Green, Matthew Demmler, Amy Demmler,
Anna Rose Demmler, and Haley Harrison
To my grandchildren, Jensen Wolfe and William Green
To my brother, Loddie Naymola
Gail Harrison

To my wife, Marsha Kaplan
To my children, Lauren Kaplan, Mindy Kaplan Langland,
and son-in-law Lance Langland
To my grandchildren, Reece and Macy Langland
Sheldon Kaplan

To my wife, Sandy Steinbach
To my children, Amelia Steinbach, Aidan Steinbach, and Conner Franzen
To my parents, Charles and Kathy Steinbach
William Steinbach

To my wife, Ann Hotez
To my children, Matthew, Emily, Rachel, and Daniel Hotez
To my mother, Jean Hotez, and mother-in-law, Marcia Frifield
To the memories of my father, Ed Hotez, and father-in-law, Don Frifield
Peter Hotez

Ralph D. Feigin, MD
April 3, 1938–August 14, 2008

This eighth edition of the *Textbook of Pediatric Infectious Diseases* is dedicated to Ralph D. Feigin. As everyone in pediatrics and, in particular, pediatric infectious diseases, knows, Ralph was an extraordinary individual, and his untimely death in 2008 leaves a void that will never be filled.

Ralph Feigin was born in New York City on April 3, 1938. He graduated from Columbia College in New York City in 1958 and received his M.D. from Boston University School of Medicine in 1962. He married Judith S. Zobel, a childhood friend, in 1960 while in medical school. Ralph completed his first two years of pediatric residency at Boston City Hospital and his third year at the Massachusetts General Hospital. He then fulfilled his military service requirement at the United States Army Research Institute of Infectious Diseases, Ft. Detrick, Frederick, Maryland. While at the United States Army Research Institute, he participated in significant studies relating to circadian periodicity and susceptibility to infections, as well as other studies that resulted in eight publications for which he was the first author. After completing his service commitment, he was Chief Resident at Massachusetts General Hospital during the 1967-68 academic year.

Ralph was recruited to Washington University in St. Louis by Phil Dodge in 1968, and soon thereafter he and one of us (JDC), who was then at St. Louis University, got together and forged an academic and personal friendship that continued until the time of his death. Over 40 years ago, Ralph and Jim recognized the need for a comprehensive book on pediatric infectious diseases, but because of their busy schedules the plan was put on hold, and in 1973 Jim moved to California. In 1976, the pediatric research meetings were held in St. Louis, and at this time Jim and Ralph met with W. B. Saunders representatives, and the book was conceived. The first edition of the textbook was published 5 years later in the fall of 1981. In comparison with this 8th edition, it was a modest effort, with 44 chapters and 124 contributors.

At Washington University and St. Louis Children's Hospital, Ralph developed one of the finest infectious diseases divisions in the country. His "Feigin Rounds" were an unparalleled learning experience and were legendary among medical students and residents. In 1977, Ralph moved to Houston, Texas, to accept the challenge of being the Chair of Pediatrics for Baylor College of Medicine and the Physician-in-Chief at Texas Children's Hospital. During the ensuing 30 years, the Department grew from 43 faculty members to almost 500. One of us (SLK) came under Ralph's spell in St. Louis and moved to Houston with him. Another one of us (GJH), an intern in Houston in 1977, was waiting for Dr. Feigin when he arrived.

In Houston, Ralph served as the Chair of Pediatrics for Baylor College of Medicine and the Physician-in-Chief at Texas Children's Hospital for 31 years. For 7 years of his tenure, he also served as President and CEO of Baylor College of Medicine. In addition to his commitments in Houston, Ralph served in leadership roles on more than 100 local, regional, and national committees and professional societies. His efforts in persuading government officials of all ranks helped children in Texas, the United States, and in all parts of the world. Many consider him to have been the foremost pediatrician in the world.

Not only was Dr. Feigin a powerhouse of energy, speed, and unsurpassed accomplishments, but he also was a gentleman, full of compassion, warmth, and kindness, and a man who kept people and patients first in his heart and mind. He was a loving husband to his wife, Judy, and a proud father to his three children, Susan, Debra, and Michael; doting grandfather to his six grandchildren, Rebecca, Matthew, Sarah, Rachel, Jacob, and Eli; and a mentor to so many in the field of pediatrics and pediatric infectious diseases. Ralph Feigin is missed by everyone who knew him, particularly by Judy Feigin and the family as well as by the present editors of this eighth edition of Feigin and Cherry.

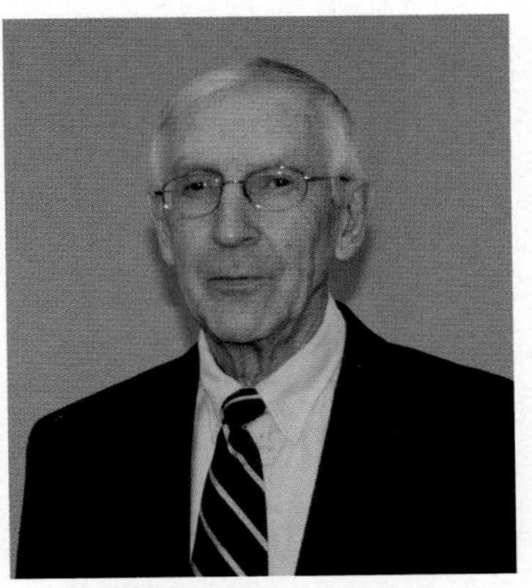

James D. Cherry, MD, MSc
Distinguished Research Professor of Pediatrics
David Geffen School of Medicine at UCLA;
Attending Physician
Pediatric Infectious Diseases
Mattel Children's Hospital UCLA
Los Angeles, California

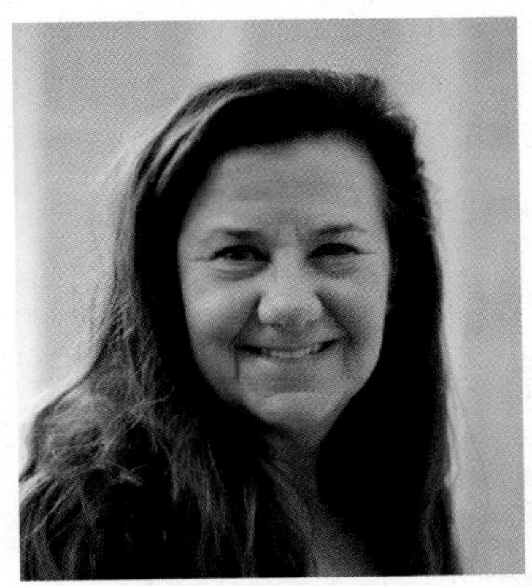

Gail J. Harrison, MD
Professor
Department of Pediatrics
Section of Infectious Diseases
Baylor College of Medicine;
Attending Physician
Infectious Diseases Service
Texas Children's Hospital
Houston, Texas

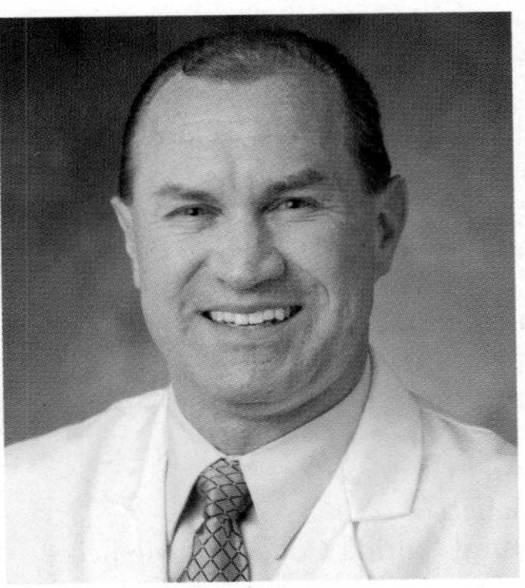

William J. Steinbach, MD
Professor of Pediatrics
Professor in Molecular Genetics and Microbiology
Chief, Pediatric Infectious Diseases
Director, Duke Pediatric Immunocompromised Host Program
Director, International Pediatric Fungal Network
Duke University School of Medicine
Durham, North Carolina

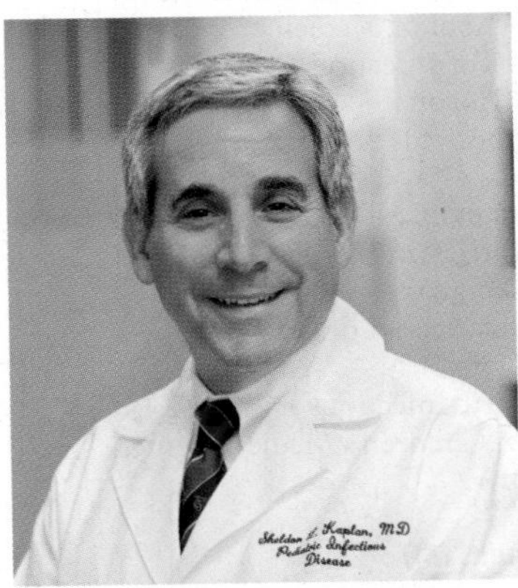

Sheldon L. Kaplan, MD
Professor and Executive Vice-Chair
Head, Section of Infectious Diseases
Department of Pediatrics
Baylor College of Medicine;
Chief, Infectious Disease Service
Head, Department of Pediatric Medicine
Texas Children's Hospital
Houston, Texas

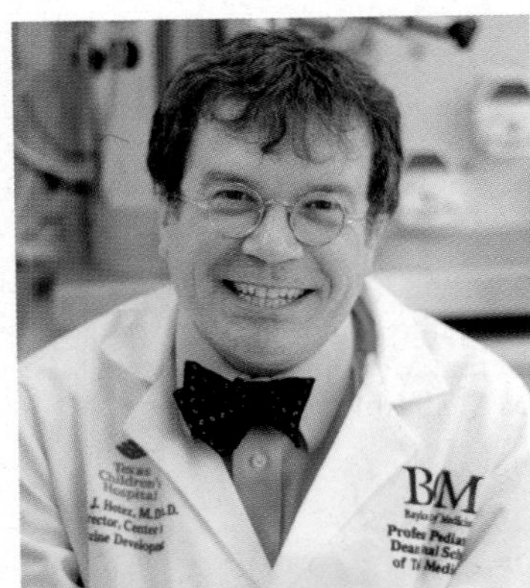

Peter J. Hotez, MD, PhD
Dean, National School of Tropical Medicine
Professor, Pediatrics and Molecular & Virology and Microbiology
Head, Section of Pediatric Tropical Medicine
Baylor College of Medicine;
Endowed Chair of Tropical Pediatrics
Center for Vaccine Development
Texas Children's Hospital;
Professor, Department of Biology
Baylor University
Waco, Texas;
Baker Institute Fellow in Disease and Poverty
Rice University
Houston, Texas;
Co-Editor-in-Chief, *PLoS Neglected Tropical Diseases*

Contributors

John Aaskov, BSc, PhD, FRCPath
World Health Organization Collaborating Centre for Arbovirus Reference and Research
Institute of Health and Biomedical Innovation
Queensland University of Technology
Brisbane, QLD, Australia

Kristina Adachi, MD, MA
Clinical Instructor
Department of Pediatrics
Division of Infectious Diseases
David Geffen School of Medicine at UCLA
Los Angeles, California

Christoph Aebi, MD
Professor of Pediatrics and Infectious Diseases
Chairman, Department of Pediatrics
University of Bern
Bern, Switzerland

Kenneth A. Alexander, MD, PhD
Chief
Division of Allergy, Immunology, Rheumatology, and Infectious Diseases
Nemours Children's Hospital;
Professor of Pediatrics
University of Central Florida College of Medicine
Orlando, Florida

Ghada N. Al-Rawahi, MD, DTM&H (London), D(ABMM), FRCPC
Medical Microbiologist
Children's and Women's Health Centre of British Columbia;
Medical Lead, Infection Prevention & Control
BC Cancer Agency;
Clinical Associate Professor
University of British Columbia
Vancouver, BC, Canada

Duha Al-Zubeidi, MD
Children's Mercy Hospital
Kansas City, Missouri

Seher Anjum, MD
Professor, Division of Infectious Disease
Department of Internal Medicine
University of Texas Medical Branch
Galveston, Texas

Monica I. Ardura, DO, MSCS
Associate Professor
Department of Pediatrics
Ohio State University;
Medical Director, Host Defense Program
Department of Pediatrics, Infectious Diseases, and Immunology
Nationwide Children's Hospital
Columbus, Ohio

Stephen S. Arnon, MD, MPH
Founder and Chief
Infant Botulism Treatment and Prevention Program
California Department of Public Health
Richmond, California

Amy Arrington, MD, PhD
Section Chief, Global Biologic Preparedness
Department of Pediatrics
Baylor College of Medicine and Texas Children's Hospital;
Assistant Professor
Department of Pediatric Critical Care Medicine
Baylor College of Medicine
Houston, Texas

Ann M. Arvin, MD
Lucile Salter Packard Professor of Pediatrics
Professor of Microbiology and Immunology
Stanford University School of Medicine
Stanford, California

Robert L. Atmar, MD
Professor
Department of Medicine
Baylor College of Medicine
Houston, Texas

Amira Baker, MD
Fellow, Pediatric Infectious Diseases
Mattel Children's Hospital
University of California–Los Angeles
Los Angeles, California

Carol J. Baker, MD
Professor
Departments of Pediatrics and Molecular Virology & Microbiology
Baylor College of Medicine
Houston, Texas

Robert S. Baltimore, MD
Professor
Departments of Pediatrics and Epidemiology
Yale University School of Medicine;
Associate Director of Infection Control
Yale-New Haven Hospital
New Haven, Connecticut

Stephen J. Barenkamp, MD
Professor of Pediatrics and Molecular Microbiology
Department of Pediatrics
St. Louis University School of Medicine;
Director
Division of Pediatric Infectious Diseases
Cardinal Glennon Children's Medical Center
St. Louis, Missouri

Elizabeth D. Barnett, MD
Attending Physician
Boston Medical Center
Boston, Massachusetts

Theresa Barton, MD
Associate Professor
Department of Pediatrics
Baylor College of Medicine
Houston, Texas

Gil Benard, MD, PhD
Medical Researcher
Departamento Dermatologia
Faculdade de Medicina;
Laboratorio de Micologia Medica
Instituto de Medicina Tropical
Universidade de São Paulo
São Paolo, Brazil

Jeffrey M. Bender, MD
Assistant Professor
Department of Pediatrics
Division of Pediatric Infectious Diseases
Children's Hospital Los Angeles;
Assistant Professor of Pediatrics and Pediatric Infectious Diseases
University of Southern California
Los Angeles, California

Gregory J. Berry, PhD, D(ABMM)
Assistant Medical Director
Division of Infectious Disease Diagnostics
Northwell Health Laboratories;
Assistant Professor of Pathology and Laboratory Medicine
Hofstra Northwell School of Medicine
Lake Success, New York

Amit Bhatt, MD
Assistant Professor
Department of Ophthalmology
Baylor College of Medicine;
Pediatric Ophthalmology Subsection
Texas Children's Hospital
Houston, Texas

Charles D. Bluestone, MD
Distinguished Professor Emeritus of Otolaryngology
University of Pittsburgh School of Medicine
Pittsburgh, Pennsylvania

Jeffrey L. Blumer, PhD, MD
Professor and Chairman
Department of Pediatrics
The University of Toledo
Toledo, Ohio

Claire Bocchini, MD, MS
Texas Children's Hospital
Houston, Texas

Kenneth M. Boyer, MD
Professor and Woman's Board Chair
Department of Pediatrics
Rush Medical College of Rush University;
Clinical Associate
Department of Pediatrics
University of Chicago
Chicago, Illinois

John S. Bradley, MD
Professor and Chief
Division of Infectious Diseases
Department of Pediatrics
University of California–San Diego School of Medicine
San Diego, California

Patricia Brasil, MD, PhD
Clinical Researcher
Instituto Nacional de Infectologia
Fundação Oswaldo Cruz
Rio de Janeiro, Brazil

William J. Britt, MD
Charles A. Alford Professor of Pediatric Infectious Diseases
Department of Pediatrics
University of Alabama
Birmingham, Alabama

David E. Bronstein, MD, MS
Department of Pediatrics
Southern California Permanente Medical Group
Palmdale, California

David A. Bruckner, ScD
Professor Emeritus
Department of Pathology & Laboratory Medicine
David Geffen School of Medicine at UCLA
Los Angeles, California

Kristina A. Bryant, MD
Professor of Pediatric Diseases
Department of Pediatrics
University of Louisville
Louisville, Kentucky

Steven C. Buckingham, MD, MA[†]
Associate Professor
Department of Pediatrics
University of Tennessee Health Science Center
Memphis, Tennessee

Carrie L. Byington, MD
Vice Chancellor, Health Services
Senior Vice President, Health Sciences Center
Jean and Thomas McMullin Professor and Dean
College of Medicine
Texas A&M University and System
Bryan, Texas

Miguel M. Cabada, MD, MSc
Assistant Professor
Department of Internal Medicine
Division of Infectious Diseases
University of Texas Medical Branch
Galveston, Texas

Adriana Cadilla, MD
Physician
Department of Pediatric Infectious Disease
Nemours Children's Hospital
Orlando, Florida

Judith R. Campbell, MD
Professor
Department of Pediatrics
Section of Infectious Diseases
Baylor College of Medicine;
Attending Physician
Infectious Disease Service
Texas Children's Hospital
Houston, Texas

Justin E. Caron, MD
Pathology Resident
Department of Pathology
University of Utah School of Medicine
Salt Lake City, Utah

[†]Deceased.

Maria Carrillo-Marquez, MD
Assistant Professor
Department of Pediatrics
University of Tennessee Health Science Center
Memphis, Tennessee

Janet R. Casey, MD
Director of Research
Legacy Pediatrics;
Clinical Associate Professor of Pediatrics
Department of Pediatrics
University of Rochester
Rochester, New York

Luis A. Castagnini, MD, MPH
Assistant Professor
Department of Pediatrics
Baylor College of Medicine/Children's Hospital of San Antonio
San Antonio, Texas

Mariam R. Chacko, MBBS
Professor
Department of Pediatrics
Section of Adolescent Medicine and Sports Medicine
Baylor College of Medicine and Texas Children's Hospital;
Medical Director, Adolescent Medicine
Baylor Teen Health Clinics
Houston, Texas

Lakshmi Chandramohan, PhD, D(ABMM)
Senior Scientist
Biopharma Division
NeoGenomics Laboratories
Houston, Texas

Louisa E. Chapman, MD, MSPH[†]
Medical Epidemiologist
Centers for Disease Control and Prevention
Atlanta, Georgia

Remi N. Charrel, MD, PhD
UMR "Emergence des Pathologies Virales"
Aix Marseille Université;
Fondation IHU Mediterranée Infection
APHM Public Hospitals of Marseille
Marseille, France

Elsa Chea-Woo, MD
Professor
Department of Pediatrics
Universidad Peruana Cayetano Heredia
Lima, Peru

Ira M. Cheifetz, MD, FCCM, FAARC
Chief Medical Officer
Children's Services
Duke Children's Hospital;
Associate Chief Medical Officer
Duke University Hospital;
Division Chief, Pediatric Critical Care Medicine
Professor, Departments of Pediatrics and Anesthesiology
Duke University Medical Center
Durham, North Carolina

Tempe K. Chen, MD
Assistant Clinical Professor
Department of Pediatrics
University of California Irvine School of Medicine
Irvine, California

James D. Cherry, MD, MSc
Distinguished Research Professor of Pediatrics
David Geffen School of Medicine at UCLA;
Attending Physician
Pediatric Infectious Diseases
Mattel Children's Hospital UCLA
Los Angeles, California

Javier Chinen, MD, PhD
Associate Professor
Pediatrics, Allergy, and Immunology
Baylor College of Medicine and Texas Children's Hospital
Houston, Texas

Natascha Ching, MD
Assistant Clinical Professor
Department of Pediatrics
John A. Burns School of Medicine at the University of Hawaii;
Physician
Department of Pediatric Infectious Diseases
Kapiolani Medical Center for Women and Children
Kapiolani Medical Specialists
Honolulu, Hawaii

Ivan K. Chinn, MD
Assistant Professor
Department of Pediatrics
Baylor College of Medicine and Texas Children's Hospital
Houston, Texas

John C. Christenson, MD
Professor of Clinical Pediatrics
Ryan White Center for Pediatric Infectious Disease and Global Health
Indiana University School of Medicine
Indianapolis, Indiana

Susan E. Coffin, MD, MPH
Professor of Pediatrics
Associate Chief
Division of Infectious Diseases
UPENN School of Medicine;
Associate Hospital Epidemiologist
Children's Hospital of Philadelphia
Philadelphia, Pennsylvania

Armando G. Correa, MD
Assistant Professor
Department of Pediatrics
Baylor College of Medicine;
Attending Physician
Texas Children's Hospital
Houston, Texas

Elaine G. Cox, MD
Professor of Clinical Pediatrics
Ryan White Center for Pediatric Infectious Disease and Global Health
Indiana University School of Medicine
Indianapolis, Indiana

[†]Deceased.

Jonathan D. Crews, MD, MS
Assistant Professor
Department of Pediatrics
Baylor College of Medicine;
Attending Physician
Pediatric Infectious Diseases
Children's Hospital of San Antonio
San Antonio, Texas

Andrea T. Cruz, MD, MPH
Assistant Professor
Department of Pediatrics
Baylor College of Medicine
Houston, Texas

Zev Davidovics, MD
Department of Pediatric Gastroenterology, Digestive Diseases, Hepatology, and Nutrition
Connecticut Children's Medical Center
Hartford, Connecticut;
Assistant Professor of Pediatrics
University of Connecticut School of Medicine
Farmington, Connecticut

Walter N. Dehority, MD, MSc
Associate Professor
Department of Pediatrics
University of New Mexico Health Sciences Center
Albuquerque, New Mexico

Xavier de Lamballerie, MD
Professor
Emergence des Pathologies Virales
Aix-Marseille Université;
IRD French Institute of Research for Development
EHESP French School of Public Health
Laboratory of Virology
IHU Mediterranée Infection
APHM Public Hospitals of Marseille
Marseille, France

Penelope H. Dennehy, MD
Director
Division of Pediatric Infectious Diseases
Hasbro Children's Hospital;
Professor and Vice Chair for Academic Affairs
Department of Pediatrics
Alpert Medical School of Brown University
Providence, Rhode Island

Minh L. Doan, MD, COL, MC, USA
Chief, Division of Pediatric Pulmonology
Brooke Army Medical Center
San Antonio, Texas

Simon R. Dobson, MD, FRCPC
Medical Director, Infection Prevention and Control
Antimicrobial Stewardship Consultant
Sidra Medical and Research Center
Qatar Foundation
Doha, Qatar

Jan E. Drutz, MD
Professor
Department of Pediatrics
Baylor College of Medicine and Texas Children's Hospital
Houston, Texas

Kara A. Dubray, MD
Clinical Instructor
Pediatric Infectious Disease
Lucile Packard Children's Hospital
Palo Alto, California

Andrea Duppenthaler, MD
Pediatric Infectious Diseases
Children's University Hospital
Bern, Switzerland

Christopher C. Dvorak, MD
Professor & Chief
Department of Pediatric Allergy, Immunology, & Bone Marrow Transplant
University of California–San Francisco Benioff Children's Hospital
San Francisco, California

Paul H. Edelstein, MD
Professor Emeritus of Pathology and Laboratory Medicine
University of Pennsylvania Perelman School of Medicine
Philadelphia, Pennsylvania

Kathryn M. Edwards, MD
Sarah H. Sell and Cornelius Vanderbilt Chair in Pediatrics
Department of Pediatrics
Vanderbilt University School of Medicine
Nashville, Tennessee

Morven S. Edwards, MD
Professor of Pediatrics
Baylor College of Medicine;
Attending Physician
Pediatric Infectious Diseases Section
Texas Children's Hospital
Houston, Texas

Samer S. El-Kamary, MBChB, MS, MPH
Associate Professor
Department of Epidemiology and Public Health
University of Maryland School of Medicine;
Associate Professor
Department of Pediatrics
University of Maryland School of Medicine
Baltimore, Maryland

Janet A. Englund, MD
Professor
Department of Pediatrics
University of Washington/Seattle Children's Hospital
Seattle, Washington

Jessica Ericson, MD, MPH
Assistant Professor
Department of Pediatrics
Division of Pediatric Infectious Diseases
Pennsylvania State University College of Medicine
Hershey, Pennsylvania

Leland L. Fan, MD
Professor Emeritus
Department of Pediatrics
University of Colorado School of Medicine
Aurora, Colorado

Myke Federman, MD
Associate Professor of Pediatrics
Division of Pediatric Critical Care
University of California–Los Angeles
Los Angeles, California

Pedro Fernando da C. Vasconcelos, MD, PhD
Chief, Department of Arbovirology and Hemorrhagic Fevers
Coordinator, National Reference Laboratory of Arboviruses
Director, National Institute of Science and Technology for Viral Hemorrhagic Fevers
Director, PAHO-WHO CC for Research and Diagnostic Reference on Arbovirus
Instituto Evandro Chagas
SVS/Ministry of Health
Ananindeua, Brazil

Philip R. Fischer, MD
Professor of Pediatrics
Mayo Clinic
Rochester, Minnesota

Brian T. Fisher, DO, MPH, MSCE
Assistant Professor of Pediatrics and Epidemiology
Perelman School of Medicine at the University of Pennsylvania;
Division of Infectious Diseases
Children's Hospital of Philadelphia
Philadelphia, Pennsylvania

Randall G. Fisher, MD
Professor
Department of Pediatrics
Eastern Virginia Medical School;
Medical Director
Division of Pediatric Infectious Diseases
Children's Hospital of The King's Daughters
Norfolk, Virginia

Douglas S. Fishman, MD
Director of Gastrointestinal Endoscopy and Pancreaticobiliary Program
Texas Children's Hospital;
Associate Professor of Pediatrics
Baylor College of Medicine
Houston, Texas

Anthony R. Flores, MD, MPH, PhD
Assistant Professor
Department of Pediatrics
Section of Infectious Diseases
Texas Children's Hospital
Baylor College of Medicine
Houston, Texas

Catherine Foster, MD
Clinical Postdoctoral Fellow
Pediatrics, Section of Infectious Diseases
Baylor College of Medicine
Houston, Texas

Ellen M. Friedman, MD
Professor
Department of Otolaryngology
Texas Children's Hospital;
Director
Center for Professionalism in Medicine
Baylor College of Medicine
Houston, Texas

Claudia Raja Gabaglia, MD, PhD
Assistant Professor
Biomedical Research Institute of Southern California
Oceanside, California

Lynne S. Garcia, MS, CLS, BLM, FAAM
Director
LSG & Associates
Santa Monica, California

Gregory M. Gauthier, MD, MS
Associate Professor
Department of Medicine
University of Wisconsin
Madison, Wisconsin

Anne A. Gershon, MD
Professor
Department of Pediatrics
Columbia University College of Physicians and Surgeons
New York, New York

Francis Gigliotti, MD
Professor and Chief of Infectious Diseases
Department of Pediatrics
Associate Chair for Academic Affairs
University of Rochester School of Medicine and Dentistry
Rochester, New York

Mark A. Gilger, MD
Pediatrician-in-Chief
Children's Hospital of San Antonio;
Professor and Vice Chair
Department of Pediatrics
Baylor College of Medicine
Houston, Texas

Susan L. Gillespie, MD, PhD
Associate Professor
Department of Pediatrics
Baylor College of Medicine
Houston, Texas

Carol A. Glaser, DVM, MPVM, MD
Pediatric Infectious Diseases
Permanente Medical Group
Oakland Medical Center
Oakland, California

David L. Goldman, MD
Associate Professor
Department of Pediatrics
Children's Hospital at Montefiore/Albert Einstein College of Medicine
New York, New York

Jennifer L. Goldman, MD
Department of Pediatrics
Children's Mercy Hospitals and Clinics
Kansas City, Missouri

Nira A. Goldstein, MD, MPH
Professor and Attending Physician
Department of Otolaryngology
State University of New York Downstate Medical Center
New York, New York

Blanca E. Gonzalez, MD
Assistant Professor of Pediatrics
Cleveland Clinic Lerner College of Medicine of Case Western Reserve University
Center for Pediatric Infectious Diseases
Cleveland Clinic Children's
Cleveland, Ohio

Michael D. Green, MD, MPH
Professor
Department of Pediatrics, Surgery, & Clinical and Translational Research
University of Pittsburgh School of Medicine
Division of Pediatric Infectious Diseases
Children's Hospital of Pittsburgh of UPMC
Pittsburgh, Pennsylvania

Andreas Groll, MD
Professor
Department of Pediatric Hematology/Oncology
University Children's Hospital
Muenster, Germany

Charles Grose, MD
Professor
Department of Pediatrics
Director of Infectious Diseases
Children's Hospital
University of Iowa
Iowa City, Iowa

Duane J. Gubler, ScD, FAAAS, FIDSA, FASTMH
Emeritus Professor
Programme in Emerging Infectious Diseases
Duke-NUS Medical School
Singapore;
Chair, Global Dengue and Aedes Transmitted Diseases Consortium
International Vaccine Institute
Seoul, Korea

Javier Nieto Guevara, MD, MPH
Infectious Diseases Specialist
Panama City, Panama

Caroline B. Hall, MD†
Formerly Professor
Department of Pediatrics and Medicine
University of Rochester School of Medicine and Dentistry
Rochester, New York

Roy A. Hall, BSc(Hons), PhD
Professor
School of Chemistry and Molecular Biosciences
University of Queensland
St Lucia, QLD, Australia

Scott B. Halstead, MD
Adjunct Professor
Preventive Medicine and Biostatistics
Uniformed Services University of the Health Sciences
Bethesda, Maryland

Shinjiro Hamano, MD, PhD
Professor
Department of Parasitology
Institute of Tropical Medicine
Nagasaki University
Nagasaki, Japan

Margaret R. Hammerschlag, MD
Professor of Pediatrics and Medicine
SUNY Downstate Medical Center
New York, New York

Nicole L. Hannemann, MD
Chief Resident and Clinical Instructor
Department of Pediatrics
Baylor College of Medicine and Texas Children's Hospital
Houston, Texas

I. Celine Hanson, MD
Professor
Department of Pediatrics
Baylor College of Medicine
Houston, Texas

Nada Harik, MD
Associate Professor
Department of Pediatrics
Division of Pediatric Infectious Diseases
George Washington University School of Medicine and Health Sciences
Children's National Medical Center
Washington, DC

Kathleen H. Harriman, PhD, MPH, RN
Chief
Vaccine Preventable Diseases Epidemiology Section
Immunization Branch
California Department of Public Health
Richmond, California

Gail J. Harrison, MD
Professor
Department of Pediatrics
Section of Infectious Diseases
Baylor College of Medicine;
Attending Physician
Infectious Diseases Service
Texas Children's Hospital
Houston, Texas

C. Mary Healy, MB BCh, BAO, MD
Associate Professor
Department of Pediatrics
Division of Infectious Diseases
Baylor College of Medicine and Texas Children's Hospital
Houston, Texas

Ulrich Heininger, MD
Chair, Pediatric Infectious Diseases
University of Basel Children's Hospital;
Member, Medical Faculty
University of Basel
Basel, Switzerland

Maria Hemming-Harlo, MD, PhD
Medical Researcher
Vaccine Research Center
University of Tampere
Tampere, Finland

Sheryl L. Henderson, MD, PhD
Assistant Professor
Department of Pediatrics
University of Wisconsin School of Medicine and Public Health
American Family Children's Hospital
Madison, Wisconsin

†Deceased.

Gloria P. Heresi, MD
Professor
Department of Pediatrics
University of Texas Medical School at Houston
Houston, Texas

Peter W. Hiatt, MD
Associate Professor of Pediatrics
Section Head, Pediatric Pulmonology
Baylor College of Medicine;
Chief, Pulmonary Medicine
Texas Children's Hospital
Houston, Texas

Harry R. Hill, MD
Professor
Departments of Pediatrics, Pathology, and Internal Medicine
University of Utah
Salt Lake City, Utah

David C. Hilmers, MD, EE, MPH
Professor
Departments of Internal Medicine and Pediatrics
Baylor Global Initiatives
Baylor Center for Space Medicine
Baylor College of Medicine
Houston, Texas

Jill A. Hoffman, MD
Associate Professor
Department of Pediatrics
Keck School of Medicine
University of Southern California;
Attending Physician
Division of Infectious Diseases
Children's Hospital Los Angeles
Los Angeles, California

Peter J. Hotez, MD, PhD
Dean, National School of Tropical Medicine
Professor, Pediatrics and Molecular & Virology and Microbiology
Head, Section of Pediatric Tropical Medicine
Baylor College of Medicine;
Endowed Chair of Tropical Pediatrics
Center for Vaccine Development
Texas Children's Hospital;
Professor, Department of Biology
Baylor University
Waco, Texas;
Baker Institute Fellow in Disease and Poverty
Rice University
Houston, Texas;
Co-Editor-in-Chief, *PLoS Neglected Tropical Diseases*

Leigh M. Howard, MD, MPH
Assistant Professor
Department of Pediatric Infectious Diseases
Vanderbilt University Medical Center
Nashville, Tennessee

Kristina G. Hulten, PhD
Assistant Professor
Department of Pediatrics
Baylor College of Medicine
Houston, Texas

Romney M. Humphries, PhD
Chief Scientific Officer
Accelerate Diagnostics
Tucson, Arizona

David A. Hunstad, MD
Associate Professor
Departments of Pediatrics and Molecular Microbiology
Washington University School of Medicine
St. Louis, Missouri

W. Garrett Hunt, MD, MPH, DTM&H, FAAP
Associate Professor
Department of Pediatrics
Section of Infectious Diseases
Nationwide Children's Hospital/Ohio State University
Columbus, Ohio

W. Charles Huskins, MD, MSc
Professor of Pediatrics
Mayo Clinic School of Medicine;
Chair, Division of Pediatric Infectious Diseases
Mayo Clinic;
Vice Chair of Quality and Health Care Epidemiologist
Mayo Clinic Children's Center
Rochester, Minnesota

David Y. Hyun, MD
Senior Officer
Antibiotic Resistance Project
Pew Charitable Trusts
Philadelphia, Pennsylvania

Mary Anne Jackson, MD
Director, Infectious Diseases
Children's Mercy Kansas City
Professor of Pediatrics
UMKC School of Medicine
Kansas City, Missouri

Michael R. Jacobs, MB BCh, PhD
Professor of Pathology and Medicine
Department of Pathology
Case Western Reserve University;
Director of Clinical Microbiology
Department of Pathology
University Hospitals Cleveland Medical Center
Cleveland, Ohio

Richard F. Jacobs, MD, FAAP
Robert H. Fiser Jr, MD, Endowed Chair in Pediatrics
Pediatrician-in-Chief
Department of Pediatrics
Arkansas Children's Hospital;
Chairman and Professor
Department of Pediatrics
University of Arkansas for Medical Sciences
Little Rock, Arkansas

Ravi Jhaveri, MD
Associate Professor
Department of Pediatrics
University of North Carolina at Chapel Hill School of Medicine
Chapel Hill, North Carolina

Audrey R. Odom John, MD, PhD
Associate Professor
Departments of Pediatrics and Molecular Microbiology
Washington University School of Medicine
Saint Louis, Missouri

Samantha H. Johnston, MD, MPH
Associate Physician
Pediatric Infectious Diseases
UCSF Benioff Children's Hospital Oakland
Oakland, California

Meena R. Julapalli, MD
Assistant Professor
Department of Dermatology
University of Colorado
Denver, Colorado

Sheldon L. Kaplan, MD
Professor and Executive Vice-Chair
Head, Section of Infectious Diseases
Department of Pediatrics
Baylor College of Medicine;
Chief, Infectious Disease Service
Head, Department of Pediatric Medicine
Texas Children's Hospital
Houston, Texas

Gregory L. Kearns, PharmD, PhD
President
Arkansas Children's Research Institute
Senior Vice President and Chief Research Officer
Arkansas Children's;
Ross and Mary Whipple Family Distinguished Research Scientist
Professor of Pediatrics
University of Arkansas for Medical Sciences
Little Rock, Arkansas

Jessica M. Khouri, MD
Senior Medical Officer
Infant Botulism Treatment and Prevention Program
California Department of Public Health
Richmond, California

Kwang Sik Kim, MD
Professor and Director
Department of Pediatric Infectious Diseases
Johns Hopkins University School of Medicine;
Professor
Department of Molecular Microbiology and Immunology
Johns Hopkins University Bloomberg School of Public Health
Baltimore, Maryland

Yae-Jean Kim, MD, PhD
Associate Professor
Department of Pediatrics
Samsung Medical Center
Sungkyungkwan University School of Medicine
Seoul, Korea

Katherine Y. King, MD, PhD
Assistant Professor
Department of Pediatric Infectious Diseases
Baylor College of Medicine
Houston, Texas

Louis V. Kirchhoff, MD, MPH
Professor
Department of Internal Medicine (Infectious Diseases), Psychiatry, and Epidemiology
Carver College of Medicine and College of Public Health
University of Iowa
Iowa City, Iowa

Martin B. Kleiman, MD
Ryan White Professor Emeritus of Pediatrics
Ryan White Center for Pediatric Infectious Disease and Global Health
Indiana University School of Medicine
Indianapolis, Indiana

Bruce S. Klein, MD
Gerard B. Odell and Shirley S. Matchette Professor of Pediatrics
Professor of Internal Medicine and Medical Microbiology and Immunology
University of Wisconsin–Madison
Madison, Wisconsin

Stephan A. Kohlhoff, MD
Associate Professor
Departments of Pediatrics and Medicine
State University of New York Downstate Medical Center
New York, New York

Tobias R. Kollmann, MD, PhD
Professor of Pediatrics
Interim Head, Division of Infectious Diseases
University of British Columbia
Vancouver, BC, Canada

Poonum S. Korpe, MD
Assistant Scientist
Department of Epidemiology
Johns Hopkins Bloomberg School of Public Health
Baltimore, Maryland

Margaret Kosek, MD
Assistant Professor
Department of International Health
Johns Hopkins University Bloomberg School of Public Health
Baltimore, Maryland

Michael P. Koster, MD
Division of Pediatric Hospital Medicine
Hasbro Children's Hospital;
Associate Professor, Clinical Educator
Department of Pediatrics
Alpert Medical School of Brown University
Providence, Rhode Island

Peter J. Krause, MD
Senior Research Scientist
Yale School of Public Health
Yale School of Medicine
New Haven, Connecticut

Leonard R. Krilov, MD
Chairman, Department of Pediatrics
Chief, Pediatric Infectious Disease
Children's Medical Center
NYU Winthrop Hospital
Mineola, New York;
Professor of Pediatrics
State University of New York Stony Brook School of Medicine
Stony Brook, New York

Paul Krogstad, MD
Professor
Departments of Pediatrics and Molecular and Medical Pharmacology
David Geffen School of Medicine at UCLA
Los Angeles, California

Damian J. Krysan, MD, PHD
Associate Professor
Departments of Pediatrics and Microbiology/Immunology
University of Rochester School of Medicine and Dentistry
Rochester, New York

Edward Kuan, MD, MBA
Resident Physician
Department of Head and Neck Surgery
David Geffen School of Medicine at UCLA
Los Angeles, California

Thomas Kuhls, MD
Department of Pediatrics
Norman Pediatric Associates
Norman, Oklahoma

Sarah M. Labuda, MD, MPH
Pediatric Infectious Diseases Fellow
Tulane School of Medicine
New Orleans, Louisiana

Paul M. Lantos, MD
Assistant Professor
Division of Pediatric Infectious Diseases
Division of General Internal Medicine
Duke University School of Medicine
Duke Global Health Institute
Durham, North Carolina

Timothy R. La Pine, MD
Professor
Department of Pediatrics and Pathology
University of Utah;
Director of Neonatology
St. Mark's Hospital
Salt Lake City, Utah

Suvi Heinimäki, PhD
Project Researcher
Vaccine Research Center
University of Tampere
Tampere, Finland

Jerome M. Larkin, MD
Division of Infectious Diseases
Rhode Island Hospital
Associate Professor, Clinical Educator
Department of Medicine
Alpert Medical School of Brown University
Providence, Rhode Island

Matthew B. Laurens, MD, MPH
Associate Professor
Institute for Global Health
University of Maryland School of Medicine
Baltimore, Maryland

Charles T. Leach, MD
Professor and Chief of Infectious Diseases
Department of Pediatrics
Baylor College of Medicine/Children's Hospital of San Antonio
San Antonio, Texas

Amy Leber, PhD
Director, Clinical Microbiology and Immunoserology
Department of Pathology and Laboratory Medicine
Nationwide Children's Hospital
Columbus, Ohio

Robert J. Leggiadro, MD
Adjunct Professor
Departments of Biology and Geography and the Environment
Villanova University
Villanova, Pennsylvania;
Adjunct Clinical Professor
Department of Pediatrics
Donald and Barbara Zucker School of Medicine at Hofstra/Northwell
Hempstead, New York;
Adjunct Attending Physician
General Pediatrics
Cohen Children's Medical Center
New Hyde Park, New York

Deborah Lehman, MD
Professor
Department of Pediatrics
David Geffen School of Medicine at UCLA
Los Angeles, California

Diana R. Lennon, MB CHB, FRACP
Professor of Population Health, Child, and Youth
Department of Pediatrics
University of Auckland;
Pediatrician in Infectious Diseases
Department of Pediatrics
Starship and KidzFirst Children's Hospital
Auckland, New Zealand

Daniel H. Leung, MD
Associate Professor of Pediatrics
Division of Gastroenterology, Hepatology, and Nutrition
Baylor College of Medicine;
Director of Clinical Research
Medical Director, Viral Hepatitis Program
Texas Children's Hospital
Houston, Texas

Moise L. Levy, MD
Chief, Pediatric/Adolescent Dermatology
Dell Children's Medical Center;
Professor of Pediatrics and Medicine (Dermatology)
Dell Medical School
University of Texas
Austin, Texas;
Clinical Professor of Dermatology and Pediatrics
Baylor College of Medicine
Houston, Texas

W. Matthew Linam, MD, MS
Medical Director of Infection Prevention and Hospital Epidemiology
Associate Professor, Department of Pediatrics
Division of Pediatric Infectious Diseases
Arkansas Children's Hospital
University of Arkansas for Medical Sciences
Little Rock, Arkansas

Latania K. Logan, MD
Chief, Pediatric Infectious Diseases
Department of Pediatrics
Rush University Medical Center
Associate Professor
Rush Medical College
Chicago, Illinois

Timothy E. Lotze, MD
Associate Professor of Pediatrics and Neurology
Division of Child Neurology
Baylor College of Medicine and Texas Children's Hospital
Houston, Texas

Yalda C. Lucero, MD, PhD
Pediatric Gastroenterologist
Assistant Professor
Microbiology and Mycology Program
Institute of Biomedical Sciences
Faculty of Medicine
University of Chile and Northern Campus Department of Pediatrics
Santiago, Chile

Debra J. Lugo, MD
Fellow, Pediatric Infectious Diseases
Mattel Children's Hospital
University of California–Los Angeles
Los Angeles, California

Berkley Luk, BSc
PhD Candidate
Program in Integrative Molecular and Biomedical Sciences
Baylor College of Medicine;
Department of Pathology
Texas Children's Hospital
Houston, Texas

Susan A. Maloney, MD, MHSc
Global Tuberculosis Coordinator
Division of Global Migration and Quarantine
National Center for Infectious Diseases
Centers for Disease Control and Prevention
Atlanta, Georgia

Michelle C. Mann, MD
Assistant Professor
Department of Pediatrics
Baylor College of Medicine
Houston, Texas

Lucila Marquez, MD, MPH
Assistant Professor of Pediatrics, Section of Infectious Diseases
Associate Medical Director, Infection Control and Prevention
Baylor College of Medicine and Texas Children's Hospital
Houston, Texas

Kimberly C. Martin, DO, MPH
Assistant Professor of Pediatrics
Division of Pediatric Infectious Diseases
University of Oklahoma School of Community Medicine
Tulsa, Oklahoma

Laurene Mascola, MD, MPH, FAAP
Epidemiology Consultant
Acute Communicable Disease Program
Los Angeles County Department of Public Health
Los Angeles, California

Edward O. Mason Jr, PhD
Professor
Department of Pediatrics
Baylor College of Medicine
Houston, Texas

Aldo Maspons, MD
CEO/Cofounder
VeMiDoc, LLC;
Maspons Pediatric Gastro
Pediatric Gastroenterology
El Paso, Texas

Marc A. Mazade, MD
Consultant
Pediatric Infectious Disease
Cook Children's Medical Center
Fort Worth, Texas

Holly E. McBride, MPH, MHS, PA-C
Physician Assistant
Internal Medicine
University of Colorado Health
Loveland, Colorado

Jonathan A. McCullers, MD
Chair
Department of Pediatrics
University of Tennessee Health Science Center
Memphis, Tennessee

Kenneth McIntosh, MD
Professor
Department of Pediatrics
Harvard Medical School;
Senior Physician
Department of Medicine
Children's Hospital
Boston, Massachusetts

James E. McJunkin, MD
Professor of Pediatrics
Department of Pediatrics
West Virginia University Health Sciences Center
Charleston, West Virginia

Kelly T. McKee Jr, MD, MPH
Vice President
Department of Public Health and Government Services
QuintilesIMS
Durham, North Carolina

Ross McKinney Jr, MD
Professor Emeritus
Department of Pediatrics
Duke University School of Medicine
Durham, North Carolina;
Chief Scientific Officer
Association of American Medical Colleges
Washington, DC

J. Chase McNeil, MD
Assistant Professor
Department of Pediatrics
Section of Infectious Diseases
Baylor College of Medicine
Houston, Texas

Rojelio Mejia, MD
Assistant Professor of Infectious Diseases and Pediatrics
National School of Tropical Medicine
Baylor College of Medicine
Houston, Texas

Asuncion Mejias, MD, PhD
Associate Professor of Pediatrics
Ohio State University College of Medicine
Department of Pediatrics
Division of Infectious Diseases
Nationwide Children's Hospital
Columbus, Ohio

Maria José Soares Mendes Giannini, PhD
Full Professor
Department of Clinical Analysis
Laboratory of Clinical Mycology
São Paulo State University-UNESP
Araraquara, São Paulo, Brazil

Marian G. Michaels, MD, MPH
Professor
Department of Pediatrics and Surgery
University of Pittsburgh School of Medicine
Division of Pediatric Infectious Diseases
Children's Hospital of Pittsburgh of UPMC
Pittsburgh, Pennsylvania

Ian C. Michelow, MD, DTM&H
Division of Pediatric Infectious Diseases
Hasbro Children's Hospital
Associate Professor
Department of Pediatrics
Alpert Medical School of Brown University
Providence, Rhode Island

Marjorie J. Miller, DrPH
Senior Specialist, Virology
Department of Pathology and Laboratory Medicine
UCLA Medical Center
Los Angeles, California

James N. Mills, PhD
Adjunct Faculty
Population Biology, Ecology, and Evolution Group
Emory University
Atlanta, Georgia

Leena B. Mithal, MD, MSCI
Attending Physician
Department of Pediatric Infectious Diseases
Ann & Robert H. Lurie Children's Hospital of Chicago;
Instructor, Department of Pediatrics
Northwestern University Feinberg School of Medicine
Chicago, Illinois

Kathryn S. Moffett, MD
Professor of Pediatrics
Section Chief, Infectious Diseases
Department of Pediatrics
West Virginia University
Morgantown, West Virginia

Martin Montes, MD
Assistant Professor
Instituto de Medicina Tropica "Alexander von Humboldt"
Universidad Peruana Cayetano Heridia
Lima, Peru;
Assistant Professor
Department of Medicine
Division of Infectious Diseases
University of Texas Medical Branch
Galveston, Texas

Martha Muller, MD
Associate Professor
Department of Pediatrics
University of New Mexico
Albuquerque, New Mexico

Randy George Mungwira, MBBS, MPH
Blantyre Malaria Project
Blantyre, Malawi

James R. Murphy, PhD
Professor
Department of Pediatrics
University of Texas
Houston, Texas

Santhosh M. Nadipuram, MD
Postdoctoral Fellow
Department of Microbiology, Immunology, & Molecular Genetics
University of California–Los Angeles
Los Angeles, California

James P. Nataro, MD, PhD, MBA
Benjamin Armistead Shepherd Professor and Chair
Department of Pediatrics
University of Virginia School of Medicine;
Physician-in-Chief
University of Virginia Children's Hospital
Charlottesville, Virginia

Heather Needham, MD, MPH
Assistant Professor of Pediatrics
Section of Adolescent Medicine & Sports Medicine
Baylor College of Medicine and Texas Children's Hospital
Houston, Texas

Karin Nielsen-Saines, MD, MPH
Professor of Clinical Pediatrics
Division of Pediatric Infectious Diseases
David Geffen School of Medicine at UCLA;
Director, Center for Brazilian Studies
Los Angeles, California

Delma J. Nieves, MD
Assistant Clinical Professor
Department of Pediatric Infectious Diseases
University of California–Irvine School of Medicine
Children's Hospital of Orange County
Orange, California

Richard Oberhelman, MD
Professor and Chair
Global Community Health & Behavioral Sciences
Tulane School of Public Health and Tropical Medicine;
Professor of Pediatrics
Tulane School of Medicine
New Orleans, Louisiana

Theresa J. Ochoa, MD
Associate Professor
Department of Pediatrics
Instituto de Medicina Tropical "Alexander von Humboldt"
Universidad Peruana Cayetano Heredia
Lima, Peru;
Associate Professor
Division of Epidemiology, Human Genetics, and Environmental Sciences
Center for Infectious Diseases
School of Public Health
University of Texas Health Science Center at Houston
Houston, Texas

Rosemary M. Olivero, MD
Clinical Associate Professor of Pediatrics and Human Development
Michigan State College of Human Medicine;
Attending Physician
Section of Pediatric Infectious Diseases
Helen DeVos Children's Hospital
Grand Rapids, Michigan

Miguel O'Ryan, MD
Professor, Pediatric Infectious Disease
Millennium Institute of Immunology and Immunotherapy
Faculty of Medicine
Microbiology and Mycology Program
Institute of Biomedical Sciences
University of Chile
Santiago, Chile

Gary D. Overturf, MD
Professor Emeritus
Departments of Pediatrics and Pathology
University of New Mexico School of Medicine;
Medical Director, Infectious Diseases
TriCore Reference Laboratories
Albuquerque, New Mexico

Debra L. Palazzi, MD, MEd
Associate Professor of Pediatrics
Section of Infectious Diseases
Baylor College of Medicine;
Chief, Infectious Diseases Clinic
Texas Children's Hospital
Houston, Texas

Pia S. Pannaraj, MD, MPH
Associate Professor
Pediatrics and Molecular Microbiology and Immunology
University of Southern California/Children's Hospital Los Angeles
Los Angeles, California

Janak A. Patel, MD
Professor and Division Director
Department of Pediatrics
Division of Pediatric Infectious Disease and Immunology
University of Texas Medical Branch
Galveston, Texas

Mary E. Paul, MD
Associate Professor
Department of Pediatrics
Baylor College of Medicine
Chief, Retrovirology and Global Health
Texas Children's Hospital
Houston, Texas

Stephen I. Pelton, MD
Professor of Pediatrics and Epidemiology
Department of Pediatrics
Boston University Schools of Medicine and Public Health;
Chief, Section of Pediatric Infectious Diseases
Department of Pediatrics
Boston Medical Center
Boston, Massachusetts

Morgan A. Pence, PhD, D(ABMM)
Clinical Microbiologist
Department of Laboratory and Pathology
Cook Children's Medical Center
Fort Worth, Texas

John R. Perfect, MD
James B. Duke Professor of Medicine
Duke University Medical Center
Durham, North Carolina

C.J. Peters, MD
Department of Microbiology and Immunology
University of Texas Medical Branch
Galveston, Texas

William A. Petri Jr, MD, PhD
Chief
Division of Infectious Disease and International Health
University of Virginia Health System;
Wade Hampton Frost Professor of Epidemiology
University of Virginia
Charlottesville, Virginia

Yen H. Pham, MD
Assistant Professor
Department of Pediatric Gastroenterology, Hepatology, and Nutrition
Baylor College of Medicine and Texas Children's Hospital
Houston, Texas

Francisco P. Pinheiro, MD
Department of Arbovirus
Instituto Evandro Chagas
FNS
Ministry of Health
Belem, Brazil

Benjamin A. Pinsky, MD, PhD
Associate Professor
Departments of Pathology and Medicine (Infectious Diseases)
Stanford University School of Medicine;
Medical Director
Clinical Virology Laboratory
Stanford Health Care and Stanford Children's Health
Stanford, California

Alice Pong, MD
Department of Pediatric Infectious Diseases
University of California–San Diego;
Department of Pediatric Infectious Diseases
Rady Children's Hospital San Diego
San Diego, California

Eric A. Porsch, PhD
Department of Pediatrics
Children's Hospital of Philadelphia
Philadelphia, Pennsylvania

Joan S. Purcell, MD
Adolescent Medicine and Pediatrics
STEP Pediatrics
Woodlands, Texas

Natalie M. Quanquin, MD, PhD
Research Fellow
Department of Microbiology, Immunology, and Molecular Genetics
University of California–Los Angeles
Los Angeles, California

Kevin K. Quinn, MD
Physician
Department of Pediatric Infectious Diseases
Southern California Permanente Medical Group
Fontana, California

Susan M. Abdel-Rahman, PharmD
Chief, Section of Therapeutic Innovation
Clinical Pharmacology, Medical Toxicology & Therapeutic Innovation
Children's Mercy–Kansas City;
Professor of Pediatrics
University of Missouri–Kansas City School of Medicine
Kansas City, Missouri

Octavio Ramilo, MD
Henry G. Cramblett Chair in Medicine
Professor of Pediatrics
Ohio State University College of Medicine
Department of Pediatrics
Chief, Division of Infectious Diseases
Nationwide Children's Hospital
Columbus, Ohio

Ramya Ramraj, MD, MBBS
Affiliate Assistant Professor
Oregon Health and Sciences University;
Attending Pediatrician and Pediatric Gastroenterologist
Doernbecher Children's Hospital and Kaiser NW Permanente
Portland, Oregon

Paula A. Revell, PhD
Assistant Professor
Departments of Pathology and Immunology and Pediatrics
Baylor College of Medicine;
Director of Microbiology and Virology
Texas Children's Hospital
Houston, Texas

Anne W. Rimoin, PhD, MPH
Associate Professor
Department of Epidemiology
UCLA Fielding School of Public Health
Los Angeles, California

José R. Romero, MD
Horace C. Cabe Professor of Infectious Diseases
Department of Pediatrics
University of Arkansas for Medical Sciences;
Director, Pediatric Infectious Diseases Section
Department of Pediatrics
Arkansas Children's Hospital;
Director, Clinical Trials Research
Arkansas Children's Hospital Research Institute
Little Rock, Arkansas

Lawrence Ross, MD, DTM&H
Professor Emeritus
Division of Pediatric Infectious Diseases
Children's Hospital of Los Angeles
Keck School of Medicine at the University of Southern California
Los Angeles, California

Anne H. Rowley, MD
Professor
Department of Pediatrics and Microbiology/Immunology
Northwestern University Feinberg School of Medicine
Attending Physician, Division of Infectious Diseases
Department of Pediatrics
Ann & Robert H. Lurie Children's Hospital of Chicago
Chicago, Illinois

Charles E. Rupprecht, VMD, MS, PhD
Chief Executive Officer
LYSSA, LLC
Atlanta, Georgia

Xavier Saez-Llorens, MD
Professor of Pediatrics
Head of Infectious Diseases
Hospital del Niño "Dr. José Renán Esquivel"
Distinguished Investigator, SNI, Senacyt
Panama City, Panama

Julia Shaklee Sammons, MD, MSCE
Assistant Professor of Clinical Pediatrics
Division of Infectious Diseases
Perelman School of Medicine at the University of Pennsylvania;
Medical Director and Hospital Epidemiologist
Infection Prevention and Control
Children's Hospital of Philadelphia
Philadelphia, Pennsylvania

Pablo Sánchez, MD
Prinicipal Investigator
Center for Perinatal Research
Fellow, Infectious Diseases
Fellow, Neonatology
Nationwide Children's Hospital
Columbus, Ohio

Linette Sande, MD
Assistant Professor of Pediatrics
Department of Pediatric Infectious Diseases
Loma Linda University;
Attending Physician
Department of Pediatric Infectious Diseases
Loma Linda University Children's Hospital
Loma Linda, California

Javier Santisteban-Ponce, MD
Attending Physician
Pediatric Infectious Disease Unit
Department of Pediatrics
Hospital Nacional Edgardo Rebagliati Martins-EsSalud;
Lima, Peru

Laura A. Sass, MD
Assistant Professor
Department of Pediatrics
Eastern Virginia Medical School;
Attending Physician
Department of Pediatric Infectious Diseases
Medical Director, Infection Prevention and Control, Antiobiotic Stewardship
Children's Hospital of The King's Daughters
Norfolk, Virginia

Stephen J. Scholand, MD
Associate Professor
Department of Medicine
Frank Netter School of Medicine
Quinnipiac University
North Haven, Connecticut

Danica J. Schulte, MD
Assistant Professor in Residence
Department of Pediatrics
University of California–Los Angeles;
Assistant Professor
Departments of Pediatrics, Pediatric Infectious Diseases, Immunology and Allergy
Cedars-Sinai Medical Center
Los Angeles, California

Jennifer E. Schuster, MD, MSCI
Assistant Professor
Department of Pediatrics
Children's Mercy Kansas City
Kansas City, Missouri

Gordon E. Schutze, MD, FAAP
Professor of Pediatrics
Executive Vice Chairman
Martin I. Lorin, MD, Endowed Chair in Medical Education
Department of Pediatrics
Baylor College of Medicine;
Vice President, International Programs
Baylor International Pediatric AIDS Initiative at Texas Children's Hospital
Houston, Texas

Patrick C. Seed, MD, PhD
Assistant Professor
Department of Pediatrics/Pediatric Infectious Diseases
Duke University School of Medicine;
Assistant Professor
Department of Molecular Genetics and Microbiology
Duke University School of Medicine
Durham, North Carolina

Jose A. Serpa, MD, MS
Associate Professor
Department of Medicine
Baylor College of Medicine
Houston, Texas

Samir S. Shah, MD, MSCE
Professor
Department of Pediatrics
University of Cincinnati College of Medicine;
Director, Division of Hospital Medicine
Attending Physician
Divisions of Infectious Diseases and Hospital Medicine
James M. Ewell Endowed Chair
Cincinnati Children's Hospital Medical Center
Cincinnati, Ohio

Eugene D. Shapiro, MD
Professor
Departments of Pediatrics, Epidemiology of Microbial Diseases, and Investigative Medicine
Yale University
New Haven, Connecticut

Nina L. Shapiro, MD
Professor, Department of Head and Neck Surgery
Director, Division of Pediatric Otolaryngology
David Geffen School of Medicine at UCLA
Los Angeles, California

William T. Shearer, MD, PhD
Professor of Pediatrics and Pathology and Immunology
Distinguished Service Professor
Baylor College of Medicine;
Allergy and Immunology Service
Texas Children's Hospital
Houston, Texas

Robyn Shimizu-Cohen, CLS(ASCP)
Specialist
Department of Pathology and Laboratory Medicine
University of California–Los Angeles
Los Angeles, California

Stanford T. Shulman, MD
Chief Emeritus, Division of Infectious Diseases
Ann & Robert H. Lurie Children's Hospital of Chicago
Virginia H. Rogers Professor of Pediatric Infectious Diseases
Northwestern University Feinberg School of Medicine
Chicago, Illinois

Kareem W. Shehab, MD
Assistant Professor
Department of Pediatrics
Section of Infectious Disease
University of Arizona
Tucson, Arizona

Ziad M. Shehab, MD
Professor of Pediatrics and Pathology
University of Arizona
Tucson, Arizona

Constantine Simos, DMD
Attending Surgeon
Oral and Maxillofacial Surgery
Robert Wood Johnson University Hospital
Saint Peter's University Hospital
New Brunswick, New Jersey;
Assistant Clinical Professor
Oral and Maxillofacial Surgery
Columbia University College of Dental Medicine
New York, New York

Michael A. Smit, MD, MSPH
Division of Pediatric Infectious Diseases
Hasbro Children's Hospital
Assistant Professor
Department of Pediatrics
Alpert Medical School of Brown University
Providence, Rhode Island

P. Brian Smith, MD, MPH, MHS
Professor of Pediatrics
Duke University Medical Center
Duke Clinical Research Institute
Durham, North Carolina

Priya R. Soni, MD
Fellow, Pediatric Infectious Disease
Mattel Children's Hospital
University of California–Los Angeles
Los Angeles, California

Sunil K. Sood, MBBS, DCH, MD
Professor
Departments of Pediatrics and Family Medicine
Hofstra Northwell School of Medicine
Hempstead, New York;
Chair of Pediatrics
Southside Hospital, Northwell Health
Bay Shore, New York;
Attending Physician
Pediatric Infectious Diseases
Cohen Children's Medical Center
New Hyde Park, New York

Mary Allen Staat, MD, MPH
Professor
Department of Pediatrics
University of Cincinnati College of Medicine;
Director
International Adoption Center
Cincinnati Children's Hospital Medical Center
Cincinnati, Ohio

Damien Stark, MSc, PhD, FASM, FACTM
Associate, Department of Medical and Molecular Biosciences
University of Technology Sydney
Broadway, NSW, Australia;
Senior Hospital Scientist
Department of Microbiology
St. Vincent's Hospital
Darlinghurst, NSW, Australia

Jeffrey R. Starke, MD
Professor
Department of Pediatrics
Baylor College of Medicine
Houston, Texas

Victoria A. Statler, MD, MSc
Assistant Professor
Department of Pediatric Infectious Diseases
University of Louisville
Louisville, Kentucky

Barbara W. Stechenberg, MD
Pediatric Infectious Diseases Specialist
Department of Pediatrics
Baystate Children's Hospital
Springfield, Massachusetts;
Professor Emerita of Pediatrics
Department of Pediatrics
Tufts University School of Medicine
Boston, Massachusetts

William J. Steinbach, MD
Professor of Pediatrics
Professor in Molecular Genetics and Microbiology
Chief, Pediatric Infectious Diseases
Director, Duke Pediatric Immunocompromised Host Program
Director, International Pediatric Fungal Network
Duke University School of Medicine
Durham, North Carolina

Joseph W. St. Geme III, MD
Professor of Pediatrics and Microbiology
Chair, Department of Pediatrics
Perelman School of Medicine at the University of Pennsylvania;
Chair, Department of Pediatrics
Physician-in-Chief
Children's Hospital of Philadelphia
Philadelphia, Pennsylvania

Jeffrey Suen, MD
Private Practice
Bakersfield, California

Lillian Sung, MD, PhD
Professor
Division of Haematology/Oncology
Hospital for Sick Children
Toronto, ON, Canada

Douglas S. Swanson, MD
Associate Professor of Pediatrics
Department of Pediatric Infectious Diseases
Children's Mercy Kansas City;
Associate Professor of Pediatrics
University of Missouri–Kansas City
Kansas City, Missouri

Tina Q. Tan, MD
Professor
Department of Pediatrics
Feinberg School of Medicine
Northwestern University;
Infectious Diseases Attending Physician
Department of Pediatrics
Ann & Robert H. Lurie Children's Hospital
Chicago, Illinois

Ruston S. Taylor, PharmD
Department of Pharmacy
Legacy Community Health
Houston, Texas

Michael A. Tolle, MD, MPH
Assistant Professor
Department of Pediatrics
Retrovirology and Global Health Section
International Pediatrics AIDS Initiative (BIPAI)
Baylor College of Medicine Children's Foundation
Texas Children's Hospital
Houston, Texas;
Tanzania Buganda Medical Centre
Mwanza, Tanzania

Philip Toltzis, MD
Professor
Department of Pediatrics
Rainbow Babies and Children's Hospital
Cleveland, Ohio

Stuart R. Tomko, MD
Division of Child Neurology
Texas Children's Hospital
Houston, Texas

Michael F. Tosi, MD
Professor of Pediatrics
Division of Pediatric Infectious Diseases
Mount Sinai School of Medicine
New York, New York

Leidy J. Tovar Padua, MD
Fellow
Division of Pediatric Infectious Diseases
Mattel Children's Hospital of UCLA
Los Angeles, California

Amelia P.A. Travassos da Rosa, BSc
Research Associate
Center for Tropical Diseases
Department of Pathology
University of Texas Medical Branch
Galveston, Texas

Theodore F. Tsai, MD, MPH
Senior Vice President, Scientific Affairs
Novartis Vaccines
Cambridge, Massachusetts

Andrew M. Vahabzadeh-Hagh, MD
Resident
Department of Head and Neck Surgery
David Geffen School of Medicine at UCLA
Los Angeles, California

Jorge J. Velarde, MD, PhD
Instructor
Division of Infectious Diseases
Boston Children's Hospital
Boston, Massachusetts

Jesus G. Vallejo, MD
Associate Professor
Department of Pediatric Infectious Diseases
Baylor College of Medicine
Houston, Texas

John A. Vanchiere, MD, PhD
Professor and Chief
Section of Pediatric Infectious Diseases
Louisiana State University Health Sciences Center
Shreveport, Louisiana

Robert S. Venick, MD
Associate Professor
Departments of Pediatrics and Surgery
David Geffin School of Medicine at UCLA
Los Angeles, California

Sanjay Verma, MBBS, MD
Additional Professor of Pediatrics
Advanced Pediatrics Centre
Postgraduate Institute of Medical Education and Research
Chandigarh, India

James Versalovic, MD, PhD
Pathologist-in-Chief
Department of Pathology
Texas Children's Hospital;
Milton J. Finegold Professor
Department of Pathology and Immunology
Baylor College of Medicine
Houston, Texas

Timo Vesikari, MD, PhD
Director
Vaccine Research Center
University of Tampere
Tampere, Finland

Ellen R. Wald, MD
Chair, Department of Pediatrics
University of Wisconsin School of Medicine & Public Health;
Pediatrician-in-Chief
American Family Children's Hospital
Madison, Wisconsin

Thomas J. Walsh, MD
Director, Transplantation-Oncology Infectious Diseases Program
Weill Cornell Medical Center of Cornell University
New York, New York

Mark A. Ward, MD
Associate Professor
Department of Pediatrics
Baylor College of Medicine
Houston, Texas

Rachel L. Wattier, MD, MHS
Assistant Clinical Professor
Department of Pediatrics
University of California–San Francisco
San Francisco, California

Sing Sing Way, MD, PhD
Professor of Pediatrics
Pauline and Lawson Reed Chair
Division of Infectious Diseases
Cincinnati Children's Hospital
University of Cincinnati College of Medicine
Cincinnati, Ohio

Jill Weatherhead, MD
Assistant Professor of Infectious Diseases and Pediatrics
National School of Tropical Medicine
Baylor College of Medicine
Houston, Texas

Michelle Weinberg, MD, MPH
Medical Epidemiologist
Immigrant, Refugee, and Migrant Health Branch
Division of Global Migration and Quarantine
Centers for Disease Control and Prevention
Atlanta, Georgia

Nicholas Weinberg, MD
Assistant Professor
Department of Emergency Medicine
Geisel School of Medicine
Dartmouth-Hitchcock Medical Center
Hanover, New Hampshire

Melanie Wellington, MD, PhD
Associate Professor
Department of Pediatrics
University of Rochester Medical Center
Rochester, New York

Robert C. Welliver Sr, MD
Professor of Pediatrics
Division of Pediatric Infectious Diseases
University of Oklahoma Health Sciences Center
Oklahoma City, Oklahoma;
Emeritus Professor of Pediatrics
Division of Pediatric Infectious Diseases
SUNY at Buffalo and Children's Hospital
Buffalo, New York

J. Gary Wheeler, MD, MPS
Professor of Pediatrics
Division of Infectious Diseases
University of Arkansas for Medical Sciences
Little Rock, Arkansas

A. Clinton White Jr, MD
Professor, Division of Infectious Disease
Department of Internal Medicine
University of Texas Medical Branch
Galveston, Texas

Suzanne Whitworth, MD
Medical Director
Department of Pediatric Infectious Diseases
Cook Children's Healthcare System
Fort Worth, Texas

Bernhard L. Wiedermann, MD, MA
Professor
Department of Pediatrics
George Washington University School of Medicine and Health Sciences;
Attending Physician
Division of Infectious Diseases
Children's National Health System
Washington, DC

John V. Williams, MD
Professor and Chief
Pediatric Infectious Diseases
Henry L. Hillman Chair in Pediatric Immunology
Children's Hospital of Pittsburgh of UPMC
Pittsburgh, Pennsylvania

Natalie M. Williams-Bouyer, PhD, D(ABMM)
Associate Professor, Department of Pathology
Associate Director, Division of Clinical Microbiology
University of Texas Medical Branch;
Clinical Consultant, Clinical Laboratory Services
Shriners Hospitals for Children
Galveston, Texas

Charles R. Woods Jr, MD, MS
Professor and Vice Chair for Faculty Development
Department of Pediatrics
University of Louisville School of Medicine
Louisville, Kentucky

Terry W. Wright, PhD
Associate Professor
Department of Pediatrics
University of Rochester Medical Center
Rochester, New York

Nave Yeganeh, MD, MPH
Assistant Professor
Department of Pediatrics
Division of Pediatric Infectious Diseases
David Geffen School of Medicine at UCLA
Los Angeles, California

Edward J. Young, MD
Professor of Medicine
Baylor College of Medicine
Houston, Texas

Ramia Zakhour, MD
Clinical Instructor
Department of Pediatrics and Adolescent Medicine
Division of Pediatric Infectious Diseases
American University of Beirut
Beirut, Lebanon

Theoklis Zaoutis, MD, MSCE
Professor of Pediatrics and Epidemiology
Perelman School of Medicine at the University of Pennsylvania;
Associate Chief
Division of Infectious Diseases
Children's Hospital of Philadelphia
Philadelphia, Pennsylvania

Preface

Morbidity and mortality rates related to infectious diseases decreased dramatically during the first half of the 20th century in the developed world because of major improvements in public health (e.g., clean water, adequate sanitation, and vector control) and personal health. Further major reductions occurred in the second half of that century following the introduction of antimicrobial therapy, as well as active and passive immunization efforts. Despite these advances, infectious diseases in the developed world remain the leading cause of morbidity in infants and children in the 21st century. Children in the United States continue to experience three to nine respiratory infections and one to three gastrointestinal illnesses annually, requiring visits to physicians that outnumber the visits made for the purpose of well-child care. Infectious diseases are also the most common cause of school absenteeism.

Children in low and middle income countries also experience high rates of respiratory and gastrointestinal infections, which are often more severe and more frequent than those in children in the developed world. In addition, in the developing world there are great morbidity and mortality due to parasitic and vector-borne diseases. Also of importance are "spillover" infectious diseases such as Ebola, which because of increased urbanization resulted in an extensive epidemic in three African countries in 2014–15. In addition, mosquito-borne diseases such as Zika and Chikungunya have increased in prevalence in the Americas.

In more recent years, the emergence of resistance to multiple antibiotics by a large number of bacterial microorganisms (e.g., community-associated methicillin-resistant *Staphylococcus aureus*) has contributed to this infection-related morbidity and mortality, as have new infectious agents (e.g., SARS and MERS coronaviruses) and changes in the clinical manifestations and severity of established infectious agents (e.g., enterovirus 71, swine influenza).

The first edition of *Textbook of Pediatric Infectious Diseases* was written because Drs. Feigin and Cherry and many of their colleagues were concerned that no single reference text existed that comprehensively covered infectious diseases in children and adolescents. With each subsequent edition, including this one, the goal has been to provide comprehensive coverage of all subjects pertinent to the study of infectious diseases in children. Any attempt to summarize our present understanding of infectious diseases for serious students of the subject is a formidable task. In many areas, new information continues to accrue so rapidly that material becomes dated before it can appear in a text of this magnitude. Nevertheless, in this edition the editors and their author colleagues have endeavored to provide the most comprehensive and up-to-date discussion of pediatric infectious diseases ever compiled. This new edition is available online as well as in print. Purchasers can access the online version by registering their personal identification number (PIN) (found on the inside front cover of the book) at expertconsult.inkling.com. Online access includes not only fully searchable text, photos, illustrations, and tables, but also references linked to PubMed.

To provide a text as comprehensive and authoritative as possible, we, the editors, have enlisted contributions from a large number of individuals whose collective expertise is responsible for whatever success we may have had in meeting our objective. We offer our most profound appreciation to the 307 fellow contributors from nearly 100 universities or institutions in 18 countries for their professional expertise and devoted scholarship. Their cooperation and willingness to work with us leave us deeply in their debt. Of note is the fact that 10 authors (Carol Baker, Ken Boyer, Jim Cherry, Morven Edwards, Chuck Grose, Scott Halstead, Maggie Hammerschlag, Shelly Kaplan, Ed Mason, and Barbara Stechenberg) have contributed to all eight editions of *Textbook of Pediatric Infectious Diseases*.

Once again, infectious diseases are discussed according to organ systems that may be affected, as well as individually by microorganisms. In all sections in which diseases related to specific agents are discussed, emphasis has been placed, to the greatest extent possible, on the specificity of clinical manifestations that may be related to the organism causing the disease. Detailed information regarding the best means to establish a diagnosis and explicit recommendations for therapy are provided. In the present era of instant information, we have noted that historical perspectives relating to disease categories, as well as specific agents, are ignored. Because history is an important teacher, we have retained relevant historical details in this eighth edition.

Throughout the 37 years and eight-edition history of the *Textbook of Pediatric Infectious Diseases*, a number of classic chapters exist (e.g., measles, rubella, enteroviruses, and mycoplasma infections). The data in these chapters are unavailable in any other single-source publication.

The entire text of this eighth edition has been revised extensively. The seventh edition contained almost 4000 pages even though we included only new references in the print edition, which is close to the maximum that can be included in a two-volume book. Therefore, with this eighth edition, we were faced with a major dilemma: specifically, how to include new important material that had become available since the seventh edition but not to substantially increase the size of the book. We approached this dilemma in two ways. One problem in previous editions was redundancy, which we have addressed by combining information in some previous separate chapters into more concise single presentations and by shortening some chapters. The second way, which we introduced in the last edition, is to print only new references. The electronic version of the text contains all references.

This edition continues the format that was initiated in the fourth edition, in that infections with specific microorganisms have been organized to provide appropriate emphasis on the common features that may relate specific microorganisms to one another. Thus, all gram-positive coccal organisms are presented sequentially and are followed by gram-negative cocci, gram-positive bacilli, enterobacteria, gram-negative coccobacilli, Treponemataceae, anaerobic bacteria, and so forth. In addition, special sections of the text have been devoted to discussions of each of the following: molecular determinants of microbial pathogenesis; immunologic and phagocytic responses to infection; metabolic response of the host to infections; interaction of infection and nutrition; pathogenesis and treatment of fever; the human microbiome; epidemiology and biostatistics of infectious diseases; infections of the compromised host; Kawasaki disease; chronic fatigue syndrome; international travel issues for children; infectious disease problems of international adoptees and refugees; nosocomial infections; prevention and control of infections in hospitalized children; pharmacology and pharmacokinetics of antibacterial, antiviral, antifungal, and antiparasitic agents; immunomodulating agents; active and passive immunizing agents; public health considerations; infections in day care environments; and use of the bacteriology, mycology, parasitology, virology, and serology laboratories. The section on infections in the compromised host has again been expanded. This expansion has been necessitated by the large number of children, particularly transplant recipients, who have many infectious disease problems and constitute a large part of the consulting practice of many pediatric infectious disease physicians.

With some sadness, we have retained a section on bioterrorism, which is necessitated by the current state of world affairs. The section on immunomodulating agents and their potential use in the treatment of infectious diseases has been expanded because information on this subject has become more extensive since the publication of the last edition. We have also expanded the section on Ebola virus and included a new chapter on Zika virus.

This project could not have been brought to fruition without the help and assistance of many people whose names do not appear in the text. No words are sufficient to adequately convey our gratitude appropriately; we hope that they know they have our heartfelt thanks.

We would like to single out certain individuals for specific mention. First and foremost, we convey our appreciation to Laura Wennstrom Sheehan for the many hours she devoted to this edition. In her spare time between her position as Manager of Research Administration for the UCLA Department of Family Medicine and raising her young daughter, she coordinated the overall process of moving the book forward. She tended to numerous details relating to copyediting, transcribing, references, timing, and communication between the editors and Elsevier. Her expertise in EndNote was invaluable to the authors, editors, and publishing team for the organization of countless references throughout this edition. We are extremely grateful to have her as a part of our team. We would also like to acknowledge the hard work of Jordan Mann who assisted Laura throughout this process.

The following students at UCLA played a key role in processing chapters and in particular helping with references: Lauren M. Nguyen, David Dang, and Jewel Powe. We would also like to thank Nathaniel Wilder Wolf at Baylor who coordinated all the parasite chapters.

Of course this eighth edition of *Textbook of Pediatric Infectious Diseases* would not have been possible without Elsevier. We have been particularly fortunate to have been able to work with Kate Dimock, Executive Content Strategist, Clinical Solutions at Elsevier throughout the whole process relating to this eighth edition. In addition, the initial planning contribution by Lauren Elise Boyle, Content Development Specialist, was invaluable. This was followed-up by the day-to-day contributions of Margaret Nelson, also a Content Development Specialist at Elsevier. Margaret kept everyone on track in meeting deadlines.

Finally, we thank the Baylor College of Medicine and Texas Children's Hospital in Houston, Texas, the David Geffen School of Medicine at UCLA and the Mattel Children's Hospital UCLA in Los Angeles, California, and Duke University School of Medicine in Durham, North Carolina for providing an environment that is supportive of intellectual pursuits.

James D. Cherry, MD
Gail J. Harrison, MD
Sheldon L. Kaplan, MD
William J. Steinbach, MD
Peter J. Hotez, MD

Contents

VOLUME ONE

PART I Host-Parasite Relationships and the Pathogenesis of Infectious Diseases

PART II Infection of Specific Organ Systems

SECTION 1 Upper Respiratory Tract Infections

SECTION 2 Lower Respiratory Tract Infections

SECTION 3 Infections of the Heart

SECTION 4 Central Nervous System Infections

SECTION 5 Genitourinary Tract Infections

PART

I

Host-Parasite Relationships and the Pathogenesis of Infectious Diseases

1 Molecular Determinants of Microbial Pathogenesis

David A. Hunstad • Ravi Jhaveri • Audrey R. Odom John • Joseph W. St. Geme III

Despite the availability of a wide variety of antimicrobial agents and expansion of vaccination programs, infectious diseases remain a leading cause of childhood morbidity and mortality worldwide. A number of factors contribute to the increasing importance of infectious agents: rates of antimicrobial resistance continue to rise, global travel has become routine, and the number of individuals with altered immunity has increased. Furthermore, in recent years, microorganisms have been implicated in diseases previously considered noninfectious, and a variety of new, emerging, and reemerging pathogens have been recognized.

Pathogens are defined as microorganisms that are capable of causing disease. However, not all pathogens are equal with respect to their pathogenic potential (i.e., their virulence). Many pathogens are, in fact, commensal organisms that live in harmony with their host under most conditions, causing disease only when normal immune mechanisms are disrupted or absent. Other pathogens produce disease even in the setting of intact host defenses and almost always cause symptoms.

For a given microbe, pathogenic potential is often determined by the genomic content and regulation of virulence-associated genes. Some bacterial species are capable of natural transformation and readily acquire fragments of DNA from other organisms, thus expanding or altering their genetic composition, occasionally with consequences related to virulence or antimicrobial resistance. A number of microorganisms carry virulence-associated genes on mobile genetic elements, including plasmids, transposons, and bacteriophages. These elements may equip the organism with genetic information that facilitates rapid adaptation to an unfavorable or changing environment. Comparison of genomes from pathogenic and nonpathogenic bacteria within a single genus or species has led to the identification of *pathogenicity islands*, which are large blocks of chromosomal DNA that are present in pathogens and absent from related nonpathogens. These blocks are flanked by insertion sequences or repeat elements and differ in nucleotide composition relative to the surrounding genome, suggesting acquisition by horizontal exchange. Pathogenicity islands in bacteria encode a variety of virulence factors, including protein secretion systems, secreted effector molecules, adhesins, and regulatory proteins. In an analogous way, some viral pathogens such as influenza virus are capable of exchanging nucleic acid segments with other viruses, leading to changes in pathogenicity, host tropism, and transmissibility.

To be successful, a pathogen must enter the host, occupy an appropriate niche, and then multiply. Sometimes the pathogen will induce damage to the host and then spread to other tissues, either near the initial site of infection or more distant. Often the pathogen will stop short of causing death to the host, maintaining latent infection or producing symptoms such as cough or diarrhea that facilitate spread to another host. This chapter addresses several key steps in the pathogenic process, each illustrated with examples of pathogens and paradigms of relevance to infectious diseases in children.

COLONIZATION

Most bacterial infections begin with microbial colonization of a host surface, typically the skin, the respiratory tract, the gastrointestinal tract, or the genitourinary tract. Although colonization is not sufficient for an organism to produce disease, it is a necessary prerequisite. The process of bacterial colonization requires specialized microbial factors, called adhesins, that promote adherence to host structures and enable these organisms to overcome local mechanical defenses such as mucociliary function, peristalsis, and urinary flow. The cognate receptors for these interactions are generally either carbohydrate or protein structures, in some cases expressed on host cells and in other instances present in mucosal secretions or in submucosal tissue.

Pilus Adhesins

Perhaps most common among bacterial adhesins are hairlike fibers called pili (also called fimbriae). Pili are heteropolymeric protein structures comprised largely of a major subunit usually ranging in size from 15 to 25 kDa. Because of their size and morphology, most pili can be visualized by negative-staining transmission electron microscopy.

The prototype example among adhesive pili is the P (or Pap) pilus, which is expressed by uropathogenic *Escherichia coli* (UPEC) and has been strongly associated with pyelonephritis. P pili recognize globoseries glycolipids, which are host molecules that are characterized by a core structure consisting of Gal-α1,4-Gal. The globoseries glycolipids are especially abundant in renal epithelium,[25] thus accounting for the predilection of P-piliated *E. coli* to adhere to kidney tissue and cause pyelonephritis. Type 1 pili are analogous fibers expressed by UPEC and bind mannosylated uroplakin proteins in the mammalian bladder to initiate cystitis.[153] As shown in Fig. 1.1, P pili are composite structures and consist of two subassemblies, including a thick rod that emanates from the bacterial surface and a thin tip fibrillum that extends distally.[173,270] The pilus rod is a right-handed helical cylinder and is composed of repeating PapA subunits, whereas the tip fibrillum has an open helical configuration and contains mostly repeating PapE subunits. The two subassemblies are joined to each other by the PapK adaptor protein. PapG contains the adhesive moiety and is located at the distal end of the tip fibrillum, joined to PapE by the PapF adaptor.[150]

P pili are assembled through a canonical process termed the *chaperone-usher pathway* that involves a periplasmic chaperone (PapD) and an outer membrane usher (PapC) (see Fig. 1.1).[65,174] Subunit proteins (e.g., PapA) are translated in the bacterial cytoplasm, enter the periplasm through the inner membrane Sec machinery, and are stabilized by interaction with the chaperone, which ferries them to the usher. Extrusion of the nascent fiber is controlled by a "plug" domain in the usher pore; because the periplasm is devoid of adenosine triphosphate (ATP), the assembly process is energetically driven by the entropically favorable final conformation of the incorporated subunits.[189,259] More than 30 different bacterial adhesive structures are assembled via this chaperone-usher pathway, with distinct PapD-like chaperones and PapC-like ushers. The PapD-like chaperones can be divided into two distinct subfamilies based on conserved structural differences that occur near the subunit binding site.[138] One subfamily is involved in the assembly of rod-like pili similar to P pili, whereas the second subfamily participates in the biogenesis of more atypical filamentous structures, such as Caf1 of *Yersinia pestis* (the plague bacterium), which forms an amorphous "mat" on the bacterial surface. Thus the nature of the chaperone is directly correlated with the architecture of the adhesive appendage that it helps to assemble.[285]

Type 4 pili represent a second class of pili and are distinguished by a methylated first amino acid (usually phenylalanine); a short, positively charged leader sequence; a conserved hydrophobic N-terminal domain; and a tendency to form bundle-like structures. Type 4 pili have been identified in a number of gram-negative bacterial pathogens, including *Neisseria gonorrhoeae, N. meningitidis*, enteropathogenic *E. coli* (EPEC), *Vibrio cholerae, Pseudomonas aeruginosa, Kingella kingae, Eikenella corrodens, Haemophilus influenzae*, and *Moraxella* species.[32,99,193,208,250,256,272,296,323] Although the mechanism of

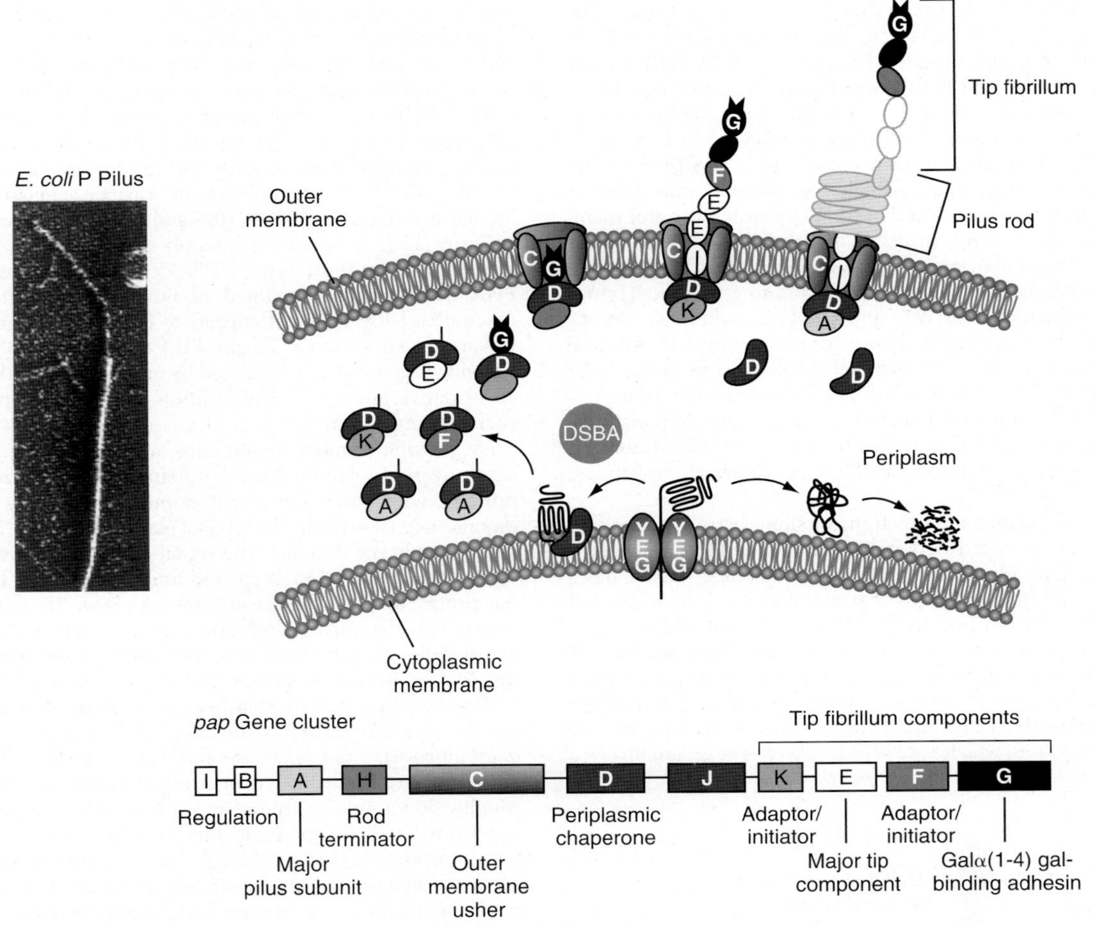

FIG. 1.1 Biogenesis and structure of *Escherichia coli* P pili. The *pap* gene cluster and the function of each of the gene products are indicated in the lower portion of the figure. Nascent pilin subunits are complexed with the PapD chaperone and added to the base of the developing pilus via the PapC usher. The mature pilus rod is composed of repeating units of PapA; the tip fibrillum contains the adhesin PapG. The ultrastructure of the pilus is shown in the electron micrograph at the left side of the figure. (Courtesy S.J. Hultgren and F.J. Sauer.)

assembly of type 4 pili is still being elucidated, existing data suggest that the process is complex. For example, between 20 and 40 gene products are required for the assembly of *P. aeruginosa* type 4 pili, and at least 15 plasmid-encoded proteins are involved in the biogenesis of EPEC type 4 pili.[127,294] Based on studies of *P. aeruginosa*, EPEC, *Neisseria*, and *V. cholerae*, the presence of an inner membrane prepilin peptidase appears to be a general prerequisite for type 4 pilus biogenesis.[161,176,226] Type 4 pili are often glycosylated, with carbohydrate decoration affecting function in at least some cases and perhaps serving to obscure antigenic epitopes.[33,190,278,319] However, despite marked differences in the assembly pathways for type 4 pili and P pili, shared structural themes exist. For example, gonococcal type 4 pili are composed predominantly of PilE structural subunits polymerized into a helical rod.[235] A minor phase-variable adhesive protein called PilC is displayed at the tip of gonococcal pili and is essential for pilus-mediated binding to epithelial cells.[154,267] These observations suggest that *N. gonorrhoeae* pili may be composite structures with a tip-associated adhesin, analogous to P pili and other pili assembled by the chaperone-usher pathway.

Although adhesive pili are more prevalent in gram-negative bacteria, they are also found in some gram-positive species. One example is *Streptococcus parasanguinis*, an oral pathogen and a member of the *S. sanguinis* family. This organism binds to calcium phosphate (the primary mineral component of tooth enamel) and also to other oral bacteria, epithelial cells, platelets, and fibronectin. Several adhesins mediate these binding functions, including pili referred to as *long fimbriae*. Based on studies of *S. parasanguinis* strain FW213, long fimbriae are fashioned primarily from Fap1, a 200-kDa protein that includes an unusually long (50 amino acids) signal sequence and a cell-wall sorting signal typical of other gram-positive bacterial surface proteins.[338,339] Specific glycosylation of Fap1 appears critical to the adhesive function of this fimbrial protein.[27,293,337] Interestingly, similar to gram-negative bacterial pili, long fimbriae appear to have a composite structure with a pilus tip. The tip contains an additional adhesin called FimA, which in purified form is capable of blocking bacterial adherence to saliva-coated hydroxyapatite.[81,231] In work by Burnette-Curley and coworkers, disruption of the *fimA* gene resulted in a 7- to 20-fold reduction in the incidence of endocarditis after intravenous inoculation of rats.[29] Other gram-positive organisms capable of expressing pili include *Streptococcus pneumoniae* (a common cause of respiratory tract and invasive disease),[11,216] *Streptococcus agalactiae* (group B streptococcus; a common cause of neonatal pneumonia, sepsis, and meningitis),[73,264] and *Enterococcus faecalis* (a cause of endocarditis and urinary tract infections).[215,277]

Nonpilus Adhesins

Beyond pili, a variety of nonpilus adhesins exist. In most cases, nonpilus adhesins are surface-expressed monomeric or oligomeric proteins, although isolated examples of carbohydrate- and lipid-containing adhesive structures have been identified. In general, these molecules are more difficult to visualize by electron microscopy, reflecting their smaller size. Similar to pili, for the most part nonpilus adhesins can be classified according to their mechanism of secretion and presentation on the bacterial surface.

Among the best-characterized bacterial nonpilus adhesins is filamentous hemagglutinin (FHA), a surface protein expressed by *Bordetella pertussis* and other *Bordetella* species. The export of FHA to the surface of the organism occurs via the so-called two-partner secretion (TPS) *pathway*, a conserved strategy in which a secreted protein (TpsA) interacts with a cognate outer membrane transporter (TpsB).[128] In *B. pertussis*, the TpsA-type protein FHA is transported by a TpsB-type outer membrane protein called FhaC, which has β-barrel pore-forming properties and facilitates translocation of FHA across the outer membrane.[333] Homologous TpsB proteins in other species export the hemolysins of *Serratia marcescens, Proteus mirabilis*, and *Haemophilus ducreyi*; the *H. influenzae* heme:hemopexin binding protein (HxuA); and the *H. influenzae* HMW1 and HMW2 adhesins, among others.[9,46,234,249,287,316] The crystal structure of FhaC reveals a 16-stranded β-barrel that is occluded by an N-terminal α-helix and an extracellular loop and a periplasmic module composed of two polypeptide-transport-associated (POTRA) domains. Functional studies have demonstrated that the N terminus of FHA interacts with the FhaC POTRA 1 domain, illuminating what appears to be a general feature of interactions between TpsA and TpsB proteins.[39,104]

Examination of purified FHA by transmission electron microscopy and circular dichroism spectroscopy showed that the FHA molecule is 50 nm in length and adopts the shape of a horseshoe nail. It has a globular head, a 37-nm-long shaft that averages 4 nm in width but tapers slightly from the head end, and a small flexible tail (Fig. 1.2).[157,188] In the crystal structure of the N terminus of FHA (the so-called TPS domain that interacts with FhaC), a series of 19-residue repeat motifs form a β-helix that is central to the overall structure of full-length FHA.[40] Consistent with its large size, FHA contains at least five separate binding domains, four of which have been localized. The region involved in adherence to sulfated saccharides has been mapped to the N terminus of the FHA molecule.[206] Sulfated saccharides such as heparin and heparan sulfate are a major component of mucus and extracellular matrix in the respiratory tract and are also found on the surface of epithelial cells.[195,342] The region that recognizes lactosylceramides and promotes adherence to ciliated respiratory epithelial cells and macrophages has been localized to amino acids 1141 to 1279 (the carbohydrate recognition domain).[251] An arginine-glycine-aspartic acid (RGD) tripeptide is located at amino acids 1097 to 1099 and interacts with leukocyte response integrin (LRI), a leukocyte integrin that stimulates upregulation of complement receptor type 3 (CR3).[146] The C terminus of mature FHA has been demonstrated to interact with epithelial cells and macrophage-like cells and appears to modulate the immune response to *Bordetella* infection.[155] Finally, FHA recognizes CR3 (CD11b/CD18), allowing organisms to be ingested by macrophages without stimulating an oxidative burst.[258,336] The location of the CR3-binding domain is currently unknown.

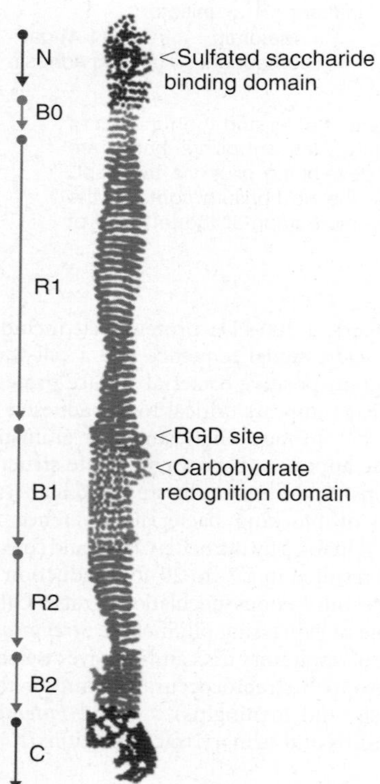

FIG. 1.2 Ribbon representation model structure of filamentous hemagglutinin from *Bordetella pertussis.* There are five regions that are assigned β-helical coils, designated B0, R1, B1, R2, and B2. The N terminus of the protein is designated with "N," and the C terminus of the protein is designated with "C." The locations of the sulfated saccharide binding domain, the carbohydrate recognition domain, and the RGD tripeptide are noted. (From Kajava AV, Cheng N, Cleaver R, et al. Beta-helix model for the filamentous haemagglutinin adhesin of *Bordetella pertussis* and related bacterial secretory proteins. *Mol Microbiol.* 2001;42:279–92.)

A growing number of nonpilus adhesins belong to the so-called autotransporter family. These proteins are synthesized as precursor proteins with three functional domains, including an N-terminal canonical signal sequence, an internal passenger domain, and a C-terminal outer membrane domain. The signal sequence directs the protein to the Sec machinery and is cleaved after it facilitates transport of the polypeptide from the cytoplasm to the periplasm. The C-terminal domain inserts into the outer membrane and forms a β-barrel with a central hydrophilic channel. Ultimately, the passenger domain is presented on the surface of the organism and influences interaction with host molecules.[120] Recent studies have established that autotransporter proteins can be separated into two distinct groups, designated *conventional autotransporters* and *trimeric autotransporters* (Fig. 1.3).[52] In conventional autotransporters, the C-terminal outer membrane domain contains roughly 300 amino acids and is a monomeric β-barrel with a single N-terminal α-helix spanning the pore (Fig. 1.4A).[232,299] In trimeric autotransporters, the C-terminal outer membrane domain contains approximately 70 amino acids and forms heat- and detergent-resistant trimers in the outer membrane. Each trimer forms a β-barrel with four strands from each of the three subunits and with three N-terminal α-helices spanning the pore (Fig. 1.4B).[204]

One example of a conventional autotransporter adhesin is the *H. influenzae* Hap protein, which was discovered based on its ability to promote adherence and low-level invasion in assays with cultured human epithelial cells.[286] Hap also promotes bacterial binding to extracellular matrix proteins and bacterial microcolony formation.[83,121] Examination of chimeric proteins and studies with purified protein have demonstrated that the adhesive activity responsible for Hap-mediated adherence, invasion, binding to extracellular matrix proteins, and microcolony formation localizes to the passenger domain, referred to as Hap_S.[83,121] More detailed characterization of Hap_S has established that the region responsible for interaction with host epithelial cells and microcolony formation resides in the C-terminal 311 amino acids and may have utility as a vaccine antigen.[57,82,183] This region folds into a triangular prism-like structure that can mediate Hap-Hap dimerization and higher degrees of multimerization, thus facilitating interbacterial interaction and microcolony formation.[202] A prototype member of the trimeric autotransporter subfamily is the *H. influenzae* Hia adhesin. This protein is expressed in a subset of nontypable *H. influenzae* strains and contains two homologous high-affinity trimeric binding domains, creating the potential for stable multivalent interaction with respiratory epithelial cells.[175,203,343]

Another group of nonpilus adhesins is typified by intimin, a protein expressed by enteropathogenic *E. coli* (EPEC), enterohemorrhagic *E. coli* (EHEC), and the murine pathogen *Citrobacter rodentium.* Intimin contains a flexible N terminus, a central β-barrel domain that integrates into the outer membrane, and a C-terminal binding domain that interacts with the translocated intimin receptor (Tir).[311] Tir is an interesting example of a pathogen-derived receptor that is inserted into target host cells. After initial cell attachment mediated by type 4 pili, EPEC employs a type III secretion system (discussed in detail later in this chapter) to inject Tir into the host cell cytoplasm,[164,335] from where it is then inserted into the host cell membrane.[254] The subsequent interaction between

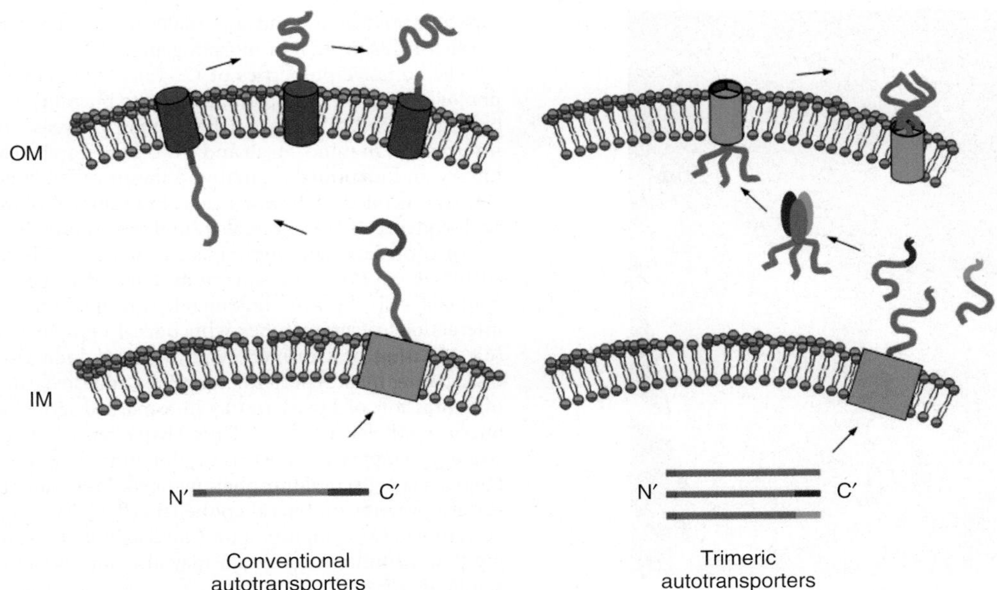

FIG. 1.3 Autotransporter protein secretion pathway. Conventional autotransporter secretion is shown on the left, and trimeric autotransporter secretion is shown on the right. Autotransporter proteins are synthesized as preproteins with three functional domains, including an N-terminal signal sequence (shown in green), an internal passenger domain (shown in red), and a C-terminal outer membrane β-barrel domain (shown in blue). IM indicates inner membrane, and OM indicates outer membrane. Protein secretion begins with export of the protein from the cytoplasm via the inner membrane Sec machinery (Sec). Most conventional autotransporters are cleaved on the bacterial surface. (From Cotter SE, Surana NK, St Geme JW III. Trimeric autotransporters: a distinct subfamily of autotransporter proteins. *Trends Microbiol.* 2005;13:199–205.)

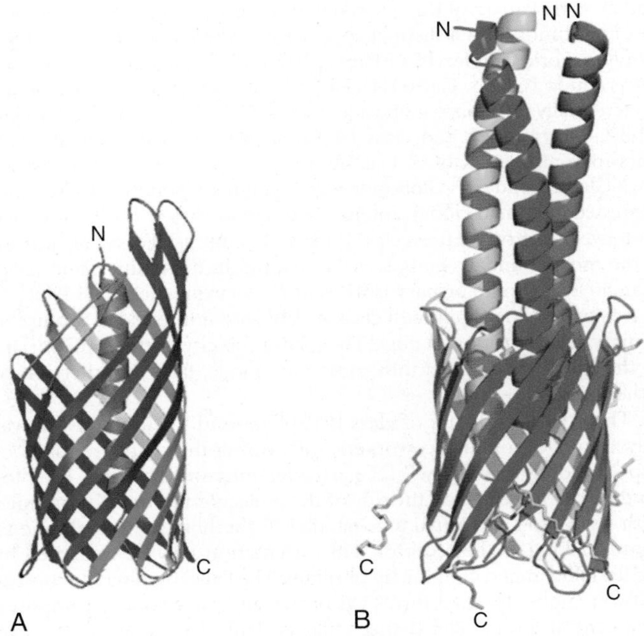

FIG. 1.4 Crystal structures of the C-terminal outer membrane β-barrel of autotransporter proteins. (A) Crystal structure of NalP, a conventional autotransporter; β strands are shown in shades of blue, and the α-helix that crosses the channel is shown in red. (B) Crystal structure of Hia, a trimeric autotransporter; individual subunits are shown in red, green, and yellow. (A, From Surana NK, Cotter SE, Yeo HJ, et al. Structural determinants of *Haemophilus influenzae* adherence to host epithelium: variations on type V secretion. In: Waksman G, Caparon MG, Hultgren SJ, editors. *Structural Basis of Bacterial Pathogenesis.* Washington, DC: American Society for Microbiology; 2005:129–148. B, From Meng G, Surana NK, St Geme JW III, et al. Structure of the outer membrane translocator domain of the *Haemophilus influenzae* Hia trimeric autotransporter. *EMBO J.* 2006;25:2297–304.)

intimin (on the bacterial surface) and Tir (now present on the host cell surface) triggers receptor clustering, dramatic rearrangement of the actin cytoskeleton, and formation of a distinctive pedestal referred to as an *attaching and effacing (A/E) lesion* (Fig. 1.5).[164,263] The bacterial genes essential for formation of A/E lesions reside within a 35-kb region of the EPEC chromosome called the locus of enterocyte effacement (LEE), an example of a pathogenicity island.[70,196] This locus is highly conserved in content and organization across all A/E pathogens and contains the genes encoding intimin, Tir, and the requisite type III secretion system. The interactions of Tir and other type III secreted effectors with host proteins influencing actin polymerization are beginning to be understood.[265,344] Tir contains domains analogous to host immunoreceptor tyrosine-based inhibition motifs (ITIM) important for regulation of eukaryotic signaling. On this basis, Tir recruits certain host proteins to regulate actin dynamics and inhibit proinflammatory signaling pathways.[61,266,280,328] Given its central role in EHEC/EPEC pathogenesis and its immunogenicity, intimin is also being examined as a target for the development of antivirulence therapeutics or vaccines in A/E diseases.

In recent years, investigators have identified a large family of nonpilus adhesins involved in adherence to host extracellular matrix proteins including fibronectin, laminin, vitronectin, collagen, fibrinogen, and a variety of proteoglycans. These adhesins have been classified as microbial surface components recognizing adhesive matrix molecules (MSCRAMMs) and are especially prevalent among gram-positive bacteria.[238] In gram-positive organisms these proteins are covalently anchored to the cell wall peptidoglycan and have a characteristic primary amino acid sequence. In particular, the C terminus contains a segment rich in proline and glycine residues, an LPXTG motif (involved in sorting and covalently anchoring the protein to the cell wall), a hydrophobic membrane-spanning domain, and a short positively charged segment that resides in the cytoplasm and serves as a cell wall retention signal. Adhesive functions are typically located near the N terminus.[85]

Staphylococcus aureus is a common gram-positive pathogen in children and is capable of producing a variety of MSCRAMMs, including collagen-binding protein (CNA), fibronectin-binding proteins A and B, and clumping factors A and B. Recent work indicates that although

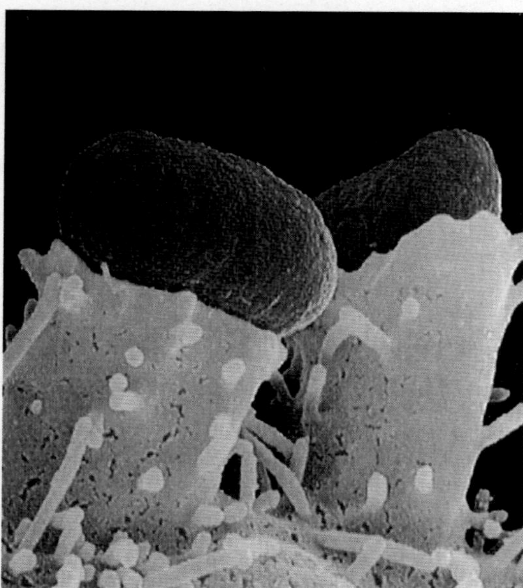

FIG. 1.5 Enteropathogenic *E. coli* are perched on pedestals in the attaching and effacing lesion. (Courtesy B.B. Finlay; from Rosenshine I, Ruschkowski S, Stein M, et al. A pathogenic bacterium triggers epithelial signals to form a functional bacterial receptor that mediates actin pseudopod formation. *EMBO J.* 1996;15:2613–24.)

these proteins mediate typical binding interactions with host proteins, they are not monospecific, and a given MSCRAMM may bind multiple host connective tissue components or multiple motifs within a single host fiber type.[284] In addition, many are capable of provoking platelet activation. *S. aureus* strains recovered from patients with septic arthritis commonly express CNA, which mediates binding to cartilage in vitro and appears to play a key role in the pathogenesis of septic arthritis in experimental mice.[237,239,300] Fibronectin-binding protein A (FnBPA) shares homology with *S. pyogenes* protein F and mediates binding to fibronectin and the γ chain of fibrinogen, as well as to elastin and tropoelastin.[162,262,322] Accordingly, this protein is important in *S. aureus* endocarditis[247] and in infections of implanted biomaterials, which become coated with fibrinogen and fibrin soon after implantation. Clumping factor (ClfA) was named based on the observation that it mediates bacterial clumping in the presence of soluble fibrinogen.[197] Similar to FnBPA, ClfA mediates binding to fibrinogen-coated surfaces in vitro and probably contributes to infections of artificial surfaces.

Other Mechanisms of Adherence

Candida albicans is a common inhabitant of mucosal surfaces and an important cause of systemic disease, especially in patients with compromised immunity. *Candida* blastospores are capable of efficient adhesion to epithelial cells, leading to budding and division. In addition, germ tube formation occurs, facilitating penetration through the epithelial barrier and then dissemination to distant sites.[135] In recent years, several candidate *C. albicans* adhesins have been identified.[10,134,180,346] Of particular interest is a protein called INT1, which shares functional homology with the vertebrate integrin family. Integrins are normally expressed by cells of the human immune system (neutrophils, monocytes, macrophages) and mediate cellular binding and shape-changing functions. Each integrin is a heterodimer of an α chain and a β chain. There are a number of distinct α and β chains, and each combination displays a unique binding specificity. INT1 is an α integrin–like protein that recognizes the RGD sequence of the C3 fragment iC3b on epithelial cells. In in vitro assays, short peptides encompassing the RGD sequence are capable of inhibiting *C. albicans* adherence by 50%, confirming that INT1 plays a significant role as an adhesin and suggesting that other adhesins also exist.[135] Beyond promoting adherence to epithelium, INT1 disguises organisms as leukocytes, allowing evasion of phagocytosis. Of note, introduction of INT1 into *Saccharomyces cerevisiae* confers a capacity for adherence and also results in germ tube formation, indicating a role for this protein in morphogenesis.[95,94]

The adhesive properties of *C. albicans* are closely tied to its morphologic state. For example, adherence to buccal epithelial cells is greater by organisms bearing germ tubes than by yeast forms.[169] With this information in mind, Staab and coworkers searched a germ tube cDNA library and identified a putative adhesin called hyphal wall protein 1 (Hwp1) encoded by the *hwp1* gene. Examination of the predicted amino acid sequence of Hwp1 revealed similarity to proteins that are substrates for mammalian transglutaminase enzymes.[290] These enzymes form a cornified envelope on squamous epithelial cells (including buccal epithelial cells) by cross-linking relevant substrates.[302] Interestingly, the interactions of germ tubes with buccal epithelial cells resist stresses (e.g., heating or treatment with sodium dodecylsulfate) capable of dissociating most typical microbe-host adhesive pairs, and elimination of expression of Hwp1 results in a marked reduction in adhesion to buccal epithelial cells.[23,289] Thus Hwp1 represents a unique adhesive strategy, employing host transglutaminase enzymes to cross-link Hwp1 (via a glycosylphosphatidylinositol remnant anchor) directly to surface proteins on buccal epithelial cells.[288] More recently, Hwp1 has been shown to be important for *Candida* biofilm formation,[77,220] indicating that a similar mechanism may also support interactions between candidal cells.

TISSUE TROPISM

Most microorganisms demonstrate restriction in the range of hosts, tissues, and cell types that they colonize. This restriction is referred to as *tropism* and generally reflects the specificity of the interaction between a given microbial adhesin and its cognate receptor. Accordingly, tropism is determined by the distribution of the relevant host receptor.

P pili of uropathogenic *E. coli* serve as the platform for presentation of one of three different PapG variants, referred to as class I, class II, and class III PapG. All three variants recognize globoseries glycolipids, but each binds with a distinct specificity to the globoseries glycolipid isotypes. For example, class I PapG preferentially recognizes globotriosylceramide (GbO3, Gal-α1,4-Gal-β1,3-Glc-ceramide), class II PapG preferentially recognizes globoside (GbO4, GalNAc-β1,3-Gal-α1,4-Gal-β1,3-Glc-ceramide), and class III PapG preferentially interacts with Forssman antigen (GbO5, GalNAc-α1,3-GalNAc-β1,3-Gal-α1,4-Gal-β1,3-Glc-ceramide).[297] Globoside is the dominant globoseries glycolipid expressed in human kidney, and most human isolates of *E. coli* associated with pyelonephritis express class II PapG. In contrast, Forssman antigen is the most abundant globoseries glycolipid in dog kidney, and more than 50% of canine urinary isolates of *E. coli* express class III PapG.[341] *E. coli*–expressing P pili with class II PapG are not found as a cause of urinary tract infection in dogs. Thus the specificity of the PapG variant at the tip of the P pilus influences host range, favoring infection of either human or dog.

The crystal structure of class II PapG bound to Gal-α1,4-Gal was solved by Dodson and coworkers, uncovering the structural basis of PapG binding specificity.[66] Of particular interest, the PapG receptor binding site is located on the side of the molecule and must be oriented with its N- to C-terminal axis parallel to the host cell membrane to allow docking to the receptor. This orientation may be facilitated by the flexibility inherent in the tip fibrillum. The PapG binding site consists of two regions. The first forms a β-barrel, and the second is composed of a central antiparallel β-sheet that is flanked on one side by two 2-stranded β-sheets and on the other side by an α-helix. When class II PapG interacts with GbO4, the arginine residue at position 170 in PapG makes contact with the GbO4 side chain. Interestingly, in class I PapG, a histidine residue occupies position 170, interfering with potential contact with the GbO4 side chain. Similarly, class II PapG and class III PapG differ in amino acids required for interaction with the GbO5 side chain.[66]

Group A streptococcus (*S. pyogenes*) is a common cause of infections of skin and soft tissue, including impetigo, cellulitis, and necrotizing fasciitis. Adherence to host cells by *S. pyogenes* is influenced by nonpilus adhesins called M protein and protein F. M protein forms a fiber and consists of a C-terminal region that anchors the protein in the cell wall, a coiled-coil rod region extending approximately 50 nm from the cell wall, and a short nonhelical domain extending more distally.[84] Protein F is a 120-kDa protein that is notable for a tandem repeat element consisting of up to six repeats of 32 to 44 amino acids adjacent to the C terminus.[112,233] M protein promotes adherence to human keratinocytes via interaction with the CD46 molecule (also called membrane cofactor protein, or MCP), whereas protein F mediates adherence to epidermal Langerhans cells, which are located in the basal layer of the epidermis.[229,230] Thus both M protein and protein F contribute to group A streptococcal adherence to the skin, but each protein directs interaction with a different population of epidermal cells.

Early studies demonstrated that human immunodeficiency virus type 1 (HIV-1) infects CD4$^+$ cells and interacts with the CD4 molecule but that CD4 alone is not sufficient to permit infection. More recent observations have established that a number of host cell chemokine receptors, especially CCR5 and CXCR4, serve as coreceptors for HIV-1 and are required for viral entry into CD4$^+$ target cells. These coreceptors appear to influence the cellular tropism displayed by different HIV-1 variants.[62] All HIV variants are able to replicate in primary T cells, but only some can also replicate in primary macrophages or in immortalized T-cell lines. Asymptomatic HIV-infected individuals carry strains that generally use CCR5 as a coreceptor (termed *M5 strains*) and are non–syncytium-inducing in vitro. Such strains have classically been described as macrophage tropic (M-tropic), but recent experiments have demonstrated that these M5 strains can also infect CD4$^+$ T cells and peripheral blood mononuclear cells.[245] Rapid viral mutation due to the error-prone HIV polymerase and HIV reverse transcriptase leads to the production within the host of syncytium-inducing, T-cell–tropic (T-tropic) HIV-1 strains, which predominate in the circulation of patients with acquired immunodeficiency syndrome.[62] These variants are generally restricted to CXCR4 (expressed on T cells) as a coreceptor, although some primary syncytium-inducing variants can use both CCR5 and CXCR4.[71,79,276] T-tropic, syncytium-inducing strains are characterized by positively charged residues at fixed positions of the V3 loop and changes in charge and length of the V2 region of the viral envelope glycoprotein gp120, which binds to CD4 and coreceptors before viral entry into host cells.[86,87,106] Thus cellular tropism is closely aligned, but not synonymous, with HIV coreceptor usage.

New HIV-1 infection is selectively established by M-tropic HIV-1 strains, even if the transmitting host harbors more pathogenic non–M-tropic strains as well.[317,352] CCR5 is also expressed on the surface of rectal and vaginal epithelial cells, which may be sites of initial encounter between HIV-1 and the human host.[349] The importance of CCR5 in HIV-1 binding to CD4$^+$ cells is underscored by the observation that individuals homozygous for a 32-bp deletion in CCR5 (the Δ32 allele) are resistant to infection with HIV-1.[137,184] The Δ32 heterozygous state does not necessarily protect against HIV-1 acquisition, although HIV disease in heterozygous patients may follow an attenuated course. This allele is surprisingly frequent (10%–14%) in white populations, leading to speculation that it provided a survival advantage during one or more historical epidemics of infectious diseases.[225] However, more recent data suggest that the Δ32 allele may actually confer immune deficiency in the presence of challenge with certain viral pathogens, such as West Nile virus.[100,101] Of note, CCR5 may have a role in controlling the development of malignancy, including lymphoma, raising some concern about developing anti-HIV pharmacologic agents that target CCR5 function.[178] Finally, co-evolution of viral determinants and host cell receptors may determine the spectrum of tissue and organ involvement within the host. For example, the chemokine receptor CCR8 may facilitate the entry of neurotropic HIV-1 strains into brain cells,[152] and envelopes derived from brain isolates of HIV are adapted to infect cells with low-level CD4/CCR5 expression, such as neuroglia and brain macrophages.[244]

Other viruses also demonstrate tropism for specific cells or tissues within the host. Hepatitis C virus (HCV) has been demonstrated to use multiple cell surface molecules in sequence to locate and gain entry into target cells. HCV is bound to low-density lipoprotein (LDL) in serum and first binds to scavenger-receptor B1 (SR-B1), which is enriched on liver cells and serves to bind lipoprotein molecules.[34] After this initial binding event, HCV E2 protein interacts with the CD81 molecule, the critical receptor for free virus.[159,321,351] Once virus has bound to CD81, this virus-receptor complex traffics to the gap junction, where the virus interacts with two key gap junction proteins, claudin-1 and occludin-1, to enter cells.[78,114,172] Human occludin-1 recently has been shown to be necessary for HCV entry into mouse cells, an advance that will facilitate disease modeling in the laboratory.[248] Although the liver does not exclusively express any of these four molecules, the combination of these four, the structural organization of liver cells, and other yet-undetermined intracellular factors account for the tropism of HCV for the liver.[246]

Similar observations have been made for coxsackievirus isolates, which bind to the coxsackie-adenovirus receptor (CAR) molecule located in the tight junction for entry into cells.[12,42,53,158] Brain, heart, and muscle cells are enriched for CAR in the fetal and neonatal period, whereas adult cells from these tissues express significantly lower levels of the receptor.[131,147] This developmental difference in CAR density is the likely explanation for severe coxsackievirus infections that are disproportionately seen in infants and young children compared with adults. CAR then allows for an interaction with the tight junction that is mediated by occludin-1, which allows for viral co-opting of host trafficking pathways.[53]

Among eukaryotic pathogens, tissue tropism can also be a major determinant of virulence. Cerebral malaria is a life-threatening consequence of infection with the protozoan parasite *Plasmodium falciparum* and results from adherence of parasite-infected erythrocytes to cerebral vascular endothelium.[209] During erythrocyte infection, the malaria parasite exports a variety of surface receptors to the host plasma membrane. The *P. falciparum* erythrocyte membrane protein 1 (PfEMP1) multigene family represents a highly variable set of such receptors, only one variant of which is expressed at any given time. A substantial body of work has established that different forms of PfEMP1 possess distinct tissue adherence patterns.[171] Specific classes of PfEMP1 types (Group A DC8 and DC13) are associated with cerebral vascular adherence in vitro and are correlated with severe malaria in clinical populations.[7,38,177] More recent studies suggest that these PfEMP1 forms mediate adherence through interaction with the endothelial protein C receptor.[314]

BIOFILMS

After attachment to a particular surface, a number of pathogens are capable of forming *biofilms*, which can be defined as structured communities of microbial cells enclosed in a self-produced exopolysaccharide matrix. Although most studies of biofilms have involved a single species, it is likely that biofilms relevant to human infection often involve multiple species sharing the advantages of biofilm existence. Human infections associated with biofilms include dental caries, lower airway infection with *P. aeruginosa* and other organisms in patients with cystic fibrosis, and foreign body infections in patients with prostheses and implanted devices. In addition, biofilm formation likely occurs during osteomyelitis and endocarditis.[49]

P. aeruginosa is a model organism for the study of biofilms and forms pillars of stationary (sessile) bacteria held together by an extracellular polysaccharide called alginate. Interposed among these pillars are channels that facilitate the flow of nutrients and provide pathways for motile (planktonic) organisms to move about (Fig. 1.6A). In experiments directed at defining the early steps of *P. aeruginosa* biofilm formation, O'Toole and Kolter established that flagella are required for initial bacterial attachment, presumably because these appendages promote movement toward the relevant surface. After attachment, type 4 pili and pilus-mediated twitching motility promote formation of microcolonies[227] in which transcription of *algC*, *algD*, and *algU* is activated, resulting in synthesis of alginate.[59] Pulmonary isolates from patients with cystic fibrosis often form highly mucoid colonies (reflecting expression of alginate) or can form tiny colonies on agar plates, the so-called small-colony variant (SCV) phenotype associated with biofilm formation and increased antibiotic resistance.[115,116,291]

Development of the complex community present within a biofilm requires intercellular communication to coordinate the metabolic and other activities of members of the community. *P. aeruginosa* employs several identified *quorum-sensing* systems, which involve the production

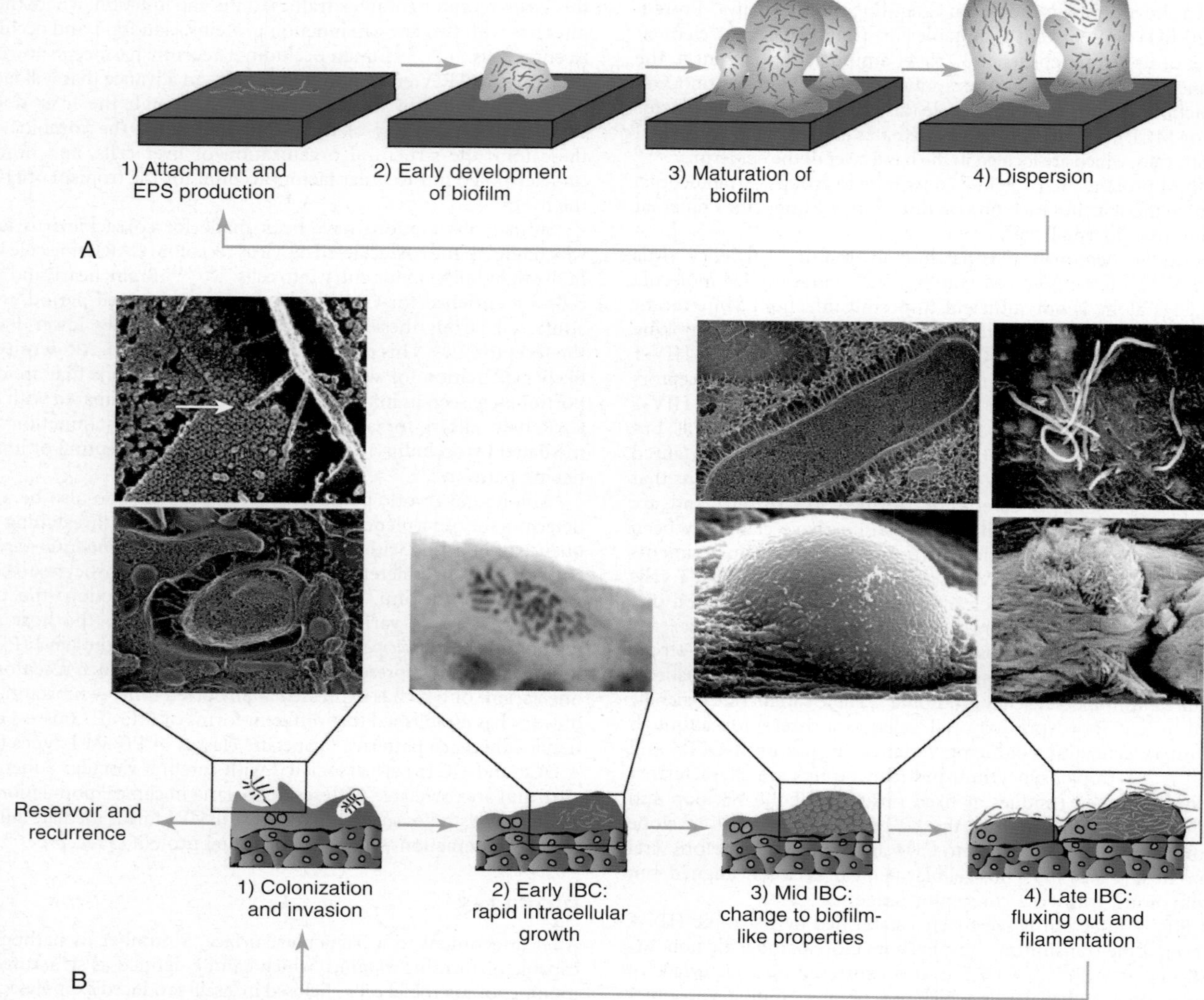

FIG. 1.6 In vitro *Pseudomonas* biofilm formation and parallel stages of formation of uropathogenic *Escherichia coli* intracellular bacterial communities (IBCs). (A) Dynamics of *P. aeruginosa* biofilm formation on an inert surface. Keys to the formation of the biofilm include flagella-mediated attachment, production of exopolysaccharide (EPS), type 4 pilus–based twitching motility, and a quorum sensing system. (B) Composite representation of the stages of IBC formation and maturation. (A, From Costerton JW, Stewart PS, Greenberg EP. Bacterial biofilms: a common cause of persistent infections. *Science.* 1999;284:1318–22, copyright 1999 American Association for the Advancement of Science. B, From Kau AL, Hunstad DA, Hultgren SJ. Interaction of uropathogenic *Escherichia coli* with host uroepithelium. *Curr Opin Microbiol.* 2005;8:54–9.)

of small molecules that are sensed by neighboring organisms and regulate gene expression in these neighbors. One well-studied system is based on the acyl-homoserine lactone called *N*-(3-oxododecanoyl)-L-homoserine lactone (3OC12-HSL).[60,236] 3OC12-HSL is synthesized in a reaction catalyzed by LasI and accumulates with increases in population density. Ultimately, 3OC12-HSL reaches a critical concentration and then interacts with LasR, serving to activate transcription of a number of genes. Host inflammatory pathways are also induced directly by accumulated 3OC12-HSL.[279] Organisms with a mutation in *lasI* are capable of attachment and microcolony formation, but the resulting microcolonies remain thin, undifferentiated, and sensitive to dispersion by detergents. Addition of the missing lactone signal to the *lasI* mutant restores development into structured, thick, biocide-resistant biofilms, as are observed with wild-type organisms.[60] In vivo, mutation in *lasI* impedes establishment of pulmonary infection in mice.[242,340]

Biofilms also play a prominent role in human infections with *Candida* species, with examples including oral thrush and catheter-associated infections. Although several pathogenic *Candida* species can form biofilms in the host, the ultrastructure and the molecular strategies underlying biofilm formation vary from one species to another. *C. albicans* is the best studied *Candida* species and relies on the expression of certain cell wall proteins (including Hwp1),[219] a regulated yeast-to-hyphal switch described earlier, and quorum-sensing molecules such as *E,E*-farnesol, which represses filamentation and can suppress the growth of other nearby bacterial and fungal species.[63,133,275]

Biofilms constitute a protected mode of growth that allows survival in a hostile environment—for example, in the presence of host immune mechanisms or antimicrobial agents.[49] Based on studies of *P. aeruginosa*, sessile bacteria release antigens and stimulate production of antibodies, but these antibodies are ineffective in killing organisms within biofilms.[41] Similarly, sessile *P. aeruginosa* stimulate a diminished oxidative burst and are relatively refractory to phagocytic uptake. In addition, fungi and bacteria within biofilms are resistant to the effects of a number of antimicrobial agents, in part because these agents are unable to diffuse into the biofilm and in part because these organisms may exist in a slow-growing or otherwise protected phenotypic state.[49] Biofilm-like microbial communities have also been described within host epithelial cells, as with uropathogenic *E. coli* in the mammalian bladder.[6] Recently, new approaches to antimicrobial therapy include novel natural products and other small molecules that inhibit quorum-sensing and biofilm formation.[36,96]

CELL ENTRY AND INTRACELLULAR LIFE

After adherence to a host surface, many pathogenic bacteria are able to invade and survive inside epithelial cells and other nonprofessional phagocytes (i.e., M cells in intestinal Peyer's patches). In addition, some pathogens are able to survive inside professional phagocytes (macrophages and neutrophils). Invasion may represent a mechanism to breach host mucosal barriers and gain access to deeper or more distant tissues. Alternatively, invasion may provide the organism with a special niche (e.g., protecting it from host immune mechanisms). In the case of viruses, cell entry ensures access to the cell machinery required for viral replication.

Generally the process of bacterial invasion involves a class of molecules called invasins that mediate adherence and entry. For many bacteria, invasion is an active event that relies on underlying host cell functions and is associated with rearrangement of the host cell cytoskeleton. Once inside the host cell, the invading or internalized organism usually is localized within a membrane-bound vacuole that contains lysosomal enzymes. In some cases the pathogen escapes from this vacuole and enters the cytoplasm, a more permissive environment. In other cases, the pathogen remains in the vacuole and neutralizes lysosomal enzymatic activity. The processes of invasion into cells, survival within cells, cell-to-cell spread, and entry into the circulation define the extent of infection and dissemination.

Invasion

In considering the molecular mechanism of bacterial invasion, perhaps best characterized are the enteropathogenic *Yersinia* species—namely, *Y. pseudotuberculosis* and *Y. enterocolitica*. These organisms are usually acquired by ingestion of contaminated food or water and typically cause self-limited enteritis or mesenteric adenitis. In infants and other individuals with compromised immunity, they sometimes produce systemic disease. The primary determinant of *Y. pseudotuberculosis* and *Y. enterocolitica* invasion is an adhesive outer membrane protein called invasin, which is encoded by a chromosomal locus called inv and binds tightly to a family of β1 integrins expressed on host cells, including α3β1 integrin on the surface of intestinal M cells.[145] The interaction between invasin and β1 integrins initiates a cascade of signaling steps in the host cell, resulting in actin rearrangement and formation of large complexes of cytoskeletal elements (talin, vinculin, α-actinin, and others) termed *focal adhesions.*[144] Bacterial entry into the host cell occurs via a "zipper-like" mechanism, with the plasma membrane zippering around the invading organism.

Beyond invasin, two additional proteins called YadA and Ail also influence invasion by enteropathogenic *Yersinia* species. YadA is a 45-kDa surface protein that is encoded by the 70-kb *Yersinia* virulence plasmid. It is highly expressed under environmental conditions (e.g., temperature of 37°C) in which invasin is repressed.[75] YadA reaches the bacterial surface via the autotransporter pathway and exists in a trimeric form that is essential for its adhesive activity.[51] Like invasin, YadA promotes invasion through binding to β1 integrins on the host cell surface, but its binding occurs indirectly via extracellular matrix molecules, including collagens, laminin, and fibronectin.[76] Based on studies using a mouse oral infection model, in *Y. enterocolitica* YadA is essential for survival and multiplication in Peyer's patches, whereas in *Y. pseudotuberculosis* YadA is dispensable for full virulence.[22] Ail is a 17-kDa outer membrane protein that also is encoded by a chromosomal locus *(ail)* and mediates high levels of adherence and low levels of invasion in assays with cultured epithelial cells. In addition, Ail mediates resistance to complement-mediated serum killing, independent of an effect on invasion.[19]

Similar to these pathogenic *Yersinia* species, *Listeria monocytogenes* invades epithelial cells via a zipper-like mechanism. Invasion is mediated by proteins called internalin A (InlA) and internalin B (InlB), which are required for virulence in animal models. InlA interacts with E-cadherin, a host cell transmembrane protein with an intracellular domain that interacts with the cytoskeleton.[205] InlB interacts with C1q on host cells and promotes invasion by activating the PI-3 kinase pathway.[24] Uropathogenic strains of *E. coli* also invade epithelial cells via a zipper-like mechanism mediated by the FimH adhesin expressed on the tip of type 1 pili. In experiments with cultured bladder epithelial cells, FimH is both necessary and sufficient for entry, as demonstrated by examination of a *fimH⁻* mutant and of latex beads coated with purified FimH.[194] In vitro experiments further suggest that FimH-mediated bacterial binding to a mannose-coated surface may be strengthened by shear forces, such as fluid flow over the surface.[307,308] After FimH-dependent invasion into superficial epithelial cells of the murine bladder, UPEC multiply rapidly to form intracellular bacterial communities, which display some features of biofilms, including community behavior, differential gene expression, and protection from antimicrobial agents (see Fig. 1.6B).[6,156,160] A subset of internalized bacteria ultimately form a quiescent bacterial reservoir within the uroepithelium that resists immune clearance and antibiotic therapy and may serve as a seed for recurrent infections.[139,213,214]

Salmonella enterica serovar *typhimurium (S. typhimurium)* is an example of a pathogen that invades cells by a mechanism distinct from zippering. On contact with the epithelial cell surface, *S. typhimurium* triggers a dramatic host cell response characterized by actin rearrangement, calcium and inositol phosphate fluxes, and a "splash" of membrane ruffling surrounding the point of entry. Bacterial internalization into the cell occurs rapidly, with organisms appearing in membrane-bound vacuoles within a few minutes of initial contact with the host cell. The determinants of *S. typhimurium* invasion are encoded by a pathogenicity island called SPI-1, located at centisome 63 on the bacterial chromosome.[92] Especially important in this region is a prototypical *type III secretion system,* which forms a needle-like complex on the bacterial surface that breaches the host cell membrane and serves to translocate bacterial proteins directly into the host cell, altering the host cell cytoskeleton[43,186] and influencing immune responses. The base of the needle complex spans both the inner and outer membranes and is about 40 nm in diameter, whereas the needle itself is 8 nm in width and approximately 80 nm in length (Fig. 1.7).[45,93]

The proteins secreted through the *S. typhimurium* needle complex (and other type III secretion systems) and into the host cell are referred to as *effector proteins.* SopE is an effector protein that mediates the initial rearrangement of actin and ruffling of the host cell membrane. It functions as a guanyl-nucleotide exchange factor (GEF) and activates two host cell Rho GTPase proteins called Rac and Cdc42.[35,111,113] SptP is an effector protein that functions as an antagonist of SopE, mediating reversal of actin rearrangement by converting Rac and Cdc42 to the inactive forms (GDP forms). Consistent with these functions, SopE and SptP directly antagonize each other when coinjected into cells.[91] Other effector proteins secreted by the *S. typhimurium* SPI-1 type III secretion system include the inositol phosphate phosphorylase SopB, which disrupts normal host cell signaling mechanisms,[224] and AvrA, which interferes with the nuclear factor κB (NF-κB) signaling pathway in host cells, thereby downregulating host inflammatory responses.[44]

Important accessory and regulatory genes are also present within SPI-1. As an example, the *sicA* gene is just upstream of the *sipB* and *sipC* genes and encodes an accessory protein with chaperone activity essential for stabilization and translocation of SipB, SipC, and SopE.[313] Other chaperones encoded by SPI-1 are involved in the stabilization and translocation of other effector proteins. The genetic and environmental factors that regulate the expression of type III secretion machinery and secreted proteins represent an area of ongoing study.[5]

In *Plasmodium falciparum*, the mechanisms of both host erythrocyte invasion and immune evasion are tightly linked. A mature parasite may release as many as 32 daughter parasites, called merozoites, into the bloodstream. In less than 30 seconds, merozoites attach to and invade new erythrocytes. High-titer antibodies to invasion proteins, as are present in the serum of semi-immune individuals living in endemic areas, can block these processes. For this reason, the molecular invasion machinery of *P. falciparum* is of considerable interest for vaccine development.[240,303] The initial contact between *Plasmodium* merozoites and host erythrocytes is weak and is thought to be mediated through

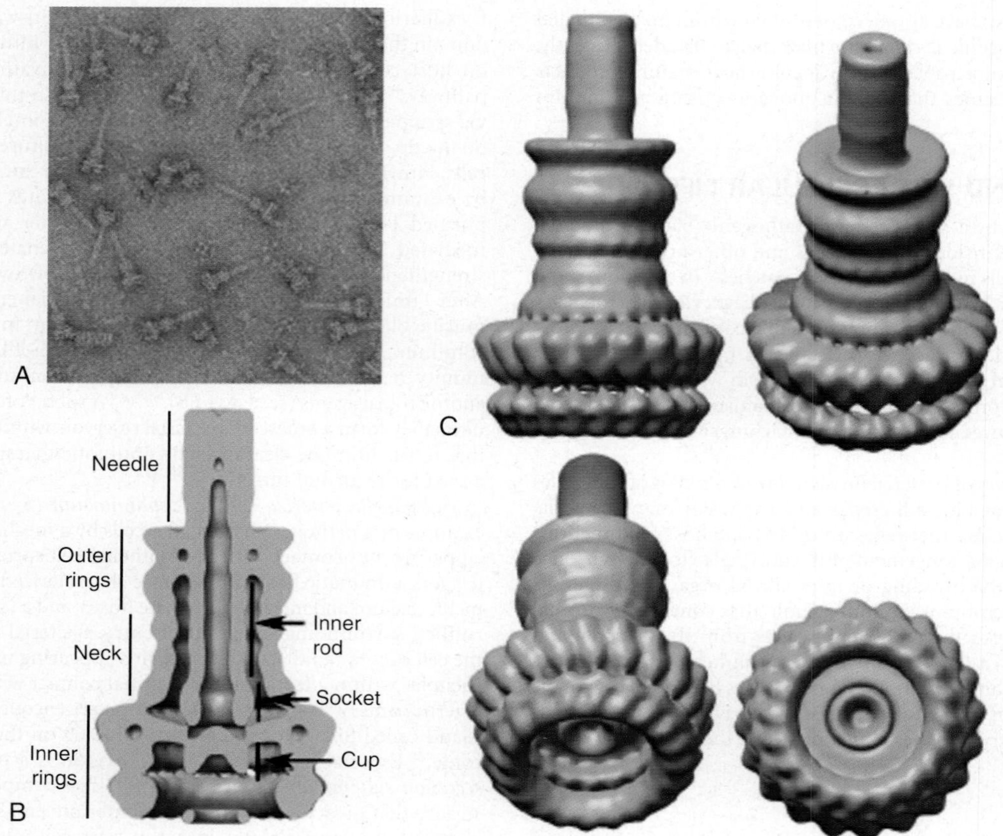

FIG. 1.7 General structure of the gram-negative type III secretion system, according to electron micrographic and other data. Represented are (A) electron micrographs of isolated needle complexes, (B) cross-sectional schematic of the components of the needle complex, and (C) surface views of the assembly. (From Galan JE, Wolf-Watz H. Protein delivery into eukaryotic cells by type III secretion machines. *Nature.* 2006;444:567–73.)

merozoite surface proteins (MSPs) present along the entire merozoite surface. Stronger interactions are mediated by several additional receptors, notably the erythrocyte binding antigens EBA-175 and EBA-140, which engage the erythrocyte-specific receptors glycophorin A and glycophorin B, respectively. Recently, an additional parasite protein called PfRH5 was recognized as an indispensible mediator of parasite invasion via interaction with the human receptor basigin.[54] Anti-RH5 antisera have potent invasion-inhibiting activities,[312] and an RH5-based vaccine showed efficacy in an *Aotus* monkey infection model.[72] On the basis of these data, PfRH5 has emerged as a strong candidate vaccine antigen to prevent severe malaria.

Intracellular Survival

Once an organism invades a nonprofessional phagocyte or is ingested by a professional phagocyte, several potential outcomes exist. Often, the organism is killed. However, some pathogens have developed strategies to survive and replicate inside host cells, in some cases within a vacuole and in others by escaping from the vacuole.

There is general agreement that *S. typhimurium* resides within a membrane-bound vacuole in both professional and nonprofessional phagocytes. However, the vacuole lacks several lysosomal markers typical of the main endocytic pathway (the mannose-6-phosphate receptor pathway) and appears to be distinct from this pathway. Insight into the molecular determinants of intravacuolar survival came when two independent groups reported the discovery of a second *Salmonella* pathogenicity island, now called SPI-2.[122,228] This island maps to centisome 31 and encodes another type III secretion system, including structural proteins (*ssa* locus),[122] effector proteins (*sse* locus), and accessory proteins (*ssc* locus). In addition, this region encodes a *two-component regulatory system* consisting of a membrane-located sensor kinase (SsrA) and a transcriptional regulator (SsrB).[228] Mutations in SPI-2 result in reduced survival inside macrophages, with no effect on adherence and invasion in assays with intestinal epithelial cells.[228] *Salmonella* SPI-2 mutants demonstrate reduced virulence in experimental mice (up to a 104-fold reduction in 50% lethal dose), suggesting that survival inside macrophages is a key factor in the pathogenesis of disease.[273] Expression of SPI-2 genes within the macrophage vacuole depends at least in part on the acidic intravacuolar environment. Inhibition of macrophage vacuolar acidification using bafilomycin A1 (an inhibitor of the vacuolar proton ATPase) results in a sharp attenuation in transcription of SPI-2 genes. This effect is not reproduced by low pH alone outside the vacuole, suggesting that other environmental effects within the vacuole influence SPI-2 expression.[37] Recent work indicates that *Salmonella* SPI-2 transcription is activated before invasion, apparently preparing the pathogen for the hostile intracellular environment.[26] As a group, the SPI-2 genes appear to modulate host endocytic and exocytic transport mechanisms and inflammatory signaling.[1,142]

A third *Salmonella* pathogenicity island called SPI-3 also promotes survival inside macrophages. This island is located at centisome 82 and was discovered by examining the *Salmonella selC* locus, a tRNA gene where pathogenicity islands reside in some strains of *E. coli.*[15,17] SPI-3 contains the *mgtBC* operon, which permits *S. typhimurium* growth in environments with low concentrations of Mg^{2+}, including macrophages. In particular, mutation of the *mgtBC* operon abolishes the ability of *S. typhimurium* to replicate in low-Mg^{2+} liquid media and in macrophages, and addition of Mg^{2+} to the medium after phagocytosis restores the ability to survive intracellularly. Homologous *mgtBC* genes have been found in other organisms with intracellular lifestyles, such as *Brucella melitensis* and *Yersinia pestis.*[16] In *Salmonella,* the *mgtBC* genes are expressed after internalization into host cells under control of the

PhoP-PhoQ two-component regulatory system, a complex that directs expression of a number of virulence determinants.[191]

The ability to survive within phagocytic cells may provide *Salmonella* with a means to exploit an intrinsic host pathway and disseminate to distant sites. In particular, certain phagocytes express the β2 integrin CD18, which mediates leukocyte migration in response to various stimuli. During *S. typhimurium* infection, CD18-expressing phagocytes carry organisms from the intestine to the spleen. Indeed, bacterial loads in the liver and spleen are reduced after oral inoculation in CD18-deficient mice when compared with infection in wild-type mice.[318] On the one hand, this function of CD18 facilitates initiation of a systemic immune response and benefits the host. However, at the same time, it provides bacteria with a mechanism of transit from the gut to organs of the reticuloendothelial system and elsewhere.

Mycobacterium tuberculosis is another intracellular pathogen, and it uses an array of mechanisms to ensure intracellular survival. The *M. tuberculosis* vacuole lacks the usual amounts of the vesicular proton ATPase responsible for mediating acidification and fails to acidify to normal levels.[298] In addition, *M. tuberculosis* blocks fusion of the vacuole with acidic lysosomes, further preventing acidification.[268] Similar to intracellular gram-negative bacterial pathogens, *M. tuberculosis* contains an *mgtC* gene, and mutation of this gene results in impaired virulence in cultured human macrophages and in mouse spleen and lung. Low Mg^{2+} concentration and mildly acidic pH inhibit the growth of the *mgtC* mutant, suggesting that the gene is important for survival in the phagosome, where such conditions may exist.[28] Another factor that influences *M. tuberculosis* survival within macrophages is isocitrate lyase, an enzyme of the glycolytic shunt that is essential for metabolism of fatty acids. Expression of isocitrate lyase is upregulated during infection of activated macrophages and is required for full virulence in a murine model of infection, independent of an effect on bacterial growth.[198] The crystal structure of *M. tuberculosis* isocitrate lyase has been solved and may provide a target for new drug therapies against persistent infection because this enzyme is absent from vertebrates.[271,282]

During the course of interaction with macrophages, *M. tuberculosis* (at a low to moderate multiplicity of infection) is capable of stimulating caspase-1 and inducing macrophage apoptosis. Interestingly, less virulent strains of *M. tuberculosis* are more potent inducers of apoptosis, perhaps resulting in benefit to the host by preventing systemic spread of infection.[163] At the same time *M. tuberculosis* possesses at least two anti-apoptotic mechanisms that further influence the outcome of macrophage encounters. First, *M. tuberculosis* infection enhances host macrophage production of soluble TNFR2, a protein that binds to tumor necrosis factor alpha (TNFα) and interferes with apoptosis.[8] Second, *M. tuberculosis* infection activates production of NF-κB, a transcriptional regulator that activates anti-apoptotic pathways within the host cell.[97] Of note, higher multiplicities of infection with virulent strains of *M. tuberculosis* can induce caspase-independent cell death in macrophages, a mechanism proposed to contribute to the formation of necrotic lesions during tuberculous disease.[179]

L. monocytogenes is an example of an organism that escapes from the phagocytic vacuole in macrophages and epithelial cells and moves into the cytoplasm. This organism causes meningitis and focal brain abscesses in humans and exhibits tropism for the fetoplacental unit. In pregnant women, listeriosis results in fetal loss in 30% of cases. Intravacuolar replication and escape from the vacuole are dependent on listeriolysin O, a hemolysin encoded by the *hly* gene.[13] Listeriolysin O interacts with cholesterol in host cell membranes and forms pores, leading to lysis of the phagosome.[90] Host enzymatic activities may also contribute to *Listeria* escape from the phagosome. In human epithelial cells the contributions of a broad-range phospholipase C (called PC-PLC) and a metalloproteinase called Mpl are most important for vacuolar escape in the absence of listeriolysin O.[107,192,281]

Intracellular survival of the protozoan parasite *Toxoplasma gondii* is thought to rely on parasite virulence factors that directly counter innate host defenses. In mice, interferon gamma (IFNγ) production is required to limit replication of *T. gondii*, in part through induction of immunity-related GTPases (IRGs). In mammalian cells, successful *T. gondii* strains replicate within a protected parasitophorous vacuole (PV) that does not fuse to the host lysosome. During infection with relatively nonpathogenic parasites, recruitment of IRGs to the PV results in disruption of the PV and parasite death. In contrast, highly pathogenic *T. gondii* express an active serine-threonine kinase called ROP18, which is exported into the host cytoplasm and prevents the recruitment of IRGs.[140,301] The ROP kinase family is highly expanded in *T. gondii*, comprising 44 other proteins, many of which lack critical catalytic residues and are thought to function as regulatory "pseudokinases." Interestingly, ROP kinases are absent from the related apicomplexan *Plasmodium* spp., presumably because prevention of IRG recruitment is unnecessary within the protected niche of the host erythrocyte.

Viral Cell Entry

Viruses have developed a specialized family of proteins that specifically function to engage host cell proteins and fuse with cell membranes and that allow for transfer of viral genetic material. The details regarding structure and function of these proteins are reviewed elsewhere.[168] There are two known classes of viral fusion proteins: class I proteins form a hairpin structure with a known α-helix domain (e.g., HIV gp41, influenza HA2), and class II proteins exist in β-sheets and transition from a moderately stable dimeric form to a very stable trimer (e.g., dengue E protein). These fusion proteins undergo conformational changes when transitioning from the prefusion to the postfusion state, resulting in a more stable form that favors the process of viral fusion and entry.

Cell-to-Cell Spread

Movement from one cell to another may help an organism gain a stronger foothold in host tissues. *L. monocytogenes* is one example of a pathogen capable of cell-to-cell spread. Once this organism is free in the cytoplasm, actin begins to polymerize on the bacterial surface. Eventually the condensed actin forms a polar tail or comet, which propels the organism through the cytoplasm and into adjacent cells. The rate of bacterial movement within a cell correlates with actin tail length.[305] Actin accumulation and condensation is mediated by the *L. monocytogenes* ActA protein, which is tightly anchored to the bacterial surface and is expressed asymmetrically over the length of the organism.[283,304] ActA is the sole *Listeria* factor required for actin polymerization because actin tails form in *Xenopus* cytoplasmic extracts containing ActA-coated beads. However, in these experiments, motility occurs only when ActA is distributed asymmetrically on the beads.[30] ActA appears to interact directly with actin and also with a variety of other host cytoskeletal proteins.[90,306] Cytochalasin D is an inhibitor of actin polymerization and inhibits the cell-to-cell spread of *L. monocytogenes* in epithelial monolayers.[58,210]

On reaching the plasma membrane, bacteria protrude from the cell in filopodium-like structures (called listeriopods), which are then engulfed by neighboring cells. This engulfment may be part of a normal host process because MDCK cells demonstrate low-level endocytosis of adjacent cell membrane fragments even in the absence of bacteria.[261] The formation of listeriopods and the engulfment of these structures by neighboring cells are independent of listeriolysin O, PI-PLC, and PC-PLC.[98] Once inside a nascently infected cell, *Listeria* escapes from the double-membrane vacuole via the action of PI-PLC, PC-PLC, and Mpl.[90] On arrival in the cytosol, bacteria can enter another cycle of actin-based motility and cell-to-cell spread, although one or two bacterial generations may be necessary to regain motility.[261]

A second pathogen capable of actin-based motility and cell-to-cell spread is *Shigella flexneri.* In *Shigella,* a single protein called IcsA is sufficient to induce formation of an actin tail, similar to that observed in *L. monocytogenes.* IcsA is an autotransporter protein that is encoded on the *Shigella* virulence plasmid and is distributed on the bacterial surface in a polarized fashion, possibly as a result of specialized machinery for autotransporter protein secretion near the poles of some gram-negative bacteria.[151] Initially, IcsA is distributed over the whole bacterial surface, with a predominance at one pole. However, over time a secreted bacterial protease called IcsP cleaves roughly half of the surface IcsA, mostly at the opposite pole, further polarizing distribution.[74,292] Elimination of expression of IcsP leads to increased quantities of IcsA and increased actin-based motility, suggesting that IcsA (rather than host factors) is rate limiting in the motility process.[274] Like ActA, IcsA is necessary and sufficient to induce polymerization of the actin tail, and the tail forms at the end where IcsA concentration is highest.[102] Despite the functional similarities between IcsA and ActA, there is no significant sequence homology between the two proteins. In contrast to ActA, no direct interaction between IcsA and actin has been demonstrated, and IcsA is found throughout the actin tail, not only at the bacterial pole–actin tail junction.

When considering cell-to-cell spread of viruses, it is helpful to return to the example of HCV. Claudin-1 and occludin-1 are the gap junction proteins that serve as the final entry point for this virus.[78,248] It has been demonstrated that HCV can infect neighboring liver cells directly via these gap junction proteins, likely bypassing the extracellular release of virus and subsequent SR-B1 and CD81 binding steps.[309] Experiments have demonstrated that antibodies blocking the E2–CD81 interaction inhibit infection from virus-infected media but do not affect infection of naïve cells when co-cultured with previously HCV-infected cells.[309] It has also been shown that after infecting a liver cell, HCV promotes breakdown of typical apical to basal organization of liver cells, exposing the gap junction complexes and presumably facilitating cell-to-cell spread.[199,200]

DAMAGE TO THE HOST

Damage to host cells and host tissues represents a fundamental mechanism by which a pathogen is able to survive at a given site and then spread within a host. Generally, damage is induced by microbial toxins. Most toxins are released extracellularly and are capable of inducing damage at very low concentrations *(exotoxins)*. Microbial attachment and invasion facilitate toxin delivery to target cells and target tissues and serve to enhance toxicity.

Historically, microbial toxins have been classified according to a variety of criteria, including cellular target of action (e.g., enterotoxins, leukotoxins, neurotoxins), mechanism of action (e.g., adenosine diphosphate [ADP]–ribosylating toxins, adenylate cyclase toxins, pore-forming toxins, proteolytic toxins), and major biologic effect (e.g., hemolytic toxins, edema-producing toxins). In recent years the term *toxin* has been applied more broadly to include enzymes that mediate damaging effects via phospholipase or hyaluronidase activity.

Bordetella pertussis Toxins

Whooping cough (*B. pertussis* infection) is a classic example of a toxin-mediated disease and involves the interplay of multiple toxins.[165] The pathogenesis of whooping cough begins with *B. pertussis* colonization of the trachea, which is facilitated by a molecule called tracheal cytotoxin (TCT). TCT is a naturally occurring disaccharide-tetrapeptide fragment of peptidoglycan and belongs to the family of muramyl peptides.[103] Many gram-negative organisms produce an analogous fragment during normal turnover of cell wall components, but significant extracellular release appears to occur only in *Bordetella* species and gonococci. In most other species an inner membrane protein called AmpG recycles this fragment back into the bacterial cell.[50] TCT is toxic to tracheal epithelial cells in vitro, stimulating nitric oxide synthase and local production of interleukin-1 and causing inhibition of ciliary motility, inhibition of DNA synthesis, and cell death.[117–119,124] During natural infection, TCT is thought to paralyze the mucociliary escalator and thereby interfere with clearance of *B. pertussis* and respiratory mucus.

Pertussis toxin is believed to be a key determinant of the clinical manifestations of whooping cough. This toxin belongs to a family of bacterial ADP-ribosyltransferase enzymes. The target of pertussis toxin is host cell G proteins, resulting in disruption of normal signaling processes. A number of biologic effects have been ascribed to pertussis toxin, including induction of lymphocytosis, stimulation of insulin release, sensitization to histamine, and disruption of phagocytic cell function; however, the specific relationship between the effects of pertussis toxin and the symptoms of whooping cough remains unclear.[125] Of note, *B. parapertussis* is closely related to *B. pertussis* and produces a similar cough illness but fails to produce pertussis toxin because of mutations in the *ptx* promoter region.[218]

B. pertussis also elaborates a toxin called adenylate cyclase toxin (CyaA), a member of the RTX (repeat-in-toxin) family of bacterial cytolysins whose prototype is the *E. coli* hemolysin HlyA.[50] These toxins cause target cell lysis by creating pores in the host cell plasma membrane, but at sublytic concentrations many of these toxins also manipulate host enzymatic and signaling pathways within the host cell. In the case of *B. pertussis,* CyaA inhibits host adenylate cyclase, resulting in accumulation of cyclic adenosine monophosphate (cAMP); elevated levels of cAMP within phagocytic cells inhibit oxidative activity and induce apoptosis, thus disabling this arm of the immune system.[166,167,243] In respiratory epithelial cells, elevated cAMP may result in increased fluid and mucus secretion, further impairing mucociliary function.

Among other examples of these dual-function RTX toxins, the prototypic HlyA of uropathogenic *E. coli* induces the degradation of host actin-associated proteins, resulting in exfoliation of the superficial epithelial layer in the bladder.[64] The α-hemolysin of contemporary community-associated *S. aureus* strains activates a host epithelial cell surface molecule called ADAM10, which cleaves E-cadherin at cell–cell junctions to permit access of the pathogen across the epithelial layer.[143,332]

Hemolytic-Uremic Syndrome and Shiga Toxins

A number of intestinal pathogens produce Shiga toxins, including *Shigella dysenteriae,* enterohemorrhagic *E. coli* (including *E. coli* O157:H7), and *Citrobacter freundii,* among others. Shiga toxins are classic A-B toxins, consisting of an A subunit that has toxic activity and five B subunits arranged in a pentameric ring-like structure that promotes binding to host cells and delivery of the A subunit. The B subunits interact with host cell globoseries glycolipids, especially the Pk trisaccharide moiety of globotriaosylceramide (GbO3). The A subunit is endocytosed by the host cell and traverses the cytoplasm in membrane-bound vesicles. Some of these vesicles travel in a retrograde fashion to the Golgi apparatus and then to the endoplasmic reticulum.[269] Shiga toxin then co-opts the function of the endoplasmic reticulum proteins HEDJ and BiP to enter the cytosol, where it enzymatically inhibits host 28S ribosomal RNA by cleaving a single adenine residue, resulting in inhibition of protein synthesis and cell death.[269,347]

In humans, *E. coli* O157:H7 is an important cause of hemorrhagic colitis and sometimes produces hemolytic-uremic syndrome. Infection begins with adherence to epithelial cells via intimin and other proteins encoded by the locus of enterocyte effacement (LEE), resulting in formation of attaching and effacing lesions analogous to those observed in EPEC infection.[196] After adherence, the organism releases Shiga toxin, which traverses the intestinal epithelial cell and enters the bloodstream.[2] Toxin circulates to distant organs and mediates damage via toxicity to endothelium. Diarrhea likely results from damage to endothelium in small mesenteric vessels, leading to ischemia and sloughing of the intestinal mucosa. The renal effects observed in human hemolytic-uremic syndrome arise from microvascular and glomerular damage with luminal occlusion by fibrin and platelets.[353] Hemolysis and thrombocytopenia likely develop as a consequence of microangiopathy.

Tissue-Degrading Toxins

A number of toxins have enzymatic activity and are capable of degrading tissue components. One example is hyaluronidase, which degrades hyaluronic acid, a repeating disaccharide glycosaminoglycan involved in cell motility, adhesion, and proliferation in normal hosts. Hyaluronic acid contains alternating *N*-acetylglucosamine and glucuronic acid moieties, connected by β linkages. It is prominent in extracellular matrix when cell turnover and tissue repair are prominent—for example, in embryogenesis, wound healing, and carcinogenesis.[55] The primary host receptor for hyaluronic acid is CD44, which undergoes post-translational modification that varies according to host cell type. Interactions between hyaluronic acid and CD44 are critical to T- and B-cell stimulation, growth of certain lymphoid malignancies, and propagation of certain inflammatory responses.[207]

In *S. pyogenes,* hyaluronidase is a 96-kDa protein that is encoded by the *hylA* gene and is released extracellularly. It is proposed to promote invasion through cell layers and tissue planes and is considered one of several *S. pyogenes* spreading factors.[141] Interestingly, *S. pyogenes* also produces a thick "capsule" of hyaluronic acid that can interact with other host cellular and extracellular matrix proteins to contribute to tissue invasion by the organism. Other pathogens that produce a hyaluronidase include *S. agalactiae* (group B streptococcus),

Treponema pallidum, Candida spp., *Entamoeba histolytica,* and *Ancylostoma braziliense.*[55]

EVASION OF IMMUNITY

To survive and replicate within the host, a pathogen must evade the host immune system. Initially the organism must circumvent innate immune mechanisms, including mechanical forces, resident phagocytes, and complement activity. Over time the organism must overcome adaptive immunity as well, including the presence of specific antibodies.

Antiphagocytic Factors

As described earlier in this chapter, invasin-mediated entry into M cells plays an important role in the early stages of *Yersinia* infection. At the same time, evasion of phagocytosis is critical to the pathogenesis of *Yersinia* disease. The ability to avoid phagocytosis is dependent on the *Yersinia* virulence plasmid, which encodes a number of proteins called Yops.[48,295] Both YopE and YopH interfere with ingestion by macrophages and neutrophils via slightly different mechanisms. YopE shares sequence homology with the *Salmonella typhimurium* SptP protein and downregulates all three of the Rho GTPases (Rho, Cdc42, and Rac), thus inhibiting actin rearrangement and blocking formation of membrane ruffles (lamellipodia) and spikes (filopodia).[3,19] YopH is a protein tyrosine phosphorylase that appears to act on a host cell cytosolic protein called Cas, interfering with recruitment of Rho, Cdc42, and Rac and preventing formation of actin stress fibers, focal complexes, and focal adhesions.[14,18] YopJ is an acetyltransferase that covalently modifies and inactivates intermediate kinases in the mitogen-activated protein kinase and NF-κB signaling pathways, leading to host cell apoptosis.[212,345] Importantly some Yop effectors also represent important immunogens; for example, the immunodominant epitope of YopE represents a major $CD8^+$ T-cell antigen in experimental plague and may facilitate a new direction in *Yersinia* vaccine development.[182,350]

Shigella employs another strategy to induce apoptosis in phagocytic cells. This pathogen produces hemorrhagic enterocolitis and is an important cause of bloody diarrhea in children. Infection begins with ingestion of organisms, which attach to intestinal M cells and then cross the intestinal epithelium.[356] On entry into the subepithelial space, organisms are engulfed by resident macrophages and contained in membrane-bound vacuoles. However, they quickly escape from macrophage vacuoles and move to the cytosol of the cell, where they induce apoptosis.[355] The mechanism of apoptosis involves a protein called IpaB, which is encoded by the *Shigella* virulence plasmid and is injected into host cell membranes via the *Shigella* type III secretion system.[20] Work by Zychlinsky and coworkers showed that IpaB binds to cytosolic interleukin-1β converting enzyme (caspase-1), a cysteine protease that cleaves IL-1β to its active form.[126] Of note, the *S. typhimurium* SipB protein shares homology with IpaB and also induces apoptosis by interacting with caspase-1.[123] Interestingly, recent work has shown that IpaB has contrasting effects in epithelial cells, binding to the cell-cycle regulator Mad2L2 to inhibit epithelial turnover and promoting epithelial colonization with *Shigella.*[148]

Evasion of Complement Activity

S. pyogenes expresses at least three factors that interfere with host complement activity. Perhaps best known is M protein, which inhibits activation of the alternative complement pathway. This effect is mediated at least in part by the ability of M protein to bind complement factor H, a regulatory protein that inhibits assembly and accelerates decay of C3bBb. Recent studies indicate that serotype M1 and M57 strains express an extracellular protein called Sic (streptococcal inhibitor of complement-mediated lysis), which associates with human plasma proteins called clusterin and histidine-rich glycoprotein (HRG) and apparently blocks formation of the membrane attack complex (C5b-C9).[4] Studies of epidemic waves of M1 infection demonstrate that Sic undergoes significant variation over time, perhaps in response to the selective pressure associated with specific antibodies.[129,130,201] Of note, nonpolar inactivation of *sic* results in reduced mucosal colonization of mice.[185] In addition, *S. pyogenes* produces a serine protease called C5a peptidase, which cleaves and inactivates C5a.[330] C5a is a cleavage product of C5 and serves as a powerful chemoattractant for neutrophils; thus, streptococcal C5a peptidase serves to attenuate the neutrophil response to infection.

N. gonorrhoeae is a common cause of cervicitis, urethritis, and pelvic inflammatory disease and is also capable of producing disseminated disease. Recent spread of antibiotic resistance in this pathogen highlights the need for understanding its pathogenic mechanisms to develop new mitigating strategies. Resistance to complement-mediated killing is important in gonococcal pathogenesis and is due in part to sialylation of lipo-oligosaccharide (LOS), which involves addition of host-derived cytidine monophospho-*N*-acetylneuraminic acid (CMP-NANA) by a bacterial sialyltransferase. Given the requirement for CMP-NANA, subcultivation in the absence of human serum or human neutrophils is associated with loss of sialylation and loss of resistance. Sialylated LOS binds factor H, resulting in downregulation of activity of the alternative pathway C3 convertase. In addition, sialylated LOS interferes with neutrophil phagocytosis and with the normal oxidative burst in neutrophils.[260,329] A second determinant of resistance to complement-mediated killing is Por1, an outer membrane porin protein that binds both factor H and C4b binding protein (C4b BP).[255] C4b BP binds C4b and serves to inhibit assembly and accelerate decay of C4b2a, the classical pathway C3 convertase. Gonococci also produce a third factor that influences resistance to complement—namely, an outer membrane-expressed nitrite reductase called AniA.[21,31]

Evasion of Humoral Immunity

A number of pathogens have evolved mechanisms to vary surface-exposed immunogenic molecules, thus facilitating evasion of a specific antibody response. *Antigenic variation* represents one such mechanism and is characterized by the emergence of modified molecules with novel antigenic properties. *Phase variation* represents a second such mechanism and is typified by the reversible loss or gain of a given molecule or structure.

N. gonorrhoeae is capable of producing recurrent infection, reflecting the fact that the antibody response to infection fails to provide lasting immunity. In this context, it is noteworthy that *N. gonorrhoeae* pili are an important target of serum antibody and undergo frequent antigenic variation. Gonococcal pilin expression is controlled by the *pilE* locus (the expression locus), which contains an intact pilin gene along with promoter sequences. In addition to *pilE,* the gonococcal chromosome contains numerous copies of variant *pil* sequences, called *pilS* loci.[110] These loci are transcriptionally inactive because they lack a promoter and 5′ coding sequence. However, they can be introduced into the expression locus by RecA-dependent recombination, resulting in an altered structural subunit and antigenically variant pili.[136] Because *N. gonorrhoeae* is naturally transformable, horizontal exchange of species-specific DNA may also give rise to new *pil* sequences.

The African trypanosomes (including *Trypanosoma brucei*) are parasites that cause sleeping sickness in sub-Saharan Africa and account for more than 50,000 deaths per year. These organisms are able to avoid humoral immunity by antigenic variation of a large family of proteins called variable surface glycoproteins (VSGs), which coat the entire surface of the trypanosome. VSGs are highly immunogenic and stimulate antibodies that lead to efficient and rapid clearing of parasites from the bloodstream. However, at any given point in time, the organism is able to express a new VSG, allowing some organisms to escape the antibody response against the previous VSG. Each parasite can express more than 100 different VSGs, with variation in expression occurring spontaneously at a rate of up to 10^{-2} per cell per generation. Overall, the genome of *T. brucei* contains more than 1000 *vsg* genes, including so-called expression sites (ESs) located near telomeres on mini-chromosomes and silent loci in nontelomeric sites on large chromosomes.[241,310] In general, VSG antigenic variation occurs by two different mechanisms. The first is called in situ activation and involves the simultaneous activation of a new ES and inactivation of the old ES, occurring independently of DNA rearrangement. The second involves DNA recombination, either between the expressed *vsg* and another telomeric ES (reciprocal recombination) or between the expressed *vsg* and a silent *vsg* locus (gene conversion).[310]

In the case of *H. influenzae,* lipopolysaccharide (LPS) is likely a key factor in facilitating colonization and is also a major target of the antibody response to infection. Interestingly, *H. influenzae* LPS undergoes phase variation. LPS biosynthesis involves multiple enzymatic steps and a number of genes. Among these genes, *lic1A, lic2A, lic3A, lex-2, lgtC,* and an *oafA*-like gene contain long stretches of tandem four-base pair repeats within their 5′ coding region. In studies of the *lic* loci, Weiser and coworkers observed that the number of repeats varies spontaneously, generating translational frameshifts with different ATG start codons falling in or out of frame.[324] Such frameshifts result in synthesis of a protein with a different N terminus or eliminate protein production altogether (when no in-frame start codon exists). The mechanism of variation in repeat number is presumed to be slipped-strand mispairing, which occurs during DNA replication and involves a single repeat looping out on either the template or the replicating strand. Changes in *lic2A* and *lic3A* influence glycotransferase activity and alter reactivity with monoclonal antibodies directed against specific LPS oligosaccharide epitopes.[108] The *lic2A* gene product is responsible for the addition of a Gal-α1,4-Gal moiety, which resembles the globoseries glycolipids and protects *H. influenzae* from antibody-mediated killing, possibly by molecular mimicry.[325] *lgtC* may be involved in formation of a Gal-β1,4-Glu moiety.[132] Variation in the *lic1A* gene affects production of a choline kinase responsible for addition of phosphorylcholine to the LPS molecule, a physical change that enhances binding of C-reactive protein and results in susceptibility to serum bactericidal activity.[187,326,327] Expression of *lex2* results in addition of a tetrasaccharide (Gal-α1,4-Gal-β1,4-Glc-β1,4-Glc) to the proximal heptose in LPS and increases resistance to complement-mediated serum killing.[105] Similarly, expression of the *oafA*-like gene results in LPS *O*-acetylation, which facilitates resistance to serum killing.[88]

Recent studies of hepatitis A virus (HAV) have identified a novel mechanism by which viruses can evade humoral responses. HAV was long considered to be nonenveloped, a characteristic that seemed well suited to promote fecal-oral transmission. However, elegant centrifugation studies demonstrated that HAV features an envelope as it exits an infected cell.[80] The enveloped HAV particle (eHAV) is fully infectious. Formation of eHAV requires proteins involved in host cell exosome formation (VPS4B and ALIX), suggesting that HAV has co-opted these pathways to facilitate spread. While temporary, this enveloped form of HAV is fully protected from neutralizing antibodies and likely facilitates cell-to-cell spread in the liver. Following these studies of HAV, additional viruses have been observed to generate a temporary envelope, indicating an established strategy for viruses to evade humoral responses.[253]

Encapsulation

Expression of an extracellular capsule represents a common strategy to evade phagocytosis, complement activity, and humoral immunity among pathogenic bacteria, fungi, and parasites. One example is *H. influenzae,* a common cause of childhood bacteremia and meningitis in underdeveloped countries. Among isolates of *H. influenzae,* six structurally and antigenically distinct capsular types are recognized, designated serotypes a to f. Historically, serotype b isolates accounted for more than 95% of all *H. influenzae* invasive disease, reflecting the distinct virulence properties of the type b capsule, which is a polymer of ribose and ribitol-5-phosphate (PRP) and is encoded by the *cap*b locus.[211] In animal studies comparing derivatives of *H. influenzae* strain Rd expressing type a, b, c, d, e, or f capsule, the strain expressing the type b capsule was associated with the highest incidence of bacteremia after intranasal inoculation of infant rats. Similarly, this strain was associated with the highest magnitude of bacteremia and incidence of meningitis after intraperitoneal inoculation of experimental rats.[354]

In considering the mechanism by which the type b capsule promotes intravascular survival and invasive disease, in vitro studies using mouse peritoneal macrophages and human peripheral blood monocytes provide some insights. The type b capsule inhibits bacterial binding to macrophages in the absence of complement and a source of C3.[223] In addition, the type b capsule interferes with ingestion by macrophages when anti-PRP antibody is lacking.[223,222] Furthermore the type b capsule blocks complement deposition on the bacterial surface and resultant complement-mediated bacteriolysis. In almost all isolates of *H. influenzae* type b, the *cap*b locus is a tandem repeat of 18-kb *cap*b gene sequences.[221] As a consequence of this arrangement, the *cap*b locus serves as a template for further amplification of capsule gene sequences in vivo, resulting in increased capsule production. In a study by Corn and colleagues, 23 of 66 minimally passaged invasive isolates had between three and five copies of the 18-kb repeat.[47] Further analysis demonstrated that amplification of the repeat results in augmented resistance to phagocytosis and complement-mediated bacterial killing.[221] The importance of the type b capsule in disease pathogenesis was recognized in vaccine development efforts, and the routine implementation of the Hib polysaccharide-conjugate vaccine in many countries has sharply curtailed the incidence of invasive Hib disease.

Capsule production is also a critical virulence determinant for a number of disease-causing fungi, including the opportunistic pathogen *Cryptococcus neoformans,* which causes infections primarily in HIV-infected and other immunocompromised hosts. *C. neoformans* elaborates a thick polysaccharide capsule that is the basis for the classic "halo" appearance of the organism upon India ink staining of cerebrospinal fluid in patients with cryptococcal meningitis. The capsule comprises a complex polymer with a galactose backbone modified by xylose, mannose, and glucuronic acid. The enzymes responsible for assembly have begun to be identified, suggesting new possible targets for new antifungal development.[170,257] However, several elements required for capsule biosynthesis remain to be elucidated, and major questions persist regarding the spatial organization of capsule components and the basis for interstrain variation in the chemical structure and antibody reactivity of the galactoxylomannan backbone.[68]

Viral Immune Suppression and Latency

Infection with HCV is a potent inducer of interferon-stimulated gene expression (as with other viruses).[331] However, HCV has evolved several mechanisms to evade host innate immune responses. The viral protease NS3-NS4A interferes with nuclear localization of interferon regulatory factor-3 (IRF-3) in response to interferon in HCV-infected hepatocytes.[89] This disruption of IRF-3 signaling, which prevents cells from activating antiviral genes downstream of IRF-3, results from specific cleavage of the molecule IPS-1.[181] Similar observations regarding evasion of innate immunity have been made with the influenzavirus NS1 protein and with West Nile virus and HIV.[67,69,334]

Among some other viral pathogens, *latency* represents an important mechanism for persistence in the presence of host immunity, especially in the case of viruses belonging to the herpesvirus family. Herpes simplex viruses (HSV types 1 and 2) commonly establish latency after either gingivostomatitis or genital tract infection. After infection of a host cell, HSV replication begins. Eventually cell death occurs, resulting in cell lysis and release of viral particles, which can then infect adjacent cells. This so-called lytic replication cycle is under control of a small number of immediate early (IE) genes, which must be transcribed in moderate amounts to allow expression of the remainder of the viral genome. IE gene expression is activated by VP16, a viral protein that binds to a sequence common to IE gene promoters.[252] After lysis of the host cell, new virions enter local nerve termini and travel up the long axon to sensory ganglia, where latency is established within days. In the latent state, viral DNA can be detected in the neuron, but infectious virions cannot be isolated. During latency,[217] IE genes are repressed and only one fragment of viral DNA is actively transcribed, yielding several latency-associated transcripts (LATs) via alternative splicing.[348] No protein product has been definitively attributed to the LAT; instead, recent work has demonstrated HSV-1 production of microRNAs, transcribed from LAT exons, that promote latency by inhibiting transforming growth factor-β signaling, favoring survival of infected cells and regulating the expression of activation-associated viral genes.[56,109,315] LAT-deficient mutants are still able to establish initial latency, suggesting that IE gene expression may be under multiple controls.[320] The mechanism by which HSV is reactivated is an area of intense study and some controversy. Host cellular mechanisms may provide the inciting signals, and the actions of viral thymidine kinase and the protein ICP0 are required for a return to lytic replication.[217]

CONCLUSION

With the proliferation of molecular techniques in recent years, our understanding of the specific microbial and host factors involved in the pathogenesis of a variety of infectious diseases continues to expand remarkably. As a consequence of this understanding, we have witnessed the development of new vaccines and potential targets for antivirulence therapeutics. In the coming years, it is likely that advances in immunology and microbial pathogenesis will inform novel approaches for treating and preventing human infections. Examples might include inhibitors of type III protein secretion systems,[149] antagonists of periplasmic chaperones, analogs of important host cell receptors, and vaccine adjuvants that direct polarization of T-cell responses. However, given the impressive adaptability of human pathogens, as new therapeutic agents become available, we must remain vigilant for new microbial strategies allowing evasion of our interventions.

NEW REFERENCES SINCE THE SEVENTH EDITION

7. Avril M, Tripathi AK, Brazier AJ, et al. A restricted subset of var genes mediates adherence of *Plasmodium falciparum*-infected erythrocytes to brain endothelial cells. *Proc Natl Acad Sci USA*. 2012;109:E1782-E1790.
11. Barocchi MA, Ries J, Zogaj X, et al. A pneumococcal pilus influences virulence and host inflammatory responses. *Proc Natl Acad Sci USA*. 2006;103:2857-2862.
32. Carruthers MD, Tracy EN, Dickson AC, et al. Biological roles of nontypeable *Haemophilus influenzae* type IV pilus proteins encoded by the pil and com operons. *J Bacteriol*. 2012;194:1927-1933.
38. Claessens A, Adams Y, Ghumra A, et al. A subset of group A-like var genes encodes the malaria parasite ligands for binding to human brain endothelial cells. *Proc Natl Acad Sci USA*. 2012;109:E1772-E1781.
54. Crosnier C, Bustamante LY, Bartholdson SJ, et al. Basigin is a receptor essential for erythrocyte invasion by *Plasmodium falciparum*. *Nature*. 2011;480:534-537.
72. Douglas AD, Baldeviano GC, Lucas CM, et al. A PfRH5-based vaccine is efficacious against heterologous strain blood-stage *Plasmodium falciparum* infection in Aotus monkeys. *Cell Host Microbe*. 2015;17:130-139.
80. Feng Z, Hensley L, McKnight KL, et al. A pathogenic picornavirus acquires an envelope by hijacking cellular membranes. *Nature*. 2013;496:367-371.
104. Grass S, Rempe KA, St. Geme JW III. Structural determinants of the interaction between the TpsA and TpsB proteins in the *Haemophilus influenzae* HMW1 two-partner secretion system. *J Bacteriol*. 2015;197:1769-1780.
140. Hunter CA, Sibley LD. Modulation of innate immunity by *Toxoplasma gondii* virulence effectors. *Nat Rev Microbiol*. 2012;10:766-778.
171. Kraemer SM, Smith JD. A family affair: var genes, PfEMP1 binding, and malaria disease. *Curr Opin Microbiol*. 2006;9:374-380.
177. Lavstsen T, Turner L, Saguti F, et al. *Plasmodium falciparum* erythrocyte membrane protein 1 domain cassettes 8 and 13 are associated with severe malaria in children. *Proc Natl Acad Sci USA*. 2012;109:E1791-E1800.
209. Milner DA Jr, Whitten RO, Kamiza S, et al. The systemic pathology of cerebral malaria in African children. *Front Cell Infect Microbiol*. 2014;4:104.
216. Nelson AL, Ries J, Bagnoli F, et al. RrgA is a pilus-associated adhesin in *Streptococcus pneumoniae*. *Mol Microbiol*. 2007;66:329-340.
240. Paul AS, Egan ES, Duraisingh MT. Host-parasite interactions that guide red blood cell invasion by malaria parasites. *Curr Opin Hematol*. 2015;22:220-226.
253. Qi Y, Zhang F, Zhang L, et al. Hepatitis E virus produced from cell culture has a lipid envelope. *PLoS ONE*. 2015;10:e0132503.
301. Taylor S, Barragan A, Su C, et al. A secreted serine-threonine kinase determines virulence in the eukaryotic pathogen *Toxoplasma gondii*. *Science*. 2006;314:1776-1780.
303. Tham WH, Healer J, Cowman AF. Erythrocyte and reticulocyte binding-like proteins of *Plasmodium falciparum*. *Trends Parasitol*. 2012;28:23-30.
312. Tran TM, Ongoiba A, Coursen J, et al. Naturally acquired antibodies specific for *Plasmodium falciparum* reticulocyte-binding protein homologue 5 inhibit parasite growth and predict protection from malaria. *J Infect Dis*. 2014;209:789-798.
314. Turner L, Lavstsen T, Berger SS, et al. Severe malaria is associated with parasite binding to endothelial protein C receptor. *Nature*. 2013;498:502-505.

The full reference list for this chapter is available at ExpertConsult.com.

Normal and Impaired Immunologic Responses to Infection

2

Michael F. Tosi

This chapter provides an overview of immunologic responses to infection and considers host interactions with different classes of pathogens, normal innate and adaptive immune mechanisms, the developing host responses of neonates, specific primary and secondary immunodeficiencies, and approaches to the evaluation of children suspected of having impaired immunity. Human immunodeficiency virus (HIV) and acquired immunodeficiency syndrome (AIDS) are not considered here because they are addressed fully in Chapter 192B. This chapter is intended to supply a basic understanding of mechanisms involved in normal host responses to infection, an appreciation of the underlying basis and clinical presentation of important immunodeficiencies, and familiarity with general principles of evaluation and management of patients with suspected or documented disorders of immunity.

HOST-PATHOGEN INTERACTIONS

General Features of Host-Pathogen Interactions

Humans are constantly exposed to a daunting number and diversity of microorganisms that can cause infection. Many organisms that usually coexist harmoniously with the human host on the skin or on mucous membranes of the oral cavity, upper airways, or lower gastrointestinal tract may invade and become pathogens only if the balance of the commensal relationship is disrupted. Other organisms are more virulent, and they overtly challenge the host's normal surface barriers and internal defense mechanisms. The human host has evolved a complex array of protective mechanisms designed to defend itself against these continuous microbial challenges.[592] To understand the pathogenesis, pathology, and natural history of infectious diseases, familiarity with the features of infectious agents that confer virulence is necessary; these topics are addressed elsewhere in this book. However, it is equally important to understand the elements of the host's response that contribute to containment, elimination, and protection against subsequent infection with these agents. Furthermore, it is important to recognize that host responses to infections also may contribute to the pathophysiology of infectious diseases and may injure the host in other ways.

The characteristic features of specific infectious diseases are determined by the interactions of structural components and released products of microbial pathogens with host tissue, cells, and their products. Virulence tactics commonly employed by organisms include adherence to host cell surfaces, internalization within or invasion of host cells, production of toxins, elaboration of surface barriers such as bacterial polysaccharide capsules, usurpation of host synthetic mechanisms, and direct inhibition of specific defense mechanisms within host cells. The successful evolution of host strategies to protect against microbial attack has resulted in defenses designed to interfere with or to counteract many of these modes of microbial virulence.[592] In recent decades, some of humanity's oldest microbial adversaries (e.g., smallpox, poliomyelitis, measles) systematically have been, or are being, eradicated with aggressive implementation of immunization programs. In the meantime, previously unrecognized human pathogens such as human immunodeficiency virus–1 (HIV-1) and Ebola virus have emerged as new adversaries. Moreover, many of our oldest nemeses (e.g., tuberculosis, malaria) continue to elude our efforts to bring them under control, and they remain serious problems worldwide. Continued research at the interface between microbial pathogenesis and immunologic mechanisms is essential for the development of innovative approaches that can support and augment human immune responses to both old and new infectious diseases.

Main Features of Host Responses to Specific Classes of Infectious Agents

Viruses

Viruses are obligate intracellular parasites that consist of genetic material in the form of either DNA or RNA that usually is surrounded by a protein coat and may or may not be bound by a lipid envelope.[372] Diseases caused by viruses are remarkably diverse, ranging from mild and merely inconvenient to rapidly fatal, and from acute or brief to chronic or lifelong. However, certain features are common to the pathogenesis of most viral infections. First, viruses must enter host cells to replicate. Viral entry ordinarily is initiated by attachment of a viral surface protein to a specific receptor molecule on the host cell. The specific viral ligands or their corresponding host cell receptors have been identified for some viruses. For example, rhinovirus has evolved a capsid protein that binds to human intercellular adhesion molecule–1 (ICAM-1) on respiratory epithelium[245]; the envelope glycoproteins of HIV-1 interact with CD4 on T lymphocytes and distinct chemokine receptors on lymphocytes or macrophages[154,308,589]; and internalization of adenoviruses depends on interaction between a specific peptide sequence in the penton base complex of the viral capsid and α_V integrins on host cell surfaces.[584] After the virus has entered the host cell, the cellular synthetic machinery is redirected to the synthesis of viral components. As with many native proteins synthesized by the host cell, a portion of newly synthesized viral protein is processed into peptides and presented on the infected cell surface by major histocompatibility complex (MHC) class I molecules (see later discussion). The host mechanisms most important in defense against the majority of viral pathogens include the production of specific neutralizing antibodies against viral surface proteins, the development of specific CD8$^+$ cytotoxic T-cell responses that eliminate infected cells, and the production by different immune cells of type 1 interferons (IFNs) that disrupt viral replication.[38,345,347,476,536] Natural killer (NK) cells appear to mediate the destruction of some virus-infected host cells,[120,513] and antibody-dependent cellular cytotoxicity (ADCC) may ensue after immunoglobulin (Ig)G antibodies bind to viral antigens on the infected cell, permitting subsequent attachment of either NK cells or cytotoxic T cells via IgG Fc receptors.[200] IFNs and other cytokines may enhance NK and ADCC activity, and cytokines such as tumor necrosis factor-α (TNF-α) may exert cytotoxic actions on cells infected with certain viruses.[347] Additionally, opsonic complement components bound to viral surfaces can interfere with cell attachment, and the complement-derived membrane attack complex can lyse enveloped viruses.[60]

Bacteria

The human host is colonized with a large variety of bacteria at skin and mucous membrane surfaces.[108,404] The integrity of these mechanical barriers ordinarily prevents systemic invasion of local commensal bacteria.[89] The epithelial cells that constitute these barriers, on recognition of an organism as a pathogen, also can release defensins and other microbicidal molecules.[225] In healthy hosts, circulating polymorphonuclear leukocytes (PMNs) help keep the resident flora in check by leaving the bloodstream at the mucosal sites containing the highest bacterial burdens, such as the lower intestine and the gingival crevices of the oral cavity.[28] This phenomenon helps account for the increased risk for local and systemic infection caused by oral and intestinal organisms in patients with severe neutropenia, including those who receive prolonged chemotherapy for malignancies, and in patients with phagocyte migration disorders such as leukocyte adhesion deficiency syndromes.[28] Important host defenses against most bacteria that invade the human host systemically include the complement system, specific antibodies that promote both the opsonic and the bacteriolytic functions of complement, and phagocytes.[1,28,60,293]

Fungi

Host mechanisms critical for defense against fungi are less well understood than those directed at bacteria and viruses, but phagocytes and cell-mediated immunity appear to be most important.[187,215] The relative importance of these factors appears to depend on the specific organisms involved, as is demonstrated by clinical observations in patients with isolated defects of one or the other. Severe mucosal infections caused by *Candida* spp. are common in patients with acquired or primary cell-mediated immune deficits, such as HIV infection, thymic aplasia (see later discussion), chronic mucocutaneous candidiasis, and some forms of severe combined immunodeficiency, as well as in patients with disorders of leukocyte migration.[28,187] In contrast to *Candida, Aspergillus* infections are not as great a problem for patients with cell-mediated immune defects as they are for patients with defects in phagocytic host defenses, such as neutropenia associated with cancer chemotherapy or stem cell transplantation, or genetic defects in phagocyte killing such as chronic granulomatous disease.[58,588] Fungi such as *Histoplasma* and *Cryptococcus,* like *Candida,* tend to cause severe infections in patients with defects in cell-mediated immunity, although phagocytes clearly are required for optimal clearance of these organisms.[170,290,582] The main role of antibodies and complement in protection from fungi probably is to provide opsonic activity to enhance phagocyte function.[172]

Parasites

Parasites such as protozoa and helminths comprise such a widely varying group of pathogenic organisms that it is difficult to generalize about mechanisms of immunity to these organisms as a group. However, the importance of specific host mechanisms in defense against certain parasites may be appreciated by considering the characteristic host responses mobilized by parasitic infection or infestations. Some helminths induce production by host cells of chemokines that recruit eosinophils and stimulate their production. This suggests a likely role for these cells in antiparasitic defenses, and eosinophils have been shown to be important in protection against helminths such as *Strongyloides* and other parasites in this group that can invade tissues. IgE, among the immunoglobulins, appears to play a special role, often in concert with eosinophils, in anthelmintic defenses. IgG also may be important based on the susceptibility of individuals with hypogammaglobulinemia to hyperinfection with *Strongyloides*. Patients with hypogammaglobulinemia also are at risk for chronic or severe infestations with the flagellate intestinal parasite *Giardia lamblia*, suggesting a role for some degree of antibody-mediated protection in normal hosts. Patients with primary or acquired disorders of cell-mediated immunity are prone to development of serious central nervous system and ocular manifestations of infection with the protozoan *Toxoplasma gondii,* an obligate intracellular parasite, as well as hyperinfection with *Strongyloides*.[299,429]

FEATURES OF NORMAL IMMUNE FUNCTION

The immune system can be viewed as consisting of two broad response categories: innate immunity and adaptive immunity. The former encompasses the more rapid and phylogenetically primitive, nonspecific responses to infection, such as surface defenses, cytokine elaboration, complement activation, and phagocytic responses. The latter involves more slowly developing, persistent, and highly evolved antigen-specific responses, such as cell-mediated immunity and antibody production that exhibit extraordinarily diverse ranges of specificities. The various arms of the immune system engage in a wide range of interactions that may enhance or regulate functions of other components of immunity, adding to the already remarkable complexity of the human immune response, and numerous examples of such interactions will be provided.

Innate Immune Responses

Epithelia, Defensins, and Other Antimicrobial Peptides

The epithelium of skin and mucosal tissue functions as a mechanical barrier to the invasion of microbial pathogens. In recent decades, it has become clear that epithelial cells also are a major source of antimicrobial peptides that play important roles in local host defense.[48,224,223,421] Studies of their structure, sources, expression, and actions also have revealed an unexpected range of immunologic activities for these molecules whose functions once were considered mainly antimicrobial in nature.[2,33]

Epithelial cells of mucous membranes of the airways and intestines, as well as keratinocytes, express the human β-defensins (HBD)-1, HBD-2, HBD-3, and HBD-4. These small cationic peptides are similar to the α-defensins stored in the azurophilic granules of neutrophils, and they display antimicrobial activity against a broad range of bacteria, fungi, chlamydiae, and enveloped viruses.[48,223,225,421] Their production by epithelial cells may be constitutive, as for HBD-1, or inducible as for HBD-2, HBD-3, and HBD-4. For example, recent evidence indicates that epithelial cells of the airway or intestine can produce HBD-2 in response to activation by bacterial products via the Toll-like receptors TLR2 or TLR4 (see later discussion) on the epithelial cells.[263,568,574] Stimulation of epithelium by cytokines, including interleukin (IL)-1 or TNF-α also can induce defensin production.[48,225] Defensins have been reported to exert their antimicrobial action either by the creation of membrane pores or by membrane disruption resulting from electrostatic interaction with the polar head groups of membrane lipids, with more evidence now favoring the latter mechanism.[48,275] Some microorganisms have evolved mechanisms for evading the action of defensins. For example, bacterial polysaccharide capsules may limit access of microbial peptides to the cell membrane,[112] and an exoprotein of *Staphylococcus aureus,* staphylokinase, neutralizes the microbicidal action of neutrophil α-defensins.[288]

Several immunoregulatory properties of defensins and related peptides, distinct from their antimicrobial actions, have been documented.[223] Several such peptides have been shown to facilitate post-translational processing of IL-1β.[439] Some of the β defensins have been shown to function as chemoattractants for neutrophils, memory T cells, and immature dendritic cells by binding to the chemokine receptor CCR-6.[274,403,421] Separately, HBD-2 has been shown to act, via a mechanism that requires TLR4, to activate immature dendritic cells and promote their maturation.[69,591] The β-defensins also act as chemoattractants for mast cells and can induce mast cell degranulation.[402] HBD-2 and several other antimicrobial peptides can interfere with binding between bacterial lipopolysaccharide (LPS) and LPS-binding protein (LBP), a process important in activating inflammatory cells via TLR4 (see later discussion).[493]

Additional antimicrobial peptides of epithelial cells include lysozyme and cathelicidin. Lysozyme, an antimicrobial peptide also found in neutrophil granules, attacks the peptidoglycan cell walls of bacteria and may be released from cells by mechanisms that involve TLR activation.[431] Cathelicidin, or LL37, like lysozyme, is released from both neutrophils and epithelial cells. It exhibits broad antimicrobial activity and can inhibit lentiviral replication.[274,527] Cathelicidin also exhibits chemotactic activity for neutrophils, monocytes, and T lymphocytes. This activity is mediated via a formyl peptide receptor–like molecule (FPRL-1), rather than the chemokine receptor (CCR)6 bound by β-defensins.[590]

The release of defensins in response to activation of TLRs and the various actions of these peptides, including their direct antimicrobial activities, their chemoattractant actions for a wide range of immune cells, and their activation of dendritic cell maturation, already suggest a highly complex and regulatory role in the development of host defense and immunity. Genomic evidence for the possible existence of many additional human defensins that have not yet been characterized suggests that current knowledge describes but a small sample of the overall contribution of these peptides to immune responses.[48,490]

Toll-Like Receptors

Mononuclear phagocytes, including circulating monocytes and tissue macrophages, other phagocytic cells, and many epithelial cells, express a family of receptors that is highly homologous to the *Drosophila* receptor called Toll.[95,263,370,568,574] These receptors mediate a phylogenetically primitive, nonclonal mechanism of pathogen recognition based on binding, not to specific antigens, but to structurally conserved pathogen-associated molecular patterns.[8,412,413,595] At least 10 human TLRs with a range of microbial ligands have been identified, such as gram-negative bacterial LPS, bacterial lipoproteins, lipoteichoic acids of gram-positive bacteria, bacterial cell wall peptidoglycans, cell wall components of yeast and mycobacteria, unmethylated CpG dinucleotide motifs in bacterial DNA, some viral particles, and viral RNA.[8,412,413,595] Gram-positive cell wall components bind mainly to TLR2, and TLR2 also can bind components of herpes simplex virus.[323,538] TLR2 forms dimers with either TLR1 or TLR6 when bound jointly by their ligands.[288,342] Gram-negative LPS activates TLR4 indirectly by first binding to LBP, which transfers the LPS to the host accessory protein CD14 at the cell surface. The bound CD14 has no transmembrane domain but associates directly with an extracellular domain of TLR4.[413,538] MD-2, an additional accessory protein associated with TLR4, also plays a role in binding LPS.[434] TLR5 has been identified as the receptor for bacterial flagellin, TLR9 recognizes CpG motifs of bacterial and viral DNA, and TLR3 has been shown to bind synthetic and viral double-stranded RNA.[56,255,319,323] A listing of known human TLRs with their major ligands and cellular distribution is summarized in Table 2.1.

Signaling by TLRs occurs via a well-described pathway in which receptor binding generates a signal via an adaptor molecule, myeloid differentiation factor 88 (MyD88), that leads to intracellular association with IL-1 receptor–associated kinase (IRAK). In turn, this leads to activation of TNF receptor–associated factor–6 (TRAF-6), which results in nuclear translocation of nuclear factor-κB (NF-κB).[133] NF-κB is an important transcription factor that activates the promoters of the genes for a broad range of cytokines and other proinflammatory products, such as TNF-α, IL-1, IL-6, and IL-8. This signaling pathway, based on studies with TLR4, is similar but not identical to the signaling pathways activated by other TLRs.[133] The activation of cytokine production by TLRs plays an important role in recruiting other components of innate host defense against bacterial pathogens. However, with large-scale cytokine release, the deleterious effects of sepsis or other forms of the systemic inflammatory response syndrome demonstrate that these

TABLE 2.1 Human Toll-Like Receptors: Their Ligands and Cellular Distribution

TLR	Ligands	Cellular Distribution
TLR1 (+TLR2) TLR2 (+TLR6)	Mycobacterial lipoarabinomannans, bacterial lipoproteins, bacterial lipoteichoic acids, bacterial and fungal β-glucans	Mo, DC, MC, Eos, Bas, AEC
TLR3	Viral double-stranded RNA	NK cell
TLR4 (+CD14, MD-2)	Bacterial lipopolysaccharide	MΦ, DC, MC, Eos, AEC
TLR5	Bacterial flagellin	AEC, IEC
TLR7	Viral single-stranded RNA	PDC, NK, Eos, BL
TLR8	Viral single-stranded RNA	NK cell
TLR9	Unmethylated CpG dinucleotides	PDC, Eos, BL, Bas (bacteria, herpesvirus)
TLR10	Unknown ligands	PDC, Eos, BL, Bas

AEC, Airway epithelial cell; *Bas,* basophil; *BL,* B lymphocyte; *DC,* dendritic cell; *Eos,* eosinophil; *IEC,* intestinal epithelial cell; *MΦ,* macrophage; *MC,* mast cell; *Mo,* monocyte; *NK,* natural killer; *PDC,* plasmacytoid dendritic cell; *TLR,* Toll-like receptor.

pathways have both beneficial and potentially harmful effects for the host.[133] Genetic polymorphisms in TLRs may play a role in determining the balance of these effects in certain individuals responding to the challenge of systemic infection.[133,352,353]

In addition to their "first responder" roles in generating an inflammatory response to invading pathogens, TLRs may network with other components of innate and adaptive immunity. TLR4 function is suppressed by activation of cells via the chemokine receptor CXCR4.[307] Activation of some TLRs also can induce expression of the costimulatory molecule B7 on antigen-presenting cells, which is required for activation of naïve T cells.[370]

Cytokines

A heterogeneous group of soluble small polypeptide or glycoprotein mediators, often collectively called cytokines, forms part of a complex network that helps regulate immune and inflammatory responses. Included in this group of mediators, whose molecular weights range from about 8 to about 45 kDa, are the ILs, IFNs, growth factors, and chemokines (see separate discussions later). Most cells of the immune system and many other host cell types release cytokines, respond to cytokines via specific cytokine receptors, or both. A list of cytokines and related molecules that play a role in immune function, with selected characteristics, is provided in Table 2.2.[322,422,443] Excellent general reviews are available,[321,322,347,422,443] and the use of cytokines as immunomodulating agents is discussed in Chapter 242. However, two cytokines, IL-1 and TNF-α, are of such fundamental importance in acute host responses to infection that they warrant specific attention here.

IL-1 and TNF-α are small polypeptides, each with a molecular weight of approximately 17 kDa, that exhibit a broad range of effects on immunologic responses, inflammation, metabolism, and hematopoiesis.[66,422] IL-1 originally was described as "endogenous pyrogen," referring to its ability to produce fever in experimental animals, and TNF-α, which produces some of the same effects produced by IL-1, was originally named "cachectin" after the wasting syndrome it produced when injected chronically in mice.[66,422] Many of the physiologic changes associated with gram-negative sepsis can be reproduced by injecting experimental animals with these cytokines, including fever, hypotension, and either neutrophilia or leukopenia.[66,422] In the development of endotoxic shock resulting from gram-negative sepsis, IL-1 and TNF-α are produced by mononuclear phagocytes in response to activation of TLRs by bacterial LPS. They in turn activate the production of other cytokines and chemokines, lipid mediators such as platelet-activating factor and prostaglandins, and reactive oxygen species. They also induce expression of adhesion molecules of both endothelial cells and leukocytes, stimulating recruitment of leukocytes by inducing release of the chemokine IL-8 and activating neutrophils for phagocytosis, degranulation, and oxidative burst activity.[66,133] These are all important, usually beneficial host responses to infection. However, at very high levels of activation,

TABLE 2.2 Features of Selected Human Cytokines and Growth Factors

Cytokines and Growth Factors	Main Cellular Sources	Biologic Effects
IL-1	Mo, TL, BL, NK, PMN, others	Broad range of cellular activation in inflammatory and immune responses
IL-2	TL, BL, NK	TL, BL proliferation and activation; enhances TL and NK cytotoxicity
IL-3	TL	General stimulation of hematopoiesis
IL-4	TL, BL, Mast, Mo	TL, BL proliferation; BL isotype switching; stimulates IgE synthesis; enhances MHC class II expression
IL-5	TL	Stimulation of Eos production
IL-6	TL, BL, Mo	Broad inflammatory activity; stimulates BL differentiation and megakaryocyte production
IL-7	Marrow and thymus stromal cells	TL, BL growth and differentiation
IL-8	Mac, Mo, Endo, Epi, PMN, Eos	Activation and chemotaxis of PMN, Eos
IL-9	TL	Mast growth and differentiation; growth of activated TL
IL-10	TL, BL, Mast, Mac	Broad antiinflammatory actions; inhibits synthesis of several other cytokines (TNF, IL-2, IL-3, IFN-γ)
IL-11	Marrow stromal cells	General stimulation of hematopoiesis; BL growth and differentiation
IL-12	BL, Mo	Stimulation of TL growth; induction of IFN-γ production; enhancement of TL and NK cytotoxicity
IL-13	TL	BL proliferation and isotype switching; enhances MHC class II expression; inhibits production of cytokines by Mac
IL-14	TL, malignant BL	Induces BL growth
IL-15	Epi, Endo, Mo, Mac, marrow stromal cells	Enhances NK growth, development, function; enhances TL growth and migration
IL-17	TL	Enhances TL growth; induces Mac cytokine release
IL-18	Kupffer cells, Epi, spleen, Mac	Promotes TL, BL, NK cytokine release; promotes TL, BL cytotoxicity
IL-21	TL	Promotes BL, TL proliferation; NK cytoxicity
IL-23	Dendritic cells, Mac	Similar to IL-12
IL-25	TL (T_H2), Mast	TL, Mac T_H2 cytokine secretion
IL-27	Dendritic cells, Mac	TL responsiveness to IL-12
IFN-α	Mo, TL	Interference with viral replication; increases MHC class I expression
IFN-β	Epi, Fibro	Similar to IFN-α
IFN-γ	TL, NK	Similar to IFN-α, IFN-β; stimulates Mac inflammatory functions
TNF-α	Mo, Mac, TL, NK	Broad inflammatory effects; fever; cachexia; stimulates catabolism; activation of leukocytes and Endo
GM-CSF	TL, BL, Mo, PMN, Eos, Fibro, Mast, Endo	Growth of PMN, Eos, Mo, and Mac precursors; enhances leukocyte function
G-CSF	Mo, Epi, Fibro	Enhances production and function of granulocytes
M-CSF	Mo, TL, BL, Endo, Fibro	Promotes Mo production; stimulates Mo and Mac function

BL, B lymphocyte; *Endo,* endothelial cell; *Eos,* eosinophil; *Epi,* epithelial cell; *Fibro,* fibroblast; *G-CSF,* granulocyte colony-stimulating factor; *GM-CSF,* granulocyte-macrophage colony-stimulating factor; *IFN,* interferon; *IL,* interleukin; *Mac,* macrophage; *Mast,* mast cell; *M-CSF,* macrophage colony-stimulating factor; *MHC,* major histocompatibility complex; *Mo,* monocyte; *NK,* natural killer cell; *PMN,* polymorphonuclear leukocyte; *TL,* T lymphocyte; *TNF,* tumor necrosis factor.

pathologic effects of this proinflammatory cascade may occur, including vascular instability, decreased myocardial contractility, capillary leak, tissue hypoperfusion, coagulopathy, and multiple organ failure.[133,569] For some systemic actions, notably the production of hemodynamic shock, IL-1 and TNF-α are synergistic. Both IL-1 and TNF-α also induce production of IL-6, a somewhat less potent cytokine that exhibits some of the actions of IL-1 and TNF-α.[422] The human host produces several soluble antagonists of IL-1 and TNF-α that can modulate their effects, including IL-1 receptor antagonist (IL-1ra), soluble TNF-α receptor (sTNF-αR), and antiinflammatory cytokines, especially IL-10.[133]

The importance of effects mediated by IL-1 and TNF-α in the pathophysiology of septic shock has prompted much active research aimed at blocking their direct and downstream effects to reduce sepsis morbidity and mortality. To date, despite promise and progress, clinical strategies to interfere with the cytokine-induced cascade that leads to endotoxin shock have continued, overall, to meet with limited success.[29,43,96,133,212,422,456,562,572]

Chemokines

A specialized group of small cytokine-like polypeptides, chemokines, which all share the feature of being ligands for G-protein–coupled, seven-transmembrane-segment receptors, play a complex role in the immune response as cellular activators that induce directed cell migration mainly of immune and inflammatory cells.[44,285,304,363,393,472] The chemokines and their receptors have been classified into four families based on the motif displayed by the first two cysteine residues of the respective chemokine peptide sequence. Each of at least 16 CXC chemokines binds to one or more of the CXCRs, CXCR1 to -6. Examples of CXC chemokines include IL-8 and Gro-α. Similarly, at least 28 CC chemokines, such as macrophage inflammatory protein (MIP)-1α; regulated and normal T cell expressed and secreted (RANTES); and eotaxin-1, -2, and -3 bind to one or more of the CCRs, CCR1 to -10. The sole CX3C chemokine, fractalkine (neurotaxin), binds to CX3CR1, currently the only receptor in its family. The two XC chemokines, including lymphotaxin, bind to the sole receptor in this family, XCR1. A chemokine nomenclature currently designates each of the chemokines as a numbered ligand for its respective receptor family. In this system, Gro-α is CXC ligand (L)-1 (or CXCL-1), and IL-8 now becomes CXCL-8. Similarly, RANTES becomes CCL-5, fractalkine is CX3CL-1, and lymphotactin is XCL-1.[285,472] A review of this nomenclature system tabulates the members of each family with their respective ligands and receptors, as well as with the traditional names in both human and murine systems.[285]

Virtually every cell type of the immune system expresses receptors for one or more of the chemokines. The cells of virtually any inflamed tissue can release a range of chemokines, and tissues infected with different bacteria or viruses release chemokines that recruit characteristic sets of immune cells.[235,304] For example, whereas rhinoviruses induce the release of chemokines that result mainly in recruitment of neutrophils (early in the course of infection), Epstein-Barr virus induces a set of chemokines that result in recruitment of B cells, NK cells, and both $CD4^+$ and $CD8^+$ T cells.[235] It is of interest that almost mutually exclusive sets of chemokines are induced by cytokines associated with T_H1 (IFN-γ) versus T_H2 (IL-4, IL-13) versus T_H17 (IL-17) immune responses (see later discussion), indicating a tight interplay between cytokines and chemokines in determining the type of immune response to specific infectious challenges generated under differing conditions.[71] The specificity of such responses is strongly influenced by the type of chemokines released by specific tissues, the vascular adhesion molecules expressed in those tissues, the chemokine receptors expressed by different leukocyte populations, and the specific adhesion molecules expressed by leukocytes.[71,235,304]

Modulation of chemokine functions may occur by several mechanisms. Chemokines themselves may be potentiated or inactivated by tissue proteases including tissue peptidases and matrix metalloproteases.[369] Heparin sulfate–related proteoglycans on endothelial cell surfaces tether chemokines locally, where they can most efficiently activate circulating leukocytes for adhesion (see later discussion). However, similar proteoglycans free in the extracellular environment may act to bind and sequester chemokines, keeping them from interacting with their cellular receptors.[136,324] Finally, in addition to the well-described use of chemokine receptors as coreceptors for viral entry by HIV-1, other viruses, especially members of the herpesvirus family, encode soluble decoy receptors that compete with native host receptors for chemokine binding, thereby disrupting normal host responses.[136,469]

Natural Killer Cells

NK cells are an important cellular component of innate immunity. They are lymphoid cells found in the peripheral circulation, spleen, and bone marrow that do not express clonally distributed receptors, such as T-cell receptors or surface immunoglobulin, for specific antigens.[387,388,513] They respond in an antigen-independent manner to aid in the control of malignant tumors and to help contain viral infections, especially those caused by members of the herpesvirus family, before the development of adaptive immune responses.[513,514] Activated NK cells are an important source of IFN-γ, which limits tumor angiogenesis and promotes the development of specific protective immune responses.[387,388,513,514]

Regulation of NK cell activity involves a complex balance between activating and inhibitory signals. Several cytokines can activate NK cell proliferation, cytotoxicity, or IFN-γ production, including IL-12, IL-15, IL-18, IL-21, and IFN-αβ.[514] Activating signals via other receptors on NK cells, such as NKG2D, may lead either to cytotoxicity or cytokine production or both, depending on the receptor's association with distinct intracellular adaptor proteins that signal via different kinases.[514,566] Other molecules on NK cells may act as either costimulatory or adhesion receptors, including CD27, CD28, CD154 (CD40 ligand), and lymphocyte function–associated (LFA)-1 (CD11a/CD18).[50,514] Additionally, FcγRIII (CD16) can contribute to NK cell–mediated antibody-dependent cell cytotoxicity.[200,387] NK cells are able to distinguish normal cells of self-origin via receptors that recognize specific MHC class I molecules. Activation of such receptors provides an inhibitory signal that protects healthy host cells from NK cell–mediated lysis. Virus-infected cells and malignant cells may express MHC class I molecules at reduced levels, rendering them more susceptible to attack by NK cells.[120,513] NK cell inhibitory receptors, some of which have been characterized, appear to contain intracytoplasmic tyrosine-based inhibition motifs and antagonize NK cell activation pathways via protein tyrosine phosphatases.[454,514]

NK cells kill virus-infected or malignant cells by the release of perforin and granzymes from granular storage compartments and by binding of the death receptors Fas and TRAIL-R on target cells via their respective NK cell ligands.[485,513,514] The mechanisms by which perforin and granzymes mediate target cell death are not fully understood. One or more of the granzymes appear to activate intracellular pathways leading to target cell apoptosis via pathways that involve the mitochondria or caspases or both.[300,553] Separately, binding of the death receptors also activates caspases, causing target cell apoptosis.[494,514] NK cells engage in several kinds of interactions with other cells of the immune system, including dendritic cells and other antigen-presenting cells. Dendritic cells can influence the proliferation and activation of NK cells both by release of cytokines, including IL-12, and by cell surface interactions, including CD40/CD40L, LFA-1/ICAM-1, and CD27/CD70.[164] In return, NK cells can provide signals that result in either dendritic cell maturation or apoptosis.[120,513]

Complement System

The complement system consists of more than 30 different free and membrane-bound activation and regulatory proteins. It has multiple key roles in the clearance of invading microbes, including opsonization, recruitment of phagocytic cells, and lytic destruction of pathogens.[59,168,169,188,189,208,290,289,292,392]

Approximately 90% of complement proteins are synthesized in the liver, but some components can be produced locally at sites of infection by tissue mononuclear phagocytes and fibroblasts.[134,438] In healthy persons the majority of complement is found in the circulation. Circulating complement levels vary over time, particularly in the presence of inflammation. The inflammatory response may lead to increases in levels of those complement components such as C3 that are acute-phase reactants or to decreases in individual components and total complement activity as a result of consumption.

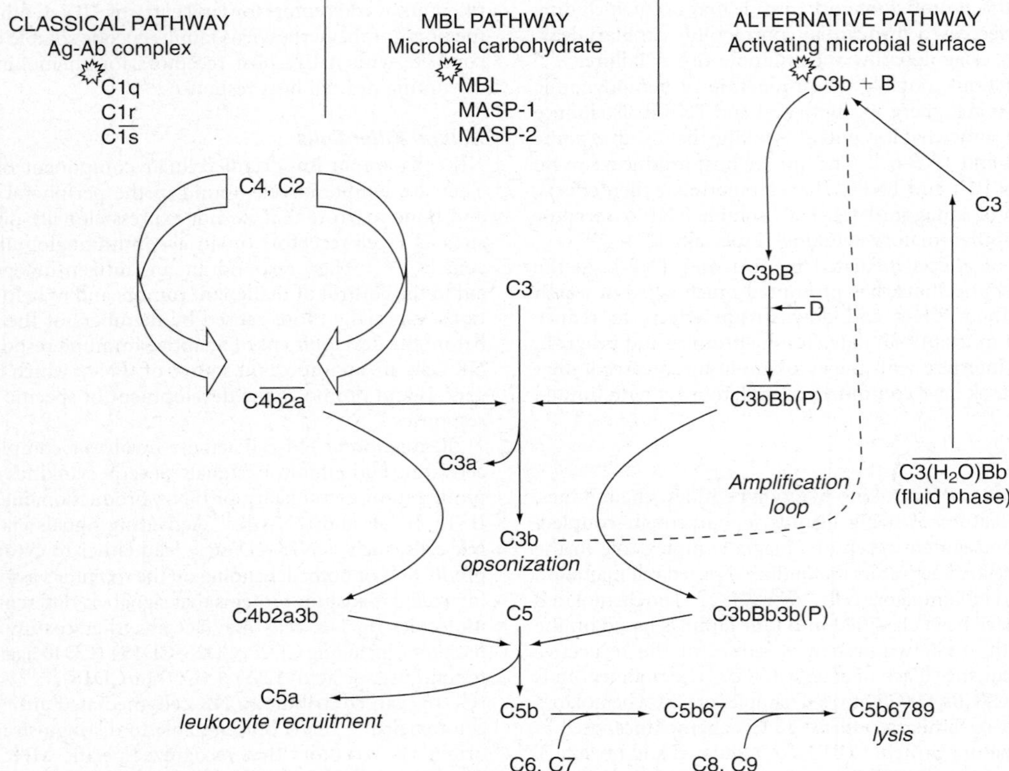

FIG. 2.1 The complement cascade. The initial binding events of the classical, mannan-binding lectin (MBL) and alternative pathways are indicated by a *starburst*. These pathways intersect at the conversion of *C3* to *C3b*. This is followed by activation of the terminal components, beginning with the binding and cleavage of *C5*, releasing *C5a* and leaving bound *C5b* to initiate assembly of the remaining components to form the membrane attack complex *(C5b6789)*. Enzymatically active proteases of the classical and alternative pathways that cleave and activate subsequent components are, by convention, shown with an *overbar*. The alternative pathway *C3* and *C5* convertases are shown associated with properdin (P), which increases their stability. *B*, Complement factor B; *D*, complement factor D; *MASP*, MBL-associated serine proteases.

The importance of normal complement component levels and activity in host defense has been well established and is based primarily on the increased susceptibility of patients with specific complement component deficiencies to recurrent or severe bacterial infections.[166,168,188,289,290] Although the complement response to infection usually is beneficial to the host, it also may be associated with adverse clinical manifestations such as septic shock and acute respiratory distress syndrome.[158,203,576]

Complement activation. Complement proteins are activated in a specific sequence or "cascade" via one or more of three pathways: the classical pathway, the alternative pathway, and the more recently described MBL pathway, as shown in Fig. 2.1. These pathways converge at C3, and the complement cascade downstream from C3 proceeds identically, irrespective of the pathway by which activation occurs. The C3 convertases, C4b2a for the classical and MBL pathways and C3bBb for the alternative pathway, cleave the C3 molecule at exactly the same location, producing C3b, which binds to the target surface, and C3a, which is released into the fluid phase. Cleavage and activation of C3 lead to a conformational change in C3b that transiently renders its reactive thioester group capable of forming covalent ester or amide bonds with acceptor molecules on the target surface.[276,331] Surface-bound C3b can act as an opsonin to promote phagocytosis, or it can bind with the classical and alternative pathway C3 convertases to form the C5 convertases C4b2a3b and C3bBb3b, respectively.[452] C5 convertases bind and then cleave C5, with release of the chemoattractant C5a fragment into the fluid phase. The bound C5b fragment then can initiate formation of the membrane attack complex by the sequential incorporation of the remaining terminal components, C6, C7, C8, and multiple molecules of C9. The membrane attack complex can insert into the outer membrane of target cells, such as erythrocytes or gram-negative bacteria, and cause cell lysis and death.[292]

Classical pathway. Ordinarily the classical pathway is activated by IgM or IgG bound to microbial antigenic targets or by other kinds of antigen-antibody complexes.[169] IgM activates complement more efficiently than IgG because only one molecule of polymeric IgM is required in contrast to at least two molecules of IgG.[141] Activation typically is initiated when C1q binds directly to an immunoglobulin molecule on the surface of an organism. C1r and C1s are activated and bound to C1q sequentially, forming C1qrs. The enzymatic activity of this complex, which resides in the C1s molecule, can cleave multiple molecules of C4 and C2 into two fragments each. The C4a and C2b fragments are released into the environment, whereas C4b and C2a remain bound to each other on the target surface to form the classical pathway C3 convertase, C4b2a. C4bC2a can cleave and activate C3 and localize C3b binding to nearby sites on the target surface. As noted earlier, some C3b binds with C4b2a to form the classical pathway C5 convertase, C4b2a3b.

Alternative pathway. Alternative pathway activation of C3 is the principal means by which a nonimmune host can activate the effector functions of complement until a specific antibody response can be mounted.[167,205]

A spontaneous low level of hydrolysis of the thioester of C3 in the fluid phase results in an activated form of C3, C3(H_2O). This activated form of C3 can bind factor B, and the latter is then cleaved by factor D to form the fluid phase C3 convertase C3(H_2O)Bb. The constitutive presence of small amounts of this convertase in the fluid phase ensures that a small amount of C3b always is available to bind to microbial surfaces and initiate the alternative pathway.[432] The alternative pathway protein factor B can bind to surface-bound C3b, after which factor B undergoes proteolytic cleavage by factor D to release a small soluble fragment, Ba, while the larger fragment, Bb, remains associated with

C3b. C3bBb, the alternative pathway C3 convertase, is analogous to the classical pathway C3 convertase, C4b2a. Properdin stabilizes the C3 convertase C3bBb, permitting more efficient activation of C3 to form more C3b, creating the C3 amplification loop (see Fig. 2.1).[202,205]

The most important factor in determining whether a specific microbial pathogen will activate the alternative pathway is the biochemical nature of its surface. On surfaces rich in sialic acid, bound C3b is less able to bind factor B because another molecule, factor H, has a strong competitive advantage over factor B under these conditions. When bound by factor H, C3b becomes highly susceptible to further cleavage by factor I (C3b inactivator), resulting in C3bi (or iC3b). Although C3bi is an effective opsonin, it cannot bind factor B. Thus no alternative pathway convertases can be formed, and no amplification loop is established.[59,325,392] Organisms whose surfaces do not support activation of the alternative pathway, such as K1 *Escherichia coli,* groups A and B streptococci, *Streptococcus pneumoniae, Neisseria meningitidis, Haemophilus influenzae* type b, and some salmonellae are some of the most successful pathogens in infants and young children who lack specific protective antibodies.[115,292]

Mannan-binding lectin pathway. The most recently described complement activation pathway is the MBL pathway. It is similar to the classical pathway but does not involve antibodies. MBL is a serum protein of the collectin family that has structural and functional similarities to those of C1q. However, it does not require antigen-antibody complexes to initiate its complement-activating function. MBL binds to mannose-containing carbohydrates on microbial surfaces, leading to its association at the microbial surface with activated MBL-associated serine proteases (MASP-1 and -2). These latter proteases have structural and functional similarities to C1r and C1s, respectively, and result in activation of C4, with sequential binding of C4b and C2a and formation of C4b2a, the C3 convertase of the classical pathway. C3 is activated, and the cascade proceeds as described. A more detailed characterization of the MBL pathway and its role in immune responses to infection may be found in an excellent review.[440]

Effector functions of complement in host defense. The principal complement effector functions in host defense include opsonization via bound fragments of C3; phagocyte recruitment, especially via release of C5a; lysis of microorganisms, especially gram-negative bacteria, via the membrane attack complex (C5b–C9); and immune regulation via interactions with host cells involved in adaptive immunity. Complement sometimes may be activated and bound to microbial surfaces but unable to carry out these functions if it is bound at a disadvantageous location; for example, C3b bound to a pneumococcal cell wall beneath a thick polysaccharide capsule or C5b–C9 bound to long lipopolysaccharide molecules distant from the gram-negative bacterial outer membrane.[93,240,277,292]

Opsonic activity. Complement opsonic activity is essential for effective phagocytic removal of organisms from the circulation by macrophages in the liver and spleen and from other sites by local macrophages and neutrophils.[78] Opsonins facilitate recognition, binding, ingestion, and killing of microorganisms by phagocytes. Opsonization particularly is important for protection against gram-positive bacteria and fungi because their thick cell walls prevent them from being killed by the membrane attack complex.

The major complement-derived opsonins are the C3 fragments C3b and iC3b. Surface-bound C3b and iC3b permit microbes to be recognized by circulating and tissue phagocytes by interacting with the phagocyte surface complement receptors CR1 (CD35) and CR3 (CD11b/CD18), respectively. These interactions lead to binding, ingestion, and intracellular killing of the organisms.[117,240,277,276,331]

Antibodies, especially of the IgG class, are important opsonins in their own right, but they also facilitate more rapid complement activation via the classical pathway and more effective localization of C3b binding to the surface of encapsulated organisms, where it is accessible to phagocyte receptors.[93,277,294]

Inflammation. The cleavage products of several complement proteins contribute to the development of inflammatory responses. C3a stimulates an increase in the number of circulating granulocytes, and C5a serves as a potent stimulus for monocyte, neutrophil, and eosinophil migration toward the source of C5a gradients being produced at infected tissue sites. C5a also upregulates phagocyte expression of CR1 and CR3 and stimulates these cells to release granule contents that also are important mediators of inflammation and microbicidal activity. C5a-induced neutrophil aggregation and stasis in the pulmonary circulation can be an important feature of the respiratory distress syndrome associated with sepsis.[576]

The anaphylatoxins, C4a, C3a, and especially C5a, induce release of histamine from mast cells and basophils, causing increased vascular dilation and permeability, which, in turn, permit local diffusion of other inflammatory mediators.[279,576] When large quantities of anaphylatoxins are produced rapidly, they can contribute to septic shock.[203]

Microbicidal activity. As noted earlier, C5b and the terminal complement proteins C6, C7, C8, and C9 form the membrane attack complex, which can lyse gram-negative bacteria by penetrating their outer membranes.[292] The C5b-C8 complex serves as a polymerization site for several molecules of C9, which increases the efficiency of lysis.[68,539] As has been noted, the membrane attack complex cannot penetrate the thick cell walls of gram-positive bacteria and fungi and therefore cannot kill these organisms directly. The membrane attack complex can lyse some virus-infected host cells and some enveloped viruses themselves.[143]

Immune regulation. Complement components and fragments can modulate immune responses, both directly by binding to CR1, CR2, and CR3 on the surfaces of T cells, B cells, and other cells involved in antigen recognition and indirectly by stimulating the synthesis and release of cytokines.[195] For example, the C3b cleavage product, C3dg, when covalently bound to antigen, brings the antigen close to B cells by binding to B-cell CR2 (CD21).[70,84,113] C3 influences antigenic localization within germinal centers, and it is involved in anamnestic responses and isotype switching. Additionally, C1-, C2-, C4-, and C3-deficient animals have decreased antibody responses that can be restored by providing the missing protein,[70,84,113] and C2 deficiency in humans also has been associated with antibody deficiencies.[15,113]

Phagocytes

PMNs, the most abundant circulating phagocytes in the human host, will serve as a model for discussing phagocyte functions. These cells constitute a major line of defense against invading bacteria and fungi. The proliferation of myeloid marrow progenitors and their differentiation into mature progeny are regulated by specific growth factors and cytokines.[45,345,346,547] The normal half-life of circulating PMNs is approximately 8 to 12 hours.[365,570] In the absence of active infection, most PMNs leave the circulation via the gingival crevices and the lower gastrointestinal tract, where the resident flora stimulate ongoing local extravasation of PMNs, a process that helps maintain the integrity of these tissues.[29] In response to invasive bacterial infection, circulating PMNs engage in three major functions: (1) migration to the site of infection, (2) recognition and ingestion of invading microorganisms, and (3) killing and digestion of these organisms.

Phagocyte recruitment to infected sites. Activation of endothelial cells that line the microvessels of acutely infected tissue occurs via locally produced cytokines, eicosanoid compounds, and microbial products.[110,505] As a result, the endothelial cells rapidly upregulate their surface expression of P-selectin from preformed intracellular storage pools and, subsequently, of E-selectin by new synthesis.[344,509] These selectins interact with the fucosylated tetrasaccharide moiety sialyl Lewis X, which is presented on constitutively expressed glycoproteins on PMNs including L-selectin and P-selectin glycoprotein ligand–1 (PSGL-1).[328,344,598] These early interactions slow the PMNs in this first adhesive phase of leukocyte recruitment, sometimes described as "slow rolling."[67,110,505] Within several hours, newly synthesized ICAM-1 is expressed at the endothelial surface.[110,505,508] The slowly rolling PMNs are activated by transient selectin-mediated interactions and locally produced mediators, especially endothelium-derived chemokines such as IL-8.[343] These chemokines are most effective in PMN activation when they are bound by complex proteoglycans at the endothelial cell surface.[324,573] The activated PMNs then signal the conformational activation of binding function of their surface β_2 integrins LFA-1 and Mac-1,[171,563] as well as translocating an additional large quantity of Mac-1 from intracellular storage pools to the cell surface.[60,80,82] This newly translocated Mac-1 also may undergo conformational activation as the PMN is exposed to increasing

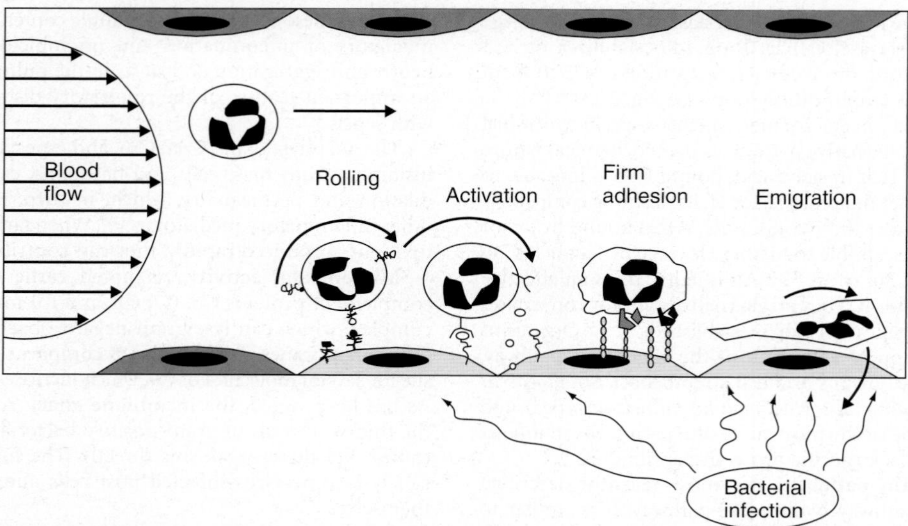

FIG. 2.2 Events during leukocyte (polymorphonuclear leukocytes [PMNs]) recruitment to infected sites. Interactions between microorganisms in infected tissue and host cells and proteins result in elaboration of mediators that diffuse to the local microcirculation and stimulate the endothelial cells. This induces new surface expression of P-selectin and E-selectin, release of interleukin-8 and other chemokines, and new surface expression of intercellular adhesion molecule 1 (ICAM-1). The endothelial selectins bind to constitutively expressed carbohydrate ligands on circulating PMNs and slow the passage of the PMNs through the microvessels. As the PMNs slow further, they become activated by interaction with chemokines bound to complex glycopeptides on the endothelial surface. This activation of PMNs increases their expression and binding activity of the β_2 (CD11/CD18) integrins, Mac-1 and lymphocyte function–associated antigen–1 (LFA-1). Interactions between these integrins and ICAM-1 (and ICAM-2 in the case of LFA-1) lead to tight adhesion and spreading on the endothelial surface. These latter adhesive interactions also are used for migration between endothelial cells and through the subjacent extracellular matrix in response to the gradient of chemoattractants, such as C5a, chemokines, and bacterial peptides, released at the infected site. Homophilic interactions between PECAM-1 on the PMNs and endothelial cells (not diagrammed) also appear to contribute to transendothelial migration. (Courtesy Scott Seo, MD.)

concentrations of mediators.[171,269] These activated β_2 integrins interact with the endothelial cell ICAM-1 in this second, firm adhesion phase, which is necessary for transendothelial migration of the PMNs.[60,110,170,343,496,505,508] Other chemoattractants, such as C5a, N-formyl bacterial oligopeptides, and leukotrienes (e.g., LTB_4) that diffuse from the site of infection further activate PMNs and provide a chemotactic gradient for PMN migration into tissue.[177,232,393] The receptors for these chemoattractants, like the chemokine receptors, are G-protein coupled and have a seven-transmembrane-domain structure.[232,393] They constitute important sensory mechanisms of the PMNs for activating adhesion, directional orientation, and the contractile protein-dependent lateral movement of adhesion sites in the PMN membrane necessary for cell locomotion.[24,232,393,531] A scheme for PMN recruitment from the microcirculation into infected tissue is presented in Fig. 2.2. Although the specific stimuli and adhesion molecules may vary, this general scheme applies to the local recruitment of virtually all circulating cells of the immune system.[71,235,304]

Phagocytosis. After PMNs reach the site of infection, they must recognize and ingest, or phagocytose, the invading bacteria. Opsonization, especially with IgG and fragments of C3, greatly enhances phagocytosis.[277,293] Although nonopsonic phagocytosis may occur, only opsonin-mediated phagocytosis is considered here.[483,546] CR1 and CR3 are the main phagocytic receptors for opsonic C3b and iC3b, respectively.[60–62,204] When PMNs are activated by chemoattractants or other stimuli, CR1 and CR3 are rapidly translocated to the cell surface from intracellular storage compartments, thus increasing surface expression up to 10-fold.[60,204] Note that CR3 is identical to the adhesion-mediating integrin Mac-1.[35,60] CR1 and CR3 act synergistically with receptors for the Fc portion of antibodies, especially IgG.[34,293] Phagocytic cells may express up to three different types of IgG Fc receptors, or FcγRs, all of which can mediate phagocytosis.[200,556] FcγRI (CD64) is a high-affinity receptor that is expressed mainly on mononuclear phagocytes.[556] The two FcγRs ordinarily expressed on circulating PMN are FcγRII (CD32) and FcγRIII (CD16).[547,556] FcγRII is conventionally anchored in the cell membrane, exhibits polymorphisms that determine preferences for binding of certain IgG subclasses, and can directly activate PMN oxidative burst activity.[547,556,557] FcγRIII is expressed on PMNs as a glycolipid-anchored protein, although it is anchored conventionally on NK cells and macrophages.[482,549,556] Many phagocytes also express IgA FcRs, which promote phagocytosis and killing of IgA-opsonized bacteria.[278,385]

The engagement of phagocyte receptors with microbial opsonins on microbes locally activates cytoskeletal contractile elements, leading to engulfment of the microbe within a sealed phagosome.[530] This is followed by fusion of the phagosome with lysosomal compartments containing the phagocyte's array of microbicidal products.

Phagocyte microbicidal mechanisms. Intracellular killing by phagocytes, usually within the fused phagolysosome, involves microbicidal weapons that can be categorized as either oxygen-dependent or oxygen-independent.[466] The oxygen-dependent microbicidal mechanisms of phagocytes depend on a complex enzyme, reduced nicotinamide adenine dinucleotide phosphate (NADPH) oxidase, which catalyzes the conversion of molecular oxygen (O_2) to superoxide anion (O_2^-), the reaction that is deficient in chronic granulomatous disease (see later discussion).[39,40,129] As the name suggests, the reaction catalyzed by this enzyme requires a supply of NADPH, which is supplied in turn by reactions of enzymes of the hexose monophosphate shunt. The NADPH oxidase is assembled at the plasma or phagolysosomal membrane of activated cells from six known components that include a cytochrome (α- and β-subunits, designated gp91*phox* and p22*phox*, respectively) and at least three cytosolic proteins, p40*phox*, p47*phox*, and p67*phox* ("phox" refers to phagocyte oxidase), along with a Rac-1 GTPase, which assemble with the membrane-associated components to form the active enzyme complex (Fig. 2.3).[40,80,129] Each of the main oxidant products derived from this enzyme's activity exhibits microbicidal activity, including the earliest

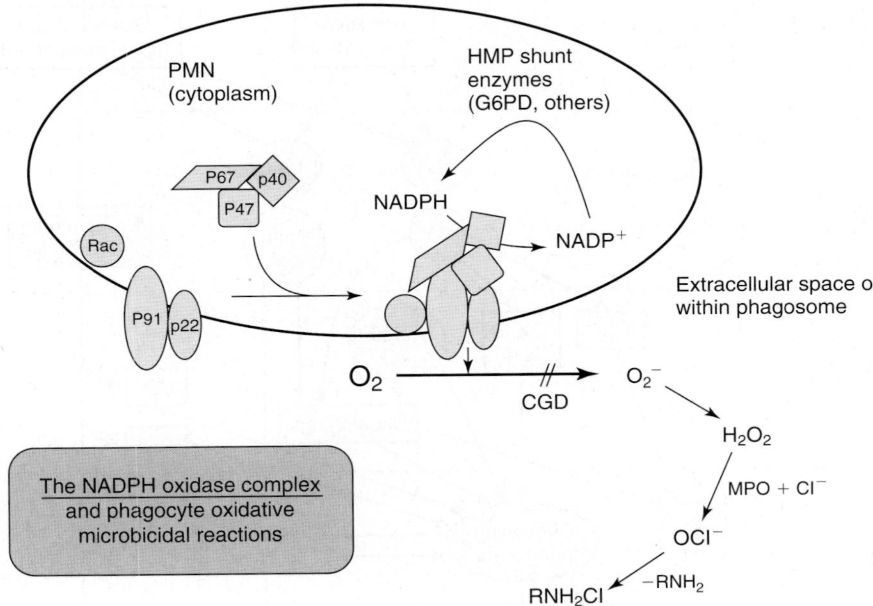

FIG. 2.3 The phagocyte reduced nicotinamide adenine dinucleotide phosphate (NADPH)-oxidase enzyme complex and the major reactions in the evolution of oxygen-dependent PMN microbicidal activity. The diagram depicts the six main components of the NADPH oxidase complex: the 91-kDa and 22-kDa subunits of the membrane-bound cytochrome; the 40-kDa, 47-kDa, and 67-kDa cytosolic components; and a Rac-1 signaling molecule. After assembly at the plasma or phagolysosome membrane, the enzyme catalyzes the conversion of molecular oxygen (O_2) to superoxide anion (O_2^-), the initial step in the sequence of production of oxidant antimicrobial products. This reaction requires a supply of NADPH, most of which is derived from activity of enzymes of the hexose monophosphate shunt (not shown). Shown in sequence are subsequent reactions for the spontaneous formation of hydrogen peroxide (H_2O_2), the myeloperoxidase-catalyzed formation of hypochlorite (OCl^-), and formation of chloramines (RNH_2Cl).

products, O_2^- and H_2O_2, and the more potent downstream products hypochlorite (OCl^-) and chloramines (NH_3Cl, RNH_2Cl), with chloramines being the most stable.[248,466]

The oxygen-independent microbicidal activity of PMNs resides mainly in a group of proteins and peptides stored within their primary (azurophilic) granules and, to a lesser extent, in their secondary (specific) granules.[80,81,83,225] Lysozyme is contained in both the primary and the secondary (specific) granules of PMN.[522] It cleaves important linkages in the peptidoglycan of bacterial cell walls and is most effective when it can act in concert with the complement MAC.[293] The primary granules contain several cationic proteins with important microbicidal activity. A 59-kDa protein, bactericidal/permeability-increasing protein, is active against only gram-negative bacteria.[578] Smaller arginine- and cysteine-rich peptides, the α-defensins, similar to the β-defensins of epithelial cells, are active against a range of bacteria, fungi, chlamydiae, and enveloped viruses; other related molecules include cathelicidin and a group of peptides called p15s.[221,224,225,337,341] Some of these PMN proteins and peptides interact with each other synergistically to enhance overall antimicrobial activity.[340]

Important Interactions Among Innate Immune Mechanisms

A schematic overview of many of the main features of innate immunity discussed earlier, along with some of their important interactions, is diagrammed in Fig. 2.4. Several levels of interactions are depicted, from initial host-pathogen contact, through a variety of activating signals, to the attack by host effector mechanisms on their respective pathogenic targets.[545]

Adaptive Immune Responses

Adaptive immunity involves the host's antigen-specific responses to infectious challenges that can provide specific protection against subsequent challenges by the same infectious agent. The major steps in the development of adaptive immunity include the processing and presentation of specific antigens to T lymphocytes (T cells) by antigen-presenting cells (APCs); the activation and differentiation of T cells for specific cytotoxic T-cell activity, T-cell cytokine production, and T-cell help in activating antigen-specific B cells; and the differentiation of activated B cells into plasma cells for the production of specific antibodies. Whereas the innate immune responses described earlier often occur in a matter of minutes to hours and may activate early cellular responses that are essential for the development of adaptive immunity, the full development of most adaptive immune responses requires days to weeks. Once developed, however, the latter often can provide durable protection. A summary of the major events in the adaptive immune response to infection is diagrammed in Fig. 2.5.

Antigen Presentation and Specific Cell-Mediated Immunity

Specific cell-mediated immunity provides T-cell help for antibody production by B cells, cytokine production for the stimulation and regulation of a range of immune responses, and cytotoxic T-cell activity against host cells infected with viruses.[175,391,436] The development of cell-mediated immunity requires complex interactions between T cells and APCs via several types of surface molecules on the respective cell surfaces. These include binding of an antigen-specific T-cell receptor on the T lymphocyte to a peptide antigen presented on the class I or II MHC by the APCs, with concurrent binding of the class I or class II MHC by CD8 or CD4, respectively,[144,543] as represented in Fig. 2.6. Other respective pairs of cell-surface molecules that enhance interactions between T cells and APCs include CD40 ligand/CD40, LFA-1/ICAM-1, and CD28/B7. An additional molecule, cytotoxic T lymphocyte antigen–4 (CTLA-4), expressed on activated T cells, also can bind to B7 molecules on APCs to generate a suppressive signal that may terminate T-cell activation.[543] The sustained physical interface between T cells and APCs at which these molecular interactions take place has been characterized as the "immunologic synapse."[32,92,242]

Class I major histocompatibility complex. Virtually all human cells except neurons express class I MHC.[152,153] The class I MHC molecule presents antigenic peptides to $CD8^+$ cytotoxic T lymphocytes.[67,407] It consists of a heavy chain that contains both the peptide-binding domain and a transmembrane domain and a smaller extracellular subunit,

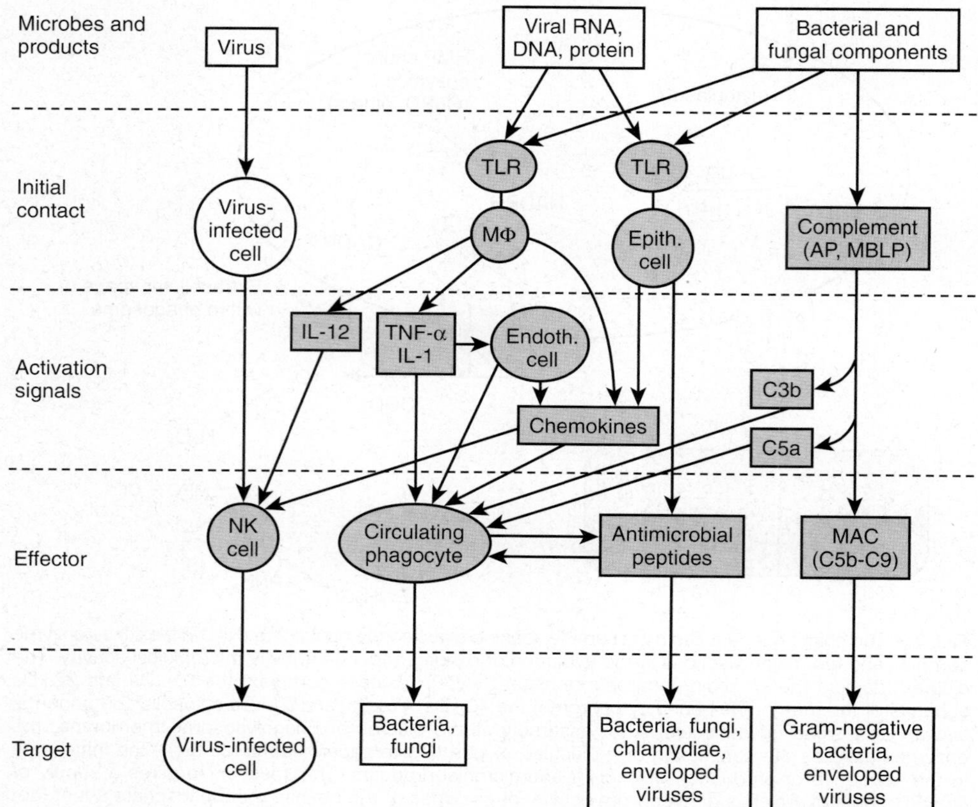

FIG. 2.4 Innate immunity: first contact, intermediate signals, and effector mechanisms. Diagrammed are important host responses to infection that are independent of specific cell-mediated immunity or antibodies. Initial contact between the host and microbes or their products may result in viral infection of cells, activation of Toll-like receptors (TLR) on macrophages (MΦ) and epithelial cells, and activation of the alternative pathway (AP) or mannose-binding lectin pathway (MBLP) of complement. The resulting activation signals, including cytokines (e.g., interleukin [IL]-12, tumor necrosis factor α [TNF-α], IL-1), chemokines, and products of the complement cascade mobilize both cellular (natural killer [NK] cells, phagocytes) and humoral (antimicrobial peptides, membrane attack complex [MAC]) effectors that attack their respective microbial targets. (From Tosi MF. Innate immune responses to infection. *J Allergy Clin Immunol* 2005;116:241–9.)

β_2-microglobulin.[73,462] The three major types of class I MHC heavy chains in humans, human leukocyte antigen (HLA)-A, HLA-B, and HLA-C, have at least 22, 31, and 12 different alleles, respectively.[597] This polymorphism permits a great diversity in the peptide-binding repertoire in individuals and within populations. A restricted degree of MHC genetic polymorphism has been invoked as a possible explanation for the predisposition of certain populations to develop infections.[74] Class I MHC molecules within the cell ordinarily bind peptides derived from recently synthesized proteins, either of self-origin or of infecting viruses.[198,199] A portion of newly synthesized proteins is processed into peptides at a cytoplasmic site, the proteasome.[236] These peptides are actively transported into the endoplasmic reticulum, where they are bound in the peptide-binding cleft of MHC class I. Suitable peptides usually are restricted to 8 to 10 amino acids in length, and they must contain certain amino acids at specific "anchor" positions on the peptide to bind.[280] Allelic variants of MHC class I may require different amino acids at these anchor positions.[218] The other amino acids of the peptide constitute the specific antigenic determinant. After trafficking of the MHC-peptide complex to the cell surface, the peptide antigen is recognized and bound by a specific T-cell receptor on CD8+ cytotoxic T cells, which concurrently bind the heavy chain of MHC class I via CD8.[67,218,280,551]

Class II major histocompatibility complex. Mononuclear phagocytes, B lymphocytes, and dendritic cells, including specialized tissue-specific dendritic cells, such as the Langerhans cells of the skin, serve the immune system as "professional" APCs.[565] Dendritic cells, the most efficient APCs for primary activation of naïve T cells, are macrophage-like cells of a distinct lineage that take up and process antigens in tissues and migrate to local lymph nodes or to the spleen, where they are likely to encounter T cells specific for the presented antigens.[182,183,253,463] A defining feature of these professional APCs is their expression of class II MHC molecules in addition to class I MHC.[153] Class II MHC molecules consist of an α and a β chain, which together form a peptide-binding cleft.[94,475] Class II MHC molecules present peptides, 13 to 17 amino acids in length, derived from proteins that are internalized by endocytosis or during phagocytosis of microorganisms.[251,281,475] The three major types of class II MHC α and β chains are HLA-DR, HLA-DP, and HLA-DQ, each exhibiting a high degree of polymorphism.[460] MHC class II, bound to a separate smaller molecule known as the "invariant chain," traffics via the Golgi to endosomal/lysosomal compartments, where it must dissociate from the invariant chain to bind antigenic peptides derived from internalized proteins.[461,541,542] The class II MHC–peptide complexes then move to the cell surface, where the peptide antigens are bound by specific T-cell receptors of CD4+ T cells, which concurrently bind class II MHC via CD4.[183,351]

Fig. 2.7 depicts the essential features of the conventional antigen presentation pathways that involve class I and class II MHC molecules, as described earlier. Alternative mechanisms have been documented by which class I MHC can present peptides derived from internalized exogenous proteins, and class II MHC may present peptides derived from newly synthesized proteins. The importance of these unconventional pathways of antigen presentation in the immune response is not fully

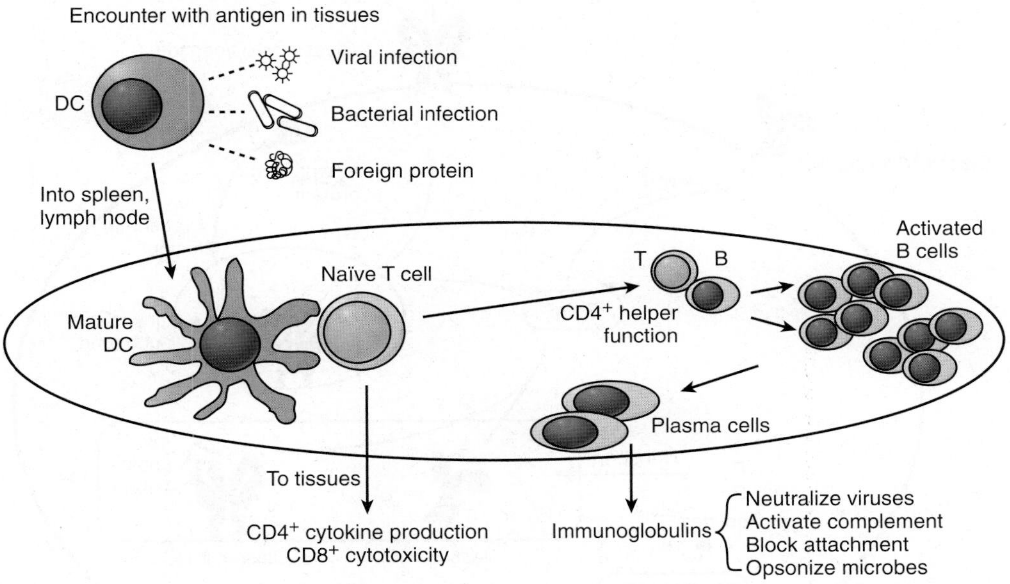

Encounter with antigen in tissues
DC
Viral infection
Bacterial infection
Foreign protein
Into spleen, lymph node
Mature DC
Naïve T cell
T
B
CD4$^+$ helper function
Activated B cells
Plasma cells
To tissues
CD4$^+$ cytokine production
CD8$^+$ cytotoxicity
Immunoglobulins
Neutralize viruses
Activate complement
Block attachment
Opsonize microbes

FIG. 2.5 A simplified scheme of major events in the development of adaptive immune responses. When antigen-presenting cells (APCs) such as dendritic cells (DCs) encounter and internalize microbes or their protein antigens in peripheral tissues, they process the microbial proteins and present the resulting antigenic peptides on either class I or class II MHC molecules. The activated APCs migrate to lymphoid tissue, where they undergo maturation. When mature dendritic cells encounter CD4$^+$ or CD8$^+$ T cells expressing T-cell receptors specific for the peptides presented in the appropriate major histocompatibility complex (MHC) context (CD4/MHC-II; CD8/MHC-I), binding between the cells occurs via TCR-peptide, MHC-CD4/8, and other pairs of accessory molecules, all necessary for stimulating the T cells to become effector cells. Cytotoxic effector CD8$^+$ T cells migrate into the periphery and kill virus-infected cells that present viral peptides via MHC class I. Effector CD4$^+$ cells either migrate to the periphery where they produce cytokines and otherwise regulate immune responses or remain in the lymphoid tissue to provide help to antigen-specific B cells, promoting their proliferation, differentiation, and eventual production by their progeny plasma cells of specific antibodies that can neutralize viruses, prevent microbial attachment, opsonize microorganisms, or activate complement.

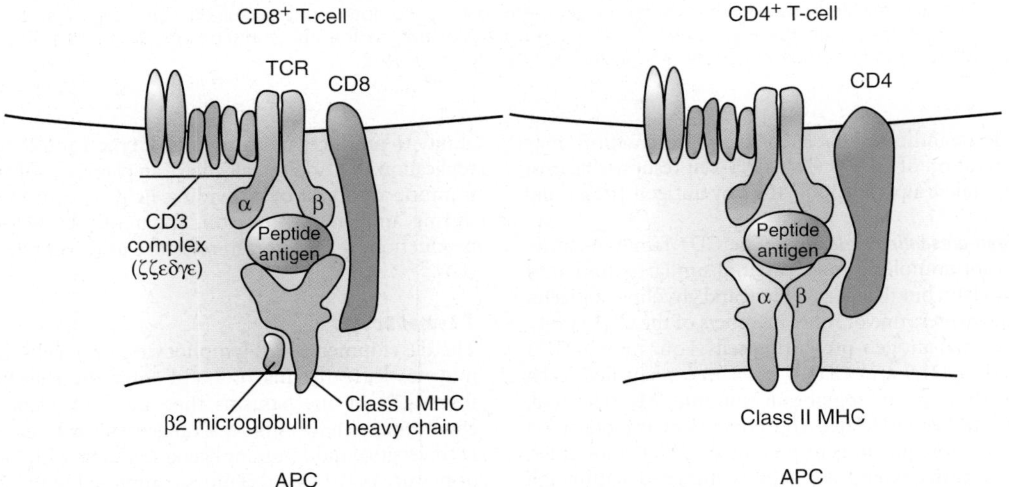

FIG. 2.6 Principal cell surface interactions between CD8 and CD4 T lymphocytes and peptide antigens complexed with major histocompatibility complex (MHC) class I and class II molecules, respectively. CD3 (composed of six subunits, ζ, ζ, ε, δ, γ, ε) is associated closely with the T-cell receptor (TCR), which recognizes a specific peptide presented on MHC molecules. Class I and class II MHC determinants are recognized by CD8 and CD4, respectively. Additional or accessory interactions are discussed in the text. *APC*, Antigen-presenting cell. (Modified from Lewis DB, Wilson CB. Developmental immunology and role of host defenses in neonatal susceptibility to infection. In: Remington JS, Klein JO, editors. *Infectious Diseases of the Fetus and Newborn Infant*. 6th ed. Philadelphia: WB Saunders; 2006:92.)

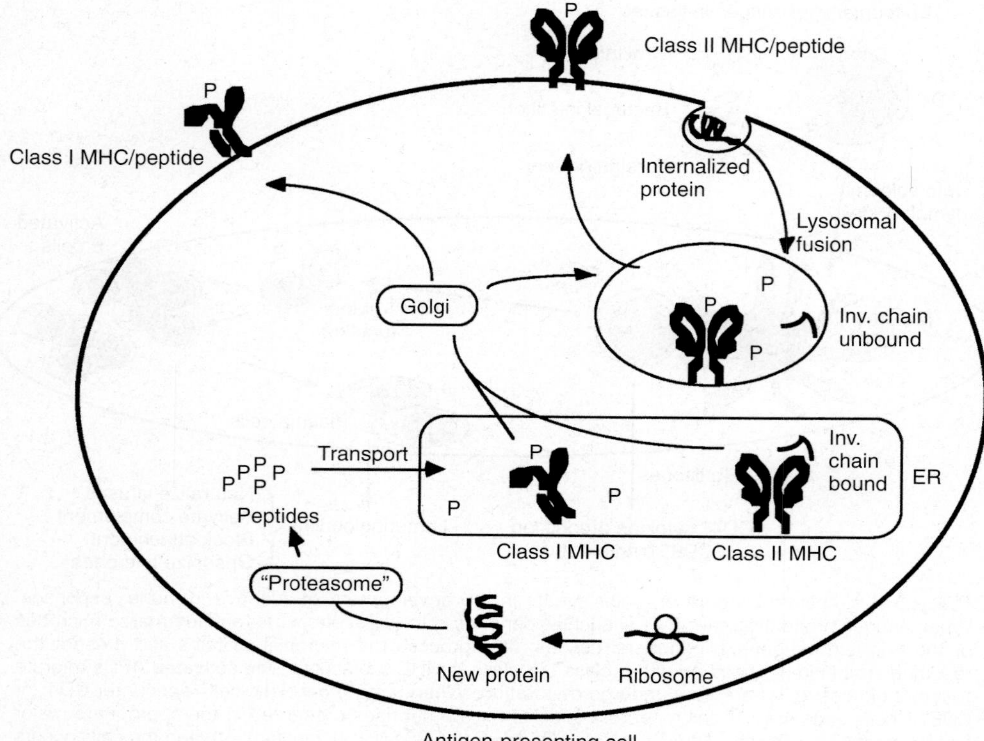

FIG. 2.7 Conventional pathways for peptide antigen presentation by class I and class II major histocompatibility complex (MHC) molecules. In the antigen-presenting cell, a proportion of newly synthesized proteins, whether of viral or host origin, undergo proteolysis into peptides by enzymes that constitute the "proteasome." The peptides are transported actively into the endoplasmic reticulum (ER), where those with the appropriate length and sequence bind to MHC class I molecules. MHC class II cannot bind peptides in the ER because of interference by the associated "invariant (inv.) chain." The class I MHC/peptide complex is transported via the Golgi to the cell surface, where it may be recognized by CD8⁺ lymphocytes. Class II MHC molecules pass via the Golgi to a lysosomal compartment, where conditions favor the release of the invariant chain. This permits class II MHC to bind peptides derived from internalized proteins that have entered the lysosomal compartment via fusion of endosomes or phagosomes with the lysosome. The lysosome translocates to the cell surface, where the class II MHC/peptide complex may be recognized by CD4⁺ lymphocytes.

understood, but evidence indicates that such "cross-presentation" may be important for generation of $CD8^+$ cytotoxic T-cell response against some viruses or fungi taken up via endocytosis by antigen-presenting cells.[36,348]

CD1 family of antigen-presenting molecules. The CD1 family includes proteins with significant homology and structural similarity to that of the MHC class I heavy chain but that present lipid and glycolipid antigens. All mammalian species express one or more members of the CD1 family, principally on professional antigen-presenting cells. Four human CD1 proteins, CD1a, CD1b, CD1c, and CD1d, have been identified, each tightly associated with a β_2-microglobulin subunit. Mycolic acid, lipoarabinomannans, and other related components of mycobacteria are the best-documented foreign antigens presented by CD1 molecules, and both internalized antigens and antigens synthesized within the antigen-presenting cells by ingested mycobacteria may be presented via distinct trafficking patterns of the CD1-antigen complexes. Antigens presented on antigen-presenting cells by CD1 molecules are recognized by a specialized subset of CD1-restricted T cells that usually lack CD4 and CD8; these are known as NK T cells. These cells share characteristics of both NK cells and T cells and exhibit a limited range of T-cell receptor specificity. Greater detail regarding the structure, function, phylogeny, trafficking, expression, and T-cell interactions for members of the CD1 family may be found in a recent review.[489]

Plasmacytoid dendritic cells. A specialized class of dendritic cells known as "plasmacytoid" dendritic cells plays a multifactorial role in both innate and adaptive immune responses. These cells are early responders to viral infections by virtue of their expression of TLR7/9 and their ability to produce large amounts of type 1 interferons that disrupt viral replication.[38,536] Additionally they can play an auxiliary role in the adaptive immune response by providing help to conventional dendritic cells during antigen presentation, apparently by helping to sustain IL-12 production by the latter in response to IFN-γ released by interacting T cells.[38,536]

T Lymphocytes

The development of T lymphocytes, or T cells, begins when prothymocytes leave the marrow and enter the subcapsular region of the thymus.[181] By mechanisms that are poorly understood, the thymic environment induces the rearrangement of T-cell receptor V (variable), D (diversity), and J (joining) gene segments with the eventual expression of mature α-β T-cell receptors complexed with CD3. The T cells, now coexpressing CD4 and CD8, migrate to the thymic cortex, where they undergo screening for T-cell receptor specificity both to optimize the repertoire for distinguishing self from nonself and to eliminate T-cell receptor rearrangements that result in undesirably high self-reactivity. Thymocytes that do not pass this dual screening procedure receive signals that induce programmed cell death (apoptosis).[373,394,567] Only about 5% of the original thymocytes pass this screening, after which they express either CD4 or CD8 but not both.[373,394,458,567] Mature thymocytes are released into the periphery, where the $CD4^+$ cells serve as the main source of IL-2 and provide help for B-cell antibody production, and the $CD8^+$ cells engage in specific cytotoxic activity.[231,391] This discussion of T cells and T-cell receptors specifically relates to T cells that express T-cell receptors composed of α and β chains, or α-β T cells. T cells of a distinct type, γ-δ T cells, are far less numerous in most tissues (intestinal epithelium is a notable exception), exhibit much less T-cell receptor diversity than do α-β T cells, may not require an intact thymus for development, and play a role in host responses to certain intracellular bacterial pathogens, including *Listeria* and mycobacteria.[106,254]

Antigen specificity of α-β T cells resides in their T-cell receptors, which are integral membrane proteins that exhibit structural homology with immunoglobulins. T-cell receptor diversity results from a rearrangement of V, (D), and J segments.[226] There are up to 100 different V segments, one (D) segment, and as many as 100 different J segments in the complete germline configuration of the T-cell receptor genes. Rearrangement of these gene segments into a mature VDJ sequence occurs by the action of a recombinase enzyme complex formed by two proteins, RAG-1 and RAG-2.[417,488] T-cell receptor diversity is generated by several factors, including the range of possible combinations of V, (D), and J segments; the imprecise action of the recombinase complex; the variability in the number of nucleotides deleted during rearrangement; and the action of another enzyme, terminal deoxytransferase, which appears to add nucleotides at random to extend segments during rearrangement.[206,504] The actions of Artemis and DNA ligase IV, two enzymes critical for the processing and joining of DNA ends, introduce additional sources of variability.[99,191,355,585] It has been estimated that as many as 10^{15} different T-cell receptor specificities theoretically could result from the preceding mechanisms.[159]

Stimulation of naïve CD4⁺ or CD8⁺ T cells occurs as they circulate through peripheral lymphoid tissue and encounter dendritic cells and other professional APCs. Localized T-cell migration is highly regulated by specific chemokines and adhesive interactions with local endothelium and involves mechanisms similar to those discussed earlier for circulating phagocytes.[185,320] When T cells engage APCs presenting specific peptide antigens on the appropriate MHC molecules, they are activated via their T-cell receptor and several costimulatory molecules, especially CD28, to produce IL-2 and proliferate and differentiate into effector T cells.[128,284]

Effector CD4⁺ T cells may be of the T_H1 or T_H2 type, and this type is influenced by several factors, including the specific cytokines elicited by a particular microbial pathogen.[395] Naïve T cells activated in the presence of IL-12 and IFN-γ are likely to develop into T_H1 cells, whereas IL-4 and IL-6 tend to drive development in the direction of T_H2 cells.[390,395,397] Preferential development of T_H1 effector cells leads mainly to macrophage activation and cell-mediated immunity, whereas T_H2 effector cells help drive certain aspects of humoral immunity, including immunoglobulin class switching to IgE in allergic responses.[395] Until recently, before the identification of the T_{FH} subset (see later discussion), T_H2 cells were thought to be the principal cell in providing T-cell help for B-cell antibody production.

A third major subset of effector CD4 T cells are T_H17 cells, whose main function appears to involve protection against extracellular bacteria and fungi by stimulating phagocytic cell responses to these pathogens.[272,349,382] Their development is favored by the presence of IL-6 and TGF-β and by the absence of IL-4 and IL-12. They are distinguished by their ability to produce IL-17 cytokines, which in turn stimulate local tissues to produce chemokines, such as IL-8, that recruit neutrophils and other phagocytic cells to tissue sites.[272,349,382] Development of T_H17 cells involves production of IL-21, which acts in an autocrine fashion to activate signal transducer and activator of transcription 3 (STAT3), a transcription factor that drives T_H17 cell development.[272,382]

In contrast to T_H1, T_H2, and T_H17 CD4 T cells, which exert their main effector functions in the periphery, a fourth T-cell subset, T follicular helper cells, or T_{FH} cells, appears to account for most of the CD4 T cells that provide help to B cells in the lymphoid follicles for antibody production.[306,411] T_{FH} cells are characterized by their location in lymphoid follicles, expression of the CXCR5 chemokine receptor, and their ability to secrete cytokines typical of both T_H1 and T_H2 cells.[306,411] The developmental origins of these cells in humans and their relationships and interactions with the other T-cell subsets are subjects of current research.

Activation of naïve CD8⁺ T cells by antigen binding, costimulation by accessory binding molecules on antigen-presenting cells, and exposure to cytokines, including IL-2, all lead to clonal proliferation of specific CD8⁺ cells and their differentiation into cytotoxic effector cells. Effector CD4⁺ T cells bound in common to an APC may play a role in activating naïve CD8⁺ T cells, either by releasing IL-2 or by activating the antigen-presenting cell to provide greater costimulation to the CD8⁺ T cell to make its own IL-2.[31] Antigenically experienced effector CD8⁺ T cells respond to specific antigenic peptides and costimulatory molecules on infected host cells by activating cytotoxic mechanisms similar to those described earlier for NK cells, including the release of both perforin and granzymes and the generation of receptor-mediated signals for target cell apoptosis.[345,476,552]

Regulatory T cells. The existence of T suppressor cells was long a subject of debate among immunologists. Within the past decade solid evidence has been developed to support the existence of suppressor T cells, now referred to as regulatory T cells, or T-regs. These cells were discovered when thymectomized mice were noted to develop autoimmune disease. Transfer of T cells that expressed CD25, the α chain of the IL-2 receptor, from normal adult mice to thymectomized mice prevented autoimmune disease. This population of CD4⁺CD25⁺ T-regs can suppress the activity of other immune cells and has been shown to prevent graft-versus-host disease and allograft rejection.[449] The mechanism of suppression by T-regs is uncertain but may involve direct contact with other cells or secretion of inhibitory cytokines, including IL-10.[349,484] These inhibitory cytokines can interfere with T-cell proliferation and inhibit the ability of antigen-presenting dendritic cells to promote T-cell activation.[349,484] The role of T-regs in immunity to infection is only beginning to be studied, but some current evidence suggests that the action of T-regs with specificity for microbial antigens may suppress protective immune responses to some infections but may also suppress excessive or injurious host responses.[449]

T-cell memory. Some proportion of activated CD4⁺ and CD8⁺ T cells become endowed with the capacity for long-term antigenic memory and can rapidly become effectors on re-exposure to specific antigen. Whether these cells develop directly from naïve T cells or previously have been effector cells, or both, is uncertain, and the mechanisms by which they become memory T cells are poorly understood. Among the features of memory T cells are high-level expression of CD45RO, the ability to suppress activation of naïve T cells of the same specificity, and a homeostatic level of ongoing proliferation in bone marrow and peripheral lymphoid organs.[296,357,481,599]

T-cell activation by superantigens. The term *superantigen* describes a class of proteins, mainly microbial exotoxins, including most staphylococcal enterotoxins, staphylococcal toxic shock syndrome toxin–1 (TSST-1), and related streptococcal TSST-1–like toxins. These bacterial toxins are potent pyrogens, can induce a potentially lethal toxic shock syndrome, and contain binding domains for both T-cell receptor V regions and MHC class II molecules. Superantigens bypass normal antigen-processing and presentation pathways by binding directly to class II MHC molecules on antigen-presenting cells and to specific variable regions on the β-chain of the T-cell antigen receptor. Through these interactions, superantigens induce a polyclonal activation of T cells at orders of magnitude above levels induced by antigen-specific activation, resulting in massive release of cytokines from T cells and antigen-presenting cells, including TNF-α and TNF-β, IL-1, IL-2, and IFN-γ, that are believed to be responsible for the most severe features of toxic shock syndromes.[14,450]

B Lymphocytes and Immunoglobulins

B lymphocytes. B lymphocytes (B cells) are the source of humoral immunity in the form of specific immunoglobulin. The earliest recognizable marrow precursors of B cells are pro-B cells whose surfaces bear the pan-B marker CD19. Further differentiation produces pre-B cells and then mature B cells, the latter expressing cell-surface immunoglobulin by which they recognize and bind antigen. B lymphocytes constitute approximately 20% of the lymphocytes in the circulation and peripheral lymphoid tissues, including the lymph nodes, spleen, bone marrow, tonsils, and intestines, and they are identified by the presence of surface immunoglobulin and the pan-B differentiation markers CD19 and CD20.[109,371]

B-cell activation is initiated by recognition and binding of specific antigens to B-cell surface immunoglobulins. Early activation leads to increased expression of receptors that either bind cytokines (e.g., IL-2, IL-4, and IL-6) or interact with T cells,[327] leading in turn to clonal proliferation and differentiation into memory B cells and plasma cells in the germinal centers of peripheral lymphoid tissue.[302] Some data suggest that B-cell differentiation into memory B cells is favored by exposure to the CD40 ligand on dendritic cells in lymphoid organs, whereas differentiation into plasma cells is favored by exposure to CD23, IL-1α, IL-6, and IL-10.[302,540] The plasma cells, later found in bone marrow and liver as well as peripheral lymphoid tissue, are responsible for most free immunoglobulin production.[540]

The B-cell response to protein antigens depends on T-cell help. B cells can process and present antigen to $CD4^+$ T_{FH} cells they encounter in the lymph nodes and spleen.[301,302,540] In the typical sequence of events, B-cell surface immunoglobulin binds to a protein antigen, which is internalized, processed, and presented to the T cell via class II MHC molecules. B cell–mediated activation of T cells during antigen presentation is much more effective for memory T cells, whereas naïve T cells are more likely to be turned off or rendered tolerant.[197,220] T-cell help is provided for B-cell proliferation and production of antibody against the specific protein antigen. This is mediated by signaling via CD40-ligand interactions with CD40 on the B cell and by the release of cytokines, which also can induce isotype switching.[163,405,526] Most B-lymphocyte responses to polysaccharide antigens proceed largely without formal T-cell help, although antibody responses to some such antigens may be enhanced in the presence of T cells.[384]

Immunoglobulin. Immunoglobulin molecules may be bound at the surface of B cells or free in the circulation, mucosal secretions, or tissues. Free immunoglobulins function in host defense against infection by binding to microbial surfaces to prevent microbial attachment, activating complement via the classical pathway, neutralizing viruses and toxins, and participating in the formation of immune complexes.[128]

Ig molecules are composed of two identical heavy and two identical light chains, as diagrammed in Fig. 2.8.[186,430] The carboxyl terminus of the immunoglobulin molecule is the heavy chain constant, or Fc, region. The amino acid sequence of this region determines the immunoglobulin isotype. The heavy chain is encoded by V, (D), J, and constant (C) regions on chromosome 14.[63,571] Each immunoglobulin molecule has a pair of either κ or λ light chains, defined by distinct constant regions.

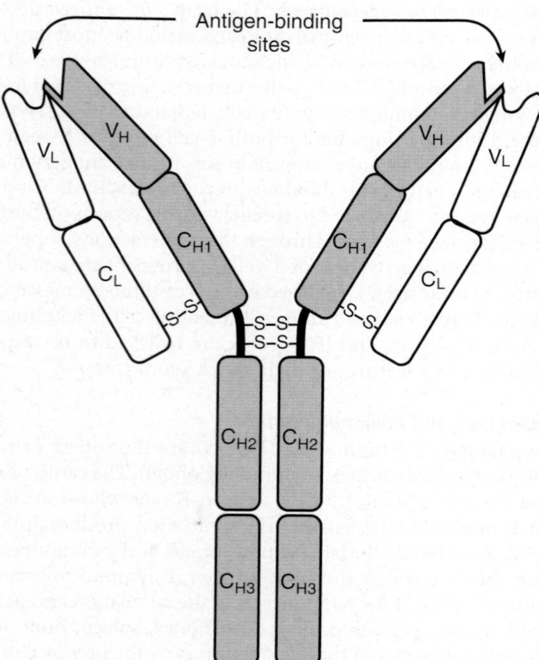

FIG. 2.8 Structure of an immunoglobulin molecule. The schematic structure of immunoglobulin G (IgG) is shown, depicting the variable (V) and constant (C) regions of both the heavy (H) and light (L) chains, the disulfide bonds that link the two heavy chains at the hinge region and the CL region with CH_1, and the antigen-binding sites formed by the complementarity-determining regions of VH and VL.

The variable region of the immunoglobulin molecule contains the antigen-binding site. Like the T-cell receptor, the Fab region consists of two identical heavy and light chain pairs; similarly, broadly diverse antigen specificity results from the variable nature of recombinase-mediated DNA rearrangements of the three hypervariable, or complementarity-determining, regions (CDR1, CDR2, and CDR3) and the four framework regions during B-cell development.[201,334,359] The imprecision inherent in this rearrangement, involving mechanisms similar to those described for the T-cell receptor, leads to the generation of more than 10^{12} potential antigenic specificities. Somatic hypermutation of variable regions after gene rearrangement adds to the repertoire, and further diversity results from differences in approximation of the three CDRs in relation to each other, affecting the three-dimensional structure of the antigen recognition site.[408,433] Thus unlike most T-cell receptors, which recognize specific peptide sequences, the antigen-binding domain of an immunoglobulin molecule recognizes the three-dimensional structure of its respective antigen.[43,156]

All immunoglobulin is derived from B cells expressing surface IgM. B cells may change immunoglobulin isotype when they differentiate into plasma cells, which produce only one class or subclass of immunoglobulin each. Isotypes other than IgM are the result of isotype switching by replacing a part of the constant region of the immunoglobulin heavy chain with another isotype-specific segment.[447,526] As already noted, isotype switching primarily depends on specific B-cell interactions with cytokines and T cells. The variable region remains unchanged during isotype switching; thus there is no change in antigen specificity. However, important features of immunoglobulins, including half-life, localization in tissues, ability to activate complement, and interactions with cellular IgG receptors, are directly determined by isotype.[91,287,556]

In addition to isotype switching, immunoglobulins undergo the process of "affinity maturation." As B cells proliferate in lymphoid tissue in response to persistent or repeated antigen exposure and T-cell help, they undergo V-region somatic hypermutation. When this mutation results in a reduced or absent affinity for antigen, B cells are less able to become activated and elicit T-cell help. Such B cells die by apoptosis, removing lower affinity immunoglobulin from the repertoire. Alternatively, B cells that undergo a mutation resulting in increased affinity for antigen are better able to bind antigen, present antigenic peptides to T cells, receive T-cell help, and survive to give rise to plasma cells, which in turn will produce immunoglobulin with higher affinity. This is a process that occurs as a result of booster doses of vaccines or during persistent infections, as with cytomegalovirus, for example.[26,444]

Immunoglobulin isotypes. IgG accounts for about 80% of circulating immunoglobulin and includes the subclasses IgG1, IgG2, IgG3, and IgG4.[64] The half-life of IgG ordinarily is about 21 days (7 days for IgG3).[287] Initial exposure to most microbial protein antigens first induces IgM and then an IgG response consisting of IgG1 and IgG3. IgG2 and IgG4 usually are produced during the secondary immune response. IgG1 usually is made in response to protein antigens.[287] In adults, the main antibody response to polysaccharides is IgG2, whereas in infants IgG1 predominates.[6,17] The functions of IgG in host defense include blocking microbial attachment, opsonization, complement activation, toxin and virus neutralization, and promoting antibody-dependent cell cytotoxicity. IgG1, IgG2, and IgG3, but not IgG4, can trigger complement activation via the classical pathway by binding to C1q.[91]

Free IgM usually exists as an immunoglobulin pentamer that has a molecular weight of approximately 950,000 and is stabilized by a single J chain.[186,314,374,433] Present mainly in the circulation, its half-life is approximately 8 to 10 days. The IgM response is the earliest of the isotype responses, appearing within the first few days of infection, but it is transient. The formation of an IgM response in the absence of an IgG response to infection is not associated with the formation of memory B cells. The main direct action of IgM in host defense is the activation of complement via the classical pathway.[374]

IgA exists in monomeric circulating and polymeric secretory forms and has a half-life of about 7 days.[287] Both forms are produced mainly by plasma cells that have migrated to mucosal sites. Secretory IgA is made up of two or three IgA molecules joined by a stabilizing J segment that is secreted by plasma cells and a secretory component produced by mucosal epithelial cells.[303,314] The secretory component permits delivery of IgA to mucosal surfaces.[406] There are two subclasses, IgA1 and IgA2, that differ in the composition of their heavy chains. Most IgA in the circulation is IgA1, whereas most IgA in secretions is IgA2. IgA1 may be cleaved at mucosal sites by bacterial proteases.[313] IgA neutralizes viruses at mucosal sites, may block bacterial adhesion, and can act directly as an opsonin to promote phagocytosis and via Fcα receptors.[278,303]

The IgE molecule has a molecular weight of 200,000 and a half-life of only 2.3 days.[287] Most IgE is produced by plasma cells in lymphoid tissue near gastrointestinal and respiratory mucosal surfaces and released into the circulation.[286,534] IgE acts via Fcε receptors to trigger activation and degranulation of mast cells and basophils, leading to immediate hypersensitivity reactions.[534] Persons with intestinal metazoan parasites often have elevated serum levels of IgE, and IgE may have a role in protecting against parasitic disease by stimulating mediator release from mast cells that can recruit eosinophils and cause intestinal smooth muscle contraction and expulsion of parasites.[534]

IgD has a molecular weight of approximately 180,000 and a half-life of 3 days.[287] It is expressed along with IgM on surfaces of naïve B cells but is present in normal adult serum and secretions in very low concentrations. Some antigenic specificity for IgD has been demonstrated, and although its function in host defense is unclear, it may serve as a secondary antigen receptor on B cells, where it may regulate the development of B-cell antibody responses.[76]

CLINICAL CONDITIONS ASSOCIATED WITH DEFICIENT HOST RESPONSES TO INFECTION

Immature Host Responses of the Newborn Infant

It is well recognized that newborn infants are much more susceptible to serious infections from many types of organisms than are older children and adults. This predisposition to infection is even more profound in infants born prematurely. The basis for this special vulnerability of the neonate is complex and encompasses all arms of the immune system.[332,342,583]

Cell-Mediated Immunity

Antigen presentation per se, via the mechanisms discussed earlier, appears to be relatively intact in the newborn infant. Expression of class I and II MHC molecules has been documented in a broad range of fetal tissues by 12 weeks' gestation,[271,419] and levels of expression are sufficient to mediate normal MHC class II–restricted antigen presentation by neonatal monocytes to maternal or paternal $CD4^+$ T cells, as well as to induce vigorous rejection of allogeneic fetal tissue by $CD8^+$ cytotoxic T cells.[258,270]

By about 20 weeks' gestation, the fetal repertoire of diversity of T-cell receptors has developed fully.[561] At the time of birth, although most basic functions of cell-mediated immunity are present, a high proportion of immature T cells are in the peripheral circulation, which can be identified by their coexpression of CD4 and CD8.[342] This phenotype typifies type II thymocytes, which usually are not found in the periphery in older persons.

Neonatal T cells appear to be relatively deficient in most of their major functions, including $CD8^+$ T cell–mediated cytotoxicity, delayed hypersensitivity, T-cell help for B-cell differentiation, and diminished cytokine production. Lack of prior antigenic exposure largely explains these defects because memory T cells are much more efficient in all of these functions.[256,342]

B Cells and Antibody

B cells. Pre-B cells are found in the fetal liver and omentum by 8 weeks' gestation and in the fetal bone marrow by 13 weeks' gestation.[228,342,516] Pre-B cells with surface IgM have been detected as early as 10 weeks' gestation. After 30 weeks' gestation and delivery, pre-B cells are seen only in the bone marrow. Mature B cells are present in the circulation by the eleventh week and have reached adult levels in the bone marrow, blood, and spleen by the twenty-second week of gestation.[161,228,516]

Fetal B cells express only IgM, whereas most adult B cells express both IgM and IgD. Neonatal B cells may express three immunoglobulin isotypes (e.g., different combinations of IgG, IgA, IgM, and IgD) on their surfaces.[228,250]

Although germinal centers are not present in lymphoid tissue at birth, they begin to develop in the first few months of life concomitant with the infant's exposure to antigens.[544] Despite conflicting in vitro data, neonatal T-cell help for B cells probably is comparable to that of adult T cells, as is reflected by the excellent T-dependent antibody response of the newborn to immunization with protein antigens.[165] In contrast to B cells of older individuals, B cells of neonates and young infants cannot respond to pure polysaccharide antigens. The recruitment of T-cell help to enhance this immature response to polysaccharides has been achieved with the advent of protein-polysaccharide conjugate vaccines. Such vaccines elicit help from T cells specific for peptides derived from the protein component as presented by polysaccharide-specific B cells that have internalized the protein-polysaccharide complex, allowing peptide-specific T cells to activate polysaccharide-specific B cells.[75]

Antibody. Maternal IgG accounts for the great majority of the newborn's circulating immunoglobulin because almost none is made by the healthy fetus and IgG is the only isotype of maternal immunoglobulin that crosses the placenta.[311,362] Maternal transport of IgG can be detected as early as 8 weeks' gestation, and the newborn's IgG level is directly proportional to gestational age, reaching 100 mg/dL by 17 to 20 weeks' gestation and 50% of the maternal level by 30 weeks' gestation (Fig. 2.9).[47,90,111] Maternal IgG is transported both passively and actively via trophoblast Fc receptors. Trophoblast Fc receptors have higher affinity for IgG1 and IgG3 than for IgG2 and IgG4, and thus more of those subclasses are transported from the mother.[336]

The concept of passive transfer of protective IgG is the basis for development of vaccines for maternal immunization before or during pregnancy so that passive transfer of vaccine-induced antibody will result in protection during the neonatal period. Examples of organisms for which such strategies have been investigated include group B streptococcus, *H. influenzae* type b, meningococcus, pneumococcus, rotavirus, and respiratory syncytial virus.[46,194,282]

By about 2 months of chronologic age, approximately half of the term infant's quantitative IgG is of maternal and half is of infant origin. The physiologic nadir of IgG in all infants is about 3 to 4 months of age and ranges from less than 100 mg/dL in preterm infants with very-low-birth weight to about 400 mg/dL in term infants (see Fig. 2.9).[47,593] Maternal IgG usually has waned completely by about 12 months of age, at which time infant levels are approximately 60% of adult levels. Production of IgG1 and IgG3 matures more rapidly than that of IgG2 and IgG4, reaching adult levels by approximately 8 years of age, versus 10 and 12 years of age, respectively.[416]

Little IgM, IgA, IgE, or IgD normally is produced by the fetus, and none is transported from the mother.[311,362] The presence of total IgM levels greater than 20 mg/dL at birth suggests an intrauterine infection, and documentation at birth of specific serum IgM or IgA against relevant organisms, such as *T. gondii* and others, would be diagnostic.[192,398,418] Serum IgA levels at birth in both preterm and term infants usually are less than 5 mg/dL and consist of both IgA1 and IgA2. Secretory IgA is not detectable until after birth but usually is present within the first few weeks of life. IgM and IgA reach approximately 60% and 20% of adult levels by 1 year of age, respectively (see Fig. 2.9). Secretory IgA reaches adult levels by 6 to 8 years of age.[342]

It has been documented that the fetus can respond to antigenic stimulation in the form of maternal immunization with tetanus toxoid vaccine and be primed for a secondary antibody response to repeat immunization after birth.[233,234] The amount of fetal antibody produced in response to intrauterine antigenic stimulation is proportional to gestational age.[162,528]

Maternal antibody inhibits the infants' ability to respond to live-virus vaccines against certain organisms, such as measles, but it does not prevent them from mounting protective immune responses to most childhood vaccine antigens, such as tetanus, diphtheria, polio, hepatitis B, and protein-conjugated polysaccharide vaccines.[12] In general, neonates have protective responses to T-dependent antigens even though they

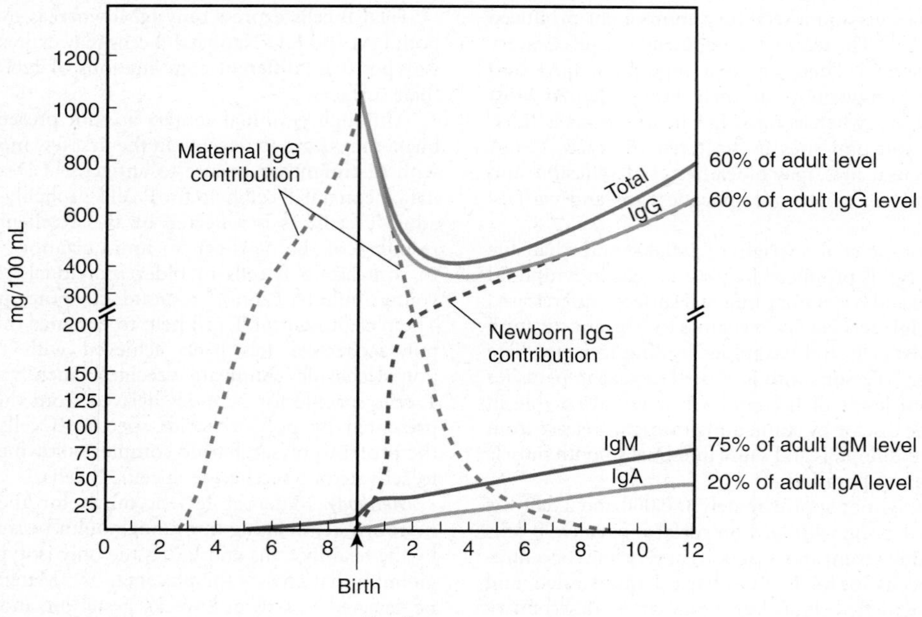

FIG. 2.9 Immunoglobulin (IgG, IgM, and IgA) levels in the fetus and infant in the first year of life. The IgG of the fetus and newborn infant solely is of maternal origin. The maternal IgG disappears by 9 months of age, by which time endogenous synthesis of IgG by the infant is well established. The IgM and IgA of the neonate are synthesized entirely endogenously because maternal IgM and IgA do not cross the placenta. (From Braun J, Stiehm ER. The B-lymphocyte system. In: Stiehm ER, editor. *Immunologic Disorders in Infants and Children.* 4th ed. Philadelphia: WB Saunders; 1996:67.)

may produce less antibody to some antigens than do older infants and adults.[11,155,165,209,506,512]

The newborn infant's response to T-independent antigens, such as polysaccharides, is poor.[237] The antibody response to most such antigens, including the polysaccharide capsules of group B streptococci, pneumococci, and *H. influenzae* type b, is not mature until 18 to 24 months of age.[510] In contrast, in the first few weeks of life, infants mount excellent antibody responses to T-independent polysaccharide antigens that have been rendered T-dependent by covalent conjugation of the polysaccharide to a protein carrier, as noted earlier.[75]

The response of premature infants to most routine childhood vaccines by 2 months of age, including diphtheria, tetanus, pertussis, and oral and inactivated polio, is comparable to that of 2-month-old term infants.[7,65,116,512] However, premature infants may not respond as well to hepatitis B vaccine for reasons that are unclear.[137,330]

Complement

Complement proteins do not cross the placenta, but there is evidence for fetal synthesis of complement beginning as early as 5.5 weeks' gestation, and most complement proteins are present by 10 weeks' gestation.[135,311] Levels of complement activity and of individual complement components vary significantly among infants, but, in general, classical pathway hemolytic activity of term neonates ranges from 60% to 90% of normal adult values.[187,594] Alternative pathway hemolytic activity is decreased to approximately 50% to 70% of normal adult values at term.[5,184,409,502] Complement activity usually is lower in premature than term infants.[409,502]

Hemolytic activity of both the classical and alternative pathways rises rapidly and reaches adult levels by 3 to 6 months of age and by approximately 6 to 18 months of age, respectively. In addition to hemolytic activity, complement-mediated opsonic and bactericidal activity is decreased in newborn sera and generally correlates with C3 and factor B levels.[187] Studies of opsonic and bactericidal activity of newborn sera have been reviewed in detail elsewhere.[187,289] Levels of individual complement proteins do not always correlate with their functional activity.[229,277] Zach and Hostetter[594] reported not only that total C3 levels in neonates were decreased but also that C3 thioester reactivity was decreased and that it correlated with gestational age.

Phagocytes

The newborn infant exhibits both quantitative and qualitative deficits in phagocytic defenses. Although the number of circulating PMNs usually does not differ greatly from that in older children and adults, under conditions of stress, including systemic infection, the availability of marrow reserves of PMNs is impaired markedly.[125] Whereas the ratio of marrow neutrophil reserves to circulating cells in older persons is nearly 15:1, in the newborn infant this ratio is more often between 2:1 and 3:1.[125] Thus, neutropenia is more likely during severe systemic infections in the newborn than in older children and adults.[125] Distinct from this quantitative deficiency in marrow reserves of PMNs, functional impairments of PMNs also are important in understanding neonatal phagocytic defenses.

The most important and best-documented functional impairments of neonatal PMNs are related to defective adhesion and migration.[3,4,23–25,27,317,367,375,376] Specific structural, functional, and biochemical abnormalities have been documented, any or all of which may contribute to the overall impairment in adhesion and migration of these cells.[267] Impaired adhesion of neonatal PMNs to endothelial cells and other biologic substrates has been linked with deficiencies in the expression or function of the β_2 integrins Mac-1 (CD11b/CD18) and LFA-1 (CD11a/CD18).[3,26,95,295,367] Perhaps the best documented of these is the diminished level of surface expression of Mac-1 on activated neonatal PMNs, although expression on resting PMNs is similar to that of adults.[95,295] The total cell content of Mac-1 in PMN at the time of birth is related directly to gestational age, and cell lysates of PMNs from very early premature infants (less than 30 weeks' gestation) have been found to contain less than 20% of the Mac-1 content of an equal number of adult PMNs, increasing to about 60% by term.[367] The PMN content of LFA-1, which is normal at term, appears to be reduced in infants born before 35 weeks' gestation.[367] In addition to reduced integrin expression, reduced adhesive function of the β_2 integrin molecules themselves at the surface of activated PMN has been documented.[26] Several other defects of neonatal relative to adult PMNs that might influence chemotaxis have been documented. These include defective redistribution of surface adhesion sites,[24] impaired uropod formation during stimulated shape change,[25] reduced cell deformability,[293] impaired microtubule assembly,[25] deficient F-actin polymerization,[252,479] reduced lactoferrin content and release,[23] reduced ability to effect membrane depolarization and intracellular calcium ion flux,[478] and impaired uptake of glucose during stimulation by chemoattractants.[4]

Evidence suggests that the number and binding efficiencies of neonatal PMN receptors for chemoattractants are normal.[24,478,532] In some studies in which assay conditions are designed to expose a potential defect (e.g., limiting concentrations of opsonins and high bacterial inocula), defects in phagocytosis and killing have been demonstrated.[376,377]

Primary and Heritable Immunologic Deficiencies

The infant or toddler who experiences even six to eight presumed viral upper respiratory tract infections during the course of a winter season, without other complications, ordinarily would not be considered likely to have an immunodeficiency. In contrast, a child who had experienced several episodes of acute otitis media in the previous 4 months, perhaps some accompanied by sinusitis or pneumonia, has displayed reasonable cause to suspect a humoral immunodeficiency.[140] For certain organisms, infection in the healthy host is so decidedly uncommon that even a single episode should prompt a high suspicion of impaired host defenses. *Pneumocystis jiroveci* pneumonia strongly suggests a severe defect of T-cell number or function.[140] Similarly, lymphadenitis or osteomyelitis caused by gram-negative enteric bacilli suggests a defect of phagocytic killing, such as chronic granulomatous disease.[291,448]

The International Union of Immunological Societies, through an expert committee on primary immunodeficiency diseases, periodically publishes an updated classification of all known primary immunodeficiency disorders based on phenotypic features.[85] The following discussion of specific immunologic defects, their genetic basis (if known), and their infectious consequences focuses on well-characterized prototypic disorders within most major classes of defects but also will address other related disorders.

Antibody Deficiencies

Humoral immunity is provided by specific antibody and plays an important role in host defense against most pathogens, as is illustrated by the finding that patients with significant antibody deficiencies develop recurrent and sometimes life-threatening infections.[139,147] They characteristically are prone to recurrent otitis media, sinusitis, pneumonia, and, less often, sepsis and meningitis.

X-linked agammaglobulinemia. X-linked agammaglobulinemia (XLA), first described by Bruton, is a primary immunodeficiency disorder of the B-cell lineage and is the most serious disorder of humoral immunity.[98,335,468] It is characterized by absent or severely decreased numbers of circulating B lymphocytes and absent or extremely low levels of all classes of circulating immunoglobulins. It is caused by several different mutations in the gene encoding for a B-cell–specific tyrosine kinase, *Btk*, which maps to the long arm of the X chromosome at Xq22.[554,564] This abnormality in kinase activity results in an arrest in the development of B cells, usually at the pre-B stage, and thus few B cells or their progeny (e.g., plasma cells) are in the circulation or lymphoid tissues.[239]

Most persons with XLA develop chronic or recurrent pyogenic bacterial respiratory or gastrointestinal tract infections, and some may have recurrent skin infections.[98,335] Sepsis and serious focal infections resulting from bacteremia do not occur as frequently but are more common and more severe than in normal hosts. The causative agents of most of these infections are *Streptococcus pneumoniae, Haemophilus influenzae,* and *Moraxella catarrhalis*, but *Staphylococcus aureus* and *Pseudomonas aeruginosa,* as well as other gram-negative organisms, may be implicated. The most troublesome gastrointestinal tract infections in XLA are caused by *Salmonella, Campylobacter,* and chronic infestation with *G. lamblia*. These patients have been found to have unusually severe or chronic enterovirus infections that can be manifested by chronic arthritis, meningoencephalitis, dermatomyositis, hepatitis, or a combination thereof, and several patients with XLA have developed vaccine-related paralytic poliomyelitis after receiving the live oral polio vaccine.[335]

The only typical abnormality on physical examination in XLA that is not related directly to infections is the absence or a paucity of normal B-cell–containing lymphoid tissues, such as tonsils, adenoids, and peripheral lymph nodes.

The diagnosis of XLA can be confirmed by studying lymphocyte markers and demonstrating a lack of circulating cells that stain for surface immunoglobulin or with B-cell–specific monoclonal antibodies against CD19, CD20, or both. The number and function of T lymphocytes are normal in XLA. It may be difficult to establish the diagnosis based on immunoglobulin levels in the newborn period because of the presence of maternally derived IgG. However, if suspected, the diagnosis can be made in the newborn period by documenting a paucity of circulating B cells by flow cytometry.

Although individuals with XLA ordinarily are thought of as having a "pure" B-cell disorder, recent evidence reveals that the absence of B cells in XLA is associated with a contracted T-cell receptor repertoire and that mice that lack B cells are unable to prime $CD4^+$ T cells for their effector function in clearing *Pneumocystis* infection, findings that are consistent with the important role of B cells in presenting antigen to $CD4^+$ T cells.[420,451]

In contrast to carriers of some other X-linked diseases examined later (see discussion of chronic granulomatous disease), circulating B lymphocytes of XLA carriers express only one population of B cells, those with the normal allele on the X chromosome, presumably because B cells with the mutant allele are at a selective disadvantage and do not develop. Advances in genetic techniques have enabled detection of maternal carriers of XLA.[139] Prenatal diagnosis can be made by genetic studies of amniotic fluid cells or quantitation of fetal circulating B cells.[139]

The prognosis for patients with XLA has improved markedly with earlier diagnosis, high-dose intravenous immunoglobulin (IVIG) therapy, and aggressive use of antibiotics. Before the availability of IVIG, most patients who survived to the third decade of life had chronic lung disease from recurrent pulmonary infections and hearing loss from recurrent otitis media.[335]

IgG subclass deficiency. Persons with IgG subclass deficiencies have levels of one or more IgG subclass that are more than two standard deviations below normal for age, normal to slightly decreased total IgG, normal levels of other immunoglobulin isotypes, and, often, a poor antibody response to certain antigens.*

Patients with IgG subclass deficiency who also have IgM and IgA deficiency may have another immunodeficiency disorder such as common variable immunodeficiency (CVID).

The most common kinds of infections in patients with any clinically significant IgG subclass deficiency include otitis media, sinusitis, and pneumonia. Ordinarily, these patients do not have life-threatening systemic infections.

Deficiency of IgG1 is likely to be associated with subnormal levels of total IgG because this subclass accounts for about 60% of total IgG, and it often is associated with other subclass deficiencies.[16,17,492,498–500]

IgG2 deficiency usually is associated with normal total serum IgG levels and is more likely to be clinically significant if accompanied by IgG4 or IgA deficiency. Patients with IgG2 deficiency typically have poor antibody responses to polysaccharide antigens but normal responses to protein antigens. Like most patients with deficiencies of humoral immunity, their infections primarily are due to encapsulated bacteria and are localized to the respiratory tract.[498,500]

IgG3 deficiency has been associated with low total levels of serum IgG and recurrent respiratory infections, which also may lead to chronic pulmonary disease.[415]

IgG4 deficiency is difficult to diagnose because many normal persons have low serum levels of IgG4, and most normal infants have no detectable IgG4.[416] IgG4 deficiency appears to be of clinical significance, however, if it is associated with IgG2 and IgA deficiency.

The treatment for children with IgG subclass deficiency typically is individualized according to the frequency and severity of symptoms. Noninvasive infections usually can be treated successfully with appropriate antibiotics. Patients with more severe presentations may benefit from

*References 260–262, 386, 416, 425, 426, 491, 492, 497–501.

regular IVIG therapy, but those who also are completely IgA-deficient should be treated only with IgA-depleted IVIG preparations.

IgA deficiency. IgA deficiency is the most common immunodeficiency, occurring as frequently as 1/400. This disorder appears to occur sporadically, but familial cases have been described.[22,147] Most of the functions of serum IgA can be performed by IgG and IgM.[147,416] Thus, although deficiencies of secretory IgA may lead to recurrent respiratory or gastrointestinal tract infections, deficiency of serum IgA alone usually is not associated with increased susceptibility to systemic infections.[22] IgA deficiency has been associated with many other conditions, including recurrent infections, IgG2 deficiency, autoimmune disorders, and malignancy.[21] Recurrent infections are most likely to occur in the subset of IgA-deficient patients who also have IgG2 deficiency.[147,425] The infections usually are relatively mild and involve the upper respiratory and gastrointestinal tracts. Chronic gastrointestinal tract disease in these patients can be caused by *G. lamblia* infestations, nodular lymphoid hyperplasia, lactose intolerance, malabsorption, or inflammatory bowel disease. Other autoimmune diseases associated with IgA deficiency include rheumatoid arthritis, systemic lupus erythematosus, thyroiditis, myasthenia gravis, and vitiligo.[147] About 20% of IgA-deficient patients have allergy, and many have elevated levels of IgE.[147] Food allergy is common and may be the result of abnormal processing of antigen at mucosal surfaces.

Rare patients with serum IgA levels less than 5 mg/dL who receive transfusions may make antibody against donor IgA and have severe reactions when transfused again. IVIG reactions also may occur because IVIG preparations contain varying amounts of IgA. IgA-depleted preparations are available and usually are well tolerated.[150]

Transient hypogammaglobulinemia of infancy. The syndrome of transient hypogammaglobulinemia of infancy can be differentiated from the physiologic hypogammaglobulinemia in infants because immunoglobulin levels of normal infants begin to rise by about 6 months of age, whereas those of infants with transient hypogammaglobulinemia of infancy do not begin to increase until between 18 and 36 months of age.[416] Infants suspected of having this syndrome should be evaluated for XLA and CVID (see later discussion) and followed closely until their immunoglobulin levels normalize for age.

Antibody deficiency with normal or elevated levels of immunoglobulins. Some persons with normal levels of all circulating immunoglobulin isotypes are at increased risk for infections similar to those seen in specific deficiencies of immunoglobulin levels described earlier.[16,18,416] As in other forms of humoral immunodeficiency, the most common infections in these patients are recurrent bacterial respiratory tract infections, although a few patients have developed pneumococcal sepsis.[18] Such persons can be identified by their inability to make antibody in response to stimulation with specific antigens. A good way to test for this disorder is to immunize with protein antigens, such as tetanus and diphtheria toxoids, and with polysaccharide antigens, such as pneumococcal and *H. influenzae* type b capsular polysaccharide vaccines. Patients who can respond to protein but not to polysaccharide antigens usually will respond to protein-polysaccharide conjugates. Treatment with IVIG may help prevent recurrent infections in these patients, although their normal overall levels of immunoglobulin can pose difficulties in determining the appropriate doses of IVIG and intervals between infusions.

Defects of Cell-Mediated Immunity: DiGeorge Syndrome

The prototypic pure T-cell defect, DiGeorge syndrome, is characterized clinically by congenital heart disease (usually involving the aortic arch), hypocalcemic tetany, unusual facial features, and recurrent infections.[173] The classical, or complete, form of this disorder has absence or hypoplasia of the thymus and parathyroid glands, cardiac or aortic arch deformities, and a stereotypical constellation of abnormal facial features, most notably micrognathia and hypertelorism, all associated with malformation of the 4th and 5th branchial arches during embryogenesis.[173,318,350,537] Although the condition usually is considered to be associated with immunodeficiency because of the thymic hypoplasia, only about 25% of patients actually exhibit an immunologic defect.[55] The term *partial DiGeorge syndrome* sometimes has been used to describe patients with the typical constellation of anatomic findings but without immunodeficiency or similar patients with mild immunologic impairment.[273] Some sources designate this disorder as an "anomaly" or "sequence" rather than a syndrome because of confusion about its relationship to 22q11 deletion syndrome (del22q11) or the more recently defined microdeletion, del22p11.2, a deletion also associated with velocardiofacial syndrome.[97] Robin and Shprintzen[459] hold that the findings in DiGeorge sequence, although often associated with del22q11.2, are etiologically heterogeneous and have been associated with other chromosomal deletions such as del10p and del17p or del10q13. Moreover, some individuals with del22p11.2 exhibit abnormalities quite distinct from those of the DiGeorge sequence.[243,244,273,326,437,459] One candidate gene, *TBX1*, encoding a T-box transcription factor and located in 22q.11.2, has been a recent focus of research into the underlying genetic defect in DiGeorge syndrome. Although mice with mutations in *TBX1* exhibit some features consistent with DiGeorge syndrome, data remain insufficient to confirm the precise role of *TBX1* in human patients with this disorder.[249]

Because of the serious nature of the cardiovascular defect, many patients with DiGeorge syndrome in earlier decades have not survived long enough for the immune defect to become a clinical problem.[273] However, with improvements in surgical treatment of the heart defects, more of these infants now survive long enough to display manifestations of the immunodeficiency that results in an increased frequency or severity of viral and fungal infections, as well as *Pneumocystis* pneumonia. In such patients, management often has included prophylaxis against *Pneumocystis,* avoidance of live virus vaccines, and, because antibody production is poor as a result of lack of T-cell help, periodic IVIG infusions.[273] HLA-matched bone marrow transplantation has been successful in some cases.[83,238,273] Earlier work with transplantation of fetal or postnatal thymic tissue provided some long-term success in correcting the immunologic defect.[238,273] Recently, a highly promising large series of cases of transplantation with postnatal cultured thymic tissue in patients with complete DiGeorge syndrome yielded immune reconstitution with 73% survival at 2 years.[361]

Combined Defects of Cellular and Humoral Immunity

Severe combined immunodeficiency disease. Severe combined immunodeficiency (SCID) describes a heterogeneous group of heritable immunodeficiencies that involve serious impairments of both cellular and humoral immunity, thus leading to recurrent severe infections by a wide range of viral, bacterial, and fungal organisms. SCID has multiple forms, which have been reviewed in greater detail elsewhere.[102,103,123] At this writing, at least 10 genes have been identified with abnormalities known to result in SCID. X-linked SCID, the most common form, is due to a mutation in the common γ chain of the receptor for IL-2 and several other cytokines (γ_c).[103,339] The other known forms of SCID are either known or presumed to be autosomal recessive. These include a deficiency of adenosine deaminase, a purine salvage pathway enzyme; a deficiency in Janus kinase 3 (Jak3), a cytokine receptor signaling molecule; and a defect in the α chain of the IL-7 receptor, IL-7Rα.[103,297,555] Mutation of one of at least six different genes whose products play a role in T-cell receptor or immunoglobulin gene recombination or T-cell receptor signaling, including RAG1, RAG2, Artemis, DNA ligase IV, CD3-δ, and CD3-ε, also results in SCID.[103,123,191,210,297,356,457] Additionally, SCID is caused by a mutation in CD45, a phosphatase that regulates signaling thresholds in immune cells.[297] Flow cytometry analysis of lymphocyte markers reveals very low to absent B- and T-cell numbers in patients with most forms of SCID.

Long-term management of patients with SCID involves modalities employed in both B- and T-cell disorders, including prophylaxis against *P. jiroveci* pneumonia, avoidance of live viral vaccines, and immunoglobulin replacement therapy.[103] Bone marrow transplantation from HLA-matched siblings has corrected the defect successfully in some cases and is considered the current treatment of choice.[101] Adenosine deaminase deficiency is of historical interest in that it is the first heritable disorder for which gene therapy was attempted, although early success was limited.[101] Approaches using retroviral-based gene therapy for X-linked SCID initially appeared to be successful. However, at least three patients developed lymphoproliferative disorders similar to lymphocytic leukemia, with malignant cells demonstrating insertion of the vector into the promoter or first intron of a proto-oncogene, *LMO2*.[79,102,118,211,446]

Because the earliest possible treatment with stem cell transplantation often is the key to meaningful survival in patients with SCID, newborn screening programs for SCID based on assays of bloodspots have been introduced in several states and in some countries. These assays are based on quantitation of T-cell receptor excision circles—circular fragments of DNA that are a by-product of T-cell receptor rearrangement during fetal development.[46,121,445]

Common variable immunodeficiency. CVID is a heterogeneous group of combined immunodeficiencies that differ from most other primary immunodeficiencies in that they often present in the second or third decade of life, although they may present at any age.[146,148] Patients with CVID characteristically have normal or only modestly decreased numbers of circulating B cells; low, but not absent, levels of IgG, IgM, and IgA; poor responsiveness to antigens; and abnormal T-lymphocyte function.[149]

Although both T- and B-cell abnormalities often can be demonstrated, the clinical presentation usually is most like that in patients with humoral or B-cell defects (i.e., recurrent bacterial otitis media and sinopulmonary infections).[146,259,468] Occasionally, these patients also have infections with organisms more common in persons with T-lymphocyte abnormalities, such as *Pneumocystis,* recurrent herpes simplex virus, and herpes zoster virus infections. Chronic gastrointestinal problems may be due to *G. lamblia* or other intestinal pathogens. CVID patients are prone to nodular lymphoid hyperplasia, autoimmune diseases, and malignancies.

Several gene mutations have been found in patients with CVID. These include the genes encoding for CD19, transmembrane activator and CAML interactor (TACI), receptor for B-cell activating factor of the TNF receptor family (BAFF-R), and inducible costimulatory molecule (ICOS).[114,487,596]

Patients with CVID usually can benefit from therapy with IVIG, which reduces the incidence of acute infections. However, most patients with CVID, even some of those who undergo long-term treatment with IVIG, develop chronic sinopulmonary disease.[148,424]

Hyper–immunoglobulin M syndrome. Immunoglobulin deficiency with increased IgM is characterized by low levels of IgG, IgA, and IgE but normal to increased levels of IgM in the circulation and normal numbers of circulating B cells.[12,37,157] The disorder is caused by an intrinsic T-cell abnormality that impairs class switching from IgM to other isotypes. The basis for the various genetic forms of this defect is in one of several possible defects that involve interactions between CD40 on B cells and CD40 ligand (CD40L) on T cells. B cells from patients with the hyper-IgM syndrome only make IgM antibody, and their B cells only express surface IgM and IgD. The originally described and most common form of the defect is X-linked recessive and results from a mutation in the gene encoding CD40L, a protein expressed transiently on activated T cells.[12,37,157] More recently described autosomal recessive forms of this disorder involve mutations either in CD40 itself[157,207] or in a CD40-activated RNA editing enzyme, activation-induced cytidine deaminase.[455] Other cells express surface CD40, thus neutropenia and the increased incidence of infections caused by *Pneumocystis* and of malignancies in patients with hyper-IgM syndrome also may be the result of impaired cell interactions via CD40.

Clinically, hyper-IgM syndrome is manifested by recurrent bacterial infections, especially of the respiratory tract.[157] Such persons are susceptible to the same kinds of recurrent pyogenic infections associated with other immunoglobulin deficiencies, as well as to infections with organisms more commonly encountered in patients with T-cell defects (e.g., *P. jiroveci*).[49] Some patients with this syndrome have recurrent diarrhea as a result of *G. lamblia* and *Cryptosporidium* infection that is severe enough to require parenteral nutrition. About half of patients have persistent or recurrent neutropenia. Those with autoantibodies may have thrombocytopenia, hemolytic anemia, nephritis, hypothyroidism, or arthritis.

The diagnosis of X-linked hyper-IgM syndrome may be established by using immunofluorescence to document absent expression of CD40L on activated T cells, absent CD40 expression on B cells, or demonstrating a mutation in one of the genes encoding CD40, CD40L, or the enzyme activation-induced cytidine deaminase.

Treatment of patients with the hyper-IgM syndrome with IVIG usually results in significant clinical benefit.[49]

Wiskott-Aldrich syndrome. Wiskott-Aldrich syndrome is a rare X-linked disorder characterized by thrombocytopenia, small platelets, eczema, recurrent infections, autoimmune disease, and hematologic malignancy. Although both T- and B-cell compartments are affected, it presents phenotypically more like a B-cell or humoral deficiency, with recurrent otitis media, sinusitis, and pneumonia. The defect involves a mutation in the gene encoding a signaling molecule, Wiskott-Aldrich syndrome protein, which regulates "immune synapse" formation and IL-2 production.[414,415]

Ataxia-telangiectasia. Ataxia-telangiectasia is a rare autosomal recessive disorder characterized by progressive cerebellar dysfunction with ataxia, oculocutaneous telangiectasias, recurrent bacterial respiratory infections such as those seen in humoral deficiencies, and a predilection to hematologic malignancy and breast cancer. Serum immunoglobulins often are low, as are lymphocyte counts. The disorder is due to a mutation in the *ATM* gene, located on chromosome 11. This gene encodes a serine-threonine kinase that is important in cell cycle regulation and double-stranded DNA repair, and it influences expression of *BRCA1* genes associated with breast cancer. The risk for breast cancer in patients with ataxia-telangiectasia is increased 15- to 20-fold over that in the general population. Heterozygotes for missense mutations of the *ATM* gene can be affected because copies of the abnormal protein can interfere with function of the wild-type protein.[368,410]

Defects of the Interferon-Gamma (IFN-γ) and Interleukin-12 (IL-12) Pathways

Macrophages infected by intracellular pathogens, especially *Mycobacterium* or *Salmonella* spp., are stimulated via a TLR4-dependent mechanism to release IL-12, along with IL-18, IL-23, and IL-27. These cytokines stimulate T and NK cells to produce IFN-γ via interactions with cellular receptors for the aforementioned cytokines. The released IFN-γ, in turn, further stimulates the macrophage to release more IL-12 and to activate killing. The mechanism by which this intracellular killing occurs is unknown. This cycle of mutual activation is essential for normal defense against mycobacterial pathogens, and some genetic defects of these cytokines, their cellular receptors, or related molecules critical for receptor-mediated signaling have been associated with increased susceptibility to mycobacterial infections. Deficiencies in this system have resulted from mutations in either of the two receptors for IFN-γ, IFN-γR1 and IFN-γR2, as well as mutations in STAT1, a molecule critical for transducing signals from both IFN-γ receptors. Mutations also have been described in the 40-kDa subunit of IL-12, IL-12p40, and the IL-12 receptor, IL-12Rβ1. These disorders are rather uncommon, all involving fewer than 100 known patients.[423,470]

Mutation of either of the IFN-γRs is associated with increased risk for mycobacterial infections. Deficiencies of IFN-γR1 may be either autosomal recessive or dominant and either complete or partial. Most recessive defects are complete and result in absent IFN-γ responsiveness. Dominant IFN-γR1 deficiency results from heterozygous truncations of the cytoplasmic domain of the receptor with excessive accumulation of nonfunctional receptors at the cell surface. Patients with the recessive complete form of this deficiency have a much more severe clinical phenotype than those with the dominant partial form, although the latter have a fivefold greater frequency of nontuberculous mycobacterial osteomyelitis. Defects in IFN-γR2, much less common, also may be recessive or dominant in inheritance and either complete or partial. Rare deficiencies in the receptor signaling molecule STAT1 have led to increased mycobacterial infections in a partial deficiency or, in two patients with a recessive complete form, to postvaccination disseminated bacille Calmette-Guérin (BCG) disease followed later by death from severe viral infections. The latter probably relates to the additional role of STAT1 in development of IFN-α/β-mediated antiviral activity.[470]

Deficiencies of IL-12p40 or its receptor IL-12Rβ1 are associated with disseminated nontuberculous mycobacterial infections, tuberculosis, and *Salmonella* infections. The receptor deficiency results in unresponsiveness to IL-12. This defect is apparently autosomal recessive with variable clinical penetrance. Deficiency of IL-12p40 also is variable in its clinical phenotype and has resulted in deaths from severe mycobacterial infections.[427,470,525]

The approach to specific diagnosis of defects of the IFN-γ pathway has been well systematized, but such studies should be undertaken only in a highly specialized reference laboratory.[470]

Complement Deficiencies

Approximately 0.03% of the general population have complement deficiencies resulting from acquired or congenital abnormalities of single or multiple complement components or regulatory proteins. Excellent reviews of complement deficiencies are available elsewhere.[166,167,169,176,265,289,471,580]

Congenital or hereditary deficiencies of complement more often are manifested by abnormality or complete absence of a single complement protein, and most of these have been well documented to predispose to potentially life-threatening infections. Most primary complement abnormalities (C1q dysfunction and C1rs, C4, C2, C3, C5, C6, C7, C8, and C9 deficiencies) are inherited as autosomal codominant traits.[166]

Patients with homozygous or heterozygous deficiency of the early classical pathway proteins C1, C2, and C4 are more prone to develop autoimmune disease than difficulty with infections. However, approximately 20% of patients with homozygous deficiency of early components have problems with recurrent or severe infections that are similar to those seen in C3 deficiency.[166,208,471] Their predilection for autoimmune disease probably is due, at least in part, to abnormal solubilization and removal of immune complexes. C2 deficiency has been associated with antibody deficiencies in individuals with recurrent infections.[15,113]

Deficiencies of alternative pathway proteins predispose to serious, often fatal, infections because of the lack of ability to respond promptly to organisms not previously encountered.[167] Properdin deficiency, the only X-linked complement deficiency, has been associated with fulminant, usually fatal, meningococcal infection.[167] Factor D deficiency is rare and appears to predispose to recurrent neisserial infection.[309]

Mutations or variants in the gene for MBL, the initiator of the MBL pathway (see earlier discussion), have been associated with an increased risk for recurrent infections.[176,265] In particular, homozygosity for such mutations or variants was found to be associated with an increased risk for systemic meningococcal disease.[214]

Because all three complement activation pathways converge at the activation of C3, patients who are deficient in C3 are unable to mobilize any of the three main effector functions of complement in host defense—opsonization, phagocyte recruitment, or bacteriolysis. Thus it is not surprising that the most serious complement deficiency state is the rare total absence of C3.[166,208,471] Patients with deficiencies or mutations of factors H and I have low but detectable levels of C3 because absence of either of these regulatory factors allows continuous activation of the alternative pathway and uncontrolled C3 consumption. Patients with C3 deficiency caused by any of these mechanisms have increased susceptibility to infections caused by encapsulated bacteria such as *S. pneumoniae, N. meningitidis,* and *H. influenzae* type b. Most of these infections involve the respiratory tract (otitis, sinusitis, bronchitis, and pneumonia), but C3-deficient patients also are predisposed to sepsis and meningitis.[166,208,471] In addition, some C3-deficient persons develop autoimmune diseases.[166,208,471]

Deficiencies of terminal complement proteins C5, C6, C7, and C8 greatly increase the risk for developing systemic infections with *N. meningitidis* or *Neisseria gonorrheae.*[72] C9 deficiency increases the risk for infection to a lesser degree than do deficiencies of other terminal components. In one study, the risk for meningococcal disease was increased 5000-fold in C7-deficient persons and about 700-fold in C9-deficient persons.[396]

The risk for infection is higher in patients with C5 deficiency than in those with deficiencies of other terminal proteins because, in addition to the role of C5 in initiating assembly of the membrane attack complex, the free C5 fragment, C5a, is important for leukocyte recruitment to sites of microbial invasion.[15,53]

At least one episode of meningococcal disease occurs in approximately 60% of persons who have been identified as having C5, C6, C7, C8, or properdin deficiency, and 75% to 85% of documented bacterial infections in complement-deficient persons are meningococcal.[166,208,471] Conversely, approximately 14% of patients presenting with sporadic meningococcal disease have a defect in one of the late complement components, and this percentage rises to about one third among individuals with two or more meningococcal infections. The mortality due to meningococcal infection in such patients is lower than in normal persons, probably because patients with these deficiencies often have antibodies to meningococci that can activate the classical pathway leading to normal opsonization and phagocyte activation, which are effector functions upstream in the cascade from the membrane attack complex. In contrast, individuals with normal complement levels who develop meningococcal infection usually do so because they do not have specific antibodies with which to mobilize any effector functions via the classical pathway, and, as noted earlier, meningococci are poor activators of the alternative pathway.

Currently no specific treatment exists for patients with hereditary complement deficiencies. Replacement of missing complement proteins is not practical because of the short half-life of most of the components.[52,329,474] Immunization of complement-deficient patients and their close household contacts against encapsulated organisms, especially *N. meningitidis,* is important.

Disorders of Phagocyte Function

General features of phagocyte disorders. The most frequently encountered reminder of the importance of an adequate supply of well-functioning phagocytes comes from patients who develop chemotherapy-associated neutropenia and are thus at high risk for bacterial and fungal infections.[442] The qualitative disorders of phagocyte function discussed in this section result in similar susceptibilities to these infections, either because the circulating cells are unable to migrate to an infected site or because, once having migrated to the infected tissue, they are unable to effect normal microbicidal activity. There is some overlap among the types of infectious complications associated with disorders of migration versus killing. However, as a rule, defects of neutrophil migration tend to be associated with infections at skin, subcutaneous tissue, and mucous membrane sites. In contrast, killing defects are more likely to result in infections of deeper soft tissues and internal organs, although skin infections are not uncommon.

Intrinsic disorders of cell migration

Type 1 leukocyte adhesion deficiency. In the late 1970s and the first half of the ensuing decade, several reports described patients with recurrent bacterial infections, diminished neutrophil motility, and delayed separation of the umbilical cord.[1,28–30,34,145,213,257] The neutrophils of these patients were discovered to be markedly deficient in adherence to both natural and artificial surfaces, response to complement-opsonized particles, and expression of members of a family of heterodimeric glycoproteins: LFA-1, Mac-1, and pl50,95, each defined by its own unique α subunit, CD11a, CD11b, and CD11c, respectively, but sharing a common 95-kDa β subunit designated CD18.[29,30,34,35,523] A fourth α subunit, CD11d, whose importance remains poorly understood, has been described more recently. The defective expression of these proteins, also called the β_2 leukocyte integrins, appeared to be directly responsible for the striking adherence-dependent defects that characterized the function of leukocytes from patients with this disorder.[28–30,34,35,523] Variously called Mac-1 deficiency, MO1 deficiency, LFA-1 deficiency, CD11/CD18 deficiency, or CR3 deficiency, this disorder, now usually called type 1 leukocyte adhesion deficiency (LAD-1), is an autosomal recessive disorder with one of numerous mutations in the β_2 integrin subunit, CD18, localized to chromosome 21.[30,35,523,524] It has been identified in more than 150 persons worldwide and encompasses a broad ethnic diversity.[30,35] Patients may exhibit a moderate or severe phenotype, depending on the extent of the defect in protein expression.[29,30] The documented mutations of the β_2 subunit (CD18) range from complete absence of the protein to extensions of the molecule, truncations of the extracellular portion or of the cytoplasmic domain of the molecule, small deletions, and point mutations.[31,35,269]

Patients with LAD-1 develop recurrent necrotic skin and soft tissue infections with poor or absent pus formation, and they exhibit poor wound healing.[20,29] They develop severe periodontitis, often losing their primary and secondary dentition along with alveolar bone.[29,30,558] They may develop enterocolitis much like that seen in neutropenic patients.[26,29] Delayed separation of the umbilical cord, presumably resulting from an impaired inflammatory response, is a common feature of the more severe phenotype of this disorder,[29,30] but this finding alone in infants without infectious complications or other characteristic features is of doubtful significance.[586] Pronounced leukocytosis is a common feature of LAD-1, even in the absence of active infection.[29,30] Recent studies in CD18-null LAD-1 mice reveal abnormally high circulating granulocyte colony-stimulating factor (G-CSF) levels and suggest the absence of a negative feedback mechanism on G-CSF production that occurs during normal transendothelial migration of leukocytes and involves IL-17. Absent ongoing transendothelial migration results in failure of this putative feedback mechanism, resulting in elevated G-CSF levels and higher circulating granulocyte counts.[216]

Functional studies of neutrophils from patients with LAD-1 reveal a marked impairment of all adherence-dependent functions that require the β_2 integrins.[28–30,107,227,269] PMNs and NK cells from patients with LAD-1 exhibit impaired ADCC for virus-infected target cells, suggesting that CD11/CD18-mediated cell-cell adhesion is essential for normal killing of virus-infected cells by this mechanism[310] and that the increased severity of viral infections in a few of the most severely affected patients could be related to defective ADCC. Currently the diagnosis of LAD usually is made by demonstrating absent or markedly deficient expression of the CD11/CD18 family of glycoproteins on circulating leukocytes by immunofluorescence flow cytometry.[28–30,35]

Careful attention to skin and oral hygiene, aggressive management of infections, and meticulous local care of wound sites are important in the care of patients with LAD-1 or any serious disorder of neutrophil migration. The efficacy of prophylactic antibiotics has not been well established. Bone marrow transplantation with HLA-matched allogeneic marrow has had mixed results, from complete correction of the phagocytic defect to death 9 months after transplantation from graft-versus-host disease.[30,213] The human CD18 gene has been cloned and sequenced, and human LAD-1 cells have been corrected successfully in vitro with the normal CD18 complementary DNA carried by retrovirus vectors, hinting at the future promise of gene therapy for patients with LAD-1.[26,30,316]

Type 2 leukocyte adhesion deficiency. In 1992, two unrelated patients were reported, both products of consanguineous matings, who exhibited clinical characteristics virtually identical to those described for LAD-1.[219] However, expression of the β_2 (CD18) integrins on leukocytes was normal. In addition to defects in neutrophil motility, these children exhibited short stature, psychomotor retardation, and the Bombay (hh) erythrocyte phenotype (homozygous for absence of the H antigen). Phagocytosis by PMNs was normal. Recently it has been documented that this defect is due to one or more mutations of a specific guanosine diphosphate (GDP)-fucose transporter,[354] resulting in the absence of fucosyl residues on sialyl Lewis X, the tetrasaccharide moiety that serves as the principal ligand for members of the selectin family of adhesion molecules.[219,328,567] In vivo and in vitro studies comparing the adhesive functions of PMNs from LAD-1 and this new disorder, now called LAD-2, provided elegant validation of the distinct roles of selectins and integrins in the recruitment of leukocytes in vivo, with the initial selectin-mediated "rolling" stage (deficient in LAD-2) required first for the second integrin-mediated "firm adhesion and extravasation" stage (deficient in LAD-1) to occur (see Fig. 2.2).[567] The other somatic and neurologic features of LAD-2 may be related to more widespread consequences of the generalized defect in fucosylation of glycoproteins.[354]

Type 3 leukocyte adhesion deficiency (integrin activation defect). During the past decade, several patients have been reported who have a clinical phenotype that includes features of both type 1 LAD and Glanzmann thrombasthenia, a bleeding disorder associated with mutations in the $\alpha_{IIb}\beta_3$ integrin on platelets. Laboratory studies of these patients revealed markedly deficient integrin-mediated adhesive functions of both leukocytes and platelets despite normal surface expression of both leukocyte and platelet integrins. Further studies led to the conclusion that this defect in integrin function was the result of defective "inside-out" signaling pathways that normally lead to integrin activation.[196,305,366] Recent data on several kindreds with this disorder, studied in different laboratories, confirmed the presence of mutations in the gene encoding Kindlin-3, a molecule that, during cell activation, forms a critical bridge between the actin cytoskeleton and the cytoplasmic domain of the β subunit of multiple classes of integrins expressed by cells of hematopoietic lineages.[266,358,389,535] This bridging by Kindlin-3 is essential for normal integrin activation in both leukocytes and platelets.

Specific granule deficiency. Rare patients with hereditary specific granule deficiency have been reported, beginning with Spitznagel's original description in 1972.[86,222,521] These persons exhibited recurrent and severe infections, primarily of the skin and mucous membranes, sometimes involving the lung and, in one patient, the mastoid. Neutrophils from patients with this disorder exhibit absent specific granules on Wright-stained blood smears. Lactoferrin released from specific granules reduces the negative surface charge of the plasma membrane, contributing to nonspecific adhesiveness of the cell.[222] The specific granule membrane also contains some of the intracellular store of the important adhesion molecule Mac-1 (CD11b/CD18) that is mobilized to the plasma membrane upon cell activation.[60,81] Recurrent skin and mucous membrane infections resulting from *S. aureus*, gram-negative bacilli, and *Candida* spp. characterize the natural history of patients with this disorder.[86,222,521] Neutrophils in this disorder also exhibit diminished microbicidal activity, presumably because of diminished amounts of the cytochrome component of NADPH oxidase that normally reside in the membrane of specific granules. In this rare disorder, males and females are represented equally. A few patients with specific granule deficiency have a deletion in the gene encoding the myeloid cell transcription factor known as CCAAT/enhancer binding protein epsilon (*C/EBPε*) with absent expression of this transcription factor, although not all patients with this disorder have a mutation of this gene.[174,338]

Chédiak-Higashi syndrome. Chédiak-Higashi syndrome is a complex, rare autosomal recessive disorder characterized by partial oculocutaneous albinism, recurrent pyogenic infections, peripheral neuropathy, and neutropenia.[77] The illness also may involve an accelerated lymphoproliferative phase.[77] Granular cells, including neutrophils, contain giant lysosomal granules that are the apparent result of spontaneous intracellular fusion of azurophilic granules and, to a lesser extent, specific granules.[77] Corresponding disorders of intracellular pigment granules and vesicle trafficking in axons account for the albinism and other manifestations of this disease.[77] The genetic basis of the defect is now known to involve either a mutation in the gene encoding a large protein called the *lysosomal trafficking regulator (LYST)*, homologous to the "beige" gene in mice, with all mutations studied so far resulting in a truncated protein.[51,119] Patients with Chédiak-Higashi syndrome develop recurrent skin and mucosal infections, most often caused by *S. aureus*.[30,77] A cell migration defect appears to be related to abnormal regulation of microtubule polymerization upon cell activation.[77] The possible role of intracellular levels of cyclic adenosine monophosphate and guanylic acid in this microtubule abnormality has been suggested.[89] Studies of two brothers with Chédiak-Higashi syndrome demonstrated abnormally increased tyrosinylation of the α subunit of tubulin.[77,399] The diagnosis of Chédiak-Higashi syndrome usually is suspected clinically on the basis of partial oculocutaneous albinism and recurrent pyogenic infections. A Wright stain demonstrating giant lysosomal granules and laboratory studies showing defective cell migration are confirmatory, and genetic confirmation is now possible.

Neutrophil actin dysfunction. Filamentous actin constitutes the main contractile mechanism of neutrophils for migration and phagocytosis.[530] An extremely rare and apparently heterogeneous disorder, neutrophil actin dysfunction has been characterized by recurrent skin infections caused by *S. aureus* and *Candida albicans*. In vivo and in vitro studies revealed severely impaired neutrophil chemotaxis and phagocytosis.[87] The capacity for polymerization of actin from cell extracts also was diminished markedly. It is of interest that PMNs from family members of this patient also were found to be variably deficient in the CD11/CD18 family of glycoproteins that are the basis of LAD-1.[518] One similarly affected infant was found to have abnormally high levels of a 47-kDa protein, now identified as *lymphocyte-specific protein–1 (LSP-1)*, which exhibits actin-binding activity.[132]

Glycogen storage disease type 1B. Beaudet and colleagues[57] first reported the association of recurrent infection, neutropenia, and impaired neutrophil migration with glycogen storage disease type 1B, a metabolic disorder characterized by defective microsomal transport of glucose-6-phosphate. In 1985, Ambruso and coworkers[19] reviewed the features of 21 patients with glycogen storage disease type 1B, 15 of whom suffered from frequent infections, especially of the skin and subcutaneous tissues. Impaired neutrophil motility was found in 8 of 11 patients in whom this was evaluated. A specific relationship between the underlying metabolic defect in glycogen storage disease type 1B and the mechanism of impaired cell motility has not been established. However, exogenous glucose is an important energy source for chemotaxis,[577] and it is interesting to note that the uptake of glucose by PMNs in response to chemoattractant stimulation is impaired in glycogen storage disease type 1B, as well as in neonates, both examples of patients with impaired PMN migration.[4,53]

Extrinsic or secondary defects of polymorphonuclear leukocyte migration

Defective neutrophil chemotaxis associated with serum inhibitors of cell function. Investigators have reported the presence of inhibitors of PMN chemotaxis in the serum of patients with recurrent infection.[315,507,517,559,575] In each case, the patient's neutrophils exhibited diminished chemotaxis in the presence of autologous serum or plasma, whereas identical assays in the presence of control serum or plasma resulted in a normal chemotactic response. Most such inhibitors appear to be immunoglobulins or immunoglobulin-like molecules.

Hyper-immunoglobulin E syndrome. In 1966, Davis and colleagues[160] described two young girls with coarse facial features, reddish hair, fair skin, severe eczema, dystrophic nails, "cold" staphylococcal skin abscesses, and recurrent sinopulmonary infections. The term *Job syndrome* was suggested, referring to the similar biblical affliction. Additional patients were described with a similar disorder, first associated by Buckley and associates[105] with very high serum IgE levels, including a patient who exhibited a defect in neutrophil chemotaxis reported in 1973 by Clark and associates.[131] Features common to all of the patients with the disease now termed *hyper-IgE syndrome* include a history of staphylococcal infections of the skin and sinopulmonary tract beginning in infancy or early childhood and serum levels of IgE that are greater than 2000 IU/mL.[100,105,179] Based on extensive reviews, other characteristic but variable features of this disorder include coarse facies, cold abscesses of the skin and subcutaneous tissues, a chronic eczematoid rash, eosinophilia, and mucocutaneous candidiasis.[100,179,217] Consistent abnormalities of cell-mediated immune functions in patients with hyper-IgE syndrome suggest that the pathogenic basis involves a defect of T-cell regulation.[104,126,179,230] An extensive study of 19 kindreds revealed autosomal dominant inheritance with a genetic locus for hyper-IgE syndrome on chromosome 4, in the proximal 4q region.[246,247] In 2007, it ultimately was determined that this disorder can be attributed to dominant negative mutations in STAT3, a factor critical for signal transduction by at least 10 different cytokines, some with proinflammatory and others with antiinflammatory functions.[272,381,519] The immunologic defect is characterized further by a paucity of T_H17 lymphocytes, which normally promote protective leukocyte responses to bacteria and fungi.[382] Recently a rare and clinically distinct autosomal recessive form of hyper-IgE syndrome has been described, resulting from a mutation in *DOCK8*, a member of a family of atypical guanine nucleoside exchange factors highly expressed in lymphocytes.[533] Patients with this form of hyper-IgE syndrome have developed chronic viral infections, severe allergies, and early-onset malignancies.[79,246,519,533]

Although hyper-IgE syndrome might more properly belong in discussions of defective T-cell regulation, some patients with hyper-IgE syndrome may have a defect in neutrophil chemotaxis.[179] The defect sometimes has been intermittent, and, in several cases, the presence of a serum inhibitor of chemotaxis has been recognized.[178,179] Recent data suggest that keratinocytes and other epithelial cells from patients with hyper-IgE syndrome may produce reduced amounts of neutrophil-attracting chemokines, and neutrophils of these patients exhibit reduced expression of chemoattractant receptors.[382,383]

Other secondary or poorly defined disorders of polymorphonuclear leukocyte migration. Patients with protein-calorie malnutrition have defective PMN chemotaxis that appears to be based on systemic preactivation of circulating cells resulting from chronic low-level endotoxemia from impaired intestinal mucosal integrity.[122,484] Shwachman-Diamond syndrome, in addition to pancreatic insufficiency, neutropenia, and growth retardation, also is associated with defective PMN migration.[10] Two kindreds with congenital ichthyosis and an associated defect of PMN migration have been described.[380] Patients with severe thermal injuries develop an acquired form of specific granule deficiency with impaired PMN migration beginning about 14 days after injury.[222] Several reports have been published of a poorly defined disorder of neutrophil migration referred to as *lazy leukocyte syndrome*,[9,378,379] marked by recurrent staphylococcal skin infections, rhinitis, gingivitis, stomatitis, neutropenia despite adequate marrow precursors, and diminished in vivo and in vitro migration of neutrophils.

Defects in phagocyte microbicidal activity. As described earlier, the broad array of available phagocyte microbicidal mechanisms may be divided into oxygen-dependent and oxygen-independent mechanisms. To date, no specific deficiency of any oxygen-independent microbicidal mechanism has been described. Thus this section is concerned mainly with the known deficiencies of oxygen-dependent microbicidal mechanisms of phagocytes, especially chronic granulomatous disease, the prototypical defect in this group. PMNs, monocytes, and the fixed phagocytes of the reticuloendothelial system generally share in the deficient microbicidal activity observed.

Chronic granulomatous disease. Chronic granulomatous disease (CGD) was one of the earliest syndromes of phagocyte dysfunction to be characterized.[448] It is recognized now to be a family of biochemically and genetically heterogeneous disorders of distinct components of the phagocyte NADPH oxidase complex (see Fig. 2.3 and related text)[122,174] that result in the inability of phagocytes to generate superoxide anion and other reactive oxygen species.[174] Organisms that produce catalase pose a special problem for patients with this disease.[174,180,291,333] This encompasses a broad range of pathogens, including staphylococci, gram-negative enteric bacteria, *Pseudomonas* spp., yeast, fungi, *Nocardia* spp., and numerous other pathogenic species.[180,289,333,588] Most microorganisms produce H_2O_2, which might be used, even by the CGD phagocyte, as an effective microbicidal weapon because it feeds into the sequence of oxidant reactions downstream from the defective oxidase enzyme (see Fig. 2.3).[465] Organisms that produce catalase are able to survive within these deficient cells because catalase is an enzyme that degrades H_2O_2 to oxygen and water.[291,466] Infections with catalase-negative bacteria, such as *Streptococcus, Haemophilus,* and *Neisseria* spp., do not occur with increased frequency in CGD patients,[588] and these organisms are killed normally in vitro by CGD phagocytes. Phagocyte functions not directly related to oxidative mechanisms of intracellular killing, including adherence, chemotaxis, phagocytosis, and degranulation, usually are normal.[42,381,448,515]

The genetic defect in CGD may be inherited by either X-linked recessive or autosomal recessive mechanisms.[83,130,151] In the report of a registry of 368 patients with CGD in the United States,[588] more than two-thirds of the patients had the X-linked recessive form with absent $gp91^{phox}$, the larger subunit of the cytochrome b_{558}; about 12% had an autosomal recessive form with absent cytosolic $p47^{phox}$; and fewer than 5% each had autosomal recessive disease with absent cytosolic $p67^{phox}$ or absence of $p22^{phox}$, the smaller subunit of the cytochrome b_{558}. Approximately 12% had an unknown genetic form of the disease. A single individual with an autosomal recessive form of CGD due to mutations in the cytosolic $p40^{phox}$ has been reported.[364] About 5% of patients with CGD have normal levels of an abnormal protein that is inactive, and at least 410 different mutations have been reported to result in CGD.[264] These genetically diverse defects all result in defective function of the oxidase and the characteristic CGD phenotype. In the female obligate carriers of X-linked CGD, the proportion of cells that express the defect usually is between 35% and 65%, depending on the proportion of cells in which random inactivation of the normal versus the affected X chromosome occurs.[355,588] Overall, patients with X-linked disease have more severe courses and experience higher yearly death rates than patients with autosomal recessive forms of the disease.[588]

Patients with CGD experience recurrent serious bacterial and fungal infections, usually beginning in the first few months of life. *S. aureus* and gram-negative bacilli, especially *Serratia marcescens* and *Burkholderia cepacia,* are the most common causes of infection in patients with CGD. Fungi, especially *Aspergillus* spp., also are prominent etiologic agents,[333,453,588] and infections caused by *Aspergillus* are the most common cause of death in these patients.[588] Granuloma formation at infected sites is one of the histologic hallmarks of this disorder.[290,453] Pulmonary infections and their complications have been the reported cause of death in up to 50% of these patients in some series, and *Aspergillus* predominates.[588] These infections often are protracted and respond slowly to appropriate antibiotic therapy.[291,453] Progression to lung abscess, empyema, or both occurs in about 20% of patients with CGD with pneumonia.[291] Liver abscesses occur in about half of patients and may be recurrent.[59,127] The hepatosplenomegaly common in CGD may result from these infections but more likely results from chronic infections at various sites with systemic lymphoid hyperplasia.[45,291] Osteomyelitis occurs in about one third of patients.[291,453,588] In contrast to normal children, in whom this infection usually involves the metaphyseal area of long bones, patients with CGD more often develop infections of the small bones of the hands and feet. In normal children, *S. aureus* is the most common etiologic agent and causes a significant proportion of cases in CGD. However, gram-negative bacilli and *Aspergillus* appear to be the predominant etiologies, and other agents, including *Nocardia,* also may be important etiologic agents of bone infection in CGD.[437,588] Skin infections in this disorder may include pyoderma, purulent dermatitis, and cutaneous or subcutaneous abscesses and often are preceded by a chronic eczematoid skin rash.[453]

Although localized infections are the rule in patients with CGD, these patients also may develop septicemia.[291,453,588] The most common cause of septicemia in most series has been *Salmonella,* but other gram-negative enteric bacilli also have been prominent.[290,333] Of note, *S. aureus* is a proportionally less common cause of septicemia in these patients.[453,588]

Granuloma formation adjacent to hollow viscera in patients with CGD can produce clinically significant obstruction, including obstruction of the gastric outlet, esophagus, small intestine, and ureters. This complication usually responds to treatment with corticosteroids.[20,180,588]

CGD should be suspected in patients with a history of recurrent indolent infections caused by catalase-positive organisms such as those described earlier, especially if granulomas are found in biopsy specimens of lymph nodes or other tissues. Confirmation of the diagnosis usually rests on the demonstration of an absent or nearly absent oxidative metabolic burst in the patient's phagocytes. This can be detected classically by the slide NBT test or by various other measurements of oxidative burst activity, most recently by flow cytometry of PMNs loaded with oxidant-sensitive fluorescent dyes.[13,40,54,465,548] Fig. 2.10A is an example of the slide NBT test in an X-linked carrier; Fig. 2.10B is an idealized set of flow cytometry histograms with typical patterns for a normal control, a patient with CGD, and both X-linked and autosomal recessive carriers. Prenatal diagnosis has been achieved by the use of the slide NBT test with blood from placental vessels obtained at fetoscopy.[401]

The management of patients with CGD includes antibiotic prophylaxis, usually with trimethoprim-sulfamethoxazole, and an aggressive approach to the specific diagnosis and treatment of acute infections.[453] Antifungal prophylaxis with itraconazole or voriconazole that has activity against *Aspergillus* also has become standard. Bone marrow transplantation met with early limited success,[241,298,581] but allogeneic peripheral blood stem cell transplantation from HLA-identical sibling donors, with prior myeloablative conditioning, has been considerably more promising, as suggested by the European experience from 1985 to 2000, with 22 of 23 patients "cured" at median follow-up of 12 years.[495]

A multicenter study reported that daily subcutaneous injections of IFN-γ reduced the requirement for hospitalization of CGD patients for serious infections by about two-thirds.[283] The mechanism by which IFN-γ exerts its beneficial effect in CGD has not been determined. Despite some systemic side effects, such as fever, fatigue, and myalgia,[283] it generally has been well tolerated,[360] and it continues to be used in the management of many patients with this disorder.[588]

Deficiencies of glucose-6-phosphate dehydrogenase, glutathione peroxidase, and glutathione synthetase. The normal activity of the NADPH oxidase enzyme complex depends on the continued availability of NADPH to reduce molecular oxygen to form superoxide anion.[129,465] The primary source of NADPH for this enzyme is the hexose

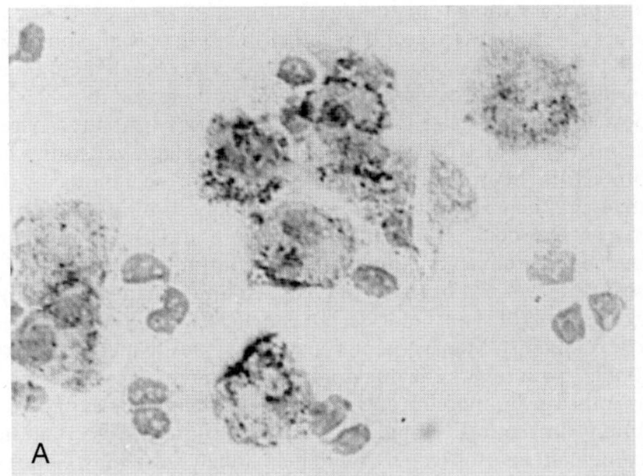

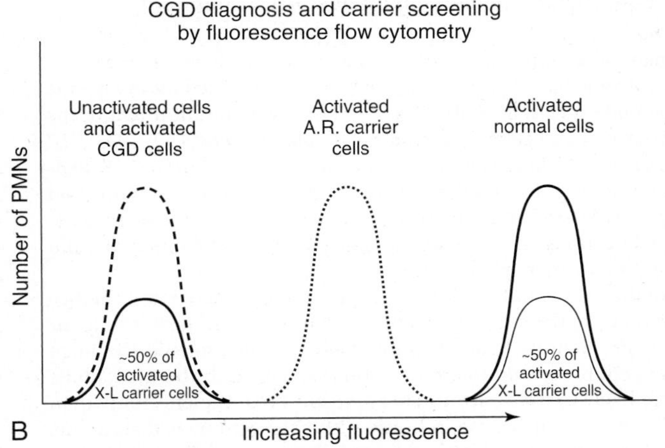

FIG. 2.10 (A) Photomicrograph of a slide nitroblue tetrazolium (NBT) test of polymorphonuclear leukocytes (PMNs) isolated from the blood of a maternal carrier of X-linked recessive chronic granulomatous disease (CGD). Because of random inactivation of either the normal or the affected X chromosome in maternal carriers of this disorder, approximately half of the PMNs exhibit the granular blue-black staining characteristic of the oxidative reduction of NBT by normal PMNs. In contrast, the remaining PMNs, which express the reduced nicotinamide adenine dinucleotide phosphate (NADPH) oxidase defect of CGD, are visible only by their nuclear counterstain. (B) Flow cytometry in CGD diagnosis and carrier testing. These idealized flow cytometry histograms demonstrate the oxidative burst activity of populations of PMNs that have been loaded with an agent such as dihydrorhodamine that becomes fluorescent when it reacts with products formed during the oxidative burst. The taller curve on the far left represents the fluorescence typical of both inactivated normal PMNs and activated PMNs from a patient with CGD with an absent oxidative burst. The taller histogram on the far right demonstrates the increased level of fluorescence exhibited by activated normal PMNs. The two smaller curves on the left and the right represent the two populations of activated PMNs from a typical maternal carrier of X-linked CGD, indicating about 50% normal PMNs and 50% expressing the defect. The taller histogram in the middle represents typical results for the cells of a carrier of autosomal recessive CGD, with all cells exhibiting an intermediate level of fluorescence.

monophosphate shunt, and this pathway is provided with the hexose substrate, 6-phosphoglucose, by the enzyme glucose-6-phosphate dehydrogenase (G6PD), which also generates NADPH in a coupled reaction.[466] The reactions of the hexose monophosphate shunt itself are coupled to two other enzymes, glutathione reductase and glutathione peroxidase, which recycle oxidized and reduced glutathione.[465] A deficiency in any of these three enzymes results in a lack of available NADPH to drive the NADPH oxidase and may result in a phagocyte killing defect similar to CGD.[41,477] G6PD deficiency usually involves erythrocytes and is associated with hemolytic anemia, especially in conjunction with the administration of sulfonamides.[142] Only when the defect also involves myeloid cells and is severe or complete (<5% of normal enzyme levels) is the CGD-like disorder manifested.[41,477] A partial deficiency of glutathione reductase has been reported, presenting with hemolytic anemia and early cataracts, but no increased incidence of infection was noted.[464]

The synthesis of an adequate supply of glutathione also is critical to these cells. Two brothers with glutathione synthetase deficiency who presented with neutropenia, hemolytic anemia, acidosis, 5-oxyprolinuria, and recurrent infection were reported by Spielberg and colleagues[520] and Boxer and associates.[88] The PMNs from these patients exhibited elevated cytosolic hydrogen peroxide levels, diminished oxidative microbicidal activity, and impaired microtubule assembly. Antioxidant therapy with vitamin E normalized the in vitro abnormalities of the patients' PMNs, with no further difficulty with recurrent infections.[88]

Myeloperoxidase deficiency. Congenital deficiency of neutrophil myeloperoxidase has come to be recognized as the single most common heritable disorder of neutrophil function, occurring in about 1/2000 persons.[400,435] The precise mode of inheritance of this defect has not been established, but myeloperoxidase is known to be a product of a single gene on chromosome 17.[560] Although PMNs from some patients with myeloperoxidase deficiency have been found to exhibit delayed killing of *C. albicans* and *S. aureus*, myeloperoxidase deficiency rarely has been associated with unusual infectious complications.

Important Examples of Secondary Immunodeficiency (Excluding Human Immunodeficiency Virus Infection)

Asplenia

Fulminant infections can occur in patients who have anatomic or functional asplenia.[78] The mortality rate from these infections in asplenic persons ranges from 40% to 80%.[78,587] The most common pathogens are encapsulated bacteria, including *S. pneumoniae* (50–70%), *H. influenzae,* and *N. meningitidis.*[587] Other streptococci, *S. aureus, Salmonella,* and other gram-negative bacilli are important but less common pathogens. Malaria and babesiosis also are more severe in asplenic persons. Infections can occur at any time but are most common within the first 2 years after splenectomy.

Both the liver and the spleen are important in phagocytic clearance of bacteria from the circulation, and the spleen is an important site for antibody production. Young children who become asplenic are much more susceptible to fulminant infection than are adults because adults are more likely to have encountered antigens before splenectomy than are children. Persons whose indication for splenectomy is thalassemia or Hodgkin disease are at higher risk for dying of overwhelming infection than are those who develop functional asplenia from sickle-cell disease. Patients who undergo spleen removal for spherocytosis or idiopathic thrombocytopenia have a lower risk for infection. The lowest risk group consists of individuals whose spleens are removed surgically after trauma.[78,138]

Congenital asplenia usually is associated with complex congenital cardiac disease and occasionally with structural abnormalities of the gastrointestinal or genitourinary tracts. Thus asplenia should be suspected in any patient with congenital heart disease and sepsis resulting from encapsulated organisms. Anatomic or functional asplenia also should be suspected in patients whose erythrocytes are found to contain Howell-Jolly bodies because these typically are removed from the circulation by the normally functioning spleen. Ultrasound or radionuclide liver and spleen scan usually can confirm asplenia or significant hyposplenia.[78]

Asplenic persons are managed using prophylactic antibiotics, usually penicillin V or amoxicillin, until at least 5 years of age.[138] They also should be immunized against encapsulated organisms at the appropriate ages (e.g., *H. influenzae* type b and pneumococcal conjugate vaccines and meningococcal conjugate vaccine beginning at 2 months), and heightened attention to clinical evaluation and treatment of febrile episodes is recommended.[138,473] Patients should be warned about the increased risk for serious infections from malaria and babesiosis.

Sickle-Cell Disease

Immunodeficiency in sickle-cell disease patients is due in large part to their functional asplenia.[484] Part of the risk for infection stems from local infarction and tissue necrosis resulting from sickling, which causes sludging and resultant tissue hypoxia. The reticuloendothelial system also may be obstructed by having to deal with chronic hemolysis. Patients with sickle-cell disease experience a high incidence of sepsis and meningitis caused by encapsulated organisms (e.g., *S. pneumoniae, H. influenzae* type b, *N. meningitidis*) and *Salmonella.*[215] *Salmonella* infections often are associated with osteomyelitis.[193]

Patients with sickle-cell disease appear to have normal antibody responses to most antigens, including age-appropriate responses to vaccines, and they usually have normal complement function.[289]

Patients with sickle-cell disease should be managed with prophylactic antibiotics until at least 5 years of age and should be immunized against *H. influenzae* type b, pneumococci, and meningococci at the appropriate ages.[138]

Cystic Fibrosis

Cystic fibrosis (CF) is an autosomal recessive disorder caused by mutations in both alleles of the gene encoding the protein called cystic fibrosis transmembrane conductance regulator (CFTR), a cyclic AMP–regulated chloride channel expressed at the luminal surface of airway epithelial cells.[579] Most patients with CF develop chronic endobronchial infection with *P. aeruginosa* of the mucoid phenotype. This infection is accompanied by an intense chronic airway inflammation with an exuberant influx of neutrophils that leads to bronchiectasis and destruction and fibrosis of lung and airway tissue and early death.[124,312] The airway inflammatory milieu, including neutrophil-derived proteases such as elastase, contributes to secondary impairments in opsonic and phagocytic host defenses by cleaving opsonic antibody and complement fragments, as well as important phagocytic receptors for these opsonins.[550] Mucociliary clearance of bacteria from the CF airway is impaired because of viscous, dehydrated epithelial lining fluid, and large quantities of DNA from dying neutrophils impair clearance of secretions by further enhancing their viscosity. The unresolved question of the relationship between the cystic fibrosis genetic defect and the pathogenesis of *Pseudomonas* chronic lung infection continues to stimulate active research.[124,441,480,511] Diagnosis of CF is classically made by documenting elevated levels of sweat chloride, but genetic diagnosis is now undertaken more frequently. Management of patients typically includes nutritional support, pancreatic enzyme replacement, frequent aggressive chest physiotherapy to mobilize secretions, intermittent courses of aerosolized tobramycin, aggressive management of pulmonary exacerbations, and recombinant aerosolized DNAse to help liquefy secretions. Gene therapy has been explored but has not resulted in correction of the defect at the clinical level. Recently a novel and promising trial of pharmacotherapy targeted the basic defect in CF. The drug ivacaftor, an orally administered potentiator of CFTR chloride channel function in CF patients with at least one G551D-CFTR mutation, resulted in sustained improvement of lung function through 48 weeks of treatment; ivacaftor is now licensed for CF patients with this mutation.[190]

Ciliary Dyskinesia

Primary ciliary dyskinesia is a rare disorder of deranged ciliary motility that predisposes patients to recurrent respiratory infections such as otitis media, sinusitis, bronchitis, and pneumonia as a result of poor clearance of secretions.[529] It is due to a mutation in one of several genes encoding for a component of either the dynein arms or radial spokes of the cilia that provide the energy, movement, and structural integrity of the specific tubulin structures that make up the normal cilia of respiratory epithelium.[529] Approximately 50% of these patients may have dextrocardia and situs inversus. In the absence of these features, this disorder should be suspected in patients who have recurrent infections, as noted earlier, but who have undergone a comprehensive evaluation of humoral immunity that has not detected an abnormality. Diagnosis ordinarily requires a brush biopsy of nasal epithelial cells, best evaluated by transmission electron microscopy, which usually will reveal an abnormality of the inner or outer dynein arm or of the radial spokes of the cilia.[503,529] Patients in whom this diagnosis is suspected should be referred to clinicians with expertise at centers with the capability to perform the necessary diagnostic studies. Long-term management can be challenging and often involves antimicrobial prophylaxis and attempts to assist in mobilization of secretions. Many of these patients develop bronchiectasis as a result of recurrent and chronic airway and lung infection. There is no specific treatment for the ciliary dysfunction.[529]

EVALUATION FOR IMMUNODEFICIENCY IN THE CHILD WITH RECURRENT OR SEVERE INFECTIONS

Most immunodeficiency disorders can be diagnosed readily by employing a methodical process that begins with careful analysis of the child's presenting history and physical examination.[140,147,167,484,486] This information serves as the foundation, when indicated, for a rational laboratory evaluation. It should be borne in mind that it is normal for children to have several infections every year. It is not unusual for normal children who are exposed to other children, particularly older school-aged siblings or classmates, to develop approximately one infection per month, especially from late fall to early spring, when respiratory viruses are most active. The overwhelming majority of infections in immunocompetent children are characterized by being mild and localized to the gastrointestinal or upper respiratory tracts, and they either are self-limited or respond rapidly to conventional therapy. Immunocompromised hosts tend to have more frequent, severe, and unusual infections that may not respond readily to appropriate therapy.

History

A detailed history alone often is sufficient to determine whether an immunologic evaluation should be pursued in many children who have recurrent or severe infections. If tests for immunity are indicated, the history also serves as a guide to the types of studies that should be performed initially.

The age of onset of suspicious infections usually helps in defining the underlying problem. For example, children with isolated immunoglobulin deficiencies tend to do well during the first few months of life because they are protected by maternal antibody. They usually start developing serious infections later in the first year of life. Those with cell-mediated or phagocytic disorders may begin developing infections in the newborn period (see earlier discussion). In contrast, healthy children who have been cared for at home by their mothers and who have no siblings often have relatively few infections in the first few years of life but may be brought to the physician for immunologic evaluation when they develop recurrent respiratory tract infections beginning the first few weeks after entering daycare, nursery school, or kindergarten because of new exposure to various respiratory viral pathogens.

The number, nature, etiology, and severity of infections help in determining how aggressively to pursue an immunologic evaluation. Certain clinical presentations of disease and causative organisms are associated with a high likelihood of an immunodeficiency. Antibody or complement deficiencies or functional asplenia should be suspected in children with recurrent or life-threatening infections such as sepsis and meningitis caused by encapsulated organisms (e.g., *S. pneumoniae, H. influenzae* type b).[98,167,289,335,467] Complement deficiencies should be considered in persons with recurrent or severe neisserial disease.[167] CGD should be suspected in the presence of recurrent or unusual deep tissue infections, such as liver abscess, lymphadenopathy, pneumonia, or osteomyelitis, especially when caused by unusual gram-negative bacteria, such as *Serratia marcescens,* or by *Aspergillus* species.[588] Bacterial skin infections in patients who have never formed pus at infected sites may suggest a leukocyte adhesion deficiency. Pneumonia caused by *Pneumocystis* suggests a T-cell deficiency, either hereditary or as a result of HIV infection. In contrast, recurrent or even severe infections with group A streptococcus have not been associated with immunodeficiency, and recurrent urinary tract infections usually are associated with anatomic abnormalities of the urinary tract rather than immunodeficiency.

Documentation of the child's growth pattern is essential because children who are thriving are much less likely to have serious immune disorders than are those with failure to thrive.

The immunization history should be documented carefully because it may prove useful in evaluating the child's ability to mount an antibody response to specific vaccine antigens. The history of recent live viral immunization should be obtained in children who have clinical presentations compatible with polio or measles because infection caused by vaccine strains of these viruses may be the first indication of immunodeficiency in some children.

Children who attend daycare facilities or preschools are constantly being exposed to common infections. Familiarity with community patterns of disease such as prevalent clinical manifestations of enterovirus infection or the beginning of croup, respiratory syncytial virus, influenza, or rotavirus seasons can be used to reassure families of normal children with frequent mild infections.

A detailed family history should be obtained that includes questions about the presence of immunodeficiency, recurrent or severe infections, contributing factors to any early deaths, the gender of affected persons, and consanguinity. A history of recurrent or severe infections in maternal male relatives should be given special attention because of the prominence of X-linked disorders among the primary immunodeficiencies. Autoimmune diseases might suggest a familial disorder of complement or cell-mediated immunity.[167]

Physical Examination

Physical examination may provide valuable clues to the nature of an immune disorder. In certain cases, such as some patients with the hyper-IgE syndrome[100,268] and the DiGeorge syndrome,[173] the characteristic facies may suggest the diagnosis.

As noted earlier, one of the most obvious signs that a child may have a serious underlying medical problem is failure to thrive. Every immunologic evaluation must include documentation of current growth parameters and comparison with past growth.

Many immunodeficiency disorders have dermatologic manifestations. Eczematoid rashes are seen in patients with the hyper-IgE syndrome and CGD.[100,268] CGD and leukocyte adhesion deficiencies also are characterized by slow wound healing and abnormal scarring patterns.[588] Patients with Chédiak-Higashi syndrome have partial albinism.[77] Severe gingival disease and early loss of teeth are prominent clinical features in disorders of neutrophil migration, such as LAD.[27,33]

The chest should be evaluated for physical signs of active disease, such as rales and rhonchi, as well as evidence of chronic infection, such as an increased anterior-posterior diameter. Pneumonia, bronchitis, bronchiectasis, and scarring can occur with many immunodeficiencies but are associated most frequently with immunoglobulin deficiencies.[98,259]

Cardiac abnormalities may be associated with primary asplenia or immunodeficiency disorders such as DiGeorge syndrome,[173] and dextrocardia with situs inversus should suggest ciliary dyskinesia as a cause of recurrent infections.[140]

Although hepatosplenomegaly may be found in many types of primary immunodeficiency diseases, it is more common in patients with disorders of phagocyte function, especially CGD.[588]

Laboratory Studies

The laboratory evaluation should be guided by the history and physical findings. Relatively simple and inexpensive screening tests often can help narrow the differential diagnosis and streamline the evaluation. One of the first tests that should be performed is a complete blood count with differential and evaluation of the blood smear. This simple test can detect several immunologic abnormalities, including neutropenia, lymphopenia associated with HIV-1 or forms of SCID, the abnormal neutrophil granules associated with the Chédiak-Higashi syndrome,

Howell-Jolly bodies found with asplenia, and some malignancies. Chest radiographs should be examined for thymic tissue, mediastinal lymphadenopathy, pneumonia, bronchiectasis, and other evidence of chronic pulmonary infections. Consideration also should be given to evaluating patients with chronic pulmonary disease for CF with a sweat chloride test.

In most patients, the specific clinical features of infections and their etiologies provide an optimal guide to choosing the most relevant and specific laboratory tests for evaluating for immunodeficiency when this is indicated. All too frequently, a comprehensive and expensive evaluation of every major aspect of immunity is undertaken for a patient whose clinical presentation suggests a more carefully considered and targeted approach.

Children with a clear history of recurrent bacterial otitis media, sinusitis, or pneumonia are candidates for evaluation of humoral immunity by measuring levels of the major classes of immunoglobulin and IgG subclasses. Enumeration of B cells and marker studies by immunofluorescence flow cytometry should be considered if more severe forms of humoral deficiency, such as XLA or some forms of CVID, are suspected. Very high IgE levels may be helpful in establishing the diagnosis of hyper-IgE syndrome; it should be noted that many laboratories do not include IgE levels in the standard Ig quantitation, and this must be ordered separately. Children who have normal quantitative Ig and IgG subclass levels but who continue to have frequent sinopulmonary infections that do not respond well to appropriate medical and surgical management (e.g., ventilation tubes) also can be evaluated by measuring antibody responses to specific antigens such as tetanus and diphtheria toxoids, *H. influenzae* type b, and meningococcal and pneumococcal capsular polysaccharides. Antibody levels can be measured before immunization and approximately 1 to 2 months after immunization to evaluate the child's ability to respond to different kinds of antigens, including T-cell–dependent antigens, such as diphtheria and tetanus toxoid, or T-cell–independent antigens such as unconjugated pneumococcal capsular polysaccharide vaccine. In a patient with recurrent bacterial respiratory infections in whom no antibody-related abnormality can be identified after a comprehensive evaluation, the possibility of ciliary dyskinesia should be considered and a brush biopsy of nasal epithelial cells performed for electron microscopic studies (see earlier discussion).

The complement system should be evaluated in persons with recurrent or life-threatening neisserial disease, including systemic gonococcal infections and sporadic meningococcal disease. The best screening test for hemolytic complement is the CH_{50}. A normal CH_{50} reflects a normal quantity and function of classical pathway proteins (C1, C4, C2), C3, and terminal components through C8, as noted earlier.[134] An abnormal CH_{50} should be confirmed, being careful that the specimen is handled correctly. If a very low CH_{50} is confirmed, it is important to determine both the serum levels of individual complement proteins and their functional activity in consultation with a reference laboratory.

In patients with infections suggesting a T-cell defect, such as *Pneumocystis, Cryptococcus,* or recurrent candidiasis, delayed hypersensitivity skin testing with antigens such as *Candida* or mumps may be useful to screen cell-mediated immunity, but results are not always reliable. Lymphocyte subset quantitation may be helpful in diagnosing such conditions as SCID, but more sophisticated testing of lymphocyte function such as mitogen and antigen stimulation should be performed in patients with recurrent or severe fungal infection or in whom CVID is suspected. Such studies ideally should be directed by a clinical immunologist.

Similarly suspected phagocyte function disorders should be evaluated in consultation with experts in phagocyte function because lack of proper standardization and expertise often produces misleading results from commercial laboratories. Phagocyte function studies should be directed toward defects of adhesion and migration in patients with recurrent skin and mucosal infections, poor or absent pus formation, and persistent leukocytosis suggestive of a leukocyte adhesion defect. Tests of oxidative metabolic activity and killing should be performed in patients with recurrent staphylococcal or unusual gram-negative or fungal tissue infections suggestive of CGD.

When clinical suspicion of an inherited immunodeficiency is confirmed by appropriate functional laboratory studies, it may be desirable to arrange for specific genetic testing to determine the precise nature of a patient's genetic mutation or variation when such testing is available. This may assist greatly in subsequent genetic counseling and will add important information to the clinical database on patients with the specific disorder.

Prevention of Infection

Patients and household members should be immunized with appropriate vaccines as soon and as fully as possible after a diagnosis of a family member with an immunodeficiency.[138] Although many immunodeficient patients, such as those with XLA or SCID, cannot respond normally to vaccines, immunization of household members and other close contacts may reduce the patients' risk for infection. Patients with complement deficiencies, asplenia, and sickle-cell disease should be immunized with vaccines directed against encapsulated organisms, such as meningococci, pneumococci, and *H. influenzae* type b. However, it should be remembered that these persons may not have normal responses to immunization and, therefore, if possible, their antibody responses to these vaccines should be measured; if responses are poor, they may benefit from additional doses of the vaccines. Live viral vaccines should not be administered to most patients with primary defects of cell-mediated immunity.

Patients with disorders characterized by recurrent or severe bacterial or fungal infections may require prophylactic antibacterial or antifungal therapy. Although this is an essential component of management for many of the more severe immunodeficiencies, such as DiGeorge syndrome, SCID, and CGD, the benefit of this approach has not been documented for all immune disorders. For many other disorders the uncertainty of the benefits of long-term antimicrobial prophylaxis must be weighed carefully along with the risk for emergence of antimicrobial resistance.

Prospects for Correction of Serious Primary Immunodeficiencies

Bone marrow or stem cell transplants have been successful in a few patients with specific immunologic disorders, including SCID,[103,118] Wiskott-Aldrich syndrome,[428] LAD, and CGD.[30,213,581] Current protocols for thymus transplantation are showing great promise in treatment of patients with DiGeorge syndrome.[361] Gene therapy has raised new possibilities for correcting certain immunologic defects, having demonstrated early promise for some forms of SCID and early success in animal models of CGD.[174,446] The development of malignancies associated with retroviral gene therapy in some cases has raised serious concerns about the ultimate feasibility of this approach,[102,446] but the means of overcoming these and other potential obstacles to gene therapy continue to be sought.

NEW REFERENCES SINCE THE SEVENTH EDITION

123. Chinn IK, Shearer WT. Severe combined immunodeficiency disorders. *Immunol Allergy Clin North Am.* 2015;35:671-694.

190. Eldredge LC, Ramsey BW. Remarkable progress toward new treatments for cystic fibrosis. *Lancet Respir Med.* 2014;2:962-964.

420. Opata MM, Hollifield ML, Lund FE, et al. B lymphocytes are required during the early priming of CD4+ T cells for clearance of *Pneumocystis* infection in mice. *Blood.* 2015;195:611-620.

444. Prince HE, Lape-Nixon M. Role of cytomegalovirus (CMV) avidity testing in diagnosing primary CMV infection during pregnancy. *Clin Vaccine Immunol.* 2014;21:1377-1384.

451. Ramesh M, Simchoni N, Hamm D, Cunningham-Rundles C. High-throughput sequencing reveals an altered T cell repertoire in X-linked agammaglobulinemia. *Clin Immunol.* 2015;161:190-196.

473. Rubin LG, Schaffner W. Clinical practice: care of the asplenic patient. *N Engl J Med.* 2014;371:349-356.

489. Schiefner A, Wilson IA. Presentation of lipid antigens by CD1 glycoproteins. *Curr Pharm Des.* 2009;15:3311-3317.

The full reference list for this chapter is available at ExpertConsult.com.

Host Response to Infections: The "-omics" Revolution

3

Asuncion Mejias • Octavio Ramilo

INTRODUCTION

There has been tremendous progress in our attempt to discern the molecular basis of infectious diseases, yet several gaps remain both in the understanding of disease processes and in the development of optimal strategies that would allow early diagnosis and targeted treatment. In addition, despite major advances in the development and implementation of vaccines and antimicrobial agents, infectious diseases continue to represent a major cause of morbidity and mortality worldwide.[128] Recent examples such as the 2009 H1N1 influenza pandemic,[30,121] the MERS coronavirus and enterovirus-D68 outbreaks, the West Africa Ebola and the Zika virus epidemics,[111,143,148,197,220] as well as the increased frequency of hospital-acquired infections caused by multiple-resistant gram-negative bacilli[78] and highly virulent strains of *Clostridium difficile*[198] highlight the challenges we encounter when managing patients with infectious diseases. In this context of outbreaks of emergent and reemergent pathogens linked to increased antimicrobial resistance, there is a clear need for improved diagnostic tools for optimal patient classification and management.[142]

HOST RESPONSES FOR IMPROVING THE DIAGNOSIS OF INFECTIOUS DISEASES

One of the most frequent challenges that physicians face in the clinical setting is the difficulty of establishing an appropriate etiologic diagnosis or even distinguishing between bacterial or viral infections in patients presenting with an acute febrile illness. These obstacles can delay initiation of appropriate therapy, which can result in unnecessary morbidity and even mortality. On the other hand, the need to promptly start appropriate antimicrobial therapy to control the infection has to be balanced with a rational use of antibiotics. Within this context there is an obvious need for improved diagnostics tools to help with patient classification, which in turn should allow appropriate use of targeted therapies.

Microbial pathogens are detected in clinically relevant specimens using a variety of assays including cultures, rapid antigen detection tests, and polymer chain reaction (PCR) assays. To date, to be able to establish causality, growing the specific pathogen (bacteria, virus, or fungus) remains the gold standard. However, this is a flawed approach, particularly if the organism is not present in the blood or from other easily accessible sites. In addition many pathogens grow slowly or require complex media, and a significant number of clinically important microbes remain unrecognized because they are resistant to cultivation in the laboratory, thus limiting clinical decision-making.[45,190] The introduction of more sensitive molecular diagnostic assays has significantly improved the diagnosis of viral infections.[99] Unfortunately this is not the case for bacterial pathogens. Moreover, in the clinical setting, it is not uncommon to encounter situations in which the sole identification of a pathogen is not sufficient to establish causality (e.g., the detection of respiratory viruses in patients with no respiratory symptoms or in patients with pneumonia who often also have a co-detected bacterial pathogen).

In view of these limitations, for almost a century, there has been a large quest to identify host-derived biomarkers indicative of infection, such as the erythrocyte sedimentation rate (ESR) or C-reactive protein (CRP).[223,231] These tests, which are useful in certain clinical scenarios, have proved to be nonspecific and are unable to differentiate between pathogen types (i.e., viral vs. bacterial) or even between infectious and noninfectious diseases. More recently, procalcitonin (PCT), a 116-amino acid protein produced in the thyroid and lungs, has shown improved sensitivity and specificity for the diagnosis of bacterial infections.[7,22,72,149] Nevertheless, there are limitations and uncertainty about its utility because serum concentrations of PCT also increase after surgery, trauma, cancer, or severe burns, thus raising the concern of false positives.[97,154] Other candidate biomarkers have been used for the diagnosis of neonates and older children with sepsis and have produced inconsistent results because data have yet to be validated in independent cohorts.[207]

There is a need for an alternative strategy that has sufficient sensitivity to differentiate infectious from noninfectious conditions, sufficient specificity to distinguish among the different types of pathogens, useful to monitor response to therapy, and, ideally, is able to predict clinical outcomes. An alternative approach to the pathogen-detection strategy is based on a comprehensive analysis of the host response to the infection caused by different pathogens (Fig. 3.1).[34,104,141,142,186,187] A wide range of molecular and cellular profiling assays are currently available for the study of the human immune system.[33] *Genomics* provide information about structural DNA changes and thus the probability of developing a condition, *epigenetics* describe the chromatin modifications that are caused by external or environmental factors and stably alter gene expression without changing the DNA sequence, *transcriptomics* study the overexpression or underexpression of genes (mRNA expression profiles) in a qualitative and quantitative manner in response to the infection, and *metabolomics* and *proteomics* analyze the structure, function, and interaction of posttranslational metabolites produced by a particular gene (Fig. 3.2). Thus the information provided by the "-omics" technologies is complementary, and their use for diagnostic, pathogenetic, or prognostic purposes is mainly limited by the available technology and complexity of the analyses (Fig. 3.3).

Independent of the -omics approach used, four tenets must be considered when using these tools for biomarker discovery to assure that the profiles are representative of the disease process and not of a confounding event: (a) selection and definition of the cases, which should be homogeneous in terms of the disease process and with limited confounders to allow interpretation of the multidimensional data; (b) need for controls, which should be also homogeneous, free of confounders, and similar in terms of the basic characteristics (i.e., demographic parameters) with the cases; (c) type of sample, which should reflect and change because of the biologic process and should be easy to obtain, ideally in a noninvasive manner; and (d) need for validation, to confirm that the profiles identified perform well in an independent cohort of patients that is different from the one used for the discovery phase. Of all these technologies, genomics and transcriptomics are moving into the clinical laboratory and are poised to become part of routine diagnostics in the next few years. In this chapter, we will review the application of analysis of host response through genomics, epigenetics, transcriptomics, proteomics, and metabolomics for diagnosis, understanding disease pathogenesis, patient classification and management, and possibly prognosis of pediatric patients with infectious diseases.

GENOMICS

The human genome, which is relatively static, is organized into 46 chromosomes consisting of 22 pairs of autosomal chromosomes shared by males and females and the sex-determining chromosomes, X and Y. One set of autosomal chromosomes is derived from each parent. Human genes are formed by *exons*, which are the coding regions, and *introns*, the noncoding regions. During transcription, the entire gene is copied into pre-mRNA, which includes exons and introns. Through the process of RNA splicing, introns are removed and exons joined to form a contiguous coding sequence. Single genes are able to generate 4 to 6 different mRNAs; thus many of the complex biological functions that characterize humans are generated by combined interactions among genes rather than a specific gene being responsible for a specific function. The genome and transcriptome consist entirely of deoxyribonucleic (DNA) and ribonucleic acids (RNA). Their uniform chemical properties have enabled efficient, low-cost, and high-throughput methods for amplification, synthesis, sequencing, and highly multiplexed analysis.

The genome represents a rich source of information about our pathophysiology. Genome analyses provide information about structural DNA changes and thus the probability of developing a condition. These analyses do not, however, provide information about whether and when a condition will manifest. Many diseases are caused by genetic mutations, and many more manifest as a genetic predisposition. More than 3000 gene mutations (www.omim.org/) have now been identified that are associated with more than 5000 human phenotypes that cause or predispose to diseases. These numbers suggest that many diseases are caused by mutations in single genes and that many more have an inheritable genetic component. The Human Genome Project (HGP) was an international research effort originated in 1990 that culminated in the identification and public release of the completed sequence of the human genome in April 2003. In the HGP, the genome was cloned first and then larger clones were divided into shorter pieces and sequenced. The HGP has revealed approximately 20,500 human genes. They are contained in more than 2.85 billion nucleotides covering more than 99% of the euchromatin (i.e., gene-containing DNA). Initial genome approaches were applied to the diagnosis of congenital birth defects and tumors. However, the introduction of next-generation DNA sequencing (NGS) has revolutionized biomedical research and promises to be of great value for the diagnosis of infectious diseases.[118]

Basics of the Genomics Approach

We now have a broad arsenal of techniques for genome analysis at our disposal, which allow the detection of gross abnormalities down to single nucleotide changes. These tools are increasingly being used for

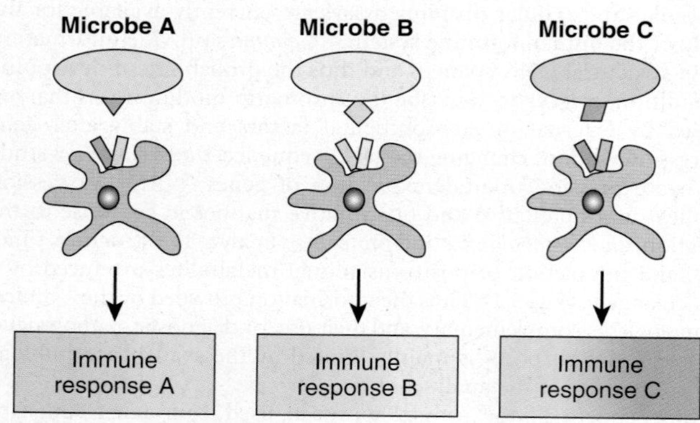

FIG. 3.1 Each pathogen induces a specific response in the host that can be measured. An alternative approach to the pathogen-detection strategy is based on a comprehensive analysis of the host response to the infection caused by different pathogens.

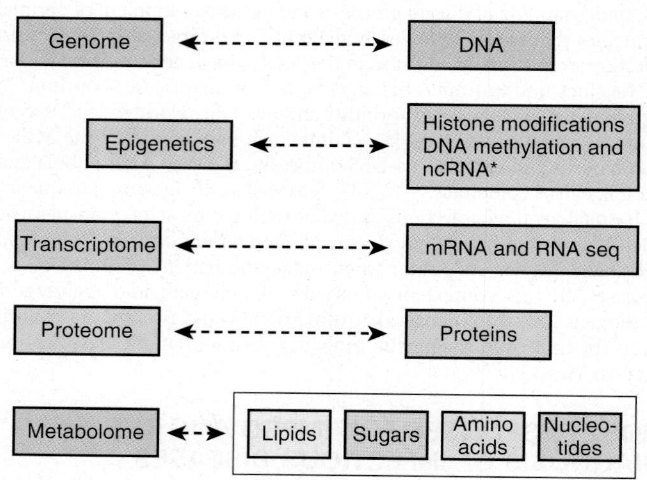

FIG. 3.2 Types of -omics approaches. *Genomics* provides information about structural DNA changes and thus the probability of developing a condition; *epigenetics* describes the chromatin modifications that are caused by external or environmental factors and stably alter gene expression without changing the DNA; *transcriptomic* approaches study the overexpression or underexpression of genes (mRNA expression profiles) in a qualitative and quantitative manner in response to the infection; and *metabolomics* and *proteomic methodology* analyze the structure, function, and interaction of posttranslational metabolites produced by a particular gene.

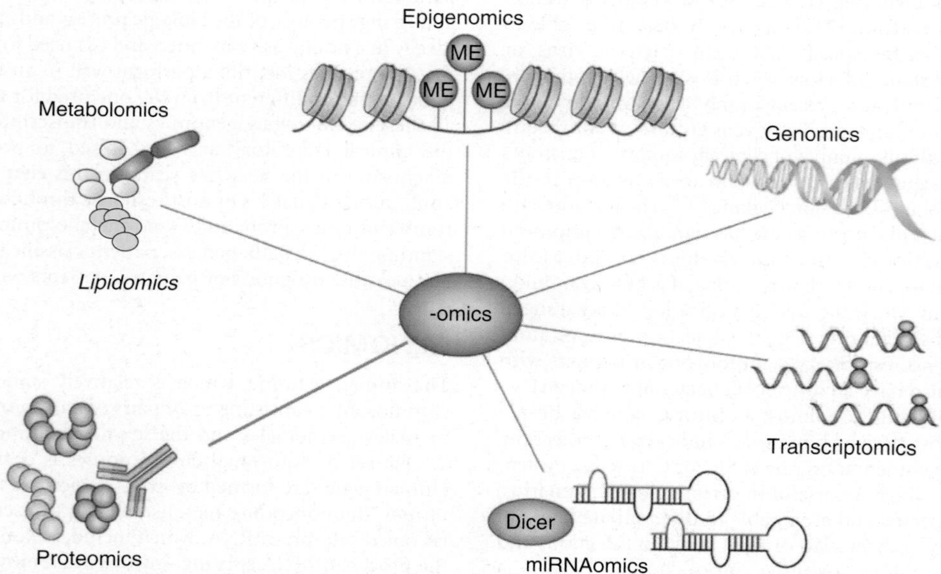

FIG. 3.3 Omics approaches are complementary. The information provided by the -omics technologies is complementary, and their use for diagnostic, pathogenesis, or prognostic purposes is mainly limited by the available technology and complexity of the analyses. *ME,* Methyl group.

clinical diagnostics. Within a few years the study of the human genome has dramatically changed and greatly improved, moving from the identification of abnormalities based on the morphology and number of chromosomes (karyotype) to the newly developed sequencing instruments that are able to generate millions of short sequences per run (NGS).

Karyotyping was the first method used for the identification of chromosomal abnormalities. Developed in the early 1960s, it is based on the identification of the banding pattern characteristic for each chromosome visible through the light microscope. Although it only reveals crude information, such as number, shapes, and gross alterations of general chromosomal architecture, it remains a mainstay of clinical genetic analysis. Trisomy 21 and chronic myelogenous leukemia were originally identified using this technique.[8,12]

Comparative genome hybridization is a cytogenetic method focused on copy number variations relative to the number of chromosomes (ploidy) in the DNA. In comparative genome hybridization, the genomes of interest, which are usually a disease genome set against a normal control genome, are labeled with different fluorescent dyes and compared. Using different colored fluorescent labels, several genes can be stained simultaneously. When the technology was developed the fluorescently labeled DNAs were hybridized to a spread of normal chromosomes and evaluated by quantitative image analysis, which was able to detect chromosome regional gains or losses with greater accuracy than conventional karyotyping.[59,105] Further improvements in resolution have been achieved using microarray-based comparative genome hybridization methods in which the probe DNA can be amplified by PCR, thus only minute amounts of starting material are required.[62,166] The labeled DNA is then hybridized to an array that can contain millions of oligonucleotides included on chips the size of a microscope slide, achieving very high resolution. Comparative genome hybridization techniques are used in prenatal screening for the detection of chromosomal defects. However, they do not provide information about balanced changes, such as inversions or balanced translocations, because they do not change the copy number and hybridization intensity. To circumvent this issue, if the gene of interest is known, the respective recombinant DNA can be labeled and used as a probe on chromosome spreads. This method, called fluorescence in situ hybridization (FISH), can detect gene amplifications, deletions, and chromosomal translocations.

DNA sequencing is the ability to identify individual genes by determining the precise order of the four nucleotides (adenine, guanine, cytosine, and thymine) within a molecule of DNA. The rapid speed of sequencing attained with modern DNA sequencing technology has been instrumental in the sequencing of the complete human genome, which culminated in 2003. Over the years different techniques have been used for DNA sequencing. Initially the Maxam-Gilbert sequencing method used chemicals to cleave specific bases. This methodology was quickly discouraged due to its complexity and the use of radioactive labeling.[139] In parallel, Sanger used small concentrations of radio- or fluorescently labeled dideoxynucleoside triphosphate (dNTP) molecules and developed a relatively reliable and less cumbersome method called chain termination. Sanger's method was soon automated and was the method used in the first generation of DNA sequencers.[200] The rapid development of novel technologies, such as NGS, has revolutionized this field. There are several NGS methods using different approaches to read DNA sequences. All these novel methods share the principle of conducting millions to billions of parallel sequencing reactions in microscopic compartments on arrays or nanobeads. Among others, DNA sequencing is used for genome-wide association studies (GWAS) using single nucleotide polymorphisms (SNPs) as high-resolution markers. SNPs are variations among individuals at a single position in a DNA sequence.[88] If more than 1% of a population does not carry the same nucleotide at a specific position in the DNA sequence, then this variation can be classified as an SNP. SNPs are associated with both genes and noncoding regions of DNA and represent the most common type of genetic variation among individuals. In 2012, more than 180 million SNPs were known. SNPs are useful to identify and assess disease risk, but it is not uncommon that they are found to have no impact on the phenotype (silent mutations).[221] Silent mutations, along with the need for extremely large cohorts of patients and for reproducibility of the studies, are among the main limitations of GWAS.

Genomics in Infectious Diseases

By 1950, using malaria as a prototype disease, the concept that genetic diversity within the host may influence the outcome of infection became apparent. In the clinical setting, the majority of infectious diseases are characterized by variation in both the disease pattern and severity, even during epidemics, thus highlighting the important role of host response on clinical manifestations and disease outcomes. Different inherited conditions, such as chronic granulomatous disease or interferon-γ receptor immunodeficiency, predispose to infectious diseases, and those conditions will be reviewed in another chapter. A number of SNPs in human leukocyte antigen (HLA) and non–major histocompatibility complex (MHC) have been found in response to a variety of bacterial and viral infections and have been associated with disease susceptibility, progression, or response to treatment. Table 3.1 illustrates examples of SNPs associated with a variety of uncommon and common viral or bacterial infections.* The main limitation of GWAS is that the same SNP can be protective or influence disease progression depending on the population and on the environment, making reproducibility of studies challenging.[251]

EPIGENETICS

In 1957, Waddington developed the idea that some heritable traits are not reflected by changes in the DNA, and this change process is now known as epigenetics. Epigenetics describe a number of chromatin modifications (phenotypic trait variations) that are caused by external or environmental factors and stably alter gene expression without changing the sequence of the DNA.[14] Thus epigenetics is able to alter the phenotype of a cell without changing the genotype and supports the idea that changes in gene expression derived from long-term exposure to a certain insult are imprinted, become independent of the activating stimulus, and persist even in its absence.[19] Epigenetics include the study of DNA methylation as well as a variety of more transient histone modifications (such as acetylation, methylation, or phosphorylation) along with the influence of SUMOylation (the addition of small ubiquitin-like modifiers [SUMOs]), ubiquitination, adenosine diphosphate (ADP) ribosylation, and microRNA. Although the epigenome is more variable than the genome, it may hold greater information on an individual basis, which will be useful for the application of personalized medicine.

Basics of the Epigenetics Approach

The methodology used to identify changes in DNA methylation are similar to that applied in genomics and include DNA sequencing of the treated versus untreated DNA, hybridization techniques, or array-based methods. These techniques may miss some incomplete modifications; however, new NGS methods that are able to detect DNA methylation directly look promising and will accelerate the field. The main epigenetic changes include histone modifications (such as acetylation and methylation that affect chromatin structure) and DNA methylation. It is important to note that although DNA methylation silences gene expression, histone modifications can enhance or suppress gene transcription. DNA methylation patterns have been associated with diseases and can be heritable by a poorly understood process called genomic imprinting. In addition, epigenetics includes the understanding of noncoding RNAs (ncRNAs), which are transcribed molecules that do not translate into proteins. In regard to epigenetic modifications, one of the long ncRNAs more recently discovered are small ncRNAs or microRNAs (miRs).[195] miRNAs are highly conserved, small noncoding RNAs that target mRNA molecules and inhibit their translation. miRNA exist intra- and extracellularly, including in blood or serum, and are resistant to boiling or repeated freezing-thawing, thus promising to be useful biomarkers in the clinical setting.[74]

Epigenetics in Infectious Diseases

There is growing evidence that histone modifications and chromatin remodeling regulate gene expression, including host immune responses,

*References 2, 5, 6, 11, 16, 17, 31, 36, 46–48, 51, 52, 57, 61, 63, 64, 70, 84–86, 95, 98, 106, 107, 114, 126, 129, 136, 138, 140, 152, 156, 159, 165, 169, 171, 179, 191, 199, 215, 226, 229, 233, 244–247.

TABLE 3.1 **Single Nucleotide Polymorphisms (SNPs)/Mutations and Associated Diseases**

Pathogen	Disease	SNPs/Mutations	Populations
Mycobacterium leprae	Leprosy	HLA-DR-DQ, TLR-1, NOD2, TNFSF15, 308 bp TNF, RIPK2, IL-23R, RAB32, LRRKW[136,165,229,244]	Adults
Mycobacterium tuberculosis	Tuberculosis	Mal/TIRAP, TLR-1, -2, -4, -6, -9, TNF-α, IFN-γ, IL-12RB1[5,6,64,191,199,226,246]	Adults
Streptococcus pneumoniae	Pneumococcal disease	MBL2, PTPN22, Mal/TIRAP[31,129,156,159]	Children
Staphylococcus aureus	*S. aureus* infection	HLA-DRA, -DRB1[51]	Adults
Neisseria meningitidis	Meningococcal disease	CFH-CFHR3, TLR-4[16,17,48]	Children and adults
Helicobacter pylori	Gastric cancer	IL-1, EPHX1[169]	Adults
HIV	AIDS	CCR5, CCR2, RANTES, CXCL12[47,85,86,95,247]	Children and adults
Norovirus, rotavirus	Gastroenteritis	FUT2[46,179]	Children
HCV	Hepatitis	IL-28B (INF-λ), IL-10R, IP-10[11,52,61,171]	Adults
Dengue virus	Dengue shock syndrome	MICB, PLCE1[107]	Children and adults
HSV	Encephalitis	TLR-3, UNC-93B[114]	Children
RSV	Bronchiolitis, severe disease	SP-A, SP-D, TLR-4, IL-8, IL-4, IL-13, IL-10, IL-1RL1, VDR[2,36,63,98,140,215,233,245]	Children
Influenza	Infection/severe disease	TNF, IL-6, IL-8, LTA, IL-1B, IL-1A, IL-10[70,106,126,138,152]	Adults
Rhinovirus	Severe bronchiolitis	IL-10, IL-6, IFN-γ[84]	Children

CCR, Chemokine receptor; *CFH*, complement factor H; *CFHR3*, CFH-related protein 3; *CXCL12*, chemokine; EPHX1, epoxide hydrolase 1, microsomal; *FUT2*, fucosyltransferase 2; *HBV*, hepatitis B virus; *HCV*, hepatitis C virus; *HIV*, human immunodeficiency virus; *HLA*, human leukocyte antigen; *HSV*, herpes simplex virus; *IFN*, interferon; *IL-1*, interleukin-1 (gene); *IL-23R*, interleukin-23 receptor (gene); *IL-28B*, interleukin-28B; *LRRK2*, leucine-rich repeat kinase 2 *(LRRK2)*; *LTA*, lymphotoxin alpha; *Mal*, myeloid differentiation primary response gene 88 (MyD88) adaptor-like protein; *MBL*, mannose-binding lectin; *MICB*, major histocompatibility complex class I polypeptide–related sequence B; *NOD2*, nucleotide-binding oligomerization domain containing 2; *PLCE1*, phospholipase C, epsilon 1; *PTPN22*, protein tyrosine phosphatase nonreceptor, type 22; *RAB32*, member RAS oncogene family; *RIPK2*, receptor-interacting serine-threonine protein kinase 2; *RSV*, respiratory syncytial virus; *TIRAP*, Toll-interleukin-1 receptor (TIR) domain adaptor protein; *TLR1*, Toll-like receptor 1 gene; *TNFSF15*, tumor necrosis factor (ligand) superfamily member 15; *VDR*, vitamin D receptor.

and thus represent key targets for pathogen manipulation during infection.[80] A variety of viral and bacterial effectors have been identified that enable a pathogen's survival by either mimicking or inhibiting host cellular machinery. Mitogen-activated protein kinase (MAPK), interferon (IFN), or transcription factor NF-κB signaling pathways, among others, are common targets of pathogen-induced posttranslational modifications on histones and chromatin-associated proteins.[91,192]

In Vitro Studies

The majority of the initial epigenetics work associated with miRNA in relation to infections was performed in vitro and mostly included viral-induced diseases. The goal of these studies was to gain a better understanding of the mechanisms of diseases or to identify markers associated with organ-specific syndromes and/or severity associated with specific pathogens. Using a laryngeal epithelial cell model of enterovirus 71, Cui and colleagues identified 64 miRNAs that target a number of genes associated with neurologic and immune responses relevant to the pathogenesis of the disease.[43] Similarly, using primary human alveolar and bronchial epithelial cells infected with influenza A virus, Buggele and colleagues identified six miRNAs targeting a number of mRNAs, including receptor-associated kinase 1 (IRAK1) or MAPK3 and other components of the innate immune response to infection.[25] Another provocative study showed that influenza H3N2 uses one of its nonstructural (NS) proteins to circumvent immune responses. Investigators showed that the influenza NS1 protein had a histone-like sequence (ARTK-histone mimic) that inhibited the host transcription elongation factor (hPAF1), selectively suppressing the host cell's production of antiviral proteins.[135] Within alveolar macrophages, Pennini and colleagues showed that *Mycobacterium tuberculosis* (TB) inhibited the expression of several interferon-γ–induced genes through histone acetylation, which appears to be a ubiquitous mechanism used by intracellular pathogens. This mechanism may help explain the protracted course and persistence of TB in some patients.[180] These studies, although descriptive, are examples of how pathogens can directly induce epigenetic changes in the host. As a diagnostic tool, a study conducted in mice infected with either *Escherichia coli*, a gram-negative bacterium, or *S. aureus*, a gram-positive bacterium, identified three circulating miRNAs predictive of gram-positive bacterial infections.[188]

In Vivo Studies

miRNA expression is a novel addition to the -omics arsenal to evaluate host responses to viral and bacterial infections. A small study in patients with dengue identified in blood samples two panels of miRNAs, one composed of 12 miRNAs and specific to dengue and another formed of 14 miRNAs common in dengue and influenza infection.[216] Another study was conducted with serum samples from children with hand-foot-and-mouth disease caused by EV-71 or Coxsackie virus 16 and included healthy controls and other infections including TB, pertussis, varicella zoster (VZV), or mumps.[44] Investigators found six miRNAs that discriminated children with EV-71 infection versus healthy controls with greater than 90% accuracy. However, only 2 of the 6 miRNAs identified were also found in their in vitro model. This emphasizes the need to perform studies in target populations because several factors, such as disease severity, age, or other parameters, may provide discordant results. A small study conducted in infants with respiratory syncytial virus (RSV) identified a distinct profile of immune-associated miRNA in respiratory samples from patients with mild or severe disease.[93] Although promising, these results will need to be validated in larger patient populations. Different studies have measured miRNA profiles in whole blood, peripheral blood mononuclear cells (PBMCs), or serum from patients infected with various strains of influenza A, including H1N1/H3N2, H7N9, or 2009 H1N1.[209,217,250] However, results could not be validated in other studies, suggesting that there may be methodologic differences that must be addressed.[243] In regard to bacterial pathogens, the majority of epigenetic studies have focused on TB or sepsis. A study that analyzed the sputum of patients with active TB versus controls found 95 miRNAs that were differentially expressed and were subsequently validated by quantitative reverse transcription PCR (RT-qPCR).[238] Other studies conducted in adult and pediatric patients, with and without HIV, found a number of whole blood miRNAs in CD4$^+$ T cells or sera that were differentially expressed in active versus latent TB or controls and had a specific role in T-cell immunity against TB.[68,108,151,184] In regard to sepsis, serum miRNAs have been used mostly as a prognostic rather than diagnostic marker in critically ill patients with negligible or no overlapping findings among studies, which may be attributed to the different levels of disease and/or the patient populations included.[131,194,213,230] Studies using miRNAs as a diagnostic tool for more common bacteria are ongoing. Nevertheless the value of miRNAs for the diagnosis of bacterial and viral infections, especially in patients with pneumonia, will be evident when studies are conducted and validated in the main target populations.

TRANSCRIPTOMICS

Major technological breakthroughs have also occurred in the field of transcriptomics, thus creating a unique opportunity for the study of humans in health and disease where inherent heterogeneity dictates that large collections of samples need to be analyzed. Among the high-throughput molecular profiling technologies available today, transcriptomic approaches are the most scalable, have the most breadth and robustness, and therefore appear to be best suited for the study of human populations. The transcriptome represents the complement of RNAs (messenger RNA) that are transcribed from the genome. Genes encode the information to make proteins, and RNA is the messenger that transports that information (hence the name mRNA). The transcription of a gene yields an average of 4 to 6 mRNA variants, which are translated into different proteins. The translation of mRNAs into proteins is highly regulated. Protein-coding genes only constitute 1% to 2% of the human genome sequence; however, more than 80% of the genome can be transcribed. Thus the largest part of the transcriptome consists of noncoding RNAs that fulfill important structural and regulatory functions, including gene transcription, mRNA processing and stability, and protein translation. One type of noncoding RNAs is the so-called small interfering (si)RNAs, which were discovered in 2006.[224] siRNAs are part of an enzyme complex that targets and cleaves mRNAs with high specificity. These types of RNAs have become a powerful tool to downregulate (or silence) the expression of selected mRNAs with high specificity and efficiency.

Different classes of pathogens trigger specific pattern-recognition receptors (PRRs) differentially expressed on peripheral blood leukocytes.[23,113,112] Blood represents both a reservoir and a migration compartment for these immune cells that become educated and implement their function by circulating between central and peripheral lymphoid organs and migrating to and from the site of infection via blood. Therefore blood leukocytes constitute an accessible source of clinically relevant information, and a comprehensive molecular phenotype of these cells can be obtained using gene expression microarrays.[33] Because they provide a comprehensive assessment of all immune-related cells and pathways, genomic studies are well suited to study the host-pathogen interaction (Fig. 3.4). In fact, studies in children and adults with acute infections have shown that different classes of pathogens induce distinct gene expression profiles that can be identified by analyses of blood leukocytes (Fig. 3.5.)[15,32,34,104,141,170,186,242]

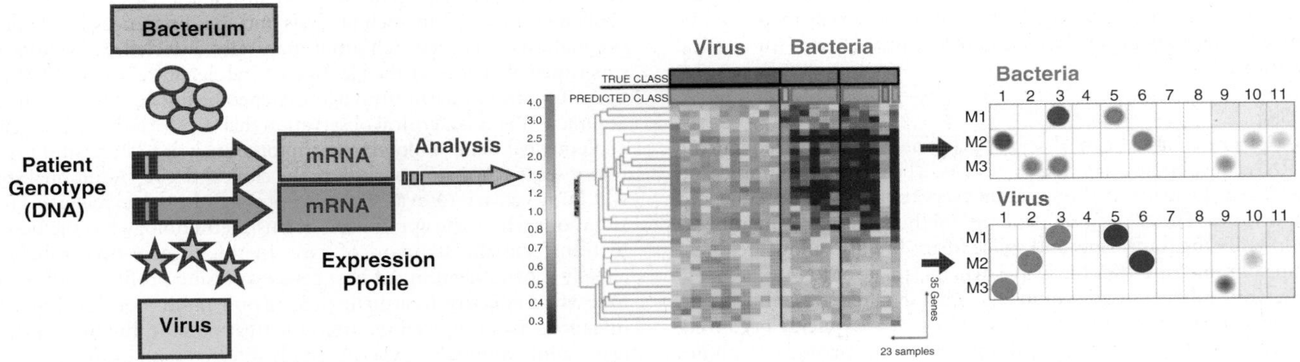

FIG. 3.4 Viral versus bacterial host responses. Microarray technology can measure the differences in gene expression patterns present in blood immune cells as induced by various types of infectious agents (viruses vs. bacteria) with a high level of specificity.

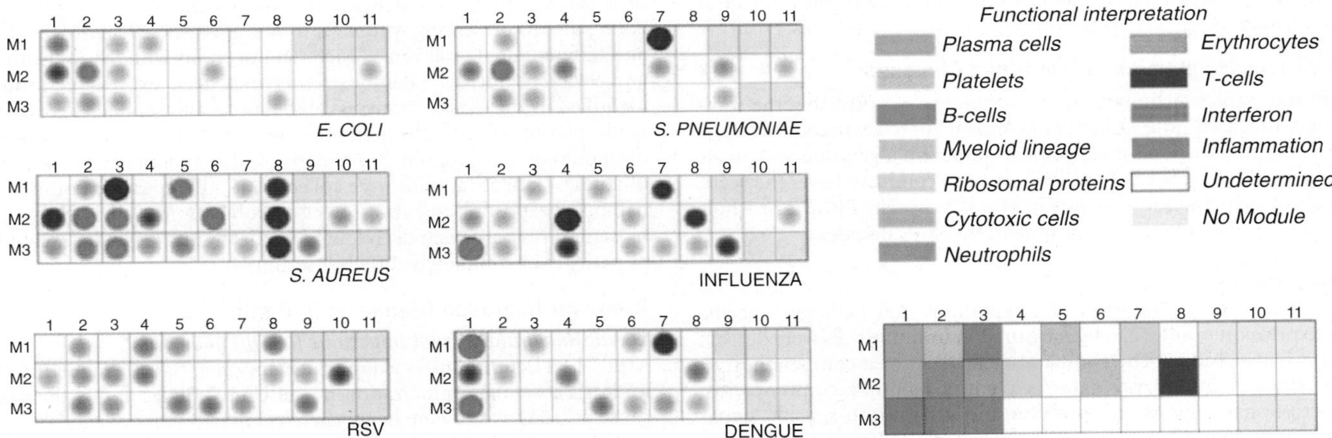

FIG. 3.5 Infectious disease fingerprints. Studies in children and adults with acute infections have shown that different classes of pathogens induce distinct gene expression profiles that can be identified by analyses of blood leukocytes. Expression levels were compared between patients and appropriately matched healthy controls on a module-by-module basis. The spots represent the percentage of significantly overexpressed (*red*) or underexpressed (*blue*) transcripts within a module (i.e., a set of coordinately expressed gene). Blank spots indicate that there are no differences in the genes included in that module between patients and healthy controls. This information is displayed on a grid, with the coordinates corresponding to one of 28 module IDs (e.g., module M3.1 is at the intersection of the third row and first column). Each pathogen induces an easily identifiable disease-specific biosignature. *RSV,* Respiratory syncytial virus.

Basics of the Transcriptomics Approach

Microarray Analyses

Microarray methods for studying global mRNA expression profiles are now well established. Microarray gene chips contain several million DNA spots arranged on a small slide in a predefined order. They allow a relative quantitation of changes in transcript abundance among different conditions. Modern arrays use unique sequences of synthetic oligonucleotides to avoid ambiguity in identifying specific RNA transcripts, and several oligonucleotides are used per gene to improve accuracy. The newer high-density arrays are able to scan the transcription of all human genesm map exon content, and splice variants of mRNAs, including noncoding RNAs (such as siRNAs and miRNAs). Briefly, RNA derived from the cells or tissue analyzed is copied first to complementary cDNA using a reverse transcriptase that can synthesize DNA from RNA templates. cDNA is transcribed back into cRNA, which is labeled with fluorescent tags, such as biotin, to improve detection. cRNA is preferred to cDNA because it hybridizes more strongly to the array oligonucleotides. After hybridization, the microarray chip is scanned and the hybridization intensities are compared using different statistical software. Thanks to a common convention for reporting microarray experiments called Minimal Information for the Annotation of Microarray Experiments (MIAME), gene array databases that have been published are publicly available free of charge and represent a valuable source for further analysis in which microarray results from different experiments can be compared. Gene array analysis is already being used for clinical applications.

RNA Seq

Transcriptome analysis can also be performed by direct sequencing once RNAs have been converted to cDNAs. The advances in rapid and cheap DNA sequencing methods permit every transcript to be sequenced multiple times. These "deep sequencing" methods not only unambiguously identify the transcripts and splice forms but also allow the direct counting of transcripts over the whole dynamic range of RNA expression, resulting in absolute transcript numbers rather than relative comparisons. Thus the sequencing methods, called RNA seq, are quickly becoming attractive alternatives to array-based transcriptomic methods.[228] Studies using RNA seq to characterize different infections are ongoing. As examples, two studies in mice, one in a model of *Staphylococcus aureus* infection[21] and the second one in a model of H5N8 avian influenza virus,[172] found transcripts associated with proinflammatory and anti-inflammatory mediators, chemotaxis, cell signaling, keratins, and TH1/TH17 cytokines.

Use of Transcriptomics in Infectious Diseases

Of all the -omics technologies, transcriptomics is probably the most popular, affordable, and easiest to implement approach because it allows measuring transcript abundance in a sample on a genome-wide scale using a single assay. Several studies have been conducted over the years, initially in vitro and subsequently in samples (usually PBMCs or whole blood) from patients with a variety of infectious diseases.

In Vitro Studies

The initial studies supporting the hypothesis that pathogen-specific gene expression profiles can be measured in immune cells were derived from in vitro studies. The comparative analysis of a compendium of host-pathogen microarray datasets identified both a common host transcriptional response to infection and a pathogen-specific signature.[20,35,94,100] Upon activation, Toll-like receptors (TLRs) trigger signaling pathways that share common components while retaining unique characteristics, accounting in part for the specificity of transcriptional responses.[214] In fact, in vitro microarray studies have shown the ability of herpes simplex virus (HSV), West Nile virus, pseudorabies virus, hepatitis C viruses (HCV), VZV, and rhinovirus to limit the ability of the host to develop effective antiviral responses by a variety of mechanisms.[90,185] However, the vast body of in vitro experimental data accumulated over the years suggests that hosts can mount pathogen-specific transcriptional responses to infections.

In Vivo Human Studies

Initial studies tested the hypothesis that leukocytes isolated from peripheral blood of patients with acute infections carry unique transcriptional signatures, which would in turn permit pathogen discrimination and classification. In those initial studies, gene expression patterns derived from PBMCs of pediatric patients hospitalized with acute infections showed that there are pathogen-specific signatures that can be measured in the blood, and these distinguished children with influenza A from *S. aureus, Streptococcus pneumoniae,* and *E. coli* acute infections with greater than 95% accuracy.[186] Analysis of PBMC samples requires processing in real time, which has limitations from a practical clinical application if there are large numbers of patients. In addition, PBMC samples do not include neutrophils, which is a relevant cell population for the pathogenesis of bacterial and viral infections. For these reasons, in recent years, there has been a shift toward whole blood samples to study transcriptional profiles in the clinical setting. Indeed whole blood signatures for several other infections have also been described from infected subjects including malaria, dengue, salmonella, melioidosis, TB, RSV, influenzavirus (including the pandemic H1N1/09), rhinovirus, adenovirus, human T-cell lymphotropic virus (HTLV-1), HIV, and neonatal sepsis (Table 3.2).*

A study performed in adult volunteers experimentally infected with RSV, rhinovirus, or influenza A identified an "acute respiratory viral signature" that was independently validated using a previously published dataset of pediatric patients with pneumonia.[186] Despite the technical challenges involved in such analysis and the differences in the patient populations analyzed (children naturally infected vs. adults with experimental infection), the identified "viral signature" classified pediatric patients with influenza from age-matched healthy controls with 100% accuracy.[242] This is a critical observation that confirms the reproducibility and potential value of blood transcriptome analysis to study host immune responses to respiratory viruses in the clinical setting. Additional studies will be necessary to evaluate this approach in other relevant clinical situations where the application of this methodology has the potential to transform the standard of care. In this regard, two studies have already shown the utility of host gene expression profiles as a diagnostic tool when effective treatment depends on rapid identification of the infectious agent or even the need for treatment. In the first study, also using adult volunteers experimentally infected with influenza A H1N1 or H3N2,[242] the authors found a blood RNA signature that was detectable more than 24 hours before the peak of clinical symptoms.[235] Subsequently, the same group of investigators used the transcriptome profiles derived from the experimental influenza signature[242] to develop a targeted host-based RT-PCR low-density array assay. This assay was applied to adult patients presenting with fever to the emergency department (ED) and differentiated viral versus bacterial infections with 89% sensitivity and 94% specificity,[241] demonstrating that gene expression profiles identified by microarray analyses can be successfully applied to custom-made platforms with the potential for a fast, point-of-care patient diagnosis and classification. It is remarkable that although in the majority of studies patient samples were collected at different time points after pathogen exposure and disease onset, robust and pathogen-specific biosignatures have been derived and validated in independent cohorts of patients in completely different settings.

Areas for Improved Diagnosis in Pediatrics

Lower Respiratory Tract Infections (LRTI)/Pneumonia

Acute LRTI/community-acquired pneumonia (CAP) represent the leading cause of hospitalization in the United States and is the main cause of death worldwide in children less than 5 years of age.[79,119,125,128] In industrialized countries, CAP has an annual incidence of 36 to 40 per 1000 children below the age of 5 years and 11 to 16 per 1000 in children 5 to 14 years of age.[103] In the United States it is second only to injuries as the most common reason for hospitalization in children less than 18 years of age.[160] In current clinical practice, establishing the precise etiologic diagnosis of pneumonia, or even simply discriminating viral from bacterial respiratory infections, remains

*References 4, 15, 53, 55, 83, 87, 92, 104, 141, 170, 173, 196, 208, 219, 222, 241.

TABLE 3.2 Studies of Pathogens in Various Populations

Country/Study Year	Pathogens	Population	Sample Type	Cohorts/Validation
US, 2007[186]	Virus vs. bacterial[a]	Children <18 yr ($n = 131$) Ctrl age matched ($n = 7$)	PBMCs	3 patient cohorts and RT-PCR
Vietnam, 2009[222]	*Salmonella typhi*	Adults ($n = 29$) Ctrl (OD, $n = 10$; HC, $n = 16$)	Whole blood	—
Thailand, 2009[170]	*Burkholderia pseudomallei*	Adults ($n = 32$) Ctrl (OD, $n = 31$; HC, $n = 29$)	Whole blood	3 patient cohorts
Cambodia, 2010[53]	Dengue	Children <15 yr ($n = 48$) DSS ($n = 19$) DF ($n = 16$) DHF ($n = 13$)	Whole blood	RT-PCR validation
UK, South Africa, 2010[15]	*Mycobacterium tuberculosis* (TB)	Adults TB ($n = 123$) Ctrl (OD = 96) HC ($n = 24$)	Whole blood	3 patient cohorts
Switzerland, 2010[196]	HIV	Adults ($n = 137$) Ctrl ($n = 19$)	$CD4^+$ T-cells	Genomewide SNP
West Africa, 2012[92]	*Plasmodium falciparum*	Children <10 yr ($n = 94$) Ctrl age matched ($n = 61$)	Whole blood	Mouse model
US, 2012[10]	*S. aureus* (invasive)	Children ($n = 99$) Ctrl ($n = 44$)	Whole blood	2 patient cohorts
UK, 2012[173]	H1N1 influenza A	Adults ($n = 11$) Ctrl (OD, $n = 28$; HC, $n = 18$)	Whole blood	2 patient cohorts Public available data sets[186,242]
US, 2012[94]	RSV, influenza	Children <2 yr ($n = 79$) Ctrl, age matched ($n = 22$)	PBMCs	Mouse model, primary human epithelial cells
US, Finland, 2013[141]	RSV, influenza, HRV	Children <2 yr ($n = 181$) Ctrl age matched ($n = 39$)	Whole blood	4 patient cohorts
UK, 2013[87]	H1N1/09 influenza, RSV, bacteria	Children <8 yr ($n = 77$) Ctrl children ($n = 33$)	Whole blood	Public available data set[173]
US, 2013[90]	Virus vs. bacterial[b]	Febrile children <3 yr ($n = 30$) Afebrile children ($n = 22$)	Whole blood	Public available data set[186]
South Africa Malawi, Kenya, UK, 2014[4]	TB ± HIV	Children TB ± HIV ($n = 193$) OD ($n = 239$) LTBI ($n = 71$)	Whole blood	3 patient cohorts
US, Australia, 2013[241]	Virus vs. bacterial[c]	Experimental infection ($n = 41$)[242] Febrile adults ($n = 102$) Ctrl ($n = 35$)	Whole blood	3 patient cohorts
UK, Australia, 2014[208]	Neonatal sepsis	Infants, confirmed inf ($n = 43$) Infants, suspected inf ($n = 30$) Controls ($n = 45$)	Whole blood	3 patient cohorts, two platforms
Scotland, Ireland, 2014[55]	Neonatal sepsis	Neonates, infected ($n = 46$) Neonates, controls ($n = 69$)	Whole blood	3 patient cohorts, two platforms
USA, Finland, Spain, 2016[83]	Rhinovirus	Children RV^+ ($n = 114$) Controls ($n = 37$)	Whole blood	3 patient cohorts and RT-PCR

Ctrl, Controls; *DF*, dengue fever; *DHF*, dengue hemorrhagic fever; *DSS*, dengue shock syndrome; *LTBI*, latent tuberculosis infection; *OD*, other diseases; *RT-PCR*, real-time polymerase chain reaction; *SNP*, single nucleotide polymorphism.

[a]Virus, influenza A; bacteria, *S. pneumoniae*, *S. aureus*, *E. coli*.

[b]Virus, human herpesevirus-6, adenovirus, and enterovirus; bacteria, *S. aureus*, *E. coli*, *Salmonella*.

[c]Virus, influenza A, human rotavirus; bacteria, *S. aureus*, *S. pneumoniae*, *E. coli*.

challenging. Unfortunately the pressure to achieve a rapid resolution of symptoms has commonly led medical practitioners to take an overcautious approach and treat many patients unnecessarily with antibiotics. Recent studies have provided an initial proof of concept of how application of blood gene expression profiles could represent an alternative approach for the diagnosis of viral and bacterial LRTI.[15,87,104,141,173,242] Two landmark studies published in 2013 have shown the potential of transcriptome analysis for diagnosis and patient classification in two completely different clinical situations in which traditional tools have been demonstrated as insufficient: TB and RSV infections.[104,141]

TB remains a major diagnostic challenge, especially in the developing world where the prevalence of HIV is high. A study conducted in Africa showed the value of whole blood transcriptome analysis for the diagnosis of TB in a large cohort of HIV-infected and uninfected patients. From the expression data, the authors developed a disease risk score that discriminated with high sensitivity and specificity (>90%) between patients with active TB and those with an alternative diagnosis but who presented initially with suspected TB and even from patients with latent TB infection.[104] In young children, respiratory viral infections and specifically RSV represent the most common cause of LRTI leading to hospitalization worldwide. In the clinical setting it is impossible to predict, based on the physical examination and available diagnostic tools, which patients with RSV infection will progress to severe disease requiring hospitalization and which patients can be discharged home safely. Hence there is a clear need to better understand the immune response to RSV and how it relates to disease pathogenesis, progression, and severity. A recent study conducted in the United States analyzed a

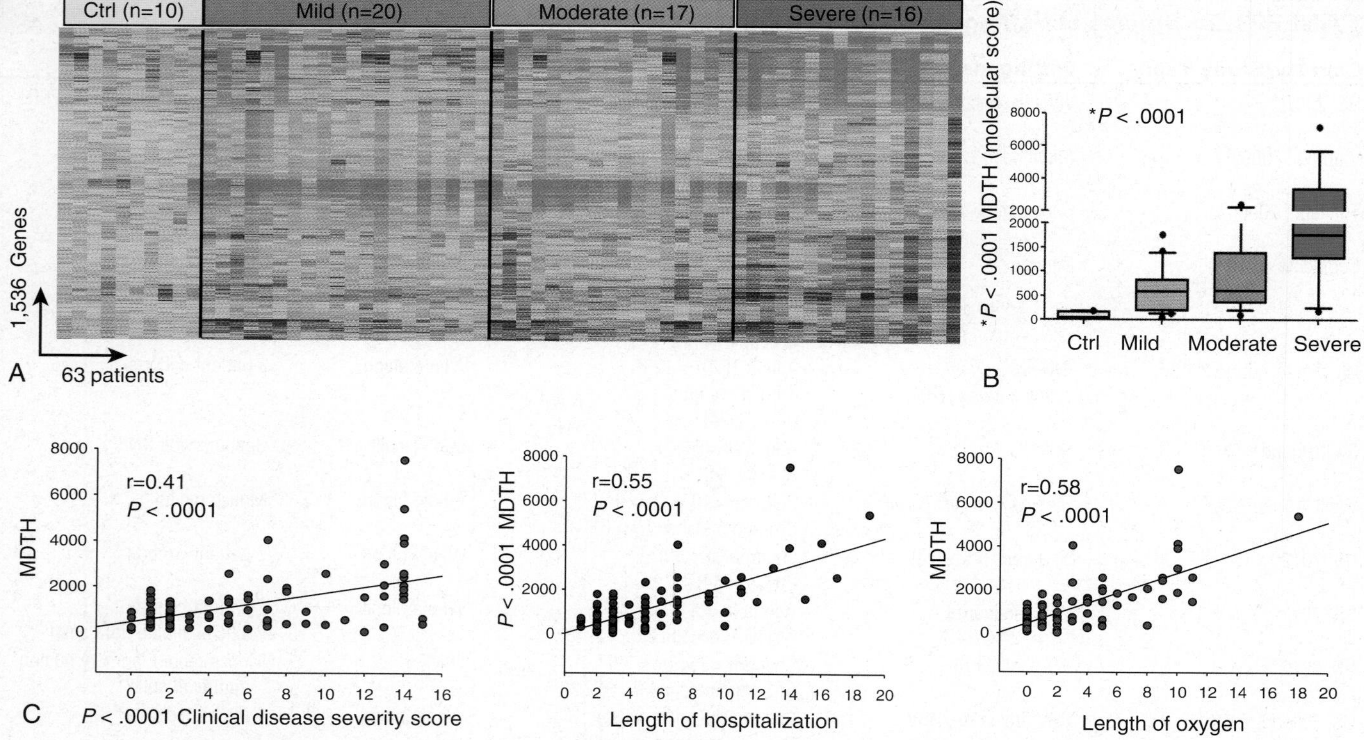

FIG. 3.6 (A) A molecular score correlates with disease severity and clinical outcomes in children. Hierarchical clustering of genes differentially expressed (Kruskal-Wallis $P < .01$, Benjamin-Hochberg multiple test correction) between infants with respiratory syncytial virus (RSV) LRTI and 10 healthy matched controls demonstrated a higher proportion of underexpressed genes in children with severe RSV ($n = 16$) that gradually declined in patients with moderate ($n = 17$) and mild RSV disease ($n = 20$). Each column represents a patient's sample and each row a transcript. (B) Using those 1536 transcripts, molecular distance to health (MDTH) scores were calculated and were higher in children with severe disease than in children with mild or moderate disease ($P < .001$). (C) The genomic MDTH score significantly correlated with the clinical disease severity score, the total length of hospitalization, and the duration of supplemental O_2 in the overall RSV cohort ($n = 91$).

cohort of 220 children younger than 2 years of age who were hospitalized with acute RSV, rhinovirus, and influenza A LRTI and showed that blood RNA profiles differentiated these three viral infections with 95% accuracy.[141] In addition, and as previously suggested,[24,94] RSV infection induced overexpression of interferon and neutrophil genes and suppression of B- and T-cell genes, which persisted beyond the acute disease and was greatly impaired in infants of less than 6 months of age. These results may explain in part the lack of protective antibody responses observed after acute RSV infection. Moreover, the authors identified a genomic score that significantly correlated with outcomes of care (Fig. 3.6). Altogether these studies demonstrate that large amount of microarray data can be translated into a biologically meaningful context that can be correlated with disease severity and applied in the relevant clinical setting to accurately classify patients. It is remarkable that blood signatures can achieve such accuracy for the diagnosis of respiratory pathogens that are thought to be mostly confined to the respiratory tract. From a practical perspective, in the majority of the clinical situations, obtaining a blood sample is more feasible than obtaining infected tissue.

Febrile Infant Without a Source

The evaluation of febrile infants, and especially those less than 2 months of age, who present to the ED continues to represent a major challenge for clinicians. Although viral infections are a common cause of fever with no apparent source in young infants, many children receive antibiotics unnecessarily due to the risk of serious bacterial infections. This is mainly due to the deceiving clinical appearance of the infant, coupled with the poor sensitivity of our current diagnostic tools. A study conducted in children 2 to 36 months of age presenting with fever to the ED showed that transcriptional profiles clearly distinguished between children with bacterial and viral infections and classified those patients with better accuracy than traditional white blood cell counts (WBC). Moreover gene expression profiles clearly differentiated symptomatic febrile from nonsymptomatic control children infected with the same virus (HHV-6 or adenovirus).[90] Currently an ongoing large multicenter study is being conducted by the Pediatric Emergency Care and Research Network (PECARN) in the United States to evaluate the application of transcriptional profiles for diagnosis of young febrile infants of less than 2 months of age in the ED.[133,252]

Differentiating Infection Versus Colonization

Whole blood RNA expression profiles represent much more than an expensive traditional WBC and have significantly superior capacity at discriminating bacterial from viral infections.[90,167,186] The readout is a combined representation of the number and cell types and the activation or suppression of all these cell types in peripheral blood. A recent study was conducted to evaluate the ability of host transcriptional profiling to differentiate between symptomatic rhinovirus infection and incidental detection of rhinovirus in a large cohort of children less than 2 years of age. Investigators found that symptomatic rhinovirus infection induced a robust and reproducible transcriptional signature, whereas identification of rhinovirus in asymptomatic children was not associated with significant systemic transcriptional immune responses.[83] These findings also demonstrate the applicability of these tools in the clinical setting where gene expression profiles can help to determine the clinical significance of detecting viral nucleic acid in individual patients.

PROTEOMICS

Proteomics is a relatively young discipline that emerged originally to complement transcriptomic studies.[40] Genomic data provide information about DNA or RNA transcription (mRNA) and thus represent the intermediate step between a given gene and its cognate protein. In contrast, the main principle underlying the use of proteomics is that proteins are the functional molecules ultimately responsible for controlling most cellular functions.[123] The main interest in proteomics is due in part to the prospects that a proteomic-based approach to disease investigation will overcome the limitations of other approaches.[181] The term *proteome* was coined by Wilkins in 1994, and it refers to the entire set of proteins expressed by a genome, cell, tissue, or organism at a certain time. Proteomics refers to the systematic analyses of these proteins, particularly their structures and functions.[177] Like genomics, proteomics is used to identify expression patterns at a specific time during the course of the disease in response to a specific stimulus. In the case of the proteome, the 22 most abundant proteins, including albumin and the immunoglobulins, account for 99% of the total proteome mass; however, many of the interesting molecules relevant to human disease occur in low abundance (in the nanomolar, picomolar, or even femtomolar range, such as tumor necrosis factor-α [TNF-α]).[3] In 2012, the Human Protein Atlas, a major resource for proteome analyses, comprised more than 14,000 proteins (approximately 70% of gene products) with ongoing efforts to include protein variants and posttranslational modifications.

Basics of the Proteomics Approach

Proteomics relies on a multistep approach including the separation of complex mixtures of proteins or peptides, quantification of protein abundance, and identification of the proteins. Proteome profiling technologies are evolving in a manner that emphasizes the need for both sensitivity and throughput. Within the past decade, mass spectrometry (MS)-based proteomics has emerged as a useful tool to better understand host-pathogen interactions,[237] allowing the identification and quantitation of large numbers of proteins with great accuracy. The measurement of the proteome and posttranslationally modified proteome dynamics using MS results in a wide array of information that can be linked to the patient's clinical picture, such as significant changes in protein expression, protein abundance, the modification status, or the functional significance of key proteins.[189] Different strategies have been developed over the years to define and quantitate proteome profiles.

Protein Separation Strategies

Separation strategies are driven by the need to reduce complexity (i.e., the number of proteins being analyzed) while retaining as much information as possible on the functional context of the protein. In its early stages, proteomics relied on high-resolution, two-dimensional polyacrylamide gel electrophoresis (2D-PAGE) to separate, identify, and quantitate single proteins present in a sample.[163] A cocktail was used to solubilize the protein contents of a biological fluid or tissue, followed by separation of the lysate protein content using two-dimensional gels. However, 2D-PAGE required that protein spots needed to be selected individually from the gels for subsequent identification by MS, allowing a limited display of relatively abundant proteins. This technology has been replaced by two-dimensional fluorescence difference gel electrophoresis (2D-DIGE) and liquid chromatography (LC), which allows multiple samples to be co-separated and can be directly coupled to MS.[218]

Nonprotein Separation Strategies

To address the different features of proteins that can be altered during the disease process, protein microarray strategies have been developed. Ideally protein chips should be able measure both the protein concentrations in biological samples as well as the protein interactions with other molecules, including other proteins, antibodies, or small ligands. Nevertheless, a major limitation of this approach is that proteins undergo numerous posttranslational modifications that may be crucial to their functions and are generally not captured using these tools.[82] Recent technological advances have made MS an indispensable technique for proteomic analyses.[176] MS is a technique used to identify the amount and types of molecules in a sample by measuring their molecular mass. There are many different types of mass spectrometers available, but the underlying principles of MS are relatively standard: ionization source, mass analyzer, and ion detector.[81] The first step in the process is to generate charged molecules, or ions, from the molecules in the sample. Molecules are then converted into gas-phase ions and separated by the mass analyzer, which uses electric or magnetic fields or time of flight (TOF) to separate ions,[26] and the matrix-assisted laser desorption/ionization (MALDI). The development of MALDI-TOF as a soft ionization technique suitable for proteins and peptides that tend to be fragile has revolutionized the applications of MS for proteomics, clinical microbiology, and biology in general.[50,60,210] Tandem MS instruments, such as the MALDI quadrupole ([Q]-TOF) have been recently developed to allow fast protein identification through database sequences.[240] For data mining and automation, which enables the accurate and fast diagnosis of human diseases, a novel approach combined two powerful techniques of chromatography and MS, and surface-enhanced laser desorption/ionization (SELDI) was developed.[96] One of the key features of SELDI-TOF MS is its ability to provide a rapid protein expression profile from a variety of clinical samples.

Proteomics in Infectious Diseases

Circulating host proteins represent an attractive alternative to monitor host responses to infection and can be used as point-of-care testing because of their fast turnaround time. Proteins that are routinely used to support the diagnosis of infections include CRP and PCT, which will be discussed separately.[206] Microbial pathogens display host specificity through a complex network of molecular interactions that help with their survival and propagation. Proteomics-based approaches and posttranslational modification analysis through MS technologies can be efficiently applied to identify and quantitate large numbers of proteins with great accuracy and to gain insight into the molecular mechanisms involved in host-pathogen interactions.[41] From a practical point of view, protein targets do not require amplification and are easily applicable to current clinical practice. An example is the rapid group A streptococcus test that relies on lateral flow immunochromatography. Thus despite the technological challenges, the potential to develop fast, simple, low-cost assays for infection diagnosis and prognosis is compelling; nevertheless, to derive meaningful conclusions using this tool, it is critical that the appropriate samples are used.

The use of proteomics in infectious diseases through MALDI-TOF MS has been mainly applied to identify causative pathogens in a time-efficient manner and to understand the mechanisms of diseases. A recent study showed that of 1660 bacterial isolates analyzed, MALDI-TOF correctly identified 95.4% of them: 84% were identified at the species level and 11.3% at the genus level. Importantly, once pathogens grew, the mean time required to identify one isolate was 6 minutes, thus significantly decreasing the cost of current methods of identification.[102,175,204]

In Vitro Studies

To better understand the pathogenesis and mechanisms of viral infections, different studies have incorporated labeled amino acids into tissue culture for MS-based quantitative proteomics in vitro. This approach, also called stable isotope labeling with amino acids in cell culture (SILAC), in conjunction with LC-MS/MS has been applied to quantify changes in the nucleolar proteome of in vitro influenza A, RSV, and adenovirus infection, among others.[116,155,248,249] Studies in different areas of infectious diseases have been conducted to discover the host-pathogen biomarkers that can help with diagnosis, assess clinical severity, and predict response to therapy. The main syndromes to which proteomics have been applied in vivo in a variety of biological fluids are lower respiratory tract infections/pneumonia including TB, hepatitis, HIV, and perinatal infections including chorioamnionitis or necrotizing enterocolitis (NEC).

Human Studies

As mentioned earlier, lower respiratory tract infections represent the global leading cause of death in children younger than 5 years.[75] Despite the frequency with which it is encountered, the diagnosis and management of pediatric lower respiratory tract infections remain a significant challenge to practitioners. First, a specific etiology is not identified in many cases,[56,103,110,144,153,225,236] making targeted therapy difficult. Additionally, the clinical features of lower respiratory tract infections are variable and overlap.[130,137] In this field, proteomics has been used mainly to identify the causative pathogen and understand the mechanisms of disease.[18,182] A limited number of studies have utilized proteomic host responses to assess disease severity and/or as a diagnostic tool to identify the causative agent. Surfactant protein A or D obtained from bronchoalveolar lavage and serum amyloid A protein have been identified as markers of lung damage in patients with a variety of respiratory diseases.[9,239] Plasma proteomic profiles from adults experimentally infected with influenza A H3N2 virus were analyzed using LC-MS tools at baseline and at the disease peak. The authors found several thousand isotope groups per sample with almost 10% mapping to known proteins; of those, AGL2 (an acute phase reactant–like protein) was greatly correlated with symptomatic disease.[243] A recent study conducted with 1000 participants, including pediatric and adult patients with a variety of infections, found that the combination of host proteins participating in viral and bacterial pathways had superior diagnostic accuracy to any of these proteins alone. In addition, the three-proteome signature (TNF-related apoptosis-inducing ligand [TRAIL], interferon γ–induced protein-10 [IP-10], and CRP) was superior to any clinical parameter used in the study.[168] The obvious next steps would be to apply this signature specifically to patients with lower respiratory tract infections to differentiate viral versus bacterial versus viral-bacterial pneumonia so appropriate management and targeted therapy can be promptly instituted.

Proteomics has also been applied to improve the diagnosis of TB. A study conducted in serum samples from 102 adult patients with culture-positive TB and 170 healthy controls found a proteomic fingerprint composed of four biomarkers (serum amyloid A protein, transthyretin, neopeptin, and CRP). This signature was able to predict the TB status in an independent cohort of 77 patients with 78% accuracy.[1] A more recent study performed in serum samples from 180 patients with active TB identified a different four-biomarker signature that was predictive of active TB versus controls also with about 80% accuracy. In addition, investigators found that patients with active TB had increased concentrations of fibrinogen and fibrinogen degradation products, which may also help to monitor response to therapy.[124]

In recent years the prevalence of hepatocellular carcinoma (HCC) associated with both hepatitis B (HBV) and HCV has significantly increased.[49] The current biomarkers used for diagnosis (α-fetoprotein) lack the appropriate sensitivity, and, until recently, the gold standard for therapy included interferon and ribavirin, whose response was variable and hard to predict. HCC usually has a poor prognosis, due in part to the fact that the disease is often diagnosed in advanced stages. Thus the discovery of host-viral biomarkers to predict response to therapy and for early detection of HCC has become a priority.[157] A study conducted in serum from treatment-naïve HCV patients and validated in a new cohort of patients identified a three-metaprotein signature that was able to predict response to therapy with high accuracy (90% in the training cohort and 88% in the validation group). Of the 105 proteins identified with two or more peptides (a total of 3768 peptides), regression modeling found vitamin D binding protein, α-2 HS glycoprotein, and complement C5 to have the best predictive area under the receiver operator (ROC) characteristic curve.[174] Unbiased protein profiling of liver tissue has also been applied to identify pathways associated with the development of HCV-related fibrosis and HCC.[54,122,158] A main limitation in these studies is the difficulty in obtaining samples and thus the inability to validate results.

HIV continues to affect millions of people worldwide and has caused more than 35 million fatalities. The virus is able to cross the blood-brain barrier, which may result in neurocognitive impairment and/or AIDS dementia. Using serum and cerebrospinal fluid (CSF), investigators have attempted to identify a proteomic fingerprint predictive of HIV-associated CNS disease, with contradictory results.[13,117] Investigators have also used proteomic approaches to diagnose damage inflicted by the antenatal or postnatal exposure of the fetus to infection/inflammation. Good examples are the studies performed by Buhimschi and colleagues in the field of chorioamnionitis; they analyzed proteomic fingerprints, including CRP and interleukin-6 (IL-6), in urine and amniotic fluid samples from pregnant women for the diagnosis of intraamniotic infections with promising results.[27,26] Similarly, Sylvester and colleagues conducted a study in 85 premature infants with suspected NEC, 17 with sepsis, and 17 controls and applied proteomics in urine samples. They found and validated a seven-proteome signature that was diagnostic of NEC and help to identify neonates at risk of developing severe or surgical disease.[212]

C-Reactive Protein

CRP is a pathogen-associated molecular pattern recognition protein of the pentraxin family synthesized by hepatocytes after IL-6 stimulation. It was first identified in 1930, when sera from patients with *Streptococcus pneumoniae* infection were found to have a protein that binds to the C-polysaccharide of the bacterial cell wall. CRP not only recognizes microbial polysaccharides but also necrotic cells, chromatin subunits, and small nuclear riboproteins, all of which are exposed at sites of tissue damage.[29] CRP bridges the gap between innate and adaptive immunity by activating the classical complement pathway and was recently found to bind cellular immunoglobulin Fc receptors as well.[58] CRP deficiency in humans has not been described. CRP induces the production of inflammatory cytokines and tissue factors and the shedding of the IL-6 receptor, all of which result in a complement-dependent increase in tissue damage.[77] Thus it is not surprising that CRP is elevated as part of the acute-phase response to inflammation or infection. After an acute inflammatory stimulus, CRP concentration increases rapidly and peaks at 2 to 3 days at levels that reflect the extent of tissue injury. If the stimulus has been removed, serum CRP levels drop rapidly, with a half-life of roughly 19 hours.[227] Persistent elevations in CRP are seen in chronic inflammatory states such as pulmonary TB. Used along with ESR, these levels are useful markers to monitor disease activity but are not as useful for differential diagnosis. Overall the value of CRP appears to be inferior to other biomarkers. CRP has shown a sensitivity of about 70% and a specificity that varies between 65% and 90% for patients with bacterial lower respiratory tract infections.[65,89] Nevertheless, as with other biomarkers, it needs to be interpreted in the appropriate clinical scenario.

Procalcitonin

PCT was discovered in the early 1960s as a peptide precursor of the hormone calcitonin. It is released by parenchymal cells (C-cells of the thyroid gland or neuroendocrine cells in the lung or intestine) in response to bacterial toxins; thus serum levels are elevated in patients with bacterial infections, whereas its production appears to be decreased in patients with viral infections. Multiple studies have shown that PCT is involved in the pathogenesis of infections and that it can be a useful diagnostic marker for bacterial infections such as bacterial pneumonia,[101] serious bacterial infections in young children, septic shock, meningitis, or urinary tract infections.[109,132,150,201] On the other hand serum PCT concentrations naturally fluctuate during the first 48 hours of life and require adjustments for the estimated gestational age of the premature newborn. Thus its value as a biomarker of early-onset sepsis appears less reliable.[127] In addition, PCT has been studied to facilitate the appropriate use of antibiotics. Two studies followed patients with lower respiratory tract infections/CAP in which clinicians were advised not to prescribe antimicrobials if patients had low PCT concentrations (<0.1 μg/L) but were encouraged to use them if PCT levels were greater than 0.25 μg/L.[37,39] These and other studies, including a meta-analysis that used individual patient data from 4221 patients with acute respiratory infections included in 14 trials, showed that information about PCT resulted in lower rates of antibiotic exposure.[202] Although PCT has been shown to have greater specificity and sensitivity than CRP as a biomarker, it should not be used without evaluation of other clinical and laboratory data in clinical decision making because the cutoffs to determine the probability of bacterial infections vary depending of the type of infection and setting and because serum PCT concentration may be normal in patients with sepsis or increased in some individuals with no clinical symptoms.[38]

METABOLOMICS

Metabolomics involves the rapid, high-throughput characterization of small metabolites. Similar to proteomics, it represents a promising approach to identify biomarkers of disease by defining metabolomics profiles. Metabolites are small chemical molecules including sugars, amino acids, or lipids that are present in a given biological sample. In 1971, it was postulated that metabolites in biologic fluids could be measured in a quantitative and qualitative manner, reflecting the functional status of those biologic systems. This approach was ultimately referred to as *metabonomics*, although today both the terms *metabonomics* and *metabolomics* are used.[161,178] More recently focused analyses of specific metabolite families or subsets, such as lipids, have given rise to "lipidomics," which is becoming a separate entity.[115] Metabolomics focuses on identifying and quantifying both the steady-state as well as the dynamic changes of metabolites, providing information regarding the activity of enzymes that in turn are modulated by substrates, cofactors, and small molecules or proteins. Since the metabolome is closely tied to the genotype of an organism, its physiology, and its environment, metabolomics offers a unique opportunity to study genotype-phenotype as well as genotype-envirotype relationships. Using MS, Millington and colleagues found that by screening for fatty acids and organic and selected amino acids in neonates, certain inborn errors of metabolism could be diagnosed.[66] This was a seminal discovery and has served as the basis for future work in this field. Since then, the application of metabolomics to gain new insights into the mechanisms of diseases, improve diagnosis, and help with prognosis has significantly increased, and it is being used in a variety of health applications including pharmacology, toxicology, transplant monitoring, and infectious diseases.[69,162,211]

In 2007, the Human Metabolome Project released the first draft of the human metabolome consisting of approximately 2900 endogenous or common metabolites that have certain specificities for given tissues or body fluids (309 metabolites in CSF, 1122 metabolites in serum, 458 metabolites in urine, and approximately 300 metabolites in other tissues/biofluids). Different tissues/biofluids have different functions and/or metabolic roles, and recent estimates suggest that the human metabolome includes approximately 5000 small molecules.[234] A key limitation to metabolomics is the fact that the human metabolome is not yet well characterized.

Basics of the Metabolomic Approach

Analyses of the metabolome are complex because of its dynamic nature and also due to the fact that many metabolites give rise to different molecules that are partially formed from products derived of food, drugs, the gut microbiome, and even the environment. Compared with proteomic techniques, metabolomic technologies focus on smaller compounds, generally less than 2 kDa in size. Metabolites are usually easily separated from proteins by simple extraction techniques and precipitation and removal of the proteins. The methods most commonly used to analyze metabolites are similar to those used for proteomic analyses and include MS, often coupled to LC, and gas chromatography (GC) MS, as well as nuclear magnetic resonance (NMR) spectroscopy. Similar to proteomics, the approach used for metabolomic analyses can be performed in a targeted manner or using a pattern discovery approach, depending on the objective of the study.

For biomarker discovery, *metabolomic fingerprinting* is commonly used because it does not require a prior knowledge of the metabolite and has less inherent bias. Using this unbiased approach investigators confront a complex pattern of peaks, many of which are anonymous, and the molecular identities of the species that give rise to the peaks are not generally known. Overall this approach is analytically more challenging.

When metabolomics is used to target a number of metabolites of known identity, it is defined as *metabolomic profiling* or *metabolite target analysis* (depending on the number of metabolites analyzed). The targeted approach is commonly used for systems biology and biomarker discovery and readily permits the assay of several hundred metabolites in as little as 10 μL of plasma. Although this approach is more limited, the analyses are more straightforward.

Metabolomics in Infectious Diseases

In Vitro and Animal Model Studies

Metabolomic studies performed in vitro and in animal models have provided insights into the mechanisms of infection and as biomarkers of disease severity. Using LC/MS and GC/MS, in vitro infection of cells with influenzavirus identified an increase of fatty acid and cholesterol metabolites, as well as intermediates of the tricarboxylic acid (TCA) pathway.[193] In the murine model, LC/MS-based metabolomics identified lipid metabolites (5-lipoxygenase and 12/15-lipoxygenase pathways) in the lungs of infected animals that were differentially regulated based on the phase of the infection and the influenza strain virulence. These markers were subsequently confirmed in nasal wash samples from actual patients with influenza infection.[243]

Human Studies

In humans, targeted and nontargeted metabolomic methods allow for the identification of more than 4000 metabolites in human biofluids, and, although increasing, the number of studies are still limited.[183] Most metabolomic studies in humans have been performed in patients with sepsis to identify early biomarkers associated with improved outcomes and survival. A study conducted in a large cohort of pediatric patients with either septic shock or systemic inflammatory response syndrome (SIRS) and healthy controls identified a circulating metabolite profile that was useful for the diagnosis and prediction of mortality in septic shock.[146,147] Other studies conducted in serum or urine samples from adult patients also with sepsis or septic shock found that metabolomic profiles had improved sensitivity and specificity over clinical scoring systems.[71,145] A small study conducted in 30 adult patients with CAP and sepsis found broad differences in 423 small metabolites related to oxidative stress, bile acid metabolism, and stress response pathways between surviving and nonsurviving patients.[205] In addition to sepsis, metabolomic studies have been performed in serum, oral washes, or bronchoalveolar samples from patients with TB and/or HIV for diagnostic purposes and to evaluate response to therapy.[42,67,73,134,232] Last, a pilot study performed in urine samples from patients with HCV identified a metabolomic fingerprint that discriminated patients with HCV infection from those with HBV with high sensitivity and specificity.[76]

Thus, overall, proteomics and metabolomics are promising tools, but there are still limitations to their application in the clinical setting from technical and practical points of view. From the technical perspective there are limitations in the ability to detect low-abundance, hydrophobic, or basic proteins or metabolites that often results in the lack of a complete proteome/metabolome coverage or the full proteome or metabolome dynamic range.[203] From the practical point of view, analytic strategies are not completely unified, and there are two main and opposite approaches for analyses that are not yet perfected: centered (or targeted) versus unbiased.[26] Despite these technical limitations, the potential to develop rapid and affordable single- or small host protein- or metabolite-derived assays for the diagnosis and management of infectious diseases in the clinical setting is promising.

FUTURE PERSPECTIVES

Each infection involves the combination of a pathogen and the host response to that pathogen. In that interaction, general but also specific molecules, pathways, cells, or tissues are activated or suppressed. The use of system immunology approaches based on analyses of host responses is transforming the research landscape in the field of infectious diseases by allowing a comprehensive molecular profiling of body fluids or tissue samples in infected versus healthy individuals. These approaches (often referred to as -omics technologies) take advantage of high-throughput methods to measure all possible parameters in a given biological system. In contrast to the more traditional approach, the -omics approach is in general inherently unbiased because investigators do not need to select the parameters that will be analyzed. As an example, system vaccinology is already using this approach to identify early after vaccination differences in immune responses to vaccines.[28,120,164] The main limitation of the -omics approach is the vast amount of data generated that need to undergo analyses and interpretation in a systematic manner. Nevertheless, as -omics bioinformatics evolves, the ability to identify biomarkers that are predictive of specific infections and/or associated with disease severity, as well as reproducible in different patient populations, will advance in parallel. These tools will also serve to truly differentiate among infection, colonization, or asymptomatic carriage, thus allowing for an optimal use of our antimicrobial armamentarium. They may even be used to identify novel outbreaks caused by less well-identified pathogens.

NEW REFERENCES SINCE THE SEVENTH EDITION

11. Mejias A, Suarez NM, Ramilo O. Detecting specific infections in children through host responses: a paradigm shift. *Curr Opin Infect Dis*. 2014;27:228-235.
19. Milcent K, Faesch S, Gras-Le Guen C, et al. Use of procalcitonin assays to predict serious bacterial infection in young febrile infants. *JAMA Pediatr*. 2015;1-8.
21. Moyer MW. New biomarkers sought for improving sepsis management and care. *Nat Med*. 2012;18:999.
26. Mejias A, Dimo B, Suarez NM, et al. Whole blood gene expression profiles to assess pathogenesis and disease severity in infants with respiratory syncytial virus infection. *PLoS Med*. 2013;10:e1001549.
35. Evangelidou P, Alexandrou A, Moutafi M, et al. Implementation of high resolution whole genome array CGH in the prenatal clinical setting: advantages, challenges, and review of the literature. *Biomed Res Int*. 2013;2013:346762.
91. Bird A. Perceptions of epigenetics. *Nature*. 2007;447:396-398.
106. Song H, Wang Q, Guo Y, et al. Microarray analysis of microRNA expression in peripheral blood mononuclear cells of critically ill patients with influenza A (H1N1). *BMC Infect Dis*. 2013;13:257.
122. Berry MP, Graham CM, McNab FW, et al. An interferon-inducible neutrophil-driven blood transcriptional signature in human tuberculosis. *Nature*. 2010;466:973-977.
125. Zaas AK, Chen M, Varkey J, et al. Gene expression signatures diagnose influenza and other symptomatic respiratory viral infections in humans. *Cell Host Microbe*. 2009;6:207-217.
126. Wang Z, Gerstein M, Snyder M. RNA-Seq: a revolutionary tool for transcriptomics. *Nat Rev Genet*. 2009;10:57-63.
146. Heinonen S, Jartti T, Garcia C, et al. Rhinovirus detection in symptomatic and asymptomatic children: value of host transcriptome analysis. *Am J Respir Crit Care Med*. 2016;193(7):772-782.
147. Anderson ST, Kaforou M, Brent AJ, et al. Diagnosis of childhood tuberculosis and host RNA expression in Africa. *N Engl J Med*. 2014;370:1712-1723.
162. Yang Y, Hu M, Yu K, Zeng X, Liu X. Mass spectrometry-based proteomic approaches to study pathogenic bacteria-host interactions. *Protein Cell*. 2015;6:265-274.
163. Ravikumar V, Jers C, Mijakovic I. Elucidating host-pathogen interactions based on post-translational modifications using proteomics approaches. *Front Microbiol*. 2015;6:1313.
178. Seng P, Drancourt M, Gouriet F, et al. Ongoing revolution in bacteriology: routine identification of bacteria by matrix-assisted laser desorption ionization time-of-flight mass spectrometry. *Clin Infect Dis*. 2009;49:543-551.
198. Agranoff D, Fernandez-Reyes D, Papadopoulos MC, et al. Identification of diagnostic markers for tuberculosis by proteomic fingerprinting of serum. *Lancet*. 2006;368:1012-1021.
209. Sylvester KG, Ling XB, Liu GY, et al. Urine protein biomarkers for the diagnosis and prognosis of necrotizing enterocolitis in infants. *J Pediatr*. 2014;164:607-12.e1–7.
220. Milcent K, Faesch S, Gras-Le Guen C, et al. Use of procalcitonin assays to predict serious bacterial infection in young febrile infants. *JAMA Pediatr*. 2016;170:62-69.
236. Mickiewicz B, Vogel HJ, Wong HR, Winston BW. Metabolomics as a novel approach for early diagnosis of pediatric septic shock and its mortality. *Am J Respir Crit Care Med*. 2013;187:967-976.
249. Obermoser G, Presnell S, Domico K, et al. Systems scale interactive exploration reveals quantitative and qualitative differences in response to influenza and pneumococcal vaccines. *Immunity*. 2013;38:831-844.

The full reference list for this chapter is available at ExpertConsult.com.

4 Fever: Pathogenesis and Treatment

Mark A. Ward • Nicole L. Hannemann

Fever is the thermoregulated increase in body temperature above normal as the result of a coordinated response to a pathologic insult. The two essential features of fever are that it represents an abnormal elevation in body temperature and that it results from a coordinated physiologic response. The first feature differentiates fever from normal regulated elevations in body temperature (e.g., elevations associated with the circadian rhythm), whereas the latter distinguishes it from conditions in which the regulatory mechanisms are overwhelmed or dysfunctional (e.g., heat stroke). In children, the pathologic insult most likely to result in fever is infection. A variety of other conditions, including malignancies and autoimmune diseases, also may result in this phenomenon, however.

NORMAL BODY TEMPERATURE

Although the general public and physicians alike often refer to "the" body temperature, the implication that a single number can represent the thermal state of the entire body is inaccurate. Depending on the site of measurement, body temperature may vary by 1°C or more.[40] These regional variations in temperature do not have a fixed relationship to each other. Although axillary temperatures are consistently lower than rectal temperatures, the absolute difference between the two varies greatly.[5] In addition, even in the healthy state, body temperature is not constant; it varies depending on numerous factors, such as time of day, level of activity, and phase of the menstrual cycle. Generally, clinicians have been most interested in the core body temperature, defined as the temperature of the internal organs of the trunk and head. Under normal circumstances, core temperature is higher than the temperature of more superficial tissues such as skin. Even within these two anatomic regions, temperature gradients exist, however.

The most widely accepted definition of normal body temperature is 37°C (98.6°F).[51] This number is derived from studies performed in the 19th century by Wunderlich.[99] He reportedly arrived at this figure based on the result of several million measurements conducted in approximately 25,000 individuals. Other more recent studies have found slightly lower mean temperatures in healthy individuals, despite the fact that these more recent studies are based on oral or rectal temperatures whereas Wunderlich's studies relied on axillary temperatures.[33] Mackowiak and colleagues[52] determined the mean oral temperature in adults to be 36.8°C (98.2°F), with the upper limit of normal ranging from 37.2°C (98.9°F) at 6:00 AM to 37.7°C (99.9°F) at 4:00 PM. Given the limitations imposed by the technology available at the time, however, perhaps the most surprising aspect of the value reported by Wunderlich is how closely it approximates these more recent determinations.

As noted previously, body temperature fluctuates depending on numerous normal physiologic factors. Core temperature shows a diurnal variation of 1°C, the nadir occurring in the early morning hours and the peak in the late afternoon.[42,52] After exercise and in the postprandial state, body temperature increases.[58] In addition, variations in the normal body temperature of women associated with the menstrual cycle are well described, with increases in baseline temperature occurring after ovulation.[16]

THERMOREGULATION

Humans, similar to other mammals, are homeothermic, indicating that they regulate body temperature within a narrow range despite wide variations in the ambient temperature. Regulation of temperature is mediated by a variety of physiologic (e.g., vasoconstriction, sweating) and behavioral (e.g., moving to a warmer environment, putting on additional clothing) responses.

The principal thermoregulatory area is located within the brain in the preoptic area and anterior hypothalamus. Although it frequently is conceptualized as a single center, no single neuronal structure seems to control all aspects of temperature regulation.[11] Rather, a complex interplay occurs among a variety of neural pathways, with the final result being the maintenance of the body's temperature within a narrow range. Regardless of the precise nature of central regulation, body temperature ultimately is a function of the balance between heat gain and heat loss.

Heat energy is a by-product of the inefficiency of the body's normal metabolic processes. It is this "waste" heat that renders the homeothermic state possible. During exercise, the increased metabolic activity in muscle tissue results in increased production of heat, leading to an increase in the body's temperature.[76] Shivering, an involuntary form of muscle activity, is the primary means by which the body generates additional heat under conditions of cold stress. Heat also may be generated by a process known as nonshivering thermogenesis. Originally described in rats, nonshivering thermogenesis has been found to occur in a variety of mammals, including humans. It seems to be of greater importance in neonates than in adults. Although this process has been shown to occur in a variety of tissues, brown adipose tissue seems to be the most important site for this phenomenon. Under the control of the adrenergic system, production of free fatty acid is increased, resulting in an uncoupling of oxidative phosphorylation and the production of large amounts of heat.[10,31]

Four mechanisms are responsible for heat transfer: radiation, conduction, convection, and evaporation. Heat loss owing to radiation occurs when heat is transferred directly between two objects not in direct contact. Conduction involves the transfer of heat energy between two objects in contact with each other. Convection is the result of the movement of a fluid or gas across the surface of the body (e.g., as the result of fanning). Evaporative heat loss occurs in association with the energy required to convert liquid to gas form.

Under normal conditions, radiation accounts for most of the body's heat loss. In contrast, conductive losses are smaller under normal circumstances. Conductive losses may become substantial, however, under conditions in which a large portion of the individual's body surface is in direct contact with a cooler object (e.g., an unclothed infant in an unheated bassinet). Convective losses are proportional to the amount of air moving over the body surface; these losses are greatest in windy conditions. Conductive and convective heat losses are particularly important in infants and children because of their relatively greater body surface area compared with that of adults. Evaporative losses occur when fluids such as sweat evaporate from the skin's surface. In addition, substantial evaporative losses are associated with respiration.

PATHOGENESIS OF FEVER

In the classic model of fever pathogenesis, exogenous pyrogens stimulate the release of circulating endogenous pyrogens, which act via prostaglandins to increase the set point of the hypothalamic thermoregulatory center.[18] In this model, exogenous pyrogens are substances extrinsic to the body, primarily various bacterial microorganisms or the products of those microorganisms. Conversely, endogenous pyrogens are a varied group of proteins produced within the human body that share the intrinsic ability to induce fever. The first endogenous pyrogen was described originally more than 60 years ago and was derived from leukocytes, primarily granulocytes, and now is known as interleukin-1 (IL-1).[19] Numerous other cytokines that qualify as endogenous pyrogens, including tumor necrosis factor, interferon-α, interferon-γ, and IL-6, have been identified.[50,100]

A variety of alternative and complementary theories of fever pathogenesis have been proposed.[59] The actual mechanisms involved likely are more varied and complex than just described. A variety of intrinsically produced substances (e.g., antigen-antibody complexes) may act as "exogenous" pyrogens.[74] Murine models suggest that neuromodulatory endocannabinoid lipids play a role in lipopolysaccharide-induced fever.[26] The classic model provides a reasonable framework, however, for understanding most of the observed phenomena associated with the febrile response.

Regardless of the precise pathogenesis, the height of fever seems to be limited. Retrospective studies of hyperpyrexia in children have found that it is unusual for the body temperature to rise above 41.1°C (106°F), and it rarely rises above 41.7°C (107°F).[68,91] Children with temperatures exceeding this range almost always have an element of heat illness.

EFFECTS OF FEVER

Attempts to treat fever often are predicated on the assumption that fever has harmful effects and that reduction in temperature would abrogate such harm. The evidence with regard to these premises is mixed, however.

Adverse Effects

Some animal studies have found that high fever may impair certain immunologic responses, including phagocytosis of staphylococci by polymorphonuclear leukocytes[6,23,25] and lymphocyte transformation in response to mitogens.[73] Whether these isolated in vitro phenomena observed in animal models are relevant to human infection is unknown.

Fever may cause seizures, a phenomenon observed most frequently in young children. The onset generally occurs in infants 6 to 30 months of age. Recurrence is common, occurring in approximately one third of children experiencing an initial febrile seizure. The primary adverse consequences of febrile seizures are the emotional distress experienced by patients and their families and the need for medical evaluation, which may involve invasive testing and substantial expense. Febrile seizures do not cause brain injury and are not associated with subsequent intellectual or neurologic deficits.[22,93] Furthermore numerous studies have failed to demonstrate that use of antipyretics is effective in preventing febrile seizures.[61,78,88]

An important nonphysiologic adverse effect of fever is caregiver anxiety, reflecting an underlying concern for harm due to untreated fevers despite a lack of supporting data.[65] The unfounded anxiety is not limited to the lay public.[66] In addition, fear phobia may be inadvertently reinforced by the actions of medical personnel; for example, it has been observed fever may routinely be treated more promptly than pain in the pediatric emergency room.[21] Caregiver distress also crosses cultural boundaries, as suggested by a recent Turkish study that revealed that 3 out of 4 parents would wake their child from sleep to administer antipyretics.[67]

Beneficial Effects

Fever may be beneficial by enhancing the host response to infection and by directly inhibiting the infecting agent. Several studies have demonstrated that the immune system responds to mildly elevated body temperature by increasing migration of leukocytes, production of interferon, and lymphocyte transformation and phagocytosis.[2,8,73,75] Studies of bacterial infection in reptiles and fish have shown an increased survival rate in groups maintained at approximately 4°C (reptiles) and 2.5°C (fish) above baseline.[15,43] Kluger and Vaughn[45] showed that rabbits infected with *Pasteurella multocida* had improved survival rates at body temperatures of approximately 4.5°C above normal. Although these data are impressive, their clinical significance with regard to humans has yet to be determined.

Fever also may inhibit the growth and survival of some infectious agents. One potential mechanism for this inhibition is the decrease in serum iron and increase in ferritin that are associated with fever, coupled with the increased iron requirement of many bacteria at higher temperatures.[6,44] Fever therapy was used historically to treat neurosyphilis and gonococcal urethritis, correlating with more recent studies that show that certain gonococci and *Treponema* are eradicated at temperatures of 40°C (104°F) and greater.[13,41] Finally, growth of some pneumococci and viruses seems to be impaired at higher temperatures.[30,86,94]

Several studies have found that the treatment of fever with antipyretics is associated with adverse consequences, providing indirect evidence of a beneficial effect of fever. Ahmady and Samadi[2] reported that the use of aspirin in children with measles prolonged the duration of the illness and was associated with an increase in prevalence of respiratory complications and diarrhea. Other investigators have reported that the length of time to total scabbing in varicella was significantly longer in children treated with acetaminophen compared with children treated with placebo.[20] Several studies in animal models and in humans have found prolongation of viral shedding, depressed neutralizing antibody response, and increased nasal symptoms in association with the use of antipyretics.[28,36,90] Although these studies establish that an association exists between reduction of fever and adverse outcomes, they do not prove a causal relationship. The adverse effects possibly are mediated by some direct physiologic effects of antipyretics rather than indirectly by their impact on fever.

CLINICAL THERMOMETRY

Types of Thermometers

For many years, glass thermometers containing mercury were the most common type of thermometer used to measure body temperature. This type of thermometer is reasonably accurate for most clinical purposes. Although they are still available, use of mercury-containing thermometers has diminished greatly because of environmental concerns about mercury exposure from broken or discarded thermometers. These thermometers have been replaced largely by digital thermometers or glass thermometers containing liquids other than mercury.

Electronic thermometers (often referred to as digital thermometers) previously were used primarily in the hospital and office setting. As their cost has decreased, they are used more frequently in the home as well. Electronic thermometers have the advantage over mercury thermometers of requiring a significantly shorter dwell time—that is, the time they must remain in situ to obtain an accurate reading. Hospital-grade electronic thermometers typically have two modes: monitor and predictive. In the monitor mode, these thermometers function similarly to mercury thermometers in that they must remain in place until equilibration occurs, a process that may require several minutes. In the predictive mode, a complex algorithm is used to estimate the final temperature based on measurements made during the first few seconds. Because the predictive mode produces a temperature reading within seconds, it is the mode used most often in clinical settings. Determinations of temperatures using these two modes have been found to correlate well.[25,60]

Infrared thermometers are a more recent addition to the clinician's armamentarium. Devices that determine the temperature by detecting infrared radiation emitted from the eardrum are used most frequently. Tympanic temperature should provide an accurate estimation of the core temperature because its blood supply is derived from the carotid artery. Additional advantages of this type of thermometer are its speed, acceptance by patients, and decreased risk of cross-contamination compared with oral or rectal thermometers. Studies of the accuracy of tympanic thermometers have yielded mixed results, with numerous studies finding tympanic thermometers inaccurate compared with mercury in glass or electronic thermometers.[14,56] A recent meta-analysis showed pooled sensitivity of 70% and specificity of 86% as compared to rectal thermometry in diagnosing pediatric fever.[101] Discrepancies seem to be particularly common in infants who are in the first few months of life.[83] Tympanic thermometers should not be used in young infants because of the importance of fever in making management decisions in these patients.[17]

Even more recently, the temporal artery thermometer has been introduced. These thermometers use an infrared sensor to determine skin temperature as the device is passed across the forehead and temporal area. The site of highest measured temperature is assumed to represent that of the temporal artery. An algorithm is applied to the measured temperature to estimate the core temperature. Studies to date suggest that temporal artery thermometer temperatures correlate significantly better with rectal and core temperatures than with temperatures determined by tympanic thermometers. The data also suggest that these thermometers are more sensitive at detecting fever in children than in adults. Temporal artery thermometers do not seem to correlate well enough with rectal or core temperature measurements, however, to replace rectal thermometry in clinical situations in which accurate measurement of fever is crucial for making decisions about management. Correlation with rectal thermometry may be particularly limited in children younger than 36 months of age, with a reported sensitivity as low as 27% to 53%.[32] The accuracy of temporal artery thermometer readings is adversely affected by sweating and may be affected by vascular constriction or dilation. In addition, data comparing temporal artery and axillary thermometry are lacking.[29,89]

Several other types of thermometers have been developed. Among them are electronic pacifier thermometers, which are used for obtaining an oral temperature in infants. Although they are appealing in theory, this type of thermometer has the disadvantage of requiring a prolonged dwell time and has not been found to be sufficiently accurate to recommend its use.[69] Another approach to measuring temperature is the use of liquid crystal thermometers that are applied to the skin of the forehead. Results generally have been disappointing when these thermometers have been compared with more standard techniques.[46,79]

Despite ready availability of thermometers, many parents continue to utilize palpation, generally of a child's forehead, to detect the presence of fever. A study of infants under the age of 3 months found the positive predictive value of this practice to be only 33%, although the negative predictive value was as high as 95%. These results support the conclusion that palpation should not be used as the sole means of fever assessment.[38]

Measurement Site

The most common locations for measuring body temperature are the mouth, rectum, axilla, and tympanic membrane. Because of the previously noted regional variations in body temperature, each of these sites has its own range of normal temperatures. The oral cavity historically has been the preferred site for measuring temperature in older children and adults. When taking a temperature orally, one should place the thermometer in the sublingual space because the blood supply for structures in this region is derived from branches of the carotid arteries and should reflect the core temperature accurately. Younger children usually are unable to cooperate adequately to permit the use of oral thermometers. In addition, the oral temperature may be affected by recent ingestion of hot or cold liquids, and it may be altered by tachypnea.

Rectal temperatures are used frequently in younger children. The rectal temperature correlates well with the core body temperature. The rectal temperature may exceed the core temperature (using the pulmonary artery temperature as the reference standard), however, possibly because of the effects of bacterial activity in the rectum. The use of rectal thermometry has the disadvantage of causing the patient discomfort and is contraindicated in patients with neutropenia because of the risks of causing invasive infection via trauma to the rectal mucosa.

Axillary temperatures are appealing because of the ready accessibility of the axillae. Considerable variability occurs in the readings obtained, however, particularly in younger children. One should not rely on axillary temperatures, particularly in neonates and young children.

TREATMENT

As noted previously, fever may have numerous beneficial effects, convincing evidence of harm owing to fever is lacking, and treatment of fever may be associated with undesirable effects. Therefore routine intervention to reduce fever is not warranted. Rather physicians should individualize the decision to treat fever and the specific method chosen to do so. This approach is in accordance with the recommendations of the American Academy of Pediatrics.[82]

Indications

Antipyretic therapy often is considered for children who have an increased risk of having febrile seizures, either because of age or because of a history of febrile seizures. Although treatment seems rational in this situation, studies of antipyretic therapy to prevent febrile seizures have repeatedly failed to demonstrate its efficacy.[12,61,78,88,92] Even this indication should be considered relative rather than absolute.

Prophylactic administration of acetaminophen prior to routine immunizations to prevent vaccine-related fever has been debated. The practice is generally not recommended due to lack of supporting evidence. While the American Academy of Pediatrics Red Book recommends considering acetaminophen administration before and after DTaP immunization for children with a personal or family history of seizures,[4] studies have generally failed to produce results to support this practice.[54]

Antipyretic therapy also should be considered for children with poorly compensated underlying cardiac or pulmonary disease, significant neurologic impairment, or sepsis and for children with significant alterations of fluid and electrolyte balance. Definitive controlled trials to support these indications are lacking. Rather the recommendations are based on the metabolic consequences of fever and their potential adverse impact on the underlying disease.

Perhaps the most frequent indication for the use of antipyretics is to improve the patient's comfort. Despite the absence of definitive studies to support this practice and the potential adverse consequences of using antipyresis, such an approach is reasonable in the absence of definitive evidence to the contrary. In some circumstances, improving the patient's comfort may enhance the ability to assess the seriousness of the patient's illness accurately.[7]

Antipyretics

A wide variety of antipyretic agents is available. In the United States, the drugs used most frequently for treatment of fever in children are acetaminophen and ibuprofen. Previously, aspirin was the antipyretic used most frequently. Aspirin has fallen into disuse for the management of fever in children, however, primarily because of its association with Reye syndrome, particularly when used in managing children with varicella or influenza.[35] In addition, aspirin has a variety of other adverse effects, including inhibition of platelet function, gastritis and gastrointestinal bleeding, and provocation of asthma exacerbations, although this third complication occurs more frequently in adults.[37,72,81] Aspirin has greater toxicity in situations of overdose than do acetaminophen and ibuprofen.

Each of these agents acts to restore normal body temperature by reducing the set point of the temperature regulatory center in the hypothalamus. The specific mechanism of action seems to be interference with prostaglandin synthesis in the preoptic anterior hypothalamus. When selecting among the available antipyretic agents, one should consider efficacy and potential toxicity.

Similar to aspirin, ibuprofen inhibits prostaglandin synthesis in a variety of tissues outside the central nervous system. It shares many of the toxicities associated with aspirin. One exception is that ibuprofen lacks the association with Reye syndrome.[70] Ibuprofen inhibits platelet function because of its effect on prostaglandin synthesis, but this effect is reversible with discontinuation of the drug, and platelet dysfunction is short lived compared with the effect of aspirin.[62] Because prostaglandins are important to the integrity of the gastrointestinal mucosa, inhibition by ibuprofen may result in gastrointestinal upset and bleeding. Although ibuprofen has been associated with exacerbations of asthma in some children, the risk seems to be small and may not be greater than that associated with the use of acetaminophen.[47,48]

Acetaminophen has a lengthy track record of safety. When used in the usual therapeutic doses, it has few adverse effects. Acetaminophen inhibits prostaglandin synthase activity, but this action is inhibited by peroxide. Because peroxide is generated at sites of inflammation, acetaminophen has little anti-inflammatory activity. It also lacks the adverse gastrointestinal and platelet effects of aspirin and ibuprofen. A growing body of evidence suggests that acetaminophen use is associated with an increased risk of subsequent asthma.[24] Despite the fact that studies have consistently found this association, evidence of a causal relationship has yet to be conclusively established. Recommended dosing of ibuprofen is 5 to 10 mg/kg every 6 hours as needed. Acetaminophen is administered at a dose of 10 to 15 mg/kg every 4 hours but no more frequently than five times per day. An important note for individuals administering these agents is that a variety of over-the-counter combination medications contain one or the other of these agents. Coadministration may result in inadvertent overdosing.

In addition, recognition that ibuprofen and acetaminophen come in a variety of formulations is important.[85] Acetaminophen, once available as infant drops (concentration 10 mg/mL) and children's liquid (concentration 32 mg/mL) is now only available in a single concentration (32 mg/mL). The voluntary removal from the market of the more concentrated formulation was prompted by reports of inadvertent overdose from substitution of infant drops for the children's liquid without adjusting the volume administered to reflect the difference in concentration. Acetaminophen also is available in suppository form. Absorption varies, however, and is delayed compared with oral administration. In addition, the medication is not distributed uniformly throughout the suppository, resulting in potential dosing errors if the suppositories are divided before use.[9] The use of acetaminophen in suppository form should be discouraged. Ibuprofen continues to be available in two concentrations: a children's liquid (20 mg/mL) and infant drops (40 mg/mL). The dual concentrations create the potential for incorrect dosing seen previously with acetaminophen.

The antipyretic efficacy of acetaminophen and ibuprofen has been the subject of numerous clinical trials.[39,95–97] These trials have shown uniformly that both are effective antipyretic agents. Ibuprofen seems to result in a greater decrease in temperature than does acetaminophen, however. In addition, the antipyretic effect of ibuprofen is more prolonged, not surprising in light of ibuprofen's longer half-life compared with acetaminophen. These observations were confirmed in a meta-analysis of trials comparing ibuprofen and acetaminophen.[64]

Acetaminophen and ibuprofen frequently are used in combination.[49] Use of alternating doses often is advocated by practicing physicians.[55,98] The pathways for metabolism of these drugs are distinct, and, theoretically, metabolism of one should not affect the metabolism of the other. Controlled trials documenting safety and efficacy of combination or alternating use are sparse, however. In one study, using alternate doses of acetaminophen (12.5 mg/kg per dose) and ibuprofen (5 mg/kg per dose) every 4 hours was found to be associated with a more rapid reduction in fever, lower mean temperature, and fewer caregiver days absent from work and infant days absent from daycare compared with use of either agent alone.[77] However, the groups assigned to a single agent received dosing that was either on the low end or infrequent compared with usual practice in the United States. In a more recent study utilizing full therapeutic doses and comparing ibuprofen alone with alternating and combined schedules of ibuprofen and acetaminophen, the alternating and combined schedules were found to provide greater antipyresis.[63] Recent systematic reviews of combination versus single-agent treatment with acetaminophen and ibuprofen concluded that the antipyretic effect of combined therapy was statistically superior but the clinical relevance was marginal at best. Furthermore the studies found no evidence of increased toxicity with combined treatment but were not designed to definitively address the issue.[71] Evidence is also lacking regarding any beneficial effects of combined therapy on child discomfort.[98]

Another approach to antipyretic treatment frequently employed is the use of a second antipyretic when the initial agent is judged to have resulted in an inadequate response. Theoretically, some individuals may have a better antipyretic response to one agent than another. Although the premise is reasonable, sequential use of acetaminophen and ibuprofen remains unproved in terms of efficacy and safety.

Acetaminophen and ibuprofen have been proved to be remarkably safe when used in the recommended doses. Although ibuprofen may be slightly more efficacious in producing and sustaining fever reduction, acetaminophen remains the antipyretic of choice because of its longer track record and more favorable side-effect profile. Because acetaminophen lacks significant antiinflammatory activity, ibuprofen or another nonsteroidal antiinflammatory drug may be preferred in febrile conditions for which antiinflammatory activity is desired (e.g., juvenile arthritis). Limited data suggest that use of acetaminophen and ibuprofen in combination may be safe and more efficacious than is either agent alone. Prudence suggests, however, that combined therapy seldom is warranted for the treatment of fever, a generally benign condition. Perhaps most important, patients and their parents should be educated about the benign nature of fever and the lack of evidence to indicate that routine treatment, particularly complete suppression, is either necessary or beneficial.

External Cooling

The use of external cooling in the management of fever has a long history. Compared with standard antipyretics, sponging with tepid water is inferior in fever reduction at 2 to 3 hours, although sponging was found to reduce the temperature more quickly than did antipyretics in one trial.[1,3] External cooling without concomitant administration of antipyretics makes little sense from a physiologic standpoint, however. In a febrile patient whose temperature regulatory center set point has not been reset by administration of an antipyretic agent, external cooling inevitably results in an increase in the body's heat-production mechanisms.

When used in conjunction with an antipyretic agent, the usual goal of external cooling is to reduce the body's temperature more rapidly or to a greater degree. Several studies have compared the use of external cooling combined with antipyretics with antipyretics alone. Results have been mixed; some studies showed no difference in efficacy of the two approaches, whereas others found combination therapy to be superior.[27,34,53,84,87] Even in the studies in which a difference was found, the superiority of combination therapy was shown primarily in the very early phase of treatment. A recent randomized controlled study performed in an adult critical care unit population concluded that external cooling decreased vasopressor requirements and early mortality in septic shock. However, it is unclear if these results can be translated to the pediatric population.[80]

In addition, the use of external cooling usually is uncomfortable for the patient. When external cooling is to be used, sponging with tepid water is preferred. Alcohol and solutions containing alcohol should not be used for this purpose. Absorption of alcohol vapors via the lungs may occur in sufficient quantities to produce toxicity and even death.[57]

SUMMARY

Fever represents an abnormal increase in body temperature resulting from a coordinated physiologic response to pyrogens. While a variety of newer modalities are available, rectal thermometry remains the preferred method for temperature measurement when accuracy is important. Routine antipyretic therapy is not recommended in the absence of patient discomfort or concern for the effects of increased metabolic demand because there are few proven adverse effects of fever. When antipyresis is desired, acetaminophen and ibuprofen are generally safe and effective agents for that purpose.

NEW REFERENCES SINCE THE SEVENTH EDITION

4. American Academy of Pediatrics. Appendix V: Guide to contraindications and precautions to immunizations. In: Kimberlin DW, Brady MT, Jackson MA, Long SS, eds. *Report of the Committee on Infectious Diseases*. 30th ed. Elk Grove Village, IL: American Academy of Pediatrics; 2015:1003.
21. Dvorkin R, Bair J, Patel H, et al. Is fever treated more promptly than pain in the pediatric emergency department? *J Emerg Med*. 2014;46(3):327-334.
26. Fraga D, Zanoni CI, Rae GA, et al. Endogenous cannabinoids induce fever through the activation of CB1 receptors. *Br J Pharmacol*. 2009;157(8):1494-1501.
32. Hoffman RJ. Response to "Comparison of rectal, axillary, tympanic, and temporal artery thermometry in the pediatric emergency room". *Pediatr Emerg Care*. 2013;29(7):876-877.
38. Katz-Sidlow RJ, Rowberry JP, Ho M. Fever determination in young infants: prevalence and accuracy of parental palpation. *Pediatr Emerg Care*. 2009;25(1):12-14.
54. Manley J, Taddio A. Acetaminophen and ibuprofen for prevention of adverse reactions associated with childhood immunization. *Ann Pharmacother*. 2007;41(7):1227-1232.
61. Offringa M, Newton R. Prophylactic drug management for febrile seizures in children (Review). *Evidence-Based Child Health*. 2013;8(4):1376-1485.
65. Poirier MP, Collins EP, McGuire E. Fever phobia: a survey of caregivers of children seen in a pediatric emergency department. *Clin Pediatr (Phila)*. 2010;49(6):530-534.
66. Poirier MP, Davis PH, Gonzalez-Del Rey JA, et al. Pediatric emergency department nurses' perspectives on fever in children. *Pediatr Emerg Care*. 2000;16(1):9-12.
67. Polat M, Kara S, Tezer H, et al. A current analysis of caregivers' approaches to fever and antipyretic usage. *J Infect Dev Ctries*. 2014;8(3):365-371.
80. Schortgen F, Clabault K, Katsahian S, et al. Fever control using external cooling in septic shock: a randomized controlled trial. *Am J Respir Crit Care Med*. 2012;185(10):1088-1095.
98. Wong T, Stang AS, Ganshorn H, et al. Combined and alternating paracetamol and ibuprofen therapy for febrile children. *Evidence-Based Child Health*. 2014;9(3):675-729.
101. Zhen C, Xia Z, Ya Jun Z, et al. Accuracy of infrared tympanic thermometry used in the diagnosis of fever in children: a systematic review and meta-analysis. *Clin Pediatr (Phila)*. 2015;54(2):114-126.

The full reference list for this chapter is available at ExpertConsult.com.

5 The Human Microbiome

Berkley Luk • Douglas S. Swanson • James Versalovic

INTRODUCTION

The human microbiome consists of different microbial communities colonizing specific body sites (Fig. 5.1) and fluctuating during several life stages. Because pediatrics is fundamentally oriented around the health and pathophysiology of the developing human, the rapid accumulation of new findings in microbiome science during the past decade provides a new frame of reference for human growth and development. Human microbes are part of the conversation regarding human physiology during fetal development even before birth, and these microbial communities continue to shift and develop during infancy and childhood. Beyond microbial composition, functional features of microbial metabolism are leading to the identification and rediscovery of potentially important bioactive compounds originating from the microbiome. Dietary changes, so prominent in early childhood, clearly impact the biology of the microbiome early in life and may have important consequences for disease risk.

Antibiotics may suppress and eliminate many commensal microbes, placing the host at risk for disorders of microbial ecology such as *Clostridium difficile* infection. Diet and antibiotics represent two major environmental factors affecting the biology of the microbiome, with potentially deleterious effects on microbial diversity and resilience of microbial communities. Commensal microbes produce a variety of antimicrobial compounds that modify microbial composition and may

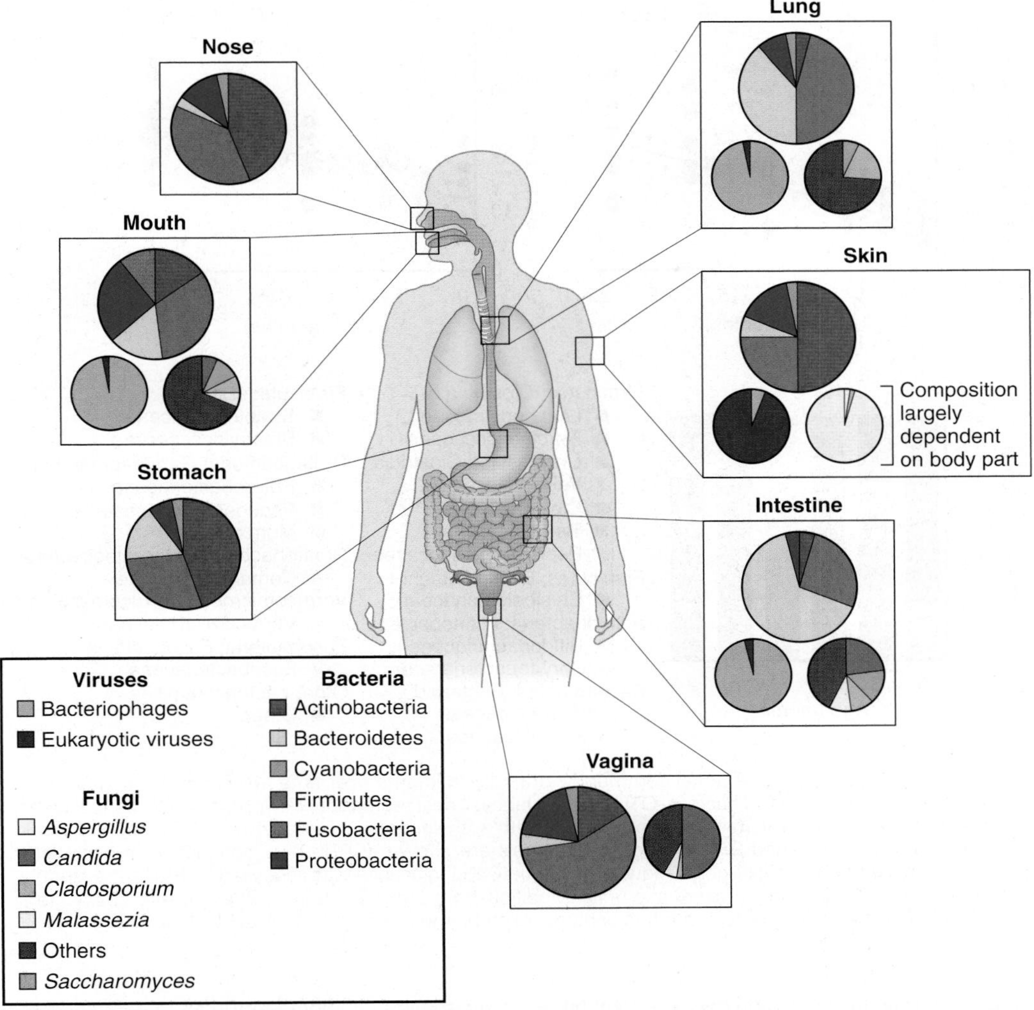

FIG. 5.1 The composition of bacterial, fungal, and viral microbiota at distinct body sites. This figure shows the distribution and relative abundance of bacterial, fungal, and viral communities at different sites on the human body that are exposed to the external environment. Bacterial composition is represented by the six most abundant phyla, fungal composition by the most prominent genera, and viral composition as bacteriophages or eukaryotic viruses. (Modified from Marsland BJ, Gollwitzer ES. Host-microorganism interactions in lung diseases. *Nat Rev Immunol.* 2014;14:827–35.)

help the host defend against pathogens. Beneficial microbial species may induce the production of antimicrobial peptides, such as defensins, by the host. During infection, bacterial and other pathogens may have a profound impact on the composition and biology of the microbiome. Humans inhabiting this microbial world must coexist and thrive with indigenous microbial communities during growth and development. This intimate partnership between microbes and infant/child may affect susceptibility to pediatric infections and modulate the course and severity of infectious diseases.

DEVELOPMENT IN EARLY LIFE THROUGH CHILDHOOD

The fetus and neonate are exposed to microbial communities during prenatal and early postnatal development.[1] Descriptions of a placental microbiome highlight the presence of functionally dynamic microbial communities at the maternal-fetal interface. Even if microorganisms do not directly contact the fetus, microbial metabolites may have an impact on fetal development. The presence of microbes in the colostrum and amniotic fluid provides evidence that placental microbes may contact the fetus via the circulation.[22,50,51] Mouse models indicate that bacterial species such as *Fusobacterium* spp. may "home" specifically to the placenta via the bloodstream.[42,82] This finding emphasizes a key point that the placental microbiome is most similar to the oral microbiome, lending support to the concept that the oral microbiome may provide founder bacterial species for the placental microbiome in the early stages of pregnancy.[1] The presence of oral pathogens may place the fetus at risk if oral pathogens can traverse the bloodstream and seed the placental microbiome. As we consider the nature of infections in utero in maternal-fetal medicine, this connection between the oral and placental microbiomes may point to new strategies to evaluate the oral microbiome before or during pregnancy and provide additional information regarding potential risks for the fetus. Additional concepts based on experimental data include differences in the placental microbiome in cases of preterm birth and whether differences in microbial composition or function may place the fetus at increased risk of preterm birth.[1,63] Microbial metabolites such as microbe-derived calcium channel blockers may affect contractility of the uterine musculature and the tendency toward premature contractions prior to childbirth.[68] Prior antimicrobial therapy has a fundamental impact on the composition of the placental microbiome, and antecedent antimicrobial exposure yields significant differences in the placental microbiome that could affect fetal development and preterm birth. All of these conceptual points highlight the rapidly emerging understanding

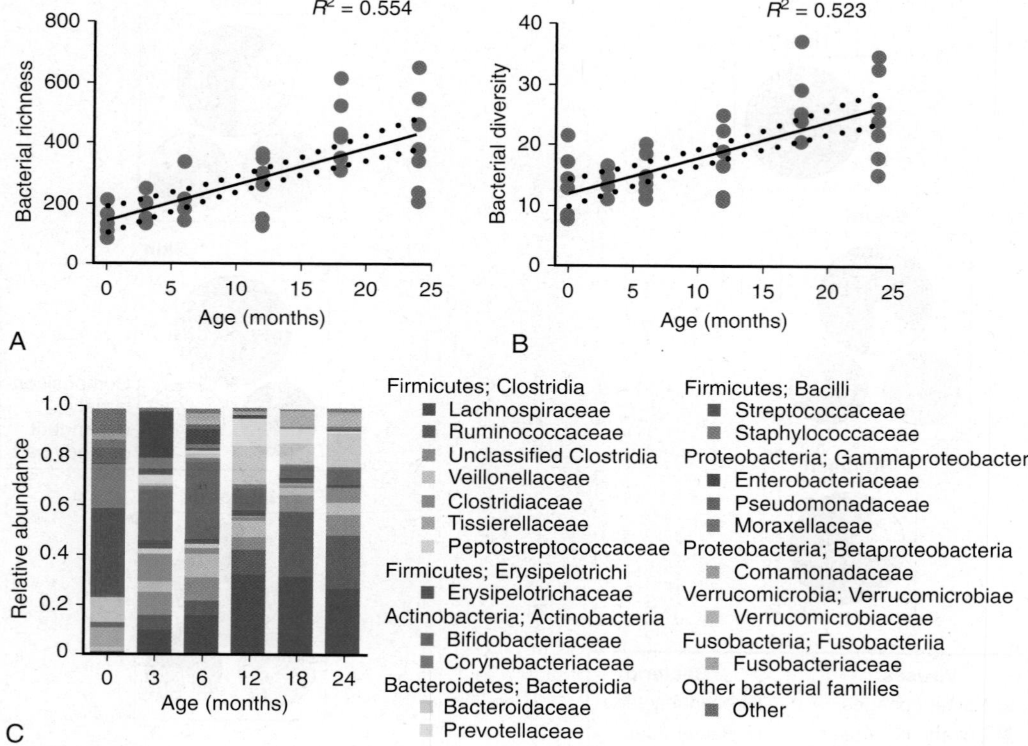

FIG. 5.2 Changes in the bacterial community structure in infants over time. (A) Richness (number of observed bacterial OTUs) of bacterial OTUs (n=8 infants). Linear regression, R^2 value, and 95% confidence intervals are shown. (B) Bacterial α diversity (Faith's phylogenetic diversity) (n = 8 infants). Linear regression, R^2 value, and 95% confidence intervals are shown. (C) Relative abundance of bacterial families based on 16S rRNA gene sequences. Statistical significance was assessed by Student's *t* test; $P < .01$. *OTU,* Operational taxonomic unit. (Modified from Lim ES, Zhou Y, Zhao G, et al. Early life dynamics of the human gut virome and bacterial microbiome in infants. *Nat Med.* 2015;21:1228–34.)

of the impact of the microbiome on the health and disease susceptibility of the fetus.

Several studies have indicated that the neonatal and infant gut microbiome develops rapidly after birth and may influence susceptibility to enteric infections and acute disease. The neonatal microbiome matures rapidly in terms of microbial acquisition, and relatively complex microbial communities form in the intestine and other body sites by the end of postnatal week 1.[24,67] Microbiome development continues at a rapid pace and with relatively large-scale fluctuations in composition and function during infancy[54,59,94] (Fig. 5.2). Immediately after birth, the neonate is colonized by various microbes belonging to different phyla at different body sites.[95] The major phyla that are established in the human body by the end of infancy include Bacteroidetes, Firmicutes, Proteobacteria, and Actinobacteria. One of the hallmarks of the early neonatal microbiome is that microbial composition does not differ significantly by body site.[24] It takes weeks or months during infancy to see evidence of "differentiation" of distinct microbial communities at each body site. Within days, different body sites are rapidly colonized, but these communities gradually change to reach a steady state of microbial communities that are highly adapted for a specific body site. This process of "microbiome differentiation" may have important consequences for infectious disease risk depending on the nature and timing of the infection.

At approximately 4 to 6 weeks age, the microbiomes at different body sites are clearly distinguishable, and the impact of mode of delivery on microbial composition is negligible.[95] By 2 to 3 years of age, it appears that the intestinal microbiome is comparable to the adult microbiome in terms of complexity.[54,94] The impact of diet on microbial composition during the first 3 years of life is dramatic, and breast milk to solid food transitions clearly change the composition and function of the intestinal microbiome.[27,54] During childhood and prior to adolescence, the pediatric intestinal microbiome continues to differentiate in terms of microbial composition and function.[46] The relative richness of the microbiome in childhood actually exceeds that of healthy young adults, so presumably bacterial species are culled during adolescence. Although the major phyla are established during infancy, the relative preponderance of different phyla differs between school-aged children and young adults. For example, children have a greater relative abundance of Firmicutes relative to Bacteroidetes, and genera such as *Bifidobacterium* and *Faecalibacterium* are enriched in children.[46] Children also contain specific functional elements, such as pathways for vitamin B_{12} and folate biosynthesis, which are enriched in the pediatric gut microbiome. These pathways may promote hematologic and central nervous system development. Firmicutes including clostridia may produce short-chain fatty acids (SCFAs) that can suppress enteric pathogenesis, and specific commensal species may produce various antimicrobial peptides and propionaldehyde compounds that suppress enteric pathogens.

IMPACT OF ENVIRONMENTAL FACTORS: DIET AND MEDICATIONS

Various environmental factors such as dietary food intake and consumption of medications may influence and modulate the composition and function of the human microbiome in different body sites. Breast milk drives predictable changes in microbial composition, and infants receiving breast milk clearly differ by intestinal microbial composition when compared to formula-fed infants.[5,11,77] Human breast milk contains indigenous microbes including *Bifidobacterium, Lactobacillus,* and *Streptococcus* species, and these species colonize the gut microbiome of infants shortly after initiation of breastfeeding.[41] The gastrointestinal microbiome rapidly expands in terms of richness and diversity during the first weeks of life if the infant is consuming breast milk and avoiding antimicrobial agents. Breastfeeding results in changes to the microbiome and host that result in reduced susceptibility to necrotizing enterocolitis (NEC).[39,78] The addition of solid foods to the diet results in the next wave of profound changes to the gastrointestinal microbiome during the first 3 years of life, and these changes may affect relative susceptibility to enteric infections during childhood.[23,54,89] Comparisons of children from western Africa (Burkina Faso) consuming a diet rich in cereals, vegetables, and plant fiber with children from Western Europe (Italy) on a diet enriched in animal protein, sugar, and fat yielded dramatic differences in gut bacterial composition at the phylum level. Children from Italy yielded gut microbiota dominated by the Firmicutes and Proteobacteria phyla, whereas children from Burkina Faso yielded microbiota more abundant in Actinobacteria and Bacteroidetes.[20] A diet rich in plant polysaccharides and low in sugars and fats is predicted to increase microbial diversity and therefore confer protection from enteric pathogens. Although host genetics, sex, and geography are known to influence the composition of the gut microbiota, accumulating evidence suggests that diet has a relatively large impact on biodiversity within the gut ecosystem.[13,80,93]

Dietary manipulation by the addition of beneficial microbes (probiotics) or creation of highly specialized diets may prevent infectious diseases or facilitate management of chronic intestinal disease phenotypes. Consumption of probiotics may dramatically alter the microbial composition and function of the pediatric intestinal microbiome, principally by changes in microbial gene expression and microbial metabolism.[8,18] Ingestion of probiotics during infancy reduced the risk of enteric infections, and probiotics may protect children from acute gastroenteritis.[48,91] On the other side of the spectrum, a restricted elemental diet used for treating pediatric patients with Crohn's disease further reduced the biodiversity of the gastrointestinal microbiome while ameliorating symptoms.[53,70] In addition to dietary manipulation, medications may have a profound impact on microbial composition and function in the intestine. Antimicrobial agents administered in the first few days of life to neonates may delay colonization of the intestine and could increase the risk of enteric infections by reducing colonization resistance in the host[29,67,69] (Fig. 5.3). Different classes of antimicrobial agents may have different effects on the intestinal microbiome, and we are just beginning to appreciate the different risks associated with exposure to different antimicrobial agents.[34,92] A classic example is recurrent *C. difficile* infection and antimicrobial-associated diarrhea due to treatment with antimicrobial agents such as cephalosporins and fluoroquinolones.

BODY METABOLISM AND IMMUNITY

SCFAs are well-known examples of microbial metabolites affecting the intestinal epithelium. Three main SCFAs produced in the human colon are acetate, propionate, and butyrate. Propionate and acetate affect adipogenesis and leptin production. By modulating gut- and adipocyte-derived hormones, SCFAs may affect the gut-brain axis and brain function, including appetite and satiety.[26,64] Acetate is able to directly affect neuronal function in the brain, especially regions associated with appetite.[30] With respect to enteric infections, Shiga toxin–producing strains of *Escherichia coli* can produce serious, life-threatening infections in children, resulting in hemolytic uremic syndrome and renal injury. Studies in mouse models indicate that *Bifidobacterium* species can suppress translocation of Shiga toxin across the intestinal epithelium and that the organic acid acetate contributes to this effect.[31] B-complex vitamins including vitamin B_{12} are also produced by bacterial members of the intestinal microbiome, and vitamin B_{12} may suppress Shiga toxin by *E. coli.*[19,74] Bioactive compounds produced by the commensal intestinal microbiota may regulate toxin production by enteric pathogens and reduce susceptibility to enteric infections.

Beneficial microbes may convert tryptophan into bioactive indole compounds. Indole derivatives act as endogenous ligands for the arylhydrocarbon receptor (AhR)[44] and are generated from dietary tryptophan by commensal intestinal microbes.[10] By binding AhR, the microbiota may stimulate mammalian immune cells to produce the cytokine interleukin (IL)-22, thereby enhancing protective mucus production, suppressing IL-17 production, and stimulating production of antimicrobial peptides via signal transducer and activator of transcription 3 (STAT3) activation. The lesson in *Lactobacillus*-mediated indole-3-aldehyde (one example of an indole derivative) production from tryptophan is that bacterial metabolites generated by the microbiome may have a profound impact on immunity. The *metabiotic concept* refers to metabolites produced by the microbiome or probiotic species that may confer specific benefits on mammalian physiology or immunity. The mammalian tryptophan catabolic enzyme indoleamine 2,3-dioxygenase 1 (IDO1) plays a key role in the conversion of dietary or microbial tryptophan into kynurenines and promotes tolerance to commensal microbes. The capacity of IDO1-expressing dendritic cells, epithelial cells, and kynurenines to induce regulatory T cells (Tregs) and inhibit T-helper 17 cells (T_H17) has revealed their unexpected potential to control inflammation, allergy, and T_H17-driven inflammation in fungal infections.[40,71]

Amino acid decarboxylation systems, such as the glutamate decarboxylase (GAD) or histidine decarboxylase (HDC) systems, enable bacterial species to cope with acid stress in the gastrointestinal tract. These systems are providing insights into infectious diseases and intestinal inflammation as it pertains to childhood. The bacterial GAD system is enriched in the intestinal microbiome relative to other body sites of healthy adults, and γ-aminobutyric acid (GABA) is enriched in the intestines of patients with recurrent *C. difficile*–associated disease (CDAD).[96] Most intestinal GABA measured in stool is microbial in origin, and this metabolite appears to potentiate the risk of *C. difficile* infection. Individuals consuming the $GABA_A$ receptor agonist zolpidem (Ambien) have increased risk of *C. difficile* infection, adding support to the potentially pathogenic role of GABA in recurrent CDAD in children.[97] Microbial species in the human gut can also convert L-histidine to histamine. This biogenic amine may promote allergic inflammation, suppress intestinal inflammation, or function as a neurotransmitter in the central nervous system by binding to any of the four different histamine receptors found on human cells. Antihistamines function by blocking signaling through the histamine 1 or histamine 4 receptors (H_1R and H_4R), and these receptors are considered proinflammatory.[87] In contrast, histamine may promote gastric acid production and suppress intestinal inflammation via H_2R. Although H_2R blockers have been useful as adjunct medications in the treatment of *Helicobacter pylori* infection,[35] they may also promote mucosal or systemic inflammation. Studies in the pediatric literature have documented increased risk of and mortality from NEC in newborns exposed to H_2R blockers.[84,85] Gut microbes may generate histamine in the small or large intestine and serve as a checkpoint for immunoregulation in the gastrointestinal tract. These amino acid metabolites may have opposing effects in terms of mucosal immunity, and microbe-derived compounds may help modulate susceptibility to pediatric infections.

MICROBIOME AT DIFFERENT BODY SITES

Airway and Respiratory Tract Microbiome

The fetal airway is likely exposed to microbial influences in utero due to the direct contact between the respiratory tract and the surrounding environment.[1] However, bacterial niches in the airway are vastly different after birth as the respiratory tract transitions from a fluid-filled cavity to a functional organ involved in gas exchange. Upon exposure to the external environment, the human respiratory tract is rapidly colonized by a community of commensal bacteria that gradually matures and diversifies during the first year of life. Skin-associated bacterial genera including *Staphylococcus* and *Corynebacterium* species are detectable in the upper respiratory tract on the first day of life and are dominant up to 3 months of age.[83] The prevalence of these species steadily declines from birth to 6 months, and these microorganisms are succeeded by other bacterial species such as *Streptococcus pneumoniae*, *Moraxella catarrhalis*, and *Haemophilus influenzae.*[3,9,83] Geography, season of birth, environment, social interactions, and presence of older siblings are primary determinants of colonization rate and sources of bacterial acquisition.[7,12,43] The infant lung has distinct compartments with different growth conditions allowing enhanced growth of Bacteroidetes, unlike the upper respiratory tract, which is dominated by Firmicutes and Proteobacteria.[61,83] Microbiota traverse the upper and lower respiratory

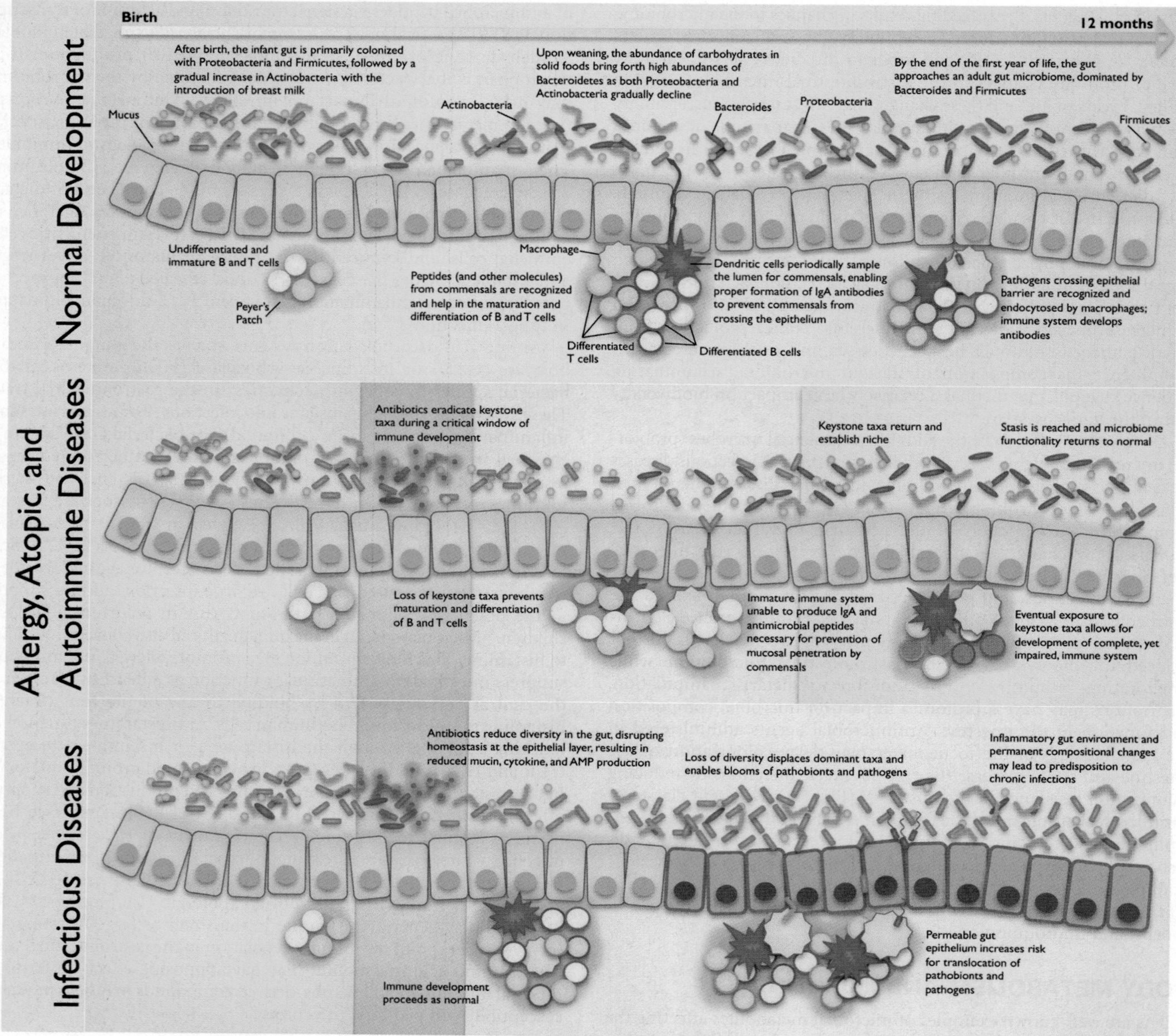

FIG. 5.3 Early host-microbiota interactions in health, antibiotic-induced dysbiosis, and disease. Interactions between early microbial colonizers of the intestinal tract and the host immune system contribute to proper immune maturation during normal development. Antibiotic-induced dysbiosis during this critical window can lead to improper immune system development resulting in allergy and atopic and autoimmune diseases. Early antibiotic use can also reduce diversity in the gut and promote blooms of potential pathogens resulting in a local inflammatory response. This inflammatory gut environment may persist and result in increased predisposition to chronic infections. (Modified from Vangay P, Ward T, Gerber JS, Knights D. Antibiotics, pediatric dysbiosis, and disease. *Cell Host Microbe.* 2015;17:553–64.)

tracts via mucosal extension, microaspiration, and ciliary transport. These factors along with local growth conditions in human airways, immunity of the respiratory tract, and microbial crosstalk contribute to the community structure at specific locations within airways. Interactions between the intestinal and respiratory microbiota have been suggested, and early nutritional exposures may also influence the developmental trajectory of the respiratory microbiome.[60]

Dynamic changes in the composition of the respiratory tract microbiome during the first year of life may affect the development of the respiratory mucosal immune system. The pattern of immune responses in the respiratory tract modulates relative susceptibilities to allergic inflammation or respiratory tract infections.[88] A diverse, homeostatic microbiome is necessary for immune priming and defense against pathogen overgrowth and invasion.[32] Microbial exposure in the lung during the first 2 weeks of life induces a programmed cell death ligand 1 (PDL1)-mediated tolerance to aeroallergens.[36] Relatively limited biodiversity and bacterial load in the airways are associated with improper development of regulatory immune cells, leaving the host susceptible to allergic inflammation lasting into adulthood.[36] The composition of the microbial community in the upper respiratory tract also influences the susceptibility of the lower airways to viral infections and affects the severity of the resulting inflammatory response.[83] Antibiotic use and inflammation resulting from viral infections can also lead to dysbiosis and the development of early allergic sensitization.[61]

Early colonization with a diverse respiratory microbiota is associated with a decreased risk of developing asthma, and overall microbial community composition appears to be a main determinant for asthma. Relative overgrowth of specific bacterial species may exacerbate the risk of developing asthma in genetically predisposed newborns.[4,61,83] Beyond allergic inflammation, physicochemical alterations in chronic lung disease may alter the airway microbiota and susceptibility to respiratory tract infections. Disruption of the microbial ecosystem can be a consequence of host factors such as cystic fibrosis in which increased mucus production and impaired mucociliary clearance result in altered local growth conditions and reduced microbial clearance favoring the growth of specific respiratory pathogens.

Gastrointestinal Microbiome

The intestinal microbiome develops rapidly after birth in both premature and full-term infants. In premature infants the succession of bacterial classes demonstrates a temporal sequence shifting from a relative abundance of Bacilli (gram-positive aerobes) to Gammaproteobacteria (gram-negative facultative anaerobes).[57] Both Clostridia and Gammaproteobacteria increase in relative abundance with increasing postconceptional age. Since the class Gammaproteobacteria contains several potential enteric pathogens, perhaps these microbes promote complete maturation of the intestinal immune system. Alternatively the gut milieu accommodates a greater variety of microbes with time during infancy, including potential pathogens. Potential pathogens lurking in the intestinal microbiome early in life may invade the bloodstream of premature infants.[16] Pathogenic bacteria such as *E. coli*, group B streptococcus (GBS), and *Serratia marcescens* were documented in the intestinal microbiomes of premature infants prior to late-onset sepsis by the same microbes (verified by molecular epidemiology/sequencing).[16] Additionally, ciprofloxacin-resistant *E. coli* were isolated from children and their mothers, and maternal colonization by drug-resistant bacteria was correlated with childhood carriage of the same organisms. Therefore, the presence of potential pathogens and drug-resistant microbes in the intestine may have important implications for familial transmission and infection risk.

A classic example of infectious disease risk associated with assaults on the intact microbiome is the category of antimicrobial-associated diarrhea (AAD) or colitis. Human patients and animal models with intestinal microbiomes of limited diversity following antimicrobial agent challenge clearly seem to be at increased risk for CDAD or related disorders.[6,17,52,86] Antimicrobial agents of various classes (cephalosporins, fluoroquinolones) are associated with development of AAD in children and adults and highlight the importance of an intact gut microbiome in resistance to infection by intestinal pathogens.[73,76] In addition to therapy by specific antimicrobial agents (e.g., metronidazole, vancomycin), microbiome supplementation or replacement by fecal microbiota transplantation (FMT) emphasizes the importance of the intestinal microbial community in resolution of CDAD.[25,47,62,90] A potential confounder is co-infection with *C. difficile* and other pathogens in cases of AAD.[21] Enteric infections result in widespread perturbations of the intestinal microbiome highlighted by the phylum Proteobacteria, a phylum that contains many enteric pathogens including *Escherichia*.[79] Resolution of infection is accompanied by distinct changes in the microbiome, with a greater abundance of the genus *Bacteroides*, as expected. Possibly rapid sequencing of the intestinal microbiome may provide valuable information regarding the condition of the microbiome in the context of undiagnosed enteric infections.

Skin and Vaginal Microbiomes

The structure of the vaginal microbiome varies in pregnancy by gestational age and is characterized by decreased bacterial diversity and species richness.[2,72] However, the genus *Lactobacillus* persistently maintains prevalence, and certain species including *L. iners, L. crispatus, L. jensenii,* and *L. johnsonii* have been demonstrated to be enriched during pregnancy.[2,72] Consequently, the dominant skin microbiota observed on vaginally delivered babies includes *Lactobacillus* spp., as well as *Prevotella*, *Atopobium*, and *Sneathia* species.[24] The transmission of the vaginal microbiota to the baby may provide protection against pathogens by occupying niches prior to the development of site-specific communities. In babies delivered via C-section, the lack of exposure to vaginal microbes results in an initial microbial community similar to the mother's skin microbiota, with an abundance of *Staphylococcus* species.[24] Premature infants are also at risk of disturbed initial bacterial colonization, and recent studies suggest that room and isolator surfaces in neonatal intensive care units are a reservoir of colonizing microbes for these infants.[14] This care environment may be detrimental to the health of these preterm newborns because they have an underdeveloped skin barrier that makes them more vulnerable to chemical damage and microbial infections.[65] However, the infant skin microbiome is dynamic, and the initial differences arising from mode of delivery do not persist as site-specific niches develop in the initial months after birth.[15]

The skin is a continuously self-renewing organ that undergoes rapid turnover and expansion during the first years of life. As a result, the infant skin microbiome continuously matures during this time frame, increasing in diversity and abundance.[15] The skin microenvironment varies greatly between infants and adults due to this rapid skin expansion and the distinct composition of infant skin microstructure, which varies in epidermal thickness and cell size.[81] Around 3 months of age, site-specific communities begin to emerge.[15] The skin microbiota consists of both commensal microbes that reestablish after perturbation and transient microbes from the surrounding environment. Distinct niches form on the body based on levels of moisture and sebum, and glands and hair follicles have their own distinct microbiota. The diversity and composition of the bacterial community at these body sites is also affected by intrinsic factors such as age and genetics, as well as by extrinsic factors such as climate and hygiene, leading to large intrapersonal variations in community composition.[56] The most abundant bacterial phylum colonizing the infant skin is Firmicutes whereas, in contrast, adults are dominated by Actinobacteria.[15,37,38] Staphylococci (Firmicutes) are abundant in infants under 1 year of age, and certain skin commensals such as *S. epidermidis* may play a protective role against pathogens. *S. epidermidis* has been demonstrated to inhibit colonization and biofilm formation of the opportunistic pathogen *Staphylococcus aureus* by competition and expression of a serine protease.[49] *S. epidermidis* also secretes small molecules that can activate Toll-like receptor TLR2 signaling and induce antimicrobial peptide expression by keratinocytes, thus enhancing the skin's defense against infection.[58] *Staphylococcus* species may promote early immune development, but their effect is predicted to decline because their abundance decreases steadily during the first year of life. However, skin barrier function and immune development are significantly affected by early microbial colonization, and microbial exposure may also affect the maturation of the systemic immune system.[75]

Shifts in microbial communities can drive some commensals to become pathogenic under certain circumstances. Although it is considered a commensal organism, *S. epidermidis* is a primary cause of nosocomial infections and can cause disease if barrier integrity is compromised and it is allowed to invade other sites.[66] Several skin disorders have also been associated with certain members of the microbiota. Atopic dermatitis (AD), or eczema, is a chronic disorder that affects approximately 15% of children in the United States.[38] AD is characterized by *S. aureus* colonization on both lesional and nonlesional skin, and it is associated with worsened disease severity in pediatric patients.[55] *Propionibacterium acnes* is well known for its role in acne vulgaris in teenagers because this species secretes enzymes that injure the tissue lining of the already inflamed pilosebaceous unit.[28,38] Although infants have limited sebum production, infantile acne begins to appear at the same time that an increase in *Propionibacterium* occurs at age 4 to 6 months.[15,45] Psoriasis is another chronic skin condition that can occur in children, and lesional skin has been demonstrated to exhibit increased bacterial diversity concurrent with a decrease in prevalence of healthy skin bacteria such as Actinobacteria.[33] These examples highlight how the skin barrier and the dynamic microbial communities that inhabit it are maintained in a delicate balance, the disturbance of which can predispose the host to cutaneous infections and other inflammatory conditions.

SUMMARY

The human microbiome influences human development and resilience in the context of challenges by infectious agents. Special considerations early in life include the unique biology of pregnancy and fetal development, age-dependent changes and differentiation of the microbiome, and the rapid shifts in microbial composition and function occurring with abrupt dietary changes. Different stages of human development and different body sites will impact microbial composition and function and affect the ability of the microbiome to modulate or prevent pediatric infections. Microbiome science provides opportunities to consider a broad menu of potential pathogens that may be present in the human microbiome prior to infection. More comprehensive diagnostic tests based on microbiome science may provide a complete list of opportunistic pathogens that pose risk of infection in children with cancer, immunodeficiencies, or chronic disease. Mining of the microbiome for bioactive compounds may lead to new microbiome-based therapeutics, and microbial manipulation by probiotics, specialized diets, or FMT may provide additional therapeutic options for diseases of microbial ecology such as CDAD.

NEW REFERENCES SINCE THE SEVENTH EDITION

1. Aagaard K, Ma J, Antony KM, et al. The placenta harbors a unique microbiome. *Sci Transl Med*. 2014;6:237ra265.
2. Aagaard K, Riehle K, Ma J, et al. A metagenomic approach to characterization of the vaginal microbiome signature in pregnancy. *PLoS ONE*. 2012;7:e36466.
3. Aniansson G, Aim B, Andersson B, et al. Nasopharyngeal colonization during the first year of life. *J Infect Dis*. 1992;165:S38-S42.
4. Arrieta MC, Stiemsma LT, Dimitriu PA, et al. Early infancy microbial and metabolic alterations affect risk of childhood asthma. *Sci Transl Med*. 2015;7:307ra152.
5. Azad MB, Konya T, Maughan H, et al. Gut microbiota of healthy Canadian infants: profiles by mode of delivery and infant diet at 4 months. *CMAJ*. 2013;185(5):386-394.
6. Bassis CM, Theriot CM, Young VB. Alteration of the murine gastrointestinal microbiota by tigecycline leads to increased susceptibility to *Clostridium difficile* infection. *Antimicrob Agents Chemother*. 2014;58:2767-2774.
7. Beck JM, Young VB, Huffnagle GB. The microbiome of the lung. *Transl Res*. 2012;160:258-266.
8. Bergmann H, Rodriguez JM, Salminen S, Szajewska H. Probiotics in human milk and probiotic supplementation in infant nutrition: a workshop report. *Br J Nutr*. 2014;112:1119-1128.
9. Bisgaard H, Hermansen MN, Buchvald F, et al. Childhood asthma after bacterial colonization of the airway in neonates. *N Engl J Med*. 2007;357:1487-1495.
10. Bjeldanes LF, Kim JY, Grose KR, Bartholomew JC, Bradfield CA. Aromatic hydrocarbon responsiveness-receptor agonists generated from indole-3-carbinol in vitro and in vivo: comparisons with 2,3,7,8-tetrachlorodibenzo-p-dioxin. *Proc Natl Acad Sci USA*. 1991;88:9543-9547.
11. Bode L. Human milk oligosaccharides: every baby needs a sugar mama. *Glycobiology*. 2012;22:1147-1162.
13. Bolnick DI, Snowberg LK, Hirsch PE, et al. Individual diet has sex-dependent effects on vertebrate gut microbiota. *Nat Commun*. 2014;5:4500.
14. Brooks B, Firek BA, Miller CS, et al. Microbes in the neonatal intensive care unit resemble those found in the gut of premature infants. *Microbiome*. 2014;2:1-16.
15. Capone KA, Dowd SE, Stamatas GN, Nikolovski J. Diversity of the human skin microbiome early in life. *J Invest Dermatol*. 2011;131:2026-2032.
16. Carl MA, Ndao IM, Springman AC, et al. Sepsis from the gut: the enteric habitat of bacteria that cause late-onset neonatal bloodstream infections. *Clin Infect Dis*. 2014;58:1211-1218.
18. Chassard C, de Wouters T, Lacroix C. Probiotics tailored to the infant: a window of opportunity. *Curr Opin Biotechnol*. 2014;26:141-147.
19. Cordonnier C, Le Bihan G, Emond-Rheault JG, et al. Vitamin B12 uptake by the gut commensal bacteria *Bacteroides thetaiotaomicron* limits the production of shiga toxin by enterohemorrhagic *Escherichia coli*. *Toxins (Basel)*. 2016;8.
20. De Filippo C, Cavalieri D, Di Paola M, et al. Impact of diet in shaping gut microbiota revealed by a comparative study in children from Europe and rural Africa. *Proc Natl Acad Sci USA*. 2010;107:14691-14696.
21. de Graaf H, Pai S, Burns DA, et al. Co-infection as a confounder for the role of *Clostridium difficile* infection in children with diarrhoea: a summary of the literature. *Eur J Clin Microbiol Infect Dis*. 2015;34:1281-1287.
22. DiGiulio DB. Diversity of microbes in amniotic fluid. *Semin Fetal Neonatal Med*. 2012;17:2-11.
23. Dominguez-Bello MG, Blaser MJ, Ley RE, Knight R. Development of the human gastrointestinal microbiota and insights from high-throughput sequencing. *Gastroenterol*. 2011;140:1713-1719.
24. Dominguez-Bello MG, Costello EK, Contreras M, et al. Delivery mode shapes the acquisition and structure of the initial microbiota across multiple body habitats in newborns. *Proc Natl Acad Sci USA*. 2010;107:11971-11975.
25. Drekonja D, Reich J, Gezahegn S, et al. Fecal microbiota transplantation for *Clostridium difficile* infection: a systematic review. *Ann Intern Med*. 2015;162:630-638.
26. Erny D, Hrabe de Angelis AL, Jaitin D, et al. Host microbiota constantly control maturation and function of microglia in the CNS. *Nat Neurosci*. 2015;18:965-977.
27. Fallani M, Amarri S, Uusijarvi A, et al. Determinants of the human infant intestinal microbiota after the introduction of first complementary foods in infant samples from five European centres. *Microbiology*. 2011;157:1385-1392.
28. Findley K, Grice EA. The skin microbiome: a focus on pathogens and their association with skin disease. *PLoS Pathog*. 2014;10:e1004436.
29. Fouhy F, Guinane CM, Hussey S, et al. High-throughput sequencing reveals the incomplete, short-term recovery of infant gut microbiota following parenteral antibiotic treatment with ampicillin and gentamicin. *Antimicrob Agents Chemother*. 2012;56:5811-5820.
30. Frost G, Sleeth ML, Sahuri-Arisoylu M, et al. The short-chain fatty acid acetate reduces appetite via a central homeostatic mechanism. *Nat Commun*. 2014;5:3611.
31. Fukuda S, Toh H, Hase K, et al. Bifidobacteria can protect from enteropathogenic infection through production of acetate. *Nature*. 2011;469:543-547.
32. Gao Z, Kang Y, Yu J, Ren L. Human pharyngeal microbiome may play a protective role in respiratory tract infections. *Genomics Proteomics Bioinformatics*. 2014;12:144-150.
33. Gao Z, Tseng CH, Strober BE, Pei Z, Blaser MJ. Substantial alterations of the cutaneous bacterial biota in psoriatic lesions. *PLoS ONE*. 2008;3:e2719.
34. Gibson MK, Crofts TS, Dantas G. Antibiotics and the developing infant gut microbiota and resistome. *Curr Opin Microbiol*. 2015;27:51-56.
35. Gisbert J. Potent gastric acid inhibition in *Helicobacter pylori* eradication. *Drugs*. 2005;65:83-96.
36. Gollwitzer ES, Saglani S, Trompette A, et al. Lung microbiota promotes tolerance to allergens in neonates via PD-L1. *Nat Med*. 2014;20:642-647.
37. Grice EA, Kong HH, Conlan S, et al. Topographical and temporal diversity of the human skin microbiome. *Science*. 2009;324:1190-1192.
39. Gritz EC, Bhandari V. The human neonatal gut microbiome: a brief review. *Front Pediatr*. 2015;3:17.
40. Grohmann U, Volpi C, Fallarino F, et al. Reverse signaling through GITR ligand enables dexamethasone to activate IDO in allergy. *Nat Med*. 2007;13:579-586.
41. Guaraldi F, Salvatori G. Effect of breast and formula feeding on gut microbiota shaping in newborns. *Front Cell Infect Microbiol*. 2012;2:94.
42. Han YW, Redline RW, Li M, et al. *Fusobacterium nucleatum* induces premature and term stillbirths in pregnant mice: implication of oral bacteria in preterm birth. *Infect Immun*. 2004;72:2272-2279.
43. Harrison LM, Morris JA, Telford DR, Brown SM, Jones K. The nasopharyngeal bacteria flora in infancy: effects of age, gender, season, viral upper respiratory tract infection and sleeping position. *FEMS Immunol Med Microbiol*. 1999;25:19-28.
44. Heath-Pagliuso S, Rogers WJ, Tullis K, et al. Activation of the Ah receptor by tryptophan and tryptophan metabolites. *Biochemistry*. 1998;37:11508-11515.
45. Hello M, Prey S, Leaute-Labreze C, et al. Infantile acne: a retrospective study of 16 cases. *Pediatr Dermatol*. 2008;25:434-438.
46. Hollister EB, Riehle K, Luna RA, et al. Structure and function of the healthy pre-adolescent pediatric gut microbiome. *Microbiome*. 2015;3:36.
47. Hourigan SK, Chen LA, Grigoryan Z, et al. Microbiome changes associated with sustained eradication of *Clostridium difficile* after single faecal microbiota transplantation in children with and without inflammatory bowel disease. *Aliment Pharmacol Ther*. 2015;42:741-752.
48. Indrio F, Di Mauro A, Riezzo G, et al. Prophylactic use of a probiotic in the prevention of colic, regurgitation, and functional constipation: a randomized clinical trial. *JAMA Pediatr*. 2014;168:228-233.
49. Iwase T, Uehara Y, Shinji H, et al. *Staphylococcus epidermidis* Esp inhibits *Staphylococcus aureus* biofilm formation and nasal colonization. *Nature*. 2010;465:346-349.
50. Jimenez E, Delgado S, Fernandez L, et al. Assessment of the bacterial diversity of human colostrum and screening of staphylococcal and enterococcal populations for potential virulence factors. *Res Microbiol*. 2008;159:595-601.
51. Jimenez E, Marin ML, Martin R, et al. Is meconium from healthy newborns actually sterile? *Res Microbiol*. 2008;159:187-193.
52. Johanesen PA, Mackin KE, Hutton ML, et al. Disruption of the gut microbiome: *Clostridium difficile* infection and the threat of antibiotic resistance. *Genes (Basel)*. 2015;6:1347-1360.
53. Kaakoush NO, Day AS, Leach ST, et al. Effect of exclusive enteral nutrition on the microbiota of children with newly diagnosed Crohn's disease. *Clin Transl Gastroenterol*. 2015;6:e71.
54. Koenig J, Spor A, Scalfone N, et al. Succession of microbial consortia in the developing infant gut microbiome. *Proc Natl Acad Sci USA*. 2011;108:4578-4585.
55. Kong HH, Oh J, Deming C, et al. Temporal shifts in the skin microbiome associated with disease flares and treatment in children with atopic dermatitis. *Genome Res*. 2012;22:850-859.
56. Kong HH, Segre JA. Skin microbiome: looking back to move forward. *J Invest Dermatol*. 2012;132:933-939.
57. La Rosa PS, Warner BB, Zhouc Y, et al. Patterned progression of bacterial populations in the premature infant gut. *Proc Natl Acad Sci USA*. 2014;111:17336.
58. Lai Y, Cogen AL, Radek KA, et al. Activation of TLR2 by a small molecule produced by *Staphylococcus epidermidis* increases antimicrobial defense against bacterial skin infections. *J Invest Dermatol*. 2010;130:2211-2221.
59. Lim ES, Zhou Y, Zhao G, et al. Early life dynamics of the human gut virome and bacterial microbiome in infants. *Nat Med*. 2015;21:1228-1234.
60. Madan JC, Koestler DC, Stanton BA, et al. Serial analysis of the gut and respiratory microbiome in cystic fibrosis in infancy: interaction between intestinal and respiratory tracts and impact of nutritional exposures. *MBio*. 2012;3(4).

61. Marsland BJ, Gollwitzer ES. Host-microorganism interactions in lung diseases. *Nat Rev Immunol.* 2014;14:827-835.
62. Mathur H, Rea MC, Cotter PD, Ross RP, Hill C. The potential for emerging therapeutic options for *Clostridium difficile* infection. *Gut Microbes.* 2014;5: 696-710.
63. Mysorekar IU, Cao B. Microbiome in parturition and preterm birth. *Semin Reprod Med.* 2014;32:50-55.
64. Nankova B, Agarwal R, MacFabe DF, La Gamma EF. Enteric bacterial metabolites propionic and butyric acid modulate gene expression, including CREB-dependent catecholaminergic neurotransmission, in PC12 cells - possible relevance to autism spectrum disorders. *PLoS ONE.* 2014;9:e103740.
65. Oranges T, Dini V, Romanelli M. Skin physiology of the neonate and infant: clinical implications. *Adv Wound Care (New Rochelle).* 2015;4:587-595.
66. Otto M. *Staphylococcus epidermidis*–the "accidental" pathogen. *Nat Rev Microbiol.* 2009;7:555-567.
68. Papatsonis D, Lok C, Bos J, Geijn HV, Dekker G. Calcium channel blockers in the management of preterm labor and hypertension in pregnancy. *Eur J Obstet Gynecol Reprod Biol.* 2001;97:122-140.
69. Preidis GA, Versalovic J. Targeting the human microbiome with antibiotics, probiotics, and prebiotics: gastroenterology enters the metagenomics era. *Gastroenterology.* 2009;136:2015-2031.
70. Quince C, Ijaz UZ, Loman N, et al. Extensive modulation of the fecal metagenome in children with Crohn's disease during exclusive enteral nutrition. *Am J Gastroenterol.* 2015;110:1718-1729.
71. Romani L, Zelante T, De Luca A, Fallarino F, Puccetti P. IL-17 and Therapeutic kynurenines in pathogenic inflammation to fungi. *J Immunol.* 2008;180:5157-5162.
72. Romero R, Hassan S, Gajer P, et al. The composition and stability of the vaginal microbiota of normal pregnant women is different from that of non-pregnant women. *Microbiome.* 2014;2:1-19.
73. Sammons JS, Toltzis P, Zaoutis TE. *Clostridium difficile* infection in children. *JAMA Pediatr.* 2013;167:567-573.
74. Santos F, Spinler JK, Saulnier DM, et al. Functional identification in *Lactobacillus reuteri* of a PocR-like transcription factor regulating glycerol utilization and vitamin B12 synthesis. *Microb Cell Fact.* 2011;10:55.
75. Scharschmidt TC, Vasquez KS, Truong HA, et al. A wave of regulatory T cells into neonatal skin mediates tolerance to commensal microbes. *Immunity.* 2015;43:1011-1021.
76. Schubert AM, Sinani H, Schloss PD. Antibiotic-induced alterations of the murine gut microbiota and subsequent effects on colonization resistance against *Clostridium difficile. MBio.* 2015;6:e00974.
77. Schwartz S, Friedberg I, Ivanov IV, et al. A metagenomic study of diet-dependent interaction between gut microbiota and host in infants reveals differences in immune response. *Genome Biol.* 2012;13:r32.
78. Shlomai ON, Deshpande G, Rao S, Patole S. Probiotics for preterm neonates: what will it take to change clinical practice? *Neonatology.* 2014;105:64-70.
79. Singh P, Teal TK, Marsh TL, et al. Intestinal microbial communities associated with acute enteric infections and disease recovery. *Microbiome.* 2015;3:45.
80. Spor A, Koren O, Ley R. Unravelling the effects of the environment and host genotype on the gut microbiome. *Nat Rev Microbiol.* 2011;9:279-290.
81. Stamatas GN, Nikolovski J, Luedtke MA, Kollias N, Wiegand BC. Infant skin microstructure assessed in vivo differs from adult skin in organization and at the cellular level. *Pediatr Dermatol.* 2010;27:125-131.
82. Stockham S, Stamford JE, Roberts CT, et al. Abnormal pregnancy outcomes in mice using an induced periodontitis model and the haematogenous migration of *Fusobacterium nucleatum* sub-species to the murine placenta. *PLoS ONE.* 2015;10:e0120050.
83. Teo SM, Mok D, Pham K, et al. The infant nasopharyngeal microbiome impacts severity of lower respiratory infection and risk of asthma development. *Cell Host Microbe.* 2015;17:704-715.
84. Terrin G, Canani RB, Passariello A, Caoci S, De Curtis M. Inhibitors of gastric acid secretion drugs increase neonatal morbidity and mortality. *J Matern Fetal Neonatal Med.* 2012;25(suppl 4):85-87.
85. Terrin G, Passariello A, De Curtis M, et al. Ranitidine is associated with infections, necrotizing enterocolitis, and fatal outcome in newborns. *Pediatrics.* 2012;129:e40-e45.
86. Theriot CM, Koenigsknecht MJ, Carlson PE Jr, et al. Antibiotic-induced shifts in the mouse gut microbiome and metabolome increase susceptibility to *Clostridium difficile* infection. *Nat Commun.* 2014;5:3114.
87. Thurmond RL, Gelfand EW, Dunford PJ. The role of histamine H1 and H4 receptors in allergic inflammation: the search for new antihistamines. *Nat Rev Drug Discov.* 2008;7:41-53.
88. Trompette A, Gollwitzer ES, Yadava K, et al. Gut microbiota metabolism of dietary fiber influences allergic airway disease and hematopoiesis. *Nat Med.* 2014;20:159-166.
89. Valles Y, Artacho A, Pascual-Garcia A, et al. Microbial succession in the gut: directional trends of taxonomic and functional change in a birth cohort of Spanish infants. *PLoS Genet.* 2014;10:e1004406.
90. van Nood E, Vrieze A, Nieuwdorp M, et al. Duodenal infusion of donor feces for recurrent *Clostridium difficile. N Engl J Med.* 2013;368:407-415.
91. Vandenplas Y, De Greef E, Devreker T, Veereman-Wauters G, Hauser B. Probiotics and prebiotics in infants and children. *Curr Infect Dis Rep.* 2013;15:251-262.
92. Vangay P, Ward T, Gerber JS, Knights D. Antibiotics, pediatric dysbiosis, and disease. *Cell Host Microbe.* 2015;17:553-564.
93. Xu Z, Knight R. Dietary effects on human gut microbiome diversity. *Br J Nutr.* 2015;113(suppl):S1-S5.
94. Yatsunenko T, Rey FE, Manary MJ, et al. Human gut microbiome viewed across age and geography. *Nature.* 2012;486:222-227.
95. Chu DM, Ma J, Prince AL, et al. Maturation of the infant microbiome community structure and function across multiple body sites and in relation to mode of delivery. *Nat Med.* 2017;23:314-326.
96. Pokusaeva K, Johnson C, Luk B, et al. GABA-producing *Bifidobacterium dentium* modulates visceral sensitivity in the intestine. *Neurogastroenterol Motil.* 2017;29:1.
97. Strom J, Tham J, Mansson F, et al. The Association between GABA modulators and *Clostridium difficile* infection: a matched retrospective case-control study. *PLoS ONE.* 2017;12:e0169386.

The full reference list for this chapter is available at ExpertConsult.com.

Epidemiology and Biostatistics of Infectious Diseases 6

Eugene D. Shapiro • Robert S. Baltimore

Clinicians care for individual patients, each of whom has certain unique problems. Clinicians base their decisions on a panoply of factors that include features of the acute and chronic medical problems of the patients as well as features of both their personalities (e.g., How likely are they to comply with a certain therapeutic regimen? Do they resist conventional medical care?) and their private lives (e.g., Can they afford a certain medication? Are they planning to travel out of the country in the next few days?).

In contrast, epidemiologists study groups of people. They draw conclusions from studies of large numbers of patients and usually base conclusions on probabilities and biostatistical analyses of average (mean) outcomes.

Fortunately, these two approaches—the individualistic approach of the clinician and the probabilistic approach of the classic epidemiologist—are not incompatible. Indeed, each can illuminate the other. So it is that a chapter on epidemiology and biostatistics is included in a clinical textbook of pediatric infectious diseases. The goal of this chapter is not to make the reader an expert in these fields—courses and textbooks are designed for that purpose.[17,29,31,33,34,58,59,62] Instead, the goal is to summarize how selected key aspects of epidemiology and biostatistics can be applied to understand studies that will improve our ability to evaluate and treat children with infectious diseases. Readers concerned with the epidemiology of a particular infection or syndrome should consult the appropriate chapter.

EPIDEMIOLOGIC STUDIES

Design of Studies

Overview and Definitions

Epidemiologic studies generally are designed to be either descriptive or analytic. In *descriptive* studies, the goal is to describe a population (e.g., the clinical manifestations and prognosis of children with tuberculosis). In *analytic* studies, the goal is to assess associations between two or more variables (e.g., whether children who receive an experimental vaccine are less likely to develop the infection that the vaccine is intended to prevent than are controls). Indeed, analytic studies usually are designed to assess whether a causal association exists among the variables (e.g., Is a vaccine efficacious? Do children who attend daycare centers have a higher risk of acquiring infections caused by certain bacteria or viruses?). Of course, categorizing a study so easily may not be possible. In a study that is primarily descriptive, causal associations within subgroups may be assessed. For instance, in a study of the clinical epidemiology of tuberculosis in children, the investigators may compare the mortality rates of younger children with those of older children or the mortality rates of children with tuberculous meningitis with those of children who have infection at other sites.

Most studies, whether descriptive or analytic, seek to reach conclusions about the particular group that is being assessed (e.g., children with tuberculosis). However, because studying all persons with the condition of interest is not possible, investigators inevitably study a *sample* of persons and hope that the conclusions drawn from studying the sample apply to the entire population of interest (the *target population*). The *validity* of a study refers to the extent to which the results are true (accurate). The extent to which the conclusions drawn from the study sample (e.g., children with tuberculosis at a certain hospital) are valid for the target population (e.g., all children with tuberculosis in the same city) is a measure of the study's *internal validity.* The extent to which the conclusions drawn from the study sample are valid for a less restrictively defined, larger population (e.g., all children with tuberculosis in the United States) is a measure of the study's *external validity,* which also is called its *generalizability.* To ensure that a study is both valid and generalizable, investigators must take steps to protect against a variety of potential biases that may distort the results of a study.

Elements of an Analytic Study

Epidemiologists refer to the major elements of an analytic study as the *exposure* and the *outcome.* The *exposure* is the factor that the investigator hypothesizes is related causally to the outcome of interest. In this context, the term *exposure* is not used in the classic sense of potential contact with an infectious agent; rather, it is any factor (e.g., living at a certain altitude, race, receipt of either a vaccine or a medication, smoking cigarettes) that may be associated causally with the outcome. The *outcome* is the effect (e.g., cancer) that putatively is related causally to the exposure. The putative association may be one in which the exposure either causes or prevents the outcome of interest.

Before the specific type of study is defined, several additional elements of a study must be considered. One is how the *sample* for the study is selected. In general, investigators select a sample of the population either on the basis of exposure (e.g., patients who either received or did not receive a vaccine or who either attend or do not attend group daycare) or on outcome (e.g., patients who either had or did not have pneumococcal bacteremia or patients who either died or survived). Another key element is the *timing* of the study in relation to the timing of exposure and outcome. In studies in which the timing is *historical,* both the exposure and the outcome occurred before the study was initiated (e.g., a case-control study of a vaccine's efficacy in which cases with disease are identified from historical logbooks and antecedent receipt of the vaccine is determined from medical records). Timing may be *concurrent*—that is, both the exposure and the outcome occur after the study is initiated (e.g., a randomized clinical trial of the efficacy of a new antibiotic). Timing also may be *mixed,* a mixture of historical and concurrent (e.g., a study of the current IQ of children who previously had aseptic meningitis).

A final important element of a study is its *direction.* Direction is used to describe the order in which outcome and exposure are assessed. It may be done in a *forward* direction, from exposure to outcome (e.g., in a clinical trial of a vaccine's efficacy, the exposure [receipt or nonreceipt of the experimental vaccine] occurs first, and the occurrence of the outcome [the infection that the vaccine is designed to prevent] is determined subsequently). Alternatively, a study's direction may be *backward,* from outcome to exposure (e.g., in a case-control study, the outcome [e.g., pneumococcal bacteremia] is determined first, and exposure [e.g., previous receipt of pneumococcal vaccine] is determined subsequently). Alternatively, exposure and outcome may be determined simultaneously (e.g., a survey in which determination of whether subjects have sickle-cell disease and whether they are taking penicillin occurs at the same time). A study's direction can have important implications for inferences about causal associations; for example, even though a strong statistical association may exist between sickle-cell disease and the use of penicillin, concluding that the penicillin caused the sickle-cell disease would be erroneous. Although such an inference obviously is not plausible in this instance, the dangers of making erroneous inferences about causality are very real when exposures and outcomes that are less well understood are studied, and these types of errors have occurred many times in the history of medical research.

Although the terms *prospective* and *retrospective* are used widely, substantial variability exists in how they are applied. The term *prospective* is used to describe studies in which selection of the sample is based on the exposure, in which the timing is concurrent, or in which the direction of the study is forward (from exposure to outcome). The term *retrospective* is used to describe studies in which selection of the sample is based on the outcome, in which the timing is historical, or in which the direction of the study is backward (from outcome to exposure). Referring to the specific elements of the study is preferable to using the terms *prospective* and *retrospective,* which are applied so imprecisely.

Types of Studies

Epidemiologic studies may be classified as either experimental or observational. In *experimental studies,* the exposure is assigned by the investigators (e.g., in a clinical trial of an experimental vaccine, the investigator assigns subjects to receive either the experimental vaccine or a placebo). In *observational studies,* the exposure occurs naturally (e.g., rainfall in a study that assesses the effect of the amount of rainfall on rates of mosquito-borne infections), is selected by the subjects or their parents (e.g., attendance at group daycare in a study that assesses the frequency of infectious illnesses in children who attend and others who do not attend group daycare), or is assigned in the course of regular medical care (e.g., receipt of an approved vaccine in a case-control study of the effectiveness of the vaccine). Observational studies also are called *surveys.*

Experimental Studies

The paradigm for an experimental study is the *randomized clinical trial,* which is a special type of *longitudinal cohort study* in which the exposure is assigned randomly to the subjects by the investigators. In randomized trials, the direction of the study always is forward, selection (or categorization) of subjects always is based on exposure (i.e., exposure is determined at the time of randomization), and timing always is concurrent (both exposure and outcome are determined during the real period of the study). Randomized trials are the sine qua non for evaluating the effect of new agents designed either to prevent (e.g., vaccines, prophylactic drugs) or to treat (e.g., antimicrobial agents) diseases. By randomly allocating subjects to either receive or not receive the agent that is being tested, potential bias is minimized. Theoretically, if the size of the sample is adequate, the only difference between the groups is whether they received the experimental agent. Consequently, if the study is conducted properly, inferring that statistically significant differences in outcomes between the groups were related causally to the experimental agent is reasonable. For this reason, in most instances, the efficacy of new therapeutic agents or new vaccines must be demonstrated in clinical trials before the U.S. Food and Drug Administration (FDA) will approve them (although in some instances new products are approved if criteria for safety and for some surrogate end point, such as a serologic correlate of immunity, are met).

The advantages and disadvantages of randomized trials are summarized in Box 6.1. Although clinical trials are the gold standard for

BOX 6.1 Randomized Clinical Trials

Advantages

Gold standard for scientific validity

Randomization ensures unbiased allocation of the exposure (e.g., a new drug or an experimental vaccine)

Blinding ensures unbiased assessment of outcomes

Disadvantages

Poor statistical power for rare diseases

Requires large samples

Requires longitudinal follow-up

Logistically complex and expensive

Impaired generalizability when the study population differs from the ultimate target population

Ethical issues

Requires informed consent

Difficult to use to evaluate approved (presumably efficacious) products

investigators who wish to design a scientifically valid study, they do have numerous limitations. A major problem is that clinical trials usually are expensive. Subjects need to be selected, enrolled, and monitored longitudinally to detect the outcomes. When the outcome is a disease that is relatively rare (e.g., pneumococcal bacteremia), large samples are necessary to provide adequate statistical power. Because sponsors of clinical trials usually want to test a new drug or an experimental vaccine under conditions that will maximize the chance that it will be found to be efficacious, patients with comorbid conditions (e.g., sickle-cell disease, asplenia, metastatic cancer) that might negatively affect their response to the new agent often are excluded from the study. If the subjects who are excluded are an important part of the target population for the new agent (e.g., the patients with comorbid conditions are likely to be at high risk for serious complications of the disease and thus potentially could benefit greatly from an effective new intervention), the generalizability of the results of the clinical trial may be impaired.

Most randomized clinical trials are conducted in a *double-blind* manner; that is, neither the investigators nor the subjects know whether they received the experimental intervention (e.g., a new drug) or the comparison agent (e.g., either a placebo or an agent used in the standard manner). Double-blinding helps ensure lack of bias in ascertainment of the outcome because neither the subject nor the investigator can be influenced either to (or not to) seek medical care or undergo diagnostic tests on the basis of which of the interventions was received.

Randomized clinical trials may pose difficult ethical problems because the new (and potentially efficacious) agent is not given to the controls. By the time that clinical trials are begun, usually some evidence suggests that the agent is efficacious (e.g., preliminary studies in a limited group of subjects showing that a new vaccine induces antibodies). Accordingly some patients and patient advocates might suggest that withholding a potentially efficacious therapeutic agent or a vaccine from persons at risk is not ethical; consequently, it may be difficult to have persons agree to be potential controls in studies of a promising new therapy.

Problems also may arise when approval of a product for the target population is based on studies that are conducted in a different population. For example, polyvalent pneumococcal polysaccharide vaccine was approved in the United States for the elderly and for adults with chronic conditions, such as chronic obstructive pulmonary disease and congestive heart failure, that put them at increased risk of acquiring serious pneumococcal infections. However, the data on which approval was based were derived from clinical trials conducted among young gold miners in South Africa who were at risk largely not because of their age or underlying illnesses but because of the conditions in which they lived and worked. Reports of vaccine failure and poor antibody response to the vaccine in the target population in the United States led to questions about the vaccine's efficacy. However, once the vaccine was approved, conducting a randomized clinical trial in the target population was difficult ethically because it would mean withholding, on a random basis, an approved (and presumably efficacious) vaccine from patients at risk. Consequently all but one of the post-licensure studies of this vaccine's efficacy were observational studies.

Conducting an experimental study in which the exposure is not assigned randomly is possible. For example, one might conduct an experimental cohort study in which volunteers receive a certain intervention (e.g., a new drug) while controls receive no intervention. Both groups would be monitored forward in time while undergoing surveillance for the outcome event. Although such a study incorporates some of the features of a randomized clinical trial, because the intervention is not assigned randomly, such studies are subject to significant biases.

There are also situations in which special kinds of clinical trials are needed. For example, *cluster randomized clinical trials* are now common. In this type of experimental study, the unit of randomization is not the individual but rather a group or "cluster" (e.g., randomization by community). This can be important in trials of, for example, experimental vaccines or other interventions that may induce herd immunity, so that unimmunized individuals in a community in which many individuals received the vaccine may be at lower risk than unimmunized individuals in the general population. However, this type of study also presents special challenges in its design and statistical analysis.[9] Another special kind of clinical trial is a *noninferiority* or an *equivalence trial*, designed to show that the effectiveness of a new agent is not inferior to a standard agent (by a specified amount) or that its effect is equivalent (with specified parameters). These kinds of trials also present special problems in design and analysis.[52,60,68]

Observational Studies

Cohort studies. The direction of cohort studies always is forward, and the selection (or categorization) of subjects is always based on exposure; however, the timing may be concurrent, historical, or mixed. Thus, a cohort study may identify a cohort of subjects at a point (or at several points) in time in the recent or remote past, categorize them regarding their status with respect to the exposure (e.g., receipt of either a vaccine or a drug), and then monitor them forward in time for the occurrence of the outcome event (e.g., an infection or an unpleasant complication) until a certain point in time, which could be in the past, present, or future. As in a clinical trial, subjects must not have the outcome at the time of enrollment in the study.

Cohort studies share many of the disadvantages of randomized clinical trials (see Box 6.1) but have the additional disadvantage that, because they are not experimental, they are subject to many potential biases. On the other hand, cohort studies have many practical advantages (e.g., the timing can be historical, so conducting a 30-year follow-up study in just months is possible), and, because they are observational studies, they usually have fewer potential ethical problems than does a randomized trial. In addition, for rare exposures, a critical factor is to be able to base selection of subjects on exposure.

Case-control studies. In both clinical trials and observational cohort studies, the selection of subjects is based on their exposures, and they are monitored in a forward direction until the outcome is determined. In case-control studies, the process is reversed. Subjects are selected on the basis of outcomes. The cases have the outcome, usually a disease; the controls do not have the outcome. The direction of the study is backward—the previous exposure is ascertained after the subjects are selected. The timing of case-control studies usually is historical, but it may be mixed; the timing of the exposure always is historical, but the timing of the outcome may be either historical or concurrent. For example an investigator may conduct a case-control study of a vaccine's effectiveness in which persons who are infected (cases) are identified concurrently through active surveillance of a microbiology laboratory (incident cases). Because case-control studies are nonexperimental and the exposure (and, sometimes, the outcome) occurred in the past, the potential for bias is great both in selection of the sample and in ascertainment of both the exposure and the outcome. The advantages and disadvantages of case-control studies are shown in Box 6.2. Use of "sham" outcomes and/or exposures in addition to the true outcomes or exposures of interest has been suggested as a means of assessing the internal validity of case-control studies.[65]

BOX 6.2 Case-Control Studies

Advantages

Statistically powerful method to assess outcomes that are rare or delayed
Logistically easier and more efficient than large experimental or observational cohort studies
No longitudinal follow-up, so it can be completed relatively quickly and inexpensively
Ethically acceptable because it is an observational study

Disadvantage

Subject to many potential biases

TABLE 6.1 Analysis of Experimental or Observational Cohort Studies

	Outcome Present	Outcome Absent	Total
Exposed	a	b	a + b
Unexposed	c	d	c + d
Total	a + c	b + d	

Risk in exposed subjects: a/(a + b).
Risk in unexposed subjects: c/(c + d).
Relative risk: (a/a + b) ÷ (c/c + d).
Attributable risk: (a/a + b) − (c/c + d).

Cross-sectional studies. Unlike cohort studies (both experimental and observational), in which timing is forward from exposure to outcome, and case-control studies, in which timing is backward from outcome to exposure, in cross-sectional studies, outcome and exposure are determined at the same time. In cohort studies, causal inference is made from cause to effect, whereas in case-control studies, causal inference is made from effect to cause. In cross-sectional studies, determining whether the exposure preceded the outcome may not be possible. Consequently making valid causal inferences from a cross-sectional study also may not be possible.

Selection of subjects for a cross-sectional study may be based on outcome, exposure, or neither. However, because cross-sectional studies include only persons with prevalent outcomes, they are particularly problematic for studies of infectious diseases because patients whose illnesses (outcomes) either resolved or resulted in death before the study is conducted are not counted as having the outcome. Consequently, cross-sectional studies are more suitable to the study of chronic conditions and rarely are used in studies of infectious diseases.

Analysis of Epidemiologic Studies

The results of epidemiologic studies with dichotomous exposures and outcomes often are displayed in a *2 × 2 contingency table.* However the way that the results are analyzed statistically depends on the type of study.

Cohort Studies

Analysis of longitudinal cohort studies (both experimental trials and observational studies) is shown in Table 6.1. The measure of association between the exposure and the outcome is the *relative risk* (sometimes called the *risk ratio*), which is an expression of the *magnitude* of this association in the study sample and represents an *estimate* of the association in the population from which the study sample was drawn. A relative risk of 1 indicates that no association exists between the exposure and the outcome, a relative risk greater than 1 indicates that the exposure is associated with an increased risk of the outcome, and a relative risk less than 1 indicates that the exposure is associated with a decreased risk of the outcome. The *attributable risk* (the risk of the outcome that is attributable to the exposure) is calculated as the risk in exposed subjects minus the risk in unexposed subjects. Of course, testing the statistical significance of any association is necessary because the relative risk could be greater than 1 or less than 1 by chance (see later sections on stochastic statistics and confidence intervals).

These analyses assume that no attrition exists among the subjects in the study. However, because of death, migration out of the study area, and loss to follow-up, as well as variation in the time of enrollment (enrollment in either a clinical trial or an observational cohort study may occur over a prolonged period or, indeed, throughout a study), variation virtually always exists among subjects in the duration of time that they are at risk for the outcome. If the average time at risk among the exposed and the unexposed subjects is equal, the analysis shown in Table 6.1 is likely to be valid. However, if a great deal of irregular attrition or new enrollment occurs during the study, the denominator is expressed better as person-time at risk (e.g., person-months, person-years) rather than as the number of persons in the group. When this method is used, the rate then is called the *incidence density rate* and the index of comparison is called the *incidence density ratio.*

In studies of infectious diseases, the outcome event often is the occurrence of an infection. Frequently, persons who become infected recover and may remain at risk for the outcome event again. Nonetheless, a subject usually should be censored (i.e., removed from the study) once the outcome event occurs. The fact that the outcome occurred may indicate that the subject has an increased risk for the outcome, independent of the exposure that is being assessed. For example, consider a study of the protective efficacy of a conjugate pneumococcal vaccine in which one of the subjects (whether the subject is a vaccinee or a control does not matter) experiences three or four episodes of invasive infection caused by pneumococci (perhaps because the subject has a previously unrecognized underlying condition, such as an acquired immunodeficiency syndrome or a congenital immunoglobulin deficiency). The estimate of the vaccine's efficacy would be distorted substantially if each of the outcome events was counted. Generally, in a primary analysis, only the initial event should be counted. Another reason to censor the subject is that, in some instances, the outcome event may be fatal. If some subjects die of the outcome (and, therefore, must be censored), not censoring subjects with the outcome who survive is, in effect, allowing prognosis of the infection to affect the estimate of the vaccine's efficacy on the risk of the outcome event.

Using a different method to adjust for unequal durations of follow-up in a study may be necessary, particularly when a long latent period exists between exposure and outcome (a condition that often is met when the study involves the effect of a potential carcinogen). In such instances, simply to sum the total person-times of exposure may be misleading because the outcome is more likely to occur many years after exposure. For example, although the total person-time at risk would be the same (1000 person-years), the risk of an outcome developing clearly may be substantially different for 500 persons, each of whom is monitored for 2 years after exposure, than it may be for 40 persons, each of whom is monitored for 25 years after exposure. In such situations, the analyses must be adjusted for variation in the length of follow-up, which can be done with the use of *survival analysis* (also known as *life-table analysis*). The two basic methods of survival analysis, the *actuarial* method and the *Kaplan-Meier (product-limit)* method, are described in detail elsewhere.[37]

Case-Control and Cross-Sectional Studies

Analysis of a case-control study (with dichotomous outcomes and exposures) is shown in Table 6.2. Because selection of subjects is based on their outcomes, one cannot calculate the risk of development of the outcome, as one would in a longitudinal study (such as a clinical trial). Instead, one calculates the proportion of each group (cases and controls) that is exposed. The measure of association in a case-control study is the *odds ratio.* The *odds* of some occurrence is the probability that it will occur divided by the probability that it will not occur. In a case-control study, we are interested in the odds of exposure. The odds ratio is the ratio of the odds of exposure among cases (a/c) divided by the odds of exposure among controls (b/d). For rare events, the odds ratio closely approximates the relative risk of exposure that would be found in a longitudinal study of the same association. Use of a method known as *risk set sampling* allows odds ratios from case-control studies to approximate a risk ratio even if the outcome is not rare.[4] Cross-sectional

TABLE 6.2 Analysis of Case-Control Studies

	Cases (Outcome Present)	Controls (Outcome Absent)
Exposed	a	b
Unexposed	c	d

Proportion of exposed cases: a/(a + c).
Proportion of exposed controls: b/(b + d).
Odds of exposure among cases: a/c.
Odds of exposure among controls: b/d.
Odds ratio: (a/c) ÷ (b/d) or (ad) ÷ (bc).

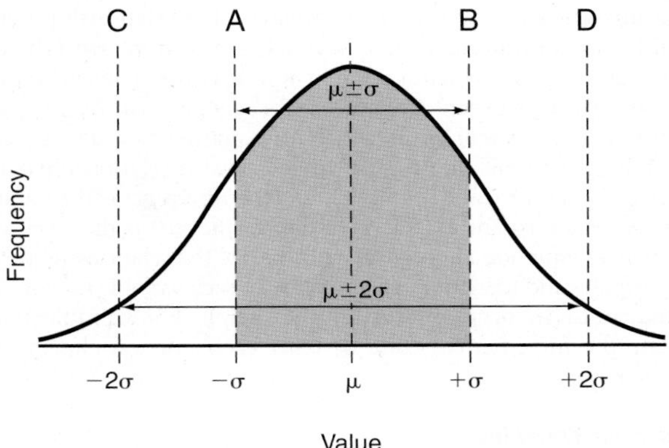

FIG. 6.1 Theoretic normal (Gaussian) distribution showing where 1 and 2 standard deviations (SD) above and below the mean would fall. The Greek letter mu (μ) stands for the mean in the theoretic distribution, and the Greek letter sigma (σ) stands for the SD in the theoretic population. In this figure, the area under the curve represents all the observations in the distribution. One SD above and below the mean, shown in dark gray and represented by the distance from point A to point B, is equivalent to 68% of the area under the curve; 68% of the observations in a normal distribution therefore fall within this range. Two SDs above and below the mean, represented by the area under the curve between lines C and D, are equivalent to 95.4% of the area of the curve or 95.4% of the observations in a normal distribution. (From Jekel JF, Elmore JG, Katz DL. *Epidemiology, biostatistics, and preventive medicine.* Philadelphia: WB Saunders; 1996:118.)

studies are analyzed either like a case-control study (if the selection of subjects was based on their outcomes) or like a cohort study (if the selection of subjects was based on their exposures).

Summary Statistics

Perhaps the most basic use of statistical analysis is to summarize data. This type of statistical analysis often is called either *summary* or *descriptive* statistics. The specific summary measures that are used depend in part on whether the variables being summarized are *continuous* (variables with equal distance between intervals) or *categorical* (variables with two or more discrete categories). Age, weight, height, temperature, concentration of creatinine in serum, and the number of hours spent in group daycare all are examples of continuous variables (sometimes called *dimensional* or *quantitative* variables). Race, sex, country of residence, and whether a patient is being ventilated artificially are examples of categorical variables (sometimes called *discrete* variables). Of course, continuous variables can be analyzed categorically (e.g., age can be divided into either a *dichotomous* variable [<45 years or ≥45 years] or a *polychotomous* variable [20 to 44 years, 45 to 59 years, and ≥60 years]).

Continuous Variables

A *frequency distribution* is classification of the values of a sample of continuous variables into successive categories (e.g., for a sample of different ages, one might place each value into different 5-year [birth to 4 years, 5 to 9 years, etc.], 3-year [birth to 2 years, 3 to 5 years, etc.], or 1-year [0 year, 1 year, 2 years, 3 years, etc.] categories) and expressed as the frequency of values within each category.

A sample of values of a continuous variable also can be summarized mathematically by describing its central tendency, shape, and spread. The *central tendency* can be expressed as a *mean* (or *average*), a *median* (the middle value of the sample), or a *mode* (the most frequent value in the sample). The mean value is calculated by summing all the individual values in the sample and dividing by the number of individual values. Thus, for a sample that is composed of subjects aged 1, 1, 2, 2, 2, 3, 3, 4, 10, and 12 years, the mean age is 4 years (40/10), the median age (the age for which half the subjects are older than and half are younger than its value—if the number of subjects is even, the median is the mean of the two middle values) is 2.5 years [(2 + 3)/2], and the mode is 2 years. These summary measures provide only a limited view of the data. For example, the mean of a distribution can be shifted in the direction of extreme outlying values; in the example, the mean is 4 years even though 70% of the subjects are younger than 4 years. Likewise, from the median value alone, one would not know whether outlying values exist. Consequently, describing the spread of a distribution is important.

The *spread* of a sample may be expressed by its *range* and by its *standard deviation.* The range of a sample is the interval between the highest and lowest value in its distribution. In the previous example, the range is from 1 to 12 years. Another useful way of mathematically summarizing the spread of a distribution is to express the interval between each individual value and the mean value of the sample. To summarize these values, one cannot simply sum all the differences because the sum always equals zero (the sum of the positive differences equals the sum of the negative differences). To avoid this problem, the standard deviation of a sample is used. This parameter is calculated by taking the square root of the *variance* of the sample. The variance is the sum of the squares of the differences from the mean of each individual value divided by the number of *degrees of freedom* of the sample (which is equal to the number of values in the sample minus one, or $N - 1$). The sum of the squares is divided by the number of degrees of freedom of the sample ($N - 1$) rather than by N (the actual number in the sample) because this calculation is thought to represent more accurately the true variance of the population from which a sample is taken.

To calculate the standard deviation of the sample in the example, one must determine the variance, which is the sum of the squares of the difference of each individual value from the mean of the sample divided by the degrees of freedom (number of values minus one):

$$(2[4-1]^2+3[4-2]^2+2[4-3]^2+[4-4]^2+[4-10]^2+[4-12]^2)\div(10-1)$$

which equals 132 ÷ 9, or 14.6667 years. The standard deviation is simply the square root of the variance, which is 3.8297 years.

In the medical literature, investigators often use the *standard error of the mean* (which is the square root of the variance divided by the square root of the number in the sample) to express the spread of the frequency distribution of a sample. However, the standard error actually is designed to be a measure of the standard deviation of the means of repeated samples from a single source population. Because the standard error always is smaller than the standard deviation of a single sample, it gives the erroneous impression that the spread of a sample is smaller than it actually is. A large sample with a large spread (and a large standard deviation) may have a small standard error. The standard error should not be used to describe the spread of a single sample.

The general shape of the frequency distribution can be inferred from the parameters given earlier. The characteristics of the most important distribution in statistics, the familiar bell-shaped curve of the normal distribution, are shown in Fig. 6.1 and are discussed in a later section about diagnostic tests. The peak value of any distribution is the mode. A distribution may be bimodal, trimodal, and so on if it has two or more modes. A frequency distribution may be asymmetric, or *skewed.* If the mean is greater than the median (as in the example), the distribution is skewed to the right; conversely, if the mean is less than the median, the distribution is skewed to the left.

An investigator may want to summarize the relationship between two different continuous variables, which can be done with the use of linear regression, in which a straight line is constructed to represent the relationship between a continuous *dependent variable* (y) and a continuous *independent variable* (x). An equation ($y = a + bx$) can be created that represents the best "fit" to describe the relationship between the actual values of y and x, in which a (the *intercept*) is the value of y when x equals zero and b (the *regression coefficient*) is the slope of the line. Such an equation allows us to summarize the relationship between these variables and to extrapolate the value of each variable for conditions that may not have been observed in the sample. For example, one can calculate the incremental value of y for each interval change in the value of x.

Categorical Variables

The measure generally used to summarize categorical data is called a *rate* or a *proportion*. Rates consist of a numerator and a denominator. The numerator represents the actual number of persons in the sample who have the characteristic of interest (e.g., those with fever, those with tuberculosis, those who received a vaccine), and the denominator is the total number of persons in the sample. The persons in the numerator must be included in the group that the denominator represents, and the persons in the denominator must be able to have the characteristic that the numerator represents. For example, if one were interested in the rate of testicular cancer in the population, women should not be included in the denominator because they cannot have testicular cancer. Some experts believe that rates, by definition, should include a time factor (e.g., incident cases per person-months or per year). However, the term is used widely to refer to a proportion of a sample, as described earlier.

One of the most important rates that is calculated in epidemiologic studies is the *incidence rate* or *attack rate*, which is the number of persons in whom a certain outcome develops divided by the number of persons in whom the outcome could have developed during a specified period. For example, a comparison may be made of the incidence rates of an infection over time in two groups in which the interventions given to prevent an infection differed (e.g., vaccine, placebo).

Another important rate, the *prevalence rate*, is the number of persons in whom a certain outcome develops divided by the total number of persons in the group at a specific point in time. In calculating the incidence rate, persons who at *zero time* (before the study begins) already have the outcome (e.g., prevalent cases) are excluded from both the numerator and the denominator. At time zero, the numerator of the incidence rate is zero. Thus, if one were interested in the incidence rate of lung cancer, persons who had lung cancer at the beginning of the study period would be excluded. The prevalence rate, by contrast, is measured at one point in time, and the numerator includes all persons with the outcome at that time.

Certain features of many infectious diseases affect both the prevalence rate and the incidence rate as measures of the occurrence of disease. The prevalence rate of any condition is related to its chronicity and the mortality rate associated with it; conditions that are common and chronic but are not associated necessarily with immediate mortality (e.g., atherosclerotic heart disease) have a relatively high prevalence rate. On the other hand, the prevalence rates are relatively low for conditions that either have a low mortality rate and resolve completely (e.g., many infectious illnesses) or have a high short-term mortality rate. To get a reliable estimate of the importance of such conditions, one must determine their incidence rates.

To describe variations in occurrence of infections over limited periods within a single population, such as a city or a state, a simple *numerical frequency* (e.g., number of cases of infection) often is used—daily or weekly (during an epidemic), monthly (to reflect seasonal patterns), or annually (to compare successive years). Comparisons among different populations or subgroups within a population or at widely separated times in the same population require use of the *incidence rate*, or *attack rate*.

For infections transmitted by contact, the frequency with which infection or disease occurs among exposed susceptible individuals provides a measure of the infectivity of the agent. This frequency, called the *secondary attack rate*, is defined as the number of contacts who become infected (or who develop disease) within the maximal incubation period of the infectious agent divided by the number of susceptible persons in the exposed group or population in question. The secondary attack rate is applied most usefully only to closed groups, households, or classrooms, where exposure safely can be presumed for all members. The first, or primary, case is the presumed source of exposure; other initial cases that occur within the minimal incubation period or since presumed exposure of the primary cases are called *co-primary cases*. In calculating the secondary attack rate, primary and co-primary cases are excluded from the numerator and the denominator. Cases that occur subsequently within the maximal incubation period constitute the secondary cases. Cases that develop later are excluded because it is presumed they occurred from either a different exposure or from tertiary spread. The exclusion of immune individuals from the denominator usually is feasible only for diseases sufficiently characteristic clinically that the history serves to identify them (e.g., measles, chickenpox). Moreover, one may not want to exclude immune individuals (who may not be easily identifiable) in calculating primary or secondary attack rates. Although immune individuals are not readily identifiable in the case of common respiratory diseases, the secondary attack rate based on all exposed members of the group still may be a useful measure. Its utility decreases, however, when the period of communicability of the primary case (as with *Mycoplasma pneumoniae* infections) is longer than the incubation period because distinguishing between secondary and tertiary cases becomes difficult.

Finally the occurrence of death caused by a specific disease typically is expressed in two different ways. One, the *cause-specific mortality rate*, is defined as the number of deaths from the disease during a specified period of time divided by the total number of persons in the population. It is a measure of the consequences of the disease in the population. The effect of the disease among infected individuals is reflected by the *case-fatality rate*, which is defined as the number of deaths due to the infection in a specified period of time divided by the number of persons infected during the same period.

Bias

Bias occurs when the estimate of the association between the exposure and the outcome in the sample differs systematically from the true value in the population. Bias in the estimate of the association is different from bias in the measurement of individual variables. The latter bias (which may occur, for example, if an instrument such as a thermometer is calibrated incorrectly) may or may not affect the estimate of association in an epidemiologic study. Biased measurements usually affect the exposed and the unexposed groups equally. By contrast, *analytic bias* is the effect of *differential error (nonrandom error)* on the assessment of the relationship between exposure and outcome. Analytic bias can occur because of *information bias* (as a result of differential error in ascertainment of either the exposure or the outcome), *sample distortion bias* (because the joint distribution of the exposure and the outcome in the sample chosen for the study is not representative of the distribution of these factors in the target population), and *confounding bias* (because the joint distribution of one or more variables that independently are related both to the exposure and to the outcome is unequal in the groups that are being compared). Ensuring that bias does not affect a study is critical to its validity. Furthermore, although using statistical methods to adjust for certain sources of bias (particularly for confounding bias) in analysis of the results of a study sometimes is possible, adjustment for bias after the fact may be impossible.

An example of information bias is *detection bias*, which occurs when there is differential detection of the outcome in the exposed and the unexposed groups. For example, numerous studies in which clinical scales to assess whether children with fever have a serious illness have been developed.[41] Often, however, the "serious illness" may include certain abnormal laboratory test results (e.g., an abnormal radiograph of the chest or a low concentration of sodium in serum). Because children with high scores on these scales were more likely to undergo diagnostic tests, detection bias may have occurred because similar abnormalities (e.g., a "silent" pneumonia or a decreased concentration of sodium in serum) might go undetected in the "unexposed" group (children with lower scores on the clinical scale), a much smaller proportion of whom underwent a diagnostic test to detect a possible outcome. The best way to avoid information bias is to use standardized, consistent methods to ascertain both the exposure and the outcome and to blind subjects and investigators to ensure that no differential ascertainment of either the outcome (in longitudinal studies) or the exposure (in case-control studies) occurs.

Sample distortion bias occurs when the sample in a study is not representative of the target population. However, a nonrepresentative sample does not lead to bias necessarily; bias in assessment of the association between exposure and outcome occurs only if differential distribution of the exposure (or differential risk of the outcome) occurs in the subjects who are selected for the study versus the overall target population. This distribution can be the result of *selection bias.* For example, consider a case-control study of the effectiveness of an approved vaccine in which the control subjects (the uninfected patients) were chosen from private practices in affluent suburbs, whereas the case subjects (the infected patients) were any patients in whom a serious infection developed and who were hospitalized. The association between antecedent vaccination and infection probably is biased because the controls are not a representative sample of the population from which the cases emerged and because the proportion of them likely to have been vaccinated is higher than in the group of all uninfected persons in the population. Another possible source of sample distortion bias is differential loss to follow-up in a longitudinal study. The potential for sample distortion bias can be minimized by maximizing the probability that a representative sample will be selected, ideally by random sampling (or some other kind of unbiased sampling), and by minimizing loss to follow-up in longitudinal studies.

Confounding bias occurs when the association between exposure and outcome is distorted by a variable (a *confounder*) that is distributed unequally between the groups, is associated independently with both the exposure and the outcome, and is not in the causal pathway from exposure to outcome. One example of confounding bias is *susceptibility bias,* which occurs when the risk of the subjects (to development of the outcome) differs in the exposed and unexposed groups, independent of the exposure. For example, imagine a longitudinal study of the protective efficacy of a vaccine against *Haemophilus influenzae* type b in infants. Ensuring that an equal proportion of subjects in the vaccinated and the unvaccinated groups attended group daycare is important because attendance at group daycare is associated with an increased risk of developing infection with *H. influenzae* type b. If a substantially higher proportion of vaccinees than of controls attended group daycare, their attendance might confound assessment of the vaccine's efficacy and result in a biased estimate of the effect of the vaccine (lower than the true effect). By contrast, if a disproportionate number of controls attended group daycare, the estimate of the vaccine's efficacy might be biased in the opposite direction (it would be erroneously high because controls would have a disproportionately higher risk of acquiring infection with *H. influenzae* type b than would vaccinees).

In the previous example, adjusting for the effect of the confounder might be possible by either stratification or multivariable analysis (see later discussion). However, identifying confounders may not always be possible. Random allocation of subjects is the best strategy to protect against confounding, especially if there is uncertainty about the ability to identify all important potential confounders.

CAUSES OF DISEASE

Historical Perspectives

Although the previously discussed principles apply to all epidemiologic studies, in studies of infectious diseases three additional factors contribute uniquely to who is and who is not affected: (1) the cause is a specific external agent (the infecting organism), (2) transmission of the organism to the host is required, and (3) certain host factors, such as immunity to infection or disease or genetic determinants of susceptibility or resistance to infection may affect both risk of and outcome of infection. Recognition of these factors (the infecting agent, transmission, and immunity) evolved gradually over many years.[25]

The discipline of epidemiology evolved from the study of great epidemic diseases such as plague, cholera, and smallpox. The periodic waves of these diseases, which were associated with high mortality rates, stimulated the first serious efforts to explain the occurrence of disease on the basis of factors other than supernatural or divine forces.

Fundamental to such explanations was the concept of *contagion.* This factor long had been implicit in attitudes toward victims of leprosy, as exemplified by such early Christian practices as conducting antemortem funerals for lepers, who then were given a bell and cup and forbidden further human contact or, more drastically, were buried alive or burned at the stake.[57] The English physician Thomas Sydenham (1624–89) introduced laudanum (derived from opium) as a painkiller, recognized the efficacy of Peruvian bark (quinine) in malaria, and revived the Hippocratic idea of "epidemic constitutions" (of atmospheric nature), which, by grafting onto existing illness, gave all concurrent illnesses the character reflecting the then prevailing "constitution." These views persisted in colonial America, where they were expounded by such eminent individuals as Noah Webster *(Webster's Dictionary)* and Dr. Benjamin Rush of Philadelphia.[76]

Nonetheless, by the mid-18th century, the theory of contagion had gained acceptance for particular diseases, including measles, syphilis, and smallpox. The theory is alleged to have been exploited in an early act of biologic warfare: Massachusetts colonists reportedly presented the blankets of smallpox victims as gifts to the Indians, who then suffered a decimating epidemic.[20]

The true origin of the concept of immunity is uncertain, but it was applied first in relation to smallpox. *Variolation* (inoculation of people with material from pox lesions that was expected to induce modified, but immunizing, disease) was practiced in the 11th or 12th century in China and in the early 18th century in both England and the American colonies. Also popular in rural England at this time was the theory that cowpox, a minor disease acquired from afflicted cattle, induced immunity to smallpox. This theory was verified by Edward Jenner (reported in 1798) and resulted, years later, in general acceptance of cowpox vaccine (vaccinia) to protect against smallpox.

The germ theory of disease was stated explicitly in 1855 by John Snow, an English anesthesiologist who took up cholera epidemiology as an avocation. Snow argued that the causative agent of cholera was a living cell that multiplied with great rapidity but was too small to be seen under the microscopes then in use.[70] Louis Pasteur (1822–95) formally validated the germ theory by showing that the microorganisms responsible for fermentation were not generated spontaneously but came from the air.[47] On this basis, Joseph Lord Lister revolutionized surgery by using carbolic acid to combat atmospheric germs and minimize "putrification" in surgical procedures.[67]

In Pasteur's wake, bacteria were cultured with great frequency from ill individuals and often were identified erroneously as causal agents. Robert Koch (1843–1910), who first isolated the bacterial causes of tuberculosis and cholera, also was the first to introduce scientific rigor into the proof of primary causation. His famed "postulates," to be satisfied before a causal relationship between a bacterium and a disease could be accepted, required that (1) the presence of the agent be shown in every case by its recovery in pure culture; (2) the agent not be found in cases of other disease; (3) the agent, when isolated, be capable of reproducing the disease in experimental animals; and (4) the agent be recovered in pure culture from such experimental disease.[23]

Koch's postulates since have been modified, largely to meet problems posed by viruses. As obligate intracellular parasites, viruses cannot be "cultivated in pure culture." In addition, they often are host specific and do not produce disease in an animal model. Other considerations that were invoked as elements of proof included the significance of recovery of the agent from diseased tissues, the demonstration of an increase in titer of specific antibody in temporal relation to the disease, and, most conclusive, the specific preventive effect of vaccines containing the viral antigen.[28] One further situation not recognized by Koch is that infections with true pathogens do not always cause disease. We now recognize pathogenicity (defined as the proportion of infections that result in disease) as an important characteristic of infectious disease agents.

General Concepts

Causation of infectious diseases is defined in terms of the *primary cause* and *contributing factors* (or secondary causes). The former is the specific microorganism (the agent of disease) without which the particular disease cannot occur. Contributing factors affect the likelihood that infection will occur and help determine that disease will result, given infection. Identification of the causative agent may lead to the development of effective means for providing specific protective immunization (e.g., diphtheria and tetanus toxoids, vaccines against polio and measles). Finding the cause of a disease also may lead to other means of control. An example is the discovery of *Legionella pneumophila* as the cause of Legionnaires' disease. The discovery of the organism led to the understanding of how the disease is transmitted—via aerosols from cooling towers, which serve as reservoirs for the bacteria.[16,42] Disinfection of these towers has helped to control Legionnaires' disease.

Infection and *disease* are not synonymous, although infection is necessary for an infectious disease to occur. *Infection* denotes replication of organisms in the tissues of a host, usually with an associated immune response; infection may be either subclinical (asymptomatic), or, if it results in development of overt clinical manifestations, it is denoted as *disease.* There are many examples of infections, such as poliomyelitis, other enteroviral infections, and mumps, that may be either asymptomatic or the cause of serious disease in the host. When disease occurs, it may vary in severity among infected individuals. Some infections produce full-blown disease in all infected susceptible individuals; measles is an example. Simple *colonization,* in contrast to infection and disease, is a state in which the organism parasitizes the host at a given site, replicates, and may persist, but it does not proceed further to cause infection or disease or to induce an immune response in the host. The *carrier state,* in which the organism persists over time and may be transmitted to others, may occur after colonization, infection, or disease. Examples of organisms that behave in this way include group A streptococcus and *Neisseria meningitidis.*

Many factors, largely related to the host and to the conditions of exposure, determine whether colonization occurs and whether the subsequent processes of infection and disease occur. These contributing or risk factors in the host are extensive and varied and may include but are not limited to age, sex, race, immune status, genetic constitution, and general state of health, including underlying diseases. Similarly, contributing factors unrelated to the host may include climate, the presence of vectors, quality of sanitation, intimacy of exposure, and socioeconomic conditions. These contributing factors vary among infectious diseases and are discussed in chapters about specific infectious agents in this textbook.

Factors Related to the Infectious Agent

What characteristics of infectious agents are significant epidemiologically? Factors associated with the occurrence of disease include factors related to perpetuation of the infectious agent, factors that govern the type of contact required to infect humans, and factors that determine the occurrence of disease. Also important are characteristics useful in classification and specific identification of agents. Some important characteristics are *intrinsic,* in that they can be described after appropriate direct examination of the agent. *Host-related* characteristics can be described only on the basis of the behavior of the agents in the host.

Intrinsic Properties

Precise classification and identification of agents are basic to the specific recognition of infections and related disease. Both depend on intrinsic properties, including morphology (which alone provides the basis for identifying most higher organisms), chemical composition (the type of nucleic acid being important in viral classification), and antigenic character, which is related to chemical composition. The last is central to specific identification of agent isolates and antibodies induced by infection. Requirements for growth or replication provide keys to the identification of some bacteria (e.g., fermentation of different sugars) and many viruses that replicate optimally or only in cultures of certain types of cells incubated at specified temperatures. For example, rhinoviruses replicate best in human diploid cells incubated at 33°C.

In recent years, we have gained the ability to rapidly detect and classify many infectious agents by identification of their genomes. The use of whole-genome analysis, molecular analysis of gene fragments, and various methods of polymerase chain reaction (PCR) has resulted in reclassification of some microorganisms and of rapid identification of pathogens, including microorganisms that cannot be cultivated by conventional means. Developments in this field are shifting the focus of clinical microbiology laboratories from morphologic and biochemical testing to molecular testing.

Several intrinsic properties relate to transmission and long-term survival of infectious agents. Persistence outside the host depends on requirements for replication (viruses replicate only within the cells of their host, whereas bacteria often can grow in food or milk) and on viability under natural conditions of temperature, moisture, and radiation. The ability of agents to persist determines whether transmission requires direct contact, as with influenzaviruses, or can involve indirect mechanisms operating over longer periods. Examples include polioviruses, typhoid bacilli, and the bacteria that cause Legionnaires' disease.

The spectrum of animals and arthropods that an agent can infect (the host range) helps determine the possibilities for the transmission of and the reservoirs for that agent. The broader the range, the greater the possibilities. Agents that are transmitted by arthropod vectors include St. Louis encephalitis virus and *Borrelia burgdorferi,* the cause of Lyme disease. The former can be transmitted by a wide variety of mosquitoes, whereas the latter is transmitted by a limited number of species of ticks. Among agents that do not require a vector, many infect only humans (diphtheria bacillus, the meningococcus, and measles virus), whereas others have multiple natural hosts (rabies virus, most *Salmonella* bacteria).

Elaboration of exotoxins is an intrinsic attribute of many bacteria and in many instances contributes in varying degrees to the pathogenesis of disease and indirectly to immunity. Another factor is susceptibility to chemotherapeutic agents or antibiotics. Successful treatment may shorten the period of communicability, as in group A streptococcal and *Bordetella pertussis* infections, but it may lead to relaxed vigilance for infection; syphilis, gonorrhea, and HIV (since the development of highly active anti-retroviral therapy) are notable examples.

The instability of some intrinsic characteristics as a result of the emergence of genetically different populations because of mutations, selective pressure, transfer of genes or plasmids between bacteria, or genetic recombination can be important. One example is the resistance to chemotherapeutic or antibiotic agents that may result from selective pressure (the probable explanation for the rapid acquisition of multiple antibiotic resistance by gonococci and in human immunodeficiency virus [HIV] or plasmid transfer of resistance to antibiotics among enteric bacteria). Antibiotic resistance is of increasing importance, as exemplified by the appearance of multidrug-resistant *Mycobacterium tuberculosis,* penicillin-resistant pneumococci, methicillin-resistant staphylococci, and carbapenem-resistant *Klebsiella pneumoniae.*[13]

Change in antigenic character can diminish the effectiveness of immunity and complicate specific recognition of infection. Influenza A virus is the classic example, with periodic major changes *(shift)* occurring in either or both crucial surface antigens, hemagglutinin and neuraminidase, associated with pandemic disease and progressive minor changes in hemagglutinin in the interpandemic period. Finally, the emergence of new diseases, such as St. Louis encephalitis, which first affected humans in Paris, Illinois, in 1932, or the appearance of a known disease in a new reservoir, possibly exemplified by the emergence of West Nile virus in North America in the early 2000s, can be the result of adaptation of the agent to a new host.[3]

Epidemiologic Properties Relating to the Host

Some epidemiologically important properties of infectious agents can be defined only with reference to specific hosts. Such properties include infectivity, pathogenicity, virulence, and immunogenicity.

Infectivity. Infectivity (ability to invade and multiply in a host) is measured conceptually in terms of the minimal number of infective particles required to establish an infection. This number, which can vary from one host to another and within the same host depending on the portal of entry, host age, and, in some cases, medications, can be determined only experimentally. Except for benign agents with which challenge of human volunteers is permissible, the infectivity of agents for humans must be inferred from the facility with which they spread in populations or, more directly, from the frequency with which infection

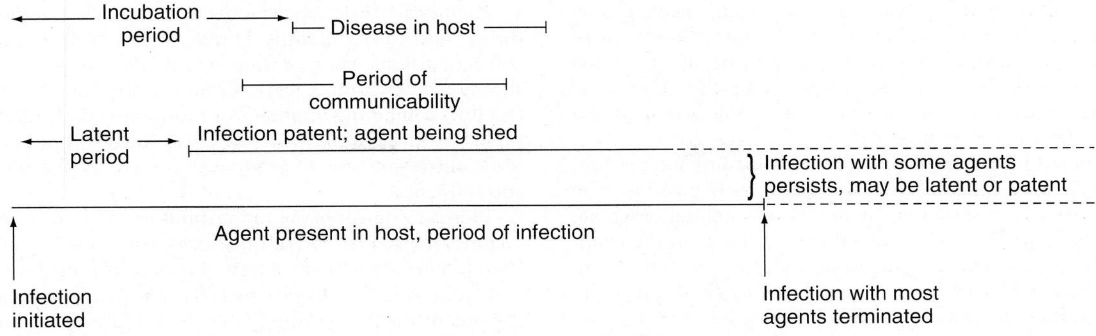

FIG. 6.2 Important phases of infection in vertebrate hosts.

develops in exposed susceptible individuals within a reasonable incubation period *(secondary attack rate).* Some researchers have used prisoners to study infectivity of *Salmonella* and *Shigella,* but the ethics of such studies has now been questioned.[38] Measles, varicella, and polioviruses are highly infective because they require few infective particles to cause infection; rubella, mumps, and rhinoviruses have intermediate infectivity; and salmonellae and tubercle bacilli have low infectivity. Infectivity and pathogenicity may vary among strains of the same organism. The infectivity of group A streptococci is related directly to the amount of M protein in the cell wall, and strains of *Staphylococcus aureus* that appear identical in the laboratory may differ strikingly in infectivity and virulence. Additionally, some evidence indicates that strains of influenza A may vary in infectivity and virulence independent of preexisting immunity in the host. Contemporary studies show that variation in certain genes that are not ordinarily expressed in the clinical diagnostic laboratory are responsible for these variations in infectivity.

Pathogenicity. Pathogenicity (ability to induce disease) is measured in terms of the proportion of infections that result in disease. It ordinarily can be determined readily by studies of the incidence and outcome of naturally occurring infections in humans. This proportion may be affected by the size of the infecting dose and numerous host factors, including age. Highly pathogenic agents include typhoid bacilli, rabies, measles, varicella, and rhinoviruses. Agents of intermediate pathogenicity include rubella, mumps, and adenoviruses; polioviruses and the tubercle bacillus have low pathogenicity.

Virulence. Virulence may sometimes be a synonym for *pathogenicity* but is defined more usefully as a measure of the severity of the disease that does occur. Various criteria may be used: days confined to bed, hospitalization rate, serious sequelae that require life support such as dialysis and mechanical ventilation and others such as persisting paralysis, and death. The measure of virulence is the number of severe cases over the total number of cases, which, when death is the criterion, becomes the familiar *case-fatality rate.* With this as our measure, the viral agents previously mentioned fall into a different gradient from that based on pathogenicity. Rabies virus (with a case-fatality rate of nearly 100%) qualifies as highly virulent, and poliovirus (with a case-fatality rate of 7% to 10% for paralytic disease) can be classed as moderately virulent. Measles, with an occasional death from encephalitis or pneumonia, is far down the scale but is still ahead of mumps, varicella, nonfetal rubella, and rhinoviruses, for which the case-fatality rates are very low. Outcomes of severity short of death such as days of intensive care utilization or of requirement for supplemental oxygen can be used in a similar fashion.

Immunogenicity. Immunogenicity (ability to induce specific immunity) is measured best functionally in terms of the degree and duration of resistance conferred by infection. Although agents may differ with respect to the immunogenicity of their intrinsic "protective antigens," more important factors are the sites of primary infection and disease and the amount of antigen formed during infection to stimulate a host response. Superficial sites, such as the respiratory mucosa, are guarded chiefly by secretory antibody, which is poorly persistent; agents such as rhinoviruses, which replicate only at such sites, are ineffective stimulants of the systemic immune response. The amounts of the respective toxins released during clinical tetanus and diphtheria usually do not induce satisfactory immunity. In contrast, systemic viral infections, such as with measles and yellow fever viruses, induce solid and long-lasting immunity.

Factors Related to Relationship Between Infectious Agent and Host

The infected host provides a shelter in which the agent can multiply and from which it may spread. Key questions involve how long the agent can persist in the host and over what period and by what avenues it can escape. The time relationships and descriptive terms of different phases of infection are suggested schematically in Fig. 6.2.

When the agent is not readily recoverable but perhaps is hidden within host cells or at some other site, infection is termed *latent.* Conversely, when the agent is being shed, as in feces or respiratory secretions, or can be recovered from blood or tissues, infection is said to be *patent.* Infections are necessarily latent at first (the *latent period*) and become patent when the agent has multiplied sufficiently for shedding to begin. The *period of communicability* commonly starts soon after initial shedding begins and continues as long as the level of shedding is sufficient for transmission. The rapidity with which disease is spread is related to the length of the latent period, which almost always is shorter (sometimes much shorter) than the better known *incubation period* (time until disease develops). The period of communicability has no consistent relationship to either the occurrence or the duration of disease.

Persistence in the host is important to the agent for as long as escape remains possible. The period of persistence (see Fig. 6.2) varies widely among agents. Infection terminates completely within 2 to 3 weeks with many agents, such as most respiratory viruses, and after a few months with some agents, such as polioviruses or adenoviruses. Truly persistent lifelong infections may become permanently latent, as with some herpesvirus group (Epstein-Barr virus, cytomegalovirus) infections. Infection may remain permanently patent (approximately 3% of typhoid cases, numerous hepatitis B virus infections), may be intermittently patent (herpes simplex virus infections [HSV]), or, after years of latency, may recrudesce with patency and associated disease (tuberculosis, Brill disease caused by *Rickettsia prowazekii,* varicella zoster virus [herpes zoster]).

Reservoirs of infectious agents. *Reservoir* is defined as any entity (living [e.g., animal or plant] or not [e.g., soil]) in which the infectious agent can survive. The reservoir may also serve as the site from which the agent can be transmitted to living hosts or to vectors. The reservoir may be a continuing chain of transmission from one host to another (including vertebrate and invertebrate species). Chains with long links requiring infrequent transmission are especially favorable to survival of agent species.

Among agents for which humans are the only natural vertebrate host, many contrasting patterns exist. The most common is exemplified by infections with most respiratory viruses, which are characterized by short latent periods (1 to several days) and short periods of communicability (rarely >1 week). The links are short, and frequent transmission is necessary. At the other extreme are long-persisting infections associated with continuous (typhoid carriers, hepatitis B virus, HIV) or intermittent (HSV) *patency* or shedding. The links in this case may be as long as the postinfection life of the host and render generation-to-generation transmission possible. Such transmission also may occur via congenital infection, as in mice infected with lymphocytic choriomeningitis virus. Examples in humans include cytomegalovirus and hepatitis B virus infections. Long links also occur in persistent infections that, after many years of latency, recrudesce to cause disease and renewed shedding (varicella zoster virus and *R. prowazekii*).

When infection of invertebrate hosts (vectors) is a link in the chain of transmission, a wide range of reservoir patterns is possible. The simplest involves agents for which humans are the only natural vertebrate hosts (malarial parasites, *R. prowazekii,* dengue virus), with the chain consisting of alternating links of human and vector infection. More commonly, the basic reservoir is a similar alternating chain primarily involving lower vertebrate hosts, with humans being an opportunistic and usually blind-end host. Examples include murine typhus rickettsiae and plague bacillus (both cycling primarily in rats and rat fleas), Lyme disease, and various arboviruses (yellow fever, St. Louis encephalitis). In the case of the latter, the broad vertebrate (numerous avian and mammalian species) and invertebrate (various mosquito species) host range results in very complex patterns that in a given area are defined by the prevalent susceptible host species. The links in these chains are defined temporally by the persistence of patent infection in the vertebrate host and the short life span of the invertebrate host.

Several aspects of infection of the invertebrate (vector) host are important. Typically, infection is acquired in a blood meal and endures for (and does not influence) the life span of the arthropod. Hibernating arthropods may be the long link in the chain by which the agent survives the winter. In at least two instances, infection kills the vector: *R. prowazekii* in the body louse and plague bacilli in the rat flea. As with malaria, infection of the arthropod also may permit completion of an essential stage in the developmental cycle of the agent. Finally, transmission of infection from arthropod to arthropod may be alternate or necessary links in the chain. Transovarial transmission of *Rickettsia tsutsugamushi* (scrub typhus) in mites is essential because the individual mite feeds only once, during the larval stage, on vertebrate hosts. Transovarial transmission also occurs in ticks infected with *Rickettsia rickettsii* (Rocky Mountain spotted fever) and in *Aedes triseriatus* mosquitoes infected with La Crosse virus (California encephalitis), in both cases affording an overwintering mechanism. Venereal transmission of La Crosse virus between mosquitoes has also been shown.[71]

Finally, the inanimate environment can play a role in the reservoir mechanism. Examples are bacteria that can multiply in the free state (salmonellae and staphylococci in food) and agents endowed with unusual survival capacity (tetanus bacillus and *Histoplasma capsulatum,* both of which form highly resistant spores). It also occurs when a brief sojourn under proper environmental conditions is required for a necessary stage in the life cycle (e.g., hookworm eggs from human feces must hatch into larvae to become infectious).

Mechanisms of transmission. *Transmission,* in this context, is defined as the transport of an agent from one vertebrate host to another. It involves escape from the source host and conveyance to and entry into the recipient host. The basic interdependence of these sequential steps is illustrated in Table 6.3, which also presents specific examples of diseases. Although humans are the usual or only source for most agents of human disease, lower vertebrates serve as the major or only (rabies virus) source for some pathogens.

Fomites are intimate personal articles, such as handkerchiefs, playthings, and eating utensils. *Direct contact* includes not only physical contact (shaking hands, kissing, sexual intercourse) but also, in practice, short-range (within 3 feet), airborne transmission by large droplets (>5 μm) containing hundreds or thousands of organisms that descend rapidly to the ground or floor. These heavy droplets are the primary route of transmission of group A streptococcal pharyngitis,[73] pertussis, and influenza.

Indirect transmission for respiratory and some other infections includes the acquisition of organisms from dust (e.g., tubercle bacilli), from fomites (inanimate objects in the environment such as bedding[51]), and from airborne droplet nuclei (<5 μm) containing only one or a few organisms that promptly dry, float in the air for long periods, and may be wafted for moderately long distances, and even between rooms or floors in a hospital. Transmission by airborne droplet nuclei is limited to highly infectious agents such as varicella virus. Because respiratory colonization with group A streptococci requires a large inoculum, airborne droplet nuclei play no role in their transmission. Other forms of indirect transmission include inanimate vectors such as food, milk, and water, which are frequent vehicles for spread, particularly of intestinal infections. Another source of indirect transmission is animate vectors, which either may function as a vehicle for transport (as with flies that carry organisms from feces to food) or may be infected. In the latter case, multiplication and transformation in the vector are required for transmission, as with African trypanosomiasis and the tsetse fly.

Conveyance ends when the agent reaches a portal of entry, which to be effective must provide ready access to a tissue in which the pathogen can lodge and multiply. For a given agent, a particular portal (nasal, genital, or oral mucosa) often is obligatory or usual, but alternative portals may be possible. Rhinoviruses replicate only in nasal mucosa, whereas typhus rickettsiae typically enter through skin broken by a louse bite but also can infect via ocular or respiratory mucous membranes.

Factors Related to the Host

Many biologic and behavioral characteristics of the human host influence the occurrence of infection and subsequent disease. Although the host characteristics to be considered are of widely differing nature, they operate by influencing one or more of the following: degree of exposure, innate susceptibility to infection, and the likelihood of specific immunity. Although much of the following discussion focuses on the individual human host, factors that influence individuals also affect whole human populations. A key principle to be emphasized is the usual existence of a gradient of response to exposure to an infectious agent. Because of this gradient, the occurrence of characteristic overt disease is a notably unreliable measure of the extent of activity of a disease agent. Given a particular exposure, infection may not occur, disease may not result, or the consequences may range from trivial to the fully developed syndrome "characteristic" of the agent. Accumulating data indicate that specific host genes may be responsible for differences in host susceptibility.

An inadequate challenge dose, an unsuitable portal of entry, or specific host immunity also may explain failure of infection to develop. Whether infection causes disease and the extent, nature, and outcome of the resulting disease are determined partly by host-related properties

TABLE 6.3 Typical Modes of Transmission From Host, Conveyance, and Portal of Entry

Agent Shed via	How Conveyed	Portal of Entry	Disease Example
Respiratory secretions	Airborne droplets, fomites, or direct contact	Respiratory	Common cold, influenza, respiratory syncytial virus
Feces	Food, fomites, water, flies	Oral	Poliomyelitis, typhoid, rotavirus
Blood	Arthropod vector, transfusion, needle stick	Skin—via insect bite, intravenous device	Typhus, dengue, malaria, human immunodeficiency virus, hepatitis B and C
Lesion exudate	Direct contact, sexual intercourse, fomites, flies	Skin, genital, or ocular mucous membrane	Syphilis, trachoma, staphylococcal abscess
Aerosols	Droplet nuclei, direct inhalation	Respiratory	Tuberculosis, varicella

of the agent (pathogenicity and virulence) and partly by host defense mechanisms, a variety of which confront an infectious agent that has reached a site of primary infection. Bacteria and other extracellular parasites stimulate an inflammatory response at the site that is an effort to localize the invaders by a retaining fibrin network, as well as cytokines that are produced by the host; the invaders are destroyed by congregating numerous phagocytic cells. Invader organisms may meet sinusoidal passages lined by phagocytic cells in regional (lymph nodes) and bloodstream (bone marrow, spleen, and liver) filters. In addition, clinicians are beginning to understand the importance of innate immunity. This complex network of receptors and responders prevents invader microorganisms from gaining access to tissues. In addition to physical barriers already mentioned, the innate immune system includes a family of receptors known as the Toll-like receptors. These recognition molecules signal the host to activate numerous protective mechanisms. Discussion of this system is beyond the scope of this chapter.

Several aspects of the outcome of infection are important, the first being survival of the host. Death is an unsatisfactory outcome not only for the host but also for the many agents for which survival as a species depends on continued transmission by the host. The remaining aspects relate to the surviving host. Was recovery from disease complete, or were permanent sequelae present? If the latter, were they stationary (as in paralysis resulting from polioviruses) or potentially progressive (rheumatic heart disease resulting from streptococcal infection, pulmonary tuberculosis)? Another aspect, persistence of the agent, was discussed previously (see "Factors Related to Relationship Between Infectious Agent and Host"). The final aspect is the state of postinfection resistance. If it is incomplete, the recovered host may experience reinfection, with or without disease, and may again become a source of infection for others.

Biologic Factors

Biologic factors include characteristics such as age, sex, and race (ethnic group), which are so important and easily ascertained that determining their relationship to occurrence of disease is a usual first step in an epidemiologic description. Biologic factors also include genetic makeup, general health status, and specific immunity.

Age

The influence of age is illustrated best by patterns of common diseases such as varicella, measles, and mumps before the advent of vaccines. All three diseases occur predominantly in young children who are affected because of their usual lack of immunity and their high risk of exposure to other children, among whom most infections occur. Older individuals are likely to be immune and, unless they are parents of young children, are less likely to be exposed to infected individuals. Vaccines that provide only temporary immunity could cause a shift to an older age at presentation in the population.

Age is also often related to the outcome of infections in nonimmune individuals. Demonstration of the influence of age requires that all infections be recognized and classified according to the severity of the resulting disease (if any). When many or most infections are subclinical (as with polioviruses and other enteroviruses), the increase in the case-fatality rate with age is apparent immediately, but special studies to document asymptomatic or mild infections are required to show that the proportion of infections that resulted in clinical disease also increased with age. In contrast, the case-fatality rate for pertussis is highest in young infants. With measles and varicella zoster virus, initial infection at any age usually results in characteristic disease, but the frequency of serious disease increases with age.

Sex, Race, and Ethnicity

That sex may be a factor is illustrated by the fact that most infectious diseases typically occur more frequently in males than females. The question, with respect to any particular disease, is whether these differences between sexes reflect innate differences in susceptibility to disease or can be attributed to sex-associated differences in behavior, occupation, or stress. The increased rate and poorer outcome of infection in male neonates suggests a true biologic difference.

The incidence of many diseases varies greatly among groups defined by race or ethnic group. This variation may be explained by differences in behavior or environment for which socioeconomic status is a marker. Ethnic groups share many genetically determined traits, however, which may include either heightened susceptibility or increased resistance to specific infectious agents. Selective evolutionary pressure may be invoked to explain the greater resistance of whites to tuberculosis and the heightened resistance of blacks to malaria.[1] Differences in host susceptibility based on race, familial clustering, and ethnicity are being investigated at the genomic level now that the code for the whole human genome has been elucidated. Current investigations are directed at discovering polymorphisms of genes that involve the immune response.

General Health Status

General health status includes the physiologic state, nutritional status, presence of intercurrent disease, and stress. The importance of such factors is commonly accepted in many cases but rarely documented by well-controlled studies. Infancy, during which immune mechanisms are immature, is a period of special vulnerability to many infectious diseases. HSV, enteroviruses, and group B streptococci manifest as disseminated infections in neonates, in marked contrast to their presentation in older individuals. Puberty, associated with rapid growth and change in endocrine balance, is a period of vulnerability to acne and tuberculosis. Pregnancy predisposes to more severe and life-threatening influenza, tuberculosis, paralytic poliomyelitis, and varicella.

Gross protein malnutrition causes definite impairment in the cell-mediated immune response,[32] a correspondingly increased susceptibility to bacterial and parasitic infections, and increased morbidity and mortality in many viral infections. Viral infections may depress cell-mediated immunity (and increase susceptibility further) to other concurrent infections. In the developing world, where malnutrition may be epidemic, the consequences of diarrhea, measles, and other respiratory virus infections are many times more devastating. Diarrheal diseases also may be the cause and the consequence of malnutrition. Patients with diabetes are especially vulnerable to bacterial infections; measles and pertussis may reactivate quiescent tuberculosis; and, perhaps of greatest importance, otherwise benign respiratory viral infections, notably influenza, may pave the way for development of serious bacterial pneumonia. Infection with HIV enhances the susceptibility to and severity of tuberculosis, toxoplasmosis, and many other infections.

Finally, stress induced by widely divergent stimuli (including strong emotions, physical exertion, trauma, or excessive heat or cold), according to Selye,[63] may operate through a pituitary-adrenocortical hormonal path to decrease resistance to infections. Widely accepted examples include physical exertion, child bearing, and rearing of children as factors predisposing to paralytic poliomyelitis and pregnancy and rapid growth during puberty as causes of reactivation of quiescent tuberculosis. The living conditions and stresses of military training are associated with an increased rate of respiratory tract infections, including invasive meningococcal disease.

Immunity and Immune Response

Immunity and immune response to viruses warrant special attention. Although important in recovery from bacterial infection, antibody response is of questionable significance in viral infections because viruses within cells are inaccessible to antibody, and, by the time antibody appears, many or most susceptible cells have been infected already. Nonetheless, the importance of antibody in viral infections is suggested by the great vulnerability of immunodeficient children to vaccine strains of poliovirus, other enteroviruses, and varicella and by the sometimes beneficial effect of passive immunoprophylaxis in preventing measles and hepatitis B. The benefits of previous experience with viruses can be seen with the decreased severity of rotavirus infections following the first bout of rotavirus and the protection afforded by varicella zoster immunoglobulin in highly vulnerable children.

At its maximum (exemplified by postinfection immunity to measles), protection against infection is virtually absolute. At the other extreme (exemplified by many respiratory viral infections), susceptibility to infection persists or wanes, as with pertussis, although the severity of related disease may be reduced. In most instances, protection seems to be mediated by antibody, but cell-mediated immunity also may be important. Children with defects in cell-mediated immunity are at particular risk for acquiring infection with varicella, *Pneumocystis carinii*, and otherwise noninvasive fungi.

To the extent that immunity protects the individual against infection or acts to minimize shedding of the agent when infection occurs, an immune host can play little or no part in the spread of an infectious agent in the population. If a sufficient proportion of a population is immune, an agent transmitted via contact cannot spread, and nonimmune members of the population would be spared exposure. The concept of *herd immunity* assumes that a nonimmune individual is protected from a communicable infection by being surrounded by immune individuals. The same concept is now referred to as *cocooning* when referring to protection of young infants in a family. What proportion must be immune to achieve effective herd immunity usually is unknown.[21] This concept is valid only in homogeneous, randomly mixing populations in which all possible pairs of individuals have the same probability of making effective contact. Although measles vaccine has been used extensively in the United States, outbreaks of measles continue to occur in segments of the population who group together in small communities and fail to accept vaccine; these groups are often defined by beliefs, race, economic status, and social behavior.

Human Behavior

Governed largely by habits of the individual and the customs and culture of groups, human behavior greatly influences exposure to and modes of transmission of infectious agents. Cultural factors also underlie attitudes toward preventive and curative practices.

Water is a potential vehicle for many agents. When commonly imbibed without boiling, as in the United States, community water systems constitute potential channels for transmission that usually are well guarded. Occasional operational failures occur, as exemplified by failure of a water quality–monitoring device in a filtration plant that resulted in an outbreak of *Cryptosporidium* diarrhea affecting an estimated 403,000 individuals in Milwaukee in 1993.[39] Foods and milk, especially items that are consumed raw or after minimal cooking, likewise are excellent vehicles for transmission of disease. Well-known examples include trichinosis from undercooked pork; bacterial enteritis from unpasteurized milk; fish tapeworm from raw fish; and various forms of food poisoning caused by bacterial contamination during handling, poor refrigeration, and inadequate cooking. In recent years, outbreaks of hemorrhagic diarrhea caused by *Escherichia coli* O157:H7, sometimes associated with hemolytic-uremic syndrome, have occurred as a result of improperly prepared products of bovine origin, particularly ground beef, but also vegetables and fruits.[53]

Closely related to water and foods is the disposal of human excreta. Casual defecation near habitations or in or near running water leads to dissemination of enteric pathogens by filth flies and by water. The use of human feces (night soil) to fertilize crops commonly eaten raw, such as strawberries and lettuce, has an obvious similar potential.

Many more individual types of behavior also are important. Infrequent bathing and laundering of clothes favors infestation with body lice. Inadequate clothing increases exposure to arthropod vectors and, as in young children lightly clad for summer weather, facilitates the exchange of feces. Going barefoot provides exposure to hookworm larvae. Hand washing minimizes the role of hands in indirect transmission of enteric (fecal) and respiratory (nasal secretion) pathogens. Rhinovirus infections result from inserting contaminated fingers into the nose and eyes.[27] Intimate personal contact such as hand shaking, kissing, and play among young children fosters the spread of a wide variety of agents. Even recreation, such as travel, picnics, and camping, may lead to unusual exposure to infectious agents. Sexual behavior is associated with the transmission of numerous infections, including HIV, syphilis, gonorrhea, group B streptococci, and hepatitis B.

Factors Related to the Environment

The environment in concept embraces all that is external to the individual human host. There are three broad environmental areas: *physical*, which includes geologic and climatologic or meteorologic features; *biologic*, which consists of all flora and fauna and all living microbial pathogens; and *socioeconomic*, which encompasses the interrelationships of humans.

Environmental factors often act through indirect paths, and some have the potential to affect the agent, the host, and the agent–host relationship. Solar radiation is lethal for many pathogens in the free state, helps humans synthesize vitamin D, and can provoke recrudescence of a latent HSV infection and result in recurrent fever blisters. The capacity of humans to modify adverse environmental conditions beneficially is another important factor.

Geographic and Geologic Factors

Spread of infectious agents on a global scale requires their transport, which is influenced by distance alone and by geographic features—mountain ranges, oceans, rivers—that assist or impede travel. The importance of these factors declines as the extent and speed of travel increase, but it remains substantial, especially in developing countries. The minimal effect of geographic barriers in containing highly infective agents is overcome by modern travel, and rapid spread by airline travel is exemplified by epidemics of severe acute respiratory syndrome (SARS), which spread from China throughout the world in a matter of weeks.[48]

The natural paths of travel (including waterways), natural harbors, and the location of mineral deposits help determine where populations concentrate. Water supply, dependent in part on geologic formations, is a factor limiting population size and, together with fossil fuels and mineral deposits, influences the type, extent, and location of industrial development. Soil types vary greatly in their ability to hold and purify water and in their capacity to support vegetation, which influences the type and abundance of animal life. Soil is a determinant of the type and importance of agriculture and a major factor influencing the biologic environment.

Climate

The term *climate* describes the typical annual pattern, along with its seasonal variation, of weather conditions in a specified region. Such conditions (climatologic factors) include solar radiation, temperature, humidity, barometric pressure, winds, precipitation (and drought), and lightning. These factors can affect infectious disease agents directly. Many microbial agents in the free-living state are vulnerable to excessive heat and radiation and uncontrolled drying. The life cycles and reservoir mechanisms of many pathogens, including higher parasites, depend on appropriate temperature and humidity. Maturation and hatching of hookworm larvae from ova deposited in the soil require warmth and reasonable humidity, and the multiplication of malarial parasites and arboviruses in their mosquito vectors and the abundance of the vectors are favored by warm temperatures.

The usual seasonal variation in the incidence of specific infectious diseases suggests important influences of climatologic factors, but how they operate may be hard to determine. Overall, respiratory tract infections occur more frequently in colder months, but within this period (roughly October through mid-May in the Northern Hemisphere) the prevalence of the many respiratory pathogens varies greatly. Rhinoviruses peak in the early fall and spring, and influenza viruses are most active in midwinter. Parainfluenza virus type 1 and 2 infections usually peak in the fall. Increased congregation of people indoors facilitates transmission, and fluctuations in temperature and humidity not only affect the viability of agents in airborne droplet nuclei or on fingers or fomites but also may affect host susceptibility to infection.

Enterically transmitted infections occur most frequently in the warmer months, presumably largely because of season-related changes in host behavior. The outdoor play of scantily clad children facilitates the spread of skin infection and fecally shed agents such as enteroviruses. Rotavirus infections are an exception in that they occur most frequently in colder months. More completely understood are the seasonal patterns of infections spread by arthropod vectors; these patterns reflect seasonal variations in the abundance and activity of the vectors and the various lower vertebrate host species, which together constitute the reservoir mechanisms of the specific infectious agents. Climate overall, as a major determinant of the biologic environment, helps determine the abundance and the particular species of flora and fauna in a given area. In the 2000s, there has been considerable interest in the effects of global warming on rates of infectious diseases.

Longer term changes in climate have been associated with changes in patterns of infection. The hantavirus outbreak in the southwestern United States in 1993 has been attributed to unusually heavy precipitation in the spring of 1993 after 6 years of drought. This precipitation resulted in marked proliferation of the deer mouse population, the reservoir of the virus.[74]

Socioeconomic Conditions

Socioeconomic factors depend on the density and distribution of populations; the available natural resources; the level of social, political, cultural, and scientific development; and, most important, the interrelationships of people. These factors typically affect health by indirect means, and, because they often are interrelated closely, the impact of individual factors is very difficult to determine.

The relationship of population distribution and density to the occurrence of infectious diseases is substantial. Increasing density favors the spread of infectious agents to humans from human and nonhuman sources and the occurrence of related disease and development of immunity. In large and dense populations, agents such as measles virus typically infect in early childhood and persist because a sufficient number of new susceptible individuals are added continuously by birth. In smaller populations, the agents are unable to persist and are reintroduced at unpredictable intervals; as a result, manifestations of "childhood" diseases may be delayed for long periods. Populations of urban and rural areas differ not only in relative density but also in other important ways. Exposure to zoonotic agents, especially agents prevalent in wildlife and livestock, is greater in rural areas, although rats and stray dogs may abound in city slums. Environmental sanitation (protection of water and milk supplies, safe disposal of sewage) often is a personal problem for rural residents but is handled by cooperative effort in wealthier urban populations. In addition, the importance of schools and school buses in facilitating exchange of infectious agents is greater in rural areas, where isolation of farm residents otherwise restricts contact among young children.

The basic population unit is the *household,* membership in which has similar implications for health in rural and urban areas. Family members are similar genetically; share a common diet and economic status; are subject to the same cultural, religious, and educational influences; and are exposed to a common local physical and biologic environment. Most important for contact-transmitted diseases, intrafamilial contact is prolonged and increases in intimacy with household crowding. In the winter, many homes are insulated and the windows are closed so that air exchange is poor and exposure to airborne organisms is great. Prolonged contact is especially important for persisting infections such as HSV infection and tuberculosis. Family size, regardless of the degree of crowding, is particularly important for acute infections because it determines the number of potential introducers who bring home infections acquired elsewhere. The likelihood of exposure in early childhood increases with family size. Except for early infancy, a period of special vulnerability to some agents (e.g., respiratory syncytial virus, pertussis), early exposure is beneficial because most resulting infections are less likely to have serious consequences.

A population with a highly developed *social and political structure,* through its capacity for cooperative action, enjoys many advantages that directly or indirectly benefit health, including provision of preventive and curative health services, effective environmental sanitation, and well-developed educational facilities. Education closely relates to personal health practices that are based on understanding what individuals should do to minimize disease hazards. Schools, where the educational process begins, are important factors in the exchange of infectious agents among children, especially agents spread by contact and airborne droplet nuclei. This matter is offset partly by the benefits derived from school-based immunization programs.

Economic status affects the occurrence of diseases indirectly through its relationship to adequacy of housing, nutrition, level of education, sanitation, and availability and use of health services. It is also related closely to occupation, which may be associated with exposure to specific infections, such as Rocky Mountain spotted fever (forest workers and hikers in the south Atlantic coast states) and ornithosis (workers in poultry-processing plants).

Occurrence of Disease in Populations

Patterns of occurrence of disease that are not random but instead reflect the influence of underlying causes (risk factors) not only help predict future occurrence of disease but also provide important clues to understanding causation. Describing the pattern of occurrence of disease begins with definition and classification of disease in the individual so that cases can be identified and counted reliably. The occurrence of disease in defined populations can be expressed quantitatively.

Infection and Disease in the Individual

Epidemiologic interest focuses on the specific etiologic identification of *infection* and *disease,* terms that are not synonyms. Technically, any deviation from normal function or state constitutes *disease.* Because virtually all infections cause at least some deviation from the normal state (e.g., a change in the white blood cell pattern and mobilization of such cells at the site of infection), they cause disease. In practice, many infections result in no clinical evidence of disease and are important to the individual only for the reason that they induce immunity. Because subclinical infections help define the overall pattern of occurrence of infection and often play a significant role in its spread, their recognition is important epidemiologically. Subclinical infections go unrecognized except when healthy individuals are observed for infection in longitudinal or case-control studies.

Only infections resulting in disease usually come to the attention of the medical community. To the extent that they are recognized etiologically, they provide the earliest and most available indicator of the pattern of infection in the population.

With few exceptions, such as measles and chickenpox, typical clinical syndromes are not pathognomonic and require the clinician to develop a differential diagnosis. Basically, clinical manifestations depend more on the site or sites of disease than on the infecting agent. Because the number of possible disease targets in the body is small and the number of potential agents is large, reasonably distinct clinical entities may be caused by any of several agents. Notable examples include "common colds," approximately 40% of which are caused by rhinoviruses and 60% by any of many other viruses, and aseptic meningitis, which may be caused by such agents as mumps virus, many enteroviruses, or *B. burgdorferi.*

Infection with a specific agent may have several possible clinical outcomes. Infection with polioviruses usually is (perhaps 80%) subclinical but can result in brief febrile illness (approximately 15%), aseptic meningitis (4% to 5%), or classic paralytic disease (<1%). The response to agents with multiple potential targets varies even more widely. Group B Coxsackie viruses can cause such disparate entities as acute upper respiratory tract disease, aseptic meningitis, polio-like paralytic disease, myocarditis, and epidemic pleurodynia (Bornholm disease).

Knowledge of the agents active in the community when a given illness occurs helps narrow the differential diagnosis, but confirming etiologic diagnosis requires laboratory assistance by culturing the agent, direct visualization in specimens, antigen detection, genome identification using molecular techniques, or demonstration of a specific antibody response in tests of "acute" and "convalescent" serum pairs.[2] The diagnosis is most secure when both approaches suggest infection with the same agent. Although demonstration of the agent in relation to the disease site carries special weight (e.g., in a pharyngeal swab specimen from a respiratory illness), its presence could be the result of preexisting persisting infection unrelated to the current illness. A significant antibody response in paired serum (acute and convalescent) indicates a newly acquired infection.

Infection and Disease in Populations

Sources of information. Many sources provide data regarding the incidence of infectious diseases, including U.S. Vital Statistics, which tabulates only fatal cases; the Centers for Disease Control and Prevention (CDC), which receives reports of specific notifiable diseases from state health departments and summarizes them in the *Morbidity and Mortality Weekly Report*; and state and local health departments. In the absence of a focused surveillance project, these data vary in their completeness by source and by disease because of underreporting, subjects who are not seen, and errors in diagnosis.

Among the different states, reporting requirements vary, and adherence to these requirements by providers also varies. Reporting is most complete for uncommon but characteristic disorders of unusual interest, particularly if they are severe or fatal and require hospitalization, such as rabies, anthrax, trichinosis, plague, and diphtheria. Reporting is enhanced by outbreaks, as with measles, mumps, and classic pertussis in recent years. Some notifiable infections, such as leptospirosis and atypical pertussis in partially immune individuals, often are unrecognized and are underreported. Reporting requirements may change from year to year based on CDC or state interests (e.g., neonatal sepsis and West Nile infection) or concerns about bioterrorism. Another source of data often useful in certain areas is state health department laboratories, which perform specific microbiologic or serologic tests for providers.

Infectious diseases that are not notifiable by law pose a difficult problem. Although necessarily limited in scale, longitudinal studies of defined populations of families have yielded valuable information. Finally, researchers now can use well-designed serosurveys to make reliable estimates of rates of previous infection with agents that induce long-persisting antibody.

International data on the incidence of infectious diseases are less precise except in well-developed countries. For the developing world, the World Health Organization (WHO) and the United Nations International Children's Emergency Fund provide estimates of the incidence of morbidity and mortality from various infectious diseases in different nations based on local reports, which are not always collected systematically. Continuing collection of such data is important for monitoring the effects of the Expanded Program of Immunization, which is directed at controlling the major vaccine-preventable diseases of childhood. More difficult to develop are definitive data about the incidence and causation of the respiratory and diarrheal diseases, which are estimated to kill 6 million children annually in the developing world (approximately 5% of the yearly birth cohort).

For developing these kinds of statistics, it is important to have a definition of disease that is as useful as possible, which means that the sensitivity and specificity of the definition should be so balanced that as many cases of the disease as possible are identified while avoiding the confusion that occurs when other disorders with overlapping manifestations meet criteria that are too nonspecific. A well-known example of a useful definition of disease is the Jones criteria for the diagnosis of rheumatic fever, established in 1944 at the request of the National Research Council in an effort to bring order out of chaos at a time when the disease was a major problem in the civilian and military populations.[30] These criteria subsequently have been modified to enhance their specificity by making evidence of a previous group A streptococcal infection a sine qua non for the reason that too many cases of polyarthritis of other causes met the original criteria.[18] Recently the Jones Criteria were revised. A less specific set of criteria were developed for areas of the world where acute rheumatic fever is common and the "pretest probability" is greater; a more specific set of criteria were developed for use where acute rheumatic fever is rare and less specific symptoms would be more likely to be due to another cause.[24] Similarly, the criteria for the diagnosis of Kawasaki disease were revised more recently to avoid missing some episodes in infants and missing the opportunity to prevent coronary artery aneurysms by using intravenous immunoglobulin.[44]

Recognizing the importance of standardized diagnostic criteria for surveillance of infectious diseases of public health importance, the CDC published in 1990 case definitions for reportable infections.[75] Optimal use of these criteria and reporting of confirmed and probable cases to the proper authorities are of particular importance currently, when, for a variety of reasons, some formerly well-controlled contagious diseases are becoming recrudescent (e.g., mumps, measles, pertussis). All states mandate reporting contagious diseases of major public health importance, particularly diseases affecting children.

Relating infection and disease to personal characteristics. Multiple characteristics may serve to distinguish one individual from another. Some factors are determined at conception—age, sex, ethnicity, genetic makeup, and birth order. Others, far more numerous, are acquired subsequently. They may be biologic (specific immunity, nutritional state), behavioral (smoking, dietary, recreational habits), or socioeconomic (occupation, educational level, marital status). Many of these characteristics relate to exposure to infectious agents or to susceptibility or resistance to the effects of such agents and to the occurrence and severity of disease.

Relative usefulness and importance of characteristics. Although almost any potentially relevant characteristic of an individual patient can be identified, it is not useful for purposes of description unless we can estimate how many people in the population also possess the characteristic. From census data or other accessible records, numbers of people in groups defined by age, sex, race, occupation, or marital status can be estimated easily. Special surveys would need to be conducted to estimate the prevalence of specific immunity or possibly significant exposure, such as to household pets.

The importance of personal characteristics to the description of a disease varies in two ways. One is in the degree of association that exists between a characteristic and a specific disease. Age is associated strongly with disease caused by prevalent contagious agents, whereas sex usually is not. The second way is in the independence or relative interdependence of characteristics as variables. Inherent characteristics, such as age, sex, and ethnic origin, are independent of one another, whereas acquired characteristics rarely are. The nature of interpersonal contacts, degree of personal hygiene, and usual forms of recreation are associated closely with age or sex or both. The common interdependence of characteristics means that before making an inference from a particular association, one should explore association with other, possibly correlated, characteristics.

Age patterns. The occurrence of infection and disease generally is related so strongly to age that until possible differences in age distribution are taken into account, differences in occurrence among population subgroups defined by other characteristics cannot be interpreted meaningfully. Age as a characteristic is ascertained easily and reliably for affected individuals and the total membership of the relevant population. Description of the age pattern involves computing a series of *age-specific rates* for sequential age groups, usually defined in intervals of 5 years or multiples thereof (e.g., birth to 4, 5 to 9, 10 to 19). For conditions of pediatric concern, the use of single-year intervals (<1, 1, 2, 3, and 4 years) to cover early childhood may be more informative. In some cases, especially in the first 2 years of life, a breakdown by months of age would be informative.

Affected individuals in an age group form the numerator, and all individuals in the population in that age group serve as the denominator. Rates so computed describe the age profile of immunity at a specified point in time (age-specific antibody prevalence rates), the age profile of new infections or disease (age-specific incidence rates), or the age profile of deaths caused by a disease (disease-specific and age-specific mortality rates). Age-specific incidence rates for acute infectious diseases indicate the risk of disease occurring in each age group and, depending on the disease agent, more or less accurately reflect the underlying age-specific infection rates.

Age adjustment of rates. The need to take age distribution into account when comparing disease in different populations is indicated when (1) the rates vary with age and (2) the distribution of the populations by age differs substantially. From published U.S. mortality data for 1983 and 1984, one can compare pneumonia and influenza mortality rates for Alaska and Florida. During those years, 89 deaths were recorded among 986,000 Alaskans at risk, for an annual mortality rate of 9/100,000. In contrast, in Florida, 4703 deaths occurred from pneumonia and influenza among the 21,792,000 residents at risk for those 2 years, for a rate of 21.6/100,000, nearly 2.5 times that of Alaska. These rates are called *crude mortality rates.* In this instance, these rates are misleading for the reasons that the likelihood of death occurring from pneumonia and influenza increases with age, and the age distributions of the populations of these two states differ markedly. National death rates from these infections are nearly 10-fold greater in people 65 to 74 years of age than in people 55 to 64 years of age. For those years, 17.5% and 3% of the Florida and Alaska populations, respectively, were 65 years or older.

To make a valid comparison of the pneumonia and influenza mortality rates for these two states, one must perform an age adjustment; this is a simple process that can be found in available texts of biostatistics and epidemiology. Briefly, one determines mortality rates for specific age groups (usually categorized within 5 or 10 years) for the two populations and calculates the deaths that would be expected in a common (or standard) population for the same age groupings by using the age-specific rates of the populations being compared, in this instance those of Alaska and Florida. Summation of these expected deaths permits calculation of the rates that would have occurred in the standard population if the age-specific rates of Alaska applied and if the age-specific rates of Florida applied. In this example, the age-adjusted mortality rate for pneumonia and influenza for Alaska is 35.2/100,000, and that for Florida is 21.8/100,000, nearly the reverse of the crude rates. (The combined population of the two states was used as the standard.)

These age-adjusted rates are not true rates; they are used for comparison. Although often applicable to infectious diseases, age-adjusted rates almost always are required for comparisons of morbidity and mortality from chronic diseases.

Sex patterns. Because sex is a readily ascertained characteristic of the membership of populations, the occurrence of infections and disease in relation to sex is described easily. Its simplest form is the *sex ratio,* or the ratio of cases in males to cases in females. This ratio is meaningful only when, as in childhood, the population is divided approximately equally by sex. Although the number of males exceeds the number of females at birth (106:100), the death rate for males exceeds that for females at all ages (average, 1.5:1). From approximately age 20 years on, females outnumber males, the difference increasing with age, which means that when comparing sex-specific rates, age adjustment must be made, or, better yet, the age profiles for the sexes should be compared directly so that important differences in the contour can be seen.

Ethnic or racial patterns. A third characteristic by which members of the population can be grouped in describing occurrence of disease is race or ethnic origin, the usefulness of which has decreased with the increasing frequency of mixed marriages. The U.S. census classification is based on information collected regarding race and native origin. Individuals of mixed racial parentage are classified by the race of the nonwhite parent or, if both are nonwhite, by that of the father. People of foreign birth are classified by country. Native-born children of foreign-born parents are identified as "foreign stock" and grouped according to parental origin. Census data provide estimates of population subgroups belonging to several "races" (white, black, Native American, Chinese, Japanese) or to "foreign stocks" (including foreign born and first generation). The U.S. Census further asks about ethnicity as a separate category and also separately asks whether the respondent is Hispanic or Latino.

Although controversial currently, this method yields differences in the occurrence of many infections and other diseases among such population subgroups. Knowledge of such differences is useful in case finding and organizing the application of specific preventive measures. Subgroups defined by ethnicity possess some similarity in genetic constitution that may determine susceptibility or resistance to specific agents. They also may be affected distinctively by environmental factors because of voluntary or involuntary differences in behavior and patterns of living.

Disease patterns in kinships. Genetically determined susceptibility and resistance to specific infectious agents have not yet been associated clearly with recognized genetic markers that could serve as a basis for defining population subgroups. Most efforts to look for genetic influences have been studies of occurrence of diseases in individuals of differing degrees of relationship within kinships or in the total memberships of different kinships. With rapid advancement in the database of the human genome, considerable interest has been generated in polymorphisms at loci that may define susceptibility to infectious diseases on a genetic basis. Populations with a high prevalence of certain alleles and known to have an increased risk of certain infections could be studied to determine whether the risk is due to abnormal function of the specified gene.

Family episodes of infection and disease. With respect to contact-transmitted infectious diseases, the family is more important as the basic epidemiologic subgroup of a population than for its shared genes. Observation of family units for episodes of infection and related illnesses has contributed significantly to knowledge of the epidemiology of widely prevalent infectious agents. The situation in all family studies begins with one member's infection, acquired from outside the house. That member then exposes the other family members. The introductory infection and any infections in family members who are exposed constitute a *family episode,* which is described basically in terms of the times of onset of the related infections and the identities (age, sex, position in the family) of the introducer and the infected and uninfected contacts.

Analysis of cumulated episodes of common respiratory illness, observed in the early studies, identified children as the most frequent introducers (important in community spread). Analysis also yielded estimates of the risk of cross-infection occurring within the family, expressed in terms of secondary attack rates among specified members (e.g., younger children) exposed to specified introducers (e.g., a schoolchild or a parent). Generally, the risk in contacts was related inversely to age overall, as a result of the influence of immunity, and to intimacy of within-family contact (ready exchange between spouses and between children nearest in age). Finally, the relationship of time between the onset of illness in the introducer and onset in family members exposed serves to define the range of incubation periods.

Analysis of the episodes can yield additional information concerning such crucial aspects as mode and duration of the agent's shedding; the spectrum of clinical response to infection, including the proportion that is subclinical; and the significance of previous immunity in the presence of close exposure, as measured by the frequency and clinical consequences of the reinfections that result. The results of the analysis of adenovirus episodes in the Virus Watch program are illustrative.[22] Virus appears regularly in the feces and less often (approximately 50%) in the pharynx, and shedding may be abortive (a few days only) or continue intermittently for many months. Overall, 50% of infections are subclinical, and illness, typically febrile and respiratory, occurs more commonly with pharyngeal excretion (65%) than with only fecal shedding (31%). Immunity is 85% protective against infection; reinfections that do occur usually are subclinical. Young children and especially infants younger than 2 years of age are the usual introducers, and within-family spread depends more on duration than on the mode of virus excretion by the introducer.

Socioeconomic patterns. *Socioeconomic status* covers a complex of characteristics, including levels of education and income and, less tangibly, "social standing." The problem is to discover a useful single indicator. One possibility is area of residence as classified by median income or measures that reflect housing standards, such as type of plumbing and average number of individuals per room. Relevant data are available for census tracts, which have proved useful when the tracts are homogeneous.

Occupation of the head of a household seems to be the one attribute most closely reflecting socioeconomic status. On this basis, the British have defined five broad social classes that directly apply to employed adults and can be extended to cover their dependents. These classes, in descending order, are professional, intermediate, skilled, partly skilled, and unskilled occupations. For use in the United States, based on census-recorded occupations, these terms have been translated as follows:

- Professional workers
- Non-farm technical, administrative, and managerial workers
- Clerical, sales, and skilled workers
- Semiskilled workers
- Non-farm laborers
- Farm workers of whatever level are included in a sixth group as agricultural workers

Relating Infection and Disease to Place

Place is of interest epidemiologically when occupied by humans and, unless indicated as relating to work, recreation, or travel, refers here to residence. Place usually is classified geographically (hemisphere, continent, nation) but also can be classified usefully by environmental characteristics such as climate, altitude, stage of economic development, population density, and urban or rural nature. Variations in occurrence of disease with place reflect parallel variations in the operation of causative factors and raise the question of whether these factors are to be found in the characteristics of the physical and biologic environment inherent to the place or in the characteristics of the inhabitants. The former is suggested when the age-adjusted risk of disease increases for immigrants and decreases for emigrants, when risk does not vary among the ethnic groups present, and when similar ethnic groups in other places enjoy a lower risk. One also must consider possible differences in reliability and completeness of recognition and reporting of disease.

Global variation. On the global scale, the WHO collects and publishes information concerning the occurrences of diseases derived from statistics compiled routinely within nations for morbidity from notifiable infectious diseases and for causes of death. The great variations among nations in the quality and availability of medical care and other health services result in corresponding variations in the reliability and completeness of the data collected by the WHO. Generally basic demographic data and the quality and availability of health services are equally good in well-developed countries, so specific disease rates can be compared. In less developed countries, demographic data may be inaccurate and medical services may be inconsistent in quality and concentrated in urban populations, within which their availability varies with economic status. Many illnesses and deaths are unattended medically, especially in rural areas, and births commonly are attended by midwives. Because infant deaths are reported more completely than births are, infant mortality rates may be unreliable.

With respect to infectious and parasitic diseases, knowledge of the frequency of disease is less important than is qualitative knowledge of the distribution and spread of disease. Such knowledge guides the application and enforcement of international control measures and is the basis for advice given by physicians to prospective foreign travelers. Important diseases, such as yellow fever, plague, and cholera, because of their high case-fatality rate and characteristic clinical picture, are almost certain to come to attention when substantial numbers of cases occur. Such knowledge may not be publicized, however, or may not be promptly available. Some countries, in the hope that a new outbreak (perhaps of cholera) will be controlled soon, may withhold information to avoid discouraging economically important tourists.

Two additional considerations are relevant to evaluating the disease hazards of foreign travel. One is the fact that recognized occurrence of disease in the indigenous population may be an inaccurate index of risk to a newcomer. Particular agents, such as polioviruses in the past and hepatitis A virus and Epstein-Barr virus at present, may be so prevalent that infections in natives occur so early in life that they usually are subclinical. The second consideration is the nature of the proposed travel. The usual tourist or business traveler visits chiefly larger population centers and popular tourist attractions, where the most important hazards are pathogens transmitted by food or water. Travelers whose activities bring them into more intimate contact with the people and the biologic environment (Peace Corps workers, global health researchers, military personnel) may encounter additional hazards, such as rabies and the locally prevalent arthropod-transmitted pathogens.

As suggested in considering geographic influences on occurrence of disease, the distribution of many diseases is influenced by relevant environmental factors rather than political boundaries. In depicting (or predicting) the global distribution of a particular disease, identifying regions defined by the presence of factors thought to be important to disease occurrence is useful.

For most agents pathogenic for humans, the chief environmental requisite is a susceptible human population, and most such agents already exist wherever the size and density of the population are sufficient for them to persist. Concern about global spread is limited to a few important pathogens, such as *Vibrio cholerae* (cholera) and the influenzavirus. Cholera is a special case in that its spread also depends on poor sanitation. Recent experience in Haiti demonstrated that transmission of this agent can occur by having disaster aid workers from foreign countries introduce cholera, which can then spread because sanitation is poor.[14] Neither persistence nor even limited spread should occur after its introduction into highly developed areas. Influenza A virus continues to be a major and so far unstoppable threat by virtue of its ability to emerge at irregular intervals in a new antigenic coat that largely negates the preexisting widespread immunity.

Local patterns of infection and disease. "Local" units of population for which demographic data are readily available in the United States include "large" units, such as counties, metropolitan areas, and large cities, which contain smaller units (smaller cities and towns [within counties] and census tracts [within metropolitan areas and large cities]). The smaller units, including unincorporated areas within counties, often can be characterized by variables (urban or rural nature, population density, socioeconomic status, racial or ethnic group) that may help explain observed differences in the occurrence of specific infections and related diseases.

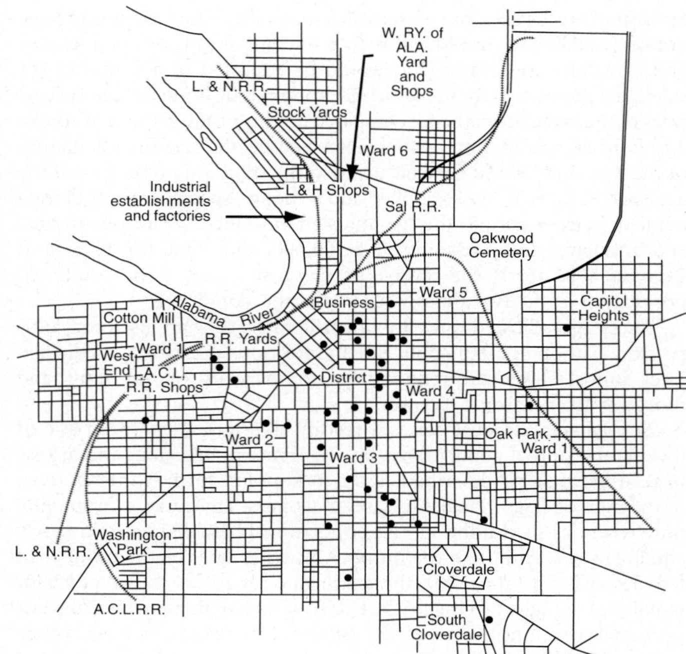

FIG. 6.3 Cases of mild typhus (Brill disease) in Montgomery, Alabama, 1922–25, recorded according to residence. (From Maxcy KF. An epidemiological study of endemic typhus [Brill disease] in the southeastern United States. *Public Health Rep.* 1926;41:2967–95.)

Particularly in relation to outbreaks of acute infectious diseases, spot maps commonly are used to show the local distribution of individual cases. Placing new pins (a different color each week) to mark the residences of newly reported cases serves to visualize the outbreak's geographic progression. The final distribution of the pins may help identify a major source of infection. A classic example is the 1854 outbreak of cholera in the Golden Square district of London, in which the clustering of residences of fatal cases helped Snow incriminate the Broad Street pump as the source.[70] Sometimes, place of work is a better guide to the source of infection than place of residence. In another classic study, that of endemic typhus in Montgomery, Alabama, in the early 1920s, the residences of cases (Fig. 6.3) were scattered widely, whereas the workplaces (Fig. 6.4) were concentrated in relation to feed stores and food-handling businesses, all heavily rat infested. This finding led Maxcy[40] to perform studies showing the basic role of rats and rat fleas in this disease.

Temporal Patterns of Infection and Disease

Definitions. The unit of time used can vary from hours to decades to centuries. In describing acute outbreaks, the units are short—hours for food poisoning, days or weeks for most infectious diseases—whereas long-term time trends are described in longer units of years or decades. Comparisons extending over 1 or more decades may be complicated by changes in diagnostic standards and reporting.

Finally, the meanings of two words commonly used to describe the occurrence of disease over time in a given area should be defined clearly. *Endemic* refers to diseases regularly present. The usual frequency, including expected seasonal variations, is called the *endemic level.* The term *epidemic* applies to any number of cases, small or large, that is a significant increase over the usual, or endemic, level (although just what constitutes a "significant increase" is not clearly defined).

This principle underlies the monitoring of many infectious diseases, deaths, and pneumonia caused by influenza by the CDC. Such monitoring is illustrated in Fig. 6.5, in which the weekly ratios of deaths caused by pneumonia and influenza to the total deaths observed from 2011 to 2015 are compared with the ratios expected from use of the time series method[15] and the "epidemic threshold," which depicts the upper 95% confidence limit. When the observed value exceeds the expected one (an increase of 1.645 standard deviations from the seasonal baseline) for 2 successive weeks, an influenza epidemic is indicated. On this basis, epidemics began in approximately the first week of 2013, 2014, and 2015.

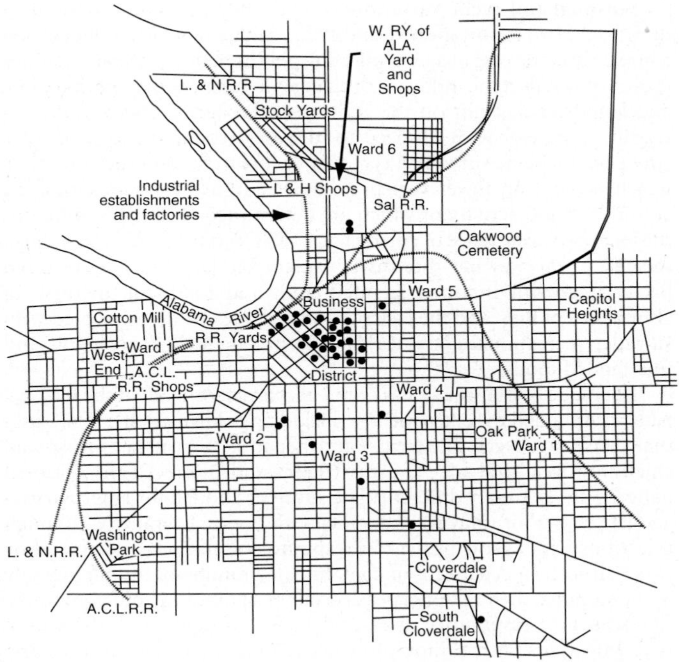

FIG. 6.4 Cases of mild typhus (Brill disease) in Montgomery, Alabama, 1922–25, recorded according to place of employment or, if unemployed, according to place of residence. (From Maxcy KF. An epidemiological study of endemic typhus [Brill disease] in the southeastern United States. *Public Health Rep.* 1926;41:2967–95.)

In practice, especially at the local level, health authorities use the term *outbreak*, rather than *epidemic* (unless the number of cases is very large), to minimize public alarm. The term *pandemic* is used to describe excess disease occurring in many countries, as influenza did in 1957, 1968, and 2009.

Time clusters. Time clusters relate to the recognition and interpretation of events (infections and disease) that occur with some increased frequency within a limited period or clustering in time. An important determinant of clustering of infections is the incubation period. Infection resulting from a known exposure is manifested within a predictable range of time by the initiation of shedding of the agent and the onset of disease (if it occurs). Although the average incubation period of a given disease is remarkably constant, the usual range broadens as the incubation period increases. This range can be estimated by accumulating cases for which the time of exposure is known precisely or approximately and, with this point as day 0 on the time axis, plotting the day of onset of each subsequent case. The width of the resulting cluster provides an estimate of the range of the incubation period. The best estimate is obtained by using only cases with single, clearly timed exposure, such as when contact with the source case occurred only once, as during a playmate's birthday party.

A more readily obtained but less precise estimate is that derived from the cumulative analysis of family episodes of a disease based on the assumption that the initial or primary case is the source of subsequent disease in family contacts. Because the primary case is infectious for several days, on any of which effective exposure may occur, the onset of secondary cases would cluster over a range that theoretically may reflect the true range plus the period of infectivity of the primary case.

Knowledge of the range of incubation periods has several practical implications. For contagious diseases, it can be used to distinguish true secondary cases that occur in families from others arising as a result of extrafamilial sources (cases with onset too soon after that of the

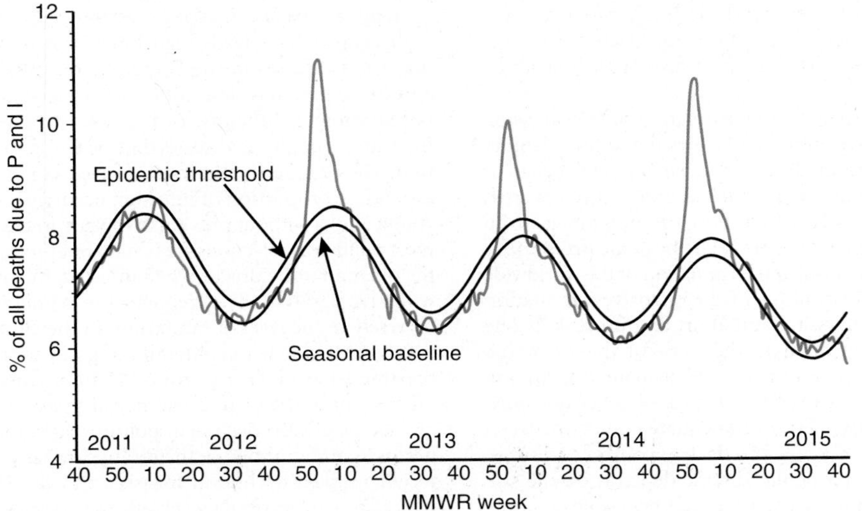

FIG. 6.5 Percentage of all deaths attributed to pneumonia and influenza reported by the 122 Cities Mortality Reporting System, by week and year—United States, week ending October 31, 2015. *I*, Influenza; *P*, pneumonia. (From Centers for Disease Control and Prevention. Available at http://www.cdc.gov/flu/weekly/.)

primary case are called *co-primary cases*) or representing a second generation of spread within the family (i.e., *tertiary cases*). Knowledge of the range of incubation periods also determines the length of time after known exposure that contacts should be observed or possibly held in quarantine for the subsequent development of disease. For poorly contagious diseases, such as typhoid fever, or for noncontagious diseases, such as food poisoning, the distribution of onset in an outbreak can be used to distinguish between "point" epidemics (common time and place of exposure) and outbreaks reflecting exposure to a possibly continuing source. In the former case, onset would fall within the usual range of incubation periods. When the point source is not obvious, investigation can be focused on the interval defined by subtracting the shortest incubation period from the date of onset of the first case and the longest period from the date of onset of the last case.

Short-term patterns

Epidemics. "Point" epidemics have a duration limited by the range of the period of incubation of the particular disease because no secondary spread of the agents occurs. Much more commonly, outbreaks or epidemics extend over longer periods. On the basis of the causative agents and the mechanisms of transmission, three distinct types can be recognized.

The first type typically consists of outbreaks of poorly contagious or noncontagious diseases; such outbreaks reflect the new but persisting activity of a source that must be identified and terminated quickly. One example of such a "continuing source" type of outbreak was a community-wide outbreak of salmonellosis in Madera, California, in 1965, which was traced quickly to the water supply.[55] Unrecognized typhoid carriers working as food handlers and shellfish harvested from sewage-polluted waters contaminated with hepatitis A virus are other examples of outbreaks requiring prompt epidemiologic investigation to identify the source. One of the major causes of point epidemics is food contaminated with *E. coli* O157:H7. More recent outbreaks, such as the contamination of spinach at the growing source, have been reported by the CDC.[11] Often the CDC posts interim reports of investigations on its website (www.cdc.gov) before publication in *Morbidity and Mortality Weekly Reports.*

The element of contagion distinguishes the second type of epidemic, in which disease spreads from person to person. Such epidemics generally are self-limited, and the curve describing them often resembles the bell-shaped curve of a normal distribution. Modification of this curve, as in an abrupt decline from the peak, is the expected result of successful efforts to control the epidemic.[43] Epidemics of contagious diseases occur when the population in which the agent persists or is newly introduced contains a sufficient number of susceptible individuals with contact with one another that is adequate to permit transfer of infection from each new case to, on average, more than one susceptible individual. When this average falls below 1, the curve declines, and when the probability of successful transfer of infection approaches zero, the epidemic stops (typically well before the supply of susceptible individuals has been exhausted).

Reasons that underlie this decline and termination of transmission include seasonal changes in environmental factors that affect viability of the agent, such as temperature and humidity; changes in the behavior of hosts that affect the intimacy of contact, such as indoor school versus outdoor play; and the progressive conversion of individuals from susceptible to immune. Institution of appropriate hygienic precautions likely was an important facet of control and termination of the worldwide outbreak of SARS in 2003.[10] Institution of an intensive vaccination program may also reduce transmission and abort an outbreak. If one assumes constant units on the time axis, the slope of the ascending limb of the epidemic curve is determined by the incubation period (interval between successive cases) and by factors that influence transmission (infectivity of the agent, frequency of adequate contact between susceptible individuals). In the absence of effective control measures, the duration of epidemics of a particular disease depends on the size of the susceptible population and the persistence of favorable environmental factors.

Epidemics of "diseases in nature" constitute the third type. Because susceptible individuals usually are abundant in the human population, these epidemics typically reflect increases in the number of sources of infection in nature. With zoonoses such as arbovirus encephalitis, the initiation, slope of the curve, and duration of the epidemic are determined by the number of susceptible lower vertebrate hosts, the seasonally determined abundance of the vector mosquitoes, and the length of the extrinsic incubation period in the vector. The occurrence of West Nile virus in the United States, which began in August 1999 and has continued with outbreaks in the late summer of each succeeding year in mosquitoes and humans, is an example.[3,12]

Seasonal and cyclic variations. Predictable periodic variations in disease take two forms, seasonal and cyclic, neither of which is understood completely in the case of agents infecting only humans. *Seasonal* variations presumably reflect the influence of changes in temperature, precipitation, and length of daylight on the activity of the agent. This variation is readily apparent with respect to diseases, such as Lyme disease (the peak incidence of which typically occurs in the summer months), which depend on lower vertebrate hosts and arthropod vectors, the abundance and activity of which are determined seasonally. Similarly, the increased occurrence of enteric bacterial infections (spread by indirect means) in the warmer months is explainable largely by more rapid bacterial growth in unrefrigerated milk and food, the increase in abundance of flies, and the lack of sanitary precautions associated with summer recreational activities such as private swimming pools and unattended foods.

The mode of transmission is only a partial determinant of the seasonal pattern. Although the enteroviruses (including poliovirus), the rotaviruses that cause acute gastroenteritis, and hepatitis A virus all are spread chiefly by fecal-oral mechanisms (direct and indirect), the seasonal patterns are distinctly different (late summer and fall for enteroviruses and late winter for rotaviruses and hepatitis A virus). Similarly, although infections with agents present in respiratory secretions and spread by either airborne mechanisms or contaminated fomites occur infrequently in the summer, their seasonal peaks occur at significantly different times. The season of respiratory diseases coincides roughly with the school year. Infections with rhinoviruses occur most frequently in the early fall and late spring, and infections with parainfluenza virus types 1 and 2 occur most frequently in the fall. The annual peaks of RSV vary among fall, winter, and spring. Mumps peaks in late fall, influenza in late winter or early spring, and measles typically in the spring.

Plotting variation over a series of years reveals a roughly regular cyclic variation for some diseases. In larger metropolitan areas, the usual biennial measles epidemic appears as an enlarged annual wave. Before 1950, deaths caused by meningococcal meningitis occurred on a nationwide basis in cycles of 7 to 9 years, a phenomenon presumably terminated by the advent of prophylactic antibiotics. Pandemic influenza A, which provides the most dramatic example of cycling, is explainable by a major change in the antigenic character of the agent.

Long-term trends. Except for poliomyelitis during the first half of the 20th century, clearly defined long-term trends in the occurrence of infectious diseases in the United States usually have been downward, and in no case has description or understanding of the mechanisms posed a major difficulty. In the case of poliomyelitis, the increase in the rate of paralytic disease that began about 1880 is attributable to numerous factors, including improved sanitation, which resulted in an expanding proportion of infection occurring among older children and young adults without previous exposure to the viruses. In young infants, most poliovirus infections are benign but produce long-lasting immunity; the older an individual is when infected, the more likely that individual will have paralysis. The frequency of paralytic poliomyelitis is related inversely to the level of sanitation. In the United States, the increase in paralytic disease with epidemics of polio continued unabated (with an apparent sharp increase around 1940 because of changes in reporting criteria) until the widespread use of polio vaccines.

The post-1955 decline in poliomyelitis; the much earlier decline in pertussis and diphtheria; the disappearance of smallpox; and the more recent marked decline in measles, rubella, *H. influenzae* type b, and varicella all are attributable chiefly to widespread use of effective specific vaccines. Similarly, the disappearance of indigenous malaria and the decline of rabies to a negligible level in humans in certain areas reflect the application of a variety of effective control measures. Unfortunately, with the exception of smallpox, these measures are not permanent, and loss of infrastructure for delivery of vaccines or of environmental controls will cause a recrudescence of disease.

Emerging infections. Although in the 1980s one might have said that most infectious disorders had been explored thoroughly epidemiologically and that little was left to do, this clearly is not the case. Infectious disease epidemiology has become increasingly challenging, and in many ways the problems are more complex and necessitate greater cooperation with additional disciplines, such as microbiology and molecular biology.

In part this increased complexity is due to so-called emerging infections, a term that has come into vogue in recent years and refers to two different groups of disorders. The first is associated with the appearance of previously unrecognized or possibly heretofore nonexistent infections in humans. Well-known examples are legionellosis, hantavirus pulmonary disease, acquired immunodeficiency syndrome, Lyme disease, hemorrhagic colitis caused by *E. coli* O157:H7, and Ebola virus infection. The other group includes previously recognized human infections that exhibit changes in epidemiologic behavior or biologic characteristics that enhance their transmission or virulence. These changes usually can be attributed to external influences, such as altered demographics including increasing population and rural-urban migration, international travel, new technology or technologic failure, changes in land use, adaptation of infecting organisms to various influences, and inadequate or underused public health measures.[36] To this list should be added changes in host factors such as immune defenses.

No clear dividing line exists between new infections and old ones that exhibit new behavior. Examples of some with new behavior include multidrug-resistant tuberculosis, penicillin-resistant pneumococcal infections, invasive group A streptococcal (popularly known as flesh-eating bacteria) infections, staphylococcal toxic shock syndrome, community-acquired methicillin-resistant staphylococcal infections, H5N1 influenza ("bird flu"), cryptosporidiosis, and numerous infections that are fostered by immunosuppression or various therapeutic measures such as antibiotics and catheters.

These emerging infections are not minor threats. Although in some instances small populations have been affected to date, the potential for widespread disease of epidemic or even of pandemic proportions exists. This potential can be expected to increase because the demographic and other conditions that have predisposed to the emergence of these infections continue to grow and intensify. Maximal efforts must be expended to reverse this process. To achieve this goal requires worldwide collaborative effort among various disciplines, including epidemiology, microbiology, entomology, immunology, clinical medicine, demography, nutrition, sanitation, and even political science.

The responsibilities of epidemiologists regarding emerging infections may be described in three categories. The first category is surveillance, including recognition of the appearance of a previously unrecognized infection or a new variant of an existing disease. Optimal surveillance requires systematic observations and specific diagnostic criteria to ensure precision. An important part of surveillance is to determine who, when, and where: who is affected (e.g., age and other personal characteristics, contact with others who are ill), when the disorder occurs (e.g., year-to-year variations, season, temporal course of the outbreak), and where it occurs (e.g., geographic locations, urban or rural, local ecology). Second, an important task is to use surveillance and other data to develop an understanding of the epidemiology of the infection, which often provides clues to its etiology and pathogenesis and to approaches to controlling the disease. The third role of epidemiologists is that of monitoring the effects of various control measures, including assessment of the safety and efficacy of new vaccines, and their effects on microbial ecology. A description of how the efficacy of vaccines is determined is provided at the end of this chapter.

The increasing magnitude and speed of international travel enhance the likelihood of global spread of disease and complicate approaches to prevent or contain epidemic infections. Many of the emerging infections are not limited geographically by their ecologic requirements. The nations of the world increasingly depend on each other for surveillance, a task not easily accomplished given the logistics; costs (in the presence of other needs and priorities, particularly of many developing countries); and the required standardization, collaboration, communication, coordination, and centralized resource for assembly and analysis of surveillance. In 2014–15, the outbreak of Ebola virus infections in Western Africa demonstrated all these issues of global spread. Although the WHO, the Pan American Health Organization, the U.S. Military and Public Health Service, and various other organizations maintain surveillance systems and laboratories in various parts of the world, these efforts at present are considered to be inadequate except for some infections and in some areas. The development of comprehensive national and worldwide surveillance systems has been urgently recommended.[36]

BIOSTATISTICS

Statistical Significance

Stochastic statistics deals with probability. Most readers are familiar with the use of *P* values to assess the *statistical significance* of a finding from a study. Usually, the threshold used to separate "significant" from "nonsignificant" results is a probability (*P* value) of <.05, which means that (arbitrarily, by convention) if a result is likely to be observed by chance fewer than 1 in 20 times, the finding is considered to be statistically significant. It must be emphasized, however, that statistical significance and clinical significance are very different. A statistically significant result means that the result is considered unlikely to be attributable to chance alone. As we shall see, the *P* value is related not only to the magnitude of the difference between the things that are being compared (e.g., a characteristic of either the exposed and the unexposed groups in a longitudinal study or the cases and controls in a case-control study) but also to the size of the sample. Consequently, differences that are clinically unimportant (e.g., a difference in mean weight of 0.2 kg between two groups, a difference of 3% in the distribution of Caucasians between two groups) can be statistically significant if the size of the sample is large. Of importance is to remember that a statistically significant finding may be of no clinical significance.

By the same token, the "magic" *P* value of .05 itself may be misleading because it is an arbitrary threshold; in fact, there usually is little difference in the results associated with a *P* value of .04 and one associated with a *P* value of .06. If the size of a sample is small, a large, clinically important difference may not be statistically significant. One should not automatically dismiss the importance of a finding for which the *P* value is .05 or higher.

Hypothesis Testing

In most epidemiologic studies, stochastic tests are used to check the validity of a hypothesis. By convention, one tests the validity of the *null hypothesis* that there is no difference in either the mean value of the characteristic (for continuous variables) or the frequency distribution of the characteristic (for categorical values) between the groups being compared. In essence, one is testing the probability that the two samples being compared (exposed subjects versus unexposed subjects or cases versus controls) emerged from the same population—that is, whether a difference between the groups could have been the result of chance if the two samples were selected randomly from the same population or whether the difference is so great that it probably (<1 chance in 20, or $P < .05$) did not occur by chance; that is, the samples probably actually represent a true difference in the populations of either exposed subjects versus unexposed subjects or cases versus controls.

Hypotheses can be either *bidirectional (nondirectional)* or *unidirectional (directional).* A nondirectional hypothesis asks whether an association exists between exposed and unexposed subjects, but it does not assume in which direction the association will occur. For example, one might ask whether an association exists between the height of fever and the outcomes of children with typhoid fever without specifying whether the association would be in the direction of better or worse outcomes (perhaps high fever indicates a more severe infection, or perhaps it indicates a more vigorous immune response). In such instances, the associated *P* value should be interpreted in a bidirectional, or *two-tailed,* manner because the distribution of the test statistic contains two "tails," one at either end of the curve; the *P* value represents the sum of the area under the two tails of the curve. In effect, one is specifying that for a result to be statistically significant, the probability of the result being in a positive direction is less than 2.5% and the probability of the result being in a negative direction is less than 2.5%. Most tables of *P* values provide results that are to be interpreted in a two-tailed manner (because this is the most conservative approach to testing a hypothesis), so the *P* value for a given test statistic can be read directly from the table.

In some instances, however, one might have good reason to suspect that an exposure is associated with an outcome in a unidirectional manner (e.g., that possession of a handgun is associated with an increased risk of sustaining a gunshot wound). If, in advance, the investigator decides to test this hypothesis in a unidirectional manner (the null hypothesis for which would be that ownership of a gun is not associated with an increased risk of incurring a gunshot wound), interpreting the results of a test statistic in a unidirectional, or *one-tailed,* manner might be appropriate. To derive a one-tailed *P* value, the two-tailed value is divided by 2. Thus, if the two-tailed *P* value is .06, the one-tailed value for the same result is .03. Clearly, obtaining statistically significant results by testing hypotheses in a unidirectional manner is easier. However it is important to specify before the study is conducted the a priori plan for how the results of statistical tests will be interpreted. Furthermore, although many hypotheses might seem to lend themselves to unidirectional analyses (e.g., one might think that an experimental vaccine that has been shown to be immunogenic could only be beneficial), in fact, unidirectional analyses are used only rarely. First, the possibility that an exposure may have an effect opposite to that expected usually cannot be ruled out in advance. For example, researchers found that persons who were immunized with a vaccine composed of inactivated respiratory syncytial virus had an increased risk of developing symptomatic infection with the virus. In addition, because two-tailed interpretation of data is more conservative, many authorities (e.g., editors of journals and such licensing agencies as the FDA) demand two-tailed analyses.

Type I Error, Type II Error, and Statistical Power

Two types of errors can be made when testing the validity of a null hypothesis. The first occurs when the null hypothesis is true but is rejected erroneously, which leads to an erroneous conclusion that a difference exists between the exposed and unexposed subjects; this kind of mistake is termed a *type I error,* or *α error.* If a test statistic with a *P* value of $\leq .05$ is accepted as statistically significant (and the null hypothesis is rejected on that basis), approximately 5% of the time a type I error is made because if no difference actually exists between the groups, that result still will occur by chance 1 in 20 times. By contrast, if the *P* value is $< .001$, a type I error will occur fewer than 1 in 1000 times if the null hypothesis is rejected.

The other kind of error, *type II error,* or *β error,* occurs when the null hypothesis erroneously is not rejected even though a difference between the two groups truly exists. If the *P* value associated with the result is .05 or greater, the probability that the null hypothesis is false is not sufficiently low to reject it (even though the probability that the observed result could have occurred by chance may be only .06).

Type I and type II errors are mutually exclusive. If one rejects the null hypothesis, one risks committing a type I error, the probability of which is equal to the *P* value. In such instances, a type II error cannot occur. If one accepts (i.e., fails to reject) the null hypothesis, one may commit a type II error (in which case a type I error cannot occur). The probability of committing a type II error is not related directly to the observed *P* value. Instead, one can estimate the probability of committing a type II error (β error) before the study begins on the basis of an assumed (clinically important) degree of association between the exposure and the outcome. Certain assumptions also must be made about the magnitude of the effect among the exposed subjects and the frequency of the outcome in the unexposed subjects. One is calculating a unidirectional probability that, by chance, the study will fail to detect an association equal to or greater than the magnitude that is specified for what is, in effect, an *alternative hypothesis* (i.e., that an association truly exists between the exposure and the outcome). The *statistical power* of a study (the unidirectional probability that the null hypothesis of no difference between groups will be rejected given a specified degree of type I error—usually <5%) is equal to $1 - \beta$.

In designing a study, adequate statistical power is critical to ensure that a true association between the exposure and the outcome is not missed erroneously. The probability of a type II error depends on the size of the sample, the degree of variance within the sample, and the magnitude of the association that one wants to be able to detect: the smaller the sample, the larger the variance, and the smaller the magnitude of the association that one wants to detect, the larger the β error (type II error) and the lower the statistical power of the study to detect an association. Of these factors, the investigator usually has control over only the size of the sample (because in the population the variance generally is a relatively fixed attribute of the characteristic being measured, and the magnitude of association that is chosen usually is the minimal association that is clinically meaningful; for example, to design a study of an experimental vaccine so that it could detect as little as 30% efficacy would not make sense because such a product would not be approved in most instances unless the magnitude of its effect was much greater).

Exactly what constitutes adequate power is debatable. Because enrolling a large number of subjects in a study often is expensive and time consuming, frequently the power that a study is designed to have depends on both the financial resources and the time available to conduct the study. A statistical power of 80% often is chosen as a reasonable compromise between ensuring that the study has a sufficient number of subjects to answer the research hypothesis and the realities of logistic and financial exigencies. On the other hand, if a pharmaceutical company has invested many years and millions (or billions!) of dollars to develop a new drug or a new vaccine, it may demand that a pivotal clinical trial of the product have at least 90% power to detect a clinically meaningful effect in an attempt to ensure that the product will be approved if it is efficacious.

Multiple Comparisons

Another more subtle problem in interpreting results arises when more than one hypothesis is assessed in a single study. If multiple tests of statistical significance are performed in a study, the probability that by chance alone the *P* value associated with any one variable will be less than .05 is substantially greater than 5%. In fact, the probability that by chance at least one test will be associated with a *P* value $< .05$ is equal to $1 - (0.95)^k$, with *k* equal to the number of independent tests of statistical significance that are performed. Thus, if 10 different hypotheses are tested, a 40% probability exists that at least one of them will be statistically significant (i.e., that at least one of the tests will have a *P* value of $<.05$). Of course, this matter violates the arbitrary rule that we consider a finding to be statistically significant only if it is likely to have occurred by chance less than 5% of the time. If multiple different associations in a study have *P* values $< .05$, determining which occurred by chance and which truly are statistically significant is difficult.

On the other hand, studies often are expensive, time consuming, and logistically difficult to conduct. Therefore, sometimes a reasonable approach is to try to increase efficiency by assessing more than one hypothesis in a single study. To address this problem, one can specify in advance the *primary hypothesis* and the *secondary* and *tertiary hypotheses.* One then might give most credence to the statistical test of the primary hypothesis. Another approach is to raise the threshold used to define statistical significance by dividing .05 by the number of different tests that are performed. Thus if five independent hypotheses are tested, any one would have to be associated with a $P < .01$ before the null hypothesis would be rejected. However, this approach might be too stringent because the different hypotheses that are being tested often are not truly independent, and the probability that two or more associations will be statistically significant may be greater than the product of their individual probabilities. For example, one might assess whether infection is associated both with diarrhea and with vomiting; if it is associated with one of these symptoms, usually a higher than chance probability exists that it also is associated with the other. At the least, an investigator should acknowledge this potential problem and its consequences before drawing conclusions from the study.

Tests of Statistical Significance

Going into detail about the many different stochastic tests that are available is beyond the scope of this chapter. However, several general comments, as well as descriptions of a few commonly used tests, are in order.

Tests of statistical significance are either parametric or nonparametric. The test statistic of a *parametric* test is based on the assumption that the frequency distribution of the characteristic being assessed in the source population follows certain parameters. For example, for certain tests, one assumes that the characteristic in the population has a normal distribution. If the assumption is violated (e.g., the characteristic is not distributed normally), the statistical test will not be valid. In such instances, an appropriate approach might be to use a test based on a different, skewed distribution, such as the *Poisson distribution* for rare events, which might reflect more accurately the distribution of the characteristic in the population.

Alternative approaches to assess the statistical significance of differences between groups, if the distribution of the characteristic in the population is known to be highly skewed, include transforming the data so that they are normalized, usually by converting the values to their logarithmic equivalent, or using a *nonparametric* test.[66] Nonparametric tests, such as the Mann-Whitney *U* test and the Wilcoxon rank sum test, do not depend directly on the numerical values of the data; instead, the individual values are ranked in order of their values, and the statistical analyses are based on the relative ranks of the values in the different groups rather than on an assumed distribution in the population or in the sample.

For large samples, parametric tests usually are valid and often are easier to calculate than are nonparametric tests. For smaller samples and for samples with highly skewed distributions, nonparametric tests or tests that use log-transformed data may be preferable.

Continuous Variables

To test the statistical significance of differences between groups in continuous variables (e.g., degree of fever, intelligence quotient, age, or a score on a standardized questionnaire), the mean values of the different groups can be compared.[69] The tests of statistical significance use the magnitude of the difference of the means and the variance in the sample to assess the probability that the difference could occur by chance. If more than two groups are being compared for a single variable, the procedure is called *one-way analysis of variance.* The null hypothesis is that the mean values from each group are the same (i.e., that the different groups are random samples from the same population). The total variance in all the subjects is separated into the amount that is attributable to differences between the groups of subjects (the *intergroup variance*) and the amount that is attributable to differences among the subjects within each group (the *intragroup variance*). The greater the quotient of the intergroup variance divided by the intragroup variance (the *F ratio*), the more likely that differences between the groups are statistically significant (i.e., that they are not due to chance variation). The statistical significance of the F ratio can be determined from the *F test* table of *P* values. When this type of test is performed to assess the statistical significance of the simultaneous effects of two factors (by stratifying into additional groups), the test is called *two-way analysis of variance.*

The familiar t *test* is just a special form of one-way analysis of variance in which the means of just two groups are compared. A *one-sample* t *test* assesses whether the mean value of the study sample is statistically significantly different from the mean value in the source population. It assumes that the mean value in the source population is known and is calculated by dividing the difference of the mean of the sample minus the mean of the population by the quotient of the variance of the sample divided by the square root of the number in the sample.

A more common use of the *t* test is to assess the statistical significance of the difference between the mean values of either a characteristic or an outcome of subjects in two different samples (e.g., of the exposed and the unexposed groups in a study). The null hypothesis of this *two-sample* t *test* is that the mean values of the two samples are not statistically significantly different (i.e., that they could be random samples from the same population). The *t* test statistic is equal to the difference in the mean values of the two samples divided by the square root of the pooled variance of the samples (the standard error of the difference of the means of the two groups). The *P* value of the result *(t)* is read from the table of the *t* distribution, with the degrees of freedom equal to the sum of the number of subjects in each sample minus 2.

TABLE 6.4 2 × 2 Contingency Table

	Outcome Present	Outcome Absent	Total
Exposed	a	b	a + b
Unexposed	c	d	c + d
Total	a + c	b + d	N

$\chi^2 = [(ad - bc)^2 N] \div [(a + b)(a + c)(b + d)(c + d)]$

Categorical Values

The chi-square statistic (χ^2) commonly is used to assess the statistical significance of differences in categorical values between groups.[6] Most often, proportions of two different groups (e.g., the proportions of the exposed and of the unexposed groups in which the outcome developed) are compared. Typically, the data are displayed in a *2 × 2 contingency table* (Table 6.4). The null hypothesis is that no association exists between the exposure and the outcome (or whatever the rows and columns represent)—that is, that the two groups could be random samples from the same population. This hypothesis is tested statistically by comparing the number of subjects who would be expected to be in a given cell by chance with the actual frequency (the observed frequency). The expected frequency can be calculated from the total number of subjects in the rows and the columns (the marginal totals) and is equal to the product of the number of subjects in the row times the number of subjects in the column divided by the total number of subjects in the sample.

The value of χ^2 (with N equal to the total number of subjects) is shown in Table 6.4. The statistical significance of χ^2 can be determined by reading the *P* values from a table of the χ^2 distribution. The larger the value of χ^2, the less likely that the observed proportions could have occurred by chance. Unfortunately, assuming that the probability that the observed proportions of a random sample of subjects will follow the χ^2 distribution is not necessarily accurate if the expected frequency of any cell is small. Consequently, many experts use a *continuity correction* (sometimes called the *Yates correction*) to adjust for the deviation from the smooth, continuous theoretic distribution of χ^2 when the discrete values of small numbers of expected subjects disrupt the validity of the assumed distribution. The equation for χ^2 with the continuity correction is

$$\chi_c^2 = [(ad - bc) - (N/2)]^2 N \div [(a+b)(a+c)(b+d)(c+d)]$$

If the expected frequency in any cell is very small (often defined as <5), the χ^2 test, even with the continuity correction, is not a valid estimate of the probability that the observed values could have occurred by chance. In such instances, the *Fisher exact test,* which is based on a hypergeometric distribution, should be used to assess the statistical significance of differences in categorical values.

Confidence Intervals

Although the validity of a null hypothesis typically is tested by stochastic tests and the use of *P* values, construction of a *confidence interval* (usually a 95% confidence interval [CI]) has the advantage of providing information about both the precision of the estimate of the association (the narrower the confidence interval, the more precise the estimate) and its statistical significance.[8] CIs have become standard components of reports of the results of epidemiologic studies.

Analyses of studies are concerned with both estimation (of the "true" value of the association between the exposure and the outcome in the population) and hypothesis testing (i.e., what is the probability that any association observed could have occurred by chance alone). A sample of the population is enrolled in any study. The association observed in the study is hoped to be an accurate estimate of the true value of the association in the entire population. However if an unbiased study were repeated many times, by chance alone the results would vary (because of random sampling error). A CI is a range of values based on the estimate and the spread of the data from a single study, within which the true value of the association in the population is likely to lie with a specified probability (i.e., 95% of the time for a 95% CI, 99% of the time for a 99% CI). CIs provide information about both the magnitude of associations (so that the clinical significance of the estimate can be assessed) and their statistical significance. If the CI is calculated for a single outcome and if the 95% CI for the difference between two groups does not include zero, the outcome is statistically significant (i.e., <5% probability that the null hypothesis of no difference existing between the groups is true). If the CI is for a risk ratio or an odds ratio, the association will be statistically significant if the 95% CI for the association does not include 1 (i.e., <5% probability that the null hypothesis that no association exists is true). CIs can be calculated with both continuous and categorical data, as well as for estimates of a single proportion and for differences (or associations) between two groups.

Adjustment for Potential Confounding Variables

The effect of confounding variables on the associations between exposure and outcome may be controlled in either the design or the analysis of a study. Random allocation of subjects to the exposed and unexposed groups is a common strategy to avoid the effect of confounding in longitudinal studies. Although randomization actually ensures only lack of bias if a confounding variable is distributed unevenly between the groups (because an uneven distribution is as likely to favor the exposed group as the unexposed group), randomization is likely to be effective in preventing confounding if the size of the sample is large (which renders substantial inequalities between groups in the distribution of an independent variable unlikely to occur). Nonetheless, an investigator must check to ensure that confounding does not occur, even in a randomized clinical trial.

Another way to ensure that a potential confounding variable does not affect the results of a study is to *match* on that variable. Subjects in the exposed and unexposed groups (or, in a case-control study, the cases and the controls) can be matched on certain variables that are known to be associated independently with both the exposure and the outcome. Such matching can be achieved either by matching subjects individually or by *frequency matching* (i.e., ensuring that the overall frequency distribution of the potential confounder is the same among the cases and the controls). Matching can ensure that the matched variable (e.g., race, age) does not affect the observed association between exposure and outcome.

One disadvantage of matching is that the effect of the matched variable on the association between exposure and outcome cannot be assessed as it might be if either stratification or multivariable analysis were used to control for confounding. If matching is used in the design of the study, analyzing the data with special tests for matched designs is necessary. For example, in a matched-pairs case-control study, only discordant pairs (matched pairs in which the cases and controls differ in their exposure status) provide information. Calculation of the matched odds ratio and the associated test of statistical significance (McNemar χ^2) is shown in Table 6.5.

Adjusting for the effect of potential confounders in the analyses also is possible. One way to accomplish this adjustment is with *stratification,* which is performed by dividing the data into different groups, or *strata,* according to the potential confounder. For example, a study may indicate that children whose parents both work were three times more likely to become febrile during the course of a study than were children whose parents both do not work. We may suspect, however, that it is not having both parents at work, per se, that results in this increased risk of fever; rather, another factor probably is related independently to the risk of fever and to the probability that both parents work. Attendance at group daycare is such a factor. If we stratified the results of the study by whether the children attended group daycare, we most likely would find that a disproportionate number of children whose parents both work also attended group daycare. When the risk ratios in the two different strata are combined (by using the Mantel-Haenszel technique), we probably would find that the apparent association between having both parents work and the risk of fever disappears when the effect of attendance of group daycare is controlled by stratification.

Advantages of stratification are that it can be understood easily and it can be performed without changing the design of the study after it is completed. One disadvantage is that it requires being able to identify and to measure accurately the potential confounders (which is not necessary if one allocates subjects to different groups randomly). In addition, if several different potential confounders exist, performing the calculations may be difficult and time consuming, and the sizes of the individual strata may be so small that the ability to make statistical inferences is poor.

Finally, one can adjust for confounding with the use of one of many multivariable statistical techniques, such as *multiple linear regression* (if both the dependent and the independent variables are continuous) or *logistic regression* (if the dependent variable is dichotomous and the independent variables are either categorical or continuous). Providing a detailed description of multivariable techniques is beyond the scope of this chapter. However, in general, these techniques involve creating a mathematical model that fits the data and then using that model to analyze various associations.[5,6,17,19,31,34,62] Although multivariable techniques are a powerful tool for both assessing the effects of and controlling for potential confounding variables, they depend on mathematical assumptions that may not always be valid and use techniques that are not intuitively obvious.

TABLE 6.5 Analysis of a Matched Case-Control Study

	CASES	
Controls	**Exposed**	**Unexposed**
Exposed	a	b
Unexposed	c	d

Matched odds ratio: b/c.
McNemar χ^2: $(b - c)^2/(b + c)$.
McNemar χ^2 (with continuity correction): $(b - c - 1)^2/(b + c)$.

Meta-Analysis

The term *meta-analysis* refers to a number of different types of analyses. The common feature of all meta-analyses is that they summarize the results of two or more different studies. The term often is used to refer to a quantitative technique in which the results of different studies are combined after they are weighted in the calculations according to the sizes of their samples and the variances of their results. The term also sometimes refers to a qualitative analysis of a group of studies, including critical analyses that rate the methodologic soundness of different studies but do not combine their results quantitatively. For example, one might review a group of studies that reached different conclusions about a topic. If the methodologically rigorous studies had similar results that differed from those of the weaker studies, one might conclude that the results of the more rigorous studies were more likely to be valid.

The concept of producing a single, statistically valid result by combining the results of different, often contradictory, studies has great appeal. However, quantitative meta-analysis has many shortcomings. Perhaps chief among them is that no distinction is made between studies that are sound methodologically and those that are not. Thus, the results of a meta-analysis may be dominated by a study that is large but is methodologically questionable, whereas a superbly performed but smaller study may fail to override the impact of the larger study in the meta-analysis. Another major problem is the selection of studies to include in a meta-analysis. Should only published, peer-reviewed studies be included? Clearly a bias exists that studies with positive results are more likely to be published than studies with negative results. Imagine that many small studies with poor statistical power are conducted and submitted to journals for publication. If the study found no association with the putative risk factor, it likely would not be published on the grounds that the statistical power of the study is poor (i.e., the risk of making a type II error and erroneously concluding there is no association when such an association truly exists is great). On the other hand, if the study did find a statistically significant association with the risk factor, it might be published and could be included in a meta-analysis. If many such small studies that found an association were published, but even more small studies that did not find an association were not published, this kind of *publication bias* could lead to erroneous conclusions in a meta-analysis. Should the analysis be limited to only those studies that meet certain basic criteria for methodologic rigor (and who should decide on the criteria and whether they are met), or should only randomized clinical trials be included? What formula should be used to weight the different studies? Is combining the results of methodologically different studies valid? Results of meta-analyses should be interpreted with great circumspection.[72]

DIAGNOSTIC TESTS

Although clinicians typically order diagnostic tests many times each day, misinterpretation and misuse of diagnostic tests are extremely common occurrences.[56] The widespread practice of interpreting continuous values (e.g., the total white blood cell count) in a dichotomous manner (so that the result is either "normal" or "abnormal") and failure to appreciate fully the difference between the accuracy of a diagnostic test (i.e., its sensitivity and specificity) and its predictive value are major factors in the misuse of diagnostic tests.

What Is Normal?

In most instances the cutoff for an abnormal test of a continuous variable, such as the total white blood cell count or the concentration of antibodies against an infectious agent, is based on the distribution of the results of the test in the population. One usually assumes that the distribution of most such results in the population will follow a Gaussian (or "normal") distribution, which is illustrated by the bell-shaped curve in Fig. 6.1. Gauss and other statisticians used the term *normal* to refer to the shape of this curve. However, in medicine, the term *normal* long has been used to mean something very different—the dichotomy between a state of health *(normal)* and one of disease *(abnormal)*. Unfortunately, the different meanings of these terms often have been used interchangeably, which has added to confusion in the interpretation of diagnostic tests.

In a normal distribution, the mode (the most frequent value) is the mean value, and 68.3%, 95.4%, and 99.7% of the values lie within (±) 1, 2, and 3 standard deviations (SD) from the mean value, respectively. The cutoff for an abnormal test result often is defined arbitrarily as any value that is more than 2 SD from the mean of a normally distributed population; thus, 5% (actually 4.6%) of the population would be categorized as abnormal. Half the people with abnormal results will be 2 SD below the mean, and half will be 2 SD above the mean. Thus, 2.5% (actually 2.3%) of the population will have abnormally high values. In some instances, 3 SD (or some other arbitrary parameter) is used to determine the cutoff. However, it is important to realize that these definitions of normal and abnormal are merely statistical models that should not necessarily be translated to mean that 2.5% of the population is "diseased." As noted earlier, with this kind of statistical logic, the diagnosis of disease may be related to the number of tests performed because if multiple tests are conducted, the likelihood that the result of any one will be abnormal is increased. If 15 independent tests are performed on a patient, the probability that any one of the test results will be abnormal by chance is 54%.

Other statistical models might be more appropriate for assessing a diagnostic test. For example, interpreting diagnostic tests would be relatively easy if two separate, nonoverlapping normal distributions of diseased and disease-free patients existed. Unfortunately, although this model may apply for some rare conditions (e.g., genetic disorders in which affected persons are missing an enzyme that metabolizes certain substances, which leads to uniquely high concentrations of the substance in persons with the disorder), the model rarely is applicable. A model that is more appropriate for most infectious illnesses is shown in Fig. 6.6. In this model (the example of which uses levels of serum calcium), the diseased and nondiseased populations have separate, partially overlapping distributions. The specificity of a diagnostic test is related directly to the degree to which the two distributions overlap.

Accuracy of a Diagnostic Test

Two important characteristics of a diagnostic test—its *reproducibility* and its *validity*—are the key components of its accuracy. The reproducibility (sometimes called *reliability* or *precision*) of a test simply is the degree to which retesting yields the same result. A test that provides results that are not reproducible is of little diagnostic value. The validity of the results of a diagnostic test may be divided into two components: *sensitivity* and *specificity* (Table 6.6). The *sensitivity* of a test is the proportion of persons with disease who are identified accurately by the test as having disease (true positives/[true positives + false negatives]). The *specificity* of a test is the proportion of persons without disease

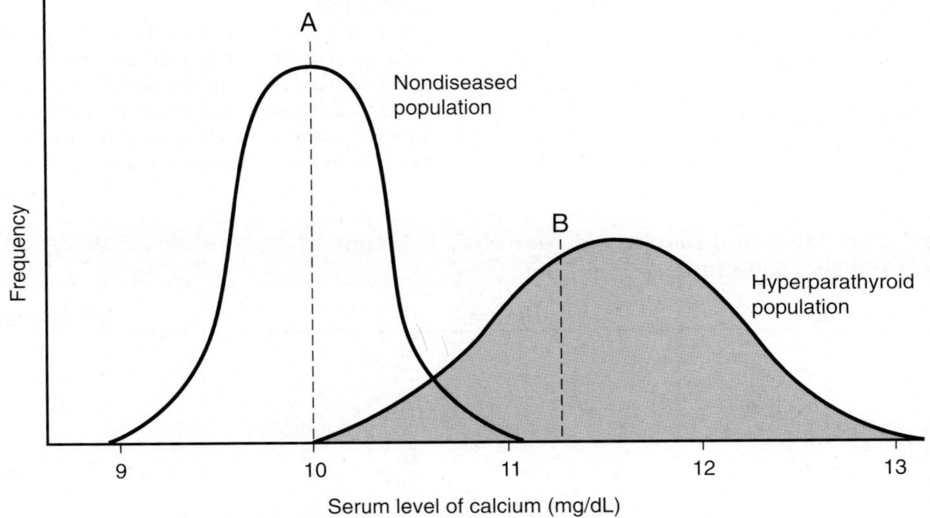

FIG. 6.6 Overlap in values of randomly performed tests in a population in which most of the people are healthy (curve on the left) but some of the people are diseased (curve on the right). A person with a level of calcium below point A would be unlikely to have hyperparathyroidism. A person with a level of calcium above point B would be likely to have an abnormality in calcium metabolism, possibly hyperparathyroidism. A person with a level of calcium between point A and point B may or may not have an abnormality in calcium metabolism. (Note: The normal range of calcium depends on the method used in a specific laboratory. In some laboratories, the range is from 8.5 to 10.5 mg/dL. In others, as in this illustration, it is from 9 to 11 mg/dL.) (From Jekel JF, Elmore JG, Katz DL. *Epidemiology, biostatistics, and preventive medicine.* Philadelphia: WB Saunders; 1996:88.)

who are identified accurately by the test as not having disease (true negatives/[true negatives + false positives]). The *diagnostic accuracy* of a test is the proportion of all persons tested who are classified correctly by the test ([true positives + true negatives]/all persons tested). The ideal test has both a specificity and a sensitivity (and therefore a diagnostic accuracy) of 1. Of course, no diagnostic test is that accurate. Indeed, a tradeoff exists between sensitivity and specificity—the more sensitive a test is, the less specific it is, and vice versa.

Although the sensitivity and specificity of a given test often are considered to be absolute characteristics of a test, in fact, these characteristics do depend on the types of patients included in the studies in which the indices of the test were developed. Indeed, tests that appear to be both highly sensitive and highly specific in preliminary studies commonly prove to be much less so when used in actual clinical practice because the preliminary studies that establish a test's sensitivity and specificity frequently are affected by problems of spectrum and bias.[54] If the patients enrolled in studies used to assess the test (both those with disease and those without disease) have a relatively narrow spectrum of clinical manifestations, both the sensitivity and the specificity of a diagnostic test may appear to be better than they actually are. For example, if one were to assess the sensitivity of a differential heterophile antibody test to diagnose infection with Epstein-Barr virus (EBV), its sensitivity would appear to be far better if all the subjects infected with EBV were teenagers with severe pharyngitis (a high proportion of whom will have a positive heterophile test result) than if it included subjects with a broader spectrum of manifestations of EBV infection (e.g., toddlers with symptoms of an infection of the upper respiratory tract who are much less likely to have a positive heterophile test result when infected with EBV). Likewise, the specificity of a diagnostic test may appear to be better when only asymptomatic, healthy persons are used as nondiseased subjects instead of including patients with other illnesses that produce symptoms similar to those of the target illness. The effects of spectrum of the illness on sensitivities and specificities of a diagnostic test also have been reported for dipstick urinalyses as a diagnostic test for urinary tract infections.[35]

In addition, it is important is to realize that the cutoffs for classifying results as either normal or abnormal usually are somewhat arbitrary and may depend on how the test is used as well as the nature of the disease that one is trying to detect. If a diagnostic test is being used to screen a population for a relatively mild disorder with a low prevalence, one would want to use a cutoff that results in high specificity to avoid having a large number of false-positive results, even at the expense of lower sensitivity. On the other hand, if the diagnostic test is for a serious disorder or is used not for screening but for diagnosis in a targeted population with at least a moderate prevalence of the disorder (e.g., a white blood cell count in cerebrospinal fluid to detect possible bacterial meningitis in febrile children), one might want to err on the side of overdiagnosis and therefore use a cutoff with a high sensitivity at the expense of lower specificity.

Predictive Value of a Diagnostic Test

Sensitivity and specificity are important characteristics of a diagnostic test, but to calculate them, one must know whether the patients do or do not have the disease; clearly, if a clinician already has this knowledge, the test does not need to be performed in the first place. From the perspective of a clinician who is caring for an individual patient, the key characteristic of a diagnostic test is its *predictive value* (see Table 6.6). That is, if a test result is positive, what is the probability that the patient has the disease *(positive predictive value)*? Conversely, if a test result is negative, what is the probability that a patient does not have the disease *(negative predictive value)*? However, unlike sensitivity and specificity, the predictive value of a test depends critically on the prevalence of the disease among the subjects who are tested.

This concern is illustrated by the examples in Table 6.7. In example *a*, the prevalence of the disease in the sample is 1% and the positive predictive value of a positive test result is only 8.8%. By contrast, as shown in examples *b* and *c*, when the prevalence of disease in the sample rises to 10% and 50%, respectively, the positive predictive value of a positive test result rises to 51.4% and 90.5%, respectively, even though the sensitivity and the specificity of the test are constant. By the same token, as the prevalence of disease in the sample that is tested rises, the predictive value of a negative test result falls, although the negative predictive value remains reasonably good until the prevalence of disease becomes high.

It is important for clinicians to be aware of these epidemiologic truths when ordering diagnostic tests for patients. Sometimes a physician orders tests to "rule out" the possibility that a patient's symptoms are caused by a disease that, based on the patient's history, physical examination, and previous laboratory test results, is unlikely to be the cause of the problem (i.e., the "prior probability" that the patient has the disease

TABLE 6.6 Statistical Indices of a Diagnostic Test

Result of Test	Disease	No Disease
Positive	a	b
Negative	c	d
True positives: a	Sensitivity = a/(a + c)	
False positives: b	Specificity = d/(b + d)	
True negatives: d	Positive predictive value = a/(a + b)	
False negatives: c	Negative predictive value = d/(c + d)	

TABLE 6.7 Predictive Value of a Diagnostic Test With 95% Sensitivity and 90% Specificity With Different Prevalence of Disease in the Sample

	Test	Disease	No Disease	Total
a*	Positive	95	990	1085
	Negative	5	8910	8915
	Total	100	9900	10,000
	Positive predictive value = 8.8%	Negative predictive value = 99.9%		
b†	Positive	950	900	1850
	Negative	50	8100	8150
	Total	1000	9000	10,000
	Positive predictive value = 51.4%	Negative predictive value = 99.4%		
c‡	Positive	4750	500	5250
	Negative	250	4500	4750
	Total	5000	5000	10,000
	Positive predictive value = 90.5%	Negative predictive value = 94.7%		

*Prevalence of disease: 1%.
†Prevalence of disease: 10%.
‡Prevalence of disease: 50%.

is low). Unless the specificity of such tests approaches 100% (which is unlikely for most serologic tests), in such situations the great majority of positive test results will be falsely positive; the physician then will be in the unfortunate position of ignoring the result, ordering additional diagnostic tests, or treating the patient for a disease that probably is not the cause of the symptoms.[61] Consequently, clinicians should be selective in ordering diagnostic tests.

ASSESSMENT OF THE PROTECTIVE EFFICACY OF A VACCINE (OR OF ANY INTERVENTION)

Assessment of the protective efficacy of a vaccine is discussed in this section, but the same methods (with different outcomes specified, of course) can be applied to any intervention, such as a drug or physical therapy. The protective efficacy (PE) of a vaccine may be assessed with either experimental or observational studies. The classic way to assess a vaccine's efficacy is in an experimental, randomized, double-blind clinical trial. The major observational designs available are cohort studies and case-control studies—although a large variety of hybrid designs such as household exposure studies and indirect cohort studies are available—but complete descriptions of them are beyond the scope of this chapter.[45,46] Table 6.8 illustrates calculation of the PE of a pneumococcal vaccine with data from clinical trials, cohort studies, and case-control studies.

Clinical Trials

In a randomized clinical trial, subjects at risk of acquiring the infection in question would be assigned randomly either to receive the vaccine (vaccinees) or not to receive the vaccine (controls). Subsequently, all subjects would be observed for occurrence of the infection during an appropriate period of follow-up. At the conclusion of the study, the *protective efficacy* of the vaccine, an index devised by Greenwood and Yule[26] to indicate the proportionate reduction in the frequency of disease attributable to the vaccine, would be calculated. PE is defined as follows:

$$\text{PE} = (\text{Risk of infection in controls} - \text{Risk of infection in vaccinees}) \div \text{Risk of infection in controls}$$

A PE of 100% indicates complete protection against infection, a PE of 0% indicates no protection, and negative values indicate that a greater risk of acquiring infection existed among vaccinees than among controls. By rearranging terms, PE equals 1 minus the risk of infection in vaccinees divided by the risk of infection in controls. Because the ratio in this equation is the relative risk of infection developing in vaccinees versus controls, PE = 1 – relative risk.

TABLE 6.8 Calculation of Protective Efficacy (PE) of Pneumococcal Vaccine

Clinical Trial or Cohort Study	Pneumococcal Infection	No Pneumococcal Infection	Total
Vaccinated	A	B	a + b
Not vaccinated	C	D	c + d
PE = [(c/c + d) – (a/a + b)] ÷ (c/c + d) = 1 – [(a/a + b) ÷ (c/c + d)]*			
Case-Control Study	**Pneumococcal Infection (Cases)**	**No Pneumococcal Infection (Controls)**	
Vaccinated	A	b	
Not vaccinated	C	d	
PE = 1 – [(ad) ÷ (bc)][†]			

*The expression [(a/a +b ÷ (c/c +d)] is also known as the relative risk of infection in vaccinated versus unvaccinated persons.

[†]The expression [(ad) ÷ (bc)] is the odds ratio relating vaccination to infection. In a case-control study, the odds ratio approximates the relative risk.

Observational Cohort Studies

In a cohort study, subjects at risk would be selected on the basis of whether they had been vaccinated or had been left unvaccinated during routine clinical care. The vaccinated and unvaccinated groups then would be monitored longitudinally to assess frequencies of infection. The analysis of a vaccine's PE for cohort studies is similar to that for clinical trials, but because the study is nonexperimental, the results are more subject to bias than are those of a well-conducted, randomized clinical trial.

Case-Control Studies

In a case-control study, patients with antecedent conditions that place them at high risk for pneumococcal infection would be eligible to be subjects. Patients with serious pneumococcal infection would become subjects in the case group. The control group would consist of subjects with similar high-risk conditions but without pneumococcal infection. The two groups then would be compared for the frequency of antecedent vaccination with pneumococcal vaccine.[64]

In a case-control study, the strength of the relationship between vaccination and subsequent infection is measured by an odds ratio (the ratio of the odds of vaccination in the case subjects to the odds of vaccination in the controls). Because the odds ratio in a case-control study closely approximates the relative risk of pneumococcal infection in a longitudinal study and because PE is defined as 1 minus the relative risk, the value (1 – odds ratio) closely approximates the PE that would be calculated from a longitudinal study.

QUALITY IMPROVEMENT

There has been an upsurge of interest in efforts to improve the quality of care given to patients. Often interventions are developed that are thought to be beneficial and are very unlikely to produce harm. Consequently, they are implemented without rigorous testing (e.g., a randomized clinical trial) as would be required for either a new drug or new vaccine before it could be approved for use. Nonetheless, typically one would like to evaluate the effect of the new intervention, which might be a new policy or use of a new method to gather or disseminate information (e.g., use of an iPad). However, typically, there is no concurrent comparison group that can be used to assess the effect of implementation of the intervention, as would be done in an experimental study. Consequently, historical comparison groups usually are used. The problem is that one does not know what other changes occurred during the same period of time (or that may have begun even earlier) that might also affect the outcome that is being assessed. That is, is it valid to attribute changes over time in the frequency of the outcome to the intervention? While it is difficult to attribute a causal effect to an intervention in a nonexperimental study, techniques have been developed that provide more refined estimates of the true effect of the intervention—for example by adjusting for the trajectory of change in the frequency of the outcome that may already have begun before implementation of the intervention (e.g., an interrupted time series analysis). Extensive discussion of these methods is beyond the scope of this chapter, but there is an extensive literature on this topic.[7,49,50]

NEW REFERENCES SINCE THE SEVENTH EDITION

7. Brown CA, Lilford RJ. The stepped wedge trial design: a systematic review. *BMC Med Res Methodol.* 2006;6:54.
10. Centers for Disease Control and Prevention. Carbapenem-resistant *Enterobacteria* in healthcare settings. 2015. Available at http://www.cdc/ncidod/sars/guidance/D/pdf/d.pdf.
24. Gewitz MH, Baltimore RS, Tani LY, et al. Revision of the Jones Criteria for the diagnosis of acute rheumatic fever in the era of Doppler echocardiography: a scientific statement from the American Heart Association. *Circulation.* 2015;131(20):1806-1818.
49. Penfold RB, Zhang F. Use of interrupted time series analysis in evaluating health care quality improvements. *Acad Pediatr.* 2013;13:S38-S44.
50. Perla RJ, Provost LP, Murray SK. The run chart: a simple analytical tool for learning from variation in healthcare processes. *BMJ Qual Saf.* 2011;20:46-51.

The full reference list for this chapter is available at ExpertConsult.com.

PART

II

Infection of Specific Organ Systems

7 The Common Cold

James D. Cherry

The common cold is an acute, communicable, viral disease characterized by nasal stuffiness, sneezing, coryza, throat irritation, and no or minimal fever. Although the terms *upper respiratory tract infection (URI)* and *nasopharyngitis* are used frequently as synonyms for the common cold by physicians and other health care workers, the practice should be discouraged; the term *URI* is too broad, and pharyngitis is not present in most colds. To add to the confusion regarding terminology, "a cold" frequently has an even more diffuse connotation to the layperson.

HISTORY

Although the common cold undoubtedly has had an impact on the events of history, the specific symptom complex in ancient times was overshadowed by more severe contagious problems (influenza, plague, smallpox) and by septic diseases (otitis, sinusitis, mastoiditis, pneumonia) that were complications of upper respiratory tract viral infections. The name *common cold* most certainly arose from the fact that the onset of symptoms included the feeling of chilliness on exposure to cold. This association was perceived as a cause-and-effect relationship. More than 200 years ago, Benjamin Franklin pointed out that colds were caught from other people rather than by exposure to cold.[178]

In 1914, Kruse[140] showed that colds could be transmitted by the nasal instillation in healthy adults of Berkefeld-filtered nasal washings from ill individuals and that the causative agent was smaller than common bacteria. These findings were confirmed clearly in 1930 by Dochez and associates.[60] The way was paved for more extensive study of respiratory viral infections in 1933, when Smith and colleagues[201] reported the isolation and cultivation of an influenza A virus from a human.

The greatest contribution to the present understanding of the common cold has been the use of human volunteers under carefully controlled conditions. The Common Cold Research Unit at Salisbury, England, which was established in 1946,[6,228] and volunteer studies at this institution and studies done in the United States* are responsible for much of the present understanding of colds in adults.

Although studies of respiratory illness in children also have been extensive, controlled virus challenge trials have not been done. Pediatric studies have been most useful in delineating the spectrum of clinical manifestations by age group and seasonal prevalence rates of the respiratory viruses.

During the past decade the use of molecular methods has increased our understanding of the contributions of both newly discovered and established viruses in the etiology of the common cold and other respiratory illnesses.[77,152,193]

ETIOLOGIC AGENTS

Initial investigations into the etiology of the common cold were based on the hypothesis that only one etiologic agent needed to be discovered.[6] Subsequent studies revealed that many different groups of viruses were involved etiologically and that many types frequently existed within each group. Table 7.1 lists the agents associated with colds. Each of these agents is covered more fully in other chapters; this chapter presents an overview. As a group, rhinoviruses are the most common cause of colds in children and adults. Also of major importance in the etiology of colds are reinfections with parainfluenza viruses and respiratory syncytial virus (RSV). Although the quantitative contribution of coronaviruses to colds in children is less well known, they are significant contributors.[61,77,88,186,193,210] More recent studies also indicate that human metapneumovirus and human bocavirus cause colds in children.*

Enteroviruses and adenoviruses have been implicated frequently in upper respiratory tract illnesses, but in most instances the illnesses do not conform to strictly defined colds. Reoviruses cause colds, but their contribution to the overall incidence is unknown. *Mycoplasma pneumoniae, Chlamydophila* (formerly *Chlamydia*) *pneumoniae, Streptococcus pneumoniae,* and *Haemophilus influenzae* infections were identified serologically in one study involving young adults with colds, but, in most instances, concomitant viral infections also were noted.[153] Other agents, such as *Coccidioides immitis, Histoplasma capsulatum, Bordetella pertussis, B. parapertussis, B. bronchiseptica, B. holmesii, Chlamydophila psittaci,* and *Coxiella burnetii,* also have been associated with illnesses with initial coldlike symptoms.

EPIDEMIOLOGY

The common cold is an exceedingly frequent illness in childhood. For rhinoviruses alone, more than 100 serologically different viral types can cause this illness. Nonetheless, a general predictability of incidence and seasonal occurrence exists for the common cold. In the past numerous epidemiologic studies were conducted on the occurrence of respiratory tract illnesses, but calculating a precise incidence of the common cold from these studies is difficult because criteria of disease classification were different. The findings in three carefully performed studies are presented in Table 7.2. Two of these studies were done approximately 60 years ago, and the other was done more than 40 years ago. These studies involved a wide range of family life settings, and the average number of colds per year in children varied from three to eight.[11–14,26,84,153] Adults had on average approximately half the number of colds as their children.

In more recent times and in the era of the common use of daycare facilities, studies of the scope and magnitude of those presented in Table 7.2 have not been done. In one study published in the 1980s, the incidence of acute respiratory tract infections in daycare attendees peaked at 10 per child-year during the second 6 months of life.[55] A study by Wald and associates[236] found that children in home care had 4.7 illnesses per year, whereas the illness rate was 7.1 per year in children in daycare. Of the illnesses, 89% in daycare attendees were respiratory tract infections.

In 2008, Grüber and associates[95] reported the history of respiratory infections in a cohort of German children. The children in this cohort were seen at ages 3, 6, 12, 18, and 24 months and then annually until age 12 years. The common cold illness rates per year were 3.1 in infancy, 3.2 at year 2, 2.1 at year 3, 2.3 at year 4, 1.8 at year 5, 1.3 at year 6, 1.1 at years 7 to 9, and 1.0 at years 10 to 12. The reason for these overall decreased rates in contrast to previous studies is not apparent, but less complete data ascertainment seems likely. In addition, smaller family size and less use of daycare could be factors.

In a study in Arizona, researchers found that 52% of 2-year-old children who attended large daycare centers had six to nine colds per

*References 1, 29, 47, 50, 55–58, 96–99, 102, 104–106, 121, 122, 129, 159, 162, 221, 222, 224, 226, 227.

*References 8, 9, 15, 43, 75–77, 109, 185, 193, 239, 240.

year.[17] The conventional spread of colds has its initial focus in the school.[11,14,26] School-aged children become infected and introduce secondary infections into the home. Under these conditions, the secondary attack rate was highest in other school-aged and preschool-aged children. Generally, the secondary attack rate in adult family members was approximately half that of the children. The introduction of infection into the family by adults is unusual. In crowded settings, such as a university, infection is common and can be associated with substantial morbidity. In a cohort study of more than 3000 college students, colds and influenza-like illness were common findings and were associated with missed classes, poor performance on class assignments, missed extracurricular activities, and increases in use of medical care.[167]

As noted previously, the present trend toward the use of daycare centers and preschool programs has increased the number of primary infections in younger children and has made them the source from which secondary family infections frequently occur.[164] In a study that involved 606 children who received care at home or in a daycare program during the first 3 years of life, researchers found that children who attended a large daycare facility (six or more unrelated children) had more frequent colds at year 2 and less frequent colds at years 6 through 11 than did the children with home care only.[17]

In a national telephone survey in Australia in 2008–09 acute respiratory infections (ARI) were noted in 19.8% of families during the 4-week period prior to the telephone call.[39] Having a family member attending daycare was a significant risk factor for ARI in the family. In a daycare hand hygiene intervention study in the Netherlands, the yearly incidence of the common cold was 7.4 per child-year.[248]

Close personal contact between children is necessary for the transmission of viruses that cause colds. In the typical pediatric practice office setting, no increased risk for the acquisition of respiratory tract illnesses by well infants has been shown.[150] Among children, boys tend to have more colds than do girls.[11,26] In the conventional family setting, mothers tend to have at least one more cold per year than their spouses have.[11,26,84,85] The usual incubation period of colds is 1 to 5 days.

In all nonisolated populations, colds occur more frequently during the winter months than during the summer.[59,86,153,228] This seasonal discrepancy in incidence is as apparent in areas of high wintertime mean temperatures as it is in locations with extremely low temperatures. In the tropics, colds are more prevalent during the rainy season. Colds occur throughout the world. In isolated populations in which the number of people is few (e.g., members of Antarctic exploration teams and isolated island communities), colds do not occur unless introduced by a visiting person.[115]

Although colds can be produced regularly in volunteers, the method of transmission of viruses that results in colds under natural circumstances is unclear.* In individuals infected with respiratory viruses that cause colds, the greatest concentration of virus is in the nasal secretions. Children tend to have greater concentrations of virus than do adults, and they tend to shed virus for longer periods. Secretions related to coughing or saliva do not contain appreciable amounts of virus, and both are unlikely sources of contagion. During the process of talking, little virus is disseminated into the air. The greatest amount of virus from an infected individual is contributed to the surrounding environment by sneezing, nose blowing, and the general contamination of external surfaces (including the person's hands) with nasal secretions.

The route of acquisition of virus is by the nose and possibly the conjunctiva. With these facts in mind, one can easily see that a susceptible individual can become infected by inhalation of virus in droplet nuclei (small particles) resulting from a sneeze, by the direct nasal hit of virus containing large droplets from a sneeze, by nose blowing, or by the inoculation of virus (usually by the fingers of the recipient) from nasal secretions from disseminators that have been transmitted directly or indirectly. In children, most likely the spread either involves close contact with large droplets of nasal secretions containing virus that are applied to the nose from the hands of the future host or occurs by close-range airborne acquisition.

Considerable folklore is related to the catching of a cold. However, all available evidence to date indicates that cold weather per se, chilling, wet feet, and drafts neither cause nor increase the susceptibility of individuals to colds caused by viral infections.[62,121] A study of 180 adult subjects showed that acute cooling of the feet was associated with the onset of common cold symptoms.[128] On day 4, after the cooling of the feet or the control procedure, significantly more subjects in the chilled group thought they were suffering from a cold (14.4%) compared with the control group (5.6%). The subjects who thought they were suffering from a cold had a history of more colds each year in contrast to subjects who did not develop cold symptoms. In this study, no virologic studies were done, so no evidence exists that the cold symptoms observed were caused by viral infections.

In a study of respiratory tract infections in Finnish military recruits, it was found that cold temperature and low humidity were associated with an increased occurrence of respiratory infections; a decrease in

*References 27, 30, 47, 50, 51, 58, 96, 98, 102, 113, 121, 127, 143, 159, 190, 227, 228.

TABLE 7.1 Infectious Agents Associated With the Common Cold

Category	Agents
Common viruses that usually cause the common cold	Rhinoviruses Parainfluenza viruses Respiratory syncytial virus Coronaviruses Human metapneumovirus
Common infectious agents that occasionally cause illness with common cold symptoms	Adenoviruses Enteroviruses Influenza viruses Reoviruses
Illnesses with initial symptoms suggestive of the common cold	Human bocavirus *Coccidioides immitis* *Histoplasma capsulatum* *Bordetella pertussis, B. parapertussis, B. bronchiseptica, B. holmesii* *Chlamydophila psittaci* *Coxiella burnetii*

TABLE 7.2 Comparative Incidence of Upper Respiratory Infection by Age: London, 1952–53; Seattle, 1965–69; and Cleveland, 1948–50

LONDON		SEATTLE		CLEVELAND	
Age (y)	**Illnesses/Person/Year**	**Age (Yr)**	**Illnesses/Person/Year**	**Age (yr)**	**Illnesses/Person/Year**
0–4	5	<1	3.5	<1	6.9
5–9	3.6	1	3.8	1	8.3
10–16	4.1	2–5	3.7	2–5	8.3
Adult	2.9	6–9	2.7	6–9	6.1
		10–19	1.6	10–>11	5.5
		Adult	2.9	Adult	4.8

Data from references 11, 26, and 84.

temperature and humidity preceded the onset of the infections.[154] However no virologic data support the findings in this study.

In contrast, in controlled studies in which virologic studies were performed, no increased susceptibility to colds after exposure to chilling conditions was found.[6,62,66] In adults, risk factors for increased susceptibility to colds include stress, smoking, high basal levels of catecholamines, infrequent exercise, low intake of vitamin C, low sleep efficiencies, and lack of diverse social networks.[46,209] Physical stress, as opposed to mental stress, does not seem to be associated with increased susceptibility to colds. In a study of nine healthy men who were competitive cyclists who underwent intensive interval training, the men experienced enhanced performance but had no change in white blood cells, cytokine levels, or the frequency of upper respiratory tract infections.[67]

A fascinating volunteer study in adults by Cohen and colleagues[45] was reported in 2008. In this study the subjects were given rhinovirus 39 or influenza A/Texas/36/91 intranasally. It was found that subjects with increased subjective socioeconomic status were less susceptible to upper respiratory tract infections than subjects with decreased subjective socioeconomic status. In contrast, no relationship was found between objective socioeconomic status and susceptibility to the two challenge viruses.

PATHOPHYSIOLOGY

The pathophysiology of human infections with viruses that cause colds is presented in the sections of this book covering the individual infectious agents. A general overview is presented here. Few studies on the pathophysiology of respiratory tract infections have been done in children; the material presented in this section has been derived mainly from studies in adults.* The clinical syndrome of the common cold can occur in association with more than 100 different viral types and in many instances can occur with either a primary infection or a reinfection with a particular viral type.

Although the primary site of virus inoculation in some colds may be on the conjunctival surface, most result from inhalation or self-inoculation of virus onto the nasal mucosa. After acquisition of a virus has occurred, infection of the cells of the local respiratory epithelium develops. This infection varies in the degree of cytopathology on the basis of the viral agent. The infection spreads locally, resulting in an increase in nasal secretions with an increased protein content. Symptoms (nasal stuffiness and throat irritation followed by sneezing) begin on the second or third day and are caused by cellular damage and irritation. Virus shedding is at its maximum in 2 to 7 days, although some shedding may continue for another 2 weeks.

Hilding[114] examined biopsy specimens, scrapings, and smears of nasal secretions and noted that submucosal edema occurred initially, followed by shedding of the ciliated epithelial cells. By the fifth day, the epithelial damage had reached its maximum, with regeneration occurring during the next 10 days. Winther and associates[243] performed similar studies and noted the sloughing of epithelial cells, but they found that the epithelial lining remained continuous with normal cell borders. On the second day of disease, an increase in the number of neutrophils in the epithelium and lamina propria occurred. Epithelial mast cells were not involved in the inflammation. The nasal discharge during the second to the seventh day is mucopurulent owing to its content of desquamated epithelial cells and polymorphonuclear leukocytes.

In experimental rhinovirus colds in adults, little or no discernible damage to the nasal epithelium has been shown.[97,217,241,242] Arruda and associates[10] noted in adults infected with rhinovirus types 14 and 39 that virus replicates in ciliated and nonciliated cells in the nasopharynx and that only a very small proportion of the cells were infected.

Because damage to the nasal epithelium is not noted in rhinovirus colds, apparently cell death is not the cause of symptoms. Naclerio and colleagues[163] and Proud and associates[187] found that kinins are generated locally, and their concentrations correlate with the severity of symptoms. The cause-and-effect relationship between kinins and symptoms is questionable, however, because treatment with a bradykinin antagonist failed to lessen symptoms.[225] In addition, steroid therapy was found to reduce the concentration of kinins in nasal wash fluid, but it did not affect clinical symptoms.

In 1994, researchers noted that interleukin-1 (IL-1) may contribute to the pathogenesis of rhinovirus infections.[187] Ongoing molecular and biochemical research has provided information on methods by which rhinoviruses interfere with the host response, induce epithelial expression of IL-6 and IL-8, and mediate infection via activation of kinases and receptor binding activity.[69,135,160,177] In a human rhinovirus type 16 volunteer study it was found that IL-18 had a protective effect against colds and asthma exacerbations.[123] Conversely, it was noted that subjects with low nasal and bronchial IL-18 levels had increased respiratory symptoms. Similarly, research into the other viruses of the common cold has helped in the understanding of their similarities and differences, such as the cell-mediated immune response to human metapneumovirus and RSV.[65]

In studies in children with acute upper respiratory tract infections, IL-1β, IL-8, IL-6, and tumor necrosis factor (TNF)-α were found to be elevated markedly in nasal lavage fluid.[168] Pacifico and associates[172] found that IL-8 concentrations and white blood cell and neutrophil counts were significantly greater in children with rhinovirus colds than in well children. In an adult volunteer study, Turner and colleagues[227] noted a significant rank correlation between nasal obstruction severity, rhinorrhea severity, and nasal-wash albumin concentrations and the increase in IL-8 concentration from baseline to days 2 to 4 after virus challenge. In a study of 285 children with a parental history of asthma, other respiratory allergy, or both, blood specimens were obtained at birth and at 1 year of age.[89] The cytokine responses of mononuclear cells when incubated with phytohemagglutinin, RSV, and a rhinovirus were analyzed. Vigorous IL-13 and interferon (IFN)-γ responses to phytohemagglutinin and a marked secretion of IFN-γ in response to the viruses were associated with a reduced risk for developing wheezing with viral infections in the first year of life.

Pedersen and colleagues[176] studied nasal mucociliary transport in naturally acquired colds, noting that transport was reduced markedly during the acute illness and that slight impairment remained for approximately 1 month. They point out that because some children have four to six colds during a winter season, these children may have constantly impaired mucociliary transport.

Although viremia has been noted during infections with some of the viruses that cause colds, viremia is not known to occur during the typical common cold. The infection is restricted to the epithelial surfaces of the upper respiratory tract air passages, including the sinuses and eustachian tubes. With infection, local IFN is produced and presumably has a major role in controlling the infection.[38] Serum antibody and secretory antibody regularly result from infection. The roles of cell-mediated factors in immunity and disease pathogenesis of colds are unknown.

Levandowski and associates[145] noted in rhinovirus-challenged volunteers that total T cells, and particularly helper T cells, were depressed. The magnitude of this finding correlated with progression of infection and symptoms. In a study in which volunteers received rhinovirus type 39, Skoner and associates[200] found a slight increase in helper ($CD4^+$) and suppressor ($CD8^+$) T cells during illness. Noting that asthma exacerbations and rhinovirus infections are associated with decreased pH and ammonium levels in exhaled breath condensates, Carraro and colleagues[33] studied whether a direct rhinovirus infection, the host immune response to the infection, or both decreased the airway epithelial cell surface pH in vitro. They found that airway epithelial cell pH is affected partly by T-helper type 1 cytokines. This decrease in pH can provide an innate host defense, inhibiting viral replication in the lower airways. By mechanisms not well understood, within already infected cells, low pH is thought to trigger uncoating of rhinoviral RNA from within the endosome, thus enabling viral replication.[25]

The role of antibody (serum and secretory) in the protection against reinfection and clinical colds is complicated. High levels of secretory and serum antibodies seem to be protective against reinfections.* Clinically abortive colds probably are reinfection colds with early antibody recall. Fleet and colleagues[82] demonstrated a short-lived heterologous

*References 10, 40, 63, 132, 168, 172, 188, 200, 217, 227, 228, 242, 247.

*References 36, 37, 82, 119, 120, 122, 124, 144, 203, 216.

resistance to rhinovirus colds that probably is not caused by interferon or antibody.

Unexplained constitutional factors also seem to control the clinical manifestations of colds.[194] Although studies have shown genetic disease susceptibility patterns related to tissue types, no studies relating to common respiratory tract infections have been done.[41] In experimental coronavirus infections in adults, clinical severity correlated with detectable immunoglobulin (Ig)E in nasal secretions.[31] This finding suggests that atopy may be related to symptoms in colds caused by coronaviruses. Although clinical symptoms and virologic data suggest that colds are upper respiratory tract diseases, some studies of pulmonary function also have indicated occult lower respiratory tract involvement.[7,37,180]

In children younger than 5 years of age, primary traffic pollutants, ozone, and the organic carbon fraction of a particle size of less than 2.5 μm exacerbate upper respiratory infections.[52]

CLINICAL PRESENTATION

Because the common cold is caused by more than 100 different viral types, considerable variation in the clinical manifestations occurs. As indicated in the beginning of this chapter, the limits of illness to be considered under the diagnosis of the common cold have been set arbitrarily but rigidly. A disappointing note is that although many comprehensive studies of respiratory viral illnesses of children have been done, little attention has been given to the details of upper respiratory tract infections.

Illness in children must be considered under two categories—infants and older children. The latter is similar to illness in adults. In studies involving 100 young adults, Jackson and colleagues[119] noted that virtually all patients complained of nasal discharge, nasal obstruction, and sore throat; approximately 80% had malaise, postnasal discharge, headache, and cough; slightly fewer than 50% reported a feverish feeling and chilliness; and approximately 25% noted burning eyes and nasal membranes and muscle aching. In older children, the onset of illness is heralded by dryness and irritation in the nose and a scratchy feeling in the throat.[166] The initial symptoms are followed within a few hours by sneezing and watery nasal discharge; chilly feelings and occasionally muscular aches also are noted. Other complaints include headache, general malaise, anorexia, and low-grade fever.

After a variable period of 1 to 3 days, the illness changes; the nasal secretions become thicker and frequently develop a purulent appearance. Persistent nasal discharge, associated with the trauma of repeated blowing of the nose, leads to excoriation around the nose. Nasal obstruction leads to mouth breathing, which causes drying of the throat, increasing the discomfort in the throat. The usual duration of illness is approximately 7 days, but lingering cough and nasal discharge may persist for 2 weeks or more.[64]

A recent review of reports relating to respiratory tract infections in children by M. Thompson and associates[214] noted that in children 50% of the colds resolved by day 10 and 90% by day 15.

In infants, the manifestations of illness may be more varied. The onset of illness in infants is associated more often with fever (38°C to 39°C [100.4°F to 102.2°F]) than it is in older children. Nasal manifestations in infants are similar to manifestations in older children, but the only other manifestations are irritability and restlessness. Occasionally, coryza is the only symptom. Nasal obstruction may interfere significantly with feeding and sleeping. Vomiting and diarrhea also may occur.

DIFFERENTIAL DIAGNOSIS

Because the clinical entity of the common cold is an arbitrary grouping of signs and symptoms limited to anatomic boundaries and is caused by many different viral types, the approach to the differential diagnosis must consider clinical and etiologic criteria. Many upper respiratory tract illnesses are caused by numerous infectious agents that should not be confused with colds. A diagnosis of the common cold should not be considered if objective pharyngitis, other enanthema, or evidence of obstructive airway disease is present. Because the common cold is an acute, self-limited disease, the diagnosis should not be considered in a child who has persistent nasal signs or symptoms. Subacute or chronic illness should suggest the possibility of adenoiditis or sinusitis.

The most important differential diagnostic considerations are clinical entities of noninfectious etiology. Allergic rhinitis is a particularly important possibility in a child with "recurrent colds." Careful attention to family history, a search for allergies, the presence or absence of nasal eosinophilia, and the serum IgE value help confirm or exclude this consideration.

Although not reported particularly in pediatric patients, mental stress can lead to vasomotor responses and rhinitis in some susceptible patients. Chemical irritants can cause coldlike symptoms; the clinical response varies greatly across individuals. Early symptoms of many illnesses, such as pertussis, croup, epiglottitis, measles, and diphtheria, are those of a cold, but in a short time, the more serious nature of the actual illness becomes apparent.

SPECIFIC DIAGNOSIS

The epidemiologic history is the most important aspect of specific diagnosis. In children, if exposure history is requested, a contact usually is uncovered. If strict attention to clinical criteria of the common cold has been adopted, routine laboratory study is unnecessary. Frequently, the physician has an urge to take a throat culture to rule out the possibility of group A streptococcal infection. Usually, this is unnecessary because nasal symptoms are not characteristic of acute streptococcal illness except in infancy, and pharyngitis is not within the limits of the diagnosis of the common cold. The white blood cell count also is of little use.

A specific diagnosis can be made by isolating virus from nasopharyngeal secretions. It is performed best by a nasal-wash technique[101] or a nasopharyngeal swab or aspirate. With laboratory techniques (culture or polymerase chain reaction [PCR]) of diagnostic virologic facilities in university hospitals, public health laboratories, and in reference laboratories, all known common cold viruses can be identified.[15,61,75,76,88,109,152,193,210] (See Chapter 253.)

TREATMENT

Although literally hundreds of over-the-counter (OTC) cold remedies are available, few offer benefit to the pediatric patient, and many may be harmful.* No clinically available antiviral agents have been shown effective in the treatment of colds.

In the approach to a child with a cold, the best assumption is that no therapy is indicated in most cases. On occasion, specific symptomatic care can be added in the individual case when it appears to be needed. Many children and adults feel miserable when they have a cold, and therapy with an analgesic often is used. Because aspirin is a risk factor for Reye syndrome in children, the use of acetaminophen rather than aspirin is prudent. The dose per single administration of acetaminophen by year of age is as follows: younger than 1 year, 60 mg; 1 to 3 years, 60 to 120 mg; 3 to 6 years, 120 mg; 6 to 12 years, 150 to 300 mg; older than 12 years, 325 to 650 mg. Administration may be repeated every 6 to 8 hours in young children and every 4 hours in older children. Acetaminophen rarely should be given to infants younger than 6 months of age.

In adult volunteers with rhinovirus infections, acetaminophen was found to be associated with suppression of the serum neutralizing antibody response, and an increase in nasal symptoms was noted, in contrast to subjects who received a placebo.[93] In another adult volunteer study, administration of naproxen resulted in a reduction in headache, malaise, myalgia, and cough in contrast to placebo.[207] Choi and colleagues[42] looked at five studies to compare the efficacy and safety of nonsteroidal antiinflammatory drugs (NSAIDs) versus acetaminophen in symptom relief for the common cold. They found no difference in effectiveness between NSAIDs and acetaminophen in common cold symptom relief.

OTC cough and cold medications that contain antihistamines, antitussives, expectorants, decongestants, and antipyretics/analgesics in various

*References 4, 8, 16, 19, 21, 23, 24, 28, 35, 34, 53, 56, 68, 70, 71, 87, 90, 91, 100, 111, 116, 118, 131, 138, 141, 147, 149, 155-157, 169, 171, 173 175, 179, 182, 184, 191, 197-199, 202, 204, 208, 212, 219, 231-233, 235, 236, 246.

combinations are readily available for children.[173] Results of the Slone Survey noted that in a 1-week period, 10.1% of children in the United States received an OTC cough/cold medication.[232] Adverse events and deaths in children younger than 6 years have been observed.[53,141,173,191,197,204,232,233] In 2007, a U.S. Food and Drug Administration (FDA) advisory group recommended that OTC cough and cold medications not be used in children younger than 2 years. Unfortunately, a large number of parents and other caregivers are not aware of the FDA recommendations on OTC cough and cold medications.[156,231,245] The American Academy of Pediatrics in 2008 recommended that OTC cough and cold medications should not be used in children younger than 6 years.

Relief of nasal obstruction is the most important therapeutic consideration in young children. Locally applied or orally administered systemically active decongestants are used frequently, but neither their true efficacy nor their adverse effects have been evaluated carefully. Excessive use of sprays and drops with vasoconstrictive drugs can lead to rebound obstruction, which prolongs the illness. The associated drying effect of vasoconstrictive drugs administered orally can be expected to be deleterious to normal mechanisms of clearance. In young infants, sympathomimetic-antihistamine mixtures in oral drop dosage forms particularly are dangerous because respiratory depression may occur.[91] In addition, in a controlled trial, brompheniramine maleate–phenylpropanolamine hydrochloride was found to be no better than a placebo in relieving cold symptoms in children 6 months to 5 years of age.[44] If vasoactive drugs are used, their use should be restricted to times when maximum benefit would occur (i.e., bedtime), and they should be discontinued within 3 days.

The use of isotonic saline drops and gentle aspiration may be effective in the temporary relief of nasal obstruction in an infant. However, a Cochrane Collaboration review noted that available data were not sufficient to demonstrate efficacy of saline nasal irrigation.[131] It also noted that 40% of babies did not tolerate nasal saline drops. The general humidification of room air may be useful because this moisture tends to dilute tenacious nasal mucus and facilitate its elimination. In a Cochrane Collaboration review, steam inhalation was not shown to offer any consistent benefits in the treatment of the common cold.[198]

Antibiotics have no place in the routine therapy of common colds.[92,117,126,133,137,142,146,170,192,205] In children, persistent cough occasionally is a problem of such magnitude that it disturbs sleep. For cough, codeine and dextromethorphan often are used.[229] No well-controlled studies support either the efficacy or the safety of codeine or dextromethorphan as an antitussive in children, however. Eccles[72] suggested that the apparent efficacy of liquid cough syrups may be due to the sweetness of the products rather than their active ingredients. The proposed mechanism is that a sweet taste may affect cough at the level of the nucleus tractus solitarius by stimulating the production of endogenous opioids.

In the past, antihistamines were often given to children with colds, but efficacy had not been demonstrated.[238] In more recent years, first-generation antihistamines, but not second-generation products, have been shown to lessen rhinorrhea in adults with colds.[161,162,217,218,225] Doxylamine succinate, clemastine fumarate, chlorpheniramine maleate, and brompheniramine have been shown to offer benefit in controlled trials. The effect of these antihistamines is due to their anticholinergic properties. To date, no studies in children have been reported.

A major controversy relates to the efficacy of vitamin C in the common cold prophylactically and therapeutically. In two carefully controlled volunteer studies, the administration of 3 g of ascorbic acid per day did not prevent or alter the symptoms of experimental colds.[195,237] In addition, several large controlled trials in which vitamin C and placebo preparations were used to prevent and to treat colds were conducted.[5,32,48,49,73,112,129,181] Benefit was reported in some of these studies, whereas in others, no efficacy was noted. The reported benefits probably are a result of statistical artifacts and placebo effect owing to poor study design, rather than specific pharmacologic drug effects. The antihistaminic action of vitamin C[230,249] probably afforded relief to some patients with allergic rhinitis who thought that their illnesses were colds. Because of the many toxic effects of ascorbic acid,[18] and because its use in treating respiratory illnesses is questionable at best, giving children vitamin C in excess of normal daily requirements seems unwarranted.

For many years, efforts have been made to develop effective rhinovirus chemotherapy, but showing convincing efficacy in natural infection has been a challenge.[174] IFN alfa-2b administered intranasally has been shown to have some efficacy in the prevention of rhinovirus colds in controlled clinical trials.[206] The effect is variable, however, and adverse effects of the medication are frequent occurrences.[211] Intranasal IFN alfa-2b was ineffective in the treatment of naturally occurring colds but showed some benefit in experimental coronavirus colds.[107,222] Studies in adults using an antiviral antiinflammatory combination for treatment of the common cold showed some benefit in contrast to either agent used alone.[100] However, the irritation caused by intranasal IFN alfa-2b and the drowsiness associated with first-generation antihistamines render these drug combinations suboptimal.

Zinc lozenges have been used to treat the common cold; the Internet and lay literature are full of claims of efficacy, although in well-done, controlled studies, efficacy has not been shown.[70,71,79,125,151,183,221,236] However, a recent Cochrane Collaboration review noted that zinc administered within 24 hours of onset of symptoms reduced the duration and severity of the common cold in healthy people.[199] It also noted that prophylactic use reduced the incidence of colds and decreased school absenteeism and antibiotic use in children. The use of intranasal zinc preparations also is not well validated and raises some concern because of the possible development of the zinc-induced anosmia syndrome.[4,23] In a double-blind, placebo-controlled trial, the use of intranasal corticosteroid (fluticasone propionate) offered no clinical benefit in young adults with colds and induced prolonged shedding of rhinovirus.[189]

In a controlled trial in adults, a soluble intercellular adhesion molecule-1 product (tremacamra) reduced the severity of rhinovirus colds.[226] The antiviral pleconaril induced an early reduction in severity of symptoms in adults with colds caused by rhinovirus.[108] Pleconaril is an antipicornavirus drug that interacts directly with viral capsid proteins. It blocks attachment of virus to cells through intercellular adhesion molecule-1 and subsequent uncoating and release of viral RNA.

In another randomized, double-blind, placebo-controlled trial, the symptomatic efficacy of pleconaril was linked to its in vivo antiviral effects and to the drug susceptibility of the infecting virus.[178] In March 2002, the Antiviral Drugs Advisory Committee of the FDA voted against recommending pleconaril for approval of its use in the treatment of the common cold in adults. This decision was based on drug interactions, poor risk-to-benefit ratio, and concerns of development of resistant virus.[174]

Clarithromycin, a macrolide antibiotic, enhances mucosal immunity in mice by increasing levels of IL-12, IgA, and IgG.[134] In a controlled trial, however, clarithromycin had no effect on the severity of cold symptoms. The intranasal administration of nedocromil sodium has been observed to have a beneficial effect on rhinoviral infections in adult volunteers.[20] Mucolytics have emerged as potential therapeutics for modulating the function of airway epithelial cells and altering the course of viral infections.[9,246] Leukoprotease inhibitors and pulmonary surfactant have been shown to be upregulated by ambroxol, a mucolytic and antioxidant agent.[8,169]

In one study, adults who took sauna baths once or twice per week were found to have fewer colds than did members of a non–sauna-bathing control group.[74] In two studies, volunteers with colds did not benefit from inhaling heated vapor.[83,171]

The list of available and proposed complementary and alternative medicines thought to be useful for prevention and treatment of the common cold is long.* Most studies evaluating complementary and alternative medicines have been carried out in adults, not children. Compounds that have been studied include *Echinacea,* immune stimulants, ipratropium bromide, pine bark extracts, probiotics, derivatives from red seaweed, vitamin D, Baker's yeast β-glucan, cranberry polyphenols, *Pelargonium sidoides,* and bovine lactoferrin/whey protein. Blinding subjects in placebo-controlled trials can be difficult, and the placebo effect seems to play a significant role in the popularity of all complementary and alternative medicines.[21,24,34,56,111,219] Fluid extracts of *Echinacea* spp. are popular for the prevention and treatment of colds.[19,94,130,217,224] Because several species of *Echinacea* have been used in prevention and treatment

*References 2, 3, 19, 22, 24, 28, 54, 68, 78, 81, 103, 136, 139, 148, 149, 158, 165, 215, 234, 235, 244.

studies, criticism of the negative results in some studies has been expressed by *Echinacea* advocates.[24,35,90,138,196,208,212,219]

In a controlled trial, Taylor and associates[213] evaluated *Echinacea* for the treatment of upper respiratory tract infections in children aged 2 to 11 years. No benefit was noted, and the *Echinacea*-treated children had an increased occurrence of rash. Preparations of North American ginseng have been reported to decrease the frequency of colds in adults.[16,157,184] In a study of North American ginseng extract involving children 3 to 12 years of age, no treatment benefit was noted.[235]

In a 2010 study in children 2 to 11 years of age, Paul and associates[175] found that the application of Vicks VapoRub to the child's neck and chest at bedtime gave symptomatic relief from nocturnal cough, congestion, and sleep difficulty caused by an upper respiratory tract infection. This was a controlled study that compared the children treated with Vicks VapoRub with those who had received petrolatum to the chest and those who had no treatment.

PROGNOSIS

The prognosis of common colds in children is excellent. Secondary complications do occur, however, and frequently require careful and prolonged therapy. The most common complications are otitis media, sinusitis, bacterial adenoiditis, bacterial pharyngitis, and lower respiratory tract bacterial infections. The primary viral pathogens identified in hospitalized children with lower respiratory tract infections include RSV, influenza A and B viruses, human metapneumovirus, parainfluenza viruses, adenoviruses, rhinoviruses, and enteroviruses.[137] Infections with multiple agents also occur.

PREVENTION

Studies in isolated populations have shown that when a particular respiratory viral infection has run through the entire group, no further respiratory viral illnesses can occur until a new infected individual enters the population. This type of evidence indicates that quarantine or isolation practices could prevent colds. However, today's average urban society is so complex that prevention through isolation procedures is impractical. Efforts to control the spread of respiratory virus should be minimal and practical. For children with undue susceptibility to complications, contact with crowds or infected children and adults should be avoided.

Probiotics are considered by many to be useful for the prevention of upper respiratory infections.[2,54,103,136] In 2015, Hao and colleagues authored a Cochrane Database Systemic Review.[103] They felt that the overall data were poor but indicated that probiotics were better than placebo in preventing upper respiratory tract infections. They also felt that their use shortened illness duration, decreased school absence, and decreased antibiotic use.

In a double-blind, placebo-controlled study over a 6-month period in children 3 to 5 years of age it was found that the children receiving a probiotic twice daily had a decreased incidence of fever, coughing, and rhinorrhea with cold and influenza-like symptoms than did placebo recipients.[147] The children who received the probiotic had a significant reduction in days absent from group childcare and a reduced incidence of antibiotic use than did the placebo recipients.

The use of virucidal nasal tissues has been shown to reduce markedly the spread of rhinovirus colds in human volunteers and to reduce modestly colds in the family setting.[57,80] Heikkinen and associates[110] found that intranasal administration of an immunoglobin preparation by nasal sprays twice per day significantly reduced the occurrence of rhinitis in children attending daycare centers. If confirmed, this form of prophylaxis might be useful for selected children. A study showed that organic acids commonly used in OTC skin care and cosmetic products had substantial virucidal activity against rhinoviruses. The amount of acid applied to the hands correlated directly with the prevention of infection in the deliberate infection model.[220,223]

NEW REFERENCES SINCE THE SEVENTH EDITION

2. Ahanchian H, Jones CM, Chen YS, et al. Respiratory viral infections in children with asthma: do they matter and can we prevent them? *BMC Pediatr*. 2012;12:147.
3. AlBalawi ZH, Othman SS, Alfaleh K. Intranasal ipratropium bromide for the common cold. *Cochrane Database Syst Rev*. 2013;(6):CD008231.
4. Alexander TH, Davidson TM. Intranasal zinc and anosmia: the zinc-induced anosmia syndrome. *Laryngoscope*. 2006;116(2):217-220.
22. Belcaro G, Shu H, Luzzi R, et al. Improvement of common cold with Pycnogenol(R): a Winter registry study. *Panminerva Med*. 2014;56(4):301-308.
39. Chen Y, Williams E, Kirk M. Risk factors for acute respiratory infection in the Australian community. *PLoS ONE*. 2014;9(7):e101440.
42. Choi IK, Lee HK, Ji YJ, et al. A comparison of the efficacy and safety of non-steroidal anti-inflammatory drugs versus acetaminophen in symptom relief for the common cold: a meta-analysis of randomized controlled trial studies. *Korean J Fam Med*. 2013;34(4):241-249.
52. Darrow LA, Klein M, Flanders WD, et al. Air pollution and acute respiratory infections among children 0-4 years of age: an 18-year time-series study. *Am J Epidemiol*. 2014;180(10):968-977.
54. del Giudice MM, Leonardi S, Ciprandi G, et al. Probiotics in childhood: allergic illness and respiratory infections. *J Clin Gastroenterol*. 2012;46(suppl):S69-S72.
78. Fan Y, Ji P, Leonard-Segal A, et al. An overview of the pediatric medications for the symptomatic treatment of allergic rhinitis, cough, and cold. *J Pharmaceut Sci*. 2013;102(12):4213-4229.
81. Fazekas T, Eickhoff P, Pruckner N, et al. Lessons learned from a double-blind randomised placebo-controlled study with a iota-carrageenan nasal spray as medical device in children with acute symptoms of common cold. *BMC Complement Altern Med*. 2012;12:147.
103. Hao Q, Dong BR, Wu T. Probiotics for preventing acute upper respiratory tract infections. *Cochrane Database Syst Rev*. 2015;(2):CD006895.
112. Hemila H, Chalker E. Vitamin C for preventing and treating the common cold. *Cochrane Database Syst Rev*. 2013;(1):CD000980.
123. Jackson DJ, Glanville N, Trujillo-Torralbo MB, et al. Interleukin-18 is associated with protection against rhinovirus-induced colds and asthma exacerbations. *Clin Infect Dis*. 2015;60(10):1528-1531.
130. Karsch-Volk M, Barrett B, Linde K. Echinacea for preventing and treating the common cold. *JAMA*. 2015;313(6):618-619.
133. Kenealy T, Arroll B. Antibiotics for the common cold and acute purulent rhinitis. *Cochrane Database Syst Rev*. 2013;(6):CD000247.
136. King S, Glanville J, Sanders ME, et al. Effectiveness of probiotics on the duration of illness in healthy children and adults who develop common acute respiratory infectious conditions: a systematic review and meta-analysis. *Br J Nutr*. 2014;112(1):41-54.
139. Koenighofer M, Lion T, Bodenteich A, et al. Carrageenan nasal spray in virus confirmed common cold: individual patient data analysis of two randomized controlled trials. *Multidiscip Respir Med*. 2014;9(1):57.
143. L'Huillier AG, Tapparel C, Turin L, et al. Survival of rhinoviruses on human fingers. *Clin Microbiol Infect*. 2014;21(4):381-385.
148. Linder JA, Vitamin D. and the cure for the common cold. *JAMA*. 2012; 308(13):1375-1376.
156. Mazer-Amirshahi M, Rasooly I, Brooks G, et al. The impact of pediatric labeling changes on prescribing patterns of cough and cold medications. *J Pediatr*. 2014;165(5):1024-1028, e1021.
158. McFarlin BK, Carpenter KC, Davidson T, et al. Baker's yeast beta glucan supplementation increases salivary IgA and decreases cold/flu symptomatic days after intense exercise. *J Diet Suppl*. 2013;10(3):171-183.
165. Nantz MP, Rowe CA, Muller C, et al. Consumption of cranberry polyphenols enhances human gammadelta-T cell proliferation and reduces the number of symptoms associated with colds and influenza: a randomized, placebo-controlled intervention study. *Nutr J*. 2013;12:161.
200. Skoner DP, Whiteside TL, Wilson JW, et al. Effect of rhinovirus 39 infection on cellular immune parameters in allergic and nonallergic subjects. *J Allergy Clin Immunol*. 1993;92(5):732-743.
214. Thompson M, Vodicka TA, Blair PS, et al. Duration of symptoms of respiratory tract infections in children: systematic review. *BMJ*. 2013;347:f7027.
215. Timmer A, Gunther J, Motschall E, et al. Pelargonium sidoides extract for treating acute respiratory tract infections. *Cochrane Database Syst Rev*. 2013;(10):CD006323.
231. Varney SM, Bebarta VS, Pitotti RL, et al. Survey in the emergency department of parents' understanding of cough and cold medication use in children younger than 2 years. *Pediatr Emerg Care*. 2012;28(9):883-885.
234. Vitetta L, Coulson S, Beck SL, et al. The clinical efficacy of a bovine lactoferrin/whey protein Ig-rich fraction (Lf/IgF) for the common cold: a double blind randomized study. *Complement Ther Med*. 2013;21(3):164-171.
245. Yang M, So TY. Revisiting the safety of over-the-counter cough and cold medications in the pediatric population. *Clin Pediatr*. 2014;53(4):326-330.
248. Zomer TP, Erasmus V, Looman CW, et al. A hand hygiene intervention to reduce infections in child daycare: a randomized controlled trial. *Epidemiol Infect*. 2015;143(12):2494-2502.

The full reference list for this chapter is available at ExpertConsult.com.

8 Infections of the Oral Cavity

Constantine Simos • Blanca E. Gonzalez

Although most infections of the oral cavity in children are odontogenic and may be treated simply with local measures, the occasional spread of these infections to adjacent or distant fascial spaces or to the maxilla and mandible may result in life-threatening complications. Consequently, careful attention, including liberal use of the dental consultation, should be given to such infections.[32,78]

MICROBIOLOGIC CONSIDERATIONS IN DENTAL INFECTIONS

Normal Flora

That the oral cavity provides an environment favorable to the growth of microorganisms is substantiated by reports of bacterial counts of 10^8 to 10^{11} organisms/mL of saliva.[8,13] More than 30 species of bacteria normally can be identified in saliva in varying proportions depending on a dynamic interaction of microbial ecosystems, including the tongue, the gingival crevice, and the presence of plaque.[71,86] Age, anatomic relationships, eruption of teeth, presence of decayed teeth, diet, oral hygiene, antibiotic therapy, systemic disease, cancer chemotherapy,[73] and hospitalization can modify the microbial population. In the older literature, emphasis was placed on the role of *Streptococcus* and *Staphylococcus* spp. in producing odontogenic infections, to the exclusion of most anaerobic bacteria. This emphasis probably was the result of failure to culture satisfactorily for anaerobic organisms, and it is now well known that the ratio of anaerobic to aerobic organisms ranges from 3:1 to 10:1.[8,19]

The nomenclature of the oral flora is changing rapidly as a result of the improved understanding of the genetic makeup of these bacteria provided by molecular biology techniques. Table 8.1 summarizes changes in nomenclature among selected members of the oral flora.[20,93,92] Molecular methods based on polymerase chain reaction allow direct identification of bacterial species to be made from the oral flora and odontogenic infections by isolation of their DNA, RNA, or both. These methods have led to appreciation of the true oral flora, for which 60% of species are unculturable. In recent years, many new species and phylotypes have been identified in the normal and pathologic oral flora.

The flora of children is similar to that of adults, with several exceptions. At birth, the oral cavity is sterile, but colonization with *Streptococcus salivarius* occurs rapidly. This organism has been found in 80% of cultures taken from 1-day-old infants.[95] The percentage of *Streptococcus* spp. decreases from 98% at day 1 to 70% at 4 months[68] as other organisms become established. *Staphylococcus, Neisseria, Veillonella, Actinomyces, Nocardia, Fusobacterium, Bacteroides, Corynebacterium,* and *Candida* spp. and a variety of coliforms gradually become established by the time the child reaches 1 year of age. As the deciduous dentition erupts, anaerobic organisms become well established in the gingival crevice, yet the spirochetes *Bacteroides* and *Prevotella* spp. and related oral anaerobes, which commonly are associated with the gingival crevice in adults, seem to be present in fewer numbers in patients younger than 13 to 16 years.[13,95] Eruption of deciduous teeth also is associated with the establishment of *Streptococcus mutans* and *S. sanguinis,* which adhere to the enamel surface.

Pathogenic Organisms

Not all residents of the oral flora are pathogens. In the odontogenic infections caries and periodontal disease, a progression from initiating infections caused by oral streptococci toward a predominance of oral anaerobes in the more severe and long-standing infections apparently occurs. Caries is initiated primarily by *Streptococcus mutans,* a member of the α-hemolytic *S. viridans* group. As tooth decay progresses toward the dental pulp, *Lactobacillus* and *Actinomyces* spp. join the carious milieu. Severe pulpal infections generally are caused by a combination of these same oral facultative streptococci plus obligate anaerobes such as *Porphyromonas endodontalis,* formerly classified as *Bacteroides endodontalis.*[98]

Periodontal infections also are polymicrobial; gram-positive aerobes, primarily streptococci, predominate in gingivitis, and the gram-negative anaerobic rods predominate in bone-destroying periodontitis. Juvenile periodontitis (formerly called *periodontosis*), a particularly aggressive periodontal infection in children and adolescents, shows a predominance of *Aggregatibacter actinomycetemcomitans* (formerly known as *Actinobacillus actinomycetemcomitans*) in its cultivable flora.

Orofacial odontogenic infections that spread beyond the teeth and alveolar processes are polymicrobial, yielding on average four to six isolates per case.[12,53,66] With the use of molecular methods, even greater numbers of species can be identified in these infections, ranging from five to 18 species per case.[29] Severe orofacial infections have been associated statistically with *Fusobacterium nucleatum.*[41] The concept of the progression from aerobic streptococci to anaerobic gram-negative rods in orofacial infections is supported further by studies that have found a predominance of streptococci in early infections (in the first 3 days of symptoms) and a predominance of anaerobes in late infections.[53] Table 8.2 lists the frequency with which the major pathogens in orofacial infections were isolated in two studies.[42,57,89] Although the majority of bacterial identification studies are done with adult subjects, research indicates that odontogenic infections in children are caused by similar bacteria. In a recent study, *S. viridans* and *Neisseria* and *Eikenella* spp. were the most frequently isolated aerobic and facultative organisms. *Prevotella* and *Peptostreptococcus* spp. predominated among anaerobes.[88]

Infections originating from nonodontogenic causes (facial trauma, surgical manipulation, tonsillitis) are included in most studies of soft tissue and fascial space infections, and contamination from the skin or oropharynx might allow aerobic organisms, such as *Staphylococcus aureus* and aerobic *Streptococcus* spp., to become established.[13] In contrast, infections originating solely from the dental periapical tissues are much more likely to be predominantly anaerobic.

A pitfall in the identification of organisms as described in the older literature was the failure to culture satisfactorily for anaerobic organisms. The more current literature recognizes this fact.[58,70] The preponderance of anaerobic organisms in odontogenic infections mandates the use of anaerobic and aerobic culturing techniques in situations in which cultures are indicated.

ANATOMIC CONSIDERATIONS

Most severe orofacial infections develop consequent to dental infection—periapical, periodontal, or pericoronal. Spread occurs along anatomic pathways of least resistance.[8,19,45,56,97] Periodontal and pericoronal infections rarely have major sequelae because they generally drain from the gingival sulcus along the surface of the tooth into the oral cavity. Infections associated with the root apices generally are confined within the bony alveolar process (Fig. 8.1). Should spontaneous intraoral drainage occur through either the periodontium or the pulp chamber, further spread through the marrow spaces is unlikely. If such drainage does not occur, spread through bone (osteomyelitis) or perforation of the cortical plate of the affected jaw may occur. Infections associated with root apices close to the buccal cortical plate generally spread buccally, whereas infections close to the lingual or palatal cortical plate or maxillary

TABLE 8.1 Terminology Changes for Selected Oral Pathogens

Older Terminology	Current Terminology
Streptococcus viridans	*Streptococcus anginosus* *Streptococcus intermedius* *Streptococcus constellatus* *Streptococcus mutans* *Streptococcus sanguinis* *Streptococcus mitis* *Streptococcus salivarius* *Streptococcus vestibularis*
Streptococcus (milleri) anginosus	*Streptococcus anginosus* *Streptococcus intermedius* *Streptococcus constellatus*
Bacteroides melaninogenicus	*Prevotella melaninogenica* *Prevotella intermedia* *Prevotella oralis* *Prevotella buccae* *Prevotella denticola* *Prevotella nigrescens* *Porphyromonas asaccharolytica* *Porphyromonas gingivalis* *Porphyromonas endodontalis* *Porphyromonas salivosa* *Porphyromonas circumdentaria*
Streptococcus faecalis	*Enterococcus faecalis*
Streptococcus faecium	*Enterococcus faecium*
Peptococcus species	*Peptostreptococcus* spp. (main oral pathogen is *P. micros)*

TABLE 8.2 Most Frequent Pathogens Isolated From Orofacial Infections in Two Studies

	PERCENTAGE OF CASES	
Microorganism	**Lewis et al.**	**Sakamoto et al.**
Streptococcus milleri	50	65
Peptostreptococcus spp.	64	65
Other anaerobic streptococci	8	9
Bacteroides (Prevotella) oralis	40	74
Bacteroides (Prevotella) gingivalis	28	[a]
Bacteroides (Porphyromonas) melaninogenicus	24	17
Fusobacterium spp.	14	52

Data from Lewis MAO, MacFarlane TW, McGowan DA. Quantitative bacteriology of acute dentoalveolar abscesses. *J Med Microbiol.* 1986;21:101–4; and Sakamoto H, Kato H, Sato T, Sasaki J. Semiquantitative bacteriology of closed odontogenic abscesses. *Bull Tokyo Dent Coll.* 1998;39:103–7.

[a]This organism was not reported in this study.

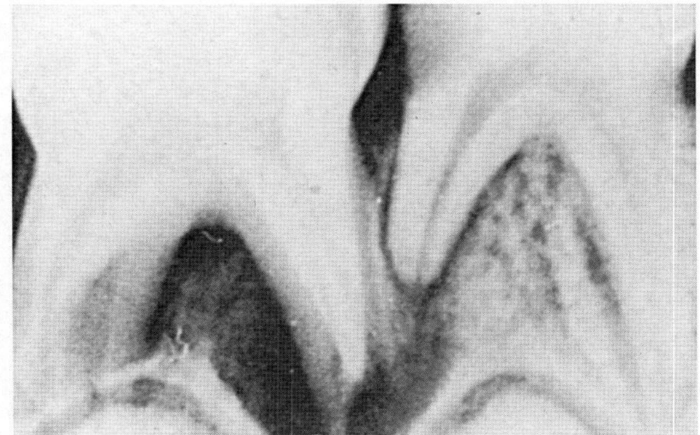

FIG. 8.1 Radiolucency representing a chronic periapical abscess involving the mesial root of the deciduous second molar and the distal root of the deciduous first molar. The developing mandibular bicuspids are seen inferior to the deciduous roots. The cause of the abscess is the deep carious lesions in both teeth, which appear to have penetrated the pulp chambers.

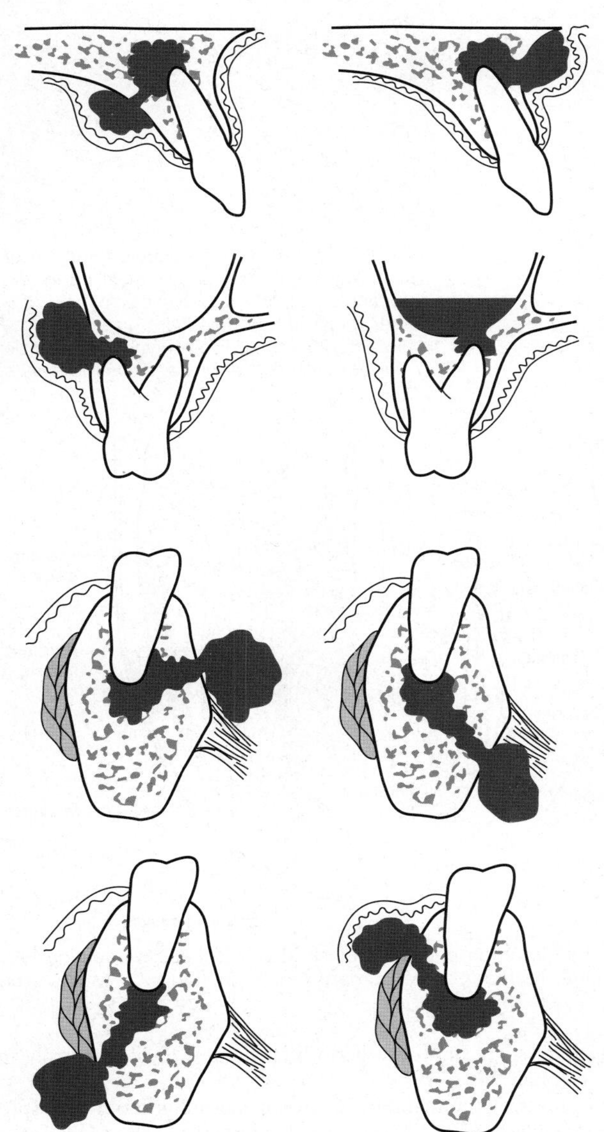

FIG. 8.2 Possible pathways of spread of periapical infection. (From Shafer WG, Hine MK, Levy BM. *Textbook of oral pathology*. 2nd ed. Philadelphia: WB Saunders; 1963.)

sinus spread in those directions (Fig. 8.2). When penetration of the cortical plate occurs, infection involves the adjacent soft tissues and may manifest as cellulitis or a soft tissue abscess, which eventually may perforate the mucous membrane or skin as a sinus tract (Fig. 8.3).

Perforation of periapical infections through bone follows a typical pattern that results from the position of the root apices in relation to the bony cortex and to muscle attachments (Fig. 8.4). Infections involving maxillary anterior teeth and buccal roots of maxillary posterior teeth generally perforate labially or buccally, whereas infections involving palatal roots of posterior teeth perforate palatally or rarely into the maxillary sinus. The presence of the buccinator muscle attachment superior to the root apices usually confines these infections and fistulas to the oral cavity. In children, maxillary root apices often are superior to the buccinator, however, and infections may spread to the buccal or

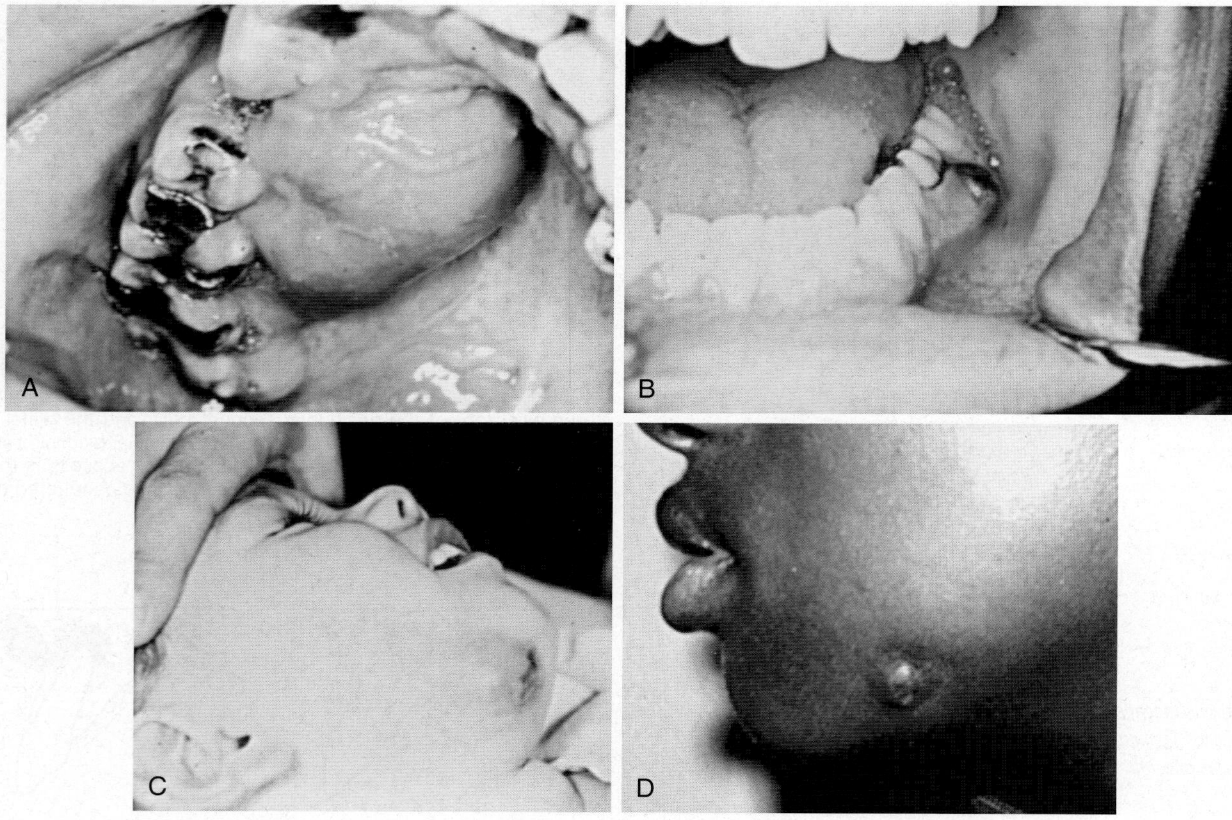

FIG. 8.3 Spread of odontogenic infection. (A) Palatal abscess resulting from infected first premolar. (B) Intraoral mucosal fistula from periapical abscess of mandibular left first molar. (C) Soft tissue infection secondary to periapical abscess. (D) Draining cutaneous sinus tract from a chronically infected lower molar in an adolescent girl. (A, From Piecuch J. Odontogenic infections. *Dent Clin North Am.* 1982;26:129–45. D, From Flynn TR, Topazian RG. Infections of the oral cavity. In: Waite DE, editor. *Textbook of practical oral and maxillofacial surgery*. Philadelphia: Lea & Febiger; 1987.)

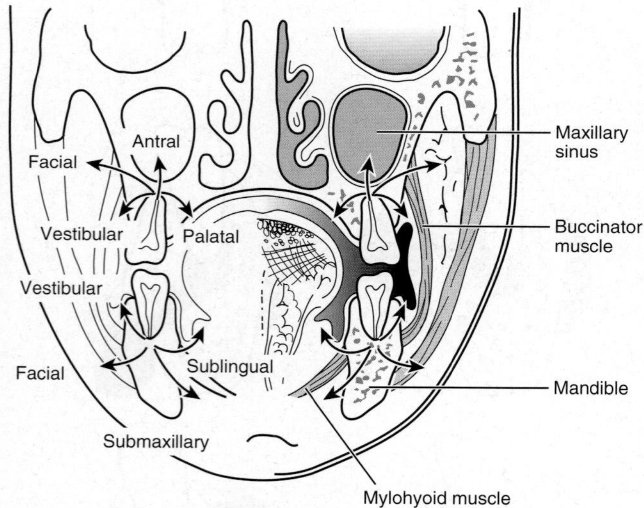

FIG. 8.4 Common pathways of spread of periapical infection. (From Kruger G. *Textbook of oral surgery*. 4th ed. St. Louis: CV Mosby; 1980.)

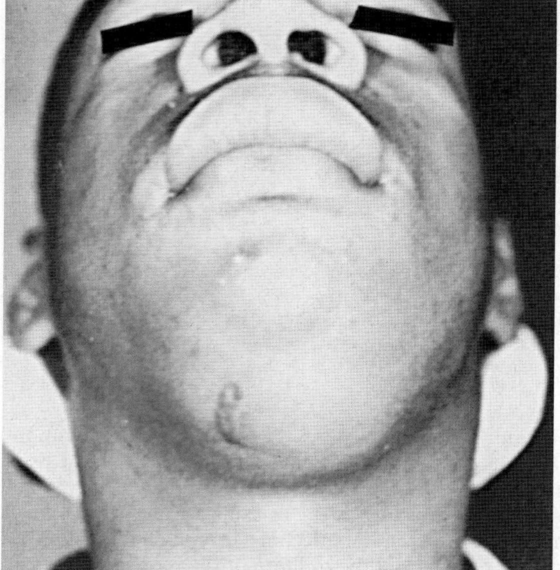

FIG. 8.5 Submental space abscess.

infraorbital space or to the periorbital tissues. They eventually may drain through the skin.

Infections of the mandibular incisor or canine tooth may spread either labially or lingually because the alveolar process is thin in this area. Labial perforation, which occurs more commonly, may be confined intraorally if the root apices are superior to the origin of the mentalis muscle but may spread extraorally if the apices are inferior to the mentalis attachment (Fig. 8.5). Infections of the mandibular premolar and first molar often perforate buccally, whereas the second and third molars perforate lingually.

When spread of mandibular infections occurs medially, the relationship of the tooth apices to the mylohyoid muscle origin is significant

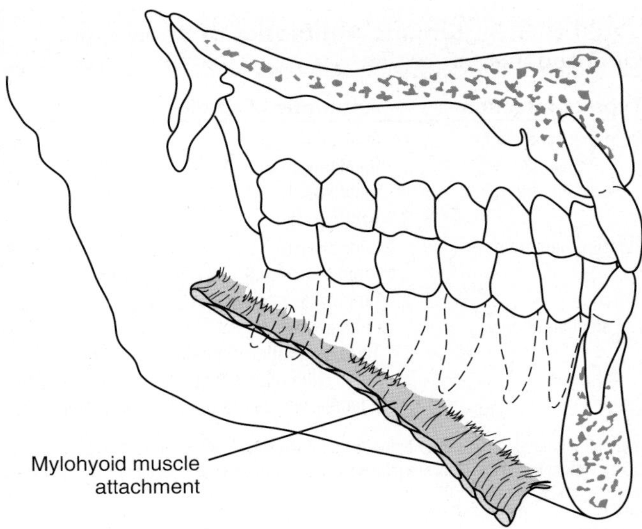

FIG. 8.6 Relation of tooth apices to the origin of mylohyoid muscle. (From Waite D. *Textbook of practical oral surgery*. Philadelphia: Lea & Febiger; 1978.)

(Fig. 8.6). From the first molar forward, the dental root apices are superior to the mylohyoid, and these infections localize intraorally in the floor of the mouth (sublingual space). The apices of the second and third molars generally are inferior to the mylohyoid and so the submandibular space is involved, with an extraoral presentation. As in maxillary infections, the relationship of the buccinator muscle to the root apices determines whether the infection spreads intraorally or extraorally.

Two fascial spaces commonly associated with odontogenic infections are the submandibular and masticator spaces.[36,37,56] The submandibular space is formed within the superficial layer of deep cervical fascia inferior to the mylohyoid muscle and inferomedial to the mandible. Anteriorly and posteriorly, it is limited by the bellies of the digastric muscle. Within this space lies the submandibular gland and portions of the facial artery and anterior facial vein. This space is closely approximated to the sublingual and masticator spaces. Infections of the submandibular space may originate in these adjacent spaces and in the mandibular posterior teeth.

The masticator space also is formed within the superficial layer of deep cervical fascia. Its name is appropriate because its contents include the masseter, internal and external pterygoid, and temporalis muscles, as well as the mandibular ramus and the inferior alveolar neurovascular bundle. The submandibular, lateral pharyngeal, and retropharyngeal spaces are adjacent. Infections of the masticator space may originate in adjacent spaces or spread to it from periapical or pericoronal infections of the mandibular second and third molars and maxillary third molar.

TREATMENT OF ODONTOGENIC INFECTIONS

Patients with odontogenic infections may present with symptoms ranging from minor to life-threatening. Too often, a patient may be given a thorough systemic and extraoral head and neck evaluation while the intraoral search for the etiologic agent is overlooked.

A thorough oral examination begins with an evaluation of the degree of mandibular opening. Interincisal distance on wide opening extends 40 mm or more, even in young children. Painful limitation of the oral opening, or trismus, is associated with inflammation of the muscles of mastication and indicates spread of the infection to the masticator space. In association with a high fever, it can represent a serious turn of events. Teeth are inspected visually for caries, by percussion for tenderness, and by electric sensitivity or hot and cold stimulation for the pulpal pain response. Gingival tissues are probed for periodontal defects, and salivary glands are palpated for tenderness and milked to observe for purulent discharge from the duct orifices.

General Therapeutic Principles

As with infections elsewhere in the body, the principles of treatment of oral infections involve surgical drainage and antibiotics. Surgical drainage may comprise standard incision and drainage of an orofacial swelling or, in the case of localized periapical infection, endodontic drainage through the pulp or extraction of the offending tooth.

Surgical treatment of odontogenic infections is primary. In a systematic review of the literature, Flynn concluded that once an abscess was drained, the usual antibiotics used for treatment of odontogenic infections worked.[27,28] Dodson and colleagues,[23] in a review of head and neck infections requiring hospitalization of children, found that facial infections of the regions at or above the level of the upper lip and teeth most frequently were upper respiratory tract– or sinus-related and that lower face infections primarily were odontogenic. Infections of the upper face resolved without surgery in 65% of cases, whereas infections of the lower face resolved without surgery in only 25% of cases. Odontogenic infections almost always required some sort of surgical intervention. This finding may be due to the fact that the portal of entry in respiratory tract infections is through the surface mucosa, whereas the tooth roots carry the invading bacterial pathogens deep into the bone of the jaw, through which the surrounding deep fascial spaces become infected.

Respiratory pathogens frequently are viral, and odontogenic infections almost uniformly are bacterial, which may explain the propensity of odontogenic infections to form abscesses that need to be drained. Odontogenic infections treated with antibiotics only almost always recur in worse form than their previous manifestation. The indications for treating with antibiotics in addition to appropriate dental surgical therapy are fever, trismus, lymphadenopathy, osteomyelitis, and compromise of the immune system. Minor infections localized to the alveolar processes can be treated by tooth extraction, gingival curettage, or root canal therapy, with or without intraoral incision and drainage, without the use of antibiotics in the nonimmunocompromised individual.

Approximately 10% of all antimicrobials prescribed in the community are for the treatment of an oral process.[18] Misuse and overuse of antimicrobials have led to increasing resistance among many bacterial species. Oral pathogens have not been the exception. In an effort to promote the judicious use of antibiotics, the American Academy of Pediatric Dentistry (AAPD) and American Dental Association have developed guidelines intended to help reduce the inappropriate use of antimicrobial therapy in oral infections.[1] Despite the guidelines, the adherence to the recommendations continue to be low, as demonstrated in a recent survey of 154 dentists revealing that adherence to guidelines was between 10% and 40%.[18] In these guidelines, consideration for treatment with antibiotics involves the assessment of certain factors such as the type of infection, location and extent of infection, risk for bacterial contamination (e.g., deep crown fractures), trauma, and immunologic status of the patient.

Selecting the appropriate antibiotic should follow the basic principles of therapeutics, which include choosing the narrowest spectrum based on cultures and susceptibilities and selecting an agent that concentrates adequately in the desired tissues and that has a good safety profile, convenient dosing, and the fewest side effects. In addition, it is important to inquire about the patient's previous antimicrobial exposures, which is a known risk factor for harboring more resistant organisms, as well as documentation of any drug allergies. In the adolescent population, asking about oral contraceptives is important because certain antibiotics used to treat dental infections, such as penicillins and tetracycline derivatives, can interfere with the efficacy of contraceptives.[1]

Antibiotic selection for odontogenic infections, although ultimately based on Gram stain and aerobic and anaerobic cultures, generally is begun empirically before culture results are available. Odontogenic infections are usually polymicrobial, with anaerobes playing an important role.[12] Penicillin and amoxicillin have been the first choice for outpatient infections on the basis of a good safety profile, bactericidal nature, and sensitivity of most streptococci and oral anaerobes to penicillin. However, there have been more reports of penicillin and amoxicillin resistance among oral pathogens that produce β-lactamases. Moreover, penicillin offers little or no coverage against *Neisseria* spp., a pathogen frequently found in odontogenic infiltrates.[88] A study of hospitalized patients with odontogenic infections found penicillin-resistant organisms in 54% of cases and therapeutic failure of empiric penicillin in 21% of cases.[28] The duration of previous therapy with β-lactam antibiotics also has been correlated with increased numbers of β-lactamase–producing bacteria in persisting infections. Patients with persisting infection after 3 days of treatment with a β-lactam antibiotic had a 50% incidence of β-lactamase–producing bacteria in the infection.[40,49] β-Lactamase inhibitors used in combination with β-lactam antibiotics may improve their effectiveness against resistant anaerobes, and using higher doses of the amoxicillin component may overcome resistance of some oral streptococci.[9]

Antibiotic susceptibility studies indicate that the oral anaerobes (especially *Fusobacterium*) and *Streptococcus* spp. now are largely resistant to erythromycin.[35,77,79] Based on these data, erythromycin should not be used as first choice in patients with odontogenic infections who are allergic to penicillin. Clindamycin, on the other hand, has an excellent track record in the treatment of odontogenic infections and can be used in patients allergic to penicillin. It concentrates well in saliva and bone and has enhanced activity against anaerobes, including bacteroides. However resistance of odontogenic flora to this lincosamide derivative is also on the rise. Poeschl and colleagues[80] tested 73 streptococci species isolated from patients with odontogenic deep-space infections and found 16% clindamycin resistance among *Streptococcus* spp. and 11% resistance among oral anaerobes (*Prevotella, Bacteroides,* and *Peptostreptococcus* spp.). *Eikenella corrodens,* an occasional pathogen in odontogenic infections, is uniformly resistant to clindamycin, which may explain the lack of effectiveness of clindamycin in some cases. A feared complication of the use of clindamycin is the development of *Clostridium difficile* colitis. This entity was first described after the use of this antibiotic and has been reported after use of clindamycin as prophylaxis for dental infections.[11] However, more cases are reported yearly of *C. difficile* after the use of penicillin and cephalosporins than with clindamycin.[12] Penetration of this drug through the blood-brain barrier is poor, and it should not be used to treat central nervous system abscesses of odontogenic origin. Azithromycin is another alternative in patients with severe penicillin allergies. It has comparable activity against oral gram positives but enhanced coverage for anaerobic gram negatives when compared to erythromycin, and it has been utilized successfully in the treatment of adult patients with periodontal disease.[43,69]

Moxifloxacin, a fluoroquinolone with a spectrum of activity similar to that of amoxicillin-clavulanate, has been studied for the treatment of odontogenic infections with very good outcomes. A double-blind, phase II randomized trial comparing moxifloxacin with clindamycin in odontogenic infections found that moxifloxacin has excellent activity against *Streptococcus* spp. and oral anaerobes and was very effective in treatment of inflammatory odontogenic infections and abscesses.[14] However, this trial did not include children. Fluoroquinolones, especially ciprofloxacin and levofloxacin, have been used more often in children in recent years, especially in those with cystic fibrosis. The concern of musculoskeletal adverse events (e.g., tendinitis or adverse cartilage effects) has always been the limiting factor for their use in children. Ciprofloxacin and levofloxacin are less active against oral pathogens. Moxifloxacin has been used successfully in the treatment of multidrug-resistant tuberculosis in children.[5,17,30,99] Yet the optimal dosing remains to be determined. A recent pharmacokinetic study of moxifloxacin in children with tuberculosis showed that using a 10 mg/kg daily dose achieved low serum concentrations when compared to the maximum 400 mg daily adult dose, suggesting that perhaps higher doses are needed.[99]

The second-line antibiotics in odontogenic infections are the cephalosporins, which, with the exception of the cephamycins (i.e., cefoxitin, cefotetan), have poor activity against oral anaerobes. Cephalosporins can be combined with metronidazole to enhance anaerobic coverage. Metronidazole has excellent activity against anaerobic bacteria but no activity against aerobic organisms. Moreover, it has no activity against organisms such as *Actinomyces* and microaerophilic streptococci, thus limiting its use as monotherapy for odontogenic infections.[54]

Tetracycline is incorporated permanently into newly formed dentin, causing permanent disfiguring discoloration of the dentition. It should not be used in children until they are at least 9 years old, when all but the third molar teeth would have full crown formation.

TABLE 8.3 Empiric Antibiotics of Choice for Odontogenic Infections

Type of Infection	Antibiotic of Choice
Outpatient infections	Penicillin Clindamycin
Penicillin allergy	Clindamycin Azithromycin
Inpatient infections	Clindamycin Ampicillin + metronidazole Ampicillin + sulbactam
Penicillin allergy	Clindamycin Third-generation cephalosporin IV (if the penicillin allergy was not the anaphylactoid type—use caution) + metronidazole

Empiric antibiotic therapy is used before culture and sensitivity reports are available. Cultures should be taken in severe infections that threaten vital structures.

Penetration into the blood-brain barrier is important when treating odontogenic infections that spread beyond the oral cavity and approach the cranial cavity. Penicillin will penetrate the barrier when the meninges are inflamed, whereas first- and second-generation cephalosporins will not. Clindamycin has poor penetration into the central nervous system and should not be used in brain abscesses. Conversely, metronidazole has excellent central nervous system penetration but needs to be combined with treatment for aerobic bacteria.[54]

The aforementioned considerations suggest that the empiric antibiotics of choice are penicillin in mild odontogenic infections and clindamycin for severe cases or in a patient with penicillin allergy. Table 8.3 lists our recommendations for empiric antibiotic therapy in odontogenic infections.

Nursing Bottle Caries

Nursing bottle caries is a pattern of tooth decay affecting mainly the primary upper incisors and frequently the upper and lower primary molars in children of bottle-feeding age. It is caused by a practice of putting the child to bed with a nursing bottle filled with a sugar-containing drink, such as milk, fruit juice, or a soft drink. The child sucks on the bottle intermittently during sleep, when salivary secretion is low, and the sugar-containing liquid stays in the mouth for extended periods. This situation provides an excellent environment for the growth of caries-producing organisms such as *S. mutans*. Nursing bottle caries can destroy virtually the entire primary dentition of a child as it erupts. Pediatric physicians and dentists should instruct parents to avoid putting their children to bed with nursing bottles or, if they must do so, to use water only in the bedtime drink.

Periapical Abscess

Extension of microorganisms through the root apex leads to the formation of an abscess. Early in this process, the acute abscess is indistinguishable clinically and radiographically from an acute pulpitis, particularly because radiographic evidence of bone destruction may take 7 to 14 days or more to develop. Sensitivity to heat stimulus (relieved by cold), exquisite sensitivity to percussion, and tenderness to finger pressure on the alveolar process are indications that the tooth has become abscessed. Electric pulp testing may be diagnostic if the tooth shows no response to the electric stimulus, but a positive pain response may be equivocal in multirooted teeth. Chronic abscesses are diagnosed more easily by looseness of the tooth, suppuration from draining sinuses or gingival crevice (see Fig. 8.3), and radiolucency on the radiographs (see Fig. 8.1). Depending on the path of least resistance, fluctuant areas may be noted in the buccal or lingual mucosa. Spread through the tissues, or cellulitis, may lead to the classic presentation of swollen face, pain, elevated temperature, and malaise.

In 1951, Krogh[49] showed a 3% complication rate when 2626 infected teeth were removed at the time of initial presentation. In 1975, Martis and Karakasis[65] published a similar study in which they treated 1376

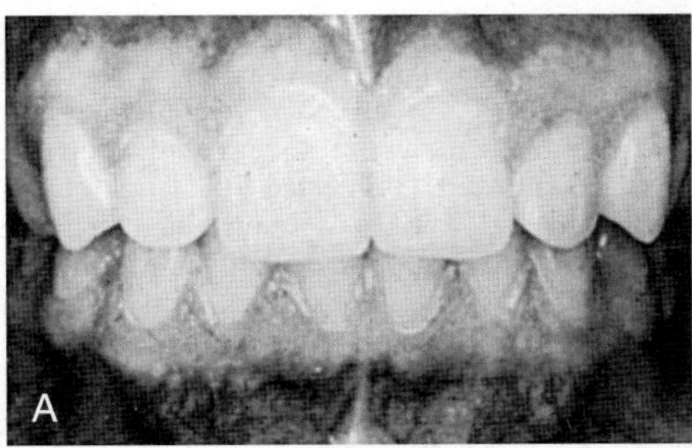

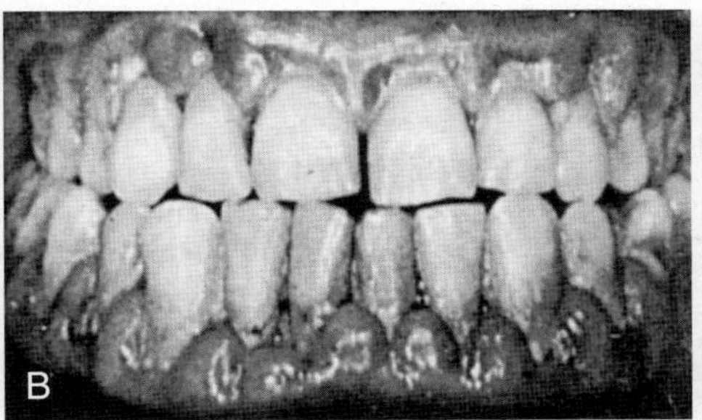

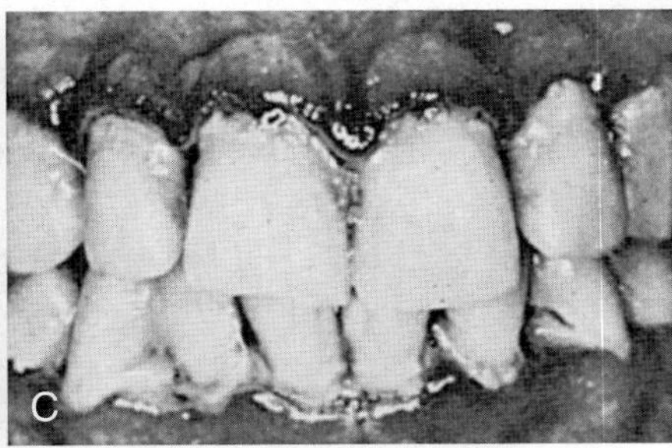

FIG. 8.7 (A) Normal gingivae. (B) Severe gingivitis. The maxillary gingivae exhibit mild inflammation; the mandibular interdental papillae are distorted grossly in form. Accumulations of plaque are prominent adjacent to the mandibular incisors. (C) Acute necrotizing ulcerative gingivitis.

BOX 8.1 Indications for Antibiotic Therapy in Odontogenic Infections

Antibiotic Therapy Is Necessary

Acute-onset facial or oral swelling
Swelling inferior to the mandible
Trismus
Dysphagia
Lymphadenopathy
Fever >38.3°C (>101°F)
Pericoronitis
Osteomyelitis

Antibiotic Therapy Is Not Necessary[a]

Asymptomatic periapical abscess
Parulis (draining sinus tract)
Dry socket (alveolar osteitis)
Periodontal disease
Dental extractions
Root canal therapy

[a]With coexisting immune system compromise, antibiotic therapy may be indicated in some of these conditions.

acute dentoalveolar abscesses by immediate extraction. A 3% complication rate was found in this study as well. A complication was defined as further extension of the infection requiring additional treatment. Hall and associates[39] published a report in 1968 in which 350 patients with odontogenic cellulitis were divided randomly into two groups. The first group had extractions performed on the day of initial presentation, whereas the second group waited (with antibiotics) until the fourth day for surgical treatment to be performed after "localization" had occurred. The investigators' observations showed that extraction did not spread the cellulitis in either group. Patients with earlier extractions recovered more rapidly, whereas patients with delayed treatment had a greater need for incision and drainage, which was twice as likely to be extraoral than intraoral. In 1978, Martis and colleagues[65] showed in a series of more than 2000 patients that extraction without antibiotics in the presence of periapical infection led to the same complication rate as did extraction of noninfected teeth. Current literature validates these earlier findings, indicating that infections in patients with poor oral health and a lack of preceding dental treatment produce a stronger systemic response. Extraction of involved teeth when indicated and other dental treatments lead to a less severe course of infection.[91]

Considering the prospect of early relief of symptoms and a 97% chance that extraction (or occasionally root canal treatment) will cure the infection, early surgical intervention is mandatory. The use of antibiotics must be determined on an individual basis according to principles outlined previously (Box 8.1).

Periodontal Infections

Surrounding the teeth is a distinctive, pink keratinized mucosa, the gingiva (Fig. 8.7A). Normal gingiva is attached firmly to the alveolar bone and extends between the teeth as the interdental papilla. A thin cuff of free (nonattached) gingiva surrounds each tooth, and the resulting crevice between the free gingiva and the tooth normally is 1 to 3 mm in depth. It is represented by a thin roll of tissue along each tooth in Fig. 8.7A.

Accumulation of food deposits and bacteria in the gingival crevice may result in gingivitis, a localized inflammation of the free gingiva that manifests as an erythematous, nonpainful swelling of the interdental papillae. In severe cases (see Fig. 8.7B), the gingival architecture may become distorted, and accumulations of plaque are evident. Although gingivitis is prevalent at all ages, affecting more than 50% of children[67] and almost all adults to some degree, it often is most severe in compromised hosts, including patients with diabetes and immunosuppressed patients. Poor oral hygiene is the usual precipitating factor for the development of gingivitis, and this condition generally responds to dental scaling and improved oral hygiene.

In adolescents and adults, gingivitis may progress to periodontitis, a progressively severe infection characterized by hypertrophied gingivae, tooth mobility caused by irreversible resorption of alveolar bone, and a purulent exudate. This insidious condition usually is painless and may progress for years before being recognized. Localized periodontal treatment and meticulous oral hygiene may arrest the condition.

A rare variant, juvenile periodontitis,[53] usually is localized to the molar and incisor regions of younger, otherwise healthy children. Deep gingival pocketing and severe bone resorption are characteristic of this process and may result in loss of the dentition in these areas. The etiology is thought to involve a gram-negative anaerobe, *A. actinomycetemcomitans*, and localized bacterial inhibition of leukocyte function. Tetracycline in older patients has been useful in combination with periodontal surgery and meticulous home care.

Acute necrotizing ulcerative gingivitis (see Fig. 8.7C) is a specific infection caused by fusiform bacilli and spirochetes. Synonyms include trench mouth and Vincent infection. Erythema at the tips of the interdental papillae soon is supplanted by frank ulceration and foci of spontaneous bleeding. A pseudomembranous necrotic exudate forms along the marginal gingivae and the interdental papillae. The papillae later become blunted. Acute necrotizing ulcerative gingivitis is characterized by pain, foul breath and taste, thick ropy saliva, malaise, and occasionally fever. Theories suggest a concomitant viral etiology. Treatment consists initially of penicillin or amoxicillin ± metronidazole therapy for 7 days followed within a few days by localized gingival curettage and oral rinses with 0.5% hydrogen peroxide or 0.12% chlorhexidine.[4,49,60]

Pericoronitis

Impaction of microorganisms and debris under the soft tissue overlying the crown of a tooth, often a mandibular third molar, or any erupting permanent tooth leads to the development of inflammation. Drainage usually occurs spontaneously from under the flap, localizing the problem.

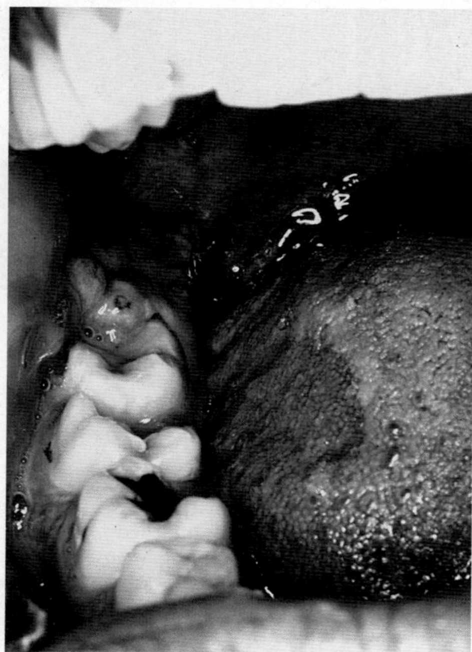

FIG. 8.8 Pericoronitis.

Blockage of natural drainage may lead to spread of infection to adjacent soft tissues and fascial spaces (Fig. 8.8).

Pericoronitis is a polymicrobial infection; the periodontal pathogens *Prevotella* and *Porphyromonas* spp. and oral spirochetes, such as *Treponema denticola,* usually are the causative organisms. The *Streptococcus milleri* group bacteria also have been found to have a significant role in acute pericoronitis.[42] These organisms usually are sensitive to penicillin or penicillin combined with metronidazole. Pericoronitis most frequently occurs around the posterior portion of the crown of the lower third molar because it erupts during adolescence. In most cases, partial eruption of the third molar is caused by insufficient length of the horizontal ramus of the mandible to house all of the teeth. Part of the third molar is trapped under the oral mucosa covering the buccinator muscle and the superior pharyngeal constrictor because they form the most anterior portion of the oropharynx. In cases in which room is insufficient for the eruption of the third molar, the pericoronitis becomes recurrent or chronic, and the impacted third molar should be removed.

Lower third molars lie in proximity to the pterygomandibular space, a portion of the masticator space. When these infections spread to involve this space, trismus results, which obscures the infection to clinical examination. The presence of trismus with a history of pain in the third molar region is an ominous sign of infection involving the masticator space, which, although not manifested by external facial swelling, may begin to involve the deeper parapharyngeal spaces. These infections may become life-threatening. The lower third molar is the most frequent offending tooth in severe odontogenic infections requiring hospitalization, and these infections occur most frequently in adolescents and young adults.[41]

Various treatment modalities, including local incision and drainage and extraction of the tooth, are applicable to pericoronitis.[64,87] Antibiotic therapy is used if fever, trismus, or lymphadenopathy is present (see Box 8.1). Resolution of symptoms should occur in less than 1 week.

Oral Manifestations of Human Immunodeficiency Virus Infection in Children

The most common oral lesions in children with human immunodeficiency virus (HIV) disease are oral candidiasis, herpes simplex virus (HSV) infections, linear gingival erythema, parotid salivary gland enlargement, and recurrent aphthous ulcerations. In contradistinction to adult HIV infection, HIV-associated periodontitis and gingivitis are much less common. Neoplastic oral manifestations of HIV infection, such as Kaposi sarcoma, non-Hodgkin lymphoma, and hairy leukoplakia, continue to be rare findings. In contrast to adults, children infected with HIV have a greater susceptibility to bacterial infections, especially with encapsulated organisms such as *Streptococcus pneumoniae* and *Haemophilus influenzae*. Septicemia from an oral focus of infection can become a life-threatening problem in an HIV-infected child, and optimal oral health must be established and vigorously maintained in these children.[51] Routine use of chlorhexidine gluconate 0.12% mouth rinse may be helpful in minimizing gingivitis, candidiasis, and bacterial superinfections of the oral cavity, although its safety and effectiveness have not been shown in children.

Oral candidiasis usually is of the pseudomembranous type, which is seen in the oral cavity as a creamy white plaque that is rubbed off easily, leaving a reddened surface mucosa exposed. Because oral candidiasis is rare in normal children older than 6 months, persistence of oral candidiasis for 2 months or more in a child older than 6 months who has not received antibiotic therapy in the past 2 weeks is suggestive of HIV infection. Persistent oral candidiasis indicates acquired immunodeficiency category P-2D3 (symptomatic infection with secondary infectious diseases) in the Centers for Disease Control and Prevention classification of HIV infection in children younger than 12 years.[48]

Oral candidiasis was associated with a decreased survival time in a study of 99 children with perinatally acquired HIV infection. The median time from birth to the manifestation of the first lesion of oral candidiasis was 2.4 years, and the median time from the appearance of lesions to death was 3.4 years, with a relative hazard rate of 14.2.[47]

Treating oral candidiasis lesions is difficult because of frequent recurrence of oral fungal infection with resistant biotypes of *Candida albicans* or colonization by related but more resistant species such as *C. krusei, C. parapsilosis,* and *C. guilliermondii*. Treatment regimens range from nystatin to clotrimazole for uncomplicated oropharyngeal candidiasis to fluconazole, other azoles, echinocandins, or amphotericin B for more severe disease depending on the extent of disease, clinical response, and culture and sensitivity results.[51,62,75,76] Sudden onset of rampant dental caries has been associated with prolonged oral use of sucrose-containing antifungal antibiotic preparations.[85]

Linear gingival erythema, formerly referred to as HIV gingivitis, is the most common form of periodontal disease seen in children with HIV infection. It is described as a fiery red, 2- to 3-mm-wide linear band of inflammation of the gingiva. Pain is not associated with the lesion, but the gingivae are likely to bleed during toothbrushing or even spontaneously. The microbiology of this lesion is unclear, but *Candida* spp. may be a possible cause.

Parotid salivary gland enlargement, which may be painful and become secondarily infected, has been reported in 14% to 30% of HIV-infected children. The enlargement apparently is caused by infiltration of the glands by T8 lymphocytes and has been associated with increased survival time. The median time was 4.6 years from birth to development of parotid enlargement and 5.4 years from development of lesions to death, with a relative hazard rate of 0.38.[47]

Herpes simplex virus infections, although common occurrences in normal children, seem to be particularly severe and recur more often in HIV-infected children. The lesions appear first as multiple clustered vesicles on the lips or keratinized oral mucosa, which soon rupture to leave painful irregular oral ulcers or crusted labial ulcers. Fever and dysphagia may warrant hospital admission for hydration, nutrition, and therapy with parenteral acyclovir. Less severe cases may be treated with oral acyclovir.

Dental caries is increased in pediatric HIV cohorts. The cause of this finding is unclear. It may be due to xerostomia secondary to parotid enlargement in some cases, prolonged use of sucrose-containing antifungal agents in others, and nursing bottle caries in still others. The association of nursing bottle caries with pediatric HIV infection may be due to their common increased prevalence in urban dwellers with limited economic resources, although nursing bottle caries also is found frequently in children with other chronic diseases.[102]

ORAL CARE OF CHILDREN WITH CANCER

Chemotherapy and other therapies such as radiation can exert a profound, detrimental, and sometimes long-lasting effect on the oral mucosa. In the presence of diminished immune function, the oral cavity becomes an important potential source of infections in these patients, and therefore careful attention to their oral and dental health is pivotal. This has been recognized by the AAPD, which adopted guidelines in 1986 regarding the dental management of patients receiving chemotherapy, radiotherapy, or a hematopoietic stem cell transplant (HSCT).[3,9] The care of the oral cavity begins before patients are subjected to these therapies. Initial evaluation by dentistry is a must to identify and eliminate any potential sources of infection and to educate the patients and parents on the importance of oral health during their cancer treatment. Patients are encouraged to brush teeth and tongue at least 2 or 3 times daily with regular soft nylon brushes, and, in cases of poor hygiene, to use alcohol-free chlorhexidine solutions. Many of these patients have indwelling central catheters at the time that dental care is being performed. Still, data at this time do not support the use of antibiotic prophylaxis in these patients when the absolute neutrophil count (ANC) is above 2000/mm^3. If the ANC falls between 1000 and 2000/mm^3 and planned dental procedures are scheduled, some authors suggest that prophylaxis at doses recommended by the American Heart Association for valvular devices may be of benefit.[3,6,44,52,74] This decision should be taken alongside the oncology team. Extractions of teeth that are found to be infected should be treated with a short course of antibiotics (7 days after extraction), ideally tailored to susceptibility of the organisms isolated in culture.

In patients undergoing HSCT, all elective procedures need to be completed before the start of the conditioning regimen because the prolonged immunosuppression that these patients face will not allow for any elective procedure until at least 100 days post transplantation.

Once patients enter those periods in which neutropenia ensues, they should continue teethbrushing at the same frequency as before. If the patient develops mucositis and cannot tolerate the soft toothbrush, foam brushes or super-soft brushes can be used, acknowledging that these alternatives do not provide optimal cleaning. Flossing may be continued if this was routine for the patient previously and care is exercised. Only emergency dental procedures should be performed when the ANC is less than 1000/mm^3 and should be performed in the inpatient setting with a multidisciplinary approach because supportive therapies such as blood products, antimicrobials, and analgesia may need to be provided.[3,6,44,52]

There is a well-established association between oral mucositis and bacteremia in cancer patients.[3,6,44,52] A recent study by Flagg et al.[26] examined the associated characteristics of bacteremia in pediatric oncology patients based on whether the organism was a commensal to the mouth, gastrointestinal tract, or skin. Having a bacteremia with oral pathogens (e.g., *S. viridans*) was associated with the presence of mucositis and with lower platelet counts, ANC, and hemoglobin. An ANC of less than 500/mm^3 was significantly associated with bacteremia with oral flora versus other organisms.[26] Palifermin is a keratinocyte growth factor that has been approved by the U.S. Food and Drug Administration for the prevention of mucositis in adult patients with hematologic malignancies; however, there are scant data at this time regarding its safety and benefit in the pediatric population.[44,21,104]

As in children with HIV, herpetic infections are common and usually are the result of reactivation. Patients who are HSV seropositive prior to HSCT are routinely started on prophylaxis at the time of conditioning and continued well into the postengraftment period. Despite prophylaxis, breakthrough infections occur and may be difficult to recognize because they are frequently confused with mucositis, graft versus host disease, or medication side effect (i.e., oral ulcers associated with foscarnet) among other. Therefore a high index of suspicion must be maintained.

Candida spp. can cause superficial and deep infections in cancer patients, especially at the time of neutropenia. Most centers will provide prophylaxis to patients undergoing HSCT because periods of prolonged neutropenia are anticipated.[100] Treatment of oral candidiasis will depend on the severity of the infection. For mild disease, topical therapy with clotrimazole troches or nystatin suspension can be used, whereas more severe symptoms require the use of systemic therapy. Updated guidelines for the treatment of *Candida* are now available.[76] Other fungal infections that may present in the oral cavity include mold infections, especially *Aspergillus*, which can extend from the sinuses into the oral cavity or by hematogenous spread. Therefore any unusual-appearing lesion (e.g., white, dark, erythematous lesions or solitary ulcers) or lesions that fail to heal in the oral cavity should be thoroughly evaluated because they may be fungal in origin.[52,74]

COMPLICATIONS OF ODONTOGENIC INFECTIONS

Fascial Space Infections

Spread of infection to the fascial spaces may result in dramatic facial swelling, high fever, and, if untreated, respiratory compromise. The characteristics of the more common fascial space infections related to odontogenic infection are described in this section.

Infraorbital space infections generally are related to maxillary anterior teeth and are well localized to the infraorbital fossa by the levator labii superioris and levator anguli oris muscles. Facial swelling lateral to the nose is prominent, as is decreased mobility of the upper lip caused by inflammation of these muscles. If the area is fluctuant, intraoral incision and drainage with placement of a small Penrose drain for 1 or 2 days generally is sufficient treatment. Antibiotics are indicated for all infections of the fascial spaces.

Trismus is the hallmark of infection of the masticator space. Trismus is caused by spasm in the muscles of mastication, which define this large potential space. The resulting inability to open the mouth hinders access to the airway for endotracheal intubation. In addition, abscesses of the masticator space may rupture into the oropharynx, causing aspiration of pus, or they may pass easily around the medial pterygoid muscle to involve the lateral pharyngeal and retropharyngeal spaces. Fig. 8.9 shows a 6-year-old boy whose lower primary molar abscesses spread to involve the buccal, pterygomandibular, and lateral pharyngeal spaces. Extraoral and intraoral drainage, prolonged intubation, and extraction of the offending teeth were required.

Infections of the submandibular space (Fig. 8.10) may be localized unilaterally or may involve bilateral structures. Treatment of submandibular space infection is via extraoral incision and drainage.

First described in 1836, Ludwig angina consists of infection of the sublingual and submandibular spaces bilaterally and is characterized by hard, brawny swelling and a minimum of suppuration. The tongue often is edematous and raised to the roof of the mouth, with little mobility (Fig. 8.11). Airway obstruction should be considered imminent; the greatest cause of death in Ludwig angina is blockage of the airway by soft tissue swelling, pus, or blood, which occurred in more than 50% of its victims in the preantibiotic era.[38] In 1940, Williams[107] published a series of 37 cases of Ludwig angina that reported a 54% mortality

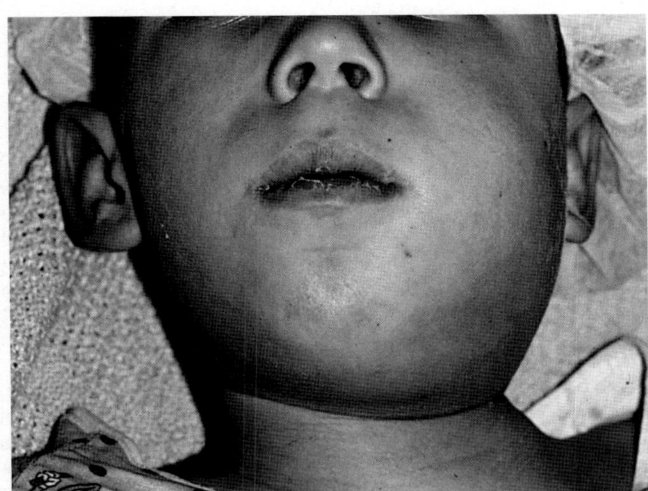

FIG. 8.9 Lateral pharyngeal space abscess in a 6-year-old boy. Note the swelling above the hyoid bone and anterior to the sternocleidomastoid muscle. Swelling also occurs in the buccal and submandibular spaces.

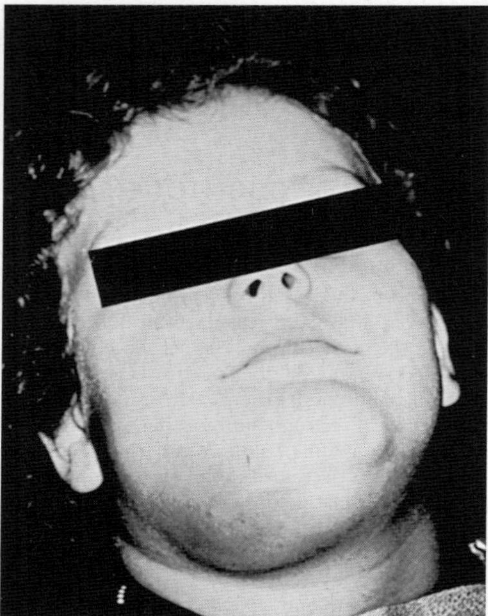

FIG. 8.10 Submandibular space abscess.

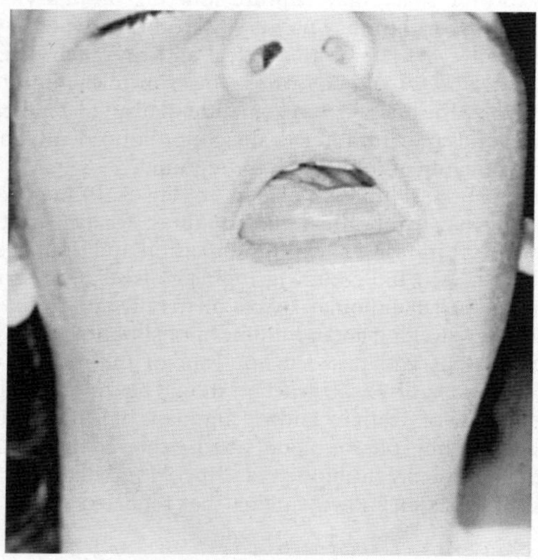

FIG. 8.11 Ludwig angina.

rate. The airway management policy at that time was emergency tracheotomy if necessary. Three years later, Williams and Guralnick[107,108] published a series of 20 cases of Ludwig angina treated with a new policy of immediate establishment of airway security by intubation or tracheotomy and aggressive incision and drainage of all anatomic spaces affected by the infection. By these measures, they were able to reduce the mortality rate of this dreaded infection to 20% only 3 years later. Antibiotics were unavailable during the course of these two studies. These studies underscore the importance of airway security and aggressive surgical management in the treatment of severe odontogenic infections.

Today death rarely occurs from severe odontogenic infections, although the need for tracheotomy or prolonged endotracheal intubation is common. The cause of this infection often is odontogenic infection but may include laceration of the floor of the mouth and mandibular fracture. Usually a disease of middle-aged adults, it is a rare occurrence in children but may occur in greater frequency in immunologically compromised children.[34] Surgical drainage of all four spaces, accompanied by vigorous antibiotic therapy, is indicated.

Necrotizing Fasciitis

Necrotizing fasciitis, which causes a frightening loss of skin and underlying tissues, has received considerable notoriety in the press. Cervicofacial necrotizing fasciitis often is odontogenic and typically causes a superficial spreading of cellulitis that follows the platysma muscle from the cheek down the entire neck to the anterior chest wall (Fig. 8.12A). Fig. 8.12B illustrates such a swelling in an 8-year-old boy. The presumptive cause was odontogenic infection of the primary molars, which caused a high fever and a rapidly progressive cellulitis extending from the cheek to the chest. The cause of these infections often is group A streptococci, but a wide variety of microorganisms may be involved.

Wide-spectrum antibiotic therapy is indicated empirically, along with hydration, transfusions if necessary, and support of electrolyte balance, especially with calcium, which may be sequestered by necrotic fat molecules.[7] Timely surgery is important in the management of necrotizing fasciitis. Incision and drainage of the involved spaces, debridement of necrotic tissue, and fasciotomy often are performed as soon as possible after the patient's admission.[106] Hyperbaric oxygen therapy has been advocated as an adjunct in the treatment of necrotizing fasciitis. A significant reduction in the mortality rate and length of hospitalization associated with necrotizing fasciitis has been shown in adults.[106] Necrotizing fasciitis is cited as an indication for hyperbaric oxygen therapy in infants and children and should be considered if available.[105]

Odontogenic Sinusitis

A significant percentage of cases of sinusitis are odontogenic, especially in adults, because the maxillary sinus follows the erupting permanent tooth roots into the alveolar process. This pneumatization of the alveolar process progresses throughout life and is accelerated by loss of the upper posterior teeth. Dental infections of the periapical upper posterior teeth occasionally rupture through the maxillary sinus floor to involve the paranasal sinuses. Dental infection should be eliminated in the complete treatment of severe recurrent sinusitis in children.

Fig. 8.13 illustrates a case in a 9-year-old boy of left pansinusitis, including ethmoiditis and a subperiosteal orbital abscess associated with infected upper primary molars. His treatment involved a team approach of the dental and otolaryngology services for tooth extraction, incision and drainage of the buccal and infraorbital spaces, endoscopic sinus surgery, and external drainage of the orbital abscess.

Buccal and Periorbital Cellulitis

A child occasionally presents with an acute buccal or periorbital space swelling and cellulitis with no clinically apparent odontogenic cause. These infections tend to occur in young children, usually younger than 36 months. They usually have a history of recent upper respiratory infection or sinusitis. *H. influenzae* type b and *S. pneumoniae* have been implicated as pathogens in these conditions, although the widespread use of conjugated vaccines has reduced dramatically the incidence of invasive disease from *H. influenzae*.[33] A possible mechanism for the inoculation of the soft tissues is migration of organisms through emissary veins piercing the thin cortical bone overlying the lateral surface of the maxillary sinus in cases with existing sinusitis. Unless the infection is severe, incision and drainage usually are unnecessary, and treatment with antibiotics is successful. Blood cultures frequently are positive in more severe cases. The role of lumbar puncture remains controversial in the overall management of infants and young children. The incidence of this infection has declined significantly as a result of the widespread use of *H. influenzae* vaccine.

Orbital and Intracranial Complications

Odontogenic infections that spread to involve the orbit and the brain are rare. Orbital and intracranial abscesses may have an odontogenic origin; however, and the dental condition of patients with these conditions should be evaluated by a dentist. Probably no more than 5% to 10% of orbital cellulitis is odontogenic in origin.[46,109] This infection generally is unilateral and is characterized by proptosis, chemosis, lid edema, and restriction of extraocular motion secondary to edema.[82] No nerve palsies or visual changes are present. Treatment includes surgical drainage, antibiotics, and elimination of the dental infection.

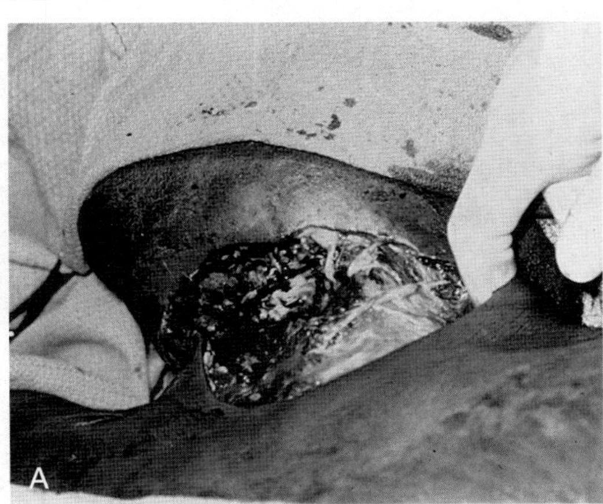

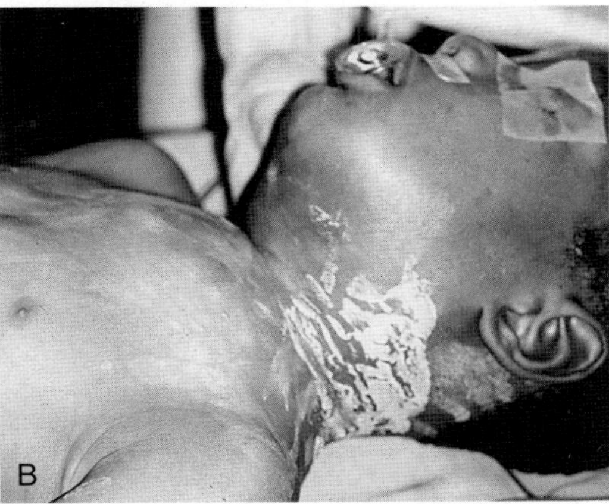

FIG. 8.12 (A) Surgical debridement of necrotic skin and platysma muscle of the left neck of a diabetic female patient with necrotizing fasciitis. Note how easily blunt finger dissection can undermine the skin in the plane of the necrotic platysma muscle. (B) Necrotizing fasciitis in an 8-year-old boy. Note the swelling extending from the buccal space down the neck and onto the anterior chest wall, following the extent of the platysma muscle. The chalky material on the posterior neck is calamine lotion placed by the patient's mother for vesicles that resembled poison ivy.

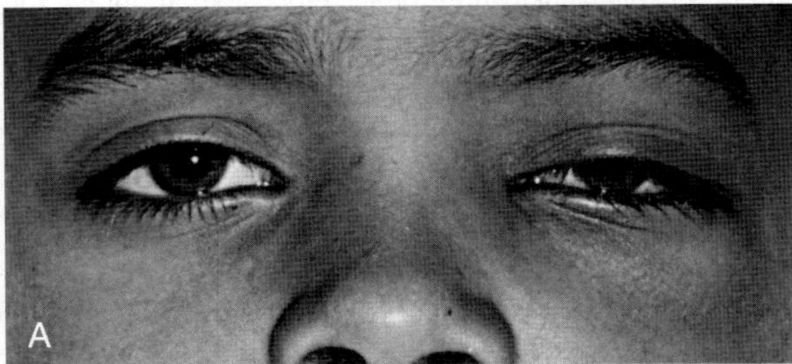

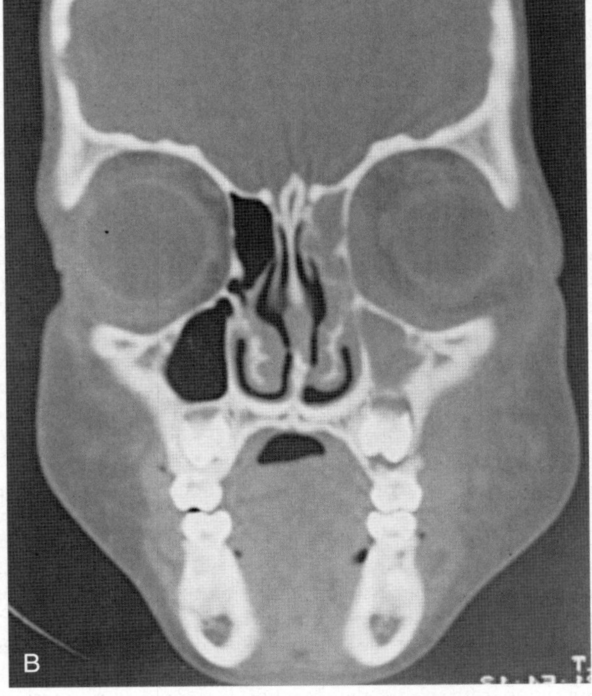

FIG. 8.13 (A) A 9-year-old boy with a left pansinusitis and an abscess of the upper left first primary molar. Note the left periorbital discoloration and swelling, with partial ptosis and displacement of the globe laterally. (B) Computed tomography scan of the same patient. Note the left maxillary sinus opacification close to the infected tooth, opacification of the ethmoid sinuses, elevation of the periosteum away from the medial orbital wall, and displacement of the globe laterally within the orbit.

Cavernous sinus thrombosis, which may be difficult to differentiate clinically from orbital cellulitis, is considerably more serious because microorganisms proliferate intracranially. The risk for death is high. Characteristics include bilateral involvement with rapid progression from one eye to the other, proptosis, chemosis, and lid edema. Extraocular movements are limited because of inflammation of the third, fourth, and sixth cranial nerves. Systemic signs of meningeal irritation and ophthalmoscopic evidence of obstruction of the retinal veins also are present.[19,82,97] Treatment includes high doses of parenteral antibiotics, elimination of the causative dental pathosis, and incision and drainage of infected fascial spaces. Odontogenic cavernous sinus thrombosis seems to be propagated by an ascending thrombophlebitis.

Brain abscess and subdural empyema are rare findings today compared with several decades ago. Dental sources of infection have been implicated in brain abscesses from less than 1% to 8.5% of cases reported.[15,81,85,94] Odontogenic brain abscesses seem to occur by direct extension through the paranasal sinuses, usually to the frontal lobe through the frontal sinuses. Typically a pansinusitis intervenes between the dental infection and the brain; however hematogenous and contiguous anatomic routes of spread are possible.[50,61,90] The literature supports the fact that oral flora are found in brain abscesses, but a correlating culture from the supposed oral source is rarely found, often making brain abscess secondary to dental infection a diagnosis of exclusion.[50]

OSTEOMYELITIS OF THE JAWS IN CHILDREN

Osteomyelitis of the jaws in children usually results from periodontal or, more commonly, periapical infection. Open fracture of the jaws with delayed treatment also is a significant cause of osteomyelitis. Extension from contiguous infections, such as otitis, parotitis, and mastoiditis, occurs much less often.

Osteomyelitis of the jaws occurring in children must be viewed with great concern because it may result in (1) loss of primary and permanent teeth; (2) sequestration of segments of the jaws; (3) growth defects, such as mandibular hypoplasia, asymmetry, and ankylosis[25]; (4) disfiguring facial scars and cutaneous fistulas; and (5) lesions suggestive of malignancy, which require open biopsy. For these reasons, osteomyelitis of the jaws in children should be diagnosed rapidly and treated aggressively. Box 8.2 presents a useful classification of this disease.[101]

Predisposing Factors

Preexisting systemic disease with accompanying alteration of host resistance plays a major role in the initiation of osteomyelitis of the jaws. It includes conditions such as uncontrolled diabetes, agranulocytosis,

BOX 8.2 Osteomyelitis of the Jaws

Suppurative	Nonsuppurative
Acute suppurative	Chronic sclerosing:
Chronic suppurative:	Facial sclerosing
Primary	Diffuse sclerosing
Secondary	Garré sclerosing
Infantile	Actinomycotic
	Radiation osteomyelitis and necrosis

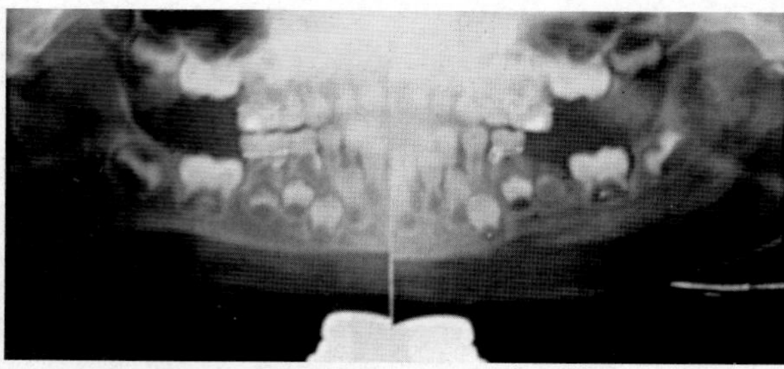

FIG. 8.14 Radiograph of the jaws of a 4-year-old girl with suppurative osteomyelitis of the left mandible. The film shows marked destruction of the body and ramus of the mandible.

leukemia, sickle-cell disease, and febrile illnesses. Conditions that alter the vascularity of bone and the ability to combat infections, including bone tumors, fibrous dysplasia, Paget disease, and radiation to the jaws, also are important predisposing conditions. Major maxillofacial injuries resulting in open fractures of the jaws, especially fractures that are not treated immediately, are an important cause of osteomyelitis.

Microbiology

Because the etiology of osteomyelitis of the jaws includes causes other than purely odontogenic infections, the bacterial spectrum is broad. Most instances of osteomyelitis of the jaws are caused by aerobic streptococci (α-hemolytic streptococci and *S. viridans* group), anaerobic streptococci, and other anaerobes, particularly *Peptostreptococcus, Fusobacterium,* and *Bacteroides* and related genera.[77] Only occasional cases are caused by *S. aureus,* with entry through the skin being the probable route. Other bacteria involved include oral anaerobes, aerobic and microaerophilic cocci, and gram-negative organisms. Specific forms of osteomyelitis are caused by *Actinomyces israelii, Treponema pallidum,* and *Mycobacterium tuberculosis. Salmonella* organisms have been associated with osteomyelitis of the jaw in patients with sickle-cell anemia.[22]

Clinical Findings

Osteomyelitis involves the mandible far more frequently than the maxilla because the poor blood supply to the mandible comes primarily from one major vessel and the periosteal blood supply. Four major forms of the disease, which may be distinguished clinically, are (1) acute suppurative; (2) secondary chronic, which begins as an acute osteomyelitis and becomes chronic; (3) primary chronic, which has no acute phase and always has seemed to be a low-grade infection; and (4) nonsuppurative osteomyelitis. The forms most often seen in children are the acute suppurative, the secondary chronic, and one nonsuppurative form: Garré sclerosing osteomyelitis. These conditions are described in some detail.

Suppurative Osteomyelitis

Suppurative osteomyelitis usually begins with deep and intense pain in the jaws, high intermittent fever, and an obvious cause, most often a deeply carious or discolored tooth. In the early stages, mental nerve paresthesia occasionally is present. During the course of several days, facial swelling develops, and in 10 to 14 days, teeth begin to loosen, pus exudes around the gingival sulcus, and multiple mucosal or cutaneous sinus tracts form. In addition to the draining sinuses, a firm cellulitis is present in the soft tissues, accompanied by trismus and cervical lymphadenopathy. A leukocytosis, ranging typically from 8000 to 15,000 cells/mm^3, is present, although it does not ordinarily reach the levels seen in acute osteomyelitis of the long bones. After 10 days to 2 weeks, radiographs may show scattered areas of bone destruction with of a moth-eaten appearance (Fig. 8.14), and periosteal reaction characterized by the laying down of new bone commonly is seen. Smears of specimens and cultures, including cultures of bone sequestra, should be taken whenever possible. Interpretation of cultures must be made with caution because of the possibility of skin and oral contaminants in the specimen.

Initially, antibiotic doses adjusted for age may be given empirically, but the selection of the antibiotic is determined by culture and sensitivity testing of specimens taken directly from the infected site.[31] The antibiotics of choice in mandibular osteomyelitis include amoxicillin-clavulanate, clindamycin, and fluoroquinolones. Fluoroquinolones are excellent choices because of their complete absorption from the gastrointestinal tract and high penetration of bone, but these drugs are generally considered second-line therapy options because of the potential of musculoskeletal adverse events in the pediatric population.[5] As results from smears and culture are obtained, antibiotics may be changed unless the infection is responding favorably, in which case no change is made. The involved tooth is removed as early as possible to allow drainage and provide material for culture.

Antibiotic therapy is continued for at least 2 to 4 weeks after all symptoms subside. If the infection persists, repeated cultures are obtained, and the antibiotic is changed if necessary. The greater vascularity of the jaws may explain their more rapid response to antibiotic therapy and surgery in contrast to that of the long bones. The duration of intravenous antibiotic therapy in osteomyelitis of the jaws may not need to be as prolonged as in that of the long bones. Consideration should be given to sequestrectomy, saucerization, or the placement of closed-wound irrigation and suction. Saucerization involves the removal of teeth in the immediate area and removal of the overlying buccal plate of bone, allowing access to the medullary portion and sequestra that may be present. Placement of catheters through an extraoral approach occasionally is necessary for closed irrigation and suction. It permits instillation of antibiotics, allowing direct contact with the bone. Hyperbaric oxygen treatment may be considered in chronic cases refractory to antibiotic treatment.[66]

Infantile Osteomyelitis

Osteomyelitis of the jaws in a newborn is an uncommon occurrence but warrants special mention because of its serious sequelae. It occurs most often a few weeks after birth and usually involves the maxilla. It is not odontogenic in origin but is thought to arise from neonatal trauma to oral tissues, hematogenous spread (from skin, middle ear, mastoid, or tonsils), or an infected nipple.[84] The patient has facial cellulitis centered around the orbit (Fig. 8.15). Irritability and malaise precede development of cellulitis and are followed by marked elevation in temperature, anorexia, and dehydration. Extraorally, inner canthal swelling, palpebral edema with closure of the eye, conjunctivitis, and proptosis may be seen, together with a purulent discharge from the nose or inner canthus. Oral examination shows swelling of the maxilla on the affected side extending to the buccal and the palatal regions, with fluctuation often present with multiple sinus tracts. *S. aureus* is the organism usually found.

Aggressive, prompt treatment must be undertaken to prevent permanent optic damage, neurologic complications, loss of tooth buds and bone, and extension to the dural sinuses. Intravenous penicillin and a penicillinase-resistant penicillin are given simultaneously with surgical drainage of all fluctuant areas, repeated Gram smears, and culture and sensitivity testing. Antibiotics are continued orally for 2 to 4 weeks after all signs of the infection have disappeared. If sequestra form, they should be removed conservatively. Tooth buds may be lost, and surviving teeth may be deformed or discolored after eruption.

Garré Sclerosing Osteomyelitis

Garré sclerosing osteomyelitis, also known as chronic nonsuppurative sclerosing osteomyelitis and proliferative osteomyelitis of Garré,[10] is notable because of the similarity of some of its characteristics to those of other neoperiostoses. It is characterized by a localized, hard, nontender

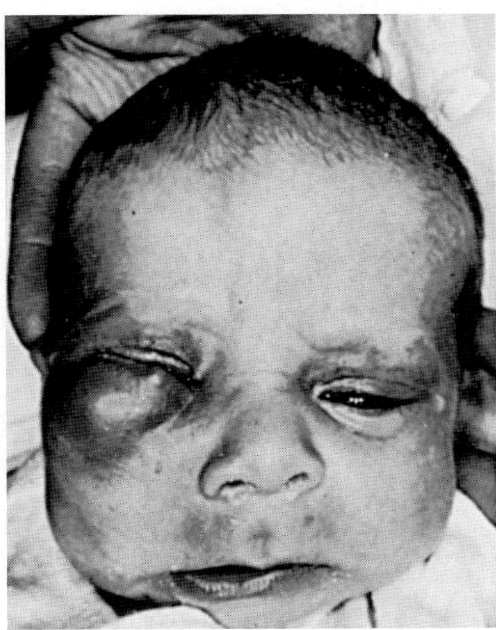

FIG. 8.15 Characteristic clinical picture of a 3-week-old child with infantile osteomyelitis. (Courtesy Dr. M. Michael Cohen Sr.)

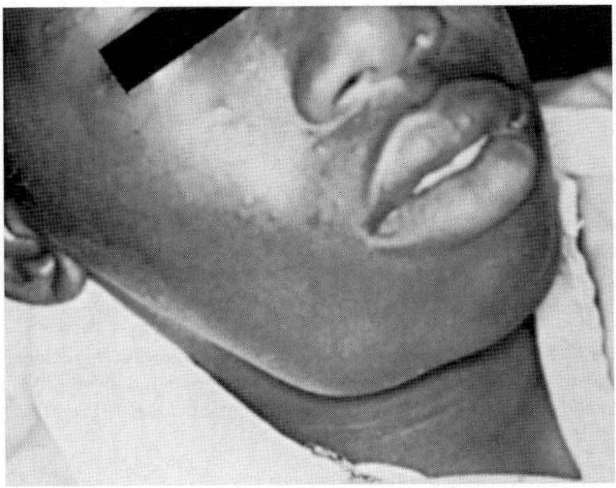

FIG. 8.16 Enlargement of the right side of the mandible in a 12-year-old patient with Garré sclerosing osteomyelitis. The swelling is hard and nontender.

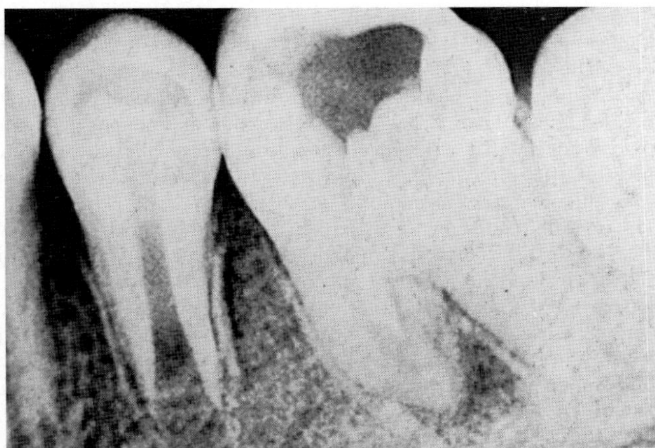

FIG. 8.17 Radiograph of a deeply carious lower first molar tooth with periapical spread of infection. It is the usual cause of Garré osteomyelitis.

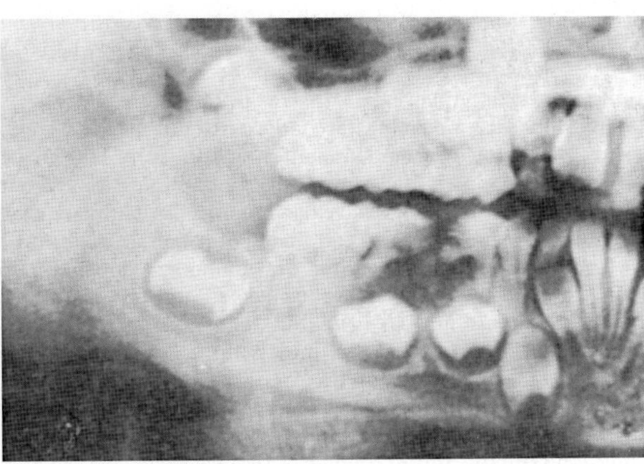

FIG. 8.18 Characteristic radiograph of Garré osteomyelitis showing the laminated or "onion peel" appearance of the mass. (Courtesy Dr. Larry J. Peterson.)

swelling of the mandible (Fig. 8.16). Lymphadenopathy, hyperpyrexia, and leukocytosis are not present. Garré osteomyelitis is associated commonly with a carious tooth, usually the lower first molar (Fig. 8.17), and a history of a past toothache. It also may be associated with a recent dental extraction or an infected flap of tissue over an erupting tooth.[59] Radiographs are impressive, showing a focal area of well-calcified, smooth bone proliferation that often has a laminated or onion-peel appearance (Fig. 8.18).

Garré osteomyelitis is thought to be a response to a low-grade stimulus, such as a dental infection, that influences the potentially active periosteum of young individuals. Its appearance resembles that of infantile cortical hyperostosis (Caffey disease), osteosarcoma, and Ewing sarcoma, and it must be distinguished from these conditions.[24] Treatment consists of extraction or endodontic treatment of the involved tooth, with continued clinical and radiographic follow-up of the patient to ensure that the new bone formation does not progress. Ordinarily, remodeling occurs over the course of time, but biopsy should be done to rule out neoplasm if the lesion does not regress. No antibiotic therapy is necessary.

HERPES SIMPLEX VIRUS INFECTIONS

HSV type 1 infections commonly are manifested as herpetic gingivostomatitis.[96] Five stages of infection have been identified: (1) primary mucocutaneous infection, (2) acute infection of ganglia, (3) establishment of latency, (4) reactivation, and (5) recurrent infection.

Primary infection is established by direct contact with individuals who have draining lesions or asymptomatic carriers who may continue to shed the virus despite the lack of symptoms. The highest incidence of primary infection appears to be in children 2 to 4 years old. Infants are protected by maternal antibodies, which may explain why this infection is not found in infants younger than 6 months. It appears to have no seasonal variation or male or female difference in incidence.

The incubation period is thought to be approximately 6 days, followed by the development of small vesicles that may coalesce to form larger lesions or ulcers. In severe cases, the lips, gingivae, oral mucosa, and pharynx may be involved. Many patients with primary herpes labialis may be asymptomatic, however, and symptoms may not develop. Healing occurs in 1 to 2 weeks, with gradual crusting of the lesions followed by re-epithelialization.

Latency is thought to continue throughout life, with reactivation occurring at various times, possibly triggered by actinic radiation and emotional or physical stress. Recurrent disease is manifested by vesicles at the mucocutaneous border, which are painful for about 2 days, followed by crusting and complete healing in 7 to 8 days.

Fifty percent of the adult population in industrialized countries and a higher percentage in less developed countries may have recurrent herpes labialis. Many, if not most, adults who have recurrent "cold sores" are not aware that they can transmit the disease and should be counseled in this regard. Likewise, medical, dental, and nursing personnel should be advised that occurrence of cutaneous lesions (herpetic whitlow) is possible after direct contact of the practitioner's fingers with lesions during the physical examination.

In treating recurrent herpes labialis in nonimmunocompromised adults, acyclovir has been shown to decrease the duration of symptoms by 12 to 24 hours, at a cost of approximately $75 per day. However, frequent use of acyclovir also may promote the spread of resistant viral strains. The use of acyclovir for treatment of recurrent herpes labialis in nonimmunocompromised individuals seems to offer little benefit at significant expense and risk.[83]

INTRAORAL AND PERIORAL PIERCINGS

Tattoos and piercings are not uncommon in the adolescent population. Forty-six percent of teenagers will receive their first piercing between the ages of 11 and 16 years.[16] The mouth and surrounding tissues are commonly pierced sites, with the tongue being the most frequently pierced.[55,72] Moreover, a lack of awareness exists among these age groups on the risks associated with these body modification practices.[72] Many times these piercings are performed by nonregulated piercing parlors and unlicensed personnel.[110]

Complications from piercing have ranged from simple local complications, such as bleeding, pain, and local infections, to severe, life-threatening infections.[103,110] Among the most severe complications, bacterial endocarditis and brain abscess have been reported. Yu and associates,[110] in a review on bacterial complications of oral piercings, found eight cases of bacterial endocarditis after oral piercings reported between 2001 and 2009, of which two were teenagers. Oral organisms such as *S. viridans*, *S. aureus*, and *Gemella* and *Neisseria* spp. were reported. Ludwig angina, glossal abscesses, and lymphadenitis, among other conditions, also were included in their report. Martinello and Cooney[63] reported a case of a solitary brain abscess in a patient 1 month after a tongue piercing. The abscess was polymicrobial with *S. viridans*, *Peptostreptococcus micros*, and *Actinomyces* and *Eikenella* spp. isolated.

Because of the risks associated with the use of oral jewelry and piercing, the AAPD has issued a statement strongly opposing the practice of piercing intraoral and perioral tissues and the use of jewelry on these tissues.[2]

NEW REFERENCES SINCE THE SEVENTH EDITION

3. American Academy of Pediatric Dentistry. Guideline on dental management of pediatric patients receiving chemotherapy, hematopoietic cell transplantation, and/or radiation. *Pediatr Dent*. 2013;35:E185-E193.
4. Atout RN, Todescan S. Managing patients with necrotizing ulcerative gingivitis. *J Can Dent Assoc*. 2013;79:d46.
5. Bacci C, Galli L, de Martino M, Chiappini E. Fluoroquinolones in children: update of the literature. *J Chemother*. 2015;27:257-265.
6. Baddour LM, Epstein AE, Erickson CC, et al. Update on cardiovascular implantable electronic device infections and their management. *Circulation*. 2010;121:458-477.
17. Chauny JV, Lorrot M, Prot-Labarthe S, et al. Treatment of tuberculosis with levofloxacin or moxifloxacin: report of 6 pediatric cases. *Pediatr Infect Dis J*. 2012;31:1309-1311.
21. Czyzewski K, Debski R, Krenska A, et al. Palifermin in children undergoing autologous stem cell transplantation: a matched-pair analysis. *Anticancer Res*. 2014;34:7379-7382.
26. Flagg A, Worley S, Foster CB. Characteristics of bacteremia in pediatric oncology patients based on pathogen classification as associated with the gastrointestinal mucosa or skin. *Infect Control Hosp Epidemiol*. 2015;36:730-733.
30. Garazzino S, Scolfaro C, Raffaldi I, et al. Moxifloxacin for the treatment of pulmonary tuberculosis in children: a single center experience. *Pediatr Pulmonol*. 2014;49:372-376.
43. Hirsch R, Deng H, Laohachai MN. Azithromycin in periodontal treatment: more than an antibiotic. *J Periodontal Res*. 2012;47:137-148.
44. Hong CH, daFonseca M. Considerations in the pediatric population with cancer. *Dent Clin North Am*. 2008;52:155-181.
52. Lerman MA, Laudenbach J, Marty FM. Management of oral infections in cancer patients. *Dent Clin North Am*. 2008;52:129-153.
69. Merriam CV, Citron DM, Tyrrell KL, et al. In vitro activity of azithromycin and nine comparator agents against 296 strains of oral anaerobes and 31 strains of *Eikenella corrodens*. *Int J Antimicrob Agents*. 2006;23:244-248.
74. Palmason S, Marty FM, Treister NS. How do we manage oral infections in allogeneic stem cell transplantation and other severely immunocompromised patients? *Oral Maxillofac Surg Clin North Am*. 2011;23:579-599.
75. Panel on Opportunistic Infections in HIV-Exposed and HIV-Infected Children. Guidelines for the Prevention and Treatment of Opportunistic Infections in HIV-Exposed and HIV-Infected Children. Department of Health and Human Services. Available at: http://aidsinfo.nih.gov/contentfiles/lvguidelines/oi_guidelines_pediatrics.pdf.
76. Pappas PG, Kauffman CA, Andes DR, et al. Clinical Practice Guideline for the Management of Candidiasis: 2016 Update by the Infectious Diseases Society of America. *Clin Infect Dis*. 2016;62:e1-e50.
99. Thee S, Garcia-Prats AJ, Draper HR, et al. Pharmacokinetics and safety of moxifloxacin in children with multidrug-resistant tuberculosis. *Clin Infect Dis*. 2015;15(60):549-556.
100. Tomblyn M, Chiller T, Einsele H, et al. Guidelines for preventing infectious complications among hematopoietic cell transplantation recipients: a global perspective. *Biol Blood Marrow Transplant*. 2009;15:1143-1238.
104. Vitale KM, Violago L, Cofnas P, et al. Impact of palifermin on incidence of oral mucositis and healthcare utilization in children undergoing autologous hematopoietic stem cell transplantation for malignant diseases. *Pediatr Transplant*. 2014;18:211-216.

The full reference list for this chapter is available at ExpertConsult.com.

9 Pharyngitis (Pharyngitis, Tonsillitis, Tonsillopharyngitis, and Nasopharyngitis)

James D. Cherry

Pharyngitis is an inflammatory illness of the mucous membranes and underlying structures of the throat. The clinical diagnostic category includes tonsillitis, tonsillopharyngitis, and nasopharyngitis; inflammation also frequently involves the uvula and soft palate. Illness usually is acute but also may be subacute or chronic. Establishing the diagnosis of pharyngitis requires objective evidence of inflammation (erythema, exudate, or ulceration). The symptom of sore throat invariably accompanies pharyngitis, but it should not be used as the sole criterion; sore throat is a common complaint of children with colds in whom no objective evidence of pharyngeal inflammation is present (see Chapter 7).

Although the clinical finding of pharyngitis suggests an almost exclusive group A streptococcal cause to many physicians, etiologic considerations should include a multitude of viruses, bacteria, and other infectious and noninfectious agents. Etiologically, pharyngitis is subdivided into two categories: illness with nasal symptoms (nasopharyngitis) and illness without nasal involvement (pharyngitis or tonsillopharyngitis).

In acute illness, nasopharyngitis nearly always is of viral origin, whereas pharyngitis without nasal signs has diverse etiologic possibilities, including bacteria, viruses, fungi, and other unidentified causes. In this chapter, nasopharyngitis and pharyngitis without nasal involvement are considered separately.

HISTORY

Although throat inflammation undoubtedly has been a physical finding of disease throughout human existence, only in more recent years has attention been given to pharyngitis as a primary complaint. The throat findings of diphtheria were mentioned in the 3rd century AD,[189] and Vincent angina was noted in the military before the Christian era,[57] but group A streptococcal infection and pharyngitis were not clearly associated until World War II.[37,158] Although Glover and Griffith[70] mentioned streptococcal tonsillitis in 1931, the major reference to streptococci in the preantibiotic era was in association with scarlet fever, erysipelas, and suppurative processes.[29]

In the early years of clinical virology large population studies of colds, pharyngitis, croup, bronchiolitis, and pneumonia were carried out.* In more recent years, studies have been mainly related to new agents, and pharyngitis is an illness category that is frequently overlooked.

NASOPHARYNGITIS

Etiologic Agents

Etiologic agents of nasopharyngitis, categorized by type of lesion, frequency, season of occurrence, and duration of illness, are listed in Table 9.1. The relative importance of nasal and pharyngeal manifestations also is presented. Although Table 9.1 shows three bacterial agents and one rickettsia, most occurrences of nasopharyngitis are caused by viral infections. The specific infectious agents are discussed fully in their respective sections of this book; only an overview is presented here.

Adenoviruses are the most common cause of nasopharyngitis; types 1, 2, 3, 4, 5, 6, 7, 7a, 9, 14, and 15 account for most illnesses.[14,27,40,41,95,131,148,173,179,194] Nasopharyngitis also commonly occurs with influenza and parainfluenza viral infections.† Although rhinoviral, respiratory syncytial viral, human metapneumovirus, and human bocavirus infections are common occurrences in children and all always have nasal manifestations (coryza), the occurrence of objective pharyngeal manifestations is less common.‡

Respiratory symptoms with cough, nasal discharge, and pharyngitis frequently occur in children with rotaviral gastroenteritis.[77,112,159]

Epidemiology

Nasopharyngitis is a common illness of childhood. It tends to be most prevalent in young children in association with primary infections with respiratory viruses. Nasal symptoms with enteroviruses occur less frequently in school-aged children than in preschool-aged children. In contrast, older children rarely have pharyngitis with respiratory syncytial viral, parainfluenza viral, and rhinoviral infections. Nasopharyngitis caused by adenoviral infection is a particularly frequent occurrence in adolescents and young adults in military training.[40,173,194]

Nasopharyngitis occurs more commonly during the cold-weather months (see Table 9.1). No apparent sex predilection has been found. The method of transmission is similar to that of other respiratory viral infections (see Chapter 7).

Pathophysiology

The pathophysiology of nasopharyngitis is discussed in Chapter 7, in the pharyngitis section of this chapter, and in the chapters discussing the individual viral agents. In nasopharyngitis associated with *Haemophilus influenzae* and *Neisseria meningitidis,* the nasal symptoms may result from a concomitant respiratory viral infection.[29]

*References 14, 26, 29, 30, 37, 39, 40, 51, 69, 83, 88, 89, 95, 131, 144, 146, 156, 164, 168, 179, 194.

†References 11, 79, 88, 89, 95, 96, 137, 144–146, 155, 156, 167, 184.

‡References 7, 26, 50, 61, 83, 86, 88, 89, 95, 126, 144, 147, 171.

Clinical Presentation

Because nasopharyngitis is caused by many different etiologic agents, a reasonable expectation is varied clinical manifestations. These differences are highlighted in Table 9.1. Fever occurs in nearly all cases of nasopharyngitis. With adenoviral and influenza viral disease, the pharyngeal findings are most prominent; with the other respiratory viruses, coryza is more notable than are pharyngeal complaints. In adenoviral infections, follicular pharyngitis is the rule, and exudate is a common manifestation. In contrast, patients with the other respiratory viral infections usually present with pharyngeal erythema only. Nasopharyngitis of a viral etiology most often is an acute, self-limited disease lasting 4 to 10 days. Generally, adenoviral illnesses tend to be more prolonged than are illnesses resulting from the other respiratory viruses. Other symptoms in nasopharyngitis are related to the causative virus. Parainfluenza and respiratory syncytial viral infections also frequently have lower respiratory tract findings (laryngotracheitis, pneumonia, or bronchiolitis), and influenza is usually associated with more severe, generalized complaints.

Although respiratory symptoms in association with rotaviral gastroenteritis have been noted frequently, little careful clinical study of the respiratory manifestations has been performed. Lewis and associates,[112] in a careful study observed a statistically significant occurrence of nasal discharge, cough, and red throat in children with rotaviral diarrhea compared with children with diarrhea caused by other agents.

Nasopharyngitis with *H. influenzae* or *N. meningitidis* infections has been noted mainly in patients with septicemia and meningitis. The nasal symptoms (coryza) usually preceded the pharyngitis and severe systemic disease by a few to several days. In Q fever, the predominant finding is pneumonia. With diphtheria, the exudative pharyngitis and constitutional symptoms are most prominent.

PHARYNGITIS, TONSILLITIS, AND TONSILLOPHARYNGITIS

Etiologic Agents

Etiologic agents of pharyngitis categorized by type of lesion, frequency of occurrence, and duration of illness are presented in Table 9.2. Numerous diverse possibilities exist for the differential diagnosis of pharyngitis. The specific agents or factors are presented in their respective sections of this book, and only an overview is given here.

As with all infectious diseases, etiologic prevalence depends on multiple factors (status of the host, age, season, environment, exposure, and type of lesion) that must be considered in each individual case. In otherwise healthy children, the following infectious agents account for more than 90% of acute infections with pharyngeal involvement: *Streptococcus pyogenes;* adenoviruses; influenza viruses A and B; parainfluenza viruses 1, 2, and 3; Epstein-Barr virus; enteroviruses; and *Mycoplasma pneumoniae.** Although group A streptococci are suggested frequently[29] as the only worthy bacterial consideration in the etiology of pharyngitis, the data in Table 9.2 indicate broader possibilities. When streptococci with β-hemolysis recovered from children and adolescents with pharyngitis are typed, group B, C, and G strains occasionally are found.[9,32,34,68,84,190,191] Turner and associates[190] found that of the group C streptococci, only *Streptococcus equisimilis* caused pharyngitis; *S. anginosus* (formerly *S. milleri*) was part of the normal oropharyngeal flora.

Laboratory accidents have provided evidence that *H. influenzae* can cause pharyngitis,[143,197] and children with systemic illnesses caused by *H. influenzae* and *N. meningitidis* frequently have an associated marked pharyngitis.[172,198,203] *Arcanobacterium haemolyticum* and *Corynebacterium ulcerans* occasionally cause an illness mimicking diphtheria.[21,76,98,103,121,149] *A. haemolyticum* also causes an illness that has been confused with streptococcal scarlet fever.[55,98,117,121]

Because anaerobic microorganisms are universal constituents of the normal throat flora, assigning etiologic significance to these agents in

*References 2, 11, 14, 15, 30, 31, 39, 40, 44, 51, 69, 73, 79, 85, 88, 89, 96, 99, 100, 119, 130–132, 137, 144–146, 155-157, 164, 167, 168, 170, 173, 177, 179, 181, 194, 195, 199, 201.

TABLE 9.1 Etiologic Agents of Nasopharyngitis

Etiologic Agent	TYPE OF PHARYNGEAL LESION[a]			RELATIVE IMPORTANCE OF NASAL AND PHARYNGEAL SYMPTOMS[b]		Frequency of Pharyngitis[c]	Main Season	Duration of Pharyngitis
	Erythematous	Follicular	Exudative	Nasal	Pharyngeal			
Bacteria								
Corynebacterium diphtheriae[165,208]	+++		++++	+	+++	+	Fall, winter, spring	Acute, subacute
Haemophilus influenzae[198]	++			++	++	+	Fall, winter, spring	Acute, subacute
Neisseria meningitidis[172]	++			+	+++	+	Fall, winter, spring	Acute, subacute
Viruses								
Adenoviruses[14,27,40,41,47,131,148,173,179,194]	++++	++++	++	+	+++	++++	All seasons	Acute
Enteroviruses[30,39,100,109,131,168,170,199]	+++		+	+	+++	+++	Summer, fall	Acute
Influenza A, B, C[43,99,145,155,167,184]	+++			+	+++	++	Fall, winter	Acute
Parainfluenza[2,5,6,8,11,79,88,89,96,137,156,164,170,172,184]	++		+	+++	+	++	Fall, winter, spring	Acute
Respiratory syncytial[26,86,89,126,144]	++			+++	+	+	Fall, winter, spring	Acute
Coronavirus[4]	+			+	++	+		Acute
Rhinoviruses[83,99,147]	+			+++	+	+	Fall, winter, spring	Acute
Human metapneumovirus[7,171]	++			+++	+	+	Fall, winter, spring	Acute
Human bocavirus[50,61]	++			+++	+	+	Fall, winter, spring	Acute
Rotaviruses[78,112,126,159]	++			++	++	++	Fall, winter, spring	Acute
Rickettsia								
Coxiella burnetii[94]	++			++	++	+	All seasons	Acute

[a]Plus signs indicate the relative degree and severity of the lesion (++++, most marked; +, minimal).
[b]Each +, 25%.
[c]++++, 76% to 100%; +++, 51% to 75%; ++, 26% to 50%; +, 1% to 25%.

TABLE 9.2 Etiologic Agents of Pharyngitis

Etiologic Agent or Factor	TYPE OF LESION[a]					Frequency of Occurrence[b]	Duration of Pharyngitis
	Erythematous	Follicular	Exudative	Ulcerative	Petechial		
Bacteria							
Streptococcus pyogenes[15,44,53,69,130,132,157,181,201]	++++	++	+++		+++	++++	Acute
Other streptococci (groups B, C, and G)[5,32-34,63,84,115,190,191]	+++	+	++			++	Acute
Brucella spp.[206]	+				+	+	Subacute
Corynebacterium diphtheriae[127,157,208]	+++		++++			+	Acute
Corynebacterium pyogenes[196]	++++		++++			+	Acute
Corynebacterium ulcerans[117,149,188]	++++		+++			+	Acute
Arcanobacterium haemolyticum[8,21,55,71,98,103,121]	++++	++	+++			+	Acute
Mixed anaerobes (*Prevotella* spp., *Peptostreptococcus, Fusobacterium* spp.)[16,17,22,51,71,120,193]	++++		+	++++		++	Subacute
Actinomyces spp.[58]	+			+		+	Chronic
Helicobacter pylori[3,97]	+					+	Chronic
Francisella tularensis[18,93,192,204]	++++		+++			+	Acute, subacute
Haemophilus influenzae[143,183,197,198,203]	++					++	Acute, subacute
Legionella pneumophila[135]	++++					+	Acute
Neisseria meningitidis[172]	++		+			++	Acute
Neisseria gonorrhoeae[92,202]	++		+			+	Acute, subacute, chronic
Leptospira spp.[90,150]	++++					+	Acute
Treponema pallidum[23,38,59,78]	+	+		+		+	Subacute
Borrelia spp.[107]	++++					+	Acute
Streptobacillus moniliformis[153]	+					+	Acute
Yersinia enterocolitica[161,185]	++++		++			+	Acute
Yersinia pseudotuberculosis[162]	+					+	Acute
Streptococcus pneumoniae[124]	+			+		+	Acute
Salmonella typhi[6,136]	+					+	Acute
Rothia dentocariosa[139]	+		+			+	Acute
Mycobacterium tuberculosis[35]				+		+	Chronic
Chlamydia pneumoniae[49,74]	++++					++	Acute
Chlamydia trachomatis[138]	++	+	+			+	Acute, recurrent

Continued

TABLE 9.2 Etiologic Agents of Pharyngitis—cont'd

Etiologic Agent or Factor	TYPE OF LESION[a]					Frequency of Occurrence[b]	Duration of Pharyngitis
	Erythematous	Follicular	Exudative	Ulcerative	Petechial		
Viruses							
Adenoviruses[14,41,131,134,148,173,194]	++++	++++	++			++++	Acute
Influenza A, B, and C[43,145,155,167,184]	+++					+++	Acute
Parainfluenza[2,5,6,8,11,79,88,89,137,144,146,156,164,184]	++					+++	Acute
Respiratory syncytial[26,86,88,89,126,144]	++					+	Acute
Enteroviruses[2,30,91,100,109,168,170,177,199,200]	+++		+	++		+++	Acute
Epstein-Barr[85,119,195]	+++	+	++++		++	+++	Acute, subacute
Reoviruses[111,207]	++					+	Acute
Cytomegalovirus[13,105]	+					+	Acute
Herpes simplex[25,29,51,131,200]	++		++	++++		++	Acute
Measles[28]	+++				+	++	Acute
Rubella[28,60]					++	+	Acute
Rhinoviruses[83]	+					+	Acute
HIV[10]	++						Acute
Mycoplasma							
Mycoplasma pneumoniae[31,49,69,73,89]	++	+	+			++	Acute
Mycoplasma hominis[133]	+		+			+	Acute
Rickettsia							
Coxiella burnetii[47,94,141]	++					+	Acute
Fungi							
Candida spp.[110,174]	+		++++			+++	Acute, subacute, chronic
Parasites							
Toxoplasma gondii[106]	+					+	Acute
Recognized Illnesses of Uncertain Etiology							
Aphthous stomatitis[72,160]	+			++++		++	Acute, recurrent
PFAPA[53,63,91,93,118,125,140,187]	++		++	++		+	Acute, recurrent
Behçet syndrome[123]	+			++++		+	Chronic, recurrent
Kawasaki disease[81,129]	++	+				+	Acute
Stevens-Johnson syndrome[28]	+		+	++++		+	Acute
Illness in which Host Factors or Therapeutic Agents are Primary Causes							
Neutropenia, other immunodeficiencies, cancer, chemotherapeutic agents, generalized neoplastic disease[28]	+			++++		++	Chronic

[a]Plus signs indicate the relative degree and severity of the lesion (++++, most marked; +, minimal).
[b]++++, 76% to 100%; +++, 51% to 75%; ++, 26% to 50%; +, 1% to 25%.
HIV, Human immunodeficiency virus; *PFAPA*, periodic fever, aphthous stomatitis, pharyngitis, and adenitis (syndrome).

throat infections frequently is difficult. Vincent stomatitis and angina seem to result from mixed infections with anaerobes.[58,71,120,193] Brook and Gober[17] noted a significant association between encapsulated organisms of the *Bacteroides melaninogenicus* group (*Prevotella melaninogenica*) and acute tonsillitis in children. My impression is that acute and subacute infections with anaerobes account for numerous pharyngeal infections in adolescents in which cultures do not reveal group A streptococci and infectious mononucleosis test results are negative. Gonococcal and treponemal infections should be considered in sexually active or known exposed teenagers and other children.[23,38,59,92,202]

Adenoviral types 1, 2, 3, 4, 5, 6, 7, 7a, 9, 11, 14, 15, and 16 are the most common causes of pharyngitis in young children, and they are prominent etiologic agents in older children and adolescents.[14,24,40,42,131,134,148,173,179,194] Pharyngeal involvement frequently is overshadowed by other respiratory symptoms (e.g., cough, coryza) in parainfluenza viral infections and by systemic complaints (e.g., fever, exanthem, meningitis) in enteroviral infections.* An enteroviral etiology should be suspected when small ulcerative lesions are noted that involve the soft palate and uvula and the posterior pharyngeal wall (see Chapter 166). Infection with Epstein-Barr virus causes infectious mononucleosis with pharyngeal involvement similar to that resulting from group A streptococcal infection.[85,195] The clinical manifestations of Epstein-Barr virus are age-related; young children rarely have marked pharyngeal involvement.

Acquired cytomegalovirus infection causes an infectious mononucleosis-like syndrome, but pharyngitis occurs less commonly than it does in Epstein-Barr virus mononucleosis.[105] Primary and recurrent herpes simplex virus (HSV) infections occasionally have pharyngeal manifestations.[25,29,51,131] Many illnesses that are ascribed clinically to HSV actually are misidentified instances of aphthous stomatitis, however. Virtually all instances of HSV infections with pharyngitis also reveal lesions in the anterior mouth and externally around the mouth. Although Koplik spots are known universally as the enanthem of measles, many physicians are unaware of the diffuse nature of the associated measles pharyngitis.[28] Primary infection with human immunodeficiency virus may cause the acute retroviral syndrome with fever, nonexudative pharyngitis, lymphadenopathy, exanthem, arthralgia, myalgia, and lethargy.[10]

The role of *Chlamydia* in the cause of pharyngitis is unclear. Grayston and associates[75,74] noted the occurrence of pharyngitis in adolescents and young adults infected with *Chlamydophila pneumoniae* (formerly *Chlamydia pneumoniae*). In a study in children, IgM antibody to *Chlamydia trachomatis* was found in children with pharyngitis.[80] Because cross-reactivity between *C. trachomatis* and *C. pneumoniae* exists, the illnesses studied were likely to be caused by *C. pneumoniae* rather than by *C. trachomatis*. Ogawa and colleagues[138] noted prolonged and recurrent tonsillitis in association with sexually transmitted *C. trachomatis*.

Mild pharyngitis occurs in young children with *M. pneumoniae* infections; in older children, pharyngeal involvement is more pronounced.[31,69,73,89] In young adult volunteers, *Mycoplasma hominis* was noted to cause pharyngitis.[116] Although lower respiratory tract findings and systemic complaints are most marked in Q fever, moderate subjective and mild objective evidence of pharyngitis also is noted.[48,94,141] Exudative pharyngeal involvement with *Candida* spp. commonly occurs.[110,174] *Candida* infection most commonly occurs in children whose normal throat flora has been disrupted and in children who have a compromised immunologic response.

Recurrent aphthous stomatitis usually involves the anterior oral cavity but occasionally is noted with extensive pharyngeal and soft palate lesions.[72,110,160,174] Although L-forms (spheroplasts) of *Streptococcus sanguinis* can be recovered consistently from the lesions of this disease,[72,110,160,174] their role in the etiology is unclear.

In Behçet syndrome, the ulcerative lesions are subacute or chronic and usually are not associated with surrounding pharyngeal inflammation.[123] In Kawasaki disease, the pharyngeal mucosa is deeply erythematous.[129]

Pharyngeal involvement is a common occurrence in noninfectious illnesses in which host resistance has been altered. The lesions usually are ulcerative, but secondary bacterial or fungal overgrowth can lead to marked erythematous and exudative findings.

*References 2, 11, 30, 39, 79, 88, 89, 96, 100, 131, 137, 144, 146, 156, 164, 170, 177, 184, 199.

Epidemiology

Pharyngitis is a common occurrence in children and, as noted in Table 9.2, is the result of many different infectious agents. Generally, bacterial pharyngitis occurs more commonly in the cold-weather seasons; an enteroviral etiology is most common in the summer and fall. In younger children, viral pharyngitis tends to occur more frequently than does bacterial disease.[42] It has no apparent sex predilection.

Most diseases associated with pharyngitis require close person-to-person contact for spread. Pathogens are transmitted directly by close-range airborne dissemination or indirectly by the hands of the future host. Several food-borne outbreaks of streptococcal pharyngitis have been reported.[52,62] Prechewing of food by adults also may be a cause of streptococcal pharyngitis in infants.[178]

Pathophysiology

The pathology and pathophysiology of diseases in which pharyngitis is prominent are presented in the chapters of this book on specific infectious agents (in particular, see Chapters 82, 156, 160, 166, and 196).

Clinical Presentation

General

The clinical findings in pharyngitis are highlighted in Table 9.2. Manifestations related to individual pathogens are detailed in the chapters of this book dealing with the specific agents. The onset of pharyngitis usually is sudden and accompanied by fever and the complaint of sore throat. Frequently, parents observe that the child's breath is not normal and that the throat and particularly the tonsils are red. Other initial complaints include headache, nausea, vomiting, and sometimes abdominal pain. Anorexia is the rule, as is some degree of lessened activity. Parents also report frequently that the child's cervical lymph nodes are enlarged and tender.

Physical examination usually substantiates the parents' observations—the child is febrile with moderate to severe pharyngeal erythema and some degree of cervical adenitis. As noted in Table 9.2, the pharyngeal response varies. With acute common infections, the basic lesion is erythema. Associated with erythema can be follicular, ulcerative, and petechial lesions and generalized or circumscribed exudative areas. Follicular lesions are most characteristic of adenoviral infections, whereas exudative lesions occur most commonly in group A streptococcal infections and in infectious mononucleosis. Meland and associates[128] noted that the absence of cough and the presence of swollen lymph nodes had the highest specificity in predicting a streptococcal cause of pharyngitis. Ulcerative lesions are observed most frequently in enteroviral infections (see Chapter 166). Petechiae on the soft palate frequently are seen in group A streptococcal infections but also commonly occur in infectious mononucleosis, measles, and rubella.

Occurrences of pharyngitis in children almost always are acute, self-limited diseases. Pharyngitis of viral origin lasts 4 to 10 days, and pharyngitis caused by group A streptococci, if untreated, lasts slightly longer. Subacute and chronic pharyngeal disease is an uncommon occurrence in children, but the etiologic possibilities are numerous (see Table 9.2).

PERIODIC FEVER, APHTHOUS STOMATITIS, PHARYNGITIS, AND ADENITIS

In 1987, Marshall and colleagues[125] described a new syndrome, periodic fever, aphthous stomatitis, pharyngitis, and adenitis (PFAPA), and it subsequently has been reported on by many others.* In 1999, Thomas and associates[187] presented an analysis of data in their PFAPA registry of 94 cases. The male-to-female ratio was 1.8 : 1, and the mean age of PFAPA onset was 2.8 years (95% confidence interval [CI], 2.4–3.3). The children had an average 11.5 febrile episodes per year, and the average symptom-free interval between episodes was 28.2 days (99%

*References 1, 18, 20, 53, 54, 63, 65, 87, 91, 93, 114, 118, 140, 182, 187, 205.

CI, 26–30.4 days). The average duration of an episode was 4.8 days, with the temperature being greater than 38.3°C (101°F) for 3.8 days. The average maximum temperature per episode was 40.5°C (104.9°F) (95% CI, 40.4–40.6°C [104.7–105°F]). Along with the periodic fevers, the children also experienced aphthous stomatitis (67%), pharyngitis (65%), cervical lymphadenopathy (77%), chills (80%), headache (65%), abdominal pain (45%), nausea (52%), diarrhea (30%), cough (20%), coryza (18%), and rash (15%). In addition to fever, 97% had one or more of aphthous stomatitis, pharyngitis, or adenopathy. The mean leukocyte count was 13,000 with 62% polymorphonuclear leukocytes, and the mean erythrocyte sedimentation rate was 41 mm/h.

Feder and Salazar[54] reported their review of 105 patients that they saw between 1998 and 2007. In this group there were 62% males. The median age at onset was 30 months (range, 3 to 144 months), the mean duration of febrile episodes was 4.1 days (range, 2 to 7 days), and the mean interval between episodes was 29.8 days (range, 14 to 50 days). It should be noted that, with any single episode of recurring fever, the patients often do not have all three of the syndrome manifestations (i.e., aphthous stomatitis, pharyngitis, and cervical adenitis).

In the Feder and Salazar[56] series the maximum temperatures ranged from 39.2°C (102.5°F) to 42.1°C (107.8°F), and other symptoms included headache, 44%; vomiting, 27%; and mild abdominal pain, 41%. The patients were said to be listless but not toxic. The parents of 46% of the children reported that their children with PFAPA were less likely to get respiratory and gastrointestinal viral illnesses that were circulating in their families and communities. Sixty-two percent of the children had a prodrome (fatigue, headache, abdominal pain, or irritability) that began 20 hours (mean) before the onset of fever. Patients in this series had normal white blood cell counts and erythrocyte sedimentation rates when afebrile. With illness the white blood cell count tended to be slightly elevated, with a preponderance of neutrophils. At the onset of illness, the C-reactive protein value was elevated.

Hofer and colleagues[87] analyzed 301 PFAPA cases in 15 centers in Europe. Of the 301 cases, 449 had the complete cluster of symptoms (pharyngitis, cervical adenitis, and oral aphthosis) with their episodes. Seventy-six percent of the patients had additional symptoms (131 gastrointestinal symptoms, 86 arthralagias and/or myalgias, 36 skin rashes, and 8 neurologic symptoms). There were 161 boys and 140 girls, the median age of onset was 1.7 years, the median interval between attacks was 4 weeks, and the median duration was 4 days.

Cochard and colleagues[36] studied the familial relationships in PFAPA syndrome. They noted a positive family history for recurrent fever in 38 of 84 (45%) children with PFAPA. The affected family member was a sibling or parent in 29 of 38 (76%) of the cases.

The etiology of the PFAPA syndrome is unknown. In extensive studies by Stojanov and associates,[182] the following were noted in PFAPA attacks: complement (C1QB, C2, SERPIN GI), interleukin-1 (IL)-related (IL-1B, IL-1RN, CASP1, IL18RAP), and interferon-induced (AIM2, IP-10/CXCL 10) genes were overexpressed, and T-cell–associated transcripts (CD3, CD8B) were downregulated. During attacks, there were increased serum levels of chemokines for activated T cells (IP-10/CXCL 10, MIG/CXCL 9), granulocyte colony-stimulating factor, and proinflammatory cytokines (IL-18, IL-6). A relative lymphopenia was noted.

In another study, Brown and colleagues[18] noted increased monocytes and decreased eosinophils during attacks and increased thrombocytes during the afebrile period. Kolly and coworkers[101] noted that IL-1β monocyte production was dysregulated in patients with PFAPA syndrome.

Wurster and associates[205] carried out a long-term follow-up study of 59 patients in a PFAPA registry. The follow-up time ranged between 12 and 21 years. Of this group 50 (85%) had complete resolution. The mean duration of the syndrome was 6.3 years (95% CI, 5.4–7.3) and none of these patients had sequelae.

Differential Diagnosis

As noted in Table 9.2, the differential diagnoses in pharyngitis are numerous, as in nasopharyngitis (see Table 9.1). Although considerable overlap exists in the spectrum of illness in pharyngeal infections, many clues help in ruling in or out certain diagnostic possibilities. The diagnosis of pharyngitis requires carefully eliciting epidemiologic and other historical data (i.e., exposure, season, incubation period, age of patient, associated clinical findings), in addition to observing pharyngeal physical findings.

Most acute instances of nasopharyngitis are of viral origin (see Table 9.1), with adenoviruses accounting for the greatest number of cases. Nasopharyngitis also occurs during epidemic influenza A and B and parainfluenza 1 and 2 infections and with sporadic parainfluenza 3 infections. In all cases, proper epidemiologic and historical data should be elicited so that early diphtheria and other unusual but treatable illnesses are not diagnosed incorrectly. Retrospective study has indicated that nasopharyngitis occasionally occurs in severe infections from *H. influenzae* and meningococci, so the possible presence of these infections should be considered when the epidemiology suggests it.

Although most cases of pharyngitis without nasal symptoms are caused by viral infections, numerous other etiologic possibilities exist. The approach taken frequently by many physicians is to consider all pharyngitis as being of bacterial origin and to treat it with antibiotics. The initial consideration in a child with pharyngitis should be the duration of illness. Subacute, chronic, and recurrent illnesses (see Table 9.2) generally suggest more unusual problems and require a more deliberate approach. In all instances of acute pharyngitis, ruling out streptococcal disease is mandatory.

PFAPA syndrome must be differentiated from *monogenic periodic fevers*, which are caused by mutations of genes involved in regulation of the inflammatory response.[65] These illnesses include familial Mediterranean fever, tumor necrosis factor receptor–associated periodic syndrome, and mevalonate kinase deficiency.

Specific Diagnosis

The epidemiologic history and careful clinical categorization are the most important aspects of specific diagnosis. The most pressing diagnostic need in upper respiratory tract infections in everyday pediatric practice is distinguishing bacterial from viral disease—who and who not to treat with antibiotics.

A child with the common cold, herpangina, or pharyngoconjunctival fever has a viral disease and does not need therapy with antibiotics. In most instances, when these clinical diagnoses are apparent, performing throat cultures for bacterial pathogens is unnecessary. A child with severe acute pharyngitis with exudate and fever and cervical lymphadenitis also is treated easily because most of these children have disease resulting from group A streptococci.

Because young children usually cry when examined by the physician, the clinical differentiation between pharyngitis/tonsillitis without nasal symptoms and nasopharyngitis is difficult. Therefore, on clinical grounds, there is no certain way to make an etiologic diagnosis and specifically to rule out infection caused by *S. pyogenes*. In the past, the usually recommended approach to management of pharyngitis and nasopharyngitis was to obtain a throat culture to determine whether group A streptococci were present. Because several rapid tests (RADTs) for the detection of group A streptococci are available, establishing the immediate diagnosis and providing treatment of streptococcal pharyngitis is recommended in the practice setting.*

Generally these rapid tests have high specificity, but sensitivity may be suboptimal. Today, a reasonable approach to establishing the diagnosis of streptococcal pharyngitis is to do an RADT. If the test result is positive, specific therapy is instituted. In the case of a negative rapid test result in children, a routine throat culture is done, and therapy is withheld pending the culture results.[46]

A common approach is to obtain two throat swabs at the time the child is examined and send both to the laboratory. The laboratory can then run the RADT and only carry out the culture if the rapid test is negative for group A streptococci.

A question exists regarding whether early treatment of streptococcal pharyngitis is desirable.[47,66,67,151,152] In the public clinic, where following up children with positive throat cultures often is difficult, providing immediate diagnosis and treatment is important. As Pichichero and associates[157] and El-Daher and colleagues[47] have shown, early treatment may result in a decreased desirable antibody response, allowing reinfection with type-specific organisms to occur. In settings in which the

*References 45, 46, 56, 104, 108, 122, 152, 154, 169, 175, 180, 186, 201.

communication between physicians and parents is satisfactory, a reasonable approach in many instances is to withhold the institution of treatment for 1 or 2 days. Gerber and associates[47,66,67] argued against this approach because providing immediate therapy can reduce the risk of transmission of infection, and they challenged the interpretation of the findings of Pichichero and associates[152] and El-Daher and colleagues.[47]

Cultures for other pathogens should be reserved for unusual situations, such as persistent symptoms, indicative epidemiology, or other pertinent historical data. Because *H. influenzae* and *Streptococcus pneumoniae* frequently are part of the normal flora, their isolation is not always etiologically significant. If cultures reveal predominant growths of either *H. influenzae* or *S. pneumoniae,* however, they are likely contributing to the disease process, and antibiotic therapy directed at the specific pathogen would benefit the patient.[29,124,203] When the possibility of disease because of anaerobic agents exists, a gram-stained smear from an exudative area may be rewarding. When the pharyngeal findings are unique, or when many cases of a similar illness are observed, a viral culture or direct antigen test from the throat is indicated.

Treatment

The specific treatments of diseases with nasopharyngitis and pharyngitis are discussed in chapters of this book that deal with the individual pathogens. That antimicrobial agents are prescribed inappropriately in children with sore throat and pharyngitis is common knowledge. Based on the etiologic agents noted in Tables 9.1 and 9.2, it is apparent that many infectious agents that are associated with nasopharyngitis and pharyngitis can be treated effectively with antimicrobial agents. However, except in rare specific circumstances, the only common pathogen that requires treatment is the group A streptococcus. The treatment of streptococcal pharyngitis is discussed in detail in Chapter 82.

Although a multitude of proprietary remedies are available for respiratory tract infections, and sore throat specifically, none has a place in the care of pediatric patients. Particularly to be condemned are throat lozenges that contain numerous useless ingredients, many potentially harmful. Antibiotic-containing lozenges particularly are to be condemned because they may allow streptococcal disease to go unrecognized. Antiseptic mouthwashes have no value, and decongestants and antihistamines have no proven efficacy and frequently lead to troublesome side effects.

Corticosteroids have been used for pain relief in acute pharyngitis, and although they appear to be modestly effective, I believe that this is a bad practice that should be discouraged.[82,102,206,163,166]

Because children with pharyngitis frequently feel ill, therapy with an analgesic is reasonable. Formerly, aspirin was the analgesic usually recommended. However, because aspirin is an etiologic factor in influenza-associated Reye syndrome and because differentiating influenza viral infections from other respiratory viral infections is difficult clinically, using acetaminophen rather than aspirin is prudent. The dose per single administration of acetaminophen by year of age is as follows: younger than 1 year, 60 mg; 1 to 3 years, 60 to 120 mg; 3 to 6 years, 120 mg; 6 to 12 years, 150 to 300 mg; older than 12 years, 325 to 650 mg. Administration may be repeated three or four times daily in young children and every 4 hours in older children. Acetaminophen rarely should be given to infants younger than 6 months old. In young children, careful attention to adequate hydration is particularly necessary.

Children with PFAPA syndrome have been treated with corticosteroids, cimetidine, tonsillectomy, and colchicine.[19,54,64,82,87,102,113,125,187,206] Most often used is prednisolone 1 mg/kg in a single dose.[56] Some patients received one or two additional doses at 12-hour intervals. This treatment is highly effective in reducing the duration of the febrile episode. However, this treatment tends to shorten the interval between febrile episodes by 7 to 14 days. Feder and Salazar[54] note that in their experience with prednisolone treatment the initially shortened cycles lengthened over time. Burton and associates[19] review two randomized tonsillectomy trials. It was noted that tonsillectomy resulted in a reduction in the frequency and severity (length of episodes) of future experiences.

Stagi and associates[176] studied 25 Italian patients and found that these children had low vitamin D serum levels. Vitamin D supplementation in these children reduced the frequency and severity of PFAPA flares.

Complications

The main bacterial complications associated with tonsillitis/pharyngitis are retropharyngeal and peritonsillar abscesses and Lemierre syndrome (see Chapter 11). Nonbacterial complications include rheumatic fever, acute glomerulonephritis, and pediatric autoimmune neuropsychiatric disorders associated with streptococcal infection (see Chapters 29 and 82).

Prognosis

Almost all occurrences of nasopharyngitis and pharyngitis are self-limited, and the overall prognosis is excellent. Keeping a constant vigil for streptococcal and other more serious diseases is necessary, however. Failure to diagnose and treat group A streptococcal infections, syphilis, and other more unusual infections can lead to serious short- and long-term difficulties.

Prevention

Because pharyngitis and nasopharyngitis are caused by infections with many different respiratory pathogens, no practical specific approach to prevention exists. Occasionally, streptococcal disease can be prevented by the judicious use of prophylactic penicillin. For young children or others with undue susceptibility to serious disease with common respiratory pathogens, reducing contact situations (e.g., daycare centers) is prudent. In the 1980s, Paradise and colleagues[142] studied the effect of tonsillectomy on the rate of recurrent throat infections in severely affected children. In this controlled study, children needed to have a history of seven or more episodes of tonsillitis in the preceding year, or five or more episodes in each of 2 preceding years, or three or more episodes in the 3 preceding years. The findings in this study indicated that children in the surgical group had significantly fewer throat infections than occurred in the nonsurgical control group during the ensuing 2 years of follow-up. In a more recent but similar study with less stringent criteria for surgery, Paradise and colleagues[147] found that tonsillectomy or adenotonsillectomy conferred a modest benefit. They concluded, however, that the modest benefit of tonsillectomy or adenotonsillectomy in children with recurrent throat infections does not justify the risks, morbidity, and cost of the operations.

Blakley and Magit[12] reviewed four randomized controlled trials in which tonsillectomy was favored over medical therapy in reducing pharyngitis and found in only one of these trials that the result was statistically significant. Their meta-analysis suggested that tonsillectomy resulted in a 43% reduction in the incidence of pharyngitis.

NEW REFERENCES SINCE THE SEVENTH EDITION

4. Amini R, Jahanshiri F, Amini Y, et al. Detection of human coronavirus strain HKU1 in a 2 year old girl with asthma exacerbation caused by acute pharyngitis. *Virol J.* 2012;9:142.
19. Burton MJ, Pollard AJ, Ramsden JD. Tonsillectomy for periodic fever, aphthous stomatitis, pharyngitis and cervical adenitis syndrome (PFAPA). *Cochrane Database Syst Rev.* 2010;(9):CD008669.
43. Dykes AC, Cherry JD, Nolan CE. A clinical, epidemiologic, serologic, and virologic study of influenza C virus infection. *Arch Intern Med.* 1980;140(10):1295-1298.
56. Felsenstein S, Faddoul D, Sposto R, et al. Molecular and clinical diagnosis of group A streptococcal pharyngitis in children. *J Clin Microbiol.* 2014;52(11):3884-3889.
87. Hofer M, Pillet P, Cochard MM, et al. International periodic fever, aphthous stomatitis, pharyngitis, cervical adenitis syndrome cohort: description of distinct phenotypes in 301 patients. *Rheumatology (Oxford).* 2014;53(6):1125-1129.
101. Kolly L, Busso N, von Scheven-Gete A, et al. Periodic fever, aphthous stomatitis, pharyngitis, cervical adenitis syndrome is linked to dysregulated monocyte IL-1beta production. *J Allergy Clin Immunol.* 2013;131(6):1635-1643.
108. Lean WL, Arnup S, Danchin M, et al. Rapid diagnostic tests for group A streptococcal pharyngitis: a meta-analysis. *Pediatrics.* 2014;134(4):771-781.
109. Lee CJ, Huang YC, Yang S, et al. Clinical features of coxsackievirus A4, B3 and B4 infections in children. *PLoS ONE.* 2014;9(2):e87391.
163. Sadowitz PD, Page NE, Crowley K. Adverse effects of steroid therapy in children with pharyngitis with unsuspected malignancy. *Pediatr Emerg Care.* 2012;28(8):807-809.
175. Spellerberg B, Brandt C. Streptococcus. In: Jorgensen J, Pfaller MA, Carroll KC, et al, eds. *Manual of Clinical Microbiology.* Vol. 1. 11th ed. Washington, DC: ASM Press; 2015.

The full reference list for this chapter is available at ExpertConsult.com.

10 Uvulitis

Ellen R. Wald

Infections of the uvula have been reported infrequently in the medical literature. When the uvula is the most inflamed structure in the posterior pharynx of a febrile child, acute infection should be suspected. Other causes of uvulitis include trauma (from instrumentation), ischemia due to pressure from an endotracheal tube or laryngeal mask airway, inhalant irritation (from use of recreational drugs, including cocaine, cannabis, and mephedrone), vasculitis, and allergy.[1,3-5,9,13,14,18]

ETIOLOGY

The main bacterial agents that cause uvulitis in children include *Haemophilus influenzae* type b and *Streptococcus pyogenes*.[8] Uvulitis caused by *H. influenzae* may occur concurrently with epiglottitis or as an isolated infection.[10,17] Uvulitis caused by *S. pyogenes* seems always to occur in concert with pharyngitis. Brook[2] reported two cases of uvulitis caused by anaerobic bacteria (*Fusobacterium nucleatum* and *Prevotella intermedia*). No search for viral agents has been conducted. Several cases of uvulitis caused by *Candida albicans* have been described in immunocompetent toddlers.[9] In adults, *Streptococcus pneumoniae* and *H. influenzae* have been reported to cause uvulitis.[6,16] In many patients, an associated epiglottitis has been present.[12,16]

EPIDEMIOLOGY

The epidemiology of uvulitis is the epidemiology of its two etiologic agents, *S. pyogenes* and *H. influenzae* type b. It occurs in school-aged children 5 to 15 years old (the so-called streptococcal age group) in association with pharyngitis. Similarly, it can be seen in the *H. influenzae* age group (3 months to 5 years) if a child has not received the now routine and universally recommended conjugate vaccine to prevent infections caused by *H. influenzae* type b. Cases of uvulitis in association with epiglottitis have been reported in the United States and in England.[2,8,15] Infections caused by *S. pyogenes* and *H. influenzae* occur primarily in the winter and spring, but both types can occur throughout the year.

PATHOGENESIS

Uvulitis is an acute cellulitis characterized by dramatic swelling and erythema. Infection of the uvula probably arises from direct invasion by *S. pyogenes* or *H. influenzae* type b; both are recognized as normal nasopharyngeal flora. In the latter case, epiglottitis also may arise by direct extension, and the bacteremia may result secondarily from either the uvula or the epiglottis as a primary site of infection.

Uvulitis that is noninfectious may result from injury, chemical irritation, or allergic inflammation. An occurrence in a child who was ultimately diagnosed to have Kawasaki disease also has been reported.[7]

CLINICAL MANIFESTATIONS

In a review of five patients with streptococcal uvulitis, all had associated pharyngitis.[8] The patients presented with low-grade fever and sore throat. Three of the five patients experienced a choking or gagging sensation in the pharynx that induced coughing and spitting; one of these patients also presented with drooling. Although pharyngitis was noted on physical examination, the swelling and erythema of the uvula were most dramatic (Fig. 10.1). None of the patients had evidence of respiratory distress.

In most children with uvulitis and epiglottitis, the presentation usually is typical for epiglottitis, with sudden onset of high fever, dysphagia, and increasing respiratory distress. Rapkin,[15] however, reported a case of uvulitis and epiglottitis in a child in which the epiglottitis initially was unsuspected. The same observation has been made in some adults with uvulitis and epiglottitis.[6,12] Lateral neck radiography (performed in one case to evaluate the possibility of a retropharyngeal abscess) belatedly alerted the clinicians to the correct diagnosis.

In patients with uvulitis and no epiglottitis, the presentation may be similar to that of epiglottitis, with acute onset of fever, odynophagia, and drooling, or, less specific, with fever and irritability or decreased appetite.[10,11,17] The diagnosis in these cases is provided by physical examination of the oropharynx, which shows a swollen and erythematous uvula (see Fig. 10.1).

DIAGNOSIS

The diagnosis of streptococcal uvulitis is suspected when a school-aged child presents with low-grade fever, pharyngitis, and uvulitis. The diagnosis is confirmed by the recovery of *S. pyogenes* from a surface culture of the throat or uvula or both.

The diagnosis of uvulitis caused by *H. influenzae* is suspected in a highly febrile infant or preschool-aged child who has uvular inflammation on physical examination. Lateral neck radiography must be performed to evaluate the possibility of epiglottitis unless obvious signs of upper respiratory tract obstruction are present, in which case immediate endoscopy is warranted. If epiglottitis is discovered, the airway must be secured, and appropriate parenteral antimicrobial agents must be initiated after blood and surface culture specimens are obtained. Any surface culture specimen obtained to search for *H. influenzae* must be plated onto chocolate agar. After appropriate culture specimens are obtained, parenteral antimicrobial agents should be initiated, as in other infections associated with bacteremia caused by *H. influenzae*.

DIFFERENTIAL DIAGNOSIS

The differential diagnosis of a patient with acute onset of fever, dysphagia, and drooling includes herpes simplex gingivostomatitis, uvulitis, epiglottitis, severe pharyngitis, and peritonsillar or retropharyngeal abscess. Although being extremely cautious in examining the pharynx of any patient with suspected epiglottitis is appropriate, some children tolerate attempted visualization of the oral cavity without becoming unduly upset. Instrumentation with a tongue blade should be avoided. If the examination does not show gingivostomatitis or peritonsillar abscess, lateral neck radiography should be performed. If epiglottitis or retropharyngeal abscess is confirmed, management of the airway and administration of antimicrobial agents are indicated for epiglottitis, and incision and drainage and administration of antimicrobial agents are indicated for retropharyngeal abscess. If the lateral neck is normal and the uvula is inflamed, uvulitis with or without pharyngitis is confirmed.

TREATMENT

Management of uvulitis is guided primarily by the associated pharyngitis or epiglottitis, if either is present. In the case of streptococcal pharyngitis, penicillin therapy for 10 days is most appropriate. These patients usually can be treated orally with penicillin V 25 to 50 mg/kg per day administered in two divided doses.

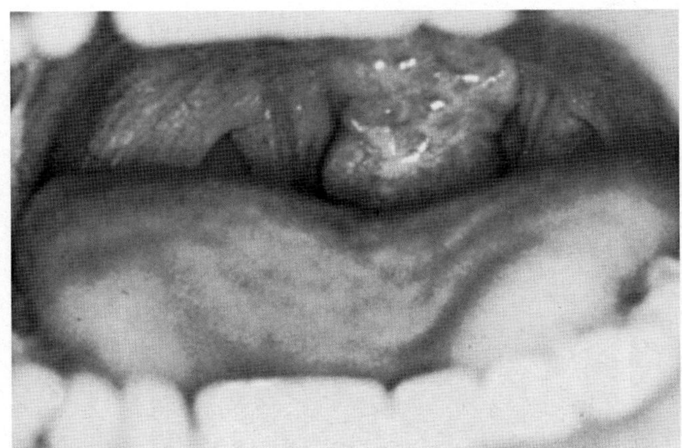

FIG. 10.1 Swollen (two to three times normal size) and erythematous uvula in a patient without epiglottitis or pharyngitis.

In the case of uvulitis and epiglottitis, management of the airway is most important and can be accomplished by performing nasotracheal intubation or tracheotomy. Appropriate parenteral antibiotic therapy usually is initiated.

In the case of uvulitis without epiglottitis in an infant or preschool-aged child, antimicrobial therapy should be planned for possible *H. influenzae* type b bacteremia. As many as 50% of respiratory isolates of *H. influenzae* produce β-lactamase. Administration of an advanced-generation cephalosporin, such as cefotaxime 200 mg/kg per day in four divided doses or ceftriaxone 100 mg/kg per day in one dose or two divided doses, is appropriate. In a patient with serious penicillin hypersensitivity, aztreonam 100 mg/kg per day in three divided doses and ciprofloxacin 30 mg/kg per day in two divided doses are also satisfactory regimens. After the patient has defervesced and has improved clinically, an oral antimicrobial agent can be substituted. The results of blood and surface cultures now can guide therapy. For an ampicillin-susceptible *H. influenzae* infection, amoxicillin 45 mg/kg per day in two divided doses should be prescribed to complete a 7- to 10-day course of treatment. For β-lactamase–producing *H. influenzae,* a variety of oral agents, including cefixime 10 mg/kg in a single daily dose, cefuroxime 30 mg/kg per day in two divided doses, or amoxicillin-potassium clavulanate (45 mg/kg per day of amoxicillin) in two divided doses, can be prescribed.

Resolution was prompt in the two cases of uvulitis allegedly caused by *C. albicans.* One child was treated with topical nystatin, and the other had spontaneous improvement.[9]

NEW REFERENCES SINCE THE SEVENTH EDITION

13. Murphy A, Haughey R. Mephedrone-induced uvulitis. *Anaesthesia.* 2014;69:189-190.
18. Ziahosseini K, Ali S, Simo R, Malhotra R. Uvulitis following general anaesthesia. *BMJ Case Rep.* 2014;doi:10.1136/bcr-2014-205038.

The full reference list for this chapter is available at ExpertConsult.com

11 Peritonsillar, Retropharyngeal, and Parapharyngeal Abscesses

Nira A. Goldstein • Margaret R. Hammerschlag

A deep neck abscess is a collection of pus in a potential space bounded by fascia.[8] These potential spaces are areas of least resistance to the spread of infection. An infection may begin with a minimal area of cellulitis and progress to a deep neck abscess, which may extend to invade adjacent potential spaces; these spaces frequently encompass vital structures in the neck. Destruction and dysfunction of these structures represent the major complications of deep neck infections.[63]

EPIDEMIOLOGY OF HEAD AND NECK SPACE INFECTIONS IN CHILDREN

Head and neck space infections in children are not uncommon. A survey of members of the American Academy of Otolaryngology found the incidence of peritonsillar abscesses to be approximately 30 per 100,000 person-years, or approximately 45,000 cases annually in the United States and Puerto Rico,[47] whereas a 3-year study in Sweden in a well-defined catchment area of 179,200 inhabitants reported an incidence of 37 per 100,000 person-years.[85] Data from the 2009 Kids' Inpatient Database (KID) that included data from 2 to 3 million pediatric hospitalizations occurring in 44 states reported an incidence of 9.4 peritonsillar abscesses per 100,000 person-years, 2.2 retropharyngeal abscesses per 100,000 person-years, and 2.0 parapharyngeal abscesses per 100,000 person-years.[80] There was a statistically significant increase in the incidence of retropharyngeal abscesses from 2000 to 2009 (1.0 to 2.2 cases per 100,000 person-years) but there was no change in the incidence of peritonsillar (8.2 to 9.4 cases per 100,000) or parapharyngeal (0.8 to 1.4 cases per 100,000) abscesses. Elsherif and associates[34] described 130 cases of retropharyngeal abscess between 2002 and 2007, and the incidence significantly increased over the study period from 13 cases in 2002 to 44 in 2007. Wright and colleagues[112] also found a doubling in the number of cases of retropharyngeal space infections from 1997 to 2001 versus 2001 to 2005. In contrast, Segal and associates[93] found no increase in the number of peritonsillar infections from 2004 to 2007.

Peritonsillar abscesses rarely occur in young children but most frequently occur in patients in their teens and early 20s. In a 5-year study of 1010 incident head and neck infections, the median (interquartile range) patient age was 13 years for peritonsillar abscesses (range, 9 to 17 years), 2 years for retropharyngeal abscesses (range, 1 to 6 years), and 6 years for parapharyngeal abscesses (range, 5 to 7 years).[92] Retropharyngeal and parapharyngeal abscesses are more common in boys,[34,42,53,60] whereas peritonsillar abscesses occur equally among boys and girls.[85] Retropharyngeal abscesses most commonly occur in the winter and spring,[42,53,60,92] whereas peritonsillar abscesses have been reported to be more common in the autumn and spring[93] and the spring and summer.[92]

PERITONSILLAR ABSCESS (QUINSY)

A peritonsillar abscess (quinsy) is circumscribed medially by the fibrous wall of the tonsil capsule and laterally by the superior constrictor muscle. Pus may be localized in the superior pole, midpoint, or inferior pole or rarely may be dispersed, with multiple loculations in the peritonsillar space. The superior pole is the most common location, with a frequency range of 41.2% to 70%; the remaining inferior locations account for the balance.[10,14,66]

The etiology of peritonsillar abscesses is not constant. The abscesses may occur after any "virulent" tonsillitis, with extension through the fibrous tonsil capsule. Results of a meta-analysis of 15 previously reported

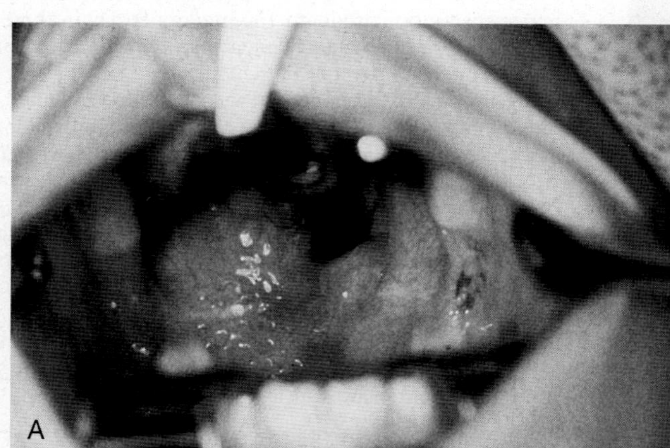

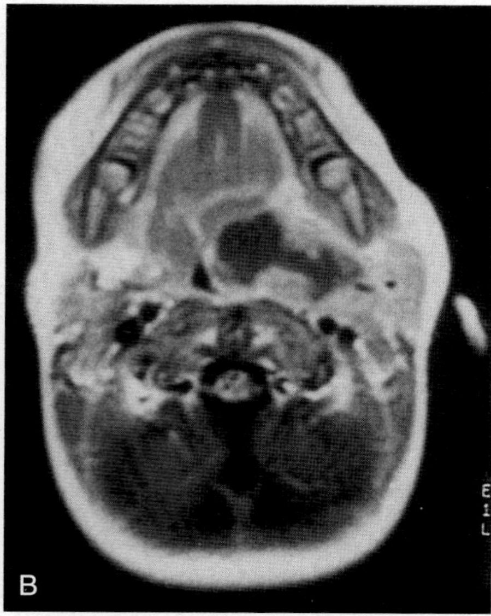

FIG. 11.1 Left peritonsillar abscess in an 18-month-old child. (From Wiatrak BJ, Woolley AL. Pharyngitis and adenotonsillar disease. In: Cummings CW, Flint PW, Harker LA, et al., editors. *Otolaryngology: head and neck surgery*. 4th ed. Philadelphia: Elsevier; 2005:4144.)

series of patients with peritonsillar abscess reported by Herzon[47] found prior tonsillar infection rates ranging from 11% to 56%, with an overall rate of 36%. Group A β-hemolytic streptococcus has a moderate role in the development of peritonsillar abscesses because throat cultures are only positive in 18% of patients,[100] rapid antigen tests are only positive in 20% to 30% of patients,[86] and abscess cultures demonstrate group A β-hemolytic streptococcus in 46%.[36]

Clinical Manifestations

The patient's recent history may include a sore throat with occasional unilateral ear pain, malaise, low-grade pyrexia, chills, diaphoresis, dysphagia, reduced oral intake, trismus, and a muffled "hot potato voice." Trismus results from irritation and reflex spasm of the internal pterygoid muscle. Impaired palatal motion from edema contributes to the muffled voice.

Physical examination reveals minimal to moderate toxicity, dehydration, and drooling. Inspection of the oropharynx may be compromised by trismus. The soft palate is displaced toward the unaffected side, swollen and red, and frequently palpably fluctuant. The edematous uvula is pushed across the midline (Fig. 11.1). The displaced tonsil and its crypts rarely are coated with exudate. The breath is fetid, and ipsilateral, tender, cervical adenopathy is present. The white blood cell count is elevated, with a predominance of polymorphonuclear leukocytes.

Brodsky and associates[15] attempted to identify the clinical signs that might distinguish peritonsillar abscess from peritonsillar cellulitis in a group of 21 children admitted to the Children's Hospital of Buffalo from 1985 through 1987. No significant difference in age, duration of sore throat, fever, or white blood cell count was noted, although a greater degree of pharyngotonsillar bulge and muffled voice was found in the patients with abscess. Patients with peritonsillar cellulitis improved after receiving 24 hours of intravenous antibiotics, whereas patients with peritonsillar abscess had no change or worsening of symptoms. Blotter and colleagues[11] confirmed these findings in 102 patients admitted to Children's Hospital of Columbus, Ohio, between 1995 and 1998.

In uncomplicated cases involving adults and older children, computed tomography (CT) has not been as useful as clinical assessment and follow-up evaluation in the management of peritonsillar abscess. CT is useful in young children with suspected peritonsillar abscess who are not cooperative with examination or children with other suspected deep neck infections.[39] In a retrospective study by Baker and associates,[4] CT was ordered in 96 (64.9%) of 148 patients presenting to the emergency department for evaluation of a potential peritonsillar abscess between 2007 and 2009. Recently ultrasonography has been investigated as a tool that avoids undue radiation exposure. Fordham and associates[37] found that transcervical ultrasonography had a sensitivity of 100% and specificity of 76.5% in diagnosing peritonsillar abscess in a study of 43 patients aged 2 through 20 years. While similar results for intraoral ultrasonography has been found in adults, the intraoral route may not be well tolerated in children due to their smaller mouth opening and lack of cooperation.[79]

Treatment

Traditionally management of peritonsillar abscess in children involved hospital admission for intravenous hydration, antibiotic therapy, analgesia, and either intraoral incision and drainage of the abscess or "acute quinsy tonsillectomy" with removal of the medial wall of the abscess. Although older children may tolerate incision and drainage under local anesthetic, the procedure is not well tolerated in young children and carries the risk of potential injury to adjacent vascular structures. The administration of a general anesthetic is required for tonsillectomy in all age groups and often is required for incision and drainage in young children. Acute tonsillectomy often was done to prevent future recurrence of the peritonsillar abscess.

Although it is a commonly accepted clinical observation, a high recurrence rate of peritonsillar abscess has not been well documented. A meta-analysis reported by Herzon[47] of 19 studies from the United States, Europe, and Israel involving 1399 patients found recurrence rates of 10% to 15% for peritonsillar abscess. The rates of recurrence seem to be lower in the United States (0% to 17%) than in the series reported from Europe and Israel (3% to 22%). A retrospective analysis of 290 patients treated for peritonsillar abscess found that patients who had a history of recurrent tonsillitis before development of the abscess had a fourfold greater rate of recurrence than patients with no history (40% vs. 9.6%).[59] The authors recommended that patients with a history of recurrent tonsillitis before admission be treated with tonsillectomy.[59] A nationwide study in Taiwan from 2001 to 2009 involving 28,837 patients found an overall recurrence rate of 5.2%, with a rate of 6.7% in patients younger than 30 years.[107] The rate increased to 13.7% in patients younger than 30 years with five or more prior episodes of tonsillitis compared to 4.4% in those with less than five episodes. Evaluation of 4199 patients with peritonsillar abscess identified in a database of hospital discharge records in Veneto, Italy, found a recurrence rate of 11.7% in patients not initially treated with tonsillectomy.[13] This rate increased to 32% and 40% after the second or third recurrence of the peritonsillar abscess, respectively.

The risks of acute tonsillectomy are not greater than the risks associated with delayed tonsillectomy.[65,73,111] In addition, the morbidity caused by two hospitalizations involving two procedures is reduced by acute tonsillectomy.[7,12,14] An additional benefit of acute tonsillectomy is the ability to evacuate inferior pole abscesses that technically are difficult to drain by needle aspiration or incision and drainage.[66] Simon and associates[96] found no significant differences in total length of hospital stay, blood loss, operative time, and postoperative complications between 23 children treated by acute quinsy tonsillectomy and 11 children treated with initial antibiotics with or without incision and drainage followed by interval tonsillectomy between 2007 and 2011.

Studies have suggested that many peritonsillar abscesses can be managed by simple needle aspiration combined with antibiotic therapy on an outpatient basis.[15,47,82,90,91,99,105,108] An extensive meta-analysis of 10 studies conducted from 1961 through 1994 involving 496 patients with peritonsillar abscesses found that needle aspiration had an overall success rate of 94% (range, 85% to 100%).[47] This success rate compares favorably with that reported for incision and drainage. Weinberg and associates[108] successfully performed needle aspiration in 41 of 43 children 7 to 18 years old (mean age, 13.9 years). All were admitted for intravenous antibiotic therapy, 2 (5%) required repeated aspiration for resolution, and 5 (12%) did not respond and required acute tonsillectomy. A pooled analysis of three prospective studies comparing needle aspiration versus incision and drainage showed no significant difference in resolution rates (93.7% for incision and drainage and 91.6% for needle aspiration), but the power was low because of the small sample size.[52] Other studies, which have included adults and children with peritonsillar abscesses, have reported that 0% to 48% of patients require hospitalization.[47,73,82,99]

Younger children often require admission to correct dehydration.[39] Younger children also are more likely than are older children to respond to intravenous antibiotics alone and to have negative findings at surgical drainage.[11] The use of conscious sedation has been reported to be a safe and effective approach for the drainage of peritonsillar abscesses in children.[68,101]

In a 10-year retrospective review of 83 children with peritonsillar abscesses by Schraff and colleagues,[91] 65% were treated by incision and drainage (51% knife vs. 14% needle aspiration), 31% had quinsy tonsillectomy, and 4% were admitted and treated with intravenous antibiotics alone. Of patients treated surgically, 51% of the procedures were done in the emergency department and 49% were done in the operating room. Forty-eight percent of the children required admission, and the average length of stay was 0.9 days (standard deviation, 1.37 days).

A suggested approach to the management of children with peritonsillar abscess is as follows.[48] Cooperative children should undergo needle aspiration of the abscess and treatment with antibiotics. Children who can tolerate liquids orally may be managed as outpatients, and the remainder should be admitted for hydration and administration of intravenous antibiotics. Approximately 4% of children require a repeated aspiration for resolution.[47] Children who remain symptomatic after undergoing needle aspiration require incision and drainage or acute quinsy tonsillectomy, depending on the prior history of recurrent tonsillitis. Children who cannot tolerate needle aspiration on initial presentation are admitted for administration of intravenous antibiotics. If no response occurs within 24 hours, incision and drainage or acute tonsillectomy is done, depending on the prior history of recurrent tonsillitis. Delayed tonsillectomy is reserved for children who recover from the peritonsillar abscess without general anesthesia but have a history of recurrent tonsillitis or prior peritonsillar abscess.

There are new data suggesting that corticosteroids may be beneficial for patients with peritonsillar abscesses. Ozbek and associates[83] randomized patients aged 16 to 65 years to antibiotics with a single dose of intravenous corticosteroid or antibiotics with a single dose of placebo after needle aspiration. The patients who received corticosteroids demonstrated significant improvements in throat pain, fever, trismus, and hospitalization time compared with control patients. Additional studies in children are needed to support their routine use.

Untreated peritonsillar abscess may point, with spontaneous rupture, or extend to the pterygomaxillary space, with potentially fatal complications. Upper airway obstruction, septicemia, and vascular catastrophe may occur. Necrotizing fasciitis also has been reported in adults with peritonsillar abscess.[41,109]

RETROPHARYNGEAL ABSCESS (POSTERIOR VISCERAL SPACE, RETROVISCERAL SPACE, AND RETROESOPHAGEAL SPACE ABSCESSES)

The anterior wall of the retropharyngeal space is the middle layer of the deep cervical fascia that abuts the posterior esophageal wall (the superior pharyngeal constrictor muscle). The deep layer of the deep cervical fascia circumscribes the posterior wall of this potential space. Inferiorly, these two fasciae fuse to limit the depth of this pocket at a level between the first and second thoracic vertebrae. A retropharyngeal abscess can erode inferiorly through the junction of these fasciae to extend posteriorly into the prevertebral space (Fig. 11.2). Subsequently, pus in the prevertebral space can descend inferiorly below the diaphragm to the psoas muscles.

The retropharyngeal space contains two paramedial chains of lymph nodes that receive drainage from the nasopharynx, adenoids, posterior paranasal sinuses, middle ear, and eustachian tube. These structures are prominent in early childhood and atrophy at puberty.[43] Retropharyngeal abscesses are common occurrences in young children and are thought to be secondary to suppurative adenitis of these retropharyngeal nodes.[6] Other sources of infection are penetrating foreign bodies, endoscopy, trauma, pharyngitis, vertebral body osteomyelitis, petrositis, dental procedures,[105] and branchial cleft anomalies.[51] In one series of 17 cases of retropharyngeal abscesses at the Children's Hospital, Denver, Colorado, seven children (41%), including two neonates (most likely associated with attempts at intubation), had perforations of the hypopharynx or esophagus.[75] In a series of 117 children with head and neck space infections treated at the Children's Hospital of Pittsburgh, 63% of the children with retropharyngeal abscesses had antecedent tonsillitis, pharyngitis, or viral upper respiratory tract infection.[105] Two children had previous trauma; however, no details on the type of trauma were given. In adults, tuberculosis and syphilis were common causes of retropharyngeal abscesses in the preantibiotic era.[78]

Clinical Manifestations

The symptoms of retropharyngeal abscess frequently begin insidiously after mild antecedent infection. Signs and symptoms include sore throat, fever, limitation of neck motion, torticollis, neck pain, neck mass, drooling, odynophagia, poor oral intake, and lethargy. Airway stridor or respiratory distress from edema, cellulitis, or an obstructing mass occasionally occurs.[26,27,30,106] Limited neck motion or torticollis is reported in 50% to 80% of patients.[27,42,84] In adults, the symptoms may be milder. Complaints of chest pain may reflect mediastinal extension.

Early in the course, midline or unilateral swelling of the posterior pharynx occurs. Later, gentle palpation may show a large fluctuant mass in the posterior pharynx. Vigorous palpation should be avoided because it may cause the abscess to rupture into the upper airway. As with other abscesses, the white blood cell count is increased, with a predominance of granulocytes.

Plain films of the neck may be performed initially but must be obtained with the patient in a true lateral position, with the neck in extension and on inspiration, or the child's retropharyngeal soft tissues may appear abnormally thickened. Widening of the prevertebral soft tissues exceeding the anteroposterior diameter of the contiguous vertebral bodies or thickening of the retropharyngeal space greater than 7 mm at C2 in children and adults or 14 mm at C6 in children or 22 mm at C6 in adults suggests retropharyngeal inflammation. Rarely a prevertebral soft tissue mass, air-fluid level, or gas may be seen. The normal cervical lordosis may be lost or reversed secondary to muscle spasm or local inflammation.

CT has rendered the diagnosis and management of deep neck space infections more precise.[16,33,57,62,103,106,110] In contrast to conventional radiologic studies, CT distinguishes cellulitis of the neck, which usually does not require surgical treatment, from a deep neck abscess, which

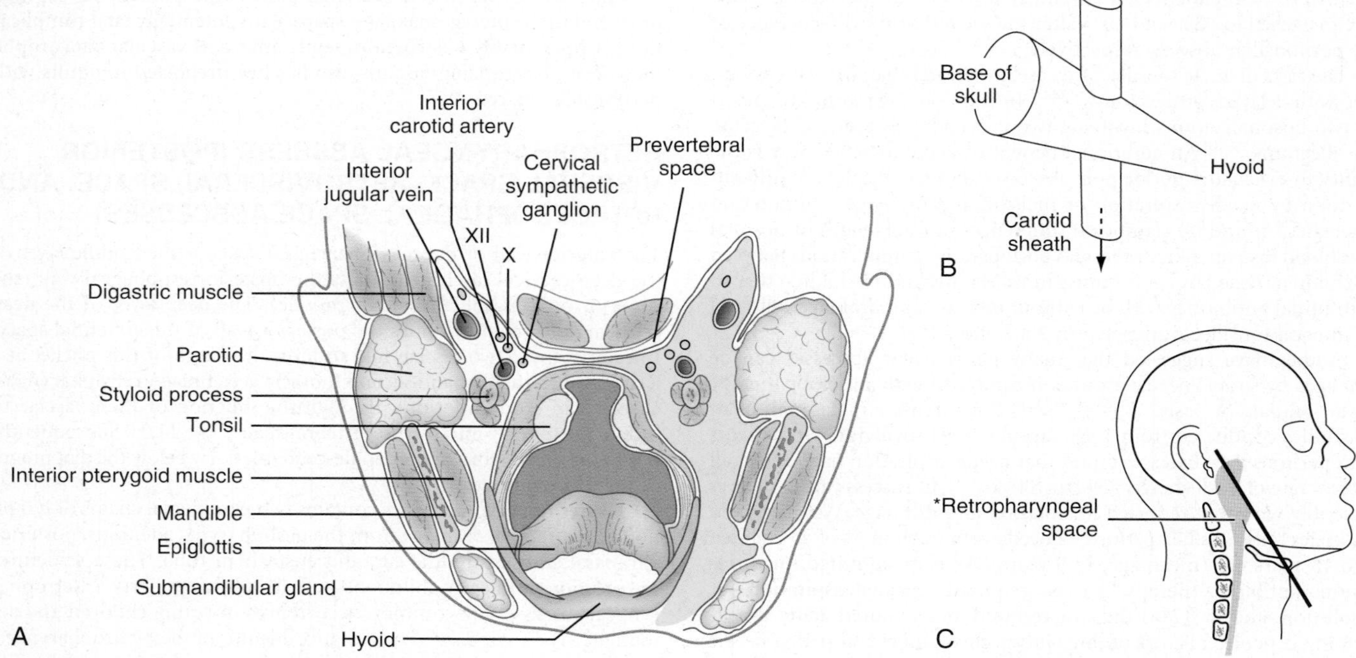

FIG. 11.2 (A) Oblique transverse section of the oropharynx posterosuperiorly and the hypopharynx anteroinferiorly. Depicted are a peritonsillar abscess on the right and a pterygomaxillary space abscess on the left. (B) The "cone" of the potential pterygomaxillary space with its carotid sheath. (C) The vertical dimensions of the retropharyngeal space *(asterisk)*. The *black oblique line* represents the level of the drawing in (A).

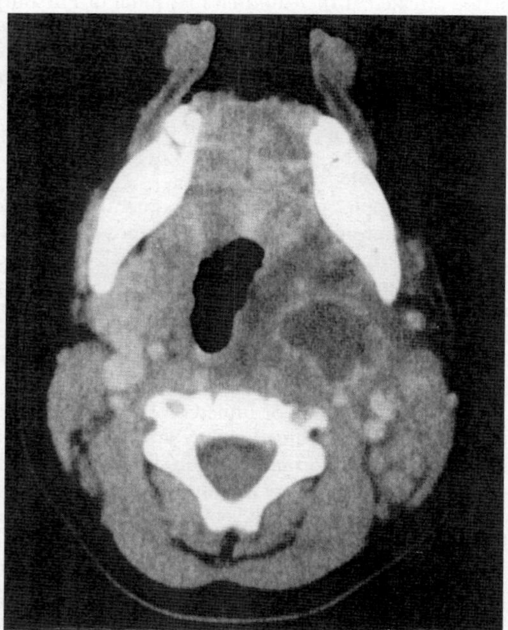

FIG. 11.3 Appearance on computed tomography scan of a focal, ring-enhancing retropharyngeal abscess with a scalloped contour to the abscess wall. (From Kirse DJ, Roberson DW. Surgical management of retropharyngeal space infections in children. *Laryngoscope.* 2001;111:1416.)

generally does require surgical drainage. With its ability to define differences in tissue density, CT permits an accurate determination of the extent of the abscess and its extension and involvement of adjacent spaces to be made. An abscess is distinguished from cellulitis by a low-attenuation homogeneous area surrounded by a ring enhancement of contrast material (Fig. 11.3). Kirse and Roberson[57] reported scalloping of the abscess wall to be a more useful predictor of the presence of pus than ring enhancement. Freling and colleagues[38] reported that the presence of air within or adjacent to the fluid collection indicated an abscess in all cases. When more than one space is involved, accurate assessment of these spaces may ensure sufficient surgical drainage. Vascular structures can be identified, as can potential complications such as venous thrombosis.

A 10-year retrospective study from the Massachusetts Eye and Ear Infirmary compared preoperative CT scans with intraoperative findings in 38 patients who underwent surgical exploration of the parapharyngeal or retropharyngeal space within 48 hours after the scans were performed.[62] Overall the intraoperative findings confirmed the CT scan interpretation in 76.3% of the patients. Of the 38 patients, five (13.2%) had CT scans indicative of abscesses that were not confirmed at surgery. Exploration of the parapharyngeal or retropharyngeal space revealed cellulitis. The false-negative rate was 10.5%. The sensitivity of CT for detection of parapharyngeal or retropharyngeal space abscess was 87.9%. Additional studies have reported that the accuracy of CT in predicting surgical findings was 63%, 69%, 73%, 76%, 76%, and 92%.[33,42,84,98,106,110]

Treatment

The treatment of choice is administration of intravenous antibiotics and incision and drainage. If the mass is small, a peroral incision with the patient in the Rose position (supine with the neck hyperextended) may provide some drainage, but a slight risk of aspiration exists. If the mass is large and extends lateral to the great vessels, or if fever persists after peroral drainage is performed, an external incision is preferred. A tracheotomy may be required if risk of compromising the airway exists. Children may need to be kept intubated postoperatively if there is significant airway obstruction. Martin and associates[70] described four patients treated successfully by CT-guided aspiration of their retropharyngeal abscesses via a percutaneous retromandibular approach in combination with intravenous antibiotics. Three aspirations were performed after failure of surgical drainage, and one was a primary aspiration.

Posterior mediastinitis can result from the spread of infection from the retropharyngeal area into the prevertebral space. The development of mediastinitis has been found to be associated with methicillin-resistant *Staphylococcus aureus* infection (MRSA), and both mediastinitis and MRSA are more common in children younger than 2 years.[1,5,19,24,112] Other complications may be seen when the abscess extends to the parapharyngeal space and involves the great vessels and cranial nerves.

Reports have documented that patients with small retropharyngeal abscesses may respond to treatment with intravenous antibiotics alone. Johnston and associates[53] treated 22 of 32 children with retropharyngeal or parapharyngeal abscesses with a trial of at least 24 hours of intravenous antibiotics. Although 13 (59%) ultimately required drainage, 9 (41%) were successfully managed medically. There were no significant differences in age or white blood cell count on admission between the two groups, but children who required drainage had significantly larger abscesses (5.38 vs. 1.53 cm^2). Cheng and Elden[24] reviewed 178 children who presented to the Children's Hospital of Philadelphia from 2007 through 2012 with retropharyngeal or parapharyngeal abscesses. Medical therapy was the initial treatment in 159 (89.3%). Of these 118 (66.3%) were treated successfully while 41 (23.0%) ultimately required surgical drainage. Risk factors for failure of medical therapy were age younger than 51 months, white blood cell count greater than 20,700/mm^3, intensive care unit admission, CT suggestive of a complete abscess, and abscess size greater than 2.2 cm. A systematic review of eight articles involving 95 patients found a pooled success rate of medical therapy of 52% (95% confidence interval [CI], 53–95%), and when children taken immediately to surgery were excluded, the success rate was 95% (95% CI, 85–100%).[21] Close clinical follow-up is mandatory for children treated with intravenous antibiotics alone. Children who do not improve within 24 to 48 hours require surgical drainage.

Similar results were found in a prospective observational study of 111 children with retropharyngeal infections managed according to a clinical practice guideline between 2001 and 2004 at the Children's Hospital of Boston.[88] Children were triaged into one of three groups at initial presentation based on clinical symptoms and CT findings: probable cellulitis, probable phlegmon, and probable abscess. Thirty-four (30.6%) children were placed in the abscess pathway and underwent prompt incision and drainage. Frank pus was found in 29 (85.3%), intensive care unit admission was required in 13 (38.2%), and 11 (32.4%) required a peripherally inserted central catheter (PICC) line due to failure to meet discharge criteria on oral antibiotics. Seventy-two (64.9%) patients were placed in the phlegmon group, and all but four required a repeat CT after 48 to 72 hours of antibiotics. Thirty-nine (54.2%) in the phlegmon group ultimately required surgical drainage, and purulence was found in 29 (74.4%). Of the 73 patients who required surgical drainage, 70 were drained transorally, two required an external approach for extension of the abscess lateral to the great vessels, and three had transcervical incisions to drain concurrent but not connected external neck abscesses. Ten patients required repeat drainage in the operating room. Presenting signs or symptoms were not significantly different between surgically and medically managed patients; however surgical patients had higher average white blood cell counts on admission and were more likely to require an intensive care unit admission, less likely to require a PICC line, and had a shorter duration of intravenous antibiotics.

PARAPHARYNGEAL ABSCESS (PTERYGOMAXILLARY, PHARYNGOMAXILLARY, LATERAL, AND PHARYNGEAL SPACE ABSCESSES)

The potential parapharyngeal or pterygomaxillary space is an inverted conical cavity (see Fig. 11.2B) lying along an oblique axis roughly parallel to the ramus of the mandible (see Fig. 11.2C). The base of the skull at the jugular foramen forms the base of the "cone," and its apex is at the hyoid bone (see Fig. 11.2B). The buccopharyngeal fascia, lateral to the superior pharyngeal constrictor, delineates the medial boundary, and the parotid gland and its partially dehiscent deep layer of the superficial cervical fascia form the lateral wall of this cone. The internal pterygoid muscle and mandible demarcate the cone on its anterolateral aspect. The parapharyngeal space is contiguous with the peritonsillar, submandibular, and retropharyngeal spaces, all of which are potential avenues of egress for an extending parapharyngeal space abscess (see Fig. 11.2A).

The posterior portion of the cone contains the contents of the carotid sheath (carotid artery and internal jugular vein), cranial nerves IX through XII, and the cervical sympathetic chain. The internal pterygoid muscle and fatty connective tissue are anterior.

Involvement of these structures determines the clinical manifestations and complications of the parapharyngeal space abscess. An abscess in the posterior compartment may show medial displacement of the lateral pharyngeal wall and parotid space induration and swelling, with variable overlying facial nerve weakness, carotid artery erosion and hemorrhage,[61] internal jugular vein thrombosis, decreased gag reflex and dysphagia, ipsilateral vocal cord paralysis, weakness of the ipsilateral trapezius muscle, ipsilateral lingual deviation, and Horner syndrome from cervical sympathetic chain involvement.[23]

Extension of the abscess into the anterior compartment causes trismus from irritation of the internal pterygoid muscle. Induration at the angle of the jaw and medial displacement of the tonsil and pharyngeal wall also occur with an anterior compartment abscess.

By the time a patient with an abscess seeks medical attention, the source of the parapharyngeal space infection may be unclear. Reports indicate variable causes, including incompletely or inadequately treated bacterial pharyngitis, tonsillitis,[6,69,84] peritonsillar abscess, dental infections, bacterial parotitis, otitis, mastoiditis (Bezold abscess from a mastoid tip infection traveling along the digastric muscles), petrositis, cervical adenitis with suppuration, cervical vertebral tubercular adenitis,[9,76] foreign bodies,[23,28] trauma, intravenous drug use,[46] branchial cleft anomalies,[102] and cat-scratch disease.[113] Parapharyngeal abscesses seem to be less common than are peritonsillar and retropharyngeal abscesses in children.

Clinical Manifestations

In addition to the symptoms noted in the preceding description, tender cervical swelling, induration and erythema of the side of the neck, torticollis, sore throat, dysphagia, trismus, hoarseness, malaise, chills, and diaphoresis may occur. Variable low-grade pyrexia with occasional temperature spikes occurs. Examination discloses variable toxicity, respiratory tract distress, laryngeal edema, medial displacement of the lateral pharyngeal wall and inferior tonsil pole, trismus, and, infrequently, drooling. Palpation of the neck reveals a tender, high cervical mass, initially diffuse and later fluctuant. Pharyngeal blood clots may presage erosion of the carotid artery. The complications of parapharyngeal abscesses are related to the structures involved: involvement of the carotid artery can produce hemiplegia from emboli, involvement of the internal jugular vein can lead to internal jugular vein thrombosis, and cephalad extension of the thrombosis may lead to cavernous sinus thrombosis. Internal jugular vein thrombosis is characterized by spiking temperature, toxicity with intense diaphoresis, headaches, and increased intracranial pressure. Septic pulmonary emboli occasionally are present. A pseudoaneurysm of the internal carotid artery may occur as a result of arteritis from contiguous infection and vessel wall erosion.[29,89] The patient may present with massive epistaxis days or weeks after the initial infection. Treatment involves airway protection, control of the epistaxis, resuscitation, intravenous antibiotics, and surgical ligation or endovascular occlusion.

Extension into the retropharyngeal region by a parapharyngeal abscess may lead to a posterior mediastinitis. Airway obstruction occurring secondary to laryngeal edema and aspiration pneumonia from suppuration of the abscess into the pharynx have been reported. Initially, the parapharyngeal abscess may be difficult to differentiate from a peritonsillar abscess, but the latter usually is less toxic and has a distinct, soft palatal fluctuation.

As described for the diagnosis of retropharyngeal abscess, CT is an extremely useful tool for distinguishing parapharyngeal abscess from cellulitis and for localizing the abscess for surgical planning. Chuang et al.[25] reported that CT had a positive predictive value of 79.6% for a drainable abscess. The CT finding most predictive was a hypodense lesion with a diameter greater than 3 cm, whereas rim enhancement alone was not a good single predictor because its presence depended on the evolution of the abscess. In a review of 47 children who presented with deep neck infections to the Children's Hospital of Buffalo during a 5.5-year period, CT showed that 34 (77%) of 44 patients who underwent CT had involvement of the parapharyngeal and retropharyngeal spaces.[77] The involvement of both spaces had implications for the approach to surgical drainage.

Treatment

Intravenous antibiotic therapy with incision and drainage is the primary treatment. An otolaryngologic consultation should be obtained for this potentially complex surgery of the neck. The conventional method of approaching this abscess is an external incision with sufficient exposure to provide immediate access to the common carotid artery for ligation should erosion of the carotid artery be present.[67] Intraoperative ultrasonography has been described as a useful modality to assist with external drainage of difficult abscesses located medial to the great vessels and close to the skull base.[32]

An intraoral drainage procedure traditionally has been condemned because rapid access to the vital structures of the neck is impossible with this approach. Nagy and associates[77] used an intraoral approach, however, to treat successfully 21 of 22 children with either parapharyngeal or combined parapharyngeal and retropharyngeal abscesses. The authors emphasized that CT with intravenous contrast enhancement showed that all of the abscesses were located medial to the great vessels and were adjacent to the pharyngeal wall. Amar and Manoukian[2] retrospectively compared 15 children with parapharyngeal abscesses who underwent intraoral drainage with 10 patients who underwent external neck drainage and found no complications or recurrences in either group. The children who underwent intraoral drainage had significantly reduced anesthesia time. The duration of intravenous antibiotics and duration of hospital stay also were shorter in the children who underwent intraoral drainage, but the differences between groups were not statistically significant. Cable and coworkers[20] described 12 children presenting to three centers with superior parapharyngeal space abscesses medial to the great vessels who were treated successfully by intraoral drainage using CT-guided systems to assist with localization of the abscess cavity. Marques and colleagues[69] successfully drained all 11 children presenting with parapharyngeal abscesses over a 5-year period via an intraoral approach with tonsillectomy. A transnasal endoscopic approach had also been used to drain an abscess located near the skull base in a 3-year-old boy.[64]

The use of CT has made it possible for some patients with parapharyngeal abscesses to be managed with intravenous antibiotics. The number of reported cases is small, however, and usually analyzed with cases of retropharyngeal abscess.[18,77] Nagy and associates[77] used intravenous antibiotics alone to treat three (13%) of 24 children with small parapharyngeal abscesses. Sichel and associates[95] used intravenous antibiotics alone to successfully treat 12 children with infection limited to the parapharyngeal space. Close clinical follow-up is necessary for children with parapharyngeal cellulitis or small parapharyngeal abscesses that are treated conservatively with intravenous antibiotics. Surgical drainage should be performed in children whose infection does not improve within 24 to 48 hours.

In another report, Sichel and colleagues[94] reviewed the CT scans of 29 patients with infections of the parapharyngeal space and divided the patients into two groups: 22 patients with posterior parapharyngeal space infections and seven patients with anterior parapharyngeal space infections. The patients with posterior infections generally were children who responded well to intravenous antibiotics and did not develop complications. The patients with anterior infections of the parapharyngeal space more commonly were adults who required external drainage in addition to intravenous antibiotics and developed complications, including septic shock, respiratory distress, mediastinitis, pericarditis, and lung empyema. The authors suggested that the location of the infection in the fat of the anterior parapharyngeal space resulted in liquefaction of the fat, with formation of pus and rapid spread of the infection to other anatomic spaces.

MICROBIOLOGY OF DEEP NECK ABSCESSES

Group A streptococci (*Streptococcus pyogenes*), viridans streptococci (including *Streptococcus anginosus* [formerly *S. milleri*]), anaerobes, and *S. aureus* are the organisms most frequently associated with pharyngeal space infections. These data have been consistent for more than 30 years.* Anaerobes and group A streptococci are responsible for the gas seen on lateral neck radiographs. This finding is not surprising because the main portals of entry for pharyngeal space infections are the nasopharynx, oropharynx, paranasal sinuses, mastoid, and lower molars, all areas colonized with anaerobes.

The most complete microbiologic data available are from studies of peritonsillar abscesses. Flödstrom and Hallander,[36] in 1976, reported the results of bacterial cultures on aspirates of pus from 37 patients with peritonsillar abscesses. The ages of the patients were not given. Group A streptococci were isolated from 17 of these patients, whereas 15 had an increase in their antistreptolysin-O or anti-DNAase titers. Anaerobes were found in 28 of the cultures, including those of 8 patients that also disclosed the presence of streptococci. The most common anaerobic species isolated were fusobacteria (13), peptostreptococci (16), and *Bacteroides* spp. (18). Among the aerobic organisms, *S. aureus* was isolated four times, and *Haemophilus influenzae* was isolated twice. No isolates of aerobic gram-negative enteric organisms were present. Jokipii and colleagues[54] performed semiquantitative cultures of aspirated pus from 42 peritonsillar abscesses and found similar results. Group A streptococci, the aerobic bacteria isolated most frequently, were isolated in pure culture four of 10 times. Anaerobes were more abundant than were aerobes; the most important species, in frequency and quantitatively, were *Bacteroides, Peptostreptococcus,* and *Fusobacterium.* Most of the infections were polymicrobial, with two to seven bacteria in 83% of the specimens. Subsequent studies from the United States and Finland have reported similar findings.[17,55,90,97]

Kieff and associates[56] found that streptococci were the most frequent isolates; group A streptococci and other non–group A β-hemolytic streptococci were present in more than 30% of patients, and α-hemolytic streptococci accounted for another 27.2%. The pathogenic role of anaerobic bacteria in peritonsillar abscesses has been reinforced by reports of complications caused by fusobacterial infection in children.[81,87] *Fusobacterium* and *Bacteroides* spp. have been associated with septic thrombophlebitis and pulmonary emboli from the jugular veins. Recent data from Aarhus, Denmark, have found *Fusobacterium necrophorum* to be the most prevalent pathogen in peritonsillar abscesses, being isolated from 41% of cultures.[58] Of the 191 *F. necrophorum* isolates detected, 81% grew as pure culture. However patients from whom *F. necrophorum* was isolated did not have a more severe presentation or outcome but tended to be younger and did have higher neutrophil counts and C-reactive protein levels than did children with other bacteria, including group A streptococci. Recent studies from other countries including Israel, Taiwan, and Japan have not found *F. necrophorum* to be an important pathogen in peritonsillar abscesses.[22,40,49]

Data on the microbiology of retropharyngeal and parapharyngeal abscesses in children are more limited. The organisms isolated are similar to those found in peritonsillar abscesses, but with a higher number of anaerobic species. Brook[16] examined aspirated pus from 14 children, 1 to 6 years old (median age, 3 years, 2 months), with retropharyngeal abscesses. Anaerobes were isolated from all patients; they were the only organisms isolated in 2 patients (14%) and were mixed with aerobes in the remainder (86%). The predominant anaerobic species were *Bacteroides, Peptostreptococcus,* and *Fusobacterium.* The predominant aerobic species were α-hemolytic and γ-hemolytic streptococci, *S. aureus, Haemophilus* spp., and group A β-hemolytic streptococci. Seventy-one percent of the isolates were β-lactamase–positive and included all isolates of the *S. aureus* group, six of 18 of the *Bacteroides melaninogenicus* group (33%), and two of three of the *Bacteroides oralis* group.

Dodds and Maniglia[31] reported the results of cultures from nine retropharyngeal and three parapharyngeal abscesses from children and adolescents. The organisms isolated were similar to those reported by Brook,[16,17] but the microbiology was not as complete because the study was retrospective and not all specimens may have been processed for anaerobic culture. Streptococcal species were the isolates that occurred most frequently, followed by *S. aureus* and *H. influenzae.* One isolate each of *Fusobacterium necrophorum, Escherichia coli,* and *Klebsiella*

*References 3, 16, 22, 36, 40, 44, 54, 55, 97, 100, 105.

pneumoniae was found. Asmar[3] performed cultures on material from 17 children with retropharyngeal abscesses; viridans streptococci were isolated from 11 of the abscesses, *S. aureus* from eight, and group A streptococci from six. The most frequently identified anaerobes were *Peptostreptococcus* spp. Overall 45 aerobic and 18 anaerobic species were identified.

Rarely retropharyngeal abscess may result from anterior extension from cervical osteomyelitis. This condition has been described with tuberculosis[78] and atypical mycobacteria causing a retropharyngeal abscess in a similar clinical setting. Barratt and colleagues[6] reported one case of retropharyngeal abscess caused by *Coccidioides immitis* in a 24-year-old woman with Hodgkin disease. The infection also was secondary to cervical vertebral osteomyelitis. Other rare and unusual causes of deep neck abscesses include cat-scratch disease (from *Bartonella*),[113] *Streptococcus pneumoniae,*[74] and Kawasaki disease.[50]

Because a large variety of organisms can be found in pharyngeal space infections, obtaining adequate culture specimens is crucial. The optimal material for culture is an aspirate of the pus obtained at operation. Throat swabs or swabs of the abscess obtained after drainage usually are inadequate because of contamination with normal oropharyngeal flora. The pus, when obtained, can be transported in a capped syringe if anaerobic transport media are unavailable. Most pathogenic obligate anaerobes can survive in a purulent exudate despite extended periods of exposure to air.[35] A Gram stain of the exudate may provide important clues to the bacterial etiology. A Gram stain showing a mixture of organisms suggests a mixed aerobic-anaerobic infection. May and associates[72] found evidence of biofilm matrices on scanning electron microscopy in 12 of 14 abscess walls of children with deep neck abscesses treated by surgical drainage. The presence of biofilms may explain the recalcitrant nature of these deep neck space infections.

Although use of a β-lactamase–resistant antibiotic may be necessary in the treatment of deep neck abscesses because of the presence of β-lactamase–producing bacteria, including *S. aureus* and *Bacteroides* spp.,[16,17,105] results of two studies suggest that penicillin alone was equivalent to broad-spectrum antibiotics for treatment of peritonsillar abscesses.[56,114] Yilmaz and colleagues[114] compared procaine penicillin with intramuscular administration of ampicillin-sulbactam in outpatient treatment of 40 patients with peritonsillar abscesses that were drained perorally. No statistical difference in duration of symptoms and clinical recovery was found between the two groups. Kieff and associates[56] retrospectively evaluated 103 patients with peritonsillar abscesses who were treated with incision and drainage. Fifty-eight patients were treated with broad-spectrum antibiotics, including ampicillin-sulbactam, clindamycin, cephalosporins, and metronidazole, alone and in combination; 45 patients were treated with penicillin alone. All patients were hospitalized after drainage, and the clinical outcomes, including duration of hospitalization and fever, did not differ significantly between the two groups. No significant difference in the organisms isolated was found, and failure and complication rates did not differ.

No comparative treatment studies for retropharyngeal or parapharyngeal abscesses have been reported. Treatment in these cases should be based on the results of cultures, as stated earlier. Drugs that may be effective include penicillin–β-lactamase inhibitor combinations such as ampicillin-sulbactam, ticarcillin-clavulanic acid, and piperacillin-tazobactam; expanded-spectrum cephalosporins such as ceftriaxone; or penicillinase-resistant penicillins, including oxacillin or nafcillin. Cephalosporins, oxacillin, or nafcillin should be used in combination with clindamycin or metronidazole for adequate anaerobic coverage. Erythromycin and other macrolides (azithromycin, clarithromycin) are less satisfactory because of increasing macrolide resistance in group A streptococci and less activity against *Bacteroides fragilis* and *Fusobacterium.*

A study by Hanna and colleagues[45] reported macrolide resistance in 26% of group A streptococcal isolates obtained from peritonsillar abscesses seen between August 2001 and July 2002. The routine use of aminoglycoside antibiotics is not indicated because aerobic gram-negative enteric rods rarely are found in these infections. More recently, community-acquired methicillin-resistant *S. aureus* (CA-MRSA) has emerged as a pathogen in deep neck abscesses in children, especially in the United States.[44,104] However there can be significant geographic variation in the prevalence of MRSA.[71] In areas where CA-MRSA is highly prevalent, including vancomycin as initial therapy may be indicated. Clindamycin may be an alternative, but resistance of CA-MRSA to clindamycin, including inducible resistance, has been increasing in some geographic areas in the United States.[71] Antibiotic therapy is effective only in conjunction with adequate surgical drainage.

NEW REFERENCES SINCE THE SEVENTH EDITION

1. Abdel-Haq N, Quezada M, Asmar BI. Retropharyngeal abscess in children: the rising incidence of methicillin-resistant *Staphylococcus aureus*. *Pediatr Infect Dis J*. 2012;31:696-699.
4. Baker KA, Stuart J, Sykes KJ, et al. Use of computed tomography in the emergency department for the diagnosis of pediatric peritonsillar abscess. *Pediatr Emer Care*. 2012;28:962-965.
13. Bovo R, Barillari MR, Martini A. Hospital discharge survey on 4,199 peritonsillar abscesses in the Veneto region: what is the risk of recurrence and complications without tonsillectomy? *Eur Arch Otorhinolaryngol*. 2016;273(1):225-230.
19. Brown NK, Hulten KG, Mason EO, et al. *Staphylococcus aureus* retropharyngeal abscess in children. *Pediatr Infect Dis J*. 2015;34:454-456.
21. Carbone PN, Capra GG, Brigger MT. Antibiotic therapy for pediatric neck abscesses: a systematic review. *Int J Pediatr Otorhinolaryngol*. 2012;78:1647-1653.
24. Cheng J, Elden L. Children with deep space neck infections: our experience with 178 children. *Otolaryngol Head Neck Surg*. 2013;148:1037-1042.
25. Chuang SY, Lin HT, Wen YS, et al. Pitfalls of CT for deep neck abscess imaging assessment: a retrospective review of 162 cases. *B-ENT*. 2013;9:45-52.
36. Fordham MT, Rock AN, Bandarkar A, et al. Transcervical ultrasonography in the diagnosis of pediatric peritonsillar abscess. *Laryngoscope*. 2015;125(12):2799-2804. doi:10.1002/lary.25354. [Epub ahead of print].
69. Martin CA, Gabrillargues J, Louvrier C, et al. Contribution of CT scan and CT-guided aspiration in the management of retropharyngeal abscess in children based on a series of 18 cases. *Eur Ann Otorhinolaryngol Head Neck Dis*. 2014; 131:277-282.
70. May JG, Shah P, Sachdeva L, et al. Potential role of biofilms in deep cervical abscess. *Int J Pediatr Otorhinolaryngol*. 2014;78:10-13.
78. Nogan S, Jandali D, Cipolla M, et al. The use of ultrasound imaging in evaluation of peritonsillar infections. *Laryngoscope*. 2015;125:2604-2607.
79. Novis SJ, Pritchett CV, Thorne MC, et al. Pediatric deep neck space infections in U.S. children, 2000-2009. *Int J Pediatr Otorhinolaryngol*. 2014;78:832-836.
87. Saluja S, Brietzke SE, Egan KK, et al. A prospective study of 113 deep neck infections managed using a clinical practice guideline. *Laryngoscope*. 2013;123:3211-3218.
88. Sankararaman S, Velayuthan S, Gonzalez-Toledo E. Internal carotid artery stenosis as the sequela of a pseudoaneurysm after methicillin-resistant *Staphylococcus aureus* infection. *Pediatr Neurol*. 2012;47:312-314.
90. da Silva PSL, Waisberg DR. Internal carotid artery pseudoaneurysm with life-threatening epistaxis as a complication of deep neck space infection. *Pediatr Emerg Care*. 2011;27:422-424.
96. Simon LM, Matijasec JW-D, Perry AP, et al. Pediatric peritonsillar abscess: quinsy versus interval tonsillectomy. *Int J Pediatr Otorhinolaryngol*. 2013;77:1355-1358.
107. Wang Y-P, Wang M-C, Lin H-C, et al. The impact of prior tonsillitis and treatment modality on the recurrence of peritonsillar abscess: a nationwide cohort study. *PLoS ONE*. 2014;9(10):e109887. doi:10.1371/journal.pone.0109887. eCollection 2014.

The full reference list for this chapter is available at ExpertConsult.com.

12 Cervical Lymphadenitis

C. Mary Healy • Carol J. Baker

Cervical lymphadenopathy is enlargement of the lymph nodes in the neck. *Cervical lymphadenitis* implies one or more nodes are inflamed. The inflammatory response by the host is triggered by some form of injury or invasion proximal to the involved lymph node or nodes. The node becomes affected secondarily by drainage through connecting afferent lymphatic channels. The injury may be acute or chronic, infectious or noninfectious. Proper anatomic definition of the inflamed node or nodes,[93] combined with knowledge of the structures of the head and neck drained by them, may allow identification of a portal of entry for infectious agents, the most common cause of cervical lymphadenitis in infants and children.

Fig. 12.1 illustrates the regional lymph nodes commonly affected in infants and children with cervical lymphadenitis. The superficial cervical lymph nodes lie on top of the sternocleidomastoid muscle along the course of the external jugular vein. They receive afferents from the superficial tissues of the neck, mastoid, superficial parotid (preauricular) nodes, and submaxillary glands. Their efferents terminate in the upper deep cervical lymph nodes. The mastoid lymph nodes overlie the mastoid process of the temporal bone and receive drainage from the parietal scalp and inner surface of the pinna. The occipital lymph nodes lie on the upper part of the trapezius and receive afferents from the occipital scalp and superficial portions of the upper posterior neck. Their efferents terminate in the deep cervical glands, as do the efferents from the mastoid nodes.

The deep cervical lymph nodes lie deep to the sternomastoid muscle along the whole length of the internal jugular vein and are divided into upper and lower groups. The jugulodigastric gland, a member of the upper group, lies at the angle of the jaw below the posterior belly of the digastric muscle. The lymphoid tissue of the palatine tonsil is drained into this gland; it frequently becomes enlarged in patients with "tonsillitis" or with tuberculous infection originating from the tonsils. The larynx, trachea, thyroid gland, and esophagus drain into the lower deep cervical glands. The submental lymph nodes, which lie between the digastric muscles below the myohyoid, receive superficial and deep drainage from the anterior tongue, lower lip, and chin, from both sides of the midline. They send efferents to the submandibular and upper deep cervical glands. The submandibular lymph nodes lie adjacent to the submandibular salivary gland and receive wide, superficial drainage from the lateral aspect of the lower lip, the vestibule of the nose, the cheeks, the medial parts of the eyelids, and the forehead. Deep drainage to these nodes arises from the posterior part of the mouth, gums, teeth, and tongue and from superficial and submental lymph nodes.

Because most of the lymphatic drainage of the head and neck goes to the submaxillary and deep cervical nodes, these glands are involved in more than 80% of cases of cervical adenitis in young children. Submental and superficial cervical lymphadenitis is observed less frequently.

EPIDEMIOLOGY

The epidemiology of infectious cervical adenitis is that of its infectious agents. Although cervical lymphadenitis can be a manifestation of focal viral infections of the oropharynx or respiratory tract, often it is part of a more generalized reticuloendothelial response to systemic infection. Viruses that commonly present with prominent cervical adenitis are Epstein-Barr virus and cytomegalovirus. In children infected with human immunodeficiency virus (HIV), prominent cervical adenopathy may either herald or be a part of more generalized lymphadenopathy associated with this infection. Although human herpesvirus–6 (HHV-6), the cause of roseola in infants (exanthem subitum), is associated with the development of a mononucleosis syndrome and cervical adenopathy in adults,[4] lymphadenitis is not a prominent feature in children with primary infection.[64] Adenoviral and enteroviral infections are causes of generalized rather than isolated cervical lymphadenopathy. The epidemiology of cervical adenitis varies by age, geographic location, and socioeconomic status. Generally, lower socioeconomic status is associated with a higher incidence of infectious etiology in younger children.

When bacterial in origin, with the exception of group A streptococci and *Mycobacterium tuberculosis,* the agents isolated from these glands are the normal inhabitants of the nose, mouth, pharynx, and skin—*Staphylococcus aureus,* anaerobes, nontuberculous mycobacteria, *Actinomyces* spp.—and person-to-person transmission does not occur. In contrast, group A streptococci and *M. tuberculosis* infection of cervical lymph nodes results from contact with human infection by way of airborne droplets. Except in neonates, for whom male dominance has been reported in cases caused by group B streptococci,[13] infectious lymphadenitis has no gender or seasonal predilection.[15,41]

Any age group can be affected by cervical lymphadenitis. In neonates, *S. aureus* and group B streptococci are the most common pathogens. Suppurative cervical lymphadenitis caused by *Staphylococcus epidermidis* in an otherwise healthy infant has been reported.[142] Nonetheless despite the high frequency of nasal colonization by *S. epidermidis,* it remains a rare etiologic agent. There are rare reports of *Streptococcus pneumoniae* causing suppurative adenitis in older children.[109] Some studies indicate that *S. aureus* has the leading role in infants,[182] whereas in children, either group A streptococci or *S. aureus* is equally likely to be pathogenic.[41,161,186] Other reports have varied regarding the relationship between age and probable etiologic agent.[15,26]

Overall, *S. aureus* and *Streptococcus pyogenes* accounted for 65% to 89% of consecutive cases in prospectively evaluated series.[15,41] Recent reviews indicate that *S. aureus* is more common in infants with cervical lymphadenitis, especially if suppuration occurs.[39,40,182] Methicillin-resistant *S. aureus* (MRSA) must be strongly considered as a possible etiology because of the increased incidence of health care–acquired MRSA and community-associated MRSA (CA-MRSA) infections in the United States and elsewhere[23,48,54,57,68,69,72,114] and recognition that the highest rates of CA-MRSA colonization and disease are found in children.[48,115] Many studies have shown that CA-MRSA strains predominantly cause skin and soft tissue infections, but a wide spectrum of illness is reported, and invasive CA-MRSA has been associated with a variety of clinical manifestations, including severe illness and death.[54,68,69,72,114] Retrospective and prospective case series report an increasing incidence of CA-MRSA infections manifesting as cervical adenitis and deep neck infections.[27,44,65,72,115,182] One single-center study found that MRSA was the infectious etiology of no head and neck abscesses from July 1999 through December 2001 but accounted for 34% of cases from January 2002 through June 2004.[123] In other reports of 76 and 185 children with neck abscess, MRSA was the etiologic agent in 33% and 42%, respectively, and was more likely to be found in abscesses located laterally in black patients and in infants and toddlers.[44,182]

The epidemiology of bacterial lymphadenitis varies by geographic location. Resurgence of infection with *Yersinia pestis* in the southwestern United States in 2015 means that, in areas where it is endemic, it also must be considered in the differential diagnosis.[79] Epidemic diphtheria, reported in the Russian Federation in 1990, subsequently spread to several newly independent states in the European region, with the number of reported cases (50,425) peaking in 1995. After the implementation

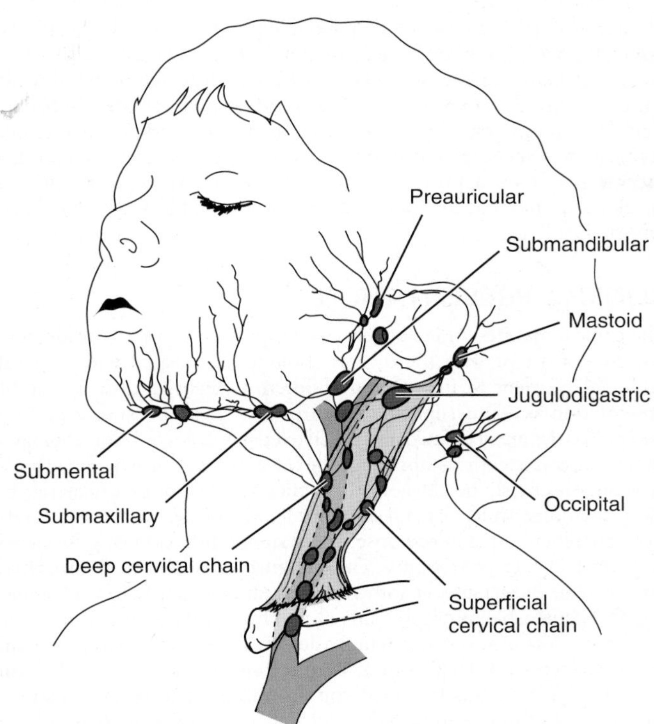

FIG. 12.1 Lymphatic drainage and lymph nodes involved in infants and children with cervical lymphadenitis.

TABLE 12.1 **Differentiation of *Mycobacterium tuberculosis* and Nontuberculous Mycobacterial Cervical Adenitis (NTM CA)**

	NTM CA	*M. tuberculosis*
Age	1–6 y	All ages
Ethnicity	White	Black, Asian, Hispanic
Exposure to tuberculosis	Absent	Present
Abnormal chest radiographs	Rare	Often
Residence	Suburban	Urban
TST >15 mm	Uncommon	Often
Positive IGRA	Unlikely[a]	Yes
Bilateral involvement	Rare	Not uncommon

IGRA, interferon-γ release assay; *TST*, tuberculin skin test.
[a]Except for infection with *M. kansasii, M. szulgai, M. marinum, M. flavescens.*

of diphtheria control measures, the number of cases declined by more than 95% from 2000 through 2009.[175] However, because circulation continues in some countries in Eastern Europe and with increasing migration between countries, sporadic cases may occur even in countries with high vaccination rates.[180] Diphtheria also must be included as a possible cause of cervical lymphadenitis in those regions of the world.

The distinctive epidemiologic features of mycobacterial infection are summarized in Table 12.1. Scrofula caused by *M. tuberculosis* is a rare disease. When it does occur, it usually affects adults and older children. In contrast, children with nontuberculous mycobacterial infection almost always are 1 to 6 years of age, live in suburban or rural communities, and have no history of contact with *M. tuberculosis.*[156] Although *M. tuberculosis* is an infection acquired primarily by inhalation, the gastrointestinal tract or respiratory tract may be the primary portal of entry for nontuberculous mycobacteria.[55,119,129,134] There seems to be an ethnic predilection for nontuberculous mycobacterial infection to occur in whites and for tuberculous infections to occur in blacks, Hispanics, Asians, and the Australian Aboriginal population.[118,159] A recent study of 139 children with confirmed *M. tuberculosis* cervical lymphadenitis in Taiwan demonstrated an association of a polymorphism in the mannose-binding lectin gene with this etiology, suggesting the potential role for innate immunity in the pathogenesis.[188]

The advent of the HIV pandemic had a major impact on the nature and frequency of mycobacterial infections. The availability of highly active antiretroviral therapy (HAART) resulted in significant decreases in the incidence of opportunistic infections, including tuberculous and nontuberculous mycobacterial infections, in HIV-infected children.[56] However, cases of tuberculous and nontuberculous infection as part of an immune reconstitution syndrome in individuals started on HAART have been reported.[1]

The presence of tuberculosis infection in the community means that all children are at risk for exposure to an infectious adult.[22] The annual tuberculosis rate in the United States decreased steadily during the years 1993 through 2014, but the annual decline has decelerated.[33,147] Drug-resistant tuberculosis also is increasingly detected in industrialized and developing countries, both multidrug-resistant (e.g., resistant to isoniazid and rifampin, first-line drugs in the treatment of tuberculosis) and extensively drug-resistant (resistant to isoniazid, rifampin, and three of the six classes of second-line antituberculosis drugs).[32,181]

The incidence of nontuberculous mycobacterial infections has increased since the 1980s, although some of this apparent increase most likely has resulted from improvements in diagnostic methods. Nontuberculous mycobacteria are ubiquitous and are found in food, water, animals, and soil. An association between nontuberculous cervical adenitis and cold weather is prompted by observations that 68% of cases occur in the winter and spring months.[55,98,127,178] A 10-year Canadian retrospective study reported that 70% of cases occurred in girls; however, most reports suggest no gender difference.[127]

Until the 1970s, *Mycobacterium scrofulaceum* was the usual etiologic agent in children with nontuberculous adenitis, followed by *Mycobacterium avium-intracellulare.*[178] This trend has reversed, with *M. avium-intracellulare* now accounting for 50% to 98% of culture-proven cases.[47,49,67,94,98,117,118,162,178] Previously uncommon species, such as *Mycobacterium kansasii, Mycobacterium malmoense* (found primarily in Europe), *Mycobacterium fortuitum, Mycobacterium haemophilum,* and *Mycobacterium bohemicum,* also are being detected more frequently.[8,12,126,171] Some of these uncommon species probably are responsible for many cases of culture-negative lymphadenitis because of their fastidious growth requirements. New diagnostic methods have led to increasing reports of cervical adenitis secondary to slow-growing species, such as *Mycobacterium lentiflavum* and *Mycobacterium interjectum.*[43,62,66,71,131,154] Cervical lymphadenitis caused by *Mycobacterium chelonae* is rare, usually involves the submandibular glands, and typically occurs in patients with an antecedent history of dental pathology.[6]

Cervical lymphadenopathy may be the direct result of infection with HIV per se. However, the development of acute, tender adenitis in an HIV-infected child should provoke a search for another etiology. Although the typical childhood pathogens remain the most common pathogens in this setting, as in other immunocompromised children, opportunists also should be sought.[60] Patients with HIV infection beginning therapy with potent antiretroviral agents can develop new-onset mycobacterial lymphadenitis (tuberculous and nontuberculous mycobacteria). When this lymphadenitis occurs, it is more localized, is associated with more sinus formation, and is more often caused by nontuberculous mycobacteria (*M. avium-intracellulare*) than by *M. tuberculosis.*[130]

Cat-scratch disease is a common cause of lymphadenitis in children and young adults.[7,25] In 1988, English and associates[46] first isolated a pleomorphic gram-negative bacillus, later identified as *Afipia felis,* from lymph nodes of patients with cat-scratch disease. *Bartonella henselae,* a morphologically similar but genetically distinct pleomorphic gram-negative bacillus, now is recognized as the cause of cat-scratch disease.[2,7]

The cervical nodes are the second most common site of cat-scratch disease involvement. Although unusual and severe manifestations of this infection have been described, it remains mostly a mild, self-limited infection in children and adolescents, with no ethnic predilection. Seasonal variation with an increased incidence in fall, winter, and early spring does occur in temperate zones. A history of animal contact with cats usually can be elicited.[31] The importance of bites and scratches by kittens in transmitting this disease has been well defined.[7,106,189] However, the absence of a history of traumatic contact with cats in a substantial number of cases supports the hypothesis of an alternative mode of transmission. The detection of *Bartonella* DNA by polymerase chain reaction (PCR) assay in collections of fleas from cats owned by two infected patients suggests that fleas or other arthropods may serve as vectors, but their role in human transmission is not well established.[7,187]

PATHOPHYSIOLOGY

Although cervical lymphadenitis is a common entity in pediatric clinical practice, little information exists regarding its pathogenesis. Viral cervical adenitis may be part of either a local response to viruses invading the oropharynx or respiratory tract (e.g., adenoviruses or coxsackieviruses) or a more generalized reticuloendothelial response to systemic viral infection (e.g., Epstein-Barr virus, cytomegalovirus, HHV-6, or HIV). Infection attributed to group A streptococci and *S. aureus* is presumed to enter the cervical lymphatics from the oropharynx (group A streptococci) or anterior nares (*S. aureus*). In a patient with group A streptococcal pharyngitis or tonsillitis, whether infection remains localized at the pharyngotonsillar tissues or spreads to cervical lymph nodes and results in suppuration primarily is a function of host response and probably strain virulence. Although peak attack rates for group A streptococcal pharyngitis are observed among school-age children, suppurative cervical adenitis is an uncommon occurrence. In contrast, infants and children younger than 3 years of age rarely have group A streptococci isolated from throat cultures, but this age group is more likely to develop suppurative cervical lymphadenitis.[133]

In infections attributed to *S. aureus,* colonization of the anterior nares is thought to be a prerequisite for cervical lymphadenitis. Brook and Winter[24,25] arrived at this conclusion because organisms of identical phage types were isolated from the anterior nares and the cervical abscesses of their patients. An investigation of children in St. Louis found no such correlation between isolates from nasal and cervical node cultures.[15] The role of *S. aureus* as a primary pathogen has been the subject of some debate. In most series, 30% of aspirates yield mixed cultures of *S. aureus* and group A streptococci, and frequently significant elevations of antistreptolysin O titer are found in the sera of patients whose lymph nodes yielded a pure culture of *S. aureus*.

In a California study, 65% of patients had lymph node aspirates yielding a pure culture of *S. aureus,* and 41% exhibited an immune response to one or more of the extracellular antigens of group A streptococci.[186] Similarly, the finding that many children improve with penicillin or ampicillin treatment, despite the high prevalence of penicillin resistance among *S. aureus,* suggests that, although streptococci and staphylococci may coexist in these nodes, staphylococci may sometimes play a subsidiary role as secondary invaders. However, most children with isolates of *S. aureus* from suppurative lymph nodes show no evidence of coexistent streptococcal infection or viral upper respiratory tract infection. In addition, the resurgence of *S. aureus* (often MRSA) as a single pathogen in more recent case series argues that this organism has a strong capacity to be the primary invader.[39,40,44,182]

Recovery of anaerobic bacteria from cervical nodes suggests invasion of the lymphatics by mouth flora, often as a result of local tissue destruction by periodontal disease.[26] The delineation of the pathophysiology of cervical lymphadenitis of diverse bacterial etiology requires an understanding of the interaction between a given microorganism (e.g., inoculum size, elaboration of extracellular enzymes, and ability to adhere to epithelium) and the host (e.g., humoral and surface immune capacity and degree of trauma).

Tuberculous cervical lymphadenopathy occurs within months of the initial exposure, through pulmonary infection and involvement of the regional and then more distant lymph nodes. It is a rapid process; chest radiographic evidence of active pulmonary disease often is seen.[10] Nontuberculous mycobacteria are ubiquitous in the environment, and oropharyngeal acquisition with local infection leads to lymph node involvement. Most children with nontuberculous mycobacterial cervical lymphadenitis are immunocompetent. However, some studies suggest that children who develop necrotic nodes may have deficient production of interferon (IFN)-γ,[117] and disseminated infections are almost always associated with impaired T-cell function.[8] Despite *M. avium* skin test positivity being linked with pet birds, no clear relationship with lymphadenitis has been shown.[86] Discontinuation of childhood bacille Calmette-Guérin vaccination has been associated with an increase in atypical mycobacterial infection in many countries, suggesting that this vaccine may have a protective effect.[172] Progressive cervical adenitis developing after bacille Calmette-Guérin vaccination also has been reported.[120]

CLINICAL PRESENTATION

The clinical manifestations of cervical lymphadenitis vary considerably but are consistent with the diverse etiologies associated with cervical node enlargement in infants and children. Categorizing the mode of presentation as acute, subacute, or chronic is useful because, although the boundaries are ill defined and much overlap exists, common etiologies tend to fall consistently within one of the categories. Cervical lymphadenitis of acute onset may be categorized further as bilateral or unilateral. In most situations, acute, bilateral cervical adenitis is either part of a generalized reticuloendothelial response to a systemic infection or a localized reaction to acute pharyngitis. The presence or absence of associated features (e.g., pharyngitis, enanthems or exanthems, generalized adenopathy, and hepatosplenomegaly) aids in making the differentiation.

Acute unilateral cervical lymphadenitis is caused by streptococcal or staphylococcal infection in 53% to 89% of cases.[15,41,44,70,170,186,182] In newborns, *S. aureus* is the most common cause, and clinical features are similar to those seen in older children. Group B streptococci have been described as causative in a "cellulitis-adenitis" syndrome in infancy.[13] These infants differ from infants with staphylococcal adenitis in that they are younger, are more often male, and have a greater incidence of systemic symptoms, irritability, and anorexia; 94% have associated bacteremia. The typical patient has fever, facial or submandibular cellulitis, and ipsilateral otitis media.[13] Isolated cervical adenitis caused by group B streptococci also has been described.[50]

Patients with disease attributed to *S. aureus* or group A streptococci can become ill at any age but typically are 1 to 4 years old (70–80% of cases), and the male-to-female ratio is equal. Clinically, little differentiates streptococcal from staphylococcal infections. Cervical adenitis can occur as part of the "streptococcosis" syndrome of infancy, with an onset heralded by coryza, an irregular low-grade fever, nasal discharge with excoriation and crusting around the nares, vomiting, and loss of appetite. Lymph node enlargement occurs within a few days of onset and resolves, as do other symptoms, without treatment within 6 to 8 weeks.[133] Suppuration of cervical glands can occur at any time during this interval but seldom does so if effective antimicrobial therapy is given early in the illness. Group A streptococci also should be suspected as a cause of cervical adenitis in a patient with typical vesiculopustular or crusted lesions of impetigo involving the face or scalp.

Systemic symptoms in children with staphylococcal or streptococcal cervical adenitis usually are minimal or absent unless associated with cellulitis, metastatic foci of infection, or bacteremia. The primary site of lymph node involvement by frequency is submandibular (50–60%), upper cervical (25–30%), submental (5–8%), occipital (3–5%), and lower cervical (2–5%).[15,41,179] Involved nodes generally vary in size from 2 to 6 cm in diameter, and one-fourth to one-third suppurate. Patients with lymphadenitis caused by *S. aureus* are more likely to develop suppuration and a longer duration of symptoms and signs before diagnosis than are patients with disease caused by other bacterial agents (Fig. 12.2).[15,137,141,161] Among patients who develop suppurative adenitis, the majority do so within 2 weeks of onset.

Approximately one-third of patients in one study had concomitant lymphadenopathy at other anatomic sites.[15] A history of recent upper respiratory tract symptoms, including sore throat (40%), earache or coryza (16%), and impetigo (32%), is a frequent finding, as are signs of pharyngitis, tonsillitis, or otitis media.[15,41] These factors do not help delineate the etiology, however. Hepatomegaly or splenomegaly is a rare occurrence and, if present, should suggest bacteremia or generalized disease processes (e.g., Epstein-Barr infection, reticuloendotheliosis, tuberculosis, or HIV infection).

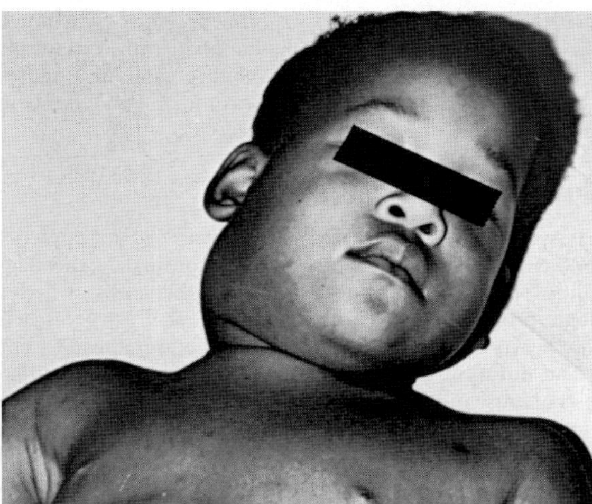

FIG. 12.2 A 2-year-old boy with fever and unilateral inflammation of the cervical lymph nodes of 2 days' duration. Needle aspirate culture of this nonfluctuant node grew *Staphylococcus aureus.* Antistaphylococcal therapy resulted in complete resolution of adenitis without surgical drainage.

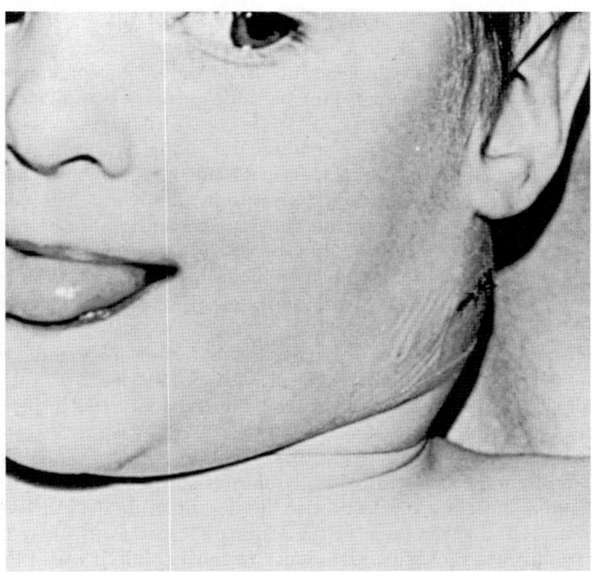

FIG. 12.3 A 4-year-old boy who had bilateral nontender enlargement of lymph nodes of 6 weeks' duration, without other symptoms. Placement of a tuberculin skin test resulted in 18-mm induration, excisional biopsy acid-fast stain was positive, and cultures grew *Mycobacterium tuberculosis.*

Kawasaki disease may manifest as a febrile illness associated with bilateral or unilateral cervical lymphadenopathy and may be confused with more common acute pyogenic infections.[174] Other features (e.g., conjunctivitis, oral manifestations, changes in the peripheral extremities, and polymorphic erythematous rash) are required criteria for the diagnosis.[9,110] Although originally termed *mucocutaneous lymph node syndrome,* unilateral lymph node enlargement of at least 1.5 cm is the most inconsistent feature.[9,17,110] Lymphadenopathy usually subsides when the fever subsides, although in some cases it may follow a more chronic course.

The rapid development of painful lymphadenitis, quickly succeeding the sudden onset of fever, chills, weakness, and headache, is a classic presentation of infection caused by *Y. pestis* (bubonic plague). The groin is the site most often involved. Other locations, including the cervical area, may be affected, however. Establishing the diagnosis and providing treatment quickly are crucial because infection can be fulminant.

In cases of diphtheria, cervical adenopathy develops secondary to infection of the posterior structures of the mouth and proximal pharynx. A whitish gray membrane covers the mucosal surfaces. In severe cases, the cervical adenopathy, which typically is bilateral, can result in a "bull neck" appearance.

Careful physical examination of the head and neck, particularly areas drained by affected lymph nodes, may yield important clues about etiology. The presence of periodontal disease is associated with a higher incidence of anaerobic organisms causing adenitis,[26] the history or presence of tick bites suggests the possibility of tularemia,[153] and the presence of papular or pustular lesions suggesting an inoculation site raises the possibility of other causes of infection, including *Nocardia* and *Bartonella* spp., actinomycosis, sporotrichosis, plague, and cutaneous diphtheria.

Mycobacterial and *Bartonella* spp. infections and toxoplasmosis are more common entities presenting as subacute or chronic lymphadenitis. The epidemiologic and clinical features that aid in the differentiation of tuberculous and nontuberculous mycobacterial infections are summarized in Table 12.1. The clinical manifestations virtually are identical (Fig. 12.3).[8,10,21,33,112] Typically a child presents with a history of painless (so-called cold) cervical node swelling. The submandibular cervical nodes usually are involved in nontuberculous mycobacterial infection, whereas other cervical nodes are involved more frequently with *M. tuberculosis.*[5,21,74,105,144] As the infection progresses, the skin overlying the node may develop a pinkish or violaceous discoloration caused by increased vascularity, although the skin temperature usually is not increased. This finding may be followed by adherence of the skin to the underlying mass. If left untreated, fluctuance and spontaneously draining sinus tracts may develop.

A patient with *M. tuberculosis* is more likely than one with atypical mycobacterial disease to be older than 4 years of age and to have generalized lymphadenopathy (10–20% of cases), bilateral node enlargement (10% of cases), a history of exposure to tuberculosis (93% of cases), and an urban residence.[21,80,105,122] No differences have been noted, however, with regard to duration of adenopathy, fever, and presence or absence of constitutional symptoms. An abnormal chest radiograph has been noted in 28% to 71% of cases caused by *M. tuberculosis,*[144,145,158,170] contrasting with the 98% to 100% of normal chest radiographs found in patients with nontuberculous mycobacterial adenitis.[55,143,144,162,169]

In a summary of 447 reported childhood cases of nontuberculous mycobacterial infections from 15 countries, Lincoln and Gilbert[85] detected only six cases of bilateral cervical node involvement, four with abnormal chest radiographs, and none with nodal enlargement other than cervical. Similar findings have been reported by other investigators.[143,169] Intradermal tuberculin skin testing with purified protein derivative uncommonly produces more than 15 mm of induration at 48 hours in a child with nontuberculous mycobacterial infection, but reactions between 5 and 15 mm are common.[90,101] Reactions of 10 to 20 mm can occur with *Mycobacterium marinum* and *M. fortuitum* infection.[129] Tuberculin skin test positivity may persist, even when children are retested many years after infection.[178] Unlike the findings with tuberculosis, IFN-γ release assays generally are negative with nontuberculous mycobacterial infections unless the infecting organism is *M. kansasii, Mycobacterium szulgai, M. marinum,* or *Mycobacterium flavescens,* which share some antigens that react in the assay and may cross react.[10,157]

Bartonella infection may manifest days to weeks after the initial inoculation. Characteristically a history of contact with a cat or kitten or a scratch is present.[7,189] Later, when the primary small papular lesion may have healed, tender regional adenopathy appears. Although axillary nodes most frequently are affected, 25% of children have isolated cervical node involvement. Middle cervical and parotid nodes are involved more often than submandibular nodes.[138] Constitutional symptoms, present early in the course of the illness, usually are mild and may have resolved by the time the adenitis appears. Fever is observed in one-fourth of patients and, if present, has a mean duration of 5 to 7 days.[100] Fever prolonged beyond this time should prompt evaluation for characteristic hepatosplenic granulomatous lesions defined by high-resolution ultrasonography with disseminated cat-scratch disease. Nodes suppurate in one-tenth to one-third of patients.[31,32] Rare manifestations include Parinaud oculoglandular syndrome,[29] encephalopathy,[97] exanthems[31] (usually of the erythema nodosum type), and osteolytic lesions.[30]

Acquired toxoplasmosis may manifest as regional lymphadenopathy, frequently with posterior cervical node involvement.[108,136,167] Most children exhibit few, if any, constitutional symptoms. If present, fatigue and generalized myalgia are prominent. The characteristic location combined with a history of exposure to cats or of eating undercooked meats should raise this diagnostic possibility, and the diagnosis can be confirmed by serologic testing. It is an uncommon etiology for cervical adenopathy in children living in the United States.

Chronic, recurrent cervical adenitis forms part of the periodic fever, aphthous ulcers, pharyngitis, cervical adenitis (PFAPA) syndrome, a chronic syndrome first described in 1987.[107] It is characterized by periodic episodes of high fever, greater than 39°C (102.2°F), lasting 3 to 6 days and recurring every 3 to 8 weeks in association with aphthous ulcers, pharyngitis, and cervical adenitis. Symptoms such as abdominal pain, nausea, diarrhea, and headache also are described in 20% to 73% of children,[168] but if any of these are the dominant features, other hereditary fever syndromes should be excluded.[53] In most children with PFAPA, the onset of disease occurs before they reach 5 years of age, the syndrome is self-limited, and recovery without long-term sequelae is the rule.[185] Although there appears to be a familial predisposition for PFAPA, to date no single gene trait has been found, suggesting that this condition may have a heterogeneous, polygenic, or complex inheritance.[77] Oral corticosteroids are effective in aborting an attack.[83,124,168]

Kikuchi-Fujimoto disease, also called *subacute necrotizing lymphadenitis,* is an uncommon disorder of uncertain etiology that also may manifest as cervical adenopathy, with or without fever. This disorder was described first in 1972 and seems to have a predilection for Asian women 25 to 30 years of age, who generally have a benign course with spontaneous resolution over 3 to 4 months.[52,173] Kikuchi-Fujimoto disease also has been reported in children, typically adolescents, although cases in children as young as 2 years old are documented.[38,82,84,176]

In contrast to the 4:1 female predominance documented in adult series, pediatric Kikuchi-Fujimoto disease occurs more commonly in boys (male-to-female ratio ranges from 1.2:1 to 1.9:1). The most common presentation is unilateral or bilateral lymphadenopathy of multiple nodes. In most cases, posterior cervical chain nodes are involved, and affected nodes can be painful and tender. Fever is an inconsistent symptom. Extranodal manifestations include malaise, night sweats, weight loss, maculopapular skin rashes, gastrointestinal symptoms, hepatosplenomegaly, arthritis, and aseptic meningitis. Associated laboratory findings include leukopenia (33% to 100% of cases with prolonged fever), elevated erythrocyte sedimentation rate, mild anemia, elevated C-reactive protein, and elevated liver enzymes.

Diagnosis is established by biopsy of the lymph nodes (not by fine-needle aspiration cytology) which shows lymphadenitis with focal proliferation of reticular cells accompanied by histiocytes and extensive nuclear debris. Lymph node biopsy also has been associated with prompt resolution of fever.[38] Treatment generally is supportive, although steroids are reported to provide more rapid resolution of symptoms. The prognosis is favorable; most cases of Kikuchi-Fujimoto disease resolve within 6 months, although a recurrence rate of 3% to 4% is recorded. Some children subsequently develop autoimmune disorders, most commonly systemic lupus erythematosus; thus clinical follow-up looking for signs of evolving autoimmune disorder is recommended.[37,116,150,176] Whether Kikuchi-Fujimoto disease is infectious or genetic, perhaps the result of infection with a single novel agent or a nonspecific host response to any of a variety of agents, remains to be determined.

Another rare but important cause of cervical lymphadenitis in association with generalized lymphadenopathy or hepatosplenomegaly is hemophagocytic lymphohistiocytosis, also known as hemophagocytic syndrome. This diagnosis should be considered if the aforementioned features occur with prolonged fever, cytopenia in at least two cell lines, low fibrinogen, and high ferritin and triglyceride serum levels.[125] Other features include rash, respiratory distress, hypotension, and coagulopathy. The diagnosis is confirmed by the presence of hemophagocytosis in bone marrow or lymph node biopsy specimens. Finally, when presented with a history of subacute or chronic lymphadenitis, careful physical examination should be undertaken to exclude obvious local causes (e.g., seborrhea, head lice, tinea capitis, and chronic otitis media) before an extensive diagnostic evaluation is initiated.

DIFFERENTIAL DIAGNOSIS

Cervical swellings are encountered frequently in pediatric practice, and most of them represent lymph nodes. When considering the diagnostic possibilities in patients with cervical lymphadenitis, whether the pathologic process involves a lymph node first must be ascertained, then whether its cause is infectious, and, if infectious, the likely etiologic agent. The duration of the cervical swelling aids in the differential diagnosis because most tumors or developmental anomalies have been noted for weeks. Rapid enlargement may occur in the latter entities but usually as a result of secondary infection. Location is a helpful clue because midline masses rarely represent lymph nodes, and the most common neck masses of congenital origin (thyroglossal duct cyst, branchial cleft cyst, and cystic hygromas) have characteristic anatomic locations.

Of the midline masses, thyroglossal duct cysts are the most common.[75,132] These cysts occur from the foramen cecum to the thyroid, are midline, and move on protrusion of the tongue. They may have an associated sinus tract, midline or just lateral to it, from which cloudy mucus sometimes can be expressed. They can become infected secondarily, but in the noninfected state these cysts are nontender, smooth, and round, with well-defined margins. Thyroglossal duct cysts must be differentiated from other midline masses, including epidermoid cysts, lipomas, thyroid tumors, and the rare midline lymph node.

The second most common benign congenital neck mass is the branchial cleft cyst. It usually arises from the second branchial cleft and lies at the anterior border of the sternocleidomastoid muscle. Although such cysts usually manifest as skin dimples, they may become infected secondarily and manifest as inflammatory swellings or draining sinus tracts. A careful examination should detect a sinus tract. Branchial cleft cysts can manifest in individuals of any age but usually occur in school-aged children.

Cystic hygromas, considerably less common than thyroglossal duct or branchial cleft cysts, are the third most frequent cause of congenital neck masses. These arise from lymphatics derived from the jugular vein or the mesenchymal tissue. They can occur elsewhere but usually are found posterior to the sternocleidomastoid muscle in the supraclavicular fossa. Most cystic hygromas appear in the first 2 years of life, many being noted at birth or soon thereafter. They are soft, compressible tumors that transilluminate well, and, although benign in themselves, they may cause symptoms through pressure exerted on surrounding structures. Confusion may arise when cystic hygromas increase in size in association with an upper respiratory tract infection. The latter process causes increased lymph flow so that the hygroma persists while other lymph nodes decrease in size after resolution of the infection. In most circumstances, palpation and transillumination readily distinguish these congenital malformations.

These four cervical masses—thyroglossal duct cysts, thyroid tumors, branchial cleft cysts, and cystic hygromas—accounted for 63.7% of lesions in children with persistent cervical masses reported by Moussatos and Baffes.[112] Other lesions included neurogenic tumors, parotid tumors, and miscellaneous benign tumors (12.3%). The remainder of masses represented lymph nodes. As a rule, masses located completely anterior to the sternocleidomastoid muscle are benign. The exception is the thyroid tumor.[112] Malignancies that mimic cervical lymph nodes usually are located in the posterior triangle or are multiple masses extending across the anterior and the posterior triangles. In contrast, approximately 50% of masses in the posterior triangle represent malignancies, most of which are of lymphoid origin. Although most cysts and tumors manifest as solitary, unilateral, nontender masses, lymph nodes of noninfectious etiology frequently are multiple and bilateral and may be mildly tender.

Noninfectious chronic inflammatory involvement of cervical lymph nodes may represent a variety of uncommon, usually benign, but sometimes malignant entities (Table 12.2). Fifty percent of malignant

TABLE 12.2 Noninfectious Etiology of Cervical Adenitis

	Isolated Cervical	Cervical Associated With Generalized Adenopathy
Malignancy		
Hodgkin disease	+	+
Non-Hodgkin lymphomas	+	+
Rhabdomyosarcoma	+	–
Neuroblastoma	+	+
Leukemia	+	+
Metastatic carcinoma	+	–
Thyroid tumors	+	–
Drugs		
Isoniazid	–	+
Phenytoin (Dilantin)	–	+
Serum sickness	–	+
Collagen Vascular Disease		
Juvenile rheumatoid arthritis	–	+
Systemic lupus erythematosus	–	+
Miscellaneous		
Sarcoidosis	–	+
Reticuloendotheliosis	–	+
Sinus histiocytosis with massive lymphadenopathy	+	+
Histiocytosis X	–	+
Postvaccinial	+	–
Storage disorders	–	+
Kawasaki disease	+	+
Hemophagocytic syndrome	–	+
PFAPA syndrome	+	–
Kikuchi-Fujimoto disease	+	+
Masses Simulating Adenopathy		
Cystic hygroma	+	–
Branchial cleft cyst	+	–
Thyroglossal duct cyst	+	–
Epidermoid cyst	+	–
Sternocleidomastoid tumor	+	–

PFAPA, Periodic fever, aphthous ulcers, pharyngitis, cervical adenitis.

TABLE 12.3 Infectious Etiology of Cervical Adenitis

	Isolated	Associated With Generalized Adenopathy
Bacterial		
Staphylococcus aureus	+	–
Group A streptococci	+	+
Mycobacterium tuberculosis	+	+
Nontuberculous mycobacteria	+	–
Bartonella henselae	+	–
Gram-negative enterics	+	–
Anaerobes	+	–
Haemophilus influenzae	+	–
Yersinia pestis	–	+
Actinomyces israelii	+	–
Diphtheria	+	–
Tularemia	+	–
Brucellosis	–	+
Syphilis	+	+
Viral		
Measles	+	+
Rubella	+	+
Epstein-Barr virus	+	+
Herpes simplex	+	–
Human herpesvirus–6	+	+
Cytomegalovirus	+	+
Mumps	+	–
Varicella	+	+
HIV	+	+
Fungal		
Histoplasmosis	+	+
Cryptococcus	+	–
Aspergillosis	+	–
Candida	+	–
Sporotrichosis	+	–
Parasitic		
Toxoplasma gondii	+	+

HIV, Human immunodeficiency virus.

neck masses in children are caused by Hodgkin and non-Hodgkin lymphomas. Neuroblastoma is the second most common malignancy, accounting for 15%. The likelihood of a given diagnosis is age dependent, with neuroblastoma being more common than Hodgkin disease in younger age groups.[70] Thyroid tumors are the third most frequent neck malignancies. Other entities to be included in the differential diagnosis include leukemia,[28] metastatic carcinoma,[112] phenytoin-induced pseudolymphoma,[28] serum sickness,[28] storage disorders (Gaucher disease and Niemann-Pick disease), collagen vascular disease,[28] sarcoidosis,[73] sinus histiocytosis with massive lymphadenopathy,[14,140] and reticuloendotheliosis or histiocytosis X. Except for malignancies, these disease entities almost always are associated with lymphadenopathy that is not limited to the cervical region and have a variety of clinical and laboratory findings that allow the correct diagnosis to be made.

Numerous infectious agents have been reported in association with cervical adenitis in infants and children (Table 12.3). Among patients evaluated prospectively with needle aspirate cultures or cultures from incision and drainage specimens of affected lymph nodes, *S. aureus* or group A streptococci are the organisms most frequently isolated.[15,26,41,44,161,186] No significant difference has been reported that distinguishes between patients with adenitis caused by streptococci or staphylococci with respect to sex, dental problems, symptoms, presence of fever, or site or size of lymph nodes. In patients from whom *S. aureus* is isolated, a longer duration of disease before diagnosis is established, and a larger percentage of fluctuant lymph nodes[15,161] and tendency toward slower resolution often are found. Two recent studies reported that *S. aureus* was more common in infants younger than 12 and younger than 16 months of age, respectively, than in older children with neck abscesses and also noted a predominance of CA-MRSA among black children.[44,182] Most patients with bacterial cervical lymphadenitis, including patients with mycobacterial infection, are 1 to 6 years of age. Older children are more likely to have negative lymph node aspirate cultures.[15,152,161]

In early studies, anaerobes rarely were associated with cervical adenitis.[15,41,183] Proper bacteriologic techniques for the isolation of these fastidious organisms allowed Brook[26] to report anaerobes alone in 18% and mixed anaerobic and aerobic bacteria in 20% of patients, suggesting that anaerobic organisms play a more significant role in the etiology of cervical lymphadenitis than recognized previously. An older child with "negative" cultures, especially a child with poor dental hygiene or periodontal disease, may have anaerobic infection, as did the 9-year-old boy in Fig. 12.4. Needle aspiration of this cervical mass yielded *Peptococcus* and *Peptostreptococcus* spp., *Bacteroides fragilis,* and viridans streptococci. Resolution of the lymphadenitis occurred promptly after incision and drainage and penicillin therapy.

Dental disease or manipulation, or oral trauma, also should suggest the possibility of cervicofacial actinomycosis (lumpy jaw), an uncommon

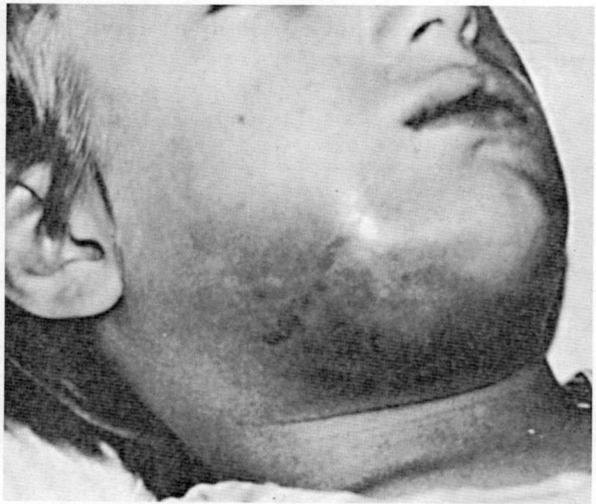

FIG. 12.4 A 9-year-old boy who developed high fever and markedly tender submental lymph node inflammation after a tooth extraction. Cultures from this fluctuant mass grew three anaerobes and viridans streptococci.

entity in children.[166] These patients may be older and have an indolent presentation, chronic submandibular mass, and frequently a fistula from the skin to the oral cavity.[18] Less frequently occurring bacteria,[81] viruses, fungi, and parasites can cause cervical lymphadenitis in children, but these patients usually have less evidence of acute inflammation, with or without adenopathy at additional sites, and historical and physical findings that suggest unusual causes of cervical lymph gland enlargement.

SPECIFIC DIAGNOSIS

A detailed history to ascertain preceding dental problems, presence of skin lesions, animal exposure (including exposure to fleas and ticks), duration of illness, presence of associated symptoms, contact with tuberculosis, presence of risk factors for HIV infection, drug usage (especially phenytoin), unusual ingestions (e.g., undercooked meat or unpasteurized dairy products), recent travel outside the geographic region of residence, and sites of occult infection drained by the affected node may yield important diagnostic clues in a patient with cervical lymphadenitis. Physical examination should include careful inspection for the presence of dental disease, noncervical lymphadenopathy, hepatosplenomegaly, and oropharyngeal or skin lesions.

Radiologic evaluation of adenitis is unnecessary in most mild to moderate cases. Ultrasonography often is performed when the presenting neck mass is very large, is increasing in size, or has not responded to initial antibiotic therapy. It is useful in diagnosing suppuration and expediting incision and drainage. High-resolution and color Doppler ultrasonography (with or without contrast enhancement) defining longitudinal to transverse nodal ratio and vascularity patterns has had some success in differentiating benign and malignant lymph nodes in adults.[3,111,113,184,187]

In children in whom most adenopathy is infectious or reactive in etiology, ultrasonography is less discriminating. In one study of 35 children, ultrasonography showed significant differences in lymph nodes in 22 children with a diagnosis of Kawasaki disease in contrast to 8 children with bacterial lymphadenitis, but findings were similar to those in children with lymphadenitis caused by Epstein-Barr virus infection.[164]

In another study of 146 children, unilateral lymph nodes and cystic necrosis were found only in lymphadenitis caused by cat-scratch disease or bacterial or tuberculous infection.[128] Individual sonographic findings were nonspecific for diagnosis, although these findings combined with clinical signs were helpful. No patients with nontuberculous mycobacterial adenitis were evaluated in this study. Nodal calcifications and spread of nodal masses into the subcutaneous tissues by ultrasonography and characteristic low-density, ring-enhancing lesions with minimal or absent inflammatory stranding of subcutaneous fat seen on computed tomography and magnetic resonance imaging have been reported with nontuberculous mycobacterial adenitis in children.[63,67,92,139] These findings may be helpful in differentiating this etiology from other bacterial causes when the diagnosis is not suspected clinically or early in the course. Differences in clinical presentation between the two entities, however, should obviate the need for such imaging in all but the most complicated of cases.

In the acute stage of cervical lymphadenitis where the etiology is not clinically obvious, needle aspiration of the affected node is a valuable diagnostic approach. Of patients with acute cervical lymphadenitis subjected to needle aspiration of the affected node for bacterial and mycobacterial culture, 50% to 88% have an etiologic agent recovered.[15,26,74,156,185] Only inflamed nodes should be aspirated. The largest or most fluctuant node should be selected, and the skin should be cleansed and anesthetized. Skin anesthesia can be induced effectively using a topical anesthetic cream (e.g., lidocaine-prilocaine [EMLA]) placed on the selected aspiration site under an occlusive dressing 30 to 45 minutes before the procedure. An 18- or 20-gauge needle attached to a 20-mL syringe is used. If no material is aspirated, sterile *nonbacteriostatic* saline 1 to 2 mL is injected into the node and reaspirated. The aspirate should be inoculated directly from the syringe onto aerobic (including chocolate agar) and anaerobic media, onto Sabouraud agar (fungi), and into a broth medium suitable for the early detection of mycobacteria, such as the Bactec radiometric assay. In the latter system, the release of labeled carbon dioxide in an automated ion chamber system can detect mycobacteria 12 to 17 days (and sometimes even sooner) after inoculation of the broth.[157] When mycobacterial infection is suspected, consultation with the laboratory is helpful to ensure that cultures are handled correctly because some species, such as *M. haemophilum,* require that the culture be kept at a temperature of 30°C (86°F) and that heme-containing medium is added for isolation.[10,151] Gram and acid-fast stains are mandatory and serve as a guide to initial antimicrobial therapy. However, a negative acid-fast stain does not rule out mycobacterial infection, as cultures may still be positive, especially when the etiologic agent is nontuberculous mycobacteria.

PCR assays have successfully confirmed the presence of tuberculous and nontuberculous mycobacteria in gastric aspirates and specimens obtained from lymph nodes by aspiration or biopsy.[45,51,61,62,149,154] This technique shows great promise in rapidly providing a specific diagnosis.

Thioglycolate broth and anaerobically incubated blood agar plates are incapable of providing optimal conditions for the isolation of many anaerobic bacteria.[15] Optimal methods for cultivation of fastidious anaerobes should be employed because anaerobic organisms may be recovered in 20% of cases.[26] Cultures of infected skin lesions and exudates on tonsils also should be done but not to the exclusion of needle aspiration.

Isolation of group A streptococci from the throat or skin cultures of a patient with lymphadenitis does *not* confirm the etiology of the lymph node inflammation. Patients have been noted to have isolation of group A streptococci from throat and of *S. aureus* from lymph node aspirate cultures.[15,133] Tuberculin skin tests should be performed in children less than 4 years of age, but inteferon-γ release assays are more useful in older children.[10] Induration of 15 mm or greater suggests infection with *M. tuberculosis,* whereas reactions of 5 to 14 mm may be caused by either a tuberculous or a nontuberculous mycobacterial infection, because the purified protein derivative preparation shares some antigens with nontuberculous species.[8,101]

Intradermal skin testing, using a crude extract from affected nodes, historically was used to establish the diagnosis of cat-scratch disease.[31] A diagnosis usually is reached, however, based on the presence of regional adenopathy, a history of cat exposure (particularly if the patient has a history of a scratch or a primary skin lesion), and negative laboratory studies for other causes of lymphadenopathy. Serologic methods for the detection of immunoglobulin (Ig)G antibodies to *Bartonella* spp. are available[2,7,189] and should be considered the gold standard for diagnosis. However, sensitivity varies among laboratories. PCR assays are available in some commercial and research laboratories and at the

Centers for Disease Control and Prevention.[7] In a few cases, a lymph node biopsy should be undertaken to exclude other, more serious pathologies.

If the etiology of adenitis remains uncertain or lymphadenopathy has persisted with no detectable response to antimicrobial therapy, a more intense diagnostic evaluation is indicated. Studies may include a complete blood count; serology for Epstein-Barr virus, cytomegalovirus, HHV-6, HIV, histoplasmosis, coccidioidomycosis, toxoplasmosis, tularemia, *B. henselae,* and *Brucella;* and a radiograph of the chest. If the diagnosis remains in doubt, and the node persists, enlarges, is hard, or is fixed to the adjacent structures, biopsy *should* be performed. Biopsy material should be submitted for the studies outlined earlier for lymph node aspirate cultures and routine histology; Giemsa, periodic acid–Schiff, and methenamine silver stains; and, in select cases only, PCR for viruses and other etiologies. If the histologic examination reveals noncaseating granulomas and the child has a history of cat exposure, the most likely diagnosis is cat-scratch disease.[100,102] Sarcoidosis involving lymph nodes would have a similar histology but is rare in children and a condition in which isolated cervical node involvement has not been observed.[73,148]

Older children are more likely to have negative cultures of lymph node aspirates[15,161] and to be more frequent candidates for excisional lymph node biopsy. They also are more likely to have lymphomas. It is important that appropriate tissue be excised, especially from adolescents, so that precise diagnostic interpretation can be done. This interpretation can be facilitated by the proper selection of a lymph node for a biopsy to be performed; intact removal of the node chosen; and proper fixation, cutting, and staining of the specimen. If only one node or one anatomic group of nodes is enlarged, the largest node should be excised. If several groups of lymph nodes are involved, the site for biopsy should be selected according to the likelihood of diagnostic yield. Biopsy specimens from the lower neck and supraclavicular area have the highest yields.[76] Other areas, including the upper cervical, submandibular, axillary, and parotid lymph nodes, are much more likely to be affected by reactive hyperplasia, which may or may not be related to the underlying disease process. If lymphoma is suspected, needle biopsies or frozen sections are contraindicated.[20,28]

Even under optimal conditions, many reactive processes, including rheumatoid arthritis, toxoplasmosis, phenytoin-induced adenopathy, dermatopathic adenitis, and infectious mononucleosis, have been noted to simulate lymphoma.[28] Obtaining a thorough history and performing appropriate serologic studies should provide sufficient information for the physician to exclude reactive processes known to simulate lymphoma.

TREATMENT

Optimal management of a child with cervical lymphadenitis depends on an accurate assessment of the underlying etiology. Because almost all cases are associated with infectious agents, every effort should be made to ascertain the etiologic agent so that specific therapy can be initiated. Aspiration of the affected lymph node for Gram and acid-fast stains is a guide for initial therapy, and culture and antimicrobial susceptibility form the basis for prescribing specific treatment in patients with bacterial lymphadenitis.[15,41] When the patient has findings typical of acute bacterial lymphadenitis, however, empiric therapy may be undertaken without prior needle aspiration. In this situation, close follow-up is essential because failure to show some clinical response after 48 hours of therapy is an indication for further diagnostic procedures to be done.

Acute suppurative cervical lymphadenitis most frequently is caused by infection with *S. aureus* or group A streptococci.[15,24,41,146,161,186] In nodes that progress to abscess formation, *S. aureus* is the most frequent agent isolated,[15,41,44,146,182] and drainage is mandatory. Because of the frequency of infection caused by *S. aureus* or group A streptococci, empiric antimicrobial therapy should be directed against these two agents. Penicillinase-resistant penicillins or cephalexin should be used. If the patient requires parenteral therapy and CA-MRSA is uncommon in the geographic area, oxacillin or nafcillin 150 mg/kg per day or cefazolin 75 to 100 mg/kg per day may be used.

When oral therapy is deemed adequate, dicloxacillin 25 mg/kg per day, or cephalexin 25 to 50 mg/kg per day is recommended. The fixed combination of amoxicillin and clavulanic acid provides good activity against methicillin-susceptible staphylococci and streptococci and has an expanded spectrum of activity against the oral anaerobic organisms. These features, combined with its palatability, render it an attractive alternative to the traditional penicillinase-resistant penicillins. Clavulanate-associated diarrhea can be problematic in some children. In children with mild penicillin allergies, cephalosporins can be used. Ceftriaxone 50 to 100 mg/kg per day is an attractive and effective alternative to the parenteral antibiotics that require more frequent administration if group A streptococcus is the etiologic agent.

In areas where CA-MRSA is prevalent and clindamycin resistance is low, clindamycin 30 to 40 mg/kg per day for parenteral or oral use is appropriate for empiric or alternative therapy. In addition to its good activity against anaerobes and methicillin-susceptible *S. aureus,* clindamycin is effective against most CA-MRSA isolates. However, clindamycin resistance is increasing among community *S. aureus* isolates, so close clinical follow-up to ensure a therapeutic response has been achieved is mandatory when this option is chosen.[48,68,69,72,115] In a severely ill child needing hospitalization or with signs of deep neck infection (e.g., airway compromise), vancomycin 60 mg/kg per day divided every 6 hours is appropriate in combination with another agent until culture results are obtained. Trimethoprim-sulfamethoxazole 10 mg/kg per day of the trimethoprim component or doxycycline 2 to 4 mg/kg per day if the child is aged 8 years or older are alternative choices for oral therapy of CA-MRSA infections[48,68,69,115] but should not be used initially because they are not active against group A streptococci. Linezolid is active against MRSA and group A streptococci, but because of concerns regarding cost and bacterial resistance, use should be reserved for cases in which a microbiological need has been confirmed or clinical failure of first-line therapies has occurred. Other parenteral agents active against MRSA and group A streptococci, such as ceftaroline, which is an advanced-generation cephalosporin, are being studied for use in children, but their use cannot be recommended until more pharmacokinetic and efficacy data are available.

Antibiotic therapy may need to be modified if an obvious primary focus of infection suggests a different etiologic agent. In a patient with periodontal or dental disease, adequate anaerobic activity is mandatory, and therapy with penicillin V 50 mg/kg per day, amoxicillin-clavulanate 45 mg/kg per day, or clindamycin 30 to 40 mg/kg per day should be initiated, pending results of cultures.

Patients with marked lymph node enlargement, moderate to severe systemic symptoms, or concomitant cellulitis frequently require parenteral therapy for the first few days. This therapy allows for a high concentration of the antimicrobial agent within the inflamed tissue and may promote more rapid localization, especially in patients with staphylococcal adenitis. Although the use of parenteral drugs has to be individualized, most infants and children with staphylococcal or streptococcal lymphadenitis respond to orally administered antimicrobials.

Adenitis caused by group A streptococci should be treated with penicillin G 100,000 to 150,000 IU/kg per day or penicillin V 50 mg/kg per day for a total of 10 days. In a child with penicillin allergy, azithromycin 10 mg/kg per day on day 1, then 5 mg/kg per day on days 2 through 5, or cephalexin 25 to 50 mg/kg per day can be used. These drugs have been shown effective in the treatment of cervical lymphadenitis.[15,24] Treatment should be continued for at least 10 days or approximately 5 days after signs of local inflammation and systemic toxicity have disappeared, whichever is longer. If required, analgesics should be given and not overlooked in infants and children too young to verbalize their discomfort. The average duration of antibiotic therapy is 10 days, unless abscess formation occurs late in the first or early in the second week of treatment.[15] In this situation, incision and drainage is indicated,[15,25,41] and therapy should be continued until resolution of the acute process occurs, usually within another 5 to 7 days.

Some clinical improvement is to be expected within 48 hours after initiation of therapy and is manifested by a decrease in inflammation and tenderness of the lymph node and a decrease in the maximum daily temperature. The size of the lymph node may not show evidence of regression at this stage, and total resolution of fever should not be expected. It is important to record accurate measurements of the node at the time of presentation because a subjective evaluation is an unreliable indicator of lymph node evolution during therapy. If no clinical improvement is noted by 48 hours, needle aspiration is recommended. The history and physical examination should be reassessed, and a more detailed laboratory evaluation should be initiated.

In a study of 284 children admitted to the hospital with acute cervical adenitis, age younger than 1 year and node involvement for more than 48 hours before admission predicted the need for node aspiration.[96] Regression of the size of a lymph node is slow, usually requiring 4 to 6 weeks or more. Persistence of significant enlargement beyond 6 to 8 weeks, even in the face of good initial response to antimicrobial therapy, demands that an underlying disorder be excluded. When signs of acute inflammation have resolved, prolonged antimicrobial therapy is of little value because penetration of antimicrobials through the fibrous capsule of the node is poor.[24] Spontaneous regression occurs in most patients, although it may require several weeks. Uncommonly, reactivation of inflammation may occur, and a meticulous search for an untreated primary source of bacterial infection, such as secondarily infected dermatitis, infestation, foreign body, or dental abscess, should be undertaken. Retreatment should include specific measures to eliminate the predisposing condition.

If Gram stain of the lymph node aspirate suggests a microorganism other than *S. aureus* or group A streptococci, initial antimicrobial therapy should include therapy for the most likely agents until culture results are known. Because attempts to perform careful Gram stains and anaerobic cultures of lymph node aspirates in most reported series have been limited, the large number of infants and children with sterile aspirates may be attributed partly to a failure to isolate fastidious anaerobes indigenous to the mouth. These microorganisms should respond to penicillin G therapy. For penicillin-resistant organisms, clindamycin is a useful alternative drug.

For infants in the first 2 months of life, group B streptococci and *S. aureus* are important pathogens to consider in selecting initial therapy. Penicillinase-resistant penicillins are active against both agents, unless the occurrence of CA-MRSA is frequent, in which case clindamycin or vancomycin should be considered for initial therapy. If group B streptococci are isolated, penicillin G can be substituted. Final bacteriologic identification and antimicrobial susceptibility tests should be the ultimate guide to selecting specific antimicrobial therapy in all patients. Treatment of cervical lymph node infections associated with rarely encountered bacteria, fungi, and parasites listed in Table 12.3 is discussed under those specific disease entities.

Although controversy exists as to whether cervical adenitis associated with *M. tuberculosis* in a child is truly a localized process, only rarely do patients have disseminated infection.[42,60,121] When infection is not localized, pulmonary or hilar lymph node involvement is a common finding.[10,42,74,122] A 2-month regimen of isoniazid 10 mg/kg per day, rifampin 10 to 20 mg/kg per day, pyrazinamide 30 mg/kg per day, and ethambutol 20 mg/kg per day is recommended for the treatment of uncomplicated pulmonary tuberculosis or isolated cervical lymphadenitis in children. This therapy is given for 2 months, daily for at least the first 2 weeks, and then 2 to 3 times per week, after which isoniazid and rifampin are administered 2 to 3 times per week for the ensuing 4 months. Twice weekly therapy is not recommended for HIV-infected people.[10]

In areas where multidrug resistance in *M. tuberculosis* is prevalent, streptomycin 20 to 40 mg/kg per day or another aminoglycoside (kanamycin, amikacin, or capreomycin) is added for initial treatment until drug susceptibilities are known.[10,34,35] The addition of a fifth drug should occur after consultation with an expert in the field because these drugs may have toxic effects, and careful assessment of the risks and benefits is warranted. Detailed discussion of the treatment of tuberculosis in children is provided in Chapter 96. Response to antituberculous therapy is usual, with rapid resolution of symptoms and marked regression of lymph nodes within 3 months. Nodes remain palpable for months, however, because scarring and fibrosis are regular accompaniments to resolution of disease. Draining sinuses, a common complication of lymph node aspiration or incision, and drainage before the advent of effective antituberculosis chemotherapy no longer develop.

Cervical lymphadenitis attributed to nontuberculous mycobacteria is much more common in a young child than that caused by *M. tuberculosis*. These microorganisms exhibit in vitro resistance to commonly employed antituberculosis drugs. Resistance particularly is common among *M. scrofulaceum* and *M. intracellulare*. Surgical excision remains the treatment of choice for nontuberculous mycobacterial lymphadenitis, and total removal of all the visibly affected nodes is recommended.* Early (within 1 month of onset) removal of affected nodes was associated significantly with better aesthetic results.[98] Thorough curettage has been found effective[88,99,121] but results in delayed healing, higher relapse rates, and less favorable aesthetic result.[49,88,190]

Antimicrobial therapy alone is less effective.[89,105,190] The macrolides clarithromycin and azithromycin, rifampin and its analogue rifabutin, ethambutol, amikacin, and cefoxitin show activity against nontuberculous mycobacteria.[8,59,163] Retrospective case series with small cohorts of patients showed that clarithromycin monotherapy and combination therapy with clarithromycin and ethambutol or rifampin (or rifabutin) had some success in the treatment of nontuberculous lymphadenitis and a relatively low rate of recurrence.[19,58,67,94,95,99,165] The regimens used generally were well tolerated. Rifabutin resulted in adverse effects in four of seven patients treated for 6 months in one study (neutropenia and yellow skin pigmentation), which disappeared after dose reduction.[94] In HIV-infected children receiving protease inhibitors, rifabutin generally is contraindicated, but it can be given at a much reduced dosage if deemed necessary.[8]

In one randomized controlled clinical trial, 100 children (median age, 45.5 months; range, 9 to 168 months) with microbiologically proven nontuberculous lymphadenitis received either surgical resection or clarithromycin 15 mg/kg per day and rifabutin 5 mg/kg per day orally for 12 weeks.[89] There was a 30% higher cure rate (96% vs. 66%) for patients treated surgically in contrast to those who received antibiotics alone. The cure rate was not influenced by lymph node stage of infection or infecting mycobacterial species. Postoperative wound infection and facial nerve weakness occurred in 12% and 14% of children, respectively, and, in one child, facial nerve weakness was permanent. In the two patients in whom surgical resection was not curative, the lesions responded to 3 months of the antibiotic regimen. In a follow-up study of this cohort 1 year later, aesthetic outcome also was significantly better in the surgical group.[91] In another study of 50 patients with advanced nontuberculous mycobacterial adenitis who received either the previously mentioned antibiotic regimen or no treatment, the median time to resolution was only 4 weeks earlier (36 vs. 40 weeks) in the treated group.[87]

Zimmermann and associates recently performed a meta-analysis of 60 publications in children with cervical lymphadenitis caused by nontuberculous mycobacteria and found an adjusted cure rate of 98% for complete surgical excision versus 73.1% for medical therapy and 70.4% for no intervention.[190] Complete excision was associated with a 10% risk of facial palsy, and 2% of cases had permanent palsy. The authors conclude that the decision to perform complete excision should be dependent on location. Regarding medical therapy, studies to date suggest that regimens of a macrolide (clarithromycin or azithromycin) plus either ethambutol and/or rifampin (or rifabutin) are options for the treatment of nontuberculous mycobacterial adenitis for which complete excision of the affected node would endanger the facial nerve or its branches if a reduction in size of the swelling would facilitate a complete and aesthetic excision at a later stage, for recurrent disease or if surgery is refused.[8] Macrolide monotherapy is not recommended because of the risk for inducing resistant organisms. The optimal duration of therapy is unknown, but regimens of 4 to 6 months or longer are usual. Expert opinion should be sought, especially as new mycobacterial species are described.[8]

Cat-scratch disease usually is a benign, self-limited disorder requiring no specific therapy, but the use of antimicrobials may relieve symptoms and hasten recovery. Rifampin, azithromycin, trimethoprim-sulfamethoxazole, doxycycline, ciprofloxacin (the latter two agents in older children), and parenteral gentamicin may be useful in promoting fever defervescence and in clinical resolution of systemic cat-scratch disease.[7,11,16,104] If the lymph node progresses to fluctuance, needle aspiration may hasten resolution and relieve discomfort. Surgical excision may be required in a few patients who have persistent problems despite having needle aspiration or who develop draining sinuses.

*References 5, 8, 33, 47, 65, 88, 89, 103, 119, 127, 135, 143, 156, 178, 190.

PROGNOSIS

With effective antimicrobial therapy, complete resolution of cervical lymphadenitis caused by *S. aureus*, group A streptococci, and *M. tuberculosis* is the rule. Delay in establishing the diagnosis or initiating therapy can prolong the clinical course and result in complications or sequelae, such as sinus tracts (mycobacteria),[21,36,122] abscess formation,[25,44] cellulitis or bacteremia (*S. aureus* and *S. pyogenes*),[15] acute glomerulonephritis (group A streptococci),[40] disseminated disease (*M. tuberculosis*),[74] or mycotic carotid artery aneurysm.[177] Except for abscess formation, these complications are rare events. Although lymph node infection caused by *S. aureus* is more likely to result in abscess formation, at least one study has noted a significantly greater duration of infection before treatment in patients in whom *S. aureus* was isolated from the abscess cavity cultures.[15] The extracellular products of this organism (e.g., coagulase, fibrinolysin, and hyaluronidase) partly explain its propensity for abscess formation, which occurs in 50% to 70% of patients.[25,41]

Even in patients whose course is complicated by suppuration, appropriate drainage in conjunction with specific antimicrobial therapy results in prompt resolution of signs and symptoms, and relapse occurs only rarely. Today, surgical excision of affected nodes seldom is recommended except when the disease is caused by nontuberculous mycobacteria, in which case surgical excision remains the treatment of choice.[190] Antimicrobial therapy has been responsible for the disappearance of the events commonly associated with cervical adenitis historically, including thrombosis of the internal jugular vein, rupture of the carotid artery, generalized septic embolic phenomena, mediastinal abscess, purulent pericarditis, and even death.[78,160]

With the advent of effective antituberculous agents, the prognosis for tuberculous cervical adenitis also is excellent. When surgical excision is performed early in the course of lymphadenitis caused by nontuberculous mycobacterial infection, resolution can be anticipated.[49,98,127,135,143,155,190] Persistent and recurrent disease is the most frequent complication encountered.[178] Macrolide monotherapy and combination therapy are useful in ameliorating these complications or in cases for which surgery is not feasible.[8,129,155] Cat-scratch disease usually is a benign, self-limited disorder in which therapeutic intervention, such as needle aspiration to relieve pain, is uncommonly needed, but antibiotic therapy can hasten recovery.

PREVENTION

Providing appropriate medical and, occasionally, surgical therapy of predisposing conditions (e.g., dental caries, abscess, group A streptococcal pharyngitis or nasopharyngitis, purulent otitis media, impetigo, other infections involving the face and scalp) and minimizing the exposure of infants and children to adults with active tuberculosis should reduce the incidence of cervical lymphadenitis. Some authors suggest that decreased exposure to animals may result in fewer infections,[16] especially for adenitis attributed to toxoplasmosis or *Bartonella*.[32,136]

NEW REFERENCES SINCE THE SEVENTH EDITION

1. Ablanedo-Terrazas Y, Alvarado-de la Barrera C, Ruiz-Cruz M, Reyes-Terán G. Mycobacterial cervicofacial lymphadenitis in human immunodeficiency virus-infected individuals after antiretroviral therapy initiation. *Laryngoscope*. 2015;125:2498-2502.
7. American Academy of Pediatrics. Cat-scratch disease. In: Kimberlin DW, Brady MT, Jackson M, Long SS, eds. *Red Book: 2015 Report of the Committee on Infectious Diseases*. 30th ed. Elk Grove Village, IL: American Academy of Pediatrics; 2015:280-283.
8. American Academy of Pediatrics. Diseases caused by nontuberculous mycobacteria. In: Kimberlin DW, Brady MT, Jackson M, Long SS, eds. *Red Book: 2015 Report of the Committee on Infectious Diseases*. 30th ed. Elk Grove Village, IL: American Academy of Pediatrics; 2015:831-839.
9. American Academy of Pediatrics. Kawasaki disease. In: Kimberlin DW, Brady MT, Jackson M, Long SS, eds. *Red Book: 2015 Report of the Committee on Infectious Diseases*. 30th ed. Elk Grove Village, IL: American Academy of Pediatrics; 2015: 494-500.
10. American Academy of Pediatrics. Tuberculosis. In: Kimberlin DW, Brady MT, Jackson M, Long SS, eds. *Red Book: 2015 Report of the Committee on Infectious Diseases*. 30th ed. Elk Grove Village, IL: American Academy of Pediatrics; 2015: 805-831.
39. Cmejrek RC, Coticchia JM, Arnold JE. Presentation, diagnosis, and management of deep-neck abscesses in infants. *Arch Otolaryngol Head Neck Surg*. 2002;128: 1361-1364.
40. Coticchia JM, Getnick GS, Yun RD, Arnold JE. Age-, site-, and time-specific differences in pediatric deep neck abscesses. *Arch Otolaryngol Head Neck Surg*. 2004;130:201-207.
71. Jiménez-Montero B, Baquero-Artigao F, Saavedra-Lozano J, et al. Comparison of *Mycobacterium lentiflavum* and *Mycobacterium avium-intracellulare* complex lymphadenitis. *Pediatr Infect Dis J*. 2014;33:28-34.
77. Kraszewska-Głomba B, Matkowska-Kocjan A, Szenborn L. The pathogenesis of periodic fever, aphthous stomatitis, pharyngitis, and cervical adenitis syndrome: a review of current research. *Mediators Inflamm*. 2015;2015:563876. doi:10.1155/2015/563876. [Epub 2015 Sep 17].
79. Kwit N, Nelson C, Kugeler K, et al. Human plague-United States, 2015. *MMWR Morb Mortal Wkly Rep*. 2015;64:918-919.
137. Rajasekaran K, Krakovitz P. Enlarged neck lymph nodes in children. *Pediatr Clin North Am*. 2013;60:923-936.
141. Rosenberg TL, Nolder AR. Pediatric cervical lymphadenopathy. *Otolaryngol Clin North Am*. 2014;47:721-731.
147. Scott C, Kirking HL, Jeffries C, et al. Tuberculosis trends–United States, 2014. *MMWR Morb Mortal Wkly Rep*. 2015;64:265-269.
157. Starke JR, Committee on Infectious Diseases. Interferon-γ release assays for diagnosis of tuberculosis infection and disease in children. *Pediatrics*. 2014;134:e1763-e1773.
166. Thacker SA, Healy CM. Pediatric cervicofacial actinomycosis: an unusual cause of head and neck masses. *J Pediatric Infect Dis Soc*. 2014;3:e15-e19.
171. Tortoli E. Epidemiology of cervico-facial pediatric lymphadenitis as a result of nontuberculous mycobacteria. *Int J Mycobacteriol*. 2012;1:165-169.
179. World Health Organization. Biologicals: diphtheria. Available at: http://www.who.int/biologicals/vaccines/diphtheria/en/.
180. World Health Organization. Diphtheria detected in Spain. Available at http://www.euro.who.int/en/health-topics/disease-prevention/vaccines-and-immunization/news/news/2015/06/diphtheria-detected-in-spain.
181. World Health Organization. Global tuberculosis report 2015. Available at http://www.who.int/tb/publications/global_report/en/.
182. Worley ML, Seif JM, Whigham AS, et al. Suppurativecervical lymphadenitis in infancy: microbiology and sociology. *Clin Pediatr (Phila)*. 2015;54:629-634.
188. You HL, Lin TM, Wang JC, et al. Mannose-binding lectin gene polymorphisms and mycobacterial lymphadenitis in young patients. *Pediatr Infect Dis J*. 2013;32:1005-1009.
190. Zimmermann P, Tebruegge M, Curtis N, Ritz N. The management of non-tuberculous cervicofacial lymphadenitis in children: a systematic review and meta-analysis. *J Infect*. 2015;71:9-18.

The full reference list for this chapter is available at ExpertConsult.com.

13 Parotitis

Judith R. Campbell

Parotitis, inflammation of the parotid gland, is caused by a variety of infectious agents and noninfectious systemic illnesses. Several terms are used to describe the clinical presentations and etiologic processes that lead to parotid gland swelling and inflammation. *Suppurative parotitis,* first described in the 1800s, is a serious bacterial infection in neonates and postsurgical patients.[51] *Epidemic parotitis,* particularly prevalent in the prevaccine era, was caused primarily by mumps virus infection.[58] In the postvaccine era, this form of parotitis also is caused by other viral pathogens and is referred to as *viral parotitis.* Rarely a more indolent, slowly progressive, granulomatous infection may occur that is referred to as *granulomatous parotitis. Recurrent parotitis of childhood* is a unique illness characterized by multiple episodes of acute and subacute parotid gland swelling. The histologic findings in this disease include architectural changes in the ducts and chronic inflammation. Many noninfectious systemic illnesses cause persistent or recurrent parotid gland swelling and inflammation, which is referred to as *chronic parotitis.* Bilateral parotid enlargement is a frequent presentation of human immunodeficiency virus (HIV) infection as part of the *diffuse infiltrative lymphocytosis syndrome.*

PATHOPHYSIOLOGY

Despite the various agents that cause parotitis, involvement of the gland occurs mainly by three mechanisms. The most common mechanism is a localized infection limited to the gland and surrounding structures. Parotitis may be a manifestation of a systemic infection, as in mumps, or rarely may develop secondary to hematogenous seeding during periods of transient bacteremia. Several common contributing factors and pathophysiologic mechanisms lead to swelling of the gland. The parotid is well encapsulated and consists of superficial and deep lobes separated by the facial nerve. The parotid duct (Stensen duct) traverses the buccal soft tissue anteriorly and exits opposite the second upper molar. Thin, watery secretions from the parotid gland cleanse the ductal system and have some bacteriostatic properties, preventing accumulation of bacteria and debris.[38] Factors that predispose individuals to the development of parotitis include side effects of certain drugs and diseases that lead to dehydration, xerostomia, or ductal obstruction (Box 13.1).[38,51] Decreased salivary flow allows retrograde migration of bacteria. Stasis in the ductal system, caused by ductal ectasia, inflammation, calculi, or strictures, allows proliferation of bacteria and inflammation within the gland.

ETIOLOGY

Infectious parotitis may be caused by aerobes, anaerobes, mycobacteria, and viruses (Box 13.2). In all age groups, *Staphylococcus aureus* is the organism most commonly associated with suppurative parotitis.[49,51] Gram-negative pathogens (e.g., *Escherichia coli* and *Klebsiella* and *Pseudomonas* spp.) also may cause suppurative parotitis, particularly in neonates and debilitated or hospitalized patients.[12,33,50,51] The role of anaerobic organisms in this infection has become apparent, especially when poor oral hygiene and oral pathology are associated features.[4,5,41] In cases of recurrent parotitis of childhood, *Streptococcus* spp. are the bacteria most commonly isolated.[23,44,48] Granulomatous parotitis most often is caused by *Mycobacterium tuberculosis* and may occur in the absence of systemic or disseminated tuberculous disease.[38,46,54] Other causes of granulomatous parotitis include *Mycobacterium avium-intracellulare, Actinomyces* spp., and gram-negative intracellular organisms (*Francisella tularensis* and *Brucella* spp.).[27,38,61]

In the postvaccine era, the most common viral cause of parotitis still is the paramyxovirus mumps virus. coxsackieviruses, Epstein-Barr virus, influenza A virus, parainfluenza viruses, adenovirus, human herpesvirus–6, herpes simplex virus, cytomegalovirus, and lymphocytic choriomeningitis virus all have been implicated in cases of parotitis.[1,2,17,30,32,34,37,38]

CLINICAL PRESENTATION AND DIAGNOSIS

A detailed history and physical examination are crucial in assisting the clinician in determining the most likely etiology of parotid gland swelling. One should determine the onset and duration of symptoms, their periodicity, and the character of salivary secretions. In addition, the presence of a systemic disease must be excluded. Examination of the parotid gland is achieved best by simultaneous palpation of the intraoral and extraoral salivary structures. Gentle external pressure should be applied to the gland, and the parotid duct should be examined for evidence of purulent secretions or surrounding erythema.

Suppurative parotitis occurs most commonly in neonates or patients with dehydration, poor oral hygiene, malnutrition, immunosuppression, oral trauma, sepsis, or any medication or disease that decreases salivary secretions.[20] Usually, the disease is unilateral; however, bilateral suppurative parotitis may occur in 17% of cases.[44] The disease is characterized by acute onset of pain, swelling, warmth, and induration of the involved gland and purulent discharge from the Stensen duct. Associated physical findings include fever, trismus, malaise, and cervical adenitis. In suppurative parotitis, Gram stain and culture (aerobic and anaerobic) of purulent material from the duct can provide a specific microbiologic diagnosis. In addition, elevation of the white blood cell count with a neutrophil predominance may help differentiate this form of parotitis from viral parotitis and parotid disease of a noninfectious etiology.

Mumps is the most common form of viral parotitis and is characterized by a prodrome of fever, malaise, anorexia, and headache. Usually, the following day, unilateral or bilateral earache and parotid tenderness develop. The gland or glands enlarge during the subsequent 2 to 3 days, and the orifice of the Stensen duct is erythematous and swollen, yet secretions from the duct are clear. At the point of maximal swelling, the angle of the jaw is obliterated and the earlobe is lifted upward and outward. The other salivary glands are involved in 10% of cases.[44] Rare systemic manifestations of mumps infection include epididymo-orchitis, meningitis, meningoencephalitis, and oophoritis. More recent outbreaks of confirmed and probable mumps emphasize that this infection may occur in highly immunized populations.[6,18] In 2006, the United States had the largest mumps epidemic in two decades, involving more than 6000 patients. Most cases occurred in Midwestern states (Iowa, Kansas, Wisconsin, Illinois, Nebraska, and South Dakota). The highest incidence was among college-aged students, most of whom had received two doses of measles-mumps-rubella (MMR) vaccine.[6,18] The largest U.S. mumps outbreak since 2006 began at a summer camp in New York in June 2009. This outbreak included 1521 cases. Vaccination status was known for 1115, of which 976 (88%) had received at least one dose of mumps-containing vaccine.[7] Other viral agents may produce similar clinical manifestations and can be differentiated from mumps only by culture and hemagglutination inhibition, complement fixation, or enzyme-linked immunosorbent assay serology.[17] In viral parotitis, the white blood cell count may be normal, slightly elevated, or depressed, with a lymphocytic predominance.

Granulomatous parotitis typically manifests as a painless, slowly enlarging mass without surrounding inflammation. It may be

BOX 13.1 Predisposing Factors for Parotitis

Drug-Induced Xerostomia
Anticholinergics
Antihistamines
Antidepressants
Phenothiazines
β-Blockers
Diuretics
General anesthesia

Disease-Related Xerostomia
Sjögren syndrome
Diabetes mellitus
Chronic liver disease
Cystic fibrosis

Obstruction
Dental appliances
Oral tumors
Radiation therapy
Trauma

BOX 13.2 Reported Infectious Etiologies of Parotitis

Aerobic Bacteria
Staphylococcus aureus
Streptococcus pneumoniae
Streptococcus pyogenes
Viridans streptococci
Francisella tularensis
Haemophilus spp.
Moraxella catarrhalis
Pseudomonas aeruginosa
Escherichia coli
Proteus spp.
Salmonella spp.
Klebsiella spp.
Brucella spp.

Anaerobic Bacteria
Peptostreptococcus spp.
Prevotella spp.
Fusobacterium spp.
Actinomyces spp.

Mycobacteria
Mycobacterium tuberculosis
Mycobacterium avium-intracellulare
Other mycobacteria

Viruses
Mumps
Coxsackieviruses A and B
Echoviruses
Epstein-Barr virus
Influenza A
Parainfluenza viruses 1 and 3
Cytomegalovirus
Herpes simplex virus type 1
Human herpesvirus–6
Lymphocytic choriomeningitis virus
Human immunodeficiency virus

misdiagnosed as a slow-growing tumor until the correct diagnosis is made by biopsy and culture. *M. tuberculosis* and *M. avium-intracellulare* may cause infection in the parenchyma of the gland or in intraglandular or periglandular lymph nodes.[45,61] Clinical evidence of systemic tuberculous disease usually is absent. Parotitis has been observed as an extension of nontuberculous cervical adenitis.[61] Actinomycosis of the parotid gland causes a slowly enlarging, nodular, nontender gland; associated oral or cervicofacial infection usually is present. Fistulas draining yellow or white material with sulfur granules are common findings.[27]

Recurrent parotitis of childhood is rare, with onset typically occurring before the child reaches 10 years of age and a peak incidence at approximately 6 years of age.[19,44] Some authors hypothesize that an underlying congenital abnormality, such as sialectasis, is a common predisposing feature.[35,45] Others suggest that selective IgA deficiency may be a contributing variable.[21] Clinically, these children experience repeated episodes of fever, pain, and unilateral swelling of the parotid gland. Purulent material can be expressed from the Stensen duct and, when cultured, often yields streptococcal organisms. Sialography and ultrasound reveal multiple areas of sialectasis throughout the parotid glands bilaterally, even if only one side is symptomatic. The frequency of attacks varies, and each episode of parotitis may last 2 weeks, when it resolves spontaneously.[11] Several authors have noted that recurrences become less frequent with increasing age and that the disease tends to cease at the onset of puberty or early adulthood.[19,44]

HUMAN IMMUNODEFICIENCY VIRUS AND PAROTID ENLARGEMENT

Salivary gland enlargement has been recognized as a common finding in children infected with HIV since before the era of highly active antiretroviral therapy (HAART).[36] The prevalence of this manifestation in HIV-infected individuals is 0% to 58%.[48] More recently, in a retrospective report of oral lesions in a cohort of HIV-infected children from Brazil, Miziara and colleagues[42] noted the prevalence of parotid gland enlargement to be 7.6%. Although parotid enlargement occurred more commonly in children older than 5 years of age, the prevalence did not differ between children who were receiving antiretroviral therapy without protease inhibitors and children who were receiving HAART.

The exact pathophysiology is unknown, but proposed mechanisms include lymphoepithelial cysts, lymph node enlargement within the gland, cytomegalovirus or Epstein-Barr virus infection, and diffuse infiltrative lymphocytosis syndrome of the gland.[48] This entity in HIV-positive children possibly is associated with the HLA-DR5 and HLA-DR11 phenotypes, but the significance of this finding is unclear.[29,48,57] Bilateral parotid enlargement frequently is seen as part of diffuse infiltrative lymphocytosis syndrome, which is characterized by proliferation of $CD8^+$ lymphocytes within the circulation and is of unclear etiology. Growth of the parotid is secondary to infiltration of CD8 lymphocytes into the gland, follicular hyperplasia of intraparotid lymphoid tissue (as occurs in lymph nodes throughout the body in HIV infection), and development of diffuse intraparotid, lymphoepithelial cysts.[9,39] Epstein-Barr virus has been proposed as an impetus for CD8 lymphoproliferation because the virus has been isolated from parotid tissue of some affected patients.[10] The absence of positive serology for the virus renders it an unlikely causative agent, however. HIV, which may be the inciting agent, has been detected in dendritic cells, macrophages, and lymphocytes isolated from the parotid glands of affected patients.[10]

Parotid enlargement may be present in 20% to 50% of children with HIV infection and acquired immunodeficiency syndrome (AIDS).[31,35,56,59] The median time from birth to development of parotid enlargement is 4.6 years, and often it is the first manifestation of HIV infection acquired during the perinatal period in an otherwise healthy older child.[29,31,36] HIV-positive children with enlarged parotid glands tend to have a slower progression to death than do HIV-positive children with oral herpes or candidiasis.[31] Usually, both parotid glands are involved, and an affected patient presents with enlarged, tender parotid glands, xerostomia, and increased serum amylase level.[8] Severity of pain and size of the gland tend to fluctuate without apparent cause. This manifestation of HIV infection and AIDS is still commonly seen in developing countries where access to antiretroviral therapy is limited.

The differential diagnoses for parotid enlargement in an HIV-positive patient include viral and bacterial parotitis. Some patients have preexisting xerostomia that may increase their susceptibility to parotitis. In addition, the immunocompromised state of patients with AIDS may predispose them to development of infection of the parotid gland with other agents, such as cytomegalovirus, Epstein-Barr virus, bacteria, mycobacteria, and fungi.[25,53,60,63] Noninfectious etiologies, such as non-Hodgkin lymphoma or Kaposi sarcoma, also should be included in the differential diagnosis of parotid gland enlargement in an HIV-infected patient, although these manifestations usually are observed in adults.

DIFFERENTIAL DIAGNOSIS

Parotitis most often is diagnosed based on clinical presentation, microbiology, serology, and response to empiric therapy. Ultrasound may be useful as a screening tool to prompt more sensitive modalities if the ultrasound scan is abnormal.[43] Computed tomography is most useful in the presence of anatomic defects, radiolucent calculi, or abscess formation in the parotid gland.[52] X-ray sialography is the gold standard in examining the parotid gland ducts; however, sialography is contraindicated in the setting of acute infection. Magnetic resonance sialography is a promising alternative and has several advantages. In contrast to x-ray sialography, magnetic resonance sialography is not contraindicated during acute parotitis and does not require injection of contrast material or involve manipulation of the Stensen duct.[22] Nonetheless, experience with magnetic resonance sialography is limited, and this mode alone may not be sufficiently sensitive to detect tertiary salivary ductules or calculous disease.[22,64]

Noninfectious causes of parotid swelling and inflammation include collagen vascular diseases (Sjögren syndrome and systemic lupus erythematosus), metabolic disorders (hepatic disease, hyperlipoproteinemia, and hyperuricemia), endocrine disorders (diabetes mellitus and hypothyroidism), tumors, leukemic infiltration, drugs (antineoplastic chemotherapy), and poisons (iodine).[38,44,49] Sjögren syndrome, the most common cause of noninfectious parotitis, is caused by lymphocyte-mediated destruction of the exocrine glands.[26,49] Patients with this disease have diminished or absent glandular secretions and mucosal dryness; xerostomia and keratoconjunctivitis sicca are prominent clinical features. In addition, the parotid glands are enlarged bilaterally, are firm, and have an irregular contour. Sialography reveals sialectasia, and saliva from these patients has unique biochemical characteristics. Antibodies to nuclear antigens SS-A and SS-B can be detected in the sera of patients with Sjögren syndrome.[49] Patients with chronic noninfectious parotitis have changes in the ductular architecture or strictures that can predispose them to episodes of infectious parotitis.

TREATMENT

Treatment of parotitis includes rehydration, parotid massage, discontinuation of any medications that diminish salivary flow, and sialagogues (e.g., lemon drops, hard candy, and chewing gum), which increase salivary flow.[3,38,49,51] In cases of suspected suppurative parotitis, a broad-spectrum antibiotic regimen that is effective against *S. aureus, Streptococcus* spp., gram-negative organisms, and anaerobes should be administered empirically, pending specific culture results. Antibiotic regimens frequently employed include penicillinase-resistant penicillins, first-generation cephalosporins, and clindamycin in combination with an aminoglycoside.[3] Vancomycin should be used if methicillin-resistant *S. aureus* (MRSA) is the likely pathogen. If the patient has been hospitalized for a prolonged period, or if the predominant organisms on Gram stain of the purulent discharge are gram-negative, ceftazidime should be considered as initial empiric therapy.[49,51]

Surgical incision and drainage of purulent fluid are indicated if there is slow or no response to medical therapy or if fluctuance increases.[55] The treatment of viral parotitis consists of antipyretics, analgesia, and hydration. In cases of mycobacterial infection, excision of the gland may be required, in addition to administration of specific antimycobacterial therapy.[46,54] Reports have described successful treatment with clarithromycin and azithromycin of parotitis caused by atypical mycobacteria.[24] In contrast, actinomycosis of the parotid gland is managed medically with penicillin G.[27] Children with recurrent parotitis should be treated with antibiotics during acute episodes, but chronic suppressive antimicrobial therapy is not recommended.

Tympanic neurectomy involves severing the parasympathetic secretomotor fibers of the tympanic plexus to the parotid. This procedure attenuates secretion from the gland and relieves sialectasis and further episodes of parotitis in more than 70% of patients.[16,47] Only 10% to 20% of these patients require parotidectomy for persistence of symptoms beyond puberty.[14] Although it is the optimal treatment for complete resolution of recurrent parotitis, parotidectomy carries a risk for facial nerve injury. Nahlieli and colleagues[45] described the use of endoscopy to diagnose and endoscopic irrigation to treat children with recurrent parotitis.

COMPLICATIONS

With improved fluid management of postsurgical patients and the use of broad-spectrum antimicrobial agents, complications secondary to infectious parotitis now are rare events. In neonates or immunocompromised patients, sepsis may be a severe complication of this infection. Abscess formation may result from delayed or ineffective therapy. Compromise of the facial nerve may occur and can resolve with successful treatment of the infected gland.[40] The most serious and rare complication is extension to other structures of the head and neck and along fascial planes to the face, external auditory canal, jugular vein, mandible, and mediastinum.

PREVENTION

Suppurative parotitis can be prevented in postsurgical patients by maintaining adequate hydration and good oral hygiene. The most common form of viral parotitis, mumps, can be prevented by appropriate vaccination. Between 1968 and 1993, a 99% reduction in the incidence of new cases of mumps occurred.[62] In the mid-1980s and more recently in 2006, a resurgence of the incidence of mumps in previously vaccinated populations was noted.[6,13,18,28] The most recent outbreaks occurred among college students and young adults in several states, raising concern of waning immunity in this highly vaccinated population.[6,18] The current recommendation is to provide two doses of live mumps vaccine for school-age children (i.e., grades kindergarten through 12) with MMR vaccine and to ensure that students in college or other post–high school educational institutions also have received two doses of MMR vaccine.[6,15,18]

NEW REFERENCE SINCE THE SEVENTH EDITION

7. Centers for Disease Control and Prevention. Update: mumps outbreak—New York and New Jersey, June 2009–January 2010. *MMWR Morb Mortal Wkly Rep.* 2010;59:125-129.

The full reference list for this chapter is available at ExpertConsult.com.

14 Rhinosinusitis

James D. Cherry • Edward C. Kuan • Nina L. Shapiro

Rhinosinusitis (commonly referred to as "sinusitis") is inflammation of the mucosal lining of one or more of the paranasal sinuses. Although inflammation of sinus mucosa most probably occurs to some degree with every upper respiratory tract infection that produces rhinitis, most of these episodes apparently have a spontaneous resolution.[106] Studies during the past 3 decades estimate that 5% to 10% of upper respiratory tract infections are complicated by acute sinusitis.[2,207,228] This rate range represents a significant increase from earlier reports,[45] possibly because of a greater awareness of the illness and improved imaging techniques. The growing number of children in daycare has led to an actual increase in the incidence of upper respiratory tract infections.[226,228] In addition, recognition that sinus infection can have a negative effect on the health of children with chronic pulmonary disease has increased interest in this disease.[123]

When considering a diagnosis of sinusitis in a child, the major problem is to distinguish simple upper respiratory tract infection or allergic inflammation from secondary bacterial infection of the sinuses.[151,181] Unless complications such as periorbital cellulitis or cavernous sinus thrombosis render the diagnosis obvious, the clinician has no reliable way to establish a diagnosis of acute sinusitis in the office setting. Sometimes symptoms and signs of sinusitis occur simultaneously with rhinitis, but most often they occur after an episode of rhinitis. Infection in the sinuses usually persists after the preceding rhinitis has resolved. Sinusitis is classified by the duration of clinical symptoms: acute (≤3 weeks), subacute (3 to 12 weeks), and chronic (>12 weeks). Available data comparing acute and subacute sinusitis are sparse; both entities may have a similar etiology, diagnosis, and prognosis; the distinction seems to be arbitrary and to have no clinical significance.

HISTORY

Purulent sinusitis and its relationship to orbital inflammation have been known for more than 2000 years.[80] Highmore, a 17th-century English physician and anatomist, is given credit for the separation of dental and antral disease.[156] Hunter indicated the importance of surgical drainage in purulent sinusitis and suggested perforating the partition between the maxillary antrum and the nose.[156] During the first half of the 20th century, sinusitis was responsible for considerable morbidity and mortality, and surgical care of sinusitis frequently was lifesaving. Since the advent of antibiotics, sinusitis has had a lower medical profile. Interest in this topic has increased, however. Some factors involved in this increased interest include the advent of the newer surgical techniques of functional endoscopic sinus surgery that yield comparable results to sinus puncture and aspiration,[204] which now have been applied to children; improved diagnostic imaging studies, especially thin-cut computed tomography (CT) imaging; and the greater social importance of upper respiratory tract infections for parents who must be absent from work to seek treatment for their children.[123]

ANATOMY

All the paranasal sinuses develop as outpouchings of the nasal cavity. Three shelflike structures—the inferior, middle, and superior turbinates—are on the lateral nasal wall. The superior turbinate is not well developed in the first year of life.[240] Beneath each turbinate is the corresponding meatus into which various drainage pathways open. Specifically, the nasolacrimal duct drains tears into the inferior meatus; the frontal, maxillary, and anterior ethmoidal sinuses drain into the middle meatus; and the sphenoidal and posterior ethmoidal cells open high in the nasal vault in the proximity of the superior meatus.[216]

The maxillary sinuses develop early in the second trimester of fetal life as lateral outpouchings in the posterior aspect of the middle meatus. They are present at birth,[7,131,174,240] with floors being barely below the attachment of the inferior turbinates.[216] They expand rapidly by the time the child is 4 years of age.[240] Ultimately, at full size, the lateral borders of the maxillary sinuses reach the lateral orbital rims. The position of the floors of the sinuses is determined by the eruption of the dentition.[216] The ostia of the maxillary sinuses are located high on the medial walls of the sinuses, which impedes gravitational drainage of secretions; ciliary activity is required to move secretions from the body of the maxillary sinuses through the ostia into the nose.[216]

The ethmoidal sinuses develop in the fourth month of gestation[216] and are present at birth.[131,174,240] They are not a single large cavity but a grouping of cells, three to 15 in number, each with its own opening or ostium. They have a honeycombed radiographic appearance and are small anteriorly and large posteriorly. The walls of the ethmoidal labyrinth, especially the lateral walls bordering on the orbits (and forming its medial walls), are thin and referred to as the *lamina papyracea*.[216]

Development of the frontal sinuses is variable. In adults, 80% have bilateral frontal sinuses, 1% to 4% have agenesis of the frontal sinuses, and the remainder have unilateral hypoplasia. The position of the frontal sinuses is supraorbital after the child reaches 4 years of age, but they are not distinguished radiographically from the ethmoidal sinuses until the child is 6 to 8 years old. The frontal sinuses do not reach adult size for another 8 to 10 years.[216]

The onset of development of the sphenoidal sinuses occurs during the child's first 2 years of life, but they remain rudimentary until the child is approximately 6 years of age. They have reached their permanent size, although not their permanent shape, by the time the child is 12 years old.[240]

Although the full development of the sinuses may take 20 years, by the time the child is 12 years old the nasal cavity and the paranasal sinuses have nearly completed their development and have reached adult proportions.[240] Sinus disease in postpubertal adolescents is similar to that in adults.

The mucosal lining of all the paranasal sinuses is composed of ciliated columnar epithelium and goblet cells.[177] It is continuous and similar to the lining of the nasal cavity except that the mucosa in the nose is thicker and contains more glands. The epithelium of all the paranasal sinuses and nasal cavity is covered in part by a blanket of mucus.

PATHOPHYSIOLOGY

The pathogenesis of sinus infection undoubtedly is similar to that of otitis media.[222] The middle ear, with its extension, the eustachian tube, and the paranasal sinuses normally are sterile, but their contiguous areas (nasopharynx and nose) have a dynamic microbial flora. Under normal conditions, ciliary function with mucus flow can be expected to keep the sinuses clear of pathogens. The cilia within the sinuses propel the mucus toward their respective ostia and, from there, nasociliary action moves the mucus blanket posteriorly toward the pharynx. Insults that damage the ciliary epithelium and affect the morphology, number, and function of cilia and insults that alter the production or viscosity of the mucus blanket lead to obstruction of the flow of mucus, however, which allows the inoculation of numerous microorganisms into the sinuses that can lead to infection. In a study in adults in whom sneezing, coughing, and nose blowing were stimulated or initiated voluntarily, intranasal pressures were measured, and the deposition of contrast medium (which before the initiation of the event had been inoculated into the nasopharynx) was determined by CT.[74] Results of this study showed that nose blowing introduced viscous fluid into the maxillary sinuses, whereas coughing or sneezing did not generate enough pressure to propel fluid into the sinuses. When instituted, sinus infection is complicated further by inflammatory obstruction of the ostium leading to the nose.

The most important factor leading to purulent sinus infection in children and in adults is upper respiratory tract viral infection.[24,52,123,228] Wald and colleagues[228] in a large prospective study involving children younger than 3 years of age showed a doubling of the rate of sinusitis (defined as upper respiratory tract symptoms persisting >15 days) among children in a daycare setting compared with children not in daycare. The differences presumably were due to increased exposure to viral respiratory illnesses. Radiographic studies in children with acute colds regularly indicate abnormalities of the maxillary sinuses, suggesting that the infection involves these areas.[126] These asymptomatic sinus opacifications may persist for 2 weeks after the symptoms of the upper respiratory tract illness have resolved.[49,104,216] Viral infection that involves the sinuses rarely is differentiated from its primary manifestations, such as the common cold, nasopharyngitis, and influenza, and recovery is the rule. If the effect of the viral infection on the mucosal surface is severe and is associated with the inoculation of one or more pathogenic bacterial agents and obstruction of an ostium, disease occurs.

The mechanisms by which upper respiratory tract viral infections set the stage for secondary bacterial infection in the sinuses are complex. Using in situ hybridization, rhinovirus RNA was shown inside epithelial cells of maxillary sinus in 50% of a small number of adults with acute sinusitis.[153] This finding is remarkable because in experimental rhinovirus infections, only a small percentage of nasal epithelial cells were noted to contain rhinovirus RNA.[8] These differences may reflect only differences in inoculum between experimental and natural infection, but they may indicate heavier infection in the sinuses than in the nose. Symptoms in upper respiratory tract viral infections are not caused by extensive damage to ciliated nasal epithelium but rather to aspects of the host response (see Chapter 7).[8,75,138,140,149,157,158,239]

Other irritants can set the stage for sinus infection. Swimming in ocean, lake, or chlorinated pool water can lead to sinus involvement. Drying of the nasal mucosa, which occurs commonly during the winter in cold climates, may be a precipitating factor.

Dental infections or extractions also can lead to maxillary sinusitis if the tooth root is adjacent to, or sometimes penetrating, the maxillary sinus floor.[39] Sudden change in pressure, as with diving or during descent in an airplane, physically can overcome local mucociliary defense mechanisms and lead to the sudden onset of acute sinusitis.[137]

A number of host factors and perhaps microbiologic factors are associated with recurrent and chronic sinusitis.*

Recurrent chronic sinusitis implies a problem with local mucociliary defense, a defect in systemic immunity, or a fixed anatomic sinus obstruction. Often, the predisposing factors work in tandem, as in a child with a septal deformity and a viral illness.[123] In chronic sinusitis, the mucosa is thickened, and marked edema, vessel dilation, and infiltration of inflammatory cells are present.[205] Goblet cells are decreased in density, and seromucous glands are increased in density compared with their presence in normal sinuses.

Children with respiratory allergies are prone to sinusitis,[60,112,162,161,163] and allergy is the second most prevalent predisposing factor in childhood sinusitis, acting through mucosal congestion and perhaps depressing local and systemic immune responses.[114,169] The treatment of respiratory allergies may contribute to sinusitis because ciliary damage occurring after the administration of nasal decongestants has been shown in organ culture and animal studies.[44,45,124] Richards and colleagues[169] reported a diagnosis of atopy in 62% of a selected cohort of pediatric patients who had documented recurrent sinusitis and were referred to allergy clinics in Los Angeles.

Defects of ciliary function, such as those occurring in cystic fibrosis, immotile cilia syndrome, and Kartagener syndrome, predispose a child to chronic sinusitis.[54,89,100,163,174,192] Refractory sinusitis also occurs commonly in children with primary and acquired immunodeficiency diseases.[33,123,135,175,186,208,219] Immunocompromised children undergoing treatment for malignancies and organ transplantations constitute a growing population with a potential for developing sinusitis that is difficult to manage. Finally, anatomic obstruction caused by septal and turbinate deformities, craniofacial anomalies, foreign bodies, adenoidal hypertrophy, or nasal masses or polyps predisposes children to sinusitis. Nasal polyps in young children usually are not caused by allergies and should be an indication for evaluation for cystic fibrosis.[123] In addition, biofilms may play an important role in chronic sinusitis and are thought to produce persistent disease despite maximal medical and surgical therapy.[137,185]

Immunologic mechanisms are important in the pathogenesis of sinus infections, as indicated by the high prevalence of chronic sinus infections in children with immunodeficiencies.[33,36,123,135,175,186,190,208] Sinonasal mucus contains IgA, IgG, IgM, and lysozymes.[28,173] Secretory IgA, which is produced locally, is the predominant immunoglobulin in nasal mucus.[78] IgG antibodies in nasal mucus result from passive leakage from plasma cells in the epithelium and submucosa and from the serum.[19] Generally, with the patient's increasing age and as a result of previous exposures, these immunoglobulins develop species-specific and type-specific antibodies that block epithelial colonization by specific microorganisms.

Shapiro and associates[186] studied 61 children with refractory sinusitis and found that 34 had abnormal immunologic studies. Abnormal findings included poor response to pneumococcal type 7 antigen after immunization, IgG3 subclass deficiency, low serum IgA or IgG values, and elevated serum IgE values.

ETIOLOGY

Table 14.1 lists etiologic agents of sinusitis by age of patient and type of illness. In all age groups and in acute, subacute, and chronic disease, *Haemophilus influenzae* and *Streptococcus pneumoniae* are the principal pathogens in most cases. Also, a large number of different bacterial species have been recovered from the sinuses of affected patients. In young children, more than 90% of all cases of sinusitis are caused by five organisms: *H. influenzae, S. pneumoniae, Moraxella catarrhalis, Staphylococcus aureus,* and *Streptococcus pyogenes.* Concern has been raised as to whether *S. aureus* is a cause of sinusitis in children.[223] This concern is based on the fact that *S. aureus* is common in the noses of all children, and therefore there is likely contamination at the time of maxillary sinus puncture or endoscopic surgery. Similar concern should also be raised regarding α-hemolytic streptococci, coagulase-negative *Staphylococcus,* and various anaerobes because they also are part of the nasal flora. In adolescents, the same organisms, plus largely penicillin-sensitive anaerobes, account for most cases. As noted in Table 14.1, a variety of gram-negative enteric and other bacilli have been recovered from patients with sinusitis, in most instances from patients who have had various forms of antibiotic therapy before culture. Organisms previously considered to be nonpathogens, such as *Staphylococcus epidermidis,* have been implicated etiologically.

Although clinically recognized sinusitis has occurred rarely in patients with *Mycoplasma pneumoniae* infection, Griffin and Klein[69] noted radiographic evidence of sinusitis in approximately two-thirds of a group of U.S. Navy recruits with *M. pneumoniae* pneumonia. In adults with chronic suppurative maxillary sinusitis, mycoplasmas have been sought but not recovered.[16,67,199] Bhattacharyya and colleagues[16] noted L-forms in 21% of all sinuses in patients with chronic disease.

In a study of 25 adults with chronic rhinosinusitis, *Chlamydophila pneumoniae* was recovered from nasopharyngeal samples in 2 patients but not from any of 10 healthy controls.[53] In addition, the patients were more likely than control subjects (20%) to have serum IgG antibody titers to *C. pneumoniae* of 1:64 or greater (72%). IgA antibody titers to *C. pneumoniae* of 1:32 or greater also were more prevalent in the patients (48%) than in the controls (10%). In a study involving 20 children with chronic sinusitis, Cultrara and colleagues[38] cultured material from 13 bilateral endoscopic ethmoidectomies with maxillary antrostomies, 10 adenoidectomies, and 3 bilateral maxillary sinus lavages. They isolated *C. pneumoniae* from a nasopharyngeal swab and adenoid tissue from a 6-year-old child.

*References 13, 33, 36, 49, 50, 54, 60, 89, 100, 112, 123, 133, 135, 148, 161, 163, 169, 174, 175, 184, 186, 190, 192, 201, 205, 208, 219, 245.

TABLE 14.1 Etiologic Agents in Sinusitis Analyzed by Patient Age and Type of Illness

	FREQUENCY				AGE GROUP (Y)		
	Overall	**Acute**	**Subacute**	**Chronic**	**≤5**	**6–12**	**>12**
Aerobic Bacteria							
Haemophilus influenzae	++++	++++	++++	++++	++++	++++	++++
Streptococcus pneumoniae	++++	++++	++++	++++	++++	++++	++++
Moraxella catarrhalis	+++	+++	++	+	+++	+	++
Staphylococcus aureus	++	+	+	++	++	++	++
Streptococcus pyogenes	++	++	++	++	+	++	++
α-Hemolytic and nonhemolytic streptococci	+		+	+			++
Staphylococcus epidermidis	+		+	+		+	++
Alcaligenes spp.	+			+			++
Escherichia coli	+			+			++
Klebsiella pneumoniae	+			+			++
Pseudomonas aeruginosa	+			+			++
Other[a]	+			+			++
Anaerobic Bacteria							
Peptostreptococcus spp.	++	+	+	+++		+	++
Prevotella and Porphyromonas spp.	++			++		+	++
Fusobacterium spp.	++			++			
Propionibacterium spp.	++			++			
Bifidobacterium spp.	+			+			
Bacteroides fragilis	+	+	+	+			+
Veillonella spp.	+	+	+	+			+
Fungi							
Scopulariopsis spp.	+			+			+
Aspergillus spp.	+	+		+	+	++	++
Alternaria spp.	+	+		+	+	+	+
Penicillium spp.	+			+	+	+	+
Curvularia spp.	+		+	+	+	+	+
Drechslera spp.	+			+	+	+	+
Bipolaris spp.	+			+	+	+	+
Mucor spp. and other Zygomycetes	+	+		+	+	+	+
Candida spp.	+			+			+
Mycoplasma and Chlamydophila							
Mycoplasma pneumoniae	+	+					+
Chlamydophila pneumoniae[b]				+	+	+	+
Other							
L-forms	+			+			++
Mixed aerobes and anaerobes	++	+	+	++			++
Mixed *Haemophilus influenzae* with other organisms	++	+	+	++		+	++
Rhinovirus, adenovirus, cytomegalovirus	+	+		+		+	+

[a]*Serratia* spp., diphtheroids, *Enterococcus* spp., *Neisseria* spp., *Haemophilus* spp., *Proteus* spp., *Acinetobacter* spp., *Citrobacter* spp., *Eikenella corrodens, Arcanobacterium haemolyticum.*
[b]Formerly *Chlamydia pneumoniae.*
Data from references 9, 16, 21–23, 27, 30, 33, 38, 51, 53, 57, 58, 66, 67, 90, 96, 97, 101, 105, 114, 115, 121, 132, 145, 163, 165, 211, 214, 215, 225, 229, 230, 237.

Fungal diseases of the sinuses have been well described in adults.[233] *Aspergillus* spp. are the most common fungal causes of sinusitis. Many cases of chronic sinusitis from which a microorganism is not recovered have been thought to be caused by *Aspergillus* spp. infections.[99] The presence of eosinophils, Charcot-Leyden crystals, and hyphae found retrospectively, and not noted on the original examination, in mucus recovered from sinuses suggests that some cases of chronic sinusitis may represent *Aspergillus* hypersensitivity. This allergic aspergillosis in the sinuses is similar to allergic bronchopulmonary aspergillosis. In a series of six patients who were 8 to 16 years of age and had allergic aspergillosis sinusitis, all presented with nasal polyposis and facial deformity, indicating advanced disease.[125] Acute fulminant fungal sinusitis, such as mucormycosis, which is caused by Zygomycetes (formerly Phycomycetes), is seen in immunosuppressed individuals and is associated with high morbidity and mortality rates.[42,95,196] *Drechslera* spp., *Bipolaris* spp., *Scopulariopsis* spp., *Candida* spp., and *Curvalaria lunata* can cause sinusitis in children.[15,27,58,66,115,194]

Although sinusitis has been reported as a complication of Epstein-Barr virus infection, the sinus infections seem to be a complication of corticosteroid treatment and not specifically the viral infection.[63] *Nocardia* spp. have been reported as a cause of acute sinusitis in an adult transplant recipient[170] and of chronic sinusitis in immunocompetent and immunocompromised individuals.[210]

EPIDEMIOLOGY

Although sinus involvement occurs commonly with viral infection of the respiratory tract, sinusitis seldom is identified as a specific illness in previously healthy children. In a survey of a total of 2613 office visits, Breese and colleagues[20] noted only six children (0.23%) in whom the initial diagnosis was sinusitis. The true incidence of sinusitis in childhood is unknown. In 1989, Wald and colleagues[225] estimated that 0.5% to 5% of upper respiratory tract infections are complicated by acute sinusitis. More recent estimates by the same authors have been 10%.[228] The most recent estimates of greater incidence could be related to a heightened awareness and concern for lost work days by working parents, a possible correlation between pulmonary problems in an increasing number of children with chronic lung disease, better imaging techniques, increased interest in endoscopic sinus surgery,[204] more disease because of more exposure as a result of more children being in daycare,[123] and an increased recognition or perhaps incidence of allergy-related illness.[168,169] Seasonal prevalence has not been studied, but a reasonable assumption is that disease would increase during the cold weather months because it is the time of greatest respiratory viral activity. Cases in older children also can be expected to occur more frequently in association with swimming.

Shapiro and colleagues[185] used data from the National Ambulatory Medical Case Survey and National Hospital Ambulatory Medical Case Survey between 1998 and 2007 and found that the annual visit rate for acute sinusitis for children younger than 18 years of age ranged between 11 and 14 visits per 1000.

Although it is not well documented, sinusitis seems to be more of a problem in geographic areas where marked temperature changes occur. In children, sinusitis seems to occur more commonly in boys than in girls.[81,131] Ueda and Yoto[207] found abnormal findings in the maxillary sinuses in 135 (6.7%) of 2013 children who presented to an outpatient department with upper respiratory symptoms; of this group, 65% were boys and 35% were girls. Manning and associates[124] found similar distribution in a group of 60 children diagnosed by CT or magnetic resonance imaging (MRI). Host factors are important in sinusitis because the illness occurs more commonly in allergic children; in children with chronic ear infections; and in patients with cystic fibrosis, primary humoral immunodeficiencies, and Kartagener syndrome.[25,89,139,174] Although an association between sinus disease and asthma exists, controversy continues regarding whether sinusitis and other upper airway stimuli can induce asthma.[59,169,180,243] A review of hospital admissions of patients with status asthmaticus at the Children's Hospital of Los Angeles showed a marked increase in admissions, and sinusitis was diagnosed in 23%.[168]

Sinusitis is noncontagious from person to person, but point-source outbreaks are possible from swimming in heavily contaminated water. A cluster of seven cases of invasive nosocomial fungal sinusitis in severely neutropenic patients has been described. It was caused by the release of airborne fungal spores from soil reservoirs that were distributed during hospital construction during a 2-year period.[117]

TABLE 14.2 Clinical Findings in Acute, Subacute, and Chronic Sinusitis in Children

	OCCURRENCE (%)	
	Acute and Subacute	**Chronic**
Symptoms		
Fever	50	20
Rhinorrhea	80	80
Cough (persistent and evening)	50	90
Pain/headache	30	30
Sore throat	20	20
Periorbital swelling	30	0
Vomiting	20	10
Allergic history	20	40
Malodorous breath	20	20
Signs		
Rhinorrhea	80	80
Temperature ≥38.3°C (≥101°F)	20	0
Sinus tenderness	20	10
Otitis media	40	60
Posterior pharyngeal pus	0	10
Transillumination positive	30	10
Periorbital swelling	30	0
Malodorous breath	20	20
Laboratory Findings		
Abnormal radiographs	100	100
Maxillary	90	90
Ethmoidal	40	40
Frontal and sphenoidal	10	10
Unilateral	70	10
Bilateral	30	90
Erythrocyte sedimentation rate elevation	50	10
White blood cell count elevation with an increased percentage of band form neutrophils	40	10

Data from references 3, 11, 81, 85, 94, 100, 103, 131, 139, 169, 174, 198, 220, 231.

CLINICAL PRESENTATION

The clinical symptoms of sinusitis vary by age. Older children and adolescents have localized complaints similar to those of adults, whereas in young children the findings are related less clearly to the sinuses.[217] The overall frequencies of symptoms, signs, and laboratory findings for acute, subacute, and chronic disease are presented in Table 14.2.

In young children, disease involves only the ethmoidal and maxillary sinuses. In these children, illness frequently has its onset after they have had an upper respiratory tract viral infection. A period of general improvement may occur, however, between the acute respiratory illness and the onset of symptoms related to sinus infection. The most prominent symptom in all children, and particularly in children younger than 10 years of age, is persistent rhinorrhea. The discharge frequently is purulent, but it occasionally can be serous or watery. Associated with rhinorrhea is cough, which becomes more prominent with increasing duration of disease. The cough particularly is troublesome at night because it is caused by the stimulation of the sinus drainage as it traverses the pharyngeal wall. The posterior drainage also occasionally causes vomiting. Fever is a variable occurrence in sinusitis and generally is related inversely to age and duration of illness. Malodorous breath often is reported by parents. The first evidence of illness in some children is fever and periorbital swelling. In most instances, periorbital cellulitis is a manifestation of ethmoidal sinusitis.

Although facial pain and headache are frequent complaints of sinus disease in adults, they have been noted in only approximately one-third of the cases in children and are unusual occurrences in young children. The main symptom in older children and adolescents is rhinorrhea. In older patients with more chronic disease, the nasal symptoms may be minimal or absent. Troublesome postnasal drip is a frequent complaint.

Acute isolated sphenoidal sinusitis in children is rare but often misdiagnosed because the symptoms are vague and there are no specific physical findings.[26,127] Findings include fever, headache, postnasal drip, and neurologic symptoms. Swimming and diving are possible predisposing factors.

Physical signs in sinusitis also differ by age. Nasal discharge is the most frequent finding in all age groups. Young children are more likely to have a serous or watery discharge, however, than are adolescents. Elevation of temperature occurs more commonly in acute disease and in association with orbital cellulitis. Sinus tenderness, a common finding in older patients, is noted only rarely in children. Particularly significant is tenderness with percussion of the upper molars. Examination of the throat frequently reveals free exudate. Occasionally the breath is malodorous.

The ears are abnormal in almost half of all patients with sinusitis. In acute disease in young children, it can be acute otitis media, but usually the findings are more suggestive of serous disease. Acute sinusitis frequently is unilateral, whereas chronic disease more often is bilateral.

Children with chronic sinusitis frequently have only minimal complaints. The parent notes that the child does not feel well and frequently reports that the child has had a persistent respiratory tract infection for months. In a series of children with chronic (>3 months) upper respiratory tract complaints who were referred to allergy clinics, 60% had sinusitis.[139] In this study, the combination of moderate to severe rhinorrhea and cough with minimal sneezing was reported to have a specificity of 95% and a sensitivity of 38% in predicting the presence of chronic sinusitis. In the referred children in this study, sinusitis was found in 63% of atopic children and in 75% of nonatopic children.

Laboratory studies other than cultures and radiography are not useful in the evaluation of a child with sinusitis. Herz and Gfeller[85] noted that in their study erythrocyte sedimentation rates were elevated in only approximately half of the patients, and leukocytosis occurred in only one-third. Generally, younger children with orbital cellulitis and ethmoidal sinusitis are more likely to have elevated sedimentation rates and white blood cell counts. The American Academy of Pediatrics (AAP) Subcommittee of Sinusitis and Committee on Quality Improvement has recommended that the diagnosis of acute bacterial sinusitis be based on clinical criteria in children who present with upper respiratory symptoms that are either persistent (nasal or postnasal discharge of any quality with or without daytime cough for >10 to 14 days) or severe (temperature >39°C [102.2°F] and purulent nasal discharge present concurrently for at least 3 or 4 consecutive days in a child who appears ill).[5]

COMPLICATIONS

Serious complications, including meningitis, osteomyelitis, cavernous sinus thrombosis, and epidural, subdural, brain, and orbital abscesses, occur in untreated sinusitis.* Ethmoidal sinusitis tends to present with orbital complications, while frontal sinusitis tends to produce intracranial complications. Classically, orbital complications of sinusitis follow a progression described by Chandler, evolving in the order of periorbital/preseptal cellulitis, orbital cellulitis, subperiosteal abscess, orbital abscess, and cavernous sinus thrombosis.[32] Clinically, these complications can present in any order or skip stepwise progression. Signs and symptoms of neurologic involvement in sinusitis frequently call for aggressive surgical management of the sinusitis and the intracranial and paracranial lesions. Osteomyelitis of the frontal bone may be a complication of frontal sinusitis and may manifest as a Pott puffy tumor if a subperiosteal abscess also is present.

DIFFERENTIAL DIAGNOSIS

Differential considerations in sinusitis are few and are more concerned with whether sinus involvement in a particular child is the primary event or a secondary problem related to a more general host defect. Children with recurrent and chronic sinusitis should be evaluated for respiratory allergy, cystic fibrosis, immunologic deficiency, and Kartagener and other immotile cilia syndromes.

Foreign bodies in the nose can be mistaken for sinusitis, as can cysts in the maxillary antra. Nasal structural defects (congenital and acquired), such as palatal clefts, unilateral choanal atresia, nasal polyps, and septal deviation, can be confused with sinusitis, but more commonly these problems are predisposing factors in sinus infections.

Dental infections frequently are mistaken for maxillary sinus disease. Dental infections can lead by direct extension to sinus involvement. Primary infections in the region of the eye also occur without sinus disease. In young children, a chronic infection of the adenoids can be confused clinically with sinusitis. Infections with *Bordetella pertussis* can be confused with subacute sinusitis.

SPECIFIC DIAGNOSIS

Although persistent nasal symptoms and the presence of other clinical findings as listed in Table 14.2 indicate a diagnosis of sinusitis, the only certain way to make the diagnosis is by obtaining radiographs and cultures reflecting sinus content. Although it has been suggested that maxillary sinus radiographs frequently are abnormal for normal children,[126,191] other data indicate that normal children older than 1 year of age seldom have abnormal radiographs.[104] During infancy, the maxillary sinuses are so small that minimal mucosal edema may "opacify" a sinus on a radiograph. Radiographs in acute upper respiratory viral infections as a rule are abnormal; these radiographs are not false-positive ones but are the result of viral infections. From a therapeutic point of view, sinus radiographs usually should not be obtained unless nasal symptoms in an upper respiratory tract illness have not shown signs of improvement after 5 to 7 days.[6]

Plain film radiographic examination has been supplanted mainly by CT and MRI for the diagnosis of sinusitis. Many endoscopic sinus surgeons consider CT to be a mandatory part of the preoperative evaluation. MRI is useful in cases that may be complicated by orbital or intracranial extension. The high prevalence of incidental sinus opacification in asymptomatic infants and children noted radiographically has been confirmed by CT studies.[44,64,87] Since the advent of MRI, researchers have realized that many incidental sinus abnormalities also occur in adults. These findings in children and adults may be from subclinical or resolving respiratory infections or may be due to unrecognized allergies.[44]

CT has been recognized widely as the standard for the diagnosis of paranasal sinus disease.[14] In particular, coronal thin-section images offer excellent delineation of lesions in the osteomeatal complex.[244] Obtaining axial images is useful for evaluating periorbital and intraorbital complications.[56] In some institutions, a so-called screening CT of the sinuses is performed with a limited number of slices.[72] It can be offered at a cost and radiation exposure that are similar to those associated with plain film studies but with much greater accuracy. Some young children and infants require sedation for CT, which limits its suitability.

The AAP Subcommittee of Sinusitis and Committee on Quality Improvement has recommended that imaging studies are not necessary to confirm a diagnosis of clinical sinusitis in children aged 1 to 18 years.[5,224] The need for radiographic evidence as a confirmatory test in children older than 6 years with severe symptoms is controversial. The American College of Radiology considers that the diagnosis of acute uncomplicated sinusitis should be made only on clinical grounds.[129]

Which radiographic technique (plain radiography, CT, or MRI) is selected for evaluation of a child with presumed sinusitis should be determined by availability of techniques and the expertise of the radiologist and by clinical symptoms. Radiography is indicated for children with continuing symptoms of sinusitis after extensive medical therapy or for children with possible complications of sinusitis. CT is optimal.[6,224] A limited CT scan with axial cuts may be obtained. It allows for excellent visualization of sinus anatomy and pathology while limiting the radiation exposure to the child. A limited sinus CT scan has radiation similar to that of a sinus plain film series. In the absence of low-cost screening CT, plain radiography should be the initial imaging study in most children who have symptoms of sinus disease.[43] Children who have periorbital swelling or proptosis should undergo immediate contrast-enhanced CT studies in axial and coronal planes. If symptoms or CT findings suggest intracranial extension, MRI should be performed.[6,43]

Although ultrasonography would seem to offer an alternative to sinus radiography, some question remains about its dependability unless one normal air-filled maxillary sinus or one opacified maxillary sinus is present for comparison.[215,222] The hallmark of specific diagnosis in sinusitis is similar to that of other infectious diseases—the culture of infected material.

The definitive method for culture requires puncture of the sinus cavity. As noted in the section on etiology, false-positive findings may occur because of contamination by the nasal flora. Nevertheless, sinus puncture and drainage are imperative in immunocompromised patients who may have fungal or other life-threatening infections. Sinus puncture for culture is not necessary for children who have uncomplicated sinus infections. However, evidence of etiology can be obtained by bacterial culture from the nose at the level of the maxillary ostium in the middle meatus. Although many experts do not believe in the usefulness of this procedure, there is considerable evidence to support the culture findings

*References 1, 17, 40, 62, 63, 76, 86, 102, 108, 128, 134, 143, 144, 147, 150, 160, 176, 179, 187, 197, 206, 234, 236.

and etiology. Although the normal flora of the nasopharynx often contains the most common causes of sinusitis (i.e., *S. pneumoniae, H. influenzae, M. catarrhalis,* and *S. pyogenes*), the anterior nose does not.* Therefore we believe that properly performed nasal cultures will reveal the causative organism in many instances. This is particularly useful in the recovery of *S. pneumoniae,* which may be resistant to usual antimicrobial treatment.

Nasal culture should be taken from the region of the maxillary ostium in the middle meatus. Culture specimens should be obtained from this area and not from the nasopharynx. Best results are obtained when a vasoconstrictor, such as 0.25% phenylephrine hydrochloride, is administered first and the culture specimen is obtained with a cotton-tipped wire swab under direct vision. With this technique, material frequently can be obtained as it comes from the sinus ostium. Bilateral cultures always should be obtained. In serious cases, such as in children with neurologic complications or in treatment failures, performing antral puncture for culture can be lifesaving. Anaerobic and aerobic cultures should be performed on any material recovered by antral puncture.

TREATMENT

Acute and Subacute Sinusitis

The successful treatment of acute and subacute sinusitis in children depends primarily on the administration of an appropriate antibiotic in adequate dosage for a sufficient period.[5,34,41,151,221,224,227] In most instances, therapy should be instituted before obtaining the results of cultures. Antibiotic selection in this situation is not a great problem in children because the etiologic agent is *H. influenzae, S. pneumoniae, M. catarrhalis, S. aureus,* or *S. pyogenes* in more than 90% of acute cases. Respiratory anaerobes are rarely the cause of acute bacterial sinusitis in children.[224]

Initial selection of an antibiotic should be based on the severity of the clinical illness and must take into consideration the antibiotic resistance patterns of the common causative organisms and the cost and ease of administration of the treatment regimen. Today, between 10% and 42% of nontypeable *H. influenzae* and close to 100% of *M. catarrhalis* strains produce β-lactamases and are resistant to amoxicillin.[46,47,224] In addition, 15% to 38% of *S. pneumoniae* strains have either intermediate (7–19%) or complete (5–19%) penicillin resistance.[12,29,48,224]

In 2012, the Infectious Diseases Society of America (IDSA) published its clinical practice guidelines for acute bacteria rhinosinusitis,[34] and in 2015, the AAP updated its guidelines for acute bacterial sinusitis in children.[224] These two guidelines often present challenges in pediatric practice because of the overemphasis of their "guideline definitions for evidence based statements." The current AAP committee recommendations are very similar to the recommendations in 2001.[5,224] The AAP committee states that "amoxicillin remains the antimicrobial agent of choice for first-line treatment of uncomplicated acute bacterial sinusitis in situations in which antimicrobial resistance is not suspected." The dose recommended is 45 mg/kg/day in two divided doses. In communities with a high prevalence of nonsusceptible *S. pneumoniae,* an amoxicillin dose of 80 to 90 mg/kg per day in two divided doses is suggested.

The committee qualifies the preceding recommendations for children with moderate to severe illness, children younger than 2 years of age, children attending daycare, and children who had recently been treated with an antimicrobial agent. For this group, high-dose amoxicillin-clavulanate (80 to 90 mg/kg per day of the amoxicillin component and 6.4 mg/kg per day of clavulanate in two divided doses with a maximum of 2 g per dose).[224]

For children who are vomiting, who are unable to tolerate oral medication, or where adherence to the oral regime could be a problem, a single 50 mg/kg dose of ceftriaxone (either IV or IM) is suggested.[224]

In contrast with the AAP committee guidelines, the IDSA suggests that amoxicillin-clavulanate rather than amoxicillin alone be the empiric antimicrobial therapy for acute bacterial sinusitis in the children.[34]

*References 18, 52, 61, 68, 77, 79, 80, 82, 88, 89, 92, 93, 97, 121, 131, 142, 188, 211, 214, 215, 225, 229, 230, 235, 241.

In contrast to the AAP committees' recommendations, we consider that an approach as noted by the IDSA, to use amoxicillin-clavulanate 90 mg/kg per day in two divided doses, would be more suitable.[5,34,224] The duration of treatment in the outpatient setting has not been studied adequately. Wald[220] suggests that therapy should be continued for 7 days after the child becomes symptom free.

The AAP committee carefully looked at treatment for children who have a history of "penicillin allergy."[224] It is noted that the risk of a serious reaction to a second- or third-generation cephalosporin in a child with reported penicillin allergy is almost nil. Therefore it is suggested that these patients can be safely treated with cefdinir, cefuroxime, or cefpodoxime. It is also suggested that a child who had a past type 1 immediate or accelerated (anaphylactoid) reaction to amoxicillin can also safely be treated with the same cephalosporins. However, they indicated that the clinician may want to seek consultation with an allergist in the latter situation.

A seriously ill child should be hospitalized, and therapy for β-lactamase–producing staphylococci and highly resistant pneumococci should be implemented in addition to coverage for amoxicillin-resistant *H. influenzae* and *M. catarrhalis.* This coverage is achieved with vancomycin 40 mg/kg per 24 hours every 6 hours and cefotaxime 100 to 200 mg/kg per 24 hours every 6 hours or ceftriaxone 100 mg/kg per 24 hours every 12 hours. Therapy should be adjusted on the basis of clinical response and culture results. The dosage and duration of antimicrobial therapy in sinusitis are crucial considerations. Penicillins penetrate the sinuses poorly.[10,55,73,95,118] The duration of therapy should be a minimum of 10 days.

The relief of obstruction at the sinus ostia and the establishment of drainage are time-honored principles of therapy. To achieve these goals, locally applied and systemically active vasoconstrictive drugs are used. To date, no evidence supports their therapeutic effectiveness, however.[182,183] The beneficial effects of oral, systemically active, vasoconstrictive drugs are hampered by the fact that their drying effect may be deleterious to the mucus blanket. Topical vasoconstrictor drugs (e.g., phenylephrine hydrochloride and oxymetazoline) are plagued by rebound vasodilation. We consider that these drugs should be used rarely in acute disease; their main use is to relieve pain caused by obstruction, and they should be used only for 2 to 3 days.

Systemic and intranasal corticosteroids have been used in acute sinusitis as monotherapy and in conjunction with antimicrobial agents.[83,213,242] Data on corticosteroid use mainly involve adult patients, and the onset of action is generally on the order of weeks. It is our opinion that corticosteroid use in acute sinusitis in children should be discouraged.

Chronic and Recurrent Sinusitis

Allergic disorders are common in chronic and recurrent sinusitis.[123,151,218] Children should be evaluated for allergy, and, when identified, specific treatment should be employed. Specific allergens and irritants should be avoided (e.g., through air filtering, removal of pets, avoidance of tobacco smoke), and pharmacologic management should be implemented.

Nasal saline irrigations (twice daily in each nostril) are useful because they liquefy secretions, dilute antigens and environmental toxins, and enhance mucociliary transport, which improves sinus drainage and ventilation.[232] Antihistamines may be useful if allergic rhinitis is a contributing factor to the chronic sinus infection. Antiinflammatory agents also may be useful. In selected cases, use of either topically applied corticosteroids or cromolyn sodium may be beneficial. Corticosteroids should be used carefully because their use occasionally can lead to superinfection in the sinuses with *Pseudomonas* spp., other highly resistant gram-negative bacilli, or fungi. For effective corticosteroid use, Wald[218] suggests using a topical decongestant first so that the corticosteroid preparation can reach the affected areas better.

In chronic or recurrent disease, antimicrobial treatment should be based on culture and sensitivity data. Specific antimicrobial agents are the same as the agents used in acute and subacute disease, but treatment should be prolonged for 3 weeks or more and for 7 days after the resolution of symptoms. In 2004, Kuhn and Swain[107] defined allergic fungal sinusitis in adults by five major criteria: (1) type I IgE-mediated hypersensitivity, (2) nasal polyps, (3) characteristic CT imaging, (4) allergic mucin within the sinuses, and (5) positive fungal smear. McClay and colleagues[130] and Campbell and associates[27] have further characterized allergic fungal sinusitis in the pediatric population. It typically presents in atopic children with recurrent sinusitis and nasal polyps. Children, when compared with adults with allergic fungal sinusitis, typically present with more facial abnormalities, including proptosis, and they present more frequently with unilateral disease or asymmetric disease. Surgical intervention is a mainstay of treatment for acute fungal sinusitis, with nearly half the patients requiring multiple procedures.[27] Allergic fungal sinusitis is typically refractory to medical management until the fungal allergic mucin is first debrided and the sinus cavities are marsupialized for postoperative irrigation.

Aspergillus and *Bipolaris* spp. and other fungal infections require prolonged therapy with an antifungal agent to which the specific agent is susceptible. Itraconazole, ketoconazole, fluconazole, and amphotericin B all have been effective in selected cases. Allergic fungal sinusitis can be treated with endoscopic sinus debridement of all fungal and polypoid disease, followed by topical and systemic corticosteroids and close follow-up, including frequent endoscopic cleaning.[37,108,109,159] Allergic aspergillosis of the sinuses can be managed with topical corticosteroids without specific antifungal therapy (see Chapter 23).

In the past, surgical therapy for sinusitis in children was of questionable benefit. Surgical therapy included diagnostic and therapeutic irrigation; permanent drainage procedures in children with complications of sinusitis and in children who had immune defects; and such procedures as adenoidectomy,[111,209] septoplasty, and turbinate reduction to relieve anatomic obstructions to improve nasal and sinus ventilation. In one uncontrolled study of children with otitis media with effusion and sinusitis, the sinusitis was improved 6 months after adenoidectomy in 56% of children, whereas only 24% of similar children who did not undergo surgery had similar improvement.[202]

Historically, creating nasoantral windows was the most common major surgical procedure for treating chronic sinusitis in children.[70,136] Long-term success with this procedure was poor, however, because of the high rate of closure of the windows. A new interest in sinus surgery has resulted from the introduction of endoscopic techniques. Several studies have found endoscopic surgery to be safe and effective.[71,110,120,154,171] Pediatric endoscopic sinus surgery now is recognized as a viable option for children with chronic recurrent sinusitis refractory to medical therapy.[31,113,164] A meta-analysis of 832 children who underwent endoscopic sinus surgery from 1986 to 1996 revealed an overall 88.4% positive outcome after surgery,[84] with a complication rate of 1.4%.[122]

The goal of functional endoscopic sinus surgery is to remove obstruction at the osteomeatal complex where the mucociliary flow from the frontal, maxillary, and ethmoidal sinuses converges.[110,171] This process results in improved drainage and restoration of normal physiologic function of the frontal, maxillary, and ethmoidal sinuses. Surgery generally involves a maxillary antrostomy, or surgical enlargement of the natural ostium of the maxillary sinus, anterior ethmoidectomy, and depending on the extent of disease, posterior ethmoidectomy as well. The sphenoid and frontal sinuses are often not yet developed in young children; surgical treatment of these sinuses should only occur if the sinus is present and if there is evidence of disease. Follow-up debridement performed 2 to 3 weeks after the initial surgery sometimes is necessary to remove crusts, blood clots, any stenting material, granulation tissue, and adhesions.[231]

In a study of 210 children with a history of chronic sinusitis for 3 months or longer, functional endoscopic sinus surgery resulted in successful outcomes in 165 (79%).[110] The follow-up period was 3 to 36 months (mean, 18 months), and all of the infections in these children had failed to respond to prior extensive medical management. In this series, no major complications occurred.

Functional endoscopic sinus surgery should be considered for children with chronic or recurrent sinusitis that has failed extensive, prolonged, and adequate medical management.[113] There have been recent advancements in image guidance for pediatric sinus surgery. Image-guided surgery was first introduced for neurosurgical procedures and was quickly adapted by otolaryngologists in the 1990s for revision sinus surgery. The indications for image-guided surgery were expanded by the American Academy of Otolaryngology–Head and Neck Surgery (AAO-HNS) to include patients with any distorted sinus anatomy, those with extensive sinonasal polyposis, pathologic processes in the frontal, posterior ethmoidal, or sphenoidal sinuses, and patients undergoing skull base surgery.[4,98,178] Image-guided surgery has not been as well studied in the pediatric population as it has in the adult population[119]; however, the largest series to date, by Postec and coworkers[155] suggests a similar utility in the pediatric population to that of the adult population. A recent literature review by Parikh and associates[146] showed that image-guided surgery can be safely utilized in children with chronic sinusitis, in those undergoing revision surgeries, and in any patient in whom the anatomy may be distorted, without increasing the rate of intraoperative complications.

Balloon catheter sinuplasty is another recent advancement in the treatment of sinus disease. This technology was first introduced in 2006 and provides a less invasive technique for enlargement of the sinus ostium. It involves the placement of a guide wire under fluoroscopic or fiberoptic light confirmation into a sinus cavity and the inflation of an oblong balloon to dilate the natural ostium by approximately 5 mm.[200] The main advantage of this technology is that, unlike traditional functional endoscopic sinus surgery, balloon catheter sinuplasty provides a mucosal sparing technique without inadvertent removal of tissue. To date, there are no published prospective trials comparing functional endoscopic sinus surgery to balloon catheter sinuplasty in the pediatric population. The major limitation of balloon catheter sinuplasty is the inability to address other anatomic abnormalities such as a malpositioned uncinate or ethmoidal disease. A limited number of studies demonstrate that balloon catheter sinuplasty is safe and efficacious in reducing sinus symptoms up to 1 year post procedure.[165-167] However, Ramadan and Terrell[167] also showed that the same reduction in symptoms was also accomplished with standard maxillary sinus irrigation plus adenoidectomy performed in children with chronic or recurrent sinusitis.

Many pediatric otolaryngologists have resumed performing adenoidectomy as a surgical intervention before proceeding with functional endoscopic sinus surgery.[195] It is thought that adenoidectomy removes a reservoir of bacteria that contributes to chronic or recurrent sinus infections.[189,193] Recently there has been a renewed interest in evaluating both endoscopic sinus surgery and adenoidectomy and clarifying indications for each. In 2004, Ramandan[164] performed a prospective nonrandomized study evaluating endoscopic sinus surgery and adenoidectomy. In this study, 202 children were divided into three groups, with group 1 receiving endoscopic sinus surgery with an adenoidectomy, group 2 receiving endoscopic sinus surgery alone, and group 3 receiving only an adenoidectomy. After 1-year follow-up, it was found that group 1 had 87% improvement in symptoms, compared with 75% and 52% in groups 2 and 3, respectively. After multivariate analysis of risk factors such as asthma, smoke exposure, and age, Ramadan concluded that adenoidectomy alone is recommended for children younger than 6 years without asthma. Children with asthma at any age or children older than 6 years with significant disease on the CT scans benefit from endoscopic sinus surgery at the time of the adenoidectomy. Other studies examining the efficacy of adenoidectomy alone in alleviating symptoms of chronic or recurrent sinusitis have demonstrated a range from 50% to 70%.[203,212] A meta-analysis of pediatric patients treated with endoscopic sinus surgery found symptomatic improvement in nearly 90% of patients.[75]

In conjunction with endoscopic sinus surgery, specific antimicrobial therapy for organisms identified by culture is carried out. In addition, other contributing conditions, such as cystic fibrosis, asthma, or immunologic disorders, need to be addressed.

Orbital and intracranial abscesses and cavernous sinus thrombosis secondary to sinus infection require emergent surgery, which often is lifesaving, to evacuate the source of infection.[172,176,234,236] Within the spectrum of orbital complications, management of subperiosteal abscess is more controversial. In a combined review of 134 patients with subperiosteal abscess of the orbit, medial abscesses (adjacent to the lamina papyracea) are most likely curable by antimicrobial therapy alone, but surgery may be indicated in cases of abscesses in other locations, those with loss of visual acuity, and abscesses refractory to 48 to 72 hours of medical therapy.[35] Cellulitis, osteomyelitis, and meningitis also frequently require surgery if they do not respond to antimicrobial therapy.[172] Surgery in these cases involves endoscopic drainage of the sinuses and abscesses. Endoscopic techniques may allow for intranasal drainage and avoidance of the development of facial scars.[7] If an intracranial complication involves an intracranial empyema or abscess, concomitant craniotomy along with functional endoscopic sinus surgery may be required.[65] Surgical procedures also may be indicated for a child with acute or chronic disease resulting from an identified underlying problem, such as an immunologic deficiency.[238]

PROGNOSIS

The prognosis for identified and adequately treated sinusitis in otherwise normal children is excellent. Frequently children have subnormal health because sinusitis goes unrecognized; it may be treated only partially because of other clinical impressions, which contributes to the chronicity of the problem. Sinusitis is likely to be recurrent in children with a history of previous chronic disease and in children with repeated adverse exposure, such as swimming in contaminated or irritating water. Children with allergic respiratory disease also are likely to have frequent recurrences. Sinusitis in an immunocompromised child frequently is resistant to cure; long-term continuous therapy can be beneficial in such patients. Signs and symptoms of neurologic involvement in sinusitis frequently call for aggressive surgical management of the sinusitis and the intracranial and paracranial lesions, and timely management is highly impactful.

Paranasal sinusitis also has been noted occasionally to be associated with bronchial asthma.[152,162] Its successful treatment has resulted in clearing of the asthma.[91,180]

PREVENTION

Sinusitis is not preventable in most instances. In some individuals, change of lifestyle can do much to improve the situation, however. Sinusitis in some children is related to their swimming habits and can be controlled by elimination of swimming or perhaps by the use of nose plugs. Good allergic management, including intranasal corticosteroid or cromolyn therapy, prevents sinus disease in certain atopic children. Relief of nasal airway obstruction caused by allergic rhinitis, enlarged adenoids, or other anatomic problems also should help to prevent sinusitis. Early attention given to persistent nasal discharge also can be expected to lessen the damage associated with sinus infection.

In Sweden, the universal use of pneumococcal conjugate vaccine decreased the risk of hospitalization for sinusitis by 66%.[116] At Texas Children's Hospital, the use of 13-valent pneumococcal vaccine resulted in a decrease in *S. pneumoniae* isolations from children with chronic sinusitis.[141]

NEW REFERENCES SINCE THE SEVENTH EDITION

26. Caimmi D, Caimmi S, Labo E, et al. Acute isolated sphenoid sinusitis in children. *Am J Rhinol Allergy*. 2011;25(6):e200-e202.
32. Chandler JR, Langenbrunner DJ, Stevens ER. The pathogenesis of orbital complications in acute sinusitis. *Laryngoscope*. 1970;80(9):1414-1428.
34. Chow AW, Benninger MS, Brook I, et al. IDSA clinical practice guideline for acute bacterial rhinosinusitis in children and adults. *Clin Infect Dis*. 2012;54(8):e72-e112.
35. Coenraad S, Buwalda J. Surgical or medical management of subperiosteal orbital abscess in children: a critical appraisal of the literature. *Rhinology*. 2009;47(1):18-23.
41. DeMuri GP, Wald ER. Complications of acute bacterial sinusitis in children. *Pediatr Infect Dis J*. 2011;30(8):701-702.
83. Hayward G, Heneghan C, Perera R, et al. Intranasal corticosteroids in management of acute sinusitis: a systematic review and meta-analysis. *Ann Fam Med*. 2012;10(3):241-249.
102. Kinis V, Ozbay M, Bakir S, et al. Management of orbital complications of sinusitis in pediatric patients. *J Craniofac Surg*. 2013;24(5):1706-1710.
116. Lindstrand A, Bennet R, Galanis I, et al. Sinusitis and pneumonia hospitalization after introduction of pneumococcal conjugate vaccine. *Pediatrics*. 2014;134(6):e1528-e1536.
122. Makary CA, Ramadan HH. The role of sinus surgery in children. *Laryngoscope*. 2013;123(6):1348-1352.
141. Olarte L, Hulten KG, Lamberth L, et al. Impact of the 13-valent pneumococcal conjugate vaccine on chronic sinusitis associated with *Streptococcus pneumoniae* in children. *Pediatr Infect Dis J*. 2014;33(10):1033-1036.
147. Patel RG, Daramola OO, Linn D, et al. Do you need to operate following recovery from complications of pediatric acute sinusitis? *Int J Pediatr Otorhinolaryngol*. 2014;78(6):923-925.
151. Peters AT, Spector S, Hsu J, et al. Diagnosis and management of rhinosinusitis: a practice parameter update. *Ann Allergy Asthma Immunol*. 2014;113(4):347-385.
150. Pena MT, Preciado D, Orestes M, et al. Orbital complications of acute sinusitis: changes in the post-pneumococcal vaccine era. *JAMA Otolaryngol Head Neck Surg*. 2013;139(3):223-227.
179. Sedaghat AR, Wilke CO, Cunningham MJ, et al. Socioeconomic disparities in the presentation of acute bacterial sinusitis complications in children. *Laryngoscope*. 2014;124(7):1700-1706.
181. Shaikh N, Hoberman A, Kearney DH, et al. Signs and symptoms that differentiate acute sinusitis from viral upper respiratory tract infection. *Pediatr Infect Dis J*. 2013;32(10):1061-1065.
182. Shaikh N, Wald ER. Decongestants, antihistamines and nasal irrigation for acute sinusitis in children. *Cochrane Database Syst Rev*. 2013;(10):CD007909.
187. Sharma PK, Saikia B, Sharma R. Orbitocranial complications of acute sinusitis in children. *J Emerg Med*. 2014;47(3):282-285.
213. Venekamp RP, Thompson MJ, Hayward G, et al. Systemic corticosteroids for acute sinusitis. *Cochrane Database Syst Rev*. 2014;(3):CD008115.
224. Wald ER, Applegate KE, Bordley C, et al. Clinical practice guideline for the diagnosis and management of acute bacterial sinusitis in children aged 1 to 18 years. *Pediatrics*. 2013;132(1):e262-e280.
227. Wald ER, DeMuri GP. Commentary: antibiotic recommendations for acute otitis media and acute bacterial sinusitis in 2013–the conundrum. *Pediatr Infect Dis J*. 2013;32(6):641-643.
242. Zalmanovici Trestioreanu A, Yaphe J. Intranasal steroids for acute sinusitis. *Cochrane Database Syst Rev*. 2013;(12):CD005149.

The full reference list for this chapter is available at ExpertConsult.com.

15 Otitis Externa

Ellen M. Friedman • Maria Carrillo-Marquez

Otitis externa is an inflammation of the external ear canal commonly caused by infection. It constitutes one of the most common otolaryngologic encounters in the emergency department. This condition is addressed commonly as *swimmer's ear* or *tropical ear* because it often occurs after a history of repeated water exposure and occurs more commonly in warm and humid environments. This condition became of significant interest during World War II because of its high incidence among the troops in the South Pacific. During World War II, otitis externa accounted for 50% to 70% of the caseload for otolaryngologists in the South Pacific.[31]

Today, otitis externa accounts for 7.5 million annual ototopical prescriptions in the United States and is a significant cause of ear pain and conductive hearing loss.[63] This chapter discusses the basic anatomy of the external canal, different etiologies of otitis externa, and treatment and prevention that are needed by the pediatric practitioner managing this condition.

EPIDEMIOLOGY

According to the Centers for Disease Control (CDC), in 2007, the burden of acute otitis externa in the United States was 2.4 million health care visits (8.1 visits/1000 population), an estimated 1/123 persons affected during that year. Estimated annual rates of ambulatory care visits for acute otitis externa between 2003 and 2007 were highest among children 5 to 9 (18.6%) and 10 to 14 years of age (15.8%). Approximately 3% of emergency department visits for acute otitis externa in 2007 led to hospitalization. Incidence peaked during summer months, and the regional rate was highest in the South. Direct health care costs were approximately $0.5 billion annually and nearly 600,000 hours annually of clinician's time.[15] In a retrospective analysis of the Nationwide Emergency Department Sample from 2009 through 2011, more than 8.6 million visits were due to an otologic diagnosis, which represented 2.2% of all emergency department and 6.7% of all pediatric emergency department encounters. Otitis externa accounted for 11.8% of all the cases.[43]

Otitis externa was the most common cause of outpatient visits for waterborne disease between 2005 and 2006.[24] Outbreaks of otitis externa have been identified in competitive swimmers in association with insufficiently chlorinated pools,[56] in divers,[3] and in association with swimming in recreational fresh water lakes.[80]

NORMAL ANATOMY

The external ear is composed of the auricle and external auditory canal. The auricle of the ear is a skin-covered cartilaginous structure on the temporal region of the head and is an extension of the external auditory canal. The external auditory canal is divided into two regions: a lateral cartilaginous portion and a medial bony portion that ends at the tympanic membrane.

The cartilaginous portion of the external auditory canal makes up approximately 40% of its 2.5 cm total length and typically is directed slightly upward and backward. This shape and the presence of cerumen help to prevent water and foreign objects from entering the canal.[41] In the anterior portion of the cartilaginous canal are the fissures of Santorini, which provide a route for the spread of infection from the canal into the adjacent parotid and surrounding tissues. The bony canal makes up the remainder of the canal length and is directed slightly downward and anterior. The isthmus, which is the narrowest portion of the canal, corresponds to the bony-cartilaginous junction.

The sensory innervation of the external auditory canal is complex and includes contributions from cranial nerves V, VII, IX, and X. This robust sensory innervation is responsible for the exquisite pain associated with otitis externa.[41] The skin of the entire external auditory canal consists of keratinizing stratified squamous epithelium. It is the only keratinizing epithelium that lacks eccrine sweat glands.

Differences exist in the canal skin of the cartilaginous canal and the skin covering the bony canal. The cartilaginous canal skin is thicker and contains rete pegs, dermis, dermal papillae, hair follicles, and sebaceous and cerumen glands, which are absent in the bony canal. The thinner skin of the bony canal lacks dermal papillae and rete pegs. The lack of subcutaneous tissue in the bony canal allows the tight attachment of the skin to the underlying periosteum, rendering the bony canal wall more vulnerable to trauma.

PROTECTIVE MECHANISMS OF THE EXTERNAL EAR

Three major defense mechanisms protect the external auditory canal and lateral surface of the tympanic membrane: the tragus and antitragus, the skin with its cerumen coat, and the isthmus of the canal. The tragus and antitragus provide a partial barrier to the entrance of the foreign bodies into the external auditory canal.

BOX 15.1 Predisposing Factors for Otitis Externa

Hot and humid environment
Water exposure
Instrumentation of ear canal
Previous radiation therapy
Draining ear
Contact dermatitis

The skin of the cartilaginous canal contains many hair cells and sebaceous and apocrine glands, such as cerumen glands. Together, these three adnexal structures are termed the *pilosebaceous unit* and provide a protective function in the external auditory canal. Migration of the skin of the external auditory canal also helps keep the canal free of debris. The pattern of migration is from the tympanic membrane laterally and radially away from the umbo.[2] Glandular secretions combine with sloughed squamous epithelium to form an acidic coat of cerumen, one of the primary barriers to infection of the canal. Cerumen is composed of lipids that are hydrophobic, and its major function is to waterproof the canal. The acidic nature of cerumen has been shown to inhibit bacterial and fungal growth.[16,26,37] This acidic pH also helps maintain the cohesion and integrity of the stratum corneum.[32]

Racial and gender differences that are noted in the characteristics of cerumen do not seem to have major clinical significance. Whites and blacks produce cerumen with higher levels of lipids in contrast to Asians, who produce cerumen with higher levels of proteins. Cerumen in males also has been shown to have a higher pH level than that in females.[26] The canal normally is a self-protecting and self-cleansing structure. The cerumen coat gradually works its way to the lateral part of the canal and sloughs externally. Instrumentation and excessive cleansing of the canal can alter this primary protective barrier and may lead to infection (Box 15.1).

NORMAL BACTERIAL FLORA

The normal bacterial flora of the external auditory canal is a combination of aerobic (80%) and anaerobic (20%) organisms.[12] Aerobic bacteria include *Staphylococcus epidermidis, Pseudomonas aeruginosa*, α-hemolytic streptococci, and diphtheroids.

The bacteriology of the cerumen and the external auditory canal is essentially the same. In a study by Stroman and colleagues[79] of 291 bacteria isolated from cerumen and 302 bacteria isolated from the canal, 99% and 96%, respectively, were gram-positive. Staphylococci accounted for 63% of bacteria. *Staphylococcus auricularis* is the isolate found most frequently (23% in cerumen and 21% in the canal), followed by *S. epidermidis* (14% from cerumen and 17% from the canal, respectively). After staphylococci, the coryneform bacteria (diphtheroids) are the organisms most frequently isolated. The third most frequently recovered bacteria belong to the streptococci and enterococci groups. *Alloiococcus otitidis* was isolated with the greatest frequency (>95%).[79]

In addition, seven species of *Bacillus* were isolated. From the Micrococcaceae family, *Micrococcus luteus* was isolated most frequently. *Turicella otitidis* was the primary coryneform recovered—58% from cerumen and 65% from the canal. *Corynebacterium auris* was the second most frequently isolated coryneform, accounting for approximately 12% of bacteria. Twenty-one other species of coryneform bacteria (including 10 previously undefined species of *Corynebacterium* and 4 of *Microbacterium*) were isolated as well. Coryneform bacteria represented approximately 20% of the bacteria isolated. *Propionibacterium acnes* and a variety of *Peptococcus* spp. make up the anaerobic flora.[79]

ACUTE OTITIS EXTERNA

Acute otitis externa is an infection of the external auditory canal that often is the end result of a combination of factors. Bacterial and fungal infections of the external auditory canal occur when the natural defenses break down, resulting in a significant reduction in the amount of cerumen, an injury to the skin of the canal, or a shift of the normal canal flora. Humidity, heat, and maceration all produce itching, which often leads to manipulation and instrumentation of the canal, which in turn leads to additional trauma. Otitis externa may be caused by insults that result in the removal of the protective lipid film from the canal, allowing the entrance of organism to the apopilosebaceous unit. Rapid proliferation of bacteria occurs as a result of the warm, dark, and moist canal environment.

Inflammation and infection can cause canal edema or complete obstruction of the canal in severe cases, with purulent discharge. If the infectious process goes untreated, it leads to cellulitis of the auricle and surrounding area.

Symptoms of otitis externa, in addition to pruritus and drainage, include pain and tenderness on palpation or manipulation of the external ear. Pain arises as the soft tissues and skin of the canal distract the periosteal lining of the bony canal. Pain is severe and may interfere with daily activities and is the major reason for medical consultation.

History and Physical Examination

Otitis externa is a clinical diagnosis. The evaluation often reveals exposure to water, previous auricular instrumentation, or trauma. The physician should inquire about predisposing factors, such as diabetes, immunosuppression, history of eczema, or previous radiation therapy, all of which may predict a more complicated course.

Symptoms of acute otitis externa include otalgia (70%), itching (60%), fullness (22%), with or without hearing loss (32%) or ear canal pain on mastication.[64]

On physical examination, the pinna may appear swollen or erythematous with eczematization (Fig. 15.1) or may be protruding. Primary care practitioners and emergency department personnel may erroneously consider the diagnosis of mastoiditis based on auricular protrusion. On manipulation of the auricle, the patient often experiences severe pain. Tragal tenderness is another key feature of this disease. A handheld otoscope often suffices to establish the diagnosis, but the microscope is recommended for full cleaning of the ear canal. The canal appears swollen, with various grades of patency, depending on the severity of the infection. Purulent discharge combined with keratin debris usually fills the canal. It is important to attempt to visualize the tympanic membrane if the canal is not completely obstructed. Absence of drainage from the middle ear confirms the diagnosis of otitis externa.

Pathogens in Acute Otitis Externa

Common bacterial pathogens that cause otitis externa include *P. aeruginosa, Staphylococcus aureus, Escherichia coli,* and *Proteus* spp. (Box 15.2). *Pseudomonas* spp. have been found to be the predominant organism in various studies.[8,11,62,72] Historically, *Pseudomonas* spp. have accounted for 50% to 80% of bacteria isolated from cases of chronic otitis externa.[7,52,54,62,72] In a study by Roland and Stroman,[62] gram-negative bacteria accounted for 53% of recovered organisms; 45.3% were gram positive. In this study, *P. aeruginosa* accounted for 37.7% of the total number of isolates, whereas *Pseudomonas otitidis* accounted for 2.3% of recovered organisms.

Staphylococci are the most common gram-positive organisms recovered in cases of otitis externa, accounting for 25% of the cases. *S. epidermidis* is the most common staphylococcal species recovered, followed by *S. aureus.* Coryneform bacteria are the second largest group of gram-positive bacteria isolated from cases of otitis externa.[62] Reports of methicillin-resistant *S. aureus* as an increasing pathogen isolated from otorrhea resulting from otitis externa showed variable prevalence: 0.3%,[62] 5.3%,[50] 6.3%,[82] and up to 9.8% of cases.[36]

Other organisms identified as pathogens include *Enterobacter, Klebsiella, Serratia,* and *Proteus* spp. and *E. coli.* Although *Microbacterium* spp. previously were considered normal flora, more recently they have been identified at a 10 times higher rate in infected ears in contrast to normal controls. *Microbacterium* also has been the single recovered isolate in treatment failures and reinfections.[62]

Management of Acute Otitis Externa

No consensus exists about the most effective treatment for otitis externa; however, evidence-based guidelines have been published with strong recommendations issued for acute uncomplicated infection in patients older than 2 years of age including pain assessment and appropriate analgesic prescription and avoidance of systemic antibiotics for initial therapy unless there is extension outside the ear canal or the presence of specific host factors that would indicate a need for systemic therapy. In addition there is continued strong support for treatment to include meticulously cleaning the external auditory canal. It is also important to differentiate acute otitis externa from other pathologies with similar symptoms, identify factors that modify management (i.e., nonintact tympanic membrane, tympanostomy tube, diabetes, immunocompromised state, prior radiotherapy), implement strategies to improve the delivery of topical drops (aural toilet, wick placement, drop administration instructions, etc.), consider use of a nonototoxic preparation in patients with known or suspected tympanic membrane perforation or tympanostomy tubes, and reassess if the patient fails to respond to treatment within 48 to 72 hours to either confirm the diagnosis or to exclude other causes of illness.[64]

Treatment usually includes thorough cleaning and suctioning of the purulent debris and application of topical agents. Topical treatment has been shown effective and is the mainstay of treatment. A wick may be placed in the canal to provide adequate delivery of the topical solution when significant swelling of the external auditory canal occurs. Although no clinical trials have assessed the effectiveness of aural toilet alone,[40] without the wick and adequate cleaning of the canal, the topical drops may not achieve adequate penetration and are ineffective. Available options for topical therapy include multiple topical antibiotics, antiseptics, steroids, and combination agents.[13,27,60,64] Topical antimicrobial therapy

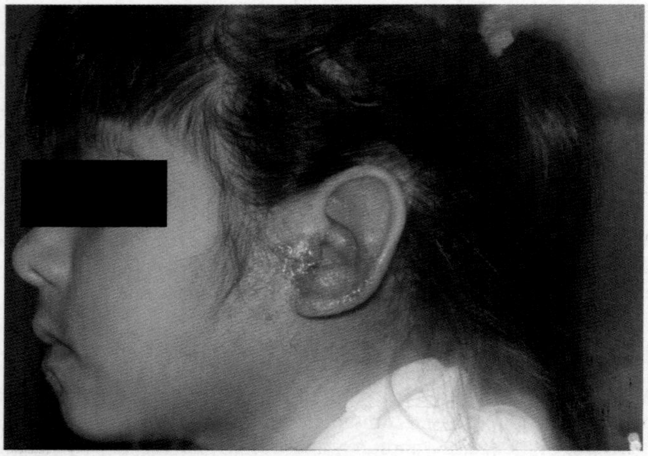

FIG. 15.1 Patient with acute otitis externa, with purulent drainage from the ear canal and mild edema and erythema of the pinna.

BOX 15.2 Common Pathogens in Otitis Externa

Gram-Negative Organisms

Pseudomonas aeruginosa
Pseudomonas spp. Nov. "otitidis"
Proteus mirabilis
Serratia marcescens

Gram-Positive Organisms

Staphylococcus aureus
Staphylococcus epidermidis
Corynebacterium auris
Enterococcus faecalis

Fungi and Yeasts

Aspergillus fumigatus
Candida albicans
Candida parapsilosis

increased absolute clinical cure rates of acute otitis externa by 46% and bacteriologic cure rates by 61% in contrast to placebo.[64] Freedman[28] compared topical neomycin/colistin/hydrocortisone with topical placebo and found less severe edema and itching by day 3 and less severe edema, itching, redness, scaling, and weeping by day 7.[64] Without treatment, only 15% of patients with acute otitis externa have clinical cure within 10 days; however, the cure rate increases to 65% to 85% when topical antimicrobial therapy is administered.[28,64]

Rosenfeld and colleagues[64] performed a meta-analysis to assess topical antiseptics and antibiotics and found comparable clinical cures at 7 to 14 days. The most common antiseptics used in the treatment of otitis externa include acetic acid, boric acid/ethyl alcohol and aluminum acetate, and *N*-chlorotaurine. Acetic acid and aluminum acetate solution at pH 3.0, commonly known as modified Burow solution, has been found to inactivate in vitro *Pseudomonas* spp., gram-positive organisms (including MRSA, but excluding *Enterococcus*), and *Candida albicans* within 5 minutes and all gram-negative bacteria within 20 minutes.[39]

Topical antibiotic preparations usually are divided into two groups: quinolones and nonquinolone antibiotics. Nonquinolone antibiotics, such as polymyxin, neomycin, gentamicin, tobramycin, and oxytetracycline, have been the mainstay of treatment for otitis externa for several decades. Most of these agents have some degree of ototoxicity, however, which renders them undesirable in the case of a tympanic membrane perforation or a patent pressure-equalizing tube.[45,57] The introduction of quinolones in the late 1980s for management of otitis externa and necrotizing external otitis provided a nonototoxic alternative treatment. Topical antibiotic therapy allows for the administration of high concentrations of antibiotics, which can overcome organisms with high minimal inhibitory concentrations. Rosenfeld and colleagues[64] reported comparable clinical cure rates for topical quinolone antibiotics compared with nonquinolones at 3 to 4 days, 7 to 10 days, and 14 to 28 days. This same study found no differences in adverse effects between the two antibiotic groups.

One of the most common mistakes in the treatment of otitis externa is not identifying a tympanic membrane perforation and draining middle ear as the source of the infection, which may have treatment implications because of the ototoxicity of some compounds.

Typical duration of topical treatment is 7 to 10 days. Patients with more severe infections may require 10 to 14 days of treatment. It is commonly recommended that drops be given for 3 days beyond the cessation of symptoms.[70]

Oral antibiotics are not routinely indicated for the treatment of otitis externa. A clinical trial by Roland and colleagues[59] comparing oral antibiotic plus antibiotic/steroid drop versus antibiotic/steroid drop showed that a single topical agent is equivalent to combination of topical and oral antibiotic treatment for otitis externa and has similar clinical outcomes.

Indications for systemic antibiotics in acute otitis externa are few and include complicated infection by associated cellulitis of the surrounding skin or other underlying conditions (e.g., diabetes or immunosuppression).[40] In spite of increasing awareness of inappropriate antibiotic use and its implications, prescription of systemic antibiotics in the outpatient setting remains frequent and has experienced only a modest decrease (about 4.9%) over the past few years.[23] Up to 40% of patients are prescribed systemic antibiotics in addition to or instead of topical therapy, many of which are not active against *P. aeruginosa* or *S. aureus,* the most common pathogens associated with otitis externa.[23,33,66] Use of systemic antibiotics can be only be justified when there is a concomitant diagnosis of otitis media or regional spread of infection. Oral antibiotics, when not appropriately prescribed, increase treatment cost, potential side effects, and likelihood of noncompliance and are more likely to contribute to emergence of antimicrobial resistance than is topical antimicrobial therapy. An evidence-based review concluded that no significant topical antibiotic resistance develops from the use of ototopical antibiotic treatment alone.[83]

CHRONIC OTITIS EXTERNA

Chronic otitis externa is an inflammatory condition of the ear canal skin, with symptoms lasting from 6 weeks to more than 3 months. This condition generally is caused by the loss of the protective coating of cerumen and oils secondary to constant mechanical debridement, such as with cotton applicators or repeated water exposure. Associated pruritus leading to self-cleaning perpetuates the vicious cycle. The ear canal with chronic otitis externa often is more vulnerable to bacterial superinfection.[58] *S. aureus* and *P. aeruginosa* have been shown to secrete proteases that may perpetuate pathologic skin conditions in the external auditory canal in cases of chronic otitis externa.[49] In chronic otitis externa, biofilm formation has been postulated as responsible for the pathogenesis and difficulty eradicating infection.[29] A shift in external ear canal pH from acidic to alkaline has been noted in patients with chronic otitis externa.[47] A subtype of chronic otitis externa is reported in 6% to 40% of patients secondary to ear canal maceration as a result of middle ear drainage after insertion of pressure equalization tubes.[44,46,61,83]

Treatment of chronic otitis externa involves debridement and application of topical antiinflammatory agents, such as corticosteroids. Cessation of habitual canal manipulation is necessary for achieving a positive response. For severe recalcitrant cases, surgical removal of the canal skin and replacement with skin grafts may be required. Chemical peeling of canal skin also has been used in refractory cases.[29]

OTOMYCOSIS

Otomycosis is a fungal infection of the skin of the external canal. Otomycosis often is the result of superinfection of chronic bacterial infection of the external canal or middle ear. It is often found after the use of multiple oral and ototopical antibacterial medications. All fungi have three basic growth requirements—moisture, warmth, and darkness—all of which commonly are present in the external auditory canal. The most common fungus is *Aspergillus* spp., although *Candida* spp., *Actinomyces* spp., and Zygomycetes also have been reported.[11] Pruritus is the primary clinical manifestation. Patients also complain of feeling moisture in their ears. Physical examination commonly shows a white, black, or dotted gray membrane in the external auditory canal. Diagnosis often is confirmed with a fungal culture.

Thorough cleaning with removal of the matted fungal debris and topical application of an acidifying solution, such as aluminum sulfate–calcium acetate (Domeboro), or a drying powder, such as boric acid, often is adequate treatment. Antifungals such as clotrimazole cream or solution (Lotrimin) also may be used. It is important to assess for perforation of the tympanic membrane because antifungals can be ototoxic.[45] Gentian violet usually is well tolerated in patients with mastoid cavities, but it permanently stains skin and clothing. Many patients with refractory otomycotic infections have had previous canal-wall-down mastoid surgery and require a hearing aid with a closed mold. Because the patient relies on the hearing aid virtually all day, trauma associated with placing and removing the hearing aid throughout the day can cause a significant problem. Ointments are not recommended for patients with closed hearing aids because they may promote fungal growth secondary to the accumulation of moisture.

NECROTIZING OTITIS EXTERNA

Necrotizing otitis externa is an uncommon severe infection of the external auditory canal that spreads to the surrounding subcutaneous tissues and can lead to osteomyelitis of the skull base.[20] This condition was described first by Chandler[17,19] and referred to as *malignant otitis externa*; although the disease is actually benign, aggressive extension occurs, and historically it often has a poor outcome. Survival rates have improved as a result of increased awareness, allowing earlier diagnosis and treatment.[20,21] Patients often are diabetic, immunocompromised, or undergoing postradiation therapy.[8,69,73] Incidence of infection has been reported to be on the rise as risk factors for infection increase in the population (e.g., aging, immunosuppression, diabetes).[22] The infection often begins as any other acute otitis externa involving the bony-cartilaginous junction and may extend through the fissures of Santorini to involve the parotid region. Elevation of inflammatory markers is common—in particular, the erythrocyte sedimentation rate.[68] Facial paralysis can occur as a complication of this disease and does so more commonly in children than in adults.[53] Facial nerve paralysis in necrotizing otitis externa often is permanent[18] and associated with more progressive disease but not with overall survival.[75] Other complications include cranial nerve palsy (X and XI),[1] subperiosteal abscess formation, mastoiditis, meningitis, and sinus thrombosis.[48]

P. aeruginosa is the most common pathogen in necrotizing otitis externa. *Proteus mirabilis* also has been reported as a causal agent in some cases.[20,21] *Staphylococcus aureus*, particularly MRSA, has been also implicated.[35,38] Necrotizing otitis externa should be suspected in the presence of a pseudomonal infection that does not resolve and may be associated with facial nerve paralysis. The presence of granulation in the external canal at the bony–cartilaginous junction also should raise suspicion of necrotizing otitis externa. The rare reported cases of fungal malignant external otitis were due to *Aspergillus fumigatus* but a few cases associated with *Aspergillus niger, Scedosporium apiospermum, Pseudallescheria boydii,* and *Malassezia sympodialis* have been described.[67]

Diagnostic imaging, including computed tomography or magnetic resonance imaging, of the temporal region often is required.[30] The most common finding of extension beyond the ear canal is retrocondylar fat infiltration.[42] A positive technetium-99m scan is diagnostic for acute osteolytic osteomyelitis because it measures osteoclastic activity, but it may remain positive long after the infection has subsided. For this reason, a ^{99m}Tc scan is not ideal for monitoring treatment response.[78]

Treatment of necrotizing otitis externa often involves multiple surgical debridements combined with topical and intravenous antipseudomonal antibiotics. In diabetic or immunocompromised patients, coadjuvant treatment to control the primary condition is crucial and should be initiated immediately. Transition to oral ciprofloxacin for infections with susceptible organisms has been reported with clinical improvement.[34] Duration of therapy is usually prolonged for at least 6 weeks and until clinical and radiographic improvement has been achieved.

Pseudomonal resistance to fluoroquinolones has been reported. Berenholz and colleagues[9] reported 33% ciprofloxacin resistance in cases of necrotizing otitis externa. Other studies have shown strains of *S. aureus* and *S. epidermidis* that developed quinolone resistance.[60]

Use of adjuvant hyperbaric oxygen also has been reported for intractable cases, but no there is no clear evidence to demonstrate its efficacy when compared with treatment with antibiotics and or surgery.[25,55]

DIFFERENTIAL DIAGNOSIS

Not every condition that manifests with pain and purulent discharge from the external auditory canal is otitis externa. Multiple other entities that may manifest with one or more similar symptoms include relapsing polychondritis, suppurative otitis media, and herpetic infections. In patients with suspected otitis externa who do not experience improvement after 48 to 72 hours of therapy, alternate conditions should be considered, such as noncompliance and foreign body obstruction of the canal.

Relapsing polychondritis is a progressive inflammatory disorder affecting cartilage. When it involves the ear, it usually involves the pinna and the cartilaginous portion of the external auditory canal, manifesting as swelling and erythema.[6] This condition can affect any cartilaginous structure, including the trachea, nasal septum, and larynx. Destruction of the cartilage by inflammatory infiltrates is followed by granulation, fibrosis, and calcifications. It often is accompanied by arthralgias involving one or more joints and rarely affects only one ear.

Herpes simplex and herpes zoster also can affect the external auditory canal. Both conditions manifest with painful vesicles along the canal (Fig. 15.2) and can be accompanied by facial nerve paralysis (Ramsay Hunt syndrome or herpes zoster oticus).[4,81] Treatment is with antivirals, such as acyclovir.

Dermatologic conditions can give the appearance of otitis externa. Allergic and contact dermatitis can manifest with erythema, weeping areas, and itching. Allergic dermatitis is a delayed hypersensitivity reaction resulting from substances such as poison ivy, rubber latex, and nickel compounds.[51,77] Type IV cell-mediated hypersensitivity reaction to components of ototopical agents used to treat acute otitis externa has been described.[74] Treatment is administration of topical steroids and removal of the causative agent. Dermatophytid eruptions can manifest in the ear canal in response to hematogenously spread fungal by-products from a primary focus (e.g., nails, scalp, vagina).[14,70,71,74]

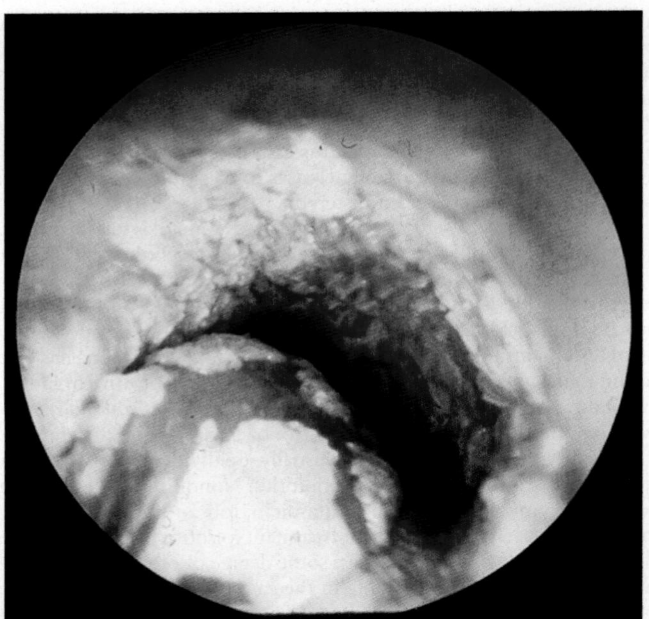

FIG. 15.2 Ear canal with multiple vesicles from herpes zoster oticus.

Furunculosis is a localized form of otitis externa usually involving the outer third of the ear canal. It is characterized by abscess development in a hair follicle, with spreading of the infection to the surrounding skin. The most common causative agent is *S. aureus*. Treatment includes incision and drainage of pointing, fluctuant abscesses and application of topical antistaphylococcal antibiotics.[10]

Ear pain without aural drainage and external canal edema may be secondary to referred pain from the pharynx, tonsils, larynx, or teeth.

PREVENTION

Avoiding ear trauma and instrumentation, minimizing exposure of the ears to water (e.g., using ear plugs or swim caps, drying ears thoroughly after water exposure, and using alcohol-based ear drying solutions after water exposure for persons with recurring episodes of acute otitis externa), and avoiding insertion of solid objects into the ear canal are the mainstay of prevention of otitis externa.[5,40,65,76] Additionally pool operators can help prevent transmission of *Pseudomonas* spp. and other common causes of infectious acute otitis externa in treated recreational water venues (e.g., pools, interactive fountains, and water parks) by maintaining proper chlorine and pH levels.[84]

Groups at high risk for infection, particularly competitive swimmers, should be the target for educational interventions. More information on preventing swimmer's ear is available at http://www.cdc.gov/healthywater/swimming/rwi/illnesses/swimmers-ear-prevention-guidelines.html.

CONCLUSION

Understanding the anatomy and physiology of the external ear allows clinicians to better comprehend the natural history of the diseases that affect this region. Despite improvements in diagnostic imaging techniques, no substitute exists for a good history and physical examination to differentiate among various conditions with a similar presentation. Treatment of otitis externa should focus on achieving pain relief, meticulous cleaning of the external auditory canal, and application of topical ear drops; at the same time, clinicians should try to help prevent recurrences in patients with higher risk factors.

NEW REFERENCES SINCE THE SEVENTH EDITION

5. American Academy of Pediatrics. Swimmer's ear/acute otitis externa. In: Kimberlin DW, Brady MT, Jackson MA, Long SS, eds. *Red Book: 2015 Report of the Committee*

on Infectious Diseases. 30th ed. Elk Grove Village, IL: American Academy of Pediatrics; 2015:218.
22. Chawdhary G, Liow N, Democratis J, et al. Necrotising (malignant) otitis externa in the UK: a growing problem. Review of five cases and analysis of National Hospital Episode Statistics trends. *J Laryngol Otol.* 2015;129:600-603.
23. Collier SA, Hlavsa MC, Piercefield EW, et al. Antimicrobial and analgesic prescribing patterns for acute otitis externa, 2004–2010. *Otolaryngol Head Neck Surg.* 2013;148:128-134.
35. Hobson CE, Moy JD, Byers KE, et al. Malignant otitis externa: evolving pathogens and implications for diagnosis and treatment. *Otolaryngol Head Neck Surg.* 2014;151(1):112-116.
38. Jacobsen LM, Antonelli PJ. Errors in the diagnosis and management of necrotizing otitis externa. *Otolaryngol Head Neck Surg.* 2010;143:506-509.
43. Kozin ED, Sethi RK, Remenschneider AK, et al. Epidemiology of otologic diagnoses in United States emergency departments. *Laryngoscope.* 2015;125: 1926-1933.
55. Phillips JS, Jones SE. Hyperbaric oxygen as an adjuvant treatment for malignant otitis externa. *Cochrane Database Syst Rev.* 2013;(5):CD004617.
64. Rosenfeld RM, Schwartz SR, Cannon CR, et al. Clinical practice guideline: acute otitis externa. *Otolaryngol Head Neck Surg.* 2014;150(1 suppl):S1-S24.
67. Rubin Grandis J, Branstetter BF 4th, Yu VL. The changing face of malignant (necrotising) external otitis: clinical, radiological, and anatomic correlations. *Lancet Infect Dis.* 2004;4(1):34-39.

The full reference list for this chapter is available at ExpertConsult.com.

16 Otitis Media

Janet R. Casey • Charles D. Bluestone

Otitis media is a broad term that includes acute otitis media (AOM), otitis media with effusion (OME), chronic otitis media with effusion (COME), and chronic suppurative otitis media (CSOM). This chapter will focus on AOM and OME.

INCIDENCE AND EPIDEMIOLOGY OF ACUTE OTITIS MEDIA

AOM primarily affects children in the first 3 years of life. Onset of AOM in the first 6 months of life is not common because infants are relatively protected from infection mediated by maternal antibodies acquired transplacentally. If a child experiences AOM in the first 6 months of life, then frequent AOM episodes are likely to occur throughout the first few years of life. Most AOM occurs between the age of 6 and 24 months of age. The peak incidence is between 9 and 15 months of age. AOM does occur with modest frequency between 2 and 3 years of age but then quickly diminishes in occurrence between 3 and 5 years of age.

The occurrence of otitis media in otherwise healthy infants is partly a reflection of their immature immune system and partly due to the fact that the eustachian tube of the young child is shorter, floppier, straighter, and more horizontal than the eustachian tube of the older child. By 3 years of age, the incidence of AOM decreases because of changes in the child's anatomy and physiology and maturing immune system. Children who have had little or no otitis media by the time they reach age 3 years are unlikely to develop problems with middle ear infections later in life unless some predisposing factor, such as allergic rhinitis, tumor or fracture of the base of the skull or a facial bone, or acquired immunodeficiency, occurs.

AOM is the most common bacterial infectious disease seen in an ambulatory pediatric practice, a leading cause of health care visits, and the most frequent reason children consume antibiotics or undergo surgery.[40,55,123] Reported AOM ambulatory visits in U.S. children younger than 2 years of age average 1244 visits per 1000 child-years,[144] and 80% of those visits resulted in an antibiotic prescription. AOM has a high socioeconomic impact worldwide.[99,139] In the United States, an estimated $4 billion is spent yearly on otitis media–related health care.[99,144]

More recently several developments have impacted AOM incidence in the United States and worldwide. First, treatment guidelines endorsed higher dose amoxicillin for the empiric treatment of AOM due to penicillin-resistant pneumococcal infections. Second, conjugate vaccines against *Streptococcus pneumoniae*, a major pathogen of AOM, were introduced. Routine use of the 7-valent pneumococcal conjugate vaccine (PCV7) in early childhood was associated with a significant reduction in AOM visit rates as well as a decrease in pressure-equalizing tube (PET) insertion due to recurrent AOM and CSOM.[26,43,46,56,113,128,129]

Three database analyses in three different countries demonstrated a positive effect of PCV7 on AOM episodes. Marom et al.[89] analyzed an insurance claims database of a U.S. nationwide managed health care plan. The authors showed a decreased trend in otitis media–related health care use in children younger than 6 years. Magnus et al.[86] studied children participating in the Norwegian Mother and Child Cohort Study and showed a decline of mother-reported AOM episodes in Norwegian children 12 to 18 months old and 18 to 36 months old of 14% and 8%, respectively. Using a national primary care database,[79] an observational cohort study investigated trends in AOM incidence and associated antibiotic utilization in children younger than 10 years during 2002 to 2012 in the United Kingdom. The authors found that the introduction of PCV7 was associated with a 22% reduction in AOM in children younger than 10 years and an additional 19% reduction following PCV13 introduction.

Otitis media in high-risk populations continues to be a significant medical problem. For example, epidemiologic studies from Bangladesh,[14] Nigeria,[3] and Australia[95] report prevalence of chronic suppurative otitis media (CSOM) of 12%, 2.5%, and 15%, respectively. Australian aboriginal children have a high rate of AOM and CSOM with tympanic membrane perforation that leads to significant long-term health impairment.[95] Native American children have a 63% incidence of AOM by 6 months of age.[41] A systematic review of population-based studies from multiple countries found the highest prevalence of OM in children to be 81% of Canadian Inuits and 84% of Australian Aborigines.[57]

Risk Factors

Many significant aspects of OM epidemiology and natural history were first characterized in 1960–1985. During those years it was shown that AOM risk increased according to the child's age at first AOM episode, male gender, Caucasian race/ethnicity (except in special high-risk populations noted earlier), low birth weight (<2500 g), preterm birth (<37 weeks' gestation), fall season of birth, bottle-feeding, daycare attendance, higher number of young siblings, lower parent's education/income/occupation, more frequent history of ear infections (plus other infectious illnesses or conditions) in siblings or parents, absent or poor health insurance coverage, and exposure to secondhand cigarette smoking.[5,6,8,9,12,13] Table 16.1 shows results of a meta-analysis of risk factors for chronic AOM and recurrent AOM.[143]

Microbiology of Acute Otitis Media in the Pneumococcal Conjugate Vaccine Era

The bacteria that cause AOM vary from country to country due to vaccination and antibiotic prescribing habits because these preventative and therapeutic interventions impact the otopathogens that predominate

TABLE 16.1 Risk Factors for Acute Otitis Media Development (Pooled Analysis)

Risk Factor	Odds Ratio	95% Confidence Interval
Allergy/atopy	1.36	1.13–1.64
Upper respiratory infection	6.59	3.13–13.89
Chronic nasal obstruction	1.19	0.84–1.69
Snoring	1.96	1.78–2.16
Male gender	1.24	0.99–1.54
Daycare center attendance	1.70	0.95–3.05
Family history of otitis media	1.40	0.86–2.28
Patient history of AOM/rAOM	11.13	1.06–116.44
Passive smoke exposure	1.39	1.02–1.89
Low socioeconomic status	3.82	1.11–13.15
Low education level of mother	1.68	0.32–8.68
Mother's smoking during pregnancy	2.34	0.64–8.54
Multiple siblings	1.57	0.93–2.63
Breastfeeding >6 mo	0.57	0.17–1.93
Any breastfeeding	0.91	0.47–1.79

rAOM, Recurrent acute otitis media.

Modified from Zhang Y, Xu M, Zhang J, et al. Risk factors for chronic and recurrent otitis media—a meta-analysis. *PLoS One.* 2014;9(1):e86397.

TABLE 16.2 Otopathogen Distribution Causing Acute Otitis Media in Rochester, NY, 2008–10

Year	Total Visits	Otopathogen Isolated From MEF	No. (%)
2008	57	*S. pneumoniae*	18 (32)
		Nontypeable *H. influenzae*	16 (28)
		M. catarrhalis	10 (18)
2009	78	*S. pneumoniae*	32 (41)
		Nontypeable *H. influenzae*	18 (23)
		M. catarrhalis	14 (18)
2010 (until September 30)	73	*S. pneumoniae*	21 (29)
		Nontypeable *H. influenzae*	25 (34)
		M. catarrhalis	5 (7)

MEF, middle ear fluid.

Modified from Casey JR, Kaur R, Friedel V, Pichichero ME. Acute otitis media otopathogens during 2008 to 2010 in Rochester, New York. *Pediatr Inf Dis J.* 2013;32(8):805–9.

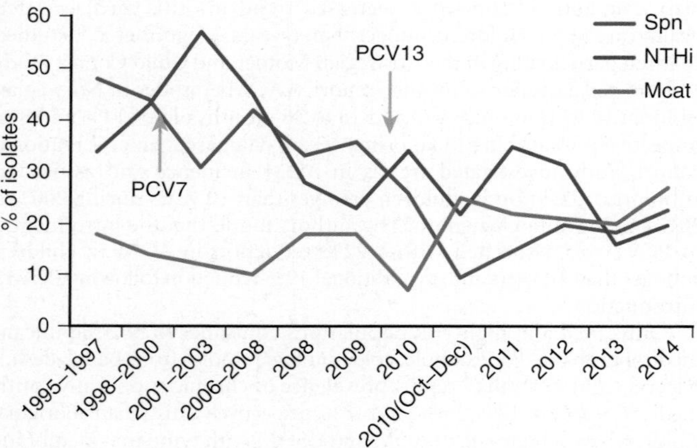

FIG. 16.1 Acute otitis media otopathogen distribution 1995– 2014. *Mcat, Moraxella catarrhalis*; *NTHi,* nontypeable *Haemophilus influenzae*; *PCV,* pneumococcal conjugate vaccine; *Spn, Streptococcus pneumoniae.* (Data from Casey JR, Pichichero ME. Changes in frequency and pathogens causing acute otitis media in 1995–2003. *Pediatr Infect Dis J.* 2004;23:824–8; Casey JR, Adlowitz DG, Pichichero ME. New patterns in the otopathogens causing acute otitis media six to eight years after introduction of pneumococcal conjugate vaccine. *Pediatr Infect Dis J.* 2010;29:304–9; and Casey JR, Kaur R, Friedel VC, Pichichero ME. Acute otitis media otopathogens during 2008 to 2010 in Rochester, New York. *Pediatr Infect Dis J.* 2013;32:805–9.)

in the nasopharynx before ascending via the eustachian tube to the middle ear space. In most developed countries virtually all children are vaccinated with the PCV7 or PCV13, discussed later in this chapter. Most children are treated with antibiotics, predominantly amoxicillin in a standard dose (40 mg/kg per day divided twice daily) or a "high" dose (80 mg/kg per day divided twice daily) for 10 days. As a consequence of PCV and amoxicillin use, the etiology of AOM continues to change over time. The dynamic changes in the otopathogen mix from 1996 to 2015, based on tympanocentesis isolations from the Rochester, New York, otitis media research center are shown in Fig. 16.1.[24]

S. pneumoniae caused approximately 30% to 60% of episodes before the PCV era. Following the introduction of PCV7, *S. pneumoniae* as a cause of AOM decreased in frequency, and nontypeable *Haemophilus influenzae* AOM increased proportionately. Two years after PCV7 introduction, *S. pneumoniae* began to increase proportionately due to nonvaccine serotypes, dominated by serotype 19A.[39,47,48,53,64,107] There was complete elimination of PCV7 serotypes and replacement with nonvaccine serotypes in the nasopharynx[36,78,90,98,104,135,138] and as a cause of AOM in the countries using PCV7.[15,21,24,26] The otopathogens causing AOM in young children in 2008 to 2010, the late PCV7 era in the Rochester otitis media research center, are shown in Table 16.2 and Fig. 16.1. After licensure of PCV13, a prompt transition from PCV7 to PCV13 occurred in 2010 in the United States. A decrease in nasopharyngeal colonization caused by *S. pneumoniae* serotypes 6A and 19A followed.[37,67,85,118,130] A decline in *S. pneumoniae* and a proportional increase in nontypeable *H. influenzae* and *M. catarrhalis* AOM occurred (Fig. 16.1). Pneumococcal otopathogens from the middle ear cultures from children from 2011 to 2013 showed a significant decrease in PCV13 serotypes and in penicillin-resistant isolates. The most common non-PCV13 serotypes were 35B; 21; 23B; 15A, B, C; 11; and 23A.[67]

Pneumococcal AOM in children younger than 2 years has been studied following the sequential introduction of PCV7 and PCV13. In the PCV7 era in Israel there was a 77% decline in pneumococcal AOM episodes. In the post-PCV13 era, there was a 51% decline in PCV13 serotypes, and the most common non-PCV13 serotypes isolated from middle ear fluid (MEF) were 15B/C, 16F, and 35B.[11] Overall the trend in AOM cases has declined since the introduction of PCVs according to other reports in the United States, the United Kingdom, and Israel.[134] In 2015, *M. catarrhalis* became the most common cause of AOM in the Rochester otitis media research center.[25]

Etiology in Neonates

Other than the more frequent occurrence of disease caused by gram-negative enteric organisms (approximately 20% of cases) and the occasional isolation of other neonatal pathogens (e.g., group B streptococci), the bacteriology of otitis media in this age group is similar to that in older children.

PATHOPHYSIOLOGY

Tympanic Membrane

As inflammation develops in the middle ear space, changes in the tympanic membrane occur rapidly. The presence of congested blood vessels, edema (which obscures normal landmarks), and bulging occurs, indicating not only a myringitis (inflammation of the tympanic membrane) but also the presence of fluid under pressure in the middle ear space. Sometimes blebs appear on the surface epithelium as a consequence of AOM and the heat of the inflammatory process (most often associated with group A streptococcal infections of the middle ear).

Inflammation may occur on outer epithelial or inner mucosal sides of the fibrous layer (middle layer) of the tympanic membrane. In severe cases, infection may involve the fibrous layer itself. The membrane thickens as a result of edema and infiltration of polymorphonuclear leukocytes. All three layers of the tympanic membrane may undergo dissolution owing to pressure necrosis resulting from the expanding middle ear abscess or thrombophlebitis of tympanic veins, with resulting perforation. With evacuation of the contents of the middle ear abscess after perforation or therapeutic tympanocentesis, healing may be rapid, and the perforation usually seals within a few days. In the process of healing, scar formation may occur.

Occasionally, when a perforation is close to the margin of the annulus or occurs in the Shrapnell membrane, the skin of the external auditory canal and the surface squamous epithelium of the tympanic membrane may grow through the aperture and invade the middle ear. This event may lead to formation of a cholesteatoma (epidermal inclusion cyst). Even if the perforation heals, a differential in gas pressure across the tympanic membrane caused by malfunction of the eustachian tube may result in resorption of gas in the middle ear cavity and negative pressure in the middle ear, which causes retraction of the Shrapnell membrane or an atrophic scar into the middle ear or mastoid attic.

Eustachian Tube

The eustachian tube is approximately 3.8 cm long in an adult. It opens in the fossa of Rosenmüller and extends upward, backward, and laterally to open in the upper anterior wall of the tympanic cavity (protympanum). At birth, the eustachian tube is immature; that is, it is much shorter and floppier than at 1 year of age. It is composed of two portions: the cartilaginous portion extending into the nasopharynx and the bony portion originating in the middle ear. The upper third of the tube is bony; the middle ear opening is the widest, and the medial end (the part joining the cartilaginous eustachian tube), or isthmus, is the narrowest. Pneumatic peritubal air cells arising from the middle ear cavity surround it and can extend to the petrous apex. The internal carotid artery courses anteromedial to this region.

The lower two-thirds of the eustachian tube is a narrow, slit-like, fibrocartilaginous passage. It makes a 160-degree angle with the bony portion at its junction.

Three muscles are associated with the eustachian tube. The tensor tympani muscle lies on top of it; the levator veli palatini muscle lies under it; and the tensor veli palatini muscle arises on the tube, scaphoid fossa, and spine of the sphenoid and then courses around the hook of the hamulus and forms an aponeurosis with its mate (from the opposite side) in the soft palate. This muscle is the only one that acts directly on the eustachian tube.[16]

The eustachian tube area, protympanum, and hypotympanum are lined by ciliated columnar epithelium with goblet cells or secretory cells. The epithelium is continuous with the upper airway system and paranasal sinuses. This area also contains a well-defined subepithelial connective tissue layer, which thins out and may be absent nearing the antrum and mastoid air cell system. The movement of the cilia and mucous blanket always is toward the eustachian tube and nasopharynx. The tube is surrounded by a plexus of lymphoid channels. It has an arterial supply from a branch of the middle meningeal or accessory meningeal artery and from branches of the artery of the pterygoid canal. The nerve supply is from the tympanic plexus (ninth cranial nerve; sensory) and sphenopalatine ganglion (sympathetics and parasympathetic palatine fiber).

The bony portion is rigid and patulous; the medial two-thirds normally is held closed by elastic recoil of the fibrocartilaginous tissue. Contraction of the tensor palatini muscle that inserts in the anterolateral wall opens the tube on swallowing. On average, an adult swallows once per minute while awake and once every 5 minutes while asleep. Suckling infants usually swallow five times per minute.

Mucus and ciliary action flow from the middle ear to the eustachian tube. The eustachian tube acts as a unidirectional valve that favors outflow from the middle ear to the pharynx. Reverse flow can be induced by an increase in pressure in the nasopharynx (Valsalva, barotrauma). During occlusion of the eustachian tube, oxygen and carbon dioxide (and other gases) are absorbed from the middle ear by diffusion into the rich vasculature, and a negative pressure is created. A patent eustachian tube is a crucial prerequisite for subsidence of middle ear disease.

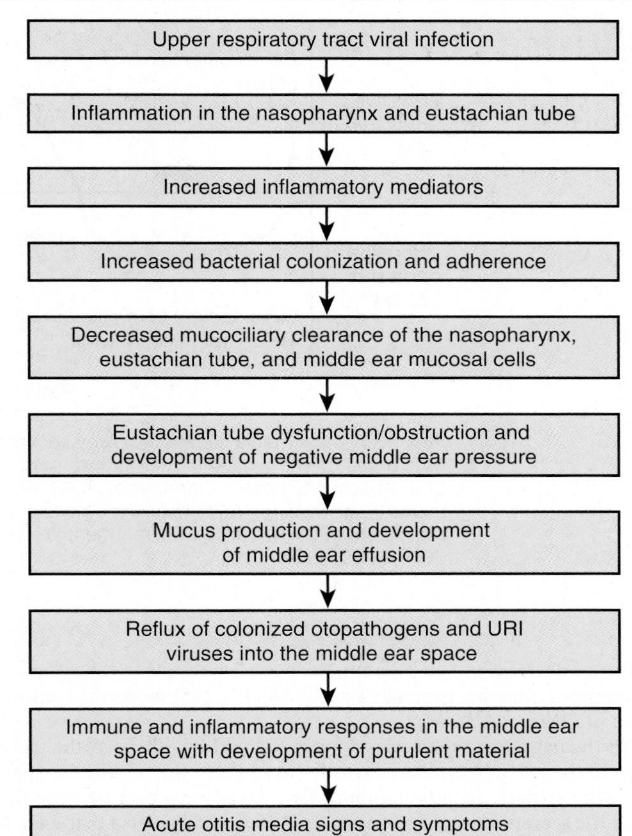

FIG. 16.2 Pathogenesis of virus-induced acute otitis media. *URI,* Upper respiratory infection.

PATHOGENESIS

Approximately 35% of upper respiratory infection (URI) episodes are complicated by AOM, which occurs usually within the first week of URI onset, and 90% to 95% of children with AOM have concurrent URI symptoms.[32,66] Disease etiology and pathogenesis are complex and begin with colonization of mucosal surfaces in the upper respiratory tract by potential AOM bacterial pathogens (Fig. 16.2). In order to colonize the nasopharynx, otopathogens must first compete with each other and with commensal bacteria in the nasopharynx. Nontypeable *H. influenzae* outcompetes *S. pneumoniae* (except serotype 19A) and *M. catarrhalis* for higher rates of colonization during AOM. The combination of respiratory bacteria, *S. pneumoniae*, nontypeable *H. influenzae*, and *M. catarrhalis,* colonizing the nasopharynx and the introduction of a viral URI results in complex interactions that set the stage for the development of AOM.[105,121,142]

Viral URI sets the stage for AOM and OME by increasing mucus production, slowing the beat of cilia in the nasopharynx, creating an inflammatory environment in the nasopharynx, and downregulating the innate and adaptive immune response (discussed later in the section "Immunology"). Next the eustachian tube closes due to inflammation caused as part of the viral URI process. Negative pressure builds in the middle ear space as the air diffuses across the tympanic membrane, resulting in a retracted tympanic membrane. The middle ear goblet cells produce mucus to keep the surface of the middle ear cells moist, and, with the eustachian tube closed, the mucous builds up and causes fluid to be visible behind the tympanic membrane. This is OME. However, when OME develops, the middle ear is still sterile, and the absence of

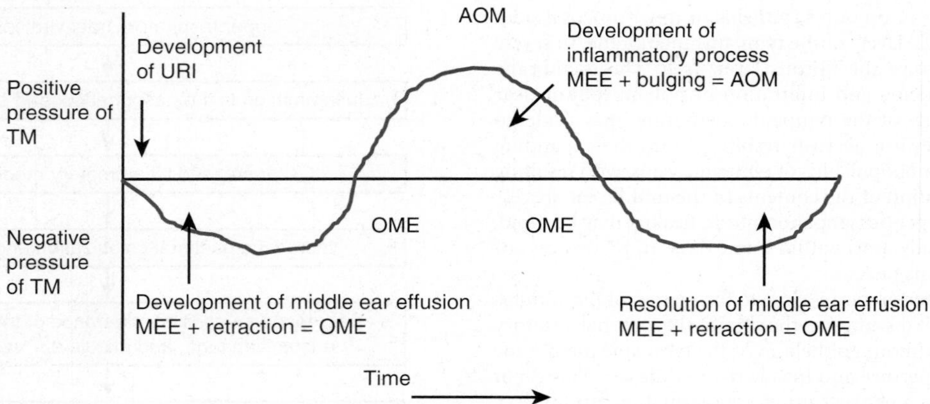

FIG. 16.3 Otitis media continuum. Area above the horizontal line represents positive pressure, bulging, or fullness of the tympanic membrane. Area below the horizontal line represents negative pressure or a retracted tympanic membrane. *AOM,* Acute otitis media; *MEE,* middle ear effusion; *OME,* otitis media with effusion; *TM,* tympanic membrane; *URI,* upper respiratory infection. (Modified from Pichichero ME. Acute otitis media: part II. Treatment in an era of increasing antibiotic resistance. *Am Fam Physician.* 2000;61:2051–56.)

a virus or bacteria and an inflammatory process results in the tympanic membrane remaining generally translucent. Fig. 16.3 shows the continuation of OME and AOM.

As the negative pressure develops in the middle ear space, the secretions in the nasopharynx are literally sucked into the middle ear space when the eustachian tube temporarily relaxes for a part of a second. Once the secretions and accompanying virus and bacteria that were in the nasopharynx gain entry to the middle ear space, the environment is free of immune-controlling factors, and the bacteria begin to divide. In response to the local bacterial invasion, the innate immune response is activated, resulting in the influx of neutrophils. The neutrophils release mediators of inflammation, and the health care provider observes that pathogenic process when glimpsing a tympanic membrane that has become thickened with edema, perhaps red, but most important bulging from the pressure of an inflammatory response (see the section "Clinical Manifestations and Diagnosis").

Bacterial otopathogens and respiratory viruses interact and play important roles in AOM development.[96,105,117] However, much confusion surrounds the role of URI viruses as an etiology of AOM and OME. While there is no doubt that viral URI plays a key role in the pathogenesis of AOM and OME, the role is more facilitation of bacterial AOM than a primary etiologic role for these viruses (see the section "Immunology").[59] Respiratory syncytial virus (RSV), influenza, parainfluenza, rhinovirus, metapneumovirus, and other viruses can be detected in the nasopharynx secretions of children with URI followed by AOM. The nasopharynx secretions can reflux from the nasopharynx via the eustachian tube into the middle ear space, so the detection of the virus in MEF by tympanocentesis does not confirm that virus is the etiology of AOM. With modern polymerase chain reaction (PCR) techniques, the DNA or RNA of viruses can be detected in the nasopharynx and MEF of many children with AOM and OME.[33,60,97,141] The presence of a respiratory virus without a bacterial otopathogen simultaneously detected is uncommon, probably around 2% to 10% of all cases of AOM.[31,116]

OME can persist for some time after an AOM. About half of children who experience AOM will have OME 1 month after initial diagnosis, one-third have OME 2 months after AOM, and 10% have OME 3 months after AOM (Fig. 16.4).

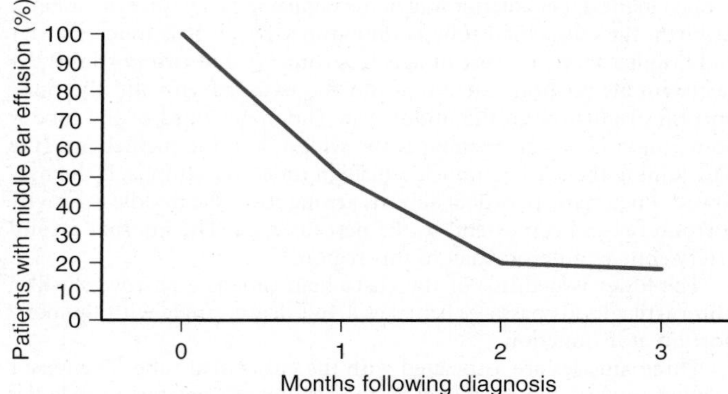

FIG. 16.4 Persistence of middle ear effusion after onset of acute otitis media. (Modified from Teele DW, Klein JO, Rosner BA. Epidemiology of otitis media in children. *Ann Otol Rhinol Laryngol.* 1980;89:5–6.)

DIAGNOSIS

Symptoms and Clinical Manifestations of AOM

Symptoms associated with AOM and its complications and sequelae include the following:

1. Otalgia, or ear pain, is the most common feature of infants and children with AOM. The symptom is suggested in young infants who are pulling at the ear or excessively irritable. Some infants do not have earache.
2. Otorrhea is drainage from the middle ear through a perforation in the tympanic membrane. Relief of the pressure on the tympanic membrane results in immediate decrease in pain. Because the tympanic membrane has a dense network of blood vessels, rapid repair of the membrane occurs, and the perforation usually closes within 24 to 72 hours. If the tympanic membrane seals and the infection still is present, fluid may reaccumulate with renewed acute signs of AOM.
3. Hearing loss occurs whenever fluid fills the middle ear space, whether the fluid is associated with acute infection or with OME. When fluid fills the middle ear space, the median hearing loss is 25 dB (the equivalent of having plugs in the ear canals).
4. Vertigo is not a common complaint of children with AOM. Vertigo occurs more commonly in unilateral than bilateral disease and may be caused by labyrinthitis. Older children describe a feeling of spinning, whereas younger children may not be able to verbalize these symptoms but manifest disequilibrium by falling or stumbling.
5. Tinnitus is an uncommon complaint in children, but when it does occur, the symptom often is caused by OME and eustachian tube dysfunction.
6. Swelling around the ear, especially in the postauricular area, may be a sign of mastoiditis.

7. Facial paralysis in children occurs as a complication of AOM or chronic otitis media with perforation of the tympanic membrane or as a result of an enlarging cholesteatoma.
8. Conjunctivitis has been associated with AOM because the organisms that cause AOM originate in the nasopharynx and may simultaneously cause AOM and conjunctival infection.

There is ample evidence to confirm that the diagnosis of AOM cannot rely on clinical manifestations. Upper respiratory viral infections and AOM occur simultaneously and share many nonspecific symptoms. Table 16.3 shows the sensitivity and specificity of a number of symptoms young children have at the time of evaluation for possible AOM. Parents who suspected that their child aged 6 to 35 months old had AOM were correct only half of the time when the clinicians used strict otoscopic criteria. Half had a URI but no AOM. Ear pain, ear rubbing, fever, irritability, restless sleep, and severe or prolonged rhinitis/cough does not increase the probability of AOM.[77]

AOM symptom scoring scales have been developed to aid in the diagnosis of AOM, to assign severity scores, and to assist in the evaluation of response to treatment or watchful waiting in young children with AOM. Table 16.4 shows AOM scoring systems and the items assessed. A 3-item score (OM-3),[119] consisting of physical symptoms including ear pain, fever, emotional distress (irritability or poor appetite), and limitation in activity, and a 5-item score (Ear Treatment Group Symptom Questionnaire, 5 Items; ETG-5), including fever, earache, irritability, decreased appetite, and sleep disturbance, have been validated. A parental assessment of symptom severity using a visual scale of faces, Acute Otitis Media–Faces Scale (AOM-FS),[112] also has been developed. None of these three scales was adequately sensitive for making the diagnosis of AOM based only on symptoms. However, the OS-8 scale,[91,92] consisting of a set of tympanic membrane photographs that the clinician could use to grade the severity of tympanic membrane inflammation and combined with the faces scale (OM-FS) to assess the parental perception of severity of symptoms, was able to show changes in the child's symptoms and signs of AOM.[50] Another validated scale included a 7-item parent-reported symptom score (Acute Otitis Media Severity of Symptom Scale–AOM-SOS) for children with AOM to aid in assessing patient-reported outcome measures during clinical trials. Symptoms included ear tugging/rubbing/holding, excessive crying, irritability, difficulty sleeping, decreased activity or appetite, and fever. The AOM-SOS scale, when compared with otoscopic diagnoses (AOM, OME, and normal), showed that it, too, changed in response to clinical improvement or deterioration similar to the OS-8 scale.[124,125]

A 30-point symptom scoring instrument (Otitis Media Clinical Severity Index, OM-CSI) was developed to determine the severity of AOM and to measure the treatment outcome of AOM in young children.[38] A shorter, easier-to-use 10-point scoring instrument was developed and compared to the 30-point scoring instrument; both the 10-point and 30-point scoring systems were able to measure treatment outcome and differentiated between clinical cure and failure at the follow-up test-of-cure visit.[23]

TABLE 16.3 Sensitivity and Specificity of Symptoms' Ability to Predict Acute Otitis Media

Symptoms	Sensitivity (%)	Specificity (%)
Cough	47–84	45–83
Ear pain	54–60	82–92
Ear rubbing	42	87
Excessive crying	55	69
Fever	40–69	23–48
Headache	9	76
Poor appetite	36	66
Restless sleep	64	51
Rhinitis	75–96	43–92
Sore throat	13	74
Upper respiratory tract infection	96	29
Vomiting	11	89

Data from Rothman R, Owens T, Simel DL. Does this child have acute otitis media? *JAMA*. 2003;290(12):1633–40.

Diagnostic Signs of Acute Otitis Media

AOM is a visual diagnosis based on viewing the tympanic membrane. The accurate diagnosis of AOM in infants and young children can be difficult. Having the proper equipment and the proper positioning of the child are critical to achieve the correct diagnosis. It is not possible to diagnose AOM accurately without complete visualization of the tympanic membrane. A glimpse of a small portion of the tympanic membrane is not sufficient to make the diagnosis of AOM. It is recommended that the clinician take the time and make the effort to clear

TABLE 16.4 Acute Otitis Media Symptom Scoring Systems Designed to Aid in Diagnosis

3-Item Otitis Media Score (OM-3)	Ear Treatment Group Symptom Questionnaire (ETG-5)	Acute Otitis Media Faces Scale (AOM-FS)	Otoscopic Severity Scale (OS-8)	Acute Otitis Media Severity of Symptom Scale (AOM-SOS)	Otitis Media Clinical Severity Index (OM-CSI) 30-Point Scale[a]	Otitis Media Clinical Severity Index (OM-CSI) 10-Point Scale[a]
Physical suffering	Ear pain	Seven facial expressions ranging from no problem to extreme problem	Eight categories of TM inflammation[b]	Ear pain	Ear pain	Ear pain
Emotional distress	Fever			Ear tugging	Fever	Fever
Limitation of activities	Irritability			Irritability	Irritability	Irritability
	Appetite			Decreased play	Fever at examination	Fever at examination
	Sleep quality			Decreased appetite	TM erythema	TM erythema
				Difficulty sleeping	TM mobility	TM mobility
				Fever	TM position	TM position
					Effusion color	Effusion color
					Otorrhea	Otorrhea

TM, Tympanic membrane.

[a]The 30-point scale used a 2- to 5-point Likert scale and the 10-point scale used a 2- to 3-point Likert scale.

[b]0 = normal; 1 = erythema only; 2 = erythema, air-fluid level, clear fluid; 3 = erythema, complete effusion, no opacification; 4 = erythema, opacification with air-fluid level or air bubbles, no bulging; 5 = erythema, complete effusion, opacification, no bulging; 6 = erythema, bulging rounded doughnut appearance of the tympanic membrane; 7 = erythema, bulging, complete effusion and opacification with bulla formation.

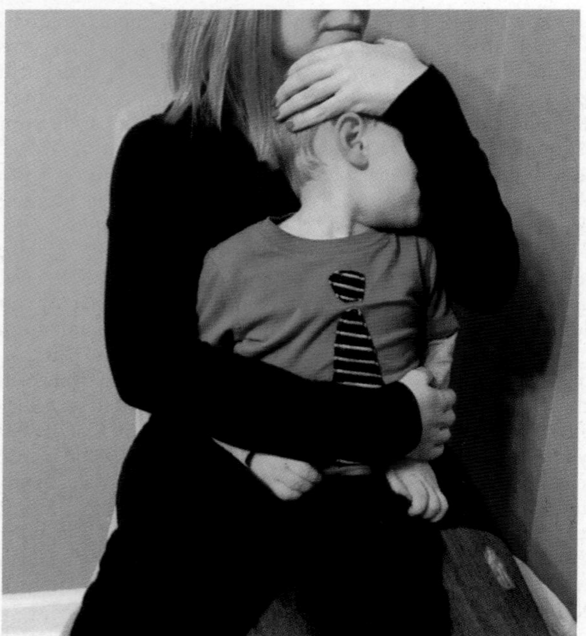

FIG. 16.5 The correct positioning of a child on the parent's lap. This position allows the child to feel secure and allows clear access to examine the ear.

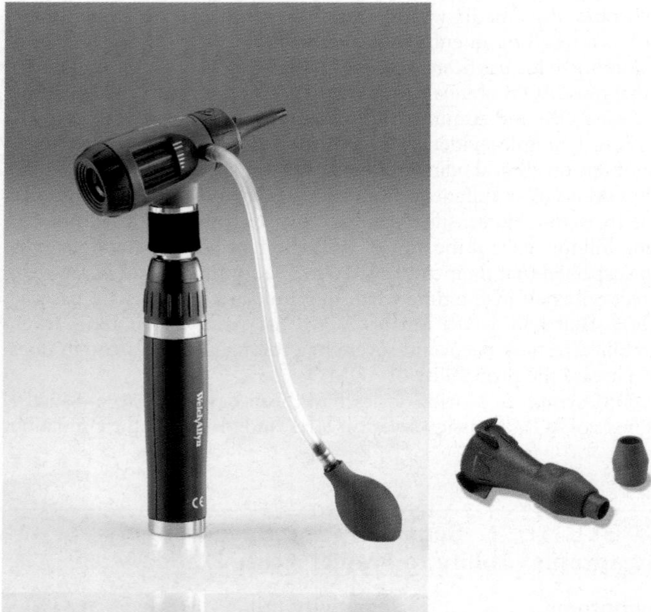

FIG. 16.6 Macroview pneumatic otoscope. (Courtesy Welch Allyn.)

all or nearly all of the ear canal cerumen, use optimal lighting, and use the largest ear speculum that can fit snuggly into the child's ear canal so that a seal can be made for pneumatic otoscopy.

EXAMINATION OF THE EAR

Otoscopy

Examination of the ear should begin with observation of the auricle and the external auditory meatus. Palpation of the periauricular areas should be done to indicate presence of periostitis or diffuse external otitis. The ear canal should be examined for inflammation or cerumen that obstructs vision of the tympanic membrane. Proper positioning of the child for optimal examination of the tympanic membrane is shown in Fig. 16.5.

For proper assessment of the tympanic membrane and its mobility, a pneumatic otoscope in which the diagnostic head has a secure seal should be used. The speculum should have the largest lumen that can fit comfortably into the child's cartilaginous external auditory meatus (Fig. 16.6). The important landmarks of the tympanic membrane that can be visualized with the otoscope are indicated in Fig. 16.7.

The otoscopic examination should include observation of the following conditions of the tympanic membrane:

- *Position:* Normal is slightly convex; bulging indicates increased pressure from positive air pressure or fluid; a retracted eardrum indicates negative pressure with or without effusion; fullness of the tympanic membrane is apparent initially in the posterosuperior portion of the pars tensa and the pars flaccida because these two areas are the most highly compliant parts of the membrane.
- *Appearance and color:* The normal color is pearly gray and translucent; any congestion of the mucous membrane of the middle ear would be reflected in congestion of the vessels of the tympanic membrane and appear pink; a blue discoloration suggests blood in the middle ear associated sometimes with basal skull fracture; the inflamed middle ear mucosa usually is reflected in a bright red tympanic membrane.
- *Integrity of the membrane:* All four quadrants of the tympanic membrane should be inspected for presence or absence of perforation, retraction pockets, or cholesteatoma.
- *Mobility:* Application of positive and negative pressures by the pneumatic otoscope enables the viewer to determine the presence of an air-filled space (rapid movement of the membrane on positive and negative pressures) or a fluid-filled space (limited or no movement of the membrane). Fig. 16.8 shows a normal tympanic membrane, a retracted tympanic membrane, and a bulging tympanic membrane.

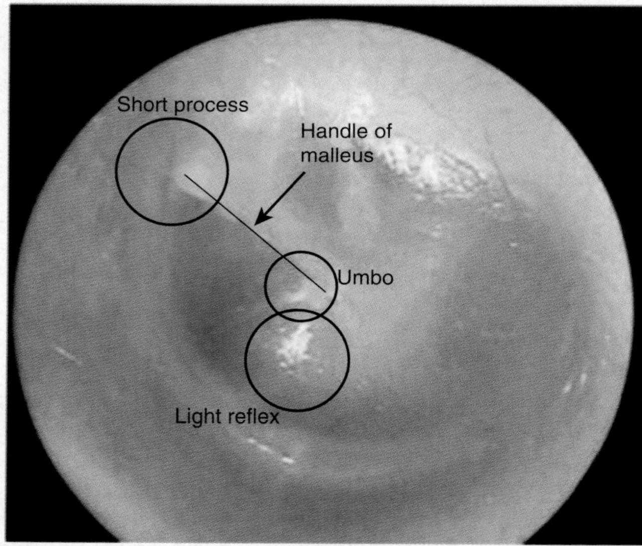

FIG. 16.7 Normal tympanic membrane with normal landmarks identified.

In 2013 the American Academy of Pediatrics (AAP) and the American Academy of Family Physicians (AAFP) released a revision and update of their 2004 AOM guidelines.[81] The 2013 updated guidelines used a more stringent diagnostic definition of AOM. Bulging of the tympanic membrane was emphasized as the most specific otoscopic sign of AOM. Three studies evaluated otoscopic signs—position, color, mobility of the tympanic membrane—and correlated the signs with the presence of middle ear effusion[68] or the isolation of an otopathogen[58,93] following myringotomy or tympanocentesis. Karma et al.[68] looked at the tympanic

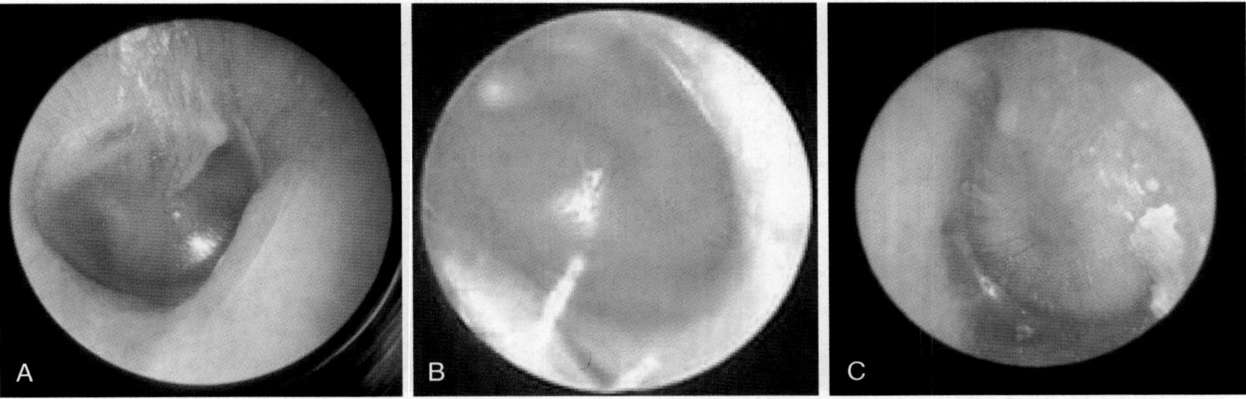

FIG. 16.8 (A) Normal tympanic membrane with a neutral position, pearly gray in color and translucent. Normal landmarks are easily visible. (B) Otitis media with effusion: a retracted tympanic membrane with a very prominent head of the malleolus, gray/yellow in color and semiopaque, with air-fluid level and air bubble visible. (C) Acute otitis media: bulging tympanic membrane with complete loss of normal landmarks, white/yellow in color, and fully opaque with injected vasculature. (Courtesy Dr. Hoberman, University of Pittsburgh.)

membrane physical findings of color, position, and mobility in children with and without acute symptoms suggestive of AOM. Of all the tympanic membrane characteristics, a bulging tympanic membrane reliably predicted the presence of middle ear effusion. Halsted et al.[58] described the likelihood of a positive tympanocentesis culture given different tympanic membrane characteristics. The authors found a positive bacterial culture in 91% of children who had a bulging tympanic membrane, in 21% with a minimally bulging or full tympanic membrane, and in 0% of children without a bulging tympanic membrane. Last, McCormick et al.[92] studied the association between certain signs and symptoms of AOM and the presence of bacterial or viral isolates from middle ear fluid. The authors concluded that the single most important clinical feature associated with a pathogen was fullness and bulging of the tympanic membrane. In all these studies, erythema or lack of mobility of the tympanic membrane was less likely to be associated with middle ear effusion or the isolation of a bacterial pathogen from the middle ear fluid. From those and other studies the key diagnostic feature of AOM was established as a bulging or full appearance to the tympanic membrane (Fig. 16.8C). The bulging of the tympanic membrane is due to positive pressure behind the tympanic membrane caused by inflammation in the middle ear space. AOM is not associated with a retracted tympanic membrane, so a determination of retraction of the tympanic membrane is a viral-mediated phenomenon or associated with OME (Fig. 16.8B). A bulging compared to a retracted tympanic membrane can be difficult to distinguish. Use of pneumatic otoscopy is very helpful in distinguishing the two because positive pressure on insufflation will result in movement backward by a bulging tympanic membrane, and negative pressure will result in movement forward by a retracted tympanic membrane.

Because of the inflammation in the middle ear space during AOM, the tympanic membrane becomes thickened and semi-translucent or completely opaque. A translucent tympanic membrane is very unlikely to be associated with AOM. A translucent or semi-translucent tympanic membrane and middle ear fluid visualized behind the tympanic membrane point to a likely diagnosis of OME (see Fig. 16.8).

Redness of the tympanic membrane is not considered a valuable diagnostic sign of AOM. Redness occurs from inflammation, but a red tympanic membrane can also occur from fever or from a crying child (and most children of the age who experience AOM cry during the examination). When an otoscope speculum is inserted into the external auditory canal, the tympanic membrane will sometimes turn red. The presence of one red tympanic membrane and the other tympanic membrane not red suggests inflammation of the tympanic membrane and is consistent with the diagnosis of AOM if there is fluid visualized behind the tympanic membrane. Such an examination most likely represents an early AOM before inflammation has persisted long enough to cause the tympanic membrane to become thickened and more yellowish and opaque.

OME is not associated with inflammation; however, a child with OME may feel discomfort and may feel popping as air gains entry via the eustachian tube into the middle ear space as well as hearing loss. This may cause the child to pull and tug at the ear or even cry. But the visual examination is distinct from AOM, as just outlined. Fig. 16.9 shows the transition from OME to AOM.

Tympanometry

The tympanogram identifies the movement of the tympanic membrane in response to positive and negative pressure. It utilizes the concept that sound energy in a closed space is diluted or concentrated as the volume increases or decreases (Fig. 16.10). The movement or compliance of the tympanic membrane that occurs following a pulse of air pressure is recorded graphically. The device sweeps pressure from 200 dekapascals (daPa, a unit of pressure equal to 1.04 mm of water) to −300 to 600 daPa. A number of different curves are generated by the tympanometer depending on the state of the middle ear and the patency of the tympanic membrane. A sharply peaked curve with maximum compliance at normal pressure is designated as an A curve and is usually seen with a normal tympanic membrane and middle ear space. A flat curve, referred to as a B curve, is found when there is no movement of the tympanic membrane, when the middle ear is full of fluid, or when there is a perforation of the tympanic membrane. A curve with a peak that occurs at an abnormal amount of negative pressure is referred to as a C curve. A C curve is often seen when there is negative pressure within the middle ear space and the tympanic membrane is retracted (Fig. 16.11). In some cases, the tympanic membrane will be full or bulging, and the tympanic reading is then called a *positive pressure tympanogram readout*. Tympanometry requires a complete seal of the inserted speculum-like device in the external auditory canal and a few seconds of patient cooperation. Children younger than 2 years of age, when AOM is most common, often move, and a seal cannot be obtained. Also if a child is crying a tympanogram reading cannot be obtained.

Acoustic Reflectometry

Spectral gradient acoustic reflectometry (SGAR) has been validated as an accurate method of testing for middle ear effusion in children and infants older than 3 months of age (Fig. 16.12). An 80-dB spectrum of sound, 1.6 to 4.7 kH, is emitted from the device and directed toward the tympanic membrane. The device measures the sum of the reflected sound energy. A normal tympanic membrane and air-filled middle ear space absorb the majority of the sound, and very little acoustic energy reflects back to the device, giving a high numeric readout. If the sound waves hit a thickened tympanic membrane and fluid in the middle ear

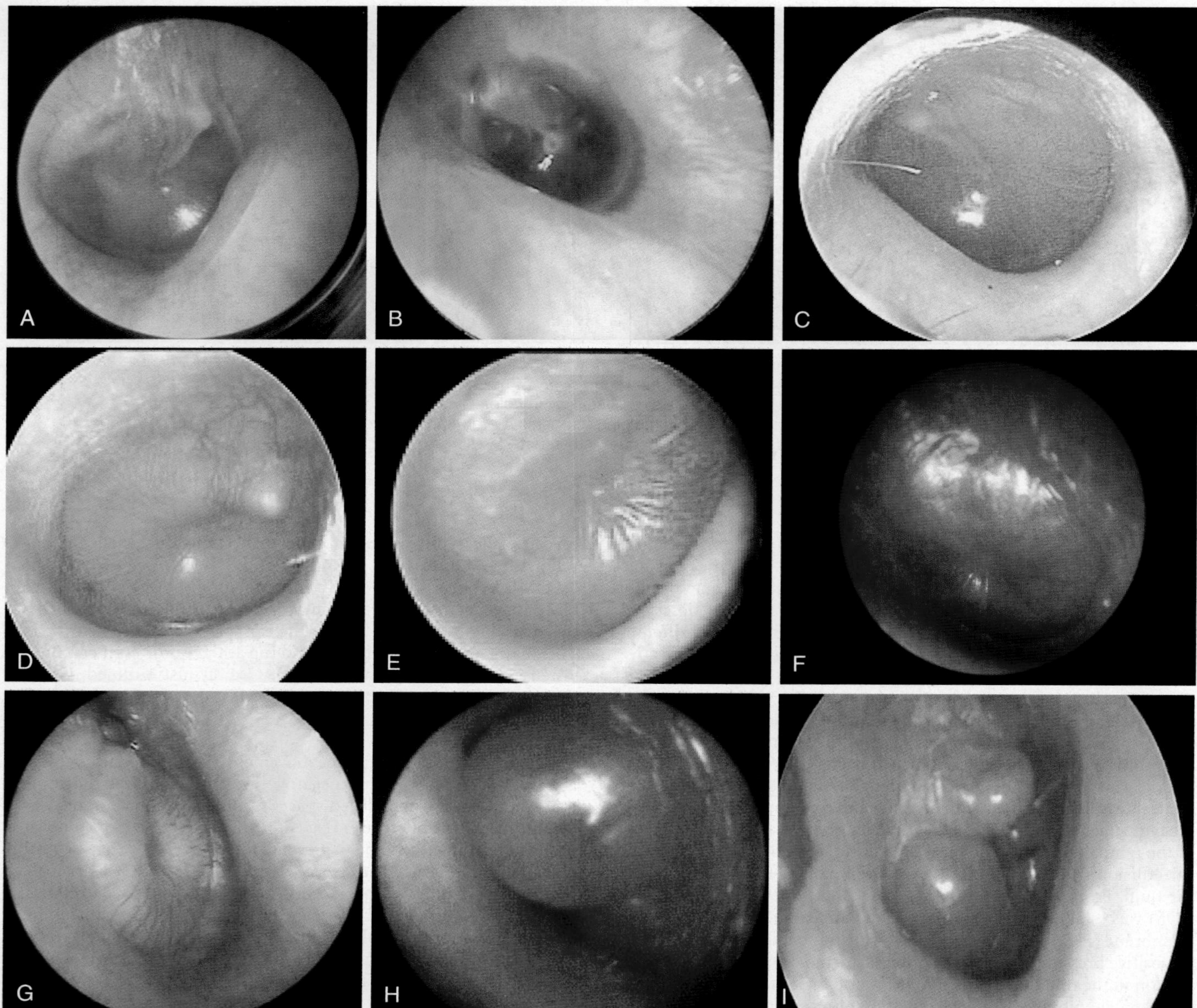

FIG. 16.9 Transition from normal to otitis media with effusion (OME) to acute otitis media. (A) Normal tympanic membrane with pearly gray translucent appearance. (B) OME with air bubbles. (C–D) OME fully filled with effusion; note retracted and translucent tympanic membrane with prominent head of the malleus. (E) Slight bulging with semiopaque white tympanic membrane. (F) Bulging semiopaque tympanic membrane. (G) Markedly bulging, donut appearance, opaque, white tympanic membrane. (H–I) Severe bulging with bullae formation. (Courtesy Dr. Hoberman, University of Pittsburgh.)

space, less sound is absorbed and more sound is reflected back to the device, giving a lower numeric readout. This instrument does not require a seal in the external auditory canal, and readings can be obtained in the crying child. The main limitation is the presence of cerumen in the external auditory canal.

A comparison of tympanometry and SGAR in the ability to assess the presence of middle ear effusion using pneumatic otoscopy as the gold standard showed an agreement between the two methods of 86%. The detection of middle ear effusion by tympanometry and SGAR compared to diagnosis by pneumatic otoscopy showed excellent agreement.[115] Table 16.5 shows the percentage of ears with middle ear effusion documented by pneumatic otoscopy versus the level of SGAR. SGAR instruments detected middle ear effusion with 67% sensitivity and 87% specificity and performed similarly to pneumatic otoscopy.[17] The ease of use, easy portability, absence of need for an airtight seal, and low cost make the use of SGAR an excellent aid in the diagnosis of middle ear effusion.

Audiometric Testing

When fluid is present in the middle ear space, it can cause diminished hearing. An audiogram can assist in establishing the extent of hearing loss for both AOM and OME. Testing the hearing of young children is difficult in clinical settings other than audiology practices that can utilize brainstem evoked responses. Thus, although a potentially useful tool to quantify hearing loss, audiometry is not often used in the first few years of life when AOM and OME most frequently occur. This paradox is problematic for compliance with national recommendations for management of OME, where the presence of unilateral hearing loss

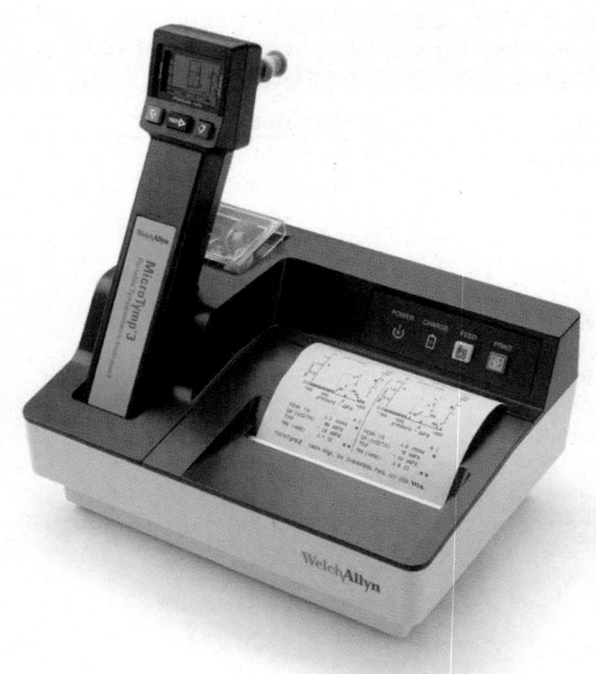

FIG. 16.10 Microtymp tympanometer. (Courtesy Welch Allyn.)

TABLE 16.5 Percent of Ears With MEE Documented by Pneumatic Otoscopy Versus Level of Spectral Gradient Acoustic Reflectometry (*N* = 870 ears)

Level	Predicted Risk of MEE	*N*	Ears With Documented MEE Based on Pneumatic Otoscopy Examination (%)
1	Low	383	3
2	Low-moderate	279	16
3	Moderate	82	34
4	Moderate-high	76	58
5	High	50	92

MEE, Middle ear effusion.
Modified from Block SL, Mandel E, McLinn S, et al. Spectral gradient acoustic reflectometry for the detection of middle ear effusion by pediatricians and parents. *Pediatr Infect Dis J.* 1998;17:560–4.

of 6 months' duration or bilateral hearing loss of 3 months' duration to greater than 30-decibel thresholds in the speech range (500–2000 Hz) is a primary criterion for the recommendation of insertion of tympanostomy tubes.

Tympanocentesis and Myringotomy

Tympanocentesis, a needle aspiration of the middle ear effusion, is used primarily for establishing the presence or absence of an effusion and for microbiologic diagnosis. The 2013 AAP/AAFP AOM guidelines endorse the use of tympanocentesis in the hands of a person skilled in the procedure for treating children with recurrent AOM or treatment failure. Because cultures of the upper respiratory tract are of limited value in providing specific microbiologic diagnosis of AOM, only bacterial cultures obtained by aspiration of the middle ear abscess can be considered a true reflection of the etiology of AOM.[72,137]

Myringotomy is an incision in the anterior lower quadrant of the tympanic membrane for therapeutic drainage. Tympanocentesis or myringotomy should be considered in patients who at onset of AOM appear toxic or are seriously ill, in patients who are not clinically responding after initiation of empiric antimicrobial therapy, in the presence of suppurative complications (including mastoiditis and meningitis), in immunologically deficient patients in whom an unusual organism may be present, and for recurrent AOM in the otitis-prone child.

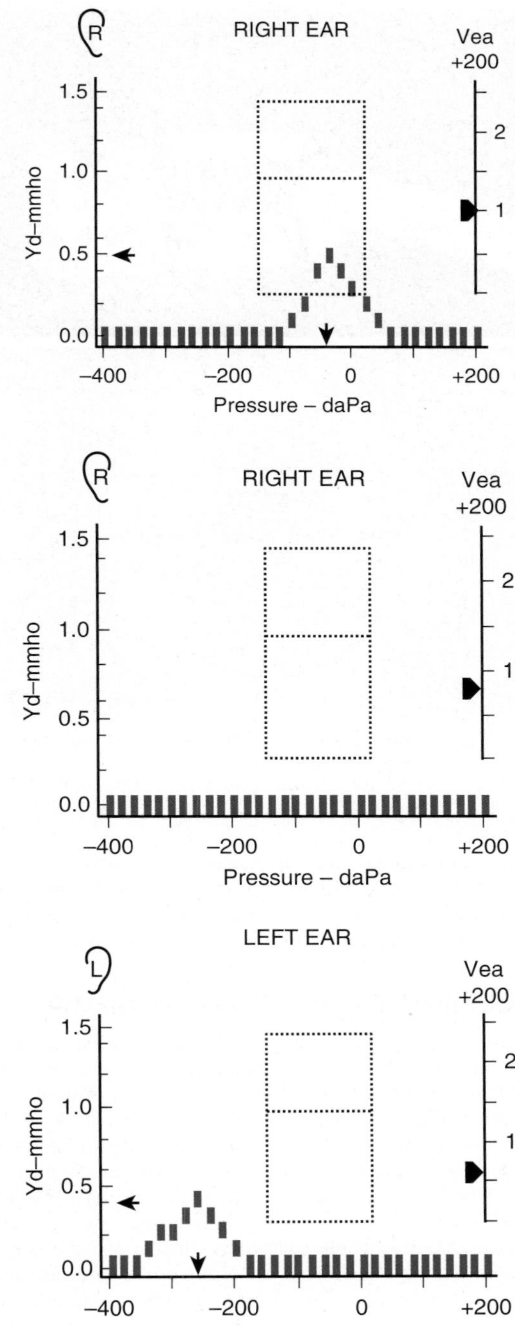

FIG. 16.11 Tympanogram curves. (Top) Normal tympanogram. Normal tympanic membrane compliance; normal tympanic membrane; no middle ear disease. (Middle) Abnormal tympanogram. Decreased compliance of the tympanic membrane; middle ear effusion (otitis media with effusion or acute otitis media). (Bottom) Abnormal tympanogram. Negative pressure in the middle ear space; retracted tympanic membrane.

Radiography

Radiographic evaluation of the temporal bone is indicated when complications or sequelae of otitis media are suspected or present. Plain

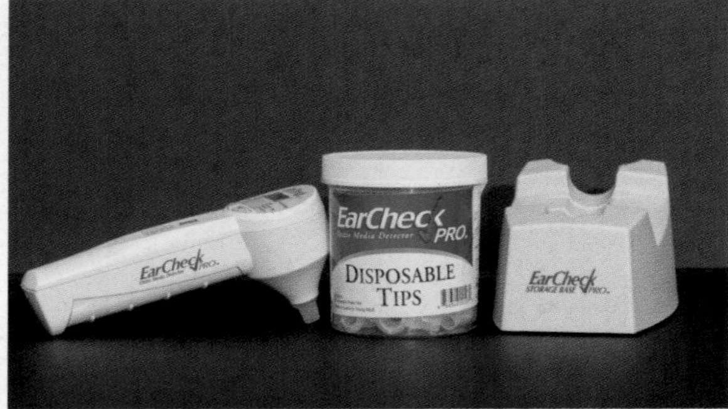

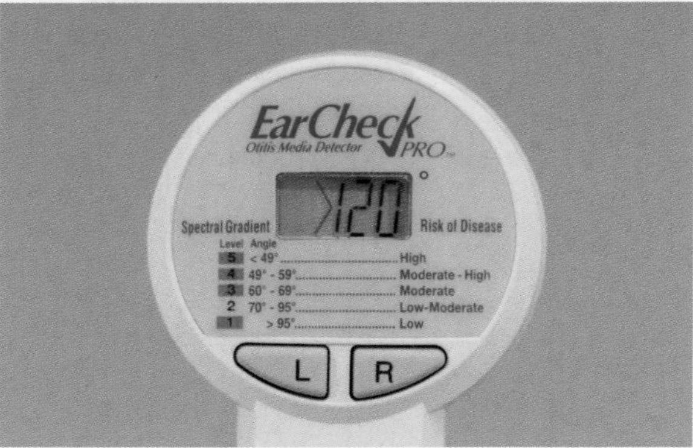

FIG. 16.12 Spectral gradient acoustic reflectometer (SGAR).

TABLE 16.6 Daily Dosage Schedule for Antimicrobial Agents With Indications for the Treatment of Acute Otitis Media

Agent	24-Hour Dosage
Amoxicillin	40–80 mg/kg in 2–3 doses
Amoxicillin-clavulanate	40–100 mg/kg in 2 doses
Cefprozil	30 mg/kg in 2 doses
Cefpodoxime	10 mg/kg in 2 doses
Cefaclor	40 mg/kg in 2–3 doses
Cefixime	8 mg/kg in 1 dose
Cefuroxime axetil	30 mg/kg in 2 doses
Loracarbef	30 mg/kg in 2 doses
Ceftriaxone	50 mg/kg in 1 dose (1–3 days)
Ceftibuten	9 mg/kg in 1 dose
Cefdinir	14 mg/kg in 1–2 doses
Erythromycin-sulfisoxazole	50 mg/kg erythromycin, 150 mg/kg sulfisoxazole in 4 doses
Clarithromycin	15 mg in 2 doses
Azithromycin	30 mg/kg in 1 dose (1 day)
	10 mg/kg in 1 dose (3 days)
	10 mg/kg in 1 dose (day 1); 5 mg/kg in 1 dose (days 2–5)
Trimethoprim-sulfamethoxazole	8 mg trimethoprim, 40 mg sulfamethoxazole in 2 doses

radiographs are of limited value in the diagnosis of osteitis of the mastoid or cholesteatoma; computed tomography and magnetic resonance imaging are more precise and should be obtained if a suppurative intratemporal or intracranial complication is suspected.

MANAGEMENT OF ACUTE OTITIS MEDIA

In the United States the principal treatment of AOM is antibiotics, whereas in other countries watchful waiting with repeat examinations for mild AOM is the norm. Table 16.6 shows the dosing schedule for the antibiotics with an indication for the treatment of AOM. The antibiotic chosen to treat AOM should have a spectrum of activity that includes coverage of the most common otopathogens *S. pneumoniae,* nontypeable *H. influenzae,* and *M. catarrhalis* and have documented clinical and microbiologic efficacy, limited side effects, availability in a convenient dosage schedule, palatability when provided in suspension, and reasonable cost. When treated with appropriate antimicrobial therapy, a patient should have substantial resolution of signs and symptoms within 72 hours and absence of signs of relapse, recurrence, or suppurative sequelae.

The 2013 AAP/AAFP AOM guidelines for initial management of uncomplicated AOM was updated. The updated guidelines differentiate treatment based on the child's age, unilateral or bilateral AOM, and severity of the child's symptoms. High-dose amoxicillin (80–100 mg/kg per day, with a maximum dose of 3 g) is the recommended first-line treatment in most patients. The selection of high-dose amoxicillin has been made on the basis of the long-term safety of the drug; a first intention to treat penicillin-resistant *S. pneumoniae* since that organism can cause the most morbidity; and the recognition that overdiagnosis of AOM is commonplace, and, as a consequence, emergence of antibiotic-resistant microbes occurs more frequently with broader spectrum antibiotics. However, the guidelines point out that a number of antibiotics are clinically effective. In children who have been treated with amoxicillin in the prior 30 days or who have purulent conjunctivitis or in those children who are more likely to have β-lactamase–producing nontypeable *H. influenzae* or *M. catarrhalis,* therapy should be initiated with high-dose amoxicillin-clavulanate (80–100 mg/kg per day of amoxicillin, with 6.4 mg/kg per day of clavulanate), a ratio of amoxicillin to clavulanate of 14 : 1, given in two divided doses, which is less likely to cause diarrhea than other amoxicillin-clavulanate preparations.

Following the introduction and wide use of PCV7 and now PCV13 in the United States, nontypeable *H. influenzae* and *M. catarrhalis* are more common causes of AOM than penicillin-nonsusceptible *S. pneumoniae.* Given the current otopathogen mix and antibiotic resistance, the best choice of antibiotic would be high-dose amoxicillin-clavulanate (90 mg/kg per day divided twice daily). Amoxicillin would not be considered the most effective antibiotic for empiric selection because it has no activity against β-lactamase–producing bacteria, currently far more common than penicillin-resistant *S. pneumoniae.* The addition of clavulanate as a β-lactamase–neutralizing product would provide anticipated efficacy against β-lactamase–producing *H. influenzae* and *M. catarrhalis* while maintaining excellent antimicrobial activity against penicillin-resistant *S. pneumoniae.* There are two disadvantages to amoxicillin-clavulanate: the suspension formulation has a marginal taste that can cause nonadherence to the prescribed regimen, and it causes more loose stools and diarrhea than amoxicillin and many cephalosporin alternatives.

The oral cephalosporins of choice for treatment of AOM, as designated by the AAP, are cefdinir, cefuroxime axetil, and cefpodoxime proxetil. Among these choices in the United States, cefdinir has emerged as the most frequently used, largely because the bitter taste of the other two drugs can be an obstacle for adherence. Cefdinir can be dosed once or divided twice daily (14 mg/kg per day). The duration of treatment with cefdinir can be 5 days with twice-daily dosing or 10 days with once-daily dosing. In a head-to-head comparison of amoxicillin-clavulanate 80 mg/kg per day divided twice daily for 10 days versus cefdinir 14 mg/kg per day divided twice daily for 5 days, amoxicillin-clavulanate demonstrated superior efficacy.[22] However, outside the context of a clinical trial, the adherence characteristics favor cefdinir (better taste and less diarrhea).

The taste of cefuroxime and cefpodoxime can be masked with chocolate syrup, but the addition of flavorings at the pharmacy should not be advised since these antibiotics have been shown to precipitate with changes in pH and chemical reactions between the active drug and the flavoring ingredients.

Ceftriaxone by injection (50 mg/kg per dose) is among the preferred antibiotics in the case of initial antibiotic treatment failure in AOM. Ceftriaxone is effective as a single injection against all penicillin-susceptible *S. pneumoniae* and against β-lactamase–producing *H. influenzae* and *M. catarrhalis*. Three doses of ceftriaxone are needed for penicillin-resistant *S. pneumoniae*.[83] In light of the long half-life of ceftriaxone, it may be possible to administer the sequential doses spaced every other day or even every third day if weekends or holidays dictate an alternative regimen.

Macrolides, such as erythromycin and azithromycin, have poor efficacy against both *S. pneumoniae* and *H. influenzae*. Clindamycin is also included as a treatment alternative for AOM following failure of other preferred first- and second-line agents. Clindamycin is ineffective against β-lactamase–producing *H. influenzae* and *M. catarrhalis* and only effective against penicillin-susceptible and penicillin-resistant *S. pneumoniae*. Its use might best be limited to cases where a tympanocentesis has been performed and the persisting bacteria and antimicrobial susceptibilities are identified.

Antibiotics not listed in the AAP/AAFP guidelines are omitted because of concerns about poor efficacy, poor adherence, or safety. Therefore, the use of alternatives not included in the guideline should be undertaken after due consideration.

Tympanocentesis as Treatment

Tympanocentesis is a treatment for AOM if performed with the intention of evacuating pus, microbes, and proinflammatory fluid from the middle ear space. Not all tympanocenteses are performed with evacuation of middle ear fluid, and that fact complicates the interpretation of available clinical studies of the therapeutic benefit of the procedure. Tympanocentesis can be performed in an office practice setting without anesthesia or conscious sedation in the hands of a person skilled in the procedure. Instillation of 8% tetracaine into the external canal and placement of an otowick to assure the anesthetic reaches the tympanic membrane are effective to allow the procedure to occur without the child experiencing pain. However, the child must be restrained to avoid head movement during the procedure, and children typically cry when they are restrained. Tympanocentesis is not a frequently performed procedure because most clinicians have not been trained how to do it, and those who have been trained become concerned about its use as a standard of care despite the AAP and U.S. Centers for Disease Control recommendation for selected use in AOM management. Tympanocentesis alone is not as effective as tympanocentesis followed by antibiotics if evacuation of middle ear pus is not achieved.[65]

Using a stringent clinical diagnosis (bulging or full tympanic membrane, cloudy or purulent effusion, and reduced or absent tympanic membrane mobility) followed by tympanocentesis for microbiologic diagnosis of AOM, the effects on recurrent AOM and tympanostomy tube placement in children younger than 3 years of age have been studied. The use of strict diagnostic criteria, tympanocentesis, and empiric antibiotic treatment using evidence-based knowledge of circulating otopathogens and their antimicrobial susceptibility profile reduces the frequency of recurrent AOM and tympanostomy tube surgery.[110]

Watchful Waiting

In 2004, the AAP/AAFP endorsed a recommendation for watchful waiting as an option for management of AOM in selected cases. The main concept was to allow observation as an option when the diagnosis is uncertain (unlikely in AOM) as long as the child was older than 2 years and reevaluation could occur if the child did not improve in 48 to 72 hours or worsened at any time. The AAP guidelines may have resulted in a reduction of AOM by establishing precise criteria for diagnosis, but a study indicated that there was no evidence that the pattern of prescribing antibiotics for AOM was altered.[34] Because of the limitations of the clinical trials that supported the strategy of watchful waiting, investigators in Pittsburgh, Pennsylvania, and Turku, Finland, independently conducted a randomized blinded trial of amoxicillin-clavulanate compared with placebo in children younger than 2 and 3 years, respectively. Amoxicillin-clavulanate showed a significant benefit in the duration of acute signs of illness as compared with placebo.[63,133] The 2013 AAP/AAFP AOM guidelines removed the "uncertain" diagnosis and encouraged practitioners to make every effort to use more stringent criteria for the diagnosis of AOM. The guidelines again endorsed the watchful waiting recommendation for children older than 2 years of age with bilateral or unilateral AOM without otorrhea and in children of any age with unilateral AOM without otorrhea and severe symptoms. Again there must be a mechanism in place for prompt reassessment if the child does not improve within 48 to 72 hours or if the child worsens at any time.[81]

Pain Management

There can be considerable pain with AOM, especially in the first 24 hours, and pain management for AOM has received more attention with the publication of the AAP's policy statement on the assessment and management of acute pain in infants, children, and adolescents.[1] A child with suspected or confirmed AOM should be given pain treatment regardless of the use of antibiotics. Various treatments of otalgia have been used; however, none has been well studied. Typically pain control is managed with oral analgesics such as acetaminophen or ibuprofen in weight-appropriate doses. The use of ototopic analgesic ear drops is also to be considered, although the evidence of efficacy is limited.[49]

Antihistamines and decongestants taken orally or intranasally are not recommended as treatment for AOM or OME because they either have been shown to be nonefficacious or have not been studied at all. They may provide some symptomatic treatment of nasal allergies or nasal congestion.

Duration of Treatment

The optimal duration of antibiotic treatment is generally considered to be 10 days in the United States; however, there is scant evidence for that recommendation. Instead, the 10-day treatment course for AOM was derived from the 10-day treatment course for streptococcal pharyngitis, which is evidence based. Treatment regimens of 1 day, 3 days, 5 days, 7 days, and 10 days are all standard in different countries. The 2013 AAP/AAFP guidelines endorse 10 days of treatment duration as the standard for most AOM but state that shorter treatment regimens may be as effective. A systematic analysis and a meta-analysis have concluded that 5 days' duration of antibiotics is as effective as 10 days of treatment for all children older than age 2 years and only marginally inferior to 10 days for children under the age of 2 years.[76] A comparison of 5-, 7-, and 10-day treatments of AOM concluded that 5-day treatment was equivalent to 7- and 10-day treatment for all ages unless the child had a perforated tympanic membrane or had been treated for AOM within the preceding month (because recently treated AOM was associated with more frequent causation of AOM by resistant bacteria and with a continued inflamed middle ear mucosa).[111]

Treatment in the Penicillin-Allergic Child

The use of cephalosporins in penicillin-allergic children has been recently reevaluated. The cephalosporins selected by the AAP took consideration of the likelihood of cross-reaction with penicillin. Second- and third-generation cephalosporins have chemical side chain structures sufficiently distinct from penicillin and amoxicillin that they may be used in penicillin- and amoxicillin-allergic children. The β-lactam ring is not the structure accountable for allergy; it is the side chain. There is some cross-reactivity among cephalosporins based on their shared chemical side chain structure (Tables 16.7 and 16.8).[4,106,108,109] The possibility of allergy to all penicillins and cephalosporins has never been confirmed as a reality, and statistically the likelihood of such a case is indeed very small.

Management of Otitis Media With Effusion

The presence of middle ear effusion without clinical signs or symptoms of inflammation is defined as OME. The two treatment options recommended for persistent OME are watchful waiting and insertion of tympanostomy tubes. Use of oral systemic steroids is not recommended because the evidence in support of their use was deemed insufficient by a US guideline review panel. When used, oral steroids in a burst similar to the burst used in the management of an acute asthma exacerbation (1 to 2 mg/kg per day in the morning for 5 to 7 days) and subsequent examination to determine if the effusion clears might be considered

TABLE 16.7 Structural Similarities of Cephalosporins to Penicillin Derivatives[a]

100% Identical R1 Side Chain	Similar R1 Structural Components
Cefaclor (second) [ampicillin]	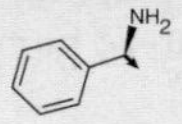 Cefamandole (second) 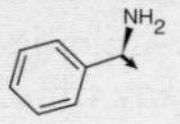
Cefadroxil (first) [amoxicillin]	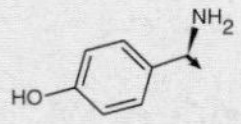 Cefonicid (second) 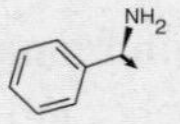
Cefatrizine (first) [amoxicillin]	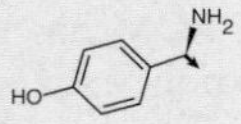
Cefprozil (second) [amoxicillin]	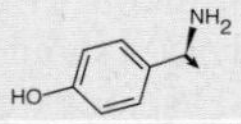
Cephalexin (first) [ampicillin]	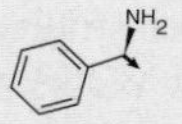
Cephaloglycin (first) [ampicillin]	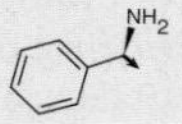
Loracarbef (second) [ampicillin]	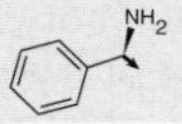

[a]The generation of the cephalosporin drug is shown in parentheses. The penicillin derivative whose R side chain is 100% identical to the cephalosporin R1 side chain is shown in brackets. These drugs are either known to elicit an allergic reaction in penicillin-allergic patients or, due to their similarity to the penicillin derivative, are suggested to be avoided in patients with known allergies to those penicillins.

From Pichichero ME, Zagursky R. Penicillin and cephalosporin allergy. *Ann Allergy Asthma Immunol.* 2014 May;112(5):404–12.

before referral to an ENT specialist for tympanostomy tube insertion. The indication to move from watchful waiting to ENT referral is persisting OME for 6 months in one ear or 3 months in both ears associated with a 30-dB hearing loss in the speech range (see the "Surgical Options" section for further discussion).

Biofilms

OME can become chronic (>3 months in duration). When this occurs, there is ample evidence to suggest that the common otopathogens form a biofilm in the middle ear and on the adenoids. Biofilms involve microbes forming a colony that reduces their process of dividing, slows their metabolism, and allows them to communicate with each other to share survival mechanisms through a process called *quorum sensing*. Biofilm colonies exist in a matrix of DNA and cover themselves with a shield of biomaterial that prevents the penetration of antibiotics and antibodies.[7] Colonies occasionally shed a few organisms from the colony, and these microbes change their biology and are termed *planktonic*. When biofilms form in chronic OME they consist of the major otopathogens as single species or as polymicrobial colonies consisting of two or even three species of otopathogens.[114] Because biofilms do not elicit an immune response, there is little clinical evidence that they exist since there is minimal inflammation in the middle ear when biofilms are present.

Recurrent Acute Otitis Media

The child who returns to the clinician within a month after an initial treatment of AOM with another AOM can be a difficult diagnostic dilemma. In the pre-PCV era, most episodes of true bacteriologic relapse occurred within 2 weeks of the initial diagnosis and were caused by nontypeable *H. influenzae*.[82] In the PCV7 era following initial treatment with amoxicillin-clavulanate, nontypeable *H. influenzae* caused true bacteriologic-recurrent AOM 77% of the time compared to 23% due to *S. pneumoniae*. A relapse of AOM with the same otopathogen most commonly occurred within 14 days of the original infection, and a new AOM episode was more likely to occur more than 14 days from the original diagnosis.[71]

Some children experience enough repeated AOM episodes that they reach a threshold at which they are termed *otitis prone*. The definition of otitis prone has varied among investigators in the field; however, the most frequently used definition currently is three episodes of AOM within 6 months or four episodes within 12 months. Children who experience their first AOM at younger than 6 months, who are male, who attend daycare, and who are exposed to passive cigarette smoke are more likely to experience recurrent AOM.[42] Children with recurrent AOM are generally treated with broader spectrum antibiotics as additional cases of infection occur. This leads to a concerning cycle of escalation of the antimicrobial resistance of bacteria causing AOM in children with recurrent infections. The 2013 AAP/AAFP guidelines address recurrent AOM for the first time. The use of prophylactic antibiotics has shown no benefit[80] in the reduction of additional episodes of AOM in children who experience recurrent AOM and has fallen into disfavor in an era of increasing antimicrobial resistance and an evolving understanding of the role of the resident microbiome of the gut and upper airways in maintaining health.[81] Insertion of tympanostomy tubes may be an option and is widely used for both OME and recurrent AOM (see "Surgical Options" for further discussion).

IMMUNOLOGY

Why do some children experience recurrent AOM while others experience infrequent AOM or no AOM at all? Anatomic dysfunction has been identified as a key element to susceptibility to frequent AOM in some children based on observations of those with poor eustachian tube function, such as children with cleft palate and Down syndrome.[45] However, in recent years the immune response to AOM has come under increased study, and new evidence has emerged to explain susceptibility to an increased frequency of AOM in otitis-prone children.[69,70,74,126,127,132]

Essentially, some of the children who experience frequent AOM have immune responses to the otopathogens causing AOM that are not as robust as the response of non–otitis-prone children. Their immune response is immature, resembling a neonatal-like immune profile.[69,70,74,126,127,132] These children have poor innate and adaptive immune responses to AOM infections. The adaptive immune system includes B cells that mature to plasma cells and plasma cells that produce antibodies. T cells help the B cells mature into plasma cells. B and T cells can also become memory cells. In otitis-prone children this adaptive response is deficient. After an AOM, the immune system of the otitis-prone child fails to generate an immune memory response.[126,127]

The antigen presenting cells (APCs) bridge the innate immune system to the adaptive immune system. APCs are also immature in their responses to the causative otopathogens and are neonatal-like in some children who are otitis prone.[132]

Therefore the otitis-prone child with these deficient immunologic responses remains susceptible to another AOM following antibiotic treatment even by the same otopathogen residing in the nasopharynx that caused a preceding AOM. These immune dysfunctions set the stage for the child to experience recurrent episodes of AOM and become otitis prone.

PREVENTION

Advising Parents

Parents of children who have severe and recurrent otitis media or risk factors for developing middle ear infections should be advised of measures that may reduce the incidence of infection, such as breastfeeding; enrolling children in small, rather than large, group daycare centers; discontinuation of bottle propping; and reducing exposure to tobacco smoke. In addition, data about the risks for developing recurrent otitis media associated with use of a pacifier may be added to the discussion with the parent. Physicians also may advise parents that the seasonal incidence of otitis media suggests that their child's condition is expected to improve in late spring and summer and that aggressive measures of management, including surgery, may be postponed until the course of disease has been determined in the next respiratory season.

TABLE 16.8 Cephalosporin Drugs With Similar R1 Side Chain Structures

Group I[a]	Group II[b]	Group III[c]	Group IV[d]	Group V[e]	Group VI[f]	Group VII[g]	Group VIII
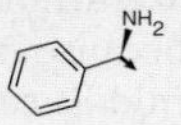	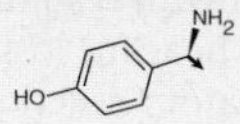	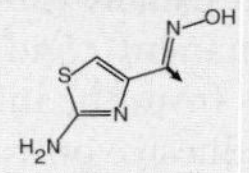	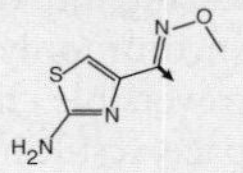	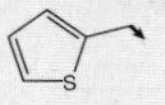	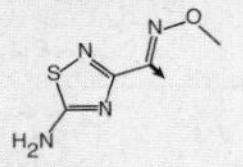	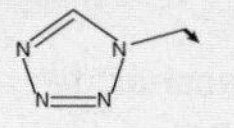	
Identical	Identical	Identical	Identical	Identical	Identical	Identical	Dissimilar
Cefaclor	Cefadroxil	Cefdaloxime	Cefepime	Cephaloridine	Cefozopran	Cefazolin	Cefazedone
Cephaloglycin	Cefatrizine	Cefdinir	Cefteram	Cephalothin	Cefclidine	Ceftezole	Cefbuperazone
Loracarbef	Cefprozil		Ceftiolene	Cefoxitin			Cefmetazole
Cephalexin			Cefditoren		Similar		Cefminox
			Cefetamet		Ceftobiprole		Cefotetan
Similar			Cefmenoxime		Cefluprenam		Cefoperazone
Cefamandole			Cefodizime				Cefpiramide
Cefonicid			Cefoselis		Less similar		Cefsulodin
			Cefotaxime		Ceftaroline fosamil		Cefuroxime
			Cefpirome				Cephacetrile
			Cefpodoxime				Cephapirin
			Ceftizoxime				Cephradine
			Ceftriaxone				Flomoxef
			Cefquinome				Moxalactam
			Similar				
			Cefixime				
			Ceftazidime				
			Less similar				
			Ceftibuten				
			Cefcapene				

[a]This group contains a benzylmethanamine core, except for cefamandole and cefonicid, which contain a core of benzylmethanol.
[b]This group contains a 4-(aminomethyl)phenol core.
[c]This group contains an (E)-2-aminothiazole-4-carbaldehyde oxime core.
[d]This group contains an (E)-2-aminothiazole-4-carbaldehyde O-methyl oxime core, except for cefixime, which contains an attached formic acid to O-methyl oxime; ceftazidime, which contains an attached propionic acid to O-ethyl oxime; ceftibuten, which contains a but-3-enoic acid moiety in place of the formaldehyde O-methyl oxime moiety; and cefcapene, which contains a but-1-en-1-yl moiety in place of the formaldehyde O-methyl oxime group.
[e]This groupi contains a 2-methylthiophene core, except for cefoxitin, which also contains a 7-methoxy group on the β-lactam ring.
[f]This group contains an (E)-5-amino-1,2,4-thiadiazole-3-carbaldehyde O-methyl oxime core, except for ceftobiprole, which contains O-methyl oxime replaced with oxime; cefluprenam, which contains O-methyl oxime replaced with O-fluoromethyl oxime; and ceftaroline fosamil, which contains the (E)-5-amino group replaced with an (E)-5-phosphonoamino group and the O-methyl oxime replaced with an O-ethyl oxime group.
[g]This group contains a 1-methyl-1H-tetrazole core.

Vaccinations to Prevent Acute Otitis Media

Pneumococcal Vaccines

The 2013 AAP/AAFP AOM guidelines recommend vaccination with the pneumococcal vaccine to help with the prevention of AOM. In developed countries, virtually all children are vaccinated with PCV13. The predecessor vaccine PCV7 was shown to be effective in preventing AOM due to the seven serotypes contained in the vaccine. Escape serotypes replaced the seven serotypes in PCV7 over time. Based on the emergence of escape serotypes the newer PCV13 was developed to include the original seven serotypes and the six additional serotypes that had emerged as fairly common.

The 10-valent pneumococcal polysaccharide vaccine (PCV10) conjugated with an outer membrane protein of nontypeable *H. influenzae* also is effective against AOM caused by *S. pneumoniae* strains expressing the capsular serotypes included in the vaccine. In the pivotal licensure trial for PCV10, a reduction of 35% of episodes caused by nontypeable *H. influenzae* was observed. The vaccine is now available in Europe, Canada, South America, and other regions but not in the United States.

The 23-valent pneumococcal polysaccharide vaccine currently available produces an antibody response in children 2 years of age or older. The polysaccharide vaccine is effective in preventing type-specific pneumococcal otitis media if an adequate immune response occurred, but the number of types producing an adequate response is limited. Administration of the polysaccharide vaccine in older children may provide protection against types not included in PCV13 and has been recommended by the AAP and the Advisory Committee on Immunization Practices of the Surgeon General for high-risk children aged 2 years and older who have received PCV13. Table 16.9 shows the currently available pneumococcal vaccines worldwide. Repeated boosting with polysaccharide vaccines has come under scrutiny since a process called "terminal B cell differentiation" may occur whereby B cells respond by producing less antibody and then die before developing into B memory cells.

Influenza Virus Vaccines

Inactivated influenza virus vaccines result in a reduction in cases of influenza-associated AOM in children.[62] A similar reduction in episodes of influenza-associated AOM was reported in children after administration of a live, attenuated cold-adapted intranasal vaccine.[10] Annual administration of influenza virus vaccines should be part of the strategy for reducing the incidence of AOM for children with recurrent and severe disease, as recommended by the 2013 AAP/AAFP guidelines.[81]

Respiratory Syncytial Virus Vaccine

Respiratory syncytial virus (RSV) is more frequently found in children with AOM than any other virus.[103] The risk of development of AOM after viral URI has been well studied. A total of 57% of children with RSV infection develop AOM as compared to 35% for influenza A virus;

TABLE 16.9 Serotypes in Pneumococcal Conjugate Vaccines (PCVs)

Serotype	Polysaccharide 23 Type (Merck)	POLYSACCHARIDE CONJUGATE PCV7 (Pfizer)	PCV13 (Pfizer)	PCV10[a] (GSK)
1	+		+	+
2	+			
3	+		+	
4	+	+	+	+
5	+		+	+
6A	–		+	
6B	+	+	+	+
7F	+			+
7V	–		+	
8	+			
9N	+			
9V	+	+	+	+
10A	+			
11A	+			
12F	+			
14	+	+	+	+
15B	+			
17F	+			
18C	+	+	+	+
19A	+		+	
19F	+	+	+	+
20	+			
22F	+			
23F	+	+	+	+
33F	+			

[a]Not available in the United States.

other viruses had lower rates of AOM.[122] An earlier study showed a somewhat lower risk of AOM (33%) following RSV infection, although it was still the most common virus associated with AOM.[61] Not all respiratory viruses may be equal in their predisposition toward AOM. An effective vaccine against RSV is likely to have the highest impact against the occurrence of AOM following URI.

COMPLICATIONS AND SEQUELAE

Otitis media, with and without its associated hearing loss, can affect a child's development, behavior, and quality of life. Intracranial suppurative complications of otitis media, including meningitis, brain abscess, and lateral sinus thrombosis, are uncommon occurrences today in developed countries but are still prevalent in developing nations. Intratemporal complications that occur within the aural cavity and adjacent structures of the temporal bone are seen more commonly. They include acute and chronic perforation of the tympanic membrane, chronic suppurative otitis media, mastoiditis, cholesteatoma and retraction pocket, adhesive otitis media, tympanosclerosis, and ossicular discontinuity and fixation. The most frequent complication is hearing loss that occurs whenever the middle ear cavity is filled with fluid, when a perforation of the eardrum occurs, and, less commonly, when the ossicles are impaired.

Hearing Loss

Fluctuating or persisting hearing loss is present in most children who have middle ear effusion; impairment of hearing is the most prevalent complication of otitis media with effusion. Audiograms of children with middle ear effusion usually reveal a mild to moderate conductive loss of 15 to 40 dB. With such deficits, the softer speech sounds and voiceless consonants may be missed. The hearing loss is not influenced by the quality of fluid in the middle ear; ears with thin fluids are impaired to the same degree as are ears with fluids of gluelike consistency. The hearing impairment usually is reversed with resolution of the effusion. Uncommonly permanent conductive hearing loss occurs because of irreversible changes from the inflammatory reaction in the middle ear space, resulting in adhesive otitis media or ossicular discontinuity. High negative pressure in the middle ear or atelectasis in the absence of effusion also may cause conductive loss.

Sensorineural hearing loss after a case of AOM is rare but may occur as a result of increased tension and stiffness of the round window membrane and is reversible. A permanent sensorineural loss may occur due to spread of infection or products of inflammation through the round window membrane.

Mastoiditis

Mastoiditis continues to be an important complication of AOM in developed countries, although at a low rate of about 1% of cases. Untreated otitis media may lead to persistent perforation of the tympanic membrane, dysarticulation of ossicles, and mastoiditis.

At birth, the mastoid consists of a single cell, the antrum, connected to the middle ear by a small channel, the aditus ad antrum. Pneumatization of the mastoid bone occurs soon after birth and usually is extensive by the time the child reaches 2 years of age. It is likely that whenever AOM occurs, some degree of mastoiditis is present. With healing of the middle ear infection, healing of the mastoid also occurs. In a few cases, mastoid disease progresses with hyperemia and edema of the mucosal lining of the pneumatized cells, accumulation of serous and then purulent exudates in the cells, demineralization of the cellular walls and necrosis of bone, and formation of abscess cavities caused by coalescence of adjacent cells after destruction of the cell walls. Pus may escape into contiguous areas, including the posterior cranial fossa, middle cranial fossa, sigmoid and lateral sinuses, canal of the facial nerve, semicircular canals, and petrous tip of the temporal bone.

Signs of acute mastoiditis with periostitis include fever, otalgia, postauricular erythema, tenderness, and slight swelling. The pinna may be displaced inferiorly and anteriorly.

Initial management of acute mastoiditis includes administration of parenteral antibiotics and myringotomy to provide drainage of the middle ear and mastoid contents. Surgical drainage of the mastoid should be performed if the symptoms of the acute infection, including fever and otalgia, persist. If the infection progresses, causing destruction of the bony trabeculae, and a mastoid empyema results, mastoidectomy should be performed to prevent spread of the infection to adjacent structures.

Petrositis

Petrositis occurs when suppurative infection extends from the middle ear and mastoid into the petrous portion of the temporal bone. Signs of petrositis include pain behind the eye, deep ear pain, persistent ear discharge, and sixth-nerve palsy. The triad of pain behind the eye, aural discharge, and sixth-nerve palsy is termed *Gradenigo syndrome.* Management is similar to that described earlier for mastoiditis.

Labyrinthitis

Spread of AOM into the cochlear and vestibular apparatus through the round (less commonly, the oval) window results in inflammation of the labyrinth. The signs of labyrinthitis include sudden, progressive, or fluctuating sensorineural hearing loss or vertigo in association with otitis media or mastoiditis. Signs of suppurative labyrinthitis (in the absence of meningitis) warrant performing aggressive otologic surgery and administering parenteral antimicrobial therapy.

Meningitis

Meningitis may be associated with middle ear infections in three circumstances:

1. *Direct invasion:* A suppurative focus in the middle ear or mastoid spreads through the dura, extends to the pia-arachnoid, and causes generalized meningitis.

2. *Inflammation in an adjacent area:* The meninges may become inflamed if there is suppuration in an adjacent area, such as the mastoid air cells.
3. *Concurrent infection:* Otitis media arises by spread of bacteria from the upper respiratory tract, and meningitis concurrently invades the blood from the upper respiratory focus.

Children with cochlear implants are at risk for development of meningitis. Imaging of the temporal bone and inner ear should be performed before cochlear implantation to identify inner ear malformations or cerebrospinal fluid fistulas or ossification of the cochlea that might increase risk of bacterial meningitis after surgery. Although the implant has been implicated in the subsequent development of meningitis, some children likely had an underlying congenital inner or middle ear malformation that provided a pathway for the bacterium to enter the cerebrospinal fluid.

Facial Paralysis

Facial paralysis may occur as a sequela of AOM because of exposure of the facial nerve in the middle ear cleft caused by a bony dehiscence. The palsy usually is unilateral. The paralysis frequently resolves with medical therapy for AOM, but a tympanocentesis (diagnosis of organism) and myringotomy for drainage may be required if the paralysis persists, and, on rare occasions, a facial nerve decompression may be necessary.

Other Suppurative Complications

The middle ear and mastoid air cells are adjacent to the dura of the posterior and middle cranial fossa, the sigmoid venous sinus of the brain, and the inner ear. Suppuration in the middle ear or mastoid may spread to these structures, producing suppurative complications such as meningitis, extradural abscess, subdural empyema, focal encephalitis, brain abscess, and lateral sinus thrombosis. Intracranial complications should be suspected when a child with acute or chronic otitis media develops persistent and severe headache, severe otalgia, and change in affect or level of responsiveness. Conversely, children with diagnosed intracranial infection, such as meningitis, should have middle ear or mastoid disease assessed as the origin of the central nervous system disease.

Intracranial extension of infection from the middle ear into the intracranial area may occur because of any of the following:

1. Progressive thrombophlebitis, permitting infection to spread through the intact bone
2. Erosion of the bony walls of the middle ear or mastoid
3. Extension along preformed pathways such as the round window, dehiscent sutures, skull fractures, and congenital or surgically acquired bony dehiscences

Vestibular Dysfunction

Middle ear effusion can cause disequilibrium and even vertigo, apparently secondary to the inflammatory process crossing the round window membrane or pressure on the oval or round windows. Tympanostomy tube placement can relieve the symptoms as long as labyrinthitis (spread of infection into the balance system of the inner ear) is not the cause.

Effects of Otitis Media on Development of the Child

Children with severe or recurrent otitis media have prolonged time spent with middle ear effusion. Hearing impairment accompanies the effusion in most children. Because language acquisition is dynamic during infancy, any problems in receiving or interpreting sound signals might have a temporary effect on development of speech and language.

Although many studies have been done and are reviewed in the clinical practice guideline "Otitis Media with Effusion in Young Children" published by the Agency for Health Care Policy and Research of the US Department of Health and Human Services, the limitations of design of many of the studies and inconsistencies of the results limit the ability to make conclusions about the effect of otitis media on development. The interested reader should consult the guideline for a valuable review and extensive bibliography. A study by Paradise and colleagues[102] indicates that early placement of ventilating tubes in children with prolonged time spent with middle ear fluid did not measurably improve developmental outcomes at age 3 years.

Perforation of the Tympanic Membrane and Chronic Suppurative Otitis Media

Acute perforation (not caused by trauma) usually is secondary to AOM. The perforation occurs because of pressure of the expanding middle ear contents on the membrane, resulting in local ischemia and tissue damage, usually in the central portion of the membrane. With rupture, the pus is discharged into the external ear canal, with instant relief of pain from the acute infection. Because the membrane is highly vascular, the perforation may seal quickly and not be evident within hours. If the mucous membrane of the middle ear remains inflamed, fluid may reaccumulate behind the resealed tympanic membrane.

Chronic perforation may occur after an acute episode, spontaneous extrusion, or removal of a tympanostomy tube. If squamous epithelium grows at the edges of the perforation, healing may be prevented, and the perforation persists. The term *chronic suppurative otitis media* is limited to a stage of ear disease in which chronic inflammation of the middle ear and mastoid occurs and in which a nonintact tympanic membrane (caused by perforation or tympanostomy tube) and otorrhea are present. Mastoiditis usually is present, and a cholesteatoma may have formed.[18] Surgical repair of a chronic perforated tympanic membrane is presented later, in the section "Surgical Options".

Cholesteatoma

A cholesteatoma usually is a cystic structure lined by squamous epithelium resting on a fibrous strand. The contents of the cyst are the products of desquamation, keratinization, and pus formation. A cholesteatoma may invade, causing local bone erosion and destruction of the ossicles. Aural cholesteatomas can be classified as congenital or acquired.

A congenital cholesteatoma is a congenital collection of epithelial tissue and appears as a white cystlike structure within the middle ear or temporal bone. Acquired cholesteatoma may be secondary to implantation of epithelial tissue or may be a sequela of otitis media, a retraction pocket, or both. Implantation cholesteatoma may develop either from epithelium that has migrated through a perforation of the tympanic membrane or from intraaural epithelium remaining after middle ear or mastoid surgery. A recent histologic study concluded that cholesteatoma can result from stimulated migration of squamous epithelium from the tympanic membrane. Initial management includes initiation of parenteral antibiotics and tympanocentesis (diagnosis of causative organism). Management of cholesteatoma is surgical removal of the entire cyst. Antimicrobial therapy may be necessary if secondary infection is present (see "Surgical Options").

Adhesive Otitis Media

Adhesive otitis media is a result of healing after chronic inflammation of the middle ear and mastoid. Fibrous tissue proliferates in the mucosal lining and may impair movement of the ossicles and result in conductive hearing loss. Adhesive changes may bind the eardrum to the ossicles and surrounding middle ear structures and cause resorption of the ossicles.

Tympanosclerosis and Tympanic Atrophy

Tympanosclerosis, or scarring of the tympanic membrane, is a common sequela following insertion of tympanostomy tubes. White plaques are present in the tympanic membrane and represent calcium deposits in the submucosal layers after blood resorption following the surgical incision of the tympanic membrane.

Tympanic atrophy, or thinning of the tympanic membrane, is also a common sequela following tympanostomy tubes. The thinned area often appears as a round area where the tube was previously inserted and subsequently extruded spontaneously or removed surgically. Tympanic atrophy is associated with mild but measurable hearing loss, depending on the total area of atrophy of the eardrum. Repeated insertions of tympanostomy tubes result in larger areas of tympanosclerosis and atrophy, with the potential for greater measurable hearing loss.

SURGICAL OPTIONS

When nonsurgical methods of prevention fail to prevent recurrent otitis media, surgery is a reasonable option.

Myringotomy and Tympanocentesis

Myringotomy is an incision in the anterior lower quadrant of the tympanic membrane for therapeutic drainage. Tympanocentesis, needle aspiration of middle ear effusion, is used primarily for establishing the presence or absence of an effusion and for microbiologic study. Because cultures of the upper respiratory tract are of limited value in providing specific microbiologic diagnosis of otitis media, only materials obtained by aspiration of the middle ear abscess can be considered a true reflection of the etiology of AOM.[44] Tympanocentesis, with or without myringotomy, should be considered in patients who at onset appear toxic or are seriously ill, in patients who are toxic after initiation of antimicrobial therapy, in the presence of suppurative complications (including mastoiditis and meningitis), and in immunologically deficient patients in whom an unusual organism may be present.

Myringotomy, Tympanostomy Tubes, and Adenoidectomy

After circumcision, myringotomy with tympanostomy tube insertion (M&T) is the most common surgical procedure performed in children that requires general anesthesia; in the United States, about 2 million tubes are inserted annually through the eardrums of probably more than 1 million individuals in this age group. Currently we now have the results of randomized controlled trials (RCTs) to arrive at criteria for tube insertion and, importantly, official guidelines for indications are now available. A shared decision-making (SDM) approach between the clinician and the patient/family to decide to operate is now preferred. A relatively new lay community, Society for Middle-Ear Disease (SMED) and its website (www.societyformiddleeardisease.org), makes available up-to-date information for the professional and caregivers related to myringotomy and tube surgery for this common malady.

Importance of Official Guidelines for Management of Middle Ear Disease

The dissemination of official guidelines on the diagnosis and management of otitis media is an important mission of SMED. One of the leading aims of the society is not only to disseminate these guidelines to health care professionals around the world but also to help lay individuals understand the issues. Most of these guidelines were developed by experts in the field who rely on outcomes of clinical trials that have complied with the scientific rigor needed to answer clinically important questions (evidence-based medicine). Unfortunately, some recent reports have revealed that noncompliance with these guidelines by physicians remains a problem.[30]

Official guidelines on the diagnosis and management of otitis media from several countries are presented on the SMED website. Most were written in language best understood by medical professionals and not lay individuals, but some use language directed at parents and other lay caregivers. Thus another important mission of SMED is to empower patients and their families when discussing management (such as M&T with or without adenoidectomy) with their primary care physician and specialist (otolaryngologist). SMED encourages patients and families to be proactive in the decision-making process when faced with options to treat or not treat and with decisions on which treatments are safe and effective. SDM is preferred over the paternalistic approach once common among many clinicians. These discussions should be in terms that the average caregiver fully understands. Dissemination of these guidelines to health care professionals as well as to patients and their caregivers will create more informed and better health care for middle ear disease in the future.

Current guidelines for otitis media from those countries that have them can be found on the SMED website under the heading Guidelines (www.societyformiddleeardisease.org).

Randomized Controlled Trials

Otitis Media With Effusion

In the past, several studies addressed the efficacy of M&T for treatment of chronic otitis media with effusion, currently the most common indication, but all had problems in design and methodology. There were, however, four relatively recent well-designed RCTs.

Gates and colleagues[51] evaluated 578 San Antonio, Texas, children in a trial that randomly assigned children aged 4 to 8 years who had chronic effusion that was unresponsive to antimicrobial therapy into one of four random arms: (1) myringotomy without tube placement, (2) M&T, (3) adenoidectomy and myringotomy, and (4) adenoidectomy and M&T. The investigators concluded that adenoidectomy and myringotomy were superior to M&T alone and, to some degree, more so than adenoidectomy and M&T. Even though they did not recommend the addition of tubes due to the associated otorrhea, after discussion with parents (i.e., SDM), We recommend both in children in this age group who are affected severely by chronic otitis media with effusion. This RCT did not include a control group of no surgery, but all three of the other treatments did statistically better than myringotomy only and were associated with too many procedures. Thus myringotomy alone is not recommended.

Mandel et al. conducted two trials that addressed M&T for this disease. The first was reported in 1989 by Mandel and coworkers[87] and was an RCT involving 109 Pittsburgh children who had chronic otitis media with effusion that had been unresponsive to antimicrobial therapy. The study randomly assigned subjects to receive (1) myringotomy, (2) myringotomy and tympanostomy tube, or (3) no surgery (control). During this 3-year trial, subjects were evaluated monthly and whenever an ear, nose, and throat illness supervened. Patients who had tympanostomy tubes inserted had less middle ear disease and better hearing than did either children who had only myringotomy or those subjects in the control group. In addition, one-half of the subjects in the myringotomy group had to have tympanostomy tubes inserted during the first year of the trial because of an excessive number of myringotomies and development of "significant" hearing loss; none of these subjects had this degree of hearing loss when they entered the trial. Myringotomy (without tube) provided no major advantage over no surgery (i.e., control) regarding percentage of time with middle ear effusion, number of bouts of AOM, and number of subsequent surgical procedures. It was concluded that myringotomy and tympanostomy tube placement provided more effusion-free time and better hearing than either myringotomy without tube insertion or no surgery, but some patients who received tubes did develop otorrhea, and perforation was a problem in one of the children. Because interpretation of this trial was difficult because of the complexities of the design, the protocol was revised and a second clinical trial was conducted.

In a second trial, reported in 1992, Mandel and colleagues[88] randomized 111 children into the same three groups as in the first study: (1) myringotomy, (2) myringotomy and tympanostomy tube insertion, and (3) no surgery (control). As in the first trial, subjects were reexamined at least every month for 3 years. Outcomes observed in this trial were similar to those reported in the first study. Again, subjects in the myringotomy and tube group had less time with middle ear effusion and better hearing than either those children who had only a myringotomy performed or the group that had no surgery.

In an RCT, Casselbrant and colleagues,[29] compared the efficacy of M&T, adenoidectomy with M&T, and adenoidectomy with myringotomy (without tubes) as the first operative procedure in reducing chronic otitis media with effusion in 2- and 3-year-old children. The investigators concluded that adenoidectomy with or without M&T provided no advantage in this age group.

On the basis of these RCTs, it is recommended that M&T be the first surgical procedure performed, as opposed to myringotomy only or adenoidectomy with M&T for children who have chronic otitis media with effusion of 3 months or longer. Even though Gates and colleagues[51] recommended an adenoidectomy and myringotomy (without tympanostomy tube insertion) as the initial surgical procedure, it is recommended to reserve adenoidectomy for those children who require another surgical procedure if otitis media recurs after extrusion of the initial tube. This recommendation is made since the study by Gates and colleagues showed that adenoidectomy in their population was only a little better than myringotomy and tympanostomy tube and since in the two Mandel trials approximately 50% of the subjects required only one M&T. The RCT conducted by Casselbrant and colleagues[29] failed to show an advantage of adenoidectomy with or without M&T as the first surgical procedure. However, if the child has significant nasal obstruction caused by obstructive adenoids, especially causing obstructive sleep apnea, adenoidectomy and myringotomy (with or without tympanostomy tube insertion) as an initial procedure is a reasonable option; this decision should be shared between the clinician and family (i.e., SDM).

Guidelines: Myringotomy, M&T, and Adenoidectomy for Chronic Otitis Media With Effusion

In 1994, Stool et al.[131] prepared the first clinical practice guideline for otitis media with effusion in young children. That guideline is now outdated. This was followed by a guideline jointly published in 2004 by the American Academy of Otolaryngology–Head and Neck Surgery, the AAP, and the AAFP.[2] That committee recommended that tympanostomy tube insertion be the preferred initial procedure when a child becomes a surgical candidate and that adenoidectomy not be performed unless another indication is present, such as nasal obstruction or chronic/recurrent acute adenoiditis. Repeat surgery should consist of adenoidectomy plus myringotomy, with or without tympanostomy tube insertion. We are in agreement with this indication but with the option of adenoidectomy for repeat surgery.

More recently, in 2013, the American Academy of Otolaryngology–Head and Neck Surgery published a Clinical Practice Guideline for tympanostomy tubes in children.[120] This committee recommended tympanostomy tube insertion in at-risk children (e.g., speech, language, or learning problems) with unilateral or bilateral otitis media with effusion that is unlikely to resolve quickly and persists for 3 months or longer.

The latest committee developing guidelines for otitis media with effusion has been convened (2015) by the American Academy of Otolaryngology–Head and Neck Surgery. Following its deliberations and the published report, we will see greater clarification for indications for tubes for this disease entity. (The guideline will be available on the SMED website.)

Recurrent Acute Otitis Media

RCTs have tested the efficacy of tympanostomy tube insertion for prevention of recurrent acute otitis media. Gebhart[52] in Columbus, Ohio, evaluated otitis-prone infants, of whom 50% had tubes inserted and 50% had no surgery. Efficacy was demonstrated, but infants with middle ear effusion were also enrolled and follow-up was limited to 6 months.

Gonzalez and coworkers[54] conducted an RCT in the U.S. Army that enrolled 65 otitis-prone infants into a trial that randomly assigned subjects into three groups: (1) sulfisoxazole prophylaxis, (2) myringotomy and tympanostomy tubes, and (3) placebo. Similar to the Gebhart trial, infants entered with and without middle ear effusion, were not stratified, and were observed for only 6 months. Infants in the tympanostomy group did significantly better if they had middle ear effusion at entry, but the attack rate of acute otitis media was not reduced in those subjects who were effusion free at the time of random assignment.

Casselbrant and colleagues[28] randomly assigned 264 Pittsburgh children aged 7 to 35 months to one of three groups: (1) amoxicillin prophylaxis (20 mg/kg per day in one dose at bedtime), (2) myringotomy and tympanostomy tube insertion, and (3) placebo. Unlike the two previously reported trials, only patients who had no middle ear effusion were randomized. The children were observed monthly and whenever an ear, nose, and throat illness supervened over the course of 2 years. The average rate of new bouts of AOM was significantly reduced in those subjects who were in the amoxicillin prophylaxis group compared with the tube or placebo group. There was no significant difference between the tympanostomy tube and placebo groups for this outcome measure. Postoperative otorrhea through a tympanostomy tube was an episode of AOM, which occurred at about the same rate as the number of episodes of AOM in the placebo group. However, the bouts of otorrhea were usually asymptomatic and less troublesome than when acute middle ear infection developed in the placebo and amoxicillin prophylaxis groups. When the average of time with otitis media of any type (i.e., acute otitis media, otorrhea, or otitis media with effusion) was evaluated, the tube group had only 6.6% compared to 10% for the amoxicillin group and 15% for subjects who received placebo; tubes had significantly less otitis media of any type than the prophylaxis and placebo groups ($P < .001$). The amoxicillin group had adverse side effects in 7%, primarily urticaria and vaginitis, and 3.9% of the tympanostomy tube group developed persistent perforation of the tympanic membrane; all of these eventually healed spontaneously. Since relatively long-term antimicrobial prophylaxis is related to the development of resistant bacteria, this question was addressed in the trial, but there were no consistent differences in percentages of β-lactamase–positive *H. influenzae* or *M. catarrhalis* found in serial nasopharyngeal cultures between those who received amoxicillin prophylaxis and those who were in the placebo group. During the 2-year trial, 70% of the subjects who were randomly assigned to the tube group required only one procedure, whereas 26% needed a second set of tubes inserted; only one child (1%) had to have three sets of tubes.

We recommended that amoxicillin prophylaxis be the first method used to prevent recurrent episodes in infants and young children, the age group included in the trial. If this failed, tympanostomy tube placement was the next option. We also recommended that children prescribed prophylaxis be reevaluated periodically even if they are symptom free since asymptomatic middle ear effusion may develop. That recommendation was made before awareness that long-term, low-dose antibiotics, especially amoxicillin, are associated with the emergence of antibiotic-resistant pathogens (e.g., *S. pneumoniae*). Thus antibiotic prophylaxis should be an option presented on an individualized basis, such as for children who are anesthetic risks or whose parents choose to withhold surgery.

More recently, Whittemore,[140] in reviewing the literature for tubes in preventing recurrent acute otitis media, cited our RCT as the only acceptable trial and concluded that the "level of evidence favoring (tube) placement is 1b given there is an individual, randomized, controlled trial." The researchers then published a letter to the editor[27] to clarify certain aspects of our trial since there had been some confusion related to its outcomes; also we wanted to provide our more current recommendations because that report was more than 20 years old. We have addressed this clarification and our recommendations earlier.

To assess the efficacy of adenoidectomy, Paradise et al.[101] conducted an RCT in children who had received an M&T in the past and again developed middle ear disease. The team concluded that adenoidectomy was warranted for children who develop recurrent otitis media after extrusion of the previously inserted tubes.

In a follow-up to that trial, Paradise and coinvestigators[100] tested the efficacy of adenoidectomy and adenotonsillectomy for recurrent acute otitis media in children who did not have an M&T in the past and concluded that neither operation was indicated as the first surgical procedure.

Guidelines: Myringotomy and Tympanostomy Tube Placement for Recurrent Acute Otitis Media

The AAP's 2013 clinical practice guideline on the diagnosis and management of acute otitis media includes this key action statement: Clinicians may offer tympanostomy tubes for recurrent acute otitis media (three episodes in 6 months or four episodes in 12 months, with one episode in the preceding 6 months).[84] The American Academy of Otolaryngology–Head and Neck Surgery (2013) in their clinical practice guideline on tympanostomy tubes in children included an action statement profile stating that clinicians should offer bilateral tympanostomy tube insertion to children with recurrent acute otitis media who have unilateral or bilateral middle ear effusion at the time of assessment for tube candidacy.[120] The committee cited the Gebhart[52] and Gonzalez et al.[54] studies to support this conclusion. Troubling is the action statement profile that "Clinicians should not perform tympanostomy tube insertion in children with recurrent acute otitis media who *do not* have MEE [middle ear effusion] in either ear at the time of assessment for tube candidacy." In the Casselbrant et al.[28] trial discussed earlier subjects were entered without middle ear disease because we believed the trials by Gebhart[52] and Gonzales et al.[54] were confounded by the inclusion of such children, and we wanted to determine the efficacy of tubes in children who present with recurrent acute otitis media who met our criteria but had no middle ear fluid at the time of the initial examination. We believe we showed efficacy in our trial given our election to include any acute infection whether the tympanic membrane was intact or not. We considered post-tube otorrhea to be not the same as acute disease when the eardrum was intact.

Tympanostomy Tube Placement and Physiologic Functions of the Eustachian Tube

As presented earlier, there are now RCT results showing that M&T can be beneficial in selected infants and children since middle ear disease is reduced and hearing is restored, although there are known complications and sequelae associated with the surgery. The rationale for the procedure may be found in certain physiologic and pathophysiologic aspects of the nasopharynx, the eustachian tube, middle ear, and mastoid gas cell system that are related to the pathogenesis of otitis media. The eustachian tube has three important physiologic functions in relation to the middle ear: (1) *pressure regulation* of the middle ear, (2) *clearance* of secretions down the eustachian tube, and (3) *protection* of the middle ear from the entry of unwanted nasopharyngeal secretions. A functioning tympanostomy tube maintains ambient pressure within the middle ear and mastoid and provides adequate drainage both down the eustachian tube and through the tympanostomy tube. Two physiologic functions of the eustachian tube are fulfilled by the tympanostomy tube. But the protective function of the eustachian tube is impaired by tympanostomy tube insertion since a patent tympanostomy tube results in an opening in the tympanic membrane, and the physiologic middle ear gas cushion is not present if the tympanic membrane is not intact. Therefore reflux of nasopharyngeal secretions into the middle ear can occur when a tympanostomy tube eliminates the middle ear gas cushion, a situation that can result in otitis media and otorrhea. The tube can result in organisms from the external canal entering the middle ear to cause tube otorrhea. The 2013 guidelines from the American Academy of Otolaryngology–Head and Neck Surgery[120] state that tube-associated otorrhea should be treated with topical antibiotic drops and not oral antimicriobial agents for children who have uncomplicated acute tube otorrhea. The ideal eustachian tube prosthesis would be a transtympanic tube that fulfills all three of the important physiologic functions of the eustachian tube: pressure regulation, drainage, and protection[19] (see the SMED website, www.societyformiddleeardisease.org).

Other Indications for Placement of Tympanostomy Tubes

Although not supported by clinical trials, other indications for tympanostomy tube placement are:

1. Recurrent otitis media with effusion in which each episode does not become chronic but the cumulative duration is excessive, such as six episodes in the previous 12 months
2. Eustachian tube dysfunction that is chronic or recurrent and unresponsive to medical management; atelectasis of the middle ear that is chronic (with or without retraction pocket)
3. Suppurative complications (e.g., facial paralysis, mastoiditis)
4. Time of tympanoplasty when eustachian tube dysfunction is chronic
5. Prevention of otic barotrauma during hypobaric chamber treatment

Acceptable clinical trials for these relatively uncommon indications are either not feasible due to the limited number of patients, or there are ethical concerns, such as when suppurative complications occur.

The rationale for tubes for middle ear infection that is persistent or when suppurative complications are present is similar to incision and drainage of an abscess in other parts of the body. A tympanostomy tube is excellent for desired drainage that is either short or long term.

When Should Tympanostomy Tubes Be Removed?

In general, once tubes are inserted they should be permitted to extrude spontaneously into the external auditory canal and not be removed too early. The rationale for such management is based on experience rather than on any RCT. In children with tympanostomy tubes in place, eustachian tube function does not change significantly, even after several months. There are differences in the life of tympanostomy tubes depending on the type: some have a short duration, whereas for others the tubes may remain in place for years, such as "permanent" long-term tubes.

Nevertheless there are indications to remove tubes in selected children. Tympanostomy tubes may be removed when still in the eardrum by an otolaryngologist as an office procedure with the aid of an operating microscope and without either local or general anesthesia, especially when the tube is partially extruded or when there is chronic infection involving the tympanic membrane. In young children, however, tympanostomy tubes are frequently removed by the otolaryngologist under general anesthesia in the operating room since the procedure can be painful, and the rim of the perforation can be denuded of epithelium and the defect closed (i.e., "paper patch" myringoplasty). Moon et al.[94] recommended tube removal in asymptomatic children when tubes are retained for more than 18 months since spontaneous extrusion seldom occurs after 18 months; removal prior to 12 months resulted in an increased possibility of recurrence, and removal after 15 months showed an increase in complications, such as a perforation of the tympanic membrane.

Removal of tympanostomy tubes depends on several factors, including:

1. Age of the child
2. Duration of time the tube has remained in place
3. Unilateral versus bilateral tubes
4. Status of the contralateral ear when that tympanic membrane is intact
5. Eustachian tube function
6. Presence or absence of recurrent or chronic otorrhea
7. Season of the year
8. Patency of the tube

Complications and Sequelae

As discussed earlier, post-tympanostomy tube otorrhea is a frequent complication but usually effectively treated with ototopical antibiotic drops; a recent study found that antibiotic-glucocorticoid ear drops were more efficacious and cost-effective than oral antibiotics.[136] However, there are other complications and sequelae. Scarring of the tympanic membrane (myringosclerosis) is present in up to half of patients after surgery and can be either localized or even result in diffuse atrophy of the eardrum, with or without a retraction pocket; tympanosclerosis is rarely present in the middle ear and ossicular chain, and thus hearing loss is rare. Atelectasis can occur in which the tympanic membrane becomes flaccid and, in the presence of middle ear negative pressures, can adhere to the medial wall of the middle ear and ossicles. Although many have questioned the presence of long-term hearing loss following tube insertion, the 25-year follow-up study after tube placement by Khodaverdi and colleagues[75] concluded that M&T had no impact on long-term hearing levels; that study also found that hearing loss associated with pathology (e.g., atrophy and myringosclerosis) was more common following tube placement than in non-tubed ears, but the levels were too small to have an impact.

Post-tympanostomy tube perforation of the eardrum can occur following spontaneous extrusion or removal, with the rate varying with the type of tube, number of insertions, and life of the tube; perforation occurs more frequently after "permanent" tubes are extruded or removed. Postoperative tympanostomy tube obstruction is common. A recent study reported a rate of 10.6% and that serous middle ear effusion at the time of surgery and an increased time to the postoperative visit were statistically significant indicators for occlusion.[35] When a tube is obstructed, usually with dried mucus, it may be opened with thin-viscosity ototopical drops. If this is unsuccessful, in older teenagers and adults, it can be opened using a thin wire under the visualization of an operating microscope; in infants, and with caregiver acceptance, it can also be opened using a thin wire procedure but with the infant restrained. When all else fails, the tube can be replaced. Very rarely an acquired cholesteatoma occurs at the site of placement, but, when identified early at postoperative follow-up visits, it can be removed with minor surgery. In general, complications and sequelae associated with tympanostomy tube placement are either transient (e.g., otorrhea) or cosmetic, such as myringoslerosis.[73]

A description of how M&T is performed is available on the SMED website (www.societyformiddleeardisease).[20]

Other Surgical Procedures

Of the other surgical operations for otitis media and its complications, procedures to repair the perforated eardrum are an option. Myringoplasty is an operation that closes the perforated tympanic membrane with a graft or other material, but the middle ear is not entered. Tympanoplasty is also a procedure to repair the tympanic membrane with graft, but the middle ear is opened to inspect the ossicles and the remainder of the middle ear. If ossicles are absent or otherwise abnormal, they can be corrected with an ossiculoplasty. Mastoidectomy for chronic suppurative otitis media and for cholesteatoma is not as common as the procedures described earlier but is still an important component of the otolaryngologist's role in providing surgical care for infants and children who have complications of otitis media.

Descriptions of how these operative procedures are performed are available on the SMED website (www.societyformiddleeardisease).[20]

NEW REFERENCES SINCE THE SEVENTH EDITION

1. AAP Committee on Psychosocial Aspects of Child and Family Health; Task Force on Pain in Infants, Children, and Adolescents. The assessment and management of acute pain in infants, children, and adolescents. *Pediatrics.* 2001;108(3):793-797.
2. American Academy of Pediatrics. Otitis media with effusion. *Pediatrics.* 2004;113(5):1412-1429.
3. Amusa YB, Ljadunota IK, Onayade OO. Epidemiology of otitis media in a local tropical African population. *West Afr J Med.* 2005;24:227-230.
4. Atanasković-Marković M, Velicković TC, et al. Immediate allergic reactions to cephalosporins and penicillins and their cross-reactivity in children. *Pediatr Allergy Immunol.* 2005;16:341-347.
7. Belfield K, Bayston R, Birchall JP, Daniel M. Do orally administered antibiotics reach concentrations in the middle ear sufficient to eradicate planktonic and biofilm bacteria? A review. *Int J Pediatr Otorhinolaryngol.* 2015;79(3):296-300.
11. Ben-Shimol S, Givon-Lavi N, Leibovitz E, et al. Near-elimination of otitis media caused by 13-valent pneumococcal conjugate vaccine (PCV) serotypes in Southern Israel shortly after sequential introduction of 7-valent/13-valent PCV. *Clin Infect Dis.* 2014;59(12):1724-1732.
14. Biswas AC, Joarder AH, Siddiquee BH. Prevalence of SCOM among rural school going children. *Mymensingh Med J.* 2005;14:152-155.
16. Block SL, Heikkinen T, Toback SL, et al. The efficacy of live attenuated influenza vaccine against influenza-associated acute otitis media in children. *Pediatr Infect Dis J.* 2011;30:203-207.
17. Block SL, Mandel E, McLinn S, et al. Spectral gradient acoustic reflectometry for the detection of middle ear effusion by pediatricians and parents. *Pediatr Infect Dis J.* 1998;17:560-564.
18. Bluestone CD, Rosenfeld RM. *Surgical Atlas of Pediatric Otolaryngology.* Hamilton, ONT: BC Decker; 2002.
22. Casey JR, Block S, Hendrick J, et al. Comparison of high dose amoxicillin-clavulanate high to cefdinir in treatment of acute otitis media. *Drugs.* 2012;72(15):1991-1997.
23. Casey JR, Block S, Puthoor P, et al. A simple scoring system to improve clinical assessment of acute otitis media. *Clin Pediatr.* 2011;50:623-629.
24. Casey JR, Kaur R, Friedel V, Pichichero ME. Acute otitis media otopathogens during 2008 to 2010 in Rochester, New York. *Pediatr Inf Dis J.* 2013;32(8):805-809.
25. Casey JR, Kaur R, Pichichero ME. Otopathogens causing AOM in the post-PCV13 era; June 2015. Alexandria, VA: International Society of Otitis Media.
27. Casselbrant ML, Bluestone CD, Kaleida PH, et al. In reference to "What is the role of tympanostomy tubes in the treatment of recurrent acute otitis media?" *Laryngoscope.* 2013;123:e127.
30. Celind J, Sodermark L, Hjalmarson O. Adherence to treatment guidelines for acute otitis media in children. The necessity of an effective strategy of guideline implementation. *Int J Pediatr Otorhinolaryngol.* 2014;78(7):1128-1132.
31. Chonmaitree T, Reval K, Grady JJ, et al. Viral upper respiratory tract infection and otitis media complication in young children. *Clin Infect Dis.* 2008;46:815-823.
32. Chonmaitree T, Ruohola A, Hendley JO. Presence of viral nucleic acids in the middle ear: acute otitis media pathogen or bystander? *Pediatr Infect Dis J.* 2012;31:325-330.
33. Chonmaitree T. Viral and bacterial interaction in acute otitis media. *Pediatr Infect Dis J.* 2000;19:S24-S30.
35. Conrad DE, Levi JR, Theroux ZA, et al. Risk factors associated with postoperative tympanostomy tube obstruction. *JAMA Otolaryngol Head Neck Surg.* 2014;140(8):727-730.
36. Dagan R, Givon-Lavi N, Porat N, et al. The effect of an alternative reduced-dose infant schedule and a second year catch-up schedule with 7-valent pneumococcal conjugate vaccine on pneumococcal carriage: a randomized controlled trial. *Vaccine.* 2012;30:5132-5140.
37. Dagan R, Juergens C, Trammel J, et al. Efficacy of 13-valent pneumococcal conjugate vaccine (PCV13) versus that of 7-valent PCV (PCV7) against nasopharyngeal colonization of antibiotic-nonsusceptible *Streptococcus pneumoniae. J Infect Dis.* 2015;211:1144-1153.
38. Dagan R, Leibovitz E, Greenberg D, et al. Early eradication of pathogens from middle ear fluid during antibiotic treatment of acute otitis media is associated with improved clinical outcome. *Pediatr Infect Dis J.* 1998;17:776-782.
39. Dagan R. Impact of pneumococcal conjugate vaccine on infections caused by antibiotic-resistant *Streptococcus pneumoniae. Clin Microbiol Infect.* 2009;15(suppl 3):16-20.
40. Daly KA, Hoffman HJ, Kvaemer KJ, et al. Epidemiology, natural history, and risk factors: panel report from the Ninth International Research Conference on Otitis Media. *Int J Pediatr Otorhinolaryngol.* 2010;74(3):231-240.
41. Daly KA, Pirie PI, Rhodes KI, Hunter LI, Davey CS. Early otitis media among Minnesota American Indians: the Little Ears Study. *Am J Public Health.* 2007;97:317-322.
42. Damoiseaux RA, Rovers MM, Van Balen FA, et al. Long-term prognosis of acute otitis media in infancy: determinants of recurrent middle ear effusion. *Fam Pract.* 2006;23:40-45.
43. De Wals P, Black S, Borrow R, Pearce D. Modeling the impact of a new vaccine on pneumococcal and nontypeable *Haemophilus influenzae* diseases: a new simulation model. *Clin Ther.* 2009;31(10):2152-2169.
45. Dinç AE, Damar M, Ugur MB, et al. Do the angle and length of the eustachian tube influence the development of chronic otitis media? *Laryngoscope.* 2015;125:2187-2192.
46. Esposito S, Lizioli A, Lastrico A, et al. Impact on respiratory tract infections of heptavalent pneumococcal conjugate vaccine administered at 3, 5 and 11 months of age. *Respir Res.* 2007;8:12.
47. Farrell DJ, Klugman KP, Pichichero ME. Increased antimicrobial resistance among nonvaccine serotypes of *Streptococcus pneumoniae* in the pediatric population after the introduction of 7-valent pneumococcal vaccine in the United States. *Pediatr Infect Dis J.* 2007;26:123-128.
48. Fenoll A, Aguilar L, Vicioso MD, et al. Increase in serotype 19A prevalence and amoxicillin non-susceptibility among paediatric *Streptococcus pneumoniae* isolates from middle ear fluid in a passive laboratory-based surveillance in Spain, 1997–2009. *BMC Infect Dis.* 2011;11:239.
49. Foxlee R, Johansson A, Wejfalk J, et al. Topical analgesia for acute otitis media. *Cochrane Database Syst Rev.* 2006;(3):CD005657.
50. Friedman NR, McCormick DP, Pittman C, et al. Development of a practical tool for assessing the severity of acute otitis media. *Pediatr Infect Dis J.* 2006;25:101-107.
52. Gebhart DE. Tympanostomy tubes in the otitis media prone child. *Larynogoscope.* 1981;91:849-866.
53. Gene A, del Amo E, Iñigo M, et al. Pneumococcal serotypes causing acute otitis media among children in Barcelona (1992–2011): emergence of the multiresistant clone ST320 of serotype 19A. *Pediatr Inf Dis J.* 2013;32(4):e128-e133.
54. Gonzales C, Arnold JE, Woody EA, et al. Prevention of recurrent acute otitis media: chemoprophylaxis versus tympanostomy tubes. *Laryngoscope.* 1986;96:1330-1334.
55. Grijalva CG, Nuorti JP, Griffin MR. Antibiotic prescription rates for acute respiratory tract infections in US ambulatory settings. *JAMA.* 2009;302(7):758-766.
56. Grijalva CG, Poehling KA, Nuorti JP, et al. National impact of universal childhood immunization with pneumococcal conjugate vaccine on outpatient medical care visits in the United States. *Pediatrics.* 2006;118:865-873.
57. Gunasekera H, Morris PS, McIntyre P, Craig JC. Management of children with otitis media: a summary of evidence from recent systematic reviews. *J Paediatr Child Health.* 2009;45:554-563.
58. Halsted C, Lepow ML, Balassanian N, et al. Otitis media clinical observations, microbiology, and evaluation of therapy. *Am J Dis Child.* 1968;115:542-551.
59. Heikkinen T, Thint M, Chonmaitree T. Prevalence of various respiratory viruses in the middle ear during acute otitis media. *N Engl J Med.* 1999;340:260-264.
60. Heikkinen T, Chonmaitree T. Importance of respiratory viruses in acute otitis media. *Clin Microbiol Rev.* 2003;16:230-241.
62. Hoberman A, Greenberg DP, Paradise JL, et al. Effectiveness of inactivated influenza vaccine in preventing acute otitis media in young children: a randomized controlled trial. *JAMA.* 2004;291:692-694.
64. Hoberman A, Paradise JL, Shaikh N, et al. Pneumococcal resistance and serotype 19A in Pittsburgh-area children with acute otitis media before and after introduction of 7-valent pneumococcal polysaccharide vaccine. *Clin Pediatr.* 2011;50:114-120.
65. Kaleida PH, Casselbrant ML, Rockett HE, et al. Amoxicillin or myringotomy or both for acute otitis media: results of a randomized clinical trial. *Pediatrics.* 1991;87:466-474.
67. Kaplan SL, Center KJ, Barson WJ, et al. Multicenter surveillance of *Streptococcus pneumoniae* isolates from middle ear and mastoid cultures in the 13-valent pneumococcal conjugate vaccine era. *Clin Infect Dis.* 2015;60(9):1339-1345.
68. Karma PH, Penttilä MA, Sipilä MM, Kataja MJ. Otoscopic diagnosis of middle ear effusion in acute and non-acute otitis media. I. The value of different otoscopic findings. *Intern J Otorhinolaryng.* 1989;17:37-49.
69. Kaur R, Casey JR, Pichichero ME. Relationship with original pathogen in recurrence of acute otitis media after completion of amoxicillin/clavulanate. *Pediatr Infect Dis J.* 2013;32:1159-1162.
70. Kaur R, Casey JR, Pichichero ME. Serum antibody response to five *Streptococcus pneumoniae* proteins during acute otitis media in otitis-prone and non-otitis-prone children. *Pediatr Infect Dis J.* 2011;30(8):645-650.

71. Kaur R, Casey JR, Pichichero ME. Serum antibody response to three non-typeable *Haemophilus influenzae* outer membrane proteins during acute otitis media and nasopharyngeal colonization in otitis prone and non-otitis prone children. *Vaccine.* 2010;29:1023-1028.
72. Kaur R, Czup K, Casey JR, Pichichero ME. Correlation of nasopharyngeal cultures prior to and at onset of acute otitis media with middle ear fluid cultures. *BMC Infect Dis.* 2014 ect;14:640.
73. Kay DJ, Nelson M, Rosenfeld RJ. Meta-analysis of tympanostomy tube sequelae. *Otolaryngol Head Neck Surg.* 2001;124(4):374-380.
74. Khan MN, Kaur R, Pichichero ME. Bactericidal antibody response against P6, protein D, OMP26 of nontypeable *Haemophilus influenzae* after acute otitis media in otitis-prone children. *FEMS Immunol Med Microbiol.* 2012;65(3):439-447.
75. Khodaverdi M, Jorgenson G, Lang T, et al. Hearing 25 years after surgical treatment of otitis media with effusion in early childhood. *Int J Pediatr Otorhinolaryngol.* 2013;77(2):241-247.
76. Kozyrsky AL, Klassen TP, Moffatt M, Harvey K. Short-course antibiotics for acute otitis media. *Cochrane Database Syst Rev.* 2010;(9):CD001095.
77. Laine MK, Tähtinen PA, Ruuskanen O, et al. Symptoms or symptom-based scores cannot predict acute otitis media at otitis-prone age. *Pediatrics.* 2010;125:e1154-e1161.
78. Lakshman R, Murdoch C, Race E, et al. Pneumococcal nasopharyngeal carriage in children following reduced doses of a 7-valent pneumococcal conjugate vaccine and a 23-valent pneumococcal polysaccharide vaccine booster. *Clin Vaccine Immunol.* 2010;17:1970-1976.
79. Lau WCY, Murray M, El-Turki A, et al. Impact of pneumococcal conjugate vaccines on childhood otitis media in the United Kingdom. *Vaccine.* 2015;8:22-30.
80. Leach AJ, Morris PS. Antibiotics for the prevention of acute and chronic suppurative otitis media in children. *Cochrane Database Syst Rev.* 2006;(4):CD004401.
81. Leiberthal AS, Carroll AE, Chonmaitree T, et al. Clinical practice guideline: the diagnosis and management of acute otitis media. *Pediatrics.* 2013;131:e964-e999.
82. Leibovitz E, Greenberg D, Piglansky L, et al. Recurrent acute otitis media occurring within one month from completion of antibiotic therapy: relationship to the original pathogen. *Pediatr Infect Dis J.* 2003;22:209-215.
83. Leibovitz E, Piglansky L, Raiz S, et al. Bacteriologic and clinical efficacy of one day vs. three day intramuscular ceftriaxone for treatment of nonresponsive acute otitis media in children. *Pediatr Infect Dis J.* 2000;19:1040-1045.
84. Liebenthal AS, Carroll AE, Chonmaitree T, et al. The diagnosis and management of acute otitis media. *Pediatrics.* 2013;131(3):e965-e999.
85. Loughlin AM, Hsu K, Silverio AL, et al. Direct and indirect effects of PCV13 on nasopharyngeal carriage of PCV13 unique pneumococcal serotypes in Massachusetts' children. *Pediatr Infect Dis J.* 2014;33:504-510.
86. Magnus MC, Vestrheim DR, Nystad W, et al. Decline in early childhood respiratory tract infections in the Norwegian mother and child cohort study after introduction of pneumococcal conjugate vaccination. *Pediatr Infect Dis J.* 2012;31(9):951-955.
87. Mandel EM, Rockette HE, Bluestone CD, et al. Efficacy of myringotomy with and without tympanostomy tubes for chronic otitis media with effusion. *Pediatr Infect Dis J.* 1992;11:270-277.
89. Marom T, Tan A, Wilkinson GS, et al. Trends in otitis media-related health care use in the United States, 2001–2011. *JAMA Pediatr.* 2014;168(1):68-75.
90. Martin JM, Hoberman A, Paradise JL, et al. Emergence of *Streptococcus pneumoniae* serogroups 15 and 35 in nasopharyngeal cultures from young children with acute otitis media. *Pediatr Infect Dis J.* 2014;33:e286-e290.
91. McCormick DP, Chonmaitree T, Pittman C, et al. Nonsevere acute otitis media: a clinical trial comparing outcomes of watchful waiting versus immediate antibiotic treatment. *Pediatrics.* 2005;115:1455-1465.
92. McCormick DP, Lim-Melia E, Saeed K, et al. Otitis media: can clinical findings predict bacterial or viral etiology? *Pediatr Infect Dis J.* 2000;19:256-258.
93. McCormick DP, Saeed KA, Pittman C, et al. Bullous myringitis: a case-control study. *Pediatrics.* 2003;112:982-986.
94. Moon IS, Kwon MO, Park CY. When should retained Paparella type 1 tympanostomy tube be removed in children? *Auris Nasus Larynx.* 2013;40(2):150-153.
95. Morris PS, Leach AJ, Silberberg P, et al. Otitis media in young Aboriginal children from remote communities in Northern and Central Australia: a cross-sectional survey. *BMC Pediatr.* 2005;5:27.
96. Nokso-Koivisto J, Pyles RB, Miller AL, et al. Viral load and acute otitis media development after human metapneumovirus upper respiratory tract infection. *Pediatr Infect Dis J.* 2012;31:763-766.
97. Nokso-Koivisto J, Räty R, Blomqvist S, et al. Presence of specific viruses in the middle ear fluids and respiratory secretions of young children with acute otitis media. *J Med Virol.* 2004;72:241-248.
98. O'Brien KL, Millar EV, Zell ER, et al. Effect of pneumococcal conjugate vaccine on nasopharyngeal colonization among immunized and unimmunized children in a community-randomized trial. *J Infect Dis.* 2007;196:1211-1220.
99. O'Brien MA, Prosser LA, Paradise JL, et al. New vaccines against otitis media: projected benefits and cost-effectiveness. *Pediatrics.* 2009;123(6):1452-1463.
100. Paradise JL, Bluestone CD, Colborn DK, et al. Adenoidectomy and adenotonsillectomy for recurrent otitis media: parallel randomized clinical trials in children not previously treated with tympanostomy tubes. *JAMA.* 1999;282:945-953.
103. Patel JA, Nguyen DT, Revai K, Chonmaitree T. Role of respiratory syncytial virus in acute otitis media: implications for vaccine development. *Vaccine.* 2007;25(9):1683-1689.
104. Pelton SI, Loughlin AM, Marchant CD. Seven valent pneumococcal conjugate vaccine immunization in two Boston communities: changes in serotypes and antimicrobial susceptibility among *Streptococcus pneumoniae* isolates. *Pediatr Infect Dis J.* 2004;23(11):1015-1022.
106. Pichichero ME, Casey JR, Almudevar A. Reducing the frequency of acute otitis media by individualized care. *Pediatr Infect Dis J.* 2013;32:473-478.
108. Pichichero ME, Casey JR. Safe use of selected cephalosporins in penicillin-allergic patients: a meta-analysis. *Otolaryngol Nead Neck Surg.* 2007;136:340-347.
109. Pichichero ME, Marsocci SM, Murphy ML, et al. A prospective observational study of 5-, 7-, and 10-day antibiotic treatment for acute otitis media. *Otolaryngol Head Neck Surg.* 2001;124(4):381-387.
110. Pichichero ME. Cephalosporins can be prescribed safely for penicillin-allergic patients. *J Fam Pract.* 2006;55:106-112.
111. Pichichero ME. Use of selected cephalosporins in penicillin-allergic patients: a paradigm shift. *Diagn Microbiol Infect Dis.* 2007;57(suppl 3):13S-18S.
112. Pittman CV, McCormick DP, Uchida T. Development, validity, reliability, and responsiveness of an acute otitis media severity faces scale. *Pediatr Res.* 2004;55:238A.
113. Poehling KA, Szilagyi PG, Grijalva CG, et al. Reduction in frequent otitis media and pressure equalizing tube insertions after introduction of pneumococcal conjugate vaccine. *Pediatrics.* 2007;119:1394-1402.
114. Post JC. Direct evidence of bacterial biofilms in otitis media. *Laryngoscope.* 2015;125:2003-2014.
115. Puhakka T, Pulkkinen J, Silvennoinen H, Heikkinen T. Comparison of spectral gradient acoustic reflectometry and tympanometry for detection of middle-ear effusion in children. *Ped Infect Dis J.* 2014;33:e183.
116. Revai K, Mamidi D, Chonmaitree T. Association of nasopharyngeal bacterial colonization during upper respiratory tract infection and the development of acute otitis media. *Clin Infect Dis.* 2008;46:e34-e37.
117. Revai K, Dobbs LA, Nair S, et al. Incidence of acute otitis media and sinusitis complicating upper respiratory tract infection: the effect of age. *Pediatrics.* 2007;119:e1408-e1412.
118. Ricketson LJ, Wood ML, Vanderkooi OG, et al. Trends in asymptomatic nasopharyngeal colonization with *Streptococcus pneumoniae* after introduction of the 13-valent pneumococcal conjugate vaccine in Calgary, Canada. *Pediatr Infect Dis J.* 2014;33:724-730.
119. Rosenfeld RM, Goldsmith AJ, Tetlus L, Balzano A. Quality of life for children with otitis media. *Arch Otolaryngol Head Neck Surg.* 1997;123:1049-1054.
120. Rosenfeld RM, Schwartz SR, Pynnonen MA, et al. Clinical practice guideline: tympanostomy tubes in children. *Otolaryngol Head Neck Surg.* 2013;149:S1-S35.
121. Ruohola A, Pettigrew MM, Lindholm L, et al. Bacterial and viral interactions within the nasopharynx contribute to the risk of acute otitis media. *J Infect.* 2013;66:247-254.
122. Ruuskanen O, Arola M, Putto-Laurila A, et al. Acute otitis media and respiratory virus infections. *Pediatr Infect Dis J.* 1989;8:94-99.
123. Schilder AG, Lok W, Rovers MM. International perspectives on management of acute otitis media: a qualitative review. *Int J Pediatr Otorhinolaryngol.* 2004;68(1):29-36.
124. Shaikh N, Hoberman A, Paradise JL, et al. Development and preliminary evaluation of a parent-reported outcome instrument for clinical trials in acute otitis media. *Pediatr Infect Dis J.* 2009;28:5-8.
125. Shaikh N, Hoberman A, Paradise JL, et al. Responsiveness and construct validity of a symptom scale for acute otitis media. *Pediatr Infect Dis J.* 2009;28:9-12.
126. Sharma SK, Casey JR, Pichichero ME. Reduced memory CD4+ T-cell generation in the circulation of young children may contribute to the otitis-prone condition. *J Infect Dis.* 2011;204(4):645-653.
127. Sharma SK, Casey JR, Pichichero ME. Reduced serum IgG responses to pneumococcal antigens in otitis-prone children may be due to poor memory B-cell generation. *J Infect Dis.* 2012;205(8):1225-1229.
128. Singleton RJ, Holman RC, Plant R, et al. Trends in otitis media and myringtomy with tube placement among American Indian/Alaska native children and the US general population of children. *Pediatr Infect Dis J.* 2009;28(2):102-107.
129. Stamboulidis K, Chatzaki D, Poulakou G, et al. The impact of the heptavalent pneumococcal conjugate vaccine on the epidemiology of acute otitis media complicated by otorrhea. *Pediatr Infect Dis J.* 2011;30(7):551-555.
130. Steens A, Caugant DA, Aaberge IS, Vestrheim DF. Decreased carriage and genetic shifts in the *Streptococcus pneumoniae* population after changing the seven-valent to the thirteen-valent pneumococcal vaccine in Norway. *Pediatr Infect Dis J.* 2015;34:875-883.
132. Surendran N, Nicolosi T, Kaur R, Pichichero ME. Peripheral blood antigen presenting cell responses in otitis-prone and non-otitis-prone infants. *Innate Immun.* 2016;22(1):63-71.
134. Tamir SO, Roth Y, Dalal I, et al. Changing trends of acute otitis media bacteriology in Central Israel in the pneumococcal conjugate vaccines era. *Pediatr Infect Dis J.* 2015;34:195-199.

135. Usuf E, Bottomley C, Adegbola RA, et al. Pneumococcal carriage in sub-Saharan Africa – a systematic review. *PLoS ONE*. 2014;9:e85001.
136. van Dongen TM, Schilder AG, Venekamp RP, et al. Cost-effectiveness of treatment of acute otorrhea in children with tympanostomy tubes. *Pediatrics*. 2015;135(5):e1182-e1189.
137. van Dongen TMA, van der Heijden GJMG, van Zon A, et al. Evaluation of concordance between the microorganisms detected in the nasopharynx and middle ear of children with otitis media. *Pediatr Infect Dis J*. 2013;332:549-552.
138. Van Gils EJ, Veenhoven RH, Hak E, et al. Effect of reduced-dose schedules with 7-valent pneumococcal conjugate vaccine on nasopharyngeal pneumococcal carriage in children: a randomized controlled trial. *JAMA*. 2009;302:159-167.
139. Vergison A, Dagan R, Arguedas A, et al. Otitis media and its consequences: beyond the earache. *Lancet Infect Dis*. 2010;10(3):195-203.
140. Whittemore KR. What is the role of tympanostomy tubes in the treatment of recurrent otitis media? *Laryngoscope*. 2013;123:9-10.
141. Wiertsema SP, Chidlow GR, Kirkham LA, et al. High detection rates of nucleic acids of a wide range of respiratory viruses in the nasopharynx and the middle ear of children with a history of recurrent acute otitis media. *J Med Virol*. 2011;83:2008-2017.
142. Xu Q, Almudevar A, Casey JR, Pichichero ME. Nasopharyngeal bacterial interactions in children. *Emerg Infect Dis*. 2012;18(11):1738-1745.
143. Zhang Y, Xu M, Zhang J, et al. Risk factors for chronic and recurrent otitis media – a meta-analysis. *PLoS ONE*. 2014;9(1):e86397.

The full reference list for this chapter is available at ExpertConsult.com.

17 Mastoiditis

James D. Cherry • Andrew M. Vahabzadeh-Hagh • Nina L. Shapiro

Mastoiditis, a suppurative infection of the mastoid air cells, is a potential complication of all cases of otitis media caused by the continuity of the mucoperiosteal lining of the mastoid with that of the middle ear.[14] The spectrum of disease in mastoiditis ranges from asymptomatic cases with apparent spontaneous resolution to progressive disease with life-threatening complications.[14] Since the advent of antibiotic therapy, mastoiditis is seen much less frequently, but the complications remain similar.[25,29,31,116] With mastoiditis occurring less commonly, physicians are less likely to consider the diagnosis, especially when the clinical picture has been masked by antibiotic therapy or when the process is chronic and of low grade. Appropriate antibiotic therapy, often accompanied by surgical drainage, can halt and prevent serious complications if mastoiditis is diagnosed early.

HISTORY

Before the advent of antibiotics, mastoiditis was a frequent complication of otitis media that could be treated only by expectant waiting or surgery.[46,53] The first surgical opening of the mastoid cavity was performed in 1736 by Petit using a trepanation system. The trepanation system gave way to the chisel and gouge, which was then replaced by the electric drill, which was introduced at the end of the 19th century.[67] When surgery was used, many patients with mastoiditis were cured by simple mastoid drainage alone, with a mortality rate quoted at 2%.[53] Intracranial complications of mastoiditis carried a very grave prognosis, however. In the preantibiotic era between 1928 and 1933, 25 of every 1000 deaths at Los Angeles County Hospital in California were caused by intracranial complications of otitis media, such as meningitis, venous sinus thrombosis, and brain abscess. In contrast, between 1949 and 1954, only 2.5 per 1000 deaths at the same hospital were caused by complications of otitis or mastoiditis. The use of antibiotics in treating mastoiditis initially led to a marked decrease in the surgical approach to treatment of this illness.[14,116] The realization that infection can persist and that complications of mastoiditis can occur even while the patient is receiving antibiotic therapy has resulted in the present-day approach of combined antibiotics and surgery, necessitating collaboration between the pediatrician and otolaryngologist.[31,32,37,57,64,70,75,102,113]

ANATOMY AND PATHOPHYSIOLOGY

The mastoid process comprises the posterior part of the temporal bone and, as such, is adjacent to many important structures. Within the mastoid is an interconnecting system of air cells divided by bony septa that drain anteriorly into the epitympanic recess of the middle ear via a narrow aditus.[14,30] Only the superior portion of the mastoid airspace, the antrum, is present at birth; pneumatization of the mastoid starts soon after birth and usually is completed by the time the child is 2 years of age.[7,53] Structures lying anteromedial to the mastoid process include the middle ear and ossicles, the facial nerve, the posterior bony wall of the external auditory canal, the jugular vein, and the internal carotid artery. Posteromedially, the mastoid borders the posterior cranial fossa and the sigmoidal sinus. Superiorly, the mastoid borders the middle cranial fossa. Medially, the mastoid cortex encases the cochlea and semicircular canals. The soft tissues and muscles of the lateral neck are located inferiorly. Any or all of these adjacent structures can be affected by extension of a suppurative process in the mastoid.

A certain amount of mastoid inflammation accompanies all cases of otitis media because the mastoid airspaces are continuous with the middle ear cavity, and both are lined by a continuous mucoperiosteum.[7,30] The first stage of an ear and mastoid infection is associated with hyperemia of the middle ear and the mastoid air cell mucosa. If the infection persists, an exudative stage develops, with serum, fibrin, polymorphonuclear cells, and red blood cells accumulating in the middle ear and mastoid. The accumulation of purulent exudate increases the middle ear pressure, eventually resulting in perforation of the tympanic membrane, followed by drainage of mucopurulent matter from the middle ear and mastoid air cells. Some children also have such marked mucoperiosteal swelling that the drainage of pus from the mastoid is blocked, causing aditus blockade. The pus under pressure creates an environment of local acidosis, hypoxia, and ischemia, causing decalcification and resorption of the bony septa. The term *coalescent mastoiditis* is applied to this process because, with the destruction of the bony septa, the mastoid air cells coalesce into large cavities. Osteomyelitis of the adjacent bone may develop, with subsequent bony erosion and eventual extension of the infection into surrounding structures.[7,30]

Congenital cholesteatomas usually manifest as a "squamous pearl" in the anterosuperior quadrant of the middle ear, abutting the tympanic membrane. They may be associated with recurrent otitis media.[61] Acquired cholesteatomas often are a result of chronic infections and tympanic membrane perforation. The perforation allows for squamous material from the external auditory canal to enter the middle ear space (medial migration or Habermann's theory).[80] This tissue contains osteolytic enzymes, leading to bony erosion or mastoid air cell obstruction.[71] Cholesteatomas also may cause slow, insidious erosion of underlying bone, predisposing the patient to extramastoid spread of infection months or years later.[30,86]

MICROBIOLOGY

The bacteriologic findings in 12 studies of acute mastoiditis and one study of chronic mastoiditis are presented in Table 17.1. These studies,

TABLE 17.1 Summary of Bacterial Isolates From the Middle Ear, Subperiosteal Abscess, or Mastoid of Children With Mastoiditis in 13 Studies

	ACUTE MASTOIDITIS										CHRONIC MASTOIDITIS		
Isolates	**Ginsburg, 1955–79**[29]	**Hoppe, 1975–92**[40]	**Ogle, 1973–84**[75]	**Nadal, 1971–88**[70]	**Ghaffar, 1983–99**[25]	**Zapalac, 1993–2000**[114]	**Bakhos, 1994–2008**[4]	**Quesnel, 2001–08**[89]	**Stenfeldt, 1996–2005**[97]	**Pang, 1996–2006**[82]	**Brook, 1976–78**[9]	**Halgrimson, 1999–2008**[34]	**Giannakopoulos, 2012–14**[28]
Streptococcus pneumoniae	14	13	5	9	20	15	19	87	19	16	1	31	17
Streptococcus pyogenes	8	4	3	4	4	10	4	20	4	3	2	22	—
Staphylococcus aureus	8	2	1	4	5	3	—	6	5	4	8	8	1
Staphylococcus spp. coagulase negative	1	2	2	6	7	12	1	13	—	—	—	—	—
Other aerobic gram-positive cocci	3	—	1	2	2	—	—	3	—	—	4	7	2
Haemophilus influenzae	1	—	2	1	—	1	—	8	1	3	—	3	4
Pseudomonas aeruginosa	2	—	—	3	5	—	—	8	5	11	7	8	—
Other aerobic gram-negative rods	1	1	1	1	4	—	—	7	—	—	7	—	—
Anaerobic cocci	1	—	—	1	—	—	—	—	—	—	23	—	—
Anaerobic gram-positive bacilli	—	—	—	1	—	—	—	—	—	—	14	—	—
Anaerobic gram-negative bacilli	1	—	1	—	—	—	1	11	—	—	24	—	—
Other	1	—	4	—	—	10	—	8	—	5	—	13	—
Total patients with cultures	49	28	30	54	49	64	31	158	42	56	24	92	24

which were all carried out in the antibiotic era, span a 61-year time period and occurred in seven countries.* In all studies the leading causative agent in acute mastoiditis is *Streptococcus pneumoniae*; surprisingly the second organism of importance is *Streptococcus pyogenes*.†

Other organisms of importance in acute mastoiditis are *Staphylococcus aureus, Haemophilus influenzae,* and *Pseudomonas aeruginosa*. Because nontypable *H. influenzae* is a very common cause of otitis media, it is surprising that this agent is not more commonly recovered in acute mastoiditis. Similarly, *Moraxella catarrhalis*, another common cause of otitis media, is rarely found in association with acute mastoiditis.[52]

Also, because neither *S. aureus* nor *P. aeruginosa* is a cause of acute otitis media it is likely that these agents, when isolated in acute mastoiditis, are secondary rather than primary pathogens. The same is likely for coagulase-negative staphylococci and various anaerobic organisms. However, in contrast to *S. aureus* and *P. aeruginosa,* if coagulase-negative staphylococci and anaerobic organisms are present they may be contaminates and may not contribute to the infectious process.

An increased incidence of penicillin-resistant *S. pneumoniae* infections has occurred during the past 25 years, leading to a higher likelihood of mastoiditis being a complication of otitis media.[13,74,76,114] The percentage of pneumococcal mastoiditis caused by penicillin-resistant strains increased from 25% to 44% between 1994 and 1998, without an increase in the total number of cases of pneumococcal mastoiditis.[43] Pneumococcal conjugate vaccine (PCV7) was introduced into the pediatric immunization schedule in 2000 and, over the ensuing decade, invasive pneumococcal disease decreased dramatically (see Chapter 85). PCV7 contains the serotypes 14, 6B, 19F, 18C, 23F, 4, and 9V. Surprisingly, in a large study performed by Choi and Lander,[13] the number of admissions for mastoiditis at an urban tertiary care children's hospital did not decrease in the PCV7 vaccine era. In fact, the post-PCV7 patients had more severe disease compared with patients seen between 1996 and 2002.

Ongkasuwan and associates[76] studied 41 cases of pneumococcal mastoiditis between 1995 and 2007. In the pre-PCV7 era (1995–99) there were 12 cases, and none was caused by the nonvaccine serotype 19A. Between April 2000 and October 2005, there were 15 cases of pneumococcal mastoiditis, and 5 of these cases were due to pneumococcal serotype 19A. In their last time period (November 2006 to June 2007), there were 14 cases, and all were due to serotype 19A. Sixty-eight percent of the serotype 19A isolates had multidrug antibiotic resistance.

In the post-PCV7 era, Giannakopoulos and associates[28] noted that nonvaccine genotype 19A was found in more than half of their mastoiditis cases. In Colorado, Halgrimson and colleagues[34] noted a significant decline in acute mastoiditis cases after the introduction of PCV7. This decline was short-lived, however, with a return to pre-PCV7 rates. In Israel, Amir and coworkers[1] noted an increase of acute mastoiditis caused by *S. pyogenes* between the early 1990s and 2003–09. In another study in Israel, it was noted that there was no overall reduction in acute mastoiditis or in pneumococcal acute mastoiditis in the era of pneumococcal conjugate vaccines.[49] PCV13, the 13-valent pneumococcal conjugate vaccine, was introduced in 2010. Most recently, Tawfik and colleagues[117] used cross-sectional data from the Healthcare Cost and Utilization Project Kids' Inpatient Database to look at the annual prevalence of hospital admission for acute otitis media and its associated complications (acute mastoiditis, suppurative labyrinthitis, or acute petrositis) for the years 2000, 2003, 2006, 2009, and 2012. They found a significant reduction in the national prevalence rates of hospital admission for acute otitis media and its associated complications for all children younger than 21 years from 3.956 to 2.618 per 100,000 persons. The most significant declines were seen between 2000 and 2003 and between 2009 and 2012.

In 2013, Yarden-Bilavsky and associates[112] noted seven cases of acute mastoiditis due to *Fusobacterium necrophorum*. The illnesses in these seven young children were quite fulminate and resulted in prolonged hospitalizations.

The bacteriologic spectrum of chronic mastoiditis differs from that of acute mastoiditis. Aerobic cultures of chronic mastoiditis and chronic otitis media show predominantly *S. aureus* and gram-negative bacilli, especially *P. aeruginosa*.[9,20,86] In addition, a wide variety of anaerobic organisms can be isolated from an infected mastoid and middle ear.[9,20] Brook[9] studied the aerobic and anaerobic bacteriology of chronic otitis media (of ≥3 months' duration) in 24 children. Anaerobic isolates alone were found in 17%, aerobic organisms alone were found in 4%, and mixed aerobic and anaerobic infections were found in 79%. All cases had from two to seven different bacterial isolates. *Peptococcus* spp., *Actinomyces* spp., and *Bacteroides melaninogenicus* (*Prevotella melaninogenica*) were the most commonly isolated anaerobic organisms. Seventeen patients were infected with β-lactamase–producing organisms (i.e., *S. aureus* or *P. melaninogenica, Bacteroides fragilis,* or other *Bacteroides* spp. that were resistant to ampicillin).

Mycobacterium tuberculosis currently is an uncommon cause of mastoiditis in the United States but continues to be a cause of chronically draining ears in lower socioeconomic groups and immigrants from endemic areas.[10,65,68] Case reports of mastoiditis implicate such organisms as nontuberculous mycobacteria,[59,73] *Turicella otitidis,*[90,96] *Aspergillus fumigatus*[35] *Paragonimus*-like trematodes,[78] *Nocardia asteroides,*[63] *Actinomyces* spp.,[101] *Blastomyces dermatitidis,*[43] and *Histoplasma capsulatum.*[63] *Pneumocystis jiroveci* otitis media and mastoiditis have occurred as the first manifestation of acquired immunodeficiency syndrome.[26]

*References 4, 9, 25, 28, 29, 34, 40, 70, 75, 82, 89, 97, 114.

†References 4, 25, 29, 34, 37, 40, 51, 52, 70, 75, 82, 89, 97, 114.

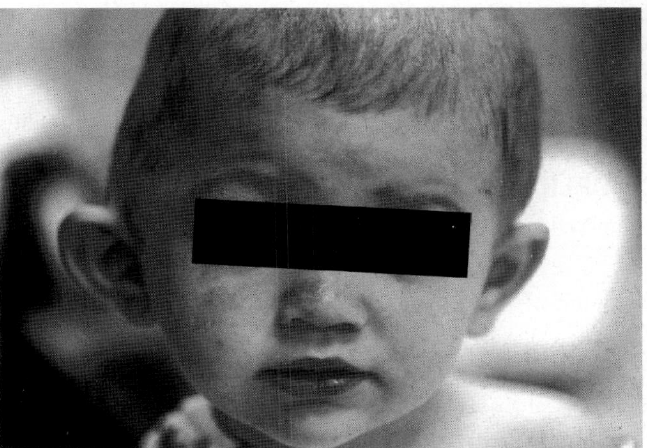

FIG. 17.1 An 18-month-old child with right-sided mastoiditis and proptotic right auricle.

CLINICAL PRESENTATION

The classic presentation of acute mastoiditis is a febrile child with ear pain, postauricular swelling, and postauricular tenderness developing days to weeks after the beginning of development of acute otitis media (Fig. 17.1).[2,25,29,33,70,75,114] If antibiotics were used to treat acute otitis media, the child may have seemed to improve only to become ill again while still receiving therapy or after the antibiotics were stopped; conversely, the inflammation may not have responded to the antibiotics at all. Examination of the tympanic membrane in acute mastoiditis usually shows that it is abnormal.[29,37,70] Early in the course of illness, periosteal inflammation produces swelling and tenderness and sometimes redness over the mastoid process.[7,29] Palpable postauricular fluctuance occurs later, when pus from the mastoid air cells breaks through the underlying bony cortex and forms a subperiosteal abscess.[36] In children older than 1 year of age, the most common area where fluctuance is felt lies behind the ear, where it pushes the earlobe up and out; however, in children younger than 1 year, the fluctuance often may occur above the ear, pushing the pinna down and out.[29]

Mastoiditis has occurred in children with cochlear implants. Zawawi and colleagues[115] reviewed all publications and noted 43 children who had cochlear implants and who subsequently developed acute mastoiditis. They observed that with proper treatment (intravenous antimicrobials and surgery) the implants did not need to be removed in all but one instance.

Chronic mastoiditis is a much more indolent disease process than acute mastoiditis. It develops when long-standing middle ear disease, usually having a duration of months to years, has been present.[86] Fever and postauricular swelling may or may not be present. Persistent or intermittent drainage of mucopurulent matter from a previously perforated eardrum suggests chronic mastoiditis. Hearing loss and ear pain also may accompany chronic mastoiditis.[86] All these symptoms can be mild enough to be ignored until serious intracranial suppuration occurs. Persistent ear drainage, persistent ear pain, or an otitis media nonresponsive to antibiotics should prompt a search for mastoiditis.

COMPLICATIONS

Complications of mastoiditis include subperiosteal abscess,[36] Bezold abscess,[22,62,92] facial nerve paralysis,[18,105,106] meningitis,[14,29] brain abscess,[12,14,29,42,93] cerebellar abscess,[7] epidural abscess,[7] subdural empyema,[8] labyrinthitis,[30,77] venous sinus thrombophlebitis,[5,17,27,47,79,85,91,108] bacteremia,[14,64,77] benign intracranial hypertension,[8] osteomyelitis of the temporal bone with occasional extension to adjacent bones,[7,30] hearing loss,[81] septic pulmonary emboli,[41] and cerebrospinal fluid otorrhea.[30] Subperiosteal abscesses appear as a postauricular fluctuant mass that obscures the postauricular sulcus. They occur when pus in the mastoid breaks through the bony cortex or extends along vascular channels and dissects under the overlying periosteum.[36]

A Bezold abscess develops when a mastoid infection erodes through the bony cortex of the inferior aspect of the mastoid tip and dissects down the tissue planes to form a deep neck abscess. Fluctuance over the mastoid is not felt. Rather, swelling and tenderness are present below the mastoid process and under the sternocleidomastoid muscle.[22]

The facial nerve runs through the mastoid and the middle ear, rendering it vulnerable to injury when extension of mastoid or middle ear infection occurs.[30] Pressure on and inflammation of the facial nerve from symptomatic or asymptomatic mastoiditis can lead to transient or permanent facial nerve paralysis that usually is unilateral, although bilateral facial palsy from mastoiditis can occur.[7,105,106]

Because the temporal bone that houses the mastoid air cells constitutes the floor of the middle and posterior cranial fossae, bony erosion from osteomyelitis, preexisting bony defects, or spread of infection along vascular channels can allow for intracranial spread of mastoid infections into the middle and posterior cranial fossae. The infection may remain confined to the extradural space as an extradural abscess, or it may penetrate the dura and produce a subdural empyema, a brain abscess, a cerebellar abscess, or meningitis.[7,30]

Invasion of infection into the bony labyrinth through the oval or round window triggers labyrinthitis. Initial tinnitus, hearing loss, nausea, and dizziness progress to severe vertigo, ear pain, vomiting, nystagmus, and difficulties with balance.[30]

Intracranial venous sinus thrombophlebitis is a rare but potentially fatal complication of mastoiditis.* The lateral aspect of the sigmoid sinus is formed by the temporal bone. Venous sinus thrombophlebitis results when an underlying mastoiditis extends through the temporal bone in close proximity to the lateral or sigmoid venous sinus. A perisinus abscess initially is formed, followed by formation of a mural thrombus in the sinus wall. The thrombus eventually may occlude the entire sinus, or it may suppurate and spread along the sinus, resulting in septicemia, increased intracranial pressure, septic emboli, and extension of infection to other intracranial structures.[17,23] The classic findings of septic thrombosis of the lateral sinus are "picket fence" spiking fevers, shaking chills, and tenderness along the jugular vein associated with acute or chronic otitis. A palpable "cord" at the jugular vein (indicating a jugular vein thrombus) also may be present. When only a perisinus abscess is present, or if the patient is being treated partially with antibiotics, the only features may be a low-grade fever and headache.[32,103]

Benign intracranial hypertension can be seen in association with lateral sinus obstruction involving the torcular and sagittal sinus secondary to mastoiditis and is termed *otitic hydrocephalus*. Rarely otitic hydrocephalus can be seen with mastoiditis in the absence of lateral sinus thrombosis. The decreased venous drainage caused by the venous sinus obstruction results in increased intracranial pressure, headache, papilledema, and sixth nerve palsy without enlarged ventricles or a space-occupying lesion.[30,32]

Permanent conductive hearing loss occurs when the middle ear mastoid infection is severe enough to damage or destroy the ossicles.

*References 5, 7, 27, 30, 47, 77, 79, 85, 91, 103, 108.

Tuberculous mastoiditis classically manifests as marked conductive hearing loss that often is irreversible.[58]

Osteomyelitis secondary to mastoiditis can spread to adjacent bones. Involvement of the petrous portion of the temporal bone produces a syndrome, described by Gradenigo in 1907, with a triad of abducens paralysis or paresis, severe pain in the distribution of the trigeminal nerve, and suppurative otitis media; this is known as Gradenigo's syndrome or petrous apicitis, and additional cranial nerve deficits also may occur.[11,57,89] Antibiotics may mask the classic signs of petrositis and allow progression to severe intracranial complications, such as meningitis and epidural abscess. Petrositis may be suspected only when antibiotic and surgical management for mastoiditis fails to control chronic ear drainage.[30]

M. tuberculosis mastoiditis is an uncommon finding but should be considered in children who have chronic ear discharge despite having received antibiotic therapy.[58,65] Children can go for months or years with chronically draining ears before the diagnosis of tuberculous mastoiditis is considered.[10,68] Children from lower socioeconomic homes, immigrants from endemic areas, and children with tuberculosis contacts in the family are at risk. The classic presentation in the preantibiotic era was an afebrile young child with painless persistent watery ear drainage, an enlarged preauricular lymph node, a history of contact with a person with tuberculosis, and often facial nerve paralysis.[94,107]

Tuberculous mastoiditis is not always painless.[111] Sometimes the diagnosis initially is suspected only when a mastoidectomy wound does not heal.[55,86] Early in the course of the disease, physical examination may reveal small yellow spots (caseating granulomas) on a thickened and hyperemic tympanic membrane. These spots coalesce early and produce multifocal tympanic membrane perforations.[55] The discharge through these perforations initially is watery, but later it becomes purulent.[54] Pale, avascular granulation tissue is abundant throughout the middle ear and mastoid and often is seen in the external auditory canal and around the tympanic membrane perforation.[10,94,111] Preauricular and postauricular nontender, enlarged lymph nodes may be present,[54,63] and early and severe hearing loss is characteristic.[111] Often, there is evidence of tuberculosis elsewhere in the body.[111] A tuberculin skin test usually, but not always, is positive.[68]

DIFFERENTIAL DIAGNOSIS

Postauricular swelling, a chronically draining ear, or radiographic evidence of mastoid abnormalities also can appear in other disease entities. Postauricular lymphadenopathy can occur secondary to a scalp infection, causing postauricular swelling. The swelling is discrete, does not displace the pinna, and does not obliterate the postauricular sulcus.[29] Severe otitis externa may lead to periauricular cellulitis, with postauricular swelling, erythema, and tenderness.[6,39] Mumps can cause parotid swelling, pushing the earlobe up and out, but the swelling is over the parotid gland rather than located postauricularly. Histiocytosis,[48,60] acute lymphocytic leukemia,[69] acute myelogenous leukemia,[48,104] Burkitt lymphoma,[109] non-Hodgkin lymphoma,[44] aneurysmal bone cysts,[16] and other benign and malignant tumors of the mastoid bone[15] also can manifest as symptoms clinically suggestive of mastoiditis. Kawasaki disease may mimic acute mastoiditis with postauricular lymph node swelling and ear pain.[88] Children with severe and recurrent ear infections may have an underlying congenital or acquired immunodeficiency.

SPECIFIC DIAGNOSIS

The diagnosis of mastoiditis can be made on clinical grounds alone when a child has an acute episode of fever, otitis media, and posterior auricular tenderness and fluctuance. Temporal bone computed tomography (CT) always is recommended to confirm the diagnosis and assess for coalescence. Mastoiditis is much less likely when swelling and tenderness over the mastoid process are absent, such as when an infection has been masked by antibiotic treatment or when it has extended to an area other than over the mastoid process. Mastoiditis needs to be considered in all cases of otitis media not responding to antibiotics and in all intracranial suppurative diseases that do not have an apparent focus.

Obtaining an aspirate from the middle ear is an important part of properly diagnosing and managing mastoiditis. Gram stains of aspirates from the middle ear are quite accurate and, as such, can help in the initial selection of antibiotic therapy for chronic mastoiditis. Brook[9] found that in 24 children with tympanocentesis, half of the Gram stains showed a complete correlation with subsequent culture results, and the other half showed a partial correlation (one bacterial species was not seen). Leukocytes were seen on all the Gram stains. In addition, cultures from the middle ear accurately reflect mastoid disease.[29,64]

Ginsburg and associates[29] compared the results of cultures of middle ear aspirates and mastoid cultures in 16 patients with acute mastoiditis and found that the same bacterial species was isolated from both sites. A sterile aspiration through an intact tympanic membrane gives the most accurate culture information. If the tympanic membrane is perforated, the purulent drainage may be contaminated by colonizing ear canal flora. An aspirate for culture generally should be obtained from the ear drainage, preferably from as close to the perforation as possible. Aspiration of postauricular fluctuance also is useful in identifying the responsible organisms.[36,75] In addition, specimens should be obtained directly from the mastoid at surgery. All of them should be sent for aerobic and anaerobic cultures with proper anaerobic transport technique. If the child has had a chronic ear infection, or if the child is in a high-risk population for acquiring tuberculosis, mycobacterial stains and cultures also should be obtained and a tuberculin skin test should be placed or a serum immunologic-based tuberculosis test should be performed.

A lumbar puncture should be performed if the clinical presentation suggests meningeal irritation. A CT scan should be obtained before performing the lumbar puncture if papilledema or a suggestion of focal intracranial extension is present. Lymphocytosis of the cerebrospinal fluid suggests a parameningeal focus of infection. An immunologic evaluation should be considered if a child has had recurrent episodes of otitis media leading to mastoiditis.

Peripheral white blood cell counts in mastoiditis may be normal or elevated, often with an increase in band-form neutrophils.[37,70] The erythrocyte sedimentation rate often is elevated in acute mastoiditis, but it usually is normal in chronic mastoiditis.[81]

When a patient is not improving on medical therapy, radiologic imaging of the temporal bone is needed. Changes in the temporal bone are seen best on a CT scan.[99] Early in the course of mastoiditis, nonspecific clouding of the middle ear and mastoid is seen. With time, necrosis and coalescence of the bony septa occur. Other CT findings in mastoiditis include hypoaeration of the mastoid and adjacent bony destruction. A CT scan of a child with unilateral mastoiditis complicated by lateral sinus thrombosis and elevated intracranial pressure is shown in Fig. 17.2. Magnetic resonance imaging is valuable to search for suppurative intracranial complications of mastoiditis.[84,98,99] In addition, sometimes magnetic resonance angiography or venography (or both) is indicated to diagnose sigmoidal sinus thrombosis.[15]

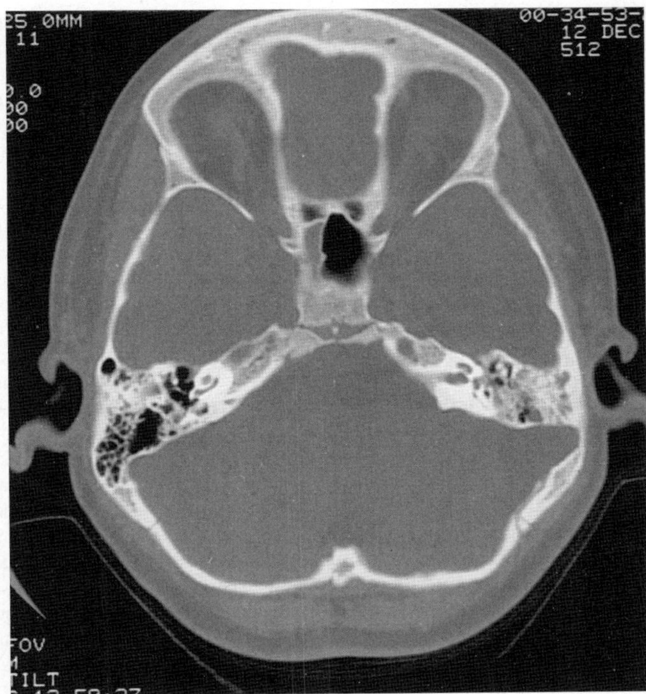

FIG. 17.2 Computed tomography scan of the head of a 12-year-old boy with left lateral sinus thrombosis and increased intracranial pressure complicating left mastoiditis. The left mastoid air cells are opacified with marked loss of the fine bony septa, in contrast to the right mastoid air cells.

TREATMENT

Medical and surgical treatments differ for acute versus chronic mastoiditis. For acute mastoiditis, the mainstay of treatment is antimicrobial therapy. The initial choice of antibiotics is made empirically after appropriate cultures have been obtained. To address the most common causes of acute mastoiditis (*S. pneumoniae, S. pyogenes, S. aureus,* and *H. influenzae*), cefepime 150 mg/kg per day given every 8 hours or cefotaxime 200 mg/kg per day divided every 6 hours or ceftriaxone 100 mg/kg per day given every 12 hours and vancomycin 60 mg/kg per day divided every 6 hours are reasonable initial choices. Antibiotic therapy for acute bacterial mastoiditis should conform to the principles of therapy for osteomyelitis in that treatment is begun with intravenous antibiotics with continuation of long-term intravenous therapy only in those cases with intracranial extension with an organism for which no effective oral antibiotic exists (e.g., *P. aeruginosa*). Otherwise, after several days to a week, most patients respond well clinically and in some instances are transferred to high-dose oral antibiotic therapy.[66] Total duration of therapy should be based on clinical response and the normalization of the white blood cell count, sedimentation rate, and the C-reactive protein value. Usually minimum therapy will be 3 weeks, but it may possibly last longer depending on severity of infection, complications, and what organism is isolated. Tailored antibiotic therapy to a specific cultured organism is ideal but not always possible, especially because many children with acute mastoiditis will have already undergone some form of outpatient antibiotic therapy.

All children with acute mastoiditis may potentially require surgical intervention in the form of myringotomy with pressure equalization tube placement and/or mastoidectomy; therefore it is imperative that pediatricians and otolaryngologists work together in treating mastoiditis.[29,37,70,75,114] The timing and degree of surgical intervention for acute mastoiditis vary by center. Traditionally the mainstay of treatment of acute mastoiditis in children has been myringotomy with or without placement of ventilation tubes in conjunction with parenteral antibiotics as described earlier.[24,56] This procedure is necessary for obtaining middle ear fluid cultures, for relieving pain, and for evacuating pus from the middle ear cavity.[100]

Mastoidectomy refers to removing the infected and inflamed mastoid air cells, thereby eliminating the further multiplication and spread of infection. In acute mastoiditis, indications for more complete surgical intervention in the form of a mastoidectomy include postauricular fluctuance; facial nerve paralysis; nausea, vomiting, and vertigo suggestive of labyrinthitis; meningitis; brain abscess; venous sinus thrombosis with or without intracranial hypertension; epidural or subdural empyema; and petrositis. In addition, patients with acute mastoiditis treated initially with parenteral antibiotics and myringotomy who have progression of postauricular swelling, fever, otalgia, or purulent otorrhea should also undergo mastoidectomy.[17,30,36,37,70,75,102] There is a growing trend toward upfront conservative management of pediatric mastoiditis with intravenous antibiotics and myringotomy and tube placement alone. Mastoidectomy is then reserved for cases that are nonresponsive to conservative measures and typically implemented within 3 to 5 days of presentation.[87] Mastoidectomy is also preferred in cases of unsuccessful drainage of a subperiosteal abscess as well as in the presence of intratemporal or intracranial complications.[100] One pediatric center in France published an algorithm for treatment of acute mastoiditis based on a series of 188 children treated between 2001 and 2008. Clinical acute mastoiditis at that center is treated initially with tympanocentesis or postauricular puncture under local anesthesia and parenteral broad-spectrum antibiotics with clinical reassessment at 48 hours. Mastoidectomy is performed only in patients who fail to improve on intravenous antibiotics alone, which in this series was necessary in only 33% of cases.[89] Another retrospective review of 167 children admitted for acute mastoiditis in Athens between 2002 and 2010 had similar conservative management with parenteral antibiotics and myringotomy on admission. If no clinical improvement was appreciated, a cortical mastoidectomy was performed within 3 to 5 days. Rate of mastoidectomy was 42%, and no child developed any additional complications under this treatment schema.[87]

Recently retroauricular puncture with tympanostomy tube placement has been advocated in lieu of a formal mastoidectomy, especially in cases of subperiosteal abscesses, because it has been shown to be effective in limiting the number of mastoidectomies performed and shortening the hospital stay.[4] Surgical treatment should always include culture of the middle ear or mastoid, which is becoming increasingly important as penicillin-resistant pneumococci and methicillin-resistant staphylococci have become more widespread.[3,21,38,45,72,83,110] In addition, during the mastoidectomy, inflammatory tissue should always be sent for histologic evaluation to exclude the rare case of eosinophilic granuloma or rhabdomyosarcoma, which can present similarly to acute mastoiditis.

In children with acute mastoiditis secondary to a cholesteatoma, modified radical mastoidectomy with removal of the cholesteatoma should be performed. In most cases, a "second-look" operation 6 to 9 months later is performed to ensure complete eradication of squamous epithelium from the middle ear cleft and mastoid.

Preoperative audiograms should also be obtained in all children with mastoiditis to assess for conductive versus sensorineural hearing loss, both of which can occur with acute and chronic mastoiditis.

The antimicrobial and surgical treatment in chronic mastoiditis differs from acute mastoiditis. By definition, symptoms have been present for longer than 1 month in children with chronic mastoiditis. In these children, *S. aureus*, gram-negative bacilli (especially *P. aeruginosa*), and anaerobes are seen more frequently (see Table 17.1). Therefore, combination broad-spectrum intravenous antibiotics are recommended. An aminoglycoside such as gentamicin 7.5 mg/kg per day divided every 8 hours can be administered for coverage of gram-negative bacilli; a semisynthetic penicillin such as piperacillin-tazobactam 200 to 300 mg/kg per day divided every 6 hours can be used to cover *P. aeruginosa* (synergistic with gentamicin), anaerobes, and methicillin-sensitive *S. aureus;* and vancomycin (60 mg/kg per day divided every 6 hours) can cover for resistant *S. aureus* and pneumococci. As with cases of acute mastoiditis, antibiotic therapy is tailored according to culture results from the middle ear or mastoid. In cases of intracranial extension caused by *P. aeruginosa*, cefepime 150 mg/kg per day divided every 8 hours is recommended because of its improved penetration of cerebrospinal fluid.

Indications for surgical intervention in patients with chronic mastoiditis include all of the indications for acute mastoiditis, with the addition of patients who have persistent chronic otorrhea with bony changes on radiographs. Complete mastoidectomy is advocated in these children because of the duration and therefore likely extent of diseased mastoid and middle ear mucosa. The presence of a middle ear cholesteatoma should always be suspected, especially in patients with chronic unremitting otorrhea.

In the unusual case of *M. tuberculosis* mastoiditis, antituberculous chemotherapy should be started in a manner similar to treatment of bony tuberculosis (see Chapter 96). It is also important to remember the possibility of underlying immunodeficiency in children with mastoiditis who demonstrate a slow response to medical and surgical therapy.

The treatment of complications of acute and chronic mastoiditis needs to be tailored to the specific complication. Treatment of subperiosteal abscesses includes postauricular needle aspiration under local anesthesia, incision and drainage under local anesthesia with placement of a surgical drain, intravenous antibiotics and myringotomy, and/or mastoidectomy. More recent series have advocated the more minimally invasive treatments under local anesthesia, citing a 92% improvement rate without the complications of mastoidectomy.[100] A Swedish retrospective study found that retroauricular needle aspiration and/or incision with intravenous antibiotics and myringotomy was an effective first-line treatment for subperiosteal abscess without any greater risk of complications and a shorter overall hospital stay compared to those treated with mastoidectomy.[19] Treatment of a Bezold abscess requires surgical drainage in addition to intravenous antibiotics.

When facial nerve paralysis occurs, treatment consists of myringotomy with pressure equalization tube placement along with parenteral antibiotics. In cases of complete facial paralysis, a mastoidectomy is thought to be beneficial.[18]

Otogenic meningitis is treated similarly to other forms of meningitis (see Chapter 31). Mastoidectomy is theoretically beneficial, although not urgent, and is infrequently performed.

In intracranial abscesses, in addition to intravenous antibiotics, surgical treatment should consist of a complete mastoidectomy because the confinement of the infection in the middle ear and mastoid allows for the disease to spread beyond the confines of the mastoid bone. Intracranial drainage either from the mastoid route or via a formal craniotomy should also be done.[50] Small, multifocal, or inaccessible intracranial lesions can be treated with antibiotics alone with a mastoidectomy[42] (see also Chapter 32).

Treatment of lateral sinus thrombosis includes long-term antibiotics, pressure equalization tube placement, and mastoidectomy to remove the nidus of infection with either needle aspiration of the sinus or thrombectomy. The use of anticoagulation for otogenic lateral sinus thrombosis is controversial and determined on an individual basis. Children who develop lateral sinus thrombosis should be evaluated for an underlying hypercoagulable state. Although rare, it is essential to consider lateral sinus thrombosis in any child with a recent history of otomastoiditis presenting with headaches and/or neurologic deficits. A retrospective case series and literature review showed that 85% of patients with acute otogenic lateral sinus thrombosis were treated with mastoidectomy, and 96% of patients received some duration of anticoagulation. Among these patients, 88% had complete clinical recovery even though clot resolution was only demonstrated in 35% of them, suggesting that venous recanalization may not be necessary for recovery.[95]

PROGNOSIS

The prognosis for mastoiditis depends on the extent of the infection and the causative organism. Mastoiditis that is treated adequately early in the course of illness before the onset of intracranial extension has a very good prognosis. Facial nerve paralysis is reversible early on,[94,105] and benign intracranial hypertension resolves with treatment of the mastoiditis.[30] Permanent neurologic deficits and death may occur if mastoiditis extends to cause meningitis, brain abscesses, epidural abscess, subdural empyema, or venous sinus thrombophlebitis. Symptoms of mastoiditis may recur if antibiotic therapy is of insufficient duration or if surgical debridement of an infected bone or of an infected cholesteatoma is inadequate. Sensorineural and conductive hearing deficits are reversible early on in mastoiditis; however, chronic infection may produce irreversible hearing loss.

PREVENTION

Early adequate antibiotic treatment of otitis media reduces significantly a child's risk for developing mastoiditis. In addition, rapid treatment of known mastoiditis along with early investigation of persistent ear drainage, persistent ear pain, or an otitis media that is not responding to antibiotic management decreases the risk for developing suppurative complications associated with mastoiditis.

NEW REFERENCES SINCE THE SEVENTH EDITION

1. Amir AZ, Pomp R, Amir J. Changes in acute mastoiditis in a single pediatric tertiary medical center: our experience during 2008–2009 compared with data for 1983–2007. *Scand J Infect Dis*. 2014;46(1):9-13.
2. Anthonsen K, Hostmark K, Hansen S, et al. Acute mastoiditis in children: a 10-year retrospective and validated multicenter study. *Pediatr Infect Dis J*. 2013;32(5):436-440.
6. Block SL. Mastoiditis mimicry: retro-auricular cellulitis related to otitis externa. *Pediatr Ann*. 2014;43(9):342-347.
19. Enoksson F, Groth A, Hultcrantz M, et al. Subperiosteal abscesses in acute mastoiditis in 115 Swedish children. *Int J Pediatr Otorhinolaryngol*. 2015;79(7):1115-1120.
28. Giannakopoulos P, Chrysovergis A, Xirogianni A, et al. Microbiology of acute mastoiditis and complicated or refractory acute otitis media among hospitalized children in the postvaccination era. *Pediatr Infect Dis J*. 2014;33(1):111-113.

33. Groth A, Enoksson F, Hultcrantz M, et al. Acute mastoiditis in children aged 0-16 years–a national study of 678 cases in Sweden comparing different age groups. *Int J Pediatr Otorhinolaryngol.* 2012;76(10):1494-1500.
34. Halgrimson WR, Chan KH, Abzug MJ, et al. Incidence of acute mastoiditis in Colorado children in the pneumococcal conjugate vaccine era. *Pediatr Infect Dis J.* 2014;33(5):453-457.
44. Kanzaki S, Saito H, Mori T, et al. Thirteen-month-old boy with malignant lymphoma having symptoms mimicking acute otitis media and mastoiditis with facial palsy. *ORL J Otorhinolaryngol Relat Spec.* 2011;73(5):266-270.
48. Kontorinis G, Psarommatis I, Karabinos C, et al. Incidence of non-infectious "acute mastoiditis" in children. *J Laryngol Otol.* 2012;126(3):244-248.
49. Kordeluk S, Orgad R, Kraus M, et al. Acute mastoiditis in children under 15 years of age in Southern Israel following the introduction of pneumococcal conjugate vaccines: a 4-year retrospective study (2009-2012). *Int J Pediatr Otorhinolaryngol.* 2014;78(10):1599-1604.
51. Laulajainen-Hongisto A, Saat R, Lempinen L, et al. Bacteriology in relation to clinical findings and treatment of acute mastoiditis in children. *Int J Pediatr Otorhinolaryngol.* 2014;78(12):2072-2078.
77. Osborn AJ, Blaser S, Papsin BC. Decisions regarding intracranial complications from acute mastoiditis in children. *Curr Opin Otolaryngol Head Neck Surg.* 2011;19(6):478-485.
84. Platzek I, Kitzler HH, Gudziol V, et al. Magnetic resonance imaging in acute mastoiditis. *Acta Radiol Short Rep.* 2014;3(2).
87. Psarommatis IM, Voudouris C, Douros K, et al. Algorithmic management of pediatric acute mastoiditis. *Int J Pediatr Otorhinolaryngol.* 2012;76(6):791-796.
95. Sitton MS, Chun R. Pediatric otogenic lateral sinus thrombosis: role of anticoagulation and surgery. *Int J Pediatr Otorhinolaryngol.* 2012;76(3):428-432.
106. Tsai TC, Yu PM, Tang RB, et al. Otorrhea as a sign of medical treatment failure in acute otitis media: two cases with silent mastoiditis complicated with facial palsy. *Pediatr Neonatol.* 2013;54(5):335-338.
112. Yarden-Bilavsky H, Raveh E, Livni G, et al. *Fusobacterium necrophorum* mastoiditis in children - emerging pathogen in an old disease. *Int J Pediatr Otorhinolaryngol.* 2013;77(1):92-96.
115. Zawawi F, Cardona I, Akinpelu OV, et al. Acute mastoiditis in children with cochlear implants: is explantation required? *Otolaryngol Head Neck Surg.* 2014;151(3):394-398.
117. Tawfik KO, Ishman SL, Altaye M, et al. Pediatric acute otitis media in the era of pneumococcal vaccination. *Otolaryngol Head Neck Surg.* 2017;156(5):938-945.

The full reference list for this chapter is available at ExpertConsult.com.

18 Croup (Laryngitis, Laryngotracheitis, Spasmodic Croup, Laryngotracheobronchitis, Bacterial Tracheitis and Laryngotracheobronchopneumonitis) and Epiglottitis (Supraglottitis)

Leidy Johana Tovar Padua • James D. Cherry

The term *croup* is used to identify several different respiratory illnesses characterized by varying degrees of inspiratory stridor, cough, and hoarseness resulting from obstruction in the region of the larynx. The etiology of croup syndromes is diverse, and the consideration of noninfectious possibilities in the differential diagnosis is of major importance. Box 18.1 classifies etiologic considerations in supraglottic, laryngeal, and infraglottic acute obstructions.

Croup is discussed under the subheadings of laryngitis, laryngotracheitis, spasmodic croup, laryngotracheobronchitis, bacterial tracheitis, and laryngotracheobronchopneumonitis. Diphtheric croup is presented in Chapter 90.

Epiglottitis (supraglottitis) is an illness characterized by inflammation and edema of the epiglottis and frequently also of the arytenoepiglottic folds and ventricular bands at the base of the epiglottis.[78] Until the present *Haemophilus influenzae* type B vaccine, era this disorder was usually caused by *H. influenzae* type B and was mainly a disease of children. The illness is characterized by rapid onset and progression, and, without treatment, death caused by obstruction of the airway occurs. Epiglottitis in children is a pediatric otolaryngologic emergency.

HISTORICAL ASPECTS

The word *croup* is derived from the Anglo-Saxon word *kropan*, "to cry aloud."[82] Until the 20th century, most crouplike illnesses were thought to be diphtheria. Diphtheritic croup is an ancient disease that has been traced to the time of Homer. The historical trail of diphtheria disappeared in the 5th century and did not reappear until 1100 years later. In the 16th century, epidemics were noted in Europe. Top[438] credits Bretonneau with differentiating diphtheritic croup from spasmodic croup in 1826. In the middle third of the 20th century, the history of croup was marked by three important events: (1) the rapid decline in incidence of diphtheria associated with the use of toxoid, (2) the introduction and widespread use of antibiotics, and (3) the advent of tissue culture techniques, resulting in the establishment of viruses as etiologic agents. After these three events occurred, a prevalent academic view was that all croup was of viral etiology, and bacteria generally were dismissed as causative agents.[83,97,133,348] However, a careful review of many publications from the first half of the 20th century indicates a causative role for several bacteria, in addition to *Corynebacterium diphtheriae,* in croup.* Bacterial croup (bacterial tracheitis) was rediscovered in 1979.†

In the 1940s, Davison[109] separated spasmodic croup from other, more severe forms of croup. The clinical and pathologic aspects of this entity were poorly defined, and today it often is not separated clinically from more severe forms of croup.

The early history of epiglottitis is obscure, probably because of the importance of diphtheritic croup.[82] In 1887, Baron[20] described in detail a 30-year-old woman with epiglottitis who recovered after treatment with hot poultices and steam with tincture of benzoin. In 1900, Theisen[437] described three cases in the United States. Not until the early 1940s did acute epiglottitis become recognized as a definite clinical entity caused by *H. influenzae* type B.[5,31,400] In 1948, Rabe,[347] in a study of 347 children with "infectious croup," presented evidence for the division of the clinical illness into three etiologic categories—diphtheritic croup, viral croup, and *H. influenzae* type B croup (acute epiglottitis). Since the early 1990s, a dramatic decrease in the number of cases of epiglottitis has occurred in many countries because of the widespread use of *H. influenzae* type B conjugate vaccines.‡

*References 28, 54, 56, 109, 110, 138, 166, 208, 221, 299, 320, 334, 356, 357.
†References 78, 81, 92, 114, 123, 126, 131, 134, 137, 173, 185, 193, 201, 227, 233, 277, 278, 297, 305, 319, 321, 411, 423, 424, 431, 458, 478.
‡References 6, 59, 140, 150, 169, 174, 276, 300, 303, 341, 448, 460, 479.

TABLE 18.1 Classification and Definition of Infectious Illnesses Involving the Larynx and Supraglottic and Infraglottic Regions

Category	Other Terms	Definitions
Supraglottitis	Epiglottitis	Infection of the epiglottis and/or arytena-epiglottic folds and ventricular bands of the base of the epiglottis resulting in swelling and upper airway obstruction
Laryngitis		Inflammation of larynx resulting in hoarseness; usually occurs in older children and adults in association with common upper respiratory viral infections
Laryngeal diphtheria	Membranous croup, true croup, diphtheritic croup	Infection involving larynx and other areas of upper and lower airway due to *Corynebacterium diphtheriae* resulting in gradually progressive obstruction of airway and associated inspiratory stridor
Laryngotracheitis	False croup, virus croup, acute obstructive subglottic laryngitis	Inflammation of larynx and trachea most often caused by infection with parainfluenza and influenza viruses
Laryngotracheobronchitis and laryngo-tracheobronchopneumonitis	Membranous laryngotracheobronchitis, pseudomembranous croup	Inflammation of larynx, trachea, and bronchi or lung or both; usually similar in onset to laryngotracheitis but more severe illness; bacterial infection frequently has causative role
Bacterial croup	Bacterial tracheitis, membranous croup, membranous tracheitis, membranous laryngotracheobronchitis, pseudomembranous croup	Severe form of laryngotracheitis, laryngotracheobronchitis, or laryngo-tracheobronchopneumonitis due to bacterial infection
Spasmodic croup	Spasmodic laryngitis, catarrhal spasm of the larynx, subglottic allergic edema	Illness characterized by sudden onset at night of inspiratory stridor; associated with mild upper respiratory infection without inflammation or fever but with edema in subglottic region

BOX 18.1 Clinical Considerations in Acute Supraglottic, Laryngeal, and Infraglottic Obstructions

Infectious

Acute epiglottitis
Laryngitis
Laryngeal diphtheria
Laryngotracheitis
Laryngotracheobronchitis
Laryngotracheobronchopneumonitis
Bacterial tracheitis
Spasmodic croup

Mechanical

Foreign body
Secondary to trauma resulting from intubation
Extrinsic or intrinsic mass

Allergic

Acute angioneurotic edema

Data from references 78, 81, 97, 142, 149, 153, 321, 346, 484.

TERMINOLOGY

The terminology and classification of infectious illnesses involving the larynx and supraglottic and infraglottic regions have evolved over time. Classifications often have mixed etiologic categories with anatomic systems and have led to confusion. Croup often has been presented in articles under the heading of *laryngotracheobronchitis* when the authors actually were discussing laryngotracheitis and spasmodic croup.[85,229,279,298,342,367,402,432] The term *membranous croup* has been used as the title for articles dealing with bacterial croup[114,185] This use is confusing because membranous croup historically was diphtheria. Many articles dealing with bacterial croup also have been titled *bacterial tracheitis*.* This term seems inappropriate because most cases of bacterial croup seen today have lower respiratory tract involvement in addition to tracheal findings. Table 18.1 lists the classifications and definitions used in this chapter.

*References 92, 123, 124, 131, 134, 137, 201, 227, 233, 277, 278, 319, 411, 458, 478.

ETIOLOGY OF CROUP SYNDROMES

The etiologic agents in laryngitis, laryngotracheitis, spasmodic croup, laryngotracheobronchitis, and laryngotracheobronchopneumonitis are presented by frequency and severity of illness in Table 18.2. Laryngitis is a common manifestation of infection with many respiratory viruses in older children, adolescents, and adults. Outbreaks of laryngitis in closed population groups (e.g., boarding schools and military training camps) most frequently are caused by adenovirus types 4 and 7, and community outbreaks most often are noted in association with epidemic influenza. Sporadic instances of laryngitis usually are caused by adenoviral infections. Laryngitis also has been reported in association with group A streptococcal infections; the incidence of this association has varied from 2% to 40%.[51,308,447] Somenek and associates[414] described an 11-month-old boy with severe membranous laryngitis caused by methicillin-resistant *Staphylococcus aureus* (MRSA).

Generally accepted today is that acute laryngotracheitis and spasmodic croup, which rarely are differentiated clinically, are caused by infection with many different viruses. Although numerous studies of respiratory viral infection exist, almost no attempt has been made to delineate the differences in etiologic spectrum by severity of illness.

Parainfluenza virus type 1 is the most common cause of acute laryngotracheitis and is responsible for frequent and clearly delineated fall and winter epidemics. Croup with parainfluenza type 2 virus seldom is severe but occasionally is related to small outbreaks. Parainfluenza virus type 3 is a frequent cause of sporadic but severe illness.

The most severe laryngotracheitis has been noted in association with influenza A viral infections. Respiratory syncytial virus and several different adenoviruses frequently are isolated in croup. Generally these illnesses are not severe, but lower respiratory tract involvement occasionally is a problem. Laryngeal, tracheal, and bronchial involvement commonly occurs in measles.[83] Although rhinoviruses, *Mycoplasma pneumoniae*, enteroviruses, herpes simplex virus, and reoviruses have been associated with croup, they generally cause only minimal distress. However, O'Niel and associates[332] reported two immunocompetent children who presented with severe acute laryngotracheitis caused by herpes simplex virus. Croup has been noted in association with infection

TABLE 18.2 Etiologic Infectious Agents in Laryngitis, Spasmodic Croup, Laryngotracheitis, Laryngotracheobronchitis, and Laryngotracheobronchopneumonitis Presented by Frequency and Severity of Illness

Category	Etiologic Agents	Frequency[a]	Associated With Outbreaks	Severity[b]	References
Laryngitis	Adenoviruses				
	Types 4 and 7	++++	Yes	+ to +++	103, 200, 447
	Types 2, 3, 5, 8, 11, 14, and 21	+++	No	+ to +++	
	Influenza viruses	++++	Yes	+ to ++++	17, 200, 336, 447
	Types A and B				
	Parainfluenza viruses				200, 447
	Type 1	++	Yes	+ to +++	
	Types 2 and 3	+	Yes	+ to ++	
	Coronavirus	++	Yes	++	24
	Rhinoviruses and respiratory syncytial virus	++	No	+ to ++	171, 308, 323, 405
	Enteroviruses	+	No	+	200, 447
	Streptococcus pyogenes	+ to +++	Yes	+ to ++	51, 308
Laryngotracheitis and spasmodic croup	Parainfluenza viruses	++++		+ to +++	37, 74-76, 79, 115, 117, 157, 161, 166, 194, 199, 202, 206, 250, 267, 282, 281, 286, 313, 336, 339, 340, 343, 361, 451, 467
	Type 1	++++	Yes		
	Type 2	++	Yes		
	Type 3	++	No		
	Influenza viruses	++			60, 74, 75, 79, 115, 117, 136, 148, 157, 166, 191, 202, 204, 206, 280, 286, 313, 336, 339, 340, 343, 361, 451, 467
	Type A	+++	Yes	+ to ++++	
	Type B	++	Yes	+ to ++	
	Respiratory syncytial virus	++	No	+ to ++	73–76, 79, 115, 117, 156, 157, 166, 202, 250, 281, 306, 339, 340, 342, 440, 457, 472, 480
	Human metapneumovirus	++	Yes	+	16
	Coronavirus	++	Yes	++	86, 269, 361, 421, 450
	Human bocavirus	+	No	+	25, 361
	Measles virus	++	Yes	+ to +++	83
	Adenoviruses	++	No	+ to ++	49, 73, 74, 76, 79, 115, 166, 199, 202, 250, 267, 280, 281, 313, 339, 340, 342, 361, 417, 440, 451, 457
	Unspecified types and types 1, 2, 3, 5, 6, and 7				
	Rhinoviruses	+	No	+	79, 157, 229, 280, 313, 361
	Mycoplasma pneumoniae	+	No	+	73, 76, 79, 115-117, 166, 202, 281, 361
	Enteroviruses	+	No	+	74, 83, 98, 156, 157, 166, 202, 217, 280, 306, 361, 418, 440, 472
	Coxsackievirus type A9	+	No	+	
	Coxsackievirus types B4 and B5	+	No	+	
	Echoviruses types 4, 11, and 21	+	No	+	
	Herpes simplex viruses	+	No	+	202, 211, 251, 313, 332, 418
	Reoviruses	+	No	+	480
	Human papillomavirus	+	No	+ to +++	484
Laryngotracheobronchitis and laryngotracheobronchopneumonitis	Parainfluenza viruses types 1, 2, and 3	+	No	+++	54, 156, 167, 199, 281, 299, 338, 340
	Influenza viruses types A and B	+	No	++++	136, 148, 204, 339
	Staphylococcus aureus, S. pyogenes, Streptococcus pneumoniae, Haemophilus influenzae, and *Moraxella catarrhalis*	++	No	++++	28, 35, 54, 56, 108, 109, 114, 126, 131, 137, 138, 165, 180, 185, 193, 201, 208, 221, 227, 233, 277, 278, 297, 298, 307, 320, 321, 334, 356, 357, 411, 478
	Other bacteria	±	No	++++	137, 185, 198, 233, 277, 305, 478
	Cryptosporidium	–	No	++	187

[a]++++, most frequent; +++, frequent; ++, occasional; +, rare; –, questionable.
[b]++++, most severe; +++, severe; ++, not severe; +, minimal distress.

with the novel coronavirus NL63, human bocavirus, and human metapneumovirus.[16,25,86,361,421,450] Lee and Storch[269] noted that coronavirus NL63 was a relatively common cause of severe croup. Recurrent croup may be due to infection with a human papillomavirus.[484]

Bacteria, other than *H. influenzae* in epiglottitis and *C. diphtheriae* in membranous croup, generally were dismissed as causative agents in croup until more recently.[97,133,348] Many publications on laryngotracheobronchitis from the first half of the 20th century indicate a role for several common bacterial pathogens.* In 1979, bacterial croup was rediscovered,[227] and numerous reports of this illness have been published since then.†

In the reports from the preantibiotic era, *Streptococcus pyogenes* was the pathogen implicated most frequently. Since 1979, *S. aureus* has been the agent implicated most commonly. Other important bacteria are *Streptococcus pneumoniae* and *H. influenzae*. More recently, *Moraxella catarrhalis* has been found to be the causative agent in several cases.[35,137,233,478] In most instances, bacterial croup is likely to be the result of bacterial superinfection in viral disease.‡ *Cryptosporidium* also has been recovered from the trachea of an infant with a subacute illness.[187]

Noninfectious causes of crouplike illnesses include airway hermangioma[240] and laryngeal or esophageal foreign bodies.[172,209]

ETIOLOGY OF SUPRAGLOTTITIS

Acute supraglottitis in children in the prevaccine era almost always was caused by *H. influenzae* type B.§ In 34 pediatric series in which blood cultures were performed in 1570 children, *H. influenzae* type B was recovered in 76%. Supraglottitis caused by other bacteria was rare. In the 1570 children with blood cultures, the following other organisms were recovered: *S. pneumoniae*, 3; *S. aureus*, 3; *Haemophilus parainfluenzae*, 2; *H. influenzae* type A, 1; *H. influenzae* nontypable, 2; and *Bacillus* spp. 1.

In countries where *H. influenzae* type B immunization is routine, supraglottitis is a rare illness in children. Nevertheless, cases still occur in association with some infectious agents. The following pathogens have been implicated in this regard: *S. pneumoniae; S. aureus; H. parainfluenzae;* groups A, B, C, and G streptococci; *Pseudomonas aeruginosa* (in a patient with severe combined immunodeficiency syndrome); untypable *H. influenzae;* and *Bacillus* spp.[19,30,34,127,212,260,262,275,282,328,366,403,408,471,481] *Candida tropicalis* was isolated from the blood of a 3½-year-old girl with supraglottitis who had been the recent recipient of an autologous bone marrow transplant.[459]

Candida albicans was noted in a case in a newborn whose mother had vaginal candidiasis and in a 6-year-old boy with chronic mucocutaneous candidiasis.[4] *Candida* spp. epiglottitis was noted in two children infected with human immunodeficiency virus (HIV),[317,398] and *C. albicans* epiglottitis was observed recently in a 2-year-old girl who was immunocompromised as a result of receiving chemotherapy for a primitive neuroectodermal tumor.[292]

Necrotizing epiglottitis in a 5-year-old boy with hemophagocytic lymphohistiocytosis associated with a mixed infection (*Enterococcus faecalis, Eikenella corrodens, Prevotella melaninogenica,* and *Neisseria* spp.) has been described.[248] Reed and colleagues[354] described a 17-year-old boy with an aryepiglottic abscess associated with a mixed infection (*Capnocytophaga ochraceae, Bacteroides stercoris,* and *P. melaninogenica*).

Since 2009 in England and Wales, there has been an increase in invasive meningococcal diseases due to capsular group W sequence type 11 complex.[263] Between 2010 and 2013, there were five cases of epiglottis due to this meningococcal complex. Lake and colleagues[265] noted necrotizing epiglottitis due to nontoxigenic *Corynebacterium diphtheriae* in a 3-year-old girl who had nondiagnosed lymphoblastic leukemia. A 14-month-old girl with prolonged stridor and epiglottitis associated with a mixed infection with herpes simplex virus type 1, *H. influenzae, S. pneumoniae,* and *S. aureus* has been reported.[394] A 16-month-old child with type 1 herpes simplex virus stomatitis complicated by stridor and respiratory distress had epiglottis; his aryteno-epiglottic folds were edematous and covered with vesicular lesions resembling those in the oral mucosa.[44] An 18-year-old girl had supraglottitis that also was caused by herpes simplex virus.[303] In addition, parainfluenza type 3 and influenza type B viruses were isolated from the nasopharynx of two children with supraglottic inflammation.[177] *Haemophilus paraphrophilus*[228] was recovered from the epiglottic surface of a single patient, as was *M. catarrhalis* in another patient.[453]

In adults, *H. influenzae* type B also has been the major cause of epiglottitis, but other organisms occur more commonly in adults than in children.* In 1992, Daum and Smith[106] reviewed 474 published cases of epiglottitis in adults, 293 of whom had blood cultures performed; 79 of those cultures (27%) yielded *H. influenzae*. Of these positive cultures, 43 were *H. influenzae* type B; 35 isolates were not typed, and 1 isolate was not *H. influenzae* type B. Trollfors and associates[443] in Sweden found that of blood cultures obtained from 185 of 356 (52%) adult patients, *H. influenzae* was isolated from 53%. Of these, 53 were *H. influenzae* type B, and the type of the remaining 45 was not known.

In Finland, Bizaki and coworkers[38] reviewed 308 adult cases of acute supraglottitis during the 2-decade period from 1989 to 2009. The incidence increased from 1.88 per 100,000 in the first decade to 4.73 in the second decade. The causative organisms were *S. pyogenes, S. pneumoniae, S. milleri,* staphylococci *Pseudomonas* spp., *H. influenzae,* and *C. albicans*.

S. pneumoniae was reported to be isolated from the blood of 18 adults with supraglottitis, 10 of whom were receiving immunosuppressive therapy or were infected with HIV-1,[42,50,214,237,239,268,347,368,371,396] and *H. parainfluenzae* was isolated from the blood of 5 patients.[87,147,287,385,463] In Denmark, between 1995 and 2002, *H. influenzae* type F was recovered from 13 cases of epiglottitis in adults.[62] Numerous other infectious agents have been implicated in case reports of adults with supraglottitis.† These agents include *S. pneumoniae, H. influenzae* type b, *Aeromonas hydrophila, Pasteurella multocida, Kingella kingae, Klebsiella pneumoniae,* group A and B streptococci, *Bacteroides* spp., *Fusobacterium necrophorum, Vibrio vulnificus, Serratia marcescens, S. aureus, Neisseria meningitidis, Aspergillus* spp., herpes simplex virus, EBV parainfluenza virus type 2, and *M. tuberculosis* and *Histoplasma* spp.[66]

Epiglottitis also can result from noninfectious causes. Hot foods and water can cause thermal epiglottitis, as can poisoning with corrosive agents, including cocaine alkaloid.[29,238,256,257,264] Tsai and Wang[444] noted acute epiglottitis in a 23-year-old man after receiving traditional Chinese *gua sha* therapy. Hereditary angioedema may manifest with findings typical of epiglottitis.[330]

EPIDEMIOLOGY OF CROUP

Croup accounts for approximately 15% of lower respiratory tract disease seen in pediatrics. In a large 11-year study in a pediatric practice in Chapel Hill, North Carolina, Denny and associates[117] noted the incidence of croup by age and sex. The highest attack rate occurred in children 7 to 36 months of age. Few cases occurred after the sixth birthday. Hoekelman[198] studied the occurrence of illness prospectively in 246 full-term, first-born, well infants during their first year of life. Three infants (1.2%) had croup during the study year. The analysis of a pediatric practice with approximately 3000 active records and approximately 10,000 yearly visits of children younger than 5 years disclosed five cases of croup in a group of 50 consecutive hospitalized patients.[52] Although croup occurs occasionally in older children, most cases occur within the first 3 years of life.[117,133,142,367,392]

---

*References 28, 54, 56, 92, 108, 123, 134, 138, 165, 173, 208, 221, 299, 320, 334, 356, 423, 431, 458.

†References 35, 114, 126, 131, 137, 185, 193, 201, 233, 277, 278, 297, 305, 319, 321, 411, 424, 478.

‡References 64, 92, 131, 185, 221, 278, 297, 318, 319, 321, 327.

§References 23, 26, 27, 31, 32, 43, 46, 50, 53, 55, 57, 61, 65, 88, 89, 125, 139, 163, 174, 197, 224, 282, 289, 290, 295, 301, 304, 309, 347, 400, 409, 410, 454, 455.

*References 20, 38, 48, 50, 78, 87, 91, 102, 128, 135, 141, 151, 152, 164, 168, 188, 190, 218, 219, 225, 239, 253, 293, 322, 324, 364, 388, 399, 407, 419, 428, 442, 443.

†References 1, 13, 45, 48, 72, 118, 128, 135, 152, 164, 168, 196, 213, 218, 219, 222, 235, 274, 283, 288, 301, 316, 322, 324, 331, 358–360, 374, 388, 404, 416, 456, 482.

Croup occurs more commonly in boys than in girls.[33,117,252,367,369,370] In a 6-year study in Alberta, Canada, involving 20,079 emergency department visits, 61.3% were boys.[369] In the Chapel Hill study, an increase was noted in the number of croup cases beginning in September, with a peak in October and November, and then a decrease during the next 7-month period.[117] In a 2-year emergency department study in Toronto involving 1700 cases, the peak month of visits and hospital admissions was found to be October.[392] Marx and associates[291] reviewed the National Hospital Discharge Survey data for hospitalizations for croup between 1979 and 1993. They also examined Centers for Disease Control and Prevention laboratory-based surveillance data and published reports with virus isolation studies. Major peaks in hospitalizations for croup occurred in October of odd-number years at the time of peak parainfluenza virus type 1 activity. Minor peaks in hospitalizations for croup occurred each year in February when influenza A, influenza B, and respiratory syncytial viral infections were common occurrences. Epidemic peaks of acute laryngotracheitis reflect community-wide activity with parainfluenza 1 and 2 viruses or influenza A or B outbreaks.[117,167,291]

In the Alberta, Canada, study in 1990 to 2000 and 2004 to 2005, biennial trends were apparent.[369,370] Peak emergency department visits for croup occurred in November for odd years and in February for the other years. For the odd years, the overall rate increased from 43.4/1000 in 1999 to 2000 to 49.6/1000 in 2003 to 2004. A similar increase was noted in the even years (30.9/1000 in 2000 to 2001 to 34.1/1000 in 2004 to 2005).

In the Toronto study, the time of the visit to the emergency department was analyzed.[392] The peak number of visits occurred between 10 PM and 4 AM. During this period, approximately 17% of the children seen were admitted to the hospital. In contrast, of children seen between noon and 6 PM, approximately 50% were admitted to the hospital. Quite similar findings were noted in Alberta in the 6-year period between 1999 and 2005.[369,370] A study of croup hospitalizations in Ontario over 14 years from 1988 to 2002 noted a biennial mid-autumn peak and an annual summer trough throughout the entire study period.[391] A striking finding in this study was a marked decrease in hospitalizations for croup after the winter of 1993 to 1994. This decrease continued in linear fashion for the remainder of the study duration. The authors suggest that the decreasing trend in croup hospitalizations was likely due to the increasing use of corticosteroid treatment in patients who presented to emergency departments with croup.

Because croup is caused by the same viruses that cause other respiratory illnesses, the method of spread probably is similar for all (see discussion of the common cold in Chapter 7). In children, most spread involves close person-to-person contact, with large droplets of virus-containing nasal secretions being applied to the nose from the hands of the future host or by close-range airborne acquisition. Parainfluenza viruses are common causes of colds in adults, so older individuals with trivial illnesses may be the source of more severe childhood croup.

EPIDEMIOLOGY OF SUPRAGLOTTITIS

In the prevaccine era, the epidemiology of invasive *H. influenzae* type B disease varied markedly among population groups.[460,461] Epiglottitis also differed by population group, but this variation was not related necessarily to the rate of overall *H. influenzae* type B invasive disease in the population. For example, among Alaskan Eskimos and Navajo Native Americans, whose risk for acquiring invasive *H. influenzae* type B disease was 4 to 10 times that of most other American populations, epiglottitis was not recognized among 295 patients with invasive *H. influenzae* type B illness.[96,461]

Of *H. influenzae* type B invasive disease, the percentage of cases of epiglottitis varied markedly among localities. For example, in Israel, only 0.3% of invasive *H. influenzae* type B infections were epiglottitis, whereas in Ireland, Wales, northeast England, Australia (Sydney), and Denmark, the percentage of epiglottitis cases varied between 16% and 32%.[101,146,203,254,296,345] In Minnesota and Dallas County, Texas, only 6% and 3%, respectively, of invasive *H. influenzae* type B infections were epiglottitis.[314] In contrast with these findings in the United States, Europe, and Australia, the most common manifestation of invasive *H. influenzae* type B infection in Sweden was epiglottitis.[88,443] In Sweden, the incidence of epiglottitis in children 14 years of age or younger in 1981 to 1983 was 10/100,000 per year. The annual incidence in Minnesota and Dallas County, Texas, in children 5 years of age or younger in 1982 to 1984 was 5.4 and 4.4 cases, respectively, per 100,000 per year.[315]

In children in the United States in the prevaccine era, the peak occurrence of epiglottitis was during the third year of life, and 72% of all cases occurred in children 1 to 5 years of age.[23,29,34,89,139,224] The disease occurred more commonly in boys than in girls; in eight studies with 611 cases, 58% of cases were in boys.[23,29-31,34,89,139,224,309]

In specific geographic areas, marked differences in the yearly percentage of cases of epiglottitis occurred, but no intercity, national, or international cycles of illness were demonstrated.[23,29,89,139,224,309] Seasonal prevalence varied by locality but was not marked. The greatest number of cases in three studies occurred in the winter and spring,[34,224,309] whereas Baxter[29] observed more cases during the summer and in November, and Cohen and Chai[89] found no seasonal pattern.

Epiglottitis is a disease that occurs most commonly in temperate climates.[143,226] In several U.S. military hospitals, a wide geographic variation in incidence was noted; no cases were found among 4625 admissions at Gorgas Hospital in Panama, whereas 1/600 admissions to Elmendorf Hospital in Alaska were for epiglottitis.[23] In the past, acute epiglottitis had not been reported in either Taiwan or Hong Kong.[220]

Epiglottitis also occurs in adults but less commonly than in children.[151,293,428,446] Annual rates in Rhode Island, Denmark, Finland, and northern California were 1.0, 0.9, 0.2, and 1.8/100,000, respectively. In both Ireland and Israel, rates of reported epiglottitis in adults appear to be increasing.[32,183] Whether these increases are true increases or are the result of increased awareness is not apparent.

In the present *H. influenzae* type B conjugate vaccine era, the incidence of epiglottitis has fallen dramatically in all countries employing routine immunization, as has the incidence of all invasive disease caused by *H. influenzae*.* In northern Finland, the incidence in children 4 years of age or younger fell from 7.6/100,000 before 1988 to 0/100,000 after 1988.[6] In Sweden, in the 10-year period from 1986 to 1996, the rate of epiglottitis in children younger than 14 years fell from 8.2/100,000 to less than 1/100,000.[160] At the Children's Hospital of Philadelphia, the average annual incidence of epiglottitis declined from 10.9/10,000 admissions before 1990 to 1.8/10,000 admissions from 1990 through 1992.[174] In this study, investigators also noted that the median age of patients increased from 35.5 months before 1990 to 80.5 months in the post-1989 period.

It should be noted that sporadic cases of epiglottitis mostly caused by non–*H. influenzae* type B bacteria continue to occur in the United States.[395] In 2006, 377 cases were reported including 369 cases in children.

In 2006, an increase in incidence of invasive *H. influenzae* type B disease, including acute epiglottitis, was reported in England.[300] Many of the cases occurred in children who had received *H. influenzae* type B conjugate vaccine at 2, 3, and 4 months of age but not a booster dose in the second year of life. This resurgence of invasive *H. influenzae* type B disease led to the implementation of a booster dose at 12 months of age, which helped to control the burden of invasive *H. influenzae* type B in all age groups.[91]

PATHOLOGY AND PATHOGENESIS OF CROUP

Laryngoscopic studies in acute laryngotracheitis reveal redness and swelling of the lateral walls of the trachea, just below the vocal cords.[110,109,426] Because the subglottic trachea is surrounded by a firm cartilaginous ring, the inflammatory swelling can occur only by encroaching on the patency of the airway; the subglottic space often is reduced to a slit 1 to 2 mm wide. As the disease progresses, the tracheal lumen becomes obstructed further by a fibrinous exudate, and its surface is covered by pseudomembranes composed of the exudative material. The vocal cords frequently are swollen, and their mobility is impaired.

Histologic study of postmortem material from the larynx and trachea reveals marked edema and cellular infiltration in the lamina propria,

*References 6, 59, 140, 154, 174, 181, 276, 300, 303, 341, 448, 460, 479.

submucosa, and adventitia. The cellular infiltrate includes histiocytes, lymphocytes, plasma cells, and polymorphonuclear leukocytes.[54,56,312,334,357] The cotton rat model of laryngotracheitis caused by human parainfluenza virus type 3 reveals pathologic findings similar to those noted in human postmortem studies.[335] This model also indicates the time course of events. Early in the course of an infection (first 2 to 4 days), moderate mucosal and submucosal inflammatory infiltrates were noted in the subglottic and proximal tracheal regions. The infiltrates initially contained lymphocytes and neutrophils, and subsequently a mononuclear infiltrate with lymphocytes and macrophages in the submucosa was noted. Cell injury was most marked on days 6 to 8 after infection. The ciliated epithelial cells were blunted, with loss of cilia in large patches. By 12 days after infection, the region reverted to a nearly normal appearance.

The older literature indicates that classic laryngotracheobronchitis and the same disease with pneumonia represent extension of disease from the trachea to the bronchi and alveoli. The progressive obstructive disease with exudate and pseudomembrane obstruction at the bronchial and bronchiolar levels usually is the result of secondary bacterial involvement. In bacterial croup, the tracheal wall is infiltrated with inflammatory cells, and ulceration, pseudomembranes, and microabscess formation occur.* In addition to the findings in laryngotracheitis of viral origin, thick pus is present within the lumen of the trachea and lower air passages.[193,233,277,297]

Spasmodic croup is an enigma because it occurs in association with respiratory viral infections similar to those that cause more severe laryngotracheitis. Using direct laryngoscopy, Davison[110] noted that the subglottic tissues in spasmodic croup showed noninflammatory edema.

Although the eventual site of clinically important pathologic change in laryngotracheitis is within the larynx and trachea, the initial acquisition of infection is similar to that of other respiratory viral infections and occurs within the upper air passages, including the nasal and pharyngeal epithelial surfaces. After acquisition of virus, infection of the cells of the local respiratory epithelium develops and spreads locally to involve the larynx and trachea. The initial symptoms of nasal stuffiness and throat irritation reflect the primary sites of involvement. Studies in organ culture systems and in the cotton rat model have shown that several respiratory viruses inhibit tracheal ciliary function and eventually lead to marked destruction of the epithelium and evidence of viral infection in the lamina propria.[246,335,353] In uncomplicated croup, failure of gas exchange within the lung, in addition to hypoxia resulting from subglottic tracheal obstruction, may occur.[323,432]

Parainfluenza virus types 1, 2, and 3 all are significant causes of respiratory infections in children (see Chapter 179). Infection with parainfluenza virus type 3 occurs in most infants, whereas infections with types 1 and 2 generally occur more frequently in older children. Only a third of children have antibodies against these two viral types by the time they reach 4 years of age.

Because parainfluenza viral infections are common occurrences in young children, and because only a few get croup, host factors probably are important in the pathogenesis. In contrast to the numerous studies of the pathogenesis of bronchiolitis and respiratory syncytial virus infection, few similar studies relating to parainfluenza viruses and croup have been reported.[84,382,485]

These pathologic data suggest that the findings in laryngotracheitis are directly virus related (parainfluenza virus types 1, 2, and 3 and influenza virus types A and B) because of the direct cytopathic effect of a virus, are related to the concomitant host response, or perhaps both.[84,382,485] In the cotton rat model, the use of topical steroid therapy led to a significant reduction in the degree of inflammatory infiltrates and cell injury, which suggests that the host response contributes to the pathologic findings.[335] Schaap-Nutt and associates[377] described the replication kinetics and cytokine secretion of the parainfluenza viruses in human tracheobronchial airway epithelium. They found serotype-specific differences of the innate immune response, suggesting that parainfluenza type 1 is able to remain undetectable for several days after infection compared to parainfluenza type 2 and 3. Parainfluenza 2 inhibits the early immune response to a lesser extent than the other serotypes, and parainfluenza 3 triggers a steady increase of the basolaterally secreted cytokines. These findings are consistent with both the epidemiology and clinical findings in croup. The pathogenesis of laryngotracheobronchitis and laryngotracheobronchopneumonitis is similar to that described previously but with the extension of infection to the lower respiratory tract and usually the occurrence of secondary bacterial infection.

Many studies suggest that allergic factors play a role in recurrent croup.[68,195,326,449,468-470,477,483] Welliver and associates[469] found that children with croup caused by parainfluenza viral infections had titers of IgE-specific antibody in their nasopharyngeal secretions that were 3.6-fold higher than titers of similarly infected children with only upper respiratory tract infections. The children with croup had a cell-mediated immune response to parainfluenza virus that was 1.6-fold greater than that of the children with only upper respiratory tract infections.

In a subsequent review, investigators noted that an atopic disposition might be associated with the development of croup.[468] Children with croup caused by a parainfluenza virus had specific IgE antibodies and released histamine into the airway more frequently than did control patients with parainfluenza viral upper respiratory tract infections. They also noted that children with recurrent croup had several atopic features, such as positive skin tests to environmental allergens, and were more likely to develop asthma when they grew older. Also, some children with a history of recurrent croup develop stridor with histamine challenge. Rennie and associates[355] found that children with C/T genotype of the CD14 G-1359T SNP were more likely to have a history of croup, and children with genotype homozygous C/C had low prevalence of croup in this study. This suggests that CD14 polymorphisms may influence the innate response to viral infections associated with croup.

The above-mentioned studies by Welliver and associates[468,469] and other reports make it easy to accept a role of atopy in recurrent croup. What is difficult to explain, however, is why many apparently primary infections result in only spasmodic croup. As one of us (JDC) suggested previously, initial sensitization may be parainfluenza virus group–specific and not type-specific.[37] This idea suggests that early infection (primary infection) with parainfluenza virus type 3 would set the stage for spasmodic croup with parainfluenza viral types 1 and 2. The primary infection itself could have been mild owing to transplacentally acquired antibody.

ANATOMY AND PATHOPHYSIOLOGY OF SUPRAGLOTTITIS

The thin, elastic, leaflike epiglottic cartilage is attached to the anterior surface of the thyroid cartilage by the thyroepiglottic ligament (Fig. 18.1). The hyoepiglottic ligament also provides support and anchors the epiglottis to the hyoid bone. The superior aspect of the epiglottis arches slightly posteriorly. Stratified squamous epithelium covers the anterior surface of the epiglottis and the superior third of the posterior portion; respiratory epithelium covers the remaining posterior surface. The stratified squamous epithelium is loosely adherent and creates a large potential space for the accumulation of inflammatory cells and edema fluid.

The arytenoepiglottic folds arise from the epiglottis and terminate posteriorly near the paired arytenoid cartilages. These structures commonly are involved in the supraglottic infection and occasionally are the site of serious disease without epiglottitis per se.[29] Immediately anterior to the epiglottis are the valleculae epiglotticae, where saliva pools before deglutition.

Supraglottic cellulitis with marked edema involving the epiglottis, arytenoepiglottic folds, ventricular bands, and arytenoids is the hallmark of this illness. As the edema increases, the epiglottis curls posteriorly and inferiorly. Inspiration tends to draw the inflamed supraglottic ring into the laryngeal inlet, whereas expiration is unopposed.[390] This "ball-valve" mechanism is thought to produce slight hypoxia without hypercapnia.[379] Diffuse infiltration with polymorphonuclear leukocytes, hemorrhage, edema, and fibrin deposition can be seen microscopically; this infiltration can progress to microabscesses, with *H. influenzae* type B occasionally seen in the tissue.[226,364] Frank abscess formation has been

*References 7, 77, 78, 81, 82, 92, 114, 123, 126, 131, 137, 173, 193, 201, 227, 233, 277–279, 321, 327, 411, 424.

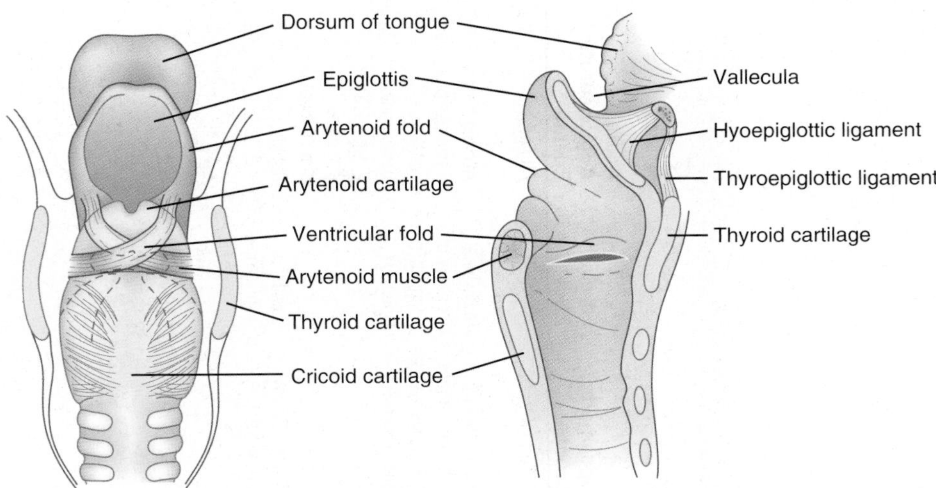

FIG. 18.1 Anatomic relationships of the supraglottic larynx. Posterior view (*left*) and sagittal view (*right*).

documented in adults.[32,274,288,360,374,416,464,475] Infection of the supraglottic larynx may spread inferiorly to involve the paraglottic space,[189] but as a rule, neither upward extension into the laryngeal lymphatics nor downward extension into the subglottic region occurs.[31,226]

Infection of the supraglottic structures probably arises from direct invasion by *H. influenzae* type B, with subsequent development of bacteremia. The bacteremia appears to be relatively short in duration and of low concentration, as suggested by several observations: (1) the serum concentration of the capsular polysaccharide is directly proportional to the concentration and duration of bacteremia,[380] (2) children with epiglottitis have less *H. influenzae* type B capsular polysaccharide in their sera than do patients with meningitis,[462] and (3) the density of *H. influenzae* type B in blood is significantly lower in patients with epiglottitis than in patients with meningitis.[259,376,420] In 23 patients with epiglottitis, the geometric mean number of organisms was 123 colony-forming units (CFUs)/mL, whereas the geometric mean number in 43 patients with meningitis was 2203 CFU/mL ($P < .001$).[259]

What predisposes the epiglottis to infection is unknown. Possibly, mild trauma to the epiglottis occurs during food intake. This trauma could result in damage to the mucosal surface, which, in turn, could allow the invasion of organisms that already were present in the upper respiratory tract. Also possible is that a viral infection damages the mucosal surface and thus predisposes the patient to secondary bacterial infection.

Acute-phase sera in most children with epiglottitis lack specific *H. influenzae* type B bactericidal and hemagglutinating antibody. Seroconversion regularly occurs after infection.[50,289]

Conflicting evidence exists relating to a possible genetic difference between patients with *H. influenzae* type B epiglottitis and other individuals.[8,176,433,475] Whisnant and associates[475] surveyed human leukocyte antigens (HLAs) and erythrocytic antigens among 30 children with epiglottitis and 20 patients with meningitis. HLA-A11 was found in 3% and 17% of the patients with epiglottitis and meningitis, respectively ($P < .01$). HLA-B5 occurred in 3% and 13% of patients with meningitis and epiglottitis, respectively ($P < .05$), whereas HLA-B40 occurred more often (23% vs. 10%) in patients with meningitis than in those with epiglottitis ($P < .05$). Moreover, the frequency of HLA-A28 and HLA-B17 was higher among the patients with epiglottitis than in uninfected control subjects.[475] However, the results of another study did not confirm these observations.[176]

The distribution and frequency of MNS erythrocyte antigens in patients with epiglottitis may differ from those observed in others. For example, the NNSS genotype occurred in 6.4% of patients with epiglottitis and in 0.5% of healthy control subjects ($P < .0002$),[475] but this difference was not confirmed.[176] However, the results of two studies suggest that the MNS genotype occurs less often in patients with *H. influenzae* type B meningitis than in patients with epiglottitis.[176,475] In one study, white children with *H. influenzae* type B meningitis lacked G2m(n), an allotype antigen of immunoglobulin (Ig) G2 subclass heavy chains, more frequently than did control subjects.[8] In another study in a white population in Finland, however, this difference was not noted.[429] The frequency of the Km(1) immunoglobulin allotype in children with epiglottitis did not differ significantly from the prevalence of that marker in blacks or whites. However, in blacks with *H. influenzae* type B meningitis, the Km(1) marker occurred less frequently in patients than in control subjects.[176] The identification of one outer membrane protein subtype of *H. influenzae* type B that was associated relatively infrequently with epiglottitis suggests that isotype-specific differences in the propensity of *H. influenzae* type B to cause epiglottitis may exist.[430]

CLINICAL PRESENTATION

Acute Laryngitis

Table 18.3 summarizes clinical characteristics of laryngitis. Laryngitis is mainly a disease of older children, adolescents, and adults that is disturbing but self-limited. The specific clinical manifestation is hoarseness. Other symptoms depend on the causative infectious agent. Adenoviruses and influenza viruses cause the most severe instances of laryngitis. With these viruses, fever usually occurs, and sore throat, headache, muscle aches and pains, and prostration are common symptoms. In contrast, patients with laryngitis resulting from rhinoviral, parainfluenza viral, or respiratory syncytial viral infections have minimal or no fever and few systemic complaints. They usually have pronounced nasal symptoms (coryza and stuffiness), however. Occasionally hoarseness may persist, which may be a result of secondary bacterial infection of the upper respiratory tract.

Acute Laryngotracheitis

Although the clinical spectrum of acute laryngotracheitis varies considerably, its manifestations usually are significantly different from the manifestations of the other acute diseases with obstruction in the region of the larynx (see Table 18.3). Onset of illness usually is not alarming and suggests the onset of a cold. Initial symptoms are nasal complaints and include dryness, irritation, and coryza. Ordinary cough and the complaint of sore throat occur frequently. Fever is a usual occurrence within the first 24 hours, which is not true of the common cold. After a period as short as a few hours, but usually after 12 to 48 hours, upper airway obstructive signs and symptoms are seen. The cough first becomes "croupy" (sounding like a barking seal), and then evidence of respiratory stridor (difficulty associated with inspiration) gradually increases. Examination at this time reveals a child with a hoarse voice, coryza, a normal or minimally inflamed pharynx, and a slightly increased

TABLE 18.3 **Differential Diagnosis of Acute Obstruction in the Region of the Larynx**

Category	Acute Epiglottitis	Laryngeal Diphtheria	Laryngitis	Acute Laryngotracheitis	Laryngotracheobronchitis and Laryngotracheobronchopneumonitis (Including Bacterial Tracheitis)	Spasmodic Croup	Foreign Body	Acute Angioneurotic Edema
Common age of occurrence	1–8 y	All ages	Older children and adults	3 mo to 3 y	3 mo to 3 y	3 mo to 3 y	All ages	All ages
Past and family history	Not contributory	No or inadequate immunization	Not contributory	Family history of croup	May be family history of croup	Family history of croup; perhaps previous attack	Occasional history of ingestion	Allergic history; perhaps previous attack
Prodrome	Occasionally coryza	Usually pharyngitis	Usually stuffy nose or coryza	Usually coryza	Usually coryza	Minimal coryza	None	Occasionally cutaneous allergic manifestations
Onset (time to full-blown disease)	Rapid; 4–12 h	Slowly for 2- to 3-day period	Variable; 12 hr to 4 days	Moderate but variable; 12–48 h	Usually gradually progressive; 12 hr to 7 days	Sudden; always at night	Usually sudden	Rapid
Symptoms on presentation								
Fever	Yes; usually 39.5°C (103°F)	Yes; usually 37.8°C to 38.5°C (100°F to 101°F)	Yes; 37.8°C to 39.4°C (100°F to 103°F) with adenoviral and influenza viral infections; usually minimal with other viruses	Yes; variable, 37.8°C to 40.5°C (100°F to 105°F)	Yes; variable, 37.8°C to 40.5°C (100°F to 105°F)	No	No, unless secondary infection	No
Hoarseness and barking cough	No	Yes	Yes	Yes	Yes	Yes	Usually no	No
Dysphagia	Yes; usually severe	Usually yes	No	No	No	No	Frequently yes	Yes
Inspiratory stridor	Yes; moderate to severe	Yes; minimal to severe	No	Yes; minimal to severe	Yes; usually severe	Yes; moderate	Variable	Yes
Toxic appearance	Severe	Usually no	No	Usually minimal	Usually moderate; may be severe	No	No	No

Signs on presentation								
Oral cavity	Pharyngitis and excessive salivation	Membranous pharyngitis	Normal or mild to moderate pharyngitis	Usually minimal pharyngitis	Usually minimal pharyngitis	Normal	Normal	Pale appearance
Epiglottis	Cherry-red and swollen	Usually normal; may contain membrane	Normal	Normal	Normal	Normal	Normal	Swollen and pale
Radiographs	Swollen epiglottis on lateral film	Not useful	Not useful	Subglottic narrowing on PA film	Subglottic narrowing on PA film; irregular soft tissue densities within trachea on lateral film	Not useful	May reveal foreign body	Swollen epiglottis on lateral film
Laboratory								
Leukocyte count	Usually markedly elevated with increased percentage of band forms	Usually elevated with increased percentage of band forms	Usually normal	Mildly elevated with >70% polymorphonuclear cells	Variable; usually mildly elevated with 70% polymorphonuclear cells; may be increased band count	Normal	Normal, unless secondary infection	Normal; sometimes eosinophilia
Bacteriology	Throat and blood cultures yield *Haemophilus influenzae* type b	Smear and culture from membrane reveal organism	Usually normal flora in throat; occasionally *Streptococcus pyogenes* in throat	Only important if secondary infection suspected	Normal throat flora; tracheal culture often yields *S. pyogenes, Staphylococcus aureus, Streptococcus pneumoniae,* or *H. influenzae*	Normal flora	Only important if secondary infection suspected	Normal flora
Clinical course	Rapidly progressive; cardiorespiratory arrest occurs within hours if not treated	Slowly progressive obstruction of airway	Hoarseness persists at a constant degree about 4–7 days; occasionally persists 2–3 wk	Variable speed of progression of obstruction; usually does not require surgical intervention	Degree of obstruction usually severe; persists 7–14 days; frequently requires surgical intervention	Symptoms of short duration with treatment; repeated attacks common	Variable depending on size and substance of foreign body	Variable; sometimes leads to rapid asphyxia without therapy

Data from references 109, 110, 114, 131, 144, 159, 193, 227, 277, 278, 302, 434.

respiratory rate with a prolonged inspiratory phase. Temperature nearly always is between 37.8°C and 40.5°C (100°F and 105°F).

The speed of progression and final degree of upper airway obstruction vary. Some children have hoarseness and barking cough but no other evidence of obstruction; in these cases, the symptoms last approximately 3 to 7 days, with a gradual return to normal. In other cases, the obstruction is progressive and leads to severe respiratory distress with supraclavicular and infraclavicular and sternal retractions, cyanosis of varying degrees, and apprehension. With hypoxia, the cardiac rate increases and the child becomes restless. Without intervention, asphyxial death occurs rapidly in some children. In others, the problem of hypoxia is more prolonged, and respiratory fatigue may lead to the patient's demise. The duration of illness in a severely affected child, regardless of therapy, is rarely less than 7 days and frequently is 14 days.

Laboratory study in acute laryngotracheitis is of only minimal value. The white blood cell count frequently is greater than 10,000 cells/mm^3, and polymorphonuclear cells predominate.[79,325] Very high white blood cell counts (>20,000/mm^3) with numerous band-form neutrophils should suggest bacterial superinfection or the possibility of acute epiglottitis. The posteroanterior chest radiograph reveals the subglottic narrowing (steeple sign), and a lateral neck radiograph indicates the size of the epiglottis.

Acute Laryngotracheobronchitis and Laryngotracheobronchopneumonitis (Bacterial Tracheitis)

Laryngotracheobronchitis and laryngotracheobronchopneumonitis are far less common occurrences than laryngotracheitis and spasmodic croup; however, these illnesses occur more commonly than generally realized.* These entities may be considered an extension of acute laryngotracheitis, as numerous descriptions in the literature suggest.† The severity of the illness is due to secondary bacterial infection. Initial signs and symptoms are similar to those of laryngotracheitis (see Table 18.3). An afflicted child usually has mild to moderately severe illness for 2 to 7 days and then suddenly becomes markedly worse. Occasionally upper and lower airway obstructions seem to occur simultaneously. In many children, the distress from tracheal obstruction is of such magnitude that the signs and symptoms of lower respiratory tract involvement go unnoticed. Signs and symptoms associated with extension of disease to the bronchi, bronchioles, and lung substance include rales, air trapping, wheezing, and a further increase in the respiratory rate. Obstruction in these illnesses usually is of such a degree that either intubation or tracheostomy is necessary.

Several instances of laryngotracheobronchopneumonitis with toxic shock syndrome have been observed.[58,77,327,412,424] Generally children with these staphylococcal infections initially have the onset of croup, then the more severe manifestations of bacterial tracheitis develop, and finally the exanthem and other manifestations of toxic shock syndrome develop. An infant with tracheitis and supraglottitis caused by *M. catarrhalis* has been described.[7] Other findings in laryngotracheobronchitis and laryngotracheobronchopneumonitis are presented in Table 18.3.

Spasmodic Croup

In recent years, the clinical entity of spasmodic croup has been incorporated by many physicians into the overall diagnosis of croup. Although distinguishing mild cases of laryngotracheitis from spasmodic croup is difficult at the onset in some instances, the delineation of the two entities is important from prognostic and therapeutic perspectives (see Table 18.3).

Spasmodic croup occurs in children 3 months to 3 years of age. The onset always is at night, and the characteristic presentation occurs in a child who previously was thought to be well or to have had a mild cold with coryza as the only symptom. The child awakens at night with sudden dyspnea, croupy cough, and inspiratory stridor but no fever. The symptoms apparently are the result of sudden subglottic edema; relief is achieved easily by general reassurance and administration of moist air. The occurrence of spasmodic croup tends to run in families, with repeated attacks occurring in some children. After one attack, the child is likely to have another attack the same evening and on three or four successive evenings. These attacks can be prevented by employing mild sedation at bedtime and ensuring that the bedroom air is adequately humidified.

*References 35, 78, 92, 114, 123, 126, 131, 137, 173, 185, 193, 201, 227, 233, 277, 278, 297, 305, 319, 424, 478.

†References 28, 54, 56, 108, 109, 138, 165, 208, 233, 299, 334, 348, 349, 356, 357.

Supraglottitis

The classic onset of epiglottitis in children is abrupt, and progression of disease is rapid; careful history on occasion reveals the occurrence of a trivial antecedent upper respiratory tract infection.* The total duration of illness before hospitalization usually is less than 24 hours and occasionally is as short as 2 hours. In one study in which 142 medical records of children with epiglottitis were reviewed, the duration of illness before tracheotomy was performed was found to be 12 hours or less in 73% and more than 24 hours in only four patients.[89]

The most common presentation of acute epiglottitis in children includes the sudden onset of fever, severe sore throat, dysphagia, and drooling. Airway obstruction always occurs and is rapidly progressive. It is manifested by distress on inspiration, a choking sensation, irritability, restlessness, and anxiety. The speech is muffled or thick sounding, but hoarseness usually does not occur. Aphonia was described in a 4-day-old infant with epiglottitis and concomitant MRSA skin and urinary tract infection.[328] The child usually insists on sitting up in a characteristic posture with the arms back, the trunk leaning forward, the neck hyperextended, and the chin pushed forward. This posture increases the diameter of the obstructed airway.

In contrast to acute laryngotracheitis, in which marked inspiratory stridor occurs, the degree of observed stridor in epiglottitis often is not severe. This apparent lack of respiratory distress often leads the unwary physician to underestimate the severity of the child's illness. With progression, the air exchange becomes progressively worse, and hypoxia, hypercapnia, and acidosis develop. These developments cause increased irritability, restlessness, and disorientation, and if an artificial airway is not established, the child will experience sudden cardiorespiratory arrest.

Fever occurs in virtually all children; most temperatures are between 38.8°C and 40.0°C (101.8°F and 104°F). Blood leukocyte counts almost always are elevated; the mean total count was approximately 20,000 cells/mm^3 in five studies.[6,34,89,224,466] The differential cell count reveals an increased percentage of neutrophils and band forms; most patients have absolute band counts of more than 500 cells/mm^3.

The clinical picture of epiglottitis in adults is more indolent than that in children.[32,188,413,487] Berger and associates[34] reviewed 118 cases of acute epiglottitis seen between 1986 and 2000. Of these patients, 33% were admitted to the hospital within 1 day of the onset of symptoms, and 77% were admitted within 3 days of onset. Symptoms on admission were as follows: sore throat, 85%; odynophagia, 83%; temperature elevation, 38%; respiratory difficulties, 34%; muffled voice, 25%; and drooling, 7%. In two other studies, an average of 1 to 3 days elapsed before medical aid was sought. The mean temperature was 38.2°C (100.7°F), and some patients were afebrile; the temperature range was 36.6°C to 40.0°C (98.0°F to 104°F). Blood leukocyte counts averaged 17,000/mm^3 (range, 8000 to 32,000/mm^3).[188,413] Sore throat and dysphagia were universal occurrences. Zwahlen and Regamy[487] reviewed the clinical features of 100 reported adult cases of epiglottitis. Of these patients, 78% had dyspnea, 49% had dysphonia, 41% had cyanosis, and 38% had stridor. Forty-six percent had edema of the neck. A precordial purring or fluttering sensation was described by one adult patient.[381] In three cases in adults, Ehara[132] noted on physical examination that all had tenderness of the anterior neck over the hyoid bone.

DIFFERENTIAL DIAGNOSIS

The therapeutic approaches to the various acute obstructions in the region of the larynx vary markedly. Establishing a correct diagnosis is essential and frequently lifesaving. Table 18.3 lists the differential points

*References 23, 26, 31, 34, 50, 57, 89, 139, 188, 224, 225, 273, 282, 289, 290, 309, 333, 347, 401, 455, 474.

of eight conditions with symptoms and signs of acute upper airway obstruction.

The most frequent serious differential diagnostic problem is the recognition of acute epiglottitis and its separation from the less fulminant laryngotracheitis. In epiglottitis (a rare disease in children today because of universal immunization with *H. influenzae* type B conjugate vaccines), the important differential points are lack of a croupy cough; the presence of a swollen, cherry-red epiglottis; the sitting posture of the child with the chin pushed forward and a reluctance or refusal to lie down; and the relatively greater apprehension and anxiety of the patient than the degree of chest retraction suggests. In contrast, a child with acute laryngotracheitis has a normal epiglottis on examination, always has a typical barking cough, is comfortable in a supine position, and frequently appears to have only minimal apprehension, despite retractions in which the sternum appears to be indenting 2 inches or more.

Early in the course of epiglottitis, the diagnosis can be confirmed only by the observation of the epiglottis, which can be done without difficulty.[249] Later in the disease, the posture of the child and the history of rapidly progressing disease render the differential from laryngotracheitis readily apparent, so examination of the epiglottis directly (a dangerous procedure if the child is forced to lie down) or indirectly by a lateral neck radiograph rarely is indicated and usually is contraindicated. A study in adults found that bedside sonography could be used as a diagnostic tool for acute epiglottitis in the emergency department.[247]

Laryngotracheobronchitis and laryngotracheobronchopneumonitis can be recognized by signs of lower respiratory involvement (rales, air trapping, wheezing, and pulmonary infiltrates on the radiograph). Bacterial disease should be suspected in laryngotracheobronchitis and laryngotracheobronchopneumonitis and when symptoms and signs become worse in laryngotracheitis. A lateral radiograph can be useful in the evaluation because it may reveal soft tissue densities within the trachea. Lateral neck and chest radiographs are regarded by many physicians as definitive tests to determine whether to rule out epiglottitis and laryngotracheitis. In a careful study by Stankiewicz and Bowes,[415] the sensitivity and specificity of both radiographs were low, however.

Although a rare occurrence today, laryngeal diphtheria always should be considered and ruled out in croup. Recently Hsia and associates[205] noted a child with Guillain-Barré syndrome who initially presented with a crouplike cough.

Spasmodic croup is rarely confused with acute laryngotracheitis, but a perusal of the literature indicates that the two entities most commonly are considered laryngotracheitis, which is unfortunate because prognostic considerations for the two entities are different. Spasmodic croup always is of sudden onset at night, occurs without fever, and is relieved by simple therapeutic modalities.

The possibility of a foreign body and angioneurotic edema always must be considered in upper airway obstructive disease. Differential points are presented in Table 18.3. Rarely acute upper airway obstruction occurs in adolescents as a result of psychogenic and emotional factors.[162,241,378]

There are many causes of recurrent croup in infants and children, and many of these cases should have operative evaluation by an otolaryngology service.[93,113,128,178,350] Diagnostic possibilities include subglottic stenosis, laryngomalacia, bronchomalacia, tracheomalacia, vascular compression of distal trachea, stenosis of left main bronchus, subglottic cyst, tracheoesophageal fistula, unilateral vocal cord immobility, tracheal bronchus, and esophagitis and gastroesophageal reflux disease.

SPECIFIC DIAGNOSIS IN CROUP SYNDROMES

The epidemiologic history frequently is an important factor in establishing a specific diagnosis. Obtaining bacterial culture specimens from the throat, laryngeal region, and blood is helpful in diagnosing epiglottitis and important in identifying laryngotracheitis, laryngotracheobronchitis, and laryngotracheobronchopneumonitis when secondary infection is suspected. The white blood cell count should be obtained because it can be helpful when secondary bacterial infection is considered.

A specific etiologic diagnosis can be made by the isolation of virus or its identification by a direct antigen test from a nasopharyngeal specimen. The diagnostic virologic facilities of many medical centers enable rapid identification of parainfluenza viruses, respiratory syncytial viruses, adenoviruses, most rhinoviruses, and influenza viruses to be established.

SPECIFIC DIAGNOSIS IN SUPRAGLOTTITIS

The clinical picture of sore throat, dysphagia, drooling, anxiety, and inspiratory distress without significant stridor and the characteristic sitting position should suggest the presumptive diagnosis in most cases. The definitive anatomic diagnosis is made by visualization of the epiglottis, and the etiologic diagnosis is confirmed by culture of an organism from the blood or the surface of the epiglottis.

In the typical case, the epiglottis is fiery red and greatly swollen. In children, the epiglottis can be seen by simple depression of the tongue with a tongue blade. In older children and adults, indirect or direct laryngoscopy usually is necessary to confirm the diagnosis. On occasion, the obstruction is caused by swelling of the ventricular bands and the arytenoepiglottic folds so that the epiglottis may appear relatively normal.

Major controversy exists concerning the safety of using a tongue depressor to examine a child with suspected epiglottitis because sudden cardiorespiratory arrest has been noted to occur. However, most instances of cardiorespiratory arrest occurred after the child was forced into a supine position rather than because of the examination itself.[80] In many instances, patients with presumptive epiglottitis can be examined while they are in an upright position by using a tongue blade or indirect laryngoscopy.

Case management should be individualized. In the child with moderate or advanced disease, the clinical diagnosis should be apparent without having to do an intraoral examination. In this situation, intraoral examination should not be performed, but the child should be prepared for the establishment of an airway. This preparation should be rapid but controlled so that intubation can be performed in an operating room.

The diagnosis of epiglottitis can be established by the classic appearance on a lateral neck radiograph (Fig. 18.2).[351,466] However radiographic procedures could lead to a delay in providing the necessary definitive therapy.[89,226,304] The use of the lateral neck radiograph should be reserved

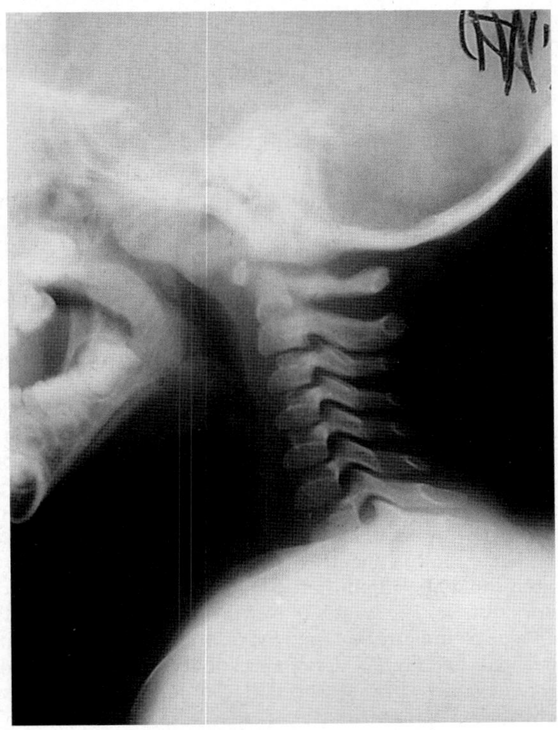

FIG. 18.2 A lateral neck radiograph from a child with acute epiglottitis shows the swollen epiglottis (thumb sign) encroaching on the airway. (Courtesy Dr. Ines Boechat.)

for subacute cases in which the specific diagnosis after completion of a clinical examination is not clear.

The lateral film of the neck, delineating the soft tissues and taken with the patient upright, gives the best view of the upper airway anatomy (see Fig. 18.2). The hypopharynx is dilated; normal cervical lordosis may be replaced by a straight or kyphotic contour. The valleculae are narrowed and may be obliterated. A thickened mass of tissue stretching from the valleculae to the arytenoids emphasizes the appropriateness of the term *supraglottitis*. In adults with epiglottitis, the widths of the epiglottis and arytenoepiglottic folds uniformly exceed 8 and 7 mm, respectively.[387]

When performed, radiography of the neck in the anteroposterior projection usually reveals that tracheal narrowing is absent. However, some children with acute supraglottitis have localized subglottic narrowing indistinguishable from that found in acute laryngotracheitis.[393,408]

All patients with suspected epiglottitis should have a blood culture, and a culture specimen should be obtained from the surface of the epiglottis when an artificial airway is established. Today, cultures are of increasing importance because of the change in epidemiology of *H. influenzae* type B infection and the resulting increased likelihood that a different organism may be causing the illness. A white blood cell count with a differential also may provide useful information. In children who have received antimicrobial treatment before cultures were obtained, performing a direct antigen test for *H. influenzae* type B on the blood and urine is worthwhile.

TREATMENT OF CROUP

During the past 70 years, the treatment of croup has created considerable controversy: tracheostomy versus no tracheostomy, intubation versus tracheostomy, warm versus cold humidification, antibiotics versus no antibiotics, corticosteroids versus no corticosteroids, sedation versus no sedation, and racemic epinephrine therapy versus mist therapy alone. Few of these controversies have been resolved scientifically, but the passage of time has lessened the importance of some of the discrepant opinions.

Of most importance in the evaluation of therapeutic modalities and the specific approach to therapy in croup is making an accurate differential diagnosis. A look at the most important controversy (the use of steroids) indicates that in most instances cases of spasmodic croup, in which a favorable outcome invariably can be expected, were not separated clinically from cases of laryngotracheitis, in which the outcome is less predictable.

Acute Laryngotracheitis and Spasmodic Croup

In managing acute laryngotracheitis and spasmodic croup, each case must be treated individually; one child may need minimal therapy, whereas another may require consideration of all modalities. In all children with acute laryngotracheitis, attention should be given to the anxiety and apprehension of the patient and parents. The parents should be reassured immediately, and it is important that the child is not separated from them. Physical examination should be done rapidly by one physician, and all but absolutely necessary procedures should be deferred.

In the past, mist therapy was the cornerstone of management of croup. In more recent years, the value of this therapy has been questioned.[47,272,310,389] It had been one of our opinions (JDC), as expressed in previous editions of this book, that mist therapy in croup was useful. However, the results of a large randomized controlled trial[389] and the extensive review by Moore and Little[310] indicate that mist treatment offers no benefit in treatment.

Oxygen should be administered to a child who is hypoxemic from respiratory distress. The studies of Newth and associates[323] and Taussig and colleagues[432] indicate that mild hypoxemia occurs more commonly than is realized clinically. The drying effect of oxygen is counterproductive to the removal of tracheal exudate, so it should not be used routinely.

Since 1952, numerous communications in the English literature have described the use of corticosteroids in croup. Nine double-blind, controlled studies were conducted before 1989.[129,130,217,249,258,271,406,422,425] In 1964, Eden and Larkin[130] noted no difference between control and methylprednisolone therapy in a study of 50 children with acute croup. In 1967, Eden and colleagues[129] studied another 50 patients and could find no benefit from dexamethasone in contrast to a control preparation. Sussman and colleagues[425] also could not show any benefit from dexamethasone therapy.

In contrast to these three studies, Skowron and coworkers[406] noted a slight benefit regarding duration of stridor, retractions, fever, and days in the hospital in a group receiving dexamethasone. They suggested, however, that steroids not be used routinely for laryngotracheitis because the overall benefits were minimal and a potential risk exists in administration of steroids. In 1969, James[217] noted that dexamethasone-treated patients recovered from obstructive symptoms more quickly than did the control group. In another study involving 30 children, Leipzig and associates[271] concluded that dexamethasone in an adequate dose (0.3 mg/kg initially and repeated in 2 hours) given intramuscularly hastens the recovery from uncomplicated croup. This study and its predecessors have major inadequacies in design.[81,445] In a study with 72 children, Koren and colleagues[249] noted that dexamethasone did not offer any benefit to patients with laryngotracheitis but did decrease significantly the respiratory rate in children with spasmodic croup in contrast to placebo-treated control subjects. Although these findings were statistically significant, the benefits were not clinically significant.

Two additional modest studies of the use of dexamethasone in croup were published in 1988 and 1989, as was a meta-analysis of the evidence from the various randomized trials and a set of related editorials and a review.[12,69,232,233,257,262,407,411,419] Kuusela and Vesikari[258] concluded that dexamethasone was beneficial in acute spasmodic croup, and Super and associates[422] concluded that dexamethasone is beneficial in reducing the overall severity of moderate to severe acute laryngotracheitis during the first day of treatment.

The 1989 meta-analysis suggested that the use of steroids in children hospitalized with croup resulted in a significantly increased number with clinical improvement 12 hours and 24 hours after treatment and a reduced incidence of endotracheal intubation than occurred in the control subjects.[232] In this analysis, improvement at 12 hours was noted to be greater in the children who received higher initial doses of steroid (≥125 mg of cortisone) than in children who received lower doses.

In the early 1990s, nebulized steroids were evaluated in the treatment of croup, which led to another round of testimonials, controlled studies, and treatment articles supporting the efficacy of steroids.* Since the 1989 meta-analysis, more than 15 additional controlled steroid treatment trials have been performed, and another meta-analysis was published in 1999.[15] Finally a large controlled trial of oral dexamethasone for mild croup was published in 2004, and a comprehensive meta-analysis was published in 2005.[40,373] Also published more recently are many articles comparing doses, types, and methods of administration of steroids and a further round of commentaries.† On the basis of the three meta-analyses and the specific studies analyzed, most reviews on the management of croup recommend the routine use of steroids (administered orally, intramuscularly, or by nebulization) in the treatment of croup.‡

A past review of the data (by JDC) on the use of steroids in croup was concerning in that the specific clinical entity being treated was poorly defined, and no evidence indicated that steroids worked in any illness other than spasmodic croup.[81] One recent meta-analysis on the effects of glucocorticoids in croup that includes 38 studies found that use of glucocorticoids improves symptoms as early as 6 hours and up to at least 12 hours after treatment. The study also showed significant improvement in the scores of croup severity, fewer return visits and/or (re)admissions, shorter length of stays, and reduced use of epinephrine.[375]

Of most concern today is that the risks of steroid use have not been evaluated and that, because of small sample sizes in all but two of the available studies, they cannot be evaluated by meta-analysis.

*References 15, 100, 171, 179, 207, 216, 223, 231, 242–245, 362, 365, 405, 468.
†References 39, 71, 84, 121, 122, 144, 145, 155, 161, 241, 285, 362, 375, 436.
‡References 10, 39, 41, 99, 111, 112, 144, 145, 171, 179, 210, 216, 217, 241–243, 245, 362, 365, 436.

Lower respiratory tract complications developed in three children receiving steroid treatment for croup. In one case, an adenoviral pneumonia worsened, and in the other cases bacterial tracheitis with pneumonia occurred. All three cases received corticosteroid treatment over the course of several days and not single-dose treatment. In the study of Super and colleagues,[422] two steroid-treated patients developed pneumonia during therapy; none of the control subjects developed pneumonia. In another trial in which 28 children received nebulized dexamethasone, two children with neutropenia developed bacterial tracheitis.[223] Burton and associates[64] reported the occurrence of *Candida* laryngotracheitis as a complication of corticosteroid and antibiotic treatment in a child with croup, and Myers and colleagues[318] reported an infant who developed multiple pulmonary abscesses caused by *Legionella pneumophila* after receiving prolonged corticosteroid treatment of severe croup.

Today the standard of care for the initial treatment of laryngotracheitis and spasmodic croup is the use of corticosteroids administered orally, intramuscularly, or by nebulization.[10,39,144] Recommended therapy is a single dose of intramuscular or oral dexamethasone. The limited use of nebulized budesonide also is effective. In the most definitive study, the treatment dose was dexamethasone 0.6 mg/kg given orally once.[40] In a subsequent review, Bjornson and Johnson[39] noted that the standard dose of dexamethasone is 0.6 mg/kg (oral or intramuscular); they suggested that oral is preferable because absorption is excellent, and peak serum concentrations are achieved as rapidly as with intramuscular administration. Recently Dobrovoljac and Geelhoed[120] reported on the effectiveness of a single 0.15 mg/kg dose of dexamethasone. They noted that this lower dose was as effective as the 0.6 mg/kg dose that they had previously used.

As noted earlier, we and others have observed bacterial and fungal infections as complications in children who have received multiple doses of steroids in croup. It is disturbing to note that in pediatric practice many children are receiving 3- to 5-day treatment courses rather than the recommended single-dose schedule. The data from the cotton rat model of human parainfluenza virus type 3 laryngotracheitis provide strong evidence supporting the limited use of steroids in croup.[335] In this model, topical steroid therapy significantly reduced the degree of inflammatory infiltrates and cell damage. The steroid therapy increased the virus load but did not prolong virus shedding.

We believe the most dramatic evidence supporting the use of steroid therapy in laryngotracheitis and spasmodic croup is the marked decrease in the number of hospitalizations for croup in Ontario, which coincided with the 1992 recommendation by the Canadian Pediatrics Society to use dexamethasone for treatment.[210,391] Steroids should not be used in laryngotracheobronchitis, laryngotracheobronchopneumonitis, or epiglottitis.

Because laryngotracheitis is a disease of viral etiology, it seems apparent that antibiotic therapy would not be indicated and consequently not employed. In an analysis of more than 200 hospitalized children with laryngotracheitis, it was noted that antibiotics had been administered to 85%.[158] A review of the records in many instances revealed that the physician had given antibiotic therapy because the possibility of epiglottitis had not been ruled out adequately. In several instances, the epiglottis had been observed and thought to be reddened or questionably enlarged.

A second consideration with regard to antibiotic therapy in croup is that the most dramatic reduction in mortality rates coincides with the introduction and widespread use of antibiotics. In our opinion, many of the deaths attributed to croup in the preantibiotic era were caused by secondary bacterial infections. Although use of antibiotics contributed to the reduction in the number of deaths caused by croup, other factors may be important. At about the same time that antibiotics were introduced, disease caused by *S. pyogenes* decreased in incidence and severity. Reasons for the decreased frequency of streptococcal disease were not clear.

Most patients with laryngotracheitis today do not need antibiotic therapy. In severe cases in which bacterial sepsis cannot be ruled out, however, antibiotic therapy should be employed. The pathogens to consider include pneumococci, group A streptococci, *S. aureus,* and *H. influenzae.* In patients with laryngotracheitis in whom fever persists or signs change, secondary infection should be considered. In these instances, appropriate culture specimens should be obtained before therapy is initiated (see the section on laryngotracheobronchitis for specific antibiotic therapy).

The use of nebulized racemic epinephrine, which was introduced by Jordan[229] in 1966 and popularized by Jordan and other members of the Utah group,[2,230] has been adopted widely throughout the United States and elsewhere.[14,41,236,255,279,302,372,402] The usual method of nebulization of racemic epinephrine is by intermittent positive-pressure breathing. This form of therapy was associated with a marked reduction in tracheostomies in several series. In a review it was found that nebulized racemic epinephrine was no better than routine L-epinephrine and that intermittent positive-pressure breathing offered no advantage over simple nebulization.[41]

In 1973, Gardner and associates[159] performed the first double-blind controlled study in which racemic epinephrine was nebulized by a compressor without intermittent positive-pressure breathing. They found that saline-treated patients responded as well to therapy as did the racemic epinephrine recipients. In retrospect, this study can be criticized because the investigators failed to differentiate spasmodic croup from laryngotracheitis. In 1975, Taussig and associates[432] reported a small but carefully conducted study with intermittent positive-pressure breathing and racemic epinephrine in which they noted acute improvement in all cases, recurrence of symptoms in 2 hours, and no change in partial pressure of oxygen with clinical improvement; 24 to 36 hours after therapy, treated and untreated children were clinically similar. In another significant study that involved children hospitalized with severe croup without improvement after admission to a high-humidity mist room, Westley and colleagues[473] showed that racemic epinephrine therapy caused definite short-term improvement in children compared with saline treatment. This study is particularly important because a parainfluenza viral etiology was documented in more than 65% of the study's subjects, and all cases were clearly laryngotracheitis and not spasmodic croup.

The following points can be made about the use of racemic epinephrine in the treatment of croup: (1) Many children with croup respond to moist air alone; (2) significant rebound occurs after racemic epinephrine therapy, so it frequently needs to be repeated many times; (3) in a hospitalized child with severe acute laryngotracheitis, racemic epinephrine should be used. Tracheotomy or endotracheal intubation can be prevented in some cases. The most important issue today regarding the use of racemic epinephrine is whether it can be used safely for outpatient therapy.[94,234,344] In the past, most experts advised against the use of racemic epinephrine in the outpatient setting because of the known rebound that occurs. Some data suggest that with careful observation for a sufficient period (at least 2 hours) after administration, patients can be managed safely, and the number of hospitalizations can be decreased.[94,234,344] In a small study, investigators found that the administration of a helium-oxygen mixture (heliox) resulted in improvement in children with croup similar to that with racemic epinephrine treatment.[465] A systemic review found some evidence that suggested that heliox in steroid-treated patients provided short-term clinical improvement.[311]

The establishment of a mechanical airway seldom is necessary today in patients with laryngotracheitis. Traditionally tracheostomy was the preferred method when a mechanical airway was needed.[18,153,486] When careful attention is given to tube size and other aspects of placement and maintenance, however, nasotracheal intubation compares favorably with tracheostomy.[18,486] The management of a child with a mechanical airway requires trained pediatric intensive care physicians and the facilities of an adequately staffed intensive care unit.[465]

Five antiviral drugs have activity against viruses that cause laryngotracheitis.[184,215,294,427,476] Amantadine and rimantadine are approved for use in treating influenza A viral infections, and ribavirin is active against parainfluenza viruses, influenza A and B viruses, and respiratory syncytial virus (see Chapters 178, 179, and 182). The neuraminidase inhibitors, zanamivir and oseltamivir, are active against influenza a and b types.[70,95] At present, consideration of therapy for severe croup that occurs during documented epidemics caused by influenza A or B viruses would seem reasonable. Because of high levels of resistance of influenza

A strains to amantadine and rimantadine, treatment with the neuraminidase inhibitors is recommended.[70]

Laryngotracheobronchitis and Laryngotracheobronchopneumonitis (Bacterial Tracheitis)

Generally all the treatment considerations discussed for laryngotracheitis except corticosteroids and racemic epinephrine by aerosol apply to laryngotracheobronchitis and laryngotracheobronchopneumonitis. Most important, however, because most patients have bacterial disease, antibiotics should be administered to all patients after appropriate culture specimens are obtained. Empiric therapy should be directed against *S. aureus, S. pyogenes, S. pneumoniae,* and *H. influenzae*. At present, initial treatment with vancomycin 40 mg/kg per day intravenously every 6 hours and a third-generation cephalosporin, such as cefotaxime 150 mg/kg per day every 6 hours intravenously, is reasonable. If methicillin-sensitive *S. aureus* is isolated, treatment should be changed to oxacillin 150 mg/kg per day every 6 hours intravenously or a similar agent.

Most children with advanced laryngotracheobronchitis or laryngotracheobronchopneumonitis need the placement of a mechanical airway. Whenever possible, this procedure should be done electively rather than as an emergency.

Laryngitis

Patients with laryngitis should rest their voices as much as possible. Increased fluid intake and perhaps the use of a vaporizer may help liquefy secretions and might provide symptomatic relief. Because group A streptococcal infection is a cause of laryngitis, culture should be performed. If it is positive, penicillin or a suitable alternative antimicrobial agent should be administered. In children and adolescents with prolonged hoarseness, sinusitis should be considered. Radiographs of the sinuses and a quantitative culture from the nose should be performed in search of a predominant abnormal bacterial flora. If either is positive, therapy with appropriate antibiotics is indicated. If laryngeal symptoms are persistent, the child should undergo laryngoscopic examination and other appropriate studies to exclude tumor, foreign body, and other chronic diseases.

TREATMENT OF SUPRAGLOTTITIS

The treatment of acute epiglottitis should be relatively simple in that it involves only two main aspects of therapy: an airway must be established, and an appropriate antimicrobial agent needs to be administered. However, in the past, the mortality rate from epiglottitis varied from 0% to 32%,[89,188] a finding suggesting major differences in the implementation of treatment.

Most deaths occur in transit to the hospital or within the first few hours after arrival. Once the diagnosis is suspected, the patient should be attended constantly by individuals skilled in resuscitation with appropriate equipment for airway stabilization and ventilatory support. Delays of 2 or 3 hours have proved fatal; every effort should be made to reduce the time needed to secure a patient's airway and to initiate antibiotic therapy, before which unnecessary stress should be avoided. In most cases, radiographic confirmation should be omitted. Blood tests, extensive history taking, and delay in transport should be eliminated.

Medical centers and pediatric services that have planned protocols for the diagnostic investigation and treatment of patients with suspected acute epiglottitis generally have better morbidity and mortality statistics than do services that do not have such protocols in place. Pediatricians, radiologists, otolaryngologists, and anesthetists may contribute to the assessment and management of a case; defining roles and responsibilities of each service in advance minimizes confusion and renders the institution of care easier.

Securing the Airway

In general, the cornerstone of all management plans is the establishment of an airway in all children in whom the diagnosis of epiglottitis is made.[82] In 1938, Sinclair[400] recognized that tracheostomy was lifesaving. Berenberg and Kevy[32] advocated hospitalization for all patients with epiglottitis but tracheostomy only "if necessary." However, Bass and associates[23] presented a compelling argument for performing routine tracheostomy. Among 83 patients with documented epiglottitis, 11 of whom were adults, these authors noted that 16 (19%) had life-threatening obstruction when they were first seen. An additional 14 (17%) progressed to this point within 6 hours of admission; 9 of the 83 (11%) required emergency tracheostomy while they were hospitalized. Of these 9, 2 died and 1 suffered anoxic brain damage. All 9 were being monitored carefully, with bedside tracheostomy equipment available and trained personnel nearby. Six of the adults required tracheostomy for survival.[23] Margolis and colleagues[290] noted that elective tracheostomy, performed at the time of diagnosis, eliminated fatalities in 15 consecutive patients. This observation was in contrast to four deaths in 20 patients observed until tracheostomy "was required."

A large body of literature attests to the safety and efficacy of nasotracheal intubation as a replacement for tracheostomy,* which has a complication rate of 50%.[435,474] Biologically inert tubes, with their decreased risk for complicating subglottic stenosis,[397] and the recollection that endotracheal tube insertion was a universal approach before tracheostomy[304] was an accepted procedure led to the routine use of nasotracheal intubation in this disease. Nasotracheal intubation requires a shorter duration of airway maintenance: 32 patients with epiglottitis managed with tracheostomy had a mean duration of intubation of 7.5 days and a mean hospitalization of 8.8 days. In contrast, a nasotracheal tube was used for a mean of 38 hours with a 6.5-day hospitalization in five patients.[304] Diaz and Lockhart[119] managed 104 patients with nasotracheal intubation. The mean intubation time was 53 ± 14.9 hours; seven patients (6.8%) extubated themselves, and two required reintubation. Laryngeal edema occurred in three patients (2.9%) who had been intubated. In two patients, subglottic granulations required excision.

Our position, as well as that of Daum and Smith,[106] is that the argument for performing elective tracheostomy or, preferably, intubation in all children with supraglottitis is compelling, and the procedure should be performed immediately after the diagnosis is established. Whether this "stimulus-response" approach is necessary for adults with epiglottitis is controversial.[21,150,188,337,390,399,413,477] MayoSmith and associates[293] compared selected clinical features in adults with epiglottitis at the time of diagnosis who died or who received an artificial airway with those of adults who recovered without airway intervention. Few differences emerged. Patients who died or who were managed with airway intervention had respiratory distress and bacteremia more often than did those who recovered without airway intervention. Obviously the presence of bacteremia was not known on presentation. Moreover the mortality rate among all adults managed expectantly was 4.6%, a figure comparable to the mortality rate (6.1%) of children in a series reported before recommendations were made for routine securing of the airway at diagnosis.[67,293] The preponderance of evidence until very recently has suggested that securing the airway in all adults with supraglottitis by nasotracheal intubation should reduce mortality rates.[11,20–22,36,239,293] However, Frantz and associates[151] reported an analysis of 129 cases of acute epiglottitis in adults in which no deaths occurred in the cohort, and 85% of these patients were managed without airway intervention.

In the large series reported by Berger and colleagues[34] involving 118 cases, 19 had airways established on admission (16 endotracheal intubation, 2 tracheotomy, 1 cricothyrotomy), and 6 other patients subsequently required either endotracheal intubation or tracheotomy. The remaining 93 patients were managed successfully without the need for airway intervention. Fifty-eight of the patients were treated with intravenous corticosteroids in addition to antibiotics, and these patients tended to have more prolonged hospital stays than those who did not receive steroids (5.7 ± 4.1 days vs. 4.7 ± 4.3 days; $P = .2$).

To aid in intubation and reduce long-term sequelae, most investigators have advocated use of a nasotracheal tube 0.5 to 1.0 mm smaller than that predicted by the patient's age.[192,304,384] Published criteria for extubation[14] include those based on duration of therapy and those based on daily examination of the epiglottis and supraglottic structures by direct laryngoscopy[107] or fiberoptic bronchoscopy.[329,452]

*References 26, 90, 192, 261, 290, 333, 352, 384, 386, 397, 435, 439.

Long-term complications of nasotracheal intubation are rare. Thirty-three children with epiglottitis who were managed with nasotracheal intubation (mean duration of intubation, 55 hours) were evaluated 1 to 8 years later. By history and measurement of peak expiratory flow rates, no complications were found.[384] Although additional long-term data are necessary to ensure absence of residua, elective nasotracheal intubation appears to be the procedure of choice.

Several reports documented the recognition of idiopathic pulmonary edema before[270] or, more commonly, after[3,105,120,148,223,386,416] insertion of an endotracheal tube to relieve laryngeal obstruction caused by epiglottitis. One hypothesis to explain this phenomenon is that airway obstruction produces markedly negative intrapleural pressure with increased venous return to the right side of the heart, with decreased left ventricular output and increased pulmonary blood volume.[266] These changes increase the pulmonary microvascular pressure and produce pulmonary hyperemia and edema. Endotoxemia may play a role in altering vascular permeability, but it is not necessary for recognition of this complication of airway obstruction because abrupt onset of pulmonary edema was described when airway obstruction caused by croup, foreign body, and malignant neoplasm was relieved acutely.[63] The frequency of pulmonary edema as a complication of intubation in supraglottitis was approximately 9%,[408] and it has occurred in an adult.[363] Continuous positive airway pressure in all intubated patients with epiglottitis probably will provide prophylaxis against this complication,[119,154] but controlled data are lacking.

Antibiotics

The mainstay of antibiotic therapy for acute epiglottitis in the recent past has been ceftriaxone 50 to 100 mg/kg per day given every 12 hours intravenously or cefotaxime 100 to 200 mg/kg per day given every 6 hours intravenously because virtually all cases in both children and adults were caused by *H. influenzae* type B. However, in the present conjugate vaccine era, the incidence of all invasive *H. influenzae* type B disease has decreased dramatically. Therefore, in children previously vaccinated, the cause is likely to be another organism. Culture results today have added significance because one possible cause that would require a change in therapy is *S. aureus*.

No controlled data exist about the duration of antimicrobial administration, but a course of 7 to 10 days seems appropriate. In the event that group A streptococci are isolated from the airway, penicillin is the drug of choice. A first-generation semisynthetic penicillinase-resistant penicillin or vancomycin (if MRSA is suspected) should be used for *S. aureus*.

Other Supportive Measures

Expert respiratory nursing care is essential. Inadvertent extubation must be avoided, particularly in the first 24 hours. Judicious use of sedatives that do not appreciably depress respiration may be appropriate.

PROGNOSIS

The prognosis of acute laryngotracheitis has improved markedly during the past 55 years. Today a child with croup only rarely requires a mechanical airway, and virtually all deaths should be preventable. The child should be observed for the following complications: hypoxemia and cardiorespiratory failure, pulmonary edema, pneumothorax and pneumomediastinum, mechanical problems caused by tracheotomies and nasotracheal tubes, and secondary bacterial infections. Children with a history of croup have a higher prevalence of increased bronchial reactivity than children without such history.[182,284,468]

The prognosis in epiglottitis after the successful establishment of an airway and the administration of specific antimicrobial agents is generally good.

Extraepiglottic complications are not common occurrences in children with acute epiglottitis. In a study involving 72 children with epiglottitis, investigators noted that 25% had pneumonia, 25% had cervical adenitis, 8% had tonsillitis, and 5% had otitis media.[309] The other common invasive manifestations of *H. influenzae* type B infections (meningitis, arthritis, and cellulitis) rarely are found in conjunction with epiglottitis.[309,383]

PREVENTION OF CROUP

At present, acute laryngotracheitis is not preventable. The widespread use of influenza vaccines could reduce the incidence of croup caused by influenza A and B viruses.

Prevention of Epiglottitis Caused by *Haemophilus influenzae* Type B

The universal use of *H. influenzae* type B vaccine in infancy with an additional dose in the second year of life has had a profound effect on the occurrence of invasive *H. influenzae* type B diseases.

In the pre–conjugate vaccine era, household contacts of patients with *H. influenzae* type B infection were at increased risk for acquiring the infection.[175] Whether an increased risk occurred in daycare contacts was unresolved.[105] Although contacts of patients with *H. influenzae* type B epiglottitis younger than 5 years of age are colonized less frequently than contacts of patients with other *H. influenzae* type B invasive infections,[104] secondary disease was described in household contacts when an index patient had epiglottitis.[3,169,170,441] Secondary *H. influenzae* type B epiglottitis was described in a child[3] and two adults who were household contacts of a patient with *H. influenzae* type B meningitis.[169,170] *H. influenzae* type B epiglottitis occurred in two siblings who presented with the condition within 1 day.[186]

Rifampin prophylaxis with 20 mg/kg per day (600 mg/dose maximum) for 4 days is recommended for all unvaccinated members of a patient's contact group when the index patient has *H. influenzae* type B epiglottitis and at least one contact in the group is 4 years of age or younger.[9,69]

The recognition that adults occasionally may acquire secondary infection, particularly epiglottitis, on exposure to children with invasive *H. influenzae* type B infection prompted some experts to extend prophylaxis to all of a patient's contact groups regardless of the presence of one or more contacts who are 4 years of age or younger. All experts, however, recommended that adults and older children be made aware of the signs and symptoms of *H. influenzae* type B disease, particularly when the patient's contact group would not receive prophylaxis under current guidelines.

NEW REFERENCES SINCE THE SEVENTH EDITION

1. Abou Zahr A, Saad Aldin E, Yunyongying P. Histoplasma epiglottitis in a patient with Crohn's disease maintained on infliximab, prednisone, and azathioprine. *Int J Infect Dis.* 2013;17(8):e650-e652.
37. Bizaki AJ, Numminen J, Vasama JP, et al. Acute supraglottitis in adults in Finland: review and analysis of 308 cases. *Laryngoscope.* 2011;121(10):2107-2113.
90. Collins S, Ramsay M, Campbell H, et al. Invasive *Haemophilus influenzae* type b disease in England and Wales: Who is at risk after 2 decades of routine childhood vaccination? *Clin Infect Dis.* 2013;57(12):1715-1721.
92. Cooper T, Kuruvilla G, Persad R, et al. Atypical croup: association with airway lesions, atopy, and esophagitis. *Otolaryngol Head Neck Surg.* 2012;147(2):209-214.
112. Delany DR, Johnston DR. Role of direct laryngoscopy and bronchoscopy in recurrent croup. *Otolaryngol Head Neck Surg.* 2015;152(1):159-164.
120. Dobrovoljac M, Geelhoed GC. How fast does oral dexamethasone work in mild to moderately severe croup? A randomized double-blinded clinical trial. *Emerg Med Australas.* 2012;24(1):79-85.
127. Durell J, Taha R, Pipi G, et al. Aspergillus epiglottitis in a non-immunocompromised patient. *BMJ Case Rep.* 2011;doi:10.1136/bcr.11.2010.3485.
128. Duval M, Tarasidis G, Grimmer JF, et al. Role of operative airway evaluation in children with recurrent croup: a retrospective cohort study. *Clin Otolaryngol.* 2015;40(3):227-233.
135. El Beltagi AH, Khera PS, Alrabiah L, et al. Case report: acute tuberculous laryngitis presenting as acute epiglottitis. *Indian J Radiol Imaging.* 2011;21(4):284-286.
155. Garbutt JM, Conlon B, Sterkel R, et al. The comparative effectiveness of prednisolone and dexamethasone for children with croup: a community-based randomized trial. *Clin Pediatr (Phila).* 2013;52(11):1014-1021.
172. Gohil R, Culshaw J, Jackson P, et al. Accidental button battery ingestion presenting as croup. *J Laryngol Otol.* 2014;128(3):292-295.
178. Greifer M, Santiago MT, Tsirilakis K, et al. Pediatric patients with chronic cough and recurrent croup: the case for a multidisciplinary approach. *Int J Pediatr Otorhinolaryngol.* 2015;79(5):749-752.
180. Griffin ES, Young TM. Bacterial tracheitis in a 9-month-old child. *J Emerg Nurs.* 2015;41(2):109-112.
191. Heininger U, Baer G, Ryser AJ, et al. Comparative analysis of clinical characteristics of pandemic influenza a/h1n1 and seasonal influenza a infections in hospitalized children. *Pediatr Infect Dis J.* 2013;32(3):293-296.

209. Ibrahimov M, Yollu U, Akil F, et al. Laryngeal foreign body mimicking croup. *J Craniofac Surg*. 2013;24(1):e7-e8.
240. King-Schultz LW, Orvidas LJ, Mannenbach MS. Stridor is not always croup. *Pediatr Emerg Care*. 2015;31(2):140-143.
247. Ko DR, Chung YE, Park I, et al. Use of bedside sonography for diagnosing acute epiglottitis in the emergency department: a preliminary study. *J Ultrasound Med*. 2012;31(1):19-22.
256. Kudchadkar SR, Hamrick JT, Mai CL, et al. The heat is on: thermal epiglottitis as a late presentation of airway steam injury. *J Emerg Med*. 2014;46(2):e43-e46.
263. Ladhani SN, Beebeejaun K, Lucidarme J, et al. Increase in endemic *Neisseria meningitidis* capsular group W sequence type 11 complex associated with severe invasive disease in England and Wales. *Clin Infect Dis*. 2015;60(4):578-585.
265. Lake JA, Ehrhardt MJ, Suchi M, et al. A case of necrotizing epiglottitis due to nontoxigenic *Corynebacterium diphtheriae*. *Pediatrics*. 2015;136(1):e242-e245.
269. Lee J, Storch GA. Characterization of human coronavirus OC43 and human coronavirus NL63 infections among hospitalized children <5 years of age. *Pediatr Infect Dis J*. 2014;33(8):814-820.
307. Miranda AD, Valdez TA, Pereira KD. Bacterial tracheitis: a varied entity. *Pediatr Emerg Care*. 2011;27(10):950-953.
311. Moraa I, Sturman N, McGuire T, et al. Heliox for croup in children. *Cochrane Database Syst Rev*. 2013;(12):CD006822.
328. Noble J, Devor R, Rogalski FJ, et al. Aphonia and epiglottitis in neonate with concomitant MRSA skin infection. *Respirol Case Rep*. 2014;2(3):116-119.
332. O'Niel MB, Chun RH, Conley SF. Ulcerative lesions as a rare cause of laryngotracheitis in the pediatric population. *Am J Otolaryngol*. 2013;34(5):541-544.
350. Rankin I, Wang SM, Waters A, et al. The management of recurrent croup in children. *J Laryngol Otol*. 2013;127(5):494-500.
355. Rennie DC, Karunanayake CP, Chen Y, et al. CD14 gene variants and their importance for childhood croup, atopy, and asthma. *Dis Markers*. 2013;35(6):765-771.
375. Russell KF, Liang Y, O'Gorman K, et al. Glucocorticoids for croup. *Cochrane Database Syst Rev*. 2011;(1):CD001955.
377. Schaap-Nutt A, Liesman R, Bartlett EJ, et al. Human parainfluenza virus serotypes differ in their kinetics of replication and cytokine secretion in human tracheobronchial airway epithelium. *Virology*. 2012;433(2):320-328.
382. Schomacker H, Schaap-Nutt A, Collins PL, et al. Pathogenesis of acute respiratory illness caused by human parainfluenza viruses. *Curr Opin Virol*. 2012;2(3):294-299.
394. Shah KM, Carswell KN, Paradise Black NM. Prolonged stridor and epiglottitis with concurrent bacterial and viral etiologies. *Clin Pediatr (Phila)*. 2016;55(1):91-92.
444. Tsai KK, Wang CH. Acute epiglottitis following traditional Chinese gua sha therapy. *CMAJ*. 2014;186(8):E298.
485. Zhang L, Bukreyev A, Thompson CI, et al. Infection of ciliated cells by human parainfluenza virus type 3 in an in vitro model of human airway epithelium. *J Virol*. 2005;79(2):1113-1124.

The full reference list for this chapter is available at ExpertConsult.com.

Acute Bronchitis

19

James D. Cherry

Bronchitis is a common diagnosis in pediatric practice, although little unanimity exists among physicians regarding its exact clinical constellation and in the true pathologic sense; it probably never occurs as an isolated entity. Acute bronchitis is a febrile illness with cough, rhonchi, and referred breath sounds.[14] Asthmatic bronchitis (infectious asthma), similar to acute bronchitis but with associated wheezing and expiratory distress, is discussed in Chapter 21. On pathologic examination, the clinical illness of acute bronchitis reflects acute inflammatory disease of the larger air passages, including the trachea and the large and medium-sized bronchi.[26]

ETIOLOGY

Table 19.1 lists various infectious agents associated with acute bronchitis. Infections with adenoviruses, influenza viruses, parainfluenza viruses, respiratory syncytial virus, and *Mycoplasma pneumoniae* account for most cases of acute bronchitis in children. These agents, plus many rhinoviruses, a few enteroviruses, and perhaps human metapneumovirus, human bocavirus, and the newer human coronaviruses, account for virtually all cases in the United States today.

Of the adenoviruses, type 7 has been associated most commonly with acute bronchitis in children. In military recruits, including adolescents, adenovirus types 4 and 7 cause epidemic acute respiratory disease, in which bronchitis is a usual occurrence.[23,67]

Influenza A virus infection is a common cause of severe acute bronchitis, particularly at the time of an antigenic shift of influenza A virus subtype and pandemic disease. Acute bronchitis caused by influenza A virus also is a regular occurrence between pandemics in new susceptible individuals (young children) in the population. In addition, influenza b virus is an important cause of bronchitis, and it was a more common causative agent than was influenza A virus in one large longitudinal study.[13]

All cases of measles involve the bronchi, but measles has been an uncommon occurrence since the advent of widespread use of vaccines. Of the parainfluenza viruses, type 3 is associated most commonly with acute bronchitis. Respiratory syncytial virus is a common cause of acute bronchitis, particularly in very young children. The more recently identified human metapneumovirus and human bocavirus are also causes of acute bronchitis.[18,59,65,74,75]

Of the bacterial agents listed in Table 19.1, only *Haemophilus influenzae* clearly can be incriminated. *Bordetella pertussis* infection involves the trachea and bronchi, but fever is an uncommon event, and the illness is outside the definition of acute bronchitis. When sought, *M. pneumoniae* is a common cause of bronchitis. *Chlamydia pneumoniae* has been found to be the cause of bronchitis in adolescents and young adults.[33]

EPIDEMIOLOGY

The epidemiology of the common viruses associated with bronchitis is presented in Sections 17 and 18 of this text. Chapman and associates[13] published the results of a study of acute bronchitis in a single private group pediatric practice in Chapel Hill, North Carolina. The study occurred during a 104-month period, during which 5489 episodes of lower respiratory tract illness occurred. Of these illnesses, 40.1% were acute bronchitis. The bronchitis attack rate was highest in children in the second year of life (6.71%), then decreased gradually to approximately 2% in teenagers. In contrast to the age-specific attack rates, the ratio of bronchitis cases to all lower respiratory illness cases increased with age. In the first year of life, the ratio was 0.29; in children 12 years old or older, it was 0.69.

During the first 6 years of life, respiratory syncytial virus and parainfluenza virus type 3 were the most common etiologic agents noted in the Chapel Hill study. During the first 2 years of life, adenoviruses also commonly were associated with bronchitis. In patients older than 6 years, *M. pneumoniae* and influenza A and B viruses were the most common etiologic agents. In a study of cough illnesses of 6 days' duration or longer in university students, investigators found that 15 of 31 students with laboratory evidence of *Bordetella* spp. infection were considered by their primary care providers to have bronchitis.[48]

The incidence of acute bronchitis peaks in the winter months, declines to midsummer, and increases again through the fall. Attack rates generally are higher in boys than in girls.[13,41,68] A sex difference is most pronounced during the first 6 years of life. Darrow and associates[22] found that primary traffic pollutants, ozone, and the organic carbon fraction of particulate matter of less than 2.5 μm in diameter exacerbate upper and lower respiratory infections in young children.

PATHOPHYSIOLOGY AND PATHOLOGY

Because acute bronchitis is an illness characterized by clinical features and one not usually associated with death, knowledge of its pathophysiology and pathology is meager. The general pathophysiology of human infections with viruses and *M. pneumoniae* that cause acute bronchitis is presented more completely in the sections of this book related to the individual infectious agents.

In virtually all cases of acute bronchitis, evidence of upper respiratory tract viral infection (pharyngitis, rhinitis) also is present. Tracheal and bronchial infection apparently is the result of distal spread. In bronchitis, the clinical features result from damage to the ciliated epithelium of the lower trachea and the large and medium-sized bronchi.[26] Although the cytopathologies of the various infectious agents is different,[76] the resulting obstruction of the air passages leads to similar symptoms. The duration of symptoms depends to some extent on the specific initial infectious agent and, in cases of prolonged illness, on secondary bacterial infection.

In acute bronchitis, the larynx and subglottic trachea are not involved prominently. Conversely, today bronchial involvement is seen only occasionally in croup.

CLINICAL PRESENTATION

Initial manifestations of acute bronchitis occur in the upper respiratory tract and, depending on the etiologic agent, are predominantly nasal, as in the common cold, or show additional objective evidence of pharyngitis, as in nasopharyngitis. Fever usually is present, and temperatures vary from 37.8°C to 39°C (100°F to 102.2°F) on most occasions. Cough is always present, and its onset can be insidious or abrupt. Initially, the cough is dry and harsh and often brassy in younger children. As the illness progresses, the cough becomes looser. In older children, purulent sputum is raised and expectorated. In younger children, the swallowing of often tenacious sputum frequently leads to gagging and

TABLE 19.1 Infectious Agents Associated With Acute Bronchitis

Agent	Importance in Causation[a]	References
Viruses		
Adenovirus types 1–7, 12	+++	1, 2, 5, 10–12, 15, 24, 30, 28, 36, 38, 44, 57, 61, 64, 68, 69, 73
Enterovirus	+	31, 36, 38, 61
Coxsackieviruses B	+	12
Echoviruses 8, 12, 14	+	66
Polioviruses	+	28, 66
Herpes simplex	+	28, 61, 66
Influenza	+++	1, 6, 8, 10–13, 16, 24, 30, 31, 63, 66
A	++	6, 10, 12, 13, 31, 36, 38, 63, 66
B	++	10, 12, 13, 31, 36
C	+	1
Measles	+	16, 26, 55
Mumps	+	66
Parainfluenza	+++	1, 6, 10–13, 16, 30, 28, 29, 31, 34, 36, 44, 61, 63, 66, 69
1	++	10–13, 24, 31, 34
2	++	6, 10–12, 31, 34
3	+++	1, 2, 6, 10-13, 24, 31, 34, 38, 63
4	+	29
Respiratory syncytial	+++	1, 2, 4, 8, 10–13, 16, 24, 30, 28, 31, 35, 36, 38, 40, 47, 58, 61, 62, 64, 66, 69
Human metapneumovirus	+	59
Human bocavirus	+	18, 39, 74, 75
Human coronavirus	+	5, 17, 27
Rhinoviruses	++	10, 12, 15, 16, 30, 28, 31, 36, 38, 54, 60, 61
Bacteria		
Bordetella pertussis	+	26, 48
Bordetella parapertussis	–	
Haemophilus influenzae	+	44, 71
Moraxella catarrhalis	–	21, 32
Streptococcus pneumoniae	–	44
Streptococcus pyogenes	–	44, 53, 61
Other		
Chlamydia psittaci	+	12
Chlamydia pneumoniae	+	33
Mycoplasma pneumoniae	+++	10–13, 16, 24, 31, 36, 43, 56, 70

[a]+++, very common; ++, common; +, rare; –, of questionable etiologic significance.

vomiting. Older children may complain of chest pain resulting from coughing.

On initial physical examination, a variable degree of rhinitis usually is present; many patients have diffuse pharyngeal erythema. As the disease progresses, these upper respiratory tract signs generally decrease. Examination of the chest reveals rhonchi and referred breath sounds. Coarse, changing rales are noted frequently.

In the usual case of acute bronchitis, the illness can be separated into three phases: (1) a 1- to 2-day prodromal period when fever and upper respiratory tract symptoms predominate, (2) a 4- to 6-day period of marked tracheobronchial symptoms with some fever and general discomfort, and (3) a recovery period that may last 1 or 2 weeks and is characterized by cough and expectoration. Occasionally the recovery period is particularly distressing and is associated with a low-grade fever, suggesting secondary bacterial infection. Bronchitis caused by *C. pneumoniae* often is insidious in onset and frequently associated with or preceded by pharyngitis.[33,42] Illness persists for several weeks but responds to appropriate antibiotic therapy.

Laboratory study in acute bronchitis is of limited use. Children in whom throat cultures reveal pathogenic bacteria in predominant growth tend to have more severe illness than do children with only viral infections.[16,49] The white blood cell count usually is greater than 10,000 cells/mm^3, and approximately one-third of the cases have a predominance of neutrophils.[49] The chest radiograph is normal unless associated pulmonary involvement is present.

DIFFERENTIAL DIAGNOSIS AND SPECIFIC DIAGNOSIS

Because acute bronchitis is a clinical entity caused by multiple etiologic agents, the most difficult differential aspect of diagnosis is the selection of the specific infectious cause. Also important is the separation of acute, self-limited bronchitis from chronic, more serious problems, such as cystic fibrosis, allergic respiratory disease, and sinusitis.

An epidemiologic history frequently can help in assigning a particular virus, *M. pneumoniae, C. pneumoniae,* or *B. pertussis,* as the presumptive etiologic agent. If epidemic bronchiolitis is occurring in the community, respiratory syncytial virus would be a likely cause. Similarly, predictions of causation by influenza virus, parainfluenza virus, adenoviruses, *M. pneumoniae, C. pneumoniae,* or *B. pertussis* can be made through clinical epidemiologic observations. Specific etiologic diagnosis can be established through the isolation of an organism or its identification by a direct antigen test or polymerase chain reaction from the nasopharyngeal secretions. Serologic study on paired sera may be useful for the diagnosis of *M. pneumoniae, C. pneumoniae,* and *B. pertussis*. Single-serum IgM studies are useful in the diagnosis of *M. pneumoniae* and *C. pneumoniae*. Single-serum study is also useful in the diagnosis of *B. pertussis* infection, specifically the demonstration of significant immunoglobulin (Ig) G or IgA values to pertussis toxin.

Children with protracted illnesses or febrile exacerbations should be examined by culture, radiograph, and perhaps further imaging studies for secondary bacterial infection of the tracheobronchial tree or the lungs or both. Children with chronic recurrent illnesses should be tested for cystic fibrosis, allergic conditions, and anatomic problems, such as gastroesophageal reflux and tracheoesophageal fistula.

TREATMENT

Treatment of acute bronchitis is distinguished more by what *not* to do than by specific modalities. In most mild cases, no specific therapy is indicated.

For children who feel miserable during the initial phases of acute bronchitis, analgesic therapy may be useful. Formerly aspirin was the recommended analgesic. Because aspirin is an etiologic factor in influenza-associated Reye syndrome and because differentiating influenza viral infections from other respiratory viral infections is difficult, it is prudent to use acetaminophen rather than aspirin. The dose per single administration of acetaminophen by year of age is as follows: younger than 1 year, 60 mg; 1 to 3 years, 60 to 120 mg; 3 to 6 years, 120 mg; 6 to 12 years, 150 to 300 mg; older than 12 years, 325 to 650 mg. Administration may be repeated three or four times daily in young children and every 4 hours in older children. Acetaminophen rarely should be given to infants younger than 6 months of age.

As a result of widespread advertising, a common practice of individuals with acute bronchitis is to use an array of cold remedies that contain various combinations of antihistamines, decongestants, and antitussives. None has been shown to be useful in acute bronchitis, and in certain stages of illness, they may aggravate the recovery process. β2-agonists are frequently used to treat acute bronchitis.[3] However, in a careful review of two trials in children, β2-agonists were not found to be beneficial. Herbal products are also used in acute bronchitis, but no controlled evidence of benefit has been demonstrated.[20,37]

Intake of fluids should be encouraged to prevent overall dehydration and decrease the viscosity of new secretions. Use of mist therapy also may help in thinning the exudate-containing respiratory secretions.[25,52]

In severe cases of acute bronchitis, treatment with specific antiviral agents should be considered. When influenza A virus is the likely etiologic agent, zanamivir or oseltamivir therapy may be beneficial.[9]

As noted in Table 19.1, most cases of acute bronchitis are caused by viruses, so antibiotic therapy would not be indicated.[50,72] In cases in which fever returns or no trend toward recovery is seen by the seventh day of illness, the possibility of a secondary bacterial infection should be considered. The association of sinusitis or a throat culture with predominant growth of a respiratory pathogen (*Streptococcus pneumoniae, Streptococcus pyogenes, Moraxella catarrhalis, H. influenzae*) is an indication for therapy. Infection with *M. pneumoniae* also should be treated, but in contrast to treatment of pneumonia, the therapy usually does not show an impressive response. Bronchitis caused by *C. pneumoniae* should be treated with erythromycin or another macrolide.[33,51]

PROGNOSIS

The prognosis in acute bronchitis usually is excellent. Although the duration of cough can be disturbing to the parent and the child, full recovery is the rule. Several studies suggest that lower respiratory tract illness in the first few years of life may be associated with persistent respiratory symptoms and with abnormalities in lung function in later life.[7,19,45,46] Although none of these studies has followed children with acute bronchitis specifically, the findings in other illnesses (bronchiolitis and croup) indicate a need to observe children with episodes of acute bronchitis carefully as well.

PREVENTION

At present, no practical method of prevention of acute bronchitis in children exists.

NEW REFERENCES SINCE THE SEVENTH EDITION

3. Becker LA, Hom J, Villasis-Keever M, et al. Beta2-agonists for acute bronchitis. *Cochrane Database Syst Rev*. 2011;(7):CD001726.
20. Cwientzek U, Ottillinger B, Arenberger P. Acute bronchitis therapy with ivy leaves extracts in a two-arm study. A double-blind, randomised study vs. an other ivy leaves extract. *Phytomedicine*. 2011;18(13):1105-1109.
22. Darrow LA, Klein M, Flanders WD, et al. Air pollution and acute respiratory infections among children 0–4 years of age: an 18-year time-series study. *Am J Epidemiol*. 2014;180(10):968-977.
37. Kamin W, Ilyenko LI, Malek FA, et al. Treatment of acute bronchitis with EPs 7630: randomized, controlled trial in children and adolescents. *Pediatr Int*. 2012;54(2):219-226.

The full reference list for this chapter is available at ExpertConsult.com.

20 Chronic Bronchitis

Celine Hanson • William T. Shearer

Chronic bronchitis is a serious and costly health problem in adults. The World Health Organization estimates 23.6 million adults have chronic obstructive pulmonary disease, representing more than 15% of the adult population, and many of these cases meet the definition for chronic bronchitis.[20] A diagnosis of chronic bronchitis without chronic obstructive pulmonary disease was present in 3.5% of 10,000 adults in a French study cohort.[13] Morbidity from chronic bronchitis in adults is significant, representing 15% to 18% of all causes for hospitalization for 20- to 44-year-old and 45- to 64-year-old adults respectively.[1] In the adult literature, the accepted definition of chronic bronchitis includes daily excessive production of sputum with manifestation of cough present on most days for 3 months in a year for not less than 2 successive years.[45]

For most pediatricians, the clinical entity of chronic bronchitis is ill defined. Acute pediatric cough lasts less than 2 weeks and typically is associated with respiratory infections.[17] Chronic cough complex in pediatrics lasts 4 weeks in contrast to the 8 to 12 weeks reported in adults. Prolonged acute cough lasting more than 4 weeks is often associated with protracted bacterial bronchitis and can be associated with significant morbidity.[8] Chronic cough complex is often diagnosed as asthma but can also be associated with other more common respiratory or cardiac diseases that must be excluded before a diagnosis of chronic bronchitis is considered.[10] The lack of uniform or standardized definitions of pediatric chronic bronchitis leads to wide discrepancies in reported childhood prevalence (Table 20.1), and a newer definition of cough lasting more than 4 weeks makes prevalence data more divergent. In affected patients, causal relationships and acute exacerbations have been linked to specific host factors (e.g., genetic predisposition) and nonspecific etiologies (e.g., noxious inhaled agents, infectious respiratory pathogens). The pathology of the disease entity varies by etiology. Bronchoscopy

TABLE 20.1 Prevalence of Childhood Bronchitis

Author	Year	Subjects	Prevalence (%)	Acute or Chronic
Bland et al.	1974	Kent schoolchildren	5.5	Acute/chronic
Burrows and Lebowitz	1975	Arizona children	7.1	Chronic
Burrows et al.	1977	Arizona retrospective	46.4	Chronic
Kubo et al.	1978	Japanese children	1.4	Chronic
Peat et al.	1980	Sydney schoolchildren	20.0	Acute/chronic

Modified from Morgan WT, Taussig LM. The chronic bronchitis complex in childhood. *Pediatr Clin. North Am* 1984;31:851–64.

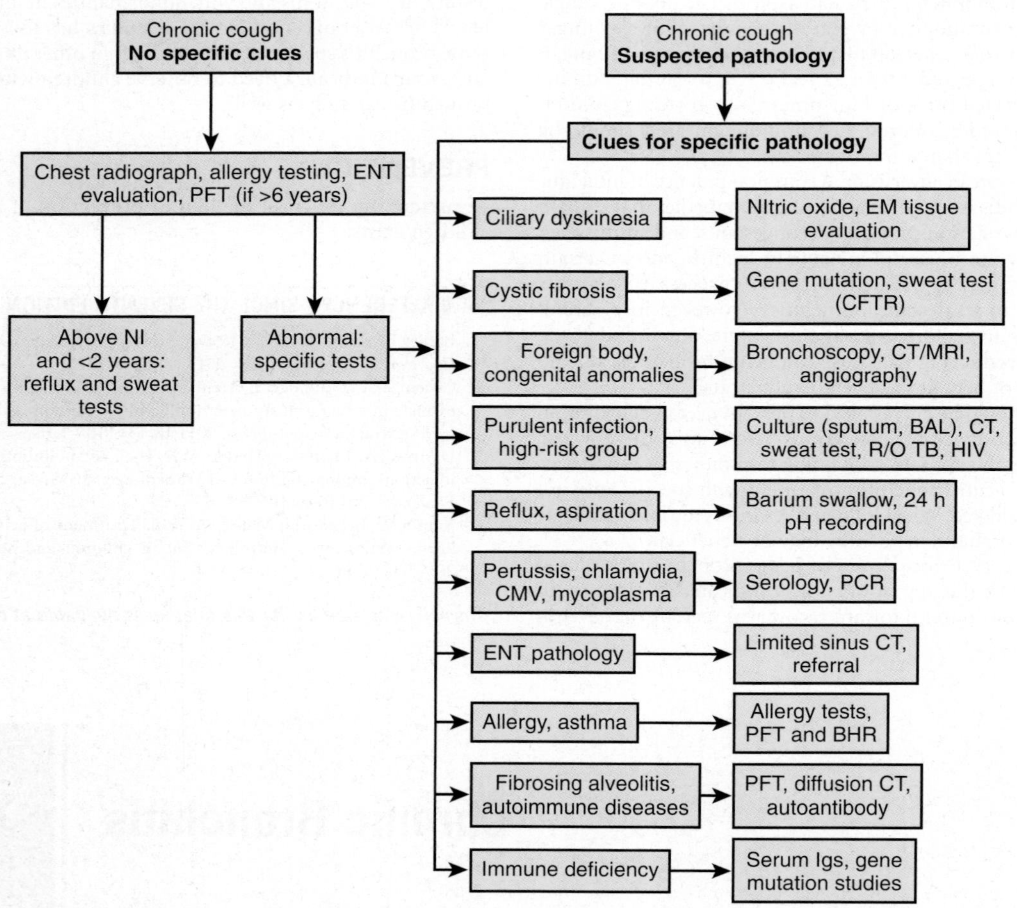

FIG. 20.1 Diagnostic evaluation of children with chronic cough. *BAL,* Bronchoalveolar lavage; *BHR,* bronchial hyperreactivity; *CFTR,* cystic fibrosis transmembrane conductance regulator; *CMV,* cytomegalovirus; *CT,* computed tomography; *EM,* electron microscopy; *ENT,* ear, nose, throat; *HIV,* human immunodeficiency virus; Igs, immunoglobulins; *MRI,* magnetic resonance imaging; *NI,* no information; *PCR,* polymerase chain reaction; *PFT,* pulmonary function test; *R/O,* rule out; *TB,* tuberculosis. (Modified from Morice AJ, Fontana GA, Sovijarvi AR, et al. Diagnoses and management of chronic cough. *Eur Respir J.* 2004;24:487.)

of pediatric patients with chronic bronchitis has revealed findings similar to those noted in children with asthma (granulocyte and mononuclear cell predominance at lavage and biopsy), which reflects the inclusion of asthma in the spectrum of the chronic bronchitis complex.[27,51] In contrast, pulmonary alveolar lavage findings in prolonged bacterial bronchitis is associated with identification of specific infectious pathogens that may in some circumstances be associated with more progressive lung disease like bronchiectasis.[28]

DIFFERENTIAL DIAGNOSIS

Because chronic bronchitis is accepted by most physicians as being a complex of symptoms characterized by persistent cough with or without wheezing, it is imperative that the physician evaluate the patient for diseases that include chronic bronchitis within their spectrum of signs and symptoms. Fig. 20.1 includes disorders that have clinical manifestations of chronic cough for longer than 3 months and provides guidelines for diagnostic evaluation of children with chronic cough.[18] Most of these disorders are accompanied with abnormal chest radiographs, including evidence of bronchiectasis.

Asthma

Heading the differential list is asthma, defined as reversible obstructive airway disease with a significant inflammatory component leading to increased edema and production of mucus. In the United States, asthma prevalence increased between 2001 and 2010 from 7.3% to 8.4%, with the highest reported prevalence of 9.5% in children between 0 and 17 years of age.[2] Asthma can be distinguished from chronic bronchitis by pulmonary function evaluation documenting reversal of airway obstruction after delivery of pulmonary bronchodilators. Recurrent episodes of acute bronchitis often can be interpreted as chronic bronchitis, although the intermittent nature of these episodes and absence of a persistent cough usually distinguish this group of patients clinically.

Acute Infections

Specific viral infections (e.g., rhinovirus, respiratory syncytial virus, human metapneumovirus) in children with or without allergic rhinitis may provoke airway hyperreactivity and late onset of asthma, which may be confused symptomatically with chronic bronchitis.[19,56] Persistent lower respiratory tract infections (i.e., *Chlamydia* spp., pertussis, *Mycoplasma* spp., and *Mycobacterium* spp.) frequently manifest with the complex of symptoms described or chronic wet cough and are evaluated best with chest radiographs in a search for enlarged hilar nodes or interstitial lung infiltrates.[37,58] Respiratory tract secretions for appropriate bacterial and viral culture and serum for determinations of antibacterial antibodies should be obtained. In the case of tuberculosis, a delayed hypersensitivity skin test for *Mycobacterium tuberculosis* antigen should be applied or, in anergic individuals with blunted skin reactivity, interferon-γ release assays can measure immune reactivity of exposed/infected individuals' white blood cells to *M. tuberculosis*. These types of assays, like the delayed hypersensitivity skin test, cannot differentiate past from active disease.[39]

Cystic Fibrosis

Cystic fibrosis is a recessively inherited illness occurring in approximately 1 in 3700 live births, with clinical manifestations of failure to thrive, steatorrhea, nasal polyps, and recurrent lower respiratory tract symptoms. The disorder is associated with mutation of the cystic fibrosis transmembrane conductance regulator *(CFTR)* gene.[42] Cystic fibrosis can be diagnosed by newborn screening, and all 50 U.S. states and the District of Columbia participate in screening but not all utilize the same methodologies. Immunoreactive trypsinogen (IRT) testing is often combined with a DNA test including identifying typical *CFTR* gene variant patterns in DNA extracted from collected blood specimens on Guthrie cards at or after birth or clinically by detecting abnormally elevated chloride levels (>60 mEq/L) as measured by the sweat iontophoresis test.[46] In clinical practice, one or both modalities may be used for establishing the diagnosis, especially for patients with genetic variations of the *CFTR* gene not typical of the classic cystic fibrosis phenotype or for patients with uninterpretable sweat test outcomes.

Ciliary Dyskinesia

Primary ciliary dyskinesia encompasses the immotile cilia disorders and Kartagener syndrome (rhinosinusitis, bronchitis or bronchiectasis, situs inversus) and affects 1 in 16,000 births in the United States.[3] Primary ciliary dyskinesia typically is inherited as an autosomal recessive disorder and is associated with defects in mucociliary transport in the respiratory tree. The symptom complex also has been associated with polycystic kidneys, hepatic disease, and central nervous system symptoms. Screening tests for primary ciliary dyskinesia include nasal nitric oxide and in vivo tests of ciliary motility, but these tests are not universally available, and standardization is problematic.[30] Genetic testing is commercially available and can detect disease-causing mutations in autonomic genes coding for outer dynein arms (present in 60% of affected individuals), radial spoke, and cytoplasm proteins involved in dynein arm assembly.[31]

Primary Immunodeficiency

The primary immune disorders associated most frequently with recurrent sinopulmonary infections include selective immunoglobulin (Ig) A deficiency, functional antibody deficiencies, hypogammaglobulinemia, and ataxia telangiectasia (AT).[29] Selective IgA deficiency is the primary immune disorder encountered most commonly, with an incidence of 1/500. It may be asymptomatic or accompanied by a propensity for atopy and an increase in associated autoimmune disease (most often rheumatoid arthritis and systemic lupus erythematosus). The diagnosis is made readily by evaluation of quantitative serum immunoglobulins defining IgA levels of less than 10 mg/dL. IgA deficiency may be associated with IgG subclass deficiencies (IgG2 deficiency was identified in 85% in a series of >150) with or without clinical symptoms. Children with normal serum Ig levels may have recurrent infections associated with specific functional antibody defects.[11] In particular, the inability to respond serologically to vaccination with polysaccharide antigens such as *Streptococcus pneumoniae* or *Haemophilus influenzae* type B has been reported in association with four separate immune phenotypes: severe (fewer than three protective titers to *S. pneumoniae*), moderate (<70% of *S. pneumoniae* titers protective), and mild (loss of response within 6 months of vaccination).[32] Clinical sinopulmonary disease has been associated with each immune phenotype, but the severe and moderate more often require clinical intervention.

Patients with hypogammaglobulinemia represent a diverse group having primary immune disorders that include but are not limited to X-linked agammaglobulinemia, common variable immune deficiency (CVID), and hyper-IgM syndrome. X-linked agammaglobulinemia typically affects boys who experience recurrent sinopulmonary infections, with onset occurring postnatally as maternal antibody wanes. X-linked agammaglobulinemia is associated with deficiency of a B-cell maturation enzyme, Bruton tyrosine kinase, and is characterized by the absence of circulating mature B lymphocytes. CVID is a disorder of young adults with immune findings of agammaglobulinemia and variable T-cell defects. Clinical classification systems for CVID have been proposed that vary by measure of B lymphocyte immune parameters and/or inclusion of autoimmune disease, but all include infections—specifically lower respiratory tract and sinus disease no matter the infectious etiology. Inherited CVID disorders have been described that include absence of B-cell markers (CD19 or CD20$^+$) in peripheral blood, defects in B-cell activating factor of the tumor necrosis factor family receptor (BAFF), inducible T-cell costimulator gene and transmembrane activator, and calcium-modulator and cyclophilin ligand interactor (TACI), but, except for the latter, they represent a small population of affected individuals with CVID.[33] Patients with TACI variant and CVID may lack circulating mature B lymphocytes. More often, patients with CVID normally express B-cell markers on circulating lymphocytes. Hyper-IgM syndrome is a rare disorder associated with elevated IgM and Ig class switch failure resulting in low IgG and IgA. The disorder can be caused by differing genetic defects with an X-linked form (CD40 ligand gene variant resulting in poor protein production) and autosomal recessive forms (CD40 antigen absence, activation-induced cytidine deaminase variant or uracil DNA glycosylase variant). Independent of genetic inheritance, all forms of hyper-IgM syndrome are associated with recurrent infections including sinopulmonary and hepatic infections.

Patients with AT have depressed serum IgA concentrations and progressive neurologic dysfunction, eventually impacting the swallowing mechanism and leading to recurrent lower respiratory tract infections probably secondary to recurrent aspiration. These patients are identified in childhood by telangiectasias of the skin and conjunctivae in association with aberrant and progressively deteriorating neurologic symptoms and immunodeficiency (depressed IgA and IgE and aberrant T-cell–mediated immunity). Some patients have depressed IgG subclasses (IgG2, IgG4) as well. The gene abnormality in AT has been identified as disruption of the ataxia telangiectasia molecules responsible for detection and implementation of DNA repair dependent on phosphatidylinositol-3-kinase signal transduction pathways.

Primary immune disorders with hypogammaglobulinemia can be diagnosed through evaluation of serum immunoglobulin levels. Further characterization includes assessment of antibody production after vaccine or neoantigen challenge, evaluation of circulating lymphocyte cell surface markers, and in vitro proliferative responses to plant lectins or specific antigens. Evaluation of associated gene variants is important for determining corrective interventions (e.g., transplantation, gene therapy) and genetic counseling. Whole exome sequencing and molecular diagnosis for patients with primary immunodeficiency disease are imperative to predict their morbidity to allow for family counseling for affected individuals or carriers and will likely impact development of therapeutic approaches.[57]

Secondary Immunodeficiency (Including HIV Infection)

Secondary immune disorders (prematurity, pediatric human immunodeficiency virus [HIV] infection, designed medical immunosuppression) also may be associated with significant sinopulmonary infections. Premature infants with attendant severe respiratory distress syndrome requiring positive-pressure ventilation may develop bronchopulmonary dysplasia. Diagnostic criteria include hypoxia requiring oxygen supplementation, characteristic diffuse interstitial markings on chest radiograph, and clinical signs of pulmonary disease (i.e., tachypnea, intercostal retractions). In one series, more than 60% of surviving children with bronchopulmonary dysplasia were documented to have significant pulmonary disease and associated morbidity (i.e., increased hospitalizations).[38] Continued improved care for premature infants and resultant decreased incidence of mortality may increase the population of infants with bronchopulmonary dysplasia.

Pediatric HIV infection has declined and is documented to affect approximately 2% of infants born to HIV-infected mothers in the United States and Europe.[54] This reduced infection rate can be attributed to (1) universal prenatal HIV counseling and testing, (2) availability and use of highly active antiretroviral therapy (HAART) in pregnant women and their newborn infants, (3) practices that minimize exposure to breast milk, and (4) obstetric practices that encourage cesarean delivery or decrease time from membrane rupture to delivery. Continued maternal-to-child infection is associated with maternal lack of knowledge about her HIV status, breastfeeding, and lack of HAART therapy during pregnancy independent of CD4 cell count or HIV RNA levels.[35]

HIV-infected infants report serious lower respiratory tract illness.[24] Lymphoid interstitial pneumonitis/hyperplasia (LIP), reported in 25% of all U.S. children with acquired immunodeficiency syndrome pre-HAART was rare, with a reported incidence rate of less than 0.5 per 100 person-years in children in 2006.[14] However, ongoing studies of HIV-infected youth in sub-Saharan Africa suggest chronic lung disease (LIP, bronchiectasis) is underrepresented and debilitating.[53] With restoration of immunocompetence with antiretroviral therapy (ARV), lower respiratory tract infections (viral, bacterial, fungal) rates in the United States lowered as compared to pre-ARV reports; the incident rate for bacterial pneumonia is 11.1 versus 123.1 (pre-/post-ARV).[14] An unexpected consequence of ARV in affected children may lead to increased risk for developing asthma through an immune reconstitution mechanism.[44]

The diagnosis of HIV infection is established by viral diagnostic assays (nucleic acid tests [NAT]) in infancy when diagnostic sensitivity of the testing is enhanced, preferably during delivery of neonatal ARV prophylaxis and then 2 to 4 weeks after cessation of prophylaxis.[35] Early diagnosis is important so that affected children may start ARV therapy early in their clinical course. HIV antibody testing (enzyme-linked immunosorbent assay and confirmation assays [Western blot analysis, indirect fluorescent antibody assay]) can confirm infection in infants presenting to care under special circumstances after 18 months or older with additional non-perinatal HIV risks. HIV serologic assays in children 18 months of age or younger with perinatal HIV exposure can confuse interpretation of such testing because passively acquired maternal HIV antibodies may persist for up to 24 months in some studies in such infants and delay diagnosis and institution of appropriate care.

Lower respiratory infections with chronic cough can be seen in individuals with autoimmune or inflammatory disorder and cancers or as a result of medical immunosuppression for the same disorders. Solid organ and stem cell transplant with immune suppression is also associated with infectious and inflammatory residual lung disease with chronic cough. Graft-versus-host disease affecting the lungs has been described in immunocompromised patients and particularly following transplantation. The lesion is caused by chronic pulmonary lymphocytic infiltrates and pulmonary fibrosis mimicking the symptom complex of chronic bronchitis and often is indistinguishable radiographically or clinically from infections that characteristically are pathogenic (i.e., *Pneumocystis jiroveci*, *Candida albicans*, *Aspergillus* spp.).

Airway Blockage

Anatomic lesions that lead to pulmonary obstructive airway disease can simulate the complex of chronic bronchitis. An infant with chronic cough, poor feeding habits, and failure to thrive should undergo evaluation for gastroesophageal reflux and tracheoesophageal fistula, which are identified most easily by upper gastrointestinal imaging studies, pH probe and impedance monitoring in older infants and adolescents, and nuclear scan. Mediastinal tumors can produce extrinsic obstruction, leading to recurrent cough and wheezing. Congenital heart disease should be considered in this patient group and can be evaluated with chest radiography, electrocardiography, and echocardiography.

Noxious Agents

Respiratory tract irritants have been implicated as a cause of chronic cough, as documented in adult populations of industrial European nations.[52] An assessment of the public health impact of pollution in Austria, France, and Switzerland concluded that air pollution caused 6% of all mortality, or 40,000 attributable cases per year.[22] Teasing out the impact of urbanization or biomass fuel smoke exposures from other noxious lung factors like smoking can be difficult in population-based studies. A recent study in Peru, a country with overall low prevalence of tobacco smoking, reported a distinct difference in the prevalence of chronic bronchitis in those living daily in urbanized communities as compared to more rural cities (8.3% vs. 1.3%, respectively).[26] In this cohort, individuals with chronic bronchitis had higher prevalence rates (PR) when they reported daily urban living (PR, 3.34) and daily exposure to biomass fuel smoke (PR, 2.0). Nonindustrial, rural communities, such as the forest zone of Nigeria, report virtually no chronic bronchitis, whereas increased risk for development of respiratory disease (i.e., persistent cough, persistent phlegm, asthma) is noted in children residing in six cities in Northern China with the highest ambient air levels of particulate air pollution.[34] After exposure to urban air particulate matter, animal models with induced chronic bronchitis (exposure to 200 ppm of sulfur dioxide for 6 weeks) have shown pathologic changes consistent with exacerbation of chronic bronchitis—changes in ventilatory capacity and marked pulmonary inflammation.[7]

A correlation between tobacco smoking and reduced ventilatory capacity in adults has been reported by many investigators. Peat and associates[38] described teenagers in Sydney, Australia, with recurrent episodes of bronchitis with worsened lung function when coupled with tobacco smoking. A meta-analysis of 21 relevant publications on relationships between exposure to environmental tobacco smoke and lower respiratory tract infection in infancy and early childhood concluded that exposure to environmental smoke resulted in adverse childhood respiratory outcomes (hospitalizations).[23] In a study of approximately 65,000 nonsmoking Canadians 12 years or older, vehicular environmental tobacco smoke was associated with chronic bronchitis for children between 12 and 19 with odds ratios of 2.3 and 2.25 for children and older teens, respectively.[12] Tashkin and colleagues[50] further found in 300 individuals followed for 10 years that both tobacco and marijuana smoking appeared to be causally associated with the development of chronic bronchitis. These data suggest that it is not only imperative to prevent smoking in individual youth to prevent respiratory disease but also to gather a smoking history (tobacco and drugs) for household members and apprise them of the impact of their smoking on their children. Newer popular practices of e-cigarette (e-cig devices or e-liquid [nicotine in a glycerol/propylene glycol vehicle with flavorings]) use or vaping cannabis may diminish individual particulate lung exposure, but data addressing whether these practices diminish lung damage have not yet been published in large population-based studies over significant exposure intervals.[43,49] These devices clearly do not reduce nicotine or cannabis exposure to the end user.

Other noxious agents associated with outdoor pollution have been associated with poor control of chronic cough complex diseases such as asthma. In Los Angeles, adults with asthma were more poorly controlled if they resided near areas of heavy traffic.[25] Similar findings of poorly controlled lung disease associated with traffic pollution have been documented in adult and pediatric patients in Lima, Peru.[4] Occupational exposures long have been cited for exacerbating pulmonary diseases and may be responsible for about 15% of chronic bronchitis and chronic obstructive pulmonary disease. Classic examples of occupational exposures leading to increased risk for developing chronic cough are described in coal dust for miners in Great Britain and recently in smoking and welding fumes in Northern European welders.[15,59]

EPIDEMIOLOGY AND ETIOLOGY

Differentiating the impact of clinical, social, and environmental factors on lower respiratory tract disease, including chronic bronchitis, has been problematic and has led to conflicting outcomes in epidemiologic assessments.[9,48] In addition, the lack of a standardized definition of chronic bronchitis in the pediatric literature leads to confusing interpretation of data when attempting to appreciate the prevalence or etiology of the disease complex. In Table 20.1, the data from Kubo and associates[21] separate acute recurrent bronchitis, asthmatic bronchitis, and chronic bronchitis, leading to a decrease in the prevalence from a proposed 46.4% (in the Arizona questionnaire) to 1.4%.

Considerable overlap also exists in evaluating etiologic agents for chronic bronchitis. The same viral agents proposed as the exacerbating factors of asthmatic bronchitis are implicated in exacerbations of chronic bronchitis[16] including rhinoviruses, parainfluenza viruses, respiratory syncytial virus, influenza A and B viruses, adenoviruses, and enteroviruses. Persistent adenovirus infection has been implicated as a cause of childhood chronic bronchitis. In a study of 11 children with chronic bronchitis, transbronchial biopsy specimens revealed no evidence of persistent adenovirus infection (culture or polymerase chain reaction),[40] suggesting that viral infections may precipitate cough, but their roles in the pathologic findings associated with chronic bronchitis should be questioned.

Table 20.2 lists predominant bacterial pathogens isolated from sputum for a group of 40 pediatric patients with chronic bronchitis and exacerbations of cough and fever; these pathogens include *H. influenzae, S. pneumoniae,* and *Staphylococcus aureus*.[21] These bacteria also are implicated as etiologic agents in the triggering of asthmatic bronchitis. Neither *Mycoplasma* nor human metapneumovirus was included in this listing, but this simply may reflect the time frame (late 1970s) when the Kubo study was conducted.[36,55] Bacterial isolates in 50 children with protracted bacterial bronchitis following flexible bronchoscopy with bronchoalveolar lavage (BAL) also included these same bacterial pathogens, but *Moraxella catarrhalis* was a not uncommon pathogen noted in 14 of 41 cases.[28] Treatment of exacerbations of chronic bronchitis with antibiotic therapy usually is effective in reducing the volume of sputum and purulence during the acute infection but shows no parallel elimination of the cultured microorganisms. Careful monitoring of affected patients is recommended because it has been suggested that prolonged bacterial wet cough and bronchiectasis may represent a continuum of the same disease process.[6]

TABLE 20.2 Predominant Pathogens in Washed Sputum of Chronic Bronchitis (40 Cases)

Pathogen	No. Cases
Haemophilus influenzae and *Streptococcus pneumoniae*	21 (52.5%)
H. influenzae	17 (42.5%)
Staphylococcus aureus	2 (5%)
Superinfection with gram-negative rods	
Pseudomonas aeruginosa	4
Klebsiella pneumoniae	2
Escherichia coli	1
Enterobacter cloacae	1

From Kubo S, Funabashi S, Uehara S, et al. Clinical aspects of "asthmatic bronchitis" and chronic bronchitis in infants and children. *J Asthma Res.* 1978;15:99–132.

TREATMENT

When a specific diagnosis is found in association with chronic cough or wheezing, therapy is directed toward the primary disease entity and the clinical presentation of cough. Bronchodilators (β-adrenergic agents), antiinflammatory agents (corticosteroids), and anticholinergic agents are used, when appropriate, for the treatment of chronic cough associated with asthma or acute exacerbations of chronic obstructive pulmonary disease.[47] Appropriate positioning techniques (prone 30 degrees), feeding schedules, and medications (e.g., gastrointestinal motility enhancers, proton pump inhibitors, or cholinergics) are indicated in the approach to infants with gastroesophageal reflux. Patients with hypogammaglobulinemia can be helped with supplemental intravenous immunoglobulin preparations currently available commercially (400 to 600 mg/kg per dose every 3 to 4 weeks) in an attempt to decrease the incidence of infections.

It is imperative that patients with chronic pulmonary diseases such as cystic fibrosis, asthma, or ciliary dyskinesias understand the pulmonary irritant effect of tobacco smoking, dust exposure, and air pollution. A change in habit or occupation may be essential for their well-being. It also is imperative to stress the irritant effect of parental smoking on the already compromised pulmonary function of the child.

Management of chronic cough in children 14 years of age or younger is outlined in Fig. 20.2. In the evidence-based guidelines for chronic cough, normal chest radiography and, as developmentally appropriate, normal spirometry suggest a "watch, wait, and review" approach to clinical management. Cough will spontaneously resolve for many children with normal chest radiographic examinations. The use of cough suppressants or over-the-counter cough medicine is discouraged, especially in very young infants who may experience significant drug-associated morbidity. Persistent cough should be reassessed clinically. For children with persistent cough (>4 weeks) without specific cough pointers, early intervention with a cough algorithm conducted at 2 weeks after physician evaluation (conducted in a multicenter randomized controlled study in 272 children [mean age 4.5 years]) resulted in a statistically significant improvement of cough resolution by 6 weeks.[5]

When considered, antibiotic therapy for chronic bronchitis usually consists of amoxicillin 45 to 90 mg/kg every 24 hours, erythromycin 40 mg/kg every 24 hours, or, in adolescents and adults, tetracycline 25 to 50 mg/kg every 24 hours or quinolones for 5 to 10 days.[45] Methylxanthine therapy is used less frequently in chronic bronchitis care. When it is used, certain antibiotics, such as erythromycin, lead to elevated serum concentrations of theophylline, which renders toxicity more likely to occur. Treatment with mucolytic agents in chronic pulmonary disease has not proved to have a significant impact except in adults with already advanced disease with multiple hospitalizations, and no evidence suggests that they are beneficial in children.[41]

As with patients with obstructive lung disease, attention must focus on careful and sequential monitoring of pulmonary function. The prognosis for chronic bronchitis varies and depends on the specific etiology of this syndrome.

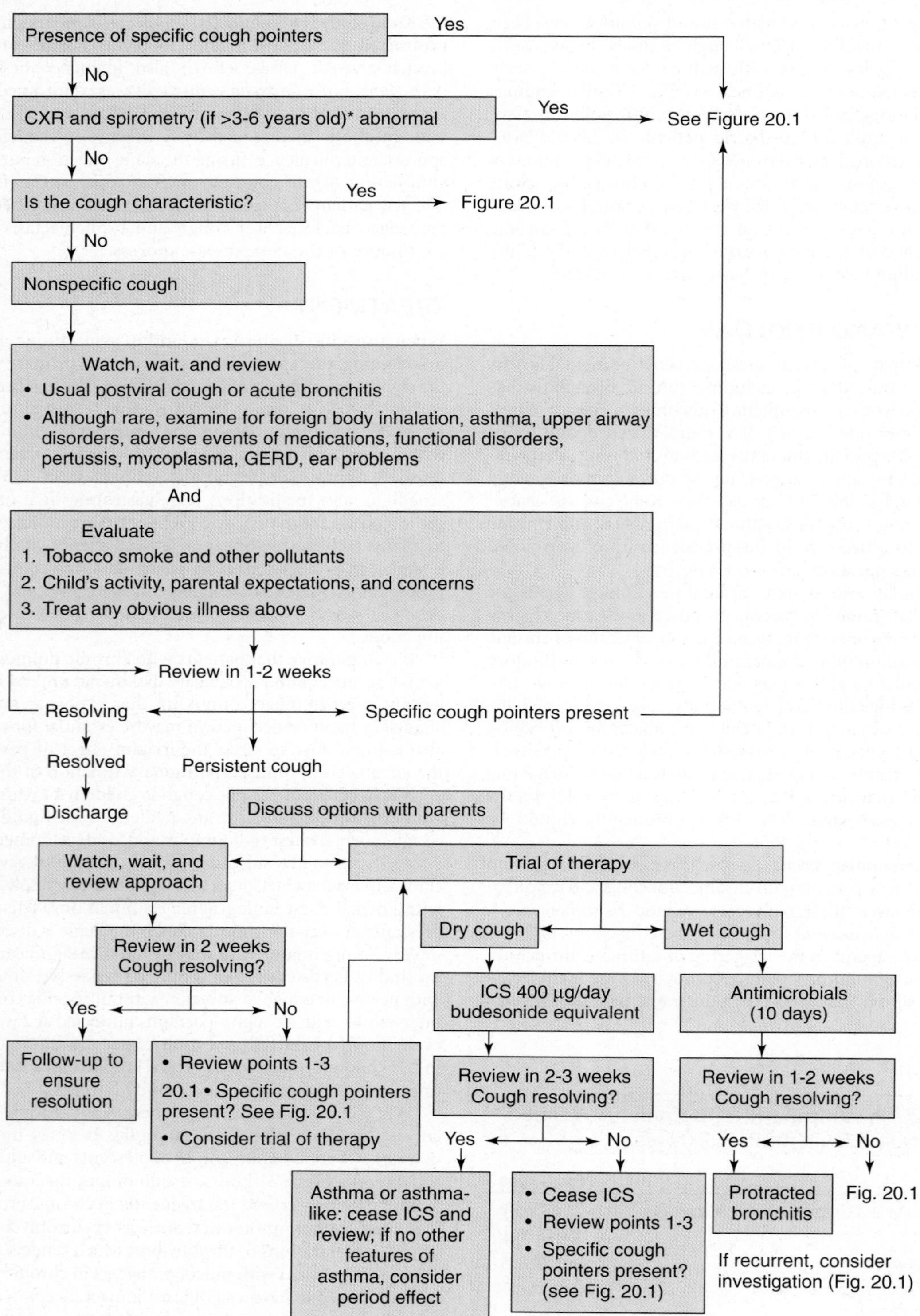

FIG. 20.2 Approach to a child <15 years with chronic cough. *CXR,* Chest radiograph; *GERD,* gastroesophageal reflux disease; *ICS,* inhaled corticosteroids. (Modified from Irwin RS, Baumann MH, Blaser DC, et al. Diagnosis and management of cough executive summary: ACCP evidence-based clinical practice guidelines. *Chest.* 2006;129:15–23S.)

NEW REFERENCES SINCE THE SEVENTH EDITION

1. Accordini S, Corsico AG, Calciano L, et al. The impact of asthma, chronic bronchitis and allergic rhinitis on all-cause hospitalizations and limitations in daily activities: a population-based observational study. *BMC Pulm Med.* 2015;15:10-19.
2. Akinbami LJ, Moorman JE, Bailey C, et al. Trends in asthma prevalence, health care use and mortality in the United States, 2001–2010. *NCHS Data Brief.* 2012;94:1-10.
5. Chang AB, Robertson OF, Van Asperen PP, et al. A cough algorithm for chronic cough in children: a multicenter, randomized controlled study. *Pediatrics.* 2013;131:e1576-e1583.
6. Chang AB, Upham JW, Masters IB, et al. Protracted bacterial bronchitis: the last decade and the road ahead. *Pediatr Pulmonol.* 2015;51:225-242.
8. Craven V, Everard ML. Protracted bacterial bronchitis: reinventing an old disease. *Arch Dis Child.* 2013;98:72-76.
13. Ferre A, Furhman C, Zureik M, et al. Chronic bronchitis in the general population; influence age, gender and socio-economic conditions. *Respir Med.* 2012;106: 467-471.
14. Gona P, Van Dyke RB, Williams PL. et a. Incidence of opportunistic and other infections in HIV-infected children in the HAART era. *JAMA.* 2006;296: 292-300.
17. Ioan I, Poussel M, Coutier L, et al. What is chronic cough in children? *Front Physiol.* 2014;5:1-7.
24. Mazurek GH, Jereb J, Vernon A, Centers for Disease Control and Prevention, et al. Updated guidelines for using interferon gamma release assays to detect mycobacterium tuberculosis infection, United States. *MMWR Recomm Rep.* 2010;59(RR-5):1-25.
26. Miele CH, Jaganath D, Miranda JJ, et al. Urbanization and daily exposure to biomass fuel smoke both contribute to chronic bronchitis risk in a population with low prevalence of daily tobacco smoking. *COPD.* 2015;9:1-10.
28. Narang R, Bakewell K, Peach J, et al. Bacterial distribution in the lungs of children with protracted bacterial bronchitis. *PLoS ONE.* 2014;9:1-3.
33. Orange JS, Glessner JT, Resnick E, et al. Genome-wide association identifies diverse causes of common variable immunodeficiency. *J Allergy Clin Immunol.* 2011;127:1360-1367.
32. Orange JS, Ballow M, Steihm ER, et al. Use and interpretation of diagnostic vaccination in primary immunodeficiency: a working group report of the Basic and Clinical Immunology Interest Section of the American Academy of Allergy, Asthma & Immunology. *J Allergy Clin Immunol.* 2012;130:21-24.
35. Panel on Antiretroviral Therapy and Medical Management of HIV-Infected Children. *Guidelines for the use of antiretroviral agents in pediatric HIV infection, August 6, 2015.* Available at: http://aidsinfo.nih.gov/contentfiles/lvguidelines/PediatricGuidelines.pdf. Accessed 1 February 2016.
43. Rowell TR, Tarran R. Will chronic e-cigarette use cause lung disease? *Am J Physiol Lung Cell Mol Physiol.* 2015;309:L1398-L1409.
44. Siberry GK, Leister E, Jacobson DL, et al. Increased risk of asthma and atopic dermatitis in perinatally HIV-infected children and adolescents. *Clin Immunol.* 2012;142:201-208.
50. Tashkin DP, Simmons MS, Tseng CH. Impact of changes in regular use of marijuana and/or tobacco on chronic bronchitis. *COPD.* 2012;9:367-374.
49. Tashkin DP. How beneficial is vaping cannabis to respiratory health compared to smoking? *Addiction.* 2015;110:1706-1707.
53. Weber HC, Gie RP, Cotton MF. The challenge of chronic lung disease in HIV-infected children and adolescents. *AIDS.* 2013;16:18633.
57. Yang Y, Muzny DM, Reid JG, et al. Clinical whole-exome sequencing for the diagnosis of Mendelian disorders. *N Engl J Med.* 2013;369:1502-1511.
58. Zgherea D, Pagala S, Mediratta M, et al. Bronchoscopic findings in children with chronic wet cough. *Pediatrics.* 2012;129:e364-e369.

The full reference list for this chapter is available at ExpertConsult.com.

21 Bronchiolitis and Infectious Asthma

Robert C. Welliver Sr

Bronchiolitis and infectious asthma, which also is called *asthmatic bronchitis, wheezy bronchitis,* or *virus-induced asthma,* are common illnesses of children, characterized by symptoms of upper respiratory tract infection and signs of obstructive airway disease, particularly wheezing. Bronchiolitis and infectious asthma often are considered to be distinct entities, and not all infants who develop bronchiolitis have infectious asthma in later life. Although the two illnesses are similar in terms of clinical presentation and have some mediators in common, the pathologic findings may contrast in most cases. Differences in terms of etiologic agents that precipitate episodes of illness or in terms of response to therapy are more a function of the patient's age (particularly older or younger than age 3 years) than of any underlying disease process. *Infectious asthma* is considered a term that defines the occurrence of repeated episodes of bronchiolitis.

DEFINITIONS

Bronchiolitis is an acute communicable disease predominantly manifesting in infancy and characterized by cough, coryza, fever, grunting, tachypnea, retractions, inspiratory crackles, expiratory wheezing, and air trapping. The first (and the most severe) episodes occur most frequently in infants aged 2 to 6 months. *Infectious asthma* is a term that generally refers to infection-induced wheezing occurring beyond infancy. Nonetheless, a patient may experience bronchiolitis during the first months of life and a recurrent episode caused by the same virus in the second year, suggesting an identical underlying nature of the two illnesses. Certain viruses (e.g., respiratory syncytial virus [RSV] and influenza viruses) seem capable of causing bronchiolitis in all children; in contrast, other agents (rhinovirus in particular) seem to induce wheezing primarily in atopic children.

HISTORY

Although all practicing pediatricians today are familiar with the term *bronchiolitis* and associate it with an acute clinical illness with the signs and symptoms of airway obstruction, it has been recognized in the medical literature for only a relatively brief period. Acute bronchiolitis finally was listed as a heading in the sixth edition of the *Textbook of Pediatrics,*[136] published in 1954; even at that time, bronchiolitis was associated with interstitial pneumonitis.

In contrast to the delayed textbook recognition of bronchiolitis, good clinical descriptions were presented in journals. In 1941, Hubble and Osborn[82] published "Acute Bronchiolitis in Children," in which they described an epidemic of bronchiolitis involving 50 hospitalized children. Pratt,[152] in 1944, and Nelson and Smith,[137] in 1945, published excellent clinical articles. Studies in the late 1950s and early 1960s established the etiologic association of RSV and other viruses with acute bronchiolitis.[9,28,29,167]

ETIOLOGIC AGENTS

RSV is the major cause of bronchiolitis in infancy and virtually the only important etiologic consideration when major epidemics are occurring. Other agents cause smaller annual outbreaks. The frequency of infectious agents in the overall cause of bronchiolitis is shown in Table 21.1. These data were compiled from 12 reports in which respiratory illness in children was observed over an extended period, and in most instances numerous clinical illness categories were being studied. During major epidemics in the colder months in temperate climates, virologic and serologic studies indicate RSV as the cause in 80% or more of the cases, especially in the more severe ones. In nonepidemic situations, more than 50% of the isolates or instances of serologic evidence of infection are infectious agents other than RSV. Human metapneumovirus becomes a prominent cause of bronchiolitis as the RSV season ends. In nonepidemic situations, more than 50% of the isolates or instances of serologic evidence of infection are infectious agents other than RSV, including parainfluenza viruses, and rhinovirus.

Children surviving infantile bronchiolitis often have recurrent episodes of wheezing that, on clinical grounds, seem to be precipitated by upper respiratory tract infections. Studies designed to determine the infectious agents responsible for these repeated wheezing episodes have yielded variable results, presumably because they involve patients of different ages observed during different seasons of the year.[13,108,127–130]

A comprehensive study based on more than a decade of observation of children from birth through 15 years of age revealed that viruses and *Mycoplasma pneumoniae* are the most common etiologic agents (Table 21.2).[133] RSV is the most common cause of recurrent, wheezing-associated respiratory illness occurring in young children, including children who previously experienced bronchiolitis, which strongly suggests the identical nature of infection-related wheezing episodes occurring in children of different ages. With increasing patient age, rhinoviruses and *M. pneumoniae* account for most infection-induced wheezing episodes. The parainfluenza viruses, metapneumoviruses, and influenza viruses are important causes of such wheezing episodes throughout childhood, whereas coronaviruses and adenoviruses are less common causes in infancy. Human bocaviruses are more recently identified causes of bronchiolitis, and their relative importance as etiologic agents is being determined. RSV remains an important cause of wheezing in adolescents and can cause airway obstruction in middle-aged and elderly individuals.[50,133]

The role of bacteria as primary agents, synergistically active participants, or secondary invaders in bronchiolitis has interested investigators for many years. No evidence has been found of a primary role for bacteria alone in bronchiolitis of infants.[9,107] The data on synergistic viral-bacterial infections also are unconvincing. Wood and colleagues[213] in 1954 and Sell[172] in 1960 reported results of studies in which bacteriologic and serologic evidence tended to associate *Haemophilus influenzae* infections with bronchiolitis. Some of the children from these studies later were shown serologically to have had RSV infection.[33] Later studies showed evidence of mixed viral-bacterial infections in bronchiolitis[111,134] and other lower respiratory tract illnesses.[139]

These serologically defined mixed infections were found no more commonly among patients with bronchiolitis than among patients with mild upper respiratory tract disease, whereas RSV was recovered 10 times as often from patients with lower respiratory tract disease as from patients with upper respiratory tract disease alone.[111] Although debate continues about whether the isolation of *H. influenzae* from the airway of infants with bronchiolitis represents secondary infection, most data indicate that a significant role for mixed viral-bacterial infection in bronchiolitis of infancy is unlikely to exist. Bacterial superinfection is an uncommon occurrence in bronchiolitis (at least in developed countries). Generally after a diagnosis of RSV or parainfluenza virus infection has been established, antibiotic courses started empirically can be safely stopped. Nevertheless while bacterial superinfection is an uncommon occurrence in bronchiolitis in developed countries, there is evidence that bacterial superinfection of RSV bronchiolitis occurs in developing countries. Initiation of pneumococcal vaccination programs has led to reduced rates of hospitalization for RSV (and influenza) infections, suggesting that superinfection with pneumococci led to more severe forms of RSV infection.[113]

The association of asthma and infectious illnesses was appreciated throughout the 20th century. Initial reports tended to relate bacterial agents to wheezing; in 1909, Carmalt-Jones[24] reported improvement of patients with asthma in association with injections of a bacterial vaccine. Throughout the first half of the 20th century, "bacterial allergy" was the main consideration in infection-related wheezing, and controversy raged about the therapeutic merits of bacterial vaccines. Despite widespread use of bacterial vaccines in the treatment of infectious asthma, no evidence exists that bacterial organisms of the normal flora precipitate asthmatic attacks.[72,81,132] More recent, large retrospective reviews have shown the rarity with which bacterial infection complicates bronchiolitis, even in severe cases.[154,158] Generally after a diagnosis of

TABLE 21.1 Infectious Agents Associated With Acute Bronchiolitis

Infectious Agent	Relative Frequency (%)
Respiratory syncytial virus	50
Parainfluenza viruses	25
Type 1	8
Type 2	2
Type 3	15
Adenoviruses	5
Mycoplasma pneumoniae	5
Rhinoviruses	5–15
Influenza viruses	5
Type A	3
Type B	2
Metapneumovirus	5–10
Enteroviruses	2
Herpes simplex virus	2
Coronavirus virus	<1

TABLE 21.2 Principal Agents Recovered From Children of Different Ages With Wheezing Precipitated by Infection

	FREQUENCY OF ISOLATION OF EACH AGE GROUP[b]			
Agent[a]	0–2 y	2–5 y	5–9 y	9–15 y
Respiratory syncytial virus	++++	+++	++	++
Adenovirus	++	++	+	0
Parainfluenza viruses	++	++	++	++
Rhinoviruses	+	++ to +++	++ to +++	+++
Metapneumovirus	++	+	+	0
Mycoplasma pneumoniae	+	++	+++	++++

Data from references 10, 48, 54, 59, 81, 83, 86, 107, 111, 119, 129, 142.

[a]Other agents that more rarely precipitate wheezing include enteroviruses, herpes simplex virus, cytomegalovirus, coronaviruses, influenza viruses, mumps virus, varicella zoster virus, *Bordetella pertussis*, and *Coxiella burnetii*.

[b]++++, very common; +++, common; ++, occasional; +, uncommon; 0, unknown.

RSV, metapneumovirus, rhinovirus, or parainfluenza virus infection has been established, antibiotic courses started empirically can be safely stopped.

EPIDEMIOLOGY

Bronchiolitis predominantly is a disease of infancy, although an identical disease occurring in older children arbitrarily may be referred to as another diagnostic entity. In a study involving 1148 children, the peak age of incidence was 2 to 6 months, with more than 80% of the cases occurring during the first year of life.[147] In a small study of families in or near Houston, Texas, rates of RSV infection were 68.8 per 100 children in the first year of life and 82.6 per 100 children in the second year, including many reinfections; larger studies have not been completed. Lower respiratory tract illness was caused by RSV in 22.4 of 100 children in the first year of life. Of all RSV infections occurring in children younger than 12 months of age, one-third were accompanied by lower respiratory tract illness. Although the attack rate of RSV decreased with age, the frequency with which lower respiratory tract disease occurred among individuals infected remained constant (Table 21.3), at least until they reached 4 years of age.[60,61] In Tucson, Arizona, a study of 1179 children enrolled in a health maintenance organization found that the rate of lower respiratory tract illness in the first year of life was 32.9 episodes per 100 children; 60% of these episodes were diagnosed as bronchiolitis.[216]

A study of the Tennessee Medicaid population found that the frequency of hospitalization for bronchiolitis was 4.4 and 1.5 per 100 child-years of observation for infants infected in the first and second 6 months of life, respectively.[17] Approximately 123,000 infants younger than 1 year of age are hospitalized annually with bronchiolitis, with RSV infection accounting for 51,000 to 82,000 of these hospitalizations. Including cases diagnosed as pneumonia, RSV infection results in 70,000 to 120,000 hospitalizations.[70,174]

The yearly incidence of hospitalization for bronchiolitis increased from 12.9 per 1000 infants in 1980 to 31.2 per 1000 in 1996, suggesting an increased severity of illness developing during this interval.[174] More frequent hospitalization may also be a result of an increased use of pulse oximetry to determine the need for hospitalization.[115] In concert with this, a subsequent study showed that the rate of RSV hospitalizations was stable from 1997 to 2006, at a rate of 132,000 to 172,000 hospitalizations annually in children younger than 5 years old in the United States.[185] More recently, however, the rate of hospitalization for RSV infection has plateaued, but the severity of illness among hospitalized cases seems to have increased.[73] This suggests that hospitalization is being progressively avoided among infants with milder forms of illness.

Epidemic bronchiolitis caused by RSV is markedly seasonal in temperate climates, with peak activity occurring from January to April (Northern Hemisphere) annually and with virtually no activity seen from August to October.[220] Sporadic bronchiolitis cases caused by other agents are seen throughout the year. Regional differences can be striking. In Miami and Puerto Rico, RSV activity occurs year round, with a peak of activity from July to October.[123,188] Epidemics usually begin in October in other southern states, although still earlier than in the Northeast. Farther north (Winnipeg, Canada, and Alaska), the duration of the RSV season again becomes longer, and cases occur essentially year round. Near the equator, temperature and humidity are positively associated with the number of bronchiolitis cases. In contrast, farther from the equator (in either direction), temperature and humidity are inversely associated with bronchiolitis cases. Ultraviolet radiation is negatively associated with bronchiolitis in several regions.[220] In contrast to yearly epidemics of RSV infection in the United States and United Kingdom, with identical peak months of occurrence each year, RSV occurs in biennial epidemic cycles in Croatia,[131] Switzerland,[44] Sweden,[162] Finland,[202] and Germany,[192] with peaks alternating between December and January in 1 year and March and April in alternate years. No explanation has been established for the biennial occurrence of these epidemics.

Bronchiolitis occurs more frequently in boys; the male-to-female ratio is approximately 1.5 : 1.[54] Crowding may be a major determinant of hospitalization rates for lower respiratory tract illness caused by RSV, with the incidence of hospitalization for infants 1 to 3 months old residing in rural, urban, and heavily industrialized areas of Great Britain being 1 in 80, 1 in 60, and 1 in 40, respectively. The figures for all children younger than 5 years of age were 1 in 714, 1 in 588, and 1 in 227, respectively.[161] Studies from Tucson, Arizona, indicate that many socioeconomic factors, including absence of breastfeeding, low level of maternal education, and exposure to cigarette smoke, are associated with an increased risk for developing lower respiratory tract infection at the time of infection with RSV. The greatest risk was conferred by sharing sleeping quarters with two or more individuals.[216]

TABLE 21.3 Attack Rates of Respiratory Syncytial Virus

Age in Months (n)	Infections per 100 Child-Years	LRTI per 100 Child-Years	LRTI per 100 Infections
0–12 (125)	68.8	22.4	32.6
13–24 (92)	82.6	13	15.8
25–36 (65)	46.2	10.8	23.3
37–48 (39)	33.3	7.7	23.1

Data from Glezen WP, Taber LH, Frank AL, Kasel JA. Risk of primary infection and reinfection with respiratory syncytial virus. *Am J Dis Child.* 1986;140:543–6.
LRTI, Lower respiratory tract infection.

CLINICAL PRESENTATION

Acute bronchiolitis occurs most commonly in infants 1 to 12 months of age. In most instances, the patient's history reveals exposure to an adult or older child with a common cold or other trivial respiratory tract infection. Occasionally, as in the daycare setting, the child is exposed to other children with more marked respiratory illness. After exposure, the incubation period is 5 to 7 days. The initial signs include copious nasal discharge (often serous in the early stage), cough, irritability, poor feeding, and vomiting in some cases. Slightly more than 50% of infants have fever, with rectal temperatures ranging from normal to 40.6°C (105.4°F) (mean, 39°C [102°F]).[160] Nasal congestion with tenacious secretions and progressive cough and dyspnea dominate the clinical picture.

Symptoms of upper respiratory tract infection persist for a few days, and the onset of lower respiratory tract infection usually is precipitous, with the time of the onset of wheezing often being recognizable from the caretaker's description of the illness. The maximum severity of illness generally is attained within 24 to 36 hours of the first signs of lower respiratory tract illness, and fewer than 2% of hospitalized infants deteriorate clinically enough to require transfer to intensive care units.[18] Apnea may occur and may be sufficiently severe to require mechanical ventilation.[19]

At the time of hospital admission, all patients have cough and evidence of respiratory distress. The pulse is rapid, and the respiratory rate usually is 40 to 80 breaths per minute. The breathing is labored, with flaring of the alae nasae; grunting; abdominal breathing; and supraclavicular, subcostal, and intercostal retractions. The degree of retraction of the lower chest wall may be an accurate indicator of the severity of the illness. Wheezing is best heard by auscultation over the upper anterior chest but often is audible without the use of a stethoscope (particularly prominent over the upper, anterior chest), and the chest is often hyperinflated. Hyperresonance may be detected on percussion, and auscultation generally reveals harsh rhonchi, high-pitched or low-pitched expiratory wheezes, or fine inspiratory crackles. Occasionally wheezing is not audible despite other evidence of airway obstruction, due to low airflows. A prolonged expiratory phase of breathing may occur, suggesting the presence of a more severe degree of illness. Cyanosis also occurs in severe cases.[2]

Other findings include a mild conjunctivitis in one-third of cases, pharyngitis of varied severity in approximately half of affected infants, and otitis media in 5% to 15% of cases. The abdomen frequently appears distended, and the liver and spleen may be palpable; the organs are not enlarged but are pushed down because of hyperexpansion of the lung.[2,144]

The duration of the hospital course of bronchiolitis varies. Significant improvement occurred in half of the cases within 2 days in one large study.[2] In the same study, approximately one-third of the cases had a gradual course without evidence of clear-cut improvement at any one time; 71% of the patients were afebrile by the third hospital day. In another study done more than 25 years later,[62] the average duration of hospitalization was 3.4 days. Longer stays were required for infants with initial oxygen saturations of less than 90% and infants younger than 6 weeks at the onset of illness. Reasonable criteria for admission in otherwise healthy infants seem to include hypoxia (i.e., oxygen saturation of <90% to 92%), age younger than 6 weeks, and a degree of respiratory distress sufficient to reduce fluid intake to inadequate levels. Other criteria include apnea, immunodeficiency, premature birth, and the presence of significant underlying heart or lung disease. Most patients can be discharged from the hospital within 2 to 3 days after admission, although mild wheezing still may be present for several days or even weeks thereafter.[14]

In 121 hospitalized patients, the total white blood cell count was less than 12,500/mm^3 in 74% and in 15 determinations had more than 60% neutrophils.[2] In another study, a mean leukocyte count of 16,000/mm^3 was determined for children with lower respiratory tract disease, including bronchiolitis, as was an increased percentage of band form neutrophils compared with that of a control group.[160] As in most infections, eosinophil counts in peripheral blood are reduced at the time of acute RSV infection.[56] Nonetheless, some patients maintain detectable eosinophilia in peripheral blood; these infants may be more likely to develop childhood asthma.[45]

Although impaired oxygenation is usually present in infants with respiratory distress, cyanosis may not be evident, even in the presence of markedly reduced oxygenation.[36,176] The respiratory rate is related inversely to the degree of oxygenation except when respiratory failure is imminent. In mild to moderate cases, carbon dioxide retention does not occur because the alveoli that are functioning can compensate for alveoli that are not ventilated. In severe disease, the blood pH is low and the $PaCO_2$ is elevated.[36,176] The technique of pulse oximetry has obviated the need for arterial blood gas sampling except perhaps in severe cases in which hypercarbia is a concern.

In certain patients, clinical findings (e.g., degree of chest wall retractions, wheezing) often are out of proportion to the degree of hypoxia as measured by pulse oximetry.[134,201] Infants with marked dyspnea must be evaluated carefully because respiratory failure may occur precipitously, despite their reassuring oximetry readings. Once infants are hospitalized and stabilized, subsequent deterioration to the point of requiring intensive care is unusual, occurring in less than 2% of cases. Respiratory rates of 63 breaths per minute and oxygen saturations less than or equal to 88% on admission were weakly associated with such eventual deterioration in one study.[18]

The radiographic appearance of the chest in bronchiolitis varies considerably.[98] Anteroposterior radiographs may be normal in mild cases or may reveal hyperinflation in the absence of hypoxia. In moderate to severe illness, radiographs often appear exceptionally clear because of hyperinflation. The diaphragms often are flattened or depressed. The costophrenic angle is less acute, and the hilar vascular shadows are stretched. Frequently areas of atelectasis may give the appearance of pneumonitis, although true consolidation is a rare occurrence. The heart usually appears small. On the lateral radiograph, the diaphragm is depressed markedly, and reversal of the normal convexity frequently may be seen. The anteroposterior diameter of the chest is increased.

With recurrent wheezing episodes, the prodrome may be considerably shorter in duration with little or no fever and minimal coryza. In these children, differentiation of infection-induced wheezing from more conventional asthma becomes essentially impossible clinically.[210]

PATHOPHYSIOLOGY

The pathophysiology of bronchiolitis deservedly has been the focus of numerous investigations. Several original theories can be discounted, whereas others warrant further study. Pathologic examinations of the lung in bronchiolitis or human airways in organ culture[76] reveal necrosis of the respiratory epithelium with destruction of the ciliated layer; mononuclear cell invasion of the peribronchial tissues and alveolar interstitium; edema of the submucosa and adventitia; and obstruction of small airways with dense plugs consisting of dying epithelial cells, fibrin, and inflammatory cells. In contrast to asthma, mucin (periodic acid–Schiff–positive material) usually is absent in fatal bronchiolitis.[204] An associated interstitial pneumonitis often is present, and patchy areas of atelectasis frequently are noted.[211]

The predominant cell types present in the lung of fatal cases are macrophages and neutrophils. Lymphocytes bearing CD4 (helper cells), CD8 (cytotoxic cells), and CD56 (natural killer cells) antigens are almost absent in fatal bronchiolitis cases.[204] In contrast to the findings in fatal cases, CD8 lymphocytes were present in the lung tissue obtained from a nonhospitalized child with a mild lower respiratory tract infection caused by RSV who died in an automobile accident.[87] Even in surviving infants, CD8 lymphocyte counts are less than 1% of the total cells in bronchoalveolar lavage fluids[49] and only appear in respiratory tract secretions of subjects with severe forms of disease after illness has largely resolved.[74,110] These findings suggest that CD8 lymphocyte responses are necessary for early control of RSV infection and that severe disease is perhaps related to an absence of CD8 responses. Cytokines characteristically released by CD4 and CD8 cells (interleukin [IL]-2, IL-4, IL-5, IL-13, and interferon [IFN]-γ) are present only in low concentrations in nasopharyngeal and tracheal secretions of infants with severe lower respiratory tract infections caused by RSV.[16,58,204] Microarray analysis of gene expression during acute RSV infection confirms these findings. Genes related to innate IFN function and neutrophil function were among the most overexpressed genes in infants infected with RSV. Genes regulating T and B cells (components of the adaptive immune response) were among the most underexpressed genes.[124]

Staining for markers of apoptosis (caspase 3 and Fas) is positive in infected epithelial cells,[204] suggesting that recovery from primary infection depends on the antiviral activity of phagocytic cells, induction of apoptosis, and perhaps the activity of other innate immune mechanisms. Strong innate immune responses occurring early in the course of infection may limit the eventual degree of illness.[12] Rhinovirus bronchiolitis appears to occur more frequently in subjects with preexisting atopic dermatitis and eosinophilia, suggesting that allergic pathways may contribute to bronchiolitis caused by this virus.[100,156]

Recovery from bronchiolitis apparently is complete histologically,[135,211] although plugging of the airway still was prominent in an infant 5 weeks after having an acute episode of bronchiolitis. This infant had experienced an apparent full clinical recovery before eventually dying of acute pneumococcal pneumonia.[135]

Infants may be particularly prone to the development of severe illness as a result of infection of the small airways for many reasons, including the small diameters of their airways. The infant lung is deficient in collateral alveolar ventilation through the pores of Kohn, which develop only in later life.[112] Atelectatic areas therefore cannot be re-expanded readily. Other studies have shown that the small airways in children younger than age 5 years contribute five- to sevenfold more to total airway resistance than do small airways of adults.[80] Viral infections involving small airways in young children are more likely to present as more serious clinical manifestations than similar infections in adults. Nonetheless, these abnormalities exist in all infants, whereas most infants infected with RSV do not develop lower respiratory tract illness. This suggests that host or environmental factors may be involved in determining the pathogenesis of RSV infection. Environmental factors are listed in Table 21.4, and potentially important host factors are described later.

Another factor that may predispose to the development of lower respiratory tract illness after RSV infection is the infecting dose of virus. Some studies show that infants with greater quantities of RSV in their nasopharyngeal secretions are more likely to exhibit severe illness,[20] although the results of other studies show no correlation with the amount of virus present in the respiratory tract with the severity of illness.[109,217] In fatal cases, abundant virus is evident in epithelial cells plugging the airway lumen by immunohistochemical staining.[204] The fact that crowding is associated with greater risk for developing lower respiratory tract

TABLE 21.4 Factors Associated With an Increased Risk and Severity of Bronchiolitis and of Postbronchiolitic Morbidity

Factor	Increase in Frequency	Increase in Severity	Increase in Later Morbidity
Crowding	+++	+++	?
Passive smoking	+++	+++	++
Male gender	+	++	++
Absence of breastfeeding	+	+	?
Family history of asthma	±	±	±
Personal atopy	–	–	+++
Congenitally small airways	++	?	–
Airway hyperreactivity	–	+	++
RSV-specific IgE responses	++	++	++

Data from references 21, 60, 67, 103, 117–119, 121, 161, 177, 187, 203, 205, 208, 209, 215, 216, 218, 221.
+++, implies strong relationship; ++, implies moderate relationship; +, implies weak relationship; ±, implies controversial relationship; –, implies no relationship; *?*, implies unknown relationship.
RSV, Respiratory syncytial virus.

infection also suggests the importance of the initial inoculum in causing disease.[215,216]

Another risk factor for the development of lower respiratory tract infection may be the relative diameter (or degree of intrinsic constriction) of the airway. When pulmonary function testing is completed on healthy infants before lower respiratory tract infection occurs, certain infants have lower air flows in smaller airways (and presumably narrower airways) than do other infants. When observed prospectively, these infants are more likely to develop wheezing early in life than are infants with better airflow.[117,119] These abnormalities of lung function no longer are associated with an increased risk for wheezing after the child reaches 3 years of age. Instead, evidence of atopy becomes the principal risk factor for recurrent wheezing.[119]

Prospective studies of infants who had bronchiolitis in infancy demonstrate reduced airflow in small airways in later childhood. Studies of adolescents reveal reversibility of this restriction of airflow after receiving bronchodilator treatment, indicating the airways were constricted, but not stenotic, in early life.[183] Several studies have shown that the airways of infants are intrinsically more reactive to bronchospastic stimuli than are airways of older children,[106,191] particularly children from families with asthma.[218] How long this increased reactivity persists is unknown, and no study has yet shown that infants with greater degrees of hereditary airway hyperreactivity are more likely to develop bronchiolitis or recurrent virus-induced wheezing. In later childhood, repeated occurrences of viral infections are necessary to sustain this increased reactivity.[199]

In addition to the hereditary airway hyperreactivity, viruses themselves may induce increases in reactivity. Viral infections that clinically appear to be restricted to the upper respiratory tract in adults and children nonetheless result in transient, increased constrictive responses of the airway to a variety of stimuli, including histamine, irritants, and other agents, and small airway dysfunction.[3,5,35,47] Whether these minor changes contribute to the airway obstruction observed in bronchiolitis is doubtful, in that they are of much lesser magnitude than is the markedly increased reactivity observed in asthmatic individuals after exposure to allergens. These virus-induced changes were observed in all infected individuals, including subjects who did not experience wheezing at the time of the virus infection. If airways already are hyperreactive in infants, on a hereditary basis or as a result of a preceding viral infection, the subsequent stimulus of RSV infection may be sufficient to cause airway obstruction.

Immunologic deficits may be expected to lead to more severe forms of virus-induced respiratory illness. Studies of the antibody response to RSV infection in serum and in respiratory secretions show, however, that the nature of responses generally is similar among patients with bronchiolitis or simple upper respiratory tract illness alone caused by this agent.[92,206] Antibody-directed cellular cytotoxicity expressed against tissue culture cells infected with RSV also is similar in patients with all forms of illness caused by RSV.[91,169] Although investigators have shown that cells infected with RSV can activate complement through classic and alternative pathways,[182] studies suggest that in vivo activation of the complement cascade occurs with equal frequency among patients with all forms of illness caused by the virus.[91] Repeated RSV infections in early life may occur because antibody formed after primary RSV exposure has a low ability to bind to neutralizing epitopes on the virus.[39,55]

The concept that serum IgG antibody to RSV, acquired by vaccination or transplacentally, might sensitize the host has been dispelled by results of studies showing that severe bronchiolitis may occur in the absence of circulating antibody[147] and that titers of maternal antibody correlate with protection against infection caused by the virus.[60,141] Circulating immune complexes appear as frequently in mild RSV-related upper respiratory infections as in RSV bronchiolitis.[91]

Lymphocyte hypersensitivity has been suggested to play a role in the development of severe bronchiolitis. Original field trials showed that a formalin-inactivated RSV (FI-RSV) vaccine induced humoral and cell-mediated immune responses to the virus. Nonetheless, vaccinated subjects manifested more severe forms of illness than did unvaccinated controls when subjects in each group subsequently were infected naturally.[94] Cell-mediated immune responses to viral antigen were greater among recipients of this FI-RSV vaccine compared with control subjects who previously had experienced natural infection.[96] The resulting disease in vaccine recipients was similar in form to bronchiolitis, and the idea that natural RSV bronchiolitis is a consequence of lymphocyte hypersensitivity to the virus has persisted.

Nonetheless, it seems unlikely that the illness that followed FI-RSV vaccination is mediated in the same way as that following natural bronchiolitis. The two FI-RSV vaccine recipients who died after having subsequent natural infection had numerous lymphocytes and eosinophils present in the lung, which is not the case after natural RSV infection.[87,94,135,204] Infants surviving RSV infection after receiving the FI-RSV vaccine had high eosinophil counts in peripheral blood, which also is unusual in natural RSV infection.[56] In addition, cytotoxic T-lymphocyte activity is not detected easily in infants after bronchiolitis,[7] and more recent autopsy studies have shown the virtual absence of CD4 and CD8 antigen-positive cells in the lung.[204] Although the development of cell-mediated cytotoxic antiviral responses may be protecting individuals with milder disease, little reason exists to contend that lymphocyte hyperresponsiveness contributes to severe bronchiolitis.

Immediate hypersensitivity to viral antigens has received much consideration as a potential contributing factor in bronchiolitis. The association of a family history of asthma with the development of bronchiolitis in infancy remains controversial.[103,178] Production of virus-specific IgE and subsequent release of mediators of bronchoconstriction have been documented, however, in infants hospitalized with bronchiolitis caused by RSV and the parainfluenza viruses.[21,205,207,208] In bronchiolitis caused by RSV, the quantities of virus-specific IgE produced and histamine present in respiratory secretions correlate with the severity of illness as measured by degree of PaO_2.[208] Leukotriene C_4 is a product of mast cells and eosinophils primarily, although also epithelial cells and macrophages, and is a potent stimulant of airway smooth muscle constriction and mucus secretion. This mediator is released into the airway in acute bronchiolitis,[197] as is the bronchoconstrictive agent histamine.[179,208] In addition, prostaglandins and metabolites can be detected in secretions and blood after bronchiolitis.[160] Thus several mediators of airway obstruction that are released in response to the interaction of IgE with antigens are released in subjects with bronchiolitis.

A possible role for eosinophils in the pathogenesis of bronchiolitis is supported by the finding of increased concentrations of eosinophil cationic protein in secretions of infants with bronchiolitis and (among high responders) an overall correlation of concentrations of this protein with the degree of hypoxia.[56,57] Peripheral blood eosinophil counts are depressed during the acute phase of most infectious diseases, including RSV infection. Nonetheless, eosinophil counts in peripheral blood are higher in infants with bronchiolitis than in infants with upper respiratory tract illness only, particularly in boys.[56] This finding is notable because boys generally have more severe forms of bronchiolitis. A contrasting viewpoint is that eosinophils contribute to the clearance of viruses after infection. This view is supported by the fact that eosinophils contain enzymes with ribonuclease activity, which inactivates RSV.[41,42] IgE-dependent and eosinophil-dependent mechanisms may be important in recovery from viral infections, much as they are in recovery from parasitic infections.[184]

The airways of asthmatic individuals are infiltrated by T lymphocytes (predominantly T-helper lymphocytes) and eosinophils. T-helper cells can be classified as type 1 (T_H1), which produce primarily IFN-γ and IL-2, or type 2 (T_H2), which produce IL-4, IL-5, IL-13, and others. This finding is important because IL-4, IL-5, and IL-13 are important factors in promoting IgE synthesis and eosinophil migration. Asthma is thought to be induced by a T_H2 bias in the airway. An attractive hypothesis is that RSV infection induces airway obstruction and wheezing by inciting the same type of T_H2 responses as observed in asthma. However, although IFN-γ and IL-4 are found in respiratory secretions of infants with RSV bronchiolitis, IL-5 and IL-13 rarely are detectable in serum or secretions,[58,197] suggesting that bronchiolitis is not characterized by a T_H2 lymphocyte bias. RSV infection in infancy does not induce a long-term Th2 lymphocyte cytokine bias lasting into later life.[26]

Chemokines are proteins released by airway epithelial cells, inflammatory cells, fibroblasts, and other cell types that are chemotactic for leukocytes. A failure to initiate strong chemokine responses at the onset of RSV infection has been linked to more severe disease outcomes, possibly because innate immune mechanisms are not activated in a timely fashion.[12] Chemokines represent an alternative to T_H2 lymphocytes in terms of initiating the inflammatory response in asthma and bronchiolitis. However, although numerous studies of the chemokine response in RSV bronchiolitis have appeared, no chemokine has been consistently associated with worse outcomes. In contrast, the release of IFN-γ has been more consistently correlated with better outcomes.[1,12,58]

DIFFERENTIAL DIAGNOSIS

A tendency exists to attribute all infantile respiratory distress occurring after the immediate neonatal period to bronchiolitis. The list of causes of infantile dyspnea consists of conditions that are associated with upper and lower airway obstruction, however. Recognition of upper airway obstructive disease should cause little difficulty because the problem is one of distress with inspiration rather than air trapping. Illnesses that cause lower airway obstructive disease and diseases that suggest this problem are listed in Box 21.1.

The differential diagnosis of allergic disease causes the most difficulty. Generally the first episode of allergic respiratory disease, when associated with infection, cannot be separated from bronchiolitis by any objective measures. Anatomic defects such as vascular rings can cause obstruction of the airway at many locations; inspiratory or expiratory distress, or a combination, can occur. Frequently a child with an anatomic defect does not have any detectable difficulty until a trivial respiratory tract infection occurs, which complicates the diagnostic picture.

BOX 21.1 Differential Diagnostic Considerations in Acute Bronchiolitis and Infectious Asthma

Allergy
Asthma
Allergic pneumonias (e.g., allergic aspergillosis)
Anatomic cause
Vascular ring, lung cysts, lobar emphysema
Pneumothorax, hydrothorax, chylothorax
Foreign body
Circulatory failure
Congenital and acquired heart disease
Anemia
Nephritis
Infections
Viral, chlamydial, rickettsial, mycoplasmal, bacterial, and fungal pneumonias
Migrating parasites
Irritants
Inhalation of toxic substances (e.g., chlorine gas)
Aspiration pneumonia
Gastroesophageal reflux
Metabolic cause
Poisons (e.g., salicylate)
Acidosis

Foreign bodies should be considered even in very young infants. Gastroesophageal reflux disease has become recognized as a frequent cause of wheezing in young infants. Because of its obvious therapeutic implications, bacterial pneumonia is the most important differential consideration, although wheezing occurs rarely in association with bacterial pneumonia.[111,122]

DIAGNOSIS

Because bronchiolitis and infectious asthma are clinical diseases with arbitrary boundaries and multiple etiologic agents, outlining a method for establishing specific diagnosis is difficult. When illness is epidemic, RSV usually is the cause. In nonepidemic situations, a careful history and appropriate laboratory studies and radiographs should be considered to exclude the other differential diagnostic possibilities that are listed in Box 21.1.

A specific etiologic diagnosis can be made by the isolation of virus from the nasopharynx. The diagnostic virologic facilities of many medical centers enable the isolation in tissue culture of RSV, parainfluenza viruses, influenza viruses, adenoviruses, rhinoviruses, enteroviruses, and herpesviruses. The use of the shell vial technique has been applied to RSV infection with success.[180] Until recently, rapid detection of viral antigen of RSV directly in nasopharyngeal secretions by commercially available (e.g., enzyme-linked immunosorbent assay) or fluorescent antibody techniques has been the method of choice in most laboratories.[193] The accuracy of these techniques often is superior to that of standard cell culture (at least in infants) because antigens remain stable under transport conditions that inactivate live virus. Gradually the technique of amplifying small quantities of RNA of respiratory viruses simultaneously from clinical specimens (polymerase chain reaction) is replacing earlier methods. This is because the sensitivity of these assays in detecting minute quantities of RSV is far greater than that of other methods, and simultaneous testing for 20 or more infectious agents is possible in a small clinical specimen.[142]

TREATMENT

The cornerstone of therapy for bronchiolitis is the administration of oxygen and correction of fluid deficits. Most patients hospitalized for bronchiolitis can be managed successfully and discharged within 48 to

72 hours when given no further therapy than supplemental oxygen and careful fluid rehydration.[40,149,200] Oxygen saturation values obtained at the time of hospitalization have been used to predict the duration of hospitalization[173,200] and eventual deterioration and need for care in a pediatric intensive care unit after hospitalization.[18] Oxygen saturation is usually maintained at 92% or higher, although it has been suggested that an overreliance on oxygen saturation values as evidence for the need for hospitalization may lead to unnecessary admissions or needlessly prolonged stays.[168] Blood gas determinations should be obtained when indicated by clinical findings (e.g., cyanosis, agitation) because pulse oximetry is less sensitive for detecting hypoxia than is arterial blood gas sampling. Oximetry cannot detect increases in P_{CO_2} that may indicate impending respiratory failure.

Although oxygen should be humidified, the use of mists and aerosols except to deliver specific antiviral therapy is discouraged; mist can act as an irritant, causing reflex bronchoconstriction, and the water usually does not reach the lower airways.[8] Although dehydration is a potential problem in children with bronchiolitis because of reduced oral intake and vomiting, care must be taken not to overhydrate such patients. Edema is an important part of the pathology of bronchiolitis, so administration of excessive amounts of intravenous fluids may contribute to obstruction of the airway.

β-Adrenergic bronchodilators have been used frequently in bronchiolitis. Slight improvements in airflow, oxygenation, and clinical illness scores have been reported,[71,97,105,166] but these effects are not meaningful clinically; hospitalization is not prevented, and hospital stays are not shortened.[40,52] Improvements observed after the administration of the first dose of these compounds usually are not sustained after administration of subsequent doses. Older individuals with infectious asthma may be more likely to respond to these agents, but viral infections remain the most common precipitant of childhood wheezing either managed on an outpatient basis or requiring hospitalization.[86,88] This suggests that children of any age with virus-induced wheezing do not respond dramatically to medications commonly used to treat asthma.

Some studies have suggested that use of aerosolized, racemic epinephrine produces greater improvement than the use of β-adrenergic aerosols alone.[166] Compounds containing epinephrine theoretically could be more effective in reversing airway edema than are β-adrenergic agents. Generally, however, the minor improvements in pulmonary function are not meaningful clinically because the length of stay in the intensive care unit or in the hospital is not reduced by the use of epinephrine.

Aerosols of ipratropium also have been administered in bronchiolitis without observable benefit.[171] Possible explanations for poor responses to bronchodilators include a paucity of β-adrenergic receptors in infancy[164]; decreased amounts of smooth muscle capable of responding to bronchodilators surrounding the terminal airways[159]; the nature of the airway obstruction itself (intense plugging with cellular debris)[204,212]; and, presumably, persistence of virus in the airway, stimulating continued inflammation or release of bronchoconstrictive mediators or both.

The general use of β-adrenergics, racemic epinephrine, and epinephrine in the management of bronchiolitis is no longer recommended,[157] and persistence with these approaches in the absence of an initial response may prove harmful.[83,144] A child treated for croup with multiple doses of racemic epinephrine developed ventricular tachycardia and a small myocardial infarction,[22] emphasizing the need to avoid the careless use of these compounds in viral respiratory tract infections.

Corticosteroids have been employed repeatedly in treating bronchiolitis. Controlled studies have failed to reveal any benefit in terms of prevention of hospitalization, reduced duration of hospitalization, reduced need for intubation, or reduced frequency of recurrent wheezing episodes after bronchiolitis.* In a child with nonrespiratory indications for the administration of corticosteroids, these drugs need not be withheld because of fear of complications, although the duration of viral shedding may be extended in individuals treated with corticosteroids. Combinations of salbutamol and dexamethasone also have been evaluated but usually show minimal benefit.[190] One study suggested some benefit for this combination, but differences observed were short of statistical significance.[150]

*References 6, 36, 37, 38, 53, 65, 104, 122, 143, 146, 150, 163.

Corticosteroids have also been used to prevent recurrent wheezing in preschool-aged children. They have been more effective in those children with atopic eczema and who were known to be sensitive to aeroallergens.[6,65] Corticosteroids have been essentially ineffective in preschool-aged children with virus-induced wheezing without atopic sensitization whose episodes are less frequent.[143,146] Long-term, sustained corticosteroid therapy has unfortunately had no effect on the course of asthma once the therapy is discontinued.[65] The use of corticosteroids in bronchiolitis is no longer recommended.[157]

Early experience with the antiviral substance ribavirin in bronchiolitis suggested that mild subjective benefits and improvement in oxygenation occurred after near-continuous aerosol administration of this compound.[68,181] The degree of improvement in patients treated with ribavirin was minimal and probably occurred because the placebo group received aerosolized water (an irritant to the airway) rather than saline.[132] No study has shown whether the administration of ribavirin could prevent deaths, avoid the need for mechanical ventilation, or shorten the duration of hospital stays.[68,132,181] Ribavirin is no longer used for RSV infection in immunologically normal infants. In immune-deficient individuals, ribavirin, when used in combination with preparations containing antibodies against RSV, may prevent the progression of lower respiratory tract disease.[32]

Other approaches to therapy for RSV infection include the use of IFN-α,[34] DNase,[125] and nitric oxide.[148] The results of these studies demonstrated no substantial benefit of any of these approaches. Infants with low serum levels of vitamin A[138,155] and vitamin D[11] are more likely to develop RSV lower respiratory tract infection than infants with normal serum levels of these vitamins. However, there is currently no evidence that supplementation with these vitamins during infection has any effect on the outcome of disease. Surfactant[93,195] has been used in very small studies of bronchiolitis or virus-induced wheezing, with positive effects that require confirmation. Several recent studies have evaluated the effect of 3% and 5% nebulized saline solutions in bronchiolitis. Some studies have demonstrated reduced length of hospitalization in subjects receiving hypertonic saline,[102,116] whereas other studies have not shown any positive effects.[63,84,89]

RSV-infected infants have elevated levels of cysteinyl leukotrienes in respiratory tract secretions.[197,198] Although initial studies of leukotriene receptor antagonists in RSV infection suggested that the use of these antagonists could reduce the magnitude of respiratory symptoms after RSV bronchiolitis,[3,95] subsequent studies demonstrated no differences in long-term complications.[4] Preparations containing a very high titer of neutralizing antibody against RSV have been tested in the prevention and treatment of RSV infection in high-risk populations. The results of the prophylaxis studies were positive (see later discussion under "Prevention"). A significant therapeutic effect of these compounds once RSV infection was established could not be identified, however.[114]

Because bronchiolitis is a viral disease, antibiotics are not useful or necessary. In many instances, the radiographic picture suggests pneumonia, and the blood leukocyte count is elevated. In these instances, a physician may feel compelled to administer antibiotics. However, bacterial infection of the lung is rare in bronchiolitis even when infiltrates are identified on chest radiographs. In one large study, secondary bacterial infection occurred in no more than 7 (1.2%) of 565 children with RSV infection.[69] In developed countries, bacterial pneumonia does not commonly complicate RSV infection and may be overdiagnosed when bacterial flora are recovered in cultures of tracheal aspirates.[158] For the vast majority of infants, antibiotics need not be prescribed once RSV infection has been diagnosed or can be stopped immediately thereafter. Institution of antibiotics should be considered during the course of therapy when a change in clinical findings suggests the possibility of secondary bacterial infection.

A child with bronchiolitis generally is more comfortable in the supine position with the head end of the crib slightly elevated. Infant seats are used frequently but are not optimal because the child's head tends to fall to the side or forward, which constricts the upper airway. The sitting position also causes a possibly deleterious upward pressure on the diaphragm. The onset of respiratory failure is usually recognized by virtue of reduced inspiratory breath sounds, severe inspiratory retractions, inability to maintain an oxygen saturation of more than 90% in 40%

ambient oxygen, cyanosis in 40% oxygen, decreased or absent response to painful stimuli, and a Pa_{CO_2} rising to 65 mm Hg or higher. Nasotracheal intubation and positive-pressure ventilation, often with neuromuscular blockade, are indicated in these circumstances.[43,144]

PREVENTION

The development of a method to prevent RSV infection is a high priority. The initial adverse experience with formalin-inactivated vaccine (described earlier) unfortunately has nearly prevented further investigation of inactivated vaccines.[94,196] Live, temperature-sensitive vaccines have been developed by adapting RSV to grow at reduced temperatures in cell culture. This attenuated vaccine was designed to grow at the lower temperatures of the upper respiratory tract but be inactive at the higher temperatures in the lung. In initial field trials, the vaccine strain caused febrile respiratory illnesses in seronegative vaccinees but did not replicate adequately in seropositive subjects.[30] Further trials of temperature-sensitive mutant RSV strains as vaccines showed improved immunogenicity and some protection, at least against rechallenge with the vaccine strain. Nasal congestion was noted in some recipients, however, and there is concern that this degree of nasal obstruction could result in apnea in infants.[89] Numerous other vaccine candidates, including RSV nucleic acid vaccines, bovine RSV strains, parainfluenza virus strains bearing RSV antigens, and human RSV strains with gene deletions or given with immunologically active adjuvants, have been developed. Many of them are in early clinical trials, but development of a successful vaccine is not imminent.[27]

Another strategy for protection of infants against RSV infection is to immunize pregnant women who will give birth shortly before or during the RSV season. It is estimated that 44% of RSV hospitalizations,[70] and most deaths,[23] occur in infants who are less than 2 months of age at the time of infection. Thus, boosting maternal antibody levels near term should provide infants with higher titers of RSV neutralizing antibody and protection against infection when severe disease is most likely to occur. Phase III clinical trials of the effect of vaccinating mothers with RSV F protein are in progress at the time of this writing.

While progress in development of an RSV vaccine has been slow, protection against serious illness caused by RSV infection has been achieved using a pooled preparation of human serum obtained from donors with very high titers of neutralizing antibody against RSV.[64] This compound, when administered during the RSV season on a monthly basis to infants and young children with a history of birth at less than 32 weeks' gestation or with bronchopulmonary dysplasia, caused a marked reduction in the rate of hospitalization related to RSV infection.

These trials have been repeated successfully using a humanized mouse monoclonal antibody (palivizumab) against the RSV fusion (F) protein.[145] The antibody is reconstructed so that it has more than 95% of the protein structure of a human antibody. This compound is approximately 50% effective in preventing RSV-related hospitalization when administered to high-risk infants, and it has received widespread use in infants born prematurely with or without lung disease of premature birth. Separate trials in infants with hemodynamically significant congenital heart disease have shown a similar reduction in the rate of hospitalization for RSV-related illness, and the compound is now used broadly in these infants as well.[51]

Because of the high cost of palivizumab, the American Academy of Pediatrics has incrementally narrowed the range of patients for whom it approves the use of palivizumab. Palivizumab is now approved only for infants born at less than 29 weeks, 0 days of gestation, or those who are less than 12 months of age at the onset of the RSV season and have bronchopulmonary dysplasia (lung disease of premature birth) or those infants with cyanotic congenital heart disease.[157] The data supporting this restriction are controversial in that no study has demonstrated that the data on which the original indications for use of palivizumab were based are flawed or inaccurate. Rather, the restriction seems to be based on cost considerations alone. While controversy continues, this action has created an opportunity for other companies to test similar monoclonal antibodies that have greater neutralizing activity or longer half-lives, with the possible long-term effect of reducing the cost of prophylaxis. One interesting study, performed in Native American tribes, demonstrated that administration of a monoclonal antibody against RSV-F to otherwise healthy full-term infants could limit the rate of subsequent RSV-related hospitalization of these infants.[140]

COMPLICATIONS AND PROGNOSIS

Nearly all cases of bronchiolitis in healthy children resolve without acute complications. Secondary bacterial infection in bronchiolitis now is a rare occurrence, at least in developed countries. Scott and colleagues[170] identified minor electrocardiographic abnormalities in 2% of 188 children with bronchiolitis. Involvement of other organs, especially the brain, apparently does not occur.

The overall mortality rate in bronchiolitis is low. Before the modern era of improved ventilatory support, mortality rates ranged from 2.0% to 5.5%.[38,77,79] A multicenter study in Great Britain published in 1978[161] estimated the mortality rate owing to RSV infection in infancy at 0.5%. Between 1979 and 1997, an average of 95 bronchiolitis-associated deaths occurred annually in the United States, with 20% occurring in infants with underlying heart disease, lung disease, or premature birth.[175] Presently deaths should occur rarely except among infants with severe underlying cardiac or pulmonary disease; even in these cases, the mortality rate should not exceed 1% of cases.[51] Current mortality rates are estimated to be 9 to 25 fatalities per 10,000 RSV hospitalizations, with nearly all deaths occurring among infants with underlying heart or lung disease.[23]

Whether bronchiolitis in infancy is causally related to the subsequent development of asthma has long been controversial. Fifty percent of patients with bronchiolitis have recurrent episodes of wheezing, although this figure decreases to approximately 10% by adolescence and may not be above that of the general population by this time.[120,121,183] Whether this recurrent wheezing is caused by RSV infection or, alternatively, suggests that RSV infection in early life is an indicator of a tendency toward airway obstruction is still being investigated. Recurrent wheezing after having a case of bronchiolitis could reflect an inherited asthmatic trait. Some studies find a strong correlation between atopic family history and postbronchiolitic wheezing,[46,165,221] whereas others, particularly studies from Great Britain,[153,177,178] do not. Studies of twins born in Denmark suggest that a hereditary predisposition to asthma is more likely to explain the development of bronchiolitis than bronchiolitis is likely to explain the development of asthma.[194] In other studies, titers of total serum IgE[151,186] and peripheral blood eosinophil counts[45,118,221] have some predictive value for the development of recurrent wheezing in infants having had bronchiolitis. Two studies showed that peripheral blood eosinophilia during viral infections, particularly RSV bronchiolitis, predicts the development of recurrent wheezing in school-aged children.[45,118] It has become apparent that rhinovirus-induced bronchiolitis has particular implications for recurrent wheezing in childhood. First, rhinovirus-induced bronchiolitis appears to be more common in infants with atopic dermatitis and eosinophilia than in other infants.[99,101,126] In addition, the occurrence of rhinovirus-induced bronchiolitis in infancy bears a much stronger relationship to the development of wheezing beyond 3 years of age than does RSV bronchiolitis, probably because rhinovirus bronchiolitis occurs more frequently in infants predisposed to develop childhood asthma.[85] Atopy seems to explain much, although not all, of the recurrent wheezing that occurs after infantile bronchiolitis.

RSV infection in early infancy could also damage the developing airway, rendering the airway more prone to obstruction in later life. Pulmonary function tests performed in former patients with bronchiolitis 12 years after an episode of bronchiolitis reveal an increased frequency of airway hyperreactivity in response to challenge with exercise or chemical agents, increased ratios of residual volume to total lung capacity, and reduced expiratory airflow at low lung volumes.* Although these abnormalities are observed commonly in individuals with asthma, they could not be explained in several of the previous studies simply by the presence of a personal or family history of atopy.[67,153,187] Some of these retrospective studies showed, however, that a single episode of RSV

*References 71, 78, 83, 90, 106, 153, 186, 187, 191, 212, 214.

bronchiolitis was not associated with long-term lung dysfunction; abnormal lung function was observed only if at least two episodes of lower respiratory tract illness had occurred before the patient had reached 2 years of age.[78,199] These studies generally suggest that atopy may explain more of the recurrent wheezing after infantile bronchiolitis than airway damage from the infection itself.

Prospective studies show that recurrent wheezing in children up to age 3 years after bronchiolitis (but not beyond) is related to abnormalities of lung function that existed before RSV infection occurred.[117] This factor may be airway hyperreactivity,[31] or at least airway constriction, as studies showed that airway dysfunction persisting beyond 3 years of age following bronchiolitis was reversed by albuterol.[183,203] Wheezing persisting beyond age 3 years was related, at least partially, to the atopic status of the host, as well as to a history of asthma in the mother.[25,85,101] Studies have not shown a clear relationship between the severity of the initial bronchiolitis episode and the degree of abnormality of long-term lung function.[66,67,153,177] Personal atopy and airway hyperreactivity are responsible for many of the long-term manifestations proposed to be sequelae of bronchiolitis.[120,203,215,216]

Some factor other than atopy, however, may determine in part the apparent lung abnormalities seen after a case of bronchiolitis.[98,186,199,200] Two intriguing studies have suggested that premature infants who are treated with palivizumab and therefore are protected against severe RSV infection in the first year of life have a reduced incidence of overall wheezing episodes from all causes possibly through the third year of life. This is the first suggestion that RSV infection itself, when it occurs in prematurely born infants, may result in an increased rate of wheezing illnesses in early life.[15,219] However, when monoclonal antibodies similar to palivizumab were given prophylactically to full-term infants, no effect on subsequent wheezing was observed.[140]

RSV infection could also account for recurrent wheezing by inducing persistent airway hyperreactivity. Retrospective studies have shown that airway reactivity is, in fact, greater in individuals one decade after having an episode of infantile bronchiolitis than in control populations without a history of bronchiolitis.[66,153] Airway reactivity in all children (even children never experiencing bronchiolitis) is greater than that in adults, however, and it is greatest in children of atopic families and in children exposed to cigarette smoke.[218] Airway hyperreactivity occurring after bronchiolitis is, therefore, not necessarily a reflection of the RSV infection itself. One prospective study found no relationship between RSV bronchiolitis and the degree of airway reactivity at age 2 years.[3]

RSV infection possibly can promote sensitization to allergens. In animal models, critically timed RSV infection can enhance temporarily the degree of airway reactivity induced after sensitization to an allergen. Whether this phenomenon occurs in humans is unknown. The absence of T_H2-like cytokine responses at the time of having RSV bronchiolitis[58] suggests, however, that RSV infection in infancy likely does not promote a persistent atopic state in the host. The results of a recent, large European study (ALSPAC) showed that hospitalization in infancy for RSV bronchiolitis was associated with subsequent childhood wheezing and asthma but not atopy.[75]

RSV infection more likely results in the release of mediators of airway obstruction, such as histamine and leukotrienes, through a mechanism other than T_H2 cytokine responses. Chemokines such as macrophage inflammatory protein (MIP)-1α, which cause mast cell and basophil degranulation, are possible candidates. Release of these mediators at the time of having RSV infection may result in wheezing in susceptible individuals. These same individuals may develop wheezing again at the time of having allergen exposure in childhood (particularly if they are atopic), but the relationship of bronchiolitis in infancy and such subsequent childhood wheezing would not be causal. Rather the association would be based on the underlying susceptibility of the airway to obstruction.

The overall outlook for infantile bronchiolitis generally is excellent. In a follow-up study,[203] severe lung disease was not observed in former bronchiolitis patients. All oxygen saturation levels were greater than 95%, and at least some of the airflow obstruction present in patients aged 7 to 9 years was reversible with a single bronchodilator treatment, as was confirmed later in other studies.[183] Single episodes of infantile bronchiolitis (in the absence of passive smoke exposure and without recurrent wheezing episodes) have not been associated with abnormalities of lung function or airway hyperreactivity in later childhood.[90,187,199]

The natural history of postbronchiolitic wheezing in childhood is for episodes of wheezing to become progressively milder,[66,121,153,177] and the frequency of postbronchiolitic wheezing apparently eventually decreases to essentially the same rate as that of children who did not experience bronchiolitis in infancy.[78,121,183] Nonetheless the overall prognosis is not entirely benign, and exposure to noxious environmental elements may result in an accelerated deterioration of lung function in later life.[186,187,210,214] The combination of respiratory tract illness in early life and subsequent cigarette smoking especially may be harmful.[189] Individuals who develop bronchiolitis in infancy should avoid smoking in later life and occupations that are associated with exposure to respiratory irritants.

NEW REFERENCES SINCE THE SEVENTH EDITION

1. Aberle JH, Aberle SW, Rebhandl W, et al. Decreased interferon gamma response in respiratory syncytial virus compared to other respiratory viral infections in infants. *Clin Exp Immunol.* 2004;137:146-150.
15. Blanken MO, Royers MM, Molenaar JM, et al. Respiratory syncytial virus and recurrent wheeze in healthy preterm infants. *New Eng J Med.* 2013;368:1791-1799.
23. Byington CL, Wilkes J, Korgenski K, et al. Respiratory syncytial virus-associated mortality in hospitalized infants and young children. *Pediatrics.* 2015;135:1-8.
31. Chawes BL, Poorisirak P, Johnston SL, et al. Neonatal bronchial hyperresponsiveness precedes acute severe bronchiolitis in infants. *J Allerg Clin Immunol.* 2012;130:354-361.
32. Chemaly RF, Ghantoji SS, Shah DP, et al. Respiratory syncytial virus infections in children with cancer. *J Pediatr Hematol Oncol.* 2014;36:e376-e381.
67. Hall CB, Weinberg GA, Blumkin AK, et al. Respiratory syncytial virus-associated hospitalizations among children less than 24 months of age. *Pediatrics.* 2013;132:e341-e348.
73. Hasegawa K, Tsugawa Y, Brown D, et al. Trends in bronchiolitis hospitalizations in the United States, 2000–2009. *Pediatrics.* 2013;132:28-36.
109. Luchsinger V, Ampuero S, Palomino MA, et al. Comparison of virological profiles of respiratory syncytial virus and rhinovirus in acute lower respiratory infections in very young Chilean infants, according to their clinical outcome. *J Clin Virol.* 2014;61:138-144.
113. Madhi SA, Klugman KP, the Vaccine Trialist Group. A role for *Streptococcus pneumoniae* in virus-associated pneumonia. *Nat Med.* 2004;10:811-813.
123. McGuiness CB, Boron ML, Saunders B, et al. Respiratory syncytial virus surveillance in the United States, 2007–2012. *Pediatr Infect Dis J.* 2014;33:589-594.
124. Mejias A, Dimo B, Suarez NM, et al. Whole blood gene expression profiles to assess pathogenesis and disease severity in infants with respiratory syncytial virus infection. *PLoS Med.* 2013;10:e1001549.
140. O'Brien KL, Chandran A, Weatherholtz R, et al. Efficacy of motavizumab for the prevention of respiratory syncytial virus disease in healthy Native American infants: a phase 3 randomised double-blind placebo-controlled trial. *Lancet Infect Dis.* 2015;15:1398-1408.
157. Ralston SL, Lieberthal AS, Meissner HC, et al. Clinical practice guideline: the diagnosis, management and prevention of bronchiolitis. *Pediatrics.* 2014;134:e1474-e1502.
188. Molinari Such M, Garcia I, Garcia L, et al. Respiratory syncytial virus-related bronchiolitis in Puerto Rico. *PR Health Sci J Neonatol.* 2005;24:137-140.
217. Wright PF, Gruber CW, Peters M, et al. Illness severity, viral shedding, and antibody responses in infants hospitalized with bronchiolitis caused by respiratory syncytial virus. *J Infect Dis.* 2002;185:1011-1018.
218. Yoshihara S, Kusuda S, Mochizuki H, et al. Effect of palivizumab prophylaxis on subsequent recurrent wheezing in preterm infants. *Pediatrics.* 2013;132:811-818.

The full reference list for this chapter is available at ExpertConsult.com.

22 Pediatric Community-Acquired Pneumonia

Samir S. Shah • John S. Bradley

Community-acquired pneumonia (CAP) is an acute lung infection that results most commonly in children from viral or bacterial pathogens. CAP remains the most important cause of death in children worldwide.[209] The World Health Organization estimates almost 1 million deaths in children younger than 5 years in 2015, accounting for 15% of deaths in this age group (http://www.who.int/mediacentre/factsheets/fs331/en/, accessed November 29, 2015). This number of deaths, most of which occur in developing countries, exceeds that of acquired immunodeficiency syndrome (AIDS), malaria, and tuberculosis combined. In the United States and other developed countries, CAP results in hundreds of thousands of medical encounters and hospitalizations.[86-88,119,129] Cumulatively, CAP ranks as the second most costly and fifth most prevalent reason for hospital admission.[112] However, death attributable to CAP is uncommon.[65,115]

In the United States, the Pediatric Infectious Diseases Society (PIDS) in collaboration with the Infectious Disease Society of America (IDSA) published current guidelines in 2011 for management of CAP in infants and children older than 3 months.[29] These guidelines define CAP as the presence of signs and symptoms of pneumonia in a previously healthy child caused by an infection acquired outside of the hospital.[29] The diagnostic, management, and prevention strategies discussed in this chapter are aligned with these published guidelines. CAP may also be caused by less typical pathogens, including mycobacteria and fungi, especially in immunocompromised children. These infections are discussed in detail in Chapter 97 and the chapters discussing fungal infections.

ETIOLOGY

Because of the difficulty of documenting the microbiology of pneumonia in infants and young children, accurate data concerning the incidence and specific agents of bacterial and viral pneumonia in children have been lacking. While viruses have historically been identified as the most common causes of CAP, etiologic studies conducted between the 1970s and 1990s indicated that two bacterial pathogens were responsible for the majority of fatal cases of childhood pneumonia—*Streptococcus pneumoniae* and *Haemophilus influenzae* type b.[80,132] In the intervening years, effective protein conjugate vaccines (PCVs) that protect against *H. influenzae* type b and *S. pneumoniae* have been introduced into the vaccine programs of many countries, including the United States, profoundly decreasing the incidence of documented bacterial pneumonia caused by these pathogens.

Recent prospective, population-based surveillance (the Centers for Disease Control and Prevention [CDC]'s Etiology of Pneumonia in the Community [EPIC] study) that included molecular diagnostic methods in addition to culture and serology, has provided invaluable data on CAP for hospitalized children.[103] Children younger than 18 years were eligible if (1) they were diagnosed with CAP between January 1, 2010, and June 30, 2012; (2) resided in 1 of 22 counties, which comprised the study catchment areas of participating children's hospitals in Nashville and Memphis, Tennessee, and Salt Lake City, Utah; and (3) had a chest radiograph performed within 72 hours before or after admission.[103]

Overall 2638 children were enrolled in the EPIC study; the final cohort included the 2358 (89%) children with radiographic evidence of pneumonia. This study had several major findings. First, a pathogen was detected in 81% of children. Viruses alone were identified in two-thirds (66%) of children overall and in half (50%) of children older than 5 years. Second, the most commonly detected pathogens were respiratory syncytial virus (RSV; 28%), rhinovirus (27%), human metapneumovirus (13%), and adenovirus (11%); adenovirus accounted for 15% of infections in younger children but only 3% of infections in children older than 5 years. Third, typical bacteria accounted for 8% of CAP overall (*S. pneumoniae* accounted for 5% of cases, *Staphylococcus aureus* and *Streptococcus pyogenes* accounted for 1% each). Fourth, atypical bacteria were quite common in older children but uncommon in younger children; *Mycoplasma pneumoniae* was detected in 19% of children older than 5 years versus 3% of young children.[103]

Children 4 years and younger had a virus as the sole pathogen in nearly half the cases and viral-viral co-detection in an additional 15% to 25% of cases depending on age subgroup.[103] Bacterial infections, either viral-bacterial coinfections or bacterial infections alone, accounted for less than 15% of infections in children younger than 4 years. In children younger than 2 years, the most common pathogens were RSV (42%), rhinovirus (29%), adenovirus (18%), and human metapneumovirus (14%), whereas influenza, parainfluenza, and coronaviruses each accounted for 6% to 7% of infections. In children 2 to 4 years of age, the most common pathogens were RSV (29%), rhinovirus (25%), human metapneumovirus (17%), and adenovirus (9%); *Mycoplasma pneumoniae*, coronaviruses, influenza, and parainfluenza were each also detected in 5% to 8% of children. Bacterial infections occurred in 5% to 6% of children younger than 4 years with CAP: *Streptococcus pneumoniae* (3% to 4%), *S. aureus* (1%), and group A *Streptococcus* (1%). *H. influenzae* type b was only rarely identified, although the majority of children were immunized.

Rhinovirus and *M. pneumoniae* were more prevalent among school-aged children. Rhinovirus was identified in 30% and 19% of children 5 to 9 years and 10 to 17 years, respectively. *M. pneumoniae* was identified in 16% and 23% of children 5 to 9 years and 10 to 17 years, respectively. Bacterial causes in these age groups included *Streptococcus pneumoniae* (3% to 4%), *S. aureus* (1%), and group A *Streptococcus* (<1%). Other studies of bacterial pathogens recovered through culture or polymerase chain reaction (PCR) of blood or pleural fluid have also identified *S. pneumoniae* as the most important bacterial cause of CAP in children, particularly CAP complicated by empyema.[23,24,38,41,68,84,124]

Internationally, the Bill and Melinda Gates Foundation is sponsoring the Pneumonia Etiology Research for Child Health (PERCH) project.[132] This case-control study involves seven countries in two geographic regions, Africa and Asia, where most cases of fatal childhood pneumonia occur. PERCH sites include Bangladesh, Gambia, Kenya, Mali, South Africa, Thailand, and Zambia.[132] The study had evaluated children aged 1 to 59 months and uses conventional and molecular methods to identify an etiology for pneumonia. Preliminary data from Kenya demonstrate an etiology in more than 75% of cases, with bacteria identified in 9% (most commonly *S. pneumoniae*), viruses in 53%, and mixed viral and bacterial infection in 15%.[94] An additional pilot study conducted in New Caledonia as part of the PERCH trial identified a pathogen in 89% of 108 hospitalized cases, with viruses representing more than 80% of the pathogens detected, similar to the findings of the EPIC study in the United States.[149]

Viral Pathogen

Of the viral pathogens, RSV generally is accepted as the agent found most frequently in pediatric pneumonias, particularly those associated with bronchiolitis. Although infection with this virus is quite common in all age groups, lower respiratory tract involvement is especially prominent in infancy.

Evidence to support the role of rhinovirus in pneumonia is increasing, with molecular diagnostic techniques now documenting rhinovirus as the most common cause of pneumonia in children aged 5 to 9 years and the second most common cause in children aged 10 to 17 years.[103]

However, rhinovirus has been detected in asymptomatic control subjects in prospective pneumonia studies in rates that are not substantially different from pneumonia subjects (17% controls, 22% CAP subjects), suggesting that not all children with CAP that is diagnosed by imaging and PCR for rhinovirus have current lower respiratory tract disease caused by rhinovirus.[103] Respiratory tract infection with the multiple serotypes of these organisms is common. Some degree of lower respiratory tract involvement by rhinoviruses has previously been shown in bronchiolitis and exacerbations of asthma.[104] Rhinovirus C has been implicated in severe pneumonia in children and neonates, as has enterovirus D68 (EV-D68), which is a structurally closely related virus.[34,44,123,222]

Human metapneumovirus (hMPV), a paramyxovirus, was first described in children with upper and lower respiratory tract infection in the Netherlands in 2001.[203] Nearly 100% of children have serologic evidence of hMPV infection by age 5 years, including the approximately 5% to 10% of children with CAP.[133,214,218] The clinical symptoms in infected children resemble those caused by RSV and influenza and may result in severe pneumonia.[203] A study conducted in Utah from 2006 to 2011 noted that the incidence of hospitalization for hMPV was 36/100,000 in those younger than 18 years of age. Rates were highest in infants younger than 2 years of age (200/100,000) and decreased sharply with increasing age; 18% required intensive care admission, and 6% required mechanical ventilation.[54]

The three parainfluenza viruses (types 1, 2, and 3) are also commonly identified as pathogens in lower respiratory tract disease in infants and younger children. Parainfluenza virus type 3 is the agent most frequently found in pneumonia[83] and has been reported as an important pathogen with significant mortality in pediatric cancer patients with lower respiratory tract infection.[138]

Influenza A and B viruses are not as prevalent overall as RSV and parainfluenza viruses, but during periods of epidemic or pandemic spread, they may become predominant isolates in children with lower respiratory tract disease.[14,72] Infection with influenza viruses predisposes children to bacterial pneumonia and empyema, particularly as a result of *S. pneumoniae* and *S. aureus*.[9,11,19,37,56,89,107,174] Additionally those with empyema in the context of influenza have more severe disease, including higher odds of mechanical ventilation and receipt of vasoactive infusions than those without influenza.[215] The threat of a pandemic of virulent influenza A, secondary to a recombination event resulting in a "human-adapted" avian or swine flu virus, keeps influenza in the forefront of concern for global public health agencies.[82]

Adenoviruses commonly are detected in children with CAP, particularly those who are hospitalized.[31,103,127] The overall impact of these viruses in the origin of nonbacterial pneumonia in children probably is somewhat less than that of the aforementioned agents; however, many fatal illnesses have been reported. Their common asymptomatic carriage and potential for endogenous activation by unrelated illnesses can render causation difficult to prove.[76] Of the 51 known adenoviruses, types 1, 2, 3, 4, 5, 7, 14, 21, and 35 clearly have been associated with pneumonia.[31,113] In certain populations, such as the Maori, Native Americans, and Inuit, adenoviruses commonly produce severe infection.[99,122] Adenovirus infections also have been reported in military recruits, some with fatal outcomes.[35,202,205]

Coronaviruses HCo-OC43 and HCo-229E have been implicated as causes of pneumonia since the 1960s, but until recently, this family of viruses was considered a rare cause of human disease.[110,148] The worldwide epidemic of severe acute respiratory syndrome (SARS) that occurred in 2002 to 2004 focused new interest on these pathogens and led to a new appreciation of their reservoirs in domestic animals and their potential to cause severe pneumonia and respiratory failure.[66,120,128,169,204,219] Two other strains of coronavirus, HCo-NL63[204] and HCo-HKU1,[219] have been discovered more recently. They appear to be among the less common causes of lower respiratory tract infections, but their clinical manifestations are similar to those caused by the other common respiratory viruses.[69,172]

HBoV is a parvovirus closely related to bovine parvovirus and canine parvovirus. The "bo" in "bocavirus" derives from "bovine" and the "ca" from canine.[6] HBoV was identified using a novel technique based on amplification of nonspecific viral nucleotide sequences, a method that holds promise for identification of other previously uncultivated human viral pathogens. Because only a few population-based studies have been performed, the contribution of HBoV to the overall epidemiology of pediatric pneumonia remains uncertain. HBoV has been identified in respiratory specimens, including sputum and bronchoalveolar lavage in children with acute respiratory tract infection,[27,33,40,92,99] and was found to be a relatively common (19%) finding in a Finnish study of children with asthma exacerbations.[5] However, bocavirus is detected far more often with another viral pathogen (up to two-thirds of cases where HBoV is identified), rather than as a sole agent.[27,45] Also reported commonly are asymptomatic respiratory tract "colonization" with bocavirus and prolonged excretion even after symptoms have resolved. Thus it is difficult to accurately assess bocavirus-attributable lower respiratory tract morbidity.[141]

Bacterial Pathogens

S. pneumoniae remains an important cause of bacterial CAP in children beyond the neonatal period in both immunized and unimmunized populations. In immunized populations, the serotype distribution changed significantly after the introduction of pneumococcal PCVs. After the introduction of the 7-valent pneumococcal conjugate vaccine (PCV7) in the United States, serotypes 3, 7F, and 19A emerged as important causes of CAP and complicated pneumonia.[10,18,41,42] Worldwide, serotype 1 also is often associated with complicated pneumonia.[24,41,68,162,166] These serotypes are included in the PCV13 formulation (serotypes 1, 3, 4, 5, 6A, 6B, 7F, 9V, 14, 18C, 19A, 19F, and 23F are included), and in the first years after introduction of PCV13 in the United States, decreases in invasive pneumococcal disease, including pneumonia, particularly for the more virulent and antibiotic resistant serotype 19A, have been reported.[57,108,109] Similar data on decreases in children less than 5 years for pediatric CAP that is presumed to be bacterial have also been reported recently from Israel, with up to a 68% reduction in outpatient visits for CAP since the introduction of PCV13.[85]

The availability of molecular diagnostics is changing our understanding of CAP and demonstrating that the presence of both viral and bacterial pathogens in children with pneumonia is common.[103] Furthermore the developing immune system from the newborn to adolescent and immunization status of children also influences the pathogens responsible for CAP in different age groups. Table 22.1 provides information regarding common pathogens seen in CAP in different age groups. Knowledge of regional data regarding pneumonia etiology, particularly the likelihood of drug-resistant pneumococci and methicillin-resistant *S. aureus* (MRSA), is vital for decision making regarding diagnostic testing and treatment. In the CDC's EPIC study that collected data in Tennessee and Utah, only 1% of CAP was caused by *S. aureus*, but of those strains, 78% were methicillin resistant.[103]

EPIDEMIOLOGY

In the developed world, CAP remains a common cause of pediatric hospitalization and ambulatory medical visits. Age is an important determinant of disease rates, with younger children more likely to have CAP and be hospitalized. In the United States, hospitalization rates published for CAP in 2010 ranged from a high of 1169/100,000 for infants younger than 1 year to a low of 44.7/100,000 for children 13 to 18 years of age.[129] Children 1 to 5 years had rates of 383/100,000 and those 6 to 12 years had rates of 69/100,000.[129] Regional data from 2010 to 2012 focused on different age groups but yielded generally comparable estimates: younger than 2 years, 620/100,000; 2 to 4 years, 238/100,000; 5 to 9 years, 101/100,000; and 10 to 17 years, 42/100,000.[103] In the outpatient setting, there are more than 1.5 million visits each year; age-specific estimates for outpatient visits (ambulatory practices and emergency departments) in 2006 and 2007 were as follows: 1 to 5 years, 48.8/1000; 6 to 10 years, 18.4/1000; and 11 to 18 years, 8.7/1000.[119] Race is also an important factor in CAP. Black children have higher rates of hospitalization for CAP in contrast to white children; however, the difference has decreased since the introduction of pneumococcal conjugate vaccines.[129] Immune status is also relevant when identifying risk for CAP. Children with congenital and acquired immune deficiency, including human immunodeficiency virus (HIV) infection, are at increased risk for lower respiratory tract infection caused by both common[7,188] and uncommon respiratory pathogens, which are described

TABLE 22.1 Etiology of Community-Acquired Pneumonia by Age

<3 Months	3 Months–5 Years	>5 Years
Viral Pathogens		
RSV	RSV	Influenza
Influenza	Influenza	Adenovirus
Parainfluenza	Parainfluenza	Human metapneumovirus
Human metapneumovirus	Human metapneumovirus	
Bacterial Pathogens		
Group B streptococcus	*Streptococcus pneumoniae*	*M. pneumoniae*
Gram-negative bacilli	*Mycoplasma pneumoniae*	*S. pneumoniae*
S. pneumoniae	*Staphylococcus aureus*	*S. aureus*
Bordetella pertussis	Group A streptococcus	Group A streptococcus
Chlamydia trachomatis	*Haemophilus influenzae* type b[a]	*H. influenzae* type b[a]

[a]In unimmunized infants.

in more detail in the chapters on immunocompromised hosts. Additionally children who are exposed to HIV in utero but are uninfected (HIV-exposed, uninfected) are also at increased risk of infectious illnesses and mortality, including pneumonia-related treatment failure, compared with unexposed children.[111]

The epidemiology of CAP in the United States changed significantly after the licensure of the *H. influenzae* type b and pneumococcal conjugate vaccines.[103] Overall, rates of invasive pneumonia have decreased in children younger than 5 years, the age group targeted for pneumococcal conjugate vaccines.[86–88,108] Decreases also have been observed in adults and suggest a likely benefit from herd immunity.[87]

PATHOGENESIS

The pathogenesis and host immune response differs significantly among viral, bacterial, and mycoplasma pathogens.[81,177,207] Detailed information regarding pathogen-specific disease can be found in chapters describing each pathogen.

For viral pneumonia, the pathologic processes associated with infection by RSV, adenoviruses, and influenza virus A have been studied most extensively in humans, aided by animal models for each pathogen.[61] For most viral lower respiratory tract pathogens, inoculation of the child starts with the upper respiratory tract after exposure to infectious secretions from others through sneezing or coughing or from fomites. Once in the lower respiratory tract, viral agents proliferate and spread by contiguity to involve the lower and more distal portions of the respiratory tract. Infected epithelium loses ciliary function, rounds up as a result of injury, and sloughs into the air passages, with subsequent stasis of mucus and accumulation of cellular and inflammatory debris. When infection extends to the terminal airways, alveolar lining cells themselves will lose structural integrity and function. As a result, surfactant production may be lost, hyaline membranes form, and pulmonary edema may develop. Mononuclear cells infiltrate submucosal and interstitial structures, further contributing to tissue edema, narrowing of air passages, and alveolar-capillary block of gas exchange.[106] With certain pathogens, particularly RSV, bronchiolar spasm in the context of accumulating airway debris gives rise to ball-valve–mediated air trapping with each inspiration, resulting in hyperinflation. Complete obstruction of an airway by debris may result in distal atelectasis. Ventilation-perfusion mismatch may compound hypoxemia that results from alveolar edema.

Histopathologic descriptions of the viral pathology can include acute bronchiolitis, necrotizing bronchiolitis, interstitial pneumonia, alveolar pneumonia, and hemorrhagic bronchopneumonia. Acute bronchiolitis is characterized by relatively superficial and reversible destruction of ciliated respiratory epithelium, along with accompanying mononuclear infiltration in submucosal tissues. Necrotizing bronchiolitis extends to the deeper submucosal layers lining the respiratory tract and may not be as readily reversible. This destructive pathology is associated particularly with adenoviral pneumonia.[164]

Interstitial pneumonia is a diffuse process in which the inflammatory mononuclear response predominantly involves the peribronchial alveolar septa. In alveolar pneumonia, the alveoli are filled with degenerating lining cells and mononuclear or polymorphonuclear inflammatory cells with or without hyaline membranes and may reflect bacterial superinfection, acute respiratory distress syndrome, or nonspecific changes associated with mechanical ventilation and oxygen toxicity. Hemorrhagic bronchopneumonia has been described in a fatal pediatric case of hMPV lower respiratory tract infection.[64] When hyaline membranes are present, the process is described as diffuse alveolar damage, the histopathologic hallmark of acute respiratory distress syndrome. Acute bronchiolitis and interstitial pneumonia have classically been observed in most cases of fatal viral pneumonia, regardless of the infecting pathogen.[1]

Both viral replication and age-specific immune responses contribute to the severity of RSV disease in infants. It appears that the severity of RSV in infants relates to a vigorous innate immune response and inadequate adaptive immune response to viral replication and destruction of the respiratory tract epithelium. RSV infection initiates tremendous innate inflammation through both chemokines and cytokines after stimulation of airway epithelial cells and phagocytic cells.[212,213]

Three important factors that influence the pathologic expression of nonbacterial pneumonia in children are anatomy, preexisting pulmonary disease, and immunity. In young infants, the small caliber of the terminal airways and the absence of interconnections between alveolar spaces (pores of Kohn) contribute to the development of wheezing and lobular atelectasis. Preexisting pulmonary disease (e.g., bronchopulmonary dysplasia) and an inability to clear the excessive secretions triggered by infection in patients with bronchopulmonary dysplasia also may lead to bronchospasm, atelectasis, and respiratory failure.

The most important factors in the pathogenesis of bacterial pneumonias are the virulence of the pathogen, the absence of specific humoral immunity, and the presence of a preceding viral respiratory tract infection. Most bacterial pneumonias are a result of colonization of the nasopharynx, followed by either bacteremia or aspiration of organisms. The lung is protected from bacterial infection by a variety of mechanisms, including entrapment and removal of organisms deposited on airways by ciliated epithelium and mucus, ingestion and killing of airway bacteria by alveolar macrophages, by reticuloendothelial system function for organisms gaining access to the lung via the bloodstream, by neutralization of invading bacteria by local and systemic nonspecific innate and specific immune substances (i.e., specific antibody, complement, opsonins), and by removal of invading organisms from the lung by lymphatic drainage. Pulmonary infection may occur when one or more of these barriers are altered, inhibited, or overwhelmed.

Animal models document that the inflammatory responses in the lung may be caused by various bacterial cell wall components, including peptidoglycans, lipoteichoic acid (of gram-positive organisms), and lipopolysaccharides (endotoxin) of gram-negative bacteria. Bacterial components stimulate a profound innate inflammatory response initiated in part by activation of pattern-recognition receptors (most notably

Toll-like receptors [TLRs]), followed by an intense inflammatory cascade mediated by cytokines and chemokines that results in upregulation of cell surface adhesion molecules in addition to multiple intracellular pathways.[43,81]

As classically described, pneumonia caused by *S. pneumoniae* begins with acute inflammation and hyperemia of the lower respiratory tract mucosa, exudation of edema fluid, deposition of fibrin, and infiltration of alveoli by polymorphonuclear leukocytes (i.e., "red hepatization"), followed by predominance of fibrin deposition and macrophage activity (i.e., "white hepatization"). Resolution subsequently occurs with absorption of exudates and return of lung morphology and physiology to normal. In contrast, when pneumonia is caused by organisms capable of inciting even more profound tissue inflammation (e.g., *S. aureus*, gram-negative enteric bacilli or pseudomonads), destruction of tissue and formation of abscesses frequently occur.

Recent animal data provide a scientific basis for the observation that signs and symptoms of a viral respiratory tract infection frequently precede development of bacterial pneumonia. The respiratory virus may act by simultaneous destruction of respiratory epithelium, cytokine-mediated exuberant local inflammatory responses, and upregulation of functional bacterial cell surface antigen receptor molecules.[143–145] Staphylococcal or pneumococcal pneumonia may occur during or shortly after infection caused by influenza virus. Severe pneumococcal pneumonia has been associated with outbreaks of influenza, and increased mortality rates from pneumonia occur during epidemics of influenza, as documented from new postmortem studies of fatalities during the influenza pandemic of 1918.[151,185] As indirect proof of the role of preceding viral infection, the use of conjugate pneumococcal vaccines appears to have decreased some of the lower respiratory tract morbidity seen with influenza infection.[114] Respiratory viruses other than influenza have also been associated with bacterial pneumonia, including RSV, parainfluenza, rhinovirus, hMPV, and adenovirus.[48,94,137,163,165,196] The pneumococcal conjugate vaccines have reduced chest radiograph–defined alveolar consolidation associated with RSV by 12%, with parainfluenza types 1 to 3 by 44%, and with hMPV by 40%, suggesting that concurrent pneumococcal infection was frequent in virus-associated pneumonias. By documenting the decrease of bacterial pneumonia in immunized patients, the conjugate pneumococcal vaccine has been valuable in identifying the role of viral and pneumococcal coinfection.[136,137] Immune compromise, anatomic defects, and neurologic comorbidities may predispose children to recurrent lower respiratory tract infection, but a detailed discussion of these risk factors is beyond the scope of this chapter.

Mycoplasma is primarily a mucosal pathogen, attaching extracellularly to the epithelial cells of the host airways. Attachment leads to the generation of an inflammatory response with production of cytokines with subsequent recruitment of lymphocytes and neutrophils to the airway mucosa, leading to the production of inflammatory infiltrates within the airways.[207] *Mycoplasma* attaches to airway cells by means of unique attachment organelles, resulting in cytopathic effects on ciliated epithelium of bronchi and bronchioles that can include loss of cilia, vacuolization, loss of metabolic function, and ultimately cell death. Edema with bronchiolar and alveolar inflammatory infiltrates containing macrophages, lymphocytes, neutrophils, and plasma cells has been described. Diffuse alveolar damage may also occur.

The nonpermanent immunity that develops with natural infection provides a vigorous cell-mediated immune response that, on reexposure to *Mycoplasma*, may lead to more severe clinical illness and pulmonary injury. This concept of immune-mediated lung disease provides the basis for increasing pulmonary disease severity with increasing age, which correlates with observed, specific cell-mediated immunity that also increases with age.[12,125] However, one study documented a similar incidence of serologic diagnosis of *Mycoplasma pneumoniae* infection in hospitalized preschool- and school-aged children with radiographic evidence of pneumonia. Although this finding suggests that *M. pneumoniae* may truly cause lower respiratory tract infection in all age groups, preschool children had clinical cure rates at 10 days into β-lactam therapy that were equivalent to cure rates in school-aged children treated with a macrolide or fluoroquinolone, raising additional questions of the natural history of mycoplasma disease in preschool children.[28]

CLINICAL MANIFESTATIONS

The clinical presentation of a child with pneumonia is most often based on symptoms directly related to decreased oxygenation of blood (hypoxemia), as well as symptoms directly related to lung inflammation, characteristically caused by a pathogen in a particular age group (from very young infants to adolescents). A benign viral lower respiratory tract infection caused by rhinovirus may produce only a cough, with no tachypnea or clinical toxicity. In contrast, a bacterial pneumonia caused by MRSA may result in tachypnea, dyspnea with grunting respirations and retractions, cyanosis, high fever, hypotension, and altered mental status. Detailed, pathogen-specific clinical presentations are provided within the chapters discussing each pathogen.

Of importance is the recent recognition of the high frequency of coinfections caused by both a virus and bacteria or caused by multiple viruses. In these situations, the clinical presentation and progression of disease may be an amalgamation of two or more pathogens. The association of influenza virus infection with subsequent bacterial pneumonia is perhaps the best studied. In these situations, the first signs of infection are those of viral disease, with coryza and sore throat. The progression of signs and symptoms and development of secondary fever may herald bacterial superinfection, which can be associated with consolidative pneumonia or necrotizing pneumonia that is characteristic of *S. pneumoniae* or *S. aureus*.[143]

Clinical manifestations of hypoxemia in children may occur after infection by either viruses or bacteria. Although these clinical presentations have been best studied in the developing world, the pathogens responsible for lower respiratory tract infection, particularly bacterial pathogens, are seldom identified in these studies, making pathogen-specific descriptions of disease presentation or clinical course difficult. Regardless of pathogen, however, those with more severe hypoxemia will have various degrees of respiratory distress (Box 22.1).

Whereas the older child and adolescent can verbalize the sensation of dyspnea, the younger child or infant may present with hypoxemia with increased respiratory effort and decreased level of attentiveness, decreased consolability, poor color, and decreased spontaneous movement, which has been best described in young infants with bronchiolitis.[140] In resource-poor areas of the world, cyanosis has been documented to be associated with severe hypoxia. A systematic review of published studies, primarily in the developing world, found that cyanosis and use of accessory muscles associated with the head tilting downward with each inspiration had a higher specificity for predicting hypoxemia in children than other signs but were not sufficiently sensitive to be able to be used in the clinical diagnosis of hypoxemia.[13]

Tachypnea is a nonspecific clinical sign that may be a result of fever, anxiety, metabolic acidosis, or the hypoxemia that accompanies respiratory failure. Whereas in the developing world rapid breathing as perceived by the mother, as well as chest retractions, nasal flaring, and crepitations, were statistically associated with hypoxemia, the sensitivity and specificity

BOX 22.1 Criteria for Respiratory Distress

Signs of Respiratory Distress in Children With Pneumonia

1. Tachypnea
    - 0–2 mo: RR >60
    - 2–12 mo: RR >50
    - 1–5 yr: RR >40
    - >5 yr: RR >20
2. Dyspnea
3. Retractions (suprasternal, intercostals, or subcostal)
4. Grunting
5. Nasal flaring
6. Apnea
7. Altered mental status
8. Pulse oximetry <90% on room air

Modified from World Health Organization criteria.

of tachypnea in diagnosing hypoxemia were both only about 70% to 75% in contrast to that of pulse oximetry.[135] Likewise among children younger than 5 years of age undergoing chest radiography for possible pneumonia at a pediatric emergency department in Boston, the respiratory rates for those with documented pneumonia by chest radiograph were not statistically higher than those whose chest radiographs were normal.[181] However, in the developing world, a high, age-specific respiratory rate (tachypnea), particularly when measured at 24 hours into antimicrobial therapy (amoxicillin or penicillin G), has been linked to clinical treatment failure in children with severe pneumonia.[139]

In the developed world, realizing that clinical presentation of pneumonia is neither sensitive nor specific for the diagnosis, pulse oximetry is widely used as the basis for management decisions, to confirm clinical suspicions of pneumonia with hypoxemia. Pulse oximetry technology is widely available, accurate in most settings, simple to perform, and has the ability to quantitate the severity of lung disease. Hypoxemia is a risk factor for poor outcome in both adults and children with lower respiratory tract infection. Although pulse oximetry is used together with clinical assessment, recommendations have been made to hospitalize a child whose SpO_2 is less than 90% in room air, although prospectively collected data to assess the risks and benefits of this particular value have not been studied in the developed world.[29,78] Given the lack of scientific data to support specific SpO_2-based recommendations, it is understandable that some practice variation exists.[36]

Viral pathogens are far more commonly associated with lower respiratory tract infection, particularly for preschool-aged children.[103] The clinical presentation generally follows a short upper respiratory tract infection prodrome (coryza, pharyngitis, mild fever) by a few days, with a gradual onset of cough, usually nonproductive. Clinical toxicity is usually mild for most viral pathogens. Some degree of bronchiolitis may occur with lower respiratory tract infection, leading to wheezing with difficult air entry and prolonged expiration with air trapping within the distal airways (primarily caused by RSV, hMPV, and rhinovirus). Lower respiratory tract disease is most often bilateral, affecting all lobes, in contrast to the more common presentation of focal, unilateral pneumonia caused by bacteria. Disease is usually benign, lasting only 3 to 5 days and resolving spontaneously. With young infants under 1 year of age, particularly those infected by RSV, increasing lung parenchymal inflammation can lead to decreasing oxygenation and respiratory failure. Hypoxemia and significant reactive airway disease may occur, not uncommonly leading to hospitalization. For the most common viral pathogens responsible for clinically significant lower respiratory tract disease, respiratory failure that leads to intubation is extremely unusual but may occur with influenza A or B viruses, particularly in children with comorbid medical conditions. Very uncommon viral pathogens, including SARS coronavirus and influenza H5N1 (avian influenza) may cause rapidly progressive respiratory failure with a high mortality rate.

In contrast, bacterial pneumonia may have a more rapid progression from cough to dyspnea and is more often associated with signs and symptoms of systemic toxicity, including high fever, hypotension, myalgias, malaise, headache, gastrointestinal complaints, restlessness, apprehension, and, on occasion, manifestations of secondary sites of infection. As with viral disease, signs and symptoms of bacterial pneumonia vary with the bacterial pathogen and the age of the child. Pleural fluid collections adjacent to infected lung may be extensive and can become infected, resulting in bacterial empyema that is a well-recognized complication of bacterial CAP (Fig. 22.1). Some bacteria are associated with a specific pattern of disease, such as the lobar pneumonia of *S. pneumoniae* (Fig. 22.2) and the empyema, abscess (Fig. 22.3), necrotizing pneumonia, and pneumatocele formation caused by *S. aureus* (Fig. 22.4); however, any of these manifestations may result from infection caused by any of the bacterial pathogens. In general, children with bacterial pneumonia have cough, tachypnea, and, with progressive disease, symptoms that are characteristic of hypoxemia, including dyspnea, shallow or grunting respirations, and flaring of the alae nasae. For lower lobe pneumonia, inflammation may be associated with gastrointestinal symptoms, including abdominal pain that may mimic that of appendicitis. Signs of pneumonia may be subtle in young infants. Percussion usually is not valuable in an infant or older child if distribution of the pneumonia is patchy. Dullness to percussion is associated more often in young children with the presence of pleural fluid than with the involvement of the parenchyma of the lung. Auscultatory findings classically include rales, or, for the child with consolidation, "tubular" breath sounds not associated with rales, lacking the normal breath sounds associated with gradual aeration and expansion of the lung with each inspiration. Abnormal findings in older children include dullness to percussion, decreased tactile and vocal fremitus on palpation, and the presence of egophony. Intercostal retraction indicates recruitment of accessory muscles, often necessary to assist respiration when hypoxemia is present.

Irritation of the pleura and accumulation of pleural fluid is accompanied by chest pain that may be severe and may limit chest movement. As the effusion enlarges, dyspnea may increase, but pleuritic pain may diminish and become a dull ache. The pain of pleural irritation may be present at the site of inflammation or may be referred. Pleural irritation

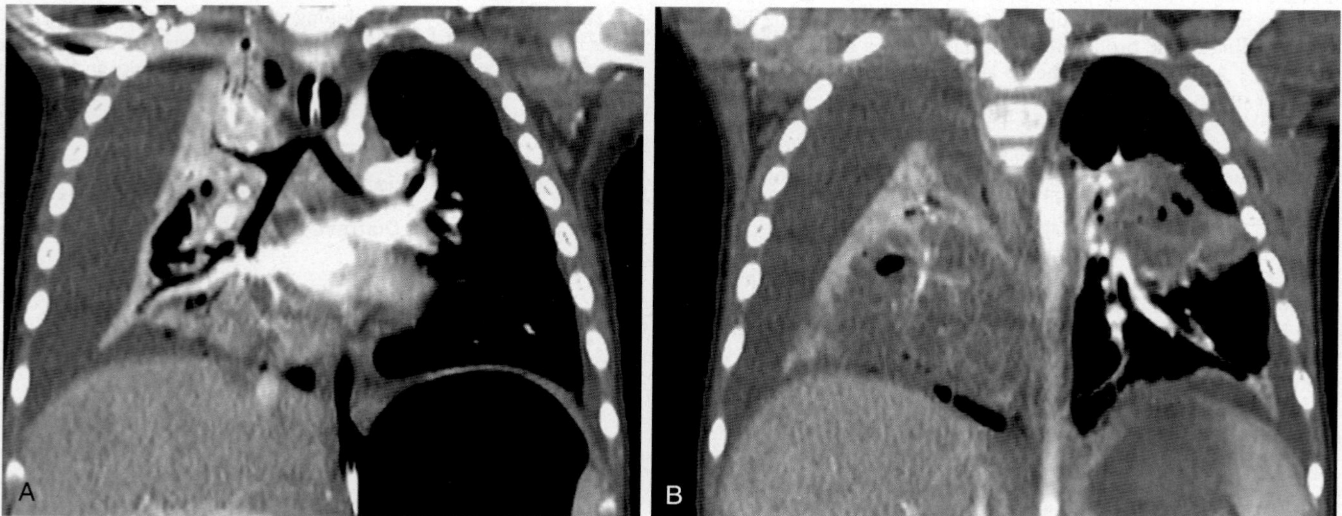

FIG. 22.1 Computed tomography scan of a 1-year-old boy with influenza complicated by an empyema caused by methicillin-resistant *Staphylococcus aureus*. (A) A large right-sided pleural effusion with compression of the adjacent lung is seen, as is pleural enhancement with areas of septation and cavitation (B).

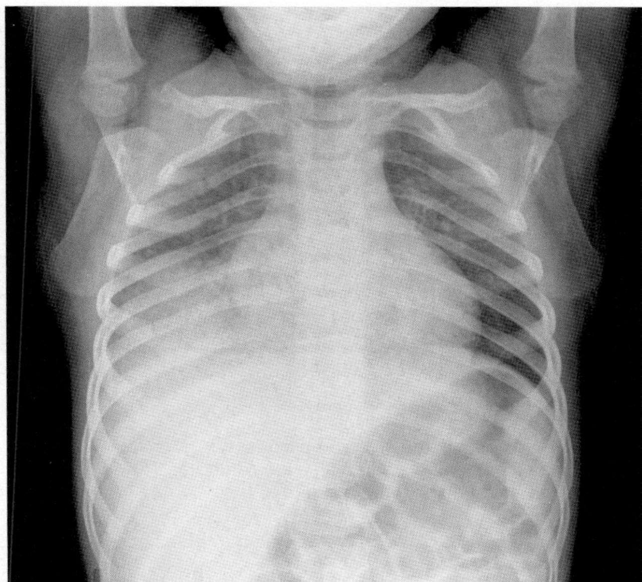

FIG. 22.2 Chest radiograph of a 2-year-old boy with pneumococcal pneumonia and bacteremia demonstrates consolidation in the right lower lobe with obliteration of the right hemidiaphragm.

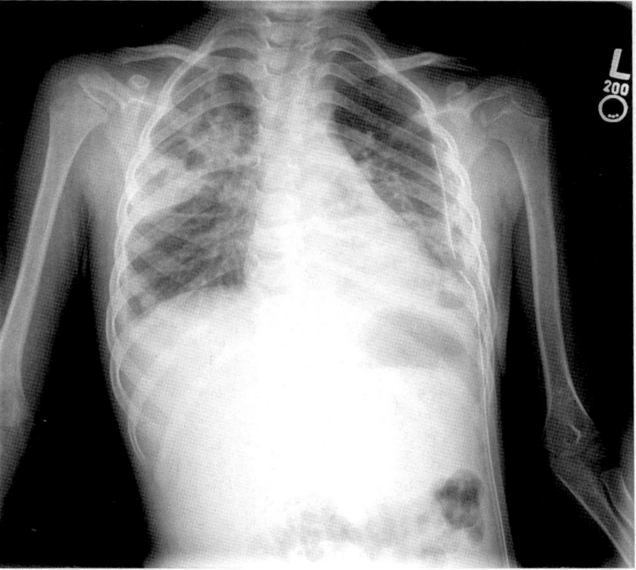

FIG. 22.4 Chest radiograph of a 6-year-old boy with multilobar pneumonia caused by methicillin-resistant *Staphylococcus aureus* reveals right upper and left lower lobe opacities with multiple areas of air-filled cavities or pneumatoceles. There is a small right pleural effusion. A chest tube appears in the left lung. The clinical picture was consistent with a necrotizing pneumonia.

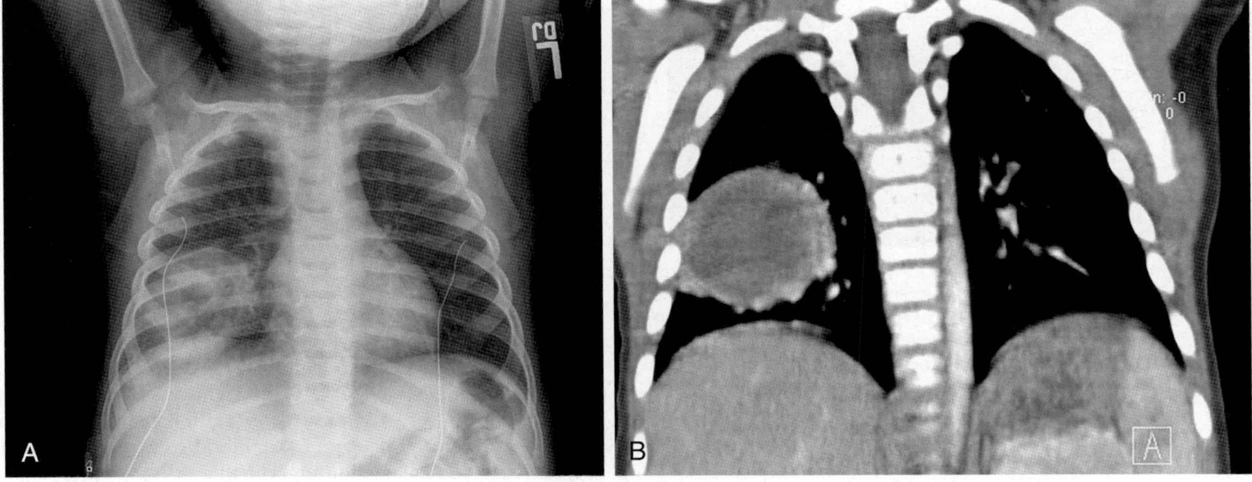

FIG. 22.3 Radiologic images of a 1-year-old boy with a lung abscess caused by methicillin-susceptible *Staphylococcus aureus*. (A) Chest radiograph reveals a cavitary right lower lobe mass consistent with lung abscess. (B) Chest computed tomography shows a rounded cavitary lesion that measures approximately 5 × 5 cm. It has minimum peripheral enhancement.

over the right upper lobe may elicit meningismus, a sign of meningeal irritation.

Atypical pneumonia in children is most often caused by *Mycoplasma pneumoniae*; disease caused by either *Legionella pneumophila* or *Chlamydophila pneumoniae* is quite rare.[29] Unfortunately, no prospective natural history studies that involve routine screening of both outpatients and inpatients for *Mycoplasma* spp. infection in all pediatric age groups have been performed.[21] Most studies of CAP in children that collected clinical information on *Mycoplasma* were retrospective, including some reporting outbreaks. Some reported data in children are derived from prospective antimicrobial therapy studies for adults, with insufficient numbers of evaluable children to allow a basic understanding of the disease in children.[154,189] *Mycoplasma* spp. clinical presentation is indistinguishable from that of viral pneumonia, prompting recommendations to clinicians to test for *Mycoplasma* before starting antimicrobial therapy.[208] Presenting complaints are generally related to slowly progressive systemic symptoms over the course of 3 to 7 days, with malaise, pharyngitis, and headache, followed by cough. Cough usually is irritative and nonproductive, reflecting tracheobronchitis, a manifestation of cell injury and host response to lung inflammation, which rarely progresses in children to hypoxemia requiring hospitalization and supplemental oxygen. Cough may last for 2 to 4 weeks or longer[55] and is associated with clinical findings of rales, rhonchi, and wheezes that may be so prominent in the context of a child who does not appear ill as to merit the common name of "walking pneumonia." Similar to certain viral pathogens, *M. pneumoniae* may be associated with increased

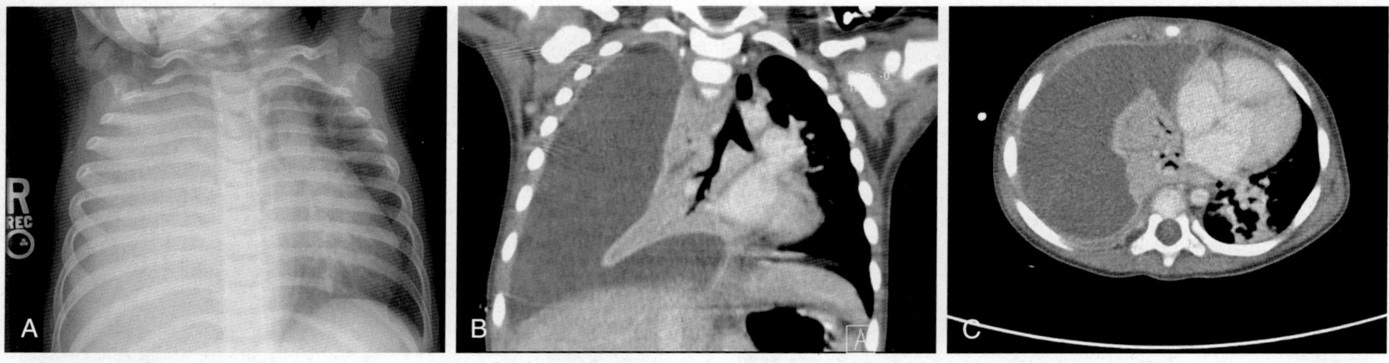

FIG. 22.5 Radiologic images of a 2-year-old girl with large parapneumonic effusion caused by *Streptococcus pneumoniae.* (A) Chest radiograph shows complete right hemithorax opacification with significant mediastinal shift to the left. (B) Computed tomography (CT) shows a massive right pleural effusion occupying the entire right hemithorax associated with leftward mediastinal shift. (C) The coronal CT view also demonstrates heterogeneous enhancement of the atelectatic right lung along with a lobulated collection of air, consistent with a mixture of compression-induced atelectasis and pneumonia.

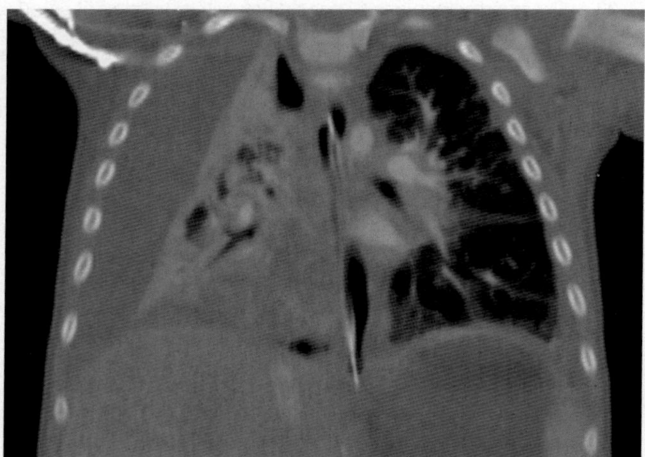

FIG. 22.6 Computed tomography image of a 1-year-old boy with influenza complicated by empyema caused by methicillin-resistant *Staphylococcus aureus.* There is a large right-sided pleural effusion with compression of the adjacent lung as well as pleural enhancement with some areas of cavitation. The left lung is hyperinflated with consolidation of the lower segment of the upper lobe.

wheezing in children with asthma,[22] particularly younger infants, although a recent meta-analysis suggested that, overall, wheezing was less likely to be present in mycoplasma infection compared with viral infection.[208] The clinical presentation in preschool children is generally less severe than in older children, presumably as a result of less immune-mediated inflammation.

DIAGNOSIS

Diagnostic testing for CAP is summarized in this section and reviewed in detail in the 2011 IDSA and PIDS guidelines.[29] Pulse oximetry is recommended in both the outpatient and inpatient settings, when feasible, to identify children with hypoxemia who may require additional testing or admission.

Outpatient Setting

In children who are immunized against common bacterial causes of CAP, including *H. influenzae* type b and *S. pneumoniae*, and who do not require admission, limited diagnostic testing is recommended. In children who do not have hypoxemia, history and physical examination are sufficient to identify signs and symptoms of pneumonia, and confirmation by chest radiography is not required at the initial visit. In children who are younger than 5 years, the majority of CAP will be due to viral pathogens, and no antibiotic treatment is indicated. In children who have a worsening course with or without antibiotic therapy, a chest radiograph to evaluate the extent of infiltrate and to identify the presence or absence of pleural fluid should be obtained. Similarly, blood culture and complete blood count rarely change the treatment course in children who are managed as outpatients and are not recommended. Testing for viral pathogens in the outpatient setting is increasingly possible with the new availability of PCR-based diagnostic techniques. Viral testing may identify children with RSV who are at low risk for secondary bacterial pneumonia and may identify children with influenza who would benefit from antiviral therapy. Antiviral therapy for influenza should be administered to all children with influenza-like illness who are also at high risk for complications during periods of influenza circulation in the community, even if rapid antigen-based influenza testing is negative, because these tests lack high sensitivity.

Inpatient Setting

For children who require hospitalization, chest radiograph to evaluate the extent of infiltrate and to identify the presence or absence of pleural fluid should be obtained (Fig. 22.5). Imaging in children with influenza and secondary fever or clinical deterioration may reveal necrotizing pneumonia or empyema (Fig. 22.6). Blood cultures are more likely to be positive in the sicker children. The rate of bacteremia ranged from 1% to 11% in published studies.[26,95,98,101,146,156,158,180,182] A systematic review reported an overall bacteremia prevalence of 5.1% in children with CAP, with rates of 4.1% and approximately 10% in nonsevere and severe CAP, respectively.[101] In the children fully immunized with PCV vaccines, blood cultures are recommended only in children with moderate to severe illness. When positive, blood culture results can guide definitive antibiotic treatment. Rapid microarray assays performed on positive blood cultures now permit rapid differentiation of *S. aureus* from other gram-positive bacteria,[192] thus minimizing the need to change the antibiotic regimen from aminopenicillins to vancomycin or antistaphylococcal penicillins in stable patients while awaiting organism identification.

Complete blood count may be useful in hospitalized children to identify anemia and thrombocytopenia associated with hemolytic uremic syndrome, a rare complication of bacterial pneumonia.[15,16,32,53,211] Sputum for Gram stain and culture is recommended in adults but rarely performed in children. For older children and adolescents with severe CAP, sputum testing should be attempted.

Urinary antigen tests for *S. pneumoniae* are not recommended for children with CAP because false-positive results are common, occurring in 15% (95% confidence interval [CI], 11% to 22%) of febrile, nonbacteremic children in one emergency department–based study.[160] The use of pneumococcal antigen testing for pleural fluid specimens, however, has been demonstrated to be reliable and improves the identification of a specific etiology for empyema, with a reported sensitivity of 83% to 96% and specificity of 95% to 100% (see Chapter 23).[124,142,168,191]

M. pneumoniae is a common cause of CAP, particularly in children aged 10 to 17 years. The role of diagnostic testing for *M. pneumoniae* is not well defined because limited studies have been conducted on the natural history of *M. pneumoniae* infection and the impact of antibiotic treatment, particularly in young children.[21,70,170,183,184] Testing may be most useful in school-aged children to guide antibiotic therapy. A variety of diagnostic tests are available. Traditional culture for *M. pneumoniae* is impractical for most clinical laboratories, given the slow growth and complex nutritional requirements of the organism. Cold-agglutinin titers greater than 1:64 are common in adults, but it is unclear how often this occurs in children. In addition, infections with other organisms may cause increases in cold-agglutinin titers, limiting the utility of this diagnostic test. Serologic diagnosis is most often used by clinical laboratories. Several serologic tests are available, including a rapid test for *M. pneumoniae* immunoglobulin (IgM), with sensitivity in published studies ranging from 74% to 96% and specificities ranging from 85% to 98%.[4,67,198,199,210,217,221] PCR technology is currently available for *M. pneumoniae* in regional reference laboratories as well as in hospital laboratories as part of a multiplex PCR test panel that is currently commercially available.[175] PCR tests have high specificity but variable sensitivity, making these tests more challenging to interpret than serology.[221] In one observational study of children 3 months to 16 years of age, the prevalence of *M. pneumoniae* by real-time PCR did not differ significantly between asymptomatic (21% of 405 children) and symptomatic (16% of 321 children, $P = .11$) children.[187] Longitudinal sampling in a subset of children found that most children with *M. pneumoniae*—15 of 21 (71%) asymptomatic children and 19 of 22 (86%) symptomatic children—tested negative after 1 month. However, 19% of all children with longitudinal follow-up demonstrated persistence of *M. pneumoniae* in the upper respiratory tract for up to 2 months.[187] Thus interpretation of positive results, including the duration of positivity, from a variety of specimens such as nasal wash fluid, throat swab, sputum, and pleural fluid will all require further validation before clinical management based on PCR can be universally realized.[199]

Pathogen-specific diagnoses for bacterial CAP remain challenging, although considerable progress has been made in the identification of pathogens through molecular testing of respiratory specimens. Both the PERCH and EPIC studies described previously use conventional and molecular diagnostics for viral and bacterial pathogens. A combination of these techniques identifies a viral or bacterial pathogen in 75% to 80% of hospitalized cases. Nucleic acid amplification techniques have been useful in identifying pathogens in culture-negative empyema.[23,24,68,84,124,155,162] The available methods and reagents are expanding rapidly and include fluorescent antibody techniques, enzyme-linked immunosorbent assay, direct DNA probes, and PCR. Clinical specimens may be tested directly or after preincubation in tissue culture systems.

Biological markers, or biomarkers, have been explored as a method to improve assessment of disease severity and prediction of etiology to facilitate management decisions, including whether to initiate antibiotic therapy or admit a child to the hospital. Currently available biomarkers, including white blood cell (WBC) count, C-reactive protein (CRP), procalcitonin (PCT), and proadrenomedullin, reflect host inflammatory response to infection. WBC counts and CRP concentrations have insufficient diagnostic accuracy to serve as biomarkers in predicting etiology in children with CAP. While the WBC count is elevated in many children with bacterial pneumonia, most children with CAP and elevated WBC counts do not have bacterial infection. Furthermore the degree of elevation does not reliably distinguish bacterial from viral infection.[63,117,171] CRP is produced by the liver in response to cytokines released at the site of inflammation. A meta-analysis that included eight studies and 1230 patients with CAP found that serum CRP concentrations exceeding 3.5 to 6.0 mg/dL weakly predicted bacterial pneumonia.[75] Furthermore there was significant variation in the sensitivity (range, 17–100%) and specificity (range, 40–88%) of elevated CRP concentrations in predicting bacterial pneumonia. Among 161 children with CAP, CRP concentrations of greater than 6 mg/dL had a sensitivity of 26% and a specificity of 83% in identifying children with pneumococcal pneumonia.[117] PCT, a non–thyroid tissue–derived precursor of the thyroid hormone calcitonin, demonstrates greater promise, but additional data, including more rigorous methods to prove or disprove bacterial infection (e.g., comparing PCT to a gold standard for bacterial infection), are necessary before PCT can be routinely recommended to inform decisions regarding antibiotic use or hospitalization. PCT concentrations in most studies are significantly higher among children with bacterial pneumonia compared with pneumonia caused by viral or atypical pathogens. Concentration cutoffs ranging from greater than 0.5 ng/mL to greater than 2 ng/mL have been proposed to distinguish bacterial from nonbacterial pneumonia, although these studies included relatively small numbers of patients with proven bacterial infection, and the PCT values lack sufficient sensitivity for routine clinical use at this time.[47,62,116,118,159,201] Among 75 children with CAP, 37 met criteria for presumed pneumococcal CAP. The authors found that a PCT of less than 0.5 ng/mL ruled out pneumococcal CAP in more than 90% of cases, suggesting that PCT may be more helpful in informing the decision to not prescribe antibiotic therapy.[79] Proadrenomedullin (ProADM), a midregion fragment of the parent precursor of adrenomedullin, demonstrates promise. ProADM improved the prognostic accuracy of the Pneumonia Severity Index, an established prediction rule in adults with CAP, in some studies[2,50] but offered only additional risk stratification among high-risk patients in another.[100] Few studies have explored its predictive value in children.[3,178] Among 88 children with CAP, Alcoba et al. found that ProADM greater than 0.16 nmol/L had 100% (95% CI, 40% to 100%) sensitivity and 70% (95% CI, 59% to 80%) specificity for bacteremia.[3] ProADM concentrations were twofold higher in complicated ($n = 11$; 0.18 nmol/L, $P = .039$) compared with uncomplicated ($n = 77$; 0.08 nmol/L) pneumonia.[3]

MANAGEMENT

Management of children with pneumonia in clinics, hospital wards, or intensive care units is based on the severity of the disease. Although severity is clearly associated with certain pathogens, significant overlap exists between the disease caused by bacterial, viral, and atypical pathogens, leading to initial management based on clinical toxicity and degree of respiratory compromise. For this discussion, management is based on access to resources available in the developed world. Significant morbidity and mortality occur in the developing world; the clinical manifestations of disease may reflect comorbidities and access to health care, and management decisions may depend on the resources available. The history, presentation, and examination of the child determine the severity of the illness and the appropriate level of care with respect to outpatient or inpatient management. The clinician's assessment of the child's respiratory status at the time of the medical encounter and the anticipated clinical course on antimicrobial therapy should determine whether hospitalization is necessary. Decision making should be based on clinical examination and pulse oximetry, supported by chest radiography and laboratory studies.

Any infant or child with respiratory distress (see Box 22.1) will demonstrate some degree of clinical toxicity, and most experts and professional societies recommend hospitalization for the "toxic" child. Although hospitalization in this setting is reasonable and represents the standard of care in the developed world, no prospective, controlled studies have been published that have quantified the degree of improved clinical outcome that results from hospitalization over management in the home.

Clinical decision rules based on initial scoring systems that incorporate a combination of clinical, laboratory, and radiographic findings have not been well defined for children as they have been for adults.[73,153] As previously noted, pulse oximetry represents a direct, simple, and widely available assessment for evaluating the degree of compromise of lower respiratory tract function. Clinical scores for critically ill children that currently exist may help determine whether a child should be hospitalized on a pediatric ward or be admitted to a pediatric intensive care unit.

Severity of illness scores built on multiple logistic regression models, such as the Pediatric Logistic Organ Dysfunction (PELOD) score,[130] the Pediatric Risk of Mortality (PRISM) score,[176] and the Pediatric Index of Mortality (PIM),[121] predict the risk for death for children admitted to a pediatric intensive care unit, including those admitted with pneumonia.

Young age (<6 months) presents additional concerns, with some degree of immunocompromise compared with school-aged children and a more compliant chest wall that impairs deep breathing and coughing as mechanisms to help clear pulmonary secretions. In the developed world, very young infants (up to 3 months of age) with pneumonia are generally admitted to the hospital for initial management. Given the increased risks for morbidity for children under 1 year of age, recommendations for hospitalization of infants up to 6 months of age with suspected bacterial pneumonia also have been made.[102,179]

Important comorbidities, including reactive airway disease, genetic syndromes, neurocognitive disorders, immune compromise, and chronic cardiac and pulmonary conditions, are also risk factors for the pneumonia requiring hospitalization.[150,194,195] Children with a comorbid condition and influenza infection are more likely to require hospitalization than otherwise healthy children.[17,52,56]

Empiric antimicrobial therapy for the hospitalized child with pneumonia depends on the suspected pathogens and their presumed susceptibilities. For the vast majority of infants with pneumonia, viral pathogens are responsible and require only supportive therapy.[177] Rapid viral diagnostic tests can assist in the diagnosis, but some children with viral disease will have a bacterial coinfection that requires antimicrobial therapy. Perhaps best documented with influenza, infection may begin with rather benign upper respiratory tract symptoms that progress to a severity of illness that is unexpected, or the infection may demonstrate a biphasic illness pattern with stable disease followed by subsequent deterioration, well documented during the 1918 influenza pandemic and in the 2009 H1N1 pandemic.

Antiviral therapy exists for influenza virus. Most influenza A strains can still be effectively treated with neuraminidase inhibitors[52,77,134]; in the past, adamantanes were effective treatment, but for the past several years, virtually all strains have been resistant. Most currently isolated strains of influenza B are susceptible to neuraminidase inhibitors. However, because substantial genetic variation occurs in influenza from year to year, resistance of influenza virus strains to any class of antiviral agents may develop and spread quickly. Globally the World Health Organization tracks and reports resistance as strains are analyzed during the influenza season. In the United States, the CDC sequences a certain proportion of all strains isolated during the season to allow rapid detection of resistance to antiviral agents. Dosages of neuraminidase inhibitor agents that are currently recommended for influenza in children were evaluated in clinical trials that mandated treatment within 48 hours of onset of symptoms. Although early initiation of treatment might provide the most benefit,[96] children with serious illness that extends beyond 48 hours are still likely to benefit from therapy and should be treated.[52,71,126,147,186]

Two recent systematic reviews challenged prior understanding of the magnitude of potential benefits of oseltamivir[105] and zanamivir.[97] These reviews were conducted with inclusion of a broader set of data, including regulatory information, than previously available. Oseltamivir modestly reduced the time to first alleviation of symptoms (by 29 hours; 95% CI, 12–47 hours) but caused significant vomiting (10.3% of oseltamivir recipients compared with 1.75% of placebo recipients) and increased the risk of headaches and renal and psychiatric syndromes (number needed to harm, 94; 95% CI, 36–1538).[105] Oseltamivir did not reduce complications such as pneumonia, although complications occurred relatively infrequently overall, even among placebo recipients. Zanamivir reduced the time to symptomatic improvement in adults (time to first alleviation of symptoms was reduced by 14 hours while total symptom duration was reduced by 10% from 6.6 to 6.0 days) but not in children with influenza-like illness, although this effect might be attenuated by symptom relief medication.[97] There was no evidence that zanamivir reduced the risk of complications of influenza, particularly pneumonia, or the risk of hospital admission or death; its harmful effects were minor except for bronchospasm. A major challenge in interpreting these reviews is that randomized trials of neuraminidase inhibitors in ambulatory patients with mild illness do not inform treatment approaches to patients with severe illness or persons at higher risk for influenza complications. Observational studies of hospitalized patients report that neuraminidase inhibitor use was associated with shorter lengths of hospital stay, fewer intensive care unit admissions, and lower mortality and that later initiation in severely ill or immunocompromised patients may still provide some clinical benefit.[51,134,157,206] In this context, the IDSA continues to recommend neuraminidase inhibitors for treatment of influenza (www.idsociety.org/influenza_Statement.aspx). Randomized trials of neuraminidase inhibitors for hospitalized and severely ill patients are needed to inform clinical practice. Available data should prompt greater consideration of the benefits and harms when making decisions for neuraminidase treatment for or prophylaxis against influenza in patients at low risk for complications.

Oseltamivir is an orally available neuraminidase inhibitor in both tablet and suspension formulations. Zanamivir is available as inhalational therapy for older children who are capable of taking a deep breath on command. Dosing guidelines are available from both the American Academy of Pediatrics (AAP)[52] and the CDC (http://www.cdc.gov/flu/professionals/antivirals/). Investigational neuroaminidase inhibitors administered intravenously (peramivir, oseltamivir, and zanamivir), were used for treatment of documented H1N1 infections during the H1N1 pandemic. Peramivir IV is now approved for adults with influenza. Zanamivir IV is still only available for compassionate investigational use and is not yet approved by the U.S. Food and Drug Administration for general use.

For RSV pneumonia, controversy exists about the efficacy of inhaled ribavirin. Ribavirin has in vitro activity against RSV, but use of this drug for RSV infection is not routinely recommended in the management of lower respiratory tract disease because of marginal efficacy, high cost, and potential toxicities to health care providers. Two new antivirals for RSV are under clinical investigation in children, but neither is likely to be available for clinical use until after 2017.[58,59] Similarly, antivirals are under investigation for some less common but potentially destructive viral pathogens causing pneumonia in immunocompromised hosts.

The etiology of bacterial pneumonia, as noted earlier, has been dramatically altered by effective PCVs for *H. influenzae* type b and *S. pneumoniae*. Disease caused by *H. influenzae* type b has been virtually eliminated in the developed world, and the susceptibility of *S. pneumoniae* to β-lactam agents such as penicillin G has improved dramatically. The increasing incidence of *S. aureus*, particularly methicillin-resistant strains, requires a more aggressive approach to diagnosis of complicated pneumonia and consideration of the addition of empiric therapy active against all strains of *S. aureus*, including those that are methicillin-resistant, in addition to that for *S. pneumoniae*. Empiric therapy is provided as the diagnostic evaluation for viral, bacterial, and atypical bacterial pathogens is in progress. Once a diagnosis is made, the most narrow-spectrum agent that is safe and well tolerated should be used.

Ampicillin or penicillin G intravenously is currently recommended for empiric therapy of acute bacterial CAP in fully immunized children who require hospitalization (Table 22.2).[29] Several prospective and retrospective observational studies conducted in the hospital setting indicate no difference in clinical outcomes between narrow-spectrum agents such as ampicillin and broad-spectrum agents such as ceftriaxone.[161,173,197,216] The use of antibiotics that are more active against penicillin-resistant pneumococci, such as ceftriaxone or vancomycin, is no longer routinely required with current low levels of β-lactam resistance following widespread use of conjugate pneumococcal vaccines. However, for children with incomplete immunization for pneumococcus, ceftriaxone or cefotaxime remain the preferred antimicrobials until more robust data on herd immunity suggests that resistance has decreased in all community isolates for children regardless of immunization status. The role of non–type b strains of *H. influenzae* in pneumonia in otherwise healthy children is difficult to define because many reports of hospitalized children with pneumonia from whom non–type b strains of *H. influenzae* are recovered have underlying comorbidities, raising the possibility that these organisms may not represent a high risk to healthy, normal children. The use of ampicillin as empiric therapy will

TABLE 22.2 **Empiric Therapy of Suspected Community-Acquired Bacterial Pneumonia in Healthy Children**

Disease	Fully Immunized	Incompletely Immunized
Uncomplicated pneumonia (lobar or bronchopneumonia, without significant pleural effusion)	Ampicillin	Ceftriaxone or cefotaxime
Complicated pneumonia (with significant pleural fluid, empyema, abscess, pneumatocele)	Ampicillin plus Vancomycin[a]	Ceftriaxone plus Vancomycin[a]
Life-threatening, complicated pneumonia (with abscesses, pneumatoceles)	Ceftriaxone plus vancomycin plus nafcillin	

[a]Clindamycin may be substituted for vancomycin if local *Staphylococcus aureus* susceptibility data document rare resistance (<5–10%).

provide activity against the majority of non–type b strains as further work clarifies the role of this organism in pediatric CAP. Since the publication of national guidelines in 2011, no reports had documented nonencapsulated β-lactamase–producing strains of *H. influenzae* causing pneumonia.

More difficult is the consideration of empiric therapy for CAP caused by *S. aureus,* particularly methicillin-resistant strains. Very little distinguishes among the clinical, laboratory, or radiographic characteristics of bacterial pneumonia caused by *S. aureus* in contrast to that caused by *S. pneumoniae.* Both can produce progressive disease associated with lung parenchymal destruction with empyema and signs and symptoms of systemic toxicity. Necrotizing pneumonia, particularly in the context of influenza coinfection, appears to be more characteristic of *S. aureus,* particularly with strains that are methicillin resistant.[46] Lung abscess formation with resulting complications may be more common with *S. aureus.*[193] With ampicillin as initial therapy of CAP, no antimicrobial activity is present against *S. aureus,* for either methicillin-susceptible or methicillin-resistant strains. Therefore a high index of suspicion should be maintained for infection caused by *S. aureus* in children who do not respond to initial empiric therapy and children who present with complicated pneumonia, including pleural effusions, empyema, abscesses, necrotizing pneumonia, and pneumatoceles. For these children with serious infection, the addition of vancomycin (or clindamycin if local susceptibility data document lack of resistance) to ampicillin while diagnostic studies are being pursued will provide adequate activity for either methicillin-susceptible or methicillin-resistant strains. With β-lactam antibiotics thought to be preferred over vancomycin for susceptible strains of *S. aureus,* the addition of nafcillin to the regimen for optimal coverage of methicillin-susceptible strains is also recommended (see Table 22.2). For children who are diagnosed with MRSA pneumonia and do not respond clinically to vancomycin, linezolid is a reasonable alternative. In prospective studies in adults, linezolid therapy of nosocomial pneumonia caused by MRSA demonstrated outcomes that were at least as good as, if not better than, those with vancomycin.[220]

Definitive therapy, in contrast to empiric therapy, may be based on susceptibilities of the organisms to antimicrobials, using the narrowest spectrum, best tolerated, and most cost-effective agent. Recent recommendations have been made for specific antimicrobial agents, by pathogen, for both first-line and alternative agents, as well as agents for children who may be allergic to preferred agents.[29] For pneumococcus, intravenous penicillin G (or ampicillin) is preferred and for oral therapy, amoxicillin (or phenoxymethyl penicillin). For methicillin-resistant strains of *S. aureus,* intravenous vancomycin (or clindamycin) is preferred and for oral therapy, clindamycin (if susceptible) or linezolid. Insufficient prospective data are available to recommend trimethoprim-sulfamethoxazole therapy for MRSA pneumonia. For methicillin-susceptible strains, nafcillin or cefazolin should provide optimal therapy, with oral cephalexin for step-down therapy.

The duration of antimicrobial therapy in children in the developed world has primarily been studied in the context of antibiotic registration trials, comparing newer agents used for 10 days with those having previously been studied for a treatment course of 10 days. A notable exception is the azalide azithromycin, which displays unusual tissue-site pharmacokinetics, with drug exposure after 3 or 5 days of therapy comparable to 10 days of β-lactam therapy. Short-course (3-day) therapy with the β-lactam amoxicillin or trimethoprim-sulfamethoxazole has been successful in the developing world for clinically defined pneumonia, but bacterial pathogen identification is infrequent in these studies, precluding conclusions about a pathogen-specific effective treatment course.[90] Although the total course of therapy is usually 7 to 10 days for uncomplicated pneumonia, longer courses of 2 to 3 weeks may be required for more severe disease, particularly associated with pleural empyema or pulmonary abscesses. All therapy does not necessarily need to occur in a hospital setting if the child's clinical condition is improved, drainage procedures and supplemental oxygen are no longer necessary, and skilled nursing care is no longer required. Transition from intravenous inpatient therapy to daily intramuscular or intravenous outpatient therapy with prolonged half-life antibiotics, particularly β-lactams such as ceftriaxone or ertapenem, provides another option for the hospitalized child who still requires parenteral therapy based on inability to tolerate oral medications, concerns about enteral drug absorption, or lack of comparable oral treatment options in the setting of antimicrobial-resistant pathogens or drug-related side effects.[200]

Depending on the response to therapy, transition to oral therapy often has been used to allow discharge from an inpatient setting. Although no prospective, controlled data are available to document the risks and benefits of this practice, clinical experience, often retrospectively documented, over several decades suggests that this practice is effective.[30,190] The duration of parenteral therapy before transition to oral therapy is based on the severity of the initial presentation and the rapidity of improvement. Improvement in fever, cough, tachypnea, and oxygen requirement with improved activity and appetite support transition to oral antibiotics. Declines in C-reactive protein or other acute-phase reactants are also often used to inform the decision to transition to oral therapy.

Management of pleural effusions and pleural empyema, primarily associated with pneumonia caused by *S. aureus* and *S. pneumoniae,* are discussed in the respective chapters (Chapters 80 and 85) on these pathogens. Algorithms for management of pleural fluid with needle aspiration, chest tube drainage, and video-assisted thoracoscopic surgery are also presented in the PIDS/IDSA Pediatric Community-Acquired Pneumonia Guidelines.[29]

Treatment for *M. pneumoniae* infection is less well studied in children than in adults.[12,21,208] Data extrapolated from adult studies suggest a modest benefit of therapy with tetracyclines and macrolides for illness of mild to moderate severity, with the assumption that children, particularly school-aged and adolescent, will respond similarly. Retrospective data from hospitalized children suggest that those who are treated have shorter inpatient admissions than those who do not receive therapy.[183] It is likely that children with moderate to severe disease will benefit from treatment with macrolides or tetracyclines (for children older than 7 years), prompting recommendations to test and treat for *Mycoplasma* spp. Azithromycin provides the shortest treatment course of the macrolides and is well tolerated, in contrast to erythromycin. Although reports have documented the existence of macrolide resistance, the rate of resistance from current epidemiologic studies in the United States is less than 5%.[60] Therapy with the respiratory fluoroquinolones has demonstrated treatment outcomes for adults not inferior to those with macrolides and tetracyclines, but fluoroquinolones are not considered agents of choice for children when other effective therapy exists. Of note, in a prospective, randomized study of preschool children with community pneumonia, for those with *Mycoplasma* lower respiratory tract infection documented serologically, amoxicillin-clavulanate demonstrated clinical outcomes equivalent to those of levofloxacin when evaluated by criteria for clinical cure at the end of therapy.[28] These results suggest the possibility of a high rate of spontaneous clinical resolution in this younger age group or that improvement may have occurred at an earlier time in the treatment course, not documented by the study design used.

Chlamydia trachomatis has been identified as an uncommon cause of afebrile pneumonia in very young infants, 2 to 12 weeks of age, after birth to a mother with genital infection. *C. pneumoniae* has been documented to cause atypical pneumonia in school-aged children and adolescents.[39,93] However, the clinical impact of antimicrobial therapy of *C. pneumoniae* lower respiratory tract infection in older children has been difficult to define, probably because of the difficulties in making an accurate diagnosis of active infection, as well as the relatively benign and self-resolving nature of infection.[25]

PREVENTION

Over the past 2 decades, great strides have been made in the prevention of CAP. The development of protein-conjugate vaccines against both *H. influenzae* type b and *S. pneumoniae* has resulted in significant declines in cases of bacterial pneumonia in countries that have introduced these vaccines.[57,85,91,109,131,152,167] Both vaccines are provided as part of the routine childhood immunization series for all children in resource-rich areas of the world and should also be made available for all children in the developing world. Children can be protected against CAP caused by viral pathogens. Influenza vaccine is recommended for all children 6 months and older and prevents CAP resulting from influenza.[52] In addition, increasing evidence shows that bacterial CAP may occur concomitantly with influenza or as a secondary infection after influenza.[20,49,74] The risk for hospitalization with CAP resulting from RSV, the most common pathogen identified in infants, can be modified by the administration of palivizumab to infants with high-risk conditions. Given the expense of this intervention, guidelines for use in high-risk infants should be followed to maximize cost-effectiveness.[8] Finally the PIDS/IDSA CAP Guidelines, the CDC, and the AAP support the immunization of parents and other caregivers against influenza, to protect children who are too young to be immunized; the AAP also recommends immunizing parents against other vaccine-preventable infections, including CAP.

NEW REFERENCES SINCE THE SEVENTH EDITION

3. Alcoba G, Manzano S, Lacroix L, et al. Proadrenomedullin and copeptin in pediatric pneumonia: a prospective diagnostic accuracy study. *BMC Infect Dis.* 2015;15:347.
8. American Academy of Pediatrics Committee on Infectious Diseases, American Academy of Pediatrics Bronchiolitis Guidelines Committee. Updated guidance for palivizumab prophylaxis among infants and young children at increased risk of hospitalization for respiratory syncytial virus infection. *Pediatrics.* 2014;134(2):e620-e638.
21. Biondi E, McCulloh R, Alverson B, et al. Treatment of mycoplasma pneumonia: a systematic review. *Pediatrics.* 2014;133(6):1081-1090.
23. Blaschke AJ, Byington CL, Ampofo K, et al. Species-specific PCR improves detection of bacterial pathogens in parapneumonic empyema compared with 16S PCR and culture. *Pediatr Infect Dis J.* 2013;32(3):302-303.
40. Byington CL, Ampofo K, Stockmann C, et al. Community surveillance of respiratory viruses among families in the Utah Better Identification of Germs-Longitudinal Viral Epidemiology (BIG-LoVE) study. *Clin Infect Dis.* 2015;61(8):1217-1224.
51. Coffin SE, Leckerman K, Keren R, et al. Oseltamivir shortens hospital stays of critically ill children hospitalized with seasonal influenza: a retrospective cohort study. *Pediatr Infect Dis J.* 2011;30(11):962-966.
52. Committee on Infectious Diseases. Recommendations for prevention and control of influenza in children, 2015–2016. *Pediatrics.* 2016;138:4.
54. Davis CR, Stockmann C, Pavia AT, et al. Incidence, morbidity, and costs of human metapneumovirus infection in hospitalized children. *J Pediatric Infect Dis Soc.* 2016;5(3):303-311.
55. Davis SF, Sutter RW, Strebel PM, et al. Concurrent outbreaks of pertussis and *Mycoplasma pneumoniae* infection: clinical and epidemiological characteristics of illnesses manifested by cough. *Clin Infect Dis.* 1995;20(3):621-628.
57. de St Maurice A, Grijalva CG, Fonnesbeck C, Schaffner W, Halasa NB. Racial and regional differences in rates of invasive pneumococcal disease. *Pediatrics.* 2015;136(5):e1186-e1194.
58. DeVincenzo JP, McClure MW, Symons JA, et al. Activity of oral ALS-008176 in a respiratory syncytial virus challenge study. *N Engl J Med.* 2015;373(21):2048-2058.
59. DeVincenzo JP, Whitley RJ, Mackman RL, et al. Oral GS-5806 activity in a respiratory syncytial virus challenge study. *N Engl J Med.* 2014;371(8):711-722.
60. Diaz MH, Benitez AJ, Cross KE, et al. Molecular detection and characterization of *Mycoplasma pneumoniae* among patients hospitalized with community-acquired pneumonia in the United States. *Open Forum Infect Dis.* 2015;2(3):ofv106.
62. Don M, Valent F, Korppi M, et al. Efficacy of serum procalcitonin in evaluating severity of community-acquired pneumonia in childhood. *Scand J Infect Dis.* 2007;39(2):129-137.
65. Dowell SF, Kupronis BA, Zell ER, et al. Mortality from pneumonia in children in the United States, 1939 through 1996. *N Engl J Med.* 2000;342(19):1399-1407.
75. Flood RG, Badik J, Aronoff SC. The utility of serum C-reactive protein in differentiating bacterial from nonbacterial pneumonia in children: a meta-analysis of 1230 children. *Pediatr Infect Dis J.* 2008;27(2):95-99.
77. Fry AM, Goswami D, Nahar K, et al. Efficacy of oseltamivir treatment started within 5 days of symptom onset to reduce influenza illness duration and virus shedding in an urban setting in Bangladesh: a randomised placebo-controlled trial. *Lancet Infect Dis.* 2014;14(2):109-118.
79. Galetto-Lacour A, Alcoba G, Posfay-Barbe KM, et al. Elevated inflammatory markers combined with positive pneumococcal urinary antigen are a good predictor of pneumococcal community-acquired pneumonia in children. *Pediatr Infect Dis J.* 2013;32(11):1175-1179.
84. Gollomp K, Rankin SC, White C, et al. Broad-range bacterial polymerase chain reaction in the microbiologic diagnosis of complicated pneumonia. *J Hosp Med.* 2012;7(1):8-13.
85. Greenberg D, Givon-Lavi N, Ben-Shimol S, et al. Impact of PCV7/PCV13 introduction on community-acquired alveolar pneumonia in children <5 years. *Vaccine.* 2015;33(36):4623-4629.
86. Griffin MR, Mitchel E, Moore MR, et al. Declines in pneumonia hospitalizations of children aged <2 years associated with the use of pneumococcal conjugate vaccines - Tennessee, 1998–2012. *MMWR Morb Mortal Wkly Rep.* 2014;63(44): 995-998.
87. Griffin MR, Zhu Y, Moore MR, et al. U.S. hospitalizations for pneumonia after a decade of pneumococcal vaccination. *N Engl J Med.* 2013;369(2):155-163.
88. Grijalva CG, Nuorti JP, Arbogast PG, et al. Decline in pneumonia admissions after routine childhood immunisation with pneumococcal conjugate vaccine in the USA: a time-series analysis. *Lancet.* 2007;369(9568):1179-1186.
91. Halasa NB, Grijalva CG, Arbogast PG, et al. Nearly complete elimination of the 7-valent pneumococcal conjugate vaccine serotypes in Tennessee. *Pediatr Infect Dis J.* 2013;32(6):604-609.
95. Heine D, Cochran C, Moore M, et al. The prevalence of bacteremia in pediatric patients with community-acquired pneumonia: guidelines to reduce the frequency of obtaining blood cultures. *Hosp Pediatr.* 2013;3(2):92-96.
97. Heneghan CJ, Onakpoya I, Thompson M, et al. Zanamivir for influenza in adults and children: systematic review of clinical study reports and summary of regulatory comments. *BMJ.* 2014;348:g2547.
101. Iroh Tam PY, Bernstein E, Ma X, et al. Blood culture in evaluation of pediatric community-acquired pneumonia: a systematic review and meta-analysis. *Hosp Pediatr.* 2015;5(6):324-336.
103. Jain S, Williams DJ, Arnold SR, et al. Community-acquired pneumonia requiring hospitalization among U.S. children. *N Engl J Med.* 2015;372(9):835-845.
105. Jefferson T, Jones M, Doshi P, et al. Oseltamivir for influenza in adults and children: systematic review of clinical study reports and summary of regulatory comments. *BMJ.* 2014;348:g2545.
108. Kaplan SL, Barson WJ, Lin PL, et al. Early trends for invasive pneumococcal infections in children after the introduction of the 13-valent pneumococcal conjugate vaccine. *Pediatr Infect Dis J.* 2013;32(3):203-207.
109. Kaplan SL, Center KJ, Barson WJ, et al. Multicenter surveillance of *Streptococcus pneumoniae* isolates from middle ear and mastoid cultures in the 13-valent pneumococcal conjugate vaccine era. *Clin Infect Dis.* 2015;60(9):1339-1345.
111. Kelly MS, Wirth KE, Steenhoff AP, et al. Treatment failures and excess mortality among HIV-exposed, uninfected children with pneumonia. *J Pediatric Infect Dis Soc.* 2015;4(4):e117-e126.
112. Keren R, Luan X, Localio R, et al. Prioritization of comparative effectiveness research topics in hospital pediatrics. *Arch Pediatr Adolesc Med.* 2012;166(12):1155-1164.
115. Kochanek KD, Murphy SL, Xu J, et al. Mortality in the United States, 2013. *NCHS Data Brief.* 2014;(178):1-8.
117. Korppi M, Heiskanen-Kosma T, Leinonen M. White blood cells, C-reactive protein and erythrocyte sedimentation rate in pneumococcal pneumonia in children. *Eur Respir J.* 1997;10(5):1125-1129.
118. Korppi M, Remes S. Serum procalcitonin in pneumococcal pneumonia in children. *Eur Respir J.* 2001;17(4):623-627.
119. Kronman MP, Hersh AL, Feng R, et al. Ambulatory visit rates and antibiotic prescribing for children with pneumonia, 1994–2007. *Pediatrics.* 2011;127(3):411-418.

129. Lee GE, Lorch SA, Sheffler-Collins S, et al. National hospitalization trends for pediatric pneumonia and associated complications. *Pediatrics.* 2010;126(2):204-213.
134. Louie JK, Yang S, Samuel MC, et al. Neuraminidase inhibitors for critically ill children with influenza. *Pediatrics.* 2013;132(6):e1539-e1545.
143. McCullers JA. The co-pathogenesis of influenza viruses with bacteria in the lung. *Nat Rev Microbiol.* 2014;12(4):252-262.
146. McCulloh RJ, Koster MP, Yin DE, et al. Evaluating the use of blood cultures in the management of children hospitalized for community-acquired pneumonia. *PLoS ONE.* 2015;10(2):e0117462.
156. Murtagh Kurowski E, Shah SS, Thomson J, et al. Improvement methodology increases guideline recommended blood cultures in children with pneumonia. *Pediatrics.* 2015;135(4):e1052-e1059.
157. Muthuri SG, Venkatesan S, Myles PR, et al. Effectiveness of neuraminidase inhibitors in reducing mortality in patients admitted to hospital with influenza A H1N1pdm09 virus infection: a meta-analysis of individual participant data. *Lancet Respir Med.* 2014;2(5):395-404.
158. Myers AL, Hall M, Williams DJ, et al. Prevalence of bacteremia in hospitalized pediatric patients with community-acquired pneumonia. *Pediatr Infect Dis J.* 2013;32(7):736-740.
159. Nascimento-Carvalho CM, Cardoso MR, Barral A, et al. Procalcitonin is useful in identifying bacteraemia among children with pneumonia. *Scand J Infect Dis.* 2010;42(9):644-649.
161. Newman RE, Hedican EB, Herigon JC, et al. Impact of a guideline on management of children hospitalized with community-acquired pneumonia. *Pediatrics.* 2012;129(3):e597-e604.
173. Queen MA, Myers AL, Hall M, et al. Comparative effectiveness of empiric antibiotics for community-acquired pneumonia. *Pediatrics.* 2014;133(1):e23-e29.
175. Ruggiero P, McMillen T, Tang YW, et al. Evaluation of the BioFire FilmArray respiratory panel and the GenMark eSensor respiratory viral panel on lower respiratory tract specimens. *J Clin Microbiol.* 2014;52(1):288-290.
178. Sarda Sanchez M, Hernandez JC, Hernandez-Bou S, et al. Pro-adrenomedullin usefulness in the management of children with community-acquired pneumonia, a preliminary prospective observational study. *BMC Res Notes.* 2012;5:363.
182. Shah SS, Dugan MH, Bell LM, et al. Blood cultures in the emergency department evaluation of childhood pneumonia. *Pediatr Infect Dis J.* 2011;30(6):475-479.
187. Spuesens EB, Fraaij PL, Visser EG, et al. Carriage of *Mycoplasma pneumoniae* in the upper respiratory tract of symptomatic and asymptomatic children: an observational study. *PLoS Med.* 2013;10(5):e1001444.
188. Steenhoff AP, Josephs JS, Rutstein RM, et al. Incidence of and risk factors for community acquired pneumonia in US HIV-infected children, 2000–2005. *AIDS.* 2011;25(5):717-720.
190. Stockmann C, Ampofo K, Pavia AT, et al. Comparative effectiveness of oral versus outpatient parenteral antibiotic therapy for empyema. *Hosp Pediatr.* 2015;5(12):605-612.
192. Sullivan KV, Turner NN, Roundtree SS, et al. Rapid detection of Gram-positive organisms by use of the Verigene Gram-positive blood culture nucleic acid test and the BacT/Alert Pediatric FAN system in a multicenter pediatric evaluation. *J Clin Microbiol.* 2013;51(11):3579-3584.
193. Taffarel P, Bonetto G, Penazzi M, et al. Severe *Staphylococcus aureus* infection in three pediatric intensive care units: analysis of cases of necrotizing pneumonia. *Arch Argent Pediatr.* 2014;112(2):163-168.
197. Thomson J, Ambroggio L, Murtagh Kurowski E, et al. Hospital outcomes associated with guideline-recommended antibiotic therapy for pediatric pneumonia. *J Hosp Med.* 2015;10(1):13-18.
201. Toikka P, Irjala K, Juven T, et al. Serum procalcitonin, C-reactive protein and interleukin-6 for distinguishing bacterial and viral pneumonia in children. *Pediatr Infect Dis J.* 2000;19(7):598-602.
206. Viasus D, Pano-Pardo JR, Pachon J, et al. Timing of oseltamivir administration and outcomes in hospitalized adults with pandemic 2009 influenza A(H1N1) virus infection. *Chest.* 2011;140(4):1025-1032.
208. Wang K, Gill P, Perera R, et al. Clinical symptoms and signs for the diagnosis of *Mycoplasma pneumoniae* in children and adolescents with community-acquired pneumonia. *Cochrane Database Syst Rev.* 2012;(10):CD009175.
214. Werno AM, Anderson TP, Jennings LC, et al. Human metapneumovirus in children with bronchiolitis or pneumonia in New Zealand. *J Paediatr Child Health.* 2004;40(9-10):549-551.
215. Williams DJ, Hall M, Brogan TV, et al. Influenza coinfection and outcomes in children with complicated pneumonia. *Arch Pediatr Adolesc Med.* 2011;165(6):506-512.
216. Williams DJ, Hall M, Shah SS, et al. Narrow vs broad-spectrum antimicrobial therapy for children hospitalized with pneumonia. *Pediatrics.* 2013;132(5):e1141-e1148.

The full reference list for this chapter is available at ExpertConsult.com.

23 Empyema and Lung Abscess

J. Gary Wheeler • Richard F. Jacobs

Most episodes of pneumonia resolve spontaneously or with limited medical therapy. Certain groups, those with underlying diseases, those with anatomic or functional abnormalities, or immunocompromised patients, are more prone to complications, but the normal host is not spared. The most concerning are those who require surgical intervention or prolonged therapy. Guideline development has provided effective management options.[16] This chapter is divided into discussions of empyema, lung abscess, and other complications (Box 23.1).

EMPYEMA

Collections of fluid in the pleural space have been described in the literature as transudates, pleural effusions, exudates, purulent pleurisy, parapneumonic effusions, empyema, and complicated empyema. A great deal of inexactitude exists in the use of these terms, and comparing methods of diagnosis and management from one study to another is difficult. The term *transudative pleural effusion* refers to fluid in the pleural space that is a nonpurulent effusion and typically nonpneumonic in origin. The term *purulent effusions* refers to effusions that are more cellular (exudative) and typically pneumonic in origin. The term *empyema* describes purulent effusions with chemical or microbial evidence of a severe process requiring drainage. *Complicated empyema* describes the processes associated with loculations or a fibropurulent rind requiring aggressive manipulations for cure. *Parapneumonic effusion* is a general term referring to any pleural exudative process resulting from an inflammatory process in the lung. Although these definitions are arbitrary and the literature is inconsistent in the use of these terms, a standard approach to the classification of these four types of effusions and their management has evolved.

The first description of parapneumonic infection is attributed to Hippocrates, who in the 4th century BCE advocated incision and drainage of empyema 2 weeks after the onset of symptoms. Since then, the physiology and microbiology of effusions have been described, and parapneumonic diseases and the management of fluid collections of the pleural space have been defined. In most cases, the directions of Hippocrates still are relevant: "set him upon a stool, which is not wobbly; someone should hold his hands, then shake him by the shoulders and listen to see on which side a noise is heard. And right at this place—preferably on the left—make an incision, and then it produces death more rarely."[97]

This description of open drainage to normal atmospheric pressures was recognized to be associated with significant mortality rates from hemodynamic instability in 1918, when the Empyema Commission of the United States Army recommended that the practice be abandoned[96];

BOX 23.1 Major Complications of Pneumonia

Abscess
Apnea or respiratory failure
Acute respiratory distress syndrome
Atelectasis
Bacteremia and sepsis
Bronchopulmonary fistula
Dissemination (skin, solid organs, joints, central nervous system)
Empyema
Hilar adenopathy
Infarction
Necrotizing pneumonia
Pericardial effusion
Pleural effusion
Pneumothorax
Pneumatocele
Recurrent pneumonia
Pneumothorax
Pericardial effusion

thereafter, closed-tube drainage was introduced and mortality rates decreased. Developments in radiology, antimicrobials, and surgery resulted in further improvements in care. Today the major cause of mortality is related to the underlying disease because the management of parapneumonic effusions in children is largely successful and without residual morbidity. The physician must understand the risks for development of pleural effusion and empyema and indications for thoracentesis, the implications of the results of pleural fluid studies, and the optimal medical and surgical management of the effusions and empyema.

Epidemiology

Parapneumonic effusions are known and expected complications in children with respiratory tract infections. The frequency of effusions may be up to 20% of patients with viral or mycoplasmal pneumonia[45,53,136] and 75% of patients with proven *Staphylococcus aureus* pneumonia.[9] Empyema has been reported to occur in 6.3 to 23 per 1000 admissions of children.[106,141] Reports before the introduction of the 13-valent pneumococcal conjugate vaccine suggested rates were increasing.[14,22,134,141]

Pathophysiology

The pleurae are mesodermally derived tissues approximately 30 to 40 μm thick and permeable to liquid and gas.[13,84] The parietal pleurae, which adhere to the chest wall, are fed from the intrathoracic and superior phrenic arteries and have sensory innervation. The visceral pleurae are splanchnic in origin, with blood flow from the pulmonic and pericardiophrenic arteries and no sensory innervation.

Parietal lymphatics absorb most of the excess fluids in pathologic situations and play an important role in normal physiology as well, removing 250 to 500 mL/day in adults.[150] They are the only mechanism for absorbing cells and other debris from the pleura.

The *raison d'être* of the pleural space is unknown. Some mammals do not have a pleural space.[164] In the normal situation, pleural fluid in small amounts is a necessary requirement for optimal lubrication of the pleural space and for mechanical coupling of the lung and chest wall.[84] The accumulation of excess fluid (i.e., effusion) occurs in a limited set of circumstances, through excess production or deficient absorption. Increased production occurs when vessels are leaky (e.g., in septic shock) or active secretion of fluid with mesothelial inflammation (e.g., pleural infection) is present. Decreased absorption occurs with decreased oncotic pressure (e.g., nephrosis), increased pulmonary hydrostatic pressure (e.g., congestive heart failure), or lymphatic obstruction (e.g., malignancy).[167]

The mechanisms behind pleural effusions may vary among different infectious diseases. Effusion can be a "sympathetic" pleural response to a bacterial infection in the lung associated with inflammatory cytokines and altered venous or lymphatic drainage because of local edema. Direct or hematogenous extension of a bacterial process can occur in the pleura. *Mycoplasma* is particularly pathogenic in patients with sickle-cell disease, presumably because of pulmonary sludging, which increases pulmonic venous drainage pressures and results in accumulation of effusions. In pneumococcal disease, effusions often develop several days after the acute infection, when bacteria no longer can be recovered. These effusions may be related to immune complex disease.[19] In patients with tuberculosis, the most common cause of pleural effusions is thought to be the rupture of an old granuloma into the pleural space, with a hypersensitivity response similar to the skin test response,[20] which partly explains the low yield in cultures.

After an inflammatory process is initiated, it tends to progress through three classic stages. The first, defined as a *purulent effusion,* is the acute exudative stage, with a thin pleural exudate characterized by normal glucose, lactate dehydrogenase (LDH), and pH. The second transitional fibropurulent stage, categorized as *empyema,* is characterized by turbid fluid, decreased glucose concentration (<60 mg/dL) and pH (7.2 to 7.35), and elevated LDH (>200 U/L). The third chronic organizing stage is notable for a very low pH (<7.2) and glucose level (<40 mg/dL), LDH concentration greater than 1000 U/L, and development of loculations and peel. This fluid is found in patients with *complicated empyema.* Intervening early (<4 days) before the organizational stages of disease has been proposed to lead to a better prognosis.[71] However a recent review concludes that, in the modern era, these data correlate poorly with management strategies and may not carry predictive weight.[68]

Analysis of the pleural fluid is most helpful when the underlying disease is unknown or when a primary pulmonic process is suspected. When patients have effusions caused by hydrostatic imbalance, the effusion is a transudate. Its protein and cell count do not exceed the range of normal pleural fluid (5000 cells/mm^3 and <2 g of protein).[9,150] Patients who have an active inflammatory process may have an exudate, defined by excess protein and cells. In children, the most common cause of exudative pleural processes is pneumonia. In adults, most pleural effusions are related to congestive heart failure or malignancy,[58,91] but pneumonia is the most common cause of empyema.[122] Table 23.1 summarizes the general differences among pleural effusions.

Box 23.2 lists causes of effusions. Some of these causes, particularly iatrogenic causes, such as invasive procedures and drugs, are important to consider in the differential diagnosis of a difficult case. Others are associated with specific syndromes, such as acute respiratory distress syndrome[154] and yellow nail lymphedema syndrome.[66,158] Motor vehicle accidents have been identified as a common cause of serosanguineous effusions when disruption of normal mechanical lung function and hematoma occur.[132]

Microbiology

Among children with parapneumonic effusions, studies continue to evolve regarding the frequency with which effusions occur and how many are associated with particular microbes. Although respiratory viruses infrequently cause symptomatic effusions, the sheer number of cases and the presence of asymptomatic cases likely would implicate viral infection as the most common cause. Definite viral disease enhanced by molecular diagnosis has been commonly associated with rhinovirus, RSV, influenza, enterovirus, cytomegalovirus, Epstein-Barr virus, measles, and adenovirus but co-infection of bacterial and viral species is also found.[48,49,73,105,111] Other pathogens, such as *Mycoplasma* and *Chlamydia,* are more difficult to diagnose but may account for a significant number of pneumonic infections in older children and adolescents.[45,49] Viral, mycoplasmal, and chlamydial organisms uncommonly are identified in patients with effusions requiring intervention.

The bacteriology of empyema is constantly changing. Several past articles have established the role of various bacterial pathogens in childhood effusions.[30] A study of 227 children by Freij and colleagues[48] published in 1984 found *S. aureus* (29%), *Streptococcus pneumoniae* (22%), and *Haemophilus influenzae* (18%) to be the three most frequent causes of parapneumonic effusions. Subsequent studies show that the frequency of these pathogens has been affected by vaccine[1,4,21,151] and antibiotic use. Pathogen frequency in different eras is shown in Table 23.2. *H. influenzae* and *S. pneumoniae* vaccines have led to a decreased incidence of vaccine-specific strains as a cause of empyema,[4] whereas

TABLE 23.1 **Characteristics of Pleural Effusions**

Characteristics	Transudative	Purulent Effusion	Empyema	Complicated Empyema
Appearance	Serous	Thin exudate	Turbid	Thick pus
Mean WBC	1000	5300	25,500	55,000
PMN (%)	50	>90	>95	>95
Protein (fluid/serum ratio)	<0.5	>0.5	>0.5	>0.5
LDH (fluid/serum ratio)	<0.6	>0.6	>0.6	>0.6
LDH (IU/L)		>200	>200	>1000
Glucose (mg/dL)	>60	<60	<60	<40
pH[a]	7.4–7.5	7.35–7.45	7.2–7.35	<7.2
Imaging	Fluid	Fluid	Fluid	Loculations, thick peel, scoliosis

[a]Should be examined immediately or stored at 0°C (32°F).
LDH, Lactate dehydrogenase; *PMN,* polymorphonuclear neutrophils; *WBC,* white blood cell count.

BOX 23.2 **Causes of Pleural Effusion**

Capillary leak
- Sepsis syndrome
- Vasculitis associated with immune complex disease
- Connective tissue diseases
- Inflammatory bowel disease
- Malignancy (lymphoreticular, sarcoma, neuroblastoma)
- Toxins (e.g., TSST-1)
- Drugs (amiodarone, bleomycin, isoniazid, methotrexate, nitrofurantoin, phenytoin)
- Myxedema
- Trauma

Increased hydrostatic pressure
- Congestive heart failure
- Sickle-cell disease
- Pulmonary venous hypertension
- Superior vena cava syndrome
- Pregnancy

Decreased oncotic pressure
- Nephrosis
- Cirrhosis
- Protein malnutrition

Obstructed lymphatics
- Congenital lymphangiectasia
- Yellow nail syndrome
- Radiation injury
- Neoplasia (metastatic disease)

Pleural inflammation
- Pneumonia
- Lung abscess with pleural fistula
- Pleural infection (e.g., tuberculosis)
- Esophageal rupture
- Pancreatitis

Iatrogenic
- Drugs
- Central line misplacement

TSST-1, Toxic shock syndrome toxin–1.

methicillin-resistant *S. aureus* (MRSA) has emerged as a frequent cause of community-acquired disease, with rates in Texas doubling from 2001 to 2009.[25,141] Among cases of *S. pneumoniae* infections, nonvaccine strains are increasing in number and severity.[21,40,47,147] Recent studies using a U.S. national hospital discharge database suggest that *S. pneumoniae* remains the most common etiology of bacterial empyema.[52] Certain groups of children (e.g., neonates,[48] immunocompromised hosts, patients with preexisting chest tubes that become infected with nosocomial pathogens, patients with a ruptured viscus, and patients with foreign body aspiration) are at higher risk for acquiring gram-negative infections.[14] Some pathogens seem to produce empyema at very high rates such as *S. aureus* and the *Streptococcus milleri* group.[25,83]

Administration of antibiotics before the diagnosis of empyema is made influences the recovery of organisms. Reports suggest 43% to 61% fewer positive cultures.[10,63] Pretreatment with antibiotics may be associated with a decrease in the number of positive blood cultures and in the number of patients from whom *S. pneumoniae* isolates are recovered.[122]

Anaerobes were sought carefully by Brook and Frazier,[18] who found them infrequently in patients younger than 6 years of age. The anaerobes rarely were found in patients with primary pneumonia, occurring most often in patients with lung abscess and aspiration pneumonia.[18] In older patients (7 to 17 years old), anaerobes were recovered as isolated pathogens in 44% of cases.[18] Virtually every bacterial organism has been associated with pleural effusion at one time or another. *Brucella,*[75] *Francisella tularensis,*[133] and *Yersinia enterocolitica*[72] may be associated with the development of pleural effusions. The diagnosis in such cases often is suggested by a unique history in the patient.

Mycobacterial effusions are uncommon in U.S. children but are well described. In four published reviews, only two patients (from Nigeria) were reported to have *Mycobacterium tuberculosis.*[48,63,98,105] In a series of 303 children younger than 2 years of age with tuberculosis, 3.3% had an effusion.[60] In adolescents with tuberculosis, the incidence of effusion likely approximates that of adult disease. In one series of adult patients with primary tuberculous disease, pleural effusion occurred in 29% of cases.[31] In another adult series, primarily of reactivation disease, pleural effusion occurred in 1% of the patients. Whether coinfection with human immunodeficiency virus (HIV) is increasing the incidence of effusion is controversial.[44]

Histoplasmosis has been associated with pleural effusion in 0% to 6% of childhood histoplasmosis cases.[124] Blastomycosis has been associated with pleural effusions in 0% to 40% of cases.[123,150] Effusions resulting from other fungi (e.g., *Coccidioides, Aspergillus*) have been described.[96] Parasitic diseases manifesting with effusions are uncommon but are found in patients with *Entamoeba histolytica* disease, most often from rupture of a hepatic abscess into the pleural space.[96] Echinococcal disease also has been reported.[46]

Pleural effusion associated with adult HIV infection has been reported in 14.6% of hospital admissions in one series in which 67 of 160 cases were infectious. Of those cases, 50 were associated with bacterial pneumonia, 10 with tuberculosis, and 5 with *Pneumocystis jiroveci* pneumonia.[2] Another report on patients infected with HIV suggested that empyema was seen primarily in patients with intravenous drug abuse.[62] We have not seen empyema in our pediatric HIV-infected patients, perhaps because of the more recent use of more effective antiretroviral therapy.

Drug resistance in community-acquired pneumonia complicates the management of parapneumonic effusions. Intermediate or fully resistant *S. pneumoniae* was found in 12.8% and 10.1% of isolates in

TABLE 23.2 **Percentage of Pathogens Recovered in Purulent Effusions From Children**

Site/Years (No. Patients)	*Staphylococcus aureus*	*Streptococcus pneumoniae*	*Haemophilus influenzae*	Other Pathogens	Sterile	Reference
Dallas/1964–82 (227)	29	22	18	8	24	48
Nashville/1977–89 (61)	11	34	3	11	39	63
Washington, DC/1973–85 (33)	15	12	21	52	Not reported	76
Israel/1972–81 (37)	14	41	Not reported	35	11	106
Dallas/1992–98 (135)	8	32	1	13	46	39
Houston/2001–02 (47)	19	9	Not reported	4	68	141
Australia/2007–09[a] (145)	9	51	3	2	35	151

[a]Polymerase chain reaction results only.

a study from multiple U.S. pediatric centers from 1993 to 2000; 7.5% were cephalosporin resistant.[155] Recent studies of nasal colonization in Israeli infants show that, post introduction of PCV13, the number of new resistant isolates has decreased,[37] as noted in other countries. A 2012–13 U.S. study in middle ear isolates showed 33% nonsusceptible strains, not a change from prior studies.[99] MRSA is a growing concern in empyema. Reports since 2000 have shown that 22% to 78% of isolates of *S. aureus* were methicillin resistant, with many being community acquired.[25,67]

Diagnosis

Clinical Presentation

Symptoms most specific for parapneumonic processes are dyspnea and pleuritic pain. Dyspnea occurs when the volume of the effusion mechanically interferes with breathing or when pain prevents adequate gas exchange. Pain occurs with irritation of the parietal pleura and on inspiration (i.e., pleurisy). Fever is generated by the inflammatory response and pathogen-specific components (e.g., lipopolysaccharide, toxins). With an acute bacterial process, the fever can be high and hectic, mimicking the fever that occurs with an abscess. Patients in the chronic organizational phase generally have less fever. Cough and malaise are secondary symptoms. Hemoptysis and purulent sputum also may occur. The onset of symptoms of a purulent effusion may be delayed in time and distinct from the symptoms found at the onset of the pneumonia in older children; infants usually have no symptom-free period[20]; in the early phases of effusions, the patient may have no symptoms.

The physical examination usually is revealing. The child is tachypneic in more than 70% of cases, but breathing is shallow as a result of the child's attempt to minimize pain. Fever and cough usually occur in more than 90% of patients with purulent effusions.[98] The patient may appear toxic, with acute infection. Patients often posture toward the affected side. Classically, auscultation reveals a decrease in breath sounds and occasionally detects a pleural rub, but pleural rubs often are absent in a very young child. Rales from an associated pneumonia may be heard. Depending on the stage of the process, percussion may reveal a level of dullness associated with free-flowing effusion. As the process organizes, it may be less evident. Empyemas can erode through the chest wall into the subcutaneous tissue (i.e., empyema necessitatis) or into a bronchus (i.e., bronchopleural fistula).

Imaging

The diagnosis most often is made by radiographic examination of the chest. Consolidation of a lobe of the lung is present, with an effusion obscuring the diaphragm. A standard posteroanterior standing view reveals blunting of the costal diaphragmatic gutter. As fluid tracks along the lateral and posterior chest wall, a meniscus configuration is seen. Distinguishing it from pleural thickening may be difficult, and in such cases, a decubitus or cross-table view of the chest allows free-flowing fluid to layer out on the dependent chest wall. In older children and adults, a decubitus layer of fluid of more than 10 mm is considered a sufficient volume of fluid to attempt to extract by thoracentesis.[16,90] With large volumes of fluid (>1000 mL),[135] compression of the lung and shift of the trachea away from the effusion (Fig. 23.1) may occur. As an empyema develops and organizes, discrete pockets of fluid (i.e., loculations) may form within the pleural cavity (Fig. 23.1C). Occasionally, loculations are confused with lung abscess. Scoliosis also is well defined by the chest radiograph and occasionally is used as an indication for surgery.[63] The observation of an air-fluid level in the pleural space signifies that air has been generated in the pleural space by gas-forming organisms or has entered through a pneumothorax, perforated viscus, or bronchopleural fistula.

Ultrasonography has shown great utility in providing better guidance for thoracentesis of pleural fluid. It is noninvasive, without ionizing radiation, allows empyema to be defined by showing internal echoes and septations (Fig. 23.2),[142,168] and is the imaging mode of choice for most pleural effusions.[23,113] Transudates uniformly are anechoic, although approximately one-third of exudates also are anechoic.[168] Ultrasonography is not as precise as computed tomography (CT) in differentiating a lung abscess from an empyema. CT and magnetic resonance imaging (MRI) occasionally are required to distinguish parenchymal from pleural disease, identify a nonopaque foreign body, or locate a fistula. CT particularly is useful in a patient whose chest radiograph shows total opacification of the lung and thus is considered by some physicians the study of choice in this situation.[63] Ultrasound can have false-negative results, and CT can have false-positive findings on examination of pleural effusions. A recent review noted that ultrasound and CT were comparable in managing pediatric effusions.[68]

Pleural Fluid Analysis

Thoracentesis can play an important role in the management of parapneumonic effusions.[33] Fluid should be obtained from the pleural cavity if the fluid is adequate in volume and anatomically accessible, if a microbial diagnosis has not been made or presumed, and if antibiotic therapy is intended or if pulmonary function is compromised by the effusion and imaging does not reveal evidence of organization to determine whether further intervention is necessary.

The volume and location of the fluid can be determined precisely by ultrasound examination. When a healthy child has a small pleural effusion, thoracentesis usually is not required because small effusions generally can resorb. Thoracentesis for microbiological diagnosis can often be avoided because a 10% to 50% chance of recovering the etiologic organism from blood cultures exists in empyema.[7,48] We suggest, however, that when the clinical presentation is atypical or a moderately sized effusion exists, thoracentesis usually is indicated to define the microbial process and choose an optimal antibiotic regimen. Atypical situations include a history of trauma, foreign body aspiration, prolonged or chronic disease, and underlying systemic diseases (e.g., congestive heart failure, malignancy).

In a classic article published in 1972, Light and associates[91] established the methodology by which transudates could be differentiated from exudates. Such criteria are valuable in determining whether antibiotic treatment is indicated, particularly in patients with underlying diseases that predispose them to sterile effusions but who may have a comorbid infectious condition. An exudate was defined by any of the following criteria: a fluid-to-serum protein ratio greater than 0.5, an LDH fluid-to-serum ratio greater than 0.6, a glucose concentration less than 50 mg/dL, or a pH less than 7.2. This study was based on the results from 150 adult patients, 103 of whom had exudates.[91] Modifications of Light's

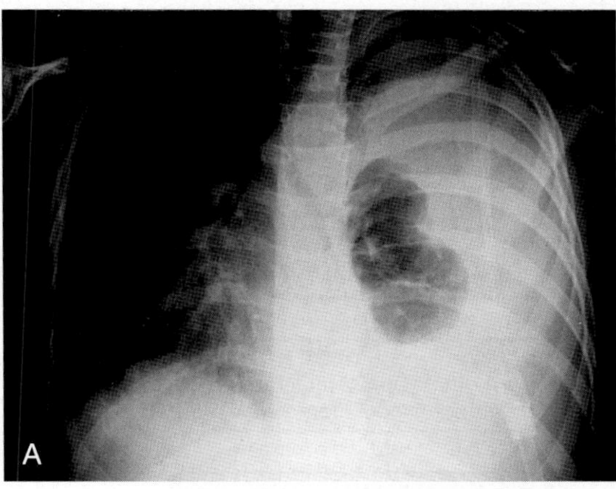

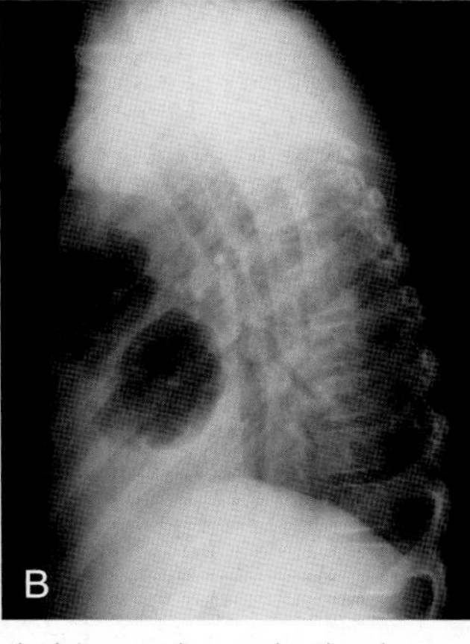

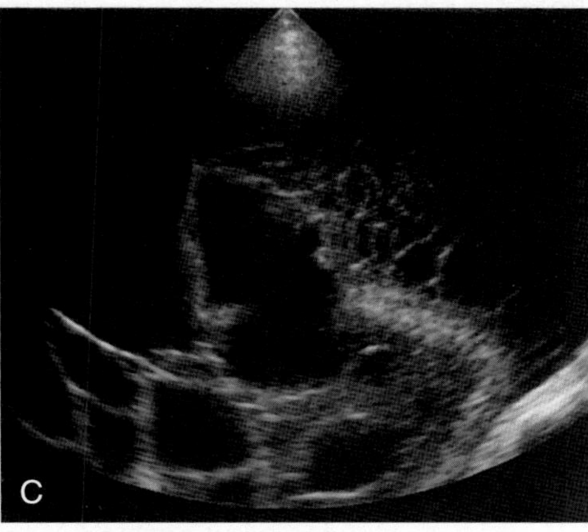

FIG. 23.1 (A–C) Chest radiograph and ultrasound examination images from a 7-year-old boy with a 5-day history of vomiting, diarrhea, and low-grade fever. He had a history of varicella 2 weeks earlier. The patient was hospitalized for dehydration and developed left-sided chest pain and a mild cough. Intravenous nafcillin was begun, but his condition deteriorated over the next 4 days, with an enlarging effusion and tracheal shift. (C) Loculations were found on ultrasound. He had a thoracotomy performed on day 6 with decortication and removal of a fibrinous rind. The patient was afebrile within 24 hours and received 1 week of intravenous antibiotics and 1 week of oral antibiotics. He was well on follow-up examination after discharge.

criteria have been made by reducing the LDH ratio threshold to 0.45.[61] A two-step process has been recommended to separate transudates from exudates using only the protein and LDH serum-to-fluid ratios in the initial evaluation. If a patient has an apparent exudate, additional studies, including cultures, stains, pH, and glucose, are indicated.[119]

The application of these criteria to children has received limited study. In one series of 61 children, patients who required chest tubes or decortication had a mean pleural fluid pH of 7.24 or 7.10 in contrast to children who were treated with antibiotics only (pH 7.35). The mean pleural fluid glucose concentration was 74 g/L in the group treated with antibiotics, 10 g/L in the group treated with chest tubes, and 24 g/L in the group treated by decortication.[63] Another more recent study confirmed that a pH less than 7.2 and low glucose concentration were predictors of reintervention.[107] The role of this analysis has been questioned, and new Infectious Diseases Society of America (IDSA) guidelines for children in 2011 do not recommend glucose, LDH, and pH studies because they rarely modify patient management.[16]

Standard Gram stain and bacterial culture (aerobic and anaerobic) are indicated when thoracentesis is performed in patients in whom diagnosis of infection is considered. The Gram stain often is positive in patients with bacterial infections and may be used to direct empiric therapy until culture or polymerase chain reaction (PCR) results are known. In one study of children, 12 of 54 sterile effusions from patients with negative blood cultures had a positive Gram stain.[48] Some experts consider that a positive Gram stain indicates a more severe process and that such patients are more likely to require more invasive surgical procedures.[20]

The total white blood cell count in empyema fluid can vary from 5000 to 625,000 cells/mm^3, with median values ranging from 5000 to 55,000 cells/mm^3.[48,63] Virtually all cells are neutrophils in bacterial infections. Marked eosinophilia may be seen in parasitic, fungal, tuberculous, or hypersensitivity disease and when blood is found in the pleural space.[20] Numerous small lymphocytes suggest malignancy, tularemia, or tuberculosis.[43,57,119,168] Other studies are required when the history suggests another underlying process. When tuberculosis is suspected by history, specific mycobacterial stains and cultures should be obtained. Identification of mycobacteria by stain and culture may be equivalent to the rate of identification of the disease process by pleural biopsy (approximately 25%).[112] Specific mycobacterial and fungal stains also should be obtained using a Ziehl-Neelsen/auramine stain and potassium hydroxide. Application of newer methods for diagnosis of pleural fluid, such as PCR, tuberculostearic acid by mass spectroscopy, and adenosine deaminase activity,[36] may be indicated. Assessment of children with interferon-γ releasing assays (IGRA) of blood specimens may not improve diagnosis of tuberculous effusions and should be used with caution for those under 5 years old.[101]

When malignancy or metastases are suspected, cytology is necessary.[57] Most effusions in children that prove to be malignant are of lymphoreticular origin. Amylase sometimes is measured and is elevated in cases of esophageal rupture, acute hemorrhagic pancreatitis, or pulmonary infarction.[89,135]

Molecular diagnostics is bringing promising advances to the bacteriologic diagnosis of empyema. PCR technology has been compared with routine culture and bacterial antigen and has shown increased sensitivity and good specificity for the diagnosis of *S. pneumoniae* with 16S rDNA or MRSA using the mec-300 gene probe.[40,134] In recently reported studies,[14,109] the sensitivity of PCR has been greater than 80%. Turnaround times can be quite rapid, exceeding traditional culture methods. PCR panels for bacterial antigens that are validated for empyema fluid are in advanced development and expected for clinical availability in the near future. The sensitivity of PCR for tuberculous effusions ranges from 20% to 81%, and specificity ranges from 78% to 100%.[44] New commercially available PCR cocktails for respiratory viruses are being widely utilized but because of expense are best reserved for difficult or critically ill patients.

Additional Diagnostic Studies

An intradermal test (PPD) or IGRA should be applied to any child with risk factors for tuberculosis with a parapneumonic effusion. One-third of patients with tuberculous effusions have a negative purified protein derivative skin test result.[12] Early morning gastric aspirates have been recommended if tuberculosis is suspected, but IGRAs are now approved for children as young as 5 years of age. Sensitivity and specificity remain problematic, however.[95,160] Bacterial blood cultures also are indicated because one-third of patients can have positive blood cultures and negative pleural fluid Gram stain and culture results.[48] Sputum is a less reliable source from which to determine the microbial cause of an effusion but may be helpful in an older patient with purulent sputum and a single predominant organism. Sputum can be diagnostic in older children with reactivation or cavitary tuberculosis and in cases of blastomycosis and histoplasmosis. Cold agglutinins, PCR, and serology for *Mycoplasma* may confirm the cause of a pleural effusion, although the nonspecificity of cold agglutinins and the delay in the increase in antibody titers render these data of marginal use in the acute management of the patient. Viral cultures are useful in only the more unusual cases and generally provide information that is not helpful in the initial

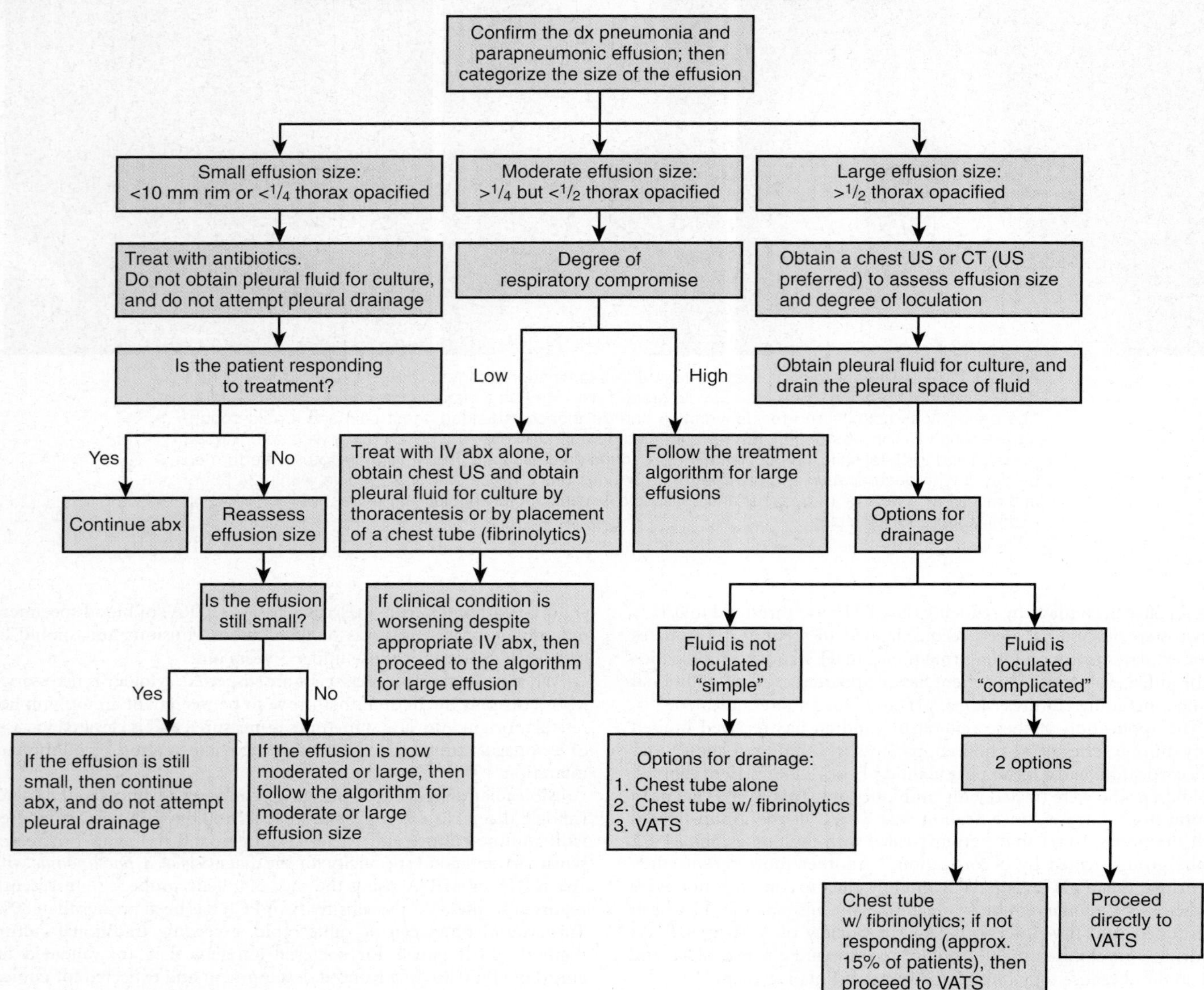

FIG. 23.2 Algorithm for the management of pneumonia with parapneumonic effusion from the Infectious Diseases Society of America guidelines. *abx,* Antibiotics; *CT,* computed tomography; *dx,* diagnosis; *IV,* intravenous; *US,* ultrasound; *VATS,* video-assisted thoracic surgery. (From Bradley JS, Byington CL, Shah SS, et al. The management of community-acquired pneumonia in infants and children older than 3 months of age: clinical practice guidelines by the Pediatric Infectious Diseases Society and the Infectious Diseases Society of America. *Clin Infect Dis.* 2011;53:e25–76.)

management of the patient. Rapid diagnostic antigen assays, such as the rapid tests for influenza A and B and other respiratory viruses, may be useful in defining the primary cause of respiratory disease but do not help exclude secondary bacterial pathogens causing pneumonia and a parapneumonic effusion. When other diseases, such as Wegener granulomatosis[8] and systemic lupus erythematosus, are suspected, disease-specific tests such as antineutrophil cytoplasmic antibody and antinucleic acid antibody are indicated.

Management

If a patient has an underlying disease process associated with pleural effusion and thoracentesis has excluded bacterial infection (e.g., normal protein and LDH fluid-to-serum ratio, normal glucose level, negative cultures, and Gram stain results), no further treatment is indicated other than treatment of the underlying disease and symptomatic drainage of large effusions. These patients continue to be at risk for developing infection of the effusion and may require repeat examination of pleural fluid later if infection is suggested clinically.

If a purulent effusion is suggested by imaging, thoracentesis, or surgical findings, empiric antibiotic therapy is indicated. Antibiotics should be adjusted with the availability of microbiological etiologies and antimicrobial susceptibilities. Pathogens of most importance are *S. pneumoniae, S. aureus,* and *Streptococcus pyogenes*. Empiric therapy choices are changing as drug resistance patterns continue to change, immunization against *H. influenzae* type b and *S. pneumoniae* has become widespread, and the ability to make a rapid diagnosis (e.g., PCR) improves. For mildly ill patients, amoxicillin orally or penicillin or ampicillin intravenously can be used. For patients who are moderately ill, unimmunized, or allergic to penicillin, or in whom *S. aureus* is suspected (because of past disease or presence of pneumatocele), clindamycin in combination with cefotaxime or ceftriaxone is used. Vancomycin is substituted for clindamycin in critically ill patients.

Imipenem-cilastatin, ticarcillin-clavulanate, imipenem-cilastatin, meropenem, and piperacillin-tazobactam are alternatives in nosocomial infections, gram-negative risk (neonates and postsurgical cases), or if anaerobes are considered, particularly if aspiration is thought to play a role, such as in patients with abnormal swallowing. Aminoglycosides are alternatives for proven gram-negative infections, and cefepime is helpful in nosocomial pneumonia and empyema because of its current efficacy for *Enterobacter* spp. In patients with renal failure or cephalosporin hypersensitivity, aztreonam is effective therapy for gram-negative infections. Ceftazidime or cefepime, broad-spectrum β-lactams with or without a β-lactamase inhibitor (i.e., ticarcillin-clavulanic acid, imipenem cilastatin, meropenem, or piperacillin-tazobactam) or aminoglycosides are indicated for *Pseudomonas* infection.

Surgical drainage is considered a crucial factor in resolving anaerobic infection. Clindamycin and metronidazole are effective, particularly when postsurgical infection or a ruptured gastrointestinal viscus is present. Upper respiratory tract anaerobes may be resistant to penicillins because of β-lactamase–producing oral flora (particularly *Prevotella* and *Porphyromonas* spp.).[18] In these situations, penicillin susceptibility should be documented before a penicillin is used as primary therapy.

Once a pathogen is isolated and susceptibility patterns are established, therapy may need to be modified. Past studies have suggested that resistant isolates of pneumococcus were treated effectively with parenteral penicillin in high doses.[17,18,85,116] Furthermore, in 2008, the Clinical Laboratory Standards Institute (CLSI) issued new standards for resistance. The net effect was to reduce the number of isolates in the community with any resistance from approximately 25% to 7%.[27] New guidelines for pediatrics now recommend amoxicillin orally or penicillin or ampicillin intravenously for *S. pneumoniae*–associated community-acquired pneumonia with a minimum inhibitory concentration (MIC) 2 μg/mL or less. When the pneumococcus is highly resistant to penicillin (>4 μg/mL), ceftriaxone is preferred, with levofloxacin, linezolid, clindamycin, and vancomycin considered alternatives.[16] New guidelines for management of MRSA were published by the IDSA in 2011.[92] These suggest that vancomycin is still the preferred treatment. The guidelines for adults suggest a non-vancomycin regimen for disease associated with a vancomycin MIC of greater than 2.0 μg/mL. A recent report notes, however, that a poor clinical outcome may be independent of antibiotic choice and directly related to an MIC of greater than 1.5 μg/mL.[65] Clindamycin or linezolid may be considered for treatment of MRSA but is discouraged as monotherapy if the patient is bacteremic or thrombosis is present. Clindamycin susceptibility should be determined because many MRSA and methicillin-susceptible *S. aureus* isolates are resistant to clindamycin.[140] Susceptibility should be confirmed with performance of a "D" test. Intravenous clindamycin can be switched to oral clindamycin later in the clinical course, offering a management advantage over vancomycin. Use of linezolid is limited at this time because of high cost and some side effects, such as neuropathy and visual changes, that may be hard to monitor in small children. Daptomycin is specifically avoided in the lung because of its inactivation by surfactant.

With appropriate antibiotic therapy, the duration of fever in uncomplicated cases of purulent effusions usually is less than 48 to 72 hours.[110] When fever persists beyond 72 hours, surgical or interventional radiologic drainage may be required. The duration of antibiotic therapy is based on the response of the patient to the medical and surgical therapy provided. In one series of pediatric patients, the total duration of parenteral antibiotic therapy for patients with severe pleural infections who did or did not have surgical drainage was comparable (approximately 12 days).[63] The duration of combined intravenous and oral therapy was 12 to 24 days in the study reported by Freij and associates,[48] with patients with *S. pneumoniae* infection receiving the shortest courses of antibiotic therapy and patients infected with *S. aureus* being treated for longer periods. The 2011 IDSA guidelines recommend treatment for a minimum of 10 days beyond the last febrile day.[16]

Drainage of the pleural space has been the standard treatment of parapneumonic effusions in four classes of patients: (1) patients in whom thick, purulent material is found at thoracentesis; (2) patients with a pleural fluid pH level less than 7.35 and glucose level less than 60 mg/dL; (3) patients for whom antibiotic therapy has not been associated with a timely clinical response (72 hours); and (4) patients in whom pulmonary function is compromised, as shown by severe hypoxemia or hypercapnia.[32] The chest tube is placed until minimal drainage is noted (usually <50 mL/day).[41] A recent small study has shown that smaller pigtail catheters may be less effective than traditional larger chest tubes in effectively draining effusions,[153] but further experience is needed.

When closed chest tube drainage is not associated with clinical improvement and defervescence, if the lung parenchyma is trapped by the fibrinopurulent peel or fever persists, video-assisted thoracoscopic surgery (VATS) or decortication may be required. If the pleural involvement is limited, a small incision (mini-thoracotomy) can be employed.[125] Ultrasonography, MRI, and CT are required to define these conditions. Decortication is rarely performed now but has shown comparable hospital length of stay to that with chest tube drainage with minimal morbidity.[50,63] Decortication seems to have an advantage in advanced disease in which fibrosis in the pleural cavity has resulted in a large peel.

VATS is done under general anesthesia, requiring two small incisions—one through the existing chest tube tract for a telescope and the second through which operating instruments are passed. This procedure allows adhesiolysis and debridement and should be performed before a thick peel develops. Proponents of VATS argue that a brief operative procedure and the attendant risks of anesthesia outweigh the child's discomfort during thoracentesis (and chest tube placement) and postoperatively. This argument has carried less weight over time as interventional radiology has stepped in to perform the tube placement under fluoroscopy and light anesthesia, thereby reducing patient discomfort. A definitive procedure is done during VATS, rather than running the risk of having to perform subsequent chest tube placements and thoracotomy. VATS tends to be the primary procedure in some facilities due to a tradition of practice, with some evidence for shorter length of stay.[74,76,138,139] Doski and colleagues[39] reported a series of 139 children who were studied from 1992 to 1998. By comparing historical cohorts, they showed a shorter length of stay (7 days vs. 11 and 12 days) for children who underwent VATS than for groups of children who had thoracentesis, chest tube drainage, or fibrinolytic therapy and rescue VATS for failure. Of 98 patients who received traditional therapy, 12 required thoracotomy, in contrast to none in the primary VATS group. A small, randomized study of 20 patients was conducted from 1994 to 1996 and showed that VATS was superior to chest tube drainage with fibrinolytic therapy. Compared with chest tube drainage with fibrinolytic therapy, VATS resulted in a higher primary success rate (91% vs. 44%), fewer hospital days (8.7 vs. 12.8 days), and lower costs (approximately $16,000 vs. $24,000).[162] Other studies have shown mixed results.[51,104]

The use of radiologist-directed thoracentesis with pigtail catheters (smaller bore than standard chest tubes) for drainage with fibrinolytic therapy was introduced as a way to reduce the number of operative procedures and achieve shorter hospital stays, and it has achieved these results in some early pediatric reports.[3,131] This approach should have value in patients with organizing pleural inflammation and inadequate drainage caused by loculations of pleural fluid without a peel.

Streptokinase was the first fibrinolytic used in children with pleural effusion as reported in 1993.[131] Urokinase is less expensive than streptokinase and has been used in children with minimal adverse effects but is not currently available in the United States.[59,77,130,152] In adults and children, these two agents seem to be equivalent.[7,15] The tissue-type plasminogen activator alteplase is the fibrinolytic therapy most commonly used at this time. It is less likely to promote allergic reactions and has a low risk for bleeding complications.[11] Early and contemporary reports have questioned the benefits of interventional radiologist-placed catheters with fibrinolytics for empyema.[129] A meta-analysis of eight evaluable reports from 2000 to 2004 of operative and nonoperative approaches to empyema suggested that the failure of primary therapy was intermediate for fibrinolytic therapy (9.4%), in contrast to simple chest tube drainage (23.6%) and either VATS (2.8%) or thoracotomy (3.1%).[6] A large retrospective review with multivariable analysis of 40 pediatric hospitals using the Pediatric Health Information Systems showed no difference in VATS, CT with fibrinolysis, CT without fibrinolysis, or thoracotomy for length of stay and only marginal differences in cost.

VATS was associated with fewer additional procedures.[144] Recent prospective studies have not shown a difference in hospital stay post intervention when comparing VATS versus tube drainage but did show increased cost.[127,149] Some emphasize the importance of early versus late operative strategies,[69] and another structured review determined that early operative procedures did shorten hospital stay.[138] Rarely are full thoracotomy and pneumonectomy required for severe pneumonic and parapneumonic disease.

The IDSA and Pediatric Infectious Diseases Society put forth consensus guidelines for clinicians for the management of pneumonia and effusions in 2011.[16] Fig. 23.2 is an algorithm from the guideline incorporating alternatives for the management of pleural collections. Other comparable guidelines exist,[68,79,120] but all emphasize the importance of local expertise and the emphasis on the individual circumstance of the patient.

In cases of chronic empyema, other approaches are used. A closed tube can be converted into an open drainage tube. This conversion is accomplished safely a minimum of 10 to 14 days into the course of an empyema when the visceral and parietal pleurae fuse, and a pneumothorax can be avoided safely.[96] Other options include open drainage by rib resection and creation of a pleural window. The window ultimately closes with lung expansion and granulation, with disappearance of the pleural space.

One frequent cause of bloody pleural effusions is motor vehicle accidents.[96,132] In one series of 100 children, 56% had pleural effusions associated with pulmonary contusions. They were treated with closed chest tube drainage, no antibiotics were used, and no infectious complications occurred.[132] Management of pleural hematoma secondary to trauma occasionally is complicated by infection because the bloody pleural fluid is an excellent growth medium. One study suggested that empyema is less common in posttraumatic effusion with closed chest tube drainage than in repeated thoracentesis.[161]

Prevention of empyema is theoretically improved by the use of vaccines against *S. pneumoniae,* the most common associated agent. One comprehensive study using national data showed an actual increase of 70% in empyema hospitalizations from 1997 to 2006, when the 7-valent pneumococcal vaccine was implemented.[87] At the same time, invasive pneumococcal disease rates decreased. After introduction of PCV13 in France, an overall 53% decrease in pleural effusions was noted.[4]

Prognosis and Long-Term Outcome

The long-term outcome of patients with effusions depends on the underlying cause. Patients with empyema or necrotizing pneumonia who previously were well recover satisfactorily in most cases.[137] Complications from closed chest tube drainage include bleeding, infection of the exit wound, bronchopleural fistula, and laceration of the lung. Because of these rare complications, chest tube placement, performed in the past by the pediatrician, now is delegated more frequently to the surgeon. Other rare complications, such as temporary paralysis of the diaphragm, have been reported.[106] In three retrospective reviews, the percentage of patients who required closed chest tube drainage or other surgical procedures ranged from 62% to 80%.[48,63,106] The rate of decortication ranged from 4% to 43%.[48,63] The immediate mortality rate for children in recent years has been 0% to 10.8%.[48,63,98,106] In one of these studies, the mortality rate was highest for children younger than 1 year old.[48] Studies conducted to evaluate long-term, specific pulmonary disability using pulmonary function tests and lung volumes have shown normalization of these study results over time.[48]

LUNG ABSCESS

A lung abscess is distinguished by liquefaction and destruction of parenchymal tissue, organization, and cavitation. Necrotizing pneumonia, which on imaging lacks the "rim" representing the organization of the abscess, has a different clinical course and management.[29] A lung abscess may erupt and form an adjacent empyema. Empyema is defined strictly by involvement of the pleural tissues, however.

In adults, lung abscess has historically been described as a disease of male alcoholics that was managed with surgery.[108] Lung abscess in children was recognized early on as having a different etiology and course than lung abscess in adults. As is true of many infectious diseases, it continues to change as the human host and the microbial environment change. The incidence of lung abscess has declined precipitously in the modern era. Smith[148] reported lung abscesses in 0.33% of pediatric admissions in 1934, and Emanuel and Shulman[42] reported a rate of 0.012% from 1985 to 1990. In major pediatric referral centers in Chicago, Houston, Dallas, and Montreal, the incidence of lung abscesses has ranged in the past 2 decades from 1.5 to 4.7 cases per year.[4,42,102,156] Many of these cases developed in compromised hosts.

Improvements in pediatric diagnosis and care have resulted in a decrease in the number of cases related to underlying diseases. The morbidity and mortality rates also have decreased with use of antibiotic therapy and modern critical care medicine. In 1920, Wessler and Schwarz reported a 33% mortality rate, with "invalidism" and hemiplegia occurring in another 27%.[165] The mortality rates in modern U.S. reports of lung abscess were 11% (1982 to 1993)[42] and 4% (1985 to 1990),[156] and 18.5% mortality was reported in Taiwan (1987 to 2003).[28]

Although lung abscesses occur in children of all ages, two studies have suggested that the trend is away from children younger than 5 years of age to an older population.[42,114] In other studies, the median age ranged from 7 to 9.5 years.[5,17,42,64,156] No consistent racial or sexual predisposition to this condition in children has been identified. In the 1950s, one series found boys to be more at risk than girls. Specific risk factors for development of lung abscess in pediatric patients include predisposition to aspiration, hematogenous spread, or compromised immunity.

Pathophysiology

Two main mechanisms explain formation of a lung abscess. The first mechanism is the introduction of pathogens directly into the air spaces, which typically results in solitary abscesses. The abscess typically follows aspiration, with a resultant neutrophilic reaction and necrosis. Lung abscesses complicated tonsillectomies in one-third of cases in a 1920 report.[165] The abscesses were theorized to result from aspiration during the operative procedure[148] and characteristically developed 13 to 14 days after the procedure.[165] Great improvements in modern pediatric anesthesia with careful efforts to prevent aspiration have rendered this complication uncommon today. Most lung abscesses related to aspiration are polymicrobial and include anaerobes. The prevalence of fluoride and the low incidence of dental disease in children may be additional factors for the reduced incidence of lung abscess in children, although aspiration pneumonia does occur in the absence of dental disease. Aspiration of a foreign body is a rarer trigger of abscess formation.[88]

The second mechanism in the formation of lung abscess is hematogenous spread. Hematogenous seeding of the lung can lead to an initial pneumonia that develops into an abscess with further organization and cavitation. Primary pneumonia rarely progresses to necrosis and abscess in modern times; this phenomenon is explained largely by the ready accessibility of antibiotics. Emboli from the venous circulation (i.e., septic thrombophlebitis) and right side of the heart (i.e., endocarditis) can cause single or multiple lung abscesses, which often are subpleural.[26] Infection in the head and neck area (e.g., Lemierre syndrome) also is a risk factor for vascular spread to the lung, with resultant lung abscess. Abscesses are found more often with sensitive tools, such as CT. Modern reviews of children suggest that single abscesses are found more frequently than multiple abscesses.[17,42,156]

A lung abscess tends to have irregular margins, with occasional bullae, and can dissect into adjacent tissues, such as the mediastinum, bronchi, and pleural space. If the abscess ruptures into a bronchus, air enters and an air-fluid level can be seen radiographically. Dissection into the pleural space creates a purulent effusion, with air noted only if an anaerobic process is present. Dissection into the mediastinum causes a widening of the mediastinum. Air is detected if communication occurs with a bronchus or in the presence of anaerobes.

Microscopically, a lung abscess is definable by a collection of necrotic material (i.e., highly neutrophilic inflammation); a surrounding irregular, fibrotic wall; and microvascular infarcts. Lymphocytes often are present and seem to play a regulatory role in the formation of the abscess.[145]

The role of preceding viral infection in undermining phagocytic host defenses is supported by the observations of preceding respiratory symptoms in patients with lung abscesses that manifest primarily in cold weather[5,42] and typically after well-defined viral illnesses, such as varicella, measles, and influenza.[86,148] The impact of chemotherapy on phagocytes also may explain the increased numbers of lung abscesses in patients with leukemia and other cancers.

On a macroscopic scale, lung abscesses tend to develop in all parts of the lung. If associated with aspiration, the anatomic site depends on whether the patient was supine or erect at the time of aspiration. Supine patients develop abscesses in the posterior upper and lower lobes, and erect patients develop infection in the middle and basilar lower lobes. Generally the tendency is for aspiration-related abscesses to develop more on the right side than on the left, presumably because of the more vertical anatomy of the right stem bronchus.[42]

Physicians have grouped lung abscesses into primary and secondary categories, presuming that primary and secondary abscesses have different microbiologic factors, management approaches, and outcomes. The arbitrary nature of this distinction is apparent when appreciating how much the microbiology, clinical course, management, and outcome of both conditions overlap. Primary abscesses occur in previously normal hosts without a history of trauma or aspiration of a foreign body. Secondary abscesses occur in the setting of underlying medical illnesses predisposing to infection, airway obstruction, embolization, or aspiration. In an earlier series, secondary abscesses were found more often in children younger than 1 year of age, but this difference was not corroborated in a later study.[42] Primary abscesses were found in 64% of patients in Chicago,[42] 33% in Houston,[156] 45% in Little Rock (1989–94) (unpublished data), 30% in Toronto (1956–65),[5] and 30% in Taiwan (1987–2003).[28]

In the modern era, lung abscess should trigger a search to exclude underlying factors that may have prognostic value and lead to treatment of the underlying disease. In children, a classic presentation would be any child with altered mental status, associated swallowing dysfunction, or both conditions. Foreign bodies can obstruct normal clearance of pathogens and precipitate the development of a lung abscess.[42,100] Obstruction predisposes to lung abscess rarely in children with metastatic disorders. Ineffective cough in patients with neurodegenerative or myopathic disorders is another risk factor for developing lung abscess, similar to that in an adult alcoholic. Patients with leukemia and patients who are receiving chemotherapy also are at increased risk. Occasionally a bronchogenic cyst can become infected and mimic a lung abscess. Tricuspid or pulmonary valve endocarditis in children with complicated congenital heart disease places them at risk for developing lung abscesses.

Immunodeficiency is another risk factor for development of a lung abscess. Patients with chronic granulomatous disease and hyperimmunoglobulin (Ig) E syndrome typically are found to have lung abscesses. Patients with hypogammaglobulinemia may develop abscesses, although bronchiectasis is the more characteristic finding. The same is true for patients with immotile cilia syndromes and cystic fibrosis, although in the latter group, large abscesses are uncommon.[24] Among pediatric patients, HIV-1 infection has not been reported as a risk factor in series from Chicago and Houston.[42,156] Studies by these authors and others of 46 reported cases of secondary lung abscesses showed associations as follows: neuropsychiatric cases (16); hematologic and oncologic disorders (11); primary pulmonary disease (8); immunodeficiency (4); congenital heart disease (2); and 1 each of solvent aspiration, foreign body aspiration, prematurity, chromosomal disorder, and endocrinopathy.[38]

Microbiology

The microbiology of lung abscesses is evolving as patients and antibiotics change. In the preantibiotic era, streptococci and *M. tuberculosis* were the most commonly reported causes of lung abscesses. After penicillin use began and tuberculosis skin testing, treatment, and control programs became widespread, staphylococci most frequently were recovered from lung abscesses. Development of better culture techniques also increased the identification of anaerobes in lung abscess material; in past eras, these organisms probably were present but not recovered. Anaerobes were suspected by the fetid odor of abscesses, the time course of postoperative aspiration infections, and Gram stains of tissue and pus, which showed fusobacteria and spirochetes.[148,165] Table 23.3 summarizes the microbiology of pediatric lung abscesses reported from 1976 to 2006.

TABLE 23.3 Microbiology of Pediatric Lung Abscess

Organism	No. Patients Reported
Staphylococcus aureus	22
Coagulase-negative staphylococci	2
Streptococcus pyogenes	5
Streptococcus pneumoniae	15
α-Hemolytic streptococcus	17
Other aerobic streptococci	7
Enterococci	2
Moraxella catarrhalis	3
Escherichia coli	10
Klebsiella	8
Pseudomonas	13
Serratia	1
Eikenella	1
Haemophilus	7
Other gram-negative organisms	2
Bacteroides	19
Peptostreptococcus	12
Other anaerobes	26
Candida	4
Aspergillus	5
Mucor	3
Mycobacterium tuberculosis	1
Total	185

Data from references 17, 42, 5, 24, 35, 70, 78, 86, 93, 100, 102, 114, 118, 146, 156, 159, 163.
These data were reported in the literature from 1976 to 2006. The isolates were recovered by direct aspiration of abscess contents, bronchoscopic aspiration, transtracheal aspiration, blood culture, or culture of surgical specimens. Data from case reports focused on procedures are included, whereas data from case reports focused on the organism recovered are not.

The primary role of anaerobes in lung abscesses has been assumed in aspiration pneumonias. Anaerobes are prominent in the oral cavity and have been recovered from the abscesses of patients with dental disease. Successful growth occurs when specimens are transported in a closed syringe, with culture inoculation beginning in less than 10 minutes.[18] In one study of developmentally delayed children with seizure disorders, poor dental care, and suspected aspiration, polymicrobial infections with aerobes were found in 9 of 10 transtracheal samples. An average of 6.2 isolates was recovered per patient. *Peptostreptococcus* and *Bacteroides* spp. were the anaerobes recovered most frequently.[17] In a larger group of 45 children, 15 of whom had primary abscesses, 14 had polymicrobial infections.[156] Older children with neurologic disorders were the primary patients with anaerobes in both studies. Anaerobes, *S. pneumoniae,* nontypeable *H. influenzae,* and *S. aureus* have been recovered from developmentally normal patients.[156] The role of tissue lysins and toxins depends on the pathogen and is thought to be crucial for the development of lung abscesses. In mixed infections, synergy probably occurs among the pathogens, as proposed by Smith in 1934.[148]

Nosocomial pathogens are becoming frequent causes of lung abscesses because of the increased numbers of patients with extended hospitalizations and use of advanced-generation antibiotics. The widespread use of third-generation cephalosporins has resulted in resistant *Enterobacter* spp. and other gram-negative organisms being recovered in secondary lung abscesses. In the report by Tan and associates,[156] fungal abscesses occurred in 6 of 34 cases and always were associated with debilitated, chronically hospitalized patients. Immunosuppression no doubt contributes to the recovery of other unsuspected organisms (e.g., *Neisseria mucosa, S. pneumoniae, Legionella, M. pneumoniae,* and *Citrobacter* spp.)[38,115] and underscores the value of obtaining specimens in chronically hospitalized patients, atypical cases, and patients not responding to empiric treatment.

Among otherwise normal hosts, tuberculosis can be a cause of single and multiple abscesses.[56] In patients with an international travel history, unusual pathogens such as parasites (e.g., hydatid cysts)[46] and regional bacteria (e.g., *Pseudomonas pseudomallei*) should be considered.

Rarely is sputum useful in defining the pathogens in a lung abscess because of three factors: (1) sputum typically is contaminated with abundant mouth flora; (2) if the lung abscess is not ruptured, no direct communication of the pathogens in the abscess occurs with the airway; and (3) sputum is difficult to obtain in preadolescent children. Obtaining cough cultures, performed by gagging a young child and culturing the coughed sputum collected on a swab before it can be swallowed, frequently is unsuccessful. A skilled clinician occasionally can acquire useful information, however.

Bronchoscopy is effective in recovering relevant organisms if the abscess has ruptured and has therapeutic value because it may assist in clearing secretions from the airway. It has been performed infrequently in pediatric practice in the past because of a lack of skilled personnel and pediatric equipment and fear of rupture of a large volume of purulent material into the airway. Rigid bronchoscopy rarely is used to drain the abscess, but, when performed, highly informative microbiologic information may be obtained. Transtracheal aspirates, likewise performed in few pediatric patients, have similar value. The upper airway frequently is colonized in debilitated patients, and microbiologic information obtained must be interpreted with care. Direct aspiration of the abscess, typically under CT or ultrasound guidance, is the most common way to provide microbiologic data and plan antimicrobial therapy. Aspiration may have therapeutic value in decompressing the abscess.

Clinical Features

Most patients with lung abscesses have had symptoms for 1 to 3 weeks before being hospitalized.[42] Fever is reported to be associated with 100% of primary abscesses[42] and 84% of a mixed group of primary and secondary abscesses.[156] All patients with secondary abscesses in a small series had fever.[17] Cough occurs in 53% to 67% of cases and initially may be nonproductive, becoming purulent when rupture into a bronchus occurs. With necrosis, hemoptysis can occur. Ipsilateral chest or shoulder pain also has been described in some patients, particularly older children.[42] Weight loss may be present if the abscess is of more than a few days' duration. Other symptoms are listed in Table 23.4.[156]

TABLE 23.4 Symptoms and Signs in Patients With Lung Abscess

Symptom	No. Cases (%)
Fever	38 (84)
Cough	24 (53)
Dyspnea	17 (38)
Chest pain	11 (24)
Anorexia	9 (20)
Purulent sputum	8 (18)
Rhinorrhea	7 (16)
Malaise/lethargy	5 (11)
Hemoptysis	4 (9)
Diarrhea	4 (9)
Nausea/vomiting	3 (7)
Irritability	3 (7)
Otitis media	2 (4)
Seizures	2 (4)
Weight loss	1 (2)
Sore throat	1 (2)
Lymphadenopathy	1 (2)

From Tan TQ, Seilheimer DK, Kaplan SL. Pediatric lung abscess: clinical management and outcome. *Pediatr Infect Dis.* 1995;14:51–55.

Some differences in presentation by age exist. Neonates and young infants typically are febrile, without localizing symptoms. Older children also are febrile but may have more cough or tachypnea and focal pain.

The clinical features of a lung abscess vary with the causative organisms and patient risk factors. Patients with bacterial pneumonia can present with dramatic onset of fever and overwhelming respiratory failure, such as in staphylococcal pneumonia. In these cases, the patient often has a recent history of influenza or varicella infection. Staphylococcal abscesses may not be noticed on chest radiographs until the patient already is on ventilatory support because of the time required for an abscess to organize. Similar presentations are typical of group A β-hemolytic streptococcus and *S. pneumoniae* infections. Often a patient has received antibiotics and a temporary defervescence occurs before the hectic fevers of an abscess reemerge. In the latter situation, the respiratory symptoms may be less notable but virtually always are present.[42] This biphasic presentation was described more than 70 years ago in postoperative aspiration[156] and continues to be typical of many lung abscesses.

Subacute presentations are typical in patients with tuberculosis or fungal abscesses and usually are associated with other chronic systemic symptoms such as anorexia, weight loss, and malaise. Cough may be prominent. Aspiration pneumonia may take an indolent or acute course, depending primarily on the organisms in the abscess, the volume of aspirated material, and the status of the host.

The physical findings in lung abscess are limited. Children usually have fever.[156] Tachypnea is a variable finding. Typically auscultation is unrevealing except in cases of very large abscesses, in which loss of normal breath sounds is perceived. Adults and older children seem to have more discrete physical findings, with rales and decreased breath sounds in approximately one-third of adult cases, but they are uncommon findings in young children.

An abscess can rupture into the bronchus, the mediastinum, or the pleura. In most cases, these complications are substantial. In children, all organisms seem capable of causing these complications, but polymicrobial and anaerobic infections are suspected most often. Rupture into the bronchus may not be harmful if the volume of the abscess cavity does not overwhelm the host's ability to cough and clear the material. In an immunocompromised host, rupture may lead to disseminated pneumonia and further abscesses or death. Among adult patients who died of lung abscess, 22% were found to have died of aspiration of the abscess contents.[22]

In an otherwise healthy individual, rupture into the bronchus can be beneficial because it decompresses the abscess and allows the affected tissues to heal more rapidly. It is associated with the sudden production of foul-smelling, abundant, and sometimes blood-stained sputum. Frank hemoptysis is uncommon. Rupture into the mediastinum can be life-threatening, can be associated with chest pain and cardiac compromise, and requires surgery to drain the resulting mediastinitis. Rupture into the pleural space results in pleuritic pain, enhancement of symptoms on inspiration, and often a more toxic presentation and may require drainage.

Routine laboratory information is of limited help. The white blood cell count, C-reactive protein (CRP), and erythrocyte sedimentation rate are elevated nonspecifically, and a left shift of the white blood cell differential count typically occurs.[42] Certain laboratory tests, such as the purified protein derivative tuberculosis skin test or IGRA, HIV serology, or sweat chloride test, may be helpful in revealing an underlying cause. Such studies should not be performed routinely and should be directed by a family history or other findings, such as chronic diarrhea or lymphadenopathy. Blood cultures are helpful but are positive in fewer than 10% of cases.[42,156]

Differential Diagnosis

The major differential diagnoses in the management of a lung abscess are anatomic. A lung abscess must be differentiated from pneumonia, necrotizing pneumonia, pneumatocele, loculated empyema, and a purulent pleural effusion with a bronchopleural fistula. CT or ultrasound may confirm an abscess by documenting central cavitation and differentiating pleural from parenchymal tissues. An abscess may be confused with a congenital cyst, pseudocyst, hydatid cyst, saccular bronchiectasis, pneumatocele, or sequestration. Chest CT allows definition of these entities in many cases by identifying the associated structures, such as the vascular supply and pleural borders.

Apart from the anatomic and infectious causes of lung abscess, the other rare cause is cancer. Unrecognized metastatic disease from Ewing sarcoma or osteosarcomas with associated central necrosis can mimic an abscess or, by obstructing a bronchus, can promote abscess formation.

Diagnosis

The diagnosis of lung abscess usually is made by imaging the lung. In most cases, the plain radiograph is adequate to define a lung abscess (Fig. 23.3), showing a thickened cavity with an air-fluid level that can be accentuated by placing the patient in the lateral decubitus or erect position. Atelectasis often occurs as an expanding abscess compressing adjacent tissues. Pleural thickening may occur if the abscess is subpleural. Hilar adenopathy occurs in subacute situations.

CT is optimal in its ability to identify smaller or multiple abscesses, document the impact of the abscess on adjacent tissues, identify cystic processes mimicking an abscess, and define an abscess for which an organized pneumonia obscures an air-fluid level on plain film.[42] CT scan of a lung abscess reveals an air-fluid level with an active rim, and the abscess is distinguished from necrotizing pneumonia, which lacks enhancement on contrast studies and lacks a distinct air-fluid level.[64] Nuclear imaging is described[34] but used rarely and adds little to the information obtained by CT. MRI is not routinely used at this time.

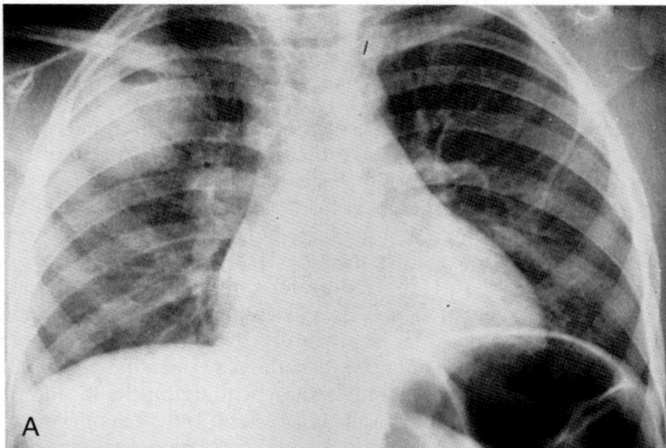

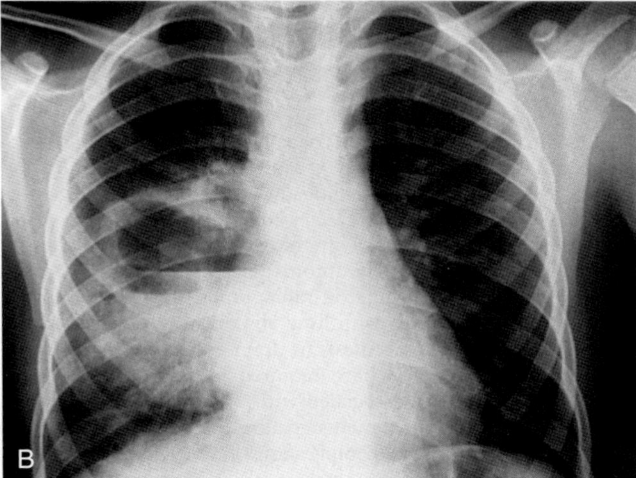

FIG. 23.3 (A) Plain chest film of a 4-year-old boy with cough and fever of 40°C (104°F) for 4 days. He was treated initially with oral cefaclor and re-presented with this radiograph showing an air-fluid level in the right upper lobe. On intravenous cefuroxime, he was afebrile in 48 hours and went home on oral cefuroxime axetil after 4 days. (B) Plain chest film of a 6-year-old boy who presented after 5 days of symptoms with high fever, productive cough, dyspnea, and abdominal pain. The plain chest film reveals multiple air-fluid levels. Nafcillin and cefotaxime were begun. On day 4, an ultrasound-guided diagnostic aspiration recovered thick purulent material, but Gram stain and all cultures, including anaerobic and fungal, were negative. He was afebrile in 7 days and went home on amoxicillin-clavulanic acid at 10 days.

After a presumed abscess is defined by imaging, needle aspiration of the abscess or bronchoscopic recovery of abscess fluid should allow confirmation and identification of the infectious cause of the process. Based on available pediatric studies, whether either procedure hastens recovery or reveals the microbiologic cause in pretreated individuals cannot be predicted. In a case report in which an infant had abscesses in both lungs, the time to recovery was equal in the abscess that was drained and the other abscesses that were treated medically. An adult study using thin-needle aspiration showed positive cultures in 92% of patients not pretreated with antibiotics and in 70% of patients pretreated.

Directly aspirating a lung abscess may be difficult or unsuccessful if the abscess is not large or peripheral, and complications such as lung laceration and sterile pleural effusions are real risks. Two groups[28,156] had satisfactory pediatric experience using direct aspiration under CT guidance (Fig. 23.4). Bronchoscopy particularly is valuable if foreign bodies are suspected or pus can be recovered. When material is obtained, a putrid quality is a clue that anaerobic organisms are present. Typically, the abscess contains pure neutrophils. Occasionally, PCR or other antigen detection systems may assist in the microbiologic diagnosis when cultures are negative.

Treatment

Although surgery has a role in specific situations, the treatment of small to moderate size lung abscesses in children is often successful when antibiotics alone are used. In most cases, the need for surgery is limited to instances of failed antibiotic therapy or to an abscess complicated by rupture into adjacent tissues.

The initial choice of antibiotics usually is presumptive because abscess material may be unavailable. For primary lung abscesses in which no risk factors are identified and in the absence of positive blood cultures, the recommended approach is to begin therapy with a regimen that covers *S. aureus, S. pneumoniae,* and the anaerobic microorganisms that normally are found in the upper respiratory tract. Clindamycin, ampicillin plus sulbactam, and ticarcillin plus clavulanate or piperacillin plus tazobactam frequently are used in this setting.

For patients at risk for aspiration or who are immunocompromised, gram-negative pathogens also must be considered. This spectrum of pathogens can be addressed with one of several drug regimens: clindamycin and cefotaxime or ceftriaxone (or an aminoglycoside); ticarcillin plus clavulanate or piperacillin plus tazobactam; or nafcillin (or cefazolin), gentamicin, and metronidazole. The possible emergence of more penicillin-resistant species, such as the milleri group of streptococci and *Klebsiella,* in community-acquired disease of adults and children supports these broad-spectrum regimens in children. Patients with cystic fibrosis are particularly vulnerable to *Pseudomonas* spp. and should receive an aminoglycoside plus an additional antipseudomonal penicillin or cephalosporin. Carbapenem therapy would be an alternative. When endocarditis is present, treatment (e.g., vancomycin plus gentamicin with or without anaerobic coverage) should be provided for staphylococci, streptococci, and enterococci while awaiting results of blood cultures.

S. pneumoniae has been isolated in lung abscesses (see Table 23.3). Most patients with isolates with reduced susceptibility are still successfully treated because achievable levels of penicillins exceed the penicillin G MICs of 0.12 to 2.0 μg/mL. Drug resistance to *S. aureus* is a concerning issue in lung abscess, and empiric therapy with vancomycin is required if MRSA is suspected while waiting for confirmation, especially if the patient is critically ill.

If culture information is available, therapy is directed specifically at the pathogens isolated. In most patients, oral or intravenous antibiotic therapy has been administered before culture results are available and may affect which organisms are recovered.[42] For this reason, coverage should be extended to include organisms that are likely to be present but are not recovered, such as anaerobes, in a setting of aspiration.

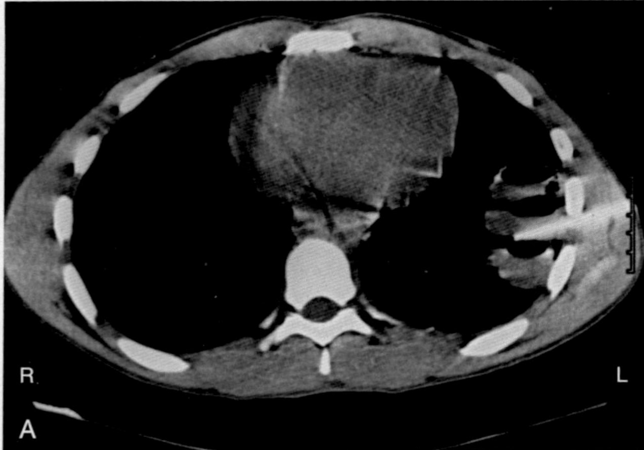

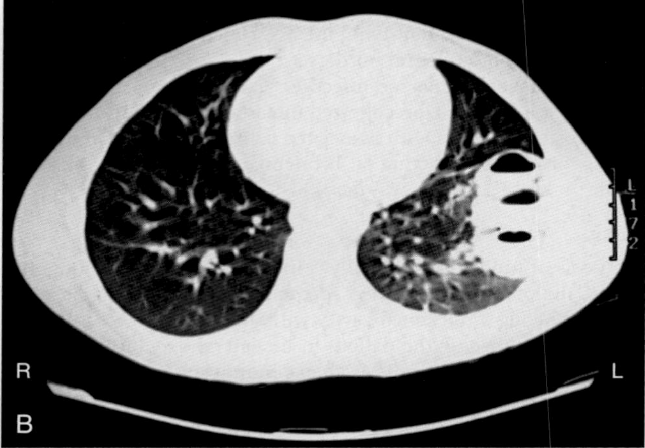

FIG. 23.4 Computed tomography (CT) scans of a 15-year-old boy who, 4 days before admission, reported a mild aspiration during fresh-water swimming. He awoke the next day with chest and back pain. He then developed low-grade fever. A plain chest film showed a large, thick-walled abscess in the left lower lobe. CT scans showed (A) insertion of a 20-gauge needle into the abscess on the first day of admission and (B) detail of the wall thickness and cavitation. *Haemophilus influenzae* grew from the aspirate. Ampicillin-sulbactam was initiated and continued for 14 days.

All bacterial lung abscesses should be treated with intravenous therapy until the patient is stable and no longer toxic. In approximately two-thirds to four-fifths of patients, this condition occurs within 3 to 7 days of instituting intravenous therapy.[42,102] After the patient has been afebrile for 48 to 72 hours, initiation of oral therapy may be considered. Certain oral drugs, such as amoxicillin plus clavulanate and clindamycin, can achieve therapeutic serum levels and are effective against the spectrum of organisms in lung abscesses.

The length of total therapy for a lung abscess should be 2 to 3 weeks. Complicated infections should be treated intravenously until fever has disappeared and no evidence of continuing inflammation exists. An additional 2 to 3 weeks of oral treatment should follow. Radiographic resolution of a lung abscess that is not drained occurs over the course of weeks. Even with drainage, resolution may not occur more rapidly. Chest radiography should be repeated every 1 to 2 weeks until complete resolution is documented.

Tuberculous lung abscesses may rupture spontaneously into the pleura. Treatment is not directed at the immediate abscess or pleuritis but at preventing spread if it erupts into a bronchus. Preventing reactivation several years later is another goal of therapy.

Clinical failure is defined by persistent fever and toxicity. The length of time treatment with intravenous antibiotics should continue before declaring therapy a failure is not clearly defined. Suggestions in the literature range from 1 to 3 weeks.[5] When clinical failure occurs, several options are available, including drainage of the abscess, which permits identification of the organisms causing the disease process.

Needle aspiration (one or more) also is possible under fluoroscopy, ultrasonography, or CT guidance.[35,64,86,93,118] Simple CT-guided needle aspiration leads to relief of symptoms in approximately two-thirds of cases within 48 hours. The risk for complications seems to be low.[64] Percutaneous transthoracic tube drainage has been used in pediatric lung abscesses. The risk is lowest if the abscess is peripheral, and adhesion of the opposing pleural surfaces is a consequence of the inflammatory process. When this adhesion occurs, the needle or catheter does not traverse the pleural space. Catheter drainage may be attempted in abscesses larger than 4 cm in diameter,[64] using 8- to 10-Fr pigtail catheters. Smaller abscesses are technically difficult to manage.

Chest tube thoracostomy previously was the standard therapy of lung abscesses; it is now recommended only when conservative therapy fails and may play a role in patients with large abscesses if the abscess abuts the parietal pleura and provides a direct path from the exterior surface to the abscess. A 25-year review of the literature found that significant complications, such as hemothorax, pneumothorax, bronchopleural fistula, empyema, and catheter occlusion, occurred in 9.7% of cases, with an overall mortality rate of 4.8%.

Surgery for lung abscess is not well described in the pediatric literature. One report that combines surgery for lung abscess and necrotizing pneumonia had no mortality in the postsurgery period and a reversible complication rate of 10%. Indications for surgery included associated pyopneumothorax, size of the abscess, and tension pneumatocele. Another possible surgical indication is proximity of a lung abscess to the mediastinum. In the face of antibiotic failure, an open lung procedure and wedge resection may be required, depending on the location of the abscess. The procedure typically is successful and often obviates the need to perform a lobectomy. In a complicated case, such as with a gangrenous lung, lobar resection may be necessary. Managing an infant with a lung abscess has required surgery more often than in older children.[146]

Prognosis

The outcome for pediatric patients usually is good when lung abscesses are uncomplicated, and recovery is more rapid than in adults. Most patients have complete symptomatic and radiographic resolution in 3 to 6 weeks, with normal pulmonary function tests at follow-up.[5,42] Complicated disease associated with thoracostomy tubes and empyema more likely leads to residual symptoms (e.g., pleurisy) and persistent effusions or pleural thickening on radiographs. In reports published since 1982, half of patients with lung abscess have required surgical intervention, such as thoracentesis to drain an empyema, lobectomy, or decortication, and 20% have required lobectomy or decortication.[5,17,42,156] Lung abscess associated with underlying disorders has a higher mortality rate.[28] If patients require lung resection, they may experience immediate surgical complications; long-term exercise tolerance may be limited, and other problems, such as scoliosis, may develop. One study found normal pulmonary functions in patients studied after undergoing lobectomy, however.[114]

Rarely a residual cavity may develop and become superinfected. The mortality rate is 4% to 11% for patients with primary and secondary lung abscesses.[42,156] Higher risk for morbidity and mortality occurs in patients with secondary abscesses who have complications caused by either a decrease in host resistance or underlying disease.[42,156]

Additional Complications

Necrotizing pneumonia is a complication of lung infection. In contrast to simple pneumonia more destruction of tissue occurs with limited purulence caused either by toxins of the pathogen or by infarction of tissue. Lung ultrasound has been utilized to diagnose necrotic lung[82] in addition to CT. The necrotizing process can be limited, requiring no special intervention, or it may require extensive surgery and have a more prolonged clinical course. The necrotizing process can lead to fistulas, pneumothorax, and pneumatocele.[64,82] Sawicki and colleagues[137] have reported an increased incidence of necrotizing pneumonia in children in the new millennium with an increased frequency of *S. aureus*. This has been noted in children of all ages, including infants.[143] However, necrotizing pneumonia is also described for diverse organisms, including *S. pneumoniae* (particularly nonvaccine strains), group A streptococcus, *Clostridium perfringens*, *M. pneumoniae*, and adenovirus. Longer therapy is often required, but resolution was seen by 6 months by chest radiograph in one series dominated by *S. pneumoniae*.[80]

The formation of a *bronchopleural fistula* can occur as a complication of the underlying pneumonia or as a complication of treatment with a chest tube or postoperatively from débridement. Rates of 55% to 67% for fistula formation have been reported associated with necrotizing pneumonia.[55,94] An increased risk was noted in the United Kingdom in 2008 to 2009 (33%) in contrast to 2002 to 2007 (1%) primarily associated with *S. pneumoniae* serotype 3[103] and in the United States from 2000 to 2009 (approximately 50% increase).[117] Thin-section CT may be required for a radiologic diagnosis.[166]

Pneumatoceles form as a result of tissue necrosis. The development occurs as an acute or delayed part of the pathologic process, with resolution occurring in some cases depending on the size of the defect. A Brazilian study reported pneumatoceles in 8.3% of 394 pediatric pneumonia cases and a spontaneous resolution rate of 85%.[81] *S. aureus* is most typically identified with this complication, although a pneumatocele represents a potential common pathway for pathologic resolution of a pneumonia and has been reported in pneumonia caused by multiple pathogens. Ramphul and colleagues[126] reported a 20% incidence of cavitary disease in patients with empyema, mostly associated with *S. pneumoniae*.

Pneumothorax is an uncommon complication of pneumonia but can occur in any setting in which lung damage creates a ball-valve effect that traps air in the pleural space. Necrotizing pneumonia is one predisposing factor. *P. jiroveci* in HIV disease has been reported as a specific cause of pneumothorax.[121] Other complications occur rarely secondary to pneumonia. Many of these represent local extension of an infected lung or pleural tissue into adjacent tissues including the airway, blood vessels (hemoptysis), bone, and nervous tissues (recurrent laryngeal nerve–Horner syndrome with apical pneumonia). Pericardial effusions are surprisingly common in patients with parapneumonic effusions. Roberts and associates reported a rate of 54.2% although a single patient in their series of 48 had hemodynamic compromise.[128] Other complications result from the hematogenous spread of pathogens causing the pneumonia including sepsis, meningitis, osteomyelitis, other solid organ abscesses, and endocarditis. Finally complications can arise from the immune response to pneumonia.

NEW REFERENCES SINCE THE SEVENTH EDITION

4. Angoulvant F, Levy C, Grimprel E, et al. Early impact of 13-valent pneumococcal conjugate vaccine on community-acquired pneumonia in children. *Clin Infect Dis*. 2014;58:918-924.
10. Becker A, Amantea SL, Fraga JC, et al. Impact of antibiotic therapy on laboratory analysis of parapneumonic pleural fluid in children. *J Pediatr Surg*. 2011;46:452-457.
25. Carillo-Marquez MA, Hulten KG, Hammerman W, et al. *Staphylococcus aureus* pneumonia in children in the era of community-acquired methicillin-resistance at Texas Children's Hospital. *Pediatr Infect Dis J*. 2011;30:545-550.
36. Da Silva CT, Behrsin RF, Cardosos GP, et al. Evaluation of adenosine deaminase activity for the diagnosis of pleural TB in lymphocytic pleural effusions. *Biomark Med*. 2013;7:113-118.
37. Dagan R, Juergens C, Trammel J, et al. Efficacy of 13-valent pneumococcal conjugate vaccine (PCV13) versus that of 7-valent PCV (PCV7) against nasopharyngeal colonization of antibiotic-nonsusceptible *Streptococcus pneumoniae*. *J Infect Dis*. 2015;211:1144-1153.
47. Fletcher MA, Schmitt HJ, Syrochkina M, et al. Pneumococcal empyema and complicated pneumonias: global trends in incidence, prevalence, and serotype epidemiology. *Eur J Clin Microbiol Infect Dis*. 2014;33:879-910.
68. Islam S, Calkins CM, Goldin AB, et al. The diagnosis and management of empyema in children: a comprehensive review from the APSA outcomes and clinical trials committee. *J Pediatr Surg*. 2012;47:2101-2110.
80. Krenke K, Sanocki M, Urbankowska E, et al. Necrotizing pneumonia and its complications in children. *Adv Exp Med Biol*. 2015;857:9-17.
82. Lai SH, Wong KS, Liao SL. Value of lung ultrasonography in the diagnosis and outcome prediction of pediatric community-acquired pneumonia with necrotizing change. *PLoS ONE*. 2015;10(6):e0130082.
83. Lee EY, Khatwa U, McAdam AJ, et al. *Streptococcus milleri* group pleuropulmonary infection in children: computed tomographic findings and clinical features. *J Comput Assist Tomogr*. 2010;34:927-932.
99. Martin JM, Hoberman A, Paradise JL, et al. Emergence of *Streptococcus pneumoniae* serogroups 15 and 35 in nasopharyngeal cultures from young children with acute otitis media. *Pediatr Infect Dis J*. 2014;33:e286-e290.
101. Mazurek GH, Jereb J, Vernon A, et al. Updated guidelines for using interferon gamma release assays to detect *Mycobacterium tuberculosis* infection - United States. *MMWR Recomm Rep*. 2010;59(RR-5):1-24.
111. Naasciemento-Carvalho CM, Oliveira JR, Cardoso MR, et al. Respiratory viral infections among children with community-acquired pneumonia and pleural effusion. *Scand J Infect Dis*. 2013;45:478-483.
115. Omae T, Matsubayashi T. Lung abscess caused by *Mycoplasma pneumonia*. *Pediatr Int*. 2015;57:773-775.
117. Pandian TK, Aho JM, Ubi DS, et al. The rising incidenc of pediatric empyema with fistula. *Pediatr Surg Int*. 2015;doi:10.1007/s00383-015-3834-5.
147. Slinger R, Hyde L, Moldovan I, et al. Direct *Streptococcus pneumoniae* real-time PCR serotyping from pediatric parapneumonic effusions. *BMC Pediatr*. 2014;14:189.
149. St. Peter SD, Tsao K, Harrison C, et al. Thoracoscopic decortication vs tube thoracostomy with fibrinolysis for empyema in children: a prospective, randomized trial. *J Pediatr Surg*. 2009;44:106-111.
153. Strutt J, Kharbanda A. Pediatric chest tubes and pigtails: an evidence-based approach to the management of pleural space diseases. *Pediatr Emerg Med Pract*. 2015;12:1-24.

The full reference list for this chapter is available at ExpertConsult.com.

24 Children's Interstitial Lung Disease and Hypersensitivity Pneumonitis

Minh L. Doan • Leland L. Fan

Children's interstitial lung disease (ILD) encompasses a heterogeneous group of uncommon lung disorders with varying clinical presentations and morbidity.[36] Because these conditions often involve the alveoli and distal airways, and not just the interstitial compartment, they are also referred to as *diffuse lung diseases*. In many of these disorders, injury to the alveolar wall gives rise to an inflammatory response with subsequent repair that potentially can lead to pulmonary fibrosis. Infections of the lung, either chronic or acute with postinfectious sequelae, form the largest category of children's ILD in both the immunocompetent and immunocompromised hosts. Diffuse lung disease can also be the presenting manifestation of certain systemic disease processes, sometimes with acute onset accompanied by fever. Therefore some of these entities may present first to the pediatric infectious disease specialist rather than the pediatric pulmonologist.

CLASSIFICATION

A recently modified classification[49] of the conditions that encompass children's ILD, based on reviews of a large number of diagnostic lung biopsies in children younger than 2 years[39] and in children between 2 and 18 years of age,[49] is presented in Box 24.1. Although a description of each disorder is beyond the scope of this chapter, certain conditions under the categories of primary lung disorders of the immunocompetent host, disorders related to systemic disease processes, and disorders of the immunocompromised host warrant brief mention because they are either caused by or associated with infection or its treatment, or they mimic community-acquired pneumonia in their presentation.

Postinfectious Bronchiolitis Obliterans

Probably the best example of postinfectious chronic lung disease is found in children who develop bronchiolitis obliterans after having severe adenoviral pneumonia.[158] Bronchiolitis obliterans is characterized by a fibrosing process of the small airways that results in severe, irreversible obstruction of the airways. Clinically patients present with tachypnea, crackles, wheezing, and a productive cough that persists for more than 8 weeks after the initial illness. Chest radiographs commonly show a mixed pattern of hyperinflation, persistent atelectasis, and peribronchial thickening; on high-resolution computed tomography (HRCT) in which both inspiratory and expiratory images are obtained, a combination of mosaic perfusion due to air trapping, central bronchiectasis, and vascular attenuation is highly specific for bronchiolitis obliterans, although not entirely sensitive.[17,102] Occasionally severe involvement of one lung leads to the development of a unilateral, small, hyperlucent lung, known as Swyer-James syndrome.[158] Pulmonary function testing demonstrates an obstructive pattern characterized by a disproportionate reduction in the midexpiratory flow (FEF_{25-75}) that is usually fixed, although a small response to bronchodilator is sometimes seen.[102]

Patients with severe adenovirus pneumonia have been shown to have immune complexes containing adenovirus antigen in the lung and increased serum levels of interleukin-6 (IL-6), IL-8, and tumor necrosis factor-α (TNF-α).[101,100] These studies suggest that abnormal or excessive host immunologic and inflammatory responses may be important in the development of chronic lung disease from adenovirus

BOX 24.1 Modified Children's Interstitial Lung Diseases Classification

Disorders of Infancy

Diffuse developmental disorders:
- Acinar/Alveolar dysgenesis/Primary pulmonary hypoplasia
- Congenital alveolar dysplasia
- Alveolocapillary dysplasia with misalignment of pulmonary veins (*FOXF1* mutations)

Growth abnormalities:
- Prenatal conditions: secondary pulmonary hypoplasia
- Postnatal conditions: chronic neonatal lung disease (in premature and term infants)
- Structural changes in chromosomal abnormalities (i.e., trisomy 21)
- Associated with congenital heart disease in chromosomally normal children
- Specific conditions of unknown/poorly understood etiology
- Pulmonary interstitial glycogenosis (primary and associated)
- Neuroendocrine cell hyperplasia of infancy/persistent tachypnea of infancy

Surfactant dysfunction disorders and related abnormalities:
- Surfactant protein B genetic mutations
- Surfactant protein C genetic mutations
- *ABCA3* genetic mutations
- *NKX2-1* genetic mutations
- Congenital GM-CSF receptor deficiency
- Others with histology consistent with surfactant dysfunction disorder without a recognized genetic disorder
- Lysinuric protein intolerance

Primary Lung Disorders of the Immunocompetent Host

Infections and postinfectious processes
Chronic airway changes with and without preceding history of viral respiratory infection
Organizing pneumonia
Specific infections identified (bacterial, fungal, mycobacterial, viral)
Disorders related to environmental agents:
- Hypersensitivity pneumonitis
- Toxic inhalation
- Aspiration syndromes
- Eosinophilic pneumonias

Acute interstitial pneumonia/Hamman-Rich syndrome/Idiopathic diffuse alveolar damage
Nonspecific interstitial pneumonia
Idiopathic pulmonary hemosiderosis
Others

Disorders Related to Systemic Disease Processes

Immune-mediated disorders
Goodpasture syndrome
Acquired pulmonary alveolar proteinosis/autoantibody to GMCSF
Pulmonary vasculitis syndromes
Nonspecific interstitial pneumonia
Pulmonary hemorrhage syndromes
Lymphoproliferative disease
Organizing pneumonia
Nonspecific airway changes
Other manifestations of collagen-vascular disease
Storage disease
Sarcoidosis
Langerhans cell histiocytosis
Malignant infiltrates
Others

Disorders of the Immunocompromised Host

Opportunistic infections (*Pneumocystis jiroveci*, fungal/yeast, bacterial, mycobacterial, viral, suspected infection)
Disorders related to therapeutic intervention (chemotherapeutic drug, radiation, drug hypersensitivity)
Disorders related to solid organ, lung, and bone marrow transplantation and rejection syndromes (rejection, graft-versus-host disease, posttransplant lymphoproliferative disorder)
Diffuse alveolar damage of undetermined etiology
Lymphoid infiltrates related to immune compromise (nontransplanted patients)

Vascular Disorders Masquerading as Interstitial Lung Disease

Arterial hypertensive vasculopathy
Congestive vasculopathy and veno-occlusive disease
Lymphatic disorders (lymphangiectasis, lymphangiomatosis)
Pulmonary edema
Thromboembolic disease
Unclassified

in infants and young children. Although lower respiratory tract infection with *Mycoplasma*,[19] respiratory syncytial virus, parainfluenza, influenza, measles, varicella,[159] and pertussis[20] also can result in bronchiolitis obliterans, adenovirus is the most common etiologic agent. The need for mechanical ventilation during the initial illness is a strong independent risk factor for the subsequent development of this disease.[26]

Organizing Pneumonia

Organizing pneumonia (OP), defined pathologically by the presence of buds of granulation tissue in the alveolar spaces that may extend into the bronchiolar lumen, is another type of inflammatory process that can result from lung injury. It can be associated with various infections, medications, malignancy, radiation therapy, and autoimmune diseases (secondary OP) or occur in isolation without a defined cause, when it is known as cryptogenic organizing pneumonia (formerly named bronchiolitis obliterans/organizing pneumonia [BOOP], although it is a distinct process from bronchiolitis obliterans).[28] Clinical descriptions of organizing pneumonia in children in the literature are rare,[155] but adults can present with fever, cough, malaise, and dyspnea,[42] with findings of bilateral, peripheral ground-glass opacities and consolidation on high-resolution CT chest scan.[56]

Infections

Chronic infections or long-term sequelae from acute infections account for many cases of ILD in children. In a prospective study of immunocompetent children with chronic diffuse infiltrates, Fan and coworkers[51] found an infectious agent as the underlying cause in 10 (20%) of 51 children with ILD. Identified agents included adenovirus alone in four children, adenovirus and cytomegalovirus in two, varicella in one, Epstein-Barr virus (EBV) in one, *Chlamydia* in one, and *Toxocara* in one. These early findings have been supported by large retrospective reviews of lung biopsies conducted by the Children's Interstitial Lung Disease Research Network. In 187 biopsies from children younger than 2 years of age, infection or postinfectious chronic lung disease was identified in 9% and infection in the immunocompromised host in 11%,[39] whereas 191 lung biopsies in children 2 to 18 years of age yielded infection or postinfectious chronic lung disease in 8% and infection in the immunocompromised host in 20%.[49]

Hypersensitivity Pneumonitis

Acute episodes of hypersensitivity pneumonitis may present as fever, cough, dyspnea, and pulmonary infiltrates (see later section for a more detailed discussion).

Toxic Inhalation

While not specific to children, inhalational exposure to metal-containing fumes generated by welding or to certain fluorinated polymer products (such as from overheating of Teflon-coated cookware) can result in metal fume fever or polymer fume fever, respectively, which are typically self-limited syndromes of acute toxic alveolitis.[64] On the other hand, outbreaks of humidifier disinfectant-associated interstitial lung disease in young Korean children, about 25% of whom presented with fevers, led to a mortality rate of 58%.[80] An acute respiratory syndrome manifesting with fever, hemoptysis, dyspnea, and pulmonary infiltrates occurring up to 48 hours after inhalation of free-base cocaine ("crack lung") has also been described.[97]

Eosinophilic Pneumonias

Acute eosinophilic pneumonia is the most severe form of the eosinophilic pneumonias. It is characterized histologically by very large numbers of eosinophils infiltrating the alveoli and interstitium, with resultant acute respiratory failure. Acute eosinophilic pneumonia can be idiopathic or result from inciting triggers such as drugs (penicillins, trimethoprim-sulfamethoxazole, minocycline, ethambutol)[61] and inhalational exposures (recent-onset cigarette smoking, cannabis). Patients present with acute onset of fever, dyspnea, and cough; pleuritic chest pain; and myalgias. On examination, crackles are present in 80% of patients; wheezing is a rare manifestation. Hypoxemia is uniformly present, and patients can progress rapidly to severe respiratory failure with a clinical picture of acute respiratory distress syndrome.[131] In contrast to patients with other eosinophilic lung diseases, patients with acute eosinophilic pneumonia generally do not have significant peripheral eosinophilia (>350 cells/mm^3) on presentation as a diagnostic clue. Chest radiographs and CT scans show bilateral infiltrates with a variable mix of interstitial and alveolar patterns; pleural effusions are present in 50% of cases. Flexible bronchoscopy to obtain a true bronchoalveolar lavage (BAL) is necessary for the diagnosis, and fluid analysis shows marked eosinophilia (>20%) in most patients. Although pleural fluid also has increased eosinophils, this finding in isolation is not specific for acute eosinophilic pneumonia. Treatment with corticosteroids (i.e., methylprednisolone 2 to 4 mg/kg per day) usually results in a rapid and complete resolution, and recurrences have not been reported.[2,62]

Pulmonary Vasculitis Syndromes

In children, the spectrum of pulmonary vasculitides includes granulomatosis with polyangiitis (GPA, formerly Wegener granuloma), eosinophilic granulomatosis with polyangiitis (EGPA, formerly Churg-Strauss syndrome), microscopic polyangiitis, and pulmonary capillaritis. These disorders can present as diffuse alveolar hemorrhage, with fever, dyspnea, hemoptysis (may not present in a third of patients), anemia, and patchy alveolar infiltrates on chest radiographs. Other patients may have fever and cavitary or nodular lesions on imaging.[71] Diffuse alveolar hemorrhage can be diagnosed with BAL when sequentially recovered aliquots of fluid show persistently bloody return. If hemosiderin-laden macrophages are seen on BAL cytology, then this suggests that the blood has been present in the alveolar spaces for at least 3 days and is not the result of the bronchoscopy itself.[45] Renal involvement may sometimes be present, with microscopic hematuria and red blood cell casts seen on urinalysis. A positive serum antineutrophil cytoplasmic antibody (ANCA) may be seen, with antiproteinase-3 antibody resulting in a cytoplasmic (c-ANCA) staining pattern being associated with GPA and with antimyeloperoxidase antibody giving a perinuclear (p-ANCA) pattern seen in EGPA and microscopic polyangiitis.[29] The presence of significant peripheral and pulmonary eosinophilia would support the diagnosis of EGPA.[9] Pulmonary capillaritis is associated with a variety of conditions and requires a surgical lung biopsy for diagnosis because it may present as an ANCA-negative, hematuria-negative diffuse alveolar hemorrhage syndrome.[60] Therapeutic options for pulmonary vasculitis include systemic corticosteroids, cyclophosphamide, intravenous immunoglobulin, and rituximab[15]; aggressive treatment is required in severe cases.

Collagen-Vascular Diseases

Pulmonary involvement can be seen at the initial presentation of systemic lupus erythematosus, juvenile idiopathic arthritis, and juvenile dermatomyositis,[37] and these patients may present with acute respiratory symptoms associated with fever.[25,82,122] In acute lupus pneumonitis, signs and symptoms include high fevers, dyspnea, tachypnea, crackles, and cyanosis. Chest radiographs may show areas of consolidation and pleural effusions or a pattern of interstitial infiltrates with elevation of the hemidiaphragms.[95] Other pulmonary manifestations of systemic lupus erythematosus include pulmonary hemorrhage, pulmonary hypertension, ILD, pneumothorax, and shrinking lung syndrome. Multisystem involvement, including renal and skin, may provide clues to the underlying diagnosis. Treatment usually requires corticosteroids and other immunosuppressive agents.[25]

Sarcoidosis

Sarcoidosis is a chronic inflammatory disease of unknown cause, characterized by the formation of noncaseating granulomas in many organs, but predominantly affecting the lung. Although uncommon, sarcoidosis can even occur in young children, with the median age at diagnosis of about 12 years in a recently reported cohort of 41 affected children; the youngest patient was diagnosed at age 1 year.[107] Fever was present at diagnosis in more than 70% of the patients under age 10 years, whereas respiratory symptoms were noted in about half of the entire cohort. Chest radiographs were reported to be normal in 44%, but high-resolution CT chest scan demonstrated abnormalities in 95% of all patients, with the predominant findings being nodules, ground-glass opacities, and hilar and mediastinal adenopathy.[107]

Drug Hypersensitivity

Several antimicrobials are known to be associated with the development of ILD, including amphotericin B, isoniazid, and nitrofurantoin.[132] In addition, certain biologics and chemotherapeutic agents may rarely induce acute pneumonitis, with associated fever.[11] Thus, in immunocompromised patients being treated with such medications, drug toxicity must also be considered in the setting of febrile respiratory illnesses. The website pneumotox.com can be a useful resource in this regard.

Nonspecific Lymphoproliferation

Well recognized because it is an acquired immunodeficiency syndrome (AIDS)-defining condition in children infected with human immunodeficiency virus (HIV),[16] lymphocytic interstitial pneumonitis (LIP) is actually a form of pulmonary lymphoproliferative disease characterized histologically by a dense interstitial infiltrate composed of T lymphocytes, plasma cells, and macrophages that diffusely expands the alveolar septa.[147] The etiology of LIP remains unknown, but EBV is thought to be important in the pathogenesis.[5,47,78] LIP also occurs in association with common variable immunodeficiency,[127] juvenile idiopathic arthritis,[90,150] and Sjögren syndrome,[83] as well as in idiopathic and familial forms.[109]

LIP occurs in 30% of children infected perinatally with HIV and typically presents between the second and third years of life as an insidious onset of cough, tachypnea, dyspnea, and hypoxemia.[77,117,125,124,135,137] Bilateral nontender parotid enlargement is frequently present and may help to differentiate LIP from other pulmonary complications of HIV infection.[135,137] Chest radiographs characteristically reveal a diffuse, symmetric reticulonodular or nodular pattern, occasionally with mediastinal or hilar adenopathy,[93] although HRCT is more sensitive and allows for the identification of the subpleural and perilymphatic distribution of the micronodules.[7] Among HIV-infected children, the incidence of acute lower respiratory tract infection is higher in children with LIP,[135] and these patients ultimately may develop bronchiectasis.[136]

CLINICAL PRESENTATION

Although some patients may present acutely, most children with ILD have insidious symptoms that may go unrecognized for years. Many have been misdiagnosed as having asthma and have been treated with bronchodilators and inhaled corticosteroids.[55] Although a history of wheezing can be elicited in half of patients, it can be documented by physical examination in only approximately 20% of cases. Clinical suspicion for children's ILD should arise when patients meet at least three of the four following criteria: (1) presenting symptoms of dyspnea, tachypnea, retractions, cough, exercise intolerance, or respiratory failure; (2) presenting signs of crackles, failure to thrive, clubbing, or respiratory failure; (3) hypoxemia; and (4) diffuse abnormality on chest radiographs or CT not attributable to other known processes.[51]

A careful history should be taken to assess the severity of the disease and to obtain information that may contribute to establishing a diagnosis. A search for precipitating factors should include a history of feeding difficulties that may suggest aspiration; any prior acute or severe respiratory tract infections; and environmental exposures, especially to birds or molds. Hemoptysis may indicate a pulmonary vascular disorder or hemosiderosis. Joint disease or rash may indicate a systemic process, such as a connective tissue disease. A family history of relatives or siblings with similar respiratory conditions may provide clues to genetic or familial lung diseases, such as inborn errors of surfactant metabolism.

On physical examination, tachypnea and retractions often are observed, and crackles commonly are heard, particularly at the bases. Chest wall deformity, in particular pectus excavatum, may be noted. In severe cases, cyanosis, clubbing, an accentuated pulmonic component of the second heart sound, and evidence of growth failure are seen. Oxygen saturation usually is normal under all conditions in most patients with mild disease, but desaturation may occur with exercise or during sleep as the disease progresses and ventilation-perfusion mismatch ensues. Patients with more advanced disease are hypoxemic at rest.

DIAGNOSTIC EVALUATION

A systematic approach to children's ILD is essential when physicians are confronted with such a large differential of rare conditions, as listed in Box 24.1.[55] In general, diagnostic studies can be divided into studies used to assess the extent and severity of disease, to identify disorders that predispose to ILD, and to identify the primary ILD (Box 24.2). However, from the perspective of the pediatric infectious disease specialist, the emphasis should be on the inclusion of specific children's ILD, such as those mentioned earlier, in the differential diagnosis when faced with difficult or atypical cases of respiratory illnesses in which infection is initially suspected. Labs to assess for immune function, autoantibodies, hypersensitivity pneumonitis, and angiotensin-converting enzyme level may have a role in selected cases; pulmonary function tests in older children may also provide clues, such as an elevated diffusion capacity for carbon monoxide as a potential indicator of pulmonary hemorrhage.[12] Most important, if a CT scan of the chest is planned as part of the evaluation, it is critical that the study be ordered in such a fashion as to also enable the evaluation for ILD—namely, with thin-section or high-resolution technique.

High-Resolution Computed Tomography

An HRCT of the chest is one of the initial recommended studies in proposed diagnostic approaches for the evaluation of possible children's ILD.[12,85] It is used to evaluate the presence, extent, and distribution of the diffuse lung disease; to select favorable sites for surgical lung biopsy; and, when classic patterns of abnormalities are seen, to either make a confident diagnosis for some conditions or to guide specific but less-invasive testing (genetic testing, autoantibody levels, bronchoscopy) for other conditions.[152] The optimal technique is a volumetric scan acquired during inspiration,[12] from which thin (usually 0.625 to 1.25 mm in

BOX 24.2 Diagnostic Studies for Pediatric Interstitial Lung Disease

To Assess Extent and Severity of Disease

- Chest radiography, high-resolution computed tomography
- Pulmonary function studies: spirometry, pulse oximetry and arterial blood gases (resting, sleeping, and with exercise), diffusion, pressure-volume curve, infant studies
- Electrocardiography, echocardiography

To Identify Primary Disorders That Predispose to Interstitial Lung Disease

- HIV test
- Immune studies: immunoglobulins including IgE, skin tests for delayed hypersensitivity, response to immunizations, T- and B-cell subsets, complement, others as indicated
- Barium swallow, pH/impedance probe
- DNA analyses for mutations in the surfactant protein B, surfactant protein C, and *ABCA3* and *TTF-1* genes

To Identify Primary Interstitial Lung Disease

- Antinuclear antibody
- Angiotensin-converting enzyme
- Antineutrophil cytoplasmic antibody
- Antiglomerular basement membrane antibody
- Hypersensitivity screen
- Infectious disease evaluation—cultures, titers, skin tests
- Cardiac catheterization (in selected cases)
- Bronchoalveolar lavage and transbronchial biopsy
- Transthoracic biopsy

HIV, Human immunodeficiency virus.

From Fan LL. Pediatric interstitial lung disease. In: Schwarz MI, King TE, eds. *Interstitial lung disease.* 4th ed. Hamilton, Ontario: BC Decker; 2003:134–51.

thickness) reformats can be constructed (on certain models of CT scanners, the bone reconstruction algorithm actually gives better lung image resolution than does the lung reconstruction algorithm, so collaboration with the radiology department may be helpful). The thin sections avoid the volume averaging that occurs with 2.5- to 5-mm sections, which obscures the fine parenchymal details and airway abnormalities, including mild bronchiectasis. At the same time, the volumetric scan allows for a complete evaluation of the central airways and mediastinum. Images obtained at end-exhalation can provide additional helpful information, especially in terms of air trapping and pulmonary vascular disease, but does entail either a second volumetric scan, or preferably, just a few spaced, successive thin-slice acquisitions to reduce the total radiation dose. If appropriate pediatric protocols are used, a volumetric pediatric chest CT scan with high-resolution reformatted images can be performed with radiation doses of less than 1.5 mSv (equivalent to 6 months of natural background radiation exposure).[67]

Obtaining high-quality CT images of the lungs also requires the avoidance of respiratory motion artifact. In younger children and infants in whom cooperation for breath-holding is impossible and in whom rapid respiratory rates especially predispose to motion artifact, a sedated controlled-ventilation CT technique can be used.[88] Giving several assisted deep breaths using mask ventilation to these sedated young children results in a short period of apnea during which the lungs can be fully inflated to obtain the routine inspiratory images. Expiratory images can be acquired after allowing for passive deflation of the lungs or with voluntary end-expiratory breath-holding. General anesthesia produces similar results, although frequent large sigh breaths are necessary to prevent dependent atelectasis, which occurs within minutes of intubation.[67]

Finally the use of intravenous contrast when evaluating for infections may be helpful in delineating hilar adenopathy but will make the assessment of ground-glass opacification seen with many interstitial lung diseases more difficult. Overall, in studies that have investigated the diagnostic accuracy of HRCT in pediatric diffuse lung disease, the first-choice diagnosis was proved correct in 38% to 61% of cases by subsequent surgical lung biopsy.[27,91,154]

Bronchoalveolar Lavage

BAL via flexible bronchoscopy allows for sampling of the alveolar lining fluid to assess its gross appearance and to send for measurement of cell count and differential, cytologic examination, and microbial cultures, as well as for molecular and biochemical analyses, all of which may be helpful in the evaluation of certain cases of children's ILD. A milky appearance of the BAL fluid with a layering of sediment strongly suggests pulmonary alveolar proteinosis, whereas the progressively bloody appearance of the fluid in sequential aliquots indicates the presence of an alveolar hemorrhage syndrome. Normal indices for pediatric BAL fluid have been described against which abnormal results can be compared.[46] Finding significant eosinophilia or lymphocytosis in the BAL would substantially narrow the differential diagnoses, and detection of lipid- or hemosiderin-laden macrophages can serve as sensitive, albeit not specific, markers for aspiration or alveolar hemorrhage syndromes. Cytologic examination can also be used to diagnose pulmonary alveolar proteinosis, lysosomal storage disorders, and histiocytosis.[54]

The most common indication for pediatric BAL has been to detect infection in the immunocompromised host. The use of quantitative bacterial cultures may help to differentiate whether recovered organisms represent true infection, colonization, or contamination, whereas polymerase chain reaction (PCR) techniques allow for increased sensitivity in detecting *Pneumocystis jiroveci* pneumonia in non–HIV-immunocompromised patients[112] and for the rapid detection of *Mycobacterium tuberculosis*.[114] Cytologic examination may identify cases of aspergillosis not otherwise detected by culture alone,[4] and measurement of galactomannan levels in BAL has also been used for early diagnosis of invasive aspergillosis.[38]

When BAL should be performed may be important because investigators have shown in a murine model that hemosiderin-laden macrophages first appear at 3 days, peak at 1 week, and persist in small numbers for 2 months after a single episode of hemorrhage.[45] In adult hematopoietic stem cell transplantation recipients with new pulmonary infiltrates, the diagnostic yield of BAL was highest when performed within 24 hours of presentation.[134]

Finally, while bronchial washings obtained via a suction catheter introduced through an endotracheal tube have proved useful in the evaluation of ventilator-associated pneumonia,[126] they do not adequately sample the alveolar lining fluid and therefore give a different cellular profile from that obtained by bronchoscopic BAL.[81] This discrepancy may result in missed detection of conditions such as acute eosinophilic pneumonia if only the former is performed.

Lung Biopsy

Lung biopsy is the gold standard for establishing the diagnosis of children's ILD because most diseases are classified in terms of previously defined histopathologic patterns. Although transbronchial or percutaneous needle biopsy may be helpful in certain conditions, a transthoracic approach, usually by video-assisted thoracoscopic surgery (VATS), remains the gold standard for obtaining tissue adequate for diagnosis. Technical advances and now widespread experience with VATS, including in infants,[123] make it the method of choice, especially in light of research demonstrating comparable diagnostic yield in the evaluation of children with ILD (54% with VATS, 57% with open-lung biopsy).[52] Selection of biopsy sites should be determined by findings on HRCT, although the tip of the right middle lobe and lingula should be avoided. Ideally biopsies should be taken from two sites and sample areas of varying disease severity.[12]

Lung biopsy material must be processed in a consistent manner to ensure optimal interpretation, and a protocol for such handling was published based on the recommendations of the Children's Interstitial Lung Disease (chILD) Pathology Group.[86] A general scheme for division of the biopsy specimen is as follows: (1) microbiology cultures, 35%; (2) snap-frozen for PCR or other molecular studies, 10%; (3) snap-frozen in cryomatrix for immunofluorescent, laser capture, or other studies requiring frozen sections, 10%; (4) fixed in glutaraldehyde for electron microscopy, less than 5%; (5) imprints for cytologic examination or rapid identification of organisms, 0%; and (6) expanded and fixed in formalin (methods previously described[34]) for light microscopy, 40%. It is crucial that the biopsy material be interpreted by a pathologist with considerable expertise in pediatric lung disease because the normal lung of an infant differs greatly from that of an older child or adolescent and any pathologic finding needs to be interpreted in light of the normal age-dependent variations of lung architecture.

TREATMENT

Supportive care is important in the management of children's ILD. Good nutrition is paramount, to the extent that gastrostomy feedings should be considered in selected patients who have poor weight gain despite maximal conventional treatment.[152] Nocturnal or continuous oxygen therapy should be provided in children who are hypoxemic to decrease the risk for the development of pulmonary hypertension. Annual influenza vaccination through the injectable route should be given. Avoiding inhalant hazards such as tobacco smoke should be stressed. Patients with underlying systemic disorders need primary treatment for that disorder, such as intravenous γ-globulin (IVIG) for hypogammaglobulinemia. Specific therapy for primary ILD should be used when possible, such as aggressive management of identified causes of aspiration syndromes, lung lavage and inhalational granulocyte-macrophage colony-stimulating factor for certain types of pulmonary alveolar proteinoses,[121,160] and interferon-α for pulmonary hemangiomatosis.[113] When environmental agents such as bird antigens are causative, avoiding contact with them is crucial (see later section on hypersensitivity pneumonia [HP]).

Generally, corticosteroids remain the treatment of choice for most patients with ILD on the presumption that suppression of inflammation may reduce the risk for developing fibrosis.[53] Although controlled clinical studies are lacking,[87] corticosteroids have been used to treat such diverse types of diffuse lung diseases as desquamative interstitial pneumonitis, nonspecific interstitial pneumonitis, acute interstitial pneumonia, cryptogenic organizing pneumonia, lymphocytic interstitial pneumonia, HP, eosinophilic pneumonia, diffuse alveolar hemorrhage, ILD associated with connective tissue diseases, and surfactant protein C mutations.[146,151] In a retrospective study of pediatric ILD by Fan and coworkers,[55] corticosteroids were judged to be effective in 40% (12 of 30) of treated children in terms of improved clinical status, decreased oxygen requirements, and improved pulmonary function. A trial of prednisone or equivalent corticosteroid in a dose of 1 to 2 mg/kg per day for at least 6 to 8 weeks probably is warranted, although it may be preferable to instead use intravenous pulses of methylprednisolone 30 mg/kg, with a maximum dose of 1 g, given for either 3 consecutive days every month or 1 day every week, based on experience that pulse intravenous therapy is at least as effective as oral therapy and has fewer side effects.[152]

Alternative immunomodulatory agents that have also been used include hydroxychloroquine, azathioprine, cyclophosphamide, methotrexate, cyclosporine, IVIG, and mycophenolate mofetil.[128] Of these, hydroxychloroquine probably has been used most frequently.[6,55,135,141] The precise mechanism of action is unknown, but chloroquine and hydroxychloroquine have shown immunosuppressive effects with the ability to inhibit the functional capabilities of monocytes and the generation of antibody-forming cells. Hydroxychloroquine is preferred over chloroquine because the former has less retinal toxicity. The recommended dose in children for the treatment of ILD is 10 mg/kg per day. Additionally there has been a case report describing the successful use of infliximab, an anti–TNF-α monoclonal antibody, in reversing bronchiolitis obliterans in a hematopoietic stem cell transplant recipient.[59] Finally treatment regimens for ILD associated with systemic sclerosis,[156] Langerhans cell histiocytosis,[99] and Wegener granulomatosis[13] have been reviewed. The fact that many alternative pharmacologic approaches are considered for children and adults with ILD implies that conventional therapy often is ineffective. New strategies are being developed based on animal models of pulmonary fibrosis and more recent advances in the cellular and molecular biology of inflammatory reactions. Such therapies would be directed against the action of certain cytokines, oxidants, and growth factors that may be involved in the fibrotic process. Two antifibrotic drugs, pirfenidone and nintedanib, have recently been shown to result in meaningful reductions in disease progression in adults with IPF.[106,108] Whether these drugs will be useful in children with fibrotic lung disease remains to be determined. The potential to deliver specific inflammatory inhibitors or inhibitors of collagen biosynthesis directly to the lung via aerosolization suggests that disease processes in the lung may be more amenable to novel therapies than are disease processes in other internal organs.

Lung transplantation can be used as a final therapeutic modality for some forms of children's ILD that progress to irreversible respiratory failure secondary to pulmonary fibrosis. Although the overall 5-year survival after lung transplantation is still disappointing at approximately 50%,[8] it appears that outcomes for children with diffuse lung disease are comparable to those undergoing transplantation for cystic fibrosis or pulmonary hypertension.[118] In certain systemic conditions, such as hereditary pulmonary alveolar proteinosis, however, transplantation may not be appropriate because the primary disease may recur in the transplanted lungs.[94,130]

OUTCOME

The prognosis of children with ILD varies. Infants with neuroendocrine cell hyperplasia of infancy generally do well, although they may be symptomatic and require oxygen for years.[41] At the other end of the spectrum, children with growth failure, pulmonary hypertension, and severe fibrosis do poorly. A survey that likely included many different types of pediatric interstitial lung diseases found an overall mortality rate of 15%.[40]

Fan and Kozinetz[50] reviewed the outcome of 99 children with chronic ILD seen in Denver, Colorado, over the course of 15 years (1980–94). As expected, a wide variety of disorders were encountered, and 15 recorded deaths occurred, with a probability that a patient would survive to 24 months, 48 months, and 60 months after onset of symptoms of 83%, 72%, and 64%, respectively. Of the clinical features present at the time of initial evaluation, weight less than the fifth percentile, crackles, clubbing, family history of ILD, and symptom duration were not associated with decreased survival rates. A severity of illness score, based on increasing levels of hypoxemia and the presence or absence of pulmonary hypertension, was related significantly to survival, with an increasing score associated with a higher probability of decreased survival rates. A simple scoring system seems to be a useful measure of outcome in children with ILD.

HYPERSENSITIVITY PNEUMONITIS

HP, also known as *extrinsic allergic alveolitis,* is a form of immune-mediated ILD that develops in response to repeated inhalation of finely dispersed organic antigens.[32] HP should be considered in the differential diagnosis of a child who presents with acute or chronic respiratory symptoms associated with fever,[10] and obtaining an environmental exposure history is essential to arrive at the proper diagnosis. A wide variety of organic particles, including mammalian and avian proteins, fungi, thermophilic bacteria, and certain low-molecular-weight volatile and nonvolatile chemical compounds, are known to induce HP in susceptible individuals.[3] Certain systemic medications, such as ciprofloxacin,[142] dapsone,[148] and methotrexate,[33] also have been reported as triggers.

In general, three forms of HP have been described: (1) acute (or episodic), with improvement between attacks; (2) insidious (gradual onset and progressive course) with superimposed acute episodes; and (3) insidious without acute attacks.[70] Although exposure to antigens capable of provoking HP occurs commonly in the home and work environment, the overall incidence of the condition in the general population is low.[10,140] It is estimated that only 5% to 15% of individuals exposed to high levels of a specific organic antigen develop clinical disease.[57,156]

Pathology and Pathogenesis

Pathologically, HP is characterized by a diffuse, lymphoplasmacytic cell infiltration of the small airways and pulmonary parenchyma, often with associated multinucleated giant cells containing cholesterol clefts and poorly formed, nonnecrotizing granulomas.[63] Foamy macrophages are seen commonly in the airspaces. With advanced disease, interstitial and intra-alveolar fibrosis develops that is indistinguishable from other causes of pulmonary fibrosis.

The mechanisms by which organic dusts induce these characteristic pathologic features of the disease are not completely understood, but it is thought that both type III (immune complex–mediated) and type IV (delayed) hypersensitivity mechanisms are involved.[115] A type III reaction is suggested by the presence of precipitating antibody to the offending antigen, immune complex deposition, and activation of complement. A type IV reaction is suggested by an increased percentage of T lymphocytes in BAL fluid, with a strong predominance of $CD8^+$ subsets and a low CD4:CD8 ratio, and the presence of granulomas on lung biopsy specimen. Considering the small proportion of exposed individuals who develop clinical symptoms, complex interactions among the nature of the antigen, the intensity and duration of the exposure, and the host response in affected individuals most likely are involved. Genetic predilection to the development of HP has been linked to polymorphisms in the genes encoding TNF-α and in those found within the major histocompatibility complex class II.[14,48] Associated viral infections may also contribute to susceptibility,[35] whereas cigarette smoking (nicotine) seems to confer a protective effect.[75] Familial cases of HP have been identified.[21,43]

Etiology

As shown in Table 24.1, HP in adults is caused by a wide variety of occupational and environmental exposures.[133] In contrast, in children, HP is caused mainly by exposure to an array of domestic birds (69%) and fungi (29%), based on a review of 191 reported pediatric cases. In HP due to bird exposure (bird fancier's lung), bird droppings and feathers are the major sources of the offending antigens.[96] Although exposure to pet birds is usually the cause,[103] even low levels of environmental exposure to wild birds in the yard or birds raised by a neighbor may be enough to induce clinical HP,[84,129] as may contact with feather-filled

TABLE 24.1 Etiologic Agents of Hypersensitivity Pneumonitis

Disease	Antigen	Source
Fungal and Bacterial		
Farmer's lung	*Faeni rectivirgula*	Moldy hay, grain, silage
Ventilation pneumonitis; humidifier lung; air conditioner lung	*Thermoactinomyces vulgaris, Thermoactinomyces sacchari, Thermoactinomyces candidus, Klebsiella oxytoca*	Contaminated forced air systems, water reservoirs
Bagassosis	*T. vulgaris*	Moldy sugarcane (i.e., bagasse)
Mushroom worker's lung	*T. sacchari*	Moldy mushroom compost
Suberosis	*T. viridis, Penicillium glabrum*	Moldy cork
Detergent lung; washing powder lung	*Bacillus subtilis* enzymes	Detergents (during processing or use)
Malt worker's lung	*Aspergillus fumigatus, Aspergillus clavatus*	Moldy barley
Sequoiosis	*Graphium, Pullularia,* and *Trichoderma* spp.; *Aureobasidium pullulans*	Moldy wood dust
Maple bark stripper's lung	*Cryptostroma corticale*	Moldy maple bark
Cheese washer's lung	*Penicillium casei, A. clavatus*	Moldy cheese
Woodworker's lung	*Alternaria* spp., wood dust	Oak, cedar, and mahogany dust; pine and spruce pulp
Paprika slicer's lung	*Mucor stolonifer*	Moldy paprika pods
Sauna taker's lung	*Aureobasidium* spp., other sources	Contaminated sauna water
Familial HP	*B. subtilis*	Contaminated wood dust in walls
Wood trimmer's lung	*Rhizopus* spp., *Mucor* spp.	Contaminated wood trimmings
Composter's lung	*T. vulgaris, Aspergillus* spp.	Compost
Basement shower HP	*Epicoccum nigrum*	Mold on unventilated shower
Hot-tub lung	*Cladosporium* spp.	Hot-tub mists, mold on ceiling
Wine maker's lung	*Botrytis cinerea*	Mold on grapes
Woodsman's disease	*Penicillium* spp.	Oak and maple trees
Thatched-roof lung	*Saccharomonospora viridis*	Dead grasses and leaves
Tobacco grower's lung	*Aspergillus* spp.	Tobacco plants
Potato riddler's lung	*Thermophilic actinomycetes, F. rectivirgula, T. vulgaris, Aspergillus* spp.	Moldy hay around potatoes
Summer-type pneumonia	*Trichosporon cutaneum*	Contaminated old houses
Dry rot lung	*Merulius lacrymans*	Rotten wood
Stipatosis	*A. fumigatus, T. actinomycetes*	Esparto dust
Machine operator's lung	*Pseudomonas fluorescens*	Aerosolized metal-working fluid
Amoebae		
Humidifier lung	*Naegleria gruberi, Acanthamoeba polyphaga, Acanthamoeba castellani*	Contaminated water
Animal Proteins		
Pigeon breeder's or pigeon fancier's disease	Avian droppings, feathers, serum	Parakeets, budgerigars, pigeons, chickens, turkeys
Pituitary snuff taker's lung	Pituitary snuff	Bovine and porcine pituitary proteins
Fish meal worker's lung	Fish meal	Fish meal dust
Bat lung	Bat serum protein	Bat droppings
Furrier's lung	Animal fur dust	Animal pelts
Animal handler's lung; laboratory worker's lung	Rats, gerbils	Urine, serum, pelts, proteins
Insect Proteins		
Miller's lung	*Sitophilus granarius*	Dust-contaminated grain (i.e., wheat weevil)
Lycoperdonosis	Puffball spores	*Lycoperdon* puffballs
Chemical		
Pauli's reagent alveolitis	Sodium diazobenzene sulfate	Laboratory reagent
Chemical worker's lung	Isocyanates, trimellitic anhydride	Polyurethane foams, spray paints, elastomers, special glues
Vineyard sprayer's lung	Copper sulfate	Bordeaux mixture
Pyrethrum HP	Pyrethrum	Pesticide
Epoxy resin lung	Phthalic anhydride	Heated epoxy resin
Dental technician's lung	Methyl methacrylate	Dental prosthesis
Unknown		
Bible printer's lung		Moldy typesetting water
Coptic lung (mummy handler's lung)		Cloth wrappings of mummies
Grain measurer's lung		Cereal grain
Coffee worker's lung		Coffee bean dust

Continued

TABLE 24.1 **Etiologic Agents of Hypersensitivity Pneumonitis** (Continued)

Disease	Antigen	Source
Tap water lung		Contaminated tap water
Tea grower's lung		Tea plants
Mollusk-shell HP		Sea-snail shell
Swimming pool worker's lung		Aerosolized endotoxin from pool water, sprays, and fountains

From Selman M. Hypersensitivity pneumonitis. In: Schwarz MI, King TE, eds. *Interstitial lung disease.* 4th ed. Hamilton, Ontario: BC Decker; 2003:452–84.

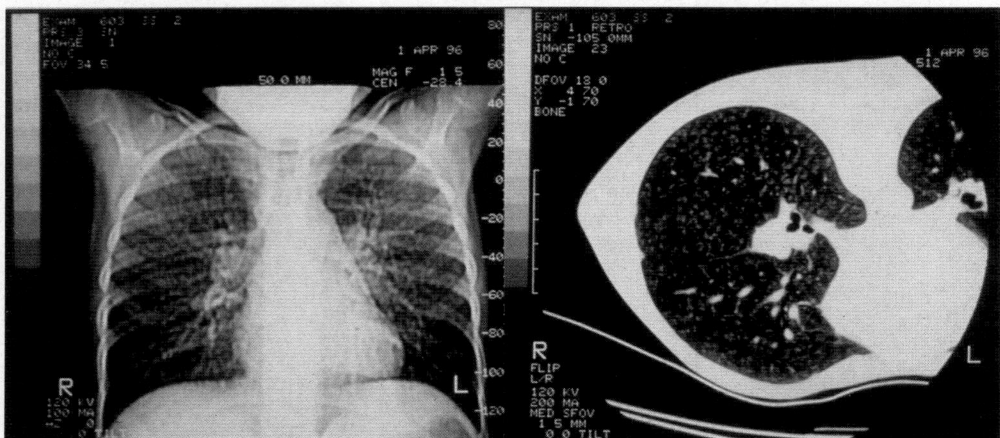

FIG. 24.1 Hypersensitivity pneumonitis from cockatiel antigens in an adolescent. Chest radiograph shows bilateral reticulonodular infiltrates. High-resolution computed tomography shows diffuse, multiple fine nodules. (Courtesy Robin Deterding, MD, University of Colorado, Denver. From Fan LL. Pediatric interstitial lung disease. In: Schwarz MI, King TE, editors. *Interstitial lung disease.* 4th ed. Hamilton, Ontario: BC Decker; 2003:134–51.)

household items such as feather pillows, down comforters, and feather duvets.[10,73,103] The onset of clinical disease typically follows months to years of continuous or intermittent exposure to the offending antigen,[70] and it has been demonstrated that bird antigens can persist for months in the home environment even after removal of the birds.[31] Possible sources of mold exposure are varied and can include contaminated air humidifiers,[116] indoor hydroponics,[44] organic compost in a play area,[1] moist hay,[145] and even wind instruments,[98] in addition to overt mold contamination in areas of water damage or in poorly ventilated spaces exposed to moisture.[72,144]

Clinical Presentation

Although a wide variety of antigens can induce HP, the immunologic response and clinical presentation are similar. In the reported pediatric cases referenced previously, the mean age (± standard deviation) was 9.7 (±4.0) years. The youngest reported patient with HP developed symptoms at 10 weeks of age.[145]

Acute episodes of HP mimic flulike illnesses, manifesting as high fevers, chills, dry cough, dyspnea, myalgias, and malaise. These symptoms begin several hours after exposure and diminish during the next 12 to 24 hours, provided that no additional exposure to the antigen occurs. Physical examination reveals a dyspneic, ill-appearing child, often with bibasilar crackles. Transient hypoxemia and nodular pulmonary infiltrates often are present. Hospitalization for presumed pneumonia often leads to resolution of symptoms due to removal from the causative environment.

More commonly, children present with more insidious and progressive symptoms, which may or may not be punctuated by intermittent acute manifestations. In the reported pediatric cases in which the following specific symptoms were recorded, exercise intolerance was present in 96% (104 of 108), cough was present in 85% (121 of 142), weight loss was present in 77% (60 of 78), and fever was present in 47% (40 of 86). On physical examination, crackles were present in 66% (67 of 102), and clubbing was present in 24% (22 of 91) of cases. Cough can be productive of thick, clear mucus, and wheezing and rhonchi are sometimes noted on examination, leading to a misdiagnosis of asthma or bronchitis, especially because there may be a partial response to a bronchodilator and temporary clearance of symptoms with systemic corticosteroids.[76]

Diagnosis

Establishing a diagnosis of HP requires maintaining a high index of suspicion, especially when patients have insidious chronic symptoms without episodic febrile illnesses. It is not uncommon that children who are eventually diagnosed with HP will have been treated with inhaled β_2 agonists and corticosteroids before referral.[10] Therefore consistently taking a careful environmental history is critical to detecting the presence of potential antigens. Compatible findings on pulmonary function testing, HRCT (Fig. 24.1), BAL, and environmental challenge then can aid in establishing the diagnosis. Surgical lung biopsy is usually reserved for atypical or advanced (fibrotic) cases.

Pulmonary function tests typically show a restrictive defect, sometimes with an obstructive component. In reported pediatric cases, the mean (± standard deviation) FEV_1 and FVC in the children tested were 54.3% (±19.4) and 52.7% (±20.0) predicted. The pressure-volume curve is shifted down and to the right, consistent with decreased compliance. Low lung volumes and diminished diffusion capacity also are present.[23] Although resting room air oxygen saturation may be normal, desaturation with exercise or sleep may occur. With long-standing disease, resting oxygen desaturation can be seen. In the pediatric cases in which oxygenation was documented, 68% (66 of 97) had hypoxemia at rest. Pulmonary hypertension may be present with advanced disease, but in contrast to other forms of children's ILD, it may reverse completely with successful treatment.

Classic features of acute HP evident on chest radiography and HRCT include poorly defined centrilobular micronodules, with predominance in the upper and middle lung zones (see Fig. 24.1). On HRCT, widespread ground-glass attenuation and air trapping (especially prominent on expiratory scans) are also characteristic features.[103,139] A small percentage of patients also may have lung cysts.[58] In the more chronic phase, diffuse interstitial infiltrates may predominate, with progression to fibrosis and honeycombing that are indistinguishable from usual interstitial pneumonia.[92] HRCT is much more sensitive for detecting these abnormalities, with the initial plain chest radiographs reported as being normal in up to 37% of cases,[10] whereas the CT was normal in only up to 2% of cases in reported series.[68,103] In the reported pediatric cases of HP, chest radiographs were abnormal at some point in 84% (134 of 160).

BAL fluid, obtained by flexible bronchoscopy, typically shows a significant lymphocytosis (>25%),[18,65] although this is not always present in patients who have insidious chronic disease without superimposed acute episodes.[110,143] In adults, a low CD4:CD8 ratio frequently accompanies the lymphocytosis. Children with HP also have marked lymphocytosis in the BAL compared with healthy pediatric controls (80% vs. 12%), although a low CD4:CD8 ratio may not be as helpful because a low ratio (0.6) is already seen in healthy children without lung disease.[120] Clinicians should be mindful, however, that the presence of BAL lymphocytosis in exposed individuals who are not symptomatic does not predict the development of HP.[30] Induced sputum does not accurately reflect the lymphocytosis seen in BAL and thus cannot be used as an alternative diagnostic step.[34] During an acute episode of HP due to avian antigen, mild BAL neutrophilia and eosinophilia may also be seen in conjunction with the lymphocytosis.[110]

Environmental challenges, in which the patient is returned to the suspected causative environment after having achieved clinical remission (usually through hospitalization or systemic corticosteroid treatment), can be helpful in establishing the exposure basis behind the condition. Signs and symptoms, spirometry, chest radiograph, and inflammatory markers are then followed for decrement. The patient's atopic status must be considered, and these challenges may be difficult to perform in patients without episodic acute manifestations.[76] Specific inhalation challenge (inhalation provocation test) performed in controlled laboratory conditions using a specific suspected antigen has been used.[69,74,103,105,110,119] However, while commercialized extracts for some fungi are available, antigen extracts from pigeon droppings or bird sera still require formulation by research laboratories.[104,110] Additionally, parameters to be monitored and the criteria for a positive test still vary in the literature, with resultant variations in reported sensitivities and specificities.[74,105] Similarly measurement of antigen-induced lymphocyte proliferation using lymphocytes gathered from BAL or blood can be a sensitive technique to confirm reaction to a specific antigen, but this test is not widely available.[110,111]

Detecting precipitating IgG antibodies to the suspected offending antigen can be useful in confirming the diagnosis in a patient with documented exposure and typical clinical features (Fig. 24.2). However, most commercial laboratory panels include only certain specific antibodies, so providers must be aware of which are tested before ordering such a panel. Ideally a sample of the suspected antigen collected directly from the original source is used to test against the patient's serum, but few laboratories can perform this technique. Precipitating antibodies should be sent only in patients who have clinical disease because 50% of individuals who are exposed to a particular antigen develop precipitating antibodies, but only a small percentage of these develop HP.[32] Long-term follow-up has shown that the simple presence of precipitins does not increase the likelihood of developing the condition.[30] Conversely not all individuals with symptomatic HP have positive precipitins for the tested antigens. In reported pediatric cases, positive precipitins were found in 94% (135 of 145) of the children tested.

Lung biopsy is typically not necessary for making the diagnosis of HP in the setting of an identified antigen exposure, typical HRCT findings, and positive serum precipitins. However, when the clinical picture is atypical or the patient is found to have an undefined ILD on CT, then lung biopsy can be useful in making the diagnosis.[149] Although transbronchial biopsies may sometimes be able to confirm the diagnosis if positive, because of the high potential for sampling error, transthoracic biopsy is usually necessary to obtain tissue to look for the characteristic histologic features described previously (Fig. 24.3). The histology in patients who underwent biopsies during the acute phase of HP has been reported to show neutrophils within the interstitium and alveoli, intra-alveolar fibrin deposits, and even capillaritis.[66] Of the 191 reported pediatric cases of HP, 31 biopsy specimens were obtained, and all showed typical histologic changes.

Treatment and Outcome

The mainstay of treatment is eliminating exposure to the offending antigen. However, there can be practical challenges to achieving this goal, especially because even small amounts of exposure can perpetuate the immunologic reaction and, as previously stated, bird antigen in the home environment can persist long after removal of the bird. The presence of markers of poor prognosis, such as traction bronchiectasis and honeycombing on HRCT[157] or fibrosis seen microscopically on a pathologic specimen,[24] would dictate much more aggressive avoidance measures. In the literature, exposure was eliminated in 98% of the pediatric cases (108 of 110), with improvement achieved in all but one fatal case.

The use of corticosteroids often results in rapid improvement of symptoms and reversal of radiographic and lung function abnormalities unless irreversible changes in the lung have occurred. Corticosteroids were used in 77% (120 of 155) of the reported pediatric cases, with a positive response occurring in all but the one fatal case. Generally, prednisone was given at 0.5 to 2 mg/kg daily for 2 to 4 weeks, followed by tapering of the dosage, although specific regimens have not been studied scientifically. Pulsed methylprednisolone also has been used, potentially with fewer side effects.[10,22] There has been a case report describing the use of rituximab in the treatment of HP that was refractory to conventional therapy.[89] The overall prognosis for children with HP is excellent, provided that a prompt diagnosis is made and appropriate treatment consisting of definitive antigen removal and the judicious

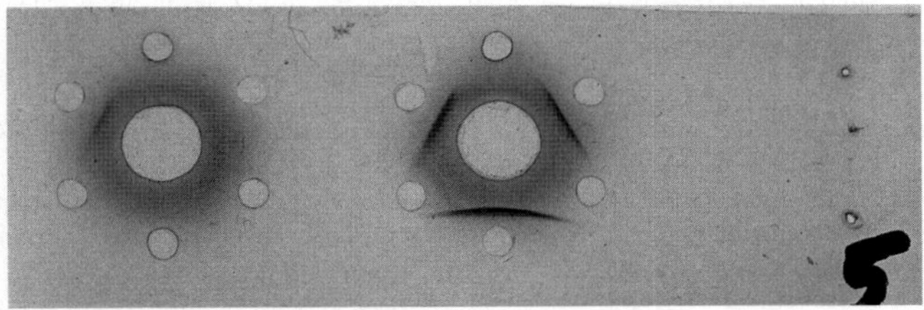

FIG. 24.2 Serum-precipitating antibodies against cockatiel antigens in the patient shown in Fig. 24.1. (Courtesy Robin Deterding, MD, University of Colorado, Denver.)

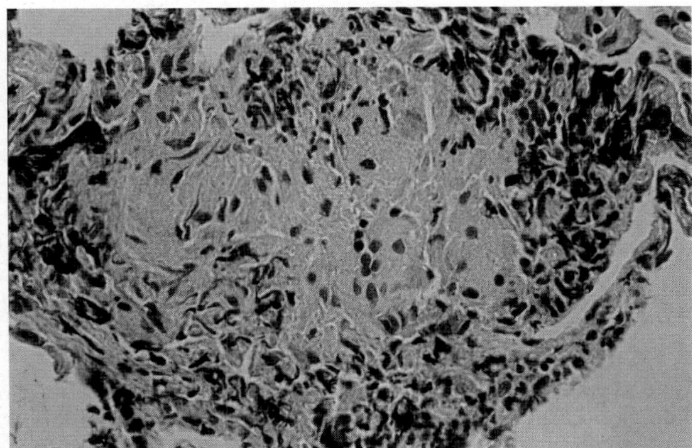

FIG. 24.3 Transbronchial biopsy specimen from the patient in Fig. 24.1 shows a poorly formed granuloma consistent with hypersensitivity pneumonitis. (Courtesy Robin Deterding, MD, University of Colorado, Denver.)

use of corticosteroids is instituted. In the 133 pediatric cases of HP with reported outcomes, 124 improved or became asymptomatic, six patients were still undergoing treatment (including two who had experienced relapse), one patient's condition remained unchanged, one had a worsening course due to continued exposures, and one patient died. In this last case, an 11-year-old girl developed classic features after several years of exposure to budgerigars and other birds.[153] Despite removal of the offending antigens and treatment with corticosteroids and penicillamine, she died of respiratory failure 13 months later. Advanced HP can lead to the need for lung transplantation in adults, and recurrence of disease in the donor lungs has been reported.[79] On the other hand, children who are diagnosed and managed appropriately seem to have minimal long-term adverse effects on their lung function.[138]

NEW REFERENCES SINCE THE SEVENTH EDITION

11. Burton C, Kaczmarski R, Jan-Mohamed R. Interstitial pneumonitis related to rituximab therapy. *N Engl J Med*. 2003;348:2690-2691.
12. Bush A, Cunningham S, de Blic J, et al. European protocols for the diagnosis and initial treatment of interstitial lung disease in children. *Thorax*. 2015;70:1078-1084.
21. Chen C, Isakow W. Identical twins, matching symptoms: hypersensitivity pneumonitis. *Am J Med*. 2015;128:1292-1295.
28. Cordier JF. Organising pneumonia. *Thorax*. 2000;55:318-328.
37. Dell S, Cernelc-Kohan M, Hagood JS. Diffuse and interstitial lung disease and childhood rheumatologic disorders. *Curr Opin Rheumatol*. 2012;24:530-540.
39. Deutsch GH, Young LR, Deterding RR, et al. Diffuse lung disease in young children: application of a novel classification scheme. *Am J Respir Crit Care Med*. 2007;176:1120-1128.
42. Drakopanagiotakis F, Paschalaki K, Abu-Hijleh M, et al. Cryptogenic and secondary organizing pneumonia: clinical presentation, radiographic findings, treatment response, and prognosis. *Chest*. 2011;139(4):893-900.
48. Falfan-Valencia R, Camarena A, Pineda CL, et al. Genetic susceptibility to multicase hypersensitivity pneumonitis is associated with the TNF-238 GG genotype of the promoter region and HLC-DRB1*04 bearing HLA haplotypes. *Respir Med*. 2014;108:211-217.
49. Fan2015 LL, Dishop MK, Galambos C, et al. Diffuse lung disease in biopsied children 2 to 18 years of age: application of the chILD classification scheme. *Ann Am Thorac Soc*. 2015;12:1498-1505.
56. Faria IM, Zanetti G, Barreto MM, et al. Organizing pneumonia: chest HRCT findings. *J Bras Pneumol*. 2015;41:231-237.
62. Giovannini-Chami L, Hadchouel A, Nathan N, et al. Idiopathic eosinophilic pneumonia in children: the French experience. *Orphanet J Rare Dis*. 2014;9:28.
61. Giovannini-Chami L, Blanc S, Hadchouel A, et al. Eosinophilic pneumonias in children: a review of the epidemiology, diagnosis, and treatment. *Pediatr Pulmonol*. 2016;51:203-216.
64. Greenberg MI, Vearrier D. Metal fume fever and polymer fume fever. *Clin Toxicol*. 2015;53:195-203.
65. Griese M, Haug M, Hartl D, et al. Hypersensitivity pneumonitis: lessons for diagnosis and treatment of a rare entity in children. *Orphanet J Rare Dis*. 2013;8:121. cases.
66. Grunes D, Beasley MB. Hypersensitivity pneumonitis: a review and update of histologic findings. *J Clin Pathol*. 2013;66:888-895.
69. Hendrick DJ, Marshall R, Faux JA, et al. Positive "alveolar" response to antigen inhalation provocation test: their validity and recognition. *Thorax*. 1980;35:415-427.
74. Ishizuka M, Miyazaki Y, Tateishi T, et al. Validation of inhalation provocation test in chronic bird-related hypersensitivity pneumonitis and new prediction score. *Ann Am Thorac Soc*. 2015;12:167-173.
79. Kern RM, Singer JP, Koth L, et al. Lung transplantation for hypersensitivity pneumonitis. *Chest*. 2015;147:1558-1565.
80. Kim KW, Ahn K, Yang HJ, et al. Humidifier disinfectant-associated children's interstitial lung disease. *Am J Respir Crit Care Med*. 2014;189:48-56.
82. Kobayashi N, Takezaki S, Kobayashi I, et al. Clinical and laboratory features of fatal rapidly progressive interstitial lung disease associated with juvenile dermatomyositis. *Rheumatology (Oxford)*. 2015;54:784-791.
83. Kreider M, Highland K. Pulmonary involvement in Sjogren syndrome. *Semin Respir Crit Care Med*. 2014;35:255-264.
85. Kurland G, Deterding RR, Hagood JS, et al. An official American Thoracic Society clinical practice guideline: classification, evaluation, and management of childhood interstitial lung disease in infancy. *Am J Respir Crit Care Med*. 2013;188:376-394.
89. Lota HK, Keir GJ, Hansell DM, et al. Novel use of rituximab in hypersensitivity pneumonitis refractory to conventional treatment. *Thorax*. 2013;68:780-781.
97. Megarbane B, Chevillard L. The large spectrum of pulmonary complications following illicit drug use: features and mechanisms. *Chem Biol Interact*. 2013;206:444-451.
104. Munozl X, Morell F, Cruz MJ. The use of specific inhalation challenge in hypersensitivity pneumonitis. *Curr Opin Allergy Clin Immunol*. 2013;13:151-158.
105. Munoz X, Sanchez-Ortiz M, Torres F, et al. Diagnostic yield of specific inhalation challenge in hypersensitivity pneumonitis. *Eur Respir J*. 2014;44:1658-1665.
106. Myllarniemi M, Kaarteenaho R. Pharmacological treatment of idiopathic pulmonary fibrosis – preclinical and clinical studies of pirfenidone, nintedanib, and N-acetylcysteine. *Eur Clin Respir J*. 2015;2:26385.
107. Nathan N, Marcelo P, Houdouin V, et al. Lung sarcoidosis in children: update on disease expression and management. *Thorax*. 2015;70:537-542.
108. Noble PW, Albera C, Bradford WZ, et al. Pirfenidone for idiopathic pulmonary fibrosis: analysis of pooled data from three multinational phase 3 trials. *Eur Respir J*. 2016;47:27-30.
110. Ohtani Y, Kojima K, Sumi Y, et al. Inhalation provocation tests in chronic bird fancier's lung. *Chest*. 2000;118:1382-1389.
118. Rama JA, Fan LL, Faro A, et al. Lung transplantation for childhood diffuse lung disease. *Pediatr Pulmonol*. 2013;48:490-496.
127. Saikia B, Gupta S. Common variable immunodeficiency. *Indian J Pediatr*. 2016;83:338-344.
131. Sauvaget E, Dellamonica J, Arlaud K, et al. Idiopathic acute eosinophilic pneumonia requiring ECMO in a teenager smoking tobacco and cannabis. *Pediatr Pulmonol*. 2010;45:1246-1249.
132. Schwaiblmair M, Behr W, Haeckel T, et al. Drug induced interstitial lung disease. *Open Respir Med J*. 2012;6:63-74.
138. Sisman Y, Buchvald F, Blyme AK. Pulmonary function and fitness years after treatment for hypersensitivity pneumonitis during childhood. *Pediatr Pulmonol*. 2016;51(8):830-837.
147. Tian X, Yi ES, Ryu JH. Lymphocytic interstitial pneumonia and other benign lymphoid disorders. *Semin Respir Crit Care Med*. 2012;33:450-461.
155. Wachowski O, Demirakca S, Muller KM, Scheurlen W. *Mycoplasma pneumoniae* associated organising pneumonia in a 10 year old boy. *Arch Dis Child*. 2003;88:270-272.

The full reference list for this chapter is available at ExpertConsult.com.

25 Cystic Fibrosis

Peter W. Hiatt • Michelle C. Mann • Kathryn S. Moffett

Cystic fibrosis (CF) is the most common inherited lethal disease of whites. It occurs primarily among individuals of Central and Western European origin and affects more than 30,000 Americans and 60,000 people worldwide.[302] The estimated incidence in the United States is 1 in 3200 whites,[318] 1 in 15,000 black, 1 in 31,000 Asian-American, and 1 in 9200 Hispanic live births.[124]

CF has an autosomal recessive mode of inheritance. Affected individuals are phenotypic homozygotes, and both parents usually are heterozygotes or carriers. The carrier frequency in whites in the United States is approximately 1 in 28, with full siblings of children with CF having a one in four chance of being affected.

Mutations in a single gene located on the long arm of chromosome 7 account for the defective protein in CF.[310] A range of different mutations at the DNA level account for the abnormal protein. The most common mutation, p.Phe508del, is the absence of three sequential nucleotides, which leads to the deletion of phenylalanine at the 508 position on the

CF transmembrane conductance regulator protein (CFTR). Approximately 80% of individuals with CF have this mutation, and half of CF patients are homozygous for p.Phe508del. To date, more than 2000 mutations in the *CFTR* gene have been identified,[36,57,59] but fewer than 25 occur with a frequency of more than 0.1%.[108] Certain populations have higher frequencies of specific mutations, such as W128X in Ashkenazi Jews[203] or G551D in French Canadians.[248]

Five to six classes of mutations have been proposed to account for reduced CFTR chloride channel function.[123,248,312,328] Class 1 mutations are mutations in which stop codons or frame shift mutations cause early termination of mRNA translation and minimal to no protein production. In class 2 mutations (p.Phe508del), protein fails to mature, resulting in little expression of CFTR at the cell membrane. Class 3 and class 4 mutations are associated with defective regulation and decreased conductance of chloride at the cell membrane. Protein production and transit to the cell surface occur, but altered chloride conductance is present or chloride conductance is nonexistent. Class 5 mutations are splice site mutations, which affect the amount of CFTR produced. Class 6 mutations are unstable and turn over rapidly.[247]

Disease expression in CF is affected by CFTR mutations, genetic modifiers, and the environment.[58,198] The presence of more than 2000 mutations for CFTR has prompted investigators to evaluate the association of genotype with clinical disease. The Cystic Fibrosis Phenotype Genotype Consortium has shown that certain mutations from classes 3 to 5 are associated with pancreatic sufficiency and lower sweat chloride levels.[57,318] However, minimal correlation of CF genotype with the severity of pulmonary disease has been observed. In general, class 1 to class 3 mutations are associated with higher sweat tests, pancreatic insufficiency, and bronchiectasis. Measurement of lung function is highly variable in patients with the same CFTR mutation (e.g., p.Phe508del), suggesting that other genetic and nongenetic factors determine the severity of lung disease. In a study of monozygotic and dizygotic twins, equal contribution of genetic and nongenetic factors contributed to the variance observed in pulmonary function; that is, approximately 50% to 60% of the variance observed in lung function was secondary to genetic factors.[46,314] Several modifier genes have been identified that affect disease severity of different organ systems in CF[48,58,69,83,156,282] (Fig. 25.1). The wide variation in pulmonary disease observed in CF reflects the effects of genetic modifiers, environment, patient compliance, and polymorphisms in CFTR.

CFTR is a glycoprotein expressed at low levels by surface epithelial cells in the lung, sweat glands, pancreas, liver, large intestine, and testes.[239] Higher levels of expression have been reported in submucosal glands. CFTR protein is a member of a group of membrane transport proteins known as the *ABC-transporter superfamily*.[140] Researchers have confirmed that CFTR functions as an apical chloride and bicarbonate channel

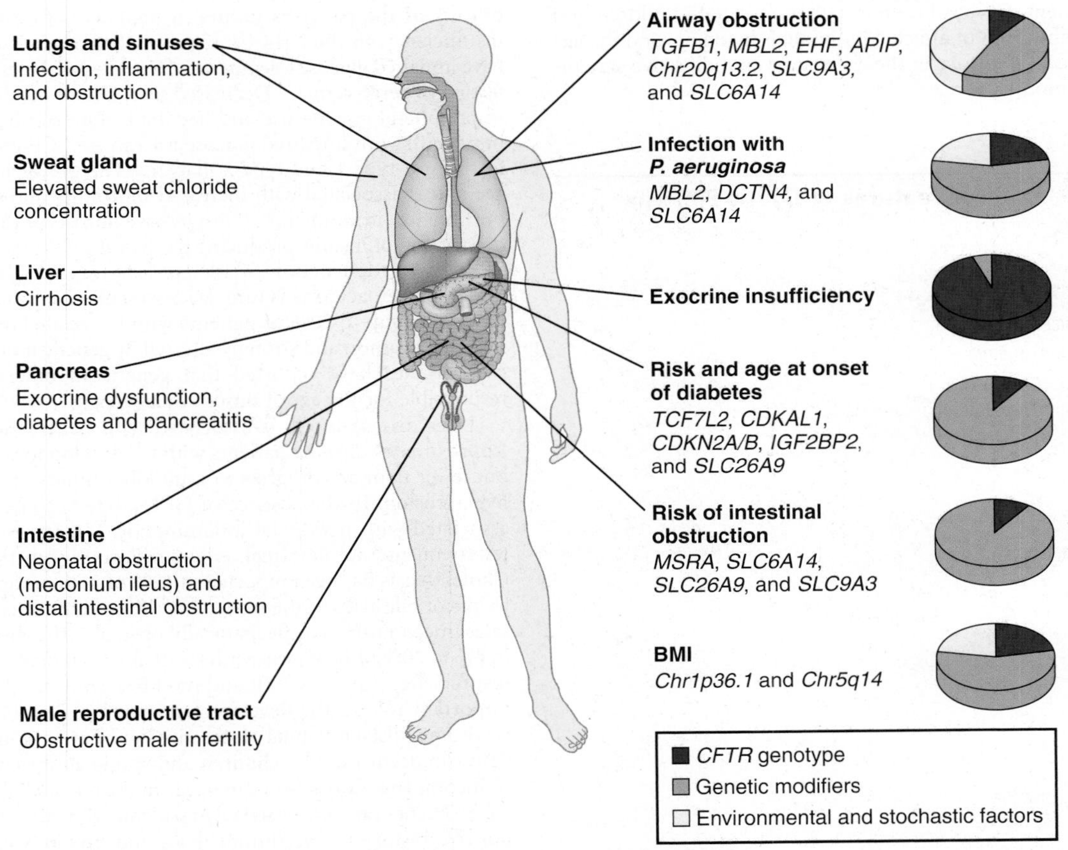

FIG. 25.1 Cardinal features of cystic fibrosis (CF) and relative contribution of genetic modifiers to variation in select cystic fibrosis traits. A diagnosis of CF is based on the presence of clinical findings shown on the left, along with an elevated sweat chloride concentration (>60 mM). The degree of organ system dysfunction varies considerably among affected individuals. Genetic modifiers and nongenetic factors both contribute to airway obstruction and infection with *Pseudomonas aeruginosa*—two traits that define lung disease in CF. CF transmembrane conductance regulator (CFTR) genotype is the primary determinant of the degree of pancreatic exocrine dysfunction. The presence of CFTR variants associated with severe pancreatic exocrine dysfunction is essentially a prerequisite for the development of diabetes and intestinal obstruction. In the setting of severe endocrine dysfunction, genetic modifiers determine when, and if, diabetes occurs and whether neonatal intestinal obstruction occurs. Genetic variation plays the predominant part in nutritional status as assessed by body mass index. (Modified from Cutting GR. Cystic fibrosis genetics: from molecular understanding to clinical application. *Nat Rev Genet.* 2015;16[1]:45–56.)

mediated by cyclic adenosine monophosphate containing 1480 amino acids. It is composed of two membrane-spanning domains, two nucleotide-binding domains that interact with adenosine triphosphate, and a regulatory domain.[5] Activation of the channel is regulated by protein kinase A, which serves as a target for phosphorylation. CFTR in epithelial cell membranes may influence the expression of other proteins important in regulating inflammation, ion transport, and cell signaling, altering the CF phenotype.[248] CFTR regulates the activity of separate calcium-activated chloride channels and downregulates sodium transport, balancing the rates of chloride secretion and sodium absorption,[108,152,165] although this view has undergone a recent challenge.[39]

CFTR is responsible for the proper hydration of secretions in the airway, pancreas, and other tissues. An inability to secrete chloride, bicarbonate, and excessive absorption of sodium and water contribute to altered luminal secretions in patients with CF. In the lung, this alteration leads to decreased airway surface liquid, decreased mucociliary clearance, and a predisposition to chronic bacterial infections.

CLINICAL MANIFESTATIONS

Individuals with CF have exocrine gland dysfunction, which results in progressive suppurative obstructive lung disease, pancreatic insufficiency (85–90%), elevated sweat electrolytes, male infertility (>95%), and female infertility. Less common manifestations include hepatobiliary disease, osteoarthropathy, diabetes mellitus, nasal polyposis, and meconium ileus (Box 25.1).[43,60,61] With the institution of newborn screening and improved treatment, CF has become a disease of both children and adults, with roughly 50% of affected individuals living beyond the age of 18 years.[90] Onset of disease in the respiratory and digestive systems begins within 6 months of age.[302]

BOX 25.1 Clinical Features of Cystic Fibrosis at Diagnosis

0–2 Years

Meconium ileus
Obstructive jaundice
Hypoproteinemia and anemia
Bleeding diathesis
Heat prostration and hyponatremia
Failure to thrive
Steatorrhea
Rectal prolapse
Bronchitis/bronchiolitis
Staphylococcal pneumonia

2–12 Years

Malabsorption
Recurrent pneumonia and bronchitis
Nasal polyps
Intussusception

>13 Years

Chronic pulmonary disease
Clubbing
Abnormal glucose tolerance
Diabetes mellitus
Chronic intestinal obstruction
Recurrent pancreatitis
Focal biliary cirrhosis
Portal hypertension
Gallstones
Aspermia

From Maclusky I, Levison H. *Kendig's disorders of the respiratory tract in children.* 5th ed. Philadelphia: WB Saunders; 1990:701.

A strong association between pancreatic function and genotype has been reported for individuals homozygous for p.Phe508del.[24] Most patients homozygous for p.Phe508del have pancreatic insufficiency.[57] Obstruction of the pancreatic duct begins in utero, resulting in fibrosis and loss of exocrine pancreatic function. Pancreatic fluid from patients with CF is low in enzyme and bicarbonate concentrations, resulting in maldigestion of fat and protein. Clinically, children can present with steatorrhea, protein-calorie malnutrition, muscle wasting, and progressive failure to thrive. A voracious appetite is characteristic, and stools are described as bulky, greasy, and foul smelling. Approximately 10% to 15% of patients have enough preservation of pancreatic function to allow for normal digestion of food (pancreatic sufficiency).[75] At least five mutations from classes 3 to 5 described earlier are associated with pancreatic sufficiency, whereas almost all patients homozygous for p.Phe508del have pancreatic insufficiency.[57]

Failure to thrive was a common complication observed at the time of diagnosis before newborn screening was implemented; however, this complication is now rare. If malnutrition is present and severe, hypoproteinemia and edema are observed. In addition, malabsorption can lead to vitamin deficiency, especially of fat-soluble vitamins A, D, E, and K. These problems can be reversed with pancreatic enzyme replacement therapy, oral nutritional supplements, and routine vitamin supplements. Infants diagnosed by newborn screening may have normal absorption of food for several months after birth; however, with time, pancreatic function is lost and symptoms of malabsorption develop.

Glucose metabolism often becomes impaired with age, because fibrosis of the pancreas occurs in patients with exocrine pancreatic insufficiency. In the 2014 CF registry, 35% of adults were reported to have impaired glucose tolerance or CF-related diabetes with and without fasting hyperglycemia.[64] Decreased secretion of insulin and reductions in peripheral glucose use and hepatic insulin sensitivity are observed in patients with impaired glucose tolerance.[197] CF-related diabetes has features of type 1 and type 2 diabetes. The prevalence increases with age and is associated with increased morbidity and mortality disproportionately in women.[194,196] Progressive fibrosis of the pancreas causes destruction of insulin-producing β cells within the islets of Langerhans. In addition, destruction of islet α cells impairs glucagon secretion; therefore, ketoacidosis is rare. Microvascular complications have been reported in up to 20% of patients with CF-related diabetes.[6] Diabetes in CF is common and strongly affected by genetic modifiers.[22] Affected-twin studies have reported that genetic modifiers were primarily responsible for the age at onset of diabetes.[56]

Liver disease in CF is associated with pancreatic insufficiency.[216] Approximately 25% of patients with CF develop focal biliary cirrhosis, but fewer than 5% progress to multilobar biliary cirrhosis and portal hypertension. In the absence of CFTR, bile becomes inspissated and associated with periductal inflammation and fibrosis. Liver function tests frequently are abnormal, as is a small, poorly functioning gallbladder. Cholelithiasis has been reported in 12% of patients and may be related to loss of bile acids in the stool.[50,97,105] Meconium ileus, the thick inspissated meconium that mechanically obstructs the distal ileum, occurs in 8% to 20% of newborns with CF. It also is associated with pancreatic insufficiency.[149] Both CFTR and modifier genes are thought to play an important role in the development of meconium ileus.[19,36] A similar syndrome (distal intestinal obstructive syndrome) mimicking meconium ileus can occur in older children and young adults with CF. Complete or incomplete obstruction can occur in the terminal ileum or proximal colon. Higher rates are observed in patients with pancreatic insufficiency, positive history of meconium ileus, and previous episodes of distal intestinal syndrome.[49]

Absence of the vas deferens with secondary aspermia renders 98% of men with CF infertile.[78] Sexual potency is normal, and with microsurgical techniques for sperm aspiration, affected men can become biologic fathers.[187] Men with congenital absence of the vas deferens can have abnormal CF alleles with little clinical expression of disease other than the reproductive system. Fertility in women with CF may be decreased secondary to amenorrhea (malnutrition) and dehydrated cervical mucus.[287] Pregnancy in women with mild to moderate disease appears to be well tolerated and not associated with an increased risk for death.[90,115,118] The live birth rate is 1.9/100.[62]

Pulmonary disease is the primary cause of morbidity and mortality in patients with CF.[318] Expression of CFTR has been localized to the airways and submucosal glands of the lung.[295] Clinical studies in young children with CF have found significant inflammatory changes in the airways in bacterial-positive and bacterial-negative patients. Large-animal models of CF suggest that infection occurs first, followed by inflammation.[284] Imaging studies using high-resolution computed tomography (CT) in infants with CF describe the presence of thickened airway walls and nonhomogeneous air trapping.[70,166,173] Smaller airways and tracheal ring abnormalities are noted at birth in the CF porcine model.[3] Human lungs are reported to be morphologically normal at birth; within weeks, they begin showing evidence of small-airway abnormalities and inflammation. Small and medium-sized airways become obstructed, and neutrophils are the inflammatory cells primarily recovered from bronchoalveolar lavage (BAL) fluid. An intense neutrophilic response leads to the release of proteases that cause chronic injury to the respiratory epithelium and supporting airway structure. The massive numbers of neutrophils subsequently release elastase, which overwhelms the antiproteases in the airway, contributing to enhanced destruction of tissue. Large amounts of neutrophil-derived DNA and cytosol proteins are released into the airway lumen, increasing sputum viscosity and worsening airway obstruction.[68]

Progressive bronchiectasis develops with time, leading to advanced destruction of the airways and parenchyma (Figs. 25.2 and 25.3).[100] Bronchiectatic cysts are prominent, especially in the upper lobes. Death eventually occurs from respiratory failure. Progressive deterioration of pulmonary function occurs despite the routine use of antiinflammatory therapy, mucolytics, airway clearance, and antimicrobial agents. Progressive destruction of the airway and increasing obstruction lead to air trapping, hyperinflation, hemoptysis, and spontaneous pneumothorax.

Many children with CF present during infancy with recurrent wheezing or persistent bronchiolitis. Most infants are asymptomatic at birth; however, many develop tachypnea, wheezing, hypoxia, and hyperinflation after having a respiratory viral infection.[129] These findings often resolve with therapy. As mucopurulent secretions increase, chronic cough develops.[43] Digital clubbing occurs gradually and correlates with severity of lung disease. Cough is the earliest symptom in infants and precedes persistent sputum production, crackles, or clubbing. It is present in half the infants in a prospective study of CF infants diagnosed by newborn screening.[97] Predictive risk factors included the presence of pancreatic insufficiency, infection with *Pseudomonas aeruginosa*, socioeconomic status, and ethnicity. On examination, evidence of crackles and decreased breath sounds secondary to mucopurulent secretions is seen. Acute exacerbations may develop, requiring intravenous antibiotic therapy and frequent hospitalization. More than a third of patients with CF in the 2014 US CF patient registry[64] experienced a pulmonary exacerbation requiring intravenous antibiotics. As lung disease progresses, tolerance for exercise is reduced, dyspnea increases, and respiratory failure develops. Marked heterogeneity occurs in the rate of progression of pulmonary disease. Some patients live to the sixth decade of life, whereas others die as a result of respiratory failure before their 20th birthday. Since newborn screening was instituted, patients are being treated at an earlier age, improving the health in children.

In 2014, the median predicted survival for individuals with CF was 39 years. Survival for children born in 2005 is expected to increase, with the median age approaching the fifth decade of life. In the United States, 50% of people with CF are 18 years old or older,[62,64] and within 5 years, half are expected to be older than 18 years.

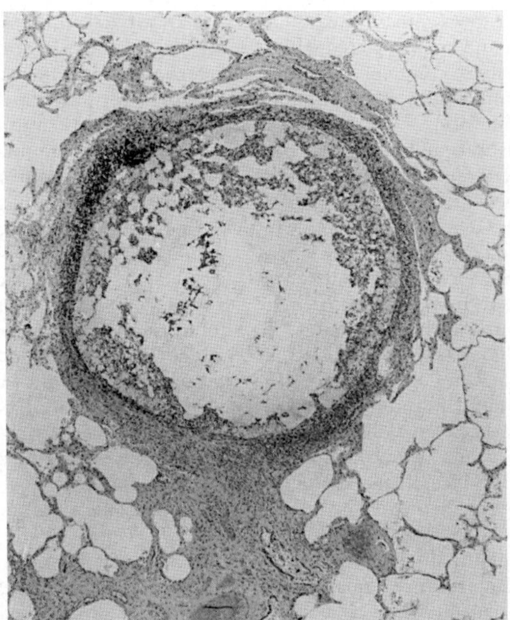

FIG. 25.2 Early stages of lung disease in cystic fibrosis are visible in this lung specimen. Airway inflammation and bronchiectasis are present. The surrounding lung parenchyma is normal.

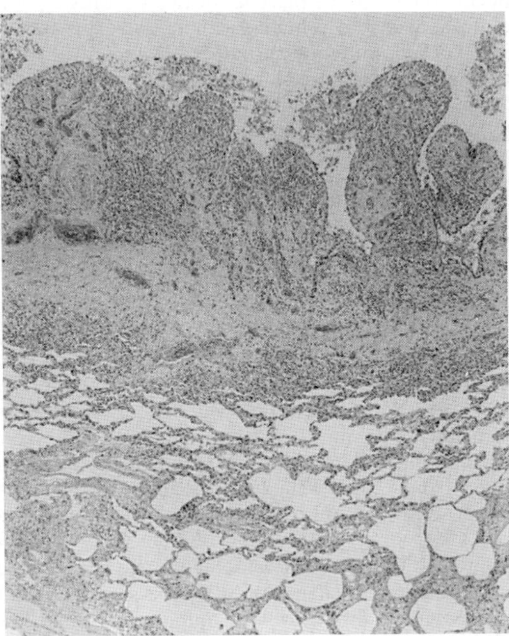

FIG. 25.3 Late stages of pulmonary disease. Epithelial ulceration of the airway, loss of smooth muscle from the airway wall, inflammation, and bronchiectasis are present in the large airway at the top of the photomicrograph. Compression of the surrounding lung parenchyma occurs as bronchiectasis increases.

DIAGNOSIS

The diagnosis of CF has changed over the past 15 years. Newborn screening for CF has been adopted by the United States, Europe, Australia, New Zealand, and many Latin American countries. The CF newborn screening program identifies patients at risk for the disease by measuring values of immunoreactive trypsinogen in dried blood spots. Trypsinogen is produced in the pancreas and is released into the serum secondary to pancreatic duct dysfunction. After an abnormal immunoreactive trypsinogen value is identified, many programs perform DNA testing to identify known CFTR mutations. Other programs repeat the immunoreactive trypsinogen testing 2 weeks after the initial test. Both programs report 90% to 95% sensitivity and identify infants with varying disease severity.[96,303] After a positive screen, infants are referred for diagnostic testing (sweat test or molecular genetic testing). For most patients, the sweat test remains the best diagnostic test to establish the diagnosis of CF. If the sweat test results are in the intermediate range, then DNA analysis may help in the diagnosis. The clinical significance of all 2000 CF mutations is unknown. Many are sequence variants without known clinical disease. Others are known to cause loss of CFTR function and are associated with clinical abnormalities in one or more organ systems. Sequence analysis of the exons, introns, and promoter regions and detection of deletions and duplications identifies 98% of CFTR mutations.[285] Infants are generally asymptomatic at the time of diagnosis, although some may be underweight. Data from the 2014 US CF registry reported that newborn screening accounted for more than 60% of newly diagnosed patients.[61,64] In the absence of newborn screening, an in utero diagnosis, or a family history of CF, a strong clinical suspicion is required for early recognition. Most children present with a history of recurrent lower respiratory tract disease and symptoms secondary to malabsorption. Approximately 15% to 20% of children have meconium ileus at birth, a family history of CF, or both. A consensus panel convened by the US Cystic Fibrosis panel recommended a combination of phenotypic features, family history of CF, or positive newborn screen and one or more laboratory tests to diagnose CF.[95,246] A new CF consensus panel was convened in 2015, but results have not been published. Laboratory tests include identification of known CF mutations, abnormal bioelectric transepithelial membrane properties, and elevated concentrations of sweat chloride. The World Health Organization adopted similar recommendations.[319]

The quantitative pilocarpine iontophoresis sweat test is the primary test to establish a diagnosis of CF.[246] A sweat chloride concentration greater than 60 mEq/L is consistent with a diagnosis of CF. Values between 40 and 60 mEq/L are considered borderline, and values less than 40 mEq/L are normal. Infants with a positive newborn screen and sweat chloride values between 30 and 59 mEq/L under 6 months of age are considered to have values in the intermediate range. Molecular genetic testing should be pursued in those infants with indeterminate sweat chloride values. In the presence of two CF-causing mutations, a diagnosis of CF can be made. Infants with intermediate sweat test values and one CF-causing mutation cannot be diagnosed definitively with CF and will need to be followed longitudinally. Infants with an elevated immunoreactive trypsinogen level and inconclusive CFTR functional and genetic testing should be designated CFTR-related metabolic syndrome (United States) or CF Screen Positive, Inconclusive Diagnosis (Europe). If the sweat test is positive, it should be repeated on two separate occasions. Identification of two CF mutations by genotype is highly specific but less sensitive and should be confirmed with a sweat test. Mutational analysis can be done by several different techniques, with commercial laboratories testing for the most common 30 to 87 mutations. These laboratories identify approximately 90% of CF mutations but leave more than 1000 mutations unidentified. Extensive screening for the remaining 10% of mutations is expensive. For rare mutations, gene sequencing is available.[245,246] The mutational classifications in the CFTR2 project (http://www.cftr2.org/index.php) should be used to help with diagnosis. The p.Phe508del mutation is found in 89% of patients with CF in the United States and a similar number of CF patients in the United Kingdom. Because each patient has two chromosomes, however, only 50% of patients are homozygous for p.Phe508del.

Nasal potential difference measurements assess the transepithelial electric potential difference that exists across nasal epithelium. Different patterns of potential difference are found in patients with CF.[318] Abnormalities in chloride transport and sodium absorption alter the transepithelial electric potential difference in CF in contrast to normal epithelia. The test can be useful in individuals with mild or atypical phenotypic features of CF, but it is not readily available and requires experienced personnel to perform.[245,246]

Newborn screening programs are associated with long-term benefits in children with CF diagnosed shortly after birth. Improved nutritional status as a result of newborn screening has been reported in a controlled, randomized trial in Wisconsin[96] as well as in countries other than the United States.[259] A total of 90% of screened infants in the Wisconsin study diagnosed with CF at birth maintained their weight greater than the 10th percentile in contrast to only 60% of unscreened controls. Children in the screened group were less likely to fall below the 10th percentile for weight and height from early childhood through 16 years of age.[30,96] In addition, cognitive function improved significantly in the screened group.[157,160] No long-term improvements in pulmonary status were observed in the Wisconsin study; however, several observational studies have reported improved pulmonary outcomes, less colonization with *P. aeruginosa,* decreased hospitalization for complications, and improved nutrition in children diagnosed by newborn screening.

In addition to improving nutritional outcomes, newborn screening may result in improved survival rates for children. A systematic literature review of mortality in children with CF reported a survival benefit for patients diagnosed by newborn screening.[55,123] A survival effect also was shown in a study from Wales.[81] Without screening, approximately 60% of patients are diagnosed by the time they reach 1 year of age and almost 90% by the time they are 5 years old. Early diagnosis through neonatal screening improves nutritional outcome, with increasing evidence that these programs are associated with improved pulmonary outcomes and improved long-term survival.

The diagnosis of CF should be based on the presence of one or more clinical features (Box 25.2), a positive newborn screening test, and laboratory evidence of abnormal CFTR function. Laboratory tests include elevated sweat chloride concentration, two identifiable CF mutations, or abnormal in vivo nasal potential difference measurements made across the nasal epithelium.

PATHOGENESIS

The CFTR protein is a cyclic adenosine monophosphate–regulated chloride channel that resides primarily in the apical membranes of epithelial cells. CFTR is highly expressed in airways; its loss of function leads to defective secretion of chloride and bicarbonate and subsequent dehydrated and acidic airway secretions.[32] Sweat glands, pancreas, liver, intestinal tract, and reproductive organs are among the other organ systems affected by dysfunctional CFTR. In affected organs, the abnormal chloride and fluid secretion impairs fluid movement and leads to ductular obstruction and organ damage. Mucociliary clearance is impeded, and a destructive cycle of inflammation and chronic infection in the airways results.

Chronic inflammation and resultant lung damage in CF results from failure of the innate immune system to protect the airways from invading pathogens. The complex process of CFTR dysfunction leading to inflammation in the airways is still not fully understood. In the CF lung, decreased volume of airway surface liquid (ASL) impairs mucociliary clearance (MCC), which is the body's primary defense against inhaled particulate matter and various microbial pathogens. The ASL is composed of a gel and sol layer that function together to help trap microbial pathogens to be propelled up and out of the lungs by beating cilia. The sol or periciliary liquid layer consists of low-viscosity fluid to hydrate mucins and allows ciliary movement to occur. The periciliary liquid layer is thin, 7 μm in height, bathes the cilia, and allows them to beat freely. The gel or mucous layer floats on top of the sol and is composed of high-molecular-weight mucins with carbohydrate side chains that bind inhaled particulate matter and pathogens.

The ASL and mucus layer is a dynamic structure that changes in response to the environment and host. ASL volume is regulated by the

BOX 25.2 Diagnosis of Cystic Fibrosis

≥1 Phenotypic Features

Chronic sinopulmonary disease
Gastrointestinal and nutritional abnormalities
Salt loss syndromes: acute salt depletion
Chronic metabolic alkalosis
Male urogenital abnormalities resulting in obstructive azoospermia

Plus Laboratory Evidence of CFTR Abnormality (≥1)

Elevated sweat chloride concentrations
Identification of two CFTR mutations
In vivo evidence of abnormal ion transport across nasal epithelium

CFTR, Cystic fibrosis transmembrane conductance regulator.

respiratory epithelium through ion transport processes by CFTR. Salt concentrations can be changed to regulate the hydration of the airway lining fluid to maintain optimal mucociliary function. The absence of CFTR in the apical cellular membrane decreases the ability of cells to secrete chloride into the periciliary fluid. CFTR inhibits the epithelial sodium channel; in its absence, excessive absorption of sodium occurs. Other channels are available for secretion of chloride (i.e., calcium-activated chloride channel) in the respiratory epithelium; however, they cannot compensate for the loss of CFTR. The net effect is increased absorption of sodium, chloride, and water, which reduces the periciliary volume, alters the composition of mucins, and decreases mucociliary clearance. The reduction in the periciliary fluid impairs ciliary movement, as they are weighed down by the heavy gel layer and mucus cannot be transported and cleared. This initiates the cycle of airway obstruction, chronic infection, inflammation, and progressive lung destruction.

Altered chloride channel function and fluid secretion also help to explain the presence of disease in the sweat gland, intestine, pancreas, and male genital tract. The epithelial cells affected by CFTR mutations in various organs represent different channel and regulatory activities of CFTR but result in deficient secretion of fluids. This deficiency causes accumulation of mucus, obstruction, and various degrees of organ damage. Plugging of pancreatic ducts leads to chronic fibrosis, pancreatic atrophy, and loss of digestive enzymes and islet cells. Similar obstruction in the biliary tract can cause inflammation and focal biliary cirrhosis. Glandular obstruction of the vas deferens causes involution of the Wolffian duct and infertility in more than 95% of men with CF. Women with CF produce abnormally tenacious cervical mucus, with reported rates of infertility of 20%.

Human cell culture models of normal and CF epithelia have shown that the airway surface liquid is decreased in CF[186,293]; this remains the primary hypothesis of the impaired MCC in the disease.[25,156,240]

Work with large-animal models of CF has revealed that there is likely a more complex pathology for early defects in MCC. CF piglets showed abnormal MCC not due to periciliary liquid depletion but rather due to abnormal CF submucosal gland secretion. Even when periciliary fluid volume was replaced, abnormal mucins remained tethered to glandular ducts, thus preventing normal upward movement on the mucociliary ladder.[131,312]

Submucosal glands have high expression of CFTR.[94,120] Loss of CFTR function alters the composition of mucins produced by the submucosal glands,[146,151,307] leading to ductular dilation with mucus and obstruction. Mucus is tightly adhered to the respiratory epithelium and prevents normal flow of the mucociliary elevator. Failure to clear mucous plugs, continued mucin secretion, and abnormal adherent mucus to the airway surface provides the focus for infection. Pili extending from the surface of the bacterium are able to bind to mucin.[272] In CF, dysfunctional bicarbonate secretion also results in ASL that is 8-fold more acidic than that of individuals without CF. This low pH can inactivate ASL and mucus antimicrobial peptides.[32]

Obstruction of small terminal airways and submucosal glands with thickened mucopurulent secretions are often the first signs of early disease in infants with CF. Ductular dilation, neutrophil infiltration, glandular hyperplasia, and peribronchiolar inflammation are classic findings of the disease. Thick mucus adherent to epithelial cell surface is seen in the lungs of even newborn CF pigs.[285] A recent study showed that CFTR activity of bicarbonate transfer is greater in small-airway epithelial cells compared with larger airways and the effect of nonfunctioning CFTR in small airways leads to more acidic, viscous ASL with impaired bacterial killing. This may help explain the vulnerability of the small airways to bacterial infection and disease.[166] Air trapping is found in infants with CF as young as a few months old even when clinically asymptomatic.[273] Also, piglets with CF have been shown to have air trapping prior to the onset of infection and inflammation in the airways. These piglets were found to have a smaller trachea and proximal airways compared with non-CF piglets. These data suggest that working CFTR is necessary for normal development of early airways.[3]

Early and exaggerated inflammation occurs in the CF airways that begins in infancy and may precede bacterial infection.[273] In CF lung disease, various immune cells migrate to the airways, contributing to the chronic unrelenting inflammation. Neutrophils predominate to fight bacterial and fungal pathogens, but the activation of these cells can lead to tissue destruction through oxidant and protease release. The serine proteases released have been shown to predict the development of bronchiectasis in CF.[282] Neutrophil elastase mediates killing of *P. aeruginosa* by degrading its outer membrane protein but also breaks down structural airway matrix proteins, cleaves proteins important for host defense, and increases mucus secretion.[32,293,297] Neutrophil elastase has a clear role in the development of bronchiectasis and tissue destruction in progressive CF lung disease. Other proteases, such as cathepsins (found to be increased in BAL samples of infants and children with CF) and matrix metalloproteinases, may play a role in early CF disease. Calgranulins are proinflammatory proteins that are also increased in CF sputum and have been shown to activate key processes of CF lung inflammation.[121,181]

The inflammatory response in CF involves different immune pathways. Neutrophils, macrophages, TLR4-dependent responses, and T lymphocytes have all been shown to have defective functioning associated with CFTR deficiency.

Lipid abnormalities, such as an accumulation of epithelial ceramide, have been suggested in CF to increase cell death, increase bacterial binding to extracellular DNA, and release inflammatory chemokines. Other investigators highlight the importance of ceramides in lipid rafts needed to clear infection. CF cell membranes are also reported to have increased arachidonic acid compared to docosahexaenoic acid. Docosahexaenoic acid has important antiinflammatory properties.[121,181] Chronic infection, with retention of the by-products of inflammation, ultimately leads to the severe bronchiectatic changes and derangements of gas exchange characteristic of end-stage CF.

A hypoxic environment develops within the thickened mucous plugs that form in the airways, which may hinder host defenses and favor bacterial growth and inflammation. *Pseudomonas aeruginosa,* after binding to mucin, is able to penetrate the thickened mucus and grow in an anaerobic environment. *P. aeruginosa* is able to grow in anaerobic conditions because of the production of nitrate reductase, which allows it to cleave oxygen from nitrate (Fig. 25.4).[270,323] When it is in the anaerobic environment, an alginate polysaccharide is formed. Biofilm-containing macrocolonies of *P. aeruginosa* are then established. The established macrocolonies remain within the airway lumen. These macrocolonies are very resistant to antibiotics and host defense and allow chronic infection, inflammation, and airway destruction to occur.[134,221,323]

Several in vivo studies have assessed the location of bacterial adherence within the lung of CF patients and the attachment of bacteria to CF and non-CF cells in vitro.[17,302] *P. aeruginosa* is found within the lumen of airways of patients with CF obtained from autopsy specimens.[17] These organisms are observed within the inflammatory exudates of the airway and not within epithelial cells lining the lung or in alveolar spaces. In vitro studies have shown adherence of *P. aeruginosa* in areas of epithelial cell destruction.[223,228,302] No adherence to the apical membrane of intact epithelial cells has been noted, however. In contrast, evidence in cell culture models indicates that defects in CFTR enhance bacterial binding to immortalized airway epithelial cells.[254] A tetrasaccharide (asialo GM_1) is expressed more on CF than on non-CF cells and promotes *P. aeruginosa* binding to the epithelial membrane. Pseudomonal exoproducts, such as neuraminidase, increase the amount of asialo GM_1 available for bacterial binding and facilitate bacterial adherence to airway epithelial cells.[29,255,259] CFTR itself can act as a receptor for *P. aeruginosa* and initiate an effective innate immune response in the initial stages of infection to clear *Pseudomonas* from the airway.[31] CFTR binding to *P. aeruginosa* induces release of IL-1β, nuclear translocation of nuclear factor-κB (NF-κB), and neutrophil influx. Endocytosis of *Pseudomonas* by the epithelial cells and subsequent clearance of infected epithelial cells by desquamation has been reported.[224,226] In the absence of CFTR, clearance of infection with *P. aeruginosa* is impaired.

Mucins also are important in binding bacteria within the airway. Sialylated and neutral forms of mucins bind *P. aeruginosa.*[235] Removal of sialylic acid from mucin by neuraminidase reduces adherence of *P. aeruginosa*. Mucus dehydration can lead to increased concentration of mucins, decreased pH, and a reduction in glutathione, which decreases mucus viscoelasticity.[249] Decreased bicarbonate secretion results in mucin cross-linking by calcium.[99] Polymeric macromolecules within the gel

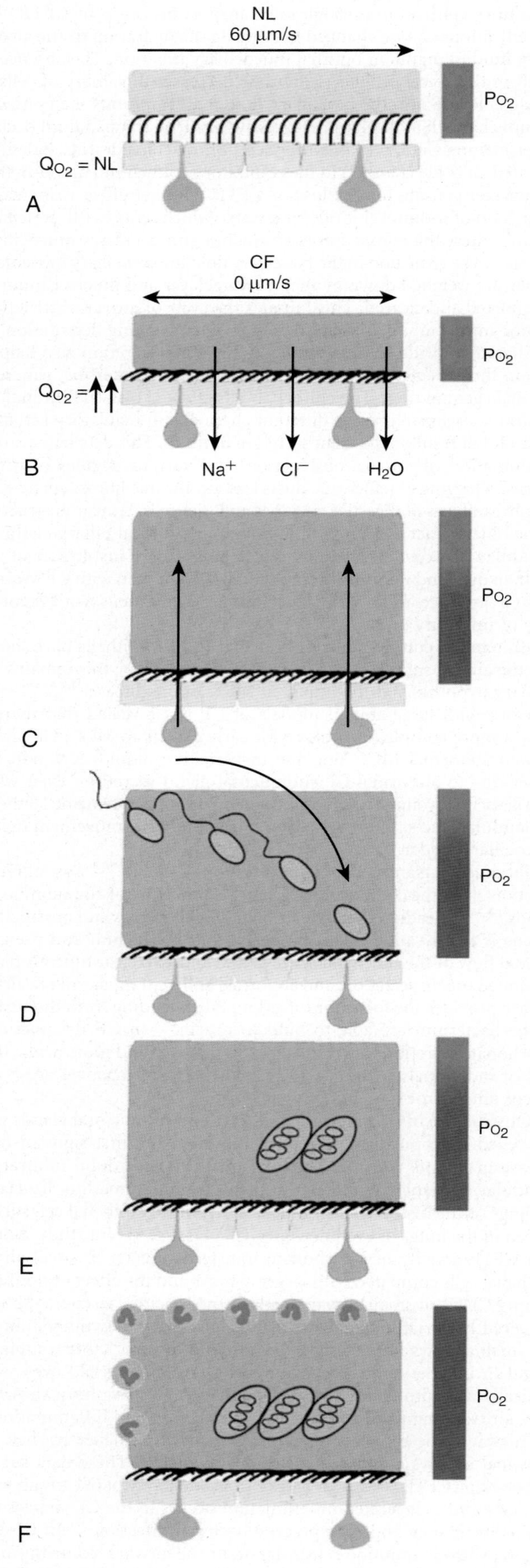

FIG. 25.4 Schematic model of the pathogenic events hypothesized to lead to chronic *Pseudomonas aeruginosa* infection in airways of patients with cystic fibrosis (CF). (A) On normal airway epithelia (NL), a thin mucous layer (*light gray*) resides atop the periciliary liquid (PCL; *clear*). The presence of the low-viscosity PCL facilitates efficient mucociliary clearance (*vector*). A normal rate of epithelial oxygen (O_2) consumption (Q_{O_2}; left) produces no O_2 gradients within this thin airway surface liquid (ASL). (B–F) CF airway epithelia. (B) Excessive CF volume depletion (*vertical arrows*) removes the PCL, mucus becomes adherent to epithelial surfaces, and mucus transport slows or stops (*bidirectional vector*). The increased O_2 consumption (*left*) associated with accelerated CF ion transport does not generate gradients in thin films of ASL. (C) Persistent mucus hypersecretion (denoted as mucus secretory gland/goblet cell units; *dark gray*) with time increases the height of luminal mucus masses and plugs. The increased CF epithelial Q_{O_2} generates steep hypoxic gradients in thickened mucus masses. (D) *P. aeruginosa* bacteria deposited on mucus surfaces penetrate actively or passively or both (as a result of mucus turbulence) into hypoxic zones within the mucus masses. (E) *P. aeruginosa* adapts to hypoxic niches within mucus masses with increased alginate formation and the creation of macrocolonies. (F) Macrocolonies resist secondary defenses, including neutrophils, setting the stage for chronic infection. The presence of increased macrocolony density and, to a lesser extent, neutrophils renders the now mucopurulent mass hypoxic. (From Worlitzsch D, Tarran R, Ulrich M, et al. Effects of reduced mucus oxygen concentration in airway *Pseudomonas* infections of cystic fibrosis patients. *J Clin Invest*. 2002;109:317–25.)

matrix reduce pore size from 500 to 150 nm, immobilizing bacteria within the mucus and inhibiting neutrophil migration and clearance.[52] The concentrated mucus impairs neutrophil migration, promotes an anaerobic environment, and reduces mucociliary transport. Mucin, a component of mucus, is decreased in CF; its decreased content may promote development of infection.[252]

The balance between oxidants and antioxidants is known as redox balance. Imbalance can lead to acute or long-term oxidative or reductive stress. Chronic redox imbalance favoring an oxidative environment is hypothesized to contribute to the disease state in CF.[329]

Increased oxidant production by neutrophils has been proposed as a mechanism of airway injury in CF. Evidence of the effects of oxidative damage in airway epithelial cells and extracellular fluids can be seen in the peroxidation of lipids and modifications of proteins.[153] Markers of reactive oxygen species increase during acute pulmonary exacerbations and improve with treatment but do not normalize.[192,295]

An intracellular imbalance in oxidant metabolism has been proposed for airway epithelial cells in CF.[267] ASL in CF is characterized by lower levels of glutathione (GSH) and nitric oxide.[17] Mucins, reduced glutathione, α-tocopherol, and metal-binding proteins function in the airway as antioxidants. The cysteine residues and carbohydrates of mucin account for its antioxidant properties.[58] Secretion of mucins is increased with oxidative stress; however, dehydration of mucins may impair its ability to scavenge reactive oxidative metabolites. Glutathione is important in regulating inflammation related to oxidative stress. GSH is reduced in ASL either from increased consumption or secondary to CFTR dysfunction.[172] GSH is found in large amounts in airway lung fluid from normal patients[33]; however, it is reduced in patients with CF.[288] CFTR may alter glutathione transport, impairing defense to oxidant injury. High-throughput metabolomic analyses of human primary airway epithelia measured decreases in GSH, glutathione disulfide, and a metabolite of *S*-nitroglutathione in CF versus non-CF cells. Also, the GSH/glutathione disulfide ratio was diminished in CF cells, suggesting oxidative stress.[313,329]

Reduced intracellular concentrations of GSH affect hydrogen peroxide content of airway cells and increase NF-κB production, contributing to airway inflammation. GSH acts to scavenge free radicals in epithelial lining. GSH is also important in the immune response with chemotaxis, phagocytosis, and oxidative burst. Impaired absorption of antioxidants from the gut in CF may contribute as well. Thus, increased production of reactive oxygen species from neutrophils and impaired antioxidant biosynthesis associated with mutant CFTR create an environment within the airway for excessive inflammation and cellular injury.[329]

There are repeated descriptions of abnormalities in oxidants and antioxidants in CF plasma, cells, and ASL. However, several studies failed to show significant clinical benefit of antioxidant therapies in CF.[121,329] Further studies using omics technology may help us to better understand redox in CF and potential therapies.

Production of cell adherence molecules and inflammatory cytokines is intact in patients with CF.[80,150] Defects in bacterial opsonization, reduction in antiinflammatory cytokines, and proinflammatory effects of bacterial DNA have been reported. Impaired phagolysosomal function and decreased respiratory burst have been found in neutrophils in CF with upregulation of Toll-like receptor 4 (TLR4) and downregulation in TLR2. These abnormalities would be expected to reduce the ability of neutrophils to clear bacteria.[18,199] Inflammation and infection can increase intracellular Ca^{2+} and affect the immune response mediated by airway epithelial cells and T-helper cells. Increased intracellular Ca^{2+} in CF mice helper T-cells affect gene expression and favor a Th2 differentiation rather than the Th1 needed for bacterial clearance.[203] Altered T-helper lymphocytes impair macrophage activation for bacterial killing. Humoral antibody responses are normal; however, increased elastase in the CF airway can alter opsonic receptors, impairing phagocytosis. Large amounts of elastase are present in lavage fluid from airways of patients with CF, overwhelming the normal antiprotease activity. This condition can lead to local impairment in phagocytosis of bacteria within the airway lumen, contributing to bacterial persistence.

Proinflammatory mediators are elevated in BAL fluid from young patients with CF, as are macrophages expressing intracellular cytokines.[148,204,325] Increased numbers of neutrophils and interleukin 8 (IL-8) in BAL fluid are seen in bacterial culture–negative and bacterial culture–positive infants with CF in contrast to controls.[136,314] Proinflammatory mediators IL-1, IL-2, tumor necrosis factor-α, and IL-8 are markedly elevated in children with advanced disease.[128,136,314] In contrast, some antiinflammatory cytokines (e.g., IL-10) are found in reduced amounts in BAL from patients with CF. These observations have prompted some investigators to assess production of IL-10 from bronchial epithelial cells in normal subjects and subjects with CF.[23] Bronchial epithelial cells from normal individuals produce significantly greater amounts of IL-10 than cells of subjects with CF. NF-κB is a transcription factor for several proinflammatory mediators and is activated persistently in CF. Inhibitors to NF-κB, including IL-10, are downregulated.[76,265,304,311]

Enhanced intracellular Ca^{2+} signaling in response to infection and inflammation in both airway epithelial and immunomodular cells may account for the hyperinflammatory response noted in CF.[237,239] Both phases of Ca^{2+} release, either by Ca^{2+} influx or endoplasmic reticulum release, can upregulate NF-κB and production of proinflammatory cytokines. Chronic airway inflammation and infection increase endoplasmic reticulum Ca^{2+} stores, enhancing the inflammatory response. Therefore, the CF gene defect may result in an inability to control airway inflammation after exposure to repeated infections, altering the innate and immune responses to specific pathogens. Although the understanding of this disease pathogenesis is incomplete, airway damage that occurs from excessive inflammation and chronic infection remains a target for new therapeutic modalities.

The range of severity of disease is related to the production of functioning CFTR. Patients with at least one "mild" mutation in CFTR have some low level of CFTR expression. They retain some degree of pancreatic function, have less severe lung disease, and have sweat chloride concentrations that are borderline normal.[55,70,318] Male patients with congenital bilateral absence of the vas deferens are pancreatic sufficient, exhibit little or no lung disease, can have normal sweat chloride concentrations, and are thought to have CFTR expression that is 10% of normal.[13] Carriers for CFTR who are heterozygotes expressing half the expected amount of CFTR are at increased risk for developing pancreatitis, allergic bronchopulmonary aspergillosis (ABPA), and sinusitis.[40,45,84,229] As we begin to see the clinical effects of pharmacologic therapies that correct and potentiate CFTR function, we are learning more about the direct effect of CFTR on the symptoms of CF. The potentiator ivacaftor has been able to show that improvement in CFTR function, evidenced by dramatic improvement in sweat chloride tests, leads to improvement in multiple clinical factors. Lung function assessed by forced expiratory volume in 1 second and MCC improved and rates of *P. aeruginosa* infection dropped by 18% in 6 months after initiation of the drug in one study.[74,217,248]

Variation in phenotype also exists in individuals with the same genotype, indicating that other factors—including modifier genes and epigenetic and environmental factors—influence the disease process.[28]

SPECIFIC CYSTIC FIBROSIS PATHOGENS

Viral Pathogens

Numerous studies have evaluated the role of nonbacterial infections with pulmonary exacerbations in CF. A clear correlation between respiratory viral infection and exacerbations of lung disease has been shown in most of these reports. Viral lower respiratory tract infections occur more often in younger children with CF and are associated with increased pulmonary disease in 40% of cases.[1,298] Respiratory syncytial virus (RSV) has been identified most often with CF pulmonary exacerbations; however, influenza, adenovirus, parainfluenza virus, rhinovirus, picornavirus, and human metapneumovirus also have been reported.[298] Respiratory viruses are isolated from patients with CF requiring hospitalization, and infection is associated with increased morbidity rates. Infants with CF infected with RSV can experience prolonged hospitalizations, mechanical ventilation, and supplemental oxygen at hospital discharge.[1] Severe viral infections in infants with CF were reported in 31 of 80 children diagnosed by newborn screening. Half of the children hospitalized had a respiratory virus identified at the time of hospitalization, and RSV infection accounted for hospitalization in 7 of the 31 children.[8]

Two studies have reported prolonged bronchiolitis-like syndromes in infants younger than 6 months of age.[106,170] These infants required intensive respiratory therapy, including bronchodilators, chest physiotherapy, and mechanical ventilation. Increased hospitalization was observed for children with CF who were infected with RSV in another study of children younger than 3 years of age.[128] Although prolonged hypoxia and respiratory failure were not observed, pulmonary function was markedly decreased after hospitalization and persisted for several months after infection.[128] Studies in older children with CF have reported reduction in pulmonary function, clinical scores, and radiographic scores and increased hospitalization after viral infection.[47,211,277,308,315] These studies show that infection with respiratory viruses results in clinical deterioration, hospitalization, and decreases in lung function.

Mechanisms to explain the enhanced disease observed with respiratory viral infections are being investigated. Normal airway epithelia use an adenosine-regulated pathway to maintain periciliary fluid volume by regulation of sodium absorption and chloride secretion. In a CF model, this regulation can be normalized by phasic motion simulating movement of the lung. Periciliary volume is restored to normal by release of adenosine triphosphate into the periciliary liquid and activation of alternative chloride channels. Viral infections, such as RSV, upregulate the extracellular adenosine triphosphatase activity, reducing periciliary fluid volume. Reduction in periciliary liquid volume promotes mucous stasis and plugging.[293] Other investigators have shown impaired innate defense manifested by reduced production of nitric oxide and impaired interferon-γ signaling pathway.[326,327] Synergism between bacteria and respiratory virus infection was suggested by Przyklenk and coworkers[227] after an increase in the number of bacterial colony-forming units was found in sputum of subjects with CF. Hordvik and associates[133] and Efthimiou and coworkers[86] noted that patients with CF and severe pulmonary disease recovered slowly from viral infection. The underlying severity of lung disease was crucial in predicting response to viral respiratory infection.

The interrelationship between the acquisition of *P. aeruginosa* and viral respiratory infection is unclear. Increased colonization with *P. aeruginosa* has been observed during the respiratory viral season,[141] and infection with *P. aeruginosa* has been associated with hospitalization for viral respiratory illness. Antipseudomonal antibodies have been reported to increase after RSV infection, and new infection with

P. aeruginosa has been observed during an acute respiratory illness.[47,220] Other investigators have not observed any change in bacterial infection or change in colonization associated with viral respiratory infection.[210] In cell culture models, RSV acts as a coupling agent between *P. aeruginosa* and enhances attachment to respiratory epithelial cells.[299] Petersen and colleagues[220] and Ong and associates[211] reported more severe pulmonary disease with viral infection in the presence of *P. aeruginosa* colonization, but Przyklenk and coworkers[227] found no correlation.

Nontypeable Haemophilus influenzae

Haemophilus influenzae is frequently the earliest pathogen isolated from patients with CF, most prevalent in the CF population during the first 5 years of life. The advent of the *H. influenzae* type b vaccine has not had an impact on the prevalence of this organism because patients with CF harbor nontypeable strains. Generally, *H. influenzae* is susceptible to a wide variety of agents and is amenable to treatment. However, recent studies suggest that more than 20% of young patients with CF are infected with *H. influenzae*, with some antibiotic resistance detected in current strains.[34] Despite the frequent recovery of this organism from infants and children, the impact of this organism on the clinical course of CF has been difficult to assess because of the frequent occurrence of coinfection with other pathogens.

Staphylococcus aureus

Staphylococcus aureus is the bacterium cultured most commonly from the respiratory tracts of children with CF; the earliest descriptions of CF lung infections focused on this species.[74] Subsequently, *P. aeruginosa* was increasingly isolated from children with CF, and studies established an association between *P. aeruginosa* and CF lung disease,[89,159] largely shifting the focus of CF microbiologic research and therapy. Recently, increases in *S. aureus* prevalence, both methicillin-susceptible (MSSA) and methicillin-resistant (MRSA), have been described in CF. Data from the Cystic Fibrosis Patient Registry shows that the overall prevalence of MSSA increased from 37% in 1995 to 54% in 2015.[62] Similarly, MRSA prevalence increased from 0.1% in 1995 to 26% in 2015, although it varied substantially from center to center (range per center, 5–48%). Causes for this variability are unclear but could reflect different laboratory practices and clinical practices or regional differences in community-acquired MRSA. Although MRSA generally infects older patients, it is associated with deterioration in both pediatric and adult patients.[193,294] Methicillin resistance is conferred by the *mecA* gene located within the staphylococcal cassette chromosome (SCC). Several SCCmec types have been described and may also carry the putative virulence factor Panton-Valentine leukocidin (PVL), which is commonly detected in the USA300 epidemic strain in the United States. A six-center observational study in the United States (STARCF) examined the clinical impact of different MRSA strains characterized by molecular typing. Of the over 200 isolates obtained from pediatric patients with chronic MRSA infection, 69.5% were SCCmec II- PVL negative, consistent with hospital associated-MRSA. The remaining isolates were 13% SCCmec IV-PVL negative and 17% SCCmec IV-PVL positive. Ongoing studies are evaluating chronic MRSA infection in CF with different SCCmec types and PVL status to determine their roles in clinical and disease outcomes.[68,87,127,144,202]

Recent studies of children with CF noted similar inflammation and lung function decline during infection with *S. aureus* compared with *P. aeruginosa*, and the pathologic consequences of MRSA infection in patients with CF have been recently determined. Chronic MRSA infection in patients with CF is associated with increased rate of lung function decline, failure to recover lung function after a pulmonary exacerbation, and decreased survival. These observations have led to a reexamination of *S. aureus* and its role in CF lung disease.[65,66,225,236,250,258]

Slow-growing, antibiotic-resistant mutants of *S. aureus* known as small-colony variants (SCVs) have been isolated from respiratory secretions in both adults and children with CF with specific but infrequently used culture techniques. Distinction of SCVs is based on colony size on the agar plate, slower growth, nonpigmentation, reduced production of alpha-toxin, and thymidine dependence. There is evidence that exoproducts of *P. aeruginosa* enhance SCV formation; conversely, SCV growth provides a survival advantage for *S. aureus* in the presence of *P. aeruginosa* infection.[130] Clinically, SCVs are associated with higher rates of antimicrobial resistance and more advanced lung disease in CF.[114] The rarity of clinical laboratory culture for SCVs indicates that physicians are frequently unaware of these highly antibiotic-resistant infections in selecting treatments for their CF patients, underestimating the presence both of all *S. aureus* and of a subtype that correlates with worse respiratory disease. Therefore, routine *S. aureus* SCV surveillance would provide more complete information to guide treatment.[316]

Pseudomonas aeruginosa

P. aeruginosa is the most common and important pathogen in patients with CF. Initial strains are nonmucoid, antibiotic-susceptible strains that express pili, flagella, and a more highly acylated lipid A component of lipopolysaccharide. *P. aeruginosa* also produces virulence factors, including exotoxin A, exoenzyme S, leukocidin, phospholipase C, elastase, and alkaline protease, which contribute to the pathogenesis of sepsis, acute lung infections, and bacteremia.[35,279,292] These factors may be chemotactic stimuli for neutrophils, and exotoxins may increase the viscosity of secretions, impair ciliary clearance, and cause small airway obstruction, thus ultimately lung destruction.

Over time, *P. aeruginosa* adapts to the CF lung and undergoes genetic and phenotypic alterations. *P. aeruginosa* initially attaches to solid surfaces (e.g., mucin or respiratory epithelial cells), using flagella and type IV pili.[53] Attachment activates genes that synthesize extracellular polysaccharide (alginate),[73] which confers the mucoid phenotype of *P. aeruginosa* unique to chronic infections in CF.[117] Strains associated with chronic infections lack pili, lack flagella, and undergo structural changes in lipopolysaccharide. These changes may render *P. aeruginosa* more resistant to host defenses, including defensins and the innate inflammatory response. The *lasR-lasI* system (quorum-sensing genes) promotes the initial formation of microcolonies, which differentiate into alginate-encased mature biofilms.[53] Bacteria in biofilms avoid ciliary clearance, evade phagocytosis, and are antibiotic resistant.[271] Biofilms are the proposed mechanism by which *P. aeruginosa* is able to infect the CF airway chronically and avoid eradication by host defenses and by antimicrobial agents. The CF lung can harbor very high concentrations of *P. aeruginosa*—10^8 to 10^9 organisms per gram of sputum may be present.[317]

In 2015, the CF Registry reported that 30.4% of patients with CF younger than 18 years of age were infected with *P. aeruginosa*.[61] Infection with *P. aeruginosa* is associated with increased morbidity and mortality rates caused by recurrent pulmonary exacerbations and a gradual deterioration in lung function.[147,214] Children who are infected with *P. aeruginosa* are more likely to have cough and lower chest radiograph scores than are uninfected children. Investigators have shown that infants younger than 2 years of age infected with *S. aureus* and *P. aeruginosa* have worse pulmonary function, chest radiograph scores, and 10-year survival rates than do uninfected children.[2,89,159,244] In a recent large, multicenter cohort of US children with CF, there was no detectable association between early acquisition of *P. aeruginosa* and more rapid decline in lung function or change in growth parameters. *P. aeruginosa* detection/acquisition was associated with an increased rate of pulmonary exacerbations, more frequent detection of crackles or wheeze on examination and increased emergence of MRSA, *S. maltophilia* and *Achromobacter xylosoxidans* on respiratory cultures.[324]

The mucoid phenotype of *P. aeruginosa* is associated with a more rapid decline in lung function.[215] Multidrug-resistant *P. aeruginosa* (MRPA) was identified in 8.6% of all patients with CF in 2014.[61] MRPA isolates are defined as resistant to all antibiotics evaluated in two or more of the following groups: aminoglycosides, fluoroquinolones, and β-lactams.[163] Infection with MRPA as opposed to *P. aeruginosa* has been shown to cause more rapid decline in pulmonary function[220] and increase in the likelihood of death or lung transplantation.[164] Additional studies have linked poor patient prognosis to a specific MRPA strain, as in the cases of the Liverpool epidemic strain and the Australian epidemic strains.[4,85,208,209]

Burkholderia cepacia *Complex*

Infection with *Burkholderia cepacia* complex (Bcc) and the associated *cepacia syndrome* was reported first in 1979 among adolescent Canadian patients with CF.[138,290] The cepacia syndrome is characterized by a virulent course, high fevers, bacteremia, rapid deterioration in lung function, and early death. Generally, patients with CF do not have bacteremia caused by other pathogens. Different clinical courses can be associated with Bcc, including transient colonization, a gradual decline in lung function, or the virulent cepacia syndrome.

Through a series of genetic and phenotypic studies, researchers have discovered that *B. cepacia* is actually a complex of several different species, previously called *genomovars*, which are indistinguishable phenotypically but distinguishable genotypically.[44] Additional genomovars are likely to be described.[44,300,301,305] Several international investigators have described the epidemiology and clinical courses associated with different genomovars, although these studies usually involved a single strain and might not be generalizable to all strains of a given genomovar.[167,177,281] Most CF isolates are *Burkholderia cenocepacia* (genomovar III) or *Burkholderia multivorans* (genomovar II). The former may be associated with a more rapidly progressive clinical course,[169] whereas *B. multivorans* is more likely to be associated with transient colonization.[177] However, patient-to-patient transmission and clinical deterioration has been associated with *B. multivorans*.[167] An outbreak of *Burkholderia dolosa* (genomovar VI) associated with increased morbidity and mortality rates in the patients following acquisition of this bacterium has also been reported.[145] Virulence factors for *Burkholderia* spp. include multidrug resistance, the ability to form biofilms, the ability to reside intracellularly, and the ability to spread from patient to patient.[177] Studies are ongoing to unravel potential environmental reservoirs of *Burkholderia* spp.

Stenotrophomonas maltophilia

Stenotrophomonas maltophilia, an intrinsically multidrug-resistant, gram-negative bacillus, is a well-known hospital-acquired pathogen in non-CF patients and is isolated with increasing frequency from the respiratory tract of patients with CF. The overall prevalence of this organism in patients with CF is 13.5% (range 0–40% in individual centers).[61,71] There is evidence that many clinical laboratories fail to identify this potential pathogen. Transient colonization also seems to be a common occurrence; Demko and colleagues[71] reported that 50% of patients with CF at their center had only a single positive culture for this microorganism. Increased use of antibiotics has been shown to be a potential risk factor for acquisition of *S. maltophilia*,[180,291] and the role of *S. maltophilia* as a pathogen in CF is still being investigated. Case-control studies have shown that *S. maltophilia* has not had a significant impact on lung function or mortality.[114,180] In contrast, Demko and colleagues[71] found that the 5-year survival of patients with *S. maltophilia* (n = 211) was 40% in contrast to patients without *S. maltophilia* (n = 471), whose 5-year survival was 70%.

Achromobacter xylosoxidans

The clinical significance of *A. xylosoxidans* in CF also is unclear; this organism was reported to the CF patient registry in 1996 when 2.7% of patients harbored this multidrug-resistant, gram-negative bacillus.[60] In 2014, *A. xylosoxidans* was found in 6.1% of patients.[61] The nationally reported prevalence most likely is underestimated; 8.7% of participants in the aerosolized tobramycin trial had positive cultures for *A. xylosoxidans*.[27] Further complicating the epidemiology of this potentially emerging pathogen is the observation that *A. xylosoxidans* may be misidentified as another nonlactose-fermenting, gram-negative bacillus, and that *P. aeruginosa*, *B. cepacia* complex, and *S. maltophilia* may be misidentified as *A. xylosoxidans*.[253] In addition, the impact of this organism is difficult to assess fully because *A. xylosoxidans* generally is cultured from patients concomitantly infected with other CF pathogens, especially *P. aeruginosa*.[162] *A. xylosoxidans* is associated with an increase in pulmonary exacerbations.[82,93]

ANAEROBIC BACTERIA

Anaerobes are organisms that do not require oxygen for growth. Steep oxygen gradients exist within CF mucus such that even at relatively shallow depths within mucus, the environment is considered to be hypoxic or even frankly anaerobic. Conventional culture-dependent approaches are not optimized for identifying anaerobes. Specific anaerobic culture methods, or culture-independent techniques, may be more appropriate.[176] Several studies on tracheal aspirates, sputum, or BAL fluid have confirmed the presence of anaerobes in the lower airways in CF in up to 80% of samples and at bacterial densities of between 10^7 and 10^9 cfu/mL in sputum. The most common genera identified were *Prevotella, Veillonella, Propionibacterium, Actinomyces, Staphylococcus saccharolyticus, Peptostreptococcus*, and *Clostridium*. No data linking anaerobes to inflammation or clinical outcomes in CF are available. Longitudinal studies are also lacking, although a comprehensive longitudinal study conducted in a single patient suggested that anaerobes of the *Streptococcus milleri* group contributed to the development of pulmonary exacerbations. Ulrich and colleagues[297] reported that 16 of 17 patients with CF produced antibodies against two immunoreactive antigens of *Prevotella intermedia* compared with 0 of 30 controls, suggesting that anaerobes are, indeed, immunogenic in CF. In studies in which anaerobes were specifically targeted during treatment for pulmonary exacerbations, the results have been conflicting. Worlitzsch and colleagues[320] did not identify any significant reduction in the density of anaerobes in sputum after treatment with antibiotics despite an increase in pulmonary function during the period of treatment. Similarly, Tunney and colleagues[296a] identified only limited reduction in the density of anaerobes at the end of 2 weeks of treatment. An important factor to consider when treating anaerobic infections is that anaerobic organisms are often resistant to the commonly administered antibiotics.[41]

Fungal Species

Oral and aerosolized antimicrobial agents are risk factors for colonization with *Aspergillus* spp.,[14,232] with 19.7% of patients with CF in the CF Registry having at least one positive culture for this mold in 2014.[61] Recent findings also confirmed the formation of biofilms and increased antifungal drug resistance by *A. fumigatus*.[268] Although *Aspergillus* spp. do not normally invade the parenchyma, the airways can become impacted with mucus-containing fibrin, eosinophils, and mononuclear cells, which can cause airway obstruction and bronchiectasis.[88] The role of *Aspergillus* colonization is unclear, and most experts do not recommend treatment.

Scedosporium spp. can be isolated from the lungs of patients with CF, but the clinical significance of this microorganism is also unknown. In the aerosolized tobramycin trial, 2.4% of patients harbored saprophytic fungi,[27] and in a single center, 8.6% of 128 patients followed for more than 5 years were colonized or infected with *Scedosporium apiospermum*.[42] Additional selective media beyond routine culture methods are necessary to recover most *Scedosporium* spp. and obtain more accurate infection rates.[21]

Candida albicans and other *Candida* spp. are frequently isolated from CF sputum; colonization rates are best predicted by features of advanced CF pulmonary disease. At present, the clinical role of *C. albicans*, if any, is unclear and there is no evidence to suggest treatment benefit.[41]

ABPA is an allergic reaction to colonization of the lungs, with the fungus *Aspergillus fumigatus* affecting approximately 5% of people with CF in 2014.[61] Several studies have also implicated *S. apiospermum* in ABPA-like reactions.[42] ABPA is associated with an accelerated decline in lung function. Of patients with CF, 2% to 10% develop APBA, which can be associated with a dramatic loss of lung function.[88,107,182,201] The diagnosis of ABPA can be difficult to establish because of variability in the application of standardized diagnostic criteria, confusion regarding these criteria, and limited recognition by physicians. This immunologically mediated syndrome is marked by a brisk immunoglobulin E (IgE) response, specific antibody to *Aspergillus fumigatus*, peripheral eosinophilia, and symptoms of reactive airway disease. Short-lived pulmonary infiltrates may be noted on chest radiograph. A workshop sponsored by the Cystic Fibrosis Foundation sought to further the understanding of the diagnostic criteria needed for ABPA in CF.[238,283] This committee established minimum criteria for the diagnosis, which include (1) new clinical deterioration not attributable to another cause; (2) asthma; (3) chest roentgenographic infiltrates—current or in the past—may be detectable on CT when chest radiography is unremarkable; (4) immediate cutaneous reactivity to *Aspergillus* species; (5) elevated total serum IgE (>417 IU/mL or >1000 ng/mL); (6) serum precipitating antibodies to

A. fumigatus; (7) central bronchiectasis on chest CT; (8) peripheral blood eosinophilia; and (9) elevated serum IgE and/or IgG to *A. fumigatus*.

Nontuberculous Mycobacteria

Since the early 1990s, appreciation has been increasing that nontuberculous mycobacteria (NTM) may be pathogens in patients with CF. Estimates of the prevalence of NTM in the CF population have ranged from 1.3% in the earliest study reported in 1984[275] to 32.7% in a review of patients with CF over the age of 40 years in Colorado.[242] In a nested case-control study from 2006 to 2010 in France, data suggested that azithromycin may be a primary prophylaxis for NTM in CF adults.[51]

The NTM species most commonly identified in individuals with CF from North America and Europe are the slow-growing *Mycobacterium avium* complex (including *M. avium*, *M. intracellulare*, and *M. chimaera*), which can be found in up to 72% of NTM-positive sputum cultures, and the rapid-growing *M. abscessus* complex (comprising the subspecies *M. abscessus* subsp. *abscessus* [*M. a. abscessus*], *M. a. bolletii*, and *M. a. massiliense* [the latter currently classified as part of *M. a. bolletii*]), which in many centers has now become the most common NTM isolated from individuals with CF. Other less commonly isolated species include *M. simiae*, *M. kansasii*, and *M. fortuitum*. There are geographic differences in both the prevalence of NTM-positive cultures and the relative frequency of different species seen between but also within countries.[102,205]

In an individual patient, determining if NTM is colonizing the lung or causing disease can be difficult. Signs and symptoms of mycobacterial disease are nonspecific and may be consistent with CF pulmonary exacerbations. Making the diagnosis of NTM does not, per se, necessitate the institution of therapy, which is a decision based on potential risks and benefits of therapy for individual patients.[104] The CF Foundation and the European Cystic Fibrosis Society recommend that (1) cultures for NTM be performed annually in spontaneously expectorating individuals with a stable clinical course, with oropharyngeal swabs not used; (2) individuals receiving azithromycin as part of their CF medical regimen who have a positive NTM culture should not continue azithromycin treatment while evaluation for NTM disease is under way, as azithromycin monotherapy may lead to resistance; (3) American Thoracic Society/Infectious Diseases Society of America diagnostic criteria,[104] which include a combination of clinical, radiographic, and microbiologic elements, be used; and (4) the potential for cross-infection of NTM (especially *M. abscessus* complex) between individuals with CF should be minimized by following national infection control guidelines. Expert consultation should be obtained when NTM is encountered or when isolates usually representing environmental contamination are recovered.[102] Recent studies focusing on *M. abscessus* have also failed to identify risk factors for infection,[306] highlighting the need to determine if NTM causes progressive deterioration in lung function and, if so, the optimal therapy.

TREATMENT OF PATHOGENS IN CYSTIC FIBROSIS PATIENTS

Airway infections are a key component of CF lung disease. Whereas the approach to common pathogens such as *P. aeruginosa* is guided by a significant body of evidence, other infections often pose a considerable challenge to the treating clinicians. A cornerstone of CF care is the aggressive use of oral, intravenous, and aerosolized antibiotics. The increasing longevity of patients with CF has paralleled the development of effective antibiotics. Antibiotics may be used during several stages of CF lung disease (1) to prevent acquisition of pathogens, most commonly MSSA; (2) to eradicate initial acquisition of pathogens, most commonly *P. aeruginosa* and MRSA, in efforts to prevent or delay chronic infection; (3) to treat pulmonary exacerbations caused by classic CF pathogens; (4) to treat patients infected with *P. aeruginosa*, as long-term suppressive therapy; and (5) to treat emerging multidrug-resistant pathogens. Newer molecular techniques have demonstrated that the airway microbiome consists of a large number of microbes, and the balance between microbes, rather than the mere presence of a single species, may be relevant for disease pathogenesis. A better understanding of this complex environment could help define optimal treatment regimens that target pathogens without affecting others. The recognition that there is a diverse microbiota in sputum samples from people with CF raises questions about how we approach antibiotic therapy. Conventional bacterial culture in aerobic conditions allows isolation of a limited number of organisms. Extended culture methods identify a much wider range of bacteria, which include more difficult to culture bacteria, such as anaerobic bacteria.[176] At present, there is no readily available methodology to identify all of these organisms in a way that makes this information valuable for clinical treatment. Studies are under way to develop technologies to allow molecular identification without prior culture.

Prophylaxis to Prevent Acquisition of *Staphylococcus aureus*

Few studies have been conducted on antibiotic prophylaxis in patients with CF, and these studies have focused exclusively on *S. aureus*. The rationale for this strategy is to prevent *S. aureus* infection and to delay acquisition of *P. aeruginosa*.[229,231] From 1985 to 1992, British investigators studied 42 newly diagnosed infants randomly assigned to 12 months of flucloxacillin versus standard care.[16,269] Infants treated with flucloxacillin had fewer infections with *S. aureus* and fewer hospitalizations, but both groups had similar pulmonary function. In a placebo-controlled trial conducted in the United States, 119 patients newly diagnosed with CF (mean age, 16 months) were randomly assigned to receive cephalexin or placebo for 5 to 7 years.[240] No significant differences were found in pulmonary function, the number of pulmonary exacerbations, nutritional status, or chest radiograph scores in the two groups. In contrast, subjects treated with cephalexin had decreased incidence of infection with *S. aureus* but increased incidence of infection with *P. aeruginosa*. Similarly, an analysis of the German national database showed that patients receiving antistaphylococcal agents had increased acquisition of *P. aeruginosa* and no improvement in lung function.[203,171]

Antistaphylococcal prophylaxis, although practiced in the United Kingdom in infants, has not been widely endorsed in the United States because of concerns about the emergence of resistance, the increased risk of acquiring *P. aeruginosa*, and the lack of impact on lung function. The different findings in these studies may reflect the different agents studied because cephalexin is broader spectrum than is flucloxacillin or the different durations of therapy, or both. In an era of increasing prevalence of MRSA, strategies to prevent MSSA may prove to be less useful. To date, no studies have been done to assess antibiotic prophylaxis for other pathogens in CF.

Early Eradication of Methicillin-Resistant *Staphylococcus aureus*

Eradication of initial *S. aureus* infection in CF represents a different approach than outlined earlier (chronic suppressive therapy). One of the earliest reports of attempts to eradicate *S. aureus* (MSSA) from the CF airways was a retrospective cohort study of a Danish CF center following 191 CF patients treated with 2349 courses of antistaphylococcal chemotherapy from 1965 to 1979. They reported eradication of *S. aureus* in 74% of these subjects after a single course of therapy and, with further treatment, only 9% of subjects were chronically infected with *S. aureus*.[289] Based on these data, the European CF Consensus group evaluating early intervention in CF lung disease has recommended an initial 2 to 4 weeks of antistaphylococcal treatment with new *S. aureus* infection and an additional 1- to 3-month course of antibiotics if the initial course fails.[79] The long-term sequelae of this treatment approach are not known and warrant further investigation. Researchers in the United Kingdom reported that patient segregation and aggressive antibiotic eradication therapy achieved *S. aureus* eradication in the majority of their patients with CF; the most successful regimens were those that included two oral antibiotics (one of which was rifampin) and nebulized vancomycin.[77] Currently, there are two ongoing studies investigating the use of inhaled vancomycin, including one accessing a novel dry powder formulation.[26,126,262] The results of these trials will help to delineate the risks and benefits of treating chronic MRSA infection.

Early Eradication of *Pseudomonas aeruginosa*

An increasingly practiced therapeutic strategy is to use antibiotics to eradicate initial acquisition of *P. aeruginosa* and prevent or delay chronic infection. This strategy was described first in Europe at the Danish Cystic Fibrosis Center.[86,121,244,260,266] The rationale for this approach is that antibiotics may be effective at eradicating initial infection and colonization with *P. aeruginosa* because the organism burden is low, organisms are largely susceptible, and a biofilm has not yet been established.

Evidence for the optimal regimen for successful eradication is emerging. In some CF centers in Europe, colistin and ciprofloxacin are administered every 3 months after the initial isolation of *P. aeruginosa* has occurred.[86] Compared with historical controls, patients treated with this approach had improved lung function, improved survival rates, decreased prevalence of *P. aeruginosa*, and increased resistance to the therapeutic regimen.[244] In Australia, investigators used intravenous antibiotics followed by ciprofloxacin or aerosolized agents and found that six of 24 children no longer had *P. aeruginosa* isolated for 12 months or longer.[7] Compared with children treated with placebo, children treated with inhaled tobramycin within 7 to 12 weeks of initial infection and colonization with *P. aeruginosa* had shorter time to conversion from a positive to negative culture.[276] All eight subjects treated with inhaled tobramycin compared with 1 of 13 subjects treated with placebo had successful eradication of *P. aeruginosa*.[92]

Despite the concerns about the potential emergence of antimicrobial resistance and lack of long-term studies that show the durability of eradication or an improvement in lung function, the growing consensus has been that early eradication for *P. aeruginosa* has merit. The Early Pseudomonal Infection Control randomized trial rigorously evaluated the efficacy of different antibiotic regimens for eradication of newly identified *Pseudomonas* in children with CF. Protocol-based therapy in the trial was provided based on culture positivity independent of symptoms and resulted in a lower rate of *Pseudomonas* recurrence but comparable hospitalization rates as compared to a historical control cohort less aggressively treated with antibiotics for new-onset *Pseudomonas*.[183]

The Cystic Fibrosis Foundation clinical care guidelines for the prevention of *P. aeruginosa* infection recommend (1) use of inhaled antibiotic therapy for the treatment of initial or new growth of *P. aeruginosa* from an airway culture, with a regimen of inhaled tobramycin (300 mg twice daily) for 28 days as the favored antibiotic; (2) against the use of prophylactic antipseudomonal antibiotics to prevent the acquisition of *P. aeruginosa*; and (3) routine oropharyngeal cultures rather than cultures obtained by bronchoscopy in individuals with CF who cannot expectorate sputum to determine if they are infected with *P. aeruginosa*.[195]

TREATMENT OF PULMONARY EXACERBATIONS

Pseudomonas aeruginosa

Much effort has been put into standardizing and validating the definition of a pulmonary exacerbation in CF. No currently accepted definition has been adopted universally, however, for use clinically, in quality improvement initiatives, or in clinical research. A combination of clinical signs and symptoms is used to define a pulmonary exacerbation in research trials; similar factors are used in the clinical setting.

Mild exacerbations often are treated with oral ciprofloxacin[35,110] with or without an inhaled agent. Treatment trials supporting the use of inhaled antibiotics for management of an exacerbation are lacking, however. Several pivotal trials have led to widely accepted principles for intravenous treatment of more severe pulmonary exacerbations. During the 1970s and early 1980s, placebo-controlled trials showed that participants in the placebo group had increased morbidity and mortality rates compared with participants treated with intravenous antibiotics.[97,113,274] Hospitalized participants treated with bronchodilators and chest physiotherapy alone had less improvement in lung function and less reduction in bacterial density compared with patients treated with these interventions plus a β-lactam and an aminoglycoside agent.[204]

Treatment with a β-lactam and an aminoglycoside agent led to a significant reduction in bacterial density and a longer time to readmission for a new exacerbation compared with treatment with a β-lactam agent alone.[227] Most studies comparing various agents, singly or in combination, enrolled small numbers of patients and concluded that the comparative treatment regimens were equivalent in efficacy, but the studies were insufficiently powered to detect differences.[20,38,98,119,136,157,189,219,222] Many studies showed the emergence of resistance to study drug at the completion of therapy, which did not correlate with clinical response to treatment.[122,185] No specific antibiotic combination can be considered to be superior to another, and neither is there evidence showing that the intravenous route is superior to the inhaled or oral routes. There remains a need to understand host-bacteria interactions and, in particular, to understand why many people fail to fully respond to treatment.[135]

Accepted treatment of a pulmonary exacerbation caused by *P. aeruginosa* consists of two parenteral agents from different antibiotic classes to potentially provide synergy and to delay the emergence of resistance.[91,164,200,214] A number of different oral and intravenous antibiotics may be combined to best tailor antibiotic therapy to particular combinations of positive bacterial culture results. The choice is largely empiric and based on the experience of the physician, patient, and previous occurrence of drug allergy. In addition, there are no data to suggest that this also applies to other bacteria cultured in CF sputum. Treatment trials for pulmonary exacerbations caused by other CF pathogens are unavailable, however.

Antibiotic dosages must be higher or more frequent (or both) in patients with CF because the volume of distribution and clearance is increased in CF.[54] Treatment is administered for 10 to 21 days; treatment outcomes include improved lung function, improved well-being or quality of life or both, and a reduction in organism burden. Examination of the safety and efficacy of single daily dosing of tobramycin versus multiple daily dosing during a pulmonary exacerbation showed that single daily dosing was associated with the same efficacy and reduced nephrotoxicity; in children, the mean percentage change in creatinine in the single daily dosing group was less than the mean change in the three-times-daily dosing group (3.7% vs. 4.5%).[230]

Data from the CF Patient Registry reports that the total median duration of intravenous antibiotic treatment for a pulmonary exacerbation in children in 2015 was 13.0 days. The Epidemiologic Study of Cystic Fibrosis analyzed the relationship between pulmonary function and treatment strategies for pulmonary exacerbations; centers with patients in the upper quartile of pulmonary function treated pulmonary exacerbations more frequently than did centers in the lower quartile.[163] It is well recognized that eradication of most pathogens does not occur.[184]

Inevitably, *P. aeruginosa* develops increasing resistance to antibiotics. Molecular studies have confirmed that resistance generally develops in the infecting strains rather than the acquisition of more resistant strains.[178] Previously, much interest existed in optimizing the treatment of pulmonary exacerbations caused by multidrug-resistant *P. aeruginosa* using in vitro synergy testing. No clinical benefits have been demonstrated from synergy testing, leading guidelines to recommend against such testing.[139,214]

CF experts have not arrived yet at a consensus regarding the efficacy of inpatient versus outpatient management of pulmonary exacerbations. Outpatient management has advantages; it is less costly, is less disruptive to patients and their families, and involves less risk of acquiring nosocomial pathogens. Patients treated at home were shown, however, to have longer treatment courses and less improvement in lung function.[168] Patients may improve more with hospitalization as a result of better compliance with antibiotics, bed rest, chest physiotherapy, and bronchodilator treatments.[22,41]

Staphylococcus aureus and Methicillin-Resistant *Staphylococcus aureus*

The clinical utility of antistaphyloccocal agents is best shown by early studies of infants with CF treated with penicillin before the nearly universal acquisition of β-lactamases by *S. aureus*.[5,158] Infants treated during that antibiotic era had markedly improved survival rates. Experts advocate the use of a first-generation cephalosporin (e.g., cephazolin) or semisynthetic penicillin (e.g., oxacillin) for treatment of a pulmonary exacerbation associated with MSSA.[91] Treatment trials justifying this approach are lacking, however.

Vancomycin generally is advocated for treatment of MRSA when this organism is considered a pathogen. Although no treatment trials in CF patients using linezolid have been conducted, a case series showed that adults with CF required 600 mg every 8 hours to provide desired pharmacokinetics.[21,218] Linezolid-resistant MRSA has been reported with frequent or prolonged use.[88,322]

Burkholderia cepacia Complex

Management of *Burkholderia cepacia* complex is more problematic because of higher levels of intrinsic antibiotic resistance and a paucity of clinical trials for this pathogen. Initial isolates may be susceptible to ciprofloxacin, β-lactam antibiotics, chloramphenicol, trimethoprim-sulfamethoxazole, meropenem, and minocycline, but with the exception of *Burkholderia gladioli*, all *Burkholderia* spp. are resistant to aminoglycosides. Temocillin has been used in Europe to treat pulmonary exacerbation caused by *B. cepacia*.[251] Resistance has developed, however, limiting therapeutic options. As described for the management of *P. aeruginosa*, combinations of two or three agents are used to treat a pulmonary exacerbation. Even more prolonged courses may be required to improve lung function. One of the new inhalation antibiotics available is tobramycin inhalation powder (TIP) delivered by the podhaler device. TIP has been shown to result in comparable increases in forced expiratory volume in 1 second and decreases in hospitalization as tobramycin inhalation solution (TIS) in the treatment of chronic *P. aeruginosa* in patients with CF. However, TIP can achieve up to 1.5- to 2-fold higher sputum tobramycin concentrations (up to 2000 mg/g) than TIS. In vitro studies of 180 Bcc and 103 *S. maltophilia* isolates demonstrated a minimum inhibitory concentration at which 50% of isolates were susceptible (MIC50) of 100 mg/mL, tested by planktonic and biofilm growth. This suggests that a maximum serum concentration/MIC ratio of up to 20 may be achievable with TIP treatment of these pathogens. Clinical trials of TIP in patients with CF with Bcc and *S. maltophilia* infection to decrease sputum bacterial densities are planned.[234]

Stenotrophomonas maltophilia and *Achromobacter xylosoxidans*

There are no published treatment trials for patients with CF who are harboring *S. maltophilia* or *A. xylosoxidans* undergoing an exacerbation. Although definitive data confirming that these organisms are pathogens in CF are unavailable, clinicians target these multidrug-resistant, gram-negative bacilli if they are consistently recovered from the respiratory tract of an individual patient. At present, the Clinical and Laboratory Standards Institute recommends testing ticarcillin-clavulanate, ceftazidime, minocycline, chloramphenicol, trimethoprim-sulfamethoxazole, and levofloxacin against *S. maltophilia*,[39] but CF strains frequently are resistant to these agents.[216]

Nonetheless, similar strategies are used to treat these organisms as described for *P. aeruginosa* or Bcc; two or more parenteral agents are chosen based on susceptibility testing and given for 10 days to 3 weeks. In a survey of 263 isolates of *S. maltophilia* from 218 patients with CF, doxycycline, ticarcillin-clavulanate, piperacillin-tazobactam, and trimethoprim-sulfamethoxazole were most active and inhibited 78%, 39%, 18%, and 13% of isolates, respectively.[216,286] A survey of 94 *A. xylosoxidans* isolates from 77 patients showed that meropenem and imipenem, or piperacillin with or without tazobactam, were most active.[212] In an in vitro study of a large number of clinical *S. maltophilia* CF isolates, levofloxacin, at levels achievable by inhalation, was the most active antibiotic alone and in combination against *S. maltophilia* grown as a biofilm or planktonically. In addition to achieving high levels of drug in the lung (4000 mg/g), levofloxacin demonstrated an antiinflammatory effect.[296,321] Inhaled levofloxacin may thus be an effective chronic suppressive antimicrobial therapy in patients with CF with chronic *S. maltophilia* infection and warrants further investigation of this multidrug-resistant organism.

Allergic Bronchopulmonary Aspergillosis

Treatment of ABPA also may be very challenging. Steroids are the treatment of choice because ABPA is immunologically mediated, although the response to steroids is varied and may have the undesirable consequence of diabetes in this vulnerable patient population. The oral antifungal therapies voriconazole[109] and itraconazole[169] have been used with reported response and toxicity, but no controlled trials have been performed.[164] Monitoring serum levels of itraconazole is desirable because this agent may be malabsorbed if the gastric pH is nonacidic.

Nontuberculous Mycobacteria

Treatment of NTM in patients with CF is challenging and guided by the clinical presentation and the mycobacterial species. Before therapy for NTM is initiated, patients should be treated aggressively for the classic CF pathogens they harbor to determine if they clinically improve without the need for specific NTM treatment. If NTM treatment is initiated, a careful history, physical examination, and pulmonary function tests should be done to determine the baseline status of the patient in efforts to monitor response to therapy. Susceptibility testing for NTM is not done routinely for patients who do not have CF. Given the increased antibiotic exposure in CF and the potential for the emergence of resistance, NTM strains isolated from patients with CF should undergo susceptibility testing at a reference laboratory. Treatment can be guided by the initial susceptibility profile.

The US Cystic Fibrosis Foundation and the European Cystic Fibrosis Society published consensus recommendations for the management and treatment of NTM in CF[102]; a lack of treatment trials have been published for NTM in CF. Treatment of NTM pulmonary disease should involve an intensive phase followed by a continuation phase and should be managed in collaboration with experts in the treatment of NTM and CF, as drug intolerance and drug-related toxicity occur frequently. Monotherapy or intermittent (three times per week) oral antibiotic therapy should never be used in the treatment of NTM. Serum levels should be monitored in patients receiving intravenous amikacin or streptomycin; serum levels of other antimycobacterial drugs are not routinely recommended. An initial course of intravenous amikacin as part of the intensive phase may be changed to inhaled amikacin in the continuation phase. Patients should be followed closely and have monthly sputum testing done for acid-fast bacillus smear and culture, and NTM antibiotic therapy should be prescribed for 12 months beyond culture conversion. Cure for *M. abscessus* is less likely; the therapeutic goal may be long-term suppression.[41,102]

Long-Term Suppressive Therapy

Inhaled Antibiotics

Long-term suppressive antibiotic therapy has been used increasingly to treat patients with CF and infected with *P. aeruginosa* to prolong the time between pulmonary exacerbations and to slow the progression of lung deterioration. The use of long-term oral antibiotics is discouraged; no clinical trials support this practice, which may contribute to antibiotic resistance.

Inhaled antibiotics are standard of care for treating chronic pseudomonal respiratory infections in CF patients; three antimicrobial agents are currently approved for intermittent management of chronic *Pseudomonas* infection in the United States: TIS and TIP, aztreonam-lysine (AZLI), and colistimethate (COL) as inhalation solution (also available as licensed dry powder in Europe).[179,195] The aerosol route delivers 100-fold higher concentrations of antibiotic without toxicity; the median concentration of tobramycin in the phase III trial was 1200 μg/g of sputum.[201] However, TIP can achieve up to 1.5- to 2-fold higher sputum tobramycin concentrations (up to 2000 mg/g) than TIS.[321] The outcomes desired from use of inhaled antibiotics in treated patients include a reduction in bacterial density, fewer days of hospitalization, and fewer days of intravenous antibiotics, with minimal systemic absorption of the drug.

Although initially approved for intermittent administration, the use of continuous alternating inhaled antibiotic regimens of differing combinations is growing. A recent double-blind trial compared continuous alternating therapy of AZLI/TIS to placebo/TIS in an intermittent treatment regimen. The AZLI/TIS treatment reduced exacerbation rates by 25.7% and rates of respiratory hospitalizations by 35.8% compared with placebo/TIS.[103] New antibiotics are in development (inhaled levofloxacin, liposomal ciprofloxacin, and liposomal amikacin), although recently two did not meet primary outcomes in large clinical trials. Although inhaled antibiotics have the advantage of being able to deliver high intrapulmonary concentrations of drug, antimicrobial resistance can still develop and is a concern in CF.

Of particular interest is the development of nonantibiotic antimicrobials, which may allow treatment of intrinsically antibiotic-resistant organisms and perhaps even mitigate antimicrobial resistance. Examples of nonantibiotic treatments being investigated in patients with CF include antibiotic adjuvants, which have activity against bacteria, such as gallium, antimicrobial peptides, anti-biofilm compounds such as alginate oligosaccharides (OligoG), and garlic. Vaccination strategies and antibody therapy (IgY) against *P. aeruginosa* have also been attempted to prevent initial infection with this organism in CF. Although aggressive and long-term use of antibiotics has been crucial in slowing lung function decline and improving survival in people with CF, it has added a significant burden of care and associated toxicities in these individuals. Careful surveillance and the use of preventive strategies for antibiotic-related toxicity (such as nephrotoxicity and ototoxicity) are essential. Continued development of effective antimicrobial agents that can function against bacterial biofilm growth and under anaerobic conditions in the conditions encountered in the CF lung is needed.[309]

Macrolide Antibiotics

Much interest has been generated in the use of macrolide agents in CF[112] as long-term suppressive therapy. The rationale for macrolide therapy in CF stems from the successful treatment of diffuse panbronchiolitis with erythromycin, azithromycin, and clarithromycin.[131,137] Diffuse panbronchiolitis is a chronic lung disease, diagnosed primarily in Asian adults, with several clinical features similar to those found in CF, including progressive lung disease caused by mucoid and nonmucoid strains of *P. aeruginosa*.[243] Long-term administration of low-dose macrolide agents to patients with diffuse panbronchiolitis has reduced morbidity and mortality rates.

In vitro studies have provided the scientific rationale for this clinical efficacy. Although macrolides are not cidal for *P. aeruginosa*, subinhibitory concentrations of macrolide agents reduce the production of several virulence factors by *P. aeruginosa*,[161,162] including the formation of biofilm.[117,133] Macrolide antibiotics also may have an antiinflammatory effect and decrease cytokine production by neutrophils, monocytes, and bronchial epithelial cells.[116,280] Four azithromycin trials have been conducted in patients with CF,[37,74,213,278] with three trials in patients chronically infected with *P. aeruginosa*.[74,213,278] All showed improvement in lung function using similar treatment regimens of azithromycin. Improvements in secondary outcomes, such as decreased hospitalization, decreased antibiotic use, and increased weight gain, also were noted. In a study performed in 82 children and adolescents, most (63 of 82; 77%) with negative cultures for *P. aeruginosa*,[37] participants in the azithromycin-treated group had fewer pulmonary exacerbations and less oral antibiotic use, with no differences in lung function or intravenous antibiotic usage. A Cochrane review concluded that short-term (i.e., 3 to 6 months) azithromycin seemed effective in CF, but long-term safety and efficacy remain unknown.[235] Patients treated with azithromycin should be screened for NTM before initiating therapy and annually thereafter because of concern about macrolide resistance in these microorganisms. A secondary analysis of a cohort of 263 subjects with CF enrolled in a recent clinical trial comparing inhaled TIS with AZLI noted that concomitant oral azithromycin may antagonize the therapeutic benefits of inhaled tobramycin in subjects, with significantly greater improvement in outcome measures noted in the AZLI-treated group. Further studies are needed to determine if this antagonism can be replicated.[206]

Lung Transplantation

Lung transplantation currently is considered a viable therapy for selected patients with end-stage pulmonary disease of CF.[281] Bilateral lung, heart-lung, and living donor lobar lung transplantation all have been performed in patients with CF, but most operations in recent years have used the bilateral lung transplant approach with lungs from deceased donors. The survival of lung transplant recipients with CF exceeds that of any other diagnostic group for all ages, with projected survival half-life of 6.2 years.[256] Patients with CF nonetheless present special challenges for successful lung transplantation. The life-threatening manifestations of CF generally are limited to the lungs except for patients with advanced liver disease with portal hypertension. Advantages of a lung transplant recipient with CF include relative young age, giving the potential of many years of productive life ahead. In addition, patients with CF have experience with complex medical regimens.

The optimal time to refer potential candidates for evaluation for lung transplant is difficult to determine because the natural history of CF cannot be predicted precisely. Although transplanted lungs do not develop CF, they can become infected with the pretransplant pathogens because the trachea and paranasal sinuses continue to manifest the pathophysiology of CF. Lung transplant recipients with CF are at risk for development of infection via pretransplant microbial flora or newly acquired pathogens.[125,143,233,237] Controversy has ensued about whether microbiologic criteria, specifically pretransplant infection with fungi, NTM, or multidrug-resistant pathogens, should be considered contraindications to performing lung transplantation in patients with CF. Several centers have published their experiences with infections that developed from lung transplantation pathogens; they include invasive aspergillosis; sepsis with *S. maltophilia*, Bcc organisms, and *B. gladioli*; and sternal wound infection.[125] Other centers have reported that morbidity and mortality caused by *P. aeruginosa* infections posttransplant are not higher in patients with CF than in patients who do not have CF.[85,175]

Patients with CF are at risk of developing invasive aspergillosis after transplant but at lower rates than patients without CF.[175,188] Many of these patients with CF were colonized with *Aspergillus* spp. or *Scedosporium* spp. before undergoing transplantations. Treatment with antifungal therapy after surgery should be considered. The decision to transplant patients infected with NTM, Bcc, or multidrug-resistant *P. aeruginosa*, or colonized with *Aspergillus* spp. or *Scedosporium* spp., should be made on a case-by-case basis. Potentially, an understanding of the microbial species infecting a patient may be a useful predictor of mortality.

Antiinflammatory Therapy

Inflammation associated with chronic bacterial colonization plays a crucial role in CF lung disease. Nonsteroidal agents and glucocorticoids have been used as potential medications for antiinflammatory therapy. A randomized trial using oral prednisone (1–2 mg/kg every other day) showed a reduction in the rate of decline in pulmonary function of patients with CF but was associated with significant steroid-related side effects.[9] Three short-term trials using inhaled steroids have led to mixed results and no clear direction for long-term use.[11,172,264] A systematic review of inhaled steroids for CF was equivocal with respect to efficacy.[10] A multicenter randomized trial of withdrawal of inhaled steroids in CF did not find a difference in pulmonary exacerbations, infection with *P. aeruginosa*, or pulmonary function after inhaled steroids were discontinued.[12] High-dose ibuprofen (20–30 mg/kg twice per day) used over a 4-year period showed a decreased rate of decline in pulmonary function with few reported side effects.[134] Macrolide antibiotics decrease inflammation by modulation of inflammatory signaling pathways and decreased cytokine production from inflammatory cells.[72] Several antiinflammatory agents—including antiproteases, statins, and antioxidants—have been proposed as potential therapies, but they remain under investigation and are not a part of routine clinical practice.

CFTR Modulators

A great deal of progress has been made over the past few years in the field of small molecule therapies targeting CFTR, the protein defective in patients with CF. Until recently, modulating CFTR dysfunction was only a research aspiration. However, greater focus placed on addressing the primary defect of CF has developed several clinical therapeutic strategies in this area to modulate CFTR and restore robust functional protein to the cell surface. This approach has now led to the licensing of two CFTR potentiator/corrector medications, which have been shown to have significant clinical improvements in a subset of CF patients. This success represents the beginning for CFTR modulation, and further research is ongoing that aims to broaden the applicability of these techniques.

Ivacaftor (Kalydeco) is the first drug licensed for clinical use in patients with a class 3 CFTR mutation, a number of mutations resulting in defective gating. For patients homozygous for delta F508, the class 2 mutation characterized by misfolding, a combination approach is required; the recently approved lumicaftor/ivacaftor (Orkambi) allows the protein to correctly localize and potentiates improved protein function. A number of other CFTR modulators are at earlier stages of clinical development. Clinicians should be aware that lumicaftor/ivacaftor has many potential drug-drug interactions. With the advent of such precision medicine, patient genotype is now highly relevant. Areas of current unmet need include drugs to cover all mutation classes, increasing access to younger children with the design of rational and tailored clinical trials, and ensuring equality of access globally.[15,67]

With the approval of ivacaftor to reverse protein defects in patients with the class 3 gating mutation, there is evidence that *P. aeruginosa* culture positivity is significantly reduced following ivacaftor treatment in persons with the G551D-CFTR mutation.[126]

Prevention

Immunizations

The use of currently available routine childhood and adolescent vaccines is strongly advocated for patients with CF. Although patients with CF are not at increased risk of developing *Streptococcus pneumoniae* infections, they should receive the pneumococcal vaccine, 13-valent (Prevnar). Annual influenza vaccination is recommended for patients with CF and household members.[78,82] One randomized controlled study comparing palivizumab (Synagis) prophylaxis against RSV infection in infants with CF failed to draw conclusions about its efficacy.[241] Most CF experts, however, agree that RSV prevention may be warranted, since viral lower respiratory disease in infants with CF puts them at risk for severe bronchiolitis and hospitalization. The results of a phase III multicenter study of a *P. aeruginosa* vaccine were published.[63] Although this bivalent antiflagella vaccine was immunogenic and was found to reduce the incidence of *P. aeruginosa* infection and serum antibody titers, it did not prevent chronic *P. aeruginosa* infection, and it did not affect lung function.

Infection Control Precautions

Although the sources of most pathogens in patients with CF are unknown, it is increasingly recognized that patient-to-patient spread and acquisition from the contaminated health care environment can occur. To date, reports of transmission of bacterial pathogens occurring between individuals with and without CF are rare.[96,111,155] Direct contact, indirect contact, and spread of droplets with infectious secretions all have been implicated as modes of transmission of CF pathogens. Risk factors for transmission were described first for Bcc.[30,101,142,190,191,252]

Perhaps of most concern have been several reports of clonal spread of *P. aeruginosa* among patients with CF.[154,221,263] These examples have involved obvious phenotypes that triggered an investigation of possible patient-to-patient spread, including an increase in ceftazidime-resistant *P. aeruginosa*[32] or initial colonization of young children with mucoid strains of *P. aeruginosa*.[7,174] These reports have led CF centers in Europe to segregate all patients, regardless of their *P. aeruginosa* or Bcc status, in hospital and clinic settings.[86,132,154] Occasional cases of patient-to-patient spread of other potential pathogens, including NTM, *S. maltophilia*, and *A. xylosoxidans*, have been reported in patients with CF.[207,261]

The U.S. Cystic Fibrosis Foundation convened an expert panel to develop revised recommendations for infection control that addressed inpatient, outpatient (i.e., CF clinic and pulmonary function test laboratories), and non–health care settings, as so much CF care is delivered in the home.[257] These recommendations have implications for treatment, transplantation, and the psychosocial well-being of patients, families, and staff (Box 25.3). The guidelines emphasized that all patients with CF could harbor potentially transmissible respiratory tract pathogens, and containing respiratory tract secretions is of paramount importance. The consensus is that all patients should be cared for apart from other patients with CF; patients are hospitalized in single rooms and seen in outpatient settings geographically or temporally apart from other patients with CF. Similarly, patients with CF should be placed in private rooms without access to common areas.

BOX 25.3 Infection Control Strategies for Cystic Fibrosis

Guideline

All patients placed into contact isolation (outpatient and inpatient settings)
Quarterly cultures of respiratory tract
Appropriate processing of CF respiratory tract cultures
Educate patients and families about proper hand hygiene
Implement contact precautions for MDROs, including MRSA
Hospitalize all patients in single-patient room
Consider all patients at risk for organisms with potential spread to/from other CF patients including, but not limited to, those with *B. cepacia* complex
Clean and disinfect respiratory therapy equipment
Avoid socialization among CF patients
Maintain at least 6 ft between CF patients to prevent droplet transmission

CF, Cystic fibrosis; *MDROs*, multidrug-resistant organisms; *MRSA*, methicillin-resistant *Staphylococcus aureus*.

CONCLUSION

The microbiology of patients with CF is complex and changing. Although the pathogenesis of lung infections is still under active investigation, the current hypothesis suggests multiple etiologies. Appropriate microbiologic processing of respiratory tract specimens is crucial to ensure an accurate understanding of the epidemiology of CF lung disease and to provide appropriate treatment and infection control. Current treatment strategies are directed largely at management of deteriorations of pulmonary function, but increasingly strategies are directed at prevention and preservation of lung function. This success from CFTR modulation and further research holds promise for a shift in outcome of this chronic progressive disease.

NEW REFERENCES SINCE THE SEVENTH EDITION

3. Adam RJ, Michalski AS, Bauer C, et al. Air trapping and airflow obstruction in newborn cystic fibrosis piglets. *Am J Respir Crit Care Med*. 2013;188:1434-1441.
15. Barry PJ, Ronan N, Plant BJ. Cystic fibrosis transmembrane conductance regulator modulators: the end of the beginning. *Semin Respir Crit Care Med*. 2015;36(2):287-298.
25. Boucher RC. Evidence for airway surface dehydration as the initiating event in CF airway disease. *J Intern Med*. 2007;261:5-16.
26. Boyle MP. Persistent methicillin resistant *Staphylococcus aureus* eradication protocol (PMEP). Clinicaltrials.Gov. NLM identifier: NCT01594827. Bethesda, MD: National Library of Medicine (US).
31. Cantin AM, Hartl D, Konstan MW, et al. Inflammation in cystic fibrosis lung disease: pathogenesis and therapy. *J Cyst Fibros*. 2015;14(4):419-430.
36. Castellani C, Cuppens H, Macek M Jr, et al. Consensus on the use and interpretation of cystic fibrosis mutation analysis in clinical practice. *J Cyst Fibros*. 2008;7(3):179-196.
41. Chmiel JF, Aksamit TR, Chotirmall SH, et al. Antibiotic management of lung infections in cystic fibrosis. II. Nontuberculous mycobacteria, anaerobic bacteria, and fungi. *Ann Am Thorac Soc*. 2014;11(8):1298-1306.
43. Clunes MT, Boucher RC. Cystic Fibrosis: the mechanisms of pathogenesis of an inherited lung disorder. *Drug Discov Today Dis Mech*. 2007;4(2):63-72.
51. Coolen N, Morand P, Martin C, et al. Reduced risk of nontuberculous mycobacteria in cystic fibrosis adults receiving long-term azithromycin. *J Cyst Fibros*. 2015;14(5):594-599.
56. Cutting GR. Cystic fibrosis genetics: from molecular understanding to clinical application. Nature reviews. *Genetics*. 2015;16(1):45-56.
62. Cystic Fibrosis Foundation. Patient Registry 2014. Bethesda, Md. 2015.
68. Davies JC. The future of CFTR modulating therapies for cystic fibrosis. *Curr Opin Pulm Med*. 2015;21(6):579-584.
70. De Boeck K, Munck A, Walker S, et al. Efficacy and safety of ivacaftor in patients with cystic fibrosis and a non-G551D gating mutation. *J Cyst Fibros*. 2014;13(6):674-680.
102. Floto RA, Olivier KN, Saiman L, et al. US Cystic Fibrosis Foundation and European Cystic Fibrosis Society consensus recommendations for the management of non-tuberculous mycobacteria in individuals with cystic fibrosis: executive summary. *Thorax*. 2016;71(1):88-90.
103. Flume PA, Clancy JP, Retsch-Bogart GZ, et al. Continuous alternating inhaled antibiotics for chronic pseudomonal infection in cystic fibrosis. *J Cyst Fibros*. 2016;15(16):30050-30059. pii: S1569-1993.
118. Griese M, Kappler M, Eismann C, et al. Inhalation treatment with glutathione in patients with cystic fibrosis. A randomized clinical trial. *Am J Respir Crit Care Med*. 2013;188:83-89.

124. Hamosh A, FitzSimmons SC, Macek M Jr, et al. Comparison of the clinical manifestations of cystic fibrosis in black and white patients. *J Pediatr*. 1998;132(2):255-259.
126. Heltshe SL, Mayer-Hamblett N, Burns JL, et al. *Pseudomonas aeruginosa* in cystic fibrosis patients with G551D-CFTR treated with ivacaftor. *Clin Infect Dis*. 2015;60(5):703-712.
127. Heltshe SL, Saiman L, Popowich EB, et al. Outcomes and treatment of chronic methicillin-resistant *Staphylococcus aureus* differs by *Staphylococcus* cassette chromosome mec (SCCmec) type in children with cystic fibrosis. *J Pediatric Infect Dis Soc*. 2015;4(3):225-231.
129. Hoegger MJ, Fischer AJ, McMenimen JD, et al. Impaired mucus detachment disrupts mucociliary transport in a piglet model of cystic fibrosis. *Science*. 2014;345(6198):818-822.
135. Hurley MN, Prayle AP, Flume P. Intravenous antibiotics for pulmonary exacerbations in people with cystic fibrosis. *Cochrane Database Syst Rev*. 2015;(7):CD009730.
146. Kang JH, Hwang SM, Chung IY. S100A8, S100A9 and S100A12 activate airway epithelial cells to produce MUC5AC via extracellular signal-regulated kinase and nuclear factor-kappaB pathways. *Immunology*. 2015;144:79-90.
150. Kleme ML, Levy E. Cystic fibrosis-related oxidative stress and intestinal lipid disorders. *Antioxid Redox Signal*. 2015;22(7):614-631.
165. Li X, Tang XX, Vargas Buonfiglio LG, et al. Electrolyte transport properties in distal small airways from cystic fibrosis pigs with implications for host defense. *Am J Physiol Lung Cell Mol Physiol*. 2016;310(7):L670-L679.
171. Lo DK, Hurley MN, Muhlebach MS, et al. Interventions for the eradication of methicillin-resistant *Staphylococcus aureus* (MRSA) in people with cystic fibrosis. *Cochrane Database Syst Rev*. 2015;(2):CD009650.
173. Lorenz E, Muhlebach MS, Tessier PA, et al. Different expression ratio of S100A8/A9 and S100A12 in acute and chronic lung diseases. *Respir Med*. 2008;102:567-573.
176. Mahboubi MA, Carmody LA, Foster BK, et al. Culture-based and culture-independent bacteriologic analysis of cystic fibrosis respiratory specimens. *J Clin Microbiol*. 2016;54(3):613-619.
179. Máiz L, Girón RM, Olveira C, et al. Inhaled antibiotics for the treatment of chronic bronchopulmonary *Pseudomonas aeruginosa* infection in cystic fibrosis: systematic review of randomised controlled trials. *Expert Opin Pharmacother*. 2013;14(9):1135-1149.
183. Mayer-Hamblett N, Rosenfeld M, Treggiari MM, et al. Standard care versus protocol based therapy for new onset *Pseudomonas aeruginosa* in cystic fibrosis. *Pediatr Pulmonol*. 2013;48(10):943-953.
192. Meyerholz DK, Stoltz DA, Namati E, et al. Loss of cystic fibrosis transmembrane conductance regulator function produces abnormalities in tracheal development in neonatal pigs and young children. *Am J Respir Crit Care Med*. 2010;182:1251-1261.
195. Mogayzel PJ Jr, Naureckas ET, Robinson KA, et al. Cystic Fibrosis Foundation pulmonary guideline. Pharmacologic approaches to prevention and eradication of initial *Pseudomonas aeruginosa* infection. *Ann Am Thorac Soc*. 2014;11(10):1640-1650.
202. Muhlebach MS, Heltshe SL, Popowitch EB, et al. Multicenter observational study on factors and outcomes associated with various methicillin-resistant *Staphylococcus aureus* types in children with cystic fibrosis. *Ann Am Thorac Soc*. 2015;12(6):864-871.
206. Nick JA, Moskowitz SM, Chmiel JF, et al. Azithromycin may antagonize inhaled tobramycin when targeting *Pseudomonas aeruginosa* in cystic fibrosis. *Ann Am Thorac Soc*. 2014;11(3):342-350.
234. Ratjen A, Yau Y, Wettlaufer J, et al. In vitro efficacy of high-dose tobramycin against Burkholderia cepacia complex and *Stenotrophomonas maltophilia* isolates from cystic fibrosis patients. *Antimicrob Agents Chemother*. 2015;59(1):711-713.
246. Rosenstein BJ. Cystic fibrosis diagnosis: new dilemmas for an old disorder. *Pediatr Pulmonol*. 2002;33:83-84.
247. Rowe SM, Heltshe SL, Gonska T, et al. Clinical mechanism of the cystic fibrosis transmembrane conductance regulator potentiator ivacaftor in G551D-mediated cystic fibrosis. *Am J Respir Crit Care Med*. 2014;190(2):175-184.
248. Rowe SM, Miller S, Sorscher EJ. Cystic fibrosis. *N Engl J Med*. 2005;352(19):1992-2001.
257. Saiman L, Siegel JD, LiPuma JJ, et al. Infection prevention and control guideline for cystic fibrosis: 2013 update. *Infect Control Hosp Epidemiol*. 2014;35(suppl 1):S1-S67.
258. Salsgiver EL, Fink AK, Knapp EA, et al. Changing epidemiology of the respiratory bacteriology of patients with cystic fibrosis. *Chest*. 2016;149(2):390-400.
262. Savara, Inc. Efficacy and safety study of AeroVanc for the treatment of persistent MRSA lung infection in cystic fibrosis patients. Clinicaltrials.Gov. NLM identifier: NCT01746095.
272. Sly PD, Brennan S, Gangell C, et al. Lung disease at diagnosis in infants with cystic fibrosis detected by newborn screening. *Am J Respir Crit Care Med*. 2009;180:146-152.
273. Sly PD, Gangell CL, Chen L, et al. Risk factors for bronchiectasis in children with cystic fibrosis. *N Engl J Med*. 2013;368(21):1963-1970.
284. Stoltz DA, Meyerholz DK, Pezzulo AA, et al. Cystic fibrosis pigs develop lung disease and exhibit defective bacterial eradication at birth. *Sci Transl Med*. 2010;2(29):29ra31.
302. VanDevanter DR, Kahle JA, O'Sullivan AK, et al. Cystic fibrosis in young children: a review of disease manifestation, progression, and response to early treatment. *J Cystic Fibros*. 2016;15:147-157.
309. Waters V, Smyth A. Cystic fibrosis microbiology: advances in antimicrobial therapy. *J Cyst Fibros*. 2015;14(5):551-560.
316. Wolter DJ, Emerson JC, McNamara S, et al. *Staphylococcus aureus* small-colony variants are independently associated with worse lung disease in children with cystic fibrosis. *Clin Infect Dis*. 2013;57(3):384-391.
321. Wu K, Yau YC, Matukas L, et al. Biofilm compared to conventional antimicrobial susceptibility of *Stenotrophomonas maltophilia* isolates from cystic fibrosis patients. *Antimicrob Agents Chemother*. 2013;57:1546-1548.
322. Yu D, Stach LM, Newland JG. Linezolid-resistant *Staphylococcus aureus* in children with cystic fibrosis. *J Pediatr Infec Dis Soc*. 2015;4(4):e163-e165.
324. Zemanick ET, Emerson J, Thompson V, et al. Clinical outcomes after initial *Pseudomonas* acquisition in cystic fibrosis. *Pediatr Pulmonol*. 2015;50(1):42-48.
325. Zemanick ET, Harris JK, Wagner BD, et al. Inflammation and airway microbiota during cystic fibrosis pulmonary exacerbations. *PLoS ONE*. 2013;8(4):e62917.
328. Ziadya AG, Hansen J. Redox balance in cystic fibrosis. *Int J Biochem Cell Biol*. 2014;52:113-123.

The full reference list for this chapter is available at ExpertConsult.com.

26 Infective Endocarditis

Sheldon L. Kaplan • Jesus G. Vallejo

Infective endocarditis results when microorganisms adhere to the endocardial surface of the heart. This process usually occurs on heart valves, although septal defects and mural surfaces can be affected. Most episodes of endocarditis begin on endocardium that has been altered by congenital defects, previous disease, surgery, or trauma. The clinical manifestations depend on the degree of compromise of cardiac function and the occurrence of embolic phenomena. Although bacteria are responsible for most cases, instances of infective endocarditis caused by fungi, chlamydiae, rickettsiae, and perhaps viruses have been described. Advances in the practice of general pediatrics and cardiology during the past three decades have contributed to changes in the predisposing conditions and etiologic agents of infective endocarditis. Before the 1950s, rheumatic fever was the major underlying condition, but its incidence has declined greatly since then.[338,463] Improvements in the medical and surgical management of children with congenital heart disease have increased survival rates. Eighty percent to 90% of children with infective endocarditis have congenital heart disease. Many cases occur after cardiac surgery, especially for replacement of valves and creation of shunts with prosthetic materials.[376] The reported incidence of infective endocarditis in neonates has been increasing, probably owing to the use of sophisticated and highly invasive techniques in neonatal intensive care nurseries.[103,178,363,446]

Infective endocarditis has been classified as acute or subacute based on the progression of untreated disease.[489] The acute form has a fulminant course, with high fever, systemic toxicity, and death from sepsis in several days to 6 weeks. The most common etiologic agents are *Staphylococcus aureus, Streptococcus pyogenes,* and *Streptococcus pneumoniae.* Children with the acute form often have no underlying cardiac lesion.[585] Subacute disease usually occurs in patients with previous valvular disease or those who have undergone cardiac surgical intervention.[66] It is characterized by a more indolent course (6 weeks to several months) and with low-grade fever, vague systemic complaints, and various embolic phenomena. Viridans streptococci are the most common etiologic agents. This classification ignores the frequent overlap in clinical manifestations caused by various organisms, especially the staphylococci and fungi, which are causes of an increasing number of subacute cases in the postcardiac surgical setting. Classification based on specific etiologic agents is preferable because it has implications for the usual clinical course, predisposing factors, and appropriate medical and surgical management.[23]

EPIDEMIOLOGY

The incidence of infective endocarditis in adults has been difficult to determine because the methods of study and criteria for diagnosis vary among series.[37,135,390] Accurate figures on the incidence of infective endocarditis in children are difficult to obtain. The most common method of reporting the incidence in pediatric series expresses the number of cases of infective endocarditis as the numerator and the total number of hospital admissions during the analyzed period as the denominator. Zakrzewski and Keith[609] reported an incidence of endocarditis of 1 in 4500 pediatric admissions at the Hospital for Sick Children in Toronto from 1952 to 1962, whereas Van Hare and colleagues[571] at Case Western Reserve in Cleveland, Ohio, found an incidence of 1 in 1280 in the period from 1972 to 1982. In a large series from Boston Children's Hospital spanning the period between 1933 and 1972, the incidence before 1963 was 1 in 4500 pediatric admissions, whereas that for 1963 to 1972 was 1 in 1800 admissions.[257] A study from a children's hospital in Australia reported an incidence of 1 in 4500 hospital admissions between 1971 and 1983.[505] One Japanese center reported an annual incidence of 0.9 cases per 1000 children seen at the cardiology clinic.[175] In a report from Canada the cumulative incidence of IE occurring in children with congenital heart disease was 6.1 per 1000 through 18 years of age.[468] Although differences in referral patterns at these centers may have introduced bias into these figures, the incidence of infective endocarditis in children appears to be rising. This rise may be explained by the increased survival rate of children with all forms of cardiovascular disease and an increase in the percentage of cases that occur after cardiac surgery[31] (especially implantation of foreign material[583]) and are related to intravascular catheters.[157,263,475] Early surgical correction of many types of congenital heart diseases, along with effective appropriate perioperative antibiotic prophylaxis regimens, ultimately may lower the incidence of postoperative infective endocarditis.[561] However, the use of invasive therapeutic modalities, especially intravenous catheters and pacemakers, has led to an increased incidence of health care–associated endocarditis.[157,163,346,447,561,584] In general children with predisposing cardiac conditions who develop infective endocarditis while hospitalized have longer hospitalizations and higher mortality than patients with community-associated endocarditis.[164,343]

The average age of children with infective endocarditis is increasing, a phenomenon that may reflect the longer life expectancy created by improved therapy for children at risk.[537] From 1930 to 1950, the mean age for children with infective endocarditis was close to 5 years.[257] Between 1960 and the present, it increased to 8.5 and then to 13 years.[175,186,291,345,475] The number of reports of infective endocarditis in children younger than 2 years of age had been small but has increased significantly since the late 1980s.[46,186,363,463,593] The clinical course of infective endocarditis in these young children often is atypical, and some cases are diagnosed at autopsy.[257,420] Before the 1950s, this disease was a rare event in neonates, with only eight autopsy cases reported.[328] Several reports suggest a rapidly increasing rate associated with the development of intensive supportive care in neonates.[54,353,363,370,404,405] Symchych and colleagues[535] found a 3% incidence of bacterial endocarditis among all neonatal autopsies. Endocarditis in neonates frequently occurs on the tricuspid valve when associated with an indwelling central venous catheter.[555] Congenital heart defects also predispose neonates to the development of infectious endocarditis.[103]

Any form of structural cardiac disease may predispose to infective endocarditis, especially disorders associated with turbulence of blood flow.[182,516] In autopsy and clinical series, children with ventricular septal defect, tetralogy of Fallot, left-sided valvular disease, and systemic-pulmonary arterial communication were at highest risk, whereas those with pulmonary stenosis, coarctation of the aorta, and secundum atrial septal defect were at low risk.[462,475] Hypertrophic obstructive cardiomyopathy rarely is associated with infective endocarditis.[85] Isolated pulmonic or tricuspid valve endocarditis can occur in "otherwise normal" children and adolescents with sepsis or focal bacterial infection,[391] but usually it is associated with congenital heart disease, intravenous catheters, or intravenous drug abuse.[76,388] A bicuspid aortic valve is recognized as an important risk factor for the development of infective endocarditis, especially in elderly men.[354] The underlying heart diseases in 266 pediatric cases of infective endocarditis are listed in Table 26.1.[263] In a large Canadian study, independent risk factors for infective endocarditis among children with congenital heart disease were cyanotic congenital

TABLE 26.1 Underlying Heart Disease in 266 Children With Infective Endocarditis

Underlying Heart Disease	Percentage Affected (%)
Congenital heart disease	78
Tetralogy of Fallot	24
Ventricular septal defect	16
Congenital aortic stenosis	8
Patent ductus arteriosus	7
Transposition of great vessel	4
Others	19
Rheumatic heart disease	14
No heart disease	8

From Kaplan EL. Infective endocarditis in the pediatric age group: an overview. In: Kaplan EL, Taranta AV, eds. *Infective endocarditis: an American Heart Association symposium.* Dallas: American Heart Association; 1977: 51–4.

heart disease, endocardial cushion defects, left-sided heart lesions, age less than 3 years, and cardiac surgery within 6 months.[468]

A cooperative study on the natural history of aortic stenosis, pulmonary stenosis, and ventricular septal defect reported data from a controlled pediatric population collected over a period of 4 to 15 years.[184] In patients not undergoing surgical correction, the risk of acquiring endocarditis by 30 years of age in those with ventricular septal defects was 9.7% versus 1.4% for aortic stenosis and 0.9% for pulmonic stenosis. Aortic valvotomy in children with aortic stenosis actually increases the relative risk, whereas successful repair of ventricular septal defect significantly decreases long-term susceptibility to infective endocarditis.[185] Similarly endocarditis is an extremely rare occurrence after ligation of patent ductus arteriosus has been performed. At present, palliative systemic-to-pulmonary shunting is the surgical procedure most often complicated by infective endocarditis.[475] In a review of 115 patients with tetralogy of Fallot, Kaplan and colleagues[264] reported an 8% incidence of infective endocarditis after placement of a Pott shunt. Transcatheter placement of prosthetic pulmonary valves (TPV) (Melody valve) has been associated with an incidence of subsequent development of infective endocarditis of 2.4% per patient-year and 0.88% per patient-year for TPV-specific endocarditis.[352,575]

The increasing use of prosthetic valves and valved conduit repairs in children with complex heart disease may lead to a larger number of cases of infective endocarditis in the future.[265,272,303,545,551] Most medical centers report an incidence of prosthetic valve endocarditis of 2% to 4% after surgery,[65,187,375,470,516] with the aortic and mitral valves affected most frequently.[244,330] Prosthetic material is also implanted for right ventricular outflow reconstruction. In such cases conduit endocarditis is more common for bovine jugular vein grafts compared to cryopreserved homografts. In a report from Canada reviewing conduits placed in almost 300 patients with a median follow-up of 3.4 years, conduit endocarditis occurred in 9.4% (23/244) of bovine jugular vein grafts implanted versus 0.7% (1/135) of the cryopreserved homografts ($P < .001$).[564]

Older studies arbitrarily divided prosthetic valve endocarditis into two categories—early and late—based on whether the infection occurred within 60 days of valve placement or later.[39] The rationale for categorizing by time was based on apparent differences in bacteriologic, pathogenetic, and prognostic associations. So-called early cases most often were caused by coagulase-negative staphylococci (CONS), gram-negative bacilli, and fungi, whereas oral and enterococcal streptococci, along with staphylococci, predominated in late cases.[269] These older reports suggested that early cases were acquired by contamination of an intraoperative valve or were secondary to postoperative extracardiac infections, whereas late cases were acquired by the same mechanisms as native-valve endocarditis. Nosocomial bacteremia that develops at any time after the patient has undergone valve placement is a significant risk factor for development of endocarditis.[145,343,566] Finally the mortality rate was thought to be higher in early versus late infection.

However, more recent studies have blurred this arbitrary time distinction between early and late prosthetic valve endocarditis.[65,244] The risk probably is highest in the first 6 to 12 months and decreases to its lowest point beyond 1 year after valve replacement. CONS are the dominant organisms both before and after the 60th postoperative day.[65,268] Clinical and epidemiologic data also suggest that prosthetic valve infection caused by staphylococci within the first year after placement probably is acquired at the time of surgery.[39] Identified risk factors for the development of prosthetic valve endocarditis in adults include native valve endocarditis, black race, male sex, a mechanical (vs. biologic) prosthesis, and prolonged cardiopulmonary bypass time[244]; no comparable information is available for children.

Mitral valve endocarditis occurs frequently on an anatomically normal valve in patients with other predisposing factors.[158] An association between mitral valve prolapse and infective endocarditis has been recognized in adults and children. This heart lesion is detected with increasing frequency in adolescent girls and may be only one component of a developmental syndrome.[495] In adults, 40% to 50% of cases of infective endocarditis associated with isolated insufficient mitral valves occur in patients with mitral prolapse.[97] In some series of native valve endocarditis, mitral valve prolapse has been the most common underlying lesion.[354] The reported incidence of infective endocarditis in patients with mitral valve prolapse has varied markedly among studies, from low rates of 14 per 100,000 per year to 5 of 58 patients monitored prospectively for 9 to 22 years.[221] A retrospective epidemiologic analysis involving matched cases and controls yielded an odds ratio of 8.2, indicative of a substantially higher risk for development of endocarditis in patients with mitral valve prolapse than in normal controls.[94]

The risk of developing infective endocarditis is not uniform for all patients with mitral valve prolapse. The risk is increased in patients with a preexisting systolic murmur (but not for those with an isolated click and no murmur), echocardiographically demonstrated regurgitation, and valvular redundancy.[105,329,340] The signs and symptoms of endocarditis associated with mitral valve prolapse may be more subtle than those of other types of left-sided endocarditis.[158,402] However, significant complications are relatively common occurrences and sometimes require valve replacement during the acute illness or during convalescence.[21,521]

Fungal endocarditis is a rare disorder in children but should be suspected in certain clinical and epidemiologic settings. It is more likely to occur after cardiac surgery and rarely occurs on native heart valves. It occurs more commonly in neonates treated in intensive care settings than in older children.[103] Other predisposing factors include (1) the presence of an indwelling vascular catheter, (2) prolonged use of antibiotics, (3) intrinsic (immunodeficiency diseases, malignancy, malnutrition) or extrinsic (corticosteroids, cytotoxic drugs) immunosuppression, (4) bowel surgery resulting in transient fungemia, (5) intravenous drug use, and (6) preexisting or concomitant bacterial endocarditis.

Many conditions other than structural heart disease predispose children to the development of infective endocarditis. The most important is the presence of an indwelling central venous catheter, especially in patients who are seriously ill or immunocompromised.[178,186,313,558,592] The catheter acts as a foreign body and presumably causes microscopic damage by abrading endocardial and valve surfaces; such damage results in nonbacterial thrombotic vegetation.[28] Infection of intracardiac pacemaker wires also can lead to endocarditis.[15] Infection acquired during the placement procedure and infection of the pacemaker pouch are most common. Infective endocarditis, usually of the tricuspid valve, has developed in children with ventriculoatrial shunts placed for the treatment of hydrocephalus.[263] In patients with arteriovenous fistulas created for hemodialysis, bacterial vegetations may develop in the fistula and on heart valves.[305,450] Rarely, penetrating wounds or foreign bodies can initiate endocarditis.[225,339] Piercings of various body parts also have been associated with endocarditis.[2,443] One important group of patients with an increased risk for development of infective endocarditis is intravenous drug users.[348,599] A predilection for involvement of the tricuspid valve, followed by the mitral and aortic valves, has been noted.[174] Radiographic evidence of septic pulmonary emboli and signs of tricuspid insufficiency dominate the clinical findings.[489] Within this group of patients, increased rates of infective endocarditis and mortality are associated with infection by human immunodeficiency virus (HIV), particularly as CD4 cell counts fall to less than 200/mm^3.[436]

Several recent studies have found an apparent shift in the epidemiology of pediatric infective endocarditis toward a higher proportion of children without preexisting heart disease, which accounted for 35% to 58% of all the infective endocarditis cases.[116,301,316] In these patients, *S. aureus* was the most common causative organism, and delay in diagnosis was common.

Although the incidence of infective endocarditis in children may be rising, the prognosis has improved dramatically during the past several decades. Current mortality rates usually are close to 10%.[379,475,494] Most survivors remain hemodynamically stable at long-term follow-up.[161,494] However, patients who experience infective endocarditis appear to be at higher risk for developing recurrent endocarditis than are those with similar cardiac abnormalities who have not had previous endocarditis.[516] The patient's functional class before treatment appears to be most predictive of long-term functional status. In one study, 22% of children who survived infective endocarditis required surgery related to the infection, including vegetectomy, evacuation of a hematoma, atrioventricular valve replacement, and placement or replacement of a graft or intracardiac shunt.[475]

PATHOPHYSIOLOGY

Clinical observations, autopsy studies, and work with experimental animal models have demonstrated that the occurrence of several independent events is required for the development of subacute infectious endocarditis. The endocardial surface usually is disrupted by stress or injury commonly caused by the turbulence of blood. This surface damage results in the deposition of fibrin and platelets, which form nonbacterial thrombotic vegetations. If bacteria adhere to these deposits, infective endocarditis will result. The surface of the infected vegetation becomes protected by a cover of fibrin and platelets. A tremendous proliferation of organisms (as many as 10^9 CFU/g) may ensue.[131] The protective sheath isolates the organisms from the action of host neutrophils and antibiotics. The clinical manifestations and complications of infective endocarditis are related to both the hemodynamic changes caused by local infection and the occurrence of embolization and metastatic infection.

In experimental animals, the valvular surface must be damaged, usually by an intravenous catheter, to produce infective endocarditis.[22] The first step in the pathogenesis of subacute infective endocarditis in humans is the development of hemodynamic factors that favor endocardial damage. In an autopsy study of 1024 patients with infective endocarditis, Lepeschkin[306] showed that the location of the endocardial lesions correlated with the impact of pressure; this finding makes a strong argument for the role of mechanical stress as a critical factor in the evolution of the lesions. When associated with valvular insufficiency, infective endocarditis usually occurs on the atrial surface of the mitral valve and the ventricular surface of the aortic valve. Injection of a bacterial aerosol into the air stream passing through a Venturi tube demonstrates how high pressure drives an infected fluid into a low-pressure sink.[457] This process establishes maximal deposition of bacteria in the low-pressure sink immediately beyond the orifice. Mitral insufficiency creates a Venturi effect when blood is driven from the high-pressure left ventricle into a low-pressure atrium; maximal deposition occurs around the mitral annulus on the atrial side. Similarly, with aortic valve insufficiency, the high-pressure source is the aorta, and the low-pressure sink is the left ventricle, which leads to deposition on the ventricular surface of the valve.

Lesions also are created more directly by a jet stream causing endocardial damage. For example, in a small, restrictive ventricular septal defect with a left-to-right shunt, a Venturi effect leads to the development of lesions on the right ventricular septal side of the defect, whereas secondary lesions created by the jet effect are located on the right ventricular wall opposite the defect.[587] Heart defects with a surface area sufficiently large to prevent a significant pressure gradient and those in which smaller volumes minimize the gradient do not create the jet and Venturi effects. This difference helps to explain the rarity of endocarditis in patients with atrial septal defects and the increased risk of infection complicating small, but not large, ventricular septal defects.

Once endocardial damage has occurred, collagen is exposed and platelet and fibrin deposition ensues in a manner analogous to formation of the primary plug of normal hemostasis after vascular injury.[253,588] The sterile platelet-fibrin thrombus that is formed subsequently is referred to as a nonbacterial thrombotic vegetation.[322,412] Formation of the vegetation reflects two pathogenic mechanisms: hypercoagulability and endothelial damage.[489] To establish experimental infective endocarditis without initial formation of the vegetation is nearly impossible. Microscopic examination demonstrates that this lesion is the one to which microorganisms attach during the early stages of experimental endocarditis. Nonbacterial thrombotic vegetations have been found in both adults and children with malignancy, chronic wasting diseases, uremia, connective tissue diseases, and congenital heart disease and after the placement of intracardiac catheters,[349,450] and they have been associated with embolism and infarction in distant organs.[50]

Once a nonbacterial thrombotic vegetation has been established, transient bacteremia or fungemia may result in colonization of the lesion. Transient bacteremias are common occurrences, especially with traumatization of a mucosal surface. The incidence of bacteremia in adults and children after various procedures is listed in Table 26.2.[143,455] The bacteremia usually is of low grade and is proportional to the amount of trauma produced by the procedure and the number of organisms inhabiting the surface. In addition, "silent" bacteremia probably occurs frequently. Many persons have circulating antibodies to their own oral flora, as well as an increase in peripheral T cells sensitized to the flora of their dental plaque.[489] Some children with congenital heart disease may be at increased risk for having gingival colonization and subsequent

TABLE 26.2 Bacteremia After Various Procedures in Adults and Children

Initiating Event	Positive Blood Cultures (%)	Predominant Organisms
Dental extraction (children)	30–65	*Streptococcus*, diphtheroids
Chewing gum, candy, paraffin	0–51	*Streptococcus, Staphylococcus epidermidis*
Tooth brushing	0–26	*Streptococcus*
Tonsillectomy	28–38	*Streptococcus, Haemophilus*, diphtheroids
Bronchoscopy (rigid scope)	15	*Streptococcus, S. epidermidis*
Bronchoscopy (fiberoptic)	0	
Orotracheal intubation	0	
Nasotracheal intubation/suctioning	16	*Streptococcus*, aerobic gram-negative rods
Sigmoidoscopy/colonoscopy	0–9.5	*Enterococcus*, aerobic gram-negative rods
Upper gastrointestinal endoscopy	8–12	*Streptococcus, Neisseria, S. epidermidis*, diphtheroids, other
Percutaneous liver biopsy	3–14	Pneumococcus, aerobic gram-negative rods, *Staphylococcus aureus*, other
Urethral catheterization	8	Not stated
Manipulation of *S. aureus* suppurative foci	54	

From Everett ED, Hirschmann JU. Transient bacteremia and endocarditis prophylaxis: a review. *Medicine (Baltimore)*. 1977;56:61–77.

development of bacteremia with organisms associated with infectious endocarditis, such as the HACEK (*Haemophilus* spp., *Actinobacillus actinomycetemcomitans, Cardiobacterium hominis, Eikenella corrodens, Kingella kingae)* microbes.[517]

The ability of microorganisms to adhere to the platelet-fibrin thrombus is a critical factor in the development of infective endocarditis.[110,209,253] In a canine model, *S. aureus* and the viridans streptococci, which frequently cause infective endocarditis, adhere more readily to normal aortic leaflets than do organisms uncommon in endocarditis.[197] Within isolates of *S. aureus,* strains devoid of microencapsulation are less capable of inducing endocarditis in an experimental model than are encapsulated strains.[21] Specific products released by these organisms, including dextran, mannan, teichoic acid, and slime, may enhance their ability to colonize the vegetation.[253,281] The amount of dextran produced by various viridans streptococci in broth correlates with both their adherence and their ability to produce endocarditis in the rabbit model.[371,491] *Candida albicans* is readily adherent and produces infective endocarditis in rabbits more easily than does *C. krusei,* a nonadherent yeast rarely implicated in human infective endocarditis.[487] In addition, endocarditis-producing strains of streptococci and staphylococci are more potent stimulators of platelet aggregation than are other bacteria that do not produce infective endocarditis.[93,218,371] This action may accelerate the formation of an infected vegetation or may increase the removal of organisms from the circulation. The importance of adherence by organisms has been studied by preincubating organisms with many classes of antibiotics. After incubation at subinhibitory concentrations, adhesion of streptococcal species to fibrin-platelet matrices and damaged canine valves is decreased.[492] Antibiotics may prevent development of infective endocarditis by both bacterial killing and inhibition of adherence to the vegetation.[191]

Host tissue factors undoubtedly play an important role in adherence of bacteria to the developing thrombus. Activation of the coagulation system ensues once bacteria become adherent to a nonbacterial thrombus. Some organisms that produce endocarditis may be able to initiate procoagulant activity through microbial enzymes. Activation of the intrinsic coagulation pathway is triggered by exposed connective tissue components and platelet aggregation.[281] However, activation of the extrinsic coagulation pathway probably is the major stimulus for growth of vegetations. Elements of the extracellular matrix, including fibronectin, laminin, and collagen, have been shown to facilitate the adherence of bacteria on fibrin-platelet matrices.[532,557] Fibronectin may be the host receptor for organisms within the nonbacterial thrombotic vegetation.[292,324] Laminin-binding proteins have been found on the cell walls of organisms recovered from patients with endocarditis.[511]

The platelet-organism interaction is complex and not understood completely. *Streptococcus sanguinis* produces two cell surface antigens that promote platelet aggregation: a class I antigen promotes adhesion of *S. sanguinis* to platelets, whereas coexpression of a class II antigen promotes platelet adhesion or aggregation.[219] The induced platelet aggregation appears to be an important determinant of further development of vegetation and progression of disease in experimental endocarditis. In addition, production of streptococcal exopolysaccharide inversely correlates with platelet adhesion while inhibiting aggregation, thus indicating that surface molecules may enhance endocarditis at only certain pathogenic steps.[529] Platelets also may be involved in host defense within the vegetation. After exposure to thrombin, platelets may release microbicidal proteins with bactericidal activity against some gram-positive cocci; resistance to these proteins may be a virulence factor for *S. aureus* in the development of endocarditis.[398,605]

As bacterial colonization of a nonbacterial thrombotic vegetation progresses, it enlarges by further bacterial proliferation and platelet-fibrin deposition (Fig. 26.1).[374] Kissane[286] described three histologic zones: (1) necrotic endocardium; (2) a broad zone of bacterial colonies, pyknotic nuclear debris, and fibrin; and (3) a thin coating on the surface of fibrin and leukocytes. The location of bacterial colonies below the surface and the minimal infiltration by phagocytic cells create an environment of impaired host resistance that results in extreme bacterial proliferation. The structure of the vegetation diminishes the penetration of antibiotics into the bacterial layer. In addition, the metabolic activity of bacteria within this lesion is slowed, thus rendering antibiotics less effective.

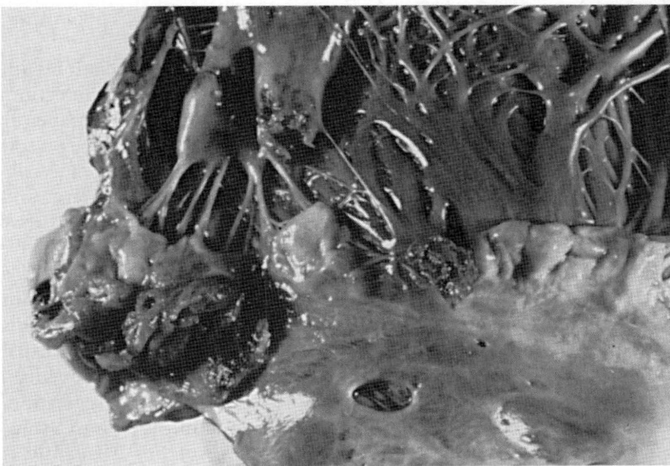

FIG. 26.1 Subacute endocarditis of the mitral valve with vegetation and rupture of the papillary muscle caused by *Staphylococcus aureus*. (Courtesy of Dr. Edith P. Hawkins, Texas Children's Hospital, Houston.)

The formation of vegetations and erosion of heart valves may cause valvular incompetence and thereby may result in cardiac failure.

Immunopathologic factors may have important roles in both the development and sequelae of infective endocarditis.[42] The susceptibility of a gram-negative bacillus to complement-mediated bactericidal activity is critical to its potential to create endocarditis.[130] Gram-positive cocci are a more frequent cause of infective endocarditis than are gram-negative bacilli. Gram-positive organisms are resistant to this bactericidal activity; phagocytosis is required for killing.

The frequent presence of hypergammaglobulinemia, splenomegaly, and monocytes in the blood of patients with infective endocarditis indicates stimulation of the humoral and cellular immune systems. Macroglobulins, cryoglobulins, and agglutinating, opsonic, and complement-fixing antibodies have been associated with infective endocarditis.[228,300] Studies in animals preimmunized with heat-killed streptococci before aortic valve trauma and infection are induced suggest that circulating antibody has a protective role.[490,567] However, antibody to *S. aureus* or *Staphylococcus epidermidis* does not prevent the development of endocarditis in immunized animals, perhaps because this antibody does not enhance opsonophagocytosis.[489] The continuous antigenic challenge created by intravascular organisms leads to increased production of specific antibody (including opsonic, agglutinating, and complement-fixing antibodies), cryoglobulins, macroglobulins, and antibodies to bacterial heat shock protein,[439] as well as to the subsequent formation of circulating immune complexes. These complexes are found with increased frequency in patients with a long duration of illness, hypocomplementemia, extravalvular manifestations, and right-sided disease.[41] Quantitative levels of circulating immune complexes may be helpful in distinguishing endocarditic from nonendocarditic sepsis and in monitoring anti-infective therapy. Effective treatment usually leads to a prompt decrease in these levels,[40] whereas relapses may be characterized by rising titers.[273] The diffuse glomerulonephritis occasionally noted with infective endocarditis is caused by subepithelial deposition of immune complexes and complement.[204] Immune complexes can be demonstrated in some diffuse purpuric lesions seen with endocarditis.[323] Bacterial antigens have been found within these complexes.[241]

Further evidence of stimulation of the immune system in infective endocarditis is the development of rheumatoid factor in approximately 50% of adults with disease lasting longer than 6 weeks.[594] Titers of rheumatoid factor correlate with hypergammaglobulinemia and, as with immune complex levels, decrease with therapy and increase during relapse. The role of rheumatoid factor in the disease process is unknown, but it may be involved by blocking immunoglobulin G opsonic activity, stimulating phagocytosis, or accelerating microvascular damage.[489] Antinuclear, antiendocardial, antisarcolemmal, and antimyolemmal antibodies also have been identified in patients with infective endocarditis; their role in pathogenesis is unclear.[332]

The pathologic changes that occur in the heart in association with infective endocarditis are secondary to local extension of the infection. The vegetations vary from a millimeter to several centimeters; frequently they are singular, but they may be multiple. Valvular stenosis may result from large lesions. Vegetations secondary to certain organisms, especially *Candida, Haemophilus,* and *S. aureus* in acute cases, often are large and friable, with a propensity for embolization.[606] Ulcerative lesions may occur and may lead to perforation of the valve and subsequent congestive heart failure. Other local complications include rupture of the chordae tendineae or papillary muscle (see Fig. 26.1), valve ring abscess with subsequent fistula formation and pericardial empyema,[55,71] aneurysms of the sinus of Valsalva or ventricle,[84,179,485] myocarditis, and myocardial infarction.[149] Persistent fever occurring during appropriate medical therapy for infective endocarditis may reflect a persistent vegetation, especially with right-sided disease, or extension of infection into a valve ring and adjacent structures.[124] In such cases, surgery frequently is required.

The pathologic changes in distant organs usually are secondary to embolization with subsequent infarction or metastatic infection. In many cases of infective endocarditis, the causative organism is of low pathogenicity; infections caused by septic emboli often are low grade because of the reduced propensity of these organisms to invade tissue. However, the emboli in acute *S. aureus* endocarditis frequently cause severe metastatic infections and overwhelming sepsis. Emboli from right-sided heart lesions lodge in the lungs and cause pulmonary infarcts and abscesses, which usually are small and multiple. Left-sided lesions may embolize to any organ but most commonly affect the brain, kidney, spleen, and skin.[287,392] Cerebral emboli have been detected in 30% of cases in adults and children and have caused infarction, abscess, mycotic aneurysm, subarachnoid hemorrhage, meningitis, and acute hemiplegia of childhood.[68,199,212,260,347,477,486,573] Kidney abscess is a rare occurrence, but infarcts are noted in most patients at autopsy.[366] Amyloidosis involving primarily the kidneys is a rare complication of chronic infective endocarditis.[217] Splenic abscess also is a rare event but can be a fatal complication if undetected.[255] The most common manifestation of embolization to the skin is petechiae. Janeway lesions are septic emboli consisting of bacteria, neutrophils, necrosis, and subcutaneous hemorrhage. Osler nodes are areas of thrombosis and necrosis. They may be related to both immune complex deposition and septic emboli.[5]

CLINICAL MANIFESTATIONS

The signs and symptoms of infective endocarditis are determined by the extent of local cardiac disease, the continuous bacteremia, and the degree of involvement of distant organs as a result of embolization, metastatic infection, and circulating immune complexes.[26] Consequently the clinical findings are highly variable and mimic those of many other diseases.[82,473] Unexplained embolic phenomena in any organ should suggest the diagnosis of endocarditis, especially in children with known heart disease. Patients with acute bacterial endocarditis initially may be seen with florid sepsis; the endocarditis is diagnosed at autopsy. The indolent manifestations of subacute endocarditis may evolve for weeks or months before medical care is sought. Endocarditis frequently occurs in children with preexisting heart disease, so subtle changes in cardiac function may be difficult to detect early in the course. The frequency of the major clinical manifestations of bacterial endocarditis in infants and children is listed in Table 26.3.

Fever is the most common symptom of infective endocarditis, but it is absent in 10% of cases. It usually is of low grade and has no specific pattern. Chills may accompany the fever, but they rarely are seen in children. Persistent fever during antimicrobial therapy is an uncommon occurrence. Prolonged (≥2 weeks) fever is associated with certain etiologic agents (*S. aureus,* gram-negative bacilli, fungi), with culture-negative endocarditis, and with complications such as embolization of major vessels, intracardiac or peripheral abscess, tissue infarction, a need for cardiac surgery, and a higher mortality rate.[56,302] Nonspecific symptoms such as malaise, anorexia, weight loss, and fatigue are common findings. Arthralgia occurs in 24% of patients. The arthralgia frequently is multiple and most commonly affects the large joints. Although adults initially may have synovitis,[91] this finding is rare in children. Osteoarticular infection in association with infective endocarditis in adults occurs almost exclusively in intravenous drug users.[484] It is seen very rarely in children except those with disseminated *S. aureus* infection. Gastrointestinal complaints are noted in 16% of cases and include nausea, vomiting, and abdominal pain. Chest pain occurs in approximately 10% of older children and generally is mild and nonspecific. Although chest pain usually is related to diffuse myalgias, it may be secondary to pulmonary complications or cardiac lesions, especially if the tricuspid valve is involved.

Heart murmurs occur in more than 90% of children with infective endocarditis, but most patients have underlying heart disease with existing murmurs. The appearance of a new murmur or appreciation of a significant change in a previous one occurs in only 25% of cases. Significant blood flow turbulence caused by compromised valvular function must have occurred for a murmur to be detected or to change. The frequent absence of changes in the cardiac examination early in the disease contributes to the long average delay in establishing the diagnosis, especially in children with preexisting heart disease. Congestive heart failure occurs in 30% of children with infective endocarditis and is especially common in those in whom a new murmur of valvular insufficiency develops. Endocarditis should be suspected in any child who has rheumatic or congenital heart disease and unexplained deterioration in cardiac function. Although valvular regurgitation is the most common hemodynamic complication of endocarditis, significant obstruction of a valve or shunt requiring rapid surgery rarely occurs.[83]

Neurologic signs and symptoms are reported in approximately 20% of children with endocarditis. These signs and symptoms may dominate the clinical findings, especially in patients with endocarditis caused by *S. aureus.*[212,477] Neurologic abnormalities also are common in children with endocarditis caused by *Kingella kingae.*[165] The sudden development of cerebral lesions in an infant or child should suggest this diagnosis. The manifestations are those that commonly accompany a cerebral infarct or abscess—namely, acute hemiplegia of childhood, seizures, ataxia, aphasia, sensory loss, focal neurologic deficits, and alterations in mental status.[68] They may be the initial features of endocarditis or may occur years after the infection has been eradicated.[610] Mycotic aneurysms of the cerebral vessels occur rarely in cases of pediatric

TABLE 26.3 Clinical Manifestations of Bacterial Endocarditis in Children

	Average (%)	Range (%)
Symptom		
Fever	90	56–100
Malaise	55	40–79
Anorexia/weight loss	31	8–83
Heart failure	30	9–47
Arthralgia	24	16–38
Neurologic findings	18	12–21
Gastrointestinal findings	16	9–36
Chest pain	9	5–20
Physical Finding		
Splenomegaly	55	36–67
Petechiae	33	10–50
Embolic phenomena	28	14–50
New or change in heart murmur	24	9–44
Clubbing	14	2–42
Osler nodes	7	7–8
Roth spots	5	0–6
Janeway lesion	5	0–10
Splinter hemorrhages	5	0–10

Data from references 57, 98, 100, 175, 257, 291, 345, 400, 473, 505, 513, 537, 546, and 571.

endocarditis.[72] They usually are single, small, and peripheral but may lead to subarachnoid hemorrhage. Whereas computed tomographic scanning of the brain is useful for delineating central nervous system involvement in patients with infective endocarditis, magnetic resonance imaging may be more sensitive for detecting small infarctions and changes secondary to cerebral edema.[47] Other neurologic manifestations associated with endocarditis include cranial nerve palsies, neuropathy, visual changes, choreoathetosis, seizures, and toxic encephalopathy.

Splenomegaly, a common manifestation of endocarditis in children, occurs in 55% of cases. It is found frequently in patients with long-standing disease and other evidence of immune system activation. The spleen generally is nontender and may be associated with mild hepatomegaly. Splenic infarction and abscess are rare events but should be suspected in patients with left upper quadrant abdominal pain that radiates to the left shoulder, a pleural friction rub, or left pleural effusion.

Skin manifestations occur less commonly in children than in adults.[323] Clubbing is found in 10% to 20% of children with endocarditis but frequently is related to underlying heart disease. Petechiae are noted in approximately one-third of patients, especially those with long-standing disease. These lesions are found most commonly on the extremities, oral mucosa, and conjunctivae. Splinter hemorrhages are linear red or brown streaks seen in the nail beds. They are present in only 5% of children with endocarditis and are associated with other conditions.[283] Three other types of lesions are more specific for infective endocarditis but occur in only 5% to 7% of patients: Osler nodes, which are small (2 to 10 mm), painful nodular lesions found in the pads of the fingers or toes[5]; Janeway lesions, which usually are painless hemorrhagic macular plaques that frequently occur on the palms and soles[147]; and Roth spots, which are small, pale retinal lesions associated with areas of hemorrhage located near the optic disk.

Other than fever and, perhaps, splenomegaly, no single sign or symptom occurs in more than 50% of children with endocarditis. That no classic clinical manifestation exists for this disease is obvious because the chance that even three or more signs will be present is extremely low. The appearance of any one of these clinical features in a child with predisposing heart disease should raise suspicion of infective endocarditis and should lead to an appropriate diagnostic evaluation.[84]

The clinical findings of infective endocarditis in infants and neonates are less specific than are those in older children. The onset more often is acute and related to overwhelming infection.[258,358] Infants with heart defects undergo corrective and palliative surgery at a younger age than in the past. Infants in whom postoperative endocarditis does develop probably will have clinical findings more similar to those in older children.

Infective endocarditis is an uncommon occurrence in neonates and frequently is associated with indwelling vascular catheters.[178,341] It may affect the tricuspid valve and have a fairly "silent" clinical manifestation. Persistent bacteremia or fungemia should lead to a search for a cardiac focus of infection. Deterioration in pulmonary function, coagulopathies, thrombocytopenia, and low-grade murmurs often develop in neonates. Skin abscesses and hepatomegaly also are common findings.

Reported series of infective endocarditis in children with prosthetic valves are scarce. In early stages of disease, fever may be the only finding because the other signs of endocarditis are masked by the medical and surgical complications occurring in the immediate postoperative period. Late infections generally produce clinical findings similar to those in native valve endocarditis. Clinical evidence of systemic embolization occurs in as many as 40% of patients.[86] Neurologic complications carry a particularly poor prognosis for survival.[279] A new or changing murmur often indicates valvular insufficiency caused by a paravalvular leak. Florid cardiac failure is the major manifestation if local infection or an abscess creates valve instability and acute, severe regurgitation.

The signs and symptoms of infective endocarditis in intravenous drug users may be similar, but these patients have several more distinctive features of their illness. Two-thirds of these patients have no predisposing heart disease. The valve most commonly affected is the tricuspid, which leads to a predominance of pulmonary signs and symptoms resulting from pleural effusion, pulmonary infarction, and lung abscesses. Signs of tricuspid insufficiency (gallop rhythm, pulsatile liver, regurgitant murmur) are found in one-third of cases.[489] Many patients have extracardiac sites of infection that are helpful in establishing the diagnosis.[544]

LABORATORY FINDINGS

The most important diagnostic procedure is the blood culture. Because many bacteria that usually are not pathogenic cause infective endocarditis, scrupulous aseptic technique must be used to distinguish causative agents from contaminants.[415] The yield of organisms is not increased by obtaining blood from arterial puncture or cardiac catheterization.[43] The bacteremia usually is of low grade and continuous. The first two cultures yield the organism 90% of the time; in two-thirds of cases, all blood cultures are positive.[591] Therefore, isolated positive cultures generally are not significant. Previous outpatient antibiotic therapy may change the yield significantly.[277] In one study, culture positivity in cases of proven endocarditis was 64% in patients who received antibiotics before blood was drawn for culture versus 100% in patients without exposure to antibiotics.[416]

When *Candida* endocarditis is suspected, several additional points should be considered. Isolation of *Candida* spp. may require incubation for 1 week or longer. All blood cultures from a patient with *Candida* endocarditis may not be positive, in contrast to the usual situation with bacterial endocarditis; several positive cultures may be interspersed among negative cultures. In patients with fungal endocarditis, *Candida* is isolated commonly from other infected sites, such as urine, sputum, synovial fluid, cerebrospinal fluid, lymph nodes, and bone marrow.[480]

Three to five samples of blood for culture should be obtained from different sites within the first 24 hours in children with suspected endocarditis. Although difficult to obtain in smaller children, 3 to 5 mL of blood per culture is desirable for optimal yield. The samples should be injected into thioglycolate and trypticase soy (or brain-heart infusion) broth and held for at least 3 weeks to detect slow-growing organisms. However, one study has shown that the method of detection and not the time of incubation is critical to detect fastidious organisms. Baron et al.[33] reported evidence that the Bactec9240 system can detect the HACEK organisms within 5 days. If gram-positive cocci grow in the broth but fail to grow on subculture, nutritionally variant streptococci should be suspected and subculture should be performed on media with either L-cysteine or pyridoxal phosphate.[69,519]

Negative blood cultures are noted in 10% to 15% of patients with clinically diagnosed endocarditis.[560] However, when patients have not received antibiotic therapy previously and blood for culture is obtained properly, these cases account for less than 5% of the total. Potential reasons for negative cultures include the following: (1) right-sided endocarditis; (2) previous administration of antibiotics; (3) fungal (especially *Aspergillus*) endocarditis; (4) endocarditis caused by *Bartonella* spp., rickettsiae, chlamydiae, or viruses; (5) mural endocarditis; (6) slow growth of organisms (*Candida, Haemophilus, Brucella,* nutritionally variant streptococci); (7) anaerobic infection; and (8) nonbacterial thrombotic endocarditis or an incorrect diagnosis.[207,211,425,560] In some instances, intraleukocytic organisms may be seen in layered peripheral blood, even when cultures are negative.[433] If surgical resection of vegetations or valve replacement is performed, a cause may be demonstrated by appropriate histologic examination and stains for bacteria and fungi.[374] Molecular testing (universal bacterial, fungal, or mycobacterial (polymerase chain reaction [PCR]) for organisms in the valvular tissue may reveal the causative organism and likely will be more widely available in the future.[506] Organisms also may be isolated from extracardiac sites (bone marrow, urine).

Many nonspecific laboratory findings are abnormal in patients with infective endocarditis (Table 26.4). The total white blood cell count rarely is helpful, but peripheral eosinophilia may be seen with Loeffler endocarditis.[227] Leukocytosis occurs in a few patients, but leukopenia is a rare finding in the absence of acute endocarditis with overwhelming sepsis. The erythrocyte sedimentation rate is elevated in 80% to 90% of cases. However, frequently it is normal or low when congestive heart failure or renal failure is present. Serum C-reactive protein levels usually are elevated initially and return to normal during the course of successful

TABLE 26.4 Selected Laboratory Findings of Bacterial Endocarditis in Children

Laboratory Finding	Average (%)	Range (%)
Positive blood culture	87	68–98
Elevated erythrocyte sedimentation rate	80	71–96
Low hemoglobin (anemia)	44	19–79
Positive rheumatoid factor	38	25–55
Hematuria	35	28–47

Data from references 56, 98, 175, 255, 291, 345, 505, 513, 546, and 571.

therapy.[350] An increase during therapy may result from treatment failure, but it can also be caused by drug allergy or intercurrent infection. Rheumatoid factor rarely has been measured in a series of pediatric patients, but when measurements have been made, they have been positive in 25% to 50% of children with endocarditis. A positive test may be a diagnostic aid in cases of culture-negative endocarditis when other causes are excluded. Serial measurements may provide evidence of efficacy of therapy, although a fall in the titer of rheumatoid factor may lag behind the clinical and bacteriologic response.[580] Hypocomplementemia is seen in association with glomerulonephritis. Anemia is present in approximately 40% of patients, especially those with long-standing disease. Although hemolysis may occur in the areas of turbulence in the heart, more often it is anemia of chronic disease. Because many patients with cyanotic heart disease normally have a compensatory polycythemia, a serial drop in hematocrit is of more significance than is a single measurement. Hematuria and proteinuria, present in 25% to 50% of cases, usually are secondary to microemboli in the kidneys and may be accompanied by "pyuria," casts, and bacteriuria.

Circulating immune complexes are present in most adults with subacute endocarditis, as measured by Raji cell radioimmunoassay[547] or the ^{125}I-Clq binding assay.[611] These immune complexes frequently are absent in acute endocarditis. Low levels of immune complexes have been found in 32% of adults with septicemia but not endocarditis, in 10% of normal controls, and in 40% of noninfected intravenous drug users.[41] However, levels higher than 100 µg/mL are correlated highly with the presence of endocarditis. Serial measurement of immune complex levels may aid in monitoring therapeutic efficacy.[40] Systematic investigation of immune complexes has been reported infrequently in children with endocarditis. When immune complexes have been sought, most patients, including two of three children with culture-negative endocarditis, have had significant levels.

When infective endocarditis is suspected but blood cultures remain negative, serologic testing for specific organisms may prove helpful. Antibodies to teichoic acid, major components of the *S. aureus* cell wall, are present in more than 85% of adults with staphylococcal endocarditis, but the false-positive rate is as high as 10%.[389] False-negative results correlate with a short (<2 weeks) duration of illness. Specific information about the accuracy of this test in children is lacking, and the tests are not readily available. Serologic testing is available or under investigation for many other organisms that cause infective endocarditis, including *Bartonella, Brucella, Candida, Aspergillus, Histoplasma, Cryptococcus, Chlamydia,* and *Coxiella.*[166,168,259,284] In general, the usefulness of these tests in children with endocarditis is unproven. Some patients with nonspirochetal bacterial endocarditis who reside in locales endemic for Lyme disease have significantly elevated levels of antibodies reactive to *Borrelia burgdorferi.*[262] Diagnostic confusion may occur because the signs and symptoms of infective endocarditis and Lyme disease can be quite similar. Other techniques, such as broad-range PCR,[68,199,212,260,347,477,486,573] have been used to identify *Bartonella* and other causative agents of endocarditis.[59,166,578]

Radiographic techniques have not been a great aid in establishing the diagnosis of infective endocarditis. The findings on plain chest radiographs are nonspecific, but evidence of complications, such as septic pulmonary emboli or congestive heart failure, may be helpful. Computed tomography may help in establishing the diagnosis of an infected shunt.[562] Immunoscintigraphy using technetium-labeled antigranulocyte antibodies has been reported as being useful in adults when the echocardiographic findings were equivocal.[372]

The electrocardiogram also is useful in the evaluation of patients with endocarditis because it detects arrhythmias and conduction disturbances that complicate the disease. Ventricular ectopy may be related to myocardial ischemia, myocarditis, or myocardial abscess. New conduction defects imply extension of infection beyond the valve ring into the myocardium. Any degree of atrioventricular block, a new left bundle branch block, or a new right bundle branch block with a left anterior hemiblock may represent extension of infection from the aortic valve into the ventricular septum. Junctional tachycardia, Wenckebach atrioventricular block, or complete heart block may be produced by extension of the infection from the mitral valve anulus into the atrioventricular node or proximal His bundle. In general, an unstable conduction block is more likely to develop in patients with aortic valve endocarditis than in those with mitral infection.[122]

Echocardiography has become a valuable adjunct to the diagnosis and treatment of endocarditis in children.[120,192,295,452,471,472,497] Color Doppler imaging is a sensitive modality for detection of valvular insufficiency, and the results may influence surgical and medical treatment decisions.[159] Echocardiography can be performed by the traditional transthoracic approach or the transesophageal approach.[430] The sensitivity and specificity of transthoracic echocardiography continue to be defined, with positive results obtained in 36% to 100% of children in various series of pediatric patients.[60,98,120,274,307,314,475]

In general, two-dimensional echocardiography is more sensitive than is the M-mode technique, especially in cases of right-sided endocarditis,[409] and it is superior in diagnosing complications of the destructive process.[26,364] The smallest vegetation detectable is approximately 2 mm, but the acoustic impedance of the mass relative to the surrounding structures is a more important factor than is size in identifying the vegetation. Echocardiography has identified vegetations in culture-negative cases.[274] Its accuracy in prosthetic valve endocarditis is diminished by the difficulty in resolution around the prosthetic device.[383,523] Serial evaluation of valvular vegetations generally does not assist in assessing the efficacy of antibiotic therapy because diminution or disappearance of vegetations may take place long after successful medical treatment has been completed.[285,460,577]

The use of transthoracic echocardiography to predict the clinical course and need for operative intervention in patients with endocarditis is controversial.[8,196] A synopsis of many reports that have assessed the role of transthoracic echocardiography in the diagnosis and management of infective endocarditis suggests the following: (1) because of variable sensitivity among studies for detection of vegetations, a negative study does not rule out endocarditis, especially when foreign material is present within the heart; (2) false-positive studies are quite rare (the specificity is high); (3) the reliability of transthoracic echocardiography depends on the experience of the examiner and the technical adequacy of the study; (4) transthoracic echocardiography is valuable in assessing local complications of endocarditis on native valves; and (5) in most but not all studies, patients with a vegetation identified by transthoracic echocardiography have an increased risk for the development of systemic emboli and congestive heart failure.[196,248,326,355,454,483,523]

Although some investigators contend that the presence of a vegetation should hasten early surgery, most suggest that a positive echocardiogram is adjunctive evidence that should be considered along with other clinical parameters when considering surgical intervention. One study suggested that the relative risk for having embolic events associated with echocardiographically visualized lesions is microorganism dependent, with a significant attributable risk seen, for instance, in patients with viridans streptococcal infection.[514] The absence of a vegetation on transthoracic echocardiography may define a subset of patients at low risk for the development of embolic complications.

Transesophageal echocardiography (TEE) has been studied extensively in adults with infective endocarditis.[109] It uses a 5-MHz phased-array transducer with Doppler and color flow encoding capabilities mounted on the tip of a flexible endoscope.[489] Biplane TEE is considered the standard technique and is superior to transthoracic echocardiography because of improved spatial resolution, lack of acoustic interference from the lungs and chest wall, and closer proximity to posterior structures, such as the mitral valve and left atrium.[108] Multiplane TEE facilitates and abbreviates the examination procedure and may be more accurate in providing the dimensions of a vegetation associated with infective endocarditis.[108,251]

TEE generally is well tolerated by children, even with the use of an adult probe (when the child's weight is more than 7 kg),[497] and rarely is associated with bacteremia.[107,298,429] TEE usually is more sensitive than is transthoracic echocardiography in the detection of intracardiac vegetations and is positive in 70% to 95% of adults with strongly suspected endocarditis.[380,504] One recent study showed that TEE significantly increased the detection of vegetations in bigger (>60 kg) children but did not improve on the results of transthoracic echocardiography in smaller children.[422] It is significantly more sensitive in the detection of vegetations and complications in infected prosthetic valves.[280,417,459,522,536] TEE is particularly useful for detecting an aortic root abscess or involvement of the sinus of Valsalva in adults, and it should be considered in children with aortic valve endocarditis and changing aortic root dimensions on a standard transthoracic echocardiogram.[159,355] It appears to be less helpful for detection of vegetations in right-sided endocarditis.[479] Although a negative transesophageal echocardiographic study does not exclude endocarditis,[510] the procedure should be considered for patients with suspected endocarditis and a negative transthoracic echocardiogram, when the transthoracic echocardiographic windows are suboptimal, and when perivalvular extension of infection is suspected.[16,237]

To aid in establishing the diagnosis of infective endocarditis, various sets of clinical criteria have been suggested.[576] The most widely used diagnostic criteria were proposed by investigators from Duke,[133] and they have been modified subsequently (Boxes 26.1 and 26.2).[297,312,360] These criteria have been validated in large series of infective endocarditis in adults and children.[117,133,222,453,482] In two pediatric series of clinically defined endocarditis, no cases were rejected by the Duke criteria, whereas 25% and 19% were rejected by older criteria.[117,524] However, one study found that 12% of pediatric endocarditis cases were not classified as "definite" by the modified Duke criteria.[549] In addition, the presence of an indwelling venous catheter causing prolonged bacteremia may cause an overestimation of the rate of infective endocarditis using the Duke criteria.[45]

MICROBIOLOGY

Many different microorganisms are capable of causing infective endocarditis in humans.[242] A list of the organisms isolated from patients in major pediatric series is presented in Table 26.5. Gram-positive cocci are the etiologic agents in 90% of cases in which an organism is isolated. Streptococci remain the bacteria isolated most frequently, although the percentage of cases caused by staphylococci and fungi has been increasing during the past two decades.[170,475,571,606] In a preliminary study, Gupta et al.[203] used the Nationwide Inpatient Sample to study the incidence, pathogens, and outcomes of infective endocarditis in children admitted to hospitals in the United States from 2000 to 2010. *Streptococcus* spp. were most common (40.1%), followed by *S. aureus* in 36.6% of the 3840 patients reported.[203] Polymicrobial infective endocarditis, especially in nosocomial settings, also appears to be increasing in incidence.[24] The characteristics of selected organisms and the type of disease that they produce are considered next.

Streptococci

Several terminologies have been used to classify streptococci. The Lancefield system defines groups (A, B, C, D, E, F, G, H) by serologic reactions. The viridans streptococci are α-hemolytic or nonhemolytic, may be Lancefield nontypeable (*Streptococcus anginosus* [formerly *S. milleri*], *S. mitior, S. salivarius,* most *S. mutans,* and *S. sanguinis*) or typeable (*S. bovis* group D, some *S. sanguinis* group H, some *S. anginosus* group F), and display similar characteristics in vivo. They are the most frequent etiologic agents in subacute infective endocarditis and cause 40% of cases in children. They may cause rapidly progressive invasive disease.[229,531]

Viridans streptococci are common pathogens in patients with underlying heart disease but are less common in postoperative patients. They are part of the indigenous flora of the human mouth and

TABLE 26.5 Etiologic Agents of Bacterial Endocarditis in Children

Organism	Average (%)	Range (%)
Streptococci		
Viridans	40.3	17–72
Enterococci	4.0	0–12
Pneumococci	3.3	0–21
β-Hemolytic	2.7	0–8
Other	1.1	0–16
Staphylococci		
Staphylococcus aureus	23.8	5–40
Coagulase-negative	4.7	0–15
Gram-negative aerobic bacilli	4.0	0–15
Fungi	1.1	0–12
Miscellaneous bacteria	2.4	0–10
Culture-negative	12.6	2–32

Data from references 57, 67, 100, 253, 255, 256, 291, 358, 475, 513, 546, and 571.

BOX 26.1 Definition of Terms Used in the Modified Duke Criteria for Infective Endocarditis

Major Criteria

1. Positive blood culture
   a. Typical microorganisms for IE from ≥2 blood cultures
      (1) Viridans streptococci, *Streptococcus bovis*, HACEK group, *Staphylococcus aureus* or
      (2) Enterococci, in the absence of another primary focus, or
   b. Persistently positive blood cultures, with recovery of a microorganism consistent with IE from
      (1) Blood cultures drawn ≥12 hours apart *or*
      (2) All of three or a majority of four or more separate blood cultures, with first and last drawn ≥1 hour apart
2. Evidence of endocardial involvement
   a. Positive echocardiogram for IE
      (1) Oscillating intracardiac mass on valve or supporting structures, in the path of regurgitant jets, or on implanted material, in the absence of an alternative anatomic explanation, *or*
      (2) Abscess *or*
      (3) New partial dehiscence of a prosthetic valve *or*
      (4) New valvular regurgitation (increase or change in preexisting murmur is not sufficient)

Minor Criteria

1. Predisposing heart condition or intravenous drug use
2. Fever ≥38°C (100.4°F)
3. Vascular phenomena: major arterial emboli, septic pulmonary infarcts, mycotic aneurysm, intracranial hemorrhage, conjunctival hemorrhages, Janeway lesions
4. Immunologic phenomena: glomerulonephritis, Osler nodes, Roth spots, rheumatoid factor
5. Microbiologic evidence: positive blood culture but not meeting major criteria as noted previously[a] or serologic evidence of active infection with organism consistent with IE

HACEK, Haemophilus spp., *Actinobacillus actinomycetemcomitans, Cardiobacterium hominis, Eikenella corrodens, Kingella kingae; IE,* infective endocarditis.

[a]Excluding single positive cultures for coagulase-negative staphylococci and organisms that do not cause IE.

From Li JS, Sexton DJ, Mick N, et al. Proposed modifications to the Duke criteria for the diagnosis of infective endocarditis. *Clin Infect Dis.* 2000;30:633–8.

BOX 26.2 Modified Duke Criteria for the Diagnosis of Infective Endocarditis

Definite

1. Pathologic criteria
   a. Microorganisms: demonstrated by culture or histology in a vegetation, in a vegetation that has embolized, or in an intracardiac abscess *or*
   b. Pathologic lesions: vegetation or intracardiac abscess present and confirmed by histology showing endocarditis
2. Clinical criteria (see Box 26.1)
   a. Two major criteria *or*
   b. One major and three minor criteria *or*
   c. Five minor criteria

Possible

1. One major criterion and one minor criterion, or
2. Three minor criteria

Rejected

1. Firm alternative diagnosis explaining evidence of IE *or*
2. Resolution of IE syndrome with antimicrobial therapy for ≤4 days *or*
3. No pathologic evidence of IE at surgery or autopsy with antibiotic therapy for ≤4 days

IE, Infective endocarditis.
From Li JS, Sexton DJ, Mick N, et al. Proposed modifications to the Duke criteria for the diagnosis of infective endocarditis. *Clin Infect Dis.* 2000;30:633–8.

gastrointestinal tract, and procedures that disrupt mucosal integrity in these areas predispose patients to development of viridans streptococcal bacteremia. In the pediatric population, most blood and cerebrospinal fluid isolates of viridans and nonhemolytic streptococci are not from patients with infective endocarditis.[210] Most strains are exquisitely susceptible to penicillin, although resistance has been increasing related to previous administration of antibiotics.[289,308] Nutritionally variant viridans streptococci, reclassified as *Abiotrophia defectiva* or *Granulicatella* spp., are recognized as one cause of culture-negative endocarditis in children and can cause endocarditis in children without congenital heart disease.[48,81,150,315,393,441,456] These organisms grow in broth but will not grow on subculture agar-based plates. Bacteriologic failure has occurred in 40% of reported cases of endocarditis caused by these organisms despite susceptibility to the antibiotics used.[26,519] Most viridans streptococci have low pathogenicity; however, the *S. anginosus* group has a predilection for suppurative complications.[385] The prognosis of endocarditis caused by nonenterococcal streptococci is excellent with good medical and surgical management; the cure rate is greater than 90%, although complications (emboli, congestive heart failure) occur in as many as 30% of cases. Enterococcal endocarditis occurs much less frequently in children than in adults[357,543,545] and accounts for only 4% of pediatric cases. The organism normally inhabits the gastrointestinal and genitourinary tracts; instrumentation of these areas may cause enterococcal bacteremia. More than 40% of adult patients have no underlying heart disease.[451] Endocarditis should be considered in all infants and children with unexplained enterococcal bacteremia. Although the incidence of enterococcal bacteremia appears to be increasing in some neonatal intensive care units, the incidence of associated endocarditis seems to be very low. Factors that may suggest endocarditis in patients with enterococcal bacteremia include (1) preexisting heart disease, (2) community acquisition, (3) a cryptogenic source, and (4) the absence of polymicrobial bacteremia.[333] Differentiation of enterococci from other group D streptococci *(S. bovis)* is important because their respective therapeutic approaches are different.

Endocarditis caused by β-hemolytic streptococci occurred more commonly in the preantibiotic era than today. Most cases are caused by Lancefield group B or G organisms,[1,18,67,177,586] whereas group C and A streptococci rarely cause endocarditis.[53,125,193,321,444] Group A, B, or C streptococcal infection may lead to large, bulky vegetations, easily seen by echocardiography, and to embolic complications.[19,369,478] Although group B streptococcal bacteremia is a common finding in neonates, endocarditis caused by this organism occurs rarely in this age group. Similarly, *S. pneumoniae* accounted for 10% to 15% of endocarditis cases in the preantibiotic era but currently causes less than 1%.[181,247,406] Pneumococcal endocarditis may involve either the aortic or the mitral valve.[139,190,553] In older studies, fewer than 50% of affected children had underlying heart disease, but in more recent series, most children have had existing heart disease.[243] The clinical course often is fulminant.[136,304,431] Concurrent meningitis or pneumonia (or both) occurs frequently. Valvular dysfunction and cardiac decompensation are common findings.[56,64,87] Early surgical intervention may be required because the mortality rate is 75% when medical management alone is used.[247]

Staphylococci

Staphylococci cause 20% to 30% of cases of infective endocarditis in children, but the relative incidence appears to be increasing, and in some series this organism has been more common than streptococci.[6,170] *S. aureus* is the etiologic agent in most cases of acute endocarditis and frequently infects normal heart valves.[171,342,378] The course often is fulminant when the mitral or aortic valve is involved, with frequent suppurative complications occurring both in the heart (myocardial abscess, pericarditis, valve ring abscess) and in other organs.[142,261,365] *S. aureus* is responsible for more than 50% of cases of endocarditis in intravenous drug users, but the disease tends to be less severe in these patients.[79,80] The origin of the infecting organism is the addict's own nose or skin, not the injection paraphernalia.[559] Endocarditis associated with indwelling vascular catheters or prosthetic valves frequently is caused by *S. aureus.*[252]

Endocarditis must be suspected in any patient with *S. aureus* bacteremia, even when a peripheral focus of infection is present.[464] However, most patients with *S. aureus* bacteremia do not have endocarditis. A risk score may help to determine which adults with *S. aureus* bacteremia should have an echocardiogram due to increased likelihood of endocarditis.[408] However, this risk score has not been evaluated in children and thus may or may not be useful in pediatric patients with *S. aureus* bacteremia. The rise of methicillin-resistant *S. aureus* (MRSA) has rendered treatment more difficult but has had little impact on the rate of local complications.[235]

CONS is a common etiologic agent of endocarditis occurring after cardiac surgery,[14,278,317] and it is occurring more frequently on native valves.[88,89] This organism is the leading agent in prosthetic valve endocarditis, for which it causes 25% to 67% of early cases and 25% to 33% of late cases.[187,244,268] CONS endocarditis also has been associated with mitral valve prolapse and the use of intravascular catheters in premature neonates.[25,401] Although metastatic infection rarely occurs, CONS can be locally invasive; the mortality rate of prosthetic valve endocarditis caused by CONS approaches 75% when valve replacement is not performed.

Gram-Negative Organisms

Although gram-negative bacteria cause 4% to 5% of cases of infective endocarditis in children, the percentage of children with gram-negative enteric bacteremia in whom endocarditis develops is extremely low. Endocarditis should be suspected in patients with gram-negative infection when bacteremia persists despite administration of usually appropriate antibiotic therapy.[74] Burn patients,[239] immunosuppressed hosts, narcotic addicts, and patients with implanted endovascular devices[373] are at an increased risk for development of gram-negative endocarditis. However, in the early postoperative period after cardiac surgery, sustained gram-negative bacillary bacteremia commonly is caused by other foci of infection and does not imply the presence of endocarditis. Many species of gram-negative enteric organisms have caused infective endocarditis in children, but no clear pattern has emerged. Among the gram-negative organisms more commonly reported are *Brucella, Escherichia coli, Serratia, Klebsiella-Enterobacter, Salmonella,* and *Pseudomonas.*[119,290,325,373,533,541] Endocarditis caused by *Salmonella* has been reported in patients with HIV infection.[156] It most often affects previously abnormal heart valves.

Endocarditis is a rare complication of tularemia.[539] Cure of left-sided endocarditis caused by the Enterobacteriaceae seldom is achieved with medical therapy alone.[489] Most information about gram-negative enteric endocarditis is limited to case reports and general medicine reviews; discussion of individual organisms is beyond the scope of this review.

Other gram-negative organisms associated with infective endocarditis are the so-called HACEK coccobacilli.[111,151,236] These organisms caused 57% of cases of gram-negative endocarditis seen at the Mayo Clinic in Rochester, Minnesota, from 1958 to 1979.[183] Endocarditis caused by *Haemophilus influenzae* has been reported in only several children.[106,337] Cases caused by *H. parainfluenzae* and *H. aphrophilus* occur slightly more commonly.[49,90,112,236,250,327,423]

They generally are seen in the setting of preexisting valvular disease and run a subacute course. However, central nervous system complications and emboli to major peripheral arteries are frequent occurrences.[90] Infective endocarditis caused by other organisms of the HACEK group is an extremely rare event in children.[13,152,331,377,413,440,590] Infection caused by *K. kingae* is being recognized more frequently due to recognition and enhanced culture techniques.[127,128,226] In one study from Israel, one clone of *K. kingae* in particular was associated with infective endocarditis compared with other invasive phenotypes.[9] All the bacteria in this group are fastidious, may require 2 to 3 weeks for primary isolation, and need subculturing onto chocolate agar in an atmosphere of 5% to 10% carbon dioxide for optimal growth. These procedures should be performed in all cases of culture-negative endocarditis.

Neisseria gonorrhoeae was responsible for 10% of cases in the preantibiotic era, but fewer episodes have been reported since 1942.[155,245] This pathogen frequently attacks previously normal heart valves and is manifested as an acute illness.[540] Valvular destruction with a need for valve replacement occurs commonly. At present, nonpathogenic *Neisseria* spp. are isolated more frequently in endocarditis than are gonococci, but they usually attack abnormal or prosthetic valves.[61,215,230,240,428,465,496] Although 1% of cases of infective endocarditis in adults are caused by anaerobic bacteria,[153] reports of anaerobic endocarditis in children are exceedingly rare.[95,394,508,527]

Gram-Positive Bacilli

Infective endocarditis caused by *Corynebacterium* spp. is an unusual finding but may occur on normal or previously abnormal valves.[44,359] Both toxigenic[115] and nontoxigenic[201,493,509,548] strains of *C. diphtheriae* cause endocarditis in children, a finding demonstrating that the toxigenic and invasive properties of the organism are independent. Infection occurs most often on native valves and may be quite aggressive and lead to major vascular complications. *Listeria monocytogenes* endocarditis rarely occurs, has a high mortality rate, and, unlike other forms of listeriosis, usually is not associated with immunocompromised hosts.[38,75] It has not been associated with listeriosis in neonates. Fewer than 40 cases of *Lactobacillus* endocarditis have been reported.[200,238,530] Endocarditis caused by *Erysipelothrix rhusiopathiae* is found predominantly in adults who are farmers or are exposed to farm animals or products.[195,213] Most cases of *Bacillus* endocarditis involve the tricuspid valve in intravenous drug users, but other patients have been affected, including those with prosthetic valves.[518] *Gemella morbillorum* (formerly *Streptococcus morbillorum*) is a gram-positive coccus that normally resides in the gastrointestinal tract and is a rare cause of endocarditis.[146,293,437]

Other Organisms

Many different bacteria, including *Acinetobacter*,[198] *Stenotrophomonas*,[458] *Nocardia*,[582] *Actinomyces*,[296] *Streptobacillus*,[467] and *Rothia*,[528] have been associated rarely with endocarditis.[63] Mycobacterial endocarditis is an exceedingly infrequent event.[176]

Infective endocarditis caused by *Coxiella burnetii*, the causative agent of Q fever, is well documented in northern Africa, Europe, and Australia.[4,62,299,311,368] Most cases are chronic (occurring over a 6- to 12-month period) and involve the aortic valve.[335] Clues to establishing the diagnosis include exposure to parturient cats or rabbits, massive splenomegaly, hypergammaglobulinemia, and thrombocytopenia.[426] The diagnosis usually is confirmed by measurement of antibodies against phase I and phase II antigens, but the organism has been isolated from leukocytes in a shell vial assay and has been demonstrated by immunohistologic techniques.[62,189] At least 20 well-documented cases of infective endocarditis caused by *Chlamydia psittaci* and *Chlamydophila pneumoniae* (formerly *Chlamydia pneumoniae*) have been reported.[223,259,344,503] Most patients have had preexisting heart disease and a subacute course.[336] *Mycoplasma* endocarditis is exceedingly rare.[123] *Legionella* has been implicated in several cases of prosthetic valve endocarditis.[554] *Bartonella quintana* and *B. henselae* have been identified as the cause of endocarditis in "culture-negative" cases.[113,126,224,249,512] Most described cases have been in immunocompetent individuals.[427] The diagnosis was established by serology, PCR, or special culture techniques.[30,154,166,445,578]

Although culture of bacteria remains the primary method for establishing the microbial cause of infective endocarditis, the number of organisms causing endocarditis that cannot be cultivated by standard culture methods is growing.[167,232] More recently, universal and species-specific primers have been designed to amplify bacterial DNA directly from resected valves. Among the organisms causing endocarditis identified by these methods are *Bartonella, Tropheryma whippelii, Coxiella, Mycoplasma, Haemophilus, Abiotrophia, Gemella, Cardiobacterium*, and *Streptococcus*.[180,194,232,319,438]

Fungi

Most cases of fungal endocarditis in children have been described as occurring after cardiovascular surgery and prolonged intravenous and antibiotic therapy.[138,144,362,550] More recently, cases have been reported in neonates[349] and after prosthetic valve placement.[397] The most common causative organism is *C. albicans*, although disease has been attributed to other *Candida* spp., including *C. krusei, C. parapsilosis, C. stellatoidea, C. tropicalis*, and *C. guilliermondii*.[435,480,498] Among intravenous drug users, *Candida* spp. other than *C. albicans* are more common causes of endocarditis.[466] The clinical manifestation usually is indolent and not specific, with symptoms occurring weeks to months before the diagnosis is established. Signs and symptoms caused by emboli to large vessels, especially those supplying the brain, kidney, spleen, and extremities, should alert the physician to the possible presence of fungal endocarditis. Large, friable vegetations occur frequently and can be detected by echocardiography.[525] Cutaneous and ocular manifestations of systemic *Candida* infection may be present.[58] The prognosis of *Candida* endocarditis is poor and is related to the propensity for septic emboli, the tendency for invasion into the myocardium, and the poor penetration of antifungal agents into the bulky vegetation. The diagnosis frequently is delayed by the tendency for negative or intermittently positive blood cultures to occur in this disease.[254] Surgical intervention usually is required.

Aspergillus spp., including *A. flavus, A. fumigatus, A. terreus*, and *A. niger*, are the second most frequent causes of fungal endocarditis.[34,35,399] Two-thirds of reported pediatric patients had underlying heart disease. *Aspergillus* endocarditis has been found in immunocompromised hosts with no previous cardiac problems.[603] The most common initial manifestations are fever and embolic phenomena, especially to the central nervous system.[579] Fewer than 25 cases have been diagnosed ante mortem, several by culture of peripheral emboli. Most cases occur after open heart surgery; the most likely source of the organism is airborne inoculation of the heart during the operation.[34,351] Surgical removal of all infected material is recommended, although only several children have been treated successfully. Other fungi that rarely cause endocarditis include *Histoplasma capsulatum, Coccidioides immitis*,[294] *Cryptococcus neoformans, Torulopsis glabrata, Trichosporon beigelii*,[276] and *Fusarium* spp.[205,233]

TREATMENT

In the preantibiotic era, infective endocarditis was a uniformly fatal disease. With the current improved methods of diagnosis and therapy, 80% to 90% of children with this disease can be expected to survive. Mortality rates are higher for acute staphylococcal infection, fungal endocarditis, and prosthetic valve endocarditis, although the tendency toward earlier surgical intervention for these entities may improve survival rates. The cornerstone of successful therapy is selection of antibiotics with specific activity against the causative organism. Better analysis of pharmacodynamic variables, such as bactericidal activity and the postantibiotic effects of various drugs, may assist in the selection of optimal therapeutic regimens.[99,282,596] Although persistent infection occasionally complicates treated endocarditis,[449] deterioration in cardiac function is the major cause of morbidity and mortality.

Several general principles provide the basis for the current recommendations for treatment of endocarditis. Parenteral administration of antibiotics is preferred because erratic absorption of oral antibiotics, especially in infants, can lead to therapeutic failure. Although patient selection criteria for the use of outpatient parenteral antibiotic therapy for endocarditis in adults have been suggested, no data have been published about this practice for children.[11] The 2015 AHA Pediatric endocarditis treatment guidelines state that home parenteral therapy can be considered after initial treatment in the hospital in selected patients who are stable, afebrile, have negative blood cultures, and are at low risk for a complication (not fungal endocarditis or young age).[29] Prolonged treatment, usually 4 to 6 weeks or longer, is necessary to sterilize the vegetations and to prevent relapse. Bacteriostatic antibiotics are not effective and lead to frequent relapses or failure to eradicate the infection, or both. Antibiotic combinations may produce a rapid bactericidal effect through synergistic mechanisms of action. When synergy exists, smaller doses of each drug may be used, thereby reducing toxic side effects.

Blood should be drawn for culture for several days to evaluate the effect of the antibiotics. Negative follow-up cultures do not guarantee the success of therapy, but persistent positive cultures usually require that a change or addition to the antibiotic regimen be made. Observation of the patient's clinical course is extremely important. When fever is present initially, the temperature often returns to normal within a few days after therapy is started. However, fever can persist for weeks in patients whose eventual outcome is good. Such patients must be monitored closely for cardiac arrhythmias and congestive heart failure, which may require intensive care observation and electrocardiographic monitoring. Evidence of major embolic phenomena must be sought diligently by physical examination.

Several laboratory tests may aid in monitoring therapy. In all cases of bacterial endocarditis, the minimal inhibitory concentration (MIC) and minimal bactericidal concentration (MBC) ideally are determined for the antibiotics being used because disk susceptibility testing may not be as reliable and is not quantitative. The role of monitoring the inhibitory and bactericidal activity of the patient's serum is highly controversial.[448] Standardization of this test is poor, with laboratories using variations in inoculum size, in composition of the broth, in timing of samples (at expected peak or trough antibiotic concentrations in serum), in methods of dilution, and in determining the bactericidal end point. In the rabbit endocarditis model, peak serum bactericidal titers greater than 1:8 correlate with therapeutic success.[73] A retrospective review of 17 reports of serum bactericidal activity in patients with endocarditis failed to show any correlation between titers greater than 1:8 and therapeutic success.[96] A prospective study suggested adjusting antibiotic doses to achieve peak titers of 1:64 or greater and trough titers of 1:32 or greater.[589] At present, no generally accepted recommendation can be made.[602]

Little information is available concerning optimal antibiotic therapy for infective endocarditis in children; most treatment regimens are adapted from studies of adults with endocarditis.[26,597] In general, these regimens have been equally successful (and generally less toxic) in children. Recommended doses of the antibiotics commonly used are listed in Table 26.6.

After performing the initial evaluation of a patient with suspected infective endocarditis, the physician must make a clinical judgment about when to initiate therapy. If the findings are strongly indicative of the diagnosis or the child is very ill, treatment should be started as soon as blood has been drawn for culture. Initial empiric therapy depends on the clinical setting in which the tentative diagnosis is made. If the infection is subacute, a combination of penicillin G and an aminoglycoside usually is recommended for its activity against viridans streptococci, enterococci, and most gram-negative organisms. If *S. aureus* endocarditis is a strong consideration (acute manifestation, narcotic addicts), vancomycin and a penicillinase-resistant penicillin should be added to this regimen. Patients who recently have undergone cardiac surgery, especially prosthetic valve placement, are treated best with an aminoglycoside and vancomycin to "cover" for health care–associated infection caused by MRSA or CONS; some physicians add penicillin G to this regimen to improve activity against streptococci. When culture and susceptibility data are known, antibiotic therapy can be changed as needed.

Most strains of viridans streptococci, *S. pyogenes*, and nonenterococcal group D streptococci are exquisitely susceptible to penicillin, with an MIC of less than 0.2 µg/mL. However, 15% to 20% of viridans streptococci have an MIC of 0.2 µg/mL or greater and are defined arbitrarily as relatively resistant.[234] In addition, some strains (particularly *S. mutans* and *S. mitior*) demonstrate tolerance; that is, an MIC to penicillin of less than 0.1 µg/mL but an MBC that is more than 10-fold higher (1.25 to 50 µg/mL). Most strains of nutritionally dependent streptococci are tolerant to penicillin.[25] Clinical failure may occur in endocarditis caused by these tolerant organisms when penicillin alone is used for treatment.[10,234] However, except for nutritionally dependent streptococci, therapy for tolerant viridans streptococci generally should be the same as for susceptible strains.

Although most experts recommend that patients with endocarditis caused by relatively resistant streptococci be treated with high doses of penicillin combined with 2 to 4 weeks of an aminoglycoside, some authorities consider that penicillin alone usually is adequate therapy.[52,121,334] Synergy in vitro between penicillin or vancomycin and streptomycin or gentamicin can be demonstrated against virtually all penicillin-susceptible streptococci.[581] This observation correlates with a faster rate of eradication of bacteria from cardiac vegetations in the rabbit endocarditis model when synergistic combinations of antibiotics are used.[131,134] However, streptomycin is not synergistic for strains with high-level streptomycin resistance; gentamicin is the preferred second drug for these rare isolates.[140] In pediatric patients, gentamicin usually is substituted for streptomycin because of its lower toxicity.

TABLE 26.6 Suggested Intravenous Antibiotic Doses and Schedules for Infective Endocarditis in Children

Antibiotic	Daily Dose/kg	Divided Doses Every:
Aqueous crystalline penicillin G sodium	200,000–300,000 U	4–6 h
Ampicillin sodium	300 mg	4–6 h
Ampicillin-sulbactam	200–300 mg	4–6 h
Cefazolin	100 mg	8 h
Ceftriaxone	100 mg[a]	12 h
	80 mg	24 h
Ciprofloxacin	20–30 mg	12 h
Daptomycin	6 mg	24 h
	<6 y: 10 mg	24 h
Doxycycline	2–4 mg	12 h
Gentamicin sulfate	3–6 mg	8 h
Imipenem/cilastatin	60–100 mg	6 h
Linezolid	30 mg for children ≤12 y	8 h
	600 mg for children >12 y	12 h
Meropenem	60 mg	8 h
Nafcillin sodium	200 mg (max, 12 g)	4–6 h
Oxacillin sodium	200 mg (max, 12 g)	4–6 h
Rifampin	20 mg	8–12 h
Vancomycin hydrochloride	40–60 mg[b]	8–12 h

[a]If dose is over 2 g, divide every 12 h; maximum is 4 g daily.

[b]Target trough usually 10–15 µg/mL although higher levels (15–20 µg/mL) when the MRSA isolate has vancomycin MIC >1 µg/mL. Both levels are difficult to achieve in children using the recommended vancomycin dose, and increasing the dose to achieve these levels can cause nephrotoxicity

From Baltimore RS, Gewitz M, Baddour LM et al. Infective endocarditis in childhood: 2015 update. A scientific statement from the American Heart Association. *Circulation.* 2015;132:1487–1515.

Several regimens have been examined in adults with penicillin-susceptible viridans streptococcal native valve endocarditis (Table 26.7). A 2-week course of penicillin alone leads to an unacceptable relapse rate. However, a 2-week course of intramuscular procaine penicillin and streptomycin cured 99% of adults with penicillin-susceptible streptococcal endocarditis in one report.[600] These results are similar to those obtained with β-lactams alone for 4 weeks[270] or with penicillin for 4 weeks combined with streptomycin for the first 2 weeks. Gentamicin may be substituted for streptomycin. The 2-week penicillin-gentamicin regimen is the least expensive and is the preferred therapy in uncomplicated cases of penicillin-susceptible streptococcal endocarditis in young adults.[489] In general, the regimen of 4 weeks of penicillin alone is preferred for patients in renal failure or at high risk for developing aminoglycoside-induced ototoxicity. Vancomycin or ceftriaxone administered for 4 weeks can be used in patients with penicillin-susceptible viridans streptococcal endocarditis who have a penicillin allergy.[172,173,499,526] A 4-week regimen of penicillin plus an initial 2 weeks of gentamicin is recommended in children with infection caused by relatively penicillin-resistant organisms (Table 26.8). Most nutritionally deficient streptococci are tolerant to penicillin and should be treated as for enterococci (Table 26.8).[26,29,597] In patients with streptococcal infection of prosthetic valves or other prosthetic materials, a 6-week regimen of penicillin usually supplemented with an aminoglycoside is recommended (Tables 26.7 and 26.8). None of the regimens discussed has been evaluated specifically in children with endocarditis.

TABLE 26.7 Suggested Regimens for 4-Week[a] Treatment of Native Valve Endocarditis Caused by Highly Penicillin-Susceptible Viridans Streptococci and *Streptococcus bovis*

Antibiotic(s)	Comments
Aqueous crystalline penicillin G sodium	Recommended
Ceftriaxone sodium	Recommended
Cefazolin	Alternative choice
Vancomycin hydrochloride	Alternative choice; recommended for patients allergic to β-lactam antibiotics

[a]Length of treatment is 6 weeks if endocarditis is related to prosthetic material.
From Baltimore RS, Gewitz M, Baddour LM, et al. Infective endocarditis in childhood: 2015 update. A scientific statement from the American Heart Association. *Circulation.* 2015;132:1487–1515.

TABLE 26.8 Suggested 4-Week[a] Therapy for Native-Valve Endocarditis Caused by Streptococci Relatively Resistant to Penicillin G (Minimum Bactericidal Concentration >0.2 μg/mL); Includes Enterococci and Less-Susceptible Viridans Streptococci

Antibiotic	Comments
Aqueous crystalline penicillin G sodium or ampicillin plus gentamicin[b]	Recommended
Vancomycin hydrochloride plus gentamicin	Alternative for enterococci
Ampicillin plus ceftriaxone	Aminoglycoside-intolerant patient or for enterococci resistant to aminoglycosides
Ceftriaxone plus gentamicin	Alternative for streptococci, not enterococci

[a]Length of therapy is 4 to 6 weeks if endocarditis is on native or prosthetic valve due to enterococcus and 6 weeks if prosthetic valve endocarditis is treated with vancomycin.
[b]Gentamicin is administered for 2 weeks for streptococci and 4 weeks for enterococcus.
From Baltimore RS, Gewitz M, Baddour LM, et al. Infective endocarditis in childhood: 2015 update. A scientific statement from the American Heart Association. *Circulation.* 2015;132:1487–1515.

Most strains of enterococci have an MIC to penicillin of 0.4 μg/mL or greater and an MBC of 6.25 μg/mL or greater.[384] All β-lactam antibiotics are bacteriostatic against enterococci and cannot be used alone. However, plasmid-mediated β-lactamase production has been found in rare strains of *Enterococcus faecalis*. Ampicillin-sulbactam overcomes the enzyme production and may be effective as therapy.[545] Although therapy with penicillin alone is ineffective, the combination of penicillin and an aminoglycoside is synergistic and produces a bactericidal effect on most enterococcal strains. Unfortunately, 20% to 50% of enterococcal strains demonstrate very high resistance (MIC >2000 μg/mL) to streptomycin, and synergy between penicillin and streptomycin does not occur.[216,488] High-level resistance to gentamicin has been found in some isolates, and the incidence is increasing in certain locales.[137,318,414] When these isolates are encountered, all aminoglycosides should be tested because the organism may be susceptible to one while resistant to others.[587] Fortunately these strains rarely cause endocarditis.[384] Although vancomycin-resistant enterococci have emerged as important nosocomial pathogens, they rarely cause endocarditis in children. Optimal therapy for these strains has not been established, but a combination of high-dose penicillin plus vancomycin and gentamicin may be effective in some cases.[70] Vancomycin-resistant enterococcal endocarditis has been treated successfully with oral linezolid.[12,17] The usual regimens for enterococcal endocarditis are listed in Table 26.8.

Most isolates of *S. aureus* are resistant to penicillin, but endocarditis caused by penicillin-susceptible (MIC <0.1 μg/mL) isolates can be treated with this agent. In general, a semisynthetic penicillinase-resistant penicillin given for 6 weeks is the drug of choice for treating methicillin-susceptible *S. aureus* endocarditis (Table 26.9).[29,320,419,515] The addition of gentamicin to nafcillin produces an enhanced bactericidal effect in vitro and in experimental staphylococcal endocarditis in rabbits.[481] However, the value of this combination in patients has not been proved, and generally it is reserved for children with overwhelming infection. In penicillin-allergic patients or in those with MRSA, vancomycin alone has been recommended, although treatment failures in children with endocarditis have been reported.[148,246,309] The addition of rifampin in patients with prosthetic material is recommended; the use of β-lactam drugs after desensitization is necessary in some cases.[36,378] Ciprofloxacin

TABLE 26.9 Suggested Therapy for Endocarditis Caused by Staphylococci in the Absence of Prosthetic Material[a]

Antibiotic	Duration	Comments
Methicillin-Susceptible Staphylococci[b]		
Nafcillin sodium or oxacillin sodium	4–6 wk	Benefit of additional aminoglycoside has not been established
with optional addition of		
Gentamicin sulfate	3–5 days	
Cefazolin	4–6 wk	For patients with non–immediate-type hypersensitivity to penicillin
with optional addition of		
Gentamicin sulfate	3–5 days	
Vancomycin	4–6 wk	For patients highly allergic to β-lactam antibiotics
Methicillin-Resistant Staphylococci		
Vancomycin hydrochloride	6 wk	Recommended
Daptomycin	6 wk	Alternative choice

[a]If prosthetic material is present, rifampin for 6 weeks and gentamicin for 2 weeks are added to the regimen.
[b]If *Staphylococcus* is penicillin susceptible (minimal inhibitory concentration ≤0.1 μg/mL), aqueous crystalline penicillin G sodium can be used for 4–6 weeks instead of nafcillin or oxacillin.
From Baltimore RS, Gewitz M, Baddour LM, et al. Infective endocarditis in childhood: 2015 update. A scientific statement from the American Heart Association. *Circulation.* 2015;132:1487–1515.

TABLE 26.10 Suggested 4-Week Therapy for Endocarditis Caused by HACEK Organisms

Antibiotic	Comments
Ceftriaxone sodium or cefotaxime	Recommended
Ampicillin-sulbactam	Recommended
Ampicillin plus aminoglycoside[a]	Alternative choice

HACEK, Haemophilus species, Actinobacillus actinomycetemcomitans, Cardiobacterium hominis, Eikenella corrodens, Kingella kingae.
[a]For susceptible organisms.
From Baltimore RS, Gewitz M, Baddour LM, et al. Infective endocarditis in childhood: 2015 update. A scientific statement from the American Heart Association. *Circulation.* 2015;132:1487–1515.

TABLE 26.11 Suggested Empiric Therapy for Culture-Negative Endocarditis

Antibiotic(s)	Duration	Comments
Native Valve		
Ampicillin-sulbactam *plus* gentamicin sulfate *plus* ciprofloxacin	4–6 wk	Ciprofloxacin can be administered IV or oral
Prosthetic Valve (early, ≤1 year)		
Vancomycin *plus*	6 wk	40 mg/kg/day in 2 or 3 divided doses
Gentamicin sulfate *plus*	2 wk	3 mg/kg/day in 3 divided doses
Cefepime *plus*	6 wk	150 mg/kg/day in 3 divided doses
Rifampin	6 wk	20 mg/kg PO/IV in 3 divided doses
Prosthetic valve (late >1 year)	6 wk	Same as for native valve endocarditis above

From Baltimore RS, Gewitz M, Baddour LM, et al. Infective endocarditis in childhood: 2015 update. A scientific statement from the American Heart Association. *Circulation.* 2015;132:1487–1515.

has been used, but treatment failures have occurred because of the emergence of resistance.[382,542] Vancomycin for at least 6 weeks is recommended for the treatment of endocarditis caused by MRSA.[29] Daptomycin and linezolid also have been used successfully to treat endocarditis caused by MRSA; only daptomycin is recommended as an alternative choice in the 2015 AHA pediatric guidelines.[29,169,367] Nosocomial infections with coagulase-negative staphylococcus usually are treated with vancomycin because of the high incidence of methicillin resistance among these isolates. The addition of rifampin and gentamicin to either nafcillin or vancomycin may increase bactericidal activity and is recommended in cases of prosthetic valve endocarditis secondary to any staphylococci (see Table 26.9).[26,29]

Therapy for endocarditis caused by gram-negative organisms must be individualized in accordance with in vitro susceptibility studies. A regimen of 6 to 8 weeks of combination therapy with two or more drugs may be required, especially with endocarditis caused by *Klebsiella* or *Pseudomonas.*[160,418] Surgical intervention frequently is necessary, especially for infection of the mitral or aortic valves. Endocarditis caused by *Haemophilus* and other fastidious gram-negative organisms usually is responsive to ampicillin-sulbactam or ceftriaxone alone[29]; the addition of an aminoglycoside is recommended if ampicillin is used as an alternative choice (Table 26.10).[26,90] Anaerobic bacilli generally are susceptible to penicillin, but infection caused by resistant *Bacteroides fragilis* is treated best by combinations including metronidazole, piperacillin-tazobactam, or meropenem.

Survival rates of only 10% to 20% in patients with fungal endocarditis are related to the poor ability of currently available antifungal agents to sterilize the vegetations. Only rare cures with medical therapy alone have been reported.[480] Most investigators contend that early surgical intervention is mandatory in every patient who has conclusive evidence of intracardiac fungal infection.[520,563,565] Neonates with fungal endocarditis can have an especially high mortality rate.[469] Eradication of fungal prosthetic valve endocarditis has been reported rarely, even when surgery was performed.[188]

Although a prolonged course of antifungal therapy before surgery does not improve the outcome, chemotherapy should be given in conjunction with operative treatment. The drug of choice is usually amphotericin B or liposomal amphotericin. This antibiotic may be either fungistatic or fungicidal, depending on the infecting organism. The optimal dosage of amphotericin B is unknown; total doses of 20 to 50 mg/kg commonly are used. 5-Fluorocytosine[356] may act synergistically with amphotericin B against many strains of fungi, but their roles in fungal endocarditis are unproven. Fluconazole is less effective than is amphotericin B for the prophylaxis or treatment of experimental *Candida* endocarditis,[601] but it has been used successfully in a few patients.[101,572] Some newer antifungal agents, such as caspofungin, have been used successfully to treat fungal endocarditis, but the reported experience in children is limited.[538] The Infectious Diseases Society of America clinical practice guidelines recommend liposomal amphotericin B (3 to 5 mg/kg per day) with or without flucytosine (25 mg/kg every 6 hours) for treatment of *Candida* native valve endocarditis.[410] Echinocandins are alternatives. Step-down therapy to fluconazole should be considered for stable patients with susceptible *Candida* isolates and with negative blood cultures.

Treatment of culture-negative endocarditis is problematic.[32] In general, the same criteria used to choose empiric therapy for infective endocarditis can be followed. Antibiotics usually are continued for 6 weeks, and ongoing surveillance for an etiologic agent must be performed. The suggested regimens for treating culture-negative endocarditis in children in the AHA 2015 Pediatric guidelines are shown in Table 26.11. In 52 adults with culture-negative endocarditis, survival correlated with the initial clinical response to antibiotics; most deaths were caused by systemic emboli or congestive heart failure.[425]

Surgery has become a valuable adjunct to medical therapy in the management of infective endocarditis.[37,407,424,432,476] The general trend has been for surgical intervention to be undertaken earlier and more frequently to prevent complications of endocarditis and lower mortality.[231,465,607] Several echocardiographic findings suggest a possible need for surgical intervention (Box 26.3).[36,159] Among the generally accepted indications for surgical intervention during active endocarditis are (1) refractory congestive heart failure,[361,552,595] (2) uncontrolled infection,[336] (3) more than one serious embolic episode, (4) fungal endocarditis, (5) most cases of prosthetic valve endocarditis,[7,114,141,386,474,608] and (6) local suppurative complications including perivalvular or myocardial abscess with conduction system abnormalities.[51,271,387,461,500,534,604] Surgical intervention should also be considered urgently for any child with acute endocarditis caused by *S. aureus.*[501] The usual indication for surgical intervention is congestive heart failure in left-sided lesions and persistent infection in right-sided disease.[116,574] Among children with endocarditis after cardiac surgery, repair or takedown of infected graft material commonly is the reason for surgery.[92,403] Recent studies have demonstrated that preservation of the child's native valve is frequently possible despite advanced clinical disease.[118,221,220,266] In general, operative mortality is low even if surgery is performed during the active infection.[381,396] The hemodynamic status of the patient, rather than the activity of the infection, is the critical factor in determining the timing of cardiac surgery or valve replacement.[3,267] The aortic valve is the site most often requiring surgical intervention.[275,434,556] Treatment with recombinant tissue plasminogen activator has been used successfully in some cases of endocarditis when surgery could not be performed safely.[202,310]

PREVENTION

Accepted medical practice has been to give prophylactic antibiotics to susceptible patients in an attempt to prevent infective endocarditis.[129,275,507] The rationale for such treatment is based on studies indicating that antibiotics can reduce the incidence of bacteremia after various

TABLE 26.12 Endocarditis Prophylaxis Regimens for a Dental Procedure to Be Considered in Children With High-Risk Conditions

Situation	Agent	REGIMEN: SINGLE DOSE 30 TO 60 min BEFORE PROCEDURE	
		Adults	**Children**
Oral	Amoxicillin	2 g	50 mg/kg
Unable to take oral	Ampicillin *or*	2 g IM or IV	50 mg/kg IM or IV
	Cefazolin *or* ceftriaxone	1 g IM or IV	50 mg/kg IM or IV
Allergic to oral penicillins	Cephalexin[a] *or*	2 g	50 mg/kg
	Clindamycin *or*	600 mg	20 mg/kg
	Azithromycin *or* clarithromycin	500 mg	15 mg/kg
Allergic to penicillins and unable to take oral	Cefazolin *or* ceftriaxone[a] *or*	1 g IM or IV	50 mg/kg IM or IV
	Clindamycin	600 mg IM or IV	20 mg/kg IM or IV

IM, Intramuscularly; *IV,* intravenously.
[a]Cephalosporins not to be used in an individual with a history of anaphylaxis, angioedema, or urticaria with penicillins.
From Wilson W, Taubert KA, Gewitz M, et al. Prevention of infective endocarditis: guidelines from the American Heart Association. *Circulation.* 2007;116:1736–54.

BOX 26.3 Echocardiographic Features Suggesting a Possible Need for Surgical Intervention in Endocarditis

Vegetation

Persistent vegetation after systemic embolization
Anterior mitral valve leaflet vegetation, particularly >10 mm
Embolic event during first 2 weeks of therapy
Increase in vegetation size after 4 weeks of therapy

Valvular Dysfunction

Acute aortic or mitral insufficiency with signs of ventricular failure
Heart failure unresponsive to medical therapy
Valve perforation or rupture

Perivalvular Extension

Valvular dehiscence, rupture, or fistula
New heart block
Large abscess or extension of abscess

Data from Bayer A., Bolger A, Taubert K, et al. Diagnosis and management of infective endocarditis and its complications. *Circulation.* 1998;98:2936–48; and Ferrieri P, Gewitz MH, Gerber MA, et al. Unique features of infective endocarditis in children. *Pediatrics.* 2002;109:931–43.

BOX 26.4 Heart Conditions With the Highest Risk for Adverse Outcome From Endocarditis for Which Prophylaxis With Dental Procedures Can Be Considered

Prosthetic heart valve
Previous infective endocarditis
Congenital heart disease

- Unrepaired cyanotic congenital heart disease, including palliative shunts and conduits
- Completely repaired congenital heart defect with prosthetic material or device, whether placed by surgery or catheter, during the first 6 months after the procedure
- Repaired congenital heart disease with residual defects at or adjacent to the site of a prosthetic patch or device

Cardiac transplantation recipients who develop cardiac valvulopathy

From Wilson W, Taubert KA, Gewitz M, et al. Prevention of infective endocarditis: guidelines from the American Heart Association. *Circulation.* 2007;116:1736–54.

procedures in humans[143] and can prevent experimental endocarditis in animals.[421] However, no controlled trials have documented the efficacy of endocarditis prophylaxis in humans.[570] Prevention of bacterial infection is most likely to be successful and cost effective when a single antibiotic is directed against a single pathogen and when the disease occurs with high frequency in the absence of prophylaxis. Prevention of endocarditis has not met these ideals because various drugs have been used against numerous organisms, and the disease rarely occurs even if prophylaxis is not given.[127] Fewer than 10% of all endocarditis cases can be attributed to bacteremia caused by previous medical, surgical, or dental procedures.[568] Many cases of prophylaxis failure have been reported,[132] but only 12% of such patients received antibiotic regimens recommended by the American Heart Association. For reasons that are not clear, mitral valve prolapse was the condition associated most frequently with failure of prophylaxis.

The most common errors in attempted prevention of endocarditis included inadequate medical histories taken by dentists and other health care professionals to identify high-risk patients, initiation of prophylactic antibiotics too early, continuation of preventive therapy too long, the use of low-dose antibiotics, lack of prophylaxis for minor dental procedures, and confusion between prevention of rheumatic fever and prevention of infective endocarditis.[162,208,214] Several studies have shown that adult patients at risk for development of infective endocarditis often have inadequate knowledge of their cardiac lesion, endocarditis, and recommended prophylaxis.[78,288,569] Several studies demonstrated that the parents of children with heart defects have a low level of knowledge about the importance of good oral health in preventing endocarditis.[27,102,206,395,442] Another study cast doubt on the cost-effectiveness of endocarditis prophylaxis for urinary catheterization in children.[77]

The American Heart Association published new and radically different guidelines for the prevention of infective endocarditis in 2007.[598] These new guidelines eliminated many of the procedures for which prophylaxis previously was recommended.[104] It is now recommended that prophylaxis be undertaken for all dental procedures that involve manipulation of gingival tissue or the periapical region of teeth or perforation of the oral mucosa. Prophylaxis also can be considered for procedures on the respiratory tract or infected skin, skin structures, or musculoskeletal tissue. Prophylaxis no longer is recommended for gastrointestinal or genitourinary tract procedures. In addition, the heart lesions for which prophylaxis is to be considered has been reduced to only those with the highest risk for adverse outcome of endocarditis (Box 26.4).[598] Finally, the specific regimens for prophylaxis have been changed and simplified to encourage more judicious use (Table 26.12). Although some experts have expressed doubt about the validity of these newer recommendations,[502] there is no evidence that the release of these guidelines has been associated with a significant change in admissions for infective endocarditis.[411]

Immunization against bacteria that commonly cause endocarditis (e.g., viridans streptococci) has been proposed, but this approach remains a theoretical possibility.[20]

NEW REFERENCES SINCE THE SEVENTH EDITION

9. Amit U, Porat N, Basmaci R, et al. Genotyping of invasive *Kingella kingae* isolates reveals predominant clones and associations with specific clinical syndromes. *Clin Infect Dis*. 2012;55:1074-1079.
29. Baltimore RS, Gewitz M, Baddour LM, et al. Infective endocarditis in childhood: 2015 update. A scientific statement from the American Heart Association. *Circulation*. 2015;132:1487-1515.
33. Baron EJ, Scott JD, Tompkins LS. Prolonged incubation and extensive subculturing do not increase recovery of clinically significant microorganisms from standard automated blood cultures. *Clin Infect Dis*. 2005;41:1677-1680.
48. Bhat DP, Nagaraju L, Asmar BI, et al. Abiotrophia endocarditis in children with no underlying heart disease: a rare but a virulent organism. *Congenit Heart Dis*. 2014;9:E116-E120.
164. Fortún J, Centella T, Martín-Dávila P, et al. Infective endocarditis in congenital heart disease: a frequent community-acquired complication. *Infection*. 2013;41:167-174.
165. Foster MA, Walls M. High rates of complications following *Kingella kingae* infective endocarditis in children. *Pediatr Infect Dis J*. 2014;33:785-786.
203. Gupta S, Sakhuja A, McGrath E, et al. Pediatric infective endocarditis in the United States over the past decade: trends and outcome. Presented at the annual meeting of the Pediatric Academic Societies April 25, 2015, San Diego, CA. (Abstract 1549.363).
342. Marom D, Ashkenazi S, Samra Z, et al. Infective endocarditis in previously healthy children with structurally normal hearts. *Pediatr Cardiol*. 2013;34:1415-1421.
352. McElhinney DB, Benson LN, Eicken A, et al. Infective endocarditis after transcatheter pulmonary valve replacement using the Melody Valve. Combined results of 3 prospective North American and European Studies. *Circ Cardiovasc Inter*. 2013;6:292-300.
408. Palraj BR, Baddour LM, Hess EP, et al. Predicting risk of endocarditis using a clinical tool (PREDICT): scoring system to guide use of echocardiography in the management of *Staphylococcus aureus* bacteremia. *Clin Infect Dis*. 2015;61:18-28.
410. Pappas PG, Kauffman CA, Andes D, et al. Clinical practice guidelines for the management of candidiasis: 2016 update by the Infectious Diseases Society of America. *Clin Infect Dis*. 2016;62:e1-e50.
463. Rosenthal LB, Jeja KN, Levasseur SM, et al. The changing epidemiology of pediatric endocarditis at a children's hospital over seven decades. *Pediatr Cardiol*. 2010;31:813-820.
468. Rushani D, Kaufman JS, Ionescu-Ittu R, et al. Infective endocarditis in children with congenital heart disease: cumulative incidence and predictors. *Circulation*. 2013;128:1412-1419.
469. Russell HM, Johnson SL, Wurlitzer KC, et al. Outcomes of surgical therapy for infective endocarditis in a pediatric population; a 21-year review. *Ann Thorac Surg*. 2013;96:171-175.
501. Shamszad P, Khan MS, Rossano JW, et al. Early surgical therapy of infective endocarditis in children: a 15-year experience. *J Thorac Cardiovac Surg*. 2013;146:506-511.
506. Shrestha NK, Ledtke CS, Wang H, et al. Heart valve culture and sequencing to identify the infective endocarditis pathogen in surgically treated patients. *Ann Thorac Surg*. 2015;99:33-37.
561. Turcotte RF, Brozovich A, Corda R, et al. Health care-associated infections in children after cardiac surgery. *Pediatr Cardiol*. 2014;35:1448-1455.
564. Ugaki S, Rutledge J, Al Aklabi M, et al. An increased incidence of conduit endocarditis in patients receiving bovine jugular vein grafts compared to cryopreserved homograft for right ventricular outflow reconstruction. *Ann Thorac Surg*. 2015;99:140-147.
575. Villafañe J, Baker GH, Austin EH III, et al. Melody valve bacterial endocarditis: experience in four pediatric patients and a review of the literature. *Catheter Cardiovasc Inter*. 2014;84:212-218.
585. Weidman DR, Al-Hashami H, Morris SK. Two cases and a review of *Streptococcus pyogenes* endocarditis in children. *BMC Pediatr*. 2014;14:227.

The full reference list for this chapter is available at ExpertConsult.com.

27 Infectious Pericarditis

Sheldon L. Kaplan

Purulent pericarditis generally refers to bacterial infection of the pericardium. Inflammation of the pericardium may result from numerous nonbacterial microorganisms, however, or may occur with a variety of noninfectious illnesses (Box 27.1). Regardless of the cause of pericarditis, the responses of the pericardium are limited to acute inflammation, effusion with or without tamponade, and fibrosis with or without constriction.[18] Because untreated purulent pericarditis is rapidly fatal, suspecting the disease early and approaching the diagnosis aggressively are important.

ANATOMY AND FUNCTION

The pericardium is composed of two loosely approximated layers: visceral and parietal. The visceral pericardium is composed of mesothelial tissue, which closely follows the contour of the heart and extends for a short distance beyond the atria and ventricles to the great vessels. The outer parietal pericardium is a more fibrous structure, composed of layers of collagen interlaced with elastic fibers. The pericardial sac is attached to the diaphragm below; to the sternum in front; and to the thoracic vertebrae, esophagus, and aorta posteriorly. It is surrounded by the lungs on either side and is related closely to the main bronchi and the mediastinal lymph nodes. The phrenic and vagus nerves supply a network of pain fibers to the parietal pericardium.

The dynamics of the pericardial fluid are poorly understood. The pericardial membrane is active in the transfer of water, electrolytes, and small molecules. Molecules of large molecular weight are absorbed poorly from the pericardial space because lymphatic channels are sparse, and drainage must occur primarily through the epicardial capillaries.[70]

Ainger[1] summarized the function of the pericardium as follows: prevention of overdistention of the heart, protection of the heart from infection and adhesions, maintenance of the heart within a fixed geometric position within the chest, and regulation of the interaction between the stroke volumes of the two ventricles.

BACTERIAL PERICARDITIS

Population and Incidence

Although purulent pericarditis is not a common infection in pediatric patients, it is an important one to recognize because of its life-threatening nature. In an extensive early review of the literature on purulent pericarditis, half of 425 cases occurred in children younger than 13 years of age.[66] In a review of 162 reported children with pericarditis from 1950 to 1977, 67% of the children were 48 months old or younger.[28] From 1962 to 1974, 67 cases were recognized at St. Louis Children's Hospital (Table 27.1).[89] During this 12-year period, pericardial disease of all causes occurred in approximately 1 of every 850 hospital admissions. Twelve (18%) of these children had purulent pericarditis.

Most cases in younger children are infectious. Acute pericarditis was found in 20 children between 1987 and 1997 in a hospital in Iran.[79] The causes of pericarditis were bacterial in eight (40%), collagen vascular disease in six (30%), viral in four (20%), and secondary to mediastinal

BOX 27.1 Causes of Pericarditis

Idiopathic
Benign
Recurrent

Infectious
Purulent
Bacterial: *Staphylococcus aureus, Haemophilus influenzae,* streptococci, *Neisseria meningitidis, Streptococcus pneumoniae,* anaerobes, *Francisella tularensis, Salmonella,* enteric bacilli, *Pseudomonas, Listeria, Neisseria gonorrhoeae, Actinomyces, Nocardia*
Tuberculosis
Fungal: *Histoplasma, Coccidioides, Aspergillus, Candida, Blastomyces, Cryptococcus*

Viral
Coxsackieviruses B
Other: influenza A and B, mumps, echoviruses, adenoviruses, Epstein-Barr virus, hepatitis, measles, influenza, human immunodeficiency virus, parvovirus B19, cytomegalovirus

Other
Rickettsial: typhus, Q fever
Mycoplasmal: *Mycoplasma pneumoniae*
Parasitic: *Entamoeba histolytica, Echinococcus*
Spirochetal: syphilis, leptospirosis
Chlamydial: psittacosis
Protozoal: toxoplasmosis

Noninfectious
Postpericardiotomy syndrome
Kawasaki disease
Rheumatic fever
Connective tissue disorders: juvenile rheumatoid arthritis, systemic lupus erythematosus, dermatomyositis, periarteritis nodosa
Trauma: blunt or penetrating
Metabolic: uremia, myxedema
Hypersensitivity: serum sickness, pulmonary infiltrates with eosinophilia, Stevens-Johnson syndrome, drugs (hydralazine, procainamide, chemotherapy)
Neoplasm: leukemia, metastatic
After irradiation

mass invasion in two (10%). In another series from Turkey, 18 children with purulent pericarditis were encountered from 1990 to 2000.[10] At the Boston Children's Hospital, fewer than 10 patients seen among more than 1700 patients in consultation by the pediatric cardiologists had pericarditis during the period July 1, 2001, to June 30, 2002.[33] Over a 21-year period, 31 children with an inflammatory large pericardial effusion requiring drainage were admitted to one tertiary care children's hospital; 12 of the effusions were caused by bacterial infections.[68] Although rare, purulent pericarditis also can occur in neonates.[53] In most series, a marked male predominance has been noted.

Etiology

Primary purulent pericarditis is a rare disease; it accounted for only seven of 50 cases of pericarditis reported by Gersony and McCracken.[34] The disease is associated most often with infection from another site, with hematogenous or direct spread to the pericardium. Feldman[28] reviewed all cases of bacterial pericarditis reported in the English language literature from 1950 to 1977. Bacteria were isolated in 146 (90%) of 162 cases. No other infection was found in 10 patients. The most common concomitant site involved was the lung, especially for *Staphylococcus aureus, Haemophilus influenzae,* and *Streptococcus pneumoniae.* When septic arthritis, osteomyelitis, or skin infections were found, *S. aureus* usually was the cause of pericarditis. *Neisseria meningitidis* and *H. influenzae* most often were responsible for concomitant meningitis and pericarditis.

TABLE 27.1 Pericarditis in Children, 1962–74 (St. Louis Children's Hospital)[a]

Etiology	No. Patients
Unknown	28
Purulent	12
Juvenile rheumatoid arthritis	9
Acute rheumatic fever	8
Uremia	5
Viral	2
Blunt chest trauma	2
Dermatomyositis	1

[a]Patients with postpericardiotomy pericarditis and patients with small exclusions at autopsy were excluded from consideration.
From Strauss AW, Santa-Maria M, Goldring D. Constrictive pericarditis in children. *Am J Dis Child.* 1975;129:822–6.

Before the introduction of antibiotics, pneumococcal and streptococcal organisms were the most frequent causes of purulent pericarditis in children. Most cases were associated with pulmonary infections. Nearly half of patients with streptococcal pericarditis had associated postinfluenzal pneumonia. Hemolytic streptococci were isolated most often; 10% were nonhemolytic streptococci, and 5% were viridans streptococci. Kauffman and colleagues[56] reviewed 113 cases of pneumococcal pericarditis reported since 1900. Preceding pneumonia was present in 93%, and empyema was present in 66%. Pericarditis was thought to be a late event resulting from delay in administering appropriate therapy for pneumonia.

S. aureus is the organism most commonly responsible for purulent pericarditis in children.[28,34,44,79] Most cases are the result of hematogenous seeding of the pericardium from staphylococcal pneumonia with empyema, acute osteomyelitis, or soft tissue abscesses. Among 117 children with *S. aureus* pneumonia at Texas Children's Hospital, 13 children had an echocardiogram; one had a large pericardial effusion.[14] Occasionally, the pericardium is infected during the course of staphylococcal endocarditis. *S. aureus* is the most frequently recovered organism when purulent pericarditis develops within 3 months after the patient has undergone open heart surgery. The clinical course of acute staphylococcal pericarditis is dominated by severe toxemia. In addition to the necrotizing infection produced by *S. aureus,* the organism may release exotoxins, which produce shock and contribute to the high mortality. Community-associated methicillin-resistant *S. aureus* isolates have been recovered from some patients with acute pericarditis.[47,64]

S. aureus was isolated from 73% of infants who died of purulent pericarditis in the series reported by Gersony and McCracken.[34] It was responsible for 50% of cases in children 1 to 4 years old in the review by Feldman.[28] In seven patients younger than 1 month of age, *S. aureus* was isolated from four. This finding is corroborated in literature from other countries.[19,50,79] Thebaud and colleagues[93] reported 19 patients with purulent pericarditis in a children's hospital in Paris between 1979 and 1994. The mean age of the children was 3 years (range, 3 months to 10 years). The organisms isolated were *S. aureus* (three cases), *H. influenzae* (four cases), group A streptococci (three cases), *S. pneumoniae* (three cases), and *N. meningitidis* (one case). Concomitant infections included pneumonia (six cases), osteomyelitis (three cases), cellulitis (one case), and sinusitis (one case). In the series from Turkey, *S. aureus* was isolated from five patients, and *S. pneumoniae* was isolated from one patient.[10] *S. aureus* pericarditis as a complication of varicella has been reported in several children.[8] *S. aureus* has also caused pericarditis associated with disseminated infection in a child with IRAK-4 deficiency.[17]

In the prevaccine era, the second most frequently encountered organism was *H. influenzae* type b.[7] It was responsible for 22% (35 of 163) of the cases in Feldman's review.[28] A single site of coexisting infection, the lung, was identified in 16 of the 35 cases. Meningitis as a single other site of infection was found in five of 35 patients, and multiple involvement was found in seven of 35. Echeverria and colleagues[24] summarized 33 cases from the literature. Pulmonary infiltrates and empyema were seen in 64% of patients. In countries where the *H. influenzae* type b conjugate vaccine is administered to infants routinely, this organism has been eliminated as a cause of pericarditis.

Pneumococcal, streptococcal, and meningococcal pericarditis have diminished in frequency since the introduction of penicillin.[6] Go and coworkers[35] summarized the 15 reported cases of pneumococcal pericarditis from 1980 to 1998. One was a child. Only four cases did not have an underlying risk factor. In a surveillance study of invasive pneumococcal infections in eight pediatric hospitals, only three cases of pericarditis have been observed in more than 2500 cases of systemic pneumococcal infection during the 6-year period of 1993 through 1999.[54] Nevertheless, *S. pneumoniae* remains an important, although rare, cause of acute bacterial pericarditis.[27] The routine administration of the pneumococcal conjugate vaccine to young children has likely resulted in *S. pneumoniae* being an even less common cause of acute pericarditis.

Pericardial involvement occurs in approximately 5% of young adults with meningococcemia.[21] The clinical course generally is milder than that observed with other types of purulent pericarditis. Pericardial involvement rarely is detected at the time of hospital admission. Pericarditis became apparent by the third day in 13 of 17 patients reported by Dixon and Sanford.[21] In some patients, it did not occur until late in the course of therapy. In a multicenter study involving 159 children with meningococcal infections in children from 2001 through 2005, pericarditis was not encountered.[55] Whether this late-onset pericardial effusion is a part of the meningococcal infection or is related to immune complexes is unclear.[21,73,84] Primary meningococcal pericarditis that occurs without clinical evidence of meningococcemia, meningitis, or any other focal infection has been reported in 16 patients, including six children 18 years old or younger (range, 2 to 18 years).[3] Meningococcal serogroup C was identified in 11 (79%) of 14 cases for which the serogroup was known. Cardiac tamponade developed in 88% of the patients. Pericarditis also has been reported in two children with W135 meningococcal infection.[25]

Occasionally, other microorganisms cause acute purulent pericarditis. Feldman[28] reported that 11 (8%) of 146 cases of pericarditis in children were caused by *Pseudomonas aeruginosa. P. aeruginosa* caused pericarditis in an immunocompetent adult with cystic fibrosis.[2] Pericarditis can occur with pneumonic tularemia, salmonellosis, sepsis from enteric bacilli, listeriosis, and disseminated gonococcal disease.[6] Anaerobic bacteria should be suspected when pericarditis develops in association with lung abscess, intraabdominal infection including ruptured appendicitis,[91] or a penetrating wound. Callanan and colleagues[12] reported the rapid development of constrictive pericarditis after purulent pericarditis caused by anaerobic streptococcal infection. The child had a history of blunt trauma to the chest with no evidence of a penetrating wound 3 weeks before cardiac tamponade developed. The incidence of anaerobic infection may be underestimated because of improper handling of specimens for culture. Prolonged symptoms related to pericarditis can be associated with *Mycoplasma pneumoniae* infection.[26]

Mycobacterium tuberculosis, previously a common cause of acute pericarditis in the United States,[5] now is responsible more often for chronic pericardial disease. This infection is a complication of miliary tuberculosis and rarely a primary infection. In the series of 2500 children with tuberculosis reported by Lincoln and Savell,[62] pericarditis was diagnosed in 0.4% and found at necropsy in 5% of patients. A review of 100 cases of tuberculous pericarditis in South Africa by Desai[20] revealed a marked male predominance (72%). The duration of symptoms, consisting of cough and peripheral edema, in most patients was 0 to 120 days. Most patients were febrile and had congestive heart failure. Generalized lymphadenopathy occurred in nearly 30% of patients, pulsus paradoxus occurred in 50%, and a friction rub was audible in 25%. Of the 52 patients who had pericardiocentesis, 40% yielded fluid, but none was positive for acid-fast bacilli. Pericardial effusion was shown in 82 patients, 16 of whom died of tamponade and another 16 of whom developed constricting pericarditis.

The four stages of tuberculous pericarditis have been described as dry, effusive, absorptive, and constrictive.[75] Granulomas usually are found in the dry stage and heal with no sequelae. The effusive stage occurs commonly with tuberculous lymphadenitis, and 15 to 200 mL of fluid usually accumulates in the pericardial space. The absorptive stage is characterized by thickening of the pericardium with fibrin deposition. Further fibrin deposition and calcification occur during the constrictive phase. The disease may progress through all stages or remain in one stage.

Latent infection in the mediastinal lymph nodes with spread directly into the pericardium is thought to be the mode of involvement with *M. tuberculosis.*[75] The lymph nodes at the tracheal bifurcation often are the source.

Histoplasma pericarditis generally occurs with pulmonary, rather than disseminated, disease.[77] Coccidioidomycosis[67] also may cause pericardial disease. *Aspergillus* and *Candida* are more serious considerations in patients who are immunosuppressed, have serious burns, or are receiving long-term, broad-spectrum antibiotics after undergoing cardiac surgery.[81]

Finally, several parasites such as *Trypanosoma cruzi* and *Toxoplasma gondii* can attack the pericardium.[42]

Pathology and Pathogenesis

Pericarditis begins with fine deposits of fibrin adjacent to the great vessels; it causes the pericardial membrane to lose its smoothness and translucency. Numerous granulocytes may extend into the myocardium.[37]

Bacterial pericarditis most commonly results from direct extension of infection from involved lung and pleura. Pulmonary infections may spread to the pericardium through the bronchial circulation.[41] Pericarditis also can develop through hematogenous dissemination from infection elsewhere, and it also may be the result of an immunologically induced response to a primary infection.

As pericardial fluid accumulates, intrapericardial pressure increases. The rate of increase is a function of the speed of accumulation and the compliance of the pericardium. With slow accumulation of fluid, large volumes can be accommodated because of the gradual expansion of the parietal pericardium. As the compliance of the pericardium reaches its maximum, however, further accumulation of even small volumes of fluid results in an abrupt increase in intrapericardial pressure. If pericardial fluid accumulates at a rapid rate, marked elevation in intrapericardial pressure may occur with much smaller volumes of fluid. In a small child, 100 mL can cause severe tamponade, whereas 3 L may accumulate slowly in an older child and not result in tamponade.[1]

The most significant hemodynamic effect of pericardial effusion is restriction of ventricular filling. Ventricular end-diastolic, atrial, and venous pressures increase on the right and left sides of the heart equally. When restriction of ventricular filling becomes more pronounced, the ventricular stroke volume and cardiac output decrease. In an attempt to maintain cardiac output, tachycardia and peripheral vasoconstriction occur. Systemic arterial blood pressure and pulse pressure are reduced markedly. Tamponade occurs when these compensatory mechanisms fail to maintain adequate cardiac output.

Clinical Manifestations

A diagnosis of purulent pericarditis should be suspected in any patient with septicemia who develops cardiomegaly. The classic signs and symptoms of pericarditis are precordial pain, pericardial friction rub, evidence of cardiac fluid, and muffled heart sounds.[15] Chest pain is not a common symptom, especially in small children; the reported rates vary from 15% to 80%.[4,6,35,45,73,77,96] However, in one study focusing on 22 children (aged 6 to 17 years old) who presented to an emergency center and ultimately were found to have acute pericarditis, 95% had chest pain.[78] Acute abdominal symptoms may be the presenting complaints of some children.[22]

The most common symptoms and signs of pericarditis are fever, tachypnea, and tachycardia, which also are presenting features of

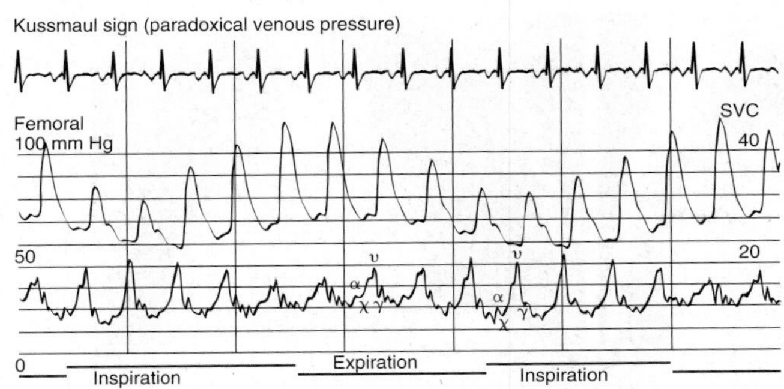

FIG. 27.1 Simultaneous recording of right atrial and femoral artery pressures. Notice the increased V wave and exaggerated decrease in the femoral artery pulse with inspiration.

associated systemic infection. If the cardiac shadow is radiographically enlarged, with or without a friction rub, and the tachypnea and tachycardia are out of proportion to the fever, myocardial dysfunction or pericarditis should be suspected.

An evanescent or ubiquitous rub may be detected. The typical sound of a rub is that of a high-frequency murmur,[76] which may have a to-and-fro or triphasic pattern but may not have any correlation with the cardiac cycle.[29] Frequently the rub is heard better with the patient leaning forward or kneeling. A rub may be differentiated from a murmur by pressing the diaphragm of the stethoscope firmly against the chest wall; this pressure amplifies the rub, and the typical scratchy quality becomes more apparent as the examiner opposes the visceral and parietal pericardium by compression of the chest. Rubs have been known to increase with inspiration.[87] Although a rub is less likely to be heard in the presence of a large effusion, it still may exist.[29] The heart sounds usually are muffled, and the palpable ventricular impulse generally is diminished. Both findings may be present in congestive heart failure, but they may be absent with tamponade.

Cardiac tamponade may be an early complication of pericarditis associated with a systemic infection. Cardiac tamponade means that there is compression of the heart by a tense pericardial sac, usually full of fluid, resulting in a decrease in venous return to the cardiac chambers and a decrease in cardiac output. During inspiration, the intrathoracic pressure decreases and venous return to the venae cavae increases. The tense pericardial sac limits the amount of blood that can enter the right atrium because of diastolic compression; a paradoxical increase in jugular venous pressure occurs during inspiration (i.e., Kussmaul sign) (Fig. 27.1).[58]

During inspiration, a small decrease in systolic blood pressure and cardiac output normally occurs and is caused by an increase in pulmonary venous capacitance. It is exaggerated with pericardial tamponade (>10 mm Hg decrease in blood pressure) because of the restricted inflow into the cardiac chambers. This clinical sign has been called *paradoxical pulse*, but it actually is an exaggeration of the normal respiratory cycle (Fig. 27.2).[36]

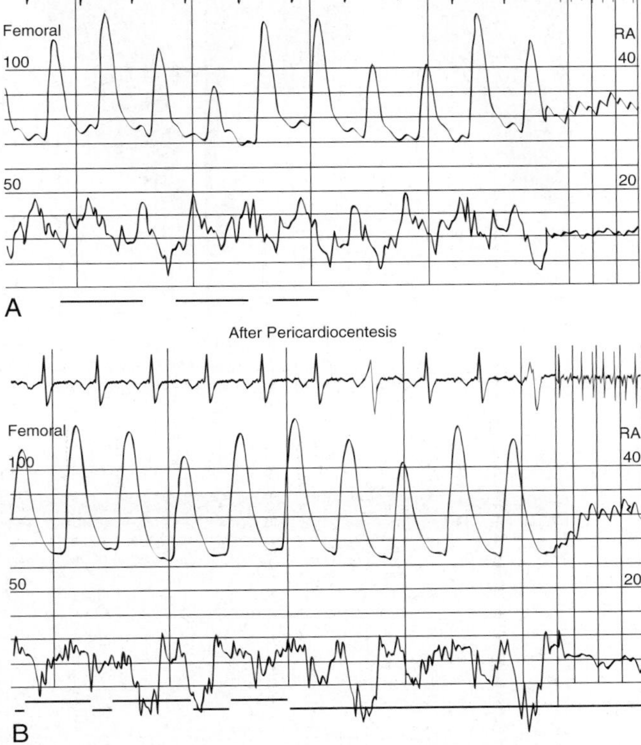

FIG. 27.2 Recordings of femoral artery and right atrial pressures (A) before and (B) after pericardiocentesis. (A) There is an exaggerated decrease in the fall of femoral artery pressure with inspiration and a sustained increase in right atrial pressure. (B) The recording shows a more normal variation of femoral pressure and a lower right atrial pressure.

Diagnosis

The radiographic appearance of a rapidly increasing cardiothoracic ratio without increasing pulmonary vascular markings is more suggestive of pericardial effusion than of congestive heart failure caused by myocardial dysfunction (Fig. 27.3). Fluoroscopy alone generally is of little value; myocardial dysfunction and pericarditis can impair cardiac contractility.

The size of the pericardial shadow does not indicate the severity of hemodynamic effects. It is a function of the rapidity of accumulation and the volume of pericardial fluid. When acute infection results in sudden cardiac tamponade, the heart size may be normal. A large, globular heart shadow with no evidence of increased pulmonary vasculature, particularly in a patient who has signs of right-sided heart failure, is strong evidence for pericardial disease. The lack of pulmonary overcirculation helps to distinguish this condition from myocarditis; however, determining whether pulmonary infiltrates also exist may be difficult.

A plain lateral chest radiograph may show findings consistent with a pericardial effusion.[59] Separation of more than 2 mm between the anterior mediastinal and subepithelial "fat stripes" suggests an effusion. Obliteration of the retrosternal space without evidence of thymic or right ventricular enlargement also indicates pericarditis.

The extent of electrocardiographic abnormalities may be explained by the amount of pericardial effusion and the presence of superficial myocardial injury or myocarditis. Pericardial effusion gives rise to low-voltage QRS complexes as a result of the damping effect of pericardial fluid between the chest wall and the myocardium. Accumulation of fluid and fibrin under pressure also may produce an injury pattern manifested by ST-segment deviation. More than 90% of patients have elevation of the ST segment, which occurs most frequently in leads I, II, V_5, and V_6. Widespread T-wave inversion indicative of epicarditis may be seen in the same leads in which ST-segment elevation occurs.

Spodick[86] described four stages of electrocardiographic changes in acute pericarditis. In stage I, ST-segment elevation is pronounced and the PR segment may be depressed. In stage II, the ST segment begins to return to the isoelectric line, the amplitude of the T wave diminishes, and the PR segment is depressed. By stage III, the ST segment has returned to the isoelectric line, and the T-wave inversion occurs. An incompletely inverted T wave (i.e., a diphasic wave or an upright T wave with a notched summit) sometimes is observed. In stage IV, these changes may resolve completely. T-wave abnormalities may persist for life, however, and do not indicate active disease.

Electrical alternans is seen in a large pericardial effusion. Electrical alternans refers to the alternation in electric amplitude of the T wave and the QRS complex with each cardiac cycle. It is thought to result from the rotational and pendular motion of the heart suspended in pericardial fluid.

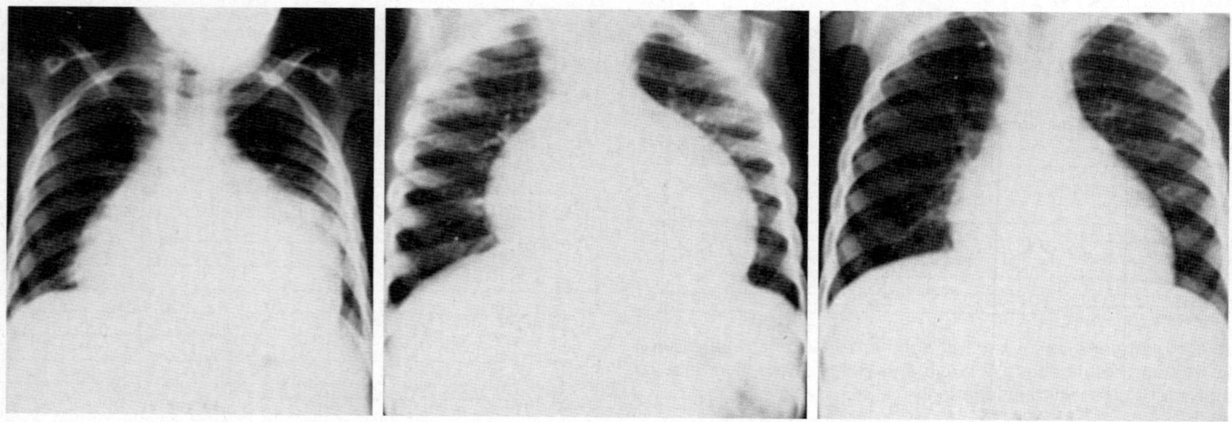

FIG. 27.3 In this patient with pericarditis, the first two radiographs show an enlarged cardiac shadow without an increase in pulmonary vascular markings. The third radiograph shows a marked decrease in apparent heart size after pericardiocentesis.

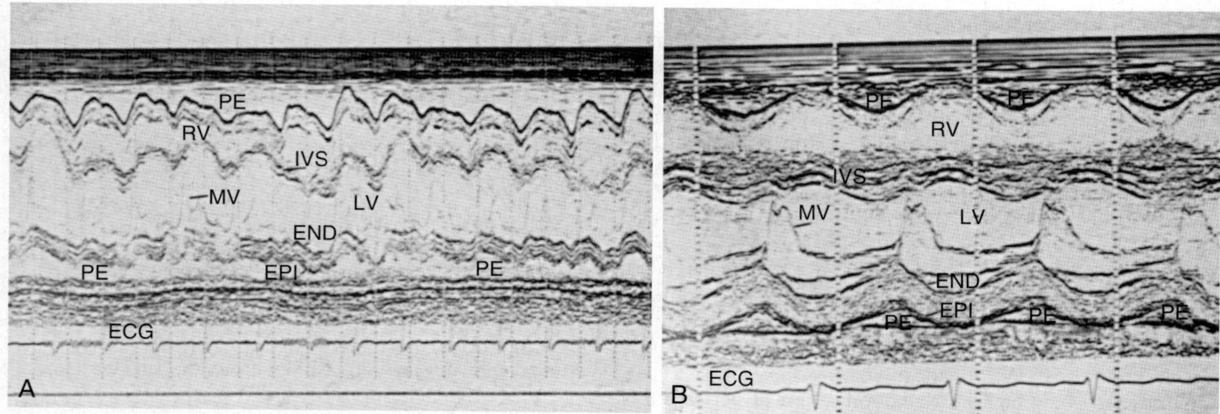

FIG. 27.4 Serial echocardiograms of a child (A) before pericardiocentesis and (B) after pericardiocentesis. (A) Note the large effusion anteriorly and posteriorly with the "swinging" movement of the septum and anterior and posterior walls. (B) The heart movement is normal, and there remains only a small effusion anteriorly and posteriorly. *ECG,* Electrocardiogram; *END,* endocardium; *EPI,* epicardium; *IVS,* interventricular septum; *LV,* left ventricle; *MV,* mitral valve; *PE,* pericardial effusion; *RV,* right ventricle.

Deviations from classic patterns occasionally occur, and single electrocardiographic changes are common findings. All 12 children reported by Okoroma and colleagues[74] had ST-segment elevation, whereas only 3 had concomitant low voltage. Dysrhythmias with pericarditis are unusual in the absence of coexisting heart disease.[88]

M-mode echocardiography is the most sensitive method for diagnosing significant pericardial effusion (Fig. 27.4).[40,45] With a small to moderate effusion, only a "fluid space" is seen posteriorly (Fig. 27.4B). With a larger effusion, fluid is seen anteriorly and posteriorly, and the septal motion becomes grossly abnormal. The heart may give the appearance of freely swinging (Fig. 27.4A). Newer echocardiographic techniques, such as two-dimensional sector scanning, are not more useful than the conventional M-mode. Pericarditis may be detected uncommonly by echocardiography in children with *S. aureus* bacteremia but without clinical evidence of pericardial or endocardial involvement.[31]

Computed tomography and magnetic resonance imaging of the chest are other modalities used to examine the pericardium.[7] They may help to differentiate a bacterial pericarditis from other conditions involving the pericardium. Occult or unsuspected pericarditis has been discerned with radionuclide techniques in immunocompromised patients and in trauma patients.[39,83]

A pericardial effusion may be diagnosed by noticing a discrepancy between the position of a catheter placed adjacent to the lateral wall of the right atrium and the right cardiac border. An injection of radiopaque contrast material into the right atrium may delineate these findings further. Pressure measurements at the time of cardiac catheterization reveal the elevated right atrial pressure and emphasize further the exaggeration of venous, systemic, and left ventricular pressures imposed by inspiration (see Fig. 27.2). Injection of carbon dioxide or air into the pericardium percutaneously may delineate further the pericardial effusion fluoroscopically and differentiate freely moving fluid from loculated areas (Fig. 27.5).

The diagnosis of purulent pericarditis is established definitively only by direct examination of pericardial fluid. Purulent fluid is characterized by a predominance of polymorphonuclear leukocytes; however, it also may occur early in the course of viral and tuberculous pericarditis. Proper handling of pericardial fluid is crucial to recovery and identification of the etiologic agent, as follows:

1. Fluid should be placed directly into broth capable of supporting aerobic and anaerobic microorganisms. The fluid should be plated directly onto agar media, such as blood agar, chocolate agar, or MacConkey agar.
2. Cultures also should be submitted for identification of *M. tuberculosis,* fungi, and viruses.
3. Several slides should be prepared for immediate examination by Gram stain and stain for acid-fast bacilli. Unstained slides should be stored in case of controversy or the need for special histochemical stains.
4. Antigen detection for *S. pneumoniae* or polymerase chain reaction for other microorganisms may be useful in selected cases, particularly when the patient has received prior antimicrobial therapy.[11,61]

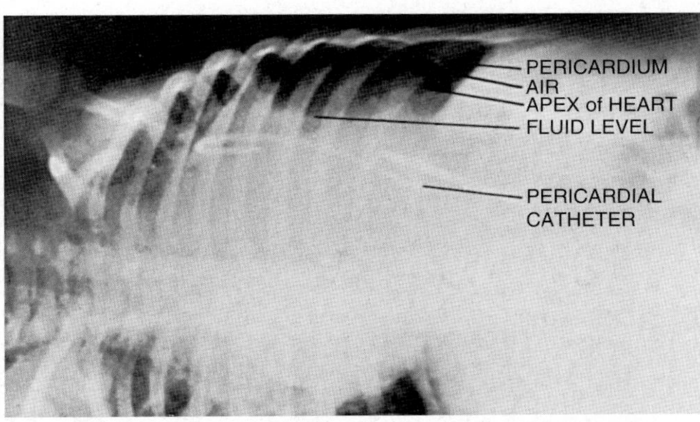

FIG. 27.5 Chest radiograph of a patient lying on the right side with a catheter in the pericardium. Air has been injected through the catheter, outlining the pericardium and fluid within the sac.

The causative microorganism is isolated from blood cultures in many patients. When indicated, cerebrospinal fluid also should be cultured. Because purulent pericarditis often occurs after infections of the lung or pleural space, thoracentesis can reveal the etiologic agent in many cases. Documentation of empyema together with evidence of pericardial disease correlates highly with purulent pericarditis.

Acid-fast bacilli are seen on stained smears of pericardial fluid from 15% to 42% of patients with tuberculous pericarditis.[5] Examination of pericardial biopsy specimens by routine methods and with special stains such as the auramine O can increase the frequency of identification of *M. tuberculosis*.[72] A negative purified protein derivative skin test does not exclude the diagnosis of tuberculous pericarditis.

Grossly bloody pericardial fluid is observed frequently in patients with *Histoplasma* pericarditis, and an aspirate of the effusion reveals a predominance of mononuclear leukocytes. Growth of *H. capsulatum* from pericardial fluid rarely is successful. Showing the typical intracellular yeast forms on special stain of pericardial tissue also is helpful. Elevation of the yeast phase of the complement-fixation titer in pericardial fluid allows one to make a more rapid diagnosis.[77] Detecting the polysaccharide of *H. capsulatum* in urine or other body fluids is a rapid and sensitive means by which to establish the diagnosis of histoplasmosis.

Differential Diagnosis

Any patient with a rapidly increasing heart size in the absence of increasing pulmonary vascular markings should be suspected to have a pericardial effusion. Purulent pericarditis must be differentiated from pericardial effusion caused by collagen diseases, other infectious agents (e.g., viral, tuberculous, rickettsial, protozoan), neoplastic disorders, metabolic disorders, and congestive heart failure.[15] Glycogen storage disease, congenital heart disease, primary myocardial disease, cardiac tumors, and coronary artery aberrations (i.e., anomalous origin from the pulmonary artery, medial wall necrosis, and Kawasaki disease) may be confused with pericardial effusion. Appropriate analysis of pericardial fluid usually permits differentiation of purulent pericarditis from pericarditis caused by other disorders. A high eosinophil count in the pericardial fluid suggests a parasite or a hypereosinophilic syndrome.[85]

Treatment

Purulent pericarditis is a potentially life-threatening illness that requires pericardial decompression and open drainage, appropriate antimicrobial therapy, and intense supportive therapy. Most children with purulent pericarditis require early or emergency drainage of the pericardium for relief of critical tamponade. Although bedside needle pericardiocentesis may be lifesaving or necessary for establishing a rapid diagnosis, deaths related to pericardiocentesis performed by inexperienced physicians can occur. Complications include arrhythmias resulting from myocardial injury, laceration of the coronary arteries leading to hemopericardium and tamponade, and pneumothorax. Ledbetter[60] described a 10-year-old girl with staphylococcal pericarditis who developed an aortic aneurysm after undergoing multiple pericardiocentesis procedures for recurrent tamponade. Ultrasound-guided pericardiocentesis is recommended.

TABLE 27.2 Influence of Pericardial Drainage on Survival in Purulent Pericarditis in Children

Treatment	Survived	Died
Antibiotics alone	5	28
Antibiotics and pericardial drainage	45	10

Data from references 4, 30, 56, and 71.

Decompression and drainage of the pericardium are safest in a controlled environment, such as in an operating room or under fluoroscopy in the catheterization laboratory. If the patient is awake and agitated, premedication may be required.

If pericardiocentesis does not relieve symptoms successfully, and evidence of tamponade continues, immediate surgical drainage is necessary. Multiple attempts may prove unsuccessful and can lead to serious complications. The pus surrounding the heart may be too thick to be aspirated.[69] Surgical creation of a pericardial window with a drain occasionally is necessary for complete removal of fluid, which accumulates rapidly. In preparation for evacuation of the pericardial fluid during tamponade, adequate cardiac output can be maintained by stimulating the heart with pharmacologic agents that cause a chronotropic and an inotropic effect.

Medications that tend to decrease heart rate and intravascular volume are contraindicated because they compromise the patient further.[95] Wyler and colleagues[95] warn against the use of halothane anesthesia because of its known depressant effect on myocardial function.

Purulent pericarditis requires some type of pericardial drainage, but the optimal approach to drainage including the extent of surgery is uncertain.[27,30,31,60,72,85] Some surgeons favor the creation of a pericardial "window"; however, others favor more extensive removal of pericardial tissue. This decision may be influenced by the severity of pericardial inflammation or the presence of bloody pericardial fluid because these conditions have greater potential for producing acute or chronic constriction.

Video-assisted thoracoscopic approaches to managing pericarditis also have been described.[65,68] For selected patients for whom surgery cannot be performed in a timely manner, the instillation of intrapericardial streptokinase or urokinase or other thrombolytic agents has been successful in draining purulent pericarditis and preventing the need for a more extensive surgical procedure.[52]

Antimicrobial therapy alone is insufficient for the successful treatment of purulent pericarditis. The survival of patients with purulent pericarditis is improved significantly when early pericardial drainage is performed (Table 27.2). In the preantibiotic era, draining the pericardium decreased the mortality rate from nearly 100% to 45%.[66] Occasionally patients with meningococcal pericarditis have been managed successfully without pericardial drainage.[18] Fyfe and colleagues[32] described 73 of 79 patients with *H. influenzae* pericarditis seen between 1928 and 1984. The mortality rate before 1960 was 64% (7 of 11 patients), although five of seven deaths were reported before the antibiotic era. From 1960 to 1969, the mortality rate was 36 percent, and from 1970 to 1979, it decreased to 11.5%. From 1980 to 1984, 25 cases with no mortality were reported.

When the etiologic agent cannot be detected rapidly, the initial antibiotic regimen should consist of two or more drugs. Because *S. aureus* is a major pathogen and community-associated methicillin-resistant *S. aureus* isolates are common in almost all areas, a penicillinase-resistant penicillin, such as nafcillin or oxacillin, in a dose of 200 mg/kg per 24 hours (maximum 12 g) plus vancomycin in a dose of 60 mg/kg per day in four divided doses is usually recommended for initial empiric therapy. Vancomycin is also recommended when strains of *S. pneumoniae* resistant to the extended-spectrum cephalosporins are present or when the infection is nosocomially acquired. Cefotaxime 200 to 300 mg/kg per day in three or four divided doses or ceftriaxone 100 mg/kg per day in one or two doses should be administered to provide protection against *S. pneumoniae* (including penicillin-resistant strains), *N. meningitidis*, and *H. influenzae* type b (for children who may be inadequately immunized).

An aminoglycoside antibiotic should be added to the just-mentioned combined drug therapy when purulent pericarditis occurs after cardiac surgery, in association with genitourinary infections, or in the immunocompromised host. The antibiotics selected for empiric therapy for acute pericarditis complicating recent cardiac surgery are influenced by the hospital's antibiogram. For patients who are allergic to penicillin, vancomycin, clindamycin, or cefazolin is substituted for the treatment of susceptible *S. aureus*.

The duration of therapy is empiric and is determined partly by the nature of concomitant infection. Generally after a pathogen is isolated and the antimicrobial susceptibilities are known, the most specific antimicrobial agent is continued intravenously for 3 to 4 weeks. Monitoring the C-reactive protein levels may help in determining the length of treatment.[49]

Using antimicrobial agents to treat tuberculous pericarditis has had a major impact on mortality. Before their use, the mortality rate in the acute phase was 80% to 90%. The other 10% to 20% of patients died of constrictive pericarditis or miliary tuberculosis.[75] The use of three or four drugs, including isoniazid, pyrazinamide, rifampin, and possibly streptomycin, for 9 to 12 months is recommended. The role of corticosteroids in preventing progression to constriction or decreasing mortality is unclear.[23,66,75] In selected cases, pericardiectomy may be indicated to prevent constrictive pericarditis. The reader is referred to Chapter 204 on histoplasmosis for details regarding treatment of pericarditis due to this organism.

As with bacterial pericarditis, open pericardiectomy is crucial for the successful treatment of *Candida* pericarditis.[71,81]

General supportive therapy in the acute stage of infection may include the administration of oxygen, volume expansion to increase ventricular filling pressure, and cardiovascular agents to facilitate systolic emptying. The input of pediatric cardiologists is critical for the optimal management of these patients. Serial electrocardiograms may indicate the presence of occult arrhythmias and alert the physician to the degree of myocardial involvement. The patient must be monitored carefully for signs of reaccumulation of pericardial fluid and for the development of acute constrictive pericarditis. Strauss and colleagues[89] reported this complication in two of 12 children with purulent pericarditis. Acute constriction may develop within weeks of the initial pericardial infection[4,9] and has been reported at 8 days.[80] Constrictive pericarditis may be suspected by increasing jugular and central venous pressure, weight gain, enlarging liver, worsening dyspnea, and decreased urinary output. The persistence of heart failure when the cardiac silhouette is becoming smaller also suggests the development of constrictive pericarditis. Complete pericardiectomy should be performed promptly when constriction is suspected.

Prognosis

Accurate mortality rates are difficult to compute from the literature because of the relative rarity of this infection as well as the nature and severity of any underlying disease. Factors that contribute to mortality are delay in recognition, absence of early surgical drainage, presence of cardiac tamponade, degree of myocardial involvement, etiologic agent (particularly *S. aureus*), and age of the patient. Long-term follow-up of children with purulent pericarditis is recommended. They should be observed carefully for the presence of a constrictive component as a sequela to the acute infection. Most children recover fully, however, and return to normal activity.

VIRAL PERICARDITIS

In 1951, Christian[16] suggested that viral infections were responsible for cases of idiopathic or benign pericarditis. A viral cause has not been substantiated in many patients, however.

Etiology

The principal viruses implicated in pericarditis are the coxsackieviruses.[71,74] Adenoviruses have been recovered less frequently.[51] Associations with varicella,[92,96] cytomegalovirus,[13] smallpox vaccinations, influenza[43] (including H1N1),[57] influenza vaccinations,[90] parvovirus B19,[38] and infectious mononucleosis[46,96] have been reported.

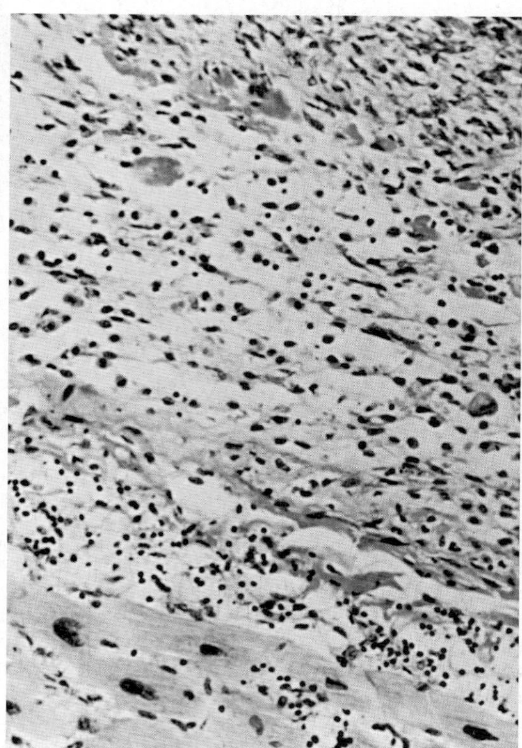

FIG. 27.6 In this case of viral pericarditis there is a layer of fibrin and fibroblasts along the pericardial surface. The mononuclear cell infiltrate in the epicardium extends into the outer myocardium (H&E, ×400). (Courtesy Edith P. Hawkins, MD, Texas Children's Hospital, Houston.)

Clinical Manifestations

In 40% to 75% of cases, the patient has a history of upper respiratory tract infection for 10 days to 2 weeks preceding the onset of symptoms. Fever and chest and abdominal pain are the most common symptoms.[16] A friction rub may be heard in 50% to 80% of cases.[94] Children with viral pericarditis generally are less toxic and experience smaller elevations in body temperature than do children with purulent pericarditis. Some appear acutely ill, however. Large amounts of pericardial fluid accumulation and tamponade are rare findings.

Investigative Techniques

The electrocardiographic, radiographic, echocardiographic, and nuclear scanning findings described for patients with purulent pericarditis also are observed in patients with viral pericarditis. Mononuclear cell infiltrates in the pericardium with extension into the myocardium may be seen (Fig. 27.6).

If obtained, pericardial fluid should be sent for cell count and viral culture. Nasopharyngeal and rectal samples also should be obtained and cultured for viruses. Molecular methods may detect evidence of a specific virus. Acute and convalescent sera should be obtained so that appropriate titers can be measured if a virus is isolated.

Course and Prognosis

Viral pericarditis generally resolves spontaneously over the course of 3 to 4 weeks.[71] Large pericardial effusions and tamponade are rare occurrences. Generally bed rest for approximately 1 week and analgesics for pain are the only therapy that is required. Constrictive pericarditis is a rare occurrence, but pericarditis may recur. In adults with recurrent pericarditis, colchicine appears to be of more benefit than corticosteroids in terms of treatment effect and decreased recurrences in adults, but the use of colchicine for this indication in children is limited.[48,63,82]

NEW REFERENCES SINCE THE SEVENTH EDITION

38. Gouriet F, Levy PY, Casalta JP, et al. Etiology of pericarditis in a prospective cohort of 1162 cases. *Am J Med*. 2015;128(7):784.e1-784.e8.

49. Imazio M, Gaita F. Diagnosis and treatment of pericarditis. *Heart.* 2015;101(14):1159-1168.
48. Imazio M, Brucato A, Cemin R, et al. A randomized trial of colchicine for acute pericarditis. *N Engl J Med.* 2013;369(16):1522-1528.
55. Kaplan SL, Schutze GE, Leake JA, et al. Multicenter surveillance of invasive meningococcal infections in children. *Pediatrics.* 2006;118(4):e979-e984.
64. Lutmer JE, Yates AR, Bannerman TL, et al. Purulent pericarditis secondary to community-acquired, methicillin-resistant *Staphylococcus aureus* in previously healthy children. A sign of the times? *Ann Am Thorac Soc.* 2013;10(3):235-238.
67. McCarty JM, Demetral LC, Dabrowski L, et al. Pediatric coccidioidomycosis in central California: a retrospective case series. *Clin Infect Dis.* 2013;56(11):1579-1585.
82. Shakti D, Hehn R, Gauvreau K, et al. Idiopathic pericarditis and pericardial effusion in children: contemporary epidemiology and management. *J Am Heart Assoc.* 2014;3(6):e001483.
96. Zakhour R, Burkholder H, Wanger A, et al. Epstein-Barr virus-associated pericarditis and pleural effusions in a 4-year-old girl. *Pediatr Infect Dis J.* 2015;34(4):458-459.

The full reference list for this chapter is available at ExpertConsult.com.

Myocarditis 28

Jesus G. Vallejo

Myocarditis is defined clinically and pathologically as inflammation of the myocardium. The clinical presentation and cause may be quite varied. This entity may go unrecognized in numerous patients whose illness may resolve spontaneously, or it may lead to significant morbidity and mortality.

In the early part of the 20th century, most cases of myocarditis were classified as idiopathic, and a diffuse or focal interstitial inflammation was identified on histologic examination. Rheumatic fever, diphtheria, and other bacterial infections were the only diseases recognized as associated with myocarditis, although some experts suspected that viruses might play a significant etiologic role in many cases.[163] After the discovery in 1947 of the coxsackievirus group and the subsequent isolation and identification of other viruses, the number of cases of myocarditis classified as idiopathic diminished rapidly.[36]

EPIDEMIOLOGY

The diverse clinical manifestations have made the true incidence of myocarditis difficult to determine. The clinical course of acute myocarditis can be insidious, with limited inflammation and cardiac dysfunction, or it can be overwhelming, leading to severe cardiac injury and cardiac failure. As a clinical entity, myocarditis is an uncommon occurrence in children. At Texas Children's Hospital, Houston, between 1954 and 1977, myocarditis represented 0.3% of the 14,322 patients seen by the Cardiology Service.

Because not all cases of myocarditis are recognized clinically, a much higher incidence is recorded in autopsy series. An autopsy incidence of 1.15% was found from 4343 studies performed between 1954 and 1977 at Texas Children's Hospital. This rate is considerably lower than the incidence of 6.83% reported by Saphir and Simon[163] in 1944 for 1420 autopsies performed on children. In Saphir's series, 32 of 97 cases had or probably had rheumatic carditis,[162] whereas only two cases occurred in the Texas Children's Hospital series. The discrepancy is even more pronounced when these observations are compared with those of Burch and colleagues,[27] who demonstrated evidence of interstitial myocarditis in the hearts of 29 of 50 infants and who showed evidence of interstitial myocarditis in the hearts of 29 of 50 infants and young children undergoing routine postmortem studies.

Recently Freedman et al.[53] reported an estimated prevalence of myocarditis of 0.5 cases per 10,000 emergency center visits to a single pediatric Canadian center. Some of the discrepancies between the clinical and autopsy series may be explained by the fact that the manifestations of myocarditis are subclinical in many cases and may be recognized only by changes on electrocardiogram (ECG) or perhaps not at all. In many instances, myocarditis is only one component of a generalized illness, and the cardiac dysfunction, if mild, may be overlooked.

ETIOLOGIES

Myocarditis may occur with many common infectious illnesses that affect infants and children (Box 28.1). In most cases of myocarditis, the etiologic agent is never identified, however. In the United States and Western Europe, viruses are the most common causes of acute myocarditis. Myocarditis generally is a sporadic disease, but epidemics have been reported. Most epidemics have been caused by coxsackievirus group B and have affected infants in the newborn period.[44,49] Gear and Measroch[62] were the first to identify coxsackievirus B in association with myocarditis after an epidemic occurred in a nursery in a maternity home in southern Rhodesia.

The association between virus infection and the development of myocardial disease also was made by Grist and Bell[72] who presented comprehensive serologic data correlating enterovirus infection with acute viral myocarditis. In the World Health Organization report during the 10-year period from 1975–85, the coxsackieviruses B represented the most frequent inflammatory agents in cardiovascular disease (34.6/1000), followed by influenza B virus (17.4/1000), influenza A virus (11.7/1000), coxsackievirus A (9.1 per 1000), and cytomegalovirus (CMV) (8/1000). Karjalainen and colleagues[91] prospectively examined 104 conscripts during the 1978 influenza A virus (H1N1) epidemic in Sweden. The incidence of myocarditis was 9% of the 67 verified cases of influenza virus infection. Randolph and colleagues[149] reported that of 838 children with pandemic H1N1 admitted to a pediatric intensive care unit, 1.4% were diagnosed with myocarditis. Although H1N1-related acute myocarditis was uncommon, it was found to be an independent risk factor for death.

The development of molecular techniques such as polymerase chain reaction (PCR) has improved the testing of endomyocardial biopsy specimens for potential viral pathogens. A study using PCR identified viral genome in 38% of endomyocardial biopsy specimens from patients diagnosed with acute myocarditis.[22] Of the positive PCR samples, 23% were positive for adenovirus, 14% for enterovirus, and 3% for CMV. Parvovirus B19, influenza A virus, Epstein-Barr virus, herpes simplex virus (HSV), and respiratory syncytial virus were detected in less than 1% of cases. In a recent retrospective study of pediatric myocarditis, viral studies (PCR of blood, myocardium, or serology) were performed in 30 of 58 patients.[159] A viral cause was identified in 17 of 30 patients (56%) and included six parvovirus B19 with influenza coinfection, seven enterovirus, one EBV, and one CMV. In a recent study of children with the diagnosis of clinical myocarditis, Simpson et al.[169] reported that blood PCR was positive at the time of presentation in 43% (9 of 21) for one of four known cardiotropic viruses (four enterovirus, two parvovirus B19, one adenovirus, and two HHV-6). The majority (89%) of the patients with clinical myocarditis and positive blood PCR were

BOX 28.1 Causes of Myocarditis

Viruses
Coxsackieviruses A and B
Echoviruses
Polioviruses
Rubella
Measles
Adenoviruses
Vaccinia
Mumps
Herpes simplex
Epstein-Barr
Cytomegalovirus
Rhinoviruses
Hepatitis viruses
Arboviruses
Influenza viruses
Varicella
Rickettsia
Rickettsia rickettsii
Rickettsia tsutsugamushi

Bacteria
Meningococcus
Klebsiella
Leptospira
Staphylococcus
Treponema pallidum
Haemophilus influenzae
Hemolytic streptococci
Mycobacterium tuberculosis
Salmonella enterica subsp. *enterica* serovar Typhi (typhoid)
Mycoplasma
Mycoplasma pneumoniae
Chlamydia psittaci

Protozoa
Trypanosoma cruzi
African trypanosomiasis
Toxoplasma
Amebiasis

Other Parasites
Toxocara canis
Trichinella spiralis

Fungi and Yeasts
Actinomyces
Coccidioides
Histoplasma
Candida

Toxin
Diphtheria
Scorpion

Drugs
Sulfonamides
Phenylbutazone
Cyclophosphamide
Neo-mercazole

Hypersensitivity/ Autoimmunity
Rheumatoid arthritis
Rheumatic fever
Ulcerative colitis
Systemic lupus erythematosus

Other
Sarcoidosis
Scleroderma
Idiopathic
Cornstarch

younger than 12 months old. In contrast, only 3.5% of healthy control children (four of 114) had a positive blood PCR for any of these four viruses. In one pediatric case series of pediatric cardiac transplant patients, parvovirus B19 genome was detected in 100 of 700 (82.6%) biopsies from 99 patients.[24] The presence of the parvovirus B19 genome did not correlate with rejection score. However, transplant coronary artery disease occurred in 20 patients, with persistent detection (>6 months) of parvovirus B19. In two retrospective studies, parvovirus B19 has been identified as a common cause of viral myocarditis in healthy children.[126,127,188] Patients with parvovirus B19 myocarditis often demonstrate persistent myocardial dysfunction requiring medical therapy and transplantation. Given the high prevalence of parvovirus B19 infection in the pediatric population, its pathogenic role in pediatric myocarditis and dilated cardiomyopathy (DCM) is still being investigated.

Investigators also have speculated for decades on the possibility that acute myocarditis is a common forerunner of idiopathic DCM. Evidence supporting this hypothesis was presented first by Orinius and Pernow[142] who found cardiac disease in humans years after an apparent uncomplicated coxsackievirus infection. Subsequently, Bowles and colleagues[23] using a slot-blot hybridization technique provided conclusive evidence for the presence of enterovirus in endomyocardial biopsy samples from patients with DCM. In another study, Bowles and associates[22] detected viral genomes in 20% of 149 patients with the diagnosis of DCM. In these patients, adenovirus was identified in 12% and enterovirus in 8% of DCM cases. In all age groups, adenovirus and enterovirus were the viruses most commonly detected in acute myocarditis and DCM.

In December 2002, the U.S. Department of Defense began mandatory smallpox vaccination for select service members and employees without contraindications to vaccination, and in January 2003, the U.S. Department of Health and Human Services implemented a voluntary civilian smallpox vaccination program. As of June 15, 2003, the Department of Defense identified more than 50 cases of suspected, probable, or confirmed myopericarditis occurring within 30 days of vaccination in these individuals, based on clinical evaluation of symptoms, electrocardiography, cardiac enzyme assays, echocardiography, and the exclusion of ischemic coronary artery disease. Myocarditis occurred in 7.8 per 100,000 primary vaccinees in the U.S. Army, an incidence that was 3.6-fold more than that in unvaccinated individuals.[74]

PATHOLOGY

Isolated or idiopathic myocarditis is a rare pathologic entity. The pathologic cardiac findings usually are nonspecific; similar gross and microscopic changes occur regardless of the causative agent.[68,138,146,156] Grossly all four chambers of the heart are enlarged, and the cardiac weight is increased. The heart usually is flabby and pale. In some instances, especially with coxsackievirus B infections, petechial hemorrhages may be seen on the epicardial surfaces; pericardial fluid may be tinged with blood. On cut section, the ventricular muscle walls may be thinned. Occasionally the ventricles are hypertrophied or increased in thickness because of edema. The valves are spared. The endocardial surface usually is unaffected but occasionally may be thickened and appear glistening white. This important observation suggested to some investigators that endocardial fibroelastosis, which manifests as congestive cardiomyopathy, represented a progression from acute viral myocarditis.[77,86] In a study of 64 hearts of children who had myocarditis or endocardial fibroelastosis, Hutchins and Vie[86] found 18 with endocardial fibroelastosis only, five with myocarditis only, and 41 with features of both diseases. When time from onset of illness to death was 2 weeks or less, only myocarditis was evident. When the time interval was 2 weeks to 4 months, a combined picture was seen, whereas only endocardial fibroelastosis with trivial myocarditis was evident when the time from onset of disease to death was more than 4 months.

These findings were supported further by Hastreiter and Miller[77] who found microscopic evidence of myocarditis after transthoracic needle biopsy of the myocardium in a child who had the classic clinical picture of endocardial fibroelastosis, including left ventricular hypertrophy on ECG. Fruhling and associates[57] extended these observations by showing coxsackievirus B3 in the myocardium of 13 of 28 infants with endocardial fibroelastosis. Ni and associates[137] analyzed 29 myocardial samples from patients with autopsy-proven endocardial fibroelastosis using specific PCR for enterovirus, adenovirus, mumps, CMV, parvovirus, influenza, and HSV. In 90% of samples, viral genome was amplified; more than 70% of the samples were positive for mumps viral RNA, whereas 28% were positive for amplified adenovirus. These data suggest that endocardial fibroelastosis also is a sequela of mumps virus infection.

The microscopic picture of acute myocarditis typically shows a focal or diffuse interstitial collection composed predominantly of mononuclear cells, lymphocytes, plasma cells, and eosinophils (Figs. 28.1 and 28.2). Polymorphonuclear leukocytes rarely are seen unless the cause of the carditis is bacterial. Virus particles and inclusion bodies rarely are recognized.[150,156] In severe infections caused by any agent, but especially coxsackieviruses and diphtheria, a loss of cross-striation in the muscle fibers, edema, and sometimes extensive necrosis of the myocardium occur.

Giant cells with or without granulomata are markers for the diagnosis of giant-cell myocarditis.[85] Granulomata have been observed in the myocardium of patients with tuberculosis, syphilis, rheumatoid arthritis,

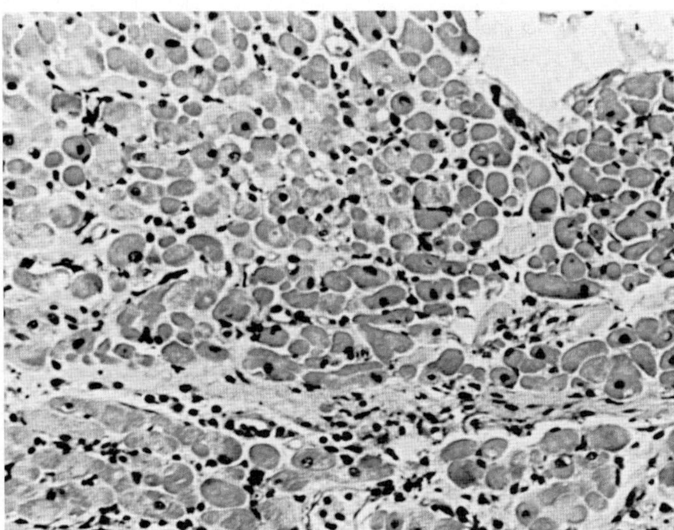

FIG. 28.1 Right ventricular biopsy specimen. The presumed viral myocarditis is characterized by focal mononuclear cell infiltrates (H&E staining, ×160). (Courtesy Edith Hawkins, MD, Houston, TX.)

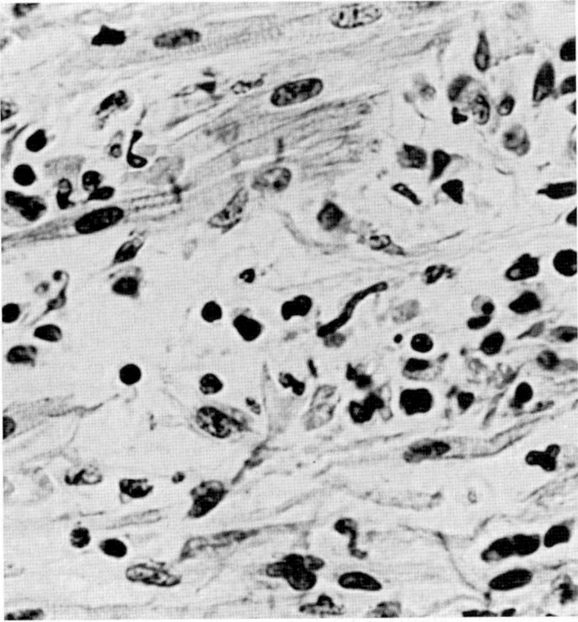

FIG. 28.2 Picornavirus myocarditis characterized by interstitial edema, mononuclear cell infiltrates, and focal myofiber disruption (H&E staining, ×400). (Courtesy Edith Hawkins, MD, Houston, TX.)

rheumatic heart disease, sarcoidosis, and certain fungal and parasitic infections. Occasionally giant cells have been seen in interstitial myocarditis (idiopathic or Fiedler). In many cases, giant-cell myocarditis occurs, but no cause is found.

PATHOGENESIS

The pathogenesis of myocarditis in humans was derived largely from experimental models of coxsackievirus infection. Liu and Mason[110] have suggested that myocarditis should be viewed as a continuum that comprises three separate phases: acute viral infection (phase I), autoimmunity (phase II), and DCM (phase III).

Phase I of the disease is triggered by the entry and proliferation in the myocardium of the causative virus. Impairment of left ventricular function in mice with histopathologically graded moderate cellular infiltration after coxsackievirus B3 infection supports the importance of direct viral damage of the myocardium.[180] Phase I concludes with activation of the cellular immune response, which attenuates viral proliferation but also may enhance cardiac injury. Ideally the immune response should downregulate to a resting state when viral proliferation is controlled. If immune activation continues unabated despite elimination of the virus, autoimmune disease may result, initiating phase II of the disease. The continuous activation of T cells long after viral clearance occurs is detrimental to the host because cytokine-mediated and direct T-cell–mediated myocyte injury leads to impairment of contractile function (Fig. 28.3). Long-term remodeling and progression to DCM characterize phase III of the disease.[82]

Numerous effector cells and molecules work in concert to restrict this initial spread of an infectious focus. The responding cells include natural killer cells, natural killer/T cells, and γδ T cells. Several lines of evidence suggest that mediators of the innate immune system, such as tumor necrosis factor (TNF) and nitric oxide, play an important role in the pathogenesis of viral myocarditis.[120,203] Elevated levels of TNF have been reported in patients with viral myocarditis, and TNF mRNA and protein are consistently upregulated in the hearts of these patients.[122,164] In mice, the exogenous administration of TNF aggravates myocarditis, and the neutralization of TNF by antibodies or soluble receptors attenuates the disease.[100,200]

More recent studies also have shown that TNF and nitric oxide are beneficial to the host by virtue of their antiviral effects. Mice with defective TNF or nitric oxide expression have increased myocardial injury, a significant increase in viral titers in the heart, and significantly higher mortality rates after infection with encephalomyocarditis virus or coxsackievirus B3.[189,203] Although the prevailing notion has been that production of cytokine in the heart during viral infection is detrimental, the host-pathogen relationship is changed fundamentally when the host is unable to produce molecules such as TNF or nitric oxide.[189,203]

An important component of the innate immune system uses pattern recognition receptors, such as the Toll-like receptors (TLRs), to recognize pathogen-associated molecular patterns present in microbes.[4] The role of TLRs in the pathogenesis of viral myocarditis is still evolving. However, recent studies suggest that cardiac inflammation during viral infection depends on TLRs. The viral genome replicates using the positive-strand RNA as its template, resulting in the formation of dsRNA intermediates. Accordingly both single-strand RNA and dsRNA are present in virally infected cells. TLR3 and TLR7/8 signaling are activated by double-stranded RNA (dsRNA) and single-stranded RNA, respectively. Thus viral infection can activate innate immune signaling in the heart through myeloid differentiation factor 88 (MyD88)-dependent (TLR 7/8) and MyD88-independent pathways (TLR3). Fairweather and colleagues[50] reported that mice with defective TLR4 signaling had decreased coxsackievirus B3 replication and less severe myocarditis 12 days after infection compared with wild-type mice. The presence of TLR4 also was associated with increased production of interleukin-1β (IL-1β) and IL-18 and increased viral replication in the heart.

In a similar study, Fuse and associates[59] reported that mice deficient in MyD88, an adapter protein involved in TLR signaling (except TLR3), also had less myocarditis and attenuated viral replication in the heart after infection with coxsackievirus B3. Coxsackievirus B3–infected, MyD88-deficient mice had significantly higher levels of interferon-β (IFN-β) but reduced expression of the coxsackievirus-adenovirus receptor in the heart. The enhanced IFN expression and lower expression of the coxsackie-adenovirus receptor in the heart could explain the attenuation of disease in the MyD88-deficient mice. Infection of TLR3-deficient mice with encephalomyocarditis virus (EMCV), a positive single-strand RNA virus, resulted in earlier mortality in TLR3-deficient mice that was associated with increased viral replication and myocardial injury when compared with wild-type mice.[75] Similar observations have been reported for coxsackievirus group B serotype 3 in TLR3-deficient mice.[136] Gorbea et al.[67] screened TLR3 in patients diagnosed with enteroviral myocarditis or DCM and identified a rare variant in one patient as well as a significantly increased occurrence of a common polymorphism compared with controls. Expression of either variant resulted in significantly reduced TLR3-mediated signaling after stimulation with

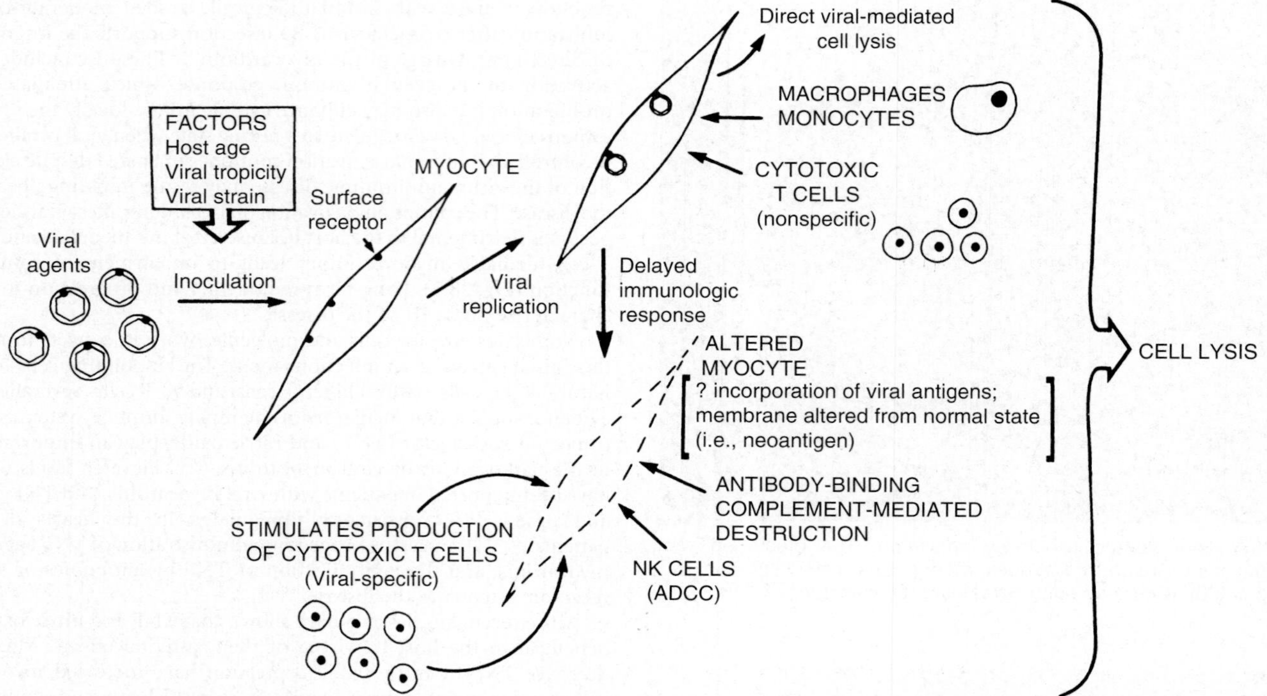

FIG. 28.3 Schema for pathogenesis of myocarditis. Viral agents attach to cells by means of surface receptors. After a cell is infected, the cell cycle is changed. Direct virus-mediated cytolysis occurs. Cellular effectors of injury (i.e., macrophages, monocytes, and nonspecific cytotoxic T cells) are involved in the primary reaction. Myocytes that survive are altered in their structure. Cytotoxic T cells specifically targeted against the altered myocyte, natural killer (NK) cells, and complement-activated, antibody-mediated cardiocytolysis or antibody-dependent cellular cytotoxicity (ADCC) participate in the secondary reaction. (From Maisch B, Trostel-Soeder R, Stechemesser E, et al. Diagnostic relevance of humoral and cell-mediated immune reactions in patients with acute viral myocarditis. *Clin Exp Immunol.* 48:533;1982.)

synthetic double-stranded RNA. Furthermore coxsackievirus B3 infection of cell lines expressing mutated TLR3 abrogated activation of the type I IFN pathway, leading to increased viral replication.

Woodruff and Woodruff,[197] using a murine model, were the first to show a role for T lymphocytes in the pathogenesis of viral myocarditis. In this study, depletion of T lymphocytes using antithymocyte serum or thymectomy and irradiation led to a decrease in mortality rates and in the inflammatory infiltrate after coxsackievirus B3 infection. Huber and associates,[84] using BALB/c mice infected with coxsackievirus B3, showed that cytolytic T cells were the agents responsible for the major part of myocardial cell injury. In addition, proinflammatory mediators, such as TNF, released by infiltration cells also adversely affect cardiac function.

Opavsky and colleagues[141] defined the specific contributions of T-cell subsets (CD4 and CD8) and the T-cell receptor β chain to the pathogenesis of viral myocarditis. When $CD4^{-/-}$ or $CD8^{-/-}$ mice were exposed to CVB3, loss of $CD8^{+/+}$ immune cells did not affect survival significantly, but viral proliferation was attenuated. In contrast, $CD4^{-/-}$ mice showed a trend toward an improvement in survival and a small but significant decrease in the inflammatory infiltrate at 14 days after infection. Mice deficient in CD4/CD8 immune cells and T-cell receptor β had the best outcome in terms of decreased mortality. A marked decrease in inflammatory infiltrate was noted in CD4/CD8 double-knockout mice. Although no significant change occurred in viral titers, a marked decrease in myocardial TNF mRNA 4 days after infection was seen in CD4/CD8 double-knockout mice. These same investigators have shown that the T-cell receptor–associated tyrosine kinase $p56^{lck}$ is crucial for coxsackievirus B3 proliferation in the heart and activation of T cells to target the heart.[109] Mice deficient in $p56^{lck}$ were protected against the development of myocarditis, providing further support for the hypothesis that T-cell activation during viral myocarditis contributes to increased inflammation and myocyte destruction in the host.

T-regulatory (T-reg) cells also are important in modulating the inflammatory response and preventing the development of autoimmunity through the production cytokines like IL-10 and tumor growth factor-β (TGF-β).[195] T-regs express CD4, but they also express the α-subunit of the IL-2 receptor, CD25. They also are high expressors of the transcription factor FoxP3. Li and associates[106] have shown that the allograft of M2 (antiinflammatory) macrophages led to improvement of virus-induced myocarditis, which was associated with enhanced levels of T-regs. Similarly, Huber and colleagues[83] have reported decreased viral titers and inflammation after adoptive transfer of a $CD4^+$ $CD25^+$ regulatory–like T-cell population into a mouse model of coxsackievirus B3 infection. Thus modulating the immune response may be critical for the prevention of chronic virus replication.

The ongoing injury that persists may be considered an autoimmune process.[84,196] At least in murine models, it is clear that both cellular and humoral autoimmunity are involved in the progression to chronic heart disease. The recently identified T helper 17 (T_H17) subset has been implicated in the onset of chronic myocarditis.[76] These cells secrete high levels of IL-17 and have been implicated in the production of autoantibodies.[76,201] In a mouse model of coxsackievirus B3 myocarditis these T_H17 cells contribute to chronic myocarditis through persistent inflammatory signaling involving the secretion of IL-17. Consistent with this, there is significant T_H17 expansion approximately 2 weeks after coxsackievirus B3 infection in mice.[202] IL-17 and its various isotypes can induce expression of TNF and T_H2 responses, which in turn leads to a prolonged inflammatory milieu that might foster the production of autoantibodies.

More recent studies also have shed light on the mechanisms by which coxsackievirus B3 may contribute directly to the development of myocarditis and DCM. Badorff and colleagues[9–11] reported that the 2A protease encoded by coxsackievirus B3 cleaves dystrophin in cultured myocytes and in infected mouse hearts, leading to disruption of dystrophin and the dystrophin-associated glycoprotein α-sarcoglycan and β-sarcoglycan complex. Dystrophin provides a structural link between the muscle cytoskeleton and extracellular matrix to maintain muscle integrity. Xiong and associates[199] compared the effects of coxsackievirus B3 infection in dystrophin-deficient (mdx) and wild-type mice. Coxsackievirus B3 infection significantly enhanced sarcolemmal disruption in the mdx mice compared with wild-type mice; the disruption was detectable 2 days postinfection and continued to increase after initial infection. Viral titers were higher in the hearts of mdx mice than in the hearts of wild-type mice, indicating greater viral replication in the absence of dystrophin. The observed differences seemed to be a result of more efficient release of coxsackievirus B3 from dystrophin-deficient myocytes. The expression of wild-type dystrophin in cultured cells decreased the cytopathic effect induced by coxsackievirus B3 and the release of virus from the cell. The expression of a cleavage-resistant mutant of the dystrophin protein inhibited coxsackievirus B3–mediated cytopathic effect and viral release further.

PATHOPHYSIOLOGY

Given the extensive interstitial inflammation, muscle cell injury, or both, myocardial contractility is reduced. Consequently the heart enlarges and the end-diastolic volume of the ventricle increases. In the normal heart, an increase in filling volume leads, by the Starling mechanism, to an increased force of contraction, ejection fraction, and cardiac output. In patients with myocarditis, the myocardium is unable to respond in this manner, and cardiac output is reduced. Systemic blood flow may be maintained, however, by use of the cardiac reserve, mediated by the sympathetic nervous system and leading to vasoconstriction of the skin vessels and an increase in heart rate. With progressive disease, the heart may be unable to meet the oxygen demands of the tissues, and the clinical picture of congestive cardiac failure may become evident. In some infants and young children, the presentation is predominantly that of right-sided heart failure.[155]

An appreciation of the disturbance of myocardial function may be gained from the angiographic frames shown in Fig. 28.4. The left ventricle is dilated considerably, and the outline is irregular in diastole and systole. The ejection fraction is reduced significantly at 35% instead of the normal 60% to 75%.

Another means of evaluating left ventricular function is the noninvasive technique of cardiac echocardiography. Gutgesell and colleagues[73] established normal standards for children. An example is shown in Fig. 28.5A.

The normal shortening fraction (i.e., percentage change in ventricular dimensions between end-diastole and end-systole) is 35% ± 4%, regardless

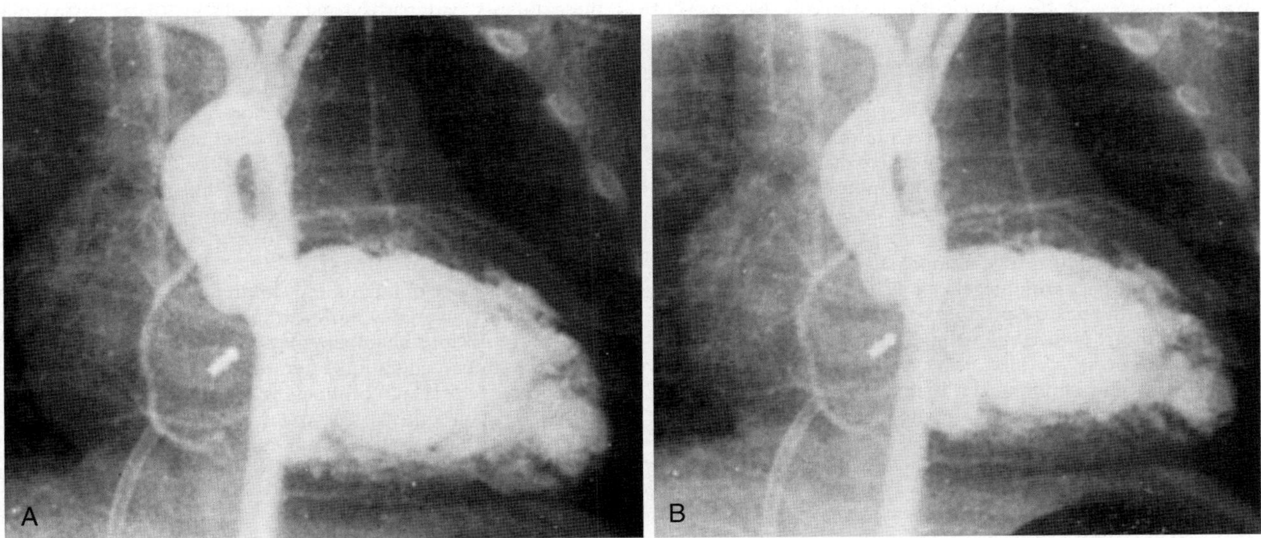

FIG. 28.4 The (A) end-diastolic and (B) end-systolic images from a left ventriculogram of a patient with idiopathic myocarditis show irregularity of the wall and poor contractility.

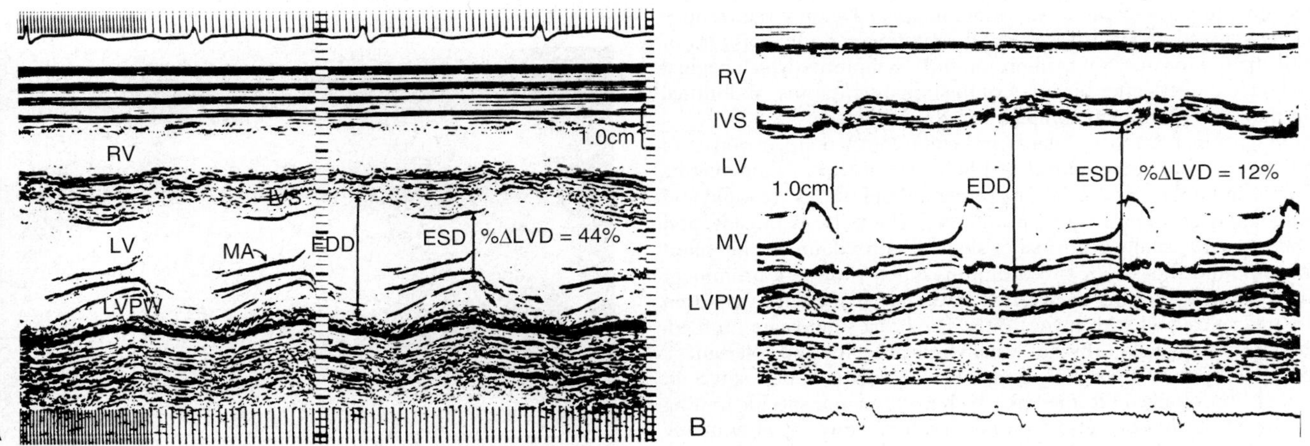

FIG. 28.5 (A) Normal echocardiogram of a 4-year-old child. (B) Echocardiogram of a 4-year-old child with idiopathic myocarditis shows left ventricular dilation and severely reduced shortening fraction. *EDD,* End-diastolic dimension; *ESD,* end-systolic dimension; *IVS,* interventricular septum; *LVPW,* left ventricular posterior wall; *MA,* mitral apparatus; *MV,* mitral valve, *%ΔLVD,* percent change in left ventricular dimension (shortening fraction).

of age (range, 28–44%). Fig. 28.5B illustrates the case of a 4-year-old child with idiopathic myocarditis and shows ventricular dilation with markedly reduced motion of the left ventricular posterior wall and septum, leading to a shortening fraction of only 12%. Further assessment of ventricular function can be achieved by measuring systolic time intervals obtained from simultaneous recording of the ECG and the semilunar valve opening and closing points on the echocardiogram.[73]

CLINICAL MANIFESTATIONS

The clinical presentation of myocarditis varies with the age of the patient and the virulence of the organism. At one end of the spectrum is a fulminant, rapidly fatal illness and, at the other, no apparent clinical disturbance at all. A newborn especially is susceptible to the severe form of myocarditis usually caused by the coxsackieviruses B,[38,93] but it also is recognized with rubella[3] and HSV[198] infections and with toxoplasmosis.[85]

In many of these infections, myocarditis is only one component of a generalized illness, often with severe hepatitis and encephalitis.[17,93] In some instances, however, infections with these organisms may produce only a mild clinical disturbance.[26,87] In the report by Brightman and colleagues,[26] a nursery epidemic of coxsackievirus B5 infection in preterm infants was recognized only by chance because a virologic survey was in progress at the time in the institution. No cases of myocarditis were documented, and all the infants recovered. Findings included lethargy, failure to gain weight, and, in some infants, evidence of aseptic meningitis.

As described in the review by Kibrick and Benirschke[93] of 25 infants with coxsackievirus B myocarditis, vague symptoms such as lethargy and anorexia may herald the onset of the severe disease, emphasizing that close attention should be paid to all symptoms, especially in a newborn, no matter how nonspecific. Four infants had episodes of vomiting, and fever was documented for more than half of the cases; occasionally, the temperature was subnormal. Cyanosis, respiratory distress, and tachycardia, cardiomegaly, or ECG changes occurred in 19 of 23 infants. Tachypnea (respiratory rate >60/min in a newborn) is an early sign of heart failure in a young infant and should alert the clinician to this diagnosis.

In older infants and children, the manifestations of myocarditis generally are less fulminant than are the manifestations in newborns.[155,161,190,194] An acute and fatal illness has been associated, however, with idiopathic myocarditis[108] and the myocarditis associated with enteroviruses,[93] adenoviruses,[78] mumps,[102] chickenpox,[143] diphtheria,[15] cytomegalovirus,[183] and many of the other causative agents listed in Box 28.1. Some older children have been reported with acute, substernal chest pain consistent with angina and have ECG changes of acute myocardial infarction.[81,124] The usual clinical picture is that of an acute or a subacute illness, which often begins with a mild upper respiratory infection and a low-grade fever.[8] Some infants have only vague, nonspecific suggestions of disease (e.g., irritability, periodic episodes of pallor) before the onset of cardiorespiratory symptoms, which begin a few days to 2 weeks after the onset of the initial symptoms. Abdominal pain may be a prominent complaint in some children.[190]

On examination, these infants and children often are anxious and apprehensive, but some appear apathetic and listless. Pallor may be striking, and mild cyanosis may be present. Respirations are rapid and labored, and grunting may be prominent. The pulse is thready, and blood pressure usually is normal or slightly reduced, unless the infant is in profound shock. The precordium is quiet, without a prominent cardiac impulse. Resting tachycardia invariably is present in children who are critically ill with myocarditis. The heart sounds are muffled, and a prominent gallop rhythm usually is heard. Fine and colleagues[52] found the most sensitive clinical sign of myocarditis to be a soft S_1 at the apex. A prolonged PR interval, which may be a nonspecific finding in many febrile illnesses, also can cause a soft S_1, however, without any other evidence of myocarditis.[168]

Almost uniformly, the liver is enlarged; edema is a rare finding. Some infants are less distressed and have signs of only mild congestive cardiac failure, without the signs of peripheral circulatory failure. Other infants have no signs of cardiac compromise, and myocarditis is recognized only as part of a generalized illness by a disturbance in the ECG pattern.

DIAGNOSIS

Myocarditis often is difficult to diagnose, but it should be suspected in any infant or child who presents with congestive heart failure and who has or recently has had a febrile illness. The history should include information regarding travel, exposure to tuberculosis, recent drug ingestion, and illnesses in other family members or schoolmates. A quiet precordium in the presence of a gallop rhythm and decreased intensity or muffling of the heart sounds are findings that strongly suggest the diagnosis. A tachycardia out of proportion to the level of fever also should be viewed with suspicion. A physiologic S_3 is a common finding in normal healthy children and in children with anemia and fever. An unusually prominent S_3 suggests a disturbance of ventricular compliance without other evidence of compromised cardiac function and should be investigated further with an echocardiogram, a chest radiograph, and an ECG.

The occurrence of an arrhythmia, especially after a febrile illness, should alert the clinician to look for other signs of myocarditis.[34,172] Lind and Hulquist[108] detected significant dysrhythmias in five infants with isolated myocarditis. Four of the five infants died, and three of these infants had paroxysmal atrial tachycardia. Paroxysmal atrial tachycardia has been reported in patients with viral myocarditis[34,172] and has been described in patients with diphtheritic myocarditis.[15] Atrial ectopic tachycardia may mimic sinus tachycardia and, if not carefully evaluated, may be the primary cause for significant myocardial dysfunction. Complete heart block has been described in children in association with acute idiopathic myocarditis[89,107] and with rubella,[111] coxsackievirus,[165] and respiratory syncytial virus[12,64] infections. In some instances, complete heart block is permanent; in others, it is temporary.[12,65,89]

Chest Radiography

Chest radiographs of infants and children who have signs of congestive cardiac failure invariably show cardiomegaly, usually of a severe degree (Fig. 28.6). All four chambers may be enlarged, and evidence of pulmonary venous congestion often is found. Sometimes, especially in newborns, the first sign of illness is acute circulatory collapse, and, in this circumstance, the cardiac size may be normal. The same is true of children who have an arrhythmia rather than congestive heart failure. Other patients may present with Stokes-Adams attacks caused by complete heart block.[107]

Electrocardiogram

The ECG is an essential diagnostic tool for all patients with suspected myocarditis. The classic ECG pattern in myocarditis is one of diffuse

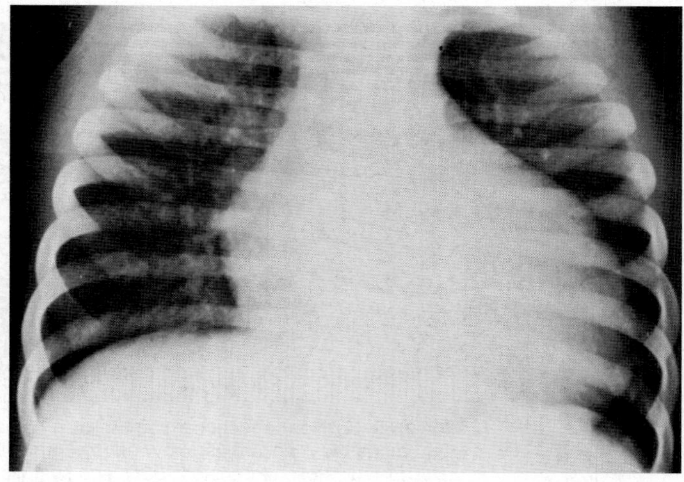

FIG. 28.6 Marked cardiomegaly with a mild increase in the pulmonary venous pattern in the upper lobes.

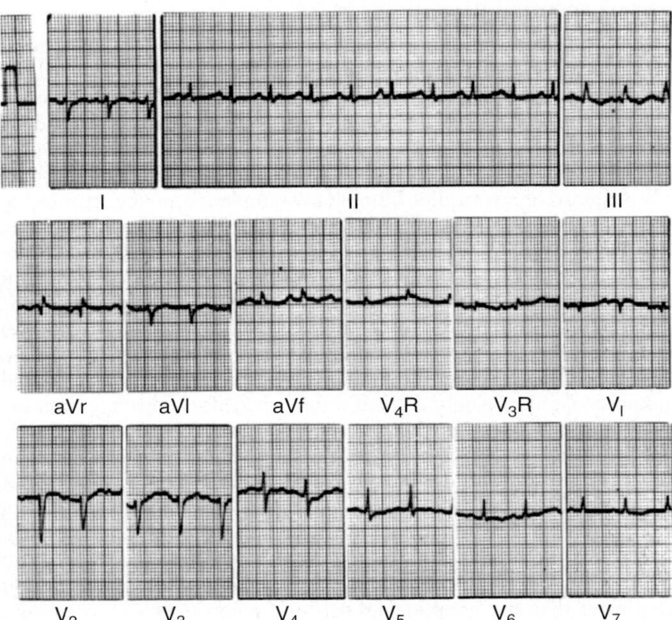

FIG. 28.7 Diffuse low-voltage or QRS complexes with T-wave flattening and 1-mm Q waves in the lateral precordial leads represents the classic pattern in myocarditis.

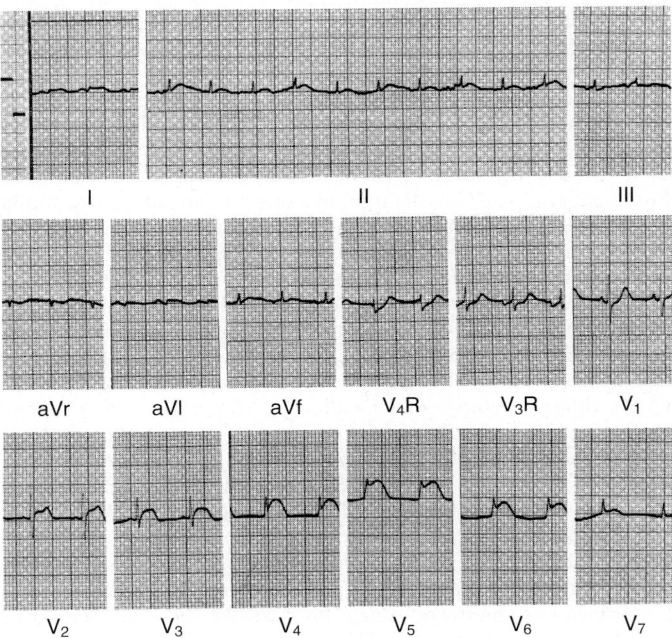

FIG. 28.8 In addition to low voltage, there is evidence of acute myocardial ischemia with 4- to 5-mm ST-segment elevation dominantly in the middle and lateral precordial leads.

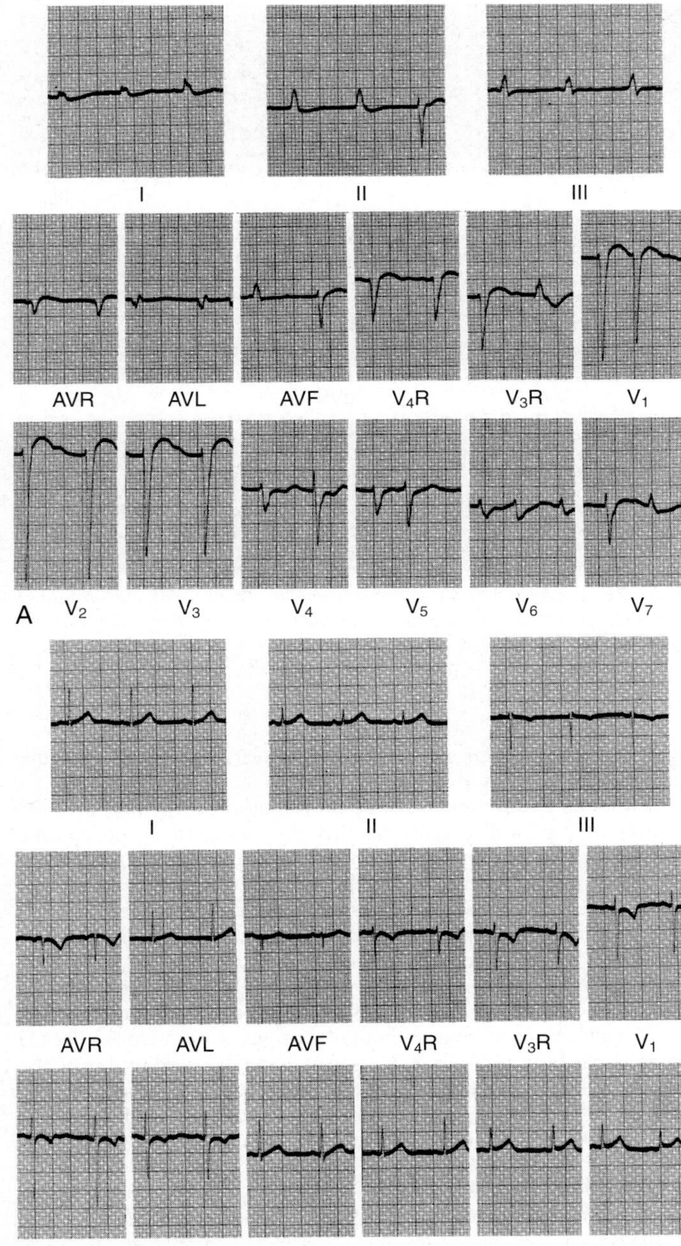

FIG. 28.9 (A) Multifocal premature beats are caused by atrioventricular dissociation and left bundle branch block resulting from diphtheritic myocarditis. (B) A normal electrocardiogram is shown for the same patient 3 months after an episode of myocarditis.

low-voltage QRS complexes (<5 mm total amplitude) with low-amplitude or slightly inverted T waves and a small or absent Q wave in leads V_5 and V_6 (Fig. 28.7). The low-voltage signal may be present in the standard leads and the precordial leads. Fig. 28.8 shows the ECG of an infant with acute myocarditis and shows a pattern of acute myocardial ischemia. Fig. 28.9A shows multifocal extrasystoles and severe intraventricular conduction delay in a patient with diphtheritic myocarditis; the ECG of this child returned to normal over the course of 3 months (see Fig. 28.9B). The ECG from a 5-month-old infant who had mild fever, diarrhea, and vomiting for 3 to 4 days before admission is shown in Fig. 28.10.

The 2:1 atrioventricular block was associated with normal QRS complexes. This abnormality persisted in the absence of clinical symptoms for 1 year.

Karjalainen and colleagues[91] studied the ECGs of 87 conscripts 18 to 30 years old, 28 of whom had myocarditis. The most frequent findings were T-wave changes of reduced amplitude or inversion in the left chest leads. Sinus tachycardia followed by premature ventricular depolarizations was the most common dysrhythmia. Take and colleagues[178] examined serial ECGs of 16 patients with confirmed viral myocarditis. They found four patterns: (1) complete normalization in the presence of severe myocardial damage in the acute stage; (2) "pseudoinfarction" patterns with Q waves and poor R-wave progression; (3) permanent conduction disturbances that might require pacemaker support; and (4) chronic

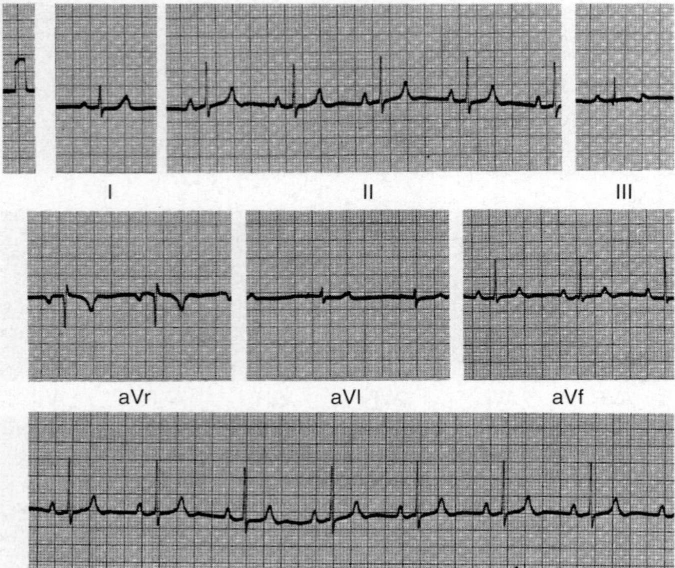

FIG. 28.10 Second-degree atrioventricular block with an effective ventricular rate of 60 beats/min. The blocked P wave is placed on top of the T wave in each cycle.

dysrhythmias, predominantly ventricular tachycardia and supraventricular tachycardia.

Although T-wave and ST-segment changes are the most sensitive indices of myocardial ischemia, they also seem to be nonspecific. Prolongation of the PR interval is another nonspecific ECG finding frequently noted in patients with febrile illnesses. Scott and colleagues[168] showed a 1.49% prevalence of these findings in a group of 737 infants and children with respiratory tract infections, but they also found a similar incidence among 108 control children without respiratory infection or other febrile illness. Abt and Vinnecour[1] recorded PR prolongation and T-wave changes in infants and children who were suffering from pneumonia without other signs of myocarditis. The QT interval has been prolonged in cases of acute myocarditis, but it also appears to be a rather nonspecific finding associated with other infectious diseases.[90,157] A diagnosis of myocarditis cannot be established with certainty on the basis of these nonspecific changes.

Echocardiography and Cardiac MRI

Noninvasive diagnostic myocardial imaging techniques that are useful in the detection of myocarditis include echocardiography and magnetic resonance imaging (MRI). Echocardiography is currently recommended in the initial diagnostic evaluation of all patients with suspected myocarditis.[160] The echocardiogram is useful in assessing ventricular function and helps to exclude pericardial effusion as the cause of the cardiomegaly. Cardiovascular magnetic resonance (CMR) imaging is a safe, noninvasive technique that can be used to assess myocardial function and tissue damage in suspected myocarditis. In particular, CMR can be used to differentiate between acute and chronic myocarditis and can be used for long-term follow-up without the use of radioactive tracers or radiation. Gagliardi et al.[60] reported the first case series on the use of cardiac MRI for the diagnosis of acute myocarditis in 11 infants and children. The authors reported 100% specificity and 100% sensitivity for T2-weighted spin echo cardiac MRI sequences when compared to endocardial biopsy. Although consensus diagnostic CMR criteria have been published for adult patients,[56] similar recommendations are not yet available for children. Interestingly, Ghelani et al.[63] reported a fivefold increase in the use CMR in cases of pediatric myocarditis (5.2% to 28.1%) over a 5-year period (2006–11) at their institution. This was accompanied by a decline in endomyocardial biopsies in cases of myocarditis from 24.7% to 14% during the same time period.

Endomyocardial Biopsy

Endomyocardial biopsy, used for establishing the diagnosis of myocarditis and possibly classifying the phase (i.e., active, healing, or healed) of viral infection, may have a direct impact on the type of therapy employed. Classification of myocarditis based on histologic evidence found on biopsy specimens has proved to be a difficult and sometimes controversial task. No widespread agreement exists on the criteria for establishing the diagnosis of myocarditis from biopsy samples. Sampling error owing to the small amounts of tissue obtained and the focal nature of sampling and the disease process may lead to misdiagnosis. Samples usually are obtained from the right ventricular septum or apex and should contain at least three and optimally five pieces of tissue. Some investigators[186] have found sampling from other areas of the heart (e.g., left ventricle) to be more sensitive, but these techniques have not been applied widely.

Cases of "borderline myocarditis" (i.e., specimens containing increased numbers of inflammatory cells but without evidence of myocyte necrosis) may require a repeat biopsy to confirm the diagnosis. Dec and colleagues[39] confirmed the diagnosis of myocarditis in four of six patients with an initial diagnosis of borderline myocarditis. These investigators did not show any significant advantage to sampling the left ventricle during the repeat study. Overinterpretation or misinterpretation has been cited as a major problem in the reading of biopsy specimens. Edwards and associates[48] looked at 170 endomyocardial biopsy samples and found that more than five lymphocytes per high-power field were consistent with a diagnosis of active lymphocytic myocarditis.

Using endomyocardial biopsy, Fenoglio and coworkers[51] diagnosed myocarditis in 34 patients presenting with congestive heart failure of unknown origin. They classified these patients on the basis of clinical and histologic findings in an attempt to establish subgroups of patients who might benefit from immunosuppressive therapy. Three groups were established: acute, rapidly progressive, and chronic. Immunosuppressive therapy was thought to be significantly beneficial for the last group only in terms of clinical improvement.

Dec and colleagues[40] studied 27 patients referred for endomyocardial biopsy because of congestive heart failure of unknown origin. Two-thirds of the patients had biopsy samples read as positive for myocarditis, but in contrast to the study of Fenoglio and coworkers,[51] in which the histologic grouping was slightly different, no correlation was found between histologic classification and outcome. Outcome did not differ between the group receiving immunosuppressives and the group not receiving immunosuppressives. Biopsy results were negative for 30% of the patients who already met all the clinical criteria of myocarditis and were positive for two of five patients without any clinical evidence of myocarditis (i.e., viral-like illness, pericarditis, or laboratory evidence of viral infection). Olsen[140] reviewed 1200 biopsy specimens from patients with a clinical diagnosis of idiopathic DCM and found that slightly more than 25% had a diagnosis of myocarditis established on the basis of critical evaluation of their tissue specimens. In a retrospective study from Italy, Brighenti et al.[25] reported that histologic examination along with PCR of myocardium yielded an etiologic diagnosis in 26 or 41 pediatric patients (63%).

In clinical practice, endomyocardial biopsy should be used in those scenarios in which the incremental prognostic and therapeutic information gained from biopsy outweighs the risks. Pophal et al.[147] described a series of 1000 endomyocardial biopsies in 194 pediatric patients. The majority (85%) of endomyocardial biopsies were performed for transplant rejection surveillance. The overall reported complication rate was 1.9%. The perforation rate was 0.9% and overall mortality rate was 0.1%. In patients with DCM being evaluated for myocarditis or in patients with new-onset arrhythmia, the incidence of complication was 9.1% (perforation rate was 5.2%) and mortality rate was 0.6%. In a recent retrospective review from five Italian centers, the overall incidence of complications reported was 15.5%, with infants younger than 12 months of age having a complication rate of 31.2%.[25] In contrast to the study by Pophal et al.,[147] this report only included 41 pediatric patients.

Most physicians would agree that many cases of idiopathic DCM probably are the sequelae of unrecognized acute viral myocarditis. The role of endomyocardial biopsy in attempting to salvage patients by selecting them for specific therapy has some validity. The hope is that early intervention in some patients, guided by this technique, would prevent them from progressing to needing transplantation or to death from intractable heart failure.

MOLECULAR DIAGNOSTIC STUDIES

Polymerase Chain Reaction

Jin and associates[88] first described the usefulness of PCR in identifying the viral genome in myocardial samples obtained from patients with suspected myocarditis. Using reverse transcription PCR, which employs RNA to amplify the corresponding complementary DNA before final DNA amplification, the researchers were able to identify an enteroviral genome from cardiac tissue samples. Patients with DCM were shown to harbor an enteroviral genome within myocardial specimens. Confirmation of the utility of PCR in the etiologic diagnosis of a viral genome in patients with clinical myocarditis and idiopathic DCM quickly followed.[33,47,69,79,134,151,191] Controversy existed, however, because reports of high levels of false-positive results,[47] contamination,[33] and low sensitivity[193] were published. The strength of this rapid (<5 hours) and powerful method of amplification of a specific viral genome is also its weakness. The method depends on the quality and quantity of nucleic acid extraction, but contamination may be commonplace in some laboratories. If any requirements are altered, amplification may not occur, leading to false-negative or false-positive (i.e., contamination) results.

Towbin and colleagues[185] used PCR to diagnose adenoviral myocarditis in a fetus with nonimmune hydrops fetalis. In this case, the adenoviral genome was amplified from fetal blood and maternal blood at 29 weeks' gestation and again at delivery at 34 weeks' gestation using blood from the infant and mother and placental specimens. Using viral primers designed to amplify enterovirus, adenovirus, CMV, and HSV nucleic acid, Martin and associates[116] reported 34 patients with suspected acute myocarditis, for whom 68% of samples analyzed were PCR-positive. In this report, samples from 17 control patients were PCR-negative. Adenovirus was the most common viral genome identified (58%), and enteroviruses were the second most common (29%). A few reported cases were PCR positive for HSV and CMV.

Lozinski and coworkers[112] confirmed the importance of adenovirus in their study of cases of myocarditis for which no cause had been found previously; in this case, 66% of the previously unidentified cases were identified as adenovirus. In a more recent study by Bowles and colleagues,[22] viral genomes were detected in 20% of 149 patients with the diagnosis of DCM. In these patients, adenovirus was identified in 12% and enterovirus in 8% of DCM cases. In all age groups, adenovirus and enterovirus were the viruses most commonly detected in acute myocarditis and DCM.

Schowengerdt and colleagues[167] showed that a variety of viruses might be the inciting cause of rejection in patients after undergoing heart transplantation. Using PCR of endomyocardial biopsy specimens, the investigators showed a direct correlation between histologic rejection and PCR-positive viral study results. Studying patients undergoing serial endomyocardial biopsies, they found that the viral genome could be amplified in transplant-rejecting patients who previously had negative PCR analyses. In these cases, as the rejection grade improved, the PCR results again became negative. The most common viruses correlated with rejection were adenoviruses, CMV, and parvovirus. The researchers postulated that this form of rejection probably is another form of myocarditis, and this hypothesis has been supported by other clinical studies.[192]

Virologic and Bacteriologic Studies

For each infant or child with a diagnosis of acute myocarditis, an attempt should be made to identify the offending organism. If the patient is seen early in the illness, isolation of the virus from throat washings, stool, blood, or the myocardium may be possible.

Lerner and colleagues[104] suggested criteria that would help define an etiologic association between a coxsackievirus infection and myocarditis. High-order associations included isolation of the virus from the myocardium, the endocardium, or pericardial fluid and localization of type-specific virus in myocardium, endocardium, or pericardium at sites of pathologic change.

Moderate-order associations are determined when virus is isolated from pharynx or feces, and a fourfold increase in type-specific, neutralizing, hemagglutination-inhibiting, or complement-fixing antibodies is shown, or when virus is isolated from pharynx or feces with a concurrent serum titer of 1:32 or greater of type-specific, IgM-neutralizing, or hemagglutination-inhibiting antibodies. In chronic illness, attempts at virologic identification are less fruitful.[71] Blood for aerobic and anaerobic cultures should be obtained from any infant with fever and signs of compromised cardiovascular function.

Serum Biomarkers

In the setting of acute myocarditis, increased levels of creatine kinase and troponin indicate inflammatory myocardial injury. However, limited myocardial necrosis during myocarditis may contribute to the limited prevalence of elevated troponin T values in biopsy-proven myocarditis cases. Although most available studies involve adult patients, it is acknowledged that cardiospecific troponins provide evidence of myocyte injury in patients with myocarditis more sensitively than do conventional cardiac enzymes. The sensitivity of cardiac biomarkers of myocardial injury varies depending on the time from symptom onset to testing and the cutoff values used. In pediatric patients with acute myocarditis, the sensitivity and specificity of troponin T (TnT) were 75% and 75% when the cutoff was set at 0.026 ng/mL and 63% and 89% with a cutoff value of 0.071 ng/mL.[170] In comparison with creatine kinase activities, TnT also provides improved sensitivity for detection of micronecrosis because of a proportionally higher and longer lasting increase in the blood.[170] The erythrocyte sedimentation rate, C-reactive protein, and leukocyte count may be elevated, but these are considered to be nonspecific.

DIFFERENTIAL DIAGNOSIS

Any cause of circulatory failure, especially when acute in onset, may mimic myocarditis. In newborns, heart failure associated with hypoxia, hypoglycemia, and hypocalcemia is well recognized, whereas circulatory collapse may occur with any infection and without direct involvement of the myocardium. A careful history may help to elucidate possible precipitating factors. Biochemical investigations to exclude hypoglycemia and hypocalcemia always should be conducted in any newborn who has signs of heart failure.

Many infants with structural cardiac defects (e.g., hypoplastic left heart syndrome, aortic valve stenosis) may not have audible murmurs when severely ill. Murmurs usually appear, however, with treatment and improvement in cardiac function. The precordium usually is hyperactive, rather than quiet, and the heart sounds are clear and increased in intensity, rather than muffled. The ECG usually shows severe right ventricular hypertrophy in the former condition and shows right ventricular or left ventricular hypertrophy in the latter; the ECG is useful in the differential diagnosis. The findings on an echocardiogram often are diagnostic.

Beyond the immediate neonatal period, the major disease entities that require differentiation from myocarditis are endocardial fibroelastosis, anomalous left coronary artery arising from the pulmonary artery, Cori type II glycogen storage disease (i.e., Pompe disease), medial necrosis of the coronary arteries, left atrial myxoma,[135] and other congestive cardiomyopathies of undetermined cause.

Common to all of these disorders is moderate to severe cardiomegaly, usually associated with congestive cardiac failure, gallop rhythm, and the infrequent occurrence or absence of murmurs. The murmurs are associated primarily with an anomalous left coronary artery and endocardial fibroelastosis. They are not more than grade 3/6 in intensity, are high pitched, are apically located, and represent some degree of mitral insufficiency. Idiopathic myocarditis occurs primarily in patients older than 6 months of age,[155,156] whereas most of the conditions described earlier manifest before the infant is 6 months old.

Endocardial fibroelastosis, a common cause of congestive cardiac failure in infants, is impossible to differentiate from acute myocarditis on the basis of clinical examination alone. An anomalous origin of the left coronary artery should be identified. The ECG usually shows left axis deviation of the QRS complex in the frontal plane, left ventricular hypertrophy, and a pattern of anterolateral myocardial infarction. It is recognized as a QR pattern with inverted T waves in standard leads I and AVL, a broad Q wave with inverted T waves in precordial leads V_5 and V_6, and loss of anterior forces in the mid-precordial leads. For definitive diagnosis, cardiac catheterization is essential.

Pericarditis, frequently caused by viruses, usually occurs in children rather than in infants. The clinical history may be identical to that of patients with myocarditis; however, considering the degree of cardiomegaly, cardiovascular function is compromised less than in patients with myocarditis, although cardiac tamponade may occur in some cases. Differentiation from myocarditis may be made clinically if the patient has a friction rub, no gallop rhythm, and a typical pattern of chest pain. Further studies may be required, however, to make a conclusive diagnosis. The echocardiogram is invaluable in establishing this diagnosis. It is the most sensitive and least traumatic technique available and easily identifies an effusion. Myocarditis and pericarditis may occur together. This combination is seen most frequently in the pancarditis of rheumatic fever, but it also may occur in coxsackievirus B infections and in many collagen vascular and autoimmune diseases. Myocarditis has been associated with rheumatoid arthritis,[125] systemic lupus erythematosus,[42] and ulcerative colitis.[54,133]

TREATMENT

Standard Approaches

Intensive medical care is required during the acute stage of the illness. Heart rate, respiratory rate, and blood pressure should be monitored frequently, and a careful assessment of urine output and fluid intake is mandatory. All patients require bed rest. Experimental studies in mice have shown that exercise increases replication of virus in the myocardium and increases the mortality rate from myocarditis by 100%.[61] Although extrapolating directly from experimental studies in animals to the human situation always is dangerous, suggesting strict bed rest during the early stages of acute myocarditis seems to be a prudent measure. For infants or children with signs of congestive cardiac failure or shock, oxygen should be administered to maintain a normal arterial blood oxygen tension.

No specific therapeutic modality is known that can reverse the myocardial injury directly, but much can be done to maintain adequate tissue perfusion, prevent metabolic disturbances, and support myocardial function. When congestive cardiac failure is identified, digitalis should be administered. This agent should be used with caution, given the increased expression of proinflammatory cytokine and increased mortality rates observed in murine myocarditis treated with high-dose digitalis.[121] Diuretics also are used frequently to treat cardiac failure. Diuretics have no direct beneficial effect on the myocardium; they should be used cautiously because rapid reduction in extracellular fluid volume may lead to shock, and the loss of potassium associated with vigorous diuresis may precipitate digitalis toxicity. The frequency of administration depends on the clinical state of the patient.

If the patient remains in shock despite administration of these high filling pressures, a positive inotropic agent is required. Dopamine exerts an inotropic effect on the heart and concomitantly dilates the renal vessels, improving urine output. Dobutamine, which is a sympathomimetic amine that stimulates β_1-adrenergic, β_2-adrenergic, and α-adrenergic receptors, may be useful when used in combination with dopamine. It has significant inotropic activity while decreasing left ventricular filling pressure.

Isoproterenol, a commonly used inotropic agent, should be avoided because it causes a significant increase in heart rate and may affect cardiac function adversely. When these drugs are used, ensuring normal acid-base balance is important because action of the agents is decreased significantly by acidosis.

Sodium nitroprusside, phentolamine, and the nitrates have been used in adults. These agents have been used less extensively in children. They improve cardiac output by indirectly reducing systemic arterial resistance or venous filling pressure, or both. One study showed a marked improvement in the reduction of inflammation, necrosis, and dystrophic calcification in mice infected with coxsackievirus B3 when they were treated with captopril, an angiotensin-converting enzyme inhibitor, early after development of infection.[153] They improve cardiac output by indirectly reducing systemic arterial resistance or venous filling pressure, or both.

Immune-Modulating Agents

The use of immunosuppressive agents in the treatment of viral or suspected viral myocarditis is controversial. Immunosuppressant therapy in animal models of viral myocarditis has not been shown to be beneficial. One reason for the lack of efficacy of immunosuppressant therapies may relate to the duality of the effects of the immune system. Corticosteroids enhanced viral titers in the early phase of viral murine myocarditis,[94,95] whereas cyclosporine caused greater mortality and cardiac insufficiency in encephalomyocarditis virus myocarditis.[128,184] A report of 13 children with biopsy-confirmed myocarditis treated with prednisone approximately 3 weeks after symptoms occurred showed a marked reduction in inflammation on the follow-up biopsy specimen.[32] This study was uncontrolled, however, and may not truly represent an accurate account of the role of immunosuppressive therapy.

Mason and colleagues[118] used endomyocardial biopsy as a means of diagnosing and following the effects of immunosuppressive therapy in 10 patients. Eight patients received a combination of prednisone and azathioprine, and two patients received prednisone alone. Four patients improved clinically and histologically while on therapy. Two patients who had medications discontinued had relapses, which were reversed with reinstitution of therapy. Only one patient worsened while on therapy, and that patient died. Although the study by Mason and colleagues[118] was uncontrolled, the reversal of congestive heart failure seen in the two patients who were restarted on therapy suggests the beneficial effect of these agents.

Kereiakes and Parmley[92] tabulated most of the studies showing the effects of immunosuppressive therapy in patients with myocarditis. Sixty percent of 82 biopsy-confirmed cases of myocarditis showed improvement with steroids alone or in combination with azathioprine. Patients with lower grade inflammatory changes seemed to do better than did patients with higher grade changes. Complications of immunosuppressive therapy, including opportunistic infections and a cushingoid state, have been reported and may limit the amount and type of therapy.[118,176]

Hobbs and associates[80] used combined prednisone and azathioprine to treat 34 adults with biopsy-confirmed myocarditis. Survival was no better for patients with histologic improvement than for patients with persistent infiltrates. Most patients experienced side effects, some of them lethal, from the corticosteroids. The potential benefits of this type of therapy must be weighed against the risks of immunosuppression in each patient with myocarditis. This therapy apparently does not prevent the observed ECG changes seen in untreated patients or the associated neuritis.[182]

Although numerous anecdotal and small case series suggested that patients with viral myocarditis might benefit from early steroid or immunosuppressive therapy, the results of the Myocarditis Treatment Trial suggested that treating patients who received a histopathologic diagnosis of myocarditis with immunosuppressive therapy for 24 weeks (prednisone plus cyclosporine or prednisone plus azathioprine) did not lead to an improvement in ejection fraction compared with conventional therapy.[119] The major limitation of this study was the unexpectedly low rate of positive biopsy specimens (<10%) and the extension of enrollment to 2 years after the initial clinical presentation. For many patients, the disease possibly already had progressed from ongoing immune-mediated cardiac injury to DCM, and any form of therapy may have been ineffective in this setting. Frustaci and colleagues[58] reported a favorable treatment response in adult patients with chronic active myocarditis. Thirty-eight out of 43 patients (88%) on immunosuppressive therapy (prednisone 1 mg/kg per day for 4 weeks followed by 0.33 mg/kg per day for 5 months and azathioprine 2 mg/kg per day for 6 months) showed an improvement in cardiac function and dimensions, defined as an increase of more than 10 percentage points in the absolute ejection fraction and a reduction of LV end-diastolic volume. None of the untreated patients showed improvement in cardiac function.

Data regarding the efficacy of immunosuppressive therapy for myocarditis in children are limited. Despite lack of consensus, Ghelani et al.[63] reported that use of steroids in acute pediatric myocarditis remained high (23–53%) in the United States between 2006 and 2011. Routine immunosuppressive therapy is not recommended for pediatric myocarditis patients with a stable clinical course. However, many clinicians still recommend aggressive immunosuppressive therapy for patients with fulminant myocarditis and/or a deteriorating clinical course.

Various immunomodulatory therapies have been proposed for the autoimmune phase of viral myocarditis. Kishimoto and colleagues[99] found that immunoglobulin therapy suppressed coxsackievirus B3–induced murine myocarditis and increased survival in C3H/He mice after infection with encephalomyocarditis virus. Intravenous immunoglobulin (IVIG) therapy reduced various proinflammatory markers, including TNF, IFN-γ, macrophage inflammatory protein-2, IL-6, plasma catecholamines, and soluble intercellular adhesion molecule-1.[99] Exogenous immunoglobulins modulate diverse immune response mechanisms; however, the exact mechanism by which IVIG modifies myocarditis remains to be determined. Drucker and associates,[45] who investigated the use of IVIG in 21 of 46 children with myocarditis, showed that patients who received this drug had better left ventricular function at follow-up. Survival tended to be higher at 1 year, although the data did not reach statistical significance because of the small number of patients in the study. More recently, in a prospective placebo-controlled trial with IVIG in adult patients with recent-onset DCM or myocarditis, treatment with IVIG did not result in an improvement in left ventricular function compared with placebo-treated patients.[123] Kim and colleagues[96] retrospectively assessed the effects of IVIG therapy in pediatric patients with presumed myocarditis on survival and recovery of ventricular function. These patients were divided into 2 groups. Group 1 consisted of 23 patients (69.6%) who received IVIG alone or IVIG in combination with steroids, and group 2 consisted of 10 patients (30.3%) who received neither IVIG nor other immunosuppressive agents. One year after the initial presentation, there was no difference between the IVIG-treated patients and the control patients in the degree of recovery of left ventricular function and survival. Although no randomized controlled trials of IVIG for the treatment of myocarditis in children have been reported, many clinicians continue to recommend its use. Ghelani et al.[63] reported that use of IVIG in acute pediatric myocarditis remained high (>70%) in the United States between 2006 and 2011. A 2015 meta-analysis of use of IVIG in acute myocarditis in children and adults did not find enough evidence to recommend its routine use in acute myocarditis.[154]

IFN-β serves as a natural defense against many viral infections. Its innate production is associated with clinical recovery from viral infection and subsequent sequelae, whereas exogenous administration may be protective. Studies have suggested that IFN-β may have a role in the treatment of chronic viral cardiomyopathy. Kuhl and colleagues[101] reported that patients with persistent enterovirus and adenovirus infections of the myocardium responded well to a 6-month course IFN-β_{1a}. Follow-up biopsies taken 3 months after completion of treatment showed complete elimination of enteroviral and adenoviral genomes. Virus clearance was associated with improvement of mean left ventricular function, a decrease in ventricular size, improvement of heart failure symptoms, and a decrease of infiltrating inflammatory cells. Patients with severely affected left ventricular dysfunction experienced the greatest improvement. Additional studies have shown that parvovirus B19 responds less well to IFN-β treatment with respect to virus clearance and hemodynamic changes.[166] Treated patients, however, do show some clinical improvement despite incomplete virus clearance. Data regarding the use of IFN-β therapy for myocarditis in children are not available.

PROGNOSIS

The prognosis of acute myocarditis caused by coxsackievirus B infection in a newborn is poor. Kibrick and Benirschke[93] reported a 75% mortality rate among 25 infants with coxsackievirus B myocarditis. The greatest number of deaths occurred in the first week of the illness. No apparent sequelae occurred in the six infants who survived, although no long-term follow-up data were available. The outlook in other infants and children with clinically recognized myocarditis is better, but mortality rates remain significant (10–25%). Hastreiter and Miller[77] observed complete recovery in 50% of patients. Another 25% became asymptomatic, but abnormal ECGs or chest radiographs persisted. An abnormality may not be evident on the ECG unless the patients are exercised.[16] Despite lack of symptoms, many adult patients have a reduced working capacity associated with exercise stress testing.

The outcome of myocarditis is related partly to the cause. Patients with diphtheritic myocarditis who have arrhythmias or conduction abnormalities have a very poor prognosis. Tahernia[177] found in his study that all patients with disturbances of conduction died. Begg[15] also reported a 100% mortality rate for patients with diphtheritic myocarditis who developed supraventricular tachycardia.

Chronic arrhythmias may persist long after the acute disease has passed. Friedman and colleagues[55] performed a retrospective analysis of 12 patients with biopsy-confirmed myocarditis and complex ventricular arrhythmias at the time of presentation (11 with ventricular tachycardia). Five of the 12 patients still were receiving antiarrhythmic therapy at a median follow-up of 50 months. Complex ventricular arrhythmias still were present in these patients (three with ventricular tachycardia and two with couplets or multiforms), requiring ongoing therapy. The investigators concluded that although the arrhythmias were controlled more easily than at presentation of the patients, ongoing surveillance was essential in ensuring the suppression of these potentially life-threatening arrhythmias. Children who recover from myocarditis, regardless of cause, should be followed indefinitely.

MYOCARDITIS IN CASES OF HUMAN IMMUNODEFICIENCY VIRUS INFECTION

Infection with human immunodeficiency virus (HIV) may affect the heart adversely. Cardiac dysfunction, including congestive heart failure, may occur; many patients who have died and undergone autopsy are shown to have myocarditis. Anderson and associates[5] retrospectively analyzed 71 consecutive necropsy patients who died of acquired immunodeficiency syndrome (AIDS) and found that 52% had evidence of myocarditis.

Another study examined autopsy specimens of 26 consecutive cases. Lymphocytic myocarditis was seen in nine patients (35%), and another seven patients had lymphocytic infiltrates without myocytolysis.[14] Acierno[2] correctly pointed out that a distinction must be made between AIDS-associated myocarditis and secondary myocarditis caused by known pathogens or idiopathic myocarditis.

Reilly and colleagues[152] found a 45% incidence of myocarditis in 58 consecutive autopsy cases. Congestive heart failure, ventricular tachycardia, and other ECG abnormalities were seen in nearly 60% of the patients. Two patients died suddenly, both with myocarditis. In a prospective study of asymptomatic HIV-infected patients, the reported mean annual incidence of progression to DCM was 15.9 cases per 1000 patients. Endomyocardial biopsy specimens revealed myocardial inflammation in 63 of 76 (83%) of these high-risk patients. HIV-infected cardiac myocytes were detected by in situ hybridization in 58 of 76 (76%) patients.

In a prospective multicenter study of 205 vertically HIV-infected children enrolled at a median age of 1.9 years and 600 HIV-exposed children enrolled prenatally or as neonates, the 5-year cumulative incidence of cardiac dysfunction ranged from 18% to 39% in HIV-infected children.[175] Myocardial inflammation, with or without cell destruction, is a frequent finding in patients infected with HIV. Whether this response is due to the virus itself or to opportunistic agents or other toxic reactions is unclear.

Another important cause of cardiomyopathy in HIV/AIDS is drug cardiotoxicity. Zidovudine is associated with diffuse destruction of cardiac mitochondrial ultrastructure and inhibition of mitochondrial DNA replication that may contribute to myocardial cell dysfunction.[105]

The use of highly active anti-retroviral therapy (HAART) regimens, by reducing the incidence of myocarditis, has reduced the prevalence of HIV-associated cardiomyopathy by about 30% in developed countries.[13]

PARASITIC MYOCARDITIS

Chagas Disease

Parasitic myocarditis is an uncommon form of heart disease in the United States. Chagas disease is caused by infection with *Trypanosoma cruzi*. It is a long-lived infection that, in 1991, affected approximately 17 million individuals in Latin America.[158] Substantial progress has been made in the control of Chagas disease in affected areas, but, in 2010, the estimated global incidence was 5.7 million.[19] This disease is endemic in Mexico and Central and South America, where vector-borne transmission of *T. cruzi* typically occurs in persons living in rural areas. Emigration from Chagas-endemic areas has changed the epidemiology of this disease in the United States and other nonendemic regions. Bern and Montgomery have estimated that 300,000 persons living in the United States are chronically infected with *T. cruzi*.[20]

After inoculation, the protozoa multiply and migrate widely throughout the body. Host control of this parasite has been shown to depend on humoral and cell-mediated adaptive responses and elements of the innate immune system.[66]

Immune-mediated cardiac injury, caused primarily by infiltrating mononuclear cells, probably is the main mechanism responsible for the development of chronic Chagas heart disease. This hypothesis is supported by several observations. Animal models of *T. cruzi* infection have shown lysis of nonparasitized cardiac myocytes by immune effector cells[6]; depletion of $CD4^+$ T-lymphocyte subpopulations abrogates myocardial injury in a murine model of chronic Chagas disease; and myocardial damage can be induced in healthy animals by passive transfer of $CD4^+$ T cells from *T. cruzi*–infected mice.[43] Although $CD4^+$ T cells seem to be crucial in myocardial injury, $CD8^+$ T cells may have a protective role. Mice depleted of $CD8^+$ T cells have a robust parasitemia, but almost no inflammatory infiltrates are seen in the parasite-infected tissues.[179] A role for TLR signaling in resistance to *T. cruzi* is suggested by the observations that mice deficient in MyD88, an adapter molecule required for signaling events by most TLRs, show enhanced susceptibility to infection with this protozoan parasite.[29]

Acute Chagas disease usually is an illness of children, but it can occur at any age.[129] Histologic examination of the heart during the acute phase reveals intracellular parasites with a marked cellular infiltrate, particularly around myocytes that have ruptured and released the parasites.[144] A well-established fact is that intracellular parasites are found in cardiac myocytes only during the acute phase of illness.

Histologic examination reveals focal but widespread areas of cellular infiltrates composed of plasma cells, eosinophils, mast cells, and macrophages.[131] Extensive fibrosis occurs, replacing previously damaged myocardial tissue. In contrast to the situation observed in acute disease, the presence of parasites (a rare finding) in tissue has little correlation with myocardial pathology. Inflammatory changes in the right bundle branch and the anterior fascicle of the left bundle branch explain the frequent occurrence of right bundle branch and left anterior fascicular block.[132]

Vector-borne acute Chagas disease is usually mild, and most acute infections are subclinical. After an incubation period of 1 to 2 weeks, a newly infected individual may develop nonspecific signs and symptoms such as fever, chills, myalgias, tachycardia, rash, and meningeal irritation. A raised inflammatory lesion at the site of parasite entry (a chagoma), unilateral periorbital edema (Romaña sign), conjunctivitis, lymphadenopathy, and hepatosplenomegaly may also be observed in acute infection.[114] The clinical manifestations of chronic Chagas disease range from isolated rhythm disturbances to advanced disease characterized by cardiomegaly, chronic congestive heart failure, and arrhythmias. Syncope also is a frequent problem of the disease. In one series of 53 patients with chronic Chagas disease, the most frequent causes of recurrent syncope were ventricular tachycardia (43%) with a poor prognosis and paroxysmal atrioventricular block (21%) with a favorable prognosis.[117] Sudden death caused by ventricular fibrillation is a constant threat and may develop before cardiomegaly or heart failure is diagnosed.[31]

Severe myocarditis develops in only a few acute cases, and most deaths are caused by the resultant congestive heart failure and pericardial effusion. Nonspecific ECG changes are seen, but the life-threatening arrhythmias that are frequent occurrences in chronic Chagas disease generally do not occur. In most patients with more acute disease (90% of cases), symptoms resolve gradually over weeks to months.

Chronic progressive Chagas disease develops in 10% to 20% of previously asymptomatically infected individuals.[46] It is manifested by a chronic, diffuse, progressive fibrosing myocarditis that involves the myocytes and the atrioventricular conduction system.[131,132] On gross examination, the heart usually is enlarged and flaccid. Thrombus formation frequently occurs, and thrombus may fill much of the apex of the left ventricle in some cases.

The diagnosis of acute *T. cruzi* infection in a patient is usually made by the detection of parasites in wet mounts of blood and in Giemsa-stained slides. Testing for anti-*T. cruzi* immunoglobulin M antibodies is not useful because tests for this antibody isotype are not well standardized. The diagnosis of chronic Chagas disease cannot be made solely on the basis of histologic examination of the heart. PCR testing is thought to be the most sensitive method for detecting acute *T. cruzi* infection. This test is available at the Centers for Disease Control and Prevention (CDC) in the United States.

Serologic testing is the method of choice for establishing the diagnosis of chronic Chagas disease. Several highly sensitive serologic tests for the detection of anti–*T. cruzi* antibodies, such as indirect hemagglutination, complement fixation, indirect immunofluorescence, and enzyme-linked immunosorbent assay, are available.[97,171] A radioimmunoprecipitation assay based on iodinated *T. cruzi* proteins is sensitive and specific and is currently being used for confirmatory testing of many U.S. blood donor samples that are positive in one of the two screening tests currently approved by the U.S. Food and Drug Administration (FDA) for donor screening.[114]

The treatment of Chagas disease involves both parasite-specific therapy and adjunctive therapy for the management of the clinical manifestations. Benznidazole and nifurtimox are the only available drugs with activity against *T. cruzi*. Neither drug is FDA-approved, but both are available under investigational use protocols (CDC Drug Service: http://www.cdc.gov/laboratory/drugservice/index.html). Although these two drugs have been thought to be ineffective and/or too toxic for treating chronic infections, in a recent report a 60-day course of benznidazole therapy eliminated infection in more than 60% of chronically infected children.[7] These drugs are most effective for the treatment of acute and congenital infection. Parasitologic cure is believed to occur in 60% to 85% of persons with acute infection who complete a full course of either drug, although there are no large-scale studies to support these data. Patients with acute infections, including congenitally acquired infections in neonates, and chronically infected children should be treated. Bern and colleagues[18,21] have described the management of persons newly diagnosed with Chagas disease as a result of screening prompted by country of origin or blood donation. Benznidazole showed sustained trypanocidal activity in 94% of patients who completed treatment and follow-up. The major problem was discontinuation of benznidazole because of allergic dermatitis in 19% of patients. The recently completed BENEFIT trial randomly assigned 2854 patients with chronic Chagas cardiomyopathy to receive either benznidazole or placebo for up to 80 days with mean 5.4-year follow-up.[130] Benznidazole reduced serum PCR parasite detection at the end of treatment compared with placebo (66.2% vs. 33.5%). At 2-year follow-up, 55.4% of the treated group versus 35.5% of the placebo group had parasitemia detected by PCR. Of note, benznidazole treatment for up to 80 days did not reduce the primary clinical outcome (death, resuscitated cardiac arrest, sustained ventricular tachycardia, insertion of a pacemaker or implantable cardioverter-defibrillator, cardiac transplantation, new heart failure, stroke, or other thromboembolic event). Based on these findings, the authors recommend antitrypanosomal therapy for patients with early chronic Chagas disease, including those with cardiomyopathy. The antifungal agent posaconazole has been reported in treatment of a patient with chronic Chagas disease.[145] However, in a recent trial that included 78 adult patients with chronic Chagas, treatment failure was most commonly associated with posaconazole treatment.[127]

Other Parasitic Causes of Myocarditis

Myocarditis is one of the most serious complications of trichinosis. The disease develops when undercooked meat contaminated with infective larvae of *Trichinella* is eaten. Myocardial invasion by *Trichinella spiralis* has been well described, but encystment within the myocardium has been reported only rarely.[98] At autopsy, the heart may be dilated and a pericardial effusion may be identified. Histologically, a prominent focal infiltrate composed of lymphocytes and eosinophils with interstitial edema and scattered hemorrhages commonly is found.[173]

Myocarditis usually is mild, with few clinical signs and symptoms. This myocarditis may range from chest pain to fatal congestive heart failure, however, and may mimic acute myocardial infarction.[35,70] The frequencies of ECG abnormalities among 154 cases of trichinellosis were determined to be 56%.[148] The abnormalities on ECG most frequently observed were a nonspecific ventricular repolarization disturbance (with ST-T–wave changes), followed by bundle branch conduction disturbances and sinus tachycardia. Despite ECG evidence of myocardial involvement, less than 0.1% of patients with trichinosis die of this complication.[70]

The definitive diagnosis of trichinosis is based on the presence of the larval forms in tissue biopsy samples, usually from a large tender area such as the gastrocnemius muscle. Serologic testing is available through state laboratories and the CDC. Typically serum antibody titers become positive during or after the third week of illness. The efficacy of mebendazole or albendazole in the treatment of myocarditis caused by *Trichinella* infection has not been evaluated adequately.

Toxocara canis, the principal cause of visceral larva migrans, is a rare cause of myocarditis. Most reported cases have occurred in children younger than 3 years of age.[37,187] The myocardial lesions noted on histologic examination have included granulomata and extensive eosinophilic infiltrates with foci of muscle necrosis. The clinical presentation may be acute respiratory distress caused by congestive heart failure, requiring administration of oxygen and diuretic therapy. Asymptomatic infection involving the heart also has been reported.[37]

The definitive diagnosis of *T. canis* infection requires microscopic identification of the larvae in biopsy specimens of the liver or heart, but this finding is infrequent. An enzyme immunoassay for *Toxocara* serum antibodies, which is available at the CDC, can provide presumptive evidence of toxocariasis.

Toxoplasma gondii may cause myocarditis as part of disseminated infection or, less frequently, as an isolated cardiac infection. In infants with congenital toxoplasmosis, the clinical manifestations usually are those of meningoencephalitis, but at autopsy, extensive myocardial involvement has been documented.[204] Outside the newborn period, infection with this intracellular parasite most commonly occurs in immunosuppressed patients with malignant diseases, patients with AIDS,[30] and patients who have undergone cardiac or bone marrow transplantation.[113] Histologic examination of the heart reveals focal interstitial infiltrates consisting of histiocytes, lymphocytes, plasma cells, eosinophils, and very few polymorphonuclear cells.[181] Toxoplasma is seen as basophilic masses within a pseudocyst in normal or damaged myocardial fibers.

Clinical manifestations may include arrhythmias (atrial and ventricular), atrioventricular block, atypical chest pain, pericarditis, and heart failure. The diagnosis of toxoplasmic myocarditis requires the exclusion of other specific forms of heart disease and the establishment of evidence of toxoplasmosis with serologic testing. The diagnosis may be aided by endomyocardial biopsy.[113] Treatment with pyrimethamine and sulfonamides (especially sulfadiazine) has been reported in patients with isolated toxoplasmic myocarditis, but the response to therapy has varied. In one series of toxoplasmic myocarditis, relapses occurred in 17% of cases after therapy.[103]

Myocardial disease also has been reported after infection with *Echinococcus granulosus* and *Plasmodium falciparum.*[98] Cardiac involvement is estimated to occur in less than 2% of cases of echinococcosis.[41] When it does occur, the cysts usually are located in the intramyocardial region and protrude into the adjacent cardiac chambers. The clinical manifestations depend primarily on the location and size of the cyst. Rupture of the cyst is the most dreaded complication because it may lead to pericarditis, anaphylactic shock, or pulmonary emboli. Two-dimensional echocardiography is the preferred imaging study to detect and localize cysts.[139] Myocardial changes also have been documented in fatal malaria, particularly when caused by *P. falciparum.* Histologically blocking of the coronary arteries and capillaries with parasites, local hemorrhage, and deposit of pigment occurs. Clinical findings suggestive of cardiac involvement are rare, however. In a series of 49 patients with falciparum malaria, no ECG evidence of cardiac involvement was found.[174]

Myocarditis also has occurred in association with primary amebic meningoencephalitis caused by *Naegleria.* In a retrospective study, focal or diffuse myocarditis was documented in more than 40% of cases.[115] Myocardial involvement is not a clinically significant manifestation of this uniformly fatal central nervous system infection.

NEW REFERENCES SINCE THE SEVENTH EDITION

4. Akira S. TLR signaling. *Curr Top Microbiol Immunol.* 2006;311:1-16.
5. Anderson DW, Virmani R, Reilly JM, et al. Prevalent myocarditis at necropsy in the acquired immunodeficiency syndrome. *J Am Coll Cardiol.* 1988;11:792-799.
12. Bairan AC, Cherry JD, Fagan LF, et al. Complete heart block and respiratory syncytial virus infection. *Am J Dis Child.* 1974;127:264-265.
16. Bengtsson E, Lamberger B. Five-year follow-up study of cases suggestive of acute myocarditis. *Am Heart J.* 1966;72:751-776.
19. Bern C. Chagas' disease. *N Engl J Med.* 2015;373:456-466.
23. Bowles NE, Richardson PJ, Olsen EG, et al. Detection of coxsackie-B-virus-specific RNA sequences in myocardial biopsy samples from patients with myocarditis and dilated cardiomyopathy. *Lancet.* 1986;1:1120-1123.
24. Breinholt JP, Moulik M, Dreyer WJ, et al. Viral epidemiologic shift in inflammatory heart disease: the increasing involvement of parvovirus B19 in the myocardium of pediatric cardiac transplant patients. *J Heart Lung Transplant.* 2010;29:739-746.
25. Brighenti M, Donti A, Giulia GM, et al. Endomyocardial biopsy safety and clinical yield in pediatric myocarditis: an Italian perspective. *Catheter Cardiovasc Interv.* 2016;87(4):762-767.
26. Brightman VJ, Scott TF, Westphal M, et al. An outbreak of coxsackie B-5 virus infection in a newborn nursery. *J Pediatr.* 1966;69:179-192.
33. Chapman NM, Tracy S, Gauntt CJ, et al. Molecular detection and identification of enteroviruses using enzymatic amplification and nucleic acid hybridization. *J Clin Microbiol.* 1990;28:843-850.
39. Dec GW, Fallon JT, Southern JF, et al. "Borderline" myocarditis: an indication for repeat endomyocardial biopsy. *J Am Coll Cardiol.* 1990;15:283-289.
47. Easton AJ, Eglin RP. The detection of coxsackievirus RNA in cardiac tissue by in situ hybridization. *J Gen Virol.* 1988;69:285-291.
56. Friedrich MG, Sechtem U, Schulz-Menger J, et al. Cardiovascular magnetic resonance in myocarditis: a JACC white paper. *J Am Coll Cardiol.* 2009;53:1475-1487.
57. Fruhling L, Korn R, Lavillaureix J, et al. Chronic fibroelastic myoendocarditis of the newborn and the infant (fibroelastosis). New morphological, etiological and pathogenic data. Relation to certain cardiac abnormalities. *Ann Anat Pathol.* 1962;7:227-303.
63. Ghelani SJ, Spaeder MC, Pastor W, et al. Demographics, trends, and outcomes in pediatric acute myocarditis in the United States, 2006 to 2011. *Circ Cardiovasc Qual Outcomes.* 2012;5:622-627.
73. Gutgesell HP, Paquet M, Duff DF, et al. Evaluation of left ventricular size and function by echocardiography. Results in normal children. *Circulation.* 1977;56:457-462.
74. Halsell JS, Riddle JR, Atwood JE. Myopericarditis following smallpox vaccination among vaccinia-naive US military personnel. *JAMA.* 2003;289:3283-3289.
75. Hardarson HS, Baker JS, Yang Z, et al. Toll-like receptors 3 is an essential component of the innate stress response in virus-induced cardiac injury. *Am J Physiol Heart Circ Physiol.* 2007;292(1):H251-H258.
98. Kirchhoff LV, Weiss LM, Wittner M, et al. B. Parasitic diseases of the heart. *Front Biosci.* 2004;9:706-723.
108. Lind J, Hulquist GT. Isolated myocarditis in newborn and young infants. *Am Heart J.* 1949;38:123.
109. Liu P, Aitken K, Kong YY, et al. The tyrosine kinase p56(lck) is essential in coxsackievirus B3-mediated heart disease. *Nat Med.* 2000;6:429-434.
114. Machado FS, Jelicks LA, Kirchhoff LV, et al. Chagas heart disease: report on recent developments. *Cardiol Rev.* 2012;20:53-65.
115. Markowitz SM, Martinez AJ, Duma RJ, et al. Myocarditis associated with primary amebic (*Naegleria*) meningoencephalitis. *Am J Clin Pathol.* 1974;62:619-628.
116. Martin AB, Webber S, Fricker FJ, et al. Acute myocarditis. Rapid diagnosis by PCR in children. *Circulation.* 1994;90:330-339.
123. McNamara DM, Holubkov R, Starling RC, et al. Controlled trial of intravenous immune globulin in recent-onset dilated cardiomyopathy. *Circulation.* 2001; 103:2254-2259.
124. Miklozek CL, Crumpacker CS, Royal HD, et al. Myocarditis presenting as acute myocardial infarction. *Am Heart J.* 1988;115:768-776.
127. Molina I, Prat J, Salvador F, et al. Randomized trial of posaconazole and benznidazole for chronic Chagas' disease. *N Engl J Med.* 2014;370:1899-1908.
126. Molina KM, Garcia X, Denfield SW, et al. Parvovirus B19 myocarditis causes significant morbidity and mortality in children. *Pediatr Cardiol.* 2013;34:390-397.
130. Morillo CA, Marin-Neto JA, Avezum A, et al. Randomized trial of benznidazole for chronic Chagas' cardiomyopathy. *N Engl J Med.* 2015;373:1295-1306.
131. Morris SA, Tanowitz HB, Wittner M, et al. Pathophysiological insights into the cardiomyopathy of Chagas' disease. *Circulation.* 1990;82:1900-1909.
147. Pophal SG, Sigfusson G, Booth KL, et al. Complications of endomyocardial biopsy in children. *J Am Coll Cardiol.* 1999;34:2105-2110.
153. Rezkalla S, Kloner RA, Khatib G, et al. Beneficial effects of captopril in acute coxsackievirus B3 murine myocarditis. *Circulation.* 1990;81:1039-1046.

154. Robinson J, Hartling L, Vandermeer B, et al. Intravenous immunoglobulin for presumed viral myocarditis in children and adults. *Cochrane Database Syst Rev.* 2015;(5):CD004370.
155. Rosenbaum HD, Nadas AS, Neuhauser EB. Primary myocardial disease in infancy and childhood. *AMA Am J Dis Child.* 1953;86:28-44.
156. Rosenberg HS, McNamara DG. Acute myocarditis in infancy and childhood. *Prog Cardiovasc Dis.* 1964;7:179-197.
157. Ross LJ. Electrocardiographic findings in measles. *AMA Am J Dis Child.* 1952;83:282-291.
159. Sachdeva S, Song X, Dham N, et al. Analysis of clinical parameters and cardiac magnetic resonance imaging as predictors of outcome in pediatric myocarditis. *Am J Cardiol.* 2015;115:499-504.
171. Spencer HC, Allain DS, Sulzer AJ, et al. Evaluation of the micro enzyme-linked immunosorbent assay for antibodies to *Trypanosoma cruzi. Am J Trop Med Hyg.* 1980;29:179-182.
172. Spencer MJ, Cherry JD, Adams FH, et al. Letter: Supraventricular tachycardia in an infant associated with a rhinoviral infection. *J Pediatr.* 1975;86:811-812.
174. Sprague WW. The effects of malaria on the heart. *Am Heart J.* 1946;31:426-430.
176. Strain JE, Grose RM, Factor SM, et al. Results of endomyocardial biopsy in patients with spontaneous ventricular tachycardia but without apparent structural heart disease. *Circulation.* 1983;68:1171-1181.
178. Take M, Sekiguchi M, Hiroe M, et al. Long-term follow-up of electrocardiographic findings in patients with acute myocarditis proven by endomyocardial biopsy. *Jpn Circ J.* 1982;46:1227-1234.
187. Vargo TA, Singer DB, Gillatte PC, et al. Myocarditis due to visceral larva migrans. *J Pediatr.* 1977;90:322-323.
188. Vigneswaran TV, Brown JR, Breuer J, et al. Parvovirus B19 myocarditis in children: an observational study. *Arch Dis Child.* 2015;101(2):177-180.
191. Weiss LM, Liu XF, Chang KL, et al. Detection of enteroviral RNA in idiopathic dilated cardiomyopathy and other human cardiac tissues. *J Clin Invest.* 1992;90:156-159.
192. Weiss LM, Movahed LA, Berry GJ, et al. In situ hybridization studies for viral nucleic acids in heart and lung allograft biopsies. *Am J Clin Pathol.* 1990;93:675-679.
193. Weiss LM, Movahed LA, Billingham ME, et al. Detection of coxsackievirus B3 RNA in myocardial tissues by the polymerase chain reaction. *Am J Pathol.* 1991;138:497-503.

The full reference list for this chapter is available at ExpertConsult.com.

29 Acute Rheumatic Fever

Diana R. Lennon

Acute rheumatic fever (ARF) is an inflammatory disease of the heart, joints, central nervous system, and subcutaneous tissues that develops after a nasopharyngeal infection by one of the group A β-hemolytic streptococci. The pathogenesis of this disease, a clinical syndrome without a specific diagnostic test, remains an enigma, and specific treatment is unavailable. Prevention of initial and recurrent attacks is possible, however, with penicillin treatment and prophylaxis. Rheumatic fever is especially important because of the heart disease that often ensues, and such disease may lead to chronic progressive damage and premature death. As succinctly stated by Lasègue many years ago, "Rheumatic fever licks the joints and bites the heart"[273]—a statement that holds true today.

The unexpected upsurge in this disease in the United States in the late 1980s and 1990s and more recently in Italy, reports of increasing invasive group A streptococcal infections in some areas,[216,317,329] the honing of echocardiography in the diagnosis of rheumatic heart disease (RHD), and increased effort in the search for a vaccine have renewed interest in group A streptococci.

Globally recognition that rheumatic fever is the leading cause of acquired heart disease in children and young adults worldwide led to action at the close of the last century.[213] Action has intensified recently after a landmark paper suggesting the global RHD burden may be considerably more than previously thought.[176]

EPIDEMIOLOGY

The overall incidence and severity of ARF have decreased in recent years in developed Western countries and in prosperous countries of Asia.[2] Reliable morbidity data on the occurrence of ARF in total populations are lacking because studies often consider only a segment of a population.[288] The trend seems clear, however. Some of the best long-term data come from Denmark, where rheumatic fever has been a reportable disease for many years.[299] A steady decline has been occurring since 1900, except for a peak during World War II (Fig. 29.1). In the United States, rheumatic fever is not a reportable disease, but mortality rates (Fig. 29.2) and hospital discharge rates (Fig. 29.3 and Table 29.1) have shown a steady decline. Although this decline was already under way, it seems to have been accelerated by the introduction of penicillin.[180]

The dramatic decline in the incidence of rheumatic fever began in the United States in the late 1940s (see Fig. 29.2). During the late 1950s, the 1960s, and the early 1970s, studies in the United States showed annual rates of 13.5 to 62.5 first attacks per 100,000 children 5 to 14 years of age; however, these studies are not strictly comparable in design.[46,67,111,220,241,255] Some of them were conducted in low-income urban areas, locations in which the incidence of rheumatic fever was thought to be higher. Secondary prevention of rheumatic fever with penicillin prophylaxis to protect against recurrent attacks probably became widespread in the 1960s. Denny and colleagues[82] showed the possibility of preventing initial attacks with injectable penicillin in 1950 in military camps after the original observation by Massell and colleagues.[187] Similar conclusive controlled studies were not repeated in the general or pediatric populations or with oral penicillin.

The most compelling evidence that appropriate medical intervention helps reduce the number of initial attacks of rheumatic fever comes from a study by Gordis[111] of health care availability in an at-risk inner-city Baltimore population. The rate of ARF was reduced by 60% over the course of a decade in only those census tracts receiving a comprehensive care program, with that reduction occurring only in patients with an identifiable preceding clinical respiratory tract infection. A similar trend with small numbers of patients was seen for the Navajo and Papago American Indian populations in school-based intervention programs[17,67] and in an Alaskan program.[42] Other school-based interventions[226] have reduced streptococcal prevalence rates but have not gone the necessary further step to show a reduction in rheumatic fever morbidity in a controlled, carefully demarcated population. A recent systematic review and meta-analysis of available evidence supports the premise that a community- or school-based initiative can reduce rheumatic fever by an estimated approximately 60% (relative risk, 0.41; 95% confidence interval [CI], 0.23–0.70), acknowledging the eligible studies are of variable quality but are unlikely to be replicated.[156]

Promising evidence is accruing with reduction of first-episode ARF in a school-based program in a well-demarcated population in New Zealand that may eventually provide evidence for primary prevention of ARF using an oral penicillin preparation outside of a military population.[161,269] Recurrences in this population had already been controlled.[269]

An unexplained high incidence of ARF persists in Hawaii, especially in Polynesian and part-Polynesian children.[61,148] Similarly, rates are higher in larger populations of Polynesian (including indigenous Maori) children in New Zealand,[159,197] although increasing evidence from that

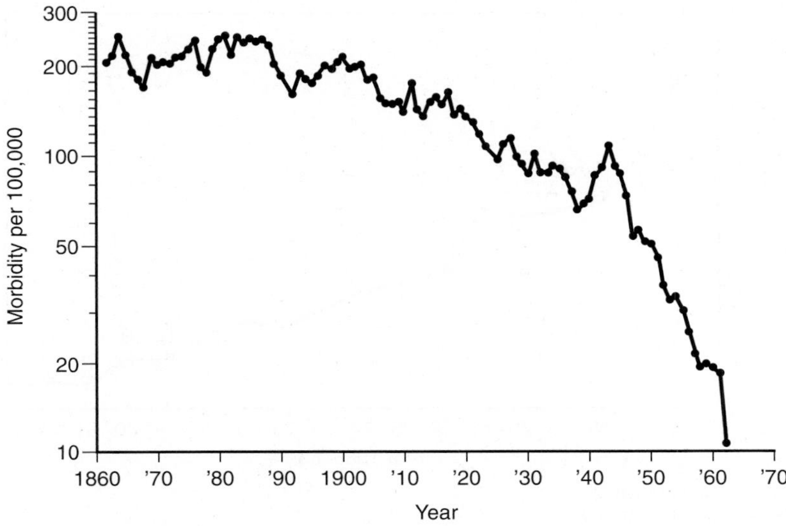

FIG. 29.1 Reported annual incidence of ARF in Denmark, 1862–1962. (Modified from Public Health Board of Denmark. Reported rheumatic fever incidence in Denmark, 1862–1962. In: Vendsborg P, Hansen LF, Olesen KH. Decreasing incidence of a history of ARF in chronic RHD. *Cardiologia.* 1968;53:332–40. Used with permission of S. Karger AG, Basel.)

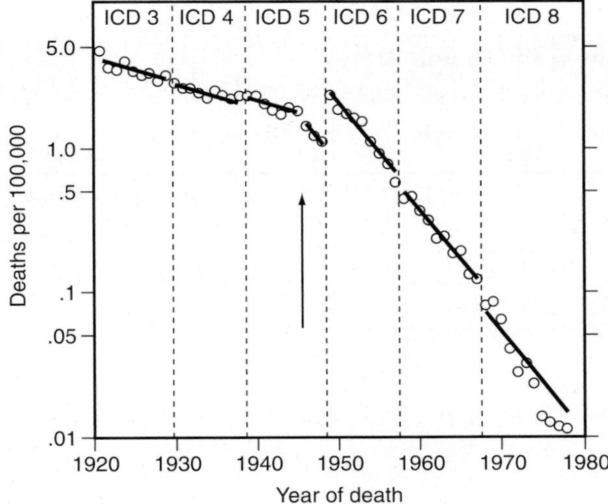

FIG. 29.2 U.S. national mortality rates from rheumatic fever in individuals 5 to 19 years old, 1921–78. Values are age adjusted to the 1950 U.S. population. Trend lines are fitted for each era (1921–45 and 1946–78) separately and take International Classification of Diseases (ICD) revisions into account. The *arrow* separates the two eras. (From Massell BF, Chute CG, Walker AM, Kurland GS. Penicillin and the marked decrease in morbidity and mortality from rheumatic fever in the United States. *N Engl J Med.* 1988;318:280–6.)

TABLE 29.1 Reported Incidence of Acute Rheumatic Fever in Studies in the United States: 1970–81

Location	Years of Study	Rate/100,000	Age Range (y)
Fairfax, VA	1970–80	1.14	0–18
Rhode Island	1976–80	0.23	5–17
Memphis, TN	1977–81	1.88	5–17
Baltimore, MD	1977–81	0.5	5–19
San Fernando, CA	1971–80	0.63	5–17

Modified from Veasy LG, Wiedmeier SE, Orsmond GS, et al. Resurgence of ARF in the intermountain area of the United States. *N Engl J Med.* 1987;316:421–7; and Markowitz M, Kaplan EL. Reappearance of rheumatic fever. *Adv Pediatr.* 1989;36:44.

country points toward low socioeconomic status, including housing and income issues, and associated factors such as a lesser degree of education playing a role.[68,132] In some areas of the continental United States, the rate of endemic rheumatic fever continues to exceed that of the general population in some children traditionally considered to be at risk (urban African Americans), although not in others (recent Hispanic immigrants).[92] In contrast, in a hospital-based study in another urban area, Hispanic children, reflecting the pediatric population being served, were the most affected.[118]

From the beginning of 1985, the number of patients with ARF in several centers on the U.S. mainland increased. Although these numbers were not large, they represented a definite increase in the outbreak areas (Table 29.2).[286] The resurgence in Utah since 1985 led to more than 600 cases.[184] Nationally, however, the number of diagnoses of ARF, in the absence of robust surveillance data, appeared to continue to decline gradually from 1984 through 1990.[286] The populations (aside from clusters in military populations)[13,303] generally did not seem to be those considered to have been at risk in the past; most patients were white and middle class and lived in suburban or rural communities with ready access to medical care. In the Utah and Tennessee outbreaks,[298,314] the families were larger than the state average. The military outbreaks[13,306] were the first in 2 decades in U.S. military personnel. Factors other than the widespread use of antibiotics and improved availability of health care are likely to be important because group A streptococci are rated moderately infectious agents in close contacts.[79,242] Overcrowded living circumstances long have been considered a risk factor.[223] This hypothesis was not substantiated as an important risk factor by conditional logistic regression in a modern (Yugoslavian) study[301] but was supported in a recent ecologic study also exploring multivariant relationships where ARF rates are high.[132] The disquieting feature in these more recent U.S. outbreaks was the severity of the illness, especially in the Salt Lake City outbreak: 72% of patients had clinical carditis (Table 29.3), 19% had severe carditis with or without congestive heart failure, and three patients required mitral valve replacement. However, this report was from a cardiology center, which is likely to reflect a referral bias. Earlier U.S. reports documented clinical carditis in initial attacks of rheumatic fever in 40% to 51% of patients (1951 through 1965).[179] Longitudinal

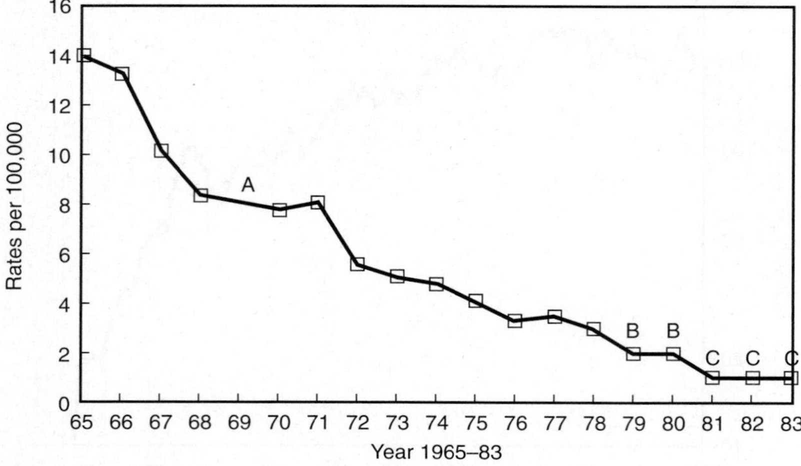

FIG. 29.3 Annual rates (per 100,000) of discharge of patients with rheumatic fever from short-stay nonfederal hospitals in the United States, 1965 to 1983. (From National Hospital Discharge Survey, NCHS. Modified from Gordis L. The virtual disappearance of rheumatic fever in the United States: lessons in the rise and fall of disease. *Circulation.* 1985;72:1155–62.)

TABLE 29.2 Reported Outbreaks of Acute Rheumatic Fever in the United States: Selected Epidemiologic Features

	Salt Lake City, UT[94,261]	Columbus, OH[59]	Akron, OH[33]	Pittsburgh, PA[329,144]	San Diego, CA[126]	Tennessee[136a]
Time	1985–92	June 1984–September 1986	1986	1987–June 1990	December 86–July 1987	January 1987–July 1988
No. cases	274	40	23	60	50	26
White (%)	93	80	96	97	50	80
Family income	80% middle	73% middle	$20,000–$40,000	3 of 17 on assistance[329]	NA	$18,000
Suburban-rural residents	Most[94]	85%	Many	75%[136]	NA	20%
History of sore throat (n^b)	77 (46)	22 (NA)	18 (NA)	4/17 (3/17)[329]; 28/43 (11/43)[144c]	6 (3)	15 (7)
Family history of rheumatic fever (%)	NA	5	16	64[329]	NA	NA
Recurrences	27	1	0	2	1	0
M types of group A streptococci isolated from:						
Patients	1 × M-1; 1 × M-5	NA	M-1, M-5, M-18	NA	[d]	Mucoid M-18/T-1; mucoid nontypeable
Families	3 × M-3; 1 × M-1; 1 × M-18; 1 × M-78	NA	M-6	NA	NA	NA
Community	9 × M-18 (8/9 mucoid); 1 × M-4, M-5, M-6, M-9, M-11, M-12; 6 nontypeable	Mucoid M-18	NA	NA	NA	Mucoid M-18

NA, Not available.
[a]Family size greater than the state average.
[b]Number who sought treatment.
[c]Respiratory illness.
[d]San Diego: Five of seven available sera positive for antibodies to M-18; three of seven, positive for M-1 antibodies; two of seven, positive for M-5 and M-6 antibodies; and one of seven, positive for M-24 antibodies.
Modified from Veasy LG, Wiedmeier SE, Orsmond GS, et al. Resurgence of ARF in the intermountain area of the United States. *N Engl J Med.* 1987;316:421–7; and Markowitz M, Kaplan EL. Reappearance of rheumatic fever. *Adv Pediatr.* 1989;36:39–68.

TABLE 29.3 Clinical Manifestations in Six Outbreaks of Acute Rheumatic Fever

Manifestation	Salt Lake City, UT, 1985–92 (*n* = 274) (%)	Columbus, OH, 1984–86 (*n* = 40) (%)	Northeastern Ohio, 1986 (*n* = 23) (%)	Pittsburgh, PA, 1985–June 1990 (*n* = 60) (%)	San Diego, CA, Naval Base, 1986–87 (*n* = 10) (%)	Tennessee, 1987–88 (*n* = 26) (%)
Arthritis	36	62	78	43	100	58
Carditis	68[a]	50	30	52	30	73
Chorea	37	17	9	37	0	31
Erythema marginatum	4	12	1	0	0	4
Subcutaneous nodules	3	0	0	0	10	0

[a]85% with Doppler ultrasound examination.
Modified from Markowitz M, Kaplan EL. Reappearance of rheumatic fever. *Adv Pediatr.* 1989;36:39–68.

observations at the same institution suggest a decreasing frequency of clinical carditis (73% from 1921 to 1930, 51% from 1951 to 1960).[40,185]

With the use of Doppler echocardiography, carditis rates in the Utah patients increased to 91% (see Table 29.3). The duration of secondary penicillin prophylaxis and endocarditis prophylaxis is an important consideration for patients with nonclinical carditis. The place of echocardiography in the diagnosis and management of rheumatic fever continues to evolve (see "Laboratory Findings"). Rheumatic fever presenting with arthritis may be misdiagnosed or not be admitted to the hospital, which is likely to affect estimates of rates of carditis in studies that are not population based.[122]

A more recent assessment of hospitalized ARF disease in the United States in children younger than 21 years of age found a low rate of 14.8/100,000 hospitalized children (503 cases).[200] The prevalence of RHD, which represents the result of many years of exposure to the risks for acquiring ARF, seems to have declined in the United States over the course of many years.[207]

Many different racial and ethnic groups have been deemed unusually susceptible to rheumatic fever. They usually have been minority groups within a given area who are of lower socioeconomic status than the general population (e.g., Malays in Singapore, Arabs in Israel, Bantus in South Africa, indigenous Maori and Pacific Polynesians in New Zealand, blacks in the United States, aborigines in Australia).[2,68,123,178] In the United States, when differences in socioeconomic status or degree of crowding were taken into account,[114] the differences in the incidence of rheumatic fever,[113] prevalence of RHD,[207] and mortality from ARF and RHD generally declined or disappeared,[233] at least in the population studied. Rates in African Americans were slow to decline, however. Rates became very low in the 1970s, at least in some areas, but cases persisted in other areas.[92,152]

Gordis and associates[112] caution that some other socioeconomically determined factor closely paralleling crowding could be the actual determinant of rheumatic fever. Most authorities agree that the reduction in the incidence and severity of rheumatic fever that has been noted in the United States and Western Europe might be due partly to a higher standard of living and less crowding. In a case-control study in the former Yugoslavia, home dampness, change of place of residence during the previous 5 years, low maternal education, body weight below normal, frequent sore throats, and a positive family history of rheumatic fever were found to be significant risk factors.[301]

A relationship between group A streptococcal throat infection and rheumatic fever was recognized in observations of the latter occurring after outbreaks of scarlet fever.[220] The attack rate noted after group A streptococcal throat infection varied widely (from 3% at Warren Air Force Base[235] to 0.39% in Chicago children).[258] Further observations in the latter study revealed that exudative pharyngitis, a positive throat culture with persistence of group A streptococci beyond 21 days, and the development of significant antibody (antistreptolysin O [ASO]) responses were associated with a higher attack rate that approached 3% in the children studied. In the New Zealand study an estimated attack rate of 0.4% was found in the school population (aged 5–17 years) studied, with approximately 60% with exudative pharyngitis from another study in the same population.[155,163]

Rheumatic fever, similar to streptococcal pharyngeal infection, occurs most commonly in children 5 to 15 years of age. First attacks of rheumatic fever rarely occur in children younger than 3 years of age or in adults older than 40 years because of the relative infrequency of streptococcal infection at these ages and perhaps other factors.

The incidence of ARF is highest in the spring and winter months in temperate zones and coincides with the seasonal variation in streptococcal pharyngitis. This incidence may be related to the greater tendency for spread of streptococcal infection by closer contact during the colder and damper months,[159,276,301] at least in some climates. In other climates, a seasonal peak for ARF is less pronounced.[38]

PATHOGENESIS

Evidence points toward ARF being preceded by a group A streptococcal upper respiratory tract infection (Fig. 29.4).[21] The events that occur after such infection and that culminate in rheumatic fever are poorly defined, suggesting a complex interaction of numerous factors. With the resurgence of interest in this disease after the outbreaks in the 1980s in the United States and more recently with increased global interest, laboratory data collected with the use of modern technologies have led to some new insights.[21,70,120,244,265,266,280] Pathogenesis involves the host, the environment (see "Epidemiology"), and group A streptococci, individually and collectively. Group A streptococci possess an enormous number of virulence factors.[204] The M protein is a major surface protein on the surface as coiled-coil fibrils. The most common method of typing currently is by nucleotide sequencing of the variable 5′ end of the M protein gene (*emm*).[28] Considering the full architecture of the M protein there are three main groups represented by the prototypic M-5, M-80, and M-77 molecules.[193] This approach may aid future epidemiology and vaccine development. So-called rheumatogenic strains of group A streptococci have been the subject of much discussion, more recently in relation to the U.S. focal upsurges in rheumatic fever in the 1980s and 1990s.[35,36,138] Because no factor has been described or isolated, however, such strains remain a hypothesis. To date, rheumatic fever has been shown to occur only after nasopharyngeal infection,[308] although debate and research continue.[72,135,218] Why the site of infection seems to predispose individuals to the development of rheumatic fever remains an enigma, perhaps related to skin lipids.[141] Acute glomerulonephritis develops after skin or throat infections with a nephritogenic type of group A streptococci (e.g., M-49 and M-12).[308]

Certain streptococcal M protein serotypes are implicated strongly and repetitively in epidemics of ARF. Serotypes M-3, M-5, M-14, M-18, and M-24 have been reported more than once in outbreaks, and M-1, M-6, M-19, M-27, and M-29 have been reported once only.[34] Distinct nucleotide sequences that determine different gene subfamilies encoding the M or M-like protein antigenic domain (*emm* gene) may be the cause of these variations in streptococcal rheumatogenic potential, depending on the site of infection.[32] Other equally prevalent M types rarely, if ever, have been associated with epidemics of the disease[34] or have failed to cause recurrences in susceptible patients.[37] The U.S. resurgence in the 1980s lends limited support for this concept. No predominance of a single serotype within a specific geographic zone

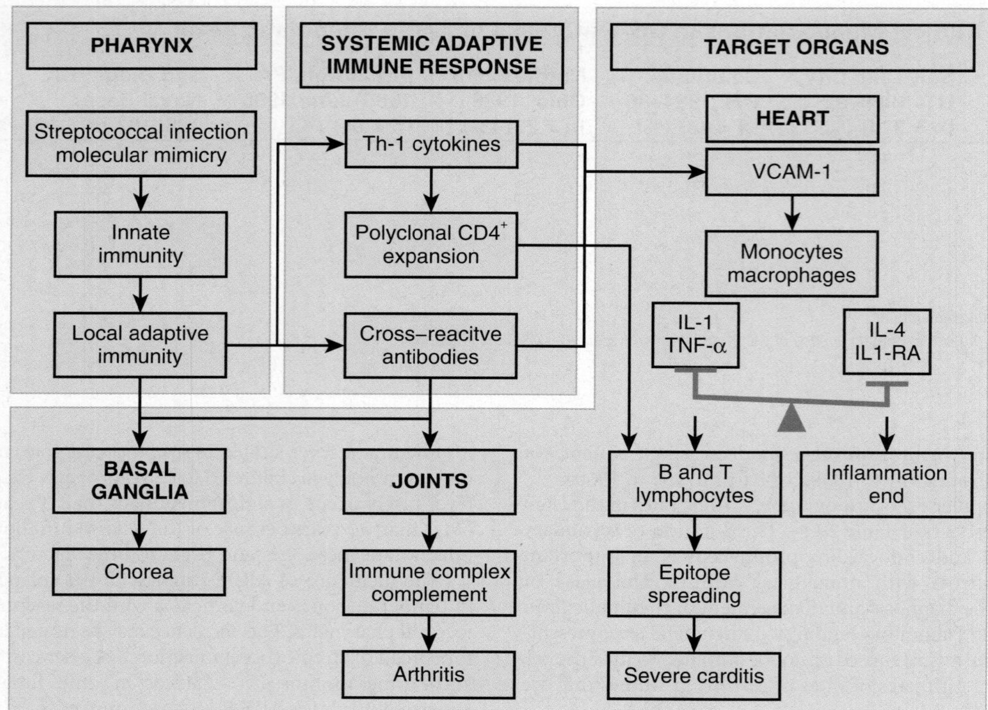

FIG. 29.4 Suggested pathophysiologic model for rheumatic fever. (Modified from Azevedo PM, Pereira RR, Guilherme L. Understanding rheumatic fever. *Rheumatol Int.* 2012;32(5):1113–20.)

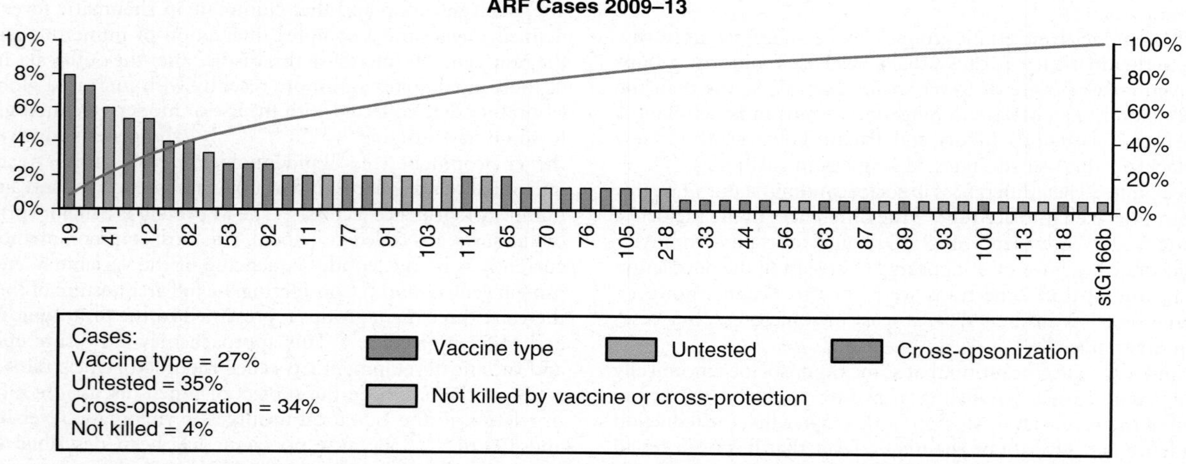

FIG. 29.5 *emm* types in acute rheumatic fever cases with potential coverage by the 30 valent vaccine and cross-reaction, Auckland 2009–12.

was identified in any of the published outbreaks (see Table 29.2). Specific M types and their production of mucoidal colonies, considered to be related to the amount of M protein and virulence,[309] may be more relevant to epidemic than to endemic rheumatic fever.

There are limited reports of endemic rheumatic fever–associated *emm* types. In Auckland, New Zealand, where rheumatic fever is endemic, in a large urbanized minority population an average of 50 highly scrutinized new cases of ARF currently occur annually in children aged 5 to 14 years of age (annual age-specific rate of 25/100,000 per year; Maori and Pacific Polynesians 60/100,000).[131,197] Nine years (1984 to 1992) of surveillance of group A streptococcal isolates from hospitalized pediatric patients (one centralized children's facility for 8 of the 9 years in question) yielded 2410 isolates. Only three of 38 throat isolates (32 from well-documented cases of rheumatic fever, six from siblings) were strains described as possibly rheumatogenic (one each of M-1, M-3, and M-6).[183] None was described as mucoidal.[183] In that series, M types 6, 53, 55, and 66 (and NZ-1437, now known as M-89, when sibling isolates were included as cases) were statistically more likely to be associated with a case of ARF. Further prospective *emm* surveillance in ARF cases in Auckland demonstrates a wide diversity of *emm* types in this population where rheumatic fever is endemic (Fig. 29.5).[128,318] Isolates associated with ARF and pharyngitis in Hawaii (Table 29.4) are rarely seen in the continental United States.[87,128,318] Of importance, the assumed link between rheumatic fever, the disease, and the disease-causing *emm* types is only temporal. It may itself not be sufficient to build a hypothesis for a possible association of initial infection site and ARF.

Strain selectivity is a further consideration. No documented evidence has shown that all members of an M type may be equally able to elicit

TABLE 29.4 Distribution of *emm* Types Among Patients With Acute Rheumatic Fever (ARF) in Hawaii Compared With Pharyngitis Isolates From Hawaii and Sterile Site Isolates From the Continental United States

emm Types Isolated From Patients With ARF in Hawaii	No. of Pharyngitis Isolates From Hawaii	No. of Isolates From Continental United States
65/69[a]	12	4
71	14	1
92	16	50
93	2	0
98	6	1
103	4	1
122	1	0

There were 1258 total pharyngitis isolates from Hawaii and 3424 isolates (from the period 1995–2001) included in the Centers for Disease Control and Prevention surveillance data from the United States.

[a]Isolated from two patients.

From Erdem G, Mizumoto C, Esaki D, et al. Group A streptococcal isolates temporally associated with ARF in Hawaii: differences from the continental United States. *Clin Infect Dis.* 2007;45:e20–4.

ARF. Some streptococci from a particular serotype may be associated with ARF and acute poststreptococcal glomerulonephritis, although the two sequelae rarely occur simultaneously.[172,182,183] M types have been shown to be composed of genetically diverse streptococci, not all of which may be established within a community.[182] This has been again demonstrated with modern tools, with analysis of the full-length sequence of 51 M proteins from Brazilian and Belgium strains of group A streptococci.[264] Genetic analysis of serotype M-18 from ARF cases in Utah separated by 12 years, however, showed strains nearly genetically identical.[265] The M type denotes possibly nothing more than a shared type-specific marker, with the property of rheumatogenicity as yet remaining elusive. Streptococcal strains that are opacity factor negative (a lipoprotein lipase) are unlikely to be rheumatogenic, according to some investigators.[138,314] This finding does not hold up in all geographic areas.[183] Surveillance of group A streptococci in multiple geographic zones will be necessary to guide M protein–based vaccine development.[84] Other vaccine options are being explored (see later discussion).

Although current evidence strongly implicates an immunologic mechanism in the pathophysiology of rheumatic fever, the details of how the disease develops are unclear.[36,69,184,274] Evidence to date strongly suggests an abnormal cell-mediated and humoral immune response to cell membrane streptococcal antigens, which, because of molecular mimicry of human tissues, may result in continued damage to the cardiovascular and nervous systems.[48,274,121] The findings of circulating immune complexes in most patients[71] and the deposition of C3 and immunoglobulin in the myocardium of patients dying of ARF support an abnormal immune response in rheumatic fever.[136]

M proteins from some rheumatogenic group A streptococcal types share antigenic determinants with myosin, with the sarcolemma of cardiac muscle,[75,76] and with antigens of articular cartilage and synovium.[22] The immune response to streptococci may mistake the host antigens as foreign and result in tissue damage. Other streptococcal antigens, such as the group A carbohydrate component, are candidates for mistaken cross-reaction with a glycoprotein in human heart valves.[110] Group A streptococci have components that can amplify or downregulate the immune response.[48] The mechanisms for molecular mimicry leading to central nervous system dysfunction are less defined.[184]

The site of the initial streptococcal infection may be important; lymphatic channels have been shown between the tonsils and the heart.[48] Unusual compartmentalization of rheumatic antigen–positive non-T cells has been shown in patients with ARF, with no positive cells detected in rheumatic tonsils but increased numbers in peripheral blood.[116]

Cell-mediated immunity to streptococcal antigens also is enhanced in patients with rheumatic fever.[274] The lymphocytic infiltrate of heart valves was found to be composed predominantly of $CD4^+$ helper cells.[234] Increased expression of human leukocyte antigen (HLA)-DR on fibroblasts, which can present antigens to $CD4^+$ lymphocytes (cytotoxic/suppressor T cells), has been observed on the heart valves of patients with acute carditis.[83] The cytotoxicity induced in normal human helper and suppressor cells in vitro by purified protein from a type M-5 group A streptococcal organism has been shown to destroy several human cell types, including cultured myocardial cells.[69] T-cell subset study results are conflicting,[205,274] but production of interleukins is reported to be enhanced.[205,206,331] The role of M protein and streptococcal pyrogenic exotoxins as superantigens is being explored and perhaps might explain the exaggeration of the streptococcal immune response.[181,289]

ARF pathogenesis is mediated by autoimmune mechanisms: the production of antibodies and T cells that react with self-antigens. Antibodies have been observed deposited in the myocardium and valves of ARF patients following death,[136] interstitial immune nodules (known as Aschoff bodies) are a hallmark of rheumatic carditis,[249] and $CD4^+$ and $CD8^+$ T cells have been shown to be attached to rheumatic heart valve endothelium.[244] Despite this relatively well-documented histopathology, there is still no consensus on which antigens initiate the autoimmune response, nor is there a clear understanding of the immune cell profile in ARF.[280] A better understanding of pathogenesis is crucial to develop interventions, both preventative and therapeutic. The application of modern immune-profiling technologies, which have been used with success in other autoimmune diseases,[166,168,251,259,294] has the potential to identify triggers of autoimmunity and characterize the immune signatures for ARF.[21]

The genetic background of the human host seems to influence susceptibility to rheumatic fever.[47] There are theories about the roles certain genes might play.[252] Aggregation of rheumatic fever cases in families has been recognized for some time.[227] Low concordance for inheritance has been reported in monozygotic twins,[284] although affected siblings have significant concordance for arthritis, residual RHD, and chorea.[267] A recent systematic review and meta-analysis of twin studies estimated heritability across all studies of 60%, suggesting whole-genome scanning might provide a clinically useful genetic risk prediction tool for rheumatic fever and RHD.[85] Patarroyo and associates[219] found that the B lymphocytes of patients with rheumatic fever have a specific marker (883 alloantigen) associated with host rheumatic susceptibility.[327,328] It seems to transcend ethnicity,[125,219] although studies in India and Africa were less supportive, and may be similar to an immune response gene.[274,304] This work has been extended with the use of monoclonal antibodies to family members of patients with rheumatic fever.[91,238] Class I HLA molecules have not been associated with ARF. Many studies in different populations have shown an association with HLA-DR but without a single HLA marker for susceptibility.[274] Genetic factors alone seem highly unlikely to be responsible for susceptibility to rheumatic fever.[180] No predictive marker for susceptibility to rheumatic fever has been defined to date. Studies in different populations have yielded conflicting results exploring the possibility that gene polymorphisms influence severity of heart disease in rheumatic fever patients.[20]

VACCINE DEVELOPMENT

Immunity to group A streptococci and to rheumatic fever is thought to depend largely on antibodies to M protein, a major virulence determinant; such antibodies can opsonize the bacteria in the presence of neutrophils.[151] Immunity is thought to be strain-specific and to depend on antibodies to the variable serotype-specific regions of the protein, and earliest vaccine development followed this pathway.[26,204] Two early landmark studies showed that vaccines containing purified M protein evoked protective immune response in humans.[27,230] Antibodies against the variable amino-terminal end of the M protein opsonize streptococci in a type-specific manner, but the results of experiments in animals suggest that the conserved carboxyl-terminal end also may be an immune target. Some human evidence suggests that this conserved epitope acts as a subunit vaccine.[231] Complexities in this area include the risk for inducing cross-reacting antibodies that could injure rather than protect.[188]

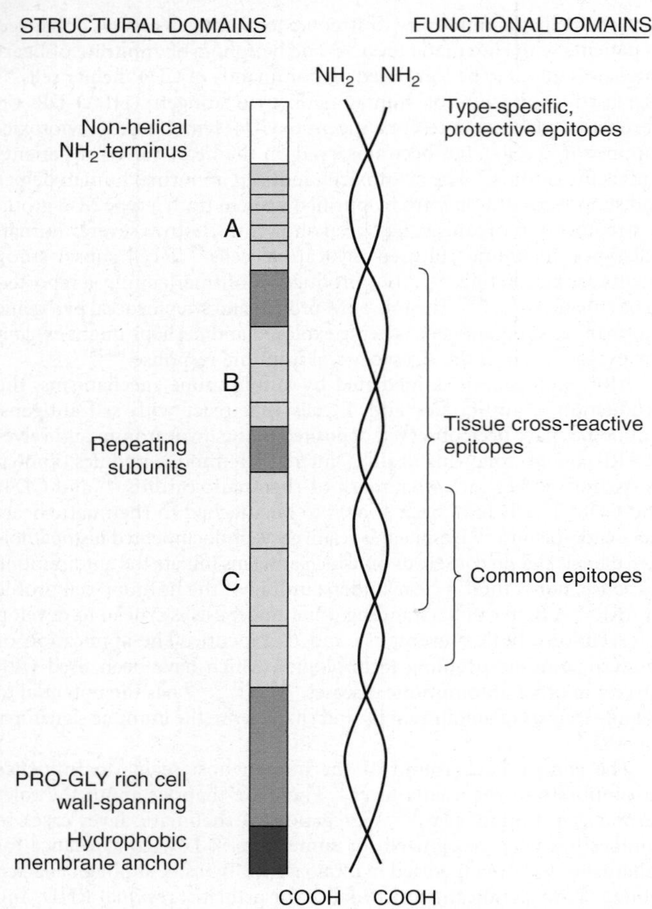

FIG. 29.6 Schematic representation of the structural and functional domains of streptococcal M protein. (From Dale J. Current status of group A streptococcal vaccine development. In: Finn A, Pollard A, eds. *Hot Topics in Infection and Immunity in Children IV: Advances in Experimental Medicine and Biology*, vol. 609. New York: Springer; 2008:53–63.)

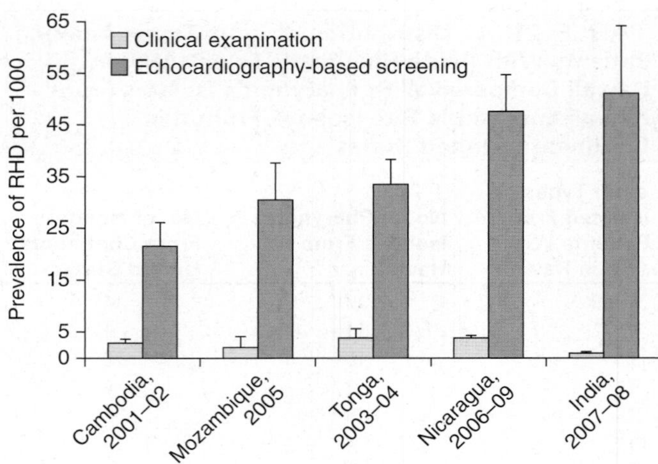

FIG. 29.7 Rheumatic heart disease prevalence rates in children: echocardiography-based screening versus clinical examination. (From Marijon E, Mirabel M, Celermajer DS, Jouven X. Rheumatic heart disease. *Lancet*. 2012;379:953–64.)

Separation of the peptide fragments of M proteins (epitopes) that evoke type-specific and not cross-reacting antibodies was an important step.[45,71] Most of the cross-reactive epitopes identified have been located in the middle of the M proteins (Fig. 29.6) and can be separated from the N-terminal, hypervariable protective epitopes that evoke antibodies with the greatest bactericidal activity.[74]

More than 200 different defined serotypes (M types) of group A streptococci have been identified. Vaccine development[36,39,204] falls into two broad approaches: vaccines based on common protective antigens of group A streptococci and multivalent vaccines based on type-specific N-terminal regions of the M protein.[74,270,119] A 26-valent vaccine with components guided by North American surveillance of ARF, invasive infections, and pharyngitis has been shown to be safe and immunogenic in adults.[194] This vaccine includes 80% to 90% of important serotypes in North America. More recent epidemiologic studies with additional data from North America and Europe, as well as some from developing countries, led to a 30-valent vaccine with broader coverage and promising animal model data against vaccine serotypes.[77,262] In addition, the researchers reported significant levels of bactericidal antibodies against a further 24 of 40 nonvaccine serotypes of group A streptococci.[78] This vaccine is now in phase I trials in North America.[204]

However, despite 98% coverage of pharyngitis isolates in North America, preliminary data from prospective studies of pharyngitis infections in Mali and South Africa indicate only 40% and 59% coverage.[77] As stated earlier there are few studies with pharyngeal *emm* typing associated with rheumatic fever cases. Epidemiologic studies of group A streptococci from low-income countries are sparse.[263,272] In general, a wider diversity of *emm* types are seen, indicating that vaccine coverage with current tools may be incomplete in other areas (see Fig. 29.6), such as in Hawaii,[87] Asia,[232] Cape Town in South Africa,[84] Mali,[78] or New Zealand,[183,318] where rheumatic fever is endemic in some populations. More comprehensive information for serotype prevalence in such areas of high endemicity is urgently needed. Cluster typing of *S. pyogenes* throat and skin isolates provides groups more likely to be associated with pharyngitis or skin infection with the latter more often seen from ARF endemic areas. However, there remains a paucity of pharyngeal isolates from these areas.[246a,246b]

RHEUMATIC FEVER IN DEVELOPING COUNTRIES

A global profile for ARF and RHD has emerged in the past decade.[53,208,252] The burden of RHD, larger than previously thought, is able to be better quantified with echocardiography (Fig. 29.7).[176] RHD is considered one of the few preventable chronic diseases.[12] Despite impressive declines in incidence in developed countries (see Figs. 29.1 and 29.3), globally RHD remains the most common form of acquired heart disease.[147,325] Four-fifths of the world's population live in developing countries where the prevalence of RHD suggests that the incidence of ARF remains at high levels in areas characterized by crowded living quarters and lower socioeconomic conditions. In Soweto, South Africa, the prevalence of RHD in the 1970s was estimated by cardiac auscultation at 7.1/1000 schoolchildren.[192] A recent estimate using echocardiography in two developing-country settings increased this estimate by nearly 10-fold.[176] Studies have been repeated in other settings (Fig. 29.7) with differing echocardiographic criteria but similar estimates of burden.[175] The true meaning of these findings in asymptomatic subjects in high-prevalence populations requires a better understanding of the natural history of subclinical carditis, standardization of the echocardiographic criteria, and cost-benefit analyses in various settings. Data on natural history is accruing.[29,33,217,250] A recent consensus standardization guideline has been published. Reliable, quality-controlled global supplies of benzathine penicillin for prevention of further attacks may need to be considered.[43,326]

An important recent prospective study in patients 14 years of age or older from Soweto highlights a significant disease burden of new-onset RHD presenting in the third and fourth decades of life,[260] suggesting a presumed unrecognized or subclinical earlier ARF episode, most likely in childhood. RHD is an important risk factor in obstetrics in low-resource settings and in other vulnerable groups.[215,261] The contribution of RHD to the burden of hospitalized disease resulting from strokes, atrial fibrillation, and other sequelae requires more elucidation.

Given the difference in medical care delivery, evaluation of the incidence of ARF must be viewed with caution. Estimates suggest, however, an annual incidence of 200 to 400 cases/100,000 population in Soweto.[147] The incidence of rheumatic fever (as judged by hospital admissions for RHD between 1966 and 1980) has remained stable in

India during this period of rapid decline in the United States and the West.[2] Some recent publications have attempted to better define the global burden of ARF (and RHD and other group A streptococcal diseases) with variable rigor.[53,252,288] Community-based secondary penicillin prophylaxis programs in developing countries are considered cost-effective and may be more achievable than is primary prevention.[147]

However, the case can be argued, even in resource-poor settings, for a comprehensive primary and secondary prevention program, particularly because benzathine penicillin is listed as a World Health Organization (WHO) essential medicine.[130,142,214,312]

PATHOLOGY

The unique pathologic lesion of rheumatic fever is the Aschoff body, which generally is considered to be a granuloma that results from injury to collagen fibers. Classically Aschoff bodies are found in the heart, usually in the left atrial appendage, but similar foci can be found in the synovia of the joints and in and around joint capsules, tendons, and fascia.[243]

The early pathologic response to rheumatic fever may be an exudative reaction with Aschoff-like bodies as an inflammatory focus. They are cardiac or extracardiac, with a central area of fibrinoid necrosis surrounded mostly by polymorphonuclear leukocytes. Clinically, this condition may be manifested as arthritis and spontaneously subside in 2 to 4 weeks. No residual joint damage results. The proliferative phase of classic Aschoff nodules, which consists of central necrosis surrounded by a rosette of large mononuclear cells, giant multinuclear cells, and other cell types, is confined to the heart and usually causes pancarditis with simultaneous involvement of all three layers (i.e., the pericardium, the myocardium, and the endocardium). This event may result in permanent valvular damage in the following order of frequency: the mitral valve, the aortic valve, the tricuspid valve, and, rarely, the pulmonary valve.

The heart disease encountered clinically usually is mitral regurgitation, aortic regurgitation, or both. The scarring that leads to valvular stenosis (mitral or aortic) typically takes decades to develop but may occur much faster in hyperendemic areas. This process is not the full story, however, because although rheumatic mitral valve stenosis occurs more commonly in India[248] and occasionally in other less advantaged populations, it was never a common occurrence in the United States or the United Kingdom at the height of rheumatic fever incidence.[285]

The presence of Aschoff bodies is not evidence of rheumatic activity because these lesions are found in biopsy specimens of the left atrial appendage many years after an acute attack of rheumatic fever. Little is known about the pathology of Sydenham chorea, and the pathologic changes cannot be related to the clinical manifestations. Patients rarely die of this form of rheumatic fever.

CLINICAL COURSE

The stage is set for the development of rheumatic fever in a susceptible host after a pharyngeal infection by one of the types of group A β-hemolytic streptococci.[108,179] Not all serotypes (M or *emm* types) appear to be equally rheumatogenic (see "Pathogenesis"). Rheumatic fever develops in approximately 1% to 3% of children with known epidemic untreated exudative pharyngitis and a culture positive for group A streptococci. The frequency decreases to less than 1%, as shown in the one controlled study involving children,[258] when patients with less severe or less precisely diagnosed streptococcal infections are included. This finding has been replicated more recently in a large community- and school-based randomized, controlled trial with high consent and retention rates in New Zealand in an area with endemic rheumatic fever. The attack rate observed was approximately 0.2%.[163]

The preceding pharyngitis is not recognized as an illness by the patient or parents in approximately 10% to 33% of cases of ARF, although 50% to 60% of patients remember having a sore throat.[111] In the New Zealand trial, episodes of sore throat (with appropriately increased streptococcal serology) in this carefully monitored series preceded development of ARF in 14 of 19 (74%) of the cases enrolled in the program at the time of presentation.[163] In some case series, this figure is lower but the methodology is less rigorous (see Table 29.2). The infection is followed by a latent period that averages 19 days in duration,[165] during which time the patient seems well. The range seems to be between 1 and 5 weeks but has been difficult to establish.[57] In the New Zealand trial, the average latent period was 27 days (range, 2 to 49 days) for seven rheumatic cases with proven group A streptococcal pharyngitis and raised streptococcal titers.[163] The average latent period is the same for recurrent attacks as for initial episodes.[57]

ARF then begins. Table 29.3 suggests a clinical profile in epidemics in the United States, although recurrent cases with their increased risk for carditis are included. The clinical profile in all settings is similar.[108] In a prospective study in India, 67% of initial episodes were associated with migrating arthritis involving one or more of the large joints[247] accompanied by a fever of 38°C to 39°C (100.4°F to 102.2°F), malaise, and anorexia. Just as the redness, swelling, and pain in a knee subside, the whole process may start again in the ankle. The elbows and wrists are likely to be involved. Arthritis of the hip also occurs.[189] The joint involved may be exquisitely tender, with the patient exhibiting extreme reluctance to move the joint or mobilize. Typically, multiple joints are involved in tandem, with overlap over the course of time, when symptoms are not suppressed by antiinflammatory therapy. The whole polyarthritic episode usually subsides over the course of 4 weeks, with no residua remaining. The joint inflammation may be of low grade in some individuals, without limitation of motion or outward manifestations of redness and swelling (arthralgia). The literature supporting monoarthritis not developing into migrating polyarthritis in ARF is unconvincing.[51,124,146,163,228,323] However, the clinician should act cautiously in an area endemic for rheumatic fever in the early phase of presentation. The development of polyarthritis in a patient with a culture-negative monoarthritis (e.g., a hip joint in a patient without prior antibiotic exposure) may be aborted by nonsteroidal antiinflammatory drugs (NSAIDs).[323] An early echocardiogram may assist in establishing the diagnosis (see "Laboratory Findings").[3,199]

In a New Zealand series 30% of sequential ARF cases ($n = 119$) in a population-based study presented with monoarthritis, 14% (5/34) of the monoarthritis cases had received an NSAID agent, and 74% (25/34) of confirmed ARF patients with monoarthritis at presentation had echocardiographic changes diagnostic of ARF.[199] At the time of the study, and according to the New Zealand diagnostic criteria, monoarthritis was allowed as a major criterion only when the patient had received an NSAID.[16,323] On the basis of this new information the New Zealand diagnostic criteria now allow monoarthritis without exhibition of an NSAID as a major criterion (www.heartfoundation.org.nz). More recently the American Heart Association (AMA) has followed suit.[108]

Carditis generally appears early in the illness (first 2 to 3 weeks) if it is going to occur.[1] It may be silent in the absence of elevated fever or symptoms of pericarditis or cardiac failure. The clinical signs are the development of a new heart murmur, cardiac enlargement, congestive cardiac failure, a pericardial friction rub, or signs of cardiac effusion. An echocardiogram early on may be diagnostic of carditis using international diagnostic criteria even in the absence of a murmur.[108,240]

However, the mode of onset of ARF can be quite variable, and access to medical care, the health knowledge of the patient or family, or the awareness of health care personnel may be factors determining when in the illness the patient initially seeks medical care. Indolent carditis, as an insidious or even subclinical presentation now recognized by the Jones criteria (Table 29.5), may present without other manifestations to fulfill the Jones criteria because the initial episode is sometime in the past. This was an uncommon but recognized presentation in the New Zealand school trial.[163]

In a classic presentation[179] on examination, the striking findings are the patient's pallor and discomfort, especially on movement of the affected joints. Carditis usually appears within 3 weeks of the start of the illness, and, in the absence of high fever or symptoms of acute pericarditis or congestive heart failure, it may be asymptomatic.[1] Examination of the heart may reveal in at least half of patients a grade 2/4 apical pansystolic murmur that is transmitted to the axilla (mitral insufficiency) with or without an apical mid-diastolic flow murmur (Carey-Coombs murmur); half of these patients also may experience an early diastolic grade 2/4 murmur at the left sternal edge (aortic insufficiency). The latter can also occur alone. The tricuspid valve is

TABLE 29.5 Revised Jones Criteria for the Diagnosis of Rheumatic Fever

A. For All Patient Populations With Evidence of Preceding GAS Infection	
Diagnosis: initial ARF	2 Major manifestations or 1 major plus 2 manifestations
Diagnosis: recurrent ARF	2 Major or 1 major and 2 minor or 3 minor
B. Major Criteria	
Low-risk populations[a]	Moderate- and high-risk populations
Carditis[b]	Carditis
Clinical and/or subclinical arthritis	Clinical and/or subclinical arthritis Monoarthritis or polyarthritis
Polyarthritis only	Polyarthralgia[c]
Chorea	Chorea
Erythema marginatum	Erythema marginatum
Subcutaneous nodules	Subcutaneous nodules
C. Minor Criteria	
Low-risk populations[a]	Moderate- and high-risk populations
Polyarthralgia	Monoarthralgia
Fever (≥38.5°C)	Fever (≥38°C)
ESR ≥60 mm in the first hour and/or CRP ≥3.0 mg/dL[d]	ESR ≥30 mm/h and/or CRP ≥3.0 mg/dL[d]
Prolonged PR interval, after accounting for age variability (unless carditis is a major criterion)	Prolonged PR interval, after accounting for age variability (unless carditis is a major criterion)

[a]Low-risk populations are those with ARF incidence ≤2 per 100,000 school-aged children or all-age RHD prevalence of ≤1 per 1000 population per year.
[b]Subclinical carditis indicates echocardiographic valvulitis as defined in reference 108.
[c]See section on polyarthralgia in reference 108, which should only be considered as a major manifestation in moderate- to high-risk populations after exclusion of other causes. As in past versions of the criteria, erythema marginatum and subcutaneous nodules are rarely "stand-alone" major criteria. Additionally, joint manifestations can only be considered in either the major or minor categories but not both in the same patient.
[d]CRP value must be greater than upper limit of normal for laboratory. Also, because ESR may evolve during the course of ARF, peak ESR values should be used.
ARF, acute rheumatic fever; *CRP*, C-reactive protein; *ESR*, erythrocyte sedimentation rate; *GAS*, group A streptococcal infection.
From Gewitz MH, Baltimore RS, Tani LY, et al.; on behalf of the American Heart Association Committee on Rheumatic Fever, Endocarditis, and Kawasaki Disease of the Council on Cardiovascular Disease in the Young. Revision of the Jones criteria for the diagnosis of ARF in the era of Doppler echocardiography: a scientific statement from the American Heart Association. *Circulation.* 2015;131:1806–18.

not usually involved and the pulmonary valve very rarely. In addition, less commonly, the child can have congestive heart failure or cardiac enlargement, indicative of active carditis. Carditis is more likely to occur in younger children. Pericarditis may be suspected with muffled heart sounds, a frictional rub, or chest pain. It becomes less common as ARF in a population becomes less severe. Ruptured chordae tendineae in a patient with fulminant carditis may present as unilateral pulmonary edema.[8] Death is a rare but well-described sequela of the acute phase of the disease. Murmurs of mitral and aortic stenosis are associated with chronic but not with acute rheumatic valve disease.

Echocardiography in ARF cases with congestive cardiac failure has shown preserved left ventricular systolic function and/or severe mitral or aortic regurgitation.[88,102,295] Serum levels of cardiac troponin I are not elevated in ARF patients with heart failure.[316]

The distinctive rash, erythema marginatum, was observed in up to 12% of patients in these case series (Fig. 29.6; see Table 29.3). It is neither pruritic nor painful. The pink, slightly raised macules, usually seen initially on the trunk and proximal ends of the extremities and never on the face, fuse centrally and coalesce to form a serpiginous pattern. The lesions may disappear after a few hours or may reappear intermittently over the course of weeks, especially after a warm shower or bath.

Subcutaneous nodules, usually associated with severe carditis, also occur uncommonly (<10% of patients). They are firm and painless and are found over bony surfaces or prominences and over tendons. ARF is not likely to be diagnosed on the basis of the latter two major criteria without another major criterion.

Sydenham chorea, or St. Vitus dance, may be the only manifestation of rheumatic fever, or it may be associated with other disease manifestations. All laboratory parameters, including streptococcal serology, may be normal. It becomes less common as ARF becomes less severe in a population, presumably as a result of improved awareness and earlier presentation of other manifestations of ARF. Chorea is characterized by purposeless (most often bilateral, uncoordinated, involuntary) movements, mostly of the hands, feet, and face, that develop over the course of weeks and are accentuated by excitement and emotional stress. They disappear during sleep. Sensation remains intact. The speech can be explosive and indistinct, and the handwriting can be clumsy. Handwriting is a useful objective means of monitoring the course of the disease. The child has difficulty counting rapidly and holding the protruded tongue still. The fingers and wrists are hyperextended when the fingers are outstretched, and the palms usually are turned outward when the arms are held above the head. Handgrip generally is weak and may consist of spasmodic contractions followed by rapid relaxation (so-called milkmaid grip). The patient may be easily irritated and quarrelsome. Chorea typically is a delayed manifestation of rheumatic fever and may develop after other signs of the disease have subsided, commonly appearing 2 to 6 months after the streptococcal infection. Historically, observers think residual heart disease occurs less commonly when chorea is the only manifestation of rheumatic fever, but in the echocardiographic era this hypothesis may prove not to be the case. The importance of prophylaxis in those with chorea to prevent recurrent attacks and possible subsequent carditis was reaffirmed in Kuwait.[171] Permanent serious residual neurologic deficits have not been observed. A 25-year review found the duration of chorea to be 1 to 22 weeks, with a median of 12 weeks.[210] Rare cases may last 2 to 3 years.[4,15,50] Recurrent attacks are common and may occur despite faithful adherence to prophylaxis with intramuscular benzathine penicillin.[31,287] The neuropsychiatric sequelae of chorea were reviewed recently.[202]

Some cases of chorea are mild or atypical and may be confused with motor tics or the involuntary jerks of Tourette syndrome. Confusion may ensue between Sydenham chorea and these conditions. The term *pediatric autoimmune neuropsychiatric disorder associated with streptococcal infection* (PANDAS) refers to a subgroup of children with tic or obsessive-compulsive disorder whose symptoms may develop or worsen after an episode of group A streptococcal infection. The following five criteria have been used to define the PANDAS subgroup[149,279]:

1. The presence of a tic disorder, obsessive-compulsive disorder, or both
2. Prepubertal age of onset (usually between 3 and 12 years of age)
3. Abrupt onset of symptoms, episodic course of symptom severity, or both
4. Temporal association between exacerbations of symptoms and streptococcal infection (approximately 7 to 14 days)
5. Presence of neurologic abnormalities during periods of exacerbation of symptoms (typically adventitious movements or motoric hyperactivity)

The evidence supporting PANDAS as a distinct disease entity has been questioned.[149] In any population with a high prevalence of ARF, clinicians should rarely (if ever) make a diagnosis of PANDAS and rather should err on the side of overdiagnosis of ARF and secondary prophylaxis. If ARF is excluded, secondary prophylaxis is not needed, but these patients should be followed carefully to ensure they do not develop carditis in the long term (see Chapter 82).

The average duration of an attack of ARF is approximately 3 months when unaltered by antiinflammatory therapy.[179] Fewer than 5% of cases persist longer than 6 months with active symptoms, so-called chronic rheumatic fever.[285]

LABORATORY FINDINGS

The degree of inflammation in patients with ARF is measured by nonspecific indicators, such as the erythrocyte sedimentation rate (ESR) and C-reactive protein (CRP).[108,179] Unless the patient has taken corticosteroids or salicylates, these test results almost always are positive in patients with polyarthritis or acute carditis but are normal in patients with chorea. The magnitude of the ESR is proportional to the intensity of the inflammatory reaction but is not site specific (i.e., it can be high with polyarthritis or carditis). The ESR is typically more than 60 mm/h in ARF.[108,164] The ESR may be decreased in congestive heart failure, whereas the CRP may be elevated in congestive heart failure attributable to any cause. The ESR may remain elevated for 6 weeks to 3 months in an untreated attack of ARF. Antiinflammatory agents may reduce the ESR, but it rebounds if the drugs are stopped before the rheumatic process has run its course. Although chronic elevation of the ESR (>6 months) is not understood, it is not a sufficient reason on its own to limit a patient's activities.[285] The CRP may reflect the patient's rheumatic activity more precisely than may the ESR.[179]

Chest radiographs are useful for detecting cardiomegaly, which may be caused by dilation, preexisting heart disease, or pericardial effusion. The degree of enlargement is helpful in judging severity. The electrocardiogram may show a prolonged atrioventricular conduction time, usually evidenced by a prolonged PR interval or even greater degrees of heart block.[237] Generally, an increase in the PR interval in tracings with comparable rates is considered significant.[179] Upper limits of normal by age are available.[164] Atrioventricular conduction abnormalities per se bear no relation to the ultimate prognosis of patients. Changes of myocarditis and pericarditis also are seen.

Every patient with suspected rheumatic fever should be considered for an echocardiogram. The AMA's recent revision of the Jones criteria allows echocardiographic changes without a concomitant murmur as a major criterion.[108] The roles of two-dimensional and Doppler echocardiography in establishing the diagnosis and determining the diagnosis and prognosis of ARF are now supported by multiple clinical studies (www.heartfoundation.org.nz).[1,93,95,108,296–298,300,320] In a prospective blinded study using febrile controls and strict color and pulsed Doppler criteria, pathologic left-sided heart regurgitation could be differentiated from physiologic regurgitation.[1] Several centers using similar strict echocardiographic guidelines have observed subclinical carditis in ARF.[97,96,108,297,298] Echocardiographic changes of ARF with usually mitral and/or aortic valvular regurgitation may be helpful in consolidating poly- or monoarthritis or chorea as true ARF.

In the New Zealand prospective randomized trial of prevention of first episode ARF (see earlier discussion), only three additional cases (3 of 59 [5%]) met the case definition for ARF using the New Zealand Rheumatic Fever diagnostic criteria, which allowed echocardiographic carditis to be a major or minor criterion in the presence of other major or minor criteria and evidence of preceding streptococcal infection.[163] Every case was scrutinized by an independent group of clinicians, including a cardiologist.[163] Monoarthritis at this time was not a major criterion in the New Zealand ARF diagnostic criteria.[16] Australia similarly incorporated echocardiographic criteria into guidelines.[49] Publications included in a systematic review found a prevalence of 17% of subclinical carditis in ARF.[292]

In 2012, an international consortium published guidelines on minimal criteria for a diagnosis of RHD with echocardiography.[240] These criteria do not address the differentiation between acute carditis and chronic RHD. The criteria for pathologic regurgitation are unlikely to be different and have been incorporated into other guidelines.[16,49,164] Morphologic changes may be different in ARF and may require further clarification. Assessment of left ventricular size and function is an important part of the evaluation of a patient with rheumatic fever, especially if surgery is being considered.[102]

A positive throat culture for group A β-hemolytic streptococci as evidence of a recent streptococcal infection seldom is found in an ARF case, although 50% of such patients could be carriers of the organism.[140] In the New Zealand randomized trial, of patients with ARF who reported sore throat episodes (n = 14), 57% (eight of 14) had a positive throat culture and appropriately increased serology.[163] A positive culture may be helpful if it can be related to the time of the acute infection.

Corroboration of a previous streptococcal infection is better determined serologically. Rising titers are preferred to raised titers.[108] Many streptococcal antibody tests are available.[253,315] Antibody titers may be elevated in the absence of clinical or bacteriologic evidence of streptococcal pharyngitis (five of 19 ARF cases in the New Zealand program).[163] The ASO titer is the most popular antibody test. It measures the inhibition of rabbit red blood cells by specific antibody to streptolysin O, an extracellular product of β-hemolytic streptococci that in its reduced form hemolyzes red blood cells. The "normal" level for an ASO titer usually is defined as the highest titer exceeded by only 20% of a population, but it is influenced significantly by age, geography, season, and other factors.[139,253] ASO titers of 500 Todd units or greater are rare findings in normal schoolchildren and are good evidence of a recent streptococcal infection. ASO titers of less than 250 Todd units could be considered normal; titers of 250 to 320 Todd units should be considered borderline elevated. Approximately 50% of patients with ARF have ASO titers in this range, and approximately 60% have titers of 500 Todd units or greater.[268] Conversely, ASO titers can be normal in 20% of patients with ARF.[275]

A recent streptococcal infection is more likely to be shown if more than one antibody titer is measured (e.g., antistreptokinase and anti-hyaluronidase).[275] Anti-deoxyribonuclease B is currently the most favored test because of its better reproducibility.

The onset of clinical ARF usually coincides with the peak of the streptococcal antibody response. It may stay elevated for many weeks. The absence of an elevated antistreptococcal titer, if three different antibodies are measured, means, however, that the clinician can be 95% certain that the patient has not had a streptococcal infection within the recent past. In patients with pure chorea or indolent carditis, antibody levels may have declined to normal because of the length of the latent period between the development of streptococcal infection and the manifestation of this symptom.

The synovial fluid in joints affected by ARF contains 10,000 to 100,000 white blood cells/mm^3, which are mostly neutrophils. The protein concentration is approximately 4 g/dL, glucose levels are normal, and a good mucin clot is present.[127] A more recent report in consecutive patients with septic arthritis (n = 111) and ARF (n = 119) found a significantly lower synovial fluid white cell count (WCC) in the latter group of patients (median 20.2 vs. 102.5/mm^3; P = .004); however, there was no significant difference in the percentage of polymorphonucleocytes (median 63.5% vs. 79.0% of synovial fluid WCC; P = .761) between the two groups.[199]

DIAGNOSIS

The American Heart Association has recently revised the Jones criteria for the diagnosis of ARF.[108,177] Important changes for the clinician are the legitimacy of echocardiographic changes of rheumatic valvitis[108] without auscultatory findings to fulfill carditis as a major criterion in any population regardless of risk, following New Zealand's lead in 2008 (www.heartfoundation.org.nz).[16] A further consideration is the risk of ARF in the population from which the patient emanates (see Table 29.5). Types of joint involvement and cutoffs for ESR and temperature are more permissive for these patients. However, the quality of evidence should be improved with the application of these newly agreed-on criteria to allow comparison of populations. Standardization of variables between publications cited has not occurred.[51,199,321,321]

An accurate diagnosis of ARF is vital because a misdiagnosis may lead to future serious cardiac disease, whereas overdiagnosis will commit the patient to a long-term and unpleasant therapy—benzathine penicillin every 4 weeks. However, a high index of suspicion is important in high-risk areas.

The signs and symptoms of rheumatic fever vary greatly depending on the stage of the disease, the epidemiology of the rheumatic fever in that place at that time, the severity of the disease, and the sites of involvement. Poor access to health care or lack of awareness of presenting symptoms may lead to late presentation. In the absence of a diagnostic test or pathognomonic sign, Jones suggested a series of criteria (major and minor; see Table 29.5) that have stood the test of time, with ongoing modifications. These are an estimate of probability of the likelihood of ARF. In the era of echocardiography up to 80% of confirmed ARF patients will have echocardiographic changes leading to the need for penicillin prophylaxis, giving this test high diagnostic status for intervention whether the Jones criteria are met or not.

The keystone on which the Jones criteria rest is the demonstration of a recent streptococcal infection. Because few patients with ARF have positive throat cultures, demonstration of a previous streptococcal infection by a rising titer or an established higher titer than the population norm of one or more of the extracellular streptococcal antibodies is crucial confirmatory evidence to establish a recent streptococcal infection. However, in the absence of the appropriate constellation of signs and symptoms for ARF, the mere presence of an elevated titer to one or more of the streptococcal antibodies (see "Laboratory Findings") means only that the subject has had a recent group A β-hemolytic streptococcal infection, site unspecified.

Clinical manifestations in outbreaks in the 1980s are summarized in Table 29.3. Before this time, during the period of declining incidence in the United States, carditis (detected clinically) was found in fewer than half of rheumatic patients and generally was less severe.[185] Joint involvement alone was the most common manifestation, so arriving at diagnostic certainty was difficult. A common avoidable error is the premature administration of NSAIDs or corticosteroids before the signs and symptoms become distinct; such therapy may leave in doubt the necessity of administering secondary prophylaxis without a firm diagnosis (unless echocardiography is helpful).[323]

Chorea is considered a stand-alone criterion for establishing the diagnosis of rheumatic fever. Recurrences of rheumatic fever in patients with a reliable history of rheumatic fever or clear-cut RHD can be diagnosed by the demonstration of a single major or several minor criteria if supporting evidence of a recent group A streptococcal infection is present.

So-called poststreptococcal arthritis has been discussed as a possible entity when the initial symptoms and signs are atypical for ARF, fail to respond to salicylate therapy, or both. In some cases, RHD has ensued.[81] In all such patients who meet the Jones criteria, a diagnosis of rheumatic fever should be considered, particularly for the purpose of administering secondary penicillin prophylaxis.[19]

Criteria have been proposed for establishing the diagnosis of poststreptococcal reactive arthritis that have yet to stand the test of time.[18] The variable response to salicylates in published series of this proposed disease entity has not often been well documented with serum salicylate levels.[109] A shorter latent period is proposed, but the latent period between a group A streptococcal throat infection in original investigations of rheumatic fever varied (mean, 18.6 days), with 10% developing disease within 8 days (see "Clinical Course").[162,235] If this diagnosis is considered and rheumatic fever per se is not supported, vigilant follow-up for cardiac sequelae should ensue, and penicillin prophylaxis should be reconsidered.[105] This diagnosis should be considered with caution in areas endemic for rheumatic fever.

A prospective epidemiologic study with rigorous application of an agreed case definition is needed to clarify this proposed disease entity.

An atypical presentation of chorea (e.g., hemichorea) warrants consideration of neuroimaging.[332]

DIFFERENTIAL DIAGNOSIS

Rheumatic fever can present in diverse ways (acute mono- or polyarthritis or arthralgia, congestive heart failure, chorea, or a combination of these), and no specific diagnostic test for the disease exists; thus, the differential diagnoses (Table 29.6) in an individual patient may be extensive. Many other diseases might be confused with ARF.[153] In polyarthritis without clinical or echocardiographic evidence of carditis and fulfilling the Jones criteria, rheumatic fever is a diagnosis of exclusion. A search for alternative diagnoses is recommended,[164] including rheumatoid arthritis, suppurative bacterial arthritis (including gonococcal arthritis in adolescents), reactive arthritis (e.g., after *Yersinia*[150] or *Mycoplasma*[203] infection), infective endocarditis, sickle-cell anemia, leukemia, Lyme disease,[229] rubella, and poststreptococcal reactive arthritis (see earlier discussion). Before presentation to medical care, the first swollen joint may be attributed to injury. A follow-up echocardiogram after 2 to 3 weeks may reveal late-presenting carditis.[1,302]

With the help of the Jones criteria and time, alternative diagnoses usually can be excluded. Heart involvement with rheumatoid arthritis is a rare occurrence. In suppurative arthritis, showing the infecting bacteria by smear and recovery by culture provide the answer.[199] However, in an area endemic for rheumatic fever, aseptic monoarthritis without previous antibiotic exposure should be considered rheumatic fever until proved otherwise.[189] Inflammatory markers may help differentiate. Treatment for possible septic arthritis may need to ensue while the diagnosis evolves. In the absence of an audible cardiac murmur, echocardiography revealing subclinical mitral or aortic valve regurgitation may be very helpful. With sickle-cell disease, the bone is affected and not the joint, and a sickle-cell preparation helps establish the diagnosis. A blood smear usually establishes the diagnosis of leukemia.

The diagnosis of isolated Sydenham chorea based on presenting symptoms may be reinforced by an abnormal echocardiogram in the absence of clinical carditis. Other, much rarer considerations, especially in an area not endemic for rheumatic fever, include systemic lupus erythematosus, Wilson disease, juvenile Huntington chorea, and various medications.[54,153]

Common errors include diagnosing ARF and prescribing NSAIDs when a single joint is involved (see "Clinical Course")[323]; when an innocent murmur is present; when a nonspecific rash, especially an urticarial or erythema multiforme rash, erroneously is identified as

TABLE 29.6 Differential Diagnosis of Arthritis, Carditis, and Chorea

Arthritis	Carditis	Chorea
Septic arthritis (including gonococcal)	Physiologic mitral regurgitation	Drug intoxication
Connective tissue and other autoimmune diseases such as juvenile idiopathic arthritis	Mitral valve prolapse	Wilson disease
Viral arthropathy	Myxomatous mitral valve	Tic disorder
Reactive arthropathy	Fibroelastoma	Choreoathetoid cerebral palsy
Lyme disease	Congenital mitral valve disease	Encephalitis
Sickle-cell anemia	Congenital aortic valve disease	Familial chorea (including Huntington disease)
Infective endocarditis	Infective endocarditis	Intracranial tumor
Leukemia or lymphoma	Cardiomyopathy	Lyme disease
Gout and pseudogout	Myocarditis, viral or idiopathic	Hormonal
Poststreptococcal reactive arthritis	Kawasaki disease	Metabolic (e.g., Lesch-Nyhan, hyperalaninemia, ataxia telangiectasia)
Henoch-Schönlein purpura		Antiphospholipid antibody syndrome
		Autoimmune: systemic lupus erythematosus, systemic vasculitis
		Sarcoidosis
		Hyperthyroidism

From Gewitz MH, Baltimore RS, Tani LY, et al.; on behalf of the American Heart Association Committee on Rheumatic Fever, Endocarditis, and Kawasaki Disease of the Council on Cardiovascular Disease in the Young. Revision of the Jones criteria for the diagnosis of ARF in the era of Doppler echocardiography: a scientific statement from the American Heart Association. *Circulation.* 2015;131:1806–18.

erythema marginatum; and when other symptoms similar to chorea (e.g., tics, phenothiazine-induced extrapyramidal syndrome) are misinterpreted.[133] Committing a child to many years of penicillin prophylaxis requires careful decision making at the time of establishing the diagnosis.

TREATMENT

Therapy for ARF is symptomatic to control the inflammation, decrease the fever, and keep cardiac failure in check.[57,73,153,192,283] Neither salicylates nor corticosteroids are thought to affect severity or outcome.[9] Cardiac drugs (e.g., diuretics, angiotensin-converting enzyme [ACE] inhibitors) may improve impaired function. The long-term benefits have not been studied systematically. Caution regarding the toxic effects of salicylates (Reye syndrome) suggests that Naprosyn (a nonselective COX inhibitor) should be considered first-line for symptomatic therapy of painful joints although there is limited supportive evidence.[126,293] There is no published evidence for other NSAIDs such as ibuprofen, although anecdotally they are effective. Breakthrough symptoms can be controlled with naproxin. If the diagnosis is uncertain, however, pain relievers, such as acetaminophen, should be used as an interim measure to allow migrating polyarthritis to occur. This approach has not been evaluated critically.

The most experience and published evidence for management of the arthritis of ARF is with salicylates. Characteristically, the joint inflammation and fever subside in 24 to 48 hours with salicylate treatment if the serum level is 10 to 20 mg/dL, which usually is achieved by a dose of 60 to 100 mg/kg/24 hr (not exceeding 6 g/day in divided doses). This dose may be increased, but the clinician is advised to measure serum salicylate levels and adjust the dose regimen accordingly. A higher dose may result in the undesirable development of salicylism (tinnitus and hyperpnea). Except for occasional patients with rheumatoid arthritis, no other forms of arthritis respond in this dramatic way to aspirin. Salicylate therapy is recommended for 1 to 2 weeks and then can be reduced gradually, keeping in mind that inflammatory markers suggesting ongoing disease activity may persist 3 months or longer. Joint symptoms may recur, obviating a more gradual withdrawal of aspirin.

Most ARF episodes subside within 6 weeks, and 90% resolve within 12 weeks. Approximately 5% of cases require 6 months or more of salicylate therapy.[276] If lengthy therapy with salicylates is contemplated, influenza and varicella vaccines are important considerations to reduce the potential for developing Reye syndrome.[65] Naproxen 10 to 20 mg/kg per day given in two divided doses (maximum dose 1250 mg) had a dramatic effect similar to that of aspirin and is well tolerated. Advantages are twice-daily administration, the availability of elixir, less hepatotoxicity, and no need to determine serum levels. No evidence has substantiated that steroid therapy is superior or that treatment with steroid or aspirin decreases the severity or prevents the development of residual heart disease.[6,9,62] Both treatments are palliative and not curative. They are, however, effective antiinflammatory agents for controlling the acute exudative manifestations of rheumatic fever. Steroids are more likely to reduce acute symptoms promptly and may be indicated for severely ill patients in whom inflammatory edema of the myocardium may be life-threatening during the acute stage of the illness.[10,62,164]

The effect of more modern NSAIDs or immune modulators has not been evaluated in this way. A randomized controlled trial of intravenous immunoglobulin, a proven immunomodulator, in ARF (excluding chorea) failed to alter the natural history. No detectable difference was noted in the clinical, laboratory, or echocardiographic parameters found during the subsequent 12 months.[302]

In the pre-penicillin era, prolonged bed rest appeared to benefit severe carditis; however, it has not been studied critically.[179] Restriction of physical activity until the rheumatic process has become quiescent is a time-honored method of treatment. It has been based on the assumption that the workload of the inflamed heart is related to the degree of residual scarring. Ambulation should be titrated according to heart disease severity. Guidelines are available (www.heartfoundation.org.nz; www.RHDAustralia.org.au).[16] All patients at diagnosis should receive penicillin, even if the throat culture does not reveal group A β-hemolytic streptococci. Patients then can be placed on the secondary preventive treatment regimen, which may be either oral penicillin V 250 mg twice per day, or injections of benzathine penicillin 1.2 million U every 4 weeks. The parenteral route has been shown to be more effective in the New Zealand setting[98,211] (Fig. 29.7) and by others (see Table 29.6).[324] In high-risk situations (e.g., after a recurrence in a fully adherent patient), administration of benzathine penicillin every 3 weeks has been advised (see "Prevention" for more detail).[66]

Rarely, a patient has congestive heart failure.[164] A diuretic, fluid restrictions, or both are recommended for mild to moderate failure. ACE inhibitors should be considered for more severe failure, particularly if aortic regurgitation is present. Experience with β-blockers in acute rheumatic carditis is very limited, and their use is not recommended.

Chorea is benign and self-limited and will resolve in most patients within weeks, with most by 6 months. Rarely chorea may last up to 2 to 3 years.[4,15,165] Mild or moderate chorea does not require any specific treatment aside from rest and a calm environment, perhaps in the hospital. Overstimulation or stress can exacerbate the symptoms. The potential toxicity of recommended medication for severe distressing or limiting chorea should be taken into consideration. Aspirin does not have a significant treatment effect.[179] A small randomized trial of prednisone in Sydenham chorea showed efficacy.[221] More studies are awaited to confirm this finding. Several case series and a larger retrospective report are supportive.[23,55,99,100,305]

Small studies of intravenous immunoglobulin have suggested more rapid recovery from chorea.[278] Immunoglobulin in a randomized trial did not show reduced incidence of long-term valve disease in ARF without chorea.[302] Until more evidence is available, intravenous immunoglobulin is not recommended except for severe chorea refractory to other treatments.

Carbamazepine and valproic acid now are preferred to haloperidol, which previously was considered the first-line medical treatment for chorea.[80,101] A small prospective comparison of these three agents concluded that valproic acid was the most effective.[222]

Because there is a small potential for liver toxicity with valproic acid, the recommendation is that carbamazepine be used initially for severe chorea requiring treatment for this self-limited disease and that valproic acid be considered for refractory cases. A response may not be seen for 1 to 2 weeks, and successful medication may reduce but not eliminate the symptoms. Medication should be continued for 2 to 4 weeks after chorea has subsided and then withdrawn gradually. Recurrences of chorea usually are mild and can be managed conservatively, but in severe recurrences, the medication can be restarted if necessary.

CARDIAC SURGERY

Severe valve lesions may need cardiac surgery. Published guidelines are based on available evidence, mostly derived from adult patients.[86,87,94,103,104,201,212,239] Mitral repair has lower morbidity and mortality than replacement and is the treatment of choice for mitral regurgitation.[86] A meta-analysis provides strong support for repair relative to replacement surgery in adult patients.[239,254] Repair offers a survival advantage and a greater freedom from valve-related morbidity (e.g., a thrombotic, embolic, or hemorrhagic event), without compromised long-term durability. In the short term, repair was associated with a higher early repeat operation rate. New Zealand data for those younger than 20 years of age found the reoperation rate for mitral valve repair is the same as for mitral valve replacement, so mitral valve repair should always be aimed for if technically feasible.[239] Less information is available for aortic valve surgery. Combined severe mitral and atrial regurgitation leads to the most deleterious long-term prognosis and such patients should be considered early for surgery.[103]

Extensive published experience in South Africa[24,59] and France[59] has challenged an older concept that congestive heart failure and death during active carditis are caused exclusively by myocarditis rather than incompetence of the valve. Studies on left ventricular mechanics support this with new evidence.[102] In addition, primary myocardial involvement as evidenced by histologic abnormalities of the myocardium has been well documented during ARF.[209,283] Careful postoperative management, including at least 4 months of physical rest, diuretics, and vasodilation with ACE inhibitors, is thought to improve the long-term outcome by avoiding increased blood pressure and myocardial contractility before the repair has consolidated.

Surgery is ideally deferred until active inflammation as best judged by CRP measurements has subsided. Rarely, valve leaflet or chordae tendineae rupture leads to severe regurgitation; this event requires emergency surgery, which can be performed safely by experienced surgeons, although the risk seems to be slightly higher than when surgery is performed after active inflammation has resolved.[5,8]

PROGNOSIS

Carditis is the most serious manifestation of ARF and is the only aspect that has well-defined permanent sequelae.[307] Up to approximately 80% of patients have cardiac involvement during their acute episode, with 20% with moderate or severe RHD in modern series using echocardiography.[163,298] The rate of progression of valvular regurgitation resulting from rheumatic carditis is subject to wide individual variation; however, many cases tend to progress over the next 5 to 10 years, particularly if ARF recurs.[195] Moderate to severe valve lesions during the initial attack of ARF are strong predictors of RHD in the long term.[52,64,195] Valve lesions of a mild nature are likely to resolve over time in the absence of recurrences of ARF.[302] According to a study conducted in Brazil by Meira and colleagues,[195] 69.5% of patients with moderate or severe carditis (in the initial attack of ARF) had clinical evidence of RHD, and all of the patients with severe carditis had persistent RHD at a mean follow-up of 5.4 years.

Before the availability of penicillin, the prognosis for patients with ARF was even more stark. In a 20-year follow-up study by Bland and Duckett Jones,[40] a patient with marked cardiomegaly, congestive heart failure, or pericarditis had about a 70% to 80% chance of dying in the 10 years before the advent of secondary prevention programs, open heart surgery, and use of prosthetic valves. The prognosis today is not as poor, although the recurrence rates (with the attendant increased risk for carditis in individual patients) reported after some outbreaks[297,330] suggest a careful look at secondary prevention and its delivery. The risk for RHD at 1-year[9] and 10-year[64] follow-up is 70% for patients with cardiomegaly or heart failure and who survive. Most of these patients have mitral insufficiency, and approximately 50% also have aortic insufficiency.

Of patients with no or questionable carditis[9] during their attack of rheumatic fever, only 6% were found to have heart murmurs when reexamined 10 years later. Heart disease was present at follow-up in 30% of the patients initially found to have only apical systolic murmurs and in 40% of patients with basal diastolic murmurs during the acute phase. Patients with chorea may have a slightly lower incidence of residual heart disease.[167] Robust data on prognosis from the echocardiographic era are required.

PREVENTION

Most (approximately two-thirds) but not all episodes of rheumatic fever have a streptococcal throat infection that comes to medical attention. Denny and associates[82] and Wannamaker and colleagues[311] made one of the most important research contributions of the past 50 years when they showed that rheumatic fever can be prevented in most susceptible subjects if the preceding pharyngeal infection by one of the group A β-hemolytic streptococci is treated adequately. These studies used intramuscular depot procaine penicillin G in oil, now replaced by benzathine penicillin. The effectiveness of other antimicrobial agents (benzathine penicillin, chlortetracycline, sulfadiazine, oxytetracycline) in the prevention of rheumatic fever also was studied. Eradication of the streptococcus was shown to be essential in the prevention of rheumatic fever.[57] A 10-day course of oral penicillin treatment was found essential for this aim.[310] From these studies, penicillin, a bactericidal agent with activity against *Streptococcus pyogenes*, became the drug of choice.[105] Group A streptococci resistant to penicillin have not been documented to date.

Efficacy studies against rheumatic fever per se were performed mainly in military populations with injectable penicillin. Only one inconclusive study was done in children.[258] These studies more recently have been subjected to meta-analysis,[245] with a relative risk of 0.20 (95% CI 0.11–0.36; $P < .00001$) favoring the intervention and demonstrating that rheumatic fever can be prevented approximately 80% of the time. The ability of oral penicillin to eradicate streptococci in throats is not equal to the ability of injectable penicillin to do so.[25]

In the absence of clear direction from the published literature for the control of rheumatic fever in children using oral penicillin, a cluster-randomized, school-based, controlled trial in an area with endemic rheumatic fever and inadequate health care access in New Zealand of sore throat clinics in schools using oral penicillin (>80,000 person-years of observation) was performed.[163] Trained and highly supervised lay workers working with public health nurses were the main workforce. Over the 4-year study period, consent, participation, antibiotic adherence (observed therapy), and retention rates remained high. The outcome suggested a clinically useful result but with uncertainty about the effect size. Possible reasons for the failure to demonstrate a statistically significant reduction in rheumatic fever were persistent house crowding,[132] an inability to follow symptomatic siblings (who may have been at a control school) because of the school-based design, use of oral rather than injectable penicillin, or other reasons. Siblings have been shown to have a nearly 50% chance of developing group A streptococcal pharyngitis.[79] Exclusion from school of streptococcal pharyngitis cases was not possible. A meta-analysis of published literature on community- and/or school-based controlled studies to prevent first attacks of rheumatic fever revealed a relative risk of 0.62 (95% CI 0.45–0.85; $P = .003$), which favors these interventions, suggesting approximately 60% efficacy.[156] The New Zealand study used supervised oral penicillin treatment, but the treatment regimen was unclear in the other studies.[60,67,109,111,225] Peer-reviewed guidelines for rheumatic fever control have led to population-based initiatives in New Zealand that are ongoing at this time as a result of these endeavors.[7,16,144,145,157,158] The New Zealand government has committed to significant investment (more than NZ$70 million) to control the first presentation ARF with an emphasis on primary school clinics and health promotion in areas where there is a concentration of ARF. Small population settlements began initiatives. This then led to government investment spear-headed by the Maori Party in coalition with the National-led coalition government in power (www.health.govt.nz).

In south Auckland, where there is the greatest concentration of first presentation ARF cases and more than 90% of 5- to 13-year-olds at high risk of ARF are in a school throat-swabbing program as described above, a significant decrease of ARF rates was demonstrated over time following the introduction of the program ($P = .008$; incident/rate ratio, 0.61 [95% CI, 0.43–0.88]). Rates dropped from 88 (95% CI, 79–111) per 100,000 before the program to 37 (95% CI, 15–83) per 100,000 after 2 years of clinics, a 58% reduction.[154a] This proof of principle for a community-based primary prevention endeavor is the first demonstration using robust methodology. Differences compared to the NZ School trial were a more intensive approach to group A streptococcal control (management of siblings with symptomatic group A streptococcal pharyngitis and geographic clustering of school clinics with once-a-day amoxicillin (and phone calls at 5 and 10 days) to ensure high adherence to a 10-day course. A reduction in annual measurement ($n = 3$) pharyngeal group A streptococcal prevalence was noted. In the study period, there were minimal housing initiatives.[197]

A comprehensive explanation for the decline in rheumatic fever in most areas of the developed world remains unclear. Improved housing after World War II, especially in Western Europe; improved access to health care; public health messages highlighting the desirability of managing sore throats appropriately; the availability of penicillin; and other factors have been cited (see "Epidemiology").

Streptococcal pharyngeal infection should be identified in most situations before treatment is started, although ARF risk in the community involved (and available laboratory backup in low-resource economies) should be taken into account. Where ARF is rare, unnecessary antibiotic use should be a consideration. Guidelines using clinical parameters have evolved[58,144,160] that have been tested in selected populations to guide rational management.[190,191] In the New Zealand school program study in an area where rheumatic fever is endemic, four prediction rules were applied to the signs and symptoms of group A streptococcal-positive and -negative cultures of 12,906 self-reported sore throat episodes. No signs or symptoms separately or in combination reliably predicted a group A streptococcal sore throat. The most sensitive rule[144] was 54% predictive, thus missing nearly half of cases.[169] Streptococcal pharyngeal infection can be diagnosed by throat culture or through a rapid diagnostic antigen-detection kit.[105,107,256] Most tests have high specificity, so a patient with acute pharyngitis and a positive test result should be treated. Many of the tests have suboptimal sensitivity and should be confirmed by a throat culture.[105] One study found that in one-third of individuals with false-negative rapid antigen-detection test results, streptococcal antibody titers increased subsequently, suggesting infection.[106] Newer molecular techniques are evolving.

One study supports the notion that primary preventive treatment with penicillin is effective even if started 9 days after the infection develops,[56] so physicians can wait 24 to 48 hours for verification of infection by recovery of group A β-hemolytic streptococci.[105] Delays should be minimized. In the New Zealand study discussed earlier, this finding has been challenged, with three students developing ARF 5, 6, and 7 days after presenting with culture-proved group A streptococcal pharyngitis.[163]

A dose of 1.2 million U of benzathine penicillin intramuscularly (0.6 million U if weight is ≤27 kg) usually is adequate treatment. Because of the discomfort and a small but possible risk associated with intramuscular penicillin,[129] oral penicillin V 250 mg two or three times per day for children ≤27 kg or 500 mg two or three times per day for adolescents and adults may be preferred. Amoxicillin,[63,89,105,155,257] 50/mg/kg once per day (maximum 1 g/day) for 10 days is the other antibiotic of choice. Although of somewhat broader spectrum, it has the advantage of once-daily dosing, is relatively inexpensive, and the suspension is considered more palatable than penicillin V suspension.[105] Erythromycin estolate 20 to 40 mg/kg per day in two to four divided doses (maximum 1 g/day) may be used in patients who are allergic to penicillin. Erythromycin ethyl succinate 40 mg/kg per day two to four times per day (maximum 1 g/day) is an alternative therapy.[73] The latter macrolides have been superseded in many countries by azithromycin 12 mg/kg per day (maximum 500 mg for 5 days) or clarithromycin 15 mg/kg per day in two divided doses (maximum 250 mg two times per day for 10 days). Clindamycin or a narrow-spectrum cephalosporin (cephalexin) 20 mg/kg twice a day, maximum 500 mg per dose, are alternatives for the penicillin allergic, though the latter should be avoided in individuals with immediate-type hypersensitivity to penicillin.[256]

All oral treatments, except azithromycin, should be given for 10 days.[105,256] Although certain new wider spectrum agents such as azithromycin have been administered in shorter courses with the desired streptococcal eradication, on the basis of penicillin's narrow spectrum of antimicrobial activity, the infrequency with which it produces adverse reactions, and its modest cost, it is the drug of choice for nonallergic patients.[105]

Careful reading of trials of new agents should take into account standards required for accurate interpretation of such trials. In particular, *emm* typing is necessary to separate recurrences, treatment failures, or a new episode.[154,224]

Reappearance of ARF in a specific geographic region should draw attention to therapeutic, preventive, and epidemiologic measures for control of the disease. A targeted approach to particularly high-risk population groups in schools may be cost-effective and efficacious.[12,42,67,226,241,291] Because treatment of pharyngitis seems likely to have contributed to the declining incidence of rheumatic fever, obtaining throat cultures (or a rapid antigen-detection test) and administering penicillin treatment, if positive, for group A streptococci are recommended in low-risk populations, although this recommendation is being challenged by some physicians.[190,191] In addition, a negative culture avoids unnecessarily prescribing antibiotics in the 70% to 80% of children with a sore throat attributable to viral pharyngitis, although clinical assessment may obviate having to obtain a throat culture.[191,255]

As the risk of ARF becomes highly unlikely after a group A streptococcal pharyngitis (e.g., in most U.S. populations), clinical prediction rules (without a throat culture) should be considered to guide judicious antibiotic use.[41] Signs and symptoms usually not associated with streptococcal infection, such as simple coryza, hoarseness, cough, conjunctivitis, anterior stomatitis, and diarrhea,[105,191] may help target the approach in a low-risk population.

Prompt administration of antibiotic therapy may shorten the duration of symptoms in patients with group A β-hemolytic streptococcal pharyngitis.[236] Cultures should be used selectively in age groups in which rheumatic fever rarely occurs (e.g., <4 years of age or >20 years). A

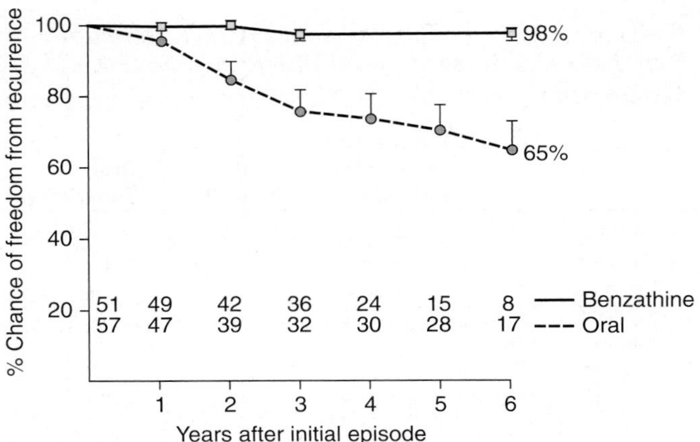

FIG. 29.8 Actuarial curves showing chance of freedom from recurrence of rheumatic fever after a first attack depending on type of penicillin prophylaxis initially instituted 1968–82. The bars on the curves refer to the standard error. The figures under the curves refer to the number of patients at risk at each time interval. (From Frankish JD. Rheumatic fever prophylaxis: Gisborne experience. *N Z Med J* 1984;97:674–5.)

follow-up throat culture taken after a course of treatment for streptococcal pharyngitis is not recommended routinely unless the patient remains symptomatic or is from a family with a rheumatic member. Such follow-up cultures probably identify long-term carriers for whom repeated courses of antibiotics generally are not indicated. Streptococcal carriers seem to pose little threat to themselves regarding the development of sequelae from streptococcal infection or dissemination of the organism to people around them. When a symptomatic viral upper respiratory tract infection develops in such a carrier, distinguishing whether the group A streptococci isolated indicate a current streptococcal infection or identify that individual as a chronic carrier is usually impossible. In one study, only 43% of children with paired sera from whom group A streptococci were recovered showed a significant antibody response to one of two different streptococcal antibodies.[140]

An often reasonable approach, especially in a population at low risk of ARF, is to administer a single course of therapy. Indications for obtaining cultures from household contacts vary according to circumstances.[73] Family contacts of high-risk patients should have a culture performed and receive treatment if the culture is positive.

In the era before penicillin, 75% of individuals developed a recurrence of ARF.[40] Continuous penicillin prophylaxis is well established in its ability to prevent recurrent attacks (Fig. 29.8), with intramuscular long-acting preparations being superior to oral twice-daily delivery.[98,174] Persistent worsening of RHD is prevented, and regression (50% to 70% over a decade) of valvular damage can occur.[170,179,290] Secondary prophylaxis, defined as the continuous administration of an antibiotic to a rheumatic fever/RHD case, is considered the most cost-effective management of ARF and its sequelae.[173,277]

The parenteral route has been shown to be more effective than oral penicillin (1.2 million U of benzathine penicillin intramuscularly at 28-day intervals) in the prevention of recurrences and reducing streptococcal throat infections.[324] In a comprehensive study, children experienced a recurrence rate of only 0.4/100 patient-years of observation (Table 29.7). A Cochrane systematic review found an 87% to 90% reduction with parenteral penicillin in four studies, including Wood et al.[324] An international study of allergic reactions to long-term benzathine penicillin prophylaxis found that the benefits of preventing recurrence far outweighed the risk for development of a serious allergic reaction.[129] In areas of particularly high risk, administration of benzathine penicillin every 21 days may be more efficacious, although this study was not performed systematically.[167] Serum levels of penicillin toward the end of treatment time can be unreliable,[43,134] although this decision should be offset against practicality, cost, and probable adherence. There is a paucity of published program evaluation.

The need for benzathine penicillin every 21 days was challenged in a carefully monitored, community-based program evaluation with high

TABLE 29.7 Prophylaxis and Attack Rates of Streptococcal Infection and Rheumatic Fever Recurrence

	Parenteral Benzathine Penicillin	Oral Penicillin	Oral Sulfadiazine
No. years	560	545	576
No./rate of all streptococcal infections, exclusive of carrier state (per 100,000)	24/4.3	101/18.5	102/17.7
No./rate of rheumatic recurrences (per 100,000)	2/0.4	30/5.5	16/2.8

Modified from Wood HF, Feinstein AR, Taranta A, et al. Rheumatic fever in children and adolescents: a long-term epidemiologic study of subsequent prophylaxis, streptococcal infections, and clinical sequelae. III. Comparative effectiveness of three prophylaxis regimens in preventing streptococcal infections and rheumatic recurrences. *Ann Intern Med.* 1964;60(suppl 5):31–45.

adherence rates.[117,269] On four weekly injections of penicillin, the penicillin failure rate per se was very low at 0.07/100 patient-years.[269] The program failure rate was 1.4/100 patient-years, with failure primarily resulting from nonadherence. This study was performed in an environment endemic for rheumatic fever, where children have a 1 : 150 chance of being hospitalized with ARF by the age of 15 years and a 1: 3 annual chance of having group A streptococci detected in their throats.[163,196] A study in Egypt[143] showed that two weekly injections of penicillin resulted in an almost 50% reduction in recurrences. This result occurred, however, in an environment in which the rate of recurrences was approximately 45% of cases in the four-weekly penicillin comparison arm, suggesting imperfect adherence to the treatment regimen. Data for adherence were not presented. Reduction of the pain of injection using lidocaine hydrochloride as a diluent for benzathine penicillin G to increase tolerability may be useful for increased program adherence.[246] Increased frequency of benzathine penicillin injections beyond those necessary will add complexity and cost to secondary prevention programs. Patients allergic to penicillin may be given erythromycin. Penicillin and sulfadiazine are oral regimens that have been studied for efficacy (Table 29.7). Sulfadiazine is not readily available in the United States.[14] The lesser efficacy of oral regimens is related at least partly to adherence difficulties.

The risk for rheumatic fever occurring after a group A streptococcal infection increases from an attack rate of 1% to 3% with the first attack of streptococcal pharyngitis to 25% to 75% with subsequent attacks.[319,82] Patients who have had carditis are at increased risk for development of further carditis.[11] Patients who have not had clinical carditis have considerably less risk for having cardiac involvement after a recurrence.[90,171] In the echocardiographic era, the dogma that a patient who escapes carditis in the first attack is highly likely to remain free of RHD, even if prophylaxis fails in subsequent attacks, has been challenged.[90,269]

The risk for recurrence depends on several other factors, such as the length of time since the most recent attack, multiple previous attacks, and the risk for acquiring streptococcal throat infections according to occupation or living circumstances.[40,282,319] If possible, the length of prophylaxis should be individualized. The suggested length ranges from a minimum of 5 years of prophylaxis to a maximum of lifelong prophylaxis.[65,105] This approach has been validated in a study from Chile.[30]

The New Zealand approach to recurrence prevention has been in place in Auckland for more than 2 decades.[16,269] All patients, regardless of cardiac status, receive at least 10 years of prophylaxis or until they reach 21 years of age (see earlier details for recurrence prevention). Evaluation of criteria for discharge from prophylaxis revealed only two recurrences in this series, which occurred in teenagers inadvertently discharged after at least 5 years of prophylaxis. It was concluded that it is safe to discharge individuals with mild or no clinically evident carditis at the time of discharge per the recommendations in this highly rheumatic fever endemic environment.[269] Recommended length of prophylaxis varies by authority.[271] Rigorous evaluation is lacking.

The AMA has recently published updated recommendations for the use of prophylactic antibiotics for prevention of infective endocarditis, most notably no longer suggesting prophylaxis for patients with RHD.[322] Some exceptions are necessary, such as those with prosthetic valves or prosthetic material used in valve repair. Some other international scientific bodies have made similar recommendations.[115] However, this approach has not been followed in New Zealand, where 12% of pediatric endocarditis cases occurred in RHD cases and where rheumatic valvular disease remains common in disadvantaged individuals who in addition have important dental and periodontal disease.[68,313]

CONCLUSION

Although having effective prophylaxis against a disease[186] for which the pathophysiology is understood incompletely and for which no pharmacologic cure exists is gratifying, rheumatic fever remains the most important cause of acquired heart disease in children and young people globally, clustering in the developing world and in disadvantaged populations in the developed world.[53,325] This rate is largely a reflection of complacency about rheumatic fever and RHD by physicians and health care funders, although it also is likely to reflect living conditions and health care access. Renewed educational efforts regarding prevention of rheumatic fever are needed among public health workers, physicians, and the public. The available preventive methods should be applied vigorously. Applying modern research tools may be beneficial.

NEW REFERENCES SINCE THE SEVENTH EDITION

7. Anderson PKJ, Moss M, Light P, et al. Nurse-led school-based clinics for rheumatic fever prevention and skin infection management—evaluation of Mana Kidz programme in Counties Manukau. *N Z Med J.* 2016;129(428):37-46.
11. Anonymous. Prophylaxis in rheumatic fever. *Br Med J.* 1972;1:64.
13. Anonymous. Acute rheumatic fever among army trainees - Fort Leonard Wood, Missouri, 1987–1988. *MMWR Morb Mortal Wkly Rep.* 1988;37:519-522.
15. Aron AM, Freeman JM, Carter S. The natural history of Sydenham's chorea. *Am J Med.* 1965;38:83-95.
21. Azevedo PM, Pereira RR, Guilherme L. Understanding rheumatic fever. *Rheumatol Int.* 2012;32(5):1113-1120.
23. Barash J, Margalith D, Matitiau A. Corticosteroid treatment in patients with Sydenham's chorea. *Pediatr Neurol.* 2005;32(3):205-207.
28. Beall B, Facklam R, Thompson T. Sequencing emm-specific PCR products for routine and accurate typing of group A streptococci. *J Clin Microbiol.* 1996; 34(4):953-958.
29. Beaton A, Okello E, Aliku T, et al. Latent rheumatic heart disease: outcomes 2 years after echocardiographic detection. *Pediatr Cardiol.* 2014;35(7):1259-1267.
30. Berrios X, del Campo E, Guzman B, et al. Discontinuing rheumatic fever prophylaxis in selected adolescents and young adults. A prospective study. *Ann Intern Med.* 1993;118(6):401-406.
33. Bhaya M, Beniwal R, Panwar S, et al. Two years of follow-up validates the echocardiographic criteria for the diagnosis and screening of rheumatic heart disease in asymptomatic populations. *Echocardiography.* 2011;28(9):929-933.
41. American Academy of Pediatrics. Group A streptococcal infections. In: Kimberlin DW, Long SS, eds. *Red Book 2015: 2015 Report of the Committee on Infectious Diseases.* Elk Grove Village, IL: Author; 2015:732-744.
43. Broderick MP, Hansen CJ, Faix DJ. Factors associated with loss of penicillin G concentrations in serum after intramuscular benzathine penicillin G injection: a meta-analysis. *Pediatr Infect Dis J.* 2012;31(7):722-725.
50. Carapetis JR, Currie BJ. Rheumatic chorea in northern Australia: a clinical and epidemiological study. *Arch Dis Child.* 1999;80(4):353-358.
51. Carapetis JR, Currie BJ. Rheumatic fever in a high incidence population: the importance of monoarthritis and low grade fever. *Arch Dis Child.* 2001;85(3):223-227.
55. Cardoso F, Maia D, Cunningham MC, et al. Treatment of Sydenham chorea with corticosteroids. *Mov Disord.* 2003;18(11):1374-1377.
70. Cunningham MW. Rheumatic fever, autoimmunity, and molecular mimicry: the streptococcal connection. *Int Rev Immunol.* 2014;33(4):314-329.
78. Dale JB, Penfound TA, Tamboura B, et al. Potential coverage of a multivalent M protein-based group A streptococcal vaccine. *Vaccine.* 2013;31(12):1576-1581.
84. Engel ME, Muhamed B, Whitelaw AC, et al. Group A streptococcal emm type prevalence among symptomatic children in Cape Town and potential vaccine coverage. *Pediatr Infect Dis J.* 2014;33(2):208-210.

86. Enriquez-Sarano M, Akins CW, Vahanian A. Mitral regurgitation. *Lancet.* 2009;373(9672):1382-1394.
94. Finucane K. Priorities in cardiac surgeery for rheumatic heart disease. *Glob Heart.* 2013;8:213-220.
99. Fusco C, Ucchino V, Frattini D, et al. Acute and chronic corticosteroid treatment of ten patients with paralytic form of Sydenham's chorea. *Eur J Paediatr Neurol.* 2012;16(4):373-378.
100. Garvey MA, Snider LA, Leitman SF, et al. Treatment of Sydenham's chorea with intravenous immunoglobulin, plasma exchange, or prednisone. *J Child Neurol.* 2005;20(5):424-429.
103. Gentles TL, Finucane KA, Mervis J, et al. Outcome of the LV in children and young adults with severe combined aortic and mitral valve regurgitation compared to isolated lesions. *J Am Coll Cardiol.* 2010;55(10A):E432.
104. Gentles TL, French JK, Zeng I, et al. Normalized end-systolic volume and pre-load reserve predict ventricular dysfunction following surgery for aortic regurgitation independent of body size. *JACC Cardiovasc Imaging.* 2012;5:626-633.
106. Gentles TL, Finucane AK, Remenyi B, et al. Ventricular function before and after surgery for isolated and combined regurgitation in the young. *Ann Thorac Surg.* 2015;100(4):1383-1389.
108. Gewitz MH, Baltimore RS, Tani LY, et al. Revision of the Jones Criteria for the diagnosis of acute rheumatic fever in the era of Doppler echocardiography: a scientific statement from the American Heart Association. *Circulation.* 2015;131(20):1806-1818.
120. Guilherme L, Kalil J. Rheumatic fever and rheumatic heart disease: cellular mechanisms leading autoimmune reactivity and disease. *J Clin Immunol.* 2010;30(1):17-23.
128. Hunter S, Jackson C, Carter P, et al. Does the 30 valent M protein-based vaccine have the potential to prevent rheumatic fever in New Zealand? Abstract for ASID 2015.
130. Irlam J, Mayosi BM, Engel M, et al. Primary prevention of acute rheumatic fever and rheumatic heart disease with penicillin in South African children with pharyngitis: a cost-effectiveness analysis. *Circ Cardiovasc Qual Outcomes.* 2013;6(3):343-351.
142. Karthikeyan G, Mayosi BM. Is primary prevention of rheumatic fever the missing link in the control of rheumatic heart disease in Africa? *Circulation.* 2009;120(8):709-713.
161. Lennon D, Stewart J, Anderson P. Primary prevention of rheumatic fever. *Pediatr Infect Dis J.* 2016;35(7):820.
165. Lessof MH, Bywaters EG. The duration of chorea. *BMJ.* 1956;1520-1523.
166. Liu M, Subramanian V, Christie C, et al. Immune responses to self-antigens in asthma patients: clinical and immunopathological implications. *Hum Immunol.* 2012;73(5):511-516.
168. Lugar PL, Love C, Grammer AC, et al. Molecular characterization of circulating plasma cells in patients with active systemic lupus erythematosus. *PLoS ONE.* 2012;7(9):e44362.
169. Kerdemelidis M, Lennon DR, Stewart J. How should sore throats be managed? Performance of four group A streptococcal sore throat prediction rules in New Zealand children. Abstract for ID Week 2015.
170. Majeed H, Batnager S, Yousof A, et al. Acute rheumatic fever and the evolution of rheumatic heart disease: a prospective 12 year follow-up report. *J Clin Epidemiol.* 1992;45(8):871-875.
173. Manji RA, Witt J, Tappia PS, et al. Cost-effectiveness analysis of rheumatic heart disease prevention strategies. *Expert Rev Pharmacoecon Outcomes Res.* 2013;13(6):715-724.
186. Massell B, Chute C, Walker A, et al. Penicillin and the marked decrease in morbidity and mortality from rheumatic fever in the United States. *N Engl J Med.* 1988;318:280-286.
193. McMillan DJ, Dreze PA, Vu T, et al. Updated model of group A streptococcus M proteins based on a comprehensive worldwide study. *Clin Microbiol Infect.* 2013;19(5):E222-E229.
196. Milne R, Lennon D, Grant CC, et al. Epidemiology and actual costs of paediatric pneumococcal infection in New Zealand. Submitted to New Zealand Ministry of Health. 2003.
199. Mistry RM, Lennon D, Boyle MJ, et al. Septic arthritis and acute rheumatic fever in children: the diagnostic value of serological inflammatory markers. *J Pediatr Orthop.* 2015;35(3):318-322.
201. Cheung MM, Sullivan ID, de Leval MR, et al. Optimal timing of the Ross procedure in the management of chronic aortic incompetence in the young. *Cardiol Young.* 2003;13:253-257.
204. Moreland NJ, Waddington CS, Williamson DA, et al. Working towards a group A streptococcal vaccine: report of a collaborative Trans-Tasman workshop. *Vaccine.* 2014;32(30):3713-3720.
208. Murray CJ, Vos T, Lozano R, et al. Disability-adjusted life years (DALYs) for 291 diseases and injuries in 21 regions, 1990–2010: a systematic analysis for the Global Burden of Disease Study 2010. *Lancet.* 2012;380(9859):2197-2223.
212. Nishimura RA, Otto CM, Bonow RO, et al. 2014 AHA/ACC guideline for the management of patients with valvular heart disease: a report of the American College of Cardiology/American Heart Association Task Force on Practice Guidelines. *J Thorac Cardiovasc Surg.* 2014;148(1):e1-e132.
213. Nordet P. WHO/ISFC global programme for the prevention and control of RH/RHD. *J Int Soc Fed Cardiol.* 1993;3:4-5.
215. North R, Sadler L, Stewart A, et al. Long-term survival and valve-related complications in young women with cardiac valve replacements. *Circulation.* 1999; 99(20):2669-2676.
216. O'Loughlin RE, Roberson A, Cieslak PR, et al. The epidemiology of invasive group A streptococcal infection and potential vaccine implications: United States, 2000–2004. [see comment]. *Clin Infect Dis.* 2007;45(7):853-862.
217. Paar JA, Berrios NM, Rose JD, et al. Prevalence of rheumatic heart disease in children and young adults in Nicaragua. *Am J Cardiol.* 2010;105(12):1809-1814.
218. Parks T, Smeesters PR, Steer AC. Streptococcal skin infection and rheumatic heart disease. *Curr Opin Infect Dis.* 2012;25(2):145-153.
224. Peter G. Streptococcal pharyngitis: current therapy and criteria for evaluation of new agents. *Clin Infect Dis.* 1992;14(suppl 2):S218-S223.
239. Remenyi B, Webb R, Gentles T, et al. Improved long-term survival for rheumatic mitral valve repair compared to replacement in the young. *World J Pediatr Congenit Heart Surg.* 2013;4(2):155-164.
244. Roberts S, Kosanke S, Terrence Dunn S, et al. Pathogenic mechanisms in rheumatic carditis: focus on valvular endothelium. *J Infect Dis.* 2001;183(3):507-511.
246. Russell K, Nicholson R, Naidu R. Reducing the pain of intramuscular benzathine penicillin injections in the rheumatic fever population of Counties Manukau District Health Board. *J Paediatr Child Health.* 2014;50(2):112-117.
248. Swedo S. Sydenham's chorea: a model for childhood autoimmune neuropsychiatric disorders. *JAMA.* 1994;272(22):1788-1791.
249. Saphir O. The Aschoff nodule. *Am J Clin Pathol.* 1959;31(6):534-539.
250. Saxena A, Ramakrishnan S, Roy A, et al. Prevalence and outcome of subclinical rheumatic heart disease in India: the RHEUMATIC (Rheumatic Heart Echo Utilisation and Monitoring Actuarial Trends in Indian Children) study. *Heart.* 2011;97(24):2018-2022.
251. Schweitzer B, Meng L, Mattoon D, et al. Immune response biomarker profiling application on ProtoArray protein microarrays. *Methods Mol Biol.* 2010;641:243-252.
256. Shulman ST, Bisno AL, Clegg HW, et al. Clinical practice guideline for the diagnosis and management of group A streptococcal pharyngitis: 2012 update by the Infectious Diseases Society of America. *Clin Infect Dis.* 2012;55(10):e86-e102.
259. Sigdel TK, Woo SH, Dai H, et al. Profiling of autoantibodies in IgA nephropathy, an integrative antibiomics approach. *Clin J Am Soc Nephrol.* 2011;6(12):2775-2784.
261. Sliwa K, Liebhaber E, Ellikott C, et al. Spectrum of cardiac disease in maternity in a low-resource cohort in South Africa. *Heart.* 2014;100:1967-1974.
262. Smeesters PR, Dramaix M, Van Melderen L. The emm-type diversity does not always reflect the M protein genetic diversity–is there a case for designer vaccine against GAS. *Vaccine.* 2010;28(4):883-885.
263. Smeesters PR, McMillan DJ, Sripraksh KS, et al. Differences among group A streptococcus epidemiological landscapes: consequences for M protein-based vaccines? *Expert Rev Vaccines.* 2009;8(12):1705-1720.
264. Smeesters PR, Vergison A, Campos D, et al. Differences between Belgian and Brazilian group A streptococcus epidemiologic landscape. *PLoS ONE.* 2006;1:e10.
280. Tandon R, Sharma N, Chandrashekhar Y, et al. Revisiting the pathogenesis of rheumatic fever and carditis. *Nat Rev Cardiol.* 2013;10:171-177.
290. Tompkins DG, Boxerbaum B, Liebman J. Long-term prognosis of rheumatic fever patients receiving regular intramuscular benzathine penicillin. *Circulation.* 1972;45(3):543-551.
294. van den Ham HJ, de Jager W, Bijlsma JW, et al. Differential cytokine profiles in juvenile idiopathic arthritis subtypes revealed by cluster analysis. *Rheumatology (Oxford).* 2009;48(8):899-905.
305. Walker AR, Tani LY, Thompson JA, et al. Rheumatic chorea: relationship to systemic manifestations and response to corticosteroids. *J Pediatr.* 2007;151(6):679-683.
312. Watkins DA, Mvundura M, Nordet P, et al. A cost-effectiveness analysis of a program to control rheumatic fever and rheumatic heart disease in Pinar del Rio, Cuba. *PLoS ONE.* 2015;10(3):e0121363.
313. Webb R, Voss L, Roberts S, et al. Infective endocarditis in New Zealand children 1994–2012. *Pediatr Infect Dis J.* 2014;33(5):437-442.
317. Williamson DA, Morgan J, Hope V, et al. Increasing incidence of invasive group A streptococcus disease in New Zealand, 2002–2012: a national population-based study. *J Infect.* 2015;70(2):127-134.
318. Williamson DA, Smeesters P, Steer A, et al. M-protein analysis of *Streptococcus pyogenes* isolates associated with acute rheumatic fever in New Zealand. *J Clin Microbiol.* 2015;53(11):3618-3620.
321. Wilson N, Voss L, Morreau J, et al. New Zealand guidelines for the diagnosis of acute rheumatic fever: small increase in the incidence of definite cases compared to the American Heart Association Jones criteria. *N Z Med J.* 2013;126(1379):50-59.
326. Wyber RTK, Markoz S, Kaplan EL. Benzathine penicillin G for the management of RHD concerns about quality and access, and opportunities for intervention and improvement. *Glob Heart.* 2013;8(3):227-234.
329. Zakikhany K, Degail MA, Lamagni T, et al. Increase in invasive *Streptococcus pyogenes* and *Streptococcus pneumoniae* infections in England, December 2010 to January 2011. *Euro Surveill.* 2011;16(5):19785.

The full reference list for this chapter is available at ExpertConsult.com.

30 Mediastinitis

Morven S. Edwards

The mediastinum is the extrapleural portion of the thoracic cavity situated between the two pleural sacs. The superior and inferior portions are separated arbitrarily by a line extending from the lower manubrium to the fourth thoracic vertebra. The superior mediastinum contains the thymus gland, trachea, esophagus, and aortic arch. The inferior mediastinum is divided into the anterior compartment, containing lymphatic tissue and fat; the middle compartment, containing the heart, pericardium, aorta, bifurcation of the trachea, main bronchi, and numerous lymph nodes; and the posterior compartment, containing the esophagus, thoracic duct, descending aorta, and vagus nerve. *Mediastinitis* refers to inflammation of the tissues located in the mediastinum. Infections of the mediastinum are uncommon, but they pose a serious threat to vital structures.

Acute mediastinitis is a fulminant, septic process, and chronic mediastinitis is an indolent process that produces late symptoms caused by compression of adjacent structures. Acute mediastinitis occurs as a consequence of trauma from perforation of the esophagus, extension of infection from adjacent structures, and postoperatively after thoracic surgery (Box 30.1).

ACUTE MEDIASTINITIS

Mediastinitis Due to Esophageal Perforation

The esophagus is a thin-walled organ, and esophageal perforation is the most common cause of acute mediastinitis.[41] Perforation usually occurs at one of the three sites of anatomic narrowing of the esophagus: (1) the proximal end, at the level of the cricopharyngeal muscle; (2) the midthoracic segment where the aortic arch and left main stem bronchus indent the esophagus; or (3) the transdiaphragmatic segment. Proximal perforations usually are caused by instrumentation or ingestion of a foreign body. The proximal segment is narrow, and perforations generally are located in the posterior wall, adjacent to the prevertebral and retrovisceral spaces. Perforations at the aortic arch usually are caused by ingested foreign objects. Transdiaphragmatic perforations usually are spontaneous. In most such cases, a longitudinal tear occurs on the left posterolateral wall just above the cardia, where the esophagus has little connective tissue support and the intrinsic musculature is weak.

Retching or vomiting can generate sufficient force to cause esophageal perforation, also known as Boerhaave syndrome. Traumatic perforation can occur after blunt trauma, from ingestion of a foreign body, or as a complication of endoscopic or open surgical procedures. Ingestion of coins, teeth, and food particles such as corn chips as well as objects such as a toy soldier or the spring from a clothespin have caused mediastinitis.[17] Children with mediastinitis from erosion of the esophagus caused by a foreign body tend to have small and well-contained perforations. Sharp objects, such as pins and bone fragments, can cause immediate transmural penetration. More commonly, and especially when a blunt object is ingested, the foreign body becomes impacted in the esophagus. Eventually, suppurative necrosis of the wall occurs, with symptoms occurring days, weeks, or months after the ingestion.[23]

Perforations from instrumentation can produce precipitous clinical deterioration from transmural laceration.[41] A superficial tear can occur from which infection subsequently extends, and hours or days can elapse between instrumentation and onset of symptoms. Repair of esophageal atresia is a common condition associated with a tear of the esophagus in childhood. In one review, 7 of 41 infants had a clinically significant esophageal disruption requiring reoperation 1 to 18 days after repair of esophageal atresia.[6] Postoperative perforations of the esophagus usually represent infectious complications of anastomotic leaks occurring after esophageal resection or of esophageal-pleural fistulas that develop after thoracic surgery. Most of these infections do not become apparent until weeks or months after surgery.

Presenting findings of acute mediastinitis after perforation of the esophagus include neck and chest pain, respiratory distress, and dysphagia. Chills, a temperature of 37.8°C to 39°C (100°F to 102°F), and leukocytosis are common. Infants can present with tachypnea, tachycardia, stridor, or a supplemental oxygen requirement. Some patients have a staccato breathing pattern characterized by an inspiratory halt with resumption of inspiration after a brief rest.[12] The onset of symptoms usually is abrupt, and the course is fulminant. Physical findings include cervical tenderness and subcutaneous emphysema in patients with proximal perforations, whereas patients with perforations of the lower esophagus are more likely to have signs suggesting an abdominal catastrophe. Examination of the lung fields often shows nonspecific abnormalities. Children with chronically retained foreign bodies can present with signs suggestive of asthma or reflux.[9]

The principal findings on chest radiographs are a widened mediastinum, subcutaneous and mediastinal emphysema, and pleural effusion. Pleural effusions occur more commonly with perforations of the lower than the upper esophagus and usually involve the left side. Basilar or retrocardiac infiltrates attributed to chemical pneumonitis can occur in the pulmonary segment adjacent to the site of perforation. Additional changes include basilar atelectasis, pneumothorax, or hydropneumothorax. Radiopaque foreign bodies can be detected with plain radiographs, but they are better visualized with mediastinal computed tomography (CT) or magnetic resonance imaging (MRI).

Gas in the soft tissues is highly suggestive of perforation of the esophagus if interpreted in the context of a compatible clinical presentation. Gas in the prevertebral tissue or superior mediastinum occurs most commonly with perforation of the upper esophagus. Other conditions, such as chest wall trauma or perforation of the trachea, also can cause mediastinal emphysema.

Clinical presentation and plain radiographic findings form the basis for the diagnosis of acute mediastinitis caused by perforation of the esophagus. Contrast-enhanced CT or MRI can provide anatomic detail and confirmation of the diagnosis.[47] Findings include esophageal thickening, fluid collections in the mediastinum adjacent to the perforation, and extraluminal air. Analysis of pleural fluid usually shows a sterile exudate early in the disease course. Pleural fluid amylase levels often are normal within the first 24 hours after perforation. After 24 hours, the pleural fluid amylase level is elevated disproportionately compared with serum levels. Esophagoscopy is unnecessary and is contraindicated except for removing a foreign body.

Surgical drainage and repair and antimicrobial therapy are indicated for large perforations, when there is communication with the pleural space or abdomen, when vascular erosion is a concern, and in the setting of underlying esophageal pathology. Nonsurgical management can be considered for children in whom the perforation is a small, well-contained lesion in the upper esophagus in the absence of an underlying esophageal pathologic process.[10,23] Supportive measures include intravenous fluid support, maintenance of an adequate airway, esophageal rest, and careful monitoring of vital functions. Blood and pleural fluid cultures should be obtained, but they usually are sterile except late in the course. Antimicrobial agents provided empirically should be directed against streptococci, staphylococci, and oral anaerobic bacteria.[5,7] Mortality rates can be high when recognition of the infection is delayed.[41]

BOX 30.1 Classification of Mediastinitis

Acute Mediastinitis

A. Due to traumatic perforation of the esophagus
   1. Spontaneous or postemetic
   2. Foreign body–associated
   3. Instrumentation or surgery
B. Due to extension of infection from adjacent structures
   1. Infection of the head and neck
   2. Infections of lungs, pleura, lymph nodes, or pericardium
   3. Subphrenic infection
   4. Vertebral osteomyelitis
   5. Hematogenous dissemination
C. Postoperative

Chronic Mediastinitis

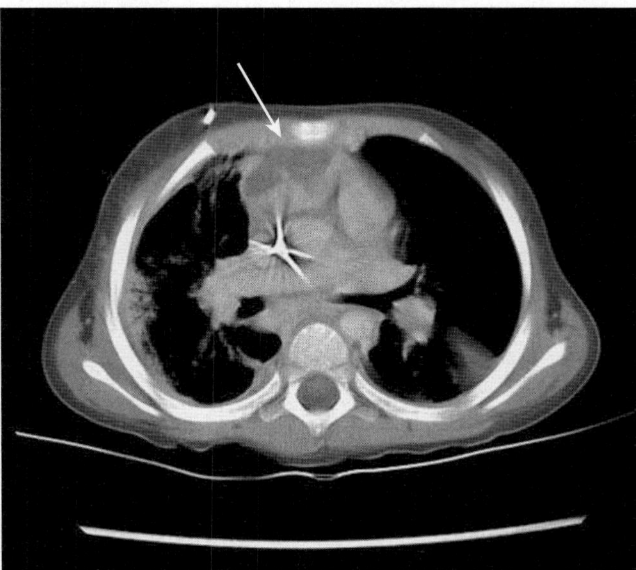

FIG. 30.1 Contrast-enhanced computed tomography scan shows a 3 × 3-cm heterogeneous enhancing abscess *(arrow)* in the anterior mediastinum of a child acutely ill with *Streptococcus pneumoniae* bacteremia and pneumonia with empyema. Cultures from the mediastinal abscess at the time of surgical drainage were sterile.

Mediastinitis Due to Extension of Infection From Adjacent Structures

The mediastinum is anatomically well situated for involvement when infection extends downward from the oropharynx. Fascial planes from the supraclavicular region and abdomen traverse the mediastinum, and the lymphatic duct is located in the mediastinum. The lung, situated laterally to the mediastinum, is a frequent locus of potentially serious infection. Despite its position as an anatomic crossroad, extension of infection to the mediastinum from adjacent structures occurs infrequently.

In the preantibiotic era, retropharyngeal or peritonsillar abscess, Ludwig angina, dental abscess, and other infections of the head and neck were common causes of acute descending mediastinitis.[14,46] Since the advent of penicillin, infections of the head and neck usually are contained at the site of origin. The principal spaces that serve as conduits to the mediastinum are the visceral division of the deep cervical fascia that envelops the esophagus, trachea, larynx, and thyroid gland and the carotid sheath, which extends from the base of the skull, passes through the posterior pharyngomaxillary space along the prevertebral fascia, and enters the chest. Mediastinitis can occur as a complication of retropharyngeal abscess, peritonsillar and dental abscesses, as well as mastoiditis, laryngectomy, mediastinotomy, tracheostomy, and surgery or trauma of the oropharynx.[44] Mediastinitis can complicate placement of airway stents for management of tracheal or bronchial stenoses in children.[21]

Children have developed mediastinitis after incurring intraoral injuries caused by falling with an object such as a toothbrush in their mouths.[25] Infection spreads to the mediastinum through the retropharyngeal space. Sharp objects, such as fish bones, can perforate the esophagus, with resultant infection.[36] A penetrating wound to the oropharynx can be caused by falling on a sharp or pointed object such as a pencil. Mediastinitis rarely complicates suppurative pleuropulmonary infection, but multiple necrotic or abscessed lymph nodes can occur with coccidioidomycosis or atypical mycobacterial infections.[31] Extension of infection from vertebrae, ribs, or sternum also is unusual. The main radiographic feature is widening of the mediastinum. Imaging by contrast-enhanced cervicothoracic CT or MRI is crucial for establishing the diagnosis and can reveal heterogeneous infiltration, gas in tissues, abscesses, and fluid collections (Fig. 30.1).

Streptococci and anaerobic oral flora are the bacteria usually responsible for suppurative infections that originate in the oral cavity and extend to the mediastinum.[7] Methicillin-sensitive and methicillin-resistant *Staphylococcus aureus* (MRSA) should be considered potential pathogens, especially in mediastinitis complicating retropharyngeal abscess.[1,42,52] Group A streptococcus is a common pathogen when the oropharynx is the original portal of entry. Other streptococci, including *Streptococcus anginosus* (formerly *S. milleri*) and group F streptococcus, are common isolates. Anaerobic bacteria, principally *Prevotella* spp., *Bacteroides* spp., *Fusobacterium* spp., and peptostreptococci, are the major anaerobic pathogens. Gram-negative aerobic bacteria, including *Pseudomonas aeruginosa*, *Serratia* spp., and *Neisseria* spp., are isolated less often.[28] Mixed infection is common. Clindamycin often is regarded as the agent of choice for streptococci and anaerobes, although some authorities prefer other regimens, including penicillin plus metronidazole, cefoxitin, cefotetan, meropenem, or a β-lactam/β-lactamase inhibitor.[7,13] Consideration should be given to including vancomycin in empiric regimens for MRSA coverage until culture results are available.

Surgical drainage combined with appropriate antibiotic therapy is the cornerstone of treatment. Transcervical incisions usually are employed when spread to the superior mediastinum has occurred. Extension of the infection below the level of the fourth thoracic vertebra requires a parasternal or paravertebral approach, depending on whether the anterior or posterior mediastinum is involved.

Postoperative Mediastinitis

Sternal wound infections are an uncommon complication of median sternotomy for cardiac surgery in children.[4] The Centers for Disease Control and Prevention classifies surgical site infections in cardiac patients as superficial or deep wound infection, sternal osteomyelitis, or mediastinitis. Mediastinitis is a serious complication, with potential involvement of contiguous structures, including prosthetic valves, grafts, pericardium, lung, and chest wall. Contemporary incidence data for mediastinitis after pediatric cardiac surgery is 0.2% to 1.4% of procedures.[2,32,48] The incidence is higher after cardiac transplantation.[27] Postoperative wound infection is more often a complication of double-outlet right ventricle repair, truncus repair, atrial switch, or valvulatory or conduit procedures than of repair of atrial septal defect, ventricular septal defect, or tetralogy of Fallot.[38] Mediastinal infection has developed from an infection of a retained epicardial pacemaker lead.[19]

Some of the risk factors for poststernotomy mediastinitis in adults are not applicable to children. Factors that are linked to risk for development of mediastinitis after median sternotomy in children are shown in Box 30.2. Obesity and diabetes mellitus, which are risk factors in adults, have not been assessed as potential risk factors in children. Factors not associated with risk for infection include emergency surgery or prior infection.[32] Intraoperative introduction of organisms is considered the source of most infections. Epidemics have been traced to operating room personnel, who can serve as the source of *S. aureus* or other bacteria.[15]

In three pediatric series, the median time to onset of mediastinitis after pediatric cardiac surgery was 10 to 14 days, with a range from

BOX 30.2 Risk Factors for Pediatric Poststernotomy Mediastinitis

Malnutrition
Preoperative respiratory tract infection
Known or possible genetic syndrome
Young age
High American Society of Anesthesiologists score
Asplenia
Prolonged duration of surgery
Cardiac transplantation
Prolonged ventilation
Intracardiac pacing wires longer than 3 days
Longer intensive care unit stay
Delayed sternal closure

Data from references 2, 22, 29, 32, and 48.

4 to 50 days.[2,27,48] The time to infection after sternotomy was longer for infections caused by gram-positive organisms than for infections caused by gram-negative bacteria or fungi in one report.[48] The presenting features include erythema, purulent drainage or tenderness of the sternal incision, wound dehiscence, sternal instability, persistent or recurrent postoperative fever, and leukocytosis. A common clinical sequence is fever and systemic toxicity followed by signs of a sternal wound infection with cellulitis or purulent drainage. Imaging abnormalities include mediastinal soft tissue swelling, pleural effusion, and sternal dehiscence or erosion, but CT does not always reveal abnormalities.[34,53] Consideration should be given to use of MRI when infection is suspected. Lack of compelling radiographic evidence of infection should not delay surgical drainage when clinical signs are evident.

Empiric antibiotic treatment should be based on the expected pathogens and modified according to results of blood and wound cultures. Approximately two-thirds of infections are caused by gram-positive bacteria, one fourth by gram-negative bacteria, and the remainder by yeasts and fungi. *Staphylococcus aureus* accounts for more than one-half of infections; coagulase-negative staphylococci and enterococci (including vancomycin-resistant isolates) constitute the remainder of the gram-positive isolates.[2,27,48] In adults, MRSA mediastinitis is associated with higher rates of overall mortality, mediastinitis-related mortality, and treatment failure than infection caused by methicillin-sensitive *S. aureus.*[33]

Approximately one-half of children have associated bacteremia, and infection with *S. aureus* is an independent risk factor for development of bacteremic postoperative mediastinitis.[43] Among gram-negative organisms, *P. aeruginosa, Serratia* spp., and *Citrobacter* are common isolates. Infection is polymicrobial in one-fourth of patients.[2,27,48] *Candida* spp. should be considered in any patient with infection of the mediastinum, particularly when broad-spectrum antimicrobial agents have been used.[8] Almost any microorganism gaining entry to the mediastinum theoretically can serve as the nidus for infection, and *Mycoplasma hominis, Ureaplasma urealyticum, Nocardia,* and *Aspergillus* all have been reported, albeit rarely.[16,26,50] Heart and lung transplant patients are prone to acquisition of infection with less common and more resistant pathogens, such as *Aspergillus fumigatus* and *Burkholderia cepacia.*[27] *M. fortuitum* can cause apparently culture-negative mediastinitis and has been reported in a child who had undergone a Fontan operation.[45]

Adequate surgical debridement is crucial to successful treatment of postoperative mediastinitis. Surgical procedures to reexplore the sternum should be undertaken and infected and devitalized tissue debrided. After wound debridement, continuous irrigation and vacuum-assisted closure and use of simple primary closed drainage have been effective management options.[3,49] Open wound packing and delayed rectus abdominis flap, pectoralis muscle flap, or omental reconstruction can be required.[37,48] Pectoralis muscle flap has been an effective treatment even in neonates.[11,48] Early consultation with plastic surgery and reconstructive teams is advisable when sternal reconstruction is anticipated. Infection superficial to the sternum can be treated simply with incision, packing, and a short course of antibiotics, usually for 10 to 14 days. Systemic antibiotics must be given for at least 3 to 6 weeks for children with postoperative mediastinitis.

CHRONIC MEDIASTINITIS

Histologically, chronic mediastinitis can be fibrosing or granulomatous. Both are rare conditions in which a definite cause often remains elusive. The clinical presentations are identical, and considerable overlap can occur in histologic findings. Fibrosing mediastinitis can be focal or diffuse; calcification within the lesion is observed more often when the process is focal. Some authors propose that mediastinal fibrosis represents the end stage of mediastinal granuloma, whereas others suggest that the two are distinct entities.[40] Fibrosing mediastinitis can be associated with a fibrotic process at another anatomic site, such as the retroperitoneum.

Chronic mediastinitis is rare in very young children but has been described in toddlers.[39] Many patients are asymptomatic, and the lesion initially is detected by routine chest radiographs showing a widened superior mediastinum near the tracheal bifurcation or the hilum with a lobulated configuration. Pulmonary parenchymal findings vary. Common clinical presentations include recurrent pneumonia and hemoptysis.[20] Symptoms can reflect compression of adjacent structures, such as the superior vena cava, pulmonary vessels, esophagus, and tracheobronchial tree. Patients can present with low-grade fever, cough, pleuritic chest pain, and dyspnea, with anemia and weight loss.[40]

When an inciting cause for chronic mediastinitis can be identified, it usually is linked to infection with *Histoplasma capsulatum.* Two types of mediastinal fibrosis caused by histoplasmosis are recognized. Mediastinal granuloma is caused by coalescence of a cluster of mediastinal lymph nodes to form an encapsulated mass that may be large and compress adjacent structures, especially the superior vena cava or esophagus. Surgical resection often is feasible but is advocated only when the obstruction is significant. Fibrosing mediastinitis is thought to represent an immune-mediated hypersensitivity response to *H. capsulatum* rather than an ongoing infectious process. Less common causes of fibrosing mediastinitis include tuberculosis, blastomycosis, cryptococcosis, aspergillosis, zygomycosis, autoimmune disease, nocardiosis, actinomycosis, and lymphoma.[18,24,30,35,39]

The diagnostic evaluation of patients with possible chronic mediastinitis should include a chest radiograph and contrast-enhanced CT or MRI. A vascular imaging study may be required if there is evidence of venous or vena caval obstruction or if arterial involvement is present. Testing for tuberculosis and histoplasmosis should be obtained. Cultures of sputum for *Mycobacterium tuberculosis* and pathogenic fungi are rarely positive. Antigen assay for *H. capsulatum* using blood and urine usually is negative, and skin tests are not helpful. Complement-fixation titers usually exceed 1:8 in patients with chronic histoplasmosis.

Surgical resection can be associated with high morbidity but can be curative. Biopsy by mediastinoscopy can exclude a malignant process and provide tissue for histopathologic evaluation. Antifungal therapy is not likely to affect resolution of the process when surgically excised tissue shows fungi consistent with *H. capsulatum* with sterile cultures, although there is some support for a 12-week course of itraconazole in patients with symptomatic mediastinal granuloma.[51] Dense fibrosis of mediastinal structures without a granulomatous component does not respond to antifungal treatment.

NEW REFERENCES SINCE THE SEVENTH EDITION

1. Abdel-Haq N, Quezada M, Asmar BI. Retropharyngeal abscess in children: the rising incidence of methicillin-resistant *Staphylococcus aureus. Pediatr Infect Dis J.* 2012;31:696-699.
29. Mangukia CV, Agarwal S, Satyarthy S, et al. Mediastinitis following pediatric cardiac surgery. *J Card Surg.* 2014;29:74-82.
31. McCarty JM, Demetral LC, Dabrowski L, et al. Pediatric coccidioidomycosis in central California: a retrospective case series. *Clin Infect Dis.* 2013;56:1579-1585.
44. Stewart E, Piteau S, Storr M, et al. Index of suspicion. *Pediatr Rev.* 2012;33:327-331.
51. Wheat LJ, Freifeld AG, Kleiman MB, et al. Clinical practice guidelines for the management of patients with histoplasmosis: 2007 update by the Infectious Diseases Society of America. *Clin Infect Dis.* 2007;45:807-825.

The full reference list for this chapter is available at ExpertConsult.com.

Bacterial Meningitis Beyond the Neonatal Period

31

Kwang Sik Kim

Bacterial meningitis is an inflammation of the meninges affecting the pia, the arachnoid, and the subarachnoid space that occurs in response to bacteria and bacterial products. A discussion of infections of neonates, including neonatal bacterial meningitis, is presented here; infections of the central nervous system (CNS) caused by mycobacteria and fungi are discussed in other chapters.

INCIDENCE AND EPIDEMIOLOGY

Before the discovery and use of antibiotics, bacterial meningitis generally was fatal. Antibiotic therapy has dramatically improved the prognosis in patients with bacterial meningitis, although bacterial meningitis continues to be a significant cause of morbidity and mortality in infants and children. The number of deaths attributed to many other infectious diseases in the United States decreased by 10- to 200-fold between 1935 and 1968, whereas the number of reported deaths caused by bacterial meningitis decreased by only half during the same period.[375,376]

The epidemiology of bacterial meningitis has been changed by several preventive measures introduced since the early 1990s, such as introduction of the *Haemophilus influenzae* type b conjugate vaccines and the pneumococcal conjugate vaccines for infants, and the screening of pregnant women for group B *Streptococcus* and intrapartum antibiotic prophylaxis since 1996.[205,243,285,331,367] The meningococcal conjugate vaccines were introduced in 2005, but the incidence of meningococcal meningitis was decreasing before the availability of conjugate vaccines.

Before the widespread use of the *H. influenzae* type b conjugate vaccines, *H. influenzae* type b was the most common cause of bacterial meningitis in children in the United States, Canada, and Scandinavia, but this pattern was not universal. Data from England from 1968 to 1977 showed that *Neisseria meningitidis* was the most common cause of bacterial meningitis for children and young adults,[93] and meningococcal meningitis accounted for 48% of meningitis in children in England.[94] A recent surveillance in England and Wales from 2004 to 2011 reports that meningococcal meningitis remains more common than pneumococcal meningitis (45% vs. 35% of bacterial meningitis, respectively).[361]

Studies in the 1970s and 1980s showed that three pathogens (*H. influenzae, Streptococcus pneumoniae,* and *N. meningitidis*) are predominant in causing meningitis in infants, children, and young adults, whereas group B *Streptococcus, Escherichia coli,* and *Listeria monocytogenes* are the most common bacteria causing meningitis in neonates. Between 1986 and 1995, the incidence of bacterial meningitis declined markedly, largely owing to the introduction of *H. influenzae* type b conjugate vaccines in infants. After the introduction of the heptavalent pneumococcal conjugate vaccine (PCV7), including pneumococcal serotypes 4, 6B, 8C, 9V, 14, 19F, and 23F, to infants in 2000, invasive pneumococcal disease in the United States declined by 75% among children younger than 5 years of age as well as by 31% among adults 65 years or older and in unvaccinated populations through herd immunity.[186,205]

In 1972, the Centers for Disease Control and Prevention (CDC) estimated that in the United States, 29,000 cases of meningitis were caused by *H. influenzae* type b, 4800 cases were caused by *S. pneumoniae,* and 4600 cases were caused by *N. meningitidis.* However, an estimate of an average of 4100 cases of bacterial meningitis, including 500 that were fatal, occurred annually in the United States during 2003 to 2007.[367] The data obtained from a population-based observational study using ICD9 coding between 1997 and 2010 indicate that the incidence of pneumococcal meningitis fell from 0.8 per 100,000 people in 1997 to 0.3 per 100,000 people by the end of 2010, while the incidence of meningococcal meningitis decreased from 0.72 per 100,000 in 1997 to 0.12 per 100,000 people in 2010, and the incidence of *H. influenzae* meningitis has remained at 0.058 per 100,000 people.[63]

Population-based studies in South Carolina, Minnesota, Vermont, and New Mexico in the 1970s suggested that the actual incidence of bacterial meningitis ranged from 5.4 to 7.3 cases per 100,000 population.[66,136–139] Studies reported from the CDC in 2011 indicated that the incidence of bacterial meningitis ranged from 6.91 cases per 100,000 population for children aged 2 to 23 months to 0.43 case per 100,000 population for adolescents aged 11 to 17 years (Table 31.1).[367]

A recent report of bacterial meningitis in the United States from 1998 to 2007 showed that the overall incidence of meningitis declined by 31% from 2.00 cases per 100,000 population in 1998 to 1999 to 1.38 cases per 100,000 population in 2006 to 2007, but the incidence remained unchanged in patients younger than 2 months of age (see Table 31.1).[367] The incidence of bacterial meningitis was highest for patients younger than 2 months of age and for black patients of any age. The median age of patients increased from 30.3 years during 1998–99 to 41.9 years during 2006–07, and this shift was significant, suggesting that the burden of bacterial meningitis is borne more by older adults. However, the case-fatality rate did not change significantly, from 15.7% in 1997–98 to 14.3% in 2006–07.[367]

In 2003 to 2007 in the United States, the most frequent cause of bacterial meningitis in children younger than 2 months of age was group B *Streptococcus* (86.1% of cases), and *N. meningitidis* caused 45.9% of cases among those 11 to 17 years of age. Among the other pediatric age groups, *S. pneumoniae* was the most common cause (Table 31.2).[367] The case-fatality rate was 6.9% among pediatric patients, and nearly 10% had underlying immunocompromising or chronic medical conditions. *E. coli* and *L. monocytogenes* are other common causes of meningitis in neonates 2 to 6 weeks of age.[367]

Epidemiology of Meningitis Caused by *Streptococcus pneumoniae*

S. pneumoniae is the most common pathogen causing bacterial meningitis in the United States. The risk for development of sepsis or meningitis caused by *S. pneumoniae* depends to some extent on the serotype with which the child is colonized and against which there is no opsonic antibody. Although more than 90 pneumococcal serotypes have been identified, invasive disease, including sepsis and meningitis, in children younger than 6 years old was associated most commonly with serotypes 14, 6B, 19F, 18C, 23F, 4, and 9V in the United States.[60] The 7-valent pneumococcal conjugate vaccine (PCV7), added to the national vaccination schedule in 2000, contains each of the just-mentioned most common serotypes.[71]

Nasopharyngeal colonization in children mainly depends on age (young age), crowding, attendance at daycare centers, and ethnicity (the Native American population). The serotype distribution of colonization isolates is by and large a reliable indicator for invasive disease, antibiotic resistance profiles, and potential vaccine coverage.[45] Daycare attendance, underlying disease, and lack of breast-feeding were risk factors for acquiring invasive pneumococcal infections in a large case-control study that included children from the United States and Canada.[233] Although cigarette smoking is a major risk factor for the development of invasive pneumococcal disease in adults, whether exposure to cigarette

TABLE 31.1 Age-Based Incidence of Bacterial Meningitis in the United States, 1998–2007, per 100,000 Population

Age	1998–99	2006–07	% Change 2006–07 vs. 1998–99
<2 mo	74.46	80.69	10
2–23 mo	14.20	6.91	−51
2–10 y	1.55	0.56	−64
11–17 y	1.03	0.43	−58
18–34 y	0.99	0.66	−33
35–49 y	1.23	0.95	−23
50–64 y	2.15	1.73	−19
≥65 y	2.64	1.92	−27
All ages	2.00	1.38	−31

From Thigpen MC, Whitney CG, Messonnier NE, et al. Bacterial meningitis in the United States 1998-2007. *N Engl J Med.* 2011;364:2016–25.

TABLE 31.2 Pathogen-Based Incidence of Bacterial Meningitis in the United States, 1998–2007, per 100,000 Population

Pathogen	1998–99	2006–07	% Change 2006–07 vs. 1998–99
S. pneumoniae	1.09	0.81	−26
N. meningitidis	0.44	0.19	−58
Group B streptococcus	0.24	0.25	4
H. influenzae	0.12	0.08	−35
L. monocytogenes	0.10	0.05	−46

From Thigpen MC, Whitney CG, Messonnier NE, et al. Bacterial meningitis in the United States 1998-2007. *N Engl J Med.* 2011;364:2016–25.

TABLE 31.3 Age–Based Incidence of Pneumococcal Meningitis in the United States, 1998–2007, per 100,000 Population

Age	1998–99	2006–07	Percent Change 2006–07 vs. 1998–99
2–23 mo	9.69	3.67	−62
2–10 y	0.54	0.36	−34
11–17 y	0.20	0.21	7
18–34 y	0.40	0.27	−33
35–49 y	0.83	0.76	−8
50–64 y	1.47	1.34	−9
≥65 y	1.88	1.43	−24
All ages	1.09	0.81	−26

From Thigpen MC, Whitney CG, Messonnier NE, et al. Bacterial meningitis in the United States 1998-2007. *N Engl J Med.* 2011;364:2016–25.

smoke increases the risk for developing systemic pneumococcal infection in children remains unclear.[280]

In the prevaccine era (before 2000 in the United States), the age-specific incidence for pneumococcal meningitis was 21, 12, 6, 2, and 0.5 cases per 100,000 for the age groups 0 to 6 months, 7 to 12 months, 13 to 24 months, 25 to 60 months, and older than 60 months, respectively.[402] The overall incidence of *S. pneumoniae* meningitis, however, decreased by 26% from 1.09 cases per 100,000 population in 1998 to 1999 to 0.81 case per 100,000 in 2006–07 in the United States.[367] This decline included a decrease of 62% among children 2 to 23 months of age (Table 31.3). The incidence of meningitis from *S. pneumoniae* PCV7 serotypes declined by 92% from 0.61 case per 100,000 population in 1998–99 to 0.05 case per 100,000 population in 2006–07. However, the incidence of meningitis from non-PCV7 serotypes increased by 62% from 0.48 case per 100,000 population in 1998–99 to 0.77 case per 100,000 population in 2006–07.[367] Pneumococcal meningitis had a case-fatality rate of 17.9% in 1998–99 and 14.7% in 2006–07.[367]

Among children aged 2 months to 10 years, *S. pneumoniae* was the most common cause of bacterial meningitis. PCV7 serotypes accounted for 15.5% of the pediatric cases overall and 13.0% of cases in the 2- to 23-month age groups. The case-fatality rates were similar among children infected with PCV7 isolates and those infected with non-PCV7 isolates (10.7% and 7.6%, respectively). Use of PCV7 also reduced invasive pneumococcal disease, including meningitis among unvaccinated populations through herd immunity (see Table 31.3).[205,367] PCV13 serotypes (PCV7 serotypes plus serotypes 1, 3, 5, 6A, 7F, and 19A) accounted for 60.0% of cases in children between 2 and 23 months of age and 57.2% in children of any age. PCV7 and PCV13 serotypes accounted for 16.0 and 41.6% of the adult meningitis cases, respectively.[367] The overall fatality rate was 16.4%, and the rate increased linearly with increasing age (8.9% among patients 18 to 34 years of age to 22.7% among those 65 years and older, $P < .001$).[367] Vaccine serotype coverages by PCV7 and PCV13 are less in European and other countries than those in the United States.[112] Surveys of nasopharyngeal carriage of *S. pneumoniae* in Australia revealed that the percentages of serotypes included in PCV13 were 40% in 2- to 15-year-old children and 29% in adults.[241]

Pneumococcal infections generally occur sporadically. Household contacts of a patient with pneumococcal disease are not considered to be at increased risk for acquiring secondary infection. The occurrence of concurrent pneumococcal disease (meningitis and bacteremia) in the household setting has been reported, however.[20,341] Although uncommon in the United States, *S. pneumoniae* has been associated with epidemics in locations such as Northern Ghana.[232]

The incidence of systemic infection with penicillin-resistant *S. pneumoniae* has been increasing steadily worldwide since it first was reported in Australia in the 1960s.[178] Systemic infection with penicillin-resistant pneumococci has become an increasing problem in the United States since the mid-1980s.[354,362] In 1995, a CDC multistate surveillance study showed that 35% of cerebrospinal fluid (CSF) isolates of *S. pneumoniae* were resistant to penicillin.[331]

The first report of meningitis caused by resistant pneumococci was published in 1974,[273] and numerous case reports appeared subsequently. Patients with systemic infections caused by penicillin-resistant pneumococci were more likely to have received a course of antibiotics within 1 month before acquiring their infection than were matched control subjects who had infections caused by pneumococci but whose isolates were susceptible to penicillin.[362]

By 1998, CDC surveillance of multiple areas around the United States found that 24% of pneumococcal isolates associated with invasive infections were nonsusceptible to penicillin; 14% of isolates were nonsusceptible to cefotaxime.[395] As with many studies, rates of resistance were higher among children younger than 5 years old. In contrast, penicillin- and cefotaxime-nonsusceptible pneumococcal isolates were 10.5% and 8.7%, respectively, in 2010.[367] In a prospective study involving eight children's hospitals nationwide during a 6-year period starting September 1993, a significant increase in the proportion of isolates nonsusceptible to penicillin or ceftriaxone was found. In the sixth year of the study ending August 1998, 37% and 11% of invasive isolates were nonsusceptible to penicillin and ceftriaxone, respectively.[197] Isolates of penicillin-resistant and third-generation cephalosporin-resistant *S. pneumoniae* have been recovered in other regions of the world as well.[98,141,259,307,386] Treatment failures in patients with *S. pneumoniae* meningitis resistant to penicillin and third-generation cephalosporins have led to changes in the empiric therapy of suspected bacterial meningitis, as discussed in the section on treatment.[144,210,344,371]

Data from the Active Bacterial Core Surveillance of the Emerging Infections Program Network after introduction of PCV7 showed an 87% decrease in rates of antibiotic-resistant disease by vaccine serotypes.[221] These results show that rates of invasive pneumococcal disease with penicillin-nonsusceptible strains and strains nonsusceptible to

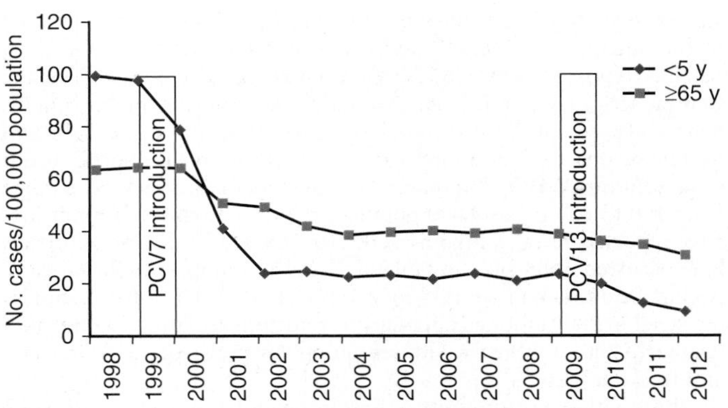

FIG. 31.1 Trends in annual incidence of invasive pneumococcal disease in children <5 years and adults ≥65 years. Active Bacterial Core Surveillance, the United States, 1998–2012. *PCV7,* 7-valent pneumococcal conjugate vaccine; *PCV13,* 13-valent pneumococcal conjugate vaccine. (Modified from Langley G, Schaffner W, Farley MM, et al. Twenty years of active bacterial core surveillance. *Emerg Infect Dis.* 2015;21(9):1520–8.)

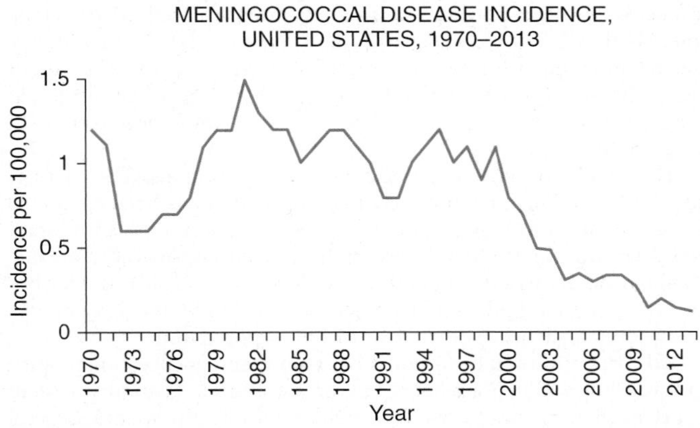

FIG. 31.2 Trends in annual incidence of invasive *N. meningitidis* disease in the United States, 1970–2013. (Data from CDC. 1970–1996 National Notifiable Diseases Surveillance System, 1997–2013. Active Bacterial Core surveillance estimated to U.S. population.)

multiple antibiotics "peaked in 1999 and decreased by 2004."[221] In children younger than 2 years old, invasive pneumococcal disease with penicillin-nonsusceptible strains decreased from 70.3 to 13.1 cases per 100,000.[221] The proportion of disease caused by penicillin-nonsusceptible strains varied by location within the United States from 9.4% in California to 29.5% in Tennessee.[221] The incidence of invasive *S. pneumoniae* disease caused by cefotaxime-resistant *S. pneumoniae* strains increased in children younger than 2 years of age, however, in the postvaccination period, from approximately 10% in 1999 to almost 15% in 2003.[221] The decreases in disease caused by vaccine-type *S. pneumoniae* strains were coupled with an increase in nonvaccine serotype *S. pneumoniae* strains, especially with serotype 19A (increased from 2.0 to 8.3 cases per 100,000).[221,370]

Recent data from 1998 to 2009 from continuous surveillance of invasive pneumococcal disease in eight geographic areas of the United States indicate that reductions in rates ranged by site from 19.0 to 29.9 cases per 100,000 population during 1998–99 to 11.2 to 18.0 cases per 100,000 population during 2009 (rate reduction of 5.1 to 15.3 cases per 100,000 population).[311] Reductions among children aged younger than 5 years ranged from 35.7 to 117.2 cases per 100,000 population across the sites. Reductions in rates due to PCV7 serotypes were seen in all age groups and at all sites, ranging from 12.0 to 21.4 cases per 100,000 population during 1998–99 to less than 2.0 cases per 100,000 population during 2009 (92% to 98% reductions). Serotype 19A rates ranged from 0.4 to 1.5 cases per 100,000 population during 1998–99 to 1.3 to 3.4 cases per 100,000 population during 2009 (rate difference of 0.9 to 2.8 cases per 100,000 population). Rates due to all other serotypes ranged from 6.3 to 10.3 cases per 100,000 population during 1998 to 1999 to 8.3 to 13.6 cases per 100,000 population during 2009 (rate difference of −0.04 to 5.67 cases per 100,000 population). Across the sites, the greatest increases were seen in the 50- to 64-year-old and older than 65-year-old age groups.[311] In February 2010, PCV13 was licensed and replaced PCV7 in the United States; PCV13 significantly reduced invasive pneumococcal disease among all age groups, including those younger than 2 years and those older than 65 years (Fig. 31.1), supporting the herd protection theme against pneumococcal disease.[261] Screening for underlying immunologic investigation maybe needed for children with invasive pneumococcal disease, particularly in those older than 2 years because immunodeficiencies have been discovered in up to 26% of cases.[149]

Epidemiology of Meningococcal Meningitis

In the United States, the incidence of *N. meningitidis* meningitis decreased by 58% from 0.44 case per 100,000 population in 1998–99 to 0.19 case per 100,000 population in 2006–07 (Fig. 31.2; also see Table 31.2).[367] Since 2005, declines have occurred among all age groups and in all vaccine-containing serogroups. The rates of meningococcal meningitis caused by serogroups B, C, and Y declined by 55%. Meningitis with *N. meningitidis* had a case-fatality rate of 10.1%, and 11% to 19% of survivors sustain long-term sequelae (e.g., neurologic disability or limb loss). *N. meningitidis* remained a major cause of bacterial meningitis among older children and young adults between 11 and 17 years of age (45.9% of cases), despite the fact that rates declined significantly between 1997 and 2007. Because the declines were similar among all major serogroups and because quadrivalent meningococcal vaccines (A, C, Y, and W135) do not include serogroup B, these declines are not likely from a vaccine effect.[367] Serogroups B, C, and Y were most common in the United States, each accounting for approximately one-third of the cases. However, the proportion of cases caused by each serogroup varies by age group. Serogroup B caused 70.5% of the cases among children younger than 11 years of age. Serogroups included in quadrivalent meningococcal vaccines accounted for 66.7% of infections among children 11 to 17 years of age. Serogroups B and C were the predominant causes of meningococcal meningitis among adults 18 to 34 years of age, accounting for 34.4% and 45.9% of cases, respectively, whereas in adults 35 years of age or older, serogroups B and Y were the most common, each serogroup accounting for 30.4% of cases.[367] As the proportion of children receiving quadrivalent meningococcal conjugate or serogroup B meningococcal conjugate vaccines continues to increase, additional reductions in the incidence of meningococcal disease are likely to occur (see Fig. 31.2).

From 1990 to 2002 in the United States, mortality rates for meningococcal disease were 0.1 death per 100,000 population per year, with 58% of deaths occurring among individuals younger than 25 years old. Infants had a higher mortality rate than that of individuals in different age groups, but they experienced a decline from 1.3 deaths per 100,000 in 1990 to 0.42 death per 100,000 population in 2002.[336] Meningococcal disease mortality rates increased each year in individuals between the ages of 10 and 19 years, which was followed by a decline in mortality rates in the years following and throughout most of adulthood.[336]

In the United States, in the 1990s, serogroup Y became more common, and the overall incidence of serogroup Y infection increased from 2% during 1989–91 to 37% during 1997–2002.[73] A study of the epidemiology of meningococcal disease in New York City from 1989 to 2000 revealed a threefold decrease in rates of serogroup B disease and almost no cases in children younger than 5 years old.[263] CDC data reveal that 75% of meningococcal infections in individuals older than 11 years of age are caused by serogroups C, Y, and W-135, all of which are included in the currently available conjugate vaccines. An increased risk for contracting meningococcal infection also exists in college students, especially freshmen who reside on campus in dormitories.[181] Following outbreaks of serogroup B meningococcal disease on two college campuses in 2013, two serogroup B conjugate vaccines have been licensed, MenB-FHbp and MenB-4C, in October 2014 and January 2015, respectively, and recommended for certain groups of persons 10 years of age or older who are at increased risk for group B meningococcal disease, as either a two-dose series of Mem-4C or a three-dose series of MenB-FHbp.[134,244]

The meningococcus is pathogenic only in humans. The carriage rate for *N. meningitidis* in the civilian population has been estimated at various times to range from 1% to 15%. Carriage rates in military personnel during epidemic periods have been considerably greater. Meningococcal carriers generally are adults (>21 years old) who harbor the organism for months, and meningococcus colonizes the nasopharynx asymptomatically in up to 40% of the adult population.[360]

No correlation has been noted between meningococcal meningitis and crowding within households, but disease seems to be more prevalent in urban than in rural areas. In a civilian population, meningococcal meningitis generally is a disease of children and young adults who have been exposed to an adult carrier, usually in the same family, or to individuals with disease or who are carrying the organism in a daycare setting. The estimated likelihood of severe meningococcal disease in family contacts occurring simultaneously with the first case is 1%.[229] The rate is 1000-fold greater than the risk in the community. The risk of meningitis being acquired in daycare center contacts of children with meningococcal disease is 1 per 1000.

Another change in the epidemiology of meningococcal disease in the United States relates to the increasing number of outbreaks (>10 cases per 100,000 population during 3 months), generally caused by serogroup C. Although these outbreaks account for only 2% to 3% of the total number of cases, they cause tremendous public concern and anxiety, which frequently result in misunderstanding of the nature of an outbreak by the media and the public.[189]

An otherwise unprecedented outbreak of meningococcal disease occurred in a sixth-grade elementary school classroom.[117] Five children from a class of 24 developed meningococcal meningitis. In addition, two siblings of one of the index patients also developed meningococcal infection. Detailed epidemiologic investigation suggested that close contact in the classroom (nose-to-nose distances of ≤34 inches) correlated with an increased rate of carriage of *N. meningitidis* and with an increased risk for development of invasive meningococcal disease.

Major outbreaks of meningococcal meningitis have occurred worldwide. In the late 1980s and early 1990s, major epidemics of meningococcal meningitis caused by a specific clone (III-1) of serogroup A *N. meningitidis* occurred throughout sub-Saharan Africa.[2,171,175,295,319] The origins of a pandemic spread of clone III-1 were traced to epidemics in Asia in the early 1980s, with spread through the Near East.[1] An outbreak occurred during the annual pilgrimage to Mecca in 1987,[260,262] with pilgrims carrying clones back to their countries of origin, including the United States and the United Kingdom. Epidemics of closely related strains of clone III-1 serogroup A meningococcal meningitis occurred in the Sudan,[319] Ethiopia,[175] and Chad in 1988[262] and in Kenya[295] in 1989. A report in 1992 described an epidemic of clone III-1 in the Central African Republic in an area traditionally outside the "meningitis belt."[171] These epidemics generally begin during the dry season and decline at onset of the rainy season. According to the World Health Organization (WHO), "in major African epidemics, attack rates range from 100 to 800 per 100,000 population, but individual communities have reported rates as high as 1000 per 100,000."[253] Major outbreaks have occurred in Brazil,[100] in Finland,[286] and at multiple sites in Africa.[395] A clonal outbreak of serogroup W135 (ET-37ST-11 clonal complex) occurred in 2000 among Hajj pilgrims returning to Europe from Saudi Arabia. In 2001, outbreaks with serogroup W135 also occurred in Niger and Burkina Faso.[359]

Shifts within a community or within a country as a whole from one serogroup to another also are associated with an increased incidence of disease for several years after the new serogroup is introduced into the community.[312] The mechanisms underlying the changing patterns of meningococcal serogroups that cause diseases are unknown.

Protection from meningococcal infection depends on a functional complement system as well as the humoral antibody response. The serum bactericidal activity assay (SBA), which measures killing of *N. meningitidis* in the presence of specific antibodies and addition of complement is the standard immunologic correlate of protection. SBA titers of 4 or higher with the use of human complement (hSBA) or 8 or higher with the use of rabbit complement (rSBA) are considered protection against subsequent diseases.[23] Meningococcal infections occur more frequently in patients with a deficiency of the terminal components (C5–C9) of the complement system, and the risk for developing meningococcal infection in persons with deficiency of complement factor C5–C9 is approximately 600-fold higher compared with the general population.[56,111,130,236,320] An increased risk for contracting meningococcal meningitis also has been reported in individuals with an inherited deficiency of C9[272] and with properdin deficiency.[349] Individuals with a complement-depleting underlying illness also are at particular risk for acquiring invasive diseases.[291] Screening for complement deficiency in pediatric patients with meningococcal disease is recommended.[230]

Epidemiology of *Haemophilus influenzae* Meningitis

The most dramatic change in the epidemiology of bacterial meningitis since the advent of antibiotics has occurred in the past two decades as a result of licensure of conjugate vaccines against *H. influenzae* type b (Fig. 31.3).[72,243,285,328,367] The first vaccine available was *H. influenzae* type b capsular polysaccharide (polyribosylribitol) phosphate [PRP], which was licensed in 1985 for use in children 18 to 59 months of age. Subsequently, vaccines with improved immunogenicity for children of younger ages were developed by covalently linking the capsular

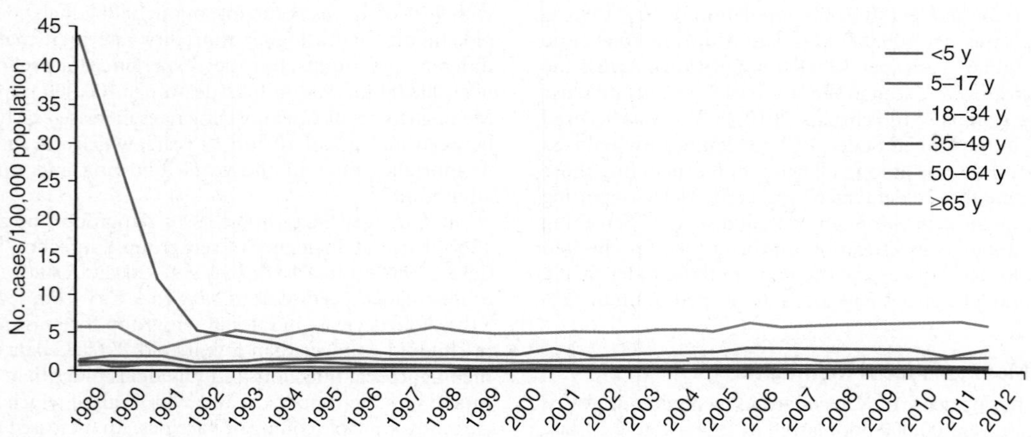

FIG. 31.3 Incidence of invasive *Haemophilus influenzae* disease by age group in the United States, 1989–2012. (Modified from Langley G, Schaffner W, Farley MM, et al. Twenty years of active bacterial core surveillance. *Emerg Infect Dis.* 2015;21[9]:1520–8.)

polysaccharide with protein antigens. In 1990, the first conjugate, PRP diphtheria CRM_{197} protein conjugate (HbOC), was approved for infant use. In 1991, the Advisory Committee on Immunization Practices (ACIP) and the American Academy of Pediatrics (AAP) recommended universal infant immunization starting at 2 months of age with either HbOC or PRP-meningococcal protein conjugate (PRP-OMP) vaccines.[8,67] Currently, two different conjugate vaccine preparations are available in the United States alone or in combination with other vaccines: PRP-OMP and PRP-T (tetanus toxoid).[361] One Hib-MenCY-TT is licensed for use in children aged 6 weeks through 18 months at increased risk of meningococcal disease (e.g., complement component deficiencies, functional or anatomic asplenia, outbreaks).[245]

Before universal vaccination was initiated, the incidence of *H. influenzae* meningitis varied worldwide. The incidence of *H. influenzae* meningitis in Scandinavian children younger than 5 years averaged 16 to 28 cases per 100,000 children from 1975 to 1984.[287] The incidence of *H. influenzae* type b meningitis in three Pacific Island countries was 70 to 84 cases per 100,000 children younger than 5 years in 2003[315] and 67 to 158 cases per 100,000 in Indonesian children younger than 5 years during 1998–2002.[158] The incidence of *H. influenzae* meningitis in The Netherlands was 22 cases per 100,000 children younger than 5 years.[378]

The incidence of *H. influenzae* meningitis is markedly higher in nonindustrialized populations. Before the vaccination era, Alaskan Eskimos had an annual incidence of 282 cases per 100,000 children younger than 5 years of age.[390] The Navajo and White Mountain Apache Native Americans had a much higher incidence compared with that of Native Americans in other regions of the United States,[87,239] and the incidence among Australian Aboriginals and among certain African populations, such as those in Gambia and Senegal, was 3 to 10 times higher than that of populations in the United States and Europe.[41,161,179] The incidence of *H. influenzae* meningitis was decreased in Gambia from more than 60 cases per 100,000 children to none per 100,000 in children younger than 5 years after implementation of *H. influenzae* type b vaccination in May 1997.[6] After the WHO recommendation in November 2006, *H. influenzae* type b vaccine was included routinely in the immunization schedule, and the impact of *H. influenzae* type b vaccination in prevention of *H. influenzae* type b meningitis has been demonstrated throughout the world. A resurgence of invasive *H. influenzae* type b disease was seen in the absence of a booster dose in the United Kingdom. Subsequently, a booster campaign with *H. influenzae* type b vaccine was introduced that offered one dose to all children aged 6 months to 4 years of age, and it resulted in decreased invasive *H. influenzae* type b disease among older children and adults in the United Kingdom.[361]

Good epidemiologic data concerning the incidence of *H. influenzae* infection are, however, lacking in many other areas of the world. Measuring the extent of *H. influenzae* disease often is difficult, time-consuming, and expensive. In an attempt to decrease complexity, cost, and time required to collect data concerning the incidence of *H. influenzae* infection, the *Haemophilus influenzae* type b Rapid Assessment Tool was developed. Increasing numbers of countries are using such tools to estimate the local *H. influenzae* disease burden and to help determine the need for implementation of a local vaccination program.[391]

In one study, the incidence of *H. influenzae* meningitis was 3.5-fold higher in blacks than in whites, but this distribution of cases seemed to be related more closely to poverty than to race.[136] In whites, no increase in incidence occurred in overcrowded households, but the incidence was higher in rural than in urban areas, which allowed the postulation that the increased incidence in rural whites and in blacks was related to lack of access to early medical care.[136] The *Haemophilus influenzae* Study Group[4] noted that the number of cases of *H. influenzae* meningitis in children younger than 5 years reported through the National Bacterial Meningitis Reporting System began declining rapidly in 1988. In another CDC surveillance project conducted from 1989 to 1997, the race-adjusted incidence of invasive *H. influenzae* type b disease among children younger than age 5 years declined from 34.0 to 0.4 per 100,000, a 99% reduction (see Fig. 31.3).[70,243]

Serotype replacement has been seen with an increase in incidence of non–type b cases. In a statewide surveillance done in Alaska from 1983 to 2011, no *H. influenzae* type a disease was identified before 2002, but from 2002 to 2011, 32 cases were identified, whereas from December 2009 to December 2011, 15 cases were identified.[361] A report from Active Bacterial Core Surveillance sites from 1998 to 2007 indicated that small increases in the incidence of serotypes a, e, and f were observed, and the largest of these increases was in serotype f and was primarily among adults aged 18 years or older.[367]

The overall incidence of *H. influenzae* meningitis decreased by 35% between 1998 and 1999 and 2006 to 2007, from 0.12 case per 100,000 population to 0.08 case per 100,000 population (see Table 31.2); 9.4% of the cases were caused by serotype b.[367] The epidemiology of invasive *H. influenzae* disease in the post–*H. influenzae* type b vaccine era seems to be shifting from *H. influenzae* type b in children toward non–type b strains in older individuals.[367] For example, among adult cases of *H. influenzae* meningitis, a majority (73.8%) of the *H. influenzae* isolates were not typable, whereas serotypes e and f were the most common serotypes identified (with each found in 11.5% of cases). The case-fatality rates were significantly higher among adults with typable *H. influenzae* than among cases from nontypable *H. influenzae* (18.8% vs. 2.2%; $P = .02$).[367]

National trends in mortality from *H. influenzae* meningitis were evaluated from 1980 to 1991.[330] From 1980 through 1987, mortality rates from *H. influenzae* meningitis decreased an average of 8.5% a year, from 1.72 per 100,000 children in 1980 to 0.94 per 100,000 children in 1987. From 1988 to 1991, mortality rates decreased an average of 48% a year, with a death rate of 0.11 per 100,000 children in 1991. The estimated case-fatality rate for *H. influenzae* meningitis was 3.3% from 1980 to 1987 and 2.3% from 1988 to 1991. In comparison, mortality rates from *S. pneumoniae* meningitis decreased 10% annually from 1980 to 1987 and 3% annually from 1988 to 1991. Similarly, mortality rates from meningococcal meningitis decreased by 13% annually from 1980 to 1987 and 12% annually from 1988 to 1991.

The dramatic decrease in the incidence of *H. influenzae* meningitis has been affected by several factors. The precipitous drop that occurred shortly after universal immunization of infants strongly suggests that this practice has affected the epidemiology of this disease. Conjugate vaccination protects against nasopharyngeal colonization,[268] decreasing the carriage rate of *H. influenzae* type b and diminishing the reservoir for transmission and providing immunity from infection. These factors would also lessen the likelihood of development of infection in unvaccinated populations through herd immunity. Other changes in medical practice, such as the widespread use of outpatient antibiotics and improvements in supportive care, may have some effect, as shown by the decrease in case-fatality rates for *H. influenzae* meningitis, the steady decrease in mortality rates before vaccination, and the decrease in instances of meningococcal and pneumococcal disease.

The risk for spread of severe *H. influenzae* illness among household contacts of patients with *H. influenzae* meningitis was studied prospectively in 19 states.[388] The risk in children younger than 1 year of age was 6%; in children younger than 4 years, 2.1%; and in children younger than 6 years, 0.5%. The risk for *H. influenzae* disease occurring in household contacts younger than 6 years is similar to the risk for secondary meningococcal disease occurring in all household contacts, indicating a need for effective antimicrobial prophylaxis. Spread of *H. influenzae* disease in daycare centers also is well documented.[31,163,252,389] The precise risk for acquiring secondary *H. influenzae* type b infection in daycare centers is unclear.

Recurrent invasive *H. influenzae* type b disease has been reported. Detailed studies suggest that age and high incidence of disease alone are not the only factors contributing to the recurrence of the disease.[55] Patients who have recurrent disease caused by *H. influenzae* type b may represent a subset of a population with unusual disease susceptibility. In addition, children who develop invasive infection caused by *H. influenzae* type b after receiving appropriate conjugate vaccine frequently have subnormal immunoglobulin concentrations and should undergo immune evaluation.[185]

PATHOPHYSIOLOGY

Organisms Encountered

Almost all microorganisms that are pathogenic to humans have the potential to cause meningitis, but a relatively small number of pathogens (i.e., group B *Streptococcus, E. coli, L. monocytogenes, H. influenzae, S. pneumoniae,* and *N. meningitidis*) account for most cases of acute bacterial meningitis in neonates and children.[204,205] The reasons for this association remain incompletely understood. In immunocompromised hosts, infection with other organisms may occur. The specific organism sometimes may be predicted on the basis of the type of deficit that is present in the host.[205]

Routes of Infection

Bacterial infection of the normally sterile leptomeningeal spaces can occur from hematogenous spread, direct extension from paranasal and dental infections as well as skull base fracture, direct implantation (e.g., after surgery, cochlear implant), or rarely secondary to infections in the epidural or subdural spaces.[203–205] Bacterial meningitis in children with otitis media generally follows bacteremia, although direct invasion of the meninges may occur as a complication of otitis media.[203]

The meninges are seeded with microorganisms during a bacteremic period. Bacterial meningitis has been induced in experimental animals (e.g., infant rats[264] and monkeys[346]) after intranasal inoculation of *H. influenzae* type b. Bacteremia developed hours before meningitis could be detected histologically, a finding that supports the concept that meningitis follows hematogenous dissemination from nasopharyngeal colonization or infection. Marginating bacteria could be detected by fluorescent staining initially in the lateral and dorsal longitudinal (sagittal) sinuses and subsequently spread to the leptomeninges. Several lines of evidence from human cases of group B *Streptococcus* and *E. coli* meningitis and animal models of experimental hematogenous meningitis, however, reveal that cerebral capillaries are the portal of entry into the brain for circulating group B *Streptococcus* and *E. coli,*[203–205] and bacterial penetration into the brain was demonstrated without exhibiting increased blood-brain barrier (BBB) permeability and accompanying host inflammatory cells.[206,207]

Meningitis can also develop after bacterial invasion from a contiguous focus of infection, as in infection of the mastoid or paranasal sinuses or as a complication of otitis media. For example, *S. pneumoniae* has been shown to enter the CNS through a nonhematogenous route in experimental animals after intranasal infection and otitis media.[203] Fracture through the paranasal sinuses as a result of head trauma may precede development of meningitis caused by *S. pneumoniae* and *H. influenzae,* which may be recurrent. Direct invasion also may occur in individuals with dermoid sinus tracts or meningomyeloceles, when a direct communication between the skin and the meninges is present. In this setting, infection usually is produced by organisms found on the skin. Recurrent meningitis has been reported in patients with basic ethmoidal encephaloceles[357] or a congenital defect in the stapedial footplate.[184] Surgical obliteration of the fistula with temporal muscle and fascia prevented the recurrence of meningitis. Meningitis also may develop subsequent to osteomyelitis of the skull or vertebral column. Rarely meningitis may develop in the normal host with commensal microorganisms after having a tooth extracted or getting dental fillings.[83,337]

Neurosurgical procedures, particularly procedures designed for diversion of CSF in children who have hydrocephalus, may lead to development of meningitis.[203] Chemical meningitis also may occur after neurosurgical procedures, especially procedures involving the posterior fossa.[135] In these patients, evidence of inflammation develops rapidly with elevation of temperature occurring on the first postoperative day.

Infection of the CNS may result from environmental contamination or manipulation. Meningeal infection may be acquired in utero transplacentally or during delivery through contact with the cervix or vaginal canal, which may be colonized with a variety of organisms, particularly group B *Streptococcus, E. coli,* and *L. monocytogenes.*[7,24,203–205] A neonate, a patient with cystic fibrosis, or a burned child may develop septicemia and meningitis as a result of persistent heavy colonization with *Staphylococcus aureus.* A humidified atmosphere promotes the colonization and growth of such organisms as *Serratia marcescens* and *Pseudomonas aeruginosa.* Placing a patient in this setting leads to an increased frequency of infection with these organisms. Indwelling catheters can predispose a patient to infection by bacterial (and fungal) organisms that generally are of low virulence in the normal host.

PATHOGENESIS

Most cases of bacterial meningitis develop through four steps: (1) colonization of the mucosal membranes such as upper respiratory or gastrointestinal tract, (2) invasion of the blood from the mucosal colonization, resulting in a threshold level of bacteremia, (3) traversal of the blood-brain barrier, and (4) inflammation of the meninges and brain.[203,204] Less commonly, infection of the leptomeninges can occur by contiguous spread or hematogenous dissemination from another remote site.

Mucosal Colonization

Most meningitis-causing bacteria colonize the mucosal membranes of the nasopharynx (*S. pneumoniae, N. meningitidis,* and *H. influenzae*) and gastrointestinal tract (*E. coli* and *L. monocytogenes*).[45,56,204,360] This attachment is mediated by specific microbial cell surface components and affected by co-colonization with other microorganisms and host immune response.

Several pneumococcal factors have been shown to enhance nasopharyngeal colonization and binding to nasopharyngeal epithelium: pneumococcal phosphorylcholine, IgA1-protease, capsular switching, pneumolysin, pneumococcal surface protein (Psp) C (also known as choline binding protein [CbpA]), pneumococcal surface adhesin A (PsaA), pneumococcal adherence and virulence factor A (PavA), neuraminidase A (NanA), and pili. Additionally, prior exposure to influenza virus has been associated with increased colonization and secondary invasive pneumococcal disease.[45,204,393] Pneumococcal phosphorylcholine binds to the platelet-activating factor (PAF) receptor on activated host epithelial cells,[45] whereas the PspC binds to epithelial polymeric immunoglobulin receptor (pIgR).[403] The pIgRs are expressed in a decreasing gradient from the upper to lower respiratory tract, whereas the opposite pattern of expression is observed for the PAF receptor, suggesting that pIgR serves mainly as a pneumococcal receptor for the nasopharynx but the PAF receptor facilitates attachment and invasion of the pulmonary epithelium.[45]

N. meningitidis strains use IgA1 protease, pili, and outer membrane proteins Opa, Opc, and porin A and B for binding to cell surface receptors on nasopharyngeal mucosal cells[56,101,204] and apparently are transported across specialized cells within phagocytic vacuoles.[358] Human embryonic antigen cell adhesion molecules (CEACAMs or CD66) are cell-surface molecules in nasopharyngeal epithelial cells that interact with meningococcal Opa proteins.[56]

Bacteremia

When in the bloodstream, the common meningitis-causing organisms (*S. pneumoniae, H. influenzae, N. meningitidis, E. coli* K1, and group B *Streptococcus*) are capable of evading host defense mechanisms,[203,204,301] which involves capsular polysaccharides and other bacterial factors, resulting in a high level of bacteremia (Table 31.4).

Several studies of humans and experimental animals suggest a relationship between the magnitude of bacteremia and development of meningitis due to *E. coli,* group B *Streptococcus, H. influenzae* type b, and *S. pneumoniae.*[203,204] For example, a significantly higher incidence of *E. coli* meningitis was noted in neonates who had bacterial counts

TABLE 31.4 Microbial Factors Contributing to a High Level of Bacteremia

Pathogens	Bacterial Factors
E. coli	Capsular polysaccharides, O-LPS, type 1 fimbriae, NlpI, SslE
Group B streptococcus	Capsular polysaccharides, C5a peptidase?, SodA
S. pneumoniae	Capsular polysaccharides, pneumolysin
N. meningitidis	Capsular polysaccharides, LOS, factor-H binding protein, PorA

LOS, Lipo-oligosaccharides; *LPS,* lipopolysaccharides; *NlpI,* new lipoprotein I; *SslE,* secreted and surface located lipoprotein from *E. coli*; *SodA,* superoxide dismutase.

in blood greater than 10^3 colony-forming units (CFU)/mL (6 of 11; 55%) compared with those with bacterial counts less than 10^3 CFU/mL (1 of 19; 5%). Similarly, meningitis due to *S. pneumoniae* was observed more frequently in patients whose bacterial counts in blood were greater than 1×10^2 to 5×10^2 CFU/mL (6 of 7; 86%) than in those with fewer bacterial counts in blood (2 of 50; 4%). For *H. influenzae* type b, the level of bacteremia is around 10^2 CFU/mL of blood. Consistent with these clinical findings, a high degree of bacteremia was a primary determinant for meningeal invasion of experimental hematogenous meningitis caused by *E. coli*, group B *Streptococcus*, *H. influenzae* type b, and *S. pneumoniae*.[203,204] All patients with *N. meningitidis* meningitis had *N. meningitidis* detected in their blood, thus also suggesting a relationship between bacteremia and development of meningitis caused by *N. meningitidis*.[91] The basis for requiring a threshold level of bacteremia for bacterial penetration into the brain is currently unknown.

Bacterial Traversal of the Blood-Brain Barrier

The bacteria in the bloodstream subsequently traverse the BBB, most likely at the cerebral capillaries (*S. pneumoniae, N. meningitidis, E. coli* K1, and group B *Streptococcus*) and choroid plexus (*H. influenzae*).[203,204,207] Meningitis-causing bacteria cross the BBB transcellularly, paracellularly, and/or by means of infected phagocytes (the so-called Trojan horse mechanism).[203,204] Transcellular traversal of the BBB has been demonstrated for most meningitis-causing bacteria in infants and children, including group B *Streptococcus*, *E. coli*, and *S. pneumoniae*, whereas *N. meningitidis* has been shown to utilize transcellular and paracellular mechanisms for traversal of the BBB, and *L. monocytogenes* penetration of the BBB has been shown to utilize transcellular and Trojan horse mechanisms.[88,203,204]

Recent studies, however, have shown that a high degree of bacteremia is necessary, but not sufficient, for the development of meningitis and that bacterial binding to and invasion of the BBB is a prerequisite for penetration into the brain.[203,204] This concept was well demonstrated with *E. coli* K1, where mutants deleted of the *E. coli* factors contributing to binding to and invasion of the BBB were significantly less able to traverse the BBB than the parent strain despite causing similar levels of bacteremia.[203,204]

Bacterial traversal of the BBB requires specific bacterial factors and their interactions with host factors (Table 31.5),[203,204] although the complete information on microbial-host factors contributing to penetration of the BBB is currently lacking for most meningitis-causing bacteria.

Recent studies have also shown that meningitis-causing bacteria exploit specific host cell signaling molecules for promoting host cell actin cytoskeleton rearrangements and bacterial invasion of the BBB (see Table 31.5).[203,204,206] *E. coli* invasion of the BBB involves focal adhesion kinase (FAK), paxillin, phosphatidylinositol 3-kinase (PI3-K), Src kinase, Rho guanosine triphosphates, signal transducers and activators of transcription (STAT)3, cytosolic phospholipase $A_2\alpha$ (cPLA2α), 5-lipoxygenase, cyteinyl leukotrienes, and protein kinase C, whereas group B *Streptococcus* invasion of the BBB is independent of Src activation and *L. monocytogenes* invasion of the BBB is independent of FAK and cPLA$_2\alpha$.[203] *N. meningitidis* has been shown to invade the BBB involving type IV pili, PilC, NadA, Opa, and Opc proteins.[56,203] The detailed information on how meningitis-causing bacteria exploit host cell signaling molecules for invasion of the BBB, however, remains incompletely understood. For example, the invasion of the BBB by unencapsulated meningococcus is mediated by Opc binding to fibronectin, which anchors the bacteria to the integrin receptor on the BBB. However, in the bloodstream, *N. meningitidis* is encapsulated and the in vivo relevance of Opc-fibronectin–mediated binding to integrin requires clarification,[203,350,374] and type IV pili have been shown to contribute to paracellular penetration of *N. meningitidis* across the BBB.[88] *S. pneumoniae* has been shown to invade the BBB via complex interaction of phosphorylcholine and CbpA proteins with receptors on activated endothelial cells.[56,204,215]

The mechanisms involved in entry of meningitis-causing bacteria into the BBB differ from those involved in the inflammation occurring in response to those bacteria. This concept has been demonstrated for *E. coli*, group B *Streptococcus*, and *N. meningitidis*.[30,147,204,228,350,374] *N. meningitidis* invasion of the BBB involves c-Jun kinases 1 and 2 (JNK1 and JNK2), but the release of interleukin (IL)-6 and IL-8 from the BBB involves the p38-mitogen–activated protein kinase (MAPK) pathways.[350]

BBB Dysfunction and Intracranial Inflammation

Once bacteria enter the CSF, because of insufficient opsonic and phagocytic activity in the CSF, organisms multiply, liberating bacterial cell wall or membrane components (lipopolysaccharide, lipoteichoic acid, peptidoglycan, lipoproteins, bacterial toxins), and induce release of inflammatory mediators and toxic compounds, which leads to CSF pleocytosis and increased BBB permeability, the hallmarks of bacterial meningitis. However, pleocytosis and increased BBB permeability can develop independently of each other in some patients with bacterial meningitis[203,204] (see later discussion).

Complement and opsonic proteins either are found at very low concentrations or are absent within normal CSF,[340] and the CSF is devoid of the factors required for enhancing bacterial killing. When bacteria first invade the meninges, the lack of complement and opsonic proteins within the sanctuary of the CNS may permit the bacteria to multiply unrestrained for some time.[39,114,159,404]

The specific pathophysiologic changes in bacterial meningitis are the result of the bacterial products and the inflammatory response of the host to those products (Fig. 31.4). Initial bactericidal antibiotic

TABLE 31.5 Microbial-Host Factors Contributing to Penetration of the Blood-Brain Barrier by Common Meningitis-Causing Bacteria

Pathogens	Bacterial Factors	Host Receptors	Host Signaling Molecules
E. coli	Type 1 fimbriae, OmpA, flagella, NlpI, IbeA, IbeB, IbeC, CNF1, AslA	CD48, gp96, 37LRP, Caspr1	FAK, paxillin, PI3-K, Src kinase, Rho GTPases, cPLA$_2\alpha$, 5-lipoxygenase, cyteinyl leukotrienes, STAT3, PKCα, VEGFR1, EGFR
Group B streptococcus	Lmb, FbsA, lagA, HvgA, PilA, LTA, β-hemolysin, ScpB, αC protein	Integrin, GAGs	FAK, Rho GTPases, cPLA$_2\alpha$, 5-lipoxygenase, and cyteinyl leukotrienes
L. monocytogenes	InlB	gC1qR, Met, gp96	PI3-K
S. pneumoniae	Phosphorylcholine, PspC (CbpA), pneumolysin, NanA	PAF receptor, 37LRP	β-Arrestin, MAPK
N. meningitidis	Type IV pili, PilC, Opa, Opc, NadA	CD46, CD66, integrin, 37LRP, β_2-adrenoreceptor	JNK1 and 2, β-arrestin

37LRP, 37 Laminin receptor precursor; *AslA,* arylsulfatase-like gene; *CNF1,* cytotoxic necrotizing factor 1; *cPLA$_2\alpha$,* cytosolic phospholipase $A_2\alpha$; *FAK,* focal adhesion kinase; *FbsA,* fibrinogen-binding protein A; *GAGs,* glycol aminoglycans; *gC1qR,* globular head of complement component C1q; *HvgA,* hypervirulent group B streptococcus adhesin; *lagA,* invasion-associated gene A; *Ibe,* invasion of brain endothelial cell; *InlB,* internalin B; *JNK,* c-Jun kinase; *Lmb,* laminin-binding protein; *LTA,* lipoteichoic acid; *MAPK,* mitogen-activated protein kinase; *Met,* Met tyrosine kinase; *NadA,* neisserial adhesin A; *NanA,* neuraminidase A; *Nlpl,* new lipoprotein I; *OmpA,* outer membrane protein A; *PI-3K,* phosphatidylinositol-3 kinase; *PilA,* pilus protein A; *PKCα,* protein kinase Cα; *PspC,* pneumococcal surface protein C; *ScpB,* C5a peptidase; *STAT3,* signal transducers and activators of transcription; *VEGFR1,* vascular endothelial growth factor receptor 1; *EGFR,* epidermal growth factor receptor kinase.

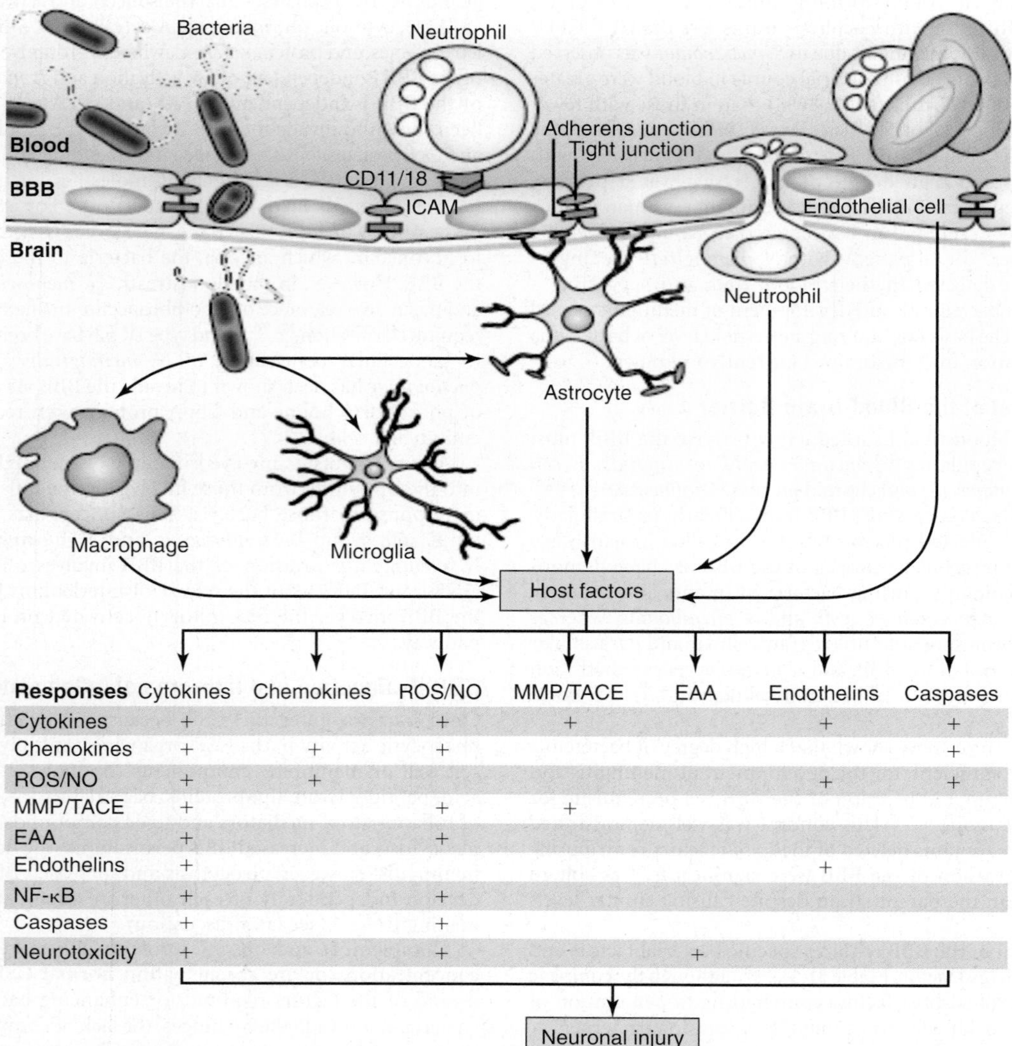

Responses	Cytokines	Chemokines	ROS/NO	MMP/TACE	EAA	Endothelins	Caspases
Cytokines	+		+	+		+	+
Chemokines	+	+	+				+
ROS/NO	+	+				+	+
MMP/TACE	+		+	+			
EAA	+		+				
Endothelins	+					+	
NF-κB	+		+				
Caspases	+		+				
Neurotoxicity	+		+		+		

FIG. 31.4 Host response during bacterial meningitis contributing to neuronal injury. Bacterial entry into the central nervous system elicits the release of many factors from host cells (macrophage, microglia, astrocyte, ependymal cell, endothelial cell, infiltrating inflammatory cell), which along with cytotoxicity of bacterial compounds exacerbate host cellular responses, resulting in neuronal injury. + denotes upregulation of specific host factors. *BBB,* Blood-brain barrier; *EAA,* excitatory amino acids; *ICAM,* intercellular adhesion molecule; *MMP,* matrix metalloproteases; *NF-κB,* nuclear factor-κB; *NO,* nitric oxide; *ROS,* reactive oxygen species; *TACE,* tumor necrosis factor-α converting enzyme. (Modified from Kim KS. Pathogenesis of bacterial meningitis: from bacteremia to neuronal injury. *Nat Rev Neurosci.* 2003;4:376–85.)

therapy results in a rapid release of bacterial products, such as lipopolysaccharides (endotoxins), teichoic acid, and peptidoglycans. For gram-positive bacterial meningitis, lipoteichoic acid and peptidoglycans are the bacterial surface elements that induce inflammation.[203,372] The threshold concentration that triggers inflammation is approximately 10^5 bacterial cell equivalents of cell wall pieces. For gram-negative meningitis, lipopolysaccharides (endotoxins) are the major inflammatory components, with peptidoglycan serving as an important cofactor.[59] The inflammatory threshold is approximately 2 pg of endotoxin, or approximately 10^5 bacterial cell equivalents.[397]

Immune activation in the CNS is initiated by the recognition of different bacterial pathogen-associated molecular patterns (PAMPs). Major pattern recognition receptors (PRRs) involved in initial sensing of bacteria in the CNS include Toll-like receptors (TLRs) 2, 4, 5, and 9 and Nod-like receptors (NLRs), which are involved in triggering an intracellular signaling pathway that leads to activation of transcription factors such as nuclear factor-κB (NF-κB) and the subsequent gene transcription of proinflammatory cytokines and chemokines such as tumor necrosis factor-α (TNF-α), IL-1, and IL-8.[56,203]

Cytokines and chemokines seem to be the primary drivers of the inflammatory response. The following cytokines and chemokines are involved in the inflammatory response noted in bacterial meningitis: IL-1, IL-3, IL-4, IL-6, IL-8, IL-10, IL-12, IL-18, interferon-γ, macrophage inflammatory protein, transforming growth factor-β, and TNF-α.[102,203,379,405]

TNF-α and IL-1β seem to be key mediators in initiation of meningeal inflammation. Both proteins stimulate vascular endothelial cells to induce adhesion and passage of leukocytes into the CNS and trigger inflammatory processes. Astrocytes and microglia are capable of producing TNF-α.[222,359] TNF-α concentrations are elevated (1) in CSF but not in serum; (2) in animal models of bacterial meningitis; and (3) in patients with bacterial meningitis caused by *H. influenzae, N. meningitidis, S. pneumoniae,* and *Streptococcus agalactiae,*[203,269] but not in patients with culture-proven viral meningitis.[303] TNF-α levels can be correlated with meningeal inflammation and severity of disease, but lack of TNF-α in the animal model is associated with increased mortality and stronger deficits in spatial memory.[153]

IL-1β can be detected in infants and children with bacterial meningitis, and its presence is correlated significantly with CSF inflammatory abnormalities, TNF-α concentrations, and adverse outcome.[269] The role of IL-1β in bacterial meningitis, however, is inconsistent. Levels of IL-1β were not associated with the degree of the BBB disruption in patients with bacterial meningitis.[203]

The chemokines are a superfamily of small chemoattractant cytokines that play an important role in the initiation and modulation of inflammation in bacterial meningitis.[353] IL-8 is one of the well-characterized chemokines in bacterial meningitis and was found to be chemotactic for neutrophils in the CSF of patients with bacterial meningitis.[147,203]

Complement factors are upregulated in bacterial meningitis. The activated complement cascade in CSF, acting on upregulated complement receptors on brain cells, potentially mediates direct brain damage.[53] Complement factors also are chemoattractants that enhance CSF leukocytosis and indirectly produce brain damage in patients with bacterial meningitis.[115]

Intracisternal administration of antibodies to TNF-α and IL-1β decreased pleocytosis and BBB permeability in response to intracisternal injection of *H. influenzae* and *S. pneumoniae,* and blockade of pleocytosis was beneficial in reducing BBB permeability in experimental meningitis induced by intracisternal inoculation of *S. pneumoniae, H. influenzae,* and *N. meningitidis.*[203] In contrast, intracisternal inoculation of *H. influenzae* and *S. pneumoniae* resulted in increased BBB permeability in both normal and leukopenic animals, indicating that increased BBB permeability in bacterial meningitis can occur in the absence of pleocytosis.[203] However, no change in BBB permeability shown as normal CSF protein concentrations and absence of pleocytosis after bacterial entry into the CNS usually reflect an early stage of bacterial meningitis.

Neuronal Injury

Neuronal damage is caused by vasculitis; focal ischemia; increased intracranial pressure; cytotoxic, vasogenic, and interstitial edema; transmigrating leukocytes; stimulation of glial cells and astrocytes; cortical necrosis and hippocampal neuronal loss stemming from an inflammatory response to bacteria or bacterial products (bacterial cell wall, teichoic and lipoteichoic acids, lipopolysaccharides, lipoproteins, bacterial DNA); and direct effects of bacterial toxins in the CNS. The various host factors contributing to neuronal injury are shown in Fig. 31.4.

Reactive oxygen species (superoxide and hydrogen peroxide) are secreted by TNF-α–stimulated macrophages, including brain microglia, and leukocytes.[203,215] Hydrogen peroxide induces extensive neuronal damage.[203,215] Nitric oxide also can be induced in brain cells in response to bacterial products.[203] Nitric oxide and superoxide radicals react to form peroxynitrite anion, which decomposes and forms nitrogen dioxide, hydroxyl radicals, and strong oxidant compounds.[34,208] Peroxynitrite seems to be an important neuronal toxin.[214] Neuronal damage caused by reactive oxygen species and reactive nitrate species occurs via at least two separate pathways—via lipid peroxidation and subsequent cell membrane instability and via DNA fragmentation and subsequent activation of poly(adenosine diphosphate ribose) polymerase (PARP) and cellular energy depletion.[203,215] Reactive oxygen species also activate NF-κB, a transcription factor affecting transcription of cytokines and chemokines, and peroxynitrite initiates activation of caspases.[215]

In addition, macrophages secrete excitatory amino acids, such as glutamate, which potentially kill *N*-methyl-D-aspartate receptor–positive cells, and glutamate concentrations in the CSF are shown to be increased in patients with bacterial meningitis.[203]

Meningitis causes damage in the cortex and the hippocampal region via different mechanisms.[203] Cortical damage is mainly via cellular necrosis surrounded by an area of caspase-3–dependent apoptosis. Damage in the hippocampus is mediated not only via the classic caspase-3–dependent pathway but also by caspase-independent apoptosis mediated by apoptosis-initiating factor.[38,40,256]

The increasing concentrations of chemotactic factors in the subarachnoid space lead to accumulation of large numbers of neutrophils in the CSF, but the growth of bacteria is not slowed significantly by this response.[114] Impaired phagocytosis by neutrophils in the meningeal spaces may be related to weak activity in fluid medium, lack of complement activity and opsonization, and poor penetration of IgM and IgG through the BBB, even during acute *H. influenzae* and *S. pneumoniae* meningitis.[160] The contribution of leukocyte entry into the CSF to bacterial meningitis remains inconsistent. Blockage of leukocyte entry into the CSF was associated with poorer prognosis (likely secondary to an increase in bacterial counts in the blood) but did not affect the risk for brain damage,[51] whereas inhibition of leukocyte migration or of products released by leukocytes is shown to interfere with the pathogenesis of bacterial meningitis.[203]

Bacterial cell wall fragments, endotoxin, or both also contribute to vascular permeability. In experimental *E. coli* meningitis, the CSF endotoxin concentration increased markedly after treatment with β-lactam antibiotics. This increase was associated with an increase in brain water content. This effect could be blocked by polymyxin or a monoclonal antibody, both of which inactivate endotoxin.[203,364]

The inflammatory and vascular events described earlier act synergistically to produce the clinical symptoms and long-term sequelae that are noted in patients with bacterial meningitis. Altered vascular permeability leads to vasogenic edema, inflammatory and electrolyte changes lead to cytotoxic edema, and alterations in production and absorption of CSF lead to interstitial edema. The cytokines also trigger increased cerebral blood flow and further formation of edema, resulting in increased intracranial pressure.[19,203,215] The increased intracranial pressure and vasculitis lead to a subsequent decrease in cerebral blood flow, and maintenance of an appropriate cerebral perfusion pressure is crucial to maintaining cerebral blood flow.[19,203,215] Activation of the coagulation cascade predisposes the patient to venous, microvascular, and, rarely, arterial thrombosis. Direct neurotoxic damage by inflammatory cells also may contribute to the neuropathologic changes seen in bacterial meningitis.[203,215]

Studies in experimental animals and human autopsy cases of bacterial meningitis reveal that neuronal injury occurs mostly as apoptosis in the dentate gyrus of the hippocampus formation and as necrosis in the neocortex and the CA1-4 region of the hippocampus.[154,203] In other regions of the brain, neurons die with necrotic morphology.[154] Not only cellular destruction but also proliferation of neuronal progenitor cells has been observed in patients after bacterial meningitis.[156] Increased neural progenitor cell proliferation and differentiation were also observed after experimental bacterial meningitis.[142,152] These findings suggest an endogenous potential of cell renewal in the hippocampal formation in bacterial meningitis. It remains to be determined whether stimulation of endogenous neurogenesis can be used as a potential option in survivors of meningitis.

In the adult brain, neural progenitor cells maintain the ability to proliferate and differentiate into new neurons. The progenitor cells are located predominantly in the subgranular zone of the dentate gyrus and the subventricular zone of the lateral ventricle. In the subgranular zone, the stem cells proliferate and differentiate into progenitor cells. The newly formed cells subsequently migrate into the granular layer of the dentate gyrus, differentiate into mature, functional neurons, and become integrated into the hippocampal network. The hippocampus is therefore potentially equipped for repair. However, because neurofunctional sequelae of bacterial meningitis related to hippocampus function persist throughout childhood and adulthood, the capacity of self-repair seems insufficient to compensate for the brain damage.[203,205,361] It remains to be determined whether the regenerative capacity of the hippocampus is compromised by bacterial meningitis.

Factors Predisposing the Host to Bacterial Meningitis

Factors that predispose the host to the development of bacterial infection in other sites also predispose the host to the development of bacterial infection of the CNS. A strong interrelationship exists among factors relating to the host, the organism, and the environment with regard to the pathogenesis and outcome of meningitis. Although presented separately, they must be considered a complex interplay of factors that leads to infection.

An increased incidence of bacterial meningitis is observed in the very young; boys are affected more frequently than girls, and the severity of disease also is increased in these groups. A neonate is predisposed to development of septicemia and meningitis by factors that reflect physiologic deficiencies or immaturity of host defense mechanisms, including (1) decreased phagocytic and bactericidal activity of polymorphonuclear leukocytes, (2) defects in the response of neonatal leukocytes to chemotactic factors, (3) a deficiency in the capacity of leukocytes to support opsonization, and (4) defects in microtubular length and number that decrease the motility of the neonatal leukocytes compared with leukocytes from older children. Deficiencies in serum complement components (C1q, C3, and C5), low levels of serum properdin, and low concentrations of serum IgM and IgA have been documented. Despite transplacental acquisition of IgG, antibodies against specific infective agents may be lacking.[205] The precise age at which each of these factors reaches the concentration and functional activity noted in older children and adults is unclear and undoubtedly varies from individual to individual. In part, meningitis in children aged 1 month to 1 year may reflect qualitative or quantitative differences of the inflammatory and immunologic responses compared with older children.

The increased risk for development of meningitis in the normal host with less than completely mature immunologic and inflammatory responses to infection may be attributable to age alone. This factor is exemplified in the report,[81] where the risk for recurrent bacteremia was studied in young children. Within 18 months of having bacteremic illness, none of 42 children older than 24 months of age had a documented additional episode of bacteremia or systemic infection. However, 15 of 135 children (11%) younger than age 24 months at the time of the initial bacteremic disease had at least one additional documented bacteremic illness. Of these 15 children, 14 contracted both infections before reaching 2 years of age. Seven of these 15 children had meningitis. Only 2 patients had documented congenital or hereditary disorders of immunoglobulin or complement concentration or function.

There is increasing evidence that genetic polymorphisms in the inflammatory response, complement system, coagulation, and fibrinolysis pathways influence the genetic predisposition and outcome in bacterial meningitis.[56] A genetic determination for the predilection of some normal children for the development of bacteremia and meningitis has been suggested.[56,366] The ability of the host to produce, within the CSF, IL-12 and TNF-α–induced interferon-γ is important in the natural immunity to various microorganisms that may cause meningitis.[56,219]

Deficiencies and polymorphisms in the PRR downstream signaling cascade have been associated with invasive pneumococcal meningitis.[294] IL-1 receptor–associated kinase 4 (IRAK-4) is an intracellular kinase that is involved in signal transduction in the TLR pathways, and MyD88 is a general adaptor molecule for TLR signaling. Individuals with IRAK-4 and MyD88 deficiency are at a high risk for developing pneumococcal meningitis, with increasing mortality.[292,293,383] IRAK-4 and MyD88, however, appear to be important at a young age because no fatal disease after 8 years of age and no invasive bacterial infection after 14 years of age have been reported.[383]

Congenital or acquired abnormalities of the immune system may predispose the host to the acquisition of bacterial infections. Congenital deficiency of the three major immunoglobulin classes may predispose the host to the acquisition of severe bacterial infection. Congenital defects of thymic-dependent, small lymphocyte function or combined T- and B-cell defects are detrimental to host defense. A deficiency of $CD4^+$ helper-inducer T cells in patients with bacterial meningitis has been reported and may contribute to the impaired antibody synthesis to bacterial capsular polysaccharides in this disease.[305] Multiple studies have shown that deficiencies of various components of the complement system and increased consumption or loss of complement have been associated with increased risk for development of bacterial meningitis caused by encapsulated organisms.[56]

In analysis of 103 children with invasive pneumococcal disease including meningitis, the proportion of primary immunodeficiencies was significantly higher in children older than 2 years of age than in younger children (26% vs. 3%; $P < .001$),[149] suggesting that immunologic investigations are warranted in children with pneumococcal meningitis, particularly in those older than 2 years.

An increased incidence of overwhelming infection, including meningitis, occurs after splenectomy, but the likelihood of developing such infection depends on the age of the child at the time of splenectomy, the time since splenectomy, and the original indication for splenectomy.[113] Congenital asplenia or polysplenia also has been associated with an increased incidence of septicemia and meningitis caused by *S. pneumoniae, H. influenzae* type b, and gram-negative enteric microorganisms. Children with sickle-cell disease and other hemoglobinopathies have meningitis caused by *S. pneumoniae, H. influenzae,* and *Salmonella* spp. more frequently than do normal children.

Children with malignant neoplasms with or without neutropenia seem to be susceptible to developing meningitis caused by organisms of low virulence that pose a minimal threat to healthy children, presumably because of abnormalities in immunologic function.[351] Decreased production of normal immunoglobulins, delayed and defective antibody responses to antigenic stimuli, production of abnormal immunoglobulins, depression in the clearance mechanisms of the reticuloendothelial system, and depression of cellular immunity have been documented in children with malignant neoplasms involving the reticuloendothelial system. In addition, the use of irradiation or immunosuppressive agents and antimetabolites predisposes the host to the development of infection in the CNS. Attributing the occurrence of bacterial meningitis in this population directly to these agents rather than to the disease for which this therapy has been provided may be difficult. Meningitis occurring after neurosurgical manipulation for tumors of the CNS in non-neutropenic children usually develops within 1 month of the neurosurgery.[351]

Malnutrition also predisposes children and adults to infectious disease. Impaired cellular immune responses, low levels of serum complement, impaired phagocytic activity of neutrophils, and decreased serum concentrations of transferrin have been documented in malnourished children.[121]

Patients with systemic diseases, such as diabetes mellitus, renal insufficiency, adrenal insufficiency, cystic fibrosis, hypoparathyroidism, and exudative enteropathy, have an increased frequency and severity of CNS infections.[45] Some type of underlying condition was noted for 21% (37 of 181) of the children with pneumococcal meningitis in a multicenter study.[17] The most common of these conditions was some disorder of the CNS, which occurred in 16 children (9%). Defective chemotaxis, phagocytosis, and bactericidal function accompany these disorders and may explain in part the increased susceptibility of these individuals to infection.[121,122]

In the normal host, bacterial infections at sites other than the leptomeninges are associated with an increased incidence of CNS infection. Infection may spread hematogenously to the meninges in children with endocarditis, pneumonia, or thrombophlebitis or by direct extension from sinusitis, mastoiditis, or osteomyelitis of the skull.[203]

An increased risk for the development of pneumococcal meningitis also occurs in children after placement of cochlear implants.[306] The incidence of meningitis caused by *S. pneumoniae* in patients after receiving cochlear implants was 138.2 cases per 100,000 person-years, which represents a more than 30-fold increase over the age-controlled general population.[306] From 1999 to 2002, some children were implanted with cochlear devices, including a positioner, which were subsequently removed from the market as a result of an associated marked increase in incidence of pneumococcal meningitis. After removing the influence of cochlear devices containing a positioner, the incidence of pneumococcal meningitis among children with cochlear implants was still 16 times higher than that of an age-matched control population.

PATHOLOGY

The most detailed account in English of the pathologic changes occurring with meningitis was written in 1948, which included the meningeal, cerebral, and vascular changes in 14 patients who died of *H. influenzae* infection 14 hours to 76 days after the onset of disease.[5] Although most patients in their series received inadequate treatment (effective antibiotic therapy was unavailable), the pathologic findings they describe differ little from the findings of subsequent reports for patients who died despite administration of antibiotics.[106,310,345]

Meningeal exudates of variable thickness may be found (Fig. 31.5). Purulent material is distributed widely but may accumulate around the veins and venous sinuses, over the convexity of the brain, in the depths of the sulci, in the sylvian fissures, within the basal cisterns, and around the cerebellum. The spinal cord may be encased in pus. Ventriculitis (purulent material within the ventricles) has been noted in children who died of their diseases (Fig. 31.6). Subsequent experience suggests that ventriculitis may be a common finding in children with bacterial meningitis who survive, particularly neonates. Loss of the ependymal lining and subependymal gliosis may be seen. In some studies, purulent exudates tended to be thicker over the convexity of the brain in patients with pneumococcal meningitis than in patients with other forms of meningitis.[106,310]

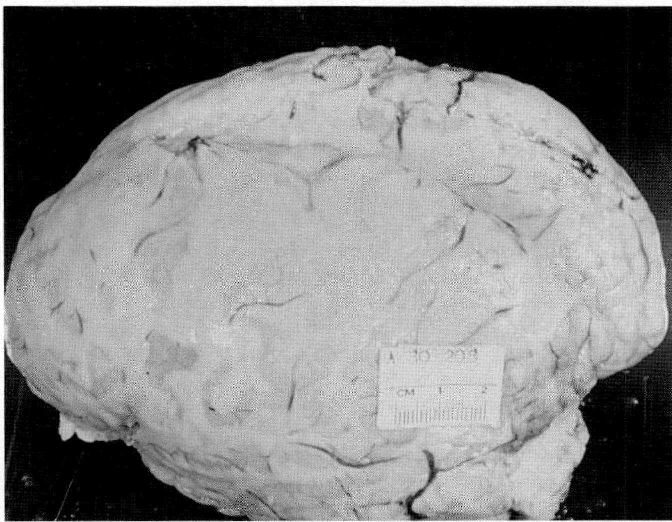

FIG. 31.5 Note extensive purulent exudates over entire cerebral cortex in a patient who died as a result of bacterial meningitis.

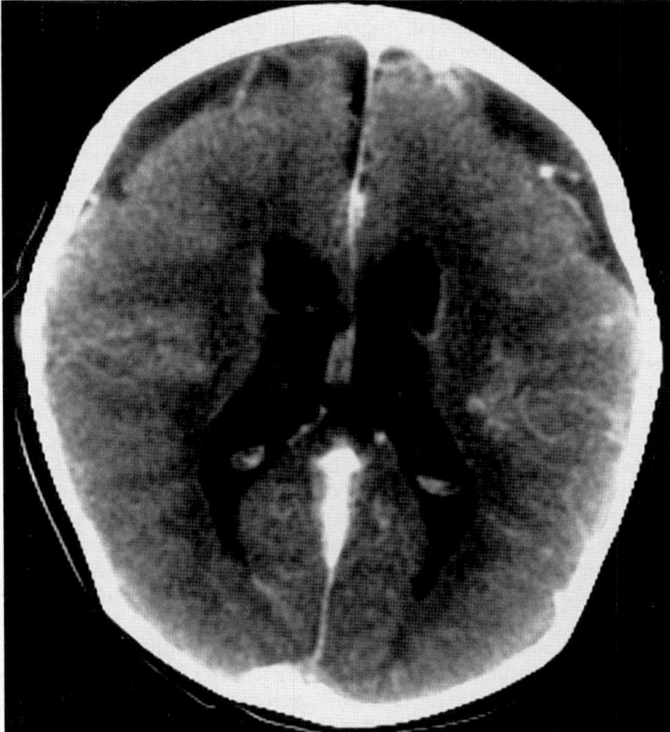

FIG. 31.6 Computed tomography scan of a 2-year-old child with bacterial meningitis. Moderately severe ventricular dilation and the presence of bilateral extracerebral fluid collections overlying the convexities of the brain (subdural effusions) are noted. Note the several prominent vessels that run through the subdural space.

Vascular and parenchymatous changes have been shown at necropsy. Polymorphonuclear infiltrates extending to the subintimal region of small arteries and veins have been associated with the exudative meningeal process. Thrombosis of small cortical veins associated with necrosis of the cerebral cortex may be noted. Occlusion of one of the major venous sinuses, subarachnoid hemorrhage secondary to necrotizing arteritis, and necrosis of the cerebral cortex in the absence of identifiable thrombosis of small vessels rarely may be observed. Reactive microglia and astrocytes may be identified in the cerebral cortex, particularly subadjacent to regions of heavy subarachnoid exudate. Because no bacteria are found in the cerebral cortex, these pathologic changes should be viewed as a noninfectious encephalopathy. "Toxic or circulatory factors" were suggested as possible causes[4] and hypoxia and fever as additional possible causes.[106] An increase in intracranial pressure might interfere with cerebral circulation.

Impaired consciousness, deficits in motor and sensory functions, seizures, and retardation may be observed. Damage to the cerebral cortex, reflecting the effects of vascular occlusion, hypoxia, toxic encephalopathy, bacterial factors, inflammatory mediators, small molecule effectors, or some combination of these factors, provides an adequate explanation for these observations.

Hydrocephalus that develops in patients beyond the newborn period is an uncommon complication of meningitis. Most often, hydrocephalus is communicating and is the result of adhesive thickening of the arachnoid around the cisterns at the base of the brain. Less frequently, the aqueduct of Sylvius or the foramina of Magendie and Luschka are obstructed by fibrosis and reactive gliosis. The ensuing ventricular dilation may be coupled with coexistent necrosis of nervous tissue because of the meningitis itself or because of occlusion of cerebral veins and, rarely, arteries.

Subdural effusions occur frequently during the course of meningitis. The exact pathogenesis is unknown. The high incidence of effusion and the fact that subdural fluid collections may be found early in the course of bacterial meningitis in children suggest, however, that subdural effusions should be considered a concomitant occurrence with meningeal inflammation rather than a complication of the disease. Numerous veins traverse the subdural space, and inflammation of these veins and of the dural capillaries could produce an increase in vascular permeability and loss of albumin-rich fluid into the subdural space. The ratio of albumin to γ-globulin is higher in the subdural fluid of children with meningitis than in serum.[165] When the inflammatory process subsides, formation of fluid generally ceases, but its presence may persist because of a continued transudation through newly formed vessels in the subdural membrane. Subdural empyema, as opposed to subdural effusion, occurs rarely.[5,106,345]

Many factors contribute to the increase in intracranial pressure in patients with meningitis. Endotoxin and fragments of the cell wall of gram-positive organisms are capable of inducing the release of IL-1β and TNF-α from macrophages, glial cells, and other sources.[203,364,368] These substances, in addition to other ILs and metabolites, affect endothelial cells, affecting the function of the vasculature and its interaction with neutrophils and other inflammatory cells. They also play an important role in the pathogenesis of increased intracranial pressure and cerebral edema in patients with meningitis by altering cerebral blood flow, intracranial blood volume, and permeability of the cerebral vasculature.[277] Experimentally, the main components of the BBB—endothelial cells, astrocyte-end feet, and pericytes—have been found to be sensitive to the effects of such inflammatory mediators.[28] Intercellular junctions, which normally are tight, are open in advanced stages of experimental meningitis, which is associated with an increased permeability to circulating albumin.[300] Pinocytotic vesicles also are noted within the cytoplasm of endothelial cells. Swelling of cellular elements (cytotoxic edema) also has been noted.

Alterations in CSF resorption exacerbate cerebral edema and increase intracranial pressure further. In experimental meningitis, resorption of CSF is diminished because an accumulation of proteins, leukocytes, and other materials interferes with the function of the arachnoid villus.[327]

During the course of meningitis, excess secretion of antidiuretic hormone (ADH) occurs, which induces water retention and exacerbates electrolyte abnormalities already created secondary to the inflammatory process occurring in the CNS. Cellular electrolyte disturbances may depolarize neuronal membranes, predisposing the host to seizure activity. Increased oxidation of glucose, increased lactate production, and depletion of high-energy compounds such as adenosine 5′-triphosphate and phosphocreatine are observed. Hypoglycorrhachia results primarily from decreased transport of glucose across the inflamed BBB and from increased use of glucose by host tissues. Use of glucose by bacteria and polymorphonuclear leukocytes is of less relative importance.[106,382]

CLINICAL MANIFESTATIONS AND PATHOPHYSIOLOGIC RELATIONSHIPS

The clinical features of bacterial meningitis in infants and children can be subtle, variable, and nonspecific, or even absent.[205] In infants, they might include fever, hypothermia, lethargy, irritability, poor feeding, vomiting, diarrhea, respiratory distress, seizures, or bulging fontanelles. In older children, clinical features might include fever, headaches, photophobia, nausea, vomiting, confusion, lethargy, or irritability. Signs of meningeal irritation are present in 75% of children with bacterial meningitis at the time of presentation.[234] In contrast, a retrospective review of 326 children presenting to a pediatric emergency department in the Netherlands between 1988 and 1998 with meningeal irritation revealed that 30% had bacterial meningitis.[284] Absence of meningeal irritation in children with bacterial meningitis was substantially more common in those younger than 12 months of age (Table 31.6).[205]

Inflammation of the meninges generally is associated with nausea, vomiting, irritability, anorexia, headache, confusion, back pain, and nuchal rigidity.[205] In many cases, Kernig and Brudzinski signs are noted. The Kernig sign is present when the leg is flexed 90 degrees at the hips and cannot be extended more than 135 degrees. The Brudzinski sign is present if the thighs and legs are flexed involuntarily when the neck is flexed. All of these findings suggest irritation of inflamed sensory nerves, which produces a reflex contraction of certain muscles in an attempt to minimize pain. These findings also can be the result of increased intracranial pressure and an associated distortion of nerve roots. These signs can be accompanied by hyperesthesia and photophobia. Currently no satisfactory pathophysiologic explanation for photophobia exists.

As indicated earlier, signs of meningeal inflammation may be minimal in the infant, but irritability, restlessness, and poor feeding may be noted.[205] Nuchal rigidity and Kernig and Brudzinski signs may occur late in a young child. Nuchal rigidity may not be elicited in comatose patients or when signs of focal or diffuse neurologic impairment are present. At the time of initial evaluation, 60% to 80% of children have a stiff neck.[205] A review of 1064 cases of bacterial meningitis in children beyond the neonatal period revealed that 16 (1.5%) had no meningeal signs during their entire period of hospitalization, despite the presence of CSF pleocytosis.[150] Fever, a hallmark of infection, generally is present; its absence in a patient with signs of meningeal inflammation, although infrequent, is not unusual.

The relative frequency with which selected findings in infants, children, and adults with bacterial meningitis occur are summarized in Table 31.6.[21,77,78,89,132,151,377]

Increased intracranial pressure is the rule; it may be reflected by complaints of headache in older children and by a bulging fontanelle and diastasis of sutures in infants. Papilledema is an uncommon finding in acute meningitis, presumably because of the brief duration of increased pressure at the time of diagnosis. When papilledema is observed, venous sinus occlusion, subdural empyema, or brain abscess should be sought.

A major contributing factor to increased intracranial pressure in bacterial meningitis is the development of cerebral edema. Vasogenic edema occurs as a consequence of increased permeability of the BBB. Interstitial edema may occur secondary to decreased clearance of CSF at the arachnoid villi and subsequent obstructive hydrocephalus. Cytotoxic cerebral edema mediated by the release of toxic factors from neutrophils, glial cells, and bacteria leads to increased concentration of intracellular water and sodium and loss of intracellular potassium. In many cases,[118] meningitis is associated with the release of ADH, causing water retention and a relative dumping of sodium by the kidney. If the patient is given excessive free water during therapy, a further increase in intracranial pressure may be noted.

Transient or permanent paralysis of cranial nerves may be noted. Deafness or disturbances in vestibular function are common findings; optic nerve involvement with blindness rarely occurs. Involvement of the eighth cranial nerve may reflect disease at the level of the cochlear and vestibular end organs, which may be related to concomitant infection of the inner ear. Paralysis of extraocular and facial nerves may be noted. Torticollis has been reported in two children with partially treated meningitis.[249] Obtundation, stupor, coma, and focal neurologic signs may be seen in children with bacterial meningitis.

Table 31.7 shows data for 235 children with bacterial meningitis in a prospective study analyzed according to the type of organism responsible for meningitis. Overall, 14.9% of children were semicomatose or comatose at the time of admission; rates for children with pneumococcal or meningococcal meningitis were higher than rates for children with *H. influenzae* disease. Focal neurologic signs were present at the time of admission in 16.5% of the total group (34.3% of children with pneumococcal meningitis). The presence of focal neurologic signs at the time of admission indicated a poor prognosis and could be correlated with persistent abnormal neurologic examinations at 1, 3, and 6 months ($P < .01$) and at 1 year after discharge ($P < .03$). The presence of focal signs at the time of admission also correlated with the presence of retardation ($P < .001$), as determined by detailed psychometric testing after discharge.

Generally when focal signs are noted in the absence of seizures, cortical necrosis, occlusive vasculitis, or thrombosis of cortical veins has occurred. Thrombosis of meningeal vessels or cortical necrosis may be associated with hemiparesis or quadriparesis and with focal seizures. These signs may appear during the first 3 or 4 days of illness or, less commonly, may be noted after the first or second week of infection. A highly significant association ($P < .001$) between neurologic signs indicative of cerebral injury and late afebrile seizures (1 to 15 years after the acute infection) has been noted.[296] Ataxia has been a presenting sign of meningitis in children and adults.[333] Adolescents with meningitis may present with behavioral abnormalities that may be confused with drug abuse or psychiatric disorders.[27]

Approximately 20% of children with bacterial meningitis experience seizures before admission, and approximately 26% have them during the first or second day in the hospital. A retrospective review[168] examined the frequency of seizures before or at the time of presentation in children with meningitis. Seizures at or before the time of diagnosis occurred in 111 of 410 (27%) children with bacterial meningitis; 88 of these children had complex seizures (focal, prolonged, or more than one in a 24-hour period). All children with bacterial meningitis who presented with seizures had other signs or symptoms of meningitis, such as

TABLE 31.6 Frequency (%) of Selected Findings in Infants, Children, and Adults With Bacterial Meningitis on Presentation

Selected Findings	Infants	Children	Adults
Underlying disorders	27–32	10–21	53–92
Headache	NA	15–92	31–87
Fever	34–98	88–97	42–97
Neck stiffness	9–54	40–80	50–88
Bulging fontanelle	14–42	NA	NA
Altered mental status	34–79	53–83	32–91
Coma	1–40	7–11	11–19
Seizures	16–62	19–41	5–21
Focal neurologic deficits	4–16	8–34	10–42
Cranial nerve palsies	10	10	10–21
Hearing loss	NA	23–34	9

NA, Not available.

TABLE 31.7 **Frequency of Selected Findings in Children With Bacterial Meningitis**

	Total Group	*H. influenzae*	*S. pneumoniae*	*N. meningitidis*
No. patients	235	151	35	26
Level of consciousness (%)				
Irritable or lethargic	184 (78.3)	117 (77.5)	24 (68.6)	21 (80.8)
Somnolent	16 (6.8)	13 (8.6)	1 (2.8)	1 (3.8)
Obtunded-semicomatose	27 (11.5)	15 (9.9)	8 (22.9)	4 (15.4)
Comatose	8 (3.4)	6 (4)	2 (5.7)	0 (0)
Focal neurologic signs on admission (%)	37 (16.5)	22 (14.6)	12 (34.3)	2 (7.7)
Seizures before admission (%)	48 (20.4)	35 (23.2)	8 (23)	3 (11.5)
Seizures in hospital (%)	61 (26)	43 (28)	12 (34)	5 (19)

altered level of consciousness, nuchal rigidity, or complex seizures and petechial rash. The frequency of seizure activity is similar for children with *H. influenzae* type b or pneumococcal meningitis; seizures occur in children with meningitis caused by these organisms approximately twice as frequently as in children with meningococcal meningitis. In a multicenter study of 181 children with pneumococcal meningitis, 41 (23%) developed seizures before admission; 74% of preadmission seizures were generalized.[17]

Overall, seizures are noted in approximately 30% of children with bacterial meningitis in the prospective study. Seizures noted before or during the first several days of hospitalization are of no particular prognostic significance. Specifically their occurrence does not herald the development of a permanent seizure disorder. Seizures that are difficult to control or that persist beyond the fourth hospital day and seizures that occur for the first time late in the hospital course may be of greater significance and have been associated with permanent sequelae of meningitis. Children with focal seizures have a greater likelihood for development of sequelae of meningitis than do children with generalized seizure activity. Focal or prolonged seizures probably indicate serious cerebral vascular disturbances or cerebral infarction. Seven percent of patients with bacterial meningitis have focal or generalized seizures 3 months to 15 years after recovery from bacterial meningitis.[296]

Collections of fluid in the subdural space can be shown in 50% of infants and children during acute illness.[106] In a prospective study of infants 1 to 18 months old with bacterial meningitis, subdural effusions were noted in 43% of infants with *H. influenzae* meningitis, 30% of infants with pneumococcal meningitis, and 22% of infants with meningococcal meningitis. Subdural effusions were found in 24% (25 of 103) of children undergoing neuroimaging in the multicenter pediatric surveillance study of pneumococcal meningitis.[17,347] No greater incidence of neurologic sequelae or developmental delay was found on long-term follow-up in patients with effusion compared with patients with bacterial meningitis who did not have effusion.[347] Subdural effusions may cause enlargement in head circumference or may be responsible for abnormal transillumination of the skull, and vomiting, seizures, a full fontanelle, focal neurologic signs, or persistent fever sometimes may be noted.

Blindness and optic atrophy may be related to optic arachnoiditis or infarction of the occipital lobe. Spastic paraparesis with sensory loss in the lower extremities may be secondary to meningomyelitis, spinal cord infarction, or both.

Shock may be associated with any form of overwhelming bacteremia, but it occurs most often in patients with fulminant meningococcemia. In a prospective study, 3.8% of children with meningococcal meningitis developed profound hypotension. In the same study, shock occurred in 5.5% of children with *H. influenzae* meningitis. Endotoxin has been detected by limulus lysate assay in the blood and CSF of children with meningococcal and *H. influenzae* meningitis.[313] Sixteen percent of the children in the multicenter pneumococcal meningitis study were in shock on admission.[17] Signs of disseminated intravascular coagulation may accompany hypotension in these patients.

Facial cellulitis (including buccal and periorbital cellulitis), epiglottitis, endophthalmitis, and other suppurative manifestations can manifest at the time of admission in any patient with bacterial meningitis. In one study of children with buccal cellulitis, less than 10% (7 of 73 children) had concomitant bacterial meningitis documented by lumbar puncture as part of their initial evaluation.[25] Five of the seven children had no clinical evidence of meningeal irritation. *H. influenzae* and *S. pneumoniae* were cultured from two patients with periorbital cellulitis, and no clinical evidence of meningeal irritation or abnormal CSF cell counts or results of chemistries was found.[321] In the largest review of facial cellulitis caused by *S. pneumoniae*,[166] 15 of 52 children had a lumbar puncture performed; 2 (13.3%) had a pleocytosis (18 white blood cells [WBCs]/mm^3—52% polymorphonuclear leukocytes, and 9 WBCs/mm^3—91% polymorphonuclear leukocytes). The Gram stain and cultures of the CSF specimens were negative. Lumbar puncture should be considered for children with facial cellulitis who are younger than 18 months of age and possibly bacteremic with *S. pneumoniae.*

Arthralgia and myalgia are noted in many patients with bacterial meningitis, reflecting the systemic nature of the disease. Arthritis also may occur and does so most commonly during the course of meningococcal disease; generally it is transient. Early findings of arthritis may be related to direct invasion of the joint by the meningococcus. Arthritis that develops late in the course of meningococcal or *H. influenzae* meningitis may be an immune complex–mediated event. Petechial or purpuric lesions may be seen in 50% of patients with meningococcal meningitis[106] but also may accompany any infectious or noninfectious disease process in which vasculitis occurs. Purpura, shock, and hypothermia indicate a poor prognosis.

Pericardial effusions may be present; they generally resolve during the course of antibiotic therapy. In some cases, pericardial effusions are the cause of persistent fever, and pericardiocentesis or an open drainage procedure may be required.

DIFFERENTIAL DIAGNOSIS

The signs and symptoms described earlier suggest meningeal or intracranial pathologic processes but are not pathognomonic of acute bacterial infection. Tuberculous meningitis, fungal meningitis, aseptic meningitis, brain abscess, intracranial or spinal epidural abscesses, cranial osteomyelitis, subdural empyema, bacterial endocarditis with embolism, ruptured dermoid cysts, ruptured spinal ependymomas, and brain tumors may show similar signs and symptoms. Differentiation of these disorders depends on careful examination of CSF obtained by lumbar puncture and additional immunologic, radiographic, and imaging studies, as delineated later.

Recurrent bacterial meningitis may be the result of a bacterial infection in the setting of an immunocompromised condition or a communication between the nasal passage or ear and the meninges from congenital anatomic defect or the result of trauma. If rhinorrhea or otorrhea is present, a leak may be suspected, but documenting that CSF is present and locating the site of leakage are difficult when the sample is small or contaminated. Sectional (2 mm) coronal cranial computed tomography (CT) is a noninvasive method for delineating anatomic abnormalities in children with recurrent meningitis.[357]

Protein electrophoresis of CSF[14,254] revealed an extra band of transferrin located in the β_2-fraction. This extra β_2-transferrin band could not be shown in serum, nasal secretions, saliva, tears, or perilymph and endolymph, suggesting that this immunochemical method is useful for documenting that fluid found draining from the nose or ear was CSF. The amount of sample required is small (<50 μL). Differential suction may permit demonstration of the site of the anatomic communication among the nose, the ear, and the meninges. Moderate contamination with other body fluids does not invalidate the method. β-trace protein has also shown to be useful for the reliable diagnosis of CSF leaks, and the method is noninvasive and safe for the patient.[251]

Noninfectious causes of meningitis include medications such as nonsteroidal antiinflammatory drugs (NSAIDs), trimethoprim-sulfamethoxazole, isoniazid, metronidazole, intravenous immune globulin treatment, Behçet syndrome, systemic lupus erythematosus, mixed connective tissue disease, Kawasaki disease, sarcoidosis, familial Mediterranean fever, Vogt-Koyanagi syndrome, procedures involving the CNS (neurosurgery, spinal anesthesia, intrathecal injection), subarachnoid hemorrhage, vein of Galen aneurysm, Mollaret meningitis, intracranial/intraspinal tumors, and cysts.

DIAGNOSIS

Early diagnosis and treatment of bacterial meningitis are imperative in reducing mortality rates and morbidity. Physicians must perform a lumbar puncture on any child in whom they suspect the diagnosis after a careful history and physical examination have been performed, unless specific contraindications to this procedure are present (e.g., clinical signs of increased intracranial pressure in a patient with a closed fontanelle and closed sutures, evidence of mass lesions, cardiopulmonary compromise).

Measurement of opening pressure, often neglected in infants and young children, is an important component of each CSF examination. When the pressure is very high, only enough fluid to permit a careful examination should be removed. Compression of the jugular vein should be avoided unless compression of the spinal cord is suspected. The CSF appearance can be cloudy, stemming from high concentrations of bacteria, protein, WBCs, and/or red blood cells (RBCs). Xanthochromic CSF derives its color primarily from bilirubin pigment. Hemorrhage, bilirubin staining in icteric patients who have meningitis (i.e., neonates, patients with leptospirosis), or an elevated protein concentration of CSF may be associated with xanthochromia.

CSF should be examined immediately. The total number of WBCs should be counted in a counting chamber, and, after cytocentrifugation, a differential cell count should be done on a Wright-stained smear of the sediment. The normal CSF of children age 3 months or older contains less than 6 WBCs/mm^3. Ninety-five percent of children older than age 3 months have no polymorphonuclear leukocytes in the CSF; the presence of a polymorphonuclear leukocyte in the CSF may be regarded as abnormal. When a lumbar puncture has been performed in a febrile child and a single polymorphonuclear leukocyte has been noted, careful clinical observation is imperative, and treatment should be considered until the results of the culture of the CSF are known.

If the lumbar puncture has been traumatic, a total cell count can be done in a counting chamber. The RBCs can be lysed by acetic acid, and a cell count can be repeated. If the total number of WBCs compared with the number of RBCs is greater than that in whole blood, one can assume the presence of CSF pleocytosis. One simple way to estimate the WBC count in the presence of RBCs is to allow 1 WBC per 1000 RBCs/mm^3. However, this adjustment cannot be reliably performed in the presence of clot. CSF protein should be measured (usually elevated in bacterial meningitis), and the CSF glucose concentration should be compared with the blood glucose concentration that has been obtained concomitantly. In patients with bacterial meningitis, depression of CSF glucose and of the ratio of CSF to blood glucose (normally 40% to 60%) is the rule (Table 31.8).

Separate smears should be made, and one smear should be Gram-stained for bacteria. A Kinyoun stain for mycobacteria is performed if tuberculous meningitis is suspected. The probability of visualizing bacteria on a Gram stain of CSF depends on the number of organisms present.[42,125] The percentage of positive smears is 25% with less than 10^3 CFU/mL, 60% in the range of 10^3 to 10^5 CFU/mL, and 97% with greater than 10^5 CFU/mL.[223] Gram stain is positive in about 90% of children with pneumococcal meningitis, about 80% of children with meningococcal meningitis, half of patients with gram-negative bacillary meningitis, and a third of patients with *Listeria* meningitis.[205] Cytospin centrifugation increases the chances of detecting organisms in Gram-stained CSF.[205] A low CSF WBC count with positive Gram stain is a risk factor for an unfavorable outcome.[17,205] Quellung and agglutination reactions can provide immediate identification of various organisms if the appropriate type of specific antisera is available.

Treating a child with bacterial meningitis with an antibiotic before performing initial lumbar puncture usually does not alter markedly the cell counts or chemical results obtained (Table 31.9). Even when children received appropriate antibiotics for meningitis intravenously for 44 to 68 hours, the bacterial character of the chemical and cellular findings could be discerned in most cases.[44] CSF culture, however, can be negative in children who receive antibiotic treatment before CSF examination. Complete sterilization of *N. meningitidis* occurred within 2 hours of giving a parenteral third-generation cephalosporin and the beginning of sterilization of *S. pneumoniae* from CSF by 4 hours into treatment.[193] In such children, pleocytosis and an increased CSF protein concentration are usually sufficient to establish the diagnosis of bacterial meningitis. Blood cultures or nonculture diagnostic tests can help in identifying the infecting organism.

The CSF should be cultured on a blood agar plate and a chocolate agar plate. The CSF specimens always should be cultured, even when the fluid appears to be crystal clear and acellular.

In the 1970s, countercurrent immunoelectrophoresis was shown to be a useful technique for rapid diagnosis (within 1 hour) and management of bacterial meningitis caused by *H. influenzae* type b, *S. pneumoniae, N. meningitidis* (serogroups A, C, W135, and D), and group B *Streptococcus*. It was also used to detect antigens from K1 strains of *E. coli* or *L. monocytogenes*.[124,205,248] Although rarely available currently, the methodology was sensitive and could detect nonviable bacteria, permitting the detection of bacterial antigen even in patients pretreated with appropriate antibiotics.[187,335]

Latex particle agglutination commercial kits are available for detecting the polysaccharide antigens of *H. influenzae* type b, *S. pneumoniae, N. meningitidis,* and group B *Streptococcus*. Nonspecific agglutination of latex particles in serum, urine, and other body fluids may result in an indeterminate test result.[92,188,326,390] In the multicenter pneumococcal meningitis surveillance study, latex agglutination was positive in 49 (66%) of 74 CSF specimens that grew *S. pneumoniae* and in 4 of 14 CSF specimens that were culture negative.[17] The U.S. Food and Drug Administration (FDA) does not recommend latex agglutination testing of urine of infants for group B *Streptococcus* as a method for inferring invasive disease with this organism. Latex agglutination of urine for group B *Streptococcus* or *N. meningitidis* should be avoided because of the high frequency of false-positive results.

The clinical utility of rapid antigen detection in CSF has been questioned in recent years since the decline in frequency of invasive infections caused by *H. influenzae* type b. A positive test response rarely alters the approach to therapy. Bacterial antigen tests should be considered for patients with suspected bacterial meningitis whose initial CSF Gram stain was negative and whose culture was negative after 48 hours of incubation.[247,290] There may be public health benefits in the early identification of the infecting organism using latex agglutination testing of CSF when the Gram stain is consistent with meningococci.[131] In the latter case, clarifying the meningococcal serogroup quickly may have implications in large outbreaks for recommending meningococcal vaccine for type A, B, C, Y, or W135 disease.

The rapidity with which results of bacterial antigen tests are obtained renders them tempting as a means to establish an early diagnosis. The degree to which they affect clinical decisions is unclear. Performing these tests is unnecessary for every patient suspected of having bacterial meningitis, but they could play a role in certain circumstances, such as when a patient's clinical presentation suggests bacterial meningitis and pretreatment with antibiotics or with a traumatic lumbar puncture. Antigen detection is useful in developing countries, where CSF culture yields are lower.[97,205]

Standard or sequential-multiplex polymerase chain reaction (PCR) has been shown to be useful in identification of infecting pathogens in patients who have previously received antibiotics or in resource-poor

TABLE 31.8 Cerebrospinal Fluid Findings in Infectious and Inflammatory Diseases of the Central Nervous System and Meninges

Condition	Pressure (mm H_2O)	Leukocytes/μL	Protein (mg/dL)	Sugar (mg/dL)	Specific Findings
Acute bacterial meningitis	Usually elevated; average 300	Several hundred to >10,000; usually a few thousand; occasionally <100 (especially meningococcal or early in disease); PMLs predominate	Usually 100–500, occasionally >1000	<40 in more than half the cases	Organism usually seen on smear or recovered on culture in >90% of cases
Subdural empyema	Usually elevated; average 300	<100 to a few thousand; PMLs predominate	Usually 100–500	Normal	No organisms on smear or by culture unless concurrent meningitis
Brain abscess	Usually elevated	Usually 10–200; fluid rarely is acellular; lymphocytes predominate	Usually 75–400	Normal	No organisms on smear or by culture
Ventricular empyema (rupture of brain abscess)	Elevated	Several thousand to 100,000; usually >90% PMLs	Usually several hundred	Usually <40	Organisms may be seen on smear or cultured
Cerebral epidural abscess	Slight to modest elevation	Few to several hundred or more cells; lymphocytes predominate	Usually 50-200	Normal	No organisms on smear or by culture
Spinal epidural abscess	Usually reduced with spinal block	Usually 10–100; lymphocytes predominate	Usually several hundred	Normal	No organisms on smear or by culture
Thrombophlebitis (often associated with subdural empyema)	Often elevated	Few to several hundred; PMLs and lymphocytes	Slightly to moderately elevated	Normal	No organisms on smear or by culture
Bacterial endocarditis (with embolism)	Normal or slightly elevated	Few to <100; lymphocytes and PMLs	Slightly elevated	Normal	No organisms on smear or by culture
Acute hemorrhagic encephalitis	Usually elevated	Few to >1000; PMLs predominate	Moderately elevated	Normal	No organisms on smear or by culture
Tuberculous infection	Usually elevated	Usually 25–100, rarely >500; lymphocytes predominate except in early stages when PMLs may account for 80% of cells	Nearly always elevated; usually 100–200; may be much higher if block in CSF flow	Usually reduced; <50 in 75% of cases	Acid-fast organisms may be seen on smear of protein coagulum (pellicle) or recovered from inoculated guinea pig or by culture
Cryptococcal infection	Usually elevated	Average 50 (0–800); lymphocytes predominate	Average 100; usually 20–500	Reduced in more than half of cases; often higher in patients with concomitant diabetes mellitus	Organisms may be seen in India ink preparation and on culture (Sabouraud medium); usually grow on blood agar; may produce alcohol in CSF from fermentation of glucose
Syphilis (acute)	Usually elevated	Average 500; usually lymphocytes; rarely PMLs	Average, 100; γ-globulin often high, with abnormal colloidal gold curve	Normal (rarely reduced)	Positive reagin test result for syphilis; spirochete not demonstrable by usual techniques of smear or by culture
Sarcoidosis	Normal to considerably elevated	0 to <100 mononuclear cells	Slight to moderate elevation	Normal	No specific findings

PMLs, polymorphonuclear leukocytes.

settings.[80,86,205,220,240] PCR analysis of CSF has been used to detect microbial DNA in patients with bacterial meningitis. Primers are available for the detection of *S. pneumoniae*, *N. meningitidis*, and *H. influenzae* type b simultaneously. Species-specific amplicons have been detected in 89% of patients with proven pneumococcal, meningococcal, or *H. influenzae* type b meningitis.[302] No false-positive results were noted.

Multiplex real-time PCR or broad-range PCR aimed at the 16S ribosomal RNA gene of eubacteria is promising for the detection of pathogens from CSF. The detection rate was substantially higher with PCR than with cultures in patients who had previously received antibiotics.[86] However, the limit of detection differs among assays. Real-time PCR has been shown to detect as few as 2 copies of *E. coli*, *N. meningitidis*, and *S. pneumoniae*; 16 copies of *L. monocytogenes*; and 28 copies of group B *Streptococcus*,[86] whereas the sensitivity for broad-range 16S ribosomal DNA PCR was 10 to 200 organisms per milliliter of CSF.[87,89] The time needed for the whole process from DNA extraction to the end of real-time PCR was 1.5 hours,[86] an attractive time frame for its application in clinical practice.

A Gram stain–specific, probe-based, real-time PCR using 16S ribosomal RNA has been shown to allow simultaneous detection and

TABLE 31.9 Comparison of Cerebrospinal Fluid Findings in Patients With Untreated and Pretreated Meningitis

	Untreated	Pretreated
No. patients	143	91
Total white blood cell count: 10^3		
Mean ± 1 SD	4.9 ± 6.5	4.1 ± 5
Range	0–55	0.006–25.5
Percentage polys		
Mean ± 1 SD	84 ± 21	81 ± 25
Range	0–100	0–100
Glucose (mg/dL)		
Mean ± 1 SD	35 ± 28	32 ± 25
Range	0–109	0–100
CSF/blood glucose (%)		
Mean ± 1 SD	29 ± 21	29 ± 21
Range	0–78	0–94
Protein (mg/dL)		
Mean ± 1 SD	226 ± 228	174 ± 193
Range	13–2290	10–1640
Culture positive	135	71
Gram positive	114	62

discrimination of clinically relevant gram-positive and gram-negative bacteria directly from blood samples,[205] which might provide more rapid and accurate diagnosis of bacterial infection in infants and children. In addition, sequential PCR-based serotyping of *S. pneumoniae* using serotype-specific primers could improve ascertainment of pneumococcal serotype distribution in settings in which prior use of antibiotics is high.[205] The approach based on amplification of 16 sDNA and hybridization with species-specific oligoprobes may be useful for the diagnosis of community-acquired meningitis.[103] No false-negative results occurred in culture-positive CSF specimens. The possible addition of gene microarray technology offers the potential to probe for multiple different bacterial species simultaneously.[180]

PCR also is useful in rapidly documenting viral antigens (e.g., enteroviruses) within CSF, thus reducing the use of antibiotics in selected patients who are treated for presumptive bacterial disease but who may have viral meningitis.[314,329,380]

Measurement of C-reactive protein (CRP) has been proposed as a test that may be valuable in distinguishing bacterial from viral meningitis. In some studies, overlap in CRP determinations among these groups of patients has been observed, and one cannot rely on the CRP result to distinguish bacterial from viral meningitis with sufficient certainty.[157] Nonetheless serum CRP was superior to CSF parameters in distinguishing gram-negative bacterial from viral meningitis.[352] Among 92 patients with viral meningitis, 93% had serum CRP levels within the normal range (<20 mg/L). Only one child with gram-negative bacterial meningitis had a serum CRP value within the normal range.

Elevated serum concentrations of the polypeptide procalcitonin were shown to be useful in differentiating between bacterial and viral meningitis. At a threshold of 0.5 ng/mL, procalcitonin had a sensitivity of 99% and a specificity of 83% by one report and has been incorporated into the Meningitest (see later discussion).[108]

Numerous metabolic changes have been reported to occur in the CSF and blood of patients with meningitis. CSF lactate has been noted to be elevated significantly in patients with bacterial meningitis. The increase in CSF lactate apparently is related to decreased cerebral blood flow, cerebral hypoxia, and a change to anaerobic metabolism in the brain. Concentration of CSF lactate tends to parallel the CSF cellular response.[316] Although the concentration of CSF lactate in patients with bacterial meningitis generally is greater than that in patients with aseptic meningitis, such is not always the case. In some patients with aseptic meningitis, CSF lactate has been in the range generally observed in patients with bacterial infections. Conversely, in patients who proved to have bacterial meningitis but who had equivocal clinical and CSF findings, measurement of CSF lactate failed to differentiate bacterial from nonbacterial infection.[316] The determination of the concentration of CSF lactate cannot be used reliably to differentiate viral from bacterial meningitis in an individual patient.[216]

Depression of the pH of CSF also has been described in patients with bacterial meningitis. The depression of pH in CSF is more transient than is the elevation of CSF lactic acid, and its measurement is of even less value in the differential diagnosis.

Lactate dehydrogenase, creatine phosphokinase, and aspartate transaminase may be elevated in patients with bacterial meningitis. In some cases, total lactate dehydrogenase activity within CSF may be similar in patients with bacterial and aseptic meningitis, but lactate dehydrogenase isoenzymic analysis may permit differentiation of bacterial from nonbacterial infection. This procedure is time-consuming and cumbersome and does not permit establishing a specific etiologic diagnosis in any patient.[275]

Despite the application of impeccable clinical judgment, examination of CSF, and use of one or more of the rapid diagnostic techniques, situations arise in which differentiation of bacterial from aseptic meningitis remains problematic. In these cases, a predominance of polymorphonuclear leukocytes generally is found in the CSF, the CSF cell counts are less than 100 cells/mm^3, the CSF glucose concentration is normal or nearly so, and the Gram stain result is negative. Most children with aseptic meningitis have a predominance of polymorphonuclear leukocytes on their initial CSF examination.[276] In addition, although patients exhibit signs and symptoms suggestive of meningitis, they do not appear acutely ill. Some investigators have advocated withholding antibiotic therapy in these patients and repeating the lumbar puncture after 6 to 12 hours of close observation.[3,120] Usually, the repeated examination of CSF either substantiates the impression of aseptic meningitis (a shift to a lymphocytic differential is noted) or points more conclusively to a bacterial process. This course of action is not recommended if the patient has been pretreated with antibiotics or is younger than 1 year. Occasionally, children have a mild CSF pleocytosis, which may have a predominance of polymorphonuclear leukocytes, after they experience seizures.[399,401] Generally CSF abnormalities should not be attributed to seizures unless other causes of CNS inflammation have been excluded.

Other approaches to differentiate bacterial from viral meningitis have been considered. For example, a number of CSF biomarkers have been examined for differentiating bacterial meningitis from viral meningitis and noninfectious etiology, and selected CSF biomarkers for predicting bacterial meningitis with their respective sensitivity and specificity are reported as follows[206,361]: TNFα (50–100% and 81–100%), IL-1β (60–97% and 92–100%), IL-6 (80–96% and 51–98%), IL-8 (50–100% and 50–92%), IL-12 (60–96% and 60–75%), IL-17 (50–60% and 50–60%), procalcitonin (68–100% and 73–96%), lactate (75–96% and 85–100%), ferritin (90–96% and 50–96%), apolipoprotein E (85% and 100%), lipocalin 2 (81% and 93%), neutrophil gelatinase-associated lipocalin (74% and 100%), S100B (91% and 82%), heparin-binding protein (100% and 99%), and soluble triggering receptor expressed on myeloid cells (73–78% and 77–100%). The validity and utilization of these biomarkers in clinical practice, however, have been limited because of the relatively small number of patients included for individual studies and use of different assays, and the results of these assays should be interpreted with caution.

The ability to distinguish between bacterial and nonbacterial aseptic meningitis in infants and children in the emergency department could contribute to limiting hospital admissions or unnecessary use of antibiotics. The bacterial meningitis score was developed for assessing infants and children with meningitis, and outpatient management might be considered for children who had pleocytosis (7 cells/μL or more) and none of the following five criteria on presentation (history of a seizure with the illness, blood neutrophil count of at least 10×10^3 cells/μL, positive CSF Gram stain, CSF protein of at least 80 mg/dL, or CSF neutrophil count of at least 1×10^3 cells/μL). This proposed diagnostic tool achieved 95% sensitivity but failed to identify five patients with bacterial meningitis.[107,278] This tool, called the Meningitest, was refined with incorporation of a serum procalcitonin level of 0.5 ng/mL or greater and was claimed to have the sensitivity of 100% and specificity of 37%.[108] The usefulness of both the bacterial meningitis score and the Meningitest for differentiating between bacterial and aseptic meningitis remains to be determined.

Additional laboratory data are helpful and should be obtained. Blood cultures should be obtained in every patient suspected to have bacterial meningitis. In one prospective study in which blood was obtained for culture from every patient, the cultures were positive in 80% of children with *H. influenzae* meningitis, in 52% of children with pneumococcal meningitis, and in 33% of children with meningococcal meningitis.[118] Forty-four percent of the entire group had received some form of antibiotic therapy before admission to the hospital and before these blood cultures were performed. If these individuals were excluded, positive blood cultures were obtained from 90%, 80%, and 91% of children with meningitis caused by *H. influenzae, S. pneumoniae,* and *N. meningitidis,* respectively.

A thorough search for foci of infection adjacent to or remote from the meninges should be conducted. Repetitive neurologic evaluation including neuroimaging (see later discussion) also should be performed, and appropriate laboratory studies should be undertaken to define the extent of neurologic dysfunction.

When the concentration of bacteria within the blood is high, a Gram-stained smear of a buffy coat obtained from the blood may reveal the presence of microorganisms. If petechial lesions are present, a smear of the lesions after puncture with a small lancet may reveal microorganisms on Gram stain. A chest radiograph may be helpful in disclosing a focus of infection.

Radioisotope scanning may be helpful in selected patients, such as patients with a leak of CSF. The pattern of distribution of radioactivity recorded by a gamma camera coincides with the accumulation of purulent material. Increased concentration of isotope may relate to the inflammatory response within the meninges or in the periventricular region or to alteration in the BBB.[162] Localized concentrations of radionuclide may be seen in children with meningitis, most likely as a result of cerebral vasculitis or infarction.[106] Confirmation of impaired cerebral circulation, including occlusion and narrowing of arteries, sluggish circulation, and retrograde flow, has been described.[145] In these studies, resolution of the arterial lesions was shown in subsequent angiograms in patients, despite the persistence of neurologic deficits; these findings prompted the authors to suspect vascular spasm at the earlier stage of disease. Hydrocephalus contributed to sluggish circulation through intracerebral vessels in patients. At least transient disturbance in the circulation of CSF was noted in 45% of patients with meningitis, but persistent hydrocephalus is a rare complication of purulent meningitis.[373]

CT and magnetic resonance imaging (MRI) are noninvasive techniques that permit the prospective and repetitive assessment of children with meningitis. These techniques permit detection of ventricular dilation, subdural effusion, decrease in brain mass, and presence of vascular lesions or of brain infarcts (see Fig. 31.6). With these procedures, ventricular dilation may be noted acutely in many children who never develop hydrocephalus after recovery from their disease.

CT is widely available and useful for rapid assessment of hydrocephalus, mass lesions, hemorrhage, or acute brain edema prior to lumbar puncture. In contrast, MRI is required to detect more subtle findings. MRI is more sensitive for assessing CSF involvement, leptomeningitis, empyema, ventriculitis, and infarctions but is not as widely available and can be logistically challenging to obtain in the acutely ill patient. Noncontrast CT and MRI can be normal in early cases of bacterial meningitis. Administration of a contrast agent may be helpful to detect meningeal enhancement, with MRI being more sensitive than CT. Meningeal enhancement, however, is not specific to the diagnosis of bacterial meningitis and can be seen with other diagnoses, such as leptomeningeal carcinomatosis. Fluid-attenuated inversion recovery (FLAIR)-weighted MRI can demonstrate high signal in the subarachnoid space, reflecting high protein content in the CSF, but high signal in the subarachnoid space can also be seen with leptomeningeal carcinomatosis and subarachnoid hemorrhage. The findings of rhombencephalitis suggest *L. monocytogenes* as the likely causative organism.

The most important role of neuroimaging is to identify potential complications of bacterial meningitis, such as cerebritis, infarction, hydrocephalus, ventriculitis, brain empyema, abscess, and venous sinus thrombosis. Neuroimaging (MRI with gadolinium contrast) may be indicated in the following situations: (1) focal neurologic signs, (2) persistently positive CSF cultures despite administration of appropriate antibiotic therapy, (3) persistent elevation of CSF polymorphonuclear leukocytes (>30–40%) after more than 10 days of therapy, and (4) recurrent meningitis.

TREATMENT

Antimicrobial Therapy

Prompt treatment of bacterial meningitis with an appropriate antibiotic is essential. Several retrospective and prospective studies showed that delay in antibiotic treatment was associated with adverse outcomes.[22,205,255] In patients with suspected bacterial meningitis for whom immediate lumbar puncture is delayed due to pending brain imaging study or the presence of disseminated intravascular coagulation or transfer to another facility, blood cultures must be obtained, and antimicrobial treatment should be initiated immediately.

Antibiotic selection should include consideration of such factors as the likely pathogens, the CSF penetration of the antibiotic, the activity of the drug in purulent CSF, the mode of administration of the drug, and the intrinsic pharmacodynamic relationships of CSF drug concentrations to bactericidal activity.[205,343,361] The initial selection always should be made before definitive cultures are available, and empiric antimicrobial regimens should cover likely pathogens based on age of the patient and specific risk factors (Table 31.10) with modification if the CSF Gram stain is positive, as well as based on incidence and susceptibility patterns in the local community.[205]

For many previous years, ampicillin and chloramphenicol were preferred as the initial empiric therapy for children older than 3 months of age and thought to have bacterial meningitis. Ampicillin and chloramphenicol continue to be effective as initial treatment of bacterial meningitis when organisms are susceptible to these agents, but they are used very infrequently, and their use is not currently recommended. Ampicillin may be given intravenously in a dose of 300 mg/kg per 24 hours in six divided doses. An initial bolus of 100 mg/kg is given. Chloramphenicol is administered intravenously in a dose of 100 mg/kg per 24 hours in four divided doses. No loading dose of chloramphenicol is required.

TABLE 31.10 Likely Pathogens for Meningitis Based on Age, Immunization Status, and Risk Factors

Age, Immunization Status, Risk Factors	Likely Pathogens
<1 mo	Group B streptococci, *E. coli, L. monocytogenes* (neonatal pathogens)
1–3 mo; no immunization or one dose of primary immunization	Neonatal pathogens, *S. pneumoniae, N. meningitidis, H. influenzae*
3–6 mo	
No immunization	*S. pneumoniae, N. meningitidis, H. influenzae*
At least two doses of Hib-OMP vaccine	*S. pneumoniae, N. meningitidis*
>7 mo to 5 yr	
No immunization	*S. pneumoniae, N. meningitidis, H. influenzae*
Primary immunization completed	*S. pneumoniae* (non-PCV serotypes), *N. meningitidis*
6–21 yr	*S. pneumoniae, N. meningitidis*
CSF leak, cochlear implant, nephrotic syndrome	*S. pneumoniae*
Complement deficiencies	*S. pneumoniae, N. meningitidis*
Asplenia, sickle-cell disease	*S. pneumoniae, N. meningitidis, H. influenzae*

The development of third-generation cephalosporins and other antibiotics that have excellent bactericidal activity against *H. influenzae* type b, *N. meningitidis,* and *S. pneumoniae* within the CSF as well as the emergence of penicillin-resistant pneumococcal isolates led to the current approaches to initial therapy of childhood meningitis. Cefotaxime and ceftriaxone are included in the empiric treatment regimen of choice in most centers.[209]

Cefotaxime is a third-generation cephalosporin that has a broad spectrum of activity against gram-positive and gram-negative organisms. It possesses a high level of resistance to hydrolysis by β-lactamase. Cefotaxime penetrates the BBB and provides bactericidal activity in the CSF equivalent to or greater than that of antibiotics that have been used conventionally for treatment of bacterial meningitis in children.[265] It is an excellent choice for inclusion in empiric therapy in children 1 month or older but must be used with ampicillin for initial therapy in children younger than 1 month because *L. monocytogenes* and enterococci are sensitive to ampicillin and cannot be treated with cefotaxime. Cefotaxime is given as a dose of 225 to 300 mg/kg per day in three or four divided doses intravenously. The high dosage is preferred by some experts because the higher CSF concentrations achieved by high-dose therapy may be beneficial for patients whose disease may be caused by *S. pneumoniae* when the organisms are of intermediate susceptibility to third-generation cephalosporins.[84]

Ceftriaxone is another third-generation cephalosporin that possesses broad antimicrobial activity against the organisms that cause bacterial meningitis. Ceftriaxone readily penetrates the CSF of patients with inflamed meninges. In patients who receive adjunctive therapy with dexamethasone, meningeal inflammation may be reduced, possibly decreasing the penetration of antibiotics into the CSF. Concentration of ceftriaxone in the CSF of children with bacterial meningitis treated with dexamethasone, however, was similar to that found in children not treated with corticosteroids.[146] The half-life of ceftriaxone in serum is approximately 4 hours; a twice-daily dose regimen provides serum and CSF concentrations far in excess of the minimal bactericidal concentrations (MBCs) of most organisms that cause bacterial meningitis. Several prospective randomized studies demonstrated that ceftriaxone is comparable to ampicillin plus chloramphenicol for the treatment of bacterial meningitis in children.[18,32,58,85,99]

Ceftriaxone therapy has been associated with an increased incidence of diarrhea, which is mild and self-limited. An increased incidence of "gallbladder sludge," or precipitation of ceftriaxone salts in the gallbladder, diagnosed by ultrasound, also occurs and generally is asymptomatic but occasionally is associated with clinical symptoms of cholecystitis.[18,325] Ceftriaxone also has a high protein-binding capacity and can displace bilirubin from albumin in vitro[172] and needs to be used cautiously in neonates.

When ceftriaxone is used for the treatment of bacterial meningitis, it can be administered in a dose of 100 mg/kg per 24 hours in two divided doses or one daily dose intravenously. Although a once-daily dose has proved to be effective,[48,140,170] is convenient, and lends itself particularly to home therapy for selected patients (after an initial period of hospitalization), single daily dosing is not advocated; dosing errors, delayed doses, or missed doses undoubtedly occur,[84] and inadequate treatment could result. Although ceftriaxone can be given intramuscularly, a single dose by this route may be impractical.[48] The solution used for intramuscular administration should contain no more than 250 mg/mL. A 15-kg child receiving a daily dose of 80 mg/kg would require 4.8 mL of fluid, a volume too large for injection in a single site in an infant.

Strains of *S. pneumoniae* that are relatively or completely resistant to penicillins and third-generation cephalosporins have been identified.[54] The Clinical and Laboratory Standards Institute established the current guidelines for interpreting the minimal inhibitory concentrations (MICs) for cefotaxime or ceftriaxone for pneumococci isolated from patients with bacterial meningitis. The guidelines indicate that strains with an MIC of 2 μg/mL or greater are considered resistant, strains with an MIC of 1 μg/mL are intermediate, and strains with an MIC of 0.5 μg/mL or less are considered fully susceptible.[274] A retrospective analysis of five children who had pneumococcal meningitis caused by strains that were penicillin resistant and that had MICs to cefotaxime or ceftriaxone of 0.5 to 2 μg/mL was compared to those infected with strains that were penicillin resistant but susceptible to cefotaxime or ceftriaxone (MIC ≤0.25 μg/mL); there was no difference in clinical outcome at the time of discharge.[363]

Vancomycin in a dose of 60 to 80 mg/kg per day (20 mg/kg every 6 hours for children older than 1 month; every-8-hour dosing is preferred for older adolescents, not to exceed 4 g/day) is recommended in addition to cefotaxime for empiric therapy of children with meningitis because of the frequency with which penicillin-resistant and cephalosporin-resistant pneumococci have been isolated in recent years worldwide. Vancomycin has been used successfully to treat penicillin-resistant pneumococcal meningitis[49] and experimental models of cephalosporin-resistant pneumococcal meningitis.[143] In eight reports of treatment failures with third-generation cephalosporins, a variety of treatment regimens were used, all successfully. Vancomycin, alone or in combination with rifampin, chloramphenicol, or both, was used most frequently. The recommendation for empiric therapy for bacterial meningitis advocated by the AAP Committee on Infectious Diseases is to include vancomycin in addition to a third-generation cephalosporin in patients aged 1 month or older.[10] If nonsusceptibility to penicillin (MIC >0.1 μg/mL) and cephalosporins (MIC >0.5 μg/mL) is documented, treatment is continued with vancomycin plus cefotaxime or ceftriaxone (a synergistic effect is achieved when they are used together) with or without rifampin to complete an appropriate course. For pneumococcal meningitis, a serum trough concentration greater than 15 to 20 μg/mL is generally recommended; monitoring of vancomycin peak concentrations is not recommended.

Antibiotic tolerance is the ability of an organism to be susceptible to inhibition of growth (MIC values show susceptibility), but resistant to the killing activity of antibiotics, which differs from conventional resistance in which resistance is shown by bacterial growth in the presence of antibiotics, resulting in high MIC.[205] Clinical isolates of *S. pneumoniae* that are tolerant to vancomycin have been reported in the United States.[279] Meningitis caused by a vancomycin-tolerant organism in a patient was treated successfully with cefotaxime (300 mg/kg per day in four divided doses) plus vancomycin (80 mg/kg per day in four divided doses) and rifampin (20 mg/kg per day in two divided doses). Chloramphenicol also may be a suitable alternative for the treatment of these organisms if the pneumococcus proves to be susceptible to this antibiotic. Chloramphenicol therapy, however, was shown to have a significantly greater unsatisfactory outcome for children with meningitis caused by penicillin-resistant pneumococci compared with those with penicillin-susceptible pneumococci, although pneumococcal isolates were susceptible to chloramphenicol with MICs of 4 μg/mL or less.[142]

Two carbapenem agents, imipenem and meropenem, have been studied in patients with bacterial meningitis. These carbapenems are active against the bacteria that cause meningitis, but the use of imipenem-cilastatin has been associated with drug-induced seizures.[400]

The safety and efficacy of meropenem were compared with those of cefotaxime in a prospective randomized trial of 190 children with bacterial meningitis.[212] Seizures occurred within 24 hours before administration of antibiotic therapy in 16% of patients randomly assigned to receive meropenem and in 7% of patients randomly assigned to receive cefotaxime. Seizures occurred in patients after administration of therapy in 6% of children receiving meropenem and in 1% of children receiving cefotaxime. None of these seizures could be attributed to drug therapy. All patients responded to therapy with clinical improvement, and bacterial eradication was proved by repeated lumbar puncture in 100% of patients in both groups. No significant difference in short-term outcomes occurred between the two groups. Similarly, the efficacy and safety of meropenem with cefotaxime were compared for the treatment of bacterial meningitis in 258 children who were randomly assigned to the meropenem or cefotaxime group.[282] Clinical cure with or without sequelae was achieved in 97% and 96% of the meropenem-treated and cefotaxime-treated patients, respectively. At 7 weeks after treatment was concluded, 54% of patients treated with meropenem and 58% of patients treated with cefotaxime had no sequelae. Seizures were noted in 12% of the patients treated with meropenem and in 17% of patients treated with cefotaxime; none of the seizures was considered to be drug related. These data suggest that meropenem is effective in the treatment of bacterial meningitis in children. Few children with pneumococcal meningitis in either study had isolates that were nonsusceptible to cefotaxime. No conclusions can be drawn regarding the usefulness of meropenem in treating pneumococcal meningitis caused by isolates with a cefotaxime or ceftriaxone MIC equal to or greater than 2 μg/mL. However, of 20 cefotaxime-resistant *S. pneumoniae* isolates, four were intermediate and 13 were resistant to meropenem, suggesting that meropenem may not be a reliable alternative agent for pneumococcal isolates that are highly resistant to penicillin and cephalosporins. Meropenem may be indicated for patients who have meningitis that is caused by organisms resistant to extended-spectrum cephalosporins (e.g., nosocomial meningitis due to extended-spectrum β-lactamases producing gram-negative bacteria), but its efficacy has not been demonstrated.

Cefepime is a fourth-generation cephalosporin that has been studied for the treatment of bacterial meningitis. In vitro, cefepime offers no advantage over cefotaxime or ceftriaxone for penicillin-resistant *S. pneumoniae*.[201] In addition, no in vitro data exist for the efficacy of cefepime against cefotaxime-resistant pneumococci. In two clinical trials, the efficacy of cefepime was found to be equivalent to the efficacy of either cefotaxime or ceftriaxone.[317,318] No penicillin-resistant or ceftriaxone-resistant pneumococci were encountered in either study, however. Cefepime has been used for the treatment of bacterial meningitis as an alternative agent.

Ceftazidime has been efficacious in the treatment of meningitis caused by *P. aeruginosa*.[182,257,308] Cefpirome concentrations in CSF of patients with bacterial meningitis were found to be significantly higher than the minimal bactericidal concentrations for *N. meningitidis, H. influenzae*, and *S. pneumoniae*,[398] but studies documenting its effectiveness in large numbers of children have not been done.

Cefoperazone and cefoxitin within CSF may fail to reach concentrations required to kill all susceptible strains of *H. influenzae* and *S. pneumoniae* and cannot be recommended for the treatment of bacterial meningitis in children.[61,128]

Cefuroxime is a second-generation cephalosporin that has been shown to be effective in vitro against *H. influenzae* type b, *S. pneumoniae*, and *N. meningitidis*. Studies showed delayed sterilization of the CSF, relapse during or after treatment was higher, and more frequent sensorineural hearing loss occurred than with use of ampicillin, chloramphenicol, cefotaxime, and ceftriaxone.[16,225,227,324] Cefuroxime should not be used to treat bacterial meningitis in children.

Aztreonam is an antimicrobial agent that belongs to the monobactam family of antibiotics. It is effective against most gram-negative organisms, including *P. aeruginosa*. Limited data suggest its efficacy in the treatment of *Pseudomonas* and *H. influenzae* meningitis, suggesting a potential role for this agent in the treatment of patients who are allergic to penicillin and who are infected with these or other gram-negative organisms.[202,226,369]

If a history of significant allergy to penicillin or cephalosporin (anaphylaxis, urticaria, exfoliative dermatitis) is documented, vancomycin plus rifampin or aztreonam may be used. A cross-reactivity of 10% to 15% has been noted for cephalosporins in penicillin-allergic patients.

When meningitis is caused by *Streptococcus pyogenes*, penicillin or ampicillin provides effective therapy. If meningitis is caused by a penicillin-resistant strain of *S. aureus*, oxacillin or nafcillin 200 mg/kg per 24 hours intravenously in four or six divided doses should be used. Vancomycin is effective against *S. aureus* strains resistant to penicillin and to semisynthetic penicillin derivatives[173] or *S. aureus* meningitis in patients who are penicillin allergic. Vancomycin also may be useful in treatment of meningitis caused by *Flavobacterium meningosepticum*.[104] Metronidazole is effective in treatment of anaerobic infection of the CNS when response to conventional therapy has been suboptimal. A dose of 30 mg/kg per 24 hours in four divided doses results in CSF concentrations of greater than 10 μg/mL.[37]

In animal models, the addition of a nonbacteriolytic antibiotic such as rifampin[155] has been associated with a neuroprotective effect, suggesting the possibility of its use as an adjunct therapy. The addition of clindamycin to standard antibiotic therapy[47] showed decreased bacterial cell wall release, a lessened proinflammatory response (including decreased leukocyte recruitment), less free radical formation, and decreased apoptosis and cellular damage in experimental pneumococcal meningitis.

Table 31.11 provides current recommendations for antibiotic treatment of meningitis caused by various microorganisms. An appropriate antibiotic should be continued until the patient is afebrile for 5 days but for at least 7 to 10 days in every patient. Although some data support a shorter course of therapy, at least 10 days of treatment is recommended for pneumococcal and *H. influenzae* type b meningitis and 7 days for *N. meningitidis* meningitis.[190,237,361] If clinical improvement is noted within 24 hours, a repeated lumbar puncture is unnecessary, in most cases, during the course of treatment or after treatment has been completed. If infection is caused by *S. pneumoniae* that is resistant to penicillin and to third-generation cephalosporins or by antibiotic-resistant bacteria, a repeated lumbar puncture is recommended at 48 to 72 hours to document bacterial sterilization of the CSF. If clinical improvement is slower than anticipated or is not noted, a repeated examination of the CSF is indicated at any time.

In the 1970s, lumbar puncture frequently was performed at the conclusion of therapy. Data from studies performed at that time (Table 31.12) reveal that WBC counts and protein concentrations within the CSF generally had not returned completely to normal and that the CSF-to-blood glucose ratios may have remained depressed. In every case, Gram stain of the CSF should reveal no organisms, and cultures should be sterile. If a lumbar puncture is performed at the conclusion of therapy, retreatment is mandatory if organisms are seen or grown. It also may be considered if more than 30% of the cells are polymorphonuclear leukocytes, or if the CSF glucose concentration is less than 20 m/dL and the CSF-to-blood ratio is less than 20% (see Table 31.12).

Bacteriologic relapse after treatment of meningitis (particularly that caused by *H. influenzae* and treated with ampicillin) was highlighted in numerous reports.[26,79,82,176,177] Precise assessment of the frequency of relapse in children who have received an appropriate antibiotic to which the organism is susceptible or an appropriate dose intravenously and for an extended period has been difficult. The relapse rate is currently less than 1%.

Some physicians have discharged children with meningitis from the hospital before the conclusion of a course of therapy and prescribed home management. Benefits of home therapy include a decreased risk for acquiring nosocomial infection, a return of the child to his or her normal environment sooner, and a decrease in the total cost of therapy.[297]

Fifty-four children with bacterial meningitis were treated as outpatients for 1 to 8 days (mean 4.6 days) with intramuscular ceftriaxone given once daily.[48] Each dose was given in conjunction with a physician's examination. Each child had to be afebrile for 24 to 48 hours before initiation of home therapy, free of neurologic dysfunction except for auditory or vestibular dysfunction, and without evidence of inappropriate secretion of ADH before being considered for outpatient therapy. No child required readmission or developed neurologic sequelae or relapse. A retrospective review of 26 patients with meningitis or other serious bacterial infections who received some portion of their therapy as an outpatient with ceftriaxone revealed that none of the patients experienced relapse or recurrence.[297]

Criteria for considering outpatient therapy for children with bacterial meningitis have been suggested,[387] which include (1) the child has received inpatient therapy for at least 6 days, (2) the child is afebrile for at least 24 to 48 hours before initiation of outpatient therapy, (3) the child has no significant neurologic dysfunction or focal findings, (4) the child has no seizure activity, (5) the child is clinically stable, (6) the child is taking all fluids by mouth, (7) the first dose of outpatient antibiotic is received in the hospital, (8) the antibiotic is administered in the office or emergency department setting or by qualified home health nursing, (9) daily examination is performed by a physician, and (10) parents are reliable and have transportation and a telephone. The dose of ceftriaxone of 100 mg/kg per 24 hours intramuscularly may need to be aliquoted to account for the volume of diluents needed to achieve a concentration of no greater than 250 mg/mL.

H. influenzae type b organisms have been recovered from the throats of patients after completion of a course of treatment for *H. influenzae* type b meningitis. When members of a household to which the patient

TABLE 31.11 **Recommendations for Antibiotic Therapy for Bacterial Meningitis**

Organism	Antibiotic(s)	Recommended Dosages (IV)
Bacteroides fragilis	Metronidazole	30 mg/kg/day in 4 dd
	Chloramphenicol	100 mg/kg/day in 4 dd
Bacteroides other than *B. fragilis*	Penicillin G	300,000 U/kg/day in 6 dd
Clostridium	Penicillin G	300,000 U/kg/day in 6 dd
Corynebacterium	Penicillin G	300,000 U/kg/day in 6 dd
	Erythromycin	50 mg/kg/day in 4 dd
Enterobacter, Klebsiella, Escherichia coli[a]	Cefotaxime	200 mg/kg/day in 4 dd
	Ceftriaxone	100 mg/kg/day in 2 dd
	Meropenem	120 mg/kg/day in 3 dd
	Ampicillin	300 mg/kg/day in 6 dd
	Gentamicin	7.5 mg/kg/day in 3 dd
	Amikacin	15 mg/kg/day in 3 dd
Haemophilus influenzae	Cefotaxime	200 mg/kg/day in 4 dd
	Ceftriaxone	100 mg/kg/day in 1 or 2 dd
	Chloramphenicol	100 mg/kg/day in 4 dd
	Ampicillin	300 mg/kg/day in 6 dd
Listeria monocytogenes	Ampicillin	300 mg/kg/day in 6 dd
	Gentamicin	7.5 mg/kg/day in 3 dd
	TMP-SMX	20 mg/kg/day in 4 dd (TMP component)
Neisseria meningitidis	Penicillin G	300,000 U/kg/day in 6 dd
	Cefotaxime	200 mg/kg/day in 4 dd
	Ceftriaxone	100 mg/kg/day in 1 or 2 dd
Proteus mirabilis (indole negative)	Ampicillin	300 mg/kg/day in 6 dd
P. mirabilis (indole positive)	Cefotaxime	200 mg/kg/day in 4 dd
	Gentamicin	7.5 mg/kg/day in 3 dd
	Amikacin	22.5 mg/kg/day in 3 dd
Pseudomonas	Ceftazidime	150–200 mg/kg/day in 3 dd
	Meropenem	120 mg/kg/day in 3 dd
	Piperacillin	300 mg/kg/day in 4 or 6 dd
	Gentamicin	7.5 mg/kg/day in 3 dd
	Amikacin	15–20 mg/kg/day in 3 dd
Salmonella	Cefotaxime	200 mg/kg/day in 4 dd
	Ampicillin	300 mg/kg/day in 6 dd
	Gentamicin	7.5 mg/kg/day in 3 dd
	Chloramphenicol	100 mg/kg/day in 4 dd
Staphylococcus aureus (penicillinase negative)[b]	Penicillin G	300,000 U/kg/day in 6 dd
S. aureus (penicillinase-positive)[b]	Oxacillin or nafcillin	200 mg/kg/day in 4 or 6 dd
S. aureus (resistant to semisynthetic penicillins)	Vancomycin *plus*	80 mg/kg/day in 4 dd
	Rifampin	20 mg/kg/day in 2 dd
Staphylococcus (coagulase negative)	Vancomycin	80 mg/kg/day in 4 dd
	Rifampin	20 mg/kg/day in 2 dd
Streptococcus pneumoniae[b]	Cefotaxime/ceftriaxone	225–300 mg/kg/day in 3 or 4 dd/100 mg/kg/day in 1 or 2 dd
	Vancomycin	60–80 mg/kg/day in 4 dd
	Rifampin[c]	20 mg/kg/day in 2 dd
	Penicillin G	300,000 U/kg/day in 6 dd
	Chloramphenicol	100 mg/kg/day in 4 dd
Unknown (<1 mo)	Ampicillin *plus*	300 mg/kg/day in 6 dd
	Cefotaxime *or*	200 mg/kg/day in 4 dd
	Gentamicin	7.5 mg/kg/day in 3 dd
Unknown (>1 mo)	Cefotaxime *or*	225–300 mg/kg/day in 4 dd
	Ceftriaxone *plus*	100 mg/kg/day in 1 or 2 dd
	Vancomycin	60–80 mg/kg/day in 4 dd
	Nafcillin or oxacillin (if question of staphylococcal infection)	200 mg/kg/day in 6 dd

dd, Divided doses.

[a]Trimethoprim-sulfamethoxazole (TMP-SMX) in a dose of 20 mg/kg per day (TMP) and 100 mg/kg per day (SMX) IV in 4 dd has been used successfully in selected patients with gram-negative enteric meningitis.

[b]Vancomycin may be provided in a dose of 80 mg/kg per day in 4 dd IV (20 mg/kg every 8 h, or 60 mg/kg per day in 3 dd in older adolescents) if patients are allergic to penicillin or penicillin derivatives or, in the case of *S. pneumoniae*, for multidrug-resistant pneumococci or pneumococci that are highly resistant to penicillin. In these cases, addition of rifampin may be considered.

[c]Should never be used alone.

TABLE 31.12 **Cerebrospinal Fluid Findings at Conclusion of Antibiotic Treatment**

	TOTAL WHITE BLOOD CELL COUNT		POLYMORPHONUCLEAR LEUKOCYTES (%)		CSF-TO-BLOOD PROTEIN RATIO (MG/DL)		GLUCOSE (MG/DL)		CSF-TO-BLOOD GLUCOSE RATIO (%)	
	Mean ± SD	**Range**	**Mean ± SD**	**Range**	**Mean ± SD**	**Range**	**Mean ± SD**	**Range**	**Mean ± SD**	**Range**
Total group	41 ± 80	0–850	5.5 ± 12	0–90	46 ± 72	7–970	47 ± 12.7	21–91	55.7 ± 17	23–156
H. influenzae	53 ± 98	0–850	5.5 ± 11	0–90	43 ± 37	10–334	47 ± 13	31–100	55 ± 17	31–100
H. influenzae (ampicillin)	56 ± 107	0–850	5.9 ± 12	0–90	44 ± 43	13–334	46 ± 14	21–91	53 ± 17	33–89
H. influenzae (chloramphenicol)	49 ± 83	0–325	5.1 ± 10.7	0–50	41 ± 26	7–127	48 ± 11	27–90	57 ± 13	30–100
S. pneumoniae	29 ± 30	0–110	5.5 ± 11.5	0–45	42 ± 39	7–211	48 ± 9	22–68	57 ± 13	22–91
N. meningitidis	16 ± 27	0–132	3.4 ± 7.9	0–27	39 ± 46	7–188	47 ± 11	29–77	47 ± 19	23–100
Others	11 ± 18	0–77	7.3 ± 19	0–75	70 ± 197	10–970	48 ± 18	37–73	70 ± 28	44–156

CSF, Cerebrospinal fluid; *SD*, standard deviation.

will return include children 4 years of age or younger, the patient should be given rifampin 20 mg/kg once daily for 4 days to prevent the occurrence of secondary cases. Children with meningococcal meningitis also should receive chemoprophylaxis to eradicate nasopharyngeal carriage before discharge unless they were treated with cefotaxime or ceftriaxone (see "Prevention").

Adjunctive Therapy

As described earlier, the pathogenesis and subsequent sequelae of bacterial meningitis are as much a consequence of the host response to infection as of the bacterial organisms themselves. Antiinflammatory agents used as adjuncts to antimicrobial therapy may decrease the degree of tissue injury during the course of the disease.

Antiinflammatory Therapy

Research studies seek additional therapies that could be used to help reduce further mortality, morbidity, or both. Five main areas serve as the targets for therapeutic development: (1) modulation of bacterial killing and the release of bacterial products by using nonbacteriolytic antibiotics such as rifampin, (2) host recognition of bacteria or its products and the initiation of the inflammatory response, (3) modulation of the inflammatory response with adjuvant dexamethasone, (4) inhibition or interruption of the host inflammatory/neurotoxic mediators, and (5) modulation of the apoptotic pathways.[153,167,203,215,361] Inhibitors of inflammatory mediators and mediator effector molecules such as TNF-α, matrix metalloproteinases, and nitric oxide and antioxidants, neuroprotective factors (melatonin and brain-derived neurotrophic factor), and other antiinflammatory therapies (triptans) are being studied in experimental animal models of bacterial meningitis.[154,203,215] Although their use is attractive theoretically because of the damage produced by the inflammatory cascade (see Fig. 31.4), none has emerged as a realistic potential candidate for general clinical use at present.

Corticosteroids

Corticosteroids have been suggested as an adjunct to therapy for bacterial meningitis because they may (1) decrease intracranial pressure by decreasing meningeal inflammation and brain water content; (2) modulate the production of cytokines, which lessens the meningeal inflammatory response; and (3) decrease the incidence of sensorineural hearing loss or other neurologic complications of meningitis.[224,281]

Corticosteroids may play a role in acute management of increased intracranial pressure and cerebral herniation, although no data specifically indicate that corticosteroids decrease cerebral edema caused by bacterial meningitis. Dexamethasone therapy in children with bacterial meningitis was shown to decrease opening lumbar CSF pressure 12 hours after administration of the first dose, but this effect was lost by 24 hours of treatment.[279] The significance of these findings is unclear because the corticosteroids were not given as specific therapy for increased intracranial pressure, and most of the subjects were not showing signs of impending herniation.

In experimental *H. influenzae* type b meningitis, administration of dexamethasone 1 hour before, but not 1 hour after, administration of ceftriaxone was associated with significantly reduced TNF-α concentration and indices of inflammation in the CSF.[270]

Administration of dexamethasone has been associated with decreased concentration in CSF of prostaglandin E_2 and decreased leakage of some proteins from serum into CSF in rabbits with experimental pneumococcal meningitis.[191] Among patients with bacterial meningitis, steroid-treated patients had significantly lower concentrations of IL-1β, TNF-α, PAF, and prostaglandin E_2 in their CSF than those of patients who received antibiotics alone.[271,281] Patients tend to become afebrile sooner when they receive dexamethasone, but they have an increased incidence of secondary fevers.[17,385]

Although the understanding of the pathophysiologic events associated with initiation of the acute inflammatory response has been enhanced by more recent data, the ability of dexamethasone to reduce long-term complications of bacterial meningitis in pediatric patients remains controversial. A prospective, randomized, double-blinded, placebo-controlled study evaluating adults in Europe with bacterial meningitis[96] showed a decrease in mortality rates in all patients and in unfavorable outcomes in patients with pneumococcal meningitis.[394] By contrast, no pediatric studies of the use of dexamethasone for treatment of bacterial meningitis have shown an overall change in mortality rates.

In randomized, placebo-controlled trials of dexamethasone as adjunctive therapy in bacterial meningitis[224,281,323,385] and in retrospective studies[164,200] published since 1988, 68% (227 of 333) of corticosteroid recipients in the six randomized trials had meningitis caused by *H. influenzae* type b; the remaining 32% had meningitis caused by *S. pneumoniae* (50 of 333) or *N. meningitidis* (56 of 333).[299] A meta-analysis of nine controlled trials published before 1991 failed to document a reduced risk for neurologic abnormality at hospital discharge or follow-up examination.[183] A more recent meta-analysis of randomized clinical trials of dexamethasone as adjunctive therapy for bacterial meningitis suggests a beneficial effect of this agent for *H. influenzae* meningitis and a possible beneficial effect in preventing severe hearing loss in *S. pneumoniae* meningitis but only if it is given early.[250]

Most patients with *S. pneumoniae* meningitis in the studies that were reviewed were not treated with vancomycin. This issue is important because the penetrance of vancomycin across the BBB is not optimal, and selected studies show that it is reduced further when dexamethasone is used concomitantly.[17,50,258] Despite the theoretical clinical concerns, CSF concentrations of vancomycin and ceftriaxone are adequate for treatment of penicillin-susceptible and penicillin-nonsusceptible *S. pneumoniae* when dexamethasone is given at recommended dosages.[116,213]

Administration of dexamethasone immediately before the initiation of cefotaxime therapy was associated with a reduced incidence of neurologic sequelae (14% compared with 38% in patients receiving cefotaxime alone).[281] These investigators found no significant difference in auditory sequelae compared with control subjects. The frequency of neurologic sequelae in placebo-treated patients, however, was significantly higher than that noted in other studies.[17,323,385]

In contrast, other studies failed to show a significant reduction in the incidence of neurologic sequelae in comparisons of corticosteroid-treated and placebo-treated patients.[224,323] A prospective, multicenter, placebo-controlled study evaluated 143 children with bacterial meningitis caused by *H. influenzae* type b (58%), *S. pneumoniae* (23%), and *N. meningitidis* (17%).[385] Patients were treated with ceftriaxone and placebo or ceftriaxone and dexamethasone administered within 4 hours of the first dose of antibiotics. No significant difference in neurologic or developmental outcome was found between patients who received dexamethasone or placebo.

Sensorineural hearing loss is a significant sequela of bacterial meningitis. In the two randomized studies,[224] patients treated with dexamethasone were significantly less likely to have moderate or severe bilateral sensorineural hearing loss; however, in one study, patients were treated with cefuroxime, which has been shown to result in delayed sterilization of CSF and a higher rate of hearing loss compared with ceftriaxone.[324] An additional 100 infants and children with bacterial meningitis were treated with ceftriaxone for 10 days and either dexamethasone or placebo for 4 days. A significant reduction in moderate to severe hearing loss in children with *H. influenzae* type b meningitis ($P < .001$) was reported. No significant differences in other neurologic sequelae were found between the two groups. In addition, two patients receiving dexamethasone developed gastrointestinal bleeding severe enough to require transfusion, and two others developed heme-positive stools.[224]

The Swiss Meningitis Group[323] found that treatment of children with dexamethasone 10 minutes before administration of ceftriaxone and then for 2 days subsequently resulted in persistent hearing loss in 5% (three) of children who had received dexamethasone and in 15% (eight) of children who received placebo, a difference that was not significant. One child treated with corticosteroid and five children treated with placebo had unilateral hearing loss only. The group also documented a transient mild to moderate hearing impairment in five children treated with dexamethasone and four children treated with placebo; in six of the nine children, the impairment was caused by a conductive disturbance. Dexamethasone did not alter the incidence or natural history of the transient hearing impairment.

In a multicenter study,[385] audiologic measurements were made early in the course of the disease (within 24 hours of admission) and 6 weeks to 12 months after recovery from disease. The authors found no significant difference in the incidence of persistent moderate or severe hearing loss between children who received dexamethasone within 4 hours of antibiotics and children who received placebo, with the exception of bilateral deafness in children with *H. influenzae* type b meningitis (5 of 72 in the placebo-treated group vs. 0 of 67 in the dexamethasone-treated group; $P = .02$). The overall incidence of moderate to severe hearing loss was 14.7% (10.3% unilateral and 4.4% bilateral) in the dexamethasone-treated group and 22.9% (13.5% unilateral and 9.4% bilateral; $P = .33$ for bilateral loss) in the placebo-treated group. These authors found that 22 children (8 in the dexamethasone-treated group and 14 in the placebo-treated group) had bilateral moderate or severe hearing loss at the initial evaluation. Only one child with *H. influenzae* meningitis and unilateral deafness at initial examination progressed to bilateral deafness. At follow-up, the resolution of hearing loss was nearly identical for each group, with 8 of the 22 children having normal hearing at follow-up, 5 having unilateral deafness, and 9 having bilateral deafness.

These results suggest that hearing loss can occur early in the course of meningitis and that early auditory brainstem response results need to be interpreted cautiously with regard to long-term audiologic sequelae. A strong relationship was noted between hearing loss early in the disease and a low concentration of CSF glucose at manifestation of meningitis, a finding that has been reported previously.[105]

Data from animal studies highlight a potential negative effect of dexamethasone therapy on neuronal injury, including hippocampal apoptosis in experimental animals with pneumococcal and *E. coli* meningitis who received dexamethasone.[231,355]

The AAP Committee on Infectious Diseases states that dexamethasone therapy should be considered for pneumococcal meningitis in infants and children 6 weeks old and older.[10] Dexamethasone also is recommended for treatment of infants and children with *H. influenzae* type b meningitis.[10] The reluctance on the part of some experts to recommend dexamethasone for pneumococcal meningitis is predicated on data that fail to show any diminution in morbidity or mortality rates from meningitis when meningitis is caused by *S. pneumoniae* and dexamethasone is used. Dexamethasone should be used cautiously when vancomycin is used to treat meningitis caused by *S. pneumoniae* that may be resistant to penicillin, third-generation cephalosporins, or both.[50] The CSF concentrations of vancomycin, ceftriaxone, cefotaxime, and rifampin when they are given in dosages recommended for meningitis in children treated with dexamethasone generally are shown to be adequate to treat meningitis caused by most nonsusceptible strains of *S. pneumoniae*. Dexamethasone plus vancomycin may decrease the transport of vancomycin into the CSF of experimental animals with pneumococcal meningitis, but this finding was not observed in nine children who were treated with vancomycin and dexamethasone (0.6 mg/kg per day).[213] Dexamethasone can lead to decreased fever and a misleading impression of clinical improvement, even though sterilization of the CSF has not been achieved.

Dexamethasone should not be used if aseptic or nonbacterial meningitis is suspected; if it is started before the diagnosis of nonbacterial meningitis is made, it should be discontinued immediately. It should not be used in "partially treated" meningitis. No data exist on which to base a recommendation for use of dexamethasone in the treatment of bacterial meningitis in infants younger than 6 weeks of age or in infants with congenital or acquired abnormalities of the CNS, with or without a prosthetic device. One prospective study in infants concluded that adjunctive dexamethasone therapy does not improve the outcome of neonatal bacterial meningitis.[90] If dexamethasone is used, it should be used in all patients, regardless of disease severity, and it should be administered as early as possible in the course of treatment in a dose of 0.15 mg/kg per dose intravenously every 6 hours for no more than 4 days. One study[323] found no difference in children treated for 2 days instead of 4 days with 0.4 mg/kg per dose every 12 hours.

Except for hearing loss after *H. influenzae* type b meningitis, no clear evidence establishes that dexamethasone significantly reduces the long-term sequelae of meningitis, and its use is not without risk for causing adverse events. The markedly decreased frequency of meningitis caused by *H. influenzae* type b and the increased frequency of meningitis caused by *S. pneumoniae* nonsusceptible to penicillin (for which therapy with vancomycin may be necessary) suggest that initiation of dexamethasone should be considered carefully and that the clinician caring for the patient should evaluate the risk-to-benefit ratio of such therapy.

Glycerol

A multicenter double-blind randomized study in six Latin American countries showed that adjunctive treatment with oral glycerol 1.5 g/kg every 6 hours for 48 hours prevents severe neurologic sequelae in childhood meningitis (odds ratio 0.31; 95% CI, 0.31 to 0.76) compared with placebo.[288] Glycerol is a hyperosmolar agent, and because of its safety, wide availability, low cost, and oral administration, its use as adjunctive treatment in children with bacterial meningitis, particularly in resource-limited settings, is attractive, but subsequent studies in experimental animals and children with bacterial meningitis did not reveal any benefits.[289]

Supportive Care

In addition to antibiotic therapy, management of bacterial meningitis includes measures that apply generally to critically ill children. Careful monitoring and attention to detail are essential. Pulse rate, blood pressure, and respiratory rate should be measured carefully every 15 minutes until stable and then every hour while the patient is in the intensive care unit. Temperature should be measured every 4 hours. A thorough neurologic examination should be done at the time of admission and at least daily thereafter. A rapid assessment of neurologic function should be done several times a day for the first several days of treatment. Body weight should be measured daily for at least the first 3 or 4 days. Head circumference should be measured in children younger than 18 months at the time of admission and repeated daily if concerns about increased intracranial pressure persist.

The following laboratory data are suggested if results of lumbar puncture indicate bacterial meningitis: (1) total peripheral WBC count and differential, (2) hemoglobin concentration, (3) hematocrit, (4) platelet count, and (5) serum electrolytes (serum and urine osmolalities may be useful in selected patients). Urine volume and specific gravity should be monitored. A low WBC count may suggest a poor prognosis. Anemia associated with *H. influenzae* type b septicemia has been reported[338,339] and has been attributed to immune hemolysis of RBCs that are coated with soluble bacterial antigens.

Every child with meningitis should be evaluated carefully to identify inappropriate secretion of ADH, recognize seizure activity, and detect the development of subdural effusions. Determinations of body weight, serum electrolytes (serum and urine osmolalities in selected patients), urine volume, and specific gravity should be made at the time of admission and observed closely (every 6 to 12 hours) for the first 24 to 36 hours that the child is in the hospital and daily for several days thereafter. Initially, the child should receive nothing by mouth because of the risk for vomiting and aspiration. In addition, delivery of all fluid intravenously ensures greater accuracy in measurement of intake and output during the critical early days of therapy. Inappropriate secretion of ADH has been documented in 88% of children enrolled in a prospective study of bacterial meningitis.[118] Elevated serum concentrations of ADH in the presence of hyponatremia have been documented by direct measurement of ADH concentration in serum obtained from the same children.[119]

An electrolyte solution containing approximately 40 mEq/L of sodium and chloride, 35 mEq/L of potassium, and 20 mEq/L of acetate or lactate should be administered at a rate of 1000 to 1200 mL/m^2 per 24 hours in a patient with lower serum sodium concentrations and without evidence of dehydration or shock. The best indicators of retention of fluid in excess of solute are body weight and serum sodium concentration. As serum sodium concentration approaches normal (135 to 140 mEq/L), fluid administration may be liberalized progressively to normal maintenance levels of 1500 to 1700 mL/m^2 per 24 hours. On the contrary, if serum sodium concentrations at admission are normal, then fluid restriction may not be needed and fluid administration is given at normal maintenance levels (see later discussion).

The syndrome of inappropriate secretion of ADH should not be diagnosed in the presence of dehydration. Decreased intravascular volume is a physiologic stimulus for the release of ADH, and its release is not inappropriate. Fluid restriction is not advocated for patients who are dehydrated; rehydration should be performed with careful and frequent assessment of fluid and electrolyte status.

The effect of fluid restriction on body water and outcome was examined in 50 consecutive children who had been hospitalized with acute meningitis.[342] These children were divided into two groups: patients with hyponatremia and patients without hyponatremia. Patients in both groups were randomly assigned to receive either normal maintenance or restricted fluids (65% to 70% of the volume of that received by the maintenance subgroup). Eleven to 15 patients were randomly assigned to any of the four subgroups in the study. No significant difference in overall outcome or intact survival was found when comparisons were made between fluid-restricted and non–fluid-restricted groups or within each group between the subgroups that received restricted fluids or maintenance fluids. After combination of the subgroups that received restricted fluids with the subgroups that received maintenance fluids, however, a trend toward higher intact survival and lower mortality rates was noted in the non–fluid-restricted groups. Nonetheless children who had an extracellular water reduction of 10 mL/kg or greater in 48 hours had a significantly lower intact survival rate (10 of 28; 36%) than that of children with less than 10 mL/kg or no reduction of extracellular water (15 of 22; 64%). The mortality rate also was higher in the former group (7 of 28; 25%) than in the latter group (2 of 22; 9%). The authors concluded that fluid restriction did not improve the outcome of acute meningitis and that a decrease in extracellular water volume at 48 hours may increase the likelihood of having an adverse outcome.

In contrast, in studies of large numbers of children with bacterial meningitis, evidence of inappropriate secretion of ADH correlated significantly ($P < .01$) with abnormal neurologic findings, even 3 months after discharge, and with low IQ scores.[123] As a result of these findings, coupled with documentation of inappropriate secretion of ADH, a recommendation was made to restrict fluids in patients who are hyponatremic at admission. Fluids are restricted only until evidence of inappropriate secretion of ADH can be excluded (usually within 2 hours). The average patient in subsequent studies[195] was fluid restricted for only 18 hours.

Because cerebral edema and increased intracranial pressure have been noted as major disturbances in seriously ill patients with meningitis and because many of the deaths and some of the sequelae have been related to the effects of cerebral edema and intracranial hypertension, it appears prudent to recommend fluid restriction in patients with hyponatremia who are not dehydrated and liberalization of fluids to normal maintenance levels when serum sodium concentration returns to normal.

Meningitis complicated by shock creates a complex fluid management problem. Shock associated with meningitis is secondary to sepsis and generally is treated with intravenous infusion of large quantities of fluid to maintain blood pressure and adequate tissue perfusion. Patients with meningitis without shock or dehydration benefit from initial fluid restriction to avoid worsening of cerebral edema and severe hyponatremia with subsequent seizures. Children with meningitis and shock should receive sufficient quantities of isotonic fluid to maintain a systolic blood pressure of 80 to 90 mm Hg, a urine output equal to or greater than 500 mL/m^2 per 24 hours, and adequate cerebral perfusion as indicated by mental status. Central venous pressure monitoring is useful to guide fluid resuscitation and to prevent fluid overload. The addition of albumin (1 g/kg) to intravenously administered fluids may decrease the total volume of fluid needed to maintain adequate perfusion. Vasopressors, such as dopamine, dobutamine, and isoproterenol, also may provide support of blood pressure and perfusion and reduce requirements for intravenously administered fluids.

When increased intracranial pressure is suggested by such signs as progressive lethargy, increased muscle tone, or bulging anterior fontanelle, elevating the head approximately 30 degrees may be helpful. Increased intracranial pressure associated with deterioration in mental status or signs of cerebral herniation may be treated more vigorously with mannitol administered intravenously at 0.5 g/kg infused during 30 minutes and repeated as necessary. If corticosteroids are used for this purpose, the recommended agent is dexamethasone in a dose of 10 to 12 mg/m^2 per day in four divided doses for no more than 4 or 5 days.[195] Other supportive measures to ensure appropriate delivery of oxygen and nutrients to the brain include a quiet environment, elective intubation, and the use of sedatives.[33]

Head circumference measurement and transillumination permit assessment of the development of subdural effusions or may suggest other causes for an enlarging head. CT may be helpful in detecting large subdural effusions or hydrocephalus. Because effusions can be considered part of the pathophysiologic changes that occur with bacterial meningitis, obtaining CT scans to evaluate effusions does not need to be part of the routine evaluation of a child with meningitis. Neuroimaging (CT or MRI with contrast) should be performed in children with focal neurologic signs. In children with hemiparesis or quadriparesis, CT or MRI may document cerebrovascular abnormalities. CT also should be performed in children with papilledema on an emergency basis before proceeding with the initial lumbar puncture. *Administration of antibiotics should not be delayed for diagnostic imaging in patients in whom bacterial meningitis is suspected, but blood culture should be obtained before administration of antibiotics.*

Subdural effusions should be treated with subdural paracentesis only when one suspects that the effusions are responsible for seizures or for prolonged fever as a result of subdural empyema. Paracentesis also may be useful if the effusion is responsible for symptoms of increased intracranial pressure or is the cause of focal neurologic signs.[118,123] In most cases, subdural taps are not required.

Seizures should be carefully monitored particularly in patients with high bacterial counts in CSF (many organisms on Gram stain) but insufficient inflammation (few polymorphonuclear leukocytes in CSF) and, when noted, are treated expeditiously. A patent airway must be maintained, and appropriate anticonvulsants must be administered. Sodium phenobarbital or phenytoin are commonly administered agents to control seizures related to acute bacterial meningitis. Phenytoin generally does not depress the respiratory center to the same extent as phenobarbital does, and it may benefit the patient by inhibiting the secretion of ADH. If the seizure activity no longer is apparent after the second hospital day and the patient has no focal neurologic signs at the time of discharge from the hospital, anticonvulsants may be discontinued. Phenytoin and phenobarbital can induce hepatic microsomal enzymes; their use may increase the metabolism rate of chloramphenicol and possibly cause a significant decrease in the serum concentration of this antibiotic if it has been used for treatment of meningitis.[298]

An electroencephalogram is indicated in patients with meningitis and seizures when focal seizures are noted, seizures persist more than 72 hours after presentation, seizures occur after the third day of hospitalization, or prolonged alteration in sensorium is present. An electroencephalogram may be valuable in distinguishing abnormal intermittent posturing from movements associated with seizure activity.

Persistent fever (>8 or 9 days' duration) has been noted.[26] In the multicenter pneumococcal study, the mean duration of fever was 4.4 ± 3.9 days.[17] Suppurative complications, including subdural or pleural empyema, septic arthritis, and pericarditis, should be sought carefully. The rare occurrence of brain abscess in association with bacterial meningitis also may lead to persistent fever. Nosocomial intercurrent infection, usually viral, may cause prolonged fever in a child with meningitis. Complications of therapy, such as suppurative thrombophlebitis or a urinary tract infection after prolonged catheterization, are additional considerations. Persistent fever may be related to the severity of the infection. Poor therapeutic response (especially in multidrug-resistant organisms) occurs, and repeated lumbar puncture must be considered on an individual basis. Drug fever often is cited but rarely is the cause of persistent fever and remains a diagnosis of exclusion.

PROGNOSIS AND SEQUELAE

The prognosis in patients with bacterial meningitis depends on many factors: (1) the age of the patient, (2) the time course or progression of illness before effective antibiotic therapy, (3) the specific microorganism causing the disease, (4) the number of organisms or the quantity of capsular polysaccharide material present in the CSF at the time of diagnosis, (5) the rapidity with which CSF is sterilized after initiation of antibiotic therapy, (6) the presence of disorders that may compromise host response to infection, and (7) the geographic location of the patient (low-income countries).[109,205,227,365]

The younger the patient and the greater the antigenic load at the time of admission, the worse the prognosis. Bacterial colony counts seem to be a more reliable indication of sequelae than is antigen concentration. Seizures, subdural effusions, bacteremia, and a more prolonged period of fever occur more frequently in children who have more than 10^7 CFUs/mL of a particular organism in the CSF at the time of admission.[126] Children with 10^7 CFUs/mL or greater also are significantly more likely to experience hearing loss and speech disturbance than children with meningitis but lower concentrations of bacteria within CSF specimens.[126] The concentration of TNF in serum has been associated with a fatal outcome in patients with meningococcal meningitis.[384] Elevated concentrations of IL-1β and TNF within the CSF of patients with bacterial meningitis also have been correlated significantly ($P < .002$) with a higher incidence of neurologic sequelae of disease.[269]

The mortality rate for bacterial meningitis in children who are beyond the neonatal period has been reduced to 1% to 5%. Although antibiotic therapy has reduced the mortality rate, up to 50% of the survivors of meningitis have some sequelae of disease.[46,106,109,123,148,205,356] Most studies from which estimates of sequelae have been derived have been retrospective.

Neurologic sequelae are common in survivors of meningitis and include hearing loss, cognitive impairment, and developmental delay.[109] For example, in 1991, the Metropolitan Atlanta Developmental Disabilities Surveillance Program identified bacterial meningitis as the leading postnatal cause of developmental disabilities, including cerebral palsy and mental retardation.[68] Hearing loss occurs in 22% to 30% of survivors of pneumococcal meningitis compared with 1% to 8% after meningococcal meningitis.[17,105,109,205,371,376,385]

A prospective cohort study reported 158 meningitis survivors, 3 months to 14 years old, who were treated in a single center between 1983 and 1986.[169] Between 1991 and 1993, 130 children (82% of the original cohort) were evaluated at a mean age of 8.4 years and a mean of 6.7 years after their meningitis. Results of blinded, audiologic, behavioral, neurologic, neuropsychologic, and sociodemographic assessments were compared with those of sex-matched and grade-matched control children. A systematic increase in the risk for abnormality or for poorer functioning was noted across all categories tested in children with meningitis versus control children. The differences reached statistical significance for tests of fine motor function, intelligence, neuropsychological function, school behavior, and auditory figure-ground differentiation. Eleven children who had experienced meningitis (8.5% of the cohort studied) had major deficits (hydrocephalus, persistent seizures, spasticity, blindness, IQ less than 70, or profound hearing loss). Twenty-four (18.5%) of the survivors of meningitis and 14 (10.8%) of the control children had minor deficits (IQ of 70–80, inability to read, abnormalities in speech discrimination possibly referable to mild to moderate hearing loss, and school behavior problems). Overall, one in four of the children in this study had either a serious disabling sequela or a functionally important behavior disorder or neuropsychologic or auditory dysfunction that adversely affected academic performance.

This prospectively followed cohort was reevaluated 12 years post meningitis; impairment, although not severe, still persisted in the postmeningitic patients compared with controls.[15] After having meningitis, the children were "more than twice as likely as controls to require special educational assistance" and "took longer to complete tasks, made more errors, were less organized, and struggled within problem-solving situations." Decreased performance in language tasks and executive skills also were seen in children whose age was younger than 12 months at onset of meningitis.

A prospective study of bacterial meningitis in children revealed that 32.8% of children had abnormalities detectable on neurologic examination at the time of discharge, but by 5 years after discharge specific deficits were noted in only 11.1% of the total group. As a result of the onset of late seizures in some of these patients, the frequency of neurologic sequelae 15 years after discharge was 14%.[296] Specific complications or sequelae of meningitis in these patients are shown in Table 31.13. Shortly after discharge, hemiparesis or quadriparesis was noted in 30 patients (12.4% of the total group), but at 1 year after discharge, paralysis was noted in only 5 patients. These data reflect the tendency for even major neurologic defects to clear unpredictably with time. This important observation suggests the need to maintain cautious optimism in discussing long-term complications of meningitis with parents.

The mean IQ (±1 standard deviation) of the entire group of patients ($n = 235$) after recovery was 94 (±23 standard deviations), with a range of 33 to 150. Twenty-nine children (17.3%) had IQs less than 80, and 22 (11.6%) had IQs less than 70. A comparison of these patients with their siblings and other control children revealed no significant difference in mean IQ. A significantly greater proportion ($P < .01$) of children who recovered from meningitis had IQs less than 80 compared with children from control groups.

The prospective nature of these studies has permitted an assessment of factors that herald a poor prognosis and that may be discernible at or near the time of admission. Evidence of inappropriate secretion of ADH was correlated significantly ($P < .01$) with abnormal neurologic examinations at 3 months after discharge and with low IQs. The age of the child correlated inversely with the development of subdural effusion ($P < .01$), the occurrence of hearing deficits ($P < .02$), and low

TABLE 31.13 Complications or Sequelae of Meningitis

	Total	*H. influenzae*	*H. influenzae* (Ampicillin)	*H. influenzae* (Chloramphenicol)	*S. pneumoniae*	*N. meningitidis*
N	235	151	90	61	35	26
Deaths <12 h in hospital	4	4	3	1	0	0
Deaths >12 h in hospital	1	0	0	0	0	1
Shock	8	6	5	1	1	1
Paralysis						
Early	30	18	7	11	7	3
Persistent	5	4	1	3	4	0
Persistent tone	5	4	1	3	1	2
Ataxia						
Early	7	5	2	3	2	0
Persistent	1	1	0	1	0	0
Visual problems	7	4	2	2	3	0
Clinically significant hearing deficit	25	17	6	11	5	2
Hydrocephalus	1	1	1	0	0	0

TABLE 31.14 Median Risk (%) of Sequelae After Bacterial Meningitis

Sequelae	All Causes	*S. pneumoniae*	*H. influenzae*	*N. meningitidis*
At least one major sequelae	12.0	24.7	9.5	7.2
Cognitive	1.1	3.1	1.0	0.4
Seizure	1.6	2.5	1.5	0.5
Hearing	4.3	6.7	3.2	2.1
Motor	1.5	3.3	1.2	0.8
Visual	0.8	1.1	0.1	2.1
At least one minor sequelae	8.6	18.6	5.7	2.3
Cognitive	2.2	3.6	2.4	0.9
Hearing	2.1	4.6	0.6	0.5
Motor	1.4	2.7	1.3	0.4
Visual	0.5	1.8	0.1	0.2
Behavioral	1.5	4.0	0.8	0.1

From a review of 90 published papers from 1980 to 2008. Edmond K, Clark A, Korczak VS, et al. Global and regional risk of disabling sequelae from bacterial meningitis: a systematic review and meta-analysis. *Lancet Infect Dis* 2010;10:317–28.

IQ ($P < .05$). The presence of focal neurologic findings in patients who were not postictal at the time of admission correlated significantly ($P < .001$) with abnormal neurologic examination, which was noted previously. Focal deficits indicating cerebral injury noted at admission or during the course of hospitalization were associated significantly ($P < .001$) with the development of late (1 to 15 years after discharge) afebrile seizures.[296] Focal neurologic findings at the time of admission proved to be a reliable predictor of permanent sequelae of bacterial meningitis. Focal deficits at admission also correlated significantly with low IQs ($P < .001$), even at 2 and 3 years after discharge from the hospital. The quantity of antigen in the initial CSF specimen and the number of organisms present also correlated significantly ($P < .01$) with sequelae of meningitis.[123] A prospective multicenter study of 180 children with pneumococcal meningitis between 1993 and 1996 revealed that 14 (7.7%) of 180 children died. No deaths were related to treatment failure by an antibiotic-resistant strain. Of the 166 surviving children, 41 (25%) developed motor defects, and 48 (32%) of 151 children had moderate to severe unilateral or bilateral hearing loss. By CT or MRI of 103 patients, brain infarcts were noted in 39 (38%), subdural effusions in 25 (24%), hydrocephalus in 22 (21%), cerebritis in 12 (12%), and brain edema in 6 (6%).[17]

The outcome of patients with pneumococcal meningitis caused by penicillin-nonsusceptible or cefotaxime-nonsusceptible isolates has not differed from that caused by susceptible strains.[17,133,199] This finding is explained in part because vancomycin has been administered empirically to most children with suspected bacterial meningitis since the mid-1990s in the United States and in other parts of the world where treatment failures have been reported as a result of antibiotic-resistant *S. pneumoniae*.[283]

Meta-analysis of 90 published reports from 1980 to 2008 revealed that the most common types of major sequelae after bacterial meningitis were hearing loss (33.6%), followed by seizures (12.6%), motor deficit (11.6%), cognitive impairment (9.1%), hydrocephalus (7.1%), and visual disturbance (6.3%) (Table 31.14). The risk for at least one major sequela was almost three times greater in the WHO African region (pooled risk estimate 25.1%) and southeast Asian region (21.6%) compared with the European region (9.4%).[109]

Other specific sequelae or complications of bacterial meningitis that have been observed include cranial nerve involvement, hemiparesis or quadriparesis, muscle hypertonia, ataxia, permanent seizure disorders, and development of obstructive hydrocephalus. Subdural effusions (as noted earlier) are so frequent in young children that they can be considered a part of the general disease process rather than a persistent or troublesome complication of the meningeal infection. Development of brain abscess after bacterial meningitis is exceedingly rare[129]; when it is found, the possibility that it preceded the development of meningeal infection must be considered, and a careful search for other sites of infections such as endocarditis should be initiated.

Significant hearing loss after bacterial meningitis has been reported frequently. The mechanisms responsible for hearing deficits include spread of infection along the auditory canal and cochlear aqueduct, serous or purulent labyrinthitis, and, with time, replacement of the membranous labyrinth with fibrous tissue and new bone.[36,192,235,238,309] Damage to inner ear structures and subsequent hearing loss also are affected by the immune response of the host.

TNF-α has been shown to produce cytolytic effects by the production of oxygen free radicals. Animal studies have shown a decreased incidence of hearing loss when animals are treated with antibody blockade of TNF-α[13] and scavenging of oxygen free radicals by antioxidant therapy.[211]

Deafness generally is noted early in the course of bacterial meningitis and is independent of the therapy provided.[105,194,267,334,381] Ataxia has been reported as a presenting sign of bacterial meningitis in children with hearing loss noted at a later date.[196,333] Presumably the insult to the vestibular and auditory systems occurred concomitantly in these children. The early loss of hearing noted by several investigators suggests that hearing loss is *not* associated specifically with the use of a particular antimicrobial agent. Early diagnosis and treatment apparently do not prevent the development of deafness in many children who develop hearing loss as a consequence of bacterial meningitis.

Estimates of the frequency of hearing loss in retrospective studies vary from 2.4% to 29%.[105,109] Overall, 48 of 151 (32%) of the children with pneumococcal meningitis in the multicenter study had unilateral or bilateral moderate to severe hearing loss.[17] Occasionally hearing loss noted early may improve over weeks to months.[309]

No correlation has been found between hearing loss and either the age of the patient at the onset of meningitis or the duration of illness before admission.[105] A significant correlation was noted between hearing loss and the presence of seizures before admission, the duration of fever in the hospital after therapy has been initiated (which presumably reflects more severe disease), treatment with antibiotics administered orally before a definitive diagnosis of bacterial meningitis was established, and a depressed CSF-to-blood glucose ratio at the time of admission.[105,198] A nomogram was developed to predict the probability of development of hearing loss using five factors[217]: (1) duration of symptoms before admission, (2) absence of petechiae, (3) CSF glucose level, (4) infection by *S. pneumoniae,* and (5) ataxia; patients at risk for developing hearing loss were effectively identified with excellent sensitivity (100%) using a cutoff of 0 on the point scale.

Because hearing deficits occur so commonly in patients with bacterial meningitis, hearing evaluation by evoked response audiometry in young, uncooperative children is recommended routinely at the time of or shortly after discharge from the hospital. Repeated audiometric evaluation is recommended after discharge if the results of the initial examination are abnormal. Pure tone audiometry can be used for older, cooperative children. Differentiation of hearing deficits resulting from conductive disturbances from deficits related to damage to the eighth cranial nerve is important. Some children who have repetitive episodes of otitis media may experience conductive loss that is unrelated to the meningitis.

Systematic review of neurocognitive impairment in children after CNS infection revealed deficits in cognition and motor function to be very common.[62,109] Childhood meningitis survivors were found to have a higher incidence of academic or behavior limitations; nonspecific symptoms, such as headaches; and significantly more symptoms of inattention, hyperactivity, and impulsiveness compared with nearest-age siblings.[35,127,218]

Only one study assessed the value of the Pediatric Risk of Mortality (PRISM) score in predicting outcomes of bacterial meningitis.[246] This study was done in a subgroup of children requiring mechanical ventilation. The best predictor of death and functional states on follow-up evaluation was the PRISM score. When the score was less than 20 within the first 24 hours of admission to the pediatric intensive care unit, a favorable outcome was noted in 82%. When the score was 20 or higher, a favorable outcome was noted in only 30% ($P < .009$).

CT of 49 children with complicated bacterial meningitis who had seizures, hemiparesis, persistent fever, persistent bulging fontanelle, or prolonged alteration in mental status revealed evidence of cerebral infarction in 13 children (27%).[348]

Plasminogen activator inhibitor-1 (PAI-1) has been shown to contribute to vascular complications and death in children with meningococcal disease and pneumococcal meningitis.[52,57]

PREVENTION

Pneumococcal Infection

Chemoprophylaxis

Antibiotic chemoprophylaxis of children exposed to pneumococcal meningitis is not recommended regardless of immunization status.[10] In asplenic patients (functional and anatomic), daily chemoprophylaxis against pneumococcal infection is recommended with oral penicillin therapy (125 mg twice a day for children younger than 2 years; 250 mg twice a day for children 2 years and older).[10] Parents should be informed that penicillin prophylaxis may not be effective in preventing all cases of invasive pneumococcal disease. In children with suspected or proven penicillin allergy, erythromycin is an alternative agent for prophylaxis.

Immunoprophylaxis

In a large randomized trial,[43] more than 37,000 infants received either the PCV7 containing polysaccharides of serotypes 4, 6B, 9V, 14, 18C, 19F, and 23F conjugated to CRM_{197} or meningococcal serogroup C oligosaccharide conjugated to the same protein. Vaccines were administered at 2, 4, 6, and 12 to 15 months of age. The PCV7 was found to be 97.4% efficacious in preventing acquisition of invasive pneumococcal infections caused by vaccine serotype isolates. As a result of this study, in 2000, the PCV7 was recommended by the ACIP and the AAP Committee on Infectious Diseases for all children younger than 24 months of age to prevent invasive pneumococcal infections.[9,71]

In February 2010, a 13-valent pneumococcal conjugate vaccine (PCV13, Prevnar 13) was licensed by the FDA for prevention of invasive pneumococcal diseases caused by the 13 pneumococcal serotypes covered by the vaccine (PCV7 serotypes plus 1, 3, 5, 6A, 7F, and 19A) and for prevention of otitis media caused by serotypes in PCV7.[74,76] PCV13 is approved for use among children aged 6 weeks to 71 months and has replaced PCV7. Use of PCV13 is recommended by the ACIP for routine vaccination for all children aged 2 to 59 months, vaccination of children aged 60 to 71 months with underlying medical conditions that increase their risk for pneumococcal disease or complications (e.g., chronic heart disease, chronic lung disease, diabetes mellitus, CSF leaks, cochlear implant, functional or anatomic asplenia, human immunodeficiency virus infection, chronic renal failure and nephrotic syndrome, diseases associated with treatment with immunosuppressive drugs or radiation therapy, congenital immunodeficiency), and children who previously received one or more doses of PCV7.[74,76]

Meningococcal Infection

Chemoprophylaxis

Chemoprophylaxis is recommended to all household members of a patient with meningococcal meningitis and in daycare and nursery school contacts, preferably within 24 hours of the diagnosis of the primary case.[12] Prophylaxis may be provided for individuals who had contact with the patient's oral secretions through kissing or sharing toothbrushes or eating utensils during the 7 days before onset of disease in the index child. Prophylaxis is not recommended routinely for health care personnel unless they have had close exposure through mouth-to-mouth resuscitation, intubation, or suctioning before antibiotic therapy was initiated. Schoolroom classmates and hospital contacts of patients usually are not given prophylactic treatment.

Minocycline and rifampin have proved to be 80% to 90% effective in eradicating carriage of meningococci.[174] Both drugs are secreted in the saliva in concentrations greater than the MICs for meningococci. The use of minocycline has been accompanied by frequent and significant vestibular reactions, even after a single dose of 100 mg, and generally should not be used.[64–66,396]

Rifampin is the drug of choice in most instances and can be used in a dose of 600 mg twice daily for four doses in adults and in doses of 10 mg/kg per dose twice daily for four doses in children 1 to 12 years of age. A dose of 5 mg/kg every 12 hours for four doses can be used in children 3 months to 1 year of age.[266] The emergence of rifampin-resistant strains in treated meningococcal carriers has been reported to occur with a frequency of 0% to 27%.[95,110,392]

A single intramuscular dose of ceftriaxone has proved to be an effective alternative to rifampin for prophylaxis in meningococcal contacts.[332] This approach to prophylaxis may be particularly useful in circumstances in which compliance with the use of oral rifampin is considered questionable. The efficacy of ceftriaxone has been confirmed for only serogroup A strains, but its effect is likely to be similar for other serogroups. Ceftriaxone has the advantage of easier dosage and administration and safety in pregnancy.[12] Ceftriaxone may be given intramuscularly in a dose of 125 mg for individuals younger than 12 years and in a dose of 250 mg for individuals 12 years and older.

Ciprofloxacin given to adults in a single oral dose of 500 mg has been effective in eradicating meningococcal carriage.[12] Ciprofloxacin presently is not recommended for individuals younger than 18 years or for pregnant women.

Immunoprophylaxis

Because secondary cases may occur several weeks or more after onset of disease in the index case, meningococcal vaccine may be used as an adjunct to chemoprophylaxis when an outbreak is caused by a serogroup contained in the vaccine. The CDC has outlined recommendations for the administration of the meningococcal serogroup C vaccine to control outbreaks.[69]

The FDA approved a quadrivalent meningococcal conjugate vaccine (MenACWY-D, Menactra) in January 2005 and a quadrivalent meningococcal conjugate vaccine (MenACWY-CRM, Menveo) in February 2010.[73,75] Both vaccines include serotypes A, C, Y, and W-135, and, in January 2011, the FDA approved the use of both vaccines to persons aged 2 through 55 years. MenACWY-D is also licensed as a two-dose series for children aged 9 through 23 months who are at increased risk for meningococcal disease; Hib-MenCY-TT (MenHibrix) is recommended for use in children aged 6 weeks through 18 months at increased risk (Table 31.15).[75]

Similar to other conjugate vaccines, meningococcal C conjugate vaccines are more immunogenic than the pure polysaccharide vaccine in infants younger than 2 years of age.[242] Because of a high incidence of meningococcal disease in the United Kingdom, a meningococcal serogroup C-CRM_{197} was administered in a phased program beginning in November 1999 to all children younger than 18 years of age.[304] Surveillance studies to assess short-term efficacy have shown a 97% efficacy for teenagers and a 92% efficacy for toddlers in the prevention of meningococcal serogroup C infection.

The FDA licensed the serogroup B meningococcal vaccines MenB-FHbp (Trumenba) as a three-dose series in October 2014 and a two-dose series in 2016, and MenB-4C (Bexsero) as a two-dose series in January 2015.[134] The two MenB vaccines are not interchangeable; the same vaccine product must be used for all doses. Both vaccines are approved for use in persons aged 10 to 25 years; they are not licensed for children aged younger than 10 years and are not currently recommended for children aged 2 months to 9 years who are at increased risk for serogroup B meningococcal disease. Both vaccines are recommended for certain groups of persons aged 10 years or older who are at increased risk for serogroup B meningococcal disease (e.g., complement component deficiencies, functional or anatomic asplenia, including sickle-cell disease) in the risk group for an outbreak for which vaccination is recommended (Table 31.15).

Haemophilus influenzae Meningitis

Chemoprophylaxis

The most comprehensive study concerning the spread of *H. influenzae* type b infection among household contacts was coordinated by the CDC.[388] Data collected from 19 states were analyzed prospectively. *H. influenzae* meningitis was reported in 1403 patients. Eighty-two percent of exposed families were investigated for the occurrence of *H. influenzae* disease within 30 days of its onset in the index patient. Systemic disease caused by *H. influenzae* type b developed in 9 of 1687 contacts (0.5%) who were younger than age 6 years. The risk for infection in patients younger than age 4 years was 2.1%; the risk in children younger than age 1 year was 6%. The risk for secondary infection of household contacts in the 30 days after onset of meningitis in the index case was 585 times greater than the age-adjusted risk in the general population and was similar to the risk for secondary meningococcal disease in household contacts. This nationwide study provided an important impetus for finding a chemoprophylactic regimen that could prevent secondary infection in household contacts.

TABLE 31.15 Recommendations for Meningococcal Vaccination of Children at Increased Risk for Meningococcal Disease

Vaccine	Age of Primary Vaccination	Booster Doses	Indicated for Infants	Not Indicated for Infants
MenACWY-CRM (Menveo)	2, 4, 6, and 12 mo	1st booster 3 y after primary series Additional boosters every 5 y	Complement component deficiencies Functional or anatomic asplenia The risk groups for an outbreak for which vaccination is recommended Traveling to or residing in epidemic or hyperendemic regions	
MenACWY-D (Menactra)	9 and 12 mo	1st booster 3 y after primary series Additional boosters every 5 y	Complement component deficiencies The risk groups for an outbreak for which vaccination is recommended Traveling to or residing in epidemic or hyperendemic regions	Functional or anatomic asplenia
Hib-MenCY-TT (MenHibrix)	2, 4, 6, and 12–15 mo	1st booster (using MenACWY-CRM or MenACWY-D) 3 y after primary series	1st booster 3 y after primary series	Traveling to or residing in epidemic or hyperendemic regions
MenB-FHbp (Trumenba)	3-dose series, with 2nd and 3rd doses after 2 and 6 mo after 1st dose; 2nd dose 6 mo after 1st dose is an option	None	≥10 y at increased risk for serogroup B disease (complement component deficiencies, functional or anatomic asplenia, the risk groups for an outbreak for which vaccination is recommended)	Children aged <10 y Traveling to or residing in epidemic or hyperendemic regions
MenB-4C (Bexsero)	2-dose series, with doses at least 1 mo apart	None	≥10 y at increased risk for serogroup B disease (complement component deficiencies, functional or anatomic asplenia, the risk groups for an outbreak for which vaccination is recommended)	Children aged <10 y Traveling to or residing in epidemic or hyperendemic regions

A nationwide, collaborative, placebo-controlled trial was conducted subsequently among household (children <6 years old) and daycare center contacts of individuals with invasive *H. influenzae* type b disease.[29] Four of 765 placebo-treated contacts experienced secondary disease versus none of 1112 rifampin-treated contacts ($P = .027$).

The AAP Committee on Infectious Diseases recommends that rifampin be provided orally once a day for 4 days in a dose of 20 mg/kg (maximum dose 600 mg/day) to all household contacts (children and adults) regardless of age in households with at least one unvaccinated contact younger than 4 years.[11] The dose for infants younger than 1 month is not established, but it may be reduced to 10 mg/kg. Rifampin prophylaxis is not required, however, when all of the household contacts younger than 4 years have been fully immunized. All members of households with a fully immunized but immunocompromised child, regardless of age, should receive rifampin because of concern that the immunization may not have been effective.

When two or more cases of invasive disease have occurred within 60 days and unimmunized or incompletely immunized children attend a daycare facility, rifampin should be administered to all personnel and attendees. When a single case has been reported, the use of rifampin is controversial, and many experts recommend *no* prophylaxis.[11] Unimmunized or incompletely immunized children should receive a dose of vaccine and should be scheduled for completion of the recommended age-specific immunization schedule.

No data document the safety of rifampin administered during pregnancy. Prophylaxis with rifampin is not recommended for pregnant women who are contacts of infected infants.

Patients receiving rifampin should be advised routinely that their urine, sweat, and tears will be stained orange. Individuals should be advised to refrain from using contact lenses while receiving rifampin therapy because the lenses may be stained permanently.

Immunoprophylaxis

The incidence of *H. influenzae* type b invasive disease and meningitis decreased dramatically after the introduction of vaccines that initially were found to be effective at 15 months of age[8] and then later found to be effective at 2 months of age.[321] (See Chapter 133 for details of *H. influenzae* type b vaccines.)

Passive immunization of infants also has been studied with use of bacterial polysaccharide immunoglobulin.[322] This preparation given in a single intramuscular dose of 0.5 mL/kg provides significant protection for infants from *H. influenzae* type b disease for 3 or 4 months.

NEW REFERENCES SINCE THE SEVENTH EDITION

14. Anani WQ, Ojerholm E, Shurin MR. Resolving transferrin isoforms via agarose gel electrophoresis. *Lab Med.* 2015;46:26-33.
52. Brandtzaeg P, Joø GB, Brusletto B, et al. Plasminogen activator inhibitor 1 and 2, alpha-2-antiplasmin, plasminogen, and endotoxin levels in systemic meningococcal disease. *Thromb Res.* 1990;57:271-278.
57. Brouwer MC, Meijers JC, Baas F, et al. Plasminogen activator inhibitor-1 influences cerebrovascular complications and death in pneumococcal meningitis. *Acta Neuropathol.* 2014;127:553-564.
63. Castelblanco RL, Lee M, Hasbun R. Epidemiology of bacterial meningitis in the USA from 1997 to 2010: a population-based observational study. *Lancet Infect Dis.* 2014;14:813-819.
134. Folaranmi T, Rubin L, Martin SW, et al. Use of serogroup B meningococcal vaccines in persons aged ≥10 years at increased risk for serogroup B meningococcal disease: recommendations of the Advisory Committee on Immunization Practices, 2015. *MMWR.* 2015;64:608-612.
149. Gaschignard J, Levy C, Chrabieh M, et al. Invasive pneumococcal disease in children can reveal a primary immunodeficiency. *Clin Infect Dis.* 2014;59:244-251.
206. Kim KS. Neonatal bacterial meningitis. *NeoReviews.* 2015;16:e535-e543.
222. Langley G, Schaffner W, Farley MM, et al. Twenty years of active bacterial core surveillance. *Emerg Infect Dis.* 2015;21:1520-1528.
244. MacNeil JR, Rubin L, Folaranmi T, et al. Use of serogroup B meningococcal vaccines in adolescents and young adults: recommendations of the Advisory Committee on Immunization Practices, 2015. *MMWR.* 2015;64:1171-1176.
245. MacNeil JR, Rubin L, McNamara L, et al. Use of MenACWY-CRM vaccine in children aged 2 through 23 months at increased risk for meningococcal disease: recommendations of the Advisory Committee on Immunization Practices, 2013. *MMWR.* 2014;63:527-530.
251. Meco C, Oberascher G, Arrer E, et al. Beta-trace protein test: new guidelines for the reliable diagnosis of cerebrospinal fluid fistula. *Otolaryngol Head Neck Surg.* 2003;129:508-517.
261. Moore MR, Link-Gelles R, Schaffner W, et al. Effect of use of 13-valent pneumococcal conjugate vaccine in children on invasive pneumococcal disease in children and adults in the USA: analysis of multisite, population-based surveillance. *Lancet Infect Dis.* 2015;15:301-309.
361. Tan YC, Gill AK, Kim KS. Treatment strategies for central nervous system infections: an update. *Expert Opin Pharmacother.* 2014;18:1-17.

The full reference list for this chapter is available at ExpertConsult.com.

32 Parameningeal Infections

Xavier Sáez-Llorens • Javier Nieto Guevara

BRAIN ABSCESS

Brain abscesses in children remain a rare entity and, as a result, their management is guided largely by clinical experience and the results of case series. Twenty-five percent of brain abscesses occur in children younger than 15 years, with a peak incidence at 4 to 7 years.[59,68] In most patients, brain abscess results from predisposing factors, such as underlying disease (e.g., infection with the human immunodeficiency virus [HIV]), a history of treatment with immunosuppressive drugs, disruption of the natural protective barriers surrounding the brain (e.g., due to an operative procedure, trauma, mastoiditis, sinusitis, or dental infection), or a systemic source of infection (e.g., endocarditis or bacteremia).[15] Bacteria enter the brain through contiguous spread in about half of cases and through hematogenous dissemination in about one-third of cases, with unknown mechanisms accounting for the remaining cases.[15]

The outcome for patients with brain abscess has improved over the past 50 years following advances in cranial imaging techniques, the use of antimicrobial treatment regimens, and the introduction of minimally invasive neurosurgical procedures.[15] Mortality has declined from 40% in 1960 to 15% in the past decade.[15] Currently, 70% of patients with brain abscess have a good outcome, with no or minimal neurologic sequelae,[15] although data on functional and neuropsychological evaluations after brain infection are lacking. Although the mortality rate seems to be decreasing, a significant percentage of children continue to have residual neurologic deficits, including epilepsy, permanent motor or sensory dysfunction, visual field defects, and personality changes.[24,27,31] Some children also require placement of a ventriculoperitoneal shunt.[18]

Pathogenesis and Pathology

Pathogenic mechanisms of infection are dependent on predisposing conditions. The first stage of brain abscess is early cerebritis,[13] which may lead to a perivascular inflammatory response surrounding the necrotic center, with increased edema in the surrounding white matter.

TABLE 32.1 **Primary Source, Usual Location of Lesion, and Associated Neurologic Findings in Children With Brain Abscess**

Primary Source	Location of Abscess	Associated Neurologic Findings
Sinusitis	Frontal lobe	Headache, behavioral changes, motor/speech disorders, depressed consciousness, forced grasping and sucking, hemiparesis
Chronic otitis/mastoiditis	Temporal lobe	Dyspraxia and aphasia (dominant hemisphere), ipsilateral third cranial nerve palsy, ipsilateral headache, upper homonymous hemianopsia, motor dysfunction of face and arm
	Cerebellum	Dizziness, vomiting, ipsilateral ataxia and tremor, sixth cranial nerve palsy, nystagmus (toward lesion)
Dental infection	Frontal lobe	
Head trauma	Related to injured site	Variable by region involved
Postoperative	At operative site	Variable by region involved
Metastatic spread	Multiple lesions	Variable by region involved
	If parietal lobe involved	Visual field defects in inferior quadrant, homonymous hemianopsia, dysphasia (dominant hemisphere), dyspraxia, and contralateral spatial neglect (no dominant hemisphere)

Subsequently, the necrotic center reaches its maximum size and a capsule is formed through the accumulation of fibroblasts and neovascularization. The capsule thickens with an abundance of reactive collagen, but inflammation and edema extend beyond the capsule. For practical purposes, brain abscesses usually are classified according to the likely entry point of the infection (Table 32.1). Ear and mastoid infections are associated with formation of an abscess at the temporal or cerebellar locations; sinus and dental infections give rise to purulent collections in the frontal lobe; and metastatic spread from distant foci in children with congenital cardiac or pulmonary right-to-left shunts commonly results in involvement of any parenchymal area, including parietal or occipital regions.[35,56]

The most common origin of microbial infection in children remains direct or indirect cranial infection arising from the middle ear, paranasal sinuses, or teeth. Seeding of the brain presumably occurs via transit of infecting microbes through the valves and emissary veins that serve these regions. A direct erosion of skull and dura by osteomyelitis-induced sinus or middle ear infection can be another mechanism of bacterial spread.[14] Resulting abscesses tend to be solitary and superficial. Metastatic inoculation of the brain from distant extracranial sources (pulmonary infection, endocarditis) tends to provoke multiple cerebral abscesses, with a distribution that reflects the regional cerebral blood flow of the area affected, usually the middle cerebral artery network.[14]

In children with cyanotic congenital heart disease, bacteria are not filtered out by the pulmonary vascular bed, which allows for systemic spread.[18] This situation rarely occurs in patients younger than 2 years, and the abscess or abscesses usually are in areas of brain perfused by the middle cerebral arteries. Evidence of associated endocarditis is rare in these cases, although acute bacterial endocarditis may be complicated by septic infarction of the brain and abscess formation.[52]

Formation of an abscess by direct bacterial implantation may complicate compound skull fractures, scalp wounds, anterior cranial fossa or temporal bone fractures, and chronic cerebrospinal fluid (CSF) fistula. Abscesses also rarely may develop during the course of bacterial meningitis.[55] Despite identification of all these potential routes, 20% to 30% of cases are classified as cryptic brain abscess for which no obvious predisposing factor can be identified.

The brain is remarkably resistant to microbial infection. Despite the common occurrence of occult bacteremia in infants and children, cerebral abscess is a quite rare disease. This resistance is attributable in part to the abundant blood supply of the brain and the relatively impermeable blood-brain barrier.[3] Although certain underlying brain morbidities, such as previous stroke, intracerebral hematoma, or underlying neoplasm, may serve as a nidus of abscess formation in adults, affected children have no apparent predisposing brain lesion. In animal models of infection, induction of abscess usually requires direct inoculation of numerous organisms into the animal's cerebrum.[44]

Experimental animal studies and use of computed tomography (CT) imaging have provided evidence of the clinical evolution of a brain abscess.[5] In the early stage of cerebritis (days 1–3), a focal area of acute

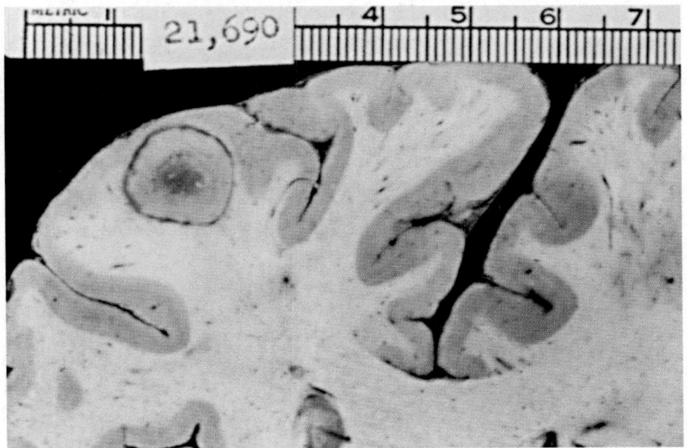

FIG. 32.1 Circumscribed cerebral abscess of hematogenous origin.

inflammation, vascular dilation, microthrombosis, rupture of small vessels, and edema is present. The center of the lesion then undergoes liquefaction. Expansion of the cerebritis and formation of a necrotic central focus are seen in the late cerebritis stage (days 4–9). Establishment of a ring-enhancing dense collagenous capsule of well-vascularized tissue with peripheral gliosis or fibrosis or both occurs at the early capsule stage (days 10–14). Finally, during the late capsule stage (>14 days), host defenses act to wall off the abscess, and a well-developed capsule results.

Death can occur if the volume of pus and surrounding edema induce a significant increase of intracranial pressure leading to brain herniation. In addition, cerebral abscesses can rupture into the ventricular system or through the cortex into the subarachnoid space, resulting in acute deterioration and a life-threatening event.[18] Fig. 32.1 shows the gross appearance of a well-defined abscess of hematogenous origin. Various microscopic features are illustrated in Figs. 32.2 through 32.4.

The spectrum of microorganisms cultured from brain abscesses has changed with time. This change reflects improved microbiologic isolation techniques, early and aggressive treatment of primary infections, and better neurosurgical procedures. In more recent series, the predominance of *Staphylococcus aureus* has decreased and identification of anaerobes has increased.[10,22,66] Nevertheless, community-acquired methicillin-resistant *Staphylococcus aureus* (CA-MRSA) has emerged as a potential etiologic agent over the past decade.[61]

Anaerobic bacteria isolated from brain abscesses include species of *Bacteroides, Peptostreptococcus, Fusobacterium, Veillonella, Propionibacterium, Prevotella,* and *Actinomyces.* Aerobic and microaerophilic streptococci, staphylococci, *Haemophilus* spp., gram-negative enteric bacilli, and *Pseudomonas aeruginosa* also are implicated frequently. In

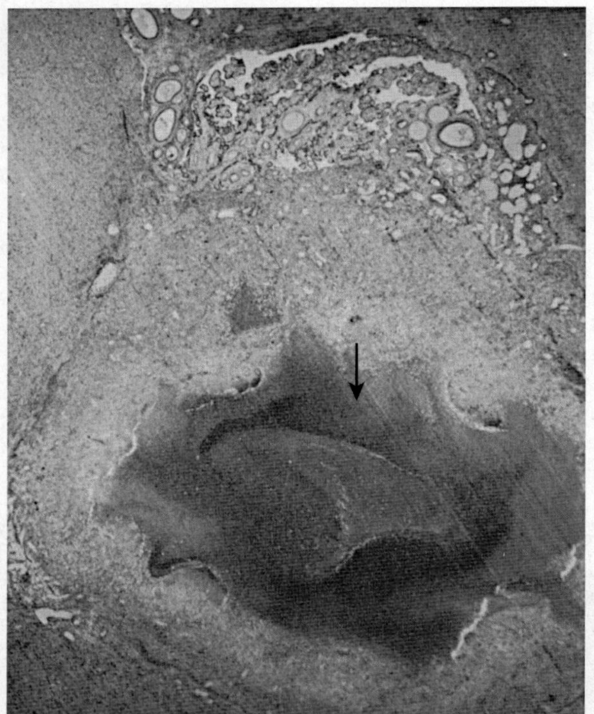

FIG. 32.2 Area of necrosis and liquefaction in a cerebral abscess *(arrow)*.

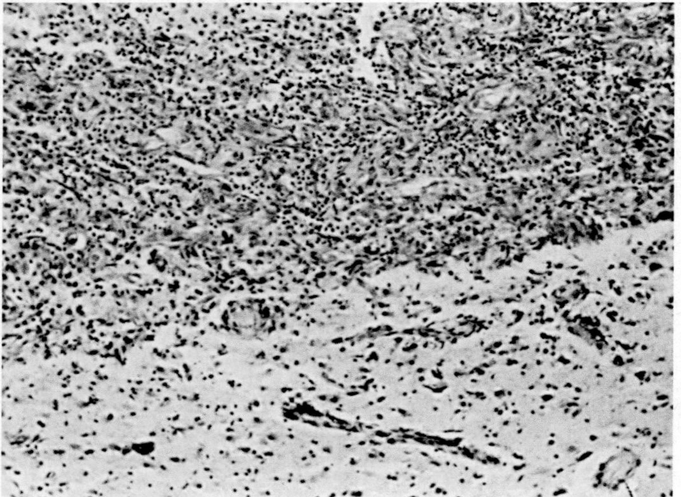

FIG. 32.3 Astroglia and fibroblasts forming the capsule of a cerebral abscess.

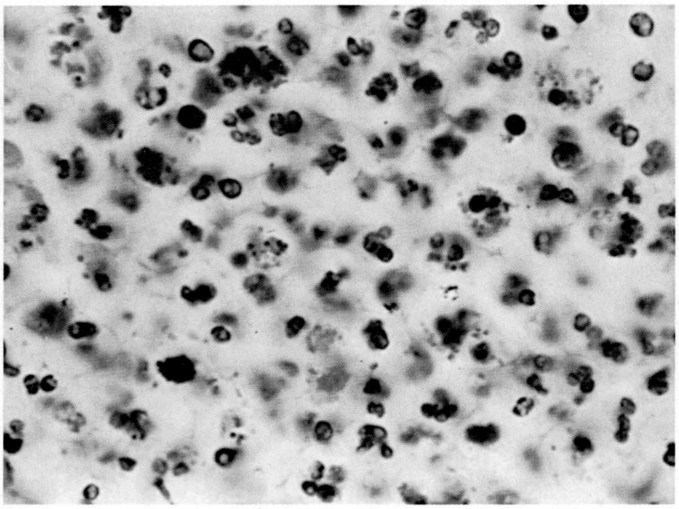

FIG. 32.4 Mononuclear and polymorphonuclear leukocytes are in the center of a cerebral abscess.

children with impaired host defenses, fungal etiology (*Candida, Aspergillus, Cryptococcus, Histoplasma, Coccidioides,* and *Mucor* spp.) or uncommon pathogens, such as *Toxoplasma, Nocardia, Mycobacterium,* and *Listeria* spp., can be identified.[24] Parasites such as amebae, *Cysticercus, Schistosoma,* or *Paragonimus* are very rare causative pathogens.[44] *Citrobacter koseri* and *Proteus* spp. are the most commonly implicated organisms causing neonatal brain abscess in most reports published to date.[53] Some reports of extended-spectrum β-lactamase (ESBL) *Klebsiella pneumoniae* in neonates have been documented.[11,65]

In order of etiologic importance, the predominant organisms causing brain abscess in children are aerobic and anaerobic streptococci (60% to 70% of cases), gram-negative anaerobic bacilli (20% to 40%), Enterobacteriaceae (20% to 30%), *S. aureus* (10% to 15%), and fungi (1% to 5%).* Multiple aerobic and anaerobic organisms are isolated in approximately one-third of patients, especially in patients with chronic otitis. No growth is reported from 30% of properly handled purulent specimens. A reasonable speculation of the likely causative microbes can be made according to the predisposing source of infection (Table 32.2).

Clinical Manifestations

The clinical presentation of a brain abscess depends on the size of the collection, its location, the multiplicity of lesions, the host's immune status, and the age of the patient. Generally symptoms and signs can be related to the effect of a space-occupying mass, to the focal neuronal dysfunction of the parenchymal region involved (see Table 32.1), or to accompanying clinical findings of the underlying predisposing infection. Because on early evaluation most children with cerebral abscess present with vague or nonspecific signs and symptoms, the physician must have a high index of suspicion to recognize the condition as early as possible (Table 32.3). When a patient develops significant alterations in mental status, the prognosis is most ominous.[18,56]

In older children and adolescents, headache is the most common initial symptom. Irritability occurs more commonly in infants and small children. Neurologic signs depend on the site of the abscess and can be subtle for days to weeks. Behavioral changes may occur in patients with abscesses in the frontal or right temporal lobes. Patients with abscesses that involve the brainstem or cerebellum may present with cranial nerve palsy, gait disorder, or either headache or altered mental status owing to hydrocephalus.[58] Up to 25% of patients present with seizures.[15]

Fever is usually a nonspecific symptom at some phase in the illness in about 50% of patients; overall it may be found in up to 80% of children.[46] Drowsiness, confusion, and vomiting occur frequently during the acute phase of disease. Lethargy, stupor, and coma usually are later events and potentially associated with adverse outcome. Papilledema is present in less than one-fourth of the cases, but its presence requires immediate neurosurgical assessment and neuroimaging.

Focal neurologic disturbances reflect the location of the abscess and can be detected in 30% to 50% of cases on presentation (see Tables 32.1 and 32.3).[67] Frontal location is characterized by development of motor speech disorders, memory deficits, personality changes, and depressed consciousness. Hemiparesis occurs with lesions in the postfrontal region or as a consequence of uncal herniation. Abscess in the temporal lobe is characterized by a contralateral homonymous upper quadrantanopia. If the dominant hemisphere is affected, nominal dysphasia and aphasia are characteristic symptoms. Patients with cerebellar abscesses classically exhibit dizziness, nystagmus, defective conjugate eye movements, ataxia, tremor, and hypotonia. Seizures occur in at least 30% to 45% of patients, may be focal or generalized, and may

*References 6, 7, 9, 10, 22, 24, 35, 44, 49, 56, 66.

TABLE 32.2 **Primary Source, Usual Etiologic Pathogens, and Recommended Empiric Antibiotic Therapy in Children With Brain Abscess**

Primary Source	Usual Etiologic Microorganisms	Recommended Empiric Antibiotic Combination
Upper Respiratory Tract Infection		
Sinusitis/dental infection	Viridans and anaerobic streptococci, *Haemophilus* spp., *Fusobacterium* spp., *Bacteroides* spp. (non-*fragilis*)	Penicillin/amoxicillin or cefotaxime/ceftriaxone + metronidazole
Chronic otitis/ mastoiditis	Aerobic and anaerobic streptococci, gram-negative enteric bacilli, *Bacteroides* spp. (including *B. fragilis*), *Pseudomonas aeruginosa*	Penicillin/amoxicillin + metronidazole + ceftazidime/ cefepime or meropenem
Head trauma	*Staphylococcus aureus*, aerobic streptococci, gram-negative enteric bacilli	Oxacillin/nafcillin/amoxicillin or vancomycin[b] + ceftazidime/cefepime or meropenem
Postoperative	*Staphylococcus epidermidis*, *S. aureus*, gram-negative rods, *P. aeruginosa*	Vancomycin[b] + ceftazidime/cefepime or meropenem[c]
Metastatic Spread		
Endocarditis	*S. aureus*, viridans streptococci	Oxacillin/nafcillin/amoxicillin or vancomycin[c] + cefotaxime/ceftriaxone/cefepime + metronidazole
Pulmonary infection	Aerobic streptococci, *Actinomyces*, *Fusobacterium*	Oxacillin/nafcillin or vancomycin[b] + cefotaxime/ ceftriaxone/cefepime + metronidazole
Congenital heart disease	Viridans streptococci, *Haemophilus* spp., *Haemophilus aphrophilus*	Cefotaxime/ceftriaxone/cefepime + metronidazole
Bacterial meningitis	*Streptococcus pneumoniae*, *Haemophilus influenzae* type b, *Salmonella* spp., *Citrobacter* (neonates), ESBL Enterobacteriaceae (*Klebsiella pneumoniae*)	Cefotaxime/ceftriaxone/cefepime ± vancomycin (resistant pneumococcal strains) Meropenem
Cryptogenic source and immunosuppression[a]	Any type of microorganism	Oxacillin/nafcillin or vancomycin[b] + ceftazidime/ cefepime + metronidazole
	Nocardia, fungi, *Mycobacterium tuberculosis*	Oxacillin/nafcillin or vancomycin[b] + ceftazidime/ cefepime + metronidazole

[a]Vancomycin + ceftazidime/cefepime should be added either in areas with significant prevalence of methicillin-resistant staphylococcal strains or for patients with penicillin allergy. Antituberculous therapy should be considered for children with exposure to tuberculosis. Antibiotic regimens are likely to vary by geographic location based on resistant organisms.
[b]If susceptibility testing reveals methicillin-susceptible *S. aureus*, vancomycin should be replaced with nafcillin *or* oxacillin.
[c]To consider in areas where extended-spectrum β-lactamase (ESBL) either has been identified or represents a high probability of isolation.
ESBL, Extended-spectrum β-lactamase.

TABLE 32.3 **Frequency of Presenting Signs and Symptoms in Children With Brain Abscess**

Symptoms	%	Signs	%
Headache	60–70	Focal neurologic deficits	35–50
Fever	50–80	Papilledema	30–40
Vomiting	35–55	Meningeal signs	25–35
Seizures	30–45	Hemiparesis	20–30
Mental changes	30–40	Nerve palsy	10–20
Coma	15–20	Ataxia	5–15

occur at any time during the course of the disease. If the parietal region is involved, visual field defects, homonymous hemianopsia, dysphasia, and dyspraxia can be present.

The rapidity with which symptoms develop can vary substantially. Most patients are symptomatic within 1 week of the onset of formation of an abscess. Immunocompromised children can have a more insidious progression of clinical findings. The presentation of brain abscess in infancy can be suspected by bulging fontanelle, vomiting, irritability, and an enlarging head circumference. Seizures occur commonly, particularly in small infants, and at any time during the course of the disease.[14] School-aged children with cyanotic congenital heart disease, notably tetralogy of Fallot or transposition of the great vessels, also can exhibit symptoms and signs related to their chronic cardiac disease.

Rupture of Brain Abscess Into the Ventricular System

Abscess rupture into the ventricular system results in ventriculitis, often leading to hydrocephalus, and is associated with a high mortality rate (27–85%). Frequently rupture occurs before the diagnosis of abscess has been established and surgical removal can occur. A sudden worsening in the patient's clinical state heralds this event. High fever, shock, meningismus, and altered consciousness are prominent clinical signs.

Rupture of the abscess into the ventricle is seen more frequently in patients with deep-seated abscesses or in immunocompromised patients.[62] Although a modest pleocytosis and elevated protein concentration in CSF may have been identified earlier, 50,000 to 100,000 polymorphonuclear leukocytes per microliter and markedly reduced glucose concentration in the CSF are usual findings. Organisms may be seen on smear of the CSF and cultured from the fluid. In other words, the patient has developed purulent meningitis, and treatment must include high doses of antibiotics and surgery (see "Treatment"). If an abscess is abutting but has not yet ruptured into the ventricular system, drainage should be considered to prevent rupture of the abscess and resulting ventriculitis.

The concurrence of abscess and meningitis in the past has led to the assumption that brain abscess can be a complication of meningitis; this rarely, if ever, is the case, although meningitis may develop during the incipient stages of abscess formation after intracranial invasion of organisms from a contiguous extracranial source. In such circumstances, the abscess may seem to be a consequence of the leptomeningitis. Given a potential source of infection in the ear or paranasal sinuses, the clinician must be wary and appreciate the possibility of this sequence of events. Abscess has been reported to complicate *Citrobacter* meningitis in infants, but careful pathologic study has shown vasculitis and liquefaction necrosis of the white matter without capsule formation.[66]

Laboratory Diagnosis

Laboratory tests frequently are not helpful in supporting the clinical diagnosis of brain abscess.[18,42,56] Children usually have unremarkable leukocyte counts, and the erythrocyte sedimentation rate can be normal. Blood cultures rarely are positive. Performance of a lumbar puncture is potentially dangerous because it can be associated with brainstem herniation.[17] In addition, CSF analysis uncommonly provides useful clinical information. Usual CSF findings include an elevated protein, mild mononuclear pleocytosis, and hypoglycorrhachia. CSF cultures usually are negative, unless the abscess has drained into the ventricular system or has been a complication of meningitis.

Culturing abscess material obtained at the time of surgical drainage provides the best opportunity to make a microbiologic diagnosis. Proper handling and processing, with attention given to optimal anaerobic and aerobic isolation techniques, can identify the causative organism in most cases, especially when antimicrobial therapy has not been instituted previously.[44] The high incidence of sterile cultures reported in the literature is probably because of the inadequacy of bacteriologic procedures. Under such conditions, sterile cultures may reach even unjustified rates higher than 32.2% or 40%.[50] If a bacterial brain abscess is strongly suspected but the culture results are negative, PCR-based 16S ribosomal DNA sequencing may provide a definitive etiologic diagnosis, allowing for targeted antimicrobial therapy.[1] When this test was performed on aspirates from brain abscesses in 71 patients, 30 (42%) of whom had positive cultures, bacterial DNA was detected in 59 patients (83%).[2] The investigators identified 80 different bacterial taxa, 44 of which had not been described previously in brain abscesses, including 37 that have not been reported to be cultured.[2] Although these data are indicative of the bacterial diversity within brain abscesses, it is unclear whether all these species are involved in the pathogenesis of abscesses and warrant treatment.

Diagnosis

Magnetic resonance imaging (MRI) is used at an increasing rate in evaluation of cerebral abscess both at the time of diagnosis and in follow-up. Similar MRI findings can be observed in infarction, demyelinating disorders, and neoplastic processes. Diffusion-weighted MRI and magnetic resonance spectroscopy have been shown to be effective methods in differentiating cerebral abscesses from tumors.[9,44] CT scanning with contrast enhancement provides a rapid means of detecting the size, number, and localization of abscess. Also, proton MRI spectroscopy and diffusion-weighted imaging are useful as additional diagnostic modalities in differentiating intracranial lesions.[38,48] Also, proton magnetic resonance spectroscopy and diffusion-weighted imaging are useful as additional diagnostic modalities in differentiating intracranial lesions.[38] Fig. 32.5 illustrates CT and MRI studies of patients with tuberculous abscess with caseous material, irregular contours, tissue edema, and the important effect of mass displacement of the ventricular system and midline. CT remains an excellent alternative if MRI is unavailable; however intravenous administration of contrast material is advised because the abscess may be missed otherwise.[21,33] Fig. 32.6 illustrates a CT scan showing a large mass in the right hemisphere causing an occupant mass effect, with tissue edema compression and displacement of the lateral ventricle and the midline, which are indirect signs of increased intracranial pressure. Serial CT or MRI performed weekly or biweekly provides evaluation of the response to therapy and of the need for repeating the surgical procedure. MRI is more accurate than CT for establishing the diagnosis of cerebritis, cerebellar abscess, edema formation, and brainstem purulent collections.[26,30] On T1-weighted sequences, brain abscesses appear hypointense and show ring enhancement after administration of intravenous gadolinium. In contrast, on T2-weighted images, the typical mature abscess has a hyperintense central area of pus surrounded by a well-defined hypointense capsule and surrounding edema.

Because specific images allow precise lesion staging, this information provides important clues for the surgeon to suspect the likelihood of encountering purulent material of a well-developed abscess at the moment of drainage. The presence of gas within the abscess cavity on head imaging suggests communication of the abscess with air outside the skull, although gas-forming bacteria in the abscess cavity rarely may be responsible.[53]

Plain skull films generally are normal in children with brain abscess. In small infants, separation of cranial sutures indicates intracranial hypertension. Conventional MRI study is useful for the identification of lesions and to determine the location and morphology, and it allows a correct hypothesis of nature in the most typical cases. The differential diagnosis from other brain lesions, such as nonpyogenic abscesses or necrotic tumors (high-grade gliomas and metastases), is often only possible through the use of functional sequences because the measurement of diffusion with apparent diffusion coefficient (DWI-ADC), proton magnetic resonance spectroscopy (H-MRS), and perfusion-weighted imaging (PWI), which complement the morphologic sequences and provide essential information of structural, metabolic, and hemodynamic characteristics, allows greater neuroradiologic confidence. Modern diagnostic MRI of pyogenic brain abscesses cannot be separated from knowledge, integration, and proper use of the morphologic and functional sequences.[45]

Abnormalities on electroencephalography may be localized and can help in excluding a more generalized, bilateral intracranial disease, such as encephalitis. Unilateral slow waves (δ, 1–3 per second) characterize the usual electroencephalographic findings in cases of cerebral abscess.

After the diagnosis of brain abscess has been established, a careful search should be made for a source of infection serving as a site of

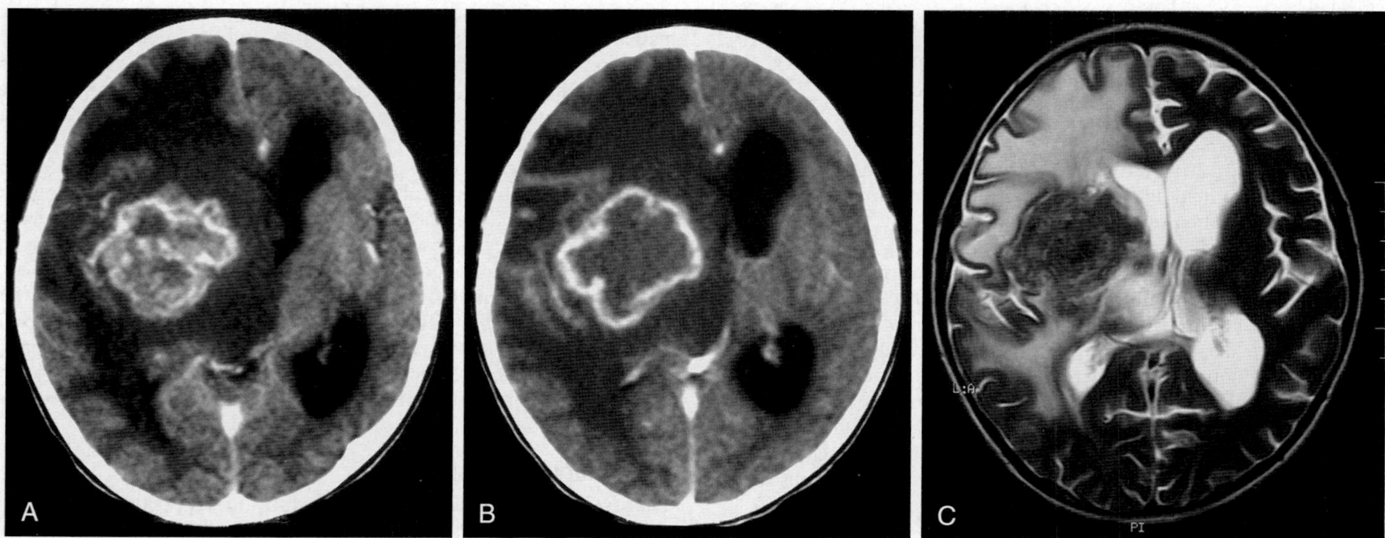

FIG. 32.5 (A–B) Computed tomography and (C) magnetic resonance imaging studies of a child with tuberculous abscess, showing caseous-like dense material, irregular contours, tissue edema, and an important mass effect with displacement of the ventricular system and the midline. (Courtesy Eric Chong, MD, and Dr. José Renán Esquivel, Hospital del Niño, Panama City, Panama.)

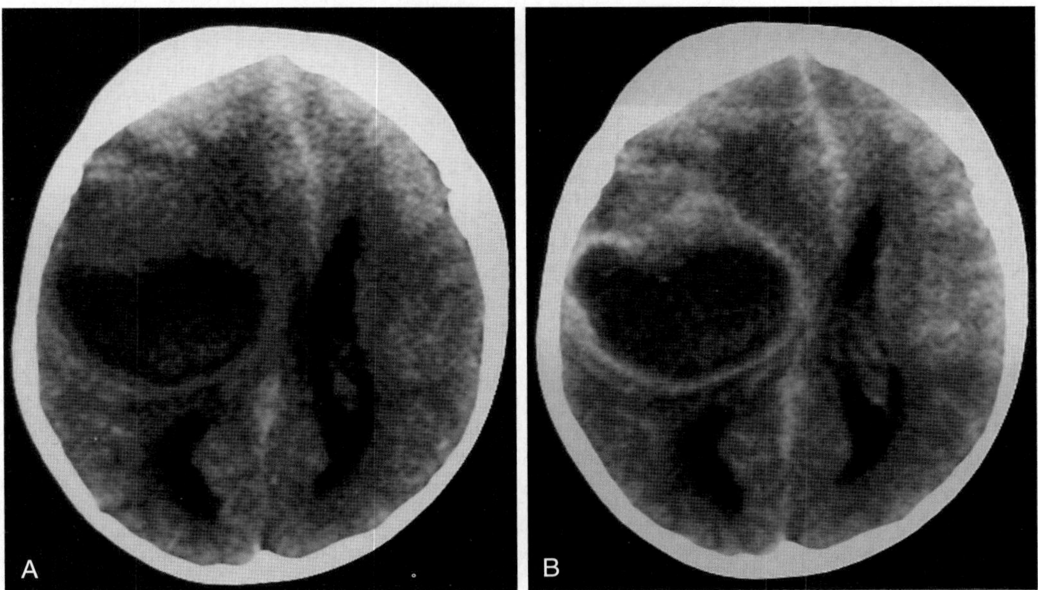

FIG. 32.6 Computed tomography scans demonstrating a large mass in the right hemisphere causing an occupant mass effect with tissue edema compression and displacement of the lateral ventricle and the midline, indirect signs of increased intracranial pressure. (Courtesy Eric Chong, MD, and Dr. José Renán Esquivel, Hospital del Niño, Panama City, Panama.)

origin for hematogenous spread or direct inoculation of organisms into the central nervous system. In addition to obtaining data from the history and physical examination, the physician should extend the MRI or CT evaluation to include the mastoids and paranasal sinuses. An echocardiogram should be obtained to assess for concurrent endocarditis. Other testing should be guided by the history and physical examination findings.

Treatment

The choice of initial antimicrobial therapy should be based on the organisms that are the most likely cause of the disease as determined on the basis of the mechanisms of infection and the patient's predisposing condition, on patterns of antimicrobial susceptibility, and on the ability of the antimicrobial agent to penetrate the abscess.

No prospective clinical trials have compared various surgical and medical treatment strategies available to guide the management of cerebral abscesses in children. Most surgical and medical treatment guidelines are based on populations consisting primarily of adult patients. Appropriate management of brain abscesses generally requires a combined surgical and medical approach,[39] with isolated medical management limited to patients who are neurologically intact and in whom the abscess is in the cerebritis stage[21] or the abscess or abscesses are small[54] or who are too unstable to undergo a surgical procedure.

The initial treatment of solitary and multiple brain abscesses relies on the aspiration of the cavity contents followed by the initiation of empiric antibiotic coverage while the cultures are being processed. CT- or MRI-guided stereotactic aspiration is accurate, minimally invasive, and associated with few complications.[25] Mamelak and colleagues[41] suggested performing head imaging biweekly or on any sign of clinical deterioration, with further aspiration if the cavity enlarges or fails to diminish after 3 to 4 weeks. Because excisions may be associated with increased risk for developing neurologic sequelae, surgery should be reserved for patients who do not respond to the strategy of repeated aspiration and medical management and when an abscess results in a significant mass effect. Madhugiri and colleagues[40] evaluated 231 children who underwent treatment for focal intradural abscess/empyema at the National Institute of Mental Health and Neurosciences in Bangalore, India. These included 57 children with cerebral abscess, 65 with supratentorial empyema, 82 with cerebellar abscess, and 27 with infratentorial empyema. All patients underwent emergency surgery (which was either burr hole and aspiration of the lesion or craniotomy/craniectomy and excision/evacuation), along with antibiotic therapy, typically 2 weeks of intravenous and 4 weeks of oral therapy. The antibiotic regimen was empiric to begin with and was altered based on the antimicrobial susceptibilities of the causative organism(s) when isolated. Hydrocephalus was managed with external ventricular drainage initially and with ventriculoperitoneal shunt if warranted. Mortality rates were 4.8% for cerebral abscess, 9.6% for cerebellar abscess, 10.8% for supratentorial subdural empyema, and 3.7% for posterior fossa subdural empyema. The choice of surgery was found to have a strong bearing on the recurrence rates and outcome in most groups, with aggressive surgery with craniotomy leading to excellent outcomes with a low incidence of residual/recurrent lesions.

While results of cultures are pending, the selection of antibiotics should be guided by the primary source of infection, pertinent patient history, and results of microscopic examination of the purulent material obtained from the abscess (see Table 32.3).

The duration of antibiotics for brain abscess is prolonged, usually 4 to 8 weeks. This recommendation derives from retrospective reports and reviews since no clinical trials have been performed.[28] United Kingdom guidelines recommend 4 to 6 weeks if the abscess has been drained or excised and 6 to 8 weeks if the abscess is treated without drainage.[32] One retrospective study reported recurrent brain abscesses in patients who received antibiotics for less than 3 weeks.[57] In a retrospective study of patients with brain abscesses, the median duration of therapy was 62 days.[28]

Some clinicians consider transitioning patients from intravenous antibiotics to oral antibiotics once the patient has improved clinically; however, there is no evidence that this approach is effective. With the exception of rifampin, linezolid, metronidazole, trimethoprim-sulfamethoxazole, and fluoroquinolones, the concentrations achieved in the abscess by administering antibiotics orally would be expected to be below the minimal inhibitory concentration for most pathogens.[4]

The duration of therapy should be guided by follow-up assessment of clinical course and imaging studies; antibiotic therapy is continued until there is a good clinical response and substantial improvement of imaging findings. CT scanning is helpful in monitoring the response to antibiotics; the size of the abscess or abscesses should decrease over time. We recommend not using MRI for follow-up because abnormalities persist for months, and clinicians utilizing MRI often continue antibiotics for unnecessarily long periods.[28] Contrast enhancement at the site of the abscess may persist for several months.[16] This finding alone is not an indication for continued antibiotic treatment or for surgical exploration.

With the advent of head imaging and the current methods of treatment employing head imaging, an overall reduction in the mortality rate has occurred; however, a high proportion of children with cerebral abscesses develop neurologic deficits. Eradication of potential sources of infection before the abscess has developed is logical preventive medicine. Early diagnosis and treatment are imperative and can be facilitated by the liberal use of MRI or CT when this diagnosis is even a remote consideration.

Antibiotic therapy, emergency surgery, and management of associated complications are the mainstays of treatment of these lesions.

Adjunctive Agents

Adjunctive glucocorticoid therapy may reduce cerebral edema and is used in about half of patients with brain abscess.[15] Since data from randomized studies are lacking and glucocorticoids may reduce passage of antimicrobial agents into the CNS, reduce the contrast enhancement on CT scan, slow capsule formation, and increase the risk of ventricular rupture, its use should be limited to patients with profound edema that is likely to lead to cerebral herniation. Randomized studies of the use of prophylactic anticonvulsant drugs in patients with brain abscess have not been performed. Anticonvulsants are recommended in children who have developed seizures potentially to prevent further episodes. Duration of anticonvulsant therapy should be individualized and guided by an electroencephalographic study in the follow-up phase of disease. Most authors recommend providing at least 3 months of prophylaxis if no more seizures have occurred.[18]

SUBDURAL EMPYEMA

Subdural empyema is defined as a collection of pus in the preformed space between the cranial dura mater and arachnoid mater, while epidural abscess is produced by suppurative infection in the potential epidural space.[63]

Pyogenic infection in the subdural space is designated as subdural empyema or sometimes, but less correctly, as subdural abscess. The sources of infection and microorganisms responsible are the same as those encountered in brain abscess. It is a rare disease; only one case was seen at St. Louis Children's Hospital during a period when 122 patients with bacterial meningitis and three patients with cerebral abscess were treated. The primary source of subdural empyema in this single case was not found, which increasingly is true for the pediatric experience. Farmer and Wise[23] and Jacobson and Farmer[34] found associated meningitis in six of eight infants with subdural empyema (seen over a 16-year period), suggesting that the latter was a complication of the former. We also have encountered this situation, albeit rarely, and the subdural fluid usually is turbid rather than frankly purulent.

In older children, the infection apparently does not follow leptomeningitis. Although leptomeningitis may complicate subdural empyema, infections of the paranasal sinuses and mastoid region, usually chronic, spread to the subdural space directly because of osteomyelitis or by way of infected veins that penetrate the skull. Extension to cortical veins and to major venous sinuses frequently is associated with subdural empyema, as discussed elsewhere in this section. There are three major pathways whereby infection can spread to the subdural space: via phlebitic bridging veins, hematogenous spread, or direct extension from adjacent structures.[12]

Clinical Manifestations

The symptoms and signs of the primary source of infection may be prominent, subtle, or absent. Increasingly severe headache, high fever, signs of meningeal irritation, and progressive neurologic deficits referable to the site of the lesion are reported in the typical untreated case.[8] Focal or generalized seizures are prominent, especially in cases of cortical injury from associated vasculitis. Signs of increased intracranial pressure become prominent as the mass of pus enlarges. In infants, a fullness of fontanelle, vomiting, and depressed responsiveness are seen. Transillumination of the skull can be positive. Older children also may develop papilledema. As the intracranial pressure increases, symptoms and signs progress, ultimately leading to temporal lobe or cerebellar herniation and the characteristic syndromes of these complications.

Diagnosis

The laboratory findings reflect the active infectious process. Peripheral leukocytosis and a predominance of polymorphonuclear leukocytes with immature cells frequently are seen. The CSF in infants reflects the common association with leptomeningitis, and the findings depend on when the fluid is examined. Before the meningitis has been treated adequately, organisms may be cultured; the glucose concentration may be low and the protein concentration high in the CSF. Later the CSF findings are the same as those for treated meningitis, but viable organisms can be recovered from the subdural collections when the CSF is sterile. Specific antigens may be shown in subdural collections by tests such as latex agglutination in the absence of viable organisms. In older children, the characteristic CSF findings include elevated pressure with a few to a few hundred or more leukocytes per microliter, with polymorphonuclear leukocytes predominating. The protein concentration frequently is elevated, the glucose concentration is normal, and the fluid is sterile.

In the past two or more decades, subdural empyema in children has become more difficult to diagnose clinically because of antimicrobial therapy. When initiated early, antimicrobial therapy may attenuate the dramatic nature of the disease, especially the symptoms and signs of acute infection. Because the diagnosis of subdural empyema often is confused with that of brain abscess, radiographic studies are necessary to establish the correct diagnosis. CT may be the most cost-effective imaging modality in epidural abscess and subdural empyema because of its accessibility and sensitivity.[8] CT scans can appear normal in up to 50% of the patients; therefore a high index of suspicion is required, coupled with subtle CT scan clues including minimal midline shift, cortical enhancement, and edema in the adjacent cerebral hemisphere.[51] The use of thin-slice coronal CT scans may help to reduce uncertainty in diagnosis.[47] In our series, the initial CT scan revealed negative findings in 10 cases, which led to delayed diagnosis (Fig. 32.7).

MRI, if available in the acute setting, may be the imaging modality of choice because it provides a better anatomic delineation of any collections that may be present than does CT, and it can adequately display areas of localized meningeal infection.[17] The use of MRI, however,

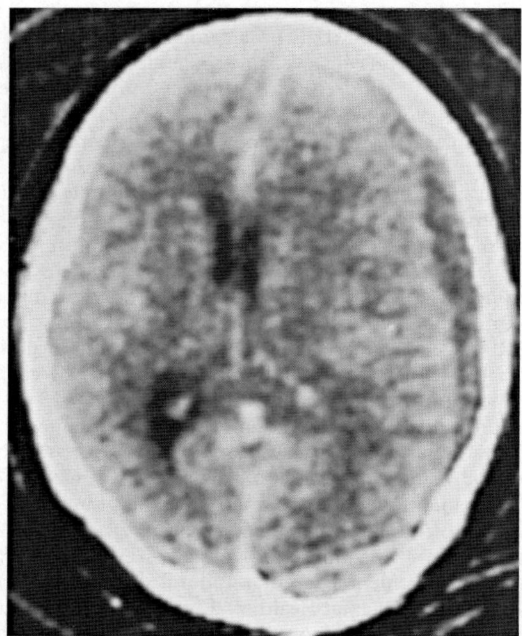

FIG. 32.7 Computed tomography scan shows a subdural empyema with marked displacement of the ventricular system.

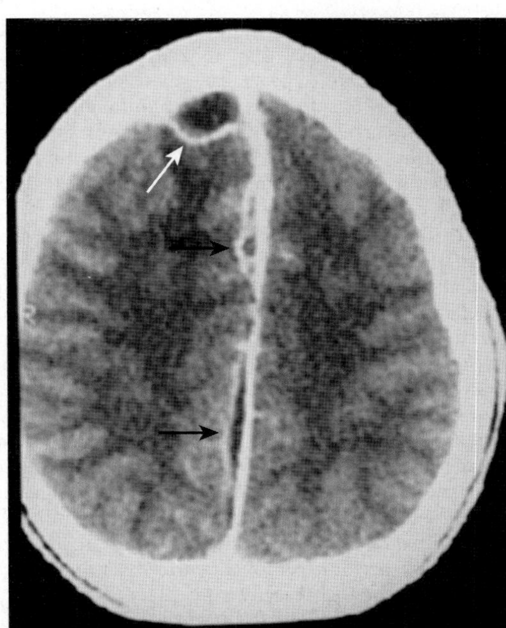

FIG. 32.8 Contrast-enhanced computed tomography scan shows a right frontal epidural abscess *(large arrow)* concurrent with an interhemispheric subdural abscess *(arrowheads)* in a 13-year-old boy who developed headache, fever, and vomiting after fracture of the right frontal sinus. (Courtesy C.D. Robson, MD, Harvard Medical School, Boston, MA, and P.D. Barnes, MD, Stanford University School of Medicine, Stanford, CA.)

must be weighed against the need for urgent diagnosis and intervention for patients in extremis (Fig. 32.8).

Treatment

The preferred treatment for subdural empyemas is surgical evacuation of the purulent collection with simultaneous treatment of the primary source and a prolonged course of high-dose intravenous antibiotics. Craniotomy is the procedure of choice because it has been shown to improve mortality and lead to better clinical improvement and lower rates of reoperation than burr hole drainage.[43]

Until a causative organism is identified, the patient should receive broad-spectrum treatment while awaiting sensitivities; this usually consists of penicillin/amoxicillin plus vancomycin plus a third- or fourth-generation cephalosporin (ceftriaxone or cefepime) and metronidazole.[8,19] After the offending organism is identified, the susceptibilities of that organism to specific antimicrobials dictate selection of more precise antibiotic therapy. In infants, antibiotic therapy may be sufficient when the fluid is cloudy only, but if thick, purulent material is obtained by subdural paracentesis or, in older children, if the clinical and radiographic evidence indicates a subdural empyema, surgery is requisite. Mortality rates have improved considerably over the past 60 years. While subdural empyemas were nearly universally fatal in the presurgical era, mortality rates currently range from 6.7% to 12.2%, reflecting the impact of early diagnosis and treatment on the prognosis of this condition.[43]

EPIDURAL ABSCESS

Because the dura mater is adherent to the inner aspect of the cranium, epidural abscesses rarely attain a large size, and they consequently do not exert significant pressure on the brain. They are important because they can serve as a focus for spread of infection into the subdural space, leptomeninges, or brain. The infection may involve local penetrating vessels and lead to their occlusion, with extension to venous sinuses and other vessels. Infection of the middle ear, mastoid bone, or ancillary air sinuses may lead to epidural abscess, as in the case of subdural empyema and brain abscess. Often epidural abscess coexists with the other lesions and presumably develops first.

Presentation can be subtle, with fever, headache, neck pain, and mental status changes developing over several days. Other findings relate to the primary site of infection and include orbital inflammation, forehead swelling, rhinitis, and otorrhea. Focal deficits and seizures are relatively uncommon.[60]

SPINAL EPIDURAL INFECTIONS

Spinal epidural infections may be acute or chronic, and they may be restricted in their extent or extend longitudinally over many segments of the spinal cord because the epidural space offers no resisting structures. Most often the process affects the posterior region of the spine, with maximal pus or granulomatous tissue found over the dorsal aspect of the cord or spinal roots. In Danner and Hartman's[20] series from the New York Hospital, however, in approximately half of the patients, the pus primarily was anterior to the cord. In spinal osteomyelitis, the pus may be more viscous ventrally. Occasionally the purulent material may encircle the neural elements. In infants and children, this condition is rare; no case was encountered at the St. Louis Children's Hospital during the 39 months in which 122 cases of bacterial meningitis were seen. In an extensive report by Baker and colleagues covering a 27-year period at the Massachusetts General Hospital, only 6 of 39 patients were younger than 20 years of age, and the youngest was 11 years old. The incidence ranged from 0.2 to 1.2 hospital admissions each year. In approximately half of the patients in this series, acute purulent material was discovered at operation or autopsy, with *S. aureus* incriminated in more than half of the cases. In the remainder, a granulomatous process was found associated with a wide variety of bacteria. No instance of tuberculous infection occurred, although in many regions of the world this organism remains an important consideration. Nonbacterial infective agents may include fungi or parasites.

The neural dysfunction probably results from direct compression of the spinal cord, roots, and nerves, but impaired circulation from associated inflammation and occlusion of vessels is at least a contributory factor in some cases. Determining with certainty the extent to which each of the previous mechanisms contributes to neural dysfunction often is difficult. Extensive necrosis of the cord may result in advanced cases in which a prompt diagnosis has not been made.

Sources of Infection

In tuberculous and other chronic infections, osteomyelitis and intervertebral disk infection are common occurrences, but adults primarily are affected. Acute spinal epidural infections usually occur after hematogenous spread from furuncles, pharyngitis, dental abscesses, decubitus ulcers, and urinary tract and wound infections.[36] They may complicate spinal surgery, and lumbar puncture rarely has been implicated as a source.[6] Osteomyelitis seldom occurs. The patient may have a history of minor trauma to the back. Presumably trauma results in local tissue injury or hemorrhage forming a nidus for the developing infection.

Clinical Manifestations

Fever is the rule, and the temperature is higher in patients with acute infections. Patients appear septic, and toxic delirium occurs frequently. Heusner,[29] in his classic article dealing primarily with acute epidural abscesses, divided the clinical phases as follows: (1) spinal ache, (2) root pain, (3) weakness, and (4) paralysis. Although certain therapeutic implications render this separation a useful way to consider the disorder, phases 3 and 4 are combined in the following discussion. That the various stages often overlap is axiomatic.

Phase 1: Spinal Ache

Spinal ache was a universal finding in Heusner's experience.[29] In a report from Baker and associates,[7] all 39 patients had backache of various degrees of severity. Local tenderness was absent in only two of their patients and should be searched for by carefully tapping over the spine.

Phase 2: Root Pain

Root pain is characteristic and is an early symptom that may assist in localization of the pathologic process. Root pain especially is prominent with lumbosacral disease, in which roots are implicated without involvement of the spinal cord. The diagnosis is suspected infrequently until functional motor and sensory losses occur, which is unfortunate because therapy is most effective during the early stages. Progression to symptoms and signs of spinal cord involvement usually occurs within a few days except when the process is granulomatous, in which case the course tends to be prolonged, extending over several or more weeks.

Phases 3 and 4: Weakness and Paralysis

After weakness and impaired sensation referable to disease of the spinal cord appear, the progression to paralysis can be rapid, and immediate surgical treatment is imperative to maximize the likelihood of reasonable functional recovery. Even appropriate therapy at this stage often is ineffective, however, in restoring normal neurologic functions. Death occurs in at least 20% of cases; this rate has not changed significantly since 1948 despite the availability of a wide range of antibiotic agents.

Diagnosis

The value of MRI in the diagnosis and differential diagnosis of pediatric spinal infection is well established.[37] Diagnostic MRI findings of spinal infection include bone marrow edema, destruction of the affected vertebrae, abnormal signal intensity of the contiguous disk, and paraspinal or epidural extension of infection (Fig. 32.9). Epidural and paravertebral soft tissue changes on short-term follow-up MRI correlated better with patients' clinical symptoms compared with bone and disk destruction. Bone and disk changes can appear to progress more so than soft tissue infection despite adequate clinical response to therapy. Although MRI is essential for initial diagnosis, serial routine follow-up MR images were not necessary for the vast majority of cases. Wang and colleagues[64] examined 35 whole-spine and 16 localized spinal scans from 17 patients (age 2 months to 16 years; 9 female, 8 male) who had 51 follow-up imaging studies done 2 weeks to 4.75 years after baseline. Seven children (41%) younger than 3 years of age underwent 33 follow-ups (65%); most required general anesthesia or conscious sedation. Short-term follow-up scans demonstrated epidural and/or paraspinal soft tissue changes correlating with clinical status and laboratory findings in all cases. However, MRI showed that bone and/or disk abnormalities continued and progressed in some cases despite clinical improvement.[64]

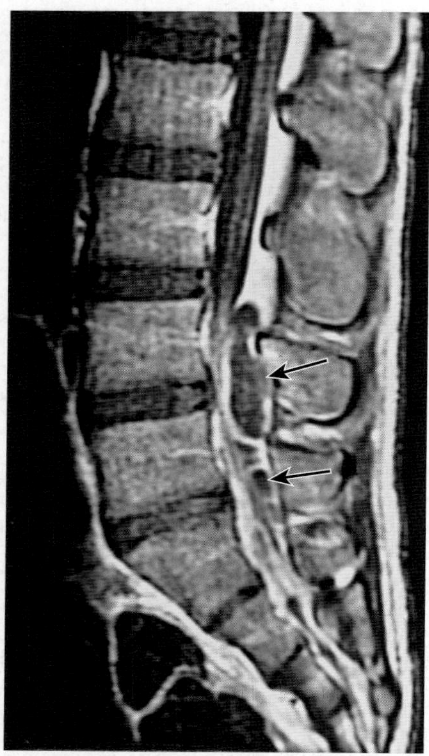

FIG. 32.9 Gadolinium-enhanced, sagittal, T1-weighted magnetic resonance image shows a rim-enhancing lumbar spinal epidural abscess *(arrows)* in a 15-year-old boy with a 3-week history of lower back pain, followed by rapidly progressing left leg numbness and decreased bowel and bladder function. *Staphylococcus aureus* was cultured from purulent fluid removed after L4–L5 laminectomy was performed. (Courtesy C.D. Robson, MD, Harvard Medical School, Boston, MA, and P.D. Barnes, MD, Stanford University School of Medicine, Stanford, CA.)

Follow-up MRI is not needed for patients with good clinical response; these patients should be observed clinically and/or have laboratory markers of inflammation tested. The segment of the pediatric population that might benefit from follow-up MRI includes those whose condition deteriorates clinically and those too young for a clinical response to be accurately assessed. If follow-up MRI is indicated, a localized spine scan rather than a whole-spine scan is recommended unless disease extension beyond the original focus is suggested. After epidural abscess is discovered, immediate neurosurgical intervention is necessary to prevent long-term neurologic sequelae. At the time of surgery, stains and cultures for aerobic and anaerobic bacteria, mycobacteria, and fungi should be obtained. If lumbar puncture is attempted when epidural abscess is suspected, the spinal needle (with stylet) is advanced slowly into the lumbar region, with periodic removal of the stylet and with suction applied gently *before* the thecal sac is entered.

If purulent material is obtained, the diagnosis is established, and the pus must be examined by a Gram-stained smear and cultured on various media under aerobic and anaerobic conditions. The leptomeninges should not be penetrated if purulent material is encountered; otherwise, CSF should be obtained. Characteristically the CSF is clear or slightly opalescent and yellow if there is a block. Pleocytosis with a few to many hundred cells (with lymphocytes predominating) reflects a contiguous infectious process, but in the absence of meningitis no organisms can be identified, and the CSF glucose concentration should be normal. The protein concentration always is elevated, and the level may be very high (several hundred to 2000 mg/dL) in the case of a partial or total manometric block.

The differential diagnosis includes myelitis caused by bacterial meningitis, syphilis, viruses, and a parainfectious process and by the syndrome of acute transverse myelopathy of unknown cause. Spinal ache is most prominent in acute transverse myelopathy, but, as a general rule, the entire illness is compressed in time, with paresis or paralysis evolving over the course of hours or a few days from the onset of disease. Impaired circulation of CSF does not occur in this or the aforementioned disorders. Rarely a lymphoma may mimic a spinal epidural abscess. Spinal cord tumors, vascular malformations, and arachnoiditis are considerations when the course of disease is prolonged and evidence of sepsis is minimal or absent, as occurs with chronic epidural infections.

Treatment

Owing to variable etiology, identification of the responsible microorganism through neurosurgical drainage followed by long-term intravenous antibiotics remains the mainstay in treating extraaxial CNS infections. Optimal outcome is achieved with early diagnosis and therapy. Initial empiric antibiotic coverage is similar to that for brain abscess, although antifungal therapy need not be included unless cultures or stains are positive for fungi. Treatment typically should be continued for 3 to 4 weeks, but it should be prolonged for twice this period if the patient has osteomyelitis. Despite advances, the morbidity and mortality rates for spinal epidural abscess remain high. One-third of children with the disease die, and another third are left with permanent neurologic sequelae, including weakness, incontinence, and sensory abnormalities. Rapid diagnosis and treatment are essential to ensure a successful outcome.

NEW REFERENCES SINCE THE SEVENTH EDITION

2. Al Masalma M, Lonjon M, Richet H, et al. Metagenomic analysis of brain abscesses identifies specific bacterial associations. *Clin Infect Dis.* 2012;54(2): 202-210.

11. Biswas B, Mondal M, Thapa R, et al. Neonatal brain abscess due to extended-spectrum beta-lactamase producing klebsiella pneumoniae. *J Clin Diagn Res.* 2014;8(11):PD1-PD2.

12. Bonfield CM, Sharma J, Dobson S. Pediatric intracranial abscesses. *J Infect.* 2015;71(suppl 1):S42-S46.
15. Brouwer MC, Coutinho JM, van de Beek D. Clinical characteristics and outcome of brain abscess: systematic review and meta-analysis. *Neurology*. 2014;82(9): 806-813.
19. Cole TS, Clark ME, Jenkins AJ, et al. Pediatric focal intracranial suppuration: a UK single-center experience. *Childs Nerv Syst*. 2012;28(12):2109-2114.
28. Helweg-Larsen J, Astradsson A, Richhall H, et al. Pyogenic brain abscess, a 15 year survey. *BMC Infect Dis*. 2012;12:332.
45. Muccio CF, Caranci F, D'Arco F, et al. Magnetic resonance features of pyogenic brain abscesses and differential diagnosis using morphological and functional imaging studies: a pictorial essay. *J Neuroradiol*. 2014;41(3):153-167.

The full reference list for this chapter is available at ExpertConsult.com.

33 Fungal Meningitis

José R. Romero • Richard F. Jacobs

Fungi are rare causes of meningitis in children. Fungal meningitis is also frequently chronic, and patients may lack obvious meningeal signs and symptoms, often causing a delay in establishing the diagnosis. Fungal central nervous system (CNS) disease generally has high morbidity and mortality rates. Making a diagnosis can be difficult due to the fastidious growth, the prolonged time needed for culture, and the requirement of special media of many fungi. Because cultivating fungi from the cerebrospinal fluid (CSF) is frequently difficult, the use of serologic tests for antibodies and antigens helps define the infection more quickly and with greater sensitivity. These tests can be performed on CSF, serum, and, in some instances, urine.[162] For most infections, lipid formulations of amphotericin B (AmB) or newer triazoles have become the drugs of choice for treatment.

EPIDEMIOLOGY

The epidemiology of fungal meningitis depends on many factors. Geographic location of the patient or travel to an endemic area can be an important diagnostic clue, and the geographic distribution of fungal meningitis varies in the United States and worldwide. Histoplasmosis generally occurs in endemic areas of the Mississippi River Valley.[161] Coccidioidomycosis occurs in the San Joaquin Valley and the southwestern United States and in Mexico.[4,107] Cryptococcosis distribution is worldwide but seems to be associated with pigeon droppings and nesting areas of other birds.[88] Blastomycosis has a sporadic pattern of infectivity but generally occurs in states bordering the Mississippi and Ohio river basins, with occasional outbreaks occurring in the Great Lakes region and Canada.[44,77,132] *Candida* spp., *Aspergillus* spp., *Sporothrix schenckii,* and other fungal pathogens generally are not defined by geographic boundaries but depend more on environmental exposures and the immunocompetence of the individual. Uncommon species of yeasts and fungi, including *Rhodotorula mucilaginosa* (formerly *Rhodotorula* rubra), *Aureobasidium mansoni, Clavispora lusitaniae, Bipolaris spicifera,* and *Exserohilum rostratum* have been reported in nosocomial or iatrogenic cases of meningitis.[60,82,140] The latter agent was associated with a multistate outbreak of nearly 750 cases of meningitis due to contaminated methylprednisolone solution used for injections.[140]

Many fungal infections (particularly those caused by *Histoplasma* and *Candida* spp.) do not usually cause meningitis unless the host is immunocompromised. A 6-year review from a large children's hospital found the incidence rate of cryptococcal infection to be 6.2 cases per 1 million hospitalizations: 20.6% were immunocompetent, 63.5% were HIV-negative with immunocompromising conditions, and 16% were HIV positive. Patients with cryptococcal meningitis comprised 38% of patients in the study.[68] Risk factors for developing *Candida* meningitis include prolonged antimicrobial therapy, indwelling venous or ventricular catheters, hyperalimentation, corticosteroid use, recent neurosurgery or intraabdominal surgery, and intravenous drug abuse.[103,125,147] Pediatric cases occur most commonly in neonates, particularly in very-low-birth-weight newborns.[10,51,62,66,138] Of neonates with candidemia, 5% to 9% have associated meningitis.[28]

DIAGNOSIS

Specific information about the diagnosis of individual organisms is provided in subsequent sections. Table 33.1 provides specific data for some fungal meningitides.

In order to improve the chances of diagnosis, as much CSF as can be removed safely should be obtained, especially at the time of ventriculography or pneumoencephalography.[39] For nonneonates, a minimum of 5 mL of CSF has been suggested, based on experimental work.[90] Repeated cultures of large volumes of CSF may be helpful.[39] The CSF should be centrifuged and the sediment saved for culture and India ink preparation with the supernatant sent for serologic tests. The India ink test should be interpreted with caution and must be followed with cultures because artifacts frequently can cause misinterpretation.[39] The cumulative efficacy of repeated lumbar punctures (LPs) for cryptococcal meningitis can improve the sensitivity of the India ink smear from 26% in one LP to 52.6% with the second.[95] If large volumes are available, membrane filtration may be used to concentrate the fungal elements. The membrane containing the fungi is placed aseptically on isolation media and incubated at 30°C for 4 weeks. The CSF that passes through the membrane can be used for serology or chemistry determinations.[95] The remaining CSF can be inoculated onto Sabouraud glucose agar, blood agar, and brain-heart infusion agar or into broth media or into both types of media. *Candida* can be cultured but may require a prolonged incubation period. CSF cultures generally are unhelpful for *Histoplasma, Blastomyces,* and other dimorphic fungi. For organisms such as *Histoplasma, Blastomyces,* and *Coccidioides,* culturing other body fluids, such as blood, urine, sputum, or draining wounds, can be helpful.

CLINICAL MANIFESTATIONS

Physical manifestations diagnostic for causes of fungal meningitis (e.g., *Cryptococcus, Blastomyces,* and *Histoplasma*) are rarely found because the infections usually are chronic. Careful examination, especially of the skin, is very important. All superficial lesions, nodules, and draining abscesses should be investigated because they may give a clue to the cause of subacute and chronic infections (e.g., *Coccidioides, Blastomyces,* and *Cryptococcus*).[56] Fungal stains, including India ink, and culture should be performed on all biopsy specimens and drainage material. Bone involvement is common with *Cryptococcus* and *Blastomyces.*

The significance of isolating a fungus from CSF cannot be overemphasized. The finding of fungal organisms should be considered a true infection, and appropriate antifungal therapy initiated. However, a single CSF culture for *Candida* in an otherwise immunocompetent host, or an unlikely meningeal pathogen with an otherwise normal CSF should lead the physician to consider the possibility of contamination.[7] Repeat CSF cultures should be sought in such cases.

TABLE 33.1 **Fungal Cerebrospinal Fluid Characteristics**

Organism	WBCs	Protein	Glucose	Smears	Serology	Cultures
Blastomyces	Variable up to 15,000 cells/mm^3 with PMNs or lymphocytes	Elevated up to 300 mg/dL	Normal or low	Rare on smear	No good serology	CSF cultures rarely positive; increased yield with ventricular taps
Candida	Mean 600 cells/mm^3 up to 1900 cells/mm^3 with lymphocytes or PMNs	Elevated	Low or normal	40% positive on smears	Serology not helpful	CSF cultures useful
Coccidioides	100–750 WBCs, mostly lymphocytes	150–2000 mg/dL	21–62% serum	Rare on smear	CSF CF antibody positive in 75–95%	CSF cultures positive in 33–60%
Cryptococcus	40–400 WBCs, mostly lymphocytes	High	Low	India ink positive in 25–50%	CSF and serum cryptococcal antigen positive in 85–90%	CSF cultures positive in 75%
Histoplasma	0–300 WBCs, lymphocytes, or PMNs; most 11–101/mm^3	Usually elevated, but can be normal	Usually low (<40 mg/dL) to normal	Rare on smear	Polysaccharide antigen in urine, blood, CSF positive in 61%	CSF cultures positive in 27–65%

CF, Complement fixation; *CSF,* cerebrospinal fluid; *PMNs,* polymorphonuclear leukocytes; *WBCs,* white blood cells.
Data from references 50, 58, 96, and 160.

Infection With Specific Organisms

Candidal Meningitis

Candidal meningitis is rare in children. In one study, 2% of all positive CSF cultures were fungal organisms, and *Candida* spp. accounted for 94.5% of the fungal isolates.[7] Risk factors for positive CSF *Candida* cultures in neonates included antimicrobial therapy, umbilical or peripherally inserted central catheterization, total parenteral nutrition, intubation, abdominal surgery, and prematurity.[42,41,168] In many cases of neonatal candidiasis, concurrent meningitis was not discovered until autopsy.[28] Extremely low-birth-weight infants with *Candida* sepsis or meningitis have an increased risk of death or neurodevelopmental impairment.[1] Risk factors in children beyond the neonatal period included concurrent bacterial infection, chronic systemic or CNS disease, and the presence of central venous catheters.

Children with human immunodeficiency virus (HIV) infection are at risk for acquiring disseminated *Candida* infections, including meningitis.[86] In one study, 27% of HIV-infected patients with disseminated *Candida* infections had CNS involvement.[86] Nearly all HIV-infected patients who develop *Candida* infection do so as a result of nosocomial infection. Predisposing factors include oral candidiasis, central venous catheters, prolonged antibiotic therapy, and total parenteral nutrition. Simultaneous pulmonary disease, particularly viral, bacterial, or *Pneumocystis jiroveci* pneumonias, exists in most HIV-infected patients with disseminated *Candida* infection. Most patients are febrile for more than 14 days, with peak temperatures of greater than 39°C (102.2°F) before the diagnosis is established.

Myeloperoxidase deficiency is also associated with the risk of developing infection.[91] A mutation in *CARD9,* a molecule that receives signals from several antifungal pattern-recognition receptors, is associated with chronic mucocutaneous candidiasis and meningitis.[49,81]

Infections caused by *Candida* spp. in very-low-birth-weight newborns can be difficult to diagnose because of the broad range of symptoms. Most infants with disseminated candidiasis with meningitis present with respiratory distress and a supplemental oxygen requirement, and most progress to require mechanical ventilation.[10] *Candida* usually is identified in endotracheal washings, urine, and blood in patients with *Candida* meningitis. Infants have symptoms on average 11 days before the diagnosis is made. Ophthalmologic examinations are very important in identifying disseminated *Candida* infections.[25] Marked abdominal distention occurs commonly in disseminated *Candida* infections in very-low-birth-weight infants and frequently is associated with guaiac-positive stools. Most patients have temperature instability, elevated white blood cell counts, and feeding intolerance. Hepatomegaly may indicate systemic infection.

Antifungal resistance in *Candida* spp. is a concern. Clinical breakpoints for antifungal agents against common *Candida* species have been published.[108] Isolates of *C. glabrata* and *C. krusei* resistant to AmB exist.[160] *C. lusitaniae* has intrinsic resistance to AmB and has been reported as a cause of meningitis.[126] *C. krusei* demonstrates near uniform azole resistance, particularly in immunocompromised patients receiving suppressive azole therapy. Isolates from patients with meningitis due to *C. glabrata* or any *Candida* spp. who are slow to clear infection, or in whom unexpected relapse occurs, should undergo antifungal susceptibility evaluation.[108]

For nonneonates the initial therapy of *Candida* meningitis is with liposomal AmB alone or in combination with oral flucytosine (FCYT).[108] Once the patient has responded, fluconazole (FCZ) is recommended if susceptible. Therapy should continue until signs, symptoms, and CSF abnormalities have resolved. In neonates, AmB deoxycholate is recommended initially.[108] Alternatively, liposomal AmB may be used.[108] Once the neonate has responded to initial therapy FCZ may be used.[108] FCYT may be considered as salvage therapy for neonates who have not responded to AmB therapy. However, it is difficult to use in neonates and low-birth-weight infants because of the immaturity of their gastrointestinal tracts and the risk for developing necrotizing enterocolitis. AmB deoxycholate for children and neonates should begin at the desired daily dose and not be preceded by smaller test doses. The use of FCYT requires careful monitoring and adjustment of dosage based on serum determinations.

Voriconazole (VCZ) has excellent penetration of the CNS and is active against most *Candida* isolates causing CNS infections; however, the clinical experience with VCZ in neonates is too limited to recommend its use at this time.[65] Caspofungin and the other echinocandins do not achieve adequate CSF concentrations[34,117] but do achieve appropriate brain parenchyma concentrations and have been successfully used for therapy.[59]

Cryptococcosis

Cryptococcosis is a systemic fungal infection, and meningitis is its most serious manifestation. Cryptococcal meningitis was rare in the United States in the pre-HIV era; however, due to HIV it has become the most common cause of fungal meningitis in immunocompromised patients, infecting 2% to 9% of adults with AIDS.[26,37,78,89,160] In the United States and worldwide it remains an uncommon finding in pediatric patients.[87,101,122,145] In adult studies, progressively severe headaches without the presence of fever were common manifestations.[150] Patients frequently have few symptoms but can present with nausea, dizziness, and irritability. Nuchal rigidity is usually absent. Cranial nerve palsies are found in approximately one-fifth of adult patients. Diplopia is one of the most common manifestations. Papilledema is seen in nearly one-third of patients.[36] Patients with coexistent AIDS frequently have very few symptoms.[37]

Pediatric patients with cryptococcal meningitis usually have signs and symptoms not referable to the CNS.[136] In a report of 13 U.S. children with AIDS[85] diagnosed with extrapulmonary cryptococcosis, meningitis was found in 62% and was the most common form of extrapulmonary disease. In eight U.S. children with acute lymphoblastic leukemia (ALL) who developed extrapulmonary cryptococcosis, 63% had meningitis.[84] Fever was the most common symptom, occurring in 60%. Headache was present in only 40% and an equal percentage were asymptomatic. In the latter, LPs performed as part of their routine management revealed unexpected growth of *C. neoformans* on culture. Treatment in this series of ALL patients included AmB (intravenous, intrathecal, or both), alone or combined with oral FCYT. Relapse was a major complication, occurring in 60% of patients thought to have been treated successfully. Relapses occurred within 2 to 6 months of completing therapy. Treatment of the relapses generally included combination therapy of AmB and FCYT, with the occasional use of intrathecal AmB.

An 18-year review of cases of *Cryptococcus* infection in Colombia identified only 41 cases (2.6%) among 1578 cases in a national database.[89] Neurocryptococcosis accounted for 87.8% of presentations. Ten children had HIV infection, 11 had other risk factors, and 19 had no identifiable risk factor. The most frequent signs and symptoms were headache (78.1%), fever (68.8%), nausea and vomiting (65.6%), and confusion (50%). Meningeal signs, alteration of vision, and seizures and other neurologic signs were found in 28.1%, 28.1%, and 18.8%, respectively. AmB alone or in combination with FCZ, FCYT, itraconazole (ITZ), or caspofungin was used for treatment in the majority of patients.

Illnesses predisposing to cryptococcal meningitis include systemic lupus erythematosus treated with corticosteroids alone or in combination with azathioprine,[3,84,87,120] chronic mucocutaneous candidiasis,[61,155] and hyper-IgE syndrome.[143] Zoonotic transmission has occurred.[132]

Direct examination of the CSF using the India ink test can provide an immediate presumptive diagnosis. The sensitivity of this test varies, but in studies of adult patients with AIDS, positive results approached 75%.[26] Other useful stains include silver, periodic acid–Schiff, and mucicarmine. Gram stain of CSF is insensitive and unreliable.

Diagnosis of cryptococcal meningitis is aided by serologic tests. The most common is the cryptococcal capsular polysaccharide antigen test, which can be performed on serum, CSF, or other sterile body fluids. Its sensitivity is nearly 100% for the serum of patients who are HIV positive.[27,78,170] The CSF antigen test in some studies seems to be less sensitive (91%).[26] In patients not infected with HIV, the sensitivity of the serologic test in the CSF approaches 90%.[58] False-positive results caused by cross-reactions of antigens in disseminated infections with *Trichosporon beigelii* have been reported.[96] Culture remains the gold standard for establishing the diagnosis and monitoring of therapy.[115]

Treatment of cryptococcal meningitis is prolonged and, in immunocompromised patients, frequently requires lifelong maintenance therapy. Practice guidelines have been published for children.[115,135] For HIV-negative, non–transplant recipient children, AmB deoxycholate plus FCYT should be given for at least 2 weeks as induction therapy if no neurologic complications are present and CSF culture performed at 2 weeks of therapy is negative. Liposomal AmB or AmB lipid complex may be substituted for AmB deoxycholate in those intolerant to the latter. In patients with neurologic complications, consideration for extension of the induction phase to 4 to 6 weeks using a lipid formulation of AmB for the final 4 weeks of therapy should be made. Consolidation using oral FCZ for 8 weeks follows, and, on completion, maintenance therapy with FCZ should be started and continued for 6 to 12 months.

For HIV-infected children, induction therapy consisting of AmB plus FCYT for 2 weeks followed by consolidation with FCZ for 8 weeks is recommended. For patients intolerant of AmB, the use of lipid formulations of AmB should be considered.[83,115,135] The combination of AmB plus FCYT results in rapid sterilization of the CSF and was associated with improved survival.[18,32] FCZ is used for maintenance therapy for 1 year or longer. Most experts would not discontinue maintenance therapy for children younger than 6 years.[135] Based on adult data, for children 6 years and older receiving highly active antiretroviral therapy with a CD4 cell count of 100 cells/μL or greater and low or undetectable viral RNA level for 3 months or more, maintenance therapy may be discontinued after a minimum of 1 year but should be restarted if the CD4 cell count falls below 100 cells/μL.[115,135]

In patients with renal compromise associated with AmB, FCYT levels must be monitored carefully. The dose of FCYT should be reduced based on glomerular filtration rate, and continuing doses should be adjusted to maintain serum FCYT levels of 25 to 60 μg/mL.[8,136] Serum cryptococcal antigens are not useful in monitoring response to therapy, and the use of CSF cryptococcal antigens to monitor response to therapy also is controversial. Therapy is best judged to be successful by the demonstration of sterility of CSF fungal cultures.

Histoplasmosis

Infection with *Histoplasma capsulatum*, usually a benign and self-limited disease, is endemic in many parts of the United States. Disseminated disease, including meningitis, is a rare occurrence in children.[72,102,104,112,128,148] Case reports of adults generally describe immunocompromised individuals.[48,153] Clinical presentations vary widely in the manifestation of meningitis. In these cases, 39% presented with meningitis associated with acute dissemination, 25% presented with single histoplasmoma that manifested as symptomatic mass lesions alone or with dissemination, 25% presented with chronic meningitis without evidence of dissemination, and the remaining patients presented with meningitis as a manifestation of recurrent disease. Rarely embolization to the brain caused by *Histoplasma* endocarditis has been associated with meningitis.[161]

Meningitis occurring in patients with AIDS has become common in endemic areas. In one report, disseminated histoplasmosis caused 8% of the AIDS-defining illnesses in children.[124] The duration of symptoms varies. In patients without AIDS, the symptoms generally last longer than 6 months and can last 7 years.[39,48,110,156] In patients with AIDS, symptoms usually manifest more acutely and within a much shorter time frame.[161] In one series, neurologic findings occurred in all but 6% of the patients.[161] The most common signs and symptoms include depressed consciousness (29%), headaches (24%), confusion (22%), cranial nerve deficits (19%), other focal deficits (16%), seizures (14%), personality changes (12%), and ataxia (11%). Findings such as meningismus, Babinski sign, or papilledema were seen in less than 8%. In adult patients without AIDS, the death rate is approximately 12%, with a relapse rate of 44%. In adult patients with AIDS, the death rate is 100% in some series.[5,164]

Diagnosis can be aided by serologic testing. High levels of anti–*H. capsulatum* antibodies were detected in the serum of 70%. CSF serology was helpful in 75% of patients who were tested. Culture of the CSF was positive for fewer than half of the cases in one review.[72] In a second series in patients with AIDS, cultures of blood, bone marrow, respiratory secretions, and brain or meninges were positive in 49%, 53%, 58%, and 75%, respectively. Ten to 25% of patients with disseminated disease lack a positive antibody response. Serology may be false positive in patients with other fungal diseases or tuberculosis. The antibody response to acute *Histoplasma* infection may remain elevated for years. The use of *Histoplasma* antigen is a useful test in immunocompromised patients with disseminated *Histoplasma*.[161]

Treatment with liposomal AmB given over 4 to 6 weeks, followed by ITZ for a minimum of 1 year and until CSF abnormalities have resolved, including *Histoplasma* antigen levels, is currently recommended.[163,164] The liposomal form provides higher CNS levels than the deoxycholate form. However, none of the AmB formulations achieves detectable concentrations in the CSF.[163] The use of intrathecal AmB is not recommended for *H. capsulatum* meningitis. A trial comparing AmB with liposomal AmB (AmBisome, LAmB) as induction therapy showed that the agents had similar efficacy for treating disseminated histoplasmosis.[67] Determination of ITZ serum trough blood levels should be performed to ensure appropriate drug levels.[165]

Patients with AIDS for whom induction therapy was successful must remain on an anti-*Histoplasma* agent indefinitely. A few cases of children with disseminated histoplasmosis and AIDS have been reported, but none with meningitis; in these children, antifungal therapy must be continued indefinitely.[20,130] A case report demonstrated that ketoconazole was ineffective for preventing recurrence of nonmeningeal disseminated disease.[130] Because of its poor CNS penetration, it is likely to be ineffective for prophylaxis of meningitis. In patients with AIDS, some success has been achieved with the use of ITZ for suppressive therapy in disseminated disease. However, few data exist on its use for suppressive therapy for meningitis or CNS disease caused by *Histoplasma*. For maintenance therapy, FCZ (high dose), ITZ, or intravenous AmB are available. In a case report, FCZ was effective in an adult with disease refractory to AmB therapy.[149]

Coccidioidomycosis

C. immitis (*Coccidioides posadasii* in Texas and Central and South America) meningitis is a more common cause of chronic meningitis than is *Histoplasma*.[64] The incidence of coccidioidomycosis has increased substantially in the past two decades.[23]

The rate of hospitalization for coccidioidal meningitis in California increased approximately twofold from 2001 to 2011.[141] Over the 12-year period, 13% of hospitalizations for coccidioidomycosis were due to meningitis.[140] Approximately 1% of children with symptomatic pulmonary disease develop disseminated disease.[69] Of patients with disseminated coccidioidomycosis, 15% to 20% develop meningitis.[69,74] History of exposure is a crucial factor in diagnosing this disease and relies on careful questioning regarding travel to or residence in an endemic area.[144,146] Exposure of wounds to colonized soil has been implicated in at least one pediatric case.[100] An association between facial cutaneous coccidioidomycosis and meningitis has been described.[9] Coccidioidomycosis in infancy was described more than 40 years ago.[151] Infants usually have severe disease with high mortality rates and morbidity.

CSF shows a mononuclear pleocytosis with an elevated protein and decreased glucose concentration. Elevated CSF pressures may herald the development of hydrocephalus. Diagnosis is made easier by the availability of reliable serologic tests. Complement-fixing antibodies appear in the CSF only in patients with meningitis and provide a sensitivity of 76%.[139] Sensitivity was increased to 96% when the complement-fixation test was incubated at 4°C.[101] Based on pooling five studies, *Coccidioides* can be cultured from the CSF of 76% of patients with meningitis but was seen on direct CSF examination in only 8%.[95] Experts in the field consider that the rate of positive CSF cultures is much lower (approximately 33%) and that visualization of the organism in CSF by direct examination rarely occurs.[142]

If untreated, *Coccidioides* meningitis is uniformly fatal. FCZ is the drug of choice for treatment of meningitis and has a success rate of 79%.[46] It is also used for sustaining remission.[114] Practice guidelines exist for the treatment of coccidioidomycosis in adults.[45] Therapy with oral FCZ is preferred; 9 to 12 months have been shown effective in adults,[46,152] but no controlled studies in pediatric patients have been published. If treatment is begun with azole therapy, it should be continued for life.[35]

ITZ is reported to be effective for the treatment of *Coccidioides* meningitis.[45] Because of its variable oral bioavailability, monitoring for adequate serum drug levels is recommended.[154] Adult patients with *Coccidioides* meningitis had high relapse rates (40–50%), which rendered them dependent on lifelong therapy with ITZ.[53]

Clinical trials with large numbers of children do not exist for the azoles; some authorities consider intravenous and intrathecal AmB to be the standard therapy for coccidioidal meningitis. It also is recommended for patients who do not respond to FCZ or ITZ treatment. Some experts initially use a combination of oral azole with intrathecal AmB with the thought that responses are more prompt with this approach. AmB can be administered intrathecally into the lumbar area or cisterna magna or by using an Ommaya reservoir.[33,47,80,169]

The initial dose of AmB administered into the CSF is 0.025 mg. The dose is increased by doubling until a maintenance dose of 0.1 to 0.5 mg is attained. After this dose has been achieved, therapy can be given every other day, alternating with intravenous administration of AmB. Therapy is continued until the child's condition has stabilized, at which point intrathecal therapy gradually can be stretched out to every 3 weeks. This program is continued until the CSF indices are normal and culture results have been negative for at least 1 year.

Use of VCZ has been successful in two case reports, and other similar anecdotal references have been reported at referral centers.[45,29,118] VCZ, posaconazole, or VCZ plus caspofungin have been used for salvage therapy alone or in combination with liposomal AmB.[29,45,75,117,118,127]

Blastomycosis

Blastomyces dermatitidis is an uncommon cause of chronic meningitis and is difficult to diagnose premortem unless the patient has other signs of systemic blastomycosis. When systemic blastomycosis occurs, it can involve the CNS in 5% to 10% of cases.[16] A review of CNS cases of blastomycosis revealed that approximately 23% were not associated with extraneural disease.[11] Common extraneural sites include bone, genitourinary tract, and skin.[12,17] Previously blastomycosis most often affected immunocompetent patients. Fifty-five percent of cases of CNS blastomycosis involve individuals with immunosuppressive conditions.[11] Patients with AIDS are at high risk for developing chronic infection.[57] Because of the difficulty in diagnosing *Blastomyces* meningitis and its similarities to tuberculous meningitis, patients usually are treated for presumptive tuberculous meningitis.[50,99] Although meningitis is the most common form of CNS blastomycosis, solitary mass lesions also can occur.[19,123] A review of 22 cases treated from 1990 to 2008 demonstrated a mortality rate of 18%.[11]

Examination of CSF obtained by LP usually is negative.[11] However, the yield from ventricular fluid seems to be higher.[79] Diagnosis relies on the characteristic histopathologic appearance in tissues and occasionally on culture of ventricular CSF. Culture isolation of *Blastomyces* from the CSF is possible in approximately half of cases.[11] Testing for the presence of *B. dermatitidis* antigen may yield better results. In one report, all CSF samples tested using a commercially available assay were found to be positive. Blastomycosis meningitis is associated with a pleocytosis that may be lymphocytic or neutrophilic in nature.[11] The CSF protein is elevated in the majority of cases.[11] Meningitis caused by *B. dermatitidis* frequently has a neutrophilic predominance.[11,57] Seeking *Blastomyces* from other sources, including sputum and urine, is indicated. In a study of AIDS patients, examination of sputum was useful for establishing the diagnosis of disseminated blastomycosis.[109]

Treatment of CNS blastomycosis relies on the administration of the lipid formulation of AmB for 4 to 6 weeks, followed by oral azole therapy (i.e., FCZ, ITZ, VCZ) for a minimum of 12 months or until CSF abnormalities have resolved.[24] For children, no specific recommendations exist for the treatment of CNS disease, although for children with severe blastomycosis AmB deoxycholate or a lipid formulation of amphotericin is recommended for initial therapy. ITZ is recommended as follow-up therapy for 12 months.[24] A review favors the use of VCZ as the azole of choice after initial therapy with lipid formulation of amphotericin.[11] Azoles should not be considered for primary treatment of CNS blastomycosis. Children respond less satisfactorily to oral azole therapy than do adults.[129] Although only a few published reports exist supporting the use of lipid formulations of AmB to treat CNS blastomycosis, these drugs are preferred because of the need of prolonged duration of therapy in these patients. Experimental animal data exist demonstrating superior penetration of liposomal AmB compared with lipid complex or the deoxycholate formulations of amphotericin.[54]

Aspergillosis

CNS infections with *Aspergillus fumigatus* and other *Aspergillus* spp. are associated with a high mortality rate. In a review containing 47 cases of *Aspergillus* meningitis alone the overall case fatality rate was 64.5%, a significant number of whom were immunocompromised.[6] The same report contained 15 cases of chronic meningitis and 5 cases of spinal arachnoiditis, among whom the mortality rates were 47% and 40%, respectively. Conditions placing patients at risk include neurosurgical procedures, spinal anesthesia, organ and bone marrow transplantation, malignancies, diabetes, and AIDS.[6] Some early reports of CNS aspergillosis were in infants who appeared to be normal.[2,92] Modes of acquisition include extension from a contiguous focus, intravenous drug abuse, hematogenous spread, and iatrogenic introduction.[119] In addition to brain abscesses, manifestations of *Aspergillus* spp. CNS infection include meningoencephalitis, isolated spinal cord lesions, aqueductal stenosis, and mycotic aneurysms.[6,22,154,162,167] Magnetic resonance imaging is superior to computed tomography for the delineation of CNS lesions.

The diagnosis of meningitis is difficult. In one review, premortem diagnosis was made in only 45% of cases of *Aspergillus* meningitis. Premortem diagnosis was greater in chronic *Aspergillus* meningitis and spinal arachnoiditis, 73% and 100%, respectively.[6] CSF antigen-based assays (galactomannan and 1,3,β-D-glucan) demonstrated a sensitivity of 86.7% compared to 31% positivity for culture in one review.[6]

Recommendations for therapy of CNS *Aspergillus* infections for children are similar to adults. Published guidelines for treatment of adults recommend the use of VCZ.[159] For those intolerant to or who fail to respond to VCZ, therapy with ITZ, posaconazole, or lipid formulations of AmB should be attempted. ITZ and VCZ have been used successfully in case reports.[97,98,157]

Sporotrichosis

Although primarily a lymphocutaneous disease, *S. schenckii* has been reported to cause meningitis.[40,43,55,76,111,134] Recent cases have occurred in adults with AIDS as an underlying risk factor.[38,55,137,158] Meningeal seeding may occur through hematogenous spread from the lungs.[40] Meningeal involvement produces CSF indices and abnormalities similar to those seen with the other fungal meningitides.[39,55] CSF fungal culture is insensitive for the diagnosis of *Sporothrix* meningitis. The use of *S. schenckii* antibody in the CSF has been effective in diagnosing meningitis in patients without other overt signs of this infection.[131]

Treatment is very difficult. Practice guidelines for adults recommend AmB given as a lipid formulation for 4 to 6 weeks as initial therapy.[73] No preference for AmB deoxycholate over a lipid formulation is provided. Step-down therapy using ITZ is recommended once response to initial therapy occurs and should be continued for at least 12 months. Monitoring of serum levels is recommended to ensure adequate drug exposure.[52] For patients with immunosuppressive diseases or conditions, ITZ suppressive therapy is recommended.

Mucormycosis

Meningitis caused by *Mucor* spp. or other Zygomycetes usually occurs as a result of direct extension from paranasal sinus disease. Infection with these organisms most commonly is seen in the immunocompromised host and particularly in patients with diabetes mellitus or patients receiving high doses of corticosteroids. Patients (particularly dialysis patients) undergoing chelation therapy with deferoxamine are at risk for developing infection.[14,15,71,162,166] The association with deferoxamine therapy is seen with *Cunninghamella*.[121] *Mucor* spp. have been reported as a cause of CNS disease in children, but very rarely.[54,63] Treatment employs AmB deoxycholate or lipid formulations. Improved survival has been seen among cancer patients with mucormycosis of the head and neck with treatment using liposomal AmB.[31] Surgical excision of rhinocerebral infection is recommended along with antifungal therapy. Isavuconazole, a broad-spectrum azole antifungal, has recently been approved by the U.S. Food and Drug Administration for the treatment of invasive mucormycosis and aspergillosis.[93] A comparison of isavuconazole to VZC demonstrated that it had fewer adverse effects than VCZ.[93]

Other Fungal Infections

Acremonium spp. are common soil fungi that may cause chronic meningitis in humans.[106] *Xylohypha bantiana*, an uncommon dematiaceous fungus, caused a fungal brain abscess in an adolescent girl; this report increases the number of cases reported in the literature to nearly 40.[105] Cerebral chromoblastomycosis also has been reported.[133] Other fungal organisms causing CNS infection include *Paracoccidioides brasiliensis* (i.e., South American blastomycosis),[113] *Prototheca wickerhamii*,[70] *Blastoschizomyces capitatus*,[21] *Rhodotorula* spp.,[94,116] *Pseudallescheria boydii*,[13] *A. mansoni*,[60] *C. lusitaniae*,[60] *B. spicifera*,[82] and *C. parapsilosis*.[30]

NEW REFERENCES SINCE THE SEVENTH EDITION

1. Adams-Chapman I, Bann CM, Das A, et al. Neurodevelopmental outcome of extremely low birth weight infants with *Candida* infection. *J Pediatr.* 2013;163:961-967.
6. Antinori S, Corbellino M, Meroni L, et al. *Aspergillus* meningitis: a rare clinical manifestation of central nervous system aspergillosis. Case report and review of 92 cases. *J Infect.* 2013;66:218-238.
19. Brown DA, Whealy MA, Van Gompel JJ, et al. Diagnostic dilemma in primary blastomyces dermatitidis meningitis: role of neurosurgical biopsy. *Case Rep Neurol.* 2015;7:63-70.
23. Centers for Disease Control and Prevention (CDC). Increase in reported coccidioidomycosis–United States, 1998–2011. *MMWR Morb Mortal Wkly Rep.* 2013;62:217-221.
30. Corti M, Solari R, De Carolis L, et al. *Candida parapsilosis* meningitis in a patient with AIDS. Report of a case and review of the literature. *Rev Iberoam Micol.* 2013;30:122-124.
68. Joshi NS, Fisher BT, Prasad PA, et al. Epidemiology of cryptococcal infection in hospitalized children. *Pediatr Infect Dis J.* 2010;29:e91-e95.
81. Lanternier F, Mahdaviani SA, Barbati E, et al. Inherited CARD9 deficiency in otherwise healthy children and adults with *Candida* species-induced meningoencephalitis, colitis, or both. *J Allergy Clin Immunol.* 2015;135:1558-1568.
89. Lizarazo J, Escandón P, Agudelo CI, et al. Cryptococcosis in Colombian children and literature review. *Mem Inst Oswaldo Cruz.* 2014;109:797-804.
90. Louria DB, Feder N, Mitchell W, et al. Influence of fungus strain and lapse on time in experimental histoplasmosis and of volume of inoculum in cryptococcosis upon recovery of the fungi. *J Lab Clin Med.* 1959;53:311-317.
93. Maertens JA, Raad II, Marr KA, et al. Isavuconazole versus voriconazole for primary treatment of invasive mould disease caused by *Aspergillus* and other filamentous fungi (SECURE): a phase 3, randomised-controlled, non-inferiority trial. *Lancet.* 2016;387:760-769.
98. Morgand M, Rammaert B, Poirée S, et al. Chronic invasive aspergillus sinusitis and otitis with meningeal extension successfully treated with voriconazole. *Antimicrob Agents Chemother.* 2015;59:7857-7861.
102. Nino-Serna L, Restrepo-Gouzy A, Garces-Samudio C, et al. Cerebral histoplasmosis in immunocompetent children. *Rev Neurol.* 2013;56:444-446.
104. Osorio N, López Y, Jaramillo JC. Histoplasmosis of the central nervous system in an immunocompetent patient. *Biomedica.* 2014;34:506-513.

The full reference list for this chapter is available at ExpertConsult.com.

34 Eosinophilic Meningitis

Jill Weatherhead • Rojelio Mejia

INTRODUCTION

Eosinophilic meningitis is a T-helper type 2 (T_H2)-mediated host immune reaction triggered by either infectious or noninfectious etiologies leading to central nervous system (CNS) disease.[13] Defined as greater than or equal to 10 eosinophils per microliter of cerebrospinal fluid (CSF) or greater than or equal to 10% of the total CSF leukocyte count, eosinophilic meningitis can be a self-limiting disease or lead to profound morbidity and/or mortality depending on the etiologic agent.[43] Eosinophils are not normally present in the CSF, and the detection of eosinophils suggests a limited differential diagnosis.[20,31] Noninfectious etiologies of eosinophilic meningitis include neoplastic diseases such as leukemia and lymphoma with CNS involvement such as Hodgkin's lymphoma, idiopathic hypereosinophilic syndrome, allergic reactions of the meninges to foreign material including ventriculoperitoneal shunts or intraventricular medications (vancomycin, gentamicin), or systemic medication allergies (ibuprofen, ciprofloxacin).[13,20,43] Viruses, bacteria, fungi (particularly coccidioidomycosis), and parasites can also cause eosinophilic meningitis (Table 34.1). The combination of increased international travel to endemic areas and importation of parasite vectors such as

TABLE 34.1 **Common Infectious Etiologies of Eosinophilic Meningitis**

Disease	Etiologic Agent	Source	Location	Symptoms	Diagnosis	Treatment	Prognosis
Angiostrongyliasis[7,13,15,17,18,20,21,38,40,43–46] (rat lung worm)	*Angiostrongylus cantonensis* *Angiostrongylus costaricensis*	Definitive host: rats Intermediate hosts: mollusks (snails, slugs) Paratenic hosts: crustaceans, frogs, vegetables	Thailand, China, South America, Caribbean Islands, United States (Hawaii, Louisiana), Australia, Egypt, Nigeria, Côte d'Ivoire	Severe headache Neck stiffness Nausea, vomiting Low-grade fever Hyperesthesia, paresthesia Rarely have focal neurologic deficits Children: more systemic symptoms (fever, abdominal pain)	CSF: eosinophilia, normal glucose, elevated protein, elevated opening pressure, symptomatic relief after lumbar puncture Peripheral blood eosinophilia ELISA (epitopes 29 kDa and 31 kDa) CT head: normal MRI brain: leptomeningeal enhancement, micronodular enhancement	Supportive interventions (repeat lumbar puncture, analgesics) Prednisolone 60 mg/day divided 3 times a day for 2 weeks Albendazole 15 mg/kg/day orally in 2 divided doses for 2 weeks	Self-limiting within 3–6 weeks Severe disease can cause coma, respiratory failure, and death (case fatality 5%) Children and elderly may have more severe disease
Gnathostomiasis[13,14,16,18–20,27,30,31,33,39] (neurognathostomiais)	*Gnathostoma spinigerum*	Definitive host: dogs, cats, pigs, fish-eating mammals Intermediate hosts: freshwater crustaceans Secondary intermediate hosts: freshwater fish, frogs Paratenic hosts: birds, reptiles, mammals	Southeast Asia (Thailand), China, India, Zambia, Botswana, Mexico, Central America, South America	Prodrome: abdominal pain, nausea, vomiting, diarrhea, cutaneous larvae migrans, fever Severe headache Neck stiffness Radicular pain Paresis Paralysis Cranial nerve deficits Seizures	CSF: eosinophilia, xanthochromia, elevated protein, normal glucose Peripheral blood eosinophilia ELISA (24 kDa epitope, immunoglobulin subclasses) CT head: nodular lesions, hemorrhage MRI brain: diffuse or segmental hyperintense micronodules, hemorrhagic tracts, intracerebral hemorrhage, subarachnoid hemorrhage, subdural hemorrhage	Supportive (repeat lumbar punctures, analgesics) Use of anthelmintics is controversial Steroids may help CNS inflammation Monitor closely for intracranial hemorrhage	Long-term neurologic disability 23–46% of survivors, including paraplegia, paresis, radicular pain, cranial nerve Case fatality rate 7–25%

	Baylisascaris procyonis	Definitive host: raccoons, domesticated dogs, kinkajou Paratenic hosts: small mammals (rabbits, rodents), birds	North America	Lethargy Seizures Sensory loss Ataxia Paralysis Spasticity Cranial nerve deficits Paresis Concurrent ocular involvement Rarely have fever More common in young children	CSF: eosinophilia, variable protein, normal glucose Variable peripheral blood eosinophilia ELISA (epitopes 33 kDa, 45 kDa, BpRAG1 protein) CT head and MRI brain: parenchyma inflammation, cerebral atrophy	Exposure: albendazole (2550 mg/kg per day orally for 1020 days) Treatment: albendazole (2550 mg/kg per day orally for 14 weeks) Corticosteroids	Fulminant eosinophilic meningoencephalitis Severe neurologic impairment Case fatality rate 38%
CNS coccidioidomycosis[10,22,36,41] (valley fever)	*Coccidioides immitis, Coccidioides posadasii*	Colonized soil in southwestern United States, Mexico, South America	Southwestern United States, Mexico, South America	Additional organ system involvement (lungs, skin, bone, soft tissue) Prodrome: febrile respiratory infection Gradual neurologic symptom onset Headache Vomiting Lethargy Fever	CSF: pleocytosis, elevated protein, decreased glucose, elevated opening pressure, culture CSF complement fixation antibodies	Lifelong fluconazole Ventriculoperitoneal shunt placement	Long-term neurologic sequelae (hydrocephalus, fatal without treatment)

CSF, Cerebrospinal fluid; *CT*, computed tomography; *ELISA*, enzyme-linked immunosorbent assay; *MRI*, magnetic resonance imaging.

rodents, snails, slugs, and mollusks to previously nonendemic areas has led to the emergence of parasitic pathogens as a leading cause of eosinophilic meningitis.[11,31,46] While neurocysticercosis, schistosomiasis, paragonimiasis, echinococcosis, trichinellosis, and toxocariasis have uncommonly been associated with eosinophilic meningitis, angiostrongyliasis, gnathostomiasis, and baylisascariasis are most commonly known to cause eosinophilic meningitis.[13,20,31,43,46]

EPIDEMIOLOGY

Angiostrongylus cantonensis (rat lung worm) is the principal pathogen of eosinophilic meningitis in humans.[43] *A. cantonensis* was first discovered in rats in 1935 in China, and the first human case was diagnosed in Taiwan in 1945.[1,46] Angiostrongyliasis is a food-borne parasite endemic in Southeast Asia, with particularly high prevalence in Thailand (47% of all reported cases) and China, including Taiwan and Hong Kong (27.22% of all reported cases).[43,46] Clustering of cases has been documented throughout the region. In 2001, an outbreak was documented in patients in Taiwan who drank raw vegetable juice.[44] More recently, geographic dispersal of *A. cantonensis* has occurred secondary to transport of infected rats and intermediate hosts on intercontinental ships. *A. cantonensis* endemicity now extends beyond Southeast Asia to regions in the Pacific basin, South Asia, the Caribbean islands, Australia, Egypt, Nigeria, Côte d'Ivoire, South America, and the United States.[15,21,40,43,45] An angiostrongyliasis outbreak in Hawaii occurred in 2004–05 and resulted in an increased incidence of eosinophilic meningitis from 0.3 per 100,000 person-years to 2.1 per 100,000 person-years during the cluster period.[15] Furthermore with increasing international travel, cases of angiostrongyliasis have been documented in returning travelers from more than 30 countries.[13,21] In 2000, 12 travelers returning to the United States from Jamaica were noted to have eosinophilic meningitis secondary to presumed *Angiostrongylus cantonensis*. Angiostrongyliasis is an emerging pathogen worldwide due to its diversifying geographic distribution.[21]

Gnathostoma spinigerum is a food-borne zoonotic parasite obtained by humans through eating raw or undercooked freshwater fish, brackish-water fish, or other intermediate hosts.[14,19] The highest prevalence of eosinophilic meningitis due to gnathostomiasis, neurognathostomiasis, occurs in Southeast Asia, particularly Thailand.[19,33] There is also increasing endemicity in Mexico, Central America, and South America.[13,14,19,31,33] Human cases of disease have been reported worldwide outside of endemic regions including Cambodia, Laos, Japan, Myanmar, Indonesia, Philippines, Malaysia, China, Sri Lanka, India, Guatemala, Peru, Ecuador, Zambia, and Botswana.[14]

Baylisascaris procyonis is a parasite highly prevalent in raccoon populations worldwide, particularly in the United States.[42] Approximately 70% of adult and 90% of juvenile raccoons in North America are infected with the parasite.[13,42] Human construction and settlements in wildlife areas have increased human and domestic animal exposure to raccoons. The proximity of raccoon habitat and human homes has led to an increased risk of human disease.[13,34] *Baylisascaris* eggs, found in raccoon feces, are durable and can contaminate the environment for years, thus serving as a long-term nidus of infection in areas with dense raccoon populations.[12] Risk factors for human infection are related to contact with infected raccoons or raccoon feces and geophagia of environmental materials contaminated with infected eggs.[12] As a result infants and young children are at particular risk of baylisascariasis due to pica behavior.[12] Human cases have been reported in the literature in California, Illinois, Louisiana, Massachusetts, Michigan, Minnesota, New York, Oregon, and Pennsylvania.[5,12,34]

PATHOGENESIS

A. cantonensis is a small, neurotropic, filiform nematode, tapering at both ends and measuring 16 to 35 mm in length.[21] Rats are the definitive hosts of *A. cantonensis*. During the life cycle, orally ingested larvae 1 (L1) stage molt a total of four times, generating L2, L3, L4, and L5 larvae, with L3 serving as the infective form in rats and in accidental hosts.[21,46] L3 larvae penetrate the intestinal tract and travel via the venous hepatoportal circulation to the right ventricle, subsequently traveling through the pulmonary capillaries to the left heart and dispersing through the systemic circulation.[21] Within days of ingestion L3 reach neural tissue. The L3 will molt into L4 and L5 in the neural parenchyma.[20,21,46] Rats can survive relatively large infective doses (150 parasites in the brain) without abnormalities.[21] Adult worms leave brain tissue and return to pulmonary arteries through the venous sinuses, superior vena cava, and right ventricle, at which time they reach sexual maturity in the pulmonary arteries 26 to 35 days after infection.[21,46] The adult worms will subsequently lay eggs in the pulmonary arteries; the eggs hatch into L1, migrate up the bronchial tree, are swallowed, and are excreted in the rodent feces 42 to 45 days postinfection.[21,46] L1 in the environment will infect intermediate hosts, mollusks (snails and slugs), through ingestion of rodent feces or penetration of the body surface.[21,46] L1 will molt into infective L3 within the intermediate host, which can also be consumed by paratenic or transport hosts.[20]

Humans are an accidental host of *A. cantonensis* and typically develop symptoms after an incubation period of a few days to several months following ingestion of raw or inadequately cooked intermediate hosts such as snails, paratenic hosts (crustaceans and frogs), or vegetables contaminated with L3.[7,15,21,38,43,46] In human disease, after oral ingestion, L3 penetrate the gastrointestinal tract and are carried via systemic blood vessels to the CNS, at which time they die and do not complete the remaining life cycle.[7,46] Neural disease is thought to be secondary to direct invasion and migration of the parasite in the neural parenchymal tissue leading to tissue damage, Th2-mediated inflammatory response with eosinophilic predominance, and eosinophilic granulomas surrounding dead worms.[7,21] Profound cellular infiltrate and cytokine release as a result of dying worms cause increased intracranial pressure within the human host.[21]

Dogs, cats, pigs, and other fish-eating mammals are definitive hosts of *G. spinigerum*, which can be up to 13 to 55 mm in length.[13,14,31] Adult worms form a tumorlike mass in the stomach wall of the definitive mammalian host.[14] The infected animal will shed eggs in its feces into freshwater; these eggs will become embryonated and hatch approximately 7 to 12 days later into L1.[14,20] Free-swimming L1 are ingested by primary intermediate freshwater crustaceans and will molt into L2.[14] L2-infected crustaceans are eaten by secondary intermediate hosts (freshwater fish, eels, frogs, birds, reptiles), leading to molting of L2 into infective L3.[14,20,31,33] L3 will migrate to muscle tissue and encyst.[14,31] The infected muscle tissue of the secondary hosts can subsequently be consumed by paratenic hosts (mammals).[13,33]

Humans are accidental hosts of *G. spinigerum* and are infected by consuming raw or undercooked primary intermediate hosts (crustaceans), secondary intermediate hosts (freshwater fish), or paratenic hosts (poultry, pigs, snakes, frogs) and less commonly by drinking contaminated water or through direct larval penetration of the skin.[13,20,31,33] In humans, L3 will migrate through subcutaneous tissue, causing intermittent cutaneous migratory skin swelling, and through internal organs including the CNS.[14,19,33] L3 will invade the CNS directly through the neural foramina at the skull base or intervertebral foramina along the cranial or spinal nerves and blood vessels.[19] *G. spinigerum* do not fully develop into adult worms in humans but cause significant disease secondary to diffuse migration.[13,19] During migration, L3 release proteolytic and hemolytic enzymes as part of the excretory-secretory (ES) product, including matrix metalloproteinases.[14,19] The incubation period is typically weeks to months, but *G. spinigerum* can remain dormant for years after initial infection, thus leading to long incubation periods and recurrences.[13,14,19]

Baylisascaris procyonis are large intestinal roundworms, range from 9 to 22 cm in length, endemic in the North American raccoon *(Procyon lotor)* population.[12,13,28] Infected adult raccoons shed an average of 20,000 to 26,000 eggs per gram of feces. As a result the host can shed millions of eggs per day into the environment and will have infective potential after 2 to 4 weeks in the environment.[12,34,42] Raccoons become infected in two different pathways. Juvenile raccoons ingest *B. procyonis* eggs, the larvae hatch within the wall of the small intestine and subsequently mature into adult worms within the lumen of small intestines within approximately 63 days.[12,13,34,42] Similarly, paratenic hosts (small birds, rodents, rabbits) become infected by ingesting eggs. Hatched larvae in the intermediate host subsequently migrate through the portal and systemic circulation to other organs, including the CNS, forming larvae encapsulated eosinophilic granulomas within tissue.[12,20] Paratenic hosts can develop significant disease from larval migration, making them easier prey for adult raccoons.[42] Adult raccoons will ingest L3 encysted tissue of the infected paratenic hosts.[12] After consumption of the cysts, the worms will mature into adult worms in small intestines within a mean of 35 days.[12,34] Unlike in intermediate hosts, *B. procyonis* typically does not cause disease in the carnivorous definitive host unless a young raccoon ingests a heavy inoculum.[34] Other carnivores, including domestic dogs and the exotic pet kinkajou, can serve as definitive hosts and are risk factors for further spread of disease to accidental hosts including humans.[4]

The risk of baylisascariasis in humans has increased as the raccoon habitat has become closer in proximity to human populations.[42] Raccoons defecate in communal latrines that are often established near residential homes.[34] *B. procyonis* eggs are particularly resistant to adverse environmental conditions, and ingestion of only a few eggs, typically less than 5000, is sufficient to cause infection in humans.[13,42] Young children are at particularly high risk due to their propensity for geophagia. The median age of baylisascariasis in humans is approximately 1 year of age.[28,40] The incubation period is unknown in humans; however, it is believed that if the inoculum is large enough neural larva migrans can present within 2 to 4 weeks after ingestion of the eggs.[12] *B. procyonis* are not specifically neurotropic, but due to significant extraintestinal migration, travel to the CNS can occur.[13] Approximately 5% to 7% of larvae migrate to the CNS, penetrating cerebral blood vessels and causing neural larva migrans, at which time the larvae can continue to migrate and grow in the tissue.[12,13,20] Because of the significant inoculum of eggs ingested and the relatively smaller brain size to parasite size, baylisascariasis neural larva migrans is particularly devastating in infants and young children.[12,28]

CLINICAL MANIFESTATIONS

Clinical symptoms of eosinophilic meningitis are most commonly a result of the host immune response to larval migration or larval death in the neural tissue. *Angiostrongylus* causes predominantly eosinophilic infiltration with associated necrosis and granulomatous reaction in the meninges and in the neural parenchyma (medulla, pons, or cerebellum). The profound inflammatory infiltration causes meningoencephalitis and increased intracranial pressure.[13] Adult patients typically present with a self-limiting severe headache without focal neurologic findings, low-grade fever, nausea, vomiting, and meningismus.[5,13,37,43,46] Occasionally patients have reported hyperesthesia, paresthesia, cranial nerve deficiencies, and radicular pain. Severe infections can lead to seizures, coma, respiratory failure, and death.[13,20,21,46] Elderly patients and young children (bimodal age distribution) may have more severe disease including encephalitis and somnolence.[21] In comparison to adults, children more commonly have systemic symptoms of fever, abdominal pain, nausea, and vomiting in combination with neck stiffness, cranial nerve abnormalities, and papilledema. Children are less likely to have paresthesia or hyperesthesia.[21,37,45,46] The constellation of headache and hyperesthesia without focal neurologic deficits in combination with eosinophilic meningitis is suggestive of angiostrongyliasis.[44]

Gnathostomiasis may present with a prodrome state of abdominal pain, nausea, vomiting, diarrhea, urticaria and cutaneous larvae migrans, and fever as the parasite migrates through the skin and viscera.[13,45] Although not considered neurotropic, larval migration through the CNS with destruction of the neural tissue causes a disease state described as neurognathostomiasis.[31] Patients with neurognathostomiasis often present with severe headache, meningismus, excruciating radicular pain, and focal neurologic deficits such as hemiparesis or hemiplegia, urinary retention, and cranial nerve palsies due to larvae ascending along nerve roots into the CNS.[13,14,31] In comparison to angiostrongyliasis, neurognathostomiasis more commonly presents with seizures.[13] Migration of the organism through the neural tissue causes necrotic tracts in the brain and spinal cord, leading to significant subarachnoid, intracerebral, intraventricular hemorrhage.[13,20] Mechanical and chemical cerebral tissue destruction by *Gnathostoma* migration elicits a strong eosinophilic, predominantly inflammatory response manifested clinically by myelitis, meningitis, meningoencephalitis, and possibly coma and death.[14,19,31]

Neural larva migrans secondary to baylisascariasis presents as an acute, rapidly progressive eosinophilic-predominant meningoencephalitis.[12] The severity of disease depends directly on the volume of the egg inoculum.[12,20] Patients may present with profound neurologic symptoms including lethargy, ataxia, paralysis, posturing, spasticity, paresis, cranial nerve involvement, sensory loss including vibration and proprioception, and seizures.[13,19,20] Fever is not a prominent symptom.[13] Unlike angiostrongyliasis and gnathostomiasis, baylisascariasis more commonly presents with concomitant ocular and neurologic disease.[13] The acute fulminant eosinophilic meningoencephalitis secondary to neural larva migrans can cause developmental milestone regression, neurologic devastation, and death, particularly in young children.[12,14]

DIAGNOSIS

Due to the lack of robust and reliable diagnostic tools, eosinophilic meningitis is commonly diagnosed based on clinical symptoms, medical history, and CSF studies.[31,33,46] Determination of the etiology of disease is challenging, and the diagnosis can be missed if a detailed history is not obtained.[15,21,31] Patients with angiostrongyliasis typically present with headaches, paresthesia, or hyperesthesia; have traveled or have residence in Southeast Asia, Australia, Africa, the Caribbean, or Hawaii; and have a history of consumption of raw mollusks, crustaceans, frogs, or raw vegetables.[20,31] Conversely patients with gnathostomiasis present with migratory cutaneous swelling, encephalitis, painful radiculomyelitis, paralysis, cranial nerve deficits, and subarachnoid hemorrhage; have traveled or have permanent residence in Southeast Asia (Thailand), Japan, China, Mexico, or Central and South America; and have consumed contaminated freshwater fish.[14,20,31] Last, patients with baylisascariasis have acute fulminant meningoencephalitis with exposure to raccoons in North America.[20] CSF typically demonstrates an eosinophilic pleocytosis exceeding 10%, more commonly between 20% and 70%, or greater than 10 eosinophils in the CSF.[13,21] Additional CSF studies, including Gram stain and cultures, acid-fast bacteria stain, India ink staining, cryptococcal antigen, and coccidioides antibody, should also be negative.[7] Isolation of the causative agent within the CSF, if of parasitic etiology, is uncommon.

In combination with CSF eosinophilia, patients with angiostrongyliasis have CSF studies consistent with elevated protein, normal to slightly reduced glucose, elevated opening CSF pressure, and symptomatic relief by lumbar puncture (LP). Patients commonly have peripheral eosinophilia as well.[13,21] Serum and CSF serologic tests may be used to support the diagnosis of angiostrongyliasis, but sensitivity and specificity of serologic testing vary and may be limited by cross-reactivity with other parasitic infections.[7,31] Monoclonal antibodies against parasite-specific antigen including excretory/secretory (ES) proteins, specifically 29 kDa and 31 kDa, have been developed with increased sensitivity and specificity.[19,46] However, these immunoassays are not globally available.[21]

Imaging may also aid in the diagnosis of angiostrongyliasis. Head computed tomography (CT) scan may be normal or show nonspecific changes including cerebral edema, ventricular dilatation, and meningeal enhancement.[21] Cerebral magnetic resonance imaging (MRI) demonstrates leptomeningeal enhancement, ventriculomegaly, and micronodular enhancement.[13,18,21,45] In comparison to other parasitic infections, *A. cantonensis* generally does not form solitary focal lesions seen on neuroimaging.[21]

In patients with neurognathostomiasis, CSF studies may demonstrate xanthochromia with increased numbers of red blood cells (RBCs), pleocytosis (<500 cells/μL) with a eosinophilia (15% to 90%), elevated protein, and normal to slightly reduced glucose.[13,19,20] Neurognathostomiasis may also cause a peripheral eosinophilia, although less commonly than in angiostrongyliasis.[13,31] Serologic studies are available for diagnostic evaluation of neurognathostomiasis, but immunoassays typically have high cross-reactivity with other helminthic infections including *Angiostrongylus*, hookworm, *Strongyloides*, *Trichuris*, and lymphatic filariasis. Immunoblot assays for detection of *Gnathostoma*-specific IgG to ES protein epitope 24 kDa in Thailand demonstrated the greatest specificity for gnathostomiasis.[14,16,19] Immunoassays also typically have poor sensitivity for total *Gnathostoma*-specific IgG detection (59–87%).[13,14,31] In comparison to total IgG,

Gnathostoma-specific IgG subclasses have shown a high sensitivity (98%) and negative predictive value (94%) for IgG1 and a higher specificity (88%) and positive predictive value (93%) for IgG2, suggesting that IgG1 and IgG2 could be useful tools for screening and confirmation of neurognathostomiasis.[14,27]

Neuroimaging is particularly useful in the diagnosis of gnathostomiasis with hallmark features of hemorrhagic tracts and subarachnoid hemorrhage.[19] Head CT scan shows nodular lesions, hemorrhage, and hydrocephalus, whereas cerebral MRI demonstrates diffuse or segmental hyperintense micronodules, hemorrhagic tracts, intracerebral hemorrhage in regions uncommon for hypertensive hemorrhage, nontraumatic subdural hemorrhage, and subarachnoid hemorrhage.[13,18,19,31,39] MRI of the cervical cord may show diffuse, linear, ill-defined lesions.[39]

Patients with baylisascariasis may have mild CSF pleocytosis (1 to 124 cells/mm^3) with extremely high eosinophilia (up to 68%), variable protein, and normal glucose. Blood eosinophilia can also be variable, ranging from 5% to 45%.[12,13] Enzyme-linked immunosorbent assay (ELISA) and Western blot immunoassays targeting ES protein epitopes 33 kDa and 45 kDa can be used for detection in serum and CSF with known high cross-reactivity with other organisms, particularly toxocariasis.[9,12,13] Recombinant *Baylisascaris procyonis* RAG1 protein (BpRAG1) ELISA showed increased sensitivity and specificity compared to using ES-based ELISA but continued to demonstrate cross-reactivity with *Toxocara* spp. (25%).[9] However, Western blot assay using BpRAG1 protein showed no cross-reactivity with *Toxocara*-positive serum, with an overall sensitivity of 88% and specificity of 98%.[32]

Neural larva migrans manifests as progressive diffuse white matter disease on neuroimaging.[24,35] Parenchyma inflammation and cerebral atrophy without predilection for a specific part of the neural tissue is common due to the random migration of the larva through the tissue.[24]

TREATMENT

Treatment options for eosinophilic meningitis are limited.[7] Symptomatic regimens with repeat LP to relieve intracranial pressure and supportive therapy including analgesics, such as acetaminophen, is critical for angiostrongyliasis, gnathostomiasis, and baylisascariasis treatment.[7,13,38,46] Corticosteroid use, prednisolone 60 mg/day in three divided doses for 2 weeks, has become more widely accepted as a supportive measure specifically for angiostrongyliasis.[8,43] Reduction in cerebral inflammation and intracranial pressure secondary to corticosteroid use has been associated with a shorter duration of headache and fewer required repeat LPs without evidence of serious adverse effects.[8,12,19,43] However, corticosteroid use remains controversial in treatment of gnathostomiasis because there are no adequate studies to demonstrate significant benefit.[6] Supportive treatment with corticosteroids for baylisascariasis may be beneficial particularly if treatment is initiated prior to onset of neurologic symptoms.[12] Of note, the use of glucocorticosteroids can induce apoptosis of eosinophils and may lower CSF levels, either decreasing concern for eosinophilic meningitis in patients previously on steroids or producing misleading laboratory values showing improvement with decreasing CSF eosinophilia.[23]

Anthelmintic therapy has been evaluated for the treatment of eosinophilic meningitis and remains controversial. The use of albendazole 15 mg/kg per day in divided doses for 2 weeks showed a trend toward reduction in mean duration of headache without evidence of serious drug events in patients with angiostrongyliasis.[17,38] However, improved outcomes using anthelmintic therapy in combination with corticosteroids may be directly a result of the corticosteroid therapy and not the anthelmintic drug.[38] Subsequent studies have shown no significant difference in clinical outcomes between patients randomized to prednisolone alone or prednisolone plus albendazole.[7] Cutaneous gnathostomiasis has been treated successfully with ivermectin or albendazole, but thorough studies have not been done to evaluate the use of anthelmintics in neurognathostomiasis.[3,2,6,25,26] A theoretical concern of catalyzing a profound inflammatory reaction secondary to larvae death and subsequent paradoxical worsening of neurologic symptoms after anthelmintic treatment has been cited as a potential risk for patients with angiostrongyliasis and neurognathostomiasis.[30,31,40] As a result, the use of anthelmintic treatment, including mebendazole, albendazole, thiabendazole, and ivermectin, remains controversial in the treatment of angiostrongyliasis and gnathostomiasis.[20,43] Conversely patients with suspected baylisascariasis should be treated immediately with albendazole (25 to 50 mg/kg per day for 1 to 4 weeks) along with corticosteroids.[5,12,34] Early initiation of albendazole is critical to reduce the risk of larval migration to the CNS.[12] Once neurologic symptoms have developed, larval invasion to the CNS has already occurred, and anthelmintic therapy has reduced benefit.[12] Due to poor prognosis associated with neural larva migrans, prophylactic anthelmintic treatment with albendazole for 10 days is recommended for asymptomatic patients with possible exposure to infected raccoons, raccoon cages, or latrines or to raccoon-contaminated environments until the possibility of baylisascariasis has been excluded.[12,13]

COURSE AND PROGNOSIS

Patients with eosinophilic meningitis secondary to angiostrongyliasis commonly have a good prognosis. Angiostrongyliasis may spontaneously resolve even without treatment in 3 to 6 weeks.[13,20] Headaches typically improve with repeat LP and corticosteroids within 1 week.[21] If patients have more severe disease, including evidence of encephalitis, or disease in young children, neurologic prognosis can be poor.[21,45] However, angiostrongyliasis has a low case fatality rate of 5%.[21,45] Despite cases of complete neurologic recovery, neurognathostomiasis more commonly causes permanent neurologic sequelae, including paraplegia, radicular pain, cranial nerve palsies, hemiparesis, or death. Long-term disability has been documented in 23% to 46% of survivors.[13,14,20] Neurognathostomiasis has a case fatality rate of 7% to 25%.[13,14,19,20] Baylisascariasis neural larva migrans causes severe neurologic disease with an overall poor prognosis in human hosts. Complete recovery, although it has been documented in case reports, is rare.[29] Cases documenting clinical recovery are thought to be secondary to a lower infective egg burden in combination with early diagnosis and aggressive treatment.[29] More commonly, neural larva migrans is rapidly fatal despite appropriate therapy, with a case fatality rate of 38% in the United States.[5,12,34] Individuals who survive typically have severe neurologic impairment including motor and cognitive deficits, seizures, and cerebral visual impairment.[12,14,29,34]

PREVENTION

Eradication of the parasitic agents that cause eosinophilic meningitis is difficult due to the worldwide distribution of the definitive, intermediate, and paratenic hosts.[14,21] Due to the persistence of the causative agents, the lack of definitive treatment regimens, the limited diagnostic tools, and poor prognosis for certain eosinophilic meningitis etiologies, preventive measures to reduce the risk of infection are critical.[20] Prevention through education may be the most successful form of treatment for eosinophilic meningitis caused by parasitic infections. Community outreach in *A. cantonensis* and *G. spinigerum* endemic areas should focus on both avoidance of raw foods as well as adequate cooking or freezing techniques to kill larvae in all potentially infected intermediate or paratenic hosts.[14] Additional education on proper washing of vegetables prior to consumption could reduce infection.[46] In areas endemic for *B. procyonis*, humans, particularly young children, and domestic animals should avoid geophagia behavior and wash hands after outdoor exposures.[34] Property owners should inspect their property for raccoon latrines.[34] Considering the geographic dispersal of *A. cantonensis*, *G. spinigerum*, and *B. procyonis*, as well as other infectious causes of eosinophilic meningitis, travelers should be educated on reducing high-risk behaviors. Furthermore, healthcare workers should have high suspicion of eosinophilic meningitis in order for early diagnosis and application of timely interventions in travelers.[13,21,46]

NEW REFERENCES SINCE THE SEVENTH EDITION

2. Bussaratid V, Desakorn V, Krudsood S, et al. Efficacy of ivermectin treatment of cutaneous gnathostomiasis evaluated by placebo-controlled trials. *Southeast Asian J Trop Med Public Health*. 2006;37:433-440.
3. Bussaratid V, Krudsood S, Silachamroon U, et al. Tolerability of ivermectin in gnathostomiasis. *Southeast Asian J Trop Med Public Health*. 2005;36:644-649.

4. Centers for Disease Control and Prevention. Raccoon roundworms in pet kinkajous. *MMWR*. 2011;60:302-305.
5. Centers for Disease Control and Prevention (CDC). Baylisascariasis. Available at: http://www.cdc.gov/parasites/baylisascariasis/. Accessed 21 November 2015.
6. Centers for Disease Control and Prevention (CDC). Gnathostomiasis. Available at: http://www.cdc.gov/parasites/gnathostoma/. Accessed 21 November 2015.
7. Chotmongkol V, Kittimongkolma S, Niwattayakul K, et al. Comparison of prednisolone plus albendazole with prednisolone alone for treatment of patients with eosinophilic meningitis. *Am J Trop Med Hyg*. 2009;8:443-445.
9. Dangoudoubiyam S, Vemulapalli R, Ndao M, et al. Recombinant antigen-based enzyme-linked immunosorbent assay for diagnosis of *Baylisascaris procyonis* larva migrans. *Clin Vaccine Immunol*. 2011;18:1650-1655.
10. Dimitrova D, Ross L. Coccidioidomycosis: experience from a children's hospital in an area of endemicity. *J Pediatric Infect Dis Soc*. 2016;5(1):89-92.
11. Eamsobhana P. Eosinophilic meningitis caused by *Angiostrongylus cantonensis* – a neglected disease with escalating importance. *Trop Biomed*. 2014;31:569-578.
14. Herman JS, Chiodini PL. Gnathostomiasis, another emerging imported disease. *Clin Microbiol Rev*. 2009;22:484-492.
16. Intapan PM, Khotsri P, Kanpittaya J, et al. Short report: immunoblot diagnostic test for neurognathostomiasis. *Am J Trop Med Hyg*. 2010;83:927-929.
17. Jitpimolmard S, Sawanyawisuth K, Morakote N, et al. Albendazole therapy for eosinophilic meningitis caused by *Angiostrongylus cantonensis*. *Parasitol Res*. 2007;100:1293-1296.
18. Kanpittaya J, Sawanyawisuth K, Intapan PM, et al. A comparative study of neuro-imaging features between human neuro-gnathostomiasis and angiostrongyliasis. *Neurol Sci*. 2012;33:893-898.
19. Katchanov J, Sawanyawisuth K, Chotmongkol V, et al. Neurognathostomiasis, a neglected parasitosis of the central nervous system. *Emerg Infect Dis*. 2011;17:1174-1180.
21. Martins YC, Tanowitz HB, Kazacos KR. Central nervous system manifestations of *Angiostrongylus cantonensis* infection. *Acta Trop*. 2015;141:46-53.
22. McCarty JM, Demetral LC, Dabrawski L, et al. Pediatric coccidioidomycosis in central California: a retrospective case series. *Clin Infect Dis*. 2013;56:1579-1585.
23. Meagher L, Cousin J, Seckl J, et al. Opposing effects of glucocorticoids on the rate of apoptosis in neutrophilic and eosinophilic granulocytes. *J Immunol*. 1996;156:4422-4428.
24. Mehta P, Boyd Z, Cully B. Raccoon roundworm encephalitis. *Pediatr Radiol*. 2010;40:1834-1836.
25. Nontasut P, Claesson BA, Dekumyoyo P, et al. Double-dose ivermectin vs albendazole for the treatment of gnathostomiasis. *Southeast Asian J Trop Med Public Health*. 2005;36:650-652.
26. Nontasut P, Bussaratid V, Chullawichit S, et al. Comparison of ivermectin and albendazole treatment for gnathostomiasis. *Southeast Asian J Trop Med Public Health*. 2000;31:374-377.
27. Nuchprayoon S, Sanprasert V, Suntravat M, et al. Study of specific IgG subclass antibodies for diagnosis of *Gnathostoma spinigerum*. *Parasitol Res*. 2003;91:137-143.
29. Peters JM, Madhavan VL, Kazacos KR, et al. Good outcome with early empiric treatment of neural larva migrans due to *Baylisascaris procyonis*. *Pediatrics*. 2012;129:e806-e811.
30. Pien FD, Pien BC. *Angiostrongylus cantonensis* eosinophilic meningitis. *Int J Infect Dis*. 1999;3:161-163.
31. Ramirez-Avila L, Slome S, Schuster FL, et al. Eosinophilic meningitis due to *Angiostrongylus* and *Gnathostoma species*. *Clin Infect Dis*. 2009;48:322-327.
32. Rascoe LN, Santamaria C, Handali S, et al. Interlaboratory optimization and evaluation of a serological assay for diagnosis of human baylisascariasis. *Clin Vaccine Immunol*. 2013;20:1758-1763.
33. Rojas-Molina N, Pedraza-Sanchez S, Torres-Bibiano B, et al. Gnathostomiasis, an emerging foodborne zoonotic disease in Acapulco, Mexico. *Emerg Infect Dis*. 1999;5:264-266.
36. Saitoh A, Homans J, Kovacs A. Fluconazole treatment of coccidioidal meningitis in children: two case reports and a review of the literature. *Pediatr Infect Dis J*. 2000;19:1204-1208.
37. Sawanyawisuth K, Chindaprasirt J, Senthong V, et al. Clinical manifestations of eosinophilic meningitis due to infection with *Angiostrongylus cantonensis* in children. *Korean J Parasitol*. 2013;51:735-738.
38. Sawanyawisuth K, Sawanyawisuth K. Treatment of angiostrongyliasis. *Trans R Soc Trop Med Hyg*. 2008;102:990-996.
39. Sawanyawisuth K, Tiamkao S, Kanpittaya J, et al. MR imaging findings in cerebrospinal gnathostomiasis. *AJNR Am J Neuroradiol*. 2004;25:446-449.
41. Sondermeyer GL, Lee LA, Gilliss D, et al. Epidemiology of pediatric coccidioidomycosis in California, 2000–2012. *Pediatr Infect Dis J*. 2016;35(2):166-171.
42. Sorvillo F, Ash LR, Berlin OGW, et al. *Baylisascaris procyonis*: an emerging helminthic zoonosis. *Emerg Infect Dis*. 2002;8:355-359.
43. Thanaviratananich S, Thanaviratananich S, Ngamjarus C. Corticosteroids for parasitic eosinophilic meningitis. *Cochrane Database Syst Rev*. 2015;(2):CD009088.
44. Tsai HC, Shin-Jung Lee S, Huang CK, et al. Outbreak of eosinophilic meningitis associated with drinking raw vegetable juice in Southern Taiwan. *Am J Trop Med Hyg*. 2004;71:222-226.
45. Tseng YT, Tsai HC, Sy CL, et al. Clinical manifestations of eosinophilic meningitis caused by *Angiostrongylus cantonensis*: 18 years' experience in a medical center in southern Taiwan. *J Microbiol Immunol Infect*. 2011;44:382-389.
46. Wang QP, Qu ZD, Wei J, et al. Human *Angiostrongylus cantonensis*: an update. *Eur J Clin Microbiol Infect Dis*. 2012;31:389-395.

The full reference list for this chapter is available at ExpertConsult.com.

Aseptic Meningitis and Viral Meningitis 35

David E. Bronstein • Carol A. Glaser

Aseptic meningitis is an inflammatory process of the meninges. It is relatively common and is caused by many different entities. The cerebrospinal fluid (CSF) is characterized by pleocytosis, normal or increased protein, and the absence of microorganisms on Gram stain and on routine culture. Usually the illnesses are self-limited; however, with some etiologies, the resulting diseases may be severe, protracted, recurrent, or progressive, and lead to disability and death. Viral meningitis, an inflammation of the leptomeninges, is the most common type of aseptic meningitis. *Serous meningitis, lymphocytic meningitis,* and *nonparalytic poliomyelitis* are terms that were used in the past to denote aseptic meningitis.

HISTORY

Aseptic meningitis is a syndrome that first was described by Wallgren in 1925.[378] Wallgren's criteria for this diagnosis included (1) an acute onset with obvious signs and symptoms of meningeal involvement; (2) alteration of CSF typical of meningitis, which may show a small or large number of cells; (3) absence of bacteria in the CSF, as shown by appropriate culture; (4) a relatively short, benign course of illness; (5) absence of local parameningeal infection (e.g., otitis, sinusitis, or trauma) or a general disease that might have meningitis as a secondary manifestation; and (6) absence from the community of epidemic disease, of which meningitis is a feature. In 1951, Wallgren[379] redefined aseptic meningitis as a syndrome likely to be encountered in many different infectious diseases.

The clinical occurrence of aseptic meningitis first was recognized in epidemic poliomyelitis and in mumps at the beginning of the 20th century.[116,386] Rivers and Scott[304] reported the recovery of lymphocytic choriomeningitis virus from the CSF of several patients with aseptic meningitis in 1935, and, in 1934, Johnson and Goodpasture[189] proved that mumps was caused by a virus. The discovery of coxsackieviruses in 1948 by Dalldorf and Sickles[93] and the introduction of tissue culture in 1949 by Enders and colleagues,[117] which resulted in the discovery of echoviruses, paved the way for the widespread investigation into the etiology of aseptic meningitis.

Rasmussen[297] reported on 374 cases evaluated at the Walter Reed Army Institute of Research laboratory between 1941 and 1946 and found the probable or definite etiology in 26% of "viral" disease of the central nervous system (CNS). Mumps and lymphocytic choriomeningitis viruses were the two etiologic agents identified in his study.

In 1953, Adair and associates[7] reviewed 480 additional cases of aseptic meningitis occurring in military personnel and their dependents from 1947 through 1952 and were able to confirm the etiology in 25% of those patients. Herpes simplex virus (HSV) and *Leptospira* spp. were added to the previously identified mumps and lymphocytic choriomeningitis viruses as causes of aseptic meningitis. Meyer and associates[248] extended these studies to include 713 more children and adults with acute CNS syndromes of "viral" etiology admitted to military and Veterans Administration hospitals between 1953 and 1958. Of these 713 patients, 430 had the clinical syndrome of aseptic meningitis. Approximately 80% of these patients were hospitalized in the United States. An etiologic diagnosis was determined in 71% of patients with aseptic meningitis. In addition to the agents identified earlier, poliovirus, coxsackieviruses of groups A and B, echoviruses, and arthropod-borne viruses were identified as causes of aseptic meningitis.

Lepow and colleagues[220,221] reported the probable viral etiology in 54% of the 407 patients they studied in Cleveland between 1955 and 1958. In 1958, Lennette and associates[219] determined a viral etiology in 65% of 511 children and adults with presumed viral CNS system disease in Los Angeles; 368 of these patients were diagnosed as having aseptic meningitis. Sköldenberg[333] analyzed 3117 patients admitted to the Hospital for Infectious Diseases in Stockholm between 1955 and 1964 with the diagnosis of aseptic meningitis, with or without encephalitis or myelitis, and a virologic or clinical diagnosis (or both) of an associated viral infection was established in 72.6%. Berlin and associates[32] performed a surveillance study of aseptic meningitis in pediatric ambulatory clinics and emergency departments of three Baltimore hospitals between July 1986 and December 1990. They identified a single viral agent in 169 (62%) of the 274 cases with laboratory study; 168 enteroviruses and 1 adenovirus were identified. Today, with the use of polymerase chain reaction (PCR) and culture and appropriate serologic study, the etiology of most cases of aseptic meningitis can be determined.

ETIOLOGY

Box 35.1 lists infectious agents and other causes of aseptic meningitis. At present, the diagnostic workup of aseptic meningitis usually is not undertaken vigorously, and the etiologic agent is identified in only approximately 10% of all cases. Epidemiologic study and intensive investigations at some centers indicate, however, that most cases result from viral infections. Enteroviruses account for approximately 85% of all cases of aseptic meningitis.[55,99-101,258] The following enteroviruses have been associated with aseptic meningitis: polioviruses 1 to 3; coxsackieviruses A 1 to 14, 16 to 18, 21, 22, and 24; coxsackieviruses B 1 to 6; echoviruses 1 to 9, 11 to 21, 24 to 27, and 29 to 33; and enterovirus 71. Recently described parechoviruses are closely related to enteroviruses and have also been associated with aseptic meningitis. Although 16 genotypes of parechoviruses have been characterized,[76] CNS infections in young infants, including meningitis, are most frequently the result of human parechovirus 3 infections.[119,302]

In recent years, multiple outbreaks of aseptic meningitis caused by enteroviruses have been described, including outbreaks caused by echovirus 30 in several countries throughout Eastern and Western Europe, China, Japan, Korea, Australia, the Arabian Gulf, the United States, and Brazil.* Echovirus 13 was responsible for reported outbreaks of aseptic meningitis in the United States, England, Wales, Germany, Belgium, Spain, France, Lithuania, Israel, Japan, Korea, and Australia.†

*References 12, 25, 33, 44, 52, 66, 63, 71, 78, 90, 110, 123, 146, 163, 193, 203, 223, 236, 238, 243, 250, 254, 268, 270, 272, 281, 285, 301, 324, 360, 370, 372, 382, 396, 401.

†References 65, 75, 79, 107, 192, 200, 204, 263, 265, 338, 360, 362.

Enterovirus 71 caused a major epidemic in Taiwan from 1998 to 1999, with multiple cases of hand, foot, and mouth syndrome associated with aseptic meningitis and other neurologic manifestations.[179,228,227,233,328,381,381,395,393] Similar outbreaks of aseptic meningitis caused by enterovirus 71 were reported in Malaysia, Japan, Hong Kong, and Australia.[72,131,172,237,247,327–329] Other enteroviruses involved in more recent outbreaks include echovirus 4 in Italy, Greece, Israel, Palestine, and Australia[160,235,241,289]; echovirus 6 in China[239]; echovirus 9 in Japan and regions of the United States[10,67]; echovirus 11 among institutionalized children in Israel[339]; echovirus 16 in Cuba[320]; echovirus 18 in Taiwan and Missouri[363,367,380]; echovirus 33 in New Zealand[177]; coxsackievirus A9 in Latvia and China[91,281]; and coxsackievirus B3 in China.[354] In the United States, the most common serotypes are coxsackievirus A6, human parechovirus 3, echovirus 11 and 18, coxsackieviruses A9 and B4, and echoviruses 30 and 6, with echoviruses 9 and 30 being the most frequently identified etiologies of aseptic meningitis since 2003.[1,68,69,66,305,355]

Sharing seasonality with the enteroviruses, several arboviruses cause CNS disease in North America. Although encephalitis is the most recognizable manifestation of many of these infections, some arboviruses commonly are associated with aseptic meningitis as well.[70,144,305,309] Since the mid-1990s, outbreaks of West Nile virus (WNV) meningitis and encephalitis have occurred in Romania, Russia, and Israel.[80,286,364] First detected in the Western Hemisphere in 1999 in New York City, WNV subsequently spread across North America from the Atlantic to the Pacific coasts and into Canada and Mexico.[47,120,181,266,283] Between 1999 and 2008, almost 29,000 cases were reported in the United States, with more than 1100 deaths.[165,231] An estimated 1/150 infections results in severe neurologic illness, with meningitis as the primary manifestation in 16% to 40% of hospitalized patients.[191] Although the incidence of neuroinvasive disease increases with age, WNV is more likely to manifest as meningitis in children than in older adults and occurred in at least one-quarter of the 150 pediatric cases diagnosed in the United States in 2002.[82,128,164,185,230] Even in regions with increased incidence of WNV, episodes of meningitis caused by enterovirus greatly outnumber those caused by WNV.[191]

Before the introduction of WNV, arboviruses accounted for approximately 5% of cases of aseptic meningitis in North America, with St. Louis encephalitis virus being the most common.[48,58,60] Infection with La Crosse encephalitis virus (a California encephalitis virus subtype) often resembles herpes encephalitis, but it may manifest as aseptic meningitis in children.[246] Unlike WNV, the majority of severe La Crosse encephalitis virus cases occur in children 15 years of age and younger, and in a study of 282 patients with La Crosse encephalitis virus infections in the Eastern United States from 2003 to 2007, 17% had aseptic meningitis.[70,157] Other California serogroup viruses, such as Jamestown Canyon virus and snowshoe hare virus, and other arboviruses, such as Colorado tick fever, result in aseptic meningitis more frequently than encephalitis.[144,305,344] Tick-borne encephalitis can manifest as aseptic meningitis in endemic areas. Tick-borne encephalitis virus cases were reported more recently in studies conducted in Poland, Slovenia, and Sweden, and, in mild cases, the clinical presentation was that of aseptic meningitis.[154,222,234,402] Toscana virus, a sandfly-transmitted phlebovirus, is an emerging pathogen and cause of CNS infection, including aseptic meningitis, during the warm season in Mediterranean countries.[13,113]

Aseptic meningitis is an occasional manifestation of acute and recurrent genital infections with herpes simplex virus type 2 (HSV-2).[22,31,88,109,334,359] In contrast to HSV-1 CNS infections, which without treatment usually are fatal, HSV-2 aseptic meningitis in otherwise immunocompetent patients is a benign, self-limited illness. Herpes family viruses other than HSV-1 and HSV-2 also are potential causes of aseptic meningitis. Although neurologic involvement in primary varicella-zoster virus (VZV) infections usually is encephalitis rather than benign meningitis, herpes zoster infection occasionally does present with concurrent meningitis.[99,159,182,183,278,290,300,384] VZV has been identified by PCR in the CSF of patients who had acute aseptic meningitis without cutaneous lesions, and meningitis associated with the VZV vaccine strain has been described.* One report detected VZV vaccine strain in a young patient with viral meningitis 11 years after vaccination.[273] A

*References 2, 74, 115, 133, 135, 138, 183, 188, 206, 216, 224, 225, 273, 342.

BOX 35.1 Etiologic Agents, Factors, and Diseases Associated With Aseptic Meningitis

Viruses

Adenoviruses (1, 2, 3, 5, 6, 7, 12, 14, 32)
Arboviruses (in the United States: West Nile, St. Louis, California, Colorado tick fever, eastern equine, western equine, Venezuelan equine, and Powassan)[a]
Coronaviruses
Cytomegalovirus
Encephalomyocarditis
Enteroviruses (echoviruses, coxsackieviruses A and B, polioviruses, enteroviruses)
Epstein-Barr
Hendra and Nipah
Herpes simplex type 1
Herpes simplex type 2
Human herpesvirus–6
Human herpesvirus–7
Human immunodeficiency virus (HIV-1)
Human parechoviruses
Human T-cell lymphotrophic virus (HTLV-1)
Influenza A and B
Lymphocytic choriomeningitis
Measles
Mumps
Parechoviruses
Parainfluenza
Parvovirus B19
Rhinoviruses
Rotaviruses
Rubella
Varicella zoster
Variola

Bacteria

Atypical Mycobacteria

Bartonella henselae
Borrelia spp. (relapsing fever)
Borrelia burgdorferi (Lyme disease)
Brucella spp.
Leptospira spp. (leptospirosis)
Mycobacterium tuberculosis
Nocardia spp. (nocardiosis)

Pyogenic: Partially Treated

Treponema pallidum (syphilis)

Rickettsia

Anaplasma phagocytophila
Coxiella burnetii
Ehrlichia chaffeensis
Rickettsia rickettsii (Rocky Mountain spotted fever)
Rickettsia prowazekii (typhus)

Mycoplasma

Mycoplasma hominis
Mycoplasma pneumoniae

Chlamydia

Chlamydia pneumoniae
Chlamydia psittaci

Ureaplasma

Ureaplasma urealyticum

Fungi

Blastomyces dermatitidis
Candida spp.
Coccidioides immitis
Cryptococcus neoformans
Histoplasma capsulatum
Other: *Acremonium* spp., *Alternaria* spp., *Aspergillus* spp., *Blastoschizomyces capitus*, *Cephalosporium* spp., *Cladosporium trichoides*, *Drechslera hawaiiensis*, *Fusarium* spp., *Paecilomyces* spp., *Paracoccidioides brasiliensis*, *Penicillium marneffei*, *Phaeohyphomycosis*, *Pseudallescheria boydii*, *Sporothrix schenckii*, *Trichosporon beigelii*, *Ustilago* spp., *Zygomycetes* spp.

Parasites (Eosinophilic Meningitis)

Flukes: *Paragonimus westermani*, schistosomiasis, fascioliasis
Roundworms: *Angiostrongylus cantonensis*, *Gnathostoma spinigerum*, *Baylisascaris procyonis*, *Strongyloides stercoralis*, *Trichinella spiralis*, *Toxocara canis*
Tapeworms: *Cysticercosis*
Protozoa and free-living amoeba (noneosinophilic meningitis)
Acanthamoeba
Naegleria fowleri
Toxoplasma gondii (toxoplasmosis)

Vaccine Associated

Measles
Mumps
Polio
Rabies
Vaccinia

Parameningeal Infection

Malignancy

Central nervous system tumor
Leukemia

Immune Diseases

Behçet syndrome
Lupus erythematosus
Sarcoidosis

Medications

Antimicrobial agents (e.g., trimethoprim-sulfamethoxazole)
Intrathecal injections (e.g., contrast media, antibiotics)
Nonsteroidal antiinflammatory drugs
Other drugs

Miscellaneous

Epidermoid, dermoid, other cysts
Foreign bodies (shunt, reservoir)
Heavy metal poisoning
Kawasaki disease

[a]In other areas of the world, many other arboviruses are important.

variety of neurologic disorders, including aseptic meningitis, are rare complications of Epstein-Barr virus infection.[121,130,150,348,366] Most non-congenital infections with cytomegalovirus in nonimmunocompromised patients are unrecognized; however, occasional instances of aseptic meningitis have been noted.[99–101,292,293]

The role of human herpesvirus–6 (HHV-6) in causing meningitis is unclear; although HHV-6 has been found in CSF samples from infants with meningitis, the virus also is detectable in the CSF of asymptomatic individuals.[15,50,394,399] Similarly PCR identified HHV-7 in the CSF of six children with neurologic diseases, including aseptic meningitis, meningoencephalitis, facial palsy, vestibular neuritis, and febrile seizures.[287] The role of HHV-7 as a causative agent in aseptic meningitis remains to be determined.

Occasionally meningitis or meningoencephalitis occurs as a manifestation of acute illness with HIV-1 infection.[23,158] Neurologic manifestations develop 3 to 6 weeks after primary infection at the same time as an infectious mononucleosis–like illness.

Lymphocytic choriomeningitis virus was an important historical cause of aseptic meningitis. In 1974, eight cases of aseptic meningitis caused by lymphocytic choriomeningitis virus were found in New York state.[102] Today it is rarely recognized as a cause of meningitis, which is likely a result of both decreasing incidence of disease and decreased detection.[11,21,24,28,35,39,102,248,340] Seroprevalence studies conducted more than 2 decades ago found seroprevalence of 4.7%, whereas more recent studies show a much lower seroprevalence of 0.4%.[77,208] Nevertheless physicians should be alert to the possibility in all situations of rodent (pet or wild) exposure and test appropriately. Encephalomyocarditis virus is another rodent virus that rarely is recognized in humans.[383] It is associated with a variety of neurologic manifestations, including aseptic meningitis.[132]

Adenoviral types 1, 2, 3, 4, 5, 6, 7, 11, 12, 14, and 32 have been associated with meningitis and meningoencephalitis.* Although they occur infrequently, adenoviral CNS infections tend to be more severe than enteroviral infections. Rarely aseptic meningitis has been noted during illnesses caused by influenza A viruses, including 2009 pandemic influenza (H1N1), influenza B, rhinoviruses, parainfluenza viruses, parvovirus B19 virus, rotaviruses, and coronaviruses.† Most infections with measles, rubella, and variola viruses that involve the CNS are encephalitic.[57,53,251]

In the prevaccine era, mumps virus was the agent responsible for the greatest number of cases of aseptic meningitis; today, in the United States, use of vaccine has rendered mumps rare, although mumps outbreaks with associated cases of aseptic meningitis occur occasionally.[67,59] Aseptic meningitis and encephalitis resulting from administration of mumps vaccine have been noted in Canada, Brazil, Japan, and Europe.‡ The Leningrad 3, Urabe Am 9, and three Japanese strains of vaccine viruses have been implicated. In the United States, where the Jeryl Lynn vaccine strain has been used exclusively, the rate of encephalitis in vaccinees has been no higher than that of the observed background incidence of similar illness in the population.[54] A preliminary analysis of the Vaccine Safety Datalink project showed a possible increased risk for developing aseptic meningitis 8 to 14 days after receiving immunization with Jeryl Lynn mumps vaccine strain. A follow-up case-control evaluation of hospitalized cases failed to show an increased risk, however.[38]

Neurologic illness is a rare complication of measles, smallpox, polio, and rabies viral vaccines. In most instances, the illnesses are complex and severe, but occasionally aseptic meningitis is the only manifestation.[32,64,57,53,253,325,343] A case of aseptic meningitis caused by vaccine-derived poliovirus was reported in the Philippines in 2001.[64] It was in association with two pediatric cases of acute flaccid paralysis that occurred during the same time period. Viral isolates from all three patients revealed type 1 poliovirus derived from the Sabin vaccine strain.

Certain bacteria are important to recognize as etiologic agents in aseptic meningitis because the illnesses are treatable and early initiation of therapy is crucial. Of greatest importance is tuberculous meningitis. Early treatment of this illness nearly always results in complete cure, whereas diagnostic delay or inadequate treatment frequently results in permanent neurologic sequelae. Lyme disease, relapsing fever, brucellosis, leptospirosis, and rickettsial infections are illnesses acquired either directly or indirectly from animals, in which aseptic meningitis may be a part of the disease process.* *Mycoplasma pneumoniae* has been implicated as a causative agent of neurologic illness.[52,115,158,293,372] Pönkä[288] noted that 8/560 hospitalized patients with *M. pneumoniae* infections had aseptic meningitis and 18 had encephalitis or meningoencephalitis. Despite numerous case reports and case series, the role of *M. pneumoniae* is thought by some experts to be unknown.[37] *Mycoplasma hominis* and *Ureaplasma urealyticum* are rare causes of neonatal meningitis.[134,240,375,376] Meningitis and meningoencephalitis have been associated with *Chlamydia pneumoniae* infections.[17,152,335,349] Partially treated common bacterial meningitides are a common cause of meningitis in which cultures of CSF fail to grow organisms. Antigen detection systems, such as latex agglutination, can be useful in identifying the causative agents in some of these cases.

Numerous fungi and yeasts cause meningitis.[317] Although many fungal meningitides occur almost exclusively in immunocompromised patients, children and adults with normal immune status may experience meningitis caused by *Blastomyces dermatitidis, Coccidioides immitis, Cryptococcus neoformans, Cladosporium* spp., *Histoplasma capsulatum, Paracoccidioides brasiliensis,* and *Aspergillus* spp.[16,27,127,244] In infants who are premature or younger than 1 month of age, *Candida albicans* is an important cause of meningitis and is associated with significant morbidity and mortality.[29,148,259]

Parasites occasionally cause aseptic meningitis. Eosinophilic meningitis is caused by *Angiostrongylus cantonensis,* a rat lungworm.[73,158,173,174,226,295,307,385] Aseptic meningitis caused by *A. cantonensis* has been observed on several islands in the Pacific, and the infection may be acquired by the consumption of freshwater shrimp.

A sterile CSF pleocytosis occurs in 12% to 13% of young infants with bacterial urinary tract infections[8,124,351] and in approximately one-third of patients with Kawasaki disease who undergo lumbar puncture.[103,143] Numerous drugs and biologics have been implicated in aseptic meningitis.† Of most importance in pediatrics are trimethoprim-sulfamethoxazole and intravenous immunoglobulin. Other causes of aseptic meningitis are listed in Box 35.1.‡

EPIDEMIOLOGY

No unified epidemiologic pattern exists because so many different types of organisms cause aseptic meningitis. The epidemiology of the specific individual infectious agents or diseases is presented in detail in the various chapters of this book, and only a brief overview is presented here.

Because approximately 85% of all cases of aseptic meningitis are caused by enteroviral infections, the basic epidemiologic pattern of aseptic meningitis reflects these agents. In temperate climates, most cases occur in the summer and fall; infection with enteroviruses is spread directly from person to person, and the incubation period usually is 4 to 6 days. Epidemiologic considerations in aseptic meningitis caused by agents other than enteroviruses depend markedly on season, geography, climatic conditions, animal exposures, and many other factors related to the specific pathogens.

CLINICAL MANIFESTATIONS

Aseptic meningitis has many causes (see Box 35.1), and clinical manifestations vary with the different diseases. In some instances, the signs and symptoms resulting from meningeal inflammation dominate the clinical illness, whereas in other instances the main signs and symptoms reflect other organ system involvement. Clinical

*References 32, 86, 99–101, 122, 178, 201, 280, 281, 330, 337.

†References 19, 51, 89, 99-101, 106, 147, 175, 199, 257, 269, 271, 274, 279, 303, 373, 392, 398.

‡References 14, 20, 83, 84, 92, 94, 111, 245, 252, 264.

*References 3, 34, 36, 40, 41, 43, 118, 142, 176, 186, 187, 190, 195, 209, 217, 275, 282, 341, 356, 358, 374, 377, 389, 391, 400.

†References 24, 45, 49, 104, 125, 145, 156, 184, 196, 242, 247, 249, 261, 262, 296, 331, 390.

‡References 61, 108, 129, 141, 167, 171, 205, 209, 211, 218, 242, 326, 350.

manifestations in aseptic meningitis, regardless of etiology, also vary markedly by patient age.

Enteroviruses

Enteroviruses are the most common cause of aseptic meningitis, and they can be considered the prototype for a description of general clinical manifestations of aseptic meningitis.* Even among the enteroviruses, however, significant differences in clinical manifestations exist among the different viral types. Some general aspects of epidemic enteroviral aseptic meningitis are presented by viral type in Chapter 165.

The onset of illness generally is acute, although it may be insidious over the course of a week or so or may be preceded by a nonspecific acute febrile illness of a few days' duration. Almost all children have fever, and most older children have headache, which most often is retro-orbital or frontal in location. Photophobia is common. Temperature elevation varies, ranging from 38°C to 40.5°C (100.4°F to 105°F), and usually lasts approximately 5 days. Occasionally, fever is biphasic, with the initial elevation occurring before the onset of neurologic signs and symptoms. Anorexia, nausea, and vomiting are common, and abdominal pain and diarrhea also are reported frequently.

Meningeal signs (i.e., stiff neck and back, tightness of the hamstring muscles, and Brudzinski and Kernig signs) usually are present, but deep tendon reflexes usually are normal or hyperactive. Seizures occur occasionally, usually when concomitant high fever is present. Muscle weakness rarely is reported, but myalgia occasionally is noted. In young children, fever, irritability, and lethargy are the most common findings. Infants may be irritable and show resentment to handling, and the fontanelle may be tense.

Other manifestations of enteroviral infections also occur in children with aseptic meningitis. The most common is pharyngitis, which may occur during infection with all of the neurotropic enteroviral types. Rash occurs commonly but varies by viral type. With echovirus 9 meningitis, 30% to 50% of children have rashes, whereas with echovirus 6, exanthem is rare. Cases of meningitis caused by enterovirus 71 and coxsackie virus A16 frequently are accompanied by hand, foot, and mouth syndrome. Enanthem, pleurodynia, pericarditis, myocarditis, and conjunctivitis are other findings noted in children with enteroviral aseptic meningitis. Illness often is biphasic, with fever, an interlude, then return of fever and neurologic manifestations.

CSF leukocyte counts vary from a few cells to a few thousand cells; the median is in the range of 100 to 500 cells/mm^3. The percentage of neutrophils also varies greatly. Initially a predominance of neutrophils commonly occurs; later, CSF examinations show a decline in the percentage of neutrophils. The CSF protein usually is elevated mildly, and the glucose concentration usually is normal; rarely hypoglycorrhachia is noted.

The duration of illness varies. Usually disability because of neurologic involvement lasts 1 to 2 weeks.

Aseptic Meningitis Caused by Other Agents

Of 1478 pediatric WNV cases reported from 1999 through 2007, 30% were classified as West Nile neuroinvasive disease (WNND).[230] Unlike in older adults who often have encephalitis, most WNND in pediatric patients manifests as meningitis. Seizures occur more commonly in arboviral meningitides than in enteroviral illnesses of otherwise comparable severity.[162] The CSF findings generally are similar to those in enteroviral disease, although some reports suggest that neutrophils are more commonly seen with WNV than with other viral entities.[96,298] Examination of the CSF in mild cases of mumps often reveals pleocytosis, and mumps is one of the few viral infections that can cause hypoglycorrhachia. When neurologic disease caused by mumps is recognized, usually evidence of brain involvement is present.

Tuberculous meningitis usually has a gradual onset over the course of 2 to 3 weeks.[202,255,306] Initially, personality changes, irritability, anorexia, listlessness, and low-grade fever may be present, followed by signs of increased intracranial pressure, such as drowsiness, stiff neck, cranial nerve palsies, inequality of the pupils, vomiting, and seizures. Finally, coma, irregular pulse and respirations, and high fever occur. In fungal diseases, the course of meningitis is similar to the course of tuberculosis. In tuberculosis and several fungal meningitides, such as those caused by *C. immitis*, *H. capsulatum*, and *C. neoformans*, historical and radiographic evidence of pulmonary disease may be present.

Aseptic meningitis associated with *M. pneumoniae* is unique in that it frequently occurs a few days to 3 weeks after a respiratory illness (i.e., pharyngitis, bronchitis, or pneumonia).[153,229,336,365] Generally the likelihood of a predominance of neutrophils is less in other aseptic meningitides, and low glucose levels are likely in parameningeal bacterial infections, partially treated bacterial meningitides, brain tumors, leukemic infiltration, *M. pneumoniae* infections, fungal infections, and tuberculosis.

Recurrent Aseptic Meningitis (Mollaret Meningitis)

In 1944, Mollaret[256] described three patients with recurrent aseptic meningitis whom he had observed over the course of 15 years. Subsequently many other cases have been reported, and some cases have been noted in children.[46,84,85,170,284,345,357] The illness is characterized by recurrent attacks of fever with meningeal signs and symptoms. The attacks last several days and are separated by symptom-free periods lasting weeks or months. In addition to a lymphocyte-predominant pleocytosis, CSF samples obtained from certain patients contain large mononuclear cells (Mollaret cells). The disease remits spontaneously. HSV-2 has been identified by PCR or DNA probes in the CSF of most patients with recurrent meningitis.[25,84,114,213,284,321,353,357,368] Other viruses, such as HSV-1 and Epstein-Barr virus, and noninfectious causes, such as systemic lupus erythematosus, intracranial cysts, antibiotics such as amoxicillin, and environmental exposures, also have been identified as less frequent etiologies of recurrent meningitis.[150,205,291,315,319,345]

DIFFERENTIAL DIAGNOSIS

Careful analysis of the history and epidemiologic circumstances may point toward one of the specific causes listed in Box 35.1. During the summer and autumn, the presence of pleurodynia, herpangina, or unexplained febrile eruptions in the community suggests the possibility of enteroviral infections. Acute paralytic disorders in other patients suggests poliomyelitis, enterovirus 71, or WNV. Exposure to mosquitoes and encephalitis in horses implicates certain arboviruses, and exposure to ticks may be suggestive of Lyme disease, relapsing fever, or rickettsial disease, depending on the geographic location and other symptoms of the illness. A history of swimming in waters contaminated by urine from infected animals and exposure to rats in urban slums suggest leptospiral infection. Knowledge of clear-cut exposure to or concurrent evidence of mumps or of one of the common exanthems is helpful in delineating the differential diagnosis. The association of pneumonia or other respiratory illness preceding aseptic meningitis strongly suggests the possibility of *M. pneumoniae* as the etiologic agent.

Most difficult from the diagnostic, therapeutic, and prognostic points of view are instances of incipient or partially treated bacterial (especially when caused by *Haemophilus influenzae*) or mycobacterial meningitis. The clinical findings; the dosage of antibiotic previously used; the spinal fluid smear, latex agglutination, or other rapid antigen identification test; the culture; and the glucose level may be helpful in diagnosing bacterial meningitis. The quantitative determination of C-reactive protein in the CSF also may be useful in differentiating bacterial from viral meningitis.[4,87,97,276,277] Lindquist and associates[232] found that the determination of CSF concentrations of lactate was the most useful test in differentiating bacterial from nonbacterial causes of meningitis. Studies suggest that the presence of tumor necrosis factor-α in the CSF is rare in viral infections but common in bacterial disease.[9,112,140] When tuberculous meningitis is suspected, a careful evaluation of contacts, a careful examination of an appropriately stained smear from the pellicle of the CSF that was allowed to settle, and a positive tuberculin reaction or positive interferon-γ release assay may confirm the diagnosis. Because combined bacterial and viral infection has occurred, examinations of CSF should be repeated if any doubt exists. The possibility that the observed meningeal reaction is of neither viral nor bacterial origin

*References 5, 8, 12, 42, 64, 65, 62, 63, 71, 95, 107, 126, 137, 151, 155, 161, 166, 168, 160, 179, 193, 197, 198, 214, 228, 299, 308, 313, 314, 316, 318, 332, 347, 352, 387.

must be considered. Finally, CNS tumor must be considered in the differential diagnosis, particularly if hypoglycorrhachia and prominent signs of increased intracranial pressure are present.[211]

SPECIFIC DIAGNOSIS

Obtaining a meticulous history is essential. The clinician must evaluate exposure of the patient in the past 2 to 3 weeks to illness in contacts; exposure to mosquitoes, ticks, and animals during recent vacations, picnics, and so on; awareness of illness in animals, especially horses and other Equidae, in the patient's environment; recent travel from the home area; recent injections or medications of any kind; and the possibility of accidental exposure to heavy metals.

The CSF must be examined carefully to exclude disorders that respond to specific therapy. Smears for bacteria, appropriate rapid antigen identification tests, and cultures of the CSF are mandatory; the history and clinical findings may indicate the need for performing acid-fast stain and culture of the sediment for mycobacteria. Other circumstances may indicate the need for excluding fungal or protozoal infection; atypical cells may require cytopathologic study to exclude neural neoplasms, which may manifest acutely.

The introduction of PCR has facilitated the etiologic diagnosis of CNS viral infections, particularly infections caused by enteroviruses and herpesviruses.[6,139,149,180,194,212,322,361,397] PCR detects enterovirus in the CSF more rapidly than does cell culture and has been shown to shorten the duration of hospitalization for children with meningitis, thus reducing costs.[18,207,267,323,346] Enterovirus PCR tests do not detect human parechoviruses; specific PCR testing for human parechoviruses should be ordered in the appropriate population (especially children younger than 3 years). The absence of pleocytosis occurs rarely in patients with enteroviral meningitis but is relatively common in infants with meningitis resulting from human parechovirus.[98,119,136,169,260,294,302,371]

PCR is the test of choice for detecting CNS infections caused by HSV, and molecular techniques also have been used to identify in CSF such causes of meningitis and meningoencephalitis as VZV, HHV-6, parvovirus B19, and rotavirus.[26,188,210,369]

For many arboviruses, serologic examination is more sensitive than molecular methods, especially for arboviruses that have a short period of viremia and presence in the CSF, such as WNV. Molecular methods may have a complementary role, as in one study in which WNV PCR analysis had a 57% sensitivity and 100% specificity.[81,215]

In any patient suspected to have viral meningitis, spinal fluid, serum, feces, and throat swabs should be collected and either held in the hospital laboratory or sent to a public health laboratory with viral diagnostic services. An additional serum specimen should be collected 10 to 21 days later so that paired sera can be examined for antibody titer increases. This pairing is particularly useful in arboviral, lymphocytic choriomeningitis, encephalomyocarditis, leptospiral, borrelial, rickettsial, mycoplasmal, and toxoplasmal infections. Although these studies may not provide an immediate diagnosis, they may give early warning of a specific epidemic, and they are useful for prognostication, particularly in very young infants.

TREATMENT

Hospitalization usually is necessary because of the possibility of treatable bacterial disease, the frequent need for fluid therapy for dehydration, and sometimes for analgesics. Headache and hyperesthesia are treated with rest; analgesics; and a reduction in room light, noise, and visitors. Antipyretics are recommended for fever. Using acetaminophen rather than aspirin is prudent because of the risk for developing Reye syndrome associated with the latter antipyretic. Codeine, morphine, and the phenothiazine derivatives often are used for pain and vomiting but are rarely necessary in children and should be avoided because they may induce misleading signs and symptoms. The investigational antiviral drug pleconaril has been shown effective in the treatment of enteroviral meningitis; however, this drug presently is unavailable.[105,310–312] Treatment for illnesses such as tuberculous meningitis, fungal meningitides, and other illnesses for which specific therapies are available is covered in specific chapters of this book.

Several weeks after the patient has apparently recovered, a careful neuromuscular assessment should be conducted to ensure that muscular weakness is not a sequela. Bilateral audiometry is recommended, especially when mumps virus was involved.

PROGNOSIS

The prognosis in aseptic meningitis depends on the etiology. Some illnesses have an ominous prognosis (i.e., tuberculous meningitis, parameningeal infections, rickettsial infections), but patients usually do well if appropriate specific therapy is instituted early in the course of the illness. In *C. immitis* meningitis, the prognosis for cure is guarded even with early optimal therapy.

In enteroviral and other viral meningitides, children usually recover completely. Some patients complain of fatigue, irritability, decreased ability to concentrate, muscle pain, muscle weakness and spasm, and incoordination for several weeks after an acute illness. Although the outcome of enteroviral meningitis most often is without residual, some infants who have enteroviral meningitis in the first few months of life have an increased risk for altered language development.[30,388] Formally evaluating such children at age 3 to 6 years is important.

PREVENTION

The universal use of polio and mumps vaccines in children clearly is effective in controlling these two diseases. Control of insect vectors by suitable spraying methods and eradication of insect breeding sites is important in the control of many arboviruses. The control of animal vectors such as mice and rats alters the incidence of infections with lymphocytic choriomeningitis and encephalomyocarditis viruses.

NEW REFERENCES SINCE THE SEVENTH EDITION

1. Abedi GR, Watson JT, Pham H, et al. Enterovirus and human parechovirus surveillance – United States, 2009–2013. *MMWR Morb Mortal Wkly Rep.* 2015;64:940-943.
3. Abhilash KP, Gunasekaran K, Mitra S, et al. Scrub typhus meningitis: an underrecognized cause of aseptic meningitis in India. *Neurol India.* 2015;63:209-214.
13. Anagnostou V, Papa A. Seroprevalence of Toscana virus among residens of Aegean Sea islands, Greece. *Travel Med Infect Dis.* 2013;11:98-102.
16. Antinori S, Corbellino M, Meroni L, et al. *Aspergillus* meningitis: a rare clinical manifestation of central nervous system aspergillosis. Case report and review of 92 cases. *J Infect.* 2013;66:218-238.
18. Archimbaud C, Ouchchane L, Mirand A, et al. Improvement of the management of infants, children and adults with a molecular diagnosis of enterovirus meningitis during two observational study periods. *PLoS ONE.* 2013;8:1-8.
39. Bonthius DJ. Lymphocytic choriomeningitis virus: an underrecognized cause of neurologic disease in the fetus, child, and adult. *Semin Pediatr Neurol.* 2012;19:89-95.
40. Boorugu H, Chrispal A, Gopinath KG, et al. Central nervous system involvement in scrub typhus. *Trop Doct.* 2014;44:36-37.
45. Bruner KE, Coop CA, White KM. Trimethoprim-sulfamethoxazole-induced aseptic meningitis – not just another sulfa allergy. *Ann Allergy Asthma Immunol.* 2014;113:520-526.
90. Croker C, Civen R, Keough K, et al. Aseptic meningitis outbreak associated with echovirus 30 among high school football players – Los Angeles County, California, 2014. *MMWR Morb Mortal Wkly Rep.* 2015;63:1228.
98. de Crom SCM, van Furth AM, Peeters MF, et al. Characteristics of pediatric patients with enterovirus meningitis and no cerebral fluid pleocytosis. *Eur J Pediatr.* 2012;171:795-800.
113. Dupouey J, Bichaud L, Ninove L, et al. Toscana virus infections: a case series from France. *J Infect.* 2014;68:290-295.
119. Esposito S, Rahamat-Langendoen J, Ascolese B, et al. Pediatric parechovirus infections. *J Clin Virol.* 2014;60:84-89.
136. Ghanem-Zoubi N, Shiner M, Shulman LM, et al. Human parechovirus type 3 central nervous system infections in Israeli infants. *J Clin Virol.* 2013;58:205-210.
149. Graham AK, Murdoch DR. Association between cerebrospinal fluid pleocytosis and enteroviral meningitis. *J Clin Microbiol.* 2005;43:1491.
169. Henquell C, Chambon M, Bailly JL, et al. Prospective analysis of 61 cases of enteroviral meningitis: interest of systematic genome detection in cerebrospinal fluid irrespective of cytologic examination results. *J Clin Virol.* 2001;21:29-53.
178. Huang YC, Huang SL, Chen SP, et al. Adenovirus infection associated with central nervous system dysfunction in children. *J Clin Virol.* 2013;57:300-304.

182. Ibrahim W, Elzouki AN, Husain A, et al. Varicella zoster aseptic meningitis: report of an atypical case and literature review. *Am J Case Rep*. 2015;16:594-597.
184. Jain RS, Kumar S, Aggarwal R, et al. Acute aseptic meningitis due to intravenous immunoglobulin therapy in Guillain-Barré syndrome. *Oxf Med Case Reports*. 2014;2014(7):132-134.
196. Karmacharya P, Mainali NR, Aryal MR, et al. Recurrent case of ibuprofen-induced aseptic meningitis in mixed connective tissue disease. *BMJ Case Rep*. 2013; 10:1-3.
207. Kleines M, Scheithauer S, Schiefer J, et al. Clinical application of viral cerebrospinal fluid PCR testing for diagnosis of central nervous system disorders: a retrospective 11-year experience. *Diagn Microbiol Infect Dis*. 2014;80:207-215.
212. Kumar A, Shukla D, Kumar R, et al. Molecular identification of enteroviruses associated with aseptic meningitis in children from India. *Arch Virol*. 2013;158:211-215.
236. Lu J, Zheng H, Guo X, et al. Elucidation of echovirus 30's origin and transmission during the 2012 aseptic meningitis outbreak in Guangdong, China, through continuing environmental surveillance. *Appl Environ Microbiol*. 2015;81:2311-2319.
238. Mantadakis E, Pogka V, Voulgari-Kokota A, et al. Echovirus 30 outbreak associated with a high meningitis attack rate in Thrace, Greece. *Pediatr Infect Dis J*. 2013;32:914-916.
243. Martinez AA, Castillo J, Sanchez MC, et al. Molecular diagnosis of echovirus 30 as the etiological agent in an outbreak of aseptic meningitis in Panama: May–June 2008. *J Infect Dev Ctries*. 2012;6:836-841.
250. Milia MG, Cerutti F, Gregori G, et al. Recent outbreak of aseptic meningitis in Italy due to echovirus 30 and phylogenetic relationship with other European circulating strains. *J Clin Virol*. 2013;58:579-583.
254. Mladenova Z, Buttinelli G, Dikova A, et al. Aseptic meningitis outbreak caused by echovirus 30 in two regions in Bulgaria, May–August 2012. *Epidemiol Infect*. 2014;142:2159-2165.
257. Moon JH, Na JY, Kim JH, et al. Neurological and muscular manifestations associated with influenza B infection in children. *Pediatr Neurol*. 2013;49:97-101.
260. Mulford WS, Buller RS, Arens MQ, et al. Correlation of cerebrospinal (CSF) cell counts and elevated CSF protein levels with enterovirus reverse transcription-PCR results in pediatric and adult patients. *J Clin Microbiol*. 2004;42:4199-4203.
261. Mullane D, Williams L, Merwick A, et al. Drug induced aseptic meningitis caused by intravenous immunoglobulin therapy. *Ir Med J*. 2012;105:182-183.
268. Nougairede A, Bessaud M, Thiberville SD, et al. Widespread circulation of a new echovirus 30 variant causing aseptic meningitis and non-specific viral illness, South-East France, 2013. *J Clin Virol*. 2014;61:118-124.
294. Ramers C, Billman G, Hartin M, et al. Impact of a diagnostic cerebrospinal fluid enterovirus polymerase chain reaction test on patient management. *JAMA*. 2000;283:2680-2685.
302. Renaud C, Harrison CJ. Human parechovirus 3: the most common cause of meningoencephalitis in young infants. *Infect Dis Clin North Am*. 2015;29:415-428.
331. Simms KM, Kortepeter C, Avigan M. Lamotrigine and aseptic meningitis. *Neurology*. 2012;78:921-927.
354. Tao Z, Song Y, Li Y, et al. Coxsackievirus B3, Shandong Province, China 1990–2010. *Emerging Infect Dis*. 2012;18:1865-1867.
371. Vergnano S, Kadambari S, Whalley K, et al. Characteristics and outcomes of human parechovirus infection in infants (2008–2012). *Eur J Pediatr*. 2015;174:919-924.
396. Yang XH, Yan YS, Weng YW, et al. Molecular epidemiology of echovirus 30 in Fujian, China between 2001–2011. *J Med Virol*. 2013;85:696-702.
402. Zielicka-Hardy A, Rosinska M, Kondrusik M, et al. Predictors for diagnosis of tick-borne encephalitis infection in Poland, 2009–2010. *Infect Dis (Lond)*. 2015;47:604-610.

The full reference list for this chapter is available at ExpertConsult.com.

36 Encephalitis and Meningoencephalitis

David E. Bronstein • Carol A. Glaser

Encephalitis is one of the most challenging syndromes for physicians to manage, especially because of the high morbidity and mortality and the vast number of causes that need to be considered. Furthermore the etiology is often not identified despite the multitudes of causal agents and entities. The focus of this chapter is on causal entities in the immunocompetent host.

Encephalitis is an inflammation of the brain, and affected patients generally have fever, headache, and altered mental status. Some patients also have an associated meningeal inflammation, thus representing an overlap with meningoencephalitis. For the purposes of this chapter, these terms are used interchangeably. The diagnosis of encephalitis can be established only by the microscopic examination of brain tissue or the recovery of a neurotropic agent. In clinical practice, however, the diagnosis is presumptive and frequently based on clinical features.

Encephalitis is often classified as primary or as postinfectious or parainfectious. In primary encephalitis, direct invasion and replication of an infectious agent in the central nervous system (CNS) occur, resulting in objective clinical evidence of cerebral or cerebellar dysfunction. Postinfectious or parainfectious encephalitis occurs after or in combination with other illnesses that are not CNS illnesses or after a vaccine or other product has been administered. Manifestations may be mediated immunologically. Clinical symptoms can result from noninfectious causes and are often indistinguishable from those of infectious encephalitis.

Frequently when encephalitis occurs, other regions of the nervous system, such as the spinal cord (myelitis), nerve roots (radiculitis), and nerves (neuritis), also are involved. When neurologic clinical findings suggest encephalitis but inflammation of the brain has not occurred (e.g., influenza encephalopathy), the condition is identified by the less specific term *encephalopathy*.

In 2012 the International Encephalitis Consortium developed diagnostic criteria for encephalitis and encephalopathy of presumed infectious or autoimmune etiology to facilitate individual case diagnostic workup, epidemiologic surveillance, clinical research, and outbreak investigations (Box 36.1).[474] According to this case definition, a diagnosis of encephalitis requires the presence of the major criterion of altered mental status lasting 24 hours or more with no alternative cause identified, in addition to two minor criteria for "possible" encephalitis or three or more for "probable or confirmed" encephalitis.

HISTORY

Rabies encephalitis was recognized in ancient times in Europe and Asia.[217] In AD 100, Celsus noted the relationship of animal rabies to human disease. "Sleeping sickness" associated with epidemic influenza was noted early in the 18th century.[485] For the past 100 years, epizootics of encephalitis in equine animals have been observed in the United States, and, in 1933, St. Louis encephalitis virus was isolated from the brains of humans dying of epidemic encephalitis.[292,318,328,354] Meningoencephalitis was recognized at the beginning of the 20th century as a complication of mumps.[143] Nonpolio enteroviruses have been known for the past 60 years to be a cause of encephalitis; during the same period, more than 400 zoonotic arthropod-borne viruses have been discovered. Of these, 100 or more cause encephalitis in humans.[36] In countries where vaccines are widely available there has been a decline in vaccine-preventable neurologic complications from measles, mumps, and rubella. However, there has been a continually expanding list of emerging or reemerging pathogens, including *Balamuthia mandrillaris*, *Baylisascaris procyonis*, human parechoviruses, Nipah virus, Chandipura virus, and Zika virus. Moreover, there has been expansion of certain agents into geographic regions.[196] West Nile virus, for instance, has expanded its geographic range from Africa to North and South America, Europe, the Middle East, western Asia, and Australia.[202] Japanese encephalitis virus has spread into India, Nepal, and northern Australia.[435]

BOX 36.1 Diagnostic Criteria for Encephalitis and Encephalopathy of Presumed Infectious or Autoimmune Etiology

Major Criterion (Required)

Patients presenting to medical attention with altered mental status (defined as decreased or altered level of consciousness, lethargy or personality change) lasting ≥24 hours with no alternative cause identified

Minor Criteria (2 Required for Possible Encephalitis; ≥3 Required for Probable or Confirmed Encephalitis)

Documented fever ≥38°C (100.4°F) within the 72 hours before or after presentation

Generalized or partial seizures not fully attributable to a preexisting seizure disorder

New onset of focal neurologic findings

CSF WBC count ≥5/mm^3

Abnormality of brain parenchyma on neuroimaging suggestive of encephalitis that is either new from prior studies or appears acute in onset

Abnormality on electroencephalography that is consistent with encephalitis and not attributable to another cause

Modified from Venkatesan A, Tunkel AR, Bloch KC, et al. Case definitions, diagnostic algorithms, and priorities in encephalitis: consensus statement of the International Encephalitis Consortium. *Clin Infect Dis.* 2013;57:1114–28.

Chikungunya is the most recent example of a striking geographic virus expansion, with outbreaks in the Indian Ocean and subsequent spread to India and Europe, and then to the Caribbean, Central, and South and North America.[395] Simultaneously the neurologic complications from Chikungunya appear to be increasing as well.[21]

ETIOLOGY

The many causes of encephalitis include both infectious and noninfectious entities. The infectious causes include viruses, bacteria, fungi, and parasites. Etiologic agents of acute encephalitis, meningoencephalitis, or illnesses that clinically resemble encephalopathy are listed in Table 36.1. Many of the infectious agents or diseases are discussed more fully and are referenced more completely elsewhere in this book.

Despite extensive testing and evaluation, the causes of many cases of encephalitis remain unexplained in recent prospective studies.[180,268,382] During the first 7 years of the California Encephalitis Project, 1570 patients were identified who met the case definition of having encephalitis (immunocompetent patients older than 6 months of age hospitalized with at least 24 hours of encephalopathy and one or more of the following characteristics: fever, seizure, focal neurologic findings, or electroencephalographic [EEG] or neuroimaging findings consistent with encephalitis). A confirmed or probable agent was identified in only 251 (16%) cases; of these agents, 69% were viral, 20% were bacterial, 3% were prion, 3% were parasitic, and 1% were fungal. An additional 13% had a possible cause identified, and a noninfectious cause was identified in 8% of cases.[181] In 2007 the California Encephalitis Project (CEP) began to test for anti–*N*-methyl-D-aspartate receptor (anti-NMDAR) encephalitis, a recently identified noninfectious cause of encephalitis. Within the CEP cohort, cases of anti-NMDAR encephalitis were identified more frequently than any viral etiology, including herpes simplex virus type 1, West Nile virus, and varicella zoster virus.[171] Overall the Centers for Disease Control and Prevention Emerging Infections Program Encephalitis Project, which represents the largest cohort of patients with encephalitis studied to date (>5000), has identified a confirmed or probable cause of encephalitis in approximately one-third of cases studied. Similar percentages of "unknown" causes have been seen in studies across the globe, such as in Australia from 1990 to 2007, with 69.8% unknown, and in England from 1989 to 1998, with 60% unknown.[42,118,233]

Viruses

Some types of viral encephalitides are an uncommon complication of a relatively common infection, such as enteroviruses and herpesviruses, whereas others are clinical manifestations of newly emerging or rare pathogens such as Hendra virus, lymphocytic choriomeningitis virus, chikungunya, or rabies.

Enteroviruses and Human Parechoviruses

Enteroviruses and human parechoviruses are small, nonenveloped single-stranded RNA viruses within the Picornaviridae. Encephalitis is a rare complication of enteroviral infection, but because enteroviruses are so common and estimated to cause 10 to 15 million illnesses per year in the United States they are a leading cause of encephalitis, particularly in children.[445] Of encephalitis cases with a cause identified, enteroviruses comprise 10% to 15% of cases.[445] Enteroviruses are now the leading viral cause of neurologic disease in children in the United States, and they are a major cause of encephalitis.* Of the 1750 patients with encephalitis enrolled in the California encephalitis project, enteroviruses were the leading causative agent.[193] Several enterovirus types have been associated with encephalitis: coxsackieviruses A2, A4 to A7, A9, A10, A16, A21, and B1 to B5; echoviruses 1 to 9, 11 to 25, 27, 30, and 33; and enteroviruses 71, 75, 76, and 89. Outside the United States, outbreaks of enterovirus 71 have been observed, often with neurologic manifestations and relatively high morbidity and mortality. In 1998, an extensive epidemic of enterovirus 71 disease occurred in Taiwan.[90,221,228,290,304,482,499] Manifestations of illness in this epidemic varied, and many children had severe neurologic events, including meningitis, encephalitis, cerebellitis, and polio-like syndrome. In particular, numerous children had brainstem encephalitis, with many fatalities occurring.

The first two human parechoviruses characterized, formerly echovirus 22 and echovirus 23, were originally described as enteroviruses. To date, 16 genotypes of human parechovirus have been characterized.[98] As a group, human parechoviruses can cause similar clinical diseases as enteroviruses, including respiratory, gastrointestinal, and sepsis-like syndromes and CNS infections. Neonates and young children have more severe clinical disease than older children. Human parechoviruses 1 and 2 are most often associated with respiratory and gastrointestinal infections, but acute flaccid paralysis and encephalitis have occasionally been associated with human parechovirus 1 (when formerly classified as echovirus 22).[150] Human parechovirus 3 has been associated with sepsis, meningitis, and encephalitis and, during the neonatal period, has been associated with white matter changes often suggestive of hypoxic-ischemia injuries.[46,52,144,176,206,213,364,392,475,476] The relative frequency of human parechovirus infections is unknown, especially in neurologic illnesses, because these viruses are often difficult to grow and molecular testing for enteroviruses would not have detected human parechoviruses.

Herpesviruses

Neurologic manifestations of herpesviruses are an uncommon complication of a common infection. Indeed, as a group, the herpesviruses are among the most frequently identified agents responsible for viral encephalitis.[190,233,243,310,457,469] Herpes simplex encephalitis is the most common cause of sporadic fatal encephalitis in the United States, with approximately one-third of cases occurring in patients younger than age 20 years but older than 6 months and with approximately half occurring in patients older than age 50 years.[328,400,468,491] Molecular analyses of paired oral or labial and brain sites have indicated that herpes simplex encephalitis can be the result of a primary infection, a reactivation of latent herpes simplex virus, or a reinfection by a second herpes simplex virus.[493] Although herpes simplex virus type 2 is a leading cause of severe and frequently fatal encephalitis in neonates,[492] type 1 is the usual cause beyond the neonatal period.[100,236,267,318,331,372,384,477]

Other herpesviruses, including varicella-zoster virus, Epstein-Barr virus, cytomegalovirus, and human herpesvirus–6, can also cause

*References 33, 77, 78, 100, 124, 125, 126, 136, 222, 252, 259, 272, 287, 328, 333, 338, 349, 366.

TABLE 36.1 **Encephalitis (With a Focus on Immunocompetent Patients and Pathogens in the United States)**

Etiology	Association With Encephalitis	Epidemiology	Clinical and Laboratory Hallmarks	Recommended Tests and "Pitfalls"
Viruses				
Adenovirus	Mostly anecdotal data; unclear neurotropic potential	Sporadic; children and immunocompromised persons at greatest risk	Respiratory symptoms common	Viral culture or PCR from respiratory site, CSF, or brain tissue
Eastern equine encephalitis virus	Proven neurotropic potential, but uncommon	Atlantic and Gulf U.S. states	Subclinical to fulminant; 50–70% mortality	Serology
Enteroviruses (include coxsackieviruses and enterovirus 71)	Most common cause of encephalitis in pediatric population	Highest incidence in late summer and early fall but can occur year round; large outbreaks of enterovirus 71 infection in Asia have occurred.	Aseptic meningitis most common but also encephalitis; hand, foot, and mouth rash may be present; enterovirus 71 can cause rhombencephalitis	CSF PCR single best test but not always sensitive; to increase sensitivity of detection add serum/plasma, throat PCR, or culture.
Epstein-Barr virus	Relatively common	During acute infection	Infectious mononucleosis during acute infection, cerebellar ataxia, sensory distortion ("Alice-in-Wonderland" syndrome)	Serology and CSF PCR. Beware of PCR false-positive results (detection of low levels may represent latent infection) and false-negative results (not all cases are CSF positive).
Hendra virus	Less common	Endemic in Australia; associated with equine exposure	Nonspecific	Contact local health department or Special Pathogens Branch at CDC.
Hepatitis C	Mostly anecdotal data; unclear neurotropic potential; neurologic symptoms may be related to vasculitis.	Hepatitis C–seropositive patients		CSF PCR
Herpes B virus	Proven neurotropic potential; rare	Transmitted by bite of Old World macaque	Vesicular eruption at site of bite followed by neurologic symptoms, including transverse myelitis	Culture and PCR of vesicles, CSF; contact CDC or Dr. Julia Hilliard.
Herpes simplex virus (HSV) types 1 and 2	Relatively common	HSV type 1 accounts for 5–10% of encephalitis; typically a reactivation disease, HSV type 2 occurs in neonates.	Temporal lobe seizures (apraxia, lip smacking), olfactory hallucinations, behavioral abnormalities, but children often have extratemporal lesions as well	CSF PCR single best test, but false-negative results can occur; if HSE strongly suspected, repeat lumbar puncture within 3–7 days and recheck HSV PCR and intrathecal antibodies.
Human herpesvirus–6	Unknown, especially owing to difficult interpretation of CSF PCR false-positive results	Young children (≤2 yr) or immunocompromised patients, particularly bone marrow transplant recipients	May be associated with "roseola rash"	CSF PCR. Beware of false-positive findings due to chromosomal integration and latent infections.
Human metapneumovirus	Anecdotal evidence only	Newly described; almost exclusively in children	Often with associated respiratory symptoms	Respiratory tract PCR (most CSF PCR negative)
Human parechoviruses	Proven neurotropic potential but frequency unknown	Children <3 yr	In young infants periventricular white matter changes resemble hypoxic ischemic encephalopathy.	Parechovirus PCR (enterovirus PCR will not detect)
Influenza virus	Unclear neurotropic potential; good data to support flu-associated encephalopathy but unclear if encephalitis and unclear mechanism	Neurologic complications occur; sporadically reported during influenza seasons; higher numbers reported in Japan and Southeast Asia	Upper respiratory tract symptoms CSF often acellular in 10% with bilateral thalamic necrosis	Respiratory tract culture, PCR, or rapid antigen; CSF and brain PCR infrequently positive
Japanese encephalitis virus	Relatively common (but only in endemic areas)	Mosquito-borne; most common worldwide cause of encephalitis; endemic throughout Asia; vaccine preventable	Seizures, parkinsonian features, acute flaccid paralysis variably seen. MRI classically shows thalamic and basal ganglia involvement.	CSF and serum antibodies

Continued

TABLE 36.1 Encephalitis (With a Focus on Immunocompetent Patients and Pathogens in the United States)—cont'd

Etiology	Association With Encephalitis	Epidemiology	Clinical and Laboratory Hallmarks	Recommended Tests and "Pitfalls"
La Crosse virus	Relatively common	Mosquito-borne; endemic in U.S. East and Midwest; highest incidence in school-aged children	Varies from subclinical illness to seizures and coma	CSF and serum antibodies
Lymphocytic choriomeningitis virus	Rare	Highest incidence in fall and winter; rodent exposure	One of few viral causes of hypoglycorrhachia	Serology
Measles virus	Less common in countries where vaccine is routinely used	Vaccine preventable; measles inclusion body encephalitis onset 1–6 mo after infection; SSPE can manifest >5 years after infection.	Measles encephalitis nonspecific. SSPE has a subacute onset with progressive dementia, myoclonus, seizures, and, ultimately, death. EEG changes are often diagnostic.	Acute form: measles IgM SSPE: measles IgG in CSF and serum
Mumps virus	Less common	Vaccine preventable; used to be leading cause of encephalitis-meningitis, now rarely seen	Parotitis, orchitis, hearing loss; one of few viral causes of hypoglycorrhachia	Serology, throat swab PCR, CSF culture, or PCR
Murray Valley encephalitis virus	Less common	Highest incidence in Aboriginal children in Australia and New Guinea	Nonspecific presentation; case fatality 15–30%	Serology (may cross-react with other flaviviruses)
Nipah virus	Less common	Epidemics in Southeast Asia; contact with pigs	Myoclonus, dystonia, pneumonitis	Serology (Special Pathogens Branch, CDC)
Parainfluenza 1-4	Unknown neurotropic potential; anecdotal evidence	Worldwide	Associated with respiratory symptoms	Respiratory DFA or PCR; CSF PCR rarely positive
Parvovirus B19	Anecdotal evidence only	Sporadic cases	Variably associated with rash	IgM antibody, CSF PCR
Powassan virus	Less common	Tick-borne; endemic to New England, Canada	Nonspecific	Serology
Rabies virus	Uncommon in developed countries; relatively common in Africa, Asia, South America	Vaccine preventable; most common vector is bat (bites often unrecognized); dogs important source in developing countries; worldwide distribution	Paresthesia at site of bite Furious form: hydrophobia, agitation, delirium, autonomic instability, coma Paralytic form: ascending paralysis in 30% Two forms sometimes overlap.	Multiple tests and assays needed for antemortem testing: antibodies (serum, CSF), PCR of saliva or CSF, IFA of nuchal biopsy, or CNS tissue. Coordinate testing with health department.
Rotavirus	Correlation with seizures in young child but unclear association with encephalitis	Typically children; winter; vaccine preventable	Usually with diarrhea	Stool antigen, CSF PCR (CDC)
Rubella virus	Less common in countries where vaccine is routinely used	Vaccine preventable	Neurologic findings typically occur at same time as rash and fever	Serology, CSF antibodies
St. Louis encephalitis virus	Relatively common	Mosquito-borne; endemic to western U.S.; occasional outbreaks in central/eastern U.S.; highest incidence in adults >50 yr	Tremors, seizures, paresis, urinary symptoms, SIADH variably present	Serology (cross reacts with other flaviviruses)
Tick-borne encephalitis virus	Relatively common in affected geographic areas	Vaccine-preventable; transmitted via tick or ingestion of unpasteurized milk; endemic to Asia, Europe, and areas of former Soviet Union	Weakness ranging from mild paresis to acute flaccid paralysis	Serology
Vaccinia	Less common	Primarily associated with vaccination	Vaccinia rash (localized or disseminated)	CSF antibodies, serum IgM (natural infection)
Venezuelan equine encephalitis virus	Less common	Central and South America; sometimes in U.S. border states (Texas, Arizona)	Myalgias, pharyngitis, upper respiratory tract infection variably present	Serology, viral cultures (blood, oropharynx), CSF antibody
Varicella zoster virus	Relatively common	Acute infection (chickenpox) or reactivation (shingles)	Vesicular rash (disseminated or dermatome), cerebellar ataxia, large vessel vasculitis	DFA or PCR of skin lesions, CSF PCR, serum IgM (acute infection)

TABLE 36.1 Encephalitis (With a Focus on Immunocompetent Patients and Pathogens in the United States)—cont'd

Etiology	Association With Encephalitis	Epidemiology	Clinical and Laboratory Hallmarks	Recommended Tests and "Pitfalls"
Western equine encephalitis virus	Less common	Onset in summer and early fall; western U.S. and Canada, Central and South America	Nonspecific	Serology
West Nile virus	Relatively common	Mosquito-borne; emerging cause of epidemic encephalitis in U.S., Europe; endemic in Middle East; highest incidence in adults >50 yr; documented transmission through organ and blood	Weakness and acute flaccid paralysis, tremors, myoclonus, parkinsonian features; MRI shows basal ganglia and thalamic lesions.	CSF IgM, serum IgM/IgG, paired serology (cross reactivity with West Nile virus and SLE)
Bacteria				
Bartonella henselae (and other *Bartonella* spp.)	Relatively common	Often occurs after scratch or bite from kitten	Encephalopathy with seizures (often status epilepticus); peripheral lymphadenopathy; CSF is usually paucicellular.	Serology (acute usually diagnostic), PCR of lymph node; CSF PCR rarely positive
Borrelia burgdorferi	Less common	Tick-borne infection; in U.S. mostly in New England and eastern Mid-Atlantic states	Facial nerve palsy (often bilateral), meningitis, radiculitis; may be associated with or follow erythema migrans rash.	Serology (serial EIA and Western blot), CSF antibody index, CSF PCR
Chlamydia spp.	Anecdotal evidence only	Associated with *C. psittaci* and *Chlamydophila pneumoniae*	Often with associated respiratory symptoms	NP swab, respiratory, or CSF PCR
Coxiella burnetti	Less common	Animal exposures, particularly placenta and amniotic fluid	Flulike symptoms	Serology
Ehrlichia/Anaplasma	Relatively common	Tick-borne bacteria causing human monocytic and human granulocytic ehrlichiosis (HME, HGE) respectively; HME endemic to southern and central U.S.; HGE endemic to northeastern U.S. and Midwest	Acute onset of fever and HA; rash seen in <30% of cases; leukopenia, thrombocytopenia, and elevated LFTs frequent manifestations	Morulae in white blood cells, PCR of whole blood, serology (seroconversion may occur several weeks after symptoms)
Mycoplasma pneumoniae	One of most frequently identified agents in case series but mostly anecdotal evidence	Worldwide distribution	Respiratory symptoms variably present, but pneumonia rare; often with white matter involvement consistent with ADEM	PCR of NP swab or respiratory culture, serum IgM; CSF PCR rarely positive
Mycobacterium tuberculosis	Relatively common	Most common in developing countries; disease of very young and very old or immunocompromised	Subacute basilar meningitis, lacunar infarcts, hydrocephalus; CSF often with low glucose, high protein levels; pulmonary findings often associated	CSF AFB smear, culture, PCR, respiratory cultures highly suggestive
Rickettsia rickettsii	Relatively common in affected geographic areas	Tick-borne infection in North America; highest incidence in southeast and south central U.S.	Acute onset of fever and headache; petechial rash in 85% of cases beginning 3 days after onset of symptoms	Serology (seroconversion may occur several weeks after symptoms), PCR or IHC on skin biopsy of rash
Treponema pallidum	Rare (especially in pediatrics)	Sexually transmitted disease; meningoencephalitis in early disseminated disease; progressive dementia in late disease	Protean manifestations including temporal lobe focality (mimics HSV), general paresis, psychosis, dementia	CSF VDRL (sensitive but not specific), serum RPR with confirmatory FTA-ABS
Tropheryma whippelii	Rare (especially in pediatrics)		Progressive subacute encephalopathy, oculomasticatory myorhythmia pathognomonic; variable enteropathy, uveitis	CSF PCR, PAS-positive cells in CSF, small bowel biopsy

Continued

TABLE 36.1 Encephalitis (With a Focus on Immunocompetent Patients and Pathogens in the United States)—cont'd

Etiology	Association With Encephalitis	Epidemiology	Clinical and Laboratory Hallmarks	Recommended Tests and "Pitfalls"
Protozoa				
Acanthamoeba spp.	Less common; more common in immunocompromised	Worldwide, inhalation of wind-blown soil	Subacute progressive	Contact CDC/Parasitology.
Balamuthia mandrillaris	Less common	Worldwide (but most case reports in US and South America), inhalation of wind-blown soil	Subacute progressive disease characterized by space-enhancing lesions, often with cranial nerve palsies and hydrocephalus (similar to tuberculosis)	Serology (research laboratories), brain histopathology, CDC laboratories Contact CDC/Parasitology for testing.
Naegleria fowleri	Less common	Summer; swimming or diving in brackish water or poorly chlorinated pools	Anosmia, progressive obtundation; CSF resembles bacterial meningitis, but sterile	Mobile trophozoites on wet mount of warm CSF, brain histopathology
Toxoplasma gondii	Rare in normal hosts	Worldwide; cats definitive hosts but humans often infected via consumption of undercooked meats, unwashed produce		
Helminths				
Angiostrongylus cantonensis	Most common cause of eosinophilic meningitis worldwide; rare in US	In the U.S. in Louisiana and Hawaii; South Pacific, Asia, Australia, and Caribbean	Meningitis or encephalitis; eosinophils in CSF; also associated with eosinophilic pneumonitis	Identification of worm in tissues
Baylisascaris procyonis	Less common	North America, Europe, and Asia; pica, particularly near raccoon latrines	Obtundation, coma; significant CSF and peripheral eosinophilia	CSF and serum antibodies; contact CDC/Parasitology for testing.
Gnasthostoma spinigerum	Relatively common in affected geographic areas	Southeast Asia, some areas of South/Central America; undercooked freshwater fish, chicken, or pork; also reported with reports of ingestion of frogs/snakes	Eosinophilic myeloencephalitis; can cause intermittent symptoms for 10–15 y because larvae are long lived	Identification of worm in tissues
Fungi				
Coccidioides spp.	Relatively common	Southwest U.S., northern Mexico, areas of Central and South America	Neurologic manifestations are result of disseminated disease; more often meningitis than encephalitis; CSF eosinophils sometimes seen	CSF fungal culture (but need to alert lab); CSF and serum antigen and antibody. EDTA-heat–treated antigen increases sensitivity of CSF and serum.
Histoplasma capsulatum	Relatively common	Eastern and central U.S., especially Mississippi, Ohio, and Missouri river valleys; grows on mold, bird, and bat droppings; especially found in caves, barns, or excavation areas	Neurologic manifestations are result of disseminated disease.	CSF fungal culture; CSF and serum antigen and antibody. EDTA-heat–treated antigen increases sensitivity of CSF and serum. Urine antigen
Blastomyces dermatitidis	Relatively common	Southeast, central, and midwestern U.S.; also in Canada, Africa, and India	Neurologic manifestations are result of disseminated disease.	CSF fungal culture; CSF and serum antigen and antibody. EDTA-heat–treated antigen increases sensitivity of CSF and serum.

ADEM, Acute demyelinating encephalomyelitis; *AFB,* acid-fast bacilli; *CDC,* Centers for Disease Control and Prevention; *CNS,* central nervous system; *CSF,* cerebrospinal fluid; *DFA,* direct fluorescent antibody test; *EDTA,* ethylenediaminetetraacetic acid; *EEG,* electroencephalogram; *EIA,* enzyme immunoassay; *FTA-ABS,* fluorescent treponemal antibody absorption test; *HA,* hemagglutination assay; *IFA,* indirect fluorescent antibody test; *IHC,* immunohistochemistry; *LFTs,* liver function tests; *MRI,* magnetic resonance imaging; *NP,* nasopharyngeal; *PAS,* periodic acid–Schiff; *PCR,* polymerase chain reaction; *RPR,* rapid plasma reagin; *SIADH,* syndrome of inappropriate secretion of antidiuretic hormone; *SLE,* systemic lupus erythematosus; *SSPE,* subacute sclerosing panencephalitis; *VDRL,* Venereal Disease Research Laboratory.

encephalitis.[404] Encephalitis can occur in association with primary infection with varicella zoster virus (chickenpox) or with endogenous recurrent disease (herpes zoster).[1,59,104,116,142,216,240,273,382,428] In a study in Finland of more than 3000 patients with acute CNS infections of suspected viral origin, varicella zoster virus constituted 29% of all confirmed or probable etiologic agents.[272] In chickenpox, the rate of encephalitis is approximately 0.3 per 1000 cases,[67] and the case-fatality rate is approximately 17%.[374] Of patients with herpes zoster, 0.5% to 5% have encephalitis.[242] This complication occurs more commonly in immunocompromised patients than immunocompetent patients.

Epstein-Barr virus encephalitis occurs in less than 1% of cases, and most patients with Epstein-Barr virus encephalitis are adolescents and young adults. Patients typically present 1 to 3 weeks after the onset of mononucleosis syndrome, but encephalitis may be the presenting complaint in Epstein-Barr virus infection.[108,114,134,222,298,317,468,316] Caruso and associates[63] reported five children with subacute and chronic neurologic deficits associated with apparent primary Epstein-Barr virus infections. Severe chronic involvement of the brain is a common finding in congenital cytomegalovirus infection.[210] Encephalitis caused by acquired cytomegalovirus infection is uncommon and usually occurs in immunocompromised children.[199,222,427]

Human herpesvirus–6 is an important cause of acute febrile illness and roseola infantum in young children and is commonly associated with febrile convulsions.[140] Encephalitis is a rare complication of this infection in children with and without roseola.[65,111,209,235,236,237,238,319,350,504] Human herpesvirus–6 increasingly has become recognized as an important cause of encephalitis in immunocompromised, posttransplant patients, occasionally manifesting as severe amnesia after they have undergone bone marrow transplantation.[48,99,106,168,308,311,409,414,477] Human herpesvirus–7 has also been implicated as a causative agent in encephalitis.[148,357,372,413,461,484]

Arboviruses

More than 400 different arboviruses exist.[36,222,253] Arboviruses that are endemic to the United States and have been associated with encephalitis include eastern equine, western equine, Venezuelan equine, St. Louis, Powassan, West Nile, California serogroup viruses including La Crosse and Jamestown canyon, and Colorado tick fever. Historically arboviruses have been cited as one of the most common causes of encephalitis; however, recent studies found arboviruses to be relatively uncommon in the pediatric age group in the United States.[181,262]

First detected in the Western Hemisphere in 1999 in New York City, West Nile virus subsequently spread across North America from the Atlantic to the Pacific coasts and into Canada and Mexico.[54,75,146,231,312,343,369] Through 2011, an estimated 2 to 4 million infections have occurred in the United States, resulting in 0.4 to 1 million illnesses and 13,000 reported cases of neuroinvasive disease.[368] Although an estimated 1 in 150 infections results in severe neurologic illness, and the incidence of neuroinvasive disease increases with age, West Nile virus has been responsible for encephalitis in young children and adolescents, occurring in 37% of the 443 pediatric cases diagnosed in the United States between 1999 and 2007.[103,164,217,301] Although West Nile virus is the most common cause of neuroinvasive arboviral disease in the United States encompassing all age groups, the most common cause among children is La Crosse virus.[18,87,207,360,390]

Outside the United States, dengue is the most common mosquito-borne viral disease in the world, responsible for 50 to 100 million infections and 25,000 deaths each year.[179] In 2009 and 2010, 89 cases of dengue virus occurred in Key West, Florida.[84,189] With the exception of a few cases that occurred along the Texas-Mexico border, the cases in Florida represented the first local transmission of dengue virus in the continental United States since 1946.[73,74] Although encephalopathy is a well-reported neurologic complication of dengue fever, there has been increasing evidence that encephalitis with direct neuronal infiltration by dengue virus can also occur.[49,473] Japanese encephalitis virus, also a mosquito-borne flavivirus, although not quite as common as dengue, is the most important cause of epidemic encephalitis worldwide, with an estimated 35,000 to 50,000 cases and 10,000 deaths annually.[433,435,465] Most cases occur in Southeast Asia, China, and the Indian subcontinent.[434]

Chikungunya, a mosquito-borne arbovirus of the Togaviridae, was first isolated in 1953 and has caused outbreaks in sub-Saharan Africa, India, and Southeast Asia.[370,470] In 2005–06, an outbreak occurred on the island of Réunion, a French territory in the Indian Ocean, involving 266,000 cases, which represented more than one-third of the island's population. During this outbreak, 25% of infected children developed neurologic symptoms, 40% to 50% of which were severe manifestations, including status epilepticus, complex seizures, and encephalitis.[395] The epidemic subsequently spread to the Indian subcontinent, where 1.4 million cases were reported in 2006. By 2013, chikungunya was reported in the Caribbean, and encephalitis was diagnosed in the United States among travelers returning from endemic areas.[62,80,284,302,397,430] The first locally acquired chikungunya cases were identified in Florida in 2014.[257,278,441]

Tick-borne encephalitis, as the name implies, is transmitted by ticks and is caused by a group of tick-borne encephalitis viruses in the Flaviviridae family. Within this group there are subtypes, including European or Western tick-borne encephalitis virus, Siberian tick-borne encephalitis virus, and Russian spring-summer encephalitis virus (also known as Far Eastern tick-borne encephalitis virus). These viruses are found in Asia, parts of Europe, and areas of the former Soviet Union, and they have become an important consideration for travelers to endemic areas.[8,45,158,161,208,219,281,334,510]

Vaccine-Preventable Viruses

Prior to the widespread availability of vaccines in the United States, measles, mumps, and rubella were a common cause of encephalitis. Although still occurring elsewhere in the world, including Europe,[16,86,151,152,155,341,379,500] measles is a relatively rare occurrence in the United States, with the exception of the recent large multistate outbreak linked to an amusement park in California in December 2014.[82,511] Approximately 30 million cases of measles occur each year worldwide. Encephalitis occurs uncommonly, at a rate of 0.74 per 1000 cases of measles; the case-fatality rate is 14%. Subacute sclerosing panencephalitis, an indolent and progressive form of encephalitis, generally occurs many years after the initial infection. Before the use of mumps vaccine became widespread, this virus was the leading cause of meningoencephalitis in the United States. Today mumps is rare, although extensive mumps outbreaks with associated cases of encephalitis occurred in 2006.[79] The incidence of encephalitis among individuals with mumps is approximately 3 per 1000 cases; the case-fatality rate is 1.4%.[71] Neurologic involvement is a common manifestation of congenital rubella virus infection,[211] and encephalitis is a rare complication of noncongenital disease.[91,204,290,331] Some data suggest a rate of encephalitis in rubella between 1 per 5000 and 1 per 10,000 cases.[69] In the prevaccine era, the encephalitis rate in one epidemic in 1964 was 1 per 5000 cases, and, in another epidemic in 1942, it was 1 per 6000 cases.[313,422] Smallpox (variola virus infection), before its worldwide eradication, was a rare cause of encephalitis. Human rabies is uncommon in the United States, but approximately 55,000 cases occur worldwide, primarily in Asia, Africa, and Latin America.[263] Since the early 1970s, approximately two cases of rabies have occurred per year in the United States, and approximately 50% of the cases have occurred in children and teenagers.[10,70,72]

Rare and/or Newly Emerging Viruses

Lymphocytic choriomeningitis virus is an arenavirus acquired from infected rodents. It was previously a relatively common cause of encephalitis in the United States but now is rarely recognized, except for occasional outbreaks.[38] Clusters of cases of lymphocytic choriomeningitis have been identified among recipients of solid organ transplants in 2003 and 2005.[154] Encephalitis caused by herpesvirus B is rare; it occurs predominantly in monkey handlers and usually after monkey bites.[232] During the 2003 monkeypox outbreak in the midwestern United States, one child developed severe acute encephalitis and seizures; no additional encephalitis cases were identified.[415]

Nipah virus, a new paramyxovirus, is the first wide-scale epizoonotic encephalitis with direct animal-to-human, rather than vectorial, transmission.[93,305] The initial outbreak of Nipah virus encephalitis occurred among pig farmers in Malaysia and Singapore in 1999, and subsequently outbreaks have been identified in Bangladesh and India.* A fatal case of encephalitis caused by Hendra virus (equine Morbillivirus), another novel paramyxovirus, was reported in an adult;[314] previously, this virus had been noted in association with fatal respiratory tract infections in horses and humans. In 2003, another emerging pathogen, Chandipura virus, was responsible for a large outbreak of acute encephalitis in 329 children in southern India, with a case-fatality rate of 56%.[1,383] This rhabdovirus, transmitted to humans by sandflies, was responsible for

*References 3, 34, 89, 184, 213, 224, 225, 226, 293, 336, 451, 452.

a second outbreak in western India in 2004, with an even higher case-fatality rate of 78%.[89]

Bacteria

Patients with acute bacterial meningitis can sometimes have signs and symptoms that are indistinguishable from those of encephalitis. For example drowsiness, coma, convulsions, and mental confusion commonly occur in *Haemophilus influenzae, Neisseria meningitidis,* and *Streptococcus pneumoniae* bacterial meningitides. Spirochetal infections are more common causes of nervous system disease, specifically encephalitis, than generally is appreciated. Encephalitis is a recognized complication of leptospirosis, Lyme disease, and relapsing fever.[53,133,362,367,436] *Brucella* spp. are infrequent causes of meningoencephalitis.[330] *Bartonella henselae* encephalopathy is an uncommon complication of cat-scratch disease.[60,160,175,326,327,348,439,505] Infection with *Listeria monocytogenes* has been shown to mimic herpetic and West Nile virus encephalitis.[112,113,375]

CNS involvement has been described in most forms of rickettsial infections. Rickettsial diseases include infections caused by organisms of the genera *Rickettsia* (spotted fever rickettsioses, typhus fever group), *Orientia* (scrub typhus), *Coxiella* (Q fever), *Ehrlichia,* and *Anaplasma.* In particular, neurologic involvement commonly occurs in Rocky Mountain spotted fever.[218,255] In one study, two-thirds of the ill children had evidence of encephalitis. Neurologic sequelae are common.[188] Neurologic involvement also occurs in non–spotted fever rickettsial infections but is generally not as severe.[138,186,277,303,363,384,387,420] *Coxiella burnetii, Ehrlichia canis, Rickettsia typhi, Rickettsia canada,* and *Rickettsia conorii* all have been implicated.

Parasites and Free-Living Amoebae

In the United States, *Baylisascaris procyonis* has been associated with severe and often fatal eosinophilic encephalitis in children.[76,102,172,173,497] *B. procyonis* is a common roundworm in raccoons, and children typically acquire the infection by ingestion of raccoon feces. Outside the United States, parasitic causes of eosinophilic meningitis/encephalitis include *Toxocara* spp., *Gnasthostoma spinigerum, Angiostrongylus cantonensis,* and neurocysticercosis.

Protozoan parasites associated with encephalitis include *Plasmodium falciparum* and *Toxoplasma gondii.* Cerebral malaria is a common complication of *P. falciparum* infection. Meningoencephalitis and enlarging cerebral mass lesions rarely occur in acute acquired toxoplasmosis.[463] The reader is referred to Section XXII, "Parasitic Diseases," for a complete review.

The free-living amoebae that cause human disease are divided into two major categories: primary amoebic meningoencephalitis and granulomatous amoebic encephalitis. *Naegleria fowleri* affects immunocompetent hosts; *Acanthamoeba* predominantly affects immunocompromised hosts, and *Balamuthia* is found in both host groups. All three pathogens are found in soil and water. Primary amoebic meningoencephalitis is caused by the free-living amoeba *N. fowleri* and is a rare but usually fatal cause of encephalitis.* Most cases occur in children and young adults and are caused by swimming or playing in contaminated water. Granulomatous amoebic encephalitis, caused by *Acanthamoeba* or *B. mandrillaris,* can be subacute or chronic. Although formerly thought to be innocuous, neurologic infections with *Acanthamoeba* and *Balamuthia* are often fatal.[274,442]

Fungi

Fungal CNS infections often present as meningitis or brain abscesses, but in some instances patients have encephalitis-like symptoms. These illnesses occur most often in immunocompromised patients, but some infections occur in apparently normal individuals. Meningitis and brain abscess are the most common pathologic events, but encephalitis is associated commonly with meningitis. The following fungal agents are the most common causes of meningoencephalitis in immunocompetent children and adults: *Blastomyces dermatitidis, Coccidioides immitis, Cryptococcus neoformans, Cladosporium* spp., *Histoplasma capsulatum,* and *Paracoccidioides brasiliensis.*[296]

*References 43, 64, 81, 131, 177, 195, 220, 250, 256, 261, 282, 314, 365, 412, 426, 429, 478.

Other Putative Agents of Encephalitis

Many other infections have been associated with encephalitis, but their relevance is unclear. This is particularly true for agents with an unclear neurotropic potential, especially when the infection is identified only outside the CNS.

Although encephalitis associated with *Mycoplasma* is identified with increasing frequency,* the true role of *Mycoplasma* in encephalitis is unknown. In most case reports and case series in which *Mycoplasma pneumoniae* is identified as a cause, there is evidence of acute infection by serology and/or from positive PCR in respiratory tract specimens.[39,101] The significance of these findings is unclear, given the high background incidence of infection. Furthermore serologic assays for *M. pneumoniae* are notoriously problematic.[32] Similar issues arise with other agents that have been associated with encephalitis cases, including parvovirus B19, human bocavirus, parainfluenza virus, respiratory syncytial virus, *Chlamydia,* adenovirus, rotavirus, human metapneumovirus, and hepatitis B and C viruses.†

Although the association of influenza and neurologic manifestations is probably better documented than the aforementioned agents, the mechanism by which influenza causes neurologic illness is not well understood. Neurologic complications associated with influenza include Guillain-Barré syndrome, Reye syndrome, myelitis, and encephalopathy/encephalitis.‡

Evidence of neurologic invasion by influenza is almost never seen, and these cases are most accurately described as an "encephalopathy" rather than an encephalitis. Influenza-associated encephalopathy is more commonly described in children than in adults and is typically characterized by a rapidly progressive encephalopathy. Although particularly notable during the 1997 to 2001 influenza A epidemics in Japan, cases of encephalitis and encephalopathy associated with influenza A and influenza B also have been described in North America and Europe.[340,344,447,458,483,503] Similarly, the 2009 influenza A H1N1 pandemic was associated with encephalitis as well as acute necrotizing encephalopathy.§

Neurologic disease is a common reported complication of pertussis. A 10-year study in the United States indicated a rate of neurologic disease in infants of approximately 9 per 1000 cases.[147] An extensive review by Miller and associates[178] suggested that the neurologic disease occurring with pertussis rarely is inflammatory and is better classified as an encephalopathy.

Postimmunization Encephalitis

Neurologic disease, including encephalitis and meningoencephalitis, has been reported after various immunizations, but establishing causality is difficult. Depending on the type of immunizing agent, the encephalitis can be the result of an immunologic reaction, a CNS infection with the vaccine virus (e.g., with live vaccines), or a combination of infection and immunologic reaction. A recent review of the immunization records from pediatric encephalitis cases referred to the California Encephalitis Project between 1998 and 2008 did not show an association between the receipt of immunizations and the subsequent development of encephalitis.[358]

Historically many of the observed neurologic reactions occurred after the administration of antisera prepared in animals in the treatment of specific diseases. Antisera to the following diseases or infectious agents have been noted in association with neurologic illness: tetanus, diphtheria, scarlet fever, tuberculosis, gas gangrene, pneumococcus, gonococcus, meningococcus, and streptococci.[5,230,258,331,398] Of 100 neurologic syndromes complicating administration of serum reviewed by Miller and Stanton,[331] only 10% were of a cerebral or meningeal type.

Neurologic disease was a common complication of rabies vaccine derived from animal nervous tissue.[331] The incidence of complications

*References 40, 66, 101, 107, 119, 120, 135, 205, 269, 300, 329, 373, 408, 423, 432, 460, 464, 466, 502.

†References 20, 24, 26, 47, 52, 61, 68, 69, 124, 126, 132, 136, 137, 165, 167, 187, 264, 271, 276, 306, 337, 339, 345, 346, 349, 355, 356, 366, 425, 440, 443, 448, 450, 479, 506.

‡References 9, 33, 69, 124, 126, 156, 182, 183, 349, 353, 360, 360, 382, 407, 444, 446, 469, 511.

§References 4,57,83,94,117,147,166,234,279,307,314,381,391,480,501.

was between 3 per 1000 and 1 per 6000 cases.[41,331] Approximately 10% of the neurologic disease attributed to this rabies vaccine was meningoencephalitic or encephalomyelitic. Five cases of CNS disease (Guillain-Barré syndrome, demyelination, meningoradiculitis) have been reported in temporal association with the administration of human diploid cell rabies vaccine.[371] This occurrence is so rare that a causal relationship with vaccine is uncertain.

Encephalitis was an important complication of smallpox vaccination.[11,51,157,192,252,288,342,437] The rate of encephalitis varied markedly from one study to another, from 1 in 4000 primary vaccinations in the Netherlands[342] to approximately 1 in 80,000 primary vaccinations in the United States.[289] After reinstatement of the vaccination among military personnel and selected civilian groups in the United States in 2002, cases of suspected encephalitis or myelitis have been identified.[325,417,472]

Neurologic disease, including encephalitis, occurs rarely after the administration of typhoid-paratyphoid vaccine.[331] Neurologic disease also rarely has been attributed to administration of tetanus toxoid and diphtheria toxoid, but the manifestations seldom are central. Two cases in children who developed acute disseminated encephalomyelitis after receiving Japanese B encephalitis vaccination have been reported.[351]

Encephalitis and encephalopathy have been observed after the administration of influenza immunization.[174,193,401,498] In the extensive surveillance that occurred in the United States during the period October 1, 1976, to December 16, 1976, when 45,651,113 people received the A/New Jersey/76 influenza vaccine, no epidemiologic evidence of an association between vaccine and encephalitis was noted.[203] More recent surveillance after the administration of 3.8 million doses of the 2012–13 influenza vaccine in the Vaccine Safety Datalink, a large US cohort of medical care organization enrollees, also did not show an increased risk of prespecified adverse events that included encephalitis.[257]

Neurologic disease developing after administration of a whole-cell pertussis vaccine has also been reported but is controversial.[95–97] Pathologic evidence in fatal cases suggests encephalopathy rather than encephalitis.[110] Because neurologic illness similar to that which occurs after the administration of pertussis vaccination is a frequent development in infants who have not been vaccinated, establishing a true rate of pertussis vaccine encephalopathy, or that such an entity exists at all, has been difficult. The analysis of studies suggests that encephalopathy caused by pertussis vaccine does not occur.[95,96,97,198,399]

Neurologic disease, including encephalitis, is a rare complication after measles immunization.[51,67,159,286] The rate in vaccinees in the United States is less than 1 per 1 million. In contrast, the finding in the National Childhood Encephalopathy Study in England, Scotland, and Wales indicated a rate of 1 per 87,000 immunizations.[2] This high rate of encephalopathy may be an artifact due to the misclassification of complicated febrile convulsions as encephalopathy. Meningoencephalitis has been shown to be a rare complication of mumps immunization with some vaccine virus strains,[212,320] although it has not been a problem in the United States. More recent studies in the United States and Finland have failed to show an association between measles-mumps-rubella vaccination and encephalitis or encephalopathy.[311,388] A fatal encephalitis occurred in a 3-year-old child after receiving 17D yellow fever vaccine.[270]

Postinfectious Encephalitis

Postinfectious or parainfectious encephalitis occurs after a demonstrated or presumed viral infection and is thought to be immune mediated rather than due to a direct effect of the virus in nerve cells.[197,246,247,405] This theory has been studied extensively by Johnson[247] and Griffin[197] in encephalitis associated with measles. These researchers have described a periventricular demyelinating disease and have not been able to isolate measles virus or identify measles antigens in nervous tissue. Other investigators have recovered measles virus from the cerebrospinal fluid (CSF) and brain of affected patients.[159,324,378,419,455] We suggest that immune mechanisms play a role in the pathogenesis of measles and perhaps other postinfectious neurologic illnesses but that the process is stimulated by the direct presence of the antigen in the nervous system. The mechanism of disease is important regarding possible treatment: corticosteroids might be useful in immune-mediated disease but could be detrimental in an acute viral infection.

In contrast to measles, other apparent postinfectious encephalitides that usually have a subacute onset are immune mediated and have multifocal white matter lesions.* Specifically acute demyelinating encephalomyelitis (ADEM) usually is subacute in onset and is usually a monophasic polysymptomatic disorder that can affect any region of the brain and/or spinal cord. Thus clinical manifestations may include optic neuritis, myelitis, ataxia, hemiparesis, cranial nerve palsies, and multifocal white matter lesions that are easily confused with multiple sclerosis. Subtle features help distinguish between the two disorders, however.[431] If solitary or unilateral lesions are present, it most likely is ADEM, whereas lesions in the corpus callosum are much more common in multiple sclerosis. Lesions of greater than 4 cm diameter suggest ADEM, and ADEM lesions have indistinct borders compared with multiple sclerosis lesions, which have sharp borders. Patients with ADEM may respond dramatically to treatment with corticosteroids and perhaps intravenous immunoglobulin or plasmapheresis.

Chronic Encephalitic or Encephalopathic Illnesses

"Slow infections" that cause encephalitic and encephalopathic illness in humans have been recognized for many years. Many of these illnesses now are recognized as viral infections or caused by prions. Viral illnesses include progressive multifocal leukoencephalopathy in primarily immunocompromised hosts (JC, SV40, and BK viruses), subacute sclerosing panencephalitis (measles virus), and acquired immunodeficiency syndrome (AIDS) (human immunodeficiency virus [HIV] type 1 [HIV-1] and HIV-2). Prion diseases, termed *transmissible spongiform encephalopathies,* include kuru, Jakob-Creutzfeldt disease, and Gerstmann-Sträussler-Scheinker disease.[376] Prion diseases are related to scrapie of sheep and bovine spongiform encephalopathy (mad cow disease), which are prion diseases of animals. These chronic illnesses are discussed in Chapter 192.

EPIDEMIOLOGY

Because of the diversity of the infectious disease agents causing encephalitis, the incidence, geographic distribution, age distribution, and seasonality vary tremendously. The specific epidemiology of each infectious agent or disease is presented in detail in the respective chapters of this book; only a brief overview is presented here.

Accurate information on the overall incidence of encephalitis is lacking owing to the vast number of agents and the imprecise case definition. Nevertheless incidence rates for encephalitis range from 1.5 to 8.8 per 100,000 population.[104,118,270] In the United States, a study of hospital discharge data from 1988 through 1997 determined a rate of 7.3 encephalitis hospitalizations per 100,000.[262] The incidence of ADEM (a form of postinfectious encephalitis) is estimated to account for 10% to 15% of encephalitis overall, with specific ADEM incidence numbers estimated to be 0.4 to 0.8 per 100,000.[27,292,454]

Although encephalitis per se does not appear to follow a seasonal pattern, specific pathogens, particularly arthropod-borne viruses, do have well-defined temporal patterns. Encephalitis caused by arboviruses can sometimes occur in localized outbreaks, and epidemics or sporadic cases may be seen. In temperate areas, most cases occur in summer and fall. The occurrence of human infection and disease is influenced by the abundance of mosquito vectors and natural reservoir in animals. Although enteroviral disease, including aseptic meningitis, occurs in epidemics, severe encephalitis caused by these agents usually is a sporadic event. Influenza-associated encephalopathy has been described sporadically, but, when it occurs, it follows a seasonal pattern with illnesses occurring primarily during the winter months in temperate climates. Sporadic cases of encephalitis occur in any season. Epidemiologic considerations that must be reviewed in a search for the causative agent include geographic area; climatic conditions; animal, water, food, soil, and personal exposures; and host factors.

For most viral agents, the incubation periods range from a few days to a few weeks. Rabies is an important exception to this. Although the

*References 6, 14, 23, 50, 115, 144, 145, 201, 260, 266, 291, 322, 326, 342, 361, 453.

incubation for rabies is typically 20 to 60 days, it can be up to 7 years.[249] Additionally, measles, which can cause an acute form of encephalitis, also can cause an indolent, slowly progressive form of encephalitis, termed subacute sclerosing panencephalitis, that can manifest years after the original infection.[35]

PATHOGENESIS

Because encephalitis has multiple causes, the lack of a unified pathogenesis is not surprising.* Clinical manifestations of encephalitis can result from a direct or an indirect effect of an infectious agent on the brain. Rabies, arboviruses, herpes simplex, and enteroviral encephalitides are examples in which the viral infections directly involve tissue cells within the brain. In contrast, agents such as measles can trigger immunologic events responsible for the pathogenesis of postinfectious or parainfectious encephalitides. Encephalitic symptoms in bacterial meningitides and in rickettsial infections may be caused by the vasculitis and liberated toxins of the surrounding infection. In addition, there is yet another group of organisms whose role and mechanism is unknown. This includes agents such as *M. pneumoniae* where there is anecdotal evidence of infection but minimal neurotropism and limited laboratory data to support direct CNS invasion.[101]

In many viral encephalitides, such as those caused by arboviruses, mumps, and enteroviruses, the CNS infection occurs after a primary viral infection elsewhere in the body. Generally the infectious agents, whether from ingestion, as in enteroviral infections, or from the bite of a mosquito, as in an arboviral infection, enter the lymphatic system. In the lymphatics, viral multiplication occurs, which results in seeding of the bloodstream and infection of other organs in the body. Viral multiplication occurs at these secondary infection sites; extensive secondary viremia occurs, and then the CNS becomes infected. The reason certain viruses are more "neurotropic" than others is not well known. One hypothesis is that the small size of arboviruses allows them to escape clearance of the reticuloendothelial system. Arboviruses may enter the CNS via the cerebral capillaries with vascular endothelial cell infection.[244] Indeed, recent studies have found that hypertension and diabetes are risk factors for the development of West Nile virus neuroinvasive disease.[241] Actual involvement of nervous tissue may result from growth across or passive diffusion through brain capillaries or centripetal axonal transport of virus from the olfactory neuroepithelium to the olfactory bulb.[335]

Infection of the brain also may occur through the peripheral nerves. This retrograde spread of virus is important in encephalitis caused by herpes simplex virus, poliovirus, and rabies virus. In the case of rabies, after the virus is introduced through the skin, usually via a bite, the rabies virus replicates in skeletal muscle and travels to the CNS via the peripheral nerves.[239] Rabies is unique among viral diseases with respect to incubation period. In some cases of prolonged incubation periods the virus likely remains close to the viral entry site.[239] Once the virus has spread to the brain via peripheral nerves, rabies virus disseminates throughout the CNS. Another mechanism organisms use to gain entry to the CNS is exemplified by free-living amoebae such as *N. fowleri*; these organisms enter transnasally, pass through the cribriform plate, and invade the frontal lobes of the brain.[478]

Postinfectious or parainfectious encephalitis is an acute demyelinating disease of the brain in which the findings suggest an autoimmune process. Usually little evidence of an active infectious process is present when symptoms occur. Viral or other agents probably invaded the CNS initially and then were cleared but were a trigger for the subsequent development of disease. An immune (T-cell) response to myelin basic protein occurs.

PATHOLOGY

The classic findings in viral encephalitis include perivascular mononuclear cell inflammation, neuronal destruction, neuronophagia, and microglial nodules,[248] with most of the abnormalities seen in the gray matter of the brain. Tissue sections of the brain generally reveal meningeal congestion and mononuclear infiltration, perivascular cuffs of lymphocytes and plasma cells, some perivascular tissue necrosis with myelin breakdown, neuronal disruption in various stages (including ultimately neuronophagia), and endothelial proliferation or necrosis. The severity and the extent of observed lesions vary with the infectious agent and with the degree of reaction of the host. The cerebral cortex, especially the temporal lobe, often is affected severely by herpes simplex virus, and arboviruses tend to affect the entire brain.[239] Intranuclear inclusions are suggestive of a member of the Herpesviridae. Rabies has a predilection for the basal structures; involvement of the spinal cord, nerve roots, and peripheral nerves varies. Negri bodies, if identified, are pathognomonic for rabies. Although rabies has one of the highest fatality rates of any infectious disease, brain tissue shows relatively benign neuropathologic changes without evidence of neuronal death. In contrast, *Naegleria* causes marked hemorrhagic necrosis, especially in the olfactory bulbs and cerebral cortex.[275] The pathologic process seen in patients with herpes simplex encephalitis is also characterized by a hemorrhagic necrosis but in different locations (i.e., the temporal and frontal lobes).[294]

In contrast to acute viral encephalitis where gray matter is predominantly affected, the white matter is most affected in postinfectious encephalitis. A marked degree of demyelination with preservation of neurons and their axons is considered to be predominantly postinfectious or parainfectious (autoimmune) encephalitis.

Finally some infectious agents such as *Mycobacterium tuberculosis* and fungi can cause encephalitis-like symptoms without parenchymal involvement. For example, tuberculosis can lead to hydrocephalus and cranial nerve palsies. Other agents, such as varicella-zoster virus and coccidioidomycosis, can cause vasculitis resulting in infarctions in the brain with resultant focal neurologic deficits mimicking encephalitis.[495]

CLINICAL MANIFESTATIONS

The clinical findings in encephalitis are determined by the severity of involvement and anatomic localization of the affected portions of the nervous system, the inherent pathogenicity of the offending agent, and the immune and other reactive mechanisms of the patient ("host factors"). Evidence of brain parenchymal involvement is the hallmark of encephalitis. Children with encephalitis may show evidence of diffuse disease, such as behavioral or personality changes; decreased consciousness; and generalized seizures or localized changes, such as focal seizures, hemiparesis, movement disorders, cranial nerve defects, and ataxia. Some children may seem to be mildly affected initially only to lapse into coma and sudden death. In others, the illness is ushered in by high fever, violent convulsions interspersed with bizarre movements, and hallucinations alternating with brief periods of clarity, and the children emerge with relatively few sequelae.

Specific forms of encephalitis or complicating manifestations of encephalitis include Guillain-Barré syndrome and related syndromes, acute transverse myelitis, acute hemiplegia, brainstem encephalitis, and acute cerebellar ataxia. Acute cerebellar ataxia is characterized by an abrupt onset of truncal ataxia resulting in varying degrees of gait disturbance and balance abnormalities. Children with this illness have tremulousness of the head and trunk when in the upright position and of the extremities when attempting to move them against gravity. The duration of illness varies from 3 to 4 days to several weeks. Acute cerebellar ataxia often follows chickenpox or other viral illnesses. In one study, 3% were related to immunization.[109] Approximately 90% of patients recovered completely from the ataxia, but 20% had transient behavioral or intellectual disturbances. Five percent had persistent learning problems.

Most commonly, the initial manifestations resemble an undifferentiated acute systemic illness with fever, headache, or, in infants, screaming spells, abdominal distress, nausea, and vomiting. Signs of an associated mild nasopharyngitis may suggest a respiratory tract infection. As the temperature increases, new findings direct attention to the nervous system: mental dullness eventuating in stupor; bizarre movements; convulsions; nuchal rigidity, often not as pronounced as in purely meningitic illness; and focal neurologic signs, which may be stationary,

*References 11, 37, 66, 107, 139, 153, 159, 178, 188, 197, 200, 211, 222, 245, 328, 329, 331, 335, 489.

progress, or fluctuate. Loss of bowel and bladder control and unprovoked emotional outbursts may occur.

A wide range of severity of clinical manifestations exists even with the same etiologic agent. Nevertheless some organisms show tropism for a specific area of the brain and consequently specific clinical characteristics are appreciated. Arboviruses often can cause diffuse brain involvement with global impairment, whereas herpes simplex virus type 1 almost universally involves the temporal lobe. The classic features of herpes simplex encephalitis include fever, altered level of consciousness, dysphagia, focal motor seizures, and hemiparesis; almost all adults with this disease exhibit these features. Children, however, may have atypical features and can have extratemporal lobe involvement.[141] One study identified up to one-fourth of children with atypical features, such as ataxia, decreased visual acuity, or tonic-clonic seizures.[141] Primary varicella infection is often associated with cerebellar inflammation, and patients present with ataxia and nystagmus and may or may not have cognitive impairment. Individuals with Epstein-Barr virus encephalitis can sometimes have micropsia, macropsia, and/or size distortion, called "Alice in Wonderland" syndrome. The occurrence of seizures is variable depending on the pathogen. In *Bartonella* encephalopathy, generalized seizures are common,[59] whereas they are unusual in West Nile virus infection.[416] Individuals with rabies often have rapidly progressive encephalitis. Paresthesia at or near the bite site is unique to rabies. Most (approximately 80%) patients with rabies have the "furious" form, characterized by agitation, hydrophobia, delirium, and seizures. Patients with the "paralytic" form (approximately 20%) have ascending paralysis, followed by confusion and coma. Although these two forms are described, it is not unusual for patients to have features of both.

Brainstem encephalitis is a rare disorder, but it is important because clinical signs appear similar to those of a brainstem glioma. The differentiation is important because treatment is radically different. The differentiation is made by the time of onset of symptoms and by the course. Brainstem glioma usually has slowly progressive symptoms developing over the course of several weeks or months. Brainstem encephalitis evolves over 1 to 7 days. Both disorders may be associated with radiographic evidence of brainstem enlargement. Brainstem encephalitis resolves after 1 to 4 weeks, whereas a tumor continues to progress until radiation therapy is given.

Most cases of brainstem encephalitis seem to be postinfectious and are similar to postinfectious cerebellar ataxia, Miller-Fisher syndrome, or Guillain-Barré syndrome. The conditions often overlap.[15] In postinfectious cases, the onset of brainstem encephalitis begins 1 to 3 weeks after a nonspecific viral infection. Brainstem encephalitis has been reported to occur, however, as a result of specific, identifiable, and some treatable infectious agents, including herpes simplex virus,[17,304,410,396,410] varicella zoster virus,[402,449] cytomegalovirus,[169,251] enterovirus 71,[228,229] West Nile virus,[121] *M. pneumoniae*,[285,438] *L. monocytogenes*,[7,12,13,19,29] *Propionibacterium acnes*,[58] and *Campylobacter jejuni*.[507]

Some patients with a typical clinical picture of brainstem encephalitis have had anti-GQ1b antibodies in the serum,[92] which may represent a subgroup of postinfectious brainstem encephalitis cases. Brainstem encephalitis may arise in HIV-infected patients and may be due to a treatable cause, such as herpes simplex encephalitis.[16] In an enterovirus outbreak in Taiwan, the most common neurologic complication was rhombencephalitis, and a 14% mortality rate was reported.[228,229]

Patients with noninfectious anti-*N*-methyl-D-aspartate receptor (NMDAR) encephalitis typically display psychiatric symptoms, seizures, cognitive dysfunction, orofacial dyskinesias, and autonomic instability.[129,235] Notably, the behavioral characteristics of a patient with anti-NMDAR encephalitis may resemble that of rabies.[170] Patients with autoimmune limbic encephalitis also present with psychiatric symptoms and seizures in addition to rapidly progressive short-term memory deficits.[191]

DIFFERENTIAL DIAGNOSIS

The evaluation of a patient with an acute CNS illness (encephalopathy) must be considered carefully, and the sequence of tests should be dictated by the specific circumstances of the individual patient. Several disease processes may have presentations similar to infectious causes.

The differential diagnosis of acute encephalopathy includes the following:

- Anti-NMDAR encephalitis has recently been found to be one of the leading causes of noninfectious encephalitis in children
- Acute demyelinating disorders, including ADEM, acute multiple sclerosis, and acute hemorrhagic leukoencephalitis
- Other postinfectious diseases, including Guillain-Barré syndrome (including Miller-Fisher variant), brainstem encephalitis, and acute cerebellar ataxia
- Status epilepticus, especially nonconvulsive status epilepticus, such as complex-partial status or absence status
- Metabolic diseases, such as hypoglycemia, uremic encephalopathy, hepatic encephalopathy, and rare genetic inborn errors of metabolism, including disorders of glucose or ammonia metabolism
- Toxic disorders, such as drug ingestion or Reye syndrome
- Mass lesions, such as tumor or abscess
- Subarachnoid hemorrhage from arteriovenous malformation or aneurysm
- Embolic lesions caused by bacterial endocarditis
- Acute confusional migraine

EVALUATION OF A PATIENT WITH ENCEPHALOPATHY OR POSSIBLE ENCEPHALITIS

Although many cases of encephalitis remain without a cause, and many of the causes are not treatable per se, a thorough diagnostic evaluation is important. For example, the identification of a specific cause may be helpful for prognosis, lead to the discontinuation of unnecessary antimicrobial therapy, and be useful for potential prophylaxis of contacts and initiation of public health interventions. Obtaining a careful history and performing a physical and neurologic examination are essential in all patients who have a history consistent with encephalitis. The differential diagnosis previously presented indicates that encephalitis is only one of many disorders that can manifest as an acute or subacute picture of encephalopathy. Although the diagnosis of encephalitis may be determined best with a lumbar puncture and evaluation of the CSF, lumbar puncture may be contraindicated in some disorders and, if performed inappropriately, may lead to serious complications and even death. A child who has a cerebellar tumor with acute obstruction of the fourth ventricle may have a decreasing level of consciousness caused by the rapidly increasing intracranial pressure. Nuchal rigidity may be present. The family may not have recognized the more subtle changes in cerebellar functions for the months before the acute obstruction developed and may give a history of acute encephalopathy. In that case, a lumbar puncture could result in herniation through the foramen magnum. It is essential that the patient be assessed for the possibility of increased intracranial pressure and the potential for herniation.

The patient's history should be reviewed carefully, questioning specifically for symptoms of neurologic problems that manifested in the days or weeks before the acute disorder occurred. The physical examination must be performed with special attention given to focal neurologic abnormalities, cerebellar signs, and evidence of increased intracranial pressure. Conducting a careful funduscopic examination is important but may be impossible in an agitated patient or young child. The presence of papilledema indicates that neuroimaging should be performed before doing the lumbar puncture. If spontaneous venous pulsations are noted on funduscopic examination, intracranial pressure is not increased and the lumbar puncture can be done without imaging.

In addition to a lumbar puncture, neuroimaging and obtaining an EEG can help in determining the cause of the encephalopathy and the most appropriate course of therapy. Results of the history and physical examination provide a guide to the most appropriate first test to perform, but generally neuroimaging is the most likely to be helpful. The exception would be a child in nonconvulsive status epilepticus. The history may suggest encephalitis as the most likely diagnosis, but, in some patients, nonconvulsive status epilepticus may be clinically indistinguishable from encephalitis.

Neuroimaging

Most patients with encephalopathy should undergo neuroimaging to aid diagnosis of treatable conditions, such as herpes simplex encephalitis. Computed tomography (CT) is helpful in the acute setting to identify abnormalities, such as tumor or abscess, and to decide whether performing a lumbar puncture is safe. However, CT is not as helpful as magnetic resonance imaging (MRI) in detecting the subtle changes associated with encephalitis.[55,56,265,296,421] In many cases of viral encephalitis, CT and MRI yield normal results or only nonspecific changes, such as swelling[488] or edema.[296] An important exception is herpes simplex encephalitis.

As previously noted, MRI is more sensitive than is CT. In a recent study of 141 children with clinically suspected encephalitis from 2005 to 2012, abnormal findings were evident on 23% of CT scans and 50% of MRI studies in the acute setting.[55] MRI in HSV encephalitis characteristically shows abnormalities in the medial temporal lobes, inferior frontal cortex, and insula.[295,490] The likelihood of finding the abnormalities may be increased by using T2-weighted imaging and fluid-attenuated inversion recovery (FLAIR) sequences[22,254] or diffusion-weighted imaging.[418,459] Diffusion-weighted MRI seems to be more sensitive than is FLAIR or T2-weighted sequences in the detection of herpes simplex virus or other encephalitides.[467] The localization of abnormalities may differ, however, from the classic pattern in young children. In neonatal herpes encephalitis, widespread changes occur in the periventricular white matter, often sparing the medial temporal and inferior frontal lobes. Another pattern has been described in children aged 4 to 13 months in whom the cortex and adjacent white matter of the hemispheres were abnormal.[295]

In addition to herpes, other encephalitides may yield abnormal neuroimaging. CT and MRI results often are abnormal in disorders caused by arbovirus or enterovirus infections. When imaging is abnormal, it usually is nonspecific, showing areas of decreased density (with CT) or increased signal intensity (with MRI) in the gray or white matter. A variety of MRI abnormalities with certain viral encephalitides have been reported. The basal ganglia, brainstem, and thalami have been reported to be abnormal on MR images of patients with eastern equine encephalitis,[128] Japanese encephalitis,[227,280] and enterovirus 71.[228,229] These differences help to distinguish herpes simplex virus from other, nontreatable causes of viral encephalitis.

Postinfectious disorders most often are associated with selective oligodendrocyte involvement.[31] Imaging shows increased signal in white matter with T2-weighted MRI or low-density white matter with CT.[28,48,215,260,352] Patients with acute hemorrhagic leukoencephalitis, a rare disease that is rapidly progressive and often fatal, may have a clinical picture similar to that of herpes simplex encephalitis. In contrast to herpes simplex virus infection, the CT results often are abnormal within the first 1 or 2 days.[403,486] If a patient with suspected herpes simplex encephalitis has abnormal CT results early in the course, acute hemorrhagic leukoencephalitis should be considered.

Another imaging technique that has been reported to be helpful in establishing the diagnosis of encephalitis is single-photon emission computed tomography (SPECT). Initial reports suggest that SPECT is more sensitive than is CT. Ackerman and colleagues[2] found that SPECT showed greater sensitivity and more precise localization than did conventional radionuclide scanning and CT. Launes and associates[291] studied 14 patients with encephalitis and found that SPECT detected temporal lobe abnormalities in all six of the patients with herpes simplex encephalitis and yielded normal results in the remaining eight whose disease had other causes. A few cases of normal MR images but abnormal SPECT scans in patients with herpes simplex encephalitis have been reported[214,315]; this is less likely to occur with newer MRI sequences such as diffusion-weighted imaging. If SPECT is performed, technetium-99m hexamethylpropyleneamine oxime seems to be superior to technetium-99m ethyl cysteinate dimer.[122,149] Generally SPECT should be reserved for cases in which the MRI results are normal and the EEG is nondiagnostic but in which herpes simplex encephalitis is still strongly suspected. Intracranial ultrasonography in neonates has been shown to be helpful in establishing the diagnosis and in follow-up of infants with herpes simplex virus or cytomegalovirus infections.[318]

Electroencephalography

Generally, an EEG should be obtained in most patients with encephalitis. Compared to a routine EEG, continuous EEG is more likely to detect both clinical and subclinical seizures.[185] The EEG results of patients with encephalitis are often nonspecifically abnormal, showing diffuse slowing. Crucial exceptions to the general rule exist, however.

In acute encephalopathy, comatose patients may be in nonconvulsive status epilepticus,[461] which requires immediate and appropriate intervention. The presence of periodic lateralized epileptiform discharges (PLEDs) on an EEG strongly suggests the possibility of herpes simplex encephalitis but also may be an indication of seizures.[30] Early in the course of herpes encephalitis, generalized slowing of the background frequencies and focal slowing over the affected temporal lobe may occur. Within a few days, the characteristic PLEDs pattern develops in most cases. Later in the course, the background activity between the bursts of PLEDs gradually may flatten. Occasionally other areas of the brain seem to be involved, primarily with herpes simplex virus. PLEDs, although strongly suggestive of herpes simplex encephalitis, are not diagnostic. PLEDs have been reported with stroke and infectious mononucleosis encephalitis,[194] and periodic complexes are characteristic of the slow virus and prion disorders, including Jakob-Creutzfeldt disease and subacute sclerosing panencephalitis.

The EEG abnormalities in neonatal herpes encephalitis are similar to those in older patients. The characteristic EEG results yield periodic or pseudoperiodic complexes, usually triangular or sharp waves, occurring in a multifocal pattern.[332] In one study of 34 infants with herpes simplex encephalitis, EEGs were obtained in 21, the results in 19 being abnormal. The results of 3 showed only focal slowing, but the other 16 showed the characteristic periodic or pseudoperiodic complexes.[406] The authors reviewed 500 other neonatal EEG records and found 20 with similar complexes; 11 patients had meningoencephalitis of unknown etiology, 3 had hemorrhage, and 2 had asphyxia. Four were placed in a miscellaneous category. Periodic or pseudoperiodic complexes on a neonatal EEG strongly suggest herpes simplex encephalitis, but they are not diagnostic.

DIAGNOSIS

A meticulous history is essential, including exposure in the previous 3 to 4 weeks of illness onset; sick contacts; exposure to mosquitoes, ticks, and animals; recent vacations or picnics or other outdoor activities; awareness of illness in animals in the patient's environment; recent travel from the home area; recent injections of any kind; and the possibility of accidental exposure to heavy metals, pesticides, or other questionable substances. The CSF must be examined carefully to exclude other disorders that respond to specific therapy. Smears for bacteria, appropriate rapid antigen-identification tests, and cultures of the CSF are mandatory; the history and clinical findings may indicate the need for acid-fast stain and culture of the sediment for mycobacteria. Although often not done because of inconvenience, opening CSF pressures should be measured. Molecular testing has advanced the diagnostics for encephalitis overall, but there are a number of important limitations of molecular diagnostics (both false-positive and false-negative findings). In particular, it is important to understand that a positive polymerase chain reaction (PCR) test in the CSF does not necessarily equate with disease and vice versa. Additionally, there is still a very important role for culture and serologic assays for the diagnosis of encephalitis. Recommended test types and "pitfalls" in testing are outlined in Table 36.1. A diagnostic algorithm is presented in Box 36.2.

Herpes simplex testing allowed for the definitive and rapid diagnosis of HSV encephalitis to be established, eliminating the need for brain biopsy.[130,283,299,471,492] If, however, testing is negative for herpes simplex virus on the first CSF specimen and herpes simplex encephalitis is strongly suspected (e.g., temporal lobe involvement on neuroimaging), a second CSF specimen should be obtained within 3 to 7 days and retested for herpes simplex virus by PCR because false-negative results can occur.[141,468,487] The etiology of encephalitis caused by other herpesviruses also has been determined by PCR assay of CSF.[116,319,468] In contrast to false negatives seen with herpes simplex virus and varicella, false

BOX 36.2 Diagnostic Algorithm

All Cases

CSF

WBC count with differential, RBC count, protein, glucose
Gram stain and bacterial culture
Herpes simplex virus–1/2 PCR (if test available, consider HSV CSF IgG and IgM in addition)
VZV PCR (sensitivity may be low; if test available, consider VZV CSF IgG and IgM in addition)
Enterovirus PCR

Blood/Serum

Routine blood culture
Epstein-Barr virus (EBV) antibodies (if positive for acute infection, check CSF EBV PCR)
Hold acute serum and collect convalescent serum 10 to 14 days later for paired antibody testing

Respiratory, Stool

Enterovirus PCR (respiratory, stool)
Enterovirus (stool)

Conditional

Host Factors

Neonate: herpes simplex virus–2 PCR (CSF), swabs of skin vesicles, mouth, nasopharynx, conjunctivae, and rectum (viral culture)
≤3 yr: parechovirus PCR (CSF and respiratory)
Immunocompromised: cytomegalovirus, human herpesvirus–6/7, JC virus, human immunodeficiency virus PCR (CSF)

Season and Exposure

Summer/fall: West Nile virus (WNV) IgM (CSF, serum), WNV IgG (paired serum), and other appropriate arboviruses as geographically relevant
Cat (particularly if with seizures and paucicellular CSF): *Bartonella* antibody (serum)
Animal bite exposure: rabies test[a]
Rodent exposure: LCM antibody (serum)
Tick and/or camping exposure: *Rickettsia* spp., antibody (serum), *Anaplasma phagocytophila* antibody (serum)
Swimming or diving in brackish water: *Naegleria fowleri* (wet mount)[a]
If history of sexual activity: herpes simplex virus–2 (CSF PCR)

Signs and Symptoms

Psychotic component or movement disorder: anti-NMDAR antibody (CSF and serum), and abdominal ultrasound evaluation for teratoma
Vesicular rash: varicella zoster virus PCR (CSF)
Rapid decompensation (especially with bite history or foreign travel): rabies test[a]
Respiratory (during influenza season): influenza PCR (respiratory)
Diarrhea and seizure (especially young child): rotavirus (check stool for antigen), if positive then rotavirus PCR (CSF)

Laboratory Features

CSF protein >100 mg/dL or CSF glucose less than two-thirds peripheral glucose and/or lymphocytic pleocytosis:
- Mycobacterial tuberculosis: culture (CSF, respiratory), place PPD, and check IGRA, chest radiograph, fungal culture (CSF)
- Fungal (specific types depend on geographic residence and/or travel to endemic areas): culture CSF *and* check antibody and antigen
- *Balamuthia mandrillaris:* contact health department/CDC for assistance with testing

CSF eosinophilia: *Baylisascaris procyonis* antibody

Travel

Consider consultation with public health department concerning specific diseases such as arboviruses, rabies, and other diseases

CDC, Centers for Disease Control and Prevention; *CSF,* cerebrospinal fluid; *IGRA,* interferon gamma release assay; *LCM,* lymphocytic choriomeningitis; *NMDAR, N*-methyl-D-aspartate receptor; *PCR,* polymerase chain reaction; *PPD,* purified protein derivative.
[a]Contact health department for assistance with testing.

positives can be seen when testing other herpesviruses. For example, because Epstein-Barr virus infections result in latency in the lymphoreticular system (including B cells), when PCR on CSF is examined for this virus, low levels can be detected when it is not necessarily the cause of encephalitis. Serology as well as Epstein-Barr virus PCR should be performed. Similarly human herpesvirus–6 PCR testing of CSF may also lead to false-positive results owing to latency. Additionally, for human herpesvirus–6 infections, the phenomenon of chromosomal integration of the virus can further confound the diagnosis.[484]

In addition to its use in herpesvirus infections, PCR can be useful for detected enteroviruses and human parechoviruses, and, in the future, it is likely to be useful to identify other encephalitides.[39,268,297,361,389] For possible enteroviral encephalitis, because the CSF PCR is not always positive, it is important to test for enteroviruses in sites outside the CNS to maximize detection, such as blood, throat, and stool.[366] Specialized PCR assays can be used in young children to detect human parechoviruses, which are not detected by routine enteroviral PCR testing.

In viral encephalitis, the CSF frequently is clear; the leukocyte count ranges from none to several thousand, often with a significant percentage of polymorphonuclear cells initially, moderate or no elevation of protein, and an initially normal level of glucose relative to the simultaneously determined blood glucose level. A nonviral entity should be considered in cases in which the CSF white blood cell count is high (particularly for values >1000 cells/mm^3), protein is greater than 100 mg/dL, and/or CSF glucose is less than two-thirds of the serum value. A lymphocytic pleocytosis with high protein and low glucose values is often found in patients with fungal or *M. tuberculosis* meningitis-encephalitis. If eosinophils are identified in the CSF, a helminthic-parasitic infection should be considered such as *B. procyonis, A. cantonensis,* or *G. spinigerum.* Eosinophils in the CSF can also be seen in patients with coccidioidomycosis and *M. tuberculosis* infection.[380]

In any patient suspected of having viral meningoencephalitis, CSF, blood, feces, and throat swabs should be collected and sent to a laboratory offering viral diagnostic services. An additional serum specimen should be collected 10 to 21 days later. Although these studies may not provide an immediate diagnosis, they may give early warning of a specific epidemic, and the use of specific antiviral chemotherapy may be indicated by the preliminary culture results.

Inquiry regarding recent illness, recent injections, and, especially, recent exposures away from the home environment sometimes is helpful. The incubation periods of some arboviruses are such that mosquito bites acquired at least 1 week earlier or insect bites now healed may give a clue. Occasionally patients who have traveled to Africa or Asia in preceding weeks have encephalitis caused by viruses, trypanosomiasis, or falciparum malaria with bizarre systemic and CNS signs and symptoms.

Rabies should be considered in any patient with a rapid progression of illness. Hydrophobia, autonomic instability, extreme agitation, and seizures are often present. Paresthesia at the site of inoculation, if present, is an important diagnostic clue unique to rabies.

For noninfectious anti-NMDAR encephalitis, CSF testing is approximately 15% more sensitive than serum testing. Furthermore anti-NMDAR encephalitis has been reported to follow herpes simplex encephalitis.[25,377,456,494,508]

TREATMENT

Acyclovir should be used to treat herpes simplex and varicella zoster virus encephalitis and perhaps encephalitis caused by Epstein-Barr virus. Cytomegalovirus encephalitis should be treated with ganciclovir, and oseltamivir should be considered for treatment of encephalitis caused by influenzaviruses A or B. If there is any suggestion of bacterial meningitis, antibiotics should be used empirically to cover for *Streptococcus pneumonia, Haemophilus influenzae,* and possibly *Listeria*. Additionally, specific antimicrobial treatment should be used for infections caused by spirochetes, *Chlamydia, Mycoplasma,* fungi, and parasites.

General treatment is nonspecific and empiric, aimed at maintaining life and supporting each involved organ system. The effectiveness of various recommended regimens in most instances has not been evaluated objectively. Until a bacterial etiology and, in particular, a brain abscess are excluded, parenteral antibiotic therapy should be administered.

Anticipating and being prepared for convulsions, cerebral edema, hyperpyrexia, inadequate respiratory exchange, disturbed fluid and electrolyte balance, aspiration and asphyxia, abrupt cardiac and respiratory arrest of central origin, cardiac decompensation, and gastrointestinal bleeding is crucial. The syndrome of disseminated intravascular coagulation may be an additional complication.

For these reasons, all patients with severe encephalitis should receive care in intensive care units. Cardiac monitoring should be maintained. Repeat CT and MRI are helpful in following the status of comatose patients and often show signs of brain swelling before the patient has the typical clinical indicators of intracranial pressure, such as Cushing triad (systolic hypertension, bradycardia, and slowing of respirations), dilated pupils, and decorticate or decerebrate posturing. The Cushing triad is an unreliable indicator of increased intracranial pressure, and, when the other signs of increased intracranial pressure occur, they often do so late in the course, when the patient's cerebral perfusion already is at risk.[321] As mentioned previously, the opening pressure should be determined when CSF is obtained. If a patient has a high opening pressure, close monitoring is advised with consideration of measures to decrease intracranial pressure. If brain swelling becomes a problem, placement of an intracranial pressure monitor may be necessary. The intracranial pressure should be maintained at less than 15 mm Hg if possible using the standard techniques for reduction of intracranial pressure, including hyperventilation, osmotic diuretics, and removal of CSF. As a last resort, inducing a barbiturate coma may be necessary. A related consequence of intracranial pressure is the syndrome of inappropriate antidiuretic hormone secretion. Careful monitoring of the fluid and electrolyte balance is essential in all seriously ill patients with encephalitis.

All fluids, electrolytes, and medications initially are given parenterally. In patients with prolonged coma, parenteral hyperalimentation is indicated. Normal blood levels of glucose, magnesium, and calcium must be maintained to minimize seizures.

Status epilepticus caused by encephalitis should be treated vigorously using a structured protocol to ensure optimal control.[424,464] The current standard initial therapy is intravenous lorazepam 0.1 to 0.2 mg/kg, up to 4 mg maximum. Seizures associated with encephalitis may be refractory to the usual therapy, and other anticonvulsants may be required to achieve and maintain control of seizures. In patients who fail initial therapy and are in medically refractory status epilepticus, continuous EEG monitoring usually is recommended to monitor the efficacy of the therapy, especially when the patient is in nonconvulsive status epilepticus.[127,462]

If, after a second attempt, lorazepam fails to control the seizures, intravenous phenytoin (preferably phosphenytoin in children) is the next drug of choice. The dose is 18 to 20 mg/kg, maximum 1000 mg, given over 20 minutes. Phosphenytoin is preferred because it can be administered faster and does not cause sclerosis of the veins as does phenytoin and is not as likely to cause cardiac arrhythmias. Virtually all patients who require therapy beyond lorazepam need to be intubated to prevent respiratory embarrassment. If phosphenytoin is unsuccessful, or as an alternative to phosphenytoin, intravenous midazolam has gained favor in recent years.[105,363] The initial dose is 0.1 to 0.2 mg/kg over 5 minutes, with a maintenance infusion starting at 0.05 mg/kg per hour up to a maximum of 0.4 mg/kg per hour. Another alternative therapy is propofol, which generally is administered by an anesthesiologist.

Many methods have been proposed to minimize cerebral edema and to diminish the consequences of cerebral anoxia. The following measures are difficult to evaluate and generally are reserved for patients with severe illness whose condition apparently is desperate.

1. Dexamethasone 0.1 to 0.2 mg/kg intravenously in an initial dose followed by 0.05 to 0.1 mg/kg intravenously every 4 to 6 hours is given. This large dose should be reduced gradually after a few days if recovery or improvement is evident. The use of steroids, however, is controversial in patients with known or suspected viral disease because of the possibility of exacerbating the viral infection.
2. Elevated intracranial pressure can also be controlled by administration of mannitol, given intravenously as a 20% solution in a dose of 0.25 to 1 g/kg over a 30- to 60-minute period (this may be repeated every 8 to 12 hours), and glycerol, given by nasogastric tube using 0.5 to 1 mL/kg diluted with twice that volume of orange juice. This regimen is nontoxic and may be repeated every 6 hours for an extended period.

For more than 40 years, corticosteroids and adrenocorticotropic hormone frequently have been used as empiric therapy for encephalitis. No controlled studies have shown any efficacy, however. In two comparative studies of measles encephalitis, corticosteroids were found to offer no benefit, and in both studies the corticosteroid recipients seemed to have had worse outcomes.[44,509] More recently, in a carefully controlled study, no benefit of high-dose dexamethasone was found in the treatment of acute encephalitis caused by Japanese encephalitis virus.[223]

In contrast to the investigations of viral encephalitis, the treatment of acute disseminated encephalomyelitis, in which MRI studies have indicated multifocal white matter lesions, are more compelling.[50,201,260,322] Patients treated with corticosteroids often have responded dramatically, with clinical improvement and resolution of the lesions as shown by MRI. Corticosteroids, along with specific antibiotic therapy, also may be beneficial in the treatment of encephalitis caused by *M. pneumoniae* infection, although, as discussed earlier, it is unknown if *M. pneumoniae* is a definitive cause of encephalitis.[269,423]

Plasmapheresis and intravenous immunoglobulin have been used empirically to treat brainstem encephalitis and other encephalitides, but no studies have been done that indicate such therapies are helpful.[347]

Equipment and personnel for handling emergencies such as cardiac and respiratory arrest always must be available. Early consultation with an anesthesiologist or intensive care specialist is useful in anticipating the need for artificially assisted respiration.

Supportive and rehabilitative efforts are important after the patient recovers. Motor incoordination, convulsive disorders, total or partial deafness, or behavioral disturbances may appear only after some time. Visual disturbances caused by chorioretinopathy and perceptual amblyopia also may make a delayed appearance.

PROGNOSIS

The prognosis in all patients with encephalitides is guarded with respect to immediate outcome and sequelae. Sequelae involving the CNS may be intellectual, motor, psychiatric, epileptic, visual, or auditory. While complete recovery does occur, up to 60% of pediatric encephalitis cases have persistent symptoms, and mortality rates range from 3% to 15%.[162,163,309,385,386] Factors associated with worse outcomes include younger age, seizures, focal neurologic signs, lower Glasgow Coma Score, and abnormal neuroimaging findings.[262,309,385,386,393,394,411,481] While the short- and long-term prognoses depend to some extent on etiology, quality data for most agents are not available, and even less is known about the "unknown" causes.

Rautonen and associates[386] examined prognostic factors in childhood acute encephalitis at the Children's Hospital, University of Helsinki, during a 20-year period from 1968 to 1987. This study comprised 462 cases with the following causes: mumps virus, measles virus, rubella virus, varicella zoster virus, herpes simplex virus, enteroviruses, respiratory viruses, *M. pneumoniae,* other agents, and cause undetermined. The investigators found that mortality was fivefold greater in infants compared with older children. Children who were disoriented or unconscious before admission had 4-fold and 25-fold greater risks for death and severe damage than did children whose level of consciousness had been normal. Patients with herpes simplex virus or (putative) *M. pneumoniae* infection had the greatest risks for death or serious residual damage compared with children with encephalitis of other causes. Generally herpes simplex virus carries a worse prognosis for survival and residual disability than do the enteroviruses.

The data on prognosis for arboviruses are more complete than for most other entities owing to the Centers for Disease Control and Prevention's excellent surveillance system. Prognosis of children affected with arboviruses is highly variable. West Nile virus tends to be less severe in children than adults; children accounted for only 4% of West Nile neuroinvasive disease in cases reported between 1999 and 2007.[301] There were only 3 fatalities (1%) in the pediatric age group compared with 45 (15%) in adults. Conversely, La Crosse virus (in the California serogroup of viruses) and eastern equine encephalitis are more severe in children than adults.[323] Eastern equine encephalitis has a high mortality rate. Infants and children younger than 5 years of age who survive usually have severe sequelae consisting of mental retardation, convulsions, and paralysis. These consequences are in contrast to adults older than 40 years of age who survive, recover completely, or have only slight damage.

St. Louis encephalitis has a low mortality rate. Although neurologic sequelae are reported, their incidence is low in the pediatric age group. The prognosis in encephalitis caused by western equine virus is guarded; 56% of infants younger than 1 month of age have had recurring seizures with marked motor and behavioral changes. After they reach 1 year of age, the sequelae appear to diminish; only 5% of adults have neurologic sequelae. Fifty-seven percent of infants who survived western equine virus infection and who were younger than 1 year of age at the time of infection had major neurologic sequelae requiring either a special school or institutionalization late in life. Severe retardation, paralysis, spasticity, recurrent convulsions, hearing deficits, and speech difficulties all were reported as complications.[140,154]

Nevertheless, progress has been made recently for some causative agents that were thought to always have a poor outcome, and the paradigm seems to be changing. For example, rabies previously was considered to be universally fatal, but in 2004 a 15-year-old girl in Wisconsin developed rabies and survived, representing the first person to survive documented clinical rabies without previous vaccination.[496] Since then, additional human rabies cases have occurred in the United States without significant neurologic sequelae.[85,88]

Correspondingly *B. mandrillaris* encephalitis was also considered to have a grave prognosis, but recent case reports described successful outcomes.[64,123,274] Similarly, all previously reported human cases of *Baylisascaris* meningoencephalitis had resulted in either severe neurologic sequelae or death; in 2007, a case report was published concerning a 4-year-old child with *Baylisascaris* meningoencephalitis who survived without any recognizable neurologic deficits.[359]

PREVENTION

The widespread use of effective attenuated viral vaccines for measles, mumps, and rubella almost has eliminated CNS complications from these diseases in the United States. The control of encephalitis caused by arboviruses is primarily through control of insect vectors. Specific vaccines for the arbovirus diseases that occur in North America are unavailable. Until we learn more about the "unknowns," it will be difficult to know how to prevent many of the causes.

NEW REFERENCES SINCE THE SEVENTH EDITION

3. Ahmad SB, Tan CT. Nipah encephalitis – an update. *Med J Malaysia.* 2014;69:103-111.
8. Amicizia D, Domnich A, Panatto D, et al. Epidemiology of tick-borne encephalitis in Europe and its prevention by available vaccines. *Hum Vaccin Immunother.* 2013;9:1163-1171.
18. Armstrong PM, Andreadis TG. Eastern equine encephalitis virus – old enemy, new threat. *N Engl J Med.* 2013;368:1670-1673.
25. Bektas O, Tanyel T, Kocabas BA, et al. Anti-N-methyl-D-aspartate receptor encephalitis that developed after herpes encephalitis: a case report and literature review. *Neuropediatrics.* 2014;45:396-401.
42. Bloch KC, Glaser CA. Encephalitis surveillance through the Emerging Infections Program, 1997–2010. *Emerg Infect Dis.* 2015;21:1562-1567.
45. Bogovic P, Strle F. Tick-borne encephalitis: a review of epidemiology, clinical characteristics, and management. *World J Clin Cases.* 2015;3:430-441.
52. Brownell AD, Reynolds TQ, Livingston B, et al. Human Parechovirus 3 encephalitis in two neonates: acute and follow-up magnetic resonance imaging and evaluation of central nervous system markers of inflammation. *Pediatr Neurol.* 2015;52:245-249.
55. Bykowski J, Kruk P, Gold JJ, et al. Acute pediatric encephalitis neuroimaging: single-institution series as part of the California Encephalitis Project. *Pediatr Neurol.* 2015;52:606-614.
62. Carter D. Chikungunya virus spreads to the United States via Caribbean travel. *Am J Nurs.* 2014;114:18.
129. DeSena AD, Greenberg BM, Graves D. Three phenotypes of anti-N-methyl-D-aspartate receptor antibody encephalitis in children: prevalence of symptoms and prognosis. *Pediatr Neurol.* 2014;51:542-549.
144. Erol I, Ozkale Y, Alkan O, et al. Acute disseminated encephalomyelitis in children and adolescents: a single center experience. *Pediatr Neurol.* 2013;49:266-273.
145. Esposito S, Di Pietro GM, Madini B, et al. A spectrum of inflammation and demyelination in acute disseminated encephalomyelitis (ADEM) of children. *Autoimmun Rev.* 2015;14:923-929.
148. Fay AJ, Noetzel MJ, Mar SS. A case of pediatric hemorrhagic brainstem encephalitis associated with HHV-7 infection. *Pediatr Neurol.* 2015;53:523-526.
155. Fisher DL, Defrez S, Solomon T. Measles-induced encephalitis. *Q J Med.* 2015;108:177-182.
158. Fomsgaard A, Fertner ME, Essbauer S. Tick-borne encephalitis virus, Zealand, Denmark 2011. *Emerg Infect Dis.* 2013;19:1171-1173.
161. Fowler A, Forsman L, Eriksson M, Wickstrom R. Tick-born encephalitis carries a high risk of incomplete recovery in children. *J Pediatr.* 2013;163:555-560.
162. Fowler A, Stodberg T, Eriksson M, et al. Long-term outcomes of acute encephalitis in childhood. *Pediatrics.* 2010;126:e828-e835.
163. Fowler A, Stoderg T, Eriksson M, et al. Childhood encephalitis in Sweden: etiology, clinical presentation and outcome. *Eur J Paediatr Neurol.* 2008;12:484-490.
170. Gable MD, Gavali S, Radner A, et al. Anti-NMDA receptor encephalitis: report of ten cases and comparison with viral encephalitis. *Eur J Clin Microbiol Infect Dis.* 2009;28:1421-1429.
171. Gable MS, Sheriff H, Dalmau J, et al. The frequency of autoimmune *N*-methyl-D-aspartate receptor encephalitis surpasses that of individual viral etiologies in young individuals enrolled in the California Encephalitis Project. *Clin Infect Dis.* 2012;54:899-904.
176. Ghanem-Zoubi N, Shiner M, Shulman LM, et al. Human parechovirus type 3 central nervous system infections in Israeli infants. *J Clin Virol.* 2013;58:205-210.
185. Gold JJ, Crawford JR, Glaser C, et al. The role of continuous electroencephalography in childhood encephalitis. *Pediatr Neurol.* 2014;50:318-323.
191. Graus F, Dalmau J. Paraneoplastic neurological syndromes. *Curr Opin Neurol.* 2012;25:795-801.
208. Haditsch M, Kunze U. Tick-borne encephalitis: a disease neglected by travel medicine. *Travel Med Infect Dis.* 2013;11:295-300.
219. Heinz FX, Stiasny K, Holzmann H, et al. Emergence of tick-borne encephalitis in new endemic areas in Austria: 42 years of surveillance. *Euro Surveill.* 2015;20:9-16.
235. Irani SR, Bera K, Waters P, et al. N-methyl-D-aspartate antibody encephalitis: temporal progression of clinical and paraclinical observations in a predominantly non-paraneoplastic disorder of both sexes. *Brain.* 2010;133:1655-1667.
243. Jeyanthi JC, Ong I, Guan YJ, et al. Epidemiology and outcome in neonatal and pediatric herpes simplex encephalitis: a 13-year experience in a Singapore tertiary children's hospital. *Pediatr Infect Dis J.* 2015;10:16-21.
257. Kawai AT, Li L, Kulldorff M, et al. Absence of associations between influenza vaccines and increased risks of seizures, Guillain-Barre syndrome, encephalitis, or anaphylaxis in the 2012–2013 season. *Pharmacoepidemiol Drug Saf.* 2014;23:548-553.
266. Koelman DL, Mateen FJ. Acute disseminated encephalomyelitis: current controversies in diagnosis and outcome. *J Neurol.* 2015;262:2013-2014.
274. Krasaelap A, Prechawit S, Chansaenroj J, et al. Fatal *Balamuthia* amebic encephalitis in a healthy child: a case report with review of survival cases. *Korean J Parasitol.* 2013;51:335-341.
278. Kuehn BM. Chikungunya virus transmission found in the United States: US health authorities brace for wider spread. *JAMA.* 2014;312:776-777.
281. Kunze U. Tick-borne encephalitis – a notifiable disease, a review after one year: report of the 16th annual meeting of the International Scientific Working Group on Tick-Borne Encephalitis. *Ticks Tick Borne Dis.* 2014;5:453-456.
302. Lindsey NP, Prince HE, Kosoy O, et al. Chikungunya virus infections among travelers – United States 2010–2013. *Am J Trop Med Hyg.* 2015;92:82-87.
309. Mailles A, De Broucker T, Costanzo P, et al. Long-term outcome of patients presenting with acute infectious encephalitis of various causes in France. *Clin Infect Dis.* 2012;54:1455-1464.
316. Mathew AG, Parvez Y. Fulminant Epstein Barr virus encephalitis. *Indian Pediatr.* 2013;50:418-419.

333. Mohareb E, Christova I, Soliman A, et al. Tick-borne encephalitis in Bulgaria, 2009 to 2012. *Euro Surveill.* 2013;18:46.
338. Mori D, Ranawaka U, Yamada K, et al. Human bocavirus in patients with encephalitis, Sri Lanka, 2009–2010. *Emerg Infect Dis.* 2013;19:1859-1862.
357. Pahud BA, Rowhani-Rahbar A, Glaser C. Lack of association between childhood immunizations and encephalitis in California, 1998–2008. *Vaccine.* 2012;30:247-253.
363. Pariani E, Pellegrinelli L, Pugni L, et al. Two cases of neonatal human parechovirus 3 encephalitis. *Pediatr Infect Dis J.* 2014;33:1191-1193.
367. Petersen LR, Fischer M. Unpredictable and difficult to control – the adolescence of West Nile Virus. *N Engl J Med.* 2012;367:1281-1284.
376. Pruss H, Finke C, Holtje M, et al. N-methyl-D-aspartate receptor antibodies in herpes simplex encephalitis. *Ann Neurol.* 2012;72:902-911.
384. Raschilas F, Wolff M, Delatour F, et al. Outcome of and prognostic factors for herpes simplex encephalitis in adult patients: results of a multicenter study. *Clin Infect Dis.* 2002;35:254-260.
391. Renaud C, Harrison CJ. Human parechovirus 3: the most common viral cause of meningoencephalitis in young infants. *Infect Dis Clin North Am.* 2015;29:415-428.
392. Rismanchi N, Gold JJ, Sattar S, et al. Epilepsy after resolution of presumed childhood encephalitis. *Pediatr Neurol.* 2015;53:65-72.
393. Rismanchi N, Gold JJ, Sattar S, et al. Neurological outcomes after presumed childhood encephalitis. *Pediatr Neurol.* 2015;53:200-206.
394. Ritz N, Hufnagel M, Gerardin P. Chikungunya in children. *Pediatr Infect Dis J.* 2015;34:789-791.
407. Sauteur PMM, Jacobs BC, Spuesens EBM, et al. Antibody responses to *Mycoplasma pneumoniae*: role in pathogenesis and diagnosis of encephalitis? *PLoS Pathog.* 2014;10:1-5.
410. Schmidt A, Buhler R, Muhlemann K, et al. Long-term outcome of acute encephalitis of unknown aetiology in adults. *Clin Microbiol Infect.* 2011;17:621-626.
412. Schwartz KL, Richardson SE, Ward KN, et al. Delayed primary HHV-7 infection and neurologic disease. *Pediatrics.* 2014;133:e1541-e1547.
429. Silverman MA, Misasi J, Smole S, et al. Eastern equine encephalitis in children, Massachusetts and New Hampshire, USA, 1970–2010. *Emerg Infect Dis.* 2013;19:194-201.
437. Stamm LV. Chikungunya: emerging threat to the United States. *JAMA Dermatol.* 2015;151:257-258.
441. Stidd DA, Root B, Weinand ME, et al. Granulomatous amoebic encephalitis caused by *Balamuthia mandrillaris* in an immunocompetent girl. *World Neurosurg.* 2012;78:715e7-715e12.
455. Titulaer MJ, McCracken L, Gabilondo I, et al. Treatment and prognostic factors for long-term outcome in patients with anti-NMDA receptor encephalitis: an observational cohort study. *Lancet Neurol.* 2013;12:157-165.
456. To TM, Soldatos A, Sheriff H, et al. Insights into pediatric herpes simplex encephalitis from a cohort of 21 children from the California Encephalitis Project, 1998–2011. *Pediatr Infect Dis J.* 2014;33:1287-1288.
468. Tunkel AR, Glaser CA, Bloch KC, et al. The management of encephalitis: clinical practice guidelines by the Infectious Diseases Society of America. *Clin Infect Dis.* 2008;47:303-327.
475. Vergnano S, Kadambari S, Whalley K, et al. Characteristics and outcomes of human parechovirus infection in infants (2008–2012). *Eur J Pediatr.* 2015;174:919-924.
480. Wang IJ, Lee PI, Huang LM, et al. The correlation between neurological evaluations and neurological outcome in acute encephalitis: a hospital-based study. *Eur J Paediatr Neurol.* 2007;11:63-69.
485. Watanabe T, Kawashima H. Acute encephalitis and encephalopathy associated with human parvovirus B19 infection in children. *World J Clin Pediatr.* 2015;4:126-134.
493. Wickstrom R, Fowler A, Cooray G, et al. Viral triggering of anti-NMDA receptor encephalitis in a child – an important cause for disease relapse. *Eur J Paediatr Neurol.* 2014;18:543-546.
505. Yu J, Chen Q, Hao Y, et al. Identification of human bocaviruses in the cerebrospinal fluid of children hospitalized with encephalitis in China. *J Clin Virol.* 2013;57:374-377.
507. Yushvayev-Cavalier Y, Nichter C, Ramirez-Zamora A. Possible autoimmune association between herpes simplex virus infection and subsequent anti-N-methyl-D-aspartate receptor encephalitis: a pediatric patient with abnormal movement. *Pediatr Neurol.* 2015;52:454-456.
509. Zielicka-Hardy A, Rosinska M, Kondrusik M, et al. Predictors for diagnosis of tick-borne encephalitis infection in Poland, 2009–2010. *Infect Dis.* 2015;48:604-610.

The full reference list for this chapter is available at ExpertConsult.com

37 Parainfectious and Postinfectious Disorders of the Nervous System

37A ▪ Parainfectious and Postinfectious Demyelinating Disorders of the Central Nervous System

Stuart R. Tomko • Timothy E. Lotze

ACUTE DISSEMINATED ENCEPHALOMYELITIS

Acute disseminated encephalomyelitis (ADEM) is a monophasic demyelinating disease of the central nervous system (CNS) that results in acute, polysymptomatic neurologic disability. It also has been termed *postinfectious encephalomyelitis*. It is related to other central inflammatory demyelinating conditions of childhood, including optic neuritis, transverse myelitis, neuromyelitis optica (NMO; Devic disease), and multiple sclerosis (MS). Certain clinical features, laboratory results, and imaging findings can be used to distinguish among these conditions to ensure a correct diagnosis. Most of these conditions are thought to be caused by autoimmune dysregulation triggered by an infectious agent in a genetically susceptible host.

Epidemiology

The estimated incidence of ADEM is 0.8 per 100,000 population per year.[38] ADEM occurs more frequently in children and has a slight male predominance.[54,53] In contrast to MS, which generally has a higher incidence at latitudes that are more northern, ADEM has no appreciable geographic distribution.

Diagnostic Criteria

Prior to the introduction of standardized diagnostic criteria in 2008, the term *acute disseminated encephalomyelitis* had been used variably in the literature in describing clinical characteristics of this disease. Discrepancies existed among descriptive studies regarding (1) the occurrence of encephalopathy, (2) the association with preceding infection, (3) symptoms that are monofocal or multifocal, and (4) the possibility for recurrence.

In 2008, the International Pediatric Multiple Sclerosis Study Group developed diagnostic criteria for ADEM, which were subsequently revised in 2013.[36] The group created working definitions for monophasic and multiphasic ADEM. Box 37A.1 lists the diagnostic criteria. An absolute criterion for a diagnosis of ADEM is the presence of encephalopathy. This is defined to include either behavioral changes, such as lethargy

BOX 37A.1 Diagnostic Criteria of Acute Disseminated Encephalomyelitis

Clinical Features

First clinical attack of demyelinating disease in CNS
Acute or subacute onset
Polysymptomatic presentation
Must include encephalopathy
- Acute behavioral change (e.g., irritability, lethargy)
- Alteration in consciousness (e.g., somnolence, coma)

Attack should be followed by improvement

Lesion Characteristics on MRI FLAIR and T2-Weighted Images

Multifocal, hyperintense, bilateral, asymmetric lesions in the white matter
At least one or more lesions >1–2 cm
Gray matter, especially basal ganglia and thalamus, may be involved
Spinal cord MRI may show confluent intramedullary lesions
- No radiologic evidence of previous destructive white matter changes

Cerebrospinal Fluid

Pleocytosis ≥50 WBCs can be observed

Other

No other etiologies can explain the event
- New or fluctuating symptoms and signs occurring within 3 months of the inciting ADEM event are part of the same acute event

Symptoms that vary during periods of steroid taper within 3 months of the inciting event or occur <30 days after discontinuation of all steroids are considered part of the initial inciting event.
ADEM, Acute disseminated encephalomyelitis; *CNS,* central nervous system; *FLAIR,* fluid-attenuated inversion recovery; *MRI,* magnetic resonance imaging; *WBCs,* white blood cells.

or irritability, or more severe alterations in level of consciousness, such as coma. The onset of the encephalopathy must correspond with the occurrence of the disease state. Magnetic resonance imaging (MRI) shows multiple lesions in both hemispheres distributed throughout the white matter (Fig. 37A.1). A distinguishing characteristic of ADEM is prominent involvement of the cortical gray matter and deep gray nuclei (basal ganglia and thalamus). Such involvement is atypical for MS and other demyelinating conditions. The lesions of ADEM are asymmetric, showing variable size, shape, and distribution between the hemispheres. MRI showing symmetric and confluent lesions should prompt the clinician to consider other diagnoses, such as leukodystrophies and inborn errors of metabolism. If MRI shows evidence of previous demyelination, the clinician should query the history further for previous attacks that would suggest either a recurrent form of the disease or a chronic demyelinating condition. Cerebrospinal fluid (CSF) analysis may show a pleocytosis of greater than 50 cells, in contrast to pediatric MS, in which only a slight pleocytosis (<50 cells) is observed.

The International Pediatric Multiple Sclerosis Study Group has defined criteria to distinguish between an evolving pattern for the initial event and multiphasic forms of ADEM. Any new and fluctuating symptoms occurring within 3 months of the initial event are considered part of the same inciting event. In addition, symptoms occurring during steroid taper or within 1 month of the patient completing a steroid taper are considered part of the same inciting event. In the 2013 revision, "recurrent ADEM" was eliminated as a diagnostic category. Multiphasic ADEM remains with an updated definition now describing patients with two episodes consistent with ADEM separated by 3 months but not followed by further events. Patients with relapsing disease extending beyond two discrete events are no longer considered to have ADEM but rather a chronic disorder such as NMO or MS.

Clinical Manifestations

A febrile illness occurs in 50% to 75% of children in the 4 weeks before the onset of typical neurologic symptoms.[43] Preceding vaccinations have been temporally associated with the occurrence of ADEM, but this is less common.[17,54] Fever, headache, vomiting, and meningismus often are present at the time of initial presentation and may persist during the hospitalization.[11] Neurologic symptoms typically appear 4 to 13 days after the infection develops or vaccination is administered.[15,46,54] New clinical symptoms may continue during hospitalization and may alter treatment. Per current diagnostic criteria, all children with ADEM have an encephalopathy at the time of presentation.[36] The degree of altered mental status varies, ranging from irritability to somnolence to coma. Encephalopathy may be the initial symptom that brings the child to medical attention. Although alteration in mental state often raises concern for the possibility of seizures, they occur in only one-third of patients.[19,54] In addition to having encephalopathy, patients exhibit various other neurologic features. The most common of these are long tract signs, acute hemiparesis, cerebellar ataxia, and cranial neuropathy.[11,19,27,46,54] Aphasia, movement disorders, and sensory deficits occur less commonly.

Demyelination of the optic nerves (optic neuritis) or spinal cord (transverse myelitis) may occur. Symptoms of optic neuritis include vision loss, pain with eye movement, and an afferent papillary defect. Inflammation of the optic disk may be seen on direct funduscopic examination if there is extensive involvement of the optic nerve. Patients with retrobulbar optic neuritis typically have a normal funduscopic examination. Optic neuritis may occur in one or both eyes, with differing degrees of involvement. Symptoms of transverse myelitis include flaccid paralysis of the legs, with a sensory level on examination. The arms can be involved as well if the demyelinating lesion is in the cervical cord. Respiratory failure may occur with high cervical lesions that extend into the brainstem. Bowel and bladder involvement secondary to spinal cord disease results in constipation and urinary retention.

The extent of demyelination in the CNS may not be recognized fully at the time of initial presentation, particularly if the patient has severe encephalopathy. Imaging of the entire CNS to include the brain, orbits, and spinal cord should be done in all patients meeting diagnostic criteria for ADEM because co-occurrence of transverse myelitis or optic neuritis can have a significant impact on rehabilitation needs and long-term outcome.

Clinical Variants

Multiphasic ADEM describes recurrent forms of the disease defined by a single reoccurrence of neurologic symptoms more than 3 months after the initial event and more than 1 month after completion of steroids. Repeated events are not consistent with an ongoing diagnosis of ADEM and should prompt assessment for a different underlying disease process, including metabolic disorders or primary inflammatory diseases such as MS.

Acute hemorrhagic leukoencephalitis is considered a severe variant of ADEM. It accounts for 2% of patients with ADEM.[54] Clinical presentation is similar to that of ADEM, including an acute onset of neurologic deficits 1 to 3 weeks after an upper respiratory tract infection or vaccination. Seizures and coma ensue within hours. The mortality rate is extremely high with fulminant disease. Survivors often have severe residual neurologic deficits. The clinical presentation and imaging features mimic those typically seen in herpes simplex virus encephalitis. Evidence of inflammatory changes and hemorrhage on MRI often is not present for the first few days in herpes simplex virus encephalitis, which may help distinguish the two conditions.[23] Early recognition with prompt institution of steroids or other immunosuppressive agents can be lifesaving.

Historically site-restricted forms of demyelination, such as optic neuritis or transverse myelitis, have been included as part of the spectrum of ADEM. Although these conditions share similar underlying pathology, clinical presentations and prognosis are different, and they should be considered separate entities. They are considered clinically isolated syndromes by the current consensus definitions for demyelinating disease.[36] Clinically isolated syndromes may carry a greater risk for

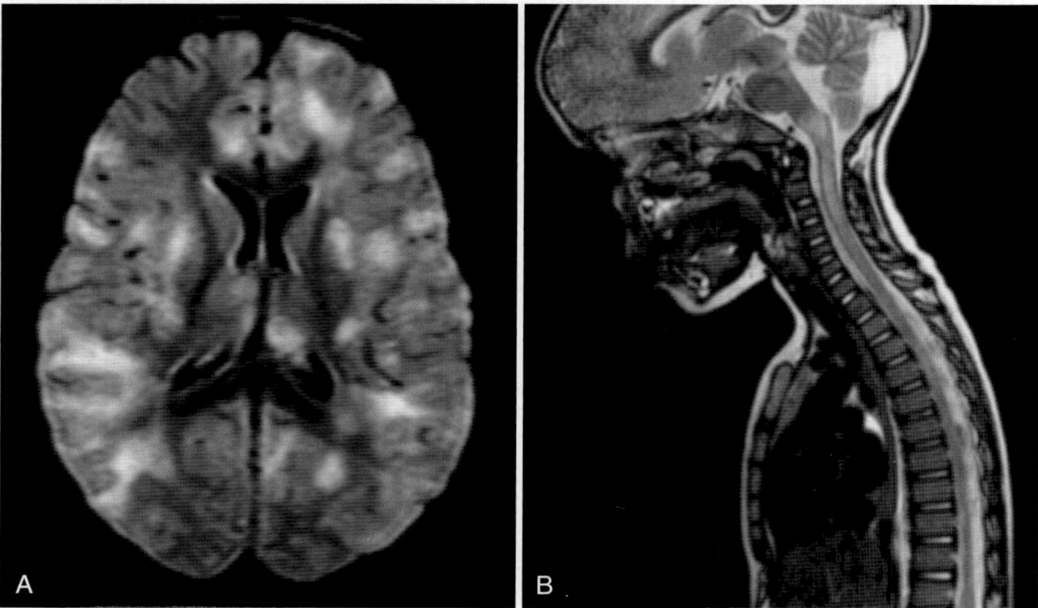

FIG. 37A.1 (A) Axial fluid-attenuated inversion recovery image showing multifocal areas of hyperintensity in both cerebral hemispheres involving cortical gray matter, centrum semiovale, and deep gray nuclei. (B) Sagittal T2-weighted spine image with increased intrinsic signal consistent with longitudinally extensive transverse myelitis in the same patient. (Courtesy Tim Lotze, MD.)

development of MS or other recurrent forms of demyelinating disease.[58] NMO, also known as Devic disease, has classically been described by coincident or sequential optic neuritis and longitudinally extensive myelitis. The discovery of NMO disease-specific antibodies directed against aquaporin-4 water channels in the CNS has further expanded the phenotypic spectrum of this disease.[13] Some patients may present with an ADEM-like event, including encephalopathy with imaging features similar to those seen in ADEM patients. The localization of NMO lesions around regions of high aquaporin-4 expression, such as the ventricular margins, diencephalon, and area postrema, can help to distinguish between the two entities. Further identification of the aquaporin-4 antibody in the serum or CSF is confirmatory for NMO.

MS is the second most common cause of acquired neurologic disability in adults. It is an uncommon finding in pediatric patients. Five percent of adults with MS had onset of disease before reaching 18 years of age.[7] Clinical phenotypes consistent with ADEM and multiphasic ADEM should not be confused with MS because the former two are time-limited in their occurrence. Although they may share some of the same initiating pathologic mechanisms, they are different diseases. However, 2% to 10% of children initially diagnosed with ADEM have subsequently been diagnosed with MS following more than one recurrence of ADEM or the occurrence of a non-ADEM event that is otherwise typical of attack findings in MS.[6,18,44,55] Thus long-term clinical monitoring of ADEM patients is necessary.

The diagnosis of MS requires clinical or radiographic evidence for demyelinating events separated in space and time in the CNS. Patients typically follow a relapsing course of neurologic attacks, with resolution or remission of disability between attacks. Evolution into a course of progressive disability occurs in 50% of patients who have had the disease for more than 15 years.[10] Treatment consists of medications that modulate the immune response by decreasing migration into the CNS, altering cytokine profiles, and interrupting antigen presentation.

Pathology and Pathogenesis

Role of Infection

ADEM is preceded by a viral or bacterial infection in 75% of cases. This infection usually is in the form of a nonspecific upper respiratory tract infection. Many different pathogens have been identified in association with the illness (Box 37A.2). No well-defined latency period has been identified in which an infection can be related to ADEM. Generally patients present within 1 month of their illness. Correlation between ADEM and an infection occurring more than 30 days earlier is more difficult because children are diagnosed with a viral infection four to six times per year, resulting in a positive infectious history in 33% to 50% of patients.[43]

BOX 37A.2 Infectious Pathogens Associated With Acute Disseminated Encephalomyelitis

Viral
Coxsackie
Cytomegalovirus
Epstein-Barr
Hepatitis A or B
Herpes simplex
Human herpesvirus–6
Human T-lymphotropic virus–1
Human immunodeficiency virus
Influenza A or B
Measles
Mumps
Rocky Mountain spotted fever
Rubella
Vaccinia
Varicella

Bacterial
Borrelia burgdorferi
Campylobacter
Chlamydia
Legionella
Leptospira
Mycoplasma pneumoniae
Rickettsia rickettsii
Streptococcus

The phenotypic presentation for ADEM varies depending on the infectious agent. Some organisms have been associated with typical clinical features. Measles virus infection is associated with ADEM in 1/1000 cases. The clinical course often is fulminating, with severe neurologic sequelae or death in most patients. Introduction of vaccination has reduced markedly the occurrence of measles in developed countries, although temporally associated cases of ADEM following vaccination have been described.

Post-varicella ADEM is characterized by ataxia in more than 90% of patients, occasionally with an explosive onset.[28] Headache and meningismus are typical constitutional signs. Pyramidal symptoms include bilateral symmetric upper motor neuron weakness. Patients also may have mood disturbances with a depressed affect or irritability.

ADEM that develops after a rubella infection is similar to measles, with an explosive onset in most children.[28] Profound lethargy, coma, and generalized seizures often occur. Most patients with explosive onset of disease have pyramidal signs and myelitis, whereas a milder phenotype is more likely to have ataxia. Both forms also have been associated with brainstem signs.

Group A β-hemolytic streptococcal infection has been associated with a dystonic extrapyramidal syndrome. Abnormal movements include dystonia, tremor, and parkinsonism. Tics and chorea have not been associated with this condition. Similar to Sydenham chorea and PANDAS, behavioral disturbances, such as emotional lability, obsessive-compulsive tendencies, and inappropriate speech, can occur. Changes in mental status can vary from irritability to coma. MRI shows a predilection for demyelination within the basal ganglia, which includes the caudate, putamen, and globus pallidus. Other deep gray structures, including the thalamus, subthalamus, and substantia nigra, may be affected as well. This finding is distinct from Sydenham chorea and PANDAS, in which imaging is unremarkable. It has been associated with anti–basal ganglia antibodies that cross-react with certain strains of *Streptococcus*.[16]

Role of Immunization

ADEM temporally associated to vaccination has been described with nearly every immunization, and such cases account for less than 5% of all published reports in the medical literature (Box 37A.3). This association does not equate to causation. The Centers for Disease Control in the United States administers the Vaccine Adverse Event Reporting System by which physicians and others voluntarily submit reports of medical events following vaccination. While limitations, such as reporting bias, in such a system exist, this system serves an important key component in detecting early warnings of possible causative links between vaccination and acquired diseases, including ADEM. At the time of this writing, the Institute of Medicine has noted inadequate medical evidence to conclude causality of vaccinations in ADEM.[1]

Historically Pasteur rabies vaccination was associated with prototypic ADEM in approximately 1/1000 individuals.[9] The inoculum was derived from rabbit spinal cord injected with fixed rabies virus. The disease was thought to result principally from the neural tissue contaminating the vaccine rather than the virus itself. This suggestion is supported further by the continued higher incidence of vaccine-associated encephalomyelitis in patients receiving the Semple or duck embryo vaccinations, both of which contain neural tissue. These forms of the vaccination usually are found in developing countries. Experimental allergic encephalomyelitis, the animal model of demyelinating disease, is induced by inoculating myelin or myelin antigens into a suitable experimental animal, further supporting a role of CNS tissue as the causal agent.

Currently measles, mumps, and rubella vaccination is associated most often with post-vaccination encephalomyelitis. A significant difference exists between the incidence of live-measles vaccination–associated ADEM (1 to 2 per 1 million) and the incidence of ADEM previously associated with the measles virus infection (1 per 1000).

Immunologic Factors

A review of the normal process of immune system regulation and surveillance of the CNS is useful when discussing immune dysfunction in the pathogenesis of ADEM. Similar to other disorders of immune dysfunction, activated $CD4^+$ T cells play a principal role in the disease process. T cells reactive against self-antigens, including myelin components, are present in the normal immune system. Several regulatory mechanisms are thought to prevent activation of these lymphocytes, and failure of such processes results in autoimmune conditions. The thymus plays a crucial role in normal T-cell development by deleting many autoreactive lymphocytes from the immune system. Other peripheral mechanisms also are needed because this thymic depletion often is incomplete. *Clonal anergy* describes the unresponsive state of T cells that have encountered their antigen without costimulatory factors.[47] A risk for failure of this mechanism exists through release of nonspecific costimulatory factors from damaged tissue. Another peripheral process is *immunologic ignorance*, in which no productive reaction exists between the T cell and its corresponding peptide/major histocompatibility complex on an antigen-presenting cell. Changes in antigen availability, such as through increased antigen presentation by an invading microorganism, can disrupt this safeguard.[39]

Active regulation is a third process by which regulatory T cells prevent expansion of self-reactive lymphocytes.[35] Regulatory T cells exert their suppressive effects through direct cell-to-cell contact with membrane-bound molecules (CTLA-4) or indirectly through soluble suppressive cytokines, such as interleukin-10 (IL-10) and transforming growth factor-β (TGF-β).[29] Natural killer cells expressing a T-cell receptor also can regulate autoimmune diseases.[42] The presence of such cells within demyelinating regions suggests that some of the inflammation associated with ADEM may have a protective effect.

Although failure of these mechanisms may result in the activation of T cells reactive against myelin antigens, migration of lymphocytes into the CNS is required to produce disease. The CNS has been considered a site of limited immunologic surveillance because of the blood-brain barrier and lack of classic lymph vessels. However, the blood-brain barrier is principally a mechanical diffusion barrier for hydrophilic molecules formed by specialized endothelial cells at the level of the capillaries. Leukocytes readily cross through endothelial cells in postcapillary venules to occupy the perivenular spaces or move on to the neuropil.[26] In addition, antigens and antigen-presenting cells drain from the brain into cervical lymph nodes via the cribriform plate and perineural sheath of the cranial nerves.[14,31] As discussed later, these factors allow for the presentation of antigen in the systemic immune compartment and passage of leukocytes into the CNS for production of disease.

Children with demyelinating disease of the CNS are thought to have a genetic predisposition for such conditions. The strongest data relate to susceptibility genes on chromosome 6p21 in the area of the histocompatibility leukocyte antigen (HLA). Much of the research into these genetic determinants has been related to adult-onset MS.[52] Limited research is available for pediatric demyelinating diseases. However, some of the findings show similarities among age groups and various demyelinating diseases. Linkage studies in Russian children found an association between ADEM and *HLA-DRB1*01* and *HLA-DRB1*017(03)* alleles.[28] Korean children with ADEM were found to have higher frequencies of *HLA-DRB4*0101* and *HLA-DRB1*1501* compared with controls. In adults with MS, the specific genes that confer the highest risk include *HLA-DRB1*1501* and *HLA-DRB5*0101*, among others. In MS, these genes have been linked to earlier disease onset, female gender, a relapsing remitting course, and optic neuritis or spinal involvement as the initial symptom. In addition, genes associated with this haplotype include TGF-β family members, CTLA-4, the tumor necrosis factor (TNF) cluster, IL-1 receptor antagonist, IL-1, and estrogen receptor. Polymorphisms in these genes also have been associated with increased risk for development of demyelinating disease.[21]

The precise mechanism by which these HLA class II genes confer risk for development of demyelinating disease is unclear. Possibilities include (1) preferential binding of self-antigens by these peptides, (2) preferential linkage of autoreactive T cells to the antigen-presenting cell expressing these peptides, (3) abnormal antigen presentation by certain DR molecules, and (4) engagement of HLA class II molecules leading to intracellular signaling events.[52]

Humoral factors also play a role in the production of demyelinating disease. This finding is based on disease-associated laboratory findings and treatment responses. Analysis of CSF in one-third of patients with ADEM shows production of oligoclonal bands, which are not found in the serum.[15] In addition, some patients with post–rabies inoculation

BOX 37A.3 Vaccines Associated With Acute Disseminated Encephalomyelitis

Diphtheria-tetanus-polio	Polio
Hepatitis B	Rabies
Hog vaccine	Smallpox
Japanese B encephalitis	Tetanus
Measles	Tick-borne encephalitis
Mumps	

ADEM have been found to have positive serum antibodies against myelin basic protein and galactocerebroside.[37]

Pathogenesis

ADEM is considered to occur in genetically susceptible individuals prone to immune system dysregulation after an encounter with an appropriate environmental stimulus. Mechanisms of disease production are based principally on two animal models that closely resemble the disease. The first is experimental autoimmune encephalomyelitis.[49] In this model, animals develop monophasic neurologic disease similar to ADEM after receiving immunization with CNS homogenate or encephalitogenic myelin peptides emulsified in Freund complete adjuvant. The second model is Theiler murine encephalomyelitis, in which susceptible mouse strains develop disease after receiving direct injection of Theiler murine encephalomyelitis virus into the cerebrum. In both of these models, increased exposure of the immune system to myelin proteins produces disease.

By comparing these models with ADEM in humans, two pathogenetic concepts have been developed. The inflammatory cascade concept implies a direct CNS infection with a neurotropic pathogen, which results in CNS tissue damage and systemic leakage of CNS-confined autoantigens through a damaged blood-brain barrier into the systemic circulation. Presentation of these antigens within systemic lymphatic organs leads to tolerance breakdown and a self-reactive encephalitogenic T-cell response. The molecular mimicry concept suggests structural amino acid homology between the invading pathogen and myelin basic protein in the host.[22] Although similar to myelin peptides, the amino acid sequence contains subtle differences that fail to prevent immune tolerance and result in activation of myelin-reactive T cells against similar "self" myelin antigens. The Epstein-Barr virus provides an example of this. The virus contains a pentapeptide sequence in its nuclear antigen (EBNA) that shares sequence homology with an epitope of myelin basic protein, a major protein of the myelin sheath.[12] Epstein-Barr virus has been implicated in the pathogenesis of MS partly based on this concept of molecular mimicry.[3] Recently antibodies to myelin oligodendrocyte glycoprotein have been shown to be present during the period of active demyelination in ADEM but quickly fall in most patients.[48] In those with persistent or rebounding of myelin oligodendrocyte glycoprotein antibody levels, a propensity was seen to develop childhood MS, suggesting this might be prognostic.

The immunopathologic events leading to ADEM can be divided into two major phases: (1) initial T-cell priming and activation and (2) subsequent recruitment and effector phase.[8] The priming phase occurs in systemic secondary lymphoid organs, in which the antigen-presenting cell presents myelin protein antigen and peptides to neuroantigen-reactive T cells. The activated T cells expand and then migrate to the CNS via the postcapillary venules into the perivascular space. In the Virchow-Robin space, the T cells reencounter their cognate antigen, in the context of HLA class II molecules expressed by dendritic cells.[24] This reactivation allows the T cells to migrate through the glial limitans and enter the brain parenchyma.

Further recruitment occurs through the production of cytokines and chemokines by antigen-presenting cells and activated T cells, promoting migration into the CNS of additional T cells and other leukocytes, such as polymorphonuclear and monomorphonuclear phagocytes.[52] Breakdown of the blood-brain barrier occurs by release of proteases from recruited mast cells, T cells, and monocytes. In addition, production of reactive oxygen radicals occurs, causing further endothelial injury, which leads to the effector phase in which T cells have more of a secondary role to other inflammatory processes that cause demyelination and axonal injury. These inflammatory processes include oxygen and nitrogen radicals, TNF-α, direct and indirect complement activation, antibody-dependent cellular toxicity, myelin phagocytosis, direct axonal injury by $CD8^+$ cytotoxic T lymphocytes, protease secretion, and oligodendrocyte apoptosis.[52] Glutamate-mediated excitotoxic injury of the oligodendrocytes also occurs.[56] The inflammatory process continues for a few days to 2 weeks, resulting in stretches of demyelinated axons, some of which may be transected.

The repair process begins with activation and proliferation of astrocytes. Clearing of debris by macrophages and increased production of antiinflammatory cytokines and various growth factors by resident cells and T cells occur. Oligodendrocyte precursors become activated and, along with surviving oligodendrocytes, begin the process of remyelination. The clinical and imaging outcome of ADEM most often shows complete recovery. Subtle differences in repaired myelin, including altered thickness and redistribution of sodium channels, may occur, however.[57] In addition, the relative composition of myelin peptides is altered to forms that may have increased vulnerability to further damage[50] and may explain recurrent forms of ADEM.

Clinical Evaluation

ADEM should be considered in a child seen several days after a febrile illness with subacute onset of encephalopathy and polysymptomatic neurologic deficits. The clinical features require ruling out other possible diagnoses, however, through additional diagnostic tests.

Diagnostic imaging is the most useful tool in establishing the diagnosis. Computed tomography (CT) scans usually are done on an emergent basis for encephalopathic patients. Areas of demyelination may appear as darker areas of hypodensity, with any hemorrhagic component being hyperdense. CT does not adequately show the full burden of disease, however, and may be completely normal. MRI is the most sensitive means for showing the widespread demyelination typical of the disease (see Fig. 37A.1). T2-weighted sequences provide the best assessment of the disease, with demyelinating areas being hyperintense and accompanied by surrounding edema. Administration of gadolinium contrast material may show breakdown of the blood-brain barrier with areas of enhancement. This enhancement may appear homogeneous throughout the lesion or show a "broken ring" appearance, with the open edge pointing toward the cortex. Lesions may be large, measuring more than 1 cm in diameter. They typically are rounded with poorly defined margins.

Of most common concern in children presenting with a febrile encephalopathy is the possibility of an underlying CNS infection. A lumbar puncture often is done to investigate this possibility. A lymphocytic pleocytosis may occur (commonly >50 cells). Elevated albumin levels also may be present. Findings of neutrophils and elevated red blood cells alternatively would raise concern for the possibility of herpes encephalitis.

Intrathecal oligoclonal bands may be positive, and IgG synthesis may be increased in 30% of patients with ADEM. Their relationship to the underlying disease pathophysiology is unclear but is thought to represent a response of B cells within the CNS to the inflammatory process.[5] Serologic studies of the CSF may be useful to uncover the causal agent, although results should be interpreted with caution because many neurotropic viruses have a high prevalence in the general population.

Rarely patients may present with very large demyelinating lesions, characteristically described as *tumefactive*. In such circumstances, a biopsy may be needed to determine the underlying etiology. Findings typical of demyelination help rule out a CNS malignancy. Before a biopsy is done, the clinician should investigate for other evidence of demyelinating disease, including imaging of the spinal cord. A comorbid transverse myelitis would provide more evidence of a demyelinating condition and reduce the need for a biopsy. In addition, normal CSF cytology helps discount an underlying malignancy.

Primary and secondary CNS vasculitis associated with collagen vascular diseases, such as systemic lupus erythematosus or antiphospholipid antibody syndrome, may manifest with a similar clinical and radiologic picture. These diseases are typified by recurrent ischemic strokes. Distinguishing features for antiphospholipid antibody syndrome include a family history of strokes or other thromboses at a young age and fetal loss. Testing for antiphospholipid antibody and lupus anticoagulant is positive. Primary CNS vasculitis with strokes is best investigated through conventional angiography showing an irregular vessel lumen. Leptomeningeal biopsy is considered the gold standard to confirm the diagnosis.

A severe course that principally affects the optic nerves, spinal cord, or other areas of high aquaporin-4 expression, including the periventricular and aqueductal regions, area postrema, diencephalon, or brainstem, should raise concern for NMO. Serum and/or CSF testing for the aquaporin-4 water channel antibody that is associated with this disease is clinically available. The test is greater than 90% specific for NMO, and up to 65% of pediatric patients meeting current diagnostic criteria will have positive antibody titers.[59,13]

Neurophysiologic studies can be useful to evaluate comorbidities and burden of disease. An electroencephalogram should be obtained in patients with seizures and severe encephalopathy to characterize the seizure focus and investigate for subclinical seizures. Findings often are consistent with a diffuse disturbance in brain function, noting slowing of the normal electric rhythms.

Treatment

To date, no controlled clinical trials have been conducted on the optimal treatment for ADEM. Based on empiric evidence, intravenous high-dose corticosteroids are accepted as first-line treatment.[51] Methylprednisolone is given at 30 mg/kg per dose (maximum 1000 mg) for five doses. Alternatively, dexamethasone, 1 mg/kg per dose for five doses, may be used. A prednisone taper typically is instituted on completion of this regimen, with an initial dosing of 1 mg/kg per day and tapering by 5 mg every 5 days. Alternative antiinflammatory and immunosuppressive therapies may be used depending on the response to the initial steroid treatment. Intravenous immunoglobulin (IVIG) has been found to be beneficial in some patients.[51] IVIG is given 2 g/kg divided over 2 to 5 days.

Plasmapheresis also may be used.[32,34] The patient receives seven treatments consisting of 1.1 to 1.4 plasma volume exchanges over a 14-day course. IVIG and plasmapheresis typically are not considered as first-line treatment for ADEM, partly related to availability of IVIG or apheresis units, cost of treatment in contrast to steroids, prolonged hospitalization, and need for adequate venous access. Nonetheless they should be considered secondary treatment options, especially in the occasional patient who continues to deteriorate during steroid treatment or who fails to show adequate recovery 7 days after completing intravenous steroids. The choice between the two agents is arbitrary. Particular consideration for plasmapheresis might be given in the setting of a comorbid myelopathy because this has been noted to be beneficial in patients presenting with transverse myelitis.[30] Severe cases failing to respond to any of these measures may require immunosuppressive agents, such as cyclophosphamide.[41] A few cases of severe ADEM with massive edema have required hemicraniectomy to prevent severe neurologic sequelae or death.[2,20]

Additional treatment that may be needed depends on the patient's neurologic deficits. Anticonvulsants should be given for management of seizures. Attention given to bowel and bladder care is important to avoid secondary complications of retention. Impaired swallowing requires adequate nutrition to be provided by gavage feedings. Transverse myelopathy can be associated with autonomic dysfunction, including orthostatic hypotension, necessitating the use of an abdominal binder. Rehabilitation should begin at the time of admission, with the assistance of physical medicine and rehabilitation specialists. During the long-term recovery period, modifications to the home and school environment may be needed, depending on residual deficits.

Outcome and Prognosis

Historically, ADEM was associated with high morbidity and mortality rates principally related to disease associated with the measles virus. Measles-associated ADEM was associated with death in 25% of affected patients, with an additional 30% of patients having severe neurologic sequelae. This dismal outcome has improved dramatically with the institution of measles vaccination. The introduction of high-dose steroid treatment in modifying the disease course also may have improved the current outcome findings. Currently a low mortality rate of between 3% and 5% remains associated with this disease, and such patients typically have a hemorrhagic form.[40]

Currently, 80% to 90% of patients show excellent recovery of functional and cognitive deficits.[4,15,28,54] Children typically have a less severe course and fewer long-term neurologic sequelae than do adults.[33] Mild neurologic disabilities, with weakness and fine motor difficulties being the most common deficits, may be present in some patients. Epilepsy may occur in 6% of patients after an episode of ADEM.[15] Neurocognitive testing of children recovering from ADEM has shown mild impairments in attention and executive function and reduced visuospatial and visuomotor skills.[25] The greatest risk for development of neurologic sequelae may be in older patients with sudden onset of severe neurologic symptoms.

Recurrent forms of the disease often raise concern for pediatric MS. The exact relationship between ADEM and MS remains to be better defined. The conditions are distinct, however, based on the clinical presentations, imaging, and clinical courses. Disease recurrence consistent with multiphasic ADEM occurs in about 30% of patients.[43] Most patients have their second attack within the first year after their initial event.[4,45] It often occurs soon after discontinuation of steroid taper or after an infection encountered shortly after the initial event. Treatment and outcome for recurrences are not different from those described for the initial event. In one study of 33 ADEM patients, 6% were eventually diagnosed with MS.[40]

NEW REFERENCES SINCE THE SEVENTH EDITION

1. Stratton KFA, Rusch E, Clayton EW, eds. *Adverse effects of vaccines: evidence and causality. Committee to Review Adverse Effects of Vaccines*. Washington, DC: National Academies Press (US); 2011.
6. Atzori M, Battistella PA, Perini P, et al. Clinical and diagnostic aspects of multiple sclerosis and acute monophasic encephalomyelitis in pediatric patients: a single centre prospective study. *Mult Scler*. 2009;15(3):363-370.
13. Chitnis T, Ness J, Krupp L, et al. Clinical features of neuromyelitis optica in children: US Network of Pediatric MS Centers report. *Neurology*. 2016;86(3):245-252.
18. Dale RC, Pillai SC. Early relapse risk after a first CNS inflammatory demyelination episode: examining international consensus definitions. *Dev Med Child Neurol*. 2007;49(12):887-893.
36. Krupp LB, Tardieu M, Amato MP, et al. International Pediatric Multiple Sclerosis Study Group criteria for pediatric multiple sclerosis and immune-mediated central nervous system demyelinating disorders: revisions to the 2007 definitions. *Mult Scler*. 2013;19(10):1261-1267.
40. Mar S, Lenox J, Benzinger T, et al. Long-term prognosis of pediatric patients with relapsing acute disseminated encephalomyelitis. *J Child Neurol*. 2010;25(6):681-688.
44. Mikaeloff Y, Caridade G, Husson B, et al. Acute disseminated encephalomyelitis cohort study: prognostic factors for relapse. *Eur J Paediatr Neurol*. 2007;11(2):90-95.
53. Tenembaum SN. Acute disseminated encephalomyelitis. *Handb Clin Neurol*. 2013;112:1253-1262.
56. Verhey LH, Branson HM, Shroff MM, et al. MRI parameters for prediction of multiple sclerosis diagnosis in children with acute CNS demyelination: a prospective national cohort study. *Lancet Neurol*. 2011;10(12):1065-1073.
57. Pitt D, Werner P, Raine CS. Glutamate excitotoxicity in a model of multiple sclerosis. *Nat Med*. 2000;6(1):67-70.
60. Wingerchuk DM, Banwell B, Bennett JL, et al. International consensus diagnostic criteria for neuromyelitis optica spectrum disorders. *Neurology*. 2015;85(2):177-189.

The full reference list for this chapter is available at ExpertConsult.com.

37B ■ Infection-Associated Myelitis and Myelopathies of the Spinal Cord

Timothy E. Lotze

ACUTE TRANSVERSE MYELITIS

The sudden and progressive onset of paresis, sensory deficits, and bowel and bladder dysfunction that characterizes acute transverse myelitis (ATM) terrifies affected children and their families. Successful management requires prompt differentiation from other myelopathic disorders to determine proper treatment. Because of the association of ATM with numerous infections, specialists in infectious diseases frequently participate in the care of children with this disease. The clinical presentation, radiologic features, differential diagnosis, pathophysiology, treatment, and prognosis of pediatric ATM are reviewed here.

TABLE 37B.1 **Transverse Myelitis Consortium Working Group Diagnostic Criteria**

Inclusion Criteria	Exclusion Criteria
Bilateral signs/symptoms (not necessarily symmetric)	Clear arterial distribution clinical deficit consistent with thrombosis of anterior spinal artery
Clearly defined sensory level	Abnormal flow voids on surface of the spinal cord consistent with AVM
Exclusion of extraaxial compressive etiology by neuroimaging (MRI or myelography; CT of spine inadequate)	Serologic or clinical evidence of connective tissue disease (sarcoidosis, Behçet disease, Sjögren syndrome, SLE, mixed connective tissue disorder)[a]
Inflammation within spinal cord shown by CSF pleocytosis or elevated IgG index or gadolinium enhancement. If no inflammatory criteria are met at symptom onset, repeat MRI and lumbar puncture evaluation 2 to 7 days after symptom onset meet criteria	CNS manifestations of syphilis, Lyme disease, HIV, HTLV-1, *Mycoplasma,* other viral infection (e.g., HSV-1, HSV-2, VZV, EBV, CMV, HHV-6, enteroviruses)[a] Brain MRI abnormalities suggestive of MS[a] History of clinically apparent optic neuritis[a]
Progression to nadir 4 hours to 21 days after onset of symptoms (if patient awakens with symptoms, symptoms must become more pronounced from point of awakening)	

Data from Transverse Myelitis Working Group. Proposed diagnostic criteria and nosology of acute myelitis. *Neurology.* 2002;59:499–505.
AVM, Arteriovenous malformation; *CMV,* cytomegalovirus; *CNS,* central nervous system; *CSF,* cerebrospinal fluid; *CT,* computed tomography; *EBV,* Epstein-Barr virus; *HIV,* human immunodeficiency virus; *HHV-6,* human herpesvirus-6; *HSV,* herpes simplex virus; *HTLV-1,* human T-cell lymphotrophic virus-1; *MRI,* magnetic resonance imaging; *MS,* multiple sclerosis; *SLE,* systemic lupus erythematosus; *VZV,* varicella zoster virus.
[a]Do not exclude disease-associated acute transverse myelitis.

DIAGNOSTIC CRITERIA

ATM is an acquired inflammatory disorder consisting of progressive signs and symptoms reflecting bilateral sensory, motor, or autonomic dysfunction attributable to the spinal cord. This constellation of signs and symptoms can be caused by a heterogeneous group of disorders, which are distinguished as either disease associated or idiopathic. Disease-associated forms, including direct spinal cord infection, can be difficult to distinguish from idiopathic disease.

Diagnostic criteria were established by the Transverse Myelitis Working Group Consortium in 2002 and consist of both inclusionary and exclusionary criteria.[55] The criteria were established to rapidly differentiate ATM from other myelopathies that require different treatment regimens. Differentiation from extramedullary compression such as that caused by extrinsic tumor, abscess, hematoma, and other intramedullary lesions such as infarction and intrinsic tumors is necessary to guide treatment and facilitate discussion of prognosis. Table 37B.1 lists both the inclusionary and exclusionary criteria for ATM.

EPIDEMIOLOGY

Two prospective studies have evaluated the incidence of acquired ATM in children.[7,16] Based on these studies, the incidence in pediatric populations is approximately 1.72 to 2 persons per 1 million. Although early case series had suggested a slight female predominance,[13,14,19,30,42,44] the more recent prospective studies have found a male predominance in the pediatric population. When stratifying for children younger than 10 years of age at onset and older than 10 years of age, one study found a striking 1:2 female to male ratio in children younger than 10 years. In children with age of onset older than 10 years, the female to male ratio was 1.2:1, similar to that of other inflammatory demyelinating disorders.[7] The mean age of onset is between 9 and 10.5 years; however, onset has been reported as early as 6 months. Of interest, one study found a bimodal distribution with peak ages of onset at 4 and 15 years.[16]

CLINICAL PRESENTATION

Three phases occur in patients with ATM: initial, plateau, and recovery. The initial phase begins with the presenting symptom and concludes with reaching the neurologic nadir. The plateau phase begins when the patient has reached the neurologic nadir and is a period during which the symptoms are more or less stable. The last phase is recovery, which is the period of slow improvement in neurologic function. The length of time in each phase has been useful for prognostication of recovery and will be discussed later. Patients typically present acutely to subacutely with a combination of sensory and motor deficits. The most common motor symptom is bilateral leg weakness (82%), with a paraplegia developing in 36% of cases, although upper extremity weakness is a rare initial feature (4%).[16] Involvement of the arms occurs in 37% of patients at some point. Approximately 70% to 90% of patients develop bowel and bladder dysfunction, ranging from urinary retention and constipation to incontinence.[14,16] A similar percentage of patients report sensory symptoms, including paresthesia and numbness. Most patients reach their neurologic nadir within 1 week, and patients rarely have worsening of symptoms more than 4 weeks after onset of symptoms.[13,14] Children with extremely rapid evolution of their symptoms (1 to 4 hours) should cause the clinician to take pause and consider a possible ischemic etiology.

The general examination, although usually unremarkable, may reveal signs suggestive of an underlying systemic infection or autoimmune disorder. Fever is not uncommon, with one study reporting its presence in 20% of children with ATM.[7] Abdominal examination may reveal a distended bladder. A diffuse or dermatomal vesicular rash or its sequelae suggest concurrent or preceding chickenpox or shingles.

The presence of any mental status changes suggests that the myelitis is a component of a more diffuse process (i.e., acute disseminated encephalomyelitis or neuromyelitis optica). In the acute stages, muscle tone is low in affected limbs but with time may become spastic. Detailed muscle strength testing with objective grading serves as a crucial baseline to compare with serial examinations to determine whether the patient is improving. All sensory modalities should be assessed carefully. In one series, 65% of children with ATM had sensory symptoms, with more than 80% of those children having a clear sensory level.[16] An early case series had suggested that severe pain is a common symptom (88%); however this is potentially skewed by selection bias of this retrospective study.[14] A spinal cord sensory level usually is located in the thoracic region (58%) and less commonly in the cervical (7%) or lumbar (31%) area.[16] In the acute phase, deep tendon reflexes are depressed in approximately 70% of patients and later become hyperactive. Similarly the Babinski sign may be negative early in the acute phase but soon becomes positive, indicating upper motor neuron dysfunction.

RADIOLOGIC FEATURES

Every patient with suspected ATM should undergo emergent gadolinium-enhanced magnetic resonance imaging (MRI) of the entire spine to confirm the diagnosis and rule out alternative diagnoses, particularly compressive lesions, such as epidural abscess, epidural hematoma, and extramedullary tumors, which are all potentially neurosurgical emergencies. T1-weighted and T2-weighted sagittal imaging of the entire spine can serve as an initial screen, followed by comparative axial imaging in areas of suspected pathology. In addition, every patient with any

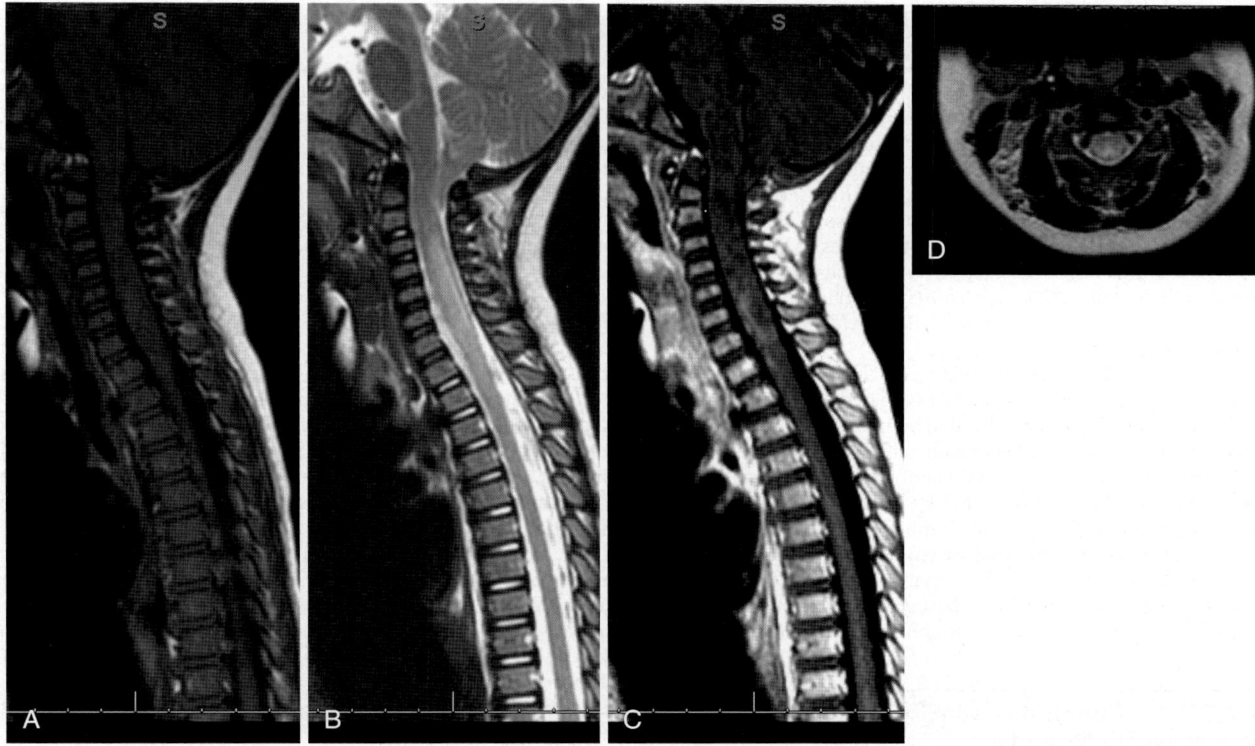

FIG. 37B.1 Acute transverse myelitis of the cervical cord. (A) Sagittal T1-weighted magnetic resonance imaging (MRI) sequence through the cervical spinal cord demonstrating swelling of the cord. (B) T2-weighted MRI sequence of same patient revealing longitudinally extensive hyperintensity through the cervical cord. (C) T1-weighted MRI sequence with gadolinium revealing patchy enhancement of the cervical cord. (D) T2-weighted axial MRI sequence through the cervical cord revealing hyperintensity of both gray and white matter.

neurologic symptoms not referable to the spinal cord should undergo MRI of the brain with gadolinium enhancement. Optimally, this should include dedicated fine sections through the orbits to evaluate for optic neuritis associated with neuromyelitis optica (NMO). The distinction between idiopathic ATM and other acquired demyelinating syndromes like multiple sclerosis (MS) and NMO is important for both treatment and prognosis. In general, it is uncommon for patients to have asymptomatic lesions outside of the spinal cord, and, in the absence of such findings, the likelihood for an eventual diagnosis of MS or NMO is low.[1]

Spinal MRI in ATM typically reveals T1-isointense (Fig. 37B.1A) and T2-hyperintense (Fig. 37B.1B) signals over several contiguous spinal cord segments[14] and may involve the entire spine.[1,2]

The most common finding is a T2-hyperintense lesion involving more than three segments, with one study finding the average length of lesion being more than six segments. The hyperintense signal can extend into the lower brainstem.[2] Spinal cord swelling with effacement of the surrounding cerebrospinal fluid (CSF) spaces may be present in severe cases (Fig. 37B.1A). Axial imaging typically reveals lesions involving both gray and white matter (Fig. 37B.1D). Contrast enhancement is variably present and may appear diffuse, patchy, or nodular (Fig. 37B.1C). In some patients with very suggestive clinical features, initial spine MRI may be normal and should be repeated several days later.[14,30,42] In rare cases, the MRI remains normal but does not rule out the diagnosis, and evidence of inflammation in the CSF is considered to meet diagnostic criteria for ATM in such cases.[55] A new modality still used exclusively in research that has been applied to ATM is diffusion tensor imaging (DTI). DTI is an MRI sequence that evaluates for the presence and integrity of white matter tracts. One study of a small number of adults with ATM revealed that those individuals with more severe disruption of white matter tracts within the lesion and distal to the lesion had a worse prognosis.[34] In the future, DTI might be useful for stratifying patients for likely prognosis and determining who might benefit from more aggressive treatment.

LUMBAR PUNCTURE

Approximately 50% of pediatric patients with ATM have CSF pleocytosis, typically with a lymphocytic predominance.[14,16] Elevated CSF protein levels, either in isolation or in conjunction with pleocytosis, also are detected in approximately 50% of patients. Glucose typically is normal. A normal CSF profile does not rule out ATM because this pattern is seen in approximately 25% of patients. Imaging evidence of an inflammatory myelopathy would be needed to meet diagnostic criteria for ATM in such cases. CSF cytology should be considered for patients with concern for neoplasm. Additional CSF testing is discussed further later.

DIFFERENTIAL DIAGNOSIS

Conditions That Mimic Acute Transverse Myelitis

ATM can be associated with more widespread central nervous system (CNS) demyelinating disorders or systemic autoimmune disorders; in such cases, the term *disease-associated transverse myelitis* has been used. Isolated ATM can be triggered by identifiable preceding infections. Alternatively, ATM can be associated with a nonspecific preceding infection or have no apparent cause; for both of these subgroups, the term *idiopathic ATM* has been used. This last group constitutes the most common category in pediatric ATM. Although the precise pathophysiology of idiopathic ATM is uncertain, the frequent association with preceding infections and accumulating immunologic data suggests an inflammatory cause for the disorder.[9,14,27,41]

Numerous disorders can affect the spinal cord and produce identical symptoms and signs that mimic idiopathic ATM (Box 37B.1). Such conditions must be ruled out through a combination of history, physical examination, neuroimaging, and laboratory evaluation.

Extramedullary Lesions

Extramedullary compressive lesions are neurosurgical emergencies that must be diagnosed rapidly for effective treatment. Spinal epidural abscesses are rare in children. In one series of eight children compiled over a 15-year period at a major children's hospital, seven had fever and all eight had back pain.[5] *Staphylococcus aureus,* some of which were methicillin-resistant, were the most common isolates in this and other series. Other species that have been isolated from spinal epidural abscesses in children include *Salmonella enteritides* (primarily in sickle-cell patients),[5] *Streptococcus pneumoniae,*[10] *Bartonella henselae,*[25] and *Mycobacterium tuberculosis.*[29]

Spinal epidural hematomas also are rare occurrences in children. They can occur spontaneously or may be associated with anticoagulant use, clotting disorders, trauma, or lumbar puncture.[46] Spinal epidural hematomas after lumbar puncture typically self-resolve with no residual sequelae.[31] The first episode of significant bleeding in individuals with hemophilia A has been reported to be a spinal epidural hematoma either forming spontaneously or after lumbar puncture.[24,58] Although they typically cause slowly progressive symptoms (Foix-Alajouainine syndrome), paraspinal arteriovenous malformations can manifest acutely as a result of hemorrhage.[28] Unruptured arteriovenous malformations (AVMs) usually can be detected as abnormal, dilated vasculature on MRI of the spine; subsequent spinal angiography can confirm the diagnosis.

Spinal cord compression resulting from metastatic disease occurred in about 6% of children with solid tumors at some point during their course in one series.[48] The most common responsible tumor types were primitive neuroectodermal tumor, soft tissue sarcoma, and neuroblastoma. When spinal cord compression is the initial manifestation of cancer, as was the case for 67% of the patients in this series, it can mimic ATM, although symptoms would in general be expected to progress more slowly than in ATM. Spinal MRI readily distinguishes spinal cord compression from ATM.

BOX 37B.1 Conditions That Mimic Idiopathic Acute Transverse Myelitis

Direct infectious myelopathies
Extramedullary compressive lesions
- Epidural abscess
- Epidural hematoma
- Extramedullary tumors

Guillain-Barré syndrome
Intramedullary spinal cord tumors
- Astrocytomas
- Ependymomas

Ischemia and infarction
Syringomyelia
Radiation injury
Traumatic spinal cord injury
Vascular malformations

Intramedullary Lesions

Spinal cord infarction is exceedingly rare in children but must be considered in the setting of acute onset of neurologic symptoms referable to the spinal cord. Clinical features and neuroimaging can be used to distinguish ATM from spinal cord infarction, although this can be difficult at initial presentation. Spinal cord infarct typically manifests in a hyperacute fashion (<4 hours from onset to severe neurologic symptoms) with dissociated sensory loss (absent temperature and pain sensation with preserved vibration and proprioception) from thrombosis of the anterior spinal artery.[43] One should inquire about recent trauma, even minor, including to the neck, because this can result in vertebral artery dissection and resultant embolic thrombi to the anterior spinal artery (Fig. 37B.2). Coagulopathies also have been associated with spinal cord ischemia and should be considered.[43] Accompanying MRI signal abnormality in the adjacent vertebral body is highly suggestive of the diagnosis but not universally present at onset of symptoms.[45] Diffusion-weighted MRI also may reveal the presence of ischemia and aid in making the diagnosis; however, diffusion restriction can be difficult to appreciate in the spinal cord.

The most common intramedullary spinal cord tumors in children are astrocytomas (60%), followed by ependymomas (30%), and finally gangliogliomas (15%).[51] Although biopsy of the tumors is necessary to establish the exact histologic diagnosis, biopsy of the spinal cord rarely is needed to distinguish tumor from ATM. Despite similarities in presenting symptoms, clinical features can help distinguish intramedullary tumors from ATM. Intramedullary spinal cord tumors manifest more subacutely or chronically than does ATM, reflecting their low cellular growth rate.[51] In one study, the mean duration of symptoms before presentation of children with intramedullary spinal cord tumors was 254 days[18] in contrast to ATM, which manifests full symptoms in about 1 week. On examination, the presence of scoliosis or torticollis suggests the presence of more longstanding tumors rather than ATM.[51]

ATM and spinal cord tumors typically are isointense on T1-weighted MRI and hyperintense on T2-weighted images. Although intramedullary

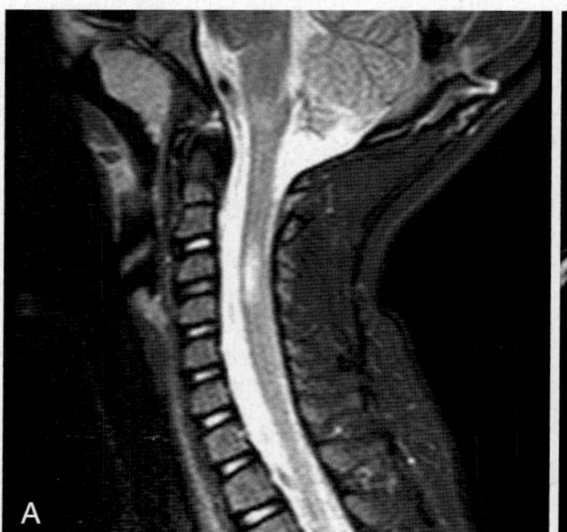

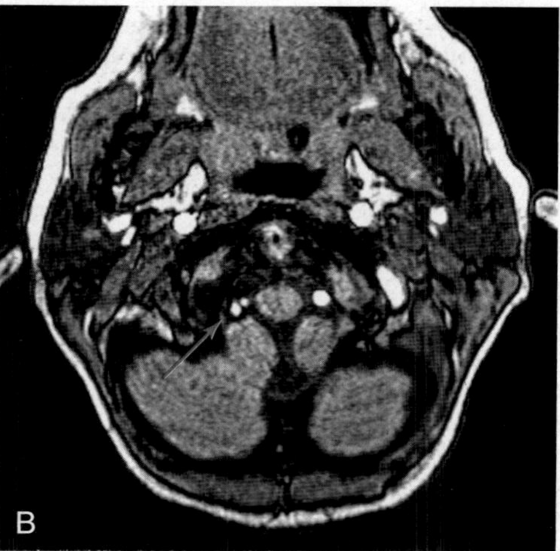

FIG. 37B.2 Ischemic infarction of the cervical cord. (A) Sagittal T2-weighted magnetic resonance imaging sequence through the cervical spinal cord revealing hyperintensity of the cord. (B) Axial magnetic resonance angiogram of the neck revealing a dissection of the vertebral artery on the right of the same patient *(arrow).*

tumors display swelling and contrast enhancement more frequently than does ATM, these features can also be seen in the latter. Other radiographic features may be used to distinguish the two entities. The eccentric location of astrocytomas within the spinal cord can be used to differentiate them from ATM, which usually produces symmetric findings.[51] Although ependymomas can produce symmetric spinal cord expansion because of their origin from the central canal, these tumors usually span three to four vertebral segments,[4] whereas pediatric ATM typically involves longer areas of the spinal cord. In addition, an area of low signal intensity reflecting hemosiderin deposits from chronic hemorrhage at the edge of ependymomas also can serve as a radiographic clue.[4] Because patients with intramedullary spinal cord tumors may be diagnosed based on CSF cytologic examination, this test should be considered in all patients with suspected ATM.

The clinical presentation of spinal cord dysfunction in the setting of prior irradiation suggests radiation-induced transverse myelitis as the most likely diagnosis. This entity typically manifests 9 to 18 months after radiotherapy, but it can occur earlier in children.[57]

Syringomyelia typically begins with pain and temperature sensory loss in a capelike distribution over the shoulders. However, if these early symptoms are missed and the syrinx grows, motor disturbances can develop that might be mistaken for ATM. The time course of developing sensory and motor dysfunction in syringomyelia is typically longer than that in ATM. The most common causes of syrinxes in children are tumors and Chiari I malformations.[52] Syringomyelia is readily distinguishable from ATM on MRI.

Peripheral Lesions

The initial clinical presentation of ATM can be quite similar to that of Guillain-Barré syndrome. Both disorders can manifest with back pain, paraparesis, and sensory abnormalities. The sensory abnormalities in Guillain-Barré syndrome are often transient and minimal in comparison to the complete sensory loss below the affected spinal cord level encountered in ATM. Preservation of deep tendon reflexes is less common in Guillain-Barré syndrome than in ATM. Likewise, bowel and bladder symptoms are more typical of ATM than Guillain-Barré syndrome. Some patients with ATM have albuminocytologic dissociation found on CSF analysis, which is indistinguishable from Guillain-Barré syndrome. In some cases, ATM and Guillain-Barré syndrome can be distinguished only with contrast-enhanced MRI. Spinal cord, nerve root, and peripheral nerve pathology can coexist in myeloradiculoneuritis, suggesting that ATM and Guillain-Barré syndrome may share a common pathophysiologic mechanism in some cases.[11,37,54]

Disease-Associated Acute Transverse Myelitis

ATM with a presumed inflammatory basis can be associated with recurrent CNS demyelinating disorders and systemic autoimmune disorders. In these cases, the term *disease-associated ATM* can be applied (Box 37B.2).[17]

The presence of encephalopathy and multifocal MRI abnormalities of cerebral white matter most often points toward acute disseminated encephalomyelitis as a possible diagnosis (Table 37B.2). Spinal cord demyelination in MS tends to be limited to fewer than two vertebral segments with partial cord involvement seen in the transverse plane, resulting in mild, asymmetric symptoms compared with the typically severe, symmetric symptoms in ATM.[23,49] In addition, evidence for dissemination of lesions in space and time in the CNS is required for establishing the diagnosis of MS.[32] Previous subtle visual or sensory symptoms suggestive of a recurrent demyelinating disorder may be elicited only with detailed questioning. Oligoclonal bands are present more commonly in MS-related myelitis, but they may occur in idiopathic ATM (Table 37B.3).

ATM is also a core feature of NMO, a severe, relapsing demyelinating disorder. Specific diagnostic criteria for NMO spectrum disorders have been developed.[60] While ATM is a core feature of this disease, it is not required for diagnosis in those who otherwise meet the diagnostic criteria. A novel biomarker (AQP4-IgG) targeting the predominant CNS water channel protein aquaporin-4 (AQP4), which is concentrated in astrocytic foot processes in the blood-brain barrier, has been detected in adult and pediatric patients with NMO.[35,36,38] It one series, it was detected in 65% of pediatric NMO patients meeting current diagnostic criteria.[12] Because of the potential lag in time from ATM to occurrence of other manifestations of NMO in some children, and the difference in recurrence risk,[59] severity, prognosis, and need for maintenance therapy, every child with ATM should have serum NMO-IgG testing and CSF testing.

ATM also can occur secondary to a variety of systemic autoimmune disorders. Involvement of other organ systems, particularly the skin, lungs, kidneys, and joints, may point to a particular diagnosis, including

BOX 37B.2 Central Nervous System and Systemic Autoimmune Disorders Associated With Acute Transverse Myelitis

Central Nervous System Disorders

Acute disseminated encephalomyelitis
Multiple sclerosis
Neuromyelitis optica

Systemic Autoimmune Disorders

Antiphospholipid antibody syndrome
Behçet disease
Mixed connective tissue disorder
Neurosarcoidosis
Sjögren syndrome
Systemic lupus erythematosus

TABLE 37B.2 Distinguishing Acute Transverse Myelitis From Other Central Nervous System Demyelinating Disorders

Finding	ATM	ADEM	MS	NMO
Myelitis	+	+/–	+/– (partial)	+
Acute mental status changes	–	+	–	+/–
Optic neuritis	–	+/–	+/–	+/–
Abnormal brain MRI	–	+	+	+/–
CSF oligoclonal bands	–	+/–	+	+/–
Serum AQP4-IgG	–	–	–	+/–
Recurrences	+/–	+/–	+	+

+, Always present; +/–, variably present; –, usually absent.
ADEM, Acute disseminated encephalomyelitis; *AQP4,* aquaporin 4; *ATM,* acute transverse myelitis; *CSF,* cerebrospinal fluid; *MRI,* magnetic resonance imaging; *MS,* multiple sclerosis; *NMO,* neuromyelitis optica.

TABLE 37B.3 Suggested Diagnostic Workup for Recurrent Central Nervous System Demyelinating Disorders and Systemic Autoimmune Disorders Associated With Acute Transverse Myelitis

All Patients	Suggestive of Neuromyelitis Optica	Also Consider
Brain MRI with gadolinium	Ophthalmology consultation	Angiotensin-converting enzyme (serum, CSF)
CSF oligoclonal bands	Visual evoked potentials	Other autoantibodies
Antinuclear antibodies	Formal visual field testing	Anti-dsDNA
Antiphospholipid antibodies		Anti-La
Serum AQP4-IgG		Anti-Ro
		Anti-Smith

CSF, Cerebrospinal fluid; *MRI,* magnetic resonance imaging; *NMO,* neuromyelitis optica.

systemic lupus erythematosus, sarcoidosis, and Sjögren syndrome. A personal or family history of recurrent miscarriages or hypercoagulability is suggestive of antiphospholipid antibody syndrome.

The long list of demyelinating and rheumatologic disorders potentially associated with ATM precludes diagnostic testing for every possible disorder. Table 37B.4 presents a schema to guide which tests should be obtained in patients with ATM.

Role of Infections in Transverse Myelitis

Infectious Myelopathies

Infectious agents can cause spinal cord dysfunction by directly infecting the spinal cord parenchyma (infectious myelopathy). The etiology of an infectious myelopathy usually is established by positive CSF culture or polymerase chain reaction (PCR) results. Biopsy or autopsy results also have provided evidence of direct CNS infection in some patients. Some authors consider elevated CSF antibody titers for specific pathogens without positive culture or PCR results to be sufficient evidence of direct CNS infection, but this issue has not been resolved. Acute and convalescent serum titers should be collected in determining the likelihood of any given pathogen being directly causative of ATM. In one prospective study, only 3 of 41 cases could be attributed directly to a specific infectious agent (influenza virus A, influenza virus B, and human herpesvirus–6).[16] Viruses constitute the most frequently reported category of infectious myelopathies, with bacteria and parasitic causes being less frequent (Box 37B.3).

Although cases of cytomegalovirus (CMV) myelitis have been reported in immunocompetent adults,[3,20] no cases have been reported in immunocompetent children. Immunocompromised children have been reported to develop CMV myelitis.[22,39] Treatment with ganciclovir or foscarnet should be considered.[8] The combined treatment of CMV-associated myelitis with ganciclovir and methylprednisolone was associated with marked recovery in an immunocompetent adult.[20] As illustrated by CMV, myelitis associated with viral infections may be produced by direct infection; accompanying secondary processes, such as vasculitis; or postinfectious immune-mediated mechanisms. Whether optimal treatment requires antiviral agents, immunomodulation, or both is unclear.

TABLE 37B.4 Diagnostic Criteria for Neuromyelitis Optica

Required	Must Have One of Two
Transverse myelitis	Longitudinally extensive (≥3 segments) transverse myelitis
Optic neuritis	Serum NMO-IgG

NMO, Neuromyelitis optica.

BOX 37B.3 Partial Listing of Microbes That Cause Infectious Myelopathies

Cytomegalovirus
Epstein-Barr virus
Echinococcus granulosus
Enteroviruses
- Coxsackieviruses
- Echoviruses
- Enterovirus 71
- Polioviruses (vaccine associated and wild type)

Herpes simplex virus–1
Herpes simplex virus–2
Human herpesvirus–6
Human immunodeficiency virus
Human T-cell lymphotrophic virus–1 and –2
Mycobacterium tuberculosis
Mycoplasma pneumoniae
Schistosoma haematobium and *Schistosoma mansoni*
Taenia solium (neurocysticercosis)
Treponema pallidum
Varicella zoster virus
West Nile virus

Postinfectious Acute Transverse Myelitis

In postinfectious cases, a specific etiology can be suggested by elevated acute or rising convalescent serum titers, isolation of the agent from systemic sources in the setting of a suggestive clinical picture, or both. In such cases, the presumptive pathophysiology entails an aberrant autoimmune response to the spinal cord via mechanisms such as molecular mimicry, rather than direct CNS invasion by the microbe. More than 50% of cases of pediatric ATM have been attributed to postinfectious or parainfectious causes.[16] A variety of bacterial and viral pathogens have been associated with postinfectious ATM. The medical literature additionally contains anecdotal reports of vaccines temporally associated with ATM (Table 37B.5). Within the postinfectious category of ATM, the preceding infection usually is a nonspecific upper respiratory tract infection without an identifiable, specific microbe.[14] Approximately 50% of patients report having had such an infection with an intervening symptom-free interval of 5 to 10 days. In instances in which the specific microbe is not identified and in cases in which no associated infection, systemic disorder, or recurrent demyelinating disorder is identified, the term *idiopathic ATM* has been applied.

The long list of potential pathogens precludes performing diagnostic testing for every possible agent. The workup instead should focus on those pathogens that are common, treatable, or suggested by particular clues in the history or examination. Table 37B.6 lists the infectious disease tests that should be performed in every patient with ATM. Additional infectious disease tests that should be considered, depending on the clinical scenario and immune status, are listed in Table 37B.7.

Role of the Immune System in Idiopathic Acute Transverse Myelitis

Several lines of evidence have implicated derangements in the immune system as the primary mechanism of damage in idiopathic ATM. First, neuropathologic studies have identified inflammatory cell invasion within the spinal cord parenchyma.[6] Both antibody-mediated damage and cell-mediated damage have been implicated, similar to findings in MS. Second, the production of interleukin-6 (IL-6) by astrocytes seems to lead to nitric oxide–induced injury to spinal cord oligodendrocytes and axons in patients with idiopathic ATM. IL-6 levels are markedly elevated in the CSF of patients with ATM and correlate with long-term disability.[27] Third, immunosuppressive therapies, including intravenous methylprednisolone, plasma exchange, and cyclophosphamide, have been used successfully as treatment for idiopathic ATM.

TABLE 37B.5 Partial Listing of Microbes and Vaccines Associated With Postinfectious or Postvaccinial Acute Transverse Myelitis

Bacteria/Spirochetes	Viruses	Vaccinations
Bartonella henselae	Adenovirus	Hepatitis B
Borrelia burgdorferi	Cytomegalovirus	Influenza
Brucellosis	Coxsackieviruses	Measles, mumps, and rubella
Chlamydia psittaci	Enterovirus 71	Poliovirus
Mycoplasma pneumoniae	Epstein-Barr virus	Rabies
	Hepatitis A	Smallpox
	Hepatitis B	
	Hepatitis C	
	Herpes simplex virus–1	
	Herpes simplex virus–2	
	Human herpesvirus–6	
	Mumps	
	Rubella	
	Varicella zoster virus	

TABLE 37B.6 Suggested Diagnostic Workup for Infections Associated With Acute Transverse Myelitis

Blood	Cerebrospinal Fluid	Other
Blood cultures Acute and convalescent titers to *Borrelia burgdorferi*, EBV, *Mycoplasma pneumoniae*	Bacterial culture Viral culture PCR testing for CMV, EBV, *Enterovirus*, HSV, *M. pneumoniae*, VZV	Viral culture of stool and respiratory secretions Consider stool ova and parasite testing and serum titers if parasitic infection is suspected

CMV, Cytomegalovirus; *EBV*, Epstein-Barr virus; *HSV*, herpes simplex virus; *PCR*, polymerase chain reaction; *VZV*, varicella zoster virus.

TABLE 37B.7 Additional Diagnostic Workup for Infections Associated With Acute Transverse Myelitis

Blood	Cerebrospinal Fluid	Other
Bartonella titers	Cryptococcal antigen	PPD placement
HIV antibody	HTLV antibody	Stool ova and parasite testing
HTLV-1 antibody	Fungal culture	
Parasitic infection titers	VDRL	
RPR		

HIV, Human immunodeficiency virus; *HTLV*, human T-cell lymphotrophic virus; *PPD*, purified protein derivative; *RPR*, rapid plasma reagin; *VDRL*, Venereal Disease Research Laboratory.

TREATMENT

All patients with ATM should be hospitalized for further monitoring and treatment. Most patients can receive care on the regular ward, although the approximately 5% of patients with respiratory involvement from cervical myelitis require intensive care monitoring and may need endotracheal tube placement and mechanical ventilation.

No randomized, controlled treatment trials of ATM in children have been done. Based on case reports and series that have suggested a beneficial effect,[13,33,50] high-dose corticosteroids have become the standard of care in ATM. In one series of 12 children with severe ATM compared with a historical control group of 17 patients, the use of high-dose intravenous methylprednisolone significantly increased the proportion of children walking independently at 1 month (66% vs. 18%) and with full recovery at 1 year (55% vs. 12%).[15] Although a variety of agents and courses has been used, we use intravenous methylprednisolone 30 mg/kg per dose for 5 days, with a maximum of 1 g per day. The need for a prednisone taper is controversial; however, we use a slow taper over 3 to 4 weeks beginning with 1 mg/kg per day. Most patients improve, often dramatically, with intravenous steroid treatment. Although some patients may improve spontaneously, the collective data suggest that high-dose intravenous methylprednisolone should be used in all patients with ATM. The use of adjunctive immunomodulating therapies has been demonstrated to be beneficial in a subset of adults with ATM—those with complete motor and sensory loss below the level of the spinal cord lesion. The adjunctive therapies include plasma exchange and cyclophosphamide. Furthermore a recent evidence-based guideline from the American Academy of Neurology cites class II evidence that plasmapheresis should be used in addition to intravenous methylprednisolone for fulminant demyelination. In our experience, any child with complete motor and sensory loss or without improvement with 1 or 2 doses of intravenous methylprednisolone should begin every other day plasma exchange with complete plasma volume exchange with each treatment for six sessions. Children who continue to have severe impairment with minimal improvement after both high-dose intravenous methylprednisolone and plasma exchange warrant consideration of immune depletion with cyclophosphamide.

The use of antimicrobial agents in patients with ATM is controversial. Because most cases are caused by secondary, immune-mediated mechanisms, such treatment may not have significant benefit. Antimicrobial therapy is indicated, however, in cases with highly suspected or proven direct or associated infections, such as doxycycline for *Mycoplasma*,[56] ganciclovir for CMV,[20] and acyclovir for herpes simplex virus and varicella zoster virus.[21] When antimicrobials are used, agents with good CSF penetration are preferred because direct invasion of the CNS may be present in some cases.

Additional treatment includes neuropathic pain management with gabapentin or pregabalin, urinary bladder catheterization, bowel regimens, and peptic ulcer and deep venous thrombosis prophylaxis. The early institution of clean intermittent catheterization may improve long-term neurourologic outcomes in children with ATM.[53] Physical and occupational therapy should be instituted early to maximize the chance for recovery and continued in inpatient rehabilitation or an outpatient setting after the patient has been discharged from the acute care hospital.

OUTCOME AND PROGNOSIS

Recurrences

In contrast to adult patients with idiopathic ATM, who have an approximately 25% likelihood of experiencing relapses,[17] most pediatric patients with idiopathic ATM do not have any recurrences. One series evaluated the recurrence risk for further episodes of demyelination after an episode of ATM and found a low risk with a hazard ratio of 0.23 (95% confidence interval [CI], 0.10–0.56).[40]

Disability

During recovery, motor function typically returns first, with an average time to independent ambulation of 56 days in one study[14] and 25 days in a group of patients treated with high-dose intravenous methylprednisolone.[15] Bowel and bladder control recovers more slowly, with an average time to recovery of normal urinary function of 7 months.[14] Another study confirmed worse prognosis for sphincter control, with more than half of children with ATM having modified or complete sphincter dependence at, on average, 8 years of follow-up.[47] Mobility and locomotion were also at least partially impaired in 36% and 33%, respectively, at follow-up, although full recovery is possible.[40]

Multiple studies have evaluated prognostic factors in children with ATM. Unfavorable outcomes have been linked with early age of onset, complete paraplegia, rapid evolution to neurologic nadir, absence or diminished deep tendon reflexes, and high rostral border of sensory level. Favorable outcomes were associated with a plateau phase of 8 days or less, normal white blood cell count in CSF, diagnosis within 7 days of symptom onset, few segments of spinal cord involved, and treatment with high-dose methylprednisolone.[14,42,47] Levels of the intracellular neuronal 14-3-3 protein in the CSF of patients with ATM may reflect the extent of neuronal injury and correlate with outcome.[26,27]

NEW REFERENCES SINCE THE SEVENTH EDITION

1. Alper G, Petropoulou KA, Fitz CR, et al. Idiopathic acute transverse myelitis in children: an analysis and discussion of MRI findings. *Mult Scler*. 2011;17(1):74-80.
3. Arslan F, Yilmaz M, Paksoy Y, et al. Cytomegalovirus-associated transverse myelitis: a review of nine well-documented cases. *Infect Dis*. 2015;47(1):7-12.
11. Carman KB, Yimenicioglu S, Ekici A, et al. Co-existence of acute transverse myelitis and Guillain-Barre syndrome associated with *Bartonella henselae* infection. *Paediatr Int Child Health*. 2013;33(3):190-192.
12. Chitnis T, Ness J, Krupp L, et al. Clinical features of neuromyelitis optica in children: US Network of Pediatric MS Centers report. *Neurology*. 2016;86(3):245-252.
23. Harzheim M, Schlegel U, Urbach H, et al. Discriminatory features of acute transverse myelitis: a retrospective analysis of 45 patients. *J Neurol Sci*. 2004;217(2):217-223.
32. Krupp LB, Tardieu M, Amato MP, et al. International Pediatric Multiple Sclerosis Study Group criteria for pediatric multiple sclerosis and immune-mediated central nervous system demyelinating disorders: revisions to the 2007 definitions. *Mult Schler*. 2013;19(10):1261-1267.
54. Topcu Y, Bayram E, Karaoglu P, et al. Coexistence of myositis, transverse myelitis, and Guillain Barre syndrome following *Mycoplasma pneumoniae* infection in an adolescent. *J Pediatr Neurosce*. 2013;8(1):59-63.
60. Wingerchuk DM, Banwell B, Bennett JL, et al. International consensus diagnostic criteria for neuromyelitis optica spectrum disorders. *Neurology*. 2015;85(2):177-189.

The full reference list for this chapter is available at ExpertConsult.com.

37C ■ Guillain-Barré Syndrome

Stuart R. Tomko • Timothy E. Lotze

Guillain-Barré syndrome (GBS) is a postinfectious immune-mediated polyneuropathy characterized by an acute and relativity symmetric areflexic paralysis. Although diagnosis can often be made clinically, albuminocytologic dissociation in the cerebrospinal fluid (CSF) is the pathologic hallmark. Originally described in 1916 by Georges Guillain, Jean-Alexandre Barré, and Andre Strohl,[7] GBS has since been understood to include a wide range of disease severity, from relativity mild to life threatening, requiring emergent management. In North America, the demyelinating form, known as acute inflammatory demyelinating polyneuropathy (AIDP), is most common, whereas in other parts of the world, especially China, acute motor axonal neuropathy (AMAN) is comparatively more common.[18]

EPIDEMIOLOGY

A systematic literature review of 16 population-based studies in North America and Europe reported an incidence of all types of Guillain-Barré syndrome from 0.89 to 1.89 cases (median, 1.11) per 100,000 person-years, with an increase after the first decade of life.[33] Another review of 63 studies from countries around the world found the overall incidence of GBS to be 1.1 to 1.8 per 100,000 and noted that the incidence was lower in children, at 0.34 to 1.34 per 100,000.[23] Two-thirds of cases are preceded by symptoms of upper respiratory tract infection or diarrhea, and antecedent infection may be more common in children.[23] However, the causative pathogen for the preceding infection is often not identified. In the setting of a preceding gastrointestinal illness, GBS has been classically associated with *Campylobacter jejuni*, and this organism has been identified in 23% to 30% of postinfectious cases of GBS.[9,30] Cytomegalovirus (CMV) has been associated with GBS in 8% of patients.[30] *C. jejuni* infection is more frequently related to the axonal subtype, whereas CMV is more frequently seen with the demyelinating subtype.[18] There are also case reports of demyelinating GBS following infection with measles.[5] In 1976, there was a reported increased risk of GBS associated with immunization against the A/New Jersey/1976/H1N1 "swine flu" in the United States.[20] In 2009, there was a small reported increase in risk of GBS for 6 weeks following H1N1 vaccination (1.6 excess cases per million people vaccinated), but the modest increased risk must be weighed against the protection offered by vaccination because influenza infection itself has a much higher risk for GBS.[38]

In addition to congenital abnormalities, Zika virus (ZIKV) has been linked to GBS. During one case-control study including 42 patients during the outbreak in French Polynesia, 98% of patients diagnosed with GBS were positive for ZIKV IgM or IgG compared to 56% of patients in an age- and sex-matched control group.[3] Nerve conduction studies were consistent with the acute motor axonal neuropathy (AMAN) subtype of GBS, and 31% of patients had some antiglycolipid antibody activity, most frequently again GA1. Assuming a 66% infection rate with ZIKV in the general population, the authors calculated the risk of GBS at 0.24 per 1000 infected patients.

CLINICAL MANIFESTATIONS

GBS often presents with some combination of weakness, numbness, paresthesia, and neuropathic-type pain in the lumbar region and limbs secondary to nerve root inflammation. These symptoms, especially the weakness, often start distally and progress proximally in a relatively symmetric manner over a period of 12 hours to 28 days.[34] There is often associated hyporeflexia or areflexia. However, normal reflexes or hyperreflexia can less frequently be seen,[41] especially in the axonal type discussed later, and the presence of hyperreflexia in an otherwise consistent presentation does not rule out GBS.[18] Up to two-thirds of patients are unable to walk during their disease course.[14] Cranial nerve involvement, especially affecting the facial nerve, can be seen. In a significant minority of cases the innervation to the diaphragm and intercostal muscles can be affected, which may lead to neuromuscular respiratory failure requiring mechanical ventilator support.[27] Dysautonomia is common and typified by sinus tachycardia, but patients may experience bradycardia, labile blood pressure, orthostatic hypotension, cardiac arrhythmias, neurogenic pulmonary edema, and abnormal sweating.[4]

SUBTYPES

Classic presentation of GBS can be broken down primarily into two variants based on the type of nerve fiber injury: AIDP and AMAN. As discussed earlier, the demyelinating subtype is more common in North America, accounting for up to 90% of cases of GBS, whereas in China the axonal type is seen more frequently.[18] A subtype of the axonal variant with a mixed sensorimotor neuropathy (AMSAN) has also been described.[4] The axonal variants are associated more frequently with *C. jejuni* infection while the demyelinating type is more frequently preceded by nonspecific viral infection, with CMV being reported in a small proportion of these patients.[9] Clinically, AMAN and AMSAN tend be associated with faster progression of weakness and an increased risk of respiratory compromise requiring mechanical ventilation.[4] Autonomic involvement is less frequently seen in AMAN compared to AIDP.[18]

The demyelinating and axonal types can also be distinguished based on serologic markers and electrophysiologic evaluation. Gangliosides, including GM1 and GD1a, are glycosphingolipids expressed on the cell surface of axons. Antibodies targeting these ganglioside antibodies are more frequently seen in AMAN,[10,19,40] which may be related to the fact that *C. jejuni* has GM1-like oligosaccharides on its surface, resulting in a molecular mimicry trigger for autoimmunity.[26] Antibodies against the ganglioside GD1a are also more frequently seen in AMAN than AIDP.[18]

Electrophysiologic evaluation with electromyography and nerve conduction studies helps to distinguish demyelinating from axonal forms of neuropathy. Demyelinating neuropathy will show slowing, dispersion, or complete blockage of an action potential propagating along the nerve. Axonal disease is characterized by an overall decrease in the number of axons contributing to the amplitude of the compound action potential and therefore demonstrates an abnormally low-amplitude action potential propagating at near normal velocities along the nerve.

Miller-Fisher syndrome is a GBS variant, representing a relativity small proportion of patients with GBS[32] clinically characterized by ophthalmoplegia, ataxia, and areflexia. Limb weakness is seen in only 5% of patients with Miller-Fisher syndrome.[24] In addition to the ophthalmoplegia, other cranial nerve involvement can be seen including ptosis and facial weakness. Miller-Fisher syndrome can be associated with ganglioside antibodies against GQ1b, which may be important in the pathophysiology and clinical presentation.[22] Similar to GM1 antibodies, GQ1b antibodies may be related to prior *C. jejuni* infection, with autoimmunity triggered by molecular mimicry.[42]

DIFFERENTIAL DIAGNOSIS

Given the myriad of presentations for GBS and its subtypes, the differential diagnosis can be extensive. In patients presenting with leg weakness and sensory changes, especially if a sensory level is felt to be present, a central cause of weakness localized to the spinal cord should be ruled out, and magnetic resonance imaging (MRI) may be considered to evaluate for extrinsic or intrinsic myelopathies, such as compressive lesions or transverse myelitis, respectively.

To evaluate for other causes of acute flaccid paralysis, a detailed history should be taken. Wakerley and Yuki (2014) recommend including the following in the history of patients with this complaint: recent travel, antecedent infective symptoms (e.g., upper respiratory tract), vaccinations, insect or animal bites (e.g., tick or snakebites), exposure to toxins (e.g., organophosphates), drugs or contaminated food (e.g., pickled sausages in the case of botulism) or water, systemic symptoms (e.g., fever, rash), trauma (e.g., neck injury), family history (e.g., familial hypokalemic periodic paralysis), and psychiatric symptoms.[39]

Infectious etiologies should also be considered in the differential. Viruses affecting the anterior horn cells, such as poliomyelitis and West Nile virus, can present similarly to GBS. Non-polio enteroviruses such as enterovirus 68, 70, and 71 can also present with acute weakness. A recent outbreak of enterovirus D68 strain was associated with an increase in reported cases of acute flaccid paralysis. In an analysis of patients presenting with acute flaccid paralysis in two states from 2012 through 2014, 48% were positive for enterovirus D68, thus supporting a causative association.[6]

Early GBS can be mistaken for functional symptoms or conversion disorder, especially when reflexes are normal or brisk. In cases where the diagnosis is unclear, the patient should be hospitalized for observation or instructed to return for further evaluation if weakness progresses or does not improve.

Differential diagnostic considerations for patients presenting primarily with bulbar symptoms include central pathologies affecting the brainstem including demyelinating disease, such as multiple sclerosis, brainstem tumor, and infectious encephalitis. Myasthenia gravis can present with bulbar symptoms. However, classically, in myasthenia the symptoms will wax and wane, worsening with exercise, while in GBS symptoms steadily progress without exercise exacerbation. Brainstem stroke can present in patients with no cardiovascular risk factors due to posterior circulation dissection, which can result from relatively minor traumas,[28] and should be considered.

PATHOGENESIS

While the exact pathogenesis of GBS has yet to be elucidated it is likely an autoimmune disorder resulting from both B- and T-cell activation leading to production of antibodies directed against proteins found in the peripheral nerves. As discussed earlier, some infections, most notably *C. jejuni*, can result in molecular mimicry, helping to explain the link between infection and GBS. The various clinical subtypes are thought to be related to distribution of the responsible antigen. The antigens targeted by antibodies seen primarily in AMAN (e.g., GM1a, GM1b, GD1a), for example, are primarily located at the node of Ranvier.[36] Antibody binding in the node of Ranvier results in complement activation causing disruption of the sodium channels and supporting structures.[35] Antibodies in AIDP likely are directed against antigens in the myelin, leading to multifocal mononuclear cell infiltration. In AIDP, activated lymphocytes attract macrophages, which invade an apparently normal myelin sheath by penetrating Schwann cell basal lamina, ultimately digesting the myelin and resulting in areas of demyelination.[12] The pattern of demyelination correlates with the type (motor vs. sensory) and distribution of neurological deficits. As the inflammation improves and the areas are remyelinated, clinical improvement can be seen.

Only a small percent of patients infected with *C. jejuni* or other organisms associated with GBS actually develop the syndrome. Patients who do develop GBS likely have some genetic predisposition, although, as of this writing, attempts to identify a specific HLA class with increased risk of developing GBS have been unsuccessful. Ongoing research is examining other potential immunogenic susceptibility factors including tumor necrosis factor (TNF).

CLINICAL EVALUATION

Several sets of diagnostic criteria exist for GBS. In 1978, while investigating the possible link between GBS and swine flu vaccination, the National Institute of Neurological Disorders and Stroke (NINDS) developed a set of diagnostic criteria, which were then updated in 1990.[1] More recently, in 2011, again while studying a link between GBS and influenza vaccination, this time against H1N1, the Brighton Collaboration published new case definitions for GBS.[34] Both sets of case definitions focus on clinical presentation, course of illness, and supporting studies including lumbar puncture and electrodiagnostic evaluation. Although both may be used clinically, they were designed for research purposes and therefore may have high specificity but lower sensitivity, which should be considered in a clinical setting.

Evaluation of a patient with suspected GBS begins with a thorough history and physical examination. The onset and course of weakness should be explored, and associated symptoms including numbness, pain, cranial neuropathies, and autonomic symptoms may be inquired about. Any preceding symptoms of infection are important to document. Symptoms of other diseases with similar presentation, such as persistent focal back pain, fevers, marked bowel or bladder dysfunction, or symptoms of central nervous system involvement may be included. Physical examination should include a thorough motor examination, which aids in diagnosis and serves as a baseline to evaluate improvement should treatment be initiated. Deep tendon reflexes are also important, although normal reflexes or hyperreflexia can less frequently be seen, especially in the axonal type, and the presence of hyperreflexia in an otherwise consistent presentation does not rule out GBS. As with the history, a thorough neurologic examination should be done to evaluate for other potential etiologies.

A lumbar puncture is often done in patients with suspected GBS both to evaluate for albuminocytologic dissociation and to rule out other possible diagnoses such as infection. Cytoalbuminologic dissociation has been defined as an elevation of CSF protein levels (above normal reference values for the laboratory doing the testing) in the relative absence of pleocytosis (elevation of CSF white blood cells). While albuminocytologic dissociation in the CSF is classically associated with GBS, it is not always present, especially if the lumbar puncture is done early in the course of illness.[29] The determination of "normal" white blood cell (WBC) count varies; the Brighton Collaboration suggest using a cutoff of less than 50 WBC/μL,[29] while the NINDS criteria suggest considering 10 or fewer mononuclear leukocytes/mm^3 normal, 11 to 50 mononuclear leukocytes/mm^3 as variant, and greater than 50 mononuclear leukocytes/mm^3 or any polymorphonuclear leukocytes in the CSF as not consistent with GBS.[1]

Clinical electrophysiology is another important aspect of diagnosis. To obtain sufficient data for interpretation, electrophysiologic studies should ideally include at least three sensory nerves, at least three motor nerves with multisite stimulation and F waves, and bilateral tibial H-reflexes.[11] While there is no definite consensus on exact values required for diagnosis, the various subtypes of GBS have distinctive patterns on electrophysiologic testing. In AIDP evidence of demyelination in motor nerves is expected. These include lowered motor conduction velocity, increased distal motor latency, and delayed F-response. Moderately depressed compound muscle action potential (CMAP) can also be seen. By contrast, in AMAN and AMSAN, the pattern would be more consistent with axonal injury, specifically, more severely depressed CMAP and generally normal conduction velocity, distal latency, and F-response. AMAN and AMSAN are distinguished by evidence of involvement of sensory nerves. As with many features of GBS, the electrophysiologic studies can be normal early in the disease course, but, with serial testing, abnormalities can often be found.[8] Isolated abnormalities in F-wave response (representing delayed proximal nerve conduction) have been reported as an early finding before more diffuse abnormalities appear.[25]

TREATMENT

The primary disease-modifying treatments used in GBS are intravenous immunoglobulin (IVIg) and plasma exchange. While no placebo-controlled studies have been conducted comparing IVIg to placebo, several small studies have compared IVIg to supportive care in children. In more severely affected children, including those requiring mechanical ventilation and a higher number of patients unable to walk even with support, treatment with IVIg demonstrated a trend toward an increase in the number of patients who recovered full strength, although this did not reach statistical significance. Treatment with IVIg did significantly decrease the time to recover unaided walking, at least in the short term, although less clearly at 1 year follow-up.[13] In more mildly affected patients who are still able to walk before treatment, IVIg did not affect disease severity at nadir of illness but did hasten recovery.[13]

Similarly, treatment with plasma exchange has been shown to reduce time to recover walking with aid in severely affected patients and time to onset of motor recovery in more mildly affected patients (those who could still walk before treatment initiation).[31] Meta-analysis of available studies revealed a statistically significant decreased risk of requiring mechanical ventilation for patients treated with plasma exchange compared to controls. For those patients requiring mechanical ventilation, treatment with plasma exchange trended toward reducing time on ventilator but did not reach statistical significance. Plasma exchange did significantly increase the chance of full muscle strength recovery at 1 year but did not significantly affect death at 1 year.

When comparing IVIg to plasma exchange, no significant differences have been demonstrated between the two in either improvement in the level of disability at 4 weeks after treatment, time until aided or unaided walking, assisted ventilation, or death.[31] Given the increased ease of administration of IVIg compared to plasma exchange and the increased safety in patients with autonomic instability, IVIg is often considered the first-line therapy. Both plasma exchange and IVIg are most effective if given within 2 weeks of symptom onset.

Steroids are generally avoided in GBS. Meta-analysis of corticosteroid use in GBS has shown either no improvement with steroids or significantly less improvement after 4 weeks with corticosteroids than without steroid treatment.[15] The lack of efficacy of steroid treatment in GBS is not completely understood, but it has been theorized that steroid treatment may counteract any beneficial antiinflammatory effects with direct, harmful effects on muscles.

In addition to immunotherapy patients with GBS often require supportive medical care. Patients in the progressive phase of GBS should be admitted to a hospital and respiratory status should be monitored closely, including frequent assessment of respiratory function to ensure timely ICU transfer when needed. All patients will require physical therapy, which may require inpatient rehabilitation. For GBS-related pain, both gabapentin and carbamazepine have been found to be effective but may require several days or weeks of treatment before a benefit is seen.[21]

OUTCOME AND PROGNOSIS

In children with GBS, at the height of illness up to 60% of patients will be unable to walk, 24% cannot use their arms, 46% show cranial nerve involvement, 51% have autonomic dysfunction, and 13% required artificial ventilation.[17] The majority of patients (up to 79%) will have neuropathic pain, which is sometimes severe. Most children, however, demonstrated good recovery, with 75% of patients becoming symptom free and 21% with residual symptoms not affecting their daily functioning. The mean time from onset to symptom freedom was 118 days. In those children without full recovery, most suffered from either chronic inflammatory demyelinating polyneuropathy (CIDP) or concurrent myelitis.

Outcomes in adults are more variable. About 5% of patients initially diagnosed with GBS are ultimately found to have CIDP.[37] Most adults with GBS will eventually become symptom free,[2] but despite current treatment, approximately a quarter of adults require artificial ventilation, and about 20% of patients are still unable to walk after 6 months, with a 3% to 10% mortality rate. Between 30% and 63% of adult patients are required to make changes in their daily lives due to sequelae of GBS.[17] Patients with GBS may also be at higher risk for psychiatric diagnoses including extreme depression, anxiety, and stress after recovery.[16]

NEW REFERENCES SINCE THE SEVENTH EDITION

1. Asbury AK, Cornblath DR. Assessment of current diagnostic criteria for Guillain-Barré syndrome. *Ann Neurol.* 1990;27(S1):S21-S24.
2. Bersano A, Carpo M, Allaria S, et al. Long term disability and social status change after Guillain–Barré syndrome. *J Neurol.* 2005;253(2):214-218.
3. Cao-Lormeau VM, Blake A, Mons S, et al. Guillain-Barre syndrome outbreak associated with Zika virus infection in French Polynesia: a case-control study. *Lancet.* 2016;387(10027):1531-1539.
4. Dimachkie MM, Barohn RJ. Guillain-Barré syndrome and variants. *Neurol Clin.* 2013;31(2):491-510.
5. Filia A, Lauria G. Guillain–Barré syndrome following measles infection: case report and review of the literature. *Neurol Sci.* 2014;35(12):2017-2018.
6. Greninger AL, Naccache SN, Messacar K, et al. A novel outbreak enterovirus D68 strain associated with acute flaccid myelitis cases in the USA (2012–14): a retrospective cohort study. *Lancet Infect Dis.* 2015;15(6):671-682.
7. Guillain G, Barré J, Strohl A. Sur un syndrome de radiculonévrite avec hyperalbuminose du liquide céphalo-rachidien sans réaction cellulaire: remarques sur les caractères cliniques et graphiques des ré- flexes tendineux. *Bull Soc Med Hop Paris.* 1916;40:1462-1470.
8. Hadden RDM, Cornblath DR, Hughes RAC, et al. Electrophysiological classification of guillain-barré syndrome: clinical associations and outcome. *Ann Neurol.* 1998;44(5):780-788.
9. Hadden RDM, Karch H, Hartung HP, et al. Preceding infections, immune factors, and outcome in Guillain-Barre syndrome. *Neurology.* 2001;56(6):758-765.
10. Ho TW, Mishu B, Li CY, et al. Guillain-Barré syndrome in northern China Relationship to Campylobacter jejuni infection and anti-glycolipid antibodies. *Brain.* 1995;118(3):597-605.
11. Hughes RAC, Cornblath DR. Guillain-Barré syndrome. *Lancet.* 2005;366(9497):1653-1666.
12. Hughes RAC, Hadden RDM, Gregson NA, et al. Pathogenesis of Guillain–Barré syndrome. *J Neuroimmunol.* 1999;100(1-2):74-97.
13. Hughes RAC, Raphaël JC, Swan AV, et al. Intravenous immunoglobulin for Guillain-Barré syndrome. *Cochrane Database Syst Rev.* 2004;(1):CD002063.
14. Hughes RAC, Swan AV, Raphael JC, et al. Immunotherapy for Guillain-Barre syndrome: a systematic review. *Brain.* 2007;130(9):2245-2257.
15. Hughes RAC, van der Meché FGA. Corticosteroids for Guillain-Barré syndrome. *Cochrane Database Syst Rev.* 2000;(1):CD001446.
16. Khan F, Pallant JF, Ng L, et al. Factors associated with long-term functional outcomes and psychological sequelae in Guillain–Barre syndrome. *J Neurol.* 2010;257(12):2024-2031.
17. Korinthenberg R, Schessl J, Kirschner J. Clinical presentation and course of childhood Guillain-Barré syndrome: a prospective multicentre study. *Neuropediatrics.* 2007;38(1):10-17.
18. Kuwabara S, Yuki N. Axonal Guillain-Barré syndrome: concepts and controversies. *Lancet Neurol.* 2013;12(12):1180-1188.
19. Kuwabara S, Yuki N, Koga M, et al. IgG Anti-GM1 antibody is associated with reversible conduction failure and axonal degeneration in guillain-barré syndrome. *Ann Neurol.* 1998;44(2):202-208.
20. Lehmann HC, Hartung H-P, Kieseier BC, et al. Guillain-Barré syndrome after exposure to influenza virus. *Lancet Infect Dis.* 2010;10(9):643-651.
21. Liu J, Wang L-N, McNicol ED. Pharmacological treatment for pain in Guillain-Barré syndrome. *Cochrane Database Syst Rev.* 2015;(10):CD009950.
22. Liu J-X, Willison HJ, Pedrosa-Domellöf F. Immunolocalization of GQ1b and related gangliosides in human extraocular neuromuscular junctions and muscle spindles. *Invest Opthamol Vis Sci.* 2009;50(7):3226.
23. McGrogan A, Madle GC, Seaman HE, et al. The epidemiology of Guillain-Barr syndrome worldwide. *Neuroepidemiology.* 2009;32(2):150-163.
24. Mori M, Kuwabara S, Fukutake T, et al. Clinical features and prognosis of Miller Fisher syndrome. *Neurology.* 2001;56(8):1104-1106.
25. Olney RK, Aminoff MJ. Electrodiagnostic features of the Guillain-Barre syndrome: The relative sensitivity of different techniques. *Neurology.* 1990;40(3 Pt 1):471.
26. Oomes PG, Jacobs BC, Hazenberg MPH, et al. Anti-GM1 IgG antibodies and Campylobacter bacteria in Guillain-Barré syndrome: evidence of molecular mimicry. *Ann Neurol.* 1995;38(2):170-175.
27. Orlikowski D, Prigent H, Sharshar T, et al. Respiratory dysfunction in Guillain-Barré syndrome. *Neurocrit Care.* 2004;1(4):415-422.
28. Ortiz J, Ruland S. Cervicocerebral artery dissection. *Curr Opin Cardiol.* 2015;30(6):603-610.
29. Paradiso G, Tripoli J, Galicchio S, et al. Epidemiological, clinical, and electrodiagnostic findings in childhood Guillain-Barré syndrome: a reappraisal. *Ann Neurol.* 1999;46(5):701-707.
30. Poropatich KO, Fischer Walker CL, Black RE. Quantifying the association between Campylobacter infection and Guillain-Barré syndrome: a systematic review. *J Health Popul Nutr.* 2010;28(6):545-552.
31. Raphaël JC, Chevret S, Hughes RAC, et al. Plasma exchange for Guillain-Barré syndrome. *Cochrane Database Syst Rev.* 2002;(2):CD001798.
32. Ropper AH. Unusual clinical variants and signs in Guillain-Barre syndrome. *Arch Neurol.* 1986;43(11):1150-1152.
33. Sejvar JJ, Baughman AL, Wise M, et al. Population incidence of Guillain-Barré syndrome: a systematic review and meta-analysis. *Neuroepidemiology.* 2011;36(2):123-133.
34. Sejvar JJ, Kohl KS, Gidudu J, et al. Guillain–Barré syndrome and Fisher syndrome: case definitions and guidelines for collection, analysis, and presentation of immunization safety data. *Vaccine.* 2011;29(3):599-612.
35. Susuki K, Rasband MN, Tohyama K, et al. Anti-GM1 antibodies cause complement-mediated disruption of sodium channel clusters in peripheral motor nerve fibers. *J Neurosci.* 2007;27(15):3956-3967.
36. Susuki K, Yuki N, Schafer DP, et al. Dysfunction of nodes of Ranvier: a mechanism for anti-ganglioside antibody-mediated neuropathies. *Exp Neurol.* 2012;233(1):534-542.
37. van Doorn PA. Diagnosis, treatment and prognosis of Guillain-Barré syndrome (GBS). *La Presse Médicale.* 2013;42(6):e193-e201.
38. Vellozzi C, Iqbal S, Broder K. Guillain-Barre syndrome, influenza, and influenza vaccination: the epidemiologic evidence. *Clin Infect Dis.* 2014;58(8):1149-1155.
39. Wakerley BR, Yuki N. Mimics and chameleons in Guillain-Barre and Miller Fisher syndromes. *Pract Neurol.* 2014;15(2):90-99.
40. Wang Y, Sun S, Zhu J, et al. Biomarkers of Guillain-Barré syndrome: some recent progress, more still to be explored. *Mediators Inflamm.* 2015;2015:1-12.
41. Yuki N, Kokubun N, Kuwabara S, et al. Guillain–Barré syndrome associated with normal or exaggerated tendon reflexes. *J Neurol.* 2011;259(6):1181-1190.
42. Yuki N, Taki T, Takahashi M, et al. Molecular mimicry between GQ1b ganglioside and lipopolysaccharides of Campylobacter jejuni isolated from patients with Fisher's syndrome. *Ann Neurol.* 1994;36(5):791-793.

The full reference list for this chapter is available at ExpertConsult.com.

Urethritis

38

Ellen R. Wald

Urethritis is an inflammation of the urethra and periurethral tissues in males and females. It may be associated with a variety of infectious and noninfectious disorders.

EPIDEMIOLOGY

The cause of urethritis varies with the age of the patient, sexual practices, and hygienic standards.[9,39] *Chlamydia* infections and gonorrhea are common occurrences in adolescents; fecal contamination or irritation caused by physical or chemical substances is a more usual occurrence in preschool-aged children. Transmission during sexual activity is the usual means of spread of *Neisseria gonorrhoeae* and *Chlamydia trachomatis* in teenagers and in sexually abused patients; nonvenereal transmission has been described in prepubertal children.[16] Manifestations after nonvenereal spread has occurred may include urethritis, vaginitis, balanitis, conjunctivitis, and complications of disseminated infection (arthritis, meningitis).[11,16]

The home and social environments of prepubertal children must be examined to identify fully the pattern of spread and infection in the patient and contacts because complex psychosocial diagnoses and therapies often are involved.[33] Children with gonorrhea and chlamydial infections are concentrated in large urban centers, usually in poor socioeconomic environments.

Although nonvenereal transmission of *N. gonorrhoeae* is well established, gonococcal infections in children 2 to 10 years of age should be considered evidence of probable sexual abuse.[1,17,19–21] Household contacts have been found to have positive cultures in 27% to 63% of such cases. Prepubertal girls infected with *N. gonorrhoeae* as a result of sexual abuse outnumber boys by a ratio of at least 3 : 1 and in one report 8 : 1.[13]

PATHOPHYSIOLOGY

Infection caused by *N. gonorrhoeae* usually is localized to the urethra in boys and to the vagina in girls; however, rectal and pharyngeal carriage sometimes occurs in the absence of urethral colonization. Gonococcal virulence factors include pili, the ability to attach to urethral epithelial cells, and production of extracellular proteases that cleave IgA. Initial attachment of gonococci to the surface of columnar epithelial cells is mediated by pili, which are filamentous outer membrane appendages composed of multiple subunits, the most important of which is pilin.[38] Local invasion involves multiple adhesins interacting with host receptors at the mucosal cell level. After attachment occurs, gonococci become internalized in a process known as membrane ruffling.[14] The organisms are able to undergo intracellular replication within phagocytic vacuoles and columnar epithelial cells, which is a successful adaptive response promoting survival.

Chlamydia infections are the most frequent cause of sexually transmitted infection in the United States.[5,8,44] Chlamydiae are structurally complex organisms that are obligate intracellular parasites and contain DNA and RNA. Attachment, which is not understood completely, is the first step in the infectious process of the susceptible host cell. It is followed by phagocytosis and then the failure of cellular lysosomes to fuse with the phagosome containing the elementary body, which may be mediated partly by macromolecules in the chlamydial cell envelope. After these two crucial events occur, the elementary bodies undergo biologic changes, and, after approximately 72 hours, they are released from the host cell as new infective elementary bodies (Fig. 38.1).

Urethritis in younger children also may be caused by the introduction of fecal bacteria or pinworms into the urethra during the early years of toilet training, particularly in girls. Inflammation may be related to bubble baths and other chemical and physical irritants. The entity of idiopathic urethritis is also observed in young boys and girls as a cause of dysuria and hematuria.[24] Edema of the mucosa and the presence of inflammation and red blood cells are common histopathologic features of urethritis that lead to dysuria, hematuria, and microscopic pyuria.

CLINICAL PRESENTATION

Gonococcal urethritis is characterized by a 2- to 7-day incubation period after sexual intercourse. The onset often is sudden, with dysuria and copious urethral discharge in boys and leukorrhea in girls. The urethral discharge often is thick, profuse, and yellow. The patient usually has no fever. In prepubertal girls, leukorrhea is more prominent as a sign of gonococcal infection (reflecting a vulvovaginitis), and urethritis occurs less commonly. This difference may be related to the method of infection and the different sensitivity of the vaginal epithelial surface to infection in a prepubertal child. Leukorrhea may be minimal in adolescent girls, and dysuria may be absent.[1]

Diagnosis often is made earlier in adolescent boys than in girls, perhaps because of the prominence of urethral discharge in boys and misinterpretation of the significance of leukorrhea in girls. Gonococcal urethritis also may cause asymptomatic pyuria in boys. Occasionally, prepubertal patients have conjunctivitis or balanitis without significant urethritis. Clinical presentations include systemic illness with fever, arthritis, and skin lesions secondary to bacteremia in 3% of untreated individuals with mucosal gonorrhea.[1] These lesions often begin on the extremities as small erythematous macules that progress to circular papules with an area of central necrosis.

The clinical presentation of nongonococcal urethritis may be similar to that described for gonorrhea, but it more commonly has a longer incubation period (often 8 to 14 days after sexual intercourse) and a scanty exudate, which may be clear and intermittent. This condition also is referred to as *nonspecific urethritis* and may be present in association with or subsequent to gonococcal urethritis. In the latter case, the scant urethral discharge may persist after the patient has been treated for gonorrhea. Asymptomatic urethral colonization with *C. trachomatis* also is reported in males.[15,42]

An equivalent syndrome, acute urethral syndrome, has been described in sexually active females. The patient experiences an acute onset of dysuria and increased frequency, and pyuria (≥10 white blood cells/mm^3 of midstream urine) is a common finding. Bacterial cultures of the urine often are sterile or show less than 10^5 bacteria/mL; coliform bacteria, *Staphylococcus saprophyticus*, and *C. trachomatis* are the most common causes. Clinical expression of infection with *C. trachomatis* in adolescent girls is characterized by a yellowish, mucopurulent secretion at the cervical os.[6] However, infection with *C. trachomatis* may be asymptomatic in both sexes, an important consideration in designing effective strategies for diagnosis and management of sexual contacts.

A patient with urethritis caused by trauma may have hematuria and dysuria without fever. The trauma may be obvious or related to masturbation or introduction of foreign bodies into the urethra. Patients with urethritis secondary to bubble bath or detergent usually have transient dysuria and no systemic signs. Fecal contamination of the urethra may be accompanied by hematuria, dysuria, and pyuria.

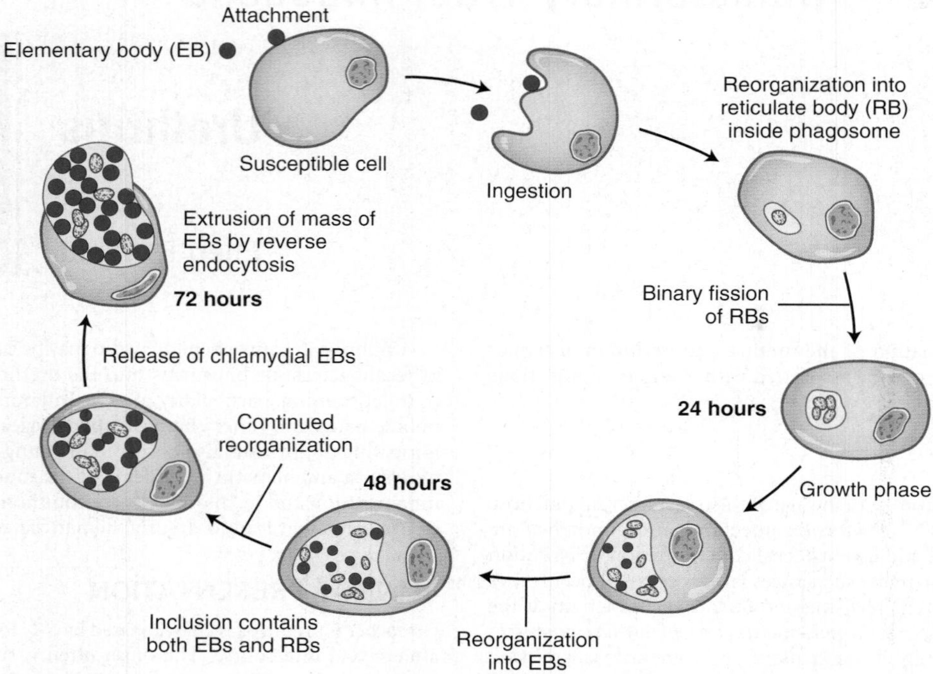

FIG. 38.1 Schematic description of the growth cycle of *Chlamydia trachomatis*. (From Batteiger BE, Jones RB. Chlamydial infections. *Infect Dis Clin North Am.* 1987;1:55–81.)

TABLE 38.1 Etiology of Urethritis

Infectious	Noninfectious
Sexually Transmitted Infections	**Vasculitides**
Neisseria gonorrhoeae	Reiter syndrome
Chlamydia trachomatis	Erythema multiforme
Trichomonas vaginalis	Kawasaki disease
Herpes simplex virus type 2	**Mechanical**
Mycoplasma spp.	Masturbation
Non–Sexually Transmitted Infections	Foreign body
Staphylococcus saprophyticus	Trauma
Enterobacteriaceae	Dysfunctional elimination
Gardnerella vaginalis	**Chemical**
Streptococcus spp.	Soaps
Enterobius vermicularis	Detergents
	Drugs

DIFFERENTIAL DIAGNOSIS

Table 38.1 lists the differential diagnoses for urethritis.

Noninfectious

Trauma, bubble bath, detergents found in shampoos, masturbation, radiation, dysfunctional elimination syndrome, and caustic substances may lead to the development of urethritis.[24] Idiopathic urethritis of childhood is characterized by blood spotting of underwear between voids or microhematuria with or without dysuria and urethral discharge.[24] Urethritis also may be a component of several systemic syndromes, including erythema multiforme (Stevens-Johnson syndrome), Kawasaki disease, and occasionally other forms of allergy. Reiter syndrome denotes the association of nongonococcal urethritis with conjunctivitis and arthritis.

Infectious

The most common forms of urethritis in sexually active adolescents and young adults are gonococcal and so-called nongonococcal urethritis. They may occur together or sequentially. Nongonococcal urethritis has been related causally to infections with *C. trachomatis* in approximately 15% to 40% of cases. *Mycoplasma genitalium* is associated with signs and symptoms of urethritis in 15% to 25% of nongonococcal urethritis in the United States.[29,37,47] In most settings it is more common than *N. gonorrhoeae* but less common than *C. trachomatis*.[8] There is increasing evidence for the role of *Ureaplasma urealyticum*.[48] The remaining cases of infectious urethritis in postpubescent, sexually active patients may be caused by a variety of pathogenic microorganisms, including *Gardnerella vaginalis, Mycoplasma hominis, Trichomonas vaginalis, Candida albicans,* herpes simplex virus type 2, *Treponema pallidum* (syphilis), and other bacteria, such as staphylococci, Enterobacteriaceae, and occasionally streptococci, including group B.[15] Studies also have implicated a causative role in *Chlamydia*-negative nongonococcal urethritis for anaerobic organisms of the *Bacteroides* spp., in particular *Bacteroides urealyticus*.

In younger children, urethritis usually has noninfectious causes as outlined earlier. Gonorrhea, *Chlamydia,* and fecal bacteria may be important as well.

SPECIFIC DIAGNOSIS

A standard method for diagnosing gonorrhea in a sexually active male is to obtain urethral discharge by manually stripping the urethra or, if that is unproductive, by gently inserting a swab 2 to 3 cm into the distal urethra. The best culture technique for isolating *N. gonorrhoeae,* a fastidious organism, is immediate inoculation of this material onto a selective growth medium, such as regular or modified Thayer-Martin agar. Any delay in inoculation of the plates necessitates the use of a transport method with growth media in a carbon dioxide environment that support the gonococcus at ambient temperatures. These media protect the organism from its marked susceptibility to the effects of drying, cold, and overgrowth by other bacteria. Urethral exudate from a male patient should be Gram stained at the same time; typical kidney bean–shaped,

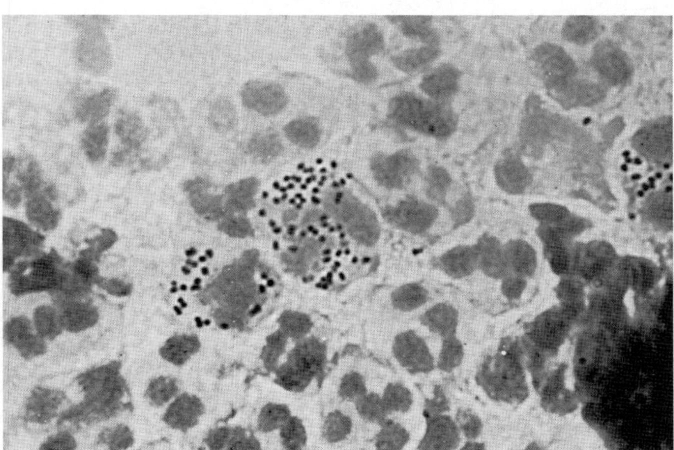

FIG. 38.2 Gram-stained smear of urethral discharge from a teenage boy with gonorrhea.

gram-negative, intracellular diplococci are presumptively diagnostic, with a sensitivity and specificity approaching 100% (Fig. 38.2).

Putative gonococcal colonies should be confirmed by oxidase reaction, Gram staining, sugar use tests, rapid enzyme tests, nucleic acid probes, or agglutination reactions with antibodies specific for *N. gonorrhoeae*. The last four tests are especially important in evaluating sites of infection (e.g., the pharynx) or populations of patients with a low prevalence of gonorrhea.

Sexually active females with urethritis also should undergo urethral culture. Although the Gram stain of cervical secretions is only 66% sensitive in detecting *N. gonorrhoeae* in adolescent girls, the finding of kidney bean–shaped, intracellular gram-negative diplococci is highly specific and helpful.[45] Vaginal, cervical, and rectal swabs are recommended. Asymptomatic colonization with gonococci seems to occur most commonly in female patients, although it has been described in adolescent boys.[1,23] Pharyngitis, conjunctivitis, balanitis, and other, less common, manifestations of gonorrhea may coexist with urethritis. Samples obtained from these sites should be handled as described earlier. Blood agar and other specialized media may be indicated to identify nongonococcal causes of urethritis.

Nucleic acid amplification tests (NAATs) are highly sensitive and specific when used on urethral swab (males), endocervical swab, patient-obtained vaginal swabs, and urine specimens.[8] These tests include polymerase chain reaction (PCR), transcription-mediated amplification, and strand displacement assays. Most commercially available products now are approved by the U.S. Food and Drug Administration (FDA) for testing male urethral swab specimens, female endocervical or vaginal swab specimens (collected by provider or patient), male or female urine specimens, or liquid cytology specimens.[1] Use of urine specimens increases the feasibility of initial testing and follow-up of hard-to-access populations such as adolescents.[1] These techniques also permit dual testing of urine for *C. trachomatis* and *N. gonorrhoeae*. NAATs are not cleared by the FDA for *N. gonorrhoeae* or *C. trachomatis* testing on rectal and pharyngeal swabs.[1] However, some noncommercial laboratories have initiated nucleic amplification testing of rectal and pharyngeal swab specimens after establishing the performance of the test to meet requirements of the Clinical Laboratory Improvement Amendments (CLIA). These tests are superior to culture, and their ease of use (i.e., for urine or self-obtained specimens) renders them extremely attractive.

Gonococcal urethritis in prepubescent boys is diagnosed as described earlier for adolescent boys. Vaginal swabs are most useful in female patients, although vaginal discharge may not be prominent. Endocervical cultures are not recommended for the diagnosis of gonorrhea in prepubescent girls. The yield of vaginal swabs seems to be adequate for most diagnostic purposes; rectal swabs also may be useful in female patients. Showing kidney bean–shaped, gram-negative intracellular diplococci in a prepubescent boy or girl is useful for establishing a presumptive diagnosis and instituting therapy. Confirmation by culture as described for a sexually active male is necessary.

Other infectious causes of urethritis may be diagnosed by specific techniques, including wet mount or nucleic acid amplification for *Trichomonas*, Gram stain, and culture on Sabouraud dextrose agar for *C. albicans*, and culture or PCR for herpes simplex virus, used in the patients and their contacts. New culture techniques for *Chlamydia*, such as the use of microtiter cell monolayers, have increased the recovery rates, decreased the cost, and shortened the turnaround time for the isolation of *C. trachomatis*.[2] The rigorous transport conditions and the small number of laboratories with cell culture techniques have limited the availability of *Chlamydia* cultures; however, nonculture methods, including direct immunofluorescence staining of smears with use of monoclonal antibodies,[2,18,25,28,40] enzyme-linked immunosorbent assay (ELISA) techniques, and NAATs, are available. The use of immunofluorescence and ELISA techniques has been surpassed in sensitivity and ease of use by NAATs.

When documentation of infection is being sought in cases of suspected child abuse, performing cultures is strongly preferred.[1] NAATs can be used as an alternative to culture with vaginal swab specimens or urine specimens from prepubertal girls. Culture remains the preferred method for urethral specimens from boys and extragenital specimens (pharynx and rectum) in boys and girls.[1] When culture is unavailable, some experts support using NAAT if a positive result can be verified by another NAAT. ELISA and fluorescent antibody tests should not be used for testing rectal, vaginal, or urethral specimens from infants and children because of low sensitivity and specificity.[1] A recent multicenter investigation showed NAATs for detection of *C. trachomatis* and *N. gonorrhoeae* in children being evaluated for child abuse were superior to culture.[4]

Ureaplasma and other genital *Mycoplasma* spp. currently can be identified only by culture. This test should be reserved for the evaluation of recurrent cases of urethritis with poor response to treatment.[25] Specimens of urethral and vaginal discharge secondary to fecal contamination and foreign bodies can be examined by conventional diagnostic bacterial techniques.

TREATMENT

Table 38.2 presents antibiotic regimens for treatment of urethritis. The treatment of urethritis should include treatment of the sexual partners of the index case to avoid reinfection and further spread of infection. Patients with urethritis frequently have mixed infections with *N. gonorrhoeae* and the pathogens linked with nongonococcal urethritis, such as *C. trachomatis*. Concurrent infection with *N. gonorrhoeae* and *C. trachomatis* is documented frequently. In a survey of adolescents admitted to juvenile detention centers throughout the United States, screening for sexually transmitted infections was performed on adolescent girls with gonorrhea. Fifty-four percent were coinfected with chlamydia; of adolescent boys infected with gonorrhea, 51% were coinfected with chlamydia.[26] A study determining chlamydia and gonorrhea co-occurrence in a high school population showed similar results: of 117 students with gonorrhea, 50 (42.7%) had chlamydia; of 451 with chlamydia, 50 (11.1%) had gonorrhea.[34] Patients with gonococcal urethritis also are at risk for development of early-incubating syphilis. One must consider these factors and the possibility of systemic infection when choosing a treatment regimen for urethritis.[31]

Sexual abuse is the most common cause of gonococcal infection among children 2 to 10 years of age. Anorectal and pharyngeal infections with *N. gonorrhoeae* are common and frequently asymptomatic occurrences among these patients.[32]

Treatment of gonorrhea is complicated by the ability of *N. gonorrhoeae* to develop resistance to antimicrobials. The epidemiology of resistance patterns guides recommendations from the Centers for Disease Control (CDC). The emergence of penicillin-resistant and tetracycline-resistant strains of *N. gonorrhoeae* led to the abandonment of penicillin and tetracycline for the treatment of gonorrhea before 2005.[12] In 2007, emergence of fluoroquinolone-resistant *N. gonorrhoeae* in the United States prompted the CDC to stop recommending fluoroquinolones for treatment of gonorrhea, leaving cephalosporins as the

TABLE 38.2 Antibiotic Regimen for Urethritis

Nongonococcal Urethritis	
Recommended regimen	Azithromycin 1 g orally in a single dose *or* Doxycycline 100 mg orally twice daily for 7 d
Alternative regimen	Erythromycin base 500 mg four times daily for 7 d *or* Erythromycin ethylsuccinate 800 mg four times daily for 7 d *or* Ofloxacin 300 mg twice daily for 7 d *or* Levofloxacin 500 mg once daily for 7 d
Chlamydial Infection	
Recommended regimen (adults and adolescents)	Azithromycin 1 g orally in a single dose *or* Doxycycline 100 mg orally twice daily for 7 d
Alternative regimen	Erythromycin base 500 mg four times daily for 7 d *or* Erythromycin ethylsuccinate 800 mg four times daily for 7 d Ofloxacin 300 mg twice daily for 7 d *or* Levofloxacin 500 mg once daily for 7 d
Children	
<45 kg	Erythromycin 50 mg/kg/day in 4 divided doses for 14 d
≥45 kg and <8 y	Azithromycin 1 g orally in a single dose
>8 y	Use same regimen as for adults
Gonococcal Infection	
Recommended regimen (adults and adolescents)	Ceftriaxone 125 mg IM in a single dose *plus* Azithromycin 1 g orally in a single dose
Children	
<45 kg	Ceftriaxone 125 mg IM in a single dose
If bacteremia, arthritis, or meningitis	Ceftriaxone 50–100 mg/kg/day (maximum 2 g/day) IV for 7–14 d
≥45 kg	Use adult regimen

IM, Intramuscularly; *IV*, intravenously.

only remaining class of antimicrobials for treatment of gonorrhea in the United States.[1,3,7,8]

Concerned about emerging gonococcal resistance, the 2010 CDC guideline for treatment of sexually transmitted disease recommended dual therapy for gonorrhea with a cephalosporin plus either azithromycin or doxycycline, even if NAAT for *C. trachomatis* was negative at the time of treatment.[8] However, during 2006–2011, the minimum concentrations of cefixime needed to inhibit in vitro growth of the *N. gonorrhoeae* strains circulating in the United States and many other countries increased, suggesting that the effectiveness of cefixime might be waning, and there were reports of treatment failures with cefixime from Asia, Europe, South Africa, and Canada.[8,43] As a result, the CDC no longer recommends the routine use of cefixime as a first-line regimen for the treatment of gonorrhea in the United States. In addition, gonococcal strains with elevated minimum inhibitory concentrations to cefixime in the United States are also likely to be resistant to tetracycline but susceptible to azithromycin. Accordingly, only one regimen, dual treatment with ceftriaxone and azithromycin, is recommended for treatment of gonorrhea in the United States.[8] Test of cure is not indicated for uncomplicated gonococcal or chlamydial infection when single-dose treatment regimens are used.[8] Current recommendations are found in Table 38.2.

When patients are symptomatic after standard treatment, it may be appropriate to repeat diagnostic testing. Particularly in males, *M. genitalium* may be resistant to azithromycin. If laboratory evidence of urethritis persists (pyuria and urethral discharge) with negative cultures and NAATs, a trial of moxifloxacin, 400 mg/day for 7 days, should be considered.[8]

PROGNOSIS

Gonococcal urethritis may subside and lead to asymptomatic carriage in female patients. Carriage may last for weeks to months in adults; this period is undefined in children. Untreated gonococcal urethritis also may lead to prostatitis and epididymitis in male patients and urethral stricture. Asymptomatic genital infections in women can progress to pelvic inflammatory disease with tubal scarring and infertility. Systemic complications of asymptomatic gonorrheal infections include arthritis, endocarditis, and necrotic skin lesions.

Chlamydial infections frequently have been associated with pelvic inflammatory disease in women, sometimes resulting in infertility or ectopic pregnancy. *Chlamydia* can be transmitted to a newborn in the birth canal, which can result in conjunctivitis, pneumonia, or both. Prenatal screening for *C. trachomatis* has limited this problem in the United States.

PREVENTION

Despite substantial efforts, a specific gonococcal vaccine has not been developed. The mainstays of prevention continue to be education and screening. Prepubescent gonorrhea can be prevented from recurring only by careful family counseling and psychosocial therapy; legal intervention may be necessary.

The availability of diagnostic tests performed on urine (a noninvasive alternative to specimens obtained from the urethra or endocervix) renders extensive screening possible in nontraditional settings such as schools and recreation centers.[21] Large-scale efforts that have implemented screening for all sexually active teens attending school-based clinics have been successful in reducing the prevalence of *Chlamydia* infection in boys.[10]

Prevention of noninfectious causes of urethritis usually depends on education and specific counseling of the family. Physical agents or allergens identified as a cause of urethritis must be removed.

NEW REFERENCES SINCE THE SEVENTH EDITION

1. American Academy of Pediatrics, et al. Gonococcal infections. In: Kimberlin DW, Brady MT, Jackson MA, eds. *2015 Red Book: Report on the Committee on Infectious Diseases*. 30th ed. Elk Grove Village, IL: American Academy of Pediatrics; 2015:356.
8. Centers for Disease Control and Prevention. Sexually transmitted diseases treatment guidelines, 2015. *MMWR Recomm Rep*. 2015;64:1-137.
47. Weinstein SA, Stiles B. A review of the epidemiology, diagnoses and evidence-based management of *Mycoplasma genitalium*. *Sex Health*. 2011;8:143-158.
48. Zhang N, Wang R, Li X, et al. Are *Ureaplasma* spp a cause of nongonococcal urethritis? A systematic review and meta-analysis. *PLoS ONE*. 2014;9(12):e113771.

The full reference list for this chapter is available at ExpertConsult.com.

Cystitis and Pyelonephritis

39

Ellen R. Wald

Urinary tract infections (UTIs) are the most common serious bacterial infections in children.[129] In several series of children evaluated for fever, UTIs accounted for 5% to 6% of infections. They are more common than occult bacteremia, bacterial pneumonia, and bacterial meningitis. UTIs are especially common as causes of infection in white female infants, and they may explain febrile episodes in nearly 20% of such infants.

EPIDEMIOLOGY

UTIs occur in all age groups and may be symptomatic or asymptomatic. Factors that affect the incidence of UTIs are associated with gender, age, race, circumcision status, and general health.[100] The site of infection may be the bladder (cystitis), ureters (ureteritis), pelvis (pyelitis), and renal parenchyma (pyelonephritis). Infections in neonates and infants are common occurrences. In the first 3 months of life, infections in uncircumcised male infants are most common.[132,144] Beyond 6 months, infections in female infants are substantially more common than are infections in male infants; the female predominance of UTIs is maintained throughout the remainder of childhood and adolescence.[33]

RISK FOR URINARY TRACT INFECTION

The risk for developing a UTI during childhood seems to have increased since early studies by Winberg and colleagues[181] in 1960. These investigations showed that the risk for developing a UTI during the first 10 years of life was 3% in girls and 1.1% in boys. In a more recent retrospective study of a cohort of 3556 school entrants, 7.8% of girls and 1.6% of boys were found to have had symptomatic UTIs as confirmed by significant bacteriuria.[50] In approximately half of these cases, the clinical presentation was consistent with acute pyelonephritis (APN).[45] Another population-based study was performed in Göteborg, Sweden, to describe the incidence of first-time symptomatic UTI in children younger than 6 years. The prevalence during the first 6 years of life was 6.6% for girls and 1.8% for boys.[101] The apparent increase in risk most likely relates to an increased awareness of the diagnosis of UTI as an explanation for fever in children and the more frequent practice of culturing the urine of children who are ill.

Several studies have investigated systematically the prevalence of UTI as the explanation for fever in febrile young children presenting to the emergency department. Although the definition of significant bacteriuria has varied among studies, the overall prevalence of UTI is 3.3% to 5.3%.[54,153] White female infants had significantly more UTIs than did black male infants. Higher prevalences occurred in uncircumcised male infants or male infants with abdominal or suprapubic tenderness on examination.[153] White female infants with a temperature of 39°C (102.2°F) or greater had a prevalence of UTIs of 17%.[61] In a large prospective study of febrile (temperature ≥38°C [100.4°F]) infants 3 months or younger evaluated in pediatric office settings, 54% of infants had urine tested and 10% had UTIs.[111]

A recent meta-analysis searched all publications on UTI in children from 1966 to 2005.[149] The overall prevalence of UTI was found to be 7%, but it varied greatly depending on age, gender, and circumcision status.[131] The prevalence was higher in white infants (8%) than black infants (4.7%) and was highest in uncircumcised male infants younger than 3 months of age and in female infants younger than 12 months of age.

RISK FACTORS FOR URINARY TRACT INFECTION

Uncircumcised Boys

The common problem of UTIs in uncircumcised boys, although suspected in the 1970s, was first documented in the 1980s by Ginsburg and McCracken.[37] The strongest evidence of a causal link between an intact foreskin and a UTI comes from several studies conducted by Wiswell and colleagues.[184] In their series, an overall 10-fold increased incidence of UTI was found in uncircumcised compared with circumcised male infants (1.12% vs. 0.11%; $P < .001$).[184] Wiswell and other investigators have continued to document this problem.[144,154,183] In the recent meta-analysis by Shaikh and associates, among febrile male infants younger than 3 months of age, 2.4% (confidence interval [CI], 1.4–3.5) of circumcised males and 20.1% (CI, 16.8–23.4) of uncircumcised males had a UTI.[149] Where and when rates of circumcision have decreased, the frequency of UTIs in boys has increased. The presence of preputial folds in uncircumcised boys encourages a high density of bacterial growth and contamination of the urethral opening.[15] Circumcision reduces meatal contamination, decreasing the ascent of bacteria into the bladder.[183] The high risk for acquiring UTIs in uncircumcised boys diminishes with age (as the foreskin becomes more retractable) but is still present in the toddler age group.[23]

Dysfunctional Voiding

Dysfunctional voiding is a risk factor for the development of a UTI and an occasional consequence of UTI. Dysfunctional voiding refers to a lack of coordination between the two functions that are essential for normal voiding to occur—relaxation of the urethral sphincter and contraction of the detrusor muscle of the bladder. Ordinarily the sphincter must relax as the detrusor contracts.[5] The failure of the sphincter to relax causes an obstruction to the outflow of urine. Consequently, voiding pressures and intravesicular pressure are high, the bladder becomes overdistended, dribbling instead of a good flow occurs, and residual urine remains in the bladder after the void. This dyscoordination is termed *dyssynergia*.[5]

Clinical manifestations typically appear after toilet training and include incontinence, enuresis, urinary urgency, and UTI.[31] Constipation is a common occurrence because of the inability to relax the musculature of the pelvic floor. The presence of dysfunctional voiding also may promote the persistence of vesicoureteral reflux (VUR) and lead to recurrence or contralateral reflux after attempts are made at surgical correction of reflux.[78]

Constipation

The distended rectum in constipated children has been suggested to press on the bladder wall and produce an obstruction to bladder outflow that may cause dysfunctional voiding and a large residual volume. Urodynamic studies have shown instability of the detrusor muscle in patients with functional constipation and associated enuresis or UTI.[185] Loening-Baucke[93] studied a group of children referred with encopresis and constipation. The history indicated that many were incontinent of urine, and 11% had histories of UTIs. When a vigorous regimen to alleviate the constipation was prescribed, a dramatic improvement occurred in the enuresis and the frequency of recurrent UTI.

Kasirga and coworkers studied 38 children with chronic functional constipation and 31 children as the control group. A detailed past and present history of UTIs or symptoms pointing to this diagnosis, enuresis, encopresis, urgency, and urge incontinence was obtained from both groups. Frequency of UTI and urgency was significantly higher in the group with constipation.[73]

Sexual Activity

The well-recognized association in women of acute cystitis with sexual intercourse is reflected in the popular, now perhaps outdated, term *honeymoon cystitis*.[113] This phenomenon is often related to the new onset of sexual activity or a recent change in sexual partners. A novel study of 15 patients with a history of recurrent UTIs involved daily monitoring for the presence of UTI with dipslides and calendars that recorded episodes of intercourse, menses, and the occurrence of symptoms.[113] Eleven patients experienced 16 infections; 12 infections occurred within 24 hours of engaging in intercourse. In 12 control subjects, three infections occurred, all within 24 hours of having intercourse. The authors concluded that in sexually active women, most UTIs are related to intercourse.

These results were reinforced by a large prospective study from Seattle, Washington, which confirmed that the incidence of symptomatic UTI is high in sexually active young women and that a strong and independent association exists between UTI and recent sexual intercourse, recent use of a diaphragm with spermicide, and a history of recurrent UTIs.[61] Most of these same risk factors, including frequency of sexual intercourse and use of spermicide, were documented as risk factors associated with development of APN in healthy women.[145]

Catheters

In the hospital, urinary catheters are major risk factors for acquisition of health care–associated infection.[26] In adults, the risk for developing an infection is approximately 5% per day of catheterization.[112] The usual infecting strains include *Escherichia coli, Proteus, Pseudomonas, Klebsiella,* and *Serratia.* Many strains of bacteria that cause infection display antibiotic susceptibilities that are more resistant than usual. The route of infection may be either intraluminal or periurethral. Bacteremia is an unusual complication of nosocomial UTI. In a study of nosocomial UTIs in a pediatric intensive care unit, catheter-associated UTI occurred at a rate of 0.95 per 100 admissions. Nosocomial UTIs were associated with previous cardiovascular surgery and with urinary tract catheterization of at least 3 days.[104] Major efforts to reduce the occurrence of catheter-associated urinary tract infections are nearly universal in both pediatric and adult care units.[26]

PATHOGENESIS

Bacteriology

Most uncomplicated UTIs are caused by members of a large family of gram-negative bacteria known as Enterobacteriaceae. In most instances, the urinary tract becomes infected by the ascending route. Bacteria derived from the fecal flora colonize the periurethral area and gain access to the urethra. The most common bacterial species in primary and recurrent infections is *E. coli.* Other gram-negative species that commonly cause UTI are *Klebsiella, Proteus, Enterobacter,* and *Citrobacter,* although virtually any enteric organism can be the cause of these infections. Gram-positive bacterial species account for approximately 5% of UTIs and primarily include *Staphylococcus saprophyticus* and enterococcal species. After *E. coli, S. saprophyticus* is the most common cause of uncomplicated UTIs in teenagers and young adults of both sexes.

Rarely the urinary tract may become infected hematogenously in the course of a bacteremic infection. This mechanism is thought to account for at least some cases of neonatal UTIs. Increasing evidence indicates that, even in neonates, most infections occur by the ascending route.

Virulence Factors

The key virulence factor for isolates of *E. coli* is the mechanism by which they attach or adhere to the uroepithelial cell.[65] Bacterial adherence is an essential initiating step in all infections. So-called uropathogenic bacteria, derived from the numerous species found in the fecal flora, can attach to specific receptor sites on the uroepithelium and can bind in a nonspecific manner by electrostatic and hydrophobic bonds.[138] The primary adherence factors encoded by uropathogenic *E. coli* and many other microbes are supramolecular, filamentous adhesive organelles known as pili or fimbriae.[176] Some of these pili are referred to as *P fimbriae* because they can recognize and agglutinate erythrocytes of the P1 blood group; this P blood group antigen also is present on human uroepithelial cells. Other common adhesive organelles elaborated by *E. coli* are types 1, 5, and F1C pili encoded by the *fim, sfa,* and *foc* operons, respectively.[176]

Evidence to support the notion of the increased pathogenicity or virulence of the P fimbriae comes from studies of *E. coli* recovered from children with infection at different levels of the urinary tract. When *E. coli* strains recovered from patients with pyelonephritis are examined, 76% to 94% are P fimbriated; in contrast, strains of *E. coli* recovered from patients with cystitis or asymptomatic bacteriuria are 19% to 23% and 14% to 18% P fimbriated, respectively.[72,167] Although P-fimbriated strains of *E. coli* are common findings in patients with pyelonephritis whose urinary tracts are completely normal, their frequency decreases considerably when strains of *E. coli* are examined from patients with pyelonephritis associated with VUR. Apparently this virulence characteristic (and others described later) is unnecessary when reflux is present.[95]

The principal adhesin on the tip of the P fimbriae that fosters adherence to the uroepithelial cell is known as the *PapG adhesin.* More recently, 153 *E. coli* organisms recovered from the urinary tracts of infants and children with pyelonephritis were analyzed by polymerase chain reaction for class I, II, and III alleles of the pyelonephritis-associated adhesin gene *papG.* Strains with any class II *papG* alleles were found significantly more often in infants with normal anatomy and function or in infants with clinically insignificant abnormalities than in infants with significant abnormalities (90 of 119 vs. 14 of 34 infants; $P < .001$).[67] This virulence factor is more important when the urinary tract is structurally normal than when anatomic features predispose the individual to infection.

Other virulence factors related to the bacterial species causing UTIs are the K antigen, lipopolysaccharides, hemolysins, colicins, resistance to the bactericidal action of serum, and increased iron-binding capacity. In addition to the immunogenic activity of lipopolysaccharides (activating an intense host response), they have been shown to have direct toxic effects on renal cells via their biologically active component lipid A.[165] The K antigen is a capsular polysaccharide that constitutes an outer surface of the *E. coli* organism. The capsule has the capacity to impede phagocytosis and to shield the bacteria from lysis induced by complement.[62] Hemolysins are cytotoxic proteins that can damage renal tubular cells in vitro.

Approximately 50% of the types of *E. coli* isolated from the urine of patients with APN produce a pore-forming toxin, α-hemolysin. α-Hemolysin damages the cell membrane and may activate apoptosis in renal tubular cells.[18] Colicins, elaborated by "uropathogenic" strains of *E. coli,* kill other bacteria that are in their vicinity. In the presence of human serum, many bacteria are killed after activation of complement. Virulent *E. coli* organisms have the capacity to resist this bactericidal effect of serum. Another virulence factor found in bacteria is their ability to acquire and bind iron. Most bacteria require iron for optimal growth and metabolism and have developed mechanisms to acquire iron when the supply is limited. One strategy to acquire iron is the use of siderophores to scavenge iron from the environment and subsequently concentrate it in the bacterial cytosol.[176] Siderophores such as enterobactin or aerobactin are secreted low-molecular-weight molecules that have a high affinity for ferric (Fe^{3+}) iron. Bacteria retrieve iron bound to siderophores through receptors that facilitate the transport of iron through the bacterial membrane.

Additional insights into the pathogenesis of *E. coli* UTI have emerged during the past decade. Models in mice and humans (including children) have shown intracellular bacterial communities in the bladder epithelium.[135] These intracellular organisms can result in more extensive infection and, because of their protected location, escape from the immune response and lead to recurrent infections.[134]

After reaching the bladder, P-fimbriated *E. coli* organisms can colonize the ureter even in the absence of VUR.[132] Bacterial colonization of the ureter affects ureteral peristalsis, leading to dilation and a physiologic obstruction. This dilation of the ureter and calyces favors a change in the shape of the renal papillae, which facilitates intrarenal reflux of colonizing bacteria at low pressure. APN develops because the receptors for the P-fimbriated *E. coli* are present in the collecting duct and proximal tubules.[114,132]

Experimental studies conducted by Roberts[132] have led to a theory of the chain of events involved in the process that ultimately leads to renal scarring. The initial event is the inoculation of the renal parenchyma with bacteria, which leads to an intense inflammatory response. Liberation of proinflammatory cytokines (interleukin-1 [IL-1], IL-6, and IL-8) is followed by recruitment of inflammatory cells and a second cytokine burst.[70] This inflammation results in the release of toxic enzymes within the granulocytes and tubular lumen. Superoxide is released simultaneously, generating oxygen radicals that are toxic to the bacteria and to the tubular cells.[133] The resultant death of the tubules intensifies and extends the inflammatory process into the interstitium. At the same time, focal ischemia results from the intravascular aggregation of granulocytes and edema.[69] The tissue damage that results from the toxic enzymes, oxygen radicals, inflammatory response, and ischemia culminates in the creation of renal scars.[65,132]

CLINICAL PRESENTATION

Cystitis

Most children older than 5 years of age with cystitis have urgency, frequency, or dysuria.[6] Children who have the urge to urinate may have a history of difficulty in initiating the urinary stream. Occasionally children may complain of abdominal or suprapubic pain. If fever is present, it is low grade. Suprapubic tenderness may be present on palpation. The urine may be foul smelling and cloudy.

Pyelonephritis

Many children who have APN have impressive chills, spiking fevers, and complaints of back pain.[150] They may have associated gastrointestinal complaints of vomiting and diarrhea, especially vomiting. Lower urinary tract symptoms, such as frequency, urgency, dysuria, and suprapubic discomfort, may or may not be present.

Other findings, such as irritability, poor feeding, vomiting, decreased urinary output, and clinical evidence of dehydration, vary. The youngest children with APN usually have high fever without other localizing features.[56,100,187]

Physical Examination

Features of the physical examination that should be emphasized include (1) an accurate measurement of blood pressure (hypertension may be present in patients who have chronic renal disease), (2) general growth and development (failure to thrive may be a sign of more chronic or recurrent UTI), and (3) a careful abdominal examination (which might reveal tenderness or a mass caused by either an enlarged bladder or an obstructed urinary tract).[163] An effort should be made to elicit the finding of costovertebral angle tenderness in children of all ages. The perineum should be inspected carefully to search for signs of irritation, scars, tears, signs of trauma, labial adhesions, or evidence of vulvovaginitis. In uncircumcised infants, the foreskin may not be retractable, leading to phimosis. A rectal examination should be considered to detect masses or poor sphincter tone, which might be associated with a neurogenic bladder.[163] The lower back should be observed for any lipoma, sinus, pigmentation, or tufts of hair that may be signs of an occult myelodysplasia.

Neurologic examination of the lower extremities and evaluation of the bulbocavernosal reflex often reflect the neurologic integrity of the lower motor neuron reflex arcs. The bulbocavernosus reflex is elicited by squeezing the glans penis or clitoris and observing or feeling a reflex contraction at the external anal sphincter. Absence of this reflex suggests a possible sacral lesion.[5]

Asymptomatic Bacteriuria

A large body of work has been produced dealing with the issue of asymptomatic bacteriuria. Data were accumulated during a long-term study by Kunin[79] of the natural history of recurrent bacteriuria among school-aged girls in a well-defined community in central Virginia. Girls were identified in the first grade and were observed prospectively for 10 years. Each year, approximately 0.5% of school-aged girls developed asymptomatic bacteriuria. The cumulative prevalence was 5% for the years between entrance to grade school and graduation from high school. Although it was billed as asymptomatic bacteriuria, approximately one-third of the girls did have symptoms, and some were known to have had infection or, rarely, abnormalities of the urinary tract before the first screening.

Just a few years after Kunin[79] began his investigations, a similar study was conducted in Göteborg, Sweden. Beginning in 1970, 19,000 girls a year were screened routinely for bacteriuria in Göteborg schools at ages 7, 11, 14, and 16 years.[91] A significant minority had a history of previous infection or symptoms that were referable to the urinary tract.

Savage and colleagues[141] also studied covert bacteriuria in school-aged girls. In their three studies, the point prevalence of bacteriuria ranged from 0.7%[91] to 1.1% to 1.6%.[141] The risks associated with asymptomatic bacteriuria are difficult to assess from these studies because patients who were truly asymptomatic were difficult to separate from patients with symptoms.

Several prospective studies of infants and school-aged girls from Scandinavia have provided important information regarding the natural history of asymptomatic bacteriuria.[45,174] Most children identified as having asymptomatic bacteriuria among a large cohort of infants ($n = 3581$) spontaneously cleared the bacteriuria within months. Only 2 of 45 went on to develop symptomatic bacteriuria. In contrast, none of 42 infants who developed symptomatic UTIs had been identified previously as having asymptomatic bacteriuria, suggesting that asymptomatic bacteriuria rarely is a precursor to symptomatic UTI. In addition, prophylactic antibiotics used to treat children with asymptomatic bacteriuria seemed to predispose them to the development of pyelonephritis, usually with microorganisms that had not been present at the outset.[45]

Currently physicians have little enthusiasm for screening children of any age to discover the presence of asymptomatic bacteriuria. The absence of pyuria in these specimens of urine provides additional evidence that the host is not perturbed by the presence of asymptomatic bacteriuria. The presence of bacteria of low virulence in the urine in asymptomatic patients seems to be protective. These strains apparently prevent invasion by other bacteria and provide a kind of biologic prophylaxis.[45,74]

Rather than screening asymptomatic populations of children, an appropriate approach is vigorous evaluation for the presence of UTIs in febrile children without an obvious focus of infection. In addition, health maintenance examinations should be used as an opportunity to screen for historical information that might suggest the need to collect a urine specimen for culture (Box 39.1). Important items include frequent episodes of unexplained fever, dribbling when urinating, enuresis, encopresis, constipation, urgency, frequency, and dysuria. In addition, it is valuable to know when toilet training was accomplished; frequency of voiding; frequency of stooling; and any apparent difficulties associated with voiding, such as in initiating the urinary stream. The practitioner also should inquire about so-called avoidance maneuvers (e.g., repetitive

BOX 39.1 Renal-Focused History and Physical Examination

History

Age at toilet training
Characteristics and frequency of voiding (urgency, dysuria, dribbling)
Frequency and characteristics of stooling
Family history of renal disease
Habitual squirming
Color and odor of urine
Unexplained episodes of fever

Physical Examination

Temperature
Blood pressure
Abdominal tenderness
Costovertebral angle tenderness
Suprapubic tenderness
Genital examination (irritation, scars, tears)
Rectal examination (sphincter tone, bulbocavernosus reflex)
Lower back (sinus, pigmentation, lipoma, tufts of hair)

habitual squirming, crossing of legs, or sitting on heels)[151] and family history of UTI.

DIFFERENTIAL DIAGNOSIS

Infectious

E. coli is the most common cause of infection in the urinary tract for primary infections (in which *E. coli* causes 85% to 90% of infections) and recurrent infections (in which *E. coli* causes approximately 75% of infections). Virtually any other gram-negative enteric bacteria may cause infection. Common etiologic agents include *Klebsiella, Proteus, Enterobacter, Serratia,* and *Pseudomonas. Proteus mirabilis* is a common cause of UTIs in some series of boys and in health care–associated UTIs associated with catheterization.[77,117] *Enterococcus* and *Pseudomonas* were the most common cause of nosocomial UTI after *E. coli* in a large series of cases reported from Austria.[127] In young women, *S. saprophyticus* is second only to *E. coli* as a cause of cystitis. Rarely *Staphylococcus epidermidis* has been reported as a cause of pyelonephritis in young boys with anatomic abnormalities of the urinary tract.[43]

Acute lobar nephronia is a localized nonliquefactive inflammatory infection of the kidney that has also been called acute focal bacterial nephritis.[20,130] It represents the midpoint in the spectrum of acute uncomplicated pyelonephritis and renal abscess. From a clinical perspective, it may be signaled by protracted fever before and after diagnosis and may warrant a longer duration of antimicrobial treatment than uncomplicated APN. The diagnosis depends on the performance of an enhanced computed tomographic (CT) scan. The bacterial etiology is the same as for other cases of APN. Occasionally the urinalysis may be misleading because of absent or diminished pyuria.

Xanthogranulomatous pyelonephritis is a rare, chronic, suppurative renal infection. Although it can occur at any age, it typically involves middle-aged women. Cases in children have been reported across all age groups, including infants.[1,42,188] The patient usually presents with what appears to be an acute UTI, caused most often by *E. coli* or *Proteus* spp. Evaluation of the patient usually reveals a unilateral enlargement of the kidney, often accompanied by urolithiasis and sometimes a staghorn calculus. The differential diagnosis of the mass lesion includes neuroblastoma, Wilms tumor, tuberculosis, and renal carcinoma. The lesion is characterized histologically by granulomas, abscesses, and lipid-laden foam cells. Nephrectomy is the usual means of management.

In the context of bacteremia or septicemia, occasionally the blood culture and the urine culture are positive for the same bacterial species. In these instances, the kidney has been seeded as part of a hematogenous dissemination. Any organism that is responsible for sepsis, such as *Haemophilus influenzae* type B, *Neisseria meningitidis, Neisseria gonorrhoeae, Staphylococcus aureus, Streptococcus pneumoniae,* or *Streptococcus pyogenes,* may be found in the urine.

Anaerobic infections of the urinary tract are rare occurrences in children despite the high density of gram-positive and gram-negative anaerobes in the fecal flora; this fact relates to the probable lack of adherence of these bacterial species to the uroepithelium. Anaerobic infections of the urinary tract should be suspected when organisms are seen on Gram stain but do not grow in conventional culture or when the urine of symptomatic children shows no bacterial growth.[13] Another unusual infecting agent that should be suspected in instances in which the Gram stain of the urine shows gram-negative rods but the urine culture is negative is *H. influenzae.*[108]

Fungal infections of the urinary tract usually are caused by *Candida* spp., but they also may be caused by *Cryptococcus neoformans, Aspergillus* spp., and the endemic mycoses.[26,161] Candiduria is an increasingly common form of health care–associated infection that may involve any level of the urinary tract.[52,123] It often occurs in immunosuppressed patients, especially patients who are receiving broad-spectrum antibiotics for treatment of documented or undocumented systemic infections. In many immunosuppressed patients, the infection is complicated by the presence of an indwelling urinary catheter.

Viruses also may cause infection of the urinary tract. For the most part, these infections involve the bladder rather than the kidney, although infection of any part of the urinary tract may occur. The principal etiologic agents are adenoviruses, enteroviruses, coxsackieviruses, and echoviruses. Mumps virus and hepatitis viruses occasionally have been implicated. Type 11 adenovirus has been the most common cause of acute hemorrhagic cystitis in school-aged boys; type 21 also has been documented to be a cause of infection in this age group. In immunosuppressed patients, especially children who have undergone bone marrow transplantation or are recipients of kidney transplants, BK polyomavirus and adenovirus may cause hemorrhagic cystitis.[21,88,118]

Granulomatous cystitis is the histopathologic description of cystitis caused by *Mycobacterium tuberculosis* and by schistosomiasis and other parasitic infections. Granulomas formed in response to certain parasites, such as *Toxocara* and microfilariae, also may contain numerous eosinophils. *Enterobius vermicularis* infection occasionally leads to signs and symptoms of cystitis and inflammatory changes of the bladder wall.

Infectious urethritis caused by *N. gonorrhoeae* or *Chlamydia trachomatis* is a common cause of symptoms suggestive of UTI. In addition, any etiologic agents of vulvovaginitis may cause inflammation of the distal urethra, with urgency, frequency, or dysuria; they include *Candida* spp., *Gardnerella vaginalis, Trichomonas vaginalis, S. pyogenes, S. pneumoniae, H. influenzae, C. trachomatis, Shigella* spp., and *Yersinia enterocolitica.*

Noninfectious

Urethral symptoms such as urgency, frequency, and dysuria may be caused by any factor or process that gives rise to inflammation in the lower urinary tract. Examples include mechanical irritation (which might result from insertion of foreign bodies, migration of pinworms, or masturbation) and chemical irritation (which might arise from bubble baths or shampoos). Chemical cystitis has been reported from the inadvertent insertion of a vaginal contraceptive suppository (nonoxynol 9) into the bladder. Pharmacologic causes of urethral symptoms include cyclophosphamide and methenamine mandelate, both of which can lead to inflammatory changes in the urinary bladder. Several other agents used in the topical treatment of bladder cancer have been noted to cause cystitis.

DIAGNOSIS

Collection of a Urine Specimen

Proper collection of a urine specimen is crucial to facilitate interpretation of the culture. In toilet-trained children, a midstream clean-catch specimen is appropriate for evaluation. When this specimen is used, the definition of significant bacteriuria is 10^5 colony-forming units (CFU)/mL or more. The child is asked to void into the toilet. Straddling the commode in a reverse position creates a natural separation between the urethra and the vulva. Cleansing of the perineum does not result in less contamination of the specimen and is no longer encouraged.[143] The child is asked to begin voiding. A second or two after the void has been initiated, a sterile cup is passed into the stream. The hope is that the initial void succeeds in washing out the distal urethra, the site from which the urine specimen is most likely to be contaminated.

If the child is not toilet trained, a specimen may be collected by urethral catheterization or suprapubic aspiration. When the urine is collected by urethral catheterization, the perineum is cleaned with 1% iodine. A properly sized catheter (10 or 12 Fr) or a size 5 feeding tube may be used. The catheter is lubricated and inserted into the urethra and threaded a short distance. The first few drops of urine should be collected outside the sterile container. This part of the specimen is the most likely to be contaminated with fecal flora from the distal urethra; these bacteria are not eliminated by the process of perineal cleansing. The remaining urine is collected in a sterile container and sent to the laboratory. When a urine specimen is collected by urethral catheterization, significant bacteriuria is defined as 50,000 CFU/mL or more.[59] This method is preferred when a small volume of urine in the bladder is anticipated and collecting a specimen of urine is necessary so that antibiotic therapy can be initiated. Unfortunately there is a high likelihood that even a urine sample obtained by catheter will be contaminated (14%), especially in infants younger than 6 months of age, when the catheterization is difficult, and in uncircumcised boys.[182] Use of bladder ultrasonography increases the success of the procedure.[19]

An alternative to urethral catheterization is suprapubic aspiration. Some physicians contend that catheterization is less traumatic than suprapubic aspiration.[163] There is modest evidence that when suprapubic aspiration is performed in very young infants it may be associated with greater discomfort than catheterization of the urine. The procedure can be done in children of any age; it has been used to obtain specimens of urine in pregnancy.[105] Urine culture specimens obtained by suprapubic aspiration are easy to interpret because the usual source of contamination, the distal urethra, has been bypassed. The presence of any bacteria in a specimen collected by suprapubic aspiration is significant, although most samples obtained from patients with infection contain 10^5 CFU/mL or more.

To perform a suprapubic aspiration, the patient is placed in a supine position with the lower extremities flexed (Fig. 39.1 and Table 39.1).[102] Iodine and alcohol are used to clean the suprapubic area. The symphysis pubis is located with the index finger. A 3-mL syringe is attached to a 1.5-inch, 22-gauge needle. A spinal needle (2.5- or 3-inch, 21-gauge) can be used in older patients. The needle is passed in the midline about 1.5 cm above the symphysis pubis. It is angled 10 to 20 degrees from the vertical, pointing in a slightly cephalad direction (Fig. 39.2). Negative pressure is applied while the needle is inserted. The procedure is most likely to be successful when the infant can be encouraged to drink and the diaper has been dry for at least 60 minutes before the procedure is done. The success rate of suprapubic aspiration can be improved with the use of a portable ultrasound device.[38,109] If the suprapubic aspiration is unsuccessful, a catheterized specimen should be obtained. Complications of suprapubic aspiration are rare and include formation of a hematoma, perforation of the bowel, and formation of a suprapubic abscess.[125] Suprapubic aspiration is contraindicated if the patient has a bleeding diathesis.

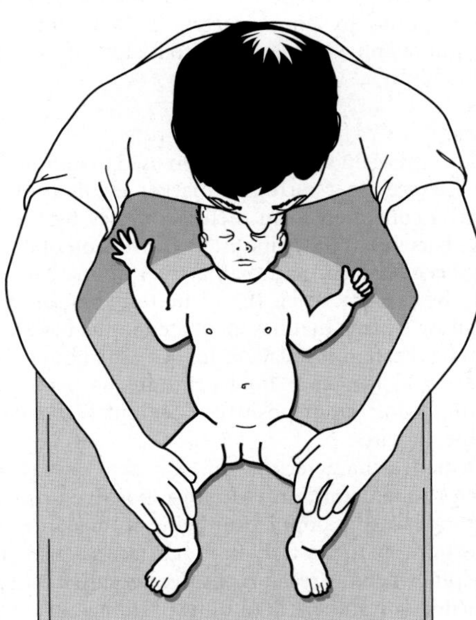

FIG. 39.1 Suprapubic aspiration technique, position of patient.

TABLE 39.1 Suprapubic Aspiration Technique

Step 1	Child should not have voided within 1 hour of the procedure.
Step 2	Restrain the infant in a supine, frog-leg position.
Step 3	Clean the suprapubic area with povidone-iodine and alcohol.
Step 4	Identify the site of puncture at 1 to 2 cm above the symphysis pubis in the midline.
Step 5	Use a 22-gauge, 1.5-inch needle (with 3-mL syringe attached to it) and puncture at 10- to 20-degree angle of the true vertical aiming cephalad; a second attempt can be made at a similar angle aiming caudad.
Step 6	Exert suction gently as the needle is advanced until urine enters syringe; aspirate urine with gentle suction. If urine is not obtained, further trials are unlikely to be successful.

The last method of urine collection is the bag technique. The perineum is washed with soap and water and allowed to dry. A sterile plastic bag is attached. The bag is removed as soon as the patient voids. If the patient has not voided in 20 minutes, the bag is removed, the perineum is cleaned again, and a new bag is attached. If this procedure is followed meticulously, a reasonable specimen can be collected. This specimen is susceptible to contamination from periurethral flora,[142] however, and the technique is not recommended if the patient appears ill and antibiotic therapy needs to be started immediately after the specimen of urine is collected. The results of the culture of a bagged specimen are useful only if they are negative. If the culture is positive, a second specimen must be collected by a more reliable method.[3]

A new noninvasive bladder stimulation technique has been described to obtain clean-catch urine in infants younger than 30 days old.[189,190] After cleaning the genital and perineal area, one clinician dangles the infant by holding under the arms, then taps the suprapubic area rapidly to provide stimulation to the bladder. Another clinician also gently massages the lumbar paravertebral area. A sterile container catches the urine. Most infants void in less than 1 minute. Although this method is labor intensive (at least three attendants are required), it is quick and effective.

Diagnosis of Urinary Tract Infection

The diagnosis of UTI hinges on the results of culture of a properly collected urine specimen. Disagreement within the literature is substantial regarding the definition of significant bacteriuria.[40] As indicated in the previous section, the definition of UTI varies according to the method by which the urine is collected. This variability in definition acknowledges that although the bladder urine is regarded as a sterile body fluid, contamination of the urine specimen may occur as it passes through the urethra. The distal urethra frequently is colonized with coliforms derived from the gastrointestinal tract. The only urine specimen that bypasses the urethra and is free of contamination is obtained by suprapubic aspiration. When a specimen is collected by this technique, any colony count of coliforms is significant.[187]

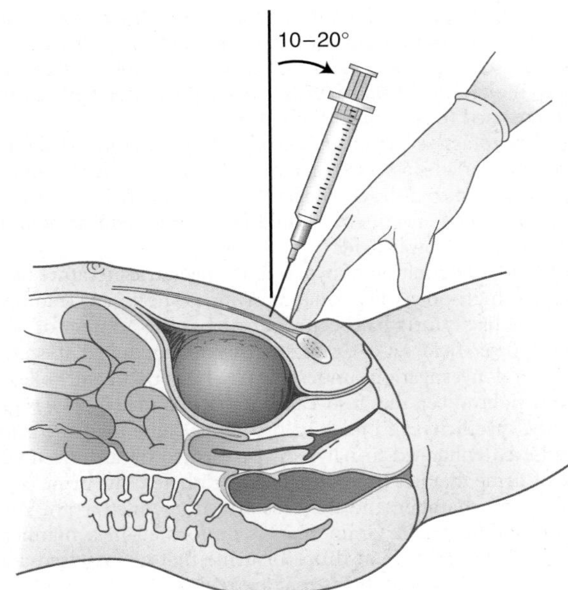

FIG. 39.2 Suprapubic aspiration technique, position of needle.

TABLE 39.2 Urinary Tract Infection: Definitions

Method of Collection	Colony Count (CFU/mL)
Clean catch	$\geq 10^5$
Catheter	$\geq 5 \times 10^4$
Suprapubic	Any

CFU, Colony-forming unit.

In urine that is collected by a midstream clean-catch method, significant bacteriuria is defined, most stringently, by the recovery of 100,000 CFU/mL or more (Table 39.2). For specimens of urine obtained by catheter, significant bacteriuria is defined as 50,000 CFU/mL or more. In each of these instances, physicians recognize that although urine specimens containing lower colony counts rarely may represent true infection, for the most part lower colony counts usually are the result of contamination of the specimen.[59]

Specimens of urine usually are inoculated onto two different kinds of solid media—one that supports the growth of only gram-negative enteric bacteria (e.g., MacConkey agar) and another that supports gram-positive and gram-negative bacteria (e.g., 5% sheep blood agar), with use of a 0.001 calibrated loop. Colonies are counted the next day (18 hours later), and the total is multiplied by 1000 to determine the colony count. The results of the urine culture are unavailable during the practitioner's first encounter with the ill child. Consequently, there is great interest in the development of a method that would predict the results of the urine culture so that appropriate antimicrobial therapy could be initiated presumptively at the time of the initial encounter. Microscopic methods (to evaluate pyuria and bacteriuria) and biochemical tests (which can be evaluated with a dipstick) have been evaluated and will be discussed. However, the performance of urine culture is mandatory because no rapid urine test is sufficiently sensitive to identify all children with UTI.[179]

Microscopy

Two surrogate markers for UTI on microscopic assessment are pyuria and bacteriuria. A problem in assessing pyuria and bacteriuria has been the issue of the definition of significant microscopic pyuria and bacteriuria. How many white blood cells (WBCs) in the urine are too many? Should the specimen of urine that is examined be centrifuged or uncentrifuged? How should the WBCs in a specimen of urine be enumerated? Should the number of WBCs on a centrifuged specimen be enumerated as the number per high-power field, or should they be enumerated on a counting chamber as the number of cells per cubic millimeter, as they would be in a sample of cerebrospinal fluid? If the urine is centrifuged, additional variables are introduced: the initial volume of urine, the duration of the spin, and the volume of urine used to resuspend the sediment. All of these variables influence substantially the enumeration of WBCs per high-power field, especially the volume used to resuspend the sediment.

Methods to assess bacteriuria also have raised issues of definition. Should bacteriuria be assessed on a centrifuged specimen or an uncentrifuged specimen, and should the bacteria be evaluated on a wet mount or a Gram-stained specimen? Should bacteria be enumerated as the number per high-power field?

The standard definition of pyuria in the pediatric literature has been 5 WBCs per high-power field on a centrifuged specimen. Traditionally, microscopic bacteriuria has been expressed as the number of bacteria per high-power field on a Gram stain of a centrifuged specimen of urine. Several investigations undertaken by Hoberman and colleagues[58] have shown, however, that a so-called enhanced urinalysis has greater sensitivity, specificity, and positive predictive value than the standard urinalysis. An enhanced urinalysis is performed on an uncentrifuged sample of urine that has been obtained by catheter. The urine is placed on a counting chamber, and the cells are enumerated as the number per cubic millimeter. A Gram stain is performed in a manner that standardizes the number of drops of urine that are assessed and the number of oil immersion fields that are reviewed.

An enhanced urinalysis is considered to be positive when 10 WBCs/mm^3 or more are present and at least one gram-negative rod in 10 oil immersion fields is present. This definition of significant pyuria is much more sensitive than were previous definitions, and it has performed well for numerous investigators and in neonates and in older infants.[51,89–91,187] A systematic review of the existing literature to assess the performance of rapid diagnostic tests for UTI concluded that use of the traditional definition of pyuria (>5 WBCs per high-power field on a centrifuged specimen) is sufficiently poor that it cannot be recommended for making a presumptive diagnosis of UTI.[40] Huicho and coworkers[64] also performed a meta-analysis of urine screening tests to determine the risk for UTI in children. This study concluded that pyuria of at least 10 WBCs/mm^3 and bacteriuria are best suited for assessing the risk for UTIs in children. The most recent meta-analysis concluded that detection of bacteriuria by microscopy with Gram stain is the single best test and, if available locally and reported rapidly, is the optimum guide to empiric treatment of children with antibiotics.[179]

Automated methods to perform urinalysis are being used in many hospitals and laboratories. The most updated automated image-based urinalysis system, the iQ200, received clearance from the U.S. Food and Drug Administration (FDA) recently. The system uses flow imaging analysis technology and so-called auto particle recognition (APR) software to classify particles found in an uncentrifuged urine specimen based on multiple parameters. Images are stored and can be viewed later on the workstation screen, thus eliminating the need for manual microscopy in most cases.[169] The iQ200 provides for a rapid turnaround time, and results correlate well with manual methods, especially for red blood cells, WBCs, and squamous epithelial cells.[80,92]

Pyuria is not specific for UTI. In several other conditions, including fever, streptococcal infections, Kawasaki disease, and after exercise, WBCs are found in the urine. Finding pyuria does not ensure that an infection of the urinary tract is present. Despite reports to the contrary, finding true UTI without pyuria is unusual.[171] Generally, inflammation is expected to accompany infection. The absence of pyuria in children with UTIs is rare; it may occur when a child is being evaluated so early in the clinical course of the infection that the inflammatory response has not yet developed. Pyuria may also be absent when a child is experiencing an episode of asymptomatic bacteriuria. However, the most likely explanation for significant bacteriuria by culture in the absence of pyuria is a contaminated specimen. In some cases when UTI has been reported to occur in the absence of pyuria, the definition of pyuria has been at fault. The requirement for 5 WBCs per high-power field on a centrifuged specimen corresponds to approximately 25 WBCs/mm^3; this is too stringent a requirement, with a low sensitivity for the detection of UTIs in infants and children.

Urine Dipsticks

Urine dipsticks (or reagent strips) have been used to indicate the presence of leukocyte esterase (as a surrogate marker for pyuria) and urinary nitrite (which is converted from dietary nitrates by the presence of gram-negative bacteria in the urine). The conversion of dietary nitrates to nitrites by bacteria takes approximately 4 hours. The test result is most likely to be positive when the urine tested is the first morning void (representing a urine that has incubated in the bladder overnight) or a urine that has been in the bladder for at least 4 hours (e.g., obtained from an older child who may hold urine in the bladder for several hours at a time). Most gram-positive cocci and *Pseudomonas* species will not produce nitrites.

The performance characteristics of leukocyte esterase and nitrites vary according to the definition used for a positive urine culture, the age and symptoms of the population being studied, and the method of urine collection. A nitrite test, although not a sensitive marker in children, is helpful when the result is positive because it is highly specific. A negative nitrite test result has little value in ruling out UTI, however.[28] The leukocyte esterase test has an average sensitivity of 83%.[29] It can have a sensitivity of 94% in settings in which UTIs are suspected clinically and a sensitivity of 52.9% when it is performed on febrile children, most of whom do not have a UTI.[59] The specificity of leukocyte esterase (average, 72%; range, 64% to 92%) generally is not as good as the sensitivity, reflecting the nonspecificity of pyuria in general. A positive leukocyte esterase test result should be interpreted with caution, depending largely on the population being evaluated.[28]

If both leukocyte esterase and nitrites are positive, the sensitivity and specificity are very high. The combination of a positive leukocyte esterase and nitrate predicts a positive urine culture very accurately; when both are negative, the likelihood of UTI is low.[129]

Determining the Site of Infection

Urinalysis is useful for detecting infection but not for determining the location of the infection within the urinary tract (i.e., upper tract vs. lower tract). To determine the site of infection (i.e., kidney vs. bladder), many investigations of the discriminatory ability of C-reactive protein, erythrocyte sedimentation rate, and total peripheral WBCs have been

BOX 39.2 Imaging Procedures in Children With Urinary Tract Infection

1. Renal ultrasonography
2. Renal scintigraphy
3. Magnetic resonance imaging
4. Voiding cystourethrography
5. Computed tomography

performed. Several studies have evaluated the accuracy of procalcitonin levels compared with C-reactive protein levels to predict renal involvement among children with febrile UTIs.[8,36,120,126,160] These studies showed that serum procalcitonin concentrations, measured with either an immunoluminetric quantitative test or a rapid semiquantitative test, diagnosed APN with a sensitivity of 70.3% to 94.1% and a specificity of 82.6% to 93.6%.

In a meta-analysis published in 2011, 12 studies representing 526 patients with UTI (10% with VUR of grade III or higher) were included.[85] The sensitivity of procalcitonin greater than or equal to 0.5 mg/mL as an indicator of VUR of grade III or higher was 83% (95% CI, 71–91) with a 43% specificity rate (95% CI, 38–47). In the subgroup of children with positive results on dimercaptosuccinic acid (DMSA) scan, procalcitonin greater than or equal to 0.5 mg/mL was also associated with high-grade VUR (adjusted odds ratio, 4.8; 95% CI, 1.3–17.6).[84]

A systematic review published in 2015 set out to determine whether procalcitonin (≥0.5 ng/mL), C-reactive protein (20 mg/L), or erythrocyte sedimentation rate (≥30 mm Hg) could replace DMSA scans in the diagnostic evaluation of UTI in children (i.e., distinguish between cystitis and APN). Six studies (434 children) included data on procalcitonin, 13 studies (1638 children) included data on CRP, and 6 studies (1737 children) included data on ESR. The summary sensitivity estimates (95% CI) for procalcitonin, CRP, and ESR were 0.86 (0.72–0.93), 0.94 (0.85–0.97), and 0.87 (0.77–0.93), respectively. The summary specificity values for procalcitonin, CRP, and ESR were 0.74 (0.55–0.87), 0.39 (0.23–0.58), and 0.48 (0.33–0.64), respectively. Although the procalcitonin looked promising, the small number of studies and marked heterogeneity does not provide enough evidence to recommend its use.[147]

Imaging

The recommendations for performing imaging procedures on children with a diagnosis of UTI have changed and remain somewhat controversial. The imaging studies that usually are considered are renal ultrasonography, contrast voiding cystourethrography (VCUG) to detect VUR, renal cortical scintigraphy, and magnetic resonance imaging (MRI) (Box 39.2).

Renal Ultrasonography

The renal ultrasound examination has replaced intravenous pyelography as a means to assess the gross anatomy of the urinary tract. Generally, ultrasonography has been performed promptly after diagnosis of the UTI has been made. It is a noninvasive test that can describe the size and shape of the urinary tract, the presence of duplication and dilation of the ureters, the presence of ureteroceles, and the existence of gross anatomic abnormalities such as a horseshoe kidney.[3] It is not sensitive enough, however, to signal consistently the presence of hydronephrosis, hydroureter, VUR, or renal scarring.[32] When ultrasonography was compared with intravenous pyelography for the detection of renal scars, wide interobserver variations were noted, with sensitivity ranging from 40% to 90%.[39]

Widespread application of prenatal ultrasonography has reduced the prevalence of previously unsuspected obstructive uropathy in infants, but the consequences of prenatal screening with respect to the risk for renal abnormalities in infants with UTIs have not yet been well defined.[3] There is considerable variability in the timing and quality of prenatal ultrasonograms, and the report of "normal" ultrasonographic results cannot necessarily be relied on to dismiss completely the possibility of a structural abnormality unless the study was a detailed anatomic survey (with measurements), was performed during the third trimester, and was performed and interpreted by qualified individuals. Unfortunately a negative prenatal ultrasound evaluation does not significantly alter

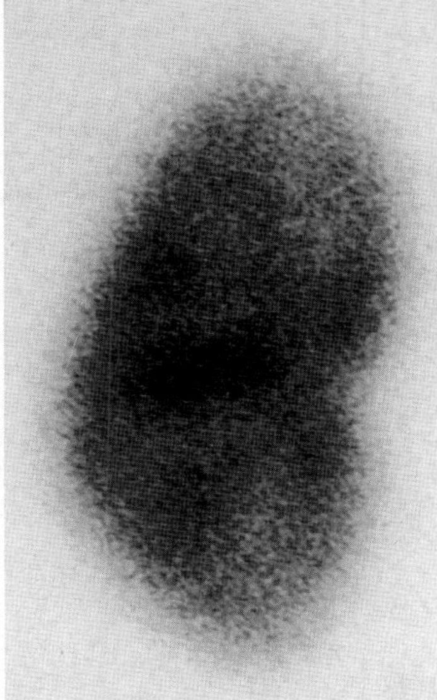

FIG. 39.3 Normal renal scintigram.

the probability of finding an abnormality on a postnatal ultrasound evaluation after a UTI.[75]

Some investigators have questioned whether routine performance of renal ultrasonography is essential.[55] Several studies of a large number ($n = 561$) of young children with their first febrile UTI disclosed that abnormalities found on ultrasound evaluation were infrequent and rarely influenced management.[57,186] In the most recent investigation of this question, the renal ultrasound study was abnormal in 23 of 155 (14.8%) children.[66] Management of four patients was changed by the results. Because of the seriousness of the uncommon but potentially correctable abnormalities in 1% to 2% of children with their first UTI and because ultrasonography is noninvasive and poses minimal risk, the American Academy of Pediatrics has recommended performance of renal and bladder ultrasonography in all febrile infants with a UTI.[3]

The timing of renal and bladder ultrasonography depends on the clinical situation. The imaging study is recommended during the first 2 days of treatment to identify serious complications such as renal or perirenal abscesses or pyonephrosis associated with obstructive uropathy when the clinical illness is unusually severe or substantial clinical improvement is not occurring. For febrile infants with UTIs who demonstrate substantial clinical improvement, however, imaging does not need to occur early during the acute infection, and the results can even be misleading. Changes in the size and shape of the kidneys and the echogenicity or renal parenchyma attributable to edema also are common during acute infection. The presence of these abnormalities makes it inappropriate to consider renal and bladder ultrasonography performed early during acute infection to be a true baseline study for later comparisons in the assessment of renal growth. An optimum time to perform the ultrasound is one week after diagnosis.

Renal Scintigraphy

In patients with presumed APN, renal scintigraphy with technetium-99m DMSA or technetium-99m glucoheptonate has been shown to be the most practical and reliable method for detecting APN.[151] DMSA and glucoheptonate are amino acids that are cleared by the renal tubules. When these amino acids are labeled with technetium and injected intravenously, they can be used to create an image of the kidney, which reflects vascular flow and tubular function (Fig. 39.3). In experimentally induced APN in piglets, the DMSA scan had a sensitivity of 87% and a specificity of 100% in showing lesions consistent with APN compared with histology as the gold standard.[139]

In most patients with APN, renal scintigraphy performed during the acute phase of the illness shows a decreased uptake of DMSA (Fig. 39.4). High-resolution pinhole images of the kidney reveal focal, multifocal, or diffuse areas of decreased uptake of isotope in the kidney without loss of volume and with maintenance of the contour of the

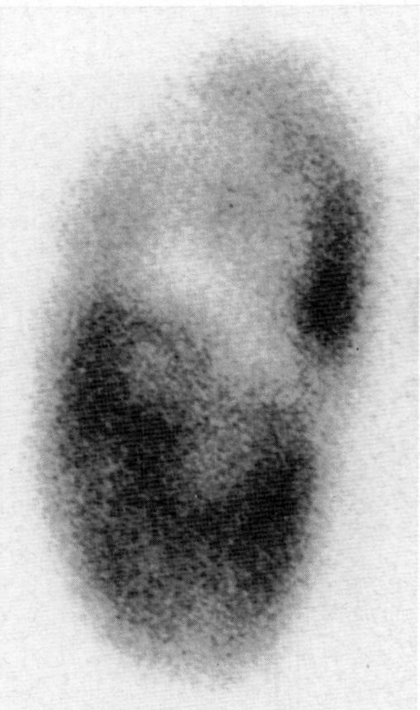

FIG. 39.4 Scintigram showing acute pyelonephritis, manifesting as a photon-deficient area in the upper pole.

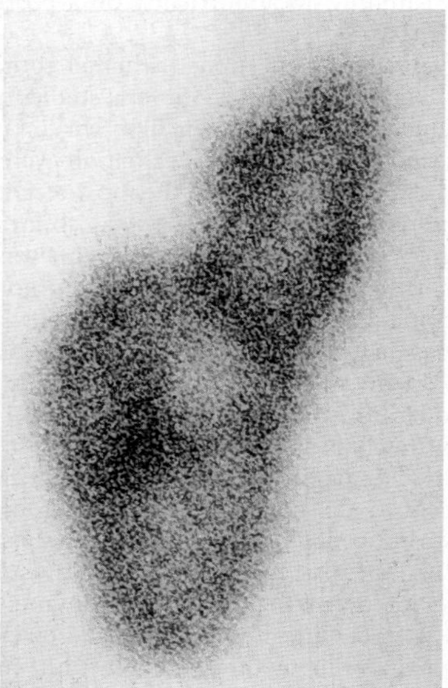

FIG. 39.5 Scintigram showing a renal scar with loss of the normal contour.

kidney.[151] DMSA renal scintigraphy can be used to localize the level at which the urinary tract is infected, specifically distinguishing between acute cystitis and APN with a sensitivity of slightly less than 90%. Rarely a patient with classic signs and symptoms of APN has a renal scan that does not show the usual findings.[34] Nonetheless, renal scintigraphy is the most sensitive study to indicate the presence of APN.

The DMSA and glucoheptonate scans also can be used to indicate the presence of renal scars that result from an episode of APN. The scar is indicated by an area in which uptake of the radioisotope is decreased (Fig. 39.5). In this case, the contour of the kidney is not preserved. Scarring also may be indicated by an overall reduction of the size of the kidney. Hoberman and colleagues[55] prospectively evaluated 309 infants who were 1 to 24 months old with their first febrile UTI. An initial DMSA scan was performed on all infants and showed that 61% (190 of 309) had findings compatible with APN and only 1 infant had evidence of previous scars. Repeat scintigraphic scanning was done 6 months after entry in 89% to detect renal scarring. A small percentage of renal parenchymal involvement (mean, 8.2%) was noted in 9.6% of the infants. All infants whose initial scans were normal had normal scans at follow-up.

DMSA scintigraphy has been suggested as the preferred imaging study to evaluate a child with a first febrile UTI rather than ultrasonography or VCUG.[44,49] A strategy to perform VCUG only in patients with an abnormal DMSA scan has been proposed. The rationale is based on the high negative predictive value of a normal DMSA for high degrees of reflux (III to V) and rarity of renal scarring when the initial DMSA is normal.[75] Reflux definitely may be present, however, when DMSA scans are normal (30 of 99 in Hoberman's data).[55] Absence of scarring may be attributable to the effect of antibiotics.

Magnetic Resonance Imaging

MRI can be used to detect the presence of APN. Two studies by Lonergan and colleagues[97,122] showed a sensitivity and a specificity of MRI that are equal to and perhaps even greater than those of renal scintigraphy with DMSA. In both instances, the best pulse sequence to show areas of APN with MRI was gadolinium-enhanced, fast spin-echo inversion recovery. These results have been confirmed by others.[17,83] Several investigators have urged, however, that MRI not become a screening test for children with UTIs until the detection of minor changes in the renal parenchyma (by either DMSA or MRI) has been proved to be of clinical importance.[83,96] The time and sedation requirements for MRI render it an unattractive choice for routine management.

Voiding Cystourethrography

Two types of cystographies are available for the diagnosis of VUR: fluoroscopic contrast VCUG and radionuclide cystography. Contrast VCUG has excellent anatomic resolution and provides detailed images of the bladder and the urethra. It can be used specifically to label the degree of reflux (according to the international classification)[81]; to look for trabeculations, diverticula, or ureteroceles of the bladder; and to outline the urethra (which is essential to identify posterior urethral valves causing obstruction). Radionuclide cystography provides less anatomic detail and is most useful when urethral disease is not suspected and when the patient has no history of voiding dysfunction. It is used to observe patients who are known to have reflux (to assess whether reflux is still present) and can be used for screening purposes in siblings of children with reflux and in children of adults known to have had reflux. Compared with conventional contrast VCUG, the amount of radiation exposure is reduced substantially when the radioisotope is used.

The international classification of reflux is a universally used system involving five degrees of reflux.[81] Grade I is reflux into the distal ureter; grade II is reflux into the proximal ureter; and grades III, IV, and V are reflux with mild, moderate, and severe dilation of the pelvis and calyces (Fig. 39.6), respectively.

VCUG is performed on children who have experienced a symptomatic UTI to determine the presence of VUR. Children who have VUR are at risk for developing reflux nephropathy—permanent renal damage secondary to the reflux of infected urine into the kidney. Because reflux often resolves spontaneously over the course of several years, the purpose of identifying a child with VUR in the past was to recommend antibiotic prophylaxis until the reflux either had resolved spontaneously or, in cases of high degrees of reflux, had been corrected surgically.

Although imaging of children with UTI has been routine, little evidence exists that diagnostic imaging of children after their first UTI results in prevention of renal scarring, hypertension, or renal failure.[22] The value of identifying abnormalities on the renal ultrasound or VCUG is predicated on the benefits of treatment for these findings, which is a subject of recent controversy.[75] If studies can show with certainty that antibiotic prophylaxis to prevent UTIs in children with VUR is superior to placebo in the prevention of renal scarring, the necessity and importance of performing VCUG would be established. Between 2006 and 2010, several studies were published that cast doubt on the effectiveness of antibiotic prophylaxis.[12,35,107,121,137] However, the results of the Randomized Intervention for Children with Vesicoureteral Reflux (RIVUR) trial, which will be discussed in detail under the management section of VUR treatment, showed modest benefit.[53]

Computed Tomography

In general, CT of the kidneys is not recommended. However, when the clinical response to treatment is sluggish, this study is occasionally

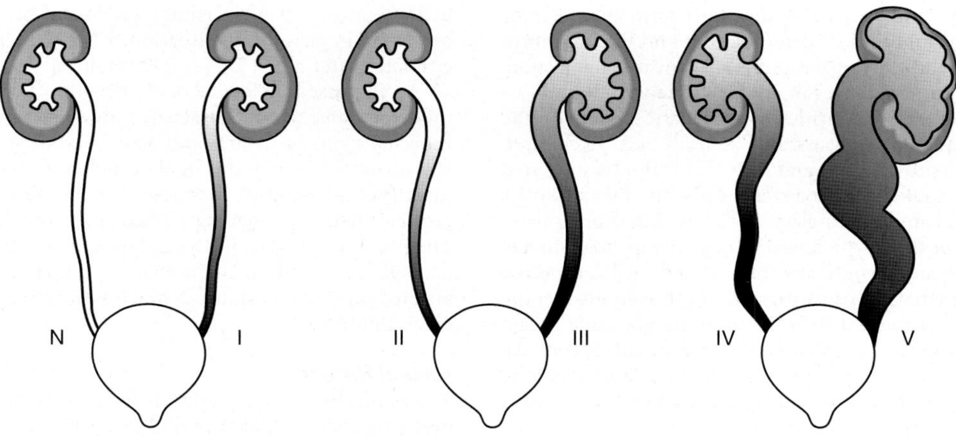

FIG. 39.6 International classification of vesicoureteral reflux.

TABLE 39.3 **Antibiotic Treatment**

Drug Name	Dosage
Oral	
Amoxicillin + potassium clavulanate	45 mg/kg/day in two divided doses
Cefuroxime	30 mg/kg/day in two divided doses
Cefprozil	30 mg/kg/day in two divided doses
Cefixime	10 mg/kg/day in one dose
Cefpodoxime	9 mg/kg/day in one dose
Ceftibuten	10 mg/kg/day in one dose
Cefdinir	14 mg/kg/day in one dose
Trimethoprim-sulfamethoxazole	10 mg/kg/day (trimethoprim) in two divided doses
Parenteral	
Ampicillin + sulbactam	200 mg/kg/day in four divided doses
Cefuroxime	150 mg/kg/day in three divided doses
Cefotaxime	200 mg/kg/day in four divided doses
Ceftriaxone	80 mg/kg/day in one dose
Ceftazidime	150 mg/kg/day in three divided doses
Cefepime	100 mg/kg/day in two divided doses
Gentamicin	7.5 mg/kg/day in three divided doses

performed. Both xanthogranulomatous pyelonephritis and lobar nephronia are best imaged with this technique.[20,42]

TREATMENT

Antibiotics for Treatment of Acute Infection

The treatment of UTI is influenced by the age of the patient, the probable site of infection (cystitis or APN), the degree of toxicity, and the likelihood of adherence to the treatment regimen. Oral antimicrobial therapy is appropriate for children with cystitis and for older children with suspected APN who are neither toxic nor vomiting. The more complex issue is the management of a young infant with high fever in whom the likely diagnosis is APN. These children traditionally have been admitted to the hospital for parenteral administration of antibiotics.

Numerous choices of oral antimicrobial agents are available for patients who have presumed cystitis (Table 39.3). Alternatives include amoxicillin + potassium clavulanate; second-generation cephalosporins, such as cefuroxime and cefprozil; third-generation cephalosporins, such as cefixime, cefpodoxime, ceftibuten, and cefdinir; and the combination agent trimethoprim-sulfamethoxazole. Generally neither amoxicillin nor first-generation cephalosporins are recommended for first-line therapy because 30% to 50% of *E. coli* now are inherently resistant to these agents. Because of some geographic variability in the prevalence of resistance, the practitioner should check with local infectious disease specialists to verify these susceptibility patterns.

In an older patient who appears ill but is not toxic, a repeat visit or telephone follow-up is indicated to ensure that recovery is progressing as predicted. If fever is present, the patient generally becomes afebrile within 1 or 2 days, although occasionally it may take longer. If other indices of recovery, such as general well-being, appetite, and playfulness, are improving appropriately, the persistence of fever is not alarming. If susceptibility test results are available and the organism causing infection is susceptible to the antimicrobial agent being used, repeating the urine culture after 24 hours is unnecessary.[57] The rapid sterilization of urine is a testimony to the fact that virtually all the antibiotics that are used to treat UTIs are concentrated in the kidney and excreted in the urine.

Duration of treatment for patients who are presumed to have cystitis has been controversial. Conventional recommendations are for 7 to 10 days of antimicrobial therapy. Short courses of therapy, varying from single-dose regimens to 3- or 4-day courses, have been evaluated with mixed results. The potential advantages of short-course therapy include the likelihood of improved adherence to the drug regimen; lower cost of drug; and fewer undesirable side effects, including less alteration of normal flora.[152] A meta-analysis (and the most comprehensive review of the data) was performed by Tran and coworkers[164] after review of 22 published trials and a total of 1279 patients. Amoxicillin in a single dose and trimethoprim-sulfamethoxazole as either a single dose or a 3-day regimen were the short-course regimens most commonly evaluated. The authors found that short-course antimicrobial therapy is less effective than therapy of conventional duration, largely because of the ineffectiveness of single-dose amoxicillin. A 3-day course of trimethoprim-sulfamethoxazole was an effective alternative to the standard course of treatment.

A more recent meta-analysis evaluated 10 trials in 652 children with lower tract UTIs.[60] No significant difference was found in the frequency of positive urine cultures between short-duration (2–4 days) and standard-duration (7–14 days) oral antibiotic therapy for UTIs in children 1 to 15 months after treatment. In children with clear evidence of cystitis without APN, short-course therapy may be acceptable.[170]

Management of a young infant with presumed APN has been controversial. A study conducted by Hoberman and colleagues[57] compared oral therapy with cefixime (for 14 days) with a combination of intravenous therapy with cefotaxime (for 3 or 4 days) plus oral cefixime for 9 to 10 days. Children were eligible for this study if they were 1 to 24 months of age and presented to the physician with temperature greater than 38.3°C (100.9°F) and were found to have a positive enhanced urinalysis (≥10 WBCs/mm^3 and 1 organism/10 oil immersion fields). After blood and urine cultures, complete blood cell count, C-reactive protein determination, and erythrocyte sedimentation rate were performed, the children were randomly assigned to treatment groups.

Outcome was evaluated with regard to the short-term measures of sterilization of the urine and time to defervescence and the long-term measures of reinfection and scarring 6 months after the initial infection. No statistically significant differences in any outcome were found.

Hodson and colleagues[106] performed a systematic review of the treatment of APN in children. They assessed 23 trials of 3295 children aged up to 18 years with proven UTIs and APN. Their results suggested that children with APN could be treated effectively with oral antibiotics (cefixime, ceftibuten, and amoxicillin-clavulanate) or with short courses (2–4 days) of intravenous therapy followed by oral therapy to complete a 10-day course. Shorter courses of treatment in patients with suspected APN have not been systematically investigated. If intravenous therapy is chosen, single-dose treatment daily with an aminoglycoside is safe and effective.[106] If the diagnosis of lobar nephronia is made secondary to a sluggish response to antimicrobial therapy, 2 or 3 weeks of antibiotic therapy (dependent on the pattern of abnormality seen on the CT scan) is recommended rather than a 10-day course.[20]

Corticosteroids

A 2011 publication examining the potential role of corticosteroid therapy as an adjunct to antibiotics in the acute phase of APN suggests a beneficial effect.[63] Nineteen patients treated with methylprednisolone were compared with 65 in the placebo group. Adjunctive oral corticosteroids reduced the occurrence and severity of renal scarring in children with APN. Larger studies must be performed before this strategy is adopted.

Dysfunctional Voiding

If a history of dysfunctional voiding is obtained, a behavioral modification approach may be helpful. The key features include frequent volitional voiding every 2 to 3 hours until the voiding pattern has been reestablished, increased water intake (1 L/day) in addition to all other fluids consumed, correction of constipation, and adequate perineal hygiene.[30] Referral to a pediatric urologist may be necessary. Children who exhibit persistent inability to relax their sphincters may require training that involves relaxation techniques reinforced with biofeedback. Pharmacologic treatment with anticholinergics may be necessary if uninhibited bladder contractions are shown with urodynamic studies.[30] Special attention must be paid to the management of constipation if anticholinergic agents are initiated because they will exaggerate the problem.

Antibiotic Prophylaxis

Although antibiotic prophylaxis commonly is recommended for children with recurrent UTIs,[86] only limited data support this position. In a review of the literature, Le Saux and colleagues[86] found sparse data of low quality to support the use of antibiotic prophylaxis in children with a normal urinary tract. A meta-analysis by Williams and colleagues[177] revealed five randomized controlled trials assessing the use of prophylactic therapy. Of these, only two trials with 71 children evaluated the effectiveness of long-term, low-dose antibiotics to prevent UTIs.[94,157] The authors concluded that well-designed, randomized, placebo-controlled trials still are required to evaluate this commonly used intervention.

Vesicoureteral Reflux

The clinical significance of VUR as a predisposing factor for UTIs in general or APN in particular and its contribution to the formation of renal scarring have been questioned recently. VUR is thought to increase the risk for UTI by increasing postvoid residual and allowing less virulent strains of bacteria to ascend into the upper tract and infect the kidney.[75] While VUR is unequivocally a risk factor in UTI and APN, at least 60% of children with APN do not have VUR.[148] The question also has been framed as to whether long-term antibiotic prophylaxis is effective in reducing reinfection, thereby preventing renal damage in patients with VUR.[12,35,53,107,121,137]

Epidemiology

The incidence of VUR in the general population is thought to be approximately 1%.[27] Children usually are tested for the possibility of VUR in one of two clinical situations—during the assessment of prenatally diagnosed hydronephrosis and in the evaluation of a UTI. Reflux is diagnosed in 10% to 20% of cases of prenatally identified hydronephrosis; it often is high grade and occurs more frequently in boys than in girls in this situation.[44,142] The incidence of reflux in girls evaluated after a first UTI is 25% to 40%.[29,168]

An increased incidence of VUR within families suggests a genetic mode of transmission.[71] Rates for prevalence of VUR in identical and fraternal twins were 80% and 35%, providing evidence that this trait is transmitted in an autosomal dominant fashion. Siblings of children identified as having VUR as part of an evaluation for UTI have a much greater chance of having reflux than the normal population.[4,119] The presence of VUR in these siblings is accompanied by silent renal damage.[16] In addition, a girl who has reflux has a 65% risk for having affected offspring.[27] Reflux is much more common among white than black children.

Natural History

The natural history of reflux is for spontaneous resolution to occur over time, with a longer period being necessary in more severe types of reflux. Other factors that may affect the rate of resolution include age at diagnosis, gender, unilaterality versus bilaterality, and whether there is dysfunctional voiding. Average figures for spontaneous resolution are 80% to 86% for grade II reflux and 40% to 46% for grade III reflux during a 5-year period.

In a report from Skoog and associates,[155] spontaneous resolution occurred within 1.65 years of diagnosis in patients with grade II reflux, but 1.97 years was required for resolution in patients with grade III reflux ($P < .04$). Ninety percent of patients with reflux grades between I and III who ultimately had resolution of reflux experienced this result within 5 years. The rate of resolution was 30% to 35% per year, although the duration of reflux was shorter for patients in whom the diagnosis was made before they reached 1 year of age compared with patients who were older at the time of diagnosis.[7]

In another study of the natural history of reflux, Schwab and coworkers[146] determined the resolution rate by patient for 179 girls and 35 boys with UTIs and diagnoses of primary VUR between 1981 and 1984. Reflux spontaneously resolved in 68% of patients during the study. Grades I to III reflux resolved at a rate of 13% per year for the first 5 years of follow-up and then at a rate of 3.5% per year during subsequent follow-up. Grades IV and V reflux resolved at a rate of 5% per year. Bilateral reflux resolved more slowly than unilateral reflux and more rapidly in boys than in girls. There is no specific age in adolescence at which one can assume reflux will not resolve. Leneghan and colleagues[82] reported cessation of reflux after 14 years of age in 27% of patients observed without surgical intervention.

Management

The optimal management of children with high grades of reflux (grades III to V) has been the subject of numerous retrospective and prospective studies.[68,172,173] Since 1970, two large prospective randomized trials, the Birmingham Reflux study[10,9,11] and the International Reflux Study in Children,[131] have been performed to compare medical therapy (antibiotic prophylaxis) with surgical therapy (reimplantation of ureters). The International Reflux Study in Children reported results from Europe and the United States. Because entry criteria were different, the results have been reported separately.

In Europe and the United States, the surgical management of VUR is neither superior nor inferior to medical treatment. In both groups, new scars were acquired during the 5-year follow-up period, some in patients who did not show scarring at the time of entry. In other children, scars present at entry worsened.[124] No detectable differences were found between study groups in either renal function or renal growth. The number of episodes of infection also was similar in both groups. The only exception was a greater frequency of episodes of febrile UTIs (presumed pyelonephritis) in children receiving medical therapy.

Wheeler and colleagues[175] conducted a systematic review of randomized trials of the effects of various interventions in patients with VUR on the development of subsequent UTI and renal parenchymal injury. The aim was to evaluate whether any intervention for reflux (surgical) is better than nonsurgical treatment. Eight trials involving 859 evaluable children were reviewed. Seven trials compared antimicrobial agents alone with surgery plus antimicrobial prophylaxis. The risk for a UTI developing by 1 or 2 and 5 years was not significantly different between surgical and medical groups, and the risk for renal scarring or progressive renal damage occurring was similar. The choice of treatment remains a value judgment governed by such local factors as preference of the parents, availability of skilled surgeons, availability of closely supervised medical treatment, and willingness to comply with prolonged periods of prophylaxis.

Does VUR predispose to pyelonephritis and renal scarring? Garin and associates[34] reviewed 10 studies of children with acute UTIs who underwent DMSA scanning and VCUG. Selection of patients in at least one of the studies was biased toward the association between reflux and APN because the VCUG often was performed after the DMSA scan was reported to be abnormal. Six of 10 studies showed statistically significant results indicating that the presence of reflux definitely was associated with the occurrence of APN; all 4 of the remaining studies showed a trend in the same direction. Kerem, in his review of imaging, endorsed the observation that children with high-grade VUR (grades IV and V) are four to six times more likely to develop scarring than those with low-grade reflux and 8 to 10 times as likely as those with no reflux.[75] Shaikh and colleagues conducted two literature reviews to assess the risk of scarring after a first UTI.[147,148] In a systematic review published in 2010, and a meta-analysis with individual patient data published in 2015, they showed that children with reflux were more likely to develop APN and renal scarring than were children without reflux and that children with VUR grades III and higher were more likely to develop scarring than were children with lower grades of VUR.

Antimicrobial Prophylaxis

Although the use of antimicrobial prophylaxis had become routine in the management of children with VUR, substantial controversy currently surrounds this approach, and an increasing amount of literature has challenged its benefit. In 2003, a Cochrane review of the effectiveness of long-term antibiotics for preventing recurrent UTIs in children indicated that most studies published before this date were poorly designed and without proper blinding.[178] Six recent randomized clinical trials have been performed to evaluate the effectiveness of antimicrobial prophylaxis in patients with VUR.[12,24,42,107,121,137] To provide comparable data from these six trials, authors of the 2011 American Academy of Pediatrics (AAP) Clinical Practice Guideline for UTIs contacted the respective researchers and requested raw data from their studies. This allowed creation of a dataset for 1091 infants, 2 to 24 months of age, according to grade of VUR. Table 39.4 and Fig. 39.7 show that there are no significant differences in the rate of recurrences of febrile UTI/APN in young infants, with or without antimicrobial prophylaxis, according to the grade of VUR.[3] This analysis lent support to the recommendation from the AAP in their 2011 guideline against the routine performance of VCUG after a first febrile UTI in children between 2 months and 2 years of age.

A large multisite randomized, placebo-controlled trial involving 607 children with VUR (diagnosed after a first or second febrile or symptomatic UTI) was conducted to determine the effectiveness of antimicrobial prophylaxis (with sulfamethoxazole-trimethoprim) in preventing recurrences of UTI.[53] Secondary outcomes were renal scarring, treatment failure (a composite of recurrences and scarring), and antimicrobial resistance. Two-thirds of enrolled children were 24 months of age or younger; 554 of 607 (91.3%) were enrolled after their first infection, and 85.8% were febrile. A total of 484 of 602 children (80.4%) had grade II or III VUR. Of 126 toilet-trained children, 71 (56.3%) had symptoms of bladder and bowel dysfunction. The overall results showed a reduction of recurrences in the group who received antimicrobial prophylaxis by about 50%; the results were most pronounced in children with lower grades of reflux and bladder and bowel dysfunction and least dramatic in those with higher grades of reflex. In children whose management might be governed by the AAP guideline, the rate of recurrence was approximately 15% in the placebo group and 10% in the prophylaxis group. Overall, eight children would have to be treated for 2 years to prevent one UTI.

No differences were noted in renal scarring between prophylaxis and placebo recipients, although the trial was underpowered to demonstrate a difference. When children in the prophylaxis group developed breakthrough infections, the likelihood of infection with an organism resistant to trimethoprim-sulfamethoxazole was 63% compared to 19% in the placebo group. The results of this study are useful in discussing long-term management of children with febrile UTI with their families and in shared decision making regarding the performance of a VCUG and prescription of prophylactic antimicrobial.

Although the RIVUR study prescribed prophylaxis for 24 months, the duration of prophylaxis is a controversial issue. VUR spontaneously remits in most cases during the first 3 to 5 years of life. Conventional wisdom is that prophylaxis should be maintained until reflux ceases, either spontaneously or with surgical intervention. Greenfield and colleagues[41] suggested that two normal VCUGs performed 12 months apart are necessary before prophylactic antibiotics are discontinued. This recommendation is based on the observation that 27% of children exhibit VUR again after a single normal study.

Greenfield and colleagues[36] maintained that administration of prophylactic antibiotics should continue until reflux resolves, no matter what the age. They supported this position by noting that older children with reflux may have new scars evolve when they become infected. In contrast, other authors suggest that prophylaxis should be discontinued in older children, even if reflux persists.[2,7,22,162,180] The only two antimicrobial agents that are recommended for prophylaxis of the urinary tract are nitrofurantoin and trimethoprim-sulfamethoxazole. Each agent is used in half the usual therapeutic dose and given before bedtime. These two agents can often be used for months to years without the emergence of antibiotic resistance. However some bacteria, such as *Pseudomonas*, are inherently resistant to both agents. In contrast, most other agents that are used for treatment of UTIs are not recommended for prophylaxis. Invariably, if agents such as amoxicillin, cephalexin, and second- and third-generation cephalosporins are used for prophylaxis, infection with resistant strains emerges within weeks.

Surgery

When antireflux surgery is undertaken, a variety of approaches are available, no one of which seems to be superior. In most cases, the surgical approach is intravesicular. Interest has been gaining in evaluation of an extravesicular approach to reimplantation of the ureters.[103] The advantage of extravesicular approaches seems to be a diminution of

TABLE 39.4 Recurrences of Febrile UTI/Pyelonephritis in Infants Aged 2–24 Months With and Without Antimicrobial Prophylaxis, According to Grade of VUR

	PROPHYLAXIS		NO PROPHYLAXIS		
Reflux Grade	*No. of Recurrences*	*Total*	*No. of Recurrences*	*Total*	*P Value*
None	7	210	11	163	.15
I	2	37	2	35	.99
II	11	133	10	124	.95
III	31	140	40	145	.29
IV	16	55	21	49	.14

UTI, Urinary tract infection; *VUR*, vesicoureteral reflux.

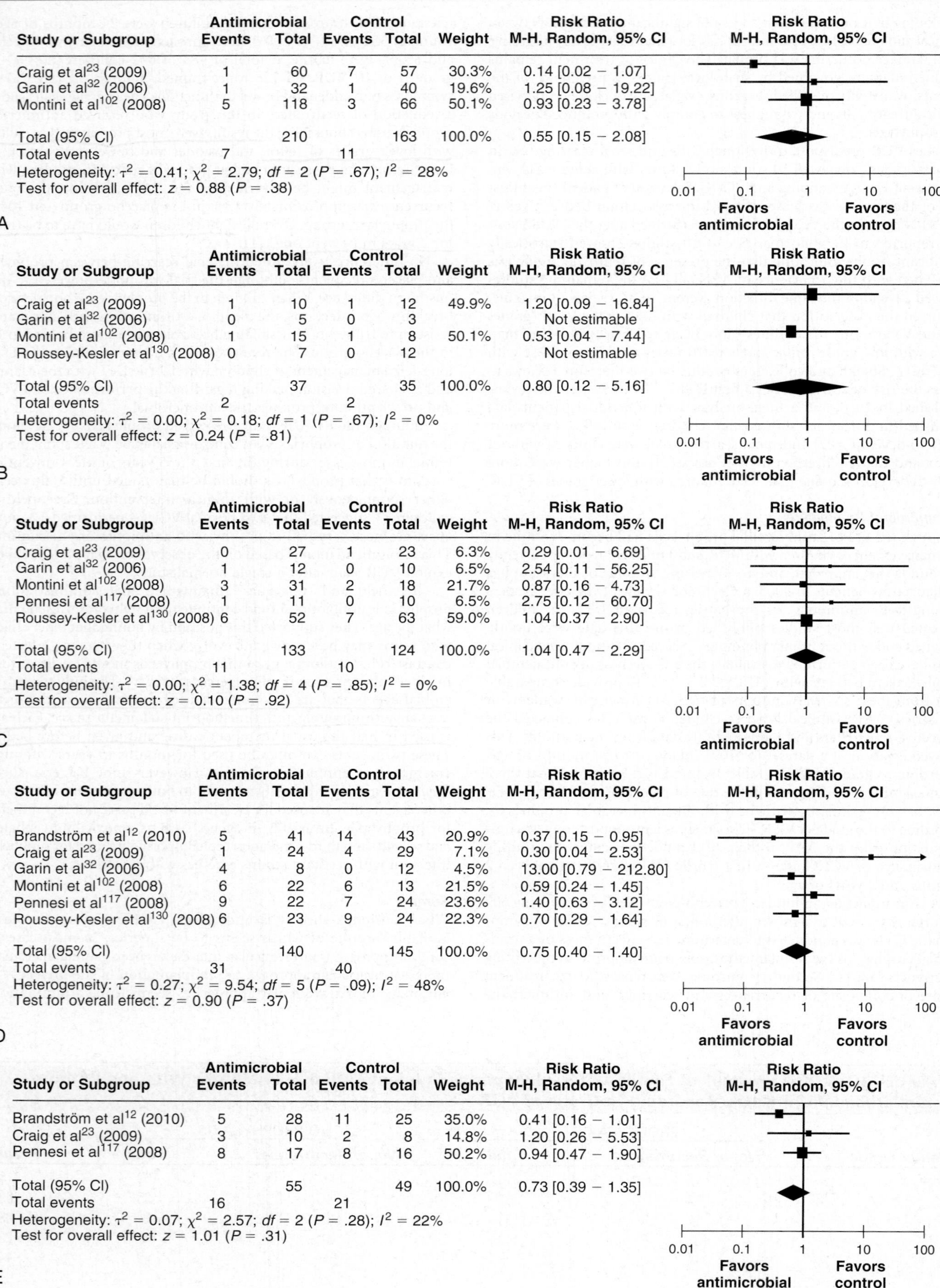
Study or Subgroup | Antimicrobial Events | Total | Control Events | Total | Weight | Risk Ratio M-H, Random, 95% CI
Craig et al[23] (2009) 1 60 7 57 30.3% 0.14 [0.02 – 1.07]
Garin et al[32] (2006) 1 32 1 40 19.6% 1.25 [0.08 – 19.22]
Montini et al[102] (2008) 5 118 3 66 50.1% 0.93 [0.23 – 3.78]
Total (95% CI) 210 163 100.0% 0.55 [0.15 – 2.08]
Total events 7 11
Heterogeneity: $\tau^2 = 0.41$; $\chi^2 = 2.79$; $df = 2$ ($P = .67$); $I^2 = 28\%$
Test for overall effect: $z = 0.88$ ($P = .38$)
Risk Ratio M-H, Random, 95% CI
0.01 0.1 1 10 100
Favors antimicrobial
Favors control
A
Study or Subgroup | Antimicrobial Events | Total | Control Events | Total | Weight | Risk Ratio M-H, Random, 95% CI
Craig et al[23] (2009) 1 10 1 12 49.9% 1.20 [0.09 – 16.84]
Garin et al[32] (2006) 0 5 0 3 Not estimable
Montini et al[102] (2008) 1 15 1 8 50.1% 0.53 [0.04 – 7.44]
Roussey-Kesler et al[130] (2008) 0 7 0 12 Not estimable
Total (95% CI) 37 35 100.0% 0.80 [0.12 – 5.16]
Total events 2 2
Heterogeneity: $\tau^2 = 0.00$; $\chi^2 = 0.18$; $df = 1$ ($P = .67$); $I^2 = 0\%$
Test for overall effect: $z = 0.24$ ($P = .81$)
Risk Ratio M-H, Random, 95% CI
0.01 0.1 1 10 100
Favors antimicrobial
Favors control
B
Study or Subgroup | Antimicrobial Events | Total | Control Events | Total | Weight | Risk Ratio M-H, Random, 95% CI
Craig et al[23] (2009) 0 27 1 23 6.3% 0.29 [0.01 – 6.69]
Garin et al[32] (2006) 1 12 0 10 6.5% 2.54 [0.11 – 56.25]
Montini et al[102] (2008) 3 31 2 18 21.7% 0.87 [0.16 – 4.73]
Pennesi et al[117] (2008) 1 11 0 10 6.5% 2.75 [0.12 – 60.70]
Roussey-Kesler et al[130] (2008) 6 52 7 63 59.0% 1.04 [0.37 – 2.90]
Total (95% CI) 133 124 100.0% 1.04 [0.47 – 2.29]
Total events 11 10
Heterogeneity: $\tau^2 = 0.00$; $\chi^2 = 1.38$; $df = 4$ ($P = .85$); $I^2 = 0\%$
Test for overall effect: $z = 0.10$ ($P = .92$)
Risk Ratio M-H, Random, 95% CI
0.01 0.1 1 10 100
Favors antimicrobial
Favors control
C
Study or Subgroup | Antimicrobial Events | Total | Control Events | Total | Weight | Risk Ratio M-H, Random, 95% CI
Brandström et al[12] (2010) 5 41 14 43 20.9% 0.37 [0.15 – 0.95]
Craig et al[23] (2009) 1 24 4 29 7.1% 0.30 [0.04 – 2.53]
Garin et al[32] (2006) 4 8 0 12 4.5% 13.00 [0.79 – 212.80]
Montini et al[102] (2008) 6 22 6 13 21.5% 0.59 [0.24 – 1.45]
Pennesi et al[117] (2008) 9 22 7 24 23.6% 1.40 [0.63 – 3.12]
Roussey-Kesler et al[130] (2008) 6 23 9 24 22.3% 0.70 [0.29 – 1.64]
Total (95% CI) 140 145 100.0% 0.75 [0.40 – 1.40]
Total events 31 40
Heterogeneity: $\tau^2 = 0.27$; $\chi^2 = 9.54$; $df = 5$ ($P = .09$); $I^2 = 48\%$
Test for overall effect: $z = 0.90$ ($P = .37$)
Risk Ratio M-H, Random, 95% CI
0.01 0.1 1 10 100
Favors antimicrobial
Favors control
D
Study or Subgroup | Antimicrobial Events | Total | Control Events | Total | Weight | Risk Ratio M-H, Random, 95% CI
Brandström et al[12] (2010) 5 28 11 25 35.0% 0.41 [0.16 – 1.01]
Craig et al[23] (2009) 3 10 2 8 14.8% 1.20 [0.26 – 5.53]
Pennesi et al[117] (2008) 8 17 8 16 50.2% 0.94 [0.47 – 1.90]
Total (95% CI) 55 49 100.0% 0.73 [0.39 – 1.35]
Total events 16 21
Heterogeneity: $\tau^2 = 0.07$; $\chi^2 = 2.57$; $df = 2$ ($P = .28$); $I^2 = 22\%$
Test for overall effect: $z = 1.01$ ($P = .31$)
Risk Ratio M-H, Random, 95% CI
0.01 0.1 1 10 100
Favors antimicrobial
Favors control
E

FIG. 39.7 (A) Recurrences of febrile urinary tract infection (UTI)/pyelonephritis in 373 infants, ages 2 to 24 months, without vesicoureteral reflux (VUR), with and without antimicrobial prophylaxis. (B) Recurrences of febrile UTI/pyelonephritis in 72 infants, ages 2 to 24 months, with grade I VUR, with and without antimicrobial prophylaxis. (C) Recurrences of febrile UTI/pyelonephritis in 257 infants, ages 2 to 24 months, with grade II VUR, with and without antimicrobial prophylaxis. (D) Recurrences of febrile UTI/pyelonephritis in 285 infants, ages 2 to 24 months, with grade III VUR, with and without antimicrobial prophylaxis. (E) Recurrences of febrile UTI/pyelonephritis in 104 infants, ages 2 to 24 months, with grade IV VUR, with and without antimicrobial prophylaxis. *CI,* confidence interval; *M-H,* Mantel-Haenszel test.

the intensity and frequency of bladder spasms and less requirement for postoperative analgesia. This technique is indicated primarily in unilateral VUR.[47] When experienced senior surgeons embark on reimplantation of ureters, the outcome usually is successful.[27] Generally all surgical techniques have a high success rate of 92% to 98%.[47] Repeated operation for persistence or recurrence of reflux seldom is required. Rarely when children younger than 2 years old undergo surgery, ureteral obstruction may result; its persistence mandates a second operation.[128]

A newer technique for the management of VUR is endoscopic injection therapy using a variety of materials. Developed as a minimally invasive approach to the treatment of VUR in 1984, dextranomer/hyaluronic acid copolymer (Deflux) has emerged as the favored bulking agent since its approval by the FDA.[46,98] A single injection of Deflux has been shown to correct VUR (decrease grade to 0 or I/V) in approximately 70% of patients, with long-term success rates of 80% to 95% for grades I and II VUR but significantly lower (43% to 73%) for grades III to IV VUR.[14,76] Furthermore, long-term outcome of the procedure has been assessed primarily for reduction in grade of VUR rather than prevention of infection or renal scarring. The bulking agent is injected beneath the ureteral orifice and effectively closes the distal ureter. The procedure is done in the outpatient setting and is associated with less pain and a quicker recovery compared with traditional reimplantation procedures.[98] The success rates are lower, however, than those of traditional therapy, and the results have questionable durability. Long-term prospective studies are necessary to evaluate endoscopic treatments critically.

PROGNOSIS

Generally the short-term prognosis for previously normal children who experience an episode of UTI is excellent. In a large cohort of 306 children experiencing their first febrile episode of UTI, 40% were found to have reflux.[57] Only five (1.6%) of the children had grade IV reflux; none had grade V reflux. Most of the children with grades I, II, and III reflux can be expected to have spontaneous resolution of the process during the subsequent several years. Although many reports indicate that recurrent UTIs are common occurrences in children who have recovered from UTIs, recurrence during the first 6 months after recovery from the index episode of UTI was an infrequent event in this cohort of children. Recurrences in general after a first UTI vary according to the degree of VUR, as shown in Table 39.4.

Recurrence is seen most commonly in the early months after a symptomatic or asymptomatic UTI has occurred.[53] Symptomatic reinfections (fever, pyuria, and positive urine culture) occurred in 7 children treated orally and in 11 children treated intravenously (for a total of 5.9% of 306 children) during the 6-month follow-up period.[57] Asymptomatic bacteriuria (positive urine culture in the absence of fever and pyuria) occurred in 1 child treated orally and in 2 children treated intravenously (1%). Renal scarring occurred in 9.5% of all children; the average percentage of renal parenchymal involvement was 8.2%. In children who had an abnormal renal scintigram at the time of diagnosis, the frequency of scarring was 15.3%. None of the children with a normal renal scintigram at the time of diagnosis developed scars. This experience, reflecting an aggressive approach to the early diagnosis of UTI in infancy, is encouraging with regard to outcome.

Two recent studies have suggested that childhood UTIs are a rare cause of chronic kidney disease.[136,140] Using data from the literature, renal registries, and medical records from a tertiary care hospital, it was concluded that, in the absence of structural kidney abnormalities evident on imaging studies performed after the first UTI, the fraction of recurrent UTI as a main cause of chronic renal disease was small, ranging from 1 in 154 to 3 in 1000 or less. In an editorial commentary, Craig and Williams estimate the risk of a child with a UTI developing end-stage renal disease at 1 in 10,000.[25]

When children with a diagnosis of UTI are found to have anomalies of the urinary tract, congenital dysplasias, or massive degrees of reflux, the prognosis is less optimistic. The most profound degrees of scarring are associated with advanced degrees of reflux. Reflux nephropathy is a major cause of severe hypertension in children and young adults. It occasionally progresses to chronic renal failure,[158] which accounts for approximately 25% of the children in the United Kingdom with end-stage renal failure requiring regular dialysis or transplantation.[87] Although surgical correction may relieve the reflux, the overall outcome for children with reflux who have undergone surgical correction has not been shown to be materially better than that for children who have been managed medically.[115,116,159]

Smellie and colleagues[156] undertook a randomized trial of medical management versus surgical correction in 53 children with bilateral severe VUR and bilateral nephropathy. The glomerular filtration rate of the children at enrollment was 20 mL/min per 1.73 m^2 body surface area. Children with this degree of severity of renal impairment are rare; recruitment to this study took 5 years. No significant differences were observed in glomerular filtration rate, renal growth, or scarring during a 10-year follow-up period. The failure to find differences may be due to the small sample size and broad heterogeneity of the study group. Nonetheless no convincing evidence that outcome for renal function is improved by surgical correction of VUR in children with bilateral disease exists.

PREVENTION

Primary prevention of UTI can be accomplished in infant boys by promoting the practice of circumcision. Whether this procedure can be justified simply to prevent UTIs in the context of social rituals is uncertain. Circumcision should be recommended, however, for selected groups of patients, including newborns with prenatal hydronephrosis who are found to have VUR in the neonatal period, boys with high grades of VUR, and boys in whom VUR is associated with unilateral renal agenesis or multicystic kidney.[15]

Other commonly recommended strategies to prevent UTI, such as the avoidance of bathing in tubs or swimming and the instruction in correct wiping techniques, are not accompanied by convincing evidence.[48] The relationship between constipation and UTI is well known. Effective treatment of constipation results in normalization of bladder function and cessation of UTIs.[93]

The role of prophylactic antibiotics for patients with VUR was discussed previously in the section on treatment. Prophylaxis has been shown in large, prospective, placebo-controlled, randomized trials to reduce by one-third to one-half the frequency of UTI in children 2 to 72 months of age with a first febrile UTI. The application of these results to the management of children and their impact on the discussion to perform a VCUG depend on many variables.[53] These might include the presence or absence of a family history of VUR, age, sex, race, the severity and course of the initial infection, bladder and bowel dysfunction, cost of VCUG, importance that parents place on preventing recurrences, perceived parental ability to adhere to prophylaxis, and parental concerns about side effects of prophylaxis or imaging procedures.[53]

An additional preventive strategy for UTI is immunization. A small pilot study was reported from Turkey.[110] Ten otherwise healthy girls aged 5 to 11 years old with recurrent UTIs were immunized with inactivated uropathogenic bacteria intramuscularly once a week for 3 consecutive weeks. A booster injection was given after 6 months. The frequency of infection was compared with that in a group of 10 age-matched girls with UTIs who were not immunized. Immunization therapy caused a significant reduction in the frequency of infection and an increase in the concentration of the secretory component of IgA in the urine. Other mucosa, such as vaginal and oral surfaces, are alternative targets for vaccine delivery.

A vaginal mucosal vaccine composed of a mixture of heat-killed bacteria from 10 human uropathic strains (six *E. coli* and four other gram-negative enteric bacteria) was developed for women with recurrent UTIs.[166] Fifty-four women completed a double-blind, placebo-controlled, phase II trial. Time until reinfection was longest for women who received primary and booster immunization compared with women receiving a placebo. This strategy has potential for further development.

Sublingual immunization with a commercial preparation of an inactivated bacterial vaccine comprised of *E. coli, Klebsiella pneumoniae, Proteus vulgaris,* and *Enterococcus faecalis* delivered by aerosolization (2 puffs/day) has been studied as a preventive strategy. When compared to antibiotic prophylaxis in an adult female population of individuals with recurrent UTI, it showed dramatically significant differences favoring immunization.[99]

NEW REFERENCES SINCE THE SEVENTH EDITION

17. Cerwinka WH, Grattan-Smith JD, Jones RA, et al. Comparison of magnetic resonance urography to dimercaptosuccinic acid scan for the identification of renal parenchyma defects in children with vesicoureteral reflux. *J Pediatr Urol.* 2014;10:344-351.
25. Craig JC, Williams GJ. Denominators do matter: it's a myth – urinary tract infection does not cause chronic kidney disease. *Pediatrics.* 2011;128:984-985.
26. Davis KF, Colebaugh AM, Eithun BL, et al. Reducing cathether-associated urinary tract infections: a quality-improvement initiative. *Pediatrics.* 2014;134:e857-e864.
53. Hoberman A (for the RIVUR trial investigators). Antimicrobial prophylaxis for children with vesicoureteral reflux. *N Engl J Med.* 2014;370:2367-2376.
99. Lorenzo-Gómez MF, Padilla-Fernández B, García-Criado FJ, et al. Evaluation of a therapeutic vaccine for the prevention of recurrent urinary tract infections versus prophylactic treatment with antibiotics. *Int Urogynecol J.* 2013;24:127-134.
102. Marin JR, Shaikh N, Docimo SG, et al. Suprapubic bladder aspiration. *N Engl J Med.* 2014;371:e13.
134. Robino L, Scavone P, Araujo L, et al. Intracellular bacteria in the pathogenesis of *Escherichia coli* urinary tract infection in children. *Clin Infect Dis.* 2014;59:e158-e164.
135. Rosen DA, Hooton TM, Stamm WE, et al. Detection of intracellular bacterial communities in human urinary tract infection. *PLoS Med.* 2007;4:1949-1957.
147. Shaikh N, Borrell JL, Evron J, et al. Procalcitonin, C-reactive protein, and erythrocyte sedimentation rate for the diagnosis of acute pyelonephritis in children. *Cochrane Database Syst Rev.* 2015;(1):CD009185.
148. Shaikh N, Ewing AL, Bhatnagar S, et al. Risk of renal scarring in children with a first urinary tract infection: a systematic review. *Pediatrics.* 2010;126:1084-1091.

The full reference list for this chapter is available at ExpertConsult.com.

40 Renal Abscess

Sheldon L. Kaplan

Although acute pyelonephritis is a common infection in children, the primary development of a renal abscess or progression of pyelonephritis to a renal or perinephric abscess is an uncommon occurrence. In one study conducted over a 10-year period, eight children with a renal abscess were found among 43,224 discharge diagnoses—approximately one case per 5400 pediatric admissions.[6] Six of the eight children were 11 years or older. In a study from a children's hospital in Taiwan, 45 children were found to have a renal abscess over a 10-year period.[7] In a third study from the Children's Medical Center of Dallas, 36 children were identified with a renal or perinephric abscess between 2000 and 2010.[21] The median age of the patients in this report was 9.3 years (range, 0.3–17 years). Although rare, renal abscesses have been reported in neonates.[12] Renal abscess may be a primary problem (i.e., one that develops in a kidney without an antecedent infection or underlying anatomic abnormality), or it may occur secondarily in a patient with previously recognized acute pyelonephritis or in a child with congenital urologic abnormalities known to predispose to the development of pyelonephritis.

A primary renal abscess is thought to develop most often after an episode of bacteremia and frequently occurs in younger children. Hematogenous spread of bacteria to the kidney usually results in a cortical abscess.[6] The most common organisms involved in these abscesses are gram-positive cocci, primarily *Staphylococcus aureus* and less often *Streptococcus* spp. In some cases, a cutaneous infection might have been present before development of the renal abscess, and this infection is thought to be the primary source for the bacteremia.[19] Most children in whom a renal abscess develops hematogenously are normal hosts.[6,14,26,28] *Bartonella henselae* has been reported to cause microabscesses in the kidney, presumably by the hematogenous route.[20]

In older children and teenagers, tuberculous abscesses and caseous necrosis of the renal parenchyma also should be included in this primary classification. These infections tend to be indolent, although renal tuberculosis may be complicated by bacterial infection because of associated ureteral strictures and severe tuberculous cystitis.

When a renal abscess occurs in association with a recognized urologic disorder, the organism responsible most often is a gram-negative bacillus or an enterococcus, bacteria usually seen in simple urinary tract infections (UTIs) and pyelonephritis.[22,25] In the Dallas study, *E. coli* alone was isolated in 44% and in combination with other organisms in another 6% of the 36 patients.[21] *Enterobacter aerogenes, Proteus mirabilis, Citrobacter* spp. and *Klebsiella* spp. together accounted for about 10% of the isolates in this study. No organism was identified in 22% of patients. Examples of urologic disorders that one might encounter with these infections include congenital and acquired obstructions (e.g., ureteropelvic and ureterovesical obstruction, retrocaval ureter, ureteral stricture after surgical intervention), calculous disease (obstructing and nonobstructing), infundibular stenosis, and renal dysplasia with cystic changes. Abscesses that occur as a result of infection of the urinary tract generally are found in a corticomedullary location.[6]

Anaerobic organisms also have been implicated as a cause of renal abscess. They often are present simultaneously with the more usual aerobic bacteria, but they can cause infections and abscesses alone. These anaerobic renal infections develop most commonly in association with infections complicating bowel injury or surgery, renal transplantation, malignancy, and orodental infections.[5] *Bacteroides fragilis* is likely to arise from an intraabdominal source, whereas an oral site is more common for *Prevotella oralis.*[5]

Children with human immunodeficiency virus infection seem to have an increased risk for development of renal abscesses from the more common traditional organisms[4] and from unusual opportunistic fungal organisms, especially *Aspergillus.*[17] As expected, these children also tend to have a more fulminant course that often requires extensive surgical intervention and drainage.

The presence of a renal abscess implies the destruction and liquefaction of tissue in a confined space. Two other infectious disorders of the kidney, xanthogranulomatous pyelonephritis and acute lobar nephropathy (acute focal bacterial nephritis), frequently are included in this general

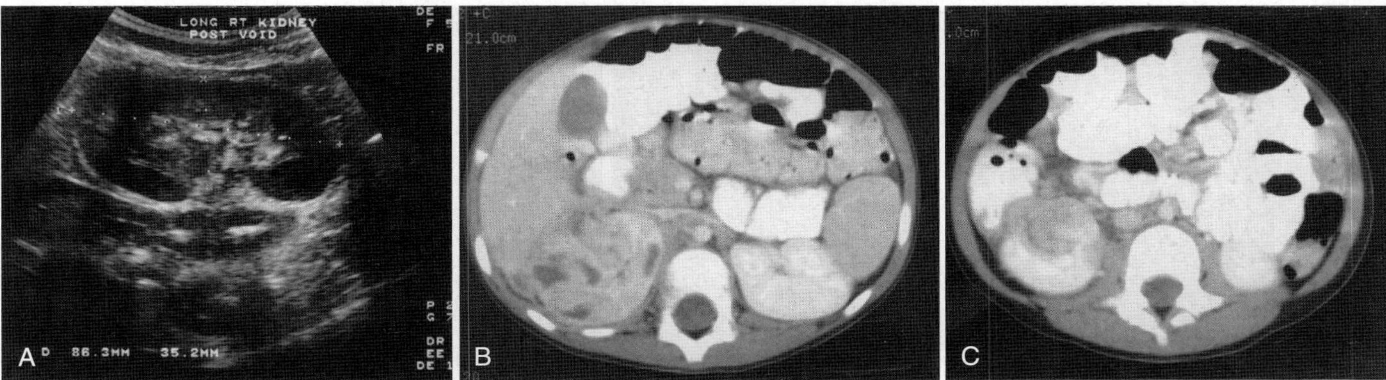

FIG. 40.1 Acute lobar nephropathy in a 3-year-old girl with fever, right flank pain, and urinary tract infection. (A) Initial renal ultrasonogram shows enlargement and swelling of the right upper pole. (B) Initial upper pole cuts by computed tomography show poor uptake of contrast media and differing tissue densities. (C) More caudal cuts reveal better function in the right lower pole. The infection and swelling resolved completely with antibiotics alone, with no evidence of postinfectious atrophy. This case was thought to represent acute lobar nephropathy.

category, although technically true abscesses do not always develop in these disorders. Acute lobar nephropathy may progress to renal abscess, however, if not treated appropriately.

Xanthogranulomatous pyelonephritis describes a more chronic form of severe renal parenchymal destruction that often is associated with chronic stone disease. The process may involve the whole kidney or may be focal. In children, the focal form occurs more commonly. The pathognomonic histologic finding is an accumulation of lipid-laden macrophages that coalesce into discrete yellow nodules. Small abscess cavities often are studded throughout the kidney. The organism most frequently recovered from the kidney is *Proteus,* and urinary calculi are common findings. Although these patients often have acute symptoms, the symptoms frequently are superimposed on more chronic manifestations, such as weight loss, failure to thrive, and anemia. Treatment is complete or partial nephrectomy because the renal destruction generally is severe.[27]

Acute lobar nephropathy describes a focal area of intense edema at the site of infection in acute pyelonephritis.[3] It usually is recognized as a mass effect on an initial screening renal ultrasonogram. Severe nephromegaly (renal length >3 standard deviations above the mean for age) is another finding on renal ultrasound suggestive of acute lobar nephropathy.[8] Computed tomography (CT) of the kidney shows poor uptake in the involved segment but no well-defined liquefaction (Fig. 40.1). Whether this edema is just an exaggerated response to infection or represents a change before an abscess is unknown. Klar and colleagues[16] described 13 children, 4 months to 8 years of age, with acute lobar nephropathy in a prospective study during a 4-year period. Bacteremia was documented in only one child. Evolution to abscess formation occurred in four (31%). In another prospective study, Cheng and associates[9] found bacteremia occurred in four of 80 children (5%) with acute lobar nephropathy. In further studies these investigators noted that patients with acute lobar nephronia who had CT findings with heterogeneously decreased nephrographic density after contrast enhancement were more likely to develop a renal abscess than those with a homogeneous decrease in density.[10] These lesions generally heal satisfactorily with administration of antibiotics alone.

CLINICAL FINDINGS

Children with acute renal or perirenal abscess typically are febrile and have localized pain in the costovertebral location.[15] Prolonged fever is a common finding, especially in older children. Most patients are febrile for longer than 7 days before the diagnosis is established. A clue to the diagnosis is persistence of symptoms and fever in a child being treated appropriately for an acute UTI. The initial findings generally do not differentiate, however, between acute pyelonephritis with and without an abscess. If the abscess has spread into the perinephric region, it may be possible to recognize psoas muscle irritation in the patient—that is, the patient is more comfortable with the ipsilateral leg in a position of flexion and experiences pain with full extension. A large abscess may be palpable as a flank mass.

Findings on urinalysis can be confusing. With a primary (hematogenous) abscess, the urine may be deceptively benign, and culture generally is negative.[19] Blood cultures may be positive, depending on the duration of the illness when blood is obtained for culture. Abscesses associated with underlying urologic disorders can be expected to contain organisms and pyuria. Generally, severe leukocytosis is present. The erythrocyte sedimentation rate and C-reactive protein typically are elevated.[21,28] All of these findings are nonspecific, however, and often further studies are needed to establish the diagnosis. If a more indolent process is encountered, appropriate testing and cultures for tuberculosis should be considered.

DIAGNOSTIC EVALUATION

All children admitted to the hospital with a febrile UTI should undergo renal ultrasonography as soon as is reasonable after admission.[23] The findings on this initial study can have a significant effect on the choice of therapeutic options. If both kidneys are normal and unobstructed, organism-specific therapy is satisfactory in most patients. If significant obstruction or stones are present, antibiotic therapy may not be as effective, and interventional drainage may become necessary if the response to antibiotics is inadequate. At the time of this initial screening study, findings may suggest the presence of a renal abscess. Such findings include a mass effect within the margins of the kidney, along with a thickened wall and material of varying sonographic density within the mass (Fig. 40.2). Similar findings can be seen in infections accompanied by severe ureteropelvic junction obstruction or infundibular stenosis with isolated calyceal dilation, in which case purulent material within the dilated collecting system layers out and can mimic a renal abscess (Figs. 40.3 and 40.4). Nephromegaly on ultrasonography also has been found to be a clue to recognizing a renal abscess with subsequent CT imaging studies.[7]

When the diagnosis of an abscess is suspected on ultrasonography, performing CT of the involved kidney may provide further information.[13] CT more clearly defines the margins of the abscess, assesses whether loss of function is significant, and can screen the remainder of the kidney for small satellite abscesses.[24] If loss of function in the affected kidney seems to be significant, a dimercaptosuccinic acid renal scan should be done because it is an even more sensitive test to quantitate overall renal function. If CT suggests the diagnosis, percutaneous aspiration can confirm clearly whether an abscess is present without having to perform additional studies and, at the same time, provide material for culture.

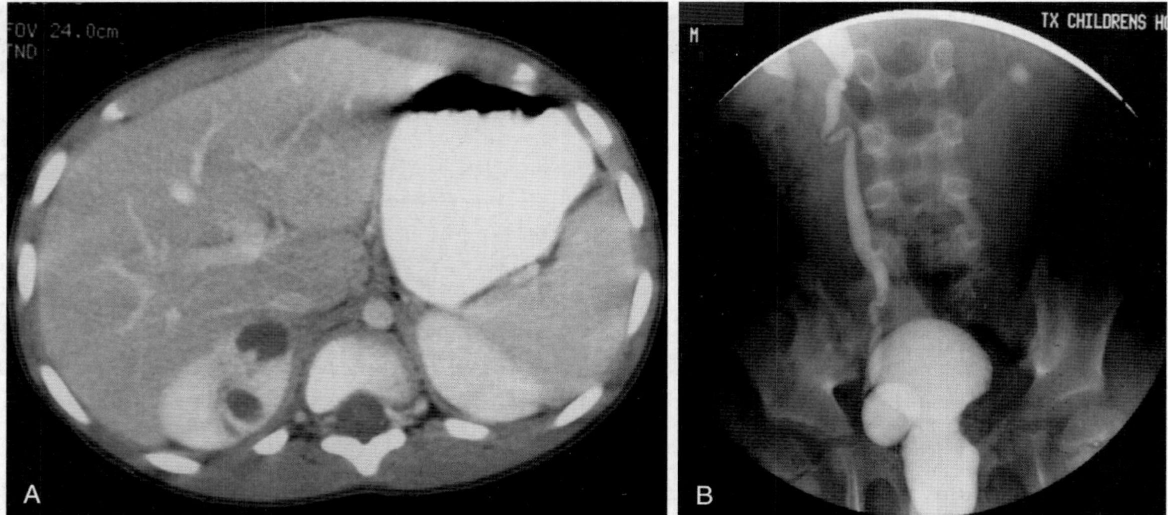

FIG. 40.2 Renal abscess (secondary) in a 6-month-old boy with urinary tract infection. A screening renal ultrasonogram showed a small mass in the right kidney. (A) Computed tomography shows two clearly defined cystic areas consistent with small parenchymal abscesses. Treatment consisted of intravenous antibiotics only. (B) Voiding cystogram revealed the presence of vesicoureteral reflux.

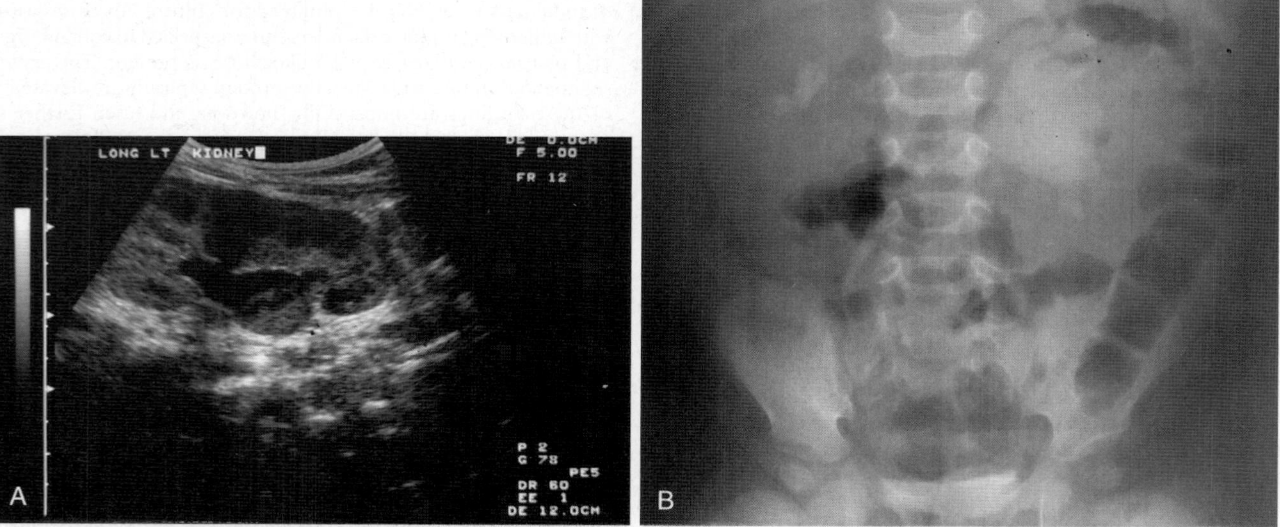

FIG. 40.3 Pyonephrosis associated with ureteropelvic junction obstruction in a 3-month-old boy with fever, left abdominal and flank tenderness, and urinary tract infection. (A) Renal ultrasonogram shows a medially placed cystic mass with layered fluids of different density consistent with purulent material. The position of the mass is most consistent with the renal pelvis. (B) Intravenous pyelogram confirms ureteropelvic junction obstruction. This infant was treated initially with percutaneous nephrostomy drainage in addition to appropriate antibiotics.

If a child with a UTI and a previously normal result on renal ultrasonogram is taking culture-specific antibiotics and a new fever subsequently develops, ultrasonography should be repeated. A previously small, unrecognized abscess may have been treated inadequately and now may be more apparent.

Occasionally imaging studies cannot distinguish between a renal abscess and severe acute lobar nephropathy. The latter condition also may show tissues of differing density by ultrasonography or CT. In these situations, ultrasonography- or CT-guided percutaneous aspiration of the lesion may be necessary to determine whether purulent material can be obtained.

THERAPEUTIC CONSIDERATIONS

When the diagnosis of an abscess is confirmed, the choice of therapeutic options is dictated by several factors including the overall status of the patient, the size and number of abscesses, whether the abscess appears to be unilocular or septate, associated uropathies, and the extent of renal function in the involved kidney. Included in these considerations is some insight into the responsible organism. If it is a solitary abscess in a child with unimpressive urinalysis findings and an otherwise normal kidney, one should suspect a staphylococcal abscess, which can be confirmed by percutaneous aspiration, Gram stain, and culture. If bacteremia caused by *S. aureus* possibly was nosocomial in origin, or

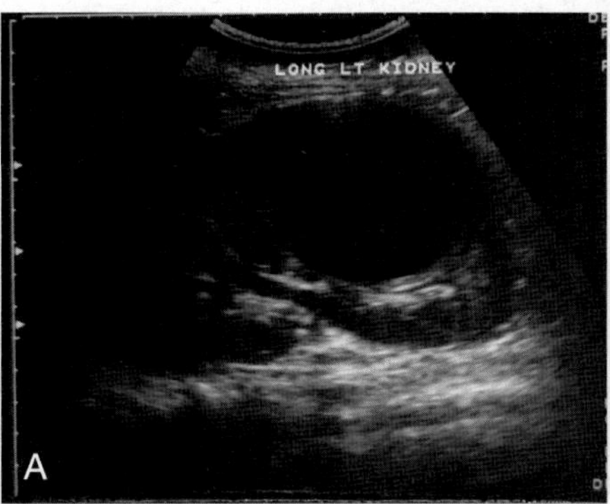

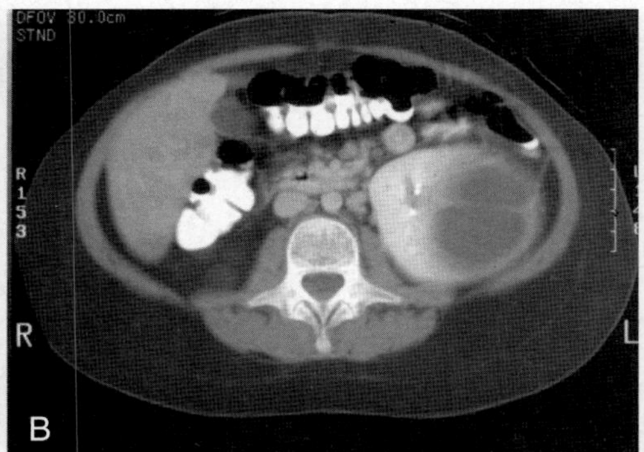

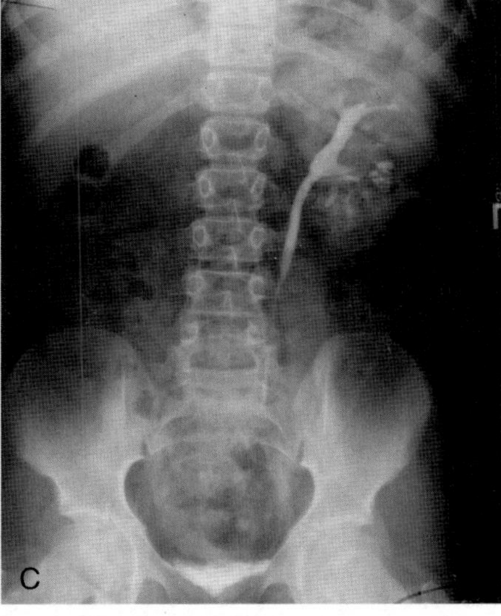

FIG. 40.4 Renal abscess complicating infundibular stenosis in a 10-year-old girl with low-grade fever, marked left costovertebral angle tenderness, leukocytosis, and pyuria but a negative urine culture (she had received outpatient antibiotics). The right kidney was absent. (A) Sonogram of the left kidney revealed a large cystic mass with septa. (B) The mass was confirmed by computed tomography. (C) Intravenous pyelogram obtained after resolution of the abscess (by percutaneous and open drainage) reveals anomalous development of the lower infundibulum and calyces.

if methicillin-resistant *Staphylococcus aureus* isolates are found commonly in the community, antibiotics such as vancomycin or clindamycin should be included in the initial empiric regimen.

Subsequent therapy is based on the antibiotic susceptibility pattern of the organism isolated. If urinalysis reveals an obvious infection, one can assume that the urine culture reflects the organism responsible for the abscess. In this situation, empiric therapy is directed against gram-negative enteric organisms. Cefotaxime, ceftriaxone, or ceftazidime would be suggested. The only caution is if the abscess is complicated by significant stone disease. In this situation, more than one organism may be in the urinary tract, and urine culture alone may be misleading. Percutaneous aspiration can identify accurately the organism responsible for the abscess. The optimal duration of antibiotic therapy for treatment of a renal abscess is not established, but 3 weeks of treatment is superior to 2 weeks for acute lobar nephropathy.[9]

Renal abscesses traditionally have been managed by open surgical drainage. With the introduction of safe percutaneous access, particularly when used with ultrasonography or CT guidance, single unilocular lesions now can be managed effectively with percutaneous placement of an indwelling catheter that allows not only for primary drainage but also for irrigation of the cavity with appropriate antibiotic solutions.[2,16] Small and moderate-sized renal abscesses have been treated successfully with antibiotics alone; some authors have commented that medical therapy alone may be more likely to result in successful treatment if the abscess size is 3 cm or smaller.[1,18,26] In the Dallas study, 20 of 22 patients with a renal or perinephric abscess of smaller than 3 cm were treated successfully with antibiotics alone.[21] Several patients in this series with an abscess of larger than 3 cm were also treated successfully with antibiotics alone. In another study from Italy, six children (median age, 31 months; range, 13–104 months) with renal abscesses were all successfully treated with antibiotics alone.[11] The median size of the abscesses in this study was 3.8 cm (range, 2.5–4.5 cm). If the child does not improve with medical therapy alone, some type of drainage procedure is indicated. When function is insufficient to justify renal salvage and ultimate nephrectomy is planned, a short course of specific antibiotics and percutaneous drainage is initiated if the abscess is large, to decrease inflammation in the perinephric tissues and to reduce the possibility of causing bacteremia at the time of surgery.

When required, surgical repair of associated congenital anomalies of the urinary tract generally is performed at a separate session after the abscess has resolved. Reconstructive surgery in the presence of active infection significantly increases the risk for development of surgical complications and the possibility that additional surgical procedures might be required.

CONCLUSION

Treatment of renal abscess today is multifaceted, and each case must be individualized. In addition to culture-specific antibiotics, treatment may include observation only, percutaneous drainage, or open surgical drainage. Diagnostic evaluation, including renal ultrasonography, CT, and percutaneous aspiration, generally can confirm that an abscess is present and assist in the decision regarding therapeutic options.

NEW REFERENCES SINCE THE SEVENTH EDITION

1. Angel C, Shu T, Green J, et al. Renal and peri-renal abscesses in children: proposed physio-pathologic mechanisms and treatment algorithm. *Pediatr Surg Int.* 2003;19:35-39.
11. Comploj E, Cassar W, Farina A, et al. Conservative management of paediatric renal abscess. *J Pediatr Urol.* 2013;9:1214-1217.
15. Jacobson D, Gilleland J, Cameron B, et al. Perinephric abscesses in the pediatric population: case presentation and review of the literature. *Pediatr Nephrol.* 2014;29:919-925.
21. Seguias L, Srinivasan K, Mehta A. Pediatric renal abscess: a 10-year single-center retrospective analysis. *Hosp Pediatr.* 2012;2:161-166.

The full reference list for this chapter is available at ExpertConsult.com.

41 Prostatitis

Sheldon L. Kaplan

Prostatitis, a major source of chronic infection and symptoms in men, occurs rarely in prepubertal children. Although prostatitis may develop in postpubertal teenagers, even in this age group the diagnosis is recognized infrequently. The disorder commonly termed *prostatitis* generally is divided into four separate clinical problems based on the National Institutes of Health Classification of prostatitis: acute bacterial prostatitis, chronic bacterial prostatitis, chronic prostatitis and chronic pelvic pain syndrome, and asymptomatic inflammatory prostatitis.[11] This chapter will focus on acute or chronic bacterial prostatitis.

Acute prostatitis is a severe infection generally associated with significant toxicity (high fever, systemic symptoms such as malaise, chills, nausea, and vomiting).[21] Marked urinary symptoms, such as frequency, suprapubic pain, dysuria, hematuria, and urinary retention, may be present. On rectal examination, the prostate is enlarged, boggy (edematous), and exquisitely tender. The urine usually is infected. Care must be taken when performing the rectal examination or when inserting a transurethral catheter because bacteremia can result. The white blood cell count and inflammatory markers are usually elevated. Urinalysis is abnormal, and urine culture is positive in the majority of cases. Bacteremia has been reported in up to 20% of patients, and blood cultures may be positive when urine cultures are negative.[6]

The organism responsible usually is one of the gram-negative pathogens that commonly causes urinary tract infection (UTI). *Escherichia coli* is most commonly isolated, but other pathogens include *Proteus mirabilis*, *Pseudomonas aeruginosa*, and *Klebsiella* and *Enterococcus* spp., among others.[3] *Neisseria gonorrhoeae* is a consideration in sexually active males. Community-associated methicillin-susceptible as well as methicillin-resistant *Staphylococcus aureus* isolates have been isolated rarely from patients with a prostatic abscess.[5,20]

The virulence factors of *E. coli* strains recovered from men with acute prostatitis and women with UTIs, such as adhesins and cytotoxins, were similar in one study.[17] Johnson and colleagues[8] found, however, that prostatitis *E. coli* isolates differed significantly from *E. coli* associated with cystitis or pyelonephritis by having a higher prevalence of the genes encoding P fimbriae structural subunits, P fimbriae assembly, fimbriae tip pilins, hemolysin, and cytotoxic necrotizing factor, and a lower prevalence of the gene encoding invasion of brain endothelium virulence factor. In a study of *E. coli* isolates from 18 previously healthy young men with acute bacterial prostatitis, Krieger and colleagues[10] reported that most isolates fell within the family of considered extraintestinal pathogenic *E. coli* (ExPEC) and carried a median of 12.5 virulence genes, characteristic of ExPEC gene clusters. Rarely *Trichomonas vaginalis* can cause prostatitis.

If the patient is not systemically ill, in adults a quinolone such as ciprofloxacin or levofloxacin or trimethoprim-sulfamethoxazole is generally recommended because these agents have been more carefully studied for this indication than oral cephalosporins.[16] These same agents also are reasonable for male adolescents. Modification of antibiotic therapy is based on the organism isolated and its antibiotic susceptibilities. The duration of treatment is generally 14 to 28 days. If the patient is more seriously ill, parenteral therapy is recommended. Empiric treatment generally begins with administration of broad-spectrum β-lactam agents, such as cefotaxime or piperacillin-tazobactam possibly combined with an aminoglycoside, that are effective against gram-negative enteric organisms pending the availability of culture-proven sensitivity results and a satisfactory clinical response. Once the patient has clearly improved and is stable, therapy can be completed with an oral agent such as a fluoroquinolone or trimethoprim-sulfamethoxazole based on susceptibility results.

Patients with suspected acute bacterial prostatitis who are receiving appropriate antibiotics but are not improving should undergo further evaluation.[9] Ultrasound may reveal evidence of abscess formation. Computed tomography or magnetic resonance imaging may provide more detailed information on the size and location of a prostate abscess. Drainage by an interventional radiology procedure or transurethral unroofing may be required to adequately treat a prostatic abscess.

Chronic bacterial prostatitis is a more indolent infection associated with intermittent UTI, bladder irritative symptoms, and perineal discomfort. Recurrent urethritis or epididymitis may be present. Ejaculation may be painful. Expressed prostatic secretions usually show an increase in the white blood cell count. Common organisms associated with chronic bacterial prostatitis are similar to those causing acute bacterial prostatitis, including *Klebsiella* spp., *E. coli*, *P. mirabilis*, *P. aeruginosa*, and *Enterococcus faecalis*.[21] *E. coli* isolates associated with chronic prostatitis possess urovirulence profiles similar to those of strains from women with acute uncomplicated pyelonephritis.[1]

The diagnosis of chronic bacterial prostatitis is related partly to detecting inflammation in expressed prostatic secretions. More precise methods of determining inflammatory parameters, such as counting the white blood cells per cubic millimeter with a hemocytometer, have been proposed.[18] In a large cohort study, the severity of symptoms in men with chronic prostatitis did not correlate with leukocyte or bacterial counts, however.[22]

Chronic bacterial prostatitis accounts for only a small fraction of men with chronic prostatitis syndromes. The cause of nonbacterial chronic prostatitis and chronic pelvic pain syndrome remains enigmatic. Prostatic secretions do not show a common organism consistently, and UTI does not recur. Culture of prostatic secretions is notoriously unreliable because of the means by which this material is collected; these secretions are contaminated easily as they pass through the urethra.[16] A specific causal relationship in nonbacterial prostatitis has not been found for either *Ureaplasma urealyticum* or *Chlamydia trachomatis,* two organisms commonly implicated in urethritis.[23] Molecular studies using polymerase chain reaction have shown DNA evidence of the presence of bacteria despite negative cultures for the typical bacteria associated with prostatitis. Using these new techniques may lead to greater understanding of the role of infection in the pathogenesis of prostatitis.

Treatment of chronic bacterial prostatitis is frustrating because few patients truly are cured, and relapse occurs commonly after discontinuation of antibiotic therapy. Several studies have confirmed satisfactory concentrations of most common antibiotics in prostatic tissues,[7,12,13,15] but no study has provided a convincing explanation for the high treatment failure rate. Levofloxacin and other fluoroquinolones penetrate well into seminal and prostatic fluids and reach concentrations equivalent to corresponding plasma levels.[4] Researchers have postulated that antibiotic concentrations may be inadequate within the acini of the prostatic glands and their secretions, but this theory has not been proved.[19] Typically, fluoroquinolones for 4 to 6 weeks of administration are the agents of choice for treating chronic bacterial prostatitis.[14]

In the older age group still seen in a pediatric practice, symptoms similar to those of the chronic form of prostatitis also might occur with urethritis. As noted earlier, *Chlamydia* and *Ureaplasma* spp. commonly are found in the urethral discharge in these patients[2] and are thought to be responsible for these specific symptoms. These organisms also have been implicated as a cause of epididymitis in young men. The organisms are transmitted sexually and are treated effectively with a tetracycline (minocycline or doxycycline) or a macrolide (erythromycin or azithromycin).[24] To prescribe these drugs empirically for sexually active young adults with lower tract irritative symptoms and clinical findings consistent with urethritis while awaiting culture results seems reasonable.

CONCLUSION

Prostatitis as it is seen and described in adults is a rare event in pediatric patients. When it does occur, it affects pubertal adolescents. Even in these patients, distinguishing true prostatitis from simple urethritis may be difficult.

Appropriate evaluation of an adolescent boy with a lower urinary tract infection generally begins with renal ultrasonography. Special attention should be directed to the region of the bladder and prostate. With this imaging modality, the presence and normalcy of both kidneys, the degree of thickening of the bladder wall, the ability of the bladder to empty, and whether any cystic masses are located behind the bladder or prostate can be assessed. Any obvious abnormality justifies obtaining a voiding cystourethrogram. A thickened detrusor or recurrence of infection suggests the possibility of urethral obstruction. Although properly performed voiding cystourethrography does image the entire urethra, other diagnostic tests might include retrograde urethrography or determination of the urinary flow rate, especially if a urethral stricture is suspected. Performing cystoscopy usually is unnecessary if all imaging study results are normal, although cystoscopy may be used to confirm, and sometimes manage, obvious urethral obstruction.

NEW REFERENCES SINCE THE SEVENTH EDITION

5. Dubose M, Barraud O, Fedou A-L, et al. Prostatic abscesses and severe sepsis due to methicillin-susceptible *Staphylococcus aureus* producing Panton-Valentine leukocidin. *BMC Infect Dis*. 2014;14:466.
9. Kiehl N, Kinsey S, Ramakrishnan V, et al. Pediatric prostatic abscess. *Urology*. 2012;80:1364-1365.

The full reference list for this chapter is available at ExpertConsult.com.

Genital Infections 42

Mariam R. Chacko • Heather E. Needham • Charles R. Woods Jr

This chapter reviews female genital tract infections in the pediatric and adolescent age groups. An initial review of normal vaginal microenvironment in the prepubertal, pubertal, and postpubertal period is followed by a section on lower genital tract infection in the prepubertal, pubertal, and postpubertal period. This section addresses infections of the external genital area, including vulvovaginitis; infections of the clitoris, urethra, and Bartholin ducts and glands; vulvovaginal lesions; ulcerative and granulomatous disorders; and infections of the cervix. Upper genital tract infections are rare in the prepubertal age group; thus, discussion of pelvic inflammatory disease (PID), tubo-ovarian abscess, and oophoritis, which follows, is predominantly addressed for the postpubertal period. Additional information on the microbes and the specific detailed treatment recommendations can be found in the respective chapters on each pathogen. Genital infections associated with pregnancy are not addressed in this chapter.

GENERAL APPROACH TO EVALUATION OF PREPUBERTAL CHILD

When genital tract symptoms are present in young girls, the history should include information about the manner and circumstances surrounding the onset of the complaint, the characteristics of any discharge, the duration of symptoms, whether the problem is recurrent, and the nature of any recent treatments or medications. Information should be elicited regarding the use of bubble baths, enuresis, history of atopic dermatitis or allergies, anal pruritus (associated with pinworm infection), recent respiratory or skin infections in family members, and hygienic practices. The possibility that the child may have had or has a systemic disorder affecting the genitalia should be explored.

Sexual abuse also must be considered when a child has a genital infection, regardless of the nature of the infection or the socioeconomic status of the family. This concern is particularly relevant when the child has a sexually transmissible disease. Sexual abuse and infection may occur without penile penetration of the vagina. The history of vaginal or penile discharge in other family members should be ascertained. Behavioral changes, nightmares, fears, abdominal pain, headaches, and enuresis can be indicators of abuse or other psychosocial stressors.[11] The possibility of nonsexual transmission of these diseases often is raised, particularly when a preliminary investigation cannot elicit a history of sexual abuse. Two or three interviews with abused children often are required to enable them to provide informative reports.[154] Forensic interviews by experts in child abuse are essential in these cases.[216]

A general physical examination should precede assessment of the genital tract. The gynecologic examination begins with abdominal inspection and palpation followed by external examination of the perineum and genitalia, including the vulva, urethral meatus, clitoris, hymen, and anus. The examination should be done with the child in the supine, frog-leg position. The labia can be retracted gently to visualize the anterior of the vagina. Speculum and bimanual examinations generally are inappropriate in prepubertal children.[74,192] Note should be made of structural abnormalities, inflammation, sores and ulcerations, and excoriations. If complaints consist only of vulvitis, and findings on external examination are limited to a scanty mucoid discharge and an erythematous introitus, further examination generally is unnecessary.[76]

If the vaginal discharge is purulent, persistent, or recurrent, a thorough gynecologic assessment is warranted. Visualization of the vagina and cervix without instrumentation is possible with the child in the prone knee-chest position.[74,129] This method is useful in children older than 2 years. In this position, with labial traction, the vaginal muscles relax and stretch the hymenal membrane open. An otoscope head or a magnifying lens with a good wall light is used to visualize the cervix. Because the vagina of a prepubertal child is short, a foreign body or a lesion may be seen.[74]

A rectal examination may be important when persistent discharge, bleeding, or pelvic or abdominal pain is present. The rectal examination may help express discharge from the vagina that previously was not recognized and can permit palpation of hard foreign bodies or abnormal masses.

Visualization with instrumentation (vaginoscopy) is required in some situations. General anesthesia may be required for girls who are small or unable to cooperate or who may experience significant anxiety or discomfort during the procedure. Conscious sedation for the procedure may be an option in some situations. When a purulent, persistent, or recurrent vaginal discharge is present, samples should be obtained for culture and Gram stain. Wet mount preparations may be useful if fungal infection (potassium hydroxide preparations) or pinworms are suspected. Saline wet mount may be indicated for trichomoniasis if sexual abuse is suspected. Urinalysis with microscopic examination should be

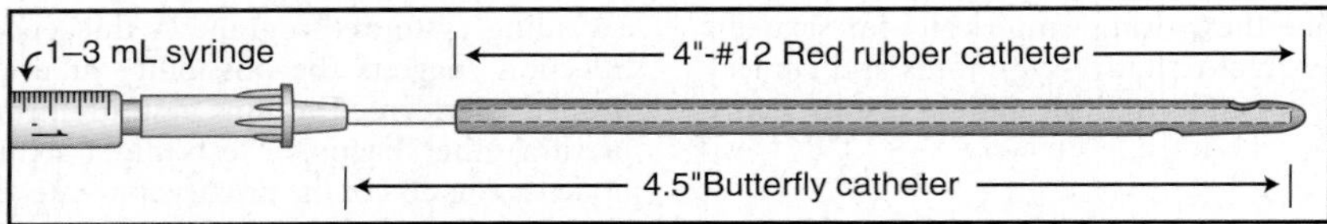

FIG. 42.1 Assembled catheter-within-a-catheter for obtaining specimens from a prepubertal child. (From Pokorny SF, Stormer J. A traumatic removal of secretions from the prepubertal vagina. *Am J Obstet Gynecol.* 1987;156:581.)

performed. A complete blood cell count may be useful when pyogenic infection is suspected or bleeding has occurred.

When cultures are indicated, separate vulvar and vaginal specimens may be necessary. The type and duration of discharge and considerations of potential sexual abuse influence this decision. Vulvar specimens alone may be appropriate when etiologies such as group A streptococci are suspected. Exudates emanating from the vagina in prepubertal girls also are adequate specimens for evaluation for gonorrhea, such that vaginal swabs or aspirates are not required. Further information on types of specimens required for specific sexually transmitted infections (STIs) such as gonorrhea or *Chlamydia trachomatis* is provided in Chapters 89 (gonorrhea) and 194 (*C. trachomatis*).

Options for obtaining vaginal specimens in young girls, when needed, include use of (1) a nasopharyngeal Dacron swab moistened in nonbactericidal saline, inserted carefully through the hymenal opening; (2) a catheter-within-a-catheter technique (Fig. 42.1)[192]; or (3) a sterile newborn suction catheter, with insertion 2 to 3 cm into the vagina.[242] For the catheter-within-a-catheter technique, the distal 4 inches of a soft, size 12 bladder catheter and the proximal 4 inches of butterfly needle intravenous tubing are excised from their parent devices by sterile technique. The catheter-within-a-catheter is inserted into the vagina, and fluid is flushed in and out of the upper part of the vagina several times before final aspiration into the syringe and removal of the device.

NORMAL VAGINAL FLORA

The lower female genital tract is colonized by nonpathogenic bacteria from birth. Throughout life, this colonization is dynamic and complex. Even in the pre-microbiome assessment era, a wide range of aerobic and anaerobic species were cultured from asymptomatic girls. The results of several modern but pre-microbiome studies of vaginal flora in childhood are summarized in Table 42.1. The majority of recent vaginal microbiome data to date has come from studies of adults and older adolescents.

The vagina and its microbial flora form an ecosystem that changes over time from infancy to childhood to adolescence and adulthood.[116] The major forces that influence these changes are fluctuations in estrogen levels and the advent of sexual activity. Hygienic practices and medications, including oral contraceptives and antimicrobial agents, also affect the complex interactions among the various flora present in the vagina in terms of persistence, predominance, and overgrowth.

Most girls harbor several organisms in the vagina at any given time. Younger adolescents have a greater prevalence of anaerobic bacteria than do women. From puberty, aerobic colonization increases with age, onset of sexual activity, and parity.[151] Vaginal specimens obtained for culture during anesthesia for elective surgery from 19 healthy girls aged 3 months to 5.7 years yielded a mean of 12 bacterial species.[117] Anaerobes predominated, with a mean of 8.7 species versus 3.4 aerobic species. In a series of 25 asymptomatic girls aged 2 months to 15 years, a mean of 8.7 different species (approximately four aerobes and five anaerobes) per vaginal specimen were detected.[102] Another series of adolescents and young adults aged 13 to 21 years in which only aerobic flora were evaluated noted a mean of approximately three organisms in non–sexually active subjects versus six in sexually active patients.[222] These numbers of culture-detected species are certainly underestimates in most instances. This heterogeneity in vaginal microflora during childhood and adolescence is similar to that found in women.[150]

TABLE 42.1 Vaginal Organisms Isolated From Asymptomatic Girls Aged 2 Months to 16 Years

Organism	%[a]
Coagulase-negative staphylococci	35–73
Diphtheroids	14–78
Streptococcus viridans	13–39
Enterococci	29–62
Group B streptococcus	5–11
Group D streptococcus	
Staphylococcus epidermidis	
Staphylococcus aureus	
Streptococcus pneumoniae	
Micrococcus spp.	
Gaffkya (Aerococcus) spp.	
Lactobacillus spp.	10–39[b]
Escherichia coli	12–67
Klebsiella spp.	15–52
Enterobacter spp.	
Proteus spp.	3–5
Pseudomonas aeruginosa	5–6.5
Citrobacter spp.	
Haemophilus influenzae	
Neisseria spp. other than gonococci	
Moraxella (Branhamella) catarrhalis	
Flavobacterium spp.	
Alcaligenes spp.	
Acinetobacter spp.	
Mycoplasma hominis	
Ureaplasma urealyticum	
Gardnerella vaginalis[c]	
Peptostreptococcus spp.	29–56
Peptococcus spp.	39–76
Veillonella spp.	
Eubacterium spp.	
Propionibacterium acnes	
Bacteroides fragilis	
Bacteroides melaninogenicus	
Other *Bacteroides* spp.	
Prevotella spp.	
Bifidobacterium spp.	
Clostridium perfringens	
Other *Clostridium* spp.	
Fusobacterium spp.	
Candida spp.	3–18
Other yeasts	
Actinomyces spp.	

[a]Percentage range when the organism was isolated from patients in at least two studies. If no range is present, the organism was isolated from 3% to 33% of patients in a single study.
[b]In one series, 88% of girls were >11 years.
[c]Isolated in numerous cases without discharge.
Data from references 50, 75, 102, 111, 117, 151, 150.

Gram-negative enteric bacteria and enterococci commonly are encountered in infants and toddlers before completion of toilet training but less frequently thereafter.[102,117] In children, lactobacilli are present more often in girls younger than 2 years than in older prepubertal girls. Lactobacilli are the predominant flora in most girls by the end of adolescence and may play a protective role in limiting the overgrowth of other flora.[116] The vaginal flora of most healthy women is dominated by one or more *Lactobacillus* spp., but a substantial minority may harbor other predominant flora, including *Atopobium vaginae, Bifidobacterium, Gardnerella, Prevotella, Pseudomonas,* or *Streptococcus,* in the absence of lactobacilli.[123,134]

Genital mycoplasmas were found in 17% of one series of young girls who were not suspected of having been sexually abused.[105,222]

Among women of reproductive age, several patterns of vaginal flora have been identified, with variation noted by race/ethnicity. These include a predominance of *L. crispatis, L. iners, L. jensenii,* and *L. vaginalis*; a predominance of *L. gasseri* and *L. vaginalis*; and a predominance of *A. vaginae* and *G. vaginalis* with none or few lactobacilli, a more bacterial vaginosis-like pattern.[134] In a study of the vaginal microbiome of 31 healthy premenarcheal girls aged 10 to 12 years, lactobacilli were dominant in most before menarche. *G. vaginalis* was found in one third of the girls.[115] As observed in adults, the vaginal flora changed over time, including variations in the relative quantities of different lactobacillus species in the same subject. Vulvar microbiota of the premenarcheal girls mirrored their vaginal flora but typically had more bacterial taxa overall.[115]

Microbes that usually behave as commensals sometimes are associated with vulvovaginitis. The difference between colonization and disease is at least partially a function of the magnitude of the replication and the quantity of a given bacterial species. For example, in women with bacterial vaginosis in which *G. vaginalis* is a predominant microbe, colony counts generally are greater than 10^7 colony-forming units (CFU)/g of vaginal fluid. Asymptomatic colonization with *G. vaginalis* usually is associated with colony counts of less than 10^5 CFU/g of vaginal fluid.[151] Alteration in the vaginal microenvironment by factors such as poor hygiene, foreign bodies, or hormonal fluctuations results in loss of environmental constraints on bacterial replication and facilitates the overgrowth of one or more commensals.

LOWER GENITAL TRACT INFECTIONS

This section includes the following topics according to anatomic areas: vulvovaginitis; infections of the clitoris, urethra, and vulvar glands; genital lesions, ulcerations, and granulomatous infections; and cervicitis. Each topic addresses the prepubertal and postpubertal aspects of infections where relevant.

Vulvovaginitis

Prepubertal

Infections and inflammation of the vulva and vagina account for 85% to 90% of all genital problems in prepubertal girls. These conditions are encountered most commonly in children 2 to 7 years old.[191,203] Infections of the vulva and vagina usually occur together and generally are considered one entity—vulvovaginitis. The various types of vulvovaginitis are differentiated by determining the presence or absence of specific microbial or other agents associated with the inflammation in a particular case. Vulvovaginitis accounts for greater than 80% of cases of recurrent vaginal discharge in prepubertal girls.[168]

Genital discharge does not always indicate infection or inflammation. Most female infants have a grayish white, mucoid discharge from the vagina during the newborn period. This discharge consists of desquamated vaginal mucosa and cervical epithelium that has undergone hypertrophy because of prenatal stimulation by placental and maternal hormones. Microscopic examination of the material reveals masses of large, superficial vaginal epithelial cells (Fig. 42.2). The condition may last for several weeks, is not pathogenic, and does not require treatment.

Similarly, a pubertal girl nearing menarche may develop a copious viscous, transparent secretion that exudes from the vagina. This normal state sometimes raises concern about possible vaginal infection. The vulvar and vaginal tissues appear thick and moist, a sign of increased estrogen stimulation, without erythema. Microscopic examination of the vaginal fluid reveals masses of estrogenized superficial vaginal epithelial cells and few leukocytes (Fig. 42.3).

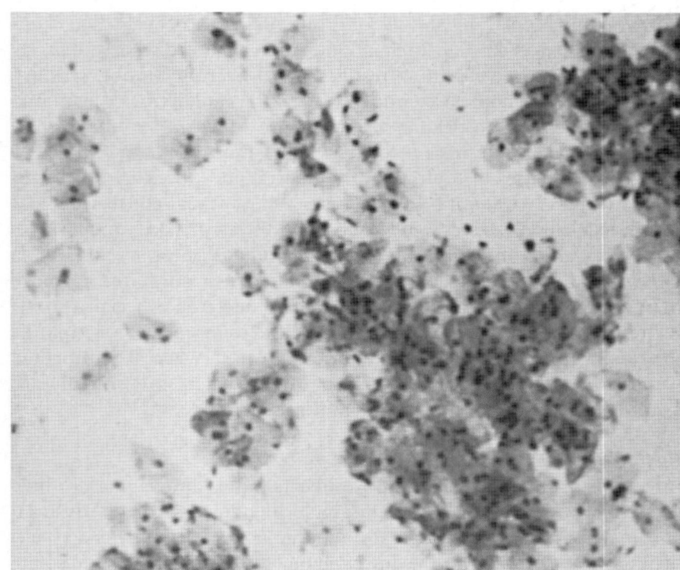

FIG. 42.2 Cytosmear from the vaginal discharge of a newborn.

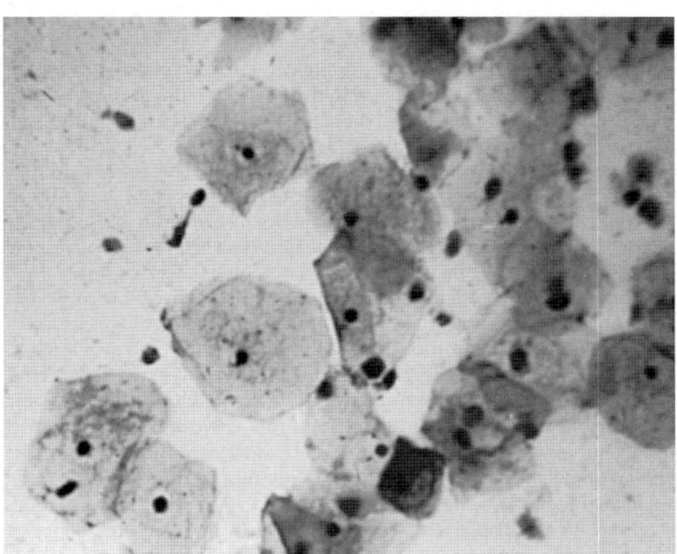

FIG. 42.3 Cytosmear from the vaginal secretion of a pubertal girl. Masses of epithelial cells and few bacteria or leukocytes attest.

Genital discharge and perineal or vulvar discomfort are the most common symptoms of vulvovaginitis.[76,191,229] The discomfort may range from minor pain or soreness to intense perineal burning or pruritus. Genital erythema is the most common sign in girls, and vulvovaginitis can be found in more than 80% of cases. Visible discharge is present in one third of cases.[191] Infections of the vulva and vagina are more likely to be accompanied by moderate or severe inflammation and prominent discharge than is nonspecific vulvovaginitis.[131] Infection can be present at times, however, with neither discomfort nor discharge.

The characteristics of the discharge frequently do not help identify a specific cause. At the onset of an infection, the discharge is often thick, purulent, and profuse. It may become scanty and seropurulent in later stages of infection.[75] Discharges that are odorless and bloody or serosanguineous may result from noninfectious conditions, such as vulvar irritation, trauma, precocious puberty, urethral prolapse, and tumor.

Vulvovaginitis caused by *Shigella* or group A streptococci also can cause bleeding, as can an eroding foreign body. Foul-smelling discharge suggests a foreign body but also may result from a necrotic tumor. Urinary leakage from an ectopic ureter opening into the genital tract may mimic a vaginal discharge. Specific diagnoses are made more often when symptoms have been present for less than 1 month.[258]

In several series of 80 to 500 prepubertal and pubertal girls up to age 12 with vulvovaginitis and no suspicion of sexual abuse, the most common bacterial isolates were groups A and B streptococci, *Staphylococcus aureus,* and nontypable *Haemophilus influenzae, Escherichia coli, P. mirabilis,* and enterococci.[38,59,168,198,242] Anaerobes were found in more than half of patients in one series.[168] These bacteria, especially group A streptococci, causing vulvovaginitis may lead to more severe symptoms that result in care being sought soon after onset, whereas pathogenic bacteria generally are less likely to be found when girls initially are examined after several weeks of symptoms.

Postpubertal

Infections of the pubertal and postpubertal vulva and vagina produce a variety of overlapping symptoms, including vulvar pruritus, dysuria, and increased or altered vaginal discharge and spotting.[21] As a result, distinguishing among various lower genital tract infections based solely on symptoms is difficult. The history, physical examination, and laboratory tests play an important role in assisting the clinician in differentiating urethritis, vaginitis, and cervicitis.

Nonspecific Vulvovaginitis

Nonspecific vulvovaginitis is a frequently encountered condition in prepubertal girls and is addressed in this section. Nonspecific vaginitis in postpubertal females is called bacterial vaginosis and is addressed in its respective section in this chapter.

Prepubertal. Nonspecific vulvovaginitis is responsible for 25% to 75% of cases of vulvovaginitis diagnosed in the prepubertal age group in referral centers.[258] In most cases, as noted in Box 42.1, identifiable secondary factors contribute to nonspecific vulvovaginitis. The presence of specific genital tract bacterial or viral pathogens excludes this diagnosis.

Poor hygiene with subsequent overgrowth of a mixed aerobic and anaerobic bacterial flora that are typically nonpathogenic on mucosal surfaces is the most common cause of premenarcheal vulvovaginitis.[188] Contact irritation and allergic reactions induced by soaps, detergents, and medications are frequent causes of vulvovaginitis. Some systemic diseases and focal skin disorders may mimic vulvovaginitis or allow it to develop as a secondary process when these conditions involve the vulvar or perineal tissues.[82] Chronic vulvitis in young girls is often associated with atopic dermatitis or psoriasis.[83] Anatomic abnormalities also may be associated with vulvovaginitis. An increased incidence of vulvovaginitis and urinary tract infections has been reported in girls with high posterior commissures.[265] Drainage from an ectopic ureter into the vagina can cause chronic vulvovaginitis and lead to the formation of a vaginal calculus. Labial adhesions were present in 7% of girls with vulvovaginitis in one series.[191] Box 42.1 outlines the causes of vulvovaginitis in premenarcheal girls.

Several factors other than those listed in Box 42.1 contribute to the occurrence of vulvovaginal infections in young children. The developing immature labia minora and majora flare outward as a young girl squats or sits. As a result, they do not protect the vestibular and vulvar mucosae from contamination, as occurs later in life. The nonestrogenized, prepubertal vulvar and vaginal epithelium, which consists of only a few layers of cells, is traumatized easily and infected readily; however, no evidence suggests that estrogen deficiency is a causative factor in premenarcheal vulvovaginitis. The alkaline vaginal reaction during childhood also is not as resistant to infection as is the acidic vaginal secretion of postmenarchal girls and women.

Vulvovaginitis secondary to poor perineal hygiene. A vulvovaginal infection is considered secondary to poor perineal hygiene when bacteria native to the lower gastrointestinal tract are found in properly obtained cultures from the vagina. In a large series of cases of vulvovaginitis subjected to culture, *E. coli* or other coliform organisms were found in 70% of patients in the series.[111] Other studies also have found a higher prevalence of *E. coli* and other enteric organisms in vaginal cultures from girls with vulvovaginitis than in asymptomatic controls.[76] Reappearance and disappearance of premenarcheal vulvovaginitis secondary to poor perineal hygiene are related directly to the appearance and disappearance of coliform organisms in vulvovaginal cultures. The primary role of vulvar and vaginal contamination with fecal material as a result of inadequate cleansing after defecation is supported by the observation that symptoms resolve in most cases when proper perineal hygiene is the only treatment recommended. In children, 15% to 20% have recurrences, usually 1 month or more after resolution of the initial episode. In most instances, recurrences can be attributed to poor perineal hygiene.[47,111]

Children with nonspecific vulvovaginitis secondary to poor perineal hygiene do not have any uniform historical findings. On examination, the vulvar mucosa and outer third of the vagina usually are hyperemic with associated scant, light gray, mucoid discharge. Many children wipe themselves from back to front after defecation. In girls, this practice easily results in fecal contamination of the vulvar area. Fecal soiling around the anus or on the perineum or in undergarments can be a clue to the etiology.

Proper cleansing of the perineum and anus after defecation and sitz baths lead to the resolution of symptoms and infection in most cases. Sitz baths (warm water with or without colloidal oatmeal or baking soda) 10 to 15 minutes in duration should be taken 2 to 6 times per day, depending on the severity of the vulvovaginal inflammation.[76] For intense inflammation, wet compresses with Burow solution (1:40) or plain water applied every 3 to 4 hours may be used instead of sitz baths.[5] In mild cases, the vulva may be washed twice per day with water or a mild, unscented, nonmedicated soap. Witch hazel pads may be used for cleansing after defecating and to provide mild analgesia.[227]

Loose-fitting clothing should be worn for several days to a few weeks after the symptoms resolve. Continued wearing of such clothing also may be helpful in preventing recurrences of vulvovaginitis, especially in warmer climates. Instructing parents on proper perineal and vulvar cleansing when girls are bathed decreases the likelihood that nonspecific vulvovaginitis will develop. Young girls should be taught proper hygiene and that they should wash their hands before and after urinating and defecating. Shampooing the hair while sitting in a bathtub and using harsh soaps, bubble baths, or other preparations that might lead to chemical irritation of the vulvar skin and vaginal mucosa should be avoided throughout the course of vulvovaginitis.[19,33] The application of powders should be avoided, at least until the acute symptoms have resolved.

As the inflammation and exudate subside over 1 to 2 days, sitz baths may be reduced in frequency and alternated two to four times per day with the application of either calamine lotion or protective ointments, such as zinc oxide. If pruritus is a significant symptom, an oral agent such as hydroxyzine or diphenhydramine may be administered. Topical application of 1% hydrocortisone cream or triamcinolone acetonide cream may be used as the inflammation resolves but should be avoided in the acute phase.[227]

Patients who do not improve after 2 to 3 days of hygienic measures should be reevaluated. Specimens taken from the vagina should be sent for aerobic and anaerobic bacterial cultures if these were not done initially. Intractable nonspecific vulvovaginal infections that are not caused by foreign bodies, intestinal parasites, or poor perineal hygiene are encountered occasionally. Reducing vaginal pH from an alkaline or neutral to an acid reaction often helps in these difficult cases and may be achieved by the local use of estrogen. Topical estrogens are not recommended for the treatment of routine cases of premenarcheal vulvovaginitis because the results do not seem to be superior to nonhormonal therapies in these cases,[111] and prolonged administration may cause isosexual pseudoprecocity. After 7 to 10 days, the vulvar and vaginal tissues usually thicken, and a mucoid vaginal secretion may appear.

Oral or parenteral antibiotics may be indicated if symptoms persist for 2 to 3 weeks or if a specific pathogen that requires antibiotic treatment is isolated. When possible, selection of antibiotic agents and the route of administration should be based on susceptibility testing of organisms isolated from vaginal cultures. Nonspecific vulvovaginal infections generally are benign, superficial, localized mucosal inflammations that usually respond to less potent chemotherapeutic agents when these are needed.

BOX 42.1 Etiologic Factors in Premenarcheal Vulvovaginitis

Bacterial Infections

Nonspecific mixed infections secondary to:
- Poor perineal hygiene
- Foreign body in vagina
- Respiratory tract infections
- Skin infections (impetigo)
- Urinary tract infection

Specific nonvenereal infection:
- Hemolytic streptococci (groups A, B, F)
- *Escherichia coli*
- *Shigella flexneri, Shigella sonnei*
- *Neisseria meningitidis, Neisseria sicca*
- *Haemophilus influenzae* type b, nontypeable strains
- *Streptococcus pneumoniae*
- *Corynebacterium diphtheriae*
- *Yersinia enterocolitica*
- *Mycobacterium tuberculosis*
- *Moraxella (Branhamella) catarrhalis*
- *Staphylococcus aureus*

Specific venereal infections:
- *Neisseria gonorrhoeae*
- *Treponema pallidum*
- *Chlamydia trachomatis*
- Chancroid (*Haemophilus ducreyi*)
- Granuloma inguinale

Bacterial vaginosis:
- *Gardnerella vaginalis*
- *Mobiluncus* species

Fungal Infections

Candida albicans
Other yeasts
Dermatophytes

Protozoan and Parasitic Infections

Trichomoniasis
Amebiasis
Enterobius vermicularis
Hirudiniasis
Schistosomiasis
Other parasitic infections (ascariasis, trichuriasis)

Viral Infections

Venereal:
- Herpes simplex
- Condyloma acuminatum (papillomavirus)
- Molluscum contagiosum

Involvement as part of systemic infection:
- Measles
- Varicella
- Mononucleosis (Epstein-Barr virus)
- Coxsackievirus
- Smallpox

Infestations

Pediculosis
Scabies

Contact Irritation or Allergic Reactions

Bubble bath preparations
Hair shampoos
Vulvar deodorant sprays
Soaps, laundry detergents
Other medications

Vulvar or Perineal Skin Diseases

Local:
- Seborrhea
- Lichen sclerosus et atrophicus
- Lichen planus
- Lichen simplex chronicus
- Premalignant leukoplakia
- Erythrasma (*Corynebacterium minutissimum*)
- Bartholinitis
- Skenitis

Involvement as part of a systemic disorder:
- Psoriasis
- Bullous pemphigoid
- Atopic dermatitis
- Drug eruption
- Generalized pruritus with excoriation
- Chronic liver disease
- Chronic renal disease
- Metabolic errors
- Psychosomatic
- Crohn disease
- Sjögren syndrome
- Henoch-Schönlein purpura
- Histiocytosis
- Kawasaki disease
- Stevens-Johnson syndrome
- Typhoid
- Zinc deficiency

Physical Factors

Sand (sandbox)
Chemical or thermal trauma
Physical trauma (accidents, abuse, masturbation)
Nylon, rayon underclothing
Tight garments (maceration in warm climates)

Anatomic abnormalities:
- Neoplasms (sarcoma botryoides)
- Polyps
- Labial agglutination, adhesion
- Prolapsed urethra
- Ectopic ureter
- Rectal fistula
- Draining pelvic abscess via fistula

Data from references 9, 25, 56, 55, 75, 82, 121, 149, 198, 229.

Vulvovaginitis secondary to intestinal parasites. Pinworms (*Enterobius vermicularis)* are the causative factor in many cases of recurrent or intractable nonspecific vulvovaginitis in children.[47,76] Infection occurs when the worms in the lower bowel crawl out of the anus onto the perineum and migrate into the vagina, where they deposit ova. The pinworms may carry *E. coli* and other coliform bacteria into the vagina, which may lead to vulvovaginitis.

Pinworm ova may be deposited in playground soil, on toys or books, and on the hands of infected individuals. Infection frequently is asymptomatic. A child with a pinworm infection and vulvovaginitis usually has a history of a chronic vaginal discharge that has recurred despite repeated attempts to eradicate it. Parents may note worms on the perineum of the child and that she awakens at night because of perineal itching.

Examination reveals a low-grade inflammation of the vulva and vagina. Excoriations from scratching may be seen on the perineum. Vaginoscopy (if indicated) shows an inflammatory reaction extending to, but not including, the cervix. Vaginal cultures produce a mixed growth of nonpathogenic bacteria, with *E. coli* and other coliform bacteria generally predominating.

The diagnosis depends on finding pinworm ova on smears from the perineum or in the vaginal discharge or a report from parents that worms are visible on the child's perianal skin. A perineal smear is most likely to show the presence of pinworms, but pinworm ova of *E. vermicularis* may be detected in a wet smear of vaginal secretions (pinworms, Fig. 42.4).

The adhesive tape test can be performed in the office or the parent asked to collect three specimens at night. The parent is given a wooden tongue blade or paddle with adhesive tape and a glass microscopic slide (Fig. 42.5). The adhesive side is applied firmly to several areas around the anus. It is removed and applied, adhesive side down, to the glass slide, which is sent to the laboratory for examination.

Treatment consists of eradicating the pinworms. All members of the family are presumed to be infected and should be treated. Recommended treatment regimens are mebendazole 100 mg orally; albendazole 400 mg orally; or pyrantel pamoate 11 mg/kg base, not to exceed 1 g. Each is given in a single dose and repeated in 2 weeks. The vulvovaginitis caused by coliform organisms carried on pinworms is treated the same as in other cases of nonspecific vulvovaginitis caused by poor perineal hygiene (see earlier discussion).

Vulvovaginitis secondary to vaginal foreign bodies. Foreign bodies account for approximately 4% of cases of vaginal discharge in premenarcheal girls.[8] When a foreign body remains in the vagina for some time, it inevitably causes nonspecific vulvovaginitis. Many types of vaginal foreign bodies, including safety pins, glass beads, coins, beans, bits of crayon, and parts of toys, have been reported. The most common objects are bits of toilet paper or shreds of cloth from nightclothes or bedding (Fig. 42.6).[113,121]

The history does not contribute to the diagnosis unless the child is known to have previously put objects in her vagina. The child usually is brought to a physician because of a profuse, foul-smelling, sometimes blood-tinged discharge. The presence of such a discharge is almost pathognomonic for the presence of a foreign body. Even without a profuse discharge or bleeding, a foul odor from the vagina suggests a foreign body. In addition a foreign body should be suspected when a recurrent discharge is reported.

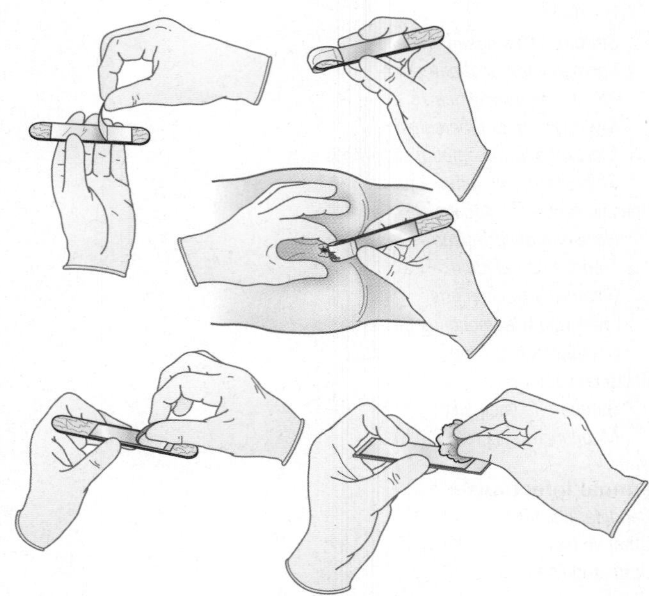

FIG. 42.5 Technique for obtaining a perianal smear for detection of pinworm ova, using adhesive tape and a tongue depressor.

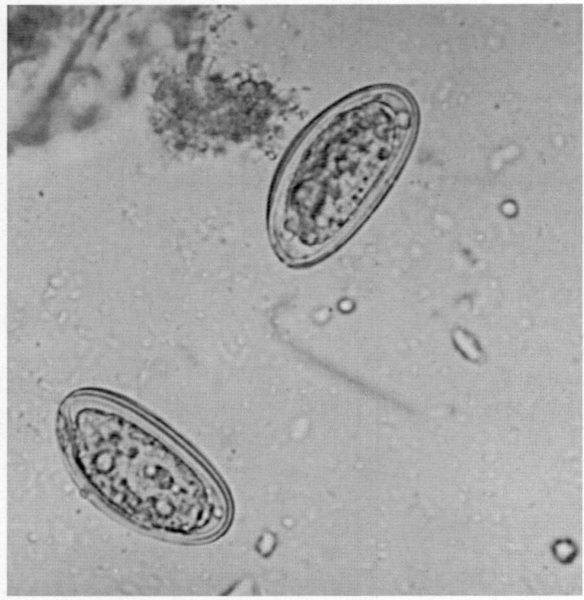

FIG. 42.4 Pinworm ova discovered in a vaginal smear from a child with intractable vulvovaginitis.

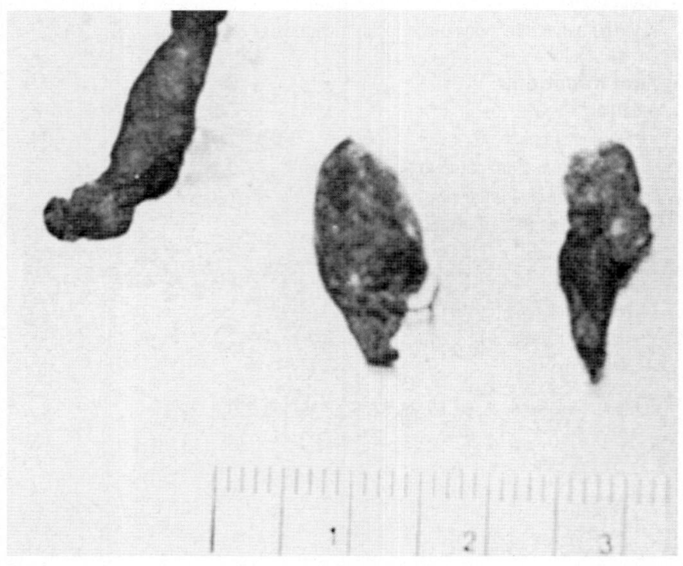

FIG. 42.6 Bits of paper or cloth are the vaginal foreign bodies most frequently found in children.

Examination reveals inflammation of the vulvar and vaginal mucosa. Soft foreign bodies, such as toilet paper, can be flushed out of the vaginal canal. Although foreign material may be seen when the labia are separated, a vaginoscopy may also be necessary to explore the full length of the vagina. A topic anesthetic agent such as xylocaine jelly can be helpful in such situations. Rarely a metallic object that has been in the vagina for some time erodes the mucosa and becomes hidden in granulation tissue. When such a condition is suspected, a radiograph should be obtained. Most foreign bodies, such as glass, plastics, paper, or cloth, are not radiopaque, however, and radiographic examination fails to detect the foreign material. An examination under anesthesia may also be necessary when a larger foreign body has to be extracted.

The nonspecific vulvovaginitis caused by a foreign body disappears gradually after removal. Recovery can be hastened by using the hygienic treatments previously described. Repeat episodes are common.

Specific Non–Sexually Transmitted Vulvovaginitis

Vulvovaginitis secondary to respiratory pathogens

***Streptococcus pyogenes* (group A *Streptococcus*) vulvovaginitis.** *Streptococcus pyogenes* is a frequent cause of vulvovaginitis in premenarcheal girls and accounted for 9% to 20% of cases in several series.[55,56,67,111,148,198,229,241] Most cases occur in girls aged 2 to 7 years, but cases in infants and teenagers have been reported.[26,67,91,241] Group B and group F streptococci also have been isolated from girls with acute vulvovaginitis.[223] A marked seasonal variation in incidence in some geographic regions, with peak rates occurring in late fall and winter, may explain the low number of cases of vulvovaginitis caused by *S. pyogenes* in some series.[81,171] The nasopharynx seems to be the primary reservoir for *S. pyogenes* in these girls. Infection may occur from self-inoculation by hand to nose to the vulvovaginal area.[218] The skin also may serve as the source of *S. pyogenes* vulvovaginitis.[91,241] Preceding or concurrent symptoms of upper respiratory tract infection are uncommon findings, but many girls with vulvovaginitis have throat cultures positive for *S. pyogenes*.[91,241] Perineal symptoms have preceded pharyngeal symptoms in some patients.[81] *S. pyogenes* vulvovaginitis may occur during the course of scarlet fever.[26,110,111]

The signs and symptoms of *S. pyogenes* vulvovaginitis often overlap those caused by other bacterial infections, but symptoms usually are abrupt in onset. Most patients seek medical care within 1 week of onset. Vaginal discharge and dysuria are the most common complaints. These girls usually are afebrile. Localized tenderness and an intense, fiery red erythema of the vulvar tissues are frequent findings, but some cases have only mild erythema. Pruritus and excoriation may be present. The discharge usually is seropurulent but may be serosanguineous. The color may be white or green. Petechiae may be present on the vaginal mucosa, and regional papular or scarlatiniform rashes can occur.[81,91,218,241] Acute poststreptococcal glomerulonephritis has been reported in association with *S. pyogenes*.[179] Labial abscesses caused by *S. pyogenes* have been noted rarely in prepubertal girls.[258]

Concomitant streptococcal proctitis and perianal skin infections have been reported.[81,144,236] Perianal pruritus, erythema, and tenderness are common findings. The diagnosis of *S. pyogenes* infection may be missed if vaginal secretions are not plated onto sheep blood agar or other media that readily support the growth of streptococci.[241] The vulvovaginitis caused by group A streptococci usually shows initial response to oral antimicrobial therapy within 24 hours. A 10-day course of oral penicillin or amoxicillin is sufficient. A cephalosporin can be prescribed when a child has a nonanaphylactic penicillin allergy. For type 1 hypersensitivity, clindamycin 30 mg/kg per day in three divided doses for 10 days can be administered. Alternative medications are erythromycin or azithromycin. A second course sometimes is necessary when perianal disease is present.[236] Adjunctive use of the hygienic measures discussed for nonspecific vulvovaginitis hastens clinical improvement.

Vulvovaginitis secondary to other nasopharyngeal bacteria. Often a history of an upper respiratory tract infection precedes the onset of vulvovaginitis by a few days. Suspicion that the two conditions are related is strengthened when vaginal cultures yield organisms that commonly colonize the nasopharynx. Vulvovaginitis is assumed to result from autoinoculation of microbes from the nasopharynx to the genitalia. The onset of vulvovaginal symptoms in these infections tends to be acute, the inflammation and discomfort marked, and the discharge less profuse and less purulent than in nonspecific vulvovaginitis.[76]

H. influenzae and *S. aureus* are the species isolated most frequently from cultures.[55,56,162,191,198,229] *Streptococcus pneumoniae* and *Neisseria meningitidis* are seen occasionally, and *Moraxella catarrhalis* has been isolated as well.[132] Labial abscesses caused by *S. aureus* have been described in prepubertal girls.[76] However, vulvovaginitis caused by *S. aureus* in prepubertal girls has not been reported in connection with toxic shock syndrome. *H. influenzae* was the organism isolated most frequently in a series of 200 girls with vulvovaginitis.[191] Acute and chronic cases of *H. influenzae* vulvovaginitis do occur, and the discharge usually is mucoid or mucopurulent, yellow, and odorless. Vulvovaginitis can be caused by *H. influenzae* serotypes a, b, and c and by nontypeable strains.[111,170] Concurrent otitis media or urinary tract infection may be present. All three of these species occasionally are found in vaginal cultures from asymptomatic children. Their isolation in pure culture from symptomatic girls is what leads to the clinical conclusion of cause and effect. One Kenyan study in toddlers has shown no change in the prevalence of *H. influenzae* in the nasopharynx after *H. influenzae* vaccine, thus indicating that this organism should continue to be suspected as a cause of vulvovaginitis.[79] Vulvovaginitis caused by *S. aureus* in prepubertal girls has not been reported in connection with toxic shock syndrome. Labial abscesses caused by *S. aureus* have been described in prepubertal girls.[76]

Neisseria meningitidis is an uncommon cause of vulvovaginitis, but the last reports were in the early 1970s.[78,96] These gram-negative intracellular and extracellular diplococci resemble *Neisseria gonorrhoeae* on stained smears. *Moraxella catarrhalis* also is identical on Gram stain. Gram-negative diplococci should be speciated completely by the microbiology laboratory to avoid misidentifying nongonococcal diplococci as gonococci and vice versa. Especially for pediatric patients, misidentification can result in serious medicolegal consequences for the family when unwarranted intervention is initiated, or it can result in failure to protect the child's welfare when appropriate measures are deemed unnecessary.[5]

Diphtheritic vulvovaginitis can be the primary site of infection, but most reported cases have been secondary to nasopharyngeal infection. Although diphtheria seldom occurs today, sporadic cases occasionally appear in areas where immunization coverage is inadequate. The vulva is the most common genital site involved in diphtheria,[85,149,190] but diphtheritic lesions may occur in the vagina without vulvar involvement. The diagnosis is suspected when a child has the severe systemic symptoms produced by upper respiratory tract diphtheria and a local ulceration covered by a gray adherent membrane; it is confirmed by finding *Corynebacterium diphtheriae* in discharge from the lesion.[73]

Vulvovaginitis caused by *H. influenzae, S. aureus,* and other nasopharyngeal organisms often resolves with hygiene measures alone (as described earlier for nonspecific vulvovaginitis secondary to poor perineal hygiene). Systemic antibiotics may be required for persistent cases or may be helpful early in severely symptomatic cases. The choice of agent depends on the anticipated or known antimicrobial susceptibilities of the specific organism.

Treatment of *N. meningitidis* vulvovaginitis, once the organism is isolated, is the same as for *N. gonorrhoeae.* The organism may not be resistant to penicillin, but decreased susceptibility has been reported. Although data are unavailable, a single dose of ceftriaxone probably should be as effective as it is for gonorrhea, pending cultures. Chemoprophylaxis, generally with rifampin, should be considered for family members and other contacts in cases of meningococcal vulvovaginitis.

Treatment of diphtheria is the same regardless of the site of the infection and is discussed in Chapter 90.

Vulvovaginitis secondary to specific enteric pathogens. *Shigella* spp., mainly *Shigella flexneri* and *Shigella sonnei,* seem to account for most of these cases.[25,29,30,64,89,177] Vaginal discharge without pain, pruritus, or dysuria is the most frequent manifestation of *Shigella* vulvovaginitis. The course can be acute, but discharge that persists for 4 weeks to several months before the diagnosis is made is common. Bloody discharge has been observed in approximately half the cases reported from developed countries, but it was not seen in any of 27 girls with *Shigella* vulvovaginitis in Rwanda between 1988 and 1991.[25,29] The discharge may be purulent and heavy; occasionally it is absent. The vulvar tissues usually appear inflamed.

In most instances, *Shigella* vulvovaginitis is not associated with current or recent diarrhea.[25,177] Local application of triple-sulfa cream (Sultrin) may clear the infection in some cases. Refractory cases have been described, however, and systemic treatment with an antibiotic to which the *Shigella* isolate is susceptible is recommended.[64,177] Trimethoprim-sulfamethoxazole and cefixime are reasonable choices for susceptible isolates; however, most *Shigella* isolates are resistant to ampicillin and trimethoprim-sulfamethoxazole. Ciprofloxacin and ceftriaxone are also effective treatment options. As with other causes of vulvovaginitis, adjunctive use of hygienic measures may help resolve the process and prevent recurrence.

One case of vulvovaginitis with *Yersinia enterocolitica* isolated as the predominant organism was reported in a 4-year-old girl who also had a positive stool culture and associated fever and abdominal pain but no diarrhea.[260] In other members of the community in which she lived diarrhea developed with cultures positive for *Y. enterocolitica.* The outbreak was linked to contaminated food. Infections with this organism may be missed because special culture techniques are required for isolation.

Rarely ulcerative vulvovaginitis caused by *Entamoeba histolytica* or related to typhoid fever has been reported. Generally specific genital infections with pathogenic organisms usually found in the gastrointestinal tract are the result of fecal contamination of the vulva and vagina. Treatment of infections caused by *E. histolytica* is described in Chapter 210.

Vulvovaginitis secondary to skin infections. Similar to a child with an upper respiratory tract infection, a child with impetigo or an infected superficial wound may transmit bacteria from the wound to the genitalia by hand contamination. Cultures in such cases usually yield hemolytic streptococci or *S. aureus*. Treatment is the same as that described for nonspecific vulvovaginitis secondary to respiratory tract infections.

Mycotic (fungal) vulvovaginitis

Prepubertal. The role of *Candida* spp. as a causative agent of vulvovaginitis in healthy prepubertal children has been controversial. While diaper dermatitis with *Candida* spp. colonization or secondary infection is common in infants, co-occurrence with vulvovaginitis is unusual.

Candida vulvovaginitis is rare in prepubertal children and is more likely to occur in girls starting with pubertal development.[119,131,223]

Risk factors for developing recurrent and persistent fungal vulvovaginitis in prepubertal children include a history of recent antibiotic use, uncontrolled diabetes mellitus, or immunosuppression. Mycotic infections are not considered STIs.

A study in Turkey among children 8 to 12 years of age with type 1 diabetes mellitus *Candida* spp. was reported in 50% of vaginal specimens; *C. albicans* in 50%, *C. glabrata* in 37%, and other *Candida* spp. in 13% (*C. dubliniensis, C. krusei*). A higher prevalence rate of *Candida* spp. was reported in postpubertal versus prepubertal children; 30% versus 6%.[14]

Mycotic vulvovaginitis in prepubertal children, when it does occur, usually causes severe persistent and/or recurrent episodes of vulvar and vaginal itching. When a discharge is present it is white, thick, and curdled and has a yeasty sour odor. The patient may have pain during and after voiding or external dysuria as a result of urine coming in contact with excoriated areas on the urethra and vulva (Fig. 42.7).

Postpubertal. Prevalence studies of *Candida* spp. in asymptomatic and symptomatic postpubertal adolescent females are few. In 198 adolescents 15 to 19 years of age at a sexually transmitted disease clinic in the northwestern United States, 30% were positive for *C. albicans.*[71] In another study of 200 sexually active adolescents (mean age, 19 years) at an adolescent health center in Sweden, a history of vulvovaginal candidiasis was reported at least once by 60% and recurrent candidiasis (at least three or more episodes) by 22%. *C. albicans* was isolated by culture in 43% and *C. glabrata* in 3 adolescents; 15% of adolescents with culture positive for *Candida* spp. were asymptomatic.[210] Several factors play roles in causing the increased incidence of vaginal candidiasis after menarche: menstruation, oral-genital sex, fecal contamination of the vulva, wearing tight-fitting underclothes, widespread use of antibiotics, and the use of oral contraceptives. Other predisposing factors include pregnancy, obesity, uncontrolled diabetes mellitus, immunosuppressive therapy, and illicit drug addiction.[21,210] *Candida* vulvovaginitis can occur concomitantly in sexually active adolescents.[272]

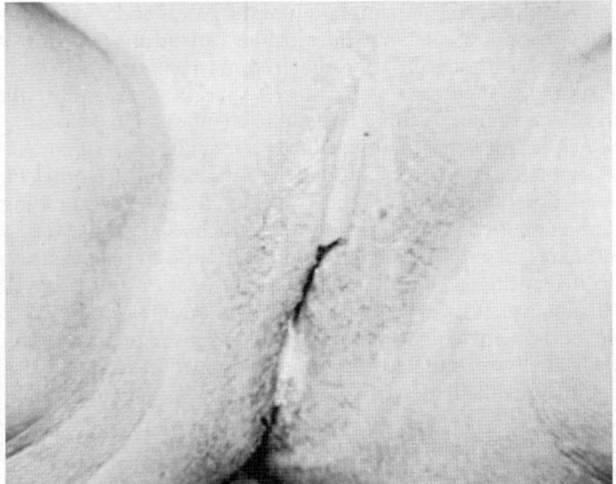

FIG. 42.7 Mycotic vulvovaginitis. The child had diabetes.

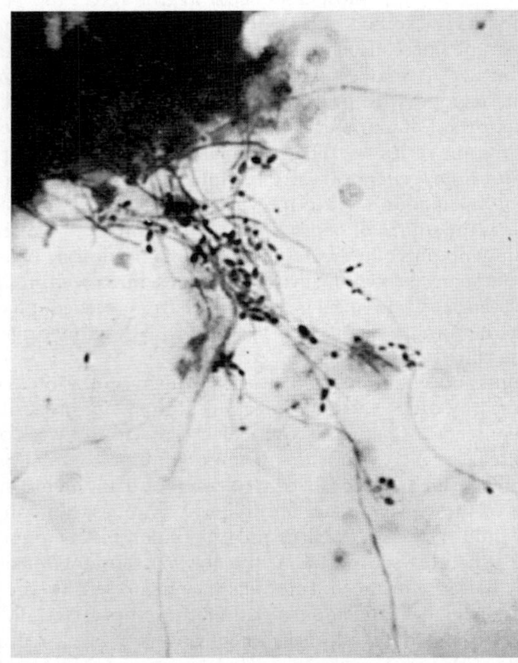

FIG. 42.8 Hyphae of *Candida albicans* discovered on a wet smear of vaginal discharge.

Mycotic vulvovaginitis in the postpubertal period causes severe vulvar and vaginal itching and external dysuria. The discharge is white, thick, and curdled and has a sour odor. Sexually active adolescents can report painful sexual intercourse.[210] Examination in the acute stage reveals intense inflammation of the vulva and vagina with shiny and beefy red mucosa with linear excoriations and edema. Long-standing infection can cause lichenification and hyperpigmentation of the perineal skin. Vaginal pH usually is less than 4.5.[21]

Diagnosis. The diagnosis in all age groups is frequently based on clinical findings. It can be established by finding hyphae and buds of the fungus in vaginal fluid by a vaginal saline wet preparation under microscopy (Fig. 42.8). If debris and cellular material render identifying the fungus difficult, a smear using 10% potassium hydroxide solution is helpful. The potassium hydroxide solution dissolves other extraneous material without affecting the fungus. Even with an experienced microscopist, this method yields a sensitivity range of 40% to 86% in symptomatic girls; however, the yield may be only 40%. Further confirmation can be obtained by identifying fungus by culture of material from the vagina or vulva on Sabouraud or Nickerson media and is helpful in recurrent candida vulvovaginitis. Culture remains the gold standard. Nucleic acid amplification tests for *Candida* spp. have not been cleared by the U.S. Food and Drug Administration (FDA). In sexually active adolescents, testing for *Chlamydia* and gonorrhea infection should be considered.

Treatment. Antifungal creams have no place in the initial treatment of vulvovaginitis in prepubertal females unless budding hyphae are seen on microscopy of vaginal fluid.[76,135] Numerous antifungal creams are available, and the topical azole creams including miconazole, clotrimazole, or terconazole are more effective than nystatin. The creams should be applied as prescribed to the affected area after cleansing.

Curing fungal infections often is difficult in prepubertal children who receive repeated courses of antibiotic therapy or with systemic risk factors for *Candida* vulvovaginitis. Fluconazole (Diflucan) can be administered as a one-time oral dose.[76]

In adolescents a variety of azoles are available as over-the-counter vaginal creams, tablets, and coated tampons. A short course of a single-dose or 3-day regimen is appropriate for an uncomplicated vaginitis. Intravaginal creams or suppositories and oral tablets (prescription) are equally effective. Over-the-counter intravaginal creams include clotrimazole (1% daily for 7 days or 2% daily for 3 days) or miconazole (2% daily for 7 days or 4% daily for 3 days) or terconazole (0.4% daily for 7 days or 0.8% daily for 3 days) or ticonazole (6.5% single application). Over-the-counter intravaginal suppositories include terconazole 80 mg daily for 3 days, miconazole 100 mg daily for 7 days, 200 mg daily for 3 days, or 1200 mg one suppository for 1 day. The cure rate with intravaginal treatment is up to 90%.[272] Oral fluconazole 150 mg as a single dose is an effective preparation for the treatment of uncomplicated vulvovaginal candidiasis.[272] If recurrent unexplainable or resistant infection occurs in children and adolescents, diabetes mellitus should be suspected.

SPECIFIC SEXUALLY TRANSMITTED VULVOVAGINITIS

Specific sexually transmitted vulvovaginitis in this section includes discussion of gonorrhea and chlamydia in prepubertal girls and trichomoniasis and bacterial vaginosis in prepubertal and postpubertal females. Gonorrhea and *Chlamydia* infections in postpubertal period females cause cervicitis instead of vulvovaginitis and are addressed under the discussion of cervicitis.

Gonorrhea

Prepubertal

Gonococcal infections of the prepubertal genital tract are manifested as vulvovaginitis.[43,76,112,220,257,271] The alkaline environment of the unestrogenized vaginal tissues of young girls apparently limits spread of infection to the upper genital tract. Gonorrhea is found less commonly in children now than in the past but must be considered whenever a girl has vulvovaginitis.

In infants, perinatal nonsexual transmission is considered the most likely cause of gonococcal infection. In 1965, Branch and Paxton[28] reported that, in 1- to 11-month-old infants, all the mothers were found to have gonococcal infection and no history of sexual contact could be elicited. The authors concluded that transmission of the infection was perinatal from freshly contaminated hands or through fomites. They also reported that 93% of children aged 1 to 9 years with gonorrhea had sexual contact with relatives in the household.

N. gonorrhoeae has been shown to survive for 20 to 24 hours in infected secretions on towels and handkerchiefs.[238] Although *N. gonorrhoeae* has survived on toilet seats for 2 hours, no gonococci were recovered from toilet seats in public restrooms or in a clinic for STIs.[90,201] Nonsexual transmission to adults is rare.

Prepubertal children with gonococcal infection frequently are found to have a history of sexual contact.[125] The rate of eliciting a history of sexual contact in prepubertal children with gonorrhea ranges from 36% to 93%.[28,84,127,128] Ingram and colleagues[127,128] found that 35% of 1- to 4-year-old children and 100% of children older than 4 years with gonorrhea reported having sexual contact with an older male family member. Folland and coworkers[84] elicited a history of sexual contact from 34% of children with gonococcal urethritis and vaginitis.

Testing of household members in an infected child's environment can detect infected adults at a rate of 18% to 29%.[4,178,195] In a retrospective study of 14 Native Alaskan children with gonococcal infection, 3 reported having sexual contact. Seven children slept with their parents, one or both of whom had gonorrhea; the authors assumed that these children acquired the infection by nonsexual means.[226] Nonsexual transmission conceivably occurs in children who sleep and bathe with their parents.

N. gonorrhoeae was the most common cause of vulvovaginal discharge among prepubertal girls in Rwanda in the late 1980s. Sexual contact was considered likely in all cases because of a cultural belief that a man with a purulent urethral discharge could be cured by rubbing his penis on the external genitalia of a prepubertal girl.[25] In a prospective study of girls 12 months to 12 years of age in the mid-1990s in Cincinnati, Ohio, who had vaginal discharge and no suspicion of sexual abuse, 4 of 43 had positive cultures for *N. gonorrhoeae*.[223] Such cases should lead to investigation for probable sexual abuse.

In summary, sexual transmission is the more common and most likely mode of transmission, and the presence of gonorrhea should be considered diagnostic of sexual abuse.[106] Thus an investigation for sexual abuse must be pursued in a child with gonorrhea by reporting the case to the appropriate legal authority.[272]

The acute stage of gonorrheal vulvovaginitis is characterized by inflammation and a purulent discharge. The child may complain of vulvar discomfort, dysuria, frequent urination, and pain on walking. The child usually is well otherwise. Asymptomatic vaginal infection is rare. On examination, the vulvar tissues are edematous, hyperemic, and covered by a profuse, thick, yellowish discharge that exudes from the vagina. The entire vaginal mucosa is inflamed.

The urethra, paraurethral glands, and major vestibular (Bartholin) glands rarely are involved in a premenarcheal gonorrheal infection. Vulvovaginal infections, including gonorrhea, in prepubertal children rarely if ever affect the upper genitalia (uterus, uterine tubes, ovaries, or pelvic peritoneum). Symptoms suggestive of pelvic peritonitis have been reported in premenarcheal children who had gonorrheal vulvovaginitis; all the patients recovered promptly after the administration of penicillin.[43,86]

Diagnosis

The diagnosis of gonorrheal vulvovaginitis and its differentiation from other types of vulvovaginitis are established by vaginal cultures. Gram stain of a vaginal specimen is not an appropriate diagnostic test. Specimens from the pharynx and rectum to test for *N. gonorrhoeae* also should be obtained. Cervical specimens are not recommended from prepubertal girls. Because of the potential medicolegal use of the test results for *N. gonorrhoeae* among children, standard culture systems should be used for the diagnosis of *N. gonorrhoeae* in children. Nucleic amplification testing for gonorrhea using urine and vaginal swabs was conducted in 485 premenarcheal girls with alleged sexual abuse from four cities in the United States. The sensitivity of urine nucleic acid amplification testing (NAAT) for gonorrhea relative to vaginal swabs was 100%.[24] The Centers for Disease Control and Prevention (CDC) states that consultation with an expert is necessary prior to obtaining a NAAT test to minimize cross-reactivity with other *Neisseria* spp. and to assure correct interpretation of positive results.[272]

Treatment

The presence of gram-negative intracellular diplococci in vaginal smears from a child with a history of exposure or with typical clinical findings is sufficient reason to start treatment, but it does not establish a definitive diagnosis. Further details on treatment are addressed in Chapter 89.

Chlamydia

Prepubertal

Although *C. trachomatis* appears to be an uncommon cause of vaginitis in prepubertal girls, vaginal infection with *C. trachomatis* can occur in children. In contrast to prepubertal gonorrhea infections, chlamydial vaginitis in children often seems to be asymptomatic. Although coinfection with *C. trachomatis* has not been studied well in prepubertal children, experience from adult populations has shown that it should be suspected in children with *N. gonorrhoeae* infection. In one study in prepubertal girls, 30% with *N. gonorrhoeae* also tested positive for *C. trachomatis.*[202]

Perinatally acquired genital *Chlamydia* infection is a strong possibility in children younger than 1 year. *C. trachomatis* has been isolated from the conjunctiva, nasopharynx, vagina, and rectum of infants born to infected mothers.[213] Subclinical infections have been reported in 14% of infants of mothers with active *C. trachomatis* infection.[215] However, perinatal transmission is possible in children up to 3 years of age. This may be due to persistence of perinatal infection. Infants infected with *C. trachomatis* at birth have remained infected for up to 372 days in the vagina; 383 days in the rectum; and 866 days in the conjunctiva, nasopharynx, and oropharynx. Thus persistent chlamydial infection of the pharynx in infants can persist for 2 years.[20] Persistence of perinatal infection for 18 months and for 6 years has been reported in other studies as well.[164,212,254]

Studies of *C. trachomatis* infection in prepubertal girls have involved mostly children being evaluated for sexual abuse or vulvovaginal symptoms, or both, and some have included a control group in an attempt to control for either a history of sexual abuse or vaginal symptoms.[87,101,108,125,126,128,188,202]

The variation in rates among studies may reflect differences in the prevalence of *C. trachomatis* in different communities. The highest rates of *C. trachomatis* infection were seen in a Los Angeles study, in which 47 prepubertal girls were examined for alleged sexual abuse and 17% had vaginal *C. trachomatis.*[87] In other studies evaluating children suspected of being sexually abused, rates of recovery (pharyngeal and rectal infection included) tend to be higher (6–8%) than those seen in children with vaginitis or controls (0–2%).[101,125,126,128] Initial evaluations of children presenting with vaginitis or in the control groups may not elicit a history of sexual abuse, but further questioning or testing of all orifices (pharyngeal and rectal) may elicit suspicion or a history of sexual abuse. For example, a history of sexual abuse was discovered in two control children only after *C. trachomatis* was identified.[101] Initially, 2% of children with a history of sexual abuse versus 4% of healthy controls had positive vaginal cultures for *C. trachomatis*. On further questioning, however, the two children in the control group with *C. trachomatis* were siblings who were sexually abused 3 years earlier, increasing the rate of *C. trachomatis* vaginal infection in the sexual abuse group to 6% and decreasing the rate in the control group to zero. This report illustrates the importance of thoroughly investigating the possibility of sexual abuse whenever a sexually transmitted pathogen is isolated in a young child.

In studies evaluating premenarcheal children presenting with vulvovaginitis, recovery of *C. trachomatis* has been low in children with symptoms and healthy control groups. In one study, none of the 35 children with symptoms had *C. trachomatis*, whereas 1 of 35 without symptoms had *C. trachomatis* isolated.[188] In another study conducted in a pediatric gynecology clinic, 4 of 29 (14%) premenarcheal girls were found to have *C. trachomatis.*[39] All four had a homogeneous white discharge, and one had a bloody discharge. Sexual abuse occurred in two of the children and was considered possible in another. In a Cincinnati study evaluating vaginitis in girls younger than 12 years in whom sexual abuse was not suspected, none of the 87 children had a positive culture for *C. trachomatis.*[223] Similarly, in a smaller study of 11 girls with vaginitis, none was found to have *C. trachomatis.*[202]

In summary, although persistence of perinatal infection can occur, when *C. trachomatis* is identified in vaginal specimens, sexual abuse as a potential mode of transmission of *C. trachomatis* infection should be considered in children older than 1 year.[87,104] There are no data demonstrating survival of *C. trachomatis* on fomites or its coexistence in family members of infected children. Thus an investigation for sexual abuse must be pursued in a child with *Chlamydia* infection by reporting the case to the appropriate legal authority.[272]

Diagnosis

Numerous diagnostic methods for *Chlamydia* are available.[23] Direct tissue culture isolation of *C. trachomatis* remains the gold standard and is the only test that should be used in prepubertal children or in cases in which sexual abuse is under consideration.[272] Culturing for *Chlamydia* requires isolation of the organism in tissue culture and confirmation of the characteristic intracytoplasmic inclusions by fluorescent monoclonal antibody staining.[272] Although the specificity of tissue culture approaches 100%, tissue culture is only 70% to 85% sensitive in contrast to DNA amplification techniques.[23] The low recovery rate in studies of prepubertal children may be due to the low sensitivity of tissue culture or the use of vaginal cultures in young children. Isolation rates from the vagina usually are lower than rates of recovery from the endocervix.[167]

Nonculture tests for *Chlamydia*, including enzyme immunoassays, direct fluorescent antibody tests, DNA hybridization, and DNA amplification tests, have not been field tested for large numbers of vaginal specimens or rectal or pharyngeal specimens from premenarcheal girls. False-positive results have been reported in vaginal specimens for some of these tests in children, and these tests should not be used in premenarcheal children.[106,193] False-positive results probably are caused by cross-reactivity with common anogenital organisms, such as group A and B streptococci, *N. gonorrhoeae, G. vaginalis, E. coli,* and *Proteus, Acinetobacter,* and *Staphylococcus* spp.[145,205,209,211,253]

However, more recently, NAAT for *C. trachomatis* using urine and vaginal swabs was conducted in 485 premenarcheal girls with alleged sexual abuse from four cities in the United States. The sensitivity of urine NAAT for *Chlamydia* relative to vaginal swabs was 100%.[24] The CDC states that consultation with an expert is necessary prior to obtaining a NAAT test to assure correct interpretation of a positive result.[272]

Treatment

Treatment for *Chlamydia* infection is addressed in Chapter 194.

Trichomoniasis

Trichomonas vaginalis is a triflagellated protozoan (Fig. 42.9). The organism, which is larger than a polymorphonuclear leukocyte, has a distinctive vibrating or whiplike movement when seen microscopically in fresh wet smears taken from the vagina. It quickly succumbs to reduction of the pH, drying, cooling, and changing the osmotic pressure of the fluid surrounding it. Most infections are encountered in sexually active adolescents and young adult women. Chapter 215 addresses trichomoniasis, including epidemiology, in more detail.

Prepubertal

Vaginal trichomoniasis is reported infrequently in prepubertal children. This low prevalence may be accurate or could be due to lack of appropriate testing or limitations of the diagnostic techniques used in studies in prepubertal children.

Trichomoniasis in newborns has been described in several case reports through the acquisition of *T. vaginalis* from the mother's vagina during

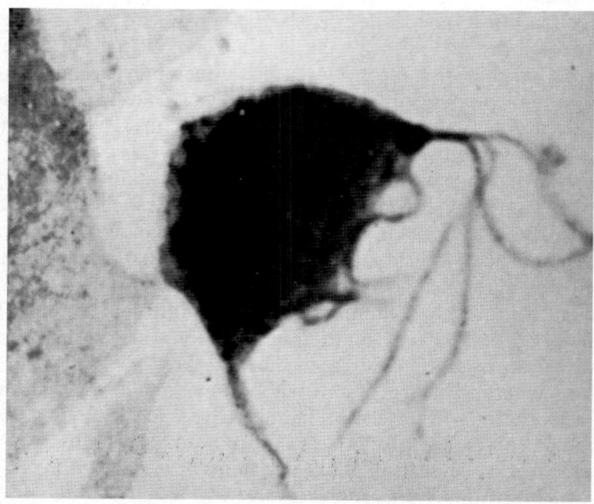

FIG. 42.9 *Trichomonas vaginalis* is a triflagellated protozoan that, when motile, is identified easily in wet smears of vaginal discharge.

delivery, with recovery of *T. vaginalis* from urine, vaginal, and respiratory tract specimens.[7,27,58,61,159,169,194,235] The prevalence of *T. vaginalis* in healthy, vaginally delivered infants of mothers with *T. vaginalis* is unknown. In one study of 868 infants, *T. vaginalis* could not be identified in any of the 14 female infants of mothers in whom *T. vaginalis* was diagnosed. The overall prevalence of *T. vaginalis* was 4%, but the denominator of mothers of female infants was not described.[27] In another study of 984 female infants, direct smear or culture (or both) of infant vaginal specimens identified three infants with *T. vaginalis,* a prevalence of 0.3%.[5] Of the three infants, two had a vaginal discharge. The overall prevalence of infection in the mothers of the 984 infants was not reported. Of the three infants with *T. vaginalis,* one mother had a history of vaginal discharge and a negative direct smear for *T. vaginalis,* and the other two mothers had no history of *T. vaginalis.* In conclusion, transmission of *T. vaginalis* in infants aged 1 year probably is perinatal.

The mode of transmission in children older than 1 year is controversial. Numerous reports confirm the occurrence of *T. vaginalis* in prepubertal girls evaluated for vaginitis but no history of sexual abuse with prevalence rates ranging from 0% to 4%.[111,131,188,223] In studies with a healthy control population,[95,111,131] *T. vaginalis* was not identified in any of the children in the asymptomatic control group.

A case report in 1985 described *T. vaginalis* in two sexually abused children with vaginal discharge[137]; however, in studies systematically evaluating children for sexual abuse regardless of symptoms, *T. vaginalis* has not been recovered.[88,228] In an Australian study evaluating 160 children younger than 10 years and 95 healthy age-matched controls, none of the children had *T. vaginalis* isolated from vaginal cultures.[88] Similarly, none of the 119 prepubertal girls evaluated for sexual abuse in a Cincinnati, Ohio, study had *T. vaginalis* identified by urinalysis or wet mount of vaginal secretions.[228] Without additional studies using culture techniques and conducted in diverse populations of prepubertal girls, determining the true prevalence of *T. vaginalis* in prepubertal girls who have vaginitis, with or without a history of sexual abuse, is difficult.

Nonsexual transmission within a family without sexual abuse or contact can conceivably occur.[2,147] In a case report, *T. vaginalis* was diagnosed in the mother, and her three prepubertal daughters were symptomatic with a vaginal discharge. Two of the three girls had *T. vaginalis* identified on wet-mount evaluation of their vaginal specimens. They had no history or evidence of sexual abuse, the father was asymptomatic, and microscopy of an early morning urine specimen was negative for *T. vaginalis.*

A study from Poland found one case of *T. vaginalis* infection in children aged 2 to 7 years and a significantly higher number of cases in 8- to 10-year-old girls. The numbers increased even further for children older than 10 years, suggesting a strong association between *T. vaginalis* and the presence of an estrogenic environment, which promotes glycogen production and decreases vaginal pH.[147]

The Polish investigation tested families of women infected with *T. vaginalis* and found that almost a third of their sexual partners and 8% of the children (mostly girls) had *T. vaginalis.* When families of men infected with *T. vaginalis* were tested, 91% of their sexual partners and 13% of the children had *T. vaginalis.* When families of children (mostly girls) infected with *T. vaginalis* were tested, 72% of the mothers and 43% of the fathers had the infection. The investigators considered that the infection in the latter group originated from mothers and that the primary mode of transmission was nonsexual (beds, sponges, towels, overcrowding). Information regarding sharing of potentially infected fomites, sexual abuse, or physically intimate behavior between parents and children was not gathered in these cases.[147]

Although *T. vaginalis* has been known to survive on fomites in controlled experiments, its ability to spread by these means is unknown. No cases of adults being infected by fomites have been documented. *T. vaginalis* has been found to survive for 6 hours on droplets of discharge and enameled surfaces of wood blocks.[141] It has been isolated from droplets of water splashed from toilets containing the urine of an infected individual.[41] *T. vaginalis* also has been found to survive in mud baths, bathing waters, and warm mineral waters and on moist bathing implements.[147,181] In rural India, a survey found that young girls who bathed in tanks or rivers had a significantly higher risk for acquiring *T. vaginalis* than did girls who used piped or well water.[50]

In summary, the likelihood of perinatal transmission of *T. vaginalis* is high in infants younger than 1 year. In a child older than 1 year, *T. vaginalis* infection may have resulted from transmission within a family without sexual abuse; however, the probability of sexual abuse must be considered highly suspicious, and the case must be investigated and reported for possible sexual abuse. Perinatal transmission and transmission through fomites should not be assumed without an investigation for sexual abuse.[272] Additionally if *T. vaginalis* is recovered from a child, the child should be evaluated for other STIs, including syphilis, *N. gonorrhoeae, C. trachomatis,* hepatitis B, and HIV infection.[76]

Postpubertal

Trichomoniasis is common and frequently is asymptomatic in sexually active adolescents (see Chapter 215). When it is symptomatic, patients complain of a profuse, irritating discharge. The discharge and the pruritus tend to be more severe just before and immediately after a menstrual period. Patients occasionally report dysuria and abdominal pain. Recurrent exacerbations of the infection occur commonly.

Examination reveals diffuse vulvitis with erythema and excoriations and copious leukorrhea that covers the vulvar tissues. The discharge typically is frothy or bubbly, grayish yellow, and watery or mucopurulent. It has a pH of 5.0 to 7.0 and an acrid or musty odor. A "strawberry" or punctate vaginal eruption with hemorrhagic spots has been described as being typical of trichomoniasis. Such eruptions frequently are not present, however, even in severe cases. More often, diffuse inflammation causes the vaginal mucosa to be brilliant red.

Diagnosis

There are numerous diagnostic methods available to diagnose trichomoniasis.[272] The diagnosis of trichomoniasis usually is confirmed clinically by finding trichomonads in a wet saline smear of vaginal fluid. It is important that the slide be viewed under the microscope (dry high power) promptly because the organisms do not remain viable for long outside the vagina and are difficult to detect when they cease to be motile. The observer sees numerous ovoid-shaped, motile organisms (see Fig. 42.9). The sensitivity of this test with immediate evaluation is 60% to 70%. A Papanicolaou (Pap) smear to detect trichomoniasis is not recommended because of the high rate of error in identifying trichomonads in stained smears. Other methods used to diagnose trichomoniasis include isolation by special culture medium, direct fluorescent immunoassay, NAAT, rapid antigen test, and nucleic acid probe. The choice of test is often based on availability. The NAATs are highly sensitive and specific and have become the gold standard for diagnosing trichomoniasis. Culture also has high sensitivity and specificity, but it is not routinely available. The NAAT is available in some clinical settings (point-of-care test); however, a false-positive result may occur in low-prevalence populations.[12,17,44,122,272]

Treatment

Treatment for trichomoniasis is addressed in Chapter 215.

Bacterial Vaginosis

Bacterial vaginosis is caused by a change in the relative proportions of bacteria in the vaginal flora: an overgrowth of anaerobes, especially *Bacteroides* and *Mobiluncus* spp., *G. vaginalis,* and *M. hominis;* and a decrease in hydrogen peroxide–producing lactobacilli.[9]

The clinical criteria used for establishing the diagnosis of bacterial vaginosis in adolescents and adults are the presence of three of four findings: a grayish homogeneous discharge, the presence of clue cells on a wet-mount evaluation (Fig. 42.10), a pH greater than 4.5, and a positive amine test result (amine or fishy odor when vaginal secretions are mixed with 10% potassium hydroxide).[272]

Prepubertal

Bacterial vaginosis is defined poorly in premenarcheal girls. The Amsel criteria used for establishing the clinical diagnosis of bacterial vaginosis are the presence of three of four findings: a grayish homogeneous discharge, the presence of clue cells on a wet-mount evaluation (Fig. 42.10), a pH greater than 4.5, and a positive amine test result

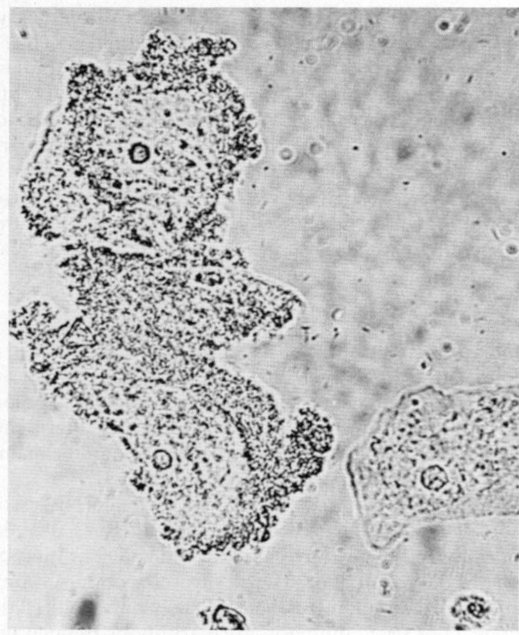

FIG. 42.10 The finding of bacteria clinging to the sides of a vaginal epithelial cell (clue cell) is significant in bacterial vaginosis. (Courtesy Herman L. Gardner, MD.)

(amine or fishy odor when vaginal secretions are mixed with 10% potassium hydroxide).[272]

No published studies using these standard diagnostic criteria in their entirety exist. A few studies have used identification of *G. vaginalis* by culture of the vaginal discharge to diagnose bacterial vaginosis. However, isolation of *G. vaginalis* must not be confused with bacterial vaginosis as it may be present in girls with or without bacterial vaginosis.[272,76] In addition, although the prevalence of *G. vaginalis* and bacterial vaginosis is reported to be higher in sexually abused children than in nonabused children, their significance in premenarcheal girls with possible sexual abuse is unclear.[18,88,103,106,125,128,131] These studies did not use the full criteria for bacterial vaginosis or only subgroups of girls or both premenarcheal and postmenarcheal girls with vaginal discharge were evaluated in these studies.[103,125,128] No data are available regarding the survival of *G. vaginalis* on fomites.

Until studies using the proper and complete criteria are done in young girls with and without a vaginal discharge, the prevalence of bacterial vaginosis will be unknown, and the significance of bacterial vaginosis as a cause of vaginal discharge in premenarcheal girls will remain unclear. Because bacterial cultures may be performed in the evaluation of a vaginal discharge in a premenarcheal girl and *G. vaginalis* may be identified, identification of *G. vaginalis* should not be considered evidence of sexual abuse or diagnostic of bacterial vaginosis. At this time, the presence of manifestations of bacterial vaginosis should prompt the health care provider to consider treatment of bacterial vaginosis. In addition, the possibility of sexual abuse should be contemplated, but a diagnosis of bacterial vaginosis does not provide evidence of sexual abuse.

Postpubertal

Bacterial vaginosis in adolescents is considered a sexually transmitted condition based on the occurrence of bacterial vaginosis with other STIs. Bacterial vaginosis also has been described in adolescent girls who are not sexually active.[40] Other risk factors are foreign bodies such as a forgotten tampon, vaginal douching,[120,269] no condom use, a new sexual partner, anal intercourse, unclean insertive sex toys, and an intrauterine device. In addition, the association among bacterial vaginosis and postpartum endometritis, premature rupture of membranes, and PID has implicated it as the cause for these gynecologic and obstetric complications.[21,272]

The primary complaint is an offensive fishy odor with moderately profuse, gray leukorrhea. A mild pruritus may be reported. Examination shows little or no vulvar or vaginal erythema. The vagina contains a thick, homogeneous, grayish-white discharge. The pH of vaginal secretions in bacterial vaginosis is 5.0 to 6.0.[272]

Diagnosis

Two methods are used to establish the diagnosis of bacterial vaginosis—Gram stain of vaginal discharge and clinical criteria,[21,76,272] with clinical criteria being used more commonly. A Gram stain of vaginal secretions is considered the most reliable diagnostic test for bacterial vaginosis in research studies but is usually not readily available.[184,225,272] A predominance of gram-variable cocci and curved rods (anaerobes) and occasional long gram-positive rods (lactobacilli) are seen.[272,33] A saline wet mount of vaginal secretions is a rapid and helpful test for clue cells in a busy clinical setting (see Fig. 42.10). The Gram stain method is used to determine the relative concentrations of bacterial morphotypes and evaluate for the overgrowth of anaerobes. This method requires an examiner with expertise in evaluating specimens for bacterial vaginosis and is less practical than is the use of clinical criteria; thus clinical criteria are used more widely.

The clinical criteria used for establishing the diagnosis of bacterial vaginosis in adolescents are the presence of any three of the four criteria[21,272]: (1) a homogeneous, gray-white malodorous discharge that smoothly coats the vaginal walls, (2) a pH of nonbloody vaginal secretions greater than 4.5, (3) a fishy odor caused by the release of amines when 10% potassium hydroxide is added to a nonbloody vaginal specimen (whiff test), and (4) the presence of clue cells in a nonbloody specimen. Microscopic examination of some of the discharge mixed with normal saline solution in a wet-mount preparation shows masses of desquamated vaginal epithelial cells and cellular debris. Clusters of bacteria adhere to the surface of many of the vaginal cells; these clue cells (see Fig. 42.10) are characteristic of the condition. Absence of erythrocytes and leukocytes in the discharge is another characteristic finding. Vaginal cultures for *G. vaginalis* and anaerobes are available; however, they are not useful clinically in children or adolescents and are not recommended.

Treatment

Numerous regimens for the treatment of bacterial vaginosis exist, but no specific recommendations are available for premenarcheal girls. Probably because bacterial vaginosis is diagnosed infrequently, clinical trials evaluating treatment of bacterial vaginosis in premenarcheal girls are lacking. The drugs recommended for use in young girls are those recommended for postmenarcheal women, with dosages based on the child's body weight. In small children (<45 kg), metronidazole can be given at 15 mg/kg per day divided two times per day for 7 days (maximum dose 1 g/day).[21,272]

The goal of therapy for symptomatic bacterial vaginosis in adolescents is to relieve vaginal symptoms and prevent an ecologic environment that predisposes to the development of PID. Treatment of asymptomatic bacterial vaginosis may be considered before performing a surgical abortion procedure to prevent postpartum PID. In most cases, bacterial vaginosis responds to metronidazole 500 mg orally twice per day for 7 days or 2% clindamycin cream intravaginally every night for 7 days or 0.75% metronidazole gel intravaginally once per day for 5 days.[272] Alternative regimens include tinidazole 2 g orally once daily for 2 days or tinidazole 1 g orally once daily for 5 days or clindamycin 300 mg orally twice per day for 7 days, or clindamycin ovules, 100 mg intravaginally once per day for 3 days.[272] These regimens provide effective coverage of anaerobes and *G. vaginalis.* Bacterial vaginosis that occurs during pregnancy generally is treated with metronidazole 500 mg orally twice daily for 7 days, metronidazole 250 mg orally three times a day for 7 days, or clindamycin 300 mg orally twice daily for 7 days.[272] The CDC no longer discourages the use of metronidazole in the first trimester, and no relationship has been found between birth defects and the use metronidazole during the first trimester of pregnancy.[31,45,158,186,204,272] Treatment of the sexual partner has not proved to be beneficial.[272]

Infections of the Clitoris

Cellulitis with induration, edema, and erythema occasionally develops in the clitoral hood in the prepubertal and pubertal period.[76] Clitoral hood piercings can cause cellulitis in older adolescents. Staphylococci and streptococci are the most common etiologies. Oral antibiotics with efficacy against these organisms usually are effective. Warm soaks or sitz baths also may provide symptomatic relief.[76]

Clitoromegaly with erythema can occur with vulvovaginitis of any etiology but usually is associated with herpes simplex virus (HSV) infections.[69] Edematous enlargement of the clitoris and the labia without erythema has been reported in patients with Crohn disease.[54,176]

Urethritis

Urethritis is manifested clinically by dysuria, urinary urgency, or both and occurs particularly in sexually active postmenarcheal girls. Urethritis with internal dysuria can occur as a result of STIs, such as *T. vaginalis, N. gonorrhoeae,* and *C. trachomatis*, and has been implicated as an important cause of dysuria in sexually active girls.[22,239] Urethral infection by *C. trachomatis* may occur with or without cervical infection; this infection was associated with sterile pyuria in 50% of girls with acute-onset dysuria and frequency, and *C. trachomatis* was isolated in 31% of these cases.[239]

When a sexually active adolescent girl has internal dysuria, in addition to being tested for conventional uropathogens, she should be screened for common STIs, such as gonorrhea, chlamydia, and trichomonas infection.[65] Urinalysis and microscopy for the presence of leukocytes and bacteria should be done in these patients as well. For treatment of urethritis caused by sexually transmitted organisms, the sections in this chapter on trichomoniasis, gonorrhea, and chlamydial infections should be reviewed.

Bartholinitis and Bartholin Abscess

Infections of the Bartholin ducts occasionally occur in adolescent girls. The Bartholin glands are small, bean-shaped glands that lie on each side of the vaginal opening, behind the hymen. Each gland opens by means of a long single duct immediately external to the hymen.

Bartholinitis, or inflammation of the Bartholin ducts, causes pain, tenderness, and a linear rope-shaped swelling, best palpated by holding the vulvar mucosa and labia majora between the fingers. Purulent or mucoid exudate can be expressed occasionally from the Bartholin duct.

The predominant pathogens isolated from a Bartholin gland abscess are *E. coli* and methicillin-resistant *S. aureus*.[32,142,252] Previously *N. gonorrhoeae* and *C. trachomatis* have been isolated almost a third of the time from ductal exudates in women with bartholinitis.[62,200] A Bartholin abscess does occur in sexually active adolescent girls. Risk factors for development of Bartholin abscess are similar to those for STIs.[3] Infection of a Bartholin cyst results in a markedly tender abscess (Fig. 42.11). The abscess can rupture spontaneously and drain foul-smelling, purulent material externally through the skin. Multiple organisms are isolated from Bartholin abscesses. An early study using percutaneous aspirates from abscesses showed predominantly anaerobes and facultative organisms. *N. gonorrhoeae* was isolated in 8% of cases, and gram-negative bacilli were isolated in 16%. Although genital Mycoplasmataceae organisms were isolated from the duct secretions, they were not isolated directly from abscesses.[155] *Porphyromonas asaccharolytica* (a black-pigmented, gram-negative anaerobe), *Salmonella panama* (after an attack of *Salmonella* enteritis), and *Mycobacterium tuberculosis* have been isolated from a Bartholin abscess.[60,66,70,121]

A Bartholin abscess should be incised and drained and not aspirated because it is likely to cause recurrent abscess formation. Incision plus drainage and primary suture of the abscess cavity along with administration of an antibiotic (clindamycin) has been found to lead to more rapid healing and decrease significantly the incidence of recurrent abscesses.[10] The cavity should be packed with sterile gauze. Alternatively, marsupialization or fistulization can be used to treat recurrent Bartholin abscesses.[262] A Word catheter inflated with water can be inserted into the cavity. Antibiotic therapy should provide coverage for staphylococcal (MRSA) and streptococcal species and gram-negative aerobes such as *E. coli*.[160] Treatment for *N. gonorrhoeae,* and *C. trachomatis* should be provided if cultures are positive.[160] Frequent sitz baths help further with drainage and healing. Close follow-up during the first week is advised. The packing or the catheter may be removed after 4 days of antibiotics. Healing should be anticipated in 2 weeks.

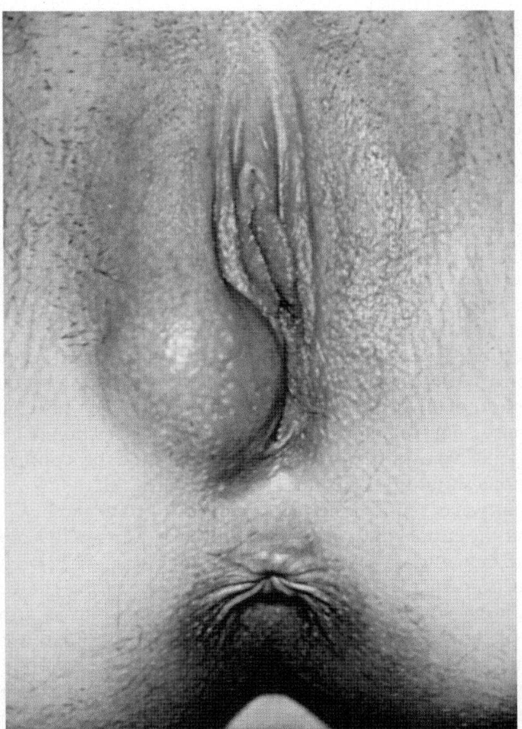

FIG. 42.11 Acute Bartholin duct abscess.

VULVOVAGINAL LESIONS, ULCERATIONS, AND GRANULOMATOUS INFECTIONS

Vulvovaginal lesions, ulcerations, and granulomatous infections include genital warts, molluscum contagiosum, herpes genitalis, syphilis, chancroid, granuloma inguinale, and tuberculosis. Human papillomavirus (HPV) and genital warts, molluscum contagiosum, and lymphogranuloma venereum will be addressed in detail in this chapter. All other conditions are described in detail in Chapters 130, 134, 144, and 158. The modes of transmission of all the previously mentioned infections and implications for child sexual abuse will also be discussed in this chapter.

Human Papillomavirus and Genital Warts

HPV is a small, slow-growing virus of the papovavirus group. HPV types 6 and 11 are responsible for 90% of genital warts (condyloma acuminata); HPV types 16, 18, 31, and 33 are associated with premalignant and malignant cervical carcinoma in women, with HPV types 16 and 18 causing 70% of premalignant and malignant lesions.[80,138]

Prepubertal

Perinatal transmission of HPV from an infected mother to her infant is well documented. The incubation period after exposure to the virus may range from 1 to 20 months.[63] Data on the presence of HPV DNA in children beyond the neonatal period are inconsistent—1.2% to 27% in three different studies.[153,196,261] In addition the relationship between the presence of HPV DNA and the ultimate development of disease in children is unclear. Because the exact incubation period for the development of genital lesions is unknown, perinatal transmission has been found to be the most likely cause of genital warts in almost 96% of patients younger than 3 years.[63] In children 3 years or older, a history of sexual abuse has been elicited in 27% to 90% with venereal warts.[51,114]

Genital warts are acquired by children as a result of close physical contact with an infected individual, by digital infection of the child's genitalia by an infected individual, or by sexual contact with an infected individual.[219,231,240] A history of genital warts in other members of the family, particularly the mother or older sisters who care for the child, sometimes may be elicited. Perinatal exposure, poor hygiene, and shared bathing have been suggested sources of infection.[243,244] HPV types 6, 11, 16, and 18 are the most common genital types detected in children. This finding has raised questions about warts in children resulting from sexual abuse. In many cases, however, the mode of transmission is unknown.[63] Transmission of HPV via fomites (underwear and towels) are possible etiologies but not a likely cause of condyloma in children.[133,232] Sexual abuse is the most common means of acquiring anogenital HPV infection and should be considered suspicious for sexual abuse and investigated and reported in all prepubertal children older than 4 years who are infected.[232] In children younger than 4 years, although perinatal transmission is likely, sexual abuse should be suspected and investigated.[231,272]

As recommended by the CDC,[272] the possibility of sexual abuse should be considered strongly if no conclusive explanation for nonsexual transmission of an STI has been identified. When the only evidence of sexual abuse is the isolation of an organism or the detection of antibodies to a sexually transmitted agent, findings should be confirmed and implications should be considered carefully.

Genital warts (condyloma acuminata) in premenarcheal children may cover the entire vulva. Most often, however, warts in this population are single or scattered cauliflower-like lesions (Fig. 42.12). They have a predilection for the smooth, moist mucosa covering the vestibular mucosa, inner surfaces of the labia minora, and mucosa around the urethral meatus. Warts seldom become ulcerative, but those arising within the vagina may become necrotic and produce a bloody vaginal discharge. Although not tumors, genital warts should be considered in the differential diagnosis of vaginal neoplasms. HIV infection should be considered in infants and children with severe, extensive warts.[51,63,80,138]

Postpubertal

The prevalence of HPV in adolescents as detected by DNA isolation techniques is far higher than the prevalence of active disease. The cell-mediated or T-cell immune system seems to play an important role in whether the presence of virus results in clinically manifested disease. Cofactors of HPV infection in adolescents are herpes, cervicitis, and tobacco use. Immunosuppression from a variety of conditions, including renal transplantation, Hodgkin disease, and HIV infection, is associated with a greater likelihood of development of HPV disease.[80,138] With regard to the natural history of HPV infection, Moscicki and colleagues[172,173] found that high-grade squamous intraepithelial lesions (HSILs) were more likely to develop in individuals with persistently positive tests showing oncogenic HPV types. During the course of a 2-year period, 70% of cases showed regression. Daily cigarette smoking was strongly linked to the development of low-grade squamous intraepithelial lesions (LSILs).[172] Regression was more likely in young women with LSIL than in those with HSIL.

In postmenarchal girls, genital warts usually form discrete, sessile, vegetative, wartlike growths covered with folded grayish-pink epithelium. They are found most frequently on the smooth mucosa of the vulvar vestibule. Vaginal and cervical lesions commonly accompany the lesions on the vulva. Usually they are accompanied by more or less vaginal discharge. Most often, associated pruritus and secondary infection are present. Contact lesions frequently appear on contiguous surfaces. Huge condylomatous masses (Fig. 42.13) that completely hide the introitus can develop in adolescents; if not treated, these huge growths may invade the rectum.

Diagnosis

Diagnosis is usually made clinically. HPV testing and biopsy of warts are not recommended in children and adolescents. A biopsy may be considered if genital warts appear necrotic or the morphologic appearance is not classic for warts.

Treatment

The goal of treatment is removal of warts and amelioration of symptoms, not eradication of HPV. No therapy has been shown to eradicate HPV. Available therapeutic options include methods that will mechanically or chemically destroy infected tissue or alter the immune response against HPV-infected cells. When only a few lesions are present, they can be treated in the outpatient setting with 85% trichloroacetic acid. In infants and children with extensive lesions, electrocautery, electrocoagulation, or laser treatment, general anesthesia may be needed and may result in deep scarring and distortion of the vulva. Older children and young adolescents usually tolerate cryotherapy without general anesthesia if they know that some tingling or burning sensation is associated with it. Liquid nitrogen may be used in the same manner as solid carbon dioxide. Reports in the international literature demonstrate successful treatment of extensive warts in children using imiquimod (topical immune modulator) 5% cream[138,80,163] and in adults using imiquimod 3.75% and 5% cream.[15,72]

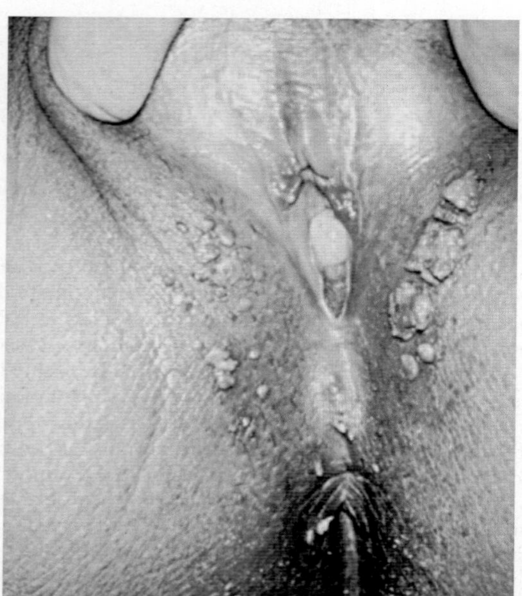

FIG. 42.12 Condylomata acuminata usually are single or scattered small warts in premenarcheal children.

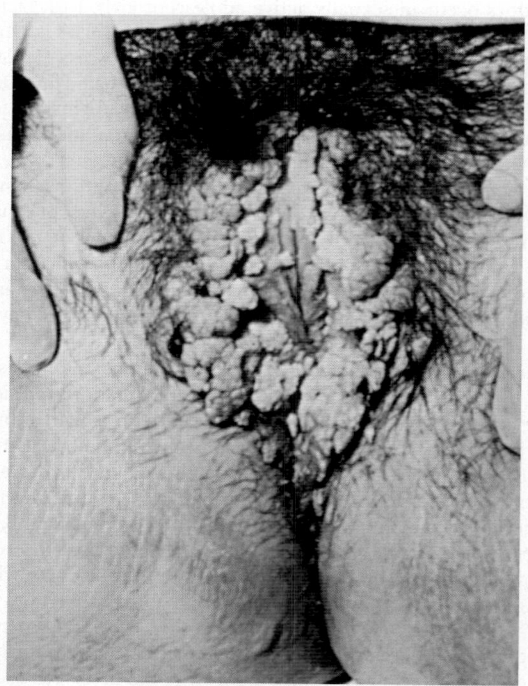

FIG. 42.13 Condylomata acuminata may form large masses covering the vulva in postmenarchal patients.

The therapeutic methods available are 22% to 94% effective in clearing exophytic genital warts, but recurrence rates are high, at least 25% within 3 months. Treatment seems to be more successful for genital warts that are small and present for less than 1 year.[272] When a few lesions are present on the vulvar and labial areas, they can be treated in the office setting with a solution of 80% to 90% trichloroacetic acid or bichloracetic acid.[272] Patient-applied treatments include imiquimod cream, which is applied to warts three times per week at bedtime, every other day for a maximum of 16 weeks. The cream should be washed off with soap and water 6 to 10 hours after application.[272] An alternative option is podophyllin (an antimitotic agent), which is applied to warts twice daily for 3 consecutive days followed by 4 days of no therapy for up to four cycles. Four hours after podophyllin has been applied, the treated area should be washed off with soap and water. Urethral, anal, vaginal, and cervical lesions should not be treated with podophyllin. The medication is applied to the wart only (not to the surrounding skin), and treatment is repeated once weekly until the lesions have disappeared (usually 3 to 4 weeks). Self-application of 0.5% podofilox gel may be considered in older nonpregnant adolescents who are comfortable using this approach and can understand the treatment regimen so as to avoid dermatologic side effects.

Laser treatment or cryocautery is recommended if the lesions do not respond to chemical cautery or if they progressively increase in size. Large perianal warts may need to be removed surgically if cryotherapy does not work. Alternative treatments for adolescents are topical 5-fluorouracil in 5% creams and intralesional interferon. 5-Fluorouracil is preferable for vaginal and intraurethral warts and seems to be more effective than the laser.

The first endocervical Pap smear is recommended at age 21 years for women who are immunocompetent and asymptomatic.[53,268] HPV testing is not recommended until age 30 years as studies have demonstrated that HPV testing in women younger than age 30 leads to detection of transient HPV infections and unnecessary colposcopies.[46,157,206] There are three HPV vaccines available in the United States. Cervarix, the bivalent (types 16, 18); Gardasil, the quadrivalent (types 6, 11, 16, and 18); and Gardasil-9 (types 6, 11, 16, 18, 31, 31, 45, 52, and 58) are approved by the FDA[165] for the prevention of HPV-related cancers. Gardasil-4 was withdrawn at the end of 2016 because almost all the vaccine being ordered is Gardasil-9.

Molluscum Contagiosum

Molluscum contagiosum is a viral infection of the skin caused by a DNA poxvirus characterized by small, discrete, translucent, grayish-pink, umbilicated, wartlike papules that sometimes are surrounded by a narrow ring of erythema. The lesions, which are asymptomatic, usually are less than 5 mm in diameter and may be missed by the patient and the examiner. The disease is transmitted by close physical contact, including sexual activity, and is encountered most often in postmenarcheal patients on the inner surfaces of the thighs, the perineum, and the lower part of the abdomen. The average incubation period is 2 to 7 weeks and can be as long as 6 months. Pediatricians frequently encounter molluscum contagiosum on the nongenital skin of children. It can be contracted from contaminated towels, bedding, and garments. Lesions of molluscum contagiosum on the lower part of the abdomen, pubis, thighs, or perineum of a child are tacit evidence of sexual contact.[52,161]

The appearance of the lesions usually is sufficient to establish the diagnosis. It can be confirmed by finding large, intracytoplasmic inclusion bodies in a smear or biopsy specimen from a lesion.

Lesions may go away on their own and usually last 6 to 8 weeks. They do not recur. A variety of treatment approaches are available if the lesions continue to spread. Curettage is the most efficacious treatment, with a low rate of side effects; however the procedure requires anesthesia and is time-consuming.[107] Cryotherapy gives good results.[6] Alternative options include cantharidin, podofilox, and imiquimod.[34,251,250] Topical imiquimod holds promise, but an optimal treatment schedule has not been determined.[52,272]

ULCERATIONS AND GRANULOMATOUS INFECTIONS

Sexually transmitted genital ulcerative and granulomatous infections occur throughout the world but are found most frequently in tropical countries. Genital ulcers are a common finding on evaluation of adolescent and adult patients with genital symptoms. They are less common findings in young children. Ulcers usually are secondary lesions that result from the breakdown of vesicles, papules, or pustules. By the time that many patients with genital infections seek medical attention for their symptoms, the primary lesion has proceeded to ulceration.[230] Microbial causes vary by geographic region and socioeconomic status: HSV is the most common cause in Western Europe and North America, whereas chancroid is the most common one in the tropics; in the United States, syphilis and chancroid are more common occurrences in urban minority groups, whereas HSV is found more commonly in more affluent groups. Complications of sexually transmitted genital ulcerative diseases also occur more commonly in developing countries and often are the reason for seeking medical care.[175]

HSV infection, syphilis, chancroid, lymphogranuloma venereum, granuloma inguinale, and tuberculosis all may have genital ulcers as a major clinical finding (Table 42.2). Although each of these diseases has a characteristic lesion and course, considerable overlap exists so a diagnosis based on the history and physical appearance alone often is inaccurate. Herpetic ulcers, contrary to classic manifestations, can be painless, and syphilis chancres can be painful at times (see Chapters 144 and 158). Secondary infection of an ulcerated area may cause pain in lesions that characteristically are painless. In addition, more than one STD may be present in at least 3% to 10% of patients with genital ulcers.

Genital ulcers also may result from infestation, fixed drug eruption, mechanical or chemical trauma, autoimmune processes (e.g., Behçet syndrome and Crohn disease),[176] and neoplasia. The presence of ulcers in sites other than the genital regions or oropharynx suggests a noninfectious etiology. The vulvar lesions of Behçet syndrome appear as destructive, deep, relatively painless ulcerations that, on recurrence, can result in scarring and distortion with progressive loss of vulvar tissue.[143,197]

In the United States, most patients with genital ulcers have genital herpes, syphilis, chancroid, or a combination thereof. Empiric treatment often must be given before diagnostic test results are available, and laboratory confirmation of a specific diagnosis is lacking in at least a quarter of patients with genital ulcer disease. Treatment of syphilis and chancroid should be considered in such circumstances, especially in geographic regions where chancroid morbidity is notable (see later discussion).[272,185]

Genital ulcers and granulomatous infections of any etiology, but especially those caused by herpes, syphilis, chancroid, and granuloma inguinale, are associated with an increased risk of acquiring HIV infection. Serologic testing for HIV infection should be considered in the management of patients with genital ulcers.[272] Improved treatment of STIs can affect the rate of HIV seroconversion in a population.[98]

Perinatal transmission of HSV types 1 and 2 in the form of stomatitis occurs in infants. HSV infection of the genitalia rarely occurs in children.[108,139] The presence of genital herpes lesions in a child or any disease that is known to be sexually transmitted in an adult should raise a question about whether the child has been subjected to some type of sexual molestation. HSV types 1 and 2 have been isolated in the genital area in children alleging sexual abuse.[88,124] The mode of acquisition of the infection is not always known, but case reports describe the possibility of autoinoculation from oral lesions, physical contact by a mother's infected finger, and sexual abuse.[139] No studies have reported the coexistence of HSV genital infection in household members and infected children. HSV has been known to survive for 2 hours on latex gloves and toilet seats, 24 hours on a speculum, and 72 hours on gauze.[152] However, transmission of HSV from fomites requires direct contact of viable virus with either a mucous membrane or a break in the skin, rendering fomite transmission unlikely. In summary a child with genital herpes infection should be considered suspicious and evaluated for sexual abuse, and the case should be reported to the authorities.[272]

Syphilis infections not found to be acquired congenitally should be considered sexually transmitted. Sexually acquired infection is a strong possibility in all prepubertal children with syphilis. The presence of syphilis should be considered diagnostic of sexual abuse, and an investigation must be pursued. In three studies, syphilis has been identified in 0%, 0.3%, and 5% of cases of alleged sexual abuse.[64,92,124]

TABLE 42.2 Diagnostic Features of Genital Ulcerations Caused by Sexually Transmitted Diseases

Feature	Primary Syphilis	Genital Herpes	Chancroid	Lymphogranuloma Venereum	Granuloma Inguinale
Incubation period	9–90 days; avg, 2–4 wk	2–7 days	1–35 days; avg, 3–7 days	3 days to 3 wk; avg, 10–14 days	Precise data unavailable; probably a few days to several months
No. lesions	Usually one; may be multiple	Multiple; may coalesce, more with primary episodes than with recurrences	Usually one to three, may be multiple	Usually single	Single or multiple
Description of genital ulcers	Sharply demarcated, round or oval ulcer with slightly elevated edges; may be irregular, symmetric "kissing chancre"	Small, superficial, grouped vesicles, erosions, or both; lesions may coalesce and form bullae or large areas of ulceration; lesions have irregular borders	Superficial, shallow, sharply demarcated ulcer; irregular, ragged, undermined edge; a few millimeters to 2 cm in diameter	Papule, pustule, vesicle, or ulcer discrete and transient; frequently overlooked	Sharply defined, irregular ulcerations or hypertrophic, verrucous, necrotic, or cicatricial granulomata
Base	Red, smooth, and shiny or crusty; oozing serous exudate when squeezed	Bright red and smooth	Rough, uneven, yellow to gray	Variable	Usually friable, rough, beefy granulations; can be necrotic, verrucous, or cicatricial
Induration	Firm; does not change shape with pressure	None	Soft; changes shape with pressure	None	Firm granulation tissue
Pain	Painless; may become tender if secondarily infected	Common; more prominent with initial infection than with recurrences	Common	Variable	Rare
Inguinal lymphadenopathy	Unilateral or bilateral, firm, movable, and nontender; does not suppurate	Usually bilateral, firm, and tender; more common in primary episodes than in recurrences	Unilateral; bilateral rarely occurs; overlying erythema; matted, fixed, and tender; suppuration may occur	Unilateral or bilateral; initially movable, firm, and tender; later indolent; fixed and matted; "sign of groove" may suppurate; fistulas	Pseudobuboes; subcutaneous perilymphatic granulomatous lesions that produce inguinal swellings
Constitutional symptoms	Rare	Common in primary episode; less likely in recurrences	Rare	Frequent	Rare
Course of untreated disease	Slowly (2–6 wk) resolves to latency	Recurrence is the rule	May progress to erosive lesions	Local lesions heal; systemic disease may progress; disfiguring; late complications	Worsens slowly
Diagnostic tests	*Treponema pallidum:* Darkfield examination, direct immunofluorescence, RPR, TPPA, FTA-ABS, VDRL	*Herpes simplex types 1 and 2:* Culture, PCR, direct immunofluorescence, Tzanck smear, electron microscopy, direct immunoperoxidase staining, serology	*Haemophilus ducreyi:* Culture, biopsy (rarely used), Gram-stained smears have low specificity	*Chlamydia trachomatis LGV 1, 2, 3:* Complement fixation, isolation of microorganism by culture	*Klebsiella granulomatis:* Donovan bodies in tissue smears; biopsy

Modified from Mroczkowski TF, Martin DH. Genital ulcer disease. *Dermatol Clin.* 1994;12:753–764.

avg, Average, *FTA-ABS,* fluorescent treponemal antibody absorption test; *RPR,* rapid plasma reagin; *TPPA,* treponema pallidum particle agglutination; *VDRL,* Venereal Disease Research Laboratory.

Syphilitic lesions and positive serologic results have been detected in alleged sexual abusers of children with syphilis.[1] No data are available on the survival of *T. pallidum* on fomites.

Lymphogranuloma venereum will be addressed in this chapter. The remaining listed infectious etiologies of genital ulcerative and granulomatous infections including herpes, syphilis, chancroid, and granuloma inguinale are described in more detail in Chapters 130, 134, 144, and 158.

Lymphogranuloma Venereum

Lymphogranuloma venereum is caused by *C. trachomatis,* subtypes L1 to L3. It is characterized by indolent inflammatory infiltration, granulomatous ulceration, abscess formation, and fibrotic cicatrization of the inguinal, perineal, and rectal lymphatics. It occurs more often in tropical than temperate climates.

Adolescents acquire lymphogranuloma venereum through sexual activity. Lymphogranuloma venereum has been reported in children[16,93,263] and always should raise suspicion for child sexual abuse. Nonsexual transmission by accidental inoculation of infected material from family members via handling of garments or towels that have been contaminated by drainage from ulcerative lesions or buboes of other household members has been postulated. Some evidence suggests that transplacental or perinatal transmission of the lymphogranuloma venereum serovars of *C. trachomatis* can occur.[93]

The primary lesion, a small papule or superficial and relatively asymptomatic ulcer (Fig. 42.14), seldom is seen in either children or older patients. A prodromal episode of fever, malaise, and joint pain accompanied by leukocytosis and anemia may precede the local signs. These symptoms often are mild and not diagnostically significant.

The most common manifestation is inguinal and/or femoral lymphadenopathy that is usually unilateral. When untreated, the adenitis may progress to abscess formation (buboes), followed by rupture with the development of draining sinuses. Spontaneous regression sometimes occurs. Rectal exposure can lead to proctocolitis that may be associated with anal pain, mucoid or hemorrhagic rectal discharge, constipation, and/or tenesmus. Fever also can occur. Untreated proctocolitis can progress to colorectal fistulas and strictures over time. Reactive manifestations, as with other forms of *C. trachomatis* infection, can occur and include arthritis, usually of the knees, and erythema nodosum.[93]

Diagnosis can be made by culture, direct immunofluorescence, or nucleic acid tests of genital or lymph node specimens for *C. trachomatis.* Swabs of ulcerative lesions or aspirates of buboes may be used. NAATs perform well on rectal specimens and are the preferred approach to testing of rectal specimens. These are not FDA approved for rectal specimens, but many laboratories have performed the required validation studies to offer these.[272] Serum complement fixation titers of greater than 1:64 or microimmunofluorescence titers of greater than 1:256 can be used to support the diagnosis of lymphogranuloma venereum in appropriate clinical contexts.

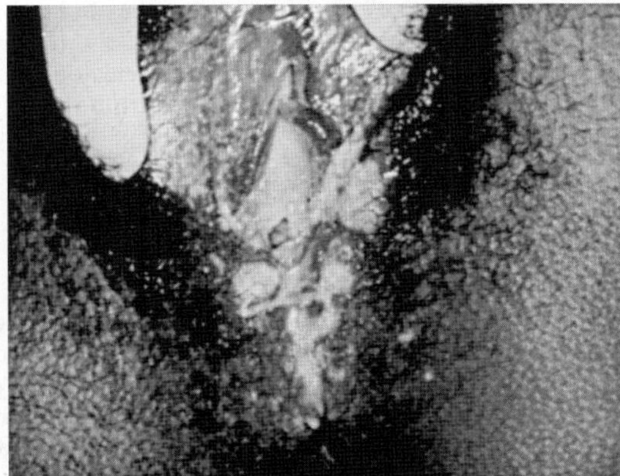

FIG. 42.14 Early lesions of lymphogranuloma venereum in the form of herpetic-like ulcers in an adolescent. The diagnosis was confirmed serologically.

Lymphogranuloma venereum may coexist with syphilis, and false-positive Venereal Disease Research Laboratory (VDRL) test results have been reported. Specific tests for antitreponemal antibodies should be obtained to confirm coinfection with syphilis when nontreponemal tests are positive. The disease is differentiated from other granulomatous and ulcerative disorders by specific tests for each, by biopsy, and by the clinical appearance of the lesions (see Table 42.2).

The preferred treatment of lymphogranuloma venereum is doxycycline, 100 mg orally twice a day for 21 days.[272] The alternative regimen is erythromycin base 500 mg orally four times a day for 21 days. Azithromycin 1 g orally once a week for 3 weeks is probably effective, but clinical data are lacking. A macrolide-based regimen is preferred for children younger than 8 years of age. Treatment is curative and can prevent progression of tissue damage but may not reverse scarring that has already occurred. Aspiration or incision and drainage of buboes may be required in some cases. Sexual contacts of patients with lymphogranuloma venereum within the 60 days prior to onset of the patient's symptoms should be evaluated and treated presumptively with a chlamydia regimen appropriate for the suspected site(s) of infection.[272]

Cervicitis

Prepubertal

The cervix is not involved when a prepubertal child has vaginitis because most vaginal infections affect only the distal half of the vagina in children; the exception is gonococcal vaginitis, which in addition usually involves the squamous epithelium over the external cervix. Cervicitis also may occur when a vaginal foreign body is present. Endocervicitis is an unusual finding in premenarcheal girls because the endocervical glands and mucosa are developed poorly before menarche, providing a poor environment for invading organisms.[21]

Postpubertal

The structure of the cervix during the reproductive years renders it vulnerable to infections induced by numerous factors. The long, narrow, deeply pocketed cervical canal, which is lined by open cryptic glands bathed in alkaline secretion and washed periodically by menstrual blood, is an excellent nidus for the growth of bacteria. Pathogenic bacteria in the vagina find ready access to the cervical canal. The use of oral contraceptive pills promotes cervical ectopy, increasing the vulnerability of endocervical cells to chlamydial infection.[21,119]

Early recognition and aggressive treatment of cervicitis in sexually active adolescents are important to prevent serious complications, including PID, tubo-ovarian abscess, ectopic pregnancy, chronic pelvic pain, and infertility. Some confusion tends to occur, however, with regard to differentiating normal ectopic columnar epithelium on the exocervix (ectopy) from cervicitis. Ectopy is not an abnormal finding. When the squamocolumnar junction is exposed on the exocervix, it is called *ectopy.* It appears bright shiny red, in contrast to the dull pearly pink appearance of the exocervix. This area does not bleed easily when touched with a swab. During adolescence, the normal cervix may exhibit no ectopy, a small area of ectopy, or sometimes 50% ectopy. When the ectopy appears edematous, raised, and friable (often with marked bleeding when touched lightly with a swab), cervicitis should be suspected.[21,166] Cervicitis primarily is endocervicitis most commonly associated with *C. trachomatis* and *N. gonorrhoeae.* However, the etiology in most cases is not determined and could be from *Mycoplasma genitalium, G. vaginalis,* group B streptococci, and *T. vaginalis.* Because of the high prevalence of coexisting infections of the cervix, associating any one organism with the clinical signs and symptoms of cervicitis often is difficult.[207,221] Cervicitis often is asymptomatic, but it should be clinically suspected if an adolescent reports a vaginal discharge and bleeding, especially after having sexual intercourse. Criteria for a clinical diagnosis of mucopurulent cervicitis include the presence of mucopurulent secretion from the endocervix, erythema of the cervix, friable ectopy, and bleeding from the cervix.[36,166] The mucopurulent secretion in chlamydial cervicitis is tenacious mucoid material mixed with yellow exudate and is difficult to remove from the endocervix. In contrast a profuse, yellowish-green, acrid discharge is present in gonococcal cervicitis. Cervical erosion ulcerations can occur in sexually active adolescents and can be caused by HSV. Rarer causes are the primary lesion of syphilis, tuberculosis, granuloma inguinale, lymphogranuloma venereum, chancroid, schistosomiasis, and actinomycosis.

Diagnosis

Tests for chlamydial and gonococcal infection should be performed in all sexually active adolescents. NAATs are considered the most sensitive and specific tests today, and testing of urine and self-obtained vaginal specimens has revolutionized screening and diagnosis. The reliability of amplification tests such as polymerase chain reaction, strand displacement amplification, and transcription-mediated amplification in detecting chlamydia and gonorrhea seems to be equivalent for vaginal, cervical, and urine specimens as long as the urine collected is a first-catch specimen; the sensitivities range from 87% to 99% and specificity from 97% to 100%.[23,214,215,227]

Other tests, including culture, direct fluorescent antibody tests, enzyme immunoassay, nucleic acid hybridization tests, enhanced optical immunoassays, and NAATs, continue to be available to diagnose *C. trachomatis* infection. The regular culture and tissue culture method was considered the gold standard for both gonorrhea and *Chlamydia*[213] but because of the high cost of this technique, it is not used widely for adolescents. In some large-volume, community-based clinics, the DNA hybridization assay or DNA probe (Gen-Probe) and enzyme immunoassay (Abbot, Wampole, Kodak, Gen-Probe) are still used for gonorrhea and *Chlamydia*.[146,217,227,234]

Commercial multiplex tests are available for *M. genitalium, U. urealyticum, T. vaginalis,* and *G. vaginalis.* However, the utility of testing for other organisms in adolescents is questioned, especially in clinical settings in which microscopy is readily available. In settings without microscopy, using commercial tests for *T. vaginalis* and *G. vaginalis* may be of value.

Although the reliability of detecting gram-negative intracellular diplococci on a Gram stain of cervical secretions is low, this test can be useful in areas where more sophisticated tests are unavailable. The presence of at least eight pairs of gram-negative intracellular diplococci in at least three polymorphonuclear cells strongly suggests gonococcal cervicitis.

Treatment

The same guidelines for the treatment of gonococcal and chlamydial cervicitis are used for the treatment of presumptive cervicitis in nonpregnant adolescents. Azithromycin 1 g orally in a single dose or doxycycline 100 mg once per day for 7 days is recommended for presumptive *C. trachomatis, M. genitalium,* and *U. urealyticum* cervicitis.[272] Current treatment of gonococcal infection is influenced by the emergence of antibiotic-resistant strains, including penicillinase-producing *N. gonorrhoeae,* fluoroquinolone-resistant strains, tetracycline-resistant strains, and chromosomally resistant strains.[272] The high frequency of chlamydial infection in individuals with gonorrhea (45% in certain populations) and the serious complications resulting from untreated gonorrhea and chlamydial infections also have influenced the treatment approach. Treatment options include intramuscular ceftriaxone 250 mg in a single dose plus azithromycin 1 g orally in a single dose. An alternative regimen if ceftriaxone is unavailable is cefixime 400 mg orally as a single dose plus azithromycin 1 g orally in a single dose.[272] In the case of penicillin allergy, cephalosporins are not contraindicated unless the patient has a history of a severe reaction (e.g., anaphylaxis, Stevens-Johnson syndrome, and toxic epidermal necrolysis). Spectinomycin is an alternative but is unavailable in the United States.[272] Pregnant adolescent girls or women should be treated with one dose of ceftriaxone 250 mg intramuscularly plus one dose of azithromycin 1 g orally. If pharyngeal or rectal gonorrhea is suspected, the recommended treatment is intramuscular ceftriaxone 250 mg plus azithromycin 1 g orally.[272] When *T. vaginalis* vaginitis is diagnosed or HSV is suspected strongly, the appropriate treatment for these infections should be given (see discussions on trichomoniasis and genital herpes). Currently no CDC consensus exists on the treatment of asymptomatic individuals with positive tests for *M. genitalium* and *U. urealyticum*.[272]

Integral to treating the patient is notification, examination, and expedited treatment of the patient's sexual partners if gonococcal or chlamydial infection, or both, is confirmed. Direct notification by the patient should be encouraged, and, based on state laws, a prescription for partner therapy can be given. Written information should be provided with names of diseases and medication side effects to assist with this process. When tests are positive for gonorrhea or chlamydial infection, retesting for these infections is recommended in 3 months if treated with other regimens to detect reinfection from an untreated or new partner.[272]

Chlamydia

Chlamydia infections are the most frequently reported STIs in the United States, and the highest rates are reported in adolescents and young adults between 15 and 24 years old.[48] Prevalence rates of chlamydial cervicitis in adolescents range from 8% to 25% in urban clinics located in hospital, community, family planning, and juvenile detention centers. It is three to four times more common than gonococcal cervicitis. *C. trachomatis* causes cervicitis by infecting the columnar and transitional epithelium of the cervix. Cervical ectopy seems to be a predisposing factor for acquisition of *C. trachomatis* infection.[13,48] *C. trachomatis* cervicitis is predominantly an asymptomatic disease in adolescent girls.[49] A clinical diagnosis is made when friable ectopy with a mucopurulent cervical discharge (mucopus) is noted. Chlamydial cervicitis is suspected when a Gram stain of an adequate endocervical smear shows more than 5 to 10 polymorphonuclear cells per oil immersion field in the absence of gram-negative intracellular diplococci.[36,174]

Treatment of chlamydial cervicitis was discussed in the earlier section on cervicitis.

Gonorrhea

The highest rates of gonorrhea infections are reported in young adults 20 to 24 years old.[48] The risk for acquiring infection varies with the population. Adolescents seen in private practices in the suburbs have a significantly lower rate of gonococcal cervicitis than that noted in adolescents seen in large outpatient hospital clinics or community clinics serving inner-city populations. The prevalence rate of gonorrhea in adolescent girls in urban hospital settings ranges from 3% to 12% in hospital, community, family planning, and juvenile detention centers.[48] Anal gonorrhea usually is secondary to discharge from gonococcal cervicitis infecting the anus. Primary anal gonorrhea as a result of anal intercourse should be suspected in a sexually active adolescent with anal discomfort. In addition, gonococcal infection should be considered in the differential diagnosis of pharyngitis in sexually active adolescents. Gonococcal endocarditis, arthritis, and dermal abscesses occur, but they are beyond the scope of this chapter.

Gonococcal cervicitis may be symptomatic or asymptomatic. Although gonococcal cervicitis is reported to be predominantly an asymptomatic condition in girls and women, many patients, after careful questioning, are found to have symptoms. The discharge is profuse and prevalent. On examination, the vulvar tissues may be inflamed and edematous. Discharge also may be seen exuding out of the urethra and paraurethral ducts in severe cases. On speculum examination, the patient has a normal-appearing cervix or the cervix appears erythematous and friable, with a foul-smelling purulent discharge draining from the cervical os.

Treatment of gonococcal cervicitis was discussed in the earlier section on cervicitis.

UPPER GENITAL TRACT INFECTIONS

Pelvic Inflammatory Disease

PID is defined as an acute clinical syndrome attributed to the ascent of microorganisms from the vagina and endocervix to the endometrium, fallopian tubes, or contiguous structures that result in pelvic and generalized peritonitis. The use of terms specifically describing the anatomic sites involved is preferable (e.g., endometritis, salpingitis, salpingo-oophoritis, tubo-ovarian abscess).

PID is an extremely rare finding in prepubertal girls and often is undiagnosed until advanced infection occurs.[35,68] With the exception of gonorrhea and the inflammation caused by a foreign body, most vulvar and vaginal infections do not involve the upper third of the vagina and do not approach the cervix of premenarcheal patients. The prepubertal cervix and endometrium apparently are barriers rather than passageways for bacteria causing all types of vulvovaginitis in children.

When intrapelvic infection has been reported in prepubertal girls, it usually has been part of either generalized primary peritonitis or peritonitis secondary to a ruptured appendix or some other intra-abdominal infection.[76] Pelvic infection that is part of an intraabdominal infection characteristically affects the surfaces of the uterine tubes, uterus, and ovaries and produces perisalpingitis and periovaritis; periappendicitis also is present even if the infection did not begin as appendicitis. An ascending infection from the lower genital tract, such as that caused by gonorrhea, involves the tubal mucosa and produces endosalpingitis and pyosalpingitis. Gonococcal pelvic infection has been reported after sexual abuse has occurred. *S. pneumoniae* serotypes 1 and 2 and *E. coli* also have been reported in pubertal girls with salpingitis and peritonitis and tubo-ovarian abscess.[35]

PID in the postpubertal period occurs primarily in sexually active adolescents at risk for STIs.[77,227] Salpingitis has been reported in virgins, and, although the etiology is unknown, the organisms are thought to spread hematogenously, lymphatically, or transmurally from intestines or ascending infection from the vagina.[68] National epidemiologic data on PID specific to the adolescent age group are not available. However, the proportion of women with acute PID due to *C. trachomatis* and *N. gonorrhoeae* is declining.[42,183] This decline has been attributed to aggressive screening for chlamydia and gonorrhea infections in sexually active adolescents in a variety of health care settings that serve urban sexually active adolescents.[272]

Reasons for the development of PID in adolescents are physiologic and social and include sexual activity and multiple sexual partners. Cervical mucus is less viscous during menses and at midcycle, rendering it more permeable to ascending infection. In vitro experiments show that *N. gonorrhoeae, C. trachomatis, U. urealyticum,* and other aerobic and anaerobic agents can adhere to spermatozoa and migrate with them.[255] Whether this event can occur in vivo is unknown. Most organisms found in nongonococcal and nonchlamydial PID also are found in bacterial vaginosis, suggesting that bacterial vaginosis may be a predisposing or a precipitating factor for the development of PID. In addition, researchers have suggested that *T. vaginalis* can act as a vector for transporting bacteria.[140] Another possible factor is upward transport of bacteria from orgasmic myometrial contractions.[187] Finally vaginal douching has been reported to be a risk factor in promoting ascending infection.[182,187,269]

Oral contraceptive pills are used commonly by adolescents and may have a protective or facilitating risk factor for PID. Laparoscopic studies also have shown that women with PID who were using oral contraceptive pills have significantly milder degrees of fallopian tube inflammation than do women who do not use the pills. This finding suggests that the oral contraceptive pill may reduce potential tubal damage. Other studies report, however, that by promoting cervical ectopy, oral contraceptives are a potential risk factor for acquiring chlamydial PID.[222,249,270] In contrast, compared with other methods of contraception, women using depot medroxyprogesterone acetate (Depo-Provera) had a significantly decreased risk for developing PID.[270] Modern intrauterine devices (IUDs) are not associated with increased risk of PID.[97,156,272] The risk for PID in association with an IUD is highest the first 3 weeks after insertion secondary to instrumentation of the cervix.[97]

Women who have had one episode of PID have a 20% to 25% chance of having subsequent ones. Reasons for this susceptibility may be reinfection from untreated sexual partners, an inadequately treated first infection, or increased susceptibility of the tubal epithelium to infection.[77,187]

Endometritis

Infections of the endometrium in postmenarcheal girls and women are as rare as previously thought. The gonococcus, on its way upward to the uterine tubes, produces a fleeting asymptomatic infection of the endometrium, or the symptoms produced are overshadowed by those of the vulvar and cervical infections. Evidence also suggests that endometritis occurs in 40% of patients with asymptomatic endocervical chlamydial infection.[136] It also is called *subclinical PID,* and repeated episodes have been linked to infertility.[136,264] The role of HIV infection in the development of subclinical PID is unclear. An increased prevalence of endometritis in HIV-infected women compared with uninfected women has been noted, and altered immune function might contribute to difficulty clearing endometritis in these cases.[37]

Symptoms specific to endometritis are uncommon. It is commonly an asymptomatic condition. Symptoms include recurrent intermittent or acute suprapubic pain and tenderness with vaginal bleeding or spotting. On bimanual examination, the uterus is tender, and cervical motion tenderness may or may not be present. Endometritis in adolescent girls and young women also has been associated with postabortive and puerperal endometritis. Poor compliance with prophylactic antibiotics places an adolescent at an increased risk for development of endometritis after having an abortion. Endometrial tuberculosis is a rare occurrence in the United States and is encountered most often in patients with pulmonary tuberculosis. This entity needs to be considered in HIV-infected girls and women and in geographic areas and regions where tuberculosis is endemic. In a study from a province in Iran, tuberculous endometritis was detected in 72% of genital tuberculosis cases in women.[180] The disease may not manifest for years after initial seeding, and the infection is thought to reach the uterus via the gastrointestinal tract through hematogenous seeding and by lymphatic spread. It is not acquired as a result of an ascending infection or through coitus with an infected man. The symptoms of endometrial tuberculosis vary from none to amenorrhea, pelvic pain, dysmenorrhea, abnormal uterine bleeding, and tuberculosis. Often the patient has a history of healed or active pulmonary disease. Overall 60% of patients with pelvic tuberculosis have tuberculous endometritis.[109]

Endometrial tuberculosis is diagnosed by endometrial biopsy and demonstration of acid-fast *M. tuberculosis* in cultures of curettage material or menstrual blood. Menstrual fluid has been reported to be culture-positive more frequently than are biopsy specimens.[109] Endometrial tuberculosis and the management of tuberculosis are described further in Chapter 96.

Salpingitis

The pathogenesis of salpingitis has been studied best with *N. gonorrhoeae* and *C. trachomatis.* In the fallopian tube, gonococci attach to nonciliated epithelial cells and induce sloughing of ciliated epithelial cells into the lumen.[187,247] Gonococci also enter the subepithelial space, where a local inflammatory response, predominantly polymorphonuclear leukocytic infiltrate and anaerobic bacteria, is produced and may reach the bloodstream. A purulent exudate is produced within the tube and may cause pelvic peritonitis. Chlamydial infection produces a similar picture except that it causes a predominantly lymphocytic infiltrate in the submucosa.[187,189,247]

Salpingitis also is caused by several other microbial agents that have been isolated directly from the fallopian tubes. The organisms most commonly recovered from the upper tract in salpingitis are mixed anaerobes (25–84%), followed by *N. gonorrhoeae* (25–40%) and *C. trachomatis* (25–40%). Mixed aerobic and anaerobic infections, including *Bacteroides* and *Peptostreptococcus* spp., account for 25% to 60% of cases. These mixed infections occur more frequently in girls and women with severe, chronic, and recurrent PID. PID develops in approximately 10% to 17% of girls and women with endocervical *N. gonorrhoeae* and in 10% to 30% with endocervical *C. trachomatis.* At first researchers thought that *N. gonorrhoeae* initiated the infection and that superinfection with anaerobes followed. They now realize that apparently anaerobes and aerobes can initiate PID without *C. trachomatis* or *N. gonorrhoeae.*[187,266]

Differentiating salpingitis caused by different microbiologic organisms is difficult. *N. gonorrhoeae* has been identified most frequently within the initial 24 hours of development of symptoms. Beyond 48 hours, the most frequent isolates are anaerobes. Gonococcal or chlamydial salpingitis seems to occur most often within 1 week of menstruation.[248] The clinical presentation varies from asymptomatic to severe disease. The severity of infection depends on duration of symptoms and the etiologic agent. Chlamydial PID tends to be less symptomatic than infection from *N. gonorrhoeae.*

Diagnosis

The classic manifestation of acute PID is lower abdominal pain, which usually is bilateral and continuous and may worsen with movement or with coitus. After the onset of abdominal pain, fever, nausea, and vomiting may develop in more severe cases. The temperature may reach 39°C to 39.5°C (102°F–103°F). A chill seldom precedes the fever. Other common initial symptoms include vaginal discharge, irregular vaginal bleeding, and urinary symptoms.[208,272]

On physical examination, the patient usually looks sick and uncomfortable. Abdominal examination reveals a markedly tender and often tense lower part of the abdomen. Rebound tenderness indicates generalized peritonitis. The genital examination may show a purulent vaginal discharge in the vaginal vault. Even gentle bimanual rectovaginal abdominal palpation causes great distress. Attempted mobilization of the cervix is extremely painful. The uterus is tense and tender. The adnexa may not be outlined because of discomfort produced by the examination. Palpation of the adnexa unilaterally or bilaterally may be exceptionally painful. An adnexal swelling may be palpated, but this finding is unreliable in diagnosing an adnexal mass. In a less acutely tender patient, the examination may reveal a thickened, tender tube.

Common laboratory findings in patients with PID include a peripheral white blood cell count greater than 10,000/mm^3 and an erythrocyte sedimentation rate greater than 15 mm/h. In addition, endocervical gonorrhea and *Chlamydia* infection may be present simultaneously in 10% to 30% of cases. Ultrasonography of the pelvic cavity helps detect pelvic abscesses. A study involving the use of pelvic ultrasonography in adolescents with PID showed that the presence of fluid in the cul-de-sac was not helpful in differentiating patients with and without PID.[94] Almost 20% of patients with PID had a tubo-ovarian abscess; in the absence of a tubo-ovarian abscess, adnexal volume was significantly larger in adolescents with PID than in adolescents without it.[94] Ultrasonography (transvaginal) can be very useful in ruling out other diagnoses and defining adnexal masses and is readily available and affordable. Magnetic resonance imaging (MRI) can also be utilized. Compared to ultrasonography it is more accurate in delineating anatomic structures.[256]

The clinical diagnosis of PID is made by having a high index of suspicion for this entity. For practical reasons, the clinical criteria developed by Jacobsen and Westrom[130] and revised by the CDC[272] are recommended to aid in making the diagnosis and subsequently to increase the index of suspicion for PID (Box 42.2).

The minimum criteria recommended for empiric treatment include abdominal pain with uterine tenderness or cervical motion tenderness or adnexal tenderness.[272] The more criteria that can be met, the more likely it is that a tubal infection is present. The differential diagnosis of PID is an acute abdomen. Conditions of the urinary tract that should be considered include cystitis, pyelonephritis, and urethritis. Gastrointestinal tract conditions include appendicitis, constipation, diverticulitis, gastroenteritis, inflammatory bowel disease, and irritable bowel syndrome. Gynecologic conditions include dysmenorrhea, ectopic pregnancy, endometriosis, endometritis, mittelschmerz, torsion or rupture of an ovarian cyst, ruptured follicle, septic abortion, threatened abortion, and pyogenic sacroiliitis. As in PID, establishing an early diagnosis of acute appendicitis and ectopic pregnancy is important.

Treatment

The major goals of treatment of PID are preservation of fertility and prevention of other long-term sequelae, including ectopic pregnancy. Although some data suggest that women younger than 25 years have a better fertility prognosis overall after having PID and ectopic pregnancy, no difference exists among age groups regarding tubal infertility specifically after PID.[187] Earlier initiation of treatment results in lower risk for developing infertility. Girls and women initially evaluated after more than 3 days of abdominal pain are found to have a 2.8-fold increased risk for having impaired fertility (tubal infertility or ectopic pregnancy) compared with those evaluated within 3 days of the onset of abdominal pain.[118] Generally, more severe PID has a higher risk for future infertility. In addition, more episodes of PID result in a higher risk for future infertility. After one episode, the risk for infertility ranges from 8% to 13%; after two episodes, the risk is 20% to 35%; and after three or more episodes, it is 40% to 75%.[246]

To reduce the incidence of sequelae associated with this condition, early recognition of PID, the use of broad-spectrum antibiotics to treat polymicrobial disease, careful clinical reevaluation 48 hours after initiating antibiotic treatment to assess antibiotic response, and evaluation and treatment of sexual partners are important. Screening the patient for other STIs, such as trichomoniasis, bacterial vaginosis, and syphilis, also is important.

Patients with PID often are treated on an ambulatory basis. The primary reason to hospitalize an adolescent with PID is to ensure compliance with medication when she is unable to follow or tolerate an outpatient oral regimen because of the seriousness of the sequelae and problems with compliance in this age group. Other reasons for hospitalization are an uncertain diagnosis, the presence of a tubo-ovarian abscess, pregnancy, infection with HIV, temperature greater than 38.5°C (101.3°F), nausea and vomiting precluding the use of oral medications, and lack of improvement after 48 hours of oral antibiotic treatment.

The recommendations of the CDC for treating PID in ambulatory and hospitalized patients address antibiotic coverage for the polymicrobial etiology of this condition (Boxes 42.3 and 42.4).[272] In addition to antibiotic treatment, bed rest is recommended. Intravenous fluids are administered for hydration when necessary. When the diagnosis of PID is certain, oral analgesic agents may be prescribed. Close follow-up is recommended, with a bimanual examination performed after 48 hours of antibiotic treatment to assess the patient's response to treatment.[272] Overall most studies show that response to antibiotic regimens is similar

BOX 42.2 Clinical Criteria for the Diagnosis of Acute Pelvic Inflammatory Disease

Minimal Criteria

Lower abdominal or pelvic pain with one or more of the following: uterine or adnexal tenderness or cervical motion tenderness

Additional Criteria to Enhance Specificity

Temperature >38.3°C (>101.9°F)
Abnormal cervical or vaginal mucopurulent discharge
Presence of white blood cells on saline microscopy of vaginal secretions
Elevation of erythrocyte sedimentation rate
Elevated C-reactive protein
Laboratory documentation of cervical infection with *Neisseria gonorrhoeae* or *Chlamydia trachomatis* or both

Specific Criteria

Endometrial biopsy specimen with histopathologic evidence of endometritis
Transvaginal sonography or magnetic resonance imaging technique showing thickened fluid-filled or tubo-ovarian complex
Laparoscopic abnormalities consistent with pelvic inflammatory disease

From Workowski KA, Bolan GA. Centers for Disease Control and Prevention. Sexually transmitted diseases treatment guidelines, 2015. *MMWR Recomm Rep.* 2015;64(RR-03):1–137.

BOX 42.3 Ambulatory Management of Pelvic Inflammatory Disease

Ceftriaxone 250 mg IM in a single dose *or* cefoxitin 2 g IM in a single dose *plus* probenecid 1 g orally in a single dose *or* other parenteral third-generation cephalosporins (e.g., ceftizoxime or cefotaxime)
plus
Doxycycline 100 mg PO two times a day for 14 days
with or without
Metronidazole 500 mg PO twice a day for 14 days

From Workowski KA, Bolan GA. Centers for Disease Control and Prevention. Sexually transmitted diseases treatment guidelines, 2015. *MMWR Recomm Rep.* 2015;64(RR-03):1–137.

BOX 42.4 Inpatient Treatment of Pelvic Inflammatory Disease

Regimen A

Cefoxitin 2 g IV every 6 h *or* cefotetan 2 g IV every 12 h

plus

Doxycycline 100 mg every 12 h PO or IV

Regimen B

Clindamycin 900 mg IV every 8 h

plus

Gentamicin loading dose 2 mg/kg IV or IM, followed by a maintenance dose 1.5 mg/kg every 8 h

From Workowski KA, Bolan GA. Centers for Disease Control and Prevention. Sexually transmitted diseases treatment guidelines, 2015. *MMWR Recomm Rep.* 2015;64(RR-03):1–137.

These regimens are given for at least 24 h after the patient improves. After discharge from the hospital, the patient is continued on doxycycline 100 mg PO two times per day for a total of 14 days.

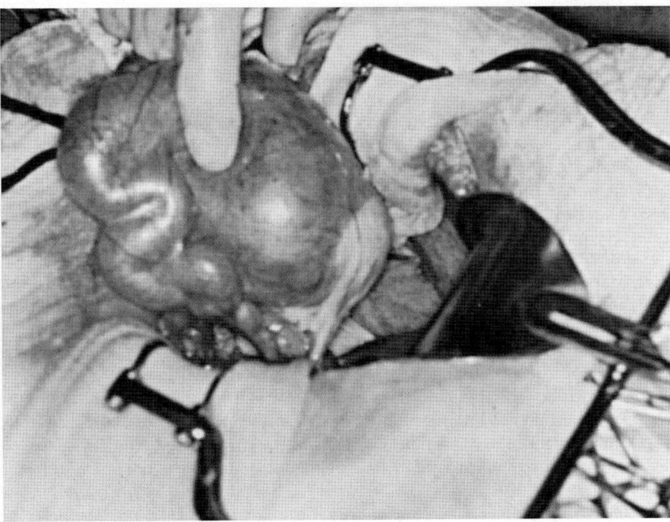

FIG. 42.15 Large hydrosalpinx, the result of gonorrheal salpingitis in an older teenage girl who had repeated gonorrheal infections. The other tube also was diseased.

between HIV-positive and HIV-negative patients. The treatment recommendations for HIV-positive patients are no different.[272]

Complications associated with PID are perihepatitis, tubo-ovarian abscess, hydrosalpinx (obstruction of the tube caused by scarring [Fig. 42.15]), chronic abdominal pain from adhesions surrounding the fallopian tubes and ovaries, recurrent PID, ectopic pregnancy, and infertility.[259]

Perihepatitis

The classic manifestation of perihepatitis, or Fitz-Hugh–Curtis syndrome,[187] is severe right upper abdominal pain that often radiates to the shoulder. Concurrent left upper abdominal pain also may be present. Lower abdominal pain and evidence of acute or subacute PID are frequent findings. The right upper quadrant pain lasts about 48 hours. Nausea, fever, and leukocytosis are common manifestations. Elevation of the erythrocyte sedimentation rate and liver enzymes may be present. The pathogenesis of perihepatitis is thought to be from direct spread of *N. gonorrhoeae* and *C. trachomatis* from the fallopian tubes into the peritoneal cavity, along the paracolic sulci. From there, they reach the subphrenic space and hepatic surface. Spread from the reproductive tract also is possible via the retroperitoneal lymphatics.[187]

The diagnosis is made by having a high index of suspicion. Perihepatitis frequently mimics cholelithiasis, hepatitis, pleuritis, subphrenic abscess, perforated peptic ulcer, nephrolithiasis, appendicitis, ectopic pregnancy, abdominal trauma, and pancreatitis. Treatment of this condition is similar to treatment of PID.

Tubo-ovarian Abscess

The formation of a tubo-ovarian abscess is a late manifestation of PID. The incidence of tubo-ovarian abscess ranges from 14% to 38% in hospital-based adolescents and adults with salpingitis.[94,99,148,233] Tubo-ovarian abscesses rarely are seen in adolescents and young women who are not sexually active, and alternative diagnoses involving congenital anomalies must be considered.[68,224] Organisms isolated from tubo-ovarian abscesses in adolescents who do not report sexual activity include *E. coli*, α-hemolytic streptococci, and *Pasteurella multocida*. The actual cause for ascending infection in these cases is unknown. Alterations in cervical secretions, which usually serve as a barrier, have been hypothesized. The abscess typically results from a mixture of facultative and anaerobic bacteria, with facultative bacteria dominating the early phase of infection, and bacterial metabolic products producing an environment of low oxygen tension that favors the growth of anaerobic bacteria.[187]

The most common organisms recovered from tubo-ovarian abscesses in sexually active women include *E. coli*, *Bacteroides fragilis*, other *Bacteroides* spp., *Peptostreptococcus*, *Peptococcus*, and aerobic streptococci.[199,267] Diagnosing the presence of a tubo-ovarian abscess clinically usually is difficult. Adolescents with a tubo-ovarian abscess tend to seek care later in their menstrual cycle than do girls without a tubo-ovarian abscess.[233] Bimanual examination frequently does not reveal a pelvic mass.[57] Four potentially useful clinical features that suggest the presence of a pelvic abscess are pain, persistent fever, adnexal tenderness (for 7 days), and an erythrocyte sedimentation rate greater than 30 mm/hr.[57] Ultrasonography of the pelvis is valuable in confirming the presence of an abscess.[94]

The prompt administration of antibiotics has reduced greatly the incidence of pelvic abscess. Most of those encountered today are in adolescents who have not had adequate care and have delayed seeking treatment.[100,237]

A conservative approach is favored for the treatment of a tubo-ovarian or ovarian abscess (i.e., bed rest, supportive care, intravenous antibiotics, and nonsteroidal analgesics).[233] This approach is appropriate when the adolescent (including an immunocompromised adolescent) is hemodynamically stable and the abscess is 9 cm or less in diameter. An abscess larger than 10 cm has a 60% chance, a 7- to 9-cm abscess has a 35% chance, and a 4- to 6-cm abscess has a 20% chance of requiring surgical intervention.[199] Surgical intervention may be needed during the initial period if hemodynamic instability and sepsis with imminent rupture is suspected. The choice of antibiotics should be based on effectiveness against lactamase-producing anaerobes, adequate coverage against resistant *Bacteroides* spp., penetration into the abscess, and ability to remain stable in an abscess environment. The antibiotic regimens for inpatient treatment of PID fulfill these considerations and are appropriate for the treatment of tubo-ovarian abscess (see Box 42.4). As is the case with cefoxitin, cefotetan, and clindamycin, metronidazole provides good activity against anaerobes.[272] Many hospitals prefer the use of triple antibiotics cefoxitin and gentamicin plus clindamycin or metronidazole.

A clinical response to treatment consisting of a decrease in pain, fever, and total leukocyte count should be noted in 72 hours. Pelvic ultrasonography should be repeated at this time to note any further increase in the size of the abscess. The duration of intravenous and oral antibiotic therapy for a tubo-ovarian abscess should be at least 21 days. The patient may begin oral antibiotics when she is afebrile and asymptomatic and when the size of the abscess has stabilized. The abscess either resolves without drainage or becomes encapsulated. The latter eventually "points" either in the cul-de-sac or anteriorly in the abdominal wall.

The fertility rate after treatment of tubo-ovarian abscesses may be 20% to 50% with conservative medical and surgical approaches.

Oophoritis

Oophoritis is a rare condition today and refers to inflammation of the substance of the ovaries, the oocytes in particular. Viral exanthems such as mumps and cytomegalovirus can be complicated by oophoritis, especially in immunosuppressed children and adolescents. Improved immunization practices have decreased the prevalence of mumps and its complications including oophoritis. However, an outbreak of mumps in children occurred in Centerville, Ohio, in 1981.[245] The severity of mumps disease (including oophoritis) was higher in children who had not been previously immunized compared to those who were immunized against mumps.[245] The presence of an enlarged, tender, boggy, smooth mobile ovary in a child with mumps or one of the exanthems suggests oophoritis. Treatment is palliative, with analgesics given for discomfort and fever.

NEW REFERENCES SINCE THE SEVENTH EDITION

6. Al-Mutairi N, Al-Doukhi A, Al-Farag S, et al. Comparative study on the efficacy, safety, and acceptability of imiquimod 5% cream versus cryotherapy for molluscum contagiosum in children. *Pediatr Dermatol*. 2010;27:388-394.
11. Anderson B, Thimmesch I, Aardsma N, et al. The prevalence of abnormal genital findings, vulvovaginitis, enuresis and encopresis in children who present with allegations of sexual abuse. *J Pediatri Urol*. 2014;10:1216-1221.
12. Andrea SB, Chapin KC. Comparison of Aptima *Trichomonas vaginalis* transcription-mediated amplification assay and BD affirm VPIII for detection of *T. vaginalis* in symptomatic women: performance parameters and epidemiological implications. *J Clin Microbiol*. 2011;49:866-869.
14. Atabek ME, Akyurek N, Eklioglu BS. Frequency of vaginal candida colonization and relationship between metabolic parameters in children with type 1 diabetes mellitus. *J Pediatr Adolesc Gynecol*. 2013;26:257-260.
15. Baker DA, Ferris DG, Martens MG, et al. Imiquimod 3.75% cream applied daily to treat anogenital warts: combined results from women in two randomized, placebo-controlled studies. *Infect Dis Obstet Gynecol*. 2011;1–11:2011.
17. Baron EJ, Miller JM, Weinstein MP, et al. A guide to utilization of the microbiology laboratory for diagnosis of infectious diseases: 2013 recommendations by the Infectious Diseases Society of America (IDSA) and the American Society for Microbiology (ASM)(a). *Clin Infect Dis*. 2013;57:e22-e121.
21. Berlan ED, Emans SJ, O'Brien RF. Vulvovaginal complaints in the adolescent. In: Emans SJ, Laufer MR, Goldstein DP, eds. *Pediatric & Adolescent Gynecology*. Philadelphia, PA: Lippincott Williams & Wilkins; 2012:305-324.
22. Best D, Ford CA, Miller WC. Prevalence of *Chlamydia trachomatis* and *Neisseria gonorrhoeae* infection in pediatric private practice. *Pediatrics*. 2001;108:E103.
31. Brocklehurst P, Gordon A, Heatley E, et al. Antibiotics for treating bacterial vaginosis in pregnancy. *Cochrane Database Syst Rev*. 2013;(1):CD000262.
32. Brook I. Aerobic and anaerobic microbiology of Bartholin's abscess. *Surg Gynecol Obstet*. 1989;169:32-34.
33. Brown JL. Hair shampooing technique and pediatric vulvovaginitis. *Pedatrics*. 1989;83:146.
38. Bumbuliene Z, Venclaviciute K, Ramasauskaite D, et al. Microbiological findings of vulvovaginitis in prepubertal girls. *Postgrad Med J*. 2014;90:8-12.
42. Burnett AM, Anderson CP, Zwank MD. Laboratory-confirmed gonorrhea and/or chlamydia rates in clinically diagnosed pelvic inflammatory disease and cervicitis. *Am J Emerg Med*. 2012;30:1114-1117.
44. Campbell L, Woods V, Lloyd T, et al. Evaluation of the OSOM *Trichomonas* rapid test versus wet preparation examination for detection of *Trichomonas vaginalis* vaginitis in specimens from women with a low prevalence of infection. *J Clin Microbiol*. 2008;46:3467-3469.
45. Caro-Paton T, Carvajal A, Martin de Diego I, et al. Is metronidazole teratogenic? A meta-analysis. *Br J Clin Pharmacol*. 1997;44:179-182.
46. Castle PE, Katki HA. Benefits and risks of HPV testing in cervical cancer screening. *Lancet Oncol*. 2010;11:214-215.
47. Cemek F, Odabas D, Senel U, et al. Personal hygiene and vulvovaginitis in prepubertal children. *J Pediatr Adolesc Gynecol*. 2016;29(3):223-227.
53. Committee on Practice Bulletins. The American College of Obstetricians and Gynecologists. Practice bulletin No. 127: Cervical cancer screening and prevention. *Obstet Gynecol*. 2016;127(1):el-e20.
54. Corbett SL, Walsh CM, Spitzer RF, et al. Vulvar inflammation as the only clinical manifestation of Crohn disease in an 8-year-old girl. *Pediatrics*. 2010;125:e1518-e1522.
71. Eckert LO, Hawes SE, Stevens CE, et al. Vulvovaginal candidiasis: clinical manifestations, risk factors, management algorithm. *Obstet Gynecol*. 1998;92:757-765.
72. Edwards L, Ferenczy A, Eron L, et al. Self-administered topical 5% imiquimod cream for external anogenital warts. HPV Study Group. Human PapillomaVirus. *Arch Dermatol*. 1998;134:25-30.
79. Feazel LM, Santorico SA, Robertson CE, et al. Effects of vaccination with 10-valent pneumococcal non-typeable *Haemophilus influenzae* protein D conjugate vaccine (PHiDCV) on the nasopharyngeal microbiome of Kenyan toddlers. *PLoS ONE*. 2015;10:1-11.
80. Feldman S, Kahn JA, Hillard PA. Human papillomavirus infection and cervical cancer screening and prevention in adolescents. In: Emans SR, Laufer MR, Goldstein DP, eds. *Pediatric & Adolescent Gynecology*. Philadelphia, PA: Lippincott Williams & Wilkins; 2012:368-380.
89. Gardner AR, Shetty AK, Goodpasture M. A 6-year-old girl with chronic vaginal discharge. *Clin Pediatr*. 2012;51:801-803.
97. Grimes DA. Intrauterine device and upper-genital-tract infection. *Lancet*. 2000;356:1013-1019.
107. Hanna D, Hatami A, Powell J, et al. A prospective randomized trial comparing the efficacy and adverse effects of four recognized treatments of molluscum contagiosum in children. *Pediatr Dermatol*. 2006;23:574-579.
115. Hickey RJ, Zhou X, Settles ML, et al. Vaginal microbiota of adolescent girls prior to the onset of menarche resemble those of reproductive-age women. *MBio*. 2015;6:e97-15.
122. Huppert JS, Batteiger BE, Braslins P, et al. Use of an immunochromatographic assay for rapid detection of *Trichomonas vaginalis* in vaginal specimens. *J Clin Microbiol*. 2005;43:684-687.
129. Jacobs AM, Alderman EM. Gynecologic examination of the prepubertal girl. *Pediatr Rev*. 2014;35:97-104.
131. Jaquiery A, Stylianopoulos A, Hogg G, et al. Vulvovaginitis: clinical features, aetiology, and microbiology of the genital tract. *Arch Dis Child*. 1999;81:64-67.
142. Kessous R, Aricha-Tamir B, Sheizaf B, et al. Clinical and microbiological characteristics of Bartholin gland abscesses. *Obstet Gynecol*. 2013;122:794-799.
154. Leander L. Police interviews with child sexual abuse victims: patterns of reporting, avoidance and denial. *Child Abuse Negl*. 2010;34:192-205.
156. Lee NC, Rubin GL, Borucki R. The intrauterine device and pelvic inflammatory disease revisited: new results from the Women's Health Study. *Obstet Gynecol*. 1988;72:1-6.
157. Leinonen M, Nieminen P, Kotaniemi-Talonen L, et al. Age-specific evaluation of primary human papillomavirus screening vs conventional cytology in a randomized setting. *J Natl Cancer Inst*. 2009;101:1612-1623.
158. Leitich H, Brunbauer M, Bodner-Adler B, et al. Antibiotic treatment of bacterial vaginosis in pregnancy: a meta-analysis. *Am J Obstet Gynecol*. 2003;188:752-758.
160. Liu C, Bayer A, Cosgrove SE, et al. Clinical practice guidelines by the Infectious Diseases Society of America for the treatment of methicillin-resistant *Staphylococcus aureus* infections in adults and children. *Clin Infect Dis*. 2011;52:e18-e55.
165. Markowitz LE, Dunne EF, Saraiya M, et al. Human papillomavirus vaccination: recommendations of the Advisory Committee on Immunization Practices (ACIP). *MMWR Recomm Rep*. 2014;63(RR-05):1-30.
166. Marrazzo JM, Handsfield HH, Whittington WL. Predicting chlamydial and gonococcal cervical infection: implications for management of cervicitis. *Obstet Gynecol*. 2002;100:579-584.
168. McGreal S, Wood P. Recurrent vaginal discharge in children. *J Pediatr Adolesc Gynecol*. 2013;26:205.
182. Ness RB, Soper DE, Holley RL, et al. Douching and endometritis: results from the PID evaluation and clinical health (PEACH) study. *Sex Trasm Dis*. 2001;28:240-245.
184. Nugent RP, Krohn MA, Hillier SL. Reliability of diagnosing bacterial vaginosis is improved by a standardized method of gram stain interpretation. *J Clin Microbiol*. 1991;29:297-301.
186. Okun N, Gronau KA, Hannah ME. Antibiotics for bacterial vaginosis or *Trichomonas vaginalis* in pregnancy: a systematic review. *Obstet Gynecol*. 2005;105:857-868.
198. Randelović G, Mladenović V, Ristić L, et al. Microbiological aspects of vulvovaginitis in prepubertal girls. *Eur J Pediatr*. 2012;171:1203-1208.
204. Riggs MA, Klebanoff MA. Treatment of vaginal infections to prevent preterm birth: a meta-analysis. *Clin Obstet Gynecol*. 2004;47:796-807, discussion 81–2.
206. Ronco G, Giorgi-Rossi P, Carozzi F, et al. Efficacy of human papillomavirus testing for the detection of invasive cervical cancers and cervical intraepithelial neoplasia: a randomised controlled trial. *Lancet Oncol*. 2010;11:249-257.
208. Ross J, Judlin P, Jensen JS. International union against sexually transmitted infections. *Int J STD AIDS*. 2014;25:1.
210. Rylander E, Berglund AL, Krassny C, et al. Vulvovaginal candida in a young sexually active population: prevalence and association with oro-genital sex and frequent pain at intercourse. *Sex Transm Infect*. 2004;80:54-57.
216. Schaeffer P, Leventhal JM, Asnes AG. Children's disclosures of sexual abuse: learning from direct inquiry. *Child Abuse Negl*. 2011;35:343-352.
225. Sherrard J, Donders G, White D, et al. European (IUSTI/WHO) guideline on the management of vaginal discharge, 2011. *Int J STD AIDS*. 2011;22:421-429.
231. Sinclair KA, Woods CR, Kirse DJ, et al. Anogenital and respiratory tract human papillomavirus infections among children: age, gender, and potential transmission through sexual abuse. *Pediatrics*. 2005;116:815-825.
232. Sinclair KA, Woods CR, Sinal SH. Venereal warts in children. *Pediatr Rev*. 2011;32:115-121, quiz 21.
240. Stefanaki C, Barkas G, Valari M, et al. Condylomata acuminata in children. *Pediatr Infect Dis J*. 2012;31:422-424.
249. Svensson L, Westrom T, Mardh PA. Contraceptives and acute salpingitis. *JAMA*. 1984;251:2553-2555.
251. Syed TA, Lundin S, Ahmad M. Topical 0.3% and 0.5% podophyllotoxin cream for self-treatment of molluscum contagiosum in males. A placebo-controlled, double-blind study. *Dermatology*. 1994;189:65-68.

252. Tanaka K, Mikamo H, Ninomiya M, et al. Microbiology of Bartholin's gland abscess in Japan. *J Clin Microbiol.* 2005;43:4258-4261.
256. Tukeva TA, Aronen HJ, Karjalainen PT, et al. MR imaging in pelvic inflammatory disease: comparison with laparoscopy and US. *Radiology.* 1999;210: 209-216.
267. Wiesenfeld HC, Sweet RL. Progress in the management of tuboovarian abscesses. *Clin Obstet Gynecol.* 1993;36:433-444.
268. Wilt TJ, Harris RP, Qaseem A, et al. Screening for cancer: advice for high-value care from the American College of Physicians. *Ann Intern Med.* 2015;162:718-725.
272. Workowski KA, Bolan GA, Centers for Disease Control and Prevention. Sexually transmitted diseases treatment guidelines, 2015. *MMWR Recomm Rep.* 2015;64(RR-03):1-137. http://www.cdc.gov/std/tg2015/default.htm.

The full reference list for this chapter is available at ExpertConsult.com.

43 Esophagitis

Paul Krogstad • Robert S. Venick

Esophagitis is usually caused by gastroesophageal reflux and other noninfectious processes. Infectious esophagitis is distinct from other gastrointestinal infections in that it generally occurs in immunocompromised children and adults and is most often caused by *Candida* species, either alone or in combination with viral pathogens. When infectious esophagitis occurs in nonimmunocompromised children, it is usually associated with conditions that compromise the esophageal defense mechanisms.[53]

In view of the numerous predisposing conditions, the incidence of infectious esophagitis in children is difficult to quantify. *Candida* and herpes simplex virus (HSV) esophagitis has been reported in 2% to 4% in immunocompromised patients.[37] Before the availability of combination antiretroviral therapy (cART), 8% to 10% of children infected with human immunodeficiency virus (HIV) developed *Candida* esophagitis.[6,10,43] *Candida* esophagitis remains one of the most common opportunistic infections in HIV-infected children and generally is associated with low CD4$^+$ T-cell count (<100/μL), prior episodes of oropharyngeal candidiasis, high HIV-1 plasma viral load, and neutropenia (<500/μL).[10,11,52] *Candida* esophagitis is also reported frequently in those who have undergone chemotherapy or radiation therapy for hematologic malignancies; after solid organ and hematopoietic stem cell transplantation; in those with chronic exposure to inhaled, oral, or parenteral corticosteroid medications; and in the setting of poorly controlled diabetes mellitus.[37]

PATHOPHYSIOLOGY AND CAUSATIVE ORGANISMS

The defense mechanisms of the esophagus against infection include motility (the continuous flow of luminal contents discourages colonization by microbes), a mucosal lining of stratified squamous epithelium that is resistant to microbial invasion, and local and systemic immune responses. Disruption of any of these protective factors may lead to esophageal infections. Immunosuppression (as seen with HIV infection or after organ transplantation), chronic mucocutaneous candidiasis, ataxia-telangiectasia, malignancy, chemotherapy, and prolonged corticosteroid treatment are the most common predisposing factors for fungal and viral infection of the esophagus.[9–11,24,31,33,43] In immunocompetent children, dysmotility of the esophagus or mucosal injury secondary to gastroesophageal reflux can render the esophagus vulnerable to infections.

Most esophageal infections are caused by fungi and viruses.[5] *Candida* spp. (especially *Candida albicans*), herpes simplex virus (HSV), and cytomegalovirus (CMV) are the major pathogens and may be present at the same time in immunocompromised individuals.[5] The esophagus can be infected by local invasion (*Candida*, HSV, bacteria), as a result of systemic infection (CMV, *Candida*, *Pneumocystis*), or by contiguous spread from the mediastinum or neck (tuberculosis, retropharyngeal abscess).[6,43,53] Infections with fungi such as *Pneumocystis*, *Aspergillus*, and *Histoplasma* spp.; viruses such as varicella-zoster virus (VZV), human papillomaviruses, Epstein-Barr virus (EBV), and HIV; and protozoa such as *Cryptosporidium* and *Leishmania donovani* are less frequent yet well-documented causes of esophagitis.[13,19,20,22,23,28,34,39,47]

Bacterial infections of the esophagus are probably underreported. Ten percent to 16% of esophageal infections can have a bacterial etiology, mostly in granulocytopenic patients and as a secondary infection in fungal or viral esophagitis. *Mycobacterium tuberculosis* and gram-positive and gram-negative organisms that are part of the oropharyngeal microbiome are most commonly identified.[17,51]

CLINICAL FEATURES

Patients with infectious esophagitis can present with systemic, esophageal, or abdominal signs and symptoms (Box 43.1). Fever is generally found in the setting of systemic or secondary infection, such as tuberculosis or disseminated CMV infection, or complications that occur after esophageal perforation. In HSV-associated esophagitis, retrosternal pain and fevers are commonly found (all cases in one series of children).[40,41] Fever does not occur commonly in bacterial esophagitis. Cough is characteristic of tuberculosis, tracheobronchial fistulas, or high-grade esophageal obstruction. A maculopapular truncal rash and fever may be present in patients with idiopathic esophageal ulceration during acute HIV infection.[8,39]

Gastrointestinal complaints are the most common complaints. In adults, 59% to 79% of patients with documented esophageal infection have dysphagia and odynophagia,[5] These may not be apparent in small children who may instead describe a sensation of food "sticking" behind the sternum or a feeling of a food or liquid bolus passing through the chest.[10,11,37] Nausea and vomiting are associated more commonly with CMV esophagitis. The abdominal pain in esophagitis may be caused by referred pain from inflammation of the distal one-third of the esophagus, associated gastritis (as in CMV infection), or concomitant intraabdominal infections in immunocompromised hosts. Diarrhea may also be present in CMV infection (due to diffuse involvement of the gastrointestinal tract) or HIV infection (either opportunistic enteral infections or HIV enteropathy). In one report of fungal esophagitis in children, hematemesis was the most common initial symptom.[53] Drooling is an unusual manifestation in esophagitis per se (except perhaps in HSV esophagitis[40]) but may be present when there is concomitant pharyngeal involvement by the infectious agent.

Thrush (oropharyngeal candidiasis) and ulcers suggestive of HSV or acute HIV infection may serve as a clue that esophageal involvement is also present. Indeed nearly all patients with untreated HIV infection and oral candidiasis and odynophagia have endoscopic evidence of esophageal candidiasis.[7,10,45] Similarly recurrent cold sores, vesicular lesions on the nasolabial folds, and esophageal symptoms sometimes may also be seen as initial features of HSV esophagitis in immunocompetent adults and children, but their absence does not exclude HSV infection.[5,40] By contrast, oral lesions are usually absent in cases of esophagitis with CMV infection and tuberculosis, and the absence of oral thrush does not rule out *Candida* esophagitis.[41] HIV-infected children who develop esophageal candidiasis despite cART are less likely to have typical symptoms (e.g., odynophagia and retrosternal pain) or to have concomitant oropharyngeal candidiasis.[7,11]

Finally it is important to note that some cases of infectious esophagitis are asymptomatic and identified incidentally. For example, asymptomatic *Candida* esophagitis has been identified during follow-up endoscopy after topical corticosteroid therapy has been given for eosinophilic esophagitis.[48] Moreover because physicians seldom seek evidence of esophagitis in the absence of dysphagia or odynophagia, infectious esophagitis may be underdiagnosed in infants and children. Consequently the true incidence of *Candida* esophagitis in infants with thrush is unknown.

BOX 43.1 Signs and Symptoms of Infectious Esophagitis

Gastrointestinal Symptoms
Dysphagia
Odynophagia
Oral lesions
Nausea/vomiting
Hematemesis
Abdominal pain
Diarrhea

Systemic Symptoms
Fever
Cough
Rash reflecting underlying disease

DIFFERENTIAL DIAGNOSIS

Noninfectious esophagitis can be caused by a variety of mechanisms. Pathologic gastroesophageal reflux is the most common cause of esophageal symptoms. Other causes include chemical irritation (including medications or caustic ingestions), immunologic factors (e.g., cow's milk protein allergy), trauma (e.g., presence of nasogastric tube), radiation therapy, cancer chemotherapy, systemic disease (e.g., Crohn disease or chronic granulomatous disease), eosinophilic esophagitis, and motility disorders.

"Pill" esophagitis may be identified by history; nonsteroidal antiinflammatory drugs, potassium chloride supplements, and tetracyclines are the most commonly implicated medications.[1] Secondary bacterial or fungal infections can be present in reflux esophagitis and Chagas disease, especially when severe inflammation and obstruction are present. Absence of reflux symptoms (long-standing heartburn, a water brash taste in the mouth, vomiting, spitting up [in infants], pillow wetting, or coughing) tends to exclude reflux esophagitis. Achalasia, diffuse esophageal spasm, foreign body impaction, and mediastinal or retropharyngeal abscesses can cause esophageal symptoms and may result in secondary infection. In addition to imaging and endoscopy (see later discussion), other available tools include 24-hour intraesophageal pH probe, esophageal impedance, and manometry.

DIAGNOSIS

Establishing a specific diagnosis is essential for management of infectious esophagitis, particularly because fungal and bacterial superinfections occur commonly in the setting of viral esophagitis. Although the clinical profile, barium esophagogram, and endoscopic appearance can provide some clue to the etiology of esophagitis, histopathology, immunohistochemistry, and culture of endoscopic and brush biopsy specimens are essential for confirmation of specific pathogens. Serology for HSV, CMV, or EBV may help establish the diagnosis in some cases by providing evidence of acute infection. DNA detection methods also may provide evidence of viremia with these herpesviruses. Detection of fungal or viral esophagitis in an ostensibly healthy host should prompt an evaluation for the presence of primary or secondary immunodeficiency states, including HIV infection.

Barium Esophagography

The usefulness of an esophagogram in diagnosing infectious esophagitis is limited because it does not generally aid in differentiating among infectious etiologies; normal or nonspecific findings also can be found in some cases of esophagitis. Barium esophagograms are useful for assessing dysmotility, which can be a predisposing factor for esophagitis and for excluding obstruction, perforation, and fistulas of the esophagus. However, barium studies are generally not needed if endoscopy is planned.

Candida esophagitis generally is found throughout the esophagus, whereas HSV or CMV lesions are found more frequently in its mid to distal portions. Discrete longitudinal plaques, a grossly irregular or "shaggy" appearance, or tiny nodular lesions with a granular radiographic appearance are characteristic of *Candida* esophagitis (Fig. 43.1). The presence of discrete superficial stellate ulcers in the mid esophagus with normal-appearing surrounding mucosa is characteristic of HSV esophagitis, whereas CMV lesions may mimic HSV lesions in barium esophagograms. Oval or elongated large ulcers are found mostly in CMV infection. Idiopathic esophageal ulceration is found in HIV infection.[29,50] Esophagograms of patients with tuberculosis can show intramural pseudodiverticula, extrinsic compression, or esophageal displacement by mediastinal lymph nodes and sinus tracts.[14]

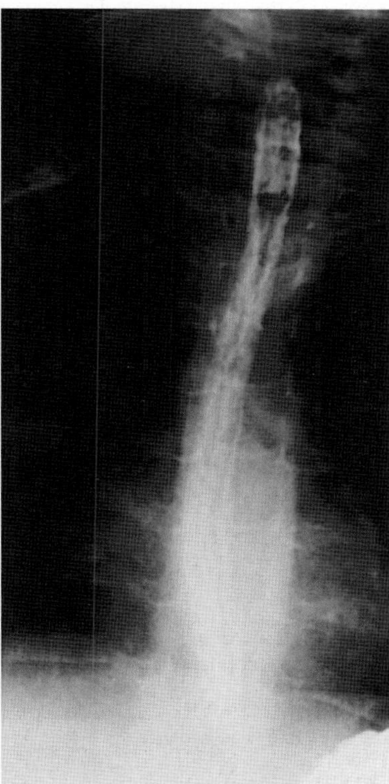

FIG. 43.1 *Candida* esophagitis. Barium esophagogram shows diffuse mucosal irregularity suggestive of inflammation and longitudinal filling defects suggestive of plaques. (Courtesy Sjirk Westra, MD, David Geffen School of Medicine at UCLA.)

Esophagoscopy

The diagnosis of esophagitis can be made by upper endoscopy with biopsies, although esophageal brushings often are of greater diagnostic yield. The technique for performing endoscopy with videoendoscope miniaturized to a diameter of 4.8 mm has made the procedure far more tolerable in immunocompromised patients, infants, and small children, and these instruments have biopsy capabilities.

Characteristic macroscopic lesions are associated with some infectious agents, but the features of these lesions overlap considerably, and histopathologic or immunohistochemical analysis (or both) of endoscopic and brush biopsy specimens is essential for specific diagnosis. A diffuse esophageal lesion is characteristic of *Candida* infection, whereas CMV and HSV infections mainly involve the distal part of the esophagus. White, longitudinal plaques that resemble cottage cheese and adhere to the esophageal mucosa are characteristic of *Candida* infection (Fig. 43.2).[25] The endoscopic severity of fungal esophagitis, which ranges from a few small raised lesions to large plaques, mucosal friability, and luminal narrowing, can be staged using Kodsi's classification.[4] Plaques from oral thrush, common findings in infants and immunocompromised children, can be washed away to reveal a nonulcerated underlying mucosa. Similar-appearing plaques also may be seen in CMV, HSV, bacterial, and "pill" esophagitis and after sucralfate ingestion.

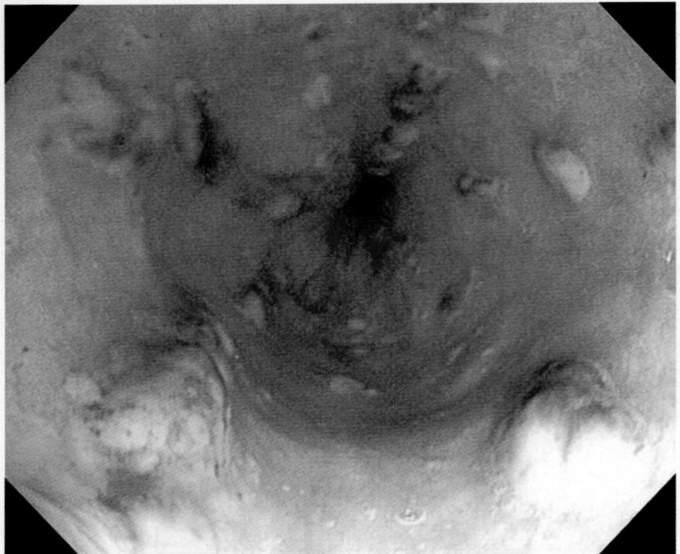

FIG. 43.2 Endoscopic image of *Candida* esophagitis. Examination of the distal one-third of the esophagus reveals whitish plaques with superficial ulceration of the esophageal mucosa.

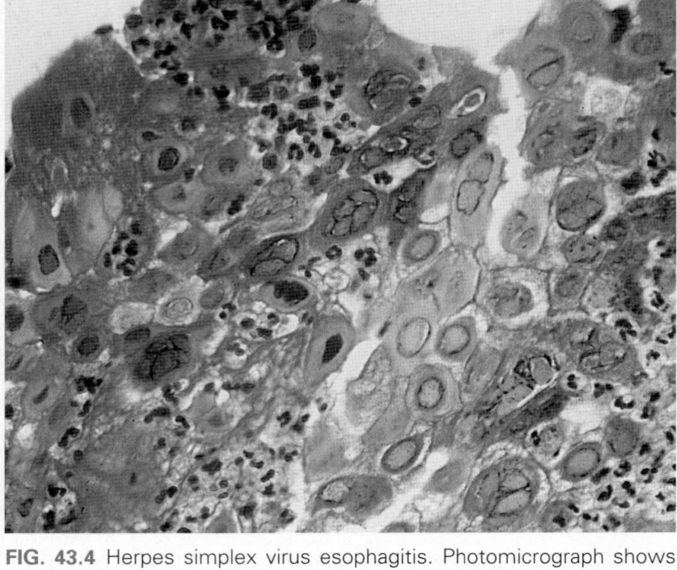

FIG. 43.4 Herpes simplex virus esophagitis. Photomicrograph shows viral inclusions in squamous epithelium (hematoxylin-eosin). (Courtesy Klaus Lewin, MD, UCLA Department of Pathology.)

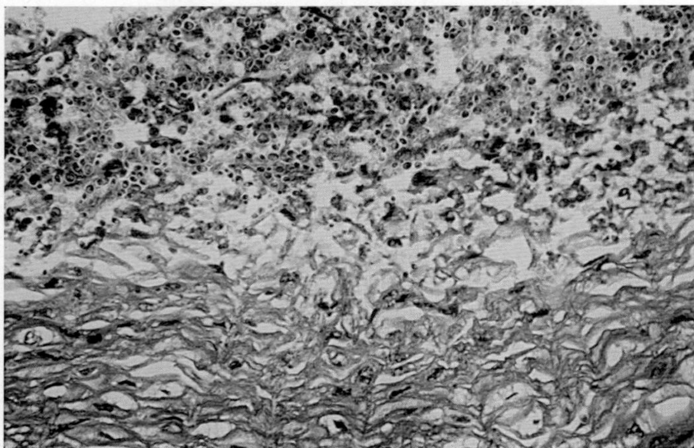

FIG. 43.3 *Candida* esophagitis. Photomicrograph shows yeastlike organisms in the esophageal mucosa (methenamine silver stain). (Courtesy Klaus Lewin, MD, UCLA Department of Pathology.)

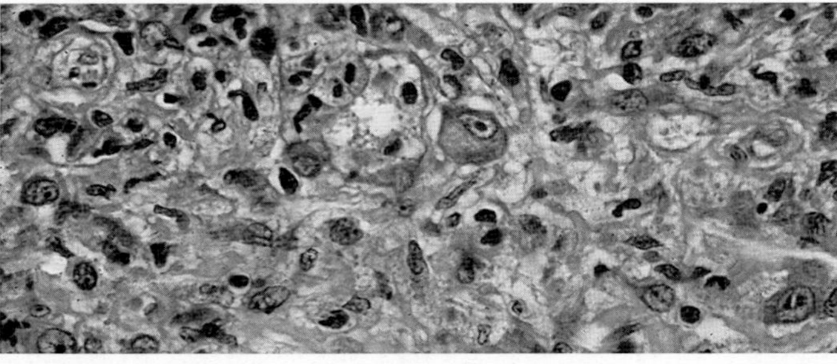

FIG. 43.5 Cytomegalovirus esophagitis. Photomicrograph shows intracytoplasmic inclusion bodies in the lamina propria (hematoxylin-eosin). (Courtesy Klaus Lewin, MD, UCLA Department of Pathology.)

Small, 1- to 3-mm vesicles are characteristic of HSV esophagitis, but by the time endoscopy is done these vesicles usually slough off and reveal sharply demarcated "volcano-like" ulcers in the distal esophagus with a raised edge, necrotic base, and normal-appearing surrounding mucosa.[37,40] In progressive disease, these ulcers may coalesce to resemble *Candida* esophagitis.[2] Multiple superficial ulcers in the distal portion of the esophagus often are seen in CMV esophagitis. Large elongated ulcers also are typical manifestations of CMV infection, but they may occur in idiopathic esophageal ulcerations in HIV infection as well.[29] Complete denudation of the mucosa is an unusual finding with CMV infection.[46] Endoscopy done in patients with VZV esophagitis can show vesicles, discrete ulcers, or necrotizing esophagitis, depending on the stage of the disease. Tubercular ulcers of the esophagus usually are of varying size, distinct, and shallow with a necrotic base.[14]

Endoscopic biopsy specimens should be obtained from the edge and the base of the lesions. The pathologist should be alerted to the possibility of fungal, viral, and polymicrobial infection. Appropriate fixatives should be used for routine hematoxylin and eosin stain, Gram stain, and special stains for fungi and bacteria such as *Mycobacterium. Candida* and *Aspergillus* can be shown by silver stain, periodic acid–Schiff stain, or Gram stain (Fig. 43.3). Diagnostic histopathologic changes, such as multinucleated giant cells, ballooning degeneration, intranuclear Cowdry type A inclusion bodies, and margination of chromatin in HSV infection (Fig. 43.4) and amphophilic intranuclear inclusions and small multiple cytoplasmic inclusion bodies in CMV infection (Fig. 43.5), can be diagnostic. Immunohistochemical studies and DNA hybridization techniques often are required to establish the diagnosis, however.

Viral culture, with or without immunohistochemical techniques, may aid in confirmation. Material obtained by endoscopy-guided brush biopsy can reveal the features of *Candida* or viral infection described earlier. If abdominal pain, fever, or other unusual symptoms are present, the possibility of disseminated or abdominal infection should be excluded by appropriate investigations.

PREVENTION

Much of the recent literature in infectious esophagitis has centered on identifying strategies to prevent illness in high-risk populations.[35] In pediatric solid organ transplantation, children are treated prophylactically with nystatin swish and swallow and intravenous ganciclovir in the early posttransplant period. Such strategies may reduce the incidence of fungal- and CMV-associated esophagitis in these children. Reports of an association between *Candida* esophagitis and acid suppression, in particular among those taking proton pump inhibitors, also highlight the possibility of iatrogenic risk factors and preventive measures that can be taken to prevent illness.[12,31]

TREATMENT

Candida Esophagitis

Treatment of esophageal candidiasis requires systemic antifungal therapy. Topical therapy may produce an initial response, but early treatment failures are common.[38] Systemic therapy with triazole medications (fluconazole, itraconazole solution, or voriconazole) is now the preferred initial approach.[36] Numerous trials have compared the azole agents, most often in adults with AIDS. Patients are less likely to respond and more likely to experience drug-related toxicity when treated with ketoconazole compared with fluconazole.[15] Oral fluconazole and itraconazole suspension seem comparable in efficacy for initial therapy, and some patients whose disease fails to respond to fluconazole may see improvement with subsequent itraconazole therapy.[16,18,42] Regardless of the initial severity of esophagitis, voriconazole and fluconazole were comparable in efficacy in one study, although toxicity occurred more commonly with voriconazole.[3]

Overall experience with the triazole medications supports recommendations for the initial use of oral fluconazole therapy for *Candida* esophagitis. Therapy generally is given for 14 to 21 days. Intravenous administration of azole medications may be used for patients with severe dysphagia.[30,36] However, the pharmacologic interactions between triazole antifungal medications with immunosuppressive medications and other drugs may be problematic in some patients, and infection with azole-resistant variants of *Candida* may occur, including species with intrinsic or acquired resistance to fluconazole (e.g., *Candida krusei*).[3,11] Although pediatric data currently are limited, large-scale studies in adults have shown that intravenous therapy with echinocandin agents (caspofungin, anidulafungin, or micafungin) is an alternative to azole therapy.[30,36,49]

Intravenous amphotericin B deoxycholate remains an alternative for patients with disease that is refractory to treatment with azole medications.[26,36] Nephrotoxicity is a major toxic effect of amphotericin B, but brief, low-dose therapy (7 to 14 days, 0.3 to 0.7 mg/kg per day) generally is sufficient to treat esophagitis. Lipid-conjugate formulations of amphotericin B also may be useful for treating refractory disease, but they are more expensive and not known to be superior in efficacy or lower in toxicity for the treatment of *Candida* esophagitis than low doses of deoxycholate formulation.

OTHER CAUSES OF FUNGAL ESOPHAGITIS

Cases of esophagitis caused by *Aspergillus, Mucor, Cryptococcus,* and *Histoplasma* spp. have been described. Optimal therapy has not been established, but systemic therapy, as for other manifestations of invasive infection with these organisms, has been successful. Currently this approach would involve the use of intravenous or oral triazole agents or an amphotericin B preparation. Echinocandins (micafungin, caspofungin, or anidulafungin) may be useful for *Aspergillus* or *Histoplasma* infections, but they have no activity against cryptococci.

VIRAL ESOPHAGITIS

Although spontaneous resolution of HSV esophagitis may occur in some individuals, antiviral therapy for HSV esophagitis generally is advised. Immunocompromised patients usually are treated with intravenous acyclovir, but in older patients valacyclovir and famciclovir may be useful alternatives because of their clinical efficacy and convenient dosing schedule.[32] Ganciclovir is used for CMV infection.[5,44] Acyclovir is the treatment of choice for VZV infection, and the prophylactic use of acyclovir has reduced effectively the rate of VZV infection after transplant surgery. Foscarnet is an alternative treatment for patients with HSV, VZV, or CMV who cannot tolerate or do not respond to initial therapy with acyclovir or ganciclovir. Therapy for 14 to 21 days usually is recommended for esophagitis caused by these herpesviruses. HIV-associated idiopathic ulcers do not respond to empiric antiviral or antifungal therapy, but they may respond to treatment with thalidomide.[21]

BACTERIAL ESOPHAGITIS

Bacterial esophagitis typically occurs in immunocompromised hosts and may involve gram-positive or gram-negative bacteria or a mixture of both. In immunocompromised hosts, esophagitis may be associated with bacteremia. Consequently empiric therapy should include broad-spectrum antibacterial agents active against *Staphylococcus aureus,* viridans streptococci, and aerobic gram-negative organisms. Blood cultures always should be performed to exclude bacteremia.[51]

Esophageal infections with *M. tuberculosis* or atypical mycobacteria are treated with regimens appropriate for other systemic infections with these organisms. Lack of response to appropriate therapy may indicate concomitant superinfection by other organisms or resistance to the drugs used. Repeat endoscopy is indicated for documenting eradication of infection.

PROGNOSIS

Candida esophagitis historically carried a poor prognosis for HIV-infected individuals. Prior to the advent of cART, survival was approximately 1 year after an episode of *Candida* esophagitis in children with untreated HIV infection.[6,39] Fungal and mycobacterial esophagitis, if not treated successfully, can lead to esophageal strictures, obstruction, perforation, and fistulas.[14,27,31] Viral esophagitis usually does not have any significant long-term sequelae.

NEW REFERENCES SINCE THE SEVENTH EDITION

1. Abid S, Mumtaz K, Jafri W, et al. Pill-induced esophageal injury: endoscopic features and clinical outcomes. *Endoscopy*. 2005;37(8):740-744.
4. Asayama N, Nagata N, Shimbo T, et al. Relationship between clinical factors and severity of esophageal candidiasis according to Kodsi's classification. *Dis Esophagus*. 2014;27(3):214-219.
8. Braun DL, Kouyos RD, Balmer B, et al. Frequency and spectrum of unexpected clinical manifestations of primary HIV-1 infection. *Clin Infect Dis*. 2015;61(6):1013-1021.
12. Daniell HW. Acid suppressing therapy as a risk factor for *Candida* esophagitis. *Dis Esophagus*. 2015;29(5):479-483.
18. Graybill JR, Vazquez J, Darouiche RO, et al. Randomized trial of itraconazole oral solution for oropharyngeal candidiasis in HIV/AIDS patients. *Am J Med*. 1998;104(1):33-39.
35. O'Rourke A. Infective oesophagitis: epidemiology, cause, diagnosis and treatment options. *Curr Opin Otolaryngol Head Neck Surg*. 2015;23(6):459-463.
36. Pappas PG, Kauffman CA, Andes DR, et al. Clinical practice guideline for the management of candidiasis: 2016 update by the Infectious Diseases Society of America. *Clin Infect Dis*. 2016;62(4):e1-e50.
37. Patel NC, Caicedo RA. Esophageal infections: an update. *Curr Opin Pediatr*. 2015;27(5):642-648.
41. Rosołowski M, Kierzkiewicz M. Etiology, diagnosis and treatment of infectious esophagitis. *Prz Gastroenterol*. 2013;8(6):5.
48. von Arnim U, Malfertheiner P. Eosinophilic esophagitis–treatment of eosinophilic esophagitis with drugs: corticosteroids. *Dig Dis*. 2014;32(1-2):126-129.

The full reference list for this chapter is available at ExpertConsult.com.

44 Approach to Patients With Gastrointestinal Tract Infections and Food Poisoning

Theresa J. Ochoa • Elsa Chea-Woo

Gastrointestinal infections can be caused by a wide array of pathogens, including bacteria, viruses, and parasites. Chemical food poisoning further broadens the spectrum of diseases. The cardinal symptoms of enteric infections/intoxications are diarrhea, emesis, and abdominal cramps in various combinations, but some enteropathogens cause less specific systemic syndromes and neurologic disorders that are the hallmark of a few food intoxications. A high degree of suspicion is necessary in these cases to formulate the correct diagnosis.

Irrespective of the underlying cause, the approach to a patient with suspected gastrointestinal infection or food poisoning starts with the assessment of patient dehydration status and need for immediate clinical intervention: the timely correction of fluid loss is the single most important intervention to decrease mortality. The next step consists of a thorough interview and physical examination aimed at formulating a presumptive differential diagnosis: circumstances of disease onset, constellation of symptoms and signs, characteristics of stools, geographic location and season of the year, and presence of other sick contacts normally are sufficient to orient the physician toward the correct cause of infection. A careful choice of diagnostic tests will not only confirm the diagnosis and establish a plan of treatment but also provide grounds for infection control actions and prevention of outbreaks.

This chapter reviews the essential information regarding epidemiology and epidemiologic classifications of enteric diseases, characteristics of common pathogens, general management of patients with diarrhea, laboratory diagnosis, and updated recommendations for treatment and prevention.

EPIDEMIOLOGY

Gastrointestinal infections represent a major cause of morbidity and mortality among children. Worldwide it is estimated that 1.6 billion episodes occur per year among children younger than 5 years.[70,267,406] The World Health Organization (WHO) and United Nations International Children's Emergency Fund (UNICEF) Child Health Epidemiology Reference Group (CHERG) have estimated the annual number of diarrhea deaths in children younger than 5 years at 0.578 million, representing 9.2% of all deaths in 2013.[408] This number is significantly lower than the 1.8 million estimated in 2003.[406] Important differences, however, exist among geographic areas related to age, race, household income, access to health care, and sanitation level. Diarrheal diseases accounted for 4% of deaths among children younger than age 5 years in the Americas, Europe, and western Pacific regions, whereas in Africa, Southeast Asia, and the eastern Mediterranean they caused up to 12% of deaths.[406] In the United States, diarrhea-associated morbidity and mortality among children younger than 5 years significantly decreased over the past century owing to improved living standards and sanitation systems, access to clinical care, clinical management, and vaccination. In the United States, risk factors for diarrhea-associated mortality are low birth weight, low 5-minute Apgar score, male sex, black race, unmarried maternal status, and young maternal age.[204,430] Racial and geographic differences likely reflect disparities in socioeconomic status and access to quality health care. Since rotavirus vaccination was included in the US vaccination program in 2006, a substantial reduction in gastroenteritis among young children has been observed in all-cause diarrhea hospitalizations and rotavirus-associated hospitalizations compared with the prevaccination era.[168,172,241,430] Similar declines in all-cause gastroenteritis and rotavirus-enteric infections rates were observed in other high- and middle-income countries where vaccination programs were implemented.[168,171,348,635] It is hoped that vaccine use in low-income countries, as endorsed by the WHO, will have a substantial impact on overall diarrheal burden of disease.[168,618,619]

There is also growing awareness of potential long-term disability caused by repeated episodes of diarrheal disease, especially in children living in developing countries: malnutrition, failure to thrive, and impaired cognition have all been described as consequences of protracted diarrhea.[266,378,512] The Etiology, Risk Factors, and Interactions of Enteric Infections and Malnutrition and the Consequences for Child Health (MAL-ED) Study is being conducted in eight countries to determine the contribution of enteric infections to malnutrition.[419]

Gastrointestinal infections are fundamentally acquired in two ways: by fecal-oral transmission and by contaminated food or water ingestion. The relative importance of the two routes, the risk for a child to be infected, and the types of microbes involved vary with age, immune status, and types of environmental exposures. Most cases of sporadic diarrhea occur in children younger than 5 years, although all age groups can be affected. The average diarrhea incidence in children younger than 5 years is three episodes per child per year, with higher rates among children age 6 to 24 months and in children from rural settings. Breastfed infants are less likely to acquire gastrointestinal infections because of the lower exposure to contaminated food and water and the protection granted by human milk components such as secretory antibodies, glycans, lactoferrin, leukocytes, cytokines, and other components produced by the mother's immune system.[634] During and after weaning the risk of diarrhea increases. In developing countries, suboptimal breastfeeding is associated with increased risk in diarrhea incidence and mortality, especially in infants younger than 6 months.[379]

Epidemiologic Categories of Diarrhea

Information regarding host immune status and environmental exposures normally allows for classification of disease into broad epidemiologic categories helpful to narrow the differential diagnosis: (1) diarrhea acquired in institutional settings, (2) antimicrobial-associated diarrhea, (3) diarrhea in immunosuppressed hosts, (4) traveler's diarrhea, and (5) foodborne or waterborne diarrhea (food poisoning).

Diarrhea Acquired in Institutional Centers: Childcare Centers

Gastrointestinal infections acquired in institutional settings are normally caused by highly contagious pathogens transmitted either by person-to-person contact, fomites, or ingestion of contaminated food. A typical setting for the pediatric population is daycare centers. Rotavirus, norovirus, astrovirus, *Giardia*, and *Cryptosporidium* are the most common pathogens reported.[196] However, a number of other pathogens have been implicated, including *Shigella*, enteric adenovirus, hepatitis A, sapovirus, *Escherichia coli* O157:H7, and *Salmonella*.[152,197,388,640] Rigorous hygiene practices, exclusion or cohorting of sick children from daycare, and judicious use of antimicrobial agents are all effective strategies for infection control.[370] Criteria for child exclusion from daycare attendance and duration of exclusion have been published.[79,196,388]

Antimicrobial-Associated Diarrhea

Intestinal microbiota play a major role in gastrointestinal function and immune system homeostasis. Antimicrobial agents induce significant modification of enteric flora both in terms of diversity and bacterial biomass.[649] Such modification, which can persist long after the inciting agent has been discontinued, can result in altered gastrointestinal function and increased susceptibility to opportunistic pathogens such as *Clostridium difficile* or *Candida albicans*.[668] Diarrhea is a common side effect of antibiotics, occurring in 11% to 40% of the children treated with antimicrobial agents.[335] *C. difficile* is the most common bacterial agent associated with severe antimicrobial-associated diarrhea. The spectrum of disease ranges from a mild self-resolving illness to pseudomembranous colitis, toxic megacolon, and possibly death.[53,72,390] Type and dose of antibiotic and host characteristics affect the severity of clinical manifestations.

The epidemiology of *C. difficile* has changed dramatically in recent years; *C. difficile* is increasingly recognized as an important pathogen among children.[577] Rates and severity of *C. difficile* infections have been increasing among adults and to a lesser extent in children, in part owing to the emergence of a hypervirulent strain called BI/NAP1/027.[428] This strain produces higher amounts of toxins A and B and a third toxin called binary toxin, and it is associated with more severe disease. In the United States, *C. difficile* was responsible for almost half a million infections and was associated with approximately 29,000 deaths in 2011.[395]

Prior use of antibiotics is the single most important risk factor for *C. difficile* disease. Nearly all the antibiotics have been implicated, but penicillins, cephalosporins, clindamycin, and fluoroquinolones are the most frequently involved.[354] Additional risk factors for *C. difficile* infection in children include gastrostomy or jejunostomy tubes, use of proton pump inhibitors, altered intestinal mobility, and prolonged hospitalization.[558] Certain underlying diseases, such as immunodeficiency, malignancy, cystic fibrosis, and inflammatory bowel disease also predispose to *C. difficile* infection.[163,356,425] Risk factors for recurrent *C. difficile* infection in children include malignancy, recent surgery, and the number of antibiotic exposures.[470] Guidelines for diagnosis and treatment of *C. difficile* infection have been published by the Infectious Diseases Society of America (IDSA), Society for Health Care Epidemiology of America (SHEA), and the American Academy of Pediatrics.[577]

Diarrhea in Immunosuppressed Host

Enteric infections are often a major problem in people with primary and secondary immunologic disorders.[34,377,559,684] The spectrum of disease and the types of involved pathogens can vary with the type of underlying deficit and the degree of immunosuppression. Patients with defects in cellular immunity (e.g., solid organ or bone marrow recipients, patients on chemotherapy for malignancies, children infected by human immunodeficiency virus [HIV] or born with congenital disorders) are mainly susceptible to pathogens with partial or predominant intracellular localization. Among common enteric pathogens, *Salmonella* and *Listeria* infections can result in disseminated, life-threatening diseases.[258,312] Viral infections by routine enteric pathogens such as rotavirus or norovirus can become chronic and debilitating.[215,361,502,678] Opportunistic agents such as cytomegalovirus can cause severe colitis in patients with advanced immune suppression, whereas cryptosporidiosis and microsporidiosis have been associated with persistent diarrhea.[441]

HIV-infected children represent a major group of immunosuppressed hosts, especially in some developing countries.[507] Gastrointestinal dysfunction is common in these patients and can be related to a number of causes: concomitant infections, HIV enteropathy, malignancy, or highly active antiretroviral therapy (HAART) medicines. In addition to the conventional enteric pathogens, opportunistic agents can cause significant disease in patients with advanced disease. In addition to protozoal infections like microsporidiosis and cryptosporidiosis, *Mycobacterium avium* complex is a common cause of persistent diarrhea and mainly affects the small intestine.[441] Cytomegalovirus can cause diffuse and severe ileocolitis and dysentery-like illness. *C. difficile* can play a role, especially in children previously treated with antibiotics. *Salmonella* infection is associated with a high risk of septicemia and should be treated aggressively.[205] A description of enteropathogens causing infections in HIV-infected patients is provided in Table 44.1.

The advent of antiretroviral treatment has dramatically changed the epidemiology of opportunistic infections in HIV-infected children.[463,535] HAART can result in complete clinical, microbiologic, and histologic responses in patients with AIDS infected with *Cryptosporidium parvum* and *Enterocytozoon bieneusi*[96] and in patients with HIV enteropathy.[371]

Severe defects in humoral immunity, such as X-linked agammaglobulinemia or common variable immunodeficiency, are often associated with persistent diarrhea and malabsorption syndrome; rotavirus and *Giardia lamblia* can be etiologic factors.[502] Enteric infections caused by *Campylobacter jejuni* and *Salmonella* spp. are more frequent and can be more severe and prolonged than in immunocompetent individuals.

TABLE 44.1 Organisms That Cause Gastrointestinal Tract Infections in Patients With HIV/AIDS

	Organisms
Esophagus	*Candida albicans*[a]
	Cytomegalovirus[a]
	Herpes simplex virus[a]
Hepatobiliary	Cytomegalovirus
	Cryptosporidium[a]
	Hepatotropic viruses
	Mycobacterium avium complex[a]
Small intestine	*Campylobacter* species
	Cytomegalovirus[a]
	Cryptosporidium[a]
	Giardia lamblia[a]
	Isospora belli[a]
	Mycobacterium avium complex[a]
	Microsporidia[a] (*Enterocytozoon bieneusi* and *Encephalitozoon intestinalis*)
	Salmonella species[a]
	Enteroaggregative *E. coli*
	Strongyloides stercoralis
Large intestine	*Campylobacter* species
	Clostridium difficile
	Cytomegalovirus[a]
	Entamoeba histolytica
	Herpes simplex virus[a]
	Salmonella species[a]
	Enteroaggregative *E. coli*
	Shigella species

[a]Diseases of the gastrointestinal tract that fulfill the Centers for Disease Control and Prevention surveillance case definition of AIDS.

Traveler's Diarrhea

Traveler's diarrhea is the most common illness reported by individuals traveling from high-income countries to middle- and low-income areas: occurrence as high as 40% to 60% is reported.[138,184,250,287,300,301,498,604] The most important determinant of risk is travel destination: high-risk areas include most of Asia, Africa, Middle East, and Central and South America.[138,498,604]

Half of travelers experience diarrhea within the first few weeks after arrival. A variety of intestinal pathogens can be responsible for traveler's diarrhea.[69,300,483,498,576] Bacteria account for 80% to 90% of the cases: enterotoxigenic *E. coli* (ETEC) is the most common pathogen, followed by *Campylobacter, Shigella, Salmonella,* and enteroaggregative *E. coli* (EAEC). Parasites account for 10% of the cases: *Giardia lamblia* and *Cryptosporidium* are the most common pathogens; *Cyclospora, Entamoeba,* and *Dientamoeba* are occasionally encountered. Viruses represent 5% to 10% of cases: rotavirus, norovirus, and calicivirus are the most frequently reported.[138] However, based on the GeoSentinel Surveillance Network, the main pathogens isolated from international travelers with gastroenteritis are parasites (65%), followed by bacteria (31%) and viruses (3%).[610]

Clinical illness varies, reflecting the diversity of causative agents. Typically illness presents as loose stools over a 24-hour period, accompanied by fever, nausea, vomiting, and abdominal cramping. Tenesmus and bloody diarrhea are less common. An incubation period of 6 to 48 hours normally suggests a bacterial or viral etiology, whereas parasites tend to have longer incubation periods and rarely present in the first week after travel; an exception is *Cyclospora cayetanensis,* which can present as an acute illness resembling bacterial pathogens. Traveler's diarrhea is normally a mild, self-limited illness that can resolve spontaneously in 3 to 5 weeks; protozoal diarrhea, however, can persist for months if untreated.

Children who travel are at risk of developing the same well-known illnesses that affect adult travelers.[277] The etiology, treatment, and actual risk of these illnesses are not as well defined as in adults.[416] Treatment of traveler's diarrhea in children consists of fluid replacement and antibiotics.[177] Antidiarrheal agents are not recommended for young children, although they can be considered for older children and adults, provided there is no gross blood in the stool or fever higher than 38.5°C (101.3°F).[25,138,198,301,416] Because access to good-quality health care can be problematic in certain regions, travelers should be advised to take with them medications with expected activity against the prevalent bacteria. Antibiotic therapy has been shown to reduce duration of disease from several days to approximately 1 day. Recommended antibiotics for empiric treatment of traveler's diarrhea in adults and children are fluoroquinolones, azithromycin, and rifaximin, which is an alternative for afebrile nondysenteric diarrhea.[1,3,185,186,198,604]

Traveler's diarrhea is mainly a food- or waterborne disease: poor hygiene practices of food handlers, inadequate food storage and refrigeration, and high levels of environment contamination by fecal flora due to poor sanitation infrastructure are risk factors for acquiring enteric infections in developing countries. Travelers should be advised on safe practices regarding food and beverage consumption. No effective vaccinations are currently available for traveler's diarrhea. Similarly chemoprophylaxis with antibiotics is not recommended in healthy travelers. Prophylactic treatment can be taken into consideration for hosts at increased risk of acquiring severe diarrhea, including patients with immunodeficiencies, malignancies, or chronic intestinal illnesses.[301,604]

Food- and Waterborne Diseases: Food Poisoning

Food- or waterborne diseases can result from ingestion of food or water contaminated with bacteria, viruses, parasites, or other types of chemical poisoning.[27,103] They can present either as sporadic cases or as outbreaks; the latter are defined as clusters of two or more individuals experiencing a similar illness after ingesting common food or water.[193,400,414] Food- and waterborne diseases represent major public health concerns and are subject to different degrees of surveillance across countries. In the United States, several surveillance systems coordinated by the Centers for Disease Control and Prevention (CDC) are in place to monitor food- and waterborne disease occurrence, track sources of contaminated food, identify emerging pathogens, and provide administrative guidance.

The Foodborne Disease Active Surveillance Network (FoodNet), coordinated by the CDC, conducts population-based, active surveillance investigation of foodborne disease in the United States.[569] The surveillance includes laboratory-confirmed infections for nine common pathogens (*Campylobacter* spp., *Listeria* spp., *Salmonella* spp., *Shigella* spp., Shiga toxin–producing *E. coli* [STEC], *Vibrio* spp., *Yersinia* spp., *Cryptosporidium* spp., and *Cyclospora* spp.). Although some other important pathogens known to be transmitted by food are not actively tracked by the system, the control measures triggered by FoodNet inputs will likely have an impact on all foodborne infection. The National Notifiable Disease Surveillance System (NNDSS) is a passive surveillance database. Reportable foodborne diseases include botulism, listeriosis, salmonellosis, STEC infections, hemolytic-uremic syndrome (HUS), and vibriosis. A complete list of other CDC surveillance systems is available at the CDC website (http://cdc.gov/foodborneburden/surveillance-systems.html).

In 2014, FoodNet reported 19,542 infections, 4445 hospitalizations, and 71 deaths in the United States. The most common isolated pathogens were *Salmonella, Campylobacter,* and *Shigella*. The incidence of STEC O157 and *Salmonella enterica* serotype Typhimurium infections declined in 2014 compared with 2006–2008, and the incidence of infection with *Campylobacter*, *Vibrio*, and *Salmonella* serotypes Infantis and Javiana was higher. Compared with 2011–2013, the incidence of STEC O157 and *Salmonella* Typhimurium infections was lower, and the incidence of STEC non-O157 and *Salmonella* serotype Infantis infections was higher in 2014.[150,455,530] Population at extremes of age were the most affected, with highest incidence for *Salmonella, Campylobacter, Shigella,* STEC O157 and non-O157, and *Cryptosporidium* being reported among children younger than 5 years, whereas individuals older than 65 years had the highest rates for infection with *Salmonella* and *Campylobacter.* Case-fatality rate is higher for *Listeria, Vibrio, Yersinia,* and STEC O157. The highest number of deaths was reported among the elderly (http://www.cdc.gov/foodnet/trends/tables-2014.html).[119,120] Data from modeling based on different surveillance systems estimates around 9.4 million foodborne illnesses, with viral infections accounting for 59% of the cases, bacterial infections 39%, and parasites 2%. Norovirus, nontyphoidal *Salmonella, Clostridium perfringens,* and *Campylobacter* were estimated to be the pathogens most commonly involved.[51,571] Norovirus, nontyphoidal *Salmonella, Campylobacter,* and *Toxoplasma* were responsible for the most hospitalizations. *Salmonella, Toxoplasma,* and *Listeria* accounted for the majority of documented deaths.[571] When modeling included foodborne illnesses caused by unspecified pathogens—either microbes or toxins for which there are no surveillance systems in place or pathogens yet to be discovered—the number of expected foodborne diseases rose to 48 million per year, leading to 128,000 hospitalizations and 3000 deaths annually.[570]

The WHO has recently estimated the number of foodborne illnesses globally at 2 billion cases, over 1 million deaths, and 78 million disability-adjusted life years (DALYs) in 2010; 29% of cases were transmitted by contaminated food. Norovirus was the leading cause of foodborne illness, causing 125 million cases, while *Campylobacter* caused 96 million foodborne illnesses.[359,369]

Clinical manifestations of foodborne disease can affect the gastrointestinal tract and the central nervous system or cause systemic symptoms with little or no intestinal tract involvement. Incubation period and type of consumed food are helpful tools for establishing a presumptive diagnosis (see Box 44.1).

Foodborne disease due to bacteria, viruses, and parasites. Table 44.2 illustrates clinical characteristics and confirmatory tests for the diagnosis of common food- and waterborne diseases. Detailed guidelines for clinical diagnosis and instructions for collecting stool specimens are available on the CDC website (http://www.cdc.gov/foodsafety/outbreaks/index.html).

A long list of foods have been associated with enteric infections:

- Unpasteurized milk and dairy products have been associated with salmonellosis and campylobacteriosis and, less frequently, infections with *Brucella* spp., *E. coli, L. monocytogenes, Mycobacterium* spp., *Staphylococcus aureus, Streptococcus* spp., *Streptobacillus moniliformis,* and *Yersinia enterocolitica.*[415] A nationwide outbreak of *Salmonella*

BOX 44.1 Foodborne Diseases: Presumptive Diagnosis Based on Clinical Manifestations and Incubation Period

- Incubation time <1 hour: chemical poisoning from mushrooms or marine biotoxins, inorganic toxins such as monosodium glutamate (Chinese restaurant syndrome) or metals.
- Nausea, vomiting, and diarrhea within 1 to 7 hours after food ingestion: preformed bacterial toxins, mainly from *Staphylococcus aureus* and *Bacillus cereus*. Biotoxins less frequent (seafood or mushroom consumption).
- Abdominal cramps and diarrhea within 8 to 14 hours: *Clostridium perfringens* or *B. cereus,* through the in vivo production of enterotoxins.
- Diarrhea, abdominal cramps, and fever with onset in 8 to 48 hours: bacterial infection: *Campylobacter, E. coli, Salmonella, Shigella,* and *Vibrio parahaemolyticus*. In the presence of frankly bloody diarrhea: STEC, *Shigella,* and *Campylobacter.*
- Watery diarrhea presenting more than 15 hours after consumption of suspected food: viral infection. Noroviruses are the most common.
- Prolonged diarrhea: parasites: *Giardia lamblia,* microsporidia, *Cyclospora* spp.

TABLE 44.2 Foodborne Disease Agents and Clinical Presentation

Usual Incubation Periods	Causative Agent	CLINICAL ILLNESS Fever	Diarrhea	Vomiting	Epidemiologic and Laboratory Diagnosis
5 min–6 h (usually <3 h)	Chemical or toxin—see Tables 44.3 and 44.4	Rare	Occasional (see Table 44.3)	Common	Demonstration of toxin or chemical from food or epidemiologic incrimination of food
1–6 h (usually <1 h)	*Staphylococcus aureus* enterotoxin	Rare	Occasional	Profuse	Isolation of organisms in food (>10^5/g)/vomitus/stool; detection of enterotoxin in food
	Bacillus cereus emetic toxin	Rare	Occasional	Profuse	Isolation of organisms in food (>10^5/g)/vomitus/stool
6–24 h	*Clostridium perfringens* enterotoxin	Rare	Typical	Occasional	Isolation of organisms or toxin from food (>g) or stools of ill persons, epidemiologic incrimination of food; detection of enterotoxin in food
	B. cereus enterotoxin	Rare	Typical	Occasional	
12–72 h	*Clostridium botulinum*	Clinical syndrome compatible with botulism	Constipation more common		Isolation of organism or toxin from food (10^5/g) or stools; demonstration of toxin in serum or food
16–96 h	*Shigella*	Common	Typical, often bloody	Occasional	Isolation of organism from clinical specimens from two or more ill persons; isolation of organism from epidemiologically implicated food
	Nontyphoidal *Salmonella*	Common	Typical	Occasional	
	Enteroinvasive *E. coli* (EIEC)	Common	Typical, may be bloody	Occasional	
	Enteropathogenic *E. coli* (EPEC)	Occasional	Typical	Occasional	
	Enterotoxigenic *E. coli* (ETEC)	Rare	Typical	Rare	
	Vibrio parahaemolyticus; V. cholerae enterotoxin	Occasional	Typical	Occasional	
1–3 days	Caliciviruses (noroviruses) Rotavirus	Occasional	Typical	Common	Antigen detection (enzyme immunoassay) in stool; immune electron microscopy of stool; detection of viral RNA in stool or vomitus by PCR
1–10 days	*Yersinia*	Uncommon	Typical, severe abdominal pain	Uncommon	Isolation of organisms from food or clinical specimens of ill persons
2–10 days	*Campylobacter jejuni*	Common	Typical, often bloody	Uncommon	Isolation of organisms from food or clinical specimens of ill persons
1–11 days	*Cryptosporidium*	Occasional	Common	Occasional	Demonstration of oocysts in stool or in small bowel biopsy of ill persons; demonstration of organism in epidemiologically implicated food
	Cyclospora	Occasional	Common	Occasional	Demonstration of parasite in stool or in small bowel biopsy of ill persons; demonstration of organism in epidemiologically implicated food
	Giardia intestinalis	Occasional	Common	Occasional	Demonstration of parasite in stool or in small bowel biopsy of ill persons; demonstration of organism in epidemiologically implicated food
2 days–weeks	*Bacillus anthracis*	Common	Typical	Frequent	Isolation of organism from blood or contaminated meat
1–7 days	*E. coli* O157:H7 and other Shiga toxin–producing *E. coli*	Uncommon	Typical	Frequent	Isolation of organism from food or stool or identification of toxin in stools of ill persons
3–60 days, usually 7–14	*Salmonella typhi*	Common	Diarrhea or constipation	Uncommon	Isolation of organisms from food or clinical specimens of ill persons
7–21 days	*Brucella* spp.	Common	Common	Rare	Isolation of organisms from blood or bone marrow culture of ill persons; fourfold increase in standard agglutination titer overall several weeks or single titer 1 : 160 in person with compatible clinical syndrome
1–4 wk	*Giardia lamblia*	Rare	Common	Rare	Stool for ova and parasite examination enzyme immunoassay
2 days–8 wk	*Trichinella spiralis*	Common	Common	Common	Serology, muscle biopsy

enteritidis gastroenteritis was associated with ingestion of contaminated ice cream.[291] Mexican-style soft cheese made with unpasteurized milk has been described as a source of infection among children; however, outbreaks caused by cheese made from pasteurized milk also occur, most commonly in restaurants, delis, or banquet settings.[257,647] Consumption of raw milk has been associated with a chronic diarrhea syndrome of unknown cause, referred to as *Brainerd diarrhea.*[357,438,493] Based on the burden of illness associated with consumption of raw and unpasteurized milk and milk products, the American Academy of Pediatrics (AAP) strongly recommends the consumption of only pasteurized milk and milk products for pregnant women, infants, and children.[137]

- Fresh fruit and vegetables have been linked with a number of pathogens. Norovirus and *Salmonella* are responsible for most of the fruit- and vegetable-related outbreaks in the United States and the European Union,[93] whereas *Salmonella, E. coli,* and *Shigella* are the most common in Canada.[375] Radish sprouts, lettuce, apple juice, alfalfa sprouts, and spinach have been described as sources of enterohemorrhagic *E. coli.*[101,110] Hot peppers, tomatoes, and cantaloupes have been described as potential sources of *Salmonella.*[104,117,539]

- Cold salads were described as a vehicle for *Shigella* and *Listeria* infection.[43] Homemade canned food can be associated with *Clostridium botulinum* infection in adults[597]; honey is associated with *Botulinum* intoxication in infants.
- Poultry, especially raw chicken, and eggs have been identified as sources of foodborne infection due to *Campylobacter* and *Salmonella.*[58,141,522]
- Pork and chitterlings have been associated with *Yersinia* infection.[108,271]
- Ingestion of raw fish (sushi or sashimi) has led to infection with *Vibrio parahaemolyticus* and various parasites.[157,415] *V. parahaemolyticus* outbreaks have been also associated with raw oysters and clams from coastal states of the United States.[113,594] Parasites acquired through ingestion of raw fish include larval nematodes of the family Anisakidae, fish tapeworm of the species *Diphyllobothrium,* the fluke *Nanophyetus salmincola* from salmon, and many other helminths.[462]
- Consumption of raw and lightly cooked shellfish (mussels, clams, oysters, lobsters, and other mollusks) is associated with infection by agents that are native to the marine environment or released by sewage effluents contaminating environmental waters. Viruses such as caliciviruses, mainly norovirus, and hepatitis A virus are commonly concentrated and transmitted through shellfish.[60,451] The *Vibrio* genus (specifically *V. vulnificus*), acquired either by eating shellfish or by contaminating open wounds by swimming, presents a serious problem in terms of the severity of human illness and death, especially in people with liver disease.[305,326,466]
- Turtle-associated salmonellosis is a reemerging public health issue. Eight multistate outbreaks associated with small turtles were investigated during 2011–13. Children younger than 5 years and Hispanics were mainly affected.[654]

Food poisoning by chemicals. Intoxication from seafood is caused by toxins accumulated in fish, shellfish, and crustaceans. Marine toxins are tasteless and odorless and are not inactivated by cooking: once ingested they normally cause symptoms within a few hours. Symptoms can be gastrointestinal, neurologic, or systemic. Clinical characteristics of shellfish poisoning are listed in Table 44.3. Prevention of such illness is accomplished by monitoring of toxin concentration in seafood samples.[596] Scombroid fish poisoning is caused by inadequate conservation of certain types of fish. If fish are not adequately refrigerated after being caught, marine bacteria proliferate and catalyze decarboxylation of fish tissue histidine into histamine; once the fish is consumed, patients present with symptoms of histamine toxicity.[208] Ciguatera and scombroid

TABLE 44.3 Marine Biotoxins

Syndrome	Symptoms	Incubation Period	Toxin	Mechanism of Action	Food Source	Geographic Distribution	Seasonality
Paralytic shellfish poisoning	Facial and perioral paresthesias, headache, muscular weakness, mental status changes, nausea, vomiting, death	30 min–4 h	Saxitoxin	Blocks sodium channels	Shellfish	NE and NW United States, Chile, Japan	May–November
Diarrheic shellfish poisoning	Diarrhea, nausea, vomiting, abdominal pain, chills	30 min–12 h	Okadaic acid	Inhibits protein phosphatase	Shellfish	Japan, Europe, Africa	
Amnesic shellfish poisoning	Nausea, vomiting, abdominal cramps, diarrhea, headache, visual disturbance, anterograde amnesia, confusion, coma	15 min–6 h	Domoic acid	Stimulates glutamate receptors	Shellfish	Canada, NE and NW United States	
Neurotoxic shellfish poisoning	Paresthesia, abdominal pain, dizziness, diplopia, gait disturbance, reversed temperature perception, respiratory difficulty	5 min–4 h	Brevetoxins	Opens sodium channels	Shellfish and other fish	Western Florida, Caribbean	Spring–fall
Ciguatera	Nausea, vomiting, abdominal cramps, facial and perioral paresthesias, headache, reverse temperature perception, extremity pain, arthralgia, myalgia, sharp pain in the legs and teeth	1–6 h	Ciguatoxin, maitotoxin	Opens Na^+ channels; opens Ca^{2+} channels	Predatory fish reef	Tropical areas	February–September
Scombroid fish poisoning	Pruritic rash, flushing, sweating, perioral tingling, dizziness, facial and lingual swelling, vomiting, diarrhea, urticaria, bronchospasm	Minutes–hours	Histamine	Histamine receptors	Tuna, mahi-mahi, mackerel, sardines	Worldwide	Year-round
Puffer fish	Facial paresthesia, ascending paralysis, respiratory failure, circulatory collapse, death	30 min–3 h	Tetrodotoxin, saxitoxin	Blocks Na^+ channels	Puffer fish	East Asia	

TABLE 44.4 **Fungal and Inorganic Toxins: Food Poisoning**

Type of Chemical, Toxin, or Poison	Food	Clinical Symptoms	Onset of Symptoms (h)
Heavy metals[a]	Water (through metallic container) and food	Gastrointestinal	1
Monosodium glutamate	Chinese food	Burning sensation, heavy feeling in chest, pressure over face, flushing, gastrointestinal	1
Ibotenic acid, muscimol	Mushroom	CNS: confusion, delirium, visual disturbances, lethargy	2
Coprine	Mushroom	Disulfiram-like effect: nausea, vomiting, headache, hypotension, flushing, paresthesia, and tachycardia	2
Muscarine	Mushroom	Parasympathetic: sweating, salivation, lacrimation, blurred vision, diarrhea, bradycardia, hypotension	2
Psilocybin, psilocin	Mushroom	CNS: hallucinations, anxiety, mood elevation, weakness	2
Diverse, mostly unknown	Mushroom	Gastrointestinal	2
Monomethylhydrazine, gyromitrin	Mushroom	Cellular destruction, gastrointestinal, loss of coordination, convulsion, coma, death	6–12
Amatoxins, phallotoxins	Mushroom	Cellular destruction, gastrointestinal, hepatic and renal necrosis	6–24
Vomitoxin (deoxynivalenol)	Cereals contaminated with *Fusarium* species	Vomiting acutely Altered mucosal immunity with chronic exposure	<3

CNS, Central nervous system.
[a]Includes antimony, arsenic, cadmium, copper, mercury, thallium, tin, and zinc.

fish poisonings are common causes of fish-related foodborne illness in the United States.[510] A large reported outbreak in the United States was associated with escolar fish. Puffer fish syndrome is a lethal intoxication resulting from consumption of certain specific species of puffer. It is very rare in the United States but more common in Japan.[596]

Chinese restaurant syndrome appears to be caused by excessive amounts of monosodium glutamate in foods. Symptoms include paresthesias, reversal of hot-cold sensations, loss of proprioception, flushing, weakness, and burning sensations.

Mushroom toxins produce several clinical syndromes, generally within 2 hours of ingestion (Table 44.4),[280] except for poisoning caused by amatoxins, phallotoxins, amantin, monomethylhydrazine, and gyromitrin, which may produce symptoms, including death, up to 24 hours after ingestion.[280] Mushroom poisoning is associated with acute liver injury and failure.[495]

Heavy metals, such as antimony, arsenic, cadmium, copper, mercury, thallium, tin, and zinc, cause irritation of the gastric mucosa, with nausea, vomiting, and abdominal cramps, that usually resolves 2 to 3 hours after the offending agent has been removed.[27,103]

Prevention of foodborne disease. Changes in human behavior; increased consumption of ready-to-eat food; centralization of food production, processing, and distribution; and globalization of the food market are all risk factors for foodborne disease. Among outbreaks reported from 1998 through 2002, 46% were associated with at least one pitfall in the food chain process.[415,681] Major risk factors for food contamination were food handling by a person infected or colonized by a pathogen, bare-handed contact with food, inadequate cleaning of preparation equipment or utensils, and cross-contamination from a raw ingredient of animal origin. Factors associated with bacterial proliferation in food include inadequate refrigeration, slow cooking, insufficient time or temperature during hot holding, or long delay between food preparation and consumption.

Detailed instructions regarding safe food processing can be retrieved on the website of the U.S. Department of Agriculture (USDA) and other websites (www.fisis.usda.gov/OA/pubs/consumerpubs.htm; www.ama-assn.org/foodborne; www.cdc.gov/foodsafety; and www.fightbac.org).

Waterborne disease. The waterborne disease and outbreak surveillance system in the United States is responsible for collecting data and reporting on waterborne disease. The database collects information on outbreaks associated with recreational water, drinking water, and water not intended for drinking. During 2007 to 2008, 36 outbreaks associated with drinking water were reported: of those, 61% manifested as acute gastrointestinal illnesses.[85] For 2011–12, 32 drinking water–associated outbreaks were reported, accounting for at least 400 cases of illness and 100 hospitalizations. *Legionella* was responsible for two-thirds of outbreaks. Other important agents were *Campylobacter* spp., *E. coli* O157:H7, *E. coli* O121, *Shigella sonnei,* norovirus, and *Giardia.* Outbreaks were associated with water systems that used surface water sources and untreated or inadequately treated groundwater.[57] Additional outbreaks are associated with recreational water that are treated (e.g., pools and hot tubs or spas) or untreated (e.g., lakes and oceans). During 2007–08 a total of 134 recreational-water outbreaks were reported.[306] For 2011–12, 90 outbreaks resulted in at least 1788 cases and 95 hospitalizations. Among outbreaks associated with treated recreational water (77%), half were caused by *Cryptosporidium,* and, among outbreaks associated with untreated recreational water, one-third were caused by *E. coli* (O157:H7 or O111).[307]

CLINICAL CLASSIFICATION OF DIARRHEA EPISODES

Diarrhea in children can be classified in several ways (Box 44.2). Based on duration, diarrhea can be acute (usually self-limited and lasting <7 days), prolonged (7–14 days), persistent (>14 days), or chronic (usually >30 days or relapsing).[445] The importance of this classification is that, in addition to focusing on the importance of subsequent development of undernutrition,[446] it can help to identify the most likely causes. Acute diarrhea can be associated with many bacterial and viral pathogens, whereas prolonged and persistent diarrhea is associated with parasites, especially *Giardia duodenalis, Cryptosporidium,* and other coccidia, and some bacterial pathogens including EAEC and enteropathogenic *E. coli* (EPEC).[446,468,479,483,633] On the other hand, chronic diarrhea, although it can start as an infectious diarrhea, is often the result of a postinfectious or noninfectious process (e.g., malabsorption, irritable bowel syndrome, inflammatory bowel disease).[686] Diarrhea can also be classified as inflammatory or noninflammatory and as osmotic or secretory, based on its pathogenesis. Inflammatory diarrhea can be defined by the presence of abundant leukocytes in the stools (>50–100) or by measuring other markers of inflammation, such as fecal lactoferrin.[318,486,644] Inflammatory diarrhea is associated with "invasive" bacterial pathogens such as *Shigella, Salmonella,* and *Campylobacter;* therefore identifying this type of diarrhea can help raise suspicion of these agents. On the other hand, osmotic diarrhea is important in young children. Because rotavirus, the most common cause of diarrhea in young children worldwide, can be associated with accumulation of carbohydrates in the intestinal lumen and malabsorption, measurement of reducing substance in stool may be helpful in resource-limited situations to aid in its diagnosis.[412] Based on its characteristics diarrhea can be classified as watery or dysenteric. Watery diarrhea is characterized by liquid or semiliquid stools, usually of large volume, with or without fever, vomiting, and abdominal pain. This type of diarrhea can be associated with any type of viral, bacterial, or parasitic agents. However, dysentery, a syndrome characterized by fever, abdominal cramps, and tenesmus with small, frequent bloody stools, sometimes with mucus (colitis or colonic inflammation), is associated with a narrower list of pathogens, including *Shigella, Salmonella, Campylobacter,* STEC, enteroinvasive *E. coli* (EIEC), *Yersinia, Clostridium,* and some parasites: *Entamoeba histolytica, Strongyloides,* and *Balantidium coli.* Recognition of this syndrome affects both diagnostic evaluation and empiric therapy.[513] Finally the diarrhea episode can be classified based on the severity (mild, moderate, or severe), determined by a clinical score and/or the degree of dehydration (see "Treatment" section). The most commonly use clinical score is the Vesikari score,[554] which is based on the duration and number of stools and vomiting episodes, fever, dehydration, and treatment. Two-thirds of the diarrhea episodes in children are mild and do not require professional care.[378]

BOX 44.2 Clinical Classification of Diarrheal Episodes

Based on Duration
Acute (usually <7 days)
Prolonged (7–14 days)
Persistent (>14 days)
Chronic (>30 days or relapsing)

Based on Inflammation
Inflammatory vs. noninflammatory

Based on Mechanism
Osmotic vs. secretory

Based on Stool Characteristics
Watery
Bloody/dysenteric

Based on Severity (Clinical Score and/or Degree of Dehydration)
Mild
Moderate
Severe

ORGANISMS THAT CAUSE DIARRHEA

Many viral, bacterial, and parasitic organisms produce diarrhea in children. The major enteric pathogens associated with infectious diarrhea are shown in Table 44.5. The relative frequency of pathogens varies by age group, severity, community or hospital setting, and regions of the world. Several large studies have been recently conducted to identify the etiology and population-based burden of pediatric diarrhea in developing countries.[521] The Child Health Epidemiology Reference Group (CHERG) of WHO and UNICEF has recently reviewed the distribution of pathogens in children younger than 5 years of age hospitalized with diarrhea. Based on 286 inpatient studies, the main pathogens found were rotavirus (38% age-adjusted median proportion), EPEC (15%), norovirus (14%), and ETEC (8%). It has been estimated that these four pathogens cause more than half of all diarrheal deaths worldwide in children younger than 5 years.[382] The Global Enteric Multicenter Study (GEMS) group conducted a prospective case-control study in children younger than 5 years in sub-Saharan Africa and south Asia. In children younger than 12 months, the most important pathogens, in order of

TABLE 44.5 Pathogens Associated With Infectious Diarrhea in Children

Type	Enteropathogen	Clinical and Epidemiologic Characteristics
Virus	Rotavirus	Acute watery dehydrating diarrhea with vomiting and fever, particularly in young children during winter
	Norovirus	Acute watery diarrhea with vomiting; short duration; most common cause of outbreaks of nonbacterial gastroenteritis worldwide
	Astrovirus	Short-duration mild watery diarrhea with fever and vomiting in young children
	Enteric adenovirus	Mild watery diarrhea with vomiting and low-grade fever in young children; serotypes 40 and 41
Bacteria	*Shigella*	Severe diarrhea, often dysenteric with fever; high risk of person-to-person transmission
	Salmonella	Acute watery diarrhea, occasionally dysenteric, and systemic infections; exposure to carriers, food, and animals (poultry, reptiles)
	Campylobacter	Acute watery diarrhea, often dysenteric with fever; food and animal exposure (poultry)
	Shiga toxin–producing *E. coli*	Watery diarrhea progressing to blood-streaked or grossly bloody diarrhea usually without fever; some serotypes are associated with HUS; food exposure, person-to-person spread, water, and contact with animals
	Other diarrheagenic *E. coli*	Watery diarrhea; associated with dehydrating diarrhea (ETEC); some pathotypes with bloody diarrhea (EIEC); usually acute; some pathotypes with prolonged diarrhea (EAEC, EPEC); food exposure
	Vibrio cholerae	Acute watery dehydrating diarrhea in endemic regions; food or water exposure
	Vibrio parahaemolyticus	Watery diarrhea, often dysenteric; seafood related
	Yersinia enterocolitica	Acute watery diarrhea, may cause fever, dysentery and pseudoappendicitis; most common in northern countries; food or animal exposure (swine)
	Aeromonas hydrophila	Acute watery diarrhea; water, food, or animal exposure
	Plesiomonas shigelloides	Acute watery diarrhea; water, fish, or animal exposure
	Clostridium difficile	Diarrhea often with fever and blood after administration of antimicrobial agents
	Clostridium perfringens	Foodborne outbreaks; short-duration acute watery diarrhea with abdominal pain and fever
	Staphylococcus aureus	Foodborne outbreaks; short-duration vomiting sometimes with diarrhea
	Bacillus cereus	Foodborne outbreaks; two distinct short-duration illnesses: emetic and diarrheal
	Listeria monocytogenes	Foodborne outbreaks; systemic infection or acute watery diarrhea, often with fever
Parasite	*Entamoeba histolytica*	Watery or bloody diarrhea (amebic dysentery) with fever and abdominal pain; hepatic amebiasis
	Giardia	Watery diarrhea; usually persistent or chronic diarrhea; food or water exposure
	Cryptosporidium	Watery diarrhea; usually persistent; severe diarrhea in patients with AIDS; food or water exposure; outbreaks
	Isospora belli	Watery diarrhea, usually persistent; severe diarrhea in patients with AIDS; food or water exposure
	Cyclospora	Watery diarrhea, usually persistent; severe in young children; food or water exposure
	Microsporidia	Watery diarrhea; usually persistent; severe diarrhea in patients with AIDS; food or water exposure
	Strongyloides	Watery diarrhea, often with mucus, blood, abdominal pain, and eosinophilia; hyperinfection syndrome

frequency, were rotavirus, *Cryptosporidium*, and ETEC; in children aged 12 to 23 months, rotavirus, *Shigella*, and *Cryptosporidium*; and in children aged 24 to 59 months, *Shigella*, rotavirus, and *Campylobacter*. In general, most attributable cases of moderate to severe diarrhea were due to four pathogens: rotavirus, *Cryptosporidium*, ST-ETEC, and *Shigella*.[373] Infections with ST-ETEC, atypical EPEC (aEPEC), and *Cryptosporidium* were associated with higher risk of death at follow-up. The MAL-ED birth cohort study conducted in eight sites in South America, Africa, and Asia between 2009 and 2014 in children younger than 2 years of age found that the major pathogens associated with diarrhea in the first year of life were norovirus (adjusted attributable fraction 5.2%), rotavirus (4.8%), *Campylobacter* (3.5%), astrovirus (2.7%), and *Cryptosporidium* (2.0%). The major pathogens in the second year of life were *Campylobacter* (7.9%), norovirus (5.4%), rotavirus (4.9%), astrovirus (4.2%), and *Shigella* (4.0%).[523] In summary, there is substantial variation in pathogen distribution according to geography, diarrhea severity, season, and age.

Viruses

Acute infectious diarrhea of viral origin generally is a self-limited disease characterized by various combinations of diarrhea, nausea, vomiting, abdominal cramps, headaches, myalgias, and low-grade fever.[439,489,624] Bowel movements are watery and generally do not contain mucus or blood. Vomiting is the most common manifestation of this condition. Rotavirus, norovirus, enteric adenovirus, and astrovirus are common causes of viral gastroenteritis.[166,538] Other viruses, including coronaviruses, Breda virus, parvoviruses, pestiviruses, picobirnaviruses, and toroviruses, have been linked to gastroenteritis in humans with varying degrees of certainty.[55,366,685]

Rotaviruses

Worldwide, rotavirus is the leading cause of severe gastroenteritis in children. Rotavirus is responsible for the deaths of nearly 450,000 children younger than 5 years each year, mainly in developing countries.[497,618] Rotavirus gastroenteritis affects more than 90% of children by the time they are 3 years old and may cause moderate to severe vomiting that precedes diarrhea. It accounts for 10% to 50% of the cases of diarrhea in children, is the most common cause of diarrhea in children during winter months in colder climates, and accounts for 35% to 50% of young children hospitalized for acute diarrhea. However, these rates have decreased in many countries after vaccine introduction. Stools usually are watery or soft, and the presence of blood or leukocytes is rare. Asymptomatic rotavirus infections occur frequently,[489,516] and reinfection appears to be a common event.[642,643] The mechanism of spread is fecal-oral. Shedding of virus most frequently occurs from a few days before to 10 days after the onset of illness.[516] Natural rotavirus infection efficiently protects against severe disease associated with reinfection. Two virus surface proteins with antigenic properties, VP4 and VP7, are found in various conformations and are the basis for a binary serologic classification scheme that defines the G/P type of the virus.[29,505] Five genotypes (G1 to G4 and G9) accounted for 88% of all strains, although extensive geographic and temporal differences exist.[46] Rotavirus vaccines have reduced the health burden of rotavirus gastroenteritis in both developed and developing countries[167,545] (see "Prevention" section).

Noroviruses

Noroviruses are in the family Caliciviridae and have been identified as the second most common viral cause of severe gastroenteritis in children younger than 5 years in developing and developed countries, preceded only by rotavirus.[240] Norovirus is considered the most common cause of outbreaks of nonbacterial gastroenteritis worldwide.[71,424,641,691] It accounts for 12% of severe gastroenteritis cases among children younger than 5 years of age.[503] It is estimated that each year norovirus causes 64,000 episodes of diarrhea requiring hospitalization, 900,000 clinic visits among children in industrialized countries, and up to 200,000 deaths of children younger than 5 years in developing countries.[503] Young children (<5 years) have the highest incidence of norovirus diarrhea; 6.5% higher than the population older than 5 years.[59] Approximately 70% of pediatric norovirus cases occur between 6 and 23 months of age, with less than 15% occurring before 6 months.[589] The mean incubation period for norovirus is 24 to 48 hours. The primary routes of transmission are fecal-oral, including consumption of fecally contaminated food or water; direct person-to-person contact, especially in schools, childcare centers, restaurants, summer camps, hospitals, nursing homes, and cruise ships[11,105,331,332,365,541]; and through contaminated objects or environments. A low inoculum dose is required for infection.[622] Clinical manifestations include acute onset of vomiting, nonbloody diarrhea, or both lasting 12 to 60 hours.[240] The identification of human histo-blood group antigens as norovirus receptors opens a new approach for evaluation of susceptibility and therapy of norovirus infection.[207,240,615] Noroviruses are genetically and antigenically diverse.[71] Five genogroups (G) and several subgenogroups have been assigned. Strains of three genogroups GI, GII, and GIV are found in humans; GII is the most prevalent worldwide.[424,688,690] Candidate vaccines are presently in clinical development (see "Prevention" section).

Astroviruses

Astrovirus gastroenteritis occurs worldwide and has been associated with outbreaks of mild gastroenteritis in schools, daycare centers, pediatric wards, and nursing homes.[170,239,268,298,439] Illness is restricted primarily to children younger than the age of 2 years, elderly people, and immunocompromised individuals.[329,452] Astrovirus infections can be asymptomatic[435] and associated with other enteric viruses.[546] Eighty percent or more of adults have antibodies against the virus. The incubation period is 2 to 4 days.[239,329] Symptoms include fever and malaise, followed by watery diarrhea that may last approximately 3 days; vomiting is an uncommon symptom. Classic human astroviruses contain eight serotypes and account for 2% to 9% of all acute nonbacterial gastroenteritis in children worldwide.[74,212–214,347] The virus can be detected by electron microscopy, enzyme immunoassays, or reverse transcriptase–PCR (RT-PCR).[74,239,329,653]

Enteric Adenoviruses

Human adenoviruses of subgroups A to F have been identified as etiologic agents in a wide range of human diseases, including conjunctivitis, upper respiratory tract infections, and pneumonia. A subgroup of fastidious adenoviruses (group F) with a distinct set of antigenic determinants and specific tissue culture growth characteristics has been shown to be associated with acute gastroenteritis and is referred to as enteric adenovirus.[82,372,639] Serotypes 40 and 41 (group F)[372] are responsible for approximately 5% to 10% of cases of endemic pediatric diarrhea worldwide,[174,217,586,587,409] with higher prevalence in children younger than 24 months.[174] Nonenteric adenoviruses, specially adenovirus 31, can also be found in children with diarrhea.[409] The clinical manifestations include watery diarrhea accompanied by vomiting, low-grade fever, and mild dehydration.[372] Antibody prevalence to enteric adenovirus increases from 20% during the first 6 months of life to 50% or greater by the third or fourth year of life.[588] Seasonal shifts in the predominance of types 40 and 41 may occur.[82,99] Outbreaks of enteric adenovirus diarrhea have been described in childcare centers, where asymptomatic excretion is a common occurrence.[639,659]

Bacteria

Shigella

Shigella is the principal cause of clinical dysentery and an important cause of morbidity and mortality among children in impoverished regions of the developing world.[367] In the United States, shigellosis is the third most frequent FoodNet pathogen in sentinel states but appears to be decreasing in incidence. There are four serogroups of *Shigella*, containing 46 serotypes: *S. dysenteriae, S. flexneri, S. boydii*, and *S. sonnei*. In developing countries *S. flexneri* is the predominant species, whereas *S. sonnei* predominates in industrialized regions; however, in recent years there has been an important shift in the etiology of bacillary dysentery, with *Shigella sonnei* expansion across industrializing regions in Asia, Latin America, and the Middle East.[625] Infection by *Shigella* spp. rarely occurs in the first few months of life but is a common occurrence in children between the ages of 6 months and 10 years.[116] Children exclusively breastfed have significantly lower risk of moderate and severe diarrhea due to *Shigella* compared to non-breastfed children.[403] In highly endemic areas, peak infection rates occur in the second year of life. Children infected with *Shigella* can have asymptomatic excretion, watery diarrhea, or dysentery. HUS may occur after infection with Shiga toxin 1 (Stx1)-producing strains (primarily *S. dysenteriae* serotype 1). The postinfectious complications include reactive arthritis[628] and postinfectious irritable bowel syndrome.[274] Shigellosis results from the exposure to low inoculums of the bacteria; in addition to person-to-person spread, shigellae can be transmitted through contaminated foods, sexual contact, and water used for drinking or recreational purposes.[193,415] Mild symptoms are self-limiting, but in more severe cases antibiotics are recommended for cure and preventing relapse. The progressive development of antibiotic resistance in *Shigella* isolates is a worldwide problem.[290,367]

Salmonella

Salmonella infections are associated with several clinical syndromes: asymptomatic carriage, acute gastroenteritis, bacteremia, enteric fever, and dissemination with localized suppuration, such as abscess, osteomyelitis, or meningitis.[89,127,560] Based on the current classification, the genus *Salmonella* contains only two species, *S. bongori* and *S. enterica,* but there are more than 2500 serovars of *S. enterica. S. enterica* serovar typhi *(S. typhi)* and nontyphoidal salmonellae (NTS) are important causes of infection and disease in children. Typhoid fever is particularly common in South and Southeast Asia and is estimated to cause more than half a million deaths each year. NTS are a major cause of foodborne infections including gastroenteritis worldwide.[28,251,259] HIV-infected persons and malaria-infected children are at increased risk for invasive NTS.[32] *Salmonella* gastroenteritis occurs most commonly in the first 5 years of life, decreases in frequency during childhood, and remains relatively constant throughout the adult years.[116] In the United States, in the past decade, the *Salmonella* isolates most frequently reported have been *S. enterica* serotype Typhimurium and *S. enterica* serotype Enteritidis.[107,116] Although most episodes of *Salmonella* infection are foodborne, reptiles, including turtles, snakes, lizards, and iguanas, carry certain serotypes of *Salmonella* in their intestinal tracts and have been associated with episodes of salmonellosis.[519,606] Numerous outbreaks of disease caused by *Salmonella* after ingestion of contaminated food products, including eggs, milk, ice cream, peanut butter, and fresh produce, have been reported[78,104,117,291,415,534] (see "Foodborne Disease" section).

Campylobacter

Campylobacter spp. are recognized as among the most important causes of acute diarrheal disease in humans throughout the world, including in the United States.[20,94,115,333,339] The organism is a microaerophilic, curved gram-negative rod, carried in the intestine of many wild and domestic animals, particularly avian species including poultry. Healthy animals may be intestinal carriers.[591] Water can be a direct source of human infection, although food contamination from food-producing animals is a more significant problem. The main risk factors for *Campylobacter* infection are international travel, consumption of undercooked chicken, environmental exposure, and direct contact with farm animals.[179,226] Most *C. jejuni* diarrheal illness in the United States is foodborne.[415] Currently, 26 *Campylobacter* spp. and subspecies are recognized; *C. jejuni* and *C. coli* are the two predominant species[591,179]; however, many clinical microbiology laboratories do not differentiate between them. People infected with *C. jejuni* may develop diarrhea, cramping abdominal pain, chills, and fever. Gross rectal bleeding may occur, and mucus and fecal leukocytes may be present, resembling the illness produced by *Shigella. Campylobacter fetus,* recognized as a cause of fever, bacteremia, and meningitis in immunocompromised hosts and of abortion rarely causes diarrhea. *Campylobacter* has been associated with periodontitis, inflammatory bowel disease, and several extraintestinal manifestations including reactive arthritis, Guillain-Barré syndrome, and Miller Fisher syndrome.[339,420,527,528] There is growing recognition of an association between *Campylobacter* infection and malnutrition.[524]

Diarrheagenic Escherichia coli

E. coli associated with diarrhea is referred to as diarrheagenic *E. coli.*[151,460] There are six well-described categories of diarrheagenic *E. coli* classified based on clinical, microbiologic, and epidemiologic characteristics. Current classification is based mainly on the identification of specific virulence genes associated with each pathotype (Table 44.6).[346,460] In children, diarrheagenic *E. coli* as a group are responsible for 30% to 40% of all diarrhea cases worldwide.[476,477,482,490]

***Shiga toxin–producing* E. coli.** STEC, also referred to as enterohemorrhagic *E. coli* (EHEC) or verotoxin-producing *E. coli* (VTEC), is probably the most important pathogen in this group owing to its association with HUS. STEC produces a spectrum of disease, from mild watery diarrhea, to afebrile bloody diarrhea, hemorrhagic colitis, and HUS.[346,418,434] Only a small proportion (5–10%) of children infected with STEC, usually younger than 5 years, develop HUS.[411,630] This syndrome is characterized by the triad of hemolytic anemia, thrombocytopenia, and renal insufficiency and is associated most frequently with *E. coli* O157:H7. However, strains of many other serotypes are also associated with HUS. For example, the large European outbreak that began in Germany in 2011 was produced by an O104:H4 strain.[222,328] STEC has two potent cytotoxins encoded by lambdoid bacteriophages: Shiga toxin 1 (Stx1, also called verotoxin 1) and Stx2 (or verotoxin 2). Multiple variants of Stx2 exist, as well as several uncommon variants of Stx1. Sxt1 is identical to Shiga toxin made by *S. dysenteriae* type 1.[151,334,434] These strains usually possess genes like those found in EPEC (see later discussion) for colonizing the gut, although the recent O104:H4 strain had colonization genes like those of EAEC (see later discussion).[88,328] Many STEC strains appear to be nonvirulent for humans. Most reported outbreaks result after ingestion of contaminated food or water, although person-to-person transmission is also important, particularly in families and daycare settings.[256] Healthy cattle harbor the organism as part of their intestinal flora and are the main animal reservoir for STEC. Direct transmission from animals and their environments to humans in public settings where children come in contact with farm animals, such as petting zoos, represents a public health concern.[519] The diagnosis of STEC is based on the identification of Shiga toxin by immunoassays or PCR or isolation of pathogenic STEC strains.[255,294]

***Enteropathogenic* E. coli.** EPEC is associated with both sporadic and epidemic diarrhea in children, especially in developing countries.[181,346] EPEC most commonly causes acute diarrhea and may also cause persistent diarrhea in young children. EPEC was originally serogroup defined as *E. coli* associated with infantile diarrhea. Subsequently it was defined by its characteristic localized adherence pattern in tissue cultured cells. Currently it is identified mainly based on the presence of a specific virulence gene *(eae).*[180,475] EPEC induces a distinctive histopathology known as the "attaching and effacing" lesion, which is characterized by the intimate attachment of bacteria to the epithelial surface and effacement of host cell microvilli.[181] EPEC is currently divided into two groups, typical EPEC (tEPEC) and atypical EPEC (aEPEC), based on the presence of the EPEC adherence factor plasmid, which is only found in tEPEC.[180] Recent epidemiologic studies indicate that aEPEC is more prevalent than tEPEC in both developed and developing countries.[151,475] However, the large variety of serotypes and genetic virulence properties of aEPEC strains makes it difficult to determine which strains are truly pathogenic.[295]

***Enterotoxigenic* E. coli.** ETEC is an important cause of diarrhea in infants and children living in developing countries and is the most important bacterial agent of traveler's diarrhea.[346,536,604,609] ETEC causes watery diarrhea, which can be a mild, self-limited disease or severe dehydrating diarrhea. Repeated episodes of ETEC diarrhea can be associated with diminished linear growth in children.[389] ETEC colonizes the small bowel mucosa and elaborates enterotoxins, which gives rise to intestinal secretion. Colonization is mediated by one or more colonization factors (CFs). ETEC strains express heat-labile (LT) and/or heat-stable (ST) enterotoxins. LT is closely related in structure and function to cholera enterotoxin (CT) expressed by *Vibrio cholerae.*[609] ST-ETEC (with or without co-expression of LT) is one of the most important agents associated with moderate to severe diarrhea in children in developing countries.[373] There are several candidate vaccines under development.[650]

***Enteroinvasive* E. coli.** EIEC is related antigenically and biochemically to *Shigella* and causes either a dysentery-like illness or watery diarrhea. EIEC is distinguished from *Shigella* by a few minor biochemical tests, but these pathotypes share essential virulence factors.[346] However, EIEC

TABLE 44.6 **Diarrheagenic *E. coli* Pathotypes**

Name	Abbreviation	Clinical and Epidemiologic Characteristics	Diagnosis
Shiga toxin-producing or enterohemorrhagic or verotoxin-producing *E. coli*	STEC or EHEC or VTEC	Watery diarrhea progressing to bloody diarrhea usually without fever; may develop HUS (5%–10%), especially in children <5 years, associated with specific strains including both O157 and non-O157 serotypes; food exposure, person-to-person spread, water, and contact with animals; important reservoir in cattle	Simultaneous culture for O157 STEC and non–culture assay for Shiga toxin: stool culture on sorbitol-MacConkey media to detect sorbitol-nonfermenting *E. coli* O157; detection of Shiga toxins on stool sample by enzyme immunoassays; detection of Shiga toxin genes (*stx1* and *stx2*) and intimin gene (*eae*) by PCR
Enteropathogenic *E. coli*	EPEC	Acute watery diarrhea; may cause prolonged or persistent diarrhea in young children in developing countries; associated with hospital nursery outbreaks; atypical strains (aEPEC) are more prevalent than typical strains (tEPEC) worldwide	Detection of intimin gene (*eae*) ± bundle-forming pili (*bfp*A) by PCR and absence of Shiga toxins; HEp-2 cell adherence assay and serotyping have been replaced by molecular methods; serotyping should be performed only for research or outbreak investigations.
Enterotoxigenic *E. coli*	ETEC	Acute watery dehydrating diarrhea; usually self-limited; important cause of diarrhea in young children in developing countries and most important cause of traveler's diarrhea	Detection of enterotoxins: heat-labile (LT) and heat-stable (ST) by enzyme immunoassays or PCR
Enteroaggregative *E. coli*	EAEC	Acute watery diarrhea; may cause prolonged or persistent diarrhea in young children in developing countries and in HIV-infected patients; second most important cause of traveler's diarrhea	Detection of the *agg*R regulatory gene and other virulence genes: *aap, aat*A, *ast*A by PCR. Characteristic "stacked-brick" attachment patterns on HEp-2 cells, used only in research laboratories
Enteroinvasive *E. coli*	EIEC	Acute watery diarrhea, usually dysenteric; *Shigella*-like pediatric diarrhea; an occasional cause of foodborne outbreaks in industrialized areas	Detection of invasion plasmid antigen of *Shigella* (*ipa*H) by PCR
Diffusely adherent *E. coli*	DAEC	Acute watery diarrhea, particularly in children >12 mo of age in developing countries; may be an important cause of childhood diarrhea in the United States	Detection of Dr adhesins (*daa*D) or Dr-associated genes by PCR; characteristic "diffuse" attachment patterns in HEp-2 cells, used only in research laboratories

PCR, Polymerase chain reaction.

exhibits reduced virulence compared to that of *Shigella*, which correlates with the less severe disease induced by EIEC.[151] EIEC infection is thought to represent an inflammatory colitis, although many patients seem to manifest a secretory, small bowel syndrome. Infections generally occur in adults; foodborne outbreaks have been reported.[200]

***Enteroaggregative* E. coli.** EAEC causes acute and persistent diarrhea in children in developing countries, adult traveler's diarrhea, and diarrhea in HIV-infected patients.[2,65,218,237,315,576] EAEC pathogenesis includes adherence to the intestinal mucosa, biofilm formation, production of enterotoxins and cytotoxins, and mucosal inflammation.[151] EAEC colonizes the intestinal mucosa in an aggregative, "stacked brick" pattern by means of one of several different aggregative adherence fimbriae (AAF). Some strains of EAEC may then elaborate cytotoxins, including the plasmid-encoded toxin and the enterotoxins EAST1 and ShET1. EAEC virulence factors are under the control of a global regulator, called AggR, in "typical EAEC strains."[282,459] EAEC infections elicit mucosal inflammation. Some infected subjects develop bloody diarrhea, and a subset develops chronic persistent diarrhea; persistent illness is particularly important in young children because it leads to chronic inflammation, intestinal epithelium damages, and malnutrition.[65,151,314,568] EAEC may be an important, unrecognized cause of childhood diarrhea in the United States and other industrialized countries.[136,289] Outbreaks of gastroenteritis linked to EAEC have been reported.[289]

***Diffusely adherent* E. coli.** Diffusely adherent *E. coli* (DAEC) has been implicated as a cause of diarrhea in several studies, particularly in children older than 12 months of age.[413,460,567,602] DAEC is defined by the presence of a characteristic, diffuse pattern of adherence to HEp-2 cell monolayers. DAEC strains produce fimbrial adhesins that belong to the Dr family of adhesins.[346,386] There is no universal method to detect DAEC strains in the clinical setting.[151] DAEC causes acute and persistent diarrhea in children and may be associated with persistent bloody diarrhea without fever.[506] DAEC was isolated in 13% of diarrhea cases in children younger than 5 years in the emergency department at a children's hospital in the United States, where it may be an important underrecognized cause of childhood diarrhea.[136]

***Adherent invasive* E. coli.** In the past decade a new *E. coli* pathotype has been recognized, the adherent invasive *E. coli* (AIEC).[151] This pathogen has been implicated in inflammatory bowel diseases. AIEC can increase the incidence and severity of gut inflammation in the context of Crohn disease.[8,426] The molecular bases that characterize the phenotypic properties of this pathotype are still not well resolved.[151,426]

Vibrio cholerae

Cholera is an acute, severe diarrheal disease caused by *Vibrio cholerae* that affects millions of people each year. Without prompt rehydration, death can occur within hours of the onset of symptoms. Cholera affects people of all ages, but children are involved disproportionately. Strains of *V. cholerae* are classified according to somatic or O groups. *V. cholerae* strains are separated further into two main serotypes (Ogawa and Inaba) and two biotypes (classic and El Tor). *V. cholerae* responsible for epidemic cholera belong to serogroups O1 and, in recent decades, O139.[122,128,345] It is estimated that *V. cholerae* causes 1 to 4 million cases of diarrhea and more than 100,000 deaths annually.[18,692] During the past several decades, despite advances in water sanitation technology and antibiotic treatment, the seventh cholera pandemic has spread.[692] The cholera burden has grown strikingly during the past 4 years and has spread to countries previously spared by this disease. The current spread has proved especially violent, as illustrated by the recent deadly epidemics in East Africa and Haiti.[514] Cholera emerged in Haiti in 2010, with more than 650,000 cases and over 8000 deaths, as of March 2013.[383,663] Cholera is rare in the United States. Most clinical isolates of *V. cholerae* O1 in the United States are associated with foreign travel and with ingestion of undercooked seafood,[116,450,465] and many are resistant to antimicrobial agents.[605] Crabs harvested from the U.S. Gulf Coast are a common source of cholera.[107] After Hurricane Katrina in 2005, crabs were the source of illness for certain cases of cholera.[112,116] Most *Vibrio* infections after the hurricane were *V. vulnificus, V. parahaemolyticus,* and non-toxigenic *V. cholerae. V. cholerae* O75 has caused cholera in the U.S. Gulf Coast states.[464] Since epidemic cholera began in Haiti in 2010, a total of 23 cholera cases caused by toxigenic *V. cholerae* O1 have been confirmed in the United States.[5,465,466]

V. cholerae O1 adheres to and multiplies on small intestinal mucosa. Diarrhea occurs after elaboration of several toxins, the most important of which is cholera toxin (CT) composed of one A and five B subunits.[578] The B subunits bind the toxin to the terminal galactose of G_{M1} ganglioside receptors present on intestinal mucosal cells. Inside the epithelial cell, the A subunit activates adenylate cyclase, initiating continuous cyclic adenosine monophosphate production. This results in chloride and fluid secretion into the small intestine lumen.[327,345,578] Strains of *V. cholerae* belonging to serotypes other than O1 and O139 are much less significant pathogens, although they can cause mild and occasionally profuse, watery diarrhea. Other *Vibrio* spp., including *V. fluvialis, V. mimicus, V. hollisae,* and *V. furnissii,* have been shown occasionally to cause gastrointestinal tract disease.[327]

Vibrio parahaemolyticus

V. parahaemolyticus inhabits warm estuarine waters worldwide. The organism has been found in water, shellfish, fish, and plankton[305] and has caused outbreaks of gastroenteritis after ingestion of contaminated seafood.[429,450] Although widely distributed in coastal waters, *V. parahaemolyticus* is an uncommon cause of diarrhea where consumption of raw seafood is common, usually in summer. Clinical manifestations of infection with *V. parahaemolyticus* are gastroenteritis in 59% of cases and include abdominal cramps, nausea, and, less frequently, vomiting, headache, low-grade fever, and chills; wound infections, including hemorrhagic cellulitis in 34% and septicemia in 5%.[157,397] A dysentery-like syndrome has been described in India and Bangladesh.[316] Preexisting liver disease predisposes infected patients to development of septicemia and death.[305] Three serotypes (O3:K6, O4:K68, and O1:K untypable) are extremely virulent and pathogenic to humans.[658] Surveillance data from the United States indicate that the incidence of vibriosis increased from 1996 to 2010 overall and for each of the three most commonly reported species: *V. parahaemolyticus, V. vulnificus,* and *V. alginolyticus.*[275,466]

Yersinia enterocolitica

Yersinia enterocolitica is a gram-negative bacillus that appears to be a common cause of gastroenteritis among children in Europe and Canada but is a relatively uncommon cause of enteritis in the United States.[75] Yersiniosis incidence is higher among African-American children and Hispanic people.[121] The ingestion of contaminated milk or food such as chitterlings[182,338,387] has been implicated as the mode of transmission in reported outbreaks. The clinical manifestations vary according to the age of the person involved. Illness in children younger than 5 years usually is self-limited gastroenteritis. Stools may contain blood and mucus or be watery. Associated symptoms consist of fever, vomiting, and abdominal pain. Older children may present with abdominal pain associated with mesenteric adenitis that mimics acute appendicitis. Adults develop diarrhea and abdominal pain less frequently than do children but may present with polyarthritis, arthralgia or erythema nodosum. Patients with β-thalassemia and iron overload are at an increased risk for development of severe yersiniosis.[4]

Aeromonas hydrophila

Aeromonas spp. are gram-negative bacteria found in soil and fresh and brackish water worldwide. *Aeromonas* spp. are recognized as colonizers and pathogens of cold-blooded animals, including fish, reptiles, and amphibians. *Aeromonas* spp. have been associated with a wide spectrum of human disease, most frequently gastroenteritis, soft tissue infection, and bacteremia, especially in immunocompromised hosts.[325] There are many species of *Aeromonas* associated with human diseases; however, *A. hydrophila, A. veroni,* and *A. caviae* are the major species associated with gastroenteritis. Because many clinical laboratories cannot perform precise identification, most species isolated are reported as *A. hydrophila.* The role of *A. hydrophila* in human diarrhea remains controversial; however, new evidence supports its pathogenic role.[12,325] *Aeromonas*-associated diarrhea occurs worldwide, but the exact prevalence of this infection on a global scale is unknown.[580] The GEMS study found *Aeromonas* in a significant proportion of children with moderate to severe diarrhea in some but not all countries.[373] Children with watery diarrhea associated with *Aeromonas* are significantly more likely to have organisms that possess genes for both heat-labile and heat-stable enterotoxins than do control children.[13] *Aeromonas* has been linked to cholera-like and dysentery-like illnesses.[325]

Plesiomonas shigelloides

P. shigelloides is a gram-negative bacillus that has been associated with opportunistic infections in immunocompromised hosts and with sporadic cases of diarrhea in immunocompetent hosts in a variety of countries.[125,201,310,342,351] In some case-control studies, the organism has been found to be associated with diarrhea, whereas in others it has not.[14] The organism has been isolated from surface water and the intestines of freshwater fish and many animals, including dogs and cats.[626] *Plesiomonas* occurs commonly in tropical and subtropical areas from which most stool isolates have been reported.[310] Coinfection with other pathogens is associated with diarrhea.[201] Patients with *P. shigelloides* infection describe self-limited diarrhea, occasionally characterized by blood and mucus. The organism has failed to produce illness when fed to volunteers, and its role as an enteric pathogen remains uncertain.[297]

Clostridium difficile

C. difficile is the most common bacterial agent associated with severe antimicrobial-associated diarrhea. Enterotoxin A and cytotoxin B account for most of its virulence. *C. difficile* infection is less common in children than adults, but the incidence of *C. difficile* infection in children is increasing.[173,353,558] Asymptomatic colonization is very common in neonates and young children; reported rates range from 0% to 50% in neonates and up to 70% in infants. Frequency of colonization gradually decreases with age: after 4 years of age, rates are less than 5%, similar to those of healthy adults.[87] Colonization generally persists for a few months, though it can persist for up to 12 months or longer.[6] Elevated colonization rates have been described among hospitalized children and children with malignancy or inflammatory bowel disease.[163,311,394,425] Despite the high frequency of colonization by *C. difficile,* infants rarely develop symptomatic disease. In older children, *C. difficile* disease was traditionally considered a hospital-acquired infection but community-acquired infection has been increasingly described.[118] Children with community-associated infection tend to be healthier and have lower rates of exposure to antibiotics and acid suppressants than children with health care–associated disease.[149,632] Gastrointestinal feeding devices (i.e., gastrostomy or jejunostomy tubes),[149] proton pump inhibitors, and, to a lesser extent, histamine-2 receptor antagonists, have been associated with an increased risk of *C. difficile* infection in children.[163,223,425,473]

Clostridium perfringens

C. perfringens types A, C, and D produce an enterotoxin that is implicated in the pathogenesis of a short-duration food poisoning syndrome.[578,636] Most foodborne outbreaks are caused by type A strains and are associated with meat and poultry products.[260] Within 14 hours after ingesting contaminated food, patients experience watery diarrhea and abdominal pain with minimal nausea, vomiting, or fever; illness resolves in less than 24 hours. *C. perfringens* type C also is associated with a rare destructive intestinal disease called *enteritis necroticans* or *pigbel,* characterized by vomiting, abdominal pain, bloody diarrhea, and small bowel necrosis, with peritonitis, shock, and death.[457,660] These strains produce three toxins (α-toxin, β-toxin, and an enterotoxin) of potential pathogenetic significance.[45,99,436,576] Enteritis necroticans occurs after ingestion of undercooked pork.

Staphylococcus aureus

S. aureus produces a wide variety of toxins including staphylococcal enterotoxins and staphylococcal-like proteins.[35] Staphylococcal enterotoxins are a major cause of food poisoning, which typically occurs after ingestion of processed meat or dairy products, which have been contaminated with *S. aureus* due to improper handling and subsequent storage at elevated temperatures.[61,73,341] Symptoms include nausea and vomiting, with or without diarrhea. The illness is usually self-limiting, and only occasionally is it severe enough to warrant hospitalization.[573] The severity of the illness depends on the amount of food ingested, the amount of toxin in the ingested food, and the general health of the host. Staphylococcal enterotoxin type A has been responsible for more than half of the reported outbreaks of staphylococcal food poisoning in the United States.[309,341,399]

Bacillus cereus

B. cereus is an aerobic, spore-forming, gram-positive bacillus that is widely distributed environmentally; it causes an emetic or a diarrheal food-associated illness primarily in the industrialized world.[76] *B. cereus* is associated mainly with food poisoning but can also cause potentially fatal nongastrointestinal infections.[76] *B. cereus* should be suspected as the cause of gastrointestinal tract illness if appropriate symptoms are present and if incriminated food, particularly fried rice, has been ingested.[51,100,103] Two distinct forms of gastrointestinal tract illness can be produced by this organism: (1) the emetic disease, a food intoxication caused by cereulide, a small ring-form peptide; the emetic toxin produces a syndrome that resembles illness produced by staphylococcal enterotoxin, with nausea, vomiting, and abdominal cramps that begin within 1 to 6 hours of ingestion; and (2) a diarrheal syndrome caused by vegetative cells, ingested as viable cells or spores, that produce protein enterotoxins in the small intestine. These enterotoxins produce profuse watery diarrhea and abdominal pain that begin within 6 to 24 hours, with minimal or no vomiting. Some strains produce both toxins, whereas others produce only one toxin.[607] Symptoms caused by either toxin usually resolve in less than 24 hours, and fever rarely occurs. Spores of *B. cereus* are resistant to heat and therefore may withstand a brief period of cooking or boiling.

Listeria monocytogenes

L. monocytogenes is the causative agent of listeriosis, a potentially fatal opportunistic foodborne infection. *Listeria* spp. are isolated from a diversity of environmental sources, including soil, water, foods, and the feces of humans and animals. The foods most frequently contaminated include soft cheeses and dairy products; pâtés and sausages; smoked fish; and industrially produced, refrigerated, ready-to-eat products that are eaten without cooking or reheating.[43,102,254] *L. monocytogenes* can cause gastroenteritis in otherwise healthy individuals and more severe invasive disease in immunocompromised patients. *Listeria* infection in pregnancy may cause fetal loss or a preterm delivery, and the neonate is prone to neonatal sepsis and death.[195,296] Common symptoms include fever, watery diarrhea, nausea, headache, cramps, and myalgia.[47,484]

Parasites

The most important parasites known to cause diarrhea are the protozoa (*Entamoeba histolytica, Giardia lamblia, Cryptosporidium parvum, Isospora belli, Cyclospora cayetanensis*) and the Microsporidia (*Encephalitozoon intestinalis* and *Enterocytozoon bieneusi*).[323] Among helminths, *Strongyloides stercoralis* and *Trichuris trichiura* may produce diarrhea. Data associating *Ascaris* and hookworm with diarrhea are lacking, but both cause abdominal pain. *Balantidium coli* is a cause of bloody diarrhea in humans. The roles of *Blastocystis hominis*[608] and *Dientamoeba fragilis* as causes of diarrhea are controversial.

Entamoeba histolytica

Entamoeba histolytica is the causative agent of amebiasis, a disease that is a major source of morbidity and mortality in the developing world.[537,603] The genus *Entamoeba* contains many species, six of which can reside in the human intestinal lumen. *E. histolytica* is the only species definitely pathogenic. New approaches to identifying *E. histolytica* are based on detection of *E. histolytica*–specific antigen and DNA in stool and other clinical specimens.[221] Clinical patterns that occur in patients with amebiasis consist of intestinal amebiasis with the gradual onset of colicky abdominal pain and frequent bowel movements, tenesmus, and little or no constitutional disturbance; amebic dysentery, characterized by profuse diarrhea containing blood and mucus and the presence of constitutional signs, such as fever, dehydration, and electrolyte alterations; hepatic amebiasis, which usually presents as abscess formation without gastrointestinal tract symptoms; and asymptomatic colonization.[281] In infants in developing countries most infections are asymptomatic; diarrhea is associated with both the amount of parasite and the composition of the microbiota.[235] Patients may experience tender hepatomegaly, jaundice, weight loss, fever, and anorexia. The frequency of liver abscess in patients with amebiasis is between 1% and 5%. The complications of intestinal amebiasis include perforation, ameboma, stricture, hemorrhage secondary to erosion into a blood vessel, intussusception, ischiorectal abscess, fistulas, and rectal prolapse.[281]

Giardia intestinalis

G. intestinalis (synonyms: *G. lamblia* and *G. duodenalis*) is a flagellated protozoan parasite that reproduces in the small intestine, causing giardiasis. *Giardia* is one of the most common intestinal parasites in the world; it contributes to diarrhea and nutritional deficiencies in children in developing regions.[17] In the United States it is the most common intestinal parasite identified by public health laboratories.[51,109] *Giardia* infection is transmitted by the fecal-oral route and occurs after ingestion of *Giardia* cysts in fecally contaminated food or water or through person-to-person transmission.[193,400,415] The low infectious dose of 10 cysts places people in close contact, including children in daycare, at risk of acquiring infection.[542] Children appear to be more susceptible to *Giardia* than adults. Specific conditions that predispose to giardiasis are hypogammaglobulinemia, secretory immunoglobulin A (IgA) deficiency, peptic ulcer disease, biliary tract disease, and pancreatitis. The parasite may exist in two forms: cyst and trophozoite. The trophozoites usually are seen in duodenal aspirates and loose stools, whereas cysts can be found in formed stools and can remain viable and infectious in water for longer than 3 months. Diagnostic assays using antigen detection are available.[17] *Giardia* infection can be asymptomatic or present as an acute illness with a sudden onset of explosive, watery, foul-smelling stools and flatulence, abdominal distention, nausea, and anorexia, with the absence of blood and mucus or as chronic diarrhea and malabsorption, with exacerbations and remissions of flatulence, abdominal distention, and abdominal pain often lasting for months.[132,515] A recent systematic review showed that *G. lamblia* was not associated with acute diarrhea in children in developing countries.[453] *Giardia* infections can result in chronic gastrointestinal disorders such as postinfectious irritable bowel syndrome, and symptoms may manifest at extraintestinal sites even though the parasite does not disseminate beyond the gastrointestinal tract.[52,145]

Cryptosporidium

Cryptosporidium is an intestinal coccidian protozoan parasite that causes diarrheal diseases in humans worldwide. Children and immunosuppressed individuals, especially those with HIV infection or AIDS, are disproportionately affected.[91] In developing countries there is a high prevalence of cryptosporidiosis in young children, particularly among those who are malnourished or HIV infected, with high rates of hospitalization and mortality.[123,313,447,486,564] The GEMS study identified *Cryptosporidium* as one of the four major contributors to moderate to severe diarrheal diseases during the first 2 years of life at all sites.[373] Fecal-oral transmission of *Cryptosporidium* oocysts occurs from person to person, through ingestion of contaminated drinking water or recreational water, through consumption of contaminated food, or by contact with infected animals (cattle and sheep).[114,116,193,308,400] Unlike bacterial pathogens, *Cryptosporidium* is resistant to chlorine disinfection and can survive for days in treated recreational water, including swimming pools and recreational water parks.[193] Children aged 4 years and younger appear to be at a particularly high risk for acquiring this organism.[116] *Cryptosporidium* has been implicated as a cause of diarrhea in travelers, outbreaks, and of epidemics in hospitals, daycare centers, and other institutional settings worldwide. Cryptosporidiosis can be manifested with a wide spectrum of symptoms, including asymptomatic excretion, acute diarrhea, chronic diarrhea, epidemic diarrhea, severe life-threatening watery diarrhea, and biliary tract disease.[134] Stools do not contain blood or leukocytes. Vomiting, flatulence, abdominal pain, and low-grade fever routinely accompany diarrhea.[285] Symptoms usually subside in an average of 9 days. Patients may have cholera-like illness, transient diarrhea, relapsing episodes, or a protracted clinical course with unremitting, profuse diarrhea lasting for months accompanied by profound malabsorption and weight loss. In immunocompetent individuals, infection with this parasite may be asymptomatic or cause a self-limiting diarrheal illness. However, in immunocompromised patients such as those with HIV infection or AIDS, *Cryptosporidium* spp. may cause severe, chronic, and possibly fatal diarrhea and wasting.[421] Identification of the organisms and symptoms is more frequent when the CD4 count is less than 200 cells/μL. Antiretroviral therapy is protective against disease.[96,421,480]

Isospora belli

Isospora gained importance with the advent of AIDS and, before HAART, was shown to be an important cause of severe and prolonged gastroenteritis.[178,496] Infection can occur in adults and children and has been reported in infants with severe diarrhea.[402] This organism also has been implicated as a cause of traveler's diarrhea.[236] Transmission is fecal-oral, through ingestion of oocysts contaminating food, water, or environmental surfaces.[402] The clinical spectrum of disease caused by *Isospora* is indistinguishable from that described for *Cryptosporidium.* The spectrum includes asymptomatic infection, acute diarrhea in children in developing countries, and chronic diarrhea or severe, protracted, life-threatening diarrhea in patients with AIDS.[269] Fever, malaise, abdominal pain, and headache have been reported. Stools are watery and do not contain blood or leukocytes. Malabsorption, steatorrhea, severe weight loss, and chronic diarrhea lasting months to years are the most likely occurrences in immunocompromised hosts.[165]

Cyclospora

Cyclospora cayetanensis, a coccidian protozoon, is transmitted by the fecal-oral route. Direct person-to-person transmission is unlikely to occur because excreted oocysts require days to weeks under favorable environmental conditions to sporulate and to become infectious. An animal reservoir has not been described. Outbreaks of diarrhea caused by consumption of water and fresh fruits contaminated with *Cyclospora* have been described,[299,415,417] and travelers to developing countries are at increased risk for development of diarrhea caused by *Cyclospora.* In the United States approximately half of the cases are associated with international travel, known outbreaks, or both.[279] Most of the reported cases have occurred during the spring and summer. The mean incubation period appears to be 7 days. Clinical manifestations include asymptomatic excretion, acute watery diarrhea, and diarrhea that may be protracted for days to weeks with frequent, watery stools, which may remit and relapse.[279,391] The clinical presentation is somewhat different in areas of endemicity, where asymptomatic infections are more frequent. Nevertheless, younger children have more severe clinical symptoms. In endemic settings, infections tend to be milder as children get older because the duration of the infection is shorter and the severity of disease decreases. As in young children, the elderly may also present with a more severe illness.[487]

Microsporidia

Microsporidia have emerged as causes of opportunistic infections associated with diarrhea and wasting in AIDS patients. Among non–HIV-infected but immune-suppressed individuals, microsporidia have infected organ transplant recipients, diabetics, children, the elderly, and patients with malignant disease.[7] In otherwise healthy immune-competent HIV-seronegative populations, self-limiting diarrhea occurred in travelers and as a result of a foodborne outbreaks. Greater awareness and implementation of better diagnostic methods are demonstrating that microsporidia contribute to a wide range of clinical syndromes in HIV-infected and non–HIV-infected people.[176,209] The nontaxonomic term human Microsporidia can refer to any of the order of Microsporidia known to cause disease in humans: *Enterocytozoon* spp., *Encephalitozoon* spp., *Pleistophora* spp., and *Nosema* spp. Of these *Enterocytozoon bieneusi* and *Encephalitozoon intestinalis* are the most important in gastrointestinal tract disease of humans.[41,662] Both species have been detected in intestinal biopsy specimens of patients with AIDS, with a clinical picture of prolonged diarrhea and weight loss.[144] The clinical spectrum appears to depend on the immune status of the host. The primary location of all intestinal spore-forming protozoal infection is the small intestine, but colonic infection has been reported with *E. bieneusi.*[249] Infection of the biliary tract with *E. bieneusi* and *E. intestinalis* in patients with AIDS can cause sclerosing cholangitis[526,584,540] and acalculous cholecystitis. *E. intestinalis* can infect lamina propria macrophages, fibroblasts, and endothelial cells and can disseminate to other organs, including liver, respiratory tract, and kidney.[249,540] Extraintestinal infection develops after infection with other species of the order of Microsporidia occurs.

Strongyloides stercoralis

S. stercoralis is a nematode that infects humans through the intestinal tract or through skin if either comes in contact with soil that contains larvae. About one-third of people with strongyloidiasis are asymptomatic, and the remainder may have skin, pulmonary, or, more frequently, gastrointestinal tract involvement.[590] People at risk include residents and travelers to endemic areas[572]; natives and residents of the Appalachian region in the United States; institutionalized patients; and people treated with corticosteroids, cimetidine, and antacids.[231] Epigastric abdominal pain occurs and is associated with diarrhea that contains mucus and blood. Some patients may complain of nausea, vomiting, and weight loss with evidence of malabsorption. Eosinophilia and an urticarial rash are prominent features of infection. Diagnosis of *Strongyloides* is often delayed, owing to patients presenting with nonspecific gastrointestinal complaints, a low parasite load, and irregular larval output. Novel diagnostic methods are expected to improve epidemiologic studies and control efforts for prevention and treatment of strongyloidiasis.[90,444,437,398] The hyperinfection syndrome caused by *Strongyloides stercoralis* has a high mortality rate (15–87%). Risk factors include new immunosuppressive therapies, human T-lymphotropic virus (HTLV)-1 infection, cadaveric transplantation, immune reconstitution syndrome, hematologic malignancies (especially lymphoma), tuberculosis, malnutrition secondary to chronic *Strongyloides* diarrhea, international travel, and immigration.[423,432]

DIAGNOSIS

Determination of the cause of an episode of infectious diarrhea depends on epidemiologic information, the clinical syndrome, laboratory tests, and knowledge or assessment of an organism for virulence factors. Because virulence properties determine clinical manifestations of disease, an understanding of pathophysiologic mechanisms guides the laboratory evaluation and empiric therapy. The major virulence properties of enteropathogens include adherence, epithelial cell invasion, and production of toxins. Some enteropathogens produce diarrhea by other mechanisms, and enteric pathogens may possess one or several of these virulence properties. Both host and microbiologic factors ultimately determine clinical expression in the individual patient. Not all of the recognized virulence properties of a given species are obvious clinically in a given episode of disease.

The diagnosis of gastroenteritis has traditionally been based on cultures and microscopy. However, this pattern may be changing because acute diarrhea diagnostics are moving away from culture toward rapid nonculture methods. These infections are mainly foodborne and therefore preventable, and it is of paramount importance that public health surveillance for these infections is consistent and reliable.[336] Isolation of cultured organisms is still an invaluable tool for determining sensitivity to antimicrobial agents in clinical settings and for identifying specific strains, virulence factors, or toxins during investigations of outbreaks.[508] However, for some pathogens it can be more important to identify the toxins than the organisms themselves; this is the case, for example, for Shiga toxins of STEC/EHEC or for toxins A and B for *C. difficile.* The use of molecular diagnostics is increasing; improvements include multiplex and quantitative PCR, fluorescence in situ hybridization, and metagenomic analyses.[265,336,337,485,525]

In recent years, several different multi–gastrointestinal-pathogen molecular diagnostic platforms have been developed for the simultaneous detection of pathogenic enteric viruses, bacteria, and parasites.[68,404,407,449,593] Some of these platforms have recently been FDA cleared. However, there are significant differences among these tests, including costs, workflow, and throughput differences.[648] In addition, interpretation of

TABLE 44.7 Diagnostic Evaluation of the Main Enteropathogens Associated With Pediatric Diarrhea

Type	Enteropathogen	Laboratory Test
Virus	Rotavirus	Immunoassays: ELISA (preferred method), EIA, immune-chromatography, latex agglutination; reverse transcriptase-PCR (RT-PCR)
	Norovirus	Real-time or conventional RT-PCR (preferred method); EIA (less sensitive)
Bacteria	*Shigella*	Conventional stool culture; fecal leukocytes
	Salmonella	Conventional stool culture; blood and bone marrow culture for systemic disease; serotype
	Campylobacter	Stool culture with special media, incubated at 42°C, with microaerophilia; Gram stain; EIA
	Shiga toxin–producing *E. coli*	Simultaneous culture for O157 STEC (sorbitol-MacConkey) and non-culture assay for Shiga toxin detection (ELISA and other enzyme immunoassays) (preferred method); PCR (see Table 44.6)
	Other diarrheagenic *E. coli*	Conventional stool culture for initial isolation of *E. coli* colonies, followed by a specific assay; conventional or real-time PCR; HEp-2 cell adherence assays; toxin detection by EIA (see Table 44.6)
	Vibrio cholerae	Stool culture in salt-containing media, with study of isolates for O1 serotype
	Vibrio parahaemolyticus	Stool culture in salt-containing media
	Yersinia enterocolitica	Stool culture in selective media
	Aeromonas hydrophila	Conventional stool culture
	Plesiomonas shigelloides	Conventional stool culture
	Clostridium difficile	Detection of toxins A and B in stools by enzyme immunoassay; cytotoxicity tissue-culture assay; stool culture
Parasites	Intestinal parasites associated with diarrhea	Examination of stools for ova and parasites (*Giardia, E. histolytica, Strongyloides*), and with special stains for coccidia (*Cryptosporidium, Isospora, Cyclospora*) and Microsporidia; enzyme immunoassays (*E. histolytica, Giardia, Cryptosporidium*) and PCR for all

molecular diagnostics in stool samples is challenging and should be carefully evaluated due to the high rates of asymptomatic carriage and coinfections with multiple enteric pathogens, particularly in children in developing countries.[525]

Proper identification of the causative agent of an episode of acute infectious diarrhea will help facilitate initiation of appropriate management. In this section we will discuss the basic concepts for enteropathogen identification by direct microscopic examination, stool cultures, immunologic methods, and molecular methods. Laboratory tests used to detect enteropathogens are listed in Table 44.7.

Macroscopic Stool Examination

A gross examination of the stool specimen should be routine in all patients with diarrhea, even if no laboratory studies are performed. Diarrheal stool that is watery and without mucus or blood usually is caused by an enterotoxin, virus, or protozoan organism, or it may be caused by infection outside the gastrointestinal tract. The color of stools generally conveys little information if the stool does not contain blood. Infectious causes to be considered when stools contain blood or mucus include a cytotoxin-producing bacterium, an enteroinvasive bacterium causing mucosal inflammation, and an enteric parasite associated with blood in stools, such as *E. histolytica, E. coli,* and *T. trichiura.* When it is present, blood usually is mixed evenly into the stool, except in the case of *E. histolytica* infections, in which blood often is on the surface of the stool, and some STEC infections, in which the stool may be blood streaked. Stools that are particularly foul smelling are consistent with *Salmonella* and other bacteria as well as *Giardia, Cryptosporidium,* and *Strongyloides* spp. Stools with little odor suggest an enterotoxin, such as cholera toxin or ETEC, or a viral enteropathogen.

Microscopic Examination

Fecal Leukocytes

Microscopic examination of stool specimens for evidence of fecal leukocytes provides information about the cause of diarrhea and helps determine the anatomic location and presence of mucosal inflammation.[517] Fecal leukocytes are produced in response to bacteria that diffusely invade the colonic mucosa and indicate that the patient has colitis. No inflammatory bacterial enteritis exists in which results of the fecal leukocyte examination are uniformly positive.[302] Thus results of examination are more helpful when they are positive than when negative. When results are positive (>50–100 leukocytes per high-power field), the patient probably has an invasive or cytotoxin-producing organism, such as *Shigella* spp., *Salmonella* spp.; *Campylobacter* spp., invasive *E. coli,* STEC, *C. difficile,* or *Y. enterocolitica,* although ulcerative colitis and Crohn disease also are associated with fecal leukocytes.

Diarrheagenic *E. coli* is associated with a mild inflammatory response during symptomatic infection in children.[436] Fecal leukocytes generally are not present in stools from patients with diarrhea secondary to viruses, enterotoxin-producing bacteria, or parasites. The leukocytes seen in cytotoxin-associated and invasive bacterial diarrhea syndromes are polymorphonuclear. If the fecal leukocyte examination shows evidence of inflammatory enteritis, further laboratory evaluation is indicated. Fecal lactoferrin and fecal calprotectin are newly available markers associated with intestinal inflammation. Fecal lactoferrin is a much more sensitive indicator of inflammatory diarrhea than the fecal leukocyte or occult blood test,[124,317] but it may not be useful in differentiating inflammatory from noninflammatory diarrhea in diarrhea-endemic countries.[40] Stool lactoferrin may be falsely positive in breastfed infants. Fecal calprotectin can also be used to screen for bacterial diarrhea and to differentiate between bacterial and viral pathogens in children with gastroenteritis[126,612] and in children with inflammatory bowel diseases.[494]

Ova and Parasites

Normally examination of stools for ova and parasites is unnecessary unless the patient has a history of recent travel to high-risk areas, stool cultures are negative for other enteropathogens, the patient is involved in an outbreak of parasitic diarrhea, diarrhea persists for longer than 1 week, or the patient is immunosuppressed. Both trophozoites and cysts of *G. lamblia* and larvae of *Strongyloides* spp. can be identified on direct smears of stool specimens. However, the sensitivity of stool examination for most parasites can be improved by use of a concentration technique and by placement of stools in vials containing a stool preservative. Trichrome and iron hematoxylin both are useful as permanent stains for *Giardia* spp. Pooling of preserved fecal samples is an efficient and economical procedure for detecting ova and parasites.[15] Rational use of the stool ova and parasite examination relies on communication between the clinician and laboratory personnel.[80] For patients in whom giardiasis, cryptosporidiosis, isosporiasis, or strongyloidiasis is considered and in whom stool cultures are negative, aspiration or biopsy of the duodenum or upper jejunum may be indicated. Because these organisms live in the upper intestine, this procedure is more reliable than is examination of stool specimens.[548] *E. histolytica* can be diagnosed by microscopic examination of fresh stool specimens or bowel wall scrapings for cysts or trophozoites. A concentration technique may be helpful in demonstrating amebic cysts. Examination of several stool samples by an experienced technician may be necessary because excretion of cysts often is intermittent and interpretation is difficult. Confusion in differentiating amebic cysts from fecal leukocytes may occur. Microscopy can be used only as presumptive evidence of *E. histolytica* because the nonpathogen *E. dispar* is morphologically identical.[203]

Special Stains for Coccidia

Diagnosis of *Cryptosporidium, Isospora, Cyclospora,* and the Microsporidia is based on morphologic appearance and staining of stool or histologic examination of tissue sections.[249] Among the most widely used stains to visualize these coccidia are standard acid-fast or modified acid-fast stains, which are based on the use of reagents that enhance the penetration of fuchsin into the organism without the need for heating (modified Kinyoun acid-fast stain). In a modified acid-fast stain, *Cryptosporidium* oocysts, which are 4 to 6 μm with four crescentic sporozoites, stain red and can be differentiated readily from yeasts that stain green.[292] In a study of seven microscopy-based *Cryptosporidium* oocyst detection methods, false-positive results were detected by acid-fast and auramine-rhodamine stains but not by monoclonal antibody–based methods.[37] Oocysts of *I. belli* often are visualized by wet-mount preparations because of their size, which is 20 to 30 μm with four sporozoites in two sporocysts. *Cyclospora* oocysts are 8 to 10 μm in diameter and are nonrefractile spherical organisms containing two sporozoites in two sporocysts that are seen easily on wet mount preparations and are variably acid fast. Microsporidia are difficult to differentiate from bacteria and debris because of the small size of the spores, which measure 1 to 2 μm. For detection, formalin-fixed stool or duodenal fluid can be stained with a calcofluor stain, a modified trichrome stain, or a fluorescent stain.[175,661] Gram, acid-fast, periodic acid–Schiff, and Giemsa stains also have been used to stain the organism.[581] Small bowel biopsy may be more sensitive than is stool examination for establishing the diagnosis of intestinal microsporidiosis.[56] Spores are gram positive, and parts of the internal structure are positive for acid-fast or periodic acid–Schiff stains.

Stool Cultures

Obtaining of stool cultures cannot be justified in all patients with acute diarrhea.[302] Patients with mild, self-limited illness do not need to have stool specimens cultured. When culture is indicated, the specimen should be inoculated onto culture plate media adequate to isolate *E. coli, Shigella, Salmonella,* and *Campylobacter.* Fecal specimens can be transported to the laboratory in a nonnutrient holding medium, such as Cary-Blair, when culture cannot be performed immediately. This medium prevents drying or overgrowth of specific organisms. All bloody stool specimens should be evaluated with MacConkey sorbitol medium for *E. coli* O157:H7.[77,132] Some bacterial enteropathogens require modified laboratory procedures for identification.[302] If these agents are suspected (e.g., *Vibrio* or *Yersinia*), the laboratory should be notified so that appropriate culture methods can be used.

Shigella and *Salmonella* organisms are isolated routinely by clinical microbiology laboratories. *Shigella* species are determined in most clinical laboratories. Speciation is important in salmonellosis because *Shigella* serotype *choleraesuis* and *Shigella* serotype *typhi* cause more severe disease than do other *Salmonella* spp. Serotyping of *Shigella* serotype *enteritidis* usually is not helpful in the individual case, although serotyping is crucial in evaluation of an outbreak. Because so many *Salmonella* serotypes exist, isolation of an unusual serotype can be of use in the investigation of a foodborne epidemic or identification of a potential reptile source of infection. As with *Shigella,* isolation of a species of *Salmonella,* even without demonstration of virulence properties, is considered adequate to make an etiologic diagnosis. Serologic studies are of no value in the individual patient.

Culture of *Campylobacter jejuni* from stools requires special methods and special media. It can be accomplished with media that contain antibiotics or using membrane filters. Inoculated plates should be incubated with microaerophilia at 42°C and read at 72 hours.

V. cholerae strains can be isolated from stool with use of thiosulfate–citrate–bile salt–sucrose agar, which is the most convenient and frequently used selective medium. This medium is suitable for most enteropathogenic *Vibrio* spp. except *V. hollisae.* Placement of the specimen into an enrichment broth, such as alkaline peptone water with 1% sodium chloride (pH 8.5) for 5 hours before placement on thiosulfate–citrate–bile salt–sucrose agar enhances the isolation of vibrios. Serotyping is necessary to classify organisms into those that cause typical epidemic cholera (i.e., O1 and O139 serotypes) and those that cause less severe disease (i.e., non-O1, or nonagglutinating vibrios).[345] *V. parahaemolyticus,* like other vibrios, can be cultured on thiosulfate–citrate–bile salt–sucrose agar. Strains associated with diarrhea are Kanagawa-positive on Wagatsuma agar (i.e., show hemodigestion resembling β-hemolysis), which is a marker for pathogenicity. *V. parahaemolyticus* can be serotyped on the basis of the O and K antigens.[157]

A. hydrophila can be overlooked easily on standard stool cultures. A specialized blood agar has been suggested for isolation.[21] Oxidase testing of organisms that resemble *E. coli* can select organisms as possible *Aeromonas* spp.[21] If oxidase-positive colonies are found, they can be evaluated biochemically to determine species.

C. difficile can be isolated by anaerobic stool culture on agar containing cycloserine, cefoxitin, and fructose. For establishing a definitive diagnosis, demonstration of the presence of cytotoxin in stool specimens and neutralization with antitoxin or by use of enzyme immunoassay or PCR-based assays are necessary.[16,529,557] *C. perfringens* is isolated commonly from feces of well people. Diagnosis of *C. perfringens* food poisoning requires isolation of the organisms from epidemiologically implicated food in a significant quantity (more than 10^5 organisms/g) or demonstration of 10^6 organisms/g of stool from two or more ill people or demonstration of enterotoxin in stools of two or more ill people.[415]

S. aureus may be isolated from food and may not be the cause of illness because not all strains of *Staphylococcus* produce enterotoxin. Conversely the absence of *S. aureus* from food that has been reheated just before being eaten does not exclude staphylococcal food poisoning because heating may destroy the organism without inactivating the toxin. Confirmation as a cause of foodborne disease requires isolation of the same phage-type *S. aureus* from stools or vomitus of two or more ill persons or detection of enterotoxin in epidemiologically implicated food or isolation of 10^5 organisms/g from epidemiologically implicated food, provided the specimen is properly handled.[415] *B. cereus* can be diagnosed by demonstration of greater than 10^5 organisms/g in the incriminated food or isolation of the organism from stool of two or more ill people and not from stool of control patients.[415]

Listeria is cultured on blood agar plates rather than on the usual enteric media.[637] *Y. enterocolitica* can be isolated from routine media, but a differential selective medium, such as cefsulodin-triclosan (Irgasan)–novobiocin agar, is more effective.[75] Cold-enrichment techniques may increase the yield of the organism from contaminated specimens, such as feces. Stool cultures positive for *Y. enterocolitica* only after prolonged cold enrichment may represent environmental strains of low virulence, unrelated to human disease. Biotyping and serotyping for O3, O8, and O9 are helpful in determining the clinical relevance of such isolates.

Immunologic Methods

Detection of antigens, toxins, and/or antibodies of several important enteric pathogens can be performed using commercially available kits such as enzyme-linked immunosorbent assay (ELISA), enzyme immunoassay (EIA), immune-chromatography, latex agglutination kits, and so on. The sensitivity, specificity, and associated positive and negative predictive values of antigen tests for enteric pathogens differ among them and from those of culture. Rapid tests are available for enteric viruses, bacteria, and parasites.

Among viruses, commercially available enzyme immunoassay and latex agglutination kits are available to detect rotavirus antigen in stool specimens. Assay procedures using monoclonal antibodies have improved the sensitivity and specificity to greater than 95%.[169,362] Non–group A rotaviruses are not detected by the commercially available assays. After the Norwalk virus was cloned and sequenced in 1990,[330] two major types of assays for diagnosing human noroviruses were developed. One detects the viral antigens or antibodies against the antigens by recombinant enzyme immunoassays, and the other detects the viral RNA by RT-PCR.[448] Although norovirus can be detected in rectal swabs and vomitus, whole-stool samples are the preferred clinical specimen for the detection of norovirus because they contain a higher quantity of virus. The sensitivity of EIA is typically less than 70%, while the specificity is usually greater than 90%. Thus EIA may be useful for rapid screening during an outbreak, but, because of the low sensitivity, caution should be exercised in interpreting test results from sporadic cases.[648] Diagnosis of enteric adenovirus can be established by immune electron microscopy of stool specimens, enzyme immunoassay of stool specimens, PCR, or cultured in human embryonic kidney cells.[372] Restriction enzyme analysis is the definitive method for classifying individual enteric adenovirus isolates. Commercially available assays for detection of enteric adenovirus are available.[639] For astroviruses electron microscopy, immune electron microscopy, immunofluorescence on cell culture, enzyme immunoassay, and PCR can be used as detection methods.[239]

Several rapid antigen detection tests are available for enteric bacteria, such as *Campylobacter, E. coli* O157:H7, STEC (detection of Shiga toxin 1 and 2), ETEC (detection of ST and LT enterotoxins), EPEC (EspA), *C. difficile* (detection of cytotoxin A and B), and *Yersinia*.[255,337,360,384,609,531]

Numerous serologic tests for amebiasis to detect different types and antibodies are available. Serologic test results for amebae almost always are positive in acute amebic dysentery and hepatic amebiasis. *G. lamblia* and *Cryptosporidium* antigens in feces can be detected by use of one of several rapid and sensitive diagnostic tests.[229,246,363] Enzyme immunoassays[229,350] and fluorescent monoclonal antibody–based assays[228,553] for detection of *Cryptosporidium* antigen in stool specimens are available.[123] For the Microsporidia, nonspecific fluorescence methods or enzyme immunoassay may enhance speed and sensitivity. After preliminary identification by these stains has been achieved, further examination by electron microscopy is needed to classify adequately the Microsporidia into an appropriate genus. Routine histopathologic studies can provide presumptive identification in infected biopsy tissue; diagnostic confirmation requires electron microscopy. Reliable serologic tests are not available.

Molecular Methods

Although molecular diagnostics are still used primarily in research laboratories, they are highly sensitive and specific in detecting infections in small samples and can simultaneously identify multiple pathogens.[369] Multiplex genetic assays are used to detect different toxins, pathogens, and species or genotypes of the same pathogen.[508] All enteric viruses can be detected by PCR; however, the most widely used is the RT-PCR for norovirus.[240] Several molecular techniques have been developed for detection and differentiation of *E. histolytica, E. dispar,* and *E. moshkovskii*[221] and for Microsporidia species *E. bieneusi* and *E. intestinalis.*[162,206] Among bacterial agents, there are several multiplex assay systems to detect for combinations of common enteric bacteria such as *Shigella, Salmonella, Campylobacter, Vibrio,* and other food- and waterborne pathogens.[153,224,245,355,405,469,666] However, worldwide, the most widely used are the PCR systems to detect STEC and other diarrheagenic *E. coli.*

STEC, including O157 and non-O157 serotypes, is a significant foodborne pathogen that requires sensitive and discriminatory methods for detection and characterization. In addition to available immunoassays, there are numerous PCR-based methods, conventional or real-time, for the detection of STEC virulence factors and common serotypes.[30,232–234,504] Recent technologic advancements have combined the high-throughput performance of the microarray with the specificity and sensitivity of real-time qPCR to make large-scale screening efforts both time- and cost-effective.[247]

Diarrheagenic *E. coli* were originally serogroup-defined *E. coli* associated with infantile diarrhea, defined also by their characteristic adherence pattern in tissue-cultured cells.[450] Currently they are identified mainly based on the presence of specific virulence genes for each pathotype.[346] Conventional methods such as colony-based serotyping are not routinely performed outside reference laboratories and as part of outbreak investigations. Many "classic" serotypes of each pathotype do not harbor the specific virulence genes of that particular pathotype, and, conversely, some genetically defined strains do not belong to the classic serogroups.[95,682] Therefore, O-serogroup identification of diarrheagenic *E. coli,* especially of EPEC, should not be used in clinical laboratories, except as part of outbreak investigations. One exception is STEC; because *E. coli* O157:H7 is the most virulent strain, it should always be sought in clinical laboratories. Other STEC serotypes (e.g., O104:H4) have also caused massive outbreaks of serious disease and should be defined when the epidemiology so dictates. Tissue-cultured cell methods for the identification of specific adherence patterns (e.g., EAEC and tEPEC) are done only in research laboratories; are laborious and time consuming; are not always specific for virulent strains; and are a challenge when the sample produces few colonies, such as a sample from a patient with early-phase gastroenteritis.[320] These traditional methods for differentiating *E. coli* strains have been replaced with more sensitive PCR methods performed in *E. coli*–isolated colonies or stool samples. Several multiplex PCR-based platforms have been developed and validated in different countries.[31,48,49,69,81,270,593,616,627,646]

New isothermal amplification diagnostic methods have been developed for enteric pathogens, such as the loop-mediated isothermal amplification (LAMP) and the recombinase polymerase amplification (RPA) for *Shigella, Salmonella, Vibrio,* ETEC, STEC, *Cryptosporidium, Giardia,* and *Entamoeba.*[147,148,454,599,656,657,683] The performance of these assays is comparable to PCR, without requiring the use of thermal cycling equipment.

TREATMENT

In caring for children with diarrhea and dehydration, the major therapeutic considerations include fluid and electrolyte therapy, dietary management, nonspecific therapy with antidiarrheal compounds, and specific therapy with antimicrobial agents to shorten the duration of the illness and eradicate fecal shedding of the organism. The timely replacement of fluid loss is the single most important intervention to decrease mortality (Box 44.3).

Several guidelines for the management of acute gastroenteritis in children have been developed in the United States[25,106,358] and elsewhere[66,86,262,263,272,273,283,461,671,673] as well as practice guidelines for management of infectious diarrhea in adults[267] and recommendations for

BOX 44.3 Management of Diarrhea in Children: Key Points

Rehydration

Clinical assessment of hydration status

Prevention of dehydration: continue breastfeeding and other milk feeds, encourage intake of fluids available at home

Oral rehydration therapy with low osmolarity oral rehydration salts (ORS) in mild or moderate dehydration

Intravenous therapy is required only in hypovolemic shock, obtunded mental status, or ileus

Nutrition

Start refeeding with the usual age-appropriate diet at the earliest opportunity (4–6 hours after onset of rehydration); no need of a special diet

Antibiotics

Most diarrhea cases in pediatrics do not require antibiotics

Antibiotics are recommended for dysentery *(Shigella, Salmonella, Campylobacter),* dysenteric amebiasis, cholera, bacteremia or extraintestinal spread of the infection, and in malnourished or immunocompromised children

Antibiotics are not recommended in patients with STEC infection

Additional Therapy

Zinc supplementation (10–20 mg/day) for 10 to 14 days in developing countries

Prevention

Rotavirus vaccination in all young infants

Exclusive breastfeeding for the first 6 months of age

Safe and clean weaning foods starting at 6 months of age

Hand-washing with soap, improved water quality, and adequate excreta disposal, especially in resource-limited conditions management of foodborne illnesses.[27,103] However, adherence to practice guidelines is not good.[410] The most important aspects of the management of diarrhea in children are highlighted.

Fluid and Electrolyte Therapy

Patients who develop diarrhea lose fluid and electrolytes through the gastrointestinal tract by several mechanisms: vomiting, loss of fecal fluid caused by the infecting enteropathogen, and fecal water loss in excess of sodium caused by the intraluminal osmotic effect of unabsorbed nutrients.[303] The composition and amount of lost fluid depend on the rate of stool loss and the causative agent. The higher the rate of stool loss, the greater the sodium loss, probably as a result of rapid passage of intestinal contents through the colon, where sodium-potassium exchange occurs. Stools from patients with cholera or ETEC infection contain sodium in a concentration of 80 to 120 mEq/L, whereas stools from patients with virus infection have sodium concentrations of less than 50 mEq/L.[284,358,563] In secretory diarrheal disorders, loss of fluid generally is derived from the small intestine, and colonic reabsorption is overwhelmed. In viral gastroenteritis, small bowel absorptive capacity primarily is impaired, and in dysenteric or invasive diarrhea, reabsorptive capacity of the large intestine is reduced. Continued loss of fluid or electrolytes may lead to dehydration, with potentially severe sequelae. Children, especially infants, are more susceptible to dehydration because they have greater basal fluid and electrolyte requirements per kilogram and because they depend on others to meet these needs.

Important factors to be considered in evaluating patients with diarrhea and possible dehydration include an estimation of deficiency, ongoing daily requirements, continued losses and their replacement, and correction of the underlying cause.[25,264,303] The clinical signs and symptoms that may help in estimating deficiencies and determining the severity of dehydration include thirst, dryness of the mucous membranes, decrease in urinary output, tachycardia, loss of skin elasticity and turgor, and mottling and coolness of the skin[25,106] (see Box 44.4). Various scores have been proposed for the assessment of dehydration and disease severity, but they have not been validated for the assessment of dehydration in individual patients.[262,263] These signs may be misleading in patients who are malnourished or in patients with hypertonic dehydration.[671–673] In clinical practice, a physical examination enables the clinician to classify patients into the three groups of no dehydration, mild/moderate dehydration, or severe dehydration. This general assessment can then be used to guide clinical management.

The main complication associated with gastroenteritis is dehydration; it should be prevented with appropriate fluid management. In children with gastroenteritis but without clinical dehydration, it is recommended as primary prevention of dehydration to continue breastfeeding and other milk feeds, encourage intake of fluids available at home, offer oral rehydration salt (ORS) solution as supplemental fluid to those at increased risk of dehydration, and discourage the drinking of fruit juices and carbonated drinks, especially in those at increased risk of dehydration. All these juices and drinks contain inadequate amounts of sodium and potassium and excessive carbohydrate concentrations, which may exceed the absorptive capacity of the intestine and may exacerbate diarrhea due to high osmotic activity.[358,583] The homemade sugar and salt solutions are not recommended because errors in preparing the solutions may result in dangerously high or low sodium concentrations.[579,667]

Oral rehydration should be used as first-line therapy for the management of mild to moderate dehydration in children with gastroenteritis. Oral therapy consists of rehydration with replacement of ongoing losses during the first 4 to 8 hours of therapy with a glucose-electrolyte solution.[129,358,563,673] Children with moderate dehydration should receive ORS ad libitum, approximately 75 mL/kg in 4 or 6 hours, following "plan B" of the WHO recommendations.[673] When oral rehydration is not feasible, enteral rehydration by the nasogastric route is as effective if not better than intravenous rehydration. Enteral rehydration is associated with significantly fewer major adverse events and a shorter hospital stay compared with intravenous therapy and is successful in most children.[219,286] Once the patient is rehydrated, feeding should be restarted.

The ORS solution must contain glucose, sodium, and other electrolytes that are lost in diarrhea (Table 44.8). The glucose in the ORS

BOX 44.4 Clinical Assessment of Dehydration

Sensorium: irritable, unconscious, or comatose
Thirst: drinks eagerly or drinks poorly or not able to drink
Skin turgor: goes back slowly or very slowly
Sunken eyes
Absent tears
Dry mucous membranes
Sunken fontanel
Tachycardia, tachypnea, hypotension
Peripheral vasoconstriction
Reduced capillary refill time
Sudden weight loss
Oliguria

TABLE 44.8 Compositions of Rehydration Solutions and Chemical Composition of Diarrheal Stools in Children

	Osmolarity (mOsm/L)	Glucose (mmol/L)	Sodium (mmol/L)	Chloride (mmol/L)	Potassium (mmol/L)	Citrate (mmol/L)	Bicarbonate (mol/L)
Oral Rehydration Solutions							
Original or standard WHO solution	311	111	90	80	20	10	—
New WHO reduced osmolarity solution	245	75	75	65	20	10	—
Hypotonic osmolarity solution[a]	240	90	60	60	20	10	—
ReSoMal[b]	300	125	45	70	40	7	—
Intravenous Fluids							
Ringer's lactate[c]	272	—	130	111	4	—	28
Cholera saline (Dhaka solution)[d]	432	140	133	98	13	—	48
Normal saline	300	—	154	154	—	—	—
Losses in Children							
Cholera stool		—	105	30	25	—	30
Noncholeraic stool		—	52	14	25	—	14

[a]This is one example; there are several other commercially available ORS solutions with different sodium (50 and 45 mmol/L) and glucose concentrations.
[b]ReSoMal is a modified oral rehydration solution for patients with severe malnutrition.
[c]Preferred IV therapy by WHO recommendations. The base is lactate, not bicarbonate.
[d]Some preparations do not have glucose and therefore have a lower osmolarity.[414]

solution is necessary to promote intestinal absorption of sodium and water in the small intestine. The composition of the original WHO ORS solution was selected to allow for use of a single solution that would effectively treat dehydration secondary to diarrhea caused by various infectious agents and resulting in varying degrees of electrolyte loss, such as cholera or ETEC infection.[358] However, viral gastroenteritis is common in pediatric patients and is associated with less severe salt losses, so there was concern that the sodium content of the original WHO ORS solution might be excessive.[183] The current WHO ORS formulation, the so-called reduced osmolarity solution, adopted in 2002 (see Table 44.8), has a reduced osmolar load (245 mOsm/L) compared with the original formulation (311 mOsm/L). The so-called hypotonic osmolarity solution, containing sodium 60 mmol/L, is also accepted. Both solutions have reduced the need for unscheduled intravenous fluid infusion and have less stool output and less risk of vomiting compared with the original formulation.[129,278] The reduced osmolarity ORS is also effective for the treatment of cholera diarrhea.[458] The rice-based ORS that contains glucose polymers and amino acids may be more beneficial than the glucose-based oral rehydration solution in children with cholera diarrhea.[253] Unlike reduced osmolarity ORS, rice-based ORS does not reduce the need for intravenous infusion.[220]

Intravenous therapy is required if the patient is in hypovolemic shock, has an obtunded mental status, or has an ileus. Children with severe dehydration should receive intravenous fluids immediately. If the patient can drink, ORS should be given by mouth until the drip is set up. Children should receive 100 mL/kg lactated Ringer solution divided as follows: infants (<12 months) 30 mL/kg in 1 hour, followed by 70 mL/kg in 5 hours; older children (>12 months) 30 mL/kg in 30 minutes, followed by 70 mL/kg in 2.5 hours, following "plan C" of the WHO recommendations.[673] If the child is able to tolerate orally administered fluids, intravenous infusion should be stopped and further rehydration completed with oral rehydration therapy alone.[129]

Children with severe acute malnutrition with some dehydration or severe dehydration but who are not shocked should be rehydrated slowly, orally, with either ReSoMal (oral rehydration solution for malnourished children) or half-strength standard WHO low-osmolarity oral rehydration solution with added potassium and glucose. Children with severe acute malnutrition and signs of shock or severe dehydration and who cannot be rehydrated orally or by nasogastric tube should be treated with intravenous fluids, either with half-strength Darrow's solution with 5% dextrose or Ringer's lactate solution with 5% dextrose.[670,671,674]

Nutritional Management

Adequate feeding is important to reduce the nutritional defects caused by diarrhea.[25,358] Children with diarrhea who are not dehydrated should be fed age-appropriate diets.[652] Children who require rehydration should be started on refeeding with the usual diet at the earliest opportunity, while the oral glucose-electrolyte solution is continued to replace ongoing losses from stools. It is recommended to feed starting 4 to 6 hours after the onset of rehydration. Early feeding may reduce duration of diarrhea and improve weight gain.[84,262,304]

Breastfeeding in infants should be continued at any time during an episode of diarrhea. Continuing breastfeeding during acute gastroenteritis has been shown to exert a beneficial effect by reducing the number and volume of diarrheal stools and reducing the duration of diarrhea in rotavirus gastroenteritis.[276,354] Refeeding with undiluted or full-strength nonhuman milk (cow's or formula milk) should continue. Weaned children should be fed whatever they eat normally. Full feeding of appropriate-for-age foods is well tolerated and is better than the practice of withholding food, resulting in better weight gain without increasing complication rates of treatment failures.[561] Controlled clinical trials suggest that complex carbohydrates (rice, wheat, potatoes, bread, and cereals), lean meats, yogurt, fruits, and vegetables are well tolerated in children with mild to moderate diarrhea and should be continued unrestricted as age-appropriate foods after the period of rehydration.[225,262]

Transient lactose intolerance occurs in some children with gastroenteritis. However, routine use of lactose-free formula is not necessary and only should be indicated in patients with severe and prolonged diarrhea. There is not enough evidence to support the routine use of soy-based formula or hydrolyzate formula in infants with acute gastroenteritis.[36,140] Beverages such as tea, soft drinks, and fruit juices that contain a high sugar concentration should be avoided owing to the risk of inducing further fluid losses as a consequence of increased osmotic loads.[544,638]

Antimicrobial Therapy

Because viruses are the predominant cause of acute diarrhea in children in developed and developing countries, the routine use of antimicrobial agents for treating diarrhea wastes resources and might lead to increased antimicrobial resistance. Even when a bacterial cause is suspected in an outpatient setting, antimicrobial therapy is not usually indicated in children because the majority of cases of acute diarrhea are self-limited and not shortened by administration of antimicrobial agents. Exceptions to these rules involve special needs of individual children (e.g., immune-compromised hosts, premature infants, malnourished children, or children with underlying disorders) and particular organisms and conditions.[358]

Therapy with antimicrobial agents is important in most cases of diarrhea caused by invasive or inflammatory bacterial pathogens and can be useful in other noninvasive forms of bacterial diarrhea. Recommendations for antibiotic therapy in each form of bacterial diarrhea are provided in Table 44.9. Antibiotics should be used for the treatment of children with suspected or confirmed septicemia; for those with extraintestinal spread of bacterial infection; for children younger than 6 months of age with *Salmonella* gastroenteritis; for those who are malnourished or immunocompromised with *Salmonella* gastroenteritis; and for those with *C. difficile*–associated pseudomembranous enterocolitis, giardiasis, dysenteric shigellosis, dysenteric amebiasis, or cholera.[461,488]

When antimicrobial therapy is administered to selected patients with gastroenteritis, the aim of the therapy is to abbreviate the duration of the clinical course, reduce severity and complications, and decrease excretion of the causative organisms. A stool culture specimen should be obtained when antibiotic treatment is anticipated, and antibiotic susceptibility testing of any suspected pathogen should be performed to ensure optimal therapy. Changing susceptibility patterns renders the initial selection of an antimicrobial agent difficult. Antimicrobial agents should not be used routinely for gastroenteritis of unknown cause.

Therapy for Dysentery

Dysentery is defined as acute bloody diarrhea typically with abdominal pain and fever caused by invasive microbial infection. The child with bloody diarrhea is at higher risk for complications, including sepsis and other systemic diseases; therefore the threshold for admission of such children to the hospital for close observation is lower. Stool cultures are indicated in the setting of acute bloody diarrhea and are helpful for guiding therapy.[513] The four major causes of bloody diarrhea (including both dysenteric and nondysenteric forms) in the United States, in descending order of frequency of occurrence, are *Shigella, Campylobacter,* nontyphoid *Salmonella,* and STEC.[187] Other organisms may also cause dysentery, including *Aeromonas* species, noncholeraic vibrios, and *Yersinia enterocolitica.* Once laboratory diagnosis is made, pathogen-specific antimicrobial therapy should be initiated for all forms of infectious colitis (*Shigella, Salmonella,* and *Campylobacter*) other than STEC.[188,513] Treatment of dysentery in cases in which stool culture is not available should be targeted at *Shigella.*

Shigella

Mild symptoms are self-limited, but in more severe cases antibiotics are recommended for cure and for preventing complications and relapse. The progressive development of antibiotic resistance in *Shigella* isolates is not new. Ampicillin and trimethoprim-sulfamethoxazole, once affordable mainstays of therapy, have long ago lost efficacy in most *Shigella*-endemic regions. Resistance to nalidixic acid, fluoroquinolones, ceftriaxone, and azithromycin and multidrug-resistant strains are also being reported in many countries.[39,261,290,367,368,687] Therefore regularly updated local or regional antibiotic sensitivity patterns to different

TABLE 44.9 Antimicrobial Therapy for Children With Bacterial Diarrhea

Pathogen	Antibiotic[a]	Comments
Shigella	Ciprofloxacin	First-line therapy by WHO recommendations; increasing resistance rates in some countries
	Azithromycin, ceftriaxone, pivmecillinam	Second-line therapy by WHO recommendations
	Cefixime, nalidixic acid, furazolidone	Alternative drugs for nonsevere dysentery
	TMP-SMX; ampicillin	High frequency of resistance; use only for susceptible strains
Salmonella	None	For nontyphoidal *Salmonella* diarrhea, except in special patients
	Ciprofloxacin; azithromycin, ceftriaxone	For severe diarrhea in special patients[b] or for systemic infection or typhoid fever
	TMP-SMX; chloramphenicol	High frequency of resistance; use only for susceptible strains
Campylobacter	Azithromycin; erythromycin	First-line therapy. High frequency of ciprofloxacin resistance in many countries
STEC	None	May increase the risk of hemolytic-uremic syndrome
ETEC, EAEC, EPEC	Ciprofloxacin; azithromycin; ceftriaxone	Based on recommendations from adults with traveler's diarrhea
	TMP-SMX	High frequency of resistance; use only for susceptible strains
EIEC	Treat as shigellosis	
Vibrio cholerae	Azithromycin, erythromycin	Azithromycin resistance is rare; it is the preferred therapy
	Ciprofloxacin, doxycycline, tetracycline	Alternative drugs; potential toxicity of tetracyclines, use in children >8 year
Diarrhea due to noncholeraic vibrios	None or treat as *Shigella*	
Aeromonas, Plesiomonas	Treat as shigellosis	
Clostridium difficile	Metronidazole, vancomycin	Stop offending antibiotic, if possible

TMP-SMX, Trimethoprim-sulfamethoxazole.

[a]Ceftriaxone is administered intravenously or intramuscularly; all other listed drugs are given orally.

[b]Infants <6 months of age, malnourished and immunocompromised children.

species and strains of *Shigella* are required to guide empiric therapy.[131,367] In the absence of local data, the recommendations from the WHO should be followed. First-line therapy is ciprofloxacin (in all age groups, including pediatrics), and second-line therapy is pivmecillinam (where available), ceftriaxone, or azithromycin.[672] Azithromycin has the added advantage of also treating most isolates of *Campylobacter,* a second major cause of dysenteric diarrhea in children younger than 2 years in developing countries.[368] The antibiotics recommended by the WHO are effective in reducing the clinical and bacteriologic signs and symptoms of dysentery and thus can be expected to decrease diarrhea mortality attributable to dysentery.[629,158]

Campylobacter

Isolation of *Campylobacter* from stool does not imply the need for antimicrobial therapy. In a meta-analysis of eight randomized, controlled trials of antimicrobial therapy versus placebo, antimicrobial therapy shortened the duration of intestinal symptoms by 1.3 days; the effect was more pronounced if treatment was started within 3 days of illness onset.[621] The decision concerning therapy should be individualized, but therapy should be considered in patients with high temperatures, bloody diarrhea, severe diarrhea, and in immunocompromised hosts. *Campylobacter* is increasingly resistant to antibiotics, especially fluoroquinolones and macrolides, which are the most frequently used antimicrobial agents for the treatment of campylobacteriosis.[414] Either erythromycin or azithromycin is preferred. In addition to resistance,[524] antibiotic management has also become more complex because postinfectious irritable bowel syndrome has been associated with a longer duration of untreated infection.[360]

Salmonella

The type of syndrome produced by *Salmonella* (acute gastroenteritis; bacteremia and enteric fever; dissemination with localized suppuration [e.g., abscess, osteomyelitis, or meningitis]) influences the selection and duration of antimicrobial therapy. Antibiotics should not be used in the treatment of patients who are nontyphoid *Salmonella* carriers or in most patients with mild gastroenteritis. Antibiotic therapy does not affect the duration of fever or diarrhea in otherwise healthy children or adults, when compared with placebo or no treatment.[592] Antibiotics may, on occasions, convert intestinal carriage into systemic disease with bacteremia,[547] prolong excretion of *Salmonella,*[38] produce a bacteriologic or symptomatic relapse,[38] or encourage development or selection of resistant strains.

Acute diarrheal disease caused by nontyphoid salmonellosis can be complicated with bacteremia in approximately 8% of normal healthy persons. Patients with bacteremia often present with high fever and systemic toxic effects. Risk factors for systemic *Salmonella* infection during bouts of gastroenteritis include extremes of age (<3 months and >65 years), corticosteroid use, inflammatory bowel disease, immunosuppression, hemoglobinopathy including most cases of sickle-cell disease, and hemodialysis. People with one of these risk factors and nontyphoid salmonellosis should be treated with antibacterial drugs.[187] Antibiotic treatment of *Salmonella* infection should be given to all patients with typhoid fever, bacteremia caused by nontyphoidal strains, and dissemination with localized suppuration.

Increasing occurrence of antimicrobial resistance in both typhoidal and nontyphoidal *Salmonella* infection is a major public health problem. Recent studies have documented the occurrence of resistance, with particular reference to quinolones and extended-spectrum cephalosporins. Occurrence of multidrug resistance has declined in some areas, but the incidence of decreased ciprofloxacin susceptibility has reached high levels, particularly in the Indian subcontinent, and isolates with full resistance to this antimicrobial agent are increasingly reported. Patterns of resistance in *Salmonella* are constantly changing. Continual surveillance of resistance levels is critical for clinicians to keep abreast of treatment options, but it is often lacking in resource-poor regions of the world with the highest disease burden.[89,499,560]

Several outbreaks of multiresistant *Salmonella* infection in the United States have been traced to animals.[98,230,242,344,575,611] Resistant strains of *Salmonella* are common findings in retail ground meats, possibly because of overuse of antibiotics in animals used for food.[664] Human isolates of *Salmonella* should have susceptibility testing performed to guide therapy. Recommended antimicrobial agents include chloramphenicol, third-generation cephalosporins, fluoroquinolone, and azithromycin. In the presence of multidrug resistance, a fluoroquinolone is the first line of therapy, and a third-generation cephalosporin is the second choice.[89,560]

Shiga Toxin–Producing E. coli

Some antibacterial drugs, including fluoroquinolones and trimethoprim-sulfamethoxazole, may increase the induction of phage-mediated production of Shiga toxin and may increase the risk of development of HUS.[688] However, an association between the use of these antibiotics and an increased risk of this syndrome has not been proved.[62,555,669] In one study in the United States, individuals with STEC O157 infection presenting with a more severe illness were at an increased risk of developing HUS; the use of bactericidal antibiotics to treat STEC O157 infection, particularly β-lactams, was associated with the subsequent development of HUS.[595] In a large prospective surveillance study in Argentina the main risk factor for progression to HUS was neutrophilic leukocytosis in the early course of the diarrheal episode in STEC-positive children with bloody diarrhea.[411] On the other hand, other drugs, including fosfomycin, azithromycin, and rifaximin, do not appear to increase production of Shiga toxin.[319,321,474] In a mouse model, azithromycin inhibited a Shiga toxin–induced inflammatory response and prevented death.[481] During the STEC O104:H4 outbreak in Germany in 2011,[328] STEC-infected patients were monitored and observed for approximately 40 days; treatment with azithromycin was associated with a lower frequency of long-term STEC O104:H4 carriage.[288,471] Additional studies are needed to determine the effects of azithromycin and rifaximin on reducing diarrhea and decreasing the risk of the HUS among patients with STEC colitis. Pending such data, most authorities recommend supportive treatment only; antibiotic therapy is not generally recommended.[187,617] Currently there is no cure for STEC infection; however, chimeric or humanized monoclonal antibodies have been developed that neutralize the Shiga toxins, and those therapies may be able to prevent the development of HUS in an STEC-infected patient.[434,623,679]

Therapy for Other Bacterial Agents

Diarrheagenic E. coli

Antibiotics are not used routinely for the treatment of diarrheagenic *E. coli* except in traveler's diarrhea. There are no clinical trials on the efficacy of antibiotics for the treatment of the different *E. coli* pathotypes in children because simple and rapid diagnostic methods are lacking in order to conduct proper trials. Most of the current information on therapy for diarrheagenic *E. coli* comes from case series in children or data from studies in adults. Antimicrobial agents have been employed frequently in attempts to treat infantile gastroenteritis caused by EPEC and as a means of controlling the spread of EPEC strains in hospital nurseries. Although no definitive studies support the effectiveness of these drugs, they may be useful in certain situations, particularly when life-threatening infection occurs or when epidemic spread of the strains continues despite the use of strict hand-washing and appropriate isolation. The treatment in patients with diarrhea caused by EIEC is similar to that in patients with shigellosis. Diarrhea caused by ETEC and EAEC usually is self-limited, but studies in adults have shown that antimicrobial agents such as ciprofloxacin, azithromycin, and rifaximin are effective therapies.[189,498,604] Antimicrobial resistance in diarrheagenic *E. coli* is an increasing problem worldwide[24,467,478,482,604] as well as resistance in commensal *E. coli.*[54,192] Therefore, regional antibiotic sensitivity patterns to different *E. coli* pathotypes are required to guide empiric therapy when a decision is made to treat an individual patient.

Cholera

Effective antibiotic treatment reduces the volume and duration of diarrhea in patients with cholera and reduces the number of days that symptomatic patients shed viable *V. cholerae.* WHO recommends administration of furazolidone, trimethoprim-sulfamethoxazole, or erythromycin to children younger than 8 years and tetracycline to older children.[675] Tetracyclines, quinolones, and macrolides are active against *V. cholerae;* however, antibiotic resistance occurs frequently, and resistant strains can emerge rapidly. Therefore the choice of antibiotic agent is based on results of local antibiotic resistance patterns. Stool cultures performed as part of a surveillance program are also useful for monitoring trends in antimicrobial resistance. In areas of endemicity, many strains have become resistant to tetracycline and to fluoroquinolones. In these areas, azithromycin treatment is preferred and is administered as a single dose of 1 g in adults and 20 mg/kg in children. At present, azithromycin resistance remains rare; and owing to the potential toxicity of tetracyclines and fluoroquinolones in children and pregnant women, azithromycin is also preferred for these patients.[352,393,663]

Therapy for Intestinal Parasites

Entamoeba histolytica

Metronidazole is the most commonly used medication for invasive amebiasis caused by infection with *E. histolytica.* The efficacy of available treatments was assessed in a meta-analysis: tinidazole was better than metronidazole at reducing clinical failure and was better tolerated, and combination drug therapy was more effective in reducing parasitologic failure compared with metronidazole alone.[248]

Giardia

Giardia should be treated if it is associated with symptoms. Metronidazole, tinidazole, secnidazole, and ornidazole are effective therapies for *Giardia.*[677] Occasionally the initial improvement is followed by a subsequent relapse of symptoms, which requires repeat treatment. Some patients experiencing relapse needed combination therapy. A meta-analysis has shown that albendazole was comparable to metronidazole, with fewer side effects.[598] However, tinidazole has better efficacy than albendazole in children.[202] There are new antigiardial drugs being developed.[440,620]

Cryptosporidium

Children and immunosuppressed individuals, especially with HIV infection or AIDS, are disproportionately affected. *Cryptosporidium* may be responsible for acute self-limiting diarrhea in immunocompetent children.[640] Treatment options, although only partially effective, include paromomycin and azithromycin. Nitazoxanide significantly shortens the duration of diarrhea and decreases mortality in malnourished children.[23,549] Recent research confirms the limited effectiveness of antiparasitic drugs to treat cryptosporidiosis in AIDS patients.[91,164] Potent antiretroviral combinations modify disease epidemiology and are key components of therapy in AIDS.[91] New drugs are being developed.[440]

Cyclospora

The treatment of choice for infection with *Cyclospora* is trimethoprim-sulfamethoxazole. Ciprofloxacin or nitazoxanide can be used as an alternative therapy, especially in patients who are allergic to sulfa products.[487]

Microsporidia

For microsporidial infections other than with *Enterocytozoon bieneusi,* albendazole is effective. A randomized trial showed that albendazole therapy was effective in improving the clinical manifestations and decreasing the duration of the illness of children with diarrhea caused by the Microsporidia.[631] *Encephalitozoon intestinalis* is susceptible to albendazole,[139,546] which has been reported to stop diarrhea and weight loss as well as to promote weight gain in patients infected with *E. intestinalis,*[442,631] although improvement has not been uniform. *E. bieneusi* does not respond to albendazole but does respond to fumagillin, which is more toxic.[443] For all patients with HIV/AIDS antiretroviral treatment to raise the CD4 count is a major element in management.[677]

Strongyloides

Patients infected with *S. stercoralis* should be treated with ivermectin or, alternatively, thiabendazole or albendazole. A recent meta-analysis suggests that ivermectin is more effective than albendazole and similar to thiabendazole, with fewer adverse events.[293] In immunocompromised patients and patients with *Strongyloides* hyperinfection, longer duration of therapy may be necessary[396]; however, the mortality rate is high despite therapy. In hyperinfection syndrome, rapid initiation of therapy with broad-spectrum antibiotics and anthelmintic drugs is the first step in management. A thorough examination should be performed before immunosuppressive therapy is given to a patient with a history of infection with *S. stercoralis.*[423]

Additional Therapy

Zinc

Zinc, an antioxidant and antiinflammatory agent, is an important trace element in gastrointestinal structure and function. It is involved in epithelial barrier integrity, tissue repair, and immune function.[64,532,582]

Zinc deficiency, which is common in young children in developing countries, is worse because intestinal losses of zinc are considerably increased during acute diarrhea.[97,374] Several studies and meta-analysis have shown that zinc supplementation can reduce the incidence of respiratory and diarrheal diseases.[67,83,551] In developing countries, zinc supplementation results in clinically important reduction in the duration and severity of acute diarrhea when given as an adjunct to oral rehydration therapy.[44,511,550,565] The WHO recommends zinc supplementation to all children with diarrhea. Supplements should be started at the beginning of symptoms, in a dosage of 10 mg/day in those younger than 6 months of age and 20 mg/day in older infants and children for 10 to 14 days.[673,676] Zinc decreases the severity and reduces the number of episodes of diarrhea occurring within 2 to 3 months following its intake. Recent meta-analyses have shown that in areas where the prevalence of zinc deficiency or the prevalence of moderate malnutrition is high, zinc supplementation in children is associated with a reduction in the morbidity and mortality of diarrhea,[380,401,651,680] especially among children older than 6 months of age[385,427] and malnourished children.[227] Zinc therapy is a highly cost-effective strategy[211] mainly in children with risk of persistent diarrhea and hospitalization.[431] However, the role of zinc supplements in developed countries needs further evaluation.[146,264,374]

Probiotics

Probiotics are living nonpathogenic microorganisms that have been studied for the prevention and treatment of a variety of disorders, including diarrhea, irritable bowel syndrome, and inflammatory bowel disease.[22,624] The most commonly used strains are lactic acid bacteria, such as lactobacilli or bifidobacteria, and the nonpathogenic yeast *Saccharomyces boulardii.* The rationale for the use of probiotics to treat and prevent diarrheal diseases is based on the assumption that they modify the composition of the colonic microflora and act against enteric pathogens. The possible mechanisms of action include competition with pathogens for binding sites and substrates, lowering of intestinal luminal pH, production of bacteriocins, promotion of mucin production, upregulation of genes mediating immunity, and production of trophic short-chain fatty acids to promote mucosal cell growth and differentiation.[322] Several meta-analyses have shown moderate clinical benefit of selected probiotic strains in the treatment of acute watery diarrhea (primarily rotaviral) mainly in infants and young children.[9,33,556,566,612,614] Probiotic effects are strain specific, so the efficacy and safety of each should be established.[520,472] *Lactobacillus* GG and *Saccharomyces boulardii* were found to be beneficial in meta-analyses devoted to single probiotics.[262,263] Probiotics may be effective in treating persistent diarrhea in children[63] and in preventing antibiotic-associated diarrhea in pediatric patients.[243,335,613]

Antisecretory Agents

Racecadotril (also known as acetorphan) is an antisecretory drug; it is a peripherally acting enkephalinase inhibitor that reduce intestinal water and electrolyte hypersecretion without changes in intestinal motility.[133,252,533] Racecadotril as an adjunct to oral rehydration therapy has been shown to decrease stool output, median duration of diarrhea, and intake of oral rehydration solution in children with severe watery diarrhea.[392] Racecadotril should be considered in the treatment of gastroenteritis in children.[252,262,273,520]

Bismuth subsalicylate and other bismuth salt preparations are used to control diarrhea and other gastrointestinal symptoms. Although the precise mechanism of their action remains unknown, their effect is thought to be due to intestinal antisecretory[199] and antimicrobial properties.[422] Laboratory studies showed that bismuth subsalicylate inhibited intestinal secretion caused by *E. coli* and cholera enterotoxins and reduced and prevented diarrhea in adults.[190,191] Studies supporting its use in children are limited.[601,600] Three randomized controlled trials that compared bismuth subsalicylate with placebo in infants with acute watery diarrhea found that bismuth subsalicylate only modestly reduced the duration and severity of diarrhea.[130,210,600] In addition to temporary side effects (i.e., darkening of the tongue and stool), bismuth subsalicylate has been reported to cause salicylate toxicity in children (potential risks of Reye syndrome).[244,518]

Loperamide is an opioid receptor agonist that reduces intestinal lumen motility. It is used for short-term symptomatic relief of acute diarrhea in adults; however, it should not be used in the management of diarrhea in children.[262,263]

Antiemetics

Antiemetics may be effective in young children with vomiting related to gastroenteritis.[263,574] A systematic review found that antiemetics significantly reduced the incidence of vomiting and hospitalization by 54% and reduced the intravenous fluid requirements by 60%.[159] A recent trial showed that a single oral dose of ondansetron, given before starting oral rehydration therapy to children younger than 5 years with acute diarrhea and vomiting, results in better oral rehydration.[156]

PREVENTION

Despite the continued reduction in overall disease burden with increased public health measures, enteric infections continue to cause significant morbidity and mortality in vulnerable populations.[562] The development of new enteric vaccines, breastfeeding, vitamin A and zinc supplementation, safe weaning foods, water quality, hygiene, and sanitation are critical for prevention of diarrhea in children, especially in developing countries, where the disease burden is higher.[160]

Breastfeeding is the most cost-effective intervention for protecting children against diarrhea and all causes of mortality.[336] Lack of exclusive breastfeeding among neonates from birth to 5 months of age and no breastfeeding among infants 6 to 23 months of age are associated with increased morbidity and mortality from diarrhea in developing countries. There is a large body of evidence regarding the protective effects of breastfeeding against diarrhea incidence, prevalence, hospitalizations, diarrhea mortality, and all-cause mortality.[634] These findings support the current WHO recommendation for exclusive breastfeeding during the first 6 months of life as a key child survival intervention and also highlight the importance of breastfeeding to protect against diarrhea-specific morbidity and mortality throughout the first 2 years of life.[379]

Contaminated foods, especially in the weaning groups, play a major role in the occurrence of diarrheal diseases. The frequency of contamination of weaning foods with enteropathogens is high in developing countries and is dependent on the food type, storage time, and ambient temperature of storage, the method used, and the temperature reached on rewarming before refeeding. Other considerations are the bacterial content of cooking and feeding utensils. Fruits and raw vegetables can become contaminated with pathogenic microorganisms by sewage-containing irrigation water and by washing produce and fruits with contaminated water. In most studies, the level of contamination is higher in weaning foods than in drinking water.[381] Food safety education is a critical and essential element in control and prevention of diarrheal diseases.[585]

The effect of water quality, hygiene, and sanitation in preventing diarrhea deaths has always been debated. In a systematic review, diarrhea risk reduction was estimated to be 48% with hand washing with soap, 17% with improved water quality, and 36% with excreta disposal.[92] A recent systematic review found that hand washing promotion probably reduces diarrhea episodes in both child daycare centers in high-income countries and among communities in low- and middle-income countries by about 30%.[194] A growing understanding of what drives hygiene behavior and creative partnerships are providing new approaches to change behavior.[154]

Vaccines

Vaccines play a critical role in public health efforts to control enteric infections. However, their use is limited in developing countries for multiple reasons, including financial and political constraints.[135] In populations in industrialized countries, live attenuated vaccines (e.g., poliovirus, typhoid, and rotavirus) mimic natural infection and generate robust protective immune responses. In contrast, a major challenge is to understand and overcome the barriers responsible for the diminished immunogenicity and efficacy of the same enteric vaccines in underprivileged populations in developing countries. Success in developing vaccines against some enteric pathogens has heretofore been elusive (e.g., *Shigella*).[500] Therefore, there is an urgent need for vaccines that induce effective and long-lasting intestinal immunity against diarrheal infections, especially during infancy and early childhood.[161] Mucosal vaccines would be appropriate for a number of pathogens. These include pathogens that are noninvasive, such as *Vibrio cholerae* and ETEC; pathogens that produce gut inflammation, such as *Shigella*; and pathogens that invade through the intestine and enter the systemic circulation, such as *Salmonella typhi*. Although the first category may need a mucosally administered vaccine for adequate protection, especially in immunologically unprimed individuals such as infants and young children, the latter, more invasive infections can probably be prevented by vaccines given either mucosally or parenterally or by a combination of such routes. Although 30 or more parenteral vaccines are licensed, only a handful of oral vaccines are licensed.[155,491,492] Many oral vaccines have performed poorly in developing countries when compared with industrialized countries, a finding attributed mainly to chronic environmental enteropathy, also called tropical enteropathy, which is characterized by disturbances of digestive and absorptive functions related to poor sanitation, intestinal flora overgrowth, and histologic changes characterized by inflammation and blunting of small intestinal villi leading to malabsorption. Children living under extreme poverty are especially sensitive.[155]

Rotavirus Vaccine

The first rotavirus vaccine licensed in the United States was associated with an increased rate of intussusception, resulting in its withdrawal from the market within 14 months of being licensed.[456,543] Two new vaccines have been shown to be safe and effective in protecting young children against severe rotavirus gastroenteritis and are now marketed worldwide: the pentavalent bovine-human recombinant rotavirus vaccine (RV5 [RotaTeq])[645] licensed as a three-dose vaccine administered orally at 2, 4, and 6 months of age[26,111] and the attenuated monovalent G1P[8] human rotavirus vaccine (RV1 [Rotarix])[552] licensed as a two-dose orally administered vaccine at 2 and 4 months of age.[143] Since the introduction of rotavirus vaccine, diarrhea-associated health care utilization and medical expenditures for U.S. children have decreased substantially.[142,216,238,349,509,655,665] Rotavirus vaccines have reduced the burden of disease in Europe and North, Central and South America.[169,170,164,348,545,635] Vaccine introductions in Asia and Africa have been increasing in recent years; however, experience with routine use of rotavirus vaccines in low-income countries has been limited to date. It is hoped the diffusion of the vaccine use in such countries, endorsed by the WHO, will have a substantial impact on the overall burden of diarrheal disease.[501,618,619] Long-term monitoring and strain surveillance are needed to assess the effects of rotavirus immunization programs and to determine whether changes in strain ecology will affect rotavirus vaccine effectiveness.[170,324] Several new multi- or monovalent vaccines may achieve licensure in the following years.[491]

Vaccines for Other Enteric Viruses

Norovirus is increasingly being recognized as the second most important cause of acute diarrhea in children. Norovirus candidate vaccines using virus-like particles, some in conjunction with newer adjuvants, are presently in clinical development.[19,42,364,433] A vaccine including both norovirus and rotavirus with high efficacy rates against different virus groups/types would be an attractive vaccine over the currently available vaccines options.[491]

Vaccines for Enteric Bacteria

Although an ideal vaccine against cholera has not yet been developed,[491] two orally administered formulations to prevent cholera are currently licensed: a whole-cell killed recombinant B subunit vaccine (Dukoral), and whole-cell killed bivalent vaccine (Shanchol and mORCVAX).[340] Dukoral was licensed in 1991 and has been distributed in 65 countries around the globe, whereas Shanchol, licensed in 2009, is currently distributed in India. Now, after being prequalified by the WHO, Dukoral and Shanchol can be distributed globally.[675] The WHO recommends that, in endemic areas, immunization should be implemented with the oral cholera vaccines available, together with other prevention and control strategies and should be considered in outbreak situations.[675]

Among the many causes of diarrheal disease, *Shigella* and ETEC are the two most important bacterial pathogens for which there are no currently licensed vaccines. Although several strategies have been used to develop vaccines targeting shigellosis, none has been licensed for use outside China. Owing to the wide range of *Shigella* serotypes and subtypes, there is a need for a multivalent vaccine representing prevalent species and serotypes. Strategies for *Shigella* vaccine development include cellular and subunit approaches (live attenuated, inactivated, conjugates, broad-spectrum, serotype-dependent mixture, and serotype-independent protein); these vaccines are currently at different stages of development.[161,343,650] Multiple barriers exist that prevent *Shigella* vaccine development[50]; one is the poor immune response to oral vaccines in children in developing areas who have minimal maternal antibodies.[376,650] Similarly no effective vaccine for ETEC is available. Several inactivated, live candidate and subunit vaccines consisting of toxin antigens, alone or together with colonization factors, fimbriae, and other novel proteins, are under development.[609,650,689] There is insufficient evidence to support the use of the oral cholera vaccine for protecting against ETEC diarrhea.[10]

NEW REFERENCES SINCE THE SEVENTH EDITION

5. Adams D, Fullerton K, Jajosky R, et al. Summary of notifiable infectious diseases and conditions - United States, 2013. *MMWR*. 2015;62(53):1-122.
6. Adlerberth I, Huang H, Lindberg E, et al. Toxin-producing *Clostridium difficile* strains as long-term gut colonizers in healthy infants. *J Clin Microbiol*. 2014;52(1):173-179.
7. Agholi M, Hatam GR, Motazedian MH. *Microsporidia* and *Coccidia* as causes of persistence diarrhea among liver transplant children: incidence rate and species/genotypes. *Pediatr Infect Dis J*. 2013;32(2):185-187.
8. Agus A, Massier S, Darfeuille-Michaud A, et al. Understanding host-adherent-invasive *Escherichia coli* interaction in Crohn's disease: opening up new therapeutic strategies. *Biomed Res Int*. 2014;2014:567929.
9. Ahmadi E, Alizadeh-Navaei R, Rezai MS. Efficacy of probiotic use in acute rotavirus diarrhea in children: a systematic review and meta-analysis. *Caspian J Intern Med*. 2015;6(4):187-195.
10. Ahmed T, Bhuiyan TR, Zaman K, et al. Vaccines for preventing enterotoxigenic *Escherichia coli* (ETEC) diarrhoea. *Cochrane Database Syst Rev*. 2013;(7):CD009029.
12. Albarral V, Sanglas A, Palau M, et al. Potential pathogenicity of *Aeromonas hydrophila* complex strains isolated from clinical, food, and environmental sources. *Can J Microbiol*. 2015;1-11.
19. Aliabadi N, Lopman BA, Parashar UD, et al. Progress toward norovirus vaccines: considerations for further development and implementation in potential target populations. *Expert Rev Vaccines*. 2015;14(9):1241-1253.
32. Ao TT, Feasey NA, Gordon MA, et al. Global burden of invasive nontyphoidal *Salmonella* disease, 2010. *Emerg Infect Dis*. 2015;21(6).
33. Applegate JA, Fischer Walker CL, Ambikapathi R, et al. Systematic review of probiotics for the treatment of community-acquired acute diarrhea in children. *BMC Public Health*. 2013;13(suppl 3):S16.
42. Atmar RL, Bernstein DI, Harro CD, et al. Norovirus vaccine against experimental human Norwalk virus illness. *N Engl J Med*. 2011;365(23):2178-2187.
45. Banaszkiewicz A, Kadzielska J, Gawronska A, et al. Enterotoxigenic *Clostridium perfringens* infection and pediatric patients with inflammatory bowel disease. *J Crohns Colitis*. 2014;8(4):276-281.
50. Barry EM, Pasetti MF, Sztein MB, et al. Progress and pitfalls in *Shigella* vaccine research. *Nat Rev Gastroenterol Hepatol*. 2013;10(4):245-255.
51. Barry MA, Weatherhead JE, Hotez PJ, et al. Childhood parasitic infections endemic to the United States. *Pediatr Clin North Am*. 2013;60(2):471-485.
52. Bartelt LA, Sartor RB. Advances in understanding *Giardia*: determinants and mechanisms of chronic sequelae. *F1000Prime Rep*. 2015;7:62.
57. Beer KD, Gargano JW, Roberts VA, et al. Surveillance for waterborne disease outbreaks associated with drinking water - United States, 2011–2012. *MMWR*. 2015;64(31):842-848.
58. Behravesh CB, Brinson D, Hopkins BA, et al. Backyard poultry flocks and salmonellosis: a recurring, yet preventable public health challenge. *Clin Infect Dis*. 2014;58(10):1432-1438.
59. Belliot G, Lopman BA, Ambert-Balay K, et al. The burden of norovirus gastroenteritis: an important foodborne and healthcare-related infection. *Clin Microbiol Infect*. 2014;20(8):724-730.
60. Bellou M, Kokkinos P, Vantarakis A. Shellfish-borne viral outbreaks: a systematic review. *Food Environ Virol*. 2013;5(1):13-23.
61. Bennett SD, Walsh KA, Gould LH. Foodborne disease outbreaks caused by *Bacillus cereus*, *Clostridium perfringens*, and *Staphylococcus aureus*–United States, 1998–2008. *Clin Infect Dis*. 2013;57(3):425-433.
63. Bernaola Aponte G, Bada Mancilla CA, Carreazo NY, et al. Probiotics for treating persistent diarrhoea in children. *Cochrane Database Syst Rev*. 2013;(8):CD007401.
68. Binnicker MJ. Multiplex molecular panels for diagnosis of gastrointestinal infection: performance, result interpretation, and cost-effectiveness. *J Clin Microbiol*. 2015;53(12):3723-3728.

73. Bortolaia V, Espinosa-Gongora C, Guardabassi L. Human health risks associated with antimicrobial-resistant enterococci and *Staphylococcus aureus* on poultry meat. *Clin Microbiol Infect*. 2016;22(2):130-140.
74. Bosch A, Pinto RM, Guix S. Human astroviruses. *Clin Microbiol Rev*. 2014;27(4):1048-1074.
86. Bruzzese E, Lo Vecchio A, Guarino A. Hospital management of children with acute gastroenteritis. *Curr Opin Gastroenterol*. 2013;29(1):23-30.
89. Bula-Rudas FJ, Rathore MH, Maraqa NF. *Salmonella* infections in childhood. *Adv Pediatr*. 2015;62(1):29-58.
90. Buonfrate D, Formenti F, Perandin F, et al. Novel approaches to the diagnosis of *Strongyloides stercoralis* infection. *Clin Microbiol Infect*. 2015;21(6):543-552.
93. Callejon RM, Rodriguez-Naranjo MI, Ubeda C, et al. Reported foodborne outbreaks due to fresh produce in the United States and European Union: trends and causes. *Foodborne Pathog Dis*. 2015;12(1):32-38.
99. Celik C, Gozel MG, Turkay H, et al. Rotavirus and adenovirus gastroenteritis: time series analysis. *Pediatr Int*. 2015;57(4):590-596.
121. Chakraborty A, Komatsu K, Roberts M, et al. The descriptive epidemiology of yersiniosis: a multistate study, 2005–2011. *Public Health Rep*. 2015;130(3):269-277.
123. Checkley W, White AC Jr, Jaganath D, et al. A review of the global burden, novel diagnostics, therapeutics, and vaccine targets for *Cryptosporidium*. *Lancet Infect Dis*. 2015;15(1):85-94.
125. Chen X, Chen Y, Yang Q, et al. *Plesiomonas shigelloides* infection in Southeast China. *PLoS ONE*. 2013;8(11):e77877.
132. Chui L, Couturier MR, Chiu T, et al. Comparison of Shiga toxin-producing *Escherichia coli* detection methods using clinical stool samples. *J Mol Diag*. 2010;12(4):469-475.
133. Ciccarelli S, Stolfi I, Caramia G. Management strategies in the treatment of neonatal and pediatric gastroenteritis. *Infect Drug Resist*. 2013;6:133-161.
137. Committee on Infectious Diseases, Committee on Nutrition, American Academy of Pediatrics. Consumption of raw or unpasteurized milk and milk products by pregnant women and children. *Pediatrics*. 2014;133(1):175-179.
148. Crannell Z, Castellanos-Gonzalez A, Nair G, et al. Multiplexed recombinase polymerase amplification assay to detect intestinal protozoa. *Anal Chem*. 2016;88(3):1610-1616.
147. Crannell ZA, Castellanos-Gonzalez A, Irani A, et al. Nucleic acid test to diagnose cryptosporidiosis: lab assessment in animal and patient specimens. *Anal Chem*. 2014;86(5):2565-2571.
149. Crews JD, Koo HL, Jiang ZD, et al. A hospital-based study of the clinical characteristics of *Clostridium difficile* infection in children. *Pediatr Infect Dis J*. 2014;33(9):924-928.
150. Crim SM, Griffin PM, Tauxe R, et al. Preliminary incidence and trends of infection with pathogens transmitted commonly through food - Foodborne Diseases Active Surveillance Network, 10 U.S. sites, 2006–2014. *MMWR*. 2015;64(18):495-499.
156. Danewa AS, Shah D, Batra P, et al. Oral ondansetron in management of dehydrating diarrhea with vomiting in children aged 3 months to 5 years: a randomized controlled trial. *J Pediatr*. 2016;169:105-109.
158. Das JK, Ali A, Salam RA, et al. Antibiotics for the treatment of cholera, *Shigella* and *Cryptosporidium* in children. *BMC Public Health*. 2013;13(suppl 3):S10.
159. Das JK, Kumar R, Salam RA, et al. The effect of antiemetics in childhood gastroenteritis. *BMC Public Health*. 2013;13(suppl 3):S9.
160. Das JK, Salam RA, Bhutta ZA. Global burden of childhood diarrhea and interventions. *Curr Opin Infect Dis*. 2014;27(5):451-458.
161. Das JK, Tripathi A, Ali A, et al. Vaccines for the prevention of diarrhea due to cholera, *Shigella*, ETEC and rotavirus. *BMC Public Health*. 2013;13(suppl 3):S11.
163. de Blank P, Zaoutis T, Fisher B, et al. Trends in *Clostridium difficile* infection and risk factors for hospital acquisition of *Clostridium difficile* among children with cancer. *J Pediatr*. 2013;163(3):699-705.
171. de Oliveira LH, Camacho LA, Coutinho ES, et al. Rotavirus vaccine effectiveness in Latin American and Caribbean countries: a systematic review and meta-analysis. *Vaccine*. 2015;33(suppl 1):A248-A254.
164. Debnath A, Ndao M, Reed SL. Reprofiled drug targets ancient protozoans: drug discovery for parasitic diarrheal diseases. *Gut Microbes*. 2013;4(1):66-71.
168. Dennehy PH. Rotavirus infection: a disease of the past? *Infect Dis Clin North Am*. 2015;29(4):617-635.
173. Deshpande A, Pant C, Anderson MP, et al. *Clostridium difficile* infection in the hospitalized pediatric population: increasing trend in disease incidence. *Pediatr Infect Dis J*. 2013;32(10):1138-1140.
177. Doan S, Steele RW. Advice for families traveling to developing countries with young children. *Clin Pediatr*. 2013;52(9):803-811.
179. Domingues AR, Pires SM, Halasa T, et al. Source attribution of human campylobacteriosis using a meta-analysis of case-control studies of sporadic infections. *Epidemiol Infect*. 2012;140(6):970-981.
180. Donnenberg MS, Finlay BB. Combating enteropathogenic *Escherichia coli* (EPEC) infections: the way forward. *Trends Microbiol*. 2013;21(7):317-319.
189. DuPont HL. Acute infectious diarrhea in immunocompetent adults. *N Engl J Med*. 2014;370(16):1532-1540.
194. Ejemot-Nwadiaro RI, Ehiri JE, Arikpo D, et al. Hand washing promotion for preventing diarrhoea. *Cochrane Database Syst Rev*. 2015;(9):CD004265.
195. Elinav H, Hershko-Klement A, Valinsky L, et al. Pregnancy-associated listeriosis: clinical characteristics and geospatial analysis of a 10-year period in Israel. *Clin Infect Dis*. 2014;59(7):953-961.
196. Enserink R, Mughini-Gras L, Duizer E, et al. Risk factors for gastroenteritis in child day care. *Epidemiol Infect*. 2015;143(13):2707-2720.
197. Enserink R, van den Wijngaard C, Bruijning-Verhagen P, et al. Gastroenteritis attributable to 16 enteropathogens in children attending day care: significant effects of rotavirus, norovirus, astrovirus, *Cryptosporidium* and *Giardia*. *Pediatr Infect Dis J*. 2015;34(1):5-10.
200. Escher M, Scavia G, Morabito S, et al. A severe foodborne outbreak of diarrhoea linked to a canteen in Italy caused by enteroinvasive *Escherichia coli*, an uncommon agent. *Epidemiol Infect*. 2014;142(12):2559-2566.
202. Escobedo AA, Ballesteros J, Gonzalez-Fraile E, et al. A meta-analysis of the efficacy of albendazole compared with tinidazole as treatments for *Giardia* infections in children. *Acta Trop*. 2016;153:120-127.
208. Feng C, Teuber S, Gershwin ME. Histamine (scombroid) fish poisoning: a comprehensive review. *Clin Rev Allergy Immunol*. 2016;50(1):64-69.
209. Field AS, Milner DA Jr. Intestinal microsporidiosis. *Clin Lab Med*. 2015;35(2):445-449.
211. Fink G, Heitner J. Evaluating the cost-effectiveness of preventive zinc supplementation. *BMC Public Health*. 2014;14:852.
217. Fletcher S, Van Hal S, Andresen D, et al. Gastrointestinal pathogen distribution in symptomatic children in Sydney, Australia. *J Epidemiol Glob Health*. 2013;3(1):11-21.
223. Freedberg DE, Lamouse-Smith ES, Lightdale JR, et al. Use of acid suppression medication is associated with risk for *C. difficile* infection in infants and children: a population-based study. *Clin Infect Dis*. 2015;61(6):912-917.
225. Gaffey MF, Wazny K, Bassani DG, et al. Dietary management of childhood diarrhea in low- and middle-income countries: a systematic review. *BMC Public Health*. 2013;13(suppl 3):S17.
227. Galvao TF, Thees MF, Pontes RF, et al. Zinc supplementation for treating diarrhea in children: a systematic review and meta-analysis. *Rev Panam Salud Publica*. 2013;33(5):370-377.
235. Gilchrist CA, Petri SE, Schneider BN, et al. Role of the gut microbiota of children in diarrhea due to the protozoan parasite *Entamoeba histolytica*. *J Infect Dis*. 2015;213(10):1579-1585.
241. Glass RI, Parashar U, Patel M, et al. The control of rotavirus gastroenteritis in the United States. *Trans Am Clin Climatol Assoc*. 2012;123:36-52.
243. Goldenberg JZ, Lytvyn L, Steurich J, et al. Probiotics for the prevention of pediatric antibiotic-associated diarrhea. *Cochrane Database Syst Rev*. 2015;(12):CD004827.
244. Goldman RD. Bismuth salicylate for diarrhea in children. *Can Fam Physician*. 2013;59(8):843-844.
246. Goni P, Martin B, Villacampa M, et al. Evaluation of an immunochromatographic dip strip test for simultaneous detection of *Cryptosporidium* spp, *Giardia duodenalis*, and *Entamoeba histolytica* antigens in human faecal samples. *Eur J Clin Microbiol Infect Dis*. 2012;31(8):2077-2082.
252. Gordon M, Akobeng A. Racecadotril for acute diarrhoea in children: systematic review and meta-analyses. *Arch Dis Child*. 2016;101(3):234-240.
256. Gould LH, Mody RK, Ong KL, et al. Increased recognition of non-O157 Shiga toxin-producing *Escherichia coli* infections in the United States during 2000–2010: epidemiologic features and comparison with *E. coli* O157 infections. *Foodborne Pathog Dis*. 2013;10(5):453-460.
257. Gould LH, Mungai E, Behravesh CB. Outbreaks attributed to cheese: differences between outbreaks caused by unpasteurized and pasteurized dairy products, United States, 1998–2011. *Foodborne Pathog Dis*. 2014;11(7):545-551.
260. Grass JE, Gould LH, Mahon BE. Epidemiology of foodborne disease outbreaks caused by *Clostridium perfringens*, United States, 1998–2010. *Foodborne Pathog Dis*. 2013;10(2):131-136.
261. Gu B, Zhou M, Ke X, et al. Comparison of resistance to third-generation cephalosporins in *Shigella* between Europe-America and Asia-Africa from 1998 to 2012. *Epidemiol Infect*. 2015;143(13):2687-2699.
263. Guarino A, Ashkenazi S, Gendrel D, et al. European Society for Pediatric Gastroenterology, Hepatology, and Nutrition/European Society for Pediatric Infectious Diseases evidence-based guidelines for the management of acute gastroenteritis in children in Europe: update 2014. *J Pediatr Gastroenterol Nutr*. 2014;59(1):132-152.
271. Gupta V, Gulati P, Bhagat N, et al. Detection of *Yersinia enterocolitica* in food: an overview. *Eur J Clin Microbiol Infect Dis*. 2015;34(4):641-650.
275. Haendiges J, Rock M, Myers RA, et al. Pandemic *Vibrio parahaemolyticus*, Maryland, USA, 2012. *Emerg Infect Dis*. 2014;20(4):718-720.
279. Hall RL, Jones JL, Hurd S, et al. Population-based active surveillance for *Cyclospora* infection–United States, Foodborne Diseases Active Surveillance Network (FoodNet), 1997–2009. *Clin Infect Dis*. 2012;54(suppl 5):S411-S417.
287. Harvey K, Esposito DH, Han P, et al. Surveillance for travel-related disease–GeoSentinel Surveillance System, United States, 1997–2011. *MMWR Surveill Summ*. 2013;62:1-23.
288. Hauswaldt S, Nitschke M, Sayk F, et al. lessons learned from outbreaks of Shiga toxin producing *Escherichia coli*. *Curr Infect Dis Rep*. 2013;15(1):4-9.

289. Hebbelstrup Jensen B, Olsen KE, Struve C, et al. Epidemiology and clinical manifestations of enteroaggregative *Escherichia coli*. *Clin Microbiol Rev*. 2014;27(3):614-630.
290. Heiman KE, Grass JE, Sjolund-Karlsson M, et al. Shigellosis with decreased susceptibility to azithromycin. *Pediatr Infect Dis J*. 2014;33(11):1204-1205.
293. Henriquez-Camacho C, Gotuzzo E, Echevarria J, et al. Ivermectin versus albendazole or thiabendazole for *Strongyloides stercoralis* infection. *Cochrane Database Syst Rev*. 2016;(1):CD007745.
296. Hernandez-Milian A, Payeras-Cifre A. What is new in listeriosis? *Biomed Res Int*. 2014;2014:358051.
307. Hlavsa MC, Roberts VA, Kahler AM, et al. Outbreaks of illness associated with recreational water–United States, 2011–2012. *MMWR*. 2015;64(24):668-672.
311. Hourigan SK, Chirumamilla SR, Ross T, et al. *Clostridium difficile* carriage and serum antitoxin responses in children with inflammatory bowel disease. *Inflamm Bowel Dis*. 2013;19(13):2744-2752.
323. Iyer RN, Rao J, Venkatalakshmi A, et al. Clinical and microbiology profile and outcome of diarrhea by coccidian parasites in immunocompetent children. *Pediatr Infect Dis J*. 2015;34(9):937-939.
324. Jain S, Vashistt J, Changotra H. Rotaviruses: is their surveillance needed? *Vaccine*. 2014;32(27):3367-3378.
326. Janda JM, Newton AE, Bopp CA. Vibriosis. *Clin Lab Med*. 2015;35(2):273-288.
328. Jandhyala DM, Vanguri V, Boll EJ, et al. Shiga toxin-producing *Escherichia coli* O104:H4: an emerging pathogen with enhanced virulence. *Infect Dis Clin North Am*. 2013;27(3):631-649.
339. Kaakoush NO, Castano-Rodriguez N, Mitchell HM, et al. Global epidemiology of *Campylobacter* infection. *Clin Microbiol Rev*. 2015;28(3):687-720.
340. Kabir S. Critical analysis of compositions and protective efficacies of oral killed cholera vaccines. *Clin Vaccine Immunol*. 2014;21(9):1195-1205.
341. Kadariya J, Smith TC, Thapaliya D. *Staphylococcus aureus* and staphylococcal food-borne disease: an ongoing challenge in public health. *Biomed Res Int*. 2014;2014:827965.
348. Karafillakis E, Hassounah S, Atchison C. Effectiveness and impact of rotavirus vaccines in Europe, 2006–2014. *Vaccine*. 2015;33(18):2097-2107.
349. Karvellas CJ, Tillman H, Leung AA, et al. Acute liver injury and acute liver failure from mushroom poisoning in North America. *Liver Int*. 2016;36(7):1043-1050.
353. Khanna S, Baddour LM, Huskins WC, et al. The epidemiology of *Clostridium difficile* infection in children: a population-based study. *Clin Infect Dis*. 2013;56(10):1401-1406.
359. Kirk MD, Pires SM, Black RE, et al. Correction: World Health Organization estimates of the global and regional disease burden of 22 foodborne bacterial, protozoal, and viral diseases, 2010: a data synthesis. *PLoS Med*. 2015;12(12):e1001940.
364. Kocher J, Yuan L. Norovirus vaccines and potential antinorovirus drugs: recent advances and future perspectives. *Future Virol*. 2015;10(7):899-913.
369. Kostakis ID, Cholidou KG, Vaiopoulos AG, et al. Fecal calprotectin in pediatric inflammatory bowel disease: a systematic review. *Dig Dis Sci*. 2013;58(2):309-319.
373. Kotloff KL, Nataro JP, Blackwelder WC, et al. Burden and aetiology of diarrhoeal disease in infants and young children in developing countries (the Global Enteric Multicenter Study, GEMS): a prospective, case-control study. *Lancet*. 2013;382(9888):209-222.
375. Kozak GK, MacDonald D, Landry L, et al. Foodborne outbreaks in Canada linked to produce: 2001 through 2009. *J Food Prot*. 2013;76(1):173-183.
377. Lai KK, Lamps LW. Enterocolitis in immunocompromised patients. *Semin Diagn Pathol*. 2014;31(2):176-191.
380. Lamberti LM, Walker CL, Chan KY, et al. Oral zinc supplementation for the treatment of acute diarrhea in children: a systematic review and meta-analysis. *Nutrients*. 2013;5(11):4715-4740.
382. Lanata CF, Fischer-Walker CL, Olascoaga AC, et al. Global causes of diarrheal disease mortality in children <5 years of age: a systematic review. *PLoS ONE*. 2013;8(9):e72788.
383. Lantagne D, Balakrish Nair G, Lanata CF, et al. The cholera outbreak in Haiti: where and how did it begin? *Curr Top Microbiol Immunol*. 2014;379:145-164.
384. Laporte J, Savin C, Lamourette P, et al. Fast and sensitive detection of enteropathogenic *Yersinia* by immunoassays. *J Clin Microbiol*. 2015;53(1):146-159.
389. Lee G, Paredes Olortegui M, Penataro Yori P, et al. Effects of *Shigella*-, *Campylobacter*- and ETEC-associated diarrhea on childhood growth. *Pediatr Infect Dis J*. 2014;33(10):1004-1009.
390. Leffler DA, Lamont JT. *Clostridium difficile* infection. *N Engl J Med*. 2015;373(3):287-288.
391. Legua P, Seas C. *Cystoisospora* and *Cyclospora*. *Curr Opin Infect Dis*. 2013;26(5):479-483.
393. Leibovici-Weissman Y, Neuberger A, Bitterman R, et al. Antimicrobial drugs for treating cholera. *Cochrane Database Syst Rev*. 2014;(6):CD008625.
394. Leibowitz J, Soma VL, Rosen L, et al. Similar proportions of stool specimens from hospitalized children with and without diarrhea test positive for *Clostridium difficile*. *Pediatr Infect Dis J*. 2015;34(3):261-266.
395. Lessa FC, Mu Y, Bamberg WM, et al. Burden of *Clostridium difficile* infection in the United States. *N Engl J Med*. 2015;372(9):825-834.
397. Letchumanan V, Chan KG, Lee LH. *Vibrio parahaemolyticus*: a review on the pathogenesis, prevalence, and advance molecular identification techniques. *Front Microbiol*. 2014;5:705.
398. Levenhagen MA, Costa-Cruz JM. Update on immunologic and molecular diagnosis of human strongyloidiasis. *Acta Trop*. 2014;135:33-43.
401. Liberato SC, Singh G, Mulholland K. Zinc supplementation in young children: a review of the literature focusing on diarrhoea prevention and treatment. *Clin Nutr*. 2015;34(2):181-188.
403. Lindsay B, Saha D, Sanogo D, et al. Association between *Shigella* infection and diarrhea varies based on location and age of children. *Am J Trop Med Hyg*. 2015;93(5):918-924.
404. Liu J, Gratz J, Amour C, et al. A laboratory-developed TaqMan array card for simultaneous detection of 19 enteropathogens. *J Clin Microbiol*. 2013;51(2):472-480.
407. Liu J, Kabir F, Manneh J, et al. Development and assessment of molecular diagnostic tests for 15 enteropathogens causing childhood diarrhoea: a multicentre study. *Lancet Infect Dis*. 2014;14(8):716-724.
408. Liu L, Oza S, Hogan D, et al. Global, regional, and national causes of child mortality in 2000–13, with projections to inform post-2015 priorities: an updated systematic analysis. *Lancet*. 2015;385(9966):430-440.
409. Liu L, Qian Y, Zhang Y, et al. Adenoviruses associated with acute diarrhea in children in Beijing, China. *PLoS ONE*. 2014;9(2):e88791.
410. Lo Vecchio A, Liguoro I, Bruzzese D, et al. Adherence to guidelines for management of children hospitalized for acute diarrhea. *Pediatr Infect Dis J*. 2014;33(11):1103-1108.
413. Lozer DM, Souza TB, Monfardini MV, et al. Genotypic and phenotypic analysis of diarrheagenic *Escherichia coli* strains isolated from Brazilian children living in low socioeconomic level communities. *BMC Infect Dis*. 2013;13:418.
418. Majowicz SE, Scallan E, Jones-Bitton A, et al. Global incidence of human Shiga toxin-producing *Escherichia coli* infections and deaths: a systematic review and knowledge synthesis. *Foodborne Pathog Dis*. 2014;11(6):447-455.
419. MAL-ED Network Investigators. The MAL-ED study: a multinational and multidisciplinary approach to understand the relationship between enteric pathogens, malnutrition, gut physiology, physical growth, cognitive development, and immune responses in infants and children up to 2 years of age in resource-poor environments. *Clin Infect Dis*. 2014;59(suppl 4):S193-S206.
425. Martinelli M, Strisciuglio C, Veres G, et al. *Clostridium difficile* and pediatric inflammatory bowel disease: a prospective, comparative, multicenter, ESPGHAN study. *Inflamm Bowel Dis*. 2014;20(12):2219-2225.
426. Martinez-Medina M, Garcia-Gil LJ. *Escherichia coli* in chronic inflammatory bowel diseases: An update on adherent invasive *Escherichia coli* pathogenicity. *World J Gastrointest Pathophysiol*. 2014;5(3):213-227.
427. Mayo-Wilson E, Junior JA, Imdad A, et al. Zinc supplementation for preventing mortality, morbidity, and growth failure in children aged 6 months to 12 years of age. *Cochrane Database Syst Rev*. 2014;(5):CD009384.
430. Mehal JM, Esposito DH, Holman RC, et al. Risk factors for diarrhea-associated infant mortality in the United States, 2005–2007. *Pediatr Infect Dis J*. 2012;31(7):717-721.
431. Mejia A, Atehortua S, Florez ID, et al. Cost-effectiveness analysis of zinc supplementation for treatment of acute diarrhea in children younger than 5 years in Colombia. *J Pediatr Gastroenterol Nutr*. 2015;60(4):515-520.
433. Melhem NM. Norovirus vaccines: correlates of protection, challenges and limitations. *Hum Vaccin Immunother*. 2016;12(7):1653-1669.
437. Miller A, Smith ML, Judd JA, et al. *Strongyloides stercoralis*: systematic review of barriers to controlling strongyloidiasis for Australian indigenous communities. *PLoS Negl Trop Dis*. 2014;8(9):e3141.
440. Miyamoto Y, Eckmann L. Drug development against the major diarrhea-causing parasites of the small intestine, *Cryptosporidium* and *Giardia*. *Front Microbiol*. 2015;6:1208.
449. Mori K, Hayashi Y, Akiba T, et al. Multiplex real-time PCR assays for the detection of group C rotavirus, astrovirus, and subgenus F adenovirus in stool specimens. *J Virol Methods*. 2013;191(2):141-147.
453. Muhsen K, Levine MM. A systematic review and meta-analysis of the association between *Giardia lamblia* and endemic pediatric diarrhea in developing countries. *Clin Infect Dis*. 2012;55(suppl 4):S271-S293.
454. Murinda SE, Ibekwe AM, Zulkaffly S, et al. Real-time isothermal detection of Shiga toxin-producing *Escherichia coli* using recombinase polymerase amplification. *Foodborne Pathog Dis*. 2014;11:529-536.
455. Murphree R, Garman K, Phan Q, et al. Characteristics of foodborne disease outbreak investigations conducted by Foodborne Diseases Active Surveillance Network (FoodNet) sites, 2003–2008. *Clin Infect Dis*. 2012;54(suppl 5):S498-S503.
458. Musekiwa A, Volmink J. Oral rehydration salt solution for treating cholera: <= 270 mOsm/L solutions vs >= 310 mOsm/L solutions. *Cochrane Database Syst Rev*. 2011;(12):CD003754.
464. Newton AE, Garrett N, Stroika SG, et al. Increase in *Vibrio parahaemolyticus* infections associated with consumption of Atlantic Coast shellfish–2013. *MMWR*. 2014;63(15):335-336.

470. Nicholson MR, Thomsen IP, Slaughter JC, et al. Novel risk factors for recurrent *Clostridium difficile* infection in children. *J Pediatr Gastroenterol Nutr*. 2015;60(1):18-22.
472. Nixon AF, Cunningham SJ, Cohen HW, et al. The effect of *Lactobacillus* GG on acute diarrheal illness in the pediatric emergency department. *Pediatr Emerg Care*. 2012;28(10):1048-1051.
473. Nylund CM, Eide M, Gorman GH. Association of *Clostridium difficile* infections with acid suppression medications in children. *J Pediatr*. 2014;165(5):979-84. e971.
488. O'Ryan GM, Ashkenazi-Hoffnung L, O'Ryan-Soriano MA, et al. Management of acute infectious diarrhea for children living in resource-limited settings. *Expert Rev Anti Infect Ther*. 2014;12(5):621-632.
491. O'Ryan M, Vidal R, del Canto F, et al. Vaccines for viral and bacterial pathogens causing acute gastroenteritis: Part I: overview, vaccines for enteric viruses and *Vibrio cholerae*. *Hum Vaccin Immunother*. 2015;11(3):584-600.
492. O'Ryan M, Vidal R, del Canto F, et al. Vaccines for viral and bacterial pathogens causing acute gastroenteritis: Part II: vaccines for *Shigella*, *Salmonella*, enterotoxigenic *E. coli* (ETEC) enterohemorragic *E. coli* (EHEC) and *Campylobacter jejuni*. *Hum Vaccin Immunother*. 2015;11(3):601-619.
494. Pang T, Leach ST, Katz T, et al. Fecal biomarkers of intestinal health and disease in children. *Front Pediatr*. 2014;2:6.
495. Panozzo CA, Becker-Dreps S, Pate V, et al. Direct, indirect, total, and overall effectiveness of the rotavirus vaccines for the prevention of gastroenteritis hospitalizations in privately insured US children, 2007–2010. *Am J Epidemiol*. 2014;179(7):895-909.
506. Patzi-Vargas S, Zaidi M, Bernal-Reynaga R, et al. Persistent bloody diarrhoea without fever associated with diffusely adherent *Escherichia coli* in a young child. *J Med Microbiol*. 2013;62(Pt 12):1907-1910.
507. Pavlinac PB, Tickell KD, Walson JL. Management of diarrhea in HIV-affected infants and children. *Expert Rev Anti Infect Ther*. 2015;13(1):5-8.
510. Pennotti R, Scallan E, Backer L, et al. Ciguatera and scombroid fish poisoning in the United States. *Foodborne Pathog Dis*. 2013;10(12):1059-1066.
520. Piescik-Lech M, Shamir R, Guarino A, et al. Review article: the management of acute gastroenteritis in children. *Aliment Pharmacol Ther*. 2013;37(3):289-303.
521. Pires SM, Fischer-Walker CL, Lanata CF, et al. Aetiology-specific estimates of the global and regional incidence and mortality of diarrhoeal diseases commonly transmitted through food. *PLoS ONE*. 2015;10(12):e0142927.
522. Pires SM, Vieira AR, Hald T, et al. Source attribution of human salmonellosis: an overview of methods and estimates. *Foodborne Pathog Dis*. 2014;11(9):667-676.
523. Platts-Mills JA, Babji S, Bodhidatta L, et al. Pathogen-specific burdens of community diarrhoea in developing countries: a multisite birth cohort study (MAL-ED). *Lancet Glob Health*. 2015;3(9):e564-e575.
524. Platts-Mills JA, Kosek M. Update on the burden of *Campylobacter* in developing countries. *Curr Opin Infect Dis*. 2014;27(5):444-450.
530. Powell MR. Trends in reported foodborne illness in the United States: 1996–2013. *Risk Anal*. 2015;36(8):1589-1598.
531. Praekelt U, Reissbrodt R, Kresse A, et al. Monoclonal antibodies against all known variants of EspA: development of a simple diagnostic test for enteropathogenic *Escherichia coli* based on a key virulence factor. *J Med Microbiol*. 2014;63(Pt 12):1595-1607.
539. Reddy SP, Wang H, Adams JK, et al. Prevalence and characteristics of *Salmonella* serotypes isolated from fresh produce marketed in the United States. *J Food Prot*. 2016;79(1):6-16.
549. Rossignol JF, Lopez-Chegne N, Julcamoro LM, et al. Nitazoxanide for the empiric treatment of pediatric infectious diarrhea. *Trans R Soc Trop Med Hyg*. 2012;106(3):167-173.
554. Ruuska T, Vesikari T. Rotavirus disease in Finnish children: use of numerical scores for clinical severity of diarrhoeal episodes. *Scand J Infect Dis*. 1990;22(3):259-267.
558. Sammons JS, Toltzis P, Zaoutis TE. *Clostridium difficile* infection in children. *JAMA Pediatr*. 2013;167(6):567-573.
564. Sarkar R, Tate JE, Ajjampur SS, et al. Burden of diarrhea, hospitalization and mortality due to cryptosporidial infections in Indian children. *PLoS Negl Trop Dis*. 2014;8(7):e3042.
572. Schar F, Trostdorf U, Giardina F, et al. *Strongyloides stercoralis*: global distribution and risk factors. *PLoS Negl Trop Dis*. 2013;7(7):e2288.
574. Schnadower D, Finkelstein Y, Freedman SB. Ondansetron and probiotics in the management of pediatric acute gastroenteritis in developed countries. *Curr Opin Gastroenterol*. 2015;31(1):1-6.
577. Schutze GE, Willoughby RE, Committee on Infectious Diseases, et al. *Clostridium difficile* infection in infants and children. *Pediatrics*. 2013;131:196-200.
589. Shioda K, Kambhampati A, Hall AJ, et al. Global age distribution of pediatric norovirus cases. *Vaccine*. 2015;33(33):4065-4068.
592. Sirinavin S, Garner P. Antibiotics for treating *Salmonella* gut infections. *Cochrane Database Syst Rev*. 2000;(2):CD001167.
593. Sjöling Å, Sadeghipoorjahromi L, Novak D, et al. Detection of major diarrheagenic bacterial pathogens by multiplex PCR panels. *Microbiol Res*. 2015;172:34-40.
594. Slayton RB, Newton AE, Depaola A, et al. Clam-associated vibriosis, USA, 1988–2010. *Epidemiol Infect*. 2014;142(5):1083-1088.
599. Soli KW, Kas M, Maure T, et al. Evaluation of colorimetric detection methods for *Shigella*, *Salmonella*, and *Vibrio cholerae* by loop-mediated isothermal amplification. *Diagn Microbiol Infect Dis*. 2013;77(4):321-323.
604. Steffen R, Hill DR, DuPont HL. Traveler's diarrhea: a clinical review. *JAMA*. 2015;313(1):71-80.
613. Szajewska H, Canani RB, Guarino A, et al. Probiotics for the prevention of antibiotic-associated diarrhea in children. *J Pediatr Gastroenterol Nutr*. 2016;62(3):495-506.
619. Tate JE, Parashar UD. Rotavirus vaccines in routine use. *Clin Infect Dis*. 2014;59(9):1291-1301.
623. Thomas DE, Elliott EJ. Interventions for preventing diarrhea-associated hemolytic uremic syndrome: systematic review. *BMC Public Health*. 2013;13:799.
625. Thompson CN, Duy PT, Baker S. The rising dominance of *Shigella sonnei*: an intercontinental shift in the etiology of bacillary dysentery. *PLoS Negl Trop Dis*. 2015;9(6):e0003708.
630. Trachtman H. HUS and TTP in children. *Pediatr Clin North Am*. 2013;60(6):1513-1526.
632. Tschudin-Sutter S, Tamma PD, Naegeli AN, et al. Distinguishing community-associated from hospital-associated *Clostridium difficile* infections in children: implications for public health surveillance. *Clin Infect Dis*. 2013;57(12):1665-1672.
634. Turin CG, Ochoa TJ. The role of maternal breast milk in preventing infantile diarrhea in the developing world. *Curr Trop Med Rep*. 2014;1(2):97-105.
635. Ulloa-Gutierrez R, Avila-Aguero ML. Rotavirus vaccination in Central American children. *Expert Rev Vaccines*. 2014;13(6):687-690.
636. Uzal FA, Freedman JC, Shrestha A, et al. Towards an understanding of the role of *Clostridium perfringens* toxins in human and animal disease. *Future Microbiol*. 2014;9(3):361-377.
648. Vinje J. Advances in laboratory methods for detection and typing of norovirus. *J Clin Microbiol*. 2015;53(2):373-381.
649. Walia R, Kunde S, Mahajan L. Fecal microbiota transplantation in the treatment of refractory *Clostridium difficile* infection in children: an update. *Curr Opin Pediatr*. 2014;26(5):573-578.
650. Walker RI. An assessment of enterotoxigenic *Escherichia coli* and *Shigella* vaccine candidates for infants and children. *Vaccine*. 2015;33(8):954-965.
654. Walters MS, Simmons L, Anderson TC, et al. Outbreaks of salmonellosis from small turtles. *Pediatrics*. 2016;137(1):1-9.
656. Wang L, Shi L, Su J, et al. Detection of *Vibrio parahaemolyticus* in food samples using in situ loop-mediated isothermal amplification method. *Gene*. 2013;515(2):421-425.
658. Wang R, Zhong Y, Gu X, et al. The pathogenesis, detection, and prevention of *Vibrio parahaemolyticus*. *Front Microbiol*. 2015;6:144.
657. Wang Y, Wang Y, Luo L, et al. Rapid and sensitive detection of *Shigella* spp. and *Salmonella* spp. by multiple endonuclease restriction real-time loop-mediated isothermal amplification technique. *Front Microbiol*. 2015;6:1400.
674. World Health Organization. WHO guidelines approved by the Guidelines Review Committee. Guideline: updates on the management of severe acute malnutrition in infants and children; 2013. Geneva: World Health Organization.
679. Wurzner R, Riedl M, Rosales A, et al. Treatment of enterohemorrhagic *Escherichia coli*-induced hemolytic uremic syndrome (eHUS). *Semin Thromb Hemost*. 2014;40(4):508-516.
683. Yano A, Ishimaru R, Hujikata R. Rapid and sensitive detection of heat-labile I and heat-stable I enterotoxin genes of enterotoxigenic *Escherichia coli* by loop-mediated isothermal amplification. *J Microbiol Methods*. 2007;68(2): 414-420.
687. Zhang J, Jin H, Hu J, et al. Antimicrobial resistance of *Shigella* spp. from humans in Shanghai, China, 2004–2011. *Diagn Microbiol Infect Dis*. 2014;78(3):282-286.
689. Zhang W, Sack DA. Current progress in developing subunit vaccines against enterotoxigenic *Escherichia coli*-associated diarrhea. *Clin Vaccine Immunol*. 2015;22(9):983-991.
675. World Health Organization. Cholera, 2014. *Wkly Epidemiol Rec*. 2015;90(40):517-528.

The full reference list for this chapter is available at ExpertConsult.com.

Antibiotic-Associated Colitis

45

Victoria A. Statler • Kristina A. Bryant

More than 130 million courses of antibiotics are prescribed in the United States each year, and diarrhea is a common side effect of antibiotic therapy. *Clostridium difficile* is the most common infectious cause of antibiotic-associated diarrhea, accounting for 15% to 25% of cases,[14] and *C. difficile* infection (CDI) is now the most frequently identified healthcare-associated infection in the United States.[86] According to a 2012 report from the Centers for Disease Control and Prevention, the incidence, mortality, and medical care costs of CDI have reached "historic highs," in part because of the emergence of a hypervirulent strain of *C. difficile* identified as toxinotype III, restriction endonuclease analysis group BI, North American pulsed-field type NAP1, and polymerase chain reaction (PCR) type 027.[27] The BI/NAP1/027 strain exhibits high-level fluoroquinolone resistance and produces increased amounts of protein exotoxins A and B (TcdA and TcdB).[88]

CDI is increasingly common in children, a population once thought to be at low risk of disease.[67,97,141] Emerging evidence suggests that most cases of pediatric CDI are community associated.[63,112,137]

HISTORY

In 1935, Hall and O'Toole described the identification of a new, anaerobic, gram-positive, spore-forming bacillus in the stools from four of 10 healthy, breastfed neonates. They named it *Bacillus difficilis,* in recognition of the fact that the organism was difficult to isolate and study in the laboratory. *B. difficilis* was noted to be highly pathogenic in guinea pigs and rabbits; guinea pigs inoculated subcutaneously with the bacteria commonly developed convulsions, which the investigators attributed to a soluble exotoxin isolated from broth culture filtrates.[51] A link between intestinal colonization and illness in human infants was much less clear, although the authors postulated a potential association with occult blood in the stools of neonates or convulsions of unexplained origin. Neither association was proved, and, for decades, *B. difficilis* was thought to be a harmless intestinal commensal in infants.[12] The role of *C. difficile* as a human pathogen was finally elucidated in the 1970s, when toxin-producing *Clostridia* were isolated from the stools of adult patients with clindamycin-associated pseudomembranous colitis.[13]

EPIDEMIOLOGY

The epidemiology of CDI is evolving. Since 2000, cases of CDI have increased in both frequency and severity. From 2000 to 2009, the number of hospitalized patients with CDI doubled.[27] Deaths attributable to CDI increased from 3000 deaths per year during 1999 to 2000 to 14,000 during 2006 to 2007.[50] In 2011, *C. difficile* was responsible for nearly 500,000 infections and approximately 29,000 deaths.[81] As in prior years, the highest burden of disease and the majority of deaths occurred in adults 65 years of age and older.

Nevertheless the burden of CDI in children is substantial. While CDI has historically been less common and less severe in children, since 1997 rates of pediatric CDI have increased in both hospitals[67,97,141] and the community.[15,63,137] In hospitalized children, CDI is associated with increased mortality, longer lengths of stays, and higher costs.[114] CDI has been reported in children previously thought to be at low risk for the disease, including those without prior antibiotic or hospital exposure, as well as infants.[26]

Forty to 70% of asymptomatic, healthy newborns may be colonized with *C. difficile* in the first 10 to 28 days of life.[56,59] Strain acquisition appears to be highest in the first week of life, likely as a result of exposure to spores in the hospital.[1] Colonization rates decrease to 3% to 10% by the second year of life.[56,59] Rates of *C. difficile* colonization in children older than 2 years of age approximate those in healthy adults and may be as low as 2% to 3%.[11,14,60]

Colonization occurs with both toxin-producing and nontoxigenic strains.[1,77,78] Factors associated with increased colonization rates in infants include longer duration of hospitalization, hospitalization in an intensive care setting, low birth weight, and formula feeding.[56] Even with a large number of toxigenic *C. difficile* bacteria and high levels of toxin A and B, infants usually remain asymptomatic,[84] and most studies have failed to show an epidemiologic association between colonization and disease in infants younger than 1 year. For example, in a study of outpatient children, *C. difficile* was isolated from 7% of patients with diarrhea and 14.8% of healthy controls. Children with *C. difficile* were younger than children without the organism (mean age, 8.2 to 9.8 months).[16] *C. difficile* was isolated with equal frequency in healthy Swedish children 1 week to 1 year of age (17%) and children younger than 6 years with diarrhea (18%).[122] Most controlled studies in neonatal intensive care units corroborate high rates of asymptomatic colonization in young infants. *C. difficile* toxin was recovered from the stools of 55% of patients in one neonatal intensive care unit, but signs of enteric disease, including necrotizing enterocolitis (NEC), occurred with equal frequency in both toxin-positive and toxin-negative infants.[34] Although severe CDI has occasionally been reported in young infants, especially those with underlying gastrointestinal disease, it has historically been thought to be rare.[106] Guidelines published in 2013 from the American Academy of Pediatrics recommended avoiding routine testing for *C. difficile* in children younger than 1 year and testing for other causes of diarrhea first in children 1 to 3 years of age.[6]

Recent reports challenge traditional paradigms about CDI; namely, that (1) CDI is uncommon in children, (2) that young children are spared, and (3) that most cases occur in hospitalized children. *C. difficile* is a common health care–acquired pathogen and the most common cause of health care–associated diarrhea in pediatric patients.[27,77] Outbreaks of CDI among hospitalized pediatric patients are well documented,[23,43,89] and cases of CDI in hospitalized children are increasing. In a study that included 21 free-standing children's hospitals, CDI increased 53% in hospitalized children between 2001 to 2006, from 2.6 cases to 4.0 cases per 1000 admissions.[67] Twenty-six percent of the children treated for CDI were younger than 1 year, and 5% were newborns. An analysis of two large administrative databases demonstrated a nearly twofold increase in CDI-associated hospitalization between 1997 and 2006.[141] Children younger than 1 year had the second highest rate of CDI hospitalizations. Investigators acknowledged that their study methodology precluded an assessment of whether these children had true CDI or *C. difficile* colonization in the setting of diarrhea attributable to another cause. Nevertheless significant increases in CDI in hospitalized children have been documented even when children younger than 1 year are excluded.[97]

Population-based studies also suggest significant increases in the incidence of CDI in children. In Olmsted County, Minnesota, the age- and sex-adjusted incidence of CDI in children 0 to 18 years of age increased from 2.6 per 100,000 person-years (1991–97) to 32.6 per 100,000 (2004–09). The median age of *C. difficile* cases was 2.3 years.[63] Similar findings were reported in Monroe County, New York, where the incidence of CDI in pediatric patients was 33.8 per 100,000 in 2010, rose to 45.8 in 2011, and remained stable in 2012. The highest incidence rate was in 1-year-old children.[112] In both Olmsted and Monroe Counties, more than 70% of cases were classified as community associated.

Some experts suggest that the apparent increase in CDI incidence be interpreted with caution because widespread use of sensitive polymerase chain reaction (PCR) tests may be leading to overdiagnosis and artificially inflated incidence rates, especially in community-associated disease. In a single-center study, 23% of children with community-associated CDI diagnosed by *tcdB* PCR had discordant results when stool samples were tested by other methods, including multiplex PCR.[73] Investigators reported that these children lacked traditional risk factors for CDI, had symptoms more consistent with viral illness, and may have been misdiagnosed.

The largest active population-based study of CDI in children to date analyzed data collected from 10 geographic areas in the United States during 2010 to 2011. The highest burden of disease was observed in children 12 to 23 months of age.[137] Clinical presentation, illness severity, and outcomes were similar across age groups, suggesting that isolation of *C. difficile* from young children in this study represented infection rather than colonization. Antibiotic use and outpatient health care exposures (i.e., visit to doctor's office, dental office, or emergency department) within the 12 weeks preceding the onset of diarrhea were common among the 71% of cases deemed to be community associated.

Changes in the epidemiology of CDI in children may be related to the emergence of the epidemic BI/NAP1/027 strain.[66,119,127] Although this strain is commonly isolated from children[137] it is not yet clear if it is associated with more severe disease, as it is in adults.[66,119,127] Ten percent of isolates from hospitalized children with CDI identified through the Canadian Nosocomial Infections Surveillance Program between November 1, 2004, and April 30, 2005, were the B1/NAP1/027 strain.[119] Children with the NAP1 strain were more likely to suffer complications from CDI than were children with other strains (29% vs. 6%; relative risk, 4.6; 95% confidence interval [CI], 1.1–17.2; $P = .04$), although none died. Similar rates of NAP1 isolation were identified in a prospective study of children at two US hospitals with CDI. NAP1 was not associated with increased disease severity.[66]

Antibiotic use remains a principal risk factor for the development of CDI in individuals of all ages.[66,115] The risk of CDI increases 7- to 10-fold during a course of antibiotics and for 1 month after antibiotic discontinuation.[52] Although the earliest reports of pseudomembranous colitis were associated with administration of clindamycin, nearly every antibiotic class has been implicated in the development of CDI, particularly cephalosporins, other β-lactam antibiotics, and fluoroquinolones. Diarrhea typically begins during antibiotic use or up to 30 days after antibiotic therapy, but symptoms may occur after a single dose of an antibiotic.[69,121]

In one study of hospitalized children, receipt of three or more antibiotic classes in the 30 days before diagnosis of CDI was a risk factor for severe disease.[66] Nevertheless antibiotic use is not a prerequisite for the development of CDI in children. Severe disease has been reported in the absence of antibiotic exposure,[26] and in one study of community-acquired CDI, 43% of patients lacked a history of antibiotic use.[15]

The use of gastric acid suppression medication is another potentially modifiable risk factor of CDI. Protein pump inhibitors and histamine-2 receptor antagonists increase the risk of CDI and recurrent CDI.[44,57,93,98,132] Several studies have demonstrated that CDI is more common in boys.[64,97,106] Underlying gastrointestinal disease, particularly Hirschsprung disease, is a risk factor for severe, complicated CDI. Other risk factors for CDI in children include solid organ transplant,[100] inflammatory bowel disease,[102] immune suppression, and cancer.[92,97,115] In a prospective study of 141 children undergoing chemotherapy for a solid tumor or lymphoma, nine (6%) tested positive for *C. difficile* toxin A and were symptomatic.[25] Another study suggests that rates of *C. difficile* diarrhea in children after chemotherapy are as high as approximately 15%.[40] In an analysis of 3 years of data from the Kids' Inpatient Database (2000, 2003, 2006), children with cancer accounted for 21% of all CDI cases, and rates of CDI were 15 times higher in children with cancer than in those without cancer.[123]

PATHOGENESIS

The pathophysiology of CDI is complex and multifactorial. Ingestion of *C. difficile* spores and subsequent intestinal colonization precedes the development of CDI, but not all exposures result in symptomatic infection. In older children and adults, colonization is inhibited by normal intestinal flora, which is thought to compete for intestinal nutrients and space on the mucosal surface. Antibiotics, by altering normal flora, facilitate *C. difficile* colonization. Disease manifestations are related to toxin production; most toxigenic strains produce both toxin A and toxin B.[108] Based on early animal studies, toxin A (TcdA) was thought to be the major virulence factor, but recent studies have documented severe CDI caused by toxin A–negative, toxin B–positive (TcdB) strains suggesting that TcdB plays the dominant role in human infections.[3,85] Approximately 25% of *C. difficile* isolated by culture do not produce toxins[42] and are not clinically significant.

C. difficile toxins act at the level of the epithelial cells and produce effects by two main pathophysiologic pathways.[96,108] Toxin A and B cause the disorganization of actin microfilaments of the enterocyte cytoskeleton. The change in enterocyte structure leads to epithelial cell destruction and opening of tight junctions between enterocytes.[96,108] Toxin A also induces activation of neutrophils and results in local inflammation. Release of proinflammatory cytokines, including interleukin-6 (IL-6) and IL-8, occurs from enterocytes, causing further damage to the intestinal mucosa.[58,108] Both pathways lead to increased permeability of and damage to enterocytes, resulting in the clinical symptoms of *C. difficile*.[58]

Why young infants are commonly colonized with toxin-producing *C. difficile* strains yet rarely have symptoms is not yet completely understood. Colonization density does not appear to be important because asymptomatic infants may have *C. difficile* colony counts as high as 10^8 bacteria per gram of feces; these colony counts are similar to those in adults with pseudomembranous colitis.[56] Experiments in newborn rabbits suggested that protection against disease may result from lack of receptors for toxin A.[38] The appearance of receptors with age may be a species-specific phenomenon. Toxin receptors have been identified in the intestines of neonatal pigs, and these animals are susceptible to disease.[62] The immaturity of the toxin receptor sites may also play a role in the absence of disease in neonates.[89]

Transmission of *C. difficile* is fecal-oral. The organism is generally spread by person-to-person contact or environment-to-person contact. Both modes of spread are important in health care environments, where *C. difficile* is shed in the environment by infected and colonized patients and occasionally from asymptomatic hospital personnel. Patients may acquire *C. difficile* via the unwashed hands of health care workers, but direct or indirect transmission through contaminated objects and surfaces also occurs. *C. difficile* spores can survive for up to 5 months in the environment and are difficult to eradicate through routine cleaning and disinfection.[14,42,58] Objects likely to harbor organisms are those contaminated with feces and include toilet seats, sinks, and scales, but *C. difficile* can also be isolated from the hands and feces of asymptomatic hospital personnel.[42] Stethoscopes may be vectors for *C. difficile* transmission when not effectively cleaned after use on a patient with CDI.[134] Electronic rectal thermometers have also been implicated in hospital spread of *C. difficile*.[21]

Foodborne transmission has been postulated as a source of *C. difficile* spread in the community. Although *C. difficile* spores have been recovered from retail food products, there is limited evidence to link contamination of food to human illness.[48] Likewise the role of zoonotic transmission has been explored because *C. difficile* is known to be both a pathogen and a commensal organism in domestic and food animals. To date, no study has convincingly demonstrated human *C. difficile* infection as a result of animal contact, although further research is needed.[48]

CLINICAL MANIFESTATIONS

C. difficile can cause a broad spectrum of disease from asymptomatic colonization or mild diarrhea to severe disease, pseudomembranous colitis (PMC), and even death.[7,12,129] Watery diarrhea occurs in 90% to 95% of cases of CDI and bloody diarrhea in 5% to 10%.[69] Most pediatric patients develop a self-resolving illness that is associated with low-grade fever, mild abdominal pain, and diarrhea, some of which may contain mucus or blood. However, some patients progress to PMC or severe disease.

While significant adverse outcomes are reported in children with CDI, especially those with hospital-onset disease,[114] severe disease and severe complicated disease are less common in children than in adults.[72] The Infectious Diseases Society of America guidelines define severe disease in adults as a white blood cell count of 15,000 cells/mm^3 or more or a serum creatinine of greater than 50% above baseline.[29] These criteria have poor predictive value in children, likely reflecting underlying medical complexity of the child rather than severity of CDI.[72] In general, severe disease is more likely to occur in neutropenic children with leukemia, infants with Hirschsprung disease, and children with inflammatory bowel disease.[7] Severe complicated disease, defined as sepsis, hypotension or shock, ileus, toxic megacolon, perforation, need for intensive care, surgery for a CDI-related complication, or death,[29] occurs in 2% to 5% of children with CDI.[61,116,130] Other less common complications include pneumatosis intestinalis[66] and rectal prolapse.[54] If severe disease develops, anasarca can also occur because of protein-losing enteropathy.[12]

Children with pseudomembranous colitis may not meet criteria for severe or severe complicated disease. PMC is generally associated with diarrhea and fever as well as abdominal distension, cramps, and systemic toxicity. Mucoid stools are the hallmark of PMC.[69] PMC lesions almost always affect the colon, but involvement of the small intestine has been reported in adults.[55] Focal necrosis and inflammation are initially found in PMC lesions, but these can progress to extensive involvement of the colon covered by confluent pseudomembranes.[12] Although uncommon, fulminant colitis occurs and can lead to bowel perforation, peritonitis, and a high mortality rate.[74]

Coinfection with other enteric viruses has also been described in children. Rotavirus and calicivirus have been reported in severe cases of CDI requiring intensive care.[106] In one cohort, 24% of patients with CDI had either norovirus or *Sapovirus* coinfection.[39] There were no differences in clinical severity or outcomes between those children with norovirus or *Sapovirus* and *C. difficile* coinfection compared to children with CDI alone.[39]

Recurrence of disease occurs in up to 25% of pediatric patients after treatment.[95,61,131] Risk factors for recurrent disease in children include receiving concomitant antibiotics during treatment of CDI[131] or having received multiple classes of antibiotics prior to onset of CDI,[95] presence of a tracheostomy tube,[71] community-associated CDI,[131] and malignancy.[95,71] Chronic diarrhea secondary to *C. difficile* can occur without evidence of colitis[122] and has been associated with failure to thrive.

The role of *C. difficile* in the pathogenesis of NEC among infants has been debated. Early studies reported no difference in colonization with *C. difficile* among infants with NEC and those without NEC.[138] A prospective study of 50 preterm infants also demonstrated that *C. difficile* colonization was not associated with a higher incidence of NEC.[41] In a retrospective cohort study of children with *C. difficile*–toxin-positive stool specimens, 50% of 22 patients in a neonatal intensive care unit had suspected or confirmed NEC, although causality was not proved.[15]

In adults, *C. difficile* colitis has been reported to mimic acute peritonitis with fever, leukocytosis, and signs and symptoms of peritonitis on physical examination.[35,94,111,129] Extraintestinal manifestations account for less than 0.2% of all *C. difficile* infections and can include bacteremia, sepsis, visceral abscesses, wound infections, pleural involvement, and reactive arthritis.[9,55,87] Most cases of *C. difficile* bacteremia are polymicrobial with the isolation of other bowel flora.[55] The mortality rate of bacteremia in adults is significant. In one recent study, mortality rate was 27% in those with bacteremia[49] and in up to 39% of those reported in a review of the literature.[61] Bacteremia is rare in children; one case has been reported in which the child survived.[28]

LABORATORY STUDIES

The diagnosis of CDI requires both the presence of diarrhea (or radiographic evidence of toxic megacolon) and the detection of *C. difficile* toxin or the toxin gene in a diarrheal stool specimen (or evidence of pseudomembranous colitis on colonoscopy or histopathology). Diarrhea is defined as stools that take the shape of their container, with three episodes that occur in a 24-hour period.[6,8] Only diarrheal stool should be tested in most instances because testing of formed stool may detect colonization rather than infection.[19] Occasionally a patient with CDI may have an ileus or evidence of toxic megacolon on imaging; a rectal swab may be the only available sample in this circumstance.[19]

Historically culture using a selective medium for *C. difficile* has been the gold standard for diagnosing CDI.[19] Because toxigenic and nontoxigenic strains can grow on culture, isolates must then be tested for the presence of toxin genes or gene products before the diagnosis of CDI can be confirmed.[74,79] Additionally culture is time intensive, requires special equipment and trained personnel, and is not standardized, which may introduce bias.[8,30] Stool culture is now generally reserved for epidemiologic investigations.[31]

Cytotoxicity assays detect the presence of toxin B directly in stool by visualizing its cytopathic effects on cells in cell or tissue culture.[19] These assays were reviewed and, as a reference method, best define true cases of CDI.[105] However, while this test is highly specific, its sensitivity may be as low as 67%. Other limitations of cytotoxicity assays include the need for skilled personnel to interpret the findings in tissue culture, the subjective nature of test interpretation, and an approximate 72-hour turnaround time.[24,75]

Enzyme immunoassays (EIAs) may detect toxin A or B or glutamate dehydrogenase (GDH), a product of *C. difficile*. EIAs offer the advantages of rapid turnaround time, ease of use, and lower cost.[5,89,139] Those that detect toxin were introduced in the mid-1980s and became routinely used for diagnosis. However, their reported low sensitivity resulted in the historical practice that multiple specimens on a single patient be tested before the patient could be considered truly negative.[2,24,30] This delayed diagnosis and increased the cost of testing. In children, both lower sensitivity and specificity of the EIA have been observed; positive tests alone should be interpreted with caution,[83,128] and testing for toxins A/B should not be the first diagnostic assay for CDI because of this poor sensitivity.[19]

EIAs for GDH offer improved sensitivity over EIAs for toxin A/B but lower specificity because GDH is present in both toxigenic and nontoxigenic strains of *C. difficile*, as well as in other *Clostridium* species. Its high negative predictive value makes it a useful screening tool.[19,24] However, positive results should be confirmed in a two-step algorithm that detects toxin.[6,8,19]

Nucleic acid amplification tests (NAATs) that detect toxin A (*tcdA*) or B (*tcdB*) genes or *tcdC* gene (a negative regulator of toxin A/B production), often by PCR, are FDA approved and now preferred by many laboratories. While more costly, these tests are rapid, specific, and more sensitive than EIAs and identify toxigenic *C. difficile* in a single step.[33,83] NAATs detect bacteria that carry the toxin gene, regardless of toxin production, and therefore may detect toxigenic *C. difficile* in asymptomatic patients as well as in patients with diarrhea ultimately found to have another etiology.[8,107] In children, NAATs may be positive in both hospitalized children with and without diarrhea, underscoring the ability of NAATs to detect *C. difficile* colonization.[80] Additionally, NAATs may misdiagnosis community-acquired CDI in children with few risk factors for CDI and who may have other causes of diarrhea.[73] These factors have led many to question the use of NAATs as a single diagnostic test for CDI.

Because no single diagnostic test is presently optimal for the diagnosis of CDI (Table 45.1), many laboratories have adopted a multistep diagnostic algorithm for stool testing. In one approach, stools are initially screened with a rapid immunoassay that detects GDH and toxins A and B. Specimens that test both positive or both negative for GDH and toxin are immediately reported as positive or negative for toxigenic *C. difficile*. GDH-positive but toxin-negative specimens are subject to further testing by an NAAT.[24,75] The sensitivity and specificity of this approach in adult populations have been reported to be from 91% to 100% and 92% to 98%, respectively.[24,105] In a tertiary pediatric population, the sensitivity of the GDH-based algorithms was less but still superior to screening by toxin immunoassay (81% vs. 56%).[99]

Approximately 90% of patients can be diagnosed with CDI on a single stool sample, and repeat stool testing does not increase the diagnostic yield significantly nor is it cost effective.[33] Test of cure is also not recommended. Because asymptomatic colonization is common in children younger than 1 year, testing for *C. difficile* should not be performed routinely in this age group if other risk factors such as Hirschsprung disease are not present; other causes for diarrhea should be sought.[75]

Leukocytosis, thrombocytosis, and hypoalbuminemia are commonly present in CDI. A leukocyte count greater than 15,000 cells/μL and a

TABLE 45.1 Laboratory Tests to Diagnose *Clostridium difficile* Infection[76]

Testing Method	Sensitivity	Specificity	Advantage(s)	Disadvantage(s)
Culture	High	Low	Often considered gold standard	Long turnaround time; no differentiation between toxigenic and nontoxigenic strains
Cell cytotoxicity neutralization assay (CCNA)	Moderate	Moderate to high	Highly specific	2- to 3-day turnaround time; requires skilled experts to interpret
Enzyme immunoassays for toxin detection	Low to moderate	High	Inexpensive; quick turnaround time; easy to perform	Overall low sensitivity
Enzyme immunoassay for glutamate dehydrogenase (GDH)	High	Low	Quick; useful for screening purposes	Low specificity; no differentiation between toxigenic and nontoxigenic strains
Nucleic acid amplification tests	High	High	High sensitivity and specificity; quick turnaround time; easy to perform	Expensive; increased detection of colonization; detects toxin gene but not toxin production

platelet count exceeding 400,000 cells/μL are more common in patients with CDI compared to those with diarrhea without CDI.[101] Leukocytosis may be an early finding of CDI among hospitalized patients, even in the setting of mild or absent symptoms of colitis.[22,136] The presence of fecal leukocytes is an insensitive method for CDI screening.[110]

In seriously ill children in whom CDI is suspected but cannot be proved by standard laboratory testing, colonoscopy or sigmoidoscopy may be helpful. If pseudomembranes are found in a patient with consistent clinical symptoms, the diagnosis of CDI can be made because nearly all cases of PMC are caused by *C. difficile.* On examination, PMC has a characteristic appearance of yellowish-white raised plaques, usually 2 to 10 mm in diameter.[89] Among infants with CDI, nonspecific colitis is more commonly found by endoscopy than are the characteristic pseudomembranes.[10]

Other radiographic modalities may provide supplemental data to aid in the diagnosis of CDI. Plain abdominal radiographs in patients with PMC may demonstrate colonic ileus, small bowel ileus, ascites, and/or nodular haustral thickening.[17] Abdominal computed tomography (CT) can be performed, but severity of colitis present on CT does not always correlate to clinical disease severity, and CT findings are less specific when compared with laboratory and clinical findings. Abnormalities on CT include nodular haustral thickening, colonic wall thickening, ascites, and pericolonic edema.[89] Abdominal ultrasonography has also been used to aid in the diagnosis of CDI because bowel wall thickening can be visualized.[109]

DIFFERENTIAL DIAGNOSIS

CDI must be distinguished from diarrhea that occurs as an adverse effect of antibiotics, other medications, or enteral nutrition, as well as diarrhea from other infectious causes. Viruses, for example, account for most cases of health care–associated diarrhea. *C. difficile* infection should be considered in hospitalized patients who develop diarrhea and who have had exposure to antibiotics.[77] Other bacteria that have occasionally been associated with antibiotic-associated diarrhea include *Staphylococcus aureus,* enterotoxin-producing strains of *Clostridium perfringens, Salmonella* spp., and *Klebsiella oxytoca.*[12] Cytotoxin-producing *K. oxytoca* was recently reported as a cause of antibiotic-associated hemorrhagic colitis (AAHC) in children.[53] In contrast to the diarrhea associated with CDI, the diarrhea associated with *K. oxytoca* AAHC is always bloody. Colitis is typically segmental and concentrated in the right colon; pseudomembranes are usually absent. AAHC is most commonly associated with exposure to amoxicillin-clavulanate.[53]

The differential diagnosis of community-onset diarrhea is broad compared with diarrhea with onset in the hospital setting. Bacteria, viruses, and parasites can all cause diarrhea in children, although viruses are still the most common.[32] Common causative viruses include astrovirus, adenovirus, and norovirus.[68] The incidence of rotavirus gastroenteritis has decreased with routine childhood immunization against this pathogen, but infections still occur.[125] Common bacterial causes of community-onset diarrhea, including *Escherichia coli, Campylobacter, Salmonella, Shigella,* and *Yersinia,* can be diagnosed by stool culture.[45,68] Like *C. difficile, Giardia intestinalis* can cause acute or protracted watery diarrhea. When clinical symptoms suggest CDI, testing should be considered even without a history of antibiotic use, especially in ambulatory patients. CDI in the absence of prior antibiotic exposure is more common in the community setting than the hospital setting and has been reported in 24% to 60% of patients with community-associated CDI.[37]

Inflammatory bowel disease, either Crohn disease or ulcerative colitis, should be considered in the setting of relapsing CDI or if colitis persists despite treatment.[18] In children previously diagnosed with inflammatory bowel disease, diarrhea and abdominal pain may be related to progression of inflammatory bowel disease and not CDI.[90]

TREATMENT

Among children with mild disease who do not require antimicrobial therapy, symptoms usually resolve within 7 to 10 days. Those with prolonged symptoms or more severe disease will require antimicrobial interventions.[20] Evidence-based guidelines have been published for the treatment of CDI in adults.[29] The American Academy of Pediatrics has made similar recommendations for the treatment of children and adolescents.[7,6] If possible, precipitating antibiotics should be discontinued. Antiperistaltic medications should be avoided. At least 10 days of oral or intravenous metronidazole (30 mg/kg per day in four divided doses, maximum 2 g/day) is recommended as initial treatment for most children and adolescents with CDI. Oral vancomycin (40 mg/kg per day in 4 divided doses, maximum 2 g/day) is generally reserved for patients with severe disease. Intravenous metronidazole in combination with vancomycin by mouth or nasogastric tube has been recommended for adults with severe CDI complicated by hypotension, shock, ileus, or megacolon; vancomycin may be administered rectally in cases of complete ileus.[29] These recommendations may have applicability for children with severe, complicated disease. Intravenous vancomycin is not effective for the treatment of CDI. Colectomy may be required for treatment of severe, complicated cases.

Relapse occurs in up to 25% of patients who initially improve with treatment with either metronidazole or vancomycin.[42] Most patients respond to a second course of the same treatment. Vancomycin is recommended for second and subsequent recurrences. A tapering and/or pulsed regimen of oral vancomycin has been recommended for adults who develop a second recurrence of CDI.[29]

In 2011, the US Food and Drug Administration (FDA) approved the use of fidaxomicin for the treatment of CDI in adults.[135] This monocyclic antibiotic acts as an RNA polymerase inhibitor and is bactericidal against *C. difficile.* In a large, multicenter randomized phase III trial, fidaxomicin was noninferior to vancomycin for the treatment of CDI (clinical cure 88.2% vs. 85.5%). However, recurrence of CDI within 4 weeks of clinical cure was significantly less in fidaxomicin-treated patients.[82] One case of recurrent CDI in a 10-year-old patient treated successfully with fidaxomicin has been published in the literature.[118] An abstract presented at IDWeek 2014 reported a 92% cure rate in children aged 11 months to 17 years treated with fidaxomicin. Twenty-eight percent of those with clinical response had recurrence, but all but one of those children had a history of recurrent CDI. The drug was otherwise well tolerated, demonstrating low plasma levels and high fecal concentrations.[117] A clinical trial with fidaxomicin is ongoing and may offer a promising new treatment of CDI in children in the future (https://clinicaltrials.gov/ct2/show/NCT02218372?term=fidaxomicin+and+children&rank=2). Nitazoxanide is a nitrothiazolyl-salicylamide thiazolide with broad-spectrum activity against both protozoa and anaerobic bacteria. It is approved by the FDA for the treatment of diarrhea caused by *Giardia lamblia* and *Cryptosporidium parvum* and is considered an alternative treatment for CDI in adults.[7]

Because perturbations in the normal bacterial flora of the gastrointestinal tract play a crucial role in the development of CDI, adjunctive therapies that promote the restoration of normal flora are becoming more commonplace. In fecal microbiota transplantation (FMT), stool from a healthy volunteer is administered to a patient with severe or relapsing CDI in an effort to restore normal intestinal flora.[64] FMT may be delivered by enema, colonoscopy, nasogastric tube, or nasojejunal tube. More recently, preliminary data have shown FMT administered via frozen capsules has also been efficacious and safe.[140] In an open-label, randomized, controlled trial, when compared with vancomycin, infusion of donor feces was significantly more effective for the treatment of recurrent CDI in adults.[133] Numerous other case reports and series have reported its efficacy in adults.[64] While there have been no randomized, controlled trials in children, published cases in children with recurrent CDI have reported no complications.[103,113] An overall cure rate of 90% to 100% in children has been reported in single-center case series, comparable to adult data.[103,113]

Probiotics have been studied alone or in combination with antibiotics for the treatment of CDI. One study of adults 18 years of age or older demonstrated that *Saccharomyces boulardii* administered in combination with high-dose vancomycin (2 g/day) decreased recurrences compared with vancomycin administered with placebo (16.7% vs. 50%).[120] Other clinical trials have failed to show a benefit of probiotics in treatment of CDI in adults.[104] Probiotic treatment of children with CDI has not been well studied.[126]

PREVENTION AND CONTROL

Because CDI is commonly precipitated by antibiotic therapy, judicious use of antibiotics is essential in inpatient and outpatient settings. Antimicrobial stewardship programs that reduce the use of broad-spectrum antibiotics have been linked to reductions in CDI in hospitalized patients.[124] Acid suppression medication should be prescribed for the minimum duration required for treatment or symptom control.[98]

Some evidence points to a potential role for probiotics in the prevention of CDI. A 2013 Cochrane Review assessed the efficacy and safety of probiotics in the prevention of *C. difficile*–associated diarrhea or CDI in both children and adults. Compared with placebo or no treatment, probiotics reduced the risk of *C. difficile*–associated diarrhea in all patients by 64% (23 randomized controlled trials [RCTs]; $n = 4213$; RR, 0.36; 95% CI, 0.26–0.51).[47] In three RCTs that involved children, probiotic administration reduced the risk of CDI from 5.9% to 2.3% ($n = 605$; RR, 0.40; 95% CI, 0.17–0.96). A limitation of this meta-analysis is that the studies with the greatest weight had unusually high incidences of CDI in the placebo group, potentially biasing the results to favor probiotics. In a randomized, placebo-controlled trial in older adults, probiotics did not reduce the incidence of CDI.[4] Data are lacking concerning the optimal dose and preparation of probiotics for CDI prevention, and this is not a routinely recommended strategy.

Contact precautions, in addition to standard precautions, are recommended for hospitalized patients for the duration of the illness.[3] Contact precautions include placement in a single-patient room when feasible, donning of gown and gloves by health care personnel before room entry, and hand hygiene after glove removal. The most appropriate method of hand hygiene when caring for patients with CDI has been the subject of some debate. Although alcohol-based hand hygiene products are not sporicidal, evidence-based guidance published by the Society for Healthcare Epidemiology of America (SHEA) and the Infectious Diseases Society of America (IDSA) recommend the preferential use of soap and water for hand hygiene only in hyperendemic or outbreak settings.[36] These recommendations may seem counterintuitive, but alcohol does not kill *C. difficile* spores. Additionally in several studies hand washing with soap and water was more effective than use of alcohol-based products in removing *C. difficile* spores from the hands of volunteers inoculated with the pathogen. Nevertheless there are no data to support an increase in CDI with the use of alcohol-based hand hygiene products, nor are there studies that demonstrate a decrease in CDI when soap and water are used for hand hygiene.

Appropriate environmental cleaning and disinfection of patient rooms and medical equipment are considered important measures in preventing health care–associated spread of *C. difficile*. Because quaternary compounds that are commonly used as hospital disinfectants are not sporicidal, chlorine-containing agents (e.g., household bleach diluted 1:10 in water) are recommended for cleaning in settings with increased rates of CDI.[36]

Measures to prevent the transmission of CDI in the community are less well defined, but children with *C. difficile* diarrhea should be excluded from daycare centers for the duration of illness.[7] Outbreaks in daycare centers have been reported.[65]

The observation that serum antibody levels against toxins A and B are associated with protection against recurrent CDI has fueled interest in the development of *C. difficile* vaccines.[76] Although no vaccine is currently available for the prevention of CDI, two candidate toxoid-based vaccines and a recombinant fusion protein vaccine are undergoing clinical trials in adults.[46,70] A mucosal vaccine using modified *Bacillus subtilis* spores that express a fragment of TcdA is in the early stages of clinical development.

NEW REFERENCES SINCE THE SEVENTH EDITION

1. Adlerberg I, Huang H, Lindberg E, et al. Toxin-producing *Clostridium difficile* strains as long-term gut colonizers in healthy infants. *J Clin Microbiol.* 2014;52:173-179.
2. Alcala L, Sanchez-Cambronero L, Catalan MP, et al. Comparison of three commercial methods for rapid detection of *Clostridium difficile* toxins A and B from fecal specimens. *J Clin Microbiol.* 2008;46(11):3833-3835.
3. Allen SJ, Wareham K, Eang D, et al. Lactobacilli and bifidobacteria in the prevention of antibiotic-associated diarrhea and *Clostridium difficile* diarrhea in older inpatients (PLACIDE): a randomized, double-blind, placebo-controlled, multicentre trial. *Lancet.* 2013;382:1249-1257.
6. American Academy of Pediatrics. *Clostridium difficile* infection in infants and children. *Pediatrics.* 2013;131:196-200.
7. American Academy of Pediatrics. *Clostridium difficile*. In: Kimberlin DW, Brady MT, Jackson MA, Long SS, eds. *Red Book: 2015 Report of the Committee on Infectious Diseases.* 30th ed. Elk Grove Village, IL: American Academy of Pediatrics; 2015:298-301.
8. Bagdarasarian N, Rao K, Malani P. Diagnosis and treatment of *Clostridium difficile* in adults: a systematic review. *JAMA.* 2015;313:398-408.
9. Balzan S, de Almeida Quadros C, de Cleva R, et al. Bacterial translocation: overview of mechanisms and clinical impact. *J Gastroenterol Hepatol.* 2007;22:464-471.
19. Brecher SM, Novak-Weekley SM, Nagy E. Laboratory diagnosis of *Clostridium difficile* infections: there is light at the end of the colon. *Clin Infect Dis.* 2013;57:1175-1181.
28. Cid A, Juncal AR, Aguilera A, et al. *Clostridium difficile* bacteremia in an immunocompetent child. *J Clin Microbiol.* 1998;36:1167-1168.
30. Crobach MJT, Dekkers OM, Wilcox MH, et al. European Society of Clinical Microbiology and Infectious Diseases (ESCMID): data review and recommendations for diagnosing *Clostridium difficile*-infection (CDI). *Clin Microbiol Infect.* 2009;15:1053-1066.
36. Dubberke ER, Calring P, Carrico R, et al. Strategies to prevent *Clostridium difficile* infections in acute care hospitals: 2014 update. *Infect Control Hosp Epidemiol.* 2014;35:628-645.
39. El Feghaly RE, Stauber JL, Tarr PI, et al. Viral co-infections are common and are associated with higher bacterial burden in children with *C. difficile* infection. *J Pediatr Gastroenterol Nutr.* 2013;57:813-816.
44. Freedberg DE, Lamousé-Smith ES, Lightdale JR, et al. Use of acid suppression medication is associated with the risk of *C. difficile* infection in infants and children: a population study. *Clin Infect Dis.* 2015;61:912-917.

46. Ghose C, Kelly CP. The prospect for vaccines to prevent *Clostridium difficile* infection. *Infect Dis Clin North Am.* 2015;29:145-162.
47. Goldenberg JZ, Ma SSY, Saxton JD, et al. Probiotics for the prevention of *Clostridium difficile*-associated diarrhea in adults and children. *Cochrane Database Syst Rev.* 2013;(5):CD006095.
49. Gupta A, Patel R, Baddour LM, et al. Extraintestinal *Clostridium difficile* infections: a single-center experience. *Mayo Clin Proc.* 2014;89:1525-1536.
57. Jimenez J, Drees M, Loveridge-Lenza B, et al. Exposure to gastric acid suppression therapy is associated with health care- and community-associated *Clostridium difficile* infection in children. *J Pediatr Gastroenterol Nutr.* 2015;61:208-211.
61. Kazanji N, Gjeorgjievski M, Yadav S, et al. Monomicrobial vs polymicrobial *Clostridium difficile* bacteremia: a case report and review of the literature. *Am J Med.* 2015;128:e19-e26.
63. Khanna S, Baddour LM, Huskins WC, et al. The epidemiology of *Clostridium difficile* infection in children: a population-based study. *Clin Infect Dis.* 2013;56:1401-1406.
70. Kociolek LK, Gerding DN. Breakthroughs in the treatment and prevention of *Clostridium difficile* infection. *Nature Rev.* 2016;13(3):150-160.
71. Kociolek LK, Palac HL, Patel SJ, et al. Risk factors for recurrent *Clostridium difficile* infection in children: a nested case control study. *J Pediatr.* 2015;167:384-389.
72. Kociolek LK, Patel SJ, Shulman ST, et al. Concomitant medical conditions and therapies preclude accurate classification of children with severe or severe complicated *Clostridium difficile* infection. *J Pediatr Infect Dis Soc.* 2014;4:e139-e142.
73. Kociolek LK, Patel SJ, Zheng X, et al. Clinical and microbiologic assessment of cases of pediatric community-associated *Clostridium difficile* infection reveals opportunities for improved testing decisions. *Pediatr Infect Dis J.* 2016;35:157-161.
76. Kyne L, Warny M, Qamar A, et al. Association between antibody response to toxin A and protection against recurrent *Clostridium difficile* diarrhea. *Lancet.* 2001;357:189-193.
80. Leibovitz J, Soma VL, Rosen L, et al. Similar proportions of stool specimens from hospitalized children with and without diarrhea test positive for *Clostridium difficile. Pediatr Infect Dis J.* 2015;34:261-266.
81. Lessa FC, Mu Y, Bamberg WM. Burden of *Clostridium difficile* infection in the United States. *N Engl J Med.* 2015;372:825-834.
86. Magill SS, Edwards JR, Bamber W, et al. Multistate point prevalence survey of healthcare-associated infections. *N Eng J Med.* 2014;370:1198-1208.
87. Mattila E, Arkkila P, Mattila PS, et al. Extraintestinal *Clostridium difficile* infections. *Clin Infect Dis.* 2013;57:e148-e153.
88. McDonald LC, Killgore GE, Thompson A, et al. An epidemic, toxin gene-variant strain of *Clostridium difficile. N Engl J Med.* 2005;353:2433-2441.
95. Nicholson MR, Thomsen IP, Slaughter JC, et al. Novel risk factors for recurrent *Clostridium difficile* infection in children. *J Pediatr Gastroenterol Nutr.* 2015;60:18-22.
98. Nylund CM, Eide M, Gorman GH. Association of *Clostridium difficile* infections with acid suppressive medication in children. *J Pediatr.* 2014;165:979-984.
100. Pant C, Deshpande A, Desai M, et al. Outcomes of *Clostridium difficile* in pediatric solid organ transplant recipients. *Transpl Infect Dis.* 2016;18:31-38.
103. Pierog A, Mencin A, Rizhalla Reilly N. Fecal microbiota transplantation in children with recurrent *Clostridium difficile* infection. *Pediatr Infect Dis J.* 2014;33:1198-1199.
105. Planche TD, Davies KA, Coen PG, et al. Differences in outcome according to *Clostridium difficile* testing method: a prospective multicentre diagnostic validation study of *C difficile* infection. *Lancet Infect Dis.* 2013;13:936-945.
107. Polage CR, Gyorke CE, Kennedy MA, et al. Overdiagnosis of *Clostridium difficile* infection in the molecular test era. *JAMA Intern Med.* 2015;175:1792-1801.
112. Rhee SM, TSay R, Nelson DS, et al. *Clostridium difficile* in the pediatric population of Monroe County, New York. *J Pediatr Infect Dis Soc.* 2014;3:183-188.
113. Russell GH, Kaplan JL, Youngster I, et al. Fecal transplant for recurrent *Clostridium difficile* infection in children with and without inflammatory bowel disease. *J Pediatr Gastroenterol Nutr.* 2014;58:588-592.
114. Sammons JS, Localio R, Coffc SE, et al. *Clostridium difficile* infection is associated with increased risk of death and prolonged hospitalization in children. *Clin Infect Dis.* 2013;57:1-8.
116. Schwartz KL, Darwish I, Richardson SE, et al. Severe clinical outcome is uncommon in *Clostridium difficile* infection in children: a retrospective cohort study. *BMC Pediatr.* 2014;14:28.
117. Sears P, Kaplan SL, Michaels M. A safety and pharmacokinetic study of fidaxomicin in children with *Clostridium difficile*-associated diarrhea [abstract LB-8]. Infectious Diseases Society of America annual meeting and IDWeek, Philadelphia, PA, 2014.
118. Smeltzer S, Hassoun A. Successful use of fidaxomicin in recurrent *Clostridium difficile* infection in a child. *J Antimicrob Chemother.* 2013;68:1688-1689.
129. Tschudin-Sutter S, Tamma PD, Milstone AM, et al. The prediction of complicated *Clostridium difficile* infections in children. *Infect Control Hosp Epidemiol.* 2014;35:901-903.
130. Tschudin-Sutter S, Tamma PD, Milstone AM, et al. Predictors of first recurrence of *Clostridium difficile* infections in children. *Pediatr Infect Dis J.* 2014;33:414-416.
133. van Nood E, Vrieze A, Nieuwdorp M, et al. Duodenal infusion of donor feces for recurrent *Clostridium difficile. N Engl J Med.* 2013;368:407-415.
137. Wendt JM, Cohen JA, Mu Y, et al. *Clostridium difficile* infection among children among diverse geographic locations. *Pediatrics.* 2014;133:651-658.
140. Youngster I, Russell GH, Pindar C, et al. Oral, capsulized, frozen fecal microbiota transplantation for relapsing *Clostridium difficile* infection. *JAMA.* 2014;312:1772-1778.

The full reference list for this chapter is available at ExpertConsult.com.

46 Whipple Disease

Zev Davidovics • Mark A. Gilger

Over the past 20 years there has been an explosion of knowledge about Whipple disease. It is now known that Whipple bacillus causes not only classic Whipple disease, a rare, systemic bacterial infection that can be fatal without therapy but also acute infection such as gastroenteritis, pneumonia, and bacteremia. In its most common form, Whipple disease affects white, middle-aged men, causing diarrhea, weight loss, abdominal pain, arthralgias, and fever. Although it is extraordinarily rare in children, its recognition may be crucial because simple treatment with appropriate antibiotics may be curative and lifesaving.[29]

HISTORY

Whipple disease was described in 1907 by George Hoyt Whipple,[93] at that time an instructor in pathology at the Johns Hopkins University.[7] Whipple's description probably was not the first; Allchin and Webb apparently described a patient with "Whipple disease" in 1895.[61]

In Whipple's account, a 37-year-old medical missionary was admitted to the Johns Hopkins Hospital with low-grade fever, steatorrhea, and an abdominal mass. The patient had a 5-year history of sporadic migratory polyarthritis. These attacks of arthritis were associated with a gradual loss of weight and strength. His skin was pigmented with a brownish hue. Laboratory evaluation found severe anemia and an enormous number of fatty acid crystals in the stool. Explorative laparotomy revealed large, firm mesenteric lymph nodes, and a diagnosis of either Hodgkin disease or tuberculosis was made. The patient died 1 week later, and autopsy revealed marked fatty deposition within intestinal mucosa and the mesenteric and retroperitoneal lymph nodes. Other findings included polyserositis (peritonitis, pleuritis, and pericarditis) and endocarditis. Histologic examination revealed infiltration of the lamina propria of the small intestine by large, foamy mononuclear cells that did not stain for fat. Fatty acids and triglycerides were found in dilated lymph channels. Silver stains of the mesenteric lymph nodes showed "great numbers of rod-shaped organisms" that resembled the tubercle bacillus. Whipple suggested that these bacillus-like organisms in the nodes could be the cause.

Whipple[93] reported "a hitherto undescribed disease characterized anatomically by deposits of fat and fatty acids in the intestinal and mesenteric lymphatic tissues." He concluded that the patient had "an obscure disease of fat metabolism" and proposed the term *intestinal lipodystrophy*.[23] Whipple recognized the most important features of this disease except for the involvement of the central nervous system (CNS). In 1949, Black-Schaffer showed that macrophages within the intestinal mucosa of patients with Whipple disease are stained intensely by the periodic acid–Schiff (PAS) method,[46] proving that the macrophages contained glycoprotein or mucopolysaccharide, not fat, as Whipple had suggested.

In 1992, Relman and colleagues[73] identified a gram-positive bacillus in association with Whipple disease by use of polymerase chain reaction (PCR). They reported a unique 1321-base-pair, 16S ribosomal RNA sequence amplified by PCR on intestinal and lymph node tissue from five unrelated patients with Whipple disease. They suggested that the responsible bacillus is a member of actinomycetes. Relman and colleagues[73] concluded that the phylogenetic relationships of the Whipple disease bacillus, the features of the illness, and its distinct morphologic characteristics provided sufficient grounds to propose a new genus and species name: *Tropheryma whippelii* from the Greek *trophe*, or "nourishment"; *eryma*, or "barrier," because of the malabsorption it causes; and *whippelii* (now *whipplei*), in honor of Whipple.

EPIDEMIOLOGY

Classic Whipple disease characteristically occurs in white middle-aged men. Its true incidence and prevalence are unknown because fewer than 1000 cases have been reported worldwide. It is an extremely rare disease in children,[1,2,5,12,44,89] with fewer than 10 cases reported. The youngest patient was a neonate,[17] and the oldest was 83 years old.[55] The peak age at presentation is 40 to 49 years.[28] In a literature review of 114 patients,[55] 88% were men and 12% were women. Most of these patients were white. Most patients reported as having Whipple disease are from continental Europe or the United States.[15] In an extensive review of 741 cases, Dobbins[22] found that most academic centers in the United States had records of three or four unreported cases. He estimated that for every published report at least two or three unpublished cases exist and that 1500 to 2000 individuals probably have had Whipple disease.[19]

Although classic Whipple disease is quite rare, the incidence of *T. whipplei*–related infection may be higher than previously thought. Raoult and associates[70] found stool PCR evidence of *T. whipplei* in 36 of 241 (15%) children with acute gastroenteritis but in none of 47 control subjects. Thirty-three percent of children with a positive stool PCR also had another identified diarrheal pathogen. The bacterial load in the children's stool was higher than in asymptomatic controls and more in line with numbers found in classic Whipple disease. These children showed seropositivity with IgM during the acute infection and recovered without treatment within 2 weeks. *T. whipplei* has also been identified in patients with pneumonia[10] and bacteremia.[30]

The prevalence of asymptomatic carriage of *T. whipplei* varies by country and exposure.[29,32,33] For example, in stools, prevalence estimates range from 2% to 4% of the general population, 12% in sewer workers, and 44% in healthy children in Senegal.[29,32,33] *T. whipplei* has been identified in 0.5% to 30% of healthy adults in saliva and gingival plaque.[75,79,86] Such studies confirm the existence of asymptomatic carriage.

ETIOLOGY AND PATHOGENESIS

Although humans are the only species to display clinical signs of *T. whipplei* infection, they are likely not the only reservoir. In a study of sewage water in Austria, *T. whipplei* was found by PCR in 17 of 46 (37%) of samples.[81] Transmission of *T. whipplei* is most likely fecal-oral. Among asymptomatic workers in those plants, 16 of 64 (25%) were PCR positive for *T. whipplei* in their stool. This compared to a baseline rate of 7% of PCR-positive stools in controls. A study in France identified an asymptomatic control population with PCR-positive *T. whipplei* in 4% in their stool.[32] Similar to the Austrian study, sewage workers had a higher carrier rate of 12%. The same study did not identify *T. whipplei* in the stool of monkeys or apes.

Classic Whipple disease is caused by an organism known as Whipple bacillus or *T. whipplei*.[28,55,69,93] Despite Whipple's account of "great numbers of rod-shaped organisms," culture of the organism was unsuccessful until more recently.[93] In 2000, Raoult and associates[69] reported that the bacterium *T. whipplei* had been cultured successfully from an aortic valve vegetation in a patient with prolonged endocarditis. The bacteria were isolated after inoculation in a human fibroblast cell line (HEL). Analysis by PCR confirmed that the 16S ribosomal RNA gene of the cultured bacterium was identical to the *T. whipplei* sequence. Subcultures of the bacterium also were obtained, and high-titer polyclonal antibodies against *T. whipplei* were produced. Such antibodies potentially may allow serologic diagnosis to become a reality.

T. whipplei may be a member of the actinomycetales,[73] which are gram-positive bacteria with DNA rich in guanine and cytosine.[94] The genus consists of actinomycetes, streptomycetes, and the nocardioforms.[16] *T. whipplei* seems to be related most closely to the four actinobacteria *Dermatophilus congolensis, Arthrobacter globiformis, Terrabacter tumescens,* and *Micrococcus luteus.*[73] Using so-called bootstrap analysis, some researchers have argued that the Whipple bacillus is only 67% associated with actinobacteria, far from the level needed for scientific conclusion.[83] The Whipple bacillus may represent another, separate, fourth line of descent with the actinomycetes. Amplification, cloning, and sequencing of a 620-base-pair fragment of *T. whipplei* heat shock protein led to the conclusion that *T. whipplei* is a member of the actinomycetales.[62]

Scant support exists for a primary humoral immunodeficiency in Whipple disease,[37] but stronger evidence exists for a distinct defect in the cell-mediated immune function. Dobbins[24] reviewed data of 30 patients with HLA-A and HLA-B locus typing and 47 patients with HLA-B27 typing. He found an increased incidence of patients who were positive for HLA-B27 (28%), even with absence of concomitant sacroiliitis. Other reports have failed to confirm the increased association with the HLA-B27 antigen.[3] Marth and associates[57] studied 27 patients with Whipple disease. They found a significantly reduced number of cells expressing the complement receptor 3 L-chain (CD11B), a reduced proliferation to phytohemagglutinin and to sheep red blood cells, and a hypoergic skin reaction. These findings indicated a defect of cell-mediated immunity.

In patients with active disease, the number of $CD8^+$ cells is increased, which results in a reduced CD4/CD8 ratio. Such defects of cellular immunity seem to persist in patients for several years, despite complete remission of the disease. Schoeden and associates[80] were able to culture *T. whipplei* in mononuclear phagocytes deactivated with interleukin-4 (IL-4), IL-10, and dexamethasone. IL-4 was found to be the crucial deactivating signal that rendered monocytes permissive for intracellular multiplication of *T. whipplei.* IL-4 is an immunoregulatory cytokine. Schoeden and associates[80] suggested that host factors, such as an imbalance in the T-helper 1 and T-helper 2 immune response, may contribute to the pathogenesis of Whipple disease.

Desnues and colleagues[20,21] reported a specific gene expression pattern associated with replication of *T. whipplei* in macrophages. *T. whipplei* organisms are killed by monocytes. The addition of exogenous IL-16 enabled *T. whipplei* to replicate in monocytes and increased bacterial replication in macrophages. *T. whipplei* replication in macrophages was completely prevented after blocking IL-16 activity with the use of anti–IL-16 antibodies. Untreated patients with Whipple disease were noted to have significantly higher circulating IL-16 than did control subjects and patients treated for Whipple disease. They concluded that response of monocytes and macrophages to IL-16 likely is crucial for replication of *T. whipplei* to occur in patients with Whipple disease.

Oral acquisition of the Whipple bacillus seems most likely, emphasizing greater involvement of the duodenum and proximal jejunum than the more distal small intestine.[28] Only three reports of siblings with this disease exist; contagious spread of Whipple disease seems unlikely.[42] *T. whipplei* has been identified free in the small intestine next to the glycocalyx of the enterocyte's microvilli, in epithelial cells, and in the lamina propria.[28] Even in patients with extraintestinal Whipple disease, the organism usually is identified in the small bowel.[28] The bacillus seems to spread through the lymphatics and through the systemic circulation[28,47,63] and then can involve several extraintestinal organs. *T. whipplei* can be seen faintly by light microscopy. The bacilli are seen best by transmission electron microscopy, which reveals a rod-shaped organism 0.2 μm wide and 1.5 to 2.5 μm long (Fig. 46.1). The ultrastructure of the wall of *T. whipplei* is similar to that of other gram-positive bacteria, with the exception of an additional surface membrane. This membrane is different from the outer membrane of gram-negative bacteria because

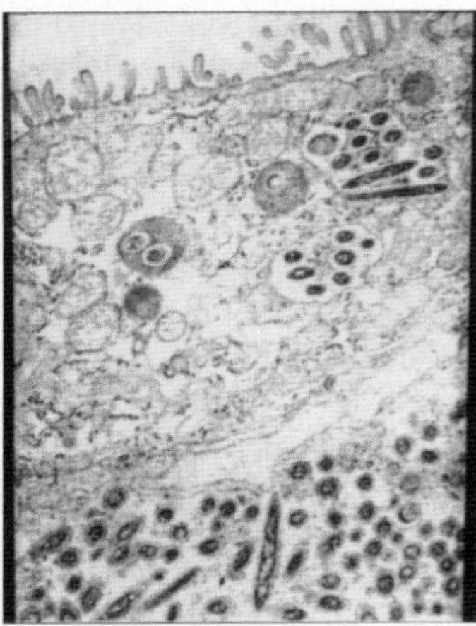

FIG. 46.1 Electron micrograph of the invasion of enterocytes by Whipple bacilli. There are numerous bacilli within the lamina propria. (×25,000.) (From Tyor MP. Whipple's disease: the Duke connection. *N C Med J.* 1994;55:237–40.)

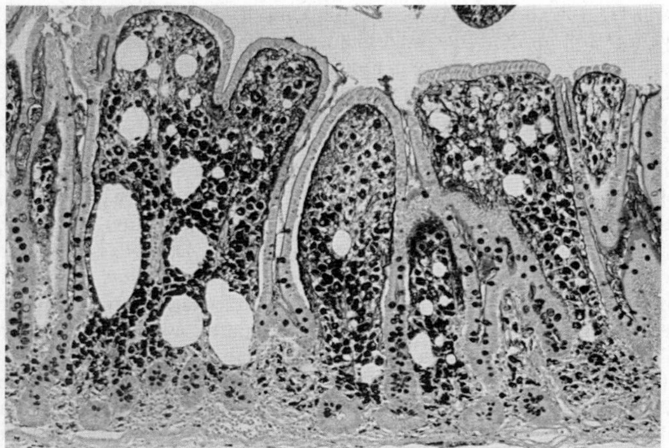

FIG. 46.2 Light microscopic photograph of intestinal mucosa from the proximal jejunum of a patient with untreated Whipple disease. The villi appear blunted and swollen with periodic acid–Schiff-positive macrophages stuffed in the lamina propria. (Courtesy Kenneth P. Batts, MD, Mayo Clinic, Rochester, MN; Jeffrey Craver, MD, DePaul Health Center, Bridgeton, MO; and Milton J. Finegold, MD, Baylor College of Medicine, Houston, TX.)

it is thinner, has a symmetric profile, and has no PAS-positive components.[83] After the bacillus has been ingested by the macrophage, the degenerative process that occurs leads to the accumulation of bacterial remnants that are resistant to degradation. The polysaccharide-containing portion of the bacillus wall correlates with these remnants, and its progressive accumulation leads to the typical intramacrophagic inclusions. These inclusions are PAS positive and one of the key features in the histologic diagnosis of Whipple disease.[7] Biopsy specimens from the small intestine in patients with Whipple disease usually show characteristic changes. The intestinal villi are preserved,[28] but distortion of the architecture occurs.[37] A clubbed appearance of the intestinal villi[55] usually is present caused by the accumulation of foamy macrophages in the lamina propria.[28] The enterocytes may appear normal,[26,55] or they may show flattening and vacuolization and occasionally appear cuboidal (Fig. 46.2).[26,55] Lipid accumulation, with large fat droplets within the lamina propria and smaller droplets within and between the absorptive cells, occurs commonly.[55] In some instances, prominent, dilated lacteals are present.[28] Ectors and associates[26] reported reduced and absent lactase and major histocompatibility complex class II (HLA-DR) expression that normalized within 3 to 6 months of starting antibiotic therapy.

The characteristic feature of Whipple disease is the presence of PAS-positive, diastase-resistant macrophages.[42] These findings are not pathognomonic, however, because intestinal PAS-positive macrophages

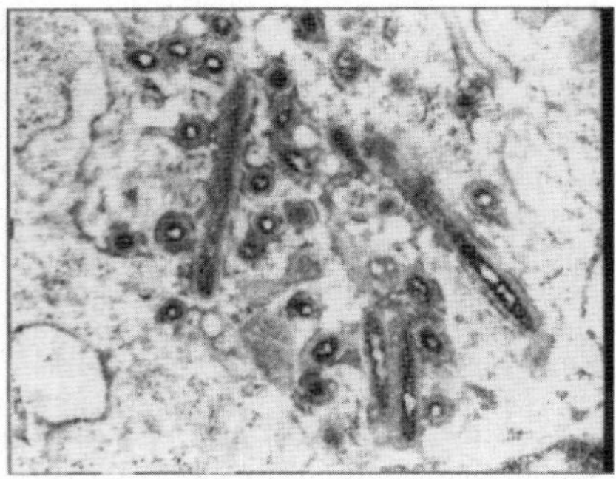

FIG. 46.3 Electron micrograph illustrating numerous rod-shaped bacilliform bodies within the cytoplasm of a macrophage. (×13,750.) (From Tyor MP. Whipple's disease: the Duke connection. *N C Med J.* 1994;55:237–40.)

can be found in other conditions,[28] such as histiocytosis, melanosis coli, and *Mycobacterium avium-intracellulare* infection, and even within macrophages in healthy individuals. The macrophages in Whipple disease do not stain with Ziehl-Neelsen.[26,42] A sickle-shaped appearance of the PAS-positive granules often is present in the macrophages of patients with Whipple disease.[55]

Sieracki and Fine[82] observed systemic involvement in the autopsies of five patients with Whipple disease. The sickle-shaped, PAS-positive macrophages were thought to be specific for Whipple disease, showing involvement of the entire gastrointestinal tract and the pancreas; diffuse involvement of the retroperitoneum and lymph nodes, the adrenals, the liver with sickle-form particles in Kupffer cells and in histiocytes, the brain, the heart, and the visceral pleura of the lungs; and minimal involvement of the genitourinary tract, skeletal muscles, and bone marrow. James and associates[47] examined the vessels of the gastrointestinal system and found abundant bacilli in the arteries of the small intestinal serosa and liver. They noted focal degeneration and fibrosis in the tunica media with arteritis and intimal proliferation. Rickman and coworkers[62] reported a case that confirmed the presence of *T. whipplei* in the vitreous of the eye.

T. whipplei produces a predominantly histiocytic inflammatory reaction, with infiltration by macrophages.[27] Noncaseating, epithelioid cell, sarcoid-like granulomas are located preferentially in peripheral lymph nodes and the liver.[19,27] These granulomas occasionally can be seen in different tissues, including three reports of granulomas in the intestinal tract.[27] Mesenteric lymph nodes often are strikingly enlarged.[15]

Electron microscopy can be useful, often revealing the presence of the rod-shaped bacterium (see Fig. 46.1).[29] Electron microscopy also shows intestinal macrophages containing bacteria with signs of lysis.[83] Silva and associates[83] described steps of a degradative process of the bacillus that starts with disorganization of the surface membrane and the thick outer wall. With the loss of intracellular material, bacterial "ghosts" composed of the three inner layers of the envelope are present. The two electron-dense layers of the cytoplasmic membrane become disorganized and solubilized, leaving the inner dense layer of the cell wall as the final bacterial remnant (Fig. 46.3).

CLINICAL MANIFESTATIONS

The manifestations of *T. whipplei* infections now include at least three forms, "classic" Whipple disease; acute infection, such as gastroenteritis and bacteremia; and asymptomatic carriage (Box 46.1).[20,21]

ACUTE INFECTION

Gastroenteritis

T. whipplei is associated with a mild acute gastroenteritis in young children.[70] Diarrhea typically lasts from 4 to 5 days and is associated with weight loss and 1 to 2 days of fever. Additional side effects include vomiting (55%), abdominal pain (25%), and bloody diarrhea (8%). The infection has no seasonality.

Bacteremia

In rural West Africa, *T. whipplei* was found by PCR in the blood of adults and children with unexplained fever.[30] Patients with *T. whipplei*

BOX 46.1 Clinical Presentations of *T. whipplei* Infection

Acute infection:
- Gastroenteritis
- Bacteremia
- Pneumonia

Asymptomatic carriage
"Classic" Whipple disease

Data from references 1–3, 12, 13.

TABLE 46.1 Major Symptoms and Signs in Classic Whipple Disease

	Cases (%)
Symptoms	
Weight loss	65–100
Chronic diarrhea	60–85
Arthralgia	65–80
Abdominal pain	60
Fever	10–55
CNS-related complaints	10–40
Signs	
Malnutrition	90–95
Hypotension	70
Lymphadenopathy	55
Hyperpigmentation	45–55
Abdominal tenderness	50
Edema	30
Abdominal mass	20
Hepatomegaly	1–14
Splenomegaly	5–10
Ascites	8

CNS, Central nervous system.
Data from references 12, 27, 28, 46, 49.

bacteremia also have associated cough and sleep disorders. The bacteremia has seasonality, occurring primarily during the months of December and January. Fevers are not commonly associated with gastrointestinal symptoms, and patients rarely have PCR-positive stool or saliva.

Pneumonia

Severe cases of pneumonia in adults and children are associated with *T. whipplei*.[10,45] PCR has detected *T. whipplei* in the bronchoalveolar lavage of mechanically ventilated patients in intensive care units. Initial presentations include aspiration pneumonia, community-acquired pneumonia, and ventilator-associated pneumonia. Duration of mechanical ventilation ranges from 3 to 81 days, and the mortality rate is high (33%).

"Classic" Whipple Disease

Whipple disease is viewed best as a multisystem illness. It usually manifests as arthralgias and then progresses to involve the gastrointestinal tract.[6] Malabsorption is the key feature of clinical disease, but no specific signs or symptoms for Whipple disease are known. The major symptoms and signs of Whipple disease are listed in Table 46.1. In children, failure to thrive, malnutrition, and chronic diarrhea appear most frequently. Abdominal distention, abdominal pain, and generalized lymphadenopathy may be found.[2] Response to antibiotic treatment may be dramatic, with rapid weight gain and resolution of symptoms.[5]

Gastrointestinal Tract

One of the most common symptoms is weight loss, which is found in 65% to 100% of patients.[15,25,28,38,55] Weight loss may be the only symptom.[12] Diarrhea is reported in 60% to 85% of patients.[15,28,38,55] The diarrhea usually is watery or fatty.[55] Several mechanisms have been proposed to explain the malabsorption and steatorrhea in Whipple disease.[28] Direct infection and secondary enterocyte dysfunction may prevent the esterification of fatty acids to triglycerides and inhibit the uptake of carbohydrates and amino acids. Blockage of transport of triglyceride-rich chylomicrons into lacteals may result from the deposition of foamy macrophages in the lamina propria. Lymphatic obstruction may occur by involvement of the mesenteric lymph nodes. Malabsorption and diarrhea tend to resolve within a few days after initiation of antibiotic treatment, whereas the lacteal dilation and PAS-positive macrophages can remain for months to years. Occult gastrointestinal bleeding frequently is found, but melena and gross gastrointestinal bleeding are rare. Hematemesis has been reported.[13] Endoscopy revealed diffuse hemorrhagic duodenitis with bleeding on contact.

Abdominal pain is experienced by 60% of patients.[15,28,38,55] The pain is nonspecific, is generally epigastric, and may be worse after meals.[55] Abdominal pain and anorexia may lead to reduced calorie intake and further weight loss.[28] Abdominal distention occurs commonly and may be secondary to intraabdominal lymphadenopathy or to thickening of loops of diseased intestine.[28,55] Ascites occasionally is seen and may be chylous, secondary to lymphatic obstruction.[12,28]

Joints

Arthralgia, the most frequent nongastrointestinal symptom in Whipple disease,[28,55] is present in 65% of adult cases.[55] Arthralgia may precede manifestation of gastrointestinal symptoms by many years or decades[28,51] and occurs less frequently in children. Generally joint symptoms continue unchanged with the onset of gastrointestinal symptoms.[28] Acute migratory arthralgia or arthritis may last days or weeks[38,42,55] and may persist as the disease progresses. The involved joints, in decreasing order of frequency, are knees, ankles, hips, fingers, wrists, elbows, hands, and spine.[28] Examination may reveal joint pain, swelling, limited range of motion, and warmth.[78] Fever sometimes is present.[28] Spondylitis, with or without sacroiliitis, may develop.[5] Permanent joint destruction and deformity are uncommon occurrences but can be severe.[28,78] Arthrocentesis may reveal an inflammatory arthritis, with cell counts of 6000 to 75,000/mm^3, often with a polymorphonuclear leukocyte predominance.[28] Synovial biopsy may show PAS-positive macrophages.[28]

Central Nervous System

Whipple disease can be confined to the brain[76] but usually is accompanied by other manifestations.[38] CNS and neurologic manifestations, such as headache, diplopia, meningoencephalitis, depression, confusion, and personality changes, are uncommon manifestations[15,28,55] but may be significant.[15,28,37,55,64,66] The spectrum of potential CNS involvement is listed in Box 46.2.

Eye

Indirect involvement of the CNS and direct involvement of the eye can produce visual problems.[28] Ophthalmoplegia and diplopia can occur with involvement of cranial nerves III, IV, and VI.[26] Reduced visual acuity and papilledema can occur with compromise of the optic nerve.[28] Numerous ophthalmologic findings, including vasculitis, vitreitis, optic atrophy, uveitis, chorioretinitis, vitreous opacities, glaucoma, keratitis, retinal hemorrhages, disk edema, and lacrimal duct obstruction, have been reported.[28,91,92] Rickman and associates[74] reported a case of ocular disease without marked CNS or gastrointestinal disease.

Skin

Hyperpigmentation of the skin in sun-exposed areas occurs in roughly half of cases.[37,55] The mechanism of hyperpigmentation is uncertain but is not related to adrenal insufficiency.[28] Subcutaneous nodules may be found and can reveal PAS-positive macrophages and bacilli on electron microscopy.[41]

Heart

The heart frequently is involved in Whipple disease. Endocarditis, myocarditis, pericarditis, pancarditis, and coronary arteritis have been found.[28,59,90] A blood culture–negative endocarditis may be caused by Whipple disease.[28] Chronic aortic regurgitation is the most common clinical finding of endocardial involvement.[28] Pericarditis with polyserositis (pleuritis, peritonitis) has been found.[36] The abnormalities on

BOX 46.2 Central Nervous System Symptoms and Signs of Classic Whipple Disease

Ataxia
Confusion
Convulsions
Dementia
Depression
Diplopia
Dizziness
Facial pain
Headache
Hearing loss
Hemiparesis
Hyperphagia
Hyperreflexia (± Babinski sign)
Incoordination
Lethargy, coma
Loss of vibratory and position sense
Meningoencephalitis
Mental and personality changes
Motor weakness
Muscle jerks and twitches
Muscle rigidity
Numbness
Nystagmus
Ophthalmoplegia
Papilledema
Polydipsia
Ptosis
Pupillary abnormalities
Sensory loss
Sleep disorders
Slurred speech
Stiff neck
Tinnitus
Visual difficulties (diplopia, blurring)

electrocardiogram are nonspecific but include first-degree atrioventricular block, left ventricular hypertrophy, sinus tachycardia, left bundle branch block, intraventricular conduction delay, old inferior wall infarct, and short PR interval.[37] Sossai and associates[85] reported a case of regression of a right bundle branch block after treatment with antibiotics, but the block spontaneously recurred 2 years later.

Skeletal Muscle

Skeletal muscle may be involved, diagnosed by electromyography or muscle biopsy.[87] Proximal muscle weakness occurs most commonly. Muscle biopsy reveals a nonspecific myopathy.

Lymph Nodes and Spleen

Whipple disease may involve any lymph node in the body.[28] Mesenteric lymph nodes frequently are involved, and splenomegaly is found in 5% to 10% of cases.[55]

Lungs

Cough, pleuritic chest pain, and dyspnea have been reported.[88] Pleural involvement may appear as a pleural rub. Pleural adhesions and granulomas have been reported at autopsy.[5,88] Chest radiography often reveals pleural thickening, parenchymal shadowing, and elevation of the diaphragm.[88] Lung function tests may show decreased lung volumes.[88]

Kidney

Renal involvement in Whipple disease is rare.[28] Granulomas have been found, however, as has focal glomerulonephritis.[49]

Blood

Anemia occurs commonly and usually is of a hypochromic, microcytic variety.[28,37,38] Macrocytic anemia caused by malabsorption of folate also may be seen. Leukocytosis, thrombocytosis,[65] and bone marrow involvement may be found.[71] Low serum iron concentration and an elevated erythrocyte sedimentation rate frequently are seen.[37] A single case of extraintestinal lymphoma in association with Whipple disease found at autopsy has been reported.[40]

DIAGNOSIS

Despite the successful culture of the organism in 2000,[69] no specific diagnostic tests have been developed. Anemia and low albumin level probably are most common, being found in approximately 90% of patients. Low serum iron and folate concentrations are seen in approximately 30% of cases. Hypokalemia, hypocalcemia, low cholesterol and carotene, prolonged prothrombin time, and increased transaminase levels are less common findings. Elevated fecal fat is found in more than 90% of cases. The D-xylose malabsorption test result frequently is abnormal.

Barium x-ray studies of the small bowel may show marked thickening of the mucosal folds and separation of bowel loops, suggesting a malabsorptive disease. These findings usually resolve completely with successful antibiotic therapy. For CNS Whipple disease, characteristic abnormalities seen on computed tomography of the brain include atrophy, focal gray matter lesions, hydrocephalus, and white matter alterations.[89]

A key feature in the histologic diagnosis of Whipple disease is the accumulation of periodic acid–Schiff-positive, diastase-resistant macrophages in the lamina propria of the small intestine.[5,37,56] These findings are not pathognomonic, and infection with *M. avium-intracellulare* must be excluded.[56] *T. whipplei* does not stain acid-fast,[56] whereas mycobacteria are identified readily. Small bowel involvement by *M. avium* complex can have endoscopic, histologic, and radiographic findings similar to those of Whipple disease.[68] Periodic acid–Schiff-positive macrophages occasionally can be seen in the mucosa of the large bowel and rectum in unrelated diseases, such as histiocytosis, and in benign conditions, such as melanosis coli and pneumatosis intestinalis.[56] Although electron microscopy can confirm the diagnosis by visualization of the characteristic bacillus,[38,83] immunohistochemistry has shown to be not only more efficient, but also more sensitive and specific than periodic acid–Schiff in the diagnosis and monitoring of *T. whipplei* infection.[4,52] Using a polyclonal rabbit antibody produced against *T. whipplei*, Baisden and associates[4] were the first to show sensitivity equal to periodic acid–Schiff without cross-reactivity with other bacterial species.

Endoscopy of the small bowel may be helpful because characteristic lesions may be seen and biopsy specimens can be obtained. No clear data suggest where the intestinal specimens should be taken[56] because intestinal involvement usually is patchy. Random biopsy samples of the small bowel are suggested, beginning at the ligament of Treitz.[60] Endoscopic findings include yellow-white plaques and an erythematous, erosive, friable mucosa.[39] Similar findings have been described on capsule endoscopy, which may aid in diagnosis as the disease can present with discontinuous changes to the small intestine.[18]

PCR amplification may be used to detect and identify bacterial pathogens. To set up a PCR, the only prerequisite information is the nucleotide sequences flanking each end of the target.[72] PCR has become an important method for establishing the diagnosis of Whipple disease. It may be especially helpful if the histopathologic examination findings are normal or in patients with unusual extraintestinal involvement. Specific identification of *T. whipplei* can be achieved by amplification of the 1321-base-pair bacterial, 16S ribosomal RNA gene isolated from infected tissue.[73] Muller and associates[63] applied this PCR technique to show *T. whipplei* in peripheral blood mononuclear cells and cells derived from pleural effusion in a patient with Whipple disease. PCR techniques have been used to detect *T. whipplei* in erythrocytes,[54] cerebrospinal fluid,[7] and resected heart valves with infective endocarditis.[12,14,63]

Sloan and colleagues[84] reported another real-time PCR method using a 213-base-pair target sequence of the heat shock protein *(hsp65)* gene of *T. whipplei.* The sensitivity, specificity, and positive and negative values of this LightCycler real-time PCR were compared with the conventional 16S rRNA gene sequence PCR assay and were 98% (sensitivity), 99% (specificity), 94% (positive), and 100% (negative). The completion time of the LightCycler assay was approximately 5 hours, which was significantly less than the 2 to 3 days required for the traditional PCR assay.[84]

The diagnostic utility of PCR in Whipple disease is clear, but it cannot be taken as the sole basis for diagnosis. Ehrbar and associates[27] studied the specificity of PCR for *T. whipplei.* They performed elective gastroscopy on patients without known Whipple disease. PCR analysis was positive in 4.8% of duodenal biopsy specimens and 11.4% of gastric juice samples. Compared with the gold standard of histology and clinical signs, the specificity of PCR for *T. whipplei* was 95.2% for duodenal biopsy specimens and 88.6% for gastric juice. These findings suggest that *T. whipplei* or a closely related bacterium may be present in some people without known Whipple disease. Street and colleagues[86] detected *T. whipplei* DNA by PCR in the saliva of 35% of 40 healthy adults tested, which suggests that this organism can be an oral commensal.

In a study by Fenollar and associates,[29] when real-time PCR detection of *T. whipplei* in saliva and stool were combined, the positive predictive value of the patient having Whipple disease was 95.2%. Additionally if the bacterial load in the stool was more than 10^4 colony-forming units (CFU)/g, the positive predictive value increased to 100%. Conversely, classic Whipple disease was unlikely in patients with saliva or stool specimens negative for *T. whipplei* by real-time PCR, having a negative predictive value of 99.2%. The authors argue that, following these negative results, additional specific investigations for classic Whipple disease could be stopped. Localized Whipple disease was poorly detected by PCR of the saliva and stool samples, with a sensitivity of only 58%.

TREATMENT

Antibiotics are the mainstay of therapy for Whipple disease.[15] In vitro antibiotic susceptibility testing using real-time PCR has identified penicillin, doxycycline, macrolides, ketolides, rifampin, aminoglycosides, teicoplanin, chloramphenicol, and trimethoprim-sulfamethoxazole (TMP-SMX) as having activity.[8,9,58] Current antibiotic treatment strategies are empirical, based only on the accumulated anecdotal experience. Generally response to antibiotics is good and often dramatic. Symptoms such as diarrhea quickly resolve, and weight gain is rapid. Several antibiotics that have been tried alone or in combination include chloramphenicol, penicillin, streptomycin, ampicillin, TMP-SMX, erythromycin, and doxycycline.[15,28,35,38] Keinath and associates[48] analyzed the antibiotic response rate of 88 patients with documented Whipple disease. Thirty-one patients experienced relapse, with a mean time to relapse of 4.2 years after initial diagnosis. CNS relapse occurred in 13 of 88, and all CNS and cardiac relapses were late (Table 46.2). In addition to diagnosis, PCR may prove useful in the monitoring of response to antibiotic therapy.[43,67] Disease relapse may be secondary to genetic mutations in *T. whipplei.* Fenollar and associates[31] discovered amino acid changes in the *T. whipplei folP* gene, which encodes dihydropteroate synthase, the target of sulfonamides. Two amino acid positions, N4S and S234F, significantly predicted treatment failure to sulfamethoxazole.

All patients with Whipple disease should receive antibiotics that penetrate the blood-brain barrier.[48,77] Tetracycline and penicillin do not penetrate the blood-brain barrier well, unless the meninges are inflamed.[77] The preferred treatment in adults and children is TMP-SMX given orally twice a day for 1 year.[77] If the small bowel is involved, repeated small bowel biopsy is suggested at least 6 months to 1 year after treatment to document the disappearance of the bacillus. For patients who do not tolerate TMP-SMX, penicillin or ampicillin is recommended. Levy and associates[53] described a case of acquired resistance to TMP-SMX that responded to oral penicillin. Feurle and Marth[35] noted that TMP-SMX was more efficacious than tetracycline in inducing clinical remission of Whipple disease. They observed the development of aqueductal stenosis with hydrocephalus in a patient receiving TMP-SMX treatment, however, and indicated that even TMP-SMX is no safeguard against cerebral recurrence.

TABLE 46.2 Treatment of Whipple Disease: Initial Antibiotic Regimen and Relapse

Antibiotics	No. Patients	Total No. Relapses	CNS Relapses
TCN[a] alone	49	21	9[b]
PCN + STM + TCN[a]	15	2	0
PCN/PCN[a]	8	3	2
PCN + STM	5	2	0
TMP-SMX[a]	3	0	0
Other	8	3	2
Total	*88*	*31*	*13*

CNS, Central nervous system; *PCN*, penicillin; *STM*, streptomycin; *TCN*, tetracycline; *TMP-SMX*, trimethoprim-sulfamethoxazole.
[a]Oral therapy.
[b]Includes two patients treated with TCN only in whom CNS relapse was the second relapse.
Data from Keinath RD, Merrell DE, Vlietstra R, et al. Antibiotic treatment and relapse in Whipple's disease: long-term follow-up of 88 patients. *Gastroenterology.* 1985;88:1867–73.

Treatment with IV antibiotics before a course of TMP-SMX may improve remission rates. In a randomized control trial, Feurle and associates[34] studied the use of ceftriaxone or meropenem IV for 2 weeks before initiating a 1-year course of TMP-SMX. At a 3-year follow-up, all 38 subjects, except for one with asymptomatic CNS infection with *T. whipplei,* had clinical and biopsy evidence of disease remission.

In 2014, Lagier and associates reported on their experience treating 29 patients with classic Whipple disease in France.[50] They report no treatment failure in 13 patients when treated with either doxycycline and hydroxychloroquine, or doxycycline, hydroxychloroquine, and TMP-SMX. However 100% of the 14 patients treated with only TMP-SMX had treatment failure. They theorize that their finding may be different from results in other studies because of differences in strain susceptibility or genetic differences in the hosts. Based on these findings, they recommend a treatment regimen of doxycycline and hydroxychloroquine for 1 year, followed by lifelong doxycycline with stringent drug monitoring. Further population-specific studies may help clarify optimal treatment regimes.

CNS relapse has a poor prognosis.[11,28,35,38,48] Feurle and Marth[35] suggested an experimental therapy for CNS recurrence with a highly active bactericidal compound, such as a third-generation cephalosporin, a quinolone, or intrathecal antibiotic therapy, that readily crosses the blood–brain barrier. In adult patients, Keinath and associates[48] recommended treatment with parenteral penicillin 1.2 million units daily plus streptomycin 1 g daily for 10 to 14 days, followed by TMP-SMX one double-strength tablet twice daily for 1 year. Because of the extreme rarity of the occurrence of Whipple disease in children, prudent management dictates long-term surveillance after resolution of symptoms.

Because Whipple disease is a malabsorptive disorder, the patient's nutritional needs must be assessed carefully. Specific attention must be paid to replacement of any vitamin or mineral deficiencies. Iron, folate, vitamin D, and calcium typically are given until the steatorrhea resolves.

CONCLUSION

T. whipplei appears ubiquitous in our environment but appears to only rarely cause disease. It is involved in not only classic Whipple disease but also in acute infection and asymptomatic carriage. These findings suggest a genetic predisposition to classic Whipple disease, but causative genes or immune factors have not yet been identified.

NEW REFERENCES SINCE THE SEVENTH EDITION

18. de Roulet J, Hassan MO, Cummings LC. Capsule endoscopy in Whipple's disease. *Clin Gastroenterol Hepatol.* 2013;11:A26.
50. Lagier J-C, Fenollar F, Lepidi H, et al. Treatment of classic Whipple's disease: from in vitro results to clinical outcome. *J Antimicrob Chemother.* 2014;69:219-227.

The full reference list for this chapter is available at ExpertConsult.com.

47 Hepatitis

Samer S. El-Kamary • Ravi Jhaveri

Hepatitis, or inflammation of the liver, may be caused by primarily hepatotropic agents such hepatitis A, B, C, D, and E viruses that produce disease almost exclusively in the liver, whereas other agents, such as cytomegalovirus (CMV), Epstein-Barr virus (EBV), adenovirus, and the hemorrhagic fever viruses, produce hepatitis as part of a systemic or disseminated illness. Hepatitis may be subclinical or silent, or symptomatic with acute or chronic clinically manifest hepatitis, and may progress to fulminant or fatal disease.[69] Both immunocompetent and immunocompromised children of all ages may contract infectious hepatitis, and their age, immune status, and history of exposure may provide clues to identification of the most likely etiologic agent. Noninfectious causes such as autoimmune disease, storage and metabolic disorders, toxins, medications, or other chemicals are also important causes of hepatitis and liver injury in children. Hepatic steatosis associated with childhood obesity and type 2 diabetes is a rapidly growing public health concern. Vasculitis, cardiac disease, hypoxic injury, or trauma also may damage the liver.

Presented in this chapter is a general approach to an infant or child with hepatitis or hepatic dysfunction from an infectious perspective. Detailed information regarding the diagnosis and management of each particular pathogen can be found in the respective chapters in the section of this textbook dedicated to infections with specific microorganisms.

HISTORY

The earliest descriptions of outbreaks of hepatitis in the ancient world most likely involved hepatitis A virus (HAV), and it was known as epidemic *jaundice* and *catarrhal jaundice* or *acute yellow atrophy of the liver* if the disease was severe or fulminant.[25] The earliest recorded outbreak in the United States occurred in Norfolk, Virginia, in 1812.[12] During wartime, outbreaks of "camp jaundice" or "field jaundice" occurred and probably were caused by HAV, yellow fever, or leptospirosis. Not until 1973 was the cause of "infectious hepatitis" determined to be a 27-nm, nonenveloped viral particle, originally designated enterovirus 72, now known as HAV.[40] Infection with hepatitis B virus (HBV) has a relatively more recent history. The earliest description was in the late 1880s in an epidemiologic study published by Luerman in 1885 in Germany, where an outbreak of prolonged hepatitis was described in shipyard and warehouse workers who received smallpox vaccine contaminated with human material.[79] Other outbreaks of "serum hepatitis" have been described in association with percutaneous therapies, such as gold for rheumatoid arthritis or contaminated vaccines stabilized with human serum.[2,15,62] In the early 1970s, the HBV infectious particle in serum was called the Dane particle. Subsequently the Australian (Au) antigen (discovered in the blood of an Australian aborigine), now known as the hepatitis B surface antigen (HBsAg), was characterized and subsequently used to diagnose HBV.[17,123,154] Soon after, parenterally transmitted "non-A, non-B hepatitis" was described and subsequently identified in 1989 as the hepatitis C virus (HCV).[22,124,146] The 1970s also marked the discovery of hepatitis delta virus (HDV), a "defective helper virus" that replicates only in the presence of HBV and is associated with chronic or fulminant hepatitis.[129,130] In the 1990s, another enterically transmitted non-A, non-B hepatitis virus was found to be associated with outbreaks of infectious hepatitis in developing parts of the world.[13,53] It was characterized originally as a calicivirus-like particle and subsequently named hepatitis E virus (HEV).[128]

CLINICAL MANIFESTATIONS AND EVALUATION

Patient History

The clinical approach to evaluating and managing a child with hepatitis includes careful attention to the age at presentation; initial signs and symptoms; history of exposure to potential pathogens, toxins, or medications; the presence of underlying conditions; travel to endemic areas; vaccination history; family history of intravenous drug use or liver or metabolic disorders; or behavioral risk factors (intravenous drug use, unprotected sexual contact [male-female, male-male]). Presenting symptoms in older children with acute hepatitis are nonspecific and may include fever, vomiting, anorexia or aversion to specific foods, change in taste and smell, lethargy and malaise, weight loss, dark urine, pale stool, jaundice, icterus, or even pruritus. Abdominal pain is a common complaint and is usually mild, dull, or aching; located in the right upper quadrant; and unaffected by meals, body position, or defecation. Often an antecedent viral syndrome or "flulike" illness is noted 7 to 14 days before the onset of hepatitis. Rarely a "serum sickness–like syndrome" may occur at the onset of the illness, before jaundice occurs, and is characterized by fever, rash, and arthritis. In contrast, neonates and young children rarely have signs and symptoms from infection with hepatotropic viruses and are more likely to have clinical disease with agents that cause congenital or perinatal infection, such as CMV, herpes simplex virus (HSV), rubella virus, parvovirus B19, or *Treponema pallidum,* especially if extrahepatic signs such as splenomegaly, skin lesions, microcephaly, or hearing loss are present. Neonates and young infants often become seriously ill with multisystem involvement that accompanies disseminated HSV, enteroviruses, or adenoviruses and show signs of acute, massive hepatocellular necrosis. These signs can include irritability or lethargy, jaundice, ascites, abdominal distention, hepatomegaly, acholic stools, anasarca, and coagulopathy. Patients from developing countries with a personal or maternal history of blood transfusions should be screened for HBV, HCV, HDV, and CMV, whereas attendance at summer camp or an institutional environment coupled with a lack of vaccination might warrant HAV screening. Recent treatment with antifungal azoles, antibiotics (macrolides, cyclines, isoniazid), antiepileptics, or even hepatotoxic over-the-counter medications such as acetaminophen may suggest drug-induced hepatitis.[100,161] Exposure of older children to feral kittens can be suggestive of infection with *Bartonella henselae* or *Toxoplasma gondii.* Children receiving cancer chemotherapy may have drug-induced hepatitis, and those who have experienced prolonged neutropenia may have fungal disease of the liver. Children with fulminant hepatitis are critically ill and initially may have persistent fever, protracted nausea and vomiting, severe abdominal pain, worsening jaundice, fluid retention with ascites, easy bruising, bleeding, and encephalopathy with seizures or coma. Patients with chronic hepatitis, on the other hand, often are clinically asymptomatic unless complications such as cirrhosis or chronic liver failure develop.

Physical Findings

Physical examination of a child with hepatitis should focus on the abdomen, liver, and spleen but also should include a careful evaluation for extrahepatic manifestations of systemic disease. Tender hepatomegaly, with or without ascites, scleral icterus, and jaundice, is often noted on physical examination of patients with acute hepatitis. Percussion over the right lower part of the thorax may produce right upper quadrant pain. Fever may or may not be present. Extrahepatic physical findings associated with the hepatotropic viruses, especially HAV, HBV, and HCV, include systemic vasculitis with rash or urticaria, polyarthralgia, and polyarthritis, similar to serum sickness or polyarteritis nodosa. A generalized papular rash, known as *Gianotti disease*, may accompany HBV infection, especially in young children. Rarely a patient with acute viral hepatitis may exhibit Raynaud phenomenon, bullous lesions, or erythema nodosa on the extensor surfaces. Skin excoriations may be present if jaundice-associated pruritus is severe, and older children and adolescents may have vascular spiders or exacerbation of acne. A child who also has conjunctivitis, pneumonitis, and a maculopapular rash may have disseminated adenoviral disease. Generalized lymphadenopathy accompanied by pharyngitis and splenomegaly, in contrast, suggests systemic infection with CMV or EBV. Idiosyncratic reactions involving the liver may occur at any time; however, drug-related hypersensitivity hepatitis occurs 1 to 5 weeks after exposure to the agent and usually is accompanied by rash and fever on examination and evidence of nephritis, eosinophilia, and neutropenia. Neonates with acute fulminant hepatitis from disseminated HSV, enteroviruses, or adenoviruses may have fever or hypothermia, respiratory distress, abdominal distention, coagulopathy, myocarditis, seizure-like activity, or a sepsis-like syndrome. Physical examination of a child with fulminant hepatitis and liver failure may actually reveal a normal or small liver with new-onset irritability, confusion, lethargy, or personality changes. As hepatic failure ensues, the patient may become deeply jaundiced, icteric, and encephalopathic with hyperreflexia, decerebrate posturing, involuntary movements, and asterixis or may even become comatose. A distinctive sweet, fecal smell (also called *fetor hepaticus*) likely from ammonia, mercaptans, and ketones shunted from the liver to the lungs of a patient also may be appreciated by an astute observer. Physical examination of a child with chronic hepatitis, on the other hand, may reveal a normal or enlarged liver with splenomegaly. Splenomegaly is often the hallmark of portal hypertension related to chronic liver disease. If the child is obese, fatty infiltration of the liver should be considered as a cause of liver inflammation and dysfunction.

Laboratory Diagnosis

Laboratory evaluation of a child with acute hepatitis should include general blood and urine chemistries (complete blood cell count with differential, electrolytes, blood urea nitrogen, creatinine, urinalysis), tests of hepatic function (albumin, glucose, ammonia, coagulopathy panel, factors V and VII), and tests of hepatic inflammation/obstruction (serum aspartate aminotransferase and alanine aminotransferase [AST/ALT], alkaline phosphatase, γ-glutamyltranspeptidase, bilirubin). Serologic tests (i.e., HAV IgM, HBsAg, HCV Ab), cultures, or detection assays (i.e., HCV RNA quantitative polymerase chain reaction [PCR]) for specific pathogens of interest according to the patient's screening laboratory results, history, or physical findings should also be pursued. Neonates with elevated aminotransferase levels should be tested for enterovirus and herpes simplex virus with PCR of blood and CSF to assess for viremia and meningoencephalitis.

In many forms of viral hepatitis, the white blood cell count may be low, usually between 3000 and 4000/mm^3.[1] Atypical lymphocytes also may be seen. Eosinophilia suggests a drug hypersensitivity reaction. If significant leukocytosis is present, sepsis or fulminant hepatitis should be considered. A rising creatinine value may indicate development of hepatorenal syndrome. Urinalysis may reveal dark urine and the presence of urobilinogen. Hematuria with casts or other signs of nephritis in an older child may signify an autoimmune disorder or a drug-induced process as the cause of the hepatitis.

The hepatic aminotransferases, including AST and ALT, will be elevated in patients with acute hepatitis, often before the onset of clinical symptoms. Most forms of acute hepatitis will be accompanied by elevations of 500 IU/mL or greater. A neonate with aminotransferase levels higher than 1000 IU/mL may have a potentially life-threatening infection with bacterial sepsis, HSV, enterovirus, or adenovirus. Similarly older children with fulminant hepatitis or hepatic necrosis may have significantly elevated aminotransferase levels. These values may begin to fall after reaching a pinnacle; however, if the γ-glutamyltranspeptidase or conjugated bilirubin level continues to rise, this may indicate disease progression with massive hepatocyte necrosis rather than improvement. Prothrombin time, international normalized ratio, and albumin and glucose levels usually are normal in cases of uncomplicated acute viral hepatitis, but if coagulation factors become prolonged and hypoalbuminemia and hypoglycemia persist, fulminant hepatitis should be considered. Direct markers of hepatic synthetic function such as factors V and VII will also be low in the setting of liver failure. Serum bilirubin, both conjugated and unconjugated, may be elevated, but it is rarely higher than 4 mg/dL unless fulminant hepatitis with hepatic failure is present. Exceptions to this rule include patients with underlying hemolytic states such as glucose-6-dehydrogenase deficiency or sickle-cell disease; such patients may exhibit marked jaundice and high indirect hyperbilirubinemia even if the viral hepatitis otherwise is mild. Some patients will have low levels of nonspecific autoantibodies, such as an elevated homogeneous pattern of antinuclear antibodies, decreased complement levels, or false-positive Venereal Disease Research Laboratory (VDRL) test reactions. The erythrocyte sedimentation rate usually is normal or slightly increased in acute viral hepatitis.

Laboratory investigation to determine the specific cause of the patient's hepatitis includes an evaluation for the hepatotropic viruses. This often includes detection of serum HBsAg and hepatitis B core antibody (HBcAb; IgM), serum hepatitis A virus antibody (HAV Ab; IgM), serum hepatitis C antibody (HCV Ab), serum hepatitis D antibody (HDV Ab) especially if the hepatitis is fulminant, and hepatitis E antibody (HEV Ab) if the travel history suggests exposure).[4,5] Because they progress to chronic infection, both HBV and HCV can be detected with real-time PCR testing. PCR-based testing is not useful for the acute hepatitis viruses because the viremia precedes clinical symptoms. Many of the nonhepatitis viruses may be identified by serologic tests that detect virus-specific IgM antibody or by fourfold rises in viral-specific IgG antibody. In certain circumstances, isolation of the specific viral agent in cell culture or detection of viral nucleic acid by PCR in blood, cerebrospinal fluid, body fluids such as saliva or stool, or liver tissue provides the confirmatory evidence. Bacterial pathogens may be detected by culture for agents associated with granulomatous hepatitis, such as *Brucella* and *Mycobacterium*, or by a variety of culture, serology, or appropriate skin tests. In neonates, gram-negative enteric organisms (e.g., *Escherichia coli*) identified from the blood or urine are common causes of jaundice and hepatic dysfunction. Noninfectious causes of hepatitis should also be considered. Autoimmune hepatitis may be identified by persistent hypergammaglobulinemia and the presence of autoantibodies, such as F-actin and anti–liver-kidney-microsome antibodies (anti-LKM). Laboratory tests that evaluate for metabolic diseases include serum amino acids and urine-reducing substances and organic acids, sweat chloride testing for cystic fibrosis, α_1-antitrypsin levels and protease inhibitor typing, serum ceruloplasmin and 24-hour urine collection for copper to rule out Wilson disease, and an iron panel for hemochromatosis. Acute hepatotoxicity from overdose of acetaminophen may be predicted from elevated acetaminophen levels. A urine or serum toxicology screen can assess for other toxic substances. Anatomic causes of hepatic dysfunction, such as biliary atresia in infants and hepatic tumors or steatosis in older children, usually require diagnostic imaging such as ultrasonography or liver biopsy for diagnosis.

INFECTIOUS CAUSES

Viruses

Hepatitis Viruses

Five hepatotropic viruses are known to cause infectious viral hepatitis in children: hepatitis A, B, C, D, and E (Box 47.1).

Hepatitis A virus. HAV (see Chapter 168) is a member of the Picornaviridae and formerly was known as enterovirus 72.[86] A small, nonenveloped RNA virus with icosahedral symmetry (Fig. 47.1), HAV is transmitted by the fecal-oral route among young and school-aged children receiving care in group settings such as daycare, summer camp, schools, and institutions.[28,45,64] The incubation period is 30 days but ranges from 15 to 50 days. HAV infection in young children often is asymptomatic, and outbreaks in children are recognized first when symptoms occur in adult caretakers. Older children are more likely to have the classic symptoms of nausea, malaise, jaundice, and tender hepatomegaly. Rarely HAV causes fulminant hepatitis. Acute HAV infection is diagnosed serologically by detecting HAV IgM antibody in serum. No licensed,

BOX 47.1 Causes of Hepatitis in Children

Infectious

Viral

Primary hepatotropic
- Hepatitis A virus
- Hepatitis B virus
- Hepatitis C virus
- Hepatitis D virus
- Hepatitis E virus

DNA viruses
- Adenovirus
- Cytomegalovirus
- Epstein-Barr virus
- Erythrovirus (human parvovirus B-19)
- Herpes B virus
- Herpes simplex viruses 1 and 2
- Human herpesviruses 6, 7, and 8
- Varicella zoster virus

RNA viruses
- Enteroviruses
- Hemorrhagic fever viruses
- Human immunodeficiency virus
- Measles virus
- Rubella virus
- Syncytial giant-cell hepatitis

Bacterial

Atypical mycobacteria
Bacille Calmette-Guérin (BCG)
Bacillus cereus toxin
Bartonella henselae and *Bartonella quintana*
Brucella spp.
Listeria monocytogenes
Mycobacterium tuberculosis
Sepsis syndrome with cholestatic jaundice
Urinary tract infection in neonates

Spirochetes
- *Leptospira* species
- *Treponema pallidum*

Rickettsiae
- *Coxiella burnetii*

Parasites

Ascaris lumbricoides
Entamoeba histolytica
Plasmodium spp.
Toxoplasma gondii

Fungal

Aspergillus spp.
Candida spp.
Cryptococcus neoformans
Histoplasma capsulatum

Noninfectious

Anoxic liver damage
Autoimmune hepatitis
Biliary atresia
Drugs and toxins
Hemophagocytic syndrome
Histiocytosis
Kawasaki disease
Lymphoma
Metabolic and genetic disorders
Obesity with hepatic steatosis (fatty infiltration)
Reye syndrome
Sarcoidosis
Sickle-cell crisis
Toxic shock syndrome
Tumors

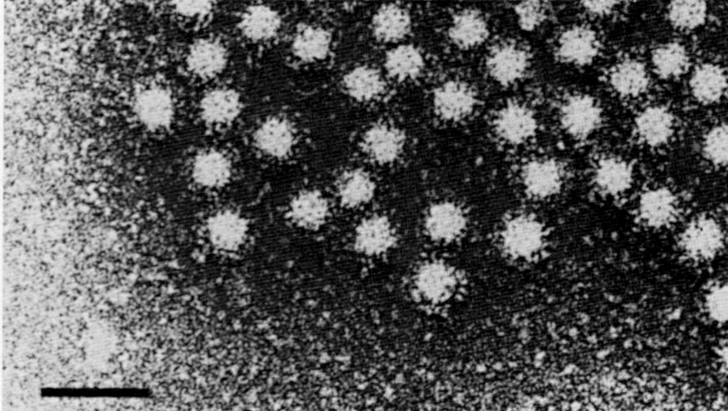

FIG. 47.1 A 27-nm hepatitis A virus (HAV) isolated from the stool filtrate of a patient with acute HAV infection. The HAV particles are aggregated by convalescent serum containing anti-HAV antibodies. The line represents 100 nm. (Courtesy Dr. Jules Dienstag, Laboratory of Infectious Diseases, National Institute of Allergy and Infectious Diseases, National Institutes of Health, Department of Health and Human Services, Bethesda, MD.)

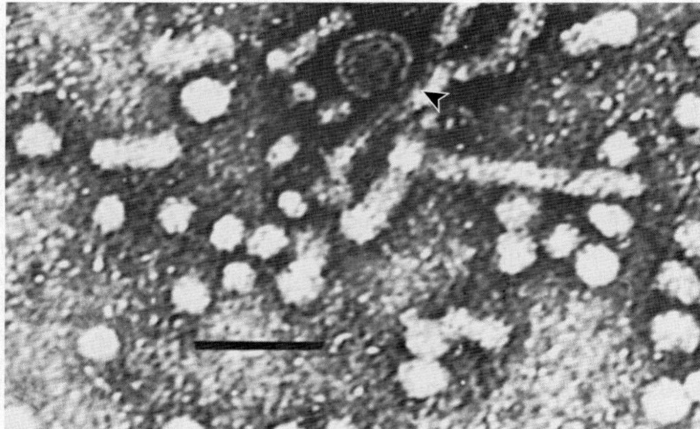

FIG. 47.2 Electron micrograph of hepatitis B virus particles. Most particles are 20 to 25 nm in diameter and consist of both spheres and tubules. A larger, 42-nm Dane particle also is present *(arrowhead)*. Hepatitis B surface antigen determinants are present on the surface of all three forms.

specific antiviral treatment is available. However, prevention may be accomplished by passive immunization with immune globulin or active immunization with licensed inactivated HAV vaccines.[44] Two monovalent HAV vaccines are approved and recommended for all children 12 months of age or older in a two-dose series in the United States.[103]

Hepatitis B virus. HBV (see Chapter 157), previously known as the *Dane particle* and *hepadnavirus type 1*, is a member of the Hepadnaviridae and is a DNA virus that is a 42-nm, nonenveloped spherical particle (Fig. 47.2).[86] There are eight known genotypes, of which A through D are the most predominant in the United States. It is highly transmissible through parenteral exposure to blood or blood products, organ transplantation, or intravenous drug use; it is also transmissible sexually and perinatally.[45] The incubation period is prolonged, usually 90 days, with a range of 45 to 180 days reported. Neonates may acquire HBV vertically from HBV-infected mothers, especially those who are positive for hepatitis Be antigen (HBeAg) and/or those with very high HBV DNA levels ($>10^7$).[72] Whereas neonates and toddlers rarely are symptomatic, older children and adults may have mild to moderate symptoms of acute hepatitis or progress to fulminant or fatal disease. HBV also is a common cause of chronic hepatitis in children, with 10% of older children and adults infected with HBV being affected. The figure rises to approximately 30% in infancy or early childhood and reaches a striking 90% to 95% in infants born to HBeAg-positive mothers.

Acute hepatitis B is diagnosed serologically by the presence of HBsAg and hepatitis B core antibody (HBcAb), which can identify infected patients in the window period. HBV DNA also may be detected and quantified in serum by PCR during acute hepatitis. Individuals with HBeAg in their serum are highly infectious. Diagnosis of chronic HBV requires a combination of persistent clinical symptoms and laboratory abnormalities and persistence of HBsAg and/or HBV DNA for at least 6 months. Primary hepatocellular carcinoma also is a long-term complication of HBV infection. Successful resolution of infection with HBV is marked serologically by the presence of antibody to HBsAg, known as hepatitis B surface antibody (HBsAb). For children with chronic HBV, the decision to treat is largely based on ALT level, HBV viral load, and liver histology.[61] Treatment of children is still controversial and should be considered for children with persistently elevated ALT levels for at least 6 months (12 months if HBeAg negative) in order to avoid treating patients who are undergoing spontaneous HBeAg seroconversion.[139] First-line therapy remains interferon-α in children with immune active chronic HBV.[24] In cases where interferon-α is not recommended, or in compensated or decompensated cirrhosis, treatment with nucleos(t)ide analogues such as entecavir for children older than 2 years of age or tenofovir for children older than 12 years of age is recommended.[24,67] Liver transplantation has been attempted in patients with end-stage HBV-associated cirrhosis, with variable results. Prevention is achieved by passive immunization with hepatitis B immune globulin (HBIG) in the delivery room and active immunization with licensed recombinant vaccines.[83] Pregnant women with chronic hepatitis B should have their HBV viral load and HBeAg status determined to assess their risk for vertical transmission. All infants born to infected women should receive hepatitis B immunoglobulin (HBIG) at delivery and a vaccination within 12 hours of birth.[83] The standard of care for prophylaxis of HBV vertical transmission is evolving, with tenofovir or telbivudine administration to mothers having HBV DNA with more than 10^5 copies continuing during pregnancy through the postpartum period to suppress HBV viremia.[112,113]

Hepatitis C virus. HCV (see Chapter 177) is a single-stranded positive-sense RNA virus in the genus *Hepacivirus,* family Flaviviridae. At least six distinct genotypes and 100 subtypes have been identified throughout the world and appear to have a variable effect on the development of clinical disease and response to antiviral therapy. It is transmitted most commonly to children and adolescents who have been exposed to blood products, clotting factor concentrates before 1987, hemodialysis, organ transplantation, intravenous drug use, cocaine snorting, or tattoos and piercing procedures performed at parlors that do not practice sterile technique. Perinatal transmission from an HCV-seropositive mother to her infant also occurs at an estimated risk of 5%, especially if the mother is HCV RNA positive at delivery.[10,66,102,108] Infection with HCV usually does not cause acute hepatitis; however, chronic hepatitis develops in more than 50% of children infected with HCV.[58] In adults, cirrhosis, end-stage liver failure, and hepatocellular carcinoma also may develop. Infection with HCV is diagnosed serologically by detecting the presence of HCV antibody and confirming with HCV RNA quantification by PCR.[75] Peginterferon-α2b (PegIntron) plus ribavirin is still the only US Food and Drug Administration (FDA)-approved therapy for children age 3 to 12 years with HCV. Achieving a sustained virologic response (SVR), defined as being HCV RNA negative 6 months after discontinuation of treatment, is the standard of care. The rates of achieving SVR with treatment in children with genotypes 2 and 3 are much higher (75–80%) than in genotype 1 (35–40%).[137,153] Treatment response, and even spontaneous clearance without treatment, seems to be strongly influenced by a genetic polymorphism near the IL28B gene.[49,135] More recently approved directly acting antiviral therapies for adults are being tested in children through currently ongoing clinical trials.[156–158] In 2017, the FDA approved two all-oral drugs, sofosbuvir alone and combined sofosbuvir/ledipasvir, for treatment of children age 12 to 17 years. With this new therapy, SVR is defined as being HCV RNA negative 12 weeks (3 months) after discontinuation of therapy. Liver transplantation may be performed in patients with end-stage liver disease. Currently no biologic products or vaccines are licensed for prevention of infection with HCV. The hypermutation rate of HCV has hindered the development of such products because a vaccine that is protective across multiple genotypes will be necessary for global protection.

Hepatitis D virus. HDV (see Chapter 157), also known as the *delta agent, delta virus, helper virus,* and *defective virus,* is a small, 37-nm RNA virus that requires the presence of HBV, especially HBsAg, to replicate.[121] HDV can coinfect a patient simultaneously or subsequent to infection with HBV. Like HBV, HDV is acquired by exposure to blood products or clotting factors, intravenous drug use, or sexual contact. It also may be transmitted by liver transplantation, and vertical transmission has been reported. Infection with HDV occurs more commonly in Europe, South America, Africa, and the Middle East and appears to be less common in the United States. The incubation period after superinfection occurs is 1 to 2 months, but it is similar to that for HBV (90 days) if coinfection occurs simultaneously. Coinfection with HDV is associated with more severe disease or progression to fulminant hepatitis in HBV-infected patients.[121] Laboratory diagnosis includes detection of HDV antibody (IgG, IgM) and HDV RNA by PCR, although this is not commercially available. Treatment with peginterferon-α2b results in sustained HDV clearance in about one-fourth of patients.[63,149] Because HDV cannot be transmitted to or infect humans without HBV, prevention of HBV infection by vaccination prevents the acquisition of HDV infection. HDV coinfection of individuals already infected with HBV, however, cannot be prevented by any licensed biologic product or vaccine.

Hepatitis E virus. HEV (see Chapter 170) is a small RNA virus that is transmitted by the fecal-oral route.[13,114,125,128] HEV infection in U.S. residents is a rare occurrence, but it may be a common cause of acute, self-limited viral hepatitis in developing countries and has been linked to outbreaks associated with contaminated water supplies and/or breakdowns in public health during times of conflict. The incubation period is an average of 6 to 7 weeks.[3] HEV appears to cause a mild to moderate acute hepatitis, especially in adults, and has a high case-fatality rate in pregnant women. Chronic hepatitis is only seen in immunosuppressed patients.[3] Laboratory diagnosis is established by detection of IgG and IgM antibody to HEV in serum or detection of HEV RNA by PCR in serum or feces performed in reference laboratories or at the Centers for Disease Control and Prevention (CDC). No antiviral agent is licensed for HEV, although ribavirin has been shown to achieve a sustained virologic response. A vaccine against HEV is licensed for use in China and has demonstrated significant protection that is durable and safe in pregnant women.[68]

Herpesviruses

Herpesviruses are large DNA viruses with icosahedral symmetry and a glycoprotein envelope, and they share the biologic properties of latency and reactivation. Infections with this family of viruses, the Herpesviridae, may be primary or recurrent. All the human herpesviruses (HHVs) and one of the primate herpesviruses (herpes B virus) can cause acute hepatitis during the course of a systemic illness, but primary hepatitis with these viral agents is an unusual event.[43]

Herpes simplex virus. HSV-1 and HSV-2 most often cause mucocutaneous vesicles or ulcers, and dissemination usually occurs during periods of relative immune compromise, such as pregnancy, the neonatal period, malnutrition, congenital or acquired immunodeficiency syndromes, or organ transplantation. Transient, subclinical hepatitis may occur during acute mucocutaneous HSV disease, but fulminant hepatitis with hepatic necrosis rarely has been documented in a normal host.[39,47,70,91] A special exception to this observation is HSV-associated primary hepatic necrosis and disseminated HSV disease in pregnant women.[47] Most cases occur during the late second or early third trimester, and most, but not all, cases are associated with primary infection with HSV-2.[152,159] Obvious skin lesions may not be present. This disease is associated with high mortality rates in both the mother and infant. Neonates, both term and preterm, are at risk for the development of neonatal HSV hepatitis as part of a disseminated HSV disease that includes viral sepsis–like syndrome, coagulopathy, abdominal distention with hepatomegaly and ascites, pneumonitis with respiratory distress, and meningoencephalitis.[19,85] Skin lesions often are absent in this form of HSV disease. Neonatal HSV hepatitis develops most often in the child's first 2 weeks of life, and aminotransferase levels may initially be slightly elevated and then rise to be more than a thousand times higher than normal as disease progresses. Recipients of solid organ, bone marrow, and stem cell transplants may have HSV infection with dissemination within the first 3 weeks after undergoing transplantation, most often as a result of reactivation.[46] Patients with hepatitis secondary to HSV infection may be shedding HSV from a mucocutaneous source or may be viremic, with virus detected in the blood by DNA PCR. Some patients may require analysis of ascites fluid or liver biopsy for confirmation. Acyclovir therapy is recommended for HSV-associated hepatitis, in preventing posttransplant HSV disease, and in preventing HSV infection of neonates born to HSV-infected mothers.[46,152] Children with HSV fulminant hepatitis have significantly better survival rates than adults before and after liver transplantation.[33,95]

Varicella-zoster virus. Varicella-zoster virus also causes mucocutaneous vesicles in both immunocompetent and immunocompromised hosts. Primary infection is known as *varicella* (also chickenpox) and is associated with primary and secondary viremias that often seed the visceral organs. Approximately one-fourth of healthy children experiencing varicella will have silent hepatitis with aminotransferase levels at least twice normal.[42,101,120] Fulminant hepatitis with varicella is rare and generally is seen in immunocompromised hosts.[6,98,115,141] Patients have severe abdominal pain with little nausea or vomiting, skin lesions may or may not be present, and aminotransferase levels may be more than a thousand times higher than normal.[97,134,136] Zoster in a normal host is not associated with fulminant hepatitis, but immunocompromised hosts may experience disseminated zoster with hepatitis and hepatic necrosis.[41] The diagnosis often is based on clinical findings, but direct PCR testing of cutaneous lesions or blood may help establish the diagnosis. Treatment with acyclovir is recommended. Varicella may be prevented or attenuated by passive immunization with varicella-zoster immune globulin or intravenous immunoglobulin (IVIG) or by active immunization with a licensed live virus vaccine.[122,20]

Cytomegalovirus. CMV infection usually is asymptomatic but can cause gastroenteritis, pneumonitis, or a mononucleosis-like syndrome that consists of fever, lymphadenopathy, and atypical lymphocytosis. Hepatitis occurs as part of these syndromes but often is silent or mild and rarely is accompanied by jaundice.[73,90] Granulomatous hepatitis also may be associated with CMV.[29] Infants born congenitally infected with CMV frequently have hepatosplenomegaly, elevated aminotransferase levels, and conjugated hyperbilirubinemia.[29,30,147] The hepatitis that neonates and infants experience with postnatal infection is self-limited and generally resolves within the first few months of life. If hepatitis with cholestasis persists, other diseases such as extrahepatic biliary atresia should be considered. Solid organ and marrow transplant recipients and patients with acquired immunodeficiency syndrome (AIDS) and other immunodeficiency states may experience persistent fever, malaise, leukopenia, and hepatitis caused by primary or recurrent infection with CMV. Severe liver disease can occur in transplant recipients and may be associated with graft-versus-host disease or graft rejection.[36,37] CMV-associated hepatitis may be diagnosed clinically and supported by evidence of high-level CMV viremia and/or demonstration of involvement of the end organ by liver biopsy.[35,105] Treatment with ganciclovir, valganciclovir, foscarnet, or cidofovir appears to be beneficial in immunocompromised hosts, and prophylaxis or preemptive therapy with antiviral agents or CMV hyperimmune globulin may prevent the development of severe CMV disease in transplant recipients.[35,38]

Epstein-Barr virus. EBV infection can be asymptomatic but is a frequent cause of a mononucleosis-like syndrome with mild hepatitis. However, in rare patients with a genetic X-linked predisposition, a severe, often fatal lymphoproliferative syndrome with prominent liver involvement may develop. Transplant recipients also may be susceptible to posttransplant lymphoproliferative disease (PTLD), in which the liver may be involved.[9,131] In addition, patients with tumors associated with EBV, such as lymphoma, may have hepatic involvement. The diagnosis of mononucleosis usually is clinical and supported by a positive heterophile or "Monospot" test in a child older than 4 years or by specific EBV serologic tests such as detection of IgM antibody to viral capsid antigen (VCA).[14] PCR testing for EBV should not be used in the diagnosis of acute mononucleosis. The immune response to EBV in immunocompromised hosts may be unusual, and the diagnosis of PTLD generally is suspected by an exponential increase in EBV DNA genome copies in peripheral blood, generalized adenopathy, visualization by positron emission tomography, and the presence of histopathologic features on biopsy. Treatment options for PTLD include reducing immunosuppression, rituximab (anti-CD20 monoclonal antibody), adoptive immunotherapy, interferon-α, and anti–interleukin-6 antibody.[27,52,55,110,135] Antiviral agents such as acyclovir or foscarnet should be used only as an adjunct therapy because they are less effective in the latent phase of PTLD.[90]

Human herpesviruses 6, 7, and 8. These viruses may involve the liver, especially in immunocompromised patients.[43] Infection with HHV-6 in recipients of liver transplants is usually a result of reactivation and has been associated with acute rejection, portal lymphocyte infiltration, and graft dysfunction. Even though HHV-6 commonly can be detected in blood and tissue, high viral loads have been associated with decreased graft survival.[119] Normal hosts with primary HHV-6 infection may have a silent hepatitis with mild elevation of aminotransferase levels. Rarely severe disseminated disease with fulminant hepatitis has been linked to HHV-6 and HHV-7.[4,11,87] HHV-8 (also known as *Kaposi sarcoma virus*) causes a complex neoplasm involving the skin, mucous membranes, and internal organs, most often in severely immunocompromised patients. Although rare, it has been reported in human immunodeficiency virus (HIV)-infected children with advanced AIDS. Recipients of solid organ transplants may be infected with HHV-8. The liver is a common site of visceral disease caused by HHV-8, which most often is associated with tumors rather than hepatitis.[26] Diagnosing infection with HHV-6, HHV-7, or HHV-8 is difficult because of the ubiquity of these viruses and their viral DNA in humans, but the diagnosis is supported by serologic evidence and by detection of viral DNA in blood, in secretions, or, more specifically, in tissue.[111] No specific licensed antiviral therapy is available, but these viruses may be inhibited by ganciclovir, foscarnet, and cidofovir. Response also may be noted after withdrawal or reduction of immunosuppression. Chemotherapy may be indicated in some cases of HHV-8.

Herpes B virus. Also known as *herpesvirus simiae* or *Cercopithecine herpesvirus 1,* herpes B virus is an α-herpesvirus of monkeys that causes severe disease in humans.[151] It can be transmitted from Asian monkeys, such as rhesus and cynomolgus monkeys, to humans through bites or contact with mucous membrane secretions from infected monkeys. The human disease associated with herpes B virus involves skin vesicles at the portal of entry, regional lymphadenitis, and hemorrhagic encephalitis. The virus also may disseminate to the liver and lungs and produce hemorrhagic necrosis, with a high mortality rate. The diagnosis is made by isolation of virus or detection of viral DNA by PCR in specialized reference laboratories, and the virus is inhibited by acyclovir and ganciclovir.

Adenoviruses

Adenoviruses are small DNA viruses that are members of the viral family Adenoviridae. They usually are respiratory or enteric pathogens, but they can cause disseminated disease with hepatitis and hepatic necrosis in both immunocompetent and immunocompromised hosts and neonates.[60,89,107] Patients often have fever, malaise or lethargy, conjunctivitis, pharyngitis, cough, respiratory distress, vomiting and diarrhea, and a viral sepsis–like syndrome. Hepatitis is marked by hepatomegaly and by elevated aminotransferases and bilirubin. A specific viral diagnosis is made by detection of adenoviral DNA by PCR from blood. Adenovirus serotype 5 generally is associated with severe hepatitis, followed in frequency by types 1 and 2.[99] For bone marrow and stem cell transplant recipients and liver transplant recipients at high risk for acquiring severe or fatal adenovirus-associated disease, surveillance blood DNA PCR testing, serotyping, and genotyping may allow early intervention before severe, disseminated disease develops.[21,89] No licensed antiviral therapy is available, but the virus is inhibited by cidofovir, an antiviral agent with broad-spectrum activity against many DNA viruses, and brincidofovir.[19,78]

Erythroviruses: Human Parvovirus B19

Erythroviruses (e.g., human parvovirus B19) are small DNA viruses. They are members of the family Parvoviridae and are responsible for a variety of illnesses, including erythema infectiosum (also called fifth disease), arthritis, and anemia. Liver involvement, often severe, may be seen in intrauterine infection with hydrops fetalis.[1,88] Fulminant liver failure with massive hepatic necrosis also has been reported in patients with aplastic anemia.[74] Pediatric patients with fulminant liver failure from the hepatotropic viruses have more severe disease and high mortality rates when coinfected with human parvovirus B19.[32] Persistent infection is seen in immunocompromised hosts. Parvovirus infection can be diagnosed by detection of virus-specific IgM antibodies or detection of viral DNA in blood, serum/plasma, bone marrow, or tissue. No specific antiviral therapy is available, but immunocompromised patients with chronic infection may benefit from receiving IVIG. Severe fetal hydrops usually requires in utero and neonatal blood transfusions for anemia.

Enteroviruses

Enteroviruses are small RNA viruses and members of the Picornaviridae, along with polioviruses and rhinoviruses. The nonpolio enteroviruses are most frequently associated with mild respiratory or gastrointestinal illnesses, often occurring in late summer or early fall, but can be a cause of more severe manifestations like myocarditis or aseptic meningitis. Significant hepatic necrosis can occur in neonates with disseminated disease, particularly with serotype echovirus 11. It often is accompanied by hepatomegaly, thrombocytopenia, viral sepsis syndrome, aseptic meningoencephalitis, myocarditis, and elevated aminotransferase and serum bilirubin levels.[92-94] Coxsackievirus B and echoviruses 9 and 30 also are associated with fatal disease. Enteroviruses may be transmitted to neonates perinatally from the mother or through contact with ill family members. Health care–associated nursery outbreaks with enteroviruses also have been reported.[105] The diagnosis is established by detection of viral RNA by PCR in throat, stool or rectal swab, urine, blood, cerebrospinal fluid, or tissue samples. Treatment is supportive; however, case reports suggest that IVIG and pleconaril may have some clinical benefit in severely ill neonates.[7,23,127]

Measles Virus

Measles virus is an RNA virus that is a member of the Paramyxoviridae, along with parainfluenza viruses, respiratory syncytial virus, metapneumovirus, and mumps virus. Of all the paramyxoviruses, measles virus is associated most often with hepatitis. Ten to twenty percent of children with measles will have subclinical hepatitis, although severe disease of the liver, lungs, and brain may occur in immunocompromised patients.[48,104,138] Rare reports of severe giant-cell hepatitis, often leading to liver failure, have implicated paramyxoviruses of undetermined type.[118] Measles and other paramyxoviruses may be identified by detection of virus-specific IgM antibody in serum and by isolation of virus or detection of RNA by PCR in secretions, blood, or tissue. No specific antiviral therapy is licensed for measles virus; however, ribavirin, a broad-spectrum antiviral agent, may have some activity against the virus. Prevention is achieved by vaccination with the live measles vaccine or by postexposure administration of IVIG.

Rubella Virus

Rubella virus is a member of the Togaviridae of RNA viruses. Clinical disease associated with infection by rubella virus generally is mild, but as many as 10% of children with rubella may have subclinical hepatitis with transient elevation of aminotransferase levels.[144] Congenital rubella syndrome caused by intrauterine infection with rubella virus, however, is associated with significant liver involvement, and hepatomegaly with jaundice is noted at birth.[34,96,143] Congenital rubella syndrome also is associated with intrauterine growth retardation, cataracts, congenital heart disease, thrombocytopenia, purpura, and hearing loss.[71] Because isolating the virus is technically challenging, the diagnosis of rubella most often is made serologically by detection of virus-specific IgM antibody or by detection of viral RNA by PCR in reference laboratories. No specific antiviral therapy is available. Rubella can be prevented, however, by vaccination with the live rubella virus vaccine.

Hemorrhagic Fever Viruses

The hemorrhagic fever viruses are a diverse group of RNA viruses from a variety of different virus families. They include arenaviruses such as Lassa fever virus, bunyaviruses such as hantavirus, filoviruses such as Marburg and Ebola, and flaviviruses such as yellow fever virus and dengue. Hemorrhagic fever is characterized by fever, malaise, lethargy, headache, retroorbital pain, myalgia, conjunctivitis, rash, and intravascular coagulation with hemorrhage. Liver involvement with these viruses is a very common event, and elevation of aminotransferase levels to 500 IU/mL occurs in almost every patient, with a thousand times the normal range seen in patients who are severely ill. Jaundice is a significant component of yellow fever.[65] The diagnosis is established by serologic means or by detection of the viral agent with electron microscopy or PCR techniques, which in most cases should be attempted only in biosafety level IV reference laboratories. Treatment of most hemorrhagic fevers is supportive; however, intravenous ribavirin reduces the mortality rate associated with Lassa fever and also may be of benefit to patients with hemorrhagic fever caused by other arenaviruses.[79,84]

Bacteria

Nonviral acute hepatitis can be caused by bacterial illnesses (see Box 47.1).[106] Sepsis with gram-positive organisms, especially pneumococci, or with gram-negative organisms, particularly gram-negative enteric bacteria, can produce hepatic dysfunction, primarily from the cholestatic effects induced by bacterial endotoxins.[106] In this form of hepatic dysfunction, the patient will appear jaundiced with mild hepatomegaly, and conjugated bilirubin levels will be elevated out of proportion to the modest elevation in aminotransferase or alkaline phosphatase levels. Neonates also may have jaundice secondary to urinary tract infection with gram-negative enteric organisms. The diagnosis is made by isolating the offending bacteria from blood, urine, or other usually sterile site. Treatment involves specific antimicrobial therapy.

Other bacterial diseases may cause chronic or granulomatous hepatitis, including actinomycosis, brucellosis, listeriosis, nocardiosis, bartonellosis (cat-scratch disease), and tuberculosis.[8,109] Diseases caused by atypical mycobacteria, especially *Mycobacterium avium-intracellulare* complex (MAC complex) or *Mycobacterium mucogenicum* may be seen, particularly in patients with congenital or acquired immunodeficiency states.[50] Rarely disseminated disease with hepatitis can occur as a complication of vaccination with bacille Calmette-Guérin (BCG) in children or, in adults, as a complication of bladder irrigation for bladder carcinoma.[8,51,77] Bacterial toxins, such as the emetic toxin of *Bacillus cereus,* also have been linked to fulminant hepatic failure in some patients.[80] A diagnosis of hepatitis caused by these unusual or indolent bacterial pathogens usually is accomplished by isolating the organism from blood or the affected organ. The diagnosis may be supported by positive skin test results in the case of tuberculosis or atypical mycobacterial disease, serologically by elevated titers to *Bartonella quintana* or *Bartonella henselae,* and by positive imaging studies that show hepatic microabscesses, as in the case of hepatic involvement with cat-scratch disease. Antimicrobial therapy is guided by the susceptibility of the offending pathogen.

Spirochetes

Acute infection with *T. pallidum,* the agent of primary or early secondary syphilis in adolescents or adults, may cause acute or granulomatous hepatitis with serum aminotransferase levels up to 5 to 10 times normal.[76] Jaundice rarely develops, but a chancre of primary disease or a rash of secondary disease often is present. Congenital syphilis also is associated commonly with hepatosplenomegaly in the neonate, along with elevated aminotransferase and bilirubin levels. Other clinical manifestations of congenital syphilis include petechiae or purpura, osteitis, and meningitis. Laboratory diagnosis is confirmed by reactive VDRL and positive fluorescent treponemal antibody tests.[59] Treatment with penicillin is recommended.

Leptospirosis, or infection with the pathogenic bacterium *Leptospira interrogans,* can cause acute hepatitis.[56] Leptospirosis usually is an abrupt, anicteric, flulike illness, but approximately 10% of patients will have an icteric or septicemic syndrome with a biphasic clinical course. Patients with the icteric or severe form will exhibit jaundice, hepatomegaly, and characteristic conjunctival injection. Usually levels of serum bilirubin are elevated out of proportion to the more modest elevations in serum aminotransferases, suggesting a defect in excretion of bilirubin rather than direct hepatic necrosis as the pathogenesis of the jaundice. Meningitis, renal failure, and even liver failure may occur in some patients. The diagnosis should be considered in older children and adolescents with a history of exposure to wild and domestic mammals, especially dogs, rats, and livestock, which may excrete *Leptospira* organisms in their urine, or with a history of exposure to contaminated water in ditches, lakes, or streams. The diagnosis is established by serology. Treatment with penicillin or doxycycline is recommended.

Rickettsiae

The rickettsial organism *Coxiella burnetii* causes Q fever, both the acute and chronic forms, in which hepatitis is a prominent feature along with persistent fever, malaise, rash, weight loss, and pneumonitis.[16] Clinical jaundice is a rare finding, and most often the hepatitis is subclinical. A history of exposure to mammals or birds suggests the diagnosis, which can be confirmed serologically by reference clinical laboratories. Treatment with antibiotics, usually doxycycline, is recommended.

Parasites and Fungi

A variety of parasites may invade the liver and occasionally cause hepatic dysfunction or disease.[106,160] Such parasites include *Plasmodium* spp. (malaria), *Entamoeba histolytica* (liver abscess), *T. gondii* (toxoplasmosis), and *Toxocara canis* (visceral larval migrans). *Ascaris lumbricoides* (roundworms) may invade the common bile duct and cause acute obstructive jaundice.

Fungi also may invade the liver, usually with only minimal elevation of aminotransferase levels and rarely causing jaundice or elevated levels of bilirubin. Patients with a compromised immune system may have hepatic abscesses with *Candida* spp. or abscesses or necrotic lesions with *Aspergillus* spp., as well as other unusual fungal species. Both immunocompromised and normal hosts may have liver involvement with *Histoplasma capsulatum* or *Cryptococcus neoformans.*[120]

NONINFECTIOUS CAUSES

An important noninfectious cause of acute hepatitis is drug-related hepatitis (see Box 47.1).[100,155,161] It can range in severity from mild, with subclinical elevation of aminotransferase levels, to fulminant hepatic failure.[69] A careful history of ingestion of prescription or over-the-counter medications, as well as exposure to toxins or herbal remedies, should be elicited. Although almost any drug can cause acute hepatitis, the most common agents associated with hepatitis in children include acetylsalicylic acid (i.e., aspirin), acetaminophen, isoniazid, rifampin, phenytoin, valproic acid, phenobarbital, β-lactam antibiotics (e.g., oxacillin, nafcillin, and third-generation cephalosporins), sulfa drugs, and antifungal agents such as ketoconazole and fluconazole. Many of these medications, including allopurinol and carbamazepine, have been implicated in the potentially life-threatening drug reaction with eosinophilia and systemic symptoms (DRESS) syndrome. The majority of patients with DRESS syndrome have hepatic involvement, and the treatment is withdrawal of the offending agent and corticosteroid therapy.[18] The anesthetic drug halothane also can cause acute hepatitis with jaundice.[126] Gold and other metals used to treat arthritis, carbon tetrachloride, and ingestion of *Amanita* mushrooms can all lead to liver injury. In addition, chronic hepatitis can develop in children, especially premature infants, who receive prolonged total parenteral nutrition (for 2 weeks or more).

Anoxic liver injury also can resemble acute viral hepatitis. It occurs in critically ill children after a period of hypotension, heart failure, or cardiopulmonary arrest. A history of such an inciting event supports the diagnosis. Anoxic liver injury is characterized by an abrupt onset of markedly elevated levels of aminotransferases, often hundreds of times higher than normal, without jaundice, and rapid recovery of enzyme levels to normal or nearly normal after the event has resolved.[57]

Other diseases such as Kawasaki syndrome and toxic shock syndrome, which have been linked to or associated with infectious pathogens, may have hepatitis as part of their manifestation. Similarly, Reye syndrome, characterized by hepatomegaly with fatty infiltration of the liver and often fatal encephalopathy, may occur after a viral syndrome such as varicella or influenza.

Metabolic disorders may manifest as hepatitis, especially in infants. Such disorders include cystic fibrosis, α_1-antitrypsin deficiency, galactosemia, hereditary fructose intolerance, glycogen storage disease, urea cycle deficiencies, organic acidemias, tyrosinemia, and lipid storage diseases such as Gaucher disease and Niemann-Pick disease.[116,145] Of note, cystic fibrosis in neonates may be associated with cholestatic jaundice in the absence of pulmonary disease, similar to biliary atresia.[140] Disorders of metal metabolism, such as Wilson disease or hereditary hemochromatosis, may cause acute, chronic, or even fulminant hepatitis in older children.[117,132] A distinct disorder, neonatal hemochromatosis, is hypothesized to be an alloimmune-mediated (maternal) hepatitis that often manifests as severe liver injury within hours of birth and notable coagulopathy.[150] In addition, patients with congenital disorders of bilirubin metabolism or transport may become jaundiced without significant elevation of aminotransferase levels, especially during an intercurrent viral illness. Of these, Rotor and Dubin-Johnson syndromes predominantly cause a conjugated hyperbilirubinemia and do not lead to hepatic injury.[142] Gilbert syndrome and Crigler-Najjar type 1 and 2 are on the same spectrum of disease causing unconjugated hyperbilirubinemia, with the complete loss of bilirubin glucuronidation being fatal.[142] Sickle-cell crisis also may manifest as hepatitis.[133]

Tumors of the liver such as hepatoblastoma and hemangioendothelioma and infiltrative diseases such as lymphoma, leukemia, and hemophagocytic lymphohistiocytosis syndrome may have hepatitis or hepatic failure as part of the initial manifestation.[54,81] Another multisystem disorder that may produce chronic granulomatous hepatitis is sarcoidosis.[31]

Anatomic causes of hepatic dysfunction in infants include extrahepatic biliary atresia, which usually develops in the first 2 months of life.[82,147]

Autoimmune hepatitis or other autoimmune disorders with liver involvement also may cause acute or chronic hepatitis, especially in older children and adolescents.[148] These disorders often are associated with rash, arthritis, inflammatory bowel disease, thyroiditis, malaise, and persistent fever. Autoimmune hepatitis may respond to corticosteroids or other immunosuppressive agents.

Hepatic steatosis (fatty infiltration) is becoming increasingly common in obese children, especially if insulin resistant. These children may have enlarged or tender livers on examination, elevated aminotransferase levels in serum, abnormal imaging studies showing fatty infiltrates of the liver, and liver biopsies that show inflammation, fibrosis, and even cirrhosis in some cases. Treatment currently includes diet and lifestyle changes with weight loss and exercise.

NEW REFERENCES SINCE THE SEVENTH EDITION

2. Aach R, Lander J, Sherman L. Transfusion-transmitted viruses: interim analysis of hepatitis among transfused and non-transfused patients. In: Vyas G, Cohen S, Schmid R, eds. *Viral Hepatitis*. Philadelphia: Franklin Institute Press; 1978:383.
10. Arshad M, El-Kamary SS, Jhaveri R. Hepatitis C virus infection during pregnancy and the newborn period–are they opportunities for treatment? *J Viral Hepat.* 2011;18(4):229-236.
20. Centers for Disease Control and Prevention. Updated recommendations for use of VariZIG–United States, 2013. *MMWR Morb Mortal Wkly Rep*. 2013;62(28):574-576.
24. Clemente MG, Vajro P. An update on the strategies used for the treatment of chronic hepatitis B in children. *Expert Rev Gastroenterol Hepatol*. 2016;1-10.
66. Jhaveri R, Hashem M, El-Kamary SS, et al. Hepatitis C virus (HCV) vertical transmission in 12-month-old infants born to HCV-infected women and assessment of maternal risk factors. *Open Forum Infect Dis*. 2015;2(2):ofv089.
67. Jonas MM, Chang MH, Sokal E, et al. Randomized, controlled trial of entecavir versus placebo in children with hepatitis B envelope antigen-positive chronic hepatitis B. *Hepatology*. 2016;63(2):377-387.
68. Kamar N, Izopet J, Tripon S, et al. Ribavirin for chronic hepatitis E virus infection in transplant recipients. *N Engl J Med*. 2014;370(12):1111-1120.
72. Kubo A, Shlager L, Marks AR, et al. Prevention of vertical transmission of hepatitis B: an observational study. *Ann Intern Med*. 2014;160(12):828-835.
85. McGoogan KE, Haafiz AB, Gonzalez Peralta RP. Herpes simplex virus hepatitis in infants: clinical outcomes and correlates of disease severity. *J Pediatr*. 2011;159(4):608-611.

103. Nelson N, Murphy T. Hepatitis A. In: *CDC Yellow Book*. Atlanta, GA: CDC; 2017. Available at: https://wwwnc.cdc.gov/travel/yellowbook/2018/infectious-diseases-related-to-travel/hepatitis-a.
107. Odio C, McCracken GH Jr, Nelson JD. Disseminated adenovirus infection: a case report and review of the literature. *Pediatr Infect Dis*. 1984;3(1):46-49.
108. Ohto H, Terazawa S, Sasaki N, et al. Transmission of hepatitis C virus from mothers to infants. The Vertical Transmission of Hepatitis C Virus Collaborative Study Group. *N Engl J Med*. 1994;330(11):744-750.
109. Oliva A, Duarte B, Jonasson O, et al. The nodular form of local hepatic tuberculosis. A review. *J Clin Gastroenterol*. 1990;12(2):166-173.
139. Sokal EM, Paganelli M, Wirth S, et al. Management of chronic hepatitis B in childhood: ESPGHAN clinical practice guidelines: consensus of an expert panel on behalf of the European Society of Pediatric Gastroenterology, Hepatology and Nutrition. *J Hepatol*. 2013;59(4):814-829.
156. Safety and efficacy of ledipasvir/sofosbuvir fixed dose combination +/−ribavirin in adolescents and children with chronic HCV-Infection. NCT02249182. https://clinicaltrials.gov/ct2/show/NCT02249182?term=harvoni+children&rank=1.
157. Safety and efficacy of sofosbuvir + ribavirin in adolescents and children with genotype 2 or 3 chronic HCV infection. NCT02175758. https://clinicaltrials.gov/ct2/show/NCT02175758?term=sofosbuvir+children&rank=1.
158. A study to evaluate treatment of hepatitis C virus infection in pediatric subjects (ZIRCON). NCT02486406. https://clinicaltrials.gov/ct2/show/NCT02486406?term=ombitasvir+paritaprevir+ritonavir+children&rank=4.

The full reference list for this chapter is available at ExpertConsult.com.

Cholangitis and Cholecystitis 48

Pia S. Pannaraj • Douglas S. Fishman

CHOLANGITIS

The term *cholangitis* refers to inflammation of the extrahepatic or intrahepatic biliary system. Acute cholangitis is most often a consequence of infection in the setting of biliary tract disease or obstruction. The diagnosis of cholangitis implies microbial colonization of the biliary tract, increased biliary pressure, and systemic signs of infection, although all of these findings are not present in all patients.

Acute biliary tract infection is rare in children and occurs most often in children with underlying disease. One specific pediatric population—children with biliary atresia and a hepatic portoenterostomy (HPE)—is particularly susceptible to cholangitis and its sequelae. This population and other patient groups at high risk of developing infectious cholangitis, such as patients with immunodeficiency states, congenital or acquired bile duct abnormalities, or liver transplants, are highlighted in this chapter. Biliary tract obstruction secondary to gallstone disease is discussed in the section on cholecystitis.

ETIOLOGY AND PATHOGENESIS

The central mechanism leading to biliary tract infection is obstruction of normal bile flow. Bile typically is sterile due to mechanical flushing with normal bile flow, the anatomic gate of the choledochal sphincter, bacteriostatic properties of bile, and biliary IgA.[35,147] When obstruction and stagnation occur, bacteria gain access either by ascending from the gut or via hematogenous spread. The exact route of bacterial invasion and spreading remains controversial. Ascent may occur from the duodenum, most commonly in the presence of abnormal function of the sphincter of Oddi. In addition, bacterial invasion may occur hematogenously via increased gut translocation across the intestine into the portal circulation,[256] followed by flow across the gallbladder wall.[60] Although the exact mechanism has not been firmly established, the consensus is that transient episodes of bactibilia combined with biliary obstruction may lead to higher concentrations of bacteria in the biliary tract. As biliary pressure increases, bacteria likely migrate from the bile ducts into lymphatic and blood vessels, resulting in bacteremia and clinical signs and symptoms of cholangitis.[35,115] Iatrogenic introduction of bacteria into the biliary tract can occur during endoscopic retrograde cholangiopancreatography (ERCP) or with indwelling stents.[147] More recently, challenges with endoscope cleaning in the duodenoscope elevator have led to infections, notably with carbapenem-resistant Enterobacteriaceae.[67,264,274]

In adults, cholangitis typically occurs in the presence of biliary tract obstruction secondary to impaction of gallstones in the common bile duct leading to bile stasis and secondary infection. In approximately 85% of cases of cholangitis in adults, evidence of a common bile duct stone is present.[19] In adults with documented gallstones in the common bile duct (choledocholithiasis), the incidence of positive bile cultures is 30% to 99%.[149,157,237] Other causes of biliary obstruction in adults possibly leading to a more chronic or recurrent presentation include neoplasm of the biliary tree or head of the pancreas, other intrinsic or extrinsic strictures, parasitic disease, inflammatory conditions (e.g., primary biliary cirrhosis, primary sclerosing cholangitis [PSC]), and congenital bile duct anomalies. More recently, with improved imaging modalities and a better understanding of the pathogenesis of biliary lithiasis, it has become accepted that biliary sludge or microcalculi may be at the root of nonobstructive cholangitis and recurrent biliary infections.

In children, acute cholangitis occurs most frequently in patients with biliary atresia who have undergone HPE surgery, also known as a Kasai operation. HPE provides a permissive setup for cholangitis: poor bile flow combined with damaged intrahepatic bile ducts and obligate bacterial colonization with enteric flora in the intestinal conduit.[109,138,154,223] In this setting, cholangitis is thought to arise from reflux of jejunal flora through the HPE (roux-en-Y loop), directly contiguous with the hepatic porta. Incidence is between 40% and 93% of patients and tends to occur more frequently within the first year after surgery.[49,68,223] Decreased biliary and duodenal motility generally are accepted as being associated with a higher incidence of cholangitis,[64,258] but most predictors and exacerbants for the development of cholangitis remain unknown.

Microbiologic evidence of biliary tract infection ideally should involve at least 10^4 organisms per milliliter of bile.[60] Table 48.1 summarizes the frequencies of specific organisms found in adult and pediatric studies.[20,29,130,152,212] *Escherichia coli, Klebsiella pneumoniae, Enterobacter* spp., and *Enterococcus* spp. are most commonly isolated from infected bile. Many cases of cholangitis are polymicrobial. Anaerobes, such as *Bacteroides fragilis* and *Clostridium perfringens,* also may play a significant role and have been identified in 40% of biliary tract infections.[30] Specifically, the latter organism has been implicated in acute emphysematous cholecystitis. Despite these findings in bile, many patients with cholangitis have negative blood cultures, thus requiring clinicians to have a high index of suspicion for cholangitis in selected circumstances and patient populations.

In addition to bacterial infection, viral, fungal, and parasitic pathogens have been reported in cases of pediatric cholangitis, particularly in immunodeficient patients (primarily patients with human immunodeficiency virus [HIV]) and patients with environmental exposure to parasites in endemic settings. Cholangitis due to viral infection is most

TABLE 48.1 **Bacterial Pathogens Isolated From Bile Cultures in Cholangitis**[a]

Organism	Keighley, 1975[130] (*n* = 231)	Boey, 1980[20] (*n* = 99)	Lewis, 1987[152] (*n* = 23)	Brook, 1989[29] (*n* = 123)	Rerknimitr, 2002[212] (*n* = 69)
Escherichia coli	65	46	15	71	16
Klebsiella/Enterobacter spp.	28	28	17	65	16
Pseudomonas spp.	1	17	0	2	6
Proteus spp.	13	8	0	15	0
Enterococcus spp.	22	14	0	42	15
Staphylococcus spp.	5	0	1	7	10
Streptococcus spp.	3	0	6	16	14
Bacteroides spp.	2	0	2	29	0
Clostridium spp.	11	0	9	27	0
Other anaerobe	7	0	0	14	4
Other species	7	23	10	8	3

[a]Pediatric and adult data.

commonly associated with hepatocellular disease with hepatotropic viruses, primarily cytomegalovirus (CMV), hepatitis C, and hepatitis B.[33,90,148] Depending on the clinical setting and age of the patient, CMV can have a markedly varied presentation, ranging from bile duct paucity seen in congenital CMV infection to hepatomegaly and jaundice in infants and children with primary CMV infection. The role of CMV hepatitis and cholangitis is significant in immunocompromised patients and solid organ transplant recipients.

Fungal cholangitis, specifically with *Cryptococcus neoformans* or *Candida albicans,* has been reported in immunocompromised and immunocompetent patients.[45,143,155] Hepatobiliary dysfunction may be the initial manifestation of disseminated infection.

The biliary tree also is susceptible to parasitic infections in normal hosts. Nematodes—*Ascaris* and, rarely, *Strongyloides*—commonly cause biliary disease in endemic regions. Migrating *Ascaris* larvae may cause either a direct inflammatory response if they pass through the biliary system, or, more commonly, a high worm burden can cause an obstruction leading to secondary pyogenic cholangitis.[134,242] Liver flukes, such as *Clonorchis* (now *Opisthorchis*) *sinensis, Opisthorchis viverrini,* and *Opisthorchis felineus,* also may pass through the biliary system through their life cycle.[167] Of these trematodes, *Clonorchis* is found frequently in cases of recurrent pyogenic cholangitis in Asian children.[291] Similar to the worms, the migration of the flukes (*Fasciola hepatica*) through the biliary tree may induce primary inflammation and, later, a secondary bacterial infection. Echinococcal cholangitis has been described in the setting of obstruction secondary to cyst formation from infection with either *Echinococcus granulosus* or *Echinococcus multilocularis.*[35,93] Although *Cryptosporidium* spp. typically are known to cause cholangitis in the immunocompromised host, one case of a child without a documented immunodeficiency has been reported.[87] A thorough travel history should be obtained in all children presenting with new-onset cholangitis, in particular in patients in whom the most common causes are ruled out rapidly.

Finally several cases of *Mycobacterium tuberculosis* cholangitis mimicking cholangiocarcinoma in immunocompromised and immunocompetent hosts have been reported in the adult literature.[14,72,139,199,208,275]

BOX 48.1 **Diagnostic Criteria for Acute Cholangitis**

Definitive Diagnosis

Clinical signs of infection and finding of purulent bile by
- ERCP
- Surgery
- Percutaneous puncture

Charcot Triad (1877)

Fever
Right upper quadrant pain
Jaundice

Reynold Pentad (1959)

Fever
Right upper quadrant pain
Jaundice
Septic shock
Altered mental status

Tokyo Guidelines (2006)

Two of three Charcot triad criteria *plus*
Evidence of inflammatory response
Abnormal white blood cell count
Elevated C-reactive protein
Abnormal liver tests
- Aspartate aminotransferase
- Alanine aminotransferase
- Alkaline phosphatase
- γ-Glutamyltranspeptidase

Imaging evidence of etiology (e.g., stone, stricture, stent)

CLINICAL PRESENTATION

The classic presentation of cholangitis first described by Charcot in 1877 and known commonly as the *Charcot triad* is reported in 50% to 70% of patients with cholangitis in most studies (Box 48.1).[20,192,257,281] It combines the clinical findings of fever, right upper quadrant pain, and jaundice.[42] The Reynold pentad added septic shock and altered mental status to the Charcot triad.[214] More recently the Tokyo guidelines updated diagnostic criteria for cholangitis to include laboratory evidence of an inflammatory response, abnormal liver test results, and imaging findings of biliary dilation or evidence of etiology of underlying disease.[281] Studies in children show that fever is the most common presenting symptom, occurring in 100% of 105 patients with cholangitis after undergoing HPE.[64] In addition, either acholic stools or an increase in serum bilirubin concentration occurs in 68% of patients. Older children and teenagers with cholangitis typically report abdominal pain that may or may not be associated with meals or localize to the right upper quadrant. Patients may report new-onset pruritus as a consequence of retained biliary constituents. Laboratory findings include elevated white blood cell count, C-reactive protein, bilirubin, and alkaline phosphatase.[294]

The findings of cholangitis may be markedly attenuated in infants and immunocompromised patients, suggesting that a low threshold for suspicion be employed in the evaluation of these children at risk.

The presentation of cholangitis in an infant with biliary atresia, status post Kasai portoenterostomy, may be as varied as lethargy, increasing jaundice, abdominal tenderness, or fever alone. Finally, patients with ongoing hemolysis (e.g., patients with hemoglobin SS disease) are at high risk for developing cholecystitis and cholangitis from bilirubin stones, yet the symptoms may readily overlap with other causes of abdominal pain.

DIAGNOSTIC EVALUATION

Physical examination may reveal a range of toxic appearances, with vital signs suggesting serious systemic infection in more advanced cases (fever, tachycardia, hypotension). Physical examination typically reveals icteric sclera and a distended abdomen, with tenderness localized to the mid or right upper quadrant. Palpation of the liver edge may reveal tenderness. Laboratory studies may reveal an elevated erythrocyte sedimentation rate (81%), leukocytosis or leukopenia (56%), and increased serum levels of conjugated bilirubin.[64] Laboratory evaluations in children should include a complete blood count with differential and liver panel (alanine aminotransferase [ALT], aspartate aminotransferase [AST], alkaline phosphatase, γ-glutamyltransferase, and fractionated bilirubin [unconjugated and conjugated]). The differential diagnosis of fever, abdominal pain, and jaundice also should include sepsis and hepatitis. No single laboratory test or combination of tests can establish a diagnosis of cholangitis.[257,294]

Attempts at identifying a microbiologic agent should be made. Blood and bile cultures should be performed at all available opportunities and drawn before antimicrobial therapy is initiated.[261] Most cases are polymicrobial, with a predominance of gut-derived organisms (see Table 48.1). Some studies report positive blood cultures in 21% to 71% of patients with acute cholangitis.[100,257,286] Other investigators have reported identification of organisms in blood in approximately 10% to 25% of patients, which is similar to our experience.[286] In patients with a history of hepatobiliary surgery, aerobic and anaerobic cultures should be considered, and in virtually all cases of young children with abdominal pain and jaundice, a urine culture should be considered. In a study of 110 patients undergoing HPE, 58.4% of patients had serum bacterial DNA detection using the 16SrDNA method compared to 14.3% using the standard culture method.[163]

The role of liver biopsy to evaluate the parenchyma for evidence of cholangitis is controversial, but occasionally this testing may have a place in the setting of negative blood cultures. When used along with blood cultures, hepatic cultures have been shown to increase the diagnostic yield of identifying a microbiologic organism to 75% of patients, whereas histologic confirmation of cholangitis may be the only firm evidence of biliary tract infection in some cases.[64] In practice, liver biopsy is performed infrequently, and patients are treated empirically. In cases of gallstone-associated biliary tract obstruction with cholangitis that requires endoscopic or surgical decompression, bile should be obtained and cultured at the time of the procedure. In an adult study, 22 of 23 patients with gallstone-associated cholangitis were found to have positive bile cultures.[152]

The initial and principal radiologic evaluation for suspected cholangitis is transabdominal ultrasound, with the primary goal being to search for evidence of biliary tract obstruction, usually associated with dilation of the common bile duct or intrahepatic ducts. Ultrasound examination may reveal anatomic biliary tract abnormalities (choledochal cyst), intrahepatic cysts or fluid collections, and hepatic or other intraabdominal masses. Other noninvasive imaging modalities include computed tomography (CT) and magnetic resonance cholangiopancreatography (MRCP), which provide increasingly detailed images of the intrahepatic and extrahepatic biliary anatomy.[75,179,219,229,238,269]

Taken together, these noninvasive imaging techniques should be able to detect the presence of biliary tract obstruction and some congenital anatomic anomalies, although even experienced ultrasonographers still may miss small stones and sludge, especially in the common bile duct. It is important to recognize the technical limitations of the methodology and the possible presence of undetected stones or sludge in the gallbladder or common bile duct (choledocholithiasis) as a cause of biliary tract dilation. The sensitivity of ultrasound for choledocholithiasis is poor, ranging from 30% to 50%.[47,48,240] Sensitivity improves to approximately 90% with CT and 95% to 99% with endoscopic retrograde cholangiopancreatography (ERCP).[209]

Newer modalities, including endoscopic ultrasound, laparoscopic ultrasound, and helical CT cholangiography, may improve detection in certain patient populations. The 2002 National Institutes of Health State-of-the-Science Consensus conference regarded endoscopic ultrasound, MRCP, and ERCP as having comparable sensitivity and specificity in detecting common bile duct stones.[190] In the hands of an experienced echoendoscopist, endoscopic ultrasound has been shown in adults to be the procedure of choice to identify small stones and sludge in the common bile duct. This method may prove useful in children as well and may prevent the unnecessary use of ERCP and the risk of its associated complications.[220,240,279]

After HPE has been performed, imaging may be able to identify lakes of retained bile (bilomas), which may be a source of infection, in a patient with biliary atresia. Nuclear medicine (hepatobiliary iminodiacetic acid [HIDA]) scans have a limited role in the evaluation of cholangitis. HIDA scans may be most helpful in determining if a patient has a complete obstruction of the common bile duct or if an isolated obstruction of the cystic duct (e.g., cholecystitis) is present.

Because of the inherent risks associated with invasive procedures in these infants, percutaneous drainage of bilomas for culture or other purposes rarely is performed. Similarly percutaneous drainage is preferred to ERCP for anatomic reasons. Invasive imaging has a role, especially when it may be coupled with therapeutic decompression of an obstructed and potentially infected biliary tree. ERCP has proved to be extremely useful in the evaluation and management of biliary tract obstruction and should be considered in the management of a child with evidence of an obstructed common bile duct.[4,77,161,241,243,247] The role of ERCP in infants and small children is limited by the number of trained pediatric gastroenterologists and also by limited availability of size-appropriate equipment. During ERCP bile for microbial and chemical analysis can be obtained and provides detailed imaging of the biliary tree. Significant technical advances have occurred in biliary endoscopy, such that direct visualization of the bile ducts (choledochoscopy) with the ability to obtain direct sampling is possible in children.[102,244] Acute cholangitis alone is an indication for ERCP when there is a suspicion for choledocholithiasis.[166]

Practically ERCP may detect (and remove) small stones and sludge that are missed by ultrasound, CT, or MRCP. ERCP is helpful in establishing the differential diagnosis of biliary tract diseases, such as PSC, which may manifest in a fashion similar to that of infectious cholangitis but have a characteristic radiographic appearance. In the future, as the use of endoscopic ultrasound in pediatrics increases, ERCP may be reserved for those patients in whom stones or sludge have been found by endoscopic ultrasound or in patients with a high pretest probability of having choledocholithiasis (e.g., patients with sickle-cell conditions).[74,78,166,240] Any child with a first episode of cholangitis warrants a detailed investigation of a possible underlying biliary tract anatomic abnormality using at least one of the available diagnostic modalities.

DIFFERENTIAL DIAGNOSIS

The differential diagnosis for an acutely ill child with fever and clinical evidence of hyperbilirubinemia is broad; a thorough workup must include consideration of infectious and noninfectious etiologies (Box 48.2). A thorough investigation for hepatic and biliary tract pathology with blood and radiologic studies must be initiated to evaluate for stones or other obstructive processes that may cause symptoms characteristic of the Charcot triad.

Acute viral hepatitis may manifest in numerous ways but often begins with nonspecific signs: fever, headache, anorexia, and jaundice.[73] Laboratory studies typically reveal a greater elevation of serum aminotransferase levels (ALT and AST) than the biliary tract enzymes alkaline phosphatase and γ-glutamyltransferase. In a child with no other evidence of biliary tract obstruction, screening assays for hepatitis infection are warranted.

Pyogenic liver abscesses and amebic abscesses tend to manifest with fever, abdominal pain, hepatomegaly, and focal right upper quadrant

BOX 48.2 Differential Diagnosis of Fever, Abdominal Pain, and Jaundice

Cholangitis
Cholecystitis
Cholelithiasis
Sepsis
Hepatitis
Choledochal cyst
Pancreatitis
Urinary tract infection
Leptospirosis and other systemic infections with hepatic involvement
Spontaneous perforation of common bile duct
Biliary cyst
Appendicitis

TABLE 48.2 Distribution of Antibiotics Used to Treat Cholangitis

Antibiotic	Blood	Bile	Tissues
Aminoglycosides	+++	+	+
Carbapenems	+++	++	+++
Cephalosporins[a]	+++	+++	++
Penicillins[b]	++	++	++
Quinolones	+++	+++	+++
Trimethoprim-sulfamethoxazole	+++	+++	++

[a]Anionic cephalosporins with molecular weight >500 such as cefpiramide, cefoperazone, ceftriaxone, cefotetan, cefixime.
[b]Ureidopenicillins such as piperacillin.
Data from references 16, 28, 110, 131, 286.

tenderness.[176] Laboratory findings vary. CT is considered to be the most sensitive technique for evaluation of these diagnoses.[179] Numerous bacterial, parasitic, and spirochetal infections also should be considered in the differential diagnosis, including but not limited to typhoid fever, brucellosis, leptospirosis, borreliosis, amebiasis, and malaria. It is beyond the scope of this chapter to expand on the systemic infections associated with hepatic involvement.[198] Recurrent pyogenic cholangitis is another consideration, although it is rare in the Western Hemisphere and even more so in the pediatric population.[228]

Jaundice may occur with sepsis of any etiology, more commonly in a critically ill infant or child. Clinical evaluation may show a predominantly direct (conjugated) hyperbilirubinemia usually accompanied by a modest elevation of γ-glutamyltransferase, although serum transaminase levels may not be elevated. These findings are caused by a hepatocellular cholestasis, owing to humoral mediators of sepsis (i.e., endotoxin and proinflammatory cytokines), but they can be exacerbated by biliary sludging that accompanies septicemia. Although sepsis-associated cholestasis historically was linked primarily to gram-negative sepsis, it can be seen in all forms of infection. In some cases, radiologic workup or biopsy is warranted to rule out ductal obstruction or biliary tract pathology. Jaundice may occur as the sole presentation of sepsis in infants and children; however, research into sepsis-induced cholestasis points to a complex, multifactorial etiopathogenesis.[41,62,83,180,271]

Drug-induced cholestasis tends to occur acutely with the onset of jaundice, pruritus, and other symptoms that may mimic cholangitis. It rarely is associated with fever, however. Among the main classes of drugs commonly used in pediatric practice that may lead to significant hepatotoxicity are antimicrobials (mainly trimethoprim-sulfamethoxazole [TMP-SMX], amoxicillin-clavulanate, clindamycin, minocycline, nitrofurantoin, erythromycin, cephalosporins, isoniazid, rifampicin, fluconazole), anticonvulsants (phenytoin, carbamazepine, valproate, felbamate), nonsteroidal antiinflammatory drugs (aspirin, ibuprofen), antihypertensive agents (propranolol, diltiazem),[31,46] and herbal remedies such as kava kava. Although rarely used in pediatric patients, statins may also lead to significant hepatotoxicity.[46] If the offending agent is identified in time, removing it typically leads to rapid improvement. Ceftriaxone has been linked directly to cholangitis and cholecystitis, possibly as a result of its biliary concentration and precipitation, leading to sludge and stones.[137,187] However, other third-generation cephalosporins also have been implicated in sludge and stone formation.[135]

Other systemic illnesses may occur with fever and evidence of biliary tract pathology, and their presentations may overlap with presentations of infectious cholangitis. PSC is defined as a chronic inflammation of the intrahepatic or extrahepatic ducts leading to a range of biliary tract pathologies from dilation to obliteration and periductal fibrosis. PSC is seen most commonly in patients with inflammatory bowel disease and affects adolescent boys with inflammatory bowel disease more commonly than girls. Symptoms include systemic findings, such as fatigue, malaise, and weight loss, and evidence of cholangitis, including fever. PSC must be suspected in a jaundiced patient with inflammatory bowel disease or in an adolescent presenting for the first time with jaundice.[151] Diagnosis is established best by ERCP or magnetic resonance cholangiography showing irregular narrowing and stricture of the hepatic and common bile ducts and the intrahepatic ducts.[164,216] Patients with PSC are at risk of developing intrahepatic and common bile duct strictures, with subsequent obstruction, sludge or stone formation, cholangitis, and ultimately cholangiocarcinoma.[117,151]

TREATMENT

Therapeutic goals in the treatment of cholangitis should include general support of the patient, early initiation of appropriate antibiotic therapy, and, in cases of obstruction by stones or stricture, decompression of biliary obstruction via ERCP or surgery. Consulting pediatric surgeons early in the course of evaluating a patient with suspected cholangitis generally is helpful. The importance of decompression and drainage of the bile tract in the face of systemic infection secondary to cholangitis cannot be overemphasized. Other potential etiologies of obstruction, such as choledochal cysts, ultimately require surgical consultation and repair.

Initial and conservative management should include appropriate inpatient monitoring, cessation of oral intake with intravenous fluid support, parenteral antibiotic therapy, and supportive management as warranted by the child's clinical status. Antimicrobials are selected to cover suspected or documented organisms based on local or documented susceptibility patterns and the ability to achieve adequate serum and tissue concentrations. Currently no single antibiotic or combination is recognized universally as being the definitive therapy for cholangitis in children. Parenteral antibiotics are indicated in almost all cases of children with suspected biliary tract sepsis. Theoretically the ability to achieve high biliary concentrations (Table 48.2) should be considered. However, clinical and experimental data are lacking to strongly support the recommendation for sole use of antimicrobials with excellent biliary penetration. Adequate serum levels may be sufficient.[2,60]

Empiric antibiotics should cover the most commonly isolated enteric pathogens, including *Escherichia coli, Klebsiella spp.*, and *Enterococcus* spp. Previously a combination of ampicillin or penicillin with an aminoglycoside was considered a standard regimen for cholangitis with a clinical cure rate of 40% to 95% in various adult studies.[40,84,182,261,267] Multiple recent studies show equivalent effectiveness of newer agents including penicillin plus β-lactamase inhibitor combinations, third- and fourth-generation cephalosporins, and carbapenems.[84,94,266,267]

The general recommendation for treatment of a pediatric patient with suspected cholangitis is a semisynthetic penicillin plus β-lactamase inhibitor combination or a third-generation cephalosporin with or without an aminoglycoside.[68,142,286] The ureidopenicillins (e.g., piperacillin plus tazobactam) exhibit broad-spectrum activity against gram-positive streptococci, gram-negative bacilli, and many anaerobes. If a cephalosporin is used in a child with clinical sepsis, it is reasonable to consider the addition of metronidazole for anaerobic species, particularly *Bacteroides* spp.[30] Rothenberg and colleagues reported a 63% success rate in the treatment of pediatric patients with cholangitis following HPE using imipenem-cilastatin or third-generation cephalosporins with or without aminoglycosides and a 58% success rate using semisynthetic penicillins with aminoglycosides.[223] As mentioned previously, ceftriaxone probably should be avoided because it has been associated with biliary sludging and cholecystitis.[120] Although carbapenems provide very broad-spectrum coverage of enteric organisms associated with bacterial cholangitis,[223,248,278] these agents should be reserved for treatment of extended-spectrum β-lactamase producers or other multidrug-resistant pathogens. Antibiotic resistance is encountered more often in patients with repeated episodes of cholangitis.[64] Empiric broad-spectrum treatment should be narrowed to target specific pathogens as soon as culture results are available to avoid emergence of antimicrobial resistance or overgrowth of flora leading to secondary infection (e.g., *Clostridium difficile*, yeast).[147,261]

Antibiotic efficacy is determined by clinical and laboratory parameters such as defervescence and improvement in biliary excretion. Duration of antibiotic treatment in adult guidelines are as short as 2 to 3 days; however, a short course may result in recurrence in pediatric patients.[223] The recommended course of therapy is 7 to 10 days,[276] with longer duration recommended in special cases, such as recurrent or refractory cholangitis, and in the case of intrahepatic abscesses or hepatic surgery. Some experts recommend 14 to 21 days. Long-term administration of antibiotics without rationale should be avoided.[261] Although oral antibiotic therapy generally has no place in the treatment of cholangitis in children, oral ciprofloxacin has been used in some adult populations.[286]

Ultimately cholangitis or the risk thereof will not resolve in the presence of ongoing biliary obstruction. Although antibiotic therapy may treat septicemia, timely establishment of biliary drainage is imperative to relieve the obstruction and to increase biliary penetration of antibiotics.[66,147] In 20% to 25% of adults with cholangitis, medical therapy is insufficient, and decompression via ERCP (or other drainage procedure) is indicated.[9,66,130,227] Furthermore almost all patients who improve with medical therapy alone will ultimately require bile duct clearance to prevent recurrence of cholangitis.[147] ERCP or percutaneous transhepatic cholangiography generally are recommended as first-line approaches because they pose a lower risk than does surgical intervention.[201] While ERCP can be diagnostic in the case of biliary obstruction, it also provides therapeutic options with sphincterotomy, stone removal or destruction, or stent placement.

Treatment of parasitic cholangitis should include appropriate treatment of biliary parasites based on regional sensitivities in addition to antibiotic coverage of secondary bacterial infections. Endoscopic or surgical intervention may be required to remove worms or cysts from the biliary tree.[88,207]

PREVENTION

Treatment of biliary obstruction is the primary means to prevent acute bacterial cholangitis. Long-term prophylactic antibiotics are not recommended. Although a few case reports and small case series have documented success with TMP-SMX, ciprofloxacin, and neomycin as prophylactic antibiotics,[32,44,113,178] there are no data showing significant benefit compared to patients without prophylaxis in controlled studies. Moreover development of highly resistant bacteria selected by continuous use of antibiotics has been documented.[36,64,232]

Antibiotics immediately prior to biliary tract surgery do play a role in prevention of wound infection rates.[174] The role for antibiotic prophylaxis before endoscopic retrograde cholangiopancreatography is less clear.[286] Antibiotics are recommended if biliary stone clearance is not anticipated during a single ERCP session; otherwise prophylaxis is unlikely to be useful.[11]

COMPLICATIONS OF CHOLANGITIS

Regardless of the patient's age at the time of presentation, cholangitis can be life-threatening. Other morbidities associated with cholangitis include biloma formation and pancreatitis. Because pediatric patients who present with cholangitis typically have underlying biliary or liver pathology, cholangitis may precipitate a rapid exacerbation of the underlying disease and potentiate cirrhosis, portal hypertension, severe gastroesophageal bleeding, or ongoing sepsis. In diseases such as biliary atresia, cholangitis may hasten the patient's course toward requiring organ replacement. Cholangitis is an important determinant of long-term survival after HPE, but it is unclear if it is a determinant of transplant survival.[54–56,287]

SPECIFIC POPULATIONS AND CHOLANGITIS

Cholangitis and Biliary Atresia

In pediatrics, cholangitis is encountered most frequently in the setting of a patient with biliary atresia who has undergone a Kasai procedure. In 1959, Kasai and Suzuki first reported relief of biliary obstruction in children with biliary atresia by HPE.[127] The procedure, a roux-en-Y hepatic portoenterostomy, is considered to be standard first-line surgical therapy for infants with biliary atresia, and it is associated with the highest success rates and long-term survival when performed early, usually by 60 days of life. Without this procedure, 90% of patients with biliary atresia die before reaching age 3 years, at an average age of 19 months.[103,126,128]

Cholangitis remains the most frequent complication of the Kasai procedure, occurring in 40% to 60% of patients.[195] A subgroup of patients with the pathologic finding of cystic dilation of the intrahepatic bile ducts seems to have the highest risk of developing postoperative cholangitis.[111] The development of cholangitis has been associated with a worsening in long-term prognosis of children with biliary atresia.[54,56,114] Complications of cholangitis are severe, ranging from inflammation and scarring, to alterations in biliary flow, and eventually to biliary cirrhosis. Repeated bouts of cholangitis are associated with worsening liver function, impaired growth, and need for early transplantation. For this reason, early detection, appropriate management, and prompt intervention and treatment of cholangitis are important in this population.

Most cases of post–Kasai procedure cholangitis occur within 1 year postoperatively. In a 1976 review of 49 cases of children who underwent the procedure, 31 achieved good bile flow restoration. Of these, 20 subsequently developed cholangitis, 15 occurring within the first postoperative month and three within the second month.[193] Likewise, in a study of 105 cases of cholangitis developing in 101 children after they underwent hepatic portoenterostomies, Ecoffey and colleagues[64] showed that 63% of the cases occurred within 3 months after surgery, and 93% occurred within 1 year. Rarely late cholangitis may occur; this has been reported to occur several years after HPE.[89]

The generally accepted mechanism for development of cholangitis after a Kasai procedure is ascending bacterial colonization. This theory is reinforced by reports of a higher incidence of cholangitis developing in patients with good or partial bile flow after the Kasai procedure (78%) than in patients with no obvious bile flow (13%).[64] A 1978 study of 19 patients concluded that all bilioenteric conduits after the procedure were colonized within 1 month, correlating with the high incidence of symptomatic infection at this early stage.[109,110] The retrograde bacterial colonization may be enhanced by overall changes in intestinal motility after the roux-en-Y loop.[258] Over time, the intestinal conduit from hepatic porta to jejunum seems to "mature," and the number of episodes of cholangitis diminishes. How this adaptation happens is unknown. Late episodes of cholangitis, occurring 1 to 2 years after a Kasai procedure, likely are related to mechanical obstruction, such as adhesions, and warrant investigation.[154]

Gram-negative enteric organisms constitute most organisms causing ascending cholangitis after HPE. *E. coli* has been found in 50% of the first and second cholangitis episodes and in decreasing frequency in subsequent episodes.[64] Anaerobes also are common findings and should be considered when selecting antibiotic treatment.[30] Refractory or recurrent cases occurring after surgery may warrant consideration of fungal disease, principally *Candida* spp.[45] Attempts to isolate an organism generally are made, but blood cultures typically have a low yield.[223] Bile cultures tend to reflect the multiple enteric organisms that colonize the conduit but may not specify the true pathogens. Percutaneous liver biopsy has been used successfully to obtain cultures, but, as in other forms of cholangitis, it rarely is used for this purpose.[194]

In the intraoperative and postoperative management of children with biliary atresia, attempts have been made to prevent the incidence of cholangitis. Various modifications in the surgical configuration of the intestinal conduit have been suggested to reduce enteric reflux. Initial studies have documented a reduced incidence of ascending cholangitis in the presence of a surgically placed antireflux valve.[25] Despite the reduction of intestinal reflux in these cases, cholangitis continues to occur.[25] Cases of refractory cholangitis may require surgical intervention, especially if obstruction of the conduit or porta hepatis is suspected. Absolute indications for reoperation after HPE are unclear; however, a recent series demonstrated positive outcomes with the primary indication of recurrent jaundice.[23]

The role of corticosteroids in improving biliary drainage is controversial. Perioperative steroid pulses, typically a 3- to 5-day course of intravenous methylprednisolone, have been shown to be clinically beneficial by decreasing temperature, increasing bile flow, and improving liver biochemistries.[146,183,223] In a recent, multicenter, randomized, double-blind, placebo-controlled study, there was no significant difference in bile drainage at 6 months between those treated with steroids and the control group. Additionally there were no differences in rates of cholangitis.[17]

In addition, some centers advocate the use of prophylactic antibiotics, typically TMP-SMX. The benefits of this practice are not well established, however (see "Prevention").[44] In adults with recurrent cholangitis secondary to fixed obstruction, as in the case of malignancy, TMP-SMX and ciprofloxacin have been shown to be helpful in preventing episodes.[277] When used, TMP-SMX is used as a first-line agent. In selected patients with recurrent episodes of cholangitis on TMP-SMX and a functional HPE, we have used oral ciprofloxacin successfully. Use of probiotics was recently studied in a Taiwanese cohort after HPE and compared to neomycin and a control group. Patients receiving *Lactobacillus casei* had fewer episodes of cholangitis compared to controls, and the probiotic was as effective at preventing cholangitis in patients with biliary atresia.[153]

In patients with post–Kasai procedure biliary atresia, each episode of cholangitis is associated with a 1% mortality risk. In a recent longitudinal series, 30% of patients who died with biliary atresia without transplant had sepsis, several with suspected or proven cholangitis.[54] Some studies suggest that no significant clinical difference exists in overall survival rates between patients who have undergone the Kasai procedure and have or have not had cholangitis.[195] Previous studies suggest, however, an 88% mortality rate among patients who develop cholangitis within 1 month after undergoing the Kasai procedure and 16% in patients who develop it more than 1 month later. More recent studies suggest that the occurrence of cholangitis is related to early postoperative mortality, and the number of repeated episodes is inversely related to survival.[292] Additionally in a series of 219 patients with biliary atresia from the Childhood Liver Disease Research and Education Network (ChiLDREN), 98% of these patients with native livers 5 or more years after HPE have evidence of chronic liver disease. Of this group, 136 patients (62.1%) experienced at least one episode of cholangitis post HPE. Multiple episodes occurred of cholangitis in 11 patients.[189] Thus patients with recurrent episodes of cholangitis are considered for liver transplantation.

Cholangitis After Liver Transplantation

Infection remains the most common reason for morbidity and mortality after pediatric liver transplantation, accounting for 20% to 30% of postoperative deaths.[225,253] Bacterial infection that develops after transplantation tends to occur within the first 2 months postoperatively and generally is of either respiratory tract or intraabdominal origin. Among patients with severe bacterial infections of intraabdominal origin, cholangitis and biliary tract infections commonly develop. Gram-negative aerobic bacteria are encountered most commonly in this setting.[230] One adult study showed that 18% of 284 patients receiving liver transplantation had confirmed episodes of cholangitis.[282] Pediatric data suggest that the rate of cholangitis after liver transplantation for biliary atresia is 5% to 11%.

Biliary tract disease frequently occurs after the post–liver transplantation complication of hepatic artery thrombosis.[162,170] This complication was more prevalent in the early days of pediatric liver transplantation but decreased owing to the use of microsurgical techniques. Hepatic artery thrombosis eventually leads to damage of the bile duct because the biliary blood supply is exclusively arterial, whereas the hepatic parenchyma is vascularized by the portal vein and the hepatic artery. Biliary injury leads to altered biliary anatomy and drainage, increasing the risk of development of infection in these patients. Although the majority of pediatric liver transplant recipients have a roux-en-Y biliary–enteric anastomosis from the donor bile duct to the recipient bowel, ascending cholangitis is rare in this population. In patients with a duct-to-duct anastomosis, cholangitis secondary to stricture formation or intraductal lithiasis can be treated by ERCP.

Cholangitis that develops after liver transplantation may manifest with fever, jaundice, elevated aminotransferases, hyperbilirubinemia, and bacteremia. The variable nature of an immunocompromised patient's response to infection renders the reliability of each of these signs and symptoms unique to each occurrence. Distinguishing these symptoms from the presentation of posttransplant rejection or infection (e.g., with CMV or Epstein-Barr virus) is important. For this reason, liver biopsy often is a necessary part of the evaluation of a posttransplant patient with fever and elevated liver tests.

Cholangitis in Immunocompromised Patients

Although biliary disease related to acquired immunodeficiency syndrome (AIDS) may be considered the most common cholangiopathy of immunocompromised hosts, it is not the most frequent one in pediatric practice. Cholangitis also may occur in children with non-AIDS immunodeficiency. Sclerosing cholangitis has been reported in cases of primary immunodeficiency, including familial T-cell deficiency, IgA/IgG deficiency, and X-linked hyper-IgM syndrome.[92,150] Patients with sclerosing cholangitis often present with superimposed bacterial cholangitis because of poor biliary drainage. Opportunistic hepatobiliary infection also has been reported in children with leukemia.[82,140,246]

AIDS-related cholangitis is a well-known complication of AIDS. It tends to occur late in the course of the illness and is more common in adults than in children. With the decline in the number of new AIDS cases in the United States, especially in pediatric patients, this diagnosis has become rare. In 1989, Cello described four distinct patterns of disease in AIDS-related cholangitis as seen on cholangiography: papillary stenosis, sclerosing cholangitis, combined papillary stenosis and sclerosing cholangitis, and long extrahepatic bile duct strictures.[39] The pathogenesis of these changes is unknown and may be related to biliary inflammation secondary to immunodeficiency, infiltration of the mucosa by HIV itself, or opportunistic infection by known gut culprits in AIDS infection.

Opportunistic agents most commonly responsible are CMV, *Cryptosporidium, Microsporida,* and, uncommonly, *Mycobacterium avium-intracellulare* and *Isospora.*[186,298] One report of unexplained cholangitis in a small cohort of HIV-positive men identified *Enterocytozoon bieneusi* in the bile of all of these patients.[204] Although AIDS cholangiopathy is extremely rare in children, these pathogens can be found in pediatric patients with primary immunodeficiencies and associated PSC and with secondary immunosuppression after undergoing solid organ transplantation.[1,58,172,217,288]

Clinical presentation is similar to that in non-HIV patients, with the exception of jaundice, which tends to be less common. In a series of 45 adults with AIDS-related cholangitis, abdominal pain was reported as the most common presenting symptom, occurring in 64% of patients, followed by diarrhea (22%), fever (20%), and jaundice (7%).[61] Twenty percent of patients were asymptomatic and identified by routine blood work alone.[61] A 1997 review reported that 90% of adults present with right upper quadrant or epigastric pain.[186] Cholangitis has been reported as the initial presentation of HIV infection in a few patients.[24,181]

Diagnostic steps include noninvasive imaging with sonography and CT, and ERCP. Abdominal ultrasound is abnormal in 75% of patients and typically shows dilation or wall thickening of the common bile duct. These findings, along with liver function studies, may be suggestive of the disease even in children.[38,224] ERCP can show further characteristic changes in the biliary tract and has the added advantage of obtaining specimens for biopsy and culture and the possibility of therapeutic intervention.[293] Although AIDS-related cholangitis typically is not directly associated with mortality, most patients with AIDS-related cholangitis die within 1 year of being diagnosed because cholangitis usually occurs in patients with end-stage disease.[159] Therapy generally is symptomatic and should include coverage of bacterial cholangitis, which often is associated because of impaired biliary drainage.

Cholangitis in Association With Congenital Anatomic Abnormalities: Choledochal Cysts and Caroli Disease

Choledochal cysts occur in 1 in 15,000 births in Western nations and 1 in 1000 live births in Japan.[65,158,249,252] Typically presenting signs suggest cholestasis and may include jaundice, dark urine, and acholic stools, or patients may present with abdominal masses with or without jaundice. If diagnosed late or left untreated, choledochal cysts may result in severe complications secondary to biliary tract obstruction, including cholangitis and pancreatitis. One series of 36 Indian patients reported 13 patients, more frequently children than infants, who presented with cholangitis.[203] Cholangitis is more likely to be the presenting sign for choledochal cyst in adult patients.[43]

Treatment of cholangitis associated with choledochal cysts involves supportive treatment of the patient, including appropriate antibiotic treatment. In the past, cyst-enteric drainage procedures were used as temporizing treatments, and this type of repair was associated with high rates of complications, including recurrent bouts of cholangitis, stones, and cholangiocarcinoma in the remnant duct.[215] The current surgical goal is complete surgical excision; compared with internal drainage procedures, this approach is associated with lower rates of postoperative cholangitis and mortality.[181] Five types of choledochal cysts have been identified, with solitary extrahepatic cysts (type I) being encountered most frequently. After this type of cyst has been excised, reconstruction of the biliary tract may involve a roux-en-Y choledochojejunostomy or hepatojejunostomy.

Patients who undergo this surgery also are at risk for developing postoperative ascending cholangitis, with an incidence of 8% to 19%.[76,233] Although recurrent cholangitis may lead to chronic liver disease in the long term, antibiotic prophylaxis is not recommended routinely.[122]

Caroli disease describes congenital dilation of the intrahepatic and extrahepatic biliary tree characterized by pure ductal ectasia.[52,53] More commonly, dilation of the intrahepatic ducts is attributed to ductal plate malformation in association with congenital hepatic fibrosis. The association of ductal ectasia with congenital hepatic fibrosis is more common than without and is termed *Caroli syndrome*. Both of these diseases may manifest with clinical signs of liver disease or renal disease secondary to the associated condition of autosomal recessive polycystic kidney disease, or both.[123,156,196] Dilation of the intrahepatic bile ducts results in biliary obstruction and places the patient at increased risk for development of intrahepatic stones and cholangitis, which significantly increases morbidity and mortality rates in Caroli disease and congenital hepatic fibrosis. Diagnosis is suspected in the case of recurrent cholangitis or portal hypertension of unknown etiology and can be confirmed by ultrasound or cholangiography (MRCP, ERCP, or PTC).[71]

Surgical shunting is considered the treatment of choice because this condition typically does not progress to liver failure. Suspicion of cholangitis, whether owing to signs of infection or sepsis or laboratory results suggesting inflammation, should be confirmed via a diagnostic liver biopsy for culture. Treatment of cholangitis in the setting of Caroli disease may be difficult. Recurrent episodes may occur even after administration of intensive intravenous antibiotic therapy.[283] In some cases, drainage procedures may be used for refractory or recurrent infections. Orthotopic liver transplantation is the treatment of choice in recurrent, life-threatening episodes of cholangitis.[101,283]

Typically patients with Caroli disease or Caroli syndrome present with cholangitis because the biliary malformation communicates with the extrahepatic biliary tree. Rarely patients are seen with hepatic cysts associated with autosomal dominant polycystic kidney disease. These lesions are noncommunicating lesions and as such are not prone to infection. In the absence of a history of cholangitis, it is advisable that these rare patients not undergo invasive procedures of the biliary tree because of the risk of microbial seeding and subsequent suppurative cholangitis.[6,133,296]

Cholangitis After Endoscopic and Other Biliary Procedures

The overall adverse event rate for pediatric ERCP is reported to be from 0% to 11%, and in adults cholangitis is a known risk of ERCP. In a series of 50 pediatric patients, low-grade fever, abdominal pain, nausea, and vomiting were reported as the most common complaints after undergoing ERCP; one patient was treated for mild cholangitis.[263] Another group reported three cases of sepsis in adults caused by multidrug-resistant *Pseudomonas aeruginosa* after ERCP, ascribed to nosocomial transmission from the endoscope despite negative surveillance cultures.[59] In adults, and rarely in children, biliary sphincterotomy with or without stent placement can be used to alleviate a common bile duct obstruction, most frequently malignant.

The major complication of biliary stents is obstruction and subsequent upstream infection. A Cochrane Review examined the role of antibiotics or ursodeoxycholic acid to maintain stent patency and demonstrated no conclusive evidence in favor of either one in the prevention of stent occlusion.[80,262] In certain children and adolescents with a history of recalcitrant cholangitis, percutaneous transhepatic biliary drainage is used by experienced centers to decompress the biliary tree upstream of the stricture or to dilate the stricture. This procedure is used primarily in patients with PSC and in transplant patients with biliary stenoses secondary to ischemia or rejection.[12,50,80,85,99,262] These patients may benefit from oral antibiotic prophylaxis, frequently ciprofloxacin for its excellent biliary penetration.

CHOLECYSTITIS

Cholecystitis and its related complications are most commonly associated with cholelithiasis (gallstones). However, it can occur without stone disease. An estimated 20 million individuals have gallbladder disease in the United States based on the National Health and Nutrition Examination Survey (NHANES) III report.[69] Although gallbladder-related diseases occur less often in children, there is a trend toward increasing rates of disease.[21,173] Gallstones accounted for 4 to 6 per 100,000 hospital discharges in children younger than 15 years.[70] Recent data suggest that the obesity epidemic and related metabolic syndrome account for a greater proportion of gallstones in children.[125,173] Despite the predominance of obesity-related disease, children with hemolytic disorders remain at high risk for gallstones and related comorbidities. Similarly, several studies have reported much higher rates of complicated gallbladder disease in children than in adults, with common bile duct obstruction and gallstone pancreatitis occurring in up to 30% of children.[21,104,173]

Cholecystitis refers to inflammation of the gallbladder, which can occur in a variety of clinical scenarios. In adults, acute cholecystitis almost always is associated with gallstones—90% of adult cases occur secondary to gallstones. In contrast, 30% to 50% of pediatric cases are acalculous.[273] Acalculous cholecystitis is discussed separately at the end of this section. The most likely cause of calculous cholecystitis is gallstone obstruction of the cystic duct, which leads to increased intraluminal pressure with gallbladder distention, mucosal damage, and release of inflammatory mediators. The end result is acute inflammation of the gallbladder. Any bacterial infection is likely a secondary occurrence to biliary obstruction.[137]

Etiology and Pathogenesis

Gallstones are divided into cholesterol or pigmented stones (black or brown), although they often are mixed in constituents. Stone formation occurs secondary to precipitation of insoluble bile content (cholesterol, bile pigments, and calcium salts). Cholesterol stones are formed when the balance of cholesterol, lecithin, and bile salts is such that cholesterol in no longer soluble and becomes supersaturated. Black pigmented stones can form when there is supersaturated bile or a decrease in the bile salt pool. This process includes an increase in bilirubin anions (as seen in unconjugated hyperbilirubinemia), an increase in unbound Ca^{2+}, or a decrease in other factors that solubilize calcium and bilirubin.[129,197] Brown pigmented stones differ from black stones in that brown stones typically are more often related to infection and form within the common bile duct rather than the gallbladder in both children and adults. *Opisthorchis sinensis* and *Ascaris lumbricoides* are major sources of brown pigmented stones in rural Asian countries.[107] Pigmented stones have been described with *E. coli*, *Pseudomonas* spp., *Staphylococcus* spp., *Enterobacter* spp., *Citrobacter* spp., and *Salmonella enterica* serovar Virchow.[15,51,272] There is also a strong relationship to urinary tract infections.[105] As discussed earlier, ceftriaxone as well as other third-generation cephalosporins have been associated with cholelithiasis and sludge in this population: up to 38% in one series of children with biliary tract disease in Israel.[135]

The majority of data on children with pigmented stones come from patients with hemolytic disease (e.g., sickle-cell anemia and thalassemia). There is a significant population of patients with biliary disease secondary to hereditary spherocytosis and other red cell membrane defects, pyruvate kinase deficiency, glucose-6-phosphate dehydrogenase deficiency, and autoimmune hemolytic anemia.[21,213,239] The prevalence of pigment gallstones in hemolytic disease increases with age. In children younger than 10 years, the frequency is 12% to 14%; the frequency increases to 36% to 42% in individuals 10 to 20 years old.[22,236]

Until recently pigmented stones were the predominant cause of gallstone disease and related morbidity in children, in which up to 72% were involved.[79] However, in a recent 3-year report of more than 400 pediatric patients with gallbladder disease, there was more than a threefold difference in obese patients with cholesterol stones compared to those with hemolytic disease.[173] This suggests a trend that children and adolescents are now more similar to adults with gallbladder disease than in years past.

Cholesterol stones are found most frequently in adults and have an increased prevalence in women from puberty to menopause and in obese patients.[231] Although boys and girls exhibit an equal incidence in gallstones at young ages, the incidence in girls increases significantly after puberty, and female predominance of gallstone disease continues through menopause.[70,191] Related risk factors for the presence of cholesterol stones in children and adolescents include ethnic background (Hispanic), obesity, pregnancy, and the use of oral contraceptives.[136,160,173,188] In addition, conditions that are associated with decreased ileal bile salt resorption predispose to stone formation. This association includes patients who have undergone ileal resection or bypass and patients with Crohn disease.[221]

Total parenteral nutrition remains a significant risk factor for children to develop biliary tract disease and in particular gallstone formation.[210] This condition occurs more commonly in premature neonates, especially neonates with enteral diseases, in which prolonged fasting, sepsis, immaturity of the enterohepatic circulation of bile acids, small bowel bacterial overgrowth, and prolonged duration of total parenteral nutrition contribute to biliary stasis and increased prevalence of gallstones and sludge.[7,132,141,202,235,259,285] The occurrence of gallstones secondary to total parenteral nutrition does not lead to increased prevalence of complications because many of these gallstones are clinically silent.

Gallstones in cystic fibrosis (CF) are common, with an estimated prevalence of gallstones in 10% to 30%. Symptomatic gallstones have been reported in 3.6% of affected pediatric patients.[250,280] Gallstones in CF are predominantly composed of a mixed pigment and smaller amounts of cholesterol. Stone formation is multifactorial but is related to altered lipid composition and altered motility.[106] Pathophysiology of pigmented stones in CF is also linked to deltaF508 mutations, with fecal bile loss and altered enterohepatic circulation as well as UGT1A1 mutations. Alterations in enterohepatic circulation have also been suggested as the mechanism for pigmented gallstone formation in Crohn disease.[27] Finally children with chronic liver disease, and in particular cholestasis, are at increased risk for gallstone formation owing to a deficit of biliary excretion.[289] Box 48.3 summarizes the pediatric patient populations at risk for the development of gallstones.

In addition to the observations made in UGT1A1 mutations, knowledge regarding the heredity of cholelithiasis continues to develop. There is likely a combination of genetic predisposition and environmental risk factors. In adults, a distinction is made between the "common" polygenic predisposition to gallstones and the rarer oligogenic predisposition. The first, polygenic, group refers to patients with evidence of increased risk of developing biliary stone formation, including lithogenic (*LITH*) genes. The oligogenic group refers to a small group of patients with known mutations in genes involved in bile synthesis and export.[96,289]

BOX 48.3 Conditions Associated With Pediatric Gallstone Disease

- Biliary tract anomaly (e.g., choledochal cyst)
- Cephalosporin use
- Cystic fibrosis
- Crohn disease
- Genetic predisposition (e.g., ABCB4, UGT1A1 mutations)
- Hispanic or Latino ancestry
- Hemolytic disorders (e.g., sickle-cell anemia, hereditary spherocytosis)
- Malabsorption
- Metabolic syndrome
- Obesity
- Parasitic disease (*Ascaris lumbricoides*)
- Pregnancy
- Rapid weight loss
- Solid organ and hematologic transplant (e.g., liver, kidney, heart, bone marrow)
- Total parenteral nutrition

From references 21, 79, 81, 144, 173.

The clearest examples to date are defects in the *ABCB4* transporter in humans and the *Mdr2* homozygous null mutant in mice.[144,145,185,222] Both conditions lead to an increased propensity toward cholelithiasis and choledocholithiasis; however, whether these subjects have a profile of biliary tract infections different from that of the polygenic group is unknown.

Clinical Presentation

Acute cholecystitis is characterized by abdominal pain with vomiting or nausea. The pain is referred to as "biliary colic" but is nonparoxysmal, with a constant, sharp pain lasting 4 to 6 hours. Pain relents only if the obstructing stone in the cystic or common bile duct mobilizes but may persist or return with gallbladder wall inflammation. In children, differentiating between other forms of acute abdomen can be difficult because pain can be in the right upper quadrant but also in the mid-epigastrium. Radiation to the left upper quadrant or the right shoulder can occur and, with peritoneal inflammation, poorly localize in the abdomen, corresponding to the gallbladder's somatic innervation.[245]

Jaundice is reported more frequently in younger children with acute cholecystitis, infrequently with acholic stools in infants. Although jaundice is typically associated in younger children, in one series of 50 children, no child younger than 6 years had jaundice.[210] If jaundice is present, choledocholithiasis or cholangitis should be strongly considered. Fever is not universally present in cholecystitis and is reported as low as 11% in pediatric patients. Similarly, in a retrospective study of 198 adults who presented to an emergency center with acute cholecystitis, 71% were afebrile; in gangrenous acute cholecystitis, 59% were afebrile.[95]

Physical examination may reveal a tender right upper quadrant. On light palpation a small mass may be appreciated, corresponding to the swollen gallbladder. Contrasting this, Murphy's sign is positive when abdominal pain is elicited upon deep palpation of the right upper quadrant corresponding to the liver's edge or gallbladder and most apparent with deep inspiration. This can be appreciated during ultrasound examination and may be reported by the ultrasonographer. With a tense abdomen, rigidity suggests cholecystitis with local peritonitis, and the patient may exhibit voluntary guarding or other peritoneal signs.

Evaluation

Laboratory evaluation may show leukocytosis, although this finding is not universally present in adults or children with cholecystitis.[95,210] Even in gangrenous cholecystitis, up to 25% of patients may fail to have leukocytosis. Bilirubin levels may be elevated, especially in the setting of hemolysis. A conjugated hyperbilirubinemia may suggest cholangitis, choledocholithiasis, or sepsis-associated cholestasis. Friesen et al. reported 38% of patients with hyperbilirubinemia in a pediatric series, and levels of bilirubin to 4 mg/dL are reported in adults.[79,245] Serum aminotransferases, alkaline phosphatase and γ-glutamyltransferase are also useful. Amylase and lipase should be obtained because of the overlap of pancreatitis with both gallstone-related disease and viral hepatitides. Pediatric surgical consultation should be obtained in patients with possible acute cholecystitis or other forms of acute abdomen. However, if common bile duct obstruction or gallstone pancreatitis is suspected, pediatric gastroenterology consultation should be obtained for possible endoscopic management with ERCP.

Abdominal ultrasound is the test of choice in establishing the diagnosis of cholecystitis and is usually the first-line examination. Findings on ultrasound include a thickened or irregular, hyperreflexive gallbladder wall with or without the presence of gallstones. Experienced sonographers may be able to elicit tenderness over the gallbladder, known as the sonographic Murphy sign. Ultrasound is useful for detecting gallstones within the gallbladder in up to 90% of cases. However, the sensitivity of common bile duct stone detection is poor, ranging from 30% to 50%.[47,48,78] The finding of gallstones alone by sonogram does not indicate cholecystitis. Other false-positive studies may occur with the finding of thickened gallbladder walls in patients with hypoalbuminemia, renal failure, or heart failure.[200] The inability to visualize the gallbladder by ultrasound may indicate the finding of a diseased, chronically obstructed gallbladder.[91]

Hepatobiliary scintigraphy (HIDA scan) can be useful in confirming the diagnosis of acute cholecystitis. The study employs a technetium-labeled iminodiacetic acid agent that is excreted into the bile ducts. Subsequent images are taken, which in a normal study should fill the gallbladder, extrahepatic ducts, and duodenum. In the case of cystic duct obstruction, a positive study fails to show the gallbladder filling. The sensitivity and specificity of this study are high, with results approaching 90% to 100% and 90% to 95%, respectively.[177,184,213] The test may be augmented by attempts to stimulate gallbladder contraction using a cholecystokinin analogue.[98] Plain abdominal radiographs and oral cholecystography are rarely used in the modern era of biliary disease.

Management

The treatment plan for patients with gallstones depends on several factors including patient symptoms, underlying conditions, and the presence of associated/concomitant choledocholithiasis. Asymptomatic patients with gallstones identified incidentally can often be managed conservatively, although guidelines in children are lacking. Symptomatic patients with large stones (>2 cm) may be considered for conservative nonoperative management or elective cholecystectomy.

Recommendations for evaluation of patients with sickle-cell disease include the evaluation with abdominal ultrasound at age 10 years.[255] When stones are detected patients should be considered for early cholecystectomy, although this plan is controversial.[5,97,121,173,284] In patients with sickle-cell anemia, the benefit of timely surgery may outweigh the morbidity of associated abdominal pain crises and the overall morbidity and mortality of surgery in these patients, which increases with age. In patients with hereditary spherocytosis, ultrasound evaluation is recommended annually beginning at age 4, but severity of disease or coexistence of Gilbert syndrome may alter this.[260]

In acute calculous cholecystitis, laparoscopic cholecystectomy is the most common surgical treatment for children and is performed in more than 95% of cases.[173] The preoperative management of patients includes hospital admission for monitoring, intravenous hydration, and pain control. Antibiotic therapy often is initiated even without clinical evidence of sepsis or perforation. The choice of antibiotics is similar to that for cholangitis and typically covers gut luminal flora (e.g., a semisynthetic penicillin/β-lactamase inhibitor combination or third- or fourth-generation cephalosporin with or without an aminoglycoside).[100,286,297] In high-risk patients in whom laparoscopic or open cholecystectomy is not feasible, cholecystotomy can be performed by interventional radiology or surgery. In adults, data suggest that early cholecystectomy should be performed in those with acute cholecystitis secondary to gallstone disease[211] and in biliary pancreatitis.[211]

The management of acalculous cholecystitis may vary based on whether it is acute or chronic, but overall limited data are available. In addition to treatment of underlying causes, options for therapy in acute acalculous cholecystitis include nonoperative therapy with nothing by mouth and intravenous hydration and nutrition, cholecystostomy, or cholecystectomy.[118,273] The majority of patients with chronic acalculous cholecystitis undergo cholecystectomy. With findings of microlithiasis by endoscopic sampling or by endoscopic ultrasound, consideration for ERCP or cholecystectomy may be appropriate to prevent cholangitis or recurrent pancreatitis.[124] The role of cholecystectomy for biliary dyskinesia, a motility disorder related to acalculous cholecystitis, is debated in children.[177]

Complications

Even with prompt recognition and therapy, acute cholecystitis may lead to complications. Perforation of the gallbladder is rare but can also occur in the cystic duct or bile duct. Mirizzi syndrome is a spectrum in which a cystic duct stone obstructs the common bile duct and, in advanced forms, can lead to fistulae and perforation. An inflamed, obstructed gallbladder may wall off to form an intraluminal abscess or empyema, although gangrenous inflammation of the gallbladder is rare in children. A localized perforation may develop into a pericholecystic abscess that is palpable as a tender right upper quadrant mass on examination. Free perforation with peritonitis is associated with a 30% mortality rate, but it is found in only a few patients, estimated at 1% to 2% of adult patients.[147] In both gangrene and perforation, intravenous fluids, antibiotic therapy, and surgical evaluation are critical.

However, the most common complication of cholecystitis is common bile duct obstruction or choledocholithiasis. Recent reports in children describe rates of obstructive jaundice and pancreatitis in up to 30% in those with symptomatic gallbladder disease.[21,104,173,210] Choledocholithiasis can lead to ascending cholangitis but is a rare cause of cholangitis in pediatric patients. Choledocholithiasis should be suspected in all patients with gallstones, along with right or left upper quadrant pain, jaundice, fever, or pancreatitis. Common bile duct stones originating from the gallbladder can be found in patients with acute cholecystitis by transabdominal ultrasound, endoscopic ultrasound, MRCP, ERCP, or intraoperative cholangiography. Although no formal recommendations are available in children, adult guidelines recommend the consideration of ERCP with stone clearance if suspicion is high for common bile duct stones. Patients with a total bilirubin of greater than 4 mg/dL or a visualized stone by abdominal ultrasound are at high risk for stones, as are patients who have both a common bile duct diameter of greater than 6 mm and a total bilirubin greater than 1.8 mg/dL.[166] In our experience, patients with a conjugated bilirubin greater than 0.5 mg/dL were 35-fold more likely to have a stone at ERCP than were those with a normal conjugated bilirubin.[74] An international multicenter study is ongoing to evaluate this in pediatric patients. Modifications are likely necessary in children owing to a smaller bile duct diameter. In patients at low risk for common bile duct stones or recently passed stones, laparoscopic cholecystectomy with or without intraoperative cholangiogram is appropriate.[211]

Acalculous Cholecystitis

Acalculous cholecystitis is a rare but important cause of cholecystitis in pediatric patients. Generally acalculous gallbladder disease in children occurs in various clinical settings ranging from congenital gallbladder abnormalities, to idiopathic gallbladder distention without inflammation (acute hydrops of the gallbladder), to acute or chronic cholecystitis (Box 48.4). The exact pathogenesis of acute acalculous cholecystitis is unclear; however, stagnation of the bile may be an important factor, as suggested by several predisposing clinical conditions that lead to bile stasis. In addition, sphincter of Oddi spasm or dysfunction, as occurs after administration of opiates, could lead to retrograde reflux of inflammatory enzymes or infectious agents. Alternatively changes in the gallbladder vascular supply may weaken the gallbladder mucosa and allow biliary components to damage the gallbladder wall.[86] Acalculous cholecystitis has been associated with many infectious and noninfectious clinical scenarios. Bacterial, viral, and parasitic agents have been implicated in the setting of acalculous cholecystitis.

BOX 48.4 Conditions Associated With Acalculous Gallbladder Disease

Biliary tract anomaly (e.g., choledochal cyst)
Bone marrow transplant
Burns
Chemotherapy in oncology patients
Critical illness in intensive care unit patients
Crohn disease, Henoch-Schönlein purpura, Kawasaki disease, systemic lupus erythematosus
Infectious agents (atypical microbes)
Microlithiasis
Postoperative state (e.g., cardiac surgery)
Sepsis
Sludge
Systemic inflammatory states
Total parenteral nutrition
Traumatic spinal cord injury

From references 116, 119, 218, 251, 268, 270.

Frequently gallstone or biliary microlithiasis missed by standard diagnostic evaluations may lead the clinician to the presumptive diagnosis of acalculous cholecystitis. One adult study revealed that 33 of 35 patients with abdominal pain and a negative transabdominal sonogram had gallbladder sludge and stones, and 21 of those patients also had common bile duct involvement.[175]

Reports of true acalculous disease have been described with systemic infection from *Salmonella* spp., *Mycoplasma pneumoniae, Leptospira* spp., *Brucella* spp., Rocky Mountain spotted fever, group A streptococci, group B streptococci, and *Staphylococcus aureus*.[8,10,57,108,171,254,265,290] Examination and culture of cholecystectomy specimens from patients with acalculous cholecystitis have revealed positive cultures for *Helicobacter* spp. and *Campylobacter jejuni*. Associations with viral disease include CMV, mumps virus, Epstein-Barr virus, and hepatitis A virus.[3,13,18,26,37,83,205] Acalculous cholecystitis has been associated with *Plasmodium falciparum* infections (malaria).[63,165,226,234,295] In immunosuppressed hosts, acalculous cholecystitis also has been described in fungal infections with *Candida* spp. or *Aspergillus* spp. or parasitic infections with *Giardia lamblia* and *Cryptosporidium parvum*.[186]

Noninfectious systemic diseases associated with acalculous cholecystitis or hydrops include neoplastic disease (i.e., leukemia), Henoch-Schönlein purpura, lupus erythematosus, and Kawasaki disease.[34,112,169,254]

Box 48.4 lists several conditions with which acalculous cholecystitis has been reported.[116,119,218,251,268,270]

Clinical presentation is similar to that of patients with calculous disease, with right upper quadrant pain, nausea, vomiting, anorexia, and fever being the most common symptoms. Leukocytosis, jaundice, or a palpable right upper quadrant mass also may be present.[273] The most common setting for acalculous disease is in critically ill or chronically ill patients with concurrent acute or chronic symptoms. A high degree of clinical suspicion is crucial in making the diagnosis in these populations because often the findings suggestive of cholecystitis are obscured by the patient's systemic disease. The most common sonographic finding is a thickened gallbladder wall and a possible sonographic Murphy sign. Gallbladder distention, sludge, or pericholecystic fluid also may be found on transabdominal ultrasound.[118] In addition to ultrasound, the HIDA scan is an important tool in the evaluation of acalculous cholecystitis. Failure to visualize the gallbladder on scintigraphy and a low ejection fraction in response to a cholecystokinin analogue are suggestive of acalculous disease.[168,184,206,299]

NEW REFERENCES SINCE THE SEVENTH EDITION

17. Bezerra JA, Spino C, Magee JC, et al. Use of corticosteroids after hepatoportoenterostomy for bile drainage in infants with biliary atresia: the START randomized clinical trial. *JAMA*. 2014;311:1750-1759.
67. Epstein L, Hunter JC, Arwady MA, et al. New Delhi metallo-β-lactamase-producing carbapenem-resistant *Escherichia coli* associated with exposure to duodenoscopes. *JAMA*. 2014;312:1447-1455.
74. Fishman DS, Chumpitazi BP, Raijman I. Endoscopic retrograde cholangiography for pediatric choledocholithiasis: assessing the need for endoscopic intervention. *World J Gastrointest Endosc*. 2016;8(11):425-432.
153. Lien TH, Bu LN, Wu JF, et al. Use of *Lactobacillus casei rhamnosus* to prevent cholangitis in biliary atresia after Kasai operation. *J Pediatr Gastroenterol Nutr*. 2015;60:654-658.
163. Luo Q, Hao F, Zhang M, et al. Serum bacterial DNA detection in patients with cholangitis after Kasai procedure. *Pediatr Int*. 2015;57:954-960.
189. Ng VL, Haber BH, Magee JC, et al. Medical status of 219 children with biliary atresia surviving long-term with their native livers: results from a North American multicenter consortium. *J Pediatr*. 2014;165:539-546. e532.
264. Terashita D, Kim M, Marquez P, et al. Los Angeles County public health response to outbreaks of carbapenem-resistant Enterobacteriaceae associated with endoscopic retrograde cholangiopancreatography. *Open Forum Infect Dis*. 2015;2(suppl 1):106.
274. U.S. Food and Drug Administration. Design of Endoscopic Retrograde Cholangiopancreatography (ERCP) duodenoscopes may impede effective cleaning: FDA safety communication. Presented at IDWeek October 7–11, 2015. San Diego CA.
276. van den Hazel SJ, Speelman P, Tytgat GN, et al. Role of antibiotics in the treatment and prevention of acute and recurrent cholangitis. *Clin Infect Dis*. 1994;19:279-286.

The full reference list for this chapter is available at ExpertConsult.com.

49 Pyogenic Liver Abscess

Sheldon L. Kaplan

Pyogenic liver abscesses are encountered infrequently in healthy children and generally have been reported more commonly in the compromised pediatric host. The rarity of liver abscesses may be explained partly by the rich blood supply, unique architecture, and extensive reticuloendothelial system of the liver, all of which present an effective barrier against bacterial invasion.

The precise incidence of pyogenic liver abscesses in children is unknown. Adult patients with hepatic abscesses constitute approximately 8 to 20 per 100,000 admissions; a 0.29% to 0.57% incidence of liver abscesses has been found in autopsies of adult patients.[11,53] In an early large series of liver abscesses in children, Dehner and Kissane[10] reported a 0.38% incidence at autopsy in patients younger than 15 years; 11 of 27 (41%) patients were younger than 2 years, and 18 of 27 (67%) patients were younger than 6 years. In a review of admissions to Milwaukee Children's Hospital, Chusid[9] found 5 children (four of whom were <6 months old) with at least one hepatic abscess and estimated an incidence of three cases per 100,000 admissions. Pineiro-Carrero and Andres[48] estimated an incidence of approximately 25 cases per 100,000 admissions in their pediatric population (11 patients >14 years old). Pyogenic liver abscess in children is encountered more frequently in developing countries than in developed countries.[56] In Taiwan the overall incidence of pyogenic liver abscesses increased from 11.2 per 100,000 population in 1996 to 17.6 per 100,000 in 2004.[60]

PATHOGENESIS

Bacteria can establish an inflammatory focus in the liver by four major routes. Direct extension from contiguous structures is the most common mode in adults, accounting for up to 60% of hepatic abscesses in adults.[7,26,49,53] Biliary tract infection (cholangitis, cholecystitis), pancreatitis, and penetrating gastric or duodenal ulcer are examples of diseases associated with liver abscesses caused by extension from a contiguous focus of infection. In a review of this problem at St. Louis Children's Hospital, three of 27 children (11%) were considered to have a liver abscess secondary to inflammation of contiguous organs.[10] Although biliary tract disease occurs infrequently in children, ascending cholangitis is a particularly frequent complication of the hepatic portoenterostomy procedure for congenital biliary atresia and may lead to infections of the liver in such patients.[14,52] Liver abscesses also may develop as a complication of liver transplantation, especially if technical problems related to vascular supply or biliary drainage develop.[32]

The portal system is the second most common route by which bacteria may reach the liver in adults; 6% to 27% of liver abscesses in adults derive from this source.[25,35,53] In newborns, solitary liver abscesses, especially abscesses caused by gram-negative organisms, have complicated the use of umbilical vein catheterization or have been secondary to omphalitis.[6] Prematurity and necrotizing enterocolitis also are important predisposing conditions.[13]

Portal vein inflammation and bacteremia can be associated with infections within the abdominal cavity. Appendicitis, diverticulitis, perirectal abscesses, regional enteritis, ulcerative colitis, and omphalitis are possible sources of portal vein sepsis.[10] In a large study conducted in Taiwan, patients with inflammatory bowel disease (IBD) had an increased risk of developing a pyogenic liver abscess compared with controls without IBD.[37] A pyogenic liver abscess may be an unusual complication of an ingested foreign body, with subsequent development of portal venous bacteremia.[42] Since antibiotics have been available, portal vein inflammation and pyelophlebitis have become less common sources of hepatic infection in children.

Systemic bacteremia with hematogenous spread of bacteria to the liver through the hepatic artery seems to be the most common source of liver abscess in children, but it is implicated in less than 20% of adult patients. In the St. Louis series, the systemic hematogenous route was responsible for 21 of 27 (78%) cases of liver abscesses.[10] Of 13 patients encountered after 1940, seven had bacteremia associated with leukemia. Anaerobic bacteremia associated with retropharyngeal or peritonsillar abscesses presumably has preceded development of anaerobic liver abscesses in several children.[8] Likewise liver abscesses in neonates may be preceded by a systemic bacteremia without evidence of portal or biliary tract involvement.[39]

Liver abscesses occur more frequently in compromised pediatric hosts, especially those with chronic granulomatous disease, than in healthy children.[27] In a registry of 368 patients with chronic granulomatous disease from the United States, a liver abscess occurred in 27% of patients.[63] Over the course of 10 years, 15 children were diagnosed with pyogenic liver abscess in a large referral center for pediatric liver disease in the United Kingdom.[40] Three children (20%) had chronic granulomatous disease. In addition to functional disorders of phagocytes, chronic neutropenia predisposes to the development of liver abscesses.[47] Wintch and colleagues[64] noted that five of 10 children with hepatic abscesses in their institution had an underlying defect in host defense. Primary hemochromatosis predisposes to multiple liver abscesses caused by *Yersinia enterocolitica* in particular.[61] Pyogenic liver abscesses also are associated with Papillon-Lefèvre syndrome, a rare autosomal recessive disease characterized by palmoplantar keratoderma and periodontitis.[1]

Penetrating and nonpenetrating trauma to the liver may lead to liver abscesses, presumably caused by bacterial proliferation within small collections of blood and bile that result from the trauma. Hepatic abscess may be a rare complication of ventriculoperitoneal shunts after penetration of a peritoneal catheter into the liver.[24,43] Liver abscess also is a complication of percutaneous liver biopsy.[16]

Unexplained or cryptogenic hepatic abscesses are encountered in most series and accounted for 40% to 50% of cases in many series.[23,26] Lee and Block[36] have proposed that these cryptogenic liver abscesses "originate from anaerobic bacterial invasion of hepatic infarcts." This theory is supported by reports that describe pyogenic liver abscesses as a complication of hepatic infarction in patients with sickle-cell anemia.[55] Normal gastrointestinal bacterial flora were isolated from nine of 11 patients with liver abscesses at the Mayo Clinic. This finding suggested to Lazarchick and associates[35] that unrecognized intraabdominal collections of pus were responsible. Although the reasons are unclear, diabetes mellitus also predisposes to the development of liver abscesses.[22,49,58] In a study from Taiwan, three of 15 children with pyogenic liver abscesses seen over a 15-year period had diabetes mellitus as an underlying condition.[23] Nematode infection with larvae migrating through the liver is thought to be another predisposing factor for the development of pyogenic abscesses in children. The larvae induce liver granulomata that trap bacteria, leading to formation of an abscess.[46] In one study from Brazil, positive serology for *Toxocara canis* was significantly more frequent for patients with pyogenic liver abscess (10 of 16) than for the 32 age-matched controls (four of 32).[51]

Biliary tract disease generally predisposes to the development of multiple liver abscesses. In contrast, blunt trauma to the liver or portal system inflammation most commonly predisposes to a single abscess. In neonates, liver abscesses may be solitary or multiple because of systemic bacteria.[39,41] Solitary abscesses are the most common findings in the right lobe of the liver.[35]

Hepatic and splenic abscesses caused by *Candida* spp. are well described in patients with cancer.[57] Multiple abscesses are typical findings. These organs presumably are infected hematogenously, usually when the host is neutropenic.

MICROBIOLOGY

Gram-negative organisms have been the predominant isolates from liver abscesses in adults. *Escherichia coli* and *Klebsiella, Aerobacter, Pseudomonas,* and *Proteus* spp. have been implicated most frequently. *Klebsiella* spp. are the most common organism isolated from children with pyogenic liver abscess in Taiwan.[23,59] *Klebsiella* spp. also predominated in Taiwan overall and in adult Asian patients in a report from New York.[50,60] Anaerobic organisms also are important; anaerobic organisms were recovered from 45% of patients with liver abscesses in the University of California–Los Angeles series.[54]

In contrast to the adult experience, Dehner and Kissane[10] reported that 33% of liver abscesses in children were caused by *Staphylococcus aureus,* whereas gram-negative organisms were found in only 32%. Two or more organisms were recovered from liver abscesses in 52% of children. In a review of 96 children (no neonates) with pyogenic liver abscesses, *S. aureus,* gram-negative enteric organisms, and anaerobes were the organisms isolated most commonly, in that order.[30] *S. aureus* is the most common isolate that causes pyogenic liver abscess in patients with chronic granulomatous disease. In neonates, gram-negative enteric organisms are isolated most commonly. Anaerobes, particularly *Fusobacterium necrophorum,* have been isolated from liver abscesses in children without underlying disease.[15] Fungi, particularly *Candida albicans,* have been associated with liver abscesses in children with leukemia and neutropenia who have received parenteral hyperalimentation.[3] Liver or splenic abscesses also may be an unusual complication of brucellosis.[62] Human rotavirus–like particles were identified in the material aspirated from a liver abscess, but they were considered a secondary phenomenon and not the primary etiology of the liver abscess.[19]

CLINICAL MANIFESTATIONS

The clinical manifestations of pyogenic liver abscesses are nonspecific. A high index of suspicion and an awareness of this illness are necessary to establish the diagnosis. A history of preceding abdominal surgery or trauma is helpful when present, as is the knowledge that the host's response to infection is compromised.

Fever, nausea, vomiting, anorexia, weakness, and malaise are prominent symptoms that may last several weeks. Abdominal or pleuritic pain, weight loss, and diarrhea are less common manifestations. A history of abdominal pain and fever of unknown origin in an otherwise healthy child suggests the diagnosis of pyogenic liver abscess.[29] In contrast, fever often is not observed in neonates.[13] Patients with a macroscopic or single abscess frequently experience a subacute to chronic course. In contrast, patients with multiple abscesses generally experience a more acute febrile illness.

Hepatomegaly occurs in 40% to 80% of patients; abdominal tenderness occurs less frequently. Right upper quadrant tenderness or even a mass may be subtle and not appreciated unless the physician specifically and carefully examines this region. Other physical findings include jaundice (generally associated with biliary tract disease and not liver abscesses), abdominal distention, and evidence of pleuropulmonary involvement (i.e., elevated or fixed hemidiaphragm, rales, and pleural effusion).

DIAGNOSIS

Routine laboratory studies are of little help in establishing a diagnosis. Anemia, leukocytosis, and an elevation in C-reactive protein are common findings. Liver function tests generally reflect underlying disease of the liver itself and usually are not caused by the abscess. When abscesses occur secondary to biliary tract obstruction, alkaline phosphatase and bilirubin concentrations generally are elevated. Transaminase concentrations usually are normal to mildly elevated in most cases. A rapidly enlarging, tender liver in a patient with normal transaminase concentrations should alert the clinician to the possibility of liver abscess. Lazarchick and colleagues[35] found that the serum albumin concentration was the most important test with regard to prognosis in adults; 14 of 16 patients with a serum albumin level of less than 2 g/dL died.

Blood cultures are positive more commonly in patients with multiple abscesses than in patients with solitary abscesses. Overall, however, blood cultures usually are sterile in children with pyogenic liver abscess.

More than 50% of adult patients have abnormalities on chest radiography. Atelectasis, pulmonary infiltrates, pleural effusion, and elevated or fixed right hemidiaphragm are the most common findings.

Computed tomography (CT) currently provides the most accurate information concerning the size, location, and number of abscesses within the liver parenchyma (Fig. 49.1).[28,34,48] Lesions measuring 1 cm in diameter can be detected by CT. Multiple small abscesses may appear in clusters in a pattern suggesting early coalescence of the abscesses.[25] Liver abscesses appear as areas of low attenuation. The target lesions of hepatic candidiasis are not visualized by CT when the patient is neutropenic, and scans may need to be repeated before these characteristic lesions are observed.[57] Structures contiguous with the liver also are shown by CT; this information is important when a surgical approach to drainage is being planned.

Magnetic resonance imaging does not have any major advantages over CT for detecting or characterizing liver abscess but may show characteristic features to distinguish an abscess from other focal liver lesions in selected patients.[2,38] Ultrasonography also is a sensitive technique for detecting liver abscesses, and, because it is noninvasive and does not require exposure to radiation, it is recommended for initial evaluation.[31,34] Hepatic angiography defines the vascular anatomy in the area of the liver abscess further and may provide information necessary for surgical management in selected cases. Nuclear medicine techniques rarely are indicated as a diagnostic method if liver abscess is suspected.

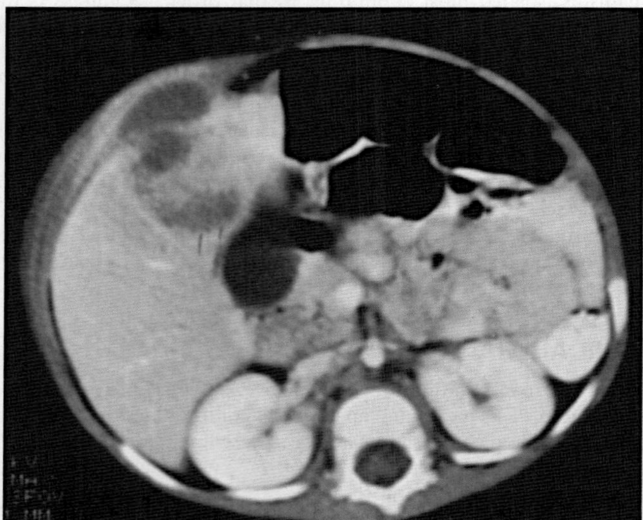

FIG. 49.1 Abdominal computed tomography scan showing a 4 × 5 cm encapsulated, septate, circular mass within the liver. A low-density soft tissue mass is noted in the abdominal wall from apparent extension from the intrahepatic mass.

TREATMENT

Numerous reports have documented that patients with undiagnosed and untreated liver abscesses generally die and that surgical drainage of the solitary pyogenic liver abscess is the key to successful treatment. The choice of extraserous or transperitoneal open drainage or percutaneous closed aspiration depends on the location and size of the abscess and the experience and preference of the surgeon.[18,26,45,53]

Numerous groups have described percutaneous catheter drainage of liver abscesses in adults.[4,5,17,31] Percutaneous drainage of liver abscesses in children should be considered as the initial approach to drainage of such abscesses, especially in the right lobe of the liver.[12,48] In one study, antibiotic administration plus percutaneous aspiration without inserting a drain was successful treatment in six of eight children considered at low risk (small abscess, within liver [rim >1 cm], very-low-level ultrasound echoes suggesting liquefaction).[56]

A catheter is placed into the cavity under CT or ultrasound guidance; material is aspirated, and, when an abscess is documented, a draining catheter is placed. The cavity can be irrigated with saline initially. Criteria for the selection of patients for percutaneous drainage have been established.[17] The optimal route of percutaneous aspiration is directly into the abscess cavity and does not involve any uninfected organs or space. Drainage may proceed for 2 weeks or more or until drainage from the cavity is decreased, the patient is afebrile and improving, and radiography shows that the cavity is becoming smaller.[21] Surgical backup is mandatory when this drainage technique is used because spillage of abscess material into the peritoneal cavity, hemorrhage, and other complications may occur. Generally percutaneous drainage is not indicated for patients with multiple large abscesses or multiloculated abscesses.[26] Heneghan and associates[20] have proposed that indications for surgical drainage of pyogenic liver abscesses are as follows:

1. No clinical response after 4 to 7 days of drainage via a percutaneous catheter placed into the abscess cavity
2. Multiple large or loculated abscesses
3. Thick-walled abscess with viscous pus
4. Concurrent intraabdominal surgical pathology

Appropriate antibiotic therapy initially is based on knowledge of the organisms most commonly involved, Gram stain of the purulent material, and culture and susceptibility to antibiotics of the organisms that are recovered. If a hematogenous source of infection is suspected or the host has an immunodeficiency disease, *S. aureus* and streptococci are more likely. Biliary tract disease and blunt trauma are associated more frequently with gram-negative aerobic and anaerobic organisms. A logical antibiotic combination for the initial therapy of children with liver abscesses includes a penicillinase-resistant penicillin, such as nafcillin, plus an extended-spectrum cephalosporin such as cefotaxime, ceftriaxone, or cefepime. Meropenem is an option if there is concern for gram-negative enterics that produce extended-spectrum β-lactamases. Vancomycin or clindamycin is selected if strains of *S. aureus* resistant to methicillin are present in the community.

The optimal duration and route of administration of antibiotics for a child with a solitary pyogenic liver abscess that has been drained have not been determined. Generally, 2 to 4 weeks of antibiotic therapy administered parenterally, followed by an appropriate oral antibiotic to complete a minimum 4-week total course, should be adequate. Penicillin, piperacillin-tazobactam, clindamycin, or metronidazole is administered for anaerobic isolates, depending on susceptibility. Meropenem is useful for polymicrobial infections, including infections caused by gram-negative aerobic and anaerobic rods or organisms that are multidrug resistant.

Multiple liver abscesses are more difficult to treat because achieving complete surgical drainage usually is impossible. Prolonged antibiotic therapy plus treatment of any underlying illnesses is the keystone to effective management. Duration of treatment can be modified depending on the evidence for resolution of the abscesses as determined by repeated ultrasound examination or CT.

Fungal liver abscesses are difficult to document by culture of the abscess material, and prolonged treatment is required. The reader is referred to Chapter 200 ("Candidiasis") and the Infectious Diseases Society of America Clinical Practice Guidelines for the Management of Candidiasis for details of management.[44]

COMPLICATIONS AND PROGNOSIS

Complications of hepatic abscesses vary and are relatively common. Twenty-eight percent of the patients described by Rubin and associates[53] and 44% of the patients studied by Pitt and Zuidema[49] had one or more complications. Possible complications include pleural and pulmonary inflammation, peritonitis, subphrenic or subhepatic abscesses, and hemobilia.[10,51] In a large case-control study from Taiwan, adults with pyogenic liver abscess were significantly more likely to develop pancreatitis at some future time point than were controls.[33]

Polymicrobial bacteremia, hypoalbuminemia, multiple liver abscesses, or the presence of any complication is associated with increased mortality rates in patients with liver abscesses. Overall mortality rates depend largely on underlying pathologic processes and are difficult to interpret. Mortality figures from more recent reports range from 2.5% to 11% in adults.[26] In children, the prognosis for pyogenic liver abscess is excellent, generally with a low chance of mortality.[40,48] An increased awareness and suspicion of liver abscesses, in conjunction with ultrasound or CT of the liver, substantially reduces the mortality rate of this disease.

NEW REFERENCES SINCE THE SEVENTH EDITION

23. Hsu Y-L, Lin H-C, Yen T-Y, et al. Pyogenic liver abscess among children in a medical center in Central Taiwan. *J Microbiol Immunol Infect.* 2015;48:302-305.
33. Lai S-W, Liao K-F, Lin C-L, et al. Pyogenic liver abscess correlates with increased risk of acute pancreatitis: a population-based cohort study. *J Epidemiol.* 2015;25:246-253.
37. Lin J-N, Lin C-L, Lin M-C, et al. Pyogenic liver abscess in patients with inflammatory bowel disease: a nationwide cohort study. *Liver Int.* 2016;36(1):136-144.
44. Pappas PG, Kauffman CA, Andes D, et al. Clinical practice guideline for the management of candidiasis: 2016 update by the Infectious Diseases Society of America. *Clin Infect Dis.* 2016;62:e1-e50.

The full reference list for this chapter is available at ExpertConsult.com.

50 Reye Syndrome

James D. Cherry

A syndrome involving the acute onset of encephalopathy associated with fatty metamorphosis of the liver and occurring primarily in children was described first by Reye and colleagues[12,13] in Australia and by Johnson and associates[11] in the United States. The similarities of these two descriptions in separate countries led to the common designation of this clinicopathologic entity as *Reye-Johnson* or *Reye syndrome.* Reye syndrome occurs most frequently after a viral illness and is characterized by the onset of severe vomiting followed by the development of encephalopathy and hepatic dysfunction. The recognition in the early 1980s that the syndrome is associated with the ingestion of aspirin during the antecedent viral illness led to public awareness of this association, a decline in aspirin use for such illnesses in children, and a dramatic decline in the occurrence of this disease in the United States.[1]

EPIDEMIOLOGY

In the United States, national surveillance for Reye syndrome was conducted first during the 1973 to 1974 nationwide outbreak of influenza B and influenza A (H1N1). Such surveillance led to the recognition of outbreaks of Reye syndrome regionally and nationally that were associated with outbreaks of influenza in these and subsequent years.[4] During the first 5 years of surveillance, 250 to 550 cases were reported nationally—an underestimate because it was based on voluntary reporting.[2] Population-based studies conducted in several geographic locations showed that the average annual incidence of the syndrome was one or two cases per 100,000 children younger than 18 years. Adults rarely were affected. Case-fatality rates reported through national surveillance, initially 40%, declined to 20% to 30% in later years when the syndrome was prevalent, although this rate undoubtedly was an overestimate because of the tendency to report more severe and fatal cases through this system.

Between 1980 and 1982, four case-control studies reported an association between Reye syndrome and the ingestion of aspirin during an antecedent respiratory or chickenpox illness.[5,14,15] The results of these studies subsequently were confirmed in the Public Health Service Pilot and Main Studies of Reye Syndrome and Medications.[6–8] In these studies, more than 90% of patients with Reye syndrome compared with 40% to 70% of controls had received aspirin for the antecedent respiratory or chickenpox illness; reported odds ratios were 11.5 to 40. After these studies were reported, publicity and recommendations from various expert panels, including recommendations issued by the US Food and Drug Administration in 1985, led to a decline in the use of aspirin and a decline in the incidence of Reye syndrome, particularly in the age group that had been affected most—children 5 to 15 years old.[1]

CLINICAL MANIFESTATIONS AND LABORATORY FINDINGS

Reye syndrome is described classically as an illness characterized by the abrupt onset of severe vomiting and progressive encephalopathy in a child who is just recovering from a viral illness, the most common of which are influenza and chickenpox. The onset of these symptoms typically occurs within several days after the onset of the viral illness and commonly during a period when the child seems to be recovering from this illness. In association with severe—often projectile—vomiting, which occurs for a transient period, are progressive encephalopathic changes that may follow stages from delirium through confusion, agitation, and lethargy to coma if untreated.

The definition used by the Centers for Disease Control and Prevention (CDC) and widely adopted for clinical purposes includes (1) evidence of acute encephalopathy manifested by alterations in consciousness and documented, when available, by cerebrospinal fluid with less than 9×10^6/L leukocytes or by biopsy or autopsy evidence of cerebral edema without perivascular or meningeal inflammation in histologic sections of the brain; (2) evidence of liver involvement, including either biopsy or autopsy findings of fatty metamorphosis of the liver if available or, in the absence of such specimens, elevations in liver enzymes (alanine aminotransaminase, aspartate aminotransaminase, or serum ammonia) that typically are more than three times normal levels; and (3) no other more reasonable explanation for the cerebral or hepatic abnormalities. The last requirement emphasizes that Reye syndrome is a diagnosis of exclusion and that every effort should be undertaken to identify other possible causes for the clinical and laboratory abnormalities.

Liver biopsy or autopsy findings are considered characteristic and include panlobular microvesicular fat and mitochondrial abnormalities on electron microscopic examination showing peroxisome swelling and enlarged pleomorphic mitochondria with loss of dense granules. Additional findings include normal bilirubin levels and absence of jaundice. Most patients also have hypoglycemia and a prolonged prothrombin time. The typically elevated cerebrospinal fluid pressure in patients leads to progressive stages of coma.

Staging criteria for Reye syndrome have been used to define the level of encephalopathy. Patients have been reported with liver involvement but without evidence of encephalopathy. These patients have been described as having stage 0 encephalopathy and, although they do not meet the CDC criteria for Reye syndrome, are considered to have mild disease. Patients with stage I encephalopathy are difficult to arouse and lethargic, whereas patients with stage II are delirious and combative, with some movement. Patients with higher stages of encephalopathy (III to V) cannot be aroused and have progressively deeper stages of coma. These patients have a poor prognosis, with a mortality rate approaching 50% for patients admitted at stage III or greater and 90% for patients admitted at stage V.

Exclusion of other diseases that may resemble Reye syndrome, such as salicylate toxicity, is essential in patients with symptoms resembling this entity. Intensive laboratory investigations should be undertaken to exclude such disorders. In young children, particularly children younger than 3 years, inherited metabolic disorders frequently may mimic Reye syndrome and must be excluded. Such metabolic disorders include disorders of fatty acid oxidation, urea cycle disorders, carnitine transport defects, and organic acidemias. Laboratory studies must be performed for the younger age group to exclude these disorders before a diagnosis of Reye syndrome is made, particularly because some of these disorders can be treated effectively. With the declining incidence of Reye syndrome in the typical age group (5 to 15 years) after virtual elimination of the use of aspirin in children, an increasing number of patients with features of Reye syndrome are in this younger age group and ultimately are found, after careful evaluation, to have one of the many metabolic disorders that mimic this syndrome.

An acute encephalopathy mimicking Reye syndrome was noted in 2010.[9] This 11-year-old boy's illness was due to the *Bacillus cereus* emetic toxin cereulide. Ikeda and Sonoda[10] noted a 26-year-old woman with Reye-like syndrome associated with suspected *Bordetella pertussis* infection and aspirin use.

TREATMENT AND PREVENTION

The mainstay of treatment of Reye syndrome is early recognition of disease and supportive care focusing on various measures to control intracranial pressure and electrolyte and other abnormalities. Patients should have glucose levels monitored, and early infusion of glucose is considered by many physicians to improve outcome. Comatose patients should be transferred to tertiary care centers that have experience in caring for such patients and can monitor and treat elevated intracranial pressure. When such measures were undertaken before the decline in incidence of this disease, they were associated with improved outcome and decreased mortality. Other therapeutic measures that have been used include efforts to reduce ammonia levels, such as exchange transfusions, peritoneal dialysis, and total-body washout via cardiopulmonary bypass. With advances in supportive care, the mortality rate declined to 10% to 20% in later years before Reye syndrome became extremely rare.

Since the association between Reye syndrome and aspirin has been recognized, aspirin no longer is recommended or used for the treatment of febrile illnesses in children. Alternative antipyretics, including nonsteroidal antiinflammatory drugs and acetaminophen (Tylenol), have replaced aspirin as the primary therapy for such illnesses. These medications have not been associated with an increased risk for development of Reye syndrome. Children with some disorders, including juvenile rheumatoid arthritis and Kawasaki disease, continue to be given aspirin to treat these disorders. Efforts to reduce the risk for development of Reye syndrome in these children have included influenza vaccination annually and vaccination against chickenpox. Careful monitoring of these children also is necessary to ensure early recognition and treatment of Reye syndrome should it occur.

A large number of over-the-counter aspirin-containing products are available in the United States as well as in other countries.[3] It is often not recognized by parents that these alternative medicine products contain aspirin, so children with respiratory illness may on occasion receive aspirin. Therefore, Reye syndrome may still occasionally occur.

NEW REFERENCE SINCE THE SEVENTH EDITION

10. Ikeda K, Sonoda K. [A case of Reye's-like syndrome due to suspected *Bordetella pertussis* infection in an adult]. *Kansenshogaku Zasshi*. 2009;83(6):658-660.

The full reference list for this chapter is available at ExpertConsult.com

Appendicitis and Pelvic Abscess

51

Thomas L. Kuhls

The ability to diagnose appendicitis accurately in a child continues to be one of the most fundamental skills that a pediatric surgeon has to master, although making the diagnosis often is difficult in young patients. The surgeon ultimately is responsible for deciding whether a child is taken to the operating room for appendectomy; however, a primary care physician often is the first person to evaluate the patient who complains of abdominal pain. Pediatricians with expertise in infectious diseases frequently are involved in the care of children who present with subtle or atypical manifestations of appendicitis, have unusual microorganisms recovered from their appendices, or have complications as a result of appendiceal rupture, such as the development of wound infections, sepsis, peritonitis, intraabdominal abscesses, and pelvic abscesses.

EPIDEMIOLOGY

Reported incidences of acute appendicitis vary widely, depending on where the studies were performed and what methodologies were used. The number of cases of acute appendicitis had been decreasing until the 1990s, when the rate began to rise.[7,90,117] It is estimated that more than 70,000 children are diagnosed with appendicitis each year in the United States.[77] Although appendicitis occurs in all age groups, the highest incidence occurs during the second decade of life.[37] Appendicitis is an uncommon event in children younger than 5 years of age and occurs extremely rarely in infants younger than 6 months old. Patients with acquired immunodeficiency syndrome (AIDS) may have a higher incidence of appendicitis than the general population.[99]

The peak rates of appendicitis occur during the summer months, whereas the lowest rates occur during the winter months.[7] Most studies show a modest increase in incidence of appendicitis in males compared with females. The rate of appendicitis in whites is higher than that of blacks and Asians.[123] Hispanics have the highest rate of appendicitis-related hospitalizations in the United States. Whether the reported racial differences are due to errors of measurement, sociodemographic factors, environmental factors, factors related to body constitution, or genetic factors remains unclear. Children with appendicitis more frequently have a history of family members who previously have had appendicitis, suggesting that genetic background plays a role in the susceptibility to appendicitis.[60] Previous breastfeeding, decreased dietary fiber, ingestion of refined carbohydrates, and atopy have all been suggested to increase the risk for developing appendicitis.[74,141] Higher perforation rates have been observed in obese individuals and tobacco smokers.[16]

PATHOPHYSIOLOGY

The initial event in the development of most cases of appendicitis is thought to be obstruction of the appendiceal lumen. Microorganisms rarely invade the appendiceal mucosa and initiate the inflammatory process. Appendiceal obstruction can be caused by inspissated feces (fecalith), hypertrophied lymphoid tissue that develops during a systemic viral infection or bacterial enterocolitis, parasitic infestation, appendiceal wall hemorrhage associated with anaphylactic purpura, inspissated barium, or ingested seeds. Continued production of mucus by the appendiceal mucosa distal to the obstruction causes the appendix to distend. Vascular congestion and ischemia occur as the increased intraluminal pressure of the appendix becomes greater than the venous pressure, and edema develops as lymphatic flow becomes obstructed.

Stasis of intestinal flow and intestinal ischemia allow the microorganisms in the appendix to invade the tissues, enhancing the already developing inflammatory response. Bacteria then may translocate across the appendiceal wall and reach the peritoneal cavity.[21] If the process is severe and arteriolar blood flow to the appendix is obstructed, transmural infarction occurs and the appendix ruptures. Microorganisms are liberated into the peritoneal cavity, causing generalized peritonitis and formation of an abscess. Animal studies have suggested that synergism occurring between enteric aerobes, such as *Escherichia coli,* and anaerobes, such as *Bacteroides fragilis,* is important in the development of intra-abdominal and pelvic abscesses after perforation.[69] An association between the development of an abscess after appendiceal perforation and the presence of *Streptococcus milleri* also exists.[73]

As the appendix distends in the early stages of appendicitis, the visceral afferent autonomic nerves that enter the spinal cord at T8 to T10 are stimulated, referring the pain to the epigastric and periumbilical areas of the abdomen. When the inflammatory response reaches the serosal surface of the appendix, the parietal peritoneum is stimulated and the pain intensifies in the right lower quadrant. If perforation occurs, the peritoneal inflammatory response causes more generalized abdominal tenderness.

Although appendiceal obstruction may play an important role in the early stages of most cases of appendicitis, not all obstructed appendices become inflamed. Ten percent of normal appendices removed during abdominal surgical procedures contain inspissated fecal material. Also, children may develop recurrent, crampy abdominal pain, possibly from intermittent appendiceal obstruction.

The classic description of the pathophysiology of appendicitis does not easily explain many epidemiologic features of this disease, including its higher incidence in males and certain races. The amount and reactivity of the lymphoid tissue in the wall of the appendix have been suggested to be key determinants to the development of appendicitis. The amount of lymphoid tissue in the appendix is greatest during adolescence when the disease process is most prevalent and the amount most likely is controlled genetically.

In a case-control study from Italy, prolonged breastfeeding during infancy was associated with a decreased risk for developing acute appendicitis later in life.[141] The investigators hypothesized that breastfeeding may have decreased the amount of stimulation to intestinal lymphocytes by microbial and food antigens early in life, so that appendiceal lymphoid tissues were less reactive to antigenic challenge during adolescence and adulthood. Appendicitis may be observed less frequently during infancy and the neonatal period because the appendix is more funnel shaped, the diet is primarily liquid, recumbent posture is maintained for prolonged periods, and gastrointestinal and respiratory tract infections develop less frequently during this time.

CLINICAL MANIFESTATIONS

In school-aged children and adolescents with appendicitis, the median duration of symptoms before the time of hospital admission is 24 to 48 hours.[147] Pain in the right iliac fossa is the most common sign of appendicitis, occurring in 88% in almost all patients.[151] Pain shifts from the periumbilical area to the right lower quadrant of the abdomen in approximately two-thirds of children with appendicitis. The pain usually worsens during movement. The characteristics of the abdominal pain do not always predict accurately which children have appendicitis. Of children found to have mesenteric adenitis at laparotomy, 25% report a shift in their abdominal pain to the right iliac fossa, and 33% experience worsening of their pain during movement.[147]

Nausea and vomiting are also commonly observed in children with appendicitis. Vomiting usually occurs after the onset of abdominal pain but may precede pain in nearly 20% of cases. Anorexia occurs less commonly in children than in adults. Complaints of diarrhea, constipation, and dysuria occasionally can be elicited from children with appendicitis.[155]

Fever is a useful diagnostic sign of appendicitis in children with right lower quadrant abdominal pain.[38,56] A temperature greater than 37.5°C (99.5°F) is found in most but not all cases. Very high temperatures (>39°C [102.2°F]) suggest that perforation already has occurred or that another intraabdominal process is present. Rarely children present with erythema and tenderness of the scrotum or a scrotal or inguinal mass as the only manifestation of acute appendicitis.[95,205]

During the physical examination, tenderness in the right iliac fossa is the most sensitive sign of appendicitis. The psoas muscle may become irritated from the inflamed appendix, causing the child to feel increased pain when the right hip is flexed actively. Likewise if the obturator internus muscle is involved, pain is elicited when the flexed thigh is rotated internally. Guarding is found in most cases of appendicitis, compared with half of cases of mesenteric adenitis and 8% of cases of nonspecific abdominal pain.[147] Similarly, rebound tenderness is found more commonly in children with appendicitis than with acute mesenteric adenitis or nonspecific abdominal pain; its presence triples the odds of the child having appendicitis.[38,56]

The development of diffuse abdominal tenderness and the absence of bowel sounds usually indicate perforation. Extremely hyperactive bowel sounds suggest that the patient may not have appendicitis. Occasionally a mass can be palpated in the right lower quadrant of the abdomen in children with appendicitis who are relaxed or well sedated. Rectal tenderness is present more commonly in children with appendicitis than with other causes of abdominal pain; however findings during the rectal examination seldom alter the clinical decision of the surgeon.[147]

In preschool-aged children, the diagnosis of appendicitis is more difficult to establish because of the inability of young children to express their symptoms and because they often do not cooperate during the physical examination.[199] Young children with appendicitis are often seen early in the course of their symptoms and are prescribed antibiotics, antihistamines, or antipyretics. By the time one realizes that the child has appendicitis, the appendix usually is perforated (50% to 90%).[20,199] In contrast to older children, vomiting is the initial symptom of appendicitis most frequently observed, and abdominal pain may be absent or may never localize in the right iliac fossa.[147] Sleep disturbances, irritability, restlessness, and crying are common manifestations of appendicitis in this age group. The preschool-aged child is more likely to have a palpable inflammatory mass at presentation.

During the newborn period, appendicitis is an extremely rare occurrence, although most cases are found when prematurity exists.[87] Symptoms of neonatal appendicitis include abdominal distention; vomiting; irritability; diarrhea; erythema, edema, or cellulitis of the abdominal wall; gastrointestinal hemorrhage; abdominal rigidity; lethargy; and jaundice. Usually the symptoms of neonatal appendicitis are indistinguishable from those of necrotizing enterocolitis. Underlying conditions such as total colonic Hirschsprung disease, meconium plugs, esophageal atresia, or hernias may predispose the neonate to develop this condition.

In children who are undergoing chemotherapy for leukemia, acute appendicitis may present as only vague abdominal pain, abdominal distention, lack of abdominal guarding, fever, dehydration, diarrhea, or unusual symptoms such as gastrointestinal bleeding.[11] Symptoms of appendicitis in immunocompromised patients may be identical to those of typhlitis.

DIAGNOSIS

A great emphasis has been placed on using various laboratory tests to help clinicians diagnose the appendicitis accurately.[97] Patients who have received prior oral antibiotics may have milder symptoms and signs of classic appendicitis, necessitating further diagnostic studies.[59]

For decades, physicians have valued peripheral blood leukocyte counts, neutrophil counts, C-reactive protein concentrations, and erythrocyte sedimentation rates to help them distinguish appendicitis from other causes of abdominal pain. When properly evaluated, these tests have been found to be too insensitive to use as reliable tools for diagnosing appendicitis.[23,137] Normal results do not rule out the possibility that the child has appendicitis, although these tests help to confirm a physician's suspicions when results are positive. When the nonspecific tests are elevated, often perforation or abscess formation has occurred.[8,135] Hyperbilirubinemia and increased serum procalcitonin levels also are signs of probable perforation.[54,66,137] Certain groups of patients commonly have normal leukocyte counts despite having acute appendicitis. African-American patients with acute appendicitis frequently do not develop leukocytosis.[83] Patients with AIDS who develop appendicitis also frequently do not have elevated white blood cell counts.[33]

Routine radiographic studies for the diagnosis of appendicitis in children no longer are suggested. Radiographs of the abdomen are neither sensitive nor specific enough for diagnosing childhood appendicitis. Graded compression ultrasonography is increasingly becoming the diagnostic procedure of choice when evaluating a patient with possible appendicitis.[18] A noncompressible, enlarged (>6 mm in diameter in adolescents) appendix or a fecalith is the major criterion used for diagnosing appendicitis by ultrasonography. Interruption in the continuity of the echogenic submucosa suggests necrosis of the appendiceal wall and impending perforation. An echogenic periappendiceal mass indicates inflammation of the mesenteric or omental fat. Loculated or generalized fluid collections suggest that perforation already has occurred.

Because graded compression ultrasonography is highly operator-dependent, a meta-analysis has demonstrated that the procedure is 88% sensitive and 94% specific in diagnosing acute appendicitis in children.[52] False-positive ultrasound results occur in obese patients who have noncompressible appendices because of overlying fat and in children who have inflamed appendices caused by Crohn disease, ulcerative colitis, or adjacent salpingitis. False-negative results occur if retrocecally located appendices are not visualized properly; if the cecum is filled with gas or feces and is not compressed adequately; or if perforation has occurred, allowing the appendix to be compressible. In one study, a noncompressible appendix was identified in only 38% of pediatric patients with perforated appendicitis, thus rendering the other ultrasound findings of appendicitis important in diagnosing the disease.[143] The examination should be directed to diagnose other causes of abdominal pain that can mimic appendicitis when a normal appendix is found during the evaluation.

The advantages of using ultrasonography over computed tomography (CT) are that it is relatively inexpensive, is safe, does not require sedation, lacks radiation exposure, and is widely available. It is especially useful in adolescent girls with abdominal pain because gynecologic causes of the pain can be evaluated easily at the time of appendiceal examination. Bedside ultrasound in the emergency department is currently being used to identify children with appendicitis.[113]

High-resolution CT has higher sensitivity (94%) and similar specificity (95%) compared to ultrasonography in diagnosing appendicitis, and it is less operator dependent.[52] Intravenous contrast agents and high-resolution, thin-section scanning techniques must be used to visualize the appendix adequately. An enlarged appendix with a circumferentially and symmetrically thickened bowel wall is the most common CT finding in appendicitis. Periappendiceal inflammatory reaction or fluid collections may be identified. If the appendix is not well visualized, the presence of a fecalith, along with pericecal inflammatory changes, strongly suggests appendicitis. Fecaliths can be visualized in normal appendices by CT, however, and are of no clinical significance unless other inflammatory changes are present.

Helical or multidetector CT techniques using rectal or no contrast have been shown to be very accurate in diagnosing appendicitis.[53,111] By using a focused right lower quadrant approach, helical CT may be completed more rapidly. Waiting for a CT scan may delay a surgical consultation and increase the rate of perforation before surgery.[105] Also CT is expensive and uses significant amounts of ionizing radiation in children who have greater radiosensitivity of organs and tissues compared with adults. Many medical centers have implemented protocols that initially use ultrasonography as the first diagnostic procedure for possible

BOX 51.1 Microorganisms Associated With Acute Appendicitis in Children

Anaerobes
Bacteroides spp.
Bilophila wadsworthia
Catabacter hongkongensis
Clostridium spp., including *C. difficile*
Fusobacterium spp.
Peptostreptococcus spp.
Pigmented bile-resistant, gram-negative rods
Turicibacter sanguinis

Enteric Aerobes and Facultative Anaerobes
Aeromonas spp.
Campylobacter spp.
Citrobacter spp.
Enterobacter spp.
Enterococcus spp.
Escherichia coli
Klebsiella spp.
Morganella morganii
Proteus spp.
Providencia rettgeri
Salmonella spp.
Shigella spp.
Streptococcus anginosus (formerly *milleri*) group
Yersinia spp.

Other Bacteria
Actinomyces spp.
Atypical mycobacteria (in patients with AIDS)
Chromobacterium violaceum
Corynebacterium appendicis
Eikenella corrodens
Haemophilus spp.
Ehrlichia chaffeensis
Kluyvera ascorbata
Pasteurella multocida
Pseudomonas spp.
Staphylococcus spp.
Streptococcus pneumoniae
Streptococcus pyogenes

Parasites
Angiostrongylus costaricensis
Anisakis spp.
Ascaris lumbricoides
Balantidium coli
Cryptosporidium parvum
Entamoeba histolytica
Enterobius vermicularis
Schistosoma spp.
Strongyloides stercoralis
Taenia spp.
Trichuris trichiura

Viruses
Adenoviruses
Coxsackievirus B
Cytomegalovirus
Epstein-Barr virus
Measles virus

Fungi
Candida albicans
Coccidioides immitis
Mucor spp.
Histoplasma capsulatum

appendicitis and only use CT when the ultrasound results are equivocal to reduce cost and radiation exposure.

Whether the increasing use of ultrasonography and CT to diagnose appendicitis in children has decreased, the misdiagnosis of the disease and subsequent negative appendectomy rate in hospitals is unclear.[45,116,207]

Radiolabeled autologous leukocyte scans also have been used to diagnose appendicitis in children; however, this modality should be reserved for atypical presentations of disease when localizing signs are not present.[78] Magnetic resonance imaging may be considered in patients with nondiagnostic ultrasound tests and concerns about radiation exposure.[154]

MICROBIOLOGY

Numerous microorganisms have been implicated as a cause of acute appendicitis; however, considerable debate has ensued as to whether simply isolating an organism from the appendiceal lumen is sufficient proof to define causation (Box 51.1).

Bacteria

In most cases of appendicitis, bacteria do not appear to be involved directly in the initial stages of the inflammatory process. Microorganisms that normally inhabit the appendix are liberated into the peritoneal cavity when appendiceal perforation occurs or when translocation through the inflamed tissues is present, and polymicrobial infections develop as a complication of the disease process. In a study of 30 adolescents and adults with nonperforated and perforated appendicitis, 223 different anaerobes and 82 aerobes were recovered from cultures of their appendiceal tissues, peritoneal fluid, and contents of abscesses.[24] An average of 10 different organisms were isolated per specimen collected. In a recent microbiome study, 12 taxa were found to be increased from inflamed appendices compared to normal appendices.[84]

In most culture-based studies of appendiceal tissues and peritoneal fluid specimens from patients with appendicitis, *B. fragilis* is the strict anaerobe isolated most frequently, occurring in more than 70% of patients.[24,149] Other anaerobes that are isolated frequently include *Bacteroides* spp., *Bilophila wadsworthia, Peptostreptococcus* spp., *Fusobacterium* spp., and *Clostridium* spp.[188,202,209] A gram-negative anaerobic rod that develops a pigment in culture and is bile resistant also has been identified frequently.[148,149] Anaerobes such as *Turicibacter sanguinis* and *Catabacter hongkongensis* continue to be newly described from patients with appendicitis.[31,101] Rarely acute appendicitis has been seen in the setting of *Clostridium difficile* colitis, although the role of the anaerobe's toxins in causing the appendiceal inflammation is unknown.[35]

E. coli is the aerobic or facultative anaerobic bacteria isolated most frequently from children with appendicitis. *E. coli* is found in more than 75% of patients.[24,149] Certain *E. coli* strains with type 1C fimbriae may contribute to the development of appendiceal inflammation.[164] Enterohemorrhagic *E. coli* O157:H7 and O111:H have been isolated infrequently from the stools and peritoneal fluid of children with appendicitis.[186,193]

Viridans streptococci of the *S. anginosus* group, especially *S. milleri*, can be found in more than 60% of cultures from children with appendicitis.[85,106,149] Group D streptococci are isolated in 20% to 30% of patients with appendicitis. *Pseudomonas* spp. are isolated slightly less frequently, although they may be found more frequently in young children.[62,149] Other aerobes or facultative anaerobes that can be isolated from appendiceal tissues, abscesses, or blood include *Citrobacter* spp., *Klebsiella* spp., *Enterobacter* spp., *Proteus* spp., *Morganella morganii, Providencia rettgeri, Eikenella corrodens*, non–group A β-hemolytic streptococci, and staphylococci.[42,76,86,145,149]

Rarely encapsulated organisms, such as *Streptococcus pneumoniae, Haemophilus influenzae, Haemophilus segnis,* and *Aggregatibacter aphrophilus* have been isolated from appendiceal tissues or peritoneal fluid of children with appendicitis, and often these organisms have been isolated in pure culture.[14,15,123,128] Very rarely organisms such as *Pasteurella multocida, Streptococcus pyogenes,* and *Actinomyces* spp. have been cultured from patients with appendicitis.[55,109,146] *Shigella, Salmonella, Campylobacter, Yersinia,* and *Aeromonas* spp. also have been isolated occasionally from appendiceal tissues or peritoneal fluid of patients with nonperforated and perforated appendicitis, but, again, whether they played a role in the pathogenesis of disease is unknown.[22,25,39,91,102,108,124] Much more commonly, these organisms cause enterocolitis or mesenteric adenitis, with symptoms mimicking appendicitis.[190]

Appendicitis has occurred during systemic infections caused by *Brucella melitensis* and *Ehrlichia chaffeensis*.[10,167] Rarely *Kluyvera ascorbata, Arcobacter butzleri,* and *Chromobacterium violaceum* have been isolated from individuals with appendicitis, as well as newly described aerobes and facultative anaerobes, such as *Corynebacterium appendicis*.[40,43,103,204]

Rarely isolated primary tuberculosis can occur in children.[26,144] The progression of disease is usually rapid; thus one should be suspicious when caseating granulomas are observed in histopathologic sections of the appendix.

Adults and children with appendicitis usually are not bacteremic at the time they are diagnosed, especially if the appendix is not perforated. Occasionally *Klebsiella pneumoniae, E. coli, B. fragilis,* and *B. wadsworthia* are isolated from the blood of patients with nonperforated appendicitis.[27,156,158] In a review of 1000 children and adults with appendicitis, 10% of patients with perforation had positive blood cultures, whereas none of the patients without perforation had bacteremia.[107] A higher rate of bacteremia may occur when laparoscopic surgery is performed because of the air that is forced into the peritoneum, although the clinical significance of the induced bacteremia is unknown.[133]

In immunocompromised patients who develop appendicitis, the microorganisms that are isolated from appendiceal tissues or peritoneal cultures usually are identical to those found in immunocompetent patients. Patients with AIDS who have gastrointestinal *Mycobacterium avium* complex or *Mycobacterium tuberculosis* infections may develop symptoms that mimic appendicitis.[49,192] Atypical mycobacteria have been isolated from an appendiceal abscess from a child with AIDS.[58]

Parasites

In Turkey, parasites were found to be the cause of appendicitis in 1.4% of cases.[203] Roundworms, such as *Ascaris lumbricoides,* may obstruct the appendiceal lumen occasionally and initiate the cascade of inflammatory events leading to perforated appendicitis.[112,134] Parasites such as *Enterobius vermicularis* can be identified in the lumen of 1% to 12% of surgically removed appendices obtained from patients living in highly endemic areas.[2,12,77] Pinworms have been found more frequently, however, in appendices with no evidence of appendiceal inflammation in some studies, suggesting that pinworms probably are a part of the normal appendiceal flora and do not play a role in the pathogenesis of appendicitis.[157,206] Whether some parasites may cause abdominal pain that mimics the symptoms of appendicitis necessitating surgical intervention remains unclear.

Scattered reports from mostly developing nations describe other worms, including *Taenia* spp., *Anisakis* spp., *Trichuris trichiura, Strongyloides stercoralis, Schistosoma* spp., and *Angiostrongylus costaricensis,* that have been identified in the lumen of appendices from patients with appendicitis.[3,13,32,129] Similarly, protozoa such as *Balantidium coli, Entamoeba histolytica,* and *Cryptosporidium parvum* have been found in inflamed appendices of immunocompromised and immunocompetent patients, but whether they play a role in the pathogenesis of disease is unknown.[36,51,136]

Viruses

The role that viruses play in causing appendicitis also has been debated. One suggestion is that a systemic viral infection may induce hypertrophied lymphoid aggregates that obstruct the appendiceal lumen. In the 1960s, elevated levels of antibodies against group B coxsackieviruses and adenoviruses were found in the sera of some children with appendicitis.[183] A later study, however, could not confirm this finding.[125] Six adolescents with infectious mononucleosis have developed appendicitis; cytomegalovirus has occasionally been observed in immunodeficient and otherwise healthy patients' inflamed appendices; and a child with acute varicella had virus demonstrated in the appendix following surgery for appendicitis.[89,110,130,142,182] Other children have had histologic evidence of measles virus or adenovirus infection in the appendix.[70,172] Because of the rarity of documented simultaneous viral infections and appendicitis, whether these viruses play a major role in the pathogenesis of acute appendicitis is doubtful.

Fungi

Rarely *Candida albicans* is isolated from inflamed appendices or abscess cultures, but its role in pathogenesis of disease is unknown.[100] Perforation of the appendix from intestinal mucormycosis has occurred in granulocytopenic patients and premature newborns.[131,181] Also, appendicitis has been described in individuals with histoplasmosis, coccidioidomycosis, and aspergillosis.[98,100,171]

TREATMENT

Nonperforated Appendicitis

In previously healthy children with signs of acute appendicitis, nasogastric suctioning should be established and imbalances in fluid and electrolyte concentrations should be corrected quickly. In the United States, most children are taken to the operating room. However, many hospitals now perform appendectomies only during day and evening hours because of limitations on resident work hours and decreased services available at night. No differences have been noted in perforation rates, lengths of stay, or complication rates in children who are diagnosed with appendicitis at night and given analgesics until a scheduled morning surgery if the delay time is less than 12 hours.[1,9] Morphine is often used to reduce the severity of abdominal pain in children with appendicitis, although there is no evidence that morphine reduces appendiceal pain compared with placebo.[5,19]

Prophylactic antibiotics given perioperatively decrease the rate of postoperative wound infection even in noncomplicated cases of childhood appendicitis.[6,168] No consensus exists concerning the appropriate antimicrobial agent or agents that should be used to reduce the complication rate. Prospective, randomized studies demonstrate that a single perioperative dose of proper antibiotic(s) with antimicrobial activity against *E. coli* and enteric anaerobes is as effective as continuing the antibiotic(s) for 1 to 5 days after surgery.[126,185] Few data support the routine intraoperative collection of peritoneal fluid or appendiceal cultures in children with nonperforated appendicitis, although immunocompromised patients should undergo intraoperative cultures, including cultures for mycobacteria and cytomegalovirus.[67]

Most surgeons are now performing laparoscopic appendectomies in children with nonperforated and perforated appendicitis. Advantages of the procedure are a reduction in wound infection, reduction in scarring, less postoperative pain at 24 hours, shorter hospital stay, and earlier return to normal activity, although the procedure must be performed by a surgeon experienced in laparoscopic technique.[162,197] The mean total cost of a laparoscopic appendectomy is higher than that of open appendectomy, and meta-analyses have determined that there is increased operative time and a small increase in the risk for developing a postoperative abscess using the laparoscopic technique.[121,162,197] Newer single-incision laparoscopic techniques reduce the length of hospital stay in children with appendicitis.[115,208] There are now some centers that discharge children with uncomplicated appendicitis on the same day as surgery.[61]

Outside the United States and in a few places within the United States, children with nonperforated appendicitis are treated initially with intravenous fluids and antibiotics. In France, a trial of oral amoxicillin-clavulanic acid versus appendectomy in adults was not inferior in outcome.[194] Proponents of initial conservative management consider that the complication rate is significantly lower than when a procedure is done during the acute stage of disease. More than 70% of patients are treated successfully without surgery.[159,191,194] When the child does not clinically improve or a walled-off abscess develops, drainage of the area and appendectomy are performed. The presence of intraluminal appendiceal fluid appears to predict recurrent appendicitis after initial nonoperative management, although many surgeons do an interval appendectomy 6 to 8 weeks after resolution of the symptoms to prevent future complications even though most children do well.[72,93]

Perforated Appendicitis

Most surgeons advocate early intervention when perforation has occurred to prevent severe complications such as fistula formation, abscess rupture, and death, despite the high chance of developing postoperative complications.[104] Surgeons are increasingly performing primary closures without drains in children.[57,65,119] A randomized prospective trial of appendiceal drains in children with perforated appendicitis showed no benefit compared with primary wound closure.[178] Appendectomy wounds can be closed with continuous, absorbable sutures even in complicated cases.[139] If incisions are not primarily closed, simple daily wound probing may decrease the incidence of wound infection.[184] Recent studies demonstrate that extensive irrigation of the peritoneum with saline or antibiotics does not reduce the rate of postoperative complications in children with perforated appendicitis who are receiving systemic antibiotics.[4,174] Ranitidine or diphenhydramine given to children with perforated appendicitis may increase the risk for developing a postoperative abscess.[176]

Antimicrobial agents should be administered routinely to children when perforation or appendiceal abscess is suggested or discovered during surgery. Antibiotics active against aerobes and anaerobes that normally inhabit the intestinal tract have been effective in treating children with perforated appendicitis. Treatment failures occur most commonly when *B. fragilis* or *Pseudomonas* spp. are isolated from intraoperative cultures and antimicrobial agents without activity against these organisms are used.[79] Controversy continues regarding the value of obtaining routine intraoperative peritoneal cultures in cases of perforated appendicitis, although most studies demonstrate that culture results seldom change the clinical management of patients.[47,67]

The antimicrobial combination of ampicillin, gentamicin, and clindamycin has been the gold standard of therapy since the 1970s. The importance of including ampicillin in the regimen for adequate enterococcal coverage continues to be controversial. Animal studies and clinical trials using antibiotics with poor enterococcal activity have shown that ampicillin probably is not required in the treatment of perforated appendicitis.[69] Because of the increasing problem of ampicillin resistance in enterococci, ampicillin probably should be reserved for the rare child with enterococcal bacteremia or with persistent intraabdominal infection in which enterococci have been isolated. Some medical centers use metronidazole instead of clindamycin because of its broader activity against enteric anaerobes, whereas other institutions substitute cefotaxime or ceftriaxone for gentamicin.[165,175] In a small study, once-daily dosing of ceftriaxone and metronidazole was comparable in efficacy to standard three-drug therapy in children with perforated appendicitis.[177]

Single-agent antibiotic therapy for perforated appendicitis may offer improvement in terms of pharmacy and hospital costs.[68] Agents that have been shown to be effective in treating children with perforated appendicitis include cefoxitin, imipenem-cilastatin, ticarcillin-clavulanate, piperacillin-tazobactam, ampicillin-sulbactam, meropenem, and ertapenem.[46,114,127,169,170,187,200] In a few medical centers, nearly 50% of *B. fragilis* isolates are resistant to cefoxitin, raising the question as to whether cefoxitin should be used routinely as a single agent in these institutions.[64] Generally, the convenience of monotherapy does not outweigh the potential development of resistance to these broad-spectrum agents. They may be useful in the treatment of appendicitis in children with renal disease or hearing loss when avoiding the use of gentamicin is prudent.

Limiting the duration of antibiotic use to 3 days after surgery does not lead to higher rates of wound infections or intraabdominal abscesses in children who are afebrile and eating.[169] Efforts have been made to shorten the hospital stay of children with perforated appendicitis. Some institutions have set criteria for hospital discharge and discontinuation of antibiotics, such as absence of fever for 24 hours, ability to eat well, and less than 3% band forms on the white blood cell differential.[80] Many surgeons will switch to oral antibiotics at home after 3 to 5 days of intravenous antibiotics in the hospital, although the benefit of adding prolonged oral antibiotics has not been shown.[63,180] Providing home single-intravenous antimicrobial therapy also can reduce costs and hasten hospital discharge in selected children with perforated appendicitis.[173]

Similar to nonperforated appendicitis, some controversy exists regarding whether immediate appendectomy should be performed on children in whom a palpable mass is associated with their appendicitis or who show evidence of appendiceal rupture with or without abscess formation at the time of presentation.[29,120] Similarly there is a lack of prospective studies to determine if interval appendectomy is required after successful nonoperative treatment of an appendiceal mass in children.[72] Families do experience more stress when nonoperative management of perforated appendicitis is implemented.[166]

PROGNOSIS AND COMPLICATIONS

Currently in the United States, the risk of dying of appendicitis is very low. The mortality rate is higher in the rare newborn or premature infant who develops appendicitis. Also, factors contributing to the death of children rarely may include delay in establishing diagnosis, inadequate fluid replacement, immunodeficiency, and postoperative vascular or infectious complications.

The most predictive factor of postoperative morbidity occurring from appendicitis is perforation.[150] Age, obesity, duration of the surgical procedure, and nutritional status also are risk factors for the development of complications. Wound infection rates in children who receive perioperative antibiotics should be less than 7%; infections generally are caused by the same organisms that are isolated in cultures obtained during the appendectomy.[168,185] Occasionally children develop peritonitis, intraabdominal abscesses, psoas abscesses, fistulas, pyelophlebitis of the portal vein, scrotal abscesses, empyema, or pneumoperitoneum during the course of treatment of appendicitis.[17,71,81,153,201,205]

CT can be successfully used to detect postoperative abscesses even in the first week after surgery. If complications occur, another surgical procedure often is performed and antibiotic treatment is prolonged. Abscesses may be treated successfully with antibiotics alone and without surgical drainage in stable patients after appendectomy.[50]

PELVIC ABSCESS

The pelvic area is a common site for development of abscesses because it is the most dependent portion of the peritoneal cavity. Pelvic abscesses most commonly occur in children who have had intestinal perforations after appendicitis, have suffered penetrating abdominal or retroperitoneal injury, or have undergone an abdominal surgical procedure. Occasionally adolescents with pelvic inflammatory disease or Crohn disease develop a pelvic abscess.

In children with perforated appendicitis, a coexisting pelvic abscess often is diagnosed at the time of surgery. In patients who recently have had penetrating trauma to the abdomen, have had pelvic inflammatory disease, or have undergone gastrointestinal surgery, a pelvic abscess should be suspected when they have continued fever or complain of abdominal pain despite receiving adequate treatment of the initial disease process. Symptoms may not develop until days to months after therapy is ended. No characteristic physical findings are associated with a pelvic abscess, although abdominal palpation or rectal examination may elicit tenderness or signs of intestinal obstruction may be present.

If a pelvic abscess is suspected, contrast CT evaluation of the pelvis should be completed. Walled-off fluid collections in the pelvis can be identified and sometimes the rectum, sigmoid colon, or bladder is compressed because of mass effect from the abscess cavity. Because most pelvic abscesses develop as complications of intestinal or pelvic infections, enteric aerobes and anaerobes are the organisms most commonly isolated from the abscess cavity. Yeasts rarely cause pelvic abscesses.[189,198] *Actinomyces*-related pelvic abscesses uncommonly are observed.[140] Tuberculous abscesses can develop as a complication of genital tuberculosis.[196]

When a pelvic abscess is identified, antibiotics covering intestinal aerobes and anaerobes, such as clindamycin and gentamicin, should be started, and the abscess contents should be drained. In most situations, reaching the abscess cavity by an anterior approach is difficult. Considerable interest has developed in using CT or ultrasonography to guide percutaneous drainage of pelvic abscesses by transgluteal, transrectal, transsacrococcygeal, transiliopsoas, or transvaginal approaches.[30,118,132,152,160] Although placement of a transgluteal catheter is easiest, the sciatic nerve and gluteal vessels must be avoided. Also an increased risk for development of a wound infection may occur because microorganisms may track along the outside of the catheter to the skin. Many surgeons prefer the transrectal approach because it often is the most direct route to the abscess. Transvaginal drainage has been used with good results in young women. Most often, drainage catheters can be removed after 7 to 10 days of treatment.

Abscesses also may develop within the muscles of the pelvic girdle, including the psoas and internal obturator muscles. Similar to true pelvic abscesses, they usually cause fever and occasionally abdominal complaints in children. Most children begin to limp, refuse to walk, or complain of pain in the buttocks, thigh, or groin. Often a suppurative hip infection is suspected initially. A pelvic muscle abscess is usually diagnosed by CT or magnetic resonance imaging. Labeled leukocyte scans sometimes are useful in localizing the infection to within the pelvis, especially when the child has no symptoms other than fever or refusing to walk.

Pelvic muscle abscesses can develop as a complication of Crohn disease or appendicitis; however, they often develop after an episode of bacteremia.[28,161] *Staphylococcus aureus* is the most common cause of a primary pelvic muscle abscess, with methicillin-resistant strains being increasingly identified.[138] *S. pneumoniae, H. influenzae* type B, *E. coli, Enterococcus faecalis, S. anginosus, Yersinia enterocolitica, Salmonella* spp., *Proteus mirabilis, Capnocytophaga sputigena,* and *Actinomyces* spp. also have been reported to cause hematogenously acquired abscesses.[34,41,44,48,82,88,92,96] Bacteremia secondary to intravenous drug abuse or the presence of central lines occasionally predisposes patients to developing this type of infection.[94,195] Rarely tuberculous psoas abscesses have been reported, often as a complication of vertebral osteomyelitis.[179]

Pelvic muscle abscesses usually are drained by a percutaneous or surgical approach, and antibiotic therapy is based on Gram stain and culture results. Successful therapy with antibiotics alone has been reported.[122] Duration of treatment is individualized and depends on the child's response and the drainage techniques that were used.

NEW REFERENCES SINCE THE SEVENTH EDITION

2. Ahmed MU, Bilal M, Anis K, et al. The frequency of *Enterobius vermicularis* infections in patients diagnosed with acute appendicitis in Pakistan. *Glob J Health Sci*. 2015;7:196-201.
4. Akkoyun I, Tuna AT. Advantages of abandoning abdominal cavity irrigation and drainage in operations performed on children with perforated appendicitis. *J Pediatr Surg*. 2012;47:1886-1890.
7. Anderson JE, Bickler SW, Chang DC, et al. Examining a common disease with unknown etiology: trends in epidemiology and surgical management of appendicitis in California, 1995–2009. *World J Surg*. 2012;36:2787-2794.
18. Bachur RG, Levy JA, Callahan MJ, et al. Effect of reduction in the use of computed tomography on clinical outcomes of appendicitis. *JAMA Pediatr*. 2015;169:755-760.
20. Bansal S, Banever GT, Katter FM, et al. Appendicitis in children less than 5 years old: influence of age on presentation and outcome. *Am J Surg*. 2012;204:1031-1035.
30. Borofsky SE, Obi C, Cahill AM, et al. Transiliopsoas approach: an alternative route to drain pelvic abscesses in children. *Pediatr Radiol*. 2015;45:94-98.
32. Botes SN, Ibirogba SB, McCallum AD, et al. Schistosoma prevalence in appendicitis. *World J Surg*. 2015;39:1080-1083.
37. Buckius MT, McGrath B, Monk J, et al. Changing epidemiology of acute appendicitis in the United States: study period 1993–2008. *J Surg Res*. 2012;175:185-190.
43. Chen CY, Chen YC, Pun HN, et al. Bacteriology of acute appendicitis and its implication for the use of prophylactic antibiotics. *Surg Infect (Larchmt)*. 2012;13:383-390.
46. Dalgic N, Karadag CA, Bayraktar B, et al. Ertapenem versus standard triple antibiotic therapy for the treatment of perforated appendicitis in pediatric patients: a prospective randomized trial. *Eur J Pediatr Surg*. 2014;24:410-418.
54. D'Souza N, Karim D, Sunthareswaran R. Bilirubin: a diagnostic marker for appendicitis. *Int J Surg*. 2013;11:1114-1117.
61. Farach SM, Danielson PD, Walford NE, et al. Same-day discharge after appendectomy results in cost savings and improved efficiency. *Am Surg*. 2014;80: 787-791.
62. Fernandez Ibieta M, Martinez Castano I, Reyes Rios P, et al. Study of bacteriology and resistances in pediatric appendicitis. *Cir Pediatr*. 2014;27:16-20.
65. Gasior AC, Marty Knott E, Ostlie DJ, et al. To drain or not to drain: an analysis of abscess drains in the treatment of appendicitis with abscess. *Pediatr Surg Int*. 2013;29:455-458.
66. Gavela T, Cabeza B, Serrano A, et al. C-reactive protein and procalcitonin are predictors of the severity of acute appendicitis in children. *Pediatr Emerg Care*. 2012;28:416-419.
85. Jackson HT, Mongodin EF, Davenport KP, et al. Culture-independent evaluation of the appendix and rectum microbiomes in children with and without appendicitis. *PLoS ONE*. 2014;9:e95414.
93. Koike Y, Uchida K, Matsushita K, et al. Intraluminal appendiceal fluid is a predictive factor for recurrent appendicitis after initial successful non-operative management of uncomplicated appendicitis in pediatric patients. *J Pediatr Surg*. 2014;49:1116-1121.
95. Kynes JM, Rauth TP, McMorrow SP. Ruptured appendicitis presenting as acute scrotal swelling in a 23-month-old toddler. *J Emerg Med*. 2012;43:47-49.
100. Larbcharoensub N, Boonsakan P, Kanoksil W, et al. Fungal appendicitis: a case series and review of the literature. *Southeast Asian J Trop Med Public Health*. 2013;44:681-689.
106. Leeuwenburgh MM, Monpellier V, Vlaminckx BJ, et al. *Streptococcus milleri* in intraabdominal abscesses in children after appendectomy: incidence and course. *J Pediatr Surg*. 2012;47:535-539.
113. Mallin M, Craven P, Ockerse P, et al. Diagnosis of appendicitis by bedside ultrasound in the ED. *Am J Emerg Med*. 2015;33:430-432.
115. Markar SR, Karthikesalingam A, Di Franco F, et al. Systematic review and meta-analysis of single-incision versus conventional multiport appendicectomy. *Br J Surg*. 2013;100:1709-1718.
118. McDaniel JD, Warren MT, Pence JC, et al. Ultrasound-guided transrectal drainage of deep pelvic abscesses in children: a modified and simplified technique. *Pediatr Radiol*. 2015;45:435-438.
121. Michailidou M, Goldstein SD, Sacco Casamassima MG, et al. Laparoscopic versus open appendectomy in children: the effect of surgical technique on healthcare costs. *Am J Surg*. 2015;210:270-275.
136. Otan E, Akbulut S, Kayaalp C. Amebic acute appendicitis: systematic review of 174 cases. *World J Surg*. 2013;37:2061-2073.
137. Panagiotopoulou IG, Parashar D, Lin R, et al. The diagnostic value of white cell count, C-reactive protein and bilirubin in acute appendicitis and its complications. *Ann R Coll Surg Engl*. 2013;95:215-221.
142. Pogorelic Z, Biocic M, Juric I, et al. Acute appendicitis as a complication of varicella. *Acta Medica (Hradec Kralove)*. 2012;55:150-152.
152. Robert B, Chivot C, Fuks D, et al. Percutaneous, computed tomography-guided drainage of deep pelvic abscesses via a transgluteal approach: a report on 30 cases and a review of the literature. *Abdom Imaging*. 2013;38:285-289.
154. Rosines LA, Chow DS, Lampl BS, et al. Value of gadolinium-enhanced MRI in detection of acute appendicitis in children and adolescents. *AJR Am J Roentgenol*. 2014;203:w543-w548.
159. Salminen P, Paajanen H, Rautio T, et al. Antibiotic therapy vs appendectomy for treatment of uncomplicated acute appendicitis: the APPAC randomized clinical trial. *JAMA*. 2015;313:2340-2348.
163. Sawyer RG, Claridge JA, Nathens AB, et al. Trial of short-course antimicrobial therapy for intraabdominal infection. *N Engl J Med*. 2015;372:1996-2005.
174. St Peter SD, Adibe OO, Iqbal W, et al. Irrigation versus suction alone during laparoscopic appendectomy for perforated appendicitis: a prospective randomized trial. *Ann Surg*. 2012;256:581-585.
203. Yabanoglu H, Aytac HO, Turk E, et al. Parasitic infections of the appendix as a cause of appendectomy in adult patients. *Turkiye Parazitol Derg*. 2014;38: 12-16.
208. Zhao L, Liao Z, Feng S, et al. Single-incision versus conventional laparoscopic appendicectomy in children: a systemic review and meta-analysis. *Pediatr Surg Int*. 2015;31:347-353.
209. Zhong D, Brower-Sinning R, Firek B, et al. Acute appendicitis in children is associated with an abundance of bacteria from the phylum Fusobacteria. *J Pediatr Surg*. 2014;49:441-446.

The full reference list for this chapter is available at ExpertConsult.com.

52 Pancreatitis

Thomas L. Kuhls

Pancreatitis was thought to be an uncommon cause of abdominal pain in children and a disease primarily of adults. Because of better recognition of symptoms in children and the more frequent use of medications that cause pancreatic inflammation, acute pancreatitis currently is being diagnosed more frequently in institutions specializing in pediatric care.[114]

Compared with causes of acute pancreatitis in adults—primarily alcoholism, cholelithiasis, and trauma—causes of childhood pancreatitis are more diverse. Microorganisms account for a significant proportion of cases of pancreatitis in children. In addition, antimicrobial agents have been associated with severe and occasionally fatal episodes of pancreatitis, and bacterial infections may complicate the natural history of acute and chronic pancreatitis. Pediatricians who care for children with pancreatitis must have expertise in the diagnosis and treatment of infectious diseases.

CLINICAL MANIFESTATIONS

More than 80% of children with acute pancreatitis complain of abdominal pain.[94] However, only 30% of pediatric patients have epigastric pain, as usually described by adults.[167] In children, other sites of focal tenderness or diffuse pain include the right upper quadrant of the abdomen, the periumbilical area, the entire abdomen, and, less commonly, the right lower quadrant of the abdomen. The onset of pain usually is rapid and increases to a maximal intensity in a few hours, but occasionally the onset may be slow and gradual. Most often the pain is sharp and excruciating. Only one-third of children complain of pain that radiates to other areas, including the back, lower part of the abdomen, upper abdominal quadrants, and anterior chest wall. In school-aged children, the pain often intensifies after meals.

Two-thirds of children with acute pancreatitis have vomiting.[16] Children younger than 5 years occasionally experience vomiting without abdominal tenderness. Fever is present in only 30% of children with pancreatitis, but temperatures greater than 38.5°C (101.3°F) are observed occasionally. Children may present with only the symptom of cough, and pleural effusions are found on radiography.[92]

On physical examination, children are classically found lying quietly on their sides with their knees flexed. They usually have epigastric tenderness to palpation and decreased or absent bowel sounds. Abdominal distention is found in 30% of children with pancreatitis and occurs more commonly in preschool-aged children.[167] Rebound tenderness, guarding of the epigastrium, jaundice, an abdominal mass, or ascites occasionally is detected. Rarely ecchymoses of the flanks (Grey Turner sign) or the umbilical area (Cullen sign) can be identified but usually only when life-threatening hemorrhagic pancreatitis is present. In severe pancreatitis, children may present with evidence of shock and multiple-organ failure.

Chronic pancreatitis occurs when irreversible damage in the pancreatic architecture causes abnormalities in the function of the pancreas.[85] Children with chronic pancreatitis often have lengthy or recurrent bouts of abdominal pain and vomiting.

LABORATORY DIAGNOSIS

The single most common useful laboratory test for the clinical diagnosis of pancreatitis in children is measurement of the serum amylase concentration, but the level correlates poorly with the severity of the disease. In most studies of childhood pancreatitis, the diagnosis is confirmed when the serum amylase level is greater than three times the normal level for the particular laboratory completing the test. The serum concentration rises quickly within hours after symptoms develop. High serum amylase concentrations can be observed, however, in numerous other illnesses, including acute cholecystitis, intestinal obstruction, perforations of abdominal organs, appendicitis, salpingitis, ruptured ectopic pregnancy, and salivary gland disease. The serum amylase concentration can return to normal in 24 to 72 hours after the onset of symptoms; thus the diagnosis of pancreatitis can be missed. In this situation, the urine amylase concentration can remain elevated for at least 1 week.

Serum amylase concentrations occasionally are not elevated during the course of pancreatitis in children.[34] Marked hyperlipidemia may interfere with the laboratory measurement of amylase.[17] Serum lipase is useful in these situations; however, high serum concentrations often are not detected until 24 hours after the beginning of the illness. Because lipase is produced only in the pancreas and intestinal cells, measurement of its serum concentration helps distinguish children with high serum amylase concentrations of pancreatic as opposed to salivary origin. Some children with pancreatitis have high amylase levels without an elevation of serum lipase.[86] Laboratory findings in children with severe and/or necrotizing pancreatitis may include leukocytosis with increased immature polymorphonuclear leukocytes, an elevated erythrocyte sedimentation rate, and elevated C-reactive protein level. In children with fulminant hemorrhagic pancreatitis, anemia develops quickly. Other associated findings include hyperglycemia, hypertriglyceridemia, hypoalbuminemia, and hypocalcemia. Scoring systems for children have been devised to predict severe pancreatitis, but these are extrapolated from adult studies or are difficult to use in clinical practice.[43,82] Procalcitonin or D-dimer plasma levels may be useful in predicting severe pancreatitis and later complications.[20,96] Elevated aminotransferase and alkaline phosphatase levels generally are observed only when the episode of pancreatitis is caused by biliary obstruction, such as in gallstone-related disease.

The radiographic features of childhood pancreatitis also are nonspecific. Radiographs of the abdomen may show localized ileus of the jejunum in the midepigastric or left upper quadrant region adjacent to the pancreas (sentinel loop), a distended transverse colon without visualization of the descending colon because of adjacent pancreatic inflammation (colon cutoff sign), duodenal distention with air-fluid levels, or loss of the left psoas shadow. Occasionally chest radiography reveals an elevated left hemidiaphragm or pleural effusion.

The ability to diagnose pancreatitis in children has been improved greatly by ultrasonography. The echodensity of the pancreas is normally equal to or greater than that of the left lobe of the liver. During acute pancreatitis, edema causes the gland to enlarge and become less dense than the liver. These two findings can aid in establishing the diagnosis of pancreatitis, and complications such as abscesses and pseudocysts can be identified. Also, ultrasonography may delineate dilations of the pancreatic ducts due to obstruction or ductal stones. Visualization of the pancreas by ultrasonography may be obscured because of overlying bowel gas. In such cases, computed tomography (CT) is useful in detecting pancreatic size and density.

CT of the pancreas should be performed in complicated cases of pancreatitis after a few days of treatment to determine the severity of disease and extent of pancreatic necrosis.[30,120] It is especially useful when surgery is being considered for drainage of abscesses and pseudocysts.

Endoscopic retrograde cholangiopancreatography (ERCP) is used in children with pancreatitis to treat gallstones, strictures, or *Ascaris* infection.[123] Because of ongoing improvement in image quality, magnetic resonance cholangiopancreatography (MRCP) is being increasingly used as a noninvasive technique for evaluating children with chronic or recurrent pancreatitis, with results similar to those from ERCP.[31,148]

CAUSES

A cause for childhood pancreatitis can be determined in more than 90% of cases if diagnostic evaluation is thorough, especially in children younger than 6 years. The frequency of each specific cause depends on the patient population of the particular medical center. The most common noninfectious causes of pancreatitis in children include trauma, medications, obstructive diseases, vasculitis, autoimmune diseases, and genetic and metabolic diseases.

Physicians with expertise in the management of infectious diseases are becoming more aware of drug-induced pancreatitis because many antimicrobial agents can cause pancreatic inflammation. Pentamidine isethionate has been used in the treatment of *Pneumocystis jejuni* pneumonia, African trypanosomiasis, and leishmaniasis. It may cause hypoglycemia because of toxicity to pancreatic islet cells and is associated with severe and occasionally fatal episodes of pancreatitis.[95,172] In children, aerosolized pentamidine prophylaxis for *P. jejuni* pneumonia also has been associated with severe cases of pancreatitis in patients with acquired immunodeficiency syndrome (AIDS).[61,95] Similarly, pentavalent antimonial agents such as sodium stibogluconate and meglumine antimonite, used for the treatment of visceral leishmaniasis, can induce pancreatic inflammation.[11,133]

Sulfonamides, including trimethoprim-sulfamethoxazole, have been implicated occasionally as a cause of acute pancreatitis in adults.[7,161] Symptoms have recurred when patients have been reexposed to the medication. The abdominal pain often is accompanied by a hypersensitivity-type rash. Tetracycline- and doxycycline-induced pancreatitis have been described in children with and without overt liver disease.[152,163] In addition, clarithromycin,[52,130] erythromycin,[146] rifampin,[118] roxithromycin,[121] linezolid,[124] dapsone,[36] nitrofurantoin,[103] isoniazid,[127] tigecycline,[119] and metronidazole[108] have been added to the list of agents that can cause pancreatitis in previously healthy individuals when given in routine doses or when high amounts are consumed. Although uncommonly used in children, quinolone antibiotics, such as gatifloxacin and ciprofloxacin, have been associated with hepatotoxicity and acute pancreatitis.[33,143] An adolescent who was receiving ceftriaxone also developed pancreatitis secondary to obstruction of the biliary tract from gallstones.[91]

Pancreatitis has been a major dose-limiting toxic effect of the human immunodeficiency virus (HIV)-inhibiting nucleoside analogue reverse transcriptase inhibitor (NRTI) class of medications because of mitochondrial toxicity, especially dideoxyinosine andstavudine.[23,47,113] Most episodes of pancreatitis associated with dideoxyinosine occur when the dose is 360 mg/m^2 per day or greater, and usually the pancreatic inflammation resolves when the medication is discontinued. Concomitant administration of pentamidine or another NRTI, such as ribavirin, used in the treatment of hepatitis C infection may increase the risk for developing pancreatitis.[98] In pediatric patients with AIDS, serum amylase concentrations often are elevated in patients without pancreatic symptoms, whereas children with pancreatitis can have normal serum amylase concentrations. The serum lipase concentration is useful in evaluating HIV-infected children for possible pancreatic inflammation.[23,95] Increased liver aminotransferase or lipase concentrations before the administration of an NRTI may be helpful in predicting those children in whom pancreatitis will develop. In all children with symptoms consistent with pancreatitis, NRTIs should be withheld pending the results of a lipase assay, and they should be discontinued if the concentration is elevated. Similarly, they should be discontinued for 1 week after treatment with pentamidine.[46] Because of increased awareness of NRTI toxicity, the incidence rate of pancreatitis in HIV-infected children in the highly active antiretroviral therapy (HAART) era appears to be decreasing.[99]

Interferon-α, which is used in the treatment of chronic hepatitis, has been associated with the development of pancreatitis.[29] The antifungal agents liposomal amphotericin B, micafungin, and itraconazole rarely cause pancreatic toxicity.[117,128,142]

INFECTIOUS CAUSES

Infections caused by various microorganisms have been shown by culture, histologic examination, or antibody titer rise during the course of acute pancreatitis (Box 52.1). A true causal relationship usually is not shown. Although not all of the following infectious agents have been shown to be associated with childhood pancreatitis, they must be considered as possible etiologic agents because adult patients with infectious pancreatitis have been described. Compared with previous decades, infectious agents are being encountered less as a cause of acute pancreatitis, most likely because of mumps vaccination.

BOX 52.1 Microorganisms Associated With Episodes of Acute Pancreatitis

Viruses
Adenoviruses
Cytomegalovirus
Epstein-Barr virus
Group B coxsackieviruses
Hepatitis A virus
Hepatitis B virus
Hepatitis E virus
Herpes simplex viruses
Human immunodeficiency virus
H1N1 influenza A virus
Measles virus
Mumps virus
Parainfluenza viruses
Rotavirus
Rubella virus
Varicella zoster virus
West Nile virus

Parasites
Ascaris lumbricoides
Clonorchis sinensis
Cryptosporidium parvum
Echinococcus granulosus
Fasciola hepatica
Plasmodium falciparum
Taenia saginata
Toxoplasma gondii
Wuchereria bancrofti

Mycoplasmas and Bacteria
Brucella melitensis
Campylobacter jejuni
Escherichia coli
Legionella spp.
Leptospira spp.
Moraxella catarrhalis
Mycobacterium tuberculosis
Mycoplasma pneumoniae
Salmonella spp.
Streptococcus pyogenes
Yersinia spp.

Fungi
Aspergillus spp.
Candida spp.
Cryptococcus neoformans

Viral Infections

Group B coxsackieviruses and mumps virus are the best documented causes of pancreatitis in children. Group B coxsackieviruses usually cause pancreatitis along with other clinical manifestations, including aseptic meningitis, mild diarrhea, rash, and myocarditis.[25,67] They rarely cause death in young infants with myocarditis and pancreatitis.[38] How commonly these enteroviruses cause pancreatic inflammation is unknown. Thirty-one percent of patients with aseptic meningitis during an epidemic of group B coxsackievirus infection had increased serum amylase concentrations.[102] Numerous studies have shown coxsackievirus B–induced damage to pancreatic acinar cells in mouse models of infection, and it is believed that the pancreas is the primary replication site for these viruses.[66,154] Coxsackievirus B strains have caused worsening bouts of pancreatic disease in children with chronic pancreatitis and the primary episode of pancreatitis in children later found to have the hereditary form of disease.[53,139] Group A coxsackieviruses have only rarely been associated with pancreatitis in humans.[5]

Usually mumps pancreatitis occurs in the presence of parotitis; however, abdominal pain and vomiting may occur for days before the development of salivary swelling.[166] Rarely mumps virus can cause pancreatitis without other common clinical manifestations.[100,159] Because more than 80% of children with mumps parotitis have elevated serum amylase concentrations, ultrasonography and serum lipase concentrations should be obtained to aid in establishing the diagnosis.[58] An estimated 15% of children with mumps virus infection have abdominal tenderness and vomiting suggestive of the diagnosis of pancreatitis. In only a single report has the pancreatitis been hemorrhagic and severe.[44] Occasionally chronic or recurring pancreatitis develops after mumps infection.[170]

Researchers previously thought that acute pancreatitis occurred in cases of viral hepatitis only when fulminant liver disease developed.

Increasingly children with mild hepatitis A infection and pancreatitis are being described.[42] In addition, a 16-year-old with acute hepatitis A infection died of severe pancreatitis with multiple-organ failure.[75] Individuals with acute hepatitis and pancreatitis have also been found to have hepatitis E viral infection.[149] Hepatitis B viral antigens have been detected in the pancreatic glandular cells of patients with severe acute hemorrhagic pancreatitis.[137] The role of hepatitis B virus in the pathogenesis of pancreatic inflammation in these patients is unknown; however, a young adult has developed three episodes of acute pancreatitis during acute exacerbations of chronic hepatitis B infection that resolved after lamivudine therapy.[32] It has been suggested that edema of the ampulla of Vater caused by biliary sludge formed during hepatitis viral infection leads to outflow obstruction of pancreatic fluid and the development of pancreatitis.[68]

Human herpesviruses are uncommon causes of childhood pancreatitis in immunocompetent patients. Occasionally pancreatitis develops in children and adolescents with infectious mononucleosis.[76] Acute pancreatitis and occasionally pseudocyst formation also have been reported in previously healthy individuals with varicella infection.[48,80,153] In addition, previously healthy adults have developed pancreatitis during primary cytomegalovirus and herpes simplex virus infections.[74,81,111]

Interstitial pancreatitis occurs relatively commonly in children with congenital rubella syndrome.[97] In addition, severe pancreatitis has been identified in immunocompetent patients with mild and fatal measles virus infection.[50,160] An adolescent has been described with measles encephalitis and pancreatitis that responded to corticosteroids.[145] Influenza A viruses have been shown to be capable of infecting human pancreatic cells, and H1N1 influenza A has caused pancreatitis in a previously healthy adult.[18,26] Rarely other viruses including adenovirus, West Nile virus, rotavirus, and dengue virus have been associated with the development of pancreatitis in previously healthy adults and children.[21,51,78,87,136]

Viral pancreatitis also occurs in immunocompromised patients. Cytomegalovirus has been identified in pancreatic specimens obtained during autopsies of patients who had AIDS, transplant recipients, individuals taking corticosteroids for autoimmune diseases, and cancer chemotherapy patients.[70,147] The symptoms of pancreatitis have resolved in a few patients with AIDS treated with ganciclovir or foscarnet.[35] Varicella zoster and herpes simplex viruses have also caused pancreatitis and death in patients with various immunodeficient conditions.[45,138]

Adenovirus has caused hemorrhagic pancreatitis and death in children with bone marrow transplants, whereas an infant with disseminated adenoviral infection and pancreatitis survived with cidofovir therapy.[15,28,107] Researchers have suggested that stool cultures for adenoviruses should be obtained when posttransplant patients develop pancreatitis. A disseminated parainfluenza virus infection in an infant with severe combined immunodeficiency was associated temporally with the development of pancreatitis; however, no attempt was made to culture the virus from postmortem pancreatic tissue.[49]

Whether HIV directly causes pancreatitis is unclear. Laboratory-diagnosed episodes of pancreatitis in adults and children with AIDS do occur, but whether the pancreatic inflammation is caused by HIV or an unrecognized opportunistic pathogen is unknown.[171] HIV-infected children frequently have elevated amylase and lipase levels with no correlation to antiviral therapy.[27] Increasing numbers of adults with primary manifestations of HIV infection have presented with acute pancreatitis, suggesting a role of HIV in the pathogenesis of the disease.[157]

Parasite Infestations and Infections

Ascaris lumbricoides can migrate in the intestines to the ampulla of Vater and subsequently to the pancreatic duct or common bile duct. Obstruction of the biliary or pancreatic duct can cause acute pancreatitis.[2,12] Ascariasis is diagnosed when adult roundworms are identified in the duodenum by radiographs of the upper gastrointestinal tract (Fig. 52.1) or more commonly by ultrasonography or ERCP. Often a history of seeing worms in the feces can be elicited. Other roundworms including hookworms and *Strongyloides stercoralis* can cause obstruction and acute pancreatitis.[89,156] The flukes *Clonorchis sinensis* and *Fasciola hepatica* and the cestode *Taenia saginata* similarly can migrate to the pancreatic and biliary drainage systems and cause pancreatitis.[73,84,140]

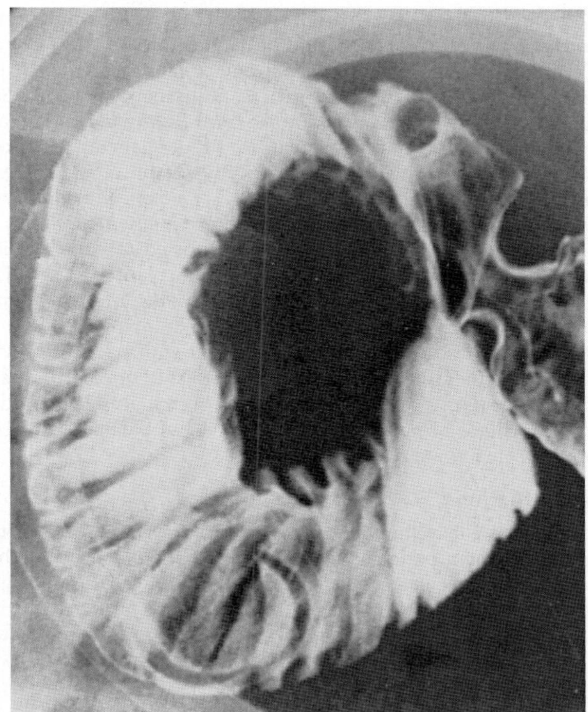

FIG. 52.1 An ascaris close to the ampulla of Vater, with the body and tail lying in the second and third parts of the duodenum. The patient was a 9-year-old girl with acute pancreatitis.

Rarely hepatic hydatid cysts caused by *Echinococcus* can obstruct biliary drainage and cause pancreatic inflammation.[71] *Wuchereria bancrofti* occasionally has been found to cause chronic pancreatitis.[69] Parasitic infestations should be considered as a cause of pancreatitis, particularly in immigrant children and patients who have traveled to developing nations.

The protozoan *Cryptosporidium parvum* has been identified in the bile of an AIDS patient with elevated serum amylase levels and right upper quadrant abdominal pain.[54] ERCP demonstrated biliary and pancreatic ductal disease, and no other opportunistic pathogens were isolated. Cryptosporidia also have been observed in the interlobular pancreatic ducts of experimentally infected immunocompromised mice.[158] Whether cryptosporidial infection causes pancreatitis in immunocompetent patients is unknown; however, a previously healthy adolescent developed pancreatitis after having cryptosporidial diarrhea.[62] *Toxoplasma gondii* cysts have been found in the postmortem pancreatic tissue of patients with AIDS.[4,65] Rarely pancreatitis occurs during acute episodes of malaria.[150] Other systemic manifestations of malaria that often are present include high fever, hepatitis, intestinal malabsorption, encephalitis, and pulmonary insufficiency.

Mycoplasmal and Bacterial Infections

In older children and adults, moderately severe symptoms of pancreatitis have occurred just before or during the course of atypical pneumonia.[6,64] Most patients have had cold agglutinins in their sera, and all have had significant changes in *Mycoplasma pneumoniae* antibody titer. Some controversy has ensued over whether *M. pneumoniae* can cause acute pancreatitis without evidence of pneumonia. Although complement-fixing IgM antibodies against *M. pneumoniae* often increase significantly during the course of acute pancreatitis, researchers have argued that pancreatic cellular antigenic components similar to *Mycoplasma* lipid antigens are exposed during the disease process and that the antibodies elicited cross-react in *Mycoplasma* serologic assays.[83] Rarely *Mycoplasma* has caused severe necrotizing pancreatitis.[101]

Along with *M. pneumoniae* infection, legionellosis must be considered when acute pancreatitis develops along with pneumonia.[94,168] Miliary tuberculosis also can cause symptoms of pancreatitis.[125] Pancreatitis may occasionally be the only manifestation of tuberculosis and is usually diagnosed by fine-needle aspiration of the pancreas.[60,104]

Common pyogenic bacteria usually do not cause acute pancreatitis. Secondary invasion of inflamed pancreatic tissue does occur. Some evidence exists that circulating endotoxin from *Escherichia coli* can cause extrahepatic cholestasis and pancreatitis.[39] Acute pancreatitis also has been seen in children with hemolytic-uremic syndrome.[122,129] Pancreatitis can occur during acute episodes of enteritis. *Salmonella typhimurium, Salmonella typhosa, Campylobacter jejuni, Yersinia enterocolitica,* and *Yersinia pseudotuberculosis* all have been reported to cause clinically evident and laboratory-confirmed cases of pancreatitis.[10,37,93,131] There have been single reports of *Moraxella catarrhalis* and *Streptococcus pyogenes* causing severe pancreatitis in young children.[1,110]

Pancreatitis has been reported in children with leptospirosis.[109,141] *Brucella melitensis* also has been added to the list of uncommon causes of acute pancreatitis.[115] *Helicobacter pylori* has been suggested to influence the clinical course of pancreatitis in humans, but data are still lacking to imply a role in pancreatic pathology.[90]

Fungal Infections

Fungal infections have not been reported to cause acute pancreatitis in immunocompetent patients. *Aspergillus* has caused fatal hemorrhagic pancreatitis, however, in an adult patient with cancer who was undergoing chemotherapy.[56] *Candida* spp. and *Cryptococcus neoformans* have been isolated from the pancreatic tissue of patients with AIDS, but whether they cause clinical symptoms of pancreatitis is unknown.[171]

PATHOGENESIS

When trypsinogen is activated prematurely to trypsin within the pancreatic acinar cells, autodigestion occurs within the pancreas, causing edema. The microcirculation may be compromised, leading to ischemia, hemorrhage, or necrosis. An inflammatory response develops, which may be mild, as occurs in episodes of infectious pancreatitis, or may be more severe with hemorrhagic necrosis. Major mediators of an intense immune response include chemoattractant chemokines and their upregulated receptors; cytokines including tumor necrosis factor, interleukin (IL)-1, IL-6, IL-8, IL-10, and IL-33; and platelet-activating factor.[55,88,116,132,134] Mast cells may also play an active role in the proinflammatory process.[112] If an imbalance of the proinflammatory response occurs within the pancreas, a systemic inflammatory response including shock may occur, leading to high morbidity and mortality. Also sepsis may occur because of extensive necrotic tissue within the pancreas and translocation of microorganisms from the intestines.

TREATMENT

Despite increasing recognition of cases of childhood pancreatitis, no major pharmacologic advances have been made in the treatment of the disease since the mid-1970s. Animal data have shown that medications such as glucagon, aprotinin, 5-fluorouracil, somatostatin, probiotics, and vitamin-based antioxidants may be useful in the treatment of pancreatitis, but human benefit is lacking.[13,40,135] Clinical trials in adults and children using high-dose octreotide or gabexate mesilate have shown no or only modest benefit.[77,164]

The continuing main objectives of treatment are to relieve abdominal pain and treat aggressively systemic manifestations, such as shock, electrolyte abnormalities, and anemia. Meperidine continues to be the medication most commonly used for controlling pain. Meta-analyses in adults and series of pediatric patients have shown that feeding with a low-fat elemental diet decreases the complication rate of patients with acute pancreatitis and now is considered the treatment of choice over total parenteral nutrition.[8,24,144] Intravenous fluids and colloids are used during the acute episode to maintain intravascular volume. During the entire course of acute pancreatitis, the hematologic and biochemical parameters of the child must be monitored closely.

If the episode of pancreatitis is drug induced, use of the medication should be curtailed immediately. Often the symptoms recur if the medication is restarted. Pancreatitis caused by *M. pneumoniae* or that involve bacteria should be treated with proper antimicrobial agents. Obstructions to pancreatic flow (e.g., gallstones, roundworms, congenital abnormalities) may have to be excised or altered either by surgery or endoscopy.[3,19,72] Overall the mortality rate of acute pancreatitis in children today is 5%, with a mean duration of hospital stay at 13 days.[57]

COMPLICATIONS

During the acute episode of pancreatitis, the systemic inflammatory response syndrome may develop, leading to renal, hematologic, central nervous system, pulmonary, and cardiovascular complications. In 12% of children with pancreatitis, an inflammatory mass develops in the first weeks after the onset of illness; however, these masses more commonly occur after trauma.[165] Continued or increasing abdominal pain, nausea, or vomiting often accompanies the development of a phlegmon, abscess, or pseudocyst. An inflammatory phlegmon usually develops into a thin-walled pseudocyst of the lesser sac but may become secondarily infected and induce the formation of an abscess. Patients in whom an inflammatory mass develops must be monitored closely with frequent physical examinations and serial CT studies. In children with pseudocysts, acute abdominal pain accompanied by hypotension often signifies bleeding into the pseudocyst or rupture of the pseudocyst into the peritoneum. Slowly leaking pseudocysts may cause pancreatic ascites. Pseudocysts should be treated conservatively but have to be resected surgically, drained externally, or drained by endoscopy when complications occur.[9] Approximately 77% of pseudocysts in children resolve spontaneously and require no surgical intervention.[126]

The development of fever and leukocytosis during the course of pancreatitis should suggest an infected pseudocyst, pancreatic abscess, or sepsis. In adults, infectious complications account for 80% of deaths associated with acute pancreatitis.[22] Isolates from pancreatic abscesses and necrotic pancreatic tissue have yielded intestinal flora, including anaerobes, in more than 90% of cases, but *Candida* spp. are being isolated more frequently in many medical centers.[41,79,155] *Candida* skin colonization appears to best predict subsequent pancreatic tissue infection in critically ill patients.[59] Rarely *Streptococcus pneumoniae* can be isolated from infected pancreatic tissues of adults with chronic pancreatitis.[151] Carbapenems, such as imipenem and meropenem, are used commonly to treat adult patients with suppurative complications of pancreatitis because these antibiotics penetrate well into pancreatic tissues and have activity against intestinal flora. Performing percutaneous catheter drainage under CT guidance may reduce the mortality rate associated with treating pancreatic abscesses.[14] Rarely fistulas from pseudocysts or abscesses to other abdominal organs may develop.[63]

The role of prophylactic antibiotics in preventing the suppurative complications of acute pancreatitis remains controversial despite three decades of debate. Most recent meta-analyses on the subject conclude that prophylactic antibiotics do not prevent pancreatic necrotic tissue from being infected and do not prevent death, although a poorly powered 2010 Cochrane review suggests that imipenem may reduce the number of pancreatic infections.[106,162,169] Infections, when they do occur after the administration of prophylactic antimicrobial agents, often are caused by multiresistant bacteria or by fungi.

Osteolytic lesions resembling osteomyelitis may develop weeks to months after an acute episode of pancreatitis.[105] Elevated systemic levels of lipase activity possibly may cause intramedullary fat necrosis in the bone. Usually the lesions are asymptomatic and resolve spontaneously without therapy.

NEW REFERENCES SINCE THE SEVENTH EDITION

3. Agarwal J, Nageshwar RD, Talukdar R, et al. ERCP in the management of pancreatic diseases in children. *Gastrointest Endosc*. 2014;79:271-278.
5. Akuzawa N, Harada N, Hatori T, et al. Myocarditis, hepatitis, and pancreatitis in a patient with coxsackievirus A4 infection: a case report. *Virol J*. 2014;11:3.
20. Boskovic A, Pasic S, Soldatovic I, et al. The role of D-dimer in prediction of the course and outcome in pediatric acute pancreatitis. *Pancreatology*. 2014;14:330-334.
26. Capua I, Mercalli A, Pizzuto MS, et al. Influenza A viruses grow in human pancreatic cells and cause pancreatitis and diabetes in an animal model. *J Virol*. 2013;87:597-610.
30. Chang YJ, Chao HC, Kong MS, et al. Acute pancreatitis in children. *Acta Paediatr*. 2011;100:740-744.

34. Coffey MJ, Nightingale S, Ooi CY. Diagnosing acute pancreatitis in children: what is the diagnostic yield and concordance for serum pancreatic enzymes and imaging within 96 h of presentation? *Pancreatology*. 2014;14:251-256.
42. El-Sayed R, El-Karaksy H. Acute pancreatitis complicating acute hepatitis A virus infection. *Arab J Gastroenterol*. 2012;13:184-185.
43. Fabre A, Petit P, Gaudart J, et al. Severity scores in children with acute pancreatitis. *J Pediatr Gastroenterol Nutr*. 2012;55:266-267.
51. Giordano S, Serra G, Dones P, et al. Acute pancreatitis in children and rotavirus infection. Description of a case and minireview. *New Microbiol*. 2013;36:97-101.
55. Gu R, Shampang A, Reilly A, et al. Dynamics of molecular responses to coxsackievirus B4 infection differentiate between resolution and progression of acute pancreatitis. *Virology*. 2012;427:135-143.
57. Guo Q, Li M, Chen Y, et al. Predictors for mortality following acute pancreatitis in children. *Pediatr Surg Int*. 2014;30:1111-1115.
59. Hall AM, Poole LA, Renton B, et al. Prediction of invasive candida infection in critically ill patients with severe acute pancreatitis. *Crit Care*. 2013;17:R49.
73. Kaya M, Bestas R, Cetin S. Clinical presentation and management of *Fasciola hepatica* infection: single-center experience. *World J Gastroenterol*. 2011;17:4899-4904.
77. Kim SC, Yang HR. Clinical efficacy of gabexate mesilate for acute pancreatitis in children. *Eur J Pediatr*. 2013;172:1483-1490.
79. Kochhar R, Noor MT, Wig J. Fungal infections in severe acute pancreatitis. *J Gastroenterol Hepatol*. 2011;26:952-959.
80. Kole AK, Roy R, Kole DC. An observational study of complications in chickenpox with special reference to unusual complications in an apex infectious disease hospital, Kolkata, India. *J Postgrad Med*. 2013;59:93-97.
82. Lautz TB, Chin AC, Radhakrishnan J. Acute pancreatitis in children: spectrum of disease and predictors of severity. *J Pediatr Surg*. 2011;46:1144-1149.
87. Majumdar R, Jana CK, Ghosh S, et al. Clinical spectrum of dengue fever in a tertiary care centre with particular reference to atypical presentation in the 2012 outbreak in Kolkata. *J Indian Med Assoc*. 2012;110:904-906.
89. Makker J, Balar B, Niazi M, et al. Strongyloidiasis: a case with acute pancreatitis and a literature review. *World J Gastroenterol*. 2015;21:3367-3375.
112. Ouziel R, Gustot T, Moreno C, et al. The ST2 pathway is involved in acute pancreatitis: a translational study in humans and mice. *Am J Pathol*. 2012;180(6):2330-2339.
113. Palmer M, Chersich M, Moultrie H, et al. Frequency of stavudine substitution due to toxicity in children receiving antiretroviral treatment in sub-Saharan Africa. *AIDS*. 2013;27:781-785.
114. Pant C, Deshpande A, Olyaee M, et al. Epidemiology of acute pancreatitis in hospitalized children in the United States from 2000–2009. *PLoS ONE*. 2014;9:e95552.
116. Park J, Chang JH, Park SH, et al. Interleukin-6 is associated with obesity, central fat distribution, and disease severity in patients with acute pancreatitis. *Pancreatology*. 2015;15:59-63.
120. Raizner A, Phatak UP, Baker K, et al. Acute necrotizing pancreatitis in children. *J Pediatr*. 2013;162:788-792.
124. Rose PC, Hallbauer UM, Seddon JA, et al. Linezolid-containing regimens for the treatment of drug-resistant tuberculosis in South African children. *Int J Tuberc Lung Dis*. 2012;16:1588-1593.
126. Russell KW, Barnhart DC, Madden J, et al. Non-operative treatment versus percutaneous drainage of pancreatic pseudocysts in children. *Pediatr Surg Int*. 2013;29:305-310.
127. Saleem AF, Arbab S, Naz FQ. Isoniazid induced acute pancreatitis in a young girl. *J Coll Physicians Surg Pak*. 2015;25:299-300.
132. Sesti-Costa R, Silva GK, Proenca-Modena JL, et al. The IL-33/ST2 pathway controls coxsackievirus B5-induced experimental pancreatitis. *J Immunol*. 2013;191:283-292.
136. Sharma V, Sharma A, Aggarwal A, et al. Acute pancreatitis in a patient with vivax malaria. *JOP*. 2012;10:215-216.
143. Sung HY, Kim JI, Lee HJ, et al. Acute pancreatitis secondary to ciprofloxacin therapy in patients with infectious colitis. *Gut Liver*. 2014;8:265-270.
144. Szabo FK, Fei L, Cruz LA, et al. Early enteral nutrition and aggressive fluid resuscitation are associated with improved clinical outcomes in acute pancreatitis. *J Pediatr*. 2015;167:397-402.
148. Thai TC, Riherd DM, Rust KR. MRI manifestations of pancreatic disease, especially pancreatitis, in the pediatric population. *AJR Am J Roentgenol*. 2013;201:W877-W892.
156. Tseng LM, Sun CK, Wang TL, et al. Hookworm infestation as unexpected cause of recurrent pancreatitis. *Am J Emerg Med*. 2014;32:1435.e3-1435.e4.
163. Wachira JK, Jensen CH, Rhone K. Doxycycline-induced pancreatitis: a rare finding. *S D Med*. 2013;66:227-229.
164. Wang R, Yang F, Wu H, et al. High-dose versus low-dose octreotide in the treatment of acute pancreatitis: a randomized controlled trial. *Peptides*. 2013;40:57-64.

The full reference list for this chapter is available at ExpertConsult.com.

53 Peritonitis and Intraabdominal Abscess

Judith R. Campbell

Intraabdominal infection can be a life-threatening condition that occurs spontaneously or as a result of intraabdominal disease, injury, or surgery. Given the compartmental anatomy and physiology of the abdominal cavity, intraabdominal infection frequently is categorized as peritonitis, intraperitoneal abscess, retroperitoneal abscess, and visceral abscess.[3] In this chapter peritonitis and intraabdominal abscess are reviewed; liver abscess, appendicitis and pelvic abscess, and retroperitoneal abscess, are reviewed in Chapters 49, 51, and 54, respectively.

PERITONITIS

Anatomy

Knowledge of the anatomic relationships within the abdomen is important for understanding the source and routes of spread of infection. The peritoneal cavity extends from the undersurface of the diaphragm to the pelvis. In males it is a closed space, whereas in females the ends of the fallopian tubes penetrate into the peritoneal cavity. The transverse mesocolon and greater omentum separate the upper and lower peritoneal cavity. Peritoneal reflections divide the intraperitoneal space further into several compartments: the lesser sac, the paracolic gutters, and the subhepatic and subphrenic spaces (Fig. 53.1). The most dependent area of the peritoneal cavity is the pelvis. Exudate can extend to any of the recesses within the peritoneal cavity distant from the original source, however, and cause diffuse inflammation.[3] When inflamed, the anterior parietal peritoneum, which is supplied by somatic afferent nerves, gives the sensation of localized pain. Stimulation of the visceral peritoneum causes dull, poorly localized pain.

Pathogenesis

Peritonitis is defined as inflammation of the serosal lining of the abdominal cavity or the peritoneum and may be caused by any chemical or infectious agent that irritates the peritoneal surfaces. Noninfectious peritonitis is caused by extravasation of irritants, such as gastric juice, bile, urine, blood, pancreatic secretions, or the contents of a ruptured cyst, into the peritoneal cavity. Although chemical peritonitis generally is aseptic, it may be an important antecedent event to the development of infectious peritonitis.

After peritoneal contamination by bacteria has occurred, the first mechanism of host defense is lymphatic clearance. In experimental peritonitis, this clearance is so efficient that peritonitis and abscess formation occur only if adjuvant substances, such as hemoglobin or necrotic tissue, are present.[24,25,48] In the first hours after bacterial contamination occurs, local resident macrophages are the predominant phagocytic cells. The macrophages then are cleared by the lymphatic system. After bacterial proliferation occurs, polymorphonuclear leukocytes become more numerous in the peritoneal cavity, and inflammation ensues. These peritoneal defense mechanisms also have adverse effects. Fibrin is deposited, which potentially entraps bacteria into a sequestered

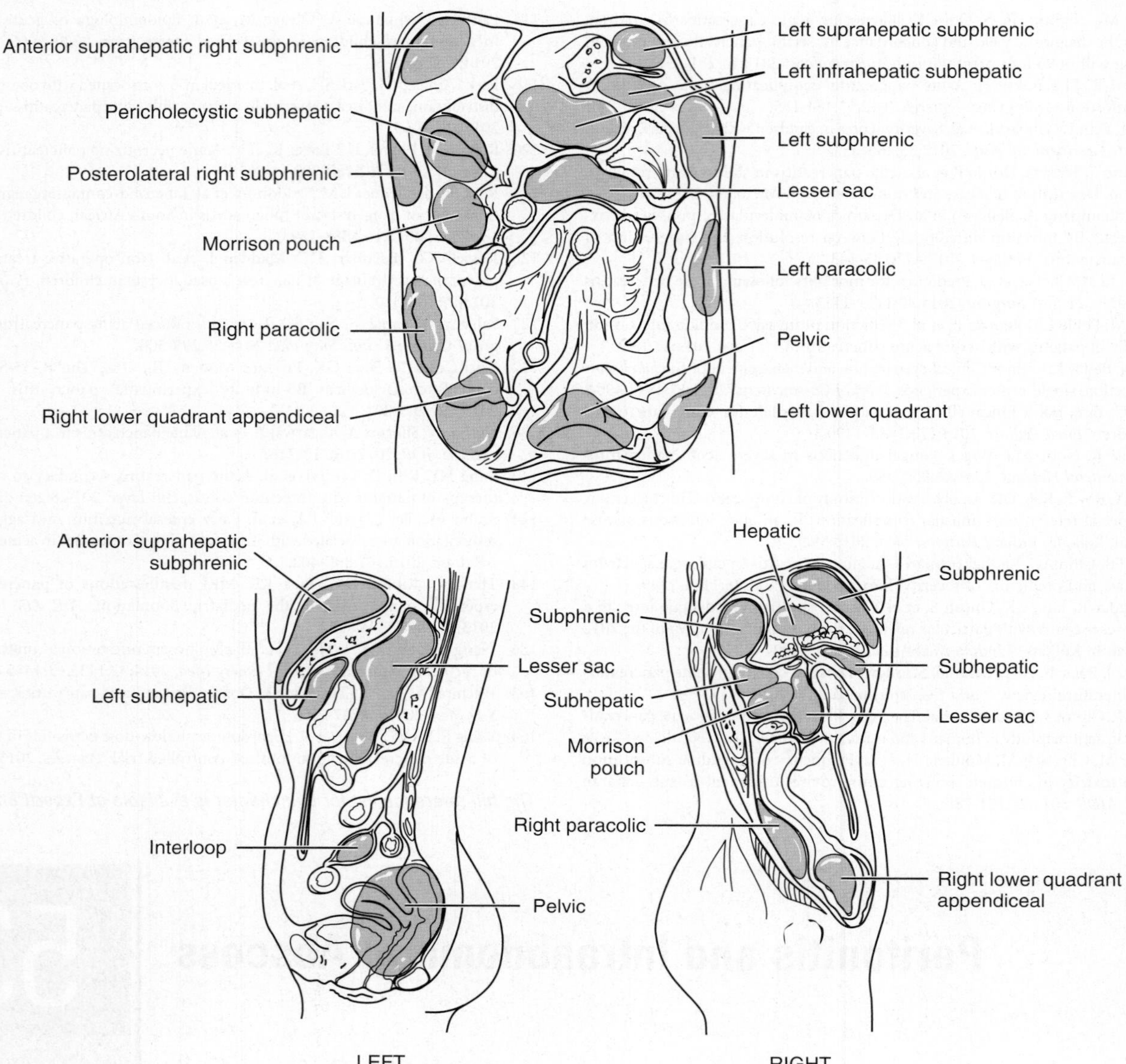

FIG. 53.1 Anterior and sagittal views of the peritoneal cavity. (From Altemeier WA, Culbertson WR, Fullen WD. Intra-abdominal sepsis. *Adv Surg.* 1971;5:281–3.)

environment. An increase in splanchnic blood flow causes exudation of fluid into the peritoneal space, further impairing host defenses by diluting important peritoneal opsonins.[24,25] These host responses serve as a means of containing infection, but they also may contribute to the formation of abscesses.

Infectious peritonitis is subdivided into primary and secondary peritonitis based on the pathophysiology of the infection. Peritonitis that is associated with peritoneal dialysis or the presence of a ventriculoperitoneal shunt is a unique form of peritonitis that also is reviewed in this chapter. The microbial causes of peritonitis vary with the underlying cause and are summarized in Table 53.1.

Primary Peritonitis

Primary, or spontaneous, bacterial peritonitis is a rare infection defined as bacterial peritonitis in the absence of intraabdominal findings, such as intestinal perforation. The incidence of spontaneous peritonitis in children is unknown; however, in the early 20th century, 8% to 10% of abdominal emergencies requiring surgical intervention were due to spontaneous peritonitis.[17,73] Freij and colleagues[30] conducted a 22-year review of children with primary peritonitis in Dallas, Texas. Primary peritonitis was diagnosed in seven previously healthy children compared with 1840 cases of appendicitis during the same period. Currently, 1% to 2% of abdominal emergencies requiring surgical intervention are due to primary peritonitis.[39,42]

Now that this condition frequently is recognized clinically with the assistance of computed tomography (CT), the diagnosis often is made without exploratory laparotomy. The peak incidence of spontaneous peritonitis in children occurs when they are 5 to 9 years of age. In children, the most common predisposing factor is nephrotic syndrome, but this form of peritonitis also occurs in children with postnecrotic cirrhosis.[3,17,33,39,43,47,73,74] Spontaneous peritonitis rarely develops in previously healthy individuals without underlying conditions.[34,49]

The exact pathophysiologic mechanism for primary peritonitis is unknown; however, hematogenous inoculation is thought to be the most likely mechanism because the same organism frequently is recovered from cultures of blood and peritoneal fluid.[17,33,39] Alternative mechanisms include peritoneal seeding via the lymphatics, transmural migration through edematous bowel, and ascending infection from the female genitourinary tract.[33,39] In certain cases, impaired host defenses allow proliferation of bacteria that invade the peritoneal cavity, but a few children with primary peritonitis have no apparent impaired defense. Ascitic fluid from patients with nephrotic syndrome or cirrhosis contains

TABLE 53.1 Most Commonly Identified Etiologic Agents

Primary Peritonitis	Secondary Peritonitis
Escherichia coli (25–40%)	Aerobes
Haemophilus influenzae type b	*Enterobacter*
Klebsiella	*Enterococcus*
Mycobacterium bovis	*E. coli*
Mycobacterium tuberculosis	*Klebsiella*
Neisseria meningitidis	*Pseudomonas aeruginosa*
Other enteric gram-negative bacilli	*Proteus mirabilis*
Other streptococci (α-hemolytic and β-hemolytic)	*Serratia*
	Anaerobes
Staphylococcus aureus (2–4%)	*Bacteroides fragilis* group
Streptococcus pneumoniae (30–50%)	*Peptostreptococcus*
	Clostridium spp.
	Prevotella spp.
	Fusobacterium spp.
	Eubacterium spp.
CAPD-Associated Peritonitis	**VP Shunt–Associated Peritonitis**
Candida	Coagulase-negative staphylococci
Coagulase-negative staphylococci	*Enterobacter*
Enteric gram-negative bacilli	*E. coli*
Mycobacterium	*Klebsiella*
Other fungi	*Pseudomonas*
Pseudomonas	*S. aureus*
S. aureus	
Stenotrophomonas	

CAPD, Continuous ambulatory peritoneal dialysis; *VP*, ventriculoperitoneal.

lower levels of complement and immunoglobulin than does peritoneal fluid from a healthy host.[17,73,81] Deficiency of these important opsonins diminishes the natural clearance of organisms from the peritoneal cavity. Proliferation of organisms triggers the influx of phagocytes, release of inflammatory mediators, and localized or diffuse peritoneal irritation that gives rise to symptoms of abdominal pain and fever.

Since the preantibiotic era, researchers have recognized that primary peritonitis frequently is caused by *Streptococcus pneumoniae,*[33] *Streptococcus pyogenes,*[34] and *Staphylococcus aureus.*[17] Rarely primary peritonitis in prepubescent girls is caused by extension of upper genital tract *S. pneumoniae* infection.[39,68] Since the 1960s, the bacteriology of primary peritonitis has shifted to include an increased proportion of infections caused by gram-negative enteric organisms, such as *Escherichia coli* and *Klebsiella* spp.[17,39,43,74,81] In some instances, primary *E. coli* peritonitis may occur concurrently with bacteremic urinary tract infection.

Tuberculous peritonitis may be caused by *Mycobacterium tuberculosis* or *Mycobacterium bovis.* It may occur as a complication of primary mycobacteremia or be caused by reactivation of latent intraabdominal infection within lymphoid tissue but only rarely does it seem to occur as a function of the ingestion of swallowed organisms from a pulmonary primary focus.[36,37,67,78] Peritoneal infection with *M. bovis,* which is clinically similar to *M. tuberculosis* peritonitis, is acquired from unpasteurized dairy products and has been reported in children living along the border between the United States and Mexico. These organisms may cause peritonitis from either mycobacteremia or erosion of organisms through the mesenteric lymph nodes or bowel wall into the peritoneal cavity.[20] *Salmonella* spp. rarely cause primary peritonitis and have been reported primarily in patients with underlying conditions.[49]

Secondary Peritonitis

Secondary peritonitis, the most common form of peritonitis, arises as a complication of intraabdominal injury or disease when microorganisms, secretions, and the particulate material of an intraabdominal organ enter the peritoneal cavity. Congenital or acquired conditions that result in ischemia, inflammation, or perforation of abdominal viscera may be complicated by secondary peritonitis.[23,48,70] In premature infants, necrotizing enterocolitis is the most common cause of secondary peritonitis.[53] In infants and children, appendicitis is the most common cause; however, it also may occur with volvulus, intussusception, incarcerated hernia, or rupture of a Meckel diverticulum.[53] Although less common in children than in adults, peritonitis also occurs as a complication of mucosal diseases, such as peptic ulcer, ulcerative colitis, Crohn disease, and pseudomembranous colitis.[53]

Rupture of or injury to an intraabdominal viscus results in spillage of the luminal contents and contamination of the peritoneal cavity with bacteria, gastrointestinal secretions, and debris. Chemical and infectious sources of inflammation are introduced. The stomach and upper gastrointestinal tract contents contain only 10^3 to 10^4 or fewer organisms per gram because of the low pH of gastric secretions. Gram-negative aerobic organisms colonize the upper gastrointestinal tract. In contrast, the colonic contents have predominantly anaerobes, with 10^{11} anaerobes and 10^8 aerobes per gram.[11,23,39,66,70]

Secondary peritonitis usually is a polymicrobial infection, with 5 to 10 different bacterial species of anaerobes and facultative gram-negative bacilli. Synergy among the various bacterial species enhances bacterial proliferation.[11,70] Members of the *Bacteroides fragilis* group and *Peptostreptococcus* spp. are the anaerobic organisms reported most commonly in secondary peritonitis. Of the aerobic organisms, *E. coli, Klebsiella* spp., *Pseudomonas aeruginosa,* and *Enterococcus* spp. are isolated most often. Several authors have noted *P. aeruginosa* was isolated from 20% to 30% of children with complicated ruptured appendicitis.[8,23,40,70] When secondary peritonitis occurs in patients with a history of prolonged hospitalization, underlying chronic conditions, or recent antibiotic therapy, the etiology may include nosocomial pathogens that have colonized the gastrointestinal tract, such as *P. aeruginosa, Enterobacter* spp., *Acinetobacter* spp., or other antibiotic-resistant organisms.

Focal suppurative infection may be present within an intraabdominal or retroperitoneal solid organ or within intraabdominal lymphoid tissue. Organisms spread from this purulent focus through the capsule of the organ or lymphoid tissue and enter the peritoneal cavity, with the subsequent development of peritonitis. The intraabdominal organ or lymphoid tissue may be inoculated either via bacteremia (e.g., *S. aureus* and renal infection) or as a complication of the normal function of the organ (e.g., *E. coli* and renal infection or *Yersinia* and mesenteric adenitis).[13,38,44]

Peritonitis and Implanted Devices

Peritonitis is the most significant infectious complication of long-term peritoneal dialysis. Contamination of the dialysis tubing, migration of skin flora from the exit site, or contamination of the dialysate may lead to peritonitis in patients undergoing continuous ambulatory peritoneal dialysis (CAPD). In each instance, a single pathogen usually is isolated.

Gram-positive organisms, coagulase-negative staphylococci, and *S. aureus* account for 30% to 45% of peritonitis episodes in children undergoing CAPD. Of CAPD-associated peritonitis episodes, 20% to 30% are caused by Enterobacteriaceae.[27] In these instances, contamination of the catheter site with fecal material most often occurs in young children who wear diapers and children with incontinence, an open urogenital sinus, or nephrostomy tubes. The waterborne pathogens *Pseudomonas* and *Acinetobacter* account for 6% and 4%, respectively, of peritonitis episodes in children receiving CAPD. *Pseudomonas* peritonitis is especially difficult to treat with the dialysis catheter in situ and may recur despite administration of appropriate antimicrobial therapy.[27]

Fungal peritonitis is another complication of CAPD that is difficult to treat successfully without removal of the catheter. Although fungal pathogens have accounted for only 2% of peritonitis episodes in children undergoing CAPD, this problem is occurring more commonly.[15,26,27,50,58,79] Most patients with fungal peritonitis have had previous episodes of bacterial peritonitis and antibiotic therapy. The most common fungal pathogens are *Candida* spp.[26,27]; however, rare fungi, such as *Curvularia* spp.,[15] *Fusarium* spp.,[27] *Trichosporon asahii,*[50] and *Aspergillus* spp.,[27] have been reported.[58,79] Other rare causes of CAPD-associated peritonitis include *Mycobacterium fortuitum* and *Mycobacterium chelonae.*[80]

Intraabdominal infectious complications develop on average in less than 5% of infants and children who undergo ventriculoperitoneal shunt placement or revision for hydrocephalus.[57,65,71] Peritonitis, peritoneal pseudocyst, or perforation of the bowel by the abdominal catheter rarely occurs in children with such shunts.[5,31,35,62,63,65,69,75] Cerebrospinal fluid (CSF) in the peritoneal cavity may be seeded during transient bacteremia or a febrile illness or after abdominal trauma. In addition, peritonitis may develop as a complication of infection within the ventricles being drained[71] as organisms descend into the peritoneal cavity via the distal tubing.

A peritoneal pseudocyst containing CSF is the most common manifestation of peritoneal inflammation in patients with ventriculoperitoneal shunts. These patients often have a history of symptoms compatible with a shunt infection before the formation of a pseudocyst and may have signs of peritoneal inflammation and a palpable abdominal mass. The microbial etiology of ventriculoperitoneal shunt–associated peritonitis varies and reflects the pathogenesis of infection. Infections occurring within months of surgery often are caused by skin flora, *Staphylococcus epidermidis,* other coagulase-negative staphylococci, and *S. aureus.*[31,62] The microbiology of late shunt-associated peritonitis is similar to that of spontaneous bacterial peritonitis and may include gram-negative enteric organisms and gram-positive cocci.[62] Peritonitis caused by colonic flora also rarely has been associated with bowel perforation by the distal end of the ventriculoperitoneal shunt.[35,62,69]

Clinical Manifestations

The initial signs and symptoms of primary bacterial peritonitis include nausea, vomiting, diarrhea, and diffuse abdominal pain.[39,42,43] These signs and symptoms are similar to those of secondary peritonitis caused by a ruptured appendix.

Rupture of the appendix is the most common cause of secondary peritonitis in children; the initial symptoms of anorexia, vomiting, and localized abdominal pain frequently precede the signs and symptoms of diffuse peritoneal inflammation. In primary and secondary peritonitis, patients typically lie very still because any movement exacerbates the abdominal pain. Physical findings include fever, tachycardia, abdominal distention, hypoactive bowel sounds, abdominal tenderness, rebound tenderness, abdominal wall rigidity, and tenderness on rectal or vaginal examination. Peritoneal inflammation is associated with an increase in splanchnic blood flow, capillary permeability, and a shift of fluid into the peritoneal space, which may lead to intravascular hypovolemia and shock, in addition to systemic absorption of endotoxin and bacteria.[48]

Fever and abdominal pain in any child undergoing peritoneal dialysis should be evaluated carefully. Turbid dialysate fluid raises the suspicion of CAPD-associated peritonitis. Similarly, symptomatic children with ventriculoperitoneal shunts should be evaluated for shunt-associated peritonitis.[63,65,71,83] In a retrospective report of 19 children with ventriculoperitoneal shunts and peritonitis, Reynolds and associates[63] noted that fever and abdominal pain were the most common symptoms in 14 of their patients. Stamos and colleagues[71] found that fever, lethargy, nausea, and vomiting were the most frequently reported symptoms in a review of 23 children with gram-negative infection of ventriculoperitoneal shunts.

Primary tuberculous peritonitis usually is gradual in onset and associated with weight loss, malaise, and night sweats.[36,37,39,67] The degree of tenderness is less than that present with acute pyogenic peritonitis and may be nonexistent. Palpation of the abdomen may reveal an extensive, irregular collection of masses, often described as "doughy," caused by widespread granulomatous inflammation.[36,39]

Diagnosis

Laboratory findings in a child with peritonitis often are nonspecific. The peripheral white blood cell count usually is elevated (16,000 to ≥25,000 cells/mm^3), with a predominance of polymorphonuclear leukocytes and an increase in immature forms.[39] The hematocrit may be elevated because of dehydration and hemoconcentration. Mild pyuria is noted occasionally because of irritation of the urinary bladder or ureters.

Diagnostic imaging studies can be useful in evaluating intraabdominal infections. Upright and lateral decubitus radiographs of the abdomen may show distended adynamic loops of bowel suggestive of ileus and obliteration of the peritoneal fat lines and psoas shadows. Free intraperitoneal air below the diaphragm indicates a ruptured viscus. The presence of a fecalith or right lower quadrant mass may be consistent with appendicitis. Abdominal ultrasonography and CT may reveal an underlying cause of the peritonitis.[49,53]

Analysis of peritoneal fluid aspirate or lavage material may be helpful in differentiating primary from secondary peritonitis. Free air, blood, or bile indicates peritonitis secondary to intestinal perforation. In peritonitis, the leukocyte count in peritoneal fluid usually is greater than 250 to 300 white blood cells/mm^3 and sometimes 3000 to 5000 white blood cells/mm^3, with granulocytes predominating in 80% of cases.[39,47,70,73] A total protein content greater than 1 g/dL, a glucose level less than 50 mg/dL, or an elevated lactate dehydrogenase concentration (>25 mg/dL) is consistent with secondary peritonitis.[17,33,39,73]

If a Gram stain of peritoneal fluid shows only gram-positive cocci, primary peritonitis is most likely. The presence of gram-negative bacilli is consistent with primary or secondary peritonitis, but the presence of many different organisms on Gram stain is diagnostic of secondary peritonitis. Bacteremia occurs in 75% of patients with primary peritonitis. Specimens of peritoneal fluid and blood should be sent for culture.[39] Similarly secondary peritonitis also can be associated with bacteremia, suggesting the need for obtaining cultures of blood in addition to peritoneal fluid. Specimens of peritoneal fluid should be processed to optimize the recovery of aerobic and anaerobic organisms, and the use of specific transport tubes or an airless, capped syringe is required.[11,39,70] The wide variety of pathogens isolated from intraabdominal infections along with the variable antibiotic susceptibility of these pathogens supports taking an aggressive approach to obtaining samples for microbiologic evaluation.

A child undergoing CAPD who is suspected of having peritonitis should have dialysate sent for cell count, Gram stain, and culture for bacterial, mycobacterial, and fungal pathogens. If a child with a ventriculoperitoneal shunt is suspected of having peritonitis, CSF from the proximal portion of the shunt should be sent for culture, cell count, and determination of glucose and protein levels in addition to Gram stain and culture of peritoneal fluid.[31] Abdominal imaging by ultrasonography or CT is useful in identifying a peritoneal pseudocyst and the location of distal tubing.

Differential Diagnosis

Other infectious diseases that may mimic primary or secondary bacterial peritonitis include mesenteric adenitis, gastroenteritis, hepatitis, streptococcal pharyngitis, lower lobe pneumonia, pyelonephritis, and pelvic inflammatory disease. Noninfectious diseases to be considered in the differential diagnosis are pancreatitis, diabetic ketoacidosis, Henoch-Schönlein purpura, ovarian torsion, sickle-cell pain crisis, and lead poisoning.[53]

Treatment

Optimal management of peritonitis involves prompt and aggressive physiologic support, surgical consultation, and antimicrobial therapy. Correction of fluid and electrolyte imbalances and hemodynamic stabilization should be initiated as soon as the diagnosis of peritonitis is suspected. Spontaneous bacterial peritonitis usually is managed medically unless the diagnosis is uncertain, in which case exploratory laparotomy or laparoscopy is performed. Before resistant strains of *S. pneumoniae* emerged, primary peritonitis in children was treated with aqueous penicillin G.[17,33] Given the increased prevalence of *S. pneumoniae* with reduced susceptibility to penicillin, third-generation cephalosporins such as cefotaxime or ceftriaxone are recommended until susceptibility results are available.[47,74] If primary peritonitis is caused by gram-negative organisms, appropriate empiric therapy includes cefotaxime or ceftriaxone, with or without an aminoglycoside, a carbapenem, ticarcillin-clavulanate, or piperacillin-tazobactam, pending completion of culture and susceptibility testing.

Patients with secondary peritonitis may require either immediate surgery to control the source of contamination and to remove necrotic tissue, blood, and intestinal contents from the peritoneal cavity or a drainage procedure if a limited number of large abscesses can be shown.[45,49,54,70,82] In cases of phlegmon, or extensive inflammatory edema, surgery usually is not performed acutely because of the child's unstable metabolic state and friable intraabdominal tissues. Surgery is delayed for several hours or weeks to allow the inflammation to resolve. Surgery also may be postponed indefinitely.[6,14,59,77]

Empiric antimicrobial therapy for secondary peritonitis should have activity against anaerobes, especially the *B. fragilis* group, and enteric gram-negative aerobes.[7] Although controversial, some regimens also include an antibiotic effective against enterococci. The gold standard for antimicrobial therapy historically has been clindamycin or metronidazole, gentamicin, and ampicillin.[7,11,28,45,48,54,64,70] Alternative efficacious regimens, as single or combination therapy, include aztreonam, cefotaxime, cefoxitin, imipenem-cilastatin, meropenem, piperacillin-tazobactam, and ticarcillin-clavulanate.[7,9,32,45,48,51,54,76,82] Rates of resistance to cefoxitin and clindamycin among the *B. fragilis* group have increased and are reported to be 49%; therefore metronidazole is now recommended, and, in some institutions, alternative regimens are used routinely.[2,48,70] Therapy for secondary peritonitis that is a health care–associated infection should be selected based on local antimicrobial susceptibility patterns at that institution.[70]

Other studies have examined the use of a single broad-spectrum antibiotic, which allows a portion of the therapy to be delivered less expensively on an outpatient basis. Fishman and coworkers[28] prospectively evaluated the clinical outcomes of 150 children with perforated appendicitis treated postoperatively with a 10-day course of piperacillin-tazobactam. They compared the outcome with that of historical controls treated with a 10-day course of ampicillin, gentamicin, and clindamycin. Rates of postoperative infectious complications were similar in both groups. Bradley and colleagues[8] prospectively identified 87 children with complicated appendicitis in five pediatric centers, also comparing costs and outcomes with historical controls. Although inpatient treatment courses were reduced by an average of 42% in meropenem-treated children, outcome measures were equivalent to those of historical controls.

Table 53.2 summarizes randomized trials of monotherapy versus combination therapy for ruptured appendicitis in children. Although no differences in outcome were observed, the potential of emerging resistance to broad-spectrum agents versus the convenience of monotherapy must be considered and balanced against the possible decreased risk for developing nosocomial infection among children who can receive a substantial component of parenteral therapy in the home.[40] Goldin and colleagues[32] retrospectively compared the use of triple antibiotic therapy versus monotherapy in a cohort of children with perforated appendicitis and found that single-agent antibiotic therapy in the treatment of perforated appendicitis was at least equal in efficacy to the traditional aminoglycoside-based combination therapy. The potential benefits of a single-agent regimen are reduced length of stay and lower pharmacy and hospital charges.

Empiric antibiotic treatment of CAPD-associated peritonitis should be effective against gram-positive and gram-negative organisms until culture results are available. Intraperitoneal antibiotics, with or without concomitant intravenous antibiotics, achieve adequate serum and dialysate concentrations. Vancomycin is used for empiric therapy for gram-positive infections, but if staphylococcal organisms are susceptible to β-lactam agents, treatment with cefazolin is effective.[27] Aminoglycosides (gentamicin or tobramycin) or cephalosporins are used for gram-negative infections; however, because most intraperitoneal antibiotics are absorbed into the systemic circulation, serum aminoglycoside or vancomycin concentrations should be monitored for possible toxicity. Therapy for fungal peritonitis usually is intravenous amphotericin B, although successful use of fluconazole or intraperitoneal amphotericin B has been reported.[27,58] Indications for removal of a dialysis catheter include persistent infection with *S. aureus* or *Pseudomonas,* tunnel infection, or fungal peritonitis.[27]

Treatment of peritonitis associated with ventriculoperitoneal shunts usually requires externalization of the distal end of the catheter in addition to institution of antibiotic therapy.[31] Empiric antibiotic therapy should include an antistaphylococcal agent active against coagulase-positive and coagulase-negative staphylococci. Coagulase-negative staphylococci are a common cause of ventriculoperitoneal shunt infection; vancomycin should be administered pending culture and susceptibility results. If Gram stain of ventricular CSF or peritoneal fluid reveals gram-negative organisms, cefotaxime, ceftriaxone, ceftazidime, or meropenem should be added.[5,63]

The duration of antibiotic therapy for peritonitis should be dictated by the clinical course of the patient because no single regimen or treatment course is accepted universally.[39,70] Indicators of sufficient therapy include resolution of fever and abdominal pain and return of the leukocyte and differential counts to normal.[39,54,70,72] Primary peritonitis caused by streptococci is treated successfully with a 10- to 14-day course of antibiotics.[17,39] Primary peritonitis with gram-negative organisms may require 10 days to 3 weeks of antibiotic treatment.[17] The duration of therapy for secondary peritonitis after adequate surgery usually is 5 to 10 days, but it depends on the clinical response to therapy.[39,54,70,72] Short-course therapy for 5 days has been shown to be efficacious in some patients,[39,54] but longer courses are required if fever persists or abdominal signs and symptoms are present. Standard therapy for tuberculous peritonitis consists of a minimum of two antituberculous drugs. As with other forms of extrapulmonary tuberculosis in children, empiric therapy with isoniazid, rifampin, and pyrazinamide is advised pending culture and susceptibility results. Although *M. bovis* is resistant to pyrazinamide, most strains are susceptible to isoniazid, rifampin, and ethambutol.

Complications

Acute complications associated with peritonitis include septic shock, adult respiratory distress syndrome, septic thrombophlebitis of the portal vein, acute renal failure, and multiorgan system failure.[48] Postoperative complications include wound infection, adhesions, bowel obstruction, formation of a fistula, and formation of an intraabdominal or retroperitoneal abscess.

Recurrent peritonitis (tertiary peritonitis) is an entity described as occurring late in the course of therapy for secondary peritonitis.[39,46,70,82]

TABLE 53.2 Monotherapy vs. Combination Therapy for Ruptured Appendicitis in Children

			NO. PATIENTS		COMPLICATIONS[a]	
Study	**Monotherapy (A)**	**Combination Therapy (B)**	**A**	**B**	**A (%)**	**B (%)**
Meller et al.[51]	Cefoxitin	Clindamycin/gentamicin	29	27	1 (3)	4 (15)
Dougherty et al.[22]	Ticarcillin-clavulanate	Clindamycin/gentamicin ± ampicillin	79	45	14 (18)	5 (11)
Uhari et al.[76]	Imipenem-cilastatin	Metronidazole/tobramycin	9	10	2 (22)	1 (10)
Collins et al.[19]	Ampicillin-sulbactam ± aminoglycoside	Ampicillin/clindamycin ± aminoglycoside	75	39	2 (1)	1 (3)
Fishman et al.,[28] Lund and Murphy[45]	Piperacillin-tazobactam	Ampicillin/gentamicin/clindamycin	150	373	14 (9)	24 (6)
Bradley et al.[9]	Meropenem	Cefotaxime ± amikacin or tobramycin, clindamycin or metronidazole	22	13	2 (9)	1 (8)

[a]Wound infections, intraabdominal abscess, or rehospitalization.

Modified from Kaplan SL. Antibiotic usage in appendicitis in children. *Pediatr Infect Dis J.* 1998;17:1047–8.

Patients with this condition continue to have symptoms despite receiving appropriate antimicrobial therapy, and peritoneal fluid reveals persistent inflammation. Bacterial cultures often are negative or may yield an organism of low virulence. Multiorgan system failure and a poor outcome frequently are associated with tertiary peritonitis. The mechanism of ongoing peritoneal inflammation is unknown; however, some investigators have proposed that immunoregulatory dysfunction and poor nutrition are contributing factors.

INTRAABDOMINAL ABSCESS

Intraabdominal abscesses often are categorized as intraperitoneal, visceral, or retroperitoneal (see Chapter 54).[4,10] In children, intraperitoneal abscesses are most common. The most common underlying conditions associated with an intraabdominal abscess in children are appendicitis and trauma.[10,53] Reviews of gangrenous or perforated appendicitis in children indicate that 2% to 20% of cases are complicated by the formation of an abscess.[54,64]

Two basic mechanisms exist for the development of an intraperitoneal abscess. In the first mechanism, diffuse peritonitis may cause loculations of purulent material to form in the areas anatomically most dependent—typically the pelvic, subphrenic, and paracolic regions (see Fig. 53.1). The second mode of formation of an abscess involves a localized focus related to contiguous disease or injury in which host defenses and the inflammatory response prevent diffuse spread and peritonitis.[4] The microbiology of intraperitoneal abscesses is polymicrobial and reflects that of the intestinal flora. In a review of intraabdominal abscess in 36 children, Brook[10,11] noted that the predominant organisms were the *B. fragilis* group, *Peptostreptococcus, E. coli,* and other Enterobacteriaceae.

The most common sites of visceral abscess in children are the liver (see Chapter 49), pancreas, and spleen. Underlying conditions that may lead to the development of a pancreatic abscess include pancreatic injury, pancreatitis, and biliary obstruction. Pancreatitis or surgical or accidental injury to the pancreas causes the release of pancreatic enzymes and focal necrosis.[29] Reflux of contaminated bile into the pancreatic duct is hypothesized to be the mechanism by which enteric organisms gain access to the injured pancreas and proliferate. A pancreatic abscess usually is a polymicrobial infection caused by aerobic (*E. coli, Klebsiella pneumoniae,* group D streptococci) or anaerobic (peptostreptococci, *B. fragilis* group) organisms that inhabit the gastrointestinal tract. Rare instances of *S. aureus* pancreatic abscess occur as a result of bacteremia.[12,13]

Splenic abscesses are unusual findings in infants and children. Before the 1970s, most reports involved solitary pyogenic abscesses. Since then, the number of reports of multiple splenic abscesses has increased.[16,41,60] Splenic abscess usually is associated with one of five underlying conditions: endocarditis, injury, hemoglobinopathy, immunodeficiency, or adjacent infection. Given the filtering function of the spleen, an abscess can form as a result of any metastatic hematogenous infection, such as endocarditis. Although rare, splenic abscess can be a delayed complication of the nonoperative management of splenic injuries. Splenic infarcts associated with hemoglobinopathies such as sickle-cell disease may become secondarily infected and form an abscess.[16] Immunodeficiency, such as malignancy or acquired immunodeficiency syndrome, is another significant risk factor for the development of multiple splenic abscesses.[41,55,60]

Rarely infection or disease in a contiguous focus may extend to the spleen. In a review of 56 children with splenic abscesses, 7 (12.5%) were cryptogenic with no apparent cause.[41] In most instances, a single pathogen is isolated, with *S. aureus,* streptococci, *E. coli,* and *Salmonella* spp. being the most common. Fungi, most often *Candida* spp., have been isolated from splenic abscesses primarily in immunocompromised hosts.[41,55,60]

Clinical Manifestations

The typical clinical features of an intraabdominal abscess include fever, abdominal pain, and tenderness over the involved area. Subphrenic abscesses also may be manifested as referred pain or pulmonary or pleuritic symptoms. Pancreatic abscess may be associated with a palpable epigastric mass and elevated serum lipase and amylase.[12] Splenomegaly or a splenic mass may be noted in approximately half of patients with splenic abscesses.[41] In postoperative patients, persistence of abdominal symptoms or fever warrants evaluation for an intraperitoneal abscess.[3] Leukocytosis (20,000 to 50,000 cells/mm^3) frequently is present in children with an intraabdominal abscess.[3,39]

Diagnosis

Imaging studies are helpful in diagnosing an intraabdominal abscess. Plain radiographs are useful as an initial procedure and may show an extraintestinal air-fluid level, right lower quadrant mass, or localized ileus.[1] Chest radiographs should be obtained because subphrenic abscesses often are associated with a pleural effusion. In a series of 27 children with splenic abscesses, chest radiographs were abnormal in 20 cases, with the most common findings being left pleural effusion and an elevated left hemidiaphragm.[41] Ultrasonography is a useful noninvasive technique that can detect abdominal and pelvic abscesses. The quality of the images depends on the examiner, however. In addition, conditions such as ileus, postoperative drains, or dressings may hinder ultrasound detection of an abscess.[1,49,52] CT is the most sensitive tool for detecting an intraabdominal abscess, and it provides good anatomic resolution. Disadvantages of CT are the radiation and, if used, exposure to intravenous, oral, or rectal contrast material.[1,49,52]

Although more recent experience with the use of magnetic resonance imaging for detecting an intraperitoneal abscess has been described in the literature,[56] this modality should be considered in children only when an abscess may not be detected more easily by other methods or in patients who should not have exposure to radiation.[56] Gallium scanning is a sensitive technique for diagnosing an abscess, but it is nonspecific, particularly in the abdomen.[1]

Treatment

Management of an intraabdominal abscess includes physiologic and nutritional support, antimicrobial therapy, and drainage. After blood cultures have been obtained, empiric antibiotic therapy should be instituted with agents effective against anaerobes, Enterobacteriaceae, and other enteric flora as discussed earlier for peritonitis. Antibiotic therapy usually is begun before surgery is done to minimize any complications of bacteremia during the procedure. Abscess material should be obtained for culture of aerobic, anaerobic, fungal, and mycobacterial pathogens. Effective surgical management depends on accurate localization of the abscess, discrimination between single and multiple abscesses, and early and adequate drainage.[3,4,48] Traditional therapy for intraperitoneal abscesses has relied on open surgical drainage, although drainage of intraperitoneal abscesses percutaneously under ultrasound or CT guidance now is used often.[1,18,21,48,52,61]

In instances of multiple intraperitoneal abscesses or if the source of peritoneal contamination has not been controlled, laparotomy is indicated.[48] Pancreatic abscesses require intensive surgical and medical therapy. Antimicrobial therapy for mixed aerobic and anaerobic infection is suggested,[12] but splenectomy remains the definitive treatment of bacterial splenic abscesses. In selected patients, percutaneous drainage or splenotomy has the advantage of preserving splenic function, however.[41,55,60] Multiple small splenic abscesses and fungal lesions generally are treated medically.[41] Antibiotic therapy for a pyogenic splenic abscess should be guided by the pathogens associated with the child's underlying condition. Therapy should include antibiotics effective against *S. aureus,* streptococci, and gram-negative enteric bacilli. Specific therapy should be revised after culture and susceptibility results are available.

Complications

Intraperitoneal and visceral abscesses, if not adequately drained, may be associated with significant complications, including ongoing spread of the infectious process and, for splenic or pancreatic abscesses, a high mortality rate. Fistula formation, adhesions, and bowel obstruction may be late complications of intraabdominal infection.

The full reference list for this chapter is available at ExpertConsult.com.

Retroperitoneal Infections

54

Alice Pong • John S. Bradley

Retroperitoneal infections consist primarily of suppurative bacterial infections that originate within the retroperitoneal structures. In children, these infections are much less common than intraabdominal infections; however, they can lead to significant morbidity if missed. Symptoms often are indolent and poorly localized. Consequently there can be a delay in diagnosis.

The retroperitoneal structures are separated from the intraabdominal organs by the posterior peritoneal fascia (Fig. 54.1). Structures posterior to this fascia layer, in the anterior retroperitoneal space, include the duodenum, pancreas, and parts of the colon. The kidneys and ureters are encased by the renal fascia. The iliopsoas and psoas muscles lie at the posterior aspect of the retroperitoneal space and are separated from the other retroperitoneal structures by the transversalis fascia. Pelvic structures, including the bladder, uterus, and rectum, that lie inferior to the pelvic peritoneum constitute the pelvic portion of the retroperitoneal space. The fascial layers limit the spread of retroperitoneal infections; however, the deep location is difficult to assess by physical examination.

ETIOLOGY AND PATHOGENESIS

Retroperitoneal infections in children arise in numerous anatomic structures. Brook[8] reviewed cases of retroperitoneal infections from five US hospitals from 1974 to 1994. Forty-one children were identified. Twenty-one had infections in the anterior retroperitoneal space related to the pancreas ($n = 4$) and intestines ($n = 13$), 6 had perinephric abscesses, 7 had iliopsoas abscesses, and 7 had pelvic retroperitoneal abscesses. Retroperitoneal infections may occur from hematogenous seeding of bacteria from another site, ascending infection from the urinary tract, or as an extension of infection from the gastrointestinal tract.

Infections of the perinephric retroperitoneal space include those involving the kidney and adrenal glands. Although renal or perinephric abscesses can result from bacteremic inoculation of renal tissue,[54,63] more recent case series report ascending urinary tract infections being a more common source.[13,16,41] Clinical presentation usually includes fever and flank or abdominal pain. Nephronia (i.e., focal renal cellulitis, focal bacterial nephritis) is thought to be an intermediate stage of renal infection between pyelonephritis and renal abscess, resulting from an ascending infection of the urinary tract.[14] Adrenal abscesses are reported more frequently in neonates than in older children and are suspected to be related to adrenal hemorrhages that become secondarily infected.[47]

Within the anterior retroperitoneal space, secondary infections occur as a direct extension from gastrointestinal perforations such as ruptured appendices or those related to Crohn disease.[8,26,28] Greenstein and associates reported retroperitoneal abscesses in 12 of 231 patients with Crohn disease.[26] Retroperitoneal infections, particularly of the pelvic space, can also develop secondary to primary infections of the vertebral spine, pelvic bones, and sacroiliac joint.[30,59] Suppurative iliac or retroperitoneal lymph nodes are another source of retroperitoneal infections. Prior surgery has been reported as a predisposing factor in perinephric abscesses[7,22] and in vascular grafts in adults.[10] Pancreatic abscesses are seen more commonly in adult patients and are associated with underlying biliary tract disease, alcoholism, surgery, and trauma.[9] Acute pancreatitis occurs less frequently in children than in adults; however, when it occurs, infections are often implicated.[32,62]

Iliopsoas abscesses may be a consequence of hematogenous seeding of the muscle, with trauma as a predisposing factor.[29,55] Although primary infection occurs most commonly,[6] the iliopsoas muscle extends from the ribs and lumbar vertebrae to its insertion on the femur and is exposed to the risk of extension of infection from numerous adjacent structures. Psoas abscesses have developed as a consequence of vertebral infections, intestinal perforations, and genitourinary sources.[29,33,34] Neonatal iliopsoas abscesses have also been reported and present with symptoms similar to those of a septic hip.[20,23,50]

Complications of retroperitoneal abscesses include both rupture into the intraperitoneal space and extension of the infection along fascial planes to adjacent muscles that extend from origins in the pelvis and trunk to insertion sites on the femur. Rupture into the thoracic cavity also has been reported.[1] Other reported complications include pneumonia, recurrent abscess, renal failure, and venous and arterial thrombosis.[17]

MICROBIOLOGY

The microbiology of retroperitoneal infections is determined by the source of the infection and the retroperitoneal compartment involved. Most primary infections thought to result from bacteremia are caused by *Staphylococcus aureus,* including methicillin-resistant *S. aureus* (MRSA).[51] Secondary infection related to the gastrointestinal tract is caused by mixed bowel flora including *Escherichia coli*, other gram-negative enteric bacteria, *Pseudomonas* spp., and gastrointestinal anaerobes, particularly *Bacteroides fragilis* and *Peptostreptococcus*.[8] Most infections in the anterior retroperitoneal space are associated with a gastrointestinal source and may be polymicrobial. *Actinomyces* infections can also present as retroperitoneal infections.[4,39]

Ascending infections from the urinary tract usually are caused by *E. coli*; however, perinephric abscesses also are reported as a complication of renal infection caused by *S. aureus*, group B *Streptococcus*, and *Salmonella*.[22,63,64]

S. aureus is the leading pathogen isolated in iliopsoas abscesses unless the infection is secondary to erosion of a primary gastrointestinal focus. In that situation, gram-negative enteric bacteria and anaerobes are more likely to be the causative agents.[6,55] Retroperitoneal necrotizing fasciitis from group A *Streptococcus* has also been reported.[19]

Tuberculosis caused by *Mycobacterium tuberculosis* or *M. bovis* may involve the retroperitoneal space as an extension of vertebral tuberculous osteomyelitis.[1,21,33,34] Abdominal tuberculosis usually manifests as an intraperitoneal infection but can produce retroperitoneal adenopathy.

The most common infectious agents associated with acute pancreatitis are viral pathogens including adenovirus, coxsackie B, mumps, and hepatitis viruses (A, B, E).[3,15,27,31,46,52,60] Varicella, herpes simplex virus (HSV), cytomegalovirus (CMV), Epstein-Barr virus (EBV), and rotavirus have also been reported as associated infections in patients with acute pancreatitis.[18,24,36,52,53] Bacterial pathogens including *Salmonella* and mycoplasma[45,48,52] are less frequently associated with pancreatitis. *Ascaris lumbricoides* can cause acute pancreatitis via obstruction of the common bile duct or other intrahepatic and pancreatic ducts.[35,52]

CLINICAL PRESENTATION

Children with retroperitoneal infections present clinically in a variety of ways, ranging from nonspecific fever to overwhelming sepsis. The most common clinical symptoms associated with retroperitoneal infections include fever and pain in the hip, back, and abdomen.[17,43] Psoas abscesses often manifest with the child limping or refusing to walk.[6] Neonates with a retroperitoneal abscess may present with an abdominal mass.[57] In children, acute pancreatitis presents most commonly with abdominal pain and vomiting, rather than back pain.[27,45,62] Symptoms associated with retroperitoneal infections can be vague, and pain is not well localized. Patients often have been evaluated previously for fevers and have been treated with antibiotics before a diagnosis has been made.[6,38,56]

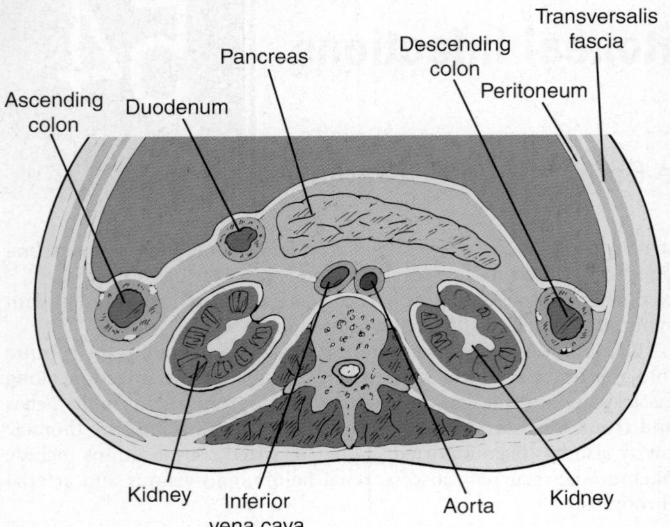

FIG. 54.1 Axial diagram of the abdomen at the level of the kidneys showing the anatomy of the retroperitoneum. (From Gore RM, Meyers MA, Rabin DN. Pathways of abdominal and pelvic disease spread. In: Gore RM, Levine MS, editors. *Textbook of Gastrointestinal Radiology*, 4th ed. Philadelphia: Saunders; 2015.)

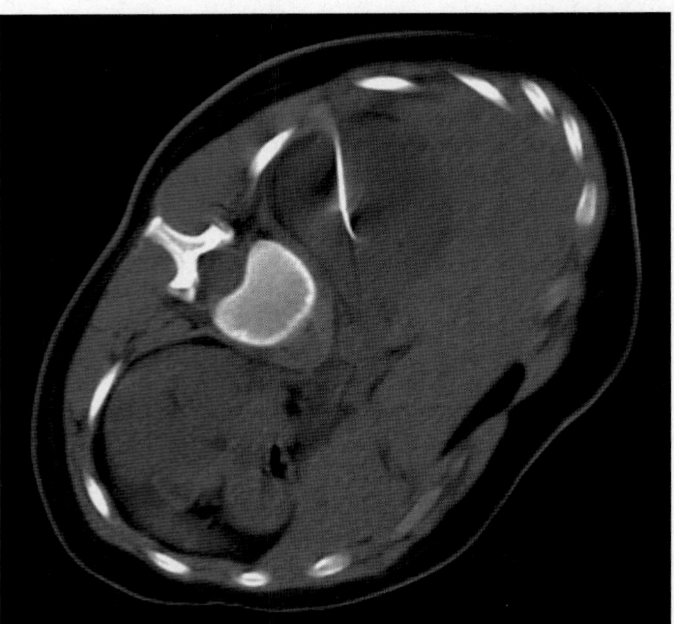

FIG. 54.2 Percutaneous drainage of a perinephric abscess by computed tomography scan.

DIFFERENTIAL DIAGNOSIS

Retroperitoneal infections can be confused with a variety of other infections. Limp and fever caused by pyogenic arthritis of the hip and infection of the sacroiliac joint and pelvic bones are more common than retroperitoneal infections. Abdominal pain and fever are more frequently seen in patients with intraabdominal infections, including appendicitis and intraabdominal abscesses. Trauma and malignant disease are more frequent causes of retroperitoneal masses compared with infectious causes and should also be considered.

SPECIFIC DIAGNOSIS

Laboratory tests often are nonspecific and of minimal benefit. Sedimentation rates and leukocyte counts often are elevated.[6,8,55,56] Pancreatic enzymes including amylase and lipase are usually elevated with acute pancreatitis. Pyuria often is absent in children with perinephric and renal abscesses, and the urine culture result may be negative.[7,13,22,61,63] However, in patients with nephronia, pyuria and positive urine cultures are more likely.[14,37] Blood cultures may be helpful in identifying a bacterial pathogen. Brook[8] reported that 40% of blood cultures were positive for the same organism isolated from abscesses in children with retroperitoneal infections who had blood cultures collected. For children with psoas abscesses, Santaella[55] reported that 71% of blood cultures were positive.

Imaging studies are the most useful diagnostic tools. Ultrasonography can be used to diagnose perinephric infections[7,61] and has been used to diagnose abscesses of the iliopsoas muscle.[28] Computed tomography (CT) with contrast enhancement can be the most helpful[12,17,55] because of superior delineation of organ involvement and the extent of infection. CT also can provide clues about the primary focus of the infection, thereby helping to guide empiric antibiotic therapy. Abscess fluid is seen on CT as areas of low attenuation, often with an enhancing rim.[12,38,63] Percutaneous drainage and biopsy of the lesions may also be accomplished with ultrasound or CT (Fig. 54.2).[13,29,41] Magnetic resonance imaging (MRI) offers the advantage over CT of superior visualization of inflamed bone and muscle tissue, although calcifications may not be as well identified.[49] Although alternative diagnoses also can be evaluated with CT,[58] hematomas and certain tumors may not be easily distinguished radiographically from infection. These noninfectious entities may be better identified by MRI. Decreased radiation exposure is an additional advantage of MRI.

TREATMENT

Although small retroperitoneal abscesses may resolve with antibiotic therapy alone,[13,16,41] percutaneous or open surgical drainage should be considered for all retroperitoneal infections for both diagnostic and treatment purposes. Culture of the aspirated fluid for aerobic and anaerobic bacteria, mycobacteria, and fungi is vital to selecting appropriate antimicrobial therapy. Treatment of patients with antibiotics alone without surgical drainage may not be effective, particularly in cases involving larger abscesses.[1,12]

Initial antimicrobial therapy of retroperitoneal infections should be directed by the presumed source of the infection, with definitive therapy guided by microbiologic culture results. Infections related to gastrointestinal perforation should include coverage directed primarily against enteric gram-negative bacteria and gastrointestinal anaerobes such as β-lactamase–producing *B. fragilis*. Coverage for *Pseudomonas* and *Enterococcus* spp. also should be considered, as these may be present in up to 25% to 30% of otherwise healthy children with complicated appendicitis. Historically antibiotic combinations such as ampicillin for enterococcus, metronidazole or clindamycin for anaerobes, and an aminoglycoside (e.g., gentamicin) or a third-generation cephalosporin for gram-negative bacteria have been used. The β-lactam and β-lactamase inhibitor combinations (e.g., ticarcillin-clavulanate, piperacillin-tazobactam), with or without an aminoglycoside, are also likely to be effective. Carbapenems such as meropenem, imipenem, or ertapenem as single agents may be more cost effective, particularly if any outpatient antibiotic therapy is being considered.

Infections of renal origin, usually caused by *E. coli* or other gram-negative enteric organisms, can be treated with extended-spectrum (third-generation) cephalosporins such as ceftriaxone, or, if abscesses have been drained successfully, with aminoglycosides such as gentamicin or tobramycin. The activity of aminoglycosides may be compromised by the anaerobic and acidic environment of abscess cavities and may lead to clinical failures despite in vitro susceptibility of the organism.[11] Resistance to ampicillin is often seen in *E. coli*,[2,5] rendering it unreliable for empiric use in severe urinary tract infections requiring the use of second- or third-generation cephalosporins. However, extended-spectrum β-lactamase (ESBL)-producing *E. coli*, *Klebsiella* spp., and other Enterobacteriaceae with resistance to third- and fourth-generation cephalosporins, are increasing in prevalence, particularly with urinary tract infections.[28,42] Carbapenems (and, in certain circumstances, fluoroquinolones) may be some of the very few options available for treatment. *Pseudomonas* is not an uncommon pathogen in children with recurrent infections caused by anatomic genitourinary abnormalities.[2] *Pseudomonas* spp. usually are resistant to ceftriaxone; extended-spectrum cephalosporins such as ceftazidime or cefepime or carbapenems may be needed. Urine or abscess culture and susceptibility results help to focus the antibiotic choice to the most narrow-spectrum agent available.

Psoas abscesses and primary perinephric abscesses caused by methicillin-susceptible strains of *S. aureus* should be treated with an antistaphylococcal agent such as nafcillin (or oxacillin) or a first-generation cephalosporin such as cefazolin. The prevalence of community-acquired MRSA (CA-MRSA) has increased significantly as a soft tissue pathogen, particularly in children.[25,44] Vancomycin or clindamycin should be considered as empiric therapy for serious infections in areas with high rates of CA-MRSA (>5% of all invasive *S. aureus* infections) until culture results are available. Recent data suggest that clindamycin resistance in *S. aureus* is also increasing in certain regions, prompting the clinician to access local susceptibility data in making empiric therapy decisions. These agents also may be effective in treating the patient who is unable to tolerate penicillin or cephalosporin antibiotics. For children unable to tolerate vancomycin due to renal compromise, newer agents including ceftaroline fosamil, daptomycin, and linezolid are also promising alternatives against MRSA infections. These agents may also be options against *S. aureus* with minimum inhibitory concentrations to vancomycin of 2 mg/dL or greater.

Infections originating in the vertebrae are most often caused by *S. aureus* or may result from tuberculosis. Empiric antistaphylococcal therapy can be started, but culture and histologic examination of tissue are needed to direct appropriate therapy. For the child with risk factors for tuberculosis, a positive tuberculin skin test or interferon-γ release assays and a negative Gram stain result, empiric therapy with three or four antituberculous antibiotics should be considered. A chest radiograph should be obtained to look for evidence of pulmonary tuberculosis.

After adequate drainage is achieved, the duration of antimicrobial therapy depends on several factors, including the organism, the site and extent of infection, and clinical improvement. Most small or drained retroperitoneal bacterial abscesses of renal or muscle origin are treated for 2 to 3 weeks with initial parenteral and follow-up oral antibiotics. Infections involving bone may require 6 to 8 weeks or longer, depending on how quickly the infection responds to treatment. Radiographic studies, erythrocyte sedimentation rate, and C-reactive protein measurements can be helpful to monitor recovery. Tuberculous infections are treated for 6 to 12 months, depending on the presence of bone involvement. *Actinomyces* infection can be difficult to treat because of lack of susceptibility to many antibiotics and the need for prolonged courses of antibiotic therapy, preferentially with penicillin.

Treatment of pancreatitis is primarily supportive with elimination of enteral feedings and pain control. There have been some reports of adenovirus treatment with cidofovir, particularly in the bone marrow transplant population.[3,40,65]

PROGNOSIS

Historically, retroperitoneal infections are reported to have high morbidity and mortality rates. However, with modern imaging techniques enabling more timely diagnoses, the overall prognosis is good, and most children with no underlying disease recover without sequelae.

NEW REFERENCES SINCE THE SEVENTH EDITION

13. Cheng CH, Tsai MH, Su LH, et al. Renal abscess in children: a 10-year clinical and radiologic experience in a tertiary medical center. *Pediatr Infect Dis J.* 2008;27:1025-1027.
16. Comploj E, Cassar W, Farina A, et al. Conservative management of paediatric renal abscess. *J Pediatr Urol.* 2013;9:1214-1217.
28. Hochreiter D, Lin J, Singh J, Shetty AK. Renal abscess due to community-acquired extended-spectrum β-lactamase-producing *Escherichia coli* in a 15-year-old girl. *Urology.* 2015;85:1480-1482.
34. Karli A, Belet N, Danaci M, et al. Iliopsoas abscess in children: report on five patients with a literature review. *Turk J Pediatr.* 2014;56:69-74.
41. Linder BJ, Granberg CF. Pediatric renal abscesses: a contemporary series. *J Pediatr Urol.* 2015;1:e1-e5.
42. Logan LK, Braykov NP, Weinstein RA, et al. Extended-spectrum β-lactamase-producing and third-generation cephalosporin-resistant Enterobacteriaceae in children: trends in the United States, 1999–2011. *J Pediatric Infect Dis Soc.* 2014;3:320-328.
54. Rote AR, Bauer SB, Retik AB. Renal abscess in children. *J Urol.* 1978;119:254-258.

The full reference list for this chapter is available at ExpertConsult.com.

55 Osteomyelitis

Paul Krogstad

INTRODUCTION

The term *osteomyelitis* denotes inflammation of bone and marrow but generally implies the presence of infection. Osteomyelitis is considered acute if diagnosed within 2 weeks of the onset of symptoms or subacute if symptoms have been present for more than 2 weeks at the time of presentation. Although bacteria are the most common cause, fungi, parasites, and other microorganisms also may cause osteomyelitis. These microorganisms can be introduced into bone in three ways: (1) by direct inoculation, usually traumatic, but also during surgery or due to the presence of orthopedic fixation devices; by local invasion from a contiguous focus of infection; and (3) by hematogenous delivery. In children, osteomyelitis is generally of hematogenous origin. Regardless of the route of infection, the goal of treatment is to arrest the infection and limit the extent of the injury to bone.

The incidence of osteomyelitis in normal children has been examined in several populations. Estimates have varied from 1 in 20,000 adolescent girls in New Zealand to 1 in 1000 Australian Aboriginals.[37,64,65,106,175] Boys contract the disease 1.2 to 3.7 times more often than do girls.[106,114,207,243] Osteomyelitis occurs most often in the first 2 decades of life. Approximately 25% of children with osteomyelitis are younger than 2 years old, and 50% are younger than 5 years.[107,153,193,270] The incidence is increased in people with sickle-cell disease and in some other immunocompromised individuals (see the section on special populations).

Although routine cultures fail to identify bacterial pathogens in approximately one-quarter to one-half of all cases of osteomyelitis in children, most microbiologically confirmed infections are caused by a single type of organism.[10,33,193,211] When polymicrobial infections are encountered, they may reflect the spread of infection from contiguous infectious foci and most often occur in the skull, face, hands, or feet. Distal extremities compromised by vascular insufficiency or immobilized because of peripheral neuropathy also are sites of polymicrobial osteomyelitis.[211]

Gram-positive bacteria are most often identified, especially *Staphylococcus aureus*[9,10,107,175,178,193,206,222,263] and *Streptococcus pyogenes*; together they account for 80% to 90% of cases in most series (Table 55.1). However, these data are largely derived from studies using traditional microbiological approaches. By contrast enhanced culture techniques and PCR studies[285] have revealed that *Kingella kingae*, a fastidious gram-negative organism, is an important cause of osteoarticular infections in young children, including osteomyelitis, diskitis, and septic arthritis. Reports demonstrating the importance of *Kingella* infections as a cause of osteoarticular infections in young children have come from countries as diverse as Israel, the United States, Australia, Switzerland, and Iceland.[66,76,112,166,175,271,286] *K. kingae* osteomyelitis has been identified at a frequency equal to *S. pyogenes* in some series,[166,175] and in several reports *Kingella* infections exceeded those of gram-positive pathogens.[50,51,54]

Streptococcus pneumoniae has been a frequent cause of osteomyelitis in the past, but protein conjugate vaccines have markedly reduced the frequency of invasive pneumococcal infections, including pneumococcal osteomyelitis. Similarly *Haemophilus influenzae* used to cause approximately 5% to 8% of cases and was found primarily in infants and younger children.[84,94,115,142,153,193,216,222,256,268] Cases of *H. influenzae* osteomyelitis are noticeably absent from case series published since 2000, likely reflecting the impact of widespread immunization against this organism.[10,107,144,206,216,289]

Even in affluent countries *Salmonella* spp. are occasionally a cause of osteomyelitis in immunocompetent patients, and *Salmonella* spp. appear to be the most common organism found in cases of osteomyelitis in patients with sickle-cell disease (see later discussion).[9,43,178,193] Osteomyelitis caused by *Escherichia coli* and other aerobic enteric gram-negative organisms is also seen, generally in neonates and young infants.[94,148] Osteomyelitis caused by *Pseudomonas aeruginosa* has been associated with injection drug use.[129,159,279]

Although rare in comparison to osteomyelitis caused by aerobic bacteria, four distinct clinical entities of osteomyelitis caused by anaerobic bacteria are recognized: (1) bacteremic seeding of previously normal bones in children and young adults[161]; superinfection of a fracture site already infected with *S. aureus*; (3) indolent (months to years after surgery) infection of a prosthetic device; and (4) contiguous chronic infection,[257] which most often occurs in the skull and the extremities. *Bacteroides* spp. are found most commonly and are associated with paranasal, sinus, or mastoid infection. In most cases, a foul odor is noted when the bone is incised or the focus is opened; trauma often has been an inciting influence.[161]

Osteomyelitis caused by fungi and other rare bacterial pathogens is discussed in greater detail later.

HEMATOGENOUS OSTEOMYELITIS

Pathogenesis

In long tubular bones, hematogenous osteomyelitis generally begins in the metaphysis, the broad cancellous end of the bone shaft adjacent to the epiphyseal growth plate. The cartilaginous epiphyseal growth plate (the physis) is nourished by diffusion of nutrients from capillaries fed by the metaphyseal branches of a nutrient artery. In a long-standing model of disease, capillaries drain into a large sinusoidal plexus that ultimately joins the large sinusoidal veins in the bone marrow (Fig. 55.1).[127] Trauma or emboli lead to occlusion of the slow-flowing sinusoidal vessels, establishing a nidus for infection. Blood-borne bacteria can seed the poorly perfused area and proliferate.[58,138,265] Others have suggested that the capillaries adjacent to the physis are open ended, permitting deposition of bacteria into this critical location.[245]

The high frequency of *S. aureus* in osteomyelitis may reflect specific pathogenic properties of the organisms, including the ability to adhere to type I collagen of bone fibrils.[44] When *S. aureus* binds to collagen, bacterial replication gives rise to microcolonies surrounded by a glycocalyx.[120] Continued injury, elicited by *S. aureus* exoproducts and the host cellular inflammatory response to the injury, causes the accumulation of exudate under pressure. The pressure compresses blood vessels of bone and produces focal bone necrosis. The low ratio of surface area to mass, combined with the blood vessel anatomy described earlier, interferes with reabsorption of necrotic cortical bone[58,138] and the effectiveness of host defense mechanisms. The very early stages of osteomyelitis may be aborted by administration of appropriate chemotherapy. In the absence of therapy, necrosis of cortical bone and marrow continues. The exudate under pressure is forced through the Haversian systems and Volkmann canals and into the cortex (see Fig. 55.1).

Beginning in the late 1990s, community-acquired methicillin-resistant *S. aureus* (CA-MRSA) isolates became a common cause of musculoskeletal infections in the United States and other countries. Most of these CA-MRSA isolates from cases of osteomyelitis carry genes encoding

TABLE 55.1 Etiology of Acute Hematogenous Osteomyelitis in Children in Microbiologically Confirmed Cases (%)

Organisms	Nelson[193] (*n* = 296)	LaMont et al.[153] (*n* = 90)	Peltola et al.[206] (*n* = 252)	Masson et al.[175] (*n* = 95)	Goegens et al.[107] (*n* = 45)	McNeil et al.[178] (*n* = 190)
Gram-Positive Bacteria						
Staphylococcus aureus	67	70	75	65	85	83
Coagulase-negative staphylococci	3	1		4		
Streptococcus pneumoniae	2	5	4	2	4	2
Other streptococci	12	16	10	10	8	10
Gram-Negative Bacteria						
Haemophilus influenzae	4	8	10	1	0	
Pseudomonas aeruginosa	3					<1
Salmonella spp.	2					4
Escherichia coli	<1					
Kingella kingae	<1			7		
Mixed or unusual organisms	4		1	10		1

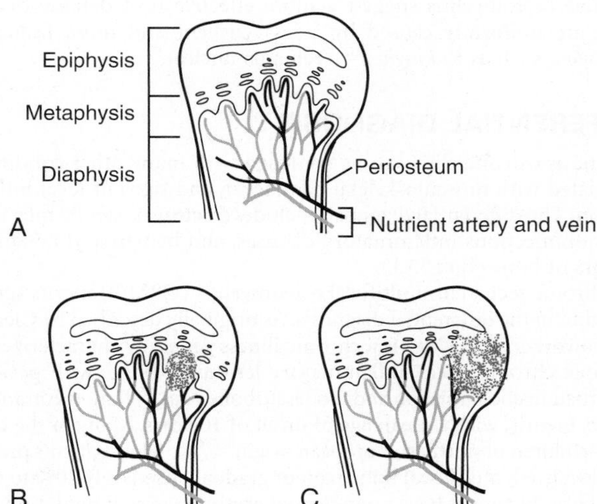

FIG. 55.1 (A) As conceived by Hobo, the sluggish blood flow in the sinusoidal venous connections located at the metaphyseal-epiphyseal junction predisposes to the development of traumatic thrombosis and infarction. (B) Bacteremic seeding of the avascular area initiates the infection, which spreads through the Volkmann canals and the haversian systems and causes septic thrombosis. (C) Infection tends to spread laterally through the cortex and elevates or ruptures through the periosteum.

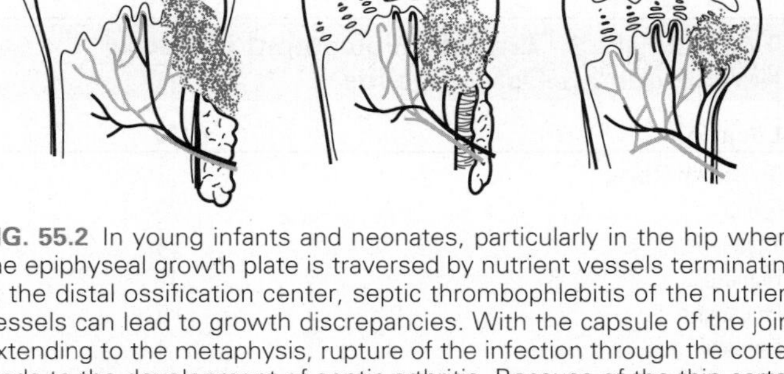

FIG. 55.2 In young infants and neonates, particularly in the hip where the epiphyseal growth plate is traversed by nutrient vessels terminating in the distal ossification center, septic thrombophlebitis of the nutrient vessels can lead to growth discrepancies. With the capsule of the joint extending to the metaphysis, rupture of the infection through the cortex leads to the development of septic arthritis. Because of the thin cortex and loose periosteum, the osteomyelitis may come to medical attention as a deep soft tissue abscess. In older infants and young children, the thicker cortex and denser periosteum are a greater barrier to infection. Local tenderness from subperiosteal edema or abscess is the rule. In late childhood and adolescence, the lesion is extremely well localized and rarely penetrates the bony cortex. In this age group, invasive procedures, such as windowing or drilling, are necessary to obtain infected material.

the Panton-Valentine leukocidin (pvl).[32] Pvl-positive CA-MRSA has been associated frequently with sepsis, venous thrombosis, adjacent myositis, and polyostotic disease, suggesting that this or other factors contribute to the development and severity of hematogenous osteomyelitis.[38,173] However, it is important to note that similar patterns of disease are seen in pvl-negative organisms.[141] Moreover multiple virulence factors are likely involved in the pathogenesis of osteomyelitis, and this remains an area of avid investigation.[100]

Signs and Symptoms

The bacteremic phase of hematogenous osteomyelitis may be entirely subclinical and associated only with malaise and low-grade fever, or it may be characterized by severe constitutional symptoms with high fevers (39°C to 40°C). Subsequent clinical manifestations of osteomyelitis are not related to the severity of initial constitutional signs of infection but are influenced by the age of the child and the etiologic agent (Fig. 55.2).

In newborns, the thin cortex and loosely attached periosteum are poor barriers to the spread of infection. Consequently the purulence rapidly ruptures through both of these structures into the contiguous muscle bed. With progression of the infection, the purulent material often dissects the muscle bundles, with the swollen, discolored limb taking the appearance of a sausage. In addition, the capsule of the diarthrodial joints frequently extends to or is slightly distal to the epiphyseal plate. These anatomic characteristics facilitate extension of infections arising from metaphysis.

In older infants, the cortex (see Fig. 55.2) is thicker, and the periosteum is slightly denser. Consequently the infection spreads less often to the soft tissues of the extremity. Subperiosteal abscess and contiguous edema readily develop, generally at the metaphysis, where the cortex is the thinnest.[116] The nutrient metaphyseal capillaries present at birth that cross the growth plate in infants are atrophic by 18 months of age, but this does not appear to alter the risk of developing septic arthritis at adjacent joints in older children, compared to infants, as once proposed.[47,206,208,224]

In children and adolescents (4 to 16 years old), the metaphyseal cortex is considerably thicker, with a dense, fibrous periosteum. The pathogenesis of the infection is the same in this age group, but the infection rarely ruptures and spreads to the outer cortical lamellae. As a result, the signs and symptoms of osteomyelitis in these older children and adolescents usually are more focal.

A newborn with osteomyelitis usually is irritable and displays evidence of pain when the affected extremity is touched or moved. Pseudoparalysis may occur, and if the disease remains untreated, massive swelling of the extremity may be seen. Obtaining a plain radiograph is particularly valuable in newborns; most have changes consistent with osteomyelitis on the initial radiograph, including soft-tissue swelling, periosteal changes, and lytic lesions of bone.[148,184,276] In infants and young children, pain is usually accompanied by limping because osteomyelitis occurs more commonly in the lower extremities. The child often refuses to use the affected extremity and displays variable constitutional symptoms.

In older children and adolescents, less restriction of function of the extremity is found compared with infants and young children. Point tenderness is often sharply circumscribed and may be found only as a small area of discomfort at rest.

Most commonly, tubular bones are involved, but osteomyelitis occurs throughout the skeleton (Table 55.2). The hallmark of the disease is the focal nature of symptoms; point tenderness and well-localized pain suggest the diagnosis. Percussion of the long bone away from the area of point tenderness may elicit pain at the site of osteomyelitis in older children and adolescents.

The clinical features of osteomyelitis are also influenced by the organisms involved. Osteomyelitis caused by CA-MRSA seems to be more complex and severe than are infections caused by methicillin-susceptible *S. aureus* (MSSA). Life-threatening infections caused by CA-MRSA have been reported in adolescents, and polyostotic disease is more common (15% in one more recent series compared with 2% in a large series that preceded the emergence of CA-MRSA).[32,193] Myositis, pyomyositis, intraosseous and subperiosteal abscesses, pathologic fractures, and septic thrombophlebitis also seem to occur more frequently with CA-MRSA than with MSSA.[10,22,100,110,111,173,216] Osteoarticular infections caused by *Kingella* spp. nearly always arise in children under 36 months of age and usually have an indolent course, with limb pain often present for longer than a week before initial medical evaluation is made; complications and sequelae of osteomyelitis are rare, but Brodie abscess and periosteal abscesses have been described with *Kingella*.[19,76,166,229,285,287] Osteomyelitis caused by *H. influenzae* seems to occur primarily in the upper extremities.[83,84,115,256]

Culture-negative osteomyelitis is generally milder than diseases with microbiologically confirmed etiologies. In one series comparing 45 culture-positive patients with 40 patients with culture-negative osteomyelitis, symptoms were of longer duration, and overlying skin changes were seen less frequently in patients with negative disease. Treatment with β-lactam antibiotics generally was successful and associated with skeletal sequelae in only one case.[92] Whether these features of culture-negative osteomyelitis suggest a more effective host defense or that these are uniformly caused by a less virulent and more fastidious pathogen, such as *K. kingae*,[51,271] remains unclear.

TABLE 55.2 Site of Involvement in Acute Hematogenous Osteomyelitis

Location	%
Tubular Bone	
Femur	25
Tibia	24
Humerus	13
Phalanges	5
Fibula	4
Radius	4
Ulna	2
Metatarsal	2
Clavicle	0.5
Metacarpal	0.5
Cuboidal	
Calcaneus	5
Talus	0.8
Carpals	0.5
Cuneiform	0.5
Cuboid	0.3
Irregular	
Ischium	4
Ilium	2
Vertebra	2
Pubis	0.8
Sacrum	0.8
Flat	
Skull	1
Rib	0.5
Sternum	0.5
Scapula	0.5
Maxilla	0.3
Mandible	0.3

Data from Nelson JD. Acute osteomyelitis in children. *Infect Dis Clin North Am.* 1990;4(3):513–22; similar distribution of affected bones is also reported in references 107 and 206.

DIFFERENTIAL DIAGNOSIS

Infectious osteomyelitis can be confused with many other conditions associated with musculoskeletal pain, fever, and signs of local inflammation. The differential diagnosis includes fracture, systemic infectious and noninfectious inflammatory diseases, and benign and malignant tumors of bone (Box 55.1).

Chronic recurrent multifocal osteomyelitis (CRMO) merits special attention in the differential diagnosis. As originally described by Giedion and coworkers[103] CRMO is a chronic illness generally characterized by multiple chronic, focal, inflammatory lesions in bone, with periodic exacerbation and remission and moderate bone pain.[269] It most commonly occurs in girls, with a mean age of onset of 10 years. Many of the cases are in children of northern European origin.[27,147,282] Most patients present with localized, multifocal bone pain of gradual onset; only 20% to 50% have fever, but most have an increased erythrocyte sedimentation rate

BOX 55.1 Differential Diagnosis of Osteomyelitis in Children

Fractures
Thrombophlebitis
Scurvy
Septicemia
Cellulitis
Septic bursitis
Myositis
Pyomyositis
Rheumatic fever
Toxic synovitis
Reactive arthritis
Complex regional pain syndrome
Chronic recurrent multifocal osteomyelitis
Osteoid osteoma
Langerhans cell histiocytosis
Leukemia
Ewing sarcoma
Malignant primary bone tumors
Bone infarction (sickle-cell or Gaucher disease)

(ESR) or increased C-reactive protein (CRP). The osseous lesions occur primarily in the distal femoral, distal tibial, and proximal tibial regions, although pelvic and clavicular lesions are common, and vertebral lesions are seen in approximately one-sixth to one-quarter of cases.[82,87,234] Patients may have 1 to 20 lesions at a time. Biopsy typically reveals a nonspecific chronic inflammatory process, and organisms seldom are identified histologically or by culture; antibiotics bring no improvement in symptoms, Approximately 10% to 20% of patients have a pustular eruption of the palms and soles at the same time that they come to medical attention with bone lesions; this condition is termed *pustulosis palmaris et plantaris.*

CRMO is a sporadic illness in most cases, but it may also be found as part of syndromic illnesses. Majeed syndrome, for example, is an autosomal recessive life-long disorder encompassing of CRMO, congenital dyserythropoietic anemia, and transient inflammatory dermatosis.[86] It may also occur in the rare patients with deficient interleukin-1 receptor antagonist[4] and in the setting of other inflammatory disorders.

The long-term outlook in children with sporadic CRMO disease generally is good, although numerous relapses may occur.[27] Glucocorticoids and nonsteroidal antiinflammatory drugs are often used as initial therapy, although recurrences are common. Treatment with interferon-γ and tumor necrosis factor-α blocking agents, bisphosphonates, and other agents have been associated with long term responses.[4,72,86,98]

Diagnosis

The diagnosis of osteomyelitis generally is suggested by the presence of fever, focal skeletal pain, warmth, swelling, and a limp or refusal to use an extremity, particularly when accompanied by elevated serum acute-phase reactants (CRP or ESR). In an otherwise healthy individual, the diagnosis is probable when a patient has fever, elevated ESR or CRP, or a positive blood culture plus one or more of the following: abnormal imaging studies (plain radiograph, magnetic resonance imaging [MRI], or computed tomography [CT]) with typical signs of inflammation, injury or repair of bone (see later discussion), scintigraphy indicative of increased bone turnover, or physical findings consistent with osteomyelitis. The diagnosis is confirmed by identification of organisms by culture or Gram stain in an aspirate of bone or by histopathologic evidence of inflammation in surgical specimens of bone.

Microbiology

The cornerstone of the diagnosis of osteomyelitis is isolation of bacteria or other microbes from bone or from anatomic structures contiguous to bone. Overall such cultures (aspirates or surgical specimens from bone debridement, subperiosteal exudate samples, or joint fluid) provide a bacteriologic diagnosis in 66% to 82% of cases. Blood cultures yield an organism in about half of cases (31% to 74% of patients in several series).[178,193,206,263,271] Recovery of *Kingella* in culture is enhanced by placing aspirates of fluid into blood cultures bottles.[285] PCR detection of bacterial DNA is likely to become more commonly used in view of its sensitivity and improved detection of fastidious pathogens such as *Kingella*.[51,54,271]

In neonates, needle aspiration of soft tissue or incision and drainage of bone may yield the offending organism. In infants and young children, subperiosteal needle aspiration can be done if the point tenderness is localized. In older children and adolescents, noninvasive culturing of the bone is less rewarding. Performing open procedures to obtain material for culture is somewhat controversial because some orthopedic surgeons consider the risk of causing epiphyseal damage and subsequent length discrepancy secondary to the procedure too great. However, in two recent reports, cultures of bony lesions were positive more than 80% of the time even when antibiotics were given prior to the diagnostic procedure and frequently led to changes in antimicrobial therapy.[178,216]

Radiology

Plain radiographs. Conventional radiographs are crucial in establishing the diagnosis of pediatric osteomyelitis and always should be obtained.[38,55,122] Because bone density must decrease 50% to be detected by radiographs,[13] changes in the less ossified bones of neonates are detected more readily than are changes in older children. In contrast, Waldvogel and Papageorgiou[272] found in adults that plain radiographs were of no diagnostic value in 23% and were misleading in an additional 16%.

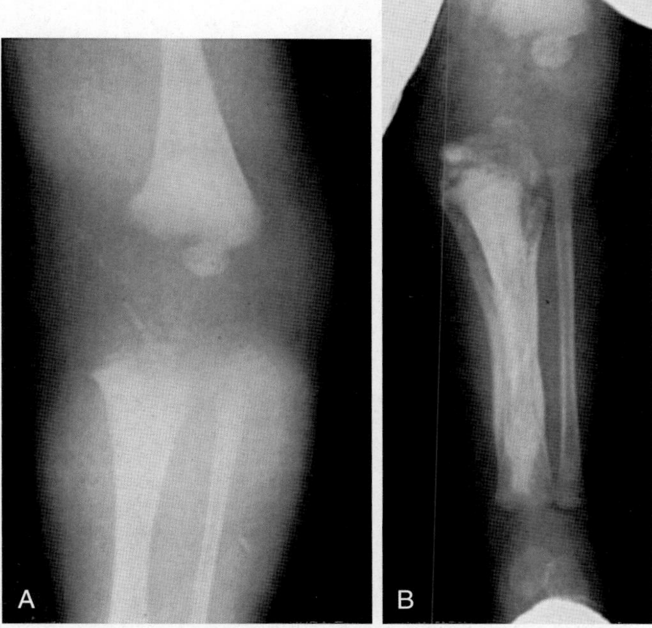

FIG. 55.3 (A) The left knee of an infant shows diffuse soft tissue swelling around the proximal ends of the tibia and fibula. (B) Six weeks later, the subcutaneous fat lines between the muscles and the skin can be seen, as well as an involucrum involving almost all of the tibia.

Radiographic changes occur in three stages.[46] The first stage, which occurs approximately 3 days after the onset of symptoms, is the formation of a small area of localized, deep soft tissue swelling, usually in the region of the metaphysis (Fig. 55.3). Consequently when diagnosis of osteomyelitis is sought soon after onset of symptoms, examination of the radiograph should be directed to the soft tissue rather than the bone. During the second stage, which occurs 3 to 7 days after the onset of symptoms, swelling of the muscles with obliteration of the interposed translucent fat planes can be noted. It is caused by continued spread of edema fluid and can progress, particularly in neonates and young infants, to superficial soft tissue edema; the skin may acquire an "orange peel" texture.

Radiographic evidence of bone destruction usually is not detected until 10 to 21 days after the onset of symptoms. The first changes detected include subperiosteal bone resorption, areas of bone destruction, and periosteal new bone formation. The variability depends on the specific bone involved; generally long tubular bones tend to show bony changes 2 to 3 weeks earlier than membranous or irregular bones.

Magnetic resonance imaging. MRI has become the imaging modality of choice when additional imaging is needed beyond plain radiographs and has sensitivity in excess of 90%.[33,38,55,88,172,176] Other major advantages over CT and plain radiographs are MRI that it accurately delineates subperiosteal or soft tissue collections of pus that might require surgical drainage without using ionizing radiation, and it can identify sinus tracts for removal (Fig. 55.4).[38,91,213,253]

In acute osteomyelitis, bone marrow edema caused by the accumulation of purulent material leads to decreased signal on T1-weighted images. On T2-weighted images of the same area, increased signal is seen. Fat-suppression sequences, including short-tau inversion recovery, decrease the signal from fat. Inversion recovery sequences allow more sensitive detection of bone marrow edema. In most cases, gadolinium contrast is not needed for the diagnosis of osteomyelitis, but enhancement may reveal small abscesses that would otherwise be missed.[139] MRI may have a particular advantage in establishing the diagnosis of spinal osteomyelitis because the vertebral body and the adjacent disk are readily

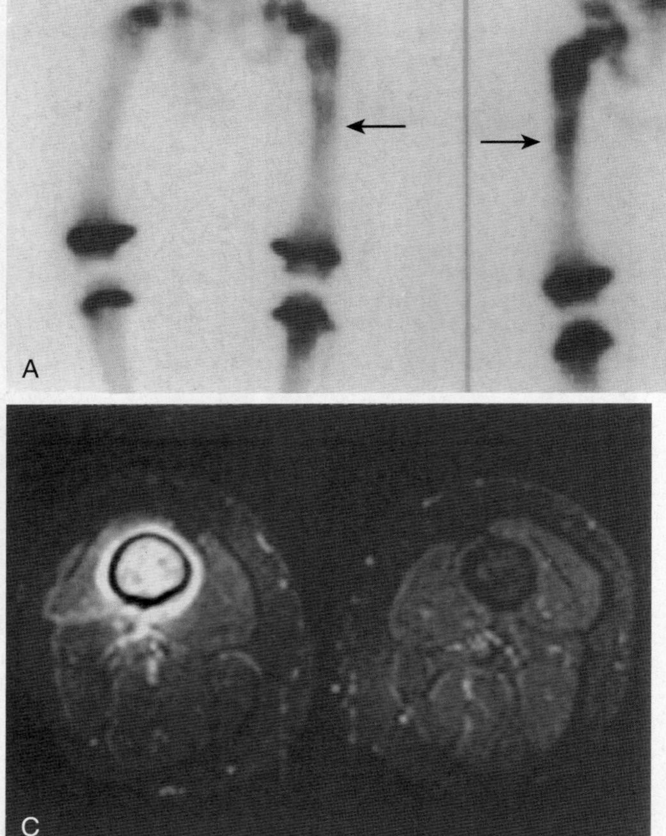

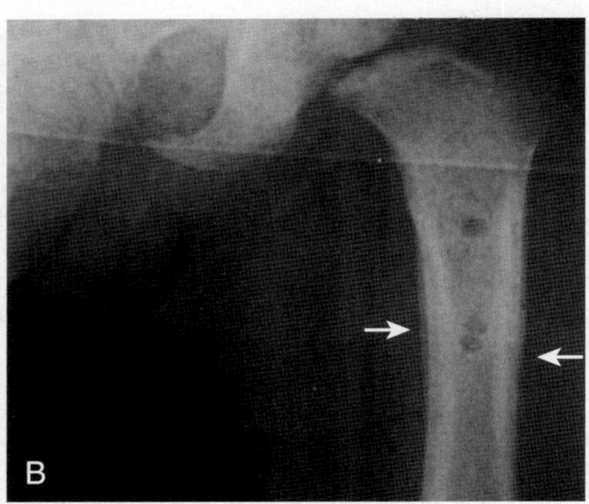

FIG. 55.4 Acute osteomyelitis. (A) Technetium 99m bone scan of a 2-year-old boy with fever and a limp. Moderately increased tracer activity is seen in the proximal end of the left femur because of the increased bone turnover *(arrows)*. (B) Plain radiograph taken 3 weeks later. Unilamellar periosteal new bone formation is seen along the femoral shaft *(arrows)*. The circular radiolucencies seen are the result of cortical drilling to allow diagnostic aspiration; the culture yielded *Streptococcus pyogenes*. (C) Axial T2-weighted magnetic resonance image of the thigh from a different patient shows abnormally high signal intensity throughout the marrow cavity. The band of high signal surrounding the cortex represents periostitis. (Courtesy Dr. Leanne Seeger.)

distinguished. Loss of this border is one of the first abnormalities detected by MRI in spinal osteomyelitis.

The need for sedation in most infants and children and the cost of MRI are the major factors that continue to impede its use. In addition, infarction and other processes can alter the appearance of bone marrow and lower the specificity of MRI and must be considered in the interpretation of the imaging study.

Radionuclide imaging. Radionuclide scanning has been used for decades in the evaluation of suspected osteomyelitis. Despite the fact that bone scanning involves exposure to ionizing radiation, it continues to be used widely because of its ready availability and utility in detecting multifocal disease.[78] Bone imaging employing technetium 99m (^{99m}Tc) diphosphonate scintigraphy is used most frequently.

Most institutions perform a three-phase bone scan for evaluation of infection. Shortly after injection (2 to 5 seconds), a nuclear angiogram (flow phase) of the area of suspected osteomyelitis is obtained. The second phase (the blood pool phase) consists of a single image obtained 5 to 10 minutes after injection. The third image is obtained 2 to 4 hours after injection. In this later phase, the specificity of the diphosphonate compounds for the bone is revealed: the phosphate adduct is adsorbed to the surface of the hydroxyapatite crystal in bone, and ^{99m}Tc becomes concentrated in the cement line located at the junction of osteoid and mineralized bone. Anything increasing local blood flow to the area, particularly if accompanied by inflammation, results in increased general uptake in the first two phases, but osteomyelitis results in focal uptake in the third phase, with the intensity of the signal detected reflecting the level of osteoblastic activity.[52,69,71,78,104,151,235]

Acute osteomyelitis in children is often diagnosed by a ^{99m}Tc scan and treated successfully before bone changes are detected by plain radiographs (see Fig. 55.4).[262] With sensitivity previously reported to be as high as 95%, bone scanning has until recently been a reliable tool in establishing the diagnosis of osteomyelitis.[46] Unfortunately, in one recent report, bone scintigraphy detected only osteomyelitis caused by CA-MRSA cases in 53% (26/49) of children.[38] This apparent lack of sensitivity for CA-MRSA may reflect the acuity of disease caused by this pathogen because changes in radionuclide scans are more characteristic when patients have had an illness of longer duration.[237] In addition to this apparent lower sensitivity for disease caused by CA-MRSA, the reported sensitivity of bone scans in neonates has varied from as little as 31% to as high as 90%.[2,11,70,80,94,148,184,276] False-negative bone scans in newborns conceivably result from limited spatial resolution, the paucity of mineralization in neonates' bones, or ischemia of bone.[184]

Older infants with osteomyelitis and a nondiagnostic ^{99m}Tc bone scan also have been described.[25,121] In such instances, scans employing gallium 67 (^{67}Ga) scan may be valuable. Gallium 67 is a transition metal that, similar to iron, is bound to plasma proteins; the unbound portion (10% to 25%) is excreted in urine. It localizes in inflammatory foci because of increased capillary permeability (leaking plasma proteins), in vivo leukocyte labeling, binding to lactoferrin in the lesion, and perhaps direct bacterial uptake. Because of slower elimination of gallium from blood, its uptake in an inflammatory focus depends less on blood flow. Delayed elimination often results in poor contrast of bone to soft tissue, however, and delays making a reliable interpretation for 24 to 72 hours after injection.[128] Combined evaluation with ^{67}Ga imaging and ^{99m}Tc bone scanning may lead to greater diagnostic certainty when the studies are not conclusively diagnostic.[241,283] Despite these successes, ^{67}Ga scans are seldom employed because repeating MRI or plain radiographs and clinical improvement during therapy usually are sufficient to resolve initial diagnostic uncertainties.

Numerous studies have been conducted to examine the utility of indium 111–labeled leukocyte scans for the diagnosis of osteomyelitis. This method involves removing leukocytes and injecting them back into the patient after in vitro labeling. It has a reported sensitivity of 86%[231] and appears to be most useful for the detection of lesions in long bones. False-positive scans can result from a variety of processes, including fracture and infarction. Enthusiasm for this modality also is limited by the higher organ absorption of the radiation dose.[96] Numerous other scintigraphic methods for the detection of osteomyelitis, including

^{99m}Tc hexamethylpropyleneamine oxime–labeled leukocytes and labeled monoclonal antibodies, have been examined. At present, these alternative methods do not offer any advantage over MRI and older radionuclide imaging approaches.

Computed tomography. CT is used occasionally in the diagnosis and management of osteomyelitis because it provides excellent definition of cortical bone and high spatial resolution. CT abnormalities commonly found in osteomyelitis include increased density of bone marrow caused by the accumulation of purulent material and periosteal new bone formation and purulence. CT is particularly useful in detecting sequestra and delineating subperiosteal abscesses. It previously has been used to define infections of the spine, but MRI has largely replaced CT for this indication.[24,88]

Treatment of Acute Hematogenous Osteomyelitis

Surgical Intervention

The need for surgical therapy must be considered immediately when osteomyelitis is diagnosed. Reports of soft tissue, subperiosteal, and intramedullary abscesses have become common in the early 21st century, mirroring the increased prevalence of skin, soft tissue, and musculoskeletal infections caused by CA-MRSA.[10,141,173] MRI, ultrasound, and CT imaging may prove useful in assessing these purulent foci.[38,139] Drainage of these sites by surgical or interventional radiology techniques also provides the opportunity to obtain cultures to confirm a microbiologic diagnosis, thus facilitating selection of the most readily tolerated antimicrobial agent. Sequestra should be removed if present. If contiguous infectious foci are present, they should be debrided adequately and treated with effective antimicrobial therapy. Immobilization of the affected extremity or splinting may afford relief from pain and sometimes is used to prevent the development of pathologic fractures when extensive bone involvement is detected by plain radiography.

Antimicrobial Therapy

The initial therapy should have potent activity against *S. aureus* and group A streptococci because these pathogens represent the primary causes of osteomyelitis. Acute bacterial hematogenous osteomyelitis should be treated initially with parenteral antiinfective agents in view of the high mortality rate in *S. aureus* osteomyelitis seen in the preantibiotic era and more recent reports of fulminant disease with CA-MRSA.[110,111,116,130,173]

The choice of initial therapy has become more complex due to the marked increase in prevalence of CA-MRSA in the United States and other countries since 2000. In areas where most (≥90%) *S. aureus* isolates remain methicillin-susceptible, initial therapy may consist of a penicillinase-resistant, semisynthetic penicillin, such as nafcillin or oxacillin, administered parenterally in a dosage of 150 to 200 mg/kg per day in four divided doses.[117,141–143,206,260] Cefazolin, a first-generation cephalosporin, and cefuroxime, a second-generation cephalosporin, have also been used for empiric therapy with good results and may be preferred in infants and young children under 36 months of age if *Kingella kingae* is strongly suspected based on clinical features.[193,284] In areas where CA-MRSA is common, either vancomycin or clindamycin (if >90% of CA-MRSA isolates are clindamycin susceptible) should be included in the initial empiric therapy for CA-MRSA.[141,174] Currently most isolates of CA-MRSA remain susceptible to clindamycin, but clinical laboratories should screen for inducible macrolide-lincosamide-streptogramin resistance using the D-test or similar methodology.[10,141,160] In children who are severely ill at presentation, some specialists advise initiating therapy with both vancomycin and oxacillin or cefazolin, in view of the superior activity of these antistaphylococcal β-lactam antibiotics compared to vancomycin for MSSA.[142]

Although protein conjugate vaccines have largely eliminated *H. influenzae* type B invasive infections in the United States, antimicrobial coverage for this possibility should be considered for younger children who have not yet completed their immunization series. In these circumstances, addition of a third-generation cephalosporin (ceftriaxone or cefotaxime) to the empiric antistaphylococcal agent (vancomycin, clindamycin, oxacillin, or nafcillin) or the use of a fourth-generation cephalosporin such as cefepime might be warranted. Other agents may be administered when epidemiologic factors suggest the possible presence of other pathogens: third- or fourth-generation cephalosporins for *P. aeruginosa*, *Salmonella* species, or other enteric gram-negative organisms, and clindamycin for suspected anaerobic infections.[85,221]

When an organism is isolated or identified by other means, antimicrobial therapy can be chosen with greater specificity. Staphylococci should be treated with penicillin G if the organisms are susceptible to this antibiotic. In most cases, staphylococci must be treated with a penicillinase-resistant penicillin (oxacillin or nafcillin), clindamycin, or vancomycin. Ceftriaxone also has proved successful in the treatment of most cases of bone infections caused by MSSA. Oxazolidinone (linezolid) and streptogramin (quinupristin-dalfopristin) drugs have been used successfully for the treatment of osteomyelitis with MRSA and MSSA and for the treatment of vancomycin-resistant enterococci, but this experience is limited.[53,75]

Trimethoprim-sulfamethoxazole (cotrimoxazole) and the lipophilic tetracyclines (minocycline and doxycycline) are readily absorbed by the oral route and have been used successfully in the treatment of osteomyelitis in children and adults. One study reported consistent success in 20 children treated with cotrimoxazole, including several children with CA-MRSA infections.[180] However, experience remains limited with cotrimoxazole or tetracycline therapy for osteomyelitis, especially for treatment of CA-MRSA infections in which pneumonia and bacteremia are common, and the potential for dental staining with tetracyclines must be kept in mind. Daptomycin, a bactericidal lipopeptide antimicrobial agent, has excellent activity against CA-MRSA, but pediatric pharmacokinetic data and clinical experience are limited.[251] Moreover daptomycin has poor activity in lung tissue, adding to concerns about the utility of daptomycin for the treatment of CA-MRSA osteomyelitis.[110,111,141]

Osteomyelitis caused by *S. pneumoniae* strains with decreased susceptibility to penicillin have been managed successfully with a variety of agents, including ceftriaxone, vancomycin, and clindamycin.[35] β-lactam antibiotics, including oxacillin, nafcillin, and cephalosporins, have been used successfully in the treatment of *K. kingae* infection, although cefazolin may be preferable to antistaphylococcal penicillins because the latter have relatively lower activity.[112,286,285]

Decades of experience and clinical investigation have led to wide acceptance of sequential use of the intravenous and oral routes of administration of antibiotics to treat pediatric osteomyelitis, which previously was controversial.[154,194,207,289] Completing treatment with oral therapy avoids the cost, pain, inconvenience, and well-known complications of long-term administration of intravenous antibiotics. The relative safety of central venous catheters has not obviated these concerns. To the contrary, local skin infections, bacteremia, and malfunctions seem to be common occurrences when centrally placed catheters are used for osteomyelitis treatment, especially for young children.[169,228,289]

Oral therapy is most likely to succeed, and oral therapy is an acceptable option when the following criteria are met: an organism has been identified, the patient has the ability to swallow and retain an appropriate medication, and the patient has a clear clinical response to intravenously administered antibiotics.[193,195] In most series in which oral therapy has been evaluated,[41,73,193,260,273] treatment was continued with intravenous antibiotics until the patient was afebrile, until local signs and symptoms of infection were reduced considerably, and until the patient was maintaining caloric and fluid balances by the oral route. Several studies have supported that success with oral therapy is highly likely when these clinical targets are achieved, the peripheral leukocyte count has normalized (if initially abnormal), and there has been a marked decrease in the serum concentration of CRP.[9,169,222,267] A review of case series employing sequential therapy affirmed these recommendations and found no evidence that a fixed period of intravenous therapy is beneficial or essential: a transition to oral therapy within 7 days of diagnosis seemed to be equal in outcome to therapy with a fixed initial period of parenteral therapy.[154]

When oral therapy is begun, most antibiotics administered orally for osteomyelitis must be given in doses higher than those used for the treatment of other infections.[194,259,260] Specific antibiotics and the recommended starting doses are listed in Table 55.3. Dosages of β-lactam antibiotics often can be increased to 150 to 200 mg/kg per day without having serious adverse side effects.[252,260] Diarrhea, an infrequent

TABLE 55.3 Initial Antibiotic Doses for Oral Treatment of Osteomyelitis

Drug	Dose
Amoxicillin	100 mg/kg/day divided into 4 doses
Cephalexin	150 mg/kg/day divided into 4 doses
Chloramphenicol	75 mg/kg/day divided into 3 doses
Clindamycin	40 mg/kg/day divided into 4 doses
Dicloxacillin	100 mg/kg/day divided into 4 doses
Linezolid	Age <12 y: 30 mg/kg per day divided into 3 doses; maximum dose 1.8 g/day Age ≥12 y: 600 mg twice per day
Penicillin V	100 mg/kg/day divided into 4 doses
Trimethoprim-sulfamethoxazole	16 mg/kg/day (for trimethoprim component)

complication of high-dose oral β-lactam therapy, can be mitigated by a reduction in dose and the administration of probenecid (40 mg/kg per day every 6 hours; maximal dose 2 g/day).[41,193,260] Clindamycin readily achieves high bone levels and does not require higher dose therapy when given orally.[143,174]

The assumption implicit in successful oral therapy is that the antibiotic reaches an effective concentration at the focus of infection. Compliance with the prescribed dose and frequency and absorption into the bloodstream are necessary to fulfill this assumption. Patient (or parent) education and a continuing time commitment by a physician or nurse are essential to maintaining the compliance required for successful treatment. Although not commonly employed, therapeutic drug monitoring (TDM) may be useful to show that adequate absorption of orally administered antibiotics is occurring.[171,194,207] This recommendation stems from the observation that rare patients have inadequate serum levels despite receiving high oral dosages. TDM also can be used to document adherence to the therapeutic regimen.[260] TDM was initially performed by measuring serum bactericidal activity, with a peak serum bactericidal titer of 1:8 or greater sought.[214,260] However, this assay is confounded by other antibiotics present in the serum sample (e.g., nafcillin administered intravenously would interfere with evaluating the oral bioavailability of oral dicloxacillin). Chemical assays that detect the specific antimicrobial agent circumvent this problem. For example, dicloxacillin can be administered orally and the dose adjusted based on dicloxacillin measurements before the intravenous administration of another β-lactam has been discontinued. This procedure avoids several days of inadequate therapy should the dosage of the oral agent need to be adjusted.

In most cases of uncomplicated disease, clinical improvement is evident within 3 to 7 days of the initiation of appropriate therapy. To help show that effective therapy is under way, it is helpful to monitor acute-phase reactants. Although CRP and ESR typically increase during the first 2 days of therapy, CRP then begins to decrease rapidly (with an approximate half-life of 1 to 2 days) and typically returns to normal in 7 to 10 days.[9,202,222] CRP returns to normal levels in blood more rapidly in children with an uneventful clinical course than in children who ultimately require repeated surgical drainage.[222] A slow decline in serum CRP to normal levels has been associated with more extensive radiographic changes or persistent symptoms 1 to 2 months after discharge from the hospital. Higher peak CRP levels may also indicate the presence of concomitant septic arthritis and adjacent osteomyelitis.[9,47,185,202] Similar to CRP, ESR generally increases during the first several days but declines in the weeks that follow.[203,267] Failure of ESR to decrease during the second week of treatment may indicate a need for surgical drainage or the development of chronic osteomyelitis.[252]

Prolonged antibiotic therapy is essential for successful treatment of acute osteomyelitis. In one early report of 45 cases of osteomyelitis, four treatment failures occurred; all had been treated for 10 days or less.[123] Likewise Dich and colleagues[73] noted a 19% failure rate in 37 patients treated for 3 weeks or less; the rate was 2% in 48 patients treated for 21 to 50 days. Blockey and Watson[31] provided similar data. Thus, 3 weeks or more appears to be the minimal duration of therapy for hematogenous osteomyelitis to achieve a low rate of recurrence. A shorter period of therapy was sufficient for most patients in one widely cited study conducted in Finland,[206] but no cases of MRSA were identified in this series of 252 patients. In contrast to this, CA-MRSA infections are common in the United States and many other countries. A conservative but individualized approach is to administer antibiotics until ESR and CRP are both within the normal range, which usually requires 4 to 6 weeks of treatment.[141,193-195,252]

Special Manifestations of Hematogenous Osteomyelitis

Brodie Abscess

Osteomyelitis occasionally is indolent in presentation. Perhaps the best-defined example is subacute osteomyelitis with the development of a localized and well-contained intraosseous abscess (Brodie abscess).[246] These lesions are most often identified in adolescents with complaints of long bone pain and tenderness and generally occur in the tibia or femur. Fever is generally absent, and the ESR usually is normal at the time of presentation. A bony defect with sclerotic margins is detected by plain radiography in most patients. A distinctive "target" lesion has been described in MRI studies of Brodie abscesses.[172] Concentric layers are seen and reflect a central abscess cavity surrounded by an inner ring of granulation tissue, an outer ring of fibrotic reaction, and a peripheral rim of endosteal reaction that is hypointense on T1-weighted images.

S. aureus and other gram-positive cocci (including β-hemolytic streptococci and *Propionibaceterium acnes*) are generally the pathogens identified, but a variety of gram-negative organisms, including *H. influenza, Pseudomonas aeruginosa, Salmonella typhi, Klebsiella* species, and *Kingella kingae* have also been isolated from these lesions.[19,152,199,229] Treatment consists of surgical drainage and curettage of the lesions followed by antimicrobial therapy, as for other forms of hematogenous osteomyelitis. Bone grafting may be needed for larger lesions.[200] The prognosis generally is good, although deformities occur in some cases.

Osteomyelitis in Patients After Closed Fractures

Acute hematogenous osteomyelitis sometimes occurs in closed fractures of tubular bones.[45,275] A clue to diagnosis is the resumption of pain after the initial postfracture pain has subsided, usually 1 to 6 weeks after the injury occurs. The pain differs from that associated with the fracture by being progressive and not being relieved by immobilization. Patients are febrile and may be thought to have another focus of infection before osteomyelitis is discovered. When the cast is removed, local erythema, fluctuance, and warmth are apparent and out of proportion to the normal healing of fracture. Although usually caused by *S. aureus*, anaerobic superinfection of staphylococcal osteomyelitis at the fracture site has been described.[257] Successful therapy requires adequate debridement, administration of appropriate antibiotics, and external fixation in some cases.

Epiphyseal and Apophyseal Osteomyelitis

Rarely, hematogenous osteomyelitis may arise in the epiphyses or, more rarely, apophyses (e.g., the greater trochanter of the femur) of the tubular bones of young children.[1,49,102,165,264] Although the pathogenesis is unclear, it may involve delivery of microorganisms to the epiphyses by transphyseal vessels in some children. After the child reaches 15 to 18 months of age, these vessels are atrophic. In older children, primary epiphyseal infections have been hypothesized to result from delivery of bacteria via venous sinusoids or by terminal branches of the epiphyseal arteries.

Hematogenous epiphyseal osteomyelitis may be acute or subacute. At the time of presentation, septic arthritis initially may be diagnosed when swelling of the related joint occurs and elevated synovial leukocytes are identified by diagnostic aspiration.

In cases with a more indolent course, pain, limp, or other symptoms prompt an evaluation for the possibility of an osteoarticular infection. In these cases, white blood cell counts are usually normal, and ESR and CRP are abnormal in about 50% of children. The correct diagnosis is usually established when a radionuclide bone scan shows evidence of increased bone turnover or plain radiographs taken weeks later reveal lytic changes characteristic of osteomyelitis.

S. aureus is the pathogen most often found; one recent series noted that *Kingella kingae* is frequently found in young children through the use of polymerase chain reaction (PCR) and more sensitive culture techniques.[49] Administration of appropriate therapy, as for other cases of acute osteomyelitis, has been followed by complete recovery without apparent sequelae 2 to 6 years after diagnosis.

Involvement of Nontubular Bones

Less than 20% of all cases of osteomyelitis involve nontubular bones. Infection of the calcaneus is the most common.[157,193,204] Osteomyelitis in the other cuboidal bones rarely occurs (Table 55.2). In patients with hematogenous infection of the calcaneus, most present after 7 days of symptoms.[157,204] Destruction occurs just under the epiphyseal line in the metaphysis posteriorly and medially, where the blood supply is greatest. It is present in all patients, in addition to destruction of the adjacent epiphysis, particularly in its middle to superior portion. Periosteal new bone formation occurs very late, with 3 to 4 months required for reossification. Osteomyelitis of the calcaneus is treated in much the same fashion as infections involving tubular bones, although complications have been frequently described, and recurrences may be more common than in osteomyelitis of other bones of children (5% in one series).[157,204,215]

Almost equal in frequency to infection of the calcaneus is infection of the bones of the pelvis.[193] Of the bones of the pelvis, the ischium is involved most commonly. The next most frequently involved bone is the ilium, followed by the sacroiliac joint. The pubis is involved in only 20% of cases of pelvic osteomyelitis.[125,190] Pelvic osteomyelitis causes an increase in the ESR in nearly all patients, and two-thirds have a peripheral leukocyte count greater than 10,000 cells/mm^3.[190] The most common organism causing pelvic osteomyelitis is *S. aureus,* which is isolated from either blood or an aspirate from the bone lesions in approximately 80% of cases.

Establishing the diagnosis of pelvic osteomyelitis is often difficult. Most patients are judged to have disease in the hip at the time that medical attention is sought. Most often, patients with pelvic osteomyelitis have hip pain and a gait abnormality but allow their hips to be put through a passive range of motion. Point tenderness at the site of the lesion can be elicited in approximately 50% of these patients. Sacroiliitis frequently is difficult to identify by clinical examination. Pressing down on the pelvis, which stresses the sacroiliac joint, produces local pain. Tenderness in the buttocks or the sciatic notch, if present, is an important diagnostic finding.[3,56,77,186,277] Pelvic osteomyelitis can mimic appendicitis and urinary tract infection.[277] It occurs more frequently in individuals with inflammatory bowel disease. In most patients, plain films of the pelvis are normal, whereas MRI is highly sensitive in identifying evidence of infection. Gadolinium enhancement improves the recognition of sacroiliac joint involvement.[139,266] Technetium 99m bone scans are also useful and indicate the diagnosis in approximately 90% of cases.[167,190] Antibiotic therapy alone is adequate in most cases of pelvic osteomyelitis. Surgery is indicated only when a lack of response to antimicrobial therapy occurs. Osteomyelitis in the pelvic bones has a uniformly good prognosis; chronic infection and sequelae are rare events.

Hematogenous osteomyelitis of flat bones occurs rarely and has been described in the skull, ribs, sternum, and scapula.[107,187,193,268]

Spinal Osteomyelitis

Spinal osteomyelitis can involve either the intervertebral disk or the vertebral bodies. Conceptualizing these infections as different entities is worthwhile because of the different pathophysiology and prognosis.[88]

Diskitis

The intervertebral disk consists of three components: the paired cartilaginous articular endplates, the fibrous ring (annulus fibrosus), and the nucleus pulposus.[60,88] The axial vessels that parallel the fetal notochord atrophy by birth, with the avascular, mucilaginous nucleus pulposus remaining. The disk has two arterial supplies: periosteal vessels and vessels descending from the central portion of the vertebral body.[60,86] The vessel from the central portion of the adjacent vertebra begins to atrophy in the first year and is obliterated completely by the time the child is 10 years old. This condition leaves only the capillary network in the annulus fibrosus, which is derived from the terminal radial ramifications of the periosteal vessels. If loss of this vascular supply is precipitous, idiopathic disk necrosis ensues, usually manifested as asymptomatic calcification.[232,249,255] If bacteremia occurs during loss of the blood supply, however, infection of an intervertebral disk may occur.

Most children with diskitis are younger than 3 years of age[88,239] and have had symptoms for several weeks.[88,233] Most cases of diskitis involve the thoracolumbar region, and the disease comes to medical attention with the patient's refusal to walk. Back pain and a progressive limp may also be present. Nonambulatory infants often become irritable and refuse to sit or crawl. On examination, the most striking feature is percussion tenderness over the contiguous spine; hip pain and stiffness with loss of lordosis of the lower part of the back are observed. Occasionally compression of the spine produces pain at the infected disk. Lesions higher in the spine (T8 to L1) can mimic gastrointestinal disease with abdominal pain, ileus, and vomiting, but the most important entities in the differential diagnosis are vertebral osteomyelitis and spinal or paraspinal tumors. Cervical diskitis has also been reported in children as well; limited neck movement or cervical pain appear to be characteristic.[233]

Fever generally is absent or low grade. Peripheral leukocytosis is present in one-third of patients, and virtually all have an increased ESR. A few patients undergoing biopsy have cultures that grow microorganisms. Most commonly, *S. aureus* is recovered, but *K. kingae* is being increasingly recognized as a cause of diskitis in children.[286] Rarely, pneumococci and gram-negative bacilli are also identified in cultures of blood or invasive sampling. Initial evaluation for suspected diskitis usually involves careful elicitation of the history and physical examination, a complete blood count, determination of the ESR and serum CRP concentrations, a blood culture, and plain lateral radiographs of the lumbosacral spine.[88]

Typical plain radiographic findings are shown in Fig. 55.5. The first finding is narrowing of the disk space, usually not detectable until 2 to 4 weeks after the onset of symptoms. Frequently this narrowing is overlooked if loss of the normal progressive (from cephalad to caudad) increase in disk width is not appreciated. It is followed by destruction of the adjacent cartilaginous vertebral endplates and may subsequently be followed by herniation of the disk into the vertebral body. Rarely compression or wedging of the vertebral body is noted. In all individuals, reactive bone proliferation is a rare finding, as are paravertebral soft tissue masses.

Because of overlap of this syndrome with noninfectious disk necrosis, investigators in the earlier literature advocated treating this disease solely by bed rest. In view of the low yield and generally favorable prognosis of diskitis, biopsy or aspiration for culture generally is unnecessary. Although controversial, oral antistaphylococcal therapy often is administered for a prolonged period (10 days to 4 weeks).[88] Other physicians have suggested giving 5 to 7 days of intravenous antistaphylococcal therapy, followed by 7 to 14 days of a similar oral agent.[63] This approach is reasonable, complicated in the current era by the increase in rates of infection caused by CA-MRSA, as discussed earlier. Very young children generally do well, and the disk space is preserved; spontaneous spinal fusion occurs commonly in older individuals.[145]

Vertebral Osteomyelitis

Vertebral osteomyelitis is rare in children, with an estimated incidence of 0.3/100,000 among those under 20 years of age.[113] Children with vertebral osteomyelitis usually are older than 8 years of age and seek medical attention because of constant back pain. They may appear toxic and have a low-grade fever (>39°C) after an indolent course (2 weeks to several months).[88] Percussion of the spinal dorsal process frequently elicits exquisite tenderness. Usually the paraspinous muscles around the involved vertebrae are in spasm, with rigidity of the area. Radiographic examination of a patient with vertebral osteomyelitis shows the earliest change to be localized rarefaction of one vertebral endplate, followed by involvement of adjacent vertebrae. Marked destruction of the bone, usually anteriorly, is followed by

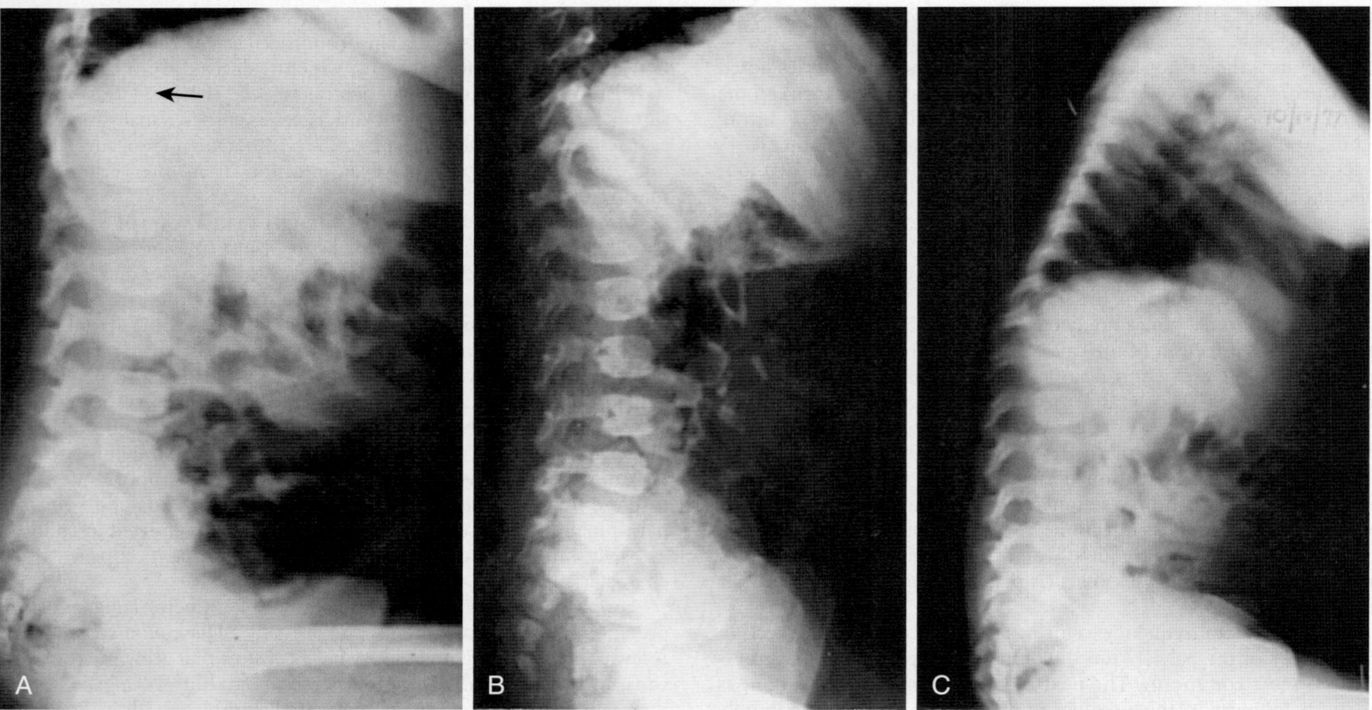

FIG. 55.5 Diskitis. (A) Lateral lumbar sacral spine of a 13-month-old child who had low-grade fever and refused to walk. The *arrow* indicates the narrow disk space. (B) Follow-up examination 2 weeks later shows almost complete collapse of the intervertebral body. (C) Two months later, destruction of the contiguous vertebra with marked kyphosis was apparent. (Courtesy Dr. Joel Blumhagen.)

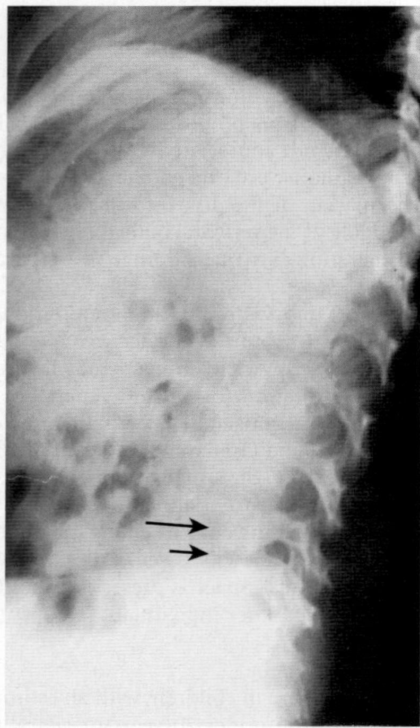

FIG. 55.6 Vertebral osteomyelitis. The *long arrow* indicates the lytic lesion with some anterior sclerosis in the lumbar vertebra. The *short arrow* indicates involvement of the adjacent lower vertebra and narrowing of the disk space. (Courtesy Dr. Joel Blumhagen.)

abundant anterior osteophytic reactions with bridging and bone sclerosis (Fig. 55.6).

In both children and adults, vertebral osteomyelitis is usually hematogenous in origin. The pathophysiology of acute hematogenous vertebral osteomyelitis reflects the unique circulation of the spine. The intervertebral disk loses its vascular supply with age, a process usually completed by 30 years of age. As a result, bacteremic pyogenic infections of the spine occur most often in the vertebral bodies. The venous drainage of the vertebral bodies is composed of three different freely communicating but valveless systems. Intraosseous vertebral veins drain the center of each body and form a large channel that exits through the nutrient foramen. They anastomose with the anterior and posterior internal plexus (between the dura mater and the vertebral body). The internal venous plexus has anastomotic connections with the external venous plexus through the vertebral ligaments. The external venous plexus communicates freely with the segmental veins on the ventral surface of the body (Batson plexus).[192]

Reversal of blood flow or thrombosis in the sluggishly flowing vertebral veins is thought to be the first event in the development of vertebral osteomyelitis. Because of the vascular communication, osteomyelitis usually involves two adjacent vertebral bodies, with the interposed disk initially skipped. The same process of septic thrombophlebitis involving the internal venous plexus can produce an epidural abscess (with cord compression) and infarction of the vertebral body. Spread along the external venous plexus can lead to a paraspinous mass. In the thoracic area, it may produce mediastinitis,[68] and in the cervical area, a retropharyngeal abscess can occur. The lumbar area is involved much more frequently than is the thoracic area, which is involved more frequently than is the cervical region.[6,137,248]

MRI is the preferred imaging approach in establishing the diagnosis of vertebral osteomyelitis[183] because the vertebral disk and the vertebral body are clearly distinguishable. Most cases of vertebral osteomyelitis begin at the margin between the disk and the anterior part of the vertebral body. In some cases, MRI has detected evidence of osteomyelitis when radionuclide imaging studies were normal.[261] Distinguishing pyogenic osteomyelitis from tuberculous lesions radiologically is impossible, but the latter usually are characterized by less bone destruction, less bone proliferation, and less sclerosis. Osteophytic bridging between adjacent vertebrae is rare in spinal tuberculosis.

Technetium 99m and gallium 67 are taken up by the lesion in vertebral osteomyelitis. A possible advantage of scanning with both isotopes is identification of paraspinous abscess with ^{67}Ga,[230] but MRI has largely supplanted these studies.

Most cases of vertebral osteomyelitis are caused by *S. aureus.* Tuberculosis and brucellosis must always be considered in the differential diagnosis[162] of vertebral osteomyelitis, though these infections are increasingly rare in developed nations.[24,113,140] Organisms causing urinary tract infection can cause osteomyelitis, presumably by local spread through the Batson plexus.[39,124,158] Urinary tract infection rarely precedes the development of vertebral osteomyelitis, however, and only approximately 2% of all cases can be shown to be related to infection of the urinary tract.[101] *P. aeruginosa* is sometimes found to cause vertebral osteomyelitis in injectable drug users, and the organisms presumably were inoculated along with the illicit drug. Young heroin addicts have been found to have *P. aeruginosa* infection in their intervertebral disks.[40,236] *Bartonella henselae* also has been found to cause vertebral osteomyelitis.[88] Fungal pathogens causing vertebral osteomyelitis include *Candida* spp. (often in immunocompromised patients) and *Coccidioides* species (in those with history of travel to in endemic areas).[26,126,181] Unless blood cultures have revealed the presence of bacteremia or serologic studies, or other noninvasive methods have implicated a pathogen, the best method of establishing the diagnosis is through examination of bone biopsy specimens and cultures.[191]

Therapy for vertebral osteomyelitis generally includes surgical debridement and stabilization, immobilization, and antimicrobial therapy. The need for surgical drainage should not be overlooked because spinal cord compression caused by an epidural or subdural abscess can lead to permanent paraplegia. A paraspinal focus of infection may rupture into the abdominal cavity or erode the aorta; both events are catastrophic complications.[95] Whether immobilization should be accomplished by simple bed rest or with a body cast is unclear, but bed rest may provide pain relief. The average duration of treatment of bacterial vertebral osteomyelitis is 2 months; however, no data are available that can be used for determining the most appropriate duration of therapy.[24,88] The optimal therapy for fungal or mycobacterial infection vertebral osteomyelitis is similarly unclear, but prolonged therapy is recommended.[99,140]

Hematogenous Osteomyelitis in Special Populations

Osteomyelitis in Newborns

Infection of the bones of newborns has distinct physiologic and clinical features that warrant emphasis.[12,70,283] Although it is rare, neonatal osteomyelitis may occur in newborns with certain risk factors, such as prematurity, prior bacterial sepsis, skin infections, and complications of delivery.[94,148,201] In newborns, polyostotic infection occurs at a higher rate compared to older children, and osteomyelitis in the long tubular bones frequently (50–70% of cases) is accompanied by contiguous septic arthritis (12–47% in several case series).[94,148,276] As indicated earlier, the epiphyseal-metaphyseal junction frequently is within the joint capsule, facilitating involvement of adjacent joints, particularly in the hip, shoulder, and knee of the newborn.

Two distinct presentations are recognized[148]: some infants are only mildly symptomatic and afebrile while others present with a septic or toxic appearance. Those with who are recognized with signs of sepsis will frequently have more complicated disease, including polyostotic disease or septic arthritis. Antecedent infections are present in half of the cases and usually are nosocomial; infections of heel puncture sites, arterial cannulas, lungs, and cut-down sites have been described.[12] Osteomyelitis often is identified when a search is instituted for the source or focus of bacteremia.[283] As noted earlier, plain radiographs often reveal evidence of osteomyelitis at the time of diagnosis (soft tissue swelling, lytic lesions, and periosteal new bone formation), whereas bone scanning may be negative. Bone scanning may be useful, however, in excluding the diagnosis of osteomyelitis; in one study, the negative predictive value was estimated at 82%.[283]

Although staphylococci, including MRSA,[150] are the most common cause of osteomyelitis in infants, group B streptococci and other gram-positive organism have been found consistently.[80] Infants with group B streptococcal osteomyelitis generally are older (2 to 4 weeks old), have no recognized preceding infection, and have only a single bone involved, often the tibia or humerus.[12] *E. coli* and other gram-negative bacteria have been reported in various case series, indicating the need for initial antibiotic coverage for common coliforms.[94,263,276]

Osteomyelitis in the skull, an uncommon disease in older children, can occur in neonates. Frequently it is associated with a cephalhematoma, with or without loss of skin integrity,[155,196] but it can be caused by fetal monitoring without a cephalhematoma.[177] Numerous bacteria have been isolated from such lesions; as one might expect, most of these bacteria are members of the vaginal microbiome, including *Gardnerella vaginalis.*[196] Radiographic changes (i.e., bony erosion) are a late finding, and CT of the skull may assist in establishing the diagnosis. Infection of a cephalhematoma should be considered if it is enlarging, if it is inflamed, or if laboratory evidence of infection is present, such as an increased CRP concentration or leukocyte count. In most cases, the lesion is drained and treated with an antibiotic appropriate for the infecting organism.

In older descriptions of neonatal osteomyelitis, sequelae were common findings. In more recent series,[148,280] approximately three-fourths of all cases have had good outcomes, even when the hip has been involved. When seen, sequelae include avascular necrosis of the femoral head, bony deformities, and shortening of the involved limb.[210]

Osteomyelitis in Children With Hemoglobinopathies

After pneumonia, osteomyelitis is the most common serious infection in children with sickle-cell disease.[16] Children at risk are children with hemoglobin SS, hemoglobin S-Thal, or hemoglobin SO-Arab and certain children with hemoglobin SC disease.[119,242] The clinical manifestations of osteomyelitis are similar to those of other children with osteomyelitis, but there is a propensity for simultaneous involvement of multiple sites, a tendency toward recurrence, and a greater frequency in children 18 to 48 months of age.

As noted earlier, the microbiology of osteomyelitis in children with sickle-cell disease is complex and dominated by *Salmonella* spp. and *S. aureus.*[16,43,81] Although *Salmonella* osteomyelitis occurs in less than 1% of normal patients with *Salmonella* bacteremia,[278] the frequency of *Salmonella* osteomyelitis in sickle-cell disease is several hundred times that occurring in the general population, with an incidence estimated at 0.36% per year.[16,74,212] While children with hemoglobinopathy with microbiological evidence of osteomyelitis have *Salmonella* spp. or *S. aureus*, many aerobic gram-negative organisms, including *Shigella sonnei,*[227] *E. coli,*[118] *Serratia* spp.,[93] and *Arizona hinshawii,*[131] have been implicated.

Many factors probably contribute to the greater incidence of osteomyelitis in patients with sickle-cell hemoglobinopathy. Injuries to the intestinal mucosa from local thrombosis during a thrombotic crisis may facilitate the entrance of *Salmonella* and other enteric organisms into the bloodstream.[43,278] When infection of the bloodstream occurs, a prolonged period or greater magnitude of bacteremia may follow due to splenic dysfunction or other immunologic abnormalities in these patients. Evidence of impaired production of opsonic antibodies also exists. Whether bacteria lodge in infarcted bone or whether a different pathogenesis exists is unclear. Infarction occurs in the capital femoral epiphysis, hands, feet, and vertebrae, whereas osteomyelitis involves the metaphyseal-diaphyseal junction of long tubular bones.[81,212]

The hand and foot syndrome seen in infants with sickle-cell disease is not easily distinguished from osteomyelitis of the phalanges of the hands or tarsal bones of the feet.[37,59,274] The radiographic changes caused by osteomyelitis are, however, usually more severe than the changes expected in uncomplicated sickle-cell disease. The most common radiographic findings are a longitudinal intracortical diaphyseal fissure and overabundant periosteal new bone formation. The cortical fissures are thought to represent a layer of purulent exudate in and between the periosteal new bone and dead bone.[74]

Acute infarction and osteomyelitis cannot always be differentiated by MRI, perhaps because of preexisting abnormalities in bone marrow. MRI may be useful, however, for presurgical evaluation. Radionuclide scans also are used frequently to help differentiate osteomyelitis from bone infarction. In theory, bone infarction should have decreased uptake of ^{99m}Tc in the early "blood pool" phase of the scan; increased uptake would be found only as the lesion healed.[146] In one series with 34 sites of infarction, increased ^{99m}Tc uptake occurred in 10, normal uptake occurred in 9, and decreased uptake surrounded by zones of increased concentration occurred in the remaining 15 sites.[105] Ultrasound imaging also has been used to distinguish osteomyelitis and sickle-cell crisis.[34]

Generally patients with bony infarcts have had dactylitis as an infant and multiple episodes; their temperature usually is less than 39°C. Children with hemoglobinopathy and osteomyelitis may lack this history and have a modest leukocytosis of immature granulocytes.[133] If fever, leukocytosis, and local symptoms persist despite provision of hydration and other supportive measures, needle aspiration of the area must be considered. Identification of an infectious pathogen is particularly important because of the large number of possible organisms involved.

Osteomyelitis in Patients With Human Immunodeficiency Virus Infection

Although recurrent invasive bacterial infections often complicate human immunodeficiency virus (HIV) infection in children and adults, osteomyelitis is not a common complication.[132,179,244] Many of the existing reports involve patients with recent intravenous drug use, which probably acted as a predisposing factor. *S. aureus* was recovered most commonly, although *E. coli, Salmonella enteritidis, Cryptococcus neoformans, Mycobacterium kansasii, Histoplasma capsulatum,* and other organisms also were seen in individual cases. One recent report, however, suggests that *S. pneumoniae* osteomyelitis may be more common than *S. aureus* infections among HIV-infected children[218] who have not received protein-conjugate pneumococcal vaccines.

Osteomyelitis in Patients With Chronic Granulomatous Disease

The phagocytes of patients with chronic granulomatous disease fail to kill intracellular organisms, and infections with catalase-positive bacteria or fungi are frequent complications. Although staphylococci are a common cause of cutaneous infection in chronic granulomatous disease, osteomyelitis is caused most often by *Serratia* and *Aspergillus* spp. Osteomyelitis is attributed less often to staphylococci, *Pseudomonas, Burkholderia, Nocardia,* and other bacterial and fungal species.[281]

NONHEMATOGENOUS OSTEOMYELITIS

Puncture Wound Osteomyelitis

Inoculation osteomyelitis most often involves either the patella or the bones of the foot. Soft tissue infections occur after puncture wounds of the foot approximately 15% of the time, and osteomyelitis occurs in 1.5% of these injuries.[90] Osteomyelitis of the foot that develops after children sustain puncture wounds may represent osteochondritis, representing infection of the articular cartilage in the metatarsals. Most patients are aged 9 to 18 years. After the initial pain of the puncture wound subsides (in 24 to 48 hours), the signs of osteochondritis appear after another 48 to 72 hours. Typically joint tenderness and localized swelling, erythema, and pain over the entrance of the puncture wound are present. Fever is an infrequent finding, and the patient seldom has any other constitutional symptoms. No peripheral leukocytosis is noted, and ESR is increased minimally.

Although the offending organism most commonly is *P. aeruginosa* (90% of the time), staphylococci, streptococci, *Stenotrophomonas maltophilia,*[14] and *Serratia marcescens*[189] also have been isolated.[36,90,134-136] In some cases (~20%), both *P. aeruginosa* and *S. aureus* are found.[135] The predominance of *Pseudomonas* can be explained partially on the basis of the mechanism of injury. *Pseudomonas* is not found commonly in surveys of the microbial flora of the skin of the feet,[109,182,254] but often it is found by culture of the spongy liner of children's sneakers.[89] In addition, many patients in whom *P. aeruginosa* osteochondritis develops have received prophylactic treatment with oral antibiotics that have activity against gram-positive bacteria. A semisynthetic penicillinase-resistant penicillin and an aminoglycoside or ceftazidime often are used as initial therapy.[134,135]

Surgical debridement of necrotic cartilage is a key element of treatment because foreign material frequently is found embedded in the soft tissue; debridement also provides the opportunity to identify organisms resistant to the initial antibiotic agents and accelerates recovery. The local signs and symptoms of infection usually resolve 4 to 5 days after adequate debridement is performed and the patient is able to bear weight on the foot. In contrast, antibiotic therapy alone after simple diagnostic aspiration may need to be continued 6 to 8 weeks before weight bearing is possible. Long-term follow-up of *P. aeruginosa* osteochondritis indicates that many patients have asymptomatic radiographic abnormalities.[18] Radiographic abnormalities are found more commonly in patients in whom a joint was involved initially.[18]

Osteomyelitis also has been described repeatedly after puncture wounds occur from stepping on wooden toothpicks. In these cases, *Eikenella corrodens,* a component of the oral microbiome, has been found with other organisms. Surgical debridement to remove toothpick fragments and drain local abscesses is essential.[219]

Osteomyelitis of the patella is frequently due to puncture wounds, although hematogenous osteomyelitis also occurs. The most common etiologic agent is *S. aureus*; signs of osteomyelitis appear 1 week after the puncture occurs. No constitutional symptoms occur, but extension of the leg produces pain over the anterior aspect of the patella. The differential diagnosis includes other cases of acute knee pain with limp and fever, including cellulitis, Lyme disease in endemic regions, prepatellar septic bursitis, reactive arthritis, cellulitis, rheumatologic conditions, and neoplasms. MRI or scintigraphy are both useful diagnostically, but the diagnosis is definitively established by isolating an organism from the patella. Treatment of this disease is similar to that for other forms of osteomyelitis.[225,226]

Osteomyelitis Caused by Spread of Infection From a Contiguous Focus

In children, osteomyelitis related to an infected contiguous focus is a rare finding. Almost all cases of osteomyelitis from a contiguous source in childhood are nosocomial or are associated with infected burn wounds. The probability of postoperative osteomyelitis developing is a function of the surgeon's experience, the technique, the length of time that the wound was open, and whether prophylactic antibiotics were administered. The interval between the precipitating event and pain and the appearance of persistent sinus drainage or ulceration is 2 to 4 weeks. The peripheral white blood cell count and ESR are often normal. More than half of cases are caused by multiple organisms. When small draining sinuses are present, correlation between sinus culture and bone biopsy findings is good. With large open areas, organisms obtained by culture of the wound may not be important etiologically, and obtaining a bone biopsy specimen is necessary for making a definitive bacteriologic diagnosis. Staphylococci and streptococci predominate, although gram-negative organisms from the hospital environment often are seen.[211,247]

Orthopedic Fixator Devices

Infection involving the wires or pins used for orthopedic stabilization represents a diagnostic and therapeutic challenge. Osteomyelitis is suspected when evidence of inflammation or infection is noted near these materials, but it seldom can be proved.[30] Plain radiographs are essential because they may reveal bone destruction or rarefaction at the site of entry of fixation pins. No controlled studies of treatment are available. Soft tissue debridement and removal of necrotic bone should be done as soon as possible. Fixation hardware should be removed if possible when extensive changes in bone are demonstrated, but fixation devices must sometimes be left in place.[15,209] Prolonged therapy usually is given, guided by the susceptibility pattern of any organisms recovered from local cultures.[209]

UNUSUAL MICROBIAL CAUSES OF OSTEOMYELITIS

Actinomyces

Cervicofacial, pulmonothoracic, and abdominopelvic forms of actinomycosis are recognized, and infections of bone may occur in all of these. More than half of all actinomycotic infections involve the facial or cervical area.[23] Poor dentition or recent dental procedures frequently precede cervicofacial disease, but some cases follow trauma or facial surgery.[17,23,156,219] The most common site of actinomycotic bone infection is the mandible, but the maxilla and, less commonly, the skull may be involved.[197,219] Local signs and symptoms of fever and discharge from a sinus often indicate the presence of the disease. Radiographically periosteal elevation is followed by lytic changes. Expansile lesions with radiographic areas of lucency and prominent bony sclerosis are characteristic, resembling "lumpy jaw" disease found in cattle and horses.[23,61] Often, "eggshell" areas of new bone are present in the mandible, representing layers of sclerosis.

Bony involvement of ribs, pelvis, and vertebral bodies is well known and is generally related to foci of infection in the gastrointestinal or pulmonary tracts or in the pelvis.[23,61,170] When disease involves vertebral bodies, patients may present with mild pain, tenderness, and some stiffness. It has been suggested that actinomycosis can be distinguished radiographically from tuberculosis by the diffuse honeycombing of the vertebral bodies, in which "suppurating channels" are bounded by bone of increased density; large lytic lesions usually are absent. Primary infections of the sternum and tibia have been described, suggesting that hematogenous infections of bone may occur.[156,219] Spinal infections can be complicated by extension to the spinal cord and brain, with devastating complications that include meningitis and vertebral collapse with spinal cord injury.

Bearing in mind that actinomycetes are usual members of the oral microbiome, a convincing diagnosis of actinomycotic osteomyelitis requires demonstration of these organisms in cultures of bone specimens; histopathologic demonstration of the organisms. *Actinomyces israelii* is most commonly identified, but other species have also been involved in osteomyelitis.[23,219] Extensive debridement is usually needed and has been linked to successful short-term treatment of mandibular actinomycosis.[17] Hemimandibulectomy may be needed in intractable cases.[220] Although no controlled trials of therapy have been done, long-term (2 to 12 months) antimicrobial therapy is generally advised.[23,219] Penicillin G and oral penicillin VK have been frequently used, as well as amoxicillin/clavulanate, clindamycin, and tetracyclines and other agents when penicillin resistance has been clinically suspected or microbiologically confirmed.[23,219]

Brucella

Although an uncommon cause of osteomyelitis in developed countries, *Brucella* spp. are well-known causes of skeletal infections, most often following the consumption of unpasteurized milk products.[5] *Brucella* spp. can produce abscesses in the vertebral bodies or long bones, although they are not striking features of the disease. The disease often is subacute in presentation, and anorexia, weight loss, sweating, adenopathy, and hepatosplenomegaly are common initial findings. Multidrug treatment with initial use of aminoglycosides for 2 to 3 weeks is generally successful. Longer (3 months or more) therapy may be needed for vertebral osteomyelitis.[24]

Fungi

Osteomyelitis may be caused by numerous endemic and opportunistic fungal agents, including various species of *Coccidioides*, *Cryptococcus*, *Candida*, *Blastomyces*, and *Aspergillus*.[149] *Sporothrix* infections occur but are particularly rare.[288]

Candida osteomyelitis may occur in people of all ages, including neonates.[99,205] *C. albicans* is identified in the majority of cases, but non-*albicans* species are encountered in approximately one-third of cases. Most patients have pain, tenderness, or edema at the time of presentation. Most cases represent hematogenous dissemination of infection, but direct inoculation and contiguous infection also occur. In children, infections of long bones (femur, humerus), ribs, and vertebrae are the most common foci. Polyostotic disease is common following hematogenous infection; careful clinical evaluation for other sites of infection should be undertaken when one focus is identified.[205] Surgical debridement of radiographically evident lesions should be undertaken. Prolonged medical therapy (6 to 12 months) brings about clinical remission in most patients, but relapses are common. Azole antifungal agents are preferred due to their tolerability over such periods, but other agents may be needed due to antimicrobial susceptibility testing and other factors.[99,205]

Coccidioidomycosis is an endemic mycosis localized to the southwestern United States (particularly California and Arizona), as well as in parts of Mexico and certain areas of Central and South America.[29,240] Skeletal coccidioidomycosis may follow a recognized earlier illness with cough, chest pain, night sweats, and anorexia, sometimes accompanied by erythema nodosum or erythema multiforme. However, most patients with skeletal coccidioidomycosis have had clinically inapparent initial infections with subsequent extrapulmonary dissemination. *Coccidioides* osteomyelitis occurs throughout the skeleton but is particularly common in vertebral bodies, the pelvis, the tibia and fibula, and the skull.[26,126,217] Approximately 40% of patients will have two or more foci of osteomyelitis at presentation. These lesions are not radiographically distinct from the lesions seen in osteomyelitis from bacterial pathogens.[238] Debridement of bone lesions often is needed initially, and months to years of therapy are required. Oral triazole agents generally are recommended.[29,97]

Blastomycosis may mimic coccidioidomycosis, but the pulmonary involvement is much more varied. A propensity for the development of verrucous, reddened, weeping skin lesions has been noted, and prostate involvement may be seen. Bone involvement occurs frequently, with the skull and vertebral bodies being infected most often. Distinguishing it from other forms of osteomyelitis is impossible by radiographic examination.

Aspergillus osteomyelitis is generally a disease of immunosuppressed patients,[48] with *Aspergillus* pneumonia seen initially followed by disseminated disease. Bone disease occurring by hematogenous spread has developed, however, in normal individuals and after injectable drug use.[62,223] *Aspergillus* osteomyelitis also has been reported following trauma.

Other fungi are infrequent causes of osteomyelitis. The medical literature contains many reports of osteomyelitis caused by *C. neoformans*, generally in immunocompromised patients and in the setting of disseminated or pulmonary infection. The few reports in pediatric patients generally have involved immunocompromised adolescents. In adolescents and adults, usually only one bone is involved. The lesions generally are slowly destructive and very discrete, occurring primarily in the long tubular bones without marginal sclerosis. This radiologic reaction is confused most commonly with tumor and occasionally with tuberculosis. Infection of the ribs and skull also has been reported. Although experience with this disease is limited, debridement of the lesions and medical therapy seem to be highly effective.[20,42,52,108,163,164] Cases of *Rhizopus* osteomyelitis have been reported intermittently and apparently are hematogenous in origin.[79]

CHRONIC OSTEOMYELITIS

Chronic osteomyelitis may develop after a surgical procedure, major trauma,[265] or unsuccessful treatment of acute osteomyelitis.[252] The diagnosis of chronic osteomyelitis usually is often straightforward; patients generally have a painful, nonfunctional extremity and may have chronically draining sinuses. Radiographs often reveal clear evidence of devitalized bone and the formation of sequestra or involucra. Surgical biopsy and debridement are generally needed; histopathologic demonstration of chronic inflammation and devitalized bone are diagnostic. Cultures of the purulent exudate or necrotic bone usually reveal *S. aureus*, although gram-negative bacteria, including *H. influenzae*,[144] may be found in some cases. Gram stains, acid-fast stains, or stains for fungi may provide the only microbiological confirmation of the organism involved. Plain radiographs, CT, and MRI all play roles in medical and surgical management by revealing details of the bony and soft tissue involvement, including the formation of abscesses and sequestra (Fig. 55.7).[57]

Treatment of chronic osteomyelitis involves the removal of devitalized bone, debridement and drainage of soft tissue disease, achieving wound closure and enhanced perfusion, stabilization of structural deficiencies, and long-term administration of appropriate antibiotics.[57] Treatment is highly individualized and based on the morbid anatomy. No controlled trials comparing different modes of therapy have been performed.

Antimicrobial regimens for chronic staphylococcal osteomyelitis that have been studied include oral cloxacillin plus probenecid for 6 to 12 months; 9 of 19 patients apparently were treated successfully.[21] In another study, the outcome of a 6-week course of nafcillin was compared with that of nafcillin and oral rifampin. No statistically significant differences were observed with the addition of rifampin, but most (10 of 17) of the patients showed no evidence of disease activity 2 years after the cessation of treatment with antibiotics.[198] The high failure rate in these and other studies has led to investigation of a variety of adjunctive

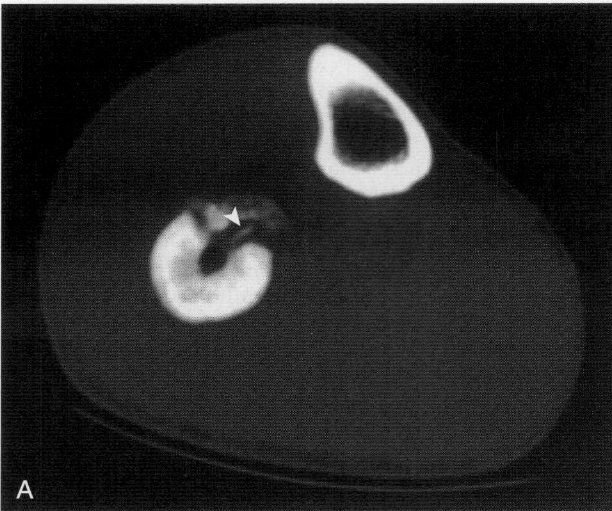

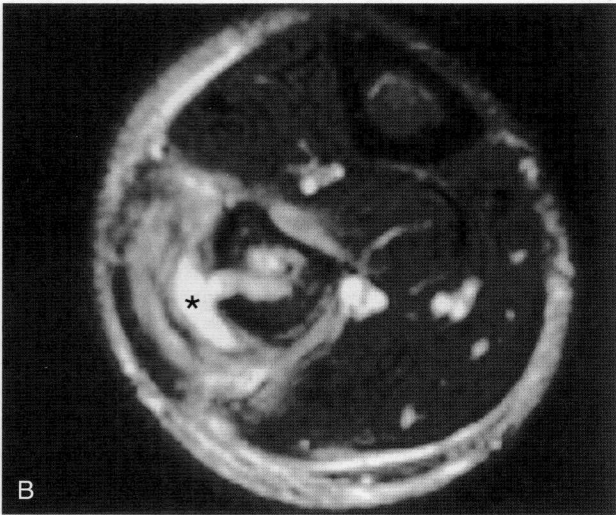

FIG. 55.7 Chronic osteomyelitis. (A) Computed tomography reveals thickening of the fibular cortex and a sinus tract that contains a sequestrum *(arrowhead)*. (B) T2-weighted axial magnetic resonance imaging from a different level shows a lateral sinus tract through the cortex communicating with a soft tissue abscess *(asterisk)*. Edema surrounds the entire fibula. (Courtesy Dr. Leanne Seeger.)

measures to improve the outcome of chronic osteomyelitis. Local irrigation with antibiotic solutions, with[168] and without[7] added detergents, has been examined. The use of surgically implanted polymethyl methacrylate beads impregnated with an antibiotic (usually gentamicin, tobramycin, and vancomycin) are sometimes used for short periods to produce high local antibiotic concentrations[67] and then removed, although the added benefit from this approach is unclear.[28] Negative-pressure wound therapy may also be used to achieve wound closure. Hyperbaric oxygen also has been suggested as an aid to therapy, but no comparative studies have been done.[188]

Because perpetuation of chronic infection seems to be caused by the presence of avascular bone and tissue, advances such as laser Doppler flowmetry ultimately may improve the outcome of this disease.[250] Surgical approaches to close open wounds after debridement and improve blood flow with mobilized tissue flaps also seem to bring about prolonged remission in some patients.[8] Meticulous surgical technique is essential to avoid thermal injury and to retain the vascular supply to compromised areas.[258] Complications of chronic osteomyelitis include secondary amyloidosis and local carcinomatous changes at the site of infection. The high likelihood of a poor outcome in chronic osteomyelitis and the complexities in its management must be kept in mind during treatment of acute hematogenous osteomyelitis.

NEW REFERENCES SINCE THE SEVENTH EDITION

2. Aigner RM, Fueger GF, Ritter G. Results of three-phase bone scintigraphy and radiography in 20 cases of neonatal osteomyelitis. *Nucl Med Commun.* 1996;17(1):20-28.
9. Arnold JC, Cannavino CR, Ross MK, et al. Acute bacterial osteoarticular infections: eight-year analysis of C-reactive protein for oral step-down therapy. *Pediatrics.* 2012;130(4):e821-e828.
19. Basmaci R, Ilharreborde B, Doit C, et al. Two atypical cases of *Kingella kingae* invasive infection with concomitant human rhinovirus infection. *J Clin Microbiol.* 2013;51(9):3137-3139.
22. Belthur MV, Birchansky SB, Verdugo AA, et al. Pathologic fractures in children with acute *Staphylococcus aureus* osteomyelitis. *J Bone Joint Surg Am.* 2012;94(1):34-42.
23. Bennhoff DF. Actinomycosis: diagnostic and therapeutic considerations and a review of 32 cases. *Laryngoscope.* 1984;94(9):1198-1217.
24. Berbari EF, Kanj SS, Kowalski TJ, et al. 2015 Infectious Diseases Society of America (IDSA) clinical practice guidelines for the diagnosis and treatment of native vertebral osteomyelitis in adults. *Clin Infect Dis.* 2015;61(6):e26-e46.
26. Bisla RS, Taber TH Jr. Coccidioidomycosis of bone and joints. *Clin Orthop Relat Res.* 1976;121:196-204.
29. Blair JE. State-of-the-art treatment of coccidioidomycosis skeletal infections. *Ann N Y Acad Sci.* 2007;1111:422-433.
47. Carrillo-Marquez MA, Hulten KG, Hammerman W, et al. USA300 is the predominant genotype causing *Staphylococcus aureus* septic arthritis in children. *Pediatr Infect Dis J.* 2009;28(12):1076-1080.
49. Ceroni D, Belaieff W, Cherkaoui A, et al. Primary epiphyseal or apophyseal subacute osteomyelitis in the pediatric population: a report of fourteen cases and a systematic review of the literature. *J Bone Joint Surg Am.* 2014;96(18):1570-1575.
61. Cope VZ. Actinomycosis of bone with special reference to infection of vertebral column. *J Bone Joint Surg Br.* 1951;33B(2):205-214.
65. Dartnell J, Ramachandran M, Katchburian M. Haematogenous acute and subacute paediatric osteomyelitis: a systematic review of the literature. *J Bone Joint Surg Br.* 2012;94(5):584-595.
82. Falip C, Alison M, Boutry N, et al. Chronic recurrent multifocal osteomyelitis (CRMO): a longitudinal case series review. *Pediatr Radiol.* 2013;43(3):355-375.
99. Gamaletsou MN, Kontoyiannis DP, Sipsas NV, et al. Candida osteomyelitis: analysis of 207 pediatric and adult cases (1970–2011). *Clin Infect Dis.* 2012;55(10):1338-1351.
100. Gaviria-Agudelo C, Aroh C, Tareen N, et al. Genomic heterogeneity of methicillin resistant *Staphylococcus aureus* associated with variation in severity of illness among children with acute hematogenous osteomyelitis. *PLoS One.* 2015;10(6): e0130415.
114. Grammatico L, Baron S, Rusch E, et al. Epidemiology of vertebral osteomyelitis (VO) in France: analysis of hospital-discharge data 2002–2003. *Epidemiol Infect.* 2008;136(5):653-660.
126. Ho AK, Shrader MW, Falk MN, et al. Diagnosis and initial management of musculoskeletal coccidioidomycosis in children. *J Pediatr Orthop.* 2014;34(5): 571-577.
139. Kan JH, Young RS, Yu C, et al. Clinical impact of gadolinium in the MRI diagnosis of musculoskeletal infection in children. *Pediatr Radiol.* 2010;40(7):1197-1205.
140. Kang HM, Choi EH, Lee HJ, et al. The etiology, clinical presentation and long-term outcome of spondylodiscitis in children. *Pediatr Infect Dis J.* 2016;35(4):e102-e106.
142. Kaplan SL. Recent lessons for the management of bone and joint infections. *J Infect.* 2014;68(suppl 1):S51-S56.
145. Kayser R, Mahlfeld K, Greulich M, et al. Spondylodiscitis in childhood: results of a long-term study. *Spine (Phila Pa 1976).* 2005;30(3):318-323.
150. Korakaki E, Aligizakis A, Manoura A, et al. Methicillin-resistant *Staphylococcus aureus* osteomyelitis and septic arthritis in neonates: diagnosis and management. *Jpn J Infect Dis.* 2007;60(2-3):129-131.
155. Lee JH, Jeon SC, Jang HJ, et al. Primary sternal osteomyelitis caused by *Actinomyces israelii. Korean J Thorac Cardiovasc Surg.* 2015;48(1):86-89.
158. Leigh W, Crawford H, Street M, et al. Pediatric calcaneal osteomyelitis. *J Pediatr Orthop.* 2010;30(8):888-892.
170. Marcus NA, Grace TG, Hodgin UG. Osteomyelitis of the sacrum and sepsis of the hip complicating pelvic actinomycosis. *Orthopedics.* 1981;4(6):645-648.
178. McNeil JC, Forbes AR, Vellejo JC, et al. Role of operative or interventional radiology-guided cultures for osteomyelitis. *Pediatrics.* 2016;137:1.
192. Nathoo N, Caris EC, Wiener JA, et al. History of the vertebral venous plexus and the significant contributions of Breschet and Batson. *Neurosurgery.* 2011;69(5):1007-1014, discussion 1014.

196. Nightingale LM, Eaton CB, Fruehan AE, et al. Cephalhematoma complicated by osteomyelitis presumed due to *Gardnerella vaginalis*. *JAMA*. 1986;256(14):1936-1937.
197. Nomura M, Shin M, Ohta M, et al. Atypical osteomyelitis of the skull base and craniovertebral junction caused by *Actinomyces* infection—case report. *Neurol Med Chir (Tokyo)*. 2011;51(1):64-66.
199. Ogbonna OH, Paul Y, Nabhani H, et al. Brodie's abscess in a patient presenting with sickle cell vasoocclusive crisis. *Case Rep Med*. 2015;2015:429876.
200. Olasinde AA, Oluwadiya KS, Adegbehingbe OO. Treatment of Brodie's abscess: excellent results from curettage, bone grafting and antibiotics. *Singapore Med J*. 2011;52(6):436-439.
201. Ono S, Fujimoto H, Kawamoto Y. A rare full-term newborn case of rib osteomyelitis with suspected preceding fracture. *AJP Rep*. 2016;6(1):e104-e107.
202. Paakkonen M, Kallio MJ, Kallio PE, et al. Sensitivity of erythrocyte sedimentation rate and C-reactive protein in childhood bone and joint infections. *Clin Orthop Relat Res*. 2010;468(3):861-866.
203. Paakkonen M, Kallio MJ, Peltola H, et al. Antibiotic treatment and surgery for acute hematogenous calcaneal osteomyelitis of childhood. *J Foot Ankle Surg*. 2015;54(5):840-843.
205. Pappas PG, Kauffman CA, Andes DR, et al. Clinical practice guideline for the management of candidiasis: 2016 update by the Infectious Diseases Society of America. *Clin Infect Dis*. 2016;62(4):e1-e50.
216. Ratnayake K, Davis AJ, Brown L, et al. Pediatric acute osteomyelitis in the postvaccine, methicillin-resistant *Staphylococcus aureus* era. *Am J Emerg Med*. 2015;33(10):1420-1424.
219. Robinson JL, Vaudry WL, Dobrovolsky W. Actinomycosis presenting as osteomyelitis in the pediatric population. *Pediatr Infect Dis J*. 2005;24(4):365-369.
224. Rosenfeld S, Bernstein DT, Daram S, et al. Predicting the presence of adjacent infections in septic arthritis in children. *J Pediatr Orthop*. 2016;36(1):70-74.
225. Roy DR. Osteomyelitis of the patella. *Clin Orthop Relat Res*. 2001;389:30-34.
226. Roy DR, Greene WB, Gamble JG. Osteomyelitis of the patella in children. *J Pediatr Orthop*. 1991;11(3):364-366.
229. Ruttan TK, Higginbotham E, Higginbotham N, et al. Invasive *Kingella kingae* resulting in a Brodie abscess. *J Pediatric Infect Dis Soc*. 2015;4(2):e14-e16.
233. Scheuerman O, Landau D, Schwarz M, et al. Cervical discitis in children. *Pediatr Infect Dis J*. 2015;34(7):794-795.
240. Sondermeyer GL, Lee LA, Gilliss D, et al. Epidemiology of pediatric coccidioidomycosis in California, 2000–2012. *Pediatr Infect Dis J*. 2016;35(2):166-171.
245. Stephen RF, Benson MK, Nade S. Misconceptions about childhood acute osteomyelitis. *J Child Orthop*. 2012;6(5):353-356.
251. Syriopoulou V, Dailiana Z, Dmitriy N, et al. Clinical experience with daptomycin for the treatment of gram-positive infections in children and adolescents. *Pediatr Infect Dis J*. 2016;35(5):511-516.
282. Wipff J, Costantino F, Lemelle I, et al. A large national cohort of French patients with chronic recurrent multifocal osteitis. *Arthritis Rheumatol*. 2015;67(4):1128-1137.
285. Yagupsky P. *Kingella kingae:* carriage, transmission, and disease. *Clin Microbiol Rev*. 2015;28(1):54-79.

The full reference list for this chapter is available at ExpertConsult.com.

56 Septic Arthritis

Paul Krogstad

Acute infection of the joints can be caused by bacteria, fungi, and viruses. Bacterial infections occur most frequently. The terms *septic arthritis, infectious arthritis,* and *acute suppurative pyarthrosis* are used interchangeably with regard to bacterial infections.

EPIDEMIOLOGY

Septic arthritis occurs most frequently in childhood, with an estimated incidence of 1 to 37 cases per 100,000 individuals.[40,62,94,116] Boys are affected more often than are girls by a ratio of 1.1 : 1.9.[12,21,40,116] Describing the age distribution of septic arthritis is difficult because of the varying age intervals selected by authors of different studies, but most cases occur below 6 years of age, and a median age of 2 years has been reported in several series.[12,45,71,74,76,98,116]

PATHOPHYSIOLOGY

Synovial joints, also termed *diarthrodial joints,* are freely movable articulations containing synovia. Synovia is a transparent viscous fluid that lubricates the joint and nourishes the avascular articular cartilage. The synovium, a connective tissue layer interposed between the fibrous joint capsule and the fluid-filled synovial cavity, is responsible for formation of the joint fluid. The synovium contains a prominent capillary supply embedded in a connective tissue network containing at least two types of cells. One morphologic type (type A) seems to be related to mononuclear phagocytes; fibroblast-like type B cells seem to be responsible for the synthesis of hyaluronic acid. Joint fluid (synovia) is formed by filtration through the capillary network (i.e., the net balance of back-diffusion into the capillary bed and diffusion into the joint space). Diarthrodial joints normally contain small amounts of fluid (e.g., 0.5 to 3 mL in the knee),[104] with glucose and electrolyte concentrations equal to those in plasma. An oxygen partial pressure of 60 to 70 mm Hg, an albumin concentration of 10 to 20 g/L, and an IgG content of 500 mg/L are typical.[27,30,42,104] Pain fibers are present in the joint capsule, accessory ligaments (e.g., cruciate ligaments of the knee), and subchondral bone,[114] but their relative contributions to the perception of pain in acute septic arthritis has yet to be elucidated.

Diffusion from the joint space is increased by any mechanism that increases pressure (distention with injected solution, active or passive motion, or external massage). Particulate material is removed from the joint space by synovial membrane macrophages and free monocytes (the latter usually are present in concentrations of $<60 \times 10^6$/L).[96] The viscosity of joint fluid is affected by the properties of hyaluronic acid; enzymatic depolymerization produces a viscosity approximately equivalent to that of water. With the loss of hyaluronidase from the synovia, the articular cartilage, with continued use, becomes eroded and sclerotic.[11]

Microorganisms can enter the joint space by hematogenous spread, direct inoculation, or extension from a contiguous focus of infection, including foci of adjacent osteomyelitis. Bacteria in blood are potentially delivered to the synovial membrane during transient bacteremia. A history of trauma often is cited as a predisposing factor for the development of bacterial arthritis,[12,112] but the significance of such a history is unclear in view of the great frequency of minor trauma in childhood. Upper respiratory tract infections frequently precede the development of septic arthritis caused by *Haemophilus influenzae* type B and *Kingella kingae,* and oral ulcers are often noted prior to *Kingella* infections. Similar to mild traumatic injuries, they are presumed to increase the likelihood of bacteremia.[12,112,115]

Coincident osteomyelitis and septic arthritis are frequently reported in studies of osteoarticular infections in children. In three recent case series, 9% to 33% of cases of acute osteomyelitis in childhood were complicated by septic arthritis.[21,40,89,91] Humeral osteomyelitis seems to be of particularly high risk; it was present in 15 of 22 cases of shoulder joint arthritis (68%) in one recent series.[38] Conversely either shoulder or elbow joint septic arthritis was present in 7 (14%) of 49 cases of humeral osteomyelitis in another case series.[105] Aside from joint involvement during osteomyelitis, extension of a contiguous infection into the

TABLE 56.1 Bacterial Etiology of Septic Arthritis in Children With Positive Cultures

	GRAM-POSITIVE BACTERIA					
Year of Report	***S. aureus***	**Streptococci**	***S. pneumoniae***	**CNS**	***H. influenzae***	***K. kingae***
1941[58]	50	45	2	10	0	0
1958[98]	18	8	5	2	3	0
1972[80]	40	20	8	5	37	0
1975[76]	37	10	0	5	14	0
1987[12]	40	8	5	0	20	0
1995[116]	0	2	3	0	8	19
1999[71]	10	5	2	2	1	3
2008[40]	19	8	5	3	1	0
Total	*195*	*98*	*25*	*24*	*83*	*22*
% of all isolates	36	18	5	4	15	4

CNS, Coagulase-negative staphylococci.
[a]Two isolates in one case each.

joint space seldom occurs. In one series, 10 of 77 patients with septic arthritis had disease resulting from extension from a contiguous soft tissue infection.[24] Eight occurred before the availability of many antibiotics (1951). This high frequency of septic arthritis caused by spread of infection from a contiguous focus has not been seen in more recent studies.

Inoculation arthritis occurs after invasion of the joint by a contaminated object, such as kneeling on sewing needles[98] or following arthroscopic surgery.[5,54]

Gram-negative organisms are the most frequent pathogens when septic arthritis occurs after other types of surgeries or instrumentation of the urinary or intestinal tract. *Salmonella* septic arthritis may develop during the course of *Salmonella* bacteremia in a normal host, but it occurs with increased frequency in patients with sickle-cell disease and related hemoglobinopathies. Although septic arthritis occurs in children and adults infected with human immunodeficiency virus (HIV),[75] as yet no data have substantiated that HIV increases the incidence of musculoskeletal infections in children. However, pneumococcal osteoarticular infections may be more common in HIV-positive children, compared with HIV-seronegative children, at least in the absence of immunization with protein-conjugate pneumococcal vacccine.[95] Septic arthritis has been described during varicella, presumably caused by bacteremia resulting from infection of skin lesions. It must be differentiated from the apparent ability of varicella zoster virus to cause joint inflammation on its own.[78,93]

ETIOLOGY

In most case series published since the mid-20th century, *Staphylococcus aureus* has been the most common cause of culture-positive septic arthritis, including methicillin-susceptible (MSSA) and methicillin-resistant *S. aureus* (MRSA). Streptococci (especially group A β-hemolytic organisms and pneumococci) have been responsible for most other gram-positive infections (Table 56.1). *K. kingae* has been recognized increasingly as a cause of septic arthritis,[33,50,71,74,115,116] perhaps because of improvements in culture methods and the use of polymerase chain reaction (PCR) detection of bacterial nucleic acids.[22,105] In one series from Israel, *Kingella* was the most common bacterial isolate (48% of cases), and *S. aureus* was not found in children less than 24 months of age.[116] In another recent report from western Europe, *Kingella* was the most common cause of both osteomyelitis and septic arthritis in children under 4 years of age.[22]

H. influenzae type B historically has been an important cause of septic arthritis in children younger than 2 years old but now is seen only rarely in areas with widespread immunization.[17,45,52,71] Arthritis caused by *Streptococcus pneumoniae* also generally occurs in children younger than 2 years old and may diminish in frequency in the era of protein conjugate vaccines. In a few cases, septic arthritis is seen with systemic *Neisseria meningitidis* infection. In neonates and sexually active adolescents with suspected septic arthritis, *Neisseria gonorrhoeae* should be considered.[4,40,46,65]

Salmonella spp. cause approximately 1% of the total cases of septic arthritis. Beyond the neonatal period, infections with other enteric gram-negative bacteria are rare occurrences in pediatric septic arthritis and often are associated with inoculation, instrumentation, or an immunocompromised state.[40,46] Infections with *Serratia, Aeromonas, Enterobacter, Bacteroides,* and *Campylobacter* generally occur in patients with malignancy who are immunosuppressed.[1,8,46,72,80,84] *Pseudomonas aeruginosa* infections are associated with arthritis in infants, with infection of puncture wounds, or with injectable drug use.[77,80,107] Discussion of Lyme arthritis is beyond the scope of this chapter, but intermittent, inflammatory arthritis is seen in many patients after *Borrelia* infection is transmitted by a tick bite.[103]

Unusual causes of septic arthritis include *Propionibacterium acnes,*[118] *Actinomyces* (formerly *Corynebacterium*) *pyogenes,*[84] *Pasteurella multocida,*[49] and *Yersinia pestis* (personal observation). *Streptobacillus moniliformis* infection of joints may become evident 2 to 3 days after a rat bite occurs; a macular rash commonly is present at initial evaluation. *Brucella,* mycobacteria (*Mycobacterium tuberculosis* and other species), and *Nocardia asteroides* may cause a chronic monarticular arthritis with granulomatous histopathology.

Although bacterial infections are the most common cause of septic arthritis, infectious arthritis is sometimes caused by viral pathogens (including varicella zoster, erythrovirus [parvovirus B19], rubella, dengue, chikungunya[68] and other togaviruses, variola, vaccinia, certain enteroviruses) as well as by mycobacteria (including *M. tuberculosis*). Septic arthritis may also be caused during disseminated fungal infections, including candidiasis, histoplasmosis,[31] coccidioidomycosis,[15] blastomycosis,[80] and cryptococcosis.[102] The knee joint is most often involved in coccidioidal and cryptococcal arthritis.[15,102]

DIAGNOSIS

Clinical Findings

Most children have fever or constitutional symptoms within the first few days of infection.[43,112,116] Table 56.2 lists the frequency of specific joint involvement in hematogenous septic arthritis of childhood. Infections of the major weight-bearing joints (hip, knee, and ankle) consistently account for approximately 80% of all cases. Focal findings in the joint involved almost always are present. In infants, in whom the hip is one of the most frequent joints involved, swelling, tenderness, and heat may be absent. Most commonly, the infant with septic arthritis lies with the involved leg abducted and externally rotated, and hip joint dislocation may occur.[82] When the capsule of the joint can be examined, swelling is noted; effusion was present in 22 of 24 cases in one series.[111] Likely because pain fibers are located in the capsule, any maneuver that increases intracapsular pressure also produces pain. In the hip, this pain can be

GRAM-NEGATIVE BACTERIA					
N. meningitidis	*Salmonella*	Non-*Salmonella* Enterobacteriaceae	*N. gonorrhoeae*	Other	Total Cases
0	0	0	14	0	121
0	0	2	0	1	38[a]
4	2	7	13	11	146[a]
0	0	2	0	7	75
4	0	2	2	9	90
1	1	1	0	5	40
3	0	4	2	1	33
0	0	2	2	4	
12	*3*	*18*	*31*	*34*	*549*
2	1	3	6	6	

TABLE 56.2 Joints Involved in Septic Arthritis of Children

Reference	Knee	Hip	Ankle	Wrist	Elbow	Shoulder	Small Diarthrodial Joints
Heberling 1941[58]	40	50	13	3	8	9	2
Samilson et al. 1958[98]	8	19	2	0	6	3	0
Nelson 1972[80]	103	48	38	12	35	10	4
Gillespie 1973[43]	37	41	13	2	3	3	0
Yagupsky et al. 1995[116]	16	6	13	1	2	3	1
Goergens et al. 2005[45]	15	15	4	2	4	1	3
Gafur et al. 2008[40]	46	51	5	1	10	3	
Total	265	230	88	21	68	32	10
% of all cases	37	32	12	3	10	4	1

elicited by compression of the head of the femur into the acetabulum. A portal of entry almost never is apparent, and bilateral hip joint infection may occur.[86] Pyogenic sacroiliitis often is accompanied by tenderness detected by pressure applied over the sacrum during a digital rectal examination and by pain experienced during simultaneous flexion, abduction, and external rotation at the hip.[2]

Gonococcal arthritis in neonates has nonspecific prodromal symptoms, including poor feeding, irritability, and fever. The exact portal of entry is unknown, and the joints below the hip usually are involved (knee, ankle, and metatarsal). During adolescence, gonococcal arthritis occurs as a manifestation of sepsis with fever, chills, rash, and multiple small joint involvement, often with tenosynovitis.[41] The illness frequently follows the onset of menses by a few days.

Radiologic Findings

Findings on plain radiography are due to capsular swelling. In the joints readily accessible to physical examination, radiographs add little to the diagnostic evaluation, but when septic arthritis of the hip is suspected in a child, they are a valuable adjunct and may identify other causes of hip pain, such as Legg-Calvé-Perthes disease, slipped capital femoral epiphysis, and fracture. Films of the hip should be made with the child in the frog-leg position and with the legs extended at the knee and slightly internally rotated. The early signs of septic arthritis of the hip are caused by swelling of the capsule, which shifts the fat lines. One of the oldest signs is the obturator sign: as the tendon of the obturator internus passes over the capsule of the hip joint, the margins of this muscle are displaced medially into the pelvis (Fig. 56.1).[59] With continued swelling of the hip joint capsule, the femoral head is displaced laterally and upward.[25] One of the most consistent findings is obliteration or lateral displacement of the gluteal fat lines (see Fig. 56.1).[113] Coincident with filling of the capsule with exudate, the femoral portion of the Shenton line is raised and its arc is widened.[113] Ultrasound evaluation has proved useful in evaluation of septic arthritis of the hip.[63,119] In a series of 96 patients, none of the 40 patients with normal ultrasound findings had septic arthritis.[119] If a technetium bone scan is performed, increased uptake on either side of the joint is seen during the "blood pool" phase of the scan.[110]

Bacterial infections causing pyogenic sacroiliitis may be particularly difficult to diagnose because bone scans and computed tomography (CT) initially may be negative. Magnetic resonance imaging (MRI) seems to be the diagnostic radiologic method of choice.[2,35] MRI may also be advisable when septic arthritis of either the shoulder or elbow joint is identified, in view of the high rate of concomitant osteomyelitis.[13,38,69,105]

Laboratory Evaluation

Diagnostic evaluation for suspected septic arthritis generally includes determination of the erythrocyte sedimentation rate (ESR) or C-reactive protein (CRP), and the peripheral blood leukocyte count and differential. These may be only mildly elevated in cases of proven infection, however.[34,119] Blood for culture always should be obtained because blood cultures sometimes may yield the pathogen when joint fluid cultures do not.[66]

Identification of organisms in joint fluid is the primary criterion for diagnosis of septic arthritis. Joint fluid should be collected in a heparinized syringe so that the large clot that usually forms in fluid obtained from patients with septic arthritis or juvenile rheumatoid arthritis does not preclude enumeration of leukocytes. A portion of

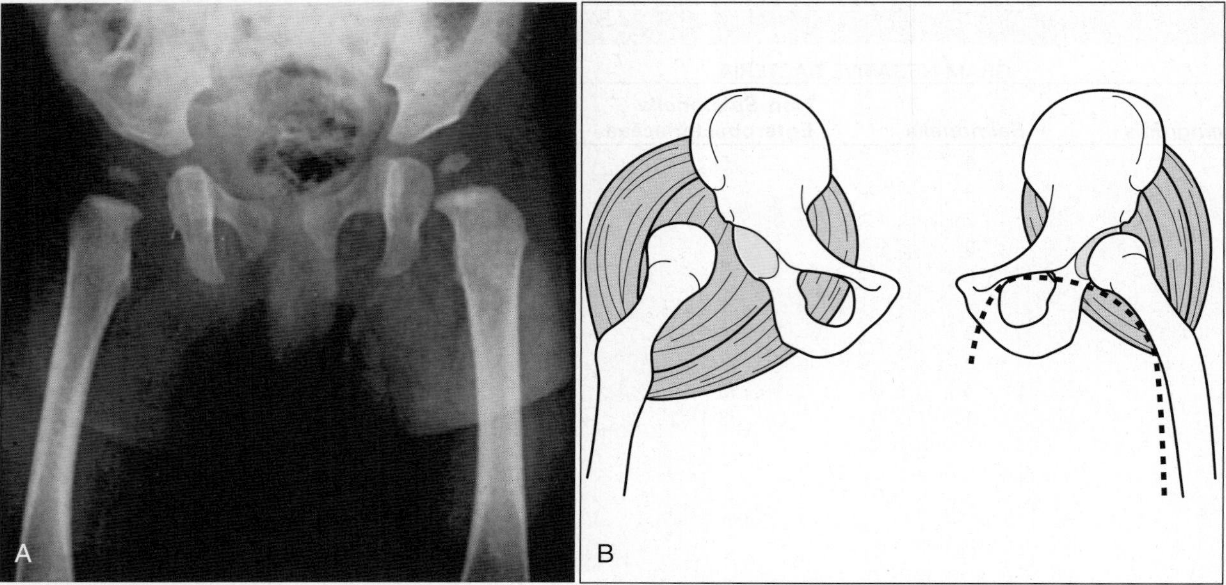

FIG. 56.1 The obturator sign in the hip is one of the oldest signs of septic arthritis. Another consistent finding is obliteration or lateral displacement of the gluteal fat lines and loss of continuity of the Shenton line. These findings are illustrated (A) radiographically and (B) schematically.

the specimen should be submitted for culture and Gram stain, and cell and differential count should also be performed. Careful examination of a Gram-stained smear of joint fluid aspirates must be emphasized because joint fluid exerts a bacteriostatic effect on microorganisms and organisms that can be seen but may not grow in culture. Approximately 35% of joint aspirates are sterile in patients with other clinical and laboratory findings of a septic joint, including positive blood cultures.[12,80] Joint fluid should be cultured aerobically and under anaerobic conditions. The use of cell lysis culture bottles may enhance the recovery of *K. kingae* and other organisms.[115,117] PCR analysis of joint fluid is likely to become a useful adjunct to the diagnosis of culture-negative disease. As noted previously, PCR had revealed that fastidious organisms, especially *K. kingae* in young children, are important causes of osteoarticular infections. However, PCR methodologies generally remain investigational and are readily available only in certain centers.[22,77,108] Specimens from other anatomic sites may implicate other pathogens. For example, oropharyngeal, rectal, and urogenital cultures or detection of gonococcal DNA in urine may confirm the diagnosis of gonococcal arthritis.

The median synovial fluid leukocyte count in bacterial arthritis in one study was 60.5×10^9 cells/L[100]; a more recent study of *S. aureus* septic arthritis in children revealed similar values (median 75×10^9 cells/L).[21] Polymorphonuclear leukocytes account for 75% to 90% of the white blood cells.[96] Cell concentrations are generally lower in fluid obtained from patients with acute rheumatic fever, juvenile rheumatoid arthritis, and other inflammatory causes of arthritis (Table 56.3).[10,96,100] However, a joint fluid leukocyte density of 0.7×10^9 cells/L has been found in joint fluid from patients ultimately proved to have septic arthritis.[21] Minimally turbid fluid with a seemingly low number of cells still should be processed for bacterial culture and Gram stain. The glucose concentration often is decreased in septic arthritis, but it may be normal and may be depressed in rheumatoid arthritis and other conditions.[100,111] Examination of the fluid for uric acid and other types of crystals should be considered in certain children (e.g., children with hyperuricemia).

DIFFERENTIAL DIAGNOSIS

The differential diagnosis of septic arthritis includes infectious and noninfectious entities. Focal infections that mimic septic arthritis include pyomyositis, obturator internus muscle abscess,[109] epiphyseal osteomyelitis, deep cellulitis and soft tissue abscesses, and, rarely, septic (suppurative) bursitis. Septic bursitis may be particularly difficult to distinguish from septic arthritis. Children with septic bursitis frequently have a history of recent trauma and fever along with limitation of joint movement.[57,88] Careful physical examination and aspiration of bursal fluid allow the entities to be differentiated. Septic arthritis and arthralgia may occur during infectious endocarditis.

Toxic (or transient) synovitis (also referred to as irritable hip and reactive synovitis) is frequently seen in children and has milder presenting features than bacterial infections of the hip. The combination of fever, elevated white blood cell count, ESR (>40 mm/h), CRP, and inability to bear weight permits septic arthritis to be distinguished from transient synovitis with high accuracy; greater than 90% sensitivity for the detection of septic arthritis has been reported when all of these factors are present.[19,34,66,119]

Other noninfectious entities to be considered in the differential diagnosis include traumatic arthritis, juvenile idiopathic arthritis, villonodular synovitis, leukemia, serum sickness, ulcerative colitis, granulomatous colitis, Schönlein-Henoch purpura, traumatic arthritis, fracture, Legg-Calvé-Perthes disease, slipped femoral capital epiphysis, and metabolic diseases affecting joints (e.g., ochronosis in adults with alkaptonuria).

TREATMENT

Surgical Treatment

In infants, septic arthritis in the hips or shoulders is a surgical emergency; these joints should be drained as soon as the diagnosis is apparent to prevent bony destruction.[85] For joints other than the hip, needle aspiration (single or multiple) may be an alternative to surgical drainage (arthrotomy or arthroscopy).[60,101] In a study in adults, the outcome of septic arthritis was better in patients treated by repeated needle aspiration than in patients treated by surgical drainage.[47] Eighty percent of the patients treated by needle aspiration were thought to have a good outcome versus 47% treated by surgical drainage. All wrist joint infections in this series were treated successfully by needle aspiration. In treatment of septic arthritis of the knee, however, the outcome was almost equivalent with either needle aspiration or open drainage.

Antibiotic Therapy

Antibiotic treatment of septic arthritis should target the most common pathogens, keeping age and other clinical factors in mind. Beyond the neonatal period, septic arthritis in immunologically normal children

TABLE 56.3 Joint Fluid Findings in Childhood Arthritides

Diagnosis	Spontaneous Clotting	Mucin Clot Appearance	Leukocytes/mL	% Polymorphonuclear Leukocytes	Glucose as Percentage of Blood Value
Septic arthritis	Rapid formation of large clot	Curdled milk	73,000	90	30
Rheumatic fever	Small to absent	Tightrope	18,000	60	75
Juvenile rheumatoid arthritis	Large clot	Small, friable masses	15,000	60	75

From Ropes M. Joint fluid findings in disease. *Bull Rheum Dis.* 1957;7(Suppl):21.

is generally caused by *S. aureus* and other gram-positive organisms.[17,71,80] Antistaphylococcal penicillins (e.g., oxacillin or nafcillin) are usually given, but vancomycin or clindamycin should be used as the empiric antistaphylococcal agent in areas where community-acquired MRSA is a common concern.[3,73] Some authorities advocate that this be done when community-acquired MRSA represents more than 10% of *S. aureus* in a geographic area.[64] Vancomycin is preferred if clindamycin resistance is common among *S. aureus* isolates (>10%). At present, no regimen is clearly preferred for the treatment of penicillin-nonsusceptible *S. pneumoniae,* but ceftriaxone, cefotaxime, and clindamycin have been used successfully.[18]

The need for coverage for gram-negative pathogens should also be considered. In children younger than 36 months,[36,115] adding empiric coverage for *Kingella* infection may also be indicated unless a cephalosporin is already being used as part of the initial empiric therapy; cefuroxime, cefotaxime, or ceftriaxone may be preferred. Ceftriaxone and cefotaxime are appropriate for the treatment of gonococcal infections in adolescents.

Although the risk of acquiring invasive *H. influenzae* type B infection is low in areas with effective immunization, rare cases continue to be reported.[3,40] Children younger than 2 years who have not been immunized against *H. influenzae* type B should be treated initially with a regimen that contains an antistaphylococcal agent, such as nafcillin, vancomycin, or clindamycin, and an agent active against this agent (e.g., cefotaxime).

All antibiotics that have been studied penetrate into joint fluid readily. Soon after administration, at the time of peak serum levels, the joint fluid concentration averages 30% of the serum value.[7,9,79,92] The efflux of antibiotic from joint fluid back to serum is slow, however. Immediately before the next systemic dose is administered, joint fluid antibiotic concentrations frequently exceed the concentrations present in serum. Antibiotics, whether administered orally or parenterally, can achieve efficacious concentrations in joint fluid. Injecting antibiotics into the joint space usually is unnecessary because of their excellent penetration. Many antibiotics (e.g., cephalothin) are capable of evoking an intense inflammatory reaction, much as they do if they are infiltrated beneath the skin.

Tetzlaff and associates[106] showed that septic arthritis can be treated for 1 week (or less) parenterally, with the balance of the drug given orally. These investigators considered the minimal duration of therapy to be 3 weeks because some cases initially thought to reflect septic arthritis alone may actually have coincident bone infection. The presence of concomitant septic arthritis and osteomyelitis remains a particular concern in areas in which osteoarticular infections due to MRSA are common.[21]

The effectiveness of antibiotic therapy can be assessed by serial joint fluid examinations, leukocyte density, and culture results.[111] The time required for resolution of joint symptoms and the time for the synovia to become sterile are proportional to the duration of symptoms before the initiation of appropriate antibiotic therapy.[61] In one study, some patients still had cultures yielding bacteria after undergoing 1 week of therapy. In these patients, cellular density ranged from 25 to 250×10^9 cells/L (mean 109×10^9 cells/L) at the beginning of therapy; 92% of the cells were polymorphonuclear leukocytes. By the end of 2 weeks of therapy, all cultures were sterile, and leukocyte density ranged from 4.9 to 23×10^9 cells/L (mean of 12.3×10^9 cells/L).[111] Similar studies of the rate of resolution of indicators of inflammation in joint fluid have suggested that after receiving 9 days of treatment patients who ultimately recovered completely had a density of 5×10^9 cells/L; however, in patients with recrudescent infection or a poor outcome, the density was 6×10^{10} cells/L.[46] When an effusion reaccumulates, one should remove it by arthrocentesis, not only to make the patient more comfortable but also to permit serial assessment of therapy.

Disease caused by *S. aureus* and Enterobacteriaceae requires longer treatment than disease caused by *H. influenzae* or meningococci. If MRI was not performed as part of the initial diagnostic evaluation, radiographs should be obtained after 14 days of therapy to seek bone changes indicating that osteomyelitis may have been present. Concomitant osteomyelitis may require surgical intervention, and antibiotic therapy must continue beyond 21 days. (See Chapter 55 for discussion of the duration of antimicrobial therapy for osteomyelitis.)

PROGNOSIS

Sequelae, including hip dislocation, are more likely to develop in infants and patients with symptoms of longer duration.[98,111] In one study, seven of eight patients in whom "permanent" hip dislocation developed had symptoms for 7 or more days before receiving treatment.[100] Similarly, patients with spontaneous ankylosis had symptoms longer than 7 days.

A detailed analysis of prognostic factors showed no significant difference when arthrotomy, with or without irrigation, was compared with repeated aspiration.[76] Likewise the specific antibiotic used had no effect on outcome as long as it was effective against the infecting organism. The literature does suggest that septic arthritis caused by Enterobacteriaceae is associated with more frequent sequelae than when caused by other pathogens.[48,81] *S. aureus* is more likely to cause sequelae than is *H. influenzae.*[12]

A randomized, placebo-controlled study was conducted in Costa Rica that examined the impact of a brief course of dexamethasone on the outcome of bacteriologically confirmed cases of septic arthritis of hematogenous origin in children.[87] Children younger than 3 months were excluded from participation, and *H. influenzae* was responsible for 13% of cases among the 100 evaluable patients. After 1 year of follow-up, limping, joint pain, and restriction of movement were found in 26% of patients who received a placebo but in only 1 of 50 patients treated with dexamethasone. A second randomized trial in Israel involved 49 children (average age of 33 months) with septic arthritis to whom adjunctive dexamethasone was given during the first 4 days of antimicrobial therapy.[56] This treatment was associated with decreased duration of fever (1.7 vs. 2.8 days), pain (7.2 vs. 10.8 days), and parenteral antibiotics (9.9 vs. 12.6 days) but no difference in long-term outcome. All *Staphylococcus aureus* isolates in these studies were methicillin susceptible, and *Kingella kingae* was the most common pathogen identified in the study performed in Israel. At present, the benefits of dexamethasone therapy in septic arthritis remain unclear in other settings.

SPECIAL PROBLEMS

Neonatal Septic Arthritis

Neonatal septic arthritis is a problem that warrants special attention because of its subtle signs and symptoms,[26] its potential for catastrophic consequences of untreated disease,[85,86] and the unusual organisms occasionally seen. Any neonate who has swelling in the region of the thigh and the buttock and holds that leg flexed with slight abduction and external rotation at the hip should be suspected to have femoral-acetabular septic arthritis. It can occur 1 to 28 days after femoral venipuncture (in most neonates, 5 to 9 days) and should not be confused with femoral vein thrombosis.[6,23]

In most neonates, no toxemia, fever, or leukocytosis is present. More than one joint may be involved when initially evaluated. The progression of disease in neonates can be so indolent that the hip spontaneously drains along the obturator internus, and the condition is manifested as a lower abdominal mass just above the inguinal canal.[39] Problems in recognizing the disease in neonates undoubtedly contribute to the poor outcome. In one series, the delay from onset to diagnosis was an average of 1 week; only two of the nine infants in this series had a normal hip examination at follow-up.[85]

In most series, the causative agents are staphylococci and streptococci,[6,16,23,26,85] but gram-negative organisms often are found. More importantly, arthritis caused by *Candida albicans* has been described,[29] and the gonococcus should not be forgotten. In gonococcal arthritis, the symptoms, which usually become apparent in infants 1 to 5 weeks of age, generally are polyarthritic (more than one joint involved).[44] As previously noted, other symptoms of neonatal gonococcal arthritis are no different from symptoms caused by other pathogens.

Initial antibiotic therapy for neonatal septic arthritis should be directed toward *S. aureus* and the nosocomial gram-negative bacteria that are prevalent in the nursery. Antibiotic therapy can be altered when the susceptibility of the causative bacterium is known. As noted earlier, the usual duration of therapy is 3 to 4 weeks, and radiography should be performed toward the end of treatment. Oral therapy has been used successfully to complete treatment of septic arthritis in neonates,[90] but absorption of antibiotics in this age range is unpredictable.[99]

Fungal Arthritis

Fungal arthritis is rare in children but may be seen with pathogens of endemic mycoses, such as *Histoplasma capsulatum, B. dermatitidis,*[80] and *Coccidioides* spp.[15] as well as with opportunistic fungal pathogens (e.g., *Candida* spp., *Cryptococcus neoformans*).[71,102] These pathogens usually manifest after an indolent course and may be misdiagnosed as juvenile idiopathic arthritis or other rheumatologic disease. The recommended medical treatment for these fungal infections is generally identical to that required for other systemic infections caused by these organisms.

Joint Infections During Rheumatologic Disease

Joint infections that develop during a case of rheumatoid arthritis seem to occur more frequently in adults with rheumatoid arthritis than in children. In one series, only 2 of 17 patients were younger than age 10 years.[8] The notable features are that the hips generally are not involved and infection of multiple joints (17 of 44 patients had more than one joint involved) frequently occurs. Because of the preexisting joint disease, the diagnosis often is delayed and the outcome usually is poor. Septic arthritis should be considered if an unusual worsening of one joint occurs during a flare of rheumatoid arthritis or other rheumatologic disease. The use of anti–tumor necrosis factor monoclonal antibodies as part of therapy for juvenile idiopathic arthritis does not appear to enhance the risk of joint infection compared to the use of methotrexate, although other significant infections increase in frequency.[32]

Reactive Arthritis

An oligoarticular arthritis may occur after infection with *Shigella* spp.,[20,83] *Chlamydia trachomatis, Salmonella* spp.,[55] and certain *Yersinia* serotypes.[67] A link to infection with *Chlamydophila pneumoniae* (formerly *Chlamydia pneumoniae*) has also been described, and rare cases of septic arthritis may follow *Clostridium difficile* colitis in children.[14,28,37,70] This postinfectious joint inflammation seems to develop with greater frequency in individuals who express the histocompatibility antigen HLA-B*27, perhaps as a result of molecular similarities between bacterial antigens and the human protein. In addition, during the initial infection, bacterial antigens apparently may be deposited in the synovium and may persist, leading to pathogenic inflammation.[51,67]

Generally the onset of joint symptoms occurs a few days to several weeks after a transient and often mild episode of diarrhea or symptoms of urethritis. The arthritis may mimic rheumatic fever and is characterized by daily low-grade fever and an increased ESR. Classic Reiter syndrome, which includes ocular inflammation, oligoarticular arthritis, and sterile urethritis, may also occur.

Reactive arthritis generally can be distinguished from septic arthritis by analysis of synovial fluid; infectious arthritis usually is associated with an increased number of white blood cells in the synovial fluid.[10] Resolution of joint symptoms in cases of reactive arthritis usually occurs several weeks to months after onset. Antiinflammatory agents are the cornerstone of therapy and may include nonsteroidal antiinflammatory drugs, corticosteroids, methotrexate, or other agents.

Reactive arthritis also may occur after acute infections with *N. meningitidis*[53] and *H. influenzae.*[97] Symptoms and signs of joint inflammation often appear 1 week or more after the acute septic episode and resolve without sequelae.

NEW REFERENCES SINCE THE SEVENTH EDITION

3. Arnold JC, Bradley JS. Osteoarticular infections in children. *Infect Dis Clin North Am.* 2015;29(3):557-574.
5. Ashraf A, Luo TD, Christophersen C, et al. Acute and subacute complications of pediatric and adolescent knee arthroscopy. *Arthroscopy*. 2014;30(6):710-714.
13. Belthur MV, Palazzi DL, Miller JA, et al. A clinical analysis of shoulder and hip joint infections in children. *J Pediatr Orthop*. 2009;29(7):828-833.
21. Carrillo-Marquez MA, Hulten KG, Hammerman W, et al. USA300 is the predominant genotype causing *Staphylococcus aureus* septic arthritis in children. *Pediatr Infect Dis J*. 2009;28(12):1076-1080.
22. Ceroni D, Kampouroglou G, Valaikaite R, et al. Osteoarticular infections in young children: what has changed over the last years? *Swiss Med Wkly*. 2014;144:w13971.
32. Davies R, Southwood TR, Kearsley-Fleet L, et al. Medically significant infections are increased in patients with juvenile idiopathic arthritis treated with etanercept: results from the British Society for Paediatric and Adolescent Rheumatology Etanercept cohort study. *Arthritis Rheumatol*. 2015;67(9):2487-2494.
38. Ernat J, Riccio AI, Fitzpatrick K, et al. Osteomyelitis is commonly associated with septic arthritis of the shoulder in children. *J Pediatr Orthop*. 2015 Dec 19. [Epub ahead of print].
40. Gafur OA, Copley LA, Hollmig ST, et al. The impact of the current epidemiology of pediatric musculoskeletal infection on evaluation and treatment guidelines. *J Pediatr Orthop*. 2008;28(7):777-785.
60. Herndon WA, Knauer S, Sullivan JA, et al. Management of septic arthritis in children. *J Pediatr Orthop*. 1986;6(5):576-578.
62. Jackson MA, Nelson JD. Etiology and medical management of acute suppurative bone and joint infections in pediatric patients. *J Pediatr Orthop*. 1982;2(3): 313-323.
64. Kaplan SL. Recent lessons for the management of bone and joint infections. *J Infect*. 2014;68(suppl 1):S51-S56.
69. Lejman T, Strong M, Michno P, et al. Septic arthritis of the shoulder during the first 18 months of life. *J Pediatr Orthop*. 1995;15(2):172-175.
74. Masson AT, Gudnason T, Jonmundsson GK, et al. [Bacterial osteomyelitis and arthritis in Icelandic children 1996–2005]. *Laeknabladid*. 2011;97(2):91-96.
91. Perlman MH, Patzakis MJ, Kumar PJ, et al. The incidence of joint involvement with adjacent osteomyelitis in pediatric patients. *J Pediatr Orthop*. 2000;20(1): 40-43.
94. Riise OR, Handeland KS, Cvancarova M, et al. Incidence and characteristics of arthritis in Norwegian children: a population-based study. *Pediatrics*. 2008;121(2):e299-e306.
101. Smith SP, Thyoka M, Lavy CB, et al. Septic arthritis of the shoulder in children in Malawi. A randomised, prospective study of aspiration versus arthrotomy and washout. *J Bone Joint Surg Br*. 2002;84(8):1167-1172.
112. Welkon CJ, Long SS, Fisher MC, et al. Pyogenic arthritis in infants and children: a review of 95 cases. *Pediatr Infect Dis*. 1986;5(6):669-676.
114. Witt KL, Vilensky JA. The anatomy of osteoarthritic joint pain. *Clin Anat*. 2014;27(3):451-454.

The full reference list for this chapter is available at ExpertConsult.com.

57 Bacterial Myositis and Pyomyositis

Sanjay Verma • Charles Grose

Myositis is not a common manifestation of bacterial infection, but, when it occurs, the consequences to the patient may be severe or even fatal. *Staphylococcus aureus* and group A streptococci are the most likely causative organisms. Myositis also has been associated with several other infectious agents, including viruses, fungi, and parasites. These pathogens are listed in Box 57.1; they are discussed briefly in this chapter and more thoroughly in the chapters on the specific microorganisms. This chapter focuses on two forms of pyogenic myositis, sometimes differentiated as *acute bacterial myositis* and classical (or *tropical*) *pyomyositis*. The former is caused primarily by group A streptococci and the latter by *S. aureus*, including methicillin-resistant *S. aureus* (MRSA). Treatment regimens are included from the United States and India.

PYOMYOSITIS

The pathologic entity termed *spontaneous acute myositis* was recognized by Virchow in the mid-19th century, but the first clinical description of suppurative myositis generally is attributed to the Japanese surgeon Scriba.[24] In 1904, another Japanese surgeon, Miyake,[18] extensively reviewed the subject of skeletal muscle abscesses and added 33 more cases. As the British and French expanded their colonial empires at the transition to the 20th century, the disease was recognized with increasing frequency in the native populations and in the soldiers who lived in the tropical areas of Asia and Africa.[3,30] It acquired the name by which it now is known widely—*tropical pyomyositis*.[9,10,15]

The suitability of this designation was confirmed by epidemiologic studies conducted in East Africa, which confirmed that the disease was found commonly in regions with a truly tropical climate (i.e., a fairly constant high temperature and high relative humidity) at an altitude below 4000 feet.[16] Pyomyositis has been described, however, in children from geographic regions of the United States as diverse as New England,[9] California,[2] Iowa,[17] and Texas.[11,21,25] Numerous reported cases within the southern half of the United States have occurred in and around San Antonio, Texas.[5] In a 10-year chart review, one or two cases of pyomyositis per 4000 pediatric admissions occurred annually. In contrast, a review of consultations at the University of Iowa Children's Hospital in the northern United States disclosed fewer cases of pyomyositis.[7] In a children's hospital in Chandigarh, India, pyomyositis was the admission diagnosis for 40 patients over the course of a decade,[33] whereas in a children's center in Brisbane, Australia, 34 patients with the diagnosis of pyomyositis were found in a 10-year retrospective review.[20]

Pathophysiology

The etiologic agent of the skeletal muscle abscesses in more than 90% of cases is *S. aureus*. An increasing percentage are caused by community-associated MRSA.[21,32] A distant second bacteriologic isolate is *Streptococcus*, including group A and nonhemolytic strains.

Miyake[18] studied extensively the experimental conditions under which *Staphylococcus* spp. cause muscle abscesses. When healthy rabbits were given boluses of *Staphylococcus* intravenously, they occasionally developed small abscesses in the kidney, liver, or spleen but never in the skeletal muscles. When specific muscles were damaged by mechanical pinching or electric current 24 or 48 hours before the intravenous injection of bacteria was administered, small abscesses developed within 2 to 28 days at some of the injured sites in nearly half of the animals. Abscesses were not found in healthy muscle tissue.

The role of trauma was supported further by a study of pyomyositis in 1963 in the British Army.[3] After physicians found this disease to be a common problem in army recruits serving in Asia, they investigated 32 cases and made several observations. Two-thirds of the men recalled having experienced trauma at the affected site, the incidence of abscesses increased as the severity of physical training increased, and the abscesses occurred three times more commonly on the dominant (right) side of the body. In an analysis of 78 cases in Uganda, abscesses also were found more commonly on the right side of the body.[16]

From experimental evidence and clinical observations, two conditions commonly are found when pyomyositis occurs: muscle injury and bacteremia, usually staphylococcal. A reported case is illustrative.[11] A 12-year-old girl caught her left foot in the wheel of a moving bicycle and tumbled to the ground. One week later, she developed a furuncle of the foot, and, within the next 2 weeks, she developed painful lumps in muscles of the thigh, shoulder, and chest wall (which had been injured during the original accident). Cultures from the furuncle and blood and from the incised muscle abscesses grew *S. aureus*. The initial episode of trauma resulted in a staphylococcal skin lesion and, presumably, a bacteremia that seeded sites of previously bruised muscle.

Seven children with pyomyositis are described in Table 57.1. An analysis of all seven cases illustrates the consistent association of pyomyositis with trauma. Sources of muscle trauma have ranged from bicycle accidents to strenuous aerobic exercises. Many of these cases explain the predilection of the disease to occur in warmer climates or warmer seasons; concomitant skin infections and muscle trauma are more likely to occur in a climate in which children can play or work outside wearing fewer clothes. An unusual cause of muscle trauma was an intramuscular inactivated influenza vaccination (case 6). One predisposing disease not listed in Table 57.1 is varicella (chickenpox), in which muscle abscesses are secondary to bacterial invasion via the skin vesicles.[12]

In older textbooks, pyomyositis is said to occur in individuals who are malnourished and who have multiple parasitic infections. However, this association has not been confirmed in children with pyomyositis seen in the United States, Australia, or India.[7,13,33] Furthermore extensive immunologic evaluations also have been normal; the tests included quantitative immunoglobulins, enumeration of T-lymphocyte subpopulations, total hemolytic complement levels, and leukocyte function as tested by reduction of nitroblue tetrazolium.

Clinical Presentation

Pyomyositis often is considered a disease of adolescents and young adults, even though it occurs in individuals of all ages, including infants and young children.[2,6,13] Boys are affected more often than girls.[6,33] As more girls enter competitive sporting activities, however, pyomyositis is being reported in female athletes.[17] Many children with pyomyositis have a solitary lesion, but multiple lesions are common findings, especially when the latest imaging technology is used (see the section on Diagnosis). The most common site of abscess formation is the thigh, followed by the calf, buttock, arm, scapula, and chest wall. The muscle lesions are firm or "woody" to palpation, with a well-defined border. The sign of fluctuation may be difficult to elicit. Erythema and warmth often are not apparent because of the deep location of the masses, although diffuse tenderness usually occurs. When a muscle in an extremity is involved, the entire limb may be swollen. Occasionally pyomyositis also can occur in muscles of the pelvis, in which case pain may be transferred to the hip.[14,21]

In case reports with a clinical history, children with pyomyositis often had similar presenting complaints.[7,11] Many had incurred a recent accidental injury (often involving a leg) that usually was not considered serious. After a few days, the children developed low-grade fever, muscle pain, and, occasionally, an impaired gait. These symptoms persisted a few days to a few weeks until a mass appeared. When first examined,

TABLE 57.1 Pyomyositis and Trauma

Case[a]	Sex	Age (y)	Source of Trauma	Circumstances of Trauma	Extent of Disease
1	F	12	Bicycle accident	Thrown from bicycle onto street after foot was caught in the wheel	Right deltoid, right chest wall, left thigh, right groin
2	M	3	Fall while running	Fell while running on street	Left calf, right scapula, right buttock
3	M	11	Hay bale accident	Struck in abdomen by bale of hay thrown from a hay baler	Abdominal wall musculature
4	M	6	Blunt trauma to abdomen	Struck in abdomen during mock fistfight with sibling	Abdominal wall musculature
5	F	17	Aerobic exercises	Injured while instructing others in aerobic exercises	Left thigh
6	M	1	Injection	Influenza vaccination into right thigh muscle	Right thigh and septicemia
7	F	13	Volleyball accident	Fell several times diving for volleyball during training exercises	Left iliopsoas

[a]Cases 1 and 2 from reference 11, cases 3 and 4 from reference 5, cases 5 from reference 7, case 6 previously unpublished, and case 7 from reference 17.

BOX 57.1 Infectious Causes of Myositis

Bacterial
Tropical pyomyositis
Acute bacterial myositis

Viral
Influenza myositis
Coxsackievirus myositis

Fungal
Disseminated candidiasis

Parasitic
Trichinosis
Cysticercosis
Toxoplasmosis

many of the patients were considered to have only a contusion or a hematoma; occasionally a child was diagnosed as having a rhabdomyosarcoma. Although the disease usually occurs in individuals who are otherwise healthy, pyomyositis has been reported in patients with malignancy. Pyomyositis also may develop in children with acquired immunodeficiency syndrome or other immunodeficiency.[13] The pathophysiology of pyogenic muscle abscess may not be the same, however, in immunodeficient individuals with increased susceptibility to bacterial infection. Most children with pyomyositis have no definable immunologic abnormalities.

An unusual clinical presentation is acute abdominal pain. Beck and Grose[5] described two children with pyomyositis whose initial complaints were confined to the abdominal wall. One patient, a 6-year-old child, had been struck in the abdomen in a mock fistfight with an older sibling. One week later, he developed a low-grade fever and began to walk with a stoop; after another week, his mother detected a "knot" in his right mid-abdominal wall. The second case involved the 11-year-old son of a rancher; the boy was struck in the abdomen by a bale of hay tossed from a hay baler. When he subsequently developed symptoms of abdominal pain, the diagnosis of appendicitis was entertained. When a mass later became palpable in his abdominal wall, rhabdomyosarcoma was suspected. A correct diagnosis was made after the use of scintigraphy and sonography (Fig. 57.1).[5] Reviews from Africa and India also included patients with muscle abscesses in the anterior abdominal wall.[2,33]

Diagnosis

The diagnosis of pyomyositis should be considered in any child with fever and acute muscle pain, especially if a recent history of trauma exists. When a child has visible masses at commonly involved sites, such as the thigh, the diagnosis of pyomyositis can be made by needle

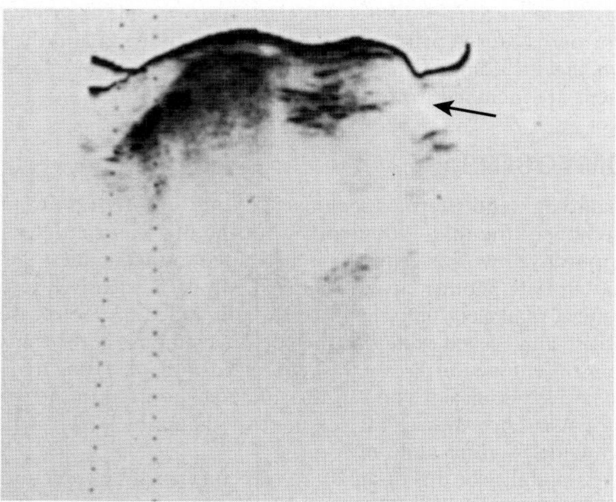

FIG. 57.1 Sonogram of the abdominal wall of a patient with pyomyositis. The transverse view of the abdomen shows an abscess cavity in the right belly of the rectus abdominis muscle *(arrow)*.

aspiration of a mass. Blood cultures occasionally are positive.[1] If a febrile child complains of myalgia in an extremity but has no palpable masses, the differential diagnosis must include more common inflammatory and infectious conditions of the bone or joint. A definitive diagnosis usually depends on one or more radiologic procedures. Plain films may show a soft tissue swelling or even a widened fascial plane suggestive of a mass lesion. Ultrasonography is used commonly in emergency treatment centers for diagnosis of muscle masses and to guide percutaneous aspiration for culture and drainage.[22,33] Ultrasonography is preferable as an initial imaging procedure because it avoids the radiation exposure from computed tomography (CT) or scintigrams (Fig. 57.1).[31]

Magnetic resonance imaging (MRI) is very helpful in delineating the extent and number of muscle abscesses. In many cases, the abscess is much larger than suspected by physical signs and symptoms. The MRI scans of an illustrative case are presented in Fig. 57.2. The patient was a 17-year-old girl with a swollen left lower thigh. She worked part-time as an attendant in an athletic club, where she participated in some of the vigorous exercise programs. Radiographs of the knee were normal, whereas a technetium bone scan showed slightly increased radionuclide uptake in the soft tissues around the distal left femur. MRI of the left and right thighs showed a large fluid collection extending from the middle to distal left femur. Surgical exploration identified extensive abscess formation around the posterior aspect of the femur; the culture grew *S. aureus*. The affected muscle groups included the vastus medialis, vastus intermedius, vastus lateralis, and biceps femoris. The bone was not involved. For the reasons described, MRI has become a preferred procedure for establishing the diagnosis of pyomyositis.[14,26,31]

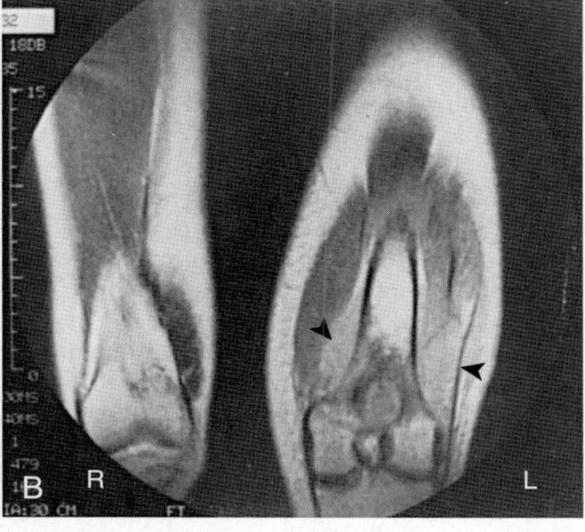

FIG. 57.2 Magnetic resonance imaging of the thighs of a patient with pyomyositis. (A) Axial images of the right *(R)* and left *(L)* thighs. (B) Coronal images around the distal femoral shafts and femoral condyles. The scans show several well-defined areas of extremely high intensity in the muscle bundles and fascial planes from the middle to distal left femur *(arrows)*. The high signal intensity suggests a fluid collection (e.g., an abscess) rather than a neoplastic process. Edema of the subcutaneous tissues also is evident in the lateral aspect of the swollen left thigh. There are no abnormal signals within the bone.

Treatment in the United States and India

Because pyomyositis is an abscess of skeletal muscle, the treatment is usually surgical incision and drainage.[2] Several physicians have observed that smaller lesions resolve spontaneously, even before the antibiotic era. An important role for systemic antibiotics is to prevent the formation of further muscle abscesses, especially in a patient with proven bacteremia. Because *S. aureus* is the most likely agent, a semisynthetic penicillinase-resistant penicillin is the preferred antibiotic in communities with relatively little MRSA. Usually, nafcillin or oxacillin 150 to 200 mg/kg per day is administered intravenously (IV), divided every 6 hours in the United States. In India, cloxacillin at similar dosages is the antibiotic of choice.[33] When pyomyositis occurs in a patient with penicillin hypersensitivity, clindamycin 40 mg/kg per day divided every 8 hours can be substituted because of its excellent coverage of gram-positive cocci. Parenteral therapy is continued until clinical improvement is evident, usually within a few days after surgical drainage. Thereafter the antibiotics can be given orally for an additional 2 to 3 weeks.[22] A cephalosporin (cephalexin 50 to 75 mg/kg per day) or clindamycin (30 to 40 mg/kg per day) is commonly prescribed in the United States, whereas oral cloxacillin is given in India.

In many cities and countries, MRSA is now a common agent.[32] In a clinical analysis of 182 patients with pyomyositis from Texas Children's Hospital in Houston, more than 50% of the isolated *S. aureus* strains were MRSA.[21] In these communities, initial antibiotic management must include either IV clindamycin (40 mg/kg per day, divided every 8 hours) or vancomycin 60 mg/kg per day divided every 6 hours. In adolescents the dosage of vancomycin is usually reduced to 45 mg/kg per day, divided every 8 hours. Serum levels of vancomycin should be closely monitored to avoid nephrotoxicity. In India, a glycopeptide antibiotic closely related to vancomycin called teicoplanin can be substituted for vancomycin at the teicoplanin loading dosage.[29]

ACUTE BACTERIAL MYOSITIS

Far less common than classical (tropical) pyomyositis is acute bacterial myositis, usually caused by group A streptococci. In this condition, the bacterial infection often is not confined to distinct abscesses within the muscle, but instead it extends diffusely through one or more muscle groups. As with pyomyositis, the disease occurs more commonly in males than in females and usually is associated with prior physical exertion and perhaps minor trauma. In contrast to pyomyositis, most published cases of acute bacterial myositis have occurred in adults and not in children.[4] The disease has been divided by Svane[28] into four main types, ranging from a fatal septicemic form to more benign subacute forms.

Clinical Presentation

The main clinical difference between the acute myositis syndrome and the pyomyositis syndrome is the virulence of streptococcal myositis. A case in a San Antonio, Texas, native is illustrative. The patient was a 23-year-old jackhammer operator who was admitted because of high fever, malaise, and pains in his arms. On examination, both upper extremities were tender to palpation, and faint erythema was visible over the same areas. He soon became incoherent, and his general condition quickly deteriorated. Death followed within 24 hours. Blood cultures drawn before death grew group A streptococcus, and cultures of the biceps muscles obtained at autopsy grew the same organism. This patient presumably incurred considerable minor trauma to the muscles of the upper arms and shoulders from his work as a jackhammer operator; these muscles were subsequently infected during a transient group A streptococcal bacteremia. This case is similar to others described in the literature.[4,28] Two reported cases of streptococcal myositis in children involved the left thigh and the left paravertebral muscles.[19] The first child developed septic shock and required intensive care for 27 days before a definitive diagnosis was made by CT imaging.

Diagnosis

Blood cultures are positive most often in patients with the most significant clinical symptoms. Cultures of muscle biopsy specimens may yield a profuse growth of bacteria. Rarely myositis has occurred as a delayed complication of chickenpox, often together with fasciitis.[12,17,23] In this situation, bacteremia may not be documented because the bacterial process usually is the result of contiguous spread from a secondarily infected pock lesion. These streptococcal complications of chickenpox often occur in an extremity, which may become swollen and painful. Under these circumstances, MRI can be an extremely valuable diagnostic tool to gauge the depth and extent of inflammation.[27]

Treatment and the Eagle Effect

The treatment of acute streptococcal myositis can become a medical emergency. As soon as the diagnosis is suspected, bacteriologic cultures should be obtained and intravenous therapy should be initiated with a high-dose semisynthetic penicillin (e.g., nafcillin or cloxacillin IV at 50 mg/kg every 6 hours) and also vancomycin in communities in which MRSA infection is common. If the cultures yield group A streptococci rather than *Staphylococcus,* the antibiotic can be switched to penicillin

G at an equivalent high dosage. Surgical consultation is required to evaluate the need for debridement and drainage. Serial imaging by ultrasonography and possibly MRI is advisable to document the extent of the disease and the response to antibiotic therapy. In severe cases of bacterial myositis, the total duration of hospitalization can exceed 4 weeks.[1,19]

An apparent resurgence of serious streptococcal infection has led to an increased interest in what has been called the *Harry Eagle effect,* named after the scientist who first described the failure of penicillin to eradicate group A streptococcal infection in a mouse model.[8] Eagle inoculated mice intramuscularly with group A streptococci and observed a markedly retarded bactericidal action of penicillin on organisms in the older abscesses, even though the bacteria remained highly sensitive to the antibiotic. Even massive doses of penicillin 10,000 times greater than the minimum inhibitory concentration were not effective at eradicating the bacteria. Subsequent studies by other investigators confirmed the existence of the Eagle effect and disclosed that clindamycin showed superior efficacy to penicillin in treatment of streptococcal myositis in the mouse model.[27] Otherwise stated, penicillin most likely fails to kill stationary-phase streptococci in muscle infections, an explanation for the Eagle effect. Under these conditions, treatment of the patient is continued with IV penicillin and IV clindamycin until both clinical and laboratory improvements have been documented.

MISCELLANEOUS CAUSES OF MYOSITIS

Viral infection occasionally leads to myositis (see Box 57.1). The most common example undoubtedly is myositis associated with influenza virus infection in children. Typically school-aged children are affected. Muscle groups of the legs often are involved, associated with a marked elevation of serum creatine phosphokinase. Clinical symptoms generally last 2 to 4 days. Another far less common myositis is caused by coxsackievirus B infection. This disease is termed *epidemic pleurodynia* because the myositis frequently involves the chest and upper abdomen. The enteroviral infection is also known as *Bornholm disease,* named after the Danish island where it was first described.

Fungal infection (e.g., *Candida albicans*) can cause myositis. Candidal myositis is uncommon, however, and usually occurs in patients who are severely immunocompromised. Frequently other sites also are involved by the disseminated fungal infection in addition to muscle.

Parasitic infection can cause myositis. The best known is trichinosis, caused by ingestion of the encysted larvae of *Trichinella spiralis.* The larvae typically are found in products containing pork or wild game, such as bear meat. The first signs of illness are fever and abdominal pain. Later muscle pain is noted in the neck and chest. Eventually calcifications form in the involved muscles. Treatment of the acute disease with mebendazole or albendazole may be beneficial. Another parasite more common in Central and South America is *Taenia solium.* Ingestion of eggs of this pork tapeworm leads to cysticercosis, with calcified densities in skeletal muscle. Finally toxoplasmosis infection can lead to symptoms of myositis. During acute infection, *Toxoplasma gondii* can encyst in the skeletal muscle and lead to an inflammatory myopathy closely resembling dermatomyositis.

NEW REFERENCES SINCE THE SEVENTH EDITION

15. Malhotra P, Singh S, Sud A, et al. Tropical pyomyositis: experience of a tertiary care hospital in northwest India. *J Assoc Physicians India.* 2000;48:1057-1059.
20. Moriarty P, Leung C, Walsh M, et al. Increasing pyomyositis presentations among children in Queensland, Australia. *Pediatr Infect Dis J.* 2015;34:1-4.
23. Sauler A, Saul T, Lewiss RE. Point-of-care ultrasound differentiates pyomyositis from cellulitis. *Am J Emerg Med.* 2015;33:482.e3-482.e5.
29. Svetitsky S, Leibovic L, Paul M. Comparative efficacy and safety of vancomycin versus teicoplanin. *Antimicrob Agents Chemother.* 2009;53:4069-4079.
33. Verma S, Singhi SC, Marwaha RK, et al. Tropical pyomyositis in children: 10 years experience of a tertiary care hospital in northern India. *J Trop Pediatr.* 2013;59:243-245.

The full reference list for this chapter is available at ExpertConsult.com.

Cutaneous Manifestations of Systemic Infections

58

James D. Cherry

Many illnesses caused by infectious agents have associated cutaneous manifestations. In some cases, the exanthem may be the hallmark of the disease; in others, it may be only a vague indicator of a more significant underlying process. When an exanthem occurs, it often offers important clues to the etiology of a patient's illness. Although most exanthematous illnesses in children are benign, their differential diagnosis is critical because the early manifestations of potentially fatal bacterial and rickettsial diseases frequently have cutaneous findings.

HISTORY

Exanthematous manifestations of infectious illnesses have been important since medical antiquity. Major epidemics of both measles and smallpox occurred in the Roman Empire and in China at the beginning of the Christian era.[26,142] Scarlet fever was recognized as a distinct entity in the 17th century, and chickenpox and rubella were identified in the 18th and 19th centuries, respectively.[50]

In the writings of the early 20th century, maculopapular exanthematous illnesses of children frequently were referred to by number. Scarlet fever and measles historically were the first two classic maculopapular exanthems of childhood. Which one had the honor of being the "first disease" is unknown today. The "third disease" was rubella, which was recognized by the beginning of the 20th century as a distinct entity.[74,94,173,179,199–201] In 1900, Dukes[68] described an exanthematous illness with the characteristics of both rubella and scarlet fever, which he suggested was a "fourth disease." The general opinion today is that his disease was not a distinct entity. Shaw[201] suggested that Dukes' cases had mild atypical scarlet fever, and Powell[173] raised the possibility that the illness resulted from epidermolytic toxin–producing staphylococci. My opinion has been that probably rubella and scarlet fever both were epidemic in the student population under Dr. Dukes' care; combined infections led to the confusion. In 1991, Morens and Katz[150] came to the same conclusion.

Erythema infectiosum (see Chapter 152) commonly is referred to as the fifth disease, and roseola infantum (see Chapter 59) qualifies as the sixth disease.[200]

During the past 65 years, interest in exanthematous diseases has been renewed because a large number of previously unknown viruses and other infectious agents that cause cutaneous manifestations have been discovered. In addition, the pattern of disease caused by classic exanthem-producing agents has changed; smallpox has been eradicated, the epidemiology of measles and rubella has been altered by immunization, and ecologic changes have resulted in differences in viral and bacterially induced rashes.

ETIOLOGIC AGENTS

Many different types of viruses, chlamydiae, rickettsiae, mycoplasmas, bacteria, fungi, and protozoan and metazoan agents cause illnesses with associated cutaneous manifestations. Although this chapter is devoted to systemic infectious diseases with cutaneous manifestations, the demarcation between exanthematous disease of systemic and local origin is not always readily apparent. For example, the recurrent cold sore caused by herpes simplex virus (HSV) infection frequently is considered a local problem, although its nature and pathogenesis involve central virus latency and host systemic immune functions. Similarly superficial fungal diseases and other local infections, such as warts, may be quite dependent on more general immunologic functions of the host. The exanthems of enteroviral infections frequently are confused with those caused by insect bites and allergic problems.

Table 58.1 presents viruses that have cutaneous manifestations in humans. Erythema infectiosum is caused by human parvovirus B19.[7,227] This virus also is an important cause of the papular-purpuric gloves-and-socks syndrome that is an uncommon occurrence and mainly affects young adults.[3,6,51,84,93,98,145,205,206] Human parvovirus B19 also has been associated with a vesiculopustular exanthem, erythema multiforme, and other petechial and purpuric rashes. In one study, an erythematous maculopapular rash was noted in 9% of children with human bocavirus infections.[9] Adenovirus types 1, 2, 3, 4, 7, and 7a have been isolated from children and young adults with exanthem.[50,118,231,232] The overall clinical expression rate of exanthem in adenovirus infection rarely has been studied. Fukumi and associates[87] noted that rash occurred in 2% of adenoviral infections, Hope-Simpson and Higgins[105] indicated a rate of approximately 8%, and Esposito and associates[76] noted an occurrence rate of 5.7%.

Eight species in the *Herpesvirus* genus have cutaneous manifestations associated with infection, but clinical expression rates vary greatly. Nearly all primary varicella infections are associated with exanthem, whereas exanthem with acquired cytomegalovirus infection is a rare manifestation.[20,23,50,185,211,231] The incidence of exanthem in Epstein-Barr virus (EBV) infection varies from 3% to 30%, depending on whether concomitant amoxicillin is administered.[16,29,57,102,112,120,162,175,219,220] EBV has been associated with a unilateral laterothoracic exanthem in a 1-year-old girl and a drug-induced hypersensitivity syndrome in an 8-year-old boy.[72,192] Although firm data are lacking, probably fewer than 10% of primary infections with HSV type 1 are associated with cutaneous manifestations. Erythema multiforme occasionally occurs with recurrent HSV infections.[37,81,115,158] Human herpesvirus–6 (HHV-6) is a major cause of roseola infantum[11,227,240] (see Chapter 59). HHV-7 also is a cause of roseola infantum[10]; in addition, some evidence suggests that this virus and HHV-6 may play a role in pityriasis rosea.[69,70,178] HHV-8 infection is necessary for the development of Kaposi sarcoma in patients with acquired immunodeficiency syndrome (AIDS) and other immunodeficiency states.[110,124,148]

At present, human illnesses with cutaneous manifestations caused by poxviruses rarely occur in the United States. Because smallpox as a disease has ceased to exist, the use of vaccinia virus for immunization has decreased dramatically. However, the terrorist events of 2001 raised concern about the possible use of smallpox virus as a terrorist weapon. Because of this potential danger, smallpox vaccines are being produced and used again. With the increased use of these vaccines, cutaneous complications of vaccinia virus infection can be expected. Monkeypox is a relatively common illness in areas of Africa (see Chapter 164). Outside of Africa, monkeypox, orf, and paravaccinia (milker's nodules) continue to occur as isolated events in exposed individuals.[190,231,232] Human infection with tanapox virus is a geographically related illness occurring in limited areas of Kenya.

In the present era, enteroviruses are the leading cause of infection-related exanthematous diseases.[52,56,117,231,232] Thirty-eight types have been associated with rash illnesses. The clinical expression rate varies greatly among the different types; it is as high as 50% in children with coxsackievirus A16 and echovirus 9 infections. Only approximately 15% of individuals infected with echovirus 4 have exanthem, and rash is a rare occurrence in echovirus 6 infection. Hope-Simpson and Higgins[105] noted exanthem in approximately 5% of patients with rhinoviral respiratory illness.

Text continued on p. 545

TABLE 58.1 Clinical Characteristics of Viral Infections With Cutaneous Manifestations

Virus	Disease or Syndrome	Incubation Period (Days)	Main Season	Clinical Characteristics	EXANTHEM Lesions	EXANTHEM Distribution	Usual Duration (Days)
Human parvovirus B19	Erythema infectiosum; gloves-and-socks syndrome	7–17	Winter and spring	Biphasic illness with mild prodromal period with headache and malaise for 2–3 days, then 7-day symptom-free period, followed by typical exanthema	Three-stage exanthema: initially, rash on cheeks (slapped-cheek appearance) and then erythematous maculopapular rash on trunk and limbs; finally, rash develops a reticular pattern	Starts on face More prominent on extensor surfaces of extremities	7–21
Human bocavirus			Fall, winter, and spring	Fever, cough, coryza, respiratory distress (bronchitis, bronchiolitis, pneumonia)	Erythematous maculopapular	Mainly face, chest, and trunk	
Human papillomaviruses	Warts		Nonseasonal	Local cutaneous disease	Papular or nodular isolated lesions	Most common on extremities	100+
Adenovirus types 1, 2, 3, 4, 7, and 7a		6–9	Winter and spring	Fever and signs and symptoms of respiratory illness Occasionally, rash occurs after defervescence (roseola-like)	Most commonly erythematous, maculopapular, and discrete (rubelliform), but occasionally confluent (morbilliform) Rarely, erythema multiforme and Stevens-Johnson syndrome	Usually starts on face and spreads downward to trunk and extremities	3–5
Herpes simplex types 1 and 2	Cold sores, genital herpes, neonatal herpes, or other	2–12	Nonseasonal	Primary disease associated with fever and systemic symptoms Recurrent disease caused by exogenous and endogenous infections	Singular or grouped vesicular lesions varying in size from 2 to 10 mm, frequently on a mildly erythematous base Occasionally, erythema multiforme, Stevens-Johnson syndrome, and erythema nodosum	Lesions in primary infection with type 1 virus are mainly in and around the mouth Recurrent type 1 lesions usually perioral Primary and recurrent type 2 lesions usually on genitals	7–14
Human herpesvirus–6 (HHV-6)	Roseola infantum		Nonseasonal	Fever 3–5 days in duration, rapid defervescence, and then the appearance of rash	Erythematous macular or maculopapular	Most prominent on neck and trunk Face and extremities may be affected	1–2
Human herpesvirus–7 (HHV-7)	Roseola infantum		Nonseasonal	Fever 3–5 days in duration, rapid defervescence, and then the appearance of rash	Erythematous macular or maculopapular	Most prominent on neck and trunk Face and extremities may be affected	1–2
Human herpesvirus–8 (HHV-8)	Kaposi sarcoma	Months to years	Nonseasonal	Asymptomatic infection Most commonly noted in AIDS patients but occurs in other immunodeficiency states	Purple to blue nodular, raised lesions	Any epidermal or mucosal surface	Months to years
Varicella zoster	Chickenpox (varicella)	12–20	Late fall, winter, and spring	Malaise and fever of 5–6 days' duration	Basic lesion is vesicular, but lesions go through stages: macules, papules, vesicles, and crusts Lesions occur in crops	Lesions more profuse on trunk than on extremities Proximal end of extremities more involved than distal end	8–10
	Herpes zoster		Nonseasonal	Endogenous infection Pain and paresthesia with dermatome distribution	Basic lesion is vesicular, but lesions go through stages: macules, papules, vesicles, and crusts	Lesions localized to area of skin innervated by a single sensory ganglion	10–28

Epstein-Barr	Infectious mononucleosis	28–49	Nonseasonal	Fever, pharyngitis, and lymphadenopathy Exanthem occurs in 3–13% of cases If amoxicillin is administered, then exanthema in 30% of cases	Most commonly erythematous, macular, maculopapular, and discrete (rubelliform) In association with ampicillin administration, the rash may be more vivid Erythema multiforme and urticaria may occur	Mainly on trunk and proximal end of extremities	2–7
Cytomegalovirus	Cytomegalovirus mononucleosis		Nonseasonal	Acquired: mild febrile illness with lymphadenopathy Congenital: disseminated disease	Erythematous, maculopapular, and discrete Vesicular or petechial in congenital infection	Located mainly on trunk and proximal end of extremities	2–7
Vaccinia	Roseola vaccinatum, eczema vaccinatum, vaccination "take," or disseminated vaccinia		Nonseasonal	Illness caused by direct exposure via vaccination or exposure to a vaccinee	Vaccination and eczema vaccinatum lesions go through stages: papule, vesicle, pustule, and scab Roseola vaccinatum: erythematous maculopapular lesions Occasionally erythema multiforme Disseminated vaccinia: papular or vesicular lesions	Lesions in roseola vaccinatum, eczema vaccinatum, and disseminated vaccinia are generalized	7–14
Variola	Smallpox	8–17	Seasonal by geographic area	Abrupt onset of high fever, headache, and muscle and joint pain Rash appears 2–4 days after onset	Basic lesion is vesicular, but lesions go through stages: macules, papules, vesicles, pustules, and crusts	Most prominent on exposed body surfaces Starts on extremities and face Spreads centripetally	12–20
Monkeypox				Similar to mild smallpox Exposure to monkeys No human-to-human spread	Similar to mild smallpox	Similar to mild smallpox	
Orf	Ecthyma contagiosum	4–7	Spring	Disease of sheep acquired by humans	Initially erythematous papule Becomes umbilicated, nodular, and then vesicular Occasionally erythema multiforme	Solitary lesion, usually on hands	30–40
Molluscum contagiosum	Molluscum contagiosum			Local cutaneous disease	Umbilicated nodular lesions: singular or clusters	Most common on face, inner aspect of thigh, breasts, and genitalia	100+
Paravaccinia	Milker's nodules	4–7		Human infection acquired from infected calves	Nodular lesion Occasionally erythema multiforme	Solitary lesion, usually on hands	30–40
Tanapox				A virus of monkeys Human infection associated with fever and regional lymphadenopathy	Umbilicated vesicular lesion	Upper part of body Solitary lesion	35–56

Continued

TABLE 58.1 Clinical Characteristics of Viral Infections With Cutaneous Manifestations—cont'd

Virus	Disease or Syndrome	Incubation Period (Days)	Main Season	Clinical Characteristics	EXANTHEM Lesions	EXANTHEM Distribution	Usual Duration (Days)
Coxsackieviruses A2, A4, A5, A6, A7, A9, A10, and A16; coxsackieviruses B1-B5; echoviruses 1–7, 9, 11–14, 16–19, 24, 25, 30, and 33; enterovirus 71; parechoviruses 1 and 3		4–7	Summer and fall	Fever and mild to moderate pharyngitis Occasionally, herpangina, meningitis, and other manifestations of systemic viral infection Exanthem occurs in 5–50% of infections, depending on virus type Rash may occur during fever or after defervescence; hand, foot, and mouth syndrome	Most commonly erythematous, maculopapular, and discrete May have macular, petechial, vesicular, and urticarial components Rarely erythema multiforme	Usually starts on face and spreads downward to trunk and extremities May have peripheral distribution (hand, foot, and mouth syndrome)	3–7
Rhinoviruses (many types)		2–4	Fall, winter, and spring	Mild fever and signs and symptoms of respiratory illness Exanthem occurs in about 5% of cases	Erythematous or maculopapular and discrete	Starts on face and spreads downward to trunk and extremities	1–4
Foot and mouth		3–4		Direct animal contact Fever, sore mouth, and lymphadenopathy Vesicles and ulcers within the mouth	Vesicular lesions	Hands and feet	3–6
Colorado tick fever		3–5	Summer	Fever, chills, eye pain, myalgia, and headache Diphasic course Rash in only about 10% of cases	Occasionally maculopapular but usually petechial	Maculopapular rash is generalized Petechial rash most prominent on arms, legs, and trunk	2–7
Reovirus 2 and 3		4–7	Summer	Fever, mild pharyngitis, and cervical adenopathy	Erythematous or maculopapular Discrete or confluent Occasionally vesicular	Starts on face and spreads downward to trunk and extremities	3–9
Rotavirus	Gianotti-Crosti syndrome; infantile acute hemorrhagic edema	2–4	Fall, winter, and spring	Gastroenteritis	Petechial and morbilliform	Generalized	7–14
Chikungunya, o'nyong-nyong, Ross River, Sindbis			During periods of arthropod prevalence	Fever, headache, eye pain, and marked myalgia, arthralgia, and arthritis Geographically localized diseases	Rubelliform and morbilliform Frequently vesicular and petechial	Starts on face and spreads downward to trunk and extremities	
Rubella	Rubella (German measles)	15–21	Winter and spring	Mild symptoms with onset 1–5 days before rash Fever usually <38.5°C (101.5°F) Headache, malaise, and suboccipital and postauricular lymphadenopathy	Erythematous, maculopapular, and discrete	Starts on face and spreads downward to trunk and extremities	4–7

West Nile				Sudden onset of fever, chills, and drowsiness Rash may appear during or after fever Geographically localized disease	Erythematous, macular, and maculopapular	Starts on trunk and spreads to extremities	3–6
Dengue and Kunjin		7	During periods of specific arthropod prevalence	Sudden onset of high fever, then severe headache, myalgia, arthralgia, abdominal pain, and marked diaphoresis Fever lasts 5–6 days and ends by crisis Rash appears within 48 hours of onset of fever Geographically localized diseases	Initially, macular, flushed appearance, then erythematous, maculopapular rash May be scarlatiniform Frequently becomes petechial and purpuric Small vesicles occur in Kunjin virus infection	Initial macular rash is more prominent centrally Maculopapular rash may start on hands and feel and spread to trunk	3–10
Influenza A and B		2–5	Fall, winter, and spring	Fever, cough, headache, and muscle aches and pains Usually in young children Rash an occasional occurrence	Erythematous, maculopapular, and discrete (rubelliform) Rarely erythema multiforme	Starts on face and trunk and spreads to extremities	1–3
Respiratory syncytial		2–5	Fall, winter, and spring	Fever, coryza, and respiratory distress (bronchitis, bronchiolitis, or pneumonia) Usually in children <2 years	Erythematous, maculopapular, and discrete (rubelliform)	Starts on face and trunk and spreads to extremities	1–3
Human metapneumovirus			Fall, winter, and spring	Fever, coryza, and respiratory distress (bronchitis, bronchiolitis, or pneumonia)	Erythematous, maculopapular		
Parainfluenza 1-3		2–5	Fall, winter, and spring	Fever, coryza, nasopharyngitis, croup, and bronchitis Usually in young children	Erythematous, maculopapular, and discrete (rubelliform)	Starts on face and trunk and spreads to extremities	1–3
Mumps	Mumps	14–21	Fall, winter, and spring	Fever, headache, and salivary gland swelling	Erythematous, maculopapular, and discrete; also, urticaria and vesicles; rarely, erythema multiforme	Most prominent on trunk	2–5
Measles	Measles	8–12	Winter and spring	Onset with fever, cough, coryza, and conjunctivitis About 2 days after onset, appearance of enanthem (Koplik spots); and 2 days later, onset of exanthem	Erythematous, maculopapular, and confluent Develops a brownish appearance, and fine desquamation occurs	Starts behind ears and on forehead Spreads downward over body Confluence most prominent on face, trunk, and proximal end of extremities	5–7
Lassa	Lassa fever			Sudden onset of fever, chills, headache, and sore throat Progresses to pneumonia and renal failure Geographically localized outbreaks	Macular and sometimes petechial	Localized or general	

Continued

TABLE 58.1 **Clinical Characteristics of Viral Infections With Cutaneous Manifestations—cont'd**

Virus	Disease or Syndrome	Incubation Period (Days)	Main Season	Clinical Characteristics	EXANTHEM		Usual Duration (Days)
					Lesions	Distribution	
Hepatitis B	Papular acrodermatitis of childhood	50–180		Insidious onset with arthralgia, arthritis, and rash occurring before jaundice	Maculopapular, macular, or urticarial In young children, papular (Gianotti-Crosti syndrome or papular acrodermatitis of childhood) Rarely, erythema multiforme	Generalized	4–10
Hepatitis C	Mixed cryoglobulinemia (not reported in children)	7–14	Nonseasonal	Acute hepatitis followed by chronic infection Skin findings occur late in disease	Palpable purpura	Mostly buttocks, lower extremities	Variable
Marburg		5–7		Headache, conjunctivitis, photophobia, myalgia, vomiting, diarrhea, and fever (biphasic) Exposure to vervet monkeys	Initially erythematous macular, then discrete maculopapular, and finally confluent maculopapular Exfoliation occurs Occasionally purpura	Generalized	2–14
Ebola	Hemorrhagic fever	5–10	Occurs in outbreaks	Febrile illness that progresses to hemorrhage, shock, and coma	Maculopapular rash that appears toward end of first week of illness	Lateral sides of trunk, groin, and axillae Can become generalized but spares the face	14–60
Hantavirus	Hemorrhagic fever with renal syndrome (nephropathia epidemica)		Spring and summer outbreaks	Febrile illness with hemorrhagic and renal manifestations	Flushing and petechial rash	Face (flushing), skin folds (petechiae)	14–28
HIV		14–60	Nonseasonal	Fever, pharyngitis, myalgia, arthralgias, adenopathy, and rash	Macular	Mainly chest and abdomen	7
Human T-lymphotropic virus	Infective dermatitis		Nonseasonal	Acute onset of eczema	Severe exudative eczema with a crusting, generalized, fine papular rash	Scalp, eyelid margins, perinasal skin, retroauricular areas, axillae, and groin	Months to years

Data from references 1, 2, 4, 6–12, 16, 19, 20, 23, 27, 37, 40, 43, 45, 47, 49–51, 53, 57, 60, 61, 63, 65, 66, 68, 81–87, 93, 98, 102, 104, 105, 108, 110, 112, 114, 120, 124, 125, 127, 130–132, 138, 148, 151–155, 158–160, 166, 168, 174, 182, 183, 185, 186, 188–190, 194–196, 205, 206, 210, 214, 219, 220, 224, 227, 228, 230–232, 239-242.

A young adult research worker had an influenza-like illness and a hand, foot, and mouth syndrome–like rash caused by infection with a calicivirus (San Miguel sea lion virus serotype 5) of oceanic origin.[204]

Two percent of patients with Colorado tick fever encephalitis have exanthem.[52] Although infection with reoviruses occurs commonly, exanthem has been noted on only nine occasions.[52,132] A morbilliform rash has been observed in one adult with a rotavirus infection, and a 4-year-old boy was noted to have a petechial rash in association with a rotaviral illness.[63,186] Di Lernia and Ricci[65] described three cases of Gianotti-Crosti syndrome and one child with infantile acute hemorrhagic edema associated with rotavirus infections.

Of the Togaviridae family of viruses, rubella virus is the most important as a worldwide cause of exanthematous disease. Several alphaviruses also frequently cause exanthems.[116,155,231,232] Each of these viruses has a marked geographic distribution. Similarly flaviviruses also have exanthem as part of their clinical expression, and they, too, have specific geographic boundaries.[231,232] In the New York City area outbreak of West Nile virus infection in 1999, 19% of patients had exanthem.[152] The rash was erythematous macular, papular, or morbilliform.

Exanthem generally is not considered to be a manifestation of influenza virus infection, but Hope-Simpson and Higgins[105] noted exanthem in approximately 8% of patients from whom influenza B virus was isolated and in 1% or 2% of those infected with influenza A virus. The occurrence of Gianotti-Crosti syndrome was noted 1 week after live H1N1 influenza virus vaccination in a 9-year-old boy.[123] Measles virus is the most notable of the Paramyxoviridae family with an associated exanthem. However, exanthem occurs rather frequently in young children infected with parainfluenza virus types 1, 2, and 3 and also in those with respiratory syncytial virus (RSV) illnesses.[89,100,101,221,224] Hope-Simpson and Higgins[105] noted a 15% incidence of rash in RSV infection and an approximately 15% incidence in parainfluenza virus infection. Rash, which was not described further, was observed in four children with respiratory illnesses caused by human metapneumovirus infections.[174] Exanthem also has been noted on rare occasion with mumps virus infection.[50]

An outbreak involving 185 cases caused by Zika virus (a flavivirus) occurred on an island in Micronesia in 2007.[73] The patients (children and adults) had fever, macular or maculopapular exanthems, arthritis or arthralgia, and nonpurulent conjunctivitis.

Lassa fever virus, Marburg virus, Ebola virus, and hepatitis B virus all have been associated with exanthem on occasion.[43,47,66,80,168,231] Rash was noted in 3 of 5 children with coronavirus OC43 lower respiratory tract infections.[215] Hepatitis B virus is the main cause of papular acrodermatitis (Gianotti-Crosti syndrome) in children.[47,189,196] Chronic hepatitis C virus infection occasionally causes systemic vasculitis and cryoglobulinemia in adults, with purpuric lesions concentrated on the lower extremities.[2,104] Other cutaneous manifestations of chronic hepatitis C virus infection include urticaria, erythema nodosum, lichen planus, and nodular prurigo.[114,239]

Hantaviruses cause two major syndromes throughout the world: hemorrhagic fever with renal syndrome and hantavirus pulmonary syndrome.[151,153,154,210] Exanthem (facial flushing and petechial lesions in skinfolds) occurs in approximately 30% of patients with hemorrhagic fever with renal syndrome, but rash is not reported in the hantavirus pulmonary syndrome. A macular rash has been noted in association with acute infection with human immunodeficiency virus type 1 (HIV-1).[151,153,154,210] Several reports have associated human T-lymphotropic virus type 1 (HTLV-1) with an atypical form of eczema termed *infective dermatitis.* This exanthem has an acute onset and is somewhat recalcitrant to treatment.[125,127,138]

Chlamydiae, rickettsiae, and mycoplasmas associated with cutaneous manifestations are listed in Table 58.2. Of the chlamydiae, only *Chlamydia psittaci* has been associated with exanthem. In contrast, all rickettsiae that infect humans, with the exception of *Coxiella burnetii,* usually display some cutaneous manifestations as part of their systemic disease.[32,75,92,126,133,157,163,193] Approximately 4% to 7% of adults with Q fever have exanthem.[41,208] Of the mycoplasmas that infect humans, only *Mycoplasma pneumoniae* is associated with exanthem.[13,52,54] In epidemics, exanthem occurs in approximately 15% of persons with respiratory illness.

In Table 58.3, bacterial agents for which cutaneous manifestations are part of the clinical illness are presented (see Chapter 60A). The clinical expression of exanthem varies tremendously among the different etiologic agents, as do the conditions associated with a specific infection. For example, infection with phage group 2 staphylococci usually results in cutaneous disease in young infants, whereas the same organisms rarely cause illness in adults. Symptomatic infection with *Streptococcus pneumoniae* is associated with cutaneous manifestations only occasionally; on the other hand, similar systemic disease with *Neisseria meningitidis* virtually always is associated with the characteristic petechial exanthem. Of the other bacterial agents listed in Table 58.3, exanthem is most important in *Neisseria gonorrhoeae, Salmonella typhi, Streptobacillus moniliformis, Spirillum minus, Pseudomonas aeruginosa,* and *Treponema pallidum.*

Fungal, protozoan, and metazoan agents associated with cutaneous manifestations in humans are listed in Tables 58.4, 58.5, and 58.6, respectively. These agents and their diseases, discussed more completely in other chapters, are included here for completeness of the differential diagnosis.

EPIDEMIOLOGY

Tables 58.1 through 58.6 clearly show that exanthematous disease has many possible etiologic agents; hence, no unified epidemiology exists. Epidemiologic events related to specific agents are considered in the appropriate sections throughout this text. Each agent with exanthem as a clinical manifestation has a unique epidemiologic pattern that, if understood, distinguishes it from many of the other agents that cause otherwise identical clinical illnesses. In the evaluation of all patients with rash, exposure, season, and incubation period are important aspects of the diagnostic process.

PATHOPHYSIOLOGY AND PATHOLOGY OF EXANTHEMS

Even though the skin can respond in only a limited number of ways, what is obvious from the extensive number of etiologic agents is that multiple pathogenic mechanisms must occur. In many sections of this book, the pathology and pathophysiology of specific agents are presented in detail. An overview is presented here.

Small vessel vasculitis (leukocytoclastic vasculitis) is a leading event in most exanthematous illnesses caused by infectious agents.[207] The cutaneous manifestations of systemic diseases can be separated into three broad categories. The first category involves dissemination of infectious agents by blood (e.g., viremia and bacteremia), which results in secondary infection at the cutaneous site. The clinical cutaneous findings in this type of infection can be the direct result of infectious agents in the epidermis, dermis, or dermal capillary endothelium or can be the result of an immune response between the organism and antibody or cellular factors in the cutaneous location. The possible events in the skin with this type of infection are presented in Fig. 58.1. Chickenpox, many enteroviral infections, and meningococcemia are examples of diseases in which infectious agents have reached the skin through the blood and are causing the cutaneous findings without the additional contribution of host immune factors. In illnesses such as measles, rubella, and gonococcemia, the timing, histologic picture, and difficulty of direct recovery of the agent by culture suggest both a direct effect and an immune-mediated response.

The second category of pathogenesis relates to the dissemination of known specific toxins of infectious agents. The infection is in a localized area of the body, but the toxin liberated by the infectious agents reaches the skin by blood-borne dissemination. Three examples of toxin-mediated exanthematous disease are streptococcal scarlet fever, staphylococcal scalded skin syndrome, and toxic shock syndrome.

The third category of pathogenesis in systemic disease with exanthem is poorly understood but appears to have an immunologic basis. Most important in this category are the clinical pictures of erythema multiforme, erythema multiforme exudativum (Stevens-Johnson syndrome), and erythema nodosum. In erythema multiforme associated with

Text continued on p. 553

TABLE 58.2 **Clinical Characteristics of Chlamydial, Rickettsial, and Mycoplasmal Infections With Cutaneous Manifestations**

Agent	Disease or Syndrome	Incubation Period (Days)	Main Season	Clinical Characteristics	EXANTHEM Lesions	EXANTHEM Distribution	Usual Duration (Days)
Chlamydia psittaci	Psittacosis	7–14	Nonseasonal	Fever, chills, headache, and cough Respiratory distress	Erythematous macules Occasionally erythema multiforme or erythema nodosum	Mainly on trunk	2–7
Rickettsia akari	Rickettsialpox	7–14	Nonseasonal	Fever, chills, headache, backache, and malaise 4–7 days after onset of primary lesion at site of mite bite Geographically localized disease	Initial lesion at site of mite bite is papular and then vesicular, and finally an eschar forms Two days after onset of fever, erythematous maculopapular discrete rash occurs Lesions progress to small vesicles and later to scabs	Most prominent on trunk and proximal end of extremities	7–10
Rickettsia typhi	Endemic, murine typhus	7–14	Nonseasonal	Fever and headache Rash appears on 4th–7th day Geographically localized disease	Initially discrete macules and then erythematous maculopapular May become purpuric	Initially upper part of trunk and axilla Progresses to entire body except face, palms, and soles	7–21
Rickettsia prowazekii	Epidemic typhus	10–14	Nonseasonal	Sudden onset of fever, chills, headache, and myalgias Rash appears on days 4–7 Geographically localized disease	Initially discrete macules and then progresses to maculopapular and petechial lesions Sometimes purpuric	Appears first on trunk and spreads to extremities Spares palms and soles	7–14
Rickettsia tsutsugamushi	Scrub typhus	7–21	Nonseasonal	Sudden onset of chills, fever, and headache	Local lesion at site of chigger bite is present at onset of symptoms; characterized by vesicle, ulcer, and eschar Maculopapular rash occurs 5–8 days after onset of fever	Maculopapular rash first occurs on trunk and then becomes generalized	7–14
Rickettsia rickettsii	Rocky Mountain spotted fever	3–12	Summer	Abrupt onset of fever, chills, and headache Rash appears 2–4 days after onset	Early maculopapular, then petechial, and sometimes purpuric	Rash starts on distal end of extremities Rarely involves the trunk	7–14
Other tick-borne rickettsiae			Tick seasons	Similar to mild Rocky Mountain spotted fever	Similar to Rocky Mountain spotted fever; eschar at site of tick bite	Similar to Rocky Mountain spotted fever	7–14

R. sibirica	North Asian tick-borne rickettsiosis						
R. australis	Queensland tick typhus						
R. conorii	Boutonneuse fever; Mediterranean spotted fever						
R. africae	African tick fever						
Coxiella burnetii	Q fever	20–40	Nonseasonal	Acute febrile illness with chills, headache, and myalgia	Fine discrete macular rash occurring during febrile illness Transient urticarial rash also noted	Mainly on trunk	2–7
Ehrlichia and *Anaplasma* spp	Ehrlichiosis; anaplasmosis	14–28	Tick seasons	Similar to Rocky Mountain spotted fever, but rash usually not on palms and soles	Similar to endemic typhus	Similar to endemic typhus	7–14
Mycoplasma pneumoniae		21	All seasons	Gradual onset of fever, malaise, headache, and cough	Maculopapular rash occurs in 5–15% of cases Vesicular and bullous lesions common (Stevens-Johnson syndrome); more common in males Papular, petechial, and urticarial lesions also noted Erythema multiforme common	Rash most prominent on trunk and proximal end of extremities	7–14

Data from references 13, 14, 18, 32, 36, 41, 52, 54, 59, 75, 92, 99, 119, 126, 133, 141, 149, 157, 163, 176, 193, 208, 233, 238.

TABLE 58.3 Bacteria Associated With Cutaneous Manifestations

Agent	Disease or Syndrome	Clinical Characteristics	EXANTHEM: Lesions	EXANTHEM: Distribution
Gram-Positive Cocci				
Staphylococcus aureus, exfoliative toxin-producing, mainly phage group 2	Bullous impetigo	Usually occurs in neonates	Rapid progression from vesicles to bullous lesions	Most common in diaper area
	Scalded skin syndrome	May be epidemic	Scarlatiniform eruption with exfoliation	Generalized
	Toxic epidermal necrolysis (Ritter disease in infants <4 months; Lyell syndrome in older children)	Usually occurs in infants and children 1 month–5 years of age Mucopurulent nasal and eye discharge	Nikolsky sign present Crusty appearance around eyes and under nose	Most marked on trunk Generalized
	Staphylococcal scarlet fever or staphylococcal scarlatiniform eruption	Fever Fever and staphylococcal infection in throat but no evidence of pharyngitis	Scarlet fever–like rash with desquamation Pastia lines present	
Staphylococcus aureus, non–exfoliative toxin producing	Septicemic disease	Severe septicemia with osteomyelitis, arthritis, endocarditis, or pneumonia	Diffuse, erythematous, confluent, and macular rash (flush) With endocarditis, may have petechiae and splinter hemorrhages, Osler nodes, Janeway spots	Trunk and proximal end of extremities
Staphylococcus aureus, toxin-1 (TSST-1) producing	Toxic shock syndrome	Fever, intense myalgias, vomiting, and diarrhea Mental confusion and hypotension	Erythematous, deep red (sunburn-like) rash Desquamation occurs	Generalized
Staphylococcus aureus, non–exfoliative toxin producing	Folliculitis, furuncles, or carbuncles	See Chapter 60A, "Bacterial Skin Infections"		
Streptococcus pyogenes	Scarlet fever	Fever, pharyngitis, and cervical lymphadenitis Rash onset within 2 days of first symptoms Incubation period 3–4 days	Diffuse erythematous and fine maculopapular (looks and feels like red sandpaper) Rash darker in skin folds (Pastia lines) Desquamation occurs	Circumoral pallor Generalized rash, with trunk and proximal end of extremities being most involved
	Erysipelas	Fever, headache, and vomiting Localized infection	Circumscribed area that is raised and erythematous Advancing edge is irregular	Anywhere
	Impetigo	Localized superficial pyoderma See Chapter 60A, "Bacterial Skin Infections"	Discrete and coalescent lesions of a vesicular nature Quickly becomes more pustular and then crusts over with a yellowish brown appearance	Forearms, legs, and face
	Septicemia	Fever and systemic foci of infection	Petechiae	Diffuse
	Miscellaneous skin manifestations of *S. pyogenes* infections		Erythema multiforme, erythema nodosum, and erythema marginatum	
Streptococcus pneumoniae	Septicemia	Fever	Petechiae	Diffuse
Enterococcal and viridans group streptococci	Endocarditis	Endocarditis	Petechiae, splinter hemorrhages, Osier nodes, and Janeway spots	
Gram-negative cocci				
Neisseria gonorrhoeae	Gonococcemia	Fever and polyarthralgias	Papular, petechial purpuric, pustular, or necrotic lesions	Most common on extremities Extensor surfaces over joints
Neisseria meningitidis	Meningococcemia	Fever and pharyngitis Sudden onset of rash	Characteristic rash is petechial or purpuric Early lesions may be erythematous maculopapular, or urticarial	Generalized
Moraxella catarrhalis	Bacteremia	Fever and pharyngitis	Maculopapular and petechial	Generalized

Gram-positive Bacilli				
Bacillus anthracis	Anthrax	Fever, headache, malaise, and joint pain	Initially, macular, pruritic lesion Later, a papule forms and then vesiculation Vesicles last 2–6 days, and then eschar forms	Usually, single lesion initially at point of exposure, secondary lesions in area develop later
Listeria monocytogenes	Listeriosis	Neonatal meningitis with hepatosplenomegaly	Maculopapular, discrete lesions Pustules	Trunk and legs
Erysipelothrix rhusiopathiae	Crab or fishnet dermatitis	Fever and local pain	Erysipeloid lesion (violet or red)	Hands
Corynebacterium diphtheriae	Cutaneous diphtheria	Secondary infection in cutaneous wounds	Impetigo- or ecthyma-like Rarely, erythema multiforme	Exposed surfaces
Arcanobacterium hemolyticum	Scarlet fever–like illness	Fever and pharyngitis	Scarlet fever–like rash Occasionally, rubelliform	Generalized rash with peripheral predominance
Enteric Gram-Negative Bacilli				
Salmonella typhi	Typhoid fever	Malaise, headache, and marked fever Rash onset 10 days after onset of fever	Rose spots, 2- to 4-mm macular lesions	Discrete lesions on abdomen
Other *Salmonella* spp.	Septicemic salmonellosis	Similar to mild typhoid fever	Similar to typhoid fever	Similar to typhoid fever
Shigella sonnei	Shigellosis	Diarrhea	Urticaria	Diffuse
Campylobacter spp.		Gastroenteritis	Skin pustules and erythema nodosum	Lower part of legs
Other Gram-Negative Bacilli				
Francisella tularensis	Tularemia	Chills, fever, headache, and localized lymphadenopathy	Initial papule that later ulcerates	Site of inoculation
Haemophilus ducreyi	Chancroid	Local pain and tenderness	Pustular lesions that ulcerate	External genitalia
Haemophilus influenzae	Septicemia	Fever	Petechiae	Diffuse
			Reddish purple cellulitis	Cellulitis mainly on cheeks and extremities
Streptobacillus moniliformis	Rat-bite fever	Fever, chills, malaise, headache, and polyarthritis	Erythematous, maculopapular rash that may become petechial	Most prominent on extremities, including palms and soles
Yersinia pestis	Septicemic plague	Sudden onset of fever	Initial generalized erythema followed by petechiae and purpura	Generalized
Yersinia pseudotuberculosis		Mesenteric lymphadenitis	Erythema nodosum and scarlatiniform eruption	Lower part of legs and generalized
Yersinia enterocolitica	Yersiniosis	Enterocolitis	Erythema nodosum and urticaria	Lower part of legs and generalized
Bartonella bacilliformis	Bartonellosis, Carrión disease, or Oroya fever	Initially intermittent fever, malaise, and myalgias 30–60 days after initial fever, exanthem appears	Erythematous maculopapular Later recurrent nodules	Face and extensor surface of extremities
Bartonella quintana	Trench fever	Usually mild fever, headache, chills, and tibial bone pain	Macular rash	Mainly on trunk
Calymmatobacterium granulomatis	Granuloma inguinale	See *Calymmatobacterium granulomatis* (Chapter 130)	Nodular, ulcerovegetative, hypertrophic, or cicatricial lesions	Genitals

Continued

TABLE 58.3 **Bacteria Associated With Cutaneous Manifestations—cont'd**

Agent	Disease or Syndrome	Clinical Characteristics	EXANTHEM	
			Lesions	**Distribution**
Pseudomonas aeruginosa	Ecthyma gangrenosa	Septicemia (usually in immunocompromised patients)	Initially vesicular and then hemorrhagic Become ulcerated with central black necrotic eschar	Anywhere
	Pseudomonas folliculitis (health spa dermatitis)	Headache, malaise, and fatigue	Papular and pustular	Generalized
Burkholderia mallei	Glanders, melioidosis	Fever, malaise, chills, arthralgia, and muscle pains	Nodule or ulcer at site of inoculation and then widespread papules, bullae, and pustules	Generalized
Brucella spp.	Brucellosis	Acute or subacute febrile illness Erythematous and maculopapular	Exanthem in 8% of urticaria, maculopapular cases Occasionally vesicles	Generalized
Legionella pneumophila	Legionnaires' disease	Severe pneumonia	Maculopapular	Anterior of trunk
Bartonella henselae	Cat-scratch fever	Subacute regional lymphadenitis	Erythematous maculopapular, morbilliform, petechial, erythema nodosum, erythema multiforme, and erythema marginatum May be pruritic	Generalized
Acid-fast Bacilli				
Mycobacterium tuberculosis	Lupus vulgaris	Usually associated with other manifestations of tuberculosis	Reddish brown nodular or scaling lesions	Mainly on face and neck
	Papulonecrotic tuberculids	Associated with disseminated tuberculosis	Initially vesicular Become pustules, umbilical, and ulcerated and then form scabs and leave scars	Single or multiple lesions anywhere
Atypical Mycobacteria			Granulomatous and ulcerative lesions at site of superficial injury	Usually on hands
Mycobacterium leprae	Erythema nodosum leprosum	General findings of lepromatous leprosy	Erythematous nodular lesions	Disseminated Most prominent on face and extremities
Spirochetes				
Treponema pallidum	Primary syphilis Secondary syphilis	Chancre	Large ulcers with indurated edges Erythematous maculopapules that frequently are scaly (psoriasiform)	Genitals Generalized, including palms and soles
Treponema pertenue	Yaws		Papular lesions at sites of inoculations Lesions ulcerate, leaving a wart-like appearance	Anywhere
Borrelia burgdorferi	Lyme disease (erythema chronicum migrans)	Skin, cardiac, neurologic, and joint abnormalities	Expanding erythematous, annular lesions	Thighs, buttocks, or axillae
Treponema carateum	Pinta		Initially, erythematous, papular lesions; increase in size during 1-month period and become scaly	Exposed surfaces of body
Spirillum minus	Rat-bite fever	Fever and chills	Discrete, macular rash	Trunk and extremities, including palms and soles
Leptospira spp.	Leptospirosis	Fever, conjunctivitis, and anorexia Rash rarely noted	Erythematous maculopapular rash	Mainly on trunk
Borrelia spp.	Relapsing fever	Relapsing fever, headache, myalgia, and photophobia	Morbilliform and petechial Erythema multiforme	Generalized

Data from references 5, 17, 22, 25, 30, 31, 33–35, 38, 39, 42, 55, 62, 67, 71, 79, 94, 95, 97, 106, 107, 109, 111, 113, 121, 122, 128, 129, 134, 136, 137, 140, 144, 156, 161, 165, 167, 169, 171, 172, 177, 180, 187, 191, 198, 209, 211–213, 216–218, 223, 226, 229, 234, 236, 237, 243.

TABLE 58.4 **Fungi Associated With Cutaneous Manifestations**

Agent	Disease or Syndrome	Clinical Characteristics	EXANTHEM Lesions	EXANTHEM Distribution
Dermatophytic fungi	Tinea capitis, tinea cruris, tinea pedis, or tinea circinata		Localized, brownish, maculopapular lesions that are scaly	
Erythema nodosum				
Candida albicans	Congenital cutaneous candidiasis	Congenital infection	Discrete vesicular lesions	Generalized
	Chronic mucocutaneous candidiasis	Immunodeficiency disease	Confluent, erythematous, and exudative lesions	Generalized, including scalp
	Acquired candidiasis		Confluent, fiery red lesions	Most common in diaper area
Candida spp.	Systemic candidiasis	Severe opportunistic infection	Erythematous nodular lesions	Generalized
Histoplasma capsulatum	Histoplasmosis	Primary respiratory infection	Erythema nodosum, erythema multiforme, and erythematous maculopapular	
Cryptococcus neoformans	Cryptococcosis	Primary respiratory infection	Erythema nodosum and acneiform eruptions	
Coccidioides immitis	Coccidioidomycosis	Primary respiratory infection	Initially, erythematous, maculopapular rash Later, erythema multiforme and erythema nodosum	Generalized maculopapular rash
Sporotrichum schenckii	Sporotrichosis	Cutaneous inoculation	Nodular lesions that ulcerate	Usually, hands, arms, and legs
Blastomyces dermatitidis	Blastomycosis	Primary respiratory infection	Nodular lesions that ulcerate Erythema nodosum	
Scedosporium spp.	No specific syndrome	Severe opportunistic infection	Nodular or necrotic skin lesions	Generalized
Fusarium spp.	No specific syndrome	Severe opportunistic infection	Nodular skin lesions, abscesses	Generalized
Aspergillus spp.	No specific syndrome	Severe opportunistic infection	Nodular and purpuric lesions	Generalized

Data from references 14, 15, 24, 28, 44, 75, 78, 88, 90, 139, 143, 181, 203, 225, 235.

TABLE 58.5 **Cutaneous Manifestations of Protozoan and Helminthic Infections**

Agent	Disease or Syndrome	Cutaneous Manifestations
Plasmodium spp.	Malaria	Occasionally generalized urticaria in chronic infection
Toxoplasma gondii	Acquired toxoplasmosis	Occasionally generalized erythematous, maculopapular rash
	Congenital toxoplasmosis	Generalized petechial rash
Giardia lamblia	Giardiasis	Rarely urticaria
Entamoeba histolytica	Amebiasis	Rarely urticaria
Leishmania tropica	Oriental sore	Red nodular lesion that ulcerates; lasts 2–3 months
Leishmania braziliensis and *mexicana*	American cutaneous leishmaniasis	Erythematous papular lesion that vesiculates and ulcerates
Trypanosoma gambiense	African trypanosomiasis	Red nodular lesion at site of bite, followed by generalized, pruritic, erythema multiforme–like rash
Trypanosoma cruzi	American trypanosomiasis or Chagas disease	Nodular lesion at site of bite; generalized recurrent erythematous, maculopapular rash
Trichomonas vaginalis	Vulvovaginalis	Rarely urticaria and erythema multiforme
Ascaris lumbricoides	Roundworm infestation	Erythema nodosum
Enterobius vermicularis	Pinworm infestation	Rarely urticaria
Necator americanus	Hookworm disease	Papules and papulovesicles on exposed surfaces (feet); generalized urticaria
Trichinella spiralis	Trichinosis	Urticaria common; also, generalized maculopapular rash may occur; petechiae frequently develop
Strongyloides stercoralis	Strongyloidiasis; also, creeping eruption (cutaneous larva migrans)	Erythematous, maculopapular lesions on feet; creeping eruption
Ancylostoma braziliense	Creeping eruption (cutaneous larva migrans)	Creeping eruption
Dermatobia hominis	Cutaneous myiasis	Creeping eruption, subacute draining lesions
Schistosoma haematobium, mansoni, and *japonicum*	Schistosomiasis	Pruritic papular eruption where exposed; generalized urticaria and granulomatous lesions
Trichobilharzia ocellata, physellae, and *stagnicolae*	Swimmer's itch or collector's itch	Initial erythema and urticaria followed by papules and vesiculation; pruritic
Wuchereria bancrofti	Filariasis	Localized erythema urticaria and erythema nodosum
Onchocerca volvulus	Onchocerciasis	Chronic, papular, scaly rash
Echinococcus granulosus and *multilocularis*	Echinococcosis	Frequent urticaria

Data from references 14, 21, 44, 58, 75, 77, 91, 96, 146.

TABLE 58.6 Cutaneous Manifestations of Arthropod Bites and Stings

Agent	Disease or Syndrome	Cutaneous Manifestations
Spiders		
Loxosceles rectus	Recluse spider bite or brown spider bite	Erythema followed by blister and necrosis
Ticks	Tick bite	Initial pruritus at site; becomes ulcerated and granulomatous
Mites		
Sarcoptes scabiei	Scabies	Pruritic burrows in body creases and generalized; become erythematous and then papular urticaria
Trombicula irritans	Chigger bite	Marked pruritus and then papular urticaria
Other mites: food, grain, murine, and fowl		Marked pruritus and then papular urticaria
Lice		
Pediculus humanus	Body lice or pediculosis	Erythematous, maculopapular, pruritic lesions; sometimes urticaria
Phthirus pubis	Crabs	Pruritus and erythema under pubic hair
Bedbugs and Kissing Bugs		
Cimex lectularius	Bedbug bite	Pruritic papular urticaria
Triatoma sanguisuga	Kissing bug bite	Papular urticaria; occasionally hemorrhagic nodular lesions
Gypsy Moth Caterpillar		
Lymantria dispar	Gypsy moth rash	Pruritic blotchy erythema and maculopapular
Moths		
Hylesia alinda	Moth-associated dermatitis	Erythema and pruritus; feeling of warmth in area of rash; may have vesicular lesions
Ants		
Solenopsis saevissima	Fire ant bite	Painful papular urticarial lesions that become pustular and then nodular
Fleas		
Pulex irritans (human flea) and fleas of many animals	Flea bite	Papular urticaria
Flies and mosquitoes	Fly and mosquito bite	Papular, nodular, and urticarial lesions in sensitive persons

Data from references 46, 48, 64, 75, 103, 164, 184, 197, 202.

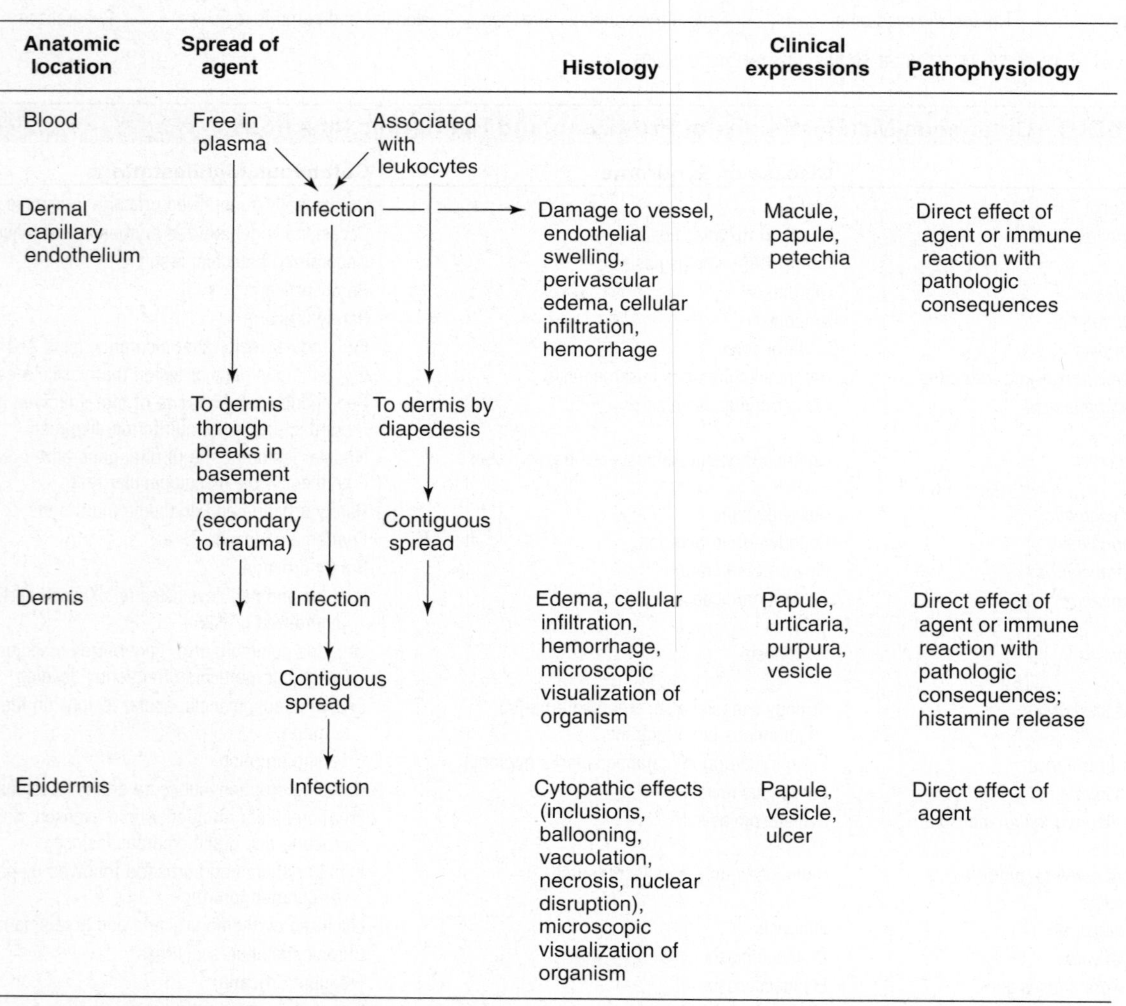

FIG. 58.1 Aspects of pathogenesis in exanthems associated with blood-borne dissemination of the infectious agent. (Modified from Cherry JD. Newer viral exanthems. *Adv Pediatr.* 1969;16:233–86.)

M. pneumoniae and HSV infection, the respective organisms have been isolated or identified at the skin site. In most instances, however, neither antigen localization nor disseminated toxin has been identified. The occurrence of erythema nodosum in a *Coccidioides immitis* infection indicates the development of cell-mediated immunity.

Important clinical aspects of exanthematous diseases are the distribution and progression of the lesions, yet little is known of the cause of these aspects. Differences in skin thickness, vascularity, proliferation rate, temperature, and metabolic activity are important in animal diseases with cutaneous manifestations.[52,80,135,147,170] In humans, similar factors must be important but obviously affect the various etiologic agents differently (e.g., the more central exanthem of chickenpox vs. that of the hand, foot, and mouth syndrome of coxsackievirus A16 infection).

CLINICAL MANIFESTATIONS

The clinical findings in exanthematous diseases resulting from systemic infections are varied and depend on the inciting pathogens. By examination of skin alone differentiating an exanthematous disease resulting from systemic infection (e.g., coxsackievirus A9, rubella virus infection) from primary cutaneous diseases of infectious and noninfectious origin (e.g., insect bites, acne, and contact with poison ivy) frequently is difficult. In Tables 58.1 through 58.6, the clinical characteristics of viral, chlamydial, rickettsial, bacterial, fungal, parasitic, and arthropod-induced illnesses with primary or secondary cutaneous manifestations are presented. In Tables 58.8 through 58.16, etiologic agents and clinical manifestations are presented on the basis of the more pronounced cutaneous manifestations or syndrome associations. The clinician must keep in mind that other aspects of an illness (e.g., exposure, season, incubation period, geographic location, patient age, and associated signs and symptoms) may be more important in determining the underlying etiologic agent. Clinical manifestations of specific exanthematous diseases are presented in greater detail in other chapters of this book.

Erythematous Macular Exanthems

When all infectious diseases with exanthems are taken into consideration, the occurrence of illnesses in which the lesions are just macular is rare. However, many important, severe diseases have a transitory erythematous macular rash early in their course, and recognition of this fact can be lifesaving. Infectious agents associated with illnesses in which macular exanthems have been observed are presented in Table 58.7.

The most common rash in infectious mononucleosis is erythematous and maculopapular, but rarely (most often in association with the administration of ampicillin) the exanthem is generalized, confluent, fiery red, and macular. Blotchy or diffuse erythematous macular rashes have been caused specifically by 12 different enterovirus types. Most of these descriptions involve neonates, other very young infants, and adults; children in the peak ages for enteroviral exanthematous diseases do not seem to have solely macular lesions. In neonates, enteroviral disease with a blotchy macular rash in association with fever and lethargy usually is confused with bacterial sepsis.

Patients with dengue, Lassa, and Marburg viral infections frequently have a macular, flushed appearance before other cutaneous manifestations develop. Similarly, in both murine and epidemic typhus, the initial skin manifestations are macular but progress rapidly to more pronounced findings.

Bacterial septicemia with both common and exotic organisms is associated frequently with a generalized flush. In staphylococcal disease, the rash is particularly apparent in endocarditis and osteomyelitis. The most famous disease with a macular rash is typhoid fever. Rose spots occur most commonly on the abdomen, but they also are seen on the chest and back. They are 2- to 4-mm erythematous, macular lesions. Lesions likewise have been noted in leptospirosis and psittacosis. In addition, rose spots are seen occasionally in septicemic illnesses caused by other *Salmonella* spp.

The slapped-cheek appearance in erythema infectiosum is caused by an erythematous macular flush of the cheeks. The full-blown rash in streptococcal scarlet fever is maculopapular, but frequently in mild cases and in those altered by antibiotic therapy the exanthem is only macular (scarlatina).

TABLE 58.7 Infectious Agents Associated With Illnesses in Which a Macular Exanthem Has Been Observed

Infectious Agent	Illness
Human herpesvirus–6, –7	Roseola infantum
Epstein-Barr virus	Infectious mononucleosis
Coxsackieviruses B1, B2, B5	—
Echoviruses 2, 4, 5, 14, 17–19, 30	—
Enterovirus 71	—
Dengue virus	Dengue fever
Lassa virus	Lassa fever
Marburg virus	Marburg fever
Parvovirus	Erythema infectiosum
HIV-1	Manifestation of acute infection
Hantavirus	Hemorrhagic fever with renal syndrome
Chlamydia psittaci	Psittacosis
Rickettsia typhi	Murine typhus
Rickettsia prowazekii	Epidemic typhus
Rickettsia quintana	Trench fever
Coxiella burnetii	Q fever
Mycoplasma pneumoniae	—
Staphylococcus aureus	Septicemia and toxic shock syndrome
Streptococcus pyogenes	Scarlatina and septicemia
Bacillus anthracis	Anthrax
Salmonella typhi	Typhoid fever
Salmonella spp.	Septicemic salmonellosis
Spirillum minus	Rat-bite fever
Leptospira spp.	Leptospirosis
Yersinia pestis	Plague

Erythematous Maculopapular Exanthems

An erythematous maculopapular rash is the most common cutaneous manifestation of systemic infection. It also is an exceedingly common occurrence in allergic conditions. However, all too frequently, the rash of an infectious illness is ascribed to an allergic reaction to an administered drug rather than correctly to the disease process. The converse—an allergic rash illness attributed mistakenly to an infectious agent—rarely occurs. Infectious agents associated with illnesses in which maculopapular exanthems occur are presented in Table 58.8.

Both by the number of possible etiologic agents and by total infections, viruses account for the vast majority of illnesses with maculopapular eruptions. Although the distribution and progression of rashes are important aspects relating to the differential diagnosis, the single most important point is whether the lesions are discrete (rubelliform) or confluent (morbilliform). Adenoviruses are not uncommon causes of erythematous maculopapular eruptions. In most instances, signs and symptoms of upper respiratory tract infection are present. Most commonly, the lesions are discrete but occasionally a confluent morbilliform rash is present. A roseola infantum picture—occurrence of rash after the fever falls by crisis—frequently occurs. As a rule, the exanthem in adenoviral infections starts on the head and spreads to the trunk and extremities.

Enteroviruses account for the greatest number of erythematous maculopapular rash illnesses; 37 different serologic types have been implicated. The enteroviral types most commonly associated with maculopapular exanthems are coxsackieviruses A9 and B5 and echoviruses 4, 9, and 16. Echovirus 9 has been the most frequent cause of enteroviral exanthem for the past 35 years. Although morbilliform rashes do occur, the more usual cutaneous manifestation is one suggestive of rubella. The exanthem usually starts on the head and upper part of the trunk and spreads to the extremities.

Although they are not common manifestations of respiratory viruses (e.g., rhinoviruses, influenza A and B viruses, RSV, and parainfluenza

TABLE 58.8 Infectious Agents Associated With Illnesses in Which Maculopapular Exanthems Occur

		CHARACTER OF RASH	
Infectious Agent	**Illness**	**Discrete**	**Confluent**
Parvovirus	Erythema infectiosum	+++	+
Human bocavirus		++++	
Adenoviruses 1, 2, 3, 4, 7, 7a		+++	+
Human herpesvirus–6	Roseola infantum	+++	+
Epstein-Barr virus	Infectious mononucleosis	+++	+
Cytomegalovirus		++++	
Vaccinia virus	Roseola vaccinatum	+++	+
Coxsackieviruses A2, A4, A5, A6, A7, A9, A10, A16		+++	+
Coxsackieviruses B1–B5		+++	+
Echoviruses 1–7, 9, 11, 13, 14, 16–19, 22, 25, 30, 33		+++	+
Enterovirus 71		++++	
Rhinoviruses (many types)		++++	
Colorado tick fever virus	Colorado tick fever	++++	
Reoviruses 2, 3		++	++
Rotavirus	Gianotti-Crosti syndrome; infantile acute hemorrhagic edema	++++	
Alphaviruses: chikungunya, Sindbis, o'nyong-nyong fever, Ross River		++	++
Rubella virus	Rubella (German measles)	+++	+
Flavivirus: dengue, Kunjin, West Nile	Dengue, Kunjin fever	++	++
Influenza viruses A, B		++++	
Respiratory syncytial virus		++++	
Parainfluenza viruses 1–4		++++	
Mumps virus	Mumps	++++	
Measles virus	Measles	+	+++
Hepatitis B virus		++++	
Marburg virus	Marburg fever	++	++
Ebola virus	Ebola hemorrhagic fever	+++	+
Rickettsia akari	Rickettsialpox	++++	
Rickettsia typhi	Murine typhus	+++	+
Rickettsia prowazekii	Epidemic typhus	+++	+
Rickettsia tsutsugamushi	Scrub typhus	+++	+
Rickettsia rickettsi	Rocky Mountain spotted fever		++++
Ehrlichia spp.	Ehrlichiosis	+++	+
Mycoplasma pneumoniae		+++	+
Staphylococcus aureus (exfoliative toxin producing)	Staphylococcal scarlet fever		++++
Streptococcus pyogenes	Scarlet fever		++++
Arcanobacterium hemolyticum		++	++
Neisseria meningitidis	Meningococcemia	++++	
Moraxella catarrhalis		++++	
Listeria monocytogenes	Listeriosis	++++	
Streptobacillus moniliformis	Rat-bite fever	+++	+
Yersinia pseudotuberculosis			++++
Bartonella bacilliformis	Bartonellosis	++++	
Brucella spp.	Brucellosis	++++	
Legionella pneumophila	Legionnaires' disease	++++	
Bartonella henselae	Cat-scratch fever	+++	+
Treponema pallidum	Secondary syphilis	+++	+
Leptospira spp.	Leptospirosis	++++	
Borrelia spp.	Relapsing fever		++++
Coccidioides immitis	Coccidioidomycosis	+++	+
Toxoplasma gondii	Toxoplasmosis	++++	
Strongyloides stercoralis	Strongyloidiasis	++++	

viruses types 1 through 4), exanthems probably occur more often than is generally realized. Because children infected with these agents frequently are given antibiotics, confusion often occurs between an allergic and an infectious etiology. With all the respiratory viruses, the signs and symptoms of respiratory illness (e.g., cough, coryza, croup, and bronchiolitis) are prominent. The exanthems virtually are always discrete and rubelliform.

In dengue, the exanthem goes through several stages. Initially, it is macular, then erythematous maculopapular, and finally hemorrhagic. Similarly the exanthems in the rickettsial diseases go through stages that vary in relation to the specific agent (see Table 58.2). In Rocky Mountain spotted fever, the rash starts on the distal ends of extremities. Although the hallmark of meningococcemia is a petechial or purpuric rash, in the initial stages, the exanthem may be erythematous and maculopapular. In addition, maculopapular eruptions are observed in chronic meningococcemia. The most notable cutaneous lesion in coccidioidomycosis is erythema nodosum, but a rubelliform rash early in infection is not an unusual manifestation.

Vesicular Exanthems

The three main categories of vesicular exanthems are single or localized lesions, generalized lesions in greatest concentration on the trunk and head, and generalized lesions with the greatest concentration on the extremities. Infectious agents associated with illnesses in which vesicular rashes develop are presented in Table 58.9. The exanthem in primary or recurrent HSV infection is localized, as it is in recurrent endogenous varicella zoster infection (herpes zoster), ecthyma contagiosum, tanapox, scrub typhus, anthrax, and papulonecrotic tuberculids.

The vesicular exanthematous disease that occurs most commonly in children today is chickenpox. It should be a readily recognizable disease but is all too frequently confused with enteroviral infections or insect bites and allergic conditions. Chickenpox has a long incubation period (16 days) and is associated with mild fever and an exanthem that starts on the head and upper part of the trunk and spreads to the extremities. The rash always is more prominent on the trunk than on the extremities. At any time during the first few days of the rash, lesions in all stages (i.e., macules, papules, and vesicles) can be seen. Individual lesions in chickenpox form scabs that persist for approximately 7 days.

In contrast to that of chickenpox, the exanthem in enteroviral infections frequently is peripheral in distribution, and the lesions generally heal without scabs. The incubation period (5 days) is much shorter than that of chickenpox. The hand, foot, and mouth syndrome is a common manifestation of enteroviral vesicular rash illnesses. Until relatively recently, the most frequent etiologic agent in the hand, foot, and mouth syndrome was coxsackievirus A16, but the syndrome also had been attributed to coxsackieviruses A5, A9, A10, B1, and B3 and enterovirus 71. In recent years, enterovirus 71 is the most common cause of this syndrome. Most recently coxsackievirus A6 has been noted in several outbreaks.[159,228]

Enteroviral infections with vesicular exanthems in which the hand, foot, and mouth distribution is not present quite frequently are diagnosed erroneously as insect bites or poison ivy.

TABLE 58.9 Infectious Agents Associated With Illnesses in Which Vesicular Exanthems Occur

Infectious Agent	Illness
Human parvovirus B19	
Herpes simplex virus types 1 and 2	Cold sores, genital herpes, or neonatal herpes
Varicella zoster virus	Chickenpox (varicella) or herpes zoster
Vaccinia virus	Disseminated vaccinia or eczema vaccinatum
Variola virus	Smallpox
Monkeypox virus	
Orf virus	Ecthyma contagiosum
Tanapox virus	
Coxsackieviruses A4, A5, A6, A8, A10, A16	
Coxsackieviruses B1–B3	
Echoviruses 6, 9,11, 17	
Enterovirus 71	
Reovirus 2	
Calicivirus of oceanic origin	
Alphaviruses: chikungunya, o'nyong-nyong fever, Ross River, Sindbis	
Kunjin virus	
Mumps virus	Mumps
Measles virus	Atypical measles
Rickettsia akari	Rickettsialpox
Rickettsia tsutsugamushi	
Mycoplasma pneumoniae	
Streptococcus pyogenes	Impetigo
Pseudomonas aeruginosa	
Brucella spp.	Brucellosis
Bacillus anthracis	Anthrax
Mycobacterium tuberculosis	Papulonecrotic tuberculids
Candida albicans	Congenital cutaneous candidiasis
Leishmania braziliensis	American cutaneous leishmaniasis
Necator americanus	Hookworm disease

Petechial and Purpuric Exanthems

A large number of infectious agents are associated with petechial and purpuric skin manifestations (Table 58.10). Infectious diseases with hemorrhagic rash can be fulminant fatal events or relatively benign illnesses. On a worldwide basis, meningococcemia is perhaps the most important and feared, although it is not the most prevalent of the petechial and purpuric exanthematous diseases. The relatively sudden onset of fever and a petechial rash must be considered and treated as meningococcemia unless another etiology can be established with absolute certainty. The most important of the differential diagnostic problems is exanthem caused by enteroviral infection. Many different enterovirus illnesses have a sudden onset with accompanying fever and petechial rash. In addition, the situation frequently is complicated further by the occurrence of meningitis. The most important enterovirus in its ability to mimic meningococcemia is echovirus 9.

Purpuric and petechial lesions in infectious illnesses can result from a direct or indirect (immunologic) effect of the infectious agent at the cutaneous site or from the occurrence of thrombocytopenia. Thrombocytopenia is noted most commonly in acquired rubella virus infections.

Urticarial Exanthems

The occurrence of urticaria all too frequently leads the physician to suspect an allergic or dermatologic condition.[221,222] However, what has become quite evident is that when urticaria develops in association with an acute febrile illness, the cutaneous reaction is a direct effect of an infectious agent, and its mediation does not require an allergic response. Listed in Table 58.11 are infectious agents associated with urticarial exanthems.

Papular urticaria occurs very commonly in children in the summer and fall and most frequently is the result of insect bites (see Table 58.6). However, virtually identical lesions occur in infections with coxsackievirus A as well as with other enteroviruses. The main point for differentiation is that fever regularly develops in the virus-induced exanthems but is not a characteristic associated with insect bites.

Early in the course of meningococcemia, the exanthem can be urticarial, so an illness of sudden onset with fever and this cutaneous manifestation never should be taken lightly.

Papular, Nodular, and Ulcerative Lesions

In many instances, the lesions in this category occur as single events at the site of primary inoculation. Specific illnesses and etiologic agents are listed in Table 58.12.

TABLE 58.10 Infectious Agents Associated With Illnesses in Which Petechial and Purpuric Exanthems Occur

Infectious Agent	Illness
Human parvovirus B19	Gloves-and-socks syndrome
Varicella zoster virus	Hemorrhagic chickenpox
Cytomegalovirus	Congenital cytomegalovirus infection
Variola virus	Hemorrhagic smallpox
Coxsackieviruses A4, A9	
Coxsackieviruses B2–B4	
Echoviruses 4, 7, 9	
Colorado tick fever virus	Colorado tick fever
Rotavirus	
Alphaviruses: chikungunya, o'nyong-nyong fever, Ross River, Sindbis	
Rubella virus	Rubella (German measles) or congenital rubella
Respiratory syncytial virus	
Measles virus	Hemorrhagic (black measles) or atypical measles
Lassa virus	Lassa fever
Marburg virus	
Hepatitis C virus	Mixed cryoglobulinemia
Hantavirus	Hemorrhagic fever with renal syndrome
Rickettsia typhi	Murine typhus
Rickettsia prowazekii	Epidemic typhus
Rickettsia rickettsii and other tick-borne rickettsiae	Rocky Mountain spotted fever
Ehrlichia spp.	Ehrlichiosis
Mycoplasma pneumoniae	
Streptococcus pyogenes	Scarlet fever or septicemia
Streptococcus pneumoniae	Pneumococcal septicemia
Enterococcal and viridans group streptococci	Endocarditis
Neisseria gonorrhoeae	Gonococcemia
Neisseria meningitidis	Meningococcemia
Moraxella catarrhalis	
Haemophilus influenzae	*H. influenzae* septicemia
Pseudomonas aeruginosa	Ecthyma gangrenosa
Streptobacillus moniliformis	
Yersinia pestis	Septicemic plague (black death)
Bartonella henselae	Cat-scratch fever
Treponema pallidum	Congenital syphilis
Borrelia spp.	Relapsing fever
Toxoplasma gondii	Congenital toxoplasmosis
Trichinella spiralis	Trichinosis

TABLE 58.11 Infectious Agents Associated With Illnesses in Which Urticarial Exanthems Occur

Infectious Agent	Illness
Epstein-Barr virus	Infectious mononucleosis
Coxsackieviruses A9, A16, B4, B5	
Echovirus 11	
Mumps virus	Mumps
Hepatitis B virus	
Hepatitis C virus	
Mycoplasma pneumoniae	
Neisseria meningitidis	Meningococcemia
Shigella sonnei	Shigellosis
Yersinia enterocolitica	Yersiniosis
Borrelia burgdorferi	Lyme disease
Plasmodium spp.	Malaria
Coxiella burnetii	Q fever
Giardia lamblia	Giardiasis
Entamoeba histolytica	Amebiasis
Trichomonas vaginalis	Vulvovaginalis
Enterobius vermicularis	Pinworm infestation
Necator americanus	Hookworm disease
Trichinella spiralis	Trichinosis
Schistosoma spp.	Schistosomiasis
Trichobilharzia spp.	Swimmer's itch or collector's itch
Wuchereria bancrofti	Filariasis
Echinococcus spp.	Echinococcosis
Sarcoptes scabiei	Scabies
Trombicula irritans	Chigger bites
Other mites	Mite bites
Pediculus humanus	Pediculosis
Bedbugs, kissing bugs, ants, fleas, flies, and mosquitoes	Bites and stings

Distinctive Clinical Features or Syndromes

Erythema Multiforme

Erythema multiforme is a self-limited skin eruption that is erythematous and characterized by distinctive target or iris lesions or both. Small vesicles and urticarial areas also may develop. On occasion, the disease is severe and associated with mucosal involvement and genital lesions. In this latter illness—Stevens-Johnson syndrome, bullous erythema multiforme, erythema multiforme exudativum major—severe ulcerative, oral, and genital lesions occur; generalized exanthems become bullous, and conjunctivitis is present. The illness is associated with fever and general distress.

Although the pathogenesis of erythema multiforme is unknown, what is clear is that multiple factors, including infectious agents, are responsible for its occurrence. Infectious agents associated with erythema multiforme are listed in Table 58.13. The single most important infectious cause of erythema multiforme and Stevens-Johnson syndrome is *M. pneumoniae*. When *M. pneumoniae* is the instigating agent, the patient nearly always has concomitant pneumonia.

HSV frequently has been recovered from the throats of persons with erythema multiforme, but the cause-and-effect relationship in many cases must be questioned. However, in a recent study, HSV DNA was found in the skin lesions of 11 of 31 patients with erythema multiforme.[61]

Erythema Nodosum

Erythema nodosum most commonly occurs on the anterior aspect of the lower part of the legs but may be seen anywhere on the body. The lesions are raised, erythematous, and painful to touch. Their usual size is approximately 2 to 4 cm, with a duration of 2 to 6 weeks.

Erythema nodosum occurs less commonly today than it did four decades ago, and the frequency of specific associated infectious agents also is different. In the past, streptococcal and mycobacterial infections were the agents most commonly related. Now, the exanthem most often is associated with respiratory tract infection with *Histoplasma capsulatum, Cryptococcus neoformans,* and *C. immitis*. Infectious agents associated with erythema nodosum are listed in Table 58.14.

Hand, Foot, and Mouth Syndrome

The hand, foot, and mouth syndrome is a clearly recognizable viral illness characterized by vesicular lesions in the anterior of the mouth and on the hands and feet in association with fever. Although several enteroviruses (i.e., coxsackieviruses A5, A6, A9, A10, A16, B1, and B3 and enterovirus 71) have been implicated, as have HSV and

TABLE 58.12 **Infectious Agents Associated With Papular, Nodular, and Ulcerative Lesions**

Agent	Illness
Wart virus	Warts (P and N)
Orf virus	Ecthyma contagiosum (N)
Molluscum contagiosum virus	Molluscum contagiosum (P and N)
Hepatitis B virus	Gianotti-Crosti syndrome (P)
Paravaccinia virus	Milker's nodules (N)
Francisella tularensis	Tularemia (U)
Haemophilus ducreyi	Chancroid (U)
Bartonella bacilliformis	Bartonellosis (N)
Calymmatobacterium granulomatis	Granuloma inguinale (N and U)
Pseudomonas aeruginosa	Ecthyma gangrenosa (U)
	Pseudomonas folliculitis (P)
Burkholderia mallei	Glanders (N and U)
Mycobacterium tuberculosis	Lupus vulgaris (N)
	Papulonecrotic tuberculids (U)
Atypical mycobacteria	(U)
Mycobacterium leprae	(N)
Treponema pallidum	Chancre (U)
Treponema pertenue	Yaws (P and U)
Sporotrichum schenckii	Sporotrichosis (U)
Blastomyces dermatitidis	Blastomycosis (N and U)
Fusarium spp.	Opportunistic infection (N)
Scedosporium spp.	Opportunistic infection (N)
Candida albicans	Systemic candidiasis (N)
Leishmania tropica	Oriental sore (N and U)
Leishmania braziliensis and *mexicana*	American cutaneous leishmaniasis (P and U)
Trypanosoma spp.	Trypanosomiasis (N)
Necator americanus	Hookworm disease (P)
Schistosoma spp.	Schistosomiasis (P)
Trichobilharzia spp.	Swimmer's itch or collector's itch (P)
Onchocerca volvulus	Onchocerciasis (P)
Loxosceles reclusa	Recluse spider bites (U)
Ticks	Tick bites (U)
Sarcoptes scabiei	Scabies (P)
Trombicula irritans	Chigger bites (P)
Other mites	Mite bites (P)
Cimex lectularius	Bedbug bites (P)
Triatoma sanguisuga	Kissing bug bites (P and N)
Solenopsis saevissima	Fire ant bites (P and N)
Fleas	Flea bites (P)
Flies and mosquitoes	Fly and mosquito bites (P)

N, Nodular; *P*, papular *U*, ulcerative.

foot-and-mouth disease virus, most of these cases today are caused by enterovirus 71 and perhaps coxsackievirus A6.

Roseola-like Illness

Roseola infantum is a classic pediatric illness characterized by fever of 3 to 5 days' duration, rapid defervescence, and then the appearance of an erythematous macular or maculopapular rash that persists for 1 to 2 days. Roseola is an age-related response to infection with many viruses. Recent studies suggest that a leading cause of roseola infantum is primary infection with HHV-6. The following other viruses have been noted in association with roseola: adenoviruses 1, 2, 3, and 14; coxsackieviruses A6, A9, B1, B2, B4, and B5; echoviruses 9, 11, 16, 25, 27, and 30; parainfluenza virus type 1; and measles vaccine virus.

Rocky Mountain Spotted Fever–like Illness

Rocky Mountain spotted fever is a clinical illness characterized by fever and a petechial rash located mainly on the distal ends of extremities. The illness is caused by *Rickettsia rickettsii* and is prevalent in many areas of North America; the infectious agent is transmitted to humans by ticks. In other areas of the world, other tick-borne rickettsiae (*Rickettsia sibirica, Rickettsia australis, Rickettsia conorii*) produce similar human illness. Infection with *Ehrlichia* spp. also can cause an illness similar to Rocky Mountain spotted fever.

The most important illness that, in the past, was confused with Rocky Mountain spotted fever was atypical measles (see Chapter 180). This illness, which has both the constitutional symptoms of Rocky Mountain spotted fever and a rash most prominent on the extremities, occurs almost exclusively after exposure to measles virus in some persons previously immunized with inactivated (killed) measles vaccine.

Rat-bite fever caused by *S. moniliformis* also has been misdiagnosed as Rocky Mountain spotted fever.[172]

TABLE 58.13 **Infectious Agents Associated With Erythema Multiforme**

Agent	Illness
Human parvovirus B19	Erythema infectiosum
Adenovirus 7	Respiratory infection
Herpes simplex virus type 1	Perioral or respiratory infection
Epstein-Barr virus	Infectious mononucleosis
Varicella virus	Chickenpox
Coxsackieviruses A10, A16, B5	Enterovirus syndrome
Echovirus 6	Enterovirus syndrome
Poliomyelitis virus	Poliomyelitis
Vaccinia virus	Smallpox vaccination
Variola virus	Smallpox
Orf virus	Ecthyma contagiosum
Paravaccinia virus	Milker's nodules
Influenza A virus	Influenza
Mumps	Mumps
Hepatitis B virus	Serum hepatitis
Chlamydia psittaci	Psittacosis
Chlamydia trachomatis	Lymphogranuloma venereum
Mycoplasma pneumoniae	Respiratory symptoms
Staphylococcus aureus	Septicemia
Streptococcus pyogenes	Respiratory symptoms
Neisseria gonorrhoeae	Gonorrhea
Corynebacterium diphtheriae	Diphtheria
Pseudomonas aeruginosa	Septicemia
Salmonella spp.	Gastroenteritis
Francisella tularensis	Tularemia
Yersinia spp.	Gastrointestinal symptoms
Vibrio parahaemolyticus	Gastroenteritis
Treponema pallidum	Syphilis
Bartonella henselae	Cat-scratch fever
Mycobacterium tuberculosis	Tuberculosis
Mycobacterium leprae	Leprosy
Coccidioides immitis	Coccidioidomycosis
Histoplasma capsulatum	Histoplasmosis
Trichomonas vaginalis	Vulvovaginalis

Exanthem and Meningitis

Aseptic and also bacterial meningitis frequently are characterized by both exanthem and symptoms and signs of neurologic involvement. Infectious agents associated with exanthem and meningitis are presented in Table 58.15. Of most importance in this category is the differential diagnosis of enteroviral syndromes and meningococcemia.

Exanthem and Pulmonary Involvement

Infectious agents associated with exanthem and pulmonary involvement are listed in Table 58.16. In patients older than 5 years, the leading cause

TABLE 58.14 Infectious Agents Associated With Erythema Nodosum

Agent	Illness
Herpes simplex virus	Perioral or respiratory infection
Epstein-Barr virus	Infectious mononucleosis
Chlamydia psittaci	Psittacosis
Chlamydia trachomatis	Lymphogranuloma venereum
Streptococcus pyogenes	Respiratory infection
Neisseria meningitidis	Meningococcemia
Corynebacterium diphtheriae	Diphtheria
Campylobacter spp.	Gastroenteritis
Haemophilus ducreyi	Chancroid
Salmonella spp.	Salmonellosis
Yersinia spp.	Gastrointestinal symptoms
Brucella spp.	Brucellosis
Treponema pallidum	Syphilis
Bartonella henselae	Cat-scratch fever
Mycobacterium tuberculosis	Tuberculosis
Mycobacterium leprae	Leprosy
Trichophyton spp.	Kerion of scalp
Histoplasma capsulatum	Histoplasmosis
Cryptococcus neoformans	Cryptococcosis
Coccidioides immitis	Coccidioidomycosis
Blastomyces dermatitidis	Blastomycosis
Ascaris lumbricoides	Roundworm infestation
Wuchereria bancrofti	Filariasis

TABLE 58.15 Infectious Agents Associated With Exanthem and Meningitis

Agent	Illness
Herpes simplex virus type 2	Recurrent genital herpes
Coxsackieviruses A2, A9, B1, B4, B5	Enterovirus syndrome
Echoviruses 4, 6, 9, 11, 14, 17, 25, 33	Enterovirus syndrome
Colorado tick fever virus	Colorado tick fever
Reovirus 2	Respiratory infection
West Nile virus	Meningoencephalitis
Neisseria meningitidis	Meningococcemia
Borrelia burgdorferi	Lyme disease
Listeria monocytogenes	Listeriosis
Toxoplasma gondii	Toxoplasmosis

of exanthem and pneumonia is *M. pneumoniae* infection. In younger children, adenoviruses are the most important etiologic agents. With the exception of enteroviral infections, which are more likely to involve young children, most of the illnesses listed in Table 58.16 occur in older children and young adults.

Gianotti-Crosti Syndrome (Papular Acrodermatitis)

Gianotti-Crosti syndrome is a distinct clinical entity characterized by a papular (lichenoid) exanthem, generalized lymphadenopathy, hepatomegaly, and acute anicteric hepatitis.[47,190,193] In most instances, this illness has been associated with hepatitis B virus infection. The syndrome also has been noted in association with EBV, cytomegalovirus, coxsackievirus B virus, and RSV infections.[68,120,191,214]

Cutaneous Manifestations Associated With Infections in Immunocompromised Patients

All infectious agents that cause exanthems in immunologically normal children can cause infections in immunocompromised children. However, the clinical manifestations may be different. For example, measles virus infection in a child who is T-cell deficient may be associated with a severe, progressive pneumonia but not the typical rash. Other viral exanthems that are self-limited in normal children, such as varicella, may be progressive and develop into hemorrhagic skin lesions with disseminated organ involvement in children with T-cell deficiency.

Of particular concern are bacterial and fungal infections, which are rarely a problem in normal children but are rapidly fatal in granulocytopenic children. These patients have characteristic skin lesions resulting from disseminated infections. Of importance are ecthyma gangrenosa resulting from *P. aeruginosa* septicemia and the nodular and purpuric lesions of disseminated fungal infections caused by *Aspergillus*, *Candida*, and other less common agents.

TABLE 58.16 Infectious Agents Associated With Exanthem and Pulmonary Involvement

Agent	Illness
Adenoviruses 7, 7a	Respiratory infection
Herpes simplex virus type 1	Respiratory infection
Varicella zoster virus	Chickenpox pneumonia
Epstein-Barr virus	Infectious mononucleosis
Coxsackievirus A9	Enterovirus syndrome
Echovirus 11	Enterovirus syndrome
Reovirus 3	Respiratory infection
Measles virus	Measles pneumonia and atypical measles
Chlamydia psittaci	Psittacosis
Mycoplasma pneumoniae	*M. pneumoniae* pneumonia
Neisseria meningitidis	Meningococcal pneumonia
Mycobacterium tuberculosis	Tuberculosis
Histoplasma capsulatum	Histoplasmosis
Cryptococcus neoformans	Cryptococcosis
Coccidioides immitis	Coccidioidomycosis

BOX 58.1 Important Aspects in the Diagnosis of Exanthematous Illness

Exposure
Type, distribution, and progression of rash
Relationship of rash with fever
Season
Incubation period
Age
Exanthem (including previous)
Adenopathy
Laboratory tests
Other associated symptoms

From Cherry JD. Newer viral exanthems. *Adv Pediatr.* 1969;16:233–86.

DIAGNOSIS

Differential Diagnosis

The diagnosis of infectious exanthems frequently is considered an impossible task by many physicians. Other physicians glibly call the first maculopapular exanthem of childhood *roseola* and the first vesicular rash *chickenpox* without consideration of more appropriate choices. The hallmark of diagnosis in exanthematous disease is careful elicitation of historical data. Differential diagnosis requires the consideration of noninfectious etiologies as well as different infectious agents. Box 58.1 lists the major considerations in the diagnosis of diseases with cutaneous manifestations.

A history of exposure is most important in making a differential diagnosis. For example, was the patient exposed to poison ivy, insects, or a person ill with a specific disease? In infectious illnesses with high clinical expression rates (e.g., measles, chickenpox, and rubella), proper questioning usually reveals a contact case or at least other cases in the community. On the other hand, in illnesses with low rates of clinical expression of exanthem, such as adenoviral and some enteroviral infections, the source may not be apparent.

Consideration of the seasonal occurrence of different infectious agents, as well as insects, is particularly useful in making a differential diagnosis. In temperate climates, enteroviral and arthropod-mediated diseases occur in the summer and fall. Exanthems with measles, varicella zoster, and rubella viruses occur most often in the winter and spring. The diagnosis of rubella is important because of fetal consequences. All too frequently rubella is overdiagnosed and underdiagnosed, both of which can be avoided if its seasonal prevalence is understood.

The incubation period is important in separating the exanthem caused by rubella, varicella zoster, or measles viruses from rash illnesses caused by enteroviruses or common respiratory viruses. The former have long incubation periods, whereas in the others, the period from exposure to the onset of illness is less than 1 week. Age can be useful. Today in the United States, measles and rubella often are illnesses of adolescents and young adults. Enteroviral exanthem frequency is related inversely to age.

Questioning to obtain a pertinent history of previous exanthems can give useful information if it is done with care. For example, if patients are asked whether they had rubella, the answer is quite unreliable. However, if the past illness is documented by year, season, and symptoms, accurate information often is obtained. The relationship of rash to fever is most significant in the diagnosis of roseola. The presence or absence of fever is important in separating exanthems of infectious and noninfectious etiology. Frequently insect bites are diagnosed as chickenpox by parents and physicians as well. Chickenpox rarely occurs without fever.

The type and distribution of exanthem obviously are important. They virtually are diagnostic in hand, foot, and mouth syndrome; Rocky Mountain spotted fever; and atypical measles. Enanthem can lead to a specific diagnosis (Koplik spots in measles) or a category diagnosis (e.g., herpangina in enteroviral infections). Other characteristics, such as those listed in Tables 58.8 through 58.16, obviously are useful in delineating a specific illness.

Specific Diagnosis

As with other infectious diseases, establishing a specific diagnosis depends on the acquisition of proper cultures, serologic tests, and microscopic study of secretions or histologic or cytologic preparations. These techniques are discussed in other chapters of this book.

Vesicular lesions always should be scraped for cytologic study or direct antigen identification (e.g., varicella and herpes simplex), and, frequently, petechial lesions should be scraped and stained in a search for infectious agents (e.g., meningococci). The etiology of viral infections can be established by isolation of virus, direct antigen detection, or serologic methods. In most instances, a virus recovered from the throat indicates acute infection and is the probable cause of a particular illness. Serologic study without culture is useful in diagnosing rickettsial diseases, some viral infections, and a few illnesses of bacterial origin. Serologic study without virus isolation generally is not useful in diagnosing enteroviral illnesses.

TREATMENT, PROGNOSIS, AND PREVENTION

The treatment, prognosis, and prevention of exanthematous diseases are presented in appropriate chapters throughout this text.

NEW REFERENCES SINCE THE SEVENTH EDITION

19. Basurko C, Alvarez EC, Djossou F, et al. The predictive value of a maculopapular rash in children hospitalized for dengue fever in Cayenne, French Guiana. *Trans R Soc Trop Med Hyg*. 2012;106(12):773-775.
57. Chovel-Sella A, Ben Tov A, Lahav E, et al. Incidence of rash after amoxicillin treatment in children with infectious mononucleosis. *Pediatrics*. 2013;131(5):e1424-e1427.
85. Fretzayas A, Moustaki M, Kotzia D, et al. Rash, an uncommon but existing feature of H1N1 influenza among children. *Influenza Other Respir Viruses*. 2011;5(4):223-224.
136. Lumbiganon P, Kosalaraksa P. Uncommon clinical presentations of melioidosis in children: 2 cases with sore throat and 1 case with urticarial rash. *Southeast Asian J Trop Med Public Health*. 2013;44(5):862-865.
195. Schneider H, Adams O, Weiss C, et al. Clinical characteristics of children with viral single- and co-infections and a petechial rash. *Pediatr Infect Dis J*. 2013;32(5):e186-e191.
242. Yermalovich MA, Semeiko GV, Samoilovich EO, et al. Etiology of maculopapular rash in measles and rubella suspected patients from Belarus. *PLoS ONE*. 2014;9(10):e111541.

The full reference list for this chapter is available at ExpertConsult.com

59 Roseola Infantum (Exanthem Subitum)

James D. Cherry

Roseola infantum (exanthem subitum, pseudorubella, exanthem criticum, sixth disease, or 3-day fever) is a common, acute illness of young children characterized by a fever of 3 to 5 days' duration, rapid defervescence, and then the appearance of an erythematous macular or maculopapular rash that persists for 1 to 2 days.

HISTORY

Zahorsky[85] generally is given credit for the original description of roseola infantum. However, in his writings, he pointed out that the syndrome was described in earlier pediatric and dermatology texts.[86–88] Altschuler[2] observed that a British dermatologist, Willan, presented a description of the illness in his 1809 book *On Cutaneous Diseases*. The descriptions in the older literature did not separate the syndrome from the known exanthematous diseases (measles, rubella, and scarlet fever), an omission that Zahorsky corrected.

In 1921, Veeder and Hempelmann[79] described the syndrome further and noted that leukopenia and relative lymphocytosis occurred. These investigators objected to the name *roseola infantum,* which in the past had been used to describe a large group of diseases with indefinite causes. They suggested the term *exanthem subitum* because it was "descriptive of the most striking clinical symptom, namely, the sudden, unexpected appearance of the eruption on the fourth day." Currently, the term *roseola* is used most commonly to describe the syndrome.

From 1920 through 1940, many excellent clinical descriptions of the syndrome were published.[7,8,11,18,19,21,25,26,38,88,89] From 1940 through 1988, articles relating to roseola were concerned with unusual manifestations and complications[9,12–14,23,33,49,51,52,56,59,66] and attempts to recover an etiologic agent.[27,31,42,47,67] In 1951 and 1954, Neva and associates[53–55] noted the association of a roseola-like illness and infection with echovirus 16. This association was noted again in 1974.[28] In 1988, Yamanishi and associates[83] identified human herpesvirus–6 (HHV-6) in the blood of infants with roseola, and, since then, the association between this virus and the disease has been confirmed on many occasions.* HHV-7 also has been found to be the cause of many cases of roseola.[4,15,32,71,74,76,78]

*References 3–6, 10, 20, 22, 28, 29, 34, 36, 37, 34, 36, 37, 41, 43–46, 57, 61, 63, 69–72, 81, 90.

EPIDEMIOLOGY

In his original article, Zahorsky[85] reported that roseola occurred most commonly in the fall. In his second article, he observed a year-round incidence[86]; in 1925, he pointed out that most cases occurred in the spring, summer, and fall.[87] Breese[11] noted that the greatest number of cases occurred in the summer and early fall. In contrast, 55% of Clemens' cases occurred in February, March, and April; 16% were seen in October.[18] In a review of 243 cases during a 10-year period, Juretic[40] observed that the peak month was May. Juretic also reviewed the seasonal incidence in 10 other studies and found only minor variations by month. Prevalence was greatest in March, April, and October and least in December. One epidemic of roseola in a maternity hospital occurred in the summer,[38] another epidemic in an infants' home occurred in the fall,[7] and a hospital outbreak occurred in the winter.[19]

Roseola predominantly is an illness of young children. It occurs rarely in infants younger than 3 months or children older than 4 years. In a review of 1462 cases, the peak age range prevalence was 7 to 13 months of age; 55% of the cases occurred within the first year of life, and 90% occurred within the first 2 years of life.[40] Occasionally cases have been seen in older children, adolescents, and young adults and in neonates and other infants younger than 6 months.[26,38]

Although Faber and Dickey[21] found twice as many girls as boys with the syndrome, the sex ratio in most large studies has been equal.[8,11,18,26,47] Although three epidemics have been reported, and cases frequently occur in groups by season, most cases occur sporadically without known exposure. The syndrome, when seen sporadically, generally is considered to be noncontagious, but secondary cases have been reported occasionally.[7,11,19,38] The incubation period range in epidemics is 5 to 15 days.[7,11,19]

The attack rate of roseola has not been well studied. Berenberg and associates[8] stated that roseola is the exanthem most commonly encountered in children younger than 2 years. Breese[11] found that 16% of a group of infants he followed for the first 12 months of life had definite roseola. He estimated that 30% of children would have clinical roseola. Juretic[40] looked at the frequency of roseola in 6735 children; the yearly attack rate during a 10-year period ranged from 1% to 10%, with a mean of 3.3%.

ETIOLOGY

In 1941, Breese[11] reported vigorous attempts to isolate a filterable virus from three children with preeruptive roseola. These studies included extensive animal inoculations, but no viral agents were uncovered. In 1950, Kempe and associates[42] reported the passage of the illness to a 6-month-old susceptible infant by the intravenous injection of serum from an 18-month-old child with preeruptive roseola. Febrile illnesses without exanthem also were produced in monkeys with serum and throat washings from a child with the syndrome. In similar experiments, Hellstrom and Vahlquist[31] produced the syndrome in three children aged 6 to 9 days after the intramuscular administration of blood from typical roseola cases.

In electron microscopy studies, Reagan and associates[64] observed uniform viruslike particles (100 to 110 nm) in the blood of an 18-month-old child with the syndrome. Febrile illness was produced in two monkeys after concentrated virus-containing material was inoculated.

Since the advent of modern diagnostic virology in the early 1950s, numerous viral agents have been recovered from children with roseola. In 1951, Neva and associates[55] studied an epidemic exanthematous illness (i.e., Boston exanthem) caused by echovirus 16, in which many of the illnesses were characteristic of roseola. In 1954, Neva[53] observed additional cases of roseola-like illness associated with echovirus 16 infection. In 1974, Hall and colleagues[27] reported four additional echovirus 16 infections with clinical manifestations of roseola. The reporting of roseola in Rochester, New York, nearly doubled during the time of echovirus 16 activity in the area. Roseola-like illnesses that also have been associated with enteroviruses are caused by coxsackievirus A6, A9, B1, B2, B4, and B5 and echovirus 9, 11, 25, 27, and 30.[17,16,28,69,82] Outbreaks of roseola that occur in the summer and fall probably are caused by enteroviral infections.

In addition to enteroviruses, adenovirus types 1, 2, 3, and 14 and parainfluenza type 1 virus have been recovered from children with roseola.[24,39,54,82] Saitoh and associates[67] detected rotavirus capsomeres in fecal specimens of nine children with roseola. In contrast to these findings, Gurwith and colleagues[27] studied fecal specimens from five children with roseola, and in none were viral particles identified. One of 13 children in this study did develop antibody to rotavirus around the time of illness, however. In addition to the occurrence of roseola associated with numerous natural viral infections, its pattern (i.e., fever and then rash with defervescence) was observed frequently in recipients of Edmonton B measles vaccine.[16]

In 1988, Yamanishi and associates[83] isolated HHV-6 from four infants with roseola, and all four had significant titer increases for this virus. Shortly after this finding was reported, several other investigators noted similar findings.[3,5,20,34,43,72,77] The implication from these studies, as suggested by the various investigators, is that HHV-6 is the cause of roseola. This viewpoint overlooks or ignores the past experience in which other viral agents have been associated with the clinical syndrome. Subsequent studies indicate that HHV-6 is a major cause of roseola and the cause of acute febrile illness without exanthem in infants.* Since 1993, HHV-7 has been accepted as an additional causative agent in roseola.[4,16,32,48,71,74,75,81]

In a study of 1653 infants and young children with acute febrile illnesses, Hall and colleagues[28] found that 160 (9.7%) had primary HHV-6 infections; 27 (17%) of the children who were infected with HHV-6 had roseola. Zerr and associates[90] identified 80 children with primary HHV-6 infections, and, of these, 30% had roseola. In the same population-based study, three of 80 (4%) children without primary HHV-6 infection also had roseola. In a study of clinical roseola, Okada and associates[57] found that 81% had serologic evidence of HHV-6 infection and that 8% had an echovirus-18 infection. In a study of roseola in Italy, Braito and Uberti[10] found serologic evidence of HHV-6 infection in only 30% of the cases. In 33% of the remaining cases, they attributed the illnesses to another infectious agent. In 1994, Hidaka and associates[32] estimated that 73.5%, 10.2%, and 16.3% of their roseola cases were caused by HHV-6, HHV-7, and other viruses, respectively. In a study of HHV-6 infections in young Brazilian children with rashes it was noted that only 21% had typical roseola.[80] In summary, HHV-6 is an important cause of roseola but not the only cause.

PATHOPHYSIOLOGY

The pathophysiology of roseola is unknown. Watson,[82] in the pre–HHV-6 era, suggested that roseola is not an infection caused by one particular pathogen but is instead the result of an immunizing reaction against many different viruses. He also suggested that the rash is caused by the neutralization of virus in the skin at the end of the period of viremia.

Viremia is common in HHV-6, HHV-7, enteroviral, and adenoviral infections; thus a reasonable conclusion (as originally suggested by Watson[82]) is that the rash in roseola is related to an immunologic event resulting from the virus that is localized in the skin. Why the pattern of fever and then rash with defervescence is so clearly age dependent is unknown. Most of the viruses that in the past have been associated with roseola cause other exanthematous manifestations in older patients.[16]

CLINICAL PRESENTATION

The basic clinical pattern of roseola is a febrile period of 3 to 5 days, defervescence, and the appearance of a rash that persists for 1 to 2 days. Because the syndrome is caused by many different viruses, the illness apparently may be associated with numerous other signs and symptoms. The major manifestations have been reviewed elsewhere.[10,17,24,38,82]

Illness usually occurs with the apparent abrupt onset of fever. Slight irritability and malaise occur frequently, but, more commonly, the child's temperature is taken because a parent notices that the child feels warm. The temperature usually is in the range of 38.9°C to 40.6°C (102.2°F to 105°F). Despite the high fever, the child usually is active, alert, and generally unfazed. The fever is constant or intermittent, with its greatest degree occurring in the early evening. Restlessness and irritability occur with higher temperatures. The usual duration of fever is 3 to 5 days,

*References 1, 5, 10, 28, 36, 44, 46, 57, 61, 63, 70, 75, 81, 90.

but it has persisted for 9 days. The temperature most often returns to normal by crisis, but, in some cases, temperature "lysis" occurs over the course of 24 to 36 hours.

Mild cough and coryza are seen frequently in cases occurring in the winter and spring. Headache and abdominal pain are reported in older children, mainly in the summer and fall. Vomiting and diarrhea occur infrequently.

On initial physical examination during the febrile period, most children appear to be happy, alert, and playful. With high temperatures, some children are irritable; occasionally a child appears to be sick, which suggests more serious illness, such as meningitis or septicemia. Examination within the oral cavity frequently reveals one or more abnormalities. Mild inflammation of the pharynx and tonsils occurs most commonly. Occasionally small exudative follicular lesions are noted on the tonsils. In other cases, small ulcerative lesions on the soft palate, uvula, and tonsillar pillars are observed. Usually the lesions on the soft palate consist of only erythematous macules and maculopapules, presumably because of lymphoid hyperplasia.

Mild injection of the tympanic membranes occurs commonly. Enlargement of the suboccipital, posterior cervical, and postauricular lymph nodes is a common finding, but the degree is not remarkable.

Berliner[9] noticed that children with roseola had palpebral edema. He suggested that the "heavy eyelids" or "droopy" or "sleepy" appearance resulting from this edema was diagnostic of the syndrome before the appearance of the rash. Bulging of the anterior fontanelle also has been observed in roseola.[59]

Appearance of the rash in roseola usually coincides with the subsidence of fever, but it may occur after an afebrile interlude of several hours to 2 days. When defervescence occurs by lysis, onset of the exanthem can occur before the temperature has returned entirely to normal. By definition, it is incorrect, however, to call an illness roseola if the fever and rash are truly concomitant.

Zahorsky[85,86] originally described the rash as morbilliform, but his use of *morbilliform* was not the same as is used today (measles-like, erythematous, maculopapular with confluence). The rash is erythematous and macular or maculopapular, and the lesions are discrete. The lesions are 2 to 5 mm in diameter and blanch on pressure. Frequently individual lesions are surrounded by a whitish ring. The rash is most prominent on the neck and trunk, but the proximal extremities and the face also may be affected. Although they have been reported,[18,25] pruritus and desquamation usually do not occur. The rash usually persists for 24 to 48 hours. In occasional cases, well-documented rashes have been observed to appear and resolve within 2 to 4 hours. Yoshida and associates[84] described a 7-month-old boy with HHV-6 infection and typical roseola initially. On the ninth day of illness, vesicular lesions appeared on the face and limbs, however. These lesions persisted for 12 days.

Except for the white blood cell count, routine laboratory studies are of little use in roseola. The total white blood cell count usually is low. Early in the febrile period, high counts occasionally are found, however. The total count reaches its nadir by the third to sixth day of illness and then gradually returns to normal over the ensuing 7 to 10 days. During the same time frame, the percentage of lymphocytes increases from a normal value of about 50% to 60% to 80% on days 3 to 10 and then returns to normal over the next 7 days. Frequently extreme counts in the range of 3000 cells/mm^3 with 90% lymphocytes are found, which raises the consideration of a granulocytic defect. Huang and Lin[35] note that sterile pyuria may occur in infants with roseola. They noted that these cases can be differentiated from bacterial urinary tract infections by the presence of leukocytosis.

CLINICAL COMPLICATIONS

The most important complications of roseola are convulsions and other neurologic symptoms.* The incidence of convulsions has varied widely among reports. Juretic[40] did not find one instance of convulsions in the 243 cases in his study. Breese[11] did not report convulsions in any of 100 roseola attacks that he studied. In contrast, Greenthal[26] noted convulsions in 6% of his cases, and Faber and Dickey[21] found seizures in eight of 26 cases of roseola. Möller[51] observed that 8% of children admitted to the hospital because of febrile convulsions eventually were diagnosed with roseola infantum.

Möller[51] also reported cerebrospinal fluid evaluations in 29 cases of roseola and febrile convulsions. In six instances, the pressure was elevated; in two, there were 5 white blood cells/mm^3; and in another instance, there were 9 white blood cells/mm^3. In most other cerebrospinal fluid examinations, the findings have been normal, but mild pleocytosis with mononuclear cells has been identified occasionally.[8,33] A surprising number of cases of encephalitis associated with roseola have been reported,[14,23,33,37] and residua have been common. Hemiplegia has occurred after illness,[14,23,62,65] and permanent paresis and mental retardation have occurred in some affected patients. The syndrome of inappropriate secretion of antidiuretic hormone has been reported in roseola associated with HHV-6 infection.[58,68] Facial nerve palsy and Guillain-Barré syndrome also have been noted after HHV-6–induced roseola.[50,60]

Thrombocytopenic purpura was noted in one report in five children with roseola; all of these patients recovered.[56] In a more recent study, Hashimoto and colleagues[30] noted five children with thrombocytopenia during the acute phase of roseola caused by HHV-6 infection. Their data suggested that the thrombocytopenia was due to bone marrow suppression, rather than immune-mediated peripheral consumption. A 14-month-old girl developed a generalized eruptive histiocytoma with rapid progression and then resolution after roseola.[73]

*References 3, 8, 12–14, 21, 23, 26, 33, 37, 45, 51, 62, 65, 66.

DIAGNOSIS

Although detecting leukopenia with relative lymphocytosis is fortuitous, the only necessity in establishing the diagnosis of roseola is to document the fever, defervescence, and exanthem pattern. Frequently the first exanthematous illness that a child has is called roseola, regardless of whether the exanthem and the fever are concomitant or the child has no febrile period at all.

The only problem in the differential diagnosis occurs when a febrile child is receiving antibiotics and a rash follows defervescence. This event occurs frequently, and the child usually is labeled allergic to the antibiotic rather than suspected of having roseola. In most instances of drug allergy, the exanthem lasts longer than roseola does, and, in allergic cases, pruritus and fever may accompany the rash.

TREATMENT AND PROGNOSIS

No specific treatment for roseola exists. When fever is a problem, it may be treated with acetaminophen. Acetaminophen can alter the temperature curve, possibly obscuring the correct diagnosis. Febrile seizures and other neurologic complications should be treated vigorously.

In most cases, the outlook is excellent. When encephalitis occurs, the prognosis must be guarded. Because roseola is the result of infection with multiple different viruses, no practical way to prevent it exists.

NEW REFERENCES SINCE THE SEVENTH EDITION

1. Agut H, Bonnafous P, Gautheret-Dejean A. Laboratory and clinical aspects of human herpesvirus 6 infections. *Clin Microbiol Rev.* 2015;28(2):313-315.
34. Huang CT, Lin LH. Differentiating roseola infantum with pyuria from urinary tract infection. *Pediatr Int.* 2013;55(2):214-218.
48. Magalhaes Ide M, Martins RV, Vianna RO, et al. Detection of human herpesvirus 7 infection in young children presenting with exanthema subitum. *Mem Inst Oswaldo Cruz.* 2011;106(3):371-373.
75. Tesini BL, Epstein LG, Caserta MT. Clinical impact of primary infection with roseoloviruses. *Curr Opin Virol.* 2014;9:91-96.

The full reference list for this chapter is available at ExpertConsult.com.

60 Skin Infections

60A ■ Bacterial Skin Infections

Duha Al-Zubeidi • Mary Anne Jackson

NORMAL SKIN

Anatomy

The epidermal skin layer provides the primary barrier to invasion by microorganisms and an interface between the body and the environment. Hair follicles, sebaceous glands, nails, and sweat glands are considered epidermal appendages and as such may be involved in skin infection. A dermal layer composed of collagen and elastic fibers gives skin its elasticity; however, other cell elements that are present, including mast cells, blood and lymph vessels, and cutaneous nerves, may be involved in the inflammatory process in response to infection. The subcutaneous fat layer is just beneath the dermis and contributes primarily to thermal stability, but it also may be involved when infection extends beyond the epidermal-dermal layer.

Flora

Colonization is defined as the presence of a microorganism on the skin without either clinical signs or symptoms of infection at the time of isolation. Normal bacterial skin colonization is divided into resident and transient flora. Resident flora predominates and includes typical nonpathogens, such as *Staphylococcus epidermidis* and *Propionibacterium acnes,* in addition to other anaerobic diphtheroids (Corynbacteriaceae) and micrococci. Transient flora include pathogenic organisms, such as *Staphylococcus aureus,* streptococci, gram-negative enteric organisms, and *Candida albicans;* these pathogens usually are present in smaller numbers than the resident flora and may be removed by skin cleansing. Fungal species such as *Malassezia* spp. can be found as part of the normal skin flora.[86] Acutely or chronically damaged skin, contact with animate and inanimate environmental sources, and exposure to antimicrobial agents or indwelling devices can modify the skin flora and predispose to infection by resident or acquired transient flora.[78,89]

CUTANEOUS INFECTION AND DERMATOLOGIC MANIFESTATIONS OF SYSTEMIC DISEASE

Dermatologic manifestations of infection can occur when the skin is infected primarily or as a secondary phenomenon. Prompt diagnosis and treatment of certain systemic or disseminated diseases may be accomplished when the secondary dermatologic manifestations are recognized. Empiric treatment of systemic diseases such as endocarditis (septic emboli) or septicemia caused by bacterial pathogens, such as *Neisseria meningitidis* or *Pseudomonas aeruginosa*, is possible when the dermatologic manifestations (i.e., purpura fulminans, ecthyma gangrenosum) are noted. Generalized viral infections may be heralded by pathognomonic skin findings, such as occur in varicella or measles. Alternatively skin manifestations may be mediated by toxin (staphylococcal scalded skin syndrome or toxic shock syndrome) or by immunologic mechanisms (gonococcemia).

The list of bacterial infectious agents associated with skin infections is extensive (Table 60A.1). This section focuses on the bacterial skin infections most frequently encountered by practicing clinicians. Viral, bacterial, and fungal systemic or disseminated diseases are categorized in Chapter 58 and are also presented in the specific chapters in Part III of this book.

IMPETIGO

Nonbullous or Simple Superficial Impetigo

The bacterial skin infection most commonly encountered in children is nonbullous impetigo, which accounts for more than 70% of impetigo cases in children. This superficial infection is seen predominantly in summer, with insect bites, cutaneous injuries, and primary dermatitis serving as the portal of entry.[45,60]

Nonbullous impetigo, sometimes called *thick crusted impetigo,* is characterized by the appearance of erythematous maculopapules that rapidly evolve from a vesicular to a pustular stage. Centrally crusted plaques range in size from a few millimeters to 1 cm and are surrounded by a distinct margin of erythema. The honey-colored crust is a classic feature, and removal of the crust results in the reaccumulation of fresh exudate. Regional lymphadenopathy can occur and often is the reason that the patient seeks medical attention. Spread to exposed areas, usually the face, neck, and limbs, occurs frequently. This form of pyoderma often is associated with a 2- to 3-week delay in establishing the diagnosis because the lesions are slow to progress, only mildly tender at the site of the lesion, and generally not associated with systemic signs or symptoms.

Nonbullous impetigo classically has been associated with infection caused by group A β-hemolytic streptococcus (GAS). More recent data underscore the importance of *S. aureus,* however, which now accounts for most cases of nonbullous impetigo in the United States.[6,49]

Primarily a disease of children, nonbullous impetigo is spread within families and by close physical contact. It is prevalent during warm, humid seasons and is seen year-round in tropical regions. Endemic disease occurs in the southeastern United States and Hawaii.

Epidemics of streptococcal impetigo have been associated with postinfectious glomerulonephritis, and streptococcal strains, including types 2, 31, 49, 53, 55, 56, 57, and 60, have been implicated in such outbreaks.[66,108] Studies published in the 1950s and 1960s from the Red Lake Indian Reservation in Minnesota first confirmed the association of impetigo in school-aged children with a postinfectious nephritis that occurred 18 to 21 days after the onset of impetigo and implicated the so-called Red Lake strain, M-type 49.[5] Further studies in this population performed in the early 1970s found that GAS was isolated from normal skin in 23 of 31 high-risk children a mean of 10 days before the development of impetigo.[33] Local trauma and other environmental factors seemed to explain the predilection of exposed skin to streptococcal infection, especially the skin of the legs, where 62% of the total lesions were noted. Secondary acquisition of streptococcal isolates in other family members occurred a mean of 5 days after the primary case, a time frame that was noted to be significantly shorter than that of secondary respiratory acquisition.[51] Rheumatic fever does not occur as a postinfectious sequela of streptococcal skin infection.

Cutaneous botryomycosis, an indolent infection reminiscent of crusted impetigo, usually is caused by *S. aureus.* Characterized by plaquelike lesions with superficial pustules and crusts, this entity has a predilection for patients with altered immune function.[22] Histologic examination may suggest the diagnosis of actinomycosis if a granulomatous lesion with granules resembling those seen with *Actinomyces* is noted. Successful treatment can be accomplished after the bacterial pathogen has been identified.

TABLE 60A.1 Bacterial Infectious Agents Associated With Cutaneous Manifestations

Anthrax	*Bacillus anthracis*
Blistering dactylitis	*Streptococcus pyogenes* *Streptococcus agalactiae* *Staphylococcus aureus*
Cellulitis	*S. pyogenes* *S. aureus* *Haemophilus influenzae* type b *Streptococcus pneumoniae*
Chancroid	*Haemophilus ducreyi*
Diphtheria	*Corynebacterium diphtheriae*
Ecthyma gangrenosum	*Pseudomonas aeruginosa*
Erysipelas	*S. pyogenes* *S. agalactiae;* groups C, G streptococci *S. pneumoniae*
Erysipeloid	*Erysipelothrix rhusiopathiae*
Folliculitis	*S. aureus* Coagulase-negative staphylococci *Klebsiella* spp. *Enterobacter* spp. *Escherichia coli* *P. aeruginosa* *Proteus* spp.
Erythrasma	*Corynebacterium minutissimum*
Furunculosis	*S. aureus*
Hidradenitis suppurativa	*S. aureus* *Streptococcus milleri* *E. coli* Anaerobic streptococci
Granuloma inguinale	*Calymmatobacterium granulomatis*
Impetigo	
Simple superficial	*S. aureus* *S. pyogenes*
Bullous	*S. aureus*
Lymphogranuloma venereum	*Chlamydia trachomatis*
Melioidosis	*Burkholderia pseudomallei*
Necrotizing fasciitis	*S. pyogenes* Polymicrobial
Nocardiosis	*Nocardia brasiliensis* *Nocardia asteroides*
Paronychia	Polymicrobial
Perianal dermatitis	*S. pyogenes*
Pitted keratolysis	Coryneform bacteria
Syphilis	*Treponema pallidum*

Entries in bold are discussed in the text.

Bullous Impetigo

Bullous impetigo is diagnosed when the primary lesion begins as small vesicles and later appears as flaccid, painless bullae, generally measuring greater than 1 cm (Fig. 60A.1). Initially filled with clear fluid, the lesions eventually may exhibit a purulent fluid level. Rupture of the thin bullae usually reveals a moist, erythematous base that dries to a shiny lacquer-like appearance, sometimes described as a varnished finish (Fig. 60A.2). Systemic toxicity is not seen except in neonates, in whom disseminated disease may occur.

In contrast to thick, crusted impetigo, in virtually all cases of bullous impetigo, staphylococci are isolated in pure culture from aspirated bulla fluid. Other bullous dermatitides of childhood, such as pemphigus or Stevens-Johnson syndrome, may be excluded by isolation of the organism. Occasionally biopsy is done in cases in which extensive bullae or an atypical clinical appearance is noted. Confirmation of a cleavage plane high in the epidermis with gram-positive organisms and polymorphonuclear leukocytes present is a definitive diagnosis of bullous staphylococcal disease.

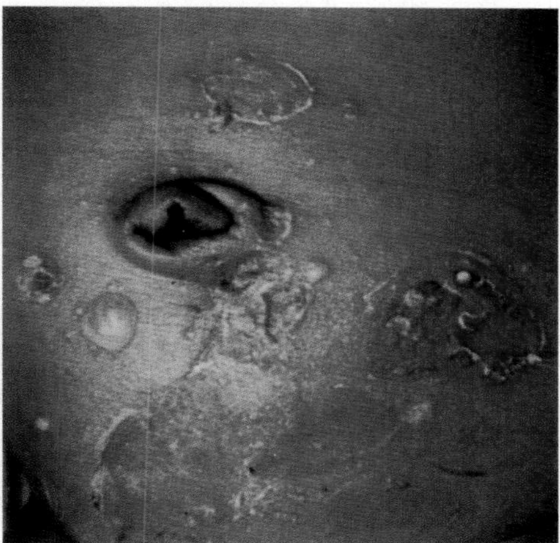

FIG. 60A.1 Bullous impetigo in a newborn infant caused by exfoliative toxin-producing *Staphylococcus aureus.*

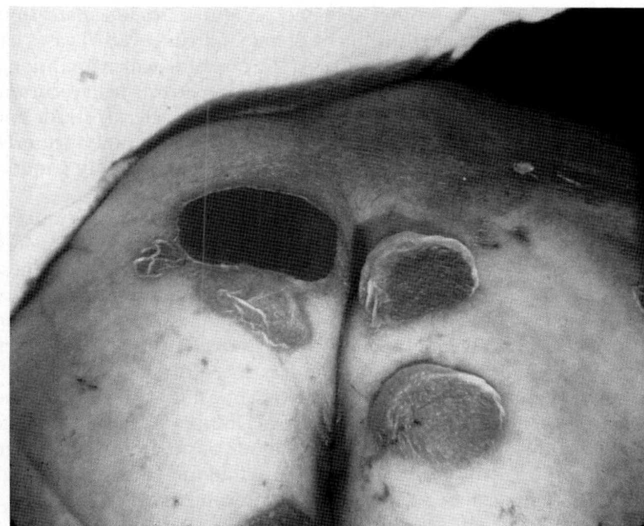

FIG. 60A.2 Flaccid bullae and shiny lacquer base of staphylococcal impetigo.

Infection generally is caused by phage group II strains, particularly phage type 71, but also 3A, 3C, and 55, which are noted to elaborate epidermolytic toxins A and B. Pathologically these toxins act by disrupting the intercellular attachment of epidermal cells of the stratum granulosum. The toxin is thought to function as a protease in separating the upper layers of the epidermis of adult and infant human skin. Production of antibody to epidermolytic toxin occurs with age; however, it does not protect against the development of new bullous lesions during the localized impetiginous stage of this staphylococcal disease.

Epidemiologically large outbreaks of bullous impetigo have been traced most notably to hospital nurseries, where identification of infected infants always occurs within the first month of life but after the infant has been sent home. A more severe, generalized form of the epidermolytic toxin–mediated disease (Ritter disease) may be seen in a few infants during one of these outbreaks, underscoring the importance of infection control surveillance practices in recognizing such an outbreak (Fig. 60A.3).

Treatment of Impetigo

Topical mupirocin 2% cream (Bactroban) may be used in cases of nonbullous impetigo in which adequate coverage of the affected sites can be ensured.[17,32,98] In other cases, systemic treatment with an oral antistaphylococcal antimicrobial agent, such as cephalexin, should be

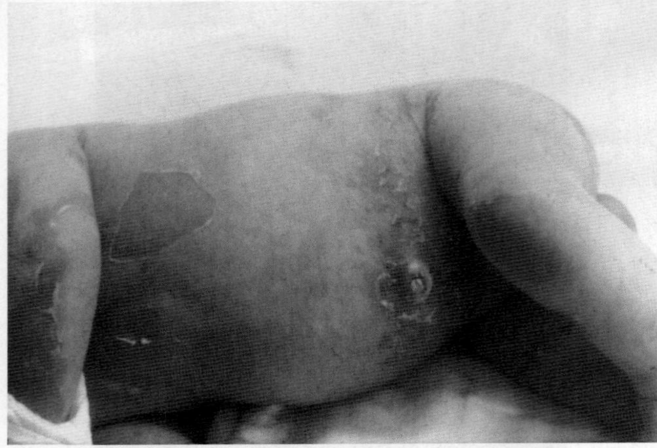

FIG. 60A.3 Typical appearance of a neonate with Ritter disease.

employed.[37,38,44,110] As in other staphylococcal diseases, an increase in community-acquired, methicillin-resistant *S. aureus* (MRSA) cases has been noted in the past decade.[61,62,71,126] In cases for which traditional antistaphylococcal agents are unsuccessful or in patients with recurrent disease, culture should be done to identify the bacterial strain and susceptibility pattern. Currently the majority of community-acquired MRSA isolates are susceptible to clindamycin, but sensitivity patterns vary throughout the United States.[16,23]

A recent study comparing clindamycin versus trimethoprim-sulfamethoxazole (TMP-SMX) for skin infections involved 524 patients; *S. aureus* was isolated from 41.4% of the patients, and 77% of these patients had MRSA. Clindamycin resistance was confirmed in 21% of the MRSA patients and in 9.9% of methicillin-susceptible *S. aureus* (MSSA) patients. Overall there was no significant difference between clindamycin and TMP-SMX for the treatment of skin infections.[101] However, one should remember that by choosing TMP-SMX, good coverage is lacking for GAS. The Infectious Diseases Society of America (IDSA) cautions the use of TMP-SMX alone as an oral option when GAS is suspected or isolated and suggests adding a β-lactam (e.g., penicillin, cephalexin, or amoxicillin) as a second agent.

PERIANAL STREPTOCOCCAL DERMATITIS

Formerly called *perianal cellulitis*, perianal streptococcal dermatitis, a commonly recognized superficial skin infection, is characterized by the presence of marked, well-demarcated, perirectal erythema with associated swelling, pruritus, and tenderness but an absence of systemic symptoms or progressive disease. Approximately half of patients complain of significant rectal pain on defecation, and a third note blood in their stools.[4,28,69,97]

Heavy growth of GAS is seen on perianal culture, and, in one study, isolation of a specific T-type *Streptococcus* (T 28) raised the question of whether certain streptococcal strains have tropism for the perineal region.[104] Asymptomatic patients were evaluated in two studies, and only sparse growth of GAS was noted in 6% of cases.

Perianal streptococcal dermatitis is treated with oral penicillin agents. Topical mupirocin also has been used successfully. Recurrences are noted commonly, however. In one large series of patients, one-third had recurrent disease.[85] Intrafamilial spread of disease frequently occurs and may provide a vector for recurrence. For patients with recurrent or persistent disease, clindamycin or a β-lactam agent plus rifampin may be used, and identification and treatment of other affected family members may be necessary.

BLISTERING DISTAL DACTYLITIS

Most commonly identified in school-aged children, blistering distal dactylitis is a distinctive superficial skin infection classically associated with GAS.[12] Bullae 2 cm in diameter develop over the anterior fat pad of the distal phalanges, sometimes extending to involve the nail folds. Involvement of the proximal phalanges or the palms occasionally is noted. Frankly pustular lesions may occur, but the lesions themselves usually are asymptomatic or only mildly tender. A thin purulent exudate generally is apparent on incision and drainage.[70]

The diagnosis is confirmed by recovery of the etiologic agent on culture, most commonly GAS, although group B streptococcus and *S. aureus* also have been noted.[57] Concurrent recovery of GAS in the pharynx has been reported in a few cases. Treatment includes a 10-day course of an oral β-lactam agent, usually penicillin or amoxicillin, in addition to incision and drainage of any tense bullae.

ERYSIPELAS

The superficial cellulitis erysipelas, referred to as *St. Anthony's fire* in the Middle Ages, is characterized by the appearance of a bright erythematous plaque with a distinct, elevated border that sharply demarcates affected from unaffected skin. The lesion most often involves the face or lower extremity, although extensive involvement of the trunk has been noted. The involved skin is warm and tender and may have a *peau d'orange* appearance. Large tension bullae may be seen in the erythematous zone.[64] The patient generally appears toxic and is highly febrile, and rapid extension of the affected skin may occur over the course of hours.[30,65,138]

Histopathologic findings include intense edema with vascular dilation of the dermis and uppermost subcutaneous tissue. Involvement of lymphatic channels and tissue spaces with polymorphonuclear leukocytes is a typical finding.

Surgical wounds, the umbilicus of the neonate, or any break in the skin may serve as the portal of entry; however, the initial lesion may be inapparent. Localized edema, such as occurs from a renal or lymphatic source, is a predisposing factor, and antecedent respiratory tract infection often is reported. An increased risk for development of erysipelas has been noted in patients with hypogammaglobulinemia, certain malignancies such as lymphoma, or lymphedema complicating radiation therapy.

The diagnosis generally is recognized on clinical grounds, and GAS traditionally has been isolated by aspiration of the advancing margin of the lesion. A few case reports have identified other streptococci (including groups B, C, and G), *Moraxella* spp., *Haemophilus influenzae*, and *Streptococcus pneumoniae* as etiologic agents.[14,29,41,87,102,125,139] A combination of intravenous penicillin and clindamycin should be used until the results of culture are available. Erysipelas has a classic clinical appearance, and appropriate diagnosis and therapy result in a prompt clinical response in most cases. Penicillin prophylaxis may be considered for patients with recurrent erysipelas, particularly patients with underlying risk factors.[15,39]

ECTHYMA

Ecthyma gangrenosa is a deep-seated infectious process that manifests as a necrotic ulcer covered by a black eschar. Usually the initial lesion, a vesicopustule, sits on an erythematous base; it eventually erodes through the epidermis to the dermis, where it forms a crusted ulcer with heaped-up borders and then becomes frankly necrotic.[63]

This process rarely occurs in an otherwise healthy child, and, if it does, an immunodeficiency workup should ensue. *Chromobacterium violaceum* has been reported to cause ecthyma and similarly should result in an immunologic evaluation focusing on neutrophil defects, including disorders such as chronic granulomatous disease.[21]

Ecthyma can occur as a primary cutaneous infection in an immunocompetent host, and other etiologic agents that have been confirmed include *S. aureus*, *Aeromonas hydrophila*, and GAS.[47,56,72,82,95,105,136] A similar-appearing lesion is seen with cutaneous anthrax; however, extensive nonpitting edema of the surrounding soft tissues is an important clue to this diagnosis. Ecthymatous-like lesions have been seen in patients with herpes simplex infection.[83] Additionally, human orf infections result in ulcerative skin lesions that appear similar to lesions of ecthyma; the clue to establishing the diagnosis is contact with an infected animal, usually sheep or goats, or a contaminated fomite.[25]

When an ecthymatous lesion is noted in a febrile neutropenic host, it generally signals disseminated infection. *P. aeruginosa* is the etiologic pathogen identified most commonly in such cases, but other gram-negative pathogens and fungi, including *Enterobacter, Escherichia coli, Morganella, Pseudomonas cepacia, Serratia marcescens, Stenotrophomonas maltophilia, Aspergillus, Mucor, Fusarium,* and *C. albicans,* have been implicated in ecthyma gangrenosum in compromised hosts.[36,50,52,96,107,113,118,124] Ecthyma has been seen as the heralding manifestation of acute lymphoblastic leukemia in children.[112] Empiric antimicrobial therapy for ecthyma gangrenosum in a neutropenic host should include intravenous therapy with an anti-*Pseudomonas* agent plus an aminoglycoside. Biopsy of the lesion may provide more specific etiologic information and allow for confirmation of antimicrobial susceptibility.

FOLLICULITIS, FURUNCULOSIS, AND CARBUNCLES

Folliculitis, furunculosis, and carbuncles represent a group of infections characterized by their origin in the hair follicles and the formation of abscesses. Virtually always caused by *S. aureus,* these infections were seen commonly in the 1950s in disease that often involved multiple family members. Outbreaks among athletes likewise have been reported.[132]

By definition, these infections involve sites where body hair is present, including the axilla, breast area, perineum, neck, and extremities. Lesions of folliculitis represent abscesses of a single hair follicle with limited surrounding tissue involvement. When deeper inflammatory nodules are associated with tissue edema, furunculosis is diagnosed. When several interconnecting furuncles are present, the lesion is referred to as a carbuncle. Generally, older children and adolescents are predisposed to the development of follicular infections, and individuals with diabetes mellitus, abnormal neutrophil chemotaxis, and impaired circulation may have recurrent disease.

Although *S. aureus* nearly always is the cause of folliculitis as in the past, outbreaks of so-called hot tub folliculitis have been described and almost always are caused by *P. aeruginosa;* rarely other gram-negative organisms have been reported.[26,27] Folliculitis in an immunocompromised host often is caused by unusual fungal pathogens.[3,116,129] Although typically associated with hot tubs and whirlpools, a large outbreak of *Pseudomonas* folliculitis reported in 1984 involved 117 individuals after swimming in an indoor pool. An incubation period of 24 to 30 hours could be ascertained, and a typical follicular, pustular eruption was noted. The mean duration of the folliculitis, 15 days, is consistent with other reports, but some patients continued to complain of rash for weeks, and recurrent pustules appearing months later have been reported in other studies.[55]

A more recent report has identified four cases of *Mycobacterium fortuitum* complex furunculosis that developed after pedicures, suggesting this pathogen may be added to the differential diagnosis in such cases when a patient presents with nonhealing furuncles on the lower legs, especially when bacterial cultures have been negative or the disease is unresponsive to antistaphylococcal therapy (including MRSA).[115] Early recognition and institution of appropriate therapy are essential, and the history of pedicures may be a clue to establishing the diagnosis. Cutaneous myiasis has been reported to manifest as a chronic boil or furuncle, but the diagnosis should be considered only in such cases in which an appropriate travel history is elicited.[31]

Recognition of the typical skin lesion usually is sufficient to establish the diagnosis. Unless the patient has a history of exposure to a hot tub or whirlpool or recently has had a pedicure, a regimen of antistaphylococcal therapy should be sufficient. In the era of MRSA infection, local susceptibility profiles should be used to confirm appropriate therapy. Isolated boils resolve with drainage alone. Systemic therapy may be considered in cases in which lesions are large or multiple. TMP-SMX is a good choice for a nontoxic patient older than 2 months. Clindamycin is a good choice for most locales, although resistance may be increasing.[80,90] Because MRSA now accounts for 75% of cases in which children present with skin and soft tissue infection, treatment should be individualized based on type of presentation, patient age, and underlying disease.[79] Systemic agents should be used for 7 to 10 days in patients who are toxic, who have extensive disease, or who have associated cellulitis. Large lesions, specifically larger than 5 cm, should be incised and drained, and culture should be done in all cases to confirm susceptibility testing. In some patients, hematogenous metastatic spread may occur, and a search for foci in the heart, bones, joints, deep tissues, or brain should be done in patients with significant systemic toxicity.

For patients in whom recurrent disease develops, chronic dermatoses, such as eczema, should be identified, and in obese adolescents, the diagnosis of diabetes mellitus should be considered.[7] The patient should be cautioned to refrain from sharing washcloths or towels, and skin trauma and use of irritants such as deodorants should be avoided.

The utility of decolonizing regimens with topical agents, such as mupirocin (nares and perianal area) and chlorhexidine or bleach baths (skin), may be considered in certain cases. *S. aureus* colonization of the nares, rectum, or skin can be detected by culture of these areas, but confirmation of carriage is likely necessary only in specific cases for which decolonization is desirable. The indications for and benefit of decolonization vary depending on host factors, underlying disease, and circumstances related to the health care setting.[128] Outbreaks of MRSA colonization or infection require a multifaceted approach, including attention given to hand washing, cohorting, barrier measures, and decolonization strategies. Implementation of a decolonization regimen should be considered in special circumstances including (1) patients who are immunosuppressed and colonized and at risk for development of systemic infections, (2) patients who are more likely to spread the organisms owing to behavior, (3) patients who have repeated infections caused by the MRSA strain they carry, or (4) patients undergoing certain surgeries (cardiac, implantable devices) in whom colonization is confirmed; in addition, targeted prophylaxis should be used preoperatively.[122] Most children with recurrent furunculosis are otherwise healthy, and no specific immunologic evaluation is necessary; however cases of recurrent furunculosis in patients with hyper-IgE syndrome and common variable immunodeficiency have been reported, and an association with mannose-binding lectin deficiency was confirmed in a family.[76,81,127] Rarely children with white blood cell defects may have recurrent staphylococcal skin abscesses, and tests of white blood cell function may be considered in specific patients. Data suggest that vitamin C may be beneficial in cases of recurrent folliculitis.[92,93]

HIDRADENITIS SUPPURATIVA

Hidradenitis suppurativa, a chronic, debilitating condition, is a disorder of the apocrine glands that involves primarily skin in the axilla and anogenital region, although scalp, umbilical, and breast involvement has been reported. Seen mainly in adolescents, this androgen-dependent condition is manifested by the development of multiple painful nodules and the formation of deep abscesses in the skin in areas where apocrine glands are present. The formation of fistulas, ulcers, and contracted scars may complicate the course, and recurrent relapses may be noted. Infection usually is polymicrobial, and pathogens to consider include *S. aureus,* gram-negative enteric organisms, and anaerobes. Drainage of abscesses and institution of systemic antimicrobial therapy may be necessary. When fistulas associated with anogenital disease develop, adjacent structures, including the urethra, bladder, and rectum, may be involved. Surgery usually is required for cure. Carbon dioxide laser treatment in some cases may be beneficial.[88]

CELLULITIS

The diagnosis of cellulitis is made when the subcutaneous tissues and dermis are involved in a clinical process manifested as localized edema, erythema, warmth, and tenderness of the tissues. The leading edge of the involved site may be notable, but it is not raised and well demarcated as in erysipelas.

Infection usually is caused by coagulase-positive staphylococci and GAS; however, infection also is caused by group B streptococcus (neonates) and *S. pneumoniae,* and, in the past, *H. influenzae* type b cellulitis was described.[133] Streptococcal and staphylococcal cellulitis can involve patients of any age and any site, although the extremity is noted most often. Frequently the patient has a history of antecedent trauma at the site of involvement, but the injury may not have appeared significant. Some researchers advocate culture of the cellulitic site, but in practice, it rarely is performed. Blood cultures are valuable in individuals with disease caused by group B streptococcus, *S. pneumoniae,* and *H. influenzae* type b.[74]

Group B streptococcal cellulitis occurs in neonates and generally is seen as part of invasive, late-onset disease. Unilateral involvement of the face or submandibular sites occurs most commonly, but inguinal, scrotal, and prepatellar involvement has been described.[10,68] When cellulitis occurs in an infant younger than 3 months, group B streptococcal bacteremia should be suspected, even in the absence of other signs of systemic infection.

Pneumococcal soft tissue infections are common findings.[111] Patients with connective tissue disorders, such as systemic lupus erythematosus, seem especially prone, although these infections can occur in healthy infants and children. Sites of involvement include the head, neck, leg, and torso.

H. influenzae type b cellulitis often involves the face of infants (Fig. 60A.4). A violaceous hue of the cellulitic area, which some researchers thought to be pathognomonic, might be observed. This process nearly always was the result of hematogenous seeding by *H. influenzae* type b, and meningitis occurred in 15% to 20% of such patients.[67,131,142] As has been the case with other forms of *H. influenzae* type b disease, almost complete eradication has been achieved in the past decade with the use of conjugate vaccine.

Treatment of simple cellulitis in patients with a clear-cut area of preceding trauma should include an agent that is active against *S. aureus* and GAS; in most locales, clindamycin remains a good choice for therapy, although resistance for *S. aureus* (10% to 15%) and GAS (2% to 3%) is noted. The aforementioned caveats for treating staphylococcal skin infections should be followed. In infants with buccal or periorbital involvement or in infants with soft tissue involvement but without a clear-cut focus of infection, a third-generation cephalosporin, such as cefotaxime or ceftriaxone, should be included with clindamycin. Vancomycin always should be included in cases of a patient who is toxic and when metastatic suppurative disease is suspected.

Antibiotic-resistant gram-negative infections should be considered in the hospitalized patient who develops cellulitis, especially in those who are immunosuppressed, and broad-spectrum therapy should be considered empirically until results of cultures are available.

NECROTIZING FASCIITIS

Necrotizing fasciitis is a rapidly progressive bacterial infection of the soft tissues associated with a fulminant course and a high mortality rate. This infection spreads rapidly in the plane between the subcutaneous tissue and superficial muscle fascia and causes widespread necrosis. Prompt and aggressive medical and surgical management is necessary to ensure a good outcome.

In children, necrotizing fasciitis usually is caused by GAS; traumatic lesions involving the skin, including varicella, burns, or eczema, may predispose to this aggressive process.[18,46,54,58,68,109,120,121,144] An association has been noted among varicella, ibuprofen use, and invasive GAS infection, although no data convincingly link this triad to necrotizing infection.[53,91,145] Patients with congenital or acquired immunodeficiencies are at greater risk for the development of necrotizing fasciitis, and in neonates, omphalitis and circumcision are predisposing conditions.

Clinical Manifestations

The child generally has a high fever and is fussy. In infants, the irritability may be profound and may not appear to be localized to an involved site, unless the clinician is meticulous in conducting the examination. An extremity most commonly is involved, and older infants and children often refuse to bear weight or move the affected extremity. Swelling of soft tissue usually is noted, but the erythema may be subtle. The hallmark tip-off on examination is the finding of intense pain on manipulation of the involved site that is out of proportion to the cutaneous signs. Skin changes that occur during the subsequent 24 to 48 hours include blistering with bleb formation, and a dusky appearance of the involved site is noted as vessels are thrombosed and cutaneous ischemia develops. Skin necrosis is a late sign and indicates a poor prognosis (Fig. 60A.5).[77,137]

Recognition of the manifestations of toxic shock syndrome (see Chapter 64) is crucial because mortality rates of 60% have been reported in patients with associated fasciitis. Multisystem complaints, including vomiting, diarrhea, and severe myalgia, are present when GAS fasciitis is associated with streptococcal toxic shock syndrome. Tachycardia out

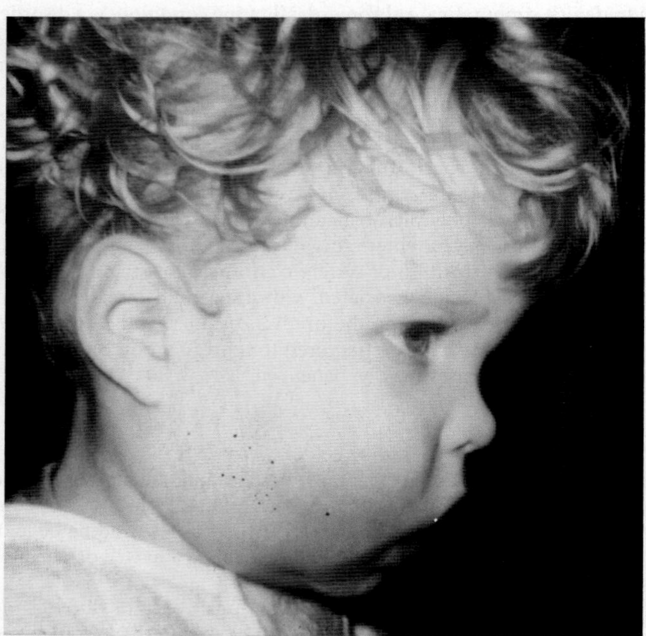

FIG. 60A.4 Buccal involvement in an infant with invasive *Haemophilus influenzae* type b disease.

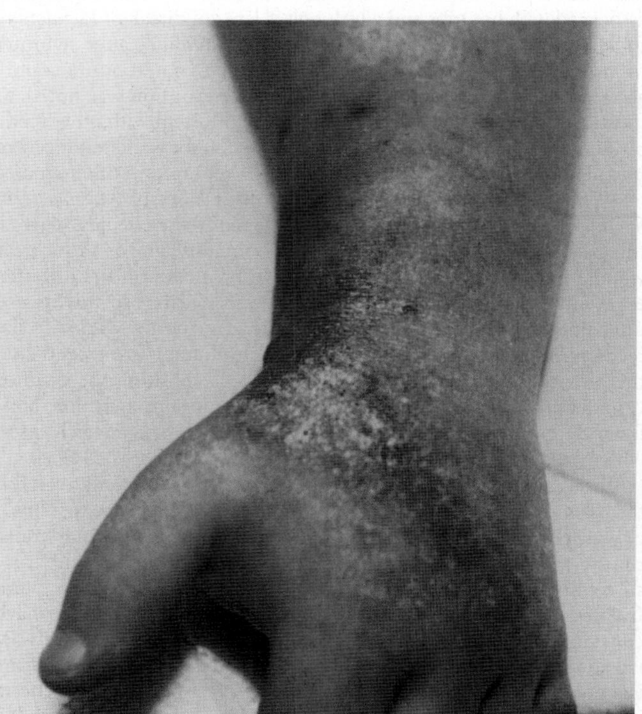

FIG. 60A.5 Necrotizing fasciitis in a toddler with varicella.

of proportion to fever and altered mental status may be early signs of toxic shock syndrome. Renal and hepatic dysfunctions occur typically, and signs and symptoms of acute respiratory distress syndrome often are identified.

Diagnosis

The diagnosis cannot be based on the appearance of the involved site because none of the early findings of necrotizing fasciitis is pathognomonic. Plain radiographs usually are normal and of no value in establishing the diagnosis. Magnetic resonance imaging (MRI) is the preferred technique to detect soft tissue involvement. MRI permits visualization of the soft tissue edema infiltrating the fascial planes.[20,114,146] Although MRI may be helpful, it should not delay performing surgical intervention. Waiting for a radiographic procedure to be performed to confirm the diagnosis may serve only to delay implementing definitive surgical therapy and to increase the risk for development of systemic complications, contributing further to the increased morbidity and mortality rates. In the typical clinical scenario in which the index of suspicion for necrotizing fasciitis is high, surgical exploration is appropriate, even in the presence of "normal" MRI findings.

Laboratory manifestations of streptococcal toxic shock syndrome should be sought in any pediatric patient with fasciitis. Typically, the white blood cell count is normal; however, most patients have a significant increase in band forms (>50%) noted on the peripheral blood smear. Thrombocytopenia and evidence of coagulopathy are found commonly, and marked hypoalbuminemia with hypocalcemia is a typical finding. Laboratory findings associated with renal failure, myocardial dysfunction, and acute respiratory distress syndrome may develop during the first 48 to 72 hours.

A microbiologic diagnosis can be made by isolating bacteria from blood, tissue, or wound culture. In some cases, a polymicrobial etiology has been noted, particularly in patients with so-called Fournier gangrene or necrotizing fasciitis of the perineum.[48,73] In these cases, *S. aureus*, GAS, and one or more anaerobes, including *Peptostreptococcus, Prevotella, Bacteroides fragilis,* and *Porphyromonas,* have been implicated in infection.[19] Fasciitis caused by *P. aeruginosa* or *Clostridium septicum* has been seen in neutropenic patients. In the past decade, GAS has been reported widely as a single pathogen and is the etiologic agent in most cases of pediatric fasciitis. As in other cases of invasive disease caused by GAS, virulence is related to certain structural characteristics of the organism and to its ability to produce biologically active substances, some of which facilitate invasion and spread of the pathogen.

Treatment

Surgical debridement of necrotic tissue is the key to managing necrotizing fasciitis, and increased mortality rates have been observed when debridement is delayed more than 24 hours.[106] Mandatory return to the operating room for examination and repeat debridement should occur during the following 24 to 48 hours. Careful management of fluids, attention to pain control, anticipation and management of multisystem organ failure, and administration of appropriate parenteral antimicrobial therapy should be initiated promptly. The use of intravenous immunoglobulin may be considered in cases of toxic shock syndrome–associated fasciitis.[24]

Appropriate therapy includes intravenous penicillin 150,000 U/kg per day divided into four to six doses, clindamycin 40 mg/kg per day divided into four doses, and vancomycin 40 mg/kg per day divided into three to four doses. The use of additional coverage with agents active against *P. aeruginosa* and gram-negative enteric organisms should be considered in neutropenic patients.

Response to therapy is assessed by careful serial examination. Control of pain is crucial in such patients, while keeping in mind that persistent, severe pain suggests ongoing tissue necrosis and may signal the need for further surgical intervention. Careful attention to nutritional support should be maintained throughout the child's hospital stay. Physical therapy is necessary for most patients, especially patients who require amputation, skin grafting, or extensive reconstructive surgery, and providing for the psychosocial needs of the child and the family is imperative.

TABLE 60A.2 Infections Associated With Animal Bites

Nature of Injury	Pathogens Involved
Human bites	Staphylococci Anaerobic and aerobic streptococci *Eikenella corrodens*
Animal bites	
Dog and cat	*Pasteurella* spp. *Staphylococcus aureus* Streptococci Anaerobes *Capnocytophaga canimorsus, Capnocytophaga cynodegmi* *Moraxella* spp. *Corynebacterium* spp. *Neisseria* spp.
Reptile	Enteric gram-negatives Anaerobes
Horse and sheep	*Actinobacillus* spp., *Pasteurella* spp.
Pig	*Flavobacterium* spp., *Actinobacillus* spp., *Pasteurella aerogenes*
Rat	*Streptobacillus moniliformis, S. aureus*

CONTAMINATED WOUNDS

Although staphylococci and streptococci are the most likely causes of infection after traumatic skin lesions, the list of causes may be extensive, depending on the nature of the injury. Specific pathogens should be considered when infections develop after human or animal bites, soil or water contamination, or various types of injuries. Management of such infections depends on recognizing infection patterns and obtaining cultures for careful identification of the specific organism or organisms involved (Table 60A.2).

Human Bites

Two types of human bites are described: occlusional and clenched fist (see also Chapter 249). Occlusional bites are related most commonly to child abuse, although in a pediatric patient, a biting toddler may be the culprit. Accidental bites may occur during sporting activities and generally involve the face of a teammate. Clenched-fist injuries are associated with the most prevalent and severe infections that occur after human bites. Rapidly progressive infection may follow despite the patient receiving early medical attention.[11] When clenched-fist injuries are associated with bite wounds, laceration and puncture wounds commonly occur along the dorsal aspect of the third metacarpophalangeal joint, and bone, joint capsule, or tendon structures may be involved.

Polymicrobial infection is the usual finding, and, in such cases, broad-spectrum empiric antimicrobial coverage should be initiated promptly after adequate drainage has been performed.[119] In a multicenter study of infected human bites, the median number of isolates per wound was four, and aerobes and anaerobes were identified. The common pathogens were *Streptococcus anginosus, S. aureus, Eikenella corrodens, Fusobacterium nucleatum,* and *Prevotella melaninogenica*. *Candida* spp. were noted less commonly.[134] Many strains of *Prevotella* and *S. aureus* are β-lactamase producers, and *E. corrodens* is intrinsically resistant to clindamycin and cephalosporins. Ampicillin with clavulanate given orally (simple infections) or ampicillin-sulbactam given intravenously for more complicated infections may be used as a single agent. Unusual pathogens rarely occur. A report of a human bite infection caused by *Mycobacterium ulcerans* is noted; this pathogen is emerging rapidly in West African countries.[35] Antimicrobial prophylaxis should be considered for patients with human bites to the hands, feet, and skin overlying joints and for patients with bites that penetrate deeper than the epidermal layer.[117]

Animal Bites

Animal bite wounds occur commonly, with more than 4 million reported annually in the United States (see also Chapter 249). Children account for more than half of patients who go to emergency departments for care of bite wounds.[2] Although one survey revealed that rodents and lagomorphs are the biting animals most commonly reported, wounds related to these bites seldom are associated with infection. By contrast, cats and dogs together account for approximately 40% of bites, and their bites are associated more frequently with morbidity. The etiology of animal bite infections often is related to the species of animal involved (see Table 60A.2).[40,43,75,94]

Approximately 1000 emergency department visits related to dog bites occur each day, at a cost of more than $100 million per year.[130] The incidence of infection related to dog bites has been estimated at 3% to 17%.[9,34] Cat bites are most likely to become infected, probably because of the puncture-like nature of the injury. One study suggests that half of cat bites result in infection, prompting recommendations for prophylaxis of such bites, especially if they involve the face or hands. In the presence of infection, exploration plus debridement of devitalized tissue is necessary, and purulent collections should be drained.

Although *Pasteurella multocida* is implicated most frequently, numerous other pathogens, including *S. aureus, Capnocytophaga canimorsus,* and other aerobic and anaerobic bacteria, are associated with dog and cat bites. Depending on the depth of the wound's penetration, underlying structures such as bones, joints, and tendons may be involved in such infections.[59] The wound itself may not appear significant, particularly in the case of puncture wounds, but several clinical features should influence treatment decisions. The presence of tissue edema and point tenderness on palpation over the site should signal that deeper structures may be involved. Soft tissue imaging may be necessary, and appropriate drainage or debridement of involved sites should be pursued.

As with human bites, oral amoxicillin-clavulanate may be used for prophylaxis or treatment of simple infections. Indications for prophylaxis of bite wounds include bites associated with a crush or puncture injury and bites involving the face, hands, feet, and genitalia. Wounds in immunocompromised, especially asplenic, individuals should be considered for prophylaxis. Intravenous ampicillin-sulbactam or ticarcillin-clavulanate can be used for more serious infections. For individuals who have a history of anaphylaxis with penicillin or cephalosporins, a combination of clindamycin plus trimethoprim-sulfamethoxazole or ciprofloxacin can be used.[114,116] Antimicrobial therapy may be modified further depending on the biting animal and suspected pathogen (see Table 60A.2).[13]

Appropriate prophylaxis against tetanus should be considered for all bites. Hepatitis B can be transmitted by human bites, and appropriate management should be ensured for susceptible patients. Rabies vaccine should be administered after bat, skunk, or raccoon bites; public health information should be accessed to decide whether rabies vaccine is indicated for other animal bites.

Soil-Contaminated and Water-Contaminated Wounds

Four factors that must be considered in the acute care of contaminated wounds include the (1) mechanism of injury, (2) the length of time that transpires from injury to treatment, (3) the types of pathogens that occur in the environment, and (4) the presence of underlying disease in the host.[42] When a traumatic wound becomes infected, a polymicrobial etiology is typical, and common pathogens such as *S. aureus,* gram-negative enteric organisms, and anaerobes characteristically are involved.[1] Unusual and rare organisms, such as nontuberculous mycobacteria; *Nocardia; Actinomyces;* fungi, including *Aspergillus* spp.; and unusual gram-negative organisms, occasionally may be encountered (Box 60A.1).[84,99,100,103,140] *A. hydrophila* has been implicated in infections associated with injuries contaminated by fresh water and may produce rapidly progressive wound infection with fascia, tendon, muscle, bone, or joint involvement.[123]

Managing wounds contaminated by soil or water is difficult, especially if the mechanism of injury is a catastrophic event with complex bone and soft tissue injuries. In the acute setting of such an event, complete exploration and thorough debridement with copious irrigation are performed primarily, and signs of infection generally are not present. Days later, the clinician often is faced with the dilemma of a patient who is receiving antimicrobial prophylaxis with broad-spectrum agents and in whom new signs or symptoms develop acutely. Separating infectious from noninfectious complications often is difficult; however, the onset of fever in such a patient, especially in the setting of an open fracture or dural tear, should prompt further evaluation. Careful serial examination of the site of injury is necessary, and more extensive evaluation generally is indicated. Such assessment may include radiographic imaging and specific evaluation of body fluids with appropriate cultures. Because open fractures are associated with an increased risk for development of infection, the utility of antibiotic-impregnated implants, which are biodegradable and osteoconductive, may prove beneficial in such cases.[135,141]

Infections associated with foreign bodies such as wood generally cannot be cured until the foreign body is identified and removed.[143] Puncture wounds should be explored carefully, and further debridement of necrotic tissue or drainage of involved sites such as joints may be necessary.[8]

Treatment of simple wound infections associated with soil or water contamination should include an agent such as ciprofloxacin, although deeper tissue infection may develop after a seemingly innocuous injury, and tissue debridement may be necessary. Determining the appropriate therapy for a patient with infection involving extensive soft tissue injury and open fractures is problematic. Administration of an empiric regimen with an agent such as piperacillin-tazobactam, imipenem, or a fluoroquinolone plus vancomycin may be reasonable after evaluation and appropriate culturing have been done.

BOX 60A.1 Infections Associated With Soil-Contaminated or Water-Contaminated Wounds

Soil-Contaminated Wounds

Staphylococcus aureus
Group A β-hemolytic streptococci
Many gram-negative enterics
Enterobacter cancerogenus
Anaerobes
Nocardia asteroides, Nocardia otitidiscaviarum
Mycobacterium fortuitum, Mycobacterium abscessus
Actinomyces
Aspergillus spp.
Enterococcus spp.

Water-Contaminated Wounds

Aeromonas hydrophila
Pseudomonas spp.
Many gram-negative enteric organisms
Edwardsiella tarda (catfish injury)
Mycobacterium marinum

NEW REFERENCES SINCE THE SEVENTH EDITION

86. Kong HH, Segre JA. Skin microbiome: looking back to move forward. *J Invest Dermatol.* 2012;132(3 Pt 2):933-939.
101. Miller LG, Daum RS, Creech CB, et al. Clindamycin versus trimethoprim-sulfamethoxazole for uncomplicated skin infections. *N Engl J Med.* 2015; 372(12):1093-1103.
122. Schweizer ML, Chiang HY, Septimus E, et al. Association of a bundled intervention with surgical site infections among patients undergoing cardiac, hip, or knee surgery. *JAMA.* 2015;313(21):2162-2171.

The full reference list for this chapter is available at ExpertConsult.com.

60B ■ Viral and Fungal Skin Infections

Meena R. Julapalli • Moise L. Levy

VIRAL INFECTIONS

Cutaneous manifestations of viral infections are common. Exanthems often accompany acute viral infections. This chapter focuses on the common viral illnesses that manifest with cutaneous manifestations. More detailed information on each of these illnesses can be found in the chapters devoted to specific viral agents.

Viruses can invade the skin indirectly as a result of viremia or directly, as with warts, molluscum, or infections due to herpes simplex virus (HSV) or varicella-zoster virus (VZV). Other mechanisms of producing exanthems include interactions between the infecting agent and humoral or cell-mediated factors, systemic immune response in the absence of viral antigen in the skin,[1,75] or medications as in the drug reaction with eosinophilia and systemic symptoms (DRESS).[1] Human herpes virus–6 (HHV-6) reactivation in DRESS appears to be associated with more severe disease.[1]

The type of exanthem encountered depends on the virus, the pathophysiologic mechanisms involved, the location of the eruption, and local and systemic immune factors. A single virus may manifest with a variety of cutaneous reactions within the same host. Clinicians caring for a patient with an exanthem usually are faced with a challenge to determine its cause. Most viral exanthems are benign and self-limited, but understanding the exact cause can be important when evaluating immunocompromised patients or in the setting of exposure of a pregnant woman. Similarly distinguishing a viral exanthem from skin eruptions caused by other infectious agents or drugs is important.

Generally children presenting with fever and a rash cannot be diagnosed accurately by the presentation of the eruption.[33] The distribution and character of exanthems, such as the often characteristic reticulated erythema after "slapped cheek" exanthem typical of parvovirus B19 infections, are helpful; however, the virus can manifest with several other cutaneous findings.[11,54,60] Typical hand, foot, and mouth syndrome is caused by coxsackievirus, although it has been related more recently to enterovirus 71 and other etiologies.[15,42,49,51,58] The concurrent administration of antibiotics in the setting of Epstein-Barr virus infection is important to know, as is the possible relationship between HHV infection and certain drugs resulting in drug rash with eosinophilia and systemic symptoms.[17]

Laboratory studies, in addition to specific viral cultures, polymerase chain reaction, and serologies, may be helpful in distinguishing between viral and bacterial diseases or drug eruptions. Coagulation studies may help clarify whether a purpuric eruption is caused by a primary coagulopathy or a viral process. Other laboratory tests, such as streptococcal screens or throat cultures or both, serum antibody titers, viral cultures, and antigen detection methods, are required for evaluating exanthems depending on the state of the patient being evaluated.

Warts

See Chapter 152.

Molluscum Contagiosum

Molluscum contagiosum represents a common viral infection of the skin (and sometimes mucous membranes) of children and adolescents. It is caused by a poxvirus and has not been grown in culture although mapping of its genome has been done recently.[55] The virus replicates within the cytoplasm[19] and is represented by four viral types based on DNA analysis: MCV-1 to MCV-4.[50] MCV-1 accounts for more than 90% of infections in the United States.[19,50] The subtypes do not show site specificity. MCV-2 was reported to be seen most commonly in patients infected with human immunodeficiency virus (HIV).[21,50]

Epidemiology

The disease is seen with increasing frequency in sexually active and immunodeficient individuals. Infection occurs at any age, with the highest frequency seen in patients younger than 5 to 10 years.[10,19] The disease is two to three times more common in school-aged and sexually active males than in females. Transmission is via close contact. Spread is reported to occur via fomites. The incidence of disease is highest in warm climates and in areas of overcrowding.

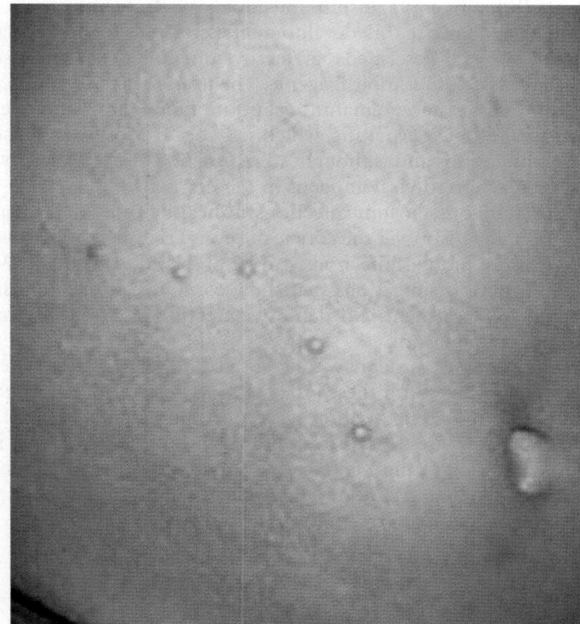

FIG. 60B.1 Grouped dome-shaped papules of molluscum contagiosum on the skin of the abdomen.

Clinical Manifestations

The incubation period for molluscum contagiosum is 2 to 7 weeks, but it has been reported to occur at 1 week of age. Typical lesions are 1 to 5 mm, dome-shaped, skin-colored or pink papules with a distinctive central umbilication (Fig. 60B.1). Giant lesions measuring 1 to 2 cm can be seen. According to an epidemiologic survey conducted at three pediatric dermatology centers, fewer than 15 lesions usually are seen.[19] In children, molluscum contagiosum is seen most frequently on the face, neck, trunk, and extremities but may be seen on any part of the body, including the mucous membranes.[10,19,45] Periocular lesions may lead to secondary keratoconjunctivitis or trachoma. In some cases, molluscum contagiosum is a sexually transmitted infection, raising the issue of sexual abuse when infection is seen in the genital area. The most common etiology of genital molluscum contagiosum is autoinoculation; however, if the lesions occur solely in the genital area or a question exists about the patient's social situation the possibility of abuse should be explored.

Atypical lesions of molluscum contagiosum are seen more commonly, particularly with the improved survival rates of patients with acquired immunodeficiency syndrome (AIDS) and other immunocompromised states. The incidence of molluscum contagiosum in HIV infection is 5% to 18%. With improved antiretroviral therapies, molluscum contagiosum has decreased in this population.[12,19]

Molluscum contagiosum lesions in immunocompromised patients often are large, are situated more deeply in the epidermis, and may number in the hundreds. HIV-positive adults usually have molluscum contagiosum on the face, neck, and trunk. In a study of immunocompromised children, molluscum contagiosum was not considered to be common or severe, however. This study included only six patients, and two were disease free and thought to be immunocompetent at the time of onset of the infection. This and other studies suggest that the presence and degree of cellular immunodeficiency are important in the presentation of molluscum contagiosum. Severe disease is known to occur in the setting of DOCK 8 deficiency.[14]

Patients with atopic dermatitis may be predisposed to develop more severe molluscum contagiosum infection. Available information is insufficient to know if this development is related to the dermatitis itself with its well-described barrier dysfunction or to the use of corticosteroids or other topical agents. The term *molluscum dermatitis* is used to describe an eczematous eruption, more commonly seen in patients with atopic dermatitis, which may occur around molluscum contagiosum lesions and is thought to represent a delayed-type hypersensitivity reaction to viral antigens in the dermis.

Molluscum contagiosum infections in healthy individuals usually resolve spontaneously over the course of several months to 3 to 5 years. For this reason, limited infections can be observed expectantly. More diffuse infections or infections that show continued extension can be considered for treatment. No definitive treatments are available for molluscum contagiosum.

Most treatments, similar to those used for warts, are destructive. Immune enhancement for these infections has been tried, but its utility has not been proved. Furthermore a recent commentary suggested that such interventions are of unproved utility.[46] Multiple treatments have been used, although utility is uncertain in all but curettage. A recent review suggested that resolution of disease was equivalent in groups of patients treated compared with those not treated.[5]

Parvovirus B19 Infections

See Chapter 152.

Gianotti-Crosti Syndrome (Papular Acrodermatitis of Childhood)

Gianotti-Crosti syndrome (papular acrodermatitis of childhood) is a viral exanthem first reported in 1955 by Gianotti,[30] who described a group of children who presented with predominantly acrally located, skin-colored, or slightly erythematous lichenoid papules (Fig. 60B.2).[80] The flexures usually were spared. Involvement of the buttocks or trunk was seen in some cases. No involvement of mucous membranes occurred. Patients generally were healthy. The initial reports showed prior infection with hepatitis B. The eruption lasted 2 weeks to 2 months.

Since the initial report, similar cases have been associated with other infections, such as Epstein-Barr virus, coxsackievirus, echovirus, other viruses, and streptococcal disease.[44,59] Most cases are thought to be viral in origin and have been reported after vaccination.[71] Topical therapies do not hasten resolution of the exanthem.

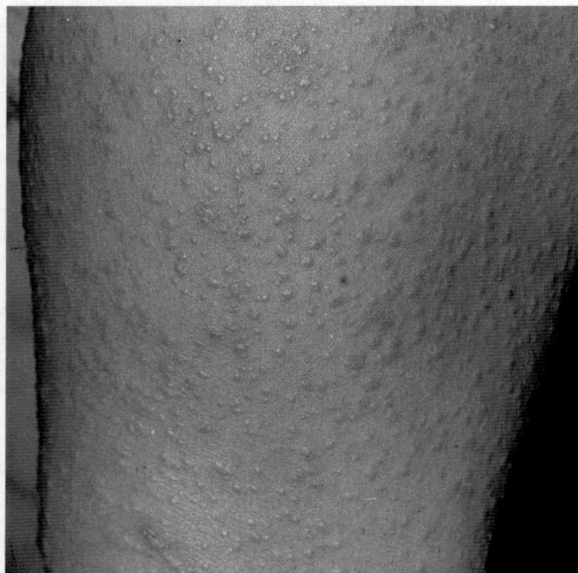

FIG. 60B.2 Diffusely distributed, isolated, monomorphous skin-colored papules on the thigh of a child typical of Gianotti-Crosti syndrome.

Asymmetric Periflexural Viral Exanthem

Some children have been described with discrete or grouped lichenoid papules or urticarial papules beginning around flexures or the torso (Fig. 60B.3).[29] The eruption generalizes over several days and can appear as a more diffuse case of the papular acrodermatitis of childhood.[16] The condition also has been described as unilateral laterothoracic viral exanthem and seems to be associated with the same infectious agents as described in papular acrodermatitis of childhood.[52] The evolution of this condition is similar to that in papular acrodermatitis of childhood.

Hand, Foot, and Mouth Syndrome

While typical cases of hand, foot, and mouth disease are usually easily recognized, there have been atypical cases with more diffuse skin findings described over the past several years. Some have been mistaken for infections due to HSV (Figs. 60B.4 and 60B.5).[13,58] When occurring in patients with atopic dermatitis, more diffuse involvement can be seen and has been called "eczema coxsackium."[49,51] While many of these

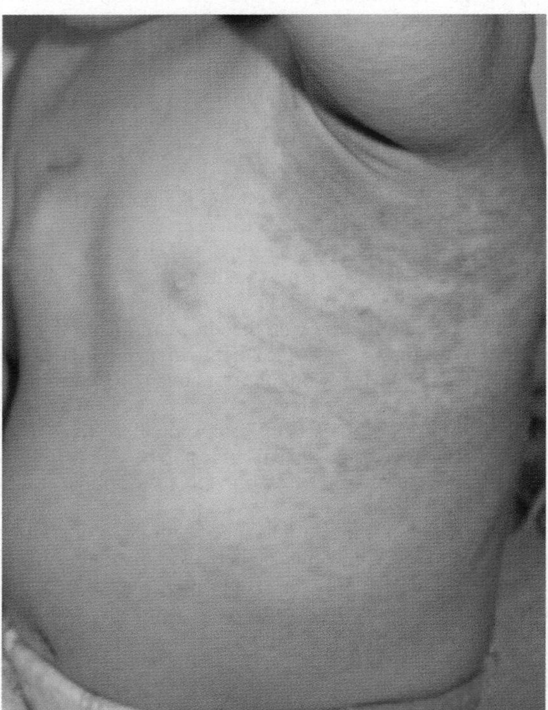

FIG. 60B.3 Lichenoid papules involving the lateral trunk typical of the unilateral periflexural viral exanthem.

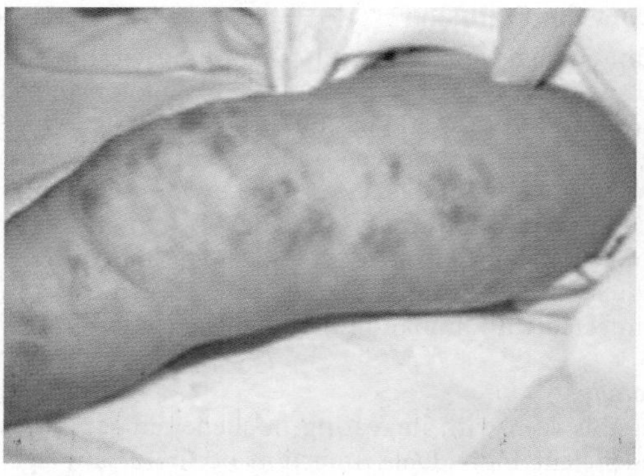

FIG. 60B.4 Inflammatory papules and plaques involving all extremities.

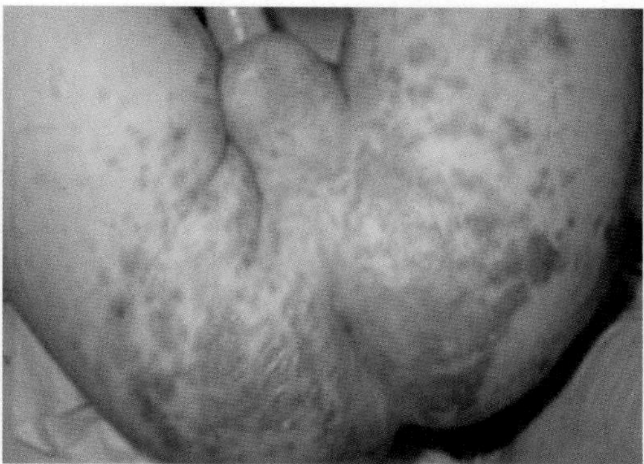

FIG. 60B.5 Erythematous papules, plaques, and erosions involving the buttocks and perineum.

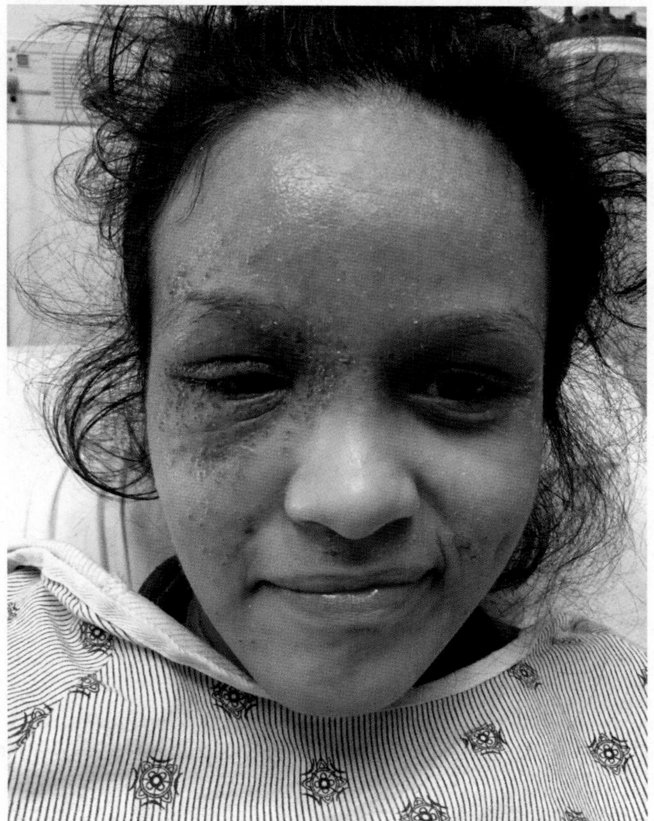

FIG. 60B.6 Healthy adolescent who presented with eye pain and grouped vesicles/erosions on face with known diagnosis of atopic dermatitis.

"atypical" hand, foot, and mouth infections have been found to be associated with coxsackievirus A6, a recent publication was unable to make a clear clinical distinction from more "classic" viral etiologies, except when perioral involvement was seen, which was more often associated with coxsackievirus A6.[42]

Herpes Simplex Virus

Infections due to HSV are completely reviewed elsewhere. The clinician should, however, be aware that skin infections due to HSV in patients with atopic dermatitis can be easily overlooked and often confused for secondary bacterial infections (Fig. 60B.6). Eczema herpeticum usually occurs without systemic involvement, but serious illness and death due to disseminated disease can occur. Younger patients and systemic symptoms are usually seen in patients requiring hospitalization.[48] Clinicians often question if management of atopic dermatitis in such patients can include topical antiinflammatory agents while treating the viral superinfection, but this can be continued.[3]

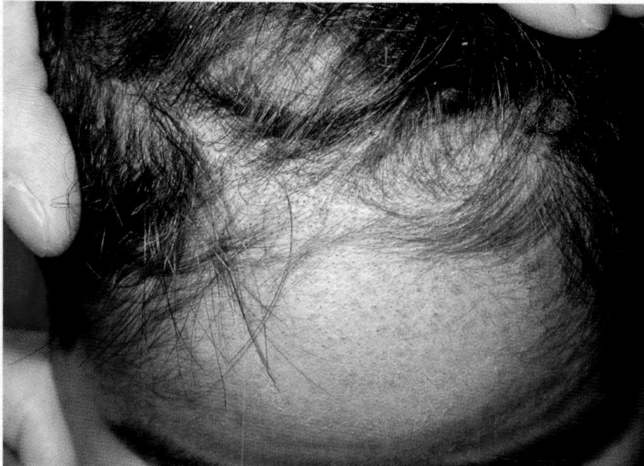

FIG. 60B.7 Nonscarring alopecia associated with tinea capitis.

Varicella-Zoster Virus

See Chapter 162.

FUNGAL INFECTIONS

Superficial fungal infections, which include dermatophytes, yeast, or dematiaceous fungi, are encountered frequently in general pediatric practice. Particularly in an immunocompromised patient, fungal infections also may involve deeper cutaneous structures and other organ systems. This section focuses on the skin manifestations, diagnosis, and treatment of pediatric superficial fungal infections.

Superficial Fungal Infections

Dermatophyte Infections

Dermatophytes invade and grow in hair, nails, and the outer layer of the skin known as the stratum corneum. These lesions vary in appearance based on the site of infection and are named accordingly.

Tinea capitis. Also known as scalp ringworm, tinea capitis is seen frequently in prepubertal children. The causative organisms vary according to country; in North America, tinea capitis is caused largely by *Trichophyton tonsurans* and less often by *Microsporum canis.*[20,68,82] *M. canis,* a zoophilic dermatophyte common to suburban and rural areas, can be transmitted to children who handle infected animals such as cats, dogs, and certain rodents; however, it does not spread between humans.[68] Thick, white patches of broken hair that fluoresce under Wood lamp examination characterize these lesions.

Human-to-human transmission of *T. tonsurans* occurs through the shedding of spores from infected skin scales and hair on items such as clothing, bed linen, combs, and hairbrushes. Lesions caused by *T. tonsurans* do not fluoresce under a Wood lamp and vary in appearance from diffuse scaling of the scalp to circumscribed areas of scaling and erythema with or without hair loss and, in dark-haired individuals, to scaly patches of hair loss that may leave small dark hairs in the follicles (black-dot ringworm) (Fig. 60B.7). Tinea capitis lesions may be associated with suboccipital or posterior cervical lymphadenopathy and may produce more inflammatory lesions, including scaly, pustular areas of hair loss and formation of a kerion—a boggy, erythematous mass with follicular pustules that may lead to permanent hair loss and scarring if left untreated (Fig. 60B.8).[20,38,82] Another hypersensitivity response to the dermatophyte infection is a dermatophytid or id reaction, which involves papulovesicular inflammatory eruptions adjacent to or distant from the site of the primary infection (Fig. 60B.9).[8]

Tinea capitis must be distinguished from alopecia areata, which consists of patches of total hair loss without scalp changes, and trichotillomania, which may be associated with excoriations, varying lengths

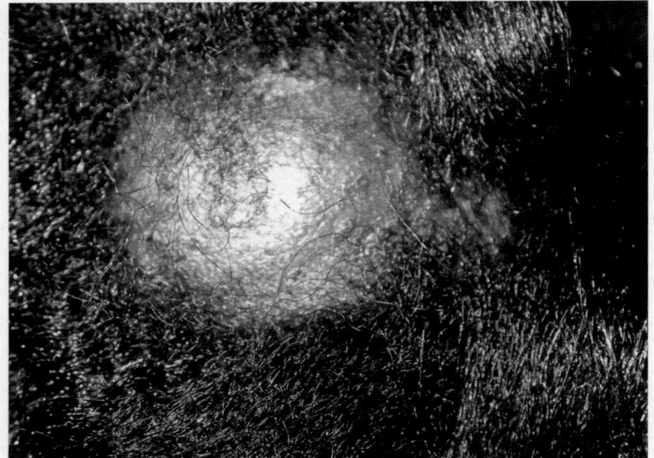

FIG. 60B.8 Indurated tumor on the scalp typical of kerion.

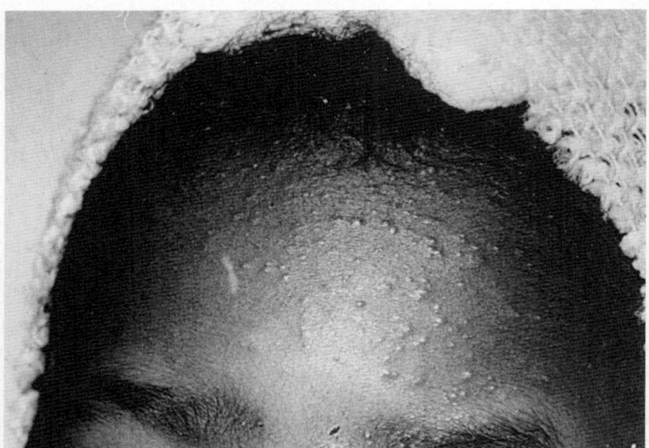

FIG. 60B.9 Multiple skin-colored papules and pustules on the forehead typical of an id reaction to tinea capitis.

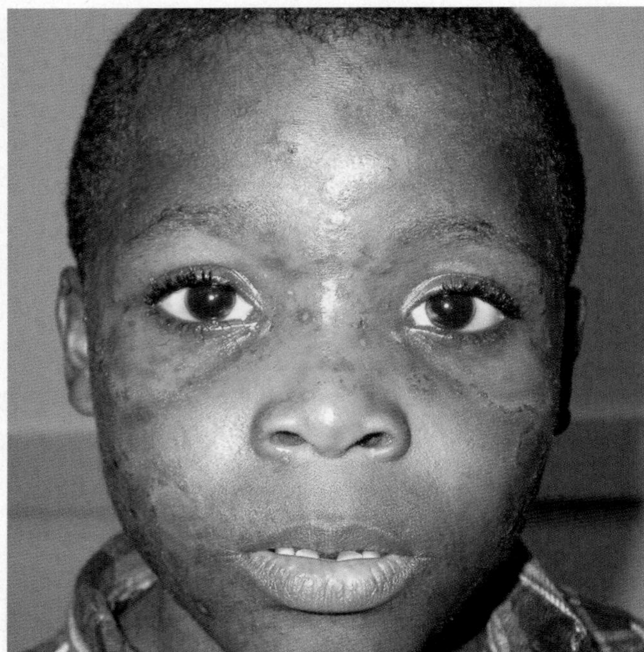

FIG. 60B.10 Diffuse scaling plaques on the face caused by tinea faciei.

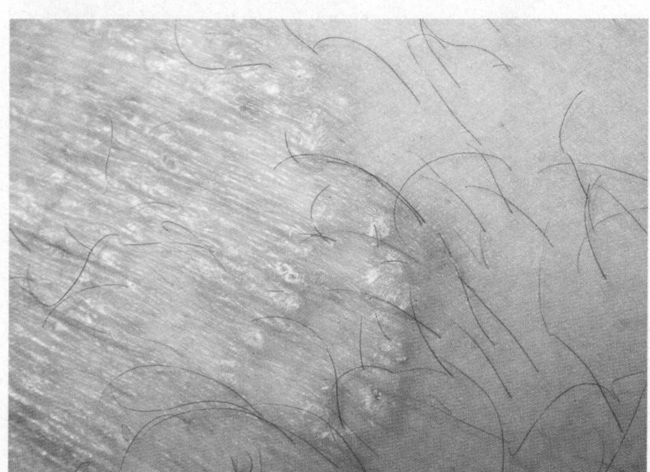

FIG. 60B.11 Annular scaling plaque on the upper inner thigh caused by tinea cruris.

of broken hairs, and ill-defined patterns of hair loss. Differential diagnosis also includes traction alopecia, seborrheic dermatitis, psoriasis, and pityriasis amiantacea. In addition, inflammatory lesions of tinea capitis may be confused with bacterial pyodermas of the scalp.[38,68,82]

Tinea corporis. Tinea corporis is a dermatophyte infection of the trunk or extremities. Lesions appear as erythematous patches or plaques with well-demarcated, annular borders that may be scaly, pustular, or vesicular.[38,68,82] The application of potent topical corticosteroids may obscure these characteristic borders, resulting in a manifestation termed *tinea incognito*.[66] The differential diagnosis includes seborrheic, atopic, and contact dermatitides; psoriasis; and granuloma annulare.[38,82]

Tinea faciei. Dermatophyte infections of the face in children are characterized by erythematous, scaly plaques that may be unilateral or occur in a "butterfly" distribution, mimicking cutaneous findings of systemic lupus erythematosus and other collagen vascular diseases (Fig. 60B.10). As with tinea corporis, differential diagnosis includes seborrheic, atopic, and contact dermatitides.[38,82]

Tinea pedis. Tinea pedis, which occurs more commonly in adolescents than in prepubertal children, is a dermatophyte infection involving the feet. Findings vary and may be vesicles or erosions over the instep of the feet, fissuring between the toes with surrounding erythema and scaling, or diffuse scaling of the soles in a "moccasin-like" distribution. Differential diagnosis includes juvenile plantar dermatosis, dyshidrotic eczema, atopic dermatitis, contact dermatitis, granuloma annulare, scabies, psoriasis, and erythrasma.[38,68,82]

Tinea cruris. Also predominantly seen in adolescents, particularly boys, tinea cruris often occurs in association with tinea pedis and is transmitted through indirect or direct contact with infected skin scales or hair. Risk factors include obesity, friction, moisture, and tight clothing. The characteristic lesions are usually symmetric, well-demarcated, erythematous, scaly eruptions in the inguinal and inner thigh area with potential spread to the buttocks and perianal region. These lesions also may have a raised papular or pustular edge and often are very pruritic, leading to lichenification in chronic disease (Fig. 60B.11). The differential diagnosis includes seborrheic dermatitis, *Candida* intertrigo, flexural psoriasis, irritant dermatitis, contact dermatitis, and erythrasma.[38,68,82]

Tinea unguium. The term *onychomycosis* refers to fungal invasion of the nail plate, which is termed *tinea unguium* when the infection is caused by dermatophytes. The lower incidence of tinea unguium in children compared with adults may be due to faster nail growth, decreased likelihood of nail trauma, and less exposure to tinea pedis, which often is seen concurrently with onychomycosis.[41,73] Clinical findings of infection include superficial white patches on the surface of the nail plate, white spots under the nail, and yellowing and thickening of the nail plate that usually extends from the distal to the proximal end (Figs. 60B.12

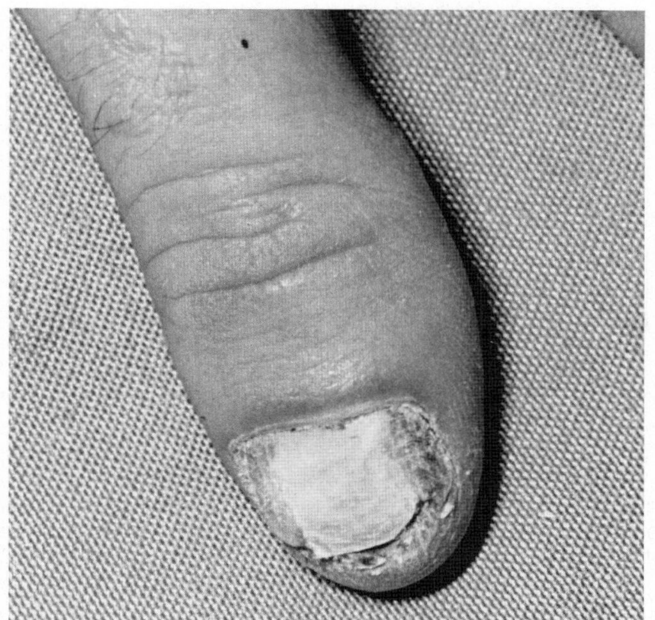

FIG. 60B.12 Onychodystrophy and subungual hyperkeratosis involving the left thumb of a child with onychomycosis.

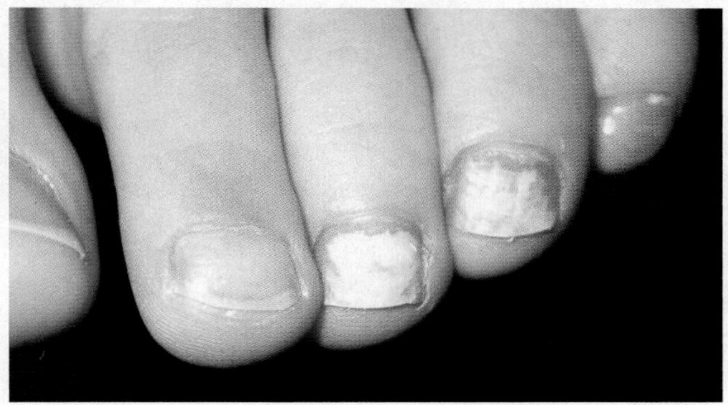

FIG. 60B.13 White superficial plaques typical of superficial white onychomycosis.

and 60B.13). The differential diagnosis includes psoriasis, lichen planus, hereditary onychodystrophy, and acquired trachyonychia, all of which may be distinguished from tinea unguium by their diffuse nail involvement as opposed to the more limited disease of a dermatophyte infection. Tinea unguium also may mimic *Candida* infection of the nails, but the latter disease differs in that it tends to spread distally from the proximal nail plate.[4,34,38,57,61,74,81]

Diagnosis

Light microscopy examination with potassium hydroxide should show spores in infected scalp hairs of tinea capitis and branching hyphae in affected nail samples or skin scrapings from advancing margins of lesions on the body (Fig. 60B.13). Fungal culture on Sabouraud dextrose agar treated with chloramphenicol and cycloheximide provides a growth medium selective for dermatophytes and may aid in differentiating various species. Rarely biopsy may be required for definitive diagnosis.[20,38,68,82]

Treatment

Localized lesions of tinea corporis, faciei, pedis, and cruris generally respond to a 2- to 4-week course of topical antifungals, such as clotrimazole, tolnaftate, ciclopirox olamine, amorolfine, or terbinafine.[20] Severe or refractory disease may require oral antifungal medications. Recurrence of tinea pedis can be prevented by avoiding occlusive footwear and keeping the feet clean and dry.[68]

Griseofulvin and terbinafine granules are the only oral antifungal medications approved by the U.S. Food and Drug Administration (FDA) for use in children. Other agents, including itraconazole and fluconazole, have been used successfully as off-label alternatives, however, despite limited data regarding their safety and efficacy in children.

Griseofulvin remains the gold standard for the treatment of tinea capitis in the United States. The approved dose of microsized griseofulvin is 11 mg/kg per day for 6 to 8 weeks; however, 20 to 25 mg/kg per day often is required to achieve an adequate response.[76] An alternative is the ultramicrosized formulation of griseofulvin at 10 to 15 mg/kg per day.[35] A 6-week course of terbinafine also has been shown to be as effective as griseofulvin, particularly in the treatment of tinea capitis caused by *Trichophyton* spp.[25,27,34,77] For *Microsporum* infections, higher doses or longer duration of therapy with terbinafine may be required.[25,27,31,34,43,47,56,72,77] Studies have shown that a regimen of fluconazole 6 mg/kg per day for 3 to 6 weeks has a cure rate comparable to that of griseofulvin.[26,31,34,43,56,72,77] Continuous or pulse itraconazole therapy of 5 mg/kg per day has been noted to result in significant improvement and even cure in *Trichophyton* and *Microsporum* tinea capitis by 6 weeks; however, infection with *Microsporum* may require a longer duration of treatment with itraconazole compared with effective courses for *Trichophyton* infection.[31,32,34,36,43,56,72] In addition, concomitant topical therapy with ketoconazole 2% shampoo or selenium sulfide 1% to 2.5% shampoo in affected individuals and household contacts reduces the number of viable spores and prevents the spread of infection.[31,43,56,72]

At present no antifungal agent is approved by the FDA for treatment of onychomycosis in children, and data are limited regarding efficacy of topical and oral antifungal agents. Topical agents have poor penetration into the nail plate, usually leading to an inadequate response rate. Treating concurrent tinea pedis infections with topical therapy may help prevent recurrences of tinea unguium, however. Although griseofulvin is the drug of choice for treating other dermatophyte infections, it is not recommended for the treatment of onychomycosis because of the lengthy course (≤18 months), inadequate response, and high recurrence rate.

Terbinafine 3 to 6 mg/kg per day for 6 to 12 weeks, continuous or pulse itraconazole 5 mg/kg per day for 3 months, and fluconazole 3 to 6 mg/kg once a week for 12 to 26 weeks have been reported as safe, effective, and well-tolerated alternatives.[32,39,62,77] Because of their keratinophilic and lipophilic natures, these agents accumulate in the stratum corneum and persist at high concentrations in the nails for months, allowing for shorter courses of therapy.[36,37,39,41,77] Terbinafine may be crushed and taken with or without food. Optimal bioavailability with itraconazole capsules occurs when taken with fatty foods, whereas itraconazole solution should be taken on an empty stomach and may be associated with a higher incidence of gastrointestinal side effects than capsules. Studies regarding use of fluconazole for treatment of onychomycosis in children are limited, but successful therapy has been reported at a pulsed dose of 3 to 6 mg/kg once a week for 3 months.[37,39,73]

Candida

The most common cause of fungal infection in healthy and immunocompromised children is *Candida,* and *C. albicans* accounts for most cases. These yeast forms have a predilection for moist, warm areas of the body such as mucosal surfaces and intertriginous regions and often colonize these areas, becoming part of the normal flora. Disease is caused by overgrowth and infiltration into the epidermis. Superficial infections may be seen in healthy individuals and individuals with predisposing risk factors, such as prematurity; low weight; diabetes mellitus; antibiotic, corticosteroid, or oral contraceptive therapy; and other immunocompromised states. These individuals also are more likely to develop systemic candidiasis.[20,28,82]

Thrush is characterized by superficial, sometimes tender, white plaques on oral mucosa that reveal denuded, erythematous bases when scraped off (Fig. 60B.14). These manifestations must be distinguished from other oral cavity lesions, such as aphthous stomatitis, epidermolysis bullosa, herpes simplex, hairy leukoplakia, lichen planus, geographic tongue, erythema multiforme, and burns.[82] Use of pacifiers in infants

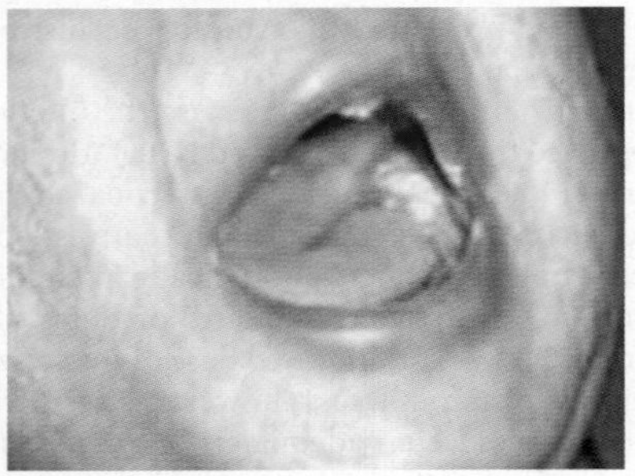

FIG. 60B.14 White patches on buccal mucosa caused by *Candida albicans*.

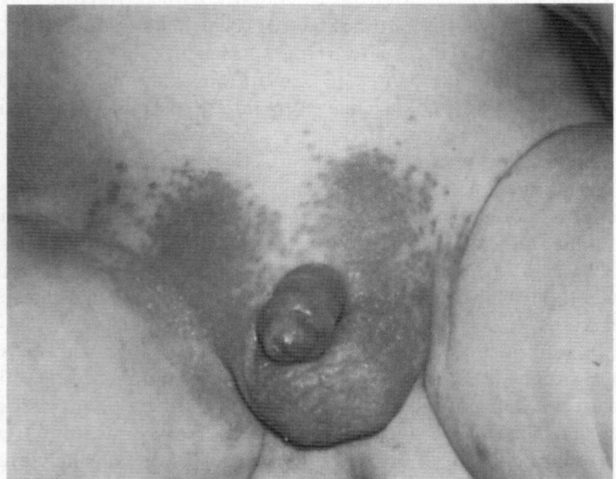

FIG. 60B.15 Infant with *Candida* diaper dermatitis. Confluent and discrete erythematous papules and plaque involve the scrotum, penis, and suprapubic and inguinal area.

may increase the risk for development of thrush and colonization of the organism.[7] Oropharyngeal candidiasis may spread to the esophagus in immunocompromised individuals and lead to difficulty with feeding.

Diaper candidiasis appears as beefy, erythematous plaques that involve the inguinal creases and perianal region and often are associated with satellite (or surrounding) erythematous papules, plaques, or pustules (Fig. 60B.15). These lesions may cause discomfort when the infant urinates onto affected skin. Superinfection with *Candida* should be suspected when irritant diaper dermatitis fails to improve within several days. Other lesions that may be confused with diaper candidiasis include psoriasis, Langerhans cell histiocytosis, and seborrheic dermatitis.[82]

Thumb-sucking or other trauma near nail beds may lead to nontender, erythematous swelling at the base of the nails termed *paronychia* (Fig. 60B.16). Some cases are complicated by *Candida* infection. Differential diagnosis of these lesions includes psoriasis, bacterial infection, lichen planus, and pachyonychia congenita. *Candida* also may produce onychomycosis, but its distribution usually involves the proximal nail plate, in contrast to dermatophytosis of the nails, which more commonly affects the distal nail plate.[82]

Adolescent girls may present with vulvovaginal candidiasis, which is characterized by thick, white discharge and white plaques on irritated, erythematous vaginal mucosa. These lesions may cause vaginal itching and dysuria.[82]

Diagnosis of localized *Candida* infection usually is made clinically. Microscopic examination of potassium hydroxide–prepared scrapings of skin and mucosal lesions reveals pseudohyphae and elongated budding yeast forms. Positive cultures of infected material on Sabouraud dextrose agar or cornmeal agar may signify infection or benign colonization. Biopsy rarely is required for establishing a definitive diagnosis.

Treatment of localized *Candida* infection depends on good hygiene practices and maintenance of a dry environment in the susceptible area.

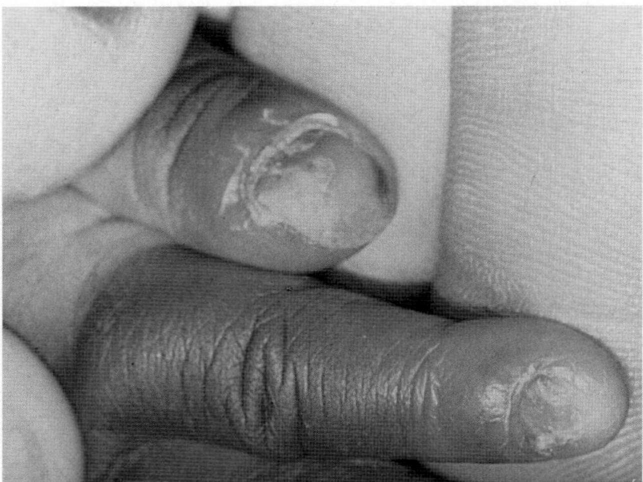

FIG. 60B.16 Onychodystrophy involving the thumb and index finger, with erythema and edema of the paronychium. These features are typical of *Candida paronychia*.

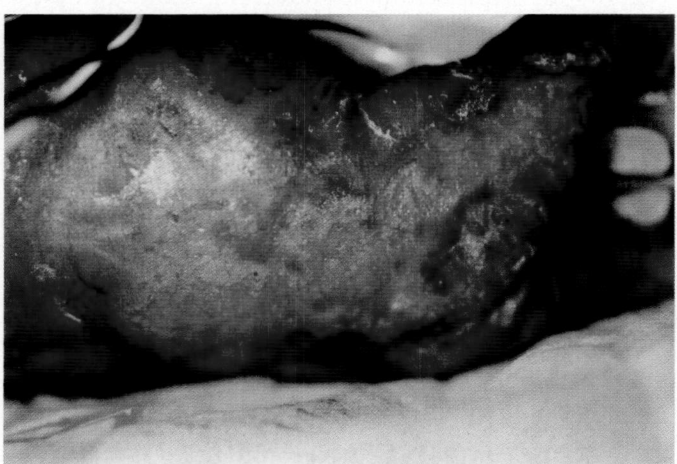

FIG. 60B.17 Dense crusting overlying the flank and buttocks of a neonate with *Candida* dermatitis. (From Rowen JL, Atkins JT, Levy ML, et al. Invasive fungal dermatitis in the 1000-gram neonate. *Pediatrics*. 1995;95:682–7.)

Localized infections usually respond well to topical antifungal therapy. Nystatin solution is the first-line agent used for thrush, but oral fluconazole or itraconazole and intravenous amphotericin B may be required to treat recurrent, refractory, or extensive disease, especially in immunocompromised children.[23] Nystatin or imidazole creams in conjunction with frequent diaper changes, barrier creams, and sometimes low-strength topical steroids are the recommended treatment for diaper candidiasis. Paronychia also is susceptible to nystatin and imidazole creams but may require oral therapy. Vulvovaginal candidiasis often can be treated successfully with topical azole medications, but oral azoles are recommended for refractory or recurrent cases. Adolescents can be treated with a single, 150-mg dose of oral fluconazole.[23,66]

Congenital candidiasis, a rare form of infection acquired in utero as a result of *Candida* chorioamnionitis, can manifest in full-term and premature neonates within the first few days of life as a diffuse, erythematous, papular eruption that progresses to formation of vesicles and pustules and subsequently crusting and desquamation (Fig. 60B.17). Palms and soles also may be affected. Term infants with congenital candidiasis rarely develop systemic manifestations, and the infection usually resolves spontaneously or with topical antifungal agents, such as nystatin, imidazoles, or allylamines. Premature neonates with very low birth weight are at risk for developing ecchymosis and necrosis of the skin with dissemination of the *Candida* infection, requiring treatment with systemic antifungal medication. Congenital candidiasis in these premature infants may manifest as sepsis or pneumonia without cutaneous findings as well.[2,20,79]

Differential diagnosis of congenital candidiasis includes epidermolysis bullosa and infection with *Listeria monocytogenes, Staphylococcus,* herpesvirus, and syphilis.[18] Early diagnosis is established by histologic examination of the placenta and umbilical cord, which shows the characteristic pseudohyphae and spores and white microabscesses.[2,18] Microscopic examination and culture of the skin lesions can confirm the diagnosis.

Malassezia

Malassezia spp., most notably *M. furfur,* are lipophilic yeast forms that are found more readily in humid, tropical environments and are part of the normal skin flora in humans. Colonization begins in the neonatal period and increases with age.[6] *Malassezia* is the organism thought to be responsible for neonatal cephalic pustulosis and tinea (or pityriasis) versicolor in older children, adolescents, and young adults. Invasion of the organism through indwelling catheters, particularly catheters being used for intralipid infusion in premature infants with very low birth weight also may lead to sepsis and death.[4,70,79]

Neonatal cephalic pustulosis is a self-limited disease characterized by scattered, erythematous papules and pustules in a head-and-neck distribution (Fig. 60B.18). Follicular accentuation and comedones are not observed. Diagnosis usually is made clinically but may be confirmed by microscopic findings.[6,20,79]

Tinea versicolor is characterized by macules with fine scales that are distributed on the upper body and neck. The macules may appear hypopigmented in dark-skinned individuals or tan or dark brown in lighter skinned individuals (Fig. 60B.19). Differential diagnosis includes vitiligo, pityriasis alba, pityriasis rosea, postinflammatory hypopigmentation, melasma, seborrheic dermatitis, contact dermatitis, and tinea corporis. Lesions of tinea versicolor are fluorescent yellow to orange under Wood lamp. Microscopic examination of potassium hydroxide–prepared scrapings of the lesions shows a "spaghetti and meatball" appearance owing to the presence of short, curved hyphae and round spores. Biopsy of the lesions, which usually is unnecessary, reveals the characteristic hyphae and spores invading the stratum corneum.

The recommended treatment is application of 2.5% selenium sulfide or ketoconazole shampoo. Other topical agents, such as ciclopirox, terbinafine solutions, sodium hypochlorite, and other azoles, also may be effective. Oral ketoconazole and itraconazole in single daily doses for 7 to 14 days or fluconazole 300 mg/week for 2 to 4 weeks have been suggested as effective treatments; however, these agents are not approved by the FDA for treating tinea versicolor in children because of their limited safety and efficacy profiles.[8,22,40,67] It is important to advise patients that skin discolorations may take months to resolve and that recurrences are very common and may require retreatment.[20,38,67,79,82] *Malassezia* sepsis responds well to removal of indwelling catheters and rarely requires systemic antifungal therapy.[79]

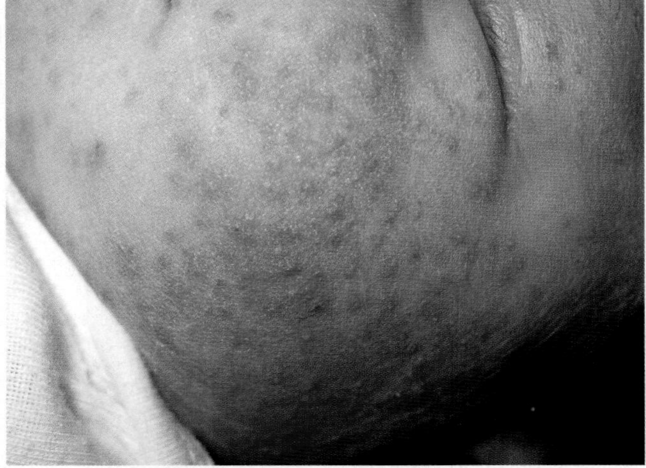

FIG. 60B.18 Pustules and papules on the face and scalp from neonatal cephalic pustulosis.

Chromoblastomycosis

Fonsecaea pedrosoi and less commonly *Cladophialophora carrionii* and *Phialophora verrucosa* are found in tropical climates and are organisms responsible for causing chromoblastomycosis, a chronic granulomatous disease affecting skin and subcutaneous tissue. Infection is acquired through traumatic inoculation into the skin. Cutaneous manifestations are described as pink papules that progressively enlarge to become tender, pruritic, hyperkeratotic nodules or verrucous plaques (Fig. 60B.20). Scratching may lead to secondary infection or result in autoinoculation of the organism to other areas of the body. Infection may lead to scarring of lymphatic vessels causing obstruction and lymphedema.[9,24,64,69]

Differential diagnosis includes tuberculosis, sporotrichosis, blastomycosis, leishmaniasis, and squamous cell carcinomas. Potassium hydroxide smears of skin scrapings reveal characteristic dark brown, round, sclerotic bodies with horizontal or vertical septa and thick, pigmented hyphae. Sclerotic bodies also are identified easily on hematoxylin and eosin stain. In addition, biopsy of the chromoblastomycosis lesions shows granulomatous inflammation with macrophages and neutrophils and a hyperkeratotic, hyperplastic epidermis with microabscesses.[9,24,69]

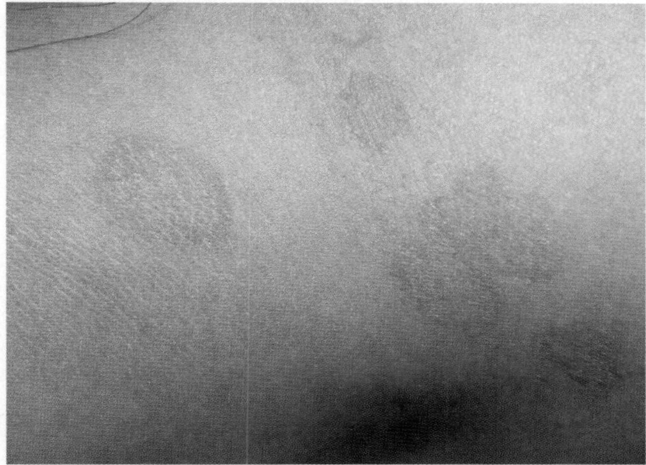

FIG. 60B.19 Well-circumscribed annular scaling plaques on the neck typical of tinea versicolor.

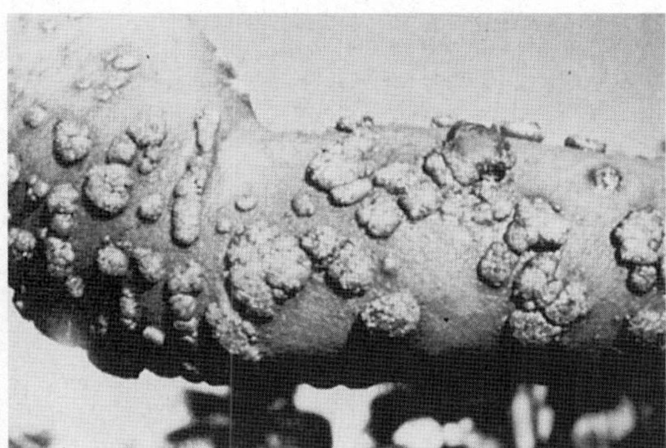

FIG. 60B.20 Chromoblastomycosis. The wart-like growth of epidermis and dermis is a result of traumatic implantation of the etiologic agent and subsequent autoinoculation from scratching. The agent was *Fonsecaea pedrosoi*.

Treatment of localized lesions involves surgical excision, cryotherapy, or heat therapy. Chemotherapy with 5-fluorocytosine and antifungal agents such as azoles, amphotericin B, and terbinafine has been used with some success in more widespread disease.[9,24,78]

Tinea Nigra

Tinea nigra, caused by the organism *Hortaea werneckii,* is a superficial fungal infection seen primarily in children and adolescents.[38,53,63] The organism is found in soil, wood, sewage, salted dried fish, and vegetation, mainly in beach environments of Central and South America, Africa, Asia, and, less frequently, in the United States and Europe. Transmission occurs by direct contact.[53,63,65] Tinea nigra usually is characterized by an asymptomatic, well-demarcated, single brown to black macule or patch primarily on the palm but may involve other areas of the body as well (Fig. 60B.21). Lesions grow slowly and usually are nonscaly.[38,63] Tinea nigra lesions may mimic melanoma, lentigines, junctional nevi, and the hyperpigmented patches of Addison disease.[38,63,65] Under microscopic examination, potassium hydroxide–prepared scrapings of the lesion show yellow to light brown, branched, septate hyphae (Fig. 60B.22).[38,65] Diagnosis is confirmed further by culture, which grows oval to spindle-shaped, moist, shiny, black colonies on Sabouraud agar.[38,63,65]

Tinea nigra has been treated successfully with keratolytic ointments or solutions, which include salicylic acid and benzoic acid and azole and allylamine creams. Scraping the lesion with a scalpel also can remove the discoloration.[65]

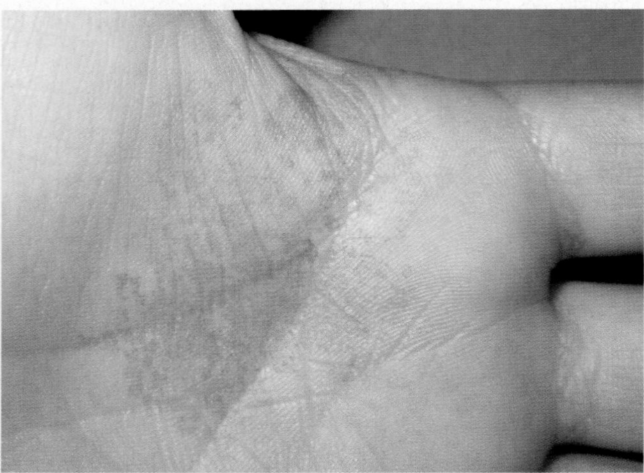

FIG. 60B.21 Brown patch on the palm of the hand caused by tinea nigra palmaris.

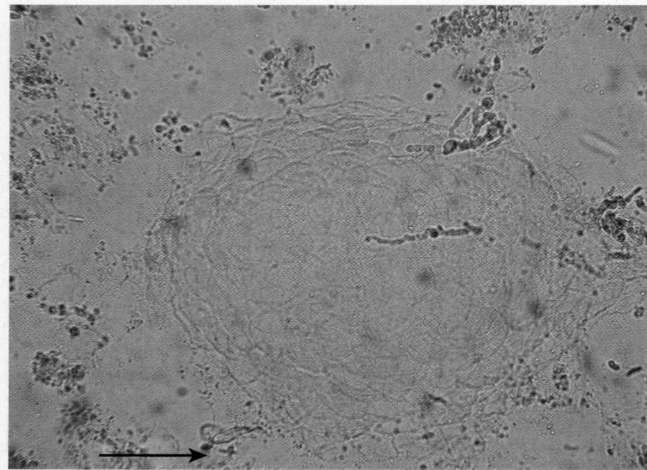

FIG. 60B.22 Septate hyphae seen by potassium hydroxide examination of scale from the patient in Fig. 60B.21.

Trichosporonosis

See Chapter 208.

Deep Fungal Infections

Aspergillosis

See Chapter 197. See Fig. 60B.23.

Blastomycosis

See Chapter 199.

Coccidioidomycosis

See Chapter 201.

Cryptococcosis

See Chapter 203.

Fusariosis

See Chapter 207.

Histoplasmosis

See Chapter 204.

Mucormycosis

See Chapter 206. See Fig. 60B.24.

Sporotrichosis

See Chapter 205. See Fig. 60B.25.

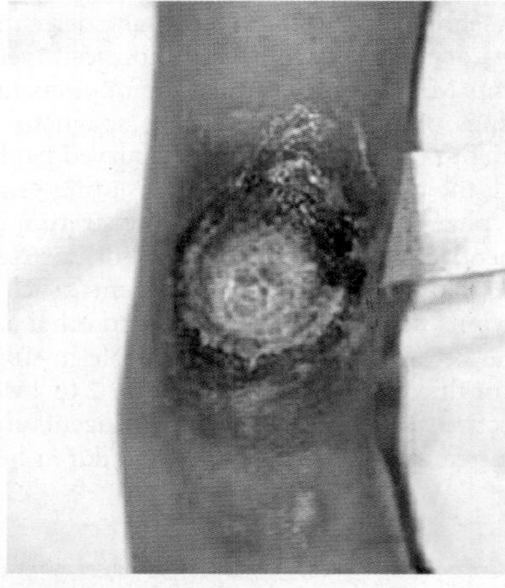

FIG. 60B.23 Eschar overlying eroded skin on a child with invasive aspergillosis.

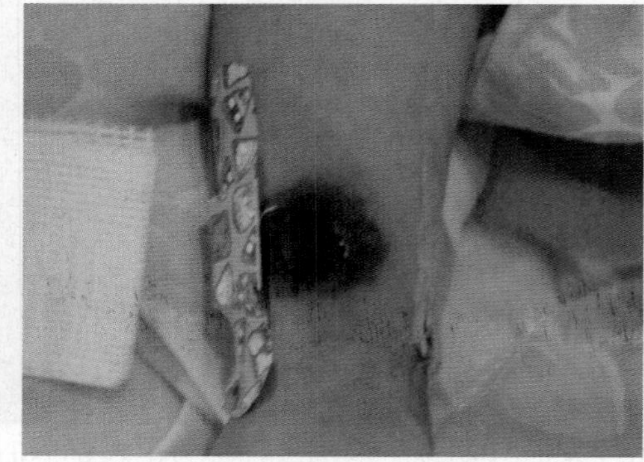

FIG. 60B.24 Purpura and ulceration in a patient with mucormycosis.

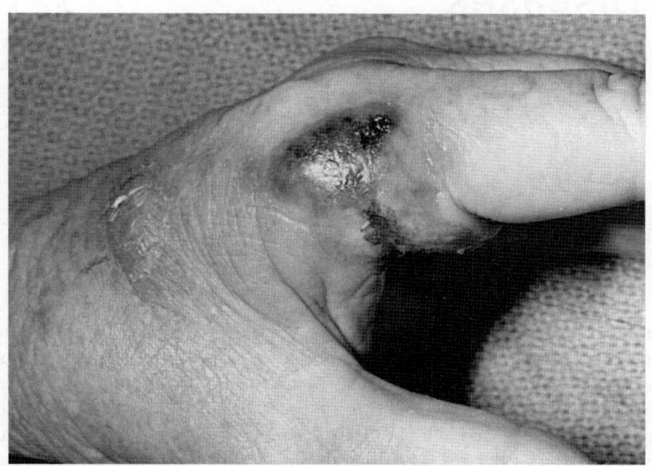

FIG. 60B.25 Two erythematous nodules on the dorsum of the left hand of a patient with sporotrichosis.

NEW REFERENCES SINCE THE SEVENTH EDITION

1. Ahluwalia J, Abuabara K, Perman MJ, et al. Human herpesvirus 6 involvement in paediatric drug hypersensitivity syndrome. *Br J Dermatol.* 2015;172(4):1090-1095.
3. Aronson PL, Shah SS, Mohamad Z, et al. Topical corticosteroids and hospital length of stay in children with eczema herpeticum. *Pediatr Dermatol.* 2013;30(2):215-221.
5. Basdag H, Rainer BM, Cohen BA. Molluscum contagiosum: to treat or not to treat? Experience with 170 children in an outpatient clinic setting in the northeastern United States. *Pediatr Dermatol.* 2015;32(3):353-357.
13. Centers for Disease Control and Prevention (CDC). Notes from the field: severe hand, foot, and mouth disease associated with coxsackievirus A6: Alabama, Connecticut, California, and Nevada, November 2011–February 2012. *MMWR Morb Mortal Wkly Rep.* 2012;61(12):213-214.
15. Chen X, Anstey AV, Bugert JJ. Molluscum contagiosum virus infection. *Lancet Infect Dis.* 2013;13(10):877-888.
16. Chuh A, Zawar V, Law M, et al. Gianotti-Crosti syndrome, pityriasis rosea, asymmetrical periflexural exanthem, unilateral mediothoracic exanthem, eruptive pseudoangiomatosis, and papular-purpuric gloves and socks syndrome: a brief review and arguments for diagnostic criteria. *Infect Dis Rep.* 2012;4(1):e12.
31. Ginter-Hanselmayer G, Seebacher C. Treatment of tinea capitis—a critical appraisal. *J Dtsch Dermatol Ges.* 2011;9(2):109-114.
35. Gupta AK, Cooper EA. Update in antifungal therapy of dermatophytosis. *Mycopathologia.* 2008;166(5-6):353-367.
40. Hu SW, Bigby M. Pityriasis versicolor: a systematic review of interventions. *Arch Dermatol.* 2010;146(10):1132-1140.
42. Hubiche T, Schuffenecker I, Boralevi F, et al. Dermatological spectrum of hand, foot and mouth disease from classical to generalized exanthema. *Pediatr Infect Dis J.* 2014;33(4):e92-e98.
43. Kakourou T, Uksal U, European Society for Pediatric Disease. Guidelines for the management of tinea capitis in children. *Pediatr Dermatol.* 2010;27(3):226-228.
44. Keighley CL, Saunderson RB, Kok J, et al. Viral exanthems. *Curr Opin Infect Dis.* 2015;28(2):139-150.
46. Levy ML. Managing molluscum with imiquimod: ignoring the evidence. *Pediatr Dermatol.* 2016;33(2):236-237.
48. Luca NJ, Lara-Corrales I, Pope E. Eczema herpeticum in children: clinical features and factors predictive of hospitalization. *J Pediatr.* 2012;161(4):671-675.
49. Lynch MD, Sears A, Cookson H, et al. Disseminated coxsackievirus A6 affecting children with atopic dermatitis. *Clin Exp Dermatol.* 2015;40:525-528.
51. Mathes EF, Oza V, Frieden IJ, et al. "Eczema coxsackium" and unusual cutaneous findings in an enterovirus outbreak. *Pediatrics.* 2013;132(1):e149-e157.
52. McCuaig CC, Russo P, Powell J, et al. Unilateral laterothoracic exanthem: a clinicopathologic study of forty-eight patients. *J Am Acad Dermatol.* 1996;34(6):979-984.
55. Mendez-Rios JD, Yang Z, Erlandson KJ, et al. Molluscum contagiosum virus transcriptome in abortively infected cultured cells and human skin lesion. *J Virol.* 2016;90(9):4469-4480.
56. Michaels BD, Del Rosso JQ. Tinea capitis in infants: recognition, evaluation, and management suggestions. *J Clin Aesthet Dermatol.* 2012;5(2):49-59.
58. Nassef C, Ziemer C, Morrell DS. Hand-foot-and-mouth disease: a new look at a classic viral rash. *Curr Opin Pediatr.* 2015;27(4):486-491.
71. Retrouvey M, Koch LH, Williams JV. Gianotti-Crosti syndrome after childhood vaccination. *Pediatr Dermatol.* 2012;29(5):666-668.

The full reference list for this chapter is available at ExpertConsult.com.

61 Ocular Infections

Amit Bhatt

The eye can be affected by infections and infestations manifested as primary diseases or as part of systemic processes. Some infections are vision threatening, whereas others may have important implications for a generalized disease process. Ocular findings can help narrow the differential diagnosis list in some systemic diseases, such as congenital viral infections. A helpful approach in this regard is to use an anatomic scheme that reflects the primary site of ocular involvement. This chapter proceeds systematically from anterior to posterior, from infections involving the eyelids and superficial ocular surface to those involving deeper tissue and intraocular structures, and concludes with a discussion of infections involving the orbit. Some disease sites overlap, and duplications are therefore unavoidable.

Most infectious processes involving the eye can be diagnosed accurately by following the standard medical protocol: history, examination, laboratory analysis, differential diagnosis. The three simple basic tools—a visual acuity chart, a pen light, and a direct ophthalmoscope—facilitate establishing a diagnosis in most instances. In some cases, however, special ophthalmologic testing such as a slit-lamp examination, indirect ophthalmoscopy, ocular ultrasound, Gram stain and culture, or a biopsy are required. One of the cardinal rules in ophthalmology is *always* to measure the vision as the very first examination step.

INFECTIONS OF THE EYELIDS

The eyelids are composed of connective tissue, hair follicles, sweat and sebaceous glands, smooth and striated muscles, sensory and motor nerves, and vascular elements. The skin covering the eyelids is the thinnest of the entire body. The inner surface of the eyelid is covered by the palpebral conjunctiva. Bulbar conjunctiva covers the surface of the globe. Connecting these two conjunctival parts is the conjunctival fornix, which designates the most posterior limit of the conjunctiva. Sebaceous glands (the glands of Zeis) are associated with eyelid hair follicles. Meibomian glands, located within the tarsal plates of the eyelids, are also sebaceous and drain at the posterior aspect of the lid margin.[115]

Infection of the eyelids may be generalized or focal. Involvement of the skin by an infectious agent is referred to as dermatoblepharitis. *Staphylococcus aureus* and *Staphylococcus epidermidis* are the main infectious agents. The exception is angular blepharitis, inflammation at the lateral canthus, which is often caused by *Moraxella* spp. Impetigo or erysipelas of the eyelids may be caused by *Streptococcus pyogenes*. A variety of parasitic infestations, including *Demodex folliculorum, Sarcoptes scabiei* (scabies), *Pediculus capitis,* and *Phthirus pubis* (the pubic louse), may involve the eyelids.[161] Infection of the lid margin is more common in adults but may occur in children. Infections of the anterior lid margin include bacterial blepharitis, molluscum contagiosum, and parasitic diseases. Infections of the posterior lid margin include those associated with chronic meibomian gland dysfunction. Herpes simplex virus (HSV) and herpes zoster virus may involve the lid and lid margin and are discussed elsewhere in this chapter.

ANTERIOR EYELID INFECTION

Staphylococcal Blepharitis

Staphylococcal eyelid infection may be acute or chronic. Typically the chronic form of the disease manifests as erythema and crusting of the lid margins, especially on awakening. Thickening of the lid margin is a frequent manifestation. Mild chronic conjunctival infection often occurs as a spillover by local reaction to material secreted by the infecting organism. A child with staphylococcal blepharitis may be asymptomatic or may complain of ocular discomfort or a burning, itching, or foreign body sensation. Lid hygiene measures are frequently all that is required to treat the condition, consisting of twice daily baby shampoo eyelid scrubs applied gently with a clean washcloth with attention given to the lid margin. Effective lid hygiene decreases the concentration of local bacterial flora and reduces or eliminates symptoms arising from chronic staphylococcal infection. A 2- to 4-week course of topical erythromycin, bacitracin, or azithromycin ophthalmic ointments applied twice daily to the eyelid margin may hasten resolution and reduce recurrences. Ophthalmologic ointments may cause significant temporary blurring of vision; therefore they often are used only at night before sleep. Severe or refractory cases can be effectively treated with a 5-day course of oral azithromycin.[47]

Molluscum Contagiosum Infection

Molluscum contagiosum is caused by members of the family *Poxviridae*. Infection of the eyelid may be unilateral or bilateral. Infection may be transmitted by skin-to-skin contact, through fomites, or by autoinoculation. Widespread development of lesions can occur as a result of autoinoculation. Epidemics in people who live in closed communities have been reported.[216] Eyelid manifestations typically include isolated nodules with mild surrounding inflammation (Fig. 61.1). The nodules are 1 to 3 mm in diameter. Older lesions frequently become umbilicated and develop a white or waxy-appearing core. Mild conjunctival injection frequently accompanies lesions on or near the margin of the eyelid. The associated conjunctivitis occasionally can be severe and chronic. In chronic cases, corneal epithelial disease may develop.

Molluscum infection is self-limited, with most lesions resolving spontaneously within a few months. However, the infection can be recalcitrant, especially in immunocompromised patients.[304,316] Chronic or atypical molluscum contagiosum lesions involving the eye have been reported in patients infected with human immunodeficiency virus (HIV).[191,253] In immunocompetent patients, treatment often is advocated to prevent autoinoculation, which can prolong the course of the disease. Treatment also may provide symptomatic relief. Mechanical treatment such as cryotherapy, expression or curettage of the central core, excision, and cautery may be effective.[56] Medical treatments effective against molluscum infection remote from the eye include 1% imiquimod cream[275] and podophyllotoxin.[276] These agents are not recommended for the treatment of periocular lesions, however, because of the possibility of injury to the eye. A newer treatment option with some proven efficacy is the use of the oral antacid cimetidine.[313]

Parasitic Eyelid Disease

Phthirus pubis *Infestation*

The crab louse *Phthirus pubis* is a tiny insect adapted to living in coarse, widely spaced hair. Infestation most commonly involves pubic, axillary, and body hair. The organism is transmitted by direct person-to-person contact and perhaps by fomites.[263] Infestation of the eyelid often is a marker for sexually transmitted infections, especially in adult patients.[263] For these reasons, infection in children should raise concern for potential sexual abuse. Affected patients typically have unilateral, chronic blepharoconjunctivitis; some patients may be asymptomatic. Although unmagnified ocular examination may rarely reveal signs of the disease, diagnosis is best facilitated by slit-lamp examination, which offers a magnified view of the eyelid margins and eyelashes (Fig. 61.2), revealing adult lice firmly adherent to the eyelashes as well as egg cases (nits)

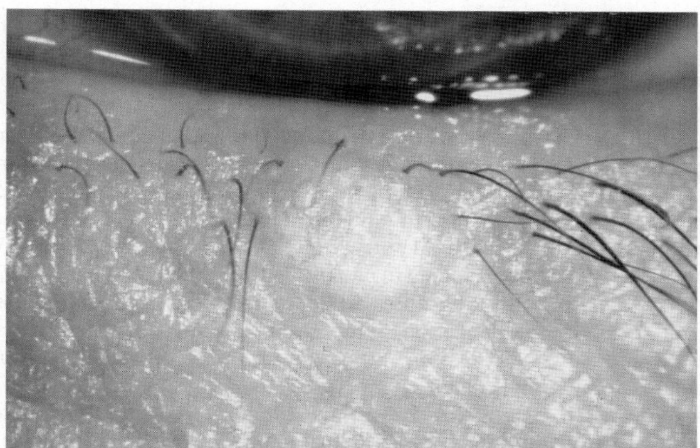

FIG. 61.1 *Molluscum contagiosum* typically is manifested as an isolated nodule or nodules approximately 1 to 3 mm in diameter. Older lesions often become umbilicated and develop a white or waxy-appearing core.

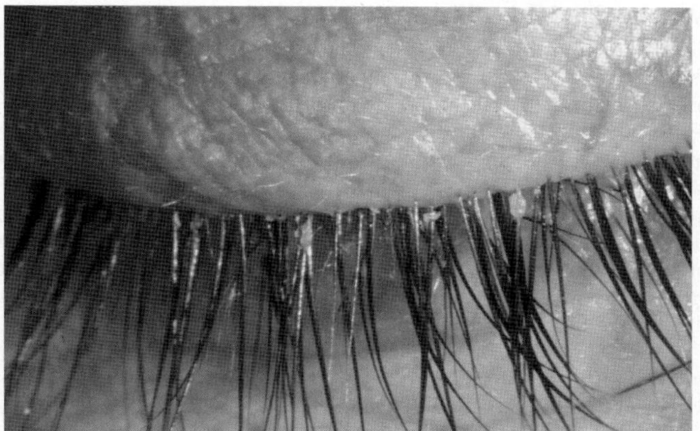

FIG. 61.2 Slit-lamp photo of *Phthirus pubis* infestation demonstrating adult lice firmly adherent to the eyelashes and egg cases (i.e., nits) attached to the proximal ends of the hair shafts.

attached to the proximal ends of the hair shafts. Reddish brown flecks of louse excreta may be found at the base of the cilia, and the cilia may be broken.[54] Treatment can be simple mechanical removal of the lice and nits under magnification (slit lamp or other devices).

Medical treatment often is preferred for young children because of their inability to tolerate or permit mechanical removal. The organisms also can be smothered by the application of a bland ointment such as petrolatum jelly applied four times each day to the eyelids. Physostigmine ointment administered twice daily can be used. This agent inhibits nerve transmission in the insect and thus is directly toxic to the insect. It should be used with caution in infants and small children. If physostigmine comes into contact with the eye, it has several significant side effects, such as stimulation of accommodation, which can produce blurred distance vision that may last for several hours. Medical treatment should be continued for 2 weeks to ensure eradication of new lice that emerge from nits during the normal life cycle.[54] Lindane shampoo scrubs of the scalp, pubic hair, and body are recommended if infestation is found in these areas. Clothing and bed linen should be laundered, and family members should be examined and treated as necessary. Follow-up 4 to 6 weeks after treatment is recommended to detect reinfestation.

Demodex *Infection*

Demodex folliculorum and *Demodex brevis* are mites that frequently infest hair follicles in humans, including the hair follicles of the eyelids (Fig. 61.3).[89,161] The organisms historically have been considered nonpathogenic parasites,[148] although it is thought they may cause increased hordeola formation as a result of obstruction of eyelid sebaceous glands.

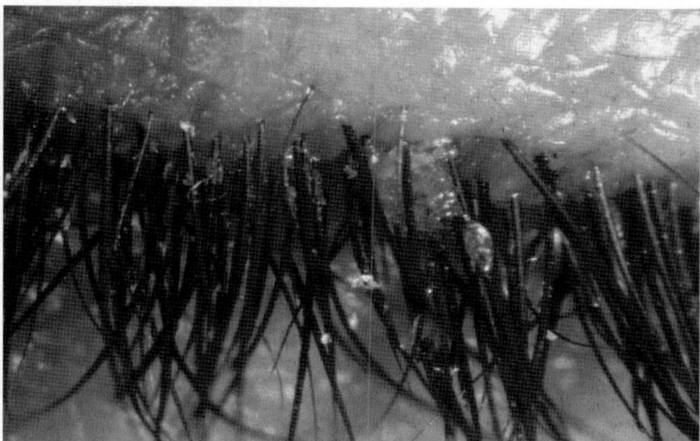

FIG. 61.3 *Demodex folliculorum* and *Demodex brevis* are mites that can infect the hair follicles of the eyelids and are found more commonly on eyelashes with cylindrical dandruff.

Demodex is found in patients with rosacea, although a causal relationship is difficult to establish.[234] Rosacea-like eruptions have been attributed to *Demodex,* and one pathologic report demonstrated a granulomatous dermal inflammation.[222] Treatment with topical pilocarpine gel may alleviate itching caused by *Demodex* infection.[99] Because of the frequency of *Demodex* infestation and the paucity of definitive disease caused by the organism, treatment often is unnecessary.

Posterior Eyelid Infection

Hordeolum

A hordeolum (i.e., stye) is an infection of the sebaceous glands in the eyelids. When the glands of Zeis are involved, the term *external hordeolum* is used. The lesion typically points to the skin surface. When the meibomian glands are involved, the term *internal hordeolum* is used. An internal hordeolum may point toward the skin or toward the palpebral conjunctiva. *S. aureus* is the most common causal agent of both internal and external hordeola.[165]

Patients with disease of the lid margin, such as those with chronic blepharitis, seborrhea, or rosacea, are prone to recurrent hordeola, especially during the first decade of life. Hordeola are manifested by erythematous, elevated, tender nodules. Nodules typically are 5 to 10 mm in diameter and usually solitary, although they may be multiple or bilateral. Patients with a history of recurrent hordeola may have them in various stages of evolution or resolution.

The lesions usually are self-limited and typically resolve within 5 to 7 days with spontaneous drainage of the abscess. Warm compresses may hasten resolution and improve comfort. Parents should be advised to place a clean washcloth soaked in warm tap water on the involved eyelid for 10 to 15 minutes several times each day. Parents should be advised to ensure that the water is not hot enough to cause a burn. For significant coexisting blepharitis, a topical antibiotic such as erythromycin ointment may prove useful by reducing the normal bacterial skin flora of the eyelid and decreasing the risk for recurrence. Systemic antibiotics rarely are indicated for acute hordeola. Children with frequent recurrences, however, may benefit from a short course of systemic antibiotics such as azithromycin,[47] erythromycin, or tetracycline (only for children older than 12 years). These agents further decrease the bacterial flora on the eyelid and may reduce the risk for recurrence even more. Lid hygiene efforts, as described for the treatment of staphylococcal blepharitis, should be instituted and maintained for children with recurrent hordeola. Surgical drainage of a hordeolum usually is unnecessary.

Chalazion

Cytologically a chalazion may represent either a mixed-cell granulomatous inflammation or a suppurating granuloma.[71] The lesion occurs in a meibomian gland as a result of a foreign body reaction to secretions produced by the gland that have been extruded into surrounding tissue. A chalazion may develop after resolution of an internal hordeolum, in which case it is preceded by an acute stage, or it may develop primarily, without a preceding acute inflammatory phase. A typical chalazion appears as a round, nontender nodule within the substance of the eyelid. Multiple and bilateral chalazia may occur in susceptible patients. Recurrent lesions are not uncommon findings. They are typically 2 to 10 mm in diameter.[206]

Spontaneous resolution of smaller chalazia can be anticipated after a period of observation without treatment, sometimes as long as several months. Larger lesions, particularly those greater than 10 mm in diameter, frequently do not resolve without specific treatment. In patients with an acute or chronic inflammatory component, application of warm compresses may be beneficial. The majority of chalazia resolve in time, but indications for earlier surgical intervention include unacceptable cosmesis, induced visually significant astigmatism, and visually significant ptosis. In rare circumstances, chalazia can result in vision loss from amblyopia.[79] The most common surgical treatment offered is incision and curettage through an internal incision on the palpebral conjunctival surface. Surgery is highly effective. It can be performed in the office, but general anesthesia is required for most young children. Because of the need for general anesthesia, we typically recommend deferring surgical treatment until several months have elapsed without spontaneous resolution. Earlier intervention may be recommended if the chalazion is particularly large, if pigmentary changes have developed in the overlying skin, or if astigmatism or ptosis is present in a young child at risk for the development of amblyopia.

Chalazia can be treated by intralesional steroid injection, surgical incision,[72] or both.[91] Dhaliwal and Bhatia[72] reported that incision plus curettage was the procedure of choice for lesions that have been present for 8.5 months or longer and for lesions 11.4 mm or larger in size, based on the results of a prospective study. The major potential drawback of intralesional steroid injection is the risk for complications developing with an otherwise relatively benign condition. Rarely steroid injection can result in sterile abscess formation or eyelid necrosis. Intralesional injections are done best with a chalazion clamp in place to protect the underlying globe from accidental needle trauma during injection. This device places a metal plate between the chalazion and the eye. If general anesthesia is required, incision and curettage is recommended over intralesional steroid injection.

Dacryoadenitis

Dacryoadenitis is an uncommon ophthalmic condition. Even in a busy ophthalmology practice, dacryoadenitis was diagnosed in approximately 1 in 10,000 patient visits.[238] The clinical manifestation is variable. Localized tenderness and swelling of the temporal aspect of the upper eyelid usually occur and often produce an S-shaped deformity of the lid margin. Pain is frequently a predominant feature. Associated signs and symptoms include fever, follicular conjunctivitis, mucopurulent discharge, limited extraocular movement, and proptosis.[238] Keratoconjunctivitis sicca has been reported as a consequence of Epstein-Barr virus (EBV)-associated dacryoadenitis in a child.[186]

Before the era of widespread immunization, mumps was a leading cause of dacryoadenitis. Today, inflammatory etiologies predominate, including idiopathic orbital inflammation (orbital pseudotumor). Bacteria such as staphylococci, streptococci, and gonococci have been occasionally implicated. Exceedingly rare organisms such as *Brucella* are involved occasionally in bacterial cases.[16] EBV has also been implicated as a causative agent in some nonsuppurative cases. Marked regional lymphadenopathy may be a distinguishing feature of EBV dacryoadenitis.[238] Other rare infectious causes include tuberculosis and Lyme disease.[207,248,251]

Appropriate laboratory evaluation includes Gram stain and culture of any mucopurulent discharge from the eye. Neuroimaging is indicated when the patient has severe inflammation, proptosis, limitation of extraocular movement, or other orbital signs to rule out a more generalized orbital process. The condition easily can be confused clinically with orbital cellulitis when signs and symptoms are severe. Biopsy of the lacrimal gland may be required to confirm the diagnosis in patients not responding to standard medical treatment or when atypical features are identified on clinical examination or radiographic studies. Blood cultures are indicated for patients with signs of systemic toxicity.

Intravenous nafcillin or vancomycin is a reasonable initial antibiotic choice for severe dacryoadenitis caused by gram-positive organisms. Oral antistaphylococcal agents may be used for less severe cases. For gram-negative cases, ceftazidime or other similar agents should be considered. For suppurative cases without Gram-stain guidance, intravenous nafcillin or vancomycin should be considered as initial therapy for severe cases and oral antistaphylococcal agents for less acute cases.

Therapy in the form of warm compresses and oral analgesics is indicated for nonsuppurative dacryoadenitis. Serum testing for evidence of EBV infection should be considered in patients with regional lymphadenopathy.[238] Other noninfectious causes of dacryoadenitis include sarcoidosis, Sjögren syndrome, leukemia, lymphoma, eosinophilic granuloma, autoimmune vasculitis (Churg-Strauss syndrome and Wegener granulomatosis), and immunoglobulin (Ig) G4-related systemic disease.[46,144,153] Noninfectious cases of dacryoadenitis sometimes can be difficult to distinguish from infectious cases. Lacrimal gland biopsy and neuroimaging usually are necessary to establish a diagnosis in noninfectious cases.[172] Steroid treatment has been shown to be effective in the management of acute idiopathic dacryoadenitis; it results in marked improvement of symptoms within 24 to 48 hours in most cases.[194]

Nasolacrimal Duct Obstruction

Simple membranous nasolacrimal duct obstruction occurs in an estimated 1% to 20% of the newborn population, and intermittent, mild, self-limited bacterial infection is a commonly associated feature.[93,113,171,209] It most commonly results from a blockage of the valve of Hasner, which is the opening from the lacrimal sac into the inferior nasal meatus. The signs of nasolacrimal duct obstruction consist of an increased tear lake, mucopurulent discharge, and epiphora. The periocular skin is sometimes mildly erythematous, with skin fissures in regions of pronounced irritation. The conjunctiva and sclera are usually white and are uninvolved. When pressure is applied over the lacrimal sac there is a reflux of mucopurulent material from the punctum.

More than 50% of congenital nasolacrimal duct obstructions resolve without surgical intervention.[205,220,224,228] Most cases can be observed with treatment limited to gentle lid hygiene and lacrimal sac massages. In more severe cases, medical treatment with a topical antibiotic is appropriate. The most common organisms identified in nasolacrimal duct obstruction cultures include *Streptococcus pneumoniae* and *Haemophilus influenzae*.[293] Most ophthalmologists prefer topical fluoroquinolones over aminoglycosides because they cause less ocular irritation and have better coverage of gram-positive organisms. When the condition fails to resolve, a probing procedure can be performed in the nasolacrimal duct system, which typically is successful in resolving the condition. This procedure is commonly performed in the operating room under general anesthesia but also can be performed in an office setting with restraint when performed in children younger than 1 year.

Dacryocystitis

Dacryocystitis may result from congenital or acquired lacrimal outflow obstruction. This condition is manifested as acute erythema, pain, and swelling in the medial canthal region. The swelling typically is located below the medial canthal tendon. Marked epiphora generally is present, and a mucopurulent discharge frequently can be expressed through the lacrimal punctum if the proximal aspect of the lacrimal drainage system is not obstructed. If the infection has resulted in or from obstruction proximal and distal to the lacrimal sac, the overlying skin may become tense as the nasolacrimal sac distends in response to the infectious process. Formation of a fistula to the overlying skin may occur as a result of dacryocystitis, and surgical excision of the fistula tract often is needed after the acute process has resolved. Dacryocystitis is a particularly common finding in neonates with a dacryocele, with dacryocystitis developing in as many as 60% of affected neonates.[221]

Aerobic and anaerobic bacteria and fungi may produce dacryocystitis.[34,35] In one study, *S. epidermidis* and *Pseudomonas* spp. were the aerobic organisms identified most frequently, and *Peptostreptococcus* spp. and *Propionibacterium* spp. were the anaerobes isolated most frequently. Less common agents include *Escherichia coli, Pseudomonas* spp., *H. influenzae, Pasteurella multocida,* and various anaerobes. Laboratory investigation should include aerobic and anaerobic culture of mucopurulent discharge from the lacrimal sac. Frequent massage of the lacrimal sac may be used to facilitate expression of material for Gram stain and culture and to aid in resolution. A sepsis workup should be considered for children who are acutely ill and for young infants.

Intravenous nafcillin, vancomycin, or both are good initial therapeutic choices for serious gram-positive infections. Mild cases in older children can be treated with oral antibiotics. Intravenous ceftazidime is a reasonable initial antibiotic choice for gram-negative dacryocystitis. Intravenous nafcillin or vancomycin typically provides good initial empiric therapy in patients when Gram-stain guidance is not available.

Ophthalmologic consultation should be requested in all cases of acute dacryocystitis. Decompression of the lacrimal sac by aspiration, incision, and drainage or probing the proximal lacrimal drainage system may be needed to hasten resolution. Probing of the distal lacrimal system often is deferred until the acute infection has subsided, as complications from probing can lead to postseptal spread and subsequent orbital cellulitis. Mucopurulent material obtained during surgical decompression should be sent for appropriate culture.

Preseptal (Periorbital) Cellulitis

The term *preseptal cellulitis* refers to an infectious process in the eyelids that is isolated to regions anterior to the orbital septum. The orbital septum is a thin layer of fascia that extends vertically from the periosteum of the orbital rim to the tarsal plate within the eyelids. Although it is penetrated by nerves and vascular structures, the septum provides a barrier that slows the spread of infectious agents into deeper orbital and retroorbital structures.[271] Typical signs and symptoms of preseptal cellulitis include erythema and edema of the eyelids. Distinctively absent are signs of deeper orbital involvement such as restricted ocular motility, pain with eye movement, and proptosis. Preseptal cellulitis may occur after trauma or be caused by spread of infection from adjacent structures, such as skin and the upper respiratory system.[302]

Posttraumatic Preseptal Cellulitis

Posttraumatic preseptal cellulitis occurs after puncture wounds on the lids, face, or scalp. It also may occur after blunt trauma with no obvious entry wound. The etiologic agents most commonly identified are *S. aureus* and *S. pyogenes,* and polymicrobial infections can occur. Other bacterial causes include non–spore-forming anaerobes such as *Peptococcus, Peptostreptococcus,* and *Bacteroides*. Infection by aerobic gram-negative bacilli is an uncommon finding.[13] *P. multocida* is a common organism that produces posttraumatic preseptal cellulitis after dog and cat bites.[160,164] Cellulitis secondary to methicillin-resistant *S. aureus* (MRSA) is increasing in frequency and is a common cause of community-acquired cellulitis in some locations.

Clinical signs and symptoms are determined in large part by the severity of the injury, the interval since injury, and the infecting organisms. The involved lids are edematous, erythematous, and typically quite tender. Fluctuation of subcutaneous tissue may be present if an abscess has developed. Swelling of the uninvolved contralateral eyelids may occur as a result of lymphedema. As with any form of isolated preseptal cellulitis, vision is unaffected, and proptosis and eye movement disturbances are absent. On rare occasions, eyelid edema may be sufficiently severe to preclude adequate evaluation of the eye. Neuroimaging is required in such cases to assess the globe and rule out involvement of structures posterior to the orbital septum. Ophthalmologic consultation is critical in cases of severe posttraumatic preseptal cellulitis because of the potential for concurrent globe injury.

Laboratory analysis includes Gram stain and aerobic and anaerobic culture of any mucopurulent material to aid in therapeutic decisions. Amoxicillin-clavulanate or a related agent is the drug of choice for treating posttraumatic cellulitis caused by a dog bite because of the high prevalence of *P. multocida*. Tetanus prophylaxis should be guided by standard recommendations. Surgical drainage of large abscesses may be required if a rapid response to antimicrobial therapy does not occur.

Nontraumatic Preseptal Cellulitis

The clinical features of nonsuppurative, nontraumatic preseptal cellulitis depend to a large degree on the causative agent. Erythema and swelling of the involved eyelids are typical and are often accompanied by pain. Signs of orbital infection such as altered vision, proptosis, and eye movement abnormalities are absent.

Before the advent of *H. influenzae* type b vaccine, this organism frequently was a cause of nonsuppurative preseptal cellulitis in children. It was a particularly dangerous agent because of a high risk for spread to the central nervous system (CNS), which occurred in as many as 2% to 3% of patients. Although rare today, *H. influenzae* type b infections still may be encountered. Like many infecting organisms, it gains access to subcutaneous tissue through infected nasal passages.

S. pneumoniae is now the most common bacterial cause of preseptal cellulitis in the pediatric age group.[78] It occurs in association with upper respiratory tract infection, although constitutional symptoms usually are less pronounced than those associated with *H. influenzae* type b infection. A variety of other bacterial agents may cause preseptal cellulitis, but they are seen less commonly. Preseptal cellulitis occasionally has been reported to be due to a variety of other organisms, including *Trichophyton* (ringworm),[296] tuberculosis,[231] and anthrax.[9,41]

Adenovirus is another particularly common cause of preseptal cellulitis in children. Adenovirus is an important consideration in the differential diagnosis of childhood preseptal cellulitis because, despite being self-limited, the condition can occasionally mimic bacterial infection and prompt unnecessary treatment with antibiotics. Adenovirus can be recognized by its characteristic copious discharge, which may be serous. Swelling of the lid may be prominent, but erythema usually is minimal. Preauricular lymphadenopathy often occurs in older children, and marked conjunctival hyperemia with or without chemosis and subconjunctival hemorrhage may be present. Photophobia may also be observed in cases of concurrent punctate keratopathy. A history of recent contact with other infected individuals frequently is noted and should be sought. Care should be taken to avoid spreading infection to family members, medical personnel, and others.

Hospital admission should be considered for children younger than 1 year of age with bacterial preseptal cellulitis. Hospitalization also is important for children with signs of systemic toxicity and those with inadequate *H. influenzae* immunization. A sepsis workup is indicated for children with signs of systemic toxicity and for extremely young children. Ophthalmologic consultation is recommended if orbital involvement is suspected or if clinical examination is inconclusive. Computed tomography (CT) usually is unnecessary for isolated preseptal cellulitis. Cultures of blood obtained from patients with preseptal cellulitis generally are negative but are more likely to be positive in children younger than 2 years. Culture of conjunctival discharge is done often but rarely has significant diagnostic benefit. A severity index for scoring preseptal cellulitis in children has been reported to help guide treatment decisions.[299]

Antibacterial treatment should include intravenous agents for infants and those with signs of serious systemic infection. Intravenous cefuroxime or a combination of nafcillin plus cefotaxime or ceftriaxone frequently is recommended for empiric therapy. When MRSA preseptal cellulitis is suspected because of poor response to treatment or through cultures, clindamycin and trimethoprim-sulfamethoxazole are often the first-line agents. In situations in which MRSA preseptal cellulitis does not respond favorably to these medications, vancomycin or linezolid with rifampin may be effective treatments.[11,270] Outpatient treatment with intramuscular or oral antibiotics is reasonable for older, less acutely ill children. Systemic antibiotics should be continued for 7 to 10 days. Patients in whom intravenous antibiotics are started initially can switch to an oral antibiotic after they have been afebrile for at least 24 hours and otherwise have improved clinically, unless the possibility of development of sepsis remains a concern. When antibiotic treatment fails, other noninfectious causes should be explored.

Orbital Cellulitis

Orbital cellulitis refers to infection of orbital structures posterior to the orbital septum and is the most frequent cause of acute orbital inflammation. Orbital cellulitis occurs more commonly in children and more frequently during cold weather, when sinusitis is more prevalent.

Initial signs and symptoms can vary from mild inflammation to severe and fulminant orbital disease. Cardinal signs and symptoms of infectious orbital cellulitis include proptosis, limited eye movement (including total ophthalmoplegia), pain with eye movement, and an abnormal pupillary response. Decreased vision or even blindness can occur as the most serious ophthalmic complication.[247] Death can result from intracranial extension of the infection if appropriate treatment is not initiated. Elevated intraocular pressure and chemosis of the conjunctiva are common ancillary signs. Preseptal cellulitis often coexists with orbital cellulitis but is not a prerequisite.

Most cases of orbital cellulitis are caused by spread of infection from an adjacent infected sinus.[49,200] Ethmoid sinusitis is the most common predisposing factor.[192] Rare cases are due to penetrating orbital trauma or skin infection involving the face, with spread of organisms into the orbit. Orbital cellulitis may occur infrequently after orbital, ocular, or periocular surgery.[7,218,310] Orbital cellulitis and cavernous sinus thrombosis have been reported to occur after dental infections and dental surgery.[38]

Comprehensive evaluation of a patient with confirmed or suspected orbital cellulitis includes ophthalmologic and systemic examination. Assessment of visual acuity individually in each eye is important for excluding vision loss and establishing a baseline to aid in monitoring progression of the disease or the effects of therapy. Evaluation of optic nerve dysfunction by examining the pupils for an afferent pupillary defect (APD) is of utmost importance throughout the course of the disease. Careful evaluation of extraocular movement should be performed in all extreme positions of gaze to identify limitation of ocular duction and to evaluate for pain on eye movement. The presence or absence of proptosis can be assessed clinically by viewing the eyes from above (bird's-eye view) or below (worm's-eye view) and by comparing their relative positions within the orbits. In severe cases of orbital cellulitis, funduscopic examination may reveal dilation of the retinal venules and signs of compressive optic neuropathy, such as optic disc edema. In severe cases, central retinal artery and vein occlusions have been reported.[60,139,214] Systemic evaluation includes determination of temperature, which usually is in the range of 39°C to 40°C (102°F to 104°F). Sinus examination, a screening neurologic examination, and evaluation for signs and symptoms of sepsis and meningitis should be performed.

In any case of clinically definite or suspected orbital cellulitis, CT of the orbit and brain is essential. CT can establish or confirm the diagnosis of orbital cellulitis and provides critical information needed to manage the patient. Imaging of the brain is important because orbital cellulitis can evolve into a brain abscess, meningitis, or cavernous sinus thrombosis. However, when a clinical response to treatment is noted, improvement in CT findings frequently is delayed. Therefore recurrent CT scanning of a child with clinically improving findings is not indicated unless new signs or symptoms of concern develop.

Microbiologic studies often are acutely unhelpful for the routine patient with orbital cellulitis. Nonetheless baseline studies remain important because critical information sometimes is acquired. Blood culture samples should be obtained at a minimum, and a lumbar puncture with culture of cerebrospinal fluid (CSF) should be considered in infants and those with signs of CNS infection. Culture of the ocular, nasal, and nasopharyngeal mucous membranes is of limited value and can be omitted. However, if surgical drainage is performed, samples of any material removed should be obtained for culture.

Optimal management of a child with orbital cellulitis requires a multidisciplinary approach. In addition to evaluation and management by an experienced pediatrician, ophthalmologic and otolaryngologic consultation should be obtained. Neurosurgical consultation is required when involvement of the CNS is diagnosed or suspected. In atypical cases and those not responding to treatment, consultation with an infectious disease specialist is warranted.

The most common offending etiologic bacteria are *S. aureus*, *Streptococcus* spp., and *Haemophilus* spp. (other than *H. influenzae*).[185] *S. pneumoniae* also is implicated frequently, and a variety of less common organisms have been reported. *H. influenzae* orbital cellulitis rarely has occurred since widespread use of the *H. influenzae* type b vaccine was implemented.[3,78] Fungal infection of the orbit occasionally is encountered, typically in immunocompromised individuals.[183]

The differential diagnosis of orbital inflammation in children includes a broad range of noninfectious conditions, including blunt trauma, idiopathic orbital inflammation (orbital pseudotumor), Wegener granulomatosis, sarcoidosis, leukemic infiltration, lymphoma, rhabdomyosarcoma, necrotic retinoblastoma, metastatic carcinoma, and histiocytosis X. Thyroid ophthalmopathy also can be manifested as an acute orbital inflammatory process, although usually its onset is slow and insidious.

Treatment of all patients with orbital cellulitis requires hospitalization and initiation of intravenous antibiotics as soon as possible. Infection with penicillin-resistant organisms is an increasingly common occurrence and must be considered during treatment.[44,265] Appropriate initial antibiotic therapy may include nafcillin, metronidazole, and cefotaxime as combination therapy. Given the increasing incidence of MRSA, initial treatment with vancomycin or clindamycin should be considered.[53,245,256] Other antimicrobial agents may be useful, and local susceptibility patterns should guide the choice of initial antimicrobial therapy. Antibiotic coverage should be modified according to the clinical course and culture results. If the patient fails to respond to antibiotic treatment within 24 to 48 hours, consultation with an infectious disease specialist and repeat CT to look for the development of an orbital abscess should be considered (Fig. 61.4). The mean hospital stay for uncomplicated cases of orbital cellulitis is 10 to 14 days, and oral antibiotics should be prescribed for 7 to 10 days after discharge. When the source of infection is believed to be from sinusitis, a nasal decongestant is commonly prescribed to aid in opening the sinus ostia, promoting drainage of the infected sinus, and speeding resolution. Nasal decongestants should be continued for 7 to 10 days after initiation.

Although treatment of orbital cellulitis with steroids remains controversial, their use in the treatment of acute and chronic sinusitis has become increasingly common. Studies have shown that steroids can reduce levels of inflammatory cytokines in the sinonasal mucosa of individuals with sinusitis.[40,301] In a study on the use of steroids in children with orbital cellulitis, Yen and Yen[314] reported no adverse effects of this adjunct treatment with systemic antibiotics. Prospective studies on the use of steroids in orbital cellulitis have been proposed to determine whether they have any clinical benefit.

Children with orbital cellulitis require diligent follow-up while in the hospital. Vision should be assessed at the bedside daily; results may be more accurate if a single examiner routinely assesses vision for a given patient. Pupillary examination for an APD should be performed at each examination. Development of an APD indicates compromise

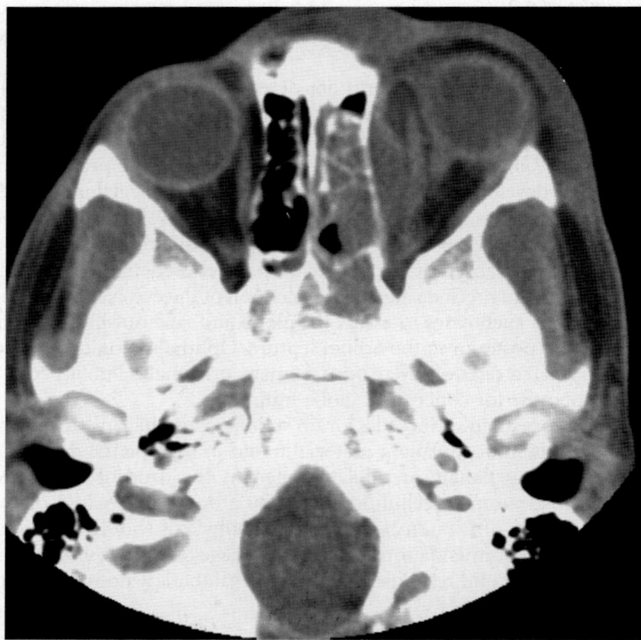

FIG. 61.4 Failure of response of orbital cellulitis to antibiotic treatment may be a sign of development of a subperiosteal orbital abscess (seen here in the right medial orbit).

BOX 61.1 Indications for Consideration of Surgical Drainage in Orbital Cellulitis

1. Age ≥9 years
2. Presence of frontal sinusitis
3. Nonmedial location of orbital abscess
4. Large orbital abscess (≥1250 mm^3)[289]
5. Suspicion of anaerobic orbital infection
   a. Presence of gas within the abscess space
   b. Infection of dental origin
6. Recurrence or abscess after prior drainage
7. Evidence of chronic sinusitis (e.g., presence of nasal polyps)
8. Acute optic nerve or retinal compromise

From Garcia GH, Harris GJ. Criteria for nonsurgical management of subperiosteal abscess of the orbit: analysis and outcomes 1988–1998. *Ophthalmology.* 2000;107(8):1454–6.

of the optic nerve, warrants escalation of treatment, and usually requires urgent surgical intervention. Worsening of extraocular motility, altered mental status, or onset of CNS signs raises the concern of progression to cavernous sinus thrombosis and should prompt emergency repeat neuroimaging of the brain and orbit, with further intervention as dictated by results of the scan. The close anatomic relationship of the orbit to the brain, with the orbital venous system freely anastomosing with the facial venous plexus and cranial venous sinus system through a series of valveless veins, seriously increases the potential for spread of infection to contiguous structures, including the brain.

Acute surgical intervention to decompress the orbit or drain an orbital or subperiosteal abscess is indicated if vision loss or an APD is identified at any point during treatment. Helpful drainage criteria have been described (Box 61.1). Immediate neurosurgical consideration is indicated if CNS involvement is documented. Most patients without evidence of vision loss, optic nerve dysfunction, or CNS involvement can be managed successfully medically.[111,244] Provided that clinical improvement continues, no worrisome signs or symptoms of CNS involvement develop, and the patient's overall clinical status does not worsen, repeat neuroimaging of patients with an orbital abscess is unnecessary. Short-term resolution of an orbital abscess often is not obvious on CT. The radiographic appearance of the abscess typically remains unchanged on early follow-up scans, although it may no longer contain viable organisms.

Sinus drainage by an otolaryngologist frequently is required to hasten resolution. Formation of an abscess is not a prerequisite for surgical intervention, and orbital cellulitis without abscess formation may progress to the point of requiring surgery. Despite prompt and appropriate treatment, serious complications such as permanent vision loss and brain abscess can occur.[36,66,122,237,247] Most patients, however, can be treated effectively with no permanent sequelae.

Orbital cellulitis caused by fungal infection has a course and prognosis markedly different from those of bacterial orbital cellulitis, particularly cellulitis caused by mucormycosis and aspergillosis. Fungal orbital cellulitis typically occurs in patients who are immunocompromised or patients with metabolic acidosis, such as those with poorly controlled diabetes. It may be manifested as a subacute or chronic process. Orbital apex syndrome is considered to be the most severe form, with loss of function of all cranial nerves traversing the orbital apex into the orbit (i.e., cranial nerves II, III, IV, V, and VI). A black eschar-like lesion may form in the oropharynx or nasopharynx in cases of fungal infection.

Aspergillus orbital infections (most commonly caused by *Aspergillus flavus, Aspergillus fumigatus,* or *Aspergillus oryzae*) are rare findings in children and may take a slow, chronic course over a period of months or years. No clear predisposing factors exist, but it has a predilection for humid climates, and most cases occur in otherwise healthy individuals. Signs and symptoms of orbital infection caused by *Aspergillus* spp. include loss of vision, constant dull pain, decreased or absent ocular motility, and proptosis with firm resistance to retropulsion. Palate and nasopharyngeal lesions occur but are rare. Biopsy is required for establishing the diagnosis.[110]

Effective treatment of orbital fungal infection requires correction of systemic and metabolic disturbances and administration of intravenous antifungal agents such as amphotericin B. Posaconazole has been shown to be effective as an alternative treatment in those who fail to respond to or cannot tolerate treatment with amphotericin B.[246] Surgical debridement of the orbit or adjacent infected sinuses frequently is required. Treatment often is unsuccessful, and fatalities are not uncommon, particularly with mucormycosis.

The larva of *Echinococcus granulosus* can produce a hydatid cyst in the orbit. The dog is the definitive host animal, although the organism also may live in the intestines of sheep, goats, cattle, pigs, and other animals. The disease is endemic in the Middle East, Africa, and Asia. Humans become infected by eating contaminated food, typically meat, and infection may occur in any age group. Affected patients have noninflammatory proptosis, decreased ocular motility, and dull orbital pain. Surgical excision is required for treatment. The cyst may be injected with hypertonic saline to kill the parasite, followed by excision.[108]

CONJUNCTIVAL INFECTIONS

The conjunctiva is the highly modified and specialized mucous membrane covering the inner surfaces of the eyelids and the anterior surface of the globe. The part that lines the inner surface of the eyelids is the *palpebral conjunctiva,* and the part covering the globe is the *bulbar conjunctiva.* The conjunctiva contains numerous small glands that produce two of the three parts of the tear film—a lower mucous layer acting as a wetting agent and a middle aqueous layer that makes up the bulk of the tear film; the third layer is oily and is produced by the sebaceous and meibomian glands of the eyelid and prevents rapid evaporation. The conjunctiva can be infected by many bacteria and viruses and by noninfectious allergic and toxic agents.

Conjunctivitis can cause mild or significant symptoms—burning, itching, or a foreign body sensation. Itching commonly signifies an allergic or viral cause. The conjunctival redness (injection and erythema) of infectious conjunctivitis is usually more severe when located away from the edge of the cornea, whereas conjunctival injection concentrated adjacent to the cornea (limbal or ciliary flush) suggests inflammation of the cornea (keratitis), inflammation of the iris (iritis), inflammation of the iris and ciliary body (iridocyclitis), or occasionally glaucoma or a corneal foreign body. When the eye is very severely infected, however, it may be so intensely red that such a differentiating pattern is not discernible.

Conjunctivitis is often accompanied by a discharge with important diagnostic properties. Thick purulence suggests a bacterial cause, a mucoid discharge suggests a viral infection, and a serous discharge may be seen with viral or allergic causes. Patients with isolated conjunctivitis usually do not have significant blurring of the vision. Apparent conjunctivitis with poor vision warrants a search for another diagnosis.[104,182]

Bacterial Conjunctivitis

Mild bacterial conjunctivitis is the most common form of infectious conjunctivitis in children. It is characterized by a purulent discharge and can be unilateral or bilateral. It is useful clinically to divide bacterial conjunctivitis into mild and severe forms because the treatments are different.[107,132]

Mild Bacterial Conjunctivitis

The agents most commonly causing mild bacterial conjunctivitis in children 5 years of age or older are *S. pneumoniae* and *Moraxella* spp.[104] *H. influenzae* was a prominent causative agent before the availability of *H. influenzae* type b vaccine. *S. aureus* conjunctivitis is seen most frequently after trauma or surgical manipulation. Conjunctival stains and cultures are usually not necessary, because the disease is almost invariably self-limited or responds rapidly to topical antibiotics.

Many topical antimicrobial agents for bacterial conjunctivitis are readily available and include ciprofloxacin, erythromycin, moxifloxacin, gatifloxacin, ofloxacin, norfloxacin, tobramycin, gentamicin, sulfacetamide, and various combinations. Aminoglycoside-containing compounds such as neomycin can occasionally cause a dramatic allergic blepharoconjunctivitis that is worse than the original disease. The choice of using either drops or ointment is best left to the person who will be instilling the medication, because neither has any proven therapeutic advantage. Newer agents, such as the fourth-generation fluoroquinolones (moxifloxacin and gatifloxacin), should not be used for routine mild bacterial conjunctivitis so as to limit antibiotic resistance. A typical regimen for treatment of mild conjunctivitis is 1 drop or a ¼-inch bead of ointment placed into the inferior conjunctival fornix three to six times daily for 5 to 7 days, depending on the medication. Persistent infection calls for a prompt return to the physician for reconsideration of the diagnosis. Mild bacterial conjunctivitis generally resolves spontaneously in 7 to 14 days even without treatment.[103,107]

Severe Bacterial Conjunctivitis

Severe bacterial conjunctivitis, characterized by ocular discomfort, pronounced redness, and copious purulent discharge, is usually caused by *Neisseria gonorrhoeae, Neisseria meningitidis, S. aureus, S. pneumoniae,* and, in children younger than 5 years, *H. influenzae*. A hyperpurulent state in which the copious purulent discharge reaccumulates in a matter of minutes is characteristic of infection with *N. gonorrhoeae*.[121,266] Severe conjunctivitis calls for stains and cultures. Samples from both eyes should be stained and cultured separately, even if only one eye is involved, to allow the uninvolved eye to serve as a control.[278] Gram stains of conjunctival scrapings should be done at the time of culture. A useful culture technique includes the use of a cotton or calcium alginate swab gently rubbed against the palpebral conjunctiva of the lower lid and inoculated onto blood and chocolate agar. If *N. gonorrhoeae* is suspected, a culture for chlamydia is also indicated, because concurrent infection with both organisms is common.[258,261]

The treatment of severe bacterial conjunctivitis is based initially on the results of the stains and later modified according to cultures and sensitivities. If *Neisseria* is strongly suspected, the patient should be treated for *Neisseria,* even if the laboratory results are not confirmatory. Ocular *N. gonorrhoeae* infection is a vision-threatening and life-threatening disease. This organism can penetrate the intact cornea and cause microbial keratitis (i.e., infection of the cornea), corneal perforation, and endophthalmitis (i.e., infection inside the eyeball), in addition to the conjunctivitis. *N. gonorrhoeae* conjunctivitis should be considered in three patient groups: neonates after passage through an infected birth canal, sexually active individuals, and victims of possible sexual abuse. For this reason, a high index of suspicion should be maintained. Pediatric infection with *N. gonorrhoeae* requires hospital admission and administration of a systemic antibiotic. Because of the prevalence of penicillin-resistant strains, a broad-spectrum (third-generation) cephalosporin, such as ceftriaxone, is the most appropriate choice of antibiotic.[117] Adjunctive treatment of *N. gonorrhoeae* conjunctivitis with topical moxifloxacin and simple saline irrigation for 5 days can be helpful, but topical agents should never be used as isolated treatment.[121] Moxifloxacin is a particularly good antibiotic choice because it is effective against chlamydia as well.

Conjunctivitis caused by gram-positive cocci can be treated with topical moxifloxacin, gatifloxacin, ciprofloxacin, or erythromycin. Systemic nafcillin, a second- or third-generation cephalosporin, or both can be added as needed for more extensive infections. Gram-negative bacterial conjunctivitis can be treated with topical erythromycin ointment or an aminoglycoside drip such as gentamicin or tobramycin. Systemic antibiotics can be added if needed.[278]

Viral Conjunctivitis

Adenoviral Conjunctivitis

Viruses are another common cause of infectious conjunctivitis in children. Many pediatric cases of viral conjunctivitis are caused by adenovirus. Serotypes 1, 2, 3, 4, 7, and 10 produce an acute form of conjunctivitis with prominent conjunctival follicles. Serotypes 3 and 7 also may cause pharyngoconjunctival fever. This entity is characterized by conjunctivitis, fever, and pharyngitis.[25] Serotypes 8, 19, and 37 can cause epidemic keratoconjunctivitis (EKC).[278] EKC is characterized by a combination of a punctate epithelial keratitis (best viewed by slit-lamp examination) and an immune response that results in subepithelial (i.e., in the corneal stroma) infiltrates. There is commonly a robust inflammatory response causing the formation of membranes on the palpebral conjunctival surface, and there can be extensive subconjunctival hemorrhages and preseptal cellulitis. Photophobia is a prominent feature of this condition, and visual acuity may be markedly decreased. Epidemic keratoconjunctivitis is often associated with pharyngitis and rhinitis, which may precede or be concurrent with the conjunctivitis.

Adenoviral conjunctivitis may be highly contagious. It is transmitted easily from an infected individual to others at home or at school. The incubation period is 5 to 10 days but may be as long as 21 days. The virus is shed from the infected conjunctiva for 7 to 12 days after the onset of infection. Frequently, a prodromal upper respiratory tract infection consisting of fever, pharyngitis, or otitis media occurs.[278] Ocular signs and symptoms include photophobia (with corneal involvement), foreign body sensation, epiphora (tearing), bulbar and palpebral conjunctival injection and chemosis (edema of the conjunctiva), and subconjunctival hemorrhage.[125] Preauricular lymphadenopathy is a common feature in older children and adults.

The diagnosis of adenoviral conjunctivitis is almost always clinical only. Only rarely is laboratory confirmation necessary. Viral cultures are possible when indicated, and a rapid enzyme immunoassay test is available.[306] Treatment of adenoviral conjunctivitis is supportive, aimed at decreasing the symptoms of irritation, photophobia, and blurred vision. Cool compresses and acetaminophen are helpful. For the more aggressive EKC, topical steroids are indicated to quiet the severe immune response. Removal of conjunctival membranes with a moistened cotton swab may relieve the foreign-body sensation. A small amount of bleeding often occurs after removal of the membranes, and they can recur after several days. The use of topical steroid preparations requires careful monitoring,[181,278] and they should only be prescribed by an ophthalmologist.[147,262]

The clinician should wear gloves when examining patients with suspected adenovirus infection. Careful hand-washing is essential after direct contact. Instruments or equipment used in examining an infected patient should be cleaned with 10% sodium hypochlorite solution or other solutions known to eradicate the adenovirus.

Mini-epidemics of adenovirus-related conjunctivitis can originate in physicians' offices.[13,100] At home, families should exercise caution and separate the towels and bedclothes of the patient from those of others in the household. Children of school age should be kept at home for 7 days or longer to reduce the risk for transmitting the infection to classmates.[278]

Herpes Simplex Virus Conjunctivitis and Complex Forms

HSV conjunctivitis may occur as a primary or secondary infection. Ocular infection usually is caused by HSV-1, except in newborns, in whom HSV-2 predominates.[51] Typical initial signs of HSV conjunctivitis include a serous discharge, scant conjunctival follicle formation on the inferior palpebral conjunctiva, and preauricular lymphadenopathy.[317] Eighty percent of cases are unilateral. Eyelid vesicles often occur in primary infections. Bulbar conjunctival ulceration is an unusual occurrence, but when present, it is virtually pathognomonic of primary HSV-1 infection. Keratitis occurs in as many as 50% of primary cases and is characterized by mild epithelial irregularities. Dendrites (branch-shaped lesions of the corneal epithelium) can occur in primary infections, but reactivated HSV keratitis frequently exhibits the characteristic dendritic pattern. Lid vesicles usually do not develop in cases of reactivated HSV infection.[146]

Primary HSV dermatoblepharitis is seen most commonly in children younger than 6 years, but it may occur at any age. The initial episode may be associated with an upper respiratory tract infection, and recurrences are common. Clinical signs include eyelid vesicular reaction, mild follicular conjunctivitis, preauricular lymphadenopathy, and, occasionally, atypical epithelial keratitis. Secondary bacterial infection can occur. Systemic acyclovir is a safe and effective treatment, although the disease itself typically is self-limited and does not require treatment.[146]

The diagnosis of HSV keratoconjunctivitis usually is made on the basis of the clinical appearance alone. Antigen detection tests or viral cultures can be used when the diagnosis is in question.[141] Viral cultures, when necessary, require special handling.[278] In culturing primary HSV cases, the skin surface is swabbed with an alcohol sponge, and a tuberculin syringe with a 30-gauge needle is used to aspirate fluid from an intact vesicle. If no vesicles are present, a Dacron swab is wiped on the palpebral conjunctiva of the lower lid. The viral transport medium is inoculated and taken to the laboratory for special handling.

Treatment of HSV conjunctivitis alone (in the absence of corneal epithelial disease) is controversial. Oral acyclovir may be used for severe cases of primary HSV infection.[254,274] Two topical antiviral agents are available: trifluridine solution and ganciclovir ointment.

When epithelial HSV keratitis is reactivated and the typical dendritic (branched) epithelial lesions are seen, the cornea usually is hypoesthetic. Iritis may be associated with HSV keratitis and is characterized by miosis, photophobia, ocular pain, and foreign-body sensation. Vision may be decreased if the epithelial disease involves the visual axis.[278] Epithelial HSV may be atypical, may be more severe, and may be more complicated in patients receiving topical steroids and in immunocompromised patients.

Treatment with topical trifluridine or ganciclovir should be strongly considered in all cases of HSV epithelial keratitis, and due to the risk of visual loss, the argument can be made to use oral acyclovir concomitantly.[114] For HSV stromal keratitis, topical steroids are effective in decreasing corneal scarring but should only be used by an ophthalmologist. When using a topical steroid, coverage with a topical antiviral agent such as trifluridine should always be included to reduce the risk for recurrent active viral proliferation. Ancillary treatments include cycloplegic eye drops to dilate the pupil and pain medications as needed.

Chronic suppression with oral acyclovir is effective in reducing the number of recurrences of HSV epithelial and stromal keratitis, especially in patients with stromal keratitis.[274,278] Interferon also significantly adds to the efficacy of topical antiviral therapy, but the adverse side effects of interferon must be weighed against its potential benefits.[274]

External Ocular Infections With Varicella-Zoster Virus

Childhood varicella infection (chickenpox) is commonly accompanied by conjunctivitis. Vesicles, ulcers, or both occur occasionally on the bulbar or palpebral conjunctiva. Conjunctivitis associated with varicella infection does not result in permanent visual sequelae. Corneal involvement rarely occurs and typically heals without sequelae. Occasionally it may result in stromal scarring and produce irregular astigmatism and reduced vision.

After primary varicella infection occurs, the virus may persist in latent form in the trigeminal nerve ganglia. Herpes zoster ophthalmicus occurs when the ophthalmic division of the trigeminal nerve is affected by reactivation of the virus. The condition occurs more commonly in immunocompromised patients, and recurrences occur infrequently except in these patients. For this reason, testing for immunocompromise, including HIV, should be considered in individuals with herpes zoster who are otherwise presumed to be immunocompetent.[157,159,166]

The diagnosis of herpes zoster ophthalmicus is almost always made on the basis of the characteristic clinical feature of a painful, tender vesicular eruption of one V-1 dermatome. Ocular involvement may include keratitis and uveitis. Corneal epithelial lesions may appear dendritiform, with or without subepithelial infiltrates. Uveitis may occur with or without associated keratitis. Usually the uveitis is mild, but occasionally it may be severe, especially in immunocompromised patients, with the formation of a hypopyon (pus in the anterior chamber) or a hyphema. Immunofluorescence testing of vesicular base scrapings or viral cultures may be helpful if the manifestation is atypical or the diagnosis is in doubt.[162]

Treatment of herpes zoster ophthalmicus involves the administration of oral or intravenous acyclovir. Treatment is most effective when initiated within 72 hours of the appearance of vesicles. The keratitis and uveitis do not respond to topical antiviral therapy.[70] Occasionally topical steroids may be helpful in treating varicella keratitis and uveitis, but such treatment should be administered under the direction of an ophthalmologist.[181]

Chlamydial Conjunctivitis and Trachoma

Chlamydia spp. can cause conjunctivitis and trachoma. *Chlamydia psittaci* rarely causes ocular disease in humans. *Chlamydia trachomatis,* however, has numerous serotypes that affect the eye. Serotypes A, B, Ba, and C cause trachoma, and serotypes B, C, D, Da, D–, E, F, G, H, I, Ia, J, and K cause inclusion conjunctivitis, including neonatal inclusion conjunctivitis. Neonatal chlamydial conjunctivitis is addressed in the discussion of neonatal conjunctivitis. Inclusion conjunctivitis in older children and adults is a subacute or chronic inflammation of the conjunctiva. The condition may be unilateral or bilateral. A mucopurulent discharge typically occurs, as do follicles on the bulbar and perilimbal conjunctiva. Preauricular lymphadenopathy is a common feature. Punctate epithelial keratitis with subepithelial infiltrates and a superior micropannus (i.e., vascular growth on the upper edge of the cornea) may develop.[63]

The differential diagnosis of inclusion conjunctivitis includes viral and bacterial conjunctivitis, molluscum contagiosum, and toxic keratoconjunctivitis from chronic administration of topical agents. Laboratory testing may be necessary to confirm the diagnosis. Giemsa staining of conjunctival scrapings may demonstrate the classic intracytoplasmic inclusions. A fluorescent antibody detection test or an enzyme immunoassay can be used for a rapid diagnosis.[278] Chlamydial cultures may be needed when the diagnosis remains in doubt.

Treatment consists of oral erythromycin or doxycycline if systemic infection is suspected. Topical erythromycin or tetracycline alone four times each day for 7 days is effective treatment of infection limited to the conjunctiva.[63,278] Moxifloxacin has been shown to be effective against chlamydia but is not yet the recommended treatment of choice.

Trachoma, a chronic blinding conjunctivitis, remains a prominent etiology of blindness worldwide, ranking sixth overall, causing 4% of all blindness. It is a disease of impoverished populations that is exacerbated by inadequate supplies of water and poor hygiene and sanitation. Trachoma seldom is seen in fully developed countries. In the United States, it is encountered on Native American reservations in the Southwest and in individuals from endemic foreign areas. Eye-seeking flies play an important role in transmission of *Chlamydia* from one person to another.[278]

Trachoma causes blindness by producing chronic inflammation of the palpebral conjunctiva of the upper eyelid with secondary scar formation. Contracture of the scars causes entropion of the eyelid and trichiasis (cilia rubbing on the cornea). After many years of infection and reinfection this leads to corneal neovascularization, opacification, and vision loss.[277,288] Less commonly, the cornea may be infected directly. The complete course of the disease from initial infection to blindness generally takes decades. Children do not become blind from trachoma, but they are the most significant constant chronic reservoir of the disease.

The diagnosis of trachoma usually is made on the basis of clinical findings alone. The disease passes through characteristic stages, from simple inflammation to scarring, entropion, and trichiasis. Multiple stages may coexist in various parts of the eyelids. The World Health Organization classifies the stages of trachoma as follows: TF, trachomatous follicular response; TI, diffuse trachomatous conjunctival inflammation; TS, trachomatous scarring of the palpebral conjunctiva; TT, trachomatous trichiasis; and CO, trachomatous corneal opacification. In the pediatric population, physicians usually encounter only stages TI and TF.[288,312] The scars on the palpebral conjunctiva, referred to as *Arlt lines,* are linear and multidirectional. Slit-lamp examination may reveal a superior limbal corneal micropannus and Herbert pits (i.e., hollowed-out areas at the superior limbus), which represent sites of resolved follicles.

Treatment of trachoma now consists of periodic dosing of susceptible populations with azithromycin or, if azithromycin is not available, topical tetracycline or erythromycin ointment instilled twice daily for 2 months, as well as improved sanitation and hygiene to prevent recurrence.[278] Trachoma can be self-limited if hygiene alone is improved.[277] In children older than 8 years of age, doxycycline should be administered orally daily for 40 days. Erythromycin can be substituted in younger children or in patients intolerant of doxycycline.

Neonatal Conjunctivitis

Neonatal conjunctivitis, or ophthalmia neonatorum, is a common vision-threatening disorder throughout the world, although it has been relegated to a position of secondary importance in the fully industrialized world, where screening and prophylactic measures are widespread. It remains a significant cause of childhood ocular morbidity in poor countries.

Dilute topical silver nitrate solution instilled just after birth for prophylaxis against ophthalmia neonatorum was the first treatment used. In the 1880s it was responsible for reducing the prevalence of gonococcal ophthalmia neonatorum from 10% to 0.17% of live births in Europe.[278] Silver nitrate has been largely supplanted by other preparations; where it is used, a mild, self-limited chemical conjunctivitis can occur.[208] It lasts 2 to 4 days and resolves with no treatment. Topical erythromycin largely has replaced silver nitrate in developed countries, because it is effective and does not produce a chemical conjunctivitis.[119] In the developing world, dilute povidone iodine solution, 2.5%, has proved to be a remarkably effective and inexpensive measure for prevention of *N. gonorrheae* neonatal conjunctivitis when instilled immediately after birth.[136]

In areas of regional conflicts, political instability, and burgeoning refugee populations, even such simple measures are often impossible.[98,119] Causes of neonatal conjunctivitis are highly variable among populations. In areas that use silver nitrate or povidone iodine drops for prophylaxis, chemical conjunctivitis is a common cause of neonatal conjunctivitis.[208] Infectious conjunctivitis occurs in 0.5% to 6.0% of live births in the United States. The leading infection is *C. trachomatis*.[18,124,259,278]

Neonatal infection is caused by ocular exposure to contaminated maternal discharge during normal birth, although it may occur in infants born by cesarean section, especially if the membranes rupture prematurely. Other important infectious agents that may cause ophthalmia neonatorum are *N. gonorrhoeae* and *S. aureus*.[97,266] Bacteria that normally reside in the vaginal or gastrointestinal tract occasionally are implicated in ophthalmia neonatorum.

Such bacteria include *Streptococcus* spp., *Haemophilus* spp., *Pseudomonas aeruginosa, Moraxella* spp. including *Moraxella catarrhalis, N. meningitidis, E. coli,* and *Enterobacter cloacae*.[249,273] Viruses occasionally produce neonatal conjunctivitis. Rarely HSV may cause keratoconjunctivitis.[98] It is associated with distinctive vesicular skin changes and systemic signs, and the diagnosis seldom is in doubt.[12]

Life-threatening HSV meningoencephalitis is a serious potential complication of HSV ophthalmia neonatorum.[201] Other viruses occasionally implicated include adenovirus, coxsackievirus A9, cytomegalovirus (CMV), and echovirus.[272]

Certain clinical features may help establish the specific etiologic diagnosis in cases of ophthalmia neonatorum (Table 61.1), but considerable overlap in findings exists, and physicians cannot rely on the history and physical examination alone to make a definitive diagnosis. Even when all appropriate investigative modalities are used, the cause may remain unknown in some cases.

Variations in the time of onset after birth, severity of inflammation, and character of the ocular discharge are common, and though none is considered pathognomonic of a specific infectious process, general considerations are worth reviewing.[249] Silver nitrate chemical conjunctivitis typically begins during the first 48 hours of life and produces a watery discharge with mild inflammation. It is self-limited and resolves within 48 to 72 hours of its appearance.[208] *C. trachomatis* conjunctivitis generally begins 1 to 21 days after birth and usually is apparent by day 7. A moderately copious mucopurulent discharge may be present but can be variable.[124,198] *S. aureus* conjunctivitis also begins during the first 3 weeks of life and can produce a moderately profuse mucopurulent discharge. Many other bacterial agents produce an overlapping clinical picture. Conjunctivitis caused by *N. gonorrhoeae* ordinarily begins somewhat earlier, usually by the third day of life, but it may appear as late as 3 weeks after birth. The hallmark is a copious, hyperpurulent discharge that can reaccumulate in a matter of minutes after it is removed. *N. gonorrhoeae* can penetrate an initially intact cornea and result in perforation of the eye and endophthalmitis.[121,252,272] Conjunctivitis caused by gastrointestinal flora often begins within a few days of birth and can produce a copious purulent discharge.

TABLE 61.1 Clinical Characteristics of Neonatal Conjunctivitis Caused by Various Agents

Agent	Day of Life at Onset	Discharge
Silver nitrate	1 (0–2)	Serous
Chlamydia trachomatis	7 (1–21)	Mucopurulent
Staphylococcus aureus	5 (1–21)	Mucopurulent
Neisseria gonorrhoeae	3 (0–21)	Purulent
Other bacteria	7 (1–21)	Mucopurulent
Herpes simplex virus	5 (0–21)	Serosanguineous
Other viruses	Not established	Probably serous

Viral causes of ophthalmia neonatorum are rarer in occurrence. HSV infection may begin during the first 3 weeks of life and usually produces a serous or serosanguineous discharge.[98,201] Other viruses have highly variable characteristics, but a serous discharge is a common finding.

The differential diagnosis of neonatal conjunctivitis includes congenital glaucoma, dacryostenosis with or without dacryocystitis, keratitis, and uveitis. Dacryostenosis is manifested as epiphora and a watery or purulent discharge. Occasionally conjunctivitis may develop. Because epiphora caused by congenital dacryostenosis ordinarily is not seen until the second or third week of life, it rarely is a serious consideration. Newborns with congenital glaucoma often are photophobic and irritable.[298] They may exhibit increased tearing, conjunctival injection, corneal edema, and enlargement of the ocular globe (buphthalmos). Both keratitis and uveitis most often are accompanied by photophobia and pain. The discharge with keratitis can vary but with bacterial causes is purulent. The discharge with uveitis, if present, is watery.

Laboratory testing is important in establishing a specific diagnosis and should include Gram and Giemsa stains, a chlamydial immunoassay, and cultures for aerobic and anaerobic bacteria. Cotton-tipped swabs should be used to obtain material for culture from the conjunctival fornices. Viral and chlamydial cultures and immunoassays can be considered but usually are unnecessary.[17,281] Gonococcal immunoassay and HSV immunochemical tests are available but not in widespread use.

The initial treatment of neonatal conjunctivitis depends on the suspected infectious agent. Broad-spectrum treatment should be considered if the diagnostic possibilities cannot be narrowed. Silver nitrate–induced conjunctivitis is self-limited and does not require treatment. *C. trachomatis* conjunctivitis is treated with tetracycline (1%) or erythromycin (0.5%) ointment four times daily for 3 weeks and with systemic erythromycin for 2 to 3 weeks to prevent or to treat chlamydial pneumonia. Sulfonamides can be used to treat chlamydial conjunctivitis if erythromycin is not tolerated. Topical antibiotics alone are insufficient for the treatment of neonatal *Chlamydia* infection.[109,120,124] Staphylococcal conjunctivitis can be treated with erythromycin ointment or a variety of other topical antimicrobial agents every 4 to 6 hours for 3 to 7 days. Appropriate systemic antibiotic treatment should be considered if the infection is particularly severe.[278]

N. gonorrhoeae infection requires systemic treatment in all cases. Aqueous penicillin G can be considered if resistant strains are unlikely. However, one dose of intramuscular ceftriaxone is the treatment of choice in the United States because it is effective against all *N. gonorrhoeae* strains.[14,233] Eyes should be irrigated with saline every hour until the discharge clears and then in reduced frequency as necessary to reduce the risk for the development of corneal infection. This interval usually is 24 to 48 hours after the initiation of systemic treatment.

Penicillin G drops are recommended by some ophthalmologists, but such drops do not appear to improve the overall prognosis or speed of recovery.

HSV neonatal conjunctivitis is treated with systemic acyclovir in appropriate doses for as long as 3 weeks.[98] Treatment should be instituted on an emergency basis because of the potential for the development of serious permanent neurologic sequelae and death if treatment is delayed. Topical ophthalmic trifluridine or ganciclovir also should be applied to the eyes four times daily for 2 to 3 weeks.

Prevention of ophthalmia neonatorum is simple and requires only instillation of an antibiotic or antiseptic agent within the first hour after birth. Silver nitrate drops (1%), erythromycin ointment (0.5%), and tetracycline ointment (1%) all are effective treatments against *N. gonorrhoeae* and *C. trachomatis*.[120,278] A 5% solution of povidone-iodine also has been effective and economical in prophylaxis against a variety of agents, including gonococcal neonatal conjunctivitis. It may be particularly useful in developing countries.[136] As with other sexually transmitted diseases, neonatal conjunctivitis caused by *N. gonorrhoeae, C. trachomatis,* or HSV should be addressed according to standard public health policies, with reporting, investigation, and case identification as required by local law.

KERATITIS: CORNEAL INFLAMMATION

The cornea, with its overlying tear film, is the major refracting component of the human eye. Keratitis means inflammation of the cornea. Microbial keratitis means inflammation of the cornea caused by infection with a microorganism.

Any irregularity of the corneal tear film, the surface of the cornea itself, or an opacity of the cornea involving the central visual axis may impair vision. The cornea is composed of five distinct layers: the epithelium, Bowman's layer, the stroma, Descemet's membrane, and the endothelium. The epithelium is several layers thick and, when healthy, can regenerate without scarring after an injury or other insult. The Bowman membrane lies beneath the epithelium. It does not regenerate, and it heals with a scar when injured. The stroma is the thickest part of the cornea. It is composed of regularly arranged collagen fibrils embedded in a matrix of mucoproteins and glycoproteins. Like the Bowman membrane, the stroma heals with scarring.

Descemet's membrane is the basement membrane of the corneal endothelium. It can regenerate after an insult and does not opacify. The innermost layer, the endothelium, is derived from neuroectoderm and consists of a single layer of cells that do not have significant regenerative capacity. The cornea is an avascular structure that is clear because of the regular arrangement of the collagen fibers in the stroma and the dehydrating pumping action of the endothelium. The cornea will become edematous and opacify if the endothelium is significantly damaged or diseased. The external corneal surface is protected from injury and exposure by the eyelids. Reflex tearing in response to mechanical irritation provides further protection. The blink response to threat and the antimicrobial properties of the tear film further protect the cornea from injury and infection.

Patients with keratitis usually have erythema of the perilimbal bulbar conjunctiva (limbal or ciliary flush) and pain. Additional complaints may include decreased vision and photophobia. The diagnosis of keratitis depends on the presence of a corneal epithelial or stromal infiltrate. The infiltrate is verified by slit-lamp examination and can be extremely difficult to see in infants and uncooperative or frightened children. Ideally the patient is examined with a slit lamp; sometimes sedation is required for this. Stains and cultures are usually required to establish the diagnosis, preferably before topical antibiotics are started, so an ophthalmologist should be consulted promptly. Rarely a biopsy of the cornea is needed to obtain material for culture. Even more rarely, a corneal transplantation is required to stop progression of an infection or to treat a corneal perforation. Exact etiologic diagnosis is based on clinical findings and on examination of stains and cultures.

Isolated Epithelial Keratitis

Keratitis can be classified according to the layer of cornea involved. Most infections involve the epithelium and/or the stroma. Isolated epithelial keratitis usually is caused by one of several viruses: HSV, varicella-zoster virus (VZV), adenovirus, EBV, and the (rubeola) measles virus. The first three organisms have been discussed in an earlier section.

EBV causes HSV-like dendritic corneal epithelial lesions; stromal disease also may occur. The lesions are self-limited and do not respond to antiviral therapy.[180] Measles keratitis usually consists of transient epithelial infiltrates, which resolve without permanent sequelae.[146] In malnourished children with vitamin A deficiency, measles represents a serious threat to life and to vision. Deep corneal ulcers may develop during the first few days of measles infection. Vitamin A deficiency remains the most common cause of pediatric blindness worldwide, almost exclusively involving children in developing countries. Measles is a common comorbidity factor. When a vitamin A–deficient child develops measles and keratitis, rapid progression leading to corneal perforation and ultimate loss of the eye may occur.[24,96] Whether the ulcers are caused by direct measles virus infection, by the keratomalacia (corneal melting) of vitamin A deficiency, or by some combination of these factors is still not entirely clear.

Measles immunization programs plus periodic mega–vitamin A dosing programs for susceptible children under 6 years of age greatly reduce childhood blindness and childhood mortality in developing countries.

Stromal Keratitis

Syphilis and certain parasitic and viral infections can cause a nonsuppurative keratitis isolated to the corneal stroma. Congenital syphilis produces interstitial (stromal) keratitis in children, although the condition usually does not become apparent until late in the first decade of life. An indolent, peripheral corneal haze develops and slowly progresses centrally. Ghost vessels devoid of blood flow are seen in the corneal stroma on slit-lamp examination.[280] The condition is manifested as a bilateral stromal process[255] in 80% of cases and is accompanied by transient iritis, iridocyclitis, or scleritis at some point in the course of the disease. When ocular syphilis is diagnosed, systemic infection is present by definition. The systemic disease must be treated according to accepted guidelines.

Bacterial Keratitis

Bacterial keratitis, usually involving a corneal ulcer, most often occurs after trauma that disrupts the normal integrity of the corneal epithelium. The trauma can be mild and occult, such as that caused by contact lens wear. *S. aureus, S. pneumoniae, P. aeruginosa,* and *Moraxella* spp. are the most common bacterial causes of severe necrotizing bacterial keratitis.[10,164,197,295] Other organisms, such as *S. epidermidis, Actinomyces* spp., viridans streptococci, *Acanthamoeba,* and a variety of others, have been implicated in less severe cases. Accurate identification of the offending organism greatly facilitates effective treatment. A specimen is obtained by scraping the edge of the ulcer with a sterile platinum spatula. Smears should be fixed in 70% methanol, not by heat, and Gram stain for bacteria and acridine orange stain for fungi and *Acanthamoeba* are recommended. The yield of culture-positive cases is higher in laboratories skilled in handling corneal cultures. Material for culture should be inoculated onto fresh media such as blood and chocolate agar (aerobes and facultative anaerobes), Sabouraud agar (fungi), and thioglycolate broth (anaerobic bacteria). Thayer-Martin agar should be plated if *N. gonorrhoeae* is suspected. Initial treatment is based on the resulting stains (Table 61.2) and modified pending cultures (Table 61.3).[20,163]

Typically patients are started on frequent fortified tobramycin and ceftazidime drops until culture results become available. Medical treatment of bacterial keratitis includes fourth-generation fluoroquinolones, fortified topical antibiotics, and, occasionally, subconjunctival antibiotic injection (see Table 61.2).[45,211,278] Antibiotics are administered as often as every 15 to 30 minutes initially and then continued hourly until there has been definite improvement, usually first manifested by improvement in pain. Systemic antibiotics are required only for gonococcal, chlamydial, and onchocercal keratitis, as well as for actual or threatened perforation of the cornea, extension of infection to the sclera, or worsening of the process during topical or periocular treatment. Topical steroids have been found to be beneficial if the resulting inflammation threatens to destroy the mechanical or optical integrity of the cornea, but steroids are never used as isolated treatment.[268,278]

Two important corneal sequelae of previously discussed eyelid blepharitis are staphylococcal marginal keratitis and phlyctenulosis. Both are thought to represent hypersensitivity reactions by the ocular surface to bacterial toxins. Symptoms include eye redness, irritation, and itching, and patients usually present late and carry the misdiagnosis of allergic conjunctivitis due to overlap of symptoms. Marginal keratitis usually affects the peripheral cornea (especially inferiorly) and appears as multiple, small, faint gray spots in the subepithelium. Phlyctenulosis is a more severe sequela and appears as a gelatinous aggregation (single or multiple) of inflammatory cells. Treatment of phlyctenulosis is particularly important due to cumulative risk of corneal scarring and its effect on vision. Combination antibiotic-steroid eye drops or ointments are effective in improving both the bacterial load and the hypersensitivity component. Consideration should also be made for using a short course of oral azithromycin for these same reasons.[47,75]

TABLE 61.2 Treatment of Keratitis Based on Smear Morphology

Organism	ANTIBIOTIC Ocular	Systemic[a]
Gram-positive cocci, gram-positive bacilli	Cefazolin[b]	Nafcillin, IV
Gram-positive filaments	Amikacin[c]	Trimethoprim-sulfamethoxazole, IV
Gram-negative cocci	Ceftriaxone[b] or ciprofloxacin[c,d]	Ceftriaxone, IV or IM
Gram-negative bacilli	Tobramycin[b]	Tobramycin, IV
Acid-fast bacilli	Amikacin[c]	
Hyphal fragments	Natamycin,[c] fluconazole[e]	Fluconazole, PO
Yeasts	Amphotericin B,[c] fluconazole[e]	Fluconazole, PO
Cysts, trophozoites	Polyhexamethylene, biguanide,[c] paromomycin,[c] and propamidine isethionate[c]	Itraconazole, PO

IM, Intramuscularly; *IV*, intravenously; *PO*, orally.
[a]Standard age-appropriate mg/kg dosages.
[b]Topical and periocular use only.
[c]Topical use only.
[d]Use in children age ≥12 years.
[e]Periocular use only.

TABLE 61.3 Treatment Based on Identification of Organisms

Organism	ANTIBIOTIC Ocular	Systemic
Micrococcus, Staphylococcus (penicillin-resistant)	Cefazolin[a]	Nafcillin, IV
Micrococcus, Staphylococcus (methicillin-resistant)	Vancomycin[a]	Vancomycin, IV
Streptococcus	Penicillin G[a]	Penicillin G, IV
Enterococcus	Vancomycin[a] and gentamicin[a]	Vancomycin, IV, and gentamicin, IV
Anaerobic gram-positive coccus	Penicillin G[a]	Penicillin G, IV
Corynebacterium spp.	Penicillin G[a]	Penicillin G, IV
Mycobacterium fortuitum-chelonae	Amikacin[b]	Amikacin, IV,[a] or clarithromycin, PO
Nocardia	Amikacin[b]	Trimethoprim-sulfamethoxazole, IV
Neisseria gonorrhoeae	Ceftriaxone[a]	Ceftriaxone, IV or IM
Pseudomonas spp.	Ceftazidime[a] Tobramycin[a]	Ceftazidime, IV or IM
Other aerobic, gram-negative bacilli	Ceftazidime[a] Tobramycin[a]	Ceftazidime, IV or IM
Filamentous fungi	Natamycin[b] Fluconazole[c]	Fluconazole, PO
Candida spp.	Amphotericin B[b] Fluconazole[c]	Fluconazole, PO
Acanthamoeba	Polyhexamethylene biguanide,[b] paromomycin,[b] and propamidine isethionate[b]	Itraconazole, PO

IM, Intramuscularly; *IV*, intravenously; *PO*, orally.
[a]Topical and periocular use.
[b]Topical use only.
[c]Periocular use only.

Fungal Keratitis

The most common causes of fungal keratitis include *Candida, Aspergillus,* and *Fusarium*. Mycotic keratitis associated with the filamentous fungi *Aspergillus* and *Fusarium* is thought to occur with trauma, whereas keratitis caused by *Candida* is associated more commonly with a preexisting ocular (e.g., dry eye) or systemic (e.g., diabetes mellitus or immunosuppression) condition.[284] Fungal keratitis tends to be relatively indolent in contrast to bacterial keratitis. Typically white stromal infiltrates with irregular and indistinct feathery borders are detected. Satellite lesions, separated from the main lesion, may be evident. Mild iritis is common. Severe iritis with hypopyon can occur but is an infrequent manifestation.[212] For possible fungal keratitis, an acridine orange stain is recommended, and culture on a Sabouraud agar plate is indicated. Hyphal fungi are treated with topical natamycin, topical fluconazole, systemic fluconazole, or some combination of these medications. Yeasts are treated with topical or systemic amphotericin B, fluconazole, or both.[95]

Protozoan Keratitis

Protozoan keratitis is a particularly serious vision-threatening process. It usually is caused by *Acanthamoeba* and occurs more frequently in wearers of soft contact lenses. Use of homemade saline solution is a significant risk factor and should be discouraged.[37] Amoebae are ubiquitous organisms in soil, water, and air. They have been identified in hot tubs and in the feces of domestic animals.[180] People living in rural areas may be at special risk.

Acanthamoeba keratitis has been reported in children without a history of contact lens use or trauma.[64] *Acanthamoeba* corneal ulcers are pleomorphic.[135] Older lesions may exhibit a ringlike infiltrate around a central ulcer. Iritis or iridocyclitis may be intense, and severe pain out of proportion to exam findings is a hallmark of the disease. Acridine orange and calcofluor white stains aid in establishing an early diagnosis.[178] Tandem scanning confocal microscopy of corneal specimens may increase diagnostic accuracy, and the organism may grow on blood and chocolate agar.[37,174,225] Treatment of *Acanthamoeba* keratitis is complex and many times unsuccessful. Topical application of polyhexamethylene biguanide (0.02%),[158] chlorhexidine (0.02%), paromomycin (0.1%), or propamidine isethionate (Brolene) drops can be attempted. Oral itraconazole (Sporanox) has been used successfully in adults.[154,174,184] Cycloplegic agents are recommended for comfort, and pain medications are often required.

Corneal transplantation is performed if the infection progresses despite treatment, if perforation occurs, or if significant corneal visual axis opacification remains after the active infection is eradicated. Infection can recur even in the transplanted cornea.[232]

Onchocerca volvulus is a filarial parasite that causes river blindness (i.e., onchocerciasis). The disease is endemic in sub-Saharan West Africa, in isolated areas of east and central Africa, and in some areas of central and northern South America. The organism is transmitted by the bite of a blackfly of the family Simuliidae.[243] Larvae migrate to subcutaneous tissue and pass through several molts to become adult worms, which encapsulate in nodules and produce microfilariae that pass into blood, skin, and other organs, including the eyes. The conjunctiva, cornea, aqueous humor, vitreous, retina, uveal tract, sclera, and optic nerve all may be infested. Corneal involvement can lead to vision loss caused by corneal opacification, but most severe vision loss is caused by choroidal, retinal, and optic nerve disease.[118] Although children are often infected, blindness usually does not occur until they reach the third or fourth decade of life.[287,298]

Treatment of onchocercal infection is administration of ivermectin every 6 to 12 months to all individuals living in endemic areas. Ivermectin kills the microfilariae but not the adult worms, which live in subcutaneous nodules and remain until their death.[283] The adult worm may live 10 or more years. Because of the long life span, ivermectin should be taken every 6 months for at least 10 years to treat microfilariae as they develop.

Microsporidia are intracellular protozoa that represent a new emerging ocular pathogen. Interest in the organism increased in the past few decades because of its association with HIV and acquired immunodeficiency syndrome (AIDS). The ocular manifestation corresponds to both the immune status of the patient and the genus of microsporidia involved.[144] Typically keratoconjunctivitis occurs in immunocompromised individuals, while stromal keratitis is more commonly seen in immunocompetent individuals. Keratoconjunctivitis is manifested as bilateral conjunctival inflammation and epithelial keratopathy, which may lead to decreased vision. Stromal keratitis is manifested as an insidious diskiform keratitis with uveitis similar to that seen in HSV stromal keratitis and may require penetrating keratoplasty because of perforation or scarring. Potassium hydroxide plus calcofluor white and acid-fast stains are thought to be the most efficient means of establishing the diagnosis of microsporidial keratitis.[143] Transmission electron microscopy provides specificity in identification of the genus and possibly the species, but it may lack sensitivity and is laborious.[144] Knowledge of the genus and species may help guide management. Albendazole, fumagillin, itraconazole, metronidazole, and topical propamidine isethionate have been used as therapeutic agents.[53,144]

INFECTIONS PRIMARILY INVOLVING THE UVEA

The uveal tract is the vascular middle coat of the eye. It is situated between the sclera and the retina. Its major function is to provide nourishment for intraocular tissues, including the retina, lens, and cornea. The uveal tract is composed of the iris, ciliary body, and choroid.

Uveitis is a nonspecific term for inflammation of the uvea. If the inflammatory process primarily affects the iris, it is called *iritis*. If the ciliary body is involved, the process is called *cyclitis*. If these two structures together are involved, the process is called *iridocyclitis* (i.e., anterior uveitis). The term *intermediate uveitis* (i.e., pars planitis) applies to inflammation in the region of the ciliary body and peripheral retina. The term *posterior uveitis* usually applies to combined inflammation of the retina and choroid, also called *chorioretinitis*. If the choroid alone is involved, it is called *choroiditis;* inflammation of the retina alone is called *retinitis*. Because of the thinness and close apposition of these two tissue layers, inflammation in one layer frequently "spills over" into the other. The vitreous body occupies the central area of the eye behind the lens. It is composed of water, mucopolysaccharides, and collagen. Although transparent in a normal, healthy eye, the vitreous is subject to inflammation or *vitreitis*, usually as a result of inflammation in adjacent retinal tissue or in the pars plana.

Causes of uveitis are numerous but can be categorized into two main groups: infectious and noninfectious. Infectious causes are discussed in this chapter. Uveitis in any area of the eye may result in pain, conjunctival or episcleral hyperemia, photophobia, tearing, and decreased vision, although these symptoms vary relative to the site and the aggressiveness of the inflammation.

With slit-lamp examination, the hallmark of anterior uveitis is the presence of leukocytes in the anterior chamber, called *cell*, and the finding of hazy, proteinaceous aqueous humor, called *flare*. The cell and flare components are graded independently on a 1+ to 4+ scale. If present in sufficiently great numbers, leukocytes can precipitate in the anterior chamber (with location dependent on gravity) and form a mass called a *hypopyon*. The cells can aggregate on the back of the cornea and create fine, medium, and large lesions known as *keratic precipitates*. The conjunctiva usually is injected or hyperemic. With chronic inflammation, the border of the pupil often adheres to the anterior surface of the lens. Such adhesions are called *posterior synechiae* and may cause the pupil to have an irregular shape and size, as well as poor reactivity to light. Chronic or recurrent anterior segment inflammation may lead to the formation of a cataract. Iris nodules or atrophy may develop with long-standing inflammation. Anterior vitreous cells may occur as a spillover phenomenon in the setting of a prolonged or vigorous anterior chamber reaction. Although inflammatory effects on the ciliary body generally compromise its production of aqueous humor and thereby reduce intraocular pressure, cellular and proteinaceous debris can occlude aqueous humor outflow channels and lead to elevated intraocular pressure.

Inflammation primarily involving the posterior segment of the eye usually leads to decreased vision, which may be the symptom for which treatment initially is sought. Pain may be minimal or absent. Inflammatory lesions of the retina and choroid also may lead to the development of cellular debris in the vitreous and cause the patient to perceive "floaters." Initially, the borders of the retinal or choroidal inflammatory foci often are indistinct and cream-colored. In the healing phase, the borders of these lesions increasingly become distinct, and a defined, partially pigmented scar results. Inflammatory perivascular sheathing of the retinal vessels may occur as well. Involvement of the macula with edema or exudates may result from inflammation of the posterior segment, and long-standing edema may evolve into a cystic configuration and cause loss of central visual acuity. The optic nerve may exhibit an inflammatory response; if the optic disc is so involved, the response is called *papillitis*. Inflammatory debris also may be found in the vitreous.[4,215,315]

Epidemiology

In the United States, most uveitis cases have noninfectious causes. Large samples demonstrate a predominance of anterior rather than posterior uveitis. The most common category of anterior uveitis is idiopathic; the most common infectious cause of anterior uveitis is herpetic keratouveitis (simplex and zoster). Posterior uveitis is caused most frequently by *Toxoplasma gondii*. In developing nations, infectious uveitis plays a larger role. In West Africa, *T. gondii* probably accounts for most cases of intraocular inflammation.[240,241]

Viral Uveitis

Herpes Simplex Virus

Most of the uveal inflammation associated with HSV (typically iridocyclitis) results from the corneal disease. Occasionally a patient will have iritis as an isolated finding, but most patients with ocular HSV demonstrate conjunctivitis, keratitis, chorioretinitis, or retinal vasculitis.[235] The iritis may require treatment with antivirals as prophylaxis against the development of corneal epithelial disease.[294,315]

Varicella-Zoster Virus

Occasionally varicella infection (i.e., chickenpox) may be associated with a transient iritis that requires no treatment. Although rare, cases of unifocal choroiditis causing visual loss but responsive to acyclovir in children with primary varicella have been reported.[195]

Herpes zoster virus may cause iridocyclitis during the acute stage of the disease; the anterior chamber reaction can persist or recur long after resolution of the cutaneous component of the condition. Herpes zoster always should be considered in the differential diagnosis of chronic unilateral iridocyclitis. Topical steroids are indicated for iritis, with the addition of oral or intravenous acyclovir for severe cases. Segmental iris atrophy is a characteristic sequela of herpes zoster uveitis. Glaucoma, hyphema, retinitis, vasculitis, and extraocular muscle palsy occasionally occur in patients with herpes zoster ophthalmicus. In a profoundly immunosuppressed patient, VZV can cause a devastating retinitis known as *progressive outer retinal necrosis*.[162] The visual prognosis is poor.

VZV and HSV-2 have been implicated as causes of acute retinal necrosis syndrome. Patients in whom this syndrome is diagnosed range from 13 to 71 years of age, with an average age of 43 years. The syndrome typically occurs in healthy patients. The virus causes a triad of acute vitreitis, retinal vasculitis, and peripheral necrotizing retinitis and is bilateral in 33% of patients. Treatment consists of intravenous acyclovir. Prophylactic laser photocoagulation may prevent retinal detachment. The visual prognosis is guarded.[26,162]

Epstein-Barr Virus

Ocular EBV involvement has been reported primarily in patients with infectious mononucleosis. Follicular conjunctivitis may be diagnosed in 2% to 40% of patients. Corneal stromal inflammation, iritis, episcleritis, optic neuritis, and chorioretinitis occur less commonly. Systemic corticosteroids and acyclovir may be useful in treating sight-threatening complications of chronic intraocular inflammation from EBV infection.[182] Postinfectious uveitis also has been described and is discussed later.

Enteroviruses

Coxsackievirus A24 and enterovirus 70 may cause a painful follicular conjunctivitis called acute hemorrhagic conjunctivitis. Rarely chorioretinitis may be diagnosed. Treatment of these infections primarily is supportive.[215]

Rubella Virus

Rubella virus can cause congenital and acquired infections. Ocular manifestations of acquired rubella include conjunctivitis in 70% of patients, superficial keratitis, and iritis. Rarely retinitis has been reported.

Congenital rubella syndrome can be manifested as cataracts, glaucoma, microphthalmos, and retinitis. Cataracts occur in 15% of patients and glaucoma in 10%. Retinal examination reveals a salt-and-pepper fundus caused by the alternating pattern of hypopigmentation and hyperpigmentation of the retinal pigment epithelium. The prognosis for patients with retinitis alone usually is good, with vision between 20/20 and 20/40. Glaucoma resulting from rubella commonly requires surgery, as do the cataracts. Iritis is reported less commonly.[142,182]

Mumps Virus

Ocular manifestations of mumps virus include dacryoadenitis, conjunctivitis, iritis, optic neuritis, and keratitis. Retinitis also has been reported. The prognosis for visual recovery from the retinitis is good, and sequelae of the iritis are rare occurrences.[95,182]

Measles Virus

Measles virus can cause congenital and acquired infections. In congenital infections, a salt-and-pepper retinopathy and cataract formation may occur, similar to that found in rubella. Ocular manifestations in acquired measles include conjunctivitis and, much less commonly, retinitis, retinal vasculitis, and optic nerve edema.[15,215]

Subacute Sclerosing Panencephalitis

Between 30% and 75% of patients with subacute sclerosing panencephalitis (SSPE or Dawson inclusion body encephalitis) have ocular findings. SSPE is caused by a variant of the measles virus; it differs from the wild-type virus by alteration or absence of viral M protein. Optic nerve edema, inflammation, and subsequent optic atrophy have been reported. Macular retinitis is a common finding, and the contiguous nonneural tissues (vitreous and choroid) almost never are involved. The visual prognosis of survivors is poor.[210,215]

Creutzfeldt-Jakob Disease

The most common ocular manifestation of Creutzfeldt-Jakob disease is cortical blindness. Optic atrophy may result from degeneration of the neurons of the optic nerve.[215]

Human Immunodeficiency Virus and Acquired Immunodeficiency Syndrome

As many as 75% of patients with advanced AIDS have ocular findings. Cotton-wool spots occur in more than 50% of patients and are bilateral in more than 80%. Cotton-wool patches represent focal infarctions of the neural layer of the retina and are the most common ocular finding in patients with AIDS. They generally produce no symptoms and do not decrease vision. These spots are white and fluffy and occur most commonly in the macular portion of the retina. They resolve in 4 to 6 weeks with no residual scars. Occasionally flame-shaped hemorrhages are detected as well. The retina and choroid in these patients may become infected with HSV, CMV, VZV, syphilis, tuberculosis, histoplasmosis, *Candida*, toxoplasmosis, and *Pneumocystis*, although in the highly active antiretroviral therapy (HAART) era, the incidence of CMV retinitis has declined, and its advance in existing cases has been slowed or halted. Symptomatic anterior uveitis in the absence of the aforementioned pathogens occurs rarely in patients with AIDS and may be caused by HIV itself.[137]

Cytomegalovirus Infection

CMV infections may occur in preterm neonates and immunosuppressed patients, especially those with AIDS. In neonates with symptoms of CMV infection (i.e., low birth weight, microcephaly, jaundice, thrombocytopenia, hepatosplenomegaly, or petechial rash), congenital CMV infection[21] (i.e., prenatal transmission) may be manifested in the fundus as chorioretinal scars (21%) and optic atrophy (7%).[50]

CMV retinitis develops in approximately 30% of adult patients with AIDS, usually those with CD4$^+$ counts less than 50/mm.[80] In the pediatric AIDS population, CD4$^+$ counts of less than 20/mm^3 may be required for appearance of the retinitis.[76] The disease is less common in pediatric patients with AIDS. Patients with CMV retinitis have no external ocular signs but may complain of loss of vision. Children may not complain of such loss, and the problem may become apparent only after bilateral severe vision loss has occurred.[76] The retinal lesions of CMV typically are yellow-white and often are associated with hemorrhage. The retinitis generally follows a perivascular distribution. The retina becomes necrotic and eventually atrophies, with a gliotic scar. CMV optic neuritis also may develop. Treatment consists of intravenous or intravitreal ganciclovir, intravenous or intravitreal cidofovir, or intravenous foscarnet[81,315] and can often be discontinued when the CD4$^+$ count rises above 100/mm.[3,286]

Parvovirus Infection

Bilateral panuveitis has been reported to be associated with parvovirus B19 infection.[173]

Human T-Cell Lymphotrophic Virus Infection

Human T-cell lymphotrophic virus is endemic in several regions of the globe: Japan, the Caribbean islands, and parts of central Africa. It probably is responsible for several cases of self-limited, occasionally recurrent uveitis in these regions.[202]

Lymphocytic Choriomeningitis Virus Infection

Lymphocytic choriomeningitis virus (LCMV) is an arenavirus endemic in mice; it is also reported in hamsters and is occasionally transmitted to humans by direct contact with the rodent or through aerosolization of its feces or urine. Postnatal exposure results in asymptomatic seroconversion or aseptic meningitis, but intrauterine infection can have devastating consequences. Spontaneous abortion, congenital hydrocephalus, psychomotor retardation, and chorioretinitis have been documented. Diffuse chorioretinal scarring identified postnatally may bode a grim visual prognosis. LCMV may be an underdiagnosed cause of unexplained congenital chorioretinitis. The diagnosis is confirmed by elevated LCMV antibody titers. A survey of severely retarded, visually disabled children revealed immunologic evidence pointing to LCMV as the cause of the visual loss in approximately half of those surveyed.[187,190]

Viruses

Rift Valley fever virus. Rift Valley fever virus is an insect-borne virus. The arthropod vector directly inoculates the virus into the bloodstream of a host, resulting in end-organ infections, including the retina. Cattle and sheep are the primary host, and mosquitoes are the vector for transmission. Outbreaks have been reported in eastern and sub-Saharan Africa and South Africa. Uveitis and conjunctivitis can occur in the acute phase of the disease.[70,260] A viral retinitis may occur 1 to 3 weeks after the illness. It may be unilateral or bilateral, affecting both the central and the peripheral fundus with hemorrhages, exudates, and retinal vasculitis.

Herpes B virus. Herpes B is an α herpes virus within the herpes virinae family. Transmission to humans occurs via bites or scratches from infected monkeys where the virus is endemic. Infection may also occur via puncture wounds from contaminated objects.[203,242]

Herpes B virus has been associated with ocular complications in persons handling monkeys.[203,242] The reports suggest that the virus can cause retinal disease indistinguishable from acute retinal necrosis syndrome, with multifocal necrotizing retinitis and panuveitis in an immunocompetent host.

Influenza A virus. Influenza A virus is a pneumotropic virus with affinity to the branchial epithelial cells. It is transmitted by droplet infection.[23] Ocular manifestations in influenza include conjunctivitis, keratitis, iritis, and dacryoadenitis during the acute phase of the disease. Retinal involvement with influenza A virus has been reported. Retinitis of influenza A is typically bilateral and predominantly affects the macula with hemorrhages, exudates, and macular edema. Fluorescein angiography reveals diffuse vascular leakage. Optic disc edema may rarely be seen. The disease is typically self-limited, with return of vision to 20/20.[230]

West Nile virus. West Nile fever is a mosquito-borne infection caused by the West Nile virus. The vast majority (~80%) of cases have few or no symptoms, while most other cases present with flu-like symptoms. Less than 1% of infections are severe and result in CNS disease, especially in people of advanced age, the very young, or those who are immunocompromised. Diagnosis is usually made by enzyme-linked immunosorbent assay (ELISA) testing of the serum or CSF.

Fundus exam can be helpful in diagnosing West Nile virus infection. The most common retinal finding is the presence of multifocal chorioretinal target lesions (69% to 85%), usually bilateral. Other findings include retinal hemorrhages, vitreitis, retinal vasculitis, and optic neuritis. Most ocular involvement is self-limited; however, less frequent lesions such as retinal vasculitis and especially optic neuritis may lead to permanent visual deficits.[43,151]

Zika virus. Zika virus is a mosquito-borne Flavivirus that was first isolated in Uganda. For many decades after its discovery, infections were only known to occur in a narrow equatorial belt from Africa to Asia; however, in 2007 the virus spread eastward and reached pandemic levels in 2015–16. Zika infections in adults usually cause no or mild symptoms, but Zika can spread from a pregnant woman to her fetus, causing devastating birth defects including microcephaly and other severe brain malformations.

Ocular findings in infected adults have not yet been reported, but those in affected infants are becoming increasingly well described. The most common retinal finding is that of a hyperpigmentary retinopathy with propensity for the macula. Hemorrhagic retinopathy can also occur. Vigilance on the part of pregnant women (or those planning to become pregnant), mainly in the form of avoiding travel to endemic areas, is the only known prevention mechanism at this time.[67,193]

Chikungunya virus. Infection by the chikungunya virus causes the sudden onset of a short fever with accompanying joint pains of long duration. Ocular manifestations are not frequent but include conjunctivitis, optic neuritis, iridocyclitis, episcleritis, retinitis, and uveitis.[179]

Bacterial Uveitis

Syphilis

Syphilis *(Treponema pallidum)* should be considered as a possible cause in all cases of intraocular inflammation. Any patient with confirmed syphilitic uveitis should undergo a lumbar puncture to rule out asymptomatic neurosyphilis.

Ocular manifestations of congenital syphilis include interstitial keratitis, a mottled salt-and-pepper fundus, and chorioretinal scarring. Acute interstitial keratitis occurs as a late manifestation of congenital syphilis (5 to 25 years of age) and is thought to be a hypersensitivity response to treponemal antigen in the cornea. Patients complain of pain and photophobia and have a diffusely opaque cornea and anterior uveitis. Blood vessels invade the inflamed cornea and eventually are obliterated, leaving "ghost vessels" in the corneal stroma. Glaucoma may occur. A unilateral manifestation of interstitial keratitis suggests postnatally acquired syphilis.

Secondary syphilis may involve any layer of the eye. Episcleritis, scleritis, iridocyclitis (acute, chronic, or recurrent), iris capillary dilation (iris roseata), vascular papules of the iris (iris papulosa), inflammatory nodules (iris nodosa), choroiditis, chorioretinitis, and retinal vasculitis all have been reported, as have optic neuritis and subsequent atrophy.

Tertiary syphilis may have associated gummata of the iris and an Argyll Robertson pupil—a miotic, irregularly shaped pupil with loss of response to light but preservation of the near response. Intraocular inflammation seldom occurs at this stage.

Ocular inflammation secondary to syphilis should be treated as neurosyphilis. With the appropriate doses of penicillin G, the inflammation typically resolves rapidly. Occasionally topical regional steroids are required to control local inflammation. Treatment of ocular syphilis may lead, at least initially, to a vigorous local and systemic self-limited febrile response, presumably caused by liberation of spirochetal antigens or toxins. Topical oral corticosteroids may be required to quell this response, which is also known as a Jarisch-Herxheimer reaction.[4,177,215]

Lyme Disease

A mild follicular conjunctivitis occurs in 11% of patients with stage 1 Lyme disease, caused by *Borrelia burgdorferi*. During the second and third stages, neuro-ophthalmic manifestations including cranial neuropathy (most often cranial nerves III, IV, VI, and VII), optic neuritis, bilateral keratitis, bilateral iridocyclitis, diffuse choroiditis, vasculitis, intermediate uveitis, and Parinaud oculoglandular syndrome may be seen. The most frequent manifestation of late Lyme disease is arthritis. Ocular inflammation occurs in approximately 4% of children with Lyme arthritis.[134] Early or localized Lyme disease may be treated with doxycycline (8 years of age and older) or amoxicillin. More advanced or persistent disease is treated best with intravenous ceftriaxone.[6] Antibiotic treatment early in the course of the disease carries a better prognosis than does therapy initiated at later stages.[22]

Leptospirosis

Leptospirosis may cause an anterior uveitis that occurs months after the acute infection. Leptospirosis is identified as an important cause of epidemic panuveitis in southern India; the most common posterior segment manifestations in this group are vasculitis and vitritis.[48]

Tuberculosis

Any structure of the eye may be affected by tuberculosis. Allergic and infectious processes have been implicated as important causes of tuberculous uveitis. Anterior uveitis with or without keratitis has been attributed to tuberculosis, and choroiditis, optic neuritis, and orbital infections have been detected in cases of miliary tuberculosis. The most frequent manifestations of ocular tuberculosis are choroidal nodules and scars (so-called tuberculomas); anterior uveitis is an uncommon occurrence.[30] Treatment should be undertaken with the appropriate antituberculous medications. Corticosteroids often are necessary in conjunction with antimicrobial therapy.

Leprosy

Because *Mycobacterium leprae*, the cause of leprosy, grows best at lower temperatures, corneal infections predominate. Corneal involvement is associated with prominence of the corneal nerves, interstitial keratitis, and corneal hypoesthesia, but corneal opacities are often peripheral and not visually significant.[58] Uveal involvement in leprosy frequently is silent and accounts for a large number of the ocular complications from the disease.[58,59]

Brucella *Infection*

Ocular manifestations of *Brucella* infection are rare but include iritis, focal nodular choroiditis, and panophthalmitis.[215]

Cat-Scratch Disease

Bartonella henselae is a gram-negative rod transmitted to humans by the bite or scratch of an infected animal, often a young cat or kitten. Regional lymphadenopathy is the predominant nonocular finding. A striking stellate neuroretinitis characterized by swelling of the optic nerves, and lipid deposition in the retina is the most easily identifiable complication of ocular infection. Other manifestations include intermediate uveitis, optic disc swelling, multifocal choroiditis, and serous macular detachment. The discrete foci of multifocal choroiditis are the most common findings in the posterior segment. The role of antibiotics in this condition is debated.[149,267]

Fungal Uveitis

Histoplasmosis

The diagnosis of presumed ocular histoplasmosis syndrome is based on the clinical picture of disseminated punched-out retinal lesions, atrophic retinal changes around the optic nerve, and a clear vitreous.[227] Later in the course of the disease, subretinal hemorrhage and retinal detachment may occur. Ocular histoplasmosis often is bilateral and can result in legal blindness from the loss of macular vision. Presumed ocular histoplasmosis syndrome may occur after an episode of benign systemic histoplasmosis during childhood. Active inflammation and vitreous cells usually are not seen in this syndrome, although case series have documented active chorioretinal inflammation as new-onset lesions and as reactivation of previously quiescent lesions.[42,145] The hallmark histoplasmosis spots appear as white, punched-out, well-demarcated chorioretinal scars and represent healed fungal lesions ("histo spots"). Generally they first appear during adolescence, do not reduce vision, and do not require treatment. Macular disease, which may reduce vision, does not develop until after the patient reaches the second decade of life. Subretinal neovascularization may develop at the site of a macular histoplasmosis spot, with fluid, blood, and lipid accumulating in the subretinal space. This process plus local scarring can result in a marked reduction in central vision.

Macular neovascularization may be treated suitably with laser photocoagulation in an attempt to salvage the remaining central vision. Antifungal drugs may play a role in the unusual setting of demonstrated active histoplasmosis choroiditis.[248]

Candidiasis

Candida spp., including *Candida albicans,* are fungi with both yeast and filamentous forms. Candidiasis is encountered in immunocompromised patients and in situations involving indwelling catheters, intravenous therapy/drug use, chronic antibiotic use, and poorly controlled diabetes. Candidal chorioretinitis develops in approximately 9% of patients with blood cultures positive for the fungus,[76] although more recent studies have demonstrated that ocular involvement (either chorioretinitis or endophthalmitis) in children is a rare occurrence.[77,94]

In the eye, *Candida* infection usually begins in the choroid and eventually causes multifocal white chorioretinal lesions. If the fungus proliferates unchecked, it may break through the retina into the vitreous and produce the classic white snowball-like "fungus ball." Candidal infection that progresses to endophthalmitis is exceedingly rare if appropriate intravenous antifungals are started promptly on notice of a positive blood culture.

Intravenous amphotericin B is the drug of choice. Other antifungal agents such as fluconazole, flucytosine, and miconazole also may be effective but none dramatically so. Surgical treatment of intraocular *Candida* disease is discussed in the section on endophthalmitis.

Aspergillosis

Aspergillus spp. can infect the choroid, retina, and vitreous of immunocompromised individuals. One group of investigators found a surprisingly high rate (7%) of these unusual infections on reviewing records of deceased liver transplant recipients.[133]

Coccidioidomycosis

Coccidioides spp. have both yeast and filamentous forms. Ocular disease consists of a multifocal chorioretinitis that develops during the course of systemic coccidioidomycosis. The lesions initially appear similar to those seen in histoplasmosis; in severe cases, endophthalmitis results, and vitrectomy may need to be performed. In less severe cases, the lesions may respond to intravenous amphotericin B. Occasionally an isolated granulomatous iridocyclitis may develop.[196]

Cryptococcosis

Cryptococcus neoformans is a yeastlike fungus that can cause multifocal chorioretinitis and endophthalmitis. Most patients with cryptococcosis are severely immunocompromised, and many have AIDS. The CNS and eye are involved commonly, and elevated intracranial pressure may cause papilledema and sixth cranial nerve palsy. Intravenous amphotericin B in combination with oral flucytosine is the treatment regimen of choice.[6,150]

Sporotrichosis

The dimorphic fungus *Sporothrix schenckii* is encountered commonly in rotting vegetable matter, wood, and soil. The fungus gains access to the host by traumatic implantation or inhalation. It has been reported to be responsible for anterior uveitis in the setting of a suggestive lesion on a finger of the dominant hand, with presumed hand-to-eye transmission.[297]

Protozoal Uveitis

Leishmaniasis

Ocular leishmaniasis has been described but is rare. Manifestations include conjunctivitis, blepharitis, and anterior uveitis. This trio of findings responds to systemic treatment with sodium stibogluconate.[87]

Protozoal Infection

Amebiasis. Humans can be infected by ingestion of the cyst form of *Entamoeba histolytica* in contaminated water and food. The primary disease manifestation in *E. histolytica* infection is dysentery. Ocular involvement is rare and includes maculopathy in the form of a transparent cyst involving the central retina with surrounding retinal hemorrhages and anterior uveitis.[31,152]

Trypanosomiasis. Trypanosoma spp. are flagellated protozoa transmitted by tsetse flies. African trypanosomiasis is caused by *Trypanosoma brucei* and *Trypanosoma cruzi.* General manifestations include headache, fever, malaise, lymphadenopathy, and then CNS involvement with sleepiness, coma, and death. Reported ocular manifestations include urticarial swelling of the eyelids, interstitial keratitis, and rarely, iritis or choroiditis.[239] In American trypanosomiasis, known as *Chagas disease,* intraocular disease has not been reported, but eye involvement may occur in the form of eyelid swelling and periorbital edema spreading to the face.

Malaria. The most serious form of malaria is caused by *Plasmodium falciparum.* Hemolytic anemia and disseminated intravascular coagulation are presumed to lead to hypoxia of the brain and other tissues, resulting in the clinical manifestations of the disease. Ocular manifestations include subconjunctival hemorrhage, retinal hemorrhages, and cranial nerve palsies. Corneal involvement and uveitis are not caused directly by malaria.[152,168–170]

Giardiasis. Giardiasis is caused by *Giardia lamblia,* which can inhabit the human jejunum. Humans are infected through ingestion of water contaminated with human sewage. Reported ocular manifestations include retinal arteritis (vasculitis) and salt-and-pepper retinal pigmentary changes.[52,176]

Helminthic Uveitis

Toxocariasis

Toxocara canis causes visceral larva migrans, which is not associated with ocular disease. In the retina, larvae get trapped in small capillaries and burrow into surrounding tissue; after dying, the dead larvae incite an intense eosinophilic abscess.

Ocular toxocariasis has three classic clinical manifestations, almost always involving one eye only. One form occurs in children 2 to 9 years of age and causes an indolent endophthalmitis and leukokoria (i.e., white pupil). Tractional retinal detachment may occur. The eye typically shows little or no external evidence of inflammation, and the patient experiences no pain.

A second form appears in children between 4 and 14 years of age. An inflammatory granuloma is seen in the macula. These patients have reduced vision but little or no external inflammation and no pain. The reduced vision may cause strabismus, which may be the first sign.

The third form of ocular toxocariasis occurs in patients between 6 and 40 years of age but may not be recognized until years later. Patients with this form of toxocariasis have good vision, but a peripheral retinal granuloma is seen on routine eye examination. Vision may be affected if a traction band from the granuloma distorts the macula.

Inactive *Toxocara* granulomas do not respond to medication. When active intraocular inflammation exists in such a magnitude that it poses a further threat to vision, administration of periocular or systemic steroids may be necessary. Anthelmintic agents eradicate migrating larvae, but their effect on "residing" larvae is questionable. When giving anthelmintics, one should combine them with a short course of corticosteroids because death of the larvae may incite vigorous inflammation. Cryotherapy and laser therapy may be useful when the *Toxocara* granuloma is located away from the macula and optic nerve. Vitrectomy may be helpful if significant traction on the retina occurs. Anthelmintic drugs should not be administered after the patient has undergone posterior segment surgery. Visual prognosis is poor if the macula is involved.[215,250,259,307]

Onchocerciasis

Onchocerciasis often causes a severe choroiditis with an overlying retinitis.[257] The various ocular manifestations of infestation with *O. volvulus* are discussed in the section on keratitis.

Loiasis

The *Loa loa* worm can migrate through the tissues of the eye and cause conjunctivitis, iridocyclitis, vitreitis, and chorioretinitis. The disease is transmitted by the bite of the mango fly.[83] Vascular obstruction with intraretinal hemorrhage and retinal exudation may occur as well. Medical treatment with diethylcarbamazine can kill the adult worms and microfilariae. Adult worms also can be removed from the eye surgically.[215]

Cysticercosis

The tapeworm *Taenia solium* causes cysticercosis. When the larva gains access to the eye, cysts form in the vitreous or subretinal space in 13% to 46% of patients. The living worm may be seen undulating in these spaces. With death of the organism, severe panuveitis can occur. Orbital and subconjunctival involvement occur less commonly. Surgical removal of the intraocular cysts may prevent the severe inflammation that occurs on the death of the worm. Praziquantel can kill the organism, but the ensuing increase in inflammation may be dramatic.[215]

Rare Causes of Parasitic Posterior Uveitis in Children

Schistosomiasis. Schistosomiasis is caused by a platyhelminth belonging to the trematode class and has three recognized species: *Schistosoma haematobium, Schistosoma mansoni,* and *Schistosoma japonicum*. Humans are infected when the larval form emerges from its snail and pierces the skin to enter the dermal lymphatics and capillaries. Reported ocular lesions include generalized cutaneous edema of the eyelids in the acute phase, dacryoadenitis, choroiditis, and rarely retinal pigment epithelium changes.[74,138,226]

Hydatid disease. Hydatid disease is caused by *Echinococcus granulosus,* for which dogs are the primary host.[309] Reported ocular lesions include painless proptosis, subretinal cysts, and rarely involvement of the choroid and the vitreous.[108,309]

Coenurosis. Coenurus infection is caused by *Multiceps multiceps,* which is a taenioid cystode. It is a parasite of dogs and related species, with sheep acting as an intermediate host. Humans may occasionally become infected. Reported ocular lesions include conjunctival cysts, intraocular cysts, and subretinal involvement. Panophthalmitis and orbital involvement have been reported.[175,308]

Ascaris. *Ascaris lumbricoides* is a species of *Ascaris* that infects humans, typically by ingestion of water contaminated with eggs containing infective larvae. Ocular lesions, which are rare, include iridocyclitis and chorioretinitis.[140]

Baylisascaris. *Baylisascaris procyonis* may cause ocular disease in humans. This is a nematode of the Ascaridida order, and humans are infected by ingestion of material contaminated with ova.[290] *B. procyonis* is a presumptive cause of diffuse unilateral subacute neuroretinitis characterized by unilateral vitreitis, papillitis, and recurrent grayish lesions affecting the outer retina and the retinal pigment epithelium.

Gnathostoma spinigerum. *Gnathostoma spinigerum* is a spiruroid nematode endemic in East Asia. The human is an accidental host, and infection occurs by eating infected food. Reported ocular lesions include eyelid swelling, orbital cellulitis, uveitis, intraocular hemorrhage, central retinal artery occlusion, and tractional retinal detachment.[154,291]

Wuchereria bancrofti. *Wuchereria bancrofti* is prevalent in many tropical areas of the world. Larvae are ingested by species of mosquito feeding on the skin. The larvae then undergo further stages of development and become capable of infecting other individuals when they are released in the saliva of the feeding insect. Reported ocular lesions include conjunctival edema, granulomatous iridocyclitis, and subretinal inflammatory lesions.[204]

Trichinosis. Trichinosis is caused by *Trichinella spiralis,* a nematode parasite of carnivorous animals of widespread distribution. Human infection results from ingestion of infected, undercooked pork or wild game. Reported ocular lesions include painful limitation of the eye movements associated with proptosis and chemosis, edema of the eyelids and the conjunctiva, and rarely retinal hemorrhages or optic disc edema.[217,279]

Rickettsial disease. *Rickettsia* are obligate intracellular parasites, possessing both RNA and DNA. Unlike viral infections, they respond to antibiotics. They are transmitted by a vector such as ticks, mites, and fleas. The organisms causing the diseases in the following section have been rarely reported as causing posterior uveitis in humans.[82]

Typhus. Murine typhus is recognized in scattered pockets worldwide. It is caused by *Rickettsia mooseri* and is transmitted by the rat louse. Ocular manifestations include chorioretinitis, conjunctivitis, and uveitis.

Spotted fever. Boutonneuse fever is recognized in the Mediterranean areas, Caspian and Black sea coastal regions, Africa, Southeast Asia, United States, Russia, and Korea. It is caused by *Rickettsia conorii* and is transmitted by ticks. Ocular manifestations include chorioretinitis, conjunctivitis, and iridocyclitis.

Q fever. Q fever is caused by *Coxiella burnetii,* which is distributed worldwide and is transmitted by ticks. Ocular manifestations include conjunctivitis, episcleritis, uveitis, and chorioretinitis.

Trench fever. Trench fever is caused by *Rochalimaea quintana* and is transmitted by the human body louse. Ocular manifestations include retinitis and conjunctivitis.

Uveitis Caused by Insect-Induced Disease

Ophthalmomyiasis is an ocular disorder caused by infestation with fly larvae, most commonly the larval form of the sheep botfly *Oestrus ovis*. Maggots may be seen in the conjunctival fornix or inside the eye. Internal ophthalmomyiasis can be diagnosed by noting a motile larva in the anterior chamber, vitreous, or subretinal space. The maggot may leave trails ("railroad tracks") throughout the retina. A mild inflammatory response in the anterior chamber or vitreous may occur. Treatment is surgical removal of the larva. Corticosteroids may be used to treat the accompanying intraocular inflammation.[84,215]

Postinfectious Uveitis

Increasingly, attention is being given to the role of bacterial and viral systemic illness in the eventual development of sterile intraocular inflammation. This type of uveitis is thought to be caused by an autoimmune response that occurs between sensitized lymphocytes and host tissues that bear some antigenic similarity to the recently cleared pathogen. Disruption of the ACAID is probably a prerequisite for the development of these postinfectious syndromes. Several reports exist of nongranulomatous anterior uveitis occurring weeks or months after streptococcal infection. These uveitides may be associated with other poststreptococcal findings (e.g., arthritis and glomerulonephritis) or may be the sole manifestation. Treatment with cycloplegics and topical corticosteroids is sufficient for the ocular manifestations.[19,292,311]

Uveitis, predominantly of the anterior type, has been reported to occur after illnesses caused by gram-negative enteric bacteria such as *Klebsiella, Salmonella,* and *Yersinia*. These gram-negative-induced uveitides are much more likely to occur in the setting of human leukocyte antigen (HLA)-B27 positivity. The ocular findings often parallel the development of arthritis, thus suggesting that parallel immunologic processes are occurring in both these mesenchymal cavities (i.e., the joint space and the anterior chamber). An association between recent EBV infection and acute tubulointerstitial nephritis and anterior uveitis has been described, with onset of the renal and ocular inflammation occurring several months after the characteristic acute EBV infection.[112]

INFECTIONS INVOLVING PRIMARILY THE RETINA

Eye Manifestations of Intrauterine Infections (TORCHES Complex)

The TORCHES complex is a group of congenital and perinatal infections that may cause severe systemic and ophthalmic abnormalities. The effect of infection with one of the TORCHES organisms—***T****oxoplasma gondii*, ***o****thers* (LCMV, parvovirus B19), ***r****ubella virus*, ***C****MV*, ***h****erpesvirus*, ***E****BV*, and ***s****yphilis*—may be evident at birth or manifest later in childhood or adulthood. All of these infections commonly cause either mild or no clinically evident disease in the mother.[188] The diagnosis cannot always be established on clinical grounds alone, and neonatal and maternal serologic tests must be performed to confirm the clinical suspicion.

Toxoplasmosis

T. gondii is an obligate intracellular parasite that has an affinity for the CNS and retina. The parasite has three forms: tachyzoite, bradyzoite, and sporozoite or oocyst. Human infection may be congenital or acquired. Acquired infection results from the ingestion of undercooked meat contaminated with oocysts or from exposure to the feces of an infected cat, the definitive host. The oocysts release tachyzoites, which multiply intracellularly and result in cell death. In adults, primary acquired infection usually is asymptomatic. The immune response then transforms the tachyzoite into a bradyzoite, which encysts and remains dormant in tissues for years. These cysts have the propensity to rupture sometime later and cause an inflammatory response resulting in recurrent infection.

Congenital infection is transmitted transplacentally. In the United States, the reported incidence of congenital toxoplasmosis is one case per 1000 to 10,000 births.[12,57] As much as 70% of the obstetric population is negative for antibodies and therefore at risk for infection and transplacental transmission to the fetus.[188] Congenital infection is most severe when acquired in the first trimester and can result in chorioretinitis, intracranial calcifications, microcephaly, mental retardation, and deafness.[57,90,92] Symptomatic neonates with disseminated disease have hepatosplenomegaly, lymphadenopathy, jaundice, fever, anemia, pneumonitis, and a poor prognosis. Other ocular manifestations include cataracts, strabismus, microcornea, vitreitis, retinal detachment, optic atrophy, microphthalmos, nystagmus, and ptosis.[188] In a prospective study, 15% of infected newborns had chorioretinal scars, indicative of infection in utero; 4% had active chorioretinitis; and in 10%, retinal lesions developed by the time the children were 1 to 2 years of age. Long-term follow-up studies found that chorioretinal lesions develop in 82% to 85% of children with subclinical *Toxoplasma* infection, some with severe visual loss. Infants with asymptomatic toxoplasmosis should undergo regular ophthalmologic examination because retinal involvement can occur later in childhood and adulthood.[32,92,155] Some researchers suggest that all neonates with toxoplasmosis should receive drug therapy, even if they are asymptomatic.[92]

Toxoplasmosis is the leading cause of acquired necrotizing retinitis and, in many cases, represents reactivation of congenitally acquired infection. Clinically, the area of active retinochoroiditis is adjacent to the border of a chorioretinal scar.[92,236] Associated choroiditis and vitreitis, sometimes severe, may be present. Primary acquired ocular toxoplasmosis manifested as retinochoroiditis is well documented also, and reports suggest that this route of infection may be more common than originally thought.[32,130] Recurrent ocular disease with postnatally acquired toxoplasmosis has been reported.[29]

T. gondii causes a focal necrotizing retinitis with secondary choroiditis and vitreitis. Patients may have floaters, blurred vision, and photophobia. Those with macular involvement can suffer significant visual loss. After the inflammation has resolved, a flat, pigmented chorioretinal scar develops. Visual loss depends on the location of the retinal lesion, with peripheral lesions resulting in little or no visual disturbance and macular lesions capable of producing profound visual loss.

Toxoplasma retinochoroiditis is an emerging problem in patients with AIDS and may be the initial manifestation of this syndrome.[303] The clinical appearance often is atypical.[264] Chronic suppressive therapy is necessary because infection recurs with discontinuation of treatment. A combination of pyrimethamine and clindamycin has been reported to be most effective as prophylaxis.[303]

The diagnosis of *Toxoplasma* retinochoroiditis usually is presumptive and is based on clinical appearance and serologic testing. Several serologic tests are available. The standard serologic diagnosis is based on the presence of anti-*Toxoplasma* IgM in any sample or demonstration of a significant rise in antibody titer in paired sera taken 4 to 6 weeks apart. However, in reactivated congenital infections, which many cases are, *Toxoplasma* IgM results are not positive. The antibody tests most commonly used are indirect immunofluorescent assay (IFA) and enzyme-linked immunosorbent assay for IgM and IgA.[106] False-positive results can occur with both tests in the presence of rheumatoid factor. If clinical infection is suspected and the initial testing results are negative, repeat testing or an alternative testing technique should be considered.

Standard treatment of *Toxoplasma* retinochoroiditis is triple therapy with sulfadiazine 100 to 200 mg/kg per day in four divided doses (maximum, 1.5 g), pyrimethamine 2 mg/kg per day for 3 days, then 1 mg/kg per day (maximum, 25 mg/day), and leucovorin (folinic acid) 10 to 25 mg given orally daily for 6 weeks. Folinic acid prevents the leukopenia and thrombocytopenia that may result from pyrimethamine therapy. Weekly complete blood counts and platelet counts are required to monitor toxicity from therapy. Alternative therapy with clindamycin 40 mg/kg per day in four divided doses (maximum, 2.4 g for 6 weeks) rather than sulfadiazine also has been effective.[282] This therapy is less toxic than triple therapy and is therefore better tolerated. In patients with severe intraocular inflammation, systemic corticosteroids can be used with concurrent antimicrobial therapy.

Preventive measures are twofold: first, avoidance of raw meat and cat feces during pregnancy, especially during the first trimester, and second, treatment of a mother known to have contracted the disease during pregnancy with spiramycin, because it has no known teratogenic effects.[55,68,69] In utero pyrimethamine and sulfadiazine treatment of a fetus known to be infected may be effective.[55,57,127]

Lymphocytic Choriomeningitis Infection

LCMV, an arenavirus discovered in 1933, was first recognized as a cause of intrauterine infection in 1955 (also see the earlier section on viral uveitis).[189] The common house mouse *Mus musculus* is the natural host and reservoir of the virus, but laboratory mice and pet hamsters also may be infected.[8,126] LCMV may be transmitted to humans by airborne means, rodent bites, or food contaminated by rodent urine, feces, or saliva; the fetus may be infected by transplacental transmission.[106] The diagnosis may be confirmed by LCMV titers.

Systemic manifestations, often devastating, include hydrocephaly, microcephaly, periventricular calcifications, neonatal meningitis, hepatosplenomegaly, cerebral palsy, mental retardation, and seizures.[106] Ocular findings include chorioretinitis, optic atrophy, nystagmus, microphthalmos, strabismus, and cataracts.[189] The chorioretinitis may mimic congenital toxoplasmosis.[33] The most common ocular findings are peripheral chorioretinal scars, although macular involvement is a common occurrence as well. At present there is no effective treatment. Prevention involves avoidance of mice and hamsters by pregnant women.[106,189]

Rubella Infection

The rubella virion is an RNA virus of the family *Togaviridae* that causes a febrile exanthem. Before the advent of rubella vaccine in 1969, rubella, or German measles, epidemics occurred every 6 to 9 years. The last major outbreak in the United States took place in 1964.[14] With preschool immunization programs, most primary cases now reported occur in individuals between 15 and 24 years of age. Transmission occurs by inhalation of aerosolized droplets in the nasopharynx. Primary infection in adults results in a mild febrile illness associated with lymphadenopathy and a rash. The proportion of susceptible nonimmunized women of child-bearing age ranges from 10% to 25%. Fetal infection occurs transplacentally, and the likelihood of transmission from mother to fetus is highest (90%) in the first trimester; transmission at this stage can produce severe fetal damage and result in spontaneous abortion, stillbirth, or multiple congenital anomalies.

The classic congenital rubella syndrome, first described by Sir Norman McAlister in Australia in 1949,[189] is characterized by cardiac defects, ocular abnormalities, and hearing deficits. The incidence of ocular and cardiac defects is higher with exposure early in the first trimester; hearing deficits appear to be associated with exposure late in the first trimester. Givens et al.[105] reported that 88% had multiorgan involvement. Hearing loss is the most frequent nonocular manifestation.[189] The most common cardiac defects are patent ductus arteriosus, pulmonary artery stenosis, and pulmonary valve stenosis. Other features include microcephaly, thrombocytopenia, hepatosplenomegaly, and mental retardation.

Ocular involvement occurs in approximately 50% of infected infants.[102] Pigmentary retinopathy (i.e., "salt-and-pepper" retinopathy) affects 22% of infected infants. The retina has a mottled appearance, most frequently observed in the posterior pole; the optic nerve and vessels usually are normal unless the patient also has glaucoma.

Nuclear cataracts, which affect between 15% and 27% of patients, are the second most frequent ocular complication. Glaucoma is seen in approximately 10% of eyes; the combination of cataracts and glaucoma is an uncommon finding.[300] Microphthalmos (which occurs in 10% to 63% of affected individuals), iris atrophy, and iritis also have been reported.[27] Live virus may persist for years in the lens, so appropriate precautions must be taken during cataract surgery to prevent transmission.[106]

The retinopathy associated with rubella usually is asymptomatic and does not necessitate treatment. In some cases, it can be complicated by subretinal neovascularization, which may require laser or macular surgery. Cataracts cause most visual morbidity. Visual rehabilitation depends on early cataract extraction to prevent deprivation amblyopia, correction of aphakia with spectacles or contact lenses, and careful follow-up. Glaucoma in infants and children can be temporized with topical medications, but most cases require glaucoma surgery.

Congenital rubella has long-term consequences for all organs involved. In nearly two thirds of infants with no manifestations at birth, hearing loss or psychomotor deficits subsequently develop. From an ophthalmic standpoint, individuals with congenital rubella need continued follow-up.[105]

Cytomegalovirus Infection

CMV is an enveloped DNA virus of the family *Herpesviridae*. An estimated 80% of adults are infected by the time they reach 40 years of age.[269] In immunocompetent adults, infection is asymptomatic or can cause a mononucleosis-like syndrome. Individuals can shed virus in saliva, urine, and other body fluids for months to years after initial infection. Transmission occurs through exposure to body fluids (sexual contact, blood transfusion) or organ transplantation, or it can occur transplacentally. Primary infection acquired in the birth canal is not likely to result in serious disease.

Congenital CMV is the most common congenital infection in humans[270] and can result from exposure to the virus in utero or in the birth canal. In utero infection produces more serious disease. CMV infection occurs in 1% of all live births, and only 5% to 10% of infants with congenital CMV infection are symptomatic. Maternal infection may be primary or recurrent, but primary infection carries the greatest risk (30% to 40%) for transmission of symptomatic CMV disease to the newborn.[269] Blood transfusions from CMV antibody–positive donors also can result in severe CMV infection in the newborn. Systemic manifestations include intrauterine growth restriction (IUGR), thrombocytopenic purpura, microcephaly with periventricular calcifications, hepatosplenomegaly, pneumonia, and sensorineural deafness.[65] In symptomatic congenital CMV infection, the retina is the primary site of ocular involvement. Cytomegalic inclusion bodies are seen in all layers of the retina. Patchy white areas of necrotic retina with hemorrhage and vascular sheathing are seen in the peripheral portion of the retina, although the posterior pole can be affected as well.[167] Nonhemorrhagic retinitis also may be seen, and most affected infants do not have active retinitis at birth, although scars may be visible as evidence of previous disease.[50] Resolution of the retinitis results in an atrophic scar with areas of hyperpigmentation. If retinitis is limited to the retinal periphery, vision may be normal. However, visual loss may occur if the posterior pole is involved or if optic atrophy or retinal detachment occurs. CMV retinopathy develops in 5% to 30% of infants with clinically apparent disease.[85] Microphthalmos, optic nerve hypoplasia, optic atrophy, optic nerve colobomata, anophthalmia, corneal opacities, and anterior segment dysgenesis also have been associated with congenital CMV infection.[128] In addition, cyclopia and anophthalmia have been reported.[167]

The diagnosis of CMV retinitis is based on the clinical appearance and the constellation of systemic symptoms and signs. Recovery of the virus from urine, maternal cervical secretions, saliva, or aqueous humor can confirm the diagnosis. Complement fixation can identify IgM antibodies to CMV that do not cross-react with other herpes viruses. Immunofluorescence techniques are more sensitive but less specific than complement fixation.[167]

Treatment of neonatal or pediatric CMV retinitis is based on the results of treatment of adults with CMV retinitis. Ganciclovir has been shown to stabilize and prevent spread of the disease in infants. Maintenance therapy is not required, but continued follow-up is necessary to detect recurrence. Leukopenia and thrombocytopenia can result. Retinal detachment requires vitrectomy, membrane peel, and silicone oil to tamponade the detached retina.[39,129]

Herpes Simplex Virus Infection

HSV is a double-stranded, enveloped DNA virus. Both subtypes, HSV-1 and HSV-2, can cause a vesicular skin eruption. HSV-1 typically is isolated from oral-facial infections; HSV-2 usually is isolated from genital infections. After primary infection occurs, HSV can maintain latency in neuronal ganglion cells and reactivate. Transmission occurs by exposure to infected body fluids such as saliva, and the risk for transmission is higher when the individual is symptomatic.[201]

Maternal-fetal transmission occurs through infected genital secretions in the birth canal (HSV-2) or exposure to infected individuals with oral-facial herpetic disease (HSV-1) in the postnatal period. In mothers with active genital disease, the risk for transmission to the neonate is 50% with vaginal delivery. Most series report that between 70% and 80% of neonatal HSV infection is caused by HSV-2. Neonatal HSV infection is life-threatening, and the mortality rate without treatment is 50% to 80%.[106,305] The diagnosis is suspected by the clinical findings—lethargy, respiratory distress, anorexia, vomiting, cyanosis, low birth weight, IUGR, microcephaly, seizures, intracranial calcifications, pneumonia, hepatosplenomegaly, and skin vesicles. The virus may be isolated from skin vesicles or from nasal or conjunctival secretions, CSF, or blood.

Ocular sequelae develop in fewer than 1% of immunocompetent adults with HSV infection. In contrast, 17% to 40% of infected neonates have ocular disease.[181,269] Thirteen percent of neonates with HSV have eye involvement. Ocular involvement can range from mild conjunctivitis to severe bilateral necrotizing retinitis and may be unilateral or bilateral. Conjunctivitis is the most common manifestation. Conjunctivitis, keratitis, and, occasionally, retinitis develop 2 to 14 days after birth. HSV retinitis causes punctate, white-yellow lesions in the periphery and the posterior pole accompanied by choroiditis, vascular sheathing, hemorrhage, and vitreitis. Chorioretinal atrophic scars with variable amounts of pigmentation around the border result after resolution of acute infection.[131,231] Visual prognosis depends on the severity of disease, presence of macular involvement, extent of optic atrophy, or CNS involvement of the visual pathways. Severe chorioretinitis and cortical blindness are the usual sequelae of HSV infection acquired through transplantation, a rare mode of transmission.

El Azazi et al.[86] examined children with serologically proven HSV infection 1 to 15 years after neonatal exposure and found a higher prevalence of chorioretinal scars than noted in previous reports (28% vs. 4%). This finding suggests that HSV remains dormant in the retina and reactivates later in childhood or adulthood. Chorioretinitis, cataracts, optic atrophy, and microphthalmos have all been reported.[116] Acute retinal necrosis from reactivation of HSV-2 has occurred as well.[285]

Ocular HSV infection can be seen in conjunction with a vesicular rash or disseminated disease. The differential diagnosis of ophthalmic complications from HSV includes infection with any of the TORCHES organisms. Identification of neonatal IgM antibody to HSV confirms the diagnosis of in utero infection. Demonstration of intranuclear inclusions and multinucleated giant cells in skin, conjunctiva, and oral and genital lesions may be diagnostic.

The drug of choice to treat neonatal HSV infection is intravenous acyclovir 60 mg/kg per day.[223] Conjunctival and corneal disease also can be treated by debridement and topical antivirals such as trifluridine drops or ganciclovir ointment. In neonatal HSV infection, systemic acyclovir should be given regardless of topical treatment. Early diagnosis and treatment can reduce ocular morbidity.

Varicella-Zoster Virus Infection

Varicella zoster is a DNA virus of the family Herpesviridae; enveloped virions are the infectious agents. Primary infection results in chickenpox, a highly communicable febrile illness with a vesicular rash that appears after 48 to 72 hours of incubation. VZV can remain dormant in sensory ganglion neurons and reactivate as herpes zoster, a painful rash in the dermatomal distribution of the sensory ganglion.

Congenital varicella syndrome is considered a rare entity, though one prospective series reported a 24% incidence of congenital varicella with serologic or clinical confirmation of maternal infection during pregnancy. Mortality rates can be high if maternal infection develops anywhere from 5 days before delivery to 2 days after delivery. Systemic complications of VZV infection include cranial nerve palsy, hemiparesis, cicatricial skin lesions, IUGR, developmental delay, seizures, neurogenic bladder, and learning difficulty.[156,219]

Ocular abnormalities in children with congenital VZV infection include chorioretinitis, cataracts, Horner syndrome, optic atrophy/optic nerve hypoplasia, retinal coloboma, and microphthalmos. The chorioretinal scars of VZV infection have a deeply pigmented center with depigmented borders or a gliotic white center with hyperpigmented edges. The neurotropic nature of VZV infection may explain the association of Horner syndrome. Ocular involvement can be unilateral or bilateral. VZV chorioretinitis affects the macula, periphery, or both.

Serologic testing for IgG and IgM antibodies to VZV, a history of maternal infection during pregnancy, and the constellation of systemic findings helps establish the diagnosis. Because active infection may occur early in pregnancy, the neonate may have IgG but no detectable IgM antibodies to VZV by the time of delivery. The persistence of elevated IgG antibodies beyond 6 months (when passive immunity through maternal antibodies has waned) without evidence of postnatal primary VZV infection is a helpful indication of infection in utero.

Syphilis

Syphilis is caused by the spirochete *Treponema pallidum*. Acquired syphilis is a sexually transmitted chronic disease and has three stages of infection. Primary infection is characterized by painless, indurated chancres of the skin or mucous membranes at the site of inoculation. The secondary stage appears as a maculopapular rash, classically involving the palms and soles. Generalized lymphadenopathy, fever, malaise, sore throat, headache, and arthralgias can accompany the rash. Hypertrophic lesions (i.e., condyloma lata) occur in moist mucous membranes. Approximately a third of untreated cases progress to the tertiary stage, which occurs after a variable latent period that may have occasional recurrences of secondary syphilis. Transmission to the fetus can occur with any stage of maternal syphilis.[280]

Pigmentary retinopathy is the most common early ocular manifestation of congenital syphilis. Diffuse mottling in the periphery ("salt-and-pepper" retinopathy) is indicative of in utero infection. Pigment clumping in the periphery usually has no effect on vision, but macular involvement can cause decreased vision. Retinal changes can appear later in adulthood, thus suggesting that inflammatory changes caused by congenital infection can occur after birth. Salt-and-pepper retinopathy is evidence of previous inflammation, and no treatment is required. Interstitial keratitis (see the previous discussion of stromal keratitis) is the hallmark of congenital syphilis and occurs in 75% of these patients.[280] It is usually not detected until late in the first decade of life. Other reported ocular manifestations include optic neuritis and iritis.

Testing the serum by nontreponemal and treponemal methods confirms the diagnosis of congenital infection. The American Academy of Pediatrics recommends physical examination, quantitative nontreponemal serologic testing, a CSF Venereal Disease Research Laboratory (VDRL) test, long-bone radiographs, and antitreponemal IgM testing, as specified by the Centers for Disease Control and Prevention (CDC). The CDC states that congenital syphilis is presumptively diagnosed with a positive VDRL and at least one of the following: physical examination evidence of congenital syphilis, characteristic radiographic long-bone findings, VDRL-positive CSF findings, an otherwise unexplained elevated CSF protein or cell count, quantitative nontreponemal serologic titer four times greater than the mother's, or a positive fluorescent treponemal antibody absorbent FTA (ABS) 19s IgM test.[5] Treatment is with intravenous penicillin G for 10 to 14 days.[6,177]

Endophthalmitis

Endophthalmitis is an infection within the eye that may arise endogenously during septicemia or exogenously from accidental or surgical trauma.[191,202] Sixty-two percent of cases occur after intraocular surgery, 20% after penetrating trauma, 10% after glaucoma surgery, and 8% result from endogenous infection.[76,229] The patient usually has severe ocular pain and visual loss at initial evaluation. Rarely patients may be asymptomatic. Signs of endophthalmitis include conjunctival injection, vitreitis, uveitis, hypopyon, and intraocular membrane formation.

Endophthalmitis is an ophthalmic emergency and necessitates immediate evaluation of aqueous and vitreous cultures and institution of intravitreal antibiotic therapy. Any significant delay in recognition and treatment of endophthalmitis can result in permanent vision loss. Vitrectomy is indicated in those patients with near-total blindness.[6,88]

Postsurgical endophthalmitis occurs in 0.086% of cataract operations.[2] The source of postsurgical infection may be from the eyelids, conjunctiva, contaminated instruments/irrigating solutions, or contamination by operating room personnel. The routine use of subconjunctival antibiotics after intraocular surgery does not prevent all cases of postoperative endophthalmitis. Vitreous loss, which may occur occasionally as a complication of cataract surgery, increases the risk for infection developing. Patients who have undergone glaucoma filtering surgery are particularly prone to endophthalmitis, primarily because sclerostomy is performed routinely as part of this procedure, and the only remaining protection the eye has from infective organisms is a thin layer of conjunctiva overlying the sclerostomy. Local antimetabolites, often used in conjunction with glaucoma filtering procedures, predispose the conjunctiva to bleb leaks that allow direct access of microorganisms to the eye.

Endogenous (metastatic) endophthalmitis should be suspected when ocular inflammation occurs in a septicemic patient, particularly if the patient is immunocompromised or has an underlying systemic illness such as diabetes or leukemia.[28,199,213]

Posttraumatic endophthalmitis should be considered in any patient with a history of injury and visual loss. A history of a high-velocity projectile presents great concern for a penetrating injury, and apparently minor accidental ocular trauma may result in perforation of the globe with or without a retained foreign body. The likelihood of posttraumatic endophthalmitis increases directly with the extent of the injury and the degree of intraocular contamination.

After the diagnosis is suspected, immediate referral to an ophthalmologist is imperative. Once the patient has been examined, a vitreous and aqueous aspirate is obtained under general anesthesia and material is evaluated with Gram and Giemsa stains. Staining with calcofluor white or acridine orange is performed if fungal infection is a concern. The material is cultured on blood and chocolate agar, thioglycolate broth, and Sabouraud agar. Vancomycin 1 mg to cover gram-positive organisms and ceftazidime 2.25 mg to cover gram-negative organisms are injected into the vitreous cavity. If fungal infection is suspected, intravitreal amphotericin B is given. Occasionally the ophthalmologist uses intravitreal dexamethasone to control associated, intense intraocular inflammation. Gram stain results often are inconsistent with cultures.

The role of vitrectomy in postoperative endophthalmitis has been addressed in the Endophthalmitis Vitrectomy Study (EVS).[6,88] In eyes with better than light perception vision at initial evaluation, outcome measurements were equal between the vitrectomy group and the vitreous tap or biopsy group. In eyes with light perception vision or worse, the EVS found that patients who underwent immediate pars plana vitrectomy did significantly better than those who underwent vitreous tap or biopsy alone.

The most common infectious agents in endophthalmitis are *S. epidermidis, Bacillus* spp., *Streptococcus* spp., *S. aureus,* and various fungi. *Bacillus cereus* is isolated in 30% to 40% of cases and can cause severe ocular morbidity.[1,61,62,73,123] *S. epidermidis* is the predominant organism in postoperative cases, and *Streptococcus* spp. with filtering blebs and *B. cereus* are the organisms associated most frequently with penetrating trauma. Approximately 65% of cases are culture positive.

Fungal endophthalmitis has become a relatively common form of endophthalmitis in childhood because of the prolonged hospital care required for severely ill immunocompromised children. The most common organism is *C. albicans*. Children with a central line catheter or receiving prolonged intravenous therapy of any type are particularly prone to infection. In patients with *Candida* endophthalmitis, the vitreous may be hazy, and small, white "snowball" localizations of infected material may appear in the vitreous or on the surface of the retina. Daily careful observation may be required during intravenous amphotericin B therapy. If the endophthalmitis clears, no ocular surgical intervention is indicated. If the infection is not adequately controlled with intravenous therapy, vitrectomy with injection of intravitreal amphotericin may be required.[88]

NEW REFERENCES SINCE THE SEVENTH EDITION

43. Chan CK, Limstrom SA, Tarasewicz DG, Lin SG. Ocular features of West Nile virus infection in North America: a study of 14 eyes. *Ophthalmology*. 2006;113(9):1539-1546.
47. Choi DS, Djalilian A. Oral azithromycin combined with topical anti-inflammatory agents in the treatment of blepharokeratoconjunctivitis in children. *J AAPOS*. 2013;17(1):112-113.
67. de Paula Fretias B, de Oliviera Dias JR, Prazeres J, et al. Ocular findings in infants with microcephaly associated with presumed Zika virus congenital infection in Salvador, Brazil. *JAMA Ophthalmol*. 2016;134(5):529-535.
75. Doan S, Gabison E, Chiambareta F, et al. Efficacy of azithromycin 1.5% eye drops in childhood ocular rosacea with phlyctenular blepharokeratoconjunctivitis. *J Ophthalmic Inflamm Infect*. 2013;3(1):38.
94. Fierro JL, Prasad PA, Fisher BT, et al. Ocular manifestations of candidemia in children. *Pediatr Infect Dis J*. 2013;32(1):84-86.
101. Deleted in review.
114. Guess S, Stone DU, Chodosh J. Evidence-based treatment of herpes simplex virus keratitis: a systematic review. *Ocul Surf*. 2007;5(3):240-250.
151. Khairallah M, Ben Yahia S, Ladjimi A, et al. Chorioretinal involvement in patients with West Nile virus infection. *Ophthalmology*. 2004;111(11):2065-2070.
157. Lai SW, Lin CL, Liao KF, et al. Herpes zoster could be an early manifestation of undiagnosed human immunodeficiency virus infection. *J Formos Med Assoc*. 2016;115(5):372-376.
159. Lee TY, Nfor ON, Tantoh DM, et al. Herpes zoster as a predictor of HIV infection in Taiwan: a population-based study. *PLoS ONE*. 2015;10(11):e0142254.
166. Liu YC, Yang YH, Hsiao HH, et al. Herpes zoster is associated with an increased risk of subsequent lymphoid malignancies—a nationwide population-based matched-control study in Taiwan. *BMC Cancer*. 2012;12:503.
179. Martinez-Pulgarin DF, Chowdhury FR, Villamil-Gomez WE, et al. Ophthalmologic aspects of chikungunya infection. *Travel Med Infect Dis*. 2016;14(5): 451-457.
193. Miranda HA 2nd, Costa MC, Frazao MA, et al. Expanded spectrum of congenital ocular findings in microcephaly with presumed Zika infection. *Ophthalmology*. 2016;123(8):1788-1794.
232. Rama P, Matuska S, Vigano M, et al. Bilateral *Acanthamoeba* keratitis with late recurrence of the infection in a corneal graft: a case report. *Eur J Ophthalmol*. 2003;13(3):311-314.
268. Srinivasan M, Mascarenhas J, Rajarama R, et al. The steroids for corneal ulcers trial (SCUT): secondary 12-month clinical outcomes of a randomized controlled trial. *Am J Ophthalmol*. 2014;157(2):327-333.
289. Todman MS, Enzer YR. Medical management versus surgical intervention of pediatric orbital cellulitis: the importance of subperiosteal abscess volume as a new criterion. *Ophthal Plast Reconstr Surg*. 2011;27(4):255-259.
313. Yashar SS, Shamiri B. Oral cimetidine treatment of molluscum contagiosum. *Pediatr Dermatol*. 1999;16(6):493.

The full reference list for this chapter is available at ExpertConsult.com.

62 Bacteremia and Septic Shock

Sheldon L. Kaplan • Jesus G. Vallejo

One of the most serious and potentially life-threatening infectious diseases in childhood is a bacteremic illness. Bacteremia may be caused by a wide variety of gram-positive or gram-negative microorganisms, and it may or may not be associated with a specific focus of infection, such as pneumonia or meningitis. Some bacteremias are transient and self-limited; they are not discussed in this chapter.

The incidence of bacteremia in children has been studied in hospital and ambulatory settings. In otherwise normal children, beyond the newborn age group, *Streptococcus pneumoniae, Escherichia coli, Staphylococcus aureus,* group A streptococcus, *Salmonella* spp., and *Neisseria meningitidis* are the most common microorganisms causing bacteremia.[92,230] The incidence of pneumococcal bacteremia has decreased substantially since the introduction of the conjugate pneumococcal vaccine.[116,165] In contrast, methicillin-resistant *S. aureus* bacteremia has increased in children in the United States since 2000.[77] Children with underlying illnesses that depress the host response to infection may develop bacteremia caused by these same microorganisms; however, in this population of children, especially when hospitalized, Enterobacteriaceae, *S. aureus,* coagulase-negative staphylococci, and fungi are the most important organisms commonly isolated from blood cultures.[5,158] Indwelling vascular lines, urinary catheters, endotracheal tubes, and other foreign material further predispose already compromised children to nosocomial infections. The incidence of diagnosed septicemia has increased over the years, partly owing to improved medical technology and the greater numbers of individuals with immunocompromising conditions who previously would not have survived.[195]

Gray and colleagues[85] reported that the incidence of bloodstream infections in a pediatric intensive care unit (ICU) during a 3-year period was 39 cases per 1000 admissions. Of the episodes, 64% were acquired in the ICU and 20.6% were community-acquired infections. Gram-positive and gram-negative organisms accounted for 62% and 31% of the isolates. Yeasts were isolated in 5.6% of episodes. The frequency of catheter-related bloodstream infections has been decreasing in many PICUs as a result of implementing insertion and maintenance bundles.[135] Children with acquired immunodeficiency syndrome or severe immunosuppression caused by human immunodeficiency virus infection also are at increased risk for developing bacteremias caused by gram-negative bacilli, especially *Pseudomonas aeruginosa*.[177]

Using a seven-state hospital discharge database, Watson and associates[230] estimated that the U.S. age-adjusted and sex-adjusted annual incidence of severe sepsis was 0.56 cases per 1000 children, or more than 42,000 cases per year. The highest age-specific incidence occurred in infants (5.16 cases per 1000), declining to 0.20 cases per 1000 for children 10 to 14 years old. Half of the children had underlying comorbidity, with neuromuscular, cardiovascular, and respiratory disorders being the most common.

One potential consequence of bacteremia is septic shock, a state characterized by inadequate tissue perfusion that is associated frequently with endotoxemia. Although most children with septic shock have infections caused by gram-negative enteric bacteria, *P. aeruginosa,* or *N. meningitidis,* organisms with endotoxin or lipopolysaccharide (LPS) within cell walls, septic shock also is associated with disease caused by gram-positive bacteria (especially *S. aureus, Streptococcus pyogenes,* and viridans streptococci), viruses, rickettsiae, and fungi. Community-acquired methicillin-resistant *S. aureus* (MRSA) in particular have been associated with severe sepsis and septic shock in young children and adolescents.[4,82] In adults, the frequency of septic shock continues to increase as the population ages, new technology including more complicated surgery and immunosuppressive agents is developed, and antibiotic resistance grows.[180]

In early studies of septic shock, Dupont and Spink[59] reviewed the cases of 172 children, age 30 days to 16 years, who were hospitalized at the University of Minnesota Medical Center with gram-negative bacteremia. Shock occurred in 25% of the children, and 98% of children with shock died. In meningococcal infections, 11% to 40% of children develop hypotension.[105,225] During a 10-month study period, Naqvi and colleagues[146] reported that shock occurred in five of 39 (13%) episodes of gram-negative bacillary sepsis, with three deaths. Jacobs and associates[98] reviewed the admissions of previously normal children to a pediatric ICU in a large children's hospital for a 30-month period. Hypotension or evidence of peripheral hypoperfusion occurred in 143 children with confirmed bacterial sepsis, mostly *Haemophilus influenzae* type b (Hib), or apparent meningococcemia. Among 1058 consecutive admissions of 916 children to a pediatric ICU in Canada from July 1, 1991, to July 31, 1992, 25 episodes (2%) of septic shock occurred.[167] During a 12-month period, 140 episodes of septicemia (135 bacterial and five fungal) were documented in 100 pediatric hematology-oncology patients.[67] Septic shock occurred in 19%.

The organisms and case-fatality rates in the study by Watson and colleagues[230] are outlined in Table 62.1. *N. meningitidis* and fungi were associated with the highest mortality rates. Early-onset group B streptococcal infections in neonates and overwhelming *S. pneumoniae* infections in children with splenic dysfunction or asplenia are associated with shock in a high percentage of cases. *S. aureus* or group A streptococcus may cause hypotension in a child with or without other manifestations of toxic shock syndrome.[189]

Using data from the Pediatric Health Information System database (2004–12; 43 hospitals), Ruth and associates[181] estimated an overall prevalence of pediatric severe sepsis of 7.7% with an associated mortality of 14.4%. Mortality was highest in patients with malignancies (22.4%), hematologic or immunologic disorders (20.3%), and cardiovascular disease (20%). The most common sites of infection were bloodstream (67.8%), respiratory tract (57.2%), and genitourinary tract (21.6%). *Staphylococcus* spp. (9.9%) and *Streptococcus* spp. (5.4%) were the most common causative agents, with fungi accounting for less than 1% of isolates. In patients in whom a bacterial pathogen was identified, the reported mortality rate was 13.2%. Although fungal infections as a cause of pediatric severe sepsis was rare, mortality in this group was high (20.1%) when compared to the overall mortality rate (14.4%).

Weiss et al.[236] described the global epidemiology of pediatric severe sepsis at 128 sites in 26 countries. The sites included 59 in North America, 39 in Europe, 10 in South America, 10 in Asia, 7 in Australia/New Zealand, and 3 in Africa. The overall point prevalence of pediatric severe sepsis was 8.2%. Point prevalence was highest in Asia (15.3%), South America (16.3%), and Africa (23.1%). The most common sites of infection were the respiratory tract (40%) and the bloodstream (19%). The proportion of infections caused by gram-positive and gram-negative organisms was similar (26.5% vs. 27.9%), with *S. aureus* accounting for most of the bacterial isolates (11.5%). Overall hospital mortality was 25% but varied across geographic regions (North America 21%, Europe 29%, Australia/New Zealand 32%, Asia 40%, and South America 11%).

Advances in understanding of the pathogenesis and pathophysiology of septic shock with respect to the host response to infection have required that more precise clinical definitions of sepsis and expanded syndromes be developed. Much of the impetus for this effort is related

TABLE 62.1 Occurrence and Case-Fatality Rates of Selected Pathogens Among Children With Severe Sepsis Based on Age[a]

	<1 Y (*N* = 4643)		1–10 Y (*N* = 2724)		11–19 Y (*N* = 2308)	
Organism	**Cases (%)**	**Case Fatality (%)**	**Cases (%)**	**Case Fatality (%)**	**Cases (%)**	**Case Fatality (%)**
Neisseria meningitidis	0.3	20	8	10.4	2.3	15.1
Haemophilus influenzae	1.6	4.2	2.4	1.6	1.9	6.8
Pseudomonas	3.6	14.6	7.7	12.4	6.9	9.4
Staphylococcus aureus	2.3	5.7	2.9	0	3.5	3.8
Group A streptococcus	0.3	0	0.7	5	0.2	0
Group B streptococcus	3.1	7.6	0.1	50	0.8	5.6
Fungus	10	10.8	13.3	16.8	10.4	11.6

[a]Represents data from a seven-state hospital discharge database in 1995.
Modified from Watson RS, Carcillo JA, Linde-Zwirble WT, et al. The epidemiology of severe sepsis in children in the United States. *Am J Respir Care Med.* 2003;167:695–701.

to the ability to more readily identify patients with infections who may benefit from administration of newer (expensive) adjunctive measures. An American College of Chest Physicians and Society of Critical Care Medicine Consensus Conference in 1991 developed new terminology to define sepsis and its sequelae.[24] This terminology has been modified for use in children by an international consensus panel of 20 experts in sepsis and clinical research (Box 62.1).[80]

In 2016, a 19-member joint task force of the Society of Critical Care Medicine and European Society of Intensive Care Medicine (ESICM) published new sepsis guidelines for adult patients.[190] According to the new guidelines, sepsis is now defined as evidence of infection plus life-threatening organ dysfunction. Organ dysfunction will be characterized clinically by a change of 2 points or greater in the Sequential (sepsis-related) Organ Failure Assessment score (SOFA). Given that SOFA is based on laboratory tests, the new guidelines recommend that clinicians use a streamlined process called quick SOFA (qSOFA) to assess patients for sepsis outside the intensive care unit.[185] The clinician will assess a patient for altered mental status, systolic blood pressure of 100 mm Hg or lower, and a respiratory rate of 22 breaths per minute or higher. Patients meeting two of the qSOFA criteria will require close monitoring.

The 2016 clinical criteria for septic shock in adults include sepsis with fluid-unresponsive hypotension, serum lactate level of greater than 2 mmol/L, and need for vasopressors to maintain a mean arterial pressure of 65 mm Hg or higher.[186] The 2016 consensus definition eliminates the use of the term systemic inflammatory response syndrome (SIRS). It should be noted that the utility of these definitions among pediatric populations is still to be determined.

BOX 62.1 Consensus Definitions of Systemic Inflammatory Response Syndrome (SIRS), Infection, Sepsis, Severe Sepsis, and Septic Shock

SIRS

The presence of two or more of the following four criteria, one of which must be abnormal temperature or white blood cell count:

1. Core temperature (rectal, bladder, oral, or central catheter probe) >38.5°C (101.3°F) or <36°C (96.8°F)
2. Tachycardia defined as more than two standard deviations above normal for age in the absence of external factors or drugs *or* otherwise unexplained persistent elevation of a 0.5- to 4-hour time period *or* for children younger than 1 year, bradycardia, defined as a mean heart rate of less than 10th percentile for age in the absence of external factors or drugs or otherwise unexplained persistent depression over a 0.5-hour period
3. Mean respiratory rate more than two standard deviations for age *or* mechanical ventilation for an acute process not related to an underlying neuromuscular disease or to general anesthesia
4. Peripheral white blood cell count elevated or depressed for age unrelated to medications or more than 10% immature neutrophils

Infection

A suspected or proven (by culture, tissue stain, polymerase chain reaction assay) infection caused by any pathogen *or* a clinical syndrome associated with a high probability of infection

Sepsis

SIRS in the presence of or caused by suspected or proven infection

Severe Sepsis

Sepsis plus one of the following: cardiovascular organ dysfunction, acute respiratory distress syndrome *or* two or more other instances of organ dysfunction as defined in the consensus statement

Septic Shock

Sepsis and cardiovascular organ dysfunction as defined in the consensus statement

Modified from Goldstein B, Giroir B, Randoph A, and the Members of the International Consensus Conference on Pediatric Sepsis. International Pediatric Sepsis Conference: definitions for sepsis and organ dysfunction in pediatrics. *Pediatr Crit Care Med.* 2005;6:2–8.

PATHOPHYSIOLOGY

The pathophysiology of bacteremia is highly variable and depends on the specific microorganism isolated, the immune status of the host, and other factors such as the locations of indwelling catheters. Highly encapsulated organisms, such as *S. pneumoniae, N. meningitidis,* and Hib, normally may reside in the nasopharynx and, for reasons that are poorly understood, are capable of invading beyond mucosal barriers into the bloodstream. A preceding viral upper respiratory tract infection may play some role in alterations in local host defense mechanisms that result in bacteremia.[106,133]

Using human columnar nasopharyngeal tissue in organ cultures, Stephens and colleagues[196] showed that *N. meningitidis* organisms were ingested by the columnar cells, then found within phagocytic vacuoles, and later observed within subepithelial tissues, suggesting that the meningococci had penetrated the epithelial layer. In this same model, Hib organisms attach to nonciliated columnar epithelial cells and subsequently are found in the intercellular spaces in association with a preceding disruption of the tight junctions of epithelial cells.[60] After passing the mucosal barriers, Hib may enter the bloodstream directly through pharyngeal blood vessels.[179] Pneumococci adhere to specific ligands on respiratory cells. The inflammatory mediators generated during viral infections upregulate platelet-activating factor receptor on respiratory cells to which the pneumococci adhere more avidly and subsequently invade.[212] Pili or adhesins of gram-negative enteric organisms seem to be important in attachment and adherence of these microorganisms to specific receptors expressed on epithelial surfaces. Pili also have been shown to be important in the pathogenesis of some gram-positive infections, such as *S. pyogenes,* group B streptococcus, and *S. pneumoniae.*[13,142]

The placement of an endotracheal tube unmasks a greater number of these receptors, presumably through increased protease activity of secretions and decreased cell-bound fibronectin, and leads to colonization of the upper respiratory tract with gram-negative organisms, which are ubiquitous in the environment of an ICU.[243] Biofilm formation on the endotracheal tube surface may contribute to colonization persisting.[117] Altered host defense mechanisms allow these organisms to move beyond epithelial surfaces and cause bacteremia.

The gastrointestinal and genitourinary tracts are major sources of gram-negative organisms responsible for bacteremia. These organisms first may cause localized abscesses or peritonitis if intestinal perforation occurs, or they may translocate the intestinal mucosa, particularly when the mucosa is affected by antineoplastic agents. Viridans streptococci can cause bacteremia in a neutropenic patient with severe mucositis that develops after the patient undergoes chemotherapy.[171] Microorganisms within the bladder may ascend the genitourinary tract and presumably enter the bloodstream through the kidneys. *S. aureus* and *S. pyogenes* are common inhabitants of the skin and skin structures. Any skin wound or foreign matter within the skin tissue renders the skin more susceptible to bacterial invasion. Staphylococci have a unique capability of adhering to solid surfaces, such as catheters, which may be an important prerequisite to colonization and subsequent catheter-related bacteremia.[162]

The pathophysiology of septic shock is very complex. Septic shock associated with gram-negative organisms has been studied most extensively, especially with respect to endotoxin or bacterial LPS, which has multiple biologic effects. Bacterial LPS has three basic components, as follows:

1. Terminal side chains consist of repeating oligosaccharides that differ from strain to strain and are responsible for the antigenic specificity of the O antigens.
2. A core LPS also consists of oligosaccharides but has less diversity in structure among strains than do the terminal side chains.
3. Lipid A is very similar among the different strains and is responsible for most of the biologic activity of endotoxin.

Endotoxin shock has been the subject of intensive animal research, and much of what is known about the pathogenesis of endotoxin shock has been derived from animal models. Although septic shock in humans is not simulated precisely in these animal models for a number of reasons, including that the animals do not have underlying host defense defects, much of what has been learned about endotoxin shock in animals has been corroborated in the human host.

Endotoxin Shock in Animals

Many animal models of endotoxin shock employ infusions of live gram-negative bacteria, usually *Escherichia coli,* or purified endotoxin, after which observations are made. The effects of purified endotoxin depend partly on the species of animal being studied. Models employing cecal ligation and puncture are thought to be more relevant to human disease than direct infusion of bacteria or endotoxin.[246] The effects of endotoxin in animal models are summarized in Table 62.2.

Numerous mediators induced by endotoxin play pivotal roles in the pathogenesis of endotoxin shock. Tumor necrosis factor (TNF), a polypeptide hormone, is a key cytokine mediating septic shock.[208] The tissue injury induced by TNF largely is a result of other mediators that are induced by TNF, including interleukin-1β (IL-1β), IL-6, eicosanoids, and platelet-activating factor.[55,96,209,206] TNF is synthesized by a wide variety of cells (including monocytes/macrophages, natural killer cells, microglial cells, hepatic Kupffer cells) after stimulation by LPS, C5a, viruses, and enterotoxins, among other agents. TNF initiates a cascade of events that leads to endothelial cell injury, an enhanced inflammatory response, and, ultimately, the characteristic findings of endotoxic shock.

Nitric oxide (i.e., endothelium-derived relaxing factor) is the final pathway by which endogenous vasodilators stimulated by endotoxin result in hypotension from altered control of microcirculation. LPS through the release of cytokines induces a form of the enzyme nitric oxide synthase II, which leads to increased production of nitric oxide.[140] Inhibitors of nitric oxide synthase, such as N^G-monomethyl-L-arginine, can reverse or prevent hypotension in animals challenged with LPS.[132]

TABLE 62.2 **Endotoxin Shock in Animal Models**

Effects	Mediators
Cardiovascular Effects	
Decreased peripheral vascular resistance[147]	Histamine, bradykinin,[136] serotonin, complement activation, prostaglandins, anaphylatoxins
Decreased cardiac output[6,9,169]	
Depressed myocardial function[130]	
Decreased systemic blood pressure[43]	
Metabolic Effects[169]	
Hyperglycemia[48]	Hypoinsulinemia
Hypoglycemia[64]	
Increased adrenocorticotropic hormone, growth hormone, and antidiuretic hormone[238]	
Decreased calcium[245]	
Increased triglycerides[107,208]	
Decreased iron, transferrin, and zinc	
Pulmonary Effects	
Congestive atelectasis[43,94]	Polymorphonuclear leukocytes
Increased capillary permeability[94]	Polymorphonuclear leukocytes
Vasoconstriction	Thromboxane, prostacyclin
Bronchoconstriction[29]	Leukotrienes
Central Nervous System Effects	
Decreased regional and total cerebral blood flow[168]	
Increased cerebral oxygen consumption[168]	

The pathophysiology of septic shock caused by gram-positive bacteria is similar to that described for gram-negative organisms.[193] Cell wall components, such as peptidoglycan and teichoic acid, promote proinflammatory activity but are less potent than endotoxin.

Endotoxin Shock in Humans

The pathophysiology of septic shock is highly complex and is related predominantly to actions of endogenous mediators released as part of the systemic inflammatory response to an infection. The cascade of events is intertwining, with production of one cytokine stimulating the synthesis of others; synergistic, in that the activities of certain cytokines act in concert; and sometimes antagonistic, with the production of other molecules to inhibit or compete with various cytokines. This complicated response to an infectious stimulus has been studied best for LPS, but a similar series of events occurs in response to gram-positive infections. Although the best understood system is the one that recognizes bacterial LPS, others exist for sensing the presence of bacterial peptidoglycan, DNA, lipopeptides, flagella, viral double-stranded RNA, and other conserved microbial molecules.

The first host protein involved in the recognition of LPS is LPS-binding protein. LPS-binding protein is an acute-phase protein; its role is to bring LPS to the cell surface by binding to LPS and forming a ternary complex with the LPS receptor molecule, CD14.[231,244] Formation of the complex between LPS and CD14 facilitates the transfer of LPS to the LPS receptor complex, which is composed of Toll-like receptor 4 (TLR4) and MD2. Studies over the course of several years led to the discovery of the TLR4/MD2 receptor complex as the signaling entity for LPS (Fig. 62.1).[19] MD2 is a secreted glycoprotein that functions as an indispensable extracellular adapter molecule for LPS-initiated signaling events, perhaps by aiding in ligand recognition. The resulting signal promotes mononuclear phagocytes to produce reactive oxygen molecules, cytokines, and arachidonic acid metabolites, including prostaglandin and leukotrienes. A counterregulatory protein is a bactericidal, permeability-increasing protein that is stored in the granules of polymorphonuclear leukocytes and inhibits the effects of LPS.[72]

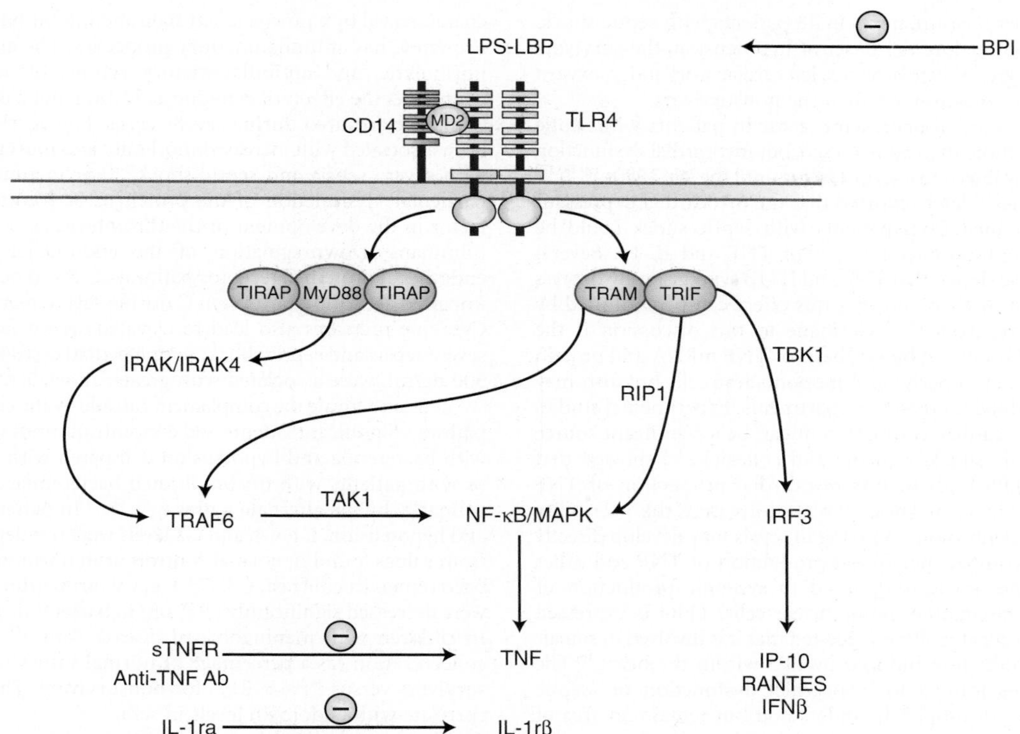

FIG. 62.1 Activation of the cytokine network by lipopolysaccharide (LPS). Circulating LPS-binding protein (LBP) recognizes LPS in the plasma and brings it to CD14. This aids the loading of LPS onto the LPS receptor complex, which is composed of dimerized Toll-like receptor 4 (TLR4) receptors and two molecules of the extracellular adapter MD2. Signals activated by TLR4 can be subdivided into signals dependent on MyD88 (and MAL [MyD88 adaptor-like protein]), which occur early (represented by the events illustrated on the left side of the diagram), and signals independent of MyD88, which occur later and use the adapters TRIF and TRAM (depicted on the right). *Ab,* Antibody; *BPI,* bactericidal/permeability increasing [protein]; *IFNβ,* interferon-β; *IL-1ra,* interleukin-1 receptor antagonist; *IP-10,* interferon-γ–induced protein 10; *IRAK,* interleukin-1 receptor–associated kinase; *IRF3,* interferon regulatory factor 3; *MAPK,* mitogen-activated protein kinase; *MyD88,* myeloid differentiation primary-response gene 88; *NF-κB;* nuclear factor-κB; *RANTES,* regulated on activation, T cell expressed and secreted; *RIP1,* receptor-interacting protein 1; *sTNFR,* soluble tumor necrosis factor receptor; *TAK1,* transforming growth factor-β–activated kinase 1; *TBK1,* TANK-binding kinase 1; *TNF,* tumor necrosis factor; *TRAF6,* TNF receptor–associated factor 6; *TRAM,* TRIF-related adaptor molecule; *TRIF,* Toll/IL-1 receptor domain–containing adaptor inducing interferon-β.

TNF is largely responsible for the biologic effects, including fever, shock, myocardial suppression, capillary leak (i.e., endothelial damage), coagulation alterations, and metabolic changes,[34,35,134,207,213] of LPS in humans. In children, including neonates, the role of cytokines in sepsis caused by a variety of organisms, but especially *N. meningitidis,* is well documented.[30,51,78,200,225] LPS and TNF each can induce the synthesis of other proinflammatory cytokines, such as IL-1β and IL-6.[56] IL-6 levels in plasma correlate with mortality. IL-8 plasma concentrations also are increased after infusion of LPS or IL-1β.[56,86] Serum IL-8 levels in children with septic shock were predictive of outcome in one study.[194]

The antiinflammatory cytokine IL-10 is produced after LPS is injected and inhibits the production of TNF, IL-1β, and IL-6.[128] Naturally occurring inhibitors of TNF or IL-1β are present in serum samples of patients with the sepsis syndrome.[79,215,216] IL-1 receptor antagonist (IL-1a) binds competitively to the IL-1 receptor to block the action of IL-1. Soluble TNF receptors bind to circulating TNF, which prevents its proinflammatory actions (see Fig. 62.1).

In adults, gram-negative bacteremia is followed by a decrease in systemic vascular resistance and mean blood pressure and an increase in cardiac output.[20,233] Decreased systemic vascular resistance may be accompanied by activation of the complement and kinin systems.[136] After this early phase, the blood pressure decreases further without change in the central venous pressure. Certain patients, especially children, are able to maintain their cardiac output and cardiac index, and this ability may be associated with increased rates of survival. When peripheral resistance is measured within 12 to 24 hours of the onset of shock, its decrease is significant in patients who survive compared with patients who die.[148] In contrast, cardiac output is reduced significantly in other patients; this decrease is associated with increased concentration of blood lactate, decreased arterial blood pH, and decreased rates of survival.

In one small study, two distinct patterns of septic shock in children admitted to the PICU of a tertiary children's hospital were described.[28] Fifteen of 16 children with bacteremia related to central venous lines had a high cardiac index and low systemic vascular resistance. This pattern was seen in only 2 of 14 children with community-onset infections in whom normal or low cardiac index with variable systemic vascular resistance was typically noted.

Depression of myocardial function has been shown in adult and pediatric patients in septic shock.[63] These patients have a reduced ejection fraction, left ventricular dilation, and significantly altered ventricular performance in response to infusion of volume.[150] This depression of myocardial function is transient in survivors, however, reverting to normal within 1 to 4 days.[153] Parker and colleagues[154] found that patients who did not survive septic shock did not have left ventricular dilation or reduction in the ejection fraction. When the systemic vascular resistance index was averaged over the course of time, nonsurvivors had a significantly lower ($P < .05$) index than that of survivors of septic shock. This study included three children who were 9 to 17 years of age. Abraham and associates[1] sequentially monitored hemodynamic and oxygen transport measurements in 33 patients with septic shock. In the 24-hour period before the onset of hypotension, the survivors showed significantly greater cardiac index, left cardiac work index, oxygen delivery, and oxygen consumption than the nonsurvivors.

A circulating myocardial depressant factor in patients with septic shock was proposed more than 50 years ago, but myocardial dysfunction was not quantitatively linked to a serum factor until the late 1980s.[130,155,170] Kumar and colleagues[113] later reported that the myocardial depressant activity of sera obtained from patients with septic shock could be eliminated by the immunoprecipitation of TNF and IL-1β. Several investigators also have shown that TNF and IL-1β synergistically depress myocardial function in vitro and that this effect can be abolished by an inhibitor of nitric oxide.[33,152] Germane to this discussion is the observation that LPS-induced biosynthesis of TNF mRNA and protein is not strictly confined to peripheral mononuclear cells but also may occur within many different tissue compartments. Experimental studies have shown that the cardiac compartment can be a significant source of TNF during septic shock. Kapadia and colleagues[102] showed that administration of LPS leads to intramyocardial production of TNF mRNA and protein in vivo. These observations raise the possibility that the myocardial depression occurring in sepsis may develop directly in response to the compartmentalized production of TNF and other cytokines within the heart, as opposed to systemic production of these mediators by circulating mononuclear cells. TLR4 is expressed in the heart, and investigators have suggested that it is involved in signaling the cytokine production induced by LPS within the heart.[16] The complex interactions leading to myocardial dysfunction or "septic cardiomyopathy" are incompletely understood but remain an area of active investigation.[70]

In children, the most comprehensive investigation of myocardial dysfunction has been in meningococcal septic shock. Thiru and coworkers[202] measured serum concentrations of the cardiac muscle–specific protein cardiac troponin I, which is released from injured cardiac myocytes, in 101 children with meningococcal septicemia. Minimum left ventricular ejection fraction was inversely related to peak cardiac troponin I levels. The degree of myocardial dysfunction, as determined by inotrope measurement, was related directly to peak cardiac troponin I concentrations. Their results suggested that myocardial cell death might contribute, at least in part, to the cardiac dysfunction associated with meningococcal septic shock.

Hematologic changes, such as leukocytosis, leukopenia, and thrombocytopenia, have been observed in human volunteers after receiving an infusion of endotoxin. Thrombocytopenia commonly occurs in association with sepsis of any cause.[45] Septic shock is one of the most common causes of disseminated intravascular coagulation in children. Hageman factor (i.e., factor XII), which initiates the coagulation cascade, can be activated directly by LPS or through endothelial damage induced by bacteria.[124] In septic shock, concentrations of Hageman factor, prekallikrein, high-molecular-weight kininogen, and factor VII are decreased partly as a result of consumption.[47,101] Similarly, levels of inactivators of clotting factors, such as C1 esterase inhibitor, α_2-macroglobulin, and antithrombin III, also are diminished. Corrigan and Jordan[47] diagnosed disseminated intravascular coagulation in 24 of 26 children with septic shock and found that improvement in coagulation parameters seemed to be related most to restoration of blood pressure. A disseminated intravascular coagulation score using four components (platelet count, fibrinogen concentration, fibrin degradation products, and prothrombin time) was found to correlate with mortality in children with sepsis or septic shock.[108] Gram-negative bacteremia may be associated with a coagulopathy that is not disseminated intravascular coagulation but is characterized by prolongation of the prothrombin and partial thromboplastin times caused by a reduction in the vitamin K–dependent coagulation factors.[46]

LPS or cell wall components of gram-positive organisms, through cytokine production, activate blood coagulation predominantly through the extrinsic pathway. The procoagulant state is enhanced further by decreased protein C activity, which is an important inhibitor of coagulation factors Va and VIIIa. The fibrinolytic system also is altered by endotoxemia and is mediated by plasminogen activator inhibitor 1–induced suppression. The coagulopathy associated with septic shock is characterized by a procoagulant state and inhibition of fibrinolysis.[118,121] Protein C has antiinflammatory properties. The antithrombotic, profibrinolytic, and antiinflammatory actions of activated protein C counteract the effects of cytokine activation, but a deficiency of protein C may be acquired during severe sepsis. Low levels of protein C have been associated with increased morbidity and mortality rates in patients with severe sepsis and septic shock.[67] For meningococcal disease in particular, dysfunction of the protein C activation pathway is a key factor in the development of the thrombosis associated with purpura fulminans. Downregulation of the endothelial thrombomodulin–endothelial protein C receptor pathway seems to be the mechanism for impaired activation of protein C during severe meningococcal sepsis.[61] Cytokine increases also lead to elevated serum ferritin levels during severe sepsis and septic shock; in one pediatric study levels higher than 500 ng/mL were associated with greater mortality.[74]

LPS can activate the complement cascade by the classic or the alternate pathway. Significantly depressed concentrations of C3 occur in patients with bacteremia and hypotension compared with normal individuals or with patients with uncomplicated bacteremia, and C3 is activated primarily by the alternate pathway.[62,101,126] In patients with bacteremia and hypotension, C1, C4, and C2 levels were not depressed significantly from values found in normal controls or in normotensive patients with bacteremia. In contrast, C3, C5, C6, C9, properdin, and factor B levels were decreased significantly ($P < .05$) in bacteremic patients with shock. In children with meningococcal disease, Tubbs[211] found a mean C3 concentration (as a percentage of normal values) of 132% ± 21% for survivors versus 91% ± 21% for nonsurvivors. The C3 levels did not correlate with endotoxin levels in sera.

Many metabolic alterations have been documented in the human host during endotoxin shock. Hyperglycemia followed by hypoglycemia can complicate the shock state induced by sepsis.[64,137] Whole-body use of glucose is increased during sepsis, which probably is cytokine mediated.[138] Glycolysis and gluconeogenesis are increased, but insulin resistance occurs in skeletal muscle. Children with underlying liver disease or with reduced glycogen stores are most likely to develop hypoglycemia during septic shock. Lactic acidosis develops as a result of poor tissue perfusion and cellular hypoxia. Lactic acid concentrations are increased in nonsurvivors and patients with poor or low-flow cardiac output during sepsis.

In clinical studies, Clowes and associates[41] identified a subgroup of patients with low-flow septic shock in whom concentrations of serum insulin were lower than concentrations in a control population. In children with meningococcal sepsis, van Waardenburg and colleagues[221] found higher blood glucose concentrations and significantly lower insulin levels on day 2 or 3 of hospitalization in children with shock compared with children without shock. Levels of plasma insulin and soluble TNF receptor 75 were inversely correlated in these children. Their findings were consistent with the inflammatory response inhibiting insulin secretion. In another study of meningococcal sepsis, both insulin resistance and β-cell dysfunction contributed to the hyperglycemia that occurred in a third of the children.[222]

Hypocalcemia and decreased serum ionized calcium concentrations occur frequently during bacterial sepsis. In one study, 12 (20%) of 60 critically ill adults with bacterial sepsis had hypocalcemia.[245] The mortality rate in the hypocalcemic patients was 50% compared with 30% in the patients who were normocalcemic. Cardenas-Rivero and associates[37] studied calcium homeostasis in 145 children admitted to an ICU. Of eight children with confirmed sepsis or meningitis (or both) not caused by Hib, seven had hypocalcemia, and six of seven had ionized hypocalcemia. Five of the six children with ionized hypocalcemia had inappropriately normal concentrations of parathyroid hormone, which suggests that transient hypoparathyroidism occurs in some children with sepsis. Hypocalcemia also occurs commonly in patients with toxic shock syndrome.[237] In women with toxic shock syndrome and hypocalcemia, serum concentrations of calcitonin are elevated by unknown mechanisms.[39] Hypocalcemia and elevated calcitonin concentrations also have been documented in children with fulminant meningococcemia.[122]

Procalcitonin levels are elevated in several conditions associated with SIRS, including sepsis, and have been proposed as adjunctive laboratory tests for the early detection of, and indicators for prognosis of, meningococcal disease and many other infections.[38,88,114] These changes in calcium levels are especially critical because the level of ionized calcium and cardiac output in septic shock can be correlated.[242] Other metabolic changes may occur during septic shock in humans, as follows:

1. Increased concentrations of cortisol and growth hormone (including in neonates)[204,226]
2. Relative adrenal insufficiency by adrenocorticotropin testing[90]
3. Depression of triiodothyronine and thyroxine levels related to poor nutrition[175]
4. Elevations in total concentrations of amino acid in plasma and the preferential use of branched-chain amino acids as an energy source for skeletal muscle[138]
5. Muscle proteolysis, possibly induced by one or more circulating agents in the plasma of patients with serious infections[40]
6. Elevations in concentrations of plasma thromboxane, which are observed in nonsurvivors of septic shock[173]
7. Elevations in concentrations of triglycerides and free fatty acid during gram-negative bacteremia[73,107]
8. Altered zinc homeostasis[240]

Liver dysfunction is an important aspect of endotoxin shock in adults. Banks and colleagues[11] found that clinical jaundice was apparent in 63% of their patients with septic shock, that it was found more commonly in nonsurvivors than in survivors, and that the degree of biochemical liver abnormalities was related to the duration of shock. Postmortem findings included focal liver necrosis, Kupffer cell hyperplasia, portal tract inflammation, venous congestion, and intrahepatic cholestasis.

Adult respiratory distress syndrome (ARDS), or shock lung, is a major complication of septic shock in children.[97,164] The lungs of children with ARDS have characteristic changes consisting of increased lung weight reflecting congestion and atelectasis, alveoli lined with hyaline membranes, microthrombi, hemorrhage, and interstitial edema.[97] Increased capillary permeability and intrapulmonary shunts have been documented in patients with ARDS.[49] C5a, a potent chemotactic factor, causes aggregation of polymorphonuclear neutrophils, is elevated in the sera of patients who ultimately develop ARDS, and is found in increased concentrations in bronchoalveolar lavage fluid obtained from patients with ARDS.[87,176] Leukocyte aggregates are thought to be trapped in lung tissue and may cause damage to the endothelium of the pulmonary microvasculature through the release of oxygen radicals, lysosomal enzymes, and products of arachidonic acid metabolism. Although neutrophils play a critical role in the pathogenesis of ARDS, other factors also are important, considering that ARDS can develop in patients who are neutropenic.[149,234] Thromboxane, platelet-activating factor, fibrin, and other substances contribute to the lung injury in ARDS.[178]

The effects of endotoxin shock on the central nervous system have not been studied carefully in humans.[84] The encephalopathy associated with sepsis seems to be caused partly by altered phenylalanine metabolism; concentrations of phenylalanine and its metabolite, phenylacetic acid, are increased in the sera and cerebrospinal fluid of septic adults who are stuporous or comatose.[139]

Endotoxin has been implicated in the pathogenesis of acute renal failure associated with sepsis. Wardle[227,228] showed that 12 of 16 patients with acute tubular necrosis had endotoxemia. Renal arterial blood flow and renal vascular resistance are decreased significantly in baboons 2 to 4 hours after infusion of endotoxin. Inadequate perfusion pressure was associated with renal ischemia and negligible urine output in these animals shortly after administration of endotoxin.[184] Pathologic examination of the kidneys revealed focal necrosis of the proximal tubular epithelium, eosinophilic casts within proximal and distal tubules, and microthrombi in the glomerular capillaries. Endothelin, a potent vasoconstrictor peptide produced by endothelial cells, is elevated in concentration in the plasma of patients with septic shock. Because endothelin contributes to the regulation of regional blood flow, elevated levels suggest that it may relate to renal vasoconstriction and dysfunction.[223]

Endotoxin can be measured in the plasma of patients with gram-negative bacteremia as well as in patients with other infections, even upper respiratory tract infections.[53] The presence of circulating endotoxin does not mean that bacteremia is present or ever has occurred because endotoxin presumably may be "absorbed or leak" into the circulation from the gastrointestinal tract.[119,199,210] Endotoxemia may be a valid indicator, however, of impending gram-negative septicemia in febrile patients.[217] Preformed antibody to LPS or lipid A is associated with protection against shock and death caused by gram-negative bacteremia in adults. McCartney and colleagues[128] detected endotoxin in the blood (after chloroform extraction) of patients with gram-negative septic shock; all 18 patients with persistently positive endotoxin assays died. In contrast, nine patients who initially had endotoxemia but subsequently had negative assays survived. Other studies confirm the association between endotoxemia and outcome.[218,123] Evidence exists that human endotoxin is cleared from the circulation by the liver and can be detoxified by neutrophil enzymes (i.e., acyloxacyl hydrolases).[125,143]

The sequence of events in the evolution of endotoxin shock has been outlined by several investigators.[147] Bacteria, endotoxin, or other bacterial products stimulate the production of TNF and other cytokines, which in concert with endotoxin set off a whole series of events. Potent mediators, including C3a, C5a, eicosanoids, platelet-activating factor, histamine, and myocardial depressant substance, are released. Potent vasodilators cause peripheral vasodilation, and decreased systemic peripheral resistance leads to pooling of blood and decreased venous return to the heart. Mean blood pressure may be low, or it may be normal if cardiac output increases sufficiently to compensate for these alterations despite depression of ventricular function. The central venous pressure, which partially depends on myocardial performance, may be low or in the normal range.

If intravascular volume is increased by the administration of sufficient fluids, shock may be prevented or corrected. Continued hypotension and diminished perfusion pressure may lead, however, to cellular hypoxia and increased production of lactic acid from pyruvate. The microcirculation is altered by local tissue acidosis. Capillary beds become congested, and intravascular fluid may leak into the interstitial spaces. Increased secretion of catecholamine leads to arteriolar and venular constriction and increased peripheral resistance. Pooling of blood is enhanced, which leads to a further diminution in venous return and a reduction of cardiac output. Oliguria, coagulation abnormalities, and additional metabolic alterations indicate multiple organ system failure and presage the death of the patient.

Wong et al.[239] have studied the genome-level expression profiles of children with sepsis and septic shock. Multiple gene networks, primarily related to inflammation and immunity, were affected over time and were differentially regulated.[187] These investigations have led to the identification of three subclasses of distinct gene expression profiles; higher mortality is associated with one of these subclasses.[241] This type of classification scheme might be able to identify patients at the time of admission who are at greater risk for poor outcomes and who would be optimal candidates for studying newer interventions or strategies for treating children in septic shock.

Genetic polymorphisms in the immune response to infection have been shown to be associated with clinical outcomes.[201] Functional and association studies involving genetic polymorphisms in essential genes, including Toll-like receptors, cytokines, and coagulation factors, have provided important insights into the mechanisms involved in the pathogenesis of sepsis-induced organ dysfunction. Precise categorization of patients based on genetic background may lead to individualized targeted treatment.

CLINICAL PRESENTATION AND DIAGNOSIS

The signs and symptoms of bacteremia vary greatly depending on the age and underlying disease of the patient, the duration of illness, and the specific microorganisms. Young, otherwise healthy children aged 3 months to 3 years may present with fever and evidence of an upper or lower respiratory tract infection or no focus of infection and yet have unsuspected bacteremia. Most studies indicated that the risk of developing bacteremia increases as the body temperature increases, and, in the unimmunized child, almost 25% of these children may be bacteremic after the temperature exceeds 41°C.[14] In a previously healthy child, the persistence of irritability and the inability to console the child despite optimal environmental conditions have been proposed as key points in the physical examination that should alert the clinician to the possibility of a serious infection such as bacteremia or meningitis.[127,191]

Underlying illnesses with splenic dysfunction place a child at increased risk for serious infections caused by encapsulated organisms, whereas children with leukemia or other immunosuppressive diseases or children in the ICU are more likely to be infected with gram-negative bacilli or *S. aureus.* A history of diarrhea may suggest *Salmonella* spp. as a possible cause of illness. Preceding skin infections or wounds are important clues to infection caused by *S. aureus* or group A streptococcus. An indwelling vascular catheter may precipitate overlying erythema in a patient with evidence of phlebitis proximally. Gram-positive cocci, gram-negative bacilli, and yeast can be associated with catheter-related sepsis. Toxic shock syndrome should be considered in a hypotensive girl or woman with a recent menstrual period and history of tampon use, although toxic shock also is associated with *S. aureus* sepsis in males and nonmenstruating females.[82,189] Evidence of osteomyelitis, with or without venous thrombosis, is a very common finding in staphylococcal sepsis. Intraabdominal sources of infection increase the likelihood of developing anaerobic bacteremia.

Petechiae may be associated with many microorganisms, especially invasive disease caused by *N. meningitidis.*[219] Purpura is an ominous finding and frequently is associated with overwhelming infection caused by *N. meningitidis, S. pneumoniae,* and Hib. *P. aeruginosa* is associated specifically with erythema gangrenosum.[57] Almost half of children presenting with erythroderma (diffuse erythema) either had shock at presentation or developed shock in one study.[32] Other skin and soft tissue manifestations of gram-negative sepsis include bullous lesions, cellulitis, fasciitis, thrombophlebitis, and symmetrical peripheral gangrene with disseminated intravascular coagulation.[144] Signs of meningeal irritation or increased intracranial pressure are important because they may modify the approach to management of fluids in a child in shock.

The onset of bacteremia may be heralded by chills, fever, nausea, vomiting, diarrhea, rashes, and petechiae. Initially, the skin feels warm and appears flushed. A change or impairment in mental status may be the first clue to the presence of shock. Hyperventilation also may develop before the onset of clinical shock occurs, which can alert the physician to impending circulatory insufficiency.[21] In time, cold, clammy extremities; a weak pulse; tachycardia; tachypnea; hypotension; and oliguria may occur. The skin over the extremities, the tip of the nose, and the earlobes especially are prone to cyanosis. Auscultation of the lungs may reveal rales, indicating pneumonia or pulmonary edema. Abnormal distention or tenderness to palpation and guarding may be evidence of peritonitis. Costovertebral angle tenderness suggests acute pyelonephritis as a source of bacteremias.

The physician must distinguish among the following three main types of shock in children:

1. *Hypovolemic shock,* such as occurs with blood loss, fluid and electrolyte loss, adrenal insufficiency, or other causes
2. *Cardiogenic shock,* which is associated with drug intoxication, cardiac surgery, arrhythmias, and pericardial tamponade, among other causes
3. *Distributive shock,* which indicates abnormal distribution of blood flow leading to inadequate tissue perfusion (e.g., septic shock, anaphylaxis)

The laboratory evaluation of a child with bacteremia, septic shock, or both conditions should provide information concerning the cause and the data required for optimal supportive management. Several studies showed that a total white blood cell (WBC) count exceeding 15,000 cells/mm^2 in a 3- to 36-month-old child who has not been immunized with conjugate vaccines and with a temperature greater than 39°C to 40°C and without a focus of infection is an indication that the child is at increased risk for having bacteremia, especially pneumococcal bacteremia.[12] Since the introduction of the pneumococcal conjugate vaccine, pneumococcal bacteremia in this scenario has been greatly reduced.[92,183,198] Elevated erythrocyte sedimentation rates and C-reactive protein levels also have been suggested as useful screening tools for detecting serious bacterial infections. A low peripheral WBC count also may suggest septicemia and commonly is observed during episodes of overwhelming bacteremic illnesses.

Procalcitonin levels are elevated in bacteremic children and are related to the severity of illness, such as organ failure and even death.[88,114] Commercial kits for the rapid measurement of concentrations of procalcitonin are available. Hemoglobin and hematocrit results should help differentiate between septic and hemorrhagic shock. Examination of the peripheral smear may disclose evidence of splenic dysfunction (i.e., Howell-Jolly bodies) or fragmented red blood cells, as seen in disseminated intravascular coagulation. Thrombocytopenia, prolongation of prothrombin time and partial prothrombin time, and the presence of fibrin split products are consistent with disseminated intravascular coagulation.

Hyponatremia is a common finding. Concentrations of serum bicarbonate may be depressed, which may signify a state of metabolic acidosis. Elevated lactic acid concentrations result from inadequate tissue perfusion and, in some reports, have been significantly greater in nonsurvivors or patients with low-flow states than in survivors or patients with high-flow shock.[41] In pediatric studies, serial lactate levels showing normalization are associated with recovery.[58] Hyperglycemia or hypoglycemia may be encountered. In one study, serum glucose levels greater than 178 mg/dL were associated with a greater risk of death caused by septic shock.[26] Transaminase levels may be elevated and presumably reflect cellular injury. Serum calcium concentrations (preferably ionized calcium levels) should be checked periodically because hypocalcemia may interfere with optimal myocardial function.

A chest radiograph may reveal a pulmonary source of infection or show a secondary pulmonary manifestation of an invasive infection such as pneumonia or septic emboli in children with staphylococcal sepsis.[81] Arterial blood gases obtained early in endotoxin shock usually reveal hypocapnia and normal to elevated pH.[21,22] At this point, the patient has a mixed metabolic acidosis and respiratory alkalosis. If the shock state progresses, the metabolic acidosis becomes so severe that respiratory compensation is ineffective, and the patient becomes acidotic. In some patients, respiratory acidosis accompanies metabolic acidosis. In either case, decompensated metabolic acidosis in a patient with septic shock is associated with a grave prognosis. A major consequence of ARDS is hypoxemia. For patients with ARDS, the chest radiograph characteristically shows bilateral and diffuse hazy infiltrates; opacification of all lung fields usually is seen during the late phases of ARDS. Positive fluid balance contributes to the pulmonary dysfunction in patients with acute lung injury, including those related to sepsis.[69]

Concentrations of blood urea nitrogen and serum creatinine may be elevated. Jones and Weil[100] found that the ratio of urine to plasma osmolality was the most valuable indicator of renal impairment in adult patients with shock. When this ratio was greater than 1.5, the likelihood of developing progressive renal failure was remote. A urine osmolality value greater than 400 mOsm/kg also indicated adequate renal function. Gene microarray studies may identify novel biomarkers that identify a patient in septic shock who is at greater risk for acute kidney injury.[15] Many WBCs or WBC casts in the urine may suggest the genitourinary tract as the source of bacteremia. If one or more gram-negative rods are seen on the Gram stain of unspun urine, more than 10^5 colony-forming units/mL of bacteria are likely to be present.

Isolating the organism responsible for bacteremia or septic shock is important for documenting the infection and for providing optimal antimicrobial therapy. With instruments that continuously monitor growth in the blood culture bottles, growth can be detected sooner than if the bottles are inspected just once or twice daily. Before the use of the pneumococcal conjugate vaccine became routine, many authorities recommended that a blood culture be obtained in a 3- to 36-month-old child with temperature greater than 39°C to 40°C and a total WBC count greater than or equal to 15,000 cells/mm^2 and without a specific focus of infection. In this way, instances of "unsuspected" or "outpatient" bacteremia could be identified. In an outpatient setting, almost 90% of blood cultures growing true pathogens were positive within 24 hours of incubation using a continuously monitored system.[131] This approach is now less useful in the era of administration of pneumococcal conjugate vaccine to young infants.[99]

In an infant who has received three or more doses of the conjugate pneumococcal vaccine, the likelihood of developing invasive pneumococcal infection is reduced approximately 90%. The proportion of children with high fever without localizing findings and a WBC count of 15,000/mm^2 or greater who might have occult pneumococcal bacteremia may be less than 1%, a level that no longer justifies this approach. Most organisms isolated from blood cultures in these patients are now more likely to be a contaminant than a true pathogen. Currently, the approach to a febrile child without a source has changed in many emergency departments such that more selective criteria for obtaining blood cultures are being developed.

When appropriate, cerebrospinal fluid, urine, and other pertinent sites should be cultured before initiating antibiotic therapy, if possible. When an intraabdominal source of infection is likely, blood and other cultures should be processed anaerobically. Gram stain or acridine orange stain of a buffy coat smear of peripheral blood may reveal evidence of the causative microorganism, especially in an overwhelming infection.[110] Gram stain of material obtained from petechial or purpuric lesions may show gram-negative diplococci suggestive of meningococcus. Polymerase chain reaction for detecting *N. meningitidis* is available in selected laboratories and may be the only method by which infection is documented when cultures are sterile. The development of newer molecular techniques hopefully will lead to a greater availability of tests to detect a wider range of pathogens rapidly.

TREATMENT

The initial selection of antibiotics for administration to a child with suspected bacteremia is based on the clinical situation (Table 62.3). If untreated initially, children with occult bacteremia are at risk of developing serious complications, such as meningitis or pneumonia.[123,145] Empiric antibiotic therapy for children who are selected carefully and followed seems reasonable.[12,14,68]

In children who have not received more than two doses of the pneumococcal conjugate vaccine, one approach may be to obtain a blood culture from children aged 3 to 36 months with a temperature of 39°C or greater who have no focal findings and whose peripheral WBC count is greater than or equal to 15,000/mm^2. In such patients, the decision to administer antibiotics expectantly may be based on several factors, especially the ability of the parents to observe the child and communicate this information back to the physician in a timely manner. Ceftriaxone given parenterally, an oral agent such as amoxicillin and amoxicillin-clavulanate, or other oral antibiotics can be administered. If treatment is initiated, a properly collected urine specimen for urinalysis or urine culture also should be obtained so that a urinary tract infection would not be treated inadvertently since UTI is now the most common serious bacterial infection in young children with fever without a source.[99]

TABLE 62.3 Empiric Antibiotic Regimens for Septic Shock in Infants and Children Under Selected Clinical Circumstances

Circumstances	Antibiotics
Normal Child	
Skin findings suggesting meningococcemia or preceding skin trauma or varicella	Cefotaxime or ceftriaxone + vancomycin ± nafcillin
Urinary tract source	Cefotaxime or ceftriaxone + aminoglycoside
Intraabdominal source	Clindamycin or metronidazole + gentamicin + piperacillin-tazobactam
Immunocompromised Child	
Malignancy or immunodeficiency or neutropenia or central line	Vancomycin + aminoglycoside + piperacillin-tazobactam or ceftazidime
Asplenia or splenic dysfunction	Vancomycin + cefotaxime or ceftriaxone

Occult bacteremia caused by *S. pneumoniae* intermediate or resistant to penicillin or intermediate to ceftriaxone in an otherwise normal child should resolve with any of the options noted earlier.[104] This approach probably is less useful in an infant or child who has received three or more doses of the conjugate pneumococcal vaccine.

Children who subsequently are determined to have *S. pneumoniae* bacteremia and who have been treated with antibiotics expectantly need to be reevaluated as soon as the results of the blood cultures are known. If the child appears well and has been afebrile for at least 24 hours and if the parents can observe the child carefully and are able to communicate frequently with the physician, outpatient management can be continued. For children who were not treated initially, who remain febrile, and who are called back to be reevaluated for a positive blood culture, a parenteral dose of antibiotics is recommended.[10] It is in this situation where rapid identification of gram-positive cocci growing in blood cultures is particularly helpful. Determining that the organism growing is coagulase-negative staphylococcus by molecular tests (GenXpert) may avoid calling the patient back because of a blood culture contaminant. Close contact with the parents and patient is mandatory no matter how these children are managed initially. Hospitalization for intravenous antibiotics is indicated if the child appears "toxic" or has other signs suggesting a serious infection.

For children with suspected bacteremia who are ill and require admission to the hospital, antibiotics are selected to cover the most serious organisms causing that infection. In normal children aged 3 months or older, a combination of nafcillin (150 to 200 mg/kg per day) or another semisynthetic antistaphylococcal penicillin plus cefotaxime (150 to 200 mg/kg per day) or ceftriaxone (75 to 100 mg/kg per day) covers most of the likely pathogens (e.g., *S. pneumoniae, S. aureus, S. pyogenes, N. meningitidis,* Hib). In areas of the world where community-acquired MRSA is a problem, an agent effective against MRSA should be included in the initial empiric regimen.[91,103] Vancomycin (45 to 60 mg/kg per day) is the gold standard for treating infections caused by MRSA. Adding an aminoglycoside or rifampin to vancomycin is not beneficial.[120] Although most community-acquired MRSA isolates are susceptible to clindamycin, this agent is not generally recommended alone for bacteremic illness since it is not bactericidal. Some experts recommend adding clindamycin to vancomycin or nafcillin theoretically to reduce toxin production. This reduction occurs in vitro, but no clinical data indicate that this approach leads to a decrease in the incidence of morbidity or mortality.[197]

Treatment of bacteremia associated with a genitourinary or gastrointestinal source requires antibiotics to which gram-negative enterics are susceptible. In such cases, initial therapy could consist of an aminoglycoside with an additional antibiotic active against anaerobes, such as clindamycin, metronidazole, or piperacillin-tazobactam, for a gastrointestinal focus of infection. Extended-spectrum cephalosporins, such as cefotaxime, ceftriaxone, or cefepime are the most commonly recommended drugs for treating serious gram-negative enteric infections. Optimal management of intraabdominal or other abscesses usually requires surgical drainage, which should be undertaken as soon as the child's condition allows.

Immunosuppressed children or children with serious illnesses in the ICU require a different initial approach to suspected bacteremia. Gram-negative enterics, *P. aeruginosa, S. aureus,* and coagulase-negative staphylococcus are likely to be isolated from these patients. Empiric therapy of nosocomial infection is based on the current antibiotic susceptibility pattern within the hospital.[205] *E. coli, Klebsiella* spp., and *Enterobacter* spp. are among the most common organisms causing bacteremia in patients in the pediatric ICU.[174] *E. coli* and *Klebsiella* spp. frequently produce β-lactamases that lead to resistance to piperacillin. Generally a combination of an antistaphylococcal semisynthetic penicillin or vancomycin (if a central line is present) or, if MRSA is a relatively common nosocomial pathogen, an aminoglycoside and an extended-spectrum penicillin (e.g., piperacillin-tazobactam), or a third- or fourth-generation cephalosporin (cefotaxime, ceftazidime, cefepime) is administered initially until a specific pathogen is isolated. Broad-spectrum penicillins and aminoglycosides frequently exhibit synergy in vitro against gram-negative organisms, especially against *P. aeruginosa.*[188] In critically ill patients, it is not clear that a synergistic combination of antibiotics is beneficial for treating bacteremia caused by *P. aeruginosa* or gram-negative enteric rods.[93,111,160] Combination therapy may be helpful in the neutropenic patient with bacteremia, especially due to *P. aeruginosa*. When administering two different classes of antibiotics directed against gram-negative organisms, it is most beneficial to have at least one antibiotic active in vitro against the causative pathogen prior to knowing the antibiotic susceptibilities.

After a specific organism is identified and antibiotic susceptibilities are known, the most appropriate agent is selected. If *E. coli* or *Klebsiella* spp. are isolated, these organisms can produce extended-spectrum β-lactamases (ESBL). With the current Clinical and Laboratory Standards Institute breakpoints, the ESBL-producing bacteria should be detected.[42,157] If an ESBL-producing organism is identified, treatment with an extended-spectrum cephalosporin (e.g., cefotaxime, ceftriaxone, ceftazidime) is not recommended.[159] In this case, a carbapenem, such as imipenem-cilastatin or meropenem, is suggested.[159]

Enterobacter spp., *Citrobacter* spp., and *Serratia marcescens* may hyperproduce β-lactamase enzymes or be induced to hyperproduce these enzymes and are resistant or can become resistant to the extended-spectrum cephalosporins.[163] In many institutions, a high percentage of these isolates are resistant to ceftazidime.[31] Cefepime may be more active than is ceftazidime or cefotaxime against *Enterobacter* spp. and other Amp C, β-lactamase enzyme–producing, gram-negative bacilli.[182] A carbapenem with an aminoglycoside is the treatment regimen recommended for treating infections caused by these isolates when resistant to the third-generation cephalosporins.

In these patients, rapidly achieving therapeutic aminoglycoside levels in the plasma is important.[141] Serum concentrations of the aminoglycoside should be measured within 24 hours of initiation of therapy to ensure that therapeutic concentrations have been reached. Higher doses of antibiotics than normally administered may be required in some patients.

Antibiotics should be administered as soon as the diagnosis of septic shock is suspected. The Surviving Sepsis Campaign (SSC) endorses administering antibiotics within 1 hour of shock recognition.[52] In adults, a delay in treatment with appropriate antibiotics is associated with increased mortality.[112] Weiss and associates[235] reported on the impact of antimicrobial timing on mortality and organ dysfunction in pediatric patients with severe sepsis or septic shock at a single institution. These investigators noted that delayed administration of initial and first appropriate antibiotic therapy beyond 3 hours from recognition of severe sepsis and septic shock were independent risk factors for mortality. This study, however, was not powered to address the SSC recommendation of administering empiric antibiotics within 1 hour of sepsis recognition. Ames and associates[7] have also evaluated the effect of empiric and appropriate antibiotic administration in the emergency department on the development of new or progressive MODS. In this study, 48% (153/321) of pediatric patients admitted to the intensive care unit received empiric antibiotics in 1 hour or less. Early (≤1 hour), appropriate antibiotics were administered to 36% (56 of 154) of patients with a documented bacterial infection. Although these patients had significantly greater PIM2 scores, rates of new or progressive MODS (15% vs. 15%) and hospital mortality (10% vs. 6%) were similar to those of patients treated at more than 1 hour. These two studies suggest that a multicenter study will be needed to determine the ideal time goal for early appropriate antibiotic treatment that will improve patient outcomes.

The selection of antibiotics is the same as that for bacteremia. If *S. aureus* is suspected among the potential causes of septic shock, antibiotic therapy is complicated by two factors: MRSA may make up more than 50% of community-acquired isolates,[103] and nafcillin or oxacillin is superior to vancomycin for the treatment of serious infections caused by methicilin-susceptible *S. aureus*.[83] Nafcillin or oxacillin plus an aminoglycoside may be synergistic against staphylococci, but adding an aminoglycoside increases the risk for nephrotoxicity to develop. Some authorities include nafcillin or oxacillin plus vancomycin plus gentamicin in the initial empiric therapy of patients with life-threatening infections possibly caused by *S. aureus*.[161] Combination empiric antibiotics appear to be advantageous because it is more likely that an antibiotic active against the causative pathogen will be administered compared with empiric monotherapy and not because of potential synergy.[54]

The management of septic shock is directed toward three main objectives: (1) control of the infectious process, (2) restoration of adequate tissue perfusion, and (3) maintenance of efficient respiratory function. Providing aggressive fluid resuscitation early in the emergency center proved to be one factor in decreasing the length of hospital stay in one study.[115] Details of management have been the subject of numerous reports.[36,109,180] The reader is referred to these reviews for expert detailed guidance in the fluid management, use of vasoactive agents, and respiratory treatments in children with septic shock.

The benefits of therapy with high doses of corticosteroids in the treatment of endotoxin shock remain unproved. Extensive experimental data document the salutary hemodynamic, metabolic, microcirculatory, and cellular effect of steroids in laboratory models of endotoxin shock.[95] High-dose steroids were never found to be efficacious, however, in randomized controlled trials conducted in adults with severe sepsis or septic shock.[25,192] In a recent meta-analysis, 35 randomized trials (4682 adult patients) were reviewed.[224] Fourteen trials evaluated high-dose steroids and 21 used low-dose steroids. The authors concluded that there was no evidence for a beneficial effect of steroids in patients with SIRS, sepsis, severe sepsis, or septic shock.

On the basis of these studies, the routine use of high-dose corticosteroids in patients with severe sepsis or septic shock is not recommended. Results of randomized studies enrolling adults suggested that lower stress doses of hydrocortisone might be beneficial in managing patients with septic shock.[23,27] However it is not clear if there is a survival benefit at 28 days.[156] The role of low-dose hydrocortisone in children with septic shock remains controversial.[8,220] In one pediatric study the addition of fludrocortisone, a mineralocorticoid given enterally, to parenteral hydrocortisone was associated with shorter duration of norepinephrine support but more hypokalemia in children with sepsis.[89] Randomized studies are needed to clarify the role of stress doses of hydrocortisone in children with septic shock.

Every effort should be made to ensure an adequate airway, which may require periodic suctioning if the patient is unable to clear pooled secretions. Humidified oxygen in concentrations required to maintain an adequate partial pressure of oxygen should be provided early. The method of oxygen administration (e.g., mask, ventilator) depends on the clinical state of the patient. Intubation and assisted ventilation are indicated if the child shows evidence of impending respiratory failure.

ARDS, usually appearing within 2 days after the onset of shock, may complicate the respiratory and fluid management.[97] Pulmonary edema, atelectasis, decreased pulmonary compliance, and ventilation-perfusion abnormalities are some factors that can lead to inadequate oxygenation. Administration of excessive fluids may contribute to ARDS. The central venous pressure may remain normal despite the presence of pulmonary edema. Positive end-expiratory pressure, oxygen, and careful attention to cardiovascular parameters are the mainstays of therapy for ARDS.[97,164,178]

The general supportive care of a child with septic shock includes attention to nutritional and metabolic requirements.[172] Parenteral alimentation may be the only means by which to provide nutrition, although the optimal amount and composition of elemental nutrients for children with septic shock are unknown. Hypocalcemia should be corrected. Platelet transfusions or fresh-frozen plasma may be necessary to correct coagulopathies. Continuous venovenous hemofiltration with or without dialysis may be instituted for complications of renal failure, such as fluid overload with pulmonary edema or hyperkalemia. Children who have acute renal failure complicating severe septic shock have a significantly higher mortality rate than that of children without acute renal failure.[166]

INVESTIGATIVE THERAPIES

Based on the evolving understanding of the pathophysiology of septic shock, many large, randomized, double-blind, multicenter trials have been conducted to assess the efficacy of agents that neutralize or counteract toxins or cytokines that are important in the evolution of septic shock. These immunomodulating strategies have been used on the basis of experimental data from animal studies. The conditions seen in experimental animal models of sepsis do not reflect the pathophysiologic situation seen in patients with severe sepsis or septic shock,

TABLE 62.4 Clinical Trials of Sepsis Medications in Adults

Trial	Agent Studied	Total Patients (N)	28-DAY MORTALITY (%)	
			Medications	Controls
CHESS	HA-1A human monoclonal antibody[129]	1578	41	37
INTERSEPT	Anti-TNF[44]	564	37.3	39.5
	Steroids[25]	1267	39	35
	IL1-RA[66]	893	31	35
	Soluble TNF receptor[65]	141	40	38
COMPASS	Platelet-activating factor acetylhydrolase[151]	1425	25	24
KyberSept	Antithrombin III[229]	2314	38.9	38.7
OPTIMIST	Tissue factor pathway inhibitor[3]	1754	34.2	33.9
PROWESS	Activated protein C[18]	1690	24.7	30.8
ADDRESS	Activated protein C[2]	2613	17	18.5

TNF, Tumor necrosis factor.

however, which has led to many negative clinical trials (Table 62.4). One interesting newer approach is the development of endotoxin removal devices that are being evaluated to assess their potential as adjunctive measures to improve the outcome of patients with septic shock.[50]

Intravenous immunoglobulin is recommended as adjunctive therapy for patients with toxic shock syndrome caused by either group A streptococcus or *S. aureus* that is not responding to aggressive therapy after several hours or after appropriate drainage of focal infections.[161] The value of intravenous immunoglobulin in the treatment of septic shock caused by *S. aureus* infection but not associated with toxic shock syndrome has not been established.[76] Investigative antibodies such as tefibazumab, a monoclonal antibody directed against clumping factor A, an adhesin on the surface of *S. aureus,* has not been shown to improve the outcome of adults with *S. aureus* bacteremia.[232] Early phase 2 clinical trials of eritoran tetrasodium, a TLR4 antagonist, for the treatment of severe sepsis seemed promising; however, a recently completed phase 3 randomized trial did not improve the primary endpoint of 28-day all-cause mortality in 2000 adult patients with severe sepsis (http://www.ukmi.nhs.uk/applications/ndo/record_view_open.asp?newDrugID=4747).[203]

Plasmapheresis, exchange transfusions, and extracorporeal membrane oxygenation are heroic measures that seem to be beneficial in selected patients not responding to standard management.[17,75,214] These procedures may be considered for such patients when, in the opinion of experienced clinicians, their use is justified and they are the last hope for a successful outcome.[71]

PROGNOSIS

The morbidity and mortality rates for septic shock in children vary with age, the presence or absence of underlying diseases, and the specific microorganisms responsible for the septicemic state. Dupont and Spink reported a 98% mortality rate in their series of children with septic shock and gram-negative bacteremia. Jacobs and colleagues reported a 9.8% case-fatality rate for otherwise normal children with septic shock. In the pediatric HA-1A study, the overall mortality rate for severe sepsis or septic shock was 31%. The overall mortality rate for children with meningococcal infection was 8% in a 10-center surveillance study. For the seven-state sepsis cohort, the overall mortality rate was approximately 10%. Much progress has been made in the treatment of sepsis and septic shock since the report of Dupont and Spink was published. As with many infections, prevention is more desirable than is treatment. Careful attention given to sterile techniques for insertion and maintenance of intravascular or other lines and other procedures is crucial and may prevent some episodes of bacteremia and septic shock.

NEW REFERENCES SINCE THE SEVENTH EDITION

7. Ames SG, Workman JK, Olson JA, et al. Infectious etiologies and patient outcomes in pediatric septic shock. *J Pediatric Infect Dis Soc.* 2017;6(1):80-86.
52. Dellinger RP, Levy MM, Rhodes A, et al. Surviving sepsis campaign: international guidelines for management of severe sepsis and septic shock: 2012. *Crit Care Med.* 2013;41(2):580-637.
112. Kumar A, Ellis P, Arabi Y, et al. Initiation of inappropriate antimicrobial therapy results in a fivefold reduction of survival in human septic shock. *Chest.* 2009;136(5):1237-1248.
120. Liu C, Bayer A, Cosgrove SE, et al. Clinical practice guidelines by the Infectious Diseases Society of America for the treatment of methicillin-resistant *Staphylococcus aureus* infections in adults and children: executive summary. *Clin Infect Dis.* 2011;52(3):285-292.
181. Ruth A, McCracken CE, Fortenberry JD, et al. Pediatric severe sepsis: current trends and outcomes from the Pediatric Health Information Systems database. *Pediatr Crit Care Med.* 2014;15(9):828-838.
185. Seymour CW, Liu VX, Iwashyna TJ, et al. Assessment of clinical criteria for sepsis: for the Third International Consensus Definitions for Sepsis and Septic Shock (Sepsis-3). *JAMA.* 2016;315(8):762-774.
186. Shankar-Hari M, Phillips GS, Levy ML, et al. Developing a new definition and assessing new clinical criteria for septic shock: for the third International Consensus Definitions for Sepsis and Septic Shock (Sepsis-3). *JAMA.* 2016;315(8):775-787.
190. Singer M, Deutschman CS, Seymour CW, et al. The third International Consensus Definitions for Sepsis and Septic Shock (Sepsis-3). *JAMA.* 2016;315(8):801-810.
201. Sutherland AM, Walley KR. Bench-to-bedside review: association of genetic variation with sepsis. *Crit Care.* 2009;13(2):210.
224. Volbeda M, Wetterslev J, Gluud C, et al. Glucocorticosteroids for sepsis: systematic review with meta-analysis and trial sequential analysis. *Intensive Care Med.* 2015;41(7):1220-1234.
235. Weiss SL, Fitzgerald JC, Balamuth F, et al. Delayed antimicrobial therapy increases mortality and organ dysfunction duration in pediatric sepsis. *Crit Care Med.* 2014;42(11):2409-2417.
236. Weiss SL, Fitzgerald JC, Pappachan J, et al. Global epidemiology of pediatric severe sepsis: the sepsis prevalence, outcomes, and therapies study. *Am J Respir Crit Care Med.* 2015;191(10):1147-1157.

The full reference list for this chapter is available at ExpertConsult.com.

63 Fever Without Source and Fever of Unknown Origin

Debra L. Palazzi

Petersdorf and Beeson[82] in 1961 proposed that the term *fever of unknown origin* (FUO) be reserved for persons with an illness persisting for 3 or more weeks and accompanied by temperatures higher than 38.4°C (101.2°F) on at least several occasions. They further specified that the cause of the fever should remain undetermined after at least 1 week of investigation in the hospital. Although this definition was arbitrary, it was useful at that time, when many of the diagnostic tests now in routine use were unknown. The purpose of their precise definition was to explore the cause of fever in this select group of adult patients and to permit comparison of data from different investigations. This exacting definition probably never was applied rigorously in pediatric practice. In children, the term *fever of unknown origin* should be reserved for fever of at least 8 days' duration and for which no diagnosis is apparent after the initial workup in the hospital or as an outpatient.

Many investigators use the term *fever without source* (FWS) for fever of recent onset with no adequate explanation determined by the history or physical examination. The distinction between FUO and FWS is of more than academic interest for several reasons. First, although overlap exists, the differential diagnoses of these clinical conditions are distinct, and the most frequent causes of one can be different from the most frequent causes of the other. Second, a child with fever of recent onset generally warrants more immediate evaluation than does a child with FUO. The latter usually does not occur as an emergency and requires timely, but not urgent, diagnostic or therapeutic intervention. Third, although expectant antibiotic treatment of children with FUO generally is not indicated, expectant treatment of infants with FWS is recommended in certain cases.

FEVER WITHOUT SOURCE

A convenient definition of FWS is the occurrence of fever for 1 week or less in a child in whom a careful history and physical examination fail to reveal a probable cause of the fever. An estimated 14% of children with fever have no localizing signs or symptoms.[103] Most children with fever of recent onset have acute infectious diseases, the majority of which are self-limited.[110] A few of these patients have serious acute infectious diseases, including meningitis, bacteremia, and urinary tract infection, and a very few have acute noninfectious diseases or chronic disorders. For example, an occasional patient with FWS is discovered to have a disorder such as heat illness, drug poisoning, Kawasaki disease, malignancy, or connective tissue disease. However, these disorders occur infrequently. A physician faced with a child with FWS should consider the possibility of a noninfectious cause or the onset of a chronic disease, but unless a clinical clue suggests one of these entities, investigation in this direction is not warranted.

Many children with FWS are in the prodromal stages of an acute infectious illness, and evidence of a specific infection, such as pharyngitis, otitis media, or pneumonia, develops within hours to days of first being evaluated by a physician. Fever can precede the appearance of specific signs and symptoms by as long as 3 days, as in measles, Rocky Mountain spotted fever, and leptospirosis. In some infections, such as roseola, viral hepatitis, infectious mononucleosis, typhus, and typhoid fever, the interval between the onset of fever and the appearance of specific findings often is more than 3 days.

Occult Bacteremia

One concern regarding a young child with FWS is the possibility that the child has occult bacteremia.[47] The patient does not appear ill, is judged clinically well enough to be managed as an outpatient, and does not have an infection commonly associated with bacteremia, such as pneumonia, but the blood culture yields pathogenic bacteria such as *Streptococcus pneumoniae, Neisseria meningitidis, Haemophilus influenzae, Escherichia coli, Salmonella,* group A streptococcus, or *Staphylococcus aureus.* Before introduction of the pneumococcal conjugate vaccines, the incidence of occult bacteremia in children with FWS was approximately 3% to 5%.[7,14,25,50,61,65,75,99,110] More recent data report an incidence of less than 1%, although this figure may vary depending on vaccine coverage rates in the population studied.[2,3,31,46,85,90,97,103,108] A large prospective study of 3571 febrile children younger than 3 years of age found that no patients who had received at least one vaccination of heptavalent pneumococcal vaccine had pneumococcal bacteremia.[26] With the introduction of the 13-valent pneumococcal conjugate vaccine, further decreases in occult bacteremia caused by pneumococci are anticipated.[27,45]

Historically occult bacteremia was found to occur more commonly in children with FWS than in febrile children of the same age with infections such as pharyngitis, otitis media, or upper respiratory tract infection. In the 1970s, investigators[65] reported the incidence of bacteremia in febrile children without an obvious source of infection to be 9.9%, as opposed to 3.3% in children with otitis media, upper respiratory tract infection, or a flulike syndrome. During the same era, Teele and colleagues[99] found a 3.9% incidence of bacteremia in children with FWS and a 1.5% incidence in comparably febrile children with otitis media or pharyngitis.

The risk for occult bacteremia developing in a child with FWS is age related, with the greatest risk occurring in the first few months of life. Numerous studies have demonstrated a higher risk for bacteremia or other serious bacterial infections in febrile infants younger than 3 months old.[63,65,89,99] In a group of children with clinically unsuspected meningococcemia, all 12 patients who initially looked well enough to be treated as outpatients were younger than 24 months of age.[34] In the 1990s, Bonadio and colleagues[21] found the incidence of positive bacterial cultures to be 12% in febrile infants younger than 4 weeks and 6% in those between 4 and 8 weeks of age. A more recent retrospective study of bacteremia in infants 1 week to 3 months of age found 2% of all blood cultures were positive for pathogens.[41] The risk for having occult bacteremia and other serious bacterial infections increases with the severity of fever.[66] In a prospective study in which blood was obtained for culture from all febrile children younger than 2 years seen in a walk-in clinic, no positive blood cultures were found in 44 children with FWS and rectal temperatures lower than 38.9°C (102°F), whereas five (3.9%) positive blood cultures were found in 129 children with FWS and rectal temperatures of 38.9°C (102°F) or higher.[87,99] Other studies have reported similar findings.[14,63,90] Several series of children with fevers of 41°C (105.8°F) or higher found a relatively high prevalence of bacteremia and other serious bacterial infections, especially meningitis and pneumonia.[20,63,87] However, even in this group of children with very high fever, most of those older than 2 or 3 months of age who looked well did not have a serious bacterial infection.

The white blood cell (WBC) count has been studied extensively as a potential tool in the diagnosis of occult bacteremia. On the basis of a study of hospitalized children, Todd[100] reported that the absolute number of polymorphonuclear leukocytes and the absolute number of nonsegmented polymorphonuclear leukocytes were more sensitive than was the total WBC count, the percentage of polymorphonuclear leukocytes, or the percentage of nonsegmented polymorphonuclear leukocytes. However, whether information based on hospitalized children—presumably all of whom had serious localized infections or looked ill enough to warrant hospitalization—can be applied to children with FWS who look well enough to be treated on an ambulatory basis is questionable.

Considerable debate continues over the usefulness of the WBC count in febrile children evaluated in the outpatient setting. McCarthy and associates[66] concluded that a WBC count of 15,000/mm^3 or greater was helpful in identifying patients at greatest risk for the development of bacteremia. Dershewitz[35] found a direct relationship between the total leukocyte count and the prevalence of bacteremia and stated that "knowledge of the count was a helpful but limited predictor of patients with positive blood cultures." Other investigators reported that the incidence of bacteremia increased with an increased WBC count[90] and that bacteremia most commonly occurred in patients with counts of 20,000/mm^3 or higher.[71]

Other studies have examined the utility of the WBC count specifically in children with FWS who look well enough to be treated on an outpatient basis. One such study found a sensitivity of 1.0 and a positive predictive value of 0.11 for a total WBC count of 15,000/mm^3.[99] Using a WBC count of 20,000/mm^3 would have decreased the sensitivity to 0.4 while increasing the positive predictive value to only 0.13. In another series, the sensitivity for a WBC count of 15,000/mm^3 was 0.87, with a specificity of 0.73.[14] Although a total WBC count of 15,000/mm^3 does not accurately predict which child is or is not bacteremic, it is helpful in dividing the population of children with FWS into high- and low-risk groups.[15,46] However, the value of the 15,000/mm^3 level has been substantially reduced in the studies conducted since the pneumococcal conjugate vaccine was introduced.

Some investigators have found the erythrocyte sedimentation rate to be no more useful than the WBC count in predicting bacteremia in ambulatory febrile patients.[66] Others have reported that the serum concentration of C-reactive protein may be more accurate than the complete blood count or erythrocyte sedimentation rate in distinguishing bacterial from viral infections.[64,81] However, recent studies reported conflicting data regarding the utility of the C-reactive protein test in screening children 3 to 36 months old for occult bacteremia.[48,88,95] An elevated serum procalcitonin level has been found by some investigators to be at least as sensitive and specific as C-reactive protein in predicting serious bacterial infection in children with fever and no localizing signs.[5,56,86,113] A meta-analysis of 881 children from developed countries with FWS found that procalcitonin in addition to WBC count and C-reactive protein tests was more accurate for detecting early meningococcal disease than WBC and C-reactive protein testing alone.[17]

Other hematologic findings that suggest bacteremia include thrombocytopenia,[30] Döhle inclusion bodies, toxic granulations, and vacuolization of neutrophils. In one study, peripheral blood smears of children younger than 24 months with acute febrile illnesses were reviewed the following day by a single investigator to determine whether vacuolization and toxic granulations were present; when both abnormalities were present, the positive predictive value for bacteremia was 0.76.[58] The presence of these findings should be considered when estimating the risk for bacteremia.[1,30,74]

Several studies have examined the response to acetaminophen and found no difference in the rate of reduction of temperature or improvement in clinical appearance between bacteremic and nonbacteremic children.[10,101,112] Mazur and associates,[62] however, found that febrile children aged 2 months to 6 years who did not respond to a dose of acetaminophen by a reduction in temperature of at least 0.8°C in 2 hours had a statistically significant increased risk for having occult bacteremia in contrast to those who did respond.

The most important aspects of assessment of a febrile child are a careful history and physical examination. Laboratory data are secondary and should be ordered on the basis of the clinical assessment. By definition, a child with FWS has no localizing signs to explain the fever or indicate a site of infection. Many physicians suggest that a general impression can indicate whether the child has occult bacteremia. Some physicians have suggested that careful clinical judgment, based on extensive experience, can identify most, if not all, children with serious illnesses.[19,79] McCarthy and colleagues,[65,67-69] in a series of carefully designed studies, elucidated the variables of history and observation that were most useful in assessing febrile children. They found that observation of the variable *playfulness* had the strongest correlation with overall assessment.[68] However, they observed that even an experienced attending pediatrician could identify only 57% of seriously ill children by initial impression before performing a full physical examination. Dershewitz[35] found that private pediatricians were no more accurate than pediatric residents in identifying children with occult bacteremia and that, in the private office, pediatricians were no better at predicting bacteremia in familiar patients than in first-time patients.

In a study of 292 consecutive febrile children seen in an emergency department, Waskerwitz and Berkelhammer[105] identified a subgroup of patients who had no localizing signs and who looked so well that they were predicted not to have bacteremia. The physicians were assisted in their assessment by a functional scale that gave 0 to 2 points for the child's eating, drinking, sleeping, and play activities, with a best possible score of 8. The group of patients who had functional scores of 5 or greater, with no localized infection and predicted clinically not to have bacteremia, were free of bacteremia, whereas 14 of 202 patients with functional scores of 4 or less were bacteremic. In this study, the physicians were not able to identify which patients had bacteremia and which did not; rather, they were able to identify one subgroup at high risk for having bacteremia and another at very low risk. Teach and Fleisher[98] found that although Yale Observation Scale scores were higher in patients with bacteremia than in those without, the difference was not clinically useful in detecting bacteremia in well-looking febrile children without a discernible focus of infection. The clinician's overall assessment of the degree of illness of the child appears to be a valuable but not infallible tool in estimating the risk for occult bacteremia in children with FWS.

Clinical Management of Fever Without Source

The clinician should not be dogmatic about the management of children with FWS. One reasonable approach, based on a careful history, thorough physical examination, and overall clinical impression, is to classify these children as being at low or high risk for the presence of occult bacteremia and other serious bacterial infections. For the low-risk group, no laboratory investigation is required routinely. For the high-risk group, a complete blood count and blood culture should be obtained, especially in young infants and children who are incompletely immunized. Many studies have shown that the most common serious bacterial infection in children with FWS is urinary tract infection.[4,103,106] Therefore, urinalysis and urine culture should be performed in febrile infants and children younger than 24 months of age. Lumbar puncture and chest radiography are considered on an individual basis. If the patient appears ill, admission to the hospital may be justified even if all test results are negative. When high-risk children look well enough to be sent home, they are reasonable candidates for expectant antibiotic therapy pending the outcome of blood and urine cultures. For patients clinically considered to be at moderate risk (not clearly high or low risk), the physician has the option of obtaining a WBC count and using the results to decide whether to obtain blood and urine for culture and prescribe antibiotics expectantly.

Table 63.1 lists risk factors for the development of occult bacteremia. Current information is not sufficient to warrant the use of scoring systems except as part of investigational series. In the final analysis, the clinician's judgment, taking into account all available clinical and laboratory data about each patient, is the guide to selecting which children require a diagnostic workup and expectant therapy with antibiotics.

If the physician elects to prescribe antibiotics while awaiting the results of blood culture, such antibiotic therapy should provide adequate coverage for *S. pneumoniae, N. meningitidis,* and *H. influenzae,* although the frequency of *H. influenzae* and *S. pneumoniae* has decreased dramatically with current immunization practice, and *N. meningitidis* is uncommon. A single injection of ceftriaxone 50 to 75 mg/kg given while awaiting the results of blood culture has been successful in resolving fever, clearing bacteremia, and preventing meningitis and was found to be superior to oral regimens in several series.[13,16,40] Children with a positive blood culture should be recalled for re-evaluation even if they are afebrile.[8] Children who have been immunized against both *H. influenzae* and *S. pneumoniae* should be considered to be at relatively low risk for the development of occult bacteremia and may require less workup unless they appear ill or have a very high fever.

Infants younger than 90 days pose a special problem because they have an increased risk for developing a serious bacterial infection, clinical evaluation is more difficult, and a broader spectrum of invading organisms (e.g., group B streptococcus, *E. coli,* and *Listeria monocytogenes*) exists. Baker and coworkers[9] showed the safety of managing selected

TABLE 63.1 Risk Factors for Occult Bacteremia

Factor	High Risk	Low Risk
Age	≤3 months	>3 months
Immunization status[a]	Incomplete	Complete
Magnitude of fever	≥40°C (104°F)	≤39.4°C (103°F)
White blood cell count	≥15,000/mm^3	<15,000/mm^3
Peripheral blood smear	Toxic granulation or vacuolization of polymorphonuclear leukocytes, thrombocytopenia	Unremarkable
Underlying chronic disorder	Sickle-cell disease, immunodeficiency, malnutrition	None
History of contact with bacterial disease	Contact with *Neisseria meningitidis* or *Haemophilus influenzae*	None
Clinical appearance	Appears ill, toxic, or unhappy; inconsolable; irritable or lethargic; not eating or drinking enough	Looks well, playful, eating normally, not irritable

[a]Vaccination status is incomplete if the child has received fewer than three doses of *Haemophilus influenzae* vaccine and fewer than three doses of conjugated pneumococcal vaccine and is complete if the child received at least three doses of each vaccine.

low-risk infants (i.e., normal WBC count, urinalysis, lumbar puncture, and chest radiograph, and, if diarrhea was present, negative smear for fecal leukocytes) 30 to 90 days of age on an outpatient basis without antibiotics. Jaskiewicz and coworkers[52] found the Rochester criteria (WBC count of 5000 to 15,000/mm^3, band count <1500/mm^3, spun urine specimen <10 WBCs/high-power field, stool specimen [if diarrhea] <5 WBCs/high-power field) to have a 98.9% negative predictive value in well-appearing, previously healthy infants younger than 90 days with no focal infections. One reasonable practice guideline for managing infants with FWS is to hospitalize and treat all who appear toxic and all younger than 28 to 30 days. Those between 30 and 90 days of age can be managed as outpatients if they look well and the blood count, urinalysis, and cerebrospinal fluid analysis (if empiric antibiotics are to be prescribed) are within normal limits.[11,12]

FEVER OF UNKNOWN ORIGIN

The exact definition of FUO is a subject of considerable disagreement, and series in the pediatric literature differ in their criteria for inclusion. Brewis[22] defined FUO in children as a temperature of 38.3°C (101°F) or higher for 5 to 7 consecutive days without localizing signs or symptoms. In sharp contrast, McClung[70] and Lohr and Hendley[59] considered children with fever for at least 3 weeks on an outpatient basis or 1 week in the hospital to have FUO. Pizzo and associates,[84] however, required only that the fever be present for 2 weeks, with no distinction made between outpatient or in-hospital status. A reasonable working definition of FUO for clinical purposes is the presence of fever for 8 or more days in a child for whom a careful and thorough history, physical examination, and preliminary laboratory data fail to reveal a probable cause of the fever.

Most cases of FUO in children are caused by relatively common diseases.[38] In four series of FUO totaling 418 children, only five patients would be considered to have rare disorders (i.e., Behçet syndrome, ichthyosis, variant of "blue diaper" syndrome, diencephalic seizure disorder, and "possible chronic lead and/or arsenic intoxication").[22,59,70,84] The adage that FUO is more likely to be caused by an unusual manifestation of a common disorder than by a common manifestation of a rare disorder certainly is true in pediatrics. The three most common discernible causes of FUO in children, in order of decreasing frequency, are infectious diseases, connective tissue diseases, and neoplasms. In approximately 10% to 20% of cases, a definitive diagnosis never is established.

In the United States, the systemic infectious diseases diagnosed most frequently in children with FUO include tuberculosis, brucellosis, tularemia, salmonellosis, cat-scratch fever and infections caused by rickettsia, spirochetes (e.g., leptospirosis), Epstein-Barr virus, cytomegalic inclusion virus, human immunodeficiency virus (HIV), hepatitis viruses, and other viruses. The most common causes of localized infection are upper respiratory tract infections (e.g., sinusitis, otitis, tonsillitis), urinary tract infection, osteomyelitis, and occult abscesses, including hepatic and pelvic abscesses.

The connective tissue disease most commonly manifested as FUO in children is juvenile idiopathic arthritis, which accounts for more than 90% of connective tissue diseases in most series, followed by systemic lupus erythematosus and then by undefined vasculitis.[59,70,73,84] Frequently a definitive diagnosis of juvenile idiopathic arthritis can be made only after an extended period of observation because physical examination may yield few findings and the results of specific serologic studies generally are normal or negative.

Malignancy is a less frequent cause of FUO in children than in adults and usually is the third-largest group, after infectious diseases and connective tissue diseases. Malignancy accounted for 7% of FUO cases in the series reported by Pizzo and associates[84] and for 13% in the Lohr and Hendley[59] series. Leukemia and lymphoma are responsible for most cases of cancer manifested as FUO in children. Other tumors less commonly reported as causing FUO include neuroblastoma, hepatoma, sarcoma, and atrial myxoma.

The prognosis for children with FUO is better than that for adults, and most children with FUO have treatable or self-limited disease. Historically mortality rates for children with FUO were 6% to 9%.[59,84] However, more contemporary studies indicate that mortality is quite low.[80]

Diagnostic Approach to a Child With Fever of Unknown Origin

A child with FUO may be admitted to the hospital for more than simply laboratory investigation. Hospitalization provides an opportunity to observe the child, repeat the history and physical examination, analyze all available data, and investigate every potential diagnostic lead. In the Lohr and Hendley[59] series of 54 children with FUO, an incomplete history delayed establishing the diagnosis in nine cases, and physical findings that were ignored delayed rendering the diagnosis in four cases. In McClung's report[70] of 99 pediatric cases of FUO, errors in the history or physical examination obscured the correct diagnosis for at least 10 patients. Failure to use existing laboratory data correctly is another common factor preventing early determination of the diagnosis in children with FUO.[59,84]

Clinical Evaluation

The first and most important step in the diagnostic workup of a child with FUO is obtaining a complete and detailed history and conducting a physical examination. The clinical evaluation must be thorough and careful, and it must be repeated frequently. Often a patient or parent eventually recalls information that was omitted or forgotten when the initial history was obtained. Physical findings change, and abnormalities not originally present can appear subsequently. Lohr and Hendley[59] noted that in more than 25% of children admitted to the hospital with FUO, significant physical findings developed that were not present at the time of admission.

A detailed history should be obtained regarding contact with infected or otherwise ill persons and any exposure to animals, including pets and wild animals. The number of children with zoonotic infections is increasing each year. History of a cat scratch or exposure to kittens may be a clue for *Bartonella henselae*. Immunization of domestic animals such as the dog against leptospirosis can prevent canine disease, but it does not prevent carriage, excretion, and transmission of this infection. A history of travel extending back to birth must be elicited. Reemergence of histoplasmosis, coccidioidomycosis, blastomycosis, leishmaniasis, or malaria years after visiting or living in an endemic area can occur. Inquiring about prophylactic immunizations, precautions taken against the ingestion of contaminated food or water, and malarial prophylaxis is important. Questioning should include the possibility that rocks, soil, or artifacts from geographically distant regions may have been brought into the home, as well as the possibility that contact with persons who have visited distant countries has occurred. Even contact with insects can be important. Tick bites can be a clue to Rocky Mountain spotted fever or tick-borne relapsing fever. North American mosquitoes and some ticks carry a variety of arboviruses.

The physician should determine whether the patient has eaten game meat, raw meat, or raw shellfish. A history of pica should be sought routinely. Ingestion of dirt can suggest a diagnosis of visceral larva migrans, toxoplasmosis, or other infectious diseases. A detailed history regarding all medications, including topical agents and nonprescription items, must be elicited. Any history of surgical procedures should be explored.

Questions designed to determine the genetic or ethnic background of the patient can reveal information that specifically suggests or largely excludes diagnoses such as nephrogenic diabetes insipidus (found in Ulster Scots), familial Mediterranean fever (found in Armenians, Arabs, and Sephardic Jews), familial dysautonomia (found in Jews), and Kikuchi-Fujimoto disease, a benign and self-limited histiocytic necrotizing lymphadenitis (found mostly in young Asian females and characterized by fever, lymphadenopathy, and malaise).

The history should be exacting regarding the duration, height, and pattern of the fever, as well as the circumstances under which temperature elevation occurs, whether the child appears ill or any signs or symptoms develop, and how well the fever responds to antipyretic drugs. A history of "fever" occurring only after exercise or late in the afternoon can indicate parental concern about normal variations in body temperature. A history of high fever occurring in the absence of malaise or other generalized signs can be a clue to factitious fever. The physician also should obtain a careful history regarding how well the fever has been documented. Has a thermometer been used, by whom, and in whose presence? A history of sweating and heat intolerance can indicate hyperthyroidism, whereas a history of heat intolerance with the absence of sweating can be a clue to ectodermal dysplasia.

Several investigators found that neither the pattern of fever nor its duration was useful in pointing to or establishing a diagnosis in children with FUO.[59,84] However occasionally the character of the fever can be helpful. *Intermittent fever* is characterized by a return of temperature to normal at least once daily. If the peak of fever is high and the rate of defervescence quick, this pattern often is referred to as *hectic* or *spiking*. Intermittent fevers suggest pyogenic infections but also occur with tuberculosis, lymphoma, and juvenile idiopathic arthritis. In *remittent fever,* the temperature fluctuates but does not return to normal. A *sustained fever* pattern is characterized by persistent fever with little or no fluctuation and can occur in typhoid fever or typhus. Antipyretic agents can make a remittent or sustained fever appear intermittent. *Relapsing fever* refers to a pattern in which the patient is afebrile for 1 or more days between episodes of fever and can be seen with malaria, rat-bite fever, infection with *Borrelia,* and lymphoma. Recurrent episodes of fever of more than a year's duration can suggest metabolic defects, central nervous system abnormalities in temperature control, and immunodeficient states.

The general activity and appearance of the patient should be observed, vital signs checked, and growth parameters measured. Weight loss is an important, though nonspecific, finding. Impairment of linear growth or short stature can be a clue to inflammatory bowel disease, an intracranial lesion involving the pituitary gland, or a long-standing chronic disease. Examining the patient during an episode of fever to observe the presence or absence of sweating, the effect of the fever on the heart and respiratory rate, the presence or absence of malaise or other symptoms, and the appearance of "toxicity" is helpful. The rash of juvenile idiopathic arthritis characteristically is evanescent and may be present only during periods of temperature elevation.

Some special aspects of the physical examination merit mention. Hypohidrosis, anomalous dentition, and sparse hair, particularly involving the eyebrows and eyelashes, suggest anhidrotic ectodermal dysplasia. Palpebral conjunctivitis can be a clue to the presence of infectious mononucleosis, Newcastle disease, or lupus erythematosus, whereas predominantly bulbar conjunctivitis can suggest leptospirosis or Kawasaki disease. Phlyctenular conjunctivitis can signal tuberculosis.

Absence of the pupillary constrictor response can be caused by a deficiency of the constrictor sphincter muscle of the eye. This muscle, derived from ectoderm rather than mesoderm, develops embryologically at the same time that hypothalamic structures and function are undergoing differentiation. Absence of this muscle can suggest that the elevation in temperature is the result of hypothalamic or autonomic dysfunction. Careful funduscopic examination can disclose evidence of miliary tuberculosis, vasculitis, or toxoplasmosis. Lack of tears, absence of corneal reflexes, and a smooth tongue with absence of the fungiform papillae suggest familial dysautonomia.

Purulent or persistent nasal discharge can be a sign of sinusitis. The physician should palpate for tenderness over the sinuses.

Hyperemia of the pharynx, even in the absence of exudate or specific symptoms, can be a clue to the diagnosis of infectious mononucleosis, cytomegalovirus, toxoplasmosis, tularemia, or leptospirosis. Gingival hypertrophy or inflammation and loosening or loss of teeth can indicate leukemia or Langerhans cell histiocytosis.

The bones and muscles should be palpated carefully. Tenderness over a bone can be found in cases of osteomyelitis or marrow invasion by neoplastic disease. The appreciation of a new heart murmur may result from infective endocarditis. Muscle tenderness can be associated with trichinosis, dermatomyositis, polyarteritis, or various arboviral infections.

The search for skin lesions and rash must be careful, extensive, and repeated. Petechiae can indicate endocarditis or other sources of bacteremia but also can occur with viral and rickettsial infections. A seborrheic rash can be a sign of histiocytosis. A small papule present for more than a week may be the inoculation site for cat-scratch disease.

A careful rectal examination can reveal pararectal tenderness or a mass indicative of a pelvic abscess or tumor. A test for occult blood should be performed on stool. Examination of the external genitalia should be completed on patients of all ages, and sexually active adolescent females should undergo a pelvic examination.

Laboratory Evaluation

The extent of laboratory investigation depends on the age of the patient, duration of the fever, and history and physical examination findings. Laboratory studies should be directed, as much as possible, toward the most likely diagnostic possibilities. The tempo of the diagnostic evaluation should be adjusted to the severity of the illness. In a critically ill child, speedy evaluation is important. If the patient is less severely ill, however, the evaluation can proceed more slowly; sometimes the fever can disappear without apparent explanation before a definitive diagnosis can be established and any invasive diagnostic procedures have been undertaken.

A complete blood count and careful examination of the peripheral smear are indicated for all patients. Anemia, thrombocytosis, and thrombocytopenia should be noted. Although mild or moderate changes in the total WBC or differential count usually are of no help, in some series, children with more than 10,000 polymorphonuclear leukocytes or 500 nonsegmented neutrophils/mm^3 were found to have a greater likelihood of having a serious bacterial infection.[100] Atypical lymphocytes generally indicate viral infection, whereas bizarre or immature forms can suggest leukemia. Although the erythrocyte sedimentation rate and C-reactive protein are of no specific diagnostic value, they are a general indicator of inflammation and can help in ruling out factitious fever, determining the need for further evaluation, and monitoring the progress of the disease process.

Blood should be obtained from all patients for aerobic and anaerobic culture. In select cases, media appropriate for the isolation of *Francisella* organisms, *Leptospira,* and *Spirillum* also should be used.

Urine analysis and culture should be completed for all patients. In one series of FUO in children, failure to perform urinalysis and failure to investigate pyuria adequately were the most common laboratory errors.[70] Radiographic study of the urinary tract, however, should be performed only when indicated.

All patients should undergo radiographic examination of the chest. Diagnostic imaging of the nasal sinuses, mastoids, and gastrointestinal tract is performed initially only for specific indications but may be done eventually in all children whose fever persists without explanation for a long period. Persistent fever and elevation of the erythrocyte sedimentation rate or C-reactive protein, with or without anemia, abdominal complaints, anorexia, and weight loss, are sufficient indications for radiographic study to evaluate for inflammatory bowel disease.

All patients should have an intradermal tuberculin skin test. Control skin tests with antigens such as *Candida* are of limited value because the anergy may be specific for tuberculosis rather than universal for all skin-testing materials.[60,72,76,77] A positive control test result and negative tuberculin test result do not rule out tuberculosis.

Bone marrow examination is most useful in diagnosing cancer (especially leukemia), histiocytic disorders, and hemophagocytic disease. It is less useful in determining infection. Hayani and associates[44] reviewed the results of 414 bone marrow examinations for FUO in children. In only one case was an organism (*Salmonella* group D) recovered from the marrow that also was not recovered from blood or another source. Noninfectious causes of FUO were found in 8% of specimens: malignancy (6.7%), hemophagocytic lymphohistiocytosis (0.7%), histiocytosis (0.5%), and hypoplastic anemia (0.2%). In most of these cases, the diagnosis had been suspected clinically before the bone marrow was examined.

Patients should undergo a serum test for HIV infection. Other appropriate serologic tests can help establish a diagnosis of cat-scratch disease, brucellosis, tularemia, Epstein-Barr virus infection, cytomegalovirus infection, other viral infections, toxoplasmosis, and certain fungal infections.

Hepatic enzymes and serum chemistry, including electrolytes, urea nitrogen, and creatinine, should be determined in all patients. Serum antinuclear antibody should be measured in those older than 5 years if family history is significant or clinical suspicion warrants it. Serum hepatitis antigens, electrocardiography, electroencephalography, echocardiography, and stool culture and examination for ova and parasites generally should be performed in selected cases. Other tests to be considered for individual patients include ophthalmologic examination by slit lamp, radiographic bone survey, technetium bone scan, abdominal imaging by ultrasonography, computed tomography (CT), or magnetic resonance imaging (MRI).[24,83] CT scanning and indium-111 scanning[39] can detect inflammatory lesions and tumors. Such scanning procedures offer a relatively noninvasive technique for screening patients with FUO for a variety of disorders. Steele and associates[94] found that radionucleotide scans seldom led to unsuspected diagnoses in children and suggested that they not be used indiscriminately. Gallium scanning has been helpful in diagnosing adult patients with FUO[43] but is not generally recommended in children. Recent evidence suggests that (18)F fluorodeoxyglucose positron emission tomography (FDG PET) imaging may be useful in select adults and children with FUO in whom the etiology of fever remains elusive despite thorough physical examination, laboratory evaluation, and basic imaging techniques.[53,92] FDG PET may be able to detect causes of FUO such as infection, tumor, and noninfectious inflammation because they all exhibit hypermetabolism of glucose. Identification of abnormalities using FDG PET could guide the next steps in clinical decision making to make the diagnosis. More invasive testing such as lymph node biopsy, liver biopsy, and exploratory laparoscopy are reserved for patients with evidence of involvement of these organs.

In general, antibiotics or other medications should not be administered empirically as a diagnostic measure in children with FUO. Exceptions include the use of nonsteroidal agents in children with presumed juvenile idiopathic arthritis and the use of antituberculosis drugs in critically ill children thought to have disseminated tuberculosis. Empiric trials of broad-spectrum antibiotics generally do more to obscure than illuminate the etiology of FUO and can mask or delay establishing the diagnosis of infections such as meningitis, parameningeal infection, endocarditis, or osteomyelitis.

Examples of disorders that can be manifested as FUO in children are listed in Box 63.1. A few of these disorders are discussed briefly in the following sections.

Infectious Causes of Fever of Unknown Origin

Infectious causes of FUO can be divided into systemic and localized. Immunodeficiency states may be considered under the general classification of infections.

Generalized Infections

Brucellosis. The manifestation of this disease as FUO is explained by the nonspecific symptoms that it engenders and by the chronicity of untreated infection. Many physicians, particularly in urban areas, tend to ignore the possibility of this disease and neglect to inquire about a history of exposure to animals or animal products, especially the consumption of unpasteurized goat's milk cheese (see Chapter 128).

Cat-scratch disease. During recent years, many children with FUO have proved to be infected with *B. henselae*. Cat-scratch disease is one of the most common causes of FUO in patients seen at the infectious disease service at Texas Children's Hospital in Houston.[6] Most of the children with this manifestation of cat-scratch disease have hepatosplenic involvement. Jacobs and Schutze[49] reported that *B. henselae* infection was the cause of 4.8% of all cases of FUO at the Arkansas Children's Hospital and 10.9% of the cases of FUO caused by infection. *B. henselae* infection is best diagnosed by serologic evaluation (i.e., immunofluorescence assay that detects serum antibody to *B. henselae*). Biopsy of lesions (e.g., lymph nodes, liver, bone marrow) may allow visualization of bacilli with the Warthin-Starry silver stain; however, this finding is not specific for *B. henselae*. Management of patients with cat-scratch disease is primarily symptomatic because the disease usually is self-limited. Antimicrobial therapy can be helpful in acutely or severely ill patients, especially those with hepatosplenic disease. Several oral antimicrobial regimens (rifampin, trimethoprim-sulfamethoxazole, and azithromycin) and parenteral gentamicin have been used successfully for the treatment of this disease. Specifically rifampin 20 mg/kg per day in two divided doses for 14 days has been particularly efficacious.[6] However, the optimal duration of therapy is not known.

Leptospirosis. Leptospirosis is caused by a single family of organisms composed of multiple serotypes; it is one of the most widespread zoonoses in the world. Transmission of infection from animal to human can occur by direct contact with the blood, tissue, organs, or urine of infected animals or indirectly by exposure to an environment that has been contaminated by leptospires. The organism also can be acquired from soil or from fresh water after ingestion. Reports indicate that leptospirosis is not a rare disease, that many infections are not associated with occupational exposure, and that urban and suburban cases are becoming more prevalent.[114] Clinical manifestations of leptospirosis usually are not specific. A variety of laboratory aids are available, but specimens must be collected and handled properly. In some cases, establishing a definitive diagnosis may be impossible; negative cultures or failure to demonstrate a rise in antibody titer does not exclude the possibility that the patient has active infection because the organism may not be present in the specimens that have been cultured, the antibody titer may have peaked before an acute-phase specimen was collected, and antibiotic therapy may suppress the development of positive titers or delay their appearance (see Chapter 142).

Toxoplasmosis. Toxoplasmosis should be considered in any child with persistent fever. Cervical or supraclavicular adenopathy is present in most cases, but occasionally fever is the only manifestation. The diagnosis is established by demonstration of a rising serologic titer; antibody to *Toxoplasma gondii* is so prevalent that demonstration of a high titer alone is not diagnostic of acute infection. Demonstration of *Toxoplasma* in tissue sections or body fluid is highly suggestive, although the organism can persist in tissue for years. Isolation of the parasite is not absolutely diagnostic of recent infection (see Chapter 224).

Malaria. Malaria also should be considered in children with FUO. In addition to fever, splenomegaly usually is present. A history of travel to endemic areas should be sought, although malaria has occurred in patients who never traveled outside the United States. Disease can occur even in persons who have taken antimalarial drugs when they visited

BOX 63.1 Causes of Fever of Unknown Origin in Children

Infectious Diseases

Bacterial

Bacterial endocarditis
Brucellosis
Cat-scratch disease
Leptospirosis
Liver abscess
Mastoiditis (chronic)
Osteomyelitis
Pelvic abscess
Perinephric abscess
Pyelonephritis
Salmonellosis
Sinusitis
Subdiaphragmatic abscess
Tuberculosis
Tularemia

Viral

Adenovirus
Arboviruses
Cytomegalovirus
Epstein-Barr virus (infectious mononucleosis)
Hepatitis viruses

Chlamydial

Lymphogranuloma venereum
Psittacosis

Rickettsial

Q fever
Rocky Mountain spotted fever

Fungal

Blastomycosis (nonpulmonary)
Histoplasmosis (disseminated)

Parasitic

Malaria
Toxoplasmosis
Visceral larva migrans

Unclassified

Sarcoidosis

Collagen Vascular Diseases

Juvenile rheumatoid arthritis
Polyarteritis nodosa
Systemic lupus erythematosus

Malignancies

Hodgkin disease
Leukemia and lymphoma
Neuroblastoma

Miscellaneous

Central diabetes insipidus
Drug fever
Ectodermal dysplasia
Factitious fever
Familial dysautonomia
Granulomatous colitis
Hemophagocytic lymphohistiocytosis
Infantile cortical hyperostosis
Kikuchi-Fujimoto disease
Nephrogenic diabetes insipidus
Pancreatitis
Periodic fever
Serum sickness
Thyrotoxicosis
Ulcerative colitis

the endemic region. A delay of several months can occur between the development of infection and the onset of symptoms. The infection can be transmitted from a person who has visited an endemic area to one who has not when an appropriate mosquito vector is present. Malaria also can be acquired by blood transfusion or by the use of needles and syringes contaminated by the parasite. Demonstration of malarial organisms on appropriately stained thin or thick smears of blood is diagnostic (see Chapter 220).

Salmonellosis. *Salmonella* organisms are contaminants in many food products. In view of the nonspecific signs and symptoms with which salmonellosis can occur, its association with FUO in children is not surprising. Repetitive blood and stool cultures are most helpful in establishing a diagnosis (see Chapter 111).

Tuberculosis. Tuberculosis is an important cause of FUO in children, as well as in adults. Nonpulmonary tuberculosis is manifested as FUO more frequently than is pulmonary tuberculosis, which usually is evident on routine chest radiographs. FUO occurs most commonly with disseminated tuberculosis or infection of the liver, peritoneum, pericardium, or genitourinary tract. Active disseminated tuberculosis has been well documented in children with negative results on chest radiography and tuberculin skin tests.[77,96] Negative interferon-γ release assay results also may occur.[32] A high index of suspicion and a careful history of possible contacts are important to make the diagnosis. Funduscopic examination can reveal choroid tubercles. Liver and bone marrow frequently are involved in children with miliary tuberculosis; liver biopsy specimens and bone marrow aspirates should be obtained and processed for morphologic evaluation and culture. If the chest radiograph yields abnormal results, cultures of gastric aspirates, sputum, or both should be obtained. Because nontuberculous mycobacteria (i.e., atypical organisms) are present in the gastric contents of normal individuals, demonstration of acid-fast organisms on smears of gastric secretion does not necessarily indicate disease. Rarely a patient with tuberculous pericarditis has fever, weight loss, and weakness but no precordial pain or other specific cardiac complaints. Disseminated infection with atypical mycobacteria generally is seen in patients infected with HIV (see Chapter 96) or those with other immunodeficiencies.

Tularemia. Generally failure to consider tularemia in children with FUO may be attributed to a lack of appreciation of the many sources of infection and the various routes of inoculation. The organism can be acquired from contact with a variety of animal species, as well as from ticks, mosquitoes, lice, fleas, flies, and contaminated water. The organism can penetrate mucous membranes and broken or unbroken skin, or it can be inhaled or swallowed. Patients and parents should be questioned about animal contact and the ingestion of rabbit or squirrel meat (see Chapter 132).

Viral infections. Infection by most viruses produces an illness that is relatively brief. Exceptions to this rule can include infections by adenovirus, cytomegalovirus, Epstein-Barr virus, hepatitis viruses, and certain arboviruses. In all of these diseases, symptoms are extremely variable, and signs and symptoms frequently are nonspecific. The diagnosis can be established by appropriate cultures and serologic studies (see Chapter 253).

Immunodeficiency. A variety of congenital and acquired immunodeficiency states can manifest as FUO. Patients with immunoglobulin deficiencies (e.g., Bruton agammaglobulinemia) may have a long history of recurrent fever, with or without evident infection, whereas patients with abnormalities in lymphocyte function are more likely to have prolonged fever caused by persistent viral or parasitic infection.

Localized Infections

Bacterial endocarditis. Infective endocarditis is an infrequent cause of FUO in children. Acute bacterial endocarditis tends to be fulminant, but the subacute form begins insidiously, generally at the site of a preexisting cardiac lesion. Subacute bacterial endocarditis is a rare occurrence in infants and increases in frequency with advancing age. The organisms most commonly encountered are viridans streptococci, enterococci, *S. aureus,* and *Staphylococcus epidermidis.* The absence of a cardiac murmur does not exclude the possibility of endocarditis, especially when the infection is limited to the right side of the heart. Endocarditis also can occur in the absence of positive blood cultures, particularly in association with the following factors: use of antibiotics for an undefined febrile illness, right-sided cardiac lesions, prolonged duration of disease, infection by unusual organisms such as *Brucella* or *Coxiella burnetii,* and inadequate culture methods for the detection of infection with anaerobic organisms. Frequently associated laboratory findings include anemia, leukocytosis, and an elevated erythrocyte sedimentation rate. Several blood cultures (aerobic and anaerobic) of adequate volume should be obtained before starting antibiotics. Echocardiography can reveal vegetations, but negative results do not rule out endocarditis (see Chapter 26).

Bone and joint infections. Infections of bones and joints usually can be diagnosed clinically but occasionally are manifested as FUO. This manifestation occurs commonly in young children who cannot explain where they hurt and is more likely to occur with osteomyelitis than with septic arthritis. Infection of the pelvic bones is implicated most often in this regard. Radioisotopic bone scan and MRI are more sensitive than are plain radiographs of the bones (see Chapters 55 and 56).

Intraabdominal abscesses. Subphrenic, perinephric, and pelvic abscesses may be manifested as FUO. A history of previous intraabdominal disease or abdominal surgery or a history of vague abdominal complaints should heighten suspicion of an intraabdominal collection of pus. The organisms involved most commonly are *S. aureus,* streptococci, *E. coli,* and anaerobic flora. Fever may be the only sign of a pelvic, perinephric, or psoas abscess. Urinalysis generally yields normal results, but the mass can be demonstrated by ultrasound examination, CT, or MRI.

Liver abscess and other hepatic infections. Pyogenic liver abscesses are encountered most frequently in immunocompromised pediatric patients but can be seen in otherwise normal children.[55] In some patients, persistent fever is the only finding. Blood cultures usually are sterile, and serum levels of liver enzymes generally are close to or within normal limits. Many patients have hepatomegaly and right upper quadrant abdominal tenderness. The diagnosis can be established by examination of the liver by ultrasonography, CT, or MRI. Bacterial hepatitis and bacterial cholangitis can occur in the absence of jaundice and other specific signs of liver dysfunction.[107,111] Granulomatous hepatitis is not a specific disease but rather a syndrome characterized by granuloma formation within the liver. A specific cause cannot be determined in every case. Although most reported cases have been in adults,[91] pediatric cases do occur, particularly with Epstein-Barr virus infection and with cat-scratch disease. The diagnosis can be made by ultrasound or other diagnostic imaging (see Chapter 49).

Upper respiratory tract infections. Frequently, infections of the upper respiratory tract and related organs manifest as FUO.[59,70,84] Although obvious signs or symptoms would be expected, the complaints often appear trivial and may be ignored. Reported cases of FUO have occurred in children with mastoiditis, sinusitis, chronic or recurrent otitis media, chronic or recurrent pharyngitis, tonsillitis, peritonsillar abscess, and nonspecific upper respiratory tract infection. A parapharyngeal inflammatory pseudotumor manifested as FUO has been reported in a 3-year-old girl in whom anemia and weight loss also developed. The cause never was discerned, but the symptoms resolved after surgical removal of the inflammatory mass.[28]

Noninfectious Causes of Fever of Unknown Origin

Central Nervous System Dysfunction

Children with severe brain damage can have dysfunctional thermoregulation, and body temperature in some of these patients can remain elevated for months. Cases of otherwise neurologically normal children who have had fever as a result of central dysfunction also have been reported. Berger[18] discussed a 16-year-old child with recurrent episodes of fever that were thought to represent a form of epilepsy but disappeared when treatment with phenytoin was begun. Wolff and associates[109] reported a 14-year-old child with cyclic episodes of fever, nausea, vomiting, and emotional disturbance caused by a central nervous system lesion.

Diabetes Insipidus

Central and nephrogenic diabetes insipidus can cause FUO in infants and young children. Polyuria and polydipsia may not be appreciated during infancy. Hyperthermia, weight loss, and peripheral vascular collapse can ensue. Signs of dehydration or an increased serum concentration of sodium suggests the diagnosis. The diagnosis is established by simultaneous measurements of urine and serum electrolytes and osmolality during periods of normal hydration and after carefully controlled periods of water deprivation. Serum levels of antidiuretic hormone also can be measured.

Drug Fever

Nearly any medication can be associated with an allergic reaction, including fever. The offending agent may be a prescribed drug, an over-the-counter preparation, or a street drug such as amphetamine or 1-[1-phenylcyclohexyl]piperidine (phencyclidine [PCP]). Atropine, whether taken systemically or used topically in the form of eye drops, can cause elevation of temperature. Phenothiazines and anticholinergic drugs can inhibit sweating and impair regulation of temperature. Epinephrine and related compounds can affect thermoregulatory control mechanisms and produce fever. Drug fever can be low-grade or high and spiking. Fever can be continuous or intermittent. Discontinuation of the drug generally is followed by disappearance of the fever within 48 to 72 hours, but it sometimes persists for as long as a month as a result of slow excretion of the offending agent.

Factitious Fever

A parent or patient may report the presence of fever that does not exist. The reading of the thermometer can be increased by immersing the bulb in hot liquid or by rinsing the mouth with hot liquid immediately before inserting the thermometer. Clues to factitious fever include absence of tachycardia, malaise, or discomfort despite a markedly elevated temperature; apparent rapid defervescence unaccompanied by diaphoresis; failure of the temperature curve to follow the normal diurnal variation of body temperature; hyperpyrexia; and normal temperature reading when the temperature is obtained rectally by someone who remains in attendance during the procedure. The presence of fever also can be confirmed or excluded by measuring the temperature of a freshly voided urine specimen. The current use of electronic thermometers in most hospitals decreases the possibility of factitious fever in that setting because the nurse or aide usually brings in the thermometer and stays in attendance during the relatively brief period of insertion. In more unusual cases, the patient or parent can induce fever by the injection of infective or foreign materials.

Familial Dysautonomia

Familial dysautonomia (Riley-Day syndrome), an autosomal recessive disorder, is characterized by autonomic and peripheral sensory nerve dysfunction. Eighty percent of patients are children of Jewish parentage, particularly Ashkenazi Jews. Defective regulation of temperature can result in hypothermia or hyperthermia.[33]

A careful history and physical examination can reveal poorly coordinated swallowing movements that lead to recurrent aspiration and pneumonia; recurrent episodes of vomiting; excessive salivation; excessive or diminished sweating; diminished formation of tears; periods of hypotension, hypertension, or both; and erythema or blanching of the skin. The fungiform papillae of the tongue are absent or diminished in number, and the sensation of taste is deficient.[93] Self-mutilation or multiple sites of skin trauma can reflect diminished or absent pain sensation peripherally. Deep tendon reflexes are diminished; corneal reflexes are impaired; and mental deficiency, dysarthria, and emotional lability are common findings.

Placement of methacholine (2.5%) into the conjunctival sac produces pupillary constriction in children with familial dysautonomia but no response in normal children. Intravenous infusion of norepinephrine is followed by an exaggerated pressor response, and the hypotensive response to infusion of methacholine is increased.

Hemophagocytic Lymphohistiocytosis

Hemophagocytic lymphohistiocytosis is characterized by prolonged fever, hepatosplenomegaly, cytopenia, and hyperferritinemia and hemophagocytosis in the bone marrow, liver, spleen, or lymph nodes.[51,78] It is a life-threatening and unusual disorder in which uncontrolled proliferation of activated lymphocytes and histiocytes results in unregulated hypersecretion of inflammatory cytokines. Hemophagocytic lymphohistiocytosis can be primarily a familial disease or can be manifested as a reactive process triggered by infection, malignancy, immunologic disease, or drugs.

The diagnosis of hemophagocytic lymphohistiocytosis is suggested by fever, hepatosplenomegaly, cytopenia in at least two cell lines, hypertriglyceridemia or hypofibrinogenemia, and an elevated ferritin level. Other laboratory abnormalities associated with hemophagocytic lymphohistiocytosis can include low or absent natural killer cell activity or elevated soluble CD25 (α chain of the interleukin-2 receptor), but these studies take time for results to return from reference laboratories.[54] Because this disorder can be manifested initially as FUO and progress to masquerade as overwhelming sepsis, a high index of suspicion is required for establishing the diagnosis. Further investigation should include evaluation of bone marrow or lymph nodes for the presence of hemophagocytosis. Therapy should include treatment of the underlying infection or trigger, if one exists, in addition to appropriate immune modulation therapies. A substantial proportion of hemophagocytic lymphohistiocytosis cases progress rapidly to death despite administration of appropriate chemotherapy.[51,54,78]

Inflammatory Bowel Disease

Fever is a prominent feature in many children with inflammatory bowel disease.[29,57,104] A greater percentage of children than adults with regional enteritis have fever. Appropriate contrast-enhanced radiographic studies of the intestines should be undertaken in children with prolonged FUO, even in the absence of findings specifically referable to the gastrointestinal tract, especially if the erythrocyte sedimentation rate is elevated and if the patient has anemia, weight loss, failure of linear growth, or a positive stool guaiac test.

Ulcerative colitis can be manifested as FUO, although less commonly than with regional enteritis. In patients with ulcerative colitis, symptoms referable to the gastrointestinal tract generally are present at the time that the patient is febrile.

Infantile Cortical Hyperostosis

The cause of infantile cortical hyperostosis (i.e., Caffey disease) is unknown. The decreased incidence in recent years suggests an infectious, possibly a viral, cause. Spontaneous hyperplasia of subperiosteal bone begins during infancy and is associated with swelling of the overlying tissues. The skull, mandible, clavicles, scapula, and ribs are affected most frequently, but in some children the long bones and even the metatarsal bones can be involved. Most patients have persistent fever, sometimes as high as 40°C (104°F). Tenderness over the affected regions, irritability, elevated erythrocyte sedimentation rate, and leukocytosis are common findings. The diagnosis is established by the clinical picture in conjunction with radiographically demonstrated periosteal involvement.

Juvenile Idiopathic (Rheumatoid) Arthritis

Juvenile idiopathic arthritis is a chronic inflammatory disorder that usually is manifested as one of three distinct syndromes: the systemic form, characterized by high, spiking temperatures (generally once or twice each day), evanescent rash, and lymphadenopathy; a polyarticular form; and a monarticular or pauciarticular form. Fever is associated with all three manifestations but occurs most commonly in the systemic form, in which case it is present in nearly 100% of patients. This form also is the one most likely to be manifested as FUO.[23] Arthritis may not develop for months to years after onset of the fever. The diagnosis often needs to be made by exclusion because no laboratory findings are specific for the diagnosis.

Periodic Fevers

The periodic fever disorders, also known as unprovoked inflammatory events that sometimes can occur without accompanying fever, are rare heritable disorders characterized by recurrent (periodic or irregular) attacks of fever and inflammation.[102] Between attacks, patients feel well. These disorders include familial Mediterranean fever and hyperimmunoglobulinemia D with periodic fever syndrome, which are autosomal recessive diseases. Familial Mediterranean fever is caused by a mutation in the *MEFV* gene, which encodes the protein pyrin. The illness is characterized by fever for 1 to 3 days accompanied by abdominal pain, pleurisy, and arthritis or arthralgia. Laboratory findings include peripheral leukocytosis and elevation of acute-phase reactants. The episodes occur irregularly. Persistent inflammation can lead to secondary amyloidosis. The disease occurs most commonly in Armenians, North Africans, Sephardic Jews, and Turks, and sometimes in Ashkenazi Jews, Italians, and Greeks or persons of other ethnicities.

Hyperimmunoglobulinemia D with periodic fever syndrome is associated with mutations in the *MVK* gene that encodes mevalonate kinase. Disease commonly presents before the age of 1 year, with episodes of fever lasting 3 to 7 days accompanied by cervical lymphadenopathy, abdominal pain, and vomiting or diarrhea.[36,42] Patients also can have aphthous ulcers, rash, splenomegaly, and arthritis or arthralgias. Attacks may occur at irregular intervals and can be triggered by stress, vaccination, and viral infections. Immunoglobulin (Ig) D levels are elevated, and most patients also have elevated IgA. Secondary amyloidosis is rare.

Other periodic fever syndromes include tumor necrosis factor receptor–associated periodic syndrome; pyogenic sterile arthritis, pyoderma gangrenosum syndrome, and acne; and Blau syndrome. These are rare disorders that are autosomal dominant in transmission. The genes associated with these disorders encode proteins that share domains involved in innate immunity and apoptosis. Muckle-Wells syndrome, familial cold autoinflammatory syndrome, and neonatal-onset multisystem inflammatory disorder are cryopyrin-associated periodic syndromes, a group of overlapping autoinflammatory disorders in which fever is an accompanying but not major feature of illness.

The syndrome of periodic fever with aphthous stomatitis, pharyngitis, and adenitis is a relatively common periodic fever syndrome. Symptoms such as fever, pharyngitis, cervical lymphadenopathy, and mild aphthous ulcers usually recur at 3- to 4-week intervals, generally beginning abruptly and resolving spontaneously in 3 to 5 days. Leukocytosis and elevation of inflammatory markers occur during the acute episode and normalize in between. The cause of this syndrome remains unknown.[37]

Acknowledgments

The author acknowledges Martin I. Lorin and the late Ralph D. Feigin as the original authors of this chapter.

NEW REFERENCES SINCE THE SEVENTH EDITION

17. Bell JM, Shields MD, Agus A, et al. Clinical and cost-effectiveness of procalcitonin test for prodromal meningococcal disease—a meta-analysis. *PLoS ONE*. 2015;10(6):e01288993.
41. Greenhow TL, Hung YY, Herz AM. Changing epidemiology of bacteremia in infants aged 1 week to 3 months. *Pediatrics*. 2012;129(3):e590-e596.
45. Hernandez-Buo S, Trenchs V, Batlle A, et al. Occult bacteraemia is uncommon in febrile infants who appear well, and close clinical follow-up is more appropriate than blood tests. *Acta Pediatr*. 2015;104(2):e76-e81.
53. Jasper N, Dabritz J, Frosch M, et al. Diagnostic value of [(18)F]-FDG PET/CT in children with fever of unknown origin or unexplained signs of inflammation. *Eur J Nucl Med Mol Imaging*. 2010;37(1):136-145.
92. Sioka C, Assimakopoulos A, Fotopoulos A. The diagnostic role of (18)F fluorodeoxyglucose positron emission tomography in patients with fever of unknown origin. *Eur J Clin Invest*. 2015;45(6):601-608.

95. Stein M, Schachter-Davidov A, Babai I, et al. The accuracy of C-reactive protein, procalcitonin, and s-TREM-1 in the prediction of serious bacterial infection in neonates. *Clin Pediatr (Phila)*. 2015;54(5):439-444.

113. Yo CH, Hsieh PS, Lee SH, et al. Comparison of the test characteristics of procalcitonin to C-reactive protein and leukocytosis for the detection of serious bacterial infections in children presenting with fever without source: a systematic review and meta-analysis. *Ann Emerg Med.* 2012;60(5):591-600.

The full reference list for this chapter is available at ExpertConsult.com.

64 Toxic Shock Syndrome

Jeffrey Suen

Illnesses resembling toxic shock syndrome (TSS) have been reported since 1927,[7,87,99,247,273] but TSS was first defined as a disease in 1978 by Dr. James K. Todd and colleagues using criteria designed for epidemiologic studies (Box 64.1).[261] TSS is characterized by fever, hypotension due to massive loss of fluid from capillaries into the interstitial space, and subsequent multisystem end-organ dysfunction. It has unique clinical manifestations not generally noted in septic shock, including diffuse erythroderma, delayed desquamation of the palms and soles, and conjunctival and pharyngeal hyperemia.

When first described, TSS was associated with menses, tampon use, and a distinctive type of *Staphylococcus aureus*. Patients with menses-associated TSS (menstrual TSS) had cervicovaginal colonization with strains of *S. aureus*[19] that made a toxin initially called *staphylococcal enterotoxin F*[20] or *pyrogenic exotoxin C*[229] but now known as *TSST-1*. Toxic shock–like syndromes were subsequently recognized in cases not associated with tampons (nonmenstrual TSS)[215] and in patients infected with toxin producing *Streptococcus pyogenes*.[282] TSST-1, staphylococcal enterotoxins, and streptococcal pyrogenic exotoxins A and B are now recognized to be "superantigens." These superantigens are potent stimuli of T-cell proliferation, causing massive release of cytokines (interleukin-1 [IL-1], IL-2, tumor necrosis factor-α [TNF-α], and TNF-β) that mediate the systemic manifestations of the disease.[146,240]

EPIDEMIOLOGY

Surveillance and Incidence

The first 12 cases of epidemic TSS were identified and reported to the Centers for Disease Control and Prevention (CDC) between July 1979 and January 1980.[37,69,238] In May 1980, shortly after surveillance for TSS began[72,123,152,199] the CDC reported findings of the first 55 cases, 95% of which occurred in women and had onset during menstruation.[37] By June 1980, case-control studies statistically linking the occurrence of menstrual TSS with tampons had been completed.[69,238,144] Superabsorbent tampons, particularly the Rely brand and those containing polyacrylate, were found to have a high association with TSS.[21,30,36,38,226] Between 1983 and 1994, the CDC received reports of 2509 confirmed cases; 95% occurred in females, 89% had an onset of TSS associated with menstruation, and 99% occurred in tampon users.[42,214]

Between 1980 and 1996, the incidence of menstrual TSS was highest in the ages 15 to 25 years (median age, 21 years, 1979–80; 20 years, 1981–86; 25 years, 1987–96).[116,121,214] Roughly one-third of cases occurred in adolescents 15 to 19 years of age (Fig. 64.1).[272] A striking 97% of cases occurred in whites, who comprise 83% of the U.S. population.[214] Although TSS cases occurred throughout the United States, the five states of Wisconsin, Minnesota, Colorado, Utah, and California accounted for 44% of the total reported cases but represented only 16% of the U.S. population.[214,264] In addition to differences in surveillance and menses-related practices, the distribution in age, race, and geography have been attributed to the prevalence of toxin-producing organisms and antibody to exotoxins.[103,204,214,215,272]

Geographic differences continued even with an increase in the relative proportion of nonmenstrual cases.[30]

The mean age of patients with nonmenstrual TSS (27 years through 1982, 30 years in 1986) is significantly higher than that for menses-associated cases.[116,215] The number of confirmed cases reported in children younger than 10 years of age is surprisingly low, particularly in light of their low antibody titers to TSST-1 and more frequent nasal colonization with TSST-1–positive strains.[30,136,272,281] The racial distribution is less pronounced, with 87% occurring in whites, who make up 83% of the U.S. population, and the ratio of males to females with nonmenstrual TSS is closer to that in the general population.[214,215]

Since 1980, when the rate of menstrual TSS was as high as 12.3 per 100,000 women of menstruating age,[69,152,199,210] the incidence has steadily declined to less than 1 case per 100,000 (Fig. 64.2).[79,116,277] The menstrual TSS–related mortality rate has decreased from 5.5% in 1979–80 to 1.8% in 1987–96.[121] The striking reduction in the incidence of menstrual TSS has been attributed to changes in composition and usage of tampons and the impact of publicity on early recognition of symptoms.[41,69,70,72,103,198,233] Since 1982, when the U.S. Food and Drug Administration (FDA) required that information on TSS risks appear on tampon packages,[83,187,269] tampon composition has changed to cotton and rayon combinations with the removal of additives.[228] Products with high absorbency decreased from 42% to 1%,[41,199] and tampons containing polyacrylate were withdrawn by major manufacturers.[191]

The incidence of postoperative cases of TSS after all types of surgeries has been estimated to be 3/100,000.[120] For ear, nose, and throat surgery, the incidence is higher (16.5 per 100,000).[135] Overall the average annual incidence of nonmenstrual TSS has been estimated to be 0.32 per 100,000 (95% confidence interval [CI], 0.12–0.67).[79] Largely due to the declining incidence of menstrual TSS, the relative proportion of nonmenstrual cases reported has increased from 14% during 1979–86 to 42% in 1994.[30,42,116,122] The case-fatality ratio for nonmenstrual cases has remained between 5.3% and 8.5%.[30,42]

Risk Factors for Toxic Shock Syndrome

The primary risk factors necessary for the development of TSS include colonization or acquisition of a toxin-producing strain of *S. aureus*, absence of protective antitoxin antibody, and an infected site with or without a foreign body. The main distinction between menstrual and nonmenstrual TSS is the nature of the infected site. While menstrual TSS–involves cervicovaginal colonization or infection associated specifically with tampon use, cases of nonmenstrual TSS reported to the CDC include nonsurgical staphylococcal cutaneous and subcutaneous infections, 22%; postsurgical infections, 15%; childbirth or abortion, 15%; vaginal infections occurring at times other than during menses, 6%; vaginal contraceptive sponge use, 5%[66]; diaphragm use, 6%; and no obvious focus (presumed vaginal or pharyngeal colonization), 31% (Box 64.2).[19,30,215]

Colonization With Exotoxin-Producing Staphylococcus Aureus

S. aureus is present in 20% to 40% of nasal cultures.[134] In menstruating women, 26% are colonized with *S. aureus* in at least one of three body sites (nose, vagina, or anus).[204] Vaginal carriage rates vary from 7% in nonmenstruating women to 33% in menstruating women[204,208] and are

BOX 64.1 Clinical Case Definition of Toxic Shock Syndrome

Clinical Findings

- Fever: Temperature of ≥38.9°C (102°F)
- Rash: Diffuse macular erythroderma
- Desquamation: 1 to 2 weeks after onset of illness, particularly on palms, soles, fingers, and toes
- Hypotension: Systolic blood pressure ≤90 mm Hg for adults; <5th percentile by age for children <16 years; orthostatic drop in diastolic blood pressure of ≥15 mm Hg from lying to sitting; orthostatic syncope or orthostatic dizziness
- Involvement of three or more of the following organ systems:
  - Gastrointestinal: Vomiting or diarrhea at onset of illness
  - Muscular: Severe myalgia or creatinine phosphokinase level greater than twice the upper limit of normal for the laboratory
  - Mucous membrane: Vaginal, oropharyngeal, or conjunctival hyperemia
  - Renal: Blood urea nitrogen or serum creatinine greater than twice the upper limit of normal or 5 or more white blood cells per high-power field in the absence of a urinary tract infection
  - Hepatic: Total bilirubin, aspartate transaminase, or alanine transaminase greater than twice the upper limit of normal for the laboratory
  - Hematologic: Platelets <100,000/mm^2
  - Central nervous system: Disorientation or alterations in consciousness without focal neurologic signs when fever and hypotension are absent
- Negative results on the following tests, if obtained:
  - Blood, throat, or cerebrospinal fluid cultures; blood culture may be positive for *Staphylococcus aureus*
  - Serologic tests for Rocky Mountain spotted fever, leptospirosis, or measles

Case Classification

- *Probable:* A case with 5 of the 6 clinical findings above
- *Confirmed:* A case with all 6 of the clinical findings above, including desquamation, unless the patient dies before desquamation could occur

From Wharton M, Chorba TL, Vogt RL, et al. Case definitions for public health surveillance. *MMWR Recomm Rep.* 1990;39(RR-13):1–43.

higher during menses than at midcycle.[161,195] In healthy individuals, 14% to 39% of *S. aureus* isolates produce TSST-1, and 7% to 14% produce staphylococcal enterotoxin B. TSST-1–positive *S. aureus* is present in 1% to 5% of vaginal cultures in women, 7% of nasal cultures in hospitalized patients, and 18% of nasal cultures in children. Overall up to 7% of healthy individuals at any given time are colonized at a mucosal site with TSST-1–positive *S. aureus.*[78,202,204] TSST-1 producing isolates has been found in 28% of patients bacteremic with *S. aureus* without TSS.[46] Presumably these patients had circulating antibody to TSST-1 that prevented the development of TSS despite *S. aureus* infection.

The majority of toxin-producing *S. aureus* isolates in both menstrual and nonmenstrual TSS cases produce TSST-1.[19,59,160] Of the strains producing TSST-1, 60.6% also produce an enterotoxin.[59,160] A clone producing both TSST-1 and staphylococcal enterotoxin A is associated with 88% of menstrual and up to 54% of nonmenstrual TSS cases.[44,108,184] Isolates that produce TSST-1 in conjunction with staphylococcal enterotoxin C have been associated with severe respiratory tract TSS-associated infections.[59] Staphylococcal enterotoxin B is never co-expressed with TSST-1.[75] TSST-1–negative strains that produce staphylococcal enterotoxin B account for 38% of nonmenstrual TSS isolates.[153,227] Patients with nonmenstrual disease infected with these TSST-1–negative strains may have a higher mortality rate.[115]

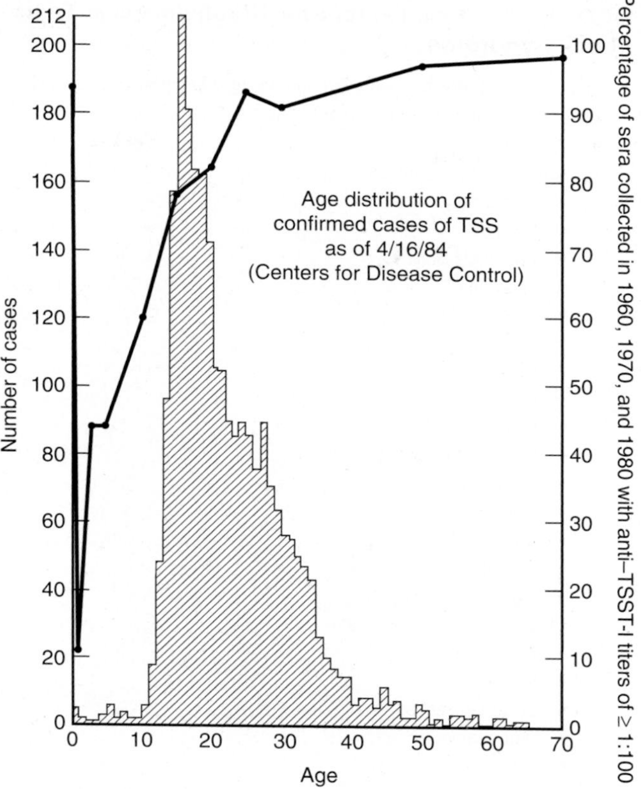

FIG. 64.1 Age distribution of patients with confirmed toxic shock syndrome (TSS) reported to the Centers for Disease Control and Prevention before April 16, 1984. The age-specific prevalence of antibodies to toxic shock syndrome toxin I (TSST-1) in a normal population in Wisconsin in the years 1960, 1970, and 1980 is indicated by the *solid connected line.* (Data from Vergeront JM, Stolz SJ, Crass BA, et al. Prevalence of serum antibody to staphylococcal enterotoxin F among Wisconsin residents: implications for toxic shock syndrome. *J Infect Dis.* 1983;148:692–8.)

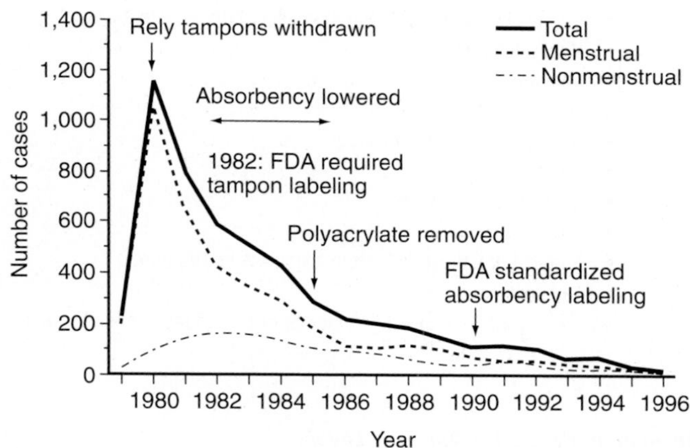

FIG. 64.2 Menstrual and nonmenstrual toxic shock syndrome cases reported to the Centers for Disease Control and Prevention by year, 1979 to 1996. (From Hajjeh RA, Reingold A, Weil A, et al. Toxic-shock syndrome in the United States: surveillance update, 1979–1996. *Emerg Infect Dis.* 1999;5:807–10.)

While toxin producing staphylococcal strains may cluster within families, living units, and hospital settings, the occurrence of TSS clusters is a rare event.[149,183] Probable TSS cases have developed within 24 hours in a husband and wife and in two mother-daughter pairs.[106] Nosocomial acquisition and transmission of TSST-1–positive organisms have been described.[9,149,183]

BOX 64.2 Risk Factors for Staphylococcal Toxic Shock Syndrome

I. Colonization of infection with toxin-producing *Staphylococcus aureus*
II. Absence of protective antitoxin antibody
III. Infected site
  A. Primary *S. aureus* infection
   - Carbuncle
   - Cellulitis
   - Dental abscess
   - Empyema
   - Endocarditis
   - Folliculitis
   - Mastitis
   - Osteomyelitis
   - Peritonitis
   - Peritonsillar abscess
   - Pneumonia
   - Pyarthrosis
   - Pyomyositis
   - Sinusitis
   - Tracheitis
  B. Postsurgical wound infection
   - Abdominal
   - Breast
   - Cesarean section
   - Dermatologic
   - Ear, nose, and throat
   - Genitourinary
   - Neurosurgery
   - Orthopedic
  C. Skin or mucous membrane disruption
   - Burns (chemical, scald, etc.)
   - Dermatitis
   - Influenza
   - Pharyngitis
   - Postpartum (vaginal delivery)
   - Superficial/penetrating trauma (insect bite, needle stick)
   - Viral infection
   - Varicella
  D. Foreign body placement
   - Augmentation mammoplasty
   - Catheters
   - Contraceptive sponge
   - Diaphragm
   - Surgical prostheses/stents/packing material/sutures
   - Tampons
  E. No obvious focus of infection (vaginal or pharyngeal colonization)

Absence of Protective Antibody Levels

Antibody formation to exotoxins is thought to result from mucosal colonization with TSST-1–positive *S. aureus* strains.[9,218]Adults and children with persistent nasal carriage of a TSST-1–positive strain have high levels of antibody to TSST-1.[204,218] Antibody titers are higher in women colonized with toxigenic *S. aureus* whether the colonization is persistent or transient.[49,205] Patients in whom TSS develops have significantly lower levels of antibody to staphylococcal exotoxins than the general population.[19,59] Following the episode of TSS, the antibody response to TSST-1 is typically absent or delayed.[202,253]

The prevalence of antibody to staphylococcal exotoxins has remained stable in studies from 1960 to 1999 and is correlated with age (see Fig. 64.1).[204,272] The increased incidence of TSS in adolescent girls is related to the lower prevalence of antibody to TSST-1 in this age group.[272]

Antibody to TSST-1 in a study of Wisconsin residents was found to be 47% at 1 year of age, 70% at 10 years, 88% at 20 years, and 96% for ages 30 to 50 years during the years 1960 to 1983.[37] A study of women across North America in 1998 to 1999 found similar results, with 85% overall and 81% of subjects aged 13 to 18 years having positive antibody to TSST-1.[204] Transplacental antibody is present in more than 90% of infants.[272]

For the staphylococcal enterotoxins, by 10 years of age, the proportion of individuals with antibody titers of 1 : 100 or higher is 15% for staphylococcal enterotoxin A, 65% for staphylococcal enterotoxin B, 30% for staphylococcal enterotoxin C, 5% for staphylococcal enterotoxin D, and 20% for staphylococcal enterotoxin E. By 22 years of age, the proportion increases to 55% for staphylococcal enterotoxin A, 77% for staphylococcal enterotoxin B, and 98% for staphylococcal enterotoxin C.[19]

Racial, sexual, and geographic differences in antibody prevalence have been noted.[272] Sera randomly selected from 87 control women were seronegative more frequently for antibody to TSST-1 (24%) than were those from 66 control men (9%).[222] A 2003 multicenter study of 3012 women from Ohio, New Jersey, Florida, Arizona, and Manitoba, Canada, found similar rates of *S. aureus* colonization, but subjects from Manitoba and Arizona were significantly more likely to have a positive antibody titer than were subjects from the other locations.[204]

Interruption of Skin or Mucosal Surface

Most cases of TSS occur in patients with an altered skin or mucosal surface. Trauma or surgery in areas of the body frequently colonized with *S. aureus* (nose, skin, vagina) places individuals at enhanced risk for infection and subsequent TSS. A wide variety of types of surgeries have been associated with TSS (see Box 64.2).[2,19,35,182,192,216,239,242,268] Primary deep-tissue staphylococcal infections (e.g., osteomyelitis, pyarthrosis, pyomyositis,[4] endocarditis,[211,278] renal carbuncles, and bacteremia) are rarely associated with TSS. Types of skin disruptions commonly associated with TSS include burns, surgical incisions, insect bites, needle sticks, tattoos, and varicella.[19,29,58] Infected abrasions under casts may be focal sites of TSST-1 production.[245]

Burn wounds provide a particularly rich environment for growth of *S. aureus* and the production of toxins.* In burn centers, TSS occurs predominantly in young children with small burns.[90] In one large pediatric burn center, *S. aureus* normally was not cultured from any site on admission but was acquired within a few days of admission and became the most common wound pathogen. Sixteen percent of wound isolates of *S. aureus* produced TSST-1. Only 50% of the children had antibodies to TSST-1 on admission. A toxic shock–like syndrome developed in 13% of children.[51] The mortality rate associated with TSS in children with burns may be as high as 57%.[111]

TSS cases following disruption of nasopharyngeal mucosa and the respiratory tract include those associated with sinusitis,[19,100] pharyngitis,[19,225] parapharyngeal and submandibular abscesses,[225] tracheitis,[19,64,85,114,188] pneumonia,[19,67] rubeola,[254] and influenza.[40,57,156,267] TSS occurring after ear, nose, and throat surgery has been associated with the use of nasal splints and packing materials that may disrupt the ciliary blanket.[3,19,110,178,284]

The vaginal mucosa may be damaged during placement of tampons or barrier contraceptives,[39,96,234] postpartum,[20,202] or after genital surgery.[97,201,220] Heavy colonization of the vagina without any other apparent risk factor has been associated with TSS.[215] Vaginal mucosal infections may provide the right conditions for production of TSST-1, including an aerobic environment, high carbon dioxide concentration, neutral pH, high protein and low glucose concentrations, and low to normal magnesium concentration.[179]

Presence of a Foreign Body

Tampon use was established as a clear risk factor for the development of TSS.[30,69,116,124,144,198,226,238] Tampons create an aerobic environment in the vagina, which normally is anaerobic.[274] Because TSST-1 production requires oxygen, the increasing concentrations of oxygen may enhance the production of toxin. Tampons may also remove vaginal substrates that normally inhibit the growth of *S. aureus.*[19] Although it has been

*References 11, 51, 55, 91, 111, 113, 117, 128, 159, 163, 265, 275.

suggested that tampons may cause vaginal ulceration leading to greater bacterial growth and toxin absorption,[61,63,276] the types of ulcerations seen are likely induced by TSST-1 because they have been found during postmortem examination in women who had never used tampons.[151]

While TSS occurs with all brands of tampons, a greater relative risk for menstrual TSS was found with brands with higher absorbency and particular compositions.[20,30,36,104,158,197,226] In one study, production of TSST-1 varied from undetectable levels to 300 μg/mL depending on the tampon studied.[19] Two studies demonstrated enhanced production of TSST-1 in vitro by the Rely tampon, which was composed of cross-linked carboxymethylcellulose and polyester foam.[207,229] The polyacrylate rayon and surfactant Pluronic L-92 included in some tampon brands also increase the production of TSST-1 under certain conditions.[178,229,259]

In addition to tampons, implanted foreign material, including sutures, central venous lines, metallic or polymeric implants, Teflon splints, and gauze packing, have been documented to enhance the risk for acquiring bacterial infection.[19,121,138] These infections are characterized by limited spread beyond the tissues in immediate contact with the implants, poor response to antibiotics, and poor healing without removal of the foreign material. The infection risk varies with the type of foreign material implanted. For example, bacterial adherence is eightfold higher for braided sutures of silk, silicone-heated blue polyester, and absorbable polyglycolic acid than for monofilament nylon.[138] Two important distinctions between TSS and other *S. aureus* infections related to foreign material are the production of exotoxin and the limited inflammation around the wound.[98]

Other Potential Risk Factors

Other factors that have been examined to identify individuals at increased risk for TSS include personal hygiene practices,[73] human leukocyte antigen type,[19] neutrophil function,[126] adherence of *S. aureus* to vaginal epithelial cells,[18] alteration of the cervicovaginal flora,[19] and hormonal factors.

Alteration of the vaginal flora, particularly co-colonization with *S. aureus* and Enterobacteriaceae, has been postulated to enhance the risk for development of TSS.[236] A prospective study found that women who were colonized with toxin-producing *S. aureus* had higher rates of colonization with *Escherichia coli* or other Enterobacteriaceae. *E. coli* isolation rates were 54% in women with TSST-1–positive isolates, 15% in women with TSST-1–negative isolates, and 11% in women with no *S. aureus*. The significance of these findings is not clear.

Hormonal control is known to be responsible for numerous cyclic changes in vaginal pH and flora. The results of early case-control studies suggested that oral contraceptives might have an effect on vaginal *S. aureus* organisms that may produce TSS-associated toxins.[69,164,198] However, one case-control study found neither protective effect nor enhanced risk associated with oral contraceptive use.[116]

HISTOPATHOLOGY

The histopathologic findings on postmortem examination support the concept that TSS is a toxin-mediated disease.[1,24,28,151,200,280] Striking histopathologic similarities exist between patients with TSS and those with "scarlet fever" reported in 1936.[28] Typically a total absence of tissue invasion by bacteria and minimal evidence of an inflammatory reaction in most organs are noted. Findings thought to be due to a direct effect of the toxin or mediators (or both) and unrelated to hypoperfusion include subepidermal ulcerations in the cervix, vagina, esophagus, and bladder; depletion of lymphocytes in lymph nodes; a subepidermal cleavage plane in the skin; and mild inflammatory changes in the kidney, liver, heart, and muscle.

Cervicovaginal ulcerations are the only characteristic lesions noted in the genital tract of patients with fatal menstrual TSS, and such ulcers have been found in a patient with menstrual TSS who had never used tampons.[151,202] The ulcerations are superficial, with separation occurring just beneath the basal layer. Capillary vasodilation and thrombosis with inflammation of the mucosa are present, but no deep-tissue bacterial invasion is seen. The same type of ulcer also has been found in the bladder and esophagus, which suggests that these ulcerations may be caused by the toxins or mediators and not by the use of tampons.

Although the myocardium was described as normal in one postmortem series of TSS, in another series of eight fatal cases, all patients had evidence of focal round-cell infiltration with variable degrees of congestion, edema, and hemorrhage.[151,200] Myxoid degeneration was found in all heart valves from four patients in one series. Sections of skeletal muscle have demonstrated only congestion, edema, focal hemorrhage or fiber necrosis, and a mild acute inflammatory infiltrate.

Varying degrees of periportal lymphocytic inflammation have been the most consistent findings in the liver; centrilobular congestion with necrosis and mild cellular degeneration also has been described.[133] In the kidney, toxin-mediated mononuclear interstitial nephritis may result from perivasculitis of the adventitia of the renal venules, lesions that probably precede the development of hypotension-induced acute tubular necrosis. The most characteristic findings in the spleen and lymph nodes have been lymphocyte depletion; inactive hypocellular, hypoplastic lymphoid follicles with edema; marked histiocytosis in the interfollicular areas; and hemophagocytosis.

Perivascular lymphocytic infiltrates and bullae that separate at the basement membrane are characteristic of the early skin changes in TSS.[8,10,126] No evidence of vasculitis has been reported.

CLINICAL SPECTRUM

Acute Phase

The manifestations in TSS are the result of release of endogenous mediators after monocyte and T-cell activation by TSST-1 or the staphylococcal enterotoxins.* The physiologic changes are striking in their rapidity of onset and progression and the involvement of almost all body tissues and organs. Endothelial damage with loss of fluid from capillaries into the interstitial space results in loss of peripheral vascular resistance, loss of intravascular volume, and interstitial edema. Prolonged hypotension, interstitial edema, and vascular congestion in turn results in ischemic organ damage. The onset of illness in patients with severe disease is abrupt, with signs and symptoms including fever, chills, malaise, headache, sore throat, myalgia, muscle tenderness, fatigue, vomiting, diarrhea, abdominal pain, and orthostatic dizziness or syncope (Figs. 64.3 and 64.4).

During the first 24 to 48 hours, diffuse erythroderma, severe vomiting and watery diarrhea (often with incontinence), decreased urine output, cyanosis, and edema of the extremities may be noted. Some patients may have purpura fulminans.[148] Cerebral ischemia and edema result in somnolence, confusion, irritability, agitation, and occasionally hallucinations, even in individuals without hypotension. Patients with TSS have had signs and symptoms of encephalopathy, cerebral infarction, meningismus,[14,23,122,155,243] and the cauda equina syndrome.[8]

On initial physical examination, fever, tachycardia, tachypnea, hypotension, erythroderma (generally not seen in patients with severe hypotension or in those without T cells)[142] (see Fig. 64.4A), and muscle tenderness are noted in conjunction with peripheral cyanosis and edema, conjunctival hyperemia, subconjunctival hemorrhages (see Fig. 64.4B), beefy red edematous mucous membranes, somnolence, disorientation, and agitation. In menstrual TSS, edema and erythema of the inner aspect of the thighs and the perineum may be noted despite normal findings on uterine and adnexal examination.

In nonmenstrual cases, another focus of infection is present. Surgical wounds and some abscesses colonized or infected with *S. aureus* and responsible for nonmenstrual TSS often have minimal or no signs of inflammation.[6,16,86,120,213,215,223] The production of TNF-α by macrophages in response to TSST-1 inhibits neutrophil mobilization in vitro,[98] which may provide an explanation for the absence of signs of inflammation. The incubation period for postoperative or postpartum TSS is usually 2 to 4 days but may be as short as 12 hours.[16] Relatively few cases have been associated with deep-tissue infection.[19] Nosocomial acquisition of TSST-1–positive organisms rarely has been documented for postoperative cases.[9,142,176] After orthopedic procedures or in association with bone and joint infections, the clinical manifestation of TSS may be confusing as a result of the intense and generalized myalgias associated with TSS, which may be misinterpreted as postoperative musculoskeletal symptoms. The wounds usually appear to be benign.[19,177,209,258]

*References 45, 53, 71, 105, 104, 125, 165, 238, 261, 262.

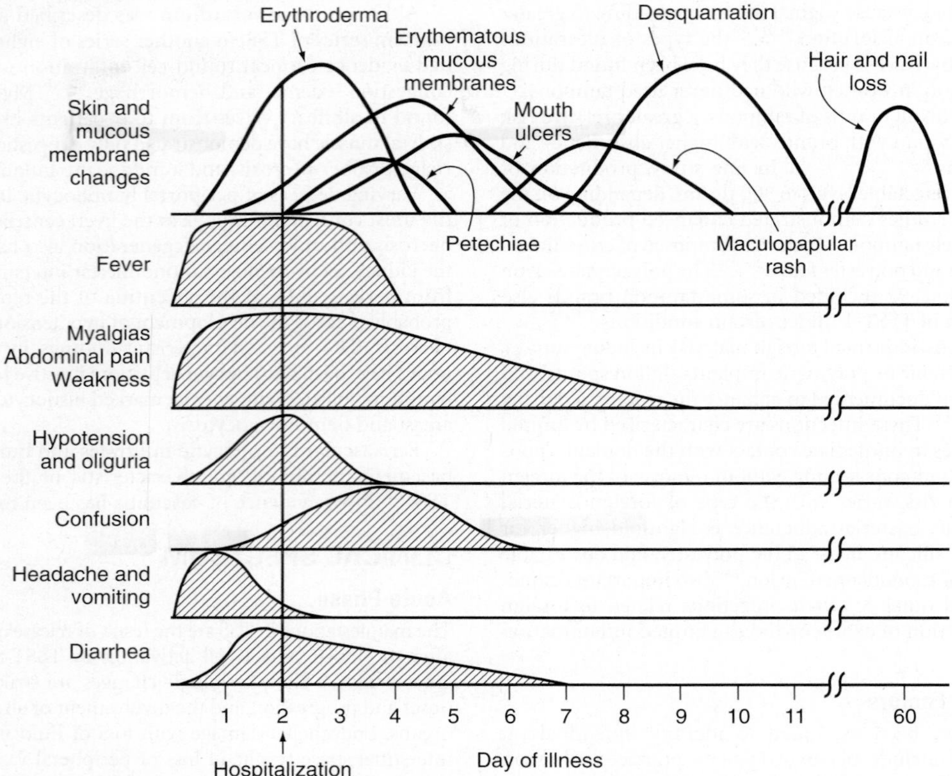

FIG. 64.3 Composite of the major systemic skin and mucous membrane manifestations of toxic shock syndrome. (From Chesney PJ, Davis JP, Purdy WK, et al. The clinical manifestations of toxic shock syndrome. *JAMA.* 1981;246:741–8.)

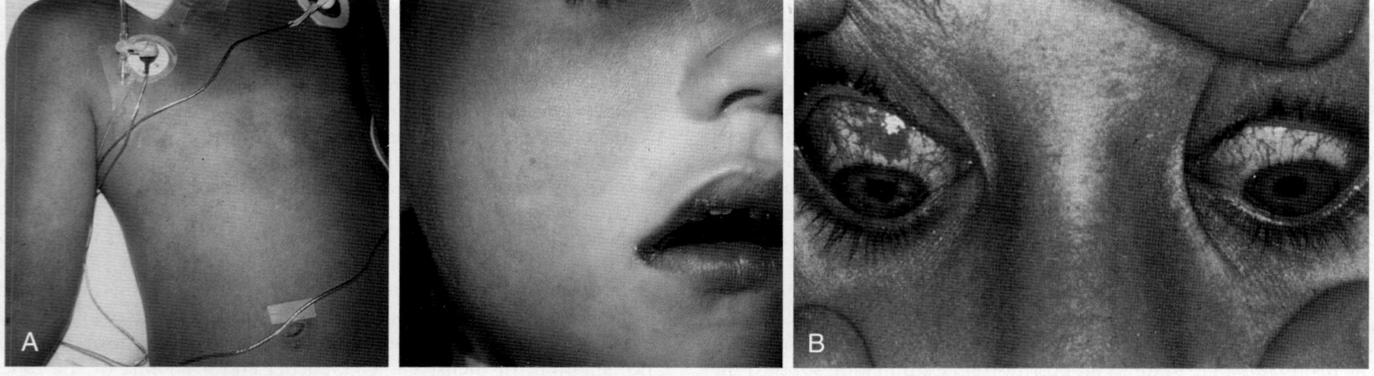

FIG. 64.4 Skin and mucous membrane manifestations present at the onset of toxic shock syndrome (TSS). (A) Diffuse erythroderma in a 7-year-old child with nonmenstrual TSS associated with osteomyelitis of the fibula. (B) Bulbar conjunctival infection and subconjunctival hemorrhage in a 24-year-old woman with nonmenstrual TSS. (B, From Bach MC. Dermatologic signs in toxic shock syndrome: clues to diagnosis. *J Am Acad Dermatol.* 1983;8:343–7.)

Laboratory Findings

Laboratory tests reflect the endogenous cytokine release, shock, and organ failure associated with TSS. Leukocytosis may not be present, but the proportion of neutrophils generally exceeds 90%. The proportion of immature neutrophils usually is 25% to 50% of the total number of neutrophils and is associated with absolute lymphopenia. Thrombocytopenia and anemia are present during the first few days and frequently are accompanied by prolonged prothrombin and partial thromboplastin times. Disseminated intravascular coagulation may be present. Sterile pyuria and cerebrospinal fluid pleocytosis are indicative of generalized involvement of the mucous membranes and serosal surfaces. Elevated blood urea nitrogen and creatinine levels reflect kidney damage,[45] and abnormalities in liver function tests reflect liver damage and acute cholestasis.[119,133] Hypoproteinemia and hypoalbuminemia reflect capillary leak, and profound hypocalcemia may reflect both hypoproteinemia and high serum levels of calcitonin.[48,246] Muscle involvement is noted by an elevated creatine phosphokinase level, and the hypophosphatemia that occurs despite impaired renal function is unexplained.[13,48] Most of these test results return to normal within 7 to 10 days of disease onset.

S. aureus is cultured from the cervix or vagina in more than 85% of patients with menstrual TSS and from the focus of infection in patients with nonmenstrual TSS. Positive blood culture results are rare findings.[62] Antibody to TSST-1 or to the staphylococcal enterotoxins is absent at the onset of disease in more than 85% of patients.[20,25,59,222,241,279]

BOX 64.3 Therapeutic Principles for Management of Toxic Shock Syndrome

1. Identify the focus of infection: debride and irrigate extensively and remove any foreign material
2. Isolate the organism for antimicrobial susceptibility studies
3. Administer parenteral antimicrobial therapy to stop toxin production and eradicate the organism
4. Manage systemic multiorgan actions of toxins or mediators
5. Administer fluid therapy to maintain adequate venous return and cardiac filling pressure and to prevent end-organ damage
6. *Consider* intravenous immunoglobulin for the following:
   - Disease refractory to initial fluid replacement and vasopressor support
   - A focus of infection that cannot be drained

Diagnosis

TSS is diagnosed clinically according to its case definition (see Box 64.1).[71,277] Aggressive attempts to find the focus of *S. aureus* include culture of the cervix and vagina in patients with menses-associated illness and culture of other potentially infected sites in patients with nonmenstrual illness. *S. aureus* isolates can be examined for their ability to produce TSST-1, although such testing seldom is indicated. This test is of limited usefulness for nonmenstrual cases because TSST-1 is produced by only 40% to 60% of *S. aureus* isolates from such patients.[115] Isolates from these patients can be examined for the presence of the other enterotoxins. Acute and convalescent sera can be tested for the presence of antibodies to TSST-1 and the other enterotoxins.[130] Elevated levels of anti–TSST-1 in the acute-phase serum of a patient with menstrual-associated TSS is highly unusual.

In most instances, toxin detection tests are of value only for research or for patients with chronic recurrent or atypical disease. Genes for TSST-1 and the enterotoxins have been detected in *S. aureus* strains by polymerase chain reaction[17,140,154,167,189,232] and hybridization techniques.[139,186,196] A noncompetitive enzyme-linked immunosorbent assay allows quantitation of TSST-1 in clinical samples.[169,180] Reversed passive latex agglutination has been used to detect TSST-1 and enterotoxins.[75,95] Research laboratories also have developed techniques for detecting the selective expansion of $V_{\beta}2$-positive T cells as evidence of host response to superantigenic toxins.[52,162]

Treatment

The four general principles of treatment of TSS (Box 64.3) are (1) identification and drainage of the focus of toxin production, (2) identification and susceptibility testing of the organism, (3) administration of antimicrobial therapy to block synthesis of the toxin and eradicate the organism, and (4) management of the systemic multiorgan actions of the toxins or mediators.*

Location and drainage of the infected site. The focus of infection should be identified rapidly, any foreign bodies should be removed, and the site should be drained or irrigated completely even if it does not appear to be inflamed. Performing this procedure is of utmost importance because perpetuation of even a small undrained focus of infection may result in serious clinical consequences. If TSS occurs in the immediate postoperative period, the wound should be assumed to be the source of infection regardless of its benign appearance.

Identification and susceptibility testing of the organism. Isolating the organism for susceptibility testing is of critical importance. The incidence of community-acquired methicillin-resistant *S. aureus* (MRSA) infections has increased dramatically during the past 10 years.[118] These MRSA strains may be acquired in the community by well individuals with no risk factors and are generally not multiresistant. MRSA strains are fully capable of producing TSST-1.[82,231] TSS may be caused by either community-acquired or multiresistant hospital-acquired strains of MRSA.[88] To date, vancomycin-resistant strains of *S. aureus* are rare findings.[43,129]

Administration of antimicrobial agents. Administration of antistaphylococcal antibiotics is indicated to stop toxin production and eradicate the organism.[69,71] The infection may be a superficial or deep-tissue infection and may be associated with bacteremia or bacteriuria. Antistaphylococcal antimicrobial agents should be administered intravenously as soon as possible. Once the patient is stable, high doses of an oral antimicrobial agent to which the organism is susceptible can be given to complete a total course of 10 to 14 days.

Subinhibitory concentrations of the protein synthesis inhibitors clindamycin, erythromycin, clarithromycin, kanamycin, gentamicin, tetracycline, and linezolid have been shown to suppress TSST-1 production in vitro.[81,206,230,251] In one study, clindamycin concentrations $\frac{1}{64}$ the minimal inhibitory concentration (MIC) were effective in totally blocking TSST-1 production.[206]

Data suggest that subinhibitory concentrations of β-lactam antibiotics actually may increase TSST-1 production by *S. aureus.* At a concentration of half the MIC, nafcillin can increase toxin production 10-fold more than under control conditions.[5] The effect is not seen with vancomycin, another cell wall–active drug, thus suggesting specificity beyond merely a cell wall effect. Coadministration of a protein synthesis inhibitor with a β-lactam antibiotic blocks the effect.[5]

The choice of initial empiric antimicrobial therapy has become more complex as a result of an increase in the number of community-acquired MRSA infections and the spread of multiresistant MRSA strains in hospitals.[143] In the past, the most effective initial empiric therapy was a combination of a β-lactamase–resistant penicillin and clindamycin. With recent concern for MRSA strains causing TSS, many experts recommend initiating therapy with vancomycin and clindamycin. As an alternative for MRSA coverage, linezolid has been used successfully for treatment of staphylococcal TSS.[251] Once the results of susceptibility testing of the organism are available, therapy can be adjusted appropriately.

Management of systemic multiorgan actions of the toxins or mediators

Fluid replacement. The most important aspect of the nonspecific treatment of symptomatic patients is fluid replacement.[260] Intravascular volume and cardiac filling pressure must be restored rapidly to achieve adequate tissue perfusion. Because of the ongoing capillary leakage, this fluid replacement may far exceed the estimated fluid requirements based on calculated maintenance and fluid deficit volumes. Some adults have required vasopressors and as much as 12 L of fluid during the first 24 hours to stabilize the circulating blood pressure. Pleural, pericardial, and peritoneal effusions and interstitial edema inevitably occur as a result of the continued vascular capillary fluid leak. Close monitoring in an intensive care unit will facilitate treatment of intravascular fluid loss, myocardial dysfunction, hemodynamic derangements, pulmonary edema, acute respiratory distress syndrome, acute renal failure, encephalopathy, and disseminated intravascular coagulation.

Intravenous immunoglobulin and toxin inhibition. High levels of antibody to TSST-1 and the staphylococcal enterotoxins are present in intravenous immunoglobulin (IVIG) preparations.[46,51,169,202,257] These antibodies may inhibit the binding of toxins to MHC class II antigen-processing cells or interfere with presentation of toxin by these cells to the T-cell receptor.[1,217] In animal models of TSS, both monoclonal antibodies to TSST-1 and human IVIG given at the time of inoculation of TSST-1–positive *S. aureus* prevent the development of TSS.[26,203,235] Even when IVIG was administered 29 hours after administration of TSST-1, the increase in survival rates in the IVIG-treated animals still was significant. No adverse reactions were noted in the treated animals, and no evidence was found of disease mediated by the formation of antigen-antibody complexes.[169–173]

Anecdotal case reports in humans have indicated a beneficial effect in treating staphylococcal TSS.[15,51,56,173,190,202] Because IVIG is expensive and most patients respond rapidly once standard therapeutic measures are initiated, some experts reserve IVIG for patients with an inaccessible focus of infection or for those who continue to deteriorate after receiving fluid and vasopressor support (see Box 64.3). The dose most often used has been 400 mg/kg given as a single dose over the course of several hours. This dose results in a serum antibody titer of greater than 1 : 100, much higher than that appearing to provide immunity to TSST-1.[202] Some studies have used IVIG doses of up to 2 g/kg.[65] Because early

*References 47, 53, 69, 71, 105, 104, 125, 165, 226, 248, 266.

administration of IVIG possibly could blunt the immune response to TSST-1 or other toxins and increase the possibility of a recurrent episode, the potential risks and benefits of this form of therapy must be considered for each patient.

The role of endotoxin in the pathogenesis of TSS is unclear. The failure of polymyxin B and anti-J5 antiserum to alter the course of TSST-1–positive TSS in a rabbit model suggests that endotoxin may not be an important mediator of TSS.[171] Early and sporadic case reports of TSS suggested therapeutic benefit with naloxone,[54] calcium,[202] and exchange transfusion in severely ill patients unresponsive to the usual forms of therapy.

Corticosteroids. Short courses of methylprednisolone or dexamethasone, if given early in the course of the disease, have been associated with a reduction in the duration of fever and the severity of illness but no reduction in mortality rates.[263] In vitro, dexamethasone has been shown to downregulate TSST-1–induced cytokine production.[147] Because no controlled prospective study has demonstrated efficacy, the use of steroids probably should be restricted to hypotensive patients unresponsive to fluid resuscitation, antimicrobial agents, and IVIG.

Subacute Phase

Once appropriate treatment is initiated, response is usually rapid with defervescence within 48 hours. The hemodynamic changes initially observed include tachycardia, decreased systemic vascular resistance, decreased central venous pressure, hypovolemia, normal pulmonary artery wedge pressure, and an increased cardiac index.[12,33,60,105,107] Once aggressive fluid therapy has been initiated, myocardial edema and potential failure, along with pulmonary and cerebral edema in the face of renal failure, become the most critical management issues.

The reasons for myocardial failure are unclear but probably are related to perivascular inflammation of the coronary vessels, edema, and postulated myocardial depressant factors.[151,200] TSST-1 has been shown to inhibit systolic function in isolated rabbit atria, although at higher than usual circulating concentrations.[194] Arrhythmias may result from myocardial damage or electrolyte abnormalities.[166,219]

During the decompensated stage of myocardial dysfunction, the cardiac index falls and pulmonary wedge pressure increases, with both left atrial and ventricular and diastolic diameters being at the upper limits of normal.[105] Reversible electrocardiographic findings include sinus tachycardia, diffuse loss of voltage, flattened T waves, and diffuse nonspecific ST-T–wave changes. If fatal arrhythmia does not occur during the decompensated stage, the toxic cardiomyopathy is reversible and rarely results in permanent changes. This process is similar to "stunned myocardium," a transient, postischemic myocardial dysfunctional state.[60]

Pulmonary edema and acute respiratory distress syndrome occur commonly in patients when massive fluid replacement is necessary and capillary leakage continues in the lungs. Pulmonary edema appears rapidly once fluid replacement is initiated and often necessitates intubation and ventilator management for several days.[260]

Forms of TSS-associated acute renal failure include prerenal azotemia and both nonoliguric and oliguric renal failure.[45] The type of renal failure manifested may depend on the degree of intravascular volume depletion. Unless severe acute tubular necrosis necessitates temporary hemodialysis, repletion of intravascular volume usually results in rapid restoration of renal function and, ultimately, diuresis. Permanent renal damage is an extremely rare event.[53]

Management of fluids, electrolytes, and metabolic acidosis in patients with TSS is complex. Although tetany is a rare occurrence, severe hypocalcemia may be life-threatening and should be corrected.[48,202,246] Most patients require potassium replacement and management of metabolic acidosis. The use of colloid for fluid replacement and removal of the toxin stimulus for capillary leakage ultimately correct the hypoproteinemia.

The typical dermatologic manifestations follow a predictable sequence (see Fig. 64.3). A flaky desquamation begins on the trunk and extremities 5 to 7 days after the onset of symptoms. From days 10 to 12 and for as long as a month, the characteristic full-thickness desquamation of the fingers, toes, palms, and soles takes place (Fig. 64.5). A variety of atypical dermatologic manifestations, including petechiae and subepidermal bullae, have been described.[10,93,131] Many patients exhibit desquamation of the mucous membranes, which is particularly painful when the oral mucous membranes are involved.[47] In addition, a small number of patients will have reactivated herpes simplex virus type 1 or 2 lesions with the acute illness.[47] A late-onset pruritic maculopapular rash with edema and low-grade fever unrelated to antimicrobial therapy occurs in more than 50% of menses-associated cases within 7 to 14 days of disease onset.[47,76] The cause of this late-onset rash is unknown.

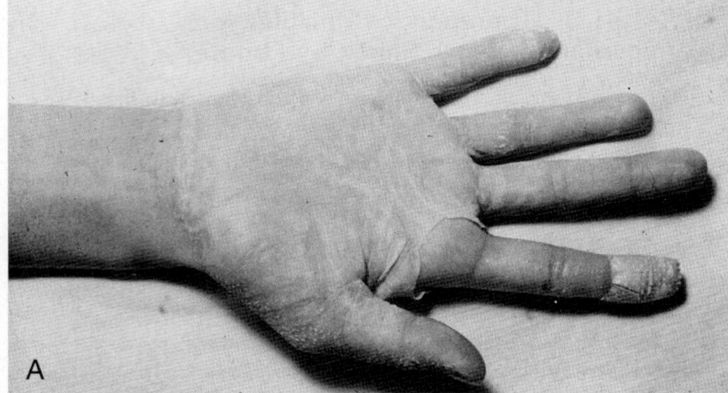

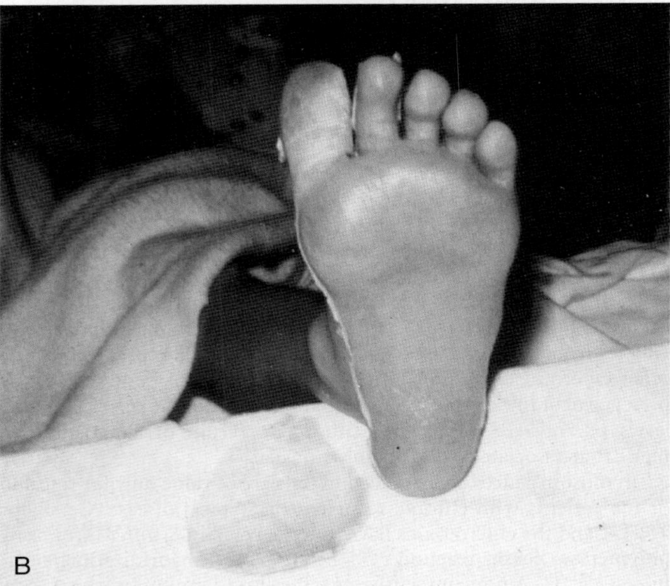

FIG. 64.5 Universal full-thickness desquamation of the (A) hands and (B) feet first noted 7 to 14 days after disease onset and persisting for up to 30 days.

The hematologic system seldom is involved with major complications in TSS. Although disseminated intravascular coagulation may be present, gastrointestinal, uterine, or cerebral bleeding rarely occurs. While thrombocytopenia may be present initially in patients with disseminated intravascular coagulation, thrombocytosis is typical in the recovery phase. Mild to moderate normocytic, normochromic anemia, likely due to a combination of hemodilution and suppressed red blood cell synthesis, develops in almost all patients with TSS and resolves during convalescence.[50,47] Hypoferrinemia occurs commonly.[50]

The relatively common toxic or ischemic encephalopathy, rarely complicated by seizures, resolves slowly during the first 4 to 5 days of hospitalization. The gastrointestinal, musculoskeletal, and hepatic changes resolve rapidly. Sequelae associated with these changes are rare, except for prolonged muscle weakness.[46,74] Joint manifestations generally are self-limited.[19,109]

Outcome and Sequelae

Death associated with TSS usually takes place within the first few days of illness, but it may occur as late as 15 days after presentation. Fatalities have been attributed to refractory cardiac arrhythmias, cardiomyopathy, irreversible respiratory failure, and, rarely, bleeding caused by coagulation defects.[151,200] The duration of circulation of toxins and mediators and the associated hypotension may be the best predictors of the severity of the end-organ damage.

Sequelae that appear to be related to a prolonged period of hypotension include chronic renal failure, gangrene, and telogen effluvium.[74,141,175,221,224] Hair and nail loss occurs 4 to 16 weeks after onset of the illness, with restoration taking place in 5 to 6 months.[19,22,47]

Other sequelae, such as neuropsychological abnormalities, prolonged myalgia and weakness, carpal tunnel syndrome, chronic dermatitis, Raynaud syndrome, and new allergies are explained less easily.[46] Impaired memory and concentration have been found in patients who did not require any therapy other than intravenous fluids to restore their blood pressure.[162,221] Fertility patterns and pregnancy outcomes were similar in controls and women with TSS, both before and after the illness.[74]

Recurrences

Recurrences for both menstrual and nonmenstrual TSS are well described, usually associated with inadequately treated disease.[6,47,69,71,164,202,253] A small number of patients with menstrual disease and repeated tampon exposure have experienced as many as 6 to 12 recurrences. In most patients the first episode is the most severe.[71] Antistaphylococcal antimicrobial therapy for 10 to 14 days and discontinuation of tampon use reduces the rate of recurrence significantly.[71]

The absent or delayed antibody response to TSST-1 found in both menstrual and nonmenstrual TSS patients probably accounts for the continued susceptibility to TSS and high recurrence rate.[19,25,157,222,241,253,279] The fact that superantigenic toxins are not processed by antigen-processing cells and T lymphocytes as conventional antigens may provide an explanation for the poor convalescent antibody response to these antigens.[146] In mice and one patient with TSS, in vivo TSST-1–induced proliferation was followed by hyporesponsiveness of TSST-1–responsive $V_{\beta}2^{+}$ T cells.[157]

Culture-negative, menses-associated recurrent episodes of TSS continue to be found in a small number of patients despite discontinuation of tampon use and administration of appropriate antimicrobial therapy during the acute episode.[71] Administration of an oral β-lactamase–resistant antistaphylococcal antimicrobial agent during menses has been tried in an attempt to prevent these recurrences but is not always successful. In recurrent cases resistant to this form of prophylaxis, consideration could be given to the empiric use of rifampin, clindamycin, erythromycin, or an oral contraceptive.[164]

Atypical Manifestations

Mild Disease

Recognition of mild episodes of menstrual TSS is particularly important because of the risk of recurrence without appropriate therapy.[49,69,71,78,165,165] Patients with mild TSS typically do not form antibody to TSST-1 during convalescence.[19,25,222,241,279] A mild episode may be recognized only in retrospect, after desquamation, a recurrent episode, or both develop.[202]

The presence of any combination of fever, headache, sore throat, diarrhea, vomiting, orthostatic dizziness, syncope, and myalgia in a menstruating woman or an individual with a potential *S. aureus* infection should raise suspicion of TSS. A positive culture for *S. aureus* is helpful but not diagnostic because *S. aureus* may be cultured from the cervix or vagina in up to 33% of menstruating women.[161,208] Other laboratory data usually do not reflect multisystem involvement in mild disease, and assays for TSST-1 in body fluids are investigational.[168,271] Support for the diagnosis of mild TSS depends on the constellation of findings present, including subsequent desquamation of the palms, soles, toes, or fingers; demonstration that *S. aureus* isolates from the site of infection produce TSST-1 or an enterotoxin; absence of antibody to TSST-1 or enterotoxins in acute-phase serum; and recurrent disease.

Recalcitrant Erythematous Desquamating Disorder

An atypical, subacute variant of TSS has been described in patients with acquired immunodeficiency syndrome (AIDS) and labeled recalcitrant erythematous desquamating disorder. *S. aureus* strains producing TSST-1 or staphylococcal enterotoxins A or B have been isolated from patients with AIDS presenting with diffuse erythema, extensive cutaneous desquamation, hypotension, and variable multiorgan involvement.[56,84,145] The illness is recalcitrant, prolonged, and characterized by multiple recurrences. In one patient, elevated levels of TNF and IL-6 were found during severe episodes. When antitoxin antibodies have been measured during recurrence, they have been undetectable. Two patients responded well to IVIG.[56,145] TSST-1 and the enterotoxins may exacerbate human immunodeficiency virus type 1 (HIV-1) infection because these toxins have been shown to activate HIV-1 gene expression in vitro.[112] Patients with the combined cellular and humoral immunodeficiencies of AIDS may be at particular risk for the development of severe, frequent, and prolonged episodes of TSS.[56,84,102,145,244]

Neonatal Toxic Shock Syndrome–like Exanthematous Disease

A toxic shock–like illness related to TSST-1–producing MRSA, labeled neonatal toxic shock syndrome–like exanthematous disease (NTED), was initially described in neonates in Japan[256] and subsequently recognized in France.[270] These infants present in the first week of life with a combination of a generalized erythematous macular rash, thrombocytopenia, elevated acute-phase reactants, and fever. Patients are colonized with a single clonal type of MRSA that produces TSST-1 and staphylococcal enterotoxin C.[144] Although no focus of infection is present and no exotoxins are detectable in serum, analysis of T cells shows the selective expansion of $V_{\beta}2$-positive T cells typically found in response to TSST-1.[255,256] Maternal IgG antibody to TSST-1 plays a protective role in preventing NTED.[255] Although complications occur in premature neonates, term infants typically recover within 5 days without active treatment. The limited disease has been attributed to the minute amount of exotoxin from colonized sites and the high susceptibility to induction of anergy in the immature T cells of neonates.[255,256]

Streptococcal Toxic Shock Syndrome

An increase in the incidence and severity of *S. pyogenes* was recognized in the 1980s. These infections included septicemia, necrotizing fasciitis, and a toxic shock–like syndrome. In 1993, the Working Group on Severe Streptococcal Infections proposed a consensus definition for streptococcal TSS based on clinical criteria including isolation of group A streptococci from a normally sterile site, hypotension, and two or more of the following: renal impairment, coagulopathy, liver dysfunction, acute respiratory distress syndrome, erythematous macular rash, and soft tissue necrosis.[282]

Since the 1990s, the rate of severe streptococcal infections has approximated 2 to 4 cases/100,000 per year. In adults, streptococcal TSS comprises 10% to 15% of severe streptococcal infections, with a mortality rate of 30% to 70%.[68,77,150] Streptococcal TSS is less common in children and carries a lower mortality rate than in adults. A multicenter study covering a US population of 29.7 million from 2000 to 2004 identified 5400 cases of invasive group A streptococcal infection (3.5 per 100,000 per year), including 572 children younger than 10 years of age. Of the 572 children with severe streptococcal infection, 26 (4.6%) developed streptococcal TSS with a 7.2% case-fatality rate.[193]

Streptococcal TSS is similar to staphylococcal TSS in that it is mediated by superantigenic toxins and results in endothelial damage, hypotension, and multisystem organ involvement. Both cell-associated and soluble streptococcal virulence factors, including M protein and pyrogenic exotoxins A and B, have been implicated as superantigens mediating the systemic effects of streptococcal TSS.[31,94,127] It differs from staphylococcal TSS in numerous respects, including severe generalized hyperesthesia; extreme pain at the site of skin involvement; a slower onset over the course of several days; typical absence of vomiting, diarrhea, and conjunctival injection; and the frequent absence of erythroderma or the presence of only a sandpaper-like rash.[56,248,250] In a multinational European study conducted from 2003–04, streptococcal TSS was most often associated with skin and soft tissue infections, particularly cellulitis and necrotizing fasciitis, followed by septic arthritis, bacteremia, sepsis, and meningitis. Notably, 50% of the cases of necrotizing fasciitis were complicated by streptococcal TSS.[150]

Treatment follows the same principles as for staphylococcal TSS: identification of the focus of toxin production, identification and susceptibility testing of the organism, administration of antibiotic therapy to kill the organism and block synthesis of the toxin, and management of the systemic multiorgan actions of the toxins. Although penicillin is the drug of choice for treatment of most group A streptococcal infections, initial broad gram-positive coverage with vancomycin and clindamycin has been advocated given the clinical overlap between streptococcal and staphylococcal TSS. The addition of clindamycin to inhibit protein synthesis is beneficial in cases of streptococcal as well as staphylococcal TSS.[248] In a mouse model of myositis caused by *S. pyogenes*, clindamycin was more efficacious than penicillin.[89,249,252]

IVIG as adjunctive therapy for streptococcal TSS has been supported by in vitro studies[218] and case reports in humans,[15,32,185,283] but clinical studies have been inconclusive.[237] Downregulation of the lymphokine production induced by streptococcal pyrogenic exotoxin A by IVIG has been demonstrated in vitro.[185,241] A multicenter, randomized, double-blind, placebo-controlled trial to study IVIG for streptococcal TSS in adults showed 3.6-fold higher mortality in the placebo group. However, statistical significance was not achieved because the study identified only 10 IVIG recipients and 11 placebo patients before premature termination due to slow patient recruitment.[65] As with staphylococcal TSS, IVIG has been advocated for cases of streptococcal TSS that are refractory to aggressive therapy or for patients with an inaccessible focus of infection.

Several patients with TSS have been reported to be simultaneously infected with *S. aureus* and *S. pyogenes*.[92] Determining which infection primarily was responsible for the manifestations or whether an amplified effect of exotoxins from both organisms was present was not possible.

DIFFERENTIAL DIAGNOSIS

The differential diagnosis of TSS includes clinical entities in which a rapid onset of fever, erythroderma-like rash, hypotension, and multisystem involvement are observed (Table 64.1).[34,101,174,181,189,202,212]

TABLE 64.1 Differential Diagnosis of Toxic Shock Syndrome Based on Clinical Manifestations

Diagnosis	Fever	Exanthem	Shock
Severe invasive *Streptococcus pyogenes* infection	+	+	+
Meningococcemia	+	+	+
Rocky Mountain spotted fever	+	+	±
Ehrlichiosis	+	+	±
Kawasaki disease	+	+	−
Staphylococcal scalded skin syndrome	+	+	−
Toxic epidermal necrolysis	+	+	−
Viral syndromes	+	+	−
Leptospirosis	+	+	−
Systemic lupus erythematosus	+	+	−
Erythema multiforme	+	+	−
Septic shock	+	−	+
Hantavirus pulmonary syndrome	+	−	+
Salmonella infections	+	−	±
Gastroenteritis	+	−	−
Urinary tract infection	+	−	−
Drug reactions			
Phenytoin (Dilantin)	+	+	±
Cocaine	+	+	±
Pseudoephedrine	+	+	±
Inhalational mercury	+	+	±
Quinidine	+	+	−
Sulfonamides	+	+	−
β-Lactam antibiotics	+	+	−
Quinolones	+	+	−

PREVENTION AND PROPHYLAXIS

To decrease the risk for development of menstrual TSS, in 1982, the Institute of Medicine Committee on TSS recommended that women, particularly adolescents, minimize their use of high-absorbency tampons.[132] The committee also recommended that women who have had TSS not use tampons. Although the frequency of changing tampons has not been associated with risk for TSS, limiting individual tampon use to less than 12 hours might decrease the risk for menstrual TSS. Women using intravaginal contraceptive devices also should be informed of the potential increase in risk for development of TSS.[234]

For prevention of nonmenstrual TSS, surgical antimicrobial prophylaxis has had limited efficacy. Perioperative systemic antistaphylococcal antibiotics did not prevent TSS in four patients[27,223] and did not eradicate nasal carriage of *S. aureus*.[137] Topical bacitracin ointment on nasal packing did not prevent the development of TSS.[27,80,135,137] Most authors contend that the rare risk for development of postoperative TSS is comparable to the risk for having a severe antimicrobial reaction and that perioperative antimicrobial prophylaxis is not indicated for clean procedures of short duration.[120,213] Effort should be intensified to recognize postoperative cases early; to open, explore extensively, and irrigate wounds; and to provide immediate antimicrobial and supportive therapy for suspected TSS. In burn patients, issues regarding the use of prophylactic antibiotics and occlusive dressings are unsettled.[91]

The full reference list for this chapter is available at ExpertConsult.com.

65 Pediatric Acute Respiratory Distress Syndrome

Jessica E. Ericson • Ira M. Cheifetz

Acute respiratory distress syndrome (ARDS) represents the final common pathway and clinical presentation of the most severe acute lung injury (ALI), which may be precipitated by various pulmonary (direct) or nonpulmonary (indirect) insults. Infections are an important cause of ARDS in children, with pneumonia and sepsis being most common.[41,118] ARDS is an important consideration in the setting of pediatric infectious diseases, given the wide range of infections that may lead to this complication and its associated morbidity and mortality.[41,118] Morbidity, mortality, and resource usage related to ARDS also increase during outbreaks of infectious diseases, as seen during the 2009–10 H1N1 influenza pandemic.[36,90] This chapter will discuss the definition, pathophysiology, presentation, and clinical management of children with ARDS, with an emphasis on aspects that may be of particular interest to pediatric infectious diseases specialists.

DEFINITION

Although first described by Ashbaugh and colleagues in 1967,[8] a formal definition of ARDS was not developed until 1994 when the American-European Consensus Conference (AECC) defined ARDS as follows[13]:

1. Acute onset of respiratory symptoms
2. Frontal chest radiograph with bilateral infiltrates
3. Partial pressure of oxygen ($Pa{O_2}$) to fraction of inspired oxygen ($Fi{O_2}$) ratio (P/F ratio) 200 mm Hg or less
4. No clinical evidence of left atrial hypertension as defined by a pulmonary capillary wedge pressure less than 18 mm Hg (if measured)

The AECC also designated the term acute lung injury (ALI) as a part of the spectrum of ARDS, and ALI is defined by a P/F ratio between 201 and 300 mm Hg. This formal definition allowed for significant research and clinical advances to occur but had important limitations related to interrater reliability of the chest radiograph interpretation and the inability of the P/F ratio to fully explain the respiratory status of the patient.

A subsequent definition that addressed these limitations is commonly referred to as the Berlin Definition of ARDS and was developed in 2011 by the European Society of Intensive Care Medicine in collaboration with the American Thoracic Society.[69,91] The term ALI was removed in favor of considering ARDS to be a single entity with three subgroups based on the severity of hypoxemia (i.e., mild, moderate, and severe). The Berlin Definition of ARDS takes into account the timing of onset, the degree of respiratory support (positive airway pressure), and the overall fluid status. This new definition also allowed for the use of either computed tomography (CT) of the chest or standard chest radiograph as part of the diagnostic criteria for ARDS.

The Berlin definition, however, failed to consider differences between adults and children in the presentation and management of ARDS. In 2015, after a 2-year process, the Pediatric Acute Lung Injury Consensus Conference (PALICC) published pediatric-specific definitions for ARDS and recommendations regarding management and suggested priorities for future research. PALICC defined pediatric ARDS (PARDS) with the use of the oxygenation index ([$Fi{O_2}$ × mean airway pressure × 100]/$Pa{O_2}$) or the oxygen saturation index ([$Fi{O_2}$ × mean airway pressure × 100]/$Sp{O_2}$) as a means of assessing severity (Table 65.1).[55] Some of the key PALICC recommendations were (1) no age criteria for the definition of PARDS in order that the pathophysiology of PARDS be better studied across the spectrum of age groups in future studies; (2) exclusion of perinatal-related lung injury; (3) inclusion of infants and children requiring noninvasive ventilation, as well as (4) inclusion of those with congenital heart disease and chronic lung disease; and (5) inclusion of patients with unilateral lung disease.

PATHOLOGY AND PATHOPHYSIOLOGY

The clinical stages of ARDS coincide with three pathologic stages: exudative stage, proliferative stage, and fibrotic stage. The exudative stage is characterized by accumulation of protein-rich edema fluid in the alveoli following direct or indirect injury to the alveolar-capillary membrane (see Table 65.1). Neutrophils play a predominant role in this stage of ARDS. Pulmonary compliance is worsened by the presence of edema, widespread atelectasis, and the inactivation of surfactant that results from the presence of fibrin and other plasma proteins and inflammatory mediators in the alveolar space.[64,97] Microthrombi develop within the pulmonary vasculature and numerous vasoactive mediators are released from inflammatory cells and the activated endothelium contributing to the development of elevated pulmonary vascular resistance and the ventilation/perfusion abnormalities characteristic of ARDS. The degree of epithelial injury and the subsequent ability to clear edema fluid, along with the reversibility of pulmonary hypertension, are important predictors of outcome in ARDS.[67,111]

The proliferative stage occurs 1 to 3 weeks after the initiation of injury and is characterized by attempted repair of the disrupted alveolar-capillary membrane. The mechanism of this repair requires not only the close coordination of numerous growth factors but also an intact basement membrane to provide a platform for cell adhesion and migration.[82] The ability of the alveolar epithelium to remove edema fluid depends on the degree of inflammation and injury in the exudative stage. Antiinflammatory cytokines such as interleukin-10 (IL-10) and lipid mediators are particularly important mechanisms aimed at limiting the degree of injury.[68] If lung injury and inflammation persist, the patient may develop severe physiologic abnormalities and may progress to the fibrotic stage of ARDS.

The fibrotic stage may be seen as early as 5 to 7 days after the onset of disease, although this degree of injury may not be clear for several weeks. Histologically the alveolar space becomes filled with mesenchymal cells, and lung tissue is replaced by collagenous tissue.[57] In addition, vascular changes in the fibrotic stage can lead to increased thickness of the pulmonary vasculature and even obliteration of small capillaries. Overall these changes markedly decrease the available surface area for gas exchange and result in decreased exercise tolerance in survivors of ARDS. In some patients, intractable respiratory failure or chronic lung disease result, necessitating prolonged ventilator support.

TABLE 65.1 Pediatric Acute Respiratory Distress Syndrome Definition From the Pediatric Acute Lung Injury Consensus Conference (2015)

Age	Exclude patients with perinatal related lung disease			
Timing	Within 7 days of known clinical insult			
Origin of Edema	Respiratory failure not fully explained by cardiac failure or fluid overload			
Chest Imaging[a]	Chest imaging findings of new infiltrate(s) consistent with acute pulmonary parenchymal disease			
Oxygenation		**Invasive Mechanical Ventilation**		
	Noninvasive Mechanical Ventilation	**Mild**	**Moderate**	**Severe**
		4 ≤OI<8	8 ≤OI<16	OI ≥16
	Full face-mask bi-level ventilation or CPAP ≥5 cm H_2O, PF ratio ≤300, SF ratio ≤264	5 ≤OSI<7.5	7.5 ≤OSI<12.3	OSI ≥12.3
	SPECIAL POPULATIONS			
Cyanotic Heart Disease	Standard preceding criteria for age, timing, origin of edema, and chest imaging with an acute deterioration in oxygenation not explained by underlying heart disease			
Chronic Lung Disease	Standard preceding criteria for age, timing, and origin of edema with chest imaging consistent with new infiltrate and acute deterioration in oxygenation from baseline that meet preceding oxygenation criteria			
Left Ventricular Dysfunction	Standard preceding criteria for age, timing, and origin of edema with chest imaging consistent with new infiltrate and acute deterioration in oxygenation that meet preceding criteria not explained by left ventricular dysfunction			

PARDS, Pediatric acute respiratory distress syndrome; *CPAP,* continuous positive airway pressure; *PF ratio,* partial pressure of oxygen ($Pa{O_2}$) to fraction of inspired oxygen ($Fi{O_2}$) ratio; *SF,* saturation fraction ($Sp{O_2}$/$Fi{O_2}$); *OI,* oxygenation index ([$Fi{O_2}$ × mean airway pressure × 100]/$Pa{O_2}$); *OSI,* oxygen saturation index ([$Fi{O_2}$ × mean airway pressure × 100]/$Sp{O_2}$).

[a]Chest x-ray or computed tomography scan.

BOX 65.1 Causes of Acute Respiratory Distress Syndrome

Direct (Pulmonary) Causes

Pneumonia

- Bacterial
- Viral: influenza, respiratory syncytial virus
- Mycobacterial
- Fungal

Aspiration
Drowning
Smoke or chemical inhalation
Pulmonary contusion

Indirect (Nonpulmonary) Causes

Severe sepsis and septic shock
Significant trauma
Severe hemorrhage
Severe pancreatitis
Transfusion reaction
Cardiopulmonary bypass
Thermal burn

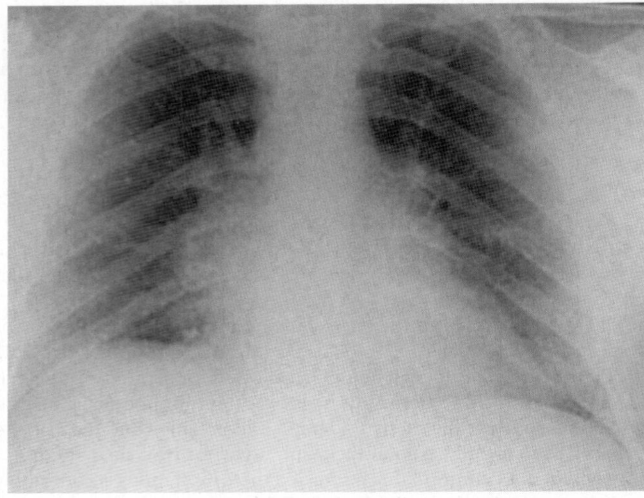

FIG. 65.1 Early stage of acute respiratory distress syndrome.

ETIOLOGY

The inflammatory cascade that ultimately results in ARDS can be triggered by a variety of insults that directly or indirectly affect the lung (Box 65.1). Direct pulmonary insults include pneumonia, aspiration, chest trauma, drowning injury, and smoke inhalation. Indirect lung injury may be the result of generalized systemic conditions, such as sepsis, closed head injury, multisystem trauma, transfusion reactions, pancreatitis, and hemorrhagic shock. A study of 146 PARDS cases found that infectious etiologies were the most common causes of ARDS: 35% had bacterial pneumonia, 20% had lung disease due to respiratory syncytial virus (RSV), and 27% had sepsis.[66] ARDS was due to trauma in only four (3%) pediatric cases.[66]

Bacterial lower respiratory tract infection is the most common inciting event in PARDS, although severe sepsis is often also present.[120] *Streptococcus pneumoniae* and *Pseudomonas aeruginosa* are bacteria commonly associated with severe pneumonia potentially leading to sepsis and, subsequently, ARDS.[12] Some bacteria may be associated with a higher risk of ARDS than other pathogens because of the production of cytotoxic and chemotactic toxin production.[78,10]

Viral pneumonia is also an important initiator of ARDS and is frequently not diagnosed due to testing limitations.[87] RSV infection is one of the most common indications for admission to the pediatric intensive care unit (PICU), especially during the winter months.[17] Although most critically ill children present as severe RSV bronchiolitis, a significant proportion (up to 27%) can present with ARDS; those with preexisting conditions are at the highest risk.[46] Influenza virus is another important cause of ARDS. In one study, 80% of children admitted to the PICU with influenza developed ARDS.[36] A single-center study found that as many as 24% of patients with the 2009 pandemic H1N1 strain developed ARDS.[92] A less common cause of viral-induced ARDS is coronavirus, particularly the strain that caused the severe acute respiratory syndrome (SARS) outbreak in 2003, which affected adults more severely than children.[62,63] Bacterial coinfection increases the risk that viral pneumonia will cause ARDS. For example, in patients with the severe pandemic H1N1 viral infection, bacterial coinfection was shown to increase the need for mechanical ventilation, duration of intensive care unit (ICU) stay, and mortality.[90,93]

In addition to lower respiratory tract infections, severe sepsis is a leading risk factor for indirect ARDS in children.[120] ARDS has been described following sepsis due to many different organisms and does not seem to be directly related to pathogen-specific factors.[56] Multiorgan dysfunction and other illnesses associated with sepsis increase the risk for ARDS, and this risk is further increased by the presence of underlying comorbidities.[50] In critically ill adults, sepsis is associated with an approximately 40% risk of developing ARDS.[80] Sepsis appears to be a less common cause of ARDS in pediatric patients; one study found that 15% of PARDS cases were attributable to sepsis.[66]

Limited data exist on the impact of the underlying etiology of ARDS on clinical outcomes in children. In a study of 736 adults with ARDS, patients with sepsis-related ARDS were more likely to have diabetes, longer pre-ICU stay, and higher APACHE III (a measure of severity of illness in critically ill adults) scores in contrast to those who had non–sepsis-related ARDS.[99] However, after accounting for differences in clinical characteristics, no difference was found in 60-day mortality between patients with sepsis-related ARDS and non–sepsis-related ARDS. Furthermore no evidence exists to suggest that the source of sepsis is an important determinant of mortality in ARDS.[98] However, genetic differences in the immune regulation underlying responses of the lungs to these precipitating factors do account for some of the differences in the degree of severity in ARDS in individual patients, even when similar risk profiles are present.[82] One such example of genetic polymorphisms is that related to nuclear factor-κB (NF-κB). A deletion polymorphism of the promoter region of this important transcription factor leads to inappropriate upregulation of proinflammatory genes, which has been shown to result in an increase in ARDS severity and mortality.[3,9]

CLINICAL MANIFESTATIONS

The initial clinical course of ARDS begins with direct or indirect acute injury to the pulmonary parenchyma. In the initial stage, the clinical symptoms and physical findings vary depending on the underlying etiology of the ALI. Children with pulmonary etiologies of ARDS will have predominantly respiratory symptoms; those with nonpulmonary etiologies of ARDS will have symptoms related to the initial insult (e.g., acute abdomen for pancreatitis). Early in the course of lung injury, patients may display mild tachypnea and dyspnea but tend to have normal radiographic findings.

After the inciting event and initial phase, a latent period of variable duration follows. During this latent period, the patient may appear to be clinically stable, but early signs of pulmonary insufficiency develop, as manifested by hyperventilation with hypocarbia and respiratory alkalosis. The chest radiograph may begin to demonstrate a fine reticular pattern related to increases in pulmonary interstitial fluid (Fig. 65.1).[33] As the degree of lung injury worsens, acute respiratory failure follows and is characterized by rapid onset of hypoxemia that is often refractory to supplemental oxygen administration. Diffuse pulmonary edema and worsening compliance cause significant atelectasis and intrapulmonary shunting. Clinically patients develop rapid, shallow tachypnea with increased work of breathing. Subcostal and supraclavicular retractions,

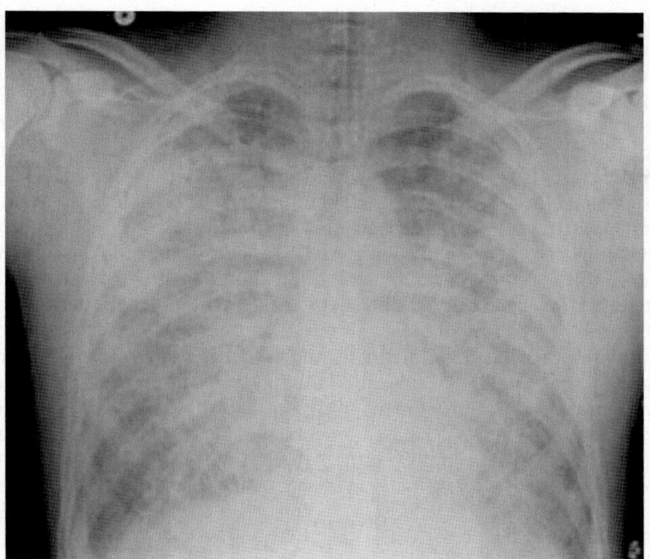

FIG. 65.2 Established acute respiratory distress syndrome.

grunting, and nasal flaring are common. Lung examination usually reveals diffuse crackles. Radiographically bilateral areas of consolidation with air bronchograms reflect alveolar filling and atelectasis (Fig. 65.2). CT may provide additional information.[102] A significant percentage of these children will require endotracheal intubation and mechanical ventilation. However, noninvasive ventilation may be an alternative for a subgroup of patients.[83]

MORTALITY

Most studies indicate that mortality associated with ARDS is due to nonrespiratory causes.[72,39] In most cases, early death (i.e., within 72 hours) is caused by the underlying illness or injury, whereas late death (i.e., beyond 72 hours) is caused by infection or multiorgan system failure. Reported mortality rates for children with ARDS vary greatly and range from 8% to 79%.[14,23,28,49,86,113,118] This variation is likely due to the myriad of underlying causes of ARDS, the differing degrees of ARDS severity, and the presence or absence of concomitant organ failures. ARDS secondary to sepsis appears to confer the highest risk of death, likely due to the systemic dysfunction present at the onset of ARDS symptoms.[118] Some of the factors that have been identified as predictors of mortality in PARDS include P/F ratio, oxygenation index, pH, Pediatric Risk of Mortality (PRISM) score (a severity index score commonly used in PICUs), and presence of multiorgan failure.[40,85] Despite the large reported variation in mortality, it is generally accepted that the overall mortality rate of PARDS is lower than that of the adult population.[120] Additionally ARDS-related mortality has decreased over the past several years, likely due to improvements in supportive care and the widespread adoption of low tidal volume ventilation strategies, the only mechanical ventilation strategy that has ever been shown to decrease mortality in ARDS in a randomized clinical study.[110] This study was conducted in adults and, although the role of low tidal volume ventilation in reducing mortality in pediatric patients in not clear, mortality rates following PARDS have fallen from 80% in the 1980s to approximately 20% in the early 2000s and are potentially under 15% now.[120]

TREATMENT

Goals of treatment of patients with ARDS include treating the underlying disease (when possible), achieving adequate tissue oxygenation, and minimizing ventilator-induced lung injury (VILI). In patients in whom ARDS is secondary to sepsis or bacterial lower respiratory tract infection, prompt administration of appropriate antibiotics is essential.[61,29] The antimicrobial approach depends on patient-specific risk factors as well as patterns of drug resistance in the community and within a given hospital. Local rates of cephalosporin-resistant *S. pneumoniae* and methicillin-resistant *Staphylococcus aureus* (MRSA) may necessitate broad-spectrum gram-positive coverage (e.g., vancomycin).[29,53] Patients with neutropenia or other risk factors for sepsis due to gram-negative pathogens may require extended-spectrum penicillins or cephalosporins as part of their empiric therapy. The mainstay of support in the ARDS patient is the provision of supplemental oxygen and mechanical ventilation. In addition, nonpulmonary organ function must be meticulously maintained to optimize the clinical care of children with ARDS.

Pulmonary Management

Modes of Mechanical Ventilation

Multiple modes of mechanical ventilation are currently used in clinical practice to provide respiratory support for patients with ARDS. Regardless of the conventional mechanical ventilation (CMV) mode used, it is paramount that VILI be minimized by paying meticulous attention to prevention of barotrauma and volutrauma.[95] Prospective, randomized multicenter studies comparing a pressure-controlled mode to a volume-control mode in the setting of ARDS are limited and have not demonstrated a single ventilatory mode as being superior.[95,35,84]

However, a landmark study of adults with ARDS published in 2000 did show that low tidal volume mechanical ventilation (6 mL/kg) decreased mortality by 22% and increased the number of ventilator-free days in contrast to a more traditional tidal volume (12 mL/kg).[110] This study is the only investigation in either adult or pediatric ARDS that has demonstrated a mortality benefit associated with a specific ventilatory approach. It is important to mention that two pediatric-focused observational studies demonstrated an inverse relationship between delivered tidal volumes and mortality.[34,54] However, a large retrospective multicenter pediatric study of acute hypoxic respiratory failure did not reveal an association between tidal volume and either mortality or ventilator-free days.[119] One must be careful not to make definitive conclusions from these pediatric-based studies, which demonstrate association rather than cause and effect. Without pediatric-specific definitive data, the low tidal volume approach has generally become standard practice in the PICU environment.

In contrast to CMV, high-frequency oscillatory ventilation (HFOV) is an alternative mode that delivers extremely small-volume "breaths" at high rates (5 to 15 Hz [equivalent to 300 to 900 breaths/min]). Although use of HFOV has become commonplace in pediatrics, the only definitive study of this method in PARDS is a crossover trial conducted more than 20 years ago that showed improved oxygenation and a reduction in the need for supplemental oxygen at 30 days.[6] The adult-based OSCAR and OSCILLATE ARDS trials of HFOV have led to a negative view of this ventilatory modality. OSCAR found no difference in mortality between HFOV and CMV.[117] OSCILLATE was prematurely stopped due to higher mortality with HFOV compared to control ventilation.[38] The RESTORE HFOV study compared the length of mechanical ventilation in pediatric subjects managed with early (within 24 to 48 hours of intubation) HFOV compared to patients receiving CMV or late HFOV by means of a propensity score analysis. After adjusting for risk category, early HFOV was associated with an increased length of ventilation but not increased mortality as compared to patients managed with CMV/late HFOV. However, this study raises an important question of whether the increased length of ventilation with early HFOV is directly related to HFOV or rather to the manner in which this modality was used.[11] Unfortunately, pediatric clinicians are left to determine whether or not to use HFOV based on their interpretation of the available data as well as their clinical experience. In general, despite the lack of definitive evidence in support of HFOV in pediatrics, it has become an often-used technique in the management of PARDS.[89]

Positive End-Expiratory Pressure

Positive end-expiratory pressure (PEEP) is the constant pressure applied to the airways and alveoli during exhalation and helps maintain alveolar patency and restore functional residual capacity. PEEP is typically titrated to a level that allows adequate oxygenation at an acceptable FiO_2.

The ARDS Network investigated the optimal PEEP-FiO_2 approach for adult patients with ARDS and showed that both "lower" and "higher"

PEEP strategies produced similar survival rates.[18] The results of this study suggest that as long as adequate PEEP is applied, higher levels are not necessary but are acceptable. Once appropriate PEEP is applied to maintain the lungs at an ideal volume, further increases in PEEP in an attempt to reduce the FiO_2 do not lead to an improved outcome.[7] A follow-up meta-analysis of almost 2300 patients demonstrated that patients with pure ALI (i.e., recruitable lung) benefited from a higher PEEP strategy, whereas those without recruitable lung did not.[14] Based on these data, a strategy that individualizes PEEP based on the specific clinical circumstances seems warranted. As long as alveolar collapse is minimized, the balance between PEEP and FiO_2 can be left to the discretion of the clinician.

Permissive Hypoxemia and Permissive Hypercapnia

Every child with ARDS is hypoxemic by definition. Prolonged administration of high concentrations of oxygen can damage lungs due to the formation of oxygen free radicals. Human and animal studies suggest that a prolonged FiO_2 of greater than 0.60 should be avoided to prevent oxygen-induced pulmonary damage.[52] However, the exact FiO_2 cutoff for oxygen toxicity in the ARDS patient, especially in children, remains unknown and may be less than 0.60. Increases in the set PEEP may allow for a reduction of the delivered FiO_2.

In the setting of ARDS, improved oxygenation has not been associated with improved outcomes. This finding was best demonstrated in the ARDS Network low tidal volume study, in which the control (12 mL/kg) group demonstrated improved oxygenation for the first 72 hours of mechanical ventilation but ultimately had a higher mortality in contrast to the lower tidal volume (6 mL/kg) group.[110] In a pediatric study of 470 children, no correlation was found between oxygenation or ventilation measured during the first 14 days of PICU admission in survivors or nonsurvivors of pediatric ALI.[108] Other studies in PARDS have demonstrated short-term improvements in oxygenation parameters with no difference in mortality.[30,31] The ideal target for oxygenation in ARDS remains controversial, but it is clinically reasonable to accept an SaO_2 of less than 90% as long as tissue oxygen delivery is adequate. This concept of accepting lower arterial oxygen saturations is termed *permissive hypoxemia*.[1,86] In general, FiO_2, PEEP, and other ventilatory parameters should be set to optimize oxygen delivery with tolerance of lower oxygen saturations to allow for minimization of VILI.[95] Specific recommendations for a lower level of acceptable oxygen saturations cannot be made.

Permissive hypercapnia is another strategy commonly used in patients with ARDS. Hypercapnia is a consequence of low tidal volume ventilation, and limited evidence suggests that low-volume, pressure-limited ventilation with permissive hypercapnia may improve outcomes in patients with ARDS.[47,48] In a 10-year study, Milberg and colleagues reported an association of permissive hypercapnia with decreased mortality.[71] Recent data from a laboratory model of ischemia-reperfusion ALI indicate that hypercapnic acidosis is protective and that buffering of the hypercapnic acidosis actually attenuates these protective effects.[60] Animal models have also suggested that permissive hypercapnia may attenuate lung damage in sepsis-induced ARDS.[22,51] Although permissive hypercapnia may inhibit the immune response to some degree,[59] this results in decreased inflammation with an associated decrease in ALI.[21] Inhibition of the immune system is of particular concern in patients with sepsis, but administration of antibiotics appears to prevent these deleterious effects.[20,76,77] These findings, along with data demonstrating worsening mortality with each hour in which antibiotics are delayed in septic patients,[58] reinforce the need for early administration of antibiotics in the management of pediatric sepsis and ARDS.[15] Despite these potential benefits and evidence suggesting that respiratory acidosis is not harmful, the exact degree of hypercapnia that can be safely tolerated remains controversial. Most of the undesirable effects of hypercapnia are reversible and minor when pH is greater than approximately 7.20.[37] Further clinical studies looking at the role of permissive hypercapnia in sepsis-related lung injury are needed given the increasing preclinical evidence of its potential therapeutic role.

Adjunctive Therapies

Corticosteroids

Given that inflammation is the cornerstone of the pathophysiology of ARDS, corticosteroids have therapeutic potential as immunomodulatory or antiinflammatory agents. An inherent difficulty in summarizing the use of corticosteroids is the significant variability in the timing and dose of steroids used in the various studies. The timing of steroids in published clinical studies of adults ranges from 72 hours to 4 weeks from the onset of ARDS, and the doses of methylprednisolone (or its equivalent) range from 1 mg/kg per day to 120 mg/kg per day.[81] Meta-analyses of corticosteroid use within the first 2 weeks in adults with established ARDS demonstrated that steroids may reduce mortality and reduce total days of mechanical ventilation.[81,106] A more recent meta-analysis of patients with ARDS due to community-acquired pneumonia found no difference in mortality for patients treated with steroids or placebo but did find that steroids reduced length of hospital stay and the duration of mechanical ventilation.[101] Although few studies evaluating steroids have included children, a recent prospective observational study of 283 PARDS patients found that steroids were associated with a longer duration of mechanical ventilation with no difference in mortality.[116] Additionally, based on current data, corticosteroids do not appear to have a role in preventing ARDS.[81] The use of steroids has not been associated with an increase in secondary infections.[81,106]

Inhaled Nitric Oxide

Pulmonary vascular dysfunction is an important component of the pathophysiologic process or ARDS.[19] The impact of ARDS on pulmonary vascular tone has led to an extensive investigation of inhaled nitric oxide, a potent vasodilator that works exclusively in the pulmonary vasculature, as a potential therapeutic option. Studies of inhaled nitric oxide for PARDS have demonstrated temporary improvement in oxygenation acutely but not improved survival.[2,31,30] The largest pediatric inhaled nitric oxide study to date involved 108 children.[31] Because of the crossover design, the study was not able to describe mortality results, but it did demonstrate that the groups of children who may acutely benefit most are immunocompromised patients and those with greater severity of hypoxemia.

A recent Cochrane Database Systematic Review looking at 14 randomized controlled trials concluded that inhaled nitric oxide cannot be recommended for either children or adults with ARDS because it resulted in transient improvement in oxygenation without mortality benefit.[4] Furthermore it appeared that inhaled nitric oxide may increase the risk for renal impairment among adults with ARDS. Except for the potential treatment of documented pulmonary hypertension and/or severe right ventricular dysfunction, the administration of inhaled nitric oxide for ARDS cannot be recommended based on the available data.[105]

Surfactant Replacement

In ARDS, injury occurs to type 2 pneumocytes, resulting in decreased production of surfactant. This injury has prompted studies examining the possibility of the effectiveness of surfactant replacement in the management of ARDS. A study of 153 pediatric patients reported that exogenous surfactant acutely improved oxygenation and significantly decreased mortality in infants and children with ALI.[113] There were no significant decreases in duration of mechanical ventilation, length of PICU admission, or length of hospital stay. The results of this study are controversial because a significantly higher number of immunocompromised patients (i.e., with a higher expected mortality) were included in the control group.[25] Randomized trials in adults found that, for 450 adults with ARDS randomized to surfactant or placebo, there was no difference in mortality and, for 308 adults randomized to calfactant or placebo, there was no improvement in oxygenation or survival.[103,115] More recent pediatric studies that included a total of 274 patients have also shown that surfactant does not improve mortality in infants and children.[107,114] Surfactant replacement is not currently recommended for the treatment of PARDS.[45]

Nonpulmonary Supportive Management

Fluid Balance

Initial aggressive fluid resuscitation is important in maintaining hemodynamics and improving clinical outcomes in patients with shock.[96] However, once hemodynamics are restored, overhydration may lead to pulmonary edema. Fluids should be carefully titrated and fluid status monitored while normalizing the patient's intravascular volume status and maintaining adequate cardiac output.[5] The ARDS Network conducted a study to investigate conservative and liberal fluid management strategies in adult patients with ARDS.[112] In this study, a difference of 6000 mL was seen in the 7-day cumulative fluid balance between the two groups, with patients in the conservative fluid management group having improved lung function and shorter duration of mechanical ventilation and ICU length of stay. In critically ill children, the role of fluid balance is less conclusive. Although some studies demonstrate that fluid balance has an impact on oxygenation and morbidity,[5,49] other prospective pediatric studies have shown otherwise.[88] The Pediatric Acute Lung Injury and Sepsis Investigators (PALISI) Network investigators showed that cumulative fluid input and output did not affect the speed of weaning from mechanical ventilation or extubation outcomes.[88]

Sedation and Neuromuscular Blockade

Appropriate sedation and analgesia are important in children who are on mechanical ventilation. Prolonged sedation and neuromuscular blockage have been associated with worse clinical outcomes, and the long-term effects of sedative medications are unknown.[7,42,65] However, a recent study demonstrated that early neuromuscular blockage improved survival in adults with ARDS.[79] In this study of 340 adults with ARDS, the use of cisatracurium for 48 hours improved 90-day survival by nearly 1.5 times compared to placebo without an increase in muscle weakness. In contrast, growing evidence in adults indicates substantial benefits associated with sedation weaning and promotion of early mobilization.[43,73] In children, a sedation weaning protocol was not found to change the duration of mechanical ventilation, PICU or hospital lengths of stay, or in-hospital mortality.[24] Given the lack of consistent evidence in both adults and children, the use of neuromuscular blockade in children with ARDS remains controversial. Overall use of sedatives and neuromuscular blocking agents should be driven by a balance between maintaining adequate gas exchange and the potential adverse effects of critical illness weakness and myopathy.

Nutrition

As a general approach, adequate nutrition should be provided to optimize caloric intake and avoid a negative nitrogen balance. However, few studies examining the effects of nutrition in children with ARDS have been conducted. Clinical guidelines with regard to nutritional support of critically ill children are, at best, supported by small, randomized trials with reasonable risk for bias in their results.[70] Although a growing number of studies are investigating the potential utility of nutritional supplementation in ARDS, the results have not been consistent or encouraging. Using bronchoalveolar and plasma biomarkers as their end points, investigators examining the effect of omega-3 oil on adults with ARDS did not note any difference in IL-8, IL-6, and leukotriene B4 levels between patients with and without supplementation.[104] This was further supported by a recent clinical study that was stopped early for futility.[94] This study of twice-daily supplementation of omega-3 fatty acids within 48 hours of onset of ARDS showed a trend toward longer duration of mechanical ventilation and higher mortality in the treatment group.[94]

Patient Isolation

Even though infectious etiologies are the most common cause of ARDS in children, routine isolation of all ARDS patients is not warranted. In certain infective etiologies such as viruses (e.g., influenza, RSV, adenovirus), resistant bacteria, and mycobacteria (e.g., tuberculosis), appropriate isolation measures should be instituted.[100]

Rescue Therapies

Some patients with severe ARDS become refractory to maximal therapies and are unable to achieve acceptable therapeutic goals while avoiding oxygen toxicity or intolerably high airway pressures. In these circumstances, extracorporeal membrane oxygenation (ECMO) has increasingly been used as a rescue modality for these patients.

ECMO involves withdrawing blood from the patient by a mechanical pump and directing it to a membrane oxygenator, where oxygenation and removal of carbon dioxide occur before the blood is returned to the patient. In refractory ARDS patients, venovenous ECMO is commonly used, which involves blood being withdrawn from the patient via a cannula placed in a central vein and returned to the venous system. Cardiac function must be sufficient to circulate this returned blood systemically to the body. ECMO has been used successfully in a wide range of clinical circumstances and is a viable treatment strategy in adults and children with refractory ARDS.[16,44] Traditionally ECMO has been implemented in patients with an anticipated mortality that is extremely high, exceeding 80% to 90% in many circumstances, but reported survival from the Extracorporeal Life Support Organization (ELSO) registry for adults and children with ARDS is currently 50% and 65%, respectively.[16,32] In the past decade, use of ECMO has continued to increase, as evidenced by reports from the 2009 H1N1 influenza A pandemic.[27,74,75,109] A more detailed discussion of ECMO support for pediatric and adult ARDS patients is beyond the scope of this chapter.[26]

CONCLUSION

ARDS represents a complex syndrome of varying pulmonary and nonpulmonary etiologies. Although much progress has been made in better understanding the pathophysiology of ARDS, the only ventilatory strategy that has been demonstrated to improve clinical outcome is low tidal volume ventilation. Effective treatment of the underlying etiology can reduce mortality related to the infectious process and likely reduces continued lung damage due to ongoing inflammation.[118,29] It is anticipated that future clinical studies will combine therapeutic strategies instead of simply focusing on a single intervention. Although meticulous balance is important in each organ system, limited data exist regarding the optimal supportive management strategies for children with ARDS. Current approaches largely represent clinical experience and extrapolation of the available data from the adult population. Hopefully the recent recommendations and comments made by the PALICC group will help to prompt future, more definitive research of the PARDS.

NEW REFERENCES SINCE THE SEVENTH EDITION

10. Bartlett AH, Foster TJ, Hayashida A. Alpha-toxin facilitates the generation of CXC chemokine gradients and stimulates neutrophil homing in *Staphylococcus aureus* pneumonia. *J Infect Dis*. 2008;198(10):1529-1535.
11. Bateman ST, Borasino S, Asaro LA, et al. Early high-frequency oscillatory ventilation in pediatric acute respiratory failure. A propensity score analysis. *Am J Respir Crit Care Med*. 2016;193(5):495-503.
24. Curley MA, Wypij D, Watson RS, et al. Protocolized sedation vs usual care in pediatric patients mechanically ventilated for acute respiratory failure: a randomized clinical trial. *JAMA*. 2015;313(4):379-389.
26. Dalton HJ, Macrae DJ, Pediatric Acute Lung Injury Consensus Conference Group (PALICC Group). Extracorporeal support in children with pediatric acute respiratory distress syndrome: proceedings from the Pediatric Acute Lung Injury Consensus Conference. *Pediatr Crit Care Med*. 2015;16(5 suppl 1):S111-S117.
29. Dellinger RP, Levy MM, Rhodes A, et al. Surviving sepsis campaign: international guidelines for management of severe sepsis and septic shock: 2012. *Crit Care Med*. 2013;41(2):580-637.
34. Erickson S, Schibler A, Numa A, et al. Acute lung injury in pediatric intensive care in Australia and New Zealand: a prospective, multicenter, observational study. *Pediatr Crit Care Med*. 2007;8(4):317-323.
38. Ferguson ND, Cook DJ, Guyatt GH, et al. High-frequency oscillation in early acute respiratory distress syndrome. *N Engl J Med*. 2013;368(9):795-805.
40. Flori H, Dahmer MK, Sapru A, et al. Comorbidities and assessment of severity of pediatric acute respiratory distress syndrome: proceedings from the Pediatric Acute Lung Injury Consensus Conference. *Pediatr Crit Care Med*. 2015;16(5 suppl 1):S41-S50.
45. PALICC Group. Pediatric acute respiratory distress syndrome: consensus recommendations from the Pediatric Acute Lung Injury Consensus Conference. *Pediatr Crit Care Med*. 2015;16(5):428-439.
54. Khemani RG, Conti D, Alonzo TA, et al. Effect of tidal volume in children with acute hypoxemic respiratory failure. *Intensive Care Med*. 2009;35(8):1428-1437.
55. Khemani RG, Smith LS, Zimmerman JJ, et al. Pediatric acute respiratory distress syndrome: definition, incidence, and epidemiology: proceedings from the Pediatric Acute Lung Injury Consensus Conference. *Pediatr Crit Care Med*. 2015;16(5 suppl 1):S23-S40.
56. Kim JS, Ko JH, Lee S, et al. *Enterobacter cloacae* sacroiliitis with acute respiratory distress syndrome in an adolescent. *Infect Chemother*. 2015;47(2):125-128.
65. Loepke AW. Developmental neurotoxicity of sedatives and anesthetics: a concern for neonatal and pediatric critical care medicine? *Pediatr Crit Care Med*. 2010;11(2):217-226.

66. López-Fernández Y, Azagra AM, de la Oliva P, et al. Pediatric acute lung injury epidemiology and natural history study: incidence and outcome of the acute respiratory distress syndrome in children. *Crit Care Med.* 2012;40(12):3238-3245.
85. Quasney MW, López-Fernández YM, Santschi M, et al. The outcomes of children with pediatric acute respiratory distress syndrome: proceedings from the Pediatric Acute Lung Injury Consensus Conference. *Pediatr Crit Care Med.* 2015;16(5 suppl 1):S118-S131.
87. Randolph AG, Agan AA, Flanagan RF, et al. Optimizing virus identification in critically ill children suspected of having an acute severe viral infection. *Pediatr Crit Care Med.* 2016;17(4):279-286.
92. Rao S, Torok MR, Bagdure D, et al. A comparison of H1N1 influenza among pediatric inpatients in the pandemic and post pandemic era. *J Clin Virol.* 2015;71:44-50.
95. Rimensberger PC, Cheifetz IM, PALICC Group. Ventilatory support in children with pediatric acute respiratory distress syndrome: proceedings from the Pediatric Acute Lung Injury Consensus Conference. *Pediatr Crit Care Med.* 2015;16(5 suppl 1):S51-S60.
100. Siegel JD, Rhinehart E, Jackson M, et al. 2007 Guideline for isolation precautions: preventing transmission of infectious agents in healthcare settings. *Am J Infect Control.* 2007;35(10 suppl 2):S65-S164.
101. Siemieniuk RA, Meade MO, Alonso-Coello P, et al. Corticosteroid therapy for patients hospitalized with community-acquired pneumonia: a systematic review and meta-analysis. *Ann Intern Med.* 2015;163(7):519-528.
102. Simon M, Braune S, Laqmani A, et al. Value of computed tomography of the chest in subjects with ARDS: a retrospective observational study. *Respir Care.* 2016;61(3):316-323.
105. Tamburro RF, Kneyber MC, PALICC Group. Pulmonary specific ancillary treatment for pediatric acute respiratory distress syndrome: proceedings from the Pediatric Acute Lung Injury Consensus Conference. *Pediatr Crit Care Med.* 2015;16(5 suppl 1):S61-S72.
107. Thomas NJ, Guardia CG, Moya FR, et al. A pilot, randomized, controlled clinical trial of lucinactant, a peptide-containing synthetic surfactant, in infants with acute hypoxemic respiratory failure. *Pediatr Crit Care Med.* 2012;13(6):646-653.
114. Willson DF, Thomas NJ, Tamburro R, et al. Pediatric calfactant in acute respiratory distress syndrome trial. *Pediatr Crit Care Med.* 2013;14(7):657-665.
115. Willson DF, Truwit JD, Conaway MR, et al. The adult calfactant in acute respiratory distress syndrome trial. *Chest.* 2015;148(2):35664.
116. Yehya N, Servaes S, Thomas NJ, et al. Corticosteroid exposure in pediatric acute respiratory distress syndrome. *Intensive Care Med.* 2015;41(9):1658-1666.
117. Young D, Lamb SE, Shah S, et al. High-frequency oscillation for acute respiratory distress syndrome. *N Engl J Med.* 2013;368(9):80613.
119. Zhu YF, Xu F, Lu XL, et al. Mortality and morbidity of acute hypoxemic respiratory failure and acute respiratory distress syndrome in infants and young children. *Chin Med J.* 2012;125(13):2265-2271.

The full reference list for this chapter is available at ExpertConsult.com.

Approach to Infections in the Fetus and Newborn

66

Gail J. Harrison

This chapter provides an overview and approach to the diagnosis and management of the more common infections that occur in the fetus and newborn infant. Details about how each organism affects the fetus and newborn, as well as information on diagnosis and management, are covered in the pathogen-specific and disease-specific chapters of this edition.

VIRAL INFECTIONS OF THE FETUS AND NEONATE

Viral infections are an important cause of fetal and neonatal morbidity and mortality. The cumulative frequency of viral infections in the fetus or newborn infant may be as high as 6% to 8% of all live births, whereas systemic bacterial disease occurs in only 1% to 2% of neonates. Viral infections of the fetus and newborn may be divided into congenital, perinatal or natal, and postnatal time periods of acquisition.

Pathogenesis

Congenital Viral Infections

Congenital viral infections are transmitted to the developing fetus during a maternal infection. Most congenital viral infections are from maternal primary infections, but some viruses (cytomegalovirus [CMV]) may be transmitted to the fetus during a recurrent (reactivation or reinfection) maternal infection.[8] Congenital viral infections can result in resorption of the embryo; spontaneous abortion or miscarriage; stillbirth; congenital malformation; prematurity; intrauterine growth restriction (IUGR); or acute disease apparent in utero, at birth, or shortly thereafter. Congenital infection with Ebola virus is uniformly fatal.[4,13,21,31] In contrast, most congenital CMV infections are asymptomatic in the fetal or neonatal period yet may be associated with persistent postnatal infection, sequelae later in life, or a normal infant with no apparent sequelae.

Most fetal infections are preceded by a systemic viral infection in the mother, with hematogenous spread of the virus to the placenta and subsequently to the fetus (Fig. 66.1). Ascending infection through amniotic membranes also may occur while the fetus is still in utero. With most viruses well known to cause fetal infection—CMV, rubella virus, herpes simplex virus (HSV), varicella zoster virus (VZV), Ebola virus, Zika virus, Dengue, and vaccinia virus—placental involvement by the virus also has been documented (Table 66.1).[4,11,31] Viruses may reach the fetal circulation by (1) replication through the layers of the placenta; (2) production of virus-induced vascular lesions in the placenta, resulting in abnormal communications between the maternal and fetal circulation; or (3) diapedesis of virus-infected maternal leukocytes through the layers of the placenta to the fetal circulation.

Developmental malformations also may occur. Rubella virus is the classic known teratogen, causing disturbances in organogenesis, cardiac disease, and cataracts.[9] VZV and Zika virus have been shown to cause limb hypoplasia and developmental malformations of the eye and brain.[11,19,20] Other viruses that result in congenital abnormalities, such as CMV and HSV, usually cause inflammatory, destructive lesions of already developed organs. Type B coxsackieviruses and other enteroviruses have been associated with a variety of congenital malformations of the heart, and mumps has been linked to endocardial fibroelastosis. Chikungunya virus also may cause congenital infection and disease.[17]

Damage to the fetus also may occur in the absence of actual fetal viral infection as a result of severe systemic illness in the mother, such as measles or influenza, or alteration of placental function.

Natal or Perinatal Viral Infections

Natal or perinatal infections are the result of exposure of the newborn to virus replicating in the maternal cervicovaginal tract (i.e., CMV, HSV, or hepatitis B virus) or perirectal area (e.g., enteroviruses). Natal or perinatal infections with some viruses can cause acute systemic illness leading to death, persistent infection with late sequelae (HSV, HBV), self-limited disease with no discernible damage (CMV), or asymptomatic infection (see Fig. 66.1 and Table 66.1). Because the incubation periods of HSV and enteroviruses are short, acute postnatal disease may appear in the neonate within 5 to 7 days of age. In contrast, the incubation periods of CMV and hepatitis B virus (HBV) are longer, and clinically apparent disease from perinatal exposure, if it occurs, may not be observed for several weeks or even months after birth. Persistent postnatal infection can occur after perinatal infection with CMV, HSV, and HBV.

Postnatal Viral Infections

Postnatal infections in the neonate may be transmitted to the neonate from the mother, family members, caretakers in extended family, health care workers, outbreaks in neonatal care units, or community exposures (see Fig. 66.1). Neonatal infections and hospital-associated outbreaks of enterovirus and parechovirus, respiratory syncytial virus (RSV), rotavirus, adenovirus, rhinovirus, parainfluenza virus, human metapneumovirus, and influenza virus infection have occurred. In addition, health care–associated HSV infections have occurred in neonates (see Table 66.1). Although the maternal respiratory and gastrointestinal tracts are the most common sites from which virus can be transmitted to the neonate postnatally, other viruses, including human immunodeficiency virus (HIV), human T-cell leukemia virus types 1 and 2 (HTLV I and II), CMV, West Nile virus, rubella virus, hepatitis C virus (HCV), Zika virus, and HBV, have been recovered from breast milk. HSV and VZV lesions on the breast of a mother also may be a source of transmission of virus for the breastfeeding neonate, even though these viruses probably are not present in the breast milk. Finally, HIV, CMV, and HBV have been transmitted to newborn infants by blood transfusion. Although most postnatal infections are acute, self-limited processes, severe disease and fatalities have been reported, especially in preterm infants infected with CMV, enteroviruses, HSV, adenoviruses, or RSV, and persistent postnatal infection may occur with CMV and HBV.[6,5]

Approach to Diagnosis

Evaluation of the Mother

Fetal viral infection may be suspected if the mother is exposed to or experiences an infection with a virus known to transmit to the fetus. A history of recent illness, travel, or exposures to the mother should be obtained to uncover circumstantial evidence for a viral infection in the fetus or newborn. For example, the occurrence of maternal viral illness with an associated maculopapular rash suggests rubella or enterovirus or Zika virus infection in the neonate, exposure to mosquitoes suggests St. Louis encephalitis virus, West Nile virus, or Zika virus, ulcerative genital lesions suggest HSV, and heterophile-negative infectious mononucleosis is suggestive of CMV.[25,26] Hemorrhagic fever after travel to Africa suggests Ebola virus.[4,11,21] Maternal rash with arthralgias also may be caused by parvovirus B19, especially if there is recent exposure to fifth disease in the community. Since viral infections in the mother may be asymptomatic, the absence of symptoms in the mother does not rule out the possibility of a viral infection in the neonate.

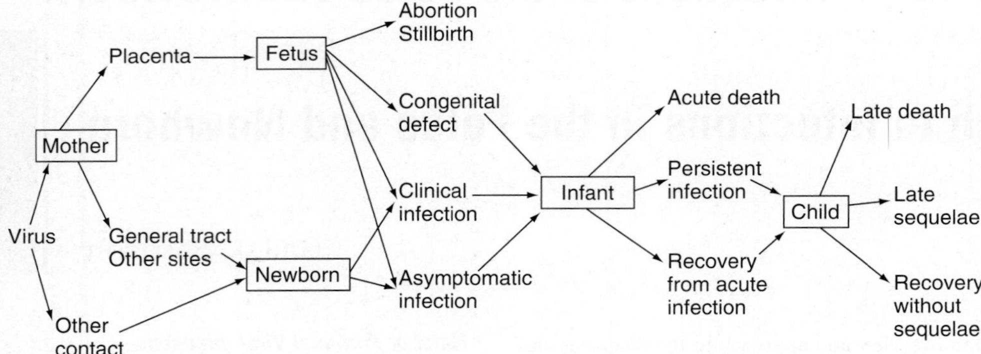

FIG. 66.1 Pathogenesis of viral infections in the fetus and newborn.

TABLE 66.1 Period of Transmission of Selected Viruses to the Fetus or Newborn Infant

Viruses	Congenital	Natal	Postnatal
Adenovirus	+	+	+
Chikungunya	++	+	–
Cytomegalovirus	++	++	++
Dengue	++	–	–
Ebola virus	++	+	+
Echoviruses	+	+	+
Epstein-Barr	+	–	+
Hepatitis A	–	++	+
Hepatitis B	+	++	+
Hepatitis C	+	++	–
Herpes simplex	+	++	+
Herpesvirus-6	+	–	+
Human immunodeficiency virus	+	++	+
Human parvovirus B19	+	–	–
Influenza	(+)	–	+
Lymphocytic choriomeningitis virus	++	–	–
Measles	+	–	+
Mumps	+	–	–
Parechovirus	–	+	+
Polioviruses	+	+	+
Rubella	++	–	–
Smallpox	+	+	+
St. Louis encephalitis	(+)	-	(+)
Type B coxsackieviruses	+	+	+
Vaccinia	+	+	+
Varicella zoster	++	+	+
West Nile virus	+	–	+
Western equine encephalitis	+	–	+
Zika virus	++	?	(+)

++, Major demonstrated route; +, minor demonstrated route; (+), suggested route, few supporting data; –, route not demonstrated.

Clinical Features in Fetus and Newborn

Abnormalities detected on routine fetal ultrasound also may suggest fetal infection. These findings include IUGR; microcephaly; cerebral ventriculomegaly or hydrocephalus; cataracts; hepatosplenomegaly; hepatic or intracranial calcifications; and cortical maldevelopment syndromes such as polymicrogyria, hydrocephalus, microcephaly, in utero central nervous system (CNS) vasculitis, echogenic bowel, fetal ascites, cardiomegaly, congestive heart failure, fetal hydrops, enlarged or swollen placenta, or polyhydramnios or oligohydramnios.[19,20] Intrauterine cardiac abnormalities, myocarditis, and heart failure may be associated with HIV, parvovirus B19, mumps virus, CMV, Zika virus, or adenovirus, and cardiac structural defects may be associated with rubella virus. Limb deformities or dysplasias, especially if they are associated with eye or CNS abnormalities, may be caused by intrauterine VZV or HSV infection and possibly Zika virus.

In more than 80% of CMV, 60% of rubella virus, and most HBV infection in the neonate are asymptomatic. In contrast, less than 1% of HSV infections and no Ebola virus infections are subclinical in the neonate.

Clinical manifestations of viral disease in the neonate may provide helpful clues to the specific etiologic agent. The presence of cataracts, congenital heart disease, bone lesions, or microphthalmos is highly suggestive of rubella, whereas chorioretinitis, cerebral calcifications, and hydrocephaly are more common with congenital infection with CMV, lymphocytic choriomeningitis virus (LCMV), Zika virus, or HSV. The features in neonates with perinatal or postnatal enterovirus, HSV, or adenovirus disease resemble those associated with bacterial sepsis: lethargy or irritability, fever or hypothermia, respiratory distress, cyanosis, anorexia or vomiting, hepatomegaly, seizures, or abnormal movements.[6,5] Laboratory abnormalities in disseminated viral disease may show neutropenia, lymphocytosis, lymphopenia, thrombocytopenia, elevated liver transaminases, hyperbilirubinemia, and cerebrospinal fluid (CSF) pleocytosis. Aseptic meningitis in the neonate may be caused by perinatal or postnatal infection with HSV1 or 2, enteroviruses, or parechoviruses. In neonates with persistent severe viral infections that are slow or minimally responsive to antiviral therapy, a primary immune deficiency disorder of T-, B-, or natural killer (NK)-cell function should be considered.

Differential Diagnosis

The differential diagnosis in a fetus or newborn infant with a suspected viral infection includes but is not limited to bacterial or fungal sepsis, toxoplasmosis, syphilis, erythroblastosis fetalis, metabolic inborn errors of metabolism, genetic chromosomal abnormalities, and other forms of congenital malformations.

Laboratory Diagnosis

Prenatal diagnosis of fetal viral infection may be established by testing amniotic fluid for viral culture and polymerase chain reaction (PCR) or by fetal blood sample for viral-specific immunoglobulin (Ig)M and PCR studies. The placenta may also be sent for histopathologic studies.

In neonates, urine, saliva, and blood for CMV; throat, cataracts, and occasionally CSF or urine for rubella; skin vesicles, blood, CSF, conjunctivae, throat, stool, and urine for HSV; throat, stool, urine, CSF, or blood for enteroviruses; and skin vesicles and blood for VZV should be sent for virus isolation or virus detection by PCR. In addition, isolation or molecular detection by PCR of virus can be attempted from biopsy or autopsy specimens. Electron-microscopic examination of vesicle fluid or tissue can demonstrate typical herpesvirus particles in both HSV and VZV infection but cannot distinguish between the two. Dried blood spots archived after completion of newborn screening for metabolic and immunodeficiency disorders may be retrieved with maternal permission from state newborn screening agencies and tested for the presence of viral DNA.[2,3] Such approaches have reliably allowed the retrospective diagnosis of congenital CMV. Research evaluating urine and saliva as screening specimens for congenital CMV infection have also been conducted.[2,3,8]

Three approaches can be used to make a serologic diagnosis of viral infection in a newborn infant: (1) assay of maternal serum and serum specimens from the infant at birth and at 5 to 6 months of age for antiviral antibody (predominantly IgG activity), (2) assay of neonatal serum for IgM antibody against a specific viral agent, and (3) assay of neonatal serum for quantitative IgM levels, a nonspecific indication of antigenic challenge in utero.[26] Maternal IgG, antibody against viruses to which the mother has been exposed, passes transplacentally, beginning at midgestation. Peak levels are reached in fetal serum at the time of birth (umbilical cord blood); they decline to undetectable levels by the time that the infant reaches 6 to 12 months of age, depending on the virus. Maternal IgM antibody normally is not passed transplacentally, but a fetus challenged in utero with a virus can have specific IgM antibodies against the viral agent as well as elevated levels of the total IgM fraction. Often a fetus with detectable virus-specific IgM will have severe in utero disease caused by the virus.

Treatment

Intravenous acyclovir followed by long-term oral suppression with oral acyclovir is the mainstay for antiviral treatment of neonatal herpes simplex virus infection.[6,5,15,23] Congenital CMV disease, especially if it is severe or involves the CNS or sensory organs such as the eye and ear, may be treated with intravenous ganciclovir or oral valganciclovir.[8,14,23] Neonates with influenza virus may receive antiviral medications such as oseltamivir, and ribavirin for severe RSV disease.

BACTERIAL DISEASES OF THE FETUS AND NEWBORN

Worldwide, millions of neonates die every year of bacterial infection.[16] In the United States, the infant mortality rate is approximately 6.85 infant deaths/1000 live births. Neonatal bacterial sepsis corresponds to the eighth leading cause of fatality. The incidence of neonatal sepsis ranges from 1 to 8/1000 live births, with the higher figures corresponding to developing countries. Low birth weight, male sex, and congenital malformation are important risk factors. Extreme prematurity is the greatest risk factor for early-onset sepsis and is associated with an increased risk for having adverse outcomes. The highest age-specific incidence of bacterial meningitis appears to occur during the first month of life.

Epidemiology and Pathogenesis

The human birth canal is host to large numbers of aerobic and anaerobic bacteria, *Mycoplasma, Ureaplasma, Chlamydia,* fungi, yeast, and viruses. *Staphylococcus epidermidis,* lactobacilli, diphtheroids, and α-hemolytic streptococci are found in 50% to 100% of vaginal cultures of pregnant women and constitute the predominant aerobic flora. Significant but less common isolates include *Gardnerella vaginalis, Proteus,* and *Klebsiella* spp. and group B and D streptococci; *Staphylococcus aureus* and miscellaneous organisms, such as *Citrobacter, Acinetobacter,* and the *Campylobacter* group, are identified even less commonly. Approximately 85% of women with genital colonization by anaerobes harbor *Bacteroides* spp., including *Bacteroides fragilis* in a third of cases. Anaerobic streptococci, *Peptostreptococcus* and *Peptococcus,* are found in approximately 40% of women, and *Clostridium* is present in 20%. Uncommon anaerobic isolates include *Veillonella, Bifidobacterium,* and *Eubacterium.*

Certain microorganisms are associated with the occurrence of stillbirths. Among these bacterial agents are *Escherichia coli,* group B streptococci (GBS), *Ureaplasma urealyticum, Listeria monocytogenes,* and *Treponema pallidum.*

Streptococcus agalactiae, or GBS, is a major pathogen for the neonate, causing both early-onset sepsis and late-onset disease, usually meningitis, but also other manifestations (Box 66.1). The acute early-onset form of GBS disease can be caused by any of the group B types (B_I to B_{VIII}), and the specific B type causing disease in the infant usually is found in the maternal vaginal tract. GBS meningitis is caused almost exclusively by the B_{III} organism. These organisms also may be acquired from nonmaternal sites. Clusters of three or four cases of GBS meningitis have occurred in nurseries during short intervals, suggesting that health care–associated outbreaks may occur. The administration of intrapartum antibiotics, such as ampicillin, has reduced the incidence of early-onset GBS disease in neonates. *E. coli* is the other important agent implicated in neonatal bacterial disease, including sepsis, meningitis, and urinary tract infection, with an annual incidence of approximately 6.8/1000 live births; it is the most common gram-negative bacterium causing meningitis during this period.[1] Ampicillin-resistant and multidrug-resistant *E. coli* strains have emerged. Neonatal colonization with *E. coli* often results from maternal transmission during delivery. *Klebsiella pneumoniae* is another important neonatal pathogen causing sepsis and meningitis, with an incidence of between 4.1 and 6.3/1000 live births and fatality rates of 18% to 68%. It is the second most frequent gram-negative organism associated with late-onset sepsis in developed nations. *L. monocytogenes* is a foodborne colonizer of the human gastrointestinal tract, and one of the host factors that increases the risk for *Listeria* infection and disease is pregnancy. Perinatal infection constituted 34% (470/1378) of cases of listeriosis. Transmission to the fetus in utero may produce granulomatous fetal disease and an early-onset sepsis syndrome or a late-onset meningitis.

S. aureus is another important bacterial neonatal pathogen, causing sepsis, meningitis, osteomyelitis, and abscesses in newborns postnatally. Since the 1980s, epidemic and endemic colonization and disease of the newborn infant with community-acquired and hospital-acquired methicillin-sensitive (MSSA) and MRSA have become commonplace. *S. epidermidis* and other coagulase-negative staphylococci also are important neonatal pathogens and a common cause of late-onset sepsis and infections associated with indwelling devices and necrotizing enterocolitis. They are the most common species of the normal flora on the skin, nasal mucosa, and umbilicus of the newborn. The ubiquitous presence of the organisms and their tolerance to drying and temperature changes contribute to the presence of coagulase-negative staphylococci in neonates. *Enterococcus faecalis* and *E. faecium* are members of the group D streptococci (enterococci), are normal inhabitants of the gastrointestinal tract, and can cause invasive disease in the neonate, usually urinary tract infections, sepsis, and meningitis. These bacteria are the third most frequent gram-positive organisms associated with late-onset sepsis. Outbreaks of bacteremia and meningitis caused by *E. faecium* resistant to ampicillin and vancomycin have also been reported in neonates.

BOX 66.1 Common Bacterial Pathogens Causing Neonatal Sepsis

Gram-Negative Organisms

Escherichia coli
Haemophilus influenzae
Citrobacter
Enterobacter spp.
Pseudomonas spp.
Acinetobacter
Neisseria meningitidis

Gram-Positive Organisms

Group B streptococci *(Streptococcus agalactiae)*
Viridans streptococci
Enterococci
Streptococcus pneumoniae
Other streptococci
Listeria monocytogenes
Coagulase-negative staphylococci
Staphylococcus aureus

Neonatal Sepsis

Sepsis neonatorum, or sepsis of the newborn, is a bacterial disease of infants 30 days of age or younger, most often in the first week of life.[22]

The major signs and symptoms of sepsis in the newborn relate to disturbances in thermoregulation, respiration, heart rate, and gastrointestinal function; abnormalities in temperature regulation, either hypothermia or hyperthermia; tachypnea; grunting respirations; cyanosis; intercostal and substernal retractions; and apnea. A heart rate persistently in excess of 160 beats per minute or above average for age and gestation can be a sensitive indicator of early-onset neonatal sepsis. Other early signs of neonatal sepsis include poor feeding, regurgitation, vomiting, weak sucking, abdominal distention, diarrhea, jaundice, and, rarely, gallbladder distention.

Neonates may have cutaneous findings with onset of sepsis neonatorum, which may provide clinical clues for the cause of the condition. Such findings include cellulitis or abscesses (*Staphylococcus* or *Streptococcus*); papular (i.e., listeriosis), vascular, or bullous lesions (i.e., *Pseudomonas*); and exfoliative dermatitis (i.e., phage group II staphylococcal disease). Jaundice develops in approximately one-third of infants with sepsis and can also occur in infants with urinary tract infection. Occasionally, jaundice is the only sign of infection and occurs in septic infants regardless of the type of bacterial pathogen.

Bacterial sepsis in the newborn may be caused by almost any gram-positive or gram-negative organism.[1,22] The most commonly identified bacteria include GBS, group A streptococcus (GAS), and group D streptococcus (GDS), including the enterococci and viridans streptococci. In addition *Streptococcus pneumoniae* may cause severe illness in the neonate. The gram-positive rod *L. monocytogenes* is also a well-recognized cause of neonatal sepsis. The staphylococci, including community-acquired and hospital-acquired MSSA and MRSA and coagulase-negative staphylococci may cause sepsis in the newborn. Gram-negative enteric organisms, such as *E. coli* and *K. pneumoniae,* are common causes of neonatal sepsis. In addition, other gram-negative organisms, such as *Enterobacter cloacae* and *Acinetobacter* spp., may cause sepsis in the neonate. *Haemophilus influenzae* also has been isolated from neonates with sepsis.

Abnormalities in the white blood cell (WBC) count may be observed, with elevation, left shift with neutrophil predominance, leukemoid reaction, or neutropenia, with thrombocytopenia. The presence of severe thrombocytopenia, or less than 50,000 cells/mL, within 72 hours of birth is an uncommon occurrence and may be caused by early bacterial infection (e.g., GBS sepsis) or congenital viral infection (CMV or HSV). Late-onset thrombocytopenia is often caused by bacterial sepsis or necrotizing enterocolitis. In these cases, platelets fall rapidly, with a nadir at 24 to 48 hours, to counts less than 50,000 cells/mL and tend to persist until the infection is controlled. Slow recovery of platelet counts over a period of 1 to 2 weeks is common.

Elevation of C-reactive protein (CRP) and erythrocyte sedimentation rate (ESR) also may occur.[24] The ESR in infected patients generally is elevated above the normal range of 1 to 2 mm/h at 12 hours of age to 17 to 20 mm/h at 14 days of age. Elevated rates usually are not observed until 24 to 48 hours after clinical signs of disease first occur.

Antimicrobial therapy, administered intravenously, directed against the usual pathogens suspected and then adjusted based on culture results is recommended. For infants whose initial bacterial cultures are sterile after 48 to 72 hours of incubation and the clinical suspicion for bacterial infection is low, antimicrobial therapy can be discontinued. If no pathogen has been isolated but bacterial sepsis cannot be excluded, a negative CRP test at 72 hours can help support the decision to discontinue antibiotics.

In addition to antibiotics, supportive care with careful attention to fluid and electrolyte balance; correcting hypoxia, acidosis, hypoglycemia, and other metabolic abnormalities; and providing nutritional support is necessary. Human immunoglobulin for intravenous use in septic neonates appears to be safe but not convincingly proved to be beneficial in randomized clinical trials. In neonates with primary immunodeficiency syndromes involving B-cell function that cause reduced levels of immunoglobulin, replacement therapy with immunoglobulin may be needed. Other supportive therapeutic options for critically ill neonates include extracorporeal membrane oxygenation and immunomodulating strategies (e.g., anticytokine agents, steroids, pentoxifylline, and nitric oxide inhibitors).

Prevention of neonatal sepsis is a priority for clinicians and physician research scientists. Intrapartum chemoprophylaxis given to women at 35 to 37 weeks' gestation with proved GBS colonization reliably prevents colonization of the newborn in the postpartum period and reduces early-onset sepsis caused by GBS. Therefore universal prophylaxis of all pregnant women with GBS colonization is now recommended and is the current cornerstone for prevention of early-onset GBS disease.[1,30] Clinical trials evaluating maternal immunization with GBS as a way to prevent neonatal GBS disease are under way. Currently, no licensed vaccine against GBS exists; however, many experts feel this strategy, when available, will be the most effective and sustainable long-term preventive strategy for neonatal GBS disease.

Prevention of early sepsis caused by gram-negative bacilli by administration of intrapartum aminoglycosides is important in developing areas of the world where these organisms are prevalent, but no standardized guidelines exist.

Prevention of late-onset infection, as opposed to early-onset disease, in neonates by the administration of intravenous immunoglobulin to preterm babies has undergone intense clinical scrutiny, but consensus of summaries of clinical trial evidence does not support its routine use at this time.[30]

Bacterial Meningitis

As many as a fourth of neonates with bacterial sepsis have a simultaneous meningeal infection.[10,27] The early signs and symptoms of neonatal meningitis frequently are indistinguishable from those of septicemia and other disorders occurring in the neonatal period. The most frequent signs of neonatal meningitis are temperature instability, respiratory distress, irritability, lethargy, and poor feeding or vomiting. GBS occasionally has been reported to manifest as hydrocephalus without other signs of infection. Signs of meningeal involvement, such as a stiff neck, bulging fontanelle, seizures, and opisthotonos, usually are not present in neonates with meningitis. Therefore newborns being evaluated for sepsis usually should undergo examination of CSF, especially if antimicrobial therapy is to be instituted.

Abnormal CSF parameters with elevated WBC count with polymorphonuclear leukocyte predominance, hypoglycorrhachia (low glucose), elevated protein concentration, and positive Gram-stained smear with a positive bacterial culture are the classic and definitive methods to diagnose bacterial neonatal meningitis. However, bacterial meningitis may be present even in the absence of these abnormalities.

Ventriculitis may complicate neonatal bacterial meningitis.[12,27] Obstructive ventriculitis is suspected when the head circumference increases dramatically, the anterior fontanelle is persistently full, CSF cultures are persistently positive, and examination of ventricular fluid shows elevation of WBCs with polymorphonuclear predominance, presence of bacteria on Gram-stained smear, and positive culture. Brain imaging by cranial ultrasound, computed tomography (CT), or magnetic resonance imaging (MRI) with contrast material may show enhancement of the lining tissue of the ventricles or brain abscess formation.

Ampicillin and gentamicin or cefotaxime, administered in meningeal doses, are recommended for initial empiric treatment of neonatal meningitis for most neonates. If there is an indwelling device, such as a ventricular-to-peritoneal shunt in place, or a Gram-stained smear shows gram-positive cocci, staphylococci should be suspected and vancomycin administered. If a multidrug-resistant gram-negative organism is suspected or present, then cefepime or meropenem may be indicated. Neonates with bacterial meningitis usually should undergo repeat CSF examination and culture 24 to 48 hours after initiation of therapy. In neonates with bacterial meningitis caused by *Citrobacter diversus* or *Cronobacter (Enterobacter) sakazakii,* cranial CT or brain MRI imaging should be obtained early because of the frequent association with brain abscess. For neonatal meningitis caused by *Flavobacterium meningosepticum* isolates, combined use of parenteral vancomycin and rifampin has been suggested as the best therapeutic option.

Penicillin G or ampicillin is preferred for GBS meningitis, ampicillin for *L. monocytogenes* and enterococci, ampicillin plus an aminoglycoside or cefotaxime for coliforms, and ceftazidime or ticarcillin-clavulanate and an aminoglycoside for *Pseudomonas* infections. The duration of systemic therapy in neonatal meningitis depends on the causative agent and the time necessary to sterilize CSF cultures. For meningitis caused by GBS or *Listeria,* approximately 2 weeks of therapy usually is satisfactory. Because delayed sterilization is a common occurrence in infants with gram-negative enteric disease, systemic therapy is given for 3 weeks and, in some babies, for additional weeks. Intraventricular therapy is not routinely recommended for management of neonatal meningitis caused by gram-negative enteric bacilli.[3] However, on an individualized basis, intraventricular therapy may be of benefit in certain patients with obstructive ventriculitis caused by persistent or resistant organisms.

Acute complications of bacterial meningitis include communicating and noncommunicating hydrocephalus, subdural effusions (~1% of patients), deafness, and blindness. Ventriculitis occurs in approximately 70% of neonates with coliform meningitis. Brain abscess is an infrequent complication, except in infants with *C. diversus* or *C. (E). sakazakii* meningitis, in whom abscess develops approximately 70% of the time. A 30% to 50% incidence in neurologic sequelae has been reported in surviving infants. Although neurologic deficits may be obvious in some infants at discharge, most babies appear "well" at this time. Only after prolonged and careful follow-up do the perceptual difficulties, behavioral problems, and other subtle neurologic signs become apparent. Within 4 to 6 weeks of recovering from meningitis, hearing should be evaluated by evoked response audiometry.

Otitis Media

Otitis media is diagnosed infrequently in neonates because of the paucity of clinical findings and the difficulty of examining an infant's tympanic membrane. The onset of illness associated with otitis media is insidious, and the most common manifestations are rhinorrhea, irritability, and failure to thrive. Fever higher than 38°C (100.4°F) is a rare finding. The presence of lethargy, hypotonia, hypothermia, high fever, or jaundice suggests the otitis media is complicated by bacteremia or meningitis.

The cause of neonatal otitis media is similar to that observed in older infants and children. *S. pneumoniae, H. influenzae,* and *Moraxella catarrhalis* account for more than 50% of cases. Approximately 10% to 15% of neonates have disease caused by coliforms, GBS, or *S. aureus.*

Diarrheal Disease

Diarrhea can be a nonspecific symptom of sepsis or urinary tract infection in a newborn infant. Bacteria that may cause diarrhea in the neonate include enteropathogenic *E. coli, Vibrio cholerae,* some *E. coli* nonenteropathogenic strains, *Vibrio parahaemolyticus, Aeromonas, Shigella, Salmonella, Campylobacter,* and *Yersinia*. Some diarrheal episodes in neonates probably can be caused by *Clostridium difficile*. Shigellosis in a newborn may occur as a diarrheic or dysenteric syndrome or may be evidenced only by a septic- or toxic-appearing infant. *Salmonella* may cause sepsis and bacterial meningitis in the neonate. Neonates with diarrhea caused by *Salmonella* should be carefully evaluated for systemic illness and treated with intravenous antibiotics.

Urinary Tract Infections

The incidence of bacteriuria and urinary tract infection in newborn infants ranges from 0.5% to 1% for term infants and is approximately 3% for premature infants. Most infants with significant bacteriuria are asymptomatic or have nonspecific signs and symptoms. The neonate may also appear septic or may have decreased activity, feeding problems, and the other constitutional signs that are seen with infections of other organ systems. Jaundice, hepatomegaly, and thrombocytopenia may be observed in a few infants with urinary tract infection; these findings are associated with septicemia or cholestatic hepatitis in some babies.

E. coli is the most common etiologic agent of urinary tract, with *Proteus, Klebsiella,* and *Pseudomonas* spp. also important pathogens. Gram-positive bacteria, with the exception of enterococci, rarely are encountered as pathogens for the urinary tract. Neonates with renal abscess caused by *S. aureus* or gram-negative enteric bacteria have been reported in the literature.

The diagnosis of urinary tract infection is confirmed by examination, urinalysis, and culture of urine. Blood and urine should be obtained for culture from all newborn infants with suspected or proved urinary tract infection before antimicrobial therapy is initiated. A repeat urine culture performed 48 to 72 hours after initiation of appropriate therapy should be sterile or show a substantial reduction in the bacterial count. Infants with persistent bacteriuria should be evaluated for the possibility of resistant organism, obstruction, or perinephric abscess. In uncomplicated disease, therapy usually is continued for a period of 7 to 10 days. Approximately 1 week after discontinuance of therapy, a repeat urine culture may be performed.

Neonates with documented infection should undergo radiologic evaluation of the urinary tract. Renal sonogram may be performed to evaluate the possibility of gross congenital abnormalities of the urinary system.

Suppurative Arthritis and Osteomyelitis

Osteomyelitis and suppurative arthritis are unusual in the first 4 weeks of life. Bone and joint infections can be difficult to detect in neonates and young infants. The predominant organisms are *S. aureus* (both MSSA and MRSA), GBS, and gram-negative enteric organisms such as *Klebsiella, Proteus,* and *E. coli*. Gonococcal arthritis and tenosynovitis were common occurrences in neonates in previous decades and still may be seen in developing countries. Other bacteria associated infrequently with newborn infection in the bones and joints are *Salmonella* and *Pseudomonas.*

Two distinct clinical syndromes that may be associated with osteomyelitis in the newborn period have been described. The first form presents as a local infection, in which the earliest sign of bone and joint infection in newborns is failure to move an extremity spontaneously or apparent pain on movement without systemic evidence of infection. Swelling, erythema, and heat localized to the affected part are late findings. Multiple bones or joints can be involved, especially when disease is caused by *S. aureus*. The second form of presentation is characterized by disseminated, systemic manifestations of sepsis; only later are multiple sites of bone and visceral involvement noted. Another unique clinical presentation of osteomyelitis in the newborn is maxillary bone involvement by osteomyelitis, usually caused by GBS or *S. aureus*. Maxillitis or osteomyelitis of the superior maxilla is an unusual form of bone infection in newborn infants. Blood should be obtained for culture from all infants with osteomyelitis or septic arthritis. A recommended sample is percutaneous needle aspiration of intraarticular pus in patients with suspected suppurative arthritis or aspiration of sequestrum, abscess, or lytic bone lesion in those with suspected osteomyelitis. If pus or tissue is obtained, the material should be Gram stained and cultured.

Selection of initial antimicrobial therapy is guided by preliminary identification of the pathogen from stained smears of material obtained by needle aspiration. Surgical removal of infected material is an integral part of treatment, even in the neonate. Open drainage is essential for managing septic hip disease. The inflammation in osteomyelitis or septic arthritis can occupy the epiphyseal and metaphyseal sides of the growth plate and result in ischemia and necrosis of the plate and permanent orthopedic damage. For other joints, repeated daily evacuation of fluid with a needle and syringe usually is adequate. In patients with osteomyelitis, the subperiosteal space and the metaphysis should be drained if pus is obtained during diagnostic aspiration. Antimicrobial treatment of neonatal musculoskeletal infections caused by *S. aureus* or gram-negative organisms is continued for a minimum of 4 to 6 weeks, depending on clinical response.

Conjunctivitis and Orbital Cellulitis

Infections of the eye of the newborn can be caused by a variety of microorganisms, including *Neisseria gonorrhoeae, Chlamydia trachomatis, S. aureus* (MSSA or MRSA), and *P. aeruginosa*. Other less frequently encountered organisms included *M. catarrhalis, Pasteurella multocida, Haemophilus,* and *Neisseria meningitides.* Nonbacterial organisms, including *Chlamydia* and HSV, should be considered in the differential diagnosis of neonatal conjunctivitis. Any infant with a conjunctival discharge should be evaluated carefully to determine the cause. Three tests should be performed: Gram and methylene blue stain of the exudate, culture of the exudate, and Giemsa stain and culture for *Chlamydia,* if available, of scrapings made from the lower palpebral conjunctiva after the exudate has been removed. The results of the stained smears and cultures determine the appropriate therapy.

Funisitis and Omphalitis

If inflammation of the cord alone is present, funisitis is diagnosed. It is characterized by a wet, malodorous umbilical cord and stump, without surrounding cellulitis. The umbilical cord may be colonized with numerous different potential bacterial pathogens, some of which, like GAS, may not only cause inflammation in the cord of the neonate but also produce nursery outbreaks of disease.

Omphalitis, or infection of the umbilicus, has many causes and occurs more frequently in low-birth-weight infants and those with complicated deliveries. The incidence is estimated to be approximately 2%, and symptoms start at an average age of 3 days. Culture and susceptibility test results are necessary for the selection of an appropriate antibiotic. *S. aureus* is the most frequent pathogen isolated, followed by GAS, GBS, and gram-negative rods. Some of the complications secondary to omphalitis reported in the literature are bacterial sepsis, spontaneous evisceration of the small bowel through the umbilical cicatrix, necrotizing fasciitis, small bowel obstruction, peritonitis, and superficial, retroperitoneal, or hepatic abscesses.

Breast Abscess

Breast abscesses are encountered most frequently during the second or third week of life and are more common findings in girls, particularly those older than 2 weeks. The disease does not appear to occur in premature infants, presumably because of underdevelopment of the mammary glands in these infants. Bilateral disease is a rare event.

The major clinical finding is swelling of the affected breast with or without accompanying erythema and warmth. Systemic manifestations are uncommon occurrences, and only a fourth of patients have low-grade fever. *S. aureus* is the major pathogen, but coliform bacteria, such as *E. coli* and *Salmonella,* and GBS have become more common causes in the past decade. Blood cultures should be obtained, but bacteremia is a rare finding in this condition. If the patient has only mild cellulitis and no discernible fluctuance, antibiotic treatment alone may suffice. Fluctuant abscesses should be drained.

Suppurative Parotitis

Suppurative parotitis of the newborn usually is easy to recognize, although occasionally it is confused with infection of a preauricular or superior anterior cervical lymph node. Infection occurs more commonly in low-birth-weight infants than in term infants and more commonly in boys. Dehydration predisposes to stasis of parotid secretions and subsequent infection. Bilateral infection is a rare event.

Although *S. aureus* (MSSA and MRSA) accounts for most cases, disease may be caused by coliform bacteria, *Pseudomonas,* pneumococci, and GAS. The clinical manifestations include fever, anorexia, irritability, and failure to gain weight. Erythema, swelling, and tenderness over the involved gland may occur. The diagnosis can be confirmed by expressing pus through the parotid duct or by needle aspiration of a fluctuant area. Gram staining of this material helps identify the causative agent. Selection of antimicrobial therapy should be based on interpretation of the Gram-stained smear of expressed pus. In most cases, antibiotic therapy alone suffices, and surgical incision and drainage are unnecessary. Response to therapy generally is rapid. Most patients require only 7 to 10 days of therapy until healing is complete.

Scalp Abscess

Scalp abscesses usually are a complication of fetal monitoring with scalp electrodes. The number of vaginal examinations, use of more than one electrode, and fetal scalp blood sampling are risk factors for the development of scalp abscesses. Pathogens incriminated include staphylococci, gonococci, and gram-negative enteric bacteria. A polymicrobial flora, including anaerobic organisms, frequently is isolated in scalp abscesses caused by electronic fetal monitoring electrodes. Incision and drainage of the infected site along with antibiotics for 7 days usually is sufficient for most term neonates with uncomplicated scalp abscesses caused by susceptible bacteria. Scalp lesions associated with scalp electrodes that do not show bacteria on Gram stain or culture may be caused by HSV and should be evaluated with viral culture of lesions and surfaces, examined by HSV DNA PCR of blood and CSF, and treated with intravenous acyclovir.

Pneumonia

Neonatal lower respiratory tract bacterial infections may be acquired congenitally or postnatally. Congenital or perinatal infection results from transplacental transfer of the agent (i.e., congenital infection) or from inhalation of infected amniotic fluid (usually associated with prolonged rupture of membranes) or infected vaginal secretions during delivery.

Common bacterial pathogens causing postnatally acquired pneumonia are *S. aureus,* coliform bacilli, and *Pseudomonas.* These infections occur sporadically or epidemically and may be acquired from the community in otherwise healthy neonates or are health care–associated in hospitalized neonates. The physical findings of pneumonia are variable. Flaring of the alae nasi, rapid respirations, and sternal and subcostal retractions are common findings. Coughing indicates lower respiratory tract involvement; brassy coughing is found frequently in viral disease. Crackles or wheezes usually can be heard on deep inspiration (or when the baby is crying) but may be absent early in disease. Cultures of blood and material from the trachea frequently help in defining the etiologic agent of neonatal pneumonia. A chest radiograph should be obtained for all babies with suspected lower respiratory tract disease. Radiographic evidence of pneumonia may exist in the absence of specific physical findings. Although the cause of neonatal pneumonia usually can be determined from a radiograph, certain radiologic patterns are associated with specific diseases. With acute-onset GBS disease, the radiograph may mimic one showing hyaline membrane disease. A consolidating bronchopneumonia with pneumatoceles, with or without empyema, suggests staphylococcal disease. When a lobar infiltrate is associated with expansion of the lobe, *K. pneumoniae* infection should be considered. A miliary type of bronchopneumonia in a septic neonate is characteristic of listeriosis or, less commonly, mycobacterial disease.

Pertussis is also an important cause of respiratory disease and pneumonia in the neonate. The onset of disease generally is in the second to sixth weeks of life; the earliest onset reported was at 10 days of age. Pertussis should be suspected when an infant has a paroxysmal cough with excessive mucus. Because apneic spells are common occurrences, newborns with pertussis should be admitted to the hospital for initial management. PCR-based methods are currently recommended to confirm the diagnosis.

YEAST AND FUNGAL INFECTIONS OF THE FETUS AND NEONATE

The improved survival of preterm infants since the early 1980s has resulted in the emergence of yeasts and fungi as significant neonatal pathogens. *C. albicans* remains the most frequently isolated pathogenic yeast overall, but other *Candida* spp., especially *C. parapsilosis, C. tropicalis, C. kruseii, C. lusitaniae, C. haemulonii,* and *C. auris*, and less common pathogenic yeasts, such as *Malassezia, Trichosporon, Rhodotorula,* and *Pichia* (formerly *Hansenula*), have increased in frequency. The incidence of invasive fungal disease, often with fatal outcomes, caused by *Aspergillus* and Zygomycetes (*Mucor, Rhizopus, Rhizomucor,* and *Absidia*) also has increased in neonates, especially infants who were born prematurely or with an inherited metabolic disorder or primary immunodeficiency.

Neonatal Candidiasis

The species isolated most frequently from neonates is *C. albicans,* which represents approximately 40% to 60% of isolates from neonates with systemic disease and is the most common *Candida* spp. associated with NICU outbreaks.[29] *Candida* spp. other than *C. albicans* have become increasingly more prevalent, however, and in some NICUs may be isolated more frequently than *C. albicans*. Among these organisms, *C. parapsilosis* is the most common, followed by *C. tropicalis;* both of them have caused outbreaks in NICUs. *C. glabrata, C. guilliermondii, C. lusitaniae,* and *C. krusei* also have caused invasive disease in neonates. Most recently, *C. haemulonii* and *C. auris* have emerged as a neonatal pathogen and caused an outbreak in an NICU.[28] Several risk factors consistently have been associated with systemic candidiasis, the most common being prematurity and very low and extremely low birth weight (VLBW and ELBW), with attendant impairment of host defense mechanisms; indwelling intravenous catheters; and prolonged use of broad-spectrum antimicrobial therapy—in particular, third-generation cephalosporins that suppress normal gastrointestinal flora. Neonatal candidiasis may be congenital or acquired and ranges from commonly encountered benign oral and cutaneous candidiasis to systemic infection with candidemia to more severe and often fatal disseminated candidiasis.

Oral candidiasis is the most common form of infection involving *Candida* spp. Cutaneous candidiasis typically is manifested by erythematous, vesiculopustular lesions found primarily on the skin of the perineum, axilla, and intertriginous areas. The periumbilical area also can be involved. In VLBW and ELBW premature infants, seemingly benign mucocutaneous lesions, including lesions in the perineum or diaper area, may progress rapidly to invasive dermatitis, producing cutaneous scales, crusting, erosions, ulcerations, or extensive maceration of skin, and result in a potentially lethal systemic candidiasis. Scattered, faint, erythematous maculopapular lesions of the skin may be an expression of a serious disseminated candidiasis. Chronic mucocutaneous candidiasis may be diagnosed in an otherwise well-appearing infant if *Candida* infections of the skin, mucous membranes, and nails persist or recur despite administration of antifungal therapy. These neonates have a congenital defect in T-lymphocyte function specific to *Candida* spp.

Congenital candidiasis may cause fetal infection with onset of premature labor or intrauterine demise; it may be evident at birth, or it may appear within the first 24 to 48 hours of life. Term and preterm neonates may be affected. Maternal risk factors include a history during pregnancy of *Candida* vaginitis, use of antibiotics, retained intrauterine contraceptive device, cervical cerclage, and prolonged rupture of fetal membranes, although none of these factors may be present in the history. Congenital systemic candidiasis may manifest as life-threatening, early-onset sepsis syndrome, especially in premature neonates with septic shock, pneumonia, or meningitis; it also may be accompanied by leukocytosis or neutropenia, or it may mimic congenital leukemia. Twins may be affected, sometimes with different *Candida* spp., manifestations, and outcomes for each twin. Premature neonates with congenital candidiasis often have more severe disease, with positive blood cultures and evidence of disseminated disease, including meningitis. The umbilical cord from a fetus or newborn with congenital candidiasis may show *Candida* funisitis with yellow-white nodules and fungal microabscesses; the placenta also may have nodules and shows chorioamnionitis on histologic examination.

Acquired systemic candidiasis includes catheter-associated sepsis, in which *Candida* is isolated from the blood of infants who have central venous catheters but no evidence of focal infection or disseminated. The organ involved most frequently in systemic candidiasis seems to be the kidney. *Candida* may be isolated from the urine of 73% of neonates with systemic candidiasis with positive blood cultures, but only 5% to 15% of such neonates have documented *Candida* pyelonephritis with renal infiltration, mycetoma, or renal abscess. The kidney seems to be particularly vulnerable to the formation of renal cortical abscesses and obstructive masses, which usually occur at the ureteropelvic junction. A neonate with persistently positive urine or blood cultures, hypertension, renal insufficiency or acute renal failure, or oliguria or anuria should undergo ultrasound imaging to determine the presence of a bezoar-associated obstructive uropathy, which requires immediate attention. Urinary catheters or nephrostomy tubes may become colonized with *Candida* and result in secondary infections that may range from asymptomatic to invasive disease with obstruction.

Candida meningitis may occur in the absence of positive blood cultures; CSF pleocytosis may be minimal or absent, and elevated protein or hypoglycorrhachia is an inconsistent finding. Gram-stained smears of CSF rarely reveal budding yeast, even when CSF cultures are positive for *Candida*. Fernandez and associates,[10] in a 10-year review of candidal meningitis in 23 infants in an NICU, reported that pleocytosis occurred in only 39% of infants and hypoglycorrhachia occurred in 25%, despite a positive CSF culture for *Candida* in 74% of infants. The remaining neonates are diagnosed when a positive blood culture occurs with an abnormal but culture-negative CSF. *Candida* also may colonize and infect external ventricular drains placed for management of hydrocephalus.

Candida endocarditis may occur in neonates with normal hearts and in neonates with structural heart disease and as a postoperative complication of cardiac surgery. It usually occurs in premature neonates with persistent candidemia associated with an indwelling vascular catheter. Most neonates with *Candida* endocarditis have structurally normal hearts, however, and not all reported cases in neonates have been associated with vascular devices. The presentation of *Candida* endocarditis in neonates may be acute and associated with an episode of persistent candidemia, or late onset, often discovered weeks or months after a presumably silent or resolved episode of candidemia. Cardiac murmurs may be absent. Intracardiac vegetations on the mitral, tricuspid, and aortic valves or the presence of a right atrial mass in association with persistently positive blood cultures for *Candida* strongly supports the diagnosis of endocarditis.

Eye disease may occur in 3% to 11% of neonates with systemic candidiasis; figures as high as 45% have been reported. Candidal eye disease may complicate systemic candidiasis in term, near-term, and preterm infants.

Osteoarthritis is a rare manifestation of systemic candidiasis in neonates. It may occur temporarily associated with persistent candidemia or as a late complication, weeks to months later, after apparent resolution of an episode of candidemia. In addition to premature infants, newborns with underlying inherited disorders of metabolism also may be at increased risk.

Intraabdominal infections, including enteritis, necrotizing enterocolitis (NEC), and peritonitis, and intraabdominal and hepatosplenic abscesses are estimated to occur in 8% of neonates with invasive systemic candidiasis. *Candida* peritonitis and sepsis may complicate surgical procedures performed on the intestine for congenital bowel atresias or bowel perforation associated with NEC. Distinct from NEC is idiopathic spontaneous focal intestinal perforation (SFIP), which occurs rarely in VLBW infants and has been associated with systemic candidiasis in half of cases.

Acquired pulmonary candidiasis with pneumonia may occur in 8% to 10% of ventilated premature neonates and must be differentiated clinically and radiographically from asymptomatic *Candida* colonization and pneumonia caused by other pathogens.

Diagnosis

Congenital or acquired cutaneous candidiasis may be diagnosed by the presence of budding yeast organisms in scrapings of skin lesions, with the species involved established by culture. Invasive dermatitis caused by *Candida* can be differentiated from benign cutaneous dermatitis by skin biopsy. Histopathologic evidence of organisms beyond the stratum corneum is evidence of more serious invasive dermatitis that leads to potentially fatal systemic candidiasis.

Congenital or acquired systemic candidiasis in a fetus or neonate is established by isolation of *Candida* spp. in culture from a normally sterile body fluid, such as amniotic fluid, urine, blood, or CSF, or from an involved site, such as joint or bone or from abscess. Culture of CSF should be performed if candidemia is documented, even if CSF indices are normal. If the urine grows *Candida*, renal or systemic infection is suggested.

Routine laboratory evaluations may support the diagnosis of systemic or invasive candidiasis. Persistent thrombocytopenia is a frequent early finding in infants with systemic candidiasis. Additional laboratory tests, such as a complete blood cell count, liver function tests, and determination of serum glucose, blood urea nitrogen, and creatinine, may be helpful in assessing the degree of systemic involvement.

Treatment

Oral candidiasis or thrush in an otherwise healthy infant is treated with oral nystatin suspension or gentian violet. Superficial cutaneous candidiasis in an otherwise healthy neonate is treated with topical nystatin cream or powder. Cutaneous candidiasis that persists or evolves into invasive candidiasis requires systemic antifungal therapy, usually with amphotericin B or fluconazole.

Congenital candidiasis usually requires only topical antifungal therapy in an otherwise healthy newborn; neonates who have pulmonary involvement or who are preterm should receive systemic antifungal therapy because they are at greater risk for dissemination and a poor outcome. In these instances, amphotericin B or fluconazole may be used for approximately 10 to 25 days, until clinical signs and symptoms have resolved.

Prompt systemic antifungal therapy, usually with amphotericin B or fluconazole, is indicated if even a single blood culture from a neonate is positive for *Candida* spp. In addition to removal of the catheter, systemic antifungal therapy should be administered for at least 10 to 14 days. If the peripheral blood culture also is positive for *Candida* spp., or end-organ disease is present, dissemination via the bloodstream may have occurred, and most experts recommend duration of antifungal therapy to be at least 25 to 30 days. Isolation of *Candida* spp. from a urine specimen obtained by sterile technique denotes invasive renal or systemic disease and requires further evaluation and systemic antifungal therapy. In some patients, medical therapy alone may eradicate the *Candida* infection, even if partial obstruction is present. Some neonates may require an urgent surgical or endoscopic procedure, however, to relieve the obstruction and restore renal function. Duration of antifungal therapy required for cure may range from 25 to 42 days or longer and should be guided by microbiologic cure and resolution of lesions by imaging studies.

Treatment of meningoencephalitis caused by *Candida* spp. in a neonate usually requires systemic therapy for at least 30 days; longer courses of treatment may be required if ventriculitis or brain abscesses or nodules are present.

Treatment of endocarditis or septic thrombophlebitis caused by *Candida* spp. requires prolonged antifungal treatment, at least 30 days and usually 42 to 60 days, depending on clearance of candidemia, clinical progress, and resolution of intracardiac vegetations or lesions as documented by echocardiography. Consultation with a cardiologist or cardiovascular surgeon is recommended. If septic thrombophlebitis with vascular abscess is present or an enlarging valvular mass obstructs blood flow, surgical intervention may be considered. Reports of resolution of endocarditis with medical therapy alone suggest, however, that it may be a valid option to consider, especially for neonates who are hemodynamically stable, with right-sided, nonvalvular lesions.

Treatment of eye disease, such as endophthalmitis, requires systemic antifungal therapy for 25 to 42 days, and consultation with an ophthalmologist is recommended to assess the extent of disease, presence or progression of comorbid retinopathy of prematurity, and response to therapy.

Treatment of osteoarthritis caused by *Candida* spp. usually requires prolonged duration of systemic antifungal therapy (≥42 days). Aspiration or surgical drainage by an orthopedic surgeon may be necessary if there is an infected joint or bone abscess.

Peritonitis associated with NEC or SFIP usually requires at least 25 days of systemic antifungal therapy, but longer duration may be required if intraabdominal abscesses develop. Surgical management of SFIP also differs from that of NEC; simple surgical procedures, such as suturing or resection with primary anastomosis, may be all that is required for treatment of SFIP, whereas NEC may require extensive bowel resection.

Duration of systemic antifungal treatment for pulmonary candidiasis is not well established. Treatment should be guided by clinical and radiographic improvement; however, 25 days is likely to be adequate for most patients.

Prevention

Single-center and cohort studies and a large, multicenter, randomized, double-blind, placebo-controlled trial have shown that fluconazole prophylaxis (administered daily, every other day, or twice weekly either orally or intravenously for 4 to 6 weeks after delivery) reduces *Candida* colonization, invasive candidiasis, or mortality rates in high-risk, VLBW premature neonates weighing less than 1500 g.[7] Emergence of fluconazole-resistant *Candida* spp., including *C. krusei* and *C. parapsilosis,* may occur. Also disease caused by invasive yeasts other than *Candida* spp. may occur. An outbreak of *Rhodotorula mucilaginosa,* a fluconazole-resistant yeast, occurred more recently in an NICU that routinely administered prophylactic fluconazole.

Invasive Yeasts Other Than *Candida*

Congenital and perinatal infections with the encapsulated yeast *Cryptococcus neoformans* have been reported. *Malassezia* spp. frequently colonize the skin of neonates and may cause invasive disease, such as skin disorders (e.g., pustulosis) and bacteremia.

Pichia (formerly *Hansenula*) *anomala* and *P. ohmeri* may cause infection in preterm VLBW neonates and infants with severe combined immunodeficiency. Invasive diseases in preterm neonates include bloodstream infections, sepsis syndrome, abscesses, and meningitis with ventriculitis. *Trichosporon beigelii* has caused invasive dermatitis, late-onset sepsis, pulmonary infiltrates, and urinary tract infections in VLBW preterm neonates with intravascular catheters. It also may cause endophthalmitis and endocarditis. *T. asahii* infection in neonates has been reported as well. *Rhodotorula* spp. are another emerging opportunistic yeast that has caused catheter-associated bloodstream infections in neonates.

Invasive Fungal Diseases

Congenital and Perinatal Transmission

Fetal demise, congenital infection, and perinatal transmission associated with the endemic dimorphic fungi *Coccidioides immitis* and *Blastomyces dermatitidis* have been described. Published case reports are very rare, however.

Acquired Invasive Fungal Disease

Invasive fungal disease acquired by VLBW or ELBW premature neonates involves primarily the skin, lungs, or gastrointestinal tract. Because many of the invasive fungi that affect neonates also are angioinvasive, sepsis syndrome with hematogenous dissemination to lung, liver, spleen, CNS, and eye may occur rapidly.

Aspergillus. *Aspergillus* spp. include *Aspergillus flavus, A. fumigatus, A. glaucus, A. nidulans, A. niger,* and *A. terreus. Aspergillus* spp. frequently are found in the environment and the hospital. Diseases associated with *Aspergillus* infection of the neonate include primary cutaneous aspergillosis or invasive dermatitis, pulmonary aspergillosis, and disseminated aspergillosis. Disseminated disease may involve the heart, liver, spleen, lungs, CNS, or eye.

***Zygomycetes* (Absidia, Rhizopus, Mucor, *and* Rhizomucor).** Zygomycosis, a term preferred now over mucormycosis, usually is caused by the following species of fungi: *Absidia (A. corymbifera), Rhizopus (R. arrhizus, R. microsporus), Mucor (M. amphibiorum, M. circinelloides, M. hiemalis, M. indicus, M. racemosus, M. ramosissimus),* and *Rhizomucor (R. pusillus, R. miehei, R. variabilis).* Zygomycosis in a neonate usually manifests during the second and third weeks of life. The Zygomycetes are angiotrophic and aggressively invade blood vessels very early in the disease process. Invasion of blood vessels leads to thrombosis, infarction, and tissue necrosis; destruction of local tissue can be extensive, and the fungus may disseminate throughout the body and CNS. The most common presentation of invasive zygomycosis in neonates is primary cutaneous disease. Cutaneous zygomycosis usually begins at an area of minor skin trauma or at the site of intravenous catheter insertion that has come in contact with adhesive tape or bandages, first appearing as a cluster of necrotic vesicles or scales that then rapidly progresses to extensive necrotizing cellulitis. Gastrointestinal zygomycosis in a premature neonate often mimics NEC clinically. Rhinocerebral zygomycosis classically manifests in diabetics with ketoacidosis, but it also may affect neonates with conditions associated with metabolic acidosis and premature infants. The fungus enters via the nasal passages and invades the sinus cavities and orbits, spreading to the CNS by fungal thrombosis of cavernous sinus and internal carotid artery. Pulmonary zygomycosis also may occur, either as a primary pneumonia with consolidation and necrosis or secondary to vascular dissemination from a cutaneous or gastrointestinal source. Disseminated zygomycosis is a fatal fungal sepsis syndrome, usually involving all major organ systems and the CNS.

Treatment

Invasive disease of the neonate caused by fungi is treated with antifungal agents. The choice of antifungal agents available to treat invasive fungal disease of the neonate include the traditional polyene antibiotics, nystatin and amphotericin B deoxycholate, and the pyrimidine analog 5-FC, as well as lipid formulations of amphotericin B, first-generation triazoles (fluconazole and itraconazole), second-generation triazoles (posaconazole, ravuconazole, and voriconazole), and echinocandins (caspofungin, micafungin, and anidulafungin). The choice of which antifungal agent to administer and the duration of treatment should be guided by the reported susceptibility pattern of the fungus, and dosages should be based on available pharmacokinetic information for neonates.

CONGENITAL TOXOPLASMOSIS

Congenital toxoplasmosis results from placental infection that develops after primary maternal infection with *Toxoplasma gondii* and subsequent hematogenous spread to the fetus.[18] Many neonates with congenital toxoplasmosis are seemingly asymptomatic at birth. The most characteristic clinical findings, frequently referred to as the classic triad of congenital toxoplasmosis, are chorioretinitis, intracranial calcifications, and hydrocephalus. They are seen in approximately 86% (chorioretinitis), 37% (intracranial calcifications), and 20% (hydrocephalus) of symptomatic infants. These conditions often are accompanied by a combination of signs and symptoms, including anemia (59%), jaundice (43%), splenomegaly (41%), seizures (41%), fever (40%), hepatomegaly (34%), lymphadenopathy (32%), microcephaly (9%), and eosinophilia (9%).

The diagnosis of congenital toxoplasmosis can be established by isolating the organism from infected body fluids and tissues, such as the placenta, amniotic fluid, fetal blood obtained by cordocentesis, umbilical cord blood, infant blood, and CSF. Alternatively a diagnosis can be established by histopathologic examination of the placenta in which tachyzoites are revealed. PCR has been used successfully to detect *Toxoplasma* DNA in amniotic fluid, placenta, CSF, and fetal and infant blood. The most practical and widely used method of establishing the diagnosis is by testing maternal and newborn blood for serologic evidence of *Toxoplasma* infection by measuring *T. gondii*–specific IgG and IgM antibodies. Consultation with a recognized reference laboratory for toxoplasmosis testing is recommended (Toxoplasmosis Serology Laboratory, Palo Alto Medical Foundation, 860 Bryant Street, Palo Alto, CA 94301; 415-326-8120).

Treatment with spiramycin of an acutely infected woman during pregnancy may prevent transmission of the infection to the fetus. Treatment during the first year of life with pyrimethamine, sulfadiazine, and leucovorin is effective for acute disease and improves long-term outcome in congenital toxoplasmosis.[18]

Routine serologic screening of women during pregnancy has been an effective means of prevention in France and Austria, and it has been advocated in other areas where the incidence of congenital toxoplasmosis remains high. Another focus of prevention should be on educating women of child-bearing age to avoid cat feces in litter boxes, outdoor sandboxes, and gardens and avoid ingestion of raw meat and mutton.

CHLAMYDIA, MYCOPLASMA, AND *UREAPLASMA* INFECTIONS IN THE NEONATE

C. trachomatis is a cause of neonatal conjunctivitis and perinatally acquired infant pneumonia. The introduction of systematic screening and treatment of pregnant women has resulted in a dramatic decrease in the number of perinatal chlamydial infections in developed countries. However, in countries in which pregnant women are not screened routinely, including many developing countries, *C. trachomatis* remains the most frequent cause of neonatal conjunctivitis.

Mycoplasma hominis, Ureaplasma urealyticum, and *U. parvum* are the genital mycoplasmas with clinical significance in neonatal disease. Vertical transmission of *Ureaplasma* spp. and *M. hominis* from a colonized mother to her newborn may occur in utero or during delivery. The roles of *Ureaplasma* spp. and *M. hominis* in neonatal disease continue to be investigated and defined.

Acknowledgments

I acknowledge the contributions of Pablo J. Sánchez, Margaret Hammerschlag, Vladana Milisavljevic, James Cherry, James McAuley, Kenneth Boyer, Dora Estripeaut, and Xavier Saez-Laurens to the contents of this chapter from the previous editions of this textbook.

NEW REFERENCES SINCE THE SEVENTH EDITION

4. Caluwaerts S, Fautsch T, Lagrou D, et al. Dilemmas in managing pregnant women with Ebola: 2 case reports. *Clin Infect Dis.* 2016;62(7):903.
11. Franca GV, Schuler-Gaccini L, Oliveria WK, et al. Congenital Zika virus syndrome in Brazil: a case series of the first 1501 livebirths with complete investigation. *Lancet.* 2016;376(10047):891.
13. Jamieson DJ, Uyeki TM, Callaghan WM, et al. What obstetrician-gynecologists should know about Ebola: a perspective from the Centers for Disease Control and Prevention. *Obstet Gynecol.* 2014;124(5):2005.
17. Lyra P, Campos G, Bandeira I, et al. Congenital Chikungunya virus infection after an outbreak in Salvador, Bahia, Brazil. *AJP Rep.* 2016;6(3):e299.
19. Moore CA, Staples JE, Dobyns WB, et al. Characterizing the pattern of anomalies in congenital Zika syndrome for pediatric clinicians. *JAMA Pediatr.* 2017;171(3):288-295.
20. Moura de Silva AA, Ganz JS, Sousa PD, et al. Early growth and neurologic outcomes of infants with probable congenital Zika virus syndrome. *Emerg Infect Dis.* 2016;22(11):1953.
21. Muehlenbachs A, de la Rosa Vazquez O, Bausch DG, et al. Ebola virus disease in pregnancy: clinical, histopathologic, and immunohistochemical findings. *J Infect Dis.* 2017;215(1):64-69.
23. Muller WJ. Treatment of perinatal viral infections to improve neurologic outcomes. *Pediatr Res.* 2017;81(1-2):162-169.
25. Pridjian G, Sirois P, McRae S, et al. Prospective study of pregnancy and newborn outcomes in mothers with West Nile illness during pregnancy. *Birth Defects Res A Clin Mol Teratol.* 2016;106(8):716.
28. Silva CM, Carvalho-Parahym A, Macedo D, et al. Neonatal candidemia caused by *Candida haemulonii*: case report and review of the literature. *Mycopathologia.* 2015;180(1):69.
31. Zavattoni M, Rovida F, Campanini G, et al. Miscarriage following dengue virus 3 infection in the first six weeks of pregnancy of a dengue virus-naïve traveler returning from Bali to Italy, April 2016. *Euro Surveill.* 2016;21(31):30308.

The full reference list for this chapter is available at ExpertConsult.com.

67 Primary Immunodeficiency Diseases

Ivan K. Chinn • Javier Chinen • William T. Shearer

Primary immunodeficiency diseases (PIDDs) can be defined as congenital disorders caused by an intrinsic molecular defect that alters the development or function of the immune system. As a consequence, patients with these conditions display increased susceptibility to infections, neoplasia, and autoimmunity. More than 300 PIDDs have been recognized, and many of the gene defects responsible for the immunologic phenotypes have been identified.[17] Previously considered to be uncommon, PIDDs have been estimated to occur at a minimum incidence of 1 per 10,000 live births. A 2007 US survey of 10,000 households, however, reported a prevalence of 1 in every 1200 people for clinically diagnosed PIDD,[18] suggesting that these conditions occur even more frequently than often suspected. A more recent survey of pediatricians in the United States demonstrated a significant lack of awareness or comfort regarding the recognition and evaluation of patients with PIDDs.[65]

In patients with immune deficiency, PIDDs must be distinguished from secondary immunodeficiency disorders. These latter conditions represent acquired immune defects that occur as either a result of exogenous factors or together with nonimmunologic primary disease processes. They are encountered much more frequently than PIDDs. Causes of secondary immunodeficiency states include infection (e.g., by human immunodeficiency virus [HIV]), medications (e.g., corticosteroids), malnutrition, and neoplastic or metabolic diseases (e.g., Hodgkin disease, diabetes mellitus, cystic fibrosis, and systemic lupus erythematosus [SLE]). These factors may also affect a fetus in utero and present in the neonatal period. Thus they must be considered in infants who exhibit signs or symptoms of immune deficiency.

An immunologic evaluation is indicated when a patient develops unusually frequent or severe infections or when infections are caused by atypical or pathognomonic organisms (Box 67.1). Most of these individuals are immunocompetent and have risk factors for increased frequency of infections, such as allergic disorders, anatomic abnormalities (e.g., eustachian tube dysfunction), or increased exposure to pathogens (e.g., attendance at daycare). They may also have a clinical condition that results in an acquired immunodeficiency state. However a number of children will have an established PIDD and will benefit from prompt referral to a clinical immunologist for early diagnosis and management.

This chapter will focus on the elements of the medical history and physical examination that suggest a diagnosis of a PIDD. Relevant laboratory tests are discussed. Representative antibody, combined (primarily T- and often B-cell) immunity, complement, phagocytic, and other innate immunity deficiencies are presented. Finally a summary of PIDDs that are known to be associated with susceptibility to certain infectious pathogens is provided.

INITIAL EVALUATION FOR SUSPECTED IMMUNODEFICIENCY

Medical History

A comprehensive medical history remains essential for identifying children with a defective immune response. Children with PIDDs often have a history of frequent or severe infections (e.g., pneumonia, meningitis, septicemia, osteomyelitis, abscesses of soft tissue or an internal organ). Although infections occur routinely throughout childhood, epidemiologic studies have established a range for the average number of infections that a normal child may develop per year. For example, otherwise healthy children younger than 5 years of age average between three and eight episodes of upper respiratory tract infections annually.[56,73,76] By 1 year of age, 62% of children have had at least one acute otitis media infection, and 17% have had three or more episodes.[145] By 3 years of age, more than 80% of children have had at least one episode of acute otitis media, and 46% have had three or more episodes. The incidence of gastroenteritis among children in the United States is approximately two to three episodes per child-year, with rates as high as five episodes per child-year among children attending daycare centers.[12,59] The frequency of these infections in normal children during infancy or early childhood can be modified by several factors, including immunologic immaturity or naïveté (i.e., lack of prior exposure to infectious agents), poor hygiene, mouthing behavior, allergic disease, exposure to tobacco smoke, and frequent exposure to ill contacts in the home, school, or daycare settings.

Other elements of the infection history may raise concern for the presence of a PIDD. Clinicians should suspect immune deficiency when the course of an infection is unusually prolonged or associated with unexpected complications (e.g., lung abscess in a child with pneumonia or osteomyelitis as a complication of sinusitis). In general, infections of multiple body sites over time more highly suggest a defective immune response than infections occurring at only one site (e.g., recurrent otitis media alone). In the latter circumstance, a mechanical or anatomic etiology (e.g., foreign body, occult tracheoesophageal fistula in a child with recurrent pneumonia, allergic inflammation, congenital fistulous tract to the middle ear in a child with recurrent bacterial meningitis) should be considered.

Identified infectious organisms may themselves suggest a defect in a particular compartment of the immune system. Several pathogens are discussed in depth at the end of this chapter. Children with primary antibody deficiencies are typically susceptible to infections caused by polysaccharide-encapsulated extracellular bacteria (e.g., *Streptococcus pneumoniae, Haemophilus influenzae*). In contrast, children with T-cell–mediated immune deficiencies often develop infections caused by unusual or opportunistic viruses, fungi, protozoa, and mycobacteria (Table 67.1). Because of impaired T-cell–dependent antibody responses, bacterial infections may also be observed. Children with primary deficiencies of complement proteins can present with a history of recurrent neisserial infections, and patients with certain phagocyte deficiencies may have invasive infections due to catalase-positive bacterial (e.g., *Staphylococcus aureus, Pseudomonas aeruginosa, Serratia marcescens*) or fungal (e.g., *Aspergillus* spp.) organisms.

Other elements of the clinical history may help to define the risk for and nature of a potential PIDD. Because young infants are afforded some protection against infections by the presence of maternal immunoglobulin (Ig) G, children with primary antibody deficiencies generally begin to develop infections between 3 and 18 months of age. In contrast, children with severe T-cell–mediated, complement, or phagocytic deficiencies may have onset of infections in the first days or weeks of life. Omphalitis, resulting in delayed detachment of the umbilical cord stump, and poor wound healing suggest phagocytic deficiency. Hypocalcemic seizures in the neonatal period and congenital heart disease should lead to suspicion for a diagnosis of DiGeorge syndrome. Severe infection from live vaccine strains after immunization (e.g., bacille Calmette-Guérin [BCG] lymphadenitis, measles, poliomyelitis, varicella, rotavirus) warrants screening for functional immunologic defects.

The family history can augment suspicion for the presence of a PIDD. A history of consanguinity, recurrent or unusual infections, or

BOX 67.1 When to Suspect an Immunodeficiency Disorder

- Frequency of infectious illnesses higher than expected
- Unusual severity or duration of infectious disease
- Poor response to conventional antibiotic therapy
- Unusual organisms or opportunistic infections causing disease
- Failure to thrive secondary to frequent illnesses
- Poor wound healing
- Noninflammatory *Staphylococcus* spp. skin infection (or absence of pus)
- Recurrent periodontitis
- Low granulocyte or lymphocyte count

BOX 67.2 X-Linked Primary Immunodeficiency Diseases

- X-linked agammaglobulinemia (Bruton disease)
- Immunodeficiency with hyper–immunoglobulin M (CD40 ligand deficiency)
- X-linked ectodermal dysplasia with immunodeficiency (NEMO deficiency)
- Immunodeficiency, polyendocrinopathy, enteropathy, X linked (IPEX)
- X-linked lymphoproliferative syndrome
- Severe combined immunodeficiency (common γ-chain deficiency)
- Properdin deficiency
- Wiskott-Aldrich syndrome
- X-linked chronic granulomatous disease

TABLE 67.1 Common Pathogens in Children With Primary Immunodeficiency Diseases

Immunodeficiency	Common Pathogens
Antibody deficiencies	*Streptococcus pneumoniae, Haemophilus influenzae, Staphylococcus aureus, Pseudomonas aeruginosa, Mycoplasma, Salmonella, Shigella, Campylobacter,* rotavirus, enteroviruses, *Giardia*
Combined immune deficiencies	Pathogens in antibody deficiencies plus: *Mycobacteria, Candida, Pneumocystis jiroveci,* herpesviruses, adenoviruses
Complement deficiencies	*Neisseria, S. pneumoniae, H. influenzae*
Phagocyte deficiencies	*S. aureus, B. cepacia, Nocardia* spp., *Serratia, Klebsiella,* enteric gram-negative bacilli, *Aspergillus, P. aeruginosa*

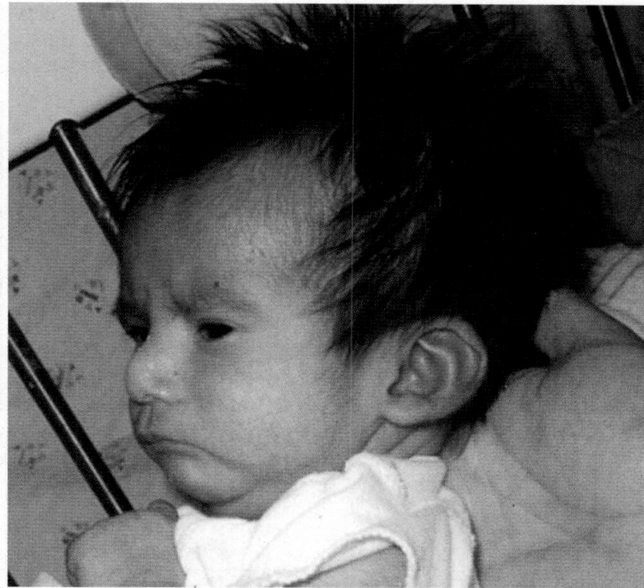

FIG. 67.1 Typical facial appearance of a child with DiGeorge syndrome. Notice the microstomia, hypertelorism, upturned nose, and posteriorly rotated and small, low-set ears.

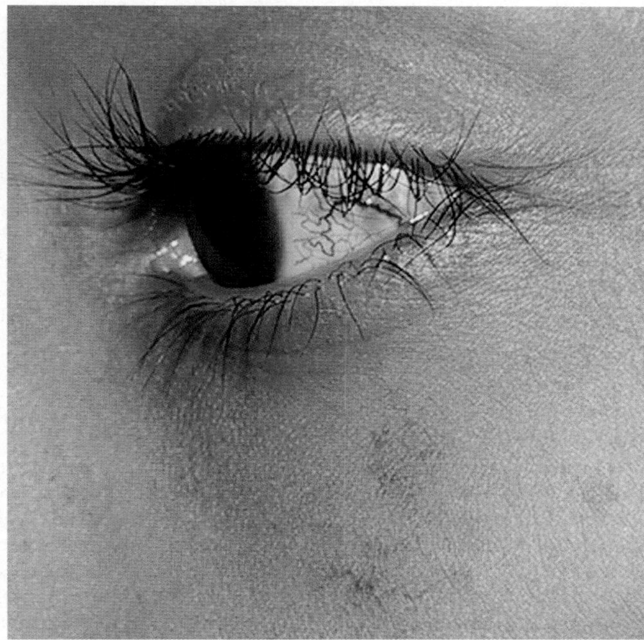

FIG. 67.2 Telangiectasias of the bulbar conjunctivae in a child with ataxia-telangiectasia.

deaths from infection or from unexplained causes during infancy or early childhood in close relatives increases the likelihood for an inheritable immunologic defect. Many PIDDs have X-linked inheritance patterns (Box 67.2), explaining the male-to-female ratio of 5:1 observed in children with PIDDs.

Physical Examination

In patients who are very young and have not been exposed to requisite pathogens to develop infections, the physical examination in many children with PIDDs often provides few clues pointing to an immune defect. A paucity of lymphoid tissues (e.g., tonsils, lymph nodes) may suggest impaired lymphocyte development at an early age. Other examples of helpful physical stigmata include the characteristic facial features (Fig. 67.1) and cardiac malformations in children with DiGeorge syndrome.

In older children, physical examination findings may help to increase suspicion for the presence of a PIDD. Short stature with wasting or failure to thrive appear frequently, likely due to recurrent infections or other chronic issues, such as intestinal malabsorption associated with persistent or frequent diarrhea. Recurrent or recalcitrant oral candidiasis, omphalitis, or multiple skin abscesses can serve as signs of immune deficiency. Severe rash, hepatomegaly, and lymphadenopathy are observed in conditions such as Omenn syndrome. Telangiectasias of the bulbar conjunctivae (Fig. 67.2), nasal bridge, ears, and flexor surfaces of the extremities, with or without ataxia, suggest a diagnosis of ataxia-telangiectasia. Chronic eczema can be observed in the hyperimmunoglobulinemia E (hyper-IgE) and Wiskott-Aldrich syndromes, and severe gingivitis with secondary loss of alveolar bone and dentition (Fig. 67.3) can occur in children with leukocyte adhesion deficiency (LAD).

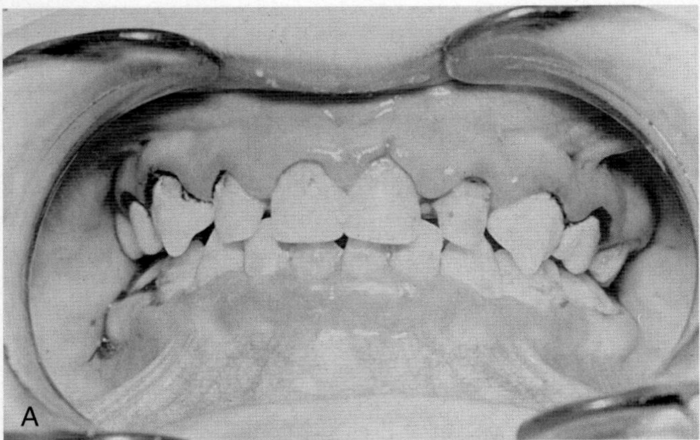

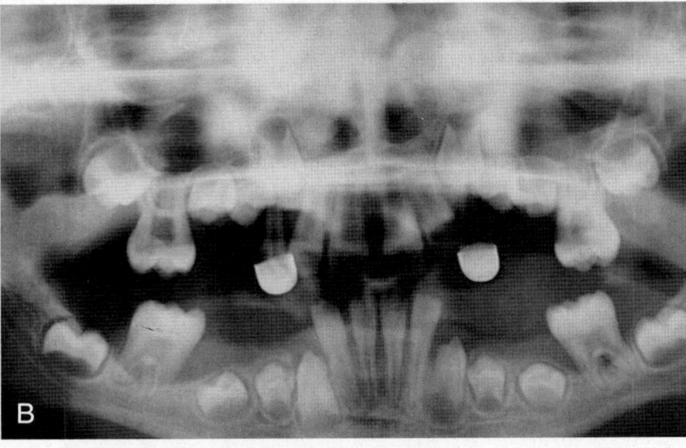

FIG. 67.3 (A) Chronic periodontitis in a boy with leukocyte adhesion deficiency. (B) Radiograph of the same patient shows extensive alveolar bone loss. (Courtesy Dr. Bruce Carter, Texas Children's Hospital, Houston, TX.)

TABLE 67.2 Screening Tests for Suspected Primary Immunodeficiency Disease

Immunodeficiency	Screening Tests
All types	Complete blood cell count Peripheral blood smear
Antibody deficiency	Quantitative serum immunoglobulins: IgG, IgA, IgM, IgE Postimmunization specific IgG antibody titers Isohemagglutinins
T-cell deficiency	Delayed hypersensitivity skin tests or lymphocyte proliferation response to mitogens Chest imaging studies for thymus size Lymphocyte subset phenotyping
Complement deficiency	Total hemolytic complement (CH50) assay
Phagocyte deficiency	Dihydrorhodamine (DHR)-1,2,3 reduction by flow cytometry Neutrophil CD18 and CD15 expression

Laboratory Tests

Widely available, relatively inexpensive laboratory tests can be used to screen for the presence of a PIDD and exclude most of the severe disorders (Table 67.2). The evaluation should be targeted to the type of immune deficiency (e.g., antibody deficiency vs. phagocyte deficiency) suspected by the medical history and physical examination findings. Laboratory test results must be interpreted against age-defined ranges because normal absolute lymphocyte counts, serum immunoglobulin levels, T-cell counts, and other immune parameters change physiologically with age.[109] Tests to exclude secondary immune deficiency caused by HIV infection, malnutrition, or metabolic disorders should always be considered.

A complete blood count with manual differential provides an excellent screening test for PIDDs. Because 50% to 70% of circulating lymphocytes consist of T cells, children with defects in T-cell production (e.g., severe combined immunodeficiency [SCID], complete DiGeorge syndrome) can typically be recognized by absolute lymphopenia. Meanwhile children with Wiskott-Aldrich syndrome are characterized by reduced numbers of platelets that are small (decreased mean platelet volume), a feature that is specific for this syndrome and the related X-linked thrombocytopenia. Large neutrophil cytoplasmic granules are observed in children with Chédiak-Higashi syndrome. Furthermore a complete blood cell count can help to exclude congenital neutropenia. Children with LAD, on the other hand, typically exhibit markedly increased baseline neutrophil and total white blood cell counts. The presence of Howell-Jolly bodies, with or without thrombocytosis, suggests anatomic or functional asplenia.

Evaluation of Humoral Immunity

Screening assessments for antibody deficiency should include quantitative measurement of serum immunoglobulin levels and functional assessment of specific antibody responses. Evaluations of serum IgG, IgA, IgM, and IgE levels help to identify children with panhypogammaglobulinemia, IgA deficiency, hyper-IgM syndrome, hyper-IgE syndrome, and so forth. Functional antibody production should be tested by measuring antibody titers generated in response to immunization with vaccines, such as *Diphtheria* and tetanus toxoids. Antibody responses to polysaccharide antigens should be assessed separately using the 23-serotype pneumococcal polysaccharide vaccine after 24 months of age.[111] Infants younger than 2 years are felt to have functional immaturity in the ability to respond to this class of antigens, although this assertion has been challenged.[10,86] Alternatively, because ABO blood group antigens are polysaccharides, and cross-reacting environmental antigen epitopes exist ubiquitously, some antipolysaccharide antibody production may be assessed by measuring serum isohemagglutinin titers, taking into consideration the fact that children with blood type AB do not form isohemagglutinins. The 13-valent conjugated pneumococcal antigen and *H. influenzae* type b vaccines do not assess antipolysaccharide antibody responses because the immune response to the conjugated protein element drives antibody production to each target antigen. Patients vaccinated with the conjugated pneumococcal vaccine can still be evaluated for antipolysaccharide antibody production to the serotype antigens in the pneumococcal polysaccharide vaccine that are not present in the conjugated vaccine, however. Assessments of children whose screening tests indicate significant humoral immune abnormalities should be followed by enumeration of B-cell subsets in the peripheral blood.

Evaluation of T-Cell–Mediated Immunity

The screening evaluation for T-cell deficiency can begin without specialized immunologic testing. Assessments include measurement of the absolute lymphocyte count, delayed hypersensitivity skin tests, and, in the young infant, posteroanterior and lateral chest radiographs to assess the size of the thymus (Fig. 67.4).

Delayed hypersensitivity skin tests are performed using vaccine or microbial antigens to which the child has had prior exposure. Commonly used antigens include tetanus toxoid and *Candida albicans.* The standard initial dilution is 1:100 for both antigens, but a *C. albicans* dilution of 1:10 may be more appropriate for children 5 years of age or younger who are less likely to have had repeated exposures to this antigen. The diluted antigen is administered intradermally, and the skin reaction is examined for the presence of wheal formation after 24 and 48 hours.

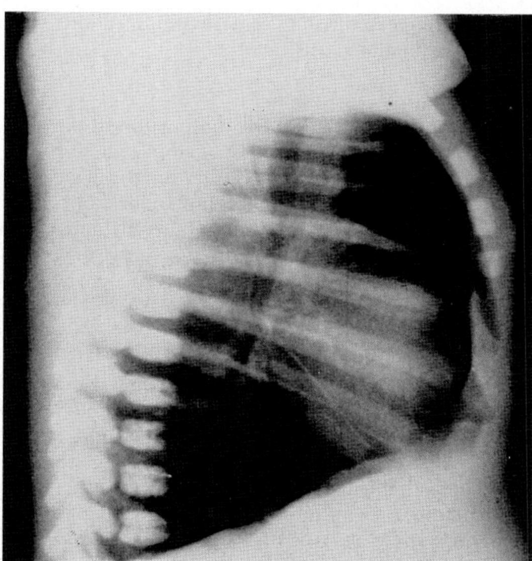

FIG. 67.4 Lateral chest radiograph of an infant with severe combined immunodeficiency disease. Note the absence of the normal thymic shadow.

Specialized tests include enumeration of peripheral blood T cells, T-cell subset phenotyping (e.g., $CD4^+$ or $CD8^+$ T-cell counts), and mitogen- and antigen-induced lymphocyte proliferation studies.[109]

Evaluation of the Complement System

Deficiencies of components of the classic complement pathway can be detected by the total serum hemolytic complement (CH50) assay. This test measures the ability of complement proteins in fresh patient serum to lyse antibody-coated sheep erythrocytes and reflects the activity of all components of the classic complement pathway from C1 through C9. Complete deficiency of any of these components results in very low CH50 values. Improper sample handling can produce low CH50 results. Thus assessments of single complement component levels and targeted functional testing should only be pursued when the CH50 value is zero or near zero.[164] Measurement of serum levels of C3 and C4 is available in most clinical laboratories. The alternate complement pathway is assessed with a similar assay (AH50).

Evaluation of Phagocyte Function

Few assays are available for the assessment of phagocyte function. Children with chronic granulomatous disease (CGD) show abnormally reduced superoxide production in phagocytes in a flow cytometry analysis that detects using dihydrorhodamine-1,2,3 (DHR) as a fluorescent indicator.[109] More sophisticated tests available in research laboratories include assays of chemotaxis, phagocytosis, and bactericidal activity, which may be performed when a high clinical suspicion of a phagocytic disorder exists. Assessment of CD18 and CD15 expression on white blood cells is indicated when a diagnosis of LAD is suspected.

Genetic Testing

More than 300 molecular defects have been identified as causes of PIDDs (Table 67.3). Gene sequence testing for many of these defects is available in a few specialized laboratories and should be pursued when a PIDD with a known genetic defect is suspected.[171] In patients for whom a PIDD is highly likely, and the clinical phenotype can be caused by a defect in one of several candidate genes, whole exome or genome sequencing may be considered.[167,172] Genetic testing is recommended for patients who have a suspicious clinical history and abnormal immune function, for prenatal diagnosis of an unborn child who has a sibling with a known PIDD, and for an individual who may have inherited or who may be a carrier of a known PIDD gene defect. For some conditions, identification of the specific genetic defect may help to determine prognosis and therapeutic options. For example, it has been established that patients with SCID due to Artemis deficiency should not be given alkylator therapy during conditioning for hematopoietic stem cell transplantation because use of such agents is associated with poor growth, abnormal dental development, and late endocrinopathies after transplantation.[130] Determination of the specific genetic defect is also necessary for genetic counseling, usually regarding the probability that the parents will have another child with the same condition.

TABLE 67.3 Examples of Gene Defects in Primary Immunodeficiencies

Immunodeficiency	Defect	Chromosome
Antibody Deficiency		
Agammaglobulinemia	Heavy-chain immunoglobulin	14q23
	Bruton tyrosine kinase	Xq22
Hyper-IgM syndrome	Activation-induced deaminase	12p13
	CD40 ligand *(CD40LG)*	Xq26
Cellular Immunodeficiency		
DiGeorge syndrome	Unknown	22q11.2, 10p13
Severe combined immunodeficiency disease	*RAG1, RAG2*	11p13
	JAK3	19p13.1
	Adenosine deaminase	20q13.11
	Common γ-chain	Xq13.1
	IL-7 receptor-α	5p13
Ataxia-telangiectasia	*ATM*	11q22.3
Wiskott-Aldrich syndrome	*WAS*	Xp11.23
Phagocyte Deficiency		
Chronic granulomatous disease	$p67^{phox}$	1q25
	$p47^{phox}$	7q11.23
	$p22^{phox}$	16q24
	$gp91^{phox}$	Xp21.1
Leukocyte adhesion deficiency type I	*ITGB2*	21q22

Neonatal Screening for T-Cell Deficiencies

In June 2010, the U.S. Department of Health and Human Services approved the addition of SCID to the list of diseases recommended for universal neonatal screening.[133] Children with severe T-cell deficiencies, such as SCID, are born with absent or very low numbers of T-cell receptor excision circles (TRECs), which are DNA byproducts of T-cell receptor recombination. In 2005, Drs. Puck and Chan demonstrated that TREC levels can be measured using blood spots from Guthrie cards.[29] Newborn screening for SCID was subsequently pioneered in Wisconsin in 2008 and continues to be rapidly implemented across the nation. As of July 2017, 44 states and the District of Columbia had active programs to screen all newborns for SCID, resulting in the testing of more than 10 million infants.[170] An additional four states committed to begin screening before the end of 2017. The programs have shown notable success in identifying children with SCID and other PIDDs, resulting in excellent treatment outcomes.[80] Thus all infants who have abnormal newborn screening results for SCID should be evaluated by a clinical immunologist according to the specific algorithm developed by the Health Department of that state. Newborn screening has also determined that the incidence of SCID in the United States is one per 58,000 live births. A similar approach for the diagnosis of B-cell deficiencies in the newborn is being developed.[15]

Management

The immunodeficient patient requires specialized care according to the specific diagnosis and clinical condition. For example, hematopoietic stem cell transplantation is indicated for many PIDDs and needs careful individualized assessment of risks and benefits to provide a treatment protocol that ensures optimal outcomes.[24,115]

BOX 67.3 Key Concepts in the Management of Primary Immunodeficiencies

Immune function: T- and B-cell number and function should be assessed periodically.

IgG replacement therapy: Infusions are indicated for patients with poor antibody responses to immunizations.

Immunizations: Live vaccines should not be administered to patients who have severe T-cell deficiencies unless they have received definitive treatment. Household contacts of children with immunodeficiency should not receive oral poliovirus vaccines because of the risk for transmission to the immunodeficient child. Other live vaccines (BCG, MMRV) may be administered to household contacts. If the vaccine recipient develops a rash, contact with the immunodeficient child should be avoided.[7]

Blood products: When needed, patients with immune deficiencies should receive only irradiated, cytomegalovirus-negative, leukocyte-depleted blood products.

Antibiotic prophylaxis: T-cell–deficient patients should be given antibiotic prophylaxis to prevent *Pneumocystis jirovecii* infection. Antibiotic prophylaxis is recommended for dental and surgical procedures and should be considered for patients with recurrent infections.

Infectious diseases: Infections should be recognized promptly, and unusual pathogens should be considered. Antibiotic therapy should be started early and discontinued cautiously.

Diet and activity: Patients with immune deficiency should have a regular diet and lifestyle but should be instructed to avoid eating raw food and playing in environments potentially highly contaminated with pathogens, including daycare centers. Strict hand-washing precautions and reverse isolation may be indicated for patients with poor T-cell function.

Administration of intravenous or subcutaneous IgG (IVIG or SCIG, respectively) serves as a common therapeutic measure for patients who lack IgG antibody responses, whether isolated or as part of combined immune deficiency.[173] Other recommendations specific to patients with PIDDs may include exclusion from contact with infectious illness and avoidance of live vaccines[6,135]; use of irradiated, leukocyte-depleted, cytomegalovirus-negative blood products when needed; antibiotic prophylaxis; and prompt diagnosis and treatment of infections. Aside from patients with severe T-cell deficiency awaiting hematopoietic stem cell transplantation, isolation in sterile environments is not recommended because the risk for infection must be balanced with the severe impact in psychosocial development induced by isolation. Instead the infection risk should be minimized using advances in the treatment and prevention of community-acquired infections (Box 67.3).

SELECTED PRIMARY ANTIBODY DEFICIENCIES

X-Linked Agammaglobulinemia

Clinical Features

Boys with X-linked agammaglobulinemia (XLA) are often healthy during the first months of life due to the protective presence of transplacentally acquired maternal IgG. As maternal immunoglobulin disappears from the infant, chronic or recurrent infections develop.[36,37,119,165] The most common findings include recurrent otitis media, sinusitis, pneumonia, and diarrhea, but infections are not limited to mucosal surfaces: bacteremia, meningitis, and osteomyelitis may also occur. In a retrospective study of 201 patients with XLA, the mean age at diagnosis was 2.5 years in patients with a family history of the disease and 3.5 years when no family history was present.[165] The most common bacterial pathogens identified in patients with XLA include *S. pneumoniae, H. influenzae, S. aureus,* and *P. aeruginosa*. *Mycoplasma* spp. infections also occur with increased frequency and have been implicated as a cause of a subacute, destructive arthritis. Gastrointestinal infections may be caused by *Salmonella, Shigella, Campylobacter,* or rotavirus. Chronic giardiasis with intestinal malabsorption has been observed. Patients with XLA also demonstrate increased risk for enteroviral infections, particularly viral meningoencephalitis.

Pathogenesis

The defective gene *(BTK)* maps to the midportion of the long arm of the X chromosome. The gene encodes a cytoplasmic tyrosine kinase, BTK, which is a signal transducer necessary for B-cell survival during maturation.[149] As a consequence, blood, lymph nodes, and bone marrow contain markedly diminished numbers of B cells and plasma cells, resulting in agammaglobulinemia. BTK also plays a role in viral immunity within macrophages and dendritic cells, perhaps explaining the enteroviral susceptibility.[81,82,90,138]

Diagnosis

Because of the presence of transplacentally acquired maternal IgG, a normal level of serum IgG in a male infant during the first 6 months of life does not exclude the diagnosis of XLA. IgA, IgM, and IgE levels may be low as well, but defining values that clearly differentiate infants with the disease from normal infants has remained difficult. Diagnosis can be better obtained by immunophenotyping, using flow cytometry analysis to demonstrate absence of B cells in peripheral blood. After an infant with XLA reaches 6 months of age, serum IgG concentrations usually fall below 100 mg/dL, and levels of other immunoglobulin isotypes remain low or undetectable. No isohemagglutinins are present, and specific antibodies are not produced in response to immunization or natural infection. Recurrent infections or early mortality in male family members may suggest the characteristic X-linked pattern of inheritance. Definitive diagnosis is obtained by identifying functionally deleterious mutations in the *BTK* gene.

Treatment and Prognosis

Lifetime IgG replacement therapy is needed for all patients with XLA.[113] It decreases the frequency of severe infections, reduces the need for hospitalization, and helps to prevent the development of chronic lung disease with progressive decline in pulmonary function. The dose and frequency of administration of IVIG or SCIG should be adjusted to minimize the frequency of infections. Some patients receiving IVIG will require serum IgG trough levels of 800 to 1300 mg/dL to achieve this goal.[91] Most patients receive IVIG at a dose of 400 to 600 mg/kg every 3 or 4 weeks or SCIG at 140 to 200 mg/kg weekly. Patients who are given SCIG should have steady-state serum IgG levels measured periodically (SCIG administration does not produce trough serum IgG levels). SCIG recipients should maintain steady state serum IgG levels higher than the serum IgG trough level targeted by IVIG administration in order to achieve a comparable pharmacokinetic area under the curve.

Infections should be treated aggressively in patients with XLA. Routine middle ear, sinus, and skin infections usually respond to oral antibiotics. Therapy for pneumonia and other significant focal or systemic infections should start with intravenously administered antibiotics. Empirical antibiotic therapy should be directed against common bacterial pathogens, including *S. pneumoniae, H. influenzae,* and *S. aureus*. If possible, a causative pathogen should be identified, particularly in severe or chronic infections. Additional doses of IVIG are indicated for treatment of pneumonia or invasive infections. Because chronic pulmonary disease with bronchiectasis represents a significant cause of mortality in patients with XLA, defined periods of antibiotic therapy, similar to strategies employed in patients with cystic fibrosis, may be helpful for certain patients.

Immunoglobulin Deficiency With Increased IgM

Clinical Features

About 70% of patients with immunoglobulin deficiency with increased IgM (i.e., hyper-IgM syndrome) are male, associated with X-linked inheritance of the condition, while the remainder display an autosomal recessive inheritance pattern.[8,83,85,103,120] Patients with this disorder develop recurrent pyogenic infections during infancy as transplacentally acquired maternal IgG wanes. Recurrent respiratory tract infections and chronic diarrhea with failure to thrive occur; patients can develop septicemia, meningitis, and other invasive infections as well. Patients who have hyper-IgM syndrome due to defects in the CD40 and NF-κB signaling

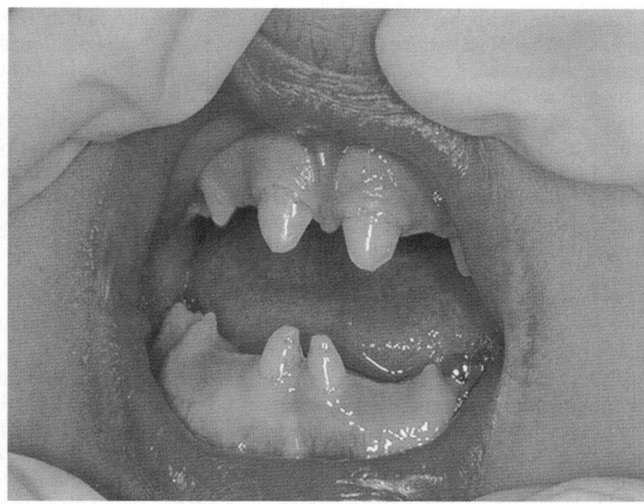

FIG. 67.5 Conical teeth characteristic of immunodeficiency due to defects in the *IKBKB* gene (NEMO deficiency).

pathways carry increased risk for opportunistic infections, such as *Pneumocystis jiroveci* pneumonia.[120]

Other clinical manifestations can also arise. Almost two-thirds of patients with hyper-IgM syndrome have a history of neutropenia, which typically appears intermittently but without the precise periodicity of cyclic neutropenia.[120] Patients frequently develop aphthous ulcers; perirectal ulcers and abscesses have also been reported. Lymphoid hyperplasia can develop in patients who have defects in enzymes responsible for isotype switching and somatic hypermutation. Intestinal nodular lymphoid hyperplasia may lead to malabsorption and protein-losing enteropathy. Patients also demonstrate increased risk for malignancy and autoimmune disease, including arthritis and nephritis, compared to normal children. Male patients with mutations in *IKBKG* may but do not necessarily have anhidrotic ectodermal dysplasia and conical teeth (Fig. 67.5).

Pathogenesis

Several genetic defects have been identified as causes of hyper-IgM syndrome. Most boys with hyper-IgM syndrome have mutations in *CD40LG*, a gene on the X chromosome that encodes the T-cell ligand for CD40.[3,8] CD40 is a signaling molecule that is expressed on the surface of B cells; several patients with hyper-IgM syndrome due to CD40 deficiency have also been reported.[120] Engagement of CD40 by CD40 ligand is essential for B-cell proliferation, isotype switching, and terminal differentiation into antibody-secreting plasma cells. Most cases of autosomal recessive hyper-IgM syndrome occur due to mutations in the activation-induced cytidine deaminase *(AICDA)* and the uracil DNA glycosylase *(UNG)* genes.[103,120] Hyper-IgM syndrome can also be caused by defects in NEMO, encoded by *IKBKG* on the X chromosome,[137,169] and IKBα, which both play key roles in modulation of NF-κB signaling.[120] Most mutations in *IKBKG* are lethal for male fetuses, and female carriers of these mutations may have incontinentia pigmenti.

Diagnosis

Various laboratory test findings can help to establish the diagnosis. Most patients with hyper-IgM syndrome have a characteristic increase in serum IgM level with low to absent concentrations of serum IgA and IgG. Serum IgM concentrations may exceed 1000 mg/dL. However, they can also exist within the normal range, especially in younger children. Patients have normal numbers of circulating IgM$^+$ B cells but few B cells that express surface IgA or IgG. Antibody responses to immunization may be present but consist predominantly or exclusively of IgM antibodies because isotype switching does not occur. Evaluation of boys with suspected hyper-IgM syndrome should include assessment of CD40 ligand expression in activated T cells by flow cytometry and genetic sequencing of *CD40LG*.[8]

BOX 67.4 Criteria for the Diagnosis of Common Variable Immunodeficiency Disease

- At least one of the following:
  - Increased susceptibility to infection
  - Autoimmune manifestations
  - Granulomatous disease
  - Unexplained polyclonal lymphoproliferation
  - Affected family member with antibody deficiency
- *And* marked decrease of IgG and marked decrease of IgA with or without low IgM levels (measured at least twice; <2 standard deviations below the normal levels for age)
- *And* at least one of the following:
  - Poor antibody response to vaccines (and/or absent isohemagglutinins)
  - Low switched-memory B cells (<70% of the age-related normal value)
- *And* secondary causes of hypogammaglobulinemia have been excluded
- *And* diagnosis is established after the fourth year of life (although symptoms may present before that age)
- *And* no evidence of severe T-cell deficiency, defined as two of the following:
  - CD4$^+$ cells/mm^3: 2–6 years old, <300; 6–12 years old, <250; >12 years, <200
  - Naive CD4$^+$ %: 2–6 years old, <25; 6–16 years old, <20; >16 years, <10
  - Significantly decreased T-cell proliferation to stimulation

Ig, Immunoglobulin.

Treatment and Prognosis

Patients with hyper-IgM syndrome must be followed closely. All affected individuals require IgG replacement therapy.[113] Patients with defects in the CD40 and NF-κB signaling pathways should receive antibiotic prophylaxes against a limited number of opportunistic pathogens, such as *Pneumocystis* or atypical mycobacteria, as well. Males with *CD40LG* defects have increased morbidity and mortality compared with patients with autosomal forms of hyper-IgM syndrome, likely related to the fact that *CD40LG* deficiency affects both T and B cells. Significant causes of long-term mortality include invasive infections, liver failure, and malignancy.[120] Hepatic diseases include sclerosing cholangitis, cirrhosis, and hepatocellular carcinoma and are associated with *Cryptosporidium parvum* infection.[120] Thus patients should be warned against trips to water parks and drinking of tap water. Human leukocyte antigen (HLA)-identical bone marrow transplantation has been successful in treating this condition and should be considered early after diagnosis before severe complications occur. Administration of recombinant CD40 ligand or agonistic anti-CD40 antibodies has also been reported to improve immune responses in these patients.[49,69]

Common Variable Immunodeficiency Disease

Clinical Features

Common variable immunodeficiency disease (CVID) includes a heterogeneous group of antibody-deficient disorders with similar clinical manifestations, such as recurrent infections and a propensity for autoimmune conditions.[14] Although the diagnosis is often given indiscriminately, CVID is strictly defined using diagnostic criteria established by the European Society for Immunodeficiencies (Box 67.4).[5] Onset can occur at any age. A study of more than 2200 European patients with CVID has demonstrated two peaks for diagnosis: during childhood and between 30 and 40 years of age.[52]

CVID typically manifests with susceptibility to infections in a similar manner to XLA and hyper-IgM syndrome.[108] Patients develop recurrent bacterial infections of the respiratory tract or invasive bacterial infections. Bronchiectasis and chronic lung disease from recurrent pneumonias remain significant causes of long-term morbidity and mortality.[52] The most common infectious organisms isolated from the respiratory tract include *S. pneumoniae* and *H. influenzae.*[108] Many individuals with CVID develop chronic diarrhea and intestinal malabsorption associated with gastrointestinal infections by *Giardia, Campylobacter,* and *Salmonella.*[108] The inflammation induced by these infections can result in protein-losing enteropathy, which may exacerbate the underlying hypogammaglobulinemia. Patients are also susceptible to infections of the genitourinary tract, joint tissues, and lungs by *Ureaplasma* spp.[14]

Patients with CVID can demonstrate increased risk for noninfectious complications.[14,52] They are known to have increased prevalence for ulcerative colitis, Crohn disease, other enteropathies, atrophic gastritis with achlorhydria, and cholelithiasis. Almost 30% of individuals with CVID develop autoimmunity, which includes chronic arthritis resembling rheumatoid arthritis, scleroderma, lupus-like disease, hypothyroidism, autoimmune chronic hepatitis, and autoimmune cytopenias.[52] Abnormal lymphoid proliferation, granulomas, and malignancies, such as lymphoma and gastric carcinoma, appear over time in some patients. They can develop a pseudolymphoma syndrome in the lungs (i.e., lymphoid interstitial pneumonia) and intestines (i.e., nodular lymphoid hyperplasia), splenomegaly, or mediastinal adenopathy.[52]

Pathogenesis

No single genetic defect has been widely identified as the cause of CVID. Instead the diagnosis of CVID encompasses a number of different genetic defects that result in loss of antibody secretion.[112] B-cell phenotyping studies have demonstrated a variety of maturational defects in patients with CVID.[44] Decreased or absent numbers of switched memory B cells is associated with disease severity and development of autoimmune disorders and malignancies.[2,125,163] A variety of T-cell functional abnormalities also have been reported. They include decreased lymphocyte proliferation to mitogens and antigens and reduced expression of cytokines. Overall, polymorphisms or mutations in the *TNFRSF13B, ICOS, MSH5, TNFRSF13C, CD27, CD81, CD19, MS4A1, CR2, NFKB2,* and *LRBA* genes have all been individually associated with disease in several families or individuals with CVID.[14,28,32,78,89,131,153,154,160]

Diagnosis

The diagnosis should be established according to defined criteria (see Box 67.4).[5] The clinical history must support a diagnosis of CVID. In terms of laboratory studies, the serum IgG and IgA levels must be less than 2 standard deviations below the normal ranges for age, and patients with CVID will typically have a serum IgG level persistently below 250 to 300 mg/dL. Patients must also demonstrate either impaired antibody responses to immunizations or low numbers of switched memory B cells; some patients will have both abnormalities. Secondary causes of hypogammaglobulinemia and severe T-cell deficiency must be excluded. The diagnosis of CVID is not generally given to patients under 4 years of age.

Treatment and Prognosis

No therapies are currently recommended for definitive treatment of CVID. Hematopoietic stem cell transplantation has been demonstrated to result in survival of less than 50%.[162] Thus patients must be given lifelong IgG replacement therapy to minimize the frequency of infections, particularly of the lungs.[113] Some patients require IVIG doses to maintain serum IgG trough levels of 500 to 1700 mg/dL or SCIG doses to achieve pharmacokinetically equivalent levels of steady-state serum IgG in order to accomplish this goal.[52,91] Patients with CVID who have enteric protein loss due to enteropathy may require remarkable doses of IVIG or SCIG to maintain protective serum IgG concentrations. Limited antibiotic prophylaxis may be needed as an adjunctive measure in patients who continue to develop infections, especially in sites primarily protected by secretory IgA (e.g., the sinuses), despite appropriate serum IgG levels. Patients who have low serum IgM levels carry significantly increased risk for developing bronchiectasis.[52] Overall, however, morbidity and mortality in patients with CVID are equally associated with either infectious (e.g., chronic lung disease with bronchiectasis) or noninfectious (e.g., autoimmunity, lymphoid hyperplasia) complications.[52]

IgA Deficiency

Clinical Features

IgA deficiency is the most common PIDD. Its prevalence varies by ethnicity but ranges from one in 155 individuals to one of every 18,550.[159] In Caucasians, it appears at a frequency of one in 300 to one in 1200 persons.[136] The vast majority of individuals with IgA deficiency are clinically asymptomatic.[136,159] Some patients develop recurrent infections of the respiratory tract, gastrointestinal tract (e.g., by *Giardia*), or other tissues.[92] IgA deficiency is associated with increased risk for autoimmunity, such as SLE, rheumatoid arthritis, pernicious anemia, autoimmune thyroid disease, type 1 diabetes, or celiac disease.[136,159] Lymphoid and gastrointestinal malignancies may occur more frequently than in the general population. An association with increased atopy has been suggested but remains controversial.[136,159]

Pathogenesis

The pathogenesis of IgA deficiency has not been determined. Of interest, some individuals with selective IgA deficiency subsequently develop CVID, and variations in *TNFRSF13B* and *ICOS* genes have been found in families with members that have either of these conditions.[28] Genetic variations within the major histocompatibility complex (MHC) III region on chromosome 6 have also been associated with the development of selective IgA deficiency and CVID, further arguing that these two disorders may be related.[157] In particular, the *MSH5* gene falls within this region, and mutations in this gene have been implicated as a cause of CVID.[159] Certain HLA haplotypes, such as 8.1, undeniably play a role, and associated candidate genes near or within the MHC class II and II regions are being investigated.[136,159] Mutations in other genes outside of MHC regions have also been proposed as causes of IgA deficiency. Associated genes include *IFIH1, CLEC16A, TNFAIP3, PVT1, FAS, CDH23,* and *TM7SF3.*[136,159]

Diagnosis

International consensus defines selective IgA deficiency as the presence of serum IgA levels of less than 7 mg/dL with normal IgG and IgM levels in individuals 4 years of age or older.[87,136,159] Normal serum IgA concentrations can vary in children under the age of 4 and can even be undetectable in healthy infants younger than 6 to 9 months of age. In fact, more than 20% of children who meet criteria for a diagnosis of IgA deficiency between 4 and 10 years of age no longer have serum IgA levels of less than 7 mg/dL when they become adolescents, arguing that the diagnosis should be given very carefully in the pediatric population.[87]

Treatment and Prognosis

IVIG and SCIG therapies are not indicated for the treatment of patients with selective IgA deficiency. Respiratory tract infections in individuals with selective IgA deficiency may require prolonged courses of antibiotic therapy. Antibiotic prophylaxis for respiratory tract infections should be considered if infections recur frequently. Parenteral antibiotics may be needed for refractory cases of sinusitis or pneumonia. IgA-deficient patients carry a small risk for development of IgE-mediated anaphylaxis if sensitized to IgA and given a blood product that contains IgA.[122] The incidence of this kind of reaction is estimated to range between one in 20,000 and one in 47,000 transfusions.[136] Broad, routine restriction of IgA-deficient patients against receiving IgA-containing blood products is not recommended.[126]

Transient Hypogammaglobulinemia of Infancy

Clinical Features

Infants with transient hypogammaglobulinemia of infancy (THI) come to medical attention because of recurrent respiratory tract infections (e.g., otitis media, sinusitis) and serum immunoglobulin levels below laboratory normal ranges. Septicemia, meningitis, skin infections, and other invasive infections very rarely occur.[114,152]

Pathogenesis

THI is caused by delayed physiologic maturation of immunoglobulin synthesis, resulting in prolongation of the relative hypogammaglobulinemia ("physiologic nadir") observed in most normal infants at 3 to 6 months of age as maternal IgG is cleared from the circulation. No molecular etiology has been identified and confirmed. Patients with THI are able to produce protective specific antibody responses.

Diagnosis

The diagnosis can be made with certainty only in retrospect. More than 80% of children with THI recover to normal immunoglobulin levels by 3 years of age.[152] In some children, however, serum immunoglobulin concentrations may remain low until the children are several years of age.[114,152] Demonstration of normal specific antibody responses can help to support the diagnosis.

Treatment and Prognosis

Infants with suspected THI should be followed clinically, and serial measurements of serum immunoglobulin levels should be performed. Initial immunoglobulin levels may help to predict which infants will recover more quickly.[152] Some children are eventually diagnosed with CVID, selective IgA deficiency, or another immunodeficiency disease. Because THI is self-limited and specific antibody production is normal, IgG replacement therapy is not indicated. Antibiotic prophylaxis may be considered in selected cases for recurrent respiratory tract infections.

IgG Subclass "Deficiency"

Four subclasses of IgG are known to exist. IgG1 constitutes 60% of total IgG, IgG2 accounts for 25%, and IgG3 and IgG4 are present in smaller quantities (10% and 5%, respectively).[23] Normal ranges of serum levels for each subclass vary by age and must be considered when interpreting clinical laboratory data. The prevalence of IgG subclass deficiency has been reported at between 4.8% and 24% for different patient groups.[140] Although various roles for each subclass have been proposed, the exact function of each subclass is not fully understood in immune processes.[23] Thus the importance of isolated IgG subclass deficiency as a PIDD remains debatable.

In general, patients gain little benefit from measurements of IgG subclass levels and assignment of a diagnosis of IgG subclass deficiency as part of the initial evaluation for suspected PIDD. First, the clinical relevance of "low" levels of IgG2, IgG3, or IgG4 remains dubious. Individuals have been reported with complete lack of various subclasses who yet remain entirely asymptomatic.[23] In fact, IgG subclass deficiencies may be present in 1% to 3% of healthy persons.[23] Patients with allergic diseases in particular can have IgG subclass deficiencies yet do not merit a diagnosis of humoral immune deficiency.[39,107] Thus inappropriate measurements of IgG subclass levels can lead to overdiagnosis or misdiagnosis and improper treatment. Second, the levels of IgG subclasses provide no information about humoral function. Most children with low IgG subclass levels demonstrate normal antibody responses against protein and polysaccharide antigens, indicating normal humoral immune function.[23] The rest may have selective antibody deficiency, a separate diagnosis that remains controversial, or another PIDD. In either case, testing of responses to vaccines is required, indicating that assessments of specific antibody function and not measurements of IgG subclass levels should be performed in the initial evaluation for suspected PIDDs.[93] Finally, some patients with IgG subclass deficiencies have other clinically relevant PIDDs (most commonly IgA deficiency) that can be identified through routine screening tests of immune function.[23,79] Measurements of IgG subclass levels play no role in establishing the proper diagnosis in these patients.

Most patients with low IgG subclass levels should be managed with reassurance. Routine bacterial infections should be treated with antibiotics. Limited antibiotic prophylaxes against sinopulmonary tract infections may be offered to some patients. Immunoglobulin replacement therapy is not indicated, except perhaps in abbreviated courses for patients who have abnormally poor antibody responses to immunizations and a demonstrated propensity for frequent or chronic infections.

SELECTED PRIMARY COMBINED IMMUNE DEFICIENCIES

Severe Combined Immunodeficiency Disease

Clinical Features

Most infants with SCID appear completely healthy at birth. Thus infants identified by newborn screening programs may not exhibit any clinical abnormalities other than lack of palpable lymph nodes and tonsils. In the absence of newborn screening, infants with SCID can typically be recognized during the first few months of life by the appearance of recurrent or severe infections.[139] These infections include recurrent otitis media or pneumonia and persistent or severe viral infections caused by respiratory syncytial virus, parainfluenza virus, adenovirus, or rhinovirus. Infants with SCID may also develop a severe, disseminated infection from cytomegalovirus, especially if accompanied by very high plasma viral load and hemolytic anemia. Infections occur from attenuated virus strains in immunizations, including disseminated varicella after varicella or measles-mumps-rubella-varicella (MMRV) vaccine administration and persistent infection with vaccine strains of rotavirus, oral poliovirus, rubella, or measles virus. Infants with SCID can also develop disseminated infection with BCG after BCG immunization. Other signs of SCID include recurrent or recalcitrant oral and cutaneous candidiasis, septicemia, and other invasive bacterial infections. Patients demonstrate increased susceptibility to routine pathogens (e.g., *S. pneumoniae, H. influenzae*), unusual organisms, and opportunistic pathogens, such as *P. jiroveci*. Other signs of SCID include chronic diarrhea and failure to thrive associated with onset of infections. In the neonatal period, a rash may appear that is produced by a graft-versus-host reaction induced by maternal T lymphocytes.

Pathogenesis

SCID represents a heterogeneous group of genetic disorders that share the ability to produce profound failure of both T and B cell function. At least 16 molecular defects have been confirmed to cause SCID (Table 67.4).[17] In the United States, the most prevalent cause of SCID is a defect in the γ chain of the IL-2 receptor, identified in 36% of patients with SCID.[115] Because the molecule is encoded by the *IL2RG* gene on the X chromosome, all of these patients are male, and the defect is inherited in an X-linked recessive pattern. This protein is a functional component of the receptors for IL-2, IL-4, IL-7, IL-9, IL-15,

TABLE 67.4 Types of Severe Combined Immunodeficiency

Type	Defect
IL2RG (common γ-chain) deficiency	Signaling for IL-2, IL-4, IL-7, IL-15, and IL-21
JAK3 (janus kinase 3) deficiency	Cytokine signaling
IL7R (IL-7 receptor-α) deficiency	Signaling for IL-7
PTPRC (CD45) deficiency	Protein tyrosine phosphatase regulation of signaling, cell activation
CD3D (CD3δ) deficiency	T-cell receptor signaling
CD3E (CD3ε) deficiency	T-cell receptor signaling
CD247 (CD3ζ) deficiency	T-cell receptor signaling
CORO1A (coronin 1A) deficiency	Defective thymic egress of T cells and T-cell actin organization, homeostasis
RAG1 (recombinase activating gene 1) deficiency	Rearrangement of B- and T-cell receptor genes
RAG2 (recombinase activating gene 2) deficiency	Rearrangement of B- and T-cell receptor genes
DCLRE1C (Artemis) deficiency	Rearrangement of B- and T-cell receptor genes
PRKDC (DNA PK_{CS}) deficiency	Rearrangement of B- and T-cell receptor genes
LIG4 (DNA ligase 4) deficiency	Rearrangement of B- and T-cell receptor genes
NHEJ1 (Cernunnos) deficiency	Rearrangement of B- and T-cell receptor genes
AK2 deficiency (reticular dysgenesis)	Defective stem cell maturation
ADA (adenosine deaminase) deficiency	Metabolite (dATP) toxicity to lymphocytes

and IL-21 and is essential for development of human T cells and natural killer cells.[74,75] All of the other known causes of SCID are inherited in an autosomal recessive pattern. IL-7 receptor α-chain deficiency produces the second most common cause of SCID in the United States and is followed in frequency by defects in recombinase activating genes 1 and 2 (RAG1 and RAG2), adenosine deaminase (ADA) deficiency, Janus kinase 3 (JAK3) deficiency, and Artemis deficiency.[115] In more than 30% of patients, the molecular cause remains unknown.[115]

Diagnosis

Specific criteria have been established to define the diagnosis of SCID. These requirements include (1) absence or very low number of T cells (less than 300 $CD3^+$ T cells/mm^3) *and* no or very low T-cell function (<10% of lower limit of normal) as measured by response to phytohemagglutinin or (2) presence of T cells of maternal origin.[134]

Other studies can help to support the diagnosis of SCID. In states that have newborn screening programs for SCID, very low levels of TRECs may suggest the diagnosis. Clinically, infants with SCID typically lack radiographic evidence of a thymus gland. They usually have absolute lymphocyte counts of less than 2000 cells/mm^3.[25] Some patients have panhypogammaglobulinemia, whereas others have depressed concentrations of only one or two immunoglobulin isotypes. Antibody responses are profoundly impaired or absent, and delayed type hypersensitivity skin test anergy is observed. X-linked or JAK3-deficient SCID may be suspected if B cells (that do not function) account for all circulating lymphocytes. Biochemical tests for adenosine deaminase and purine nucleoside phosphorylase levels and enzymatic activities are available in specialized laboratories. Testing for a specific genetic defect should be pursued, and a genetic evaluation of immediate relatives for carrier status is recommended for genetic counseling purposes. Lymphocyte enumeration and genetic testing remain especially important for identifying radiosensitive B cell–negative, natural killer (NK) cell–positive forms of SCID.

Treatment and Prognosis

In patients with SCID who have not received definitive therapy, infection risks must be minimized. Infants should be kept isolated from infected individuals as much as possible and kept in reverse isolation with respiratory and contact precautions in hospital settings. Patients with SCID should receive prophylaxis against *Pneumocystis jirovecii* and immunoglobulin replacement therapy. Candidal prophylaxis may be considered as well. Except for live polio virus (no longer available in the United States), all household members should be kept immunized, but the patient should not receive any live viral or bacterial immunizations.[117] Any acute infections must be treated aggressively, and providers should set a low threshold for hospital admission. If transfusion of blood products is needed, they must be leukocyte-reduced, irradiated, and CMV negative. Patients with radiosensitive forms of SCID should minimize exposure to sunlight, ultraviolet light, and ionizing radiation, such as γ-radiation delivered during radiologic studies. In addition, providers who perform hematopoietic stem cell transplantation must be made aware of increased sensitivity of tissues to DNA crosslinking medications and adjust any conditioning regimens accordingly.

Hematopoietic stem cell transplantation (HSCT) serves as the treatment of choice for most patients with SCID.[115] HSCT using HLA-matched related donors yields a survival rate of greater than 95%. HSCT can also be performed using HLA-haploidentical related or HLA-matched unrelated donors either with or without conditioning.[45,58,115] However overall survival falls to 58% to 79% if transplantation is performed using cells that do not come from an HLA-matched related donor—unless infants are transplanted prior to 3.5 months of age, before infections and organ damage occur.[115] Survival improves to 94% overall for transplants that are given before 3.5 months of age.[115] Use or absence of conditioning does not appear to impact survival except in infants who have infections at the time of transplantation. These patients demonstrate 65% survival after HLA-haploidentical–related HSCT performed without conditioning but only 39% to 53% survival when conditioning is used.[115]

Alternative therapies may be considered for some patients. Experimental gene therapy trials were started for X-linked SCID in 1999. Eighteen of the initial 20 recipients showed successful immune reconstitution, but 5 developed leukemia due to insertional mutagenesis of the retroviral vector within the *LMO2* oncogene.[60,63,68] A new trial has since been initiated using a self-inactivating γ-retrovirus vector, resulting in eight survivors among nine recipients. The survivors have developed appropriate gene marking in T cells, no evidence of insertional mutagenesis, and acceptable immune reconstitution 1 to 3 years after treatment.[62] For patients with ADA-deficient SCID, either enzyme replacement using bovine-derived polyethylene glycol-modified adenosine deaminase (PEG-ADA) or gene therapy has been used as an alternative form of treatment.[27,51] PEG-ADA increases lymphocyte counts and provides adequate immunity in most affected patients. Most recipients, however, ultimately develop "resistance" to the drug in the form of neutralizing anti-ADA antibodies or declining lymphocyte counts over time. Gene therapy for ADA deficiency has demonstrated marked success in all clinical trials to date with no evidence of insertional mutagenesis or treatment-related leukemia.

DiGeorge Syndrome

Clinical Features

DiGeorge syndrome is characterized by facial, cardiac, parathyroid, and thymic abnormalities that can all vary to differing degrees.[11,41,97,146] The condition may be identified early in infancy with findings unrelated to immune deficiency. Characteristic facial features include microstomia and micrognathia; hypertelorism; upturned nose; arched palate; posteriorly rotated and small, low-set ears with notched pinnae; and downward slanting of the palpebral fissures (see Fig. 67.1). Congenital heart disease, particularly truncus arteriosus and interrupted aortic arch, usually presents in the first few weeks of life and appears in almost 80% of affected children.[26] Neonatal hypocalcemia from hypoparathyroidism (in approximately 40% of DiGeorge infants[26]) can result in seizures or tetany. Other defects, such as hypothyroidism, esophageal atresia, tracheoesophageal fistula, and bifid uvula, have also been described. A significant percentage of patients meet criteria for CHARGE (***c***oloboma, ***h***eart defect, **a**tresia or stenosis of the choanae, ***r***etardation of development or growth, ***g***enitourinary abnormality, ***e***ar malformation) syndrome or VACTERL (i.e., ***v***ertebral abnormality, ***a***nal atresia, ***c***ardiac defect, ***t***racheo-***e***sophageal anomaly, ***r***enal or radial defect, ***l***imb malformation) association.[97,123] In as many as 2% of patients with DiGeorge syndrome, congenital athymia is present, resulting in the diagnosis of "complete" DiGeorge syndrome.[88] Complete DiGeorge syndrome produces a severe combined T- and B-cell deficiency that results in death from infection by 2 years of age if left untreated. However partial DiGeorge syndrome remains 50 times more prevalent and is characterized by some degree of thymic function and immune protection.

According to the degree of immune deficiency, clinical manifestations may include predisposition to a wide variety of common and opportunistic infectious diseases. Many infections are caused by neuroanatomical defects associated with DiGeorge syndrome and not by immune deficiency. Most infections tend to involve the sinopulmonary tract.[26,38] At Texas Children's Hospital, 20% of patients with DiGeorge syndrome and mild T-cell deficiency have an increased incidence of respiratory tract infections.[33] A number of patients with DiGeorge syndrome develop hypogammaglobulinemia or humoral immunity defects that require IgG replacement therapy.[26,116] Patients may also have difficulty with chronic diarrhea or mucocutaneous candidiasis. Recurrent or severe herpesviral infections (e.g., herpes simplex virus 1 [HSV1], cytomegalovirus), *P. jiroveci* pneumonia, and other opportunistic infections may be observed if immune deficiency is severe. Graft-versus-host disease can occur if infants receive blood products containing viable lymphocytes, often during surgical correction of heart defects. Most patients with partial DiGeorge syndrome develop adequate T-cell numbers and function by 1 year of age and do not have an increased incidence of opportunistic infections.

Pathogenesis

DiGeorge syndrome is caused by abnormal embryologic development of the third and fourth branchial arches and their derivatives, including the parathyroid glands, aortic arch structures, and the thymus gland.[146] The condition is most frequently associated with 22q11.2 hemizygosity, but fewer than 60% of patients with DiGeorge anomaly have microdeletions within chromosome 22q11.[97,123] Some patients have mutations in *CHD7*, which is associated with CHARGE syndrome.[38] A few patients have been reported who carry a deletion in chromosome 10p.[38] Fetal exposure to retinoic acid, fetal alcohol syndrome, and diabetic embryopathy can also produce DiGeorge syndrome.[38]

Searches for single molecular causes of DiGeorge syndrome have focused on genes located within the critical chromosomal region that is deleted in patients with 22q11.2 hemizygosity. Early studies implicated *TBX1*, since mice that bear *TBX1* deletions reproduce many of the characteristic features of DiGeorge syndrome.[166] A role for *TBX1* may be supported by the finding that the DiGeorge phenotype, including athymia, can be reproduced by homozygous deletions in *NKX26*, which encodes a protein that mediates effector functions downstream from TBX1.[143] However DiGeorge syndrome is also known to occur in patients who have 22q11.2 deletions that do not affect the *TBX1* gene, suggesting that it may not provide the sole answer.[155] *DGCR8, MAPK1,* and *CRKL* lie within the 22q11 critical region, and mutations in any of these genes have also been demonstrated to reproduce the DiGeorge phenotype in both mice and humans.[30,38,132,168] Of note, patients with partial DiGeorge syndrome have been found to display a dose-sensitive effect of CRKL protein expression despite normal levels of TBX1 protein expression.[168] In these patients, haploinsufficiency of the *CRKL* gene is sufficient for disrupting LFA-1-mediated activation and polarization of NK cells during immunologic synapse formation with target cells. Others have shown that decreased CRKL expression in patients with partial DiGeorge syndrome may be associated with decreased T-cell function.[53] It remains intriguing to observe whether the same CRKL dosage effect applies to other processes, such as cardiac outflow tract formation, in patients with DiGeorge syndrome.[121]

Diagnosis

DiGeorge syndrome remains a clinical diagnosis. It should be suspected by the presence of characteristic facial dysmorphic features, hypocalcemia, or congenital heart disease in the neonatal period. Despite the widely used practice of excluding the diagnosis based on fluorescence in situ hybridization or other genetic testing for 22q11.2 hemizygosity, the fact that approximately 40% of patients do not have 22q11 deletions indicates that many patients will be missed or inappropriately treated if only 22q11.2 hemizygosity is considered. Thus genetic testing alone cannot be used to exclude the diagnosis.

Other laboratory testing should be performed to establish the degree of immune deficiency. Lymphopenia and T-cell numbers can vary significantly.[26,38] Determination of naïve T-cell numbers and percentages and testing for lymphocyte proliferative responses to mitogens and antigens should be performed to distinguish complete from partial DiGeorge syndrome and to provide an assessment of overall thymic function. Imaging studies may support the presence of thymic hypoplasia or aplasia if they show absence of the thymic shadow. However, radiographic studies must also be considered in relation to any history of cardiac surgery, when total or partial thymectomy may be performed. Some patients may be observed to have low levels of IgG, IgA, or IgM, suggesting abnormal humoral immunity.[38] Patients should be assessed for defective specific antibody responses to immunizations to determine the potential need for IgG replacement therapy.[26,116] However, predisposition to infections due to DiGeorge syndrome–related neuroanatomical abnormalities must always be considered.

Treatment and Prognosis

Immunologic treatment strategies should be adjusted according to the degree of immune deficiency. Initial management should always focus on the treatment of hypocalcemia and the surgical correction of any congenital heart disease. Antibiotic prophylaxis may be considered for patients with recurrent infections. In patients who have recurrent infections and defective antibody responses to immunizations, IgG replacement therapy is indicated. Children with very low $CD4^+$ T-cell counts or markedly diminished T-cell responses to mitogens should receive prophylaxis against *P. jirovecii* pneumonia. Infections should be recognized early and treated promptly. Only irradiated, cytomegalovirus-negative blood products should be administered. Patients should receive all scheduled inactivated, toxoid, recombinant, and protein-conjugated vaccines. Infants should be referred for evaluation by a clinical immunologist, however, before being administered live attenuated measles, mumps, rubella, and varicella vaccines. Oral poliovirus immunization is no longer available in the United States and is not recommended; no data are available regarding live attenuated rotavirus and influenza vaccines. Several retrospective studies have suggested that children with partial DiGeorge syndrome may safely receive live MMR and varicella immunizations if $CD4^+$ T-cell counts are normal or mildly decreased but not if $CD4^+$ T-cell counts are reduced to the level at which infants with HIV infection would be considered severely suppressed (less than 750 cells/mm^3 if under 12 months of age and less than 500 cells/mm^3 between 1 and 5 years of age).[9,66,105,117,161] Thus administration of live measles, mumps, rubella, and varicella immunizations is not indiscriminately recommended for all DiGeorge syndrome patients.

For patients with complete DiGeorge syndrome, therapeutic options include either thymus transplantation or hematopoietic cell infusions. Thymus transplantation has been studied in greater depth and results in 70% survival.[38,98,99] Significantly fewer patients have been treated with hematopoietic cell infusions, demonstrating approximately 40% survival.[70] Thymus transplantation, however, is only available as an experimental procedure.

Autoimmunity represents the most significant long-term immunologic complication in all patients with DiGeorge syndrome.[26,147] It can be present in more than 10% of individuals at the time of diagnosis and increases to a prevalence of almost 25% over time. The most common manifestations include autoimmune cytopenias, thyroid disease, arthritis, hepatitis, and celiac disease.

Wiskott-Aldrich Syndrome

Clinical Features

Wiskott-Aldrich syndrome (WAS) is an X-linked disorder traditionally characterized by recurrent infections, propensity for bleeding, and eczema. However, only a minority of patients develop this classic triad of features.[22,94,101] Fewer than 5% of patients present with only infectious manifestations.[22] Recurrent otitis media (almost two-thirds of all patients) and pneumonia (25% of patients) are frequently caused by encapsulated bacteria (e.g., *S. pneumoniae, H. influenzae*). Septicemia, meningitis, and other serious systemic bacterial infections may also occur. Common opportunistic pathogens include *Candida,* cytomegalovirus, varicella, other herpesviruses, and *P. jirovecii.* Almost all individuals with WAS have microthrombocytopenia, which is nearly pathognomonic for the disease. As a result, bleeding complications occur in more than 80% of patients.[22] Bleeding diathesis may present as easy bruisability or gastrointestinal bleeding in the first months of life. Patients have increased risk for life-threatening hemorrhages, particularly intracranially.[22,94] Eczema is associated with increased serum IgE levels and can exacerbate the risk for skin infections.

Important long-term complications of WAS include autoimmunity and malignancy. Approximately 40% of patients with WAS develop autoimmunity.[22] The most common manifestations include autoimmune hemolytic anemia, vasculitis, nephropathy, arthritis, and inflammatory bowel disease.[22,94,101] Autoimmune platelet destruction can contribute toward the thrombocytopenia.[22,94] Regarding malignancy, many patients with WAS develop neoplastic disease before 10 years of age.[22] Lymphomas, particularly non-Hodgkin lymphoma, represent the most common malignancies. Other malignancies include myelodysplasia, leukemia, and myeloproliferative disorders.

Pathogenesis

The *WAS* gene is mutated in individuals with Wiskott-Aldrich syndrome and maps to the X chromosome.[40] This gene encodes a protein (Wiskott-Aldrich syndrome protein [WASP]) that is expressed in leukocytes and platelets and is important for cytoskeletal organization and formation of pseudopodia.[101] Disrupted protein expression causes immunologic synapses to form poorly, resulting in defective interactions between antigen-presenting cells and T cells, T cells and B cells, regulatory T cells and effector cells, and T and NK cells and target cells. Most mutations in *WAS* that lead to Wiskott-Aldrich syndrome consist of nonsense mutations, insertions, deletions, or complex mutations.[101] Missense mutations have been identified toward the N-terminus of *WAS* that result in X-linked thrombocytopenia without or with only mild immunodeficiency.[156] Other missense mutations near the middle of *WAS* produce X-linked neutropenia with variable myelodysplasia.[101]

Diagnosis

WAS should be suspected in a male infant with microthrombocytopenia, which is best assessed by examining a peripheral blood smear because automated cell counters report only mean values. The presence of eczema or recurrent infections can support the diagnosis. Serum immunoglobulin concentrations vary, but the serum IgE level is usually elevated. Antibody responses to protein antigens (e.g., tetanus toxoid) are typically normal but can be diminished in some patients.[22,101] Antibody responses to polysaccharide antigens (e.g., 23-valent pneumococcal polysaccharide antigen vaccine, isohemagglutinins) are characteristically absent.[22,101] T-cell lymphopenia is often present and attributed to both abnormal T-cell development in the thymus and increased apoptosis.[22,101] Patients with WAS often display anergy to delayed-type hypersensitivity skin testing. Approximately half of patients demonstrate low proliferative responses to mitogens.[22,101] Antigen-specific T-cell functions, such as activation, proliferation, and cytotoxicity, are impaired in most patients.[22,101] Neutrophils, monocytes, and other leukocytes exhibit defective chemotaxis and antibody-dependent phagocytosis. NK cell cytotoxicity is abnormally low in patients with WAS, and invariant NKT cells are notably absent. The diagnosis is ultimately confirmed by assessing WAS protein expression or sequencing of the *WAS* gene.

Treatment and Prognosis

Management strategies depend strongly on the severity of clinical disease. Patients with WAS are assigned a clinical score that ranges from 0 to 5 according to the presence of thrombocytopenia, eczema, immunodeficiency, autoimmunity, and malignancy.[22,94] Patients younger than 2 years with a score of 5 have a particularly poor prognosis associated with severe refractory thrombocytopenia, autoimmune hemolytic anemia, and vasculitis.[94] They require aggressive therapy, including HSCT using HLA-matched related, HLA-matched unrelated, or haploidentical related donors. This strategy results in 65% survival for these patients.[94] Patients who have an HLA-identical sibling or patients who have a clinical score of 3 or higher should all undergo HSCT, if possible.[22] Overall HSCT yields greater than 80% long-term survival for patients with WAS.[22] The procedure results in normalization of cellular immunity, specific antibody responses, and platelet counts. Splenectomy may be considered for severe thrombocytopenia when HSCT is not available, but splenectomy is associated with increased morbidity and mortality following HSCT.[22] Antibiotic prophylaxis directed against *S. pneumoniae* and *H. influenzae* should be given to patients who have undergone splenectomy and may be considered for patients who develop recurrent infections of the sinopulmonary tract.[22] Immunoglobulin replacement therapy is indicated in patients with recurrent infections due to absent antibody responses to polysaccharide antigens. All patients with WAS should be placed on prophylaxis against *P. jirovecii* infection. In patients who develop autoimmunity, the use of immune suppressive or modulating agents must be weighed against the risk for infection.

Prognosis remains guarded in patients with WAS, even after HSCT. Leading causes of mortality include infection, bleeding, and malignancy.[22] HSCT recipients carry an increased risk for viral reactivation.[22] Autoimmunity continues to present as a significant cause of morbidity and has been attributed to mixed chimerism in patients who have received HSCT.[16,101]

Gene therapy trials offer hope for improved definitive treatment of patients with WAS. Between 2006 and 2009, 10 patients were treated using a γ-retroviral vector.[20] Nine patients demonstrated sustained engraftment and correction of defective WAS protein expression associated with improved clinical features. However seven of nine patients developed leukemia due to insertional mutagenesis in similar fashion to the early X-linked SCID gene therapy trial.[16,20] A new WAS gene therapy trial has since been started using a lentiviral vector to treat seven patients. Six have survived (one died from herpesviral infection). The six survivors have shown successful engraftment, WAS protein expression, clinical and immunological improvement, and no evidence of insertional mutagenesis.[1,61]

Ataxia-Telangiectasia

Clinical Features

Ataxia-telangiectasia is characterized by cerebellar ataxia, oculocutaneous telangiectasias, variable immunodeficiency with frequent infections, and a high incidence of malignancy.[35,142,144] Ataxia usually becomes evident between 1 to 2 years of age. Progressive choreoathetosis, myoclonic jerking movements, and oculomotor abnormalities subsequently develop, resulting in severe disability. Telangiectasias appear on the bulbar conjunctivae, usually in patients between 2 and 5 years of age (see Fig. 67.2). They subsequently appear on the nasal bridge, ears, and other areas of sun exposure or trauma. Other cutaneous manifestations include café-au-lait spots, vitiligo, necrobiotic noninfective granulomas, and prematurely gray hair. Most patients develop recurrent infections of the sinopulmonary tract; systemic infections rarely occur despite immunologic abnormalities. Pathogens frequently identified in pediatric patients include *Staphylococcus aureus*, *Haemophilus influenzae*, and *Streptococcus pneumoniae* while older patients are susceptible to *Pseudomonas aeruginosa*.[129] Almost 25% of patients with ataxia-telangiectasia develop malignancies, of which the most prevalent include B-cell non-Hodgkin lymphoma, leukemia, and solid organ carcinomas (especially of the breast and stomach).[142,144]

Pathogenesis

Ataxia-telangiectasia is inherited in an autosomal recessive manner. The defective gene *(ATM)* responsible for the disease maps to chromosome 11.[127] Various domains of the ATM protein play different roles in cellular responses, including cytokine signaling. ATM is critically involved in DNA damage checkpoint control and repair.[31] Immune deficiency in ATM patients is attributed to impairment of DNA repair during rearrangements required for expression of the T-cell receptor genes and B-cell immunoglobulin heavy-chain genes. Abnormal repair mechanisms result in radiosensitivity. Impaired checkpoint control and defective repair activities together likely contribute to the increased risk for malignancy.

Diagnosis

Ataxia-telangiectasia can be diagnosed in a variety of manners.[144] A clinical diagnosis is possible when the disease is fully manifested. Increased serum α-fetoprotein concentrations are observed in essentially all patients older than 6 months of age. Serum IgG levels can be normal or slightly low, while IgA deficiency is frequently observed.[35] Some patients may have elevated levels of IgM, which usually exists in a monomeric 7S form rather than the usual pentameric 19S molecule. Specific antibody responses correlate with the level of ATM kinase activity.[43] They often remain intact, although they may decline in some patients as they age.[35] T- and B-cell numbers can be low in approximately two-thirds of patients.[35,77] Patients may exhibit delayed-type hypersensitivity skin test anergy, and about one-third of patients can have reduced decreased lymphocyte proliferative responses to mitogens.[77] Patients cells will typically demonstrate decreased survival in clonogenic or other radiosensitivity assays. Definitive diagnosis should be confirmed through sequencing of the *ATM* gene.

Treatment and Prognosis

No specific treatment is available for ataxia-telangiectasia because the pathologic processes involve multiple body systems. Infections should be treated with oral or parenteral antibiotics. Continuous prophylactic antibiotic therapy may benefit individual patients. Immunoglobulin replacement therapy should only be given to patients with recurrent infections and abnormal specific antibody responses. Patients should be advised to minimize exposure to ionizing radiation. Median survival ranges from 19 to 25 years of age, although patients who have less deleterious *ATM* mutations may survive into the fourth decade of life.[144] Important causes of mortality include interstitial or chronic pulmonary disease and malignancies.[142,144]

PRIMARY COMPLEMENT DEFICIENCIES

Clinical Features

Complement deficiencies are rare PIDDs that lead to increased susceptibility to infections or autoimmunity. All patients demonstrate increased susceptibility to infections by *N. meningitidis*.[57] Primary complement deficiencies can be identified in up to 20% of patients with invasive meningococcal disease, and the likelihood of having complement deficiency increases significantly to about 30% in individuals who have had more than one infection.[7,57,102] Patients who have deficiencies of early classical complement pathway components (i.e., C1, C4, C2, and C3) are also susceptible to infections by other encapsulated bacteria, including *S. pneumoniae* and *H. influenzae*.[57] C2 deficiency represents the most common complement pathway deficiency and is estimated to occur at a prevalence of one in 20,000 individuals. Fewer than 40% of patients with C2 deficiency develop autoimmunity; approximately 1% of patients with SLE have been found to have C2 deficiency.[57] C1q deficiency is the next most common early pathway complement deficiency. About 95% of patients with C1q deficiency develop severe autoimmune disease.[57] C4 and C3 deficiencies are very rarely observed. C4 deficiency is associated with increased risk for autoimmunity while C3 deficiency is not.[57] In patients with deficiencies of terminal complement components (C5 through C9), *Neisseria meningitidis* remains the most significant bacterial cause of infection.[7,57] Patients with terminal complement protein deficiencies have increased risk for recurrent episodes of septicemia and meningitis; about 40% of patients develop neisserial meningitis.[57] C5 deficiency is the most rare terminal complement pathway deficiency and is also associated with the development of SLE.[57] C9 deficiency may not be uncommon, and most affected individuals are asymptomatic.[57] Properdin is another complement component that functions in the alternative pathway. Patients with properdin deficiency demonstrate increased risk for *Neisseria meningitidis* infections, and approximately 6% develop neisserial meningitis.[57] Mannose-binding lectin deficiency has been proposed as a complement pathway defect that leads to recurrent pyogenic infections. However its essential role as a primary cause of PIDD remains controversial because a significant percentage of healthy individuals (about 5%) are known to have mannose-binding lectin deficiency.[57]

Pathogenesis

Various gene defects are responsible for the many distinct primary complement deficiencies. C3 is an important opsonin that promotes ingestion and killing of bacteria. As a consequence, patients with C3 deficiency have increased susceptibility to encapsulated bacterial infections (e.g., *S. pneumoniae, H. influenzae*), for which opsonization serves as a critical mechanism of host defense. Individuals with deficiencies of C1, C4, or C2 also have increased susceptibility to these encapsulated bacteria because these components are necessary for activation of C3 in the classical pathway. Activation of terminal complement components C5, C6, C7, C8, and C9 results in assembly of the membrane attack complex, a multicomponent macromolecule that results in membrane pore formation and lysis. Only gram-negative bacteria, such as *N. meningitidis*, are susceptible to this bactericidal effect. The gene for properdin is found on the X chromosome; properdin deficiency is the only complement pathway defect that is inherited in an X-linked recessive manner. Properdin stabilizes the C3-factor B complex in the alternative pathway. Mechanisms for increased risk for autoimmunity remain unclear. B cells express CD21, which is a receptor for activated products of C3 and plays a role in regulating transport of immune complexes in follicles. Dysregulation of this process may contribute toward development of autoimmunity.

Diagnosis

The CH50 reflects the combined activity of all numbered components of the classic complement pathway from C1 through C9. Thus a patient with a classical complement pathway deficiency will have a very low CH50. In similar fashion, the AH50 can be used to assess the alternative complement pathway. Specific immunochemical and functional testing can then be performed to identify the deficient component. Deficiency is defined as a serum level of 0 or close to zero for any given component. All of these tests, including specific component testing, can be easily affected by sample conditions, and the most common cause of an abnormal result is sample mishandling.[57]

Treatment and Prognosis

No specific therapy exists for primary complement deficiencies. Both polysaccharide and protein-conjugated meningococcal vaccines are recommended.[57] Antibiotic prophylaxis and immunizations against other encapsulated organisms may be beneficial. Close surveillance for autoimmunity is recommended for patients with C1, C2, C4, and C5 deficiencies.

BOX 67.5 Primary Phagocyte Deficiencies

Quantitative Defects
Infantile agranulocytosis
Familial granulocytopenia
Cyclic neutropenia

Qualitative Defects
Adhesion Defects
Leukocyte adhesion deficiency:
- Type I, β-integrin deficiency
- Type II, fucose-transporter deficiency
- Type III, *FERMT3* deficiency

Intracellular Killing Defects
Chronic granulomatous disease:
- X-linked
- Autosomal recessive

Glucose-6-phosphate dehydrogenase deficiency
Myeloperoxidase deficiency
Chédiak-Higashi syndrome
Griscelli syndrome

PRIMARY PHAGOCYTE DEFICIENCIES

Primary phagocyte deficiencies include a heterogeneous group of disorders sharing a common susceptibility for frequent infections due to either a decreased number of phagocytic cells (e.g., neutropenia), impaired adhesion, chemotaxis, opsonization, and phagocytosis, or defective intracellular killing (Box 67.5). Affected patients tend to have prolonged and recurrent infections with slower responses to antibiotic therapy than expected. Common pathogens include *S. aureus, P. aeruginosa*, enteric gram-negative bacteria, and certain fungi (e.g., *Aspergillus* spp.).

Quantitative Phagocyte Abnormalities

Primary quantitative phagocyte deficiencies can be observed as solitary defects or in association with other disorders (e.g., Shwachman syndrome). Severe congenital neutropenia (i.e., Kostmann syndrome[72]) is characterized by arrest of granulocyte maturation, markedly decreased numbers of circulating granulocytes, and severe infection. Severe congenital neutropenia syndromes are caused by mutations in the leukocyte elastase *(ELANE), HAX1, G6PC3, GFI1, JAGN1, CSF3R*, and *WAS* genes.[17,19] The more benign familial granulocytopenia syndrome manifests at various ages from infancy to adulthood, usually with indolent infections of the skin and soft tissues.

Cyclic neutropenia is an autosomal dominant defect of myelopoiesis in which periodic disappearance of granulocytes from the circulation occurs. The condition is caused by mutations in *ELANE*.[95] Early granulocyte precursors are present in the bone marrow during periods of neutropenia, suggesting transient maturation arrest. Periods of neutropenia usually last 5 to 7 days and occur at 14- to 35-day intervals. The length of the cycle generally remains constant for any given individual. Fever and malaise are often observed during periods of neutropenia. Patients demonstrate increased episodes of aphthous stomatitis, pneumonia, abscesses, sepsis, cellulitis, and peritonitis.[95] Certain mutations in *ELANE* appear to predispose to development of myelodysplasia or acute myeloid leukemia.[95]

Some of the primary quantitative phagocyte deficiencies, particularly familial granulocytopenia and cyclic neutropenia, respond to therapy with recombinant granulocyte colony-stimulating factor.[95]

Chronic Granulomatous Disease

Clinical Features

Patients with CGD develop infections that begin during infancy and recur throughout their lives. Occasionally, patients display a relatively mild disease course and come to medical attention only during adolescence or adulthood. Infections of the lungs, skin, lymph nodes, and liver present as the most frequent initial manifestations of CGD.[67] Patients also demonstrate susceptibility to soft tissue abscesses, perirectal abscesses, central nervous system infections, and osteomyelitis.[47] Infections in patients with CGD may progress with few symptoms, and the erythrocyte sedimentation rate and C-reactive protein levels may provide the most sensitive signs of active infection.[47] Patients with CGD are susceptible to infections caused by catalase-positive organisms. For infections in the United States in which a responsible organism can be identified, most episodes are caused by *S. aureus, Burkholderia cepacia, Serratia marcescens, Klebsiella pneumoniae, Nocardia,* and *Aspergillus* spp.[67,96] In many cases, no organism can be isolated. Outside of the United States, *Salmonella*, BCG, and *M. tuberculosis* serve as additional important pathogens.[67] Fungi, especially *Aspergillus* spp., account for 20% to 40% of all defined infections in patients with CGD (Fig. 67.6).[47] CGD is particularly characterized by infections due to unusual organisms. Examples include *Chromobacterium violaceum, Francisella philomiragia, Aspergillus nidulans, Paecilomyces variotii, Paecilomyces lilacinus, Neosartorya udagawae,* methylotrophic bacteria, and a variety of other fungi.[47,48,64,67] An infection caused by any of these organisms should be considered pathognomic for a diagnosis of CGD until proved otherwise. Of note, patients with CGD do not carry increased susceptibility to *Candida*.[64]

Patients with CGD also develop important noninfectious complications.[67] Poor wound healing can be observed. Granulomatous obstructive lesions of the urinary and gastrointestinal tracts occur frequently. More than 40% of patients with X-linked CGD develop an inflammatory bowel disease that mimics Crohn disease.[67] Hepatic dysfunction can lead to portal hypertension, splenomegaly, and splenic sequestration. A small percentage of boys with X-linked CGD have the McLeod blood phenotype, characterized by absence of the Kell antigen in red blood cells as a consequence of a contiguous gene deletion, which results in difficult crossmatching for blood transfusion and the potential for hemolytic transfusion reactions.[21] Female carriers of a mutated X-linked CGD gene can also develop inflammatory or autoimmune clinical features, such as photosensitivity, autoimmune arthritis, discoid lupus erythematosus, aphthous stomatitis, Raynaud's phenomenon, inflammatory colitis, and chorioretinitis.[13]

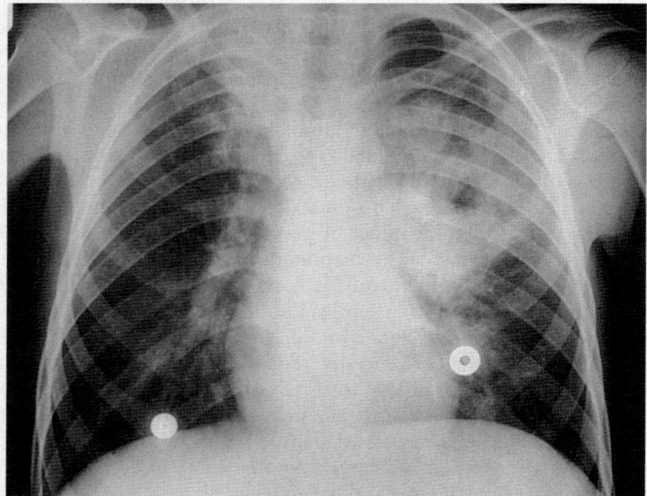

FIG. 67.6 Chest radiograph of a 10-year-old boy with chronic granulomatous disease shows a left-sided pulmonary infiltrate and cavitary lung lesion. Biopsy revealed an *Aspergillus fumigatus* infection.

Pathogenesis

CGD is caused by mutations in genes that encode membrane or cytosolic components of the nicotinamide adenine dinucleotide phosphate oxidase (NADPH oxidase) complex system. The most common defect occurs in gp91^{phox}, which is encoded by *CYBB* on the X chromosome and accounts for almost two-thirds of cases of CGD.[34,67] Mutations in genes encoding the other components (p47^{phox}, p67^{phox}, p22^{phox}, and p40^{phox}) have also been reported and are inherited in an autosomal recessive manner. p47^{phox} deficiency accounts for 25% to 30% of cases of CGD.[34,67] Defective NADPH oxidase function results in failure to generate the respiratory burst required for killing of phagocytized organisms. Inappropriate production of reactive oxygen species is also felt to contribute to dysregulated inflammation, resulting in many of the noninfectious complications.

Diagnosis

The diagnosis of CGD is made using the flow cytometry-based DHR chemiluminescence assay. Falsely abnormal DHR test results can be observed in patients who have myeloperoxidase deficiency, SAPHO syndrome, G6PD deficiency, or neutrophils that are highly activated due to significant infection.[67] The DHR assay can detect females who are carriers for X-linked CGD and is often able to differentiate X-linked CGD from autosomal recessive forms. Genotyping is not required to confirm the diagnosis but may be helpful for determining prognosis.[67]

Treatment and Prognosis

Because infectious organisms often cannot be isolated in patients with CGD, empirical antibiotic therapy is frequently used to treat infections. Still, specific microbiologic diagnoses for infections should always be established whenever possible. Due to dysregulated inflammatory processes, patients who develop infections may not present until they become very ill. Thus a low threshold should be placed for suspecting the presence of an infection. Elevated erythrocyte sedimentation rates and C-reactive protein levels should warrant concern for infection. Experience with a large cohort of patients with CGD suggests that serum galactomannan and 1,3-β-D-glucan levels may not be useful for assessing fungal infections in patients with CGD.[47] Empirical therapy should be directed against the organisms known to commonly cause infections, such as *S. aureus, S. marcescens, K. pneumoniae, Nocardia, Aspergillus* spp., and *Salmonella*. Most patients are susceptible to methicillin-sensitive *S. aureus* and do not require empirical therapy for methicillin-resistant strains. Surgical drainage or debridement of infection sites is often necessary. However surgical removal of abscesses, especially of the liver, is not recommended.[67] Hepatic abscesses can be treated with a combination of antibiotics and corticosteroid therapy.[84] Granulocyte transfusions may be helpful for treating infections that do not respond to antibiotics.

Definitive cure is provided by HSCT.[67,100] Gene therapy trials for X-linked CGD in humans have resulted in increased numbers of gene-corrected, autologous neutrophils associated with resolution of infections in all patients treated. However only three patients (25%) maintained high numbers of gene-corrected cells in the long term, and all three patients developed clonal expansions associated with insertional activation of the *EVI1* gene.[54] Thus gene therapy strategies for treatment of CGD are currently being modified.

All patients with CGD who have not received definitive therapy require continuous prophylaxis to prevent infections.[67] Antibiotic prophylaxis using cotrimoxazole reduces the frequency of bacterial infections in patients with CGD. Itraconazole prophylaxis should be given to prevent fungal infections.[47] Administration of IFN-γ to decrease the rate of infection is practiced in some centers but not others and remains controversial.[67] Patients should be educated about avoiding activities that expose them to environments containing mold spores, such as mulching or raking leaves.

Therapy for noninfectious complications remains challenging. Options usually include corticosteroid therapy or other immune modulating antiinflammatory medications. TNF-α inhibitors should not be used because they markedly increase the risk for infection and mortality.[67,150]

The prognosis for CGD has improved remarkably during the past several decades, and most patients (approximately 90%) now survive to adulthood.[67] Morbidity and mortality strongly depend on fungal infections and residual NADPH oxidase activity.[67,96] Patients with autosomal recessive forms of CGD tend to have greater superoxide production, a milder disease course, and better long-term survival.[67] Patients with p47^{phox} deficiency appear to have the best prognosis. Even among patients with X-linked CGD, rates of long-term survival are higher in those patients with greater residual superoxide production, whereas patients with no residual superoxide production demonstrate the lowest likelihood for long-term survival.[67]

Leukocyte Adhesion Deficiency

Clinical Features

Patients with LAD develop severe and recurrent bacterial infections of the skin and soft tissues, mucosal surfaces, and gastrointestinal tract, often beginning during early infancy.[151] Early presentation includes delayed separation of the umbilical cord that is associated with omphalitis. Patients later develop cutaneous infections that manifest as nonpurulent inflamed tissues that often become necrotic, resembling ecthyma gangrenosum or pyoderma gangrenosum. Absence of purulence is a hallmark feature of the disease. Poor wound healing is present. Patients can also develop severe gingivitis and periodontitis with progressive alveolar bone loss (see Fig. 67.3). Common pathogenic microorganisms include staphylococci and *Pseudomonas* spp.

Patients with LAD classically demonstrate marked leukocytosis. Circulating neutrophil counts may range between 15,000/mm^3 and 75,000/mm^3, even in the absence of infection; and counts of 100,000/mm^3 or greater can be observed during infections.

Pathogenesis

LAD type I is an autosomal recessive disorder due to mutation in *ITGB2* on chromosome 21. Neutrophils from individuals with LAD type I exhibit defective expression of surface glycoproteins known as the leukocyte-integrin complex. These molecules are critical for adhesion-dependent functions, and their absence is responsible for defects in leukocyte adherence, chemotaxis, and phagocytosis. The severity of infectious complications in LAD is related directly to the degree of CD18 expression.[148,151] Patients with the severe clinical phenotype demonstrate less than 2% expression of these complexes on their phagocytes, whereas individuals with the moderate phenotype generally have 2% to 30% expression, explained by missense gene mutations that allow surface expression of a defective protein.

Other forms of LAD have been reported. A rare second form of LAD is associated with craniofacial dysmorphism, neurologic deficits, recurrent respiratory tract infections, and marked leukocytosis.[46] Neutrophils from patients with LAD type II have normal surface expression of CD18. The molecular basis for the phagocyte dysfunction is a defect in the fucose transporter that mediates glycosylation of sialyl-Lewis X, a carbohydrate ligand for the endothelial adhesion molecules E-selectin and P-selectin. A third form of LAD has been described, characterized by deficient β-integrin–mediated activation due to mutations in *FERMT3*, which encodes a protein necessary for inside-out signaling transduction. It is associated with bleeding tendency and osteopetrosis.

Diagnosis

The diagnosis of LAD type I is made by flow cytometry using fluorescence-labeled monoclonal antibodies to CD18.[151] Supporting studies reveal abnormalities of phagocyte adherence, chemotaxis, and phagocytosis but are not required. Individuals with LAD type II have similar phagocyte function abnormalities with normal expression of CD18 but decreased expression of CD15 on leukocytes. LAD type III is characterized by altered expression of β-integrins but remains difficult to assess in clinical laboratories. Ultimately the diagnoses of LAD types I, II, or III should be confirmed by genetic mutation analyses.[151]

Treatment and Prognosis

Few therapeutic options are available for the treatment of patients with LAD.[151] Bacterial infections in patients with LAD must be treated aggressively with prolonged courses of parenteral antibiotics. Granulocyte transfusions can be used to help treat infections that do not respond to antibiotics. Antibiotic prophylaxis and universal hygiene measures are recommended. For patients with LAD type II, administration of fucose can result in enhanced leukocyte function, resolution of infections, and even improved psychomotor abilities. For patients with LAD type I who do not receive definitive therapy, survival to adulthood is possible, but almost one-half of affected individuals die before reaching the second decade of life. HSCT offers the best hope for long-term survival, demonstrating an overall survival rate of 75%.[151] Gene therapy has not yet demonstrated success for treating human LAD.

Other Primary Phagocyte Deficiencies

Other defects of phagocyte chemotaxis, phagocytosis, and intracellular killing are known and include Chédiak-Higashi syndrome, which is a rare autosomal recessive disorder characterized by partial oculocutaneous albinism, rotatory nystagmus, and peripheral neuropathy.[42] In Chédiak-Higashi syndrome, giant peroxidase-positive granules are found throughout the body in different cell types, including leukocytes. Neutrophils exhibit defective chemotaxis and abnormal bactericidal activity. Affected individuals develop recurrent infections of the lungs, skin, and gingival tissues caused by *S. aureus* and other bacteria. Chédiak-Higashi syndrome is caused by mutations in the *LYST* gene. It is a known cause of hemophagocytic lymphohistiocytosis (HLH), which is characterized by fevers, hepatosplenomegaly, lymphadenopathy, lymphocytic infiltration of multiple organs, and progressive pancytopenia.

OTHER INNATE IMMUNITY DEFICIENCY DISEASES

In addition to complement and phagocytic deficiencies, other defects in innate immunity are becoming more frequently recognized as important causes of PIDDs. Examples include NK deficiencies, hyper-IgE syndrome, and defects in the IRAK4-MyD88 signaling pathway.

NK-cell deficiencies fall into two categories: classical and functional.[110] Classical NK-cell deficiencies are identified by lack of NK cells and absence of NK-cell cytotoxicity. Affected patients are susceptible to herpesviral infections, such as varicella, cytomegalovirus, HSV1, and Epstein-Barr virus (EBV). The most common classical NK-cell deficiencies are caused by mutations in *GATA2* and *MCM4*. Functional NK-cell deficiencies, however, are defined by the presence of normal numbers of NK cells that exhibit abnormal function. Like patients with classical NK-cell deficiencies, patients with functional NK-cell deficiencies demonstrate susceptibility to infections by herpesviruses. They also have difficulty with human papillomavirus (HPV) and respiratory virus infections. The only identified associated cause is an L66H mutation in the *FCGR3A* gene that encodes CD16. NK cells from patients with this condition display abnormal natural cytotoxicity but normal antibody-dependent cellular cytotoxicity. No definitive therapies are available to cure patients who have NK-cell deficiencies. Most approaches focus on the use of acyclovir or related medications to treat herpesvirus infections. HPV immunization should be strongly considered for all patients who have NK-cell deficiency.

Hyperimmunoglobulinemia E (hyper-IgE) syndrome is a rare PIDD that is estimated to affect 1 in 100,000 individuals.[104] It is characterized by markedly elevated serum IgE levels, eczema, and recurrent infections and exists in either autosomal dominant or autosomal recessive forms. Autosomal dominant hyper-IgE syndrome is caused by mutations in the *STAT3* gene.[71] STAT3 deficiency is marked by recurrent noninflammatory staphylococcal abscesses, pneumonias that result in pneumatocele formation, and chronic mucocutaneous candidiasis. Pneumatocele formation may result in chronic infection by *Pseudomonas aeruginosa*, atypical mycobacteria, or *Aspergillus*.[104] Viral infections do not serve as a distinguishing manifestation of STAT3 deficiency.[71] Noninfectious characteristics include coarse facial features, delayed shedding of primary dentition, recurrent bone fractures, scoliosis, osteoporosis, joint hyperextensibility, and coronary artery dilatation or aneurysms.[104] Patients with STAT3 deficiency carry increased risk for developing malignancies, especially non-Hodgkin lymphoma. Laboratory studies may demonstrate an elevated serum IgE level, eosinophilia, and antibody deficiency.[71,104]

Absence of T_H17 cells is nearly pathognomonic. Autosomal recessive hyper-IgE syndrome, on the other hand, is caused by mutations in *DOCK8* or—much more rarely—*TYK2*. Patients with DOCK8 and TYK2 deficiency do not share the noninfectious manifestations present in STAT3 deficiency. DOCK8 deficiency produces marked susceptibility to viral infections of the skin, including HSV1, HPV, molluscum contagiosum, and varicella.[141] Affected patients also develop chronic mucocutaneous candidiasis, recurrent sinopulmonary infections to encapsulated bacteria, staphylococcal skin abscesses, and gastrointestinal infections. DOCK8 deficiency is further characterized by significant atopic disease, autoimmunity (i.e., hemolytic anemia or vasculitis), and increased risk for developing malignancies, particularly squamous cell carcinomas or lymphomas. No therapies have demonstrated consistent success for definitive treatment of hyper-IgE syndrome, although HSCT has been attempted in limited numbers of patients with STAT3 and DOCK8 deficiencies.[104,141] Prophylactic use of antibiotics is recommended to prevent staphylococcal infections. Bleach baths should be encouraged. Patients who have chronic mucocutaneous candidiasis may require indefinite antifungal therapy. Immunoglobulin replacement may be indicated as a therapy for patients who have recurrent infections due to defective antibody responses to immunizations.

Finally, deficiencies of IRAK-4 and MyD88 can cause PIDDs, especially in children.[118,158] IRAK-4 and MyD88 are adaptor molecules that mediate signaling downstream from all Toll-like receptors (TLRs) except TLR3 and (partially) TLR4. Patients with IRAK-4 or MyD88 deficiency are susceptible to a variety of infections, including meningitis, sepsis, arthritis, osteomyelitis, lymphadenitis, staphylococcal skin abscesses, and deep tissue upper respiratory tract infections. These infections are most commonly caused by *S. aureus*, *S. pneumoniae*, and gram-negative bacteria such as *P. aeruginosa*, *H. influenzae*, *Salmonella*, *Shigella sonnei*, and *N. meningitidis*. IRAK-4 and MyD88 deficiencies do not lead to increased susceptibility to mycobacteria, viruses, fungi, or *Pneumocystis*. No consistent laboratory findings help to identify IRAK-4 or MyD88 deficiency, although testing of TLR function may reveal some abnormalities. Some patients demonstrate defective antibody responses to polysaccharide antigens. Genetic sequencing of *IRAK4* but not *MYD88* is clinically available. Therapy focuses on aggressive treatment of infections, antibiotic prophylaxis, assiduous administration of immunizations, and immunoglobulin replacement for patients who exhibit poor antibody responses to immunizations. IRAK-4 and MyD88 deficiencies lead to high mortality in infancy and childhood, but the rate of infections interestingly decreases markedly over time in survivors for reasons that remain unclear but which may be related to enhanced adaptive immune responses.

ASSOCIATIONS BETWEEN SPECIFIC PATHOGENS AND PIDDS

In patients who demonstrate increased susceptibility to certain pathogens, a number of PIDDs may be more likely to be present than others (Table 67.5).[17]

Recurrent or recalcitrant candidal infections can occur in patients with PIDDs. Candidal susceptibility can signify the presence of a severe T-cell (e.g., SCID, complete DiGeorge syndrome) or T_H17-cell (e.g., STAT3 deficiency, DOCK8 deficiency) defect. Alternately, defects in critical innate immunity proteins (e.g., STAT1, Dectin-1, CARD9) can lead to recurrent or severe candidal infections. Finally chronic mucocutaneous candidiasis associated with autoimmune polyendocrinopathy may be due to mutations in the autoimmune regulator *(AIRE)* gene, resulting in a condition known as autoimmune polyendocrinopathy ectodermal dystrophy (APECED).[50,106]

Susceptibility to EBV often suggests deficiencies in cytotoxic ($CD8^+$) T cells or NK cells. Examples of T-cell deficiency again include SCID and complete DiGeorge syndrome. Defective NK-cell function associated with EBV susceptibility can be observed in patients who have mutations in *MCM4* and all of the genes associated with HLH or HLH-like disease (e.g., *PRF1, UNC13D, STX11, STXBP2, LYST, RAB27A, AP3B1*). The X-linked lymphoproliferative (XLP) syndrome represents a defect in control of EBV infection. Mutations in *SH2D1A*, which encodes a factor (SAP) involved in the signal transduction of T cells, have been identified as causes of XLP.[47,111] Absence of SAP affects the interaction of T and B cells,

TABLE 67.5 Key Primary Immunodeficiency Diseases Associated With Increased Susceptibility to Specific Pathogens

Pathogen	Gene Defect
Candida	Genes associated with SCID, complete DiGeorge syndrome (gene unknown), *CIITA, RFX5, RFXAP, RFXANK, STAT3, DOCK8, IL17RA, IL17RC, IL17F, ACT1, AIRE, MST1, PTPN6, SP110, DECTIN1, CARD9, RORC, STAT1* (gain of function), *MAP3K14, BCL10, ITGB2*
Epstein-Barr virus	Genes associated with SCID, complete DiGeorge syndrome, *SH2D1A, XIAP, ITK, PRKCD, CARD11, PIK3CD* (gain of function), *PIK3R1, IRF8, MALT1, MAGT1, STK4, MST1, LRBA, CD27, GATA2, MCM4, FCGR3A, PRF1, UNC13D, STX11, STXBP2, LYST, RAB27A, AP3B1, WAS, CTSC, CTPS1, STAT2*
Herpes simplex virus type 1	Genes associated with SCID, complete DiGeorge syndrome, *MCM4, FCGR3A, MALT1, TLR3, TRIF, UNC93B1, TRAF3, TBK1, DOCK8, TYK2, STAT1, WAS, IRF3*
Human papillomavirus	Genes associated with SCID, *CXCR4, RHOH, MST1, TWEAK, GATA2, MCM4, STAT2, TMC6, TMC8, CIB1, ITGB2, DOCK8*
Atypical mycobacteria	Genes associated with SCID, complete DiGeorge syndrome, *FOXN1, CIITA, RFX5, RFXAP, RFXANK, TAP1, TAP2, TAPBP, IKBKB, IKBKG, IFNGR1, IFNGR2, IL12RB1, IL12RB2, IL12B, IL23R, SPPL2A, TYK2, STAT1* (loss of function), *STAT1* (gain of function), *STAT3* (gain of function), *MAP3K14, CYBB, IRF8, ISG15, GATA2, RORC, CTPS1, NRAMP1, DOCK2*

leading to an inability to control B-cell proliferation caused by EBV infection.[55,128] At presentation, males may have severe and often fatal infectious mononucleosis or B-cell lymphoma. Defects in the closely related BIRC4 (encoded by *XIAP*) and ITK produce a similar phenotype.

Susceptibility to HSV1 is present in patients with severe T-cell deficiencies but more typically suggests a defect in NK cell or innate immunity function. An important example of NK-cell deficiency includes MCM4 deficiency. Mutations in *TLR3, TRIF, UNC93B1, TRAF3*, and *TBK1* lead to increased susceptibility to HSV1 encephalitis.

Several PIDDs are known to be associated with increased susceptibility to HPV infection. HPV infection is frequently observed in patients with SCID, especially X-linked SCID, but not in complete DiGeorge syndrome patients. NK-cell deficiencies, such as GATA2 and MCM4 deficiencies predispose to HPV infection. Disseminated cutaneous HPV infection (warts) can also develop in patients with mutations in *EVER1* or *EVER2*. Autosomal dominant gain-of-function mutations in *CXCR4* result in ***w**arts, **h**ypogammaglobulinemia, **i**nfections, and **m**yelokathexis* (WHIM) syndrome. This condition is characterized by neutropenia, B-cell lymphopenia, and hypogammaglobulinemia, leading to recurrent sinopulmonary, urinary tract, cutaneous, and invasive bacterial infections. In patients with WHIM syndrome, HPV infections can progress to malignancy.

Increased susceptibility to atypical mycobacteria is also observed in patients with certain PIDDs. Atypical mycobacterial infections have been observed in patients with severe T-cell deficiencies (e.g., SCID, complete DiGeorge anomaly, FOXN1 deficiency) in the form of disseminated BCG infection after vaccination. Defects in the IFN-γ–IL-12 pathway also result in susceptibility to severe atypical mycobacterial infections. Examples include mutations in the IFN-γ receptor genes (i.e., *IFNGR1, IFNGR2*)[124] and genes for IL-12 and the IL-12 receptor.[4]

These lists are by no means exhaustive and change rapidly as novel PIDDs are discovered or new clinical cases are reported. Thus clinicians must maintain a high index of suspicion for various PIDD diagnoses based on other clinical and laboratory findings, even if one of these infectious susceptibilities is either present or absent.

CONCLUSION

PIDDs are no longer considered rare diseases in children. Soon mutations in well over 300 genes will have been identified as causes of PIDDs, resulting in improved recognition of the pathogenesis of many of these conditions.

Scientific and medical advances have led to enhanced care of children with PIDDs, allowing them to survive well past childhood, with a quality of life that continues to improve. Early identification of these children remains critical, and medical providers must strongly suspect and investigate the presence of PIDDs in children who have infections of abnormal severity or frequency or in children who develop infections caused by unusual or highly characteristic organisms. Associated infections range from sinopulmonary tract infections that sometimes occur in patients with IgA deficiency to life-threatening opportunistic infections that appear during the first weeks of life, such as in SCID. The initial immunologic screening consists of widely available laboratory tests. Prompt referral to a clinical immunologist is warranted when any PIDD is suspected. Newborn screening for SCID has successfully identified patients who have severe T-cell deficiencies before significant infections occur, allowing for early, definitive, life-saving treatment and minimization of morbidity and mortality. Although still experimental, gene therapy has continued to progress in clinical trials for X-linked SCID, ADA-deficient SCID, WAS, and CGD, with valuable lessons learned. Successful results in these trials demonstrate continued promise for cure of many other PIDDs at some time in the future.

NEW REFERENCES SINCE THE SEVENTH EDITION

1. Aiuti A, Biasco L, Scaramuzza S, et al. Lentiviral hematopoietic stem cell gene therapy in patients with Wiskott-Aldrich syndrome. *Science.* 2013;341(6148):1233151.
5. Ameratunga R, Brewerton M, Slade C, et al. Comparison of diagnostic criteria for common variable immunodeficiency disorder. *Front Immunol.* 2014;5:415.
6. American Academy of Pediatrics. Active and passive immunization: immunization in immunocompromised children. In: Pickering LK, Baker CJ, Kimberlin DW, eds. *2015 Red Book: Report of the Committee on Infectious Diseases.* 30th ed. Elk Grove Village, IL: American Academy of Pediatrics; 2015:74-89.
7. American Academy of Pediatrics. Summaries of infectious diseases: meningococcal infections. In: Pickering LK, Baker CJ, Kimberlin DW, eds. *2015 Red Book: Report of the Committee on Infectious Diseases.* 30th ed. Elk Grove Village, IL: American Academy of Pediatrics; 2015:547-558.
10. Balloch A, Licciardi PV, Russell FM, et al. Infants aged 12 months can mount adequate serotype-specific IgG responses to pneumococcal polysaccharide vaccine. *J Allergy Clin Immunol.* 2010;126(2):395-397.
11. Barrett DJ, Ammann AJ, Wara DW, et al. Clinical and immunologic spectrum of the DiGeorge syndrome. *J Clin Lab Immunol.* 1981;6(1):1-6.
13. Battersby AC, Cale CM, Goldblatt D, et al. Clinical manifestations of disease in X-linked carriers of chronic granulomatous disease. *J Clin Immunol.* 2013;33(8):1276-1284.
14. Bonilla FA, Barlan I, Chapel H, et al. International Consensus Document (ICON): common variable immunodeficiency disorders. *J Allergy Clin Immunol Pract.* 2016;4(1):38-59.
16. Bosticardo M, Ferrua F, Cavazzana M, et al. Gene therapy for Wiskott-Aldrich syndrome. *Curr Gene Ther.* 2014;14(6):413-421.
17. Bousfiha A, Jeddane L, Al-Herz W, et al. The 2015 IUIS phenotypic classification for primary immunodeficiencies. *J Clin Immunol.* 2015;35(8):727-738.
19. Boztug K, Klein C. Genetics and pathophysiology of severe congenital neutropenia syndromes unrelated to neutrophil elastase. *Hematol Oncol Clin North Am.* 2013;27(1):43-60.
20. Braun CJ, Boztug K, Paruzynski A, et al. Gene therapy for Wiskott-Aldrich syndrome—long-term efficacy and genotoxicity. *Sci Transl Med.* 2014;6(227):227ra33.
22. Buchbinder D, Nugent DJ, Fillipovich AH. Wiskott-Aldrich syndrome: diagnosis, current management, and emerging treatments. *Appl Clin Genet.* 2014;7:55-66.
23. Buckley RH. Immunoglobulin G subclass deficiency: fact or fancy? *Curr Allergy Asthma Rep.* 2002;2(5):356-360.
25. Buckley RH. The long quest for neonatal screening for severe combined immunodeficiency. *J Allergy Clin Immunol.* 2012;129(3):597-604.
26. Cancrini C, Puliafito P, Digilio MC, et al. Clinical features and follow-up in patients with 22q11.2 deletion syndrome. *J Pediatr.* 2014;164(6):1475-1480.e1472.
29. Chan K, Puck JM. Development of population-based newborn screening for severe combined immunodeficiency. *J Allergy Clin Immunol.* 2005;115(2):391-398.
30. Chapnik E, Sasson V, Blelloch R, et al. Dgcr8 controls neural crest cells survival in cardiovascular development. *Dev Biol.* 2012;362(1):50-56.
31. Chaudhary MW, Al-Baradie RS. Ataxia-telangiectasia: future prospects. *Appl Clin Genet.* 2014;7:159-167.
32. Chen K, Coonrod Emily M, Kumánovics A, et al. Germline mutations in NFKB2 implicate the noncanonical NF-κB pathway in the pathogenesis of common variable immunodeficiency. *Am J Human Genet.* 2013;93(5):812-824.
34. Chiriaco M, Salfa I, Di Matteo G, et al. Chronic granulomatous disease: clinical, molecular, and therapeutic aspects. *Pediatr Allergy Immunol.* 2016;27(3):242-253.
35. Chopra C, Davies G, Taylor M, et al. Immune deficiency in ataxia-telangiectasia: a longitudinal study of 44 patients. *Clin Exp Immunol.* 2014;176(2):275-282.
38. Davies EG. Immunodeficiency in DiGeorge syndrome and options for treating cases with complete athymia. *Front Immunol.* 2013;4:322.
39. De Moraes Lui C, Oliveira LC, Diogo CL, et al. Immunoglobulin G subclass concentrations and infections in children and adolescents with severe asthma. *Pediatr Allergy Immunol.* 2002;13(3):195-202.
41. DiGeorge AM. Discussion of Cooper MD, Peterson RDA, Good RA. A new concept of cellular basis of immunity. *J Pediatrics.* 1965;67:907.
42. Dinauer MC. Disorders of neutrophil function: an overview. *Methods Mol Biol.* 2014;1124:501-515.
43. Driessen GJ, Ijspeert H, Weemaes CMR, et al. Antibody deficiency in patients with ataxia telangiectasia is caused by disturbed B- and T-cell homeostasis and reduced immune repertoire diversity. *J Allergy Clin Immunol.* 2013;131(5):1367-1375.e1369.
44. Driessen GJ, van Zelm MC, van Hagen PM, et al. B-cell replication history and somatic hypermutation status identify distinct pathophysiologic backgrounds in common variable immunodeficiency. *Blood.* 2011;118(26):6814-6823.
45. Dvorak CC, Hassan A, Slatter MA, et al. Comparison of outcomes of hematopoietic stem cell transplantation without chemotherapy conditioning by using matched sibling and unrelated donors for treatment of severe combined immunodeficiency. *J Allergy Clin Immunol.* 2014;134(4):935-943.e915.
47. Falcone EL, Holland SM. Invasive fungal infection in chronic granulomatous disease: insights into pathogenesis and management. *Curr Opin Infect Dis.* 2012;25(6):658-669.
48. Falcone EL, Jennifer RP, Mary Beth F, et al. Methylotroph infections and chronic granulomatous disease. *Emerg Infect Dis J.* 2016;22(3):404-409.
49. Fan X, Upadhyaya B, Wu L, et al. CD40 agonist antibody mediated improvement of chronic Cryptosporidium infection in patients with X- linked hyper IgM syndrome. *Clinical Immunology.* 2012;143(2):152-161.
50. Finnish-German APECED Consortium. An autoimmune disease, APECED, caused by mutations in a novel gene featuring two PHD-type zinc-finger domains. *Nat Genet.* 1997;17(4):399-403.
51. Gaspar H. Bone marrow transplantation and alternatives for adenosine deaminase deficiency. *Immunol Allergy Clin North Am.* 2010;30(2):221-236.
52. Gathmann B, Mahlaoui N, Gérard L, et al. Clinical picture and treatment of 2212 patients with common variable immunodeficiency. *J Allergy Clin Immunol.* 2014;134(1):116-126.e111.
53. Giacomelli M, Kumar R, Soresina A, et al. Reduction of CRKL expression in patients with partial DiGeorge syndrome is associated with impairment of T-cell functions. *J Allergy Clin Immunol.* 2016;138(1):229-240.
54. Grez M, Reichenbach J, Schwable J, et al. Gene therapy of chronic granulomatous disease: the engraftment dilemma. *Mol Ther.* 2011;19(1):28-35.
57. Grumach AS, Kirschfink M. Are complement deficiencies really rare? Overview on prevalence, clinical importance and modern diagnostic approach. *Mol Immunol.* 2014;61(2):110-117.
58. Grunebaum E, Roifman CM. Bone marrow transplantation using HLA-matched unrelated donors for patients suffering from severe combined immunodeficiency. *Hematol Oncol Clin North Am.* 2011;25(1):63-73.
60. Hacein-Bey-Abina S, Garrigue A, Wang GP, et al. Insertional oncogenesis in 4 patients after retrovirus-mediated gene therapy of SCID-X1. *J Clin Invest.* 2008;118(9):3132-3142.
62. Hacein-Bey-Abina S, Pai S-Y, Gaspar HB, et al. A modified γ-retrovirus vector for X-linked severe combined immunodeficiency. *N Eng J Med.* 2014;371(15):1407-1417.
63. Hacein-Bey-Abina S, Von Kalle C, Schmidt M, et al. *LMO2*-associated clonal T cell proliferation in two patients after gene therapy for SCID-X1. *Science.* 2003;302(5644):415-419.
61. Hacein-Bey Abina S, Gaspar H, Blondeau J, et al. Outcomes following gene therapy in patients with severe Wiskott-Aldrich syndrome. *JAMA.* 2015;313(15):1550-1563.
64. Henriet S, Verweij PE, Holland SM, et al. Invasive fungal infections in patients with chronic granulomatous disease. In: Curtis N, Finn A, Pollard AJ, eds. *Hot Topics in Infection and Immunity in Children IX.* New York: Springer; 2013:27-55.
65. Hernandez-Trujillo VP, Scalchunes C, Hernandez-Trujillo HS, et al. Primary immunodeficiency diseases: an opportunity in pediatrics for improving patient outcomes. *Clin Pediatr (Phila).* 2015;54(13):1265-1275.

66. Hofstetter AM, Jakob K, Klein NP, et al. Live vaccine use and safety in DiGeorge syndrome. *Pediatrics*. 2014;133(4):e946-e954.
67. Holland SM. Chronic granulomatous disease. *Hematol Oncol Clin North Am*. 2013;27(1):89-99.
68. Howe SJ, Mansour MR, Schwarzwaelder K, et al. Insertional mutagenesis combined with acquired somatic mutations causes leukemogenesis following gene therapy of SCID-X1 patients. *J Clin Invest*. 2008;118(9):3143-3150.
70. Janda A, Sedlacek P, Hönig M, et al. Multicenter survey on the outcome of transplantation of hematopoietic cells in patients with the complete form of DiGeorge anomaly. *Blood*. 2010;116(13):2229-2236.
71. Kane A, Deenick EK, Ma CS, et al. STAT3 is a central regulator of lymphocyte differentiation and function. *Curr Opin Immunol*. 2014;28(0):49-57.
72. Klein C, Grudzien M, Appaswamy G, et al. HAX1 deficiency causes autosomal recessive severe congenital neutropenia (Kostmann disease). *Nat Genet*. 2007;39(1):86-92.
74. Kohn LA, Seet CS, Scholes J, et al. Human lymphoid development in the absence of common γ-chain receptor signaling. *J Immunol*. 2014;192(11):5050-5058.
75. Kovanen PE, Leonard WJ. Cytokines and immunodeficiency diseases: critical roles of the γc-dependent cytokines interleukins 2, 4, 7, 9, 15, and 21, and their signaling pathways. *Immunol Rev*. 2004;202(1):67-83.
77. Kraus M, Lev A, Simon A, et al. Disturbed B and T cell homeostasis and neogenesis in patients with ataxia telangiectasia. *J Clin Immunol*. 2014;34(5):561-572.
79. Kutukculer N, Karaca NE, Demircioglu O, et al. Increases in serum immunoglobulins to age-related normal levels in children with IgA and/or IgG subclass deficiency. *Pediatr Allergy Immunol*. 2007;18(2):167-173.
80. Kwan A, Abraham RS, Currier R, et al. Newborn screening for severe combined immunodeficiency in 11 screening programs in the United States. *JAMA*. 2014;312(7):729-738.
81. Lee K-G, Kim Susana S-Y, Kui L, et al. Bruton's tyrosine kinase phosphorylates DDX41 and activates its binding of dsDNA and STING to initiate type 1 interferon response. *Cell Rep*. 2015;10(7):1055-1065.
82. Lee K-G, Xu S, Kang Z-H, et al. Bruton's tyrosine kinase phosphorylates Toll-like receptor 3 to initiate antiviral response. *Proc Natl Acad Sci USA*. 2012;109(15):5791-5796.
86. Licciardi PV, Balloch A, Russell FM, et al. Pneumococcal polysaccharide vaccine at 12 months of age produces functional immune responses. *J Allergy Clin Immunol*. 2012;129(3):794-800.e792.
87. Lim C, Dahle C, Elvin K, et al. Reversal of immunoglobulin A deficiency in children. *J Clin Immunol*. 2015;35(1):87-91.
88. Lingman Framme J, Borte S, von Döbeln U, et al. Retrospective analysis of TREC based newborn screening results and clinical phenotypes in infants with the 22q11 deletion syndrome. *J Clin Immunol*. 2014;34(4):514-519.
89. Lopez-Herrera G, Tampella G, Pan-Hammarström Q, et al. Deleterious mutations in *LRBA* are associated with a syndrome of immune deficiency and autoimmunity. *Am J Human Genet*. 2012;90(6):986-1001.
90. Lougaris V, Baronio M, Vitali M, et al. Bruton tyrosine kinase mediates TLR9-dependent human dendritic cell activation. *J Allergy Clin Immunol*. 2014;133(6):1644-1650.e1644.
92. Ludvigsson JF, Neovius M, Hammarström L. Risk of infections among 2100 individuals with IgA deficiency: a nationwide cohort study. *J Clin Immunol*. 2016;1-7.
93. Maguire GA, Kumararatne DS, Joyce HJ. Are there any clinical indications for measuring IgG subclasses? *Ann Clin Biochem*. 2002;39(Pt 4):374-377.
94. Mahlaoui N, Pellier I, Mignot C, et al. Characteristics and outcome of early-onset, severe forms of Wiskott-Aldrich syndrome. *Blood*. 2012;121(9):1510-1516.
95. Makaryan V, Zeidler C, Bolyard AA, et al. The diversity of mutations and clinical outcomes for ELANE-associated neutropenia. *Curr Opin Hematol*. 2015;22(1):3-11.
96. Marciano BE, Spalding C, Fitzgerald A, et al. Common severe infections in chronic granulomatous disease. *Clin Infect Dis*. 2015;60(8):1176-1183.
97. Markert M. Defects in thymic development: DiGeorge/CHARGE/Chromosome 22q11.2 deletion. In: Sullivan K, Stiehm E, eds. *Stiehm's Immune Deficiencies*. London: Academic Press; 2014:221-242.
98. Markert ML, Devlin BH, Alexieff MJ, et al. Review of 54 patients with complete DiGeorge anomaly enrolled in protocols for thymus transplantation: outcome of 44 consecutive transplants. *Blood*. 2007;109(10):4539-4547.
99. Markert ML, Devlin BH, McCarthy EA. Thymus transplantation. *Clin Immunol*. 2010;135(2):23646.
101. Massaad MJ, Ramesh N, Geha RS. Wiskott-Aldrich syndrome: a comprehensive review. *Ann N Y Acad Sci*. 2013;1285(1):26-43.
104. Mogensen TH. STAT3 and the hyper-IgE syndrome: clinical presentation, genetic origin, pathogenesis, novel findings and remaining uncertainties. *JAK-STAT*. 2013;2(2):e23435.
106. Nagamine K, Peterson P, Scott HS, et al. Positional cloning of the APECED gene. *Nat Genet*. 1997;17(4):393-398.
107. Ojuawo A, Milla PJ, Lindley KJ. Serum immunoglobulin and immunoglobulin G subclasses in children with allergic colitis. *West Afr J Med*. 1998;17(3):206-209.
108. Oksenhendler E, Gérard L, Fieschi C, et al. Infections in 252 patients with common variable immunodeficiency. *Clin Infect Dis*. 2008;46(10):1547-1554.
110. Orange JS. Natural killer cell deficiency. *J Allergy Clin Immunol*. 2013;132(3): 515-525.
111. Orange JS, Ballow M, Stiehm ER, et al. Use and interpretation of diagnostic vaccination in primary immunodeficiency: A working group report of the Basic and Clinical Immunology Interest Section of the American Academy of Allergy, Asthma & Immunology. *J Allergy Clin Immunol*. 2012;130(3, suppl):S1-S24.
112. Orange JS, Glessner JT, Resnick E, et al. Genome-wide association identifies diverse causes of common variable immunodeficiency. *J Allergy Clin Immunol*. 2011;127(6):1360-1367.e1366.
115. Pai S-Y, Logan BR, Griffith LM, et al. Transplantation outcomes for severe combined immunodeficiency, 2000–2009. *N Eng J Med*. 2014;371(5): 434-446.
116. Patel K, Akhter J, Kobrynski L, et al. Immunoglobulin deficiencies: the B-lymphocyte side of DiGeorge syndrome. *J Pediatr*. 2012;161(5):950-953.e951.
118. Picard C, von Bernuth H, Ghandil P, et al. Clinical features and outcome of patients with IRAK-4 and MyD88 deficiency. *Medicine (Baltimore)*. 2010;89(6):403-425.
119. Plebani A, Soresina A, Rondelli R, et al. Clinical, immunological, and molecular analysis in a large cohort of patients with X-linked agammaglobulinemia: an Italian multicenter study. *Clin Immunol*. 2002;104(3):221-230.
120. Qamar N, Fuleihan R. The hyper IgM syndromes. *Clinic Rev Allerg Immunol*. 2014;46(2):120-130.
121. Racedo Silvia E, McDonald-McGinn Donna M, Chung Jonathan H, et al. Mouse and human CRKL is dosage sensitive for cardiac outflow tract formation. *Am J Human Genet*. 2015;96(2):235-244.
122. Rachid R, Bonilla FA. The role of anti-IgA antibodies in causing adverse reactions to gamma globulin infusion in immunodeficient patients: a comprehensive review of the literature. *J Allergy Clin Immunol*. 2012;129(3):628-634.
123. Rope AF, Cragun DL, Saal HM, et al. DiGeorge anomaly in the absence of chromosome 22q11.2 deletion. *J Pediatr*. 2009;155(4):560-565.e561.
126. Sandler SG, Eder AF, Goldman M, et al. The entity of immunoglobulin A–related anaphylactic transfusion reactions is not evidence based. *Transfusion*. 2015;55(1):199-204.
129. Schroeder SA, Zielen S. Infections of the respiratory system in patients with ataxia–telangiectasia. *Pediatr Pulmonol*. 2014;49(4):389-399.
130. Schuetz C, Neven B, Dvorak CC, et al. SCID patients with ARTEMIS vs RAG deficiencies following HCT: increased risk of late toxicity in ARTEMIS-deficient SCID. *Blood*. 2013;123(2):281-289.
132. Sellier C, Hwang VJ, Dandekar R, et al. Decreased *DGCR8* expression and miRNA dysregulation in individuals with 22q11.2 deletion syndrome. *PLoS ONE*. 2014;9(8):e103884.
134. Shearer WT, Dunn E, Notarangelo LD, et al. Establishing diagnostic criteria for severe combined immunodeficiency disease (SCID), leaky SCID, and Omenn syndrome: the Primary Immune Deficiency Treatment Consortium experience. *J Allergy Clin Immunol*. 2014;133(4):1092-1098.
135. Shearer WT, Fleisher TA, Buckley RH, et al. Recommendations for live viral and bacterial vaccines in immunodeficient patients and their close contacts. *J Allergy Clin Immunol*. 2014;133(4):961-966.
136. Singh K, Chang C, Gershwin ME. IgA deficiency and autoimmunity. *Autoimmun Rev*. 2014;13(2):163-177.
138. Sochorová K, Horváth R, Rožková D, et al. Impaired toll-like receptor 8–mediated IL-6 and TNF-α production in antigen-presenting cells from patients with X-linked agammaglobulinemia. *Blood*. 2006;109(6):2553-2556.
140. Stiehm RE. The four most common pediatric immunodeficiencies. *Adv Exp Med Biol*. 2007;601:15-26.
141. Su HC, Jing H, Zhang Q. DOCK8 deficiency. *Ann N Y Acad Sci*. 2011; 1246(1):26-33.
142. Suarez F, Mahlaoui N, Canioni D, et al. Incidence, presentation, and prognosis of malignancies in ataxia-telangiectasia: a report from the French National Registry of Primary Immune Deficiencies. *J Clin Oncol*. 2015;33(2):202-208.
143. Ta-Shma A, El-lahham N, Edvardson S, et al. Conotruncal malformations and absent thymus due to a deleterious NKX2–6 mutation. *J Med Genet*. 2014;51(4):268-270.
144. Taylor AMR, Lam Z, Last JI, et al. Ataxia telangiectasia: more variation at clinical and cellular levels. *Clin Genet*. 2015;87(3):199-208.
146. Thomas RA, Landing BH, Wells TR. Embryologic and other developmental considerations of thirty-eight possible variants of the DiGeorge anomaly (DGA). *Am J Med Genetics Suppl*. 1987;3:43-66.
147. Tison BE, Nicholas SK, Abramson SL, et al. Autoimmunity in a cohort of 130 pediatric patients with partial DiGeorge syndrome. *J Allergy Clin Immunol*. 2011;128(5):1115-1117.
150. Uzel G, Orange JS, Poliak N, et al. Complications of tumor necrosis factor-α blockade in chronic granulomatous disease-related colitis. *Clin Infect Dis*. 2010;51(12):1429-1434.
151. van de Vijver E, van den Berg TK, Kuijpers TW. Leukocyte adhesion deficiencies. *Hematol Oncol Clin North Am*. 2013;27(1):101-116.
152. Van Winkle R, Hauck W, McGeady S. Phenotypic parameters predict time to normalization in infants with hypogammaglobulinemia. *J Clin Immunol*. 2013;33(8):1336-1340.

155. Verhagen JMA, Diderich KEM, Oudesluijs G, et al. Phenotypic variability of atypical 22q11.2 deletions not including TBX1. *Am J Med Genet Part A*. 2012;158A(10):2412-2420.
158. von Bernuth H, Picard C, Puel A, et al. Experimental and natural infections in MyD88- and IRAK-4-deficient mice and humans. *Eur J Immunol*. 2012;42(12):3126-3135.
159. Wang N, Hammarstrom L. IgA deficiency: what is new? *Curr Opin Allergy Clin Immunol*. 2012;12(6):602-608.
160. Warnatz K, Salzer U, Rizzi M, et al. B-cell activating factor receptor deficiency is associated with an adult-onset antibody deficiency syndrome in humans. *Proc Natl Acad Sci USA*. 2009;106(33):13945-13950.
161. Waters V, Peterson KS, LaRussa P. Live viral vaccines in a DiGeorge syndrome patient. *Arch Dis Child*. 2007;92(6):519-520.
162. Wehr C, Gennery AR, Lindemans C, et al. Multicenter experience in hematopoietic stem cell transplantation for serious complications of common variable immunodeficiency. *J Allergy Clin Immunol*. 2015;135(4):988-997.
163. Wehr C, Kivioja T, Schmitt C, et al. The EUROclass trial: defining subgroups in common variable immunodeficiency. *Blood*. 2007;111(1):77-85.
167. Yang Y, Muzny DM, Xia F, et al. Molecular findings among patients referred for clinical whole-exome sequencing. *JAMA*. 2014;312(18):1870-1879.
168. Zheng P, Noroski LM, Hanson IC, et al. Molecular mechanisms of functional natural killer deficiency in patients with partial DiGeorge syndrome. *J Allergy Clin Immunol*. 2015;135(5):1293-1302.

The full reference list for this chapter is available at ExpertConsult.com

The Febrile Neutropenic Patient 68

Brian T. Fisher • Lillian Sung

Since chemotherapeutic agents were first administered for the treatment of malignancy, infection has been a cause of significant morbidity and mortality. Initial reports documented an infection-related mortality rate among patients with acute leukemia that was greater than 70%.[65,68] In the past five and one-half decades, cancer survival rates have improved dramatically in high-income countries, with more than 80% of children with cancer surviving beyond 5 years from diagnosis.[6,168] However, the immunosuppressive consequences of chemotherapy continue to exist, and infections still account for a substantial number of deaths in children receiving intensely myelosuppressive chemotherapy,[152] especially in the 2 weeks after diagnosis.[35]

For many decades, researchers have sought to identify risk factors for infection and to devise risk-stratified therapeutic approaches to reduce infectious mortality rates in patients receiving chemotherapy. Early descriptive pediatric studies confirmed that the depth and duration of neutropenia was a risk factor for developing infection. Furthermore fever was a frequent and sometimes the only clinical sign indicating the presence of infection in this at-risk population.[68] In these early years, fever in patients with neutropenia prompted an infectious evaluation, but empiric antibiotic therapy was not considered standard of care. Because infection was the most common cause of fever in neutropenic patients and because some patients with fever and neutropenia had rapid progression to death, particularly due to *Pseudomonas aeruginosa* bacteremia, empiric therapy was explored. In 1971, Schimpff et al. published one of the sentinel experiences of combination empiric therapy with carbenicillin and gentamicin in a series of patients with fever and neutropenia.[142] Their efforts revealed a reduction in infectious mortality with this approach relative to historical controls. Specifically, in the historical control period, when empiric antibiotic therapy was not utilized, 20 of 22 *P. aeruginosa* infections ultimately resulted in death. This compared to only four deaths out of 21 *P. aeruginosa* infections during the study period. Subsequent landmark trials by Pizzo et al. supported the continuation of empiric antibiotics through the duration of neutropenia and prompted the addition of empiric antifungal therapy in the setting of prolonged fever and neutropenia despite broad-spectrum antibiotic therapy.[122,123]

In the decades that followed, empiric antibacterial and antifungal therapy has evolved into standard of care for patients with fever and neutropenia. Clinical practice guidelines from various societies have better standardized the approach to this clinical scenario.[38,54,88,102] Although these guidelines have been useful, they have primarily focused on adult patient populations. This has left pediatricians to apply guidelines that have not accounted for important differences between children and adults presenting with fever and neutropenia.[154] Fortunately, in 2012, an international group of investigators formed the Pediatric Fever and Neutropenia Guideline Panel with the objective of systematically reviewing the available literature to inform an evidence-based guideline for the management of the child with fever and neutropenia. The initial version of this guideline addressed a number of the important differences in the management of pediatric and adult patients with fever and neutropenia.[89] In addition to providing guidance on current management practices, the committee identified knowledge gaps with the goal of directing future investigation that will provide further data to improve the breadth of evidence-based clinical practice.

This chapter focuses on the epidemiology of fever and neutropenia and approaches for risk stratification that are pertinent to pediatric patients. Advances in modalities for diagnosing bacterial and fungal infections are also explored. Finally empiric, preemptive, and prophylactic therapeutic interventions are reviewed. At relevant points, areas for necessary future investigation are highlighted. There are many other etiologies of neutropenia (e.g., congenital neutropenia and autoimmune neutropenia),[129] and such patients will also incur periods of fever and neutropenia. However, the importance of fever in these settings varies substantially and thus the focus of this chapter is on fever in the setting of chemotherapy-induced neutropenia.

EPIDEMIOLOGY OF FEVER AND NEUTROPENIA

Children receiving chemotherapy are often confronted with at least one episode of fever and neutropenia during the course of their cancer care. The frequency of fever and neutropenia varies depending on factors such as type and extent of malignancy, intensity of chemotherapy, and receipt of prophylactic granulocyte colony-stimulating factor, and the incidence can range from 10% to 60%.[23,25,153] The incidence of fever and neutropenia can increase to 70% to 100% in patients receiving particularly intensive and myelosuppressive chemotherapy.[157]

Bacterial Pathogens

Fever in the setting of neutropenia is often the initial and potentially the only clinical sign of a bacterial, fungal, or viral infection. Of patients in whom a pathogen is identified, bacteria predominate. In a landmark study evaluating 793 pediatric cancer patients with fever and neutropenia, Pizzo et al. found that 87% of patients with a microbiologically documented infection had a bacterial pathogen identified.[124] Recent epidemiologic studies specific to pediatric fever and neutropenia have suggested a reduction in the proportion of episodes that are attributable to bacteria. However, despite the reduction, bacterial pathogens still accounted for the majority of all identified pathogens.[23,63]

Early reports on the epidemiology of these bacterial infections highlighted gram-negative pathogens as the predominant cause of infection in neutropenic children and adults. *Escherichia coli, Pseudomonas*

TABLE 68.1 Distribution of Bacterial Pathogens in Selected Pediatric Fever and Neutropenia Cohorts

	Ariffin[12] (2002)	Lehrnbecher[92] (2004)	Castagnola[23] (2007)	Hakim[63] (2009)	Gupta[60] (2011)
Study location	Malaysia	Germany	Italy	United States	El Salvador
Patient type	Any malignancy	Acute myeloid leukemia	Leukemia, solid tumor, or allogeneic HSCT	Any malignancy	Any malignancy
Clinical scenario	Fever and neutropenia	Fever with and without neutropenia	Fever and neutropenia	Fever and neutropenia	Fever and neutropenia
Infection episodes (total patients)	762 (513)	855 (304)	614 (NA)	337 (337)	106 (86)
Bacterial pathogen isolation; *N* (%)	270 (35.4%)	252 (29.5%)	97 (15.8%)	54 (16%)	23[b] (22%)
Gram-positive pathogens; *n* (%)	103 (38.1%)	203 (80.6%)	57 (58.8%)	31[a] (57%)	14 (61%)
Gram-negative pathogens; *n* (%)	167 (61.9%)	49 (19.4%)	40 (41.2%)	23 (43%)	11 (48%)

HSCT, Hematopoietic stem cell transplant.
[a]Includes seven episodes of *Clostridium difficile* infection.
[b]Includes polymicrobial infections.

aeruginosa, and *Klebsiella* spp. were the three most commonly isolated pathogens.[146] Subsequently, towards the end of the 1980s, gram-positive pathogens were being increasingly recognized as an important source of fever of neutropenia,[41,167] and, soon thereafter, gram-positive pathogens were found to be more common than gram-negative organisms.[175] This shift in pathogens has been attributed to increased use of central venous lines, a greater prevalence of mucositis, and prophylactic regimens with predominantly gram-negative activity. Additionally, escalation to more intensive chemotherapy regimens, such as those containing high-dose cytarabine, have resulted in more impressive mucositis, which has contributed to increases in specific pathogens such as viridans group streptococci.[152]

The spectrum of bacterial pathogens will depend on specific chemotherapy, use of antimicrobial prophylaxis, and setting. Table 68.1 displays the distribution of bacterial infections across various international pediatric oncology cohorts.[12,23,60,63,92] Variation in the frequency in isolation of a bacterial pathogen across cohorts is apparent. This is likely secondary to variation in geographic location, composition of each cohort, diagnostic testing practices, and prophylactic antimicrobial regimens. With the exception of the Malaysian cohort, the predominance of gram-positive pathogens has persisted in pediatric oncology cohorts, consistent with data published toward the end of the previous century. Among the gram-positive pathogens viridans group streptococci, *Staphylococcus aureus,* and coagulase-negative staphylococci are predominant. *E. coli, P. aeruginosa,* and *Klebsiella* spp. remain the most commonly identified gram-negative pathogens.[12,23,60,63,92]

Fungal Pathogens

As discussed in more detail later, the likelihood of invasive fungal disease (IFD) during an episode of fever and neutropenia varies depending on a number of risk factors. Generally fungal pathogens are considered as the etiology of fever and neutropenia when these two clinical signs are concurrently prolonged or when fever is recurrent during the same episode of neutropenia in the setting of broad-spectrum antibiotic therapy. Defining the epidemiology of IFD in specific patient populations can be challenging. Published consensus criteria for defining the presence an IFD have been helpful in standardizing reporting of such infections.[40] However, limitations in diagnostic modalities for identifying an IFD persist and thus published IFD rates are likely underestimated. Despite these challenges, prospective multicenter data have documented a proven or probable IFD rate ranging from 3% to 5% of children hospitalized with fever and neutropenia.[80,113,166] *Candida* spp. are the most commonly isolated fungal pathogens, likely related to the frequent existence of *Candida* as a commensal organism on the skin and mucosal surfaces.[48] Compromise of these important anatomical barriers (e.g., mucositis) can result in invasive candidiasis. Additionally *Candida* spp. can infect central venous catheters, which are commonly present in children with cancer. Although mortality data specific to candidiasis in pediatric oncology patients are limited, the attributable mortality of invasive candidiasis in all pediatric patients has been estimated to be 10%.[173]

Invasive mold disease (IMD) is less common but an extremely important complication of neutropenia, given the poor outcomes related to these pathogens. In two contemporary pediatric cases series, only 54% to 60% of patients with IMD responded to therapy in the first 12 weeks from diagnosis, and approximately 30% of patients diagnosed with an IMD died within the same time period.[56,169] Among the mold pathogens, *Aspergillus* spp. are most common, followed by organisms of the Mucorales order.[56,152,169]

Viral Pathogens

Owing to advancement in viral diagnostic methodologies, multiple publications have attempted to delineate the attribution of fever and neutropenia events to viral pathogens. Table 68.2 displays the frequency of recovered viral upper respiratory pathogens in pediatric patients presenting with fever, with or without symptoms of a viral infection.[15,30,84,94,158] Although only Torres et al. was limited to episodes of fever and neutropenia, the majority of patients in the other cohorts had fever and neutropenia at the time of their evaluation. The frequency of laboratory-confirmed viral respiratory infection ranged from 8% to 59%. A more recent publication using administrative data from the Kid's Inpatient Database suggested that up to 12.1% of fever and neutropenia episodes are the result of viral infection. However, in this study, the identification of fever and neutropenia admissions and presence of viral infection were dependent on ICD-9 discharge diagnosis codes.[107] These codes have not been validated for either fever and neutropenia or viral infection, and thus it is difficult to ascertain the accuracy of these findings.

Although some authors have suggested routine comprehensive viral testing at the time of presentation,[30,158] the utility of routine viral testing is not clear. First, ideally, the identification of a viral pathogen should allow for discontinuation of broad-spectrum antibiotics in the febrile and neutropenic patient. However, bacterial and viral infections are not mutually exclusive, with as many as 13% to 33% of patients with a viral pathogen suffering a simultaneous sterile site bacterial infection.[84,158] Second, the evolution in the availability of viral PCR testing may result in detection of virus well after clinical resolution. Finally, only a few antiviral agents are available for the treatment of some of these viral pathogens, and their effectiveness is not clearly delineated. Viral testing should be limited to patients in whom positive results would effect a change in management, such as deescalation of antibiotic therapy, initiation of an appropriate antiviral therapy (e.g., neuraminidase inhibitor for influenza), or institution of appropriate isolation precautions.

TABLE 68.2 **Frequency of Viral Respiratory Pathogens at Presentation for Fever and Neutropenia**

	Long[94] (1987)	Arola[14] (1995)	Christensen[30] (2005)	Koskenvuo[84] (2008)	Torres[158] (2012)
Study duration	5 years	17 months	12 months	5.5 years	21 months
Patient type	Leukemia, solid tumors	Any malignancy	Any malignancy	Leukemia	Any malignancy
Clinical scenario	Suspicion of virus	Fever	Fever	Fever	Fever and neutropenia
Total patients (episodes)	200 (NR)	32 (75)	66 (250)	51 (138)	193 (331)
Testing methods	Culture; immunofluroesence	Culture; antigen; and antibodies	PCR	Culture; antigen; and PCR	PCR
Respiratory virus isolation rate	148 (NA)	28 (37%)	19 (8%)[a]	61 (59%)	190 (57%)
Sterile site bacterial pathogen plus virus isolation	Not reported	None	Not reported	13%	33%

NR, Not reported; *PCR,* polymerase chain reaction; *NA,* not applicable.
[a]Mouth swabs and not nasopharyngeal swabs performed on a majority of patients.

FEVER AND NEUTROPENIA OF UNKNOWN ORIGIN

Despite evaluation, many patients have negative cultures and do not have a clinically evident site of infection. This presentation is often referred to as fever of unknown origin (FUO). Although children with FUO can have an occult infection, an infectious pathogen or clinical infection is not detected. In a combined pediatric and young adult cohort, Pizzo et al.[123] described 306 consecutive episodes of fever and neutropenia in patients cared for at the National Institute of Health. They found that only 54% of patients had an identifiable infection within 7 days from presentation. Despite advances in infectious diagnostic modalities (i.e., improved blood culture mechanisms, sensitive viral tests), the rates of unidentified etiology of fever and neutropenia in children have remained high, ranging from 33% to 79%.[12,23,63,92,158]

RISK STRATIFICATION

Risk Stratification at Initial Presentation

The risk of infection and serious morbidity is highly heterogeneous among patients with fever and neutropenia, and this heterogeneity has resulted in efforts to risk stratify patients. Most of the efforts in risk stratification have been directed toward identifying patients at low risk of bacteremia and adverse outcomes who may be managed with less aggressive interventions such as outpatient management, early discontinuation of antibiotics, or oral therapy. Some studies have focused on identifying high-risk patients to facilitate intensification of diagnostic investigation, empiric therapy, or monitoring. In adults, the predominant risk stratification schema that has emerged is the Multinational Association for Supportive Care in Cancer (MASCC) Scoring System. Unfortunately this system incorporates parameters that are not applicable to children, such as lack of chronic obstructive pulmonary disease and age less than 60 years, to determine low-risk status. The inclusion of these parameters limits the applicability of this scoring system to children.[154]

A number of both retrospective and prospective pediatric cohort studies have been performed to evaluate various clinical prediction rules for designating children as low-risk for infection in the setting of fever and neutropenia. These studies have been summarized in multiple meta-analyses.[62,120,118] Considered collectively, data from these studies support the potential success of implementing a risk stratification protocol. However, each trial used varied patient-relevant factors (e.g., age, malignancy), clinical factors (e.g., timing of chemotherapy, degree of fever, presence of hypotension), and laboratory parameters (e.g., duration and depth of neutropenia, C-reactive protein value, platelet count) and had various outcome definitions (e.g., bacteremia, serious infection, death). Furthermore attempts to validate six of the pediatric risk stratification schemas in separate populations have resulted in suboptimal performance compared to the original study.* A primary reason for suboptimal performance during validation is variation in the clinical setting between the derivation and validation cohorts. Currently centers applying a risk prediction model for children with fever and neutropenia should identify a model that is most consistent with their patient population (rules tend to perform less favorably when applied in different settings) and their local clinical practice and is most feasible to implement. Additionally, at the time of implementing a risk stratification protocol, a center should clearly delineate the goals of its risk stratification. This articulation should include a framework on how the risk stratification will inform clinical decision-making (i.e., low-risk patients can be discharged to home with outpatient follow-up). The framework should be developed by a multidisciplinary team and clearly communicated to both health care providers and patients and their families.

More recently an individual patient data meta-analysis inclusive of data from 22 datasets representing previous cohorts of children with fever and neutropenia was performed as part of a global collaboration called Predicting Infectious Complications in Children with Cancer (PICNICC).[119] The analysis considered demographic, clinical, and laboratory results in deriving a risk prediction model for likelihood of microbiologically defined infection in children with fever and neutropenia. The final model included malignancy type, temperature, clinical appearance of the child, hemoglobin level, total white blood cell count, and absolute monocyte count. The resultant prediction rates for microbiological infection closely correlated with actual estimates, and the model was robust to internal validation. Because the data that informed this model derivation were assembled from cohorts across various clinical settings, it represents a potential tool to be leveraged in various fever and neutropenia settings. Prior to widespread application, it needs to be validated externally.

As biomarkers continue to be discovered, there is always the potential to improve on current prediction rules. Investigators have studied the clinical utility of more than 170 different biomarkers, including cytokines, cell surface markers, coagulation system molecules, receptors in various inflammatory cascades, and acute phase reactants in various pediatric and adult clinical settings.[121] A number of biomarkers have emerged as potentially useful tools to guide approaches for fever and neutropenia, some of which have already been used in the aforementioned prediction rules. However, although some biomarkers are often elevated in patients with a bacterial infection, an inability to identify a threshold value for a single biomarker to accurately discriminate between infected and uninfected patients has limited their clinical applicability. Future investigations that incorporate multiple biomarkers with traditional laboratory values and clinical findings may improve the discriminating ability of a pediatric risk prediction rule.

Risk Stratification for Invasive Fungal Disease

The risk stratification prediction rules just discussed are typically relevant to risk for microbiologically documented infections at the time of presentation for fever and neutropenia. However, concern for an IFD

*References 5, 7, 8, 16, 78, 95, 96, 106, 120, 118, 128, 134, 137, 138.

is often increased when fever and neutropenia persist despite initial empiric antibiotic therapy. Unlike the risk for microbiologically documented infection at presentation, there have been no pediatric studies dedicated to deriving an IFD risk prediction rule in children with persistent fever and neutropenia. However, a number of observational studies have identified important factors that are associated with an increased risk for IFD.

Patient populations with reported IFD incidence greater than 10% include children with acute myeloid leukemia (AML),[59,151,152] relapsed acute lymphoblastic leukemia (ALL),[87] and recipients of an allogeneic stem cell transplantation.[17,47,67,82,162] Additionally increasing duration of neutropenia is a commonly identified risk factor for IFD.[47,67,72,85,170] The exact duration at which the risk significantly increases is not definitively known but observational data in children with AML suggest it is somewhere between 10 and 15 days of neutropenia.[72] Depth of neutropenia is also an important component of the neutropenia risk profile for IFD. An absolute neutrophil count (ANC) of less than 100/μL or an absolute monocyte count (AMC) of less than 100/μL during an episode of fever and neutropenia was each associated with an increased risk of IFD.[103,166] Exposure to high-dose steroids and/or prolonged steroid exposure (>10 days) have also been identified as a risk factor for IFD.[47,58,66,67,72,85,103] Finally increasing age has been associated with increasing risk for IFD. Age thresholds of 7.5 years[140] and 10 years[47,70,152] have been suggested for dichotomizing IFD risk by age. However, an optimal threshold for categorizing age related to IFD risk is unclear.

Based on these data, pediatric fever and neutropenia guidelines[90] recommend that patients with fever and neutropenia should be considered IFD high risk if they have recently received intensive chemotherapy (e.g., AML or relapsed ALL patient) with expected prolonged neutropenia and/or recent exposure to prolonged courses of steroids. This stratification for identification of IFD high-risk patients is a general guide, and it should be noted that IFD has been described in patients who would not meet this high-risk classification.[46] Additional work is necessary to establish specific prediction rules to incorporate multiple risk factors into a single risk prediction rule to more accurately discriminate between IFD high- and low-risk patients.

HISTORY AND PHYSICAL EXAM

Prior to initiating routine diagnostic testing, a complete history and physical exam should be performed. A comprehensive history can identify important exposures that could alert the physician to consider less common opportunistic infections and direct early additional diagnostic testing. The history should include details about symptoms other than fever, adherence to current medications (especially prophylactic antimicrobials), and most recent chemotherapy regimen. Additionally the clinician should ask about sick contacts at home, updates on recent travel, daycare/school/occupational exposures, animal exposures (e.g., new pets such as cats or birds, or contact with farm or wild animals), and dietary exposures (e.g., unpasteurized cheeses). A thorough history of prior dwelling locations is becoming increasingly important among pediatric oncology patients in the evolving era of country-to-country transfers. Knowledge on prior living locations may have an impact on a patient's risk for multidrug-resistant pathogens[110] and help to identify potential dietary or environmental exposures that predispose patients to rarely seen pathogens. On physical exam, specific attention should be focused on areas sometimes overlooked, such as the naso- and oropharynx, middle ears, genitalia, perineum (in particular, the perianal area), and scalp. Central venous line exit sites are also important areas for inspection.

INITIAL DIAGNOSTIC EVALUATION

Regardless of the risk designation of a pediatric patient presenting with fever and neutropenia, an infectious diagnostic evaluation is warranted in all such patients. Various testing modalities may be employed depending on the status of the presenting patient. In all patients, routine blood cultures should be performed prior to initiation of antibiotics. Because most patients have central venous access, this would include culturing all lumens of the central venous catheter.

Performing a peripheral blood culture in addition to central venous cultures is controversial. Multiple studies of paired cultures taken from pediatric and adult patients with underlying malignancy suggest a small but consistent probability of detecting true bacteremia from the peripheral culture when the central culture is negative.[1,27,43,127,141] A meta-analysis determined that 13% of bacteremias were only identified with a peripheral culture.[133] These data suggest that a peripheral blood collection should be considered concurrent with cultures from the central line to optimize detection of a causative pathogen for the fever and neutropenia episode.

The yield of repeated daily blood cultures after the initial evaluation is low. In a series of 193 consecutive fever and neutropenia episodes in 117 pediatric patients, 95 of the episodes revealed that the index culture was negative and the fever and neutropenia persisted.[111] Among these 95 episodes, 421 additional blood cultures were obtained in the ensuing 2 weeks. Only 4 of the 421 additional blood cultures were positive for a bacterial pathogen. Given the low yield of subsequent blood cultures in the setting of persistent fever and neutropenia with an initial negative culture, it is reasonable to follow the adult guideline recommendations, which suggest daily blood cultures for only the first 3 days of fever and neutropenia.[54] Any additional blood cultures should be reserved for patients with a significant clinical change (e.g., hypotension, tachypnea) or in those whose fever initially resolved but then recurred.

A urine culture is warranted if the patient presents with signs or symptoms of a urinary tract infection (UTI). The importance of routine urine cultures for children presenting with fever and neutropenia without signs or symptoms of a UTI is controversial. In a typical pediatric population, UTI is a common source of FUO.[29] Asymptomatic UTIs are likely to be more common in neutropenic children given the lack of an appropriate inflammatory response. This is evidenced by the fact that only 4% of oncology patients with a urine culture yielding a UTI pathogen will have pyuria on urinalysis.[79]

A number of observational studies have evaluated the yield of urine cultures in pediatric patients presenting with fever and neutropenia. Hakim et al. noted that of 337 patients presenting with fever and neutropenia 2 (0.6%) had a positive urine culture.[63] Data from Santolaya et al. revealed the presence of a urinary pathogen in 4.6% of fever and neutropenia episodes.[137] Urine culture was not a component of the routine diagnostic evaluation in either study, so it is possible that there were more patients with a UTI that went undetected. When urine culture is routinely performed in children presenting with fever and neutropenia, the frequency of a UTI is reported to be 8.6%.[135]

Given these data, urine culture in patients presenting with fever and neutropenia should be obtained if a mid-stream or clean catch specimen is feasible. In patients who require urinary catheterization for specimen collection, the risks of the intervention should be weighed against the benefit of potentially identifying the source of the fever. However, antibiotic administration should never be delayed if a patient is unable to provide a timely urine specimen.

In children presenting with focal respiratory signs (e.g., tachypnea or auscultatory changes) or symptoms (e.g., cough or increased work of breathing), chest radiography should be a component of the initial diagnostic workup. Additionally, in children with respiratory symptoms who are capable of producing an adequate sputum sample, the clinician should consider sputum collection for culture. The utility of chest radiography has been examined in children presenting with fever and neutropenia without respiratory symptoms. Together these studies evaluated 487 episodes of pediatric fever and neutropenia; only five chest radiographs revealed pneumonia in the absence of any respiratory signs or symptoms.[51,76,83,131] These data do not support the routine use of chest radiography in children with fever and neutropenia in the absence of signs or symptoms of respiratory issues.

Finally important findings noted on history and/or physical exam should dictate additional testing for less common sources of infection. For instance a patient presenting with fever and neutropenia and a reported history of a lovebird in the home should prompt additional testing for cryptococcosis early in the evaluation period.[161] Likewise identification of black cutaneous lesion(s) in a patient with antecedent neutropenia should prompt consideration for immediate biopsy to determine if the lesion represents a cutaneous mold infection. In the setting of exotic exposures or important clinical findings, consultation with an infectious disease physician with experience in immunocompromised patients may be warranted early in the hospitalization because early identification of less common opportunistic infections will likely translate into improved patient care.

INITIAL THERAPY FOR FEVER AND NEUTROPENIA

Traditionally the standard of care for fever and neutropenia has been hospital admission with administration of intravenous broad-spectrum antibiotics. However, employing a risk stratification rule (as discussed in the previous Risk Stratification section) offers the opportunity to differentially manage children at low risk of having bacteremia or an adverse outcome at the time of presentation for fever and neutropenia. Low-risk patients may be managed with oral antibiotics if oral therapy is feasible (e.g., absence of vomiting and malabsorption) in the inpatient or outpatient setting. If the hospital infrastructure supports an ambulatory approach, then patients may be treated as outpatients with oral or intravenous therapy.[99,132,156] Those who are not identified as low risk should be admitted for initiation of a parenteral antibiotic regimen with broad-spectrum gram-negative coverage, including *P. aeruginosa* and gram-positive coverage for organisms such as the viridans group streptococci. Antibiotic options that meet these criteria include an anti-pseudomonal penicillin (e.g., piperacillin-tazobactam), a cephalosporin (e.g., cefepime), or a carbapenem (e.g., meropenem or imipenem). Two separate pediatric meta-analyses compared anti-pseudomonal penicillins to cephalosporins,[100] as well as anti-pseudomonal penicillins to carbapenems,[101] and concluded similar effectiveness of each of these options for empiric therapy.

It is important to note that a meta-analysis of predominantly adult randomized controlled trials (RCTs) identified a significant increased risk for all-cause mortality in patients receiving cefepime compared to those receiving other β-lactam agents for fever and neutropenia.[116,172] However, in a subsequent analysis, the US Food and Drug Administration (FDA) supplemented the available published data with unpublished mortality data specific to febrile neutropenic patients and found no mortality difference between the antibiotic options. Importantly the FDA specifically reviewed the available case report forms from the fever and neutropenia trials and could not identify a biologically plausible reason for the previously identified association between cefepime and death.[77] An additional meta-analysis of fever and neutropenia trials, as well as a retrospective investigation of pediatric AML patients, did not reveal a difference in mortality risk between those exposed to cefepime compared to other antibiotics commonly used for fever and neutropenia.[52,159] Evaluating the available data, cefepime should remain as a viable option for empiric therapy for febrile neutropenia.

In general, for a child presenting with fever and neutropenia that is otherwise stable, monotherapy with an antipseudomonal penicillin, an antipseudomonal fourth-generation cephalosporin, or an antipseudomonal carbapenem is appropriate. An empiric monotherapy regimen is supported by data from recent meta-analyses in pediatric fever and neutropenia that all found no statistically significant differences in treatment failure, infection-related mortality, or overall mortality when comparing monotherapy with combination regimens.[100] Both the current pediatric[90] and adult[54] fever and neutropenia guidelines support empiric anti-pseudomonal monotherapy.

Because gram-positive organisms are an increasing cause of fever and neutropenia episodes, the utility of adding additional broad gram-positive coverage (e.g., vancomycin) to the empiric regimen has been questioned. Although pediatric-specific data do not exist, multiple adult RCTs have investigated the efficacy of adding a glycopeptide to various β-lactam–containing regimens. These trials were summarized in two separate meta-analyses, each of which failed to identify a significant benefit relative to all-cause mortality in patients receiving empiric glycopeptide therapy.[115,164] Therefore routine empiric glycopeptides are not recommended for fever and neutropenia.

As suggested by the adult and pediatric fever and neutropenia guidelines,[54,90] certain patient-specific factors should be evaluated when managing antibiotic regimens. For instance, in patients presenting or developing hemodynamic instability, broadening the coverage to include resistant gram-negative and -positive organisms, such as the addition of a second gram-negative agent (e.g., an aminoglycoside) and vancomycin, is important. Additionally broad gram-positive therapy should be considered in patients with evidence of a focal gram-positive infection (e.g., cellulitis or central access tunnel infection). Finally a history of an invasive infection with a resistance organism (e.g., methicillin-resistant *S. aureus* [MRSA]) should inform empiric antibiotic choices during subsequent fever and neutropenia episodes.

These recommendations for empiric antibiotic coverage should be considered guiding principles rather than dictums. Each center's local empiric antibiotic regimen should be customized based on information regarding pathogen resistance from the institution's antibiogram that is specific to the oncology patient population. For example, viridans group streptococci are a common group of pathogens that result in bacteremia and sepsis in AML patients. The resistance profile of these organisms is variable over time and by institution. A center may have elevated MRSA rates, and thus vancomycin would be a reasonable component to the empiric therapy regimen for fever and neutropenia until at least the initial blood culture results are available. The threshold of resistance that would trigger a change in the locally recommended empiric therapy regimen is not known. Such decisions regarding empiric regimen changes should be made with input from oncologists, infectious disease specialists, microbiologists, and pharmacists.

For low-risk patients, outpatient management with either oral or parenteral therapy for fever and neutropenia has garnered much support in recent years. A number of pediatric-specific randomized trials have noted similar safety for early hospital discharge on intravenous therapy versus continued hospitalization,[3,136] early hospital discharge on oral therapy versus continued hospitalization,[19] inpatient intravenous versus inpatient oral therapy,[21] and outpatient intravenous versus outpatient oral therapy.[61,109,114,117] Although each of these studies was limited by small sample sizes, a pediatric-stratified analysis of randomized trials and a pediatric-specific meta-analysis of prospective studies support the safety of outpatient management and oral antibiotic administration in low-risk children with fever and neutropenia.[100,132,156] In addition, outpatient management of low-risk febrile neutropenic patients is associated with a large reduction in health care costs compared with inpatient management.[136,156] Patients and parents both report that the home environment has a positive impact on physical activity, self-esteem, and family activities.[149] However, the acceptance of an outpatient management plan by patients and their caregivers is limited by the perception of reduced effectiveness of outpatient management[19,45,126] and the potential burden of outpatient care.[150] In a discrete choice experiment, Sung et al. found that an outpatient management plan that required three times a week clinic visits or a risk for readmission that was 7.5% or greater would not be tolerable to patients and families. These data highlight that as the standard of care for low-risk fever and neutropenia transitions from the inpatient to outpatient setting, it will be necessary to include families and patients in care decisions.

DIAGNOSTIC EVALUATION FOR PERSISTENT FEVER AND NEUTROPENIA

A primary concern in the patient with persistent fever and neutropenia despite broad-spectrum antibiotics is the possibility of an IFD, especially in those patients considered to be at high risk for IFD. There are often no specific clinical signs to suggest an IFD diagnosis, yield of routine blood cultures for yeasts such as *Candida* species ranges between 40% and 60%, and such cultures are not capable of reliably detecting some molds such as *Aspergillus* spp.[11] Thus there has been an increased focus on improving diagnostic modalities for detecting IFD in these patients. Two serum fungal biomarkers have received significant attention, galactomannan (GM) and β-D-glucan (BG).

The GM assay, developed to detect a cell wall component of *Aspergillus* spp., has been evaluated in a number of cohorts of patients with persistent fever and neutropenia.[13,24,28,37,44,49,71,130] Each of these cohorts had a different invasive aspergillosis incidence (i.e., pretest probability) ranging from 0% to 31%. The positive predictive value (i.e., posttest probability) from these cohorts ranged from 0% to 100%. In some reports the GM resulted in an improvement of pretest probability from approximately 4% to a posttest probability of greater than 70%.[13,24] Unfortunately, in other reports, the results of the GM assay added little diagnostic benefit over the pretest probability.[28,44,49,71,130] Interpreting the publications collectively, it is difficult to endorse routine use of the GM assay during periods of persistent fever and neutropenia. Clinicians should compare characteristics of their patient population to the cohorts studied in the aforementioned publications. If their patient population is similar to one of the cohorts in which the GM provided reasonable diagnostic improvement from pretest to posttest probability, then it would be reasonable to consider employing the GM assay as a diagnostic tool during fever and neutropenia. The other major limitation of GM is that it does not detect non-*Aspergillus* molds and thus comfort with discontinuation of mold-active antifungal therapy will vary depending on local epidemiology and provider preferences. Ultimately, prior to ordering a GM assay, a clinician needs to ask how a positive or negative result would change the provision of clinical care for the patient being tested.

The BG assay has the potential to detect a wide variety of invasive fungal pathogens with the exception of *Cryptococcus* and molds of the Mucorales order. This assay has been evaluated in three pediatric studies,[14,81,174] only one of which was exclusive to pediatric patients with persistent fever and neutropenia.[174] In this setting, the sensitivity and specificity of the BG assay were 82% with a resultant posttest probability of 49% in a cohort having a pretest probability of 16.9%.[174] It is difficult to extrapolate these results to populations in the United States because the assay used by the investigators is not the same as the assay commercially available in the United States. At this time, there are not enough data to support the routine use of the BG assay in children with persistent fever and neutropenia.

Polymerase chain reaction (PCR) testing represents another potential adjunctive diagnostic tool to detect an IFD. Both pan-fungal PCR and *Aspergillus*-specific PCR have been assessed in pediatric patients with fever and neutropenia. Similar to the GM assay, some of the reports suggest a reasonable improvement from pretest to posttest probability of disease,[48,93] whereas other studies showed little diagnostic benefit of a positive test relative to the pretest probability of an IFD.[26,42,69,86,98,130] As noted for the GM assay, these collective findings do not allow for an endorsement of routine fungal PCR analyses in children with fever and neutropenia.

Last, radiographic testing, such as systematic computed tomography (CT) imaging, has been proposed as a method to detect an infectious etiology of persistent fever and neutropenia. Evaluation of adult patients early in the course of prolonged fever and neutropenia suggested that a high-resolution CT scan of the chest with subsequent diagnostic intervention (e.g., bronchoalveolar lavage) has the potential to direct additional specific antimicrobial therapy[64] and to reduce the time to diagnosis of invasive pulmonary aspergillosis.[22] Pediatric data on the utility of systematic CT imaging of the sinuses, chest, abdomen, and pelvis in prolonged fever and neutropenia was assessed in a retrospective case series of 68 pediatric episodes. Only chest CT imaging provided clinically useful information resulting in an altered course of therapy in two patients.[2] A pilot study of a rapid protocol for magnetic resonance imaging (MRI) of the lung found comparable results of this modality to high-resolution CT scan.[148] However, the study size was too small to assess the impact of this modality on informing clinical decision making.

Regardless of the diagnostic modality, the challenge with interpreting the data on these adjunctive tools in the setting of prolonged fever and neutropenia is that, in previous studies, significant variation existed relative to patient populations, interpretations of positive assay threshold, type of test used, timing and frequency of testing, and definitions for IFD. It appears that no single diagnostic modality has proved ideal for directing the care of the pediatric patient with prolonged fever and neutropenia. It may be that a combination of diagnostic tests is necessary to best inform clinical practices. In an adult RCT, a preemptive antifungal therapy approach guided by clinical assessment, laboratory testing (e.g., GM testing), and chest imaging results was shown to be as effective as empiric antifungal therapy.[33] Future studies are necessary to confirm this as an appropriate approach for prolonged fever and neutropenia in children.

THERAPEUTIC ADJUSTMENTS FOR PROLONGED FEVER AND NEUTROPENIA

Adjustment of Empiric Antibiotic Therapy

There are few data to guide recommendations for adjusting antibiotic therapy in patients with prolonged fever and neutropenia with or without an identified source. One adult RCT found that the addition of vancomycin in patients with persistent fever and neutropenia receiving piperacillin-tazobactam monotherapy failed to provide benefit relative to fever resolution.[32] Both adult and pediatric guidelines agree that the persistence of fever alone is not an indication for expanding or modifying antibiotic coverage, assuming the patient remains clinically stable. In this setting, close monitoring is necessary to evaluate for changes in clinical status.[53,89] Signs of clinical deterioration (e.g., hypotension or respiratory distress) should prompt broadening of the antimicrobial regimen. The nature of the clinical change should dictate the specific addition or modification to the antimicrobial regimen.

An important question is the optimal time to discontinue antibiotics when fever has resolved and no pathogen has been identified. Retrospective[9,10,74,91] and prospective observational[31,108] and randomized[139] studies support the safety of antibiotic cessation after fever resolution with evidence of bone marrow recovery. However, there are limited data on stopping antibiotics prior to evidence of bone marrow recovery. In two small randomized trials of patients meeting low-risk criteria, there was no differences in the recurrence of symptoms for infection in patients continued on antibiotic therapy until neutrophil recovery versus cessation of empiric antibiotics.[78,139] However, in high-risk patients, cessation of antibiotics may be associated with worse outcomes. Pizzo et al. showed that if empiric antibiotics are stopped at 7 days in patients with resolution of fever but persistent neutropenia, there is a significant risk for return of fever and potential for death.[123] More recently, Micol et al. observed the outcomes of adults with AML and fever and neutropenia where antibiotics were discontinued after fever resolution.[105] The study was stopped after seven patients because three patients had return of fever, two had documented bacteremia, and one required intensive care monitoring. Future research is needed to compare the effectiveness of stopping antibiotics versus continuing until neutrophil recovery in both low- and high-risk populations.

In patients in whom there is documentation of an organism believed to be the source of fever, the antimicrobial regimen should be modified to target the identified organism. It is not clear whether it is necessary to retain broad-spectrum coverage appropriate for initial presentation of fever and neutropenia or whether it is possible to narrow the antibiotic regimen to the pathogen isolated while the patient is still neutropenic. Interestingly, 6% of pediatric AML patients will develop a secondary bacteremia despite continued antibiotic therapy for a bacteremia event presenting earlier in the neutropenic period.[160] Notably the second bacteremia events presented despite continued broad-spectrum antibiotic therapy. In the absence of definitive data, a reasonable approach would be to maintain broad-spectrum coverage if empiric therapy would otherwise be continued and to narrow therapy if criteria for cessation of empiric therapy are met. Future investigation of narrowing therapy in patients with an identified pathogen and clinical improvement but persistent neutropenia is necessary to determine whether this approach is safe.

Initiation of Antifungal Therapy

Initial prospective randomized data highlighted the success of empiric antifungal therapy in children with persistent fever and neutropenia despite broad-spectrum antibiotics.[122] As previously discussed, a number of publications have focused on identifying factors to assess risk for IFD and to leverage these risk factors to guide empiric antifungal therapy decisions. Current adult guidelines support the initiation of empiric antimold therapy in patients with persistent or recurrent fever lasting 4 to 7 days when the duration of neutropenia is anticipated to persist beyond 7 days.[53] Similarly the pediatric-specific guidelines have supported the initiation of empiric antifungal therapy patients after 96 hours of fever and neutropenia that is not responsive to broad-spectrum antibiotics when one of the following criteria are met: the duration of neutropenia is anticipated to last longer than 10 days; the patient has underlying AML, relapsed ALL, or is an allogeneic hematopoietic stem cell transplant (HSCT) recipient; or the patient has been exposed to high-dose steroids.[89] In patients not meeting one of these high-risk IFD criterion, it is reasonable to withhold empiric antimold therapy.

When initiating an empiric antimold agent, options include an amphotericin B product (amphotericin B deoxycholate, lipid complex amphotericin B, or liposomal amphotericin B), an echinocandin (anidulafungin, caspofungin, or micafungin), or an extended-spectrum azole (voriconazole or posaconazole). Pediatric prospective randomized trials have compared caspofungin to liposomal amphotericin B[97] and the latter to amphotericin B deoxycholate.[125] Although similar relative to efficacy outcomes, there were significantly fewer side effects associated with liposomal amphotericin B as compared to amphotericin B deoxycholate. Safety and efficacy comparisons showed no difference between caspofungin and liposomal amphotericin. Given these data, caspofungin or liposomal amphotericin are both appropriate first-line agents for empiric antifungal therapy. Second-generation triazoles represent alternative options for empiric mold therapy. However, the lack of pediatric-specific data for these agents limits the feasibility of their use. While voriconazole dosing recommendations are available for children 2 years of age and older, there is significant intra- and interpatient variability in voriconazole pharmacokinetics among the pediatric population.[75,144] Dosing recommendations for posaconazole do not exist for those younger than 13 years of age, and there are no pediatric dosing recommendations for isavuconazole. Finally, none of these azoles has been specifically studied as an empiric antimold therapeutic agent in children.

The empiric antifungal therapy approach for prolonged fever and neutropenia has been challenged because of the lack of specificity of prolonged fever and neutropenia as a marker for IFD, the potential to unnecessarily expose patients to toxicities associated with antifungal agents, and the increased costs in administering these agents for prolonged periods.[39,102] Although designation of high- and low-risk IFD status has reduced some unnecessary empiric therapy, it has not eliminated it. As noted previously, an alternate approach to empiric antifungal therapy is a preemptive strategy. In this approach, the results of a combination of adjunctive diagnostic studies (e.g., fungal biomarkers and CT scans) are utilized to inform the initiation of antifungal therapy. A retrospective analysis suggested that a preemptive approach in adult allogeneic HSCT recipients was feasible and had the potential to reduce antimold therapy exposure.[112] In an ensuing randomized trial of high-risk adult fever and neutropenia patients, Cordonnier et al. showed that a preemptive approach reduced the cost associated with antifungal therapy without a change in mortality. However, the preemptive approach was associated with a higher IFD rate.[33] Further refinement of a preemptive approach with a focus on pediatric cohorts is necessary before such a strategy can be adopted in children.

The appropriate time to discontinue empiric antifungal therapy has not been well defined. A conservative approach is to continue until resolution of neutropenia; this approach is supported by a recently published pediatric guideline, but in the absence of pediatric specific data.[89] Some clinicians perform CT scans at the time of neutropenia resolution and use this information to inform cessation of antifungal therapy. However, there are no data to document the clinical impact of this approach. Future research should focus on identifying the optimal criteria for cessation of antifungal treatment in the empiric setting.

PREVENTION MEASURES

Antibacterial Prophylaxis

Much effort has focused on determining the efficacy and safety of antibacterial prophylaxis in patients with cancer. In 2005, two large randomized placebo-controlled trials evaluated the efficacy of levofloxacin for preventing fever in patients with anticipated short and long periods of neutropenia.[20,36] These trials discovered that levofloxacin prophylaxis reduced the rates of fever and bacteremia during periods of anticipated prolonged neutropenia[20] and similarly reduced the rate of fever and infection during anticipated short periods of neutropenia.[36] Furthermore a meta-analysis of 95 randomized trials revealed a significant reduction in mortality when antibiotic prophylaxis was administered to neutropenic patients.[55] Based on these data, multiple adult guidelines support the use of fluoroquinolone prophylaxis.[53,88] However, the limited pediatric data regarding the utility of antibacterial prophylaxis[4] have precluded a similar pediatric recommendation. Furthermore potential negative consequences associated with prophylaxis, such as an increase in resistance among colonizing organisms or association with *Clostridium difficile* infection or IFD, were not adequately evaluated in the aforementioned large adult trials. Currently the Children's Oncology Group is conducting a trial to investigate the benefits of levofloxacin prophylaxis in high-risk children with neutropenia and intends to evaluate some of these important secondary outcomes.

Antifungal Prophylaxis

Prophylactic antifungal therapy has also been explored as a mechanism to reduce IFD in patients with neutropenia. The earliest adult trials showed fluconazole was efficacious as compared to placebo in reducing systemic and superficial fungal infections in bone marrow transplant recipients.[57,147] A subsequent meta-analysis suggested that the benefit of prophylactic fluconazole was realized in the setting of increased risk (>15%) for systemic fungal infection.[73] This meta-analysis appropriately highlighted the need to consider the prevalence of IFD when considering the impact of antifungal prophylaxis in a specific patient population. More recently, agents with anti-mold activity have been evaluated in the prophylactic setting. Vehreschild et al. showed, in a small cohort of adult AML patients, that voriconazole as compared to placebo was efficacious in reducing the rate of pulmonary infiltrates.[165] In additional adult-predominant clinical trials, fluconazole has been compared to posaconazole in patients with prolonged neutropenia,[34] to voriconazole in allogeneic stem cell transplant recipients,[171] and to micafungin in stem cell transplant recipients.[163] The former study revealed that posaconazole was efficacious at reducing invasive aspergillosis, whereas the latter studies suggested that voriconazole and micafungin prophylaxis trended toward improved protection against invasive aspergillosis as compared to fluconazole. Collectively these data have supported adult guideline recommendations to administer antifungal prophylaxis in patients considered high-risk for IFD. However, the different adult guidelines were not consistent as to when to administer fluconazole and when to escalate to antimold prophylaxis.[53,88]

Pediatric-specific data for antifungal prophylaxis from randomized clinical trials are not available. Based on the available adult data, pediatric guidelines support fluconazole prophylaxis during periods of neutropenia for children with AML and those receiving an allogeneic HSCT.[143] The benefits of broadening prophylaxis to include antimold coverage in a pediatric population are not yet well defined. Currently a randomized trial sponsored by the Children's Oncology Group is actively enrolling patients to compare the efficacy of caspofungin to fluconazole prophylaxis in pediatric patients with AML. The outcome of this study should inform the importance of antimold activity in a fungal prophylaxis regimen for patients at high risk for IFD.

Hospital Infection Control Practices

Children receiving chemotherapy represent a patient population at high-risk for hospital-acquired infection (HAI) because they often require prolonged hospital admissions during which they are immunosuppressed. Recently McCullers et al. documented the impact of HAIs at a single institution. Not unexpectedly, depth (<100/mm^3) and duration of neutropenia as well as prolonged length of stay were identified as risk factors for a HAI. Over the 26-year study period, they documented a decrease in the rate of HAIs that correlated with the implementation of various infection control initiatives.[104]

These data strongly support the potential impact of infection control practices in reducing HAI even in patients who are vulnerable to opportunistic infections. Important infection control practices often focus on interrupting the transmission of infectious pathogens from health care workers (HCW) to their patients. Such practices include programs to promote high compliance of hand hygiene and optimization of HCW influenza vaccination.[18,50,145] Enacting a mandatory vaccination policy has proved to result in near complete HCW vaccine coverage at a large children's hospital.[50] Furthermore devising a hospital plan to change the "working while sick culture" is of particular importance for HCWs attending to this patient population.[155] Finally, utilization of a protocol to screen visitors prior to entering the patient room can serve as a mechanism to reduce unnecessary patient exposures.

Despite the importance of infection control practices, there is likely significant variation in policies from one institution to the next, as well as variation in enforcement of policies within an institution. Enhanced efforts are needed to establish goals for reducing HAIs and to establish guidelines for standardized infection control practices specific to pediatric oncology patients in order to achieve these goals. It is also important to realize that infection control practices are important in the ambulatory setting because increasing proportions of care are being transitioned from the inpatient to the outpatient setting. Ultimately the institution of any standardized infection control practice should be accompanied by an institutional-level surveillance of HAIs to monitor the effectiveness of each intervention.

NEW REFERENCES SINCE THE SEVENTH EDITION

6. American Cancer Society. *Cancer Facts and Figures 2014*. Atlanta, GA: American Cancer Society; 2015.
15. Badiee P, Alborzi A, Karimi M, et al. Diagnostic potential of nested PCR, galactomannan EIA, and beta-D-glucan for invasive aspergillosis in pediatric patients. *J Infect Dev Ctries*. 2012;6:352-357.
24. Castagnola E, Furfaro E, Caviglia I, et al. Performance of the galactomannan antigen detection test in the diagnosis of invasive aspergillosis in children with cancer or undergoing haemopoietic stem cell transplantation. *Clin Microbiol Infect*. 2010;16:1197-1203.
25. Castelán-Martínez OD, Rodríguez-Islas F, Vargas-Neri JL, et al. Risk factors for febrile neutropenia in children with solid tumors treated with cisplatin-based chemotherapy. *J Pediatr Hematol Oncol*. 2016;38:191-196.
26. Cesaro S, Stenghele C, Calore E, et al. Assessment of the lightcycler PCR assay for diagnosis of invasive aspergillosis in paediatric patients with onco-haematological diseases. *Mycoses*. 2008;51:497-504.
28. Choi S-H, Kang E-S, Eo H, et al. *Aspergillus* galactomannan antigen assay and invasive aspergillosis in pediatric cancer patients and hematopoietic stem cell transplant recipients. *Pediatr Blood Cancer*. 2008;60:316-322.
37. de Mol M, de Jongste JC, van Westreenen M, et al. Diagnosis of invasive pulmonary aspergillosis in children with bronchoalveolar lavage galactomannan. *Pediatr Pulmonol*. 2013;48:789-796.
42. Dendis M, Horváth R, Michálek J, et al. PCR-RFLP detection and species identification of fungal pathogens in patients with febrile neutropenia. *Clin Microbiol Infect*. 2003;9:1191-1202.
44. Dinand V, Anjan M, Oberoi JK, et al. Threshold of galactomannan antigenemia positivity for early diagnosis of invasive aspergillosis in neutropenic children. *J Microbiol Immunol Infect*. 2016;49:66-73.
61. Gupta S, Bonilla M, Gamero M, et al. Microbiology and mortality of pediatric febrile neutropenia in El Salvador. *J Pediatr Hematol Oncol*. 2011;33:276-280.
62. Haeusler GM, Carlesse F, Phillips RS. An updated systematic review and meta-analysis of the predictive value of serum biomarkers in the assessment of fever during neutropenia in children with cancer. *Pediatr Infect Dis J*. 2013;32:e390-e396.
66. Hol JA, Wolfs TFW, Bierings MB, et al. Predictors of invasive fungal infection in pediatric allogeneic hematopoietic SCT recipients. *Bone Marrow Transplant*. 2014;49:95-101.
69. Hummel M, Spiess B, Roder J, et al. Detection of *Aspergillus* DNA by a nested PCR assay is able to improve the diagnosis of invasive aspergillosis in paediatric patients. *J Med Microbiol*. 2009;58:1291-1297.
70. Jain S, Kapoor G. Invasive aspergillosis in children with acute leukemia at a resource-limited oncology center. *J Pediatr Hematol Oncol*. 2015;37:e1-e5.
71. Jha AK, Bansal D, Chakrabarti A, et al. Serum galactomannan assay for the diagnosis of invasive aspergillosis in children with haematological malignancies. *Mycoses*. 2013;56:442-448.
72. Johnston DL, Lewis V, Yanofsky R, et al. Invasive fungal infections in paediatric acute myeloid leukaemia. *Mycoses*. 2013;56:482-487.
80. Kobayashi R, Kaneda M, Sato T, et al. The clinical feature of invasive fungal infection in pediatric patients with hematologic and malignant diseases: a 10-year analysis at a single institution at Japan. *J Pediatr Hematol Oncol*. 2008;30: 886-890.
81. Koltze A, Rath P, Schöning S, et al. β-D-Glucan screening for detection of invasive fungal disease in children undergoing allogeneic hematopoietic stem cell transplantation. *J Clin Microbiol*. 2015;53:2605-2610.
85. Lai H-P, Chen Y-C, Chang L-Y, et al. Invasive fungal infection in children with persistent febrile neutropenia. *J Formos Med Assoc*. 2005;104:174-179.
86. Landlinger C, Preuner S, Bašková L, et al. Diagnosis of invasive fungal infections by a real-time panfungal PCR assay in immunocompromised pediatric patients. *Leukemia*. 2010;24:2032-2038.
89. Lehrnbecher T, Phillips R, Alexander S, et al. Guideline for the management of fever and neutropenia in children with cancer and/or undergoing hematopoietic stem-cell transplantation. *J Clin Oncol*. 2012;30:4427-4438.
90. Lehrnbecher T, Phillips RS, Alexander S, et al. Guidelines for the management of fever and neutropenia in children with cancer and/or undergoing hematopoietic stem cell transplantation. *J Clin Oncol*. 2012;30:4427-4438.
93. Lin MT, Lu HC, Chen WL. Improving efficacy of antifungal therapy by polymerase chain reaction-based strategy among febrile patients with neutropenia and cancer. *Clin Infect Dis*. 2001;33:1621-1627.
98. Mandhaniya S, Iqbal S, Sharawat SK, et al. Diagnosis of invasive fungal infections using real-time PCR assay in paediatric acute leukaemia induction. *Mycoses*. 2012;55:372-379.
103. McCullers JA, Vargas SL, Flynn PM, et al. Candidal meningitis in children with cancer. *Clin Infect Dis*. 2000;31:451-457.
105. Micol J-B, Chahine C, Woerther P-L, et al. Discontinuation of empirical antibiotic therapy in neutropenic acute myeloid leukaemia patients with fever of unknown origin: is it ethical? *Clin Microbiol Infect*. 2014;20:O453-O455.
107. Mueller EL, Croop J, Carroll AE. Fever and neutropenia hospital discharges in children with cancer: a 2012 update. *Pediatr Hematol Oncol*. 2016;33:39-48.
110. Mutters NT, Günther F, Sander A, Mischnik A, Frank U. Influx of multidrug-resistant organisms by country-to-country transfer of patients. *BMC Infect Dis*. 2015;15:466.
111. Neemann K, Yonts AB, Qiu F, et al. Blood cultures for persistent fever in neutropenic pediatric patients are of low diagnostic yield. *J Pediatric Infect Dis Soc*. 2016;5:218-221.
112. Oshima K, Kanda Y, Asano-Mori Y, et al. Presumptive treatment strategy for aspergillosis in allogeneic haematopoietic stem cell transplant recipients. *J Antimicrob Chemother*. 2007;60:350-355.
113. Ozsevik SN, Sensoy G, Karli A, et al. Invasive fungal infections in children with hematologic and malignant diseases. *J Pediatr Hematol Oncol*. 2015;37:e69-e72.
120. Phillips RS, Sung L, Amman RA, et al. Predicting microbiologically defined infection in febrile neutropenic episodes in children: global individual participant data multivariable meta-analysis. *Br J Cancer*. 2016;114:623-630.
130. Reinwald M, Konietzka CAM, Kolve H, et al. Assessment of *Aspergillus*-specific PCR as a screening method for invasive aspergillosis in paediatric cancer patients and allogeneic haematopoietic stem cell recipients with suspected infections. *Mycoses*. 2014;57:537-543.
132. Robinson PD, Lehrnbecher T, Phillips R, et al. Strategies for empiric management of pediatric fever and neutropenia in patients with cancer and hematopoietic stem-cell transplantation recipients: a systematic review of randomized trials. *J Clin Oncol*. 2016;34(17):2054-2060.
135. Sandoval C, Sinaki B, Weiss R, et al. Urinary tract infections in pediatric oncology patients with fever and neutropenia. *Pediatr Hematol Oncol*. 2012;29:68-72.
140. Satwani P, Baldinger L, Freedman J, et al. Incidence of viral and fungal infections following busulfan-based reduced-intensity versus myeloablative conditioning in pediatric allogeneic stem cell transplantation recipients. *Biol Blood Marrow Transplant*. 2009;15:1587-1595.
143. Science M, Robinson PD, Macdonald T, et al. Guideline for primary antifungal prophylaxis for pediatric patients with cancer or hematopoietic stem cell transplant recipients. *Pediatr Blood Cancer*. 2013;61:393-400.
148. Sodhi KS, Khandelwal N, Saxena AK, et al. Rapid lung MRI in children with pulmonary infections: time to change our diagnostic algorithms. *J Magn Reson Imaging*. 2016;43:1196-1206.
150. Sung L, Alibhai SM, Ethier M-C, et al. Discrete choice experiment produced estimates of acceptable risks of therapeutic options in cancer patients with febrile neutropenia. *J Clin Epidemiol*. 2012;65:627-634.
153. Sung L, Nathan PC, Lange B, et al. Prophylactic granulocyte colony-stimulating factor and granulocyte-macrophage colony-stimulating factor decrease febrile neutropenia after chemotherapy in children with cancer: a meta-analysis of randomized controlled trials. *J Clin Oncol*. 2004;22:3350-3356.
155. Tanksley AL, Wolfson RK, Arora VM. Changing the "working while sick" culture: promoting fitness for duty in health care. *JAMA*. 2016;315:603-604.
158. Torres JP, Labraña Y, Ibañez C, et al. Frequency and clinical outcome of respiratory viral infections and mixed viral-bacterial infections in children with cancer, fever and neutropenia. *Pediatr Infect Dis J*. 2012;31:889-893.
160. Tran TH, Yanofsky R, Johnston DL, et al. Second bacteremia during antibiotic treatment in children with acute myeloid leukemia: a report from the Canadian Infections in Acute Myeloid Leukemia Research Group. *J Pediatr Infect Dis Soc*. 2014;3:228-233.
168. Ward E, DeSantis C, Robbins A, et al. Childhood and adolescent cancer statistics, 2014. *CA Cancer J Clin*. 2014;64:83-103.
169. Wattier RL, Dvorak CC, Hoffman JA, et al. A prospective, international cohort study of invasive mold infections in children. *J Pediatr Infect Dis Soc*. 2015;4:313-322.
170. Wiley JM, Smith N, Leventhal BG, et al. Invasive fungal disease in pediatric acute leukemia patients with fever and neutropenia during induction chemotherapy: a multivariate analysis of risk factors. *J Clin Oncol*. 1990;8:280-286.

The full reference list for this chapter is available at ExpertConsult.com.

Opportunistic Infections in Hematopoietic Stem Cell Transplantation

69

Christopher C. Dvorak • William J. Steinbach

Advances in supportive care continue to lead to improvements in hematopoietic stem cell transplant (HSCT) outcomes. The 1-year transplant-related mortality (TRM) rate for children with acute leukemia and unrelated donor HSCT performed before 1995 approached 40%. More recently, rates from 2003 to 2006 fell by more than half to approximately 15%,[137] and the 3-year TRM rate continues to fall, from 27% in 2000–04 to 21% in 2005–09.[139] Furthermore over the course of the past decade, utilization of umbilical cord blood units and haploidentical donors have become standard of care. This has led to significantly more alternative donor HSCTs performed for a wide variety of nonmalignant diseases, including T-cell and phagocyte primary immunodeficiencies, hemoglobinopathies, bone marrow failure syndromes, and metabolic syndromes. However, these children often have relatively intact immune systems at the time of HSCT and thus require increased pre-HSCT immunoablation to prevent graft rejection. This often leads to delays in post-HSCT immune reconstitution, which in turn is associated with significant opportunistic infections. In addition to causing significant morbidity and prolonged hospitalizations, opportunistic infections are directly responsible for 25% to 27% of transplant-related mortality following allogeneic HSCT.[178]

Evidence indicates that certain opportunistic infections may play a role in the triggering of alloreactivity and graft-versus-host disease (GVHD). For example, animal models suggest that administration of probiotics may alter the intestinal microflora and decrease inflammation in mesenteric lymph nodes, thereby abrogating GVHD,[72] and human studies have demonstrated that low intestinal microbial diversity at transplant is associated with poor survival, primarily due to the subsequent development of severe GVHD.[228] A randomized trial of fluconazole versus placebo demonstrated less severe GVHD of the intestinal tract in the fluconazole recipients, possibly as a result of decreased intestinal antigenic stimulation.[147] Some data suggest that both cytomegalovirus (CMV) and human herpesvirus–6 (HHV-6) reactivations can trigger the development of GVHD.[3,136,184] Because GVHD is another significant component of transplant-related mortality following allogeneic HSCT, further understanding of the interplay between opportunistic infections and initiation of GVHD may provide another avenue toward making HSCT a safer procedure with improved overall outcomes.

EPIDEMIOLOGY

Although opportunistic infections do occur after autologous HSCT, the much more profound and ongoing T-cell dysfunction that occurs before and after allogeneic HSCT makes opportunistic infections far more likely to occur in this population. Multiple therapy-induced alterations of host defenses contribute to this risk.[125] The three major contributors to the development of an opportunistic infection are (1) breakdown in natural barriers (e.g., indwelling central venous catheters and mucositis), (2) defects in cell-mediated immunity (e.g., lymphopenia from corticosteroids and other anti–T-cell cytotoxic agents), and (3) deficient numbers of phagocytes (e.g., as a result of myeloablative chemotherapy). Knowledge of the timing of the variety of infections that can occur after HSCT allows clinicians to develop rational approaches to antimicrobial prophylaxis, diagnostic monitoring for infections, and earlier treatment of proved infections. Classically three phases of risk for opportunistic infections occur after HSCT, as shown in Fig. 69.1.[231]

Phase I: Preengraftment (<30 Days)

Infections in phase I of HSCT are similar to those seen with other forms of profoundly myelosuppressive chemotherapy, and include gram-positive and gram-negative bacteremia, candidemia, invasive aspergillosis, and reactivation of herpes simplex virus contributing to oral mucositis. Administration of granulocyte-colony stimulating factor (G-CSF) during this period will shorten the time to recovery of neutrophils by several days and may decrease rates of documented infections.[55] However, less evidence exists that G-CSF improves infection-related or transplant-related mortality, and it may increase the incidence of acute GVHD.[233] Therefore only approximately 60% of HSCT centers use G-CSF routinely.[121]

Phase II: Early Postengraftment (30 to 100 Days)

Some infections in phase II are caused by a combination of persistent defects in the function of the patients' phagocytes (partly from the administration of corticosteroids to treat acute GVHD) and retention of central venous catheters, which can lead to gram-positive bacteremia and candidemia. Other infections are due to the ongoing relative and functional lymphopenia and involve reactivations of CMV and other double-stranded DNA (dsDNA) viruses, *Pneumocystis jiroveci,* or certain parasitic infections.

Phase III: Late Postengraftment (>100 Days)

Infections in phase III are generally caused by ongoing immunosuppressive therapy for the treatment of chronic GVHD, which also is associated with functional asplenia. Thus patients can develop infections with encapsulated bacteria, *P. jiroveci,* and dsDNA viruses. There is also an important second peak of invasive aspergillosis during this time.

MAJOR TYPES OF OPPORTUNISTIC INFECTIONS AFTER HEMATOPOIETIC STEM CELL TRANSPLANTATION

Bacterial

Classic Gram-Positive and Gram-Negative Bacteria

Bacterial infections after HSCT most commonly divide into gram-positive organisms originating from the skin or gastrointestinal tract and gram-negative organisms translocating from the gastrointestinal tract. The period of highest risk for bacterial bloodstream infections, especially with enteric gram-negative rods, is the pre-engraftment period,[33] during which the incidence of bacteremia can range from 21% to 34% and 21% to 58% for patients undergoing autologous and allogeneic HSCT, respectively, although some studies report no difference between the two groups.[28,30,32,34,166] In HSCT recipients, bloodstream infections before engraftment are a significant independent predictor of mortality.[1,187] Several studies have demonstrated that either host or donor polymorphisms in genes responsible for immunity may contribute to the risk for bacterial infections.[7,41,122,157,197,242]

Given the significant risk for developing bacteremia, it is surprising that there is little evidence that routine antibacterial prophylaxis plays a role in pediatric HSCT recipients. In adult patients undergoing HSCT, general consensus exists regarding the utility of a prophylactic quinolone with antipseudomonal activity[231] based on several small trials included in larger meta-analyses.[69,98] The rates of fever and bacteremia are significantly reduced in patients receiving levofloxacin, but the impact of prophylaxis on mortality is less clear.[26,69,98] Similar results have been reported using ciprofloxacin and vancomycin as a prophylactic regimen for autologous and allogeneic HSCT patients.[63,212] Few of the trials stringently evaluated rates of quinolone resistance, although one recent retrospective report suggested it has not increased in the era of routine prophylaxis.[163] All of these studies were done in adult patients; therefore

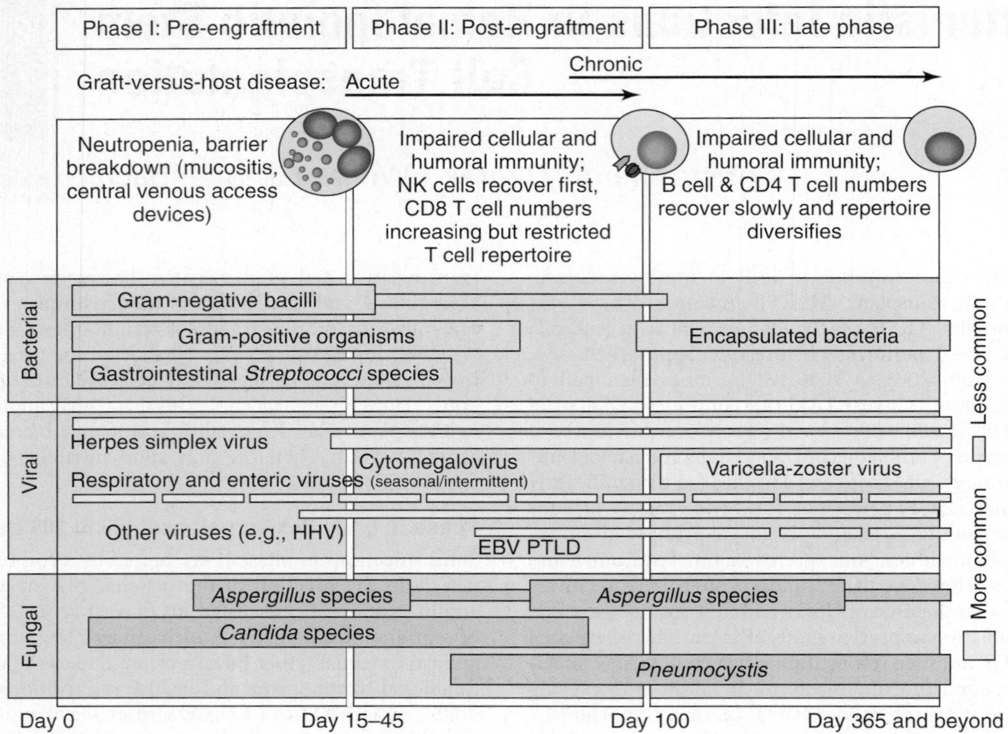

FIG. 69.1 The phases of opportunistic infections after allogeneic HSCT. *EBV*, Epstein-Barr virus; *HHV*, human herpesvirus; *NK*, natural killer; *PTLD*, posttransplant lymphoproliferative disease. (From Tomblyn M, Chiller T, Einsele H, et al. Guidelines for preventing infectious complications among hematopoietic cell transplantation recipients: a global perspective. *Biol Blood Marrow Transplant.* 2009;15:1143–238.)

caution must be used in applying the specific results to pediatric HSCT recipients. The Children's Oncology Group (COG) recently completed a large randomized trial in pediatric HSCT recipients, the pending results of which may inform future practice.

Other approaches to antibacterial prophylaxis use nonsystemic treatments to potentially spare medication toxicities and the development of resistant organisms. Chlorhexidine gluconate is an antiseptic bactericidal to gram-positive and gram-negative bacteria, including multidrug resistant organisms. The mechanism of action involves bacterial membrane disruption; its onset is relatively rapid, and the effect is persistent. A 2% chlorhexidine gluconate (CHG)–impregnated cloth product has been shown to be effective at decreasing central-line associated infections and acquisition of multidrug-resistant organisms as a skin cleansing product in the critical care setting in both adults[15,46,185,246] and children.[164] However, the effectiveness of CHG bathing outside of the critical care setting is controversial, with only one study showing a possible benefit[47] and another demonstrating increasing CHG-resistance.[227] An ongoing randomized trial by the COG may provide insight on the effectiveness and safety of CHG bathing on bloodstream infections in children undergoing HSCT. Similarly, because many cases of bacteremia are seen in the setting of central venous catheters, the use of ethanol lock solutions may potentially decrease central venous catheter colonization without the concern of resistance from antibiotic locks. However, results from randomized trials in adults receiving chemotherapy or HSCT have been controversial, with one demonstrating the benefit of ethanol locks versus heparin[204] and another showing no benefit.[265] Studies of prophylactic ethanol locks in pediatric HSCT recipients are currently lacking.

When patients develop a fever early after transplant during the neutropenic period, empirical antibacterial treatment is usually started. Although a variety of different regimens exist, they are generally tailored to cover *Streptococcus* spp. and *Staphylococcus* spp., plus enteric gram-negative organisms, based on local susceptibility patterns. Recent consensus statements have favored monotherapy, with combination therapy reserved for clinically unstable patients,[126] especially as additional reports suggest a role for anti-anaerobic antibiotics in decreasing intestinal diversity and subsequently altering immune reconstitution post-HSCT.[102]

Clostridium difficile

Although hardly unique to the pediatric HSCT population, because of the widespread use of broad-spectrum antibiotics for empirical therapy of febrile neutropenia *Clostridium difficile*–associated diarrhea is not uncommon. In adults, approximately 10% to 15% of patients may develop this complication within 30 days of HSCT,[113,257,267] although pediatric patients may behave differently, with later onset of disease.[24] The disease tends to be relatively mild, but relapses are very common.[105] Prevention of *C. difficile* may potentially be accomplished through the administration of certain strains of probiotics.[154] A small pilot trial suggests that this practice may be safe in the immediate post-HSCT phase, even during the period when a combination of neutropenia and compromised intestinal integrity could theoretically lead to the development of bacteremia from the ingested strain,[86] as long as the strain of probiotic is carefully considered.[119] Treatment of *C. difficile*–associated diarrhea in the pediatric HSCT patient is similar to that of the general population, with metronidazole or oral vancomycin, although caution must be used during the conditioning phase of HSCT, when metronidazole can enhance toxicities from radiation or busulfan.[83] Fidaxomicin is an attractive alternative due to lower rates of relapses (15% vs. 25%)[135] and potentially improved sparing of the intestinal microbiota,[134] which in turn may decrease incidence of severe GVHD. The experience with fecal microbiota transplant after HSCT is still very limited,[54] so it is unclear at this time whether that will ultimately prove to be a safe option.

Encapsulated Organisms

Patients with chronic GVHD appear to have defects in their splenic function, and thus encapsulated bacteria, such as *Streptococcus pneumoniae*, have been noted to cause significant mortality. Prophylaxis with penicillin appears to diminish this risk,[117] although the optimal duration of treatment is not yet defined. In patients with chronic GVHD (cGVHD), serum immunoglobulin G (IgG) levels should be monitored, and, for patients with levels of less than 400 mg/dL, administration of intravenous gammaglobulin should be considered.[231] When to stop penicillin prophylaxis in relation to resolution of cGVHD is unknown because robust methods to measure splenic function, such as pitted red blood cell percentage and nonswitched memory B cells,[120] have not been tested in a post-HSCT population.

Mycobacteria

Although less common than invasive fungal infections, infections with mycobacteria must always be considered in the differential diagnosis of pulmonary nodules after HSCT. In developed countries, classic *Mycobacterium tuberculosis* infections are very rare in children undergoing HSCT, although it always should be considered in patients whose households have recently immigrated.[70] More commonly encountered are environmental atypical nontuberculous mycobacteria (NTM), which can cause infections in the lungs, skin, lymph nodes, and bloodstream. Because of the relative rarity of NTM infections, a general paucity of literature exists in the HSCT population. NTM infections have been reported to occur in as many as 9.7% of T-cell depleted and 7% of conventional allogeneic HSCTs in adults, although the mortality rate was low.[256] Pediatric HSCT recipients have a somewhat lower rate of NTM infections (3.8%), which occur at a median of 115 days (range, 14 to 269 days) after HSCT,[237] while a more recent report suggests an even lower incidence (0.2%).[167]

The exact risk factors associated with the development of NTM infections after allogeneic HSCT are not well characterized. The protective immunity against NTM infections appears to be primarily driven by interferon-γ (IFN-γ) production by T cells, as evidenced by the high rate of NTM infections in patients with IFN-γ deficiency.[88] Thus T-cell depletion (ex vivo or with T-cell–depleting antibodies) or treatment of GVHD with immunosuppressants that block IFN-γ might be expected to be risk factors for the development of NTM infections. Similarly patients with an underlying T-cell immunodeficiency might be colonized with an NTM organism pre-HSCT that puts them at risk for developing NTM disease after HSCT. The optimal treatment of NTM infections is not clear. A wide variety of traditional antibiotics and antituberculosis agents have some activity against NTM organisms, but reports vary on the number of agents that must be used in combination and the duration of optimal therapy. In patients with human immunodeficiency virus (HIV) infection, the general recommendation is to treat most cases of NTM infections for 12 months after establishment of negative cultures.[82] It is not clear that such a prolonged duration is required for HSCT recipients who, in the absence of chronic GVHD, tend to have improvement in, and even normalization of, their T-cell function over time.

Fungal

Although bacteria represent the most common infection after HSCT, invasive fungal infections account for a significant amount of post-transplant mortality. Several retrospective reports on the development of invasive fungal infections in pediatric HSCT recipients have been published, with a 1-year incidence as high as 12% to 20% and a 58% to 83% mortality.[13,58,95,96,202] The most commonly identified invasive fungal organisms after HSCT are *Candida* and *Aspergillus* spp. Patients who are considered to be at the highest risk for developing an invasive fungal infection after HSCT are those who undergo transplant from either an unrelated donor (including umbilical cord blood) or a partially matched related donor or for treatment of a malignancy, bone marrow failure syndrome, or congenital immunodeficiency, and those receiving high-dose corticosteroids.[27,58,95,116,147,160,231]

Currently the use of antifungal prophylaxis is nearly universal in HSCT patients. Empirical therapy directed against resistant *Candida* or molds generally commences after approximately 72 hours of prolonged fevers despite administration of broad-spectrum antibacterials. One surprising feature to note from the original prophylactic fluconazole studies is that, even in the placebo arm, more than 80% of HSCT patients did not develop an invasive fungal infection, although these studies did include lower-risk autologous HSCT recipients.[77,218] This suggests that other explanations must exist for the development of invasive fungal infection after HSCT. Researchers are now finding that either host or donor polymorphisms in genes responsible for immunity appear to play a significant role in invasive fungal infection risk.[17,53,80,111,159,211,266] Most of these proposed genetic risk factors still require validation in a prospective multicenter cohort, but the future possibility of having different prophylactic strategies based on an a priori risk for developing an invasive fungal infection is promising.

Candida

Invasive candidiasis tends to occur during the neutropenic period immediately after HSCT, although later cases can occur in the setting of GVHD and prolonged immunosuppression, especially when central venous catheters are still in place. Typically invasive candidiasis originates from endogenous *Candida* spp. colonizing patients' gastrointestinal tracts.[49] Pediatric patients appear to have relatively more invasive infections caused by *C. parapsilosis* and fewer infections caused by *C. glabrata,* in contrast to adults.[140] Two placebo-controlled trials from the early 1990s, performed in patients older than 12 years of age undergoing autologous or allogeneic HSCT, demonstrated that prophylactic administration of fluconazole significantly decreased invasive fungal infections.[77,217] Long-term follow-up of allogeneic HSCT recipients given fluconazole prophylaxis supports a survival benefit (mortality 20% in the fluconazole arm vs. 35% in the placebo arm; $P = .004$), postulated to be at least partly due to less severe GVHD in the fluconazole recipients from decreased antigenic stimulation,[147] which may be mediated by T_H17 polarization in response to components of the fungal cell wall.[238] The classic duration of fluconazole prophylaxis administration is during the high-risk period until 75 days after HSCT.[145,147] Because fluconazole does not cover *C. krusei* and has variable activity against *C. glabrata,* alternative agents should be considered for patients known to be colonized with these species. Reasonable options include extended-spectrum triazoles, echinocandins, and lipid-formulations of amphotericin B (LFAB), all of which also have some coverage against *Aspergillus* spp.

When patients develop invasive candidiasis after HSCT, the most common site of infection is the bloodstream. In addition to initiation of appropriate antifungal agents, the standard practice is to discontinue all central venous catheters in patients with candidemia.[189] Less common, but more perplexing, disseminated *Candida* infections of the liver, spleen, or lungs can often be blood culture–negative and may require tissue biopsy to establish a diagnosis. Serum β-glucan levels may be useful for identifying cases of possible invasive candidiasis once the assay has been optimized for use in children.[220] Furthermore in patients with disseminated candidiasis, a formal ophthalmologic evaluation is recommended to rule out *Candida* endophthalmitis, which may require intravitreal injection of antifungal agents to preserve vision.[195] For treatment of invasive candidiasis, especially those cases that develop on fluconazole prophylaxis, the echinocandins are a class of antifungal agents that target β-(1,3)-D-glucan synthase and interrupt biosynthesis of the glucan polymers that make up fungal cell walls. Because mammalian cells do not possess cell walls, echinocandin administration to human patients has generally resulted in limited toxicity. Echinocandins possess fungicidal activity against most *Candida* spp.; however, *C. paraspiliosis* may be less sensitive.[5] In some settings, the echinocandins may be superior to fluconazole[191] or amphotericin B[165] for treatment of invasive candidiasis.

Aspergillus

In adult HSCT recipients, *Aspergillus* spp. time of infection has a bimodal distribution, with a first peak at a median of 16 days and the second at a median of 96 days after allogeneic HSCT.[239,241] This second peak may be less pronounced in children.[32] Invasive aspergillosis can be one of the most devastating infections to occur after allogeneic HSCT. In a multivariate analysis of risk factors for mortality among a modern cohort of pediatric patients with invasive aspergillosis, the major risk factor for death was the development of invasive aspergillosis after an allogeneic HSCT.[27] Although treatment options for invasive aspergillosis have increased in recent years, significant attention also has been paid to preventing invasive aspergillosis infections. Although fluconazole prophylaxis has been shown to reduce the risk for invasive fungal infection relative to placebo, fluconazole lacks activity against *Aspergillus* spp.

Given this lack of antimold activity, several trials have compared fluconazole to mold-active agents in hopes of decreasing rates of invasive aspergillosis. The first of these trials compared fluconazole to low-dose conventional deoxycholate amphotericin B (D-AMB).[263] However, D-AMB did not show improvement over fluconazole and resulted in a higher adverse event rate. Several trials, including one in children,[199] have evaluated the LFAB (often given only three times per week) for antifungal prophylaxis in HSCT and acute leukemia patients.[110,153,181] However, like D-AMB, LFAB has not been shown superior to fluconazole in overall success and typically demonstrates increased side effects.

Extended-spectrum triazoles such as itraconazole, voriconazole, and posaconazole do possess anti-*Aspergillus* activity[5]; however, clear limitations exist to each as a potential prophylactic agent. Several trials of itraconazole versus fluconazole have been performed, and a meta-analysis showed significantly less invasive fungal infections,[244] but because of its common gastrointestinal side effects, greater drug interactions, and poor tolerability,[145] itraconazole prophylaxis has generally been abandoned in children. The results of a multicenter, double-blinded trial showed that voriconazole was not superior to fluconazole in the prevention of invasive fungal infection, although the safety profile was similar.[260] Given voriconazole's broader spectrum of activity, this result was surprising but may have been due to an incomplete understanding of the complex pharmacokinetics of voriconazole. In adults and children over the age of 12 years, voriconazole has nonlinear pharmacokinetics with relatively well-established dosing regimens. Even in adults, however, recent studies have questioned standard dosing regimens and have proposed dosing based on serum drug levels,[177,221,232] with an optimal goal serum voriconazole level of 1 to 5.5 μg/L. Part of this variability may be due to allelic polymorphisms of the gene encoding for cytochrome (CYP)2C19, which can result in an increase or decrease in voriconazole metabolism,[177] and basing dosing on CYP2C19 genotype can improve the number of patients in the target range.[229] In children, the situation is further complicated by linear voriconazole kinetics, so that younger children may need significantly higher dosages of voriconazole.[67,107,169] Voriconazole also has significant drug interactions with commonly used agents in a pediatric HSCT population. Voriconazole is a substrate of CYP2CP (major), 2C19 (major), and 3A4 (minor) and an inhibitor of 2C9 (moderate), 2C19 (weak), and 3A4 (moderate).[52] Proton pump inhibitors increase voriconazole levels, while voriconazole increases serum levels and toxicity of corticosteroids, imatinib, and many other medications.[52] The approved voriconazole label reports that concomitant use of voriconazole can cause a 1.7- to 3-fold increase in cyclosporine or tacrolimus levels and recommends that the dosing of cyclosporine be decreased by 50% and the dosing of tacrolimus be decreased by 66% of the normal dose. Furthermore the use of voriconazole with sirolimus is officially contraindicated, and when its use has been reported, investigators have recommended dropping the levels of sirolimus by 90% of original dosing at the time of initiation of voriconazole.[150] Finally extended use of voriconazole has been linked to fluoride-induced periostitis[9] and severe phototoxicity, including development of nonmelanoma skin cancers.[216]

Posaconazole is a triazole with broad coverage of most fungi, including mucormycosis (previously called zygomycosis).[5] In a trial of adult patients with neutropenia, posaconazole prophylaxis was superior to fluconazole or itraconazole but was also associated with an increased risk for serious adverse events.[51] In a trial of teenagers and adults receiving treatment for acute or chronic GVHD, posaconazole was superior to fluconazole at preventing breakthrough and death from invasive fungal infection, with similar rates of toxicity.[236] Unfortunately this did not translate to improved overall survival. Posaconazole also shares many of the same enzymatic pathways—and therefore drug interactions—as voriconazole, albeit without the bone and skin toxicities.

Isavuconazole is the newest triazole and, like posaconazole, has broad coverage of invasive fungi. A phase 3 trial for treatment of invasive molds demonstrated noninferiority to voriconazole and lower rates of toxicities, including hepatotoxicity, visual disorders, and skin disorders.[138] It has also been used successfully as prophylaxis in neutropenic adult patients with acute myeloid leukemia (AML) in a phase II trial.[50] It has excellent bioavailability regardless of food intake and is also available intravenously, with early suggestions that therapeutic drug level monitoring may not be required. However, it still has moderate inhibition of CYP3A4, and modifications of GVHD prophylaxis agents will be required. Finally pediatric experience and dosing information is currently extremely limited. Because of the CYP interactions, azole prophylaxis when used is generally started after the conditioning regimen is complete. For patients who enter the HSCT period being treated for a preexisting invasive fungal infection, discontinuation of azoles 72 hours before the start of conditioning chemotherapy is often done to allow the CYP enzymes to return to baseline function, although some data suggest that fluconazole coadministration may actually help with cyclophosphamide metabolism and decrease toxicity.[241]

Echinocandins possess fungistatic activity against *Aspergillus* spp.[5] In a prophylactic antifungal trial, micafungin demonstrated reduced need for empirical antifungal therapy and an improved safety profile in contrast to fluconazole.[240] However, the number of pediatric subjects enrolled was small ($n = 84$), and a reduction in the incidence of proved or probable invasive fungal infection was not demonstrated. The lack of impact on invasive fungal infection may have been because the incidence of breakthrough invasive fungal infections in both groups was very low, likely as a result of the inclusion of low-risk patients (46% autologous HSCT recipients) and very few patients undergoing umbilical cord blood transplant ($n = 30$). Caspofungin has been shown to be at least equivalent to itraconazole in the setting of antifungal prophylaxis,[152] with few caspofungin-related adverse events.[45] The COG is conducting a large multicenter prospective trial in the pediatric HSCT population in North America. The major disadvantages to widespread echinocandin use are cost and the lack of an oral formulation.

If prophylaxis fails, the typical locations where invasive aspergillosis develops after an allogeneic HSCT are the lungs and sinuses, with not uncommon seeding of the brain. It should be noted that children do not always display the classic radiographic findings seen in adults with invasive aspergillosis, such as the air crescent or halo signs,[27] and a high index of suspicion must be maintained. Much attention has been focused on developing noninvasive tests for diagnosing invasive aspergillosis. Galactomannan is a polysaccharide cell-wall component released by *Aspergillus* during growth. The Platelia EIA *Aspergillus* galactomannan assay was approved by the U.S. Food and Drug Administration in 2003 for use in adult patients and, in 2006, in children.[183] Early large-scale clinical testing included few children, but available data suggest that detection values for adult patients can be extrapolated to children.[89,225] Serum β-D-glucan (found in all fungi except *Cryptococcus* spp. and mucormycosis) can be detected using an approved diagnostic serum assay and has been found to have high specificity and high positive predictive values for the detection of invasive fungal infection in adults.[173] However, data on the performance of this assay in children are limited, especially in the post-HSCT setting.[220] Ultimately obtaining cultures through bronchial alveolar washings or biopsy is the best way to be certain of what organism is being treated. Speciation of the *Aspergillus* is also important if polyene therapy is planned because of the intrinsic resistance of *Aspergillus terreus* to amphotericin B.[56]

Based on a pivotal trial performed in teenagers and adults, voriconazole has become the standard therapy for patients with invasive aspergillosis,[91] although the recent success of the apparently less toxic and erratic isavuconazole may alter this approach.[138] Because of the high mortality rate of invasive aspergillosis in post-HSCT patients, there has been great enthusiasm for potentially synergistic combination therapies, such as with a triazole and an echinocandin,[143] and a prospective trial suggested that this combination was safe and more effective than a triazole alone in some specific patients with proven infections.[146] If amenable to a surgical approach, strong consideration should be made for resection of cases of invasive aspergillosis, which has been shown to improve mortality if disease is precariously located near a major vessel.[27] During the neutropenic period in patients who develop invasive aspergillosis, transfusions of irradiated random donor granulocytes have been proposed as a method to improve outcomes, although conclusive proof that this laborious procedure is beneficial is lacking, although a recent trial suggested some benefit if the infused cell doses were high.[188] Finally exciting work has demonstrated the importance of adaptive immunity to fighting invasive aspergillosis.[90] Based on this, work has been done on creating *Aspergillus*-specific T cells for use in adoptive immunotherapy. It has been demonstrated that a cohort of patients who developed invasive aspergillosis after haploidentical HSCT and who received *Aspergillus*-specific T cells had significantly better resolution of the infection than a similar cohort not given the specific T cells.[182]

Rare Fungi

Less frequently, infections occur with the agents of mucormycosis (*Mucor, Rhizopus,* and *Absidia* spp.), *Trichosporon* spp., *Fusarium* spp., and other saprophytic fungi.[144,194,255] For these rare fungi, the key is to obtain culture identification, by biopsy if necessary, so that the optimal antifungal agent may be initiated. Posaconazole is a triazole with broad coverage of most fungi, including mucormycoses[5] and thus may be the optimal treatment for many of these organisms despite all of the caveats mentioned earlier regarding this agent. The newer agent isavuconazole also has activity against mucormycosis.[138] Recent work has demonstrated that Mucorales-specific T cells are generated after an infection with these organisms and thus might be useful as a diagnostic marker,[186] but also suggested that generation of similar cells for treatment of Mucorales infections may one day be possible.

Pneumocystis jiroveci

Previously referred to as *Pneumocystis carinii, Pneumocystis jiroveci* refers to the distinct species that infects humans. The abbreviation PCP (or now PJP) is often used to refer to pneumocystic pneumonia. PJP reactivations or infections are generally thought to be preventable after HSCT with administration of prophylaxis with trimethoprim-sulfamethoxazole (TMP-SMX). However, in the setting of alternative prophylaxis agents or TMP-SMX noncompliance, episodes of PJP may rarely occur beginning about 2 months after HSCT and continuing through recovery of T-cell functional immunity and is associated with increased mortality.[259]

TMP acts by interference with the bacterial dihydrofolate reductase, inhibiting synthesis of tetrahydrofolic acid and thus nucleic acid synthesis. Because of concerns about bone marrow toxicity, TMP-SMX is often held for several weeks after HSCT until evidence of neutrophil recovery, although this practice has been challenged.[66] The necessary amount of TMP-SMX required to prevent PJP has not been well studied, and a variety of dosing regimens exist, with administration 2 or 3 days per week being the most common.[231] Generally TMP-SMX is continued for at least 6 months after an allogeneic HSCT, although this should be lengthened for patients receiving ongoing immunosuppressive therapy.[234] In addition to possible bone marrow suppression, many patients have allergic or other reactions to TMP-SMX that induce clinicians to prematurely discontinue its use. However, the optimal second-line prophylactic agent is not well defined, and all options may be potentially less effective than TMP-SMX. Options that have been used include oral dapsone, intravenous or inhaled pentamidine, and oral atovaquone. Dapsone is inexpensive but has a high incidence of adverse events, especially in patients with glucose-6-phosphate deficiency.[205] Intravenous pentamidine given every 4 weeks also has been used, although inadequate protection has been noted in children under 2 years of age and those undergoing HSCT,[112] who may need more frequent dosing.[129] Aerosolized pentamidine is generally well tolerated, other than occasional bronchospasm, but its effectiveness has been questioned.[245] Atovaquone is generally well tolerated, but absorption can be limited in patients not eating diets containing fatty foods. In vitro, the echinocandin class of antifungal agents appear to have some activity against the cyst form of *P. jiroveci*. To date, no studies have evaluated the use of echinocandins as a solitary prophylaxis agent; however, a few case reports have described its potential utility in combination with TMP-SMX for the treatment of PJP.[2,12]

PJP must be suspected in HSCT patients presenting with hypoxemia (often disproportionally more severe than the degree of hypercapnia), dyspnea, cough, fever, and bilateral infiltrates,[215,234] especially if noncompliance is suspected or alternative prophylaxis agents have been used. Although it is highly sensitive in patients with HIV infection, measuring the serum lactate dehydrogenase level is less useful in other immunocompromised patients because of low levels of sensitivity and specificity.[250] Serum β-D-glucan levels could potentially be very useful for identifying cases of PJP once the assay has been optimized for use in children.[220] Until then, the definitive diagnosis of PJP still requires identification of the organism on special stains or polymerase chain reaction (PCR) of induced sputum or bronchoalveolar lavage fluid.[215] Once PJP is identified, the treatment of choice is high-dose TMP-SMX (15 to 20 mg TMP/kg per day divided every 6 hours).[217] This high-dose TMP-SMX may be difficult to administer to a patient recovering from HSCT with marginal bone marrow reserves. Therefore some physicians have used folinic acid "rescue," analogous to what is used after methotrexate administration, with the hypothesis that bacteria are unable to take up the folinic acid from the environment and thus only the host bone marrow cells are helped. Although no data exist in children undergoing HSCT, caution should be used with this approach because it has been associated with increased treatment failures in patients with HIV infection.[203] Although counterintuitive in a patient with poor T-cell function, TMP-SMX has been combined with a short course of corticosteroids, which appears to be beneficial in preventing temporary worsening of hypoxemia resulting from inflammation caused by dying organisms. The recommended dose is prednisone 1 mg/kg per dose twice daily (maximum 40 mg twice daily) (or the equivalent dose of methylprednisolone) tapered in half after 5 days and then again in another 5 days, then discontinued after 21 days.[106] It should be noted that these data derive solely from the HIV literature in adults, and it is unclear whether this approach is safe or beneficial in pediatric HSCT patients.

Viral

Viral infections after pediatric HSCT can be divided into two broad categories: DNA viruses that occur as a result of reactivation of a previous infection (and occasionally as a de novo infection) and community-acquired respiratory as well as enteric viruses. Other than donor and recipient serostatus, the major risk factor for reactivation of a dsDNA viral infection after HSCT is the use of T-cell depletion, either ex vivo or in vivo with serotherapy.[48,168,176] Recently a few polymorphisms in host immune response genes also have been shown to possibly contribute to the development of dsDNA viral infections after HSCT.[21,22,101]

Herpes Family Viruses

Herpes simplex virus. Herpes simplex virus–1 (HSV-1) and HSV-2 infections after HSCT usually occur as a result of reactivations from a previously acquired latent virus. Thus, pretransplant serologies are very useful in identifying at-risk patients. Because acquisition of HSV occurs as patients age, many pediatric HSCT recipients will be seronegative. In the era before routine prophylaxis of seropositive patients, reactivation rates were approximately 70% to 80% and significantly contributed to post-HSCT mucositis.[206] Dissemination of HSV to the lungs, liver, or brain is also possible. Routine acyclovir prophylaxis is usually given during the period of mucositis, and, with this, HSV reactivations are relatively rare[76] and screening of serum by PCR is likely of little benefit.[179] However, severely immunocompromised individuals can continue to develop reactivations for many months after HSCT, and thus some centers will continue prophylaxis for up to 6 months,[133] a typical period for development of T-cell reconstitution in the absence of GVHD. This is not needed for patients who receive ganciclovir for CMV prophylaxis because ganciclovir also has activity against HSV.[78] In addition, some strains of HSV have become acyclovir-resistant, and thus patients with mucositis more severe than anticipated should have a lesion swabbed for HSV culture and resistant strains treated with either foscarnet or cidofovir.[68,231]

Routine acyclovir prophylaxis does not appear to have a role in HSV-seronegative patients, although consideration of varicella zoster virus (VZV) serostatus also must be taken into account. Furthermore patients with B-cell immunodeficiencies may be unable to mount an antibody response before HSV infection and should be considered for prophylaxis, especially if close contacts such as the parents or siblings have a history of HSV infections.

Cytomegalovirus. Historically one of the most severe complications of allogeneic HSCT was CMV infection. In the modern era, the use of PCR-based detection strategies has significantly reduced the incidence of CMV disease. More than 50% of healthy adults in the United States are CMV seropositive, and the incidence increases with age, with 36% of children 6 to 11 years of age already exposed.[224] With the use of

CMV-negative blood products, the rate of de novo infection in CMV-seronegative donor and recipient (D^-R^-) pairs after HSCT is as low as 2%.[171] Thus most infections occur as a result of reactivations, likely of host CMV, because infections are much less common in donor-positive, recipient-negative (D^+R^-) transplants than in those in which the recipient is positive (D^+R^+ or D^-R^+).[171] Other factors can alter the risk for reactivation in a CMV-seropositive HSCT recipient. Data are conflicting on whether CMV-seropositive donors should be chosen for CMV-seropositive recipients in regard to decreasing mortality, although it does appear to result in lower rates of CMV reactivation and disease.[207,235] After autologous HSCT, CMV reactivations are not uncommon, but CMV disease is rare[261] except in the setting of CD34 selection. T-cell depletion of donor cells in the allogeneic HSCT setting is a major risk factor for reactivation, which may occur even before neutrophil engraftment.[92,239] GVHD and its treatment with corticosteroids, and poor T-cell reconstitution even in the absence of GVHD, are major risk factors for CMV reactivation.[20] Of interest, even in the absence of serotherapy, the choice of GVHD prophylaxis regimen may alter the risk for CMV reactivation. Sirolimus, an inhibitor of mammalian (or mechanistic) target of rapamycin (mTOR), appears to provide a protective effect against CMV when used in combination with tacrolimus and in place of other agents.[149] It remains to be determined if this effect is due to direct inhibition of CMV viral replication from sirolimus or enhanced reconstitution of anti-CMV immunity.[149] Overall as many as 65% of seropositive allogeneic HSCT recipients will develop CMV reactivation if not given specific prophylaxis.[60]

Several agents have been used for CMV prophylaxis in at-risk patients (D–R– patients are typically excluded). Because acyclovir has some in vitro activity against CMV, high-dose acyclovir (500 mg/m^2 per dose three times daily) has been shown to prevent CMV.[158,162] Because of its improved absorption, valacyclovir may be superior to high-dose acyclovir for the long-term prevention of CMV reactivation.[132] Ganciclovir is the most commonly used CMV prophylactic agent.[231] As a result of its marrow-suppressive qualities, it is typically started after neutrophil engraftment,[18,262] although some have suggested a role for a therapeutic window during the pre-HSCT conditioning.[162] In addition, ganciclovir use may partially inhibit recovery of both normal and CMV-specific T-cell function.[10] Other agents, including brincidofovir[151] and letermovir,[40] have had promising results as CMV prophylaxis in phase II studies; however, randomized phase III results are not yet available. In patients at high risk for early CMV reactivation before neutrophil recovery, foscarnet has been used because of its lack of significant marrow suppression, although it does have significant renal toxicity.[8] If prophylaxis is to be used, it is typically continued for 100 days after HSCT,[231] but longer courses may be indicated for patients with significantly impaired immune systems. All of these prophylactic strategies are generally used in combination with screening for reactivation by serum PCR.[231] An argument against CMV prophylaxis, at least in certain patient populations, is that CMV reactivation has been shown to be protective against relapse in patients with AML[64] undergoing myeloablative conditioning,[141] possibly from stimulating a graft-versus-leukemia effect. However, due to the increased risk of TRM associated with the CMV itself, this benefit does not produce any difference in overall survival.[81] Because all of the anti-CMV agents have some degree of toxicity, the alternative strategy to prophylaxis is preemptive treatment based on detection of CMV viremia. A randomized trial comparing prophylaxis versus preemptive management of CMV showed similar outcomes.[18] Patients are screened at least once weekly for CMV DNA and specific antiviral therapy begun once a threshold amount of virus has been detected. Ganciclovir is the most common first-line agent used,[231] although foscarnet can be considered in patients with poor marrow reserve.[193] Even in patients with good marrow function, ganciclovir can cause neutropenia, and its use requires monitoring of neutrophil counts and often support with G-CSF.[231] Typically ganciclovir is given twice daily for a minimum of 2 weeks, or longer for patients whose viremia is still detectable after 2 weeks.[18] Daily maintenance ganciclovir therapy also has been used in patients at high risk for a second reactivation because of poor immune recovery. The duration of maintenance therapy can vary from 4 weeks after the first negative PCR result or up to day 100. Oral valganciclovir has become more widely used for preemptive therapy, either as a first-line agent or to replace intravenous ganciclovir at the time of switching to maintenance therapy.[61] Early in the treatment course, CMV viral loads may rise, but in antiviral-naïve patients this is typically not a sign of resistance. However, continuing increases in viral loads after 2 weeks of therapy or signs of CMV disease should raise suspicion for a resistant strain of CMV. Mutations in the *CMV UL97* phosphotransferase gene typically cause resistance only to ganciclovir, so foscarnet and cidofovir remain alternative agents.[35,57] Mutations in the UL54 viral DNA polymerase will cause resistance to ganciclovir, and cidofovir, and, occasionally, foscarnet.[57] For the patient who appears be to failing or intolerant of all three drugs, leflunomide is a third-line alternative.[59] Leflunomide is an immunomodulatory agent that inhibits pyrimidine synthesis and results in both antiproliferative and antiinflammatory effects. The active metabolite appears to inhibit replication of both CMV and human polyomavirus type I, commonly referred to as BK virus.

The role of CMV-specific antibodies, either in conventional gammaglobulin products or high-titer products, is of debatable efficacy. On the other hand, efforts to produce donor-derived CMV-specific T cells have shown great promise in treating CMV disease.[62] Given the low rates of GVHD associated with these cells, they may be an upcoming preventive strategy.[182] Furthermore the techniques that enable generation of CMV-specific T cells also can be used to generate T cells active against Epstein-Barr virus (EBV) and adenoviruses,[73,87] as well as potentially HHV-6, BK virus, and others. These multivirus-specific cells represent an exciting avenue of adoptive immunotherapy in severely immunocompromised post-HSCT patients, although they are not yet available outside of single-center research protocols.

Epstein-barr virus. EBV infection after HSCT usually results from the reactivation of latent EBV in either residual host B cells or passively transferred donor B cells. As with other herpes family viruses, pre-HSCT serologies can help identify at-risk patients; however, because approximately 95% of adults are seropositive,[14] virtually all patients undergoing adult unrelated-donor HSCT are potentially susceptible. Unlike other herpes family viruses, no clearly effective antiviral agent exists against EBV and thus no post-HSCT prophylaxis strategy exists. Fortunately the rate of EBV reactivation in patients receiving T-replete grafts is quite low. Conversely patients who receive ex vivo T-cell–depleted stem cells, anti–T-cell serotherapy, and umbilical cord blood grafts have an elevated risk.[75] EBV reactivation can lead to the development of posttransplant lymphoproliferative disease (PTLD), signs and symptoms of which can include fever, lymphadenopathy, fulminate sepsis, or mass lesions in lymph nodes, spleen, or central nervous system. Several histologic subtypes exist, and all generally occur within the first 3 to 6 months of the posttransplant period. The first step to be undertaken once an EBV infection is suspected is to reduce immunosuppression when possible.[226] If that fails, because EBV proliferates primarily within B cells, administration of rituximab often is successful at eliminating the infection.[253] Copy numbers of EBV in the blood can be easily monitored after HSCT by PCR (although rare cases of PTLD without EBV viremia have been noted), and routine monitoring of high-risk patients is recommended.[231] Less clear, however, is exactly what threshold level should be used for initiation of preemptive therapy because some patients will have transient self-limited EBV viremia after HSCT.[253] Nevertheless evidence suggests that preemptive rituximab for treatment of EBV viremia is more effective than initiation once PTLD is established,[226] and mortality of PTLD in HSCT recipients is low.[71] Some groups have established methods for enriching for EBV-cytotoxic T lymphocytes, which can both prevent and treat EBV PTLD in high-risk patients with little risk for causing GVHD.[155] For centers without access to specific donor T cells, the fact that most donors are EBV seropositive allows the use of unmanipulated donor lymphocyte infusion, which is often effective, albeit with a high risk for inducing GVHD.[93,172]

Varicella zoster virus. With the advent of routine vaccination against VZV at 1 year of age, the majority of immunocompetent patients entering HSCT are seropositive for VZV. In the absence of prophylaxis, reactivations occur in approximately 30% of patients after HSCT[19] regardless of whether myeloablative or reduced intensity conditioning is used.[16] A double-blinded trial of acyclovir prophylaxis given for 1 year after HSCT demonstrated a significant reduction in VZV reactivations, although this duration of treatment was inadequate in patients who continued on immunosuppressive therapy for treatment of chronic GVHD.[19] An unresolved question is whether pediatric HSCT recipients who are VZV seropositive before HSCT as a result of prior live-attenuated vaccination, rather than exposure to wild-type VZV, are at a high enough risk for reactivation to warrant long-term prophylaxis. Several case reports suggest that the live-attenuated strain is capable of causing zoster and even disseminated disease in immunocompromised children.[38,128] Therefore, until new data are available, the recommendation for acyclovir prophylaxis should be applied to all VZV-seropositive patients.

For post-HSCT patients who are exposed to an individual with active wild-type VZV infection (including shingles) and are not receiving prophylactic acyclovir or intravenous immunoglobulin (IVIG), passive immunization with varicella zoster immunoglobulin should be initiated within 96 hours of exposure.[231] There does not appear to be a significant rate of transmission of live-attenuated vaccine strain VZV to immunocompromised individuals, and thus household contacts of HSCT recipients are allowed to receive the vaccine, although optimally it should be given before the HSCT when possible.[231]

According to the 2011 Centers for Disease Control and Prevention (CDC) recommendations, patients who underwent HSCT may be vaccinated with the live-attenuated strains of VZV on a case-by-case basis after a minimum of 24 months post-HSCT. This may place patients at risk for developing a potentially serious infection during the gap period. However, two reports have since demonstrated the safety and seroconversion rates of the live-attenuated VZV vaccine when given to this patient population after first demonstrating adequate T-cell immune reconstitution.[44,118]

Human herpesvirus–6. HHV-6 is a ubiquitous pathogen that has infected the majority of people by the age of 2 years and has been reported to reactivate in approximately 50% of HSCT recipients according to PCR-based monitoring.[268] The majority of these episodes of viremia appear to be self-limited and asymptomatic, significantly limiting recommendations regarding preemptive therapy. However, a variety of reports have linked HHV-6 reactivations to post-HSCT fevers, rashes, hepatitis, pneumonia, and delayed engraftment,[231] as well as to increased TRM and poorer overall survival,[3] although not all reports agree that HHV-6 is a major issue: thus universal PCR screening is controverial.[249] HHV-6 also appears to be a rare cause of post-HSCT encephalitis, typically manifested as memory loss, seizures, hyponatremia, cerebrospinal fluid pleocytosis, and magnetic resonance imaging (MRI) abnormalities in the mesial temporal lobe.[79,209] Patients manifesting these symptoms should have their cerebrospinal fluid examined for HHV-6 by PCR. HHV-6 replication has also been implicated in the initiation of GVHD.[3,184] When HHV-6–associated disease is diagnosed, ganciclovir is typically the first-line agent, although both foscarnet and cidofovir also have activity against HHV-6.[269] If the HHV-6 viremia does not appear to be resolving with antiviral treatment, the possibility of chromosomally integrated virus must be considered.[103] This can be determined by paired serum and whole blood PCRs demonstrating that the copy numbers in the whole blood sample are significantly higher and the serum copy numbers are generally very low.

Other Double-Stranded DNA Viruses

Adenovirus. A large number of serotypes of adenovirus have been implicated in causing human disease, and, by the age of 5 years, most individuals have been exposed to at least one serotype, thereby allowing latent virus to enter the system. Thereafter reactivation during a period of intense immunosuppression results in the majority of cases of adenoviral viremia after HSCT.[25] The major risk factor for adenoviral reactivation is the degree of immunosuppression experienced by the patient, especially among recipients of T-cell–depleted grafts or grafts from unrelated donors and those being treated for GVHD.[37,168] Of interest, for reasons that are not entirely clear, younger age also appears to be a risk factor.[25]

With the advent of PCR-based testing of blood and other body fluids, it has been demonstrated that adenoviral reactivations occur in approximately 27% to 32% of pediatric HSCT recipients.[131,168] Because of this high incidence, many centers perform routine screening of blood by PCR for early detection of adenoviral reactivations in high-risk patients.[131] When adenovirus viremia progresses to invasive disease, manifestations include pneumonia, hepatitis, enteritis, cystitis, and nephritis.[25] Adenoviral disease after HSCT has been associated with mortality rates as high as 78%.[168] The only currently available agent for treatment of adenoviral viremia or disease is intravenous cidofovir, typically given on a schedule of three times per week.[94] However, intravenous cidofovir has potentially significant toxicities to both the kidneys and bone marrow. This makes its use as a preemptive agent problematic, especially when some patients appear to spontaneously clear the viremia without treatment.[168,254] An oral liposomal formulation of cidofovir (brincidofovir) may potentially be less toxic than the intravenous formulation and may serve as a preemptive agent if FDA approved.[65] Furthermore, because the major risk factor for the development of adenoviral infection is profound immunosuppression, rapid tapering or withdrawal of immunosuppression, when possible, may potentially play a role in the treatment.[37] For patients who develop adenoviral infection after T-cell–depleted HSCT, researchers are also working on developing adenovirus-specific T cells for adoptive immunotherapy, either alone or in combination with specificity for other viruses.[123,174]

Human polyomavirus type I. Human polyomavirus type I, typically referred to as BK virus, is a common asymptomatic infection in adults, 90% of whom are seropositive.[115] Like other dsDNA viruses, it can reactivate during periods of intense immunosuppression, and between 50% and 80% of HSCT recipients will be found to shed BKV in their urine in the first several months after HSCT.[4,191] Much of the time, this viruria is asymptomatic, but BK virus reactivation can be associated with the development of hemorrhagic cystitis (HC) in approximately 5% to 15% of HSCT recipients, typically 3 to 6 weeks after HSCT.[11] The patients at highest risk for developing BK virus–associated HC appear to be those who received cyclophosphamide-based conditioning regimens and T-cell–depleted grafts.[42] Furthermore BK virus can be found in the blood of some patients after HSCT, and high levels have been associated with the development of BK virus–associated nephropathy,[84] which can be definitively diagnosed only by renal biopsy. Of interest, fluoroquinolone antibiotics inhibit BK viral replication in vitro, and some data suggest that their use as antibacterial prophylaxis after HSCT also may decrease rates of BK virus–associated HC.[127] Decreasing immunosuppression, whenever possible, is the first step toward treating BK virus disease. If the BK virus disease persists, cidofovir is the most commonly used antiviral agent, although leflunomide also appears to have some efficacy[190] and may potentially be better tolerated than cidofovir in patients with significant renal dysfunction. If approved, brincidofovir may be an attractive option for patients with severe BK virus infections.[175] Finally, T cells with BK virus specificity, among others, are also being generated for eventual clinical usage.[74]

Respiratory Viruses

In pediatric HSCT recipients, respiratory viral infections as a whole play a significant role in TRM,[97] especially in patients with low lymphocyte counts and/or high doses of corticosteroids.[264] They have also been reported to be associated with later development of alloreactive lung injury.[247] As such, it has been advocated that patients should undergo, at minimum, testing for respiratory viruses pre-HSCT and delay in HSCT whenever possible[29] and possibly even pre-HSCT detailed pulmonary screening with high-resolution CT scan and bronchoalveolar lavage (BAL).[248]

Influenza. During seasonal outbreaks (typically October to March in the northern hemisphere), HSCT recipients are at risk for developing influenza infections from close contacts. Although upper respiratory tract symptoms are common, systemic symptoms such as fever or myalgias may be absent.[180] Thus a high index of suspicion must be maintained during the peak season, because 20% to 50% of influenza infections can rapidly progress to lower respiratory tract disease with hypoxemia and a risk for mechanical ventilation and death.[43] Bronchoalveolar lavage (BAL) may be needed in patients with evidence of lower respiratory tract symptoms because highly immunosuppressed patients are at risk for harboring multiple pathogens. Early preemptive treatment with neuraminidase inhibitors (the choice depending on that year's circulating strain) appears to be relatively efficacious at preventing progress to lower respiratory tract disease.[31,114] Although the data are limited, combination regimens have been employed for patients with resistant strains or with respiratory failure. Peramivir is an available parenteral agent in the United States, and zanamivir is undergoing investigation or is available through emergency use authorization.[39] The use of moderate dosages of corticosteroids to reduce excessive inflammation is controversial but does not appear to result in worse outcomes.[23] There are limited data on whether other forms of immunosuppression should be lowered.

Prevention strategies for influenza center around strict infection control practices, including hand-washing, isolation, and eliminating potential exposures via universal vaccination of health care workers, patient family members, and caregivers. If a recent (<2 years or still immunocompromised) HSCT recipient has a significant exposure to a confirmed case of influenza, prophylactic administration of a neuraminidase inhibitor is recommended. This strategy also could be considered if a nosocomial outbreak was to occur on a HSCT unit.

Vaccination of HSCT recipients (with the inactivated strain) is highly recommended to occur for several years beginning at 6 months after HSCT, before which time the majority of adult patients are unlikely to mount a serologic response.[31] Higher doses may be required to produce significant immunogenicity.[85] However, pediatric data are limited, and a fixed 6-month rule fails to take into account the significant variation in immunologic recovery times that occurs among patients depending on stem cell source and presence of GVHD. It is not unreasonable to allow earlier vaccination for patients on tapering doses of immunosuppression,[108,231] even without documented B-cell function, because a T-cell response to influenza vaccine also may provide some protection.[6] Finally efforts are under way to create influenza-specific T cells that can be given in a prophylactic fashion following HSCT.[223]

Respiratory syncytial virus. During seasonal outbreaks, upper respiratory tract infections from the RNA virus respiratory syncytial virus (RSV) are common in HSCT recipients. Approximately 50% of those infected will progress to involve the lower respiratory tract, especially in those with GVHD or severe lymphopenia.[213] A novel "immunodeficiency" scoring system can potentially be used to determine those patients at highest risk of progressing in the absence of therapy, while lower risk patients might spontaneously resolve. Untreated RSV pneumonia in HSCT recipients has a mortality rate as high as 75% to 80%.[114,213] Ribavirin, a guanosine analog, is available in aerosolized form for the treatment of RSV. Several potential regimens exist, including a continuous 18-hour infusion and a 2- to 3-hour infusion given three times per day. Because of concerns about potential teratogenicity, it is usually administered in a scavenging tent. Respiratory side effects from inhaled ribavirin are common and include potential bronchoconstriction. Despite its problems and costs, a comprehensive review of inhaled ribavirin treatment in adult HSCT recipients suggests that initiation of ribavirin at the time of diagnosis of RSV upper respiratory tract infection can significantly decrease the risk for progression to lower respiratory tract disease and, in those with lower respiratory tract disease, can decrease the risk for death.[213] Antiviral therapy has the strongest effect in those with high-risk immunodeficiency scores, where RSV-associated mortality can potentially be lowered from 63% to 8%.[114] An oral formulation of ribavirin (used for treating hepatitis C) and an intravenous formulation (not available in the United States) have also been used for treating RSV. Newer data suggest that this formulation may as also be effective at preventing RSV-associated death, albeit with the risk of systemic side effects such as hemolytic anemia, lactic acidosis, and altered mental status.[142]

Palivizumab, an RSV-specific monoclonal antibody, is effective at preventing RSV infections in very young high-risk children. Another potential immunomodulator is IVIG, which often contains anti-RSV antibodies and may decrease RSV-mediated cytokine-induced pulmonary inflammation. A review of the available studies of immunomodulation plus inhaled ribavirin suggests that the combination may be superior at preventing progression to lower respiratory tract disease and RSV-related death than inhaled ribavirin alone.[213] However, because of the small numbers, the report was unable to separate out those who specifically received palivizumab. Once lower respiratory tract disease is established, palivizumab has not been shown to improve outcomes.[210] As a result of the lack of any controlled trial, the use of the expensive palivizumab has been questioned. Even more controversial is the prophylactic use of palivizumab. Fortunately the incidence of RSV infection in the first 100 days after HSCT is still relatively low at 5.8%.[180] However, based on decision tree analysis in children undergoing HSCT, it has been estimated that the use of prophylactic palivizumab may increase the absolute survival rate from 83% to 92%, suggesting that 12 children would need to be treated to prevent one RSV-related death.[230] Clinical confirmation of this concept is lacking.

Even with "optimal" therapy of inhaled ribavirin plus an immunomodulator, the RSV-attributable mortality in HSCT recipients with lower respiratory tract disease is approximately 25%. Therefore improved treatments are desperately needed, and work is under way on higher affinity monoclonal antibodies, high-titer RSV immune globulin, and antisense compounds.[213]

Other Respiratory Viruses

Other respiratory viruses, including parainfluenza virus,[222] human metapneumovirus,[192] rhinovirus,[161] and enterovirus D68,[251] have been implicated in causing lower respiratory tract disease in HSCT recipients. Risk factors for progression from upper respiratory tract infection to viral pneumonia include acquiring the infection early after HSCT, a low absolute lymphocyte count, and corticosteroid usage.[222] There is no FDA-approved antiviral agent with proved efficacy against these three viruses. However, identifying one of these viruses from the nasopharynx or bronchial washings can be useful in limiting empirical usage of potentially toxic agents to treat other infections, although these viruses often show up as co-pathogens. Some uncontrolled reports have suggested that inhaled ribavirin may be useful against parainfluenza[36]; however, others have questioned its utility.[170] Recently a small case series has demonstrated possible efficacy of DAS181, an inhaled sialidase fusion protein, in HSCT recipients with severe parainfluenza infection.[252] Ribavirin has in vitro activity against human metapneumovirus, and a recent report suggests that ribavirin may play a role in helping resolve lower respiratory tract disease,[214] although controlled comparisons are lacking. Clearly, the best strategy for dealing with respiratory viral infections after HSCT is to avoid them through careful respiratory isolation.

Enteric Viruses

In addition to adenovirus, other enteric viruses such as rotavirus and norovirus, which typically cause self-limited disease in healthy individuals, can be major pathogens in HSCT recipients due to longer duration of symptoms and occasionally even death.[130,198,208] Since profuse watery diarrhea may also be a symptom of gastrointestinal GVHD, careful exclusion of these viruses is critical in order to avoid potential overtreatment of that complication. Furthermore it has been suggested that these viruses may also be able to trigger the development of gastrointestinal GVHD.[243] There is no specific antiviral agent for treating either virus, although enteral administration of immunoglobulin has been reported efficacious in a small case series.[258] The antiprotozoal agent nitazoxanide has also been used with some activity against both viruses.[200]

Protozoa

Toxoplasma gondii

The majority of HSCT programs have dietary counseling in place that eliminates most undercooked meat; thus toxoplasmosis after HSCT is generally caused by reactivation of previously acquired cysts. Therefore serologic screening of HSCT candidates can identify most patients at potential risk (excepting those with deficient antibody production),[148] although reports of transmission from white blood cells do exist.[104] In seropositive patients, PJP prophylaxis with TMP-SMX also provides excellent coverage against toxoplasmosis.[148] Patients who cannot tolerate TMP-SMX need careful attention to the possibility of toxoplasmosis because most alternative PJP prophylaxis agents do not appear to provide sufficient protection.[231] A small study suggests that atovaquone may provide some protection;[156] alternatively clindamycin or pyrimethamine combinations can be used as either prophylaxis or preemptive treatment based on routine PCR screening for reactivation.[196,231]

When toxoplasmosis occurs in a post-HSCT patient the general time frame is 2 to 6 months after HSCT. Because the brain is the most commonly affected organ, fever plus focal neurologic signs, headaches, seizures, or altered mental status are the typical symptoms that should prompt evaluation for toxoplasmosis. Brain MRI may not always show the characteristic ring-enhancing lesions; therefore cerebrospinal fluid confirmation should be obtained.[99]

Strongyloides stercoralis

Strongyloides stercoralis is endemic to the tropics and subtropics, including the southeastern United States. Transmission is usually via penetration of the larvae into exposed skin, from which it migrates into the intestines and possibly the lungs. HSCT candidates with intact immune systems may be asymptomatic or have only eosinophilia, and stool testing should be considered for anyone entering HSCT with elevated eosinophil counts, especially if they have traveled to or emigrated from an endemic area.[109] If positive, treatment with ivermectin is generally effective when disease burden is low. Infected individuals may begin to show evidence of disseminated disease within 1 to 3 months after HSCT. This "hyperinfection syndrome" can manifest as respiratory failure with diffuse pulmonary infiltrates, often with blood-tinged sputum, and/or colonic wall penetration, which leads to superinfection with gram-negative enteric organisms. Despite optimal treatment, mortality rates of hyperinfection syndrome are high.[100]

Cryptosporidium parvum *and* C. hominis

Cryptosporidium spp. are enteric protozoa acquired from contaminated water supplies or livestock and infect intestinal epithelial cells. They cause seasonal transient nonbloody diarrhea and occasional systemic symptoms in healthy hosts and are frequently mistaken for a viral gastroenteritis. In immunocompromised HSCT recipients, however, cryptosporidiosis can cause a chronic severe diarrhea plus rare biliary tract disease. Multicenter incidence studies have never been performed, but, based on one single-center prospective study, it may be as high as 4% of all HSCT recipients and 10% of those with diarrhea.[124] Patients with B-cell deficiencies and CD40 ligand deficiency appear to be at especially high risk.[124] In HSCT recipients, the symptoms of a *Cryptosporidium* infection can easily be confused with that of intestinal GVHD, and testing for *Cryptosporidium* oocysts should be considered before initiation of additional immunosuppressants.[124] Therapy for *Cryptosporidium* is with paromomycin, azithromycin, or nitazoxanide. HSCT recipients may need combination therapy, and decreases in systemic immunosuppression should be performed when possible.[124]

VACCINATIONS AFTER HEMATOPOIETIC STEM CELL TRANSPLANT

HSCT, especially from an allogeneic donor, involves the creation of a new immune system that lacks protective immunity in regard to vaccines received before the HSCT. Although some memory T and B cells may be passively transferred from the donor at the time of the cell infusion, the majority of the long-term immune system derives from newly generated naïve T and B cells. Therefore all HSCT recipients require revaccination after recovery of immune function. The major HSCT and infectious disease groups, plus the CDC, have published guidelines regarding the timing of vaccine administration,[201] but it has been argued that a "one size fits all" approach, as used in generally healthy infants, is insufficient to produce protective immunity in many HSCT recipients and that the vaccine schedule should be tailored to the individual kinetics of a patient's T- and B-cell recovery and followed by titers to demonstrate adequate response.[219]

NEW REFERENCES SINCE THE SEVENTH EDITION

3. Aoki J, Numata A, Yamamoto E, et al. Impact of human herpesvirus-6 reactivation on outcomes of allogeneic hematopoietic stem cell transplantation. *Biol Blood Marrow Transplant.* 2015;21(11):2017-2022.
9. Barajas MR, McCullough KB, Merten JA, et al. Correlation of pain and fluoride concentration in allogeneic hematopoietic stem cell transplant recipients on voriconazole. *Biol Blood Marrow Transplant.* 2015;22(3):579-583.
16. Blennow O, Fjaertoft G, Winiarski J, et al. Varicella-zoster reactivation after allogeneic stem cell transplantation without routine prophylaxis—the incidence remains high. *Biol Blood Marrow Transplant.* 2014;20(10):1646-1649.
23. Boudreault AA, Xie H, Leisenring W, et al. Impact of corticosteroid treatment and antiviral therapy on clinical outcomes in hematopoietic cell transplant patients infected with influenza virus. *Biol Blood Marrow Transplant.* 2011;17(7):979-986.
24. Boyle NM, Magaret A, Stednick Z, et al. Evaluating risk factors for *Clostridium difficile* infection in adult and pediatric hematopoietic cell transplant recipients. *Antimicrob Resist Infect Control.* 2015;4:41.
29. Campbell AP, Guthrie KA, Englund JA, et al. Clinical outcomes associated with respiratory virus detection before allogeneic hematopoietic stem cell transplant. *Clin Infect Dis.* 2015;61(2):192-202.
39. Chan-Tack K, Kim C, Moruf A, et al. Clinical experience with intravenous zanamivir under an emergency IND program in the United States (2011–2014). *Antivir Ther.* 2015;20(5):561-564.
40. Chemaly RF, Ullmann AJ, Stoelben S, et al. Letermovir for cytomegalovirus prophylaxis in hematopoietic-cell transplantation. *N Engl J Med.* 2014;370(19):1781-1789.
47. Climo MW, Yokoe DS, Warren DK, et al. Effect of daily chlorhexidine bathing on hospital-acquired infection. *N Engl J Med.* 2013;368(6):533-542.
50. Cornely OA, Böhme A, Schmitt-Hoffmann A, et al. Safety and pharmacokinetics of Isavuconazole as antifungal prophylaxis in acute myeloid leukemia patients with neutropenia: results of a phase 2, dose escalation study. *Antimicrob Agents Chemother.* 2015;59(4):2078-2085.
54. de Castro CG, Ganc AJ, Ganc RL, et al. Fecal microbiota transplant after hematopoietic SCT: report of a successful case. *Bone Marrow Transplant.* 2015;50(1):145.
64. Elmaagacli AH, Steckel NK, Koldehoff M, et al. Early human cytomegalovirus replication after transplantation is associated with a decreased relapse risk: evidence for a putative virus-versus-leukemia effect in acute myeloid leukemia patients. *Blood.* 2011;118(5):1402-1412.
65. Florescu DF, Pergam SA, Neely MN, et al. Safety and efficacy of CMX001 as salvage therapy for severe adenovirus infections in immunocompromised patients. *Biol Blood Marrow Transplant.* 2012;18(5):731-738.
68. Frobert E, Burrel S, Ducastelle-Lepretre S, et al. Resistance of herpes simplex viruses to acyclovir: An update from a ten-year survey in France. *Antiviral Res.* 2014;111:36-41.
69. Gafter-Gvili A, Fraser A, Paul M, et al. Meta-analysis: antibiotic prophylaxis reduces mortality in neutropenic patients. *Ann Intern Med.* 2005;142(12 Pt 1):979-995.
71. Garcia-Cadenas I, Castillo N, Martino R, et al. Impact of Epstein Barr virus-related complications after high-risk allo-SCT in the era of pre-emptive rituximab. *Bone Marrow Transplant.* 2015;50(4):579-584.
73. Gerdemann U, Keirnan JM, Katari UL, et al. Rapidly generated multivirus-specific cytotoxic T lymphocytes for the prophylaxis and treatment of viral infections. *Mol Ther.* 2012;20(8):1622-1632.
74. Gerdemann U, Katari UL, Papadopoulou A, et al. Safety and clinical efficacy of rapidly-generated trivirus-directed T cells as treatment for adenovirus, EBV, and CMV infections after allogeneic hematopoietic stem cell transplant. *Mol Ther.* 2013;21(11):2113-2121.
81. Green ML, Leisenring WM, Xie H, et al. CMV reactivation after allogeneic HCT and relapse risk: evidence for early protection in acute myeloid leukemia. *Blood.* 2013;122(7):1316-1324.
85. Halasa NB, Savani BN, Asokan I, et al. Randomized, double blind, study of the safety and immunogenicity of standard-dose trivalent inactivated influenza vaccine versus high-dose trivalent inactivated influenza vaccine in adult hematopoietic stem cell transplant patients. *Biol Blood Marrow Transplant.* 2016;22(3):528-535.
95. Hol JA, Wolfs TFW, Bierings MB, et al. Predictors of invasive fungal infection in pediatric allogeneic hematopoietic SCT recipients. *Bone Marrow Transplant.* 2014;49(1):95-101.
97. Hutspardol S, Essa M, Richardson S, et al. Significant transplantation-related mortality from respiratory virus infections within the first one hundred days in children after hematopoietic stem cell transplantation. *Biol Blood Marrow Transplant.* 2015;21(10):1802-1807.
98. Imran H, Tleyjeh IM, Arndt CAS, et al. Fluoroquinolone prophylaxis in patients with neutropenia: a meta-analysis of randomized placebo-controlled trials. *Eur J Clin Microbiol Infect Dis.* 2008;27(1):53-63.
100. Iori AP, Ferretti A, Gentile G, et al. Strongyloides stercoralis infection in allogeneic stem cell transplant: a case report and review of the literature. *Transpl Infect Dis.* 2014;16(4):625-630.
102. Jenq RR, Taur Y, Devlin SM, et al. Intestinal Blautia is associated with reduced death from graft-versus-host disease. *Biol Blood Marrow Transplant.* 2015;21(8):1373-1383.
105. Kamboj M, Xiao K, Kaltsas A, et al. *Clostridium difficile* infection after allogeneic hematopoietic stem cell transplant: strain diversity and outcomes associated with NAP1/027. *Biol Blood Marrow Transplant.* 2014;20(10):1626-1633.
108. Karras NA, Weeres M, Sessions W, et al. A randomized trial of one versus two doses of influenza vaccine after allogeneic transplantation. *Biol Blood Marrow Transplant.* 2013;19(1):109-116.
113. Kinnebrew MA, Lee YJ, Jenq RR, et al. Early *Clostridium difficile* infection during allogeneic hematopoietic stem cell transplantation. *PLoS ONE.* 2014;9(3):e90158.
114. Kmeid J, Vanichanan J, Shah DP, et al. Outcomes of influenza infections in hematopoietic cell transplant recipients: application of an immunodeficiency scoring index. *Biol Blood Marrow Transplant.* 2016;22(3):542-548.
119. Ladas EJ, Bhatia M, Chen L, et al. The safety and feasibility of probiotics in children and adolescents undergoing hematopoietic cell transplantation. *Bone Marrow Transplant.* 2016;51(2):262-266.

120. Lammers AJJ, de Porto APNA, Bennink RJ, et al. Hyposplenism: comparison of different methods for determining splenic function. *Am J Hematol.* 2012;87(5):484-489.
126. Lehrnbecher T, Phillips R, Alexander S, et al. Guideline for the management of fever and neutropenia in children with cancer and/or undergoing hematopoietic stem-cell transplantation. *J Clin Oncol.* 2012;30(35):4427-4438.
129. Levy E, Musick L, Zinter M, et al. Safe and effective prophylaxis with bi-monthly intravenous pentamidine in the pediatric hematopoietic stem cell transplant population. *Pediatr Infect Dis J.* 2016;35(2):135-141.
130. Liakopoulou E, Mutton K, Carrington D, et al. Rotavirus as a significant cause of prolonged diarrhoeal illness and morbidity following allogeneic bone marrow transplantation. *Bone Marrow Transplant.* 2005;36(8):691-694.
135. Louie TJ, Miller MA, Mullane KM, et al. Fidaxomicin versus vancomycin for *Clostridium difficile* infection. *N Engl J Med.* 2011;364(5):422-431.
134. Louie TJ, Cannon K, Byrne B, et al. Fidaxomicin preserves the intestinal microbiome during and after treatment of *Clostridium difficile* infection (CDI) and reduces both toxin reexpression and recurrence of CDI. *Clin Infect Dis.* 2012;55(suppl 2):S132-S142.
138. Maertens JA, Raad II, Marr KA, et al. Isavuconazole versus voriconazole for primary treatment of invasive mould disease caused by *Aspergillus* and other filamentous fungi (SECURE): a phase 3, randomised-controlled, non-inferiority trial. *Lancet.* 2016;387(10020):760-769.
139. Majhail NS, Chitphakdithai P, Logan B, et al. Significant improvement in survival after unrelated donor hematopoietic cell transplantation in the recent era. *Biol Blood Marrow Transplant.* 2015;21(1):142-150.
141. Manjappa S, Bhamidipati PK, Stokerl-Goldstein KE, et al. Protective effect of cytomegalovirus reactivation on relapse after allogeneic hematopoietic cell transplantation in acute myeloid leukemia patients is influenced by conditioning regimen. *Biol Blood Marrow Transplant.* 2014;20(1):46-52.
142. Marcelin JR, Wilson JW, Razonable RR, et al. Oral ribavirin therapy for respiratory syncytial virus infections in moderately to severely immunocompromised patients. *Transpl Infect Dis.* 2014;16(2):242-250.
146. Marr KA, Schlamm HT, Herbrecht R, et al. Combination antifungal therapy for invasive aspergillosis: a randomized trial combination therapy for invasive aspergillosis. *Ann Intern Med.* 2015;162(2):81-89.
151. Marty FM, Winston DJ, Rowley SD, et al. CMX001 to prevent cytomegalovirus disease in hematopoietic-cell transplantation. *N Engl J Med.* 2013;369(13):1227-1236.
156. Mendorf A, Klyuchnikov E, Langebrake C, et al. Atovaquone for prophylaxis of toxoplasmosis after allogeneic hematopoietic stem cell transplantation. *Acta Haematol.* 2015;134(3):146-154.
163. Miles-Jay A, Butler-Wu S, Rowhani-Rahbar A, et al. Incidence rate of fluoroquinolone-resistant gram-negative rod bacteremia among allogeneic hematopoietic cell transplantation patients during an era of levofloxacin prophylaxis. *Biol Blood Marrow Transplant.* 2015;21(3):539-545.
164. Milstone AM, Elward A, Song X, et al. Daily chlorhexidine bathing to reduce bacteraemia in critically ill children: a multicentre, cluster-randomised, crossover trial. *Lancet.* 2013;381(9872):1099-1106.
167. Munoz A, Gonzalez-Vicent M, Badell I, et al. Mycobacterial diseases in pediatric hematopoietic SCT recipients. *Bone Marrow Transplant.* 2011;46(5):766-768.
174. Papadopoulou A, Gerdemann U, Katari UL, et al. Activity of broad-spectrum T cells as treatment for AdV, EBV, CMV, BKV, and HHV6 infections after HSCT. *Sci Transl Med.* 2014;6(242):242ra283.
175. Papanicolaou GA, Lee YJ, Young JW, et al. Brincidofovir for polyomavirus-associated nephropathy after allogeneic hematopoietic stem cell transplantation. *Am J Kidney Dis.* 2015;65(5):780-784.
178. Pasquini M, Wang Z Current uses and outcomes of hematopoietic stem cell transplantation. CIBMTR *Summary Slides.* 2014. Available at: http://www.cibmtr.org.
179. Patrick K, Ali M, Richardson SE, et al. The yield of monitoring for HSV and VZV viremia in pediatric hematopoietic stem cell transplant patients. *Pediatr Transplant.* 2015;19(6):640-644.
188. Price TH, Boeckh M, Harrison RW, et al. Efficacy of transfusion with granulocytes from G-CSF/dexamethasone–treated donors in neutropenic patients with infection. *Blood.* 2015;126(18):2153-2161.
192. Renaud C, Xie H, Seo S, et al. Mortality rates of human metapneumovirus and respiratory syncytial virus lower respiratory tract infections in hematopoietic cell transplantation recipients. *Biol Blood Marrow Transplant.* 2013;19(8):1220-1226.
194. Riches M, Trifilio S, Chen M, et al. Risk factors and impact of non-*Aspergillus* mold infections following allogeneic HCT: a CIBMTR infection and immune reconstitution analysis. *Bone Marrow Transplant.* 2016;51(2):322.
196. Robert-Gangneux F, Sterkers Y, Yera H, et al. Molecular diagnosis of toxoplasmosis in immunocompromised patients: a 3-year multicenter retrospective study. *J Clin Microbiol.* 2015;53(5):1677-1684.
198. Roddie C, Paul JPV, Benjamin R, et al. Allogeneic hematopoietic stem cell transplantation and norovirus gastroenteritis: a previously unrecognized cause of morbidity. *Clin Infect Dis.* 2009;49(7):1061-1068.
200. Rossignol J, El-Gohary Y. Nitazoxanide in the treatment of viral gastroenteritis: a randomized double-blind placebo-controlled clinical trial. *Aliment Pharmacol Ther.* 2006;24(10):1423-1430.
201. Rubin LG, Levin MJ, Ljungman P, et al. Executive summary: 2013 IDSA clinical practice guideline for vaccination of the immunocompromised host. *Clin Infect Dis.* 2014;58(3):309-318.
207. Schmidt-Hieber M, Labopin M, Beelen D, et al. CMV serostatus still has an important prognostic impact in de novo acute leukemia patients after allogeneic stem cell transplantation: a report from the Acute Leukemia Working Party of EBMT. *Blood.* 2013;122(19):3359-3364.
208. Schwartz S, Vergoulidou M, Schreier E, et al. Norovirus gastroenteritis causes severe and lethal complications after chemotherapy and hematopoietic stem cell transplantation. *Blood.* 2011;117(22):5850-5856.
211. Seo S, Campbell AP, Xie H, et al. Outcome of respiratory syncytial virus lower respiratory tract disease in hematopoietic cell transplant recipients receiving aerosolized Ribavirin: significance of stem cell source and oxygen requirement. *Biol Blood Marrow Transplant.* 2013;19(4):589-596.
212. Seo SK, Xiao K, Huang Y-T, et al. Impact of peri-transplant vancomycin and fluoroquinolone administration on rates of bacteremia in allogeneic hematopoietic stem cell transplant (HSCT) recipients: a 12-year single institution study. *J Infect.* 2014;69(4):341-351.
216. Sheu J, Hawryluk EB, Guo D, et al. Voriconazole phototoxicity in children: a retrospective review. *J Am Acad Dermatol.* 2015;72(2):314-320.
227. Suwantarat N, Carroll K, Tekle T, et al. High prevalence of reduced chlorhexidine susceptibility in organisms causing central line-associated bloodstream infections. *Infect Control Hosp Epidemiol.* 2014;35(9):1183-1186.
228. Taur Y, Jenq RR, Perales M-A, et al. The effects of intestinal tract bacterial diversity on mortality following allogeneic hematopoietic stem cell transplantation. *Blood.* 2014;124(7):1174-1182.
229. Teusink A, Vinks A, Zhang K, et al. Genotype-directed dosing leads to optimized voriconazole levels in pediatric patients receiving hematopoietic stem cell transplantation. *Biol Blood Marrow Transplant.* 2016;22(3):482-486.
235. Ugarte-Torres A, Hoegh-Petersen M, Liu Y, et al. Donor serostatus has an impact on cytomegalovirus-specific immunity, cytomegaloviral disease incidence, and survival in seropositive hematopoietic cell transplant recipients. *Biol Blood Marrow Transplant.* 2011;17(4):574-585.
238. Uryu H, Hashimoto D, Kato K, et al. α-Mannan induces Th17-mediated pulmonary graft-versus-host disease in mice. *Blood.* 2015;125(19):3014-3023.
243. van Montfrans J, Schulz L, Versluys B, et al. Viral PCR positivity in stool before allogeneic hematopoietic cell transplantation is strongly associated with acute intestinal graft-versus-host disease. *Biol Blood Marrow Transplant.* 2015;21(4):772-774.
248. Versluys AB, van der Ent K, Boelens JJ, et al. High diagnostic yield of dedicated pulmonary screening before hematopoietic cell transplantation in children. *Biol Blood Marrow Transplant.* 2015;21(9):1622-1626.
247. Versluys AB, Rossen JWA, van Ewijk B, et al. Strong association between respiratory viral infection early after hematopoietic stem cell transplantation and the development of life-threatening acute and chronic alloimmune lung syndromes. *Biol Blood Marrow Transplant.* 2010;16(6):782-791.
249. Violago L, Jin Z, Bhatia M, et al. Human herpesvirus-6 viremia is not associated with poor clinical outcomes in children following allogeneic hematopoietic cell transplantation. *Pediatr Transplant.* 2015;19(7):737-744.
251. Waghmare A, Pergam SA, Jerome KR, et al. Clinical disease due to enterovirus D68 in adult hematologic malignancy patients and hematopoietic cell transplant recipients. *Blood.* 2015;125(11):1724-1729.
252. Waghmare A, Wagner T, Andrews R, et al. Successful treatment of parainfluenza virus respiratory tract infection with DAS181 in 4 immunocompromised children. *J Pediatric Infect Dis Soc.* 2015;4(2):114-118.
255. Wattier RL, Dvorak CC, Hoffman JA, et al. A prospective, international cohort study of invasive mold infections in children. *J Pediatric Infect Dis Soc.* 2015;4(4):313-322.
257. Willems L, Porcher R, Lafaurie M, et al. *Clostridium difficile* infection after allogeneic hematopoietic stem cell transplantation: incidence, risk factors, and outcome. *Biol Blood Marrow Transplant.* 2012;18(8):1295-1301.
258. Williams D. Treatment of rotavirus-associated diarrhea using enteral immunoglobulins for pediatric stem cell transplant patients. *J Oncol Pharm Pract.* 2015;21(3):238-240.
259. Williams KM, Ahn KW, Chen M, et al. The incidence, mortality and timing of Pneumocystis jiroveci pneumonia after hematopoietic cell transplantation: a CIBMTR analysis. *Bone Marrow Transplant.* 2016;51(4):573-580.
264. Wolfromm A, Porcher R, Legoff J, et al. Viral respiratory infections diagnosed by multiplex PCR after allogeneic hematopoietic stem cell transplantation: long-term incidence and outcome. *Biol Blood Marrow Transplant.* 2014;20(8):1238-1241.
265. Worth LJ, Slavin MA, Heath S, et al. Ethanol versus heparin locks for the prevention of central venous catheter-associated bloodstream infections: a randomized trial in adult haematology patients with Hickman devices. *J Hosp Infect.* 2014;88(1):48-51.
267. Zacharioudakis IM, Ziakas PD, Mylonakis E. Clostridium difficile infection in the hematopoietic unit: a meta-analysis of published studies. *Biol Blood Marrow Transplant.* 2014;20(10):1650-1654.

The full reference list for this chapter is available at ExpertConsult.com.

Infections in Pediatric Heart Transplantation

70

Sheldon L. Kaplan • Claire E. Bocchini

Each year more than 500 children undergo heart transplantation around the world, and infection is an important cause of morbidity and some mortality in these patients.[44] The Registry of the International Society for Heart and Lung Transplantation (ISHLT) found that, from 2002 to 2012, infection (not including cytomegalovirus [CMV]) was the cause of death in pediatric heart transplant recipients in 8.5% of patients in the first year after transplant, 5.4% to 5.9% of patients 1 to 10 years posttransplant, and 5.5% of patients more than 10 years after transplantation.[44] Of the 9248 primary pediatric heart transplantations occurring between the years of 1998 and 2010 included in the ISHLT Registry, there were 3061 deaths, of which 9% were secondary to infection.[202]

The Pediatric Heart Transplant Study Group (PHTS) prospectively collected data from 22 pediatric centers in the United States from January 1993 to December 1994 on 332 children younger than 18 years (mean age, 5.5 years) who had undergone heart transplantation.[169] One or more infections (276 total) occurred in 41% of the patients (mean follow-up time, 11.8 months) for an average of 0.84 infections per patient; 22% had one infection, 8% had two infections, and 11% had three or more infections during the study period (Table 70.1). In an updated report from this multicenter group summarizing children who had undergone heart transplantation over the decade starting in 2000, 72% were free from infection at 1 year posttransplant.[43] In a similar multicenter study in adults who had undergone heart transplantation between January 1990 and June 1991, infections developed in 31% of 814 patients, with 22% having one infection and 9% having two or more infections.[135]

Bacterial infections were the most common type of infection occurring after transplantation in pediatric and adult patients. PHTS reported that 54% of 2038 infections in 1220 patients from January 1993 to December 2004 were bacterial, 32% were viral, 7% were fungal, 0.5% were protozoan, and 7% were unknown.[216] One single-center retrospective review of pediatric patients who underwent heart transplantation and who survived a minimum of 5 years after transplantation reported that infant transplant recipients had an increased risk of serious bacterial infections per 10 years of follow-up (mean, 2.04 ± 0.5) and chronic or recurrent bacterial infections (mean, 4.58 ± 0.67) compared with older recipients (means, 0.37 ± 0.19 and 1.87 ± 0.70, respectively).[110] Risk factors for an infectious cause of death in pediatric heart transplant recipients include pretransplant factors such as use of pretransplant extracorporeal membrane oxygenation (ECMO), presence of pretransplant infection, diagnosis of congenital heart disease, higher pretransplant creatinine, and higher sensitization levels as well as any cardiac reoperation prior to discharge and positive donor CMV serology.[202]

From 2009 to June 2014, ISHLT reported that 68% of children who underwent heart transplantation received induction immunosuppression, most commonly with antithymocyte globulin (47%) or interleukin-2 (IL-2) receptor antagonist (24%). Maintenance immunosuppressive therapy after transplant included a combination of a calcineurin inhibitor (tacrolimus in 84% and cyclosporine in 15%), an antimetabolite (mycophenolate mofetil or mycophenolic acid in 91% or azathioprine), and prednisone (70%). At 5 years posttransplant, 96% of patients were on a calcineurin inhibitor, 75% were on an antimetabolite, 36% were on a steroid, and 19% were on a mammalian target of rapamycin (mTOR) inhibitor (such as sirolimus).[44] Calcineurin inhibitors predominantly block the effect of IL-2 on T cells, an action resulting in a diminished T-cell response to mitogen stimulation.[76] The infections seen in heart transplant patients outside the postoperative period generally are a result of this block in T-cell function. Because the types of infections seen in these patients vary with the time elapsed since transplantation, this chapter is organized in such a manner.

PRETRANSPLANTATION EVALUATION

Several infectious agents may be transmitted to the patient via the transplanted organ or can become "reactivated" after transplantation. Determining the antibody status of the recipient and the donor against selected microorganisms (CMV, Epstein-Barr virus [EBV], *Toxoplasma gondii*) helps physicians anticipate, prevent, and diagnose infections that develop after transplantation. A reasonable pretransplant evaluation for children is outlined in Box 70.1 but varies depending on the patient's history and geographical location. The child's immunization status is documented, and vaccinations are completed when possible (i.e., hepatitis B vaccine, *Haemophilus influenzae* type b, or *Streptococcus pneumoniae*). The Committee on Infectious Diseases of the American Academy of Pediatrics recommends that candidates for solid organ transplantation should receive all vaccinations as appropriate for age, exposure history, and immune status.[7] The 23-valent pneumococcal polysaccharide vaccine (PPSV23) should be given to patients 2 years of age or older at least 8 weeks after the last 13-valent pneumococcal conjugate vaccine has been administered. If possible, appropriate vaccines should be administered at least 1 month before the patient undergoes transplantation. Evidence of selected active infections is a contraindication for transplantation. Chemoprophylaxis should be considered strongly for children with a positive tuberculin skin test (purified protein derivative). Dental status also is assessed.

In addition to having the routine pretransplant evaluation as outlined in Box 70.1, each patient should be screened carefully for selected infections appropriate to the individual circumstances. If surgery is planned during the respiratory disease season and the patient has respiratory symptoms just before having surgery, screening for influenza virus or respiratory syncytial virus (RSV) by rapid techniques may facilitate prescribing antiviral therapy postoperatively. In areas where community-acquired methicillin-resistant *Staphylococcus aureus* (MRSA) is an important cause of infection, performing surface cultures to detect MRSA colonization may modify the choice of antibiotics used for surgical prophylaxis.[97] Providing mupirocin intranasally as well as employing chlorhexidine baths preoperatively may decrease the rate of postoperative MRSA infections in patients colonized with MRSA.[71,142] In areas where coccidioidomycosis is endemic or for the patient with travel to endemic areas, pretransplant serology for *C. immitis* is recommended, and, if positive, antifungal prophylaxis is provided.[203] Screening for histoplasmosis is not recommended, but itraconazole prophylaxis may be considered for patients with recent history of active histoplasmosis infection.[38,134] Children from resource-poor countries may harbor *Salmonella* or intestinal parasites asymptomatically, and these organisms can cause serious infection after the child undergoes transplantation. Preoperative stool cultures for enteropathogens and examination of the stool for parasites may alert the clinician that these pathogens are present and could be the etiology of postoperative infections. Screening for *Strongyloides* is recommended for recipients in endemic areas or for patients with unexplained eosinophilia prior to transplant, and patients who are positive should be treated with ivermectin prior to transplantation.[37]

If the patient is being mechanically ventilated before undergoing transplantation, review of recent tracheal aspirate cultures may help in the selection of empirical antibiotics for initial treatment of suspected nosocomial sepsis or pneumonia. Pretransplant infections associated with procedures such as implantation of ventricular assist devices may require prolonged antibiotic therapy after transplantation is performed.[122,181] Intraoperative cultures of involved tissues including the mediastinum as well as various surfaces from the device should be obtained and the results guide therapy.[107] These infections typically are

TABLE 70.1 Types of Infections Encountered in 332 Children After Heart Transplantation in a Multiinstitutional Study[a]

Type	N
Bacterial (total)	164
Coagulase-negative staphylococci	25
Enterobacter spp.	21
Pseudomonas aeruginosa	16
Cytomegalovirus	51
Varicella zoster	11
Respiratory syncytial virus	10
Herpes simplex	6
Other viruses	8
Fungal	19
Candida spp.	12
Pneumocystis carinii	7

[a]Total of 276 infections in 136 patients.
Data from Schowengerdt KO, Naftel D, Seib PM, et al. Infection after pediatric heart transplantation: results of a multi-institutional study. *J Heart Lung Transplant.* 1997;16:1207–16.

BOX 70.1 Evaluation of Children Before Heart Transplantation

Serology:
- Cytomegalovirus[a]
- Epstein-Barr virus
- Coccidioidomycosis[b]
- *Toxoplasma gondii*
- Strongyloides[c]
- Human immunodeficiency virus
- Hepatitis A, B, and C
- Herpes simplex virus
- Parvovirus[d]
- Rubeola, mumps, rubella, varicella[e]
- Syphilis[f]

Cultures:
- Nasopharyngeal, stool, or tracheal aspirates[g]

Skin tests:
- Tuberculin skin test[h]

Consider freezing of an extra aliquot of serum
Review of the child's immunization status

[a]Urine CMV PCR for children <18 months rather than serology because maternal antibody may still be present.[153]
[b]Depends on geographic regions patient has lived in or traveled to.
[c]If from an endemic area or has eosinophilia.
[d]May help with interpretation of molecular tests of endomyocardial biopsies.
[e]For children >12 months and previously immunized.
[f]Depends on age and history.
[g]See text for an explanation.
[h]Interferon-γ release assay may be helpful in selected cases.[194]

caused by common nosocomial pathogens and are not a contraindication to undergoing heart transplantation. The reader is referred to more detailed discussions of the pretransplant assessment of the donor and recipient.[60]

SURGICAL PROPHYLACTIC ANTIBIOTICS

Prophylactic antibiotics typically are administered to patients undergoing heart transplantation surgery. For each institution, selection of prophylactic antibiotics should be based partly on the organisms isolated from postoperative wound infections in that center and the antimicrobial susceptibility of these organisms. Cefazolin is generally considered the drug of choice for perioperative prophylaxis. If MRSA is a nosocomial pathogen of concern or if the transplant recipient is colonized with MRSA, a single dose of vancomycin, in addition to cefazolin, is suggested. Both vancomycin and cefazolin are recommended because data suggest that vancomycin is less effective than cefazolin for preventing surgical site infections caused by MSSA.[23] Routine use of extended-spectrum cephalosporins is discouraged because it may lead to colonization of the patient by fungal organisms or antibiotic-resistant, gram-negative organisms that hyperproduce β-lactamase, such as *Enterobacter cloacae.* Expert guidelines recommend prophylactic antibiotics should not be administered beyond 48 hours post heart transplantation as part of a strategy to prevent the development of multidrug-resistant gram-negative bacteria and fungal pathogens.[201]

IMMEDIATE POSTOPERATIVE INFECTIONS

Common Infections

During the month after the patient undergoes heart transplantation, the types of infections encountered are the same as those complicating major thoracic surgery. Nosocomially acquired bacteria are the most common causative pathogens, and the incidence of multidrug-resistant organisms is increasing.[47] Pneumonia and bacteremia are the most common postoperative infections. The frequency of bacteremia and the distribution of organisms are similar in children and adults after undergoing heart transplantation.[135,169] In the PHTS study, the risk of development of any infection was 25% 1 month after transplantation. Overall 60 episodes of bacteremia occurred in the 136 patients who became infected, and the bloodstream was the most common site of bacterial infection.[170] Lung abscesses and mediastinitis are seen less frequently. Familiarity with the organisms and the antimicrobial susceptibility of isolates recovered from other children in the ICUs in which these patients receive care helps direct the initial empirical selection of antibiotics.

Postoperative bacteremia is related predominantly to the indwelling lines required for monitoring and infusion of medication. *S. aureus*, coagulase-negative staphylococci, *Enterococcus* spp., and gram-negative enteric organisms such as *Enterobacter* spp., *Pseudomonas aeruginosa, Klebsiella* spp., and *Escherichia coli* are the most common causes of nosocomial bacteremia in the pediatric ICU.[90,130,158] Other foci of infection, such as pneumonia, mediastinitis, or urinary tract infection also may result in bacteremia in heart transplant patients.[160,205] Vancomycin plus an extended-spectrum penicillin, third- or fourth-generation cephalosporin, or an aminoglycoside is a typical empiric antibiotic combination for suspected bacteremia in patients with central lines in place and without focal evidence of infection. Antibiotics are modified based on the organism(s) isolated and the antimicrobial susceptibilities of the isolate. Vancomycin therapy should be discontinued as soon as possible if an organism requiring the administration of vancomycin is not isolated.[155] A bacterial line infection may be eradicated successfully without removing the line, but the line should be removed if blood cultures remain positive or the patient's clinical condition deteriorates.[132] Optimally central lines are removed for *S. aureus* central line–related bloodstream infections.[30] Fungemia, generally with *Candida albicans* or other *Candida* spp., also may be associated with line-related infections. Central lines complicated by fungemia should be removed immediately.[56,132] *Candida* infections following heart transplantation are not frequent enough to warrant routine prophylaxis, but they are associated with mortality rate of up to 48% in pediatric heart transplant recipients.[180,216]

As in other critically ill children, pneumonia is a particularly common occurrence in heart transplant patients because of the operative site and requirements for intubation and mechanical ventilation. During the first postoperative week, definite bacterial pneumonia developed in three of 22 children (14%) in an early study from the University of Pittsburgh Medical Center (UPMC).[80] In the PHTS study, 56 bacterial lung infections were identified, 24 of which developed in patients maintained on a ventilator at the time of transplantation.[169] The incident rate of early nosocomial pneumonia in adult heart transplant patients has been reported to be 20% to 35%.[11,34] Nosocomial pneumonia caused by gram-negative bacilli such as *Pseudomonas* and *Enterobacter* or *S. aureus* is especially common in this setting.[158] Gram stain and culture of a tracheal aspirate or bronchoalveolar lavage (BAL) can help guide therapy for pneumonia.

A broad-spectrum combination of antibiotics, such as an extended-spectrum penicillin with a β-lactamase inhibitor (i.e., piperacillin-tazobactam) plus an aminoglycoside, usually is initiated until a pathogen or pathogens are identified. Empirical therapy should be based on the antibiotic susceptibility patterns of the common nosocomial pathogens in the specific ICU in which the patient is receiving care. Vancomycin also should be considered if MRSA is part of the resident flora in the ICU. Computed tomography (CT) of the chest may detect basilar and retrocardiac pneumonia, which may not be visualized readily by conventional chest radiographs. CT or ultrasound generally is helpful in assessing the size or characteristics of pleural effusions that may require drainage.

If interstitial pneumonitis is encountered, a more aggressive approach to determining an etiology is warranted. Bronchoscopy with BAL should be considered strongly. Lavage fluid is processed for pathogens including bacteria, mycobacteria, viruses, fungi, and protozoa by using culture techniques, special stains, and molecular techniques such as quantitative PCR. Mini-BAL are commonly employed in some pediatric centers, but how their results compare to a formal BAL procedure is not clear and has not been well studied in children.[66] *Legionella* may be an important consideration in some centers.[22,156] Noninfectious causes of pulmonary infiltrates in these children include pulmonary edema, atelectasis, hemorrhage, and acute respiratory distress syndrome.

Urinary tract infections (UTIs) also are common occurrences in the month after undergoing heart transplantation. Urinary catheterization and the immunosuppressive agents contribute to the risk for developing a UTI. Gram-negative enteric organisms (*E. coli, K. pneumoniae, P. aeruginosa,* and *Enterobacter* spp.), enterococci, and *Candida* spp. are isolated most commonly. Removal of the catheter as soon as possible minimizes the potential for development of a UTI, which has occurred in approximately 10% of adults. In the PHTS study, the urinary tract was the site of 16 bacterial infections.[169] In addition, UTIs developed in three children (14%) at UPMC during the 2 to 3 weeks after undergoing transplantation.[80]

The broad-spectrum antibiotics used to treat the bacterial complications of transplantation promote *Candida* infection of the urinary tract. Along with removal of the urinary catheter, short-course intravenous amphotericin B or fluconazole with careful dosing because of drug interactions with tacrolimus and cyclosporine is an option for treating candidal cystitis.[146] In some patients, especially infants, a urine culture positive for *Candida* is a clue that a disseminated *Candida* infection is present and that further investigation, including imaging, is necessary to exclude the involvement of other organs, especially the kidneys.

Antibiotic-associated diarrhea caused by *Clostridium difficile* is another potential complication related to antibiotics administered both pre- and posttransplant.[20,48] Toxic megacolon due to fulminant *C. difficile* infection requiring subtotal colectomy has been reported in a 10-year-old within 1 week after undergoing heart transplantation.[147]

Risk factors for early infection in the PHTS study were younger recipient age (particularly less than 6 months), mechanical ventilation at the time of transplantation, positive donor CMV serology with a CMV-negative recipient, and longer donor ischemic time.[169] Although primarily conducted among adult liver transplantation patients, studies have shown measuring procalcitonin may help distinguish infection from other causes of fever following solid organ transplantation.[214] Studies in adult heart transplant patients have shown that elevated procalcitonin levels beyond the first week after transplantation are correlated with infectious complications and that the use of serial procalcitonin measurements may be more reliable than single values.[166,190]

Sternal Wounds and Mediastinitis

Sternal wound infections and mediastinitis occur in less than 5% to 15% of adult heart transplant recipients compared with less than 5% of adult patients receiving general cardiac surgery.[29,59,99,135,136,174,218] Most of these infections occur during the first postoperative month, usually within the first 2 weeks, and are superficial. The majority of surgical site infections are caused by bacteria. Staphylococci and other gram-positive bacteria generally are responsible for 50% of cases, and the remainder are caused by a variety of gram-negative bacilli.[138] Higher incidences of fungal pathogens have been reported in heart transplant recipients compared with general cardiac surgery patients.[218] Surgical wound infections developed in eight children in the PHTS study, although the site of the infection was not noted.[169] Over a 15-year period, 15 (0.2%) children at Texas Children's Hospital (TCH), Houston, Texas, developed mediastinitis after undergoing cardiac surgery; two children had undergone heart transplantation.[195] At another children's hospital, between 1995 and 2003, 3% (5 of 165) of children undergoing heart and lung transplantation developed mediastinitis.[116]

Risk factors for surgical site infections in adult heart transplant recipients include body mass index greater than 30 kg/m^2, previous heart surgery, previous ventricular assist device implantation, inotropic support, and prolonged cardiopulmonary bypass time.[47] Immunosuppression regimens that include sirolimus have been identified as a risk factor for surgical site infection, wound dehiscence, and mediastinitis.[111,217] Postoperative bleeding requiring reexploration is also a risk factor for the development of mediastinitis. Fever, incisional pain, and an unstable sternum suggest mediastinitis; however, patients may have no specific evidence of infection, including fever. The white blood cell count may be elevated. A pericardial effusion frequently is detected with the development of mediastinitis, and pericardiocentesis may yield purulent material. CT of the chest may show a fluid collection or abscess within the mediastinum and can detect sternal osteomyelitis. Most cases of mediastinitis are caused by *S. aureus,* coagulase-negative staphylococci, or gram-negative bacteria. Median sternotomy wound infections after repair of a congenital heart lesion occur in less than 1% of children in large centers. Mediastinitis caused by gram-negative bacilli in association with pneumonia and bacteremia developed in three of the 22 children in the UPMC series; each occurred within 2 weeks postoperatively.[80] Two of the three patients died. *Candida* spp. caused both cases of mediastinitis in the two children after heart transplantation in the TCH series.[195] Long and colleagues[116] reported that mediastinitis developed in five patients who had undergone heart and lung transplantation and that the organisms identified in these children were *E. coli, Torulopsis glabrata, Aspergillus fumigatus, Burkholderia cepacia,* and vancomycin-resistant enterococcus.

A superficial median sternotomy wound infection not associated with an unstable sternum can be treated by local drainage of the infected subcutaneous tissue and administration of appropriate antibiotics.[51] Vacuum-assisted closure may be an important aid in addition to antibiotics.[1] A more aggressive approach is required for more serious infections associated with an unstable sternum, mediastinitis, or osteomyelitis of the sternum.[28,51,99] Adequate drainage and debridement of the area are crucial, and any involved wires should be removed. Mediastinal drains usually are kept in place for several days. A reoperation after the initial drainage procedure may be necessary. Pending culture results, antibiotic therapy is directed against *S. aureus* and gram-negative bacilli. A 4- to 6-week course of antibiotics usually is recommended. Antifungal therapy is initiated if a yeast or fungus is noted on Gram or special stains or isolated from cultures. Careful attention given to surgical technique to minimize postoperative bleeding and early withdrawal of chest and mediastinal tubes placed intraoperatively decrease the incidence of these potentially fatal infections.

Other Infections Encountered During the First Postoperative Month

Herpes Simplex

Herpes simplex infections of the oral mucosa and other superficial surfaces are common after heart transplantation. Oral herpes simplex was observed in 21% (11 of 53) of children undergoing transplantation at Stanford University Medical Center.[15] In the pediatric multiinstitutional PHTS study, only six episodes of herpes simplex infection were noted.[169] Visceral involvement is unusual, although it may develop.[112] Herpes simplex infection typically occurs approximately 13 days (range, 0 to 4 months) after transplantation and is secondary to reactivation, not a newly acquired infection.[152] A decrease in lymphocyte transformation in response to viral antigen in vitro may explain the increased rate of infection that occurs in the first 12 weeks posttransplantation. In a large randomized study comparing azathioprine with mycophenolate mofetil in adult heart transplant recipients who also were receiving cyclosporine and steroids, herpes simplex infection occurred more commonly in the group treated with mycophenolate mofetil (23% vs. 16%; $P < .05$).[52] Institution of antiviral therapy for herpes simplex infection is warranted in these immunocompromised patients. The most common antiviral agent for herpes simplex is acyclovir, which can be administered orally or intravenously. Valacyclovir dosing in children has been established for children older than 2 years, but a commercial suspension is unavailable.

Prophylactic acyclovir is recommended by some experts for heart transplant recipients who are seropositive for herpes simplex.[75,211] Acyclovir can be given intravenously during the perioperative period and then orally for at least a month following transplantation. Other physicians suggest that because labial or oral herpes simplex is treated so easily, a prophylactic approach after transplant is not warranted. Prophylaxis is generally used during treatment for rejection and for prolonged durations if recurrences are frequent. If the patient is receiving ganciclovir for CMV prophylaxis, additional HSV preventive measures are not necessary.

Legionella pneumophila

Legionella pneumophila infection should be included in the differential diagnosis for fever, respiratory symptoms, and pulmonary infiltrates that develop after heart transplantation.[33] *Legionella* pneumonia can develop during the first postoperative month, but the frequency with which this infection occurs varies among transplant centers. Although legionnaires' disease is an uncommon occurrence in children, nosocomial infections have been documented in a children's hospital, and immunosuppression is a risk factor.[22,27] Appropriate cultures and direct fluorescent antibody stains for *Legionella* should be performed on sputum, other respiratory secretions (obtained by invasive techniques), pleural fluid, or lung tissue to detect this pathogen in a timely fashion. A *Legionella* urinary antigen test is available for serogroup 1 antigens and is quite sensitive.[192]

Macrolides should be considered for empiric therapy if *Legionella* is a serious consideration in children with nosocomial pneumonia. A 2-week course of erythromycin or azithromycin is generally recommended. Macrolides interact with many of the immunosuppressive agents administered to these patients, however. Quinolones also are quite active against *Legionella* and avoid many of these interactions; in adult transplant patients, levofloxacin is the agent of choice.[192] The use of quinolones should be considered for pediatric organ transplant recipients in whom infection with *L. pneumophila* is suspected. In hospitals caring for patients with transplants, routine surveillance culture of the hospital water supply should be considered.

Respiratory Syncytial Virus

Ten episodes of RSV infection were noted in the multiinstitutional study by the PHTS Group.[169] RSV can be acquired in the hospital soon after undergoing transplantation or can be acquired in the community before undergoing surgery or after discharge. Too few patients in whom RSV infection developed after they underwent heart transplantation have been described to comment on the clinical features. Two children in the early UPMC study were noted to be infected with RSV, both infections occurring on postoperative day 10. Rapidly progressive patchy infiltrates on chest radiographs developed in one child after undergoing heart-lung transplantation, and the second child had only mild upper respiratory symptoms.[80] Tachypnea, cough, fever, wheezing, and the use of accessory muscles occurred commonly in the 18 pediatric liver transplant recipients from UPMC with RSV infection.[151] Radiographic changes included interstitial and lobar infiltrates, atelectasis, and pleural effusion in 12 patients. Two patients required mechanical ventilation after the onset of symptoms related to RSV infection occurred; three others were intubated before acquiring RSV infection and subsequently had complicated courses. At Boston Children's Hospital, there were 34 RSV infections in 851 solid organ transplant recipients from 1993 to 2006. Two deaths were reported: a 1-year-old with RSV 2 days after renal transplant and an 18-year-old 776 days after liver transplant who also had disseminated aspergillosis.[115]

Morbidity and mortality rates related to RSV infection are increased in otherwise immunocompetent children with congenital heart disease, especially when associated with pulmonary hypertension.[120] Because RSV can be acquired in the hospital, RSV infection should be considered in a young transplant patient with respiratory symptoms and fever, especially during the RSV season.[82] RSV infection is documented by culture or by rapid detection of RSV infection by a variety of techniques.

The decision to administer ribavirin to these patients is based primarily on the severity of the illness. In a small group of children with underlying bronchopulmonary dysplasia or congenital heart disease, aerosolized ribavirin seemed to be associated with more rapid improvement than that in patients given placebo.[83] Administration of aerosolized ribavirin to a heart transplant recipient with proved or suspected moderate to severe RSV infection is reasonable. As is the case with children requiring mechanical ventilation because of severe RSV lower respiratory tract infection, however, the efficacy of ribavirin in this situation is unknown.[185] The 2015 *Red Book* states that "ribavirin … may be considered for use in select patients with documented, potentially life-threatening RSV infection."[8]

The monoclonal antibody palivizumab was found to be safe, well tolerated, and effective in preventing serious RSV infections in young children with hemodynamically significant congenital heart disease in a large multicenter randomized, double-blind, placebo-controlled trial.[58] Palivizumab administration to children 24 months or younger who have undergone heart transplantation is reasonable, especially in children who are on medications for heart failure or pulmonary hypertension.[5] The combination of ribavirin and RSV immunoglobulin has been administered to pediatric bone marrow transplant recipients with RSV lower respiratory tract infection.[42] The outcome in these patients was improved over that of historical controls, but no randomized trials have been conducted. RSV immunoglobulin was not efficacious in treating RSV lower respiratory tract infection in children with congenital heart disease who were younger than 2 years.[159] Although palivizumab reduced the concentration of RSV in the tracheal aspirates of children with respiratory failure caused by RSV, its efficacy in treatment is unknown.[92,123] Many authorities recommend both ribavirin and an antibody product for the management of severe RSV infections in solid organ transplant patients.[125]

INFECTIONS BETWEEN THE FIRST AND SIXTH POSTOPERATIVE MONTHS

Cytomegalovirus

CMV is the most frequently identified viral infection in cardiac transplant patients. Asymptomatic or symptomatic infections are noted most commonly between the first and sixth months after undergoing transplantation but can occur late after transplant.[19] In adult series, the majority of patients have developed CMV infection at some time postoperatively.[50,78,135,187] In the multiinstitutional PHTS study, 51 episodes of CMV infection occurred in 332 patients and accounted for 60% of the viral infections, with a peak occurrence in the second month after transplantation.[169] CMV infection occurred more frequently in older children than in infants. In another study, infants younger than 120 days had CMV infection and disease less commonly than did infants older than 120 days after undergoing heart transplantation.[67] Maternal antibody to CMV may have been protective in the younger infants. In the UPMC series, seven children (32%) had CMV infections, with onset occurring at a mean of 33 days posttransplant (range, 23 to 43 days).[80]

CMV infection in transplant recipients occurs in three or four possible settings. In a seronegative recipient, primary CMV infection is acquired through the transplanted heart, through blood transfusions from seropositive donors, or from community exposure. Seropositive recipients can have reactivation of latent CMV infection or be reinfected with a second strain of CMV from the heart or from blood products derived from seropositive donors.[32,24] The exact site within the donor heart where CMV may reside in a latent form is unknown, but it may be either cardiac cells or leukocytes that remain within the donor heart.

When primary CMV infection is acquired from the donor organ, CMV disease tends to be more severe than if CMV infection is acquired from blood or blood products.[212]

Several risk factors for development of CMV infection after undergoing organ transplantation are recognized. Donor and recipient serologic status and the immunosuppressive regimen are the most significant risk factors for acquiring CMV infection after undergoing heart transplantation. Gorensek and colleagues[78] found that positive recipient CMV serology before transplantation and a larger than average dose of corticosteroids were significant risk factors for acquiring CMV infection. Among the group of patients with CMV infection, positive recipient serology was associated with asymptomatic infection, and excessive steroid dosing was a risk factor for acquiring symptomatic CMV infection. CMV tissue invasion occurred more commonly in patients receiving mycophenolate mofetil compared with azathioprine. Use of lymphocyte-depleting agents such as antilymphocyte antibodies increases the risk of CMV disease.[153]

The clinical manifestations of CMV infection vary. Patients may seroconvert or a latent infection may be reactivated, as determined by positive cultures or molecular tests, but these patients have no symptoms attributable to the CMV infection. Fever, leukopenia, and thrombocytopenia are common postoperative manifestations of systemic CMV infection. Patients may complain of arthralgias, myalgias, and nonspecific abdominal pain. Atypical lymphocytes are noted more commonly in adult than pediatric patients. CMV infection can cause hepatitis, pneumonitis, retinitis, myocarditis, and gastrointestinal disease, including colitis.[50,57,61,77,78,98,179] Invasion of organs, especially the gastrointestinal tract, can occur in the absence of detectable CMV in the blood. Retinitis may be asymptomatic or associated with complaints such as floaters or scotomata. Ophthalmologic screening for CMV retinitis is recommended by some authorities for all patients 3 to 4 months after cardiac transplantation.[61]

Of the tissues invaded by CMV, involvement of the lung leads to the greatest mortality rate—13% in one study.[103] CMV pneumonitis is characterized by fever, hypoxemia, and, usually, diffuse interstitial infiltrates, although lobar consolidation may occur.[178] Pulmonary infections with other viruses or with bacteria or *Pneumocystis jirovecii* and other pathologic processes (infarction) may coexist with CMV pneumonitis. Gastritis, gastric ulceration, duodenitis, esophagitis, pyloric perforation, and colonic hemorrhage can be documented by endoscopy. In the multiinstitutional PHTS study, the lung or gastrointestinal tract was the site of CMV infection in 13 (lung) and six (gastrointestinal tract) episodes.[80] Death related to CMV in the pediatric study occurred in 6%. In another pediatric heart transplant registry spanning 1998 to 2010, CMV was considered the cause of death in 2.7%, 0.4%, and 0.4% of patients 31 days to 1 year, after 3 to 5 years, and after 10 years post transplantation, respectively.[102] In another analysis using a multiinstitutional registry of pediatric heart transplantation patients, clinical CMV infection was uncommon in the setting of antiviral and/or CMV antibody prophylaxis.[121]

Serology is not recommended for establishing the diagnosis of CMV infection after transplantation.[106] Viral load testing by quantitative nucleic acid amplification testing (QNAT), which is the preferred test, or CMV antigenemia is recommended for the diagnosis and monitoring for CMV infection and disease.[106] Whether the CMV infection is causing a symptomatic or invasive illness is more difficult to establish. Histopathologic evidence of CMV infection, such as typical viral inclusions or detection of antigen in tissue by special stains, is required to confirm organ involvement by CMV, although this criterion often is not considered for clinical management and treatment.

In addition to the CMV infection syndromes, CMV infection itself seems to affect the transplant recipient adversely in other ways. Symptomatic or asymptomatic CMV infection is associated with a higher rate of acute rejection and graft loss, a greater risk of development of fungal infection, more frequent and earlier cardiac allograft vasculopathy, and a significantly lower survival rate than occur in patients who do not have CMV infection.[41,63,94,162] In the PHTS study, CMV-positive donor serology in conjunction with CMV-negative recipient serology was a risk factor for the acquisition of earlier infection with any organism.[169]

CMV infection of the wide variety of cells that it invades leads to the activation of protein synthesis and the production of multiple immunologically active molecules, including cytokines, especially tumor necrosis factor-α, which adds to the immune deficits induced by the immunosuppressive agents.[63,105] Allograft injury or rejection may be associated with CMV infection of the transplanted organ itself.[63]

Successful treatment or suppression of visceral CMV disease by ganciclovir, a nucleoside analogue active in vitro against CMV, requires a timely diagnosis. Ganciclovir has been shown to alter CMV disease favorably in heart transplant patients, along with reduction in immunosuppressive therapy when possible.[100] The recommended length of therapy is determined by weekly monitoring of CMV viral loads and continuing therapy until 1 or 2 consecutive negative samples. The minimum course of therapy is 2 weeks. The dose of ganciclovir is 5 mg/kg every 12 hours with careful monitoring of hematologic parameters and renal function if renal function initially is normal. Modification of the dose is necessary if renal function is impaired. The most common adverse reactions to ganciclovir are neutropenia, thrombocytopenia, impaired renal function, seizures, and other central nervous system (CNS) abnormalities. Many experts will use oral valganciclovir instead of intravenous ganciclovir in nonsevere CMV disease. Some transplant centers will use secondary prophylaxis with once daily oral valganciclovir for 1 to 3 months after completion of therapy for CMV infection.[106]

The role of CMV hyperimmunoglobulin in treating CMV infection in these patients requires further study. After bone marrow transplantation, the addition of CMV immunoglobulin to ganciclovir may be superior to ganciclovir alone in treating CMV pneumonia.[55,157]

In one pediatric study, symptomatic CMV disease developed in five children after they had undergone heart transplantation; each had blood cultures and PCR positive for CMV.[69] Four were treated with ganciclovir for 14 days; one received ganciclovir for 30 days. All received CMV-IgG (150 mg/kg) weekly for 3 weeks. Symptomatic CMV disease was treated successfully in each case. CMV-IgG may be beneficial in treating life-threatening CMV disease such as pneumonitis and enteritis.[106,153] For CMV disease in thoracic organ transplant recipients with hypogammaglobulinemia, intravenous immunoglobulin or CMV-IgG is recommended as adjunctive therapy as well.[106]

If possible, prevention of CMV infection in heart transplant recipients is optimal. Only seronegative blood should be used for transfusions when the recipient and the donor are seronegative. Careful control of immunosuppressive therapy, especially with corticosteroids, may help avoid the acquisition of some infections. Prophylactic administration of intravenous ganciclovir followed by oral valganciclovir for 3 to 6 months appears to be the strategy of choice for preventing CMV infection in adults at risk following heart transplantation.[106,153] The updated CMV consensus statement recommends 3 to 6 months for adult patients who are CMV seronegative and receive a heart from a CMV seropositive donor; 3 months is recommended if the recipient is CMV seropositive regardless of the donor's status.[106] The longer duration is determined in part by the degree of immunosuppression required. The duration of prophylaxis in children is not as well established and varies among centers. In the situation of a seronegative recipient of a heart from a seropositive donor, the addition of prophylactic administration of CMV immunoglobulin to ganciclovir may be useful.[2,154,186] If the prophylactic approach is used, routine monitoring for CMV viral load is not recommended but should be evaluated if patients have symptoms that could be caused by CMV infection.[106]

In one large randomized double-blind, placebo-controlled trial of CMV-seropositive transplant recipients, ganciclovir significantly reduced the incidence of CMV illness during the first 120 days after heart transplantation (9% vs. 46% in controls; $P < .001$).[131] No differences were noted between the study groups for seronegative recipients.

Whether the addition of CMV-IgG to antiviral therapy for prophylaxis of high-risk seronegative recipients of hearts from seropositive donors results in added benefits is still under investigation. Avery[12] found that the combination was not particularly effective; symptomatic CMV syndrome developed in 50% of patients. Gajarski and associates[69] provided CMV-IgG (150 mg/kg intravenously at weeks 0, 2, 4, 6, and 8 and 100 mg/kg intravenously at weeks 12 and 16) plus ganciclovir (5 mg/kg every 12 hours intravenously for weeks 1 and 2 and 6 mg/kg per day intravenously at weeks 3 and 4) to 19 children who were recipients of heart transplants from CMV-seropositive donors. CMV disease occurred in three of the 10 children who were CMV-seronegative and in one of the 10 recipients who were seropositive. Adverse effects of these agents were not reported. In the study from Stanford University Medical Center, high-risk recipients received CMV-IgG immediately after undergoing transplantation (150 mg/kg administered within 72 hours after transplantation, followed by 100 mg/kg at weeks 2, 4, 6, and 8 and 50 mg/kg at weeks 12 and 16).[199,200] In addition, ganciclovir was administered intravenously immediately after transplantation at a dose of 5 mg/kg every 12 hours for 14 days, followed by 6 mg/kg per day for the next 2 weeks. These patients were compared with a historical control group at the same institution that received ganciclovir in the 2 to 3 years before CMV-IgG was used. The 27 recipients treated prophylactically with ganciclovir and CMV-IgG had a higher disease-free incidence of CMV, a lower incidence of rejection, and a higher survival rate than those of the historical cohort treated with ganciclovir alone. Data from the Scientific Registry of Transplant Recipients indicated that, for children undergoing heart transplantation, CMV immune globulin with or without ganciclovir and ganciclovir with or without CMV immune globulin were associated with significant reduction in graft loss and deaths versus no prophylaxis.[186] Immunologic monitoring of CMV may be helpful in assessing the risk of patients developing CMV viremia and disease posttransplantation, although the value of this monitoring is unknown in children.[106]

CMV resistant to ganciclovir may emerge as a result of ganciclovir prophylaxis or treatment.[14,101] Foscarnet or cidofovir is an alternative agent in this situation. The reader is urged to review the "Updated International Consensus Guidelines on the Management of Cytomegalovirus in Solid-Organ Transplantation" document for expert guidance on this subject.[106]

Epstein-Barr Virus

In pediatric heart transplant recipients, EBV may cause a spectrum of diseases, including a mononucleosis-like syndrome, hepatitis, myocarditis, and hematologic abnormalities such as leukopenia, thrombocytopenia, hemophagocytic syndrome, and polyclonal or monoclonal lymphoproliferation, usually of B cells. EBV endomyocardial infection, as determined by detection of EBV viral genome in asymptomatic heart transplant recipients, has also been associated with premature graft loss as a result of premature development of advanced transplant coronary vasculopathy.[139]

In young children, the transplanted organ is thought to be the most frequent source of EBV.[3] Posttransplantation lymphoproliferative disorders (PTLDs) refer to B-cell expansion that may be localized, nodal, extranodal, or widely disseminated. The largest series of children who have undergone heart transplantation is from UPMC; in this series, PTLD developed in 7.7% (six of 78) of pediatric heart transplant recipients.[21] A major risk factor for the subsequent development of PTLD was being seronegative for EBV before undergoing transplantation. PTLD developed in one-third of seronegative recipients of thoracic organs who acquired primary EBV infection (10 of 30). PTLD developed in none of the children who were seropositive before transplantation. Almost all these cases occurred within 1 year of transplantation.

In another series, 19 children were EBV-seropositive and 31 were EBV-seronegative before undergoing heart transplantation. PTLD developed in one of 19 patients who were seropositive before undergoing transplantation and in 12 of 19 who became seropositive after transplantation.[215] It did not develop in any of the 12 recipients who remained EBV-seronegative. In contrast to the UPMC experience, the mean time to confirmation of PTLD was 29 months (range, 3 to 72 months).

Webber and associates[208,209] reviewed the experience with PTLD after heart transplantation among 1184 primary organ recipients in 19 centers from 1993 to 2002. Fifty-six patients (5%) developed PTLD a mean of 23.8 months posttransplantation. In a study from Germany, 12 of 147 (8.2%) developed PTLD a mean of 3.2 ± 2.2 years posttransplantation.[171] Among 173 heart transplant recipients at the University of Toronto Hospital, 23 (13.3%) developed PTLD within a median of 4 years posttransplantation.[124] Higher maximum EBV viral load and longer duration of induction therapy were associated with increased risk of PTLD. In a study among a multicenter group, PTLD developed in about 5% of 2374 children.[68] Pretransplant seropositivity for EBV and the receipt of induction treatment except OKT3 were associated with a reduced risk of developing PTLD. Chinnock et al. reported that, between 1993 and 2009, among 3170 pediatric heart transplant recipients at 35 institutions, 147 patients developed PTLD, with children age 1 to 10 years having the highest risk compared with children younger than 1 year or age 10 to 18 years.[31] Similarly, data from the United Network for Organ Sharing (UNOS) database from 1987 to 2013 showed that 360 out of 6818 pediatric heart transplant recipients (5169 of whom had follow-up data on posttransplant malignancy) were diagnosed with PTLD and that PTLD was associated with reduced long-term survival after heart transplant.[86]

Symptoms of PTLD may include fever, malaise, sore throat, and lymphadenopathy. Some children may have splenomegaly, CNS symptoms such as lethargy or seizures, or gastrointestinal complaints.[17,21] Concurrent opportunistic infections are common. Nodules in the lung may be noted on chest radiographs (Fig. 70.1A).

The diagnosis of PTLD requires biopsy of involved tissue showing lymphoid proliferation with an immunoblastic component (Fig. 70.1B). Molecular techniques typically detect EBV nucleic acids in tissue (Fig. 70.1C). EBV serology is not particularly helpful after transplant but is important in the pretransplant evaluation to assess risk for posttransplant infection. Quantitative measurement of EBV DNA in peripheral blood is used to detect primary infection or reactivation at a very early time point and to monitor viral loads serially over time to detect PTLD in the timeliest manner.[161] When reported as EBV copies per 10^5 peripheral blood lymphocytes, patients with PTLD typically have viral loads between 500 and 5000, which are much greater than the loads detected in normal latency.

Management generally involves decreasing the immunosuppressive regimen or discontinuing it temporarily. Anti-CD20 antibody (rituximab) is a monoclonal antibody that specifically binds to the CD20 antigen of normal and malignant B cells and results in antibody-dependent and complement-dependent cytotoxicity. Rituximab has been administered with success to children and adults with PTLD after they have undergone solid organ transplantation.[54,171,175,126] Antiviral therapy with acyclovir or ganciclovir also is administered. Some centers administer ganciclovir, acyclovir, or intravenous γ-globulin for prevention of PTLD, although no prospective studies have confirmed that such an approach is efficacious.[79] Allen et. al.[3] have provided a detailed discussion of PTLD in solid organ transplant patients.

Toxoplasma gondii

An increased incidence of toxoplasmosis is apparent in recipients of heart transplants compared with other organ transplants, although it remains an uncommon infection after heart transplantation.[189] In the multiinstitutional study by the PHTS,[169] toxoplasmosis was not mentioned. *T. gondii* has a predilection for muscle and can be transmitted to the recipient from the heart of a seropositive donor. Active *T. gondii* infections may occur in donor hearts.[164] Less commonly, reactivation of old infection occurs in the recipient. The greatest risk for acquisition of toxoplasmosis occurs in a seronegative recipient of a heart from a seropositive donor. Clinical symptoms usually develop after the first postoperative month and generally within 3 months of transplantation.[84,119,133] Fever alone may be the only clinical manifestation. Dissemination of the parasite to the CNS may lead to signs and symptoms of meningoencephalitis, such as lethargy, seizures, coma, and hemiparesis. Chorioretinitis may result in diminished visual acuity. A sepsis-like picture, pneumonia, and cutaneous lesions are unusual manifestations.[10]

CT or magnetic resonance imaging of the brain may detect ring-enhancing mass lesions, which typically are multiple and in periventricular locations. Definitive diagnosis of CNS toxoplasmosis requires the demonstration of tachyzoites or cysts in tissue on histopathology or by PCR. Serologic tests help monitor seronegative patients for seroconversion and allow a more aggressive approach to be taken with an early diagnosis of toxoplasmosis.[184] *T. gondii* has been seen on endomyocardial biopsy specimens routinely obtained to monitor for rejection.[118]

Therapy for toxoplasmosis with pyrimethamine and sulfadiazine may lead to recovery; these drugs also should be administered if the patient

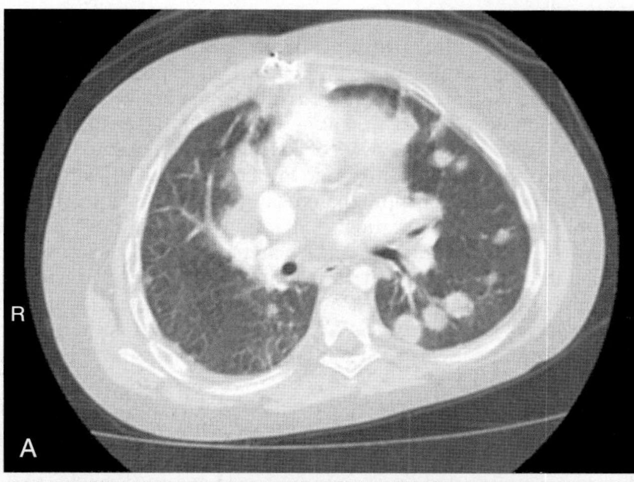

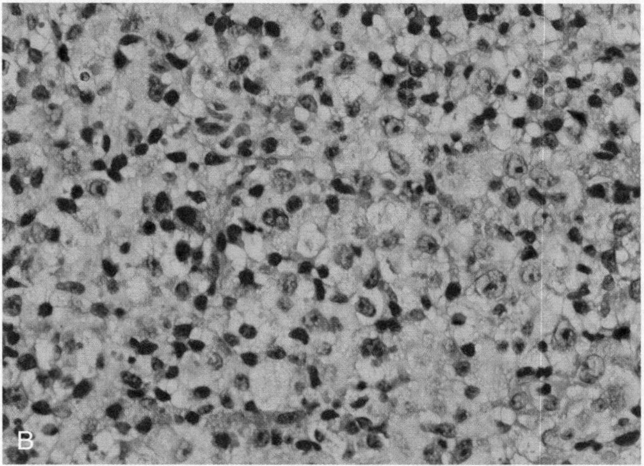

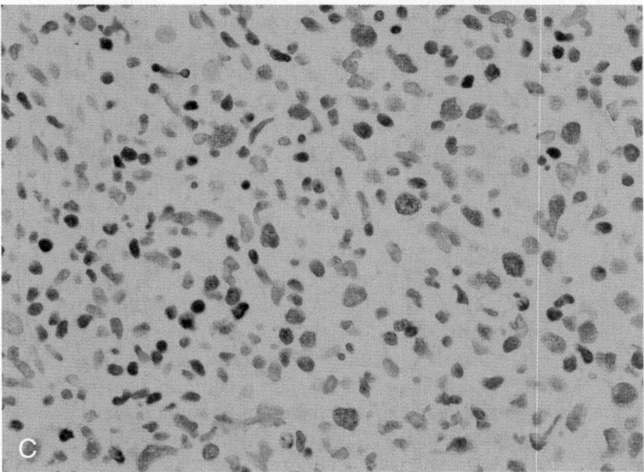

FIG. 70.1 Eight-year-old boy with history of orthotopic heart transplantation secondary to restrictive cardiomyopathy. Donor was Epstein-Barr virus (EBV) positive and recipient was EBV negative. Six months after transplantation, the patient was diagnosed with EBV-positive monomorphic posttransplant lymphoproliferative disorder (PTLD)/diffuse large B-cell lymphoma. (A) PTLD/diffuse large B-cell lymphoma involving the lungs. Computed tomography scan showing innumerable pulmonary nodules. (B–C) PTLD/diffuse large B-cell lymphoma involving the colon (B, Hematoxylin and eosin, ×400 magnification). Sheets of large, atypical B cells infiltrate the colonic mucosa (C, EBV-EBER in situ hybridization, ×400 magnification). Large B cells demonstrate very strong nuclear positivity for EBV. (Courtesy Andrea N. Marcogliese, MD, Baylor College of Medicine and Texas Children's Hospital, Houston, TX.)

seroconverts.[70] Following treatment, life-long suppressive therapy with trimethoprim-sulfamethoxazole (TMP-SMX) is suggested.[173] Prophylactic (TMP-SMX) is recommended for seronegative recipients with seropositive donors.[13,138,173] Some centers employ prophylactic administration of pyrimethamine to seronegative recipients of hearts from seropositive donors.[213] Spiramycin is not a useful prophylactic agent.[184]

Aspergillus fumigatus

A. fumigatus is the non-*Candida* fungal infection most commonly reported outside the immediate postoperative period in most series and may be noted first at necropsy.[148] In a report from Stanford University Medical Center, 54 *Aspergillus* infections developed in 620 consecutive heart transplant recipients between 1980 and 1996.[138] Most commonly, *Aspergillus* infections were in the lung ($n = 31$) or were disseminated ($n = 17$). The median time to onset was 52 days. Disseminated aspergillosis was the most common infectious episode responsible for the highest mortality rates in this series. One child in UPMC series had disseminated aspergillosis.[80] Among 1854 children in the 2011 PHTS report, 18 had infection due to *Aspergillus* spp. (including nine pulmonary and five cutaneous infections), three due to Zygomycetes, and one due to *Exserohilum* spp.[216] Thirteen (59%) of the 22 patients with mold infection died. Risk was highest in the first 6 months after transplantation; prior surgery and the need for mechanical ventilation at transplant were independent risk factors for invasive fungal infection.

CNS invasion occurs in many patients with pulmonary aspergillosis, and aspergillosis is the most common cause of brain abscess in organ transplant recipients.[84,137,183] Alterations in mental status occur most frequently, and seizures may occur in 40% of cases. Multifocal lesions are seen commonly on CT of the head and show a predilection for the junction of the gray and white matter. Mediastinitis and endocarditis are other manifestations of invasive aspergillosis.[113,176] Although isolation of *Aspergillus* from respiratory secretions in a patient with pneumonitis does not establish a diagnosis, aspergillosis is so difficult to establish firmly and is so frequently fatal that treatment should be considered seriously based on this culture alone. Measurement of serum galactomannan levels may not be as helpful in recognizing this infection in heart transplant recipients as compared to oncology patients.[140] Measuring the galactomannan in the bronchoalveolar lavage fluid may more readily detect evidence of invasive pulmonary aspergillosis in solid organ transplant patients.[35]

Voriconazole is the agent of choice for invasive aspergillosis.[87,206] The reader is referred to the Chapter 198 on aspergillosis and the Infectious Diseases Society of America clinical guidelines for recommendations regarding therapy,[206] as well as the review by Huprikar et al. on infections in solid organ transplant recipients due to less common and emerging fungi.[91] Infection due to the endemic fungi following heart transplant also occurs depending on specific geographic regions. Unlike coccidioidomycosis, pretransplant serology for histoplasmosis is not recommended.[134]

INFECTIONS AFTER THE SIXTH POSTOPERATIVE MONTH

Nocardia asteroides

A dry cough, fever, and the presence of a solitary pulmonary nodule or abscess on a chest radiograph are characteristic of infection with *N. asteroides*.[109,182] Although pulmonary nodules are characteristic of *Nocardia*, *Aspergillus* and CMV can be associated with nodules as well.[138] Some patients are asymptomatic despite having an abnormal chest radiograph. Infection with *Nocardia* was noted in only 3% of cyclosporine-treated patients in the early Stanford University Medical Center series.[88] The median time to the onset of infection was 225 days. A similar incidence of lung nodules or masses secondary to *Nocardia* was noted in a series from New York.[85] In the follow-up Stanford series, 23 episodes of *Nocardia* infection (3.7%) occurred, with 19 in the lung.[138] The median onset of infection in the second series was 147 days. *Nocardia* infections are rare in pediatric heart transplant recipients.

Nocardia is isolated best from direct lung tissue specimens, but it also may be cultured from bone, skin, or other sites of involvement as well. If a cutaneous skin lesion of *Nocardia* is recognized, other sites should be evaluated promptly for involvement.[74] The formation of single or multiple abscesses in the CNS may result from hematogenous dissemination. Seizures may develop after invasion of brain parenchyma.

For serious *N. asteroides* infection, initial treatment may be with a combination of imipenem or meropenem plus amikacin and/or (TMP-SMX) for 3 to 6 weeks followed by prolonged administration (6 to 12 months) of an oral agent.[36] The incidence of *Nocardia* infection has declined with the introduction of routine prophylaxis with (TMP-SMX).

Pneumocystis jiroveci

P. jiroveci (formally *P. carinii*) pneumonia has been reported in 3% to 4% of heart transplantation recipients during the postcyclosporine era.[62,81,88] In the early multiinstitutional study of the PHTS Group, *P. jiroveci* was noted in seven children (2.1%).[169] In the 2011 PHTS report, 18 of 1854 patients (1%) had *P. jirovecii* infection. Ninety-five percent of these infections occurred between 2 months and 2 years following transplantation.[141] Fever, a nonproductive cough, and tachypnea are typical symptoms; hypoxemia is characteristic.[216] The chest radiograph classically shows a diffuse interstitial infiltrate that can progress rapidly. The most expeditious method of documenting *P. jirovecii* pneumonia in children is methenamine silver or specific antibody staining of fluid or tissue obtained by bronchoalveolar lavage or lung biopsy. Molecular diagnostics such as *P. jirovecii* quantitative PCR on bronchoalveolar lavage fluid are also being used more frequently, although differentiating between disease and colonization is not always straightforward.[168]

Elevation in serum β-D-glucan concentration can be a clue to this infection. Coinfection with CMV or other pathogens occurs commonly.

Treatment of *Pneumocystis* pneumonia in a pediatric heart transplant recipient is identical to that for other immunocompromised children. Prophylaxis with (TMP-SMX) or some other agent is recommended for at least 6 to 12 months after transplantation.[127] Only one patient died in the PHTS study as a result of *Pneumocystis* pneumonia.[141]

Streptococcus pneumoniae

S. pneumoniae is an important community-acquired pathogen in heart transplant recipients who are at increased risk for acquiring this organism.[4] In the multiinstitutional PHTS study, two episodes of pneumococcal infection were recorded.[169] During a 10-year period, nine (11%) of 80 cardiac transplant patients in Little Rock, Arkansas, had 12 episodes of pneumococcal bacteremia.[193] Over an 11-year period, four of 105 children undergoing heart transplantation in Toronto had systemic pneumococcal infections.[196] In the follow-up series from Stanford University Medical Center, seven pulmonary infections with *S. pneumoniae* were reported.[138] In an eight-center pediatric surveillance study spanning 5 years, pneumococcal infection developed in 10 patients after a median time from transplantation of 17 months (range, 5 to 76 months).[172] Three of the 10 patients had two episodes, and one patient had three episodes of pneumococcal infection. The median age of the 10 patients at the time of the first pneumococcal infection was 26 months (range, 15 to 89 months). The pneumococcal serotypes of the isolates from these patients were the same as noted in healthy children. In a multicenter study, 15 children with invasive pneumococcal infections following solid organ transplantation were identified in eight pediatric centers from 2000 to 2014.[144] Most of the infections were bacteremia and/or pneumonia; nine isolates were not among the 13-valent pneumococcal conjugate vaccine serotypes.

Other Viruses

Influenza and parainfluenza viruses can cause serious infections at any time after transplantation, but especially in the immediate postoperative period.[9,128] Additional risk factors for development of severe disease leading to death are young age and augmentation of immunosuppression. Fever, cough, rhinorrhea, and pharyngitis are typical symptoms of upper respiratory infections. More serious manifestations include acute respiratory distress syndrome; a requirement for intubation and mechanical ventilation; a sepsis-like picture; or CNS symptoms such as headache, photophobia, and lethargy. Bacterial or fungal superinfections are possible complications. Viral infection may enhance the likelihood of allograft rejection occurring.

For influenza A infection, oseltamivir should be considered in a child of any age and zanamivir for children 7 years of age or older with a heart transplant because of their enhanced predisposition for severe or complicated influenza infection.[5] Recommendations vary depending on the susceptibility of the circulating influenza strains, and thus the treating physician needs to be aware of this information updated annually by the Centers for Disease Control and Prevention. Antiviral administration is recommended for more than 5 days in these patients who may have prolonged viral replication.[125] If intravenous administration is required, peramivir and a parenteral preparation of zanamivir are available on an investigational basis. Annual immunization with the inactivated influenza vaccine is recommended for heart transplant recipients and all family members. Additional information for respiratory viral infections in patients with solid organ transplants has been summarized by Manuel et al.[125]

Parvovirus B19 infection is recognized to cause severe anemia associated with low or no reticulocytes as well as poor response to erythropoietin in recipients of heart transplants, similar to the red blood cell suppression in other immunosuppressed patients.[143] In one child, severe pneumonia developed in association with fever and a blanching maculopapular rash involving the face, trunk, and extremities.[93] The parvovirus B19 genome also has been detected in myocardial biopsy specimens of children experiencing cardiac allograft rejection. Of six children described in one report, one had a diffuse rash and two had persistent rejection despite receiving aggressive therapy.[170] In a series of children from Loma Linda University Medical Center who underwent myocardial biopsy for possible rejection, parvovirus genome was detected in five of 553 biopsy samples taken from 149 children.[177] The parvovirus B19 genome was the most commonly detected viral genome in endomyocardial biopsies from 99 children in one study.[24] The detection of parvovirus B19 genome did not correlate with cellular rejection, but if it was present chronically there was an association with transplant coronary artery disease. Intravenous immunoglobulin is beneficial for the treatment of anemia related to parvovirus B19, but its efficacy in treating pneumonia or possible allograft rejection is unknown.[95] The dose of intravenous immunoglobulin recommended is 400 mg/kg per day for 5 consecutive days.[53]

Varicella virus infection remains a common childhood illness that can cause life-threatening disease in immunocompromised children.[150] In a group of 28 children younger than 10 years at the time of undergoing heart transplantation who had been monitored for at least 1 year between 1986 and 1999, 14 cases of primary infection with varicella zoster virus were identified.[46] The mean time posttransplant was 3 years (range, 9 months to 7.5 years). All children were seronegative at the time of transplantation. These children were treated successfully with either parenteral followed by oral acyclovir or oral valacyclovir (mean dose, 77 mg/kg per day) for 7 days. Only one child had recurrent varicella, and none had zoster. In a report of 314 adult heart transplant patients at Brigham and Women's Hospital, 51 patients had 60 episodes of herpes zoster, and cumulative zoster incidence was 0.078 at 1, 0.15 at 5, and 0.20 at 10 years.[104] Ideally pediatric heart transplant recipients should receive varicella vaccine prior to transplant if clinically feasible. Varicella vaccine is contraindicated after solid organ transplantation. Some patients do lose serologically measured immunity to varicella after undergoing transplantation, especially those children transplanted in the first 2 years of life.[198,207] Routine administration of varicella vaccine to young children does help to decrease concerns about varicella developing after organ transplantation because of herd protection.

Adenovirus has been associated with serious infections after solid organ transplantation.[64,65] Among 28 children with solid organ transplants (nine heart) and adenoviral infections, the most common symptoms were fever, diarrhea, vomiting, and abdominal pain.[40] Infection occurred a median of 1.6 months after transplantation. Only two of these patients received antiviral therapy, and all survived the infection. Cidofovir may be beneficial in some patients with disseminated infection, especially of the lungs, or with increasing viral loads determined by PCR.[45,89] In asymptomatic heart transplant children, adenovirus genome detected in endomyocardial biopsies was associated with premature graft loss.[139]

BK polyomavirus is associated with polyomavirus-associated nephropathy (PVAN) and kidney failure in kidney transplant recipients.

BOX 70.2 Effect of Various Antibiotics on Cyclosporine/Tacrolimus Levels

Increased Level	Decreased Level
Clarithromycin	Sulfadiazine
Azithromycin	Rifampin
Erythromycin	Trimethoprim-sulfamethoxazole
Ketoconazole	? Nafcillin
Fluconazole	? Isoniazid
Itraconazole	? Ciprofloxacin (counteracts immunosuppression)
Posaconazole	
Voriconazole	
Caspofungin	

PVAN has been reported with increasing frequency in nonrenal solid organ transplant recipients as well, including adult and pediatric heart transplant patients.[25,96,117,149] One systematic review identified the incidence of BK viruria and viremia in nonrenal solid organ transplant patients at 20% and 3%, respectively. Heart transplant recipients had a higher overall incidence of BK viremia than other nonrenal organ types, and the majority of cases of BK virus–associated nephropathy in nonrenal solid organ transplant recipients were in heart transplant patients.[204] A single-center study of pediatric heart transplant patients found that, out of 98 heart transplant patients, 28 had BK viruria and seven had BK viremia. One viremic patient had biopsy-proven nephropathy that progressed to end-stage renal disease.[49]

IMMUNOSUPPRESSIVE AGENTS AND ANTIBIOTICS

Cyclosporine and tacrolimus have improved the success of organ transplantation considerably. Generally the incidence of infection seems to be less since the introduction of cyclosporine than with the earlier immunosuppressive regimens, although morbidity rates remain high in heart transplant recipients. Cyclosporine and tacrolimus serum levels are monitored carefully to ensure that concentrations associated with optimal immunosuppression and minimal adverse effects are maintained. Some antibiotics interfere with the pharmacokinetics of cyclosporine or tacrolimus, which may lead to an increase or decrease in their levels.[16,26,108,145,165,167,188,191,197] These interactions are outlined in Box 70.2. Because cyclosporine and tacrolimus are nephrotoxic, the antimicrobial agents (amphotericin B, aminoglycosides, acyclovir, cidofovir, foscarnet) administered to heart transplant recipients may be additive; renal function must be monitored carefully.

IMMUNIZATIONS

Guidelines for the immunization of patients after they have received a solid organ transplant have been published, although few studies examining the immunogenicity of selected vaccines in heart transplant recipients specifically have been conducted.[39,126,163] Another prudent approach is to follow the recommendations that the Committee on Infectious Diseases of the American Academy of Pediatrics has developed for immunizing immunosuppressed children.[7] Ideally the patient will have received the recommended routine vaccines before undergoing transplantation. For patients who do not receive recommended vaccines prior to transplant, most experts recommend waiting until approximately 6 months after transplant prior to administering immunizations. Influenza vaccine can be administered as early as 2 to 8 weeks after transplant, however, if there is an influenza outbreak at that time.

Children who have received transplants before reaching 2 to 3 years of age do not respond to the pneumococcal polysaccharide vaccine as well as do children who are older when they receive a transplanted heart, even though the vaccine is administered several years after they receive the transplant.[73] An impairment in immunoglobulin isotype switching from IgM to IgG and especially IgG2 seems to result from the immunosuppressive therapy that these children are receiving.[72] In one study, the antibody response of children aged 2 to 18 months following solid organ transplantation was compared with age-matched children to the 7-valent pneumococcal conjugate vaccine (PCV7) followed by the 23-valent polysaccharide vaccine (PV23) 2 months later.[114] The antibody levels achieved were significantly higher in the controls, and a second dose of PCV7 given 2 months after the administration of the first PCV7 dose did not lead to higher antibody levels.

For previously unimmunized transplant recipients aged 2 to 18 years, the 13-valent pneumococcal conjugate vaccine is recommended, followed by the 23-valent pneumococcal vaccine at least 2 to 12 months later. Ideally children will have completed their PCV series before undergoing transplantation.[6] Ongoing immunosuppression seems to prevent maturation of the response to polysaccharide antigens in younger children, which it is hoped that the conjugate vaccine can overcome. The 23-valent pneumococcal vaccine is less immunogenic in adults after they have undergone heart transplantation than it is in healthy controls.

Antibodies to the influenza vaccine develop in most children, but previous exposure predicts a better response.[129] Annual administration of influenza vaccine seems to be safe and immunogenic in children after they have undergone solid organ transplantation. In one study, low-level histologic rejection occurred after the administration of influenza vaccine.[18] In a later study, the administration of inactivated influenza vaccine was not associated with an increased risk of rejection.[210] Depending on the time of year and the approximate date of transplantation, influenza vaccination is appropriate for the patient and all household contacts and health care workers to whom the patient might be exposed. The live-attenuated influenza vaccine is not recommended for individuals receiving immunosuppressive therapy or their close contacts.

After transplantation has been performed and after immunosuppressive therapy has been initiated, administration of live viral vaccines is contraindicated. The enhanced inactivated polio vaccine should be given to the child and to normal siblings. Measles, mumps, rubella, and varicella vaccines can be given to the siblings and adults in the household shown to have nonprotective antibody levels. Diphtheria, tetanus, and acellular pertussis inactivated vaccines should be given at the routine booster schedule, although antibody responses may not be equivalent to those observed in normal children. If varicella antibody is not detected at the pretransplant evaluation in a child aged 12 months or older, varicella vaccine should be administered at least 4 weeks before transplantation is performed if clinically feasible. Whether the antibody response data generated in children with leukemia during maintenance chemotherapy can be applied to heart transplant recipients who must continue daily immunosuppressive therapy is unclear.

NEW REFERENCES SINCE THE SEVENTH EDITION

3. Allen UD, Preiksaitis JK, Practice ASTIDCo. Epstein-Barr virus and posttransplant lymphoproliferative disorder in solid organ transplantation. *Am J Transplant*. 2013;13(suppl 4):107-120.
7. American Academy of Pediatrics. Immunization in special clinical circumstances. In: Kimberlin DW, Brady MT, Jackson MA, Long SS, eds. *Red Book: 2015 Report of the Committee on Infectious Diseases*. 30th ed. Elk Grove Village, IL: American Academy of Pediatrics; 2015:85-86.
8. American Academy of Pediatrics. Respiratory syncytial virus. In: Kimberlin DW, Brady MT, Jackson MA, Long SS, eds. *Red Book: 2015 Report of the Committee on Infectious Diseases*. 30th ed. Elk Grove Village, IL: American Academy of Pediatrics; 2015:667-676.
11. Atasever A, Bacakoglu F, Uysal FE, et al. Pulmonary complications in heart transplant recipients. *Transplant Proc*. 2006;38(5):1530-1534.
19. Blyth D, Lee I, Sims KD, et al. Risk factors and clinical outcomes of cytomegalovirus disease occurring more than one year post solid organ transplantation. *Transpl Infect Dis*. 2012;14(2):149-155.
20. Boutros M, Al-Shaibi M, Chan G, et al. *Clostridium difficile* colitis: increasing incidence, risk factors, and outcomes in solid organ transplant recipients. *Transplantation*. 2012;93(10):1051-1057.
23. Bratzler DW, Dellinger EP, Olsen KM, et al. Clinical practice guidelines for antimicrobial prophylaxis in surgery. *Am J Health Syst Pharm*. 2013;70(3):195-283.
25. Butts RJ, Uber WE, Savage AJ. Treatment of BK viremia in a pediatric heart transplant recipient. *J Heart Lung Transplant*. 2012;31(5):552-553.
28. Carrier M, Hudon G, Paquet E, et al. Mediastinal and pericardial complications after heart transplantation. Not-so-unusual postoperative problems? *Cardiovasc Surg*. 1994;2(3):395-397.

31. Chinnock R, Webber SA, Dipchand AI, et al. A 16-year multi-institutional study of the role of age and EBV status on PTLD incidence among pediatric heart transplant recipients. *Am J Transplant.* 2012;12(11):3061-3068.
34. Cisneros JM, Munoz P, Torre-Cisneros J, et al. Pneumonia after heart transplantation: a multi-institutional study. Spanish Transplantation Infection Study Group. *Clin Infect Dis.* 1998;27(2):324-331.
36. Clark NM, Reid GE, AST Infectious Diseases Community of Practice. *Nocardia* infections in solid organ transplantation. *Am J Transplant.* 2013;13(suppl 4):83-92.
37. Coster LO. Parasitic infections in solid organ transplant recipients. *Infect Dis Clin North Am.* 2013;27(2):395-427.
39. Danziger-Isakov L, Kumar D, AST Infectious Diseases Community of Practice. Vaccination in solid organ transplantation. *Am J Transplant.* 2013;13(suppl 4):311-317.
41. Delgado JF, Reyne AG, de Dios S, et al. Influence of cytomegalovirus infection in the development of cardiac allograft vasculopathy after heart transplantation. *J Heart Lung Transplant.* 2015;34(8):1112-1119.
43. Dipchand AI, Kirk R, Mahle WT, et al. Ten yr of pediatric heart transplantation: a report from the Pediatric Heart Transplant Study. *Pediatr Transplant.* 2013;17(2):99-111.
44. Dipchand AI, Rossano JW, Edwards LB, et al. The registry of the International Society for Heart and Lung Transplantation: eighteenth official pediatric heart transplantation report—2015: focus theme: early graft failure. *J Heart Lung Transplant.* 2015;34(10):1233-1243.
47. Dorschner P, McElroy LM, Ison MG. Nosocomial infections within the first month of solid organ transplantation. *Transpl Infect Dis.* 2014;16(2):171-187.
48. Dubberke ER, Burdette SD, AST Infectious Diseases Community of Practice. *Clostridium difficile* infections in solid organ transplantation. *Am J Transplant.* 2013;13(suppl 4):42-49.
49. Ducharme-Smith A, Katz BZ, Bobrowski AE, et al. Prevalence of BK polyomavirus infection and association with renal dysfunction in pediatric heart transplant recipients. *J Heart Lung Transplant.* 2015;34(2):222-226.
53. Eid AJ, Chen SF, AST Infectious Diseases Community of Practice. Human parvovirus B19 in solid organ transplantation. *Am J Transplant.* 2013;13(suppl 4):201-205.
59. Filsoufi F, Rahmanian PB, Castillo JG, et al. Incidence, treatment strategies and outcome of deep sternal wound infection after orthotopic heart transplantation. *J Heart Lung Transplant.* 2007;26(11):1084-1090.
60. Fischer SA, Lu K, AST Infectious Diseases Community of Practice. Screening of donor and recipient in solid organ transplantation. *Am J Transplant.* 2013;13(suppl 4):9-21.
64. Florescu DF, Hoffman JA, AST Infectious Diseases Community of Practice. Adenovirus in solid organ transplantation. *Am J Transplant.* 2013;13(suppl 4):206-211.
65. Florescu DF, Kwon JY, Dumitru I. Adenovirus infections in heart transplantation. *Cardiol Rev.* 2013;21(4):203-206.
71. Garzoni C, Vergidis P, AST Infectious Diseases Community of Practice. Methicillin-resistant, vancomycin-intermediate and vancomycin-resistant *Staphylococcus aureus* infections in solid organ transplantation. *Am J Transplant.* 2013;13(suppl 4):50-58.
86. Hayes D Jr, Breuer CK, Horwitz EM, et al. Influence of posttransplant lymphoproliferative disorder on survival in children after heart transplantation. *Pediatr Cardiol.* 2015;36(8):1748-1753.
91. Huprikar S, Shoham S, AST Infectious Diseases Community of Practice. Emerging fungal infections in solid organ transplantation. *Am J Transplant.* 2013;13(suppl 4):262-271.
92. Hynicka LM, Ensor CR. Prophylaxis and treatment of respiratory syncytial virus in adult immunocompromised patients. *Ann Pharmacother.* 2012;46(4):558-566.
93. Janner D, Bork J, Baum M, Chinnock R. Severe pneumonia after heart transplantation as a result of human parvovirus B19. *J Heart Lung Transplant.* 1994;13(2):336-338.
94. Johansson I, Andersson R, Friman V, et al. Cytomegalovirus infection and disease reduce 10-year cardiac allograft vasculopathy-free survival in heart transplant recipients. *BMC Infect Dis.* 2015;15(1):582.
95. Jordan SC, Toyoda M, Kahwaji J, et al. Clinical aspects of intravenous immunoglobulin use in solid organ transplant recipients. *Am J Transplant.* 2011;11(2):196-202.
96. Joseph A, Pilichowska M, Boucher H, et al. BK virus nephropathy in heart transplant recipients. *Am J Kidney Dis.* 2015;65(6):949-955.
101. Kim YJ, Boeckh M, Cook L, et al. Cytomegalovirus infection and ganciclovir resistance caused by UL97 mutations in pediatric transplant recipients. *Transpl Infect Dis.* 2012;14(6):611-617.
102. Kirk R, Edwards LB, Kucheryavaya AY, et al. The registry of the International Society for Heart and Lung Transplantation: fourteenth pediatric heart transplantation report—2011. *J Heart Lung Transplant.* 2011;30(10):1095-1103.
103. Kirklin JK, Naftel DC, Levine TB, et al. Cytomegalovirus after heart transplantation. Risk factors for infection and death: a multiinstitutional study. The Cardiac Transplant Research Database Group. *J Heart Lung Transplant.* 1994;13(3):394-404.
104. Koo S, Gagne LS, Lee P, et al. Incidence and risk factors for herpes zoster following heart transplantation. *Transpl Infect Dis.* 2014;16(1):17-25.
106. Kotton CN, Kumar D, Caliendo AM, et al. Updated international consensus guidelines on the management of cytomegalovirus in solid-organ transplantation. *Transplantation.* 2013;96(4):333-360.
107. Koval CE, Rakita R, AST Infectious Diseases Community of Practice. Ventricular assist device related infections and solid organ transplantation. *Am J Transplant.* 2013;13(suppl 4):348-354.
110. Kulikowska A, Boslaugh SE, Huddleston CB, et al. Infectious, malignant, and autoimmune complications in pediatric heart transplant recipients. *J Pediatr.* 2008;152(5):671-677.
111. Kuppahally S, Al-Khaldi A, Weisshaar D, et al. Wound healing complications with de novo sirolimus versus mycophenolate mofetil-based regimen in cardiac transplant recipients. *Am J Transplant.* 2006;6(5 Pt 1):986-992.
115. Lo MS, Lee GM, Gunawardane N, et al. The impact of RSV, adenovirus, influenza, and parainfluenza infection in pediatric patients receiving stem cell transplant, solid organ transplant, or cancer chemotherapy. *Pediatr Transplant.* 2013;17(2):133-143.
117. Lorica C, Bueno TG, Garcia-Buitrago MT, et al. BK virus nephropathy in a pediatric heart transplant recipient with post-transplant lymphoproliferative disorder: a case report and review of literature. *Pediatr Transplant.* 2013;17(2):E55-E61.
125. Manuel O, Estabrook M, AST Infectious Diseases Community of Practice. RNA respiratory viruses in solid organ transplantation. *Am J Transplant.* 2013;13(suppl 4):212-219.
126. Martin K, Drabble A, Manlhiot C, et al. Response to hepatitis A and B vaccination after pediatric heart transplant. *Pediatr Transplant.* 2012;16(7):699-703.
127. Martin SI, Fishman JA, AST Infectious Diseases Community of Practice. Pneumocystis pneumonia in solid organ transplantation. *Am J Transplant.* 2013;13(suppl 4):272-279.
130. McNeil JC, Munoz FM, Hulten KG, et al. *Staphylococcus aureus* infections among children receiving a solid organ transplant: clinical features, epidemiology, and antimicrobial susceptibility. *Transpl Infect Dis.* 2015;17(1):39-47.
135. Miller R, Assi M, AST Infectious Diseases Community of Practice. Endemic fungal infections in solid organ transplantation. *Am J Transplant.* 2013;13(suppl 4):250-261.
140. Munoz P, Ceron I, Valerio M, et al. Invasive aspergillosis among heart transplant recipients: a 24-year perspective. *J Heart Lung Transplant.* 2014;33(3):278-288.
144. Olarte L, Lin P, Barson WJ, et al. Invasive pneumococcal infections in children following transplantation in the pneumococcal conjugate vaccine era. *Transpl Infect Dis.* 2017;19.
146. Pappas PG, Kauffman CA, Andes DR, et al. Clinical practice guideline for the management of candidiasis: 2016 update by the Infectious Diseases Society of America. *Clin Infect Dis.* 2016;62(4):e1-e50.
147. Patel A, Gossett JJ, Benton T, et al. Fulminant *Clostridium difficile* toxic megacolon in a pediatric heart transplant recipient. *Pediatr Transplant.* 2012;16(1):E30-E34.
149. Pereira T, Rojas CP, Garcia-Buitrago MT, et al. A child with BK virus infection: inadequacy of current therapeutic strategies. *Pediatr Transplant.* 2012;16(7):E269-E274.
150. Pergam SA, Limaye AP, AST Infectious Diseases Community of Practice. Varicella zoster virus in solid organ transplantation. *Am J Transplant.* 2013;13(suppl 4):138-146.
153. Razonable RR, Humar A, AST Infectious Diseases Community of Practice. Cytomegalovirus in solid organ transplantation. *Am J Transplant.* 2013;13(suppl 4):93-106.
154. Rea F, Potena L, Yonan N, et al. Cytomegalovirus hyper immunoglobulin for CMV prophylaxis in thoracic transplantation. *Transplantation.* 2016;100(suppl 3):S19-S26.
159. Rodriguez C, Munoz P, Rodriguez-Creixems M, et al. Bloodstream infections among heart transplant recipients. *Transplantation.* 2006;81(3):384-391.
162. Rubin LG, Levin MJ, Ljungman P, et al. 2013 IDSA clinical practice guideline for vaccination of the immunocompromised host. *Clin Infect Dis.* 2014;58(3):e44-e100.
166. Sandkovsky U, Kalil AC, Florescu DF. The use and value of procalcitonin in solid organ transplantation. *Clin Transplant.* 2015;29(8):689-696.
168. Sasso M, Chastang-Dumas E, Bastide S, et al. Performances of four real-time PCR assays for diagnosis of pneumocystis jirovecii pneumonia. *J Clin Microbiol.* 2016;54(3):625-630.
173. Schwartz BS, Mawhorter SD, AST Infectious Diseases Community of Practice. Parasitic infections in solid organ transplantation. *Am J Transplant.* 2013;13(suppl 4):280-303.
174. Senechal M, LePrince P, Tezenas du Montcel S, et al. Bacterial mediastinitis after heart transplantation: clinical presentation, risk factors and treatment. *J Heart Lung Transplant.* 2004;23(2):165-170.
180. Silveira FP, Kusne S, AST Infectious Diseases Community of Practice. *Candida* infections in solid organ transplantation. *Am J Transplant.* 2013;13(suppl 4):220-227.
186. Snydman DR, Kistler KD, Ulsh P, et al. Cytomegalovirus prevention and long-term recipient and graft survival in pediatric heart transplant recipients. *Transplantation.* 2010;90(12):1432-1438.

187. Snydman DR, Limaye AP, Potena L, et al. Update and review: state-of-the-art management of cytomegalovirus infection and disease following thoracic organ transplantation. *Transplant Proc.* 2011;43(3 suppl):S1-S17.
190. Sponholz C, Sakr Y, Reinhart K, et al. Diagnostic value and prognostic implications of serum procalcitonin after cardiac surgery: a systematic review of the literature. *Crit Care.* 2006;10(5):R145.
194. Subramanian AK, Morris MI, AST Infectious Diseases Community of Practice. *Mycobacterium tuberculosis* infections in solid organ transplantation. *Am J Transplant.* 2013;13(suppl 4):68-76.
195. Tortoriello TA, Friedman JD, McKenzie ED, et al. Mediastinitis after pediatric cardiac surgery: a 15-year experience at a single institution. *Ann Thorac Surg.* 2003;76(5):1655-1660.
197. Trofe-Clark J, Lemonovich TL, AST Infectious Diseases Community of Practice. Interactions between anti-infective agents and immunosuppressants in solid organ transplantation. *Am J Transplant.* 2013;13(suppl 4):318-326.
201. van Duin D, van Delden C, AST Infectious Diseases Community of Practice. Multidrug-resistant gram-negative bacteria infections in solid organ transplantation. *Am J Transplant.* 2013;13(suppl 4):31-41.
202. Vanderlaan RD, Manlhiot C, Edwards LB, et al. Risk factors for specific causes of death following pediatric heart transplant: an analysis of the registry of the International Society of Heart and Lung Transplantation. *Pediatr Transplant.* 2015;19(8):896-905.
204. Viswesh V, Yost SE, Kaplan B. The prevalence and implications of BK virus replication in non-renal solid organ transplant recipients: A systematic review. *Transplant Rev.* 2015;29(3):175-180.
206. Walsh TJ, Anaissie EJ, Denning DW, et al. Treatment of aspergillosis: clinical practice guidelines of the Infectious Diseases Society of America. *Clin Infect Dis.* 2008;46(3):327-360.
210. White-Williams C, Brown R, Kirklin J, et al. Improving clinical practice: should we give influenza vaccinations to heart transplant patients? *J Heart Lung Transplant.* 2006;25(3):320-323.
211. Wilck MB, Zuckerman RA, AST Infectious Diseases Community of Practice. Herpes simplex virus in solid organ transplantation. *Am J Transplant.* 2013;13(suppl 4):121-127.
214. Yu XY, Wang Y, Zhong H, et al. Diagnostic value of serum procalcitonin in solid organ transplant recipients: a systematic review and meta-analysis. *Transplant Proc.* 2014;46(1):26-32.
217. Zucker MJ, Baran DA, Arroyo LH, et al. De novo immunosuppression with sirolimus and tacrolimus in heart transplant recipients compared with cyclosporine and mycophenolate mofetil: a one-year follow-up analysis. *Transplant Proc.* 2005;37(5):2231-2239.
218. Zuckermann A, Barten MJ. Surgical wound complications after heart transplantation. *Transpl Int.* 2011;24(7):627-636.

The full reference list for this chapter is available at ExpertConsult.com

71 Infections in Pediatric Lung Transplantation

Jill A. Hoffman

The first pediatric lung transplant was reported to the International Society for Heart and Lung Transplantation (ISHLT) in 1986 and, by June 2014, a total of 2090 pediatric lung transplants had been reported to the registry, with 124 reported in 2013.[196] Although there was a steady increase through the first decade of the 21st century in pediatric lung transplant procedures, these numbers have plateaued in the past 5 years.[578] The reasons for this are likely multifactorial, but a primary one is the increased survival of persons with cystic fibrosis (CF), which is the leading indication for pediatric lung transplantation.[4,176,542] Living lobar transplantation (LLT) has been performed at some centers as a way to address the shortage of available organs[544,557,599,621]; the number of these procedures peaked in 1999 but almost all of the pediatric lung transplants in recent years have been performed with lobes from deceased donors. At Children's Hospital Los Angeles (CHLA), the first pediatric LLT was performed in 1993 on a 13-year-old boy with CF receiving lobes from each parent, and the last of 55 LLT procedures (49% of 113 total-lung and 12 heart-lung transplants) was performed at CHLA in 2004.[347]

The primary indication for lung transplantation in the pediatric population remains CF; from 2000 to 2014, 69% of the 726 11- to 17-year-olds in the ISHLT registry who underwent lung transplantation had CF, followed by 51% of 99 6- to 10-year-olds as well. Other indications, generally for younger children, include pulmonary arterial hypertension, congenital heart disease, surfactant protein B deficiency, and idiopathic pulmonary fibrosis. Infectious morbidity and mortality remain high for lung transplant recipients (LTRs).[14] This incidence results from constant communication of the lungs and fresh bronchial anastomosis with the environment and from the high preoperative microbial burden of patients with CF. Denervation of the transplanted lung, interruption of the bronchial and lymphatic circulation, abnormal cough reflexes, and impaired mucociliary clearance also play roles.[14] In addition, these patients receive high-dose, long-term immunosuppression; at 5 years, the majority of patients are still maintained on triple immunosuppressant therapy including an antimetabolite such as mycophenolate mofetil (85%), a calcineurin inhibitor such as tacrolimus (98%), and corticosteroids (90%).[196,578]

Predisposing factors for infection after lung transplantation derive from multiple sources: (1) the recipient, (2) the donor, (3) intraoperative factors, (4) posttransplant factors.[206] An in-depth discussion of each of these issues is beyond the scope of this chapter, but rigorous screening algorithms are performed on donors and recipients using history, exposures, vaccination records, physical exam, and laboratory tests to identify infectious risks.[165] For any given solid organ transplant (SOT), the transplanted organ or organ space is the most common site of early postoperative infection, likely secondary to local immunologic and surgical factors; therefore, for LTRs, it is the lungs and the chest cavity. In addition underlying illness, such as CF, leading to organ dysfunction and, more importantly, microbial colonization and infection predispose LTRs to risk of infection. The microbiology of the CF lung has changed over the past decade, such that now *Staphylococcus aureus* (77%) (methicillin-susceptible [MSSA; 52%], and methicillin-resistant [MRSA; 26%]) is more prevalent than *Pseudomonas* spp. (50%) in CF sputum. In addition, the incidence of *Stenotrophomonas maltophilia* (14%) and *Achromobacter xylosoxidans* (6%) has increased.[122] The age of the recipient affects risk of infection, with younger children more likely to have primary and more severe viral infections (herpes family virus, respiratory viruses) and immature immunologic responses and lack full vaccine protection at the time of transplantation. Donor-derived disease transmission can be expected (cytomegalovirus [CMV], Epstein-Barr virus [EBV]) and therefore monitored and/or treated to mitigate impact, or unexpected and lead to life-threatening infections in multiple organ recipients.[264] Despite robust systems for donor risk assessment and testing (e.g., the US Organ Procurement and Transplantation Network), some donors may be asymptomatic or not tested for specific infections at the time of organ procurement. Infections with human immunodeficiency virus (HIV), hepatitis C, Chagas disease, rabies, lymphocytic choriomeningitis virus, West Nile virus, and tuberculosis have all occurred in the transplant setting (see the later section "Donor-Derived and Zoonotic Infections"). In the first year after lung transplantation at CHLA, the overall incidence of infection was 0.24 episode per patient per month, or 2.88 infections per patient per year.[327] Fifty-five percent of all infections occurred in the first month after transplantation, with infections becoming much less frequent thereafter (Table 71.1).[327] A summary of the causes of infection in this cohort during the first year after transplantation is presented in Tables 71.2 and 71.3.[327]

The additional indirect impact of infections on the outcome of LTRs is also recognized. CMV and other viruses, as well as bacterial infections, have been implicated in immunologically mediated processes leading to bronchiolitis obliterans syndrome (BOS) or chronic graft dysfunction, acute rejection, graft loss, and death (see later discussion).[14,196] The overall survival of pediatric LTRs (1990–2013; $n = 1856$) as reported to the ISHLT is 81%, 61.8%, 51%, 43%, and 36% at 1, 3, 5, 7 and 10 years, respectively. This survival is similar to that of adult recipients, with a transplant half-life (50% mortality rate in recipients) of 5.3 years.[196] There is no difference in survival according to donor lung source (i.e., living vs. deceased).[45,557,599] Infection is the single most common cause of death from 1 month (16%) to 1 year (30%) after transplantation (2000–14), and it remains a significant cause of death in all periods through 5 years after transplantation.[196] In the series of 75 pediatric lung transplants at CHLA (12 heart-lung, 18 cadaveric, 45 LLTs), the mortality rate was 18.6% at 1 year, with 50% attributed to infection.[327]

Death from graft failure has been reduced from causing a third of deaths in the first month to around 10% and up to a quarter of deaths thereafter.[196] BOS, progressive allograft dysfunction, causes 40% to 50% of deaths after the first year onward. The putative multifactorial mechanism of BOS is not completely elucidated but includes contributions from acute rejection episodes leading to chronic alloimmune injury, infections (especially viral CMV/respiratory and/or colonization with *Pseudomonas* or *Aspergillus*), and nonalloimmune factors such as primary graft dysfunction and gastroesophageal reflux.[69,184,592,603]

TABLE 71.1 Etiology of Infections in 75 Pediatric Lung Transplant Recipients in the First Postoperative Month at Children's Hospital Los Angeles

Etiology	No. of Episodes
Pseudomonas, respiratory tract	22
Candida, respiratory tract	13
Herpes stomatitis	12
Cytomegalovirus infection	10
Aspergillus infection of the respiratory tract, bronchial anastomosis	4

TABLE 71.2 Etiology of Infections in 75 Pediatric Lung Transplant Recipients in the First Year at Children's Hospital Los Angeles

Etiology	% of Total Infections
Bacterial infections	55
Pseudomonas spp.	18 (35% of bacterial infections)
Viral	27
Cytomegalovirus	12 (42% of viral infections)
Fungal	16
Candida	10
Aspergillus	4

TABLE 71.3 Timing of Infections in 75 Pediatric Lung Transplant Recipients at Children's Hospital Los Angeles

Months After Transplantation	% of Episodes
0–1	55
1–3	18
3–6	13
6–9	8
9–12	7

IMMUNOSUPPRESSION AND TIMING OF INFECTION

An understanding of the mechanisms and effects of immunosuppressive therapy is fundamental to anticipating the timing and types of infections that occur after transplantation, and several excellent reviews on these subjects are available.[110,483,489] The predictability of certain infections has facilitated establishing more timely diagnosis and determining strategies for preventive antimicrobial therapy.[170] A general timeline of the occurrence of specific infectious agents in pediatric lung transplant recipients is presented in Table 71.4.

OVERVIEW OF INFECTIONS AND ANTIBIOTIC USE IN SOLID-ORGAN TRANSPLANTATION

The "therapeutic prescription," as described by Rubin and colleagues,[489] for successful organ transplantation requires a careful balance between immunosuppression and the use of antimicrobial agents therapeutically, prophylactically, or preemptively to manage the risk for rejection versus infection. A transplant recipient's risk for developing infection is determined by multiple factors including (1) the technical skill of the surgeon; (2) the quality of perioperative care; (3) the "net state of immunosuppression"; (4) the patient's infectious exposure, including that from the community (past and present), hospital, and donor grafts; (5) the underlying condition of the patient (e.g., microbial colonization, organ dysfunction); and (6) the virulence of the organisms. Preventive/prophylactic strategies can alter these patterns, most notably for CMV and fungal infections, and delay their appearance past the expected time periods.[487] In sum, these considerations indicate that although a standard set of antimicrobial agents can be prescribed, they must be tailored closely to the risks, exposure, and immunosuppression of each individual.[490]

General principles of infection and therapy have been proposed by Rubin and Marty[490] and include the recognition that a transplant recipient is likely to have a greater microbial load and more advanced infection at the time of diagnosis, thus requiring longer therapy with greater potential for drug toxicity. Early establishment of the diagnosis and provision of therapy are paramount to a successful outcome. Furthermore a broader range of organisms must be considered. Although a common practice in medicine is to assume a single diagnosis for a given manifestation, a recognized caveat is that transplant recipients may have simultaneous and sequential infections. In fact, many infectious processes are influenced directly by proceeding or concurrent events. The prototype of this interaction is the immunomodulating effect of CMV infection such that alterations in the cytokine/chemokine milieu, T-lymphocyte subsets and function, neutrophil activity, and activation of endothelial cells emerge. The result of these derangements is further immunosuppression, enhanced production of virus, and subsequent increased susceptibility to additional infections. Other putative immunomodulating viruses include human herpesvirus–6 (HHV-6), EBV, and the hepatitis viruses.[490,520] The effects of bacterial and fungal infections is not clearly understood but may also contribute to enhanced immunosuppression.

Length of therapy depends on consideration of the degree of current immunosuppression and location of the infection. In general, experts suggest that treatment be continued until all signs and symptoms of infection are gone, followed by a buffer period of weeks to months, depending on the infection.[490] Finally drug interactions and toxicities, which may be synergistic, must be taken into consideration.[366,489]

TABLE 71.4 Timetable of Infections for Pediatric Lung Transplant Recipients

Time of Initial Evaluation	Infection/Pathogen	Comments
0–1 month	Wound, respiratory tract, line/bloodstream, and urinary tract infections	Related to the surgical procedure: *Candida, Staphylococcus* spp., *Pseudomonas* spp.
	HSV stomatitis	Reactivation
	CMV infection	
	HHV-6?	
	Bronchial anastomosis *(Aspergillus)*	
	Other: rabies, West Nile virus, lymphocytic choriomeningitis virus, endemic mycoses	Unusual pathogens preexisting in the recipient or in the donor graft
1–6 months	CMV disease	Onset of opportunistic infections from immunosuppression
	EBV	
	Aspergillus	
	Mycobacterium tuberculosis	
	Pneumocystis jiroveci	
	Endemic mycoses	
	HHV-6	
	Respiratory tract, line/bloodstream, and urinary tract infections	Continued bacterial *(Pseudomonas)* and candidal infections common through 3–4 months
	Respiratory viruses	Community-acquired infections
>6 months	Respiratory viruses	Community-acquired infections
	Persistent *Pseudomonas, Burkholderia cepacia,* and *Aspergillus* infections	Persistence of organisms from cystic fibrosis in the proximal airways and sinuses
	Opportunistic infections: *Pneumocystis jiroveci* cryptococcosis, nontuberculous mycobacteria, EBV/PTLD, herpes zoster	Patients receiving continuous high-level immunosuppression or therapy for steroid-resistant rejection, CMV infection

CMV, Cytomegalovirus; *EBV,* Epstein-Barr virus; *HHV,* human herpesvirus; *HSV,* herpes simplex virus; *PTLD,* posttransplant lymphoproliferative disease.
Modified from Rubin RH, Ikonen T, Gummert JF, Morris RE. The therapeutic prescription for the organ transplant recipient: the linkage of immunosuppression and antimicrobial strategies. *Transpl Infect Dis.* 1999;1:39.

SITES OF INFECTION

Thoracic Cavity: Respiratory Tract Infections, Including Pneumonia and Anastomotic Site Infections

The vast majority, up to 80%, of infections in LTRs occur in the thorax-lung, mediastinum, and pleural space, largely presenting as pneumonia.[6,14,296,368] Prevalence rates of pulmonary infections as high as 60% in LTRs occur in the first month posttransplant. In the CHLA cohort of patients during the first 12 months after transplantation, 62% of all infections consisted of pneumonia.[327] Organisms most frequently recovered include *Pseudomonas aeruginosa,* CMV, *Candida, Aspergillus,* and *S. aureus* (MRSA/MSSA) reflecting the high percentage of patients with CF in the transplant population.[356] The common bacterial organisms are usually successfully treated without poor outcomes; the fungal infections, non–tuberculosis-mycobacteria (particularly *M. abscessus*), multidrug-resistant (MDR) gram-negative organisms, and *Burkholderia cepacia* complex (in many centers, *B. cenocepacia* is a contraindication for transplant) are often more challenging and life-threatening.[338] The onset of pneumonia in LTRs appears in a bimodal pattern, with most cases occurring in the first few postoperative months. Surgical graft size reduction procedures to adjust for recipient/donor organ size mismatch and re-do transplantations are additional risks for early postoperative pneumonia.[368] A second albeit smaller group has late (6 to 12 months) recurrent episodes of gram-negative pneumonia associated with a poor outcome. The immunologic consequences of these infections in some patients may include bronchiolitis obliterans with organizing pneumonia (BOOP), which is characterized by inflammation and fibrotic granulation tissue of the small airways extending into the alveoli. The mortality rate of patients with BOOP is high (50%), and those who survive appear to be at an increased risk for developing BOS (41%).[14,99,203]

Unique to lung transplantation are bronchial anastomotic infections, most of which historically are fungal and caused by *Aspergillus* and *Candida.*[217,234,298,420,434] The bronchial anastomosis is susceptible to such infections for a variety of reasons. Anatomically the posttransplant bronchus is relatively devascularized, with the blood supply flowing retrograde from the pulmonary arterial circulation. Neovascularization from collateral vessels takes as long as 1 month to occur, and, in the interim, the bronchus may experience ischemia and subsequent necrosis and sloughing of bronchial epithelium. Evolving surgical techniques have diminished this risk for ischemia in recent years. This environment is optimal for developing infection caused by saprophytic flora, such as *Aspergillus,* present in ambient air to which the airways are in direct contact. In addition, local reaction to suture material, postoperative corticosteroid use, and immunosuppressive therapy have a negative impact on healing and increase the patient's susceptibility to infection. As a result of this early tenuous anatomy, infections at this site are most likely to occur within the first 2 to 3 months after surgery.[104,217,234,421] Bronchial anastomotic infections rarely can lead to early catastrophic complications, such as dehiscence and hemorrhage. They are linked to substantial late bronchial complications, including dehiscence, bronchial stenosis, malacia, and retransplantation.[408,420]

Although some studies have demonstrated that pretransplant isolation of *Aspergillus* spp. has not been found to be a risk factor for the development of *Aspergillus* infection after transplantation,[421,439] others suggest that patients with CF and perioperative *Aspergillus* colonization may be at heightened risk for the development of early bronchial anastomotic infection. Postoperative isolation of *Aspergillus* from airways appears to identify patients at risk for the later development of bronchial anastomotic abnormalities.[104,421] The overall incidence of airway infections and/or complications ranges from 5% to 25%.[104,217,408,420] The mortality rate associated with bronchial anastomotic infection and its complications is reported to be 2% to 7%.[234,420] Recent studies, including one pediatric series demonstrated airway complications of around 10%. Most were successfully treated conservatively without surgery and patient outcomes were not adversely affected.[104,627] The current common practice of perioperative antifungal agents for patients with fungal colonization has likely decreased the rate of such infections. A 2010 ISHLT consensus statement formulated standardization of thoracic site infections in cardiothoracic transplant recipients, including pneumonia, tracheobronchitis, bronchial anastomotic infections, and viral/CMV and fungal respiratory tract infections.[255] The use of standard definitions going forward will better define the epidemiology of these infections and advance the quality of research aimed at therapeutic and prophylactic interventions.

Bloodstream Infections

The second most common site of infection is the bloodstream. Data are emerging regarding the epidemiology of bloodstream infections (BSI) in pediatric and adult LTRs.[129,252,430] BSI occur in 12% to 26% of transplant recipients, with staphylococci, *Pseudomonas aeruginosa,* and *Candida* spp. being the most common organisms identified. Late infections consist of a wide range of gram-negative organisms. With increasing emphasis on reducing catheter-related BSI with infection prevention bundles for placement and maintenance of central line catheters, gram-positive BSI, especially coagulase-negative *Staphylococcus,* have decreased. Some SOT programs have reported gram-negative organisms with increasing numbers of MDR[7,66,626] and resistant *Enterococcus faecium, S. aureus, Klebsiella pneumoniae, Acinetobacter baumannii, Pseudomonas aeruginosa,* and *Enterobacter* spp. (rESKAPE) organisms, whereas other studies demonstrate a predominance of gram-positive organisms, including in a large adult population, with a high rate of vancomycin-resistant enterococci.[52] Posttransplant BSI, especially early (<30 days) infection in children and candidal infection in both adult and pediatric populations, was associated significantly with mortality. Infections are mostly related to pulmonary or vascular sites. In the pediatric population, most BSI were related to central venous catheters. These infections were most likely to occur in the first 7 days after transplantation. In adult transplant recipients, BSI largely were associated with pulmonary infections. Specifically *P. aeruginosa* bacteremia was more likely to develop in adult patients with CF (20% of the transplant cohort) than in patients with other indications for transplantation. In this study, BSI with *B. cepacia* and *S. aureus* were seen in similar frequency in non-CF patients, the former possibly related to a nosocomial outbreak.[430] In children, *Pseudomonas* BSI was not associated with the diagnosis of CF (45% of the transplant cohort) nor with any outcome measures in this study. There exists an increasing concern for the impact of MDR organisms (MDRO), which were recovered in 57% of gram-negative–resistant bacteremias in one study (see later discussion).[252] In rare cases, MDRO BSI can be transmitted from donor allografts as well,[323] with high rates of graft loss and mortality.

Empirical therapy in patients with suspected BSI should include agents active against staphylococcal and *Pseudomonas* spp. and be based on the patient's previous microbiologic susceptibilities and donor information, if available, with a low threshold for adding antifungal therapy. Furthermore the need for indwelling central catheters should be assessed routinely and catheters should be removed as soon as clinically feasible.

SELECTED PATHOGENS

Bacteria

Pseudomonas Aeruginosa *and* Burkholderia Cepacia *Complex*

P. aeruginosa and *B. cepacia* play prominent roles in postoperative infections in LTR with CF. Despite the removal of colonized lung tissue with the procedure, the proximal airways and sinuses remain colonized and a source of infection.[351] In patients with MDRO, this concern is heightened. Gram-negative MDRO have been defined as those resistant to one or more agents in three or more classes of effective drugs[349,495,575] In addition, these bacteria exist in a biofilm in the airways of patients with CF, which greatly decreases therapeutic efficacy.[117,535]

The presence of preoperative MDR *P. aeruginosa* may not have an impact on survival. Although these patients may be more likely to acquire postoperative infections, they generally respond to treatment without increases in short-term mortality rates. The most recent ISHLT guidelines for selection of LTRs list "colonization with highly resistant or highly virulent bacteria, fungi, or mycobacteria" as a relative contraindication.[427] Additionally these guidelines acknowledge that although "certain resistant pathogens may increase risk for poor outcome … it is not possible currently to identify absolute contraindications based on either the type of organisms or the pattern of antibiotic resistance." Despite the status of the immunocompromised host, the relatively low virulence of some of these organisms, the new healthy lung epithelium and improved airway function of the transplanted lungs, the aggressive use of antimicrobial agents during and after the procedure, and discordance between in vitro susceptibilities and in vivo efficacy may account for the diminished influence that MDR pseudomonads have on the outcomes of transplant recipients.[427]

B. cepacia complex represents a group of nine related species that possess variable pathogenic potential in abnormal hosts.[330] Misidentification of *B. cepacia* complex organisms at the genus (*Achromobacter/Alcaligenes, Stenotrophomonas,* and *Pseudomonas* most commonly) and species levels can occur.[329,375] This information is critical to evaluating patients considering transplantation and, in postoperative care, to assessing their risk for developing invasive disease.[329] In the United States there has been a decline in *B. cepacia* complex in the CF population, from 3.6% in 1995 to 2.5% in 2013.[122,472] In Canada, this decline has also been documented from 15%, with as many as 80% of these involving *B. cenocepacia/genomovar III,*[139] to 4.6% in 2013 (40% *B. cenocepacia*, 30% *B. multivorans*).[89] This reassuring decrease in *B. cepacia* organisms is likely multifactorial, reflecting better microbiologic techniques for identification and infection control practices.[472] Controversy continues regarding performing transplantation on patients who harbor *B. cenocepacia.* Data demonstrate increased morbidity and mortality rates associated with this organism in nontransplanted patients with CF, including the occurrence of fatal cepacia syndrome.[271,314,350] Multiple studies of LTR demonstrate an increase in mortality associated with pan-resistant *B. cenocepacia,* from 90% 1-year survival to 30%, and late deaths as a result of infection associated with BOS and possibly *Burkholderia gladiola* but not other *Burkholderia* spp. It remains a contraindication for transplantation in some centers,[12,27,71,140,329,402,407] although successful transplantation has been accomplished with aggressive multidrug antimicrobial therapy, perhaps guided by multiple combination bactericidal testing, and a reduction in immunosuppressive therapy.[139,327,407,575]

Optimal therapy for infections due to MDR *Pseudomonas* and *Burkholderia* spp. is not defined. Therapy should be tailored to susceptibility studies, with the recognition that in vitro susceptibilities may not correlate with in vivo activity and outcome.[537] A biofilm-grown model of in vitro multiple combination bactericidal testing may better inform our therapeutic choices for these MDROs and has identified a combination of high-dose tobramycin (inhaled), plus meropenem and a third antimicrobial agent (piperacillin/tazobactam, trimethoprim/sulfamethoxazole [TMP-SMX], amikacin, or ceftazidime) that inhibited the growth of most isolates.[123] How these data translate to patient care, however, has yet to be fully demonstrated, and a recent Cochran review found insufficient clinical evidence to recommend using biofilm susceptibility testing at this time.[182,602] A study that compared CF patients receiving two-drug combinations based on multiple combination bactericidal testing versus clinician preference did not find differences in outcome measures,[1] but these patients did not necessarily have multidrug-resistant/pan-resistant organisms, nor had they failed conventional therapy. Extrapolating these results to LTR with MDROs is difficult. The CHLA transplant team used multiple combination bactericidal testing from the University of Ottawa between 2001 and 2009; our experience suggests that this approach, with three or four drugs used in combination, is helpful for managing preoperative and postoperative LTRs with multidrug-resistant/pan-resistant organisms, including *B. cepacia* complex.[327] Clearly additional data are needed to assess this approach for LTRs infected with MDROs.

For LTR with susceptible *P. aeruginosa* infection, combination therapy is recommended, including an extended-spectrum, antipseudomonal β-lactam and an aminoglycoside, if renal status allows, at least for initial therapy (3 to 5 days) to limit nephrotoxicity. For MDR *Pseudomonas* spp., combinations of two and three drug classes, including antipseudomonal β-lactams + aminoglycosides ± fluoroquinolones for 10 to 14 days is current expert recommendation.[575] For resistant *B. cepacia* complex infections, combinations that include ceftazidime, meropenem, TMP-SMX, tetracyclines, quinolones, and even chloramphenicol have been used.[259,575] Aerosolized antibiotics (tobramycin, colistin, or aztreonam) can deliver drug levels above the minimal inhibitory concentrations of resistant organisms directly to the lungs and thereby reduce the bacterial burden with minimal systemic toxicity.[190,371,384,422] As a rule, aerosolized antibiotics should not be used as single therapy for infection in LTRs because they are at risk for disseminated disease. A prophylactic protocol utilizing aerosolized aztreonam has been employed at CHLA.[622] Therapy is initiated in patients identified with *B. cepacia* complex, preoperatively if possible, and continued through the first year after transplantation. Data suggest that outcomes are similar to those of patients who are colonized with susceptible *Pseudomonas* organisms. Further investigation is needed in this promising area of therapy. Colistin aerosols may also be useful for the treatment of pan-resistant organisms.[29,46] Although historically renal toxicity often precluded its systemic use, recent studies suggest that intravenous colistin can be used successfully as well.[124,160] A recent publication described a series of pediatric patients who received IV colistin for MDR gram-negative infection (mostly CF patients with *Pseudomonas*[558] spp.); 22% had renal injury, and resistance to colistin developed in 21%, possibly related to suboptimal dosing. All those with colistin resistant organisms died. Finally strategies that employ extended or continuous infusions of high-dose β-lactam antibiotics may optimize the pharmacokinetic/pharmacodynamic properties of these drugs and may improve outcome.[397,477,575] The duration of therapy for these infections requires individualization but generally is not less than 2 weeks, and treatment should be continued for a significant period after the signs and symptoms of infection have resolved.

Multidrug-Drug Resistant Gram-Negative Organisms

A full discussion of extended spectrum β-lactamase (ESBL) and carbapenamase (CR) producing organisms is beyond the scope of this chapter. MDR ESBL-producing Enterobacteriaceae *(Klebsiella pneumoniae, Escherichia coli)* and *Acinetobacter baumannii* are being increasingly recognized as causes of infection worldwide. The extent of their impact on transplant recipients in general and in pediatric LTRs is unknown and limited to case reports and small surveys, mostly in adult transplant populations,[28,53,443] and has been described in pediatric liver or intestinal transplantation, notably in outbreak situations.[208,473] Given the rise in MDROs worldwide, it is expected that this problem is increasing in scope and imposing direct effects on morbidity and mortality on transplant recipients.[94,323,575,600] Infections may originate from the recipient or donor.[197,361] Increased risk related to antimicrobial exposure, infection control practices, invasive procedures, and prolonged hospitalization, especially associated with intensive care units, is likely. Carbapenems are considered the drugs of choice for ESBL-producing organisms, especially for empirical therapy,[617] although β-lactam/β-lactam inhibitor combinations (such as piperacillin/tazobactam) may be appropriate based on in vitro susceptibilities, especially at high doses and depending on severity and site of infection.[450,480,575] Carbapenem-resistant Enterobacteriaceae (CRE)-producing organisms provide additional challenges to therapy because the number of available effective agents is limited and few new options are in development. Several hospital outbreaks have demonstrated the lethality of these organisms in transplant recipients. In a series of adult solid organ transplant recipients (SOTR), infection with *K. pneumoniae* carbapenamase producers was associated with an overall 30-day mortality rate of 42%.[54] All of four adult LTRs died from CRE *A. baumannii* infections in one study; a 91% mortality rate[419] was demonstrated in 16 adult LTR with MDR *A. baumannii* infections[511] in another. Optimal therapy is undefined; therapy should be guided by susceptibilities and possibly multiple combination bactericidal testing. Some data suggest that combination therapy may improve outcome, including the use of high-dose, prolonged infusions and dual carbapenem therapy,[78,235,619] although sufficient prospective trials are lacking, especially in children. Other drug combinations including colistin, tigecycline, doripenem, aminoglycosides, and ceftobiprole may be considered.[436,443,575] The transplant community continues to discuss the implications these organisms may have on transplant recipient and donor candidacy.[514] The basic tenet of infectious disease treatment remains important in these infections: that outcome depends not only on appropriate antimicrobials, but also on source control, such as removal of infected foreign material and drainage of fluids.

Mycobacterium Tuberculosis

Worldwide *Mycobacterium tuberculosis* (MTB) remains an important pathogen in SOTRs, and the rate of infection is associated with the endemicity of infection. As noted by many authors, MTB behaves as an opportunistic infection in these patients in that its frequency in SOTRs is greatly increased in comparison with the normal population (up to 74-fold) and presents as diverse manifestations, including high rates of extrapulmonary disease and increased mortality rates.[79,485,550] Most cases of infection with MTB in adult transplant recipients arise from reactivation of latent infection from recipient or donor; acquired cases are seen, especially in pediatric patients.[79,373,396] Multiple cases of donor-derived MTB infection, including pulmonary MTB infection in LTRs[476] and extrapulmonary MTB infection in renal and liver transplant patients, have been documented.[205,476,618] In addition, nosocomial transmission to transplant recipients has occurred.[269]

Among SOTRs, MTB infections occur most frequently after lung transplants (1% to 6.5%).[568] Studies of MTB infection in SOTR, including small numbers of children, suggest that most cases occur within the first posttransplant year, with a median time of 9 months for all SOTRs and 3.5 months for LTRs. Risk factors for MTB infection include allograft rejection; receipt of OKT3 or anti–T-cell antibodies, which also predict dissemination; previous exposure to MTB, with radiographic evidence of old infection or a history of a positive tuberculin skin test; renal failure/hemodialysis; liver disease; diabetes mellitus; and older age.[79,568] Coinfection with CMV, mycoses, *Pneumocystis jiroveci,* and *Nocardia* has been associated with the development of disease.[396,401] As would be expected, most manifestations include pulmonary disease (>70%), with interstitial infiltrates, nodules, effusion, and cavities seen on imaging studies.[532,568] Presentations that include extrapulmonary disease, in up to one-third to one-half of active cases compared to 15% of normal hosts, involve the gastrointestinal tract, skin, musculoskeletal system, genitourinary system, lymph nodes, and central nervous system (CNS). Attributable mortality from MTB infection in SOTRs is reported to be 9.5% to 29%. Significant predictors of mortality are disseminated disease, previous rejection, and receipt of OKT3 or anti–T-cell antibodies.[532]

Several studies have investigated mycobacterial infections specifically in LTRs.[73,281,353,396] Two of the studies were conducted in regions with a low endemicity of MTB infection—Australia and North America (affecting five to 15 per 100,000 population)—and two in Spain (25 to 49 per 100,000 population). Rates of MTB infection in LTRs in the two former studies were less than 1%, although still well above the national average,[281,353] but they were 2.6% and 6.4% (500-fold higher than the national average) in the Spanish studies.[73,396] Indeed nontuberculous mycobacterial infections were more common than were MTB infections in the first two reports, whereas nontuberculous mycobacterial infection was encountered only once in the Spanish study. Mortality rate ranged from 0% to 43%.[73,281,396,532]

Few data exist on MTB infections in pediatric SOTRs, and none exist in LTRs. Although children have an age-related lower accumulated risk for being infected, even immunocompetent children with MTB infection are more likely to have progression to dissemination and mortality, especially those younger than 5 years of age and again during adolescence.[119] This pattern appears to be mirrored in the transplant population. Small published series of MTB infection in SOTRs most often describe fever and pulmonary findings, with high rates of dissemination (50%); mortality ranged from 0% to 30%.[79,373,580] Pediatric patients presented later after transplant than adults (median of 8 months vs. 4 months) as a result of differences in acquisition of disease. Tuberculin skin test results were negative or minimal in all patients. Furthermore screening of family members was very useful in both series of pediatric patients, thus suggesting that, as for immunocompetent children, the index case of exposure is in the home. Invasive diagnostic procedures were needed to confirm the diagnosis in many patients. A screening risk assessment with history, including exposures, travel, receipt of bacille Calmette-Guérin (BCG) vaccine, and physical examination, as well as performing a tuberculin skin test should be documented in all pediatric transplant candidates.[79,550] A 5-mm induration should be considered positive in an immunocompromised child because positive results require intact T-cell function; false-negative results may be secondary to nutritional status, organ failure, or medication-related immunodeficient states.[16,79] Screening of household contacts should also be considered. Interferon-γ (IFN-γ) release assays (IGRA) have emerged as valuable tools for the screening/diagnosis of latent tuberculosis infection. The T-SPOT.TB test may be more sensitive in immunocompromised patients.[369,464,474] However, the use of IGRA in young children (<5 years) and immunocompromised patients is still being evaluated and may not perform optimally in children with T-cell immunodepression, although controls are contained in the testing procedure.[345,369,464,474,561] Both the tuberculin skin test and the IGRAs, along with clinical, radiologic, and microbiologic investigations, should be used to increase the sensitivity of diagnosis because discordant results in children and immunocompromised populations have been well documented.[3,79,306]

Diagnosis of active MTB infection in the transplant setting can be challenging because symptoms may be nonspecific, such as fever of unknown origin, or unusual, such as abdominal manifestations; coinfections may also modify the signs and symptoms, and immune response–based diagnostic methods lack sensitivity. Consequently a high index of suspicion is required, and, frequently, aggressive diagnostic techniques, such as bronchoscopy, laparoscopy, and tissue biopsy, are needed.[373] The American Thoracic Society and the Centers for Disease Control and Prevention (CDC) have published recommendations for diagnosis of MTB disease.[23,92,503] Several methods are available for culture-based diagnosis. Broth-based culture systems coupled with DNA probes allow more rapid establishment of a diagnosis.[503] Technologies for the rapid detection of MDROs are evolving.[30,91,96,395,503,559] Because pediatric LTRs are at heightened risk for development of progressive tuberculous infection, expert opinion supports the use of 9 months of isoniazid (INH) chemoprophylaxis for pediatric candidates or recipients with latent tuberculosis. The morbidity and mortality from MTB is high enough to warrant the risk for potential hepatotoxicity in most cases unless severe liver disease is also present.[79,401,550] Rifampin alone may also be an acceptable regimen, although drug–drug interactions are common (see later discussion). Completing therapy prior to transplant is optimal, but it can be accomplished after transplantation. An alternative strategy is active surveillance, with initiation of INH only if additional risk factors are present, such as recent conversion, exposure to active MTB, a recipient or donor with a history of MTB infection without adequate therapy, or the existence of significant abnormalities on chest radiographs.[485] All family and close contacts with latent or active tuberculosis should also be treated.[79]

Optimal therapy for pediatric LTR with active tuberculosis has not been defined, but an empirical multidrug regimen such as those recommended for active disease in other populations, modified by susceptibilities or known resistance patterns as necessary, should be initiated.[19,65,405,550] Complicating factors include liver toxicity and drug interactions. INH, especially in combination with other first-line drugs, such as rifampin and pyrazinamide, can lead to toxicity, requiring discontinuation of all or some of these drugs and the need to institute new regimens.[401,532] Liver biopsy may be necessary to distinguish drug toxicity from rejection (in liver transplantation) or hepatic granuloma from MTB infection.[401,485,532] Pediatric patients generally tolerate first-line therapy, with occasional need for reduced dosage and rarely discontinuation.[19,65] For patients with suspected or proved MDR tuberculosis, close consultation with public health services and specialists in treating this disease should be employed for optimal management.

The use of rifampin in SOTRs deserves special comment. Although rifampin-containing regimens may portend the best microbiologic outcome, significant morbidity from graft dysfunction and loss can be due to the simultaneous use of rifampin with immunosuppressant agents. Rifampin considerably lowers serum levels of cyclosporine, tacrolimus, and azole antifungals, especially fluconazole, as well as causing some decrease in corticosteroid levels via induction of cytochrome P-450.[149] Current recommendations suggest that rifampin can be used successfully with increased calcineurin inhibitor dosing and careful monitoring of calcineurin inhibitor serum levels.[353] Rifabutin may offer equivalent efficacy with less effect on drug interactions, as has been documented in tuberculosis/HIV coinfected individuals on antiretroviral therapy.[79] Others suggest that a longer duration of therapy (up to 50%) with rifampin-free/INH-containing regimens has a comparable outcome without the risk for rejection and potential graft loss.[73,401] Most authors agree that regimens should contain INH if at all possible.[73,79,401,550] If rifampin-free regimens are used, therapy should be prolonged to a minimum of 12 to 18 months.[73] Ethambutol and second-line therapies (aminoglycosides and quinolones) may be considered if a first-line drug cannot be used.[401,485] If both INH and rifampin are not used because of toxicity, drug interactions, or resistance, therapy should be continued for a prolonged period, possibly 2 to 3 years.[79,485] Patients should be monitored very closely for response to therapy, adherence to medications, drug interactions, and adverse reactions throughout the entire treatment period.[306]

Nontuberculous Mycobacterial Infections

Nontuberculous mycobacterial (NTM) infections are more common in LTRs than are MTB infections in those areas where MTB is not endemic, including the United States.[152,213] Patients with chronic lung disease and CF in particular have a high incidence of NTM colonization. More recent data suggest that 6% to 24% of patients with CF are colonized with NTM organisms, most commonly *M. abscessus (subsp abscessus, bolletii, massiliense)* or *M. avium complex* (MAC).[89,98,122,331,467] The contribution of these organisms to progression of lung disease in pretransplant patients is still being defined.[426] The impact of NTM infections on the LTR, especially from infections due to *M. abscessus,* deserves emphasis. Although there remain many gaps in knowledge regarding the epidemiology and best approaches pre- and postoperatively to patients with NTM infections, it appears to be increasingly reported in lung transplant populations and is quite therapeutically challenging.

Clinical manifestations of NTM infection in lung transplantation vary by organism and include pulmonary, surgical site infections, and cutaneous and disseminated disease.[152] In a survey of 31 transplant centers regarding *M. abscessus* infection in LTRs, 17 patients were identified (0.33%).[102] The majority had pulmonary infections, followed by skin involvement; several patients had both. Disease occurred at a median of 18.5 months after transplantation (1 to 111 months). Pulmonary disease may manifest as chronic cough, sputum production, weight loss, and fatigue. Skin infections may involve surgical sites (sternal wounds) and extremities.[98,353] Painful, erythematous cutaneous or subcutaneous nodules may develop into abscesses and ulcerate.[102] In additional single-center retrospective studies involving adult LTRs, most of whom underwent transplants because of chronic obstructive pulmonary disease (COPD), the rate of posttransplant NTM infection was 4% to 22%,[205,244,353] with progression to disease in 25% with pulmonary infection and 11% with pulmonary and surgical site infections of those colonized.[244] A study of end-stage CF patients referred for transplantation revealed 20% of patients were colonized with NTM organisms (equal numbers of MAC and *M. abscessus*); after the transplant, NTM were isolated from 14% of CF LTRs. The prevalence of posttransplant invasive disease was approximately 3% (25% of those colonized) in both pulmonary and surgical site infections, the majority being caused by *M. abscessus.*[98] Posttransplant NTM infection, disease, and even colonization has been associated with increased risk of mortality posttransplantation.[244] The presence of NTM is suggested as a marker of "overimmunosuppression"; in support of this is the higher mortality rate attributable to non-NTM infections as well, seen in LTRs with NTM. Emerging data support the association between preoperative colonization and posttransplant infections with *M. abscessus*, and, although LTRs may remain asymptomatically colonized, serious and sometimes fatal posttransplant infections are documented.[98,102,152,629]

Transmission from water and environmental sources is most common, including hospital and household plumbing systems, and health care–associated outbreaks related to laparoscopic surgery, cosmetic procedures, and surgical tourism are increasingly noted.[536] In addition, recent investigation using whole-genome sequencing, diversity analysis, resistance patterns, and epidemiologic data suggests there is evidence of person-to-person transmission of *M. abscessus* subsp. *massiliense*, albeit indirectly by way of fomites. The exact mechanism has yet to be defined, but additional data support that transmission can occur from persons with negative smears/positive cultures, suggesting that a low quantity of inoculum is required. To further define the existence of transmissible[77] *M. abscessus* clones despite current infection prevention measures will require new paradigms to protect patients from these infections.

Diagnosis requires a high level of suspicion. Cutaneous lesions should be sampled for histology, special stains, and culture. The infectious differential diagnosis includes fungal, nocardial, and other atypical infections. These organisms are ubiquitous, and differentiating respiratory tract colonization from infection may be difficult. The diagnosis of NTM infection should be entertained with a low threshold for performing bronchoalveolar lavage (BAL) or biopsy, for any unexplained or unresolving pleuropulmonary disease.[152,213] The American Thoracic Society/Infectious Diseases Society of America (ATS/IDSA) has published diagnostic criteria that include signs and symptoms present after the treatment of other possible causes of findings, such as radiologic evidence of progressive pulmonary disease, including infiltrates, cavities, nodules, or bronchiectasis, and bacteriologic evidence of NTM infection, generally on at least two respiratory or biopsy specimens.[212]

Providing therapy for NTM infection may be challenging, depends on the species isolated, and should be determined in consultation with experts and adherence to the ATS/IDSA guidelines.[213] Despite the use of seemingly adequate therapy, failures and recurrences are common.[212,213] Therapy for infection with MAC includes a macrolide, ethambutol, and rifampin, with or without an aminoglycoside, depending on the severity of disease. Susceptibility to macrolides should be performed; it is the only class of drug for MAC for which there is evidence to support an in vitro and in vivo response.[213] The optimal therapy for *M. abscessus* infection is undefined because this organism is notoriously resistant to many antimicrobial agents, and success is not always achieved using in vitro susceptibility profiles. See Chapter 97 for details of treating atypical mycobacterial infections. For SOT patients, reduction of immunosuppression, surgical excision or debridement, and treatment of coinfections, in conjunction with long-term therapy with multiple antimicrobial agents, likely improve the outcome.[102] Relapses are not uncommon. Consideration of lifelong suppression is recommended by some experts for patients with a high burden of disease and persistently high levels of immunosuppression.[244,536] Most patients (~70%) who can complete long-term therapy improve and half of these are considered cured; minimal response to therapy was seen in about a quarter of LTRs. Fatal infections occur rarely.[102,289,498] Drug interactions between macrolides and rifampin and between calcineurin inhibitors and sirolimus occur. Both can lower serum levels of immunosuppressive drugs and trigger rejection.

Most centers do not currently consider the presence of NTM infection an exclusion to transplantation, although the optimal management of these patients is debated. Clearly patients often remain colonized in respiratory tree sites above the anastomosis. Given the concern for emergence of resistance, toxicity and drug-drug interactions related to long-term therapy, prolonged antimycobacterial therapy cannot be recommended for all patients. Some centers opt for pretransplant or peritransplant prophylaxis, whereas others recommend observation for evidence of disease.[152]

Fungal Infections

Aspergillus

Aspergillus infections remain a major challenge to the success of lung transplantation. Most common presentations involve the respiratory tree (up to 90%), with manifestations ranging from semiinvasive tracheobronchitis and bronchial anastomotic infections to invasive pulmonary disease and, rarely, dissemination to extrapulmonary sites, including the CNS (10%).[187,525] The published rates of invasive aspergillosis (IA) infections vary considerably (4% to 35%) and probably reflect differences in dates of publication, patient populations, underlying disease such as CF, net state of immunosuppression, use of prophylactic measures, local issues of exposure (e.g., construction), and rates of rejection and viral infection, among others.[189,411,526] In addition, distinguishing between colonization of the airway by *Aspergillus* versus true invasive disease may be difficult. Despite these caveats, rates of IA infection in LTRs are the highest among SOTRs. Studies suggest that invasive disease occurs in 3% to 33% of LTRs, although rates of colonization/isolation of *Aspergillus* may be considerably higher. In most cases, colonization appears to be transient and does not lead to invasive disease.*

A bimodal pattern of the development of IA in transplant recipients has been recognized. Most infections develop 1 to 6 months after transplantation and are a major cause of death during this time period,[130,298,377,389,410,525] but late infections after 1 year posttransplant occur as well.[187,335,410] Infections that develop less than 3 months after transplantation are more likely to be tracheobronchitis or bronchial anastomosis site infections; patients who require retransplantation or have bronchial anastomotic infection may present in the first month.[104,217,234,389] Invasive pulmonary or disseminated aspergillosis may occur at any time.[130,335,410,525,539] Risk factors for early disease in LTRs include *Aspergillus* colonization in the 6 months before transplantation or early posttransplant colonization, a complicated postoperative period, A2 or repeated rejection, and CMV disease or receipt of CMV prophylaxis as a marker for donor/recipient seropositivity. In a study of adult CF LTRs, a positive intraoperative BAL *Aspergillus* culture from the native lung produced a fourfold higher risk of developing IA[340] compared to positive pretransplant cultures.[130,187,232,263,335,393,421] Corroboration of the importance of CMV is the observation that a significant decrease in IA was associated with the use of prophylactic ganciclovir in heart transplant recipients, reflecting the immunomodulating effects of the virus on host immune status.[486,595] Adult patients in whom IA developed later after transplantation were older and "over immunosuppressed" secondary to chronic or refractory graft rejection or dysfunction.[187,528] In both the early and late groups, IA was associated with renal failure and repeated bacterial infections.

A. fumigatus causes the majority of disease, although non–*A. fumigatus* species are becoming more common.[377] Such species include *A. flavus, A. niger, A. nodularis, A. ustus,* and *A. terreus.* Clinical findings in patients with pulmonary disease are largely nonspecific and may include cough, shortness of breath, and hypoxia, although chest pain and occasionally hemoptysis may raise clinical suspicion of infection with IA.[44] Symptoms are seen more commonly in patients with diffuse disease than in those with focal or nodular disease. Although fever is a common early manifestation of infection with IA in neutropenic patients with a hematologic disorder, it occurred in only 15% of LTRs with IA and usually more often in patients with disseminated (50%) or invasive pulmonary disease (20%) than in those with tracheobronchial or bronchial anastomotic infections (0%).[525] Lack of fever also has been documented in other studies of nonneutropenic patients with IA. Patients with disseminated disease may have involvement of the sinuses, orbits, musculoskeletal system (osteomyelitis), ophthalmologic structures, cutaneous sites, and CNS. Symptoms of CNS disease may include headache, sinus pain, cranial nerve abnormalities, seizures, changes in mental status, or other focal neurologic findings.[44,200]

The radiologic manifestations of IA in LTRs are highly variable.[147,512,564] Chest radiographs are insensitive and nonspecific. Computed tomography (CT) of the chest has become an integral part of early diagnostic strategies and has been incorporated into recent definitions of invasive fungal infections in immunocompromised hosts.[137] On chest CT scans of neutropenic adults, large nodules and cavitary lesions are common findings.[84,137] In addition, much has been made of the early halo sign, a macronodule surrounded by a perimeter of ground-glass opacity (edema and hemorrhage), and the later air crescent sign, a crescent-shaped air interface between viable lung and infarcted tissue at the periphery of a nodule that is seen with recovery and return of neutrophils. These findings are considered highly suggestive, although not pathognomonic, of IA. Unfortunately these findings are seen less commonly in LTRs and in children in general. Multiple ill-defined pulmonary nodules were the most common findings in adult LTR, with approximately half demonstrating halo signs. Cavitation was rarely seen, and no air crescent signs were observed.[147] In children, radiographic findings were highly variable and included consolidations and small nodular masses and effusions, with little evidence of cavitation or halo or crescent signs.[80,564]

The gold standard for diagnosis of IA is the demonstration of small hyaline, septate, dichotomously branched hyphae in tissue with evidence

*References 130, 187, 200, 232, 335, 377, 389, 393, 410, 421, 437, 525.

of associated tissue damage or positive cultures from a normally sterile body site in the presence of signs and symptoms of invasive disease.[137,240] Blood cultures are rarely positive. Obtaining adequate tissue specimens in a timely manner frequently is not possible. An immunocompromised patient with neutropenia or one who is on corticosteroid therapy may not exhibit obvious signs or symptoms of invasive disease until late in the course of infection.[10] Additionally these patients are often deemed too ill to undergo the invasive procedures necessary to obtain tissue for microbiologic and histopathologic evaluation.[533] Therefore the diagnosis is established late in the course of the disease or at autopsy. Indeed, frequently it is not established but is based on radiologic and host factors.

Early diagnosis is thought to be critical to improving the outcome of patients with IA, especially now with the availability of more active therapeutic agents. In addition to early CT in high-risk patients, especially those who do not respond to broad-spectrum antibacterial therapy, there have been several recent advances in molecular/non–culture-based approaches to establishing a diagnosis. The most widely used and well characterized of these modalities is the Platelia *Aspergillus* serum galactomannan antigen, detected by double-sandwich enzyme-linked immunosorbent assay (ELISA).[95,348,380,608] In SOTRs and nonneutropenic patients, galactomannan antigen testing of blood appears to be less sensitive (30% compared to 80% to 90%) for the detection of IA.[174,254,305,458,583] In addition, antifungal therapy has been shown to decrease the sensitivity of the assay.[358] However its use in BAL fluid may have a higher diagnostic yield and has been recently approved by the U.S. Food and Drug Administration (FDA) for this use.[50,141,288] Several studies in LTRs suggest that galactomannan antigen levels greater than 1.0 from BAL fluid evaluation have good sensitivity (60–100%) and specificity (90–98%) for determination of IA.[220,253,257,442,526] Galactomannan antigen values between 0.5 and 1.0 should be interpreted in clinical context.

The Fungitell (1→3)-β-D-glucan assay measures a cell wall component found in many fungi, including *Aspergillus* and *Candida* spp. and *Pneumocystis,* but, like galactomannan antigen, it does not detect Zygomycetes.[428] It is approved by the FDA to aid in the diagnosis of invasive fungal infections and has been incorporated into the definitions for these infections.[137] Cross-reacting glucan-containing material occurs commonly in the environment, and false-positive tests have been demonstrated in dialysis patients, those exposed to gauze, and those with some gram-positive bacteremia. In addition, false-positive results are associated with the use of some antimicrobial agents and with sample manipulation, thus suggesting that laboratory contamination is possible.[240,364,608] A study in LTRs suggests it has a low positive predictive value, thus limiting its use as a screening tool, and false-positive findings occurred with mold colonization and hemodialysis. Unlike serum galactomannan antigen, it does not appear to correlate with response to therapy or have prognostic value because it declines slowly, even with clinical improvement.[13,292] Most recently a point of care test for an *Aspergillus*-specific later flow device (LPD) is being developed.[237,270,381,615] This diagnostic modality detects *Aspergillus* extracellular glycoprotein antigen by monoclonal antibody JF5 on BAL fluid. Results are available in 15 minutes. The LPD has a negative predictive value of 95% to 97%, sensitivity of 64% to 100% (depending on the patient population), and a specificity of 83% to 94%. This test may be most helpful for ruling out IA, but further study is needed to determine its application in different patient populations.

Despite historically poor outcomes of IA in immunocompromised patients, new mold-active therapies appear to be associated with improving mortality figures.[418] The IDSA practice guidelines for *Aspergillus* infections published in 2016 recommends therapy with voriconazole as primary therapy for most patients[446] because it has demonstrated outcome superiority, even for CNS infection.[40,137,505,598] Data now support the use of voriconazole for IA in pediatric patients and SOTRs. ISHLT published guidelines for management of fungal infections in cardiothoracic SOTRs in 2015, giving recommendations for prophylaxis, diagnosis, and treatment as well, which corroborate those of IDSA but are transplant-specific.[260] Pediatric patients require higher doses on per kilogram basis (generally 7 to 10 mg/kg per dose twice a day).[58,76,392,409,441,446,540] In addition the importance of therapeutic drug monitoring (TDM) of voriconazole as it relates to improved outcome and decreased toxicity, with trough levels between 1 and 5 μg/mL especially in children and other patient populations, including those with CF, has been demonstrated.* Several important drug interactions occur with medications routinely used in SOTRs. The most important of these interactions involves tacrolimus and sirolimus, in which concomitant use with voriconazole can lead to decreased metabolism via cytochrome P-450 and result in greatly increased serum levels of the immunosuppressant.[492] The use of tacrolimus can be controlled safely by reducing the dose by 50% and monitoring daily levels.[492,581] The effect of voriconazole on sirolimus levels is even more pronounced, and it is labeled as an absolute contraindication by the manufacturer.[492,493] Several case reports and small series describe the use of these two drugs together, with significant dose reduction of sirolimus (up to 90%) and close follow-up of serum sirolimus levels.[363,367,493] The use of rifampin and voriconazole should be avoided if possible because voriconazole levels may be significantly decreased in this setting.[188] Posaconazole, a broad-spectrum azole with activity against many non-*Aspergillus* molds and Zygomycetes is recommended as an alternative for treatment of IA infection in patients refractory or intolerant of other therapy, including voriconazole.[11,297,446,507] It is also licensed for prophylaxis in patients 13 years of age and older with fever and neutropenia or graft-versus-host disease.[114,572] Its safety and drug interaction profile is similar, if not improved, compared to that of voriconazole, and TDM is also recommended.[510] On the other hand, optimal dosing remains an issue, especially in young children for whom no specific dose recommendations exist.[605] A new delayed-release pill formulation with improved bioavailability makes this antifungal an option for patients who can swallow pills, especially if toxicity (hepatic, dermatologic, neurologic) or achieving adequate levels limit voriconazole's use.[113,121] See Chapter 198 for complete information regarding treatment of IA.

The role of combination therapy in the treatment of IA remains undefined.[527,563,616] A survey of IA in transplant recipients documented that primary combination therapy was used in 35% of patients.[37] A study comparing voriconazole/caspofungin as primary therapy in SOT with IA (proven/probable) in a prospective multicenter study (2003 to 2005) with historical controls who had received a lipid formulation of amphotericin B (LFAB; 1999 to 2002).[527] There was a trend toward improved survival in the combination cohort and an improved 90-day survival in patients receiving combination therapy with renal failure and those with *A. fumigatus* infections. Only one only randomized, double-blind, placebo-controlled trial to date has compared voriconazole and voriconazole/anidulafungin as primary therapy for IA in adults with hematologic malignancies and stem cell transplant.[359] Unfortunately the study had limitations that reduced its power to detect treatment effect and generalizability. The results demonstrated "combination therapy was associated with a substantial, but not statistically significant reduction in overall mortality." In post hoc analysis of a dominant subgroup of patients with IA based on CT findings and galactomannan positivity, all-cause mortality at 6 weeks was improved in those patients who received combination versus monotherapy. Although these studies are not definitive, not generalizable to all patient populations, and do not include children, they do provide additional support for primary combination therapy for IA in some patients. The most recent IDSA guidelines (2016) on the treatment of IA state that "combination therapy … has been supported by generally favorable in vitro and in vivo preclinical data. … Non-randomized clinical trial data suggest the benefit" as do limited prospective randomized first-line combination therapy. For these reasons, current guidelines suggest "consideration for an echinocandin with voriconazole for primary therapy in the setting of severe disease, especially in patients with hematologic malignancy and those with profound and persistent neutropenia."[446]

No definitive data are available on the length of treatment for IA, although the natural history of disease, assessment of risk factors, and the state and length of immunosuppression, along with investigations on response to therapy and animal studies, inform us on regimens most likely to be effective. Clearly one must balance the risk for incomplete therapy and recurrent disease with the dangers of increased toxicity

*References 55, 58, 76, 150, 233, 273, 284, 341, 392, 409, 440, 540.

and expense from prolonged therapy. One thoughtful approach based on these many variables suggests use of the "most effective therapy first for 10 to 12 weeks, or for at least 4 to 6 weeks beyond resolution of all clinical and radiographic abnormalities, whichever is longer."[519] Length of therapy should be individualized, and factors such as recovery from neutropenia or other immunocompromised state, net state of immunosuppression, extent of disease, presence of graft-versus-host disease, and coinfections (e.g., with CMV) predict poorer outcome and slower response and probably will prolong duration of therapy for patients with these comorbid findings.

Adjunctive surgical therapy may be recommended for cutaneous and soft tissue infections[230] or for lesions on the great vessels or major airways to prevent massive hemoptysis.[56,83,85,429] Immunomodulatory strategies to improve host immune response, in theory, are attractive adjuvant therapies. Alveolar macrophages, polymorphonuclear neutrophils, and pulmonary dendritic cells are critical first-line defenses against IA.[481] Decreasing the use of immunosuppression and corticosteroids as much as possible should be the goal in transplant recipients with IA. Additional strategies, including enhancement of T-helper type 1 (T_H1) immune responses, exogenous administration of colony-stimulating factors (granulocyte colony-stimulating factor [G-CSF], granulocyte-macrophage colony-stimulating factor [GM-CSF]) or cytokines (IFN-γ) to activate or recruit phagocytes (or both), and G-CSF donor-primed white blood cell transfusions have been investigated and may be used in select cases.[446,545] When *Aspergillus* causes invasive disease, mortality rates are high (30–100%) and notably so for invasive and disseminated or CNS forms of the infection.[187,377,539] In a review of English-language articles on *Aspergillus* infections in adult LTRs, the overall mortality rate was 53% (59 of 112); it was 24% (nine of 38) for tracheobronchial or bronchial anastomotic infections, 82% (18 of 22) in patients with invasive pulmonary disease, and 67% (two of three) for disseminated invasive infection.[525] These published data reflect the limited therapeutic options previously available (before the advent of extended-spectrum azoles and echinocandins). Several more recent studies suggest an improvement in the mortality rate (40%) since the widespread use of voriconazole and TDM.[36,417,573]

Despite the lack of controlled trials, several surveys document that most lung transplant centers use prophylactic or preemptive systemic antifungal agents (azoles, echinocandins, or amphotericin formulations), aerosolized amphotericin formulations, or both in patients with pre- or postoperative isolation of airway *Aspergillus,* and almost 60% of the centers employed universal prophylaxis.[136,153,154,262,376,412,447] Because *Aspergillus* infections are acquired through the lungs and most infections are pulmonary, attaining high pulmonary drug levels via aerosolization and limiting systemic toxicity are attractive options for prevention.[154,376,533] Multiple trials have suggested a reduction in IA with the use of aerosolized amphotericin formulations.[68,86,154,155,159,234,389,394,431] A single retrospective study incorporating the use of universal voriconazole prophylaxis with or without inhaled amphotericin compared with targeted itraconazole in LTRs decreased the rate of IA at 1 year from 23.5% to 1.5%.[256] Abnormalities in liver enzymes were common, necessitating discontinuation of voriconazole in 14% versus 7% of the comparator. This study was performed before widespread use of voriconazole TDM, the use of which may have precluded some of this toxicity. Based on two phase II studies, posaconazole is FDA approved for prophylaxis of invasive fungal infections in certain high-risk patient populations 13 years or older.[114,573] Studies evaluating the use of posaconazole suspension prophylaxis in LTRs have demonstrated mixed results, including variability of perioperative posaconazole concentrations; serum correlating with BAL, but often both subtherapeutic; tolerability/adverse events requiring discontinuation (gastrointestinal upset, transaminase derangement); tacrolimus interactions; and IA breakthrough[478,560] (15%). A novel targeted peritransplant antifungal strategy compared sequential cohorts in which all patients received inhaled amphotericin B deoxycholate (AmBD) during hospitalization, along with 7 to 10 days of micafungin.[293] Only those with positive fungal cultures from intraoperative BAL cultures (cohort 2) received additional 3 to 6 months of targeted antifungal therapy (yeast or mold active); 19% of patients in the second cohort received additional antifungal therapy based on intraoperative cultures. Cohort 1 had 29 invasive fungal diseases, cohort 2 had 10. The rate of IA was 4%, which is similar to institutions that use universal azole prophylaxis strategies. No patient in this group experienced antifungal drug–related toxicity or fungal-associated mortality. Further randomized, multicenter studies are needed to clarify which agents and prophylactic strategies are most effective.

Prevention of IA infection through environmental controls also is important.[435,445,469,562] Infections with this fungus in transplant recipients can be nosocomial or community acquired. Most germane to prevention is air control, inasmuch as both epidemic and sporadic IA correlate with concentrations of *Aspergillus* in the air.[9] A protective hospital environment should consist of high-efficiency particulate air (HEPA) filtration, positive air pressure, high air exchange rate, properly sealed rooms, and removal of carpets, plants, and water-damaged ceiling and floor tiles.[115,156,222,445] Patients should be wearing "fit-tested" masks (N95) when leaving protected environments, efforts should be made to have construction barriers in place, and patient transport routes should be adjusted accordingly if construction is occurring in the hospital and clinics.[435] In addition, monitoring the environment and air for changes in particulates and fungal spores may be considered based on local epidemiology, rates of IA, and infection control practices. When patients are discharged home, they should be counseled to avoid certain high-risk exposure to agents such as excessive dust and molds if possible.[445]

Candida

Although *Candida* infections are the most common cause of fungal infections in SOTR recipients, those patients at highest risk are abdominal transplant recipients (liver, small bowel, and pancreas), with LTRs at intermediate risk, and renal transplants at the least risk.[410,516] The overall rate of *Candida* infections in LTRs has decreased over time, in one study from 20% (1980–86) to 1.8% (2001–04), as has attributable mortality from 39% to 15%.[502] *Candida* infections in LTRs generally occur early, within the first month after transplantation, and are associated with long-term broad-spectrum antibiotic therapy, the presence of central venous access and other indwelling foreign bodies, surgical complications, CMV infection, and renal replacement therapy.[298,516] Infections present in the form of BSI often result from catheter-associated urinary tract infections, especially if the Foley catheter remains in situ, or respiratory tract infections (tracheitis, pneumonia, and rarely bronchial anastomosis site infections).[502,516,576] Although colonization of the respiratory tract is a common occurrence, primary invasive candidal pneumonia is not. Invasion usually occurs when comorbid conditions are present.[298] In patients with a fungemia, workup for metastatic sites, including ophthalmologic examination, echocardiography, and imaging, should be performed, especially if fungemia is persistent. Rarely disseminated disease of abdominal organs and the CNS can occur in SOTRs.[438] The source of infection usually is endogenous, although contributions from donor organs and nosocomial transmission may also arise. A decline in *C. albicans* infections and a concomitant increase in non–*C. albicans* spp. has been demonstrated.[454] Mirroring these changes, the Transplant Associated Infections Surveillance Network documented an increase in non–*C. albicans* candidal species, which was the driving force increasing azole resistance in *Candida* species (overall 16%), especially for *C. glabrata* and *C. krusei.*[339,438] Of interest, the azole resistance of *C. albicans, C. tropicalis,* and *C. parapsilosis* remained relatively low (1%). In SOTRs, fluconazole resistance was associated with any fluconazole use in the 3 months before infection.

The diagnosis of *Candida* infections can be challenging and often requires differentiating colonization from infection because *Candida* spp. are ubiquitous, especially in the upper gastrointestinal and respiratory tracts. In addition, although the diagnosis is often made by culture, these techniques are insensitive, especially for invasive disease and, except for blood culture, nonspecific. If recovery of *Candida* spp. from BAL fluid is associated with respiratory symptoms or deterioration of lung function (e.g., increased sputum production), treatment should be considered, although other causes such as rejection and coinfections should be explored as well. Organisms should be identified to the species level because of species-specific susceptibility profiles.[339] Early germ tube determination can confirm the presence of *C. albicans,* and a negative test can alert the physician to the presence of non–*C. albicans* spp., which may have an impact on the choice of antifungal agent.[438]

Newer molecular probes, such as peptide nucleic acid fluorescence in situ hybridization (PNA FISH), can identify *C. albicans* rapidly from positive blood cultures.[10]

The Fungitell (1→3)-β-D-glucan assay has been FDA approved as an adjunct for the diagnosis of invasive *Candida* and[438] its role in the early diagnosis of these infections is still under investigation; it may be especially useful for the diagnosis of deep-seated candidiasis when blood cultures are known to be insensitive.[416,438] Additionally culture-independent T2MR technology can detect *Candida* spp. (*albicans, tropicalis, parapsilosis, krusei, glabrata*) directly from patient's blood by amplification of DNA and identification to species level, by T2 magnetic resonance.[403,457] Overall sensitivity in adult patients was 91%, with a mean time of 4.4 hours ± 1 hour to identification. Its use in diagnosis, specifically in pediatric patients (it requires 3 mL of blood) and in transplant recipients, requires further study. The choice of initial antifungal therapy should be based on the patient's azole exposure, dominant species and susceptibility profiles at the institution caring for the patient, comorbid conditions, sites of involvement, and the use of other medications that might have significant drug–drug interactions.[438] The IDSA guidelines for management of candidiasis recommend fluconazole or an echinocandin in most settings, the latter especially in ill patients with recent azole exposure, with transition to fluconazole when stable.[239,438] Duration of therapy, as with other infections, should be individualized, but treatment should be continued for a minimum of 2 weeks after the last positive culture has been obtained and the signs and symptoms have resolved.[438] As noted earlier for *Aspergillus* infections, issues of dosing in pediatric patients with the newer antifungal agents and drug–drug interactions should be considered. Several excellent resources are available for detailed treatment algorithms.[438,516] Susceptibility testing should be considered on non–*C. albicans* spp. and for *C. albicans* infections that are refractory to conventional therapy. Interpretive breakpoints are available for most common antifungal agents including echinocandins.[10,455,456] Although candidemia should always be treated with an antifungal agent, the issue of removal of indwelling catheters has been controversial because of the lack of randomized controlled data designed to answer this question. The 2016 IDSA guidelines for the management of candidiasis and catheter-related BSIs recommend early removal of catheters when the source is presumed to be the central venous catheter and the catheter can be removed safely; decisions to do so should be individualized.[24,424,438]

Cryptococcus Neoformans *and* Gattii

Although relatively rare, cryptococcosis is the third most common fungal infection seen in SOTRs after *Aspergillus* and *Candida,* with an overall incidence of 2.8% (0.3% to 5%).[556] Available data suggest infection is less common in pediatric patients than in adults.[38,534] This infection usually occurs late, after the first year posttransplant, but it may occur earlier in LTRs.[38,531,556] Disease can be newly acquired but most often in adults is reactivated from latent disease; cases of donor-derived infection have been documented.[38,199,261,556,625] In the latter two scenarios, presentation may be within the first few months after transplantation.[39,554,556] The overall incidence and time to onset had not changed over many decades, but there are notable shifts in the recent epidemiology. Patients with cryptococcosis are more likely to be LTRs or multivisceral transplant recipients as opposed to renal recipients. Although CNS involvement and dissemination, with or without fungemia, remains the most common presentation—in upward of one-half of SOTRs—the presentation of isolated pulmonary infection has become more common in SOTRs. This is especially true since the almost universal use of calcineurin inhibitors.[133,261,522,556,590,625] These immunosuppressants target the fungal homologs of calcineurin, resulting in synergistic interactions with antifungal therapy and increased anticryptococcal activity and thus providing some protection against disseminated disease.[201,261,291,522,523] On the other hand, steroids and T-cell–depleting antibodies, as induction therapy or especially for antirejection, are known risk factors for cryptococcal infection in SOT recipients.[590] Pulmonary infections may have a variety of nonspecific presentations, including single or multiple nodules, infiltrates, consolidation, and pleural effusion; isolated pulmonary disease may be asymptomatic and detected as an incidental finding. Cutaneous disease manifests as nodular, maculopapular ulcers or pustules or as cellulitis and may be a portal of entry but most commonly indicates disseminated disease; this finding requires a full evaluation of extent of infection including CNS involvement.[553]

The diagnosis can be made by culture, visualization of encapsulated yeast with India ink or other special stains, and testing for cryptococcal capsular polysaccharide antigen in serum or CSF.[101] Although the serum cryptococcal antigen test is most reliable for CNS and disseminated disease (83%+), and a positive test should prompt a full evaluation, it is known to have decreased sensitivity for isolated pulmonary infection; indeed, among SOTRs, those LTRs with isolated pulmonary disease appear most likely to have negative cryptococcal serum antigen.[553,590] BAL can be performed to identify yeast in the lungs. CNS imaging and lumbar puncture should also be performed with opening pressure and large-volume CSF removal on SOTRs with suspected/proved cryptococcosis.[38] The majority of infections are caused by *C. neoformans*, but *C. gattii* infections in SOTRs have also been recently described[173] and are recognized as an emerging infection in the Pacific Northwest since 2004. These infections were similar to *C. neoformans* with a high degree of dissemination/CNS at time of diagnosis, at a median time 17.8 months posttransplant. Patients with meningitis had low antigen titers (median 1:8) and less robust CSF inflammatory response. The minimum inhibitory concentration (MIC) for fluconazole was elevated (1 to 32 μg/mL) and mortality was high (36% 90-day) in this cohort.

The IDSA guidelines for management for cryptococcal disease from 2010[451] recommend that the mainstay of therapy for severe, disseminated disease with CNS involvement is a combination of an LFAB plus flucytosine, which confers a survival advantage over conventional AmBd—11% versus 40% mortality in SOTRs.[531,552] TDM should be performed for flucytosine to avoid drug toxicities of bone marrow suppression and nephrotoxicity. Combination induction therapy should continue for a minimum of 2 weeks, or 4 to 6 weeks if flucytosine is not used. An extended period of fluconazole maintenance therapy (6 to 12 months) is recommended because relapses are well documented, especially in HIV-infected patients. As noted earlier, increased MIC may be seen in *C. gattii* infections, and extended azoles may be an alternative in this setting.[38,173] The risk for relapse in SOTRs and the optimal length of therapy are not known. Duration of treatment less than 6 months has been associated with an increased rate of relapse.[451,521,531] Management of elevated intracranial pressure is essential and may require repeated, sometimes daily, lumbar punctures and, rarely, placement of a ventriculoperitoneal shunt.[101,451] For less severe disease localized to the lungs, an oral azole alone may be adequate.[173,451,531] Mortality rates for SOTRs have improved over time: the overall mortality rate for cryptococcal disease is reported as 11% to 30% and varies by site of infection, treatment regimen, type of transplant, and possibly immunosuppressive regimen. The highest mortality rates are seen in liver and kidney transplant recipients with disseminated disease or fungemia, or both (20–70%). The lowest mortality rates (3–13%) are seen in localized pulmonary disease.[133,521,522,531,552,625]

Immune reconstitution inflammatory syndrome (IRIS) or immune reconstitution syndrome (IRS) is well described in cryptococcosis in SOTRs and correlates with treatment and the evolving host response to infection. Reversal of cryptococcal induction of T_H2 responses with antifungal medication and decreasing the iatrogenic immunosuppression leads to a proinflammatory milieu as T_H1/T_H17 responses are restored.[451,521,529,530,555] This physiologic immune response can become pathologic in about 15% of transplant recipients. Criteria for IRIS in the transplant setting have been published and these include clinical findings occurring during receipt of antifungal therapy and in the absence microbiological persistence or negative cultures and without another explanation.[530] Manifestations of IRIS include fever, lymphadenopathy, and progression of pulmonary and CNS symptoms and lesions, without documentation of increased titers or positive cultures. IRIS in SOTRs presents a mean of 6 weeks after initiation of therapy and correlates with this reduction of immunosuppression, which remains a cornerstone to therapy but should be done in a gradual, stepwise fashion to avoid rapid reconstitution.[168,551] Risk factors for developing IRIS in SOTRs include disseminated/CNS disease (fungal burden), discontinuation of calcineurin inhibition (but not dose reduction or changes in other immunosuppressants), and graft rejection (greater degree of "immune reconstitution"-inadequate T_{reg} response).[168,530,551] These authors state that, based on observations including the potential benefit of calcineurin inhibitors to antifungal activity and the lack of association of the reduction of corticosteroids on the risk for developing IRIS, consideration should be given initially to tapering corticosteroids, followed by reduction but not discontinuation of calcineurin inhibitors. There is no established therapy for IRIS. Minor manifestations may resolve over time, but IRIS may be life-threatening in severe cases and can lead to graft loss.[530] Increasing doses of corticosteroids have been used. Investigational therapies include statins to promote T_H2/T_{regs} over $T_H1/17$ pathways and tumor necrosis factor-α inhibitors.[521,555]

Pneumocystis Jiroveci *(Formerly P.* Carinii*)*

Pneumocystis pneumonia (PCP) is caused by the renamed fungal pathogen *Pneumocystis jiroveci.* PCP has been associated notably with defects in T-cell immunity and with the immunosuppression used in SOTRs. In most cases, symptomatic PCP in an immunocompromised host is thought to be reactivation of latent infection, although putative nosocomial person-to-person transmission linked by molecular evidence is increasingly observed.[134,125,319,462,499,504]

Heart-lung recipients and LTRs are at increased risk for developing infection, with reported attack rates of 6.5% to 43% without prophylaxis, up to a 10-fold increase as seen in heart transplants alone.[479] Higher rates of infection in SOTR, including LTR, have been associated with CMV coinfection, use of cyclosporine and corticosteroids, and receipt of therapy for rejection; cases can occur many years after transplantation.[400,462,504,601] Therefore guidelines recommend a benefit of long-term and perhaps lifelong prophylaxis, especially if additional risk factors are ongoing.[479,504,601] The drug of choice for prophylaxis remains TMP-SMX, and its use is associated with dramatic decreases in the incidence of PCP infection. Additional benefits of this drug include prevention of many community-acquired respiratory, gastrointestinal, and urinary tract pathogens and protection against most *Toxoplasma gondii* and *Nocardia* infections. Multiple regimens exist, and dosing for 3 days per week appears to be as effective as daily dosing in all populations studied. Toxicity remains an issue for some patients and includes bone marrow suppression, decreased renal function, hepatitis, and rash (Stevens-Johnson syndrome), which may be severe. Details of alternative regimens are reviewed in Chapter 225 and elsewhere.[479,504]

PCP infection is manifested as progressive dyspnea, cough, tachypnea, chest pain, and cyanosis over the course of days to weeks. In addition, fevers, sweats, and flulike symptoms may be prominent. Hypoxia and shortness of breath, in the context of normal or minimal findings on chest radiographs, are common findings. Corticosteroids and calcineurin inhibitors may alter the signs and symptoms and render early diagnosis more difficult to establish. The diagnosis is confirmed by identification of *P. jiroveci* in a respiratory sample or lung tissue. Immunofluorescent staining of organisms with monoclonal antibodies had been the technique of choice; Gomori methenamine silver nitrate, which stains cyst forms only (5% to 10% of the total organisms), is the most reliable staining method.[479] BAL fluid and tissue obtained by open-lung biopsy have the highest diagnostic yield.[479] Polymerase chain reaction (PCR) assays on BAL specimens are now recognized as highly sensitive and specific diagnostic techniques and are commercially available. This assay may allow the distinction between colonization and low fungal burden infection.[8,70,225,497] (1→3)-β-D-Glucan is a component of the *P. jiroveci* cell wall and can be detected in the serum of patients with PCP.[116,143,292,501] This assay appears to be a reliable marker of infection, with the most convincing results shown in patients with HIV infection.[143] At this time, it cannot be recommended to supplant appropriate testing of respiratory samples, but it may be considered as an adjunct for diagnosis, especially in patients too ill to undergo invasive procedures.[398]

The mainstay of therapy for PCP infection remains high-dose TMP-SMX for 14 to 21 days.[166,362] Corticosteroids are generally recommended for severe disease, including a 5- to 7-day course with a slow taper over 7 to 14 days. For patients intolerant of TMP-SMX or those less seriously ill, alternative therapies can be considered, including dapsone with trimethoprim, atovaquone, intravenous pentamidine, trimetrexate, clindamycin/primaquine, and pyrimethamine/sulfadiazine.[166,362] Relapse in patients without HIV infection is an uncommon occurrence with TMP-SMX therapy if a reduction in immunosuppression can be accomplished and coinfections such as with CMV do not occur.

Endemic Mycoses

Endemic mycoses, or the dimorphic fungal infections histoplasmosis, blastomycosis, and coccidioidomycosis, are rare but important causes of disease in SOTRs.[279,385] There is a noted bimodal distribution in the onset of infection—within the first 6 months and again at more than 2 years after transplant (up to 11 years)—and therefore these infections should be considered in the differential at all time periods.[279] Rejection does not appear to have a major role in development of endemic mycoses, in contrast to invasive mold infections, although it may be associated with increased risk of development of coccidioidomycosis. Spores are inhaled from the environment and convert to noncontagious yeast forms at 37°C. Infection may be caused by latent reactivated disease in the recipient or donor or may be newly acquired. Donor-derived infections generally manifest within the first several weeks after transplantation. Because of the nonspecific findings, latency of these organisms, increased worldwide travel, and organ procurement strategies, infections in transplant recipients require a high index of suspicion, especially if they occur in nonendemic areas. This is important because the response to therapy is generally excellent if appropriately initiated.[279]

Coccidioidomycosis, caused by *Coccidioides immitis* and *C. posadasii,* is the endemic mycosis most commonly seen after transplantation. It occurs in up to 9% of SOTRs in endemic areas of the southwestern United States (especially California and Arizona), northern Mexico, and Central America.[63,584] Unlike histoplasmosis and blastomycosis, pretransplant infection poses an increased risk for development of serious posttransplant disease. Transplant candidates should be screened for a history of coccidioidomycosis and environmental exposure, which should prompt serologic testing for *Coccidioides.* Secondary prophylaxis is very effective and should be given to all patients with a history of *Coccidioides* infection; without its use, the mortality rate is very high (up to 70%).[63,280,385,584] Pulmonary infections may be accompanied by an acute onset of respiratory symptoms and fever and progress rapidly to respiratory failure. Nonspecific symptoms of anorexia, weight loss, and fatigue may herald extrapulmonary disease. Dissemination to bones, skin, and the CNS occurs commonly when infection occurs in transplant recipients. The time of highest risk appears to be in the first 3 months after transplantation, with the majority of infections occurring by 1 year. Donor-derived coccidioidomycosis has been documented in LTRs.[64,386,385,569,623] Recipients did not have evidence of pretransplant coccidioidomycosis, nor did they live or travel to endemic areas. Several of the donors had documented epidemiologic risk factors. Commonly these LTRs had fulminant pulmonary or disseminated infections within the first 3 weeks after transplantation, the majority of which were fatal.

The diagnosis of coccidioidomycosis can be made definitively by culture, usually from respiratory samples or urine and rarely from blood or CSF.[25] Histopathologic evaluation may reveal large spherules with the presence of endospores. Serologic tests include tube-precipitin antigen (IgM), detected early in disease, and complementation fixation or immunodiffusion (IgG), which can be titered and is helpful in monitoring response to therapy.[25,63] Coccidioides antigen testing may improve diagnostic sensitivity, especially in immunocompromised patients who may have negative serologic studies. Recent data suggest it is a useful addition to the diagnosis in meningitis as well.[274] The optimal therapy for SOTRs with coccidioidomycosis is unknown but generally follows published guidelines.[182] Patients with evidence of previous infection should receive secondary prophylaxis with azole therapy for a minimum of 6 to 12 months after undergoing transplantation.[25,63,182,385]

Histoplasma capsulatum infection is a rare occurrence after transplantation, even in patients with presumed pretransplant infection. Cases in transplant recipients have been observed in endemic areas and in conjunction with outbreaks in areas hyperendemic for histoplasmosis, the Mississippi and Ohio River valleys, and Central America.[120,577] Two cases of histoplasmosis in renal transplant recipients were linked by molecular typing to donor-derived disease.[326] Several series of histoplasmosis in SOTRs have noted a high rate of dissemination, fungemia, and severe disease, although generally with good response to prolonged therapy (12 months), although mortality rates were 10% to 13%.[35,120,279] Median time to diagnosis was 17 months after transplant, and time from onset of symptoms to diagnosis was 3 weeks, reflecting the protean nature of initial presentation. Up to 50% of cases occurred within the first 2 years. Donor-derived infection has been documented by typing and usually presents in the first month after transplantation. Relapse occurred rarely, often many years after initial infection, and was associated with mortality in some cases. Several patients were identified with evidence of histoplasmosis in explant or donor tissues and received antifungal prophylaxis without developing active infection.[609] Manifestations of infection include pulmonary, mediastinal, inflammatory, and disseminated syndromes with or without CNS involvement. The diagnosis can be made by culture, histopathology, serology, or antigen detection.[609] In immunosuppressed patients with disseminated disease, culture of appropriately obtained specimen, and antigen detection (urine, serum, BAL) appear to be the most useful (sensitivity of 80% to 100% using third-generation assays).[218,221] Antigemia and antigenuria together likely is the most sensitive diagnostic approach in SOTR.[35] Cross-reactivity with *Aspergillus* and *Blastocystis* can result in false-positive *Histoplasma* antigen tests with these infections.[582] In addition, positive galactomannan antigen assays have been reported in SOTRs with histoplasmosis.[582] New enzyme immunoassay (EIA) antibody testing appears more sensitive than previous assays and allows for detection of IgM and IgG although data on use in immunocompromised patients is not available.[475] Guidelines recommend long-term therapy (3 to 4 months) with LFAB for immunocompromised patients with disseminated or CNS involvement, followed by 6 to 12 months of itraconazole.[385,610] Voriconazole and posaconazole have good in vitro activity and have been successfully used as well.[177,178] Monitoring antigen levels is beneficial to assess response to therapy and for relapse.[219,610]

Blastomyces dermatitidis, the causative agent of blastomycosis, appears to be the least common endemic fungal infection in the posttransplant setting.[186] These infections are rare events in series of fungal infections in immunocompromised patients, including patients with acquired immunodeficiency syndrome (AIDS), even in endemic areas of the south central and north central United States, particularly in the Ohio and Mississippi River valleys and around the Great Lakes.[385] Cases of posttransplant disease most commonly present as pulmonary disease, which may lead to acute respiratory distress syndrome and a high mortality rate. Diseases of the skin and CNS are also common.[278,508] Diagnosis is made by histopathology, culture, and antigen detection.[100,111,385] Guidelines for therapy recommend that immunocompromised patients should receive LFAB until stabilized (4 to 6 weeks), followed by a prolonged course (6 to 12 months) of an azole.[100,385] Most data are available for itraconazole, although voriconazole and posaconazole also may be effective.[100,278]

Emerging Fungi

The impact of these emerging fungi for LTRs is increasingly appreciated. Published reports suggest that these infections are becoming more commonly recognized pathogens in LTRs and other SOTRs.* These organisms include non-*Aspergillus* hyalohyphomycetes or hyaline hyphae without pigment (*Scedosporium apiospermum, Fusarium* spp., *Pupureocillium/Paecilomyces* spp.); phaeohyphomycetes, or dematiaceous pigmented molds (*Cladophialophora bantiana, Alternaria* spp., *Curvularia* spp., *Scedosporium prolificans, Exophiala jeanselmei, Pyrenochaeta romeroi, Cladosporium* spp.); Zygomycetes, or nonseptated hyphae (*Rhizopus* spp., *Mucor* spp.); and yeast-like organisms (*Trichosporon, Malessezia, Rhodotorula*).[250] These infections represent upward of 10% of fungal infections in SOTRs and should be considered along with IA. Lung and liver transplant recipients are at the highest risk for these infections. Risk factors include profound immunosuppression (in donor and/or recipient), exposure to azole therapy, breaks in skin integrity, and chronic lung disease. These infections tend to present late after transplantation, often after the first year, and have been associated with donor-derived infections utilizing organs from near drowning events and "commercial transplantation/transplant tourism," which has been linked to poor posttransplant outcomes.[198] Many of these organisms are highly resistant and have unique susceptibility profiles, which include the newer azoles voriconazole and posaconazole, as well as LFAB and terbinafine. The newest azole to be FDA approved for treatment of IA and mucormycosis, isavuconazole, has demonstrated some promise in treatment of mold infections.[382] Several recent studies offer evidence that isavuconazole demonstrates noninferiority to voriconazole for *Aspergillus* infections and has greater in vitro activity against these emerging pathogens.[347,365] It is well tolerated, without dermatologic, ophthalmologic, and hepatic toxicity; has excellent PO bioavailability; and the intravenous formulation does not require solubilization by cyclodextrin. Frequent poor outcomes with mold infections has prompted the use of combination therapy as well, which is supported by some in vitro data,[277] although clinical data are lacking and/or inconclusive at present.[150,250,541] Indeed, these infections may be more likely to be disseminated and fatal than those caused by *Aspergillus* spp.[151,250,251,365,385] Surgical debridement may play an important role in therapy, in addition to medical therapy as well as decreasing immunosuppression and perhaps additional immune modulation with IFN-γ and/or GM-CSF.[250]

Donor-derived fungal infections are rare events, although well-documented serious complications can occur in SOTRs,[524] as mentioned earlier. Most commonly recognized is donor-derived candidiasis in renal transplant recipients; intestinal perforation in the donor has been identified as a risk factor. Other infections, such as cryptococcosis from unrecognized cryptococcal meningoencephalitis in donor and endemic fungal pulmonary infections in undiagnosed/asymptomatic donors, have occurred. Even less common, although with great consequence, are donor-derived mold infections such as aspergillus and mucormycosis, with high mortality rates. Source of infection can be from donor allograft or contaminated preservation fluid. Allografts should be carefully examined for granulomas or other unusual findings. All potential donor-derived infections should be reported to the Organ Procurement and Transplantation Network. This is especially important if organs from a donor have gone to multiple recipients, so the epidemiologic link can be documented and therapy or prophylaxis can be initiated to other recipients in a timely manner. The American Society of Transplantation has developed guidelines to enhance the ability to identify donors with risk factors to transmit fungal infections, although data to address all issues are lacking.

Viral Infections

Cytomegalovirus

The epidemiology of CMV infection in SOTRs has changed in recent years. Advances in diagnosis and in preemptive and prophylactic strategies and therapy have decreased the impact of early CMV infection in transplant populations. However once antiviral medication is discontinued, CMV infection is common in high-risk patients, and it remains one of the most important pathogens in SOTRs, with wide-ranging effects on morbidity and mortality.[131,248,249,391] Thus continued efforts to optimize preventative strategies are paramount.[391,433,444] The source of infection can be endogenous reactivation or from the donor graft or leukocyte-containing blood products and cause primary infection or reinfection. Rarely primary infection may be acquired from the community, especially in young children.

The effects of CMV infection have both profound direct and indirect consequences. As per published definitions, direct effects of the virus range from "asymptomatic" CMV infection, which can be detected by viremia (culture positive), antigenemia (pp65 in leukocytes), and DNAemia or RNAemia (generally by quantitative PCR methods or quantitative nucleic acid amplification testing [QNAT]); to CMV syndrome with viremia, fever, neutropenia, thrombocytopenia; to true end-organ disease, which is often found primarily in the allograft but may disseminate.[295,471] The diagnosis of end-organ disease, such as pneumonitis, enteritis/colitis, hepatitis, and encephalitis/meningitis, requires signs or symptoms of disease at that site, with detection of CMV by culture, histopathology, immunohistochemical staining, or in situ hybridization. Except for CNS disease, detection by QNAT is not sufficient for establishing the diagnosis because it is too sensitive and may signify transient viral shedding. Investigation regarding the use of CMV QNAT, including the appropriate specimen (plasma or whole blood) and establishing international standards and thresholds for

*References 151, 250, 251, 307, 370, 390, 448, 494, 509, 517, 546.

therapy are ongoing. Data support the use of plasma for testing, which is likely equivalent to whole blood in determining undetectable viremia and risk of relapse despite the increased sensitivity of the later specimen. In addition, in 2010, the first World Health Organization (WHO) International Standard for Human Cytomegalovirus for Nucleic Acid Amplification Techniques was released as a tool that can be used to standardize patient results from different sites and using different assays.[179,226,272] Data from different sites are now available to validate the use of international units (IU) in quantitative measurements of CMV DNAemia (calibrate and establish colinearity to reference material), which may help future multicenter studies to delineate testing algorithms, define relevant cutoffs and testing frequencies, and further clarify clinician guidance and patient outcome.[236,354,470,491]

The indirect, immunomodulatory effects of CMV have broad-reaching consequences and can be divided into three categories: (1) immunomodulation as it contributes to the net state of immunosuppression and increased risk for opportunistic super infections (e.g., aspergillosis, PCP); (2) increased risk for oncogenesis, such as seen with EBV-related lymphoproliferative diseases; and (3) allograft injury and dysfunction, as seen in classic rejection and vasculopathy of the allograft. In LTRs, BOS, a severe form of chronic rejection (small airways disease), has been associated with CMV infection.[336,488,631] Of interest, in a retrospective, multicenter study of almost 600 pediatric LTRs, development of BOS in the first year (14%) was not associated with CMV infection.[131]

The greatest risk factor for developing CMV infection in children, as in adults, is donor/recipient (D/R) seropositivity, most notably D^+/R^- mismatch, followed by D^-/R^+ mismatch. Infection can occur in D^+/R^+ and rarely in D^-/R^- matches.[126,131] Other risks include the use of induction therapy, antilymphocyte antibody, and blood product transfusion (performed previously).[631,633] In pediatric LTRs, the risk for CMV infection has also been associated with living donor transplant, older age at transplant, and multiple episodes of A2 rejection before CMV.[131] The incidence of CMV infection in LTRs is higher than that in other SOTRs. The reasons are multifactorial but include long-term, intense immunosuppression and high levels of CMV latency, viral load, and reactivation associated with the lung and its transplantation.[43,633] The incidence of infection and disease is reported to be 54% to 92% without prophylaxis.[631,633] The rates of CMV infection and its consequences have been considerably decreased by utilizing various preventative strategies (see later discussion), although different study design, endpoints, and follow-up periods point to the difficulty in identifying the optimal regimen and time course.[131,433,444,631]

A combination of approaches is employed to reduce the incidence of CMV infection. The use of CMV-negative or leukocyte-free blood products for CMV-negative recipients is standard practice in most transplant centers and has been shown to reduce infection rates. Matching of D/R serologic status probably would reduce infection rates but also would limit the donor pool for recipient-negative recipients significantly and is not considered to be indicated. The final strategies use different regimens of antivirals to suppress replication with or without immunoglobulin products for enhanced passive immunity.[488,631] These regimens can be prophylactic, in which all patients at risk are treated for a certain period, universal prophylaxis (UP), or preemptive therapy (PET), in which highly sensitive screening techniques, such as antigenemia (pp65) or QNAT, are used to identify patients needing therapy. The rationale of this approach is to limit drug exposure, thereby decreasing toxicity and viral resistance. To complicate matters, regimens can include multiple antiviral agents, such as intravenous ganciclovir or acyclovir and/or oral ganciclovir, acyclovir, or valganciclovir for various periods. Most of the studies discussed here are performed primarily in adult transplant populations; pediatric recommendations are extrapolated from these data. Several surveys of lung transplant centers show a preponderance of the use of UP, based on serostatus stratification, although in a recent survey one-third of centers now use a hybrid combination of early UP followed by PET based on risk.[127,196,312] Centers used a variety and combination of antiviral agents, although intravenous ganciclovir and/or valganciclovir were most commonly used; interestingly, underdosing in adults was common. Oral valganciclovir has been demonstrated to be noninferior to intravenous ganciclovir in adult SOTRs for eradication of viremia and long-term clinical outcome.[32-34] Side effects and discontinuations were also comparable. The dosing of ganciclovir and especially valganciclovir in pediatric patients is still evolving. There are now several published algorithms based on achieving the target ganciclovir area under the curve (AUC) of 40 to 60 μg × h/mL (protective for CMV infection in adults), although target levels were not initially achieved (ranging both above and below target) in up to 40% to 60% of children.[31,285,453,548,549,591] The optimal algorithm and sampling strategy are yet to be determined. TDM is suggested to improve outcome and decrease toxicity. The recommendation for the duration of prophylaxis, especially in high-risk patients, has increased over the past 5 years (see later discussion), and the most recent survey suggests that most international centers now extend UP for a median of 6 months (range, 3 to 12 months) for D^+/R^- LTR. In addition, few responding centers (16%) now use CMV intravenous immunoglobulin (IVIG) with variable schedules, although the benefits of its use remain unproved.[67,468,630,634] Methods and regimens for viral monitoring also varied greatly. These surveys highlight the need for additional data, some of which are now available, including a randomized controlled trial comparing 3 versus 12 months of valganciclovir in adult LTRs.[433,612] This study and others provide evidence that, for high-risk LTRs, UP and extending prophylaxis beyond 3 months to 12 months and possibly "indefinitely" has an overall beneficial effect in terms of CMV infection and its consequences.[131,191,248,391,433,444,612,634] A cohort of LTRs who received extended UP (12 months) were followed for an additional 3.9 years.[112] Patients who had received extended-course UP had a sustained proactive benefit with a lifetime CMV incidence of 12% versus 55% (P = .009). No long-term adverse hematologic effects were documented. Other retrospective, single-center reviews of SOTRs who received 6 months versus "indefinite" (minimum, 12 months) UP failed to show a similar long-term benefit and reported leukopenia (55% and 66%, respectively), some requiring discontinuation; ganciclovir resistance occurred in a small but notable number of patients, including fatal infections.[49,612]

Although increasing the length of prophylactic antiviral therapy may decrease the incidence of CMV infection, additional complexity relates to the resultant immature T-cell response associated with long-term and potent antiviral suppression, whereas some "escape" may allow a protective T-cell response after therapy is discontinued.[488] In addition, the concern remains for the creation of drug-resistant CMV infection in the presence of long-term antiviral exposure. Rates of resistant CMV remain relatively low in spite of broad use of antiviral agents for prophylaxis, although they are highest in LTRs among the SOTRs; this is believed to be secondary to intense immunosuppression and high viral load associated with lung tissue.[433,612] A study in high-risk adult renal transplant recipients documents a higher incidence of drug-resistant isolates in preemptive strategies designed to decrease drug exposure.[118] This supposed contradiction may be explained because the higher viral loads were seen in these patients, because by definition they were viremic before antiviral agents were initiated, and because of the use of oral valganciclovir, rather than intravenous therapy, during periods of high replication; all are risk factors for resistance.[167]

Several evidence-based consensus guidelines by expert advisory groups on the management of CMV infection in SOTRs have been published and are summarized here[295,471,633]:

1a. All D^+/R^- or R^+ LTRs should be considered for CMV prevention (UP or PET).
2a. Prophylaxis should continue for a minimum of 180 days, although some pediatric experts would limit this to 3 months given the risk for catheter-associated infection if intravenous ganciclovir is used.
2b. The drug of choice for prophylaxis is intravenous ganciclovir or oral valganciclovir.
3a. Monitoring should be performed every 2 weeks for the first 6 months after transplantation to assess for breakthrough viremia and disease and then periodically for 8 to 12 weeks after completion of prophylaxis.
3b. Whole-blood assay is the monitoring method of choice and should be validated at each center.
3c. If a PET approach is being used, CMV monitoring should be performed more frequently.
4. Breakthrough disease should be treated with ganciclovir 5 mg/kg administered intravenously every 12 hours for up to 21 days until

the viral load is below detection. Immunosuppression should be reduced if possible.

5. Infection that occurs after the initial prophylaxis has been stopped should be treated with ganciclovir or valganciclovir until the viral load is below detection.

6a. Resistance should be considered in patients with breakthrough viremia, recurrent infections, or poor response to therapy, persistent viremia at 21 days. Genotypic analysis for common mutations (UL97 [viral kinase] and UL54 [DNA polymerase]) should be performed on isolates recovered from these patients.

6b. Foscarnet is the drug of choice, with or without ganciclovir, for possible resistant strains.

7. Reinitiation of prophylaxis should be considered in patients requiring antilymphocyte antibodies or high doses of corticosteroids for rejection.

Of note, valganciclovir is not FDA approved for prophylaxis in LTRs, although it is for other SOTRs, and available data suggest that it is safe and effective in LTR as well.[248,391,433,612,633] Data in pediatric patients for the safety and efficacy of valganciclovir for prophylaxis and treatment are emerging. Some preliminary data on formulations and pharmacokinetics are available and support concerns for underdosing, leading to resistance and some hematologic toxicity.[87,360]

Epstein-Barr Virus/Posttransplant Lymphoproliferative Disorder

The disease manifestations of primary EBV infection in SOTRs range from uncomplicated mononucleosis (fever, malaise, exudative pharyngitis, lymphadenopathy, hepatosplenomegaly, atypical lymphocytosis) to conditions indistinguishable from malignant lymphoma. Organ-specific disease may include pneumonitis and hepatitis, as well as gastrointestinal, CNS, and hematologic involvement. Early lesions of EBV-driven lymphoproliferation, such as plasmacytic hyperplasia, are seen in mononucleosis-like syndromes within the context of normal tissue architecture. The term posttransplant lymphoproliferative disease (PTLD) is generally reserved for proliferation of EBV-positive immunoblasts and atypical lymphocytes associated with effacement or destruction of normal tissue architecture. The reader is referred to several excellent, in-depth reviews and guidelines.[15,211,465]

The manifestation of EBV/PTLD is varied and depends on the site of involvement, which may be intrathoracic, extrathoracic (abdominal, head and neck, CNS), or disseminated and intranodal or extranodal.[325] Often PTLD is seen in the allograft, as with lung, liver, and intestinal transplantation.[211] Signs and symptoms of PTLD can be nonspecific, such as fever of unknown origin, malaise, weight loss, and sore throat.[72] Abdominal pain, gastrointestinal bleeding, intestinal obstruction and perforation, allograft dysfunction such as changes in respiratory status in LTRs, diffuse lymphadenopathy on physical examination or CT, or hepatosplenomegaly should raise the index of suspicion for PTLD. Focal neurologic findings also can be seen with CNS disease. An additional challenge is to differentiate allograft rejection from PTLD; both entities in LTRs may be characterized by allograft dysfunction with diffuse consolidation on imaging, without obvious lymphadenopathy or a mass. Because the therapies for these two conditions are diametrically opposed, increasing or decreasing immunosuppression, this distinction obviously is critical.[15,210]

Risk factors for the development of PTLD have been identified.[15,72,109] Pretransplant EBV seronegativity (as a surrogate marker for the risk for development of posttransplant primary EBV infection) is probably the most important predisposing factor for the development of PTLD. Because primary EBV infection occurs almost universally by the time of adulthood, older individuals are already immune, and young children undergoing transplantation are therefore at greatest risk. Presumably it is the lytic phase of the primary EBV infection that sets the stage for PTLD because the delayed EBV-specific cytotoxic T lymphocyte (CTL) response observed in immunocompromised children allows for high viral loads and uncontrolled B-cell infection, latency, and reactivation.[15] In addition, concomitant CMV infection or CMV mismatch before transplantation increases the risk for developing PTLD, contributing to the "net state of immunosuppression." Certain immunosuppressive regimens, such as the use of OKT3 and polyclonal antilymphocyte antibodies and possibly tacrolimus in pediatric patients, are linked to the development of PTLD, although it is likely that the overall intensity of immunosuppression, not a specific agent, is most important in defining the risk for development of PTLD. Indeed, EBV DNAemia may be a marker for "over immunosuppression" and is associated with subsequent occurrences of other opportunistic infections in LTR.[515]

Patients at highest risk by type of transplant are small bowel recipients, followed by recipients of hearts and lungs and livers. This risk is probably multifactorial and includes more intense immunosuppressive regimens and transplantation of large amounts of lymphoid tissue with the graft, thereby increasing recipients' potential exposure to donor-derived EBV. The published incidence of PTLD in pediatric LTR ranges from 7.7% to 26.3%.[72,109,459] PTLD most often occurs within 12 months after transplantation, with median onset of primary infection at 6 weeks and symptoms presenting in the 2- to 3-month range.[15,72] When late PTLD occurs, it is associated with older recipients, long duration of immunosuppression, EBV-negative disease, and poorer prognosis.[15,109,313]

The diagnosis of PTLD requires a high index of suspicion. The gold standard is histopathologic examination of tissue. Specimens should be processed by pathologists familiar with the morphologic classifications (e.g., phenotype, lineage, clonality) and ancillary tests that may be helpful, such as tissue staining for EBV-encoded RNA 2 by in situ hybridization (EBERS), which is more sensitive than in situ targeting viral DNA or the use of immunohistochemical staining of latent antigens (EBNA-1 and 2, LMP-1) and more specific than EBV DNA amplification; the expression of CD20, which has implications for therapy, should also be determined.[15,465] Imaging also can be used for presumptive diagnosis, to guide biopsy, and for follow-up.[459,513] In LTRs, CT of the chest may reveal discrete nodules, air space consolidation, or mediastinal lymphadenopathy. Extrathoracic involvement is less common but may include abdominal lymphadenopathy, liver and spleen lesions, and a thickened bowel wall. Head and neck imaging may reveal involvement of cervical lymph nodes, pharynx, orbit, sinus, and rarely the brain. Fluorodeoxyglucose-labeled positron emission tomography combined with CT (FDG-PET/CT) in adult and pediatric SOTRs with PTLD may offer a more nuanced approach to diagnosis and staging and may be particularly helpful in management to distinguish between active versus necrotic/fibrotic lesions.[57,61,346,579]

Viral load determination (quantitative PCR) from blood should be sought in patients with a concern for PTLD. Although an elevated load may support the diagnosis, the value of a single measurement is uncertain; no diagnostic threshold level has been identified. In addition, these assays are not standardized, and many questions remain regarding their use, including which compartment is most revealing and should be sampled (peripheral blood lymphocytes, whole blood, or serum), extraction methods, thresholds for initiation of therapy, and the effect of serostatus on the sensitivity and specificity of viral loads.[15,207,210,276,309,465] Because of significant interlaboratory variability, longitudinal testing of patient samples should be performed at a single site. Finally not all patients with EBV/PTLD have elevated viral loads, and viral loads may be elevated without evidence of disease; therefore PCR assays lack sensitivity and specificity for PTLD.[15,60] Although these assays are now widely used at transplant centers, further controlled studies are necessary to optimize their use in immunocompromised patients and to establish international standardization of viral load assessments, as with CMV.

Patients at the highest risk for PTLD and mortality are those in whom primary EBV infection develops early after transplantation; therefore every effort should be made to identify these patients. Pretransplant serologic assessment of donors and recipients for both EBV and CMV can alert physicians to most of these high-risk patients because donor-recipient mismatch of either virus appears to play an important role in risk stratification.[72,109] Once identified, these patients should be monitored by PCR assay for evidence of primary infection, and careful examination and use of CT for early diagnosis of disease should be included. Several strategies have been used for the prevention of EBV/PTLD in high-risk patients.[211] The use of EBV-negative donors, although probably effective, would reduce the donor pool substantially and generally is not advocated. The use of prophylactic antiviral therapy has not been proved to prevent the development of PTLD. Although these agents are active against the lytic viral infection that precedes PTLD, they are not active against the latent viral phase that characterizes

PTLD. Theoretically antiviral agents may decrease the number of newly infected cells, thus impacting viral loads. Acyclovir and ganciclovir are often used for prevention of CMV, and comparisons of the incidence of PTLD in certain high-risk patients receiving these antiviral agents suggest some benefit; however PTLD has developed in some patients while receiving these agents.[132,180] A small prospective controlled study of high-risk (D^+/R^-) pediatric renal transplant recipients found valganciclovir prophylaxis to significantly reduce the incidence of primary EBV infection, lower viral loads in those who became infected, and less symptomatic disease associated with infection but did not investigate the link to PTLD.[243] The use of IVIG or CMV IVIG is similarly a potential but unproved strategy.[209,210,247] Given insufficient evidence, universal and routine use of antiviral agents and IVIG products for prophylaxis and preemption has not been endorsed by the American Transplant Society.[15]

Preemptive strategies aimed at identifying primary infection by blood PCR monitoring have received significant attention.* In these protocols, high-risk patients undergo EBV quantitative viral load monitoring at frequent intervals (usually weekly) to identify increases associated with infection, which is a prerequisite for the development of EBV/PTLD. Patients with a persistently high viral load should be evaluated aggressively for the presence of PTLD on examination and imaging, and suspicious lesions should be sampled. When the diagnosis of PTLD is made, immunosuppression should be decreased as much as feasible, the optimal duration of which is uncertain.[15,316] Most patients with nonmalignant lesions will respond to this maneuver alone. Return to higher levels of immunosuppression is usually prompted by rejection or clear evidence of clinical and virologic response. The use of antiviral agents in this setting has become routine, although without proven benefit.[15] Surgical resection and local radiation therapy may be beneficial for localized disease and in the event of gastrointestinal involvement. Characterization and outcome of patients with chronic high viral loads without evidence of PTLD is emerging. These studies suggest that up to 45% of patients will progress to PTLD up to 8 years after transplant.[60] Efforts to immunologically define and identify this high-risk group are ongoing.[343,344] Risk factors for poor outcomes include poor performance status, multisite disease, CNS involvement, T- or NK cell- and EBV-negative PTLD, monoclonal disease, and presence of certain oncogenes or tumor suppressor genes.[15]

Monoclonal B-cell antibody therapy has become an attractive option for $CD20^+$ lesions not responsive to a reduction in immunosuppression.[15,465] The currently available product is an anti-CD20 antibody (rituximab). Reports document initial response rates of 40% to 60%, although relapses are not uncommon.[62,105,106,207,387,423] A PTLD-specific prognostic index identified high-risk patients with a 0% 2-year survival, in contrast to 50% in intermediate and 88% in low-risk adult patients receiving rituximab for PTLD; this highlights the potential heterogeneity of the patients and outcomes.[106] These high-risk patients all required additional chemotherapy, and 55% died of PTLD. Although generally well-tolerated, long-term hypogammaglobulinemia is a common occurrence in recipients, and viral complications, such as severe CMV and hepatitis B and C infections, as well as parvovirus B19–induced aplasia and enteroviral meningoencephalitis, have been associated with its use.[465] For refractory disease, cytotoxic chemotherapy may be indicated, in consultation with oncology colleagues. Small studies on pediatric SOTRs suggest that the combination of low dose chemotherapy and rituximab may be safe and effective.[215] Unfortunately even patients who respond to reduction of immunosuppression and do not have progression of PTLD, mortality may be high, secondary to chronic allograft rejection.[399] The preliminary data on the use of adoptive immunotherapy (autologous and allogeneic EBV-specific cytotoxic T lymphocytes) show promising expansion, persistence, and efficacy of cytotoxic lymphocytes.[223,500] The generation of calcineurin-resistant T-cell clones is expected to improve the performance of cytotoxic lymphocyte therapy in the presence of ongoing immunosuppression.[74] Other investigational therapies include immunomodulatory therapy (anti–interleukin-6, T_H1 response with IFN-α), interruption of viral signaling pathways (LMP1, LMP2a), and vaccine technology.[15,207,224,465]

*References 15, 42, 51, 158, 207, 211, 465, 482, 547, 571.

Other Herpesviruses: Herpes Simplex Viruses Types 1 and 2, Varicella-Zoster Virus, Human Herpesviruses Types 6, 7, and 8

Infections with herpes simplex virus (HSV) types 1 and 2 are common occurrences in SOTRs; in older children and adults, HSV usually is a reactivation disease manifested as orolabial or genital disease. Primary disease occurs in young children who contract the infection from viral shedding of close contacts or from allograft. Serostatus of transplant candidates should be determined because symptomatic reactivation occurs in up to 68% of seropositive SOTRs not receiving prophylaxis, especially in the setting of treatment for rejection, and naïve recipients are at risk for severe and prolonged primary infections given their lack of immunologic memory. In LTRs, serious or disseminated disease such as esophagitis, hepatitis, keratitis, pneumonitis, and severe disseminated and/or CNS infection can occur.[538,613] Infections tend to occur early, within the first month after transplantation, unless prophylaxis is used. As with other herpesviruses, concomitant infection with CMV is not an uncommon event. The diagnosis can be made clinically when typical lesions are present. Culture and PCR technology can confirm the diagnosis and be helpful for unusual manifestations. PCR, which has replaced culture as the preferred test, has advantages of rapidity, increased sensitivity (fourfold higher than tissue culture), and identifying HSV in blood and other body fluids. Prophylactic strategies with acyclovir or ganciclovir used for CMV (3 to 6 months) can prevent HSV. Generally prophylaxis for HSV infection does not need to be continued past the early transplant period unless there are frequent clinical recurrences, in which case suppressive antiviral therapy should be continued until reduction of immunosuppression can occur. Occasionally lifelong suppression may be necessary. Intravenous acyclovir and oral valacyclovir or famciclovir are effective therapies for localized mucocutaneous disease. More severe disease should be treated with intravenous formulations until resolution of symptoms. Resistance of HSV in SOTRs is rare, but when it is suspected in instances of clinical failure, culture and susceptibility should be performed. Most resistance results from changes in the viral thymidine kinase gene.[461] Foscarnet, which does not require this viral gene for phosphorylization, is usually the drug of choice. Less frequent mutations with altered DNA polymerase may require cidofovir. A new lipid ester of cidofovir, CMX001(brincidofovir), which has broad and potent antiviral activity and less toxicity, is currently in phase III trials for treatment of several DNA virus infections.[138,466]

Primary varicella-zoster virus (VZV) infection can occur in pediatric LTRs, as can reactivation of previous disease leading to herpes zoster. The rates of VZV infections in SOTRs are not known, but presumably the infection rate after transplantation is low since the widespread use of varicella vaccine (Varivax), as it is in the general community.[20] Because VZV infection is a vaccine-preventable disease and complications of primary infection can be life-threatening, all patients should be screened for evidence of immunity, and seronegative transplant candidates should receive varicella vaccine.[2,128,452] Available data demonstrate that this vaccine is safe and effective in this setting, although seroconversion rates may be reduced. Optimally, two doses 4 to 6 weeks apart and a minimum of 2 to 4 weeks before transplant should be administered. If the vaccine does not prevent disease, it should mitigate development of severe disease. In addition, susceptible family members also should receive the vaccine.

Exposure in posttransplant patients should be treated with a high-titer varicella immunoglobulin preparation if available (VariZIG); IVIG is recommended based on the "best judgment of experts" if high-titer preparations are not available, although no clinical data document its efficacy. The window for benefit of administration of immunoglobulin preparations is up to 10 days after exposure.[20,93] Additionally some experts recommend the use of prophylactic acyclovir if exposure such as household or intimate contact is likely to lead to development of disease or is revealed past the window for immunoglobulin prophylaxis to be effective. Varicella vaccine, which is an attenuated live viral product, generally is not recommended in LTRs at this time.[128]

VZV infection in LTRs should be treated with intravenous acyclovir until all lesions are crusted and the patient's symptoms have lessened.[452] Patients taking corticosteroids, especially during the incubation period, are at increased risk for the development of severe disease. Hemorrhagic and disseminated disease, including encephalitis, hepatitis, and pneumonitis, can occur in immunocompromised patients. All patients admitted to the hospital with VZV infections should be placed in combined airborne precautions; immunocompromised patients may shed virus for a prolonged period. Hospitalized LTRs who have received immunoglobulin post exposure prophylaxis should remain in isolation from day 10 to day 28.[452]

Herpes zoster is a common event in adult transplant recipients; rates in children have not been determined. A study of SOTRs aged 16 to 74 years found a 15% incidence of herpes zoster in LTRs, with a mean time to onset of 14 months and a median of 9 months (9 days to 5.8 years).[204] The diagnosis is made clinically and with the use of viral culture or PCR techniques if necessary. Infections can become disseminated, as evidenced by multiple dermatomal spread, and should be treated with intravenous acyclovir and pain control. The use of corticosteroids should be decreased, if possible.

HHV-6 variants A and B, the latter of which is most commonly implicated in human disease, is an emerging opportunistic viral pathogen. Seropositivity reaches nearly 100% in early childhood and therefore disease in all but the very youngest transplant recipients probably represents reactivation. Several studies have documented HHV-6 by PCR assay or culture in a majority (66–90%) of apparently asymptomatic adult LTRs.[268,320] Infections occur early after transplantation (median, 6 and 18 days) and can occur in the setting of CMV antiviral prophylaxis. Most are without obvious clinical manifestations that could be ascribed to HHV-6 alone.[311] HHV-6 DNA can be recovered from BAL fluid in 20% of LTRs and often is found with other pathogens, including other herpesviruses.[310] In immunocompromised patients, HHV-6 may exert direct and indirect effects on the host. It probably is responsible for rare cases of encephalitis, hepatitis, pneumonitis, febrile illnesses, and bone marrow suppression.[320] The presence of HHV-6 alone or as a cofactor to CMV may augment the immunomodulatory effects and increase the risk associated with fungal and other infections, as well as allograft rejection, BOS, and mortality.[268,310,311,379,414] Many questions regarding HHV-6 in this population remain unanswered. PCR assay of peripheral blood lymphocytes is the most sensitive method for detection of virus, but it cannot differentiate between latent and active virus. Therefore detection of infection generally requires exclusion of other etiologies before causality can be ascribed to HHV-6 for clinical findings. Routine monitoring of asymptomatic patients is not recommended. Data are insufficient to recommend prophylactic or preemptive therapies, although the virus is susceptible to achievable levels of ganciclovir, foscarnet, and cidofovir. Treatment with these drugs may be considered in patients with compatible syndromes if other causes are eliminated and reduction in immunosuppression has not led to clinical improvement.[311] Whether asymptomatic patients with documented HHV-6 infection would benefit from therapy with regard to the indirect effects of the virus remains unknown. Finally HHV-6, unique in the herpesvirus family, can rarely be chromosomally integrated as a mechanism of latency (CIHHV-6).[567] It is estimated to occur in 0.8% of the normal population. Because the viral DNA integrates into every nucleated human cell, CIHHV-6 is characterized by extremely high viral loads (>1 million copies/mL blood), which may not indicate active infection. This has been described in SOTRs, although the significance of this occurrence is unclear.[315] Although some patients received antiviral therapy because of the concern of high titers, none had perceivable decline in their viral loads and those who did not receive therapy remained clinically asymptomatic. For this reason, the finding of CIHHV-6 may lead to unnecessary antiviral therapy.

The role of HHV-7 and HHV-8 in SOTRs is undefined. HHV-7 behaves in a similar manner as HHV-6 in normal hosts, although it appears to be less prevalent and occurs later in life. Symptomatic disease is less well characterized, but it may be responsible for similar syndromes seen with HHV-6 in normal children and transplant recipients.[311] Evidence of HHV-8 infection in normal children is rare. It is associated with Kaposi sarcoma in immunocompromised patients, as well as body cavity lymphomas, PTLD, and Castleman disease.[17,311] It also may be associated with fever and bone marrow suppressive syndromes of donor origin in transplant recipients.[342] Therapy includes reduction of immunosuppression and/or the use of mammalian target of rapamycin (mTOR; rapamycin/sirolimus) in the place of calcineurin inhibition for its antiproliferative effect. Surgical excision, chemotherapy, and radiation may also be necessary.[311]

Community-Acquired Respiratory Viruses: Respiratory Syncytial Virus, Parainfluenza Virus, Human Metapneumovirus, Influenza, and Adenovirus

The paramyxoviruses respiratory syncytial virus (RSV), parainfluenza virus (PIV), and human metapneumovirus (hMPV) are common causes of upper and lower respiratory tract disease in normal children; symptoms range from congestion and rhinorrhea to laryngeal tracheobronchitis (croup), bronchiolitis, and pneumonia.[17,18,21,22] Similar clinical syndromes can be caused by a variety of viruses, and LTRs may have atypical presentation; thus testing should remain broad until a diagnosis is made.[355] Data on the impact of these viruses on LTR are emerging. Respiratory viral illness is encountered commonly after pediatric lung transplantation and can be severe and persistent. Coinfection and sequential infection with other respiratory viruses, CMV, and fungal pathogens occurs.[192] A decreased 1-year survival was associated with respiratory viral illness, but not at 2 years in retrospective studies of pediatric LTRs.[333,334] Neither study found an association with BOS, in concordance with some studies, although others have found associations with viral respiratory infections and acute and chronic rejection/allograft dysfunction (BOS) in LTR,[255,301] thus this remains an area of ongoing investigation.[241,355,388,593] Risk factors for respiratory viral illness and severe courses/complications among SOTRs include young age, lung transplantation, and CMV infection. Transmission occurs person to person, from exposure to infected nasopharyngeal secretions, and from fomites. Consideration should be given to screen recipients for incubating respiratory viruses before they undergo transplantation, especially if high levels of circulating virus are present in the community or illness is present in family members. Immunocompromised patients can shed infectious virus for long periods. Strict adherence to hospital infection control practices is most important in reducing nosocomially acquired disease from infected patients, visitors, and health care workers.[355] Patients and their families should be counseled on avoidance of exposure and on good hand hygiene practices when discharged from the hospital.

RSV can cause severe lower respiratory tract infection (LRTI) in LTRs. Although most infections resolve with or without therapy, fatal cases have been reported, as have long-term declines in pulmonary function.[59,192,372,606] The diagnosis can be made from nasal washings by rapid antigen-detection kits, standard viral culture, or more rapid shell vial culture methods, although PCR-based assays, which provide sensitive detection of a broad range of viral pathogens, are now considered the preferred method.[355] Risk factors for poor outcome in immunocompromised patients include neutropenia, lymphopenia, age younger than 1 year, underlying lung disease, and augmented immunosuppression. High mortality rates in hematopoietic stem cell transplant recipients have led to prevention and treatment strategies that can serve as models for care in SOTRs,[144,194,611] although they are not without controversy.[59,195] A recent survey of centers providing adult lung transplantation documented differences in therapy. While all transplant centers treated LRTI with ribavirin, some used inhaled, some oral, with different dosing regimens, with or without steroids and/or IVIG. Some centers treated upper RTI (URTI) to prevent LRTI.[48] This heterogeneity demonstrates the need for further studies to define optimal treatment. Supportive care and reduction in immunosuppression remain the mainstay of therapy. For children with URTI and risk factors, or LRTI, aerosolized ribavirin should be considered. In addition, because outcomes, even in treated hematopoietic stem cell transplant recipients, are poor with ribavirin alone, some experts suggest combination therapy with RSV IVIG or monoclonal antibody (palivizumab) for immunocompromised patients with significant infections.[59,82] Increasingly published reports using oral ribavirin, which is considerably easier and less expensive to use, suggest successful treatment.[324,332,357,449] Several investigational drugs undergoing clinical trials show promise, including oral ALS-008176, a nucleoside analogue that inhibits viral polymerase, and ALN-RSV01, an intranasal small interfering RNA targeting RSV replication.[145,146,202,632] Effective prophylaxis with palivizumab and RSV IVIG has been achieved in young infants with lung disease.[214,378] Care must be taken when extrapolating to other patient populations, given the unexpected poor outcomes of some infants with complex congenital heart disease who were administered RSV IVIG[518] but not pavilizumab.[162] Some experts would consider the use of immunoprophylaxis in young infants undergoing organ transplantation during the RSV season.[355]

hMPV was described in healthy young children in 2001.[574] It has signs and symptoms similar to those of RSV, and almost universal infection probably occurs by 5 years of age.[614] The impact of hMPV on immunocompromised patients is as yet uncharacterized, in part because diagnostic tests have only recently become widely available. The virus can be cultured, but reverse transcriptase PCR appears to be the test of choice and is available as part of a PCR respiratory viral panel in most centers.[18] Studies on adult LTRs demonstrate that hMPV respiratory viral illnesses are common, often with coinfections and associated with graft dysfunction/acute rejection, but less likely than RSV infections to be associated with chronic graft rejection and BOS.[192,241,308,604] There is no established therapy for hMPV infections outside of supportive care and treatment of co-pathogens, although ribavirin and IVIG are sometimes utilized.[241,355]

PIV (types 1 to 4) is isolated frequently as a cause of URTIs and croup in normal children.[21] PIV can cause severe lower tract infection in immunocompromised patients, including respiratory failure in LTRs, most notably caused by serotype 3.[26,586,588,607] Although rarely fatal in adults, persistent declines in pulmonary function and acute allograft rejection are important consequences of PIV infection.[372,586,607] A retrospective study on PIV in pediatric SOTRs (after liver, small bowel, lung, heart, kidney transplants) found significant age-related morbidity and mortality.[26] Although 44% of all patients with PIV infection had URTI, only 11% of children younger than 1 year had limited disease. A 16% mortality rate was associated with PIV, and predictors of mortality included age younger than 6 months, infection occurring less than 3 months after transplantation, and augmented immunosuppression. Infection in these children occurred in the context of community outbreaks. The diagnosis can be made by PCR assays and antigen detection; culture isolation can take weeks. Respiratory secretions obtained from nasal washings or BAL fluid can be used.[59] No proven therapy for PIV in LTRs is available. Intravenous and aerosolized ribavirin has been used in immunocompromised hosts, but without randomized controlled data or clear evidence of efficacy.[59,355,372] A novel sialidase fusion protein, DAS181, which removes viral receptors from respiratory epithelial cells, shows therapeutic promise and is currently in clinical trials for PIV in immunocompromised patients.[216,496,594]

Transplant recipients are at risk for acquiring community-acquired infection during the yearly influenza A and B epidemics, as well as nosocomial infection from visitors, hospital workers, and other transplant recipients as a result of infections occurring in the inpatient setting.[183,352,484,587] Seasonal influenza infection is relatively rare in SOTRs—4.2% of adult LTRs over the course of a 10-year period and 2.6% of pediatric SOTRs over a similar period[26,59]—but LTRs appear to be at a uniquely high risk for acquiring infection. In the adult study, the incidence was 41.8 cases per 1000 person-years for adult LTR versus 2.8 and 4.3 per 1000 person-years in liver and kidney transplant recipients, respectively.[589] These authors speculate that optimal protection from influenza infection afforded by serum and secretory antibodies in the respiratory tract are altered in LTRs, thereby leading to higher attack rates. In addition, risk for disease and complications are high for pediatric transplant recipients in particular.[355] Previous data suggested that upper respiratory tract symptoms were the most common presentation of pediatric SOTRs with influenza, although 3 of 13 patients (23%) died.[26] In these children, corticosteroid bolus and OKT3 therapy given within a week of diagnosis of infection were associated with mortality. Transplant recipients may be at increased risk for acquiring secondary bacterial infections and nonpulmonary complications such as hepatitis, myocarditis, and aseptic meningitis.[59,589] Influenza was the causative agent in 8.9% of 101 respiratory viral illnesses documented in a series of pediatric LTRs observed between 1998 and 2007.[334]

Although we have an incomplete picture of the current epidemiology of influenza infections in pediatric LTRs, the H1N1 epidemic of 2009–10 has added to our understanding of its impact. Risk factors for hospitalization and severe disease included age younger than 5 years and immunosuppression.[624] Two studies on adult LTRs suggest the majority of patients did well, but with a wide range of clinical impact from upper respiratory tract symptoms, association with progression to BOS, mechanical ventilation, and mortality (0%, 21%).[175,415] In a retrospective series of SOTRs (adults and children) with H1N1 infection, children were more likely to have fever, rhinorrhea, sore throat, and headache and less likely to have chest radiographic evidence of lower tract disease.[302] Of note, almost 50% of all patients had gastrointestinal complaints. In the pediatric cohort, mortality was 0% versus 7% in adults, with similar rates of admission (66%, 73%) and intensive care unit care (12%, 17.5%). Children were more likely to receive antiviral therapy within 48 hours.

Infection with the influenza virus is unique among respiratory virus infections in that both vaccine and chemoprophylactic strategies are available. Unfortunately immunosuppressed patients may not respond well to influenza vaccine, and, if disease is not recognized promptly, the effectiveness of therapy for established disease may not be optimal. Studies on the immunogenicity of influenza vaccine in pediatric SOTRs are more encouraging than in adult reports, which have documented poor response, especially when associated with mycophenolate mofetil or sirolimus.[81,227] In pediatric renal transplant recipients, response was similar to that of normal controls, without evidence of rejection,[157,181] although in pediatric heart transplant recipients protective antibody responses were not achieved until three doses of vaccine were administered.[5] Preliminary studies using high-dose (60 μg) versus standard-dose (15 μg) trivalent inactive influenza vaccine suggest no increase in toxicity or graft dysfunction and improved immunogenity.[193] No conclusive evidence documents a link between immunization and graft dysfunction with the intramuscular trivalent inactivated influenza vaccines, which have been used routinely for decades.[299] The current recommendation is that influenza vaccine be administered yearly to all SOTRs older than 6 months of age and 3 to 6 months after transplantation and to those awaiting transplantation, as well as to household contacts and caretakers.[2,81,299] During the 2009 H1N1 pandemic, recommendations for immunization were reduced to 1 month after transplant, with the acknowledgment that only partial protection was likely.[303] Children younger than 9 years of age receiving influenza vaccine for the first time should have two doses 4 weeks apart. The use of live attenuated influenza vaccine and intradermal and adjuvant vaccines is not recommended. Oseltamivir chemoprophylaxis can be administered to patients who have not been vaccinated or who have not had sufficient time to respond to vaccination, especially if influenza is circulating in the community or if there is a known exposure. Dosing for young children and infants is now available.[266,286,303] Other agents approved for prophylaxis of influenza A in children older than 1 year include amantadine and rimantadine (M2 inhibitors), although resistance of influenza A is high and they are not active against influenza B strains.[587]

The diagnosis of influenza should be made by real-time PCR or other nucleic acid–based detection whenever possible. Multiplex PCR assays for respiratory viruses are now routinely available at most centers.[303] See Chapter 178 for additional information on laboratory diagnosis. Most experts would recommend empirical therapy with antiviral agents in an LTR with suspected (community epidemic with compatible symptoms) or proven influenza, regardless of duration of symptoms (e.g., >48 hours).[59,355] During the 2009–10 H1N1 pandemic, early therapy was associated with improved outcome (decreased hospitalization, intensive care unit, mortality) in high-risk patients as well as normal hosts.[302,624] The choice of agent depends on the type of virus (A or B) and information about resistance. The neuraminidase inhibitors oseltamivir (oral) and zanamivir (inhaled, IV) are currently favored because of their broad spectrum of activity and less reported resistance.[355,587] Oseltamivir-resistant H1N1 retained susceptibility to zanamivir.[303] In addition, higher/double doses and prolonged therapy may be necessary because the viral burden and length of shedding are increased in transplant recipients and children. Optimal length of therapy is not known, but the minimum is 5 days; consideration for continuation of therapy until PCR testing is negative must be countered by the concern for emergence of viral resistance. Two intravenous antiviral agents, peramivir and zanamivir, are available, as well as combination therapies undergoing investigation.[303] Choice of antiviral therapy should be made after consultation with the CDC and public health officials about circulating virus strains and resistance patterns.

With improved management of herpesvirus infections and better diagnostic techniques, the impact of adenoviral infections in transplant recipients is increasingly recognized. Adenoviral infections in SOTRs follow the epidemiology of infection in the general population, such that infections are more common in young pediatric than adult transplant recipients, who may remain naïve to many of the 52 recognized serotypes.[135,171,383,425] Other risk factors for infection include exposure to lytic antibodies, high levels of maintenance immunosuppression, and adenovirus serologic mismatch. Establishment of latency in lymphoid tissue has been documented, and numerous immune evasion genes have been identified.[171] Adenoviral infections have multiple putative sources, including the donor organ, reactivation from latency in host tissues, and infection acquired from the community or nosocomially.[88,290,374,383,460]

Infections in LTR may be asymptomatic, lead to recognizable syndromes of the respiratory and/or gastrointestinal tracts, or cause disseminated disease, defined as involvement in two or more organs. Often disease is most pronounced in the allograft (e.g., pneumonitis, hepatitis, enteritis, hemorrhagic cystitis).[171] Cases of acute, disseminated, and fatal disease have been described in cardiothoracic transplant recipients. In LTRs, infections occur in the early posttransplant period and often cause disease in the graft in the form of necrotizing pneumonia.[75,425] Adenoviral infection has been associated with graft dysfunction, BOS, retransplantation, and death.[75]

Available diagnostic methods for the detection of adenovirus include culture, direct identification of antigens, and serology, as well as histologic examination of tissues for the presence of adenoviral inclusions and immunohistochemical staining.[103] Direct identification of adenoviral antigens, usually performed on respiratory specimens, can be achieved by radioimmunoassay, immunofluorescence, or ELISA techniques, which are rapid and specific but less sensitive than culture.

PCR assay has emerged as a powerful tool for detection of adenovirus in body fluids (blood, nasal wash, BAL) and tissues and for serotyping.[171,246] The virus's ability to establish latency can render interpreting the presence of virus or viral DNA in clinical specimens a challenge.[185,321] A single determination of the presence of adenovirus by PCR assay in immunocompromised patients may be nonspecific and perhaps misleading and should be correlated with histopathology if available and appropriate clinical syndromes to differentiate between asymptomatic infection and disease. As with other important viruses that establish latency, quantitative viral load patterns appear to be more informative with regard to the pathogenic role of adenovirus in these patient populations. No threshold has been identified to predict progression of infection or outcome. Studies in pediatric hematopoietic stem cell transplant recipients (HSCTR) support the use of blood PCR surveillance as a method to identify patients at risk for disseminated disease.[108,171,328,597] Although routine surveillance is not recommended for LTRs, its use for early detection and monitoring in certain high-risk patients may be advocated.

The optimal therapy for adenovirus infection has not been determined. Supportive care and reduction of immunosuppression are the mainstays of therapy.[171,620] The role of immune recovery should not be underestimated, of which adenovirus-specific cytotoxic T cells are particularly critical.[97,229] Cidofovir (CDV), an acyclic nucleoside phosphonate, inhibits viral DNA polymerase with activity against all serotypes. It may be beneficial in severely ill patients with disseminated disease and rising viral loads.[90,238,318,337,596,628] Use of this agent may be associated with significant renal toxicity,[228,318,463] and use of modified dosing regimens has been investigated with some success.[90,238,404,596] CMX001 (brincidofovir) is an oral lipid ester prodrug of CDV with broad-spectrum antiviral activity that achieves very high intracellular antiviral activity and improved toxicity profile. It has been used for therapy for adenoviral infection in immunocompromised patients, mostly HSCTR, and appears promising.[171,172,620] Strategies involving adoptive immunotherapy, such as infusion of adenovirus-specific cytotoxic lymphocytes that has been investigated in adenoviral infections in HSCTR and other immunodeficient patients,[163,317,406] may also be feasible, with proof of concept for cytotoxic lymphocyte therapy published for SOTRs and EBV infections.[74,223,500]

Although a detailed discussion is beyond the scope of this chapter, the link between respiratory viruses, BOS, and chronic allograft dysfunction should be addressed briefly. BOS is a progressive condition without good treatment options and is the greatest impediment to long-term survival for LTRs. It affects upward of 50% of patients alive 5 years after transplantation and is the leading cause of death in adult and pediatric LTRs 1 year after transplantation.[570,599] Although the exact mechanisms are still being determined, the final common pathway is epithelial injury and intraluminal proliferation of fibroblasts leading to airflow obstruction.[258,282,565,585] Activation of innate immune pathways (e.g., Toll-like receptors) in response to pathogen-associated molecular patterns (PAMPs) and more recently recognized endogenous damage-associated molecular patterns (DAMPs),[566] as well as stimulation of T cells and release of cytokines and chemokines by viruses, are leading candidates for the initiation of these pathways. Not surprisingly, genetic polymorphisms in related genes such as Toll-like receptors, cytokines, mannose-binding lectin, matrix metalloproteinase 7, and others may further help to explain the variability in development in BOS and in the future may allow for risk stratification and personalized therapy.[275] Many studies have linked viral infections, such as those caused by CMV, adenovirus, RSV, PIV, and others, often working in concert, to the development of BOS.[161,301,432,586,588] The exact role of these agents has yet to be proved, although it is biologically plausible.[258] Reduction of BOS syndrome remains an incentive for the continued development of preventive strategies against these viral infections.

Donor-Derived and Zoonotic Infections: Rabies, West Nile Virus, Lymphocytic Choriomeningitis Virus, and *Bordetella*

Although most donor-derived infections are expected and CMV, HBV, and the risk to the recipient can be mitigated, the isolation of unusual pathogens often is a sign of an unexpected exposure.[41,264,489] This statement is epitomized by reports of SOTRs with uncommon zoonotic infections. In the case of donor-derived rabies, lymphocytic choriomeningitis virus, HIV, HCV, Chagas, and West Nile virus infections, multiple cases were traced to a donor or donors with retrospectively assessed exposures and risk factors.[164,231,265,267,322,543] West Nile virus in SOTRs also has been community acquired,[287,304] and cases of infection with *Bordetella bronchiseptica* in transplant recipients have been traced to sick pet dogs.[47,107] These cases are humbling in multiple respects. Many of these infections have no established therapy and, as expected, are associated with increased morbidity and mortality in SOTRs.[142,164,287,304,413] Therefore prevention is of utmost importance. These cases advise us to counsel our posttransplant recipients and families on avoidance of potentially infectious exposures, such as travel, sick pets, and arthropod vectors of diseases.[294,300,413] Undeniably they remind us of the almost limitless pathogens that may befall SOTRs, including those not yet described. These cases have newly informed the policies for reporting suspected donor-transmitted conditions and opened a new dialogue on how screening procedures of organ and blood donors are conducted.[148,164,169,245,264,283] To ensure an optimal balance of patient safety and organ utilization, new guidelines are in place to more accurately define donors with "increased risk for disease transmission."[506] A rigorous three-pronged approach can mitigate risk of donor-derived infections: risk stratification based on donor medical, behavior, and social history; physical exam/assessment of donor's body (deceased or living) and of the organ itself; and, finally, laboratory screening, including serology, culture, and nucleic acid amplification testing (NAT).[264] Going forward, an increased understanding of the epidemiology and risk of donor disease transmission is needed.

NEW REFERENCES SINCE THE SEVENTH EDITION

7. Al-Hasan MN, Razonable RR, Eckel-Passow JE, et al. Incidence rate and outcome of gram-negative bloodstream infection in solid organ transplant recipients. *Am J Transplant.* 2009;9:835-843.
15. Allen UD, Preiksaitis JK, AST Infectious Diseases Community of Practice. Epstein-Barr virus and posttransplant lymphoproliferative disorder in solid organ transplantation. *Am J Transplant.* 2013;13:107-120.
31. Asberg A, Bjerre A, Neely M. New algorithm for valganciclovir dosing in pediatric solid organ transplant recipients. *Pediatr Transplant.* 2014;18:103-111.
32. Asberg A, Humar A, Jardine AG, et al. Long-term outcomes of CMV disease treatment with valganciclovir versus IV ganciclovir in solid organ transplant recipients. *Am J Transplant.* 2009;9:1205-1213.
33. Asberg A, Humar A, Rollag H, et al. Oral Valganciclovir is noninferior to intravenous ganciclovir for the treatment of cytomegalovirus disease in solid organ transplant recipients. *Am J Transplant.* 2007;7:2106-2113.

34. Asberg A, Humar A, Rollag H, et al. Lessons learned from a randomized study of oral valganciclovir versus parenteral ganciclovir treatment of CMV-disease in solid organ transplant patients – the Victor trial. *Clin Infect Dis.* 2016;62:1154-1160.
35. Assi M, Martin S, Wheat LJ, et al. Histoplasmosis after solid organ transplant. *Clin Infect Dis.* 2013;57:1542-1549.
38. Baddley JW, Forrest GN, AST Infectious Diseases Community of Practice. Cryptococcosis in solid organ transplantation. *Am J Transplant.* 2013;13:242-249.
48. Beaird OE, Freifield A, Ison MG, et al. Current practices for treatment of respiratory syncytial virus and other non-influenza respiratory viruses in high-risk patient populations: a survey of institutions in the Midwestern Respiratory Virus Collaborative. *Transpl Infect Dis.* 2016;18:210-215.
49. Beam E, Lesnick T, Kremers W, et al. Cytomegalovirus disease is associated with higher all-cause mortality after lung transplantation despite extended antiviral prophylaxis. *Clin Transpl.* 2016;30:270-278.
52. Berenger BM, Doucette K, Smith SW. Epidemiology and risk factors for nosocomial bloodstream infections in solid organ transplants over a 10-year period. *Transpl Infect Dis.* 2016;18(2):183-190.
54. Bergamasco MD, Barroso Barbosa MB, de Oliveira Garcia D, et al. Infection with Klebsiella pneumoniae carbapenemase (KPC)-producing K. pneumoniae in solid organ transplantation. *Transpl Infect Dis.* 2012;14:198-205.
66. Bodro M, Sabé N, Tubau F, et al. Risk factors and outcomes of bacteremia caused by drug-resistant ESKAPE pathogens in solid-organ transplant recipients. *Transplantation.* 2013;96:843-849.
69. Botha P, Archer L, Anderson RL, et al. Pseudomonas aeruginosa colonization of the allograft after lung transplantation and the risk of bronchiolitis obliterans syndrome. *Transplantation.* 2008;85:771-774.
77. Bryant JM, Grogono DM, Greaves D, et al. Whole-genome sequencing to identify transmission of *Mycobacterium abscessus* between patient with cystic fibrosis: a retrospective cohort study. *Lancet.* 2013;381:1551-1561.
78. Bulik CC, Nicolau DP. In vivo efficacy of simulated human dosing regimens of prolonged-infusion doripenem against carbapenemase-producing *Klebsiella pneumoniae. Antimicrob Agents Chemother.* 2010;54:4112-4115.
82. Burrows FS, Carlos LM, Benzimra M, et al. Oral ribavirin for respiratory syncytial virus infection after lung transplantation: efficacy and cost-efficiency. *J Heart Lung Transplant.* 2015;34:958-962.
89. Canadian Cystic Fibrosis Registry. Microbiology: bacterial species and respiratory infections, annual report; 2013. Available at: www.cysticfibrosis.ca/uploads/registryreport 2013/203registryannualreporten.pdf.
91. CDC Availability of an assay for detecting Mycobacterium tuberculosis, including rifampin resistant strains, and consideration for its use-United States, 2013. *MMWR Morb Mortal Wkly Rep.* 2013;62(41):821-824.
94. Cervera C, van Delden C, Welte J, et al. Multidrug resistant bacteria in solid organ transplant recipients. *Clin Microbiol Infect.* 2014;20:49-73.
112. Copeland CAF, Davis WA, Snyder LD. Long-term efficacy and safety of 12 months of valganciclovir prophylaxis compared with 3 months after lung transplantation: a single-center, long-term follow-up analysis from a randomized, controlled cytomegalovirus prevention trial. *J Heart Lung Transplant.* 2011;30:990-996.
113. Cornely OA, Duarte RF, Haider S, et al. Phase 3 Pharmacokinetics and safety study of a posaconazole tablet formulation in patients at risk for invasive fungal disease. *J Antimicrob Chemother.* 2016;71:718-726.
121. Cumpston A, Caddell R, Shillingburg A, et al. Superior serum concentrations with Posaconazole delayed-release tablets compared to suspension formulation in hematological malignancies. *Antimicrob Agents Chemother.* 2015;59:4424-4428.
122. Cystic Fibrosis Foundation. Patient registry annual data report; 2013. Available at: www.cff.org/2013_cff_annual_data_report_to_the_center_directors.pdf.
128. Danziger-Isakov L, Kumar D, AST Infectious Diseases Community of Practice. Vaccination in solid organ transplantation. *Am J Transplant.* 2013;13:311-317.
138. De SK, Hart JCL, Breuer J. Herpes simplex virus and varicella zoster virus: recent advances in therapy. *Curr Opin Infect Dis.* 2015;28:589-595.
145. DeVincenzo J, Lambkin-William R, Wilkinson T, et al. A randomized, double-blind, placebo-controlled study of an RNAi-based therapy directed against respiratory syncytial virus. *Proc Natl Acad Sci USA.* 2010;107:8800-8805.
146. DeVincenzo JP, McClure MW, Symons JA, et al. Activity of oral ALS-008176 in a respiratory syncytial virus challenge study. *N Engl J Med.* 2015;373:2048-2058.
151. Doligalski CT, Benedict K, Cleveland AA, et al. Epidemiology of invasive mold infections in lung transplant recipients. *Am J Transplant.* 2014;14:1328-1333.
165. Fischer SA, Lu K, AST Infectious Diseases Community of Practice. Screening of donor and recipient in solid organ transplantation. *Am J Transplant.* 2013;13(4):9-21.
168. Fishman JA. Immune reconstitution syndrome: how do we tolerate our microbiome? *Clin Infect Dis.* 2015;60:45-47.
171. Florescu DF, Hoffman JA, AST Infectious Diseases Community of Practice. Adenovirus in solid organ transplantation. *Am J Transplant.* 2013;13:206-211.
173. Forrest GN, Bhalla P, DeBess EE, et al. *Cryptococcus gattii* infection in solid organ transplant recipients: description of Oregon outbreak cases. *Transpl Infect Dis.* 2015;17:467-476. ISSN 1398-2273.
179. Fryer JF, Heath AB, Anderson R, et al. *Collaborative Study to Evaluate the Proposed 1st WHO International Standard for HCMV for NAT-Based Assays.* Geneva: WHO expert Committee on Biological Standardization; 2010.
182. Galgiani JN, Ampel NM, Blair JE, et al. 2016 Infectious diseases of America guideline for the treatment of Coccidioidomycosis. *Clin Infect Dis.* 2016;63(6):e112-e146.
184. Garantziotis S, Palmer SM. An unwelcome guest: *Aspergillus* colonization in lung transplantation and its association with bronchiolitis obliterans syndrome. *Am J Transplant.* 2009;9:1705-1706.
189. Geltner C, Lass-Florl C. Invasive pulmonary aspergillosis in organ transplants-focus on lung transplants. *Respir Investig.* 2016;54:76-84.
193. GiaQuinta S, Michaels MG, McCullers JA, et al. Randomized, double-blind comparison of standard-dose vs. high-dose trivalent inactivated influenza vaccine in pediatric solid organ transplant patients. *Pediatr Transplant.* 2015;19:219-228.
196. Goldfarb SB, Benden C, Edwards LB, et al. The registry of the International Society for Heart and Lung transplantation: eighteenth official pediatric lung and heart-lung transplantation report-2015. *J Heart Lung Transplant.* 2015;34:1255-1263.
198. Gomez CA, Singh N. Donor-derived filamentous fungal infections in solid organ transplant recipients. *Curr Opin Infect Dis.* 2013;26:309-316.
202. Gottlieb J, Zamora MR, Hodges T, et al. ALN-RSV01 for prevention of bronchiolitis obliterans syndrome after respiratory syncytial virus infection in lung transplant recipients. *J Heart Lung Transplant.* 2016;35:213-221.
206. Green M. Introduction: Infections in solid organ transplantation. *Am J Transplant.* 2013;13:3-8.
215. Gross TG, Orjuela MA, Perkins SL, et al. Low-dose chemotherapy and rituximab for post-transplant lymphoproliferative disease (PTLD): a Children's Oncology Group Report. *Am J Transplant.* 2012;12:3069-3075.
216. Guzman-Suarez BB, Buckley MW, Gilmore ET, et al. Clinical potential of DAS181 for the treatment of parainfluenza-3 infection in transplant recipients. *Transpl Infect Dis.* 2012;14:427-433.
226. Haynes RL, Kline MC, Toman B, et al. Standard reference material 2366 for measurement of HCMV DNA. *J Mol Diag.* 2013;15:177-185.
235. Hirsch EB, Guo B, Chang KT, et al. Assessment of antimicrobial combinations for Klebsiella pneumoniae carbapenemase-producing *K. pneumoniae. J Infect Dis.* 2013;207:786-793.
236. Hirsch HH, Lautenschlager I, Pinsky BA, et al. An international multicenter performance analysis of cytomegalovirus load tests. *Clin Infect Dis.* 2013;56:367-373.
237. Hoenigl M, Prattes J, Spiess B, et al. Performance of galactomannan, Beta-D-glucan, *Aspergillus* lateral-flow device, conventional culture and PCR tests with bronchoalveolar lavage fluid for diagnosis of invasive pulmonary aspergillosis. *J Clin Microbiol.* 2014;52:2039-2045.
250. Huprikar S, Shoham S, AST Infectious Diseases Community of Practice. Emerging fungal infections in solid organ transplantation. *Am J Transplant.* 2013;13:262-271.
260. Husain S, Sole A, Alexander BD, et al. The 2015 International Society for Heart and Lung Transplantation guideline for the management of fungal infections in mechanical circulatory support and cardiothoracic organ transplant recipients. *J Heart Lung Transplant.* 2016;35:261-282.
264. Ison MG, Grossie P, AST Infectious Diseases Community of Practice. Donor-derived infections in solid organ transplantation. *Am J Transplant.* 2013;13:22-30.
265. Ison MG, Llata E, Gonover CS, et al. Transmission of human immunodeficiency virus and hepatitis C virus from an organ donor to four transplant recipients. *Am J Transplant.* 2011;11:1218-1225.
270. Johnson GL, Sarker SJ, Nannini F, et al. *Aspergillus* specific lateral flow device and real time PCR testing of bronchoalveolar lavage: a combination biomarker approach for clinical diagnosis of invasive pulmonary aspergillosis. *J Clin Microbiol.* 2015;53:2103-2108.
272. Jones S, Webb EM, Barry CP, et al. Commutability of CMV: WHO international standard in different matrices. *J Clin Microbiol.* 2016;54(6):1512-1519.
273. Kang HM, Jong Lee H, Cho EY, et al. The clinical significance of voriconazole therapeutic drug monitoring in children with invasive fungal infections. *Pediatr Hematol Oncol.* 2015;32:557-567.
274. Kassis C, Zaidi S, Kuberski T, et al. Role of *Coccidioides* antigen testing in the cerebrospinal fluid for the diagnosis of coccidioidal meningitis. *Clin Infect Dis.* 2015;61:1521-1526.
275. Kastelijn EA, van Moorsel CH, Ruven HJ, et al. Genetic polymorphisms and bronchiolitis obliterans syndrome after lung transplantation: promising results and recommendations for the future. *Transplantation.* 2012;93:127-135.
277. Katragkou A, McCarthy M, Meletiadis J, et al. In vitro combination of isavuconazole with micafungin or amphotericin B deoxycholate against medically important molds. *Antimicrob Agents Chemother.* 2014;58:6934-6937.
279. Kauffman CA, Freifeld AG, Andes DR, et al. Endemic fungal infections in solid organ and hematopoietic cell transplant recipients enrolled in the Transplant-Associated Infection Surveillance Network (TRANSNET). *Transpl Infect Dis.* 2014;16:213-224. ISSN 1398-2273.
284. Kim SH, Yim DS, Choi SM, et al. Voriconazole-related severe adverse events: clinical application of therapeutic drug monitoring in Korean patients. International. *J Infect Dis.* 2011;15:e753-e758.
285. Kimberlin DW, Acosta EP, Sanchez PJ, et al. Pharmacokinetic and pharmacodynamic assessment of oral valganciclovir in the treatment of symptomatic congenital cytomegalovirus disease. *J Infect Dis.* 2008;197:836-845.

293. Koo S, Kubiak W, Issa NC, et al. A targeted peritransplant antifungal strategy for the prevention of invasive fungal disease after lung transplantation: a sequential cohort analysis. *Transplantation*. 2012;94:281-286.
295. Kotton CN, Kumar D, Caliendo AM, et al. Updated international consensus guidelines on the management of *Cytomegalovirus* in solid-organ transplantation. *Transplantation*. 2013;96:333-360.
296. Kovats Z, Sutto Z, Murakozy G, et al. Airway pathogens during the first year after lung transplantation: a single center experience. *Transplant Proc*. 2011;43:1290-1291.
306. Lancella L, Galli L, Chiappini E, et al. Recommendations concerning the therapeutic approach to immunocompromised children with tuberculosis. *Clin Ther*. 2016;38:180-190.
311. Le J, Gantt S, AST Infectious Diseases Community of Practice. Human herpesvirus 6, 7 and 8 in solid organ transplantation. *Am J Transplant*. 2013;13:128-137.
312. Le Page AK, Jager MM, Kotton CN, et al. International survey of cytomegalovirus management in solid organ transplantation after the publication of consensus guidelines. *Transplantation*. 2013;95:1455-1460.
317. Leen AM, Bollard CM, Mendizabal AM, et al. Multicenter study of banked third-party virus-specific T cells to treat severe viral infections after hematopoietic stem cell transplantation. *Blood*. 2013;121:5113-5123.
322. Levi ME, Curtis DJ. West Nile infections in pediatric solid organ transplant recipients. *Pediatr Transplant*. 2016;20(6):744-746.
323. Lewis JD, Sifri CD. Multi-drug resistant bacterial donor derived infections in solid organ transplantation. *Curr Infect Dis Rep*. 2016;18:18.
324. Li L, Avery R, Budey M, et al. Oral versus inhaled ribavirin therapy for respiratory syncytial virus infection after lung transplantation. *J Heart Lung Transplant*. 2012;31:838-844.
332. Liu V, Dhillon GS, Weill D. A multi-drug regimen for respiratory syncytial virus and parainfluenza virus infections in adult lung and heart-transplant recipients. *Transpl Infect Dis*. 2010;12:38-44.
338. Lobo LJ, Noone PG. Respiratory infections in patients with cystic fibrosis undergoing lung transplantation. *Lancet Respir Med*. 2014;2:73-82.
340. Luong ML, Chaparro C, Stephenson A, et al. Pretransplant *Aspergillus* colonization of cystic fibrosis patients and the incidence of post-lung transplant invasive aspergillosis. *Transplantation*. 2014;97:351-357.
347. Maertens JA, Raad II, Marr KA, et al. Isavuconazole versus voriconazole for primary treatment of invasive mould disease caused by *Aspergillus* and other filamentous fungi (SECURE): a phase 3, randomised-controlled, non-inferiority trial. *Lancet*. 2016;387:760-769.
349. Magiorakos AP, Srinivasan A, Carey RB, et al. Multidrug resistant, extensively drug resistant and pandrug resistant bacteria: an international expert proposal for interim standard definitions for acquired resistance. *Clin Microbiol Infect*. 2012;18:68-81.
354. Mannonen L, Loginov R, Helantera I, et al. Comparison of two quantitative real-time CMV-PCR tests calibrated against the 1st WHO international standard for viral load monitoring of renal transplant patients. *J Med Virol*. 2014;86:576-584.
355. Manuel O, Estabrook M, AST Infectious Diseases Community of Practice. RNA respiratory viruses in solid organ transplantation. *Am J Transplant*. 2013;13:212-219.
356. Manuel O, Lien D, Weinkauf J, et al. Methicillin-resistant *Staphylococcus aureus* infection after lung transplantation: 5-year review of clinical and molecular epidemiology. *J Heart Lung Transplant*. 2009;28:1231-1236.
357. Marcelin JR, Wilson JW, Razonable RR, et al. Oral ribavirin therapy for respiratory syncytial virus infections in moderately to severely immunocompromised patients. *Transpl Infect Dis*. 2014;16:242-250.
359. Marr KA, Schlamm HT, Herbrecht R, et al. Combination antifungal therapy for invasive aspergillosis—a randomized trial. *Ann Intern Med*. 2015;162:81-89.
361. Martin SI, Fishman JA, AST Infectious Diseases Community of Practice. Pneumocystis pneumonia in solid organ transplantation. *Am J Transplant*. 2013;13:272-279.
365. Marty FM, Ostrosky-Zeichner L, Cornely OA, et al. Isavuconazole treatment for mucormycosis: a single-arm open-label trial and case control analysis. *Lancet Infect Dis*. 2016;16(7):828-837.
368. Mattner F, Fischer S, Weissbrodt H, et al. Post-operative nosocomial infections after lung and heart transplantation. *J Heart Lung Transplant*. 2007;26:241-249.
370. McCarty TP, Baddley JW, Walsh TJ, et al. Phaeohyphomycosis in transplant recipients: results from the Transplant Associated Infection Surveillance Network (TRANSNET). *Med Mycol*. 2015;53:440-446.
371. McCoy KS, Quittner AL, Oermann CM, et al. Inhaled aztreonam lysine for chronic airway *Pseudomonas aeruginosa* in cystic fibrosis. *Am J Respir Crit Care Med*. 2008;178:921-928.
376. Mead L, Danziger-Isakov LA, Michaels MG, et al. Antifungal prophylaxis in pediatric lung transplantation: an international multicenter survey. *Pediatr Transplant*. 2014;18:393-397.
381. Miceli MH, Goggins MI, Chander P, et al. Performance of lateral flow device and galactomannan for the detection of *Aspergillus* species in bronchoalveolar fluid of patients at risk for invasive pulmonary aspergillosis. *Mycoses*. 2015;58:368-374.
382. Miceli MH, Kauffman CA. Isavuconazole: a new broad-spectrum triazole antifungal agent. *Clin Infect Dis*. 2015;61:1558-1565.
385. Miller R, Assi M, AST Infectious Diseases Community of Practice. Endemic fungal infections in solid organ transplantation. *Am J Transplant*. 2013;13:250-261.
388. Milstone AP, Brumble LM, Barnes J, et al. A single-season prospective study of respiratory viral infections in lung transplant recipients. *Eur Respir J*. 2006;28:131-137.
399. Muchtar E, Kramer MR, Vidal L, et al. Posttransplantation lymphoproliferative disorder in lung transplant recipients: a 15-year single institution experience. *Transplantation*. 2013;96:657-663.
403. Mylonakis E, Clancy CJ, Ostrosky-Zeichner L, et al. T2 Magnetic resonance assay for the rapid diagnosis of candidemia in whole blood: a clinical trial. *Clin Infect Dis*. 2015;60:682-689.
405. Nahid P, Dorman SE, Alipanah N, et al. Official American Thoracic Society/Centers for Disease Control and Prevention/Infectious Diseases Society of America clinical practice guidelines: treatment of drug-susceptible tuberculosis. *Clin Infect Dis*. 2016;63(7):e147-e195.
406. Naik S, Micholas SK, Martinez CA, et al. Adoptive immunotherapy for primary immunodeficiency disorders with virus specific T lymphocytes. *J Allergy Clin Immunol*. 2016;137(5):1498-1505.
411. Neoh CF, Snell G, Levvey B, et al. Antifungal prophylaxis in lung transplantation. *Int J Antimicrob Agents*. 2014;44:194-202.
419. Nunley DR, Bauldoff GS, Mangino JE, et al. Mortality associated with *Acinetobacter baumannii* infections experienced by lung transplant recipients. *Lung*. 2010;188:381-385.
422. Oermann CM, Retsch-Bogart GZ, Quittner AL, et al. An 18 month study on the safety and efficacy of repeated courses of inhaled aztreonam lysine in cystic fibrosis. *Pediatr Pulmonol*. 2010;45(11):1121-1134.
436. Pankey GA, Ashcreft DS. Detection of synergy using the combination of polymyxin B with either meropenem or rifampin against carbapenemase-producing *Klebsiella pneumoniae*. *Diagn Microbiol Infect Dis*. 2011;70:561-564.
438. Pappas PG, Kauffman CA, Andes DR, et al. Clinical practice guideline for the management of candidiasis: 2016 update by the Infectious Diseases Society of America. *Clin Infect Dis*. 2016;62:e1-e50.
440. Park WB, Kim NH, Kim KH, et al. The effect of therapeutic drug monitoring on the safety and efficacy of voriconzole in invasive fungal infections: a randomized controlled trial. *Clin Infect Dis*. 2012;15:1080-1087.
446. Patterson TF, Thompson GR, Denning DW, et al. Practice guidelines for the diagnosis and management of aspergillosis: 2016 update by the Infectious Diseases Society of America. *Clin Infect Dis*. 2016;63(4):e1-e60.
447. Peghin M, Monforte V, Martin-Gomez MT, et al. 10 years of prophylaxis with nebulized liposomal amphotericin B and the changing epidemiology of *Aspergillus* spp. infection in lung transplantation. *Transpl Int*. 2016;29:51-62.
448. Peghin M, Monforte V, Martin-Gomez MT, et al. Epidemiology of invasive respiratory disease caused by emerging non-*Aspergillus* molds in lung transplant recipients. *Transpl Infect Dis*. 2016;18:70-78.
452. Pergam SA, Limaye AP, AST Infectious Diseases Community of Practice. Varicella zoster virus in solid organ transplantation. *Am J Transplant*. 2013;13:138-146.
453. Pescovitz MD, Ettenger RB, Strife CF, et al. Pharmacokinetics of oral valganciclovir solution and intravenous ganciclovir in pediatric renal and liver transplant recipients. *Transpl Infect Dis*. 2010;12:195-203.
457. Pfaller MA, Wolk DM, Lowery TJ. T2MR and T2 Candida: novel technology for the rapid diagnosis of candidemia and invasive candidiasis. *Future Microbiol*. 2015;11:103-117.
470. Razonable RR, Asberg A, Rollag H, et al. Virologic suppression measured by a cytomegalovirus (CMV) DNA test calibrated to the World Health Organization international standard is predictive of CMV disease resolution in transplant recipients. *Clin Infect Dis*. 2013;56:1546-1553.
471. Razonable RR, Humar A, AST Infectious Diseases Community of Practice. Cytomegalovirus in solid organ transplantation. *Am J Transplant*. 2013;13:93-106.
475. Richer SM, Medema JL, Durkin MM, et al. Improved diagnosis of acute pulmonary histoplasmosis by combining antigen and antibody detection. *Clin Infect Dis*. 2016;62:896-902.
478. Robinson CL, Chau C, Yerkovich ST, et al. Posaconazole in lung transplant recipients: use, tolerability and efficacy. *Transpl Infect Dis*. 2016;18:302-308.
491. Rychert J, Danziger-Isakov L, Yen-Lieberman B, et al. Multicenter comparison of laboratory performance in cytomegalovirus and Epstein-Barr virus load testing using international standards. *Clin Transpl*. 2014;28:1416-1423.
496. Salvatore M, Satlin MJ, Jacobs SE, et al. DAS181 for the treatment of parainfluenza virus infections in hematopoietic stem cell recipients at a single center. *Biol Blood Marrow Transplant*. 2016;22:957-970.
499. Sassi M, Ripamonti C, Mueller NJ, et al. Outbreaks of *Pneumocystis* pneumonia in 2 renal transplant centers linked to a single strain of pneumocystis: implications for transmission and virulence. *Clin Infect Dis*. 2012;54(10):1437-1444.
506. Seem DL, Lee I, Umscheid CA, et al. PHS guideline for reducing human immunodeficiency virus, hepatitis B virus and hepatitis C virus transmission through organ transplantation. *Public Health Rep*. 2013;128:247-343.

511. Shields RK, Kwak EJ, Potoski BA, et al. High mortality rates among solid organ transplant recipients infected with extensively drug-resistant *Acinetobacter baumannii*: using in vitro antibiotic combination testing to identify the combination of a carbapenem and colistin as an effective treatment regimen. *Diagn Microbiol Infect Dis.* 2011;70:246-252.
515. Silva JT, Lopez-Medrano F, Alonso-Moralejo R, et al. Detection of Epstein-Barr virus DNAemia after lung transplantation and its potential relationship with the development of post-transplant complications. *Transpl Infect Dis.* 2016;18(3):431-441.
516. Silveira FP, Kusne S, AST Infectious Diseases Community of Practice. *Candida* infections in solid organ transplantation. *Am J Transplant.* 2013;13:220-227.
524. Singh N, Huprikar S, Burdette SD, et al. Donor-derived fungal infections in organ transplant recipients: guidelines of the American Society of Transplantation, Infectious Diseases Community of Practice. *Am J Transplant.* 2012;12: 2414-2428.
526. Singh NM, Husain S, AST Infectious Diseases Community of Practice. Aspergillosis in solid organ transplantation. *Am J Transplant.* 2013;13:228-241.
536. Smibert O, Snell GI, Bills H, et al. *Mycobacterium abscessus* complex—a particular challenge in the setting of lung transplantation. *Expert Rev Anti Infect Ther.* 2016;14:325-333.
542. Spoonhower KA, Davis PB. Epidemiology of cystic fibrosis. *Clin Chest Med.* 2016;37:1-8.
548. Stockmann C, Roberts JK, Knackstedt ED, et al. Clinical pharmacokinetics and pharmacodynamics of ganciclovir and valganciclovir in children with cytomegalovirus infection. *Expert Opin Drug Metab Toxicol.* 2015;11:205-219.
549. Stockmann C, Sherwin CM, Knackstedt ED, et al. Therapeutic drug monitoring of Ganciclovir treatment for cytomegalovirus infections among immunocompromised children. *J Pediatric Infect Dis Soc.* 2016; [Epub ahead of print].
550. Subramanian AK, Morris MI, AST Infectious Diseases Community of Practice. *Mycobacterium tuberculosis* infections in solid organ transplantation. *Am J Transplant.* 2013;13:68-76.
551. Sun HY, Alexander BD, Huprikar S, et al. Predictors of immune reconstitution syndrome in organ transplant recipients with cryptococcosis: implications for the management of immunosuppression. *Clin Infect Dis.* 2015;60:36-44.
558. Tamma PD, Newland JG, Pannaraj PS, et al. The use of Colistin among children in the United States: results from a multicenter, case series. *Pediatr Infect Dis J.* 2013;32:17-22.
560. Thakuria L, Packwood K, Firouzi A, et al. A pharmacokinetic analysis of posaconazole oral suspension if ht serum and alveolar compartment of lung transplant recipients. *Int J Antimicrob Agents.* 2016;47:69-76.
565. Todd JL, Palmer SM. Bronchiolitis obliterans syndrome: the final frontier for lung transplantation. *Chest.* 2011;140:502-508. Abstract, PMID: 21813529.
566. Todd JL, Wang X, Sugimoto S, et al. Hyaluronan contributes to bronchiolitis obliterans syndrome and stimulates lung allograft rejection through activation of innate immunity. *Am J Respir Crit Care Med.* 2014;189:556-566.
575. van Duin D, van Delden C, AST Infectious Diseases Community of Practice. Multidrug-resistant gram-negative bacteria infections in solid organ transplantation. *Am J Transplant.* 2013;13:31-41.
578. Valapour M, Skeans MA, Heubner BM, Smith JM, et al. OPTN/SRTR 2013 annual data report: lung. *Am J Transplant.* 2015;15:1-28.
579. Vali R, Punnett A, Bajno L, et al. The value of 18F-FDG PET in pediatric patients with post-transplant lymphoproliferative disorder at initial diagnosis. *Pediatr Transplant.* 2015;19:932-939.
591. Villeneuve D, Brothers A, Harvey E, et al. Valganciclovir dosing using area under the curve calculations in pediatric solid organ transplant recipients. *Pediatr Transplant.* 2013;17:80-85.
592. Vos R, Vanaudenaerde BM, Geudens N, et al. Pseudomonal airway colonisation: risk factor for bronchiolitis obliterans syndrome after lung transplantation? *Eur Respir J.* 2008;31:1037-1045.
593. Vu DL, Bridevaux PO, Aubert JD, et al. Respiratory viruses in lung transplant recipients: a critical review and pooled analysis of clinical studies. *Am J Transplant.* 2011;11:1071-1078.
594. Waghmare A, Wagner T, Andrews R, et al. Successful treatment of parainfluenza virus respiratory tract infection with DAS181 in 4 immunocompromised children. *J Pediatric Infect Dis Soc.* 2015;4:114-118.
600. Wan QQ, Ye QF, Yuan H. Multidrug resistant gram negative bacteria in solid organ transplant recipients with bacteremia. *Eur J Clin Microbiol Infect Dis.* 2015;34:431-437.
602. Waters V, Ratjen F. Standard versus biofilm antimicrobial susceptibility testing to guide antibiotic therapy in cystic fibrosis. *Cochrane Database Syst Rev.* 2015;(3):CD009528.
603. Weigt SS, Finlen Copeland CA, Derhovanessian A, et al. Colonization with small conidia aspergillus species is associated with bronchiolitis obliterans syndrome: a two-center validation study. *Am J Transplant.* 2013;13:919-927.
613. Wilck MB, Zucherman RA, AST Infectious Diseases Community of Practice. Herpes simplex virus in solid organ transplantation. *Am J Transplant.* 2013;13: 121-127.
615. Willinger B, Lakner M, Lass-Florl C, et al. Bronchoalveolar lavage lateral flow device test of invasive pulmonary aspergillosis in solid organ transplant patients: a semiprospective multicenter study. *Transplantation.* 2014;98:898-902.
619. Wiskirchen DE, Crandon JL, Nicolau DP. Impact of various conditions on the efficacy of dual carbapenem therapy against KPC-producing *Klebsiella pneumoniae.* *Int J Antimicrob Agents.* 2013;41:582-585.
620. Wold WSM, Toth K. New drug on the horizon for treating adenovirus. *Expert Opin Pharmacother.* 2015;16:2095-2099.
626. Ye QF, Zhao J, Wan QQ, et al. Frequency and clinical outcomes of ESKAPE bacteremia in solid organ transplantation and the risk factors for mortality. *Transpl Infect Dis.* 2014;16:767-774.
627. Yserbyt J, Dooms C, Vos R, et al. Anastomotic airway complications after lung transplantation: risk factors, treatment modalities and outcome—a single-centre experience. *Eur J Cardiothorac Surg.* 2015;49:e1-e8.
632. Zamora MR, Budev M, Rolfe M, et al. RNA interference therapy in lung transplant patients infected with respiratory syncytial virus. *Am J Respir Crit Care Med.* 2011;183:531-538.

The full reference list for this chapter is available at ExpertConsult.com.

Opportunistic Infections in Liver and Intestinal Transplantation 72

Michael D. Green • Marian G. Michaels

Liver transplantation has been established as an effective treatment for children with end-stage liver disease for more than 30 years. Improving surgical techniques and the availability of new and more potent immunosuppressive regimens have led to enhanced survival rates, with 3-year survival rates approaching or exceeding 84%.[60] In response to these excellent results, children with end-stage liver disease are routinely referred for liver transplantation, and increasing numbers of pediatric centers routinely perform this procedure. Intestinal transplantation, performed as an isolated procedure or in combination with the liver or other organs, has also gained expanded acceptance as a treatment for children with refractory intestinal failure, with steadily improving survival rates over time.[102] This is particularly true for those children who experience progressive liver failure due to hyperalimentation-induced liver disease. Although this newer procedure has been routinely performed at a relatively limited number of centers, an increasing number of transplant programs are beginning to offer intestinal transplantation.

Infectious complications have been a significant cause of morbidity and mortality in children undergoing liver transplantation since this procedure gained its initial acceptance in the 1980s. However, improvements in the treatment options for and management of immune suppression along with the increasing availability of new antimicrobial agents and diagnostic tools have resulted in reductions in the impact of infectious complications on these children. Intestinal transplantation is associated with many of the same infectious complications seen after liver transplantation, as well as a number of infectious issues that appear to be unique to this procedure. Although development of increasingly effective treatment strategies for infectious complications is of great benefit to the children undergoing these procedures, emphasis has increasingly shifted to the development of strategies aimed at the prevention of infectious complications in children undergoing abdominal transplantation. A general overview of the problem of infections after liver and intestinal transplantation in children is presented in this chapter.

PREDISPOSING FACTORS

Liver and intestinal transplantation are associated with a set of technical and medical conditions that predispose to a unique set of infectious complications. The abdomen is a common site of infection in patients undergoing both of these procedures.[24,67] This is almost certainly due to the occurrence of local ischemic injury and bleeding, as well as potential soilage with contaminated material.[49] Additional factors predisposing to infection can be divided into those that exist before a transplant and those secondary to intraoperative and posttransplant activities.

Pretransplant Factors

The underlying illnesses leading to transplantation may be associated with intrinsic risk factors for infection. Some disorders may have required palliative surgery, which increases the technical difficulty of the transplant and may be associated with an enhanced risk for developing posttransplant infections.[20] For example, children undergoing liver transplantation for biliary atresia may have previously undergone a Kasai procedure (choledochojejunostomy), which may predispose to recurrent episodes of bacterial cholangitis before transplantation, increasing the likelihood of colonization with multidrug-resistant (MDR) bacteria that can cause infection after transplantation. Similarly children undergoing liver transplantation for cystic fibrosis may have an increased risk for developing invasive aspergillosis if they were colonized with this pathogen before transplantation. Complications of end-stage liver disease (as part of a primary liver disease or as a consequence of hyperalimentation in patients with intestinal insufficiency) may also predispose to infection after a transplant. A history of one or more episodes of spontaneous bacterial peritonitis before transplantation in patients with ascites has been associated with an increased rate of bacterial infections after liver transplantation[114] and could occur in patients with liver disease associated with intestinal insufficiency. Finally children awaiting intestinal transplantation experience frequent episodes of gastrointestinal-associated bloodstream infections. Recurrent exposure to antimicrobial agents to treat these episodes of bacteremia increases the likelihood of colonization and disease with MDR bacterial and fungal pathogens after transplantation. Risks for bacterial translocation after intestinal transplantation with resultant bloodstream infection include the presence of a colon graft,[18] hospitalization before transplantation, and treatment with mycophenolate mofetil (MMF).[67]

Age, another important pretransplant factor, is a major determinant of susceptibility to certain pathogens, severity of expression of infection, and immune maturation.[1] Young children undergoing abdominal transplantation may experience moderate to severe infection with certain viral (e.g., respiratory syncytial virus [RSV]) or bacterial (coagulase-negative staphylococci) pathogens compared with more mild illness experienced by adult recipients infected with these pathogens. In contrast, certain pathogens, such as *Cryptococcus neoformans,* uncommonly manifest infection before young adulthood.[117] Age is also an important factor governing clinical expression of infection with cytomegalovirus (CMV) and Epstein-Barr virus (EBV). When transplants are performed in young patients, there is a high likelihood that they will be seronegative for CMV and EBV and therefore susceptible to primary infections, which are more severe than infections due to reactivation.[9,50,92]

Donor-related issues represent another set of pretransplant factors. Transplant recipients are at risk for acquiring infections that may be active or latent within the donor at the time of organ harvesting. The most common examples of donor-associated infections are CMV and EBV.[8,10,16,92] Infections caused by CMV and EBV have been more severe after intestinal transplant compared with other organs. This may be because the intestine is an organ rich in lymphoid tissue, which may result in bringing a larger viral load of viruses from the donor compared with other graft types. Similarly adenovirus has been isolated more commonly from pediatric recipients of intestinal transplants compared with other organs, which may also be related to donor transmission in the accompanying lymphoid tissue.[29,74,87] In contrast to CMV and EBV, for which donor-derived transmission is expected, increasing attention has focused on the unexpected transmission of other pathogens such as human immunodeficiency virus (HIV), hepatitis B virus (HBV), and hepatitis C virus (HCV). Although the systematic use of donor screening has led to a decreased frequency of unexpected transmission of HIV, HBV, and HCV,[3,25,57] evidence demonstrates donor-associated transmission of West Nile virus and rabies, as well as a number of other uncommonly transmitted pathogens.[56–58,106] Because organs from a single donor often go to disparate sites, it is important for the recipient center to report back to the United Network for Organ Sharing (UNOS) any unusual infections that might possibly have come from the donor.

Intraoperative Factors

Operative factors unique to liver transplantation may predispose to infectious complications. For example, liver transplant recipients undergoing Roux-en-Y choledochoduodenostomy experience more infectious episodes than do those who undergo a choledochocholedochostomy with T-tube drainage.[62,94] However, only the former option is usually performed in children undergoing liver transplantation because of the small size of their bile ducts. For combined liver-intestinal transplantation, evolution to en bloc replacement of the liver and intestine avoids the need for additional biliary anastomosis and minimizes the risk for infection related to biliary complications. Prolonged operative time (>12 hours) during the initial transplant has been associated with an increased risk for infection after transplant[34,62] and is likely a surrogate marker for the technical difficulty of the surgery. Intraoperative events, such as contamination of the operative field, also predispose to postoperative infections. Finally the inability to close the abdomen after the transplantation due to size discrepancy or intraoperative complications appears to increase the risk for postoperative infections.

Posttransplant Factors

Technical problems, immunosuppression, presence of indwelling cannulas, and nosocomial exposures are major postoperative risk factors for infectious complications. Thrombosis of the hepatic artery is the most serious technical problem after liver transplantation and predisposes to areas of necrotic liver and development of hepatic abscesses and bacteremia.[93,94] Bile duct strictures, developing as a sequelae of thrombosed hepatic artery and ischemia or due to technical difficulties, may predispose to cholangitis.[94] Retransplantation represents a high risk for intraabdominal infection after intestinal transplantation.[67]

Immunosuppression is the critical postoperative factor predisposing to infection in all transplant recipients. Immunosuppressive regimens have evolved in an attempt to achieve more specific control of rejection with the least impairment of immunity. Thus this evolution is aimed not only at improved control of rejection but also at decreased morbidity and mortality from infections. The use of cyclosporine-based regimens resulted in a decreased incidence of infections in renal and cardiac transplant recipients.[24,51,83] The introduction of tacrolimus has allowed many patients to be managed without corticosteroids.[42,113] Although reported rates of infection have been similar in liver transplant recipients treated with tacrolimus compared with those receiving cyclosporine, an apparent decrease in morbidity and mortality, especially from viral pathogens, was noted with tacrolimus.[42] In contrast to these results, some centers reported an increased rate of EBV-associated posttransplant lymphoproliferative disease (PTLD) in patients receiving tacrolimus.[19] However, data from the University of Pittsburgh suggest that the short- and long-term incidence of EBV-associated PTLD appears to be similar in pediatric liver transplant recipients treated with either cyclosporine or tacrolimus.[12] More recently, induction immunotherapy has been used in combination with corticosteroid-free or corticosteroid-sparing immunosuppressive regimens, and newer agents also are being explored. Potential infectious risks will need to be assessed for these and other evolving immunosuppressive regimens.

Children undergoing intestinal transplantation require an increased baseline level of immunosuppression compared with patients undergoing most other solid-organ transplant procedures.[92] With this increased level of immunosuppression has come an increased risk for development of infection. In an effort to overcome this, a number of alternative immunosuppressive strategies have been explored. Looking at one such alternative strategy, Loinaz and colleagues found an increased risk for bacterial infections with both MMF and daclizumab after intestinal transplantation.[67] Another alternative approach evaluated the use of alemtuzumab induction in pediatric intestinal transplant recipients, and this was associated with a marked increased incidence of EBV-associated PTLD in one study[98] but not another.[59]

The treatment of rejection with additional or higher doses of immunosuppressant agents increases the risk for invasive and potentially fatal infection. Of particular concern is the use of antilymphocyte preparations, which are often indispensable in the management of corticosteroid-resistant rejection.[8,34,62]

The prolonged use of indwelling cannulas at any site is an important cause of infection throughout the postoperative course. The presence of central venous catheters is a cause of bacteremia after transplantation. This is particularly important for children undergoing intestinal transplantation, where maintenance of long-term central venous access has been required for prolonged periods of time after transplantation.[31] The development of urinary tract infections and bacterial pneumonia are associated with the use of urethral catheters and prolonged nasotracheal or endotracheal intubation, respectively.[34,62]

Nosocomial exposures constitute the final group of postoperative risk factors in the hospital setting. Transplant recipients, especially children, may be exposed to many common viral pathogens (e.g., rotavirus, RSV, or influenza) while hospitalized. The presence of resistant bacteria in the hospital increases the risk for nosocomial transmission and disease. Attention to infection control policies aimed at local epidemiology of circulating infections is paramount. Finally the presence in the hospital of heavy areas of contamination with pathogenic fungi, such as *Aspergillus,* may increase the risk for invasive fungal disease in these patients. The rate of fungal colonization increases during times of hospital construction. Infection control policies aimed at local epidemiology of circulating infections is paramount.

TABLE 72.1 Differential Diagnosis of Infectious Complications During the Early Period (0–30 Days) After Pediatric Liver and Intestinal Transplantation

Clinical Syndrome	Associated Pathogens
Wound infection:	
Superficial	*Staphylococcus aureus* Enterococci
Deep	Enterobacteriaceae Enterococci *Staphylococcus aureus* *Candida* spp.
Intraabdominal infection:	
Peritonitis	Enterobacteriaceae
Intraabdominal abscess	Enterococci
Intrahepatic abscess (isolated liver and liver-intestine transplants) ± bacteremia	*Candida* spp.
Bloodstream infection, associated with:	
Central venous catheters	Coagulase-negative staphylococci Enterobacteriaceae Enterococci *S. aureus* *Candida* spp.
Hepatic artery thrombosis (isolated liver transplant only)	Enterobacteriaceae Enterococci *Candida* spp.
Intestinal rejection (intestine only)	Enterobacteriaceae Enterococci *Candida* spp.
Bacterial cholangitis (isolated liver transplant only)	Enterobacteriaceae Enterococci *Candida* spp.
Urinary tract infection	Enterobacteriaceae Enterococci *Candida* spp.
Ventilator-associated pneumonia	Enterobacteriaceae Enterococci *S. aureus*
Nosocomial acquisition of common community pathogens	Respiratory syncytial virus Parainfluenza virus Influenza virus Human metapneumovirus Rotavirus Norovirus
Noninfectious etiologies	Rejection Drug fever

TIMING OF INFECTIONS

The time of onset of infection with various pathogens after transplantation tends to be predictable. The majority of clinically important infections occur within the first 180 days after transplantation,[40,62] although infections continue to occur quite frequently beyond this time after intestinal transplantation.[59] The timing of infections can be divided into three intervals: early (0 to 30 days after transplantation), intermediate (30 to 180 days after transplantation), and late (>180 days after transplantation). In addition, some infections may occur throughout the postoperative course. These divisions should be viewed with flexibility because they may be modified by prophylaxis strategies and are somewhat less applicable to recipients of intestinal transplantation. Despite this, they remain useful, giving a general approach to a patient with fever after transplantation, and can be used as a guide to differential diagnosis. An overview of the infectious complications occurring during each of these time periods is provided in Tables 72.1 to 72.3 and is summarized in the following sections.

Early Infections (0 to 30 Days)

Early infections (Table 72.1) tend to be associated with preexisting conditions and surgical manipulation. In general, they are caused by either bacteria or yeast. Bacterial infections are particularly common after intestinal transplantation, being reported in up to 90% of recipients.[67,110] As many as half of these early infectious complications may develop in the first 2 weeks after abdominal transplantation.[7] Cholangitis or spontaneous bacterial peritonitis presenting at or near the time of liver transplantation may lead to intraabdominal infection after the transplant. Technical difficulties (e.g., thrombosis of the hepatic artery or portal vein and biliary strictures) predispose to early bacterial infections. Likewise development of bile leaks and bowel perforations are associated with polymicrobial intraabdominal infections, primarily consisting of enteric bacteria and *Candida* spp., in the first month after transplantation.[35] Early bacteremia is exceptionally common in intestinal transplant recipients and is usually associated with the presence of central venous catheters.[31] Likewise early bacteremia with gram-negative pathogens in these children has been associated with intestinal rejection.[31,37] Reexploration of the abdomen is associated with increased rates of fungal infection.[62] Finally herpes simplex infection can also reactivate and cause early symptomatic disease,[62] although this is uncommon in children.

Intermediate Period (31 to 180 Days)

The intermediate period (Table 72.2) is the typical time of onset of infections associated with nonbacterial donor-associated transmission (either organ or blood products), reactivated viruses, and opportunistic infections. CMV peaks in incidence during this time.[8,62] However, the use of prophylaxis against CMV can modify the time of presentation so that the occurrence of disease from these organisms may be after 180 days. The intermediate period is also when many patients begin to present with EBV disease (including PTLD)[11,50] and *Pneumocystis jiroveci*

TABLE 72.2 Differential Diagnosis of Infectious Complications During the Intermediate Period (31–180 Days) After Pediatric Liver and Intestinal Transplantation

Clinical Syndrome	Associated Pathogens
Viral syndrome (fever, leukopenia, thrombocytopenia ± atypical lymphocytosis)	CMV EBV
Hepatitis	CMV EBV Adenovirus Hepatitis B Hepatitis C
Enteritis	CMV EBV Rotavirus Adenovirus *Clostridium difficile*
PTLD	EBV
Bacterial cholangitis[a]	Enterobacteriaceae Enterococci *Candida* spp.
Pneumonia	*Streptococcus pneumoniae* CMV Adenovirus RSV Parainfluenza virus Influenza virus Human metapneumovirus *Pneumocystis jiroveci* *Aspergillus fumigatus*
Bacteremia[b]	Enterobacteriaceae *Enterococcus* Coagulase-negative staphylococci (with central venous catheter) *Candida* spp.
Adenopathy	EBV/PTLD
Pulmonary nodules	EBV/PTLD *Aspergillus fumigatus*

CMV, Cytomegalovirus; *EBV,* Epstein-Barr virus; *PTLD,* posttransplant lymphoproliferative disease.
[a]Typically only seen in isolated liver transplant recipients and usually associated with the presence of technical complication (e.g., biliary stricture).
[b]Seen in intestinal transplant recipients in association with presence of central venous catheters, intestinal rejection, or PTLD involving intestine.

pneumonia.[62] Finally bacteremia continues to be a frequent occurrence in pediatric intestinal transplant recipients, with as many as 50% of all bloodstream infections occurring in this population being identified in this time period.[31]

Late Infections (Greater Than 180 Days)

Late infections (Table 72.3) after abdominal transplantation are less well characterized than other periods because patients have usually been discharged from the transplant center to their respective homes, which often are quite far away. This makes the accurate accumulation of data on these late infections difficult. Nonetheless problems such as recurrent episodes of bacterial cholangitis in liver transplant recipients (typically associated with underlying problems of the biliary tree) and bacteremia associated with ongoing requirement for a central venous catheter, intestinal graft rejection, and/or PTLD in intestinal transplant recipients, continue to occur in this time period.[31,67] In addition, children who are at high risk for CMV infection and have been kept on prolonged or recurrent courses of prophylaxis may develop late-onset CMV infection in the late period.[14]

TABLE 72.3 Differential Diagnosis of Infectious Complications During the Late Period (>180 Days) After Pediatric Liver and Intestinal Transplantation

Clinical Syndrome	Associated Pathogens
Bacterial cholangitis[a]	Enterobacteriaceae Enterococci *Candida* spp.
PTLD	EBV
Bacteremia[b]	Enterobacteriaceae *Enterococcus* *Candida* spp.
Varicella zoster	Varicella zoster virus
Respiratory tract infections	Community-acquired viruses[c]

EBV, Epstein-Barr virus; *PTLD,* posttransplant lymphoproliferative disease.
[a]Usually associated with the presence of technical complication (e.g., biliary stricture).
[b]Seen in intestinal transplant recipients in association with presence of central venous catheters, intestinal rejection, or PTLD involving intestine.
[c]Respiratory syncytial virus, parainfluenza virus, influenza virus A and B, human metapneumovirus, adenovirus, rhinovirus, and enterovirus.

Infections Occurring Throughout the Postoperative Course

Iatrogenic factors are an important cause of bacterial and fungal infections at all times but predominate in the early transplant period. Central venous lines are maintained for a variable time; the risk for infection persists for the entire period that the catheter remains in place. This is a particularly important problem for recipients of intestinal transplants who frequently require central line access for prolonged periods of time. Similarly the presence of urethral catheters and endotracheal tubes increases the risk for infections whenever they are in use.

Nosocomial acquisition of community viruses, such as RSV, rotavirus, and influenza A or B can occur at any time after transplant. These viruses spread easily in hospital environments from personnel or other hospitalized patients to transplant recipients. It is therefore important to modify diagnostic considerations according to local epidemiologic considerations.

BACTERIAL AND FUNGAL INFECTIONS

Bacterial and fungal pathogens are important causes of morbidity and occasional mortality in children undergoing liver and/or intestinal transplantation. With the exception of infections related to the use of indwelling catheters, sites of bacterial infection tend to occur at or near the transplanted organ. Accordingly the intraabdominal space is an important site of infection after any of the abdominal transplant procedures. Adding to the complexity of the management of bacterial infections in children undergoing abdominal transplantation is the fact that recovery of MDR bacteria is increasingly common. Outbreaks of colonization and disease due to vancomycin-resistant *Enterococcus faecium,* extended-spectrum β-lactamase (ESBL)–producing *Klebsiella pneumoniae,* and carbapenem-resistant Enterobacteriaceae have been reported among pediatric liver and intestinal transplant recipients.[17,36,107] These MDR bacteria have been transmitted from patient to patient, prompting the need for close attention to and strict compliance with infection control procedures. In some cases, effective antimicrobial agents may be unavailable to treat these complications. Knowledge of results of previous cultures and antimicrobial resistance patterns locally as well as from the home institution of the patient are critical components in choosing initial empirical antibiotic therapy for these patients to maximize their outcomes.

Liver Transplantation

Bacterial and fungal infections are a common early problem after liver transplantation.[52,116] Rates for bacterial infection of 40% to 70% have been reported from multiple series.[51,76,110] A 2008 review of the SPLIT registry for children undergoing liver transplantation between 1995 and 2006 found that around 33% of pediatric liver recipients experienced a bacterial infection, with the vast majority of these presenting in the first 30 days after transplant.[96] Similar rates have been reported following living donor liver transplantation in children. Bacteremia often occurs in association with intraabdominal infection or with use of central venous catheters, but it can occur without an obvious source. Enteric gram-negative organisms account for more than one-half of episodes.[82] Bacterial infections involving the abdomen or surgical wound are common in most series. Infectious complications of the transplanted liver also occur. The most important complication is hepatic abscess associated with hepatic artery or portal vein thrombosis, which can be accompanied by persistent bacteremia. However, the introduction of frequent surveillance Doppler studies early after transplant to monitor for development of thrombosis, coupled with the use of operative thrombectomy and thrombolysis, have markedly diminished the development of hepatic abscesses in this population.

Ascending cholangitis is relatively common after liver transplantation accounting for 7% of infections in the SPLIT series and usually associated with biliary abnormalities.[96] This diagnosis typically is made on clinical grounds in a patient with fever and biochemical evidence of biliary inflammation. Enteric gram-negative bacteria and enterococcal species predominate. However, this clinical picture can be identical to that of acute graft rejection; liver biopsy should be performed to differentiate these processes. A cholangiogram is performed to assess the status of the biliary tract for patients with proven cholangitis.

Historically as many as 40% of children undergoing liver transplantation developed a fungal infection during the first year following this procedure, with *Candida* spp. being the most common fungal pathogen and infection usually being associated with an intraabdominal focus or indwelling catheter.[116] Infections due to *Candida* spp. have been most commonly recognized in the first month after transplantation, with candidal peritonitis most likely presenting in the first 2 weeks after liver transplantation in association with a bile leak or bowel perforation. The recovery of *Candida* from a Jackson-Pratt drain in the early postoperative period may be the first indication of either of these two technical complications and may occur before the onset of clinical symptoms of intraabdominal infection.[35] Accordingly recovery of *Candida,* alone or in combination with enteric bacteria, should prompt initiation of antimicrobial therapy and an aggressive evaluation for the presence of these complications. However, rates of invasive candidiasis have markedly declined, as demonstrated by a recent study of pediatric liver transplant recipients at two different centers that found that only 2.5% of 397 children developed invasive candidiasis in the first month following transplantation[22] as compared to a rate of 21% documented in an older study evaluating invasive candidiasis during the first month posttransplant.[40] Candidemia accounted for 80% of episodes of invasive candidiasis in the recent series with the only identified risk factor associated with the development of candidal infection being ICU admission in the 2 weeks prior to transplant. Historically additional risk factors for fungal infection have included prolonged duration of intubation after transplant, hepatic artery thrombosis, volume of blood transfused, and exposure to corticosteroids within the 3 months before the transplant. Early initiation of antifungal treatment is particularly important, given an attributable mortality rate of up to 33% for candidal infections in pediatric liver transplant recipients in older literature.[35] The availability of fluconazole and echinocandin antifungal agents (e.g., caspofungin, micafungin, and anidulafungin) increases the number of therapeutic options for the treatment of candidal infections. However, acquired or inherent resistance to the azoles is an increasing concern, as are drug-drug interactions between azoles with both cyclosporine and tacrolimus and echinocandins with cyclosporine.

Episodes of invasive aspergillosis among pediatric liver transplant recipients are uncommon but can be fatal[43]; infections due to other invasive molds are rarely seen. However, children undergoing liver transplantation for cystic fibrosis (CF) are at particular risk for developing infection due to *Aspergillus* and other fungi seen in children with CF lung disease.[84] Early disseminated aspergillosis in children with CF undergoing liver transplantation at Children's Hospital of Pittsburgh of UPMC (CHP) was observed in the early era of transplantation, prompting the use of perioperative antifungal prophylaxis in liver recipients with CF and a history of recovery of *Aspergillus* before transplant. Because data defining the precise duration of prophylaxis necessary to protect against this complication are not available, prophylactic treatment has ranged from 1 month of intravenous amphotericin to prolonged use of an oral azole agent (e.g., itraconazole or voriconazole). The availability of newer antifungal agents, including the advanced-generation azoles (voriconazole and posaconazole) as well as the echinocandins, has increased the number and complexity of therapeutic options for treatment of aspergillosis in children undergoing liver transplantation.[45] A summary of a suggested approach to the diagnosis and management of fungal infections after liver transplantation in children is provided in Table 72.4.

Intestinal Transplantation

Although increasing, the numbers of children having undergone intestinal transplantation remain relatively small. Many have received combined liver and intestine or multivisceral transplants. Bacterial infection occurs frequently in these patients.[37,97] One series reported that as many as 92% of children undergoing intestinal transplantation experienced an average of 2.9 episodes of bacterial infection per patient.[67] More than 80% of these patients experienced their first bacterial infection during the first 2 months after transplant. Bacteremia, which can be explained in part by disruption of the mucosal barrier associated with harvest injury or intestinal allograft rejection, is a common finding,[37,97] with one center reporting that 69% of pediatric intestinal transplant recipients experienced at least one episode of bloodstream infection.[31] Coagulase-negative staphylococci, enterococci, and gram-negative enteric bacilli account for most episodes. As noted earlier, antibiotic resistance is commonly seen in recovered pathogens. In the CHP experience, episodes of gut-associated bacteremia frequently secondarily infect central venous catheters, producing persistent positive cultures even after resolution of clinical symptoms. Accordingly treatment strategies aimed at preserving the catheter (e.g., antibiotic lock therapy) may need to be used in combination with systemic antibiotics to accomplish a sustained clinical cure.[76]

Intraabdominal and wound infections also are seen commonly in this population, occurring in more than one-third of patients, and are typically detected during the first month after transplantation. Gram-negative enteric pathogens, which frequently demonstrate multiple-antibiotic resistance as well as enterococci (often exhibiting vancomycin resistance) are the most common organisms associated with these complications. Recurrent laparotomies have been identified as a risk factor for intraabdominal infection. One unique aspect of intestinal transplantation is the potential inability to achieve abdominal wall closure. Although failure to close the abdominal wall is an obvious risk for the development of intraabdominal infection, the use of abdominal mesh as part of efforts to resolve difficult abdominal wall closures has also been associated with the development of superficial and deep wound infection.[23]

Another important site of infection is the intestine itself. *Clostridium difficile* enteritis can present with fever, abdominal pain, and diarrhea that can easily be mistaken for graft rejection or viral infection due to CMV, EBV, and adenovirus. Accordingly the diagnosis of *C. difficile* enteritis must be considered in any child in whom fever and changes in stool output are noted. In one small series, *C. difficile* enteritis was diagnosed in nearly 10% of children undergoing intestinal transplantation.[121] The frequent exposure to antibiotics and prolonged hospital stays that children undergoing intestinal transplantation experience are major risk factors for the development of this complication. Standard treatment with oral metronidazole is the recommended first-line therapy. However, use of oral vancomycin (including prolonged tapered courses) or alternate therapies such fidaxomicin might be necessary for patients who experience relapse or recurrent episodes after primary treatment.

Invasive candidiasis and candidemia occur relatively frequently after intestinal transplantation in children, with one center reporting an incidence of approximately 23% in a series of 98 pediatric intestinal transplant recipients.[32] Candidemia accounted for 50% of the episodes of infection in this series, whereas nearly 40% involved the intraabdominal space. Although the majority of episodes of candidemia infection occur

TABLE 72.4 Overview of Diagnosis and Management of Fungal Infections After Liver and Intestinal Transplantation in Children

	***Candida*—Noninvasive (Mucositis, Dermatitis and Cystitis)**	***Candida*—Invasive**	***Aspergillus***	***Cryptococcus***	**Others (*Histoplasma, Mucor, Fusarium, Blastomycetes, Alternaria*, etc.)**
Frequency	Common[a]	Common[a]	Uncommon[a]	Rare[a]	Rare[a]
Diagnostic Tests	Clinical examination Culture Gram stain	Culture Gram stain Histology	Culture Gram stain Histology Radiographic staging[g]	Culture Antigen test India ink stain Histology CSF examination	Culture Histology Antigen testing (when appropriate)
Treatment:					
Primary	Nystatin Clotrimazole	Echinocandin[j] Lipid formulation of amphotericin B[d] Fluconazole[c,j]	Voriconazole[c] Lipid formulation of amphotericin B[d]	Lipid formulation of amphotericin B[d] Fluconazole[c,e,l]	Lipid formulation of amphotericin B[d]
Secondary	Topical amphotericin B[b] Fluconazole[c,g]	Flucytosine[h]	Echinocandin therapy[j] Itraconazole[c,h,i,k]	Flucytosine[f]	Azole therapy (for susceptible organisms)[c]
Adjunctive		Removal of central lines	Surgical resection		Surgical debridement
Duration of therapy	Dependent on rate of clearance	Dependent on the rate of clearance: minimum of 14 days	Dependent on the rate of clearance: minimum of 4 weeks, usually 8–12 weeks	Minimum of 6–8 weeks Many would continue with fluconazole indefinitely	Dependent on rate of clearance
Follow-up	Clinical examination Repeat urinalysis/ cultures	Dependent on clinical scenario	Dependent on clinical scenario	Clinical examination Antigen testing Repeat culture of appropriate source (sputum, CSF, urine) Radiographs if relevant	Clinical examination Antigen testing Repeat culture of appropriate source (sputum, CSF, urine) Radiographs if relevant

[a]Common: >5%; uncommon 1–5%; rare <1%.
[b]Topical amphotericin B for bladder wash for noninvasive candiduria; ultrasonography of kidneys recommended to confirm absence of invasive disease.
[c]Azole use must be accompanied by close follow-up of levels of cyclosporine or tacrolimus. In general, tacrolimus dosing should be cut in half when using a standard dose of fluconazole.
[d]Dose varies according to specific agent.
[e]Fluconazole is alternative first-line drug for invasive disease if the species is known to be sensitive to fluconazole and the patient is clinically stable. Dosage is 6 to 12 mg/kg per day based on severity of infection.
[f]Flucytosine should not be used alone but is synergistic when used in conjunction with amphotericin B. Dosage is 100 to 150 mg/kg per day divided every 6 hours.
[g]Radiographic staging includes computed tomography of head, chest, and abdomen.
[h]Itraconazole can be used long term for patients who have been treated for invasive *Aspergillus* but in general is not recommended as first-line therapy.
[i]Itraconazole absorption can be erratic. Accordingly, monitoring of itraconazole levels is recommended. Itraconazole is dosed at 3 to 5 mg/kg per day as a single dose. Dosing adjustment based on monitoring of levels is recommended. Adjustment of cyclosporine or tacrolimus dosing should be individualized.
[j]The use of either of the approved echinocandins (caspofungin, micafungin, or anidulafungin) may be an appropriate alternative for treatment of invasive candidiasis, candidemia, and aspergillosis. Dose adjustments may be necessary in the presence of impaired liver function. Monitoring of tacrolimus levels are indicated because these agents may decrease tacrolimus levels.
[k]Voriconazole levels should be checked for patients treated with oral therapy.
CSF, Cerebrospinal fluid.

in the first 3 to 6 months after transplant, later episodes may occur. Intraabdominal infection with *Candida* frequently present as part of a polymicrobial infection related to technical problems occurring during the initial transplant surgery or subsequent laparotomies. Specific risk factors associated with invasive candidiasis and candidemia include ongoing requirement for total parenteral nutrition and antibiotic treatment in the 7 days before diagnosis.[32]

Invasive mycoses due to fungal pathogens other than *Candida* are rarely observed. A recent report on fungal infections from the University of Nebraska identified four cases of invasive aspergillosis in 98 children undergoing intestinal transplantation,[28] whereas our experience at CHP has identified rare infections with *Aspergillus, Alternaria,* and *Scedosporium* in this population. In general, these children have been on high levels of immune suppression or have other complications such as PTLD, and outcome of these infections has been poor. Guidelines for the diagnosis and management of fungal infection in children undergoing intestinal transplantation are provided in Table 72.4.

VIRAL INFECTIONS

Viral pathogens, especially herpesviruses, are a major source of morbidity and mortality after solid-organ transplantation. Patterns of disease associated with individual viral pathogens generally are similar among all transplant recipients. However, frequency, mode of presentation, and relative severity can differ according to the type of organ transplanted and the serologic status of the recipient.

Cytomegalovirus

CMV continues to be the most common and one of the most important viral pathogens after organ transplantation in children. CMV infection can be asymptomatic or symptomatic and may be due to primary infection (either from the donor graft or blood products), reactivation of latent infection, or infection with a different CMV strain in a previously seropositive child. Prior to the use of prophylaxis, the incidence of symptomatic CMV infection was reported to be as high as 40% in pediatric liver transplant recipients.[8] Use of ganciclovir prophylaxis or viral monitoring to inform preemptive treatment has resulted in a decreased rate and severity of CMV disease. Intestinal transplantation was introduced after the availability of ganciclovir and therefore has been able to take advantage of using ganciclovir both as prophylaxis and treatment. Despite this, it is clear that CMV disease can be very severe after intestinal transplantation and may have a high rate of recurrence.[10] More recent reports identify decreased incidence and severity of CMV disease in this population, although, compared to CMV after other organ transplants, these patients continued to experience high recurrence rates of CMV infection, more severe disease, and high rates of resistance.[30,70,81,112] Primary CMV infection, typically acquired from the donor organ (or passenger donor leukocytes that accompany the organ), is associated with the greatest degree of morbidity and mortality.[32,112] Accordingly CMV-seronegative recipients of organs from CMV-seropositive donors are considered at high risk for developing CMV disease. Reactivation of or infection with a new strain of CMV tends to result in milder illness after liver transplantation but can still be severe after intestinal transplantation.[9] CMV disease appears more likely to develop in CMV-seropositive recipients of CMV-seropositive donors than in seropositive recipients of seronegative donors. Patients treated with unusually high doses of immunosuppressants, especially antilymphocyte antibody preparations, experience an increased rate of CMV disease regardless of previous immunity.[8,62]

Symptomatic CMV disease classically presented between 1 and 3 months after transplantation. It is important to note that the use of prophylactic or preemptive monitoring regimens may delay onset of CMV disease.[30] When present, a characteristic constellation of fever (which may be high-grade, prolonged, and hectic) and hematologic abnormalities (including leukopenia, atypical lymphocytosis, and thrombocytopenia) is frequently seen. This "CMV syndrome" occurs in 25% to 50% of patients with symptomatic CMV infection. Invasive CMV disease is manifest by visceral organ involvement; common sites include the gastrointestinal tract, liver, and lungs. CMV hepatitis appears to be the most common site among liver transplant recipients, whereas CMV enteritis is a frequent finding among intestinal transplant recipients. CMV chorioretinitis is rare in organ transplant recipients.

Diagnosis of CMV disease may be confirmed by detecting the presence of CMV DNA or pp65 antigen in the blood of a patient with a compatible clinical syndrome.[111] The pp65 antigenemia assay is less frequently used in recent years as nucleic acid test (NAT) assays have become more widely available. Clinicians must be aware that results of viral cultures of the urine, bronchoalveolar lavage specimens, or even a positive blood test for CMV by NAT or pp65 antigen, are difficult to interpret in previously infected patients because CMV is identified in these sites in the absence of clinical disease. Serial evaluation of quantitative determinations of the pp65 antigen or CMV DNA may add to specificity, but histologic examination of involved organs to confirm the presence of CMV remains the gold standard when the diagnosis of invasive CMV is being entertained.[61,91]

Antiviral agents with activity against CMV (e.g., ganciclovir, foscarnet, and cidofovir) have improved the survival of transplant recipients with CMV disease. Fatal disseminated CMV disease occurred in 19% of infected children[8] and 5% of infected adults undergoing liver transplantation in the era before ganciclovir was introduced.[99] For clinical CMV disease, ganciclovir therapy is given in conjunction with reduction of immunosuppression unless evidence of rejection is present.[61] Clinical response usually occurs 5 to 7 days after initiation of therapy. Baseline immunosuppression levels are typically restored at the time of initial clinical response or on recognition of rejection. Data support the use of serial monitoring of CMV load in the peripheral blood as a guide to initiation of and duration of CMV therapy.[61,91] Valganciclovir was equally efficacious in treating adult kidney transplant recipients with CMV disease but not those who had undergone liver transplantation.[5] Controlled studies in children are lacking, but many centers use valganciclovir in children once they are discharged from the hospital. The role of CMV hyperimmune globulin in combination with ganciclovir in the treatment of CMV disease is controversial, although some evidence for improved outcome has been reported in the treatment of CMV pneumonia in adult liver transplant recipients.[61] Finally because of the relatively high rates of nephrotoxicity associated with their use, foscarnet or cidofovir should be restricted to patients with apparent or proven resistance to ganciclovir, which should be suspected in patients who either fail to clinically improve or have persistent or rising CMV viral loads after 2 weeks of ganciclovir therapy.[61,91]

Historically approximately 25% of patients treated with ganciclovir for an initial episode of symptomatic CMV will develop one or more episodes of recurrent CMV disease,[108] although rates of recurrent disease may have fallen in the presence of longer initial treatment and the use of secondary prophylaxis.[61] When present, recurrences are observed about 1 month after the initial infectious episode and may be associated with invasive disease. More commonly, however, these recurrent episodes tend to be milder than the initial episode. Factors identified with an increased risk for developing recurrent CMV disease include being a CMV-seronegative recipient of a CMV-seropositive donor, having disseminated CMV disease, and having a history of multiple treatment courses for rejection and persistent elevations of the CMV load at the end of therapy.[61] Although current guidelines recommend continuing antiviral therapy until the CMV viral load becomes negative, further research is needed on duration.[61,91] A summary of our suggested approach to the diagnosis and management of CMV infection is provided in Table 72.5.

Epstein-Barr Virus

EBV infection, including EBV-associated PTLD, is an important cause of morbidity and mortality after liver transplantation and intestinal transplantation.[2,11,50,120] This is particularly true among children undergoing intestinal transplantation, who experience higher rates of EBV-related disease than any of the other organ transplant recipients.[85]

Symptomatic EBV infection in general and PTLD in particular most commonly occur among transplant recipients experiencing primary EBV infection, particularly those who receive organs from seropositive donors. Accordingly children undergoing transplantation are disproportionately affected by EBV compared with their adult counterparts.[39] As many as 80% of children who are EBV seronegative before liver transplantation will develop a primary EBV infection after this procedure.[101,105] Although primary infection occurs in the vast majority of seronegative patients, clinical disease develops in less than one-third of these children.[101,105] In one study, 4% of children undergoing solid-organ transplantation and 10% of children with primary EBV infection developed PTLD between 1 month and 5 years after transplant[50]; 75% of cases occurred during the first postoperative year in patients undergoing cyclosporine-based immune suppression. Historically cumulative occurrence rates reached as high as 12% to 20% by 7 to 12 years after pediatric liver transplantation.[68,80] Current rates of PTLD in this cohort appear lower, with an incidence of 4.4% at 5 years after liver transplant for recipients who were EBV seronegative prior to the procedure, likely owing to improvements in immune suppression and the use of preventive monitoring strategies.[60]

Pediatric recipients of intestinal transplantation appear to behave differently than children undergoing other types of organ transplantation in that the rate of EBV disease, including PTLD, occurs irrespective of EBV serostatus before transplantation. Rates of EBV disease and PTLD after intestinal transplantation as high as 30% to 40% were reported during the initial experiences with intestinal transplantation. More recently, these rates have declined to approximately 11%,[70] reflecting improved immune suppression regimens and EBV-monitoring protocols. However, these rates still remain higher than those seen among other organ recipients.

A wide spectrum of EBV disease is recognized that includes nonspecific viral illness, mononucleosis, and PTLD (including lymphoma). Histologic evaluation is important in differentiating among these categories; manifestations can evolve in individual patients. Asymptomatic seroconversion also occurs. Variation in severity and extent of disease is related to the degree of immunosuppression and adequacy of the host immune response. Although EBV disease and PTLD may present as involvement of many different clinical sites, there is a tendency for EBV disease to involve the transplanted organ. Thus EBV hepatitis and PTLD of the liver are observed more commonly among liver transplant recipients. Similarly the intestine is the most frequently observed site of involvement of EBV disease among intestinal transplant recipients.

TABLE 72.5 Overview of Diagnosis and Management of Viral Infections After Liver and Intestinal Transplantation in Children

	CMV	EBV	Respiratory Syncytial Virus	Influenza	Parainfluenza	Adenovirus
Frequency	Common[a]	Common	Uncommon	Uncommon	Uncommon	Liver: uncommon[b] Intestine: common[a]
Diagnostic tests	Culture Quantitative CMV PCR (blood) pp65 antigen Histology	Quantitative EBV PCR (blood) Histology Serology	NP aspirate for antigen detection or PCR	NP aspirate for antigen detection, PCR and/or culture	NP aspirate for culture or PCR	Viral culture or PCR Histology
Treatment:						
Primary	Ganciclovir IV (5 mg/kg bid)	Decrease immune suppression	Supportive care	Supportive care Oseltamivir Zanamivir	Supportive care	Decrease immune suppression
Secondary	Foscarnet[c] Cidofovir[c]	Rituximab Cytoxan/prednisone	Aerosolized ribavirin[d]			IV cidofovir
Adjunctive	Decrease immune suppression CMV-IVIG	Ganciclovir IVIG	Palivizumab Decrease immune suppression	Decrease immune suppression	Decrease immune suppression	IVIG[c]
Duration of therapy	Site dependent	Individualized	Individualized	Individualized	Individualized	Individualized
Follow-up	Monitor quantitative CMV PCR or pp65 (treat until negative)	Monitor quantitative EBV PCR Repeat imaging studies if positive at outset	None	None	None	None

[a]Common: frequency approximately >5%.
[b]Uncommon: frequency approximately 1–5%.
[c]Foscarnet or cidofovir used for CMV infection when ganciclovir resistance is suspected or proved. Experience from HIV-infected patients suggests that a synergistic benefit will be obtained from the combined use of both of these agents when ganciclovir resistance is present.
[d]Some experts have used oral ribavirin, but definitive data on efficacy are lacking.
CMV, Cytomegalovirus; *EBV,* Epstein-Barr virus; *HIV,* human immunodeficiency virus; *IV,* intravenous; *IVIG,* intravenous immunoglobulin; *NP,* nasopharyngeal; *PCR,* polymerase chain reaction;

Of interest, involvement of sites beyond the gastrointestinal tract is uncommon in intestinal transplant recipients.

Onset of viral syndrome, mononucleosis, and PTLD occur primarily within the first year, whereas lymphoma tends to present later. Immunosuppressive regimens based on the use of tacrolimus appear to have affected a shift in the timing of PTLD; only rare cases occur later than 18 months after liver transplant, although late cases are more likely to occur after intestinal transplantation.[13,120,102] The impact of newer immunosuppressive agents and regimens on EBV disease needs to be constantly reevaluated because unexpectedly high rates of PTLD have occurred with some new regimens.[44,98]

The diagnosis of EBV-associated PTLD is made on the basis of clinical, laboratory, and histopathologic examination and should be suspected in patients with protracted fever, exudative tonsillitis, lymphadenopathy, organomegaly, leukopenia, or atypical lymphocytosis.[39,85] Gastrointestinal involvement should be suspected in patients with persistent fever and diarrhea. Accordingly EBV must be considered in the differential diagnosis of rejection among intestinal transplant recipients. Serologic diagnosis is often confounded by the presence of passive antibody acquired at the time of transplantation or during subsequent transfusions. The detection of increased EBV viral load in peripheral blood identified by PCR has gained wide acceptance as an assay to predict risk for or presence of EBV or PTLD.[39,85] Although extremely sensitive, these assays are limited by both a lack of uniformity across different laboratories[89] and their lack of specificity; they are often elevated in asymptomatic patients.[2,39] Accordingly every effort should be made to histologically confirm the diagnosis of EBV or PTLD. Occult sites of PTLD are assessed by computed tomography of chest and abdomen. More recently, increasing interest has focused on the potential role of positron emission tomography (PET) scans as an alternative or supplemental imaging modality in the diagnostic evaluation of patients thought to have EBV disease and/or PTLD.[2,39] Palpable nodes or lesions (or both) identified by radiographic surveillance should be sampled. Endoscopic evaluation should be considered in patients with diarrheal illnesses and elevated viral loads.[15] Histologic evaluation for typical features may be augmented through the use of the Epstein-Barr–encoded RNA (EBER) probe.[90] The use of the EBER probe may be particularly useful in differentiating between the presence of rejection and EBV infection among intestinal transplant recipients.

Management of patients with PTLD is controversial.[2,39,85] Reduction of immunosuppression is recommended widely. Antiviral agents typically are used,[47] although their role has not been studied formally. Reduction of immunosuppression, alone or in combination with antiviral agents, results in an approximate 67% cure rate of EBV disease and PTLD. The potential impact of monoclonal antibodies,[27] interferon,[95] and chemotherapy[33] awaits formal clinical trials. Resection of tumor also may be of value for patients with lymphoma. Recent experience has focused on several novel approaches to the management of EBV disease and PTLD. These newer strategies have typically been used for patients who fail to respond to reduction of immune suppression (with or without the use of antiviral agents). Rituximab, an anti-CD20 antibody, has been increasingly used for the treatment of EBV disease. Experience to date suggests that as many as two-thirds of patients who fail initial withdrawal of immunosuppression will respond to a 4-week course of this agent.[41] However, relapse of EBV disease has been observed in 20% to 25% of treated patients 6 to 8 months after completion of therapy at the time the rituximab is no longer present in the body. An alternate chemotherapy-based approach for patients who fail to respond to initial reduction or withdrawal of immunosuppression has also been proposed.[46] This strategy, which uses modified doses of cyclophosphamide and prednisone, has also achieved success in approximately two-thirds of treated patients. Unfortunately, as with rituximab, relapse of PTLD has been seen in 22% of treated patients, and outright treatment failures have occurred in patients presenting with fulminant disease. Definitive studies comparing these two second-line therapies are needed to define the best option for those children who fail to respond to initial therapeutic modification of immunosuppression. A summary of our suggested approach and management of EBV/PTLD is provided in Table 72.5.

Other Herpesviruses

Other herpesviruses can also be hazardous after transplantation. Herpes simplex virus (HSV) can reactivate early after surgery or after augmentation of immunosuppression. Prophylaxis with acyclovir (or ganciclovir) has been beneficial in these situations. A summary of the suggested approach to the diagnosis and management of HSV is provided in Table 72.5. Primary varicella infection (chickenpox) in transplant recipients can lead to disseminated, fatal disease[73] and should be treated early and aggressively with intravenous acyclovir. Some centers have used valacyclovir rather than intravenous medication, but further studies are needed. Reactivation disease as shingles is more commonly seen in adults and can be prevented with antiviral prophylaxis early in the transplant period. Valacyclovir can be used for treatment if shingles is mild, but if severe or disseminated, then intravenous acyclovir use is prudent.

Interest has also focused on determining what role, if any, human herpesvirus–6 (HHV-6) and 7 (HHV-7) may play in causing disease in organ transplant recipients in general and abdominal transplant recipients in particular. Several groups of investigators have identified a potential interaction between the development of HHV-6 and HHV-7 and CMV infection in organ transplant recipients.[55,75] Reactivation of HHV-6 infection after liver transplantation has been associated with the development of an increased CMV viral load in the peripheral blood as well as a greater likelihood of developing symptomatic CMV disease.[55] In addition, it has been suggested that some or all of the symptoms typically associated with the CMV syndrome (e.g., fever, leukopenia) in patients with proven CMV infection may be attributable in part to HHV-6 or HHV-7. Studies in children have suggested that infection due to HHV-6 alone is a relatively common cause of unexplained fever in pediatric liver transplant recipients.[118,119] Interest also exists in the role, if any, that human herpesvirus–8 (HHV-8) may have in causing infection and disease in organ transplant recipients. This is particularly true for recipients who come from countries with moderate to high rates of HHV-8 prevalence such as Africa, the Middle East, and the Caribbean.[79] The full spectrum of disease of these more recently recognized herpesviruses and their potential therapies remain to be determined.

Adenovirus

Adenovirus has been reported to be the third most important virus affecting pediatric liver transplant recipients, occurring in 10% of one series of 484 children undergoing liver transplantation under cyclosporine-based immunosuppression.[78] Symptomatic disease (ranging from self-limited fever, gastroenteritis, or cystitis to devastating illness with necrotizing hepatitis or pneumonia) occurred in more than 60% of infected patients. Infection was most commonly diagnosed within the first 3 months after transplantation.[77] The frequency of invasive adenovirus infection after pediatric liver transplantation appears to have decreased markedly with the use of tacrolimus-based immunosuppression.[42] In the tacrolimus era, McLaughlin and colleagues found that only 4.2% of pediatric liver recipients experienced adenovirus disease.[74] This is in contrast to a significantly higher incidence of 20.8% of adenovirus infection in pediatric intestinal transplant recipients at the same institution. A high rate of adenovirus infection after pediatric intestinal transplantation was also reported by Florescu and colleagues, who noted that 39% of their cohort was infected, with 60% of infected patients recognized as having adenovirus-attributed disease.[29] Finally Pinchoff and colleagues found adenovirus in all 14 of their pediatric intestinal transplant recipients.[87] However, these exceptionally high rates might be attributable to the fact that viral cultures and PCRs were performed as part of routine screening of graft biopsies, and not all of the patients were symptomatic. When symptomatic, high stool output, alone or in the presence of fever, was the most common sign found.

It is difficult to presumptively diagnose infection due to adenovirus in pediatric abdominal transplant recipients because fever, hepatitis, and pneumonia may be caused by a variety of other pathogens, and high stool output after intestinal transplantation is nonspecific and can also occur with rejection. The presence of high-grade fevers and symptoms suggestive of adenovirus infection should prompt serial cultures for viruses (including adenovirus) or PCR investigation and evaluation of graft biopsies. Unexplained elevations in hepatocellular enzymes suggestive of hepatitis should warrant consideration of a liver biopsy. Similarly an increase in stool output, with or without fever, should prompt endoscopic evaluation of the intestinal allograft. Histologic examination for the presence of adenoviral inclusions as well as the use of immunohistochemical stains of biopsies specimens from either site should be undertaken to help confirm this diagnosis.

Definitive evidence evaluating potential treatments for adenoviral disease is not available at this time. The most important component of therapy is supportive care along with a decrease in immunosuppression. The role of antiviral agents is unproved,[6,77] but increasing data support the use of cidofovir in bone marrow[66] or solid-organ transplant recipients.[26,77] Current available guidelines support consideration of use of this agent for patients with proven disease.[26] Ongoing studies are investigating the potential role of brincidofovir (a lipid ester of cidofovir), which is currently in trial in bone marrow transplant recipients.[26] This drug, which is orally bioavailable, has been associated with less nephrotoxicity and may actually be more potent than the parent compound. Finally a single case report also raised the possible role of intravenous immunoglobulin as treatment for adenovirus infection.[21] A summary of a suggested approach to the diagnosis and management of adenovirus infection is provided in Table 72.5.

Common Community-Acquired Viruses

Although the course of illness has been poorly documented, most children who undergo liver and intestinal transplantation experience the usual respiratory viruses and gastrointestinal illness without significant problems. However, infections due to influenza virus, parainfluenza virus, or RSV led to more severe disease in young children, especially if infection occurs soon after transplant and/or during periods of maximal immunosuppression.[4,57,88] Likewise transplant recipients may have prolonged viral shedding even after resolution of symptoms. A summary of suggested strategies for the diagnosis and management of these community-acquired viruses can be found in Table 72.5.

Other Viruses

Other viruses, including both donor-associated viral infections (e.g., hepatitis B and hepatitis C virus) as well as community-acquired viral pathogens (e.g., rotavirus, norovirus, arboviruses) are relatively uncommon causes of clinically significant infection or disease after abdominal transplantation. Although this may be explained in part by the paucity of data describing infectious complications late after transplant, severe infection owing to these agents appears uncommon. For those patients for whom infection due to these pathogens is recognized, consultation with the primary transplant center is strongly recommended. Suggested approaches to the diagnosis and management of each of these viral pathogens are provided in Table 72.5.

OPPORTUNISTIC INFECTIONS

P. jiroveci is a well-documented cause of pneumonia in immunocompromised patients, including liver and intestinal transplant recipients. Prophylactic trimethoprim-sulfamethoxazole is safe, inexpensive, and effective.[53,54] The use of this strategy has eliminated *P. jiroveci* pneumonia in these patients at CHP, with rare breakthroughs occurring in patients who discontinued prophylaxis. Alternative prophylactic regimens for the sulfa-allergic patient include aerosolized pentamidine (for patients >5 years of age)[64] atovaquone or dapsone.[69]

Tuberculosis (TB) is a particular concern in immunosuppressed hosts, including recipients of liver and intestinal transplantation. The incidence of TB after liver transplantation in Europe and the United States has been reported to range from 0.9% to 2.3%, with most reported cases in adults.[100,115] In contrast, up to 15% of organ transplant recipients in areas of high-level endemicity may develop TB.[100] However, development of TB after pediatric liver transplantation is uncommon, with less than 20 cases reported.[71,100,115] To date, no cases have been reported among recipients of intestinal transplantation. Development of TB among solid-organ transplant recipients is associated with mortality rates ranging from 25% to 40%, with additional morbidity and mortality associated with development of rejection in patients receiving anti-TB therapy.[100,115] Diagnosis of TB in transplant recipients is complicated by the fact that extrapulmonary disease occurs frequently and purified protein derivative (PPD) testing is likely to be unreliable after transplant. Management of TB in liver transplant recipients is difficult both because of the side effects of anti-TB agents and their potential interactions with immunosuppressive agents.[100,115] Limited published experience in pediatric liver transplant recipients suggests that the majority of infections due to *Mycobacterium tuberculosis* are most likely due to a primary infection often associated with family contacts who have positive skin tests.[115] In contrast, experience with adult transplant recipients suggests that development of TB is more likely due to reactivation of latent TB.[48,100,115] Although only limited published information is available describing TB in these patients, transplant recipients known to have a positive PPD or who come from an area endemic for TB appear to be at increased risk for symptomatic reactivation after transplantation.[48,115] Similar data are not available for recipients of intestinal transplantation. Additional factors predisposing to the development of TB after transplantation include severe hepatic failure at the time of transplant, aggressive antirejection therapy, and/or concurrent HIV infection.[48,109] Experience among adult renal transplant recipients suggests that although the risk appears greatest in patients who received inadequate or no prior TB therapy,[65] it can also occur in patients who received appropriate anti-TB therapy in the pretransplant period.[65] Although TB has only rarely been encountered among pediatric liver transplant recipients,[115] and not among intestinal recipients, screening for TB by history and a PPD test or interferon-γ release assay (IGRA), along with review of a chest radiograph for lesions consistent with healed TB, is highly recommended. However, the use of IGRA assays for even immune-competent children younger than 5 years of age is not recommended at this time. Patients with a positive TB history and/or a positive screening test (either PPD or IGRA) result should receive isoniazid for 6 to 12 months after transplant, although some experts recommend continuing this agent indefinitely while patients remain on immunosuppression. Attempts at a more definitive diagnosis are indicated for patients from endemic areas with a negative PPD result but suggestive chest radiograph. Careful evaluation for evidence of side effects, particularly hepatotoxicity, is recommended, and isoniazid is discontinued if unacceptable toxicity is identified.

Additional potential opportunistic infections include cryptococcosis, coccidioidomycosis, and histoplasmosis, although the pathogens of these infections have not been frequently reported among pediatric liver or intestinal transplant recipients. Prior infection with these pathogens is common in geographic areas where they are endemic. Because patients often travel to transplant centers distant to their homes, it is imperative that transplant physicians be aware of the local environmental risks for each patient. Experience with coccidioidomycosis in transplant recipients suggests that a minimum of 4 months of antifungal therapy, such as fluconazole, should be given in transplant recipients with this history.[81] Similarities between coccidioidomycosis and other fungal pathogens suggest that similar strategies may be necessary for patients with a positive history of prior fungal infection with pathogens known to recur after resolution of primary infection.

MANAGEMENT

Pretransplant Evaluation

A pretransplant evaluation is helpful in the management of infectious complications in liver and intestinal transplant recipients. A complete history and physical examination should be performed with particular attention paid to previous infections, immunizations, and drug allergies. Attention should be paid to a history of infection with MDR bacteria, which may provide guidance for future empirical treatment that may be required after transplantation. An intermediate-strength tuberculin skin test or an IGRA for children older than 5 years of age should be performed on all patients.

The CHP pretransplant protocol includes obtaining serology for CMV; EBV; varicella; herpes simplex virus; hepatitis A, B (surface antibody, surface antigen, and core antibody), and C; and HIV for all candidates. In addition, serology to measles, mumps, and rubella is obtained to ensure that the patients have a measurable antibody response to prior immunizations. Serologic tests on the donor should include HIV, hepatitis B and C, CMV, and EBV. Donors positive for HIV should be excluded, with the rare exception of approved research protocols in the United States as prescribed under the HOPE Act. The use of organs from donors who test positive for hepatitis B or C virus would typically be contraindicated except in the circumstance in which the recipient is also positive for hepatitis B or C, respectively. Knowledge of donor and recipient status for these viruses allows one to anticipate infection, identifying patients who might benefit from prophylactic regimens and guiding in the diagnostic evaluation of fever.

Prophylactic Regimens

Prophylactic regimens vary among transplant centers. These strategies have been divided into perioperative and long-term prophylaxis and often evolve to reflect the infectious complications seen at individual institutions.

Perioperative prophylaxis is used to prevent intraoperative sepsis and wound infection. It is based on individual patient characteristics and expected normal flora. At CHP, piperacillin-tazobactam is used as the standard agent for perioperative prophylaxis. This is modified if the recipient is known to harbor antimicrobial-resistant bacteria. If sepsis is suspected in the donor, antibiotics are chosen to cover those organisms identified from the donor, and treatment is usually extended to a therapeutic course of 10 to 14 days. In the absence of proved or suspected infection in the donor, perioperative prophylaxis is usually limited to the first 48 hours after transplant.

Considerations regarding long-term prophylaxis against infections occurring beyond the perioperative period include the risk and severity of infection as well as the toxicity, cost, and efficacy of a given prophylactic strategy. Nystatin is recommended for all pediatric transplant recipients in an effort to prevent oropharyngeal candidiasis until the patients are on less than 5 mg/day of prednisone. Trimethoprim-sulfamethoxazole is used to prevent *P. jiroveci* pneumonia. Although some centers recommend using trimethoprim-sulfamethoxazole for only the first 6 months after liver transplantation, anecdotal experience with patients presenting with PCP long after transplant and the relative safety of this agent have led us to recommend its use indefinitely after liver and intestinal transplantation in children.

The frequency and severity of CMV infection in transplant recipients prompts consideration of prophylactic strategies; optimizing the target population and timing of interventions requires further study.[61,91] Current guidelines primarily focus on two approaches to the prevention of CMV: chemoprophylaxis, where all "at risk" recipients receive antiviral therapy for a defined period, and surveillance monitoring of CMV load in blood (most commonly using NAT) in those deemed to be at risk to inform preemptive initiation of antiviral therapy.[38,61,91] Data on use of monitoring and preemptive therapy after pediatric transplantation remain sparse, although sequential use of shorter courses of prophylaxis followed by monitoring (also called *hybrid method*) has been employed[61] and is currently favored by many pediatric transplant centers.

Whichever CMV prevention strategy is chosen, potential roles exist for intravenous and oral ganciclovir and oral valganciclovir as the antiviral agents for these strategies. Currently CHP protocols use intravenous ganciclovir alone (for varying durations) for liver and low-risk intestinal transplant recipients (recipient CMV positive before transplant or donor and recipient seronegative) and ganciclovir plus intravenously administered immune globulin containing a high titer of antibody against CMV[103,104] for high-risk (donor CMV positive and recipient CMV negative) intestinal transplant recipients if available. As noted earlier, at CHP, we now include sequential monitoring to inform the need for a secondary course of antiviral therapy after completion of an initial course of antiviral chemoprophylaxis. At present, the use of oral valganciclovir is an alternative to prophylaxis with intravenous ganciclovir for adolescents, although the use of this medication is not approved for liver transplant recipients because a higher rate of tissue-invasive disease was observed in liver transplant recipients receiving valganciclovir compared with oral ganciclovir in the pivotal trial evaluating this agent.[86] Nonetheless published guidelines support the use of valganciclovir for adult liver transplant recipients.[61,91] Pharmacokinetic studies for dosing oral valganciclovir suspension in children after transplantation adjusted for body surface area and renal function suggest that ganciclovir exposures similar to those established as safe and effective in adults can be achieved.

Similar to CMV, there is an interest in the prevention of EBV infections and PTLD. A number of different strategies are used, including immunoprophylaxis, viral load monitoring, and preemptive therapy[41,72]; the efficacy of these approaches has not been established. The use of viral load monitoring to inform preemptive reductions in immunosuppression appears to be the most promising of these strategies.[2,63,72] Because reduction of immune suppression is not always possible for intestinal transplant recipients with a rising EBV load, preemptive intravenous ganciclovir and intravenous immune globulin have been used in addition to reduction of immune suppression (where possible) for this cohort of patients. Although prospective comparative data are not available, the use of this strategy appears to have resulted in decreased risk for disease and improved outcome compared with historical controls who were not followed with this strategy.[37] The use of anti-CD20 monoclonal therapy has also been used by some centers when decreased immunosuppression is not possible.

CONCLUSION

Infections remain an important problem after liver and intestinal transplantation. Knowledge of the type, timing, and predisposing risk factors for these infectious complications allows for their timely and appropriate diagnosis and management.

NEW REFERENCES SINCE THE SEVENTH EDITION

22. De Luca M, Green M, Symmonds J, et al. Invasive candidiasis in liver transplant patients: incidence and risk factors in a pediatric cohort. *Pediatr Transplant.* 2016;20:235-240.
27. Florescu DF, Hoffman JA, AST Infectious Diseases Community of Practice. Adenovirus in solid organ transplantation. *Am J Transplant.* 2013;13:206-211.
39. Green M, Michaels MG. Epstein-Barr virus infection and post-transplant lymphoproliferative disorder. *Am J Transplant.* 2013;13:41-54.
60. Kim WR, Lake JR, Smith JM, et al. Special Issue: OPTN/SRTR annual data report 2014: liver. *Am J Transplant.* 2016;16(suppl 2):69-98.
61. Kotton CN, Kumar D, Caliendo AM, et al. Updated international consensus guidelines on the management of cytomegalovirus in solid organ transplantation. *Transplantation.* 2013;96:333-360.
69. Martin SI, Fishman JA, AST Infectious Diseases Community of Practice. Pneumocystis pneumonia in solid organ transplantation. *Am J Transplant.* 2013;13:272-279.
77. Michaels MG, Green M, Ison M. Adenovirus infections in solid organ transplantation. In: Bowden R, Ljungman P, Snydman D, eds. *Transplant Infections.* 4th ed. Philadelphia: Lippincott-Raven; 2016:623-630.
81. Miller R, Assi M, AST Infectious Diseases Community of Practice. Endemic fungal infections in solid organ transplantation. *Am J Transplant.* 2013;13(suppl 4):250-261.
91. Razonable RR, Humar A, AST Infectious Diseases Community of Practice. Cytomegalovirus in solid organ transplant recipients. *Am J Transplant.* 2013;13:93-106.
102. Smith JM, Skeans MA, Horslen SP, et al. Special issue: OPTN/SRTR annual data report 2014: intestine. *Am J Transplant.* 2016;16(suppl 2):99-114.
107. Stillwell T, Green M, Barbadora K, et al. Outbreak of KPC-3 producing carbapenem-resistant *Klebsiella pneumoniae* in a U.S. pediatric hospital. *J Pediatric Infect Dis Soc.* 2015;4:330-338.
112. Timpone JG, Yimen M, Cox S, et al. Resistant cytomegalovirus in intestinal and multivisceral transplant recipients. *Transpl Infect Dis.* 2016;18(2):202-209.

The full reference list for this chapter is available at ExpertConsult.com

73 Opportunistic Infections in Kidney Transplantation

Gail J. Harrison

Renal transplantation is the therapy of choice for end-stage renal disease (ESRD) in children and adolescents.[37,161,220,261] It is successful in 90% of recipients and allows most children the best opportunities for normal growth and development and an almost normal lifestyle.[87,165,255] Despite the overall success of renal transplantation, infection remains the major cause of morbidity, graft loss, and mortality in renal transplant recipients.[62,105,156,248] Effective immunosuppressive regimens have reduced the rates and hospitalizations for graft rejection after renal transplantation, but rates and hospitalizations for bacterial and viral infections seem to be unchanged or increasing.[65,166,213] Prednisone-free maintenance immunosuppressive combinations with tacrolimus, mycophenolate mofetil, and sirolimus help maintain graft function, but they also may increase the risk for development of infections, including posttransplantation lymphoproliferative disorders (PTLD), papillomaviruses, and invasive fungal diseases.[122,158]

These infections can be managed successfully if detected early and treated appropriately.[122] In this chapter a general approach to renal transplant recipients is presented from the perspective of the infectious disease specialist. Specific, detailed information regarding the diagnosis and management of each particular pathogen can be found in the respective chapters in the section of this textbook dedicated to infections with specific microorganisms.

PRETRANSPLANT EVALUATION

The role of the pediatric infectious disease specialist in the care of a renal transplant recipient ideally begins during the pretransplantation period.[195,197] Before the patient undergoes transplantation, a thorough history and physical examination should be performed, with a focus on evaluation for evidence of an active infection that may require immediate therapy or, rarely, preclude transplantation (Box 73.1). The history should be comprehensive but focus on the details of any history of previous infections that may reemerge during the posttransplant period, including urinary tract infections (UTIs); mucocutaneous diseases such as herpes simplex virus (HSV) infection; systemic illnesses such as tuberculosis; chronic infections such as those caused by hepatitis B virus (HBV), hepatitis C virus (HCV), or human immunodeficiency virus (HIV); and diarrheal diseases. Infection with HIV previously was regarded as a reason to exclude a potential recipient from undergoing renal transplantation. Patients with primary immune disorders, such as chronic granulomatous disease, may now survive long term but experience end-stage renal failure and require kidney transplantation.[35] Successes with highly active antiretroviral therapy have improved long-term survival in HIV-infected pediatric patients, however, and have led clinicians, research scientists, and family members themselves to provide renal transplantation as a treatment for ESRD.[73,196]

BOX 73.1 Guidelines for Pretransplant Evaluation in Pediatric Kidney Transplant

Candidates

History:
- Past infectious diseases
- Routine childhood illnesses
- Travel to or birth or residence in areas endemic for fungal or parasitic diseases or Zika virus transmission
- Tuberculosis exposure
- Animal exposure
- Diet preferences and water resources
- Vaccinations
- Reactions or allergies to antimicrobial agents
- Current or past immunosuppression

Physical examination:
- Search for active or latent focus of infection
- Nutritional status

Laboratory and other tests:
- Purified protein derivative
- Chest radiograph
- Urinalysis and urine culture
- Viral serology IgG and or IgM for HSV, CMV, EBV, VZV, human erythrovirus (formerly human parvovirus B19), HAV, HBV, HCV, HIV, BK virus, WNV, ZV, and others depending on the history
- Baseline HSV, CMV and EBV DNA PCR, erythrovirus, HCV, BK virus if seropositive or posttransplant monitoring is anticipated
- Fungal and parasitic testing if travel or exposure history positive; sputum or stool tests as indicated

Anticipatory guidance

Update vaccines

Counsel regarding measures to reduce infection risk

Consider antimicrobial or viral prophylaxis if at risk

CMV, Cytomegalovirus; *EBV*, Epstein-Barr virus; *HAV*, hepatitis A virus; *HBV*, hepatitis B virus; *HCV*, hepatitis C virus; *HIV*, human immunodeficiency virus; *HSV*, herpes simplex virus; *PCR*, polymerase chain reaction; *VZV*, varicella zoster virus; *WNV*, West Nile virus; *ZV*, Zika virus.

Renal transplant candidates undergo peritoneal dialysis or hemodialysis, so a history of previous dialysis catheter–associated infections should be documented and any current infection should be treated and eliminated before transplantation is performed. Another focus of the history should include an exposure history for the patient's country of origin or foreign travel, especially to areas endemic for organisms such as *Strongyloides stercoralis, Trypanosoma cruzi* (Chagas disease), *Coccidioides immitis, Blastomyces dermatitidis,* or *Histoplasma capsulatum,* Zika virus or West Nile virus, and for diseases such as malaria and tuberculosis.[101,213] Other important exposures include blood product transfusions; exposure to animals or plants; well water as a source of drinking water; and dietary habits, especially consumption of raw or undercooked eggs or meat or unpasteurized dairy products.[195,197] Patients waiting for transplantation may become colonized with resistant organisms, including methicillin-resistant *Staphylococcus aureus,* vancomycin-resistant *Enterococcus,* gram-negative–multidrug resistant bacteria, fluconazole-resistant or multidrug resistant *Candida* species, and *Clostridium difficile.* In children who are unimmunized, a careful history of routine childhood illnesses, including varicella, measles, mumps, and rubella, should be documented.[125]

The immunization history of the patient should be documented carefully and, if needed or indicated, updated before the patient undergoes transplantation. Ideally children with chronic renal disease should be fully immunized before progression to ESRD for optimal immune response and protection during outbreaks of vaccine-preventable diseases.[52,162] Vaccinations against tetanus, pertussis, and diphtheria; polysaccharide vaccines, such as those against pneumococcus and *Haemophilus influenzae* type b; inactivated vaccines against polio and hepatitis A; and recombinant vaccines, such as those for hepatitis B, may be given or updated at any time before transplantation is performed.[34,241,254] Meningococcal vaccine is indicated routinely now for specific age groups and for special outbreak situations. The live varicella vaccine is recommended for renal transplant candidates who have not had varicella; it should be given at least 2 to 4 weeks before transplantation is performed.[275] The measles-mumps-rubella vaccine should be administered even earlier, preferably months before the patient undergoes transplantation. Measles immunity and immunity from other live virus vaccines may wane over time in renal transplant recipients.[215] In addition, annual influenza vaccine and a tetanus booster every 10 years are recommended for patients who are renal transplant candidates or recipients.

If the child is unable to be fully immunized before undergoing transplantation, the routine immunization schedule for the inactivated vaccines may be reinstituted after immunosuppression is decreased, which usually occurs 6 to 12 months after an uncomplicated transplant procedure.[34,162,241,254] Live virus vaccines should be avoided in the posttransplant period in most instances. Reports of safe and effective vaccination with varicella vaccine in selected posttransplant patients have been published, however.[32,43,84,189,190] Close contacts and family members of renal transplant candidates and recipients also should be fully immunized and should receive the annual influenza vaccine.[11] Other important points in the pretransplant evaluation history include allergies or reactions to medications, especially antibiotics, and the use of immunosuppressive agents.

Pretransplant laboratory and diagnostic imaging evaluations for most renal transplant candidates should include a chest radiograph, urinalysis, and urine culture for bacteria. Baseline renal and liver function tests also should be performed.

Serologic screening of the transplant recipient's status regarding organisms that may reactivate in the recipient or infect the recipient via the donor organ should be performed; such screening should include tests for HSV; cytomegalovirus (CMV); varicella zoster virus (VZV); Epstein-Barr virus (EBV); human erythrovirus (parvovirus B19); *Treponema pallidum; Toxoplasma gondii;* hepatitis A, B, and C viruses; and HIV. Hepatitis E virus has also been shown to infect kidney transplant recipients, but the clinical significance of infection with hepatitis E virus in these patients is not clear.[226,243] Transplant recipients who are seropositive for HSV or CMV usually receive antiviral prophylaxis during the peritransplant period, whereas recipients seropositive for EBV may undergo posttransplant monitoring. It may be helpful to save an aliquot of the recipient's (and donor's) serum in case unusual circumstances occur, such as infection with West Nile virus (WNV) or Zika virus. In CMV-seropositive transplant candidates, baseline CMV quantitative DNA polymerase chain reaction (PCR) may be useful; and in EBV-seropositive candidates, detection of EBV DNA by quantitative PCR may be helpful to document pretransplant viral load especially if posttransplant virologic monitoring is to be performed.

Evaluation for active or latent tuberculosis infection should also be performed before the transplant. This evaluation should include a history of risk factors, including Bacillus Calmette–Guérin (BCG) vaccination, close contacts, country of origin, and a chest radiograph. In addition, a tuberculin skin test (TST) and interferon-γ release assay (IGR) (QuantiFERON-TB gold, QuantiFERON-TB gold in tube, or T-SPOT.TB) should be performed. Positive IGR assay results predict subsequent development of tuberculosis in adult kidney transplant recipients in whom latent tuberculosis infection cannot be detected by TST.[130] General reviews of IGR assay results in adults with ESRD and in children also suggest that IGR assays are useful, but caution should be used when interpreting IGR test results in young children, especially when results are discordant with TST.[45,216] The pretransplant evaluation also is an opportunity for the infectious disease specialist to counsel the patient and family about measures that may reduce the transplant recipient's risk for development of infectious disease complications after the transplant. Patients who have an exposure, or even a suspected exposure, to varicella (chickenpox) or zoster (shingles) should contact their physicians immediately to see whether passive immunoprophylaxis with varicella zoster immunoglobulin or postexposure antiviral therapy with acyclovir or valacyclovir is indicated. Plans for foreign travel to remote areas also should be discussed with the physician. The transplant recipient should consume only thoroughly cooked meat and seafood and thoroughly washed fresh fruits and vegetables. In addition, drinking water should be pure. Transplant recipients should avoid, if possible, changing cat litter boxes, aquariums, and birdcages and should avoid close contact with people who have viral respiratory tract illnesses. Finally, medical attention should be sought if fever occurs, especially if it is significant or persistent.

POSTTRANSPLANT INFECTIOUS COMPLICATIONS

Infections occurring in the posttransplant period can be grouped into three main time frames: the first month posttransplant (early), 2 to 6 months posttransplant (middle), and 6 months posttransplant and onward (late).[217,237] Although almost any organism or pathogen can infect a transplant recipient at any time, these time periods provide the clinician with a guide to the organisms and disease processes most commonly encountered (Box 73.2).

Infections Occurring During the Early Posttransplant Period

Infections occurring during the first month after renal transplantation usually are bacterial.[225] Common sites of early infections include the wound, urinary tract, lungs, and indwelling intravascular catheters.[202]

Wound Infections

As with any surgical procedure, wound infections may develop in a renal transplant recipient. They occur in approximately 2% of renal transplant recipients and range in severity from a superficial wound infection easily treated with wound care and antimicrobial therapy to deep perinephric abscesses that may be difficult to treat and result in transplant nephrectomy.[218,225] Wound infections are more likely to occur in patients with technical problems associated with the transplant surgery, including urinary leaks, vesicoureteral reflux, wound hematomas, or lymphoceles.[171,276] Malnutrition during the pretransplant period may impair wound healing and predispose the patient to development of wound infection.

Open Penrose drains may increase the likelihood of introducing microorganisms into the wound, whereas closed suction drainage, such as with a Jackson-Pratt drain, may reduce this risk. In addition, prompt removal of all drains, usually within 5 days in most uncomplicated cases, and administration of prophylaxis with perioperative antibiotics may decrease the incidence of wound infections; such measures are performed routinely in most renal transplant centers. The regimen usually is aimed at uropathogens and staphylococci. One dose generally is given before the transplant, and the regimen is continued for only 24 hours after the transplant.

The diagnosis of a wound infection should be suspected if erythema, warmth, or discharge is present at the wound site or if an unexplained fever develops. Fluid may drain from the wound persistently, or a fluid collection or abscess may be seen on imaging of the deeper operative sites. The patient will be receiving immunosuppressive agents, however, and the findings may be unusual or the symptoms may be blunted. Any fluid or pus obtained should be stained and cultured for bacterial, mycobacterial, and fungal organisms. Organisms most likely to be identified as causes of wound infection include staphylococci (*Staphylococcus aureus,* especially methicillin-resistant *S. aureus* [MRSA], but also coagulase-negative staphylococci), streptococci, and gram-negative enteric organisms. Unusual, multidrug-resistant, or health care–associated bacterial pathogens and yeast, such as *Candida albicans,* also may cause wound infections after the transplant. In addition, case reports of wound and perinephric fluid collections infected with *Mycoplasma hominis* have been published.[239]

Appropriate antimicrobial therapy, initially broad-spectrum and then ultimately tailored to the isolated organism and its susceptibility pattern, should be administered. The duration of appropriate antimicrobial therapy usually is 10 to 14 days or until the wound infection has resolved and the patient has been afebrile for 3 to 5 days. Deep abscesses or unusual organisms may require longer therapy.

BOX 73.2 Timetable for the Occurrence of Common Infections and Usual Pathogens After Kidney Transplantation

Early Period

Wound infections
Urinary tract infection
Bacteremia and sepsis syndrome
Pneumonia
Herpes simplex virus
Hepatitis B virus
Human erythrovirus (parvovirus B19)
West Nile virus
Zika virus?
Seasonal viruses
Drug reactions

Middle Period

Herpesviruses:
- Cytomegalovirus
- Epstein-Barr virus
- Varicella-zoster virus
- Herpesvirus types 6, 7, and 8

Polyomaviruses:
- JC virus
- BK virus

Papillomaviruses
Adenoviruses
Zika virus?
Human erythrovirus (parvovirus B19)
Listeria monocytogenes
Mycobacterium tuberculosis
Atypical mycobacteria
Nocardia
Fungal diseases
Pneumocystis jiroveci
Parasitic diseases

Late Period

Community-acquired respiratory viruses and bacterial pathogens
Urinary tract infection
Streptococcus pneumoniae
Cytomegalovirus
Epstein-Barr virus
Varicella zoster virus
Hepatitis B virus
Hepatitis C virus
Human immunodeficiency virus/acquired immunodeficiency syndrome
Zika virus?

Urinary Tract Infections

UTIs are common developments after renal transplantation and may affect 35% to 79% of renal transplant recipients.[135,276] Posttransplant UTIs are associated with acute and chronic graft dysfunction and may threaten renal graft survival.[2,14,39,60,124,176,247] They may occur during the early, middle, or late posttransplant period and should be differentiated as afebrile and febrile.[122] A UTI that is febrile and occurs during the early or early/middle posttransplant period often is a severe illness complicated by pyelonephritis, urosepsis, metastatic foci of infection, allograft dysfunction, rejection, and relapse.[178,219] UTIs occurring in the early posttransplant period are associated more often with graft loss than are UTIs that occur later.[60]

The risk for developing an invasive UTI after undergoing renal transplantation seems to be increased in patients with prolonged bladder catheterization (most catheters can be removed during the first few days after transplant), dysfunctional bladder, ureterovesical disorders with reflux, malnutrition, underlying disorders, renal stones, obstructive uropathy, or a contaminated cadaveric kidney.[2,195] The inability of the bladder to empty completely or surgical complications, such as hematoma, reflux, or obstruction at the urinary anastomosis, are associated with UTIs. In addition, young infants, especially infants who have vesicoureteral reflux, seem to have a high incidence of complicated UTIs after a transplant procedure.[178] Procedures that address the etiology and correct underlying physiologic and anatomic abnormalities of the bladder and ureters should be performed before transplantation to avoid or lessen development of complications associated with these problems.[2,14,39,247] Newer surgical techniques allow children with reconstructed bladders to undergo successful renal transplantation with minimal risk for posttransplant development of UTIs.[171,219]

The organisms most commonly isolated from patients with early onset UTIs include not only the typical gram-negative enteric bacteria but also enterococci, staphylococci, and *Pseudomonas aeruginosa.* Unusual organisms, such as *Streptococcus mitis, Serratia marcescens,* and *Corynebacterium urealyticum,* also can be found. Antimicrobial therapy should be tailored to the susceptibility pattern of the organism isolated from the urine. Because 30% of patients experiencing a UTI during the early posttransplant period may have recurrent UTIs, a prolonged 6-week course of antibiotics usually is recommended to reduce the risk for developing a relapsing kidney infection.[171,219] Antimicrobial prophylaxis may reduce the risk for developing a UTI. Trimethoprim-sulfamethoxazole administered for the first 4 months after renal transplantation is effective in preventing most UTIs and can provide cross-cover prophylaxis against *Pneumocystis jiroveci* pneumonia and other diseases.[82]

Pneumonia

Pneumonia can occur during the first month after renal transplantation and often is associated with prolonged endotracheal intubation. Gram-positive and gram-negative bacterial pathogens acquired from normal oropharyngeal flora and unusual or health care–associated multidrug-resistant organisms predominate during the early posttransplant period.[197] *Legionella pneumophila* and unusual *Legionella* spp., such as *L. micdadei, L. bozemanae,* and *L. dumoffii,* also have caused outbreaks of serious, life-threatening pneumonia in transplant recipients in some centers.[38,50,134,197] *P. jiroveci* can cause pneumonia in a transplant recipient during the early posttransplant period, but more often it is associated with disease after the first month posttransplant.[104] Rare or unusual pathogens, such as *Rhodococcus equi,* may cause pneumonia in these patients.[147]

Patients with pneumonia usually have fever, chills, chest pain, malaise, change in tracheal secretions, cough, dyspnea, tachypnea, change in ventilatory status, rales or rhonchi on auscultation of the lungs, and pulmonary infiltrates evident on a chest radiograph. Pneumonia may be complicated by pleural effusion, empyema, or pulmonary abscess, and death may occur if pneumonia is severe and not diagnosed and treated promptly. Treatment with antibiotics effective against the bacterial pathogens isolated from culture of tracheal aspirates, bronchoalveolar lavage fluid, or lung tissue is appropriate.

Bacteremia, Fungemia, and Sepsis

Bacteremia, fungemia, and sepsis occurring during the early posttransplant period often are associated with indwelling catheters.[196] The urinary tract, surgical wound, or transplanted or native kidney also may be a source.[160]

Usual bacterial organisms such as coagulase-negative staphylococci or *S. aureus,* unusual bacterial organisms, and yeasts such as *C. albicans* and other *Candida* spp. may be involved. *Listeria monocytogenes* also may cause primary bacteremia or sepsis at any time after a kidney transplantation has been performed but the greatest risk occurs during the early period. Complications include meningitis, and 10% of these patients may die.[175,232] Renal transplant recipients also are at increased risk for development of bacteremia with *Salmonella* nontyphoidal species.[58,116,196]

Complications such as UTI, graft infection, peritonitis, abscesses, and meningitis can occur, and recurrences are common. Therapy for bacteremia, sepsis, or its complications is tailored to the susceptibility pattern of the organism isolated from the patient's blood. The duration of therapy for uncomplicated bacteremia usually is 10 to 14 days, but a longer course of treatment may be indicated if abscesses occur or an unusual organism is isolated. Removal of the indwelling catheter may be necessary to clear persistent bacteremia, and abscesses and other foci of infection should be drained.

Other Bacterial Diseases

Pediatric renal transplant recipients also seem to be at increased risk for development of antibiotic-associated colitis caused by *Clostridium difficile.*[47,267] Infection of a lymphocele with *Pasteurella multocida* has been reported, as has systemic infection with *Bartonella henselae.*[3,48,64,152,196] A high index of suspicion always must be maintained when evaluating a transplant recipient for infection because the immunosuppression required to maintain the transplanted kidney predisposes the recipient to development of infection with unusual organisms.

Viral Infections

Herpes simplex virus. HSV is the most common virus encountered during the early posttransplant period, although antiviral prophylaxis significantly reduces the risk for development of this infection.[69,70] It occurs less frequently in pediatric (8%) than in adult renal transplant recipients (30%).[196,195] Most HSV infections encountered posttransplant are due to reactivation of the recipient's strain; however, primary or recurrent infection acquired from the renal allograft may occur and primary infection from person-to-person transmission has been documented.[69,196,195,219]

Posttransplant HSV infection may be asymptomatic or associated with disease, most frequently oral ulcers in pediatric patients.[97] Genital and perianal ulcers may occur in adolescents and adults. Rarely HSV may cause disseminated cutaneous lesions or zosteriform eruptions. HSV esophagitis may be manifested as dysphagia, refusal to eat, irritability, and substernal chest pain, and it may complicate oral HSV disease, especially if the oral mucosa has been traumatized by orogastric or nasogastric tubes. Acute severe hepatitis with hepatic necrosis, often accompanied by hypotension and disseminated intravascular coagulation, also can occur. Tracheobronchitis and pneumonitis may occur as a result of HSV, primarily in patients with pneumonia caused by another pathogen and whose mucosa has been traumatized by endotracheal intubation. It is often severe and life threatening, even with appropriate supportive care and antiviral therapy.[196] Encephalitis also has been reported in renal transplant recipients.[92]

The diagnosis is made by isolation of HSV in cell culture or detection of viral antigen by immunofluorescence or viral DNA by PCR in the end organ involved. Detection or isolation of HSV in body secretions may represent asymptomatic shedding or disease and should be correlated clinically. If HSV DNA by PCR is detected in blood, viremia is likely present and should be treated. Treatment with acyclovir is recommended for patients with mucocutaneous lesions, viremia, or end-organ disease, and HSV-seropositive transplant recipients should receive acyclovir or valacyclovir prophylaxis during the peritransplant period to prevent development of HSV infection. Most patients receiving ganciclovir, valganciclovir, foscarnet, or cidofovir for CMV prophylaxis also are protected against HSV.

Other viruses. Seasonal viruses, especially winter respiratory viruses such as respiratory syncytial virus, influenza viruses, parainfluenza viruses, and adenoviruses; winter diarrhea viruses, such as rotavirus; and late summer/early fall viruses, such as the enteroviruses, can infect the transplant recipient during the early posttransplant period and cause disease. Such infections may be acquired from the family or the community, or they may occur from health care–associated exposures. Transplant recipients who may not be adequately protected by routine vaccination are at risk for severe influenza and its complications. In 2012, results of a study on oseltamivir prophylaxis with once-daily dosing for 12 weeks during periods of local influenza circulation showed that it was well tolerated and reduced influenza in adult and pediatric kidney and other solid-organ transplant recipients.[119] Oseltamivir-resistant influenza A was detected during the study period.[119]

Renal transplant recipients who are chronically infected with HBV or HCV may experience liver dysfunction during the early transplant period, but the late posttransplant period, beyond the first year, carries the greatest risk for progression of liver disease to cirrhosis. If a renal transplant recipient acquires HBV soon after undergoing transplantation, acute hepatitis can develop, often with death from liver failure.[57,196]

Noninfectious Causes of Fever

The most common noninfectious cause of fever in the first posttransplant month is allograft rejection.[218] Fever often is the first sign of rejection, especially in children, and rejection should be considered if an infectious source of the fever is not identified. Another common noninfectious cause of fever early after transplantation is antilymphocyte antibody therapy (OKT3). The first two or three doses of OKT3 produce a release of cytokines, which cause fever and chills. In most patients, these symptoms resolve after the third dose. Other noninfectious causes of fever during this period include drug reactions and pulmonary emboli.

Infections Occurring During the Middle Posttransplant Period

The cumulative effects of immunosuppression begin to be revealed during the period 2 to 6 months after transplantation. If a significant amount of antirejection therapy is required for multiple episodes of rejection, the effects may be more pronounced. Such immunosuppression allows classic opportunistic pathogens, such as CMV, *P. jiroveci, Toxoplasma gondii, L. monocytogenes, Aspergillus,* and *Nocardia,* to evade immune surveillance and cause disease.[104,196,266,268] Reactivation of organisms previously infecting the transplant recipient or the donor allograft, including *Mycobacterium tuberculosis,* HBV, HCV, HIV, *H. capsulatum,* and *C. immitis,* also may cause disease. In addition, an occult bacterial focus of infection that was not adequately identified and treated before the transplant may become apparent at this time and cause significant disease.[218]

Herpesviruses

The Herpesviridae (HSV types 1 and 2, CMV, EBV, VZV, and human herpesvirus [HHV] types 6, 7, and 8) share the biologic properties of latency, reactivation, cell association, and oncogenicity, which renders them the most important group of pathogens that affect renal transplant recipients.[196,227] HSV is more important during the early posttransplant period, whereas the other herpesviruses are important causes of morbidity and mortality during the middle and late posttransplant periods.[105]

Cytomegalovirus. CMV may cause primary infection in a CMV-seronegative transplant recipient through a renal allograft or blood product transfusion from a seropositive donor.[20,56,214] Person-to-person transmission within the family or close community also is possible. Recurrent CMV infection develops in seropositive transplant recipients if the recipient's CMV strain becomes reactivated. The renal allograft from a seropositive donor also can be a source of reinfection to the recipient and produce active CMV infection or disease.[46,98] CMV infection in renal transplant recipients may cause silent or asymptomatic infection; end-organ diseases such as hepatitis, esophagitis, colitis, encephalitis, vasculitis, and retinitis; and systematic disease with persistent fever and leukopenia with thrombocytopenia. A case report also linked CMV infection with posttransplant occurrence of atypical hemolytic-uremic syndrome that resolved with plasma exchange and ganciclovir antiviral therapy.[188] It has been linked in some studies to allograft dysfunction and nephropathy.

CMV also causes depressed cell-mediated immunity and impaired alveolar macrophage function, rendering the host more vulnerable to other opportunistic infections, such as fungal disease and *P. jiroveci* pneumonia, and it serves as a cofactor for other viruses, such as EBV and HHV-6 and HHV-7.[129,191,203,250,251] In addition, CMV is associated with acute and chronic rejection and allograft nephropathy and decreased long-term patient survival.[1,71,140,196,214]

Disease caused by CMV can be documented by isolation of CMV from tissue; detection of CMV DNA by PCR or similar assays in blood, bronchoalveolar fluid, or tissue.[27,28,199,204,214] Isolation of PCR detection of CMV in urine or saliva documents active infection but has little significance in diagnosis of organ disease; serologic tests may document seroconversion in primary infections but generally should be reserved for pretransplant screening only. Most transplant patients at risk for acquiring CMV disease (i.e., CMV-seropositive recipients [D^+/R^+] or CMV-seronegative recipients [D^+/R^-] who received a renal allograft from a seropositive donor) should be monitored by viral surveillance, usually by testing blood weekly for quantitative CMV DNA by PCR.[26,110]

Detection of significant levels of the virus by quantitative or semi-quantitative assay, or an increase from baseline levels, usually predicts CMV disease.[251] Reduction of immunosuppression, along with preemptive antiviral therapy, generally is indicated and results in a decrease or resolution of CMV levels detected in blood.[7,28,51,54,90,95,148] Despite receiving adequate antiviral therapy, some patients have persistently positive low, stable levels of CMV DNA by PCR, however, which should be interpreted within the clinical context.[27] In some patients who otherwise appear well, the DNA may be fragmented and nonreplicating, whereas in other patients with persistent symptoms, and rising PCR levels, a strain of CMV resistant to one or more antiviral agents may be the cause.

The antiviral agents currently available for the treatment of CMV disease and preemptive therapy for positive CMV markers include ganciclovir, valganciclovir, foscarnet, and cidofovir.[265] For renal transplant patients with moderate to severe CMV-associated disease, 2 to 3 weeks of therapy with intravenous ganciclovir usually is adequate to treat disease; however, patients with CMV retinitis or repeat episodes of rejection may require maintenance therapy, usually with oral valganciclovir.[117,154,180] Asymptomatic or mild CMV infections may respond to oral valganciclovir administered for 1 to 3 months.[154,172] Preemptive therapy should be continued throughout the period of immunosuppression in patients who are severely immunosuppressed and at risk for development of CMV disease and recurrence (D^+/R^-).[95,110,155,172] Foscarnet and cidofovir have significant renal toxicity and should be used with caution in renal transplant recipients. Prophylaxis for CMV disease is indicated in high-risk transplant recipients (D^+/R^-); options include intravenous CMV immune globulin and oral valganciclovir.[31,79,90,143,180,223,231,238,260]

Epstein-barr virus. EBV infection in children who have received a renal transplant may be asymptomatic or may be associated with a variety of different syndromes, including a nonspecific viral syndrome, mononucleosis, smooth muscle tumors (leiomyoma), posttransplant PTLD, and lymphoma.[29,30,66,100,102,112] Infection and disease may occur after primary and recurrent EBV infection, but primary infection is more likely to occur and produce PTLD in younger children than in adults who have received solid-organ transplants.[39,102] EBV disease may affect 10% of pediatric renal transplant recipients and may develop 1 month to 5 or more years posttransplant, with the risk accumulating every year of posttransplant survival. Recurrence of posttransplant PTLD may also occur years after transplant and may involve unusual sites.[13,62,233]

Knowledge about posttransplant EBV infection and disease is evolving; as graft survival has improved through more intense immunosuppressive regimens that preserve graft function and other opportunistic infections, such as HSV, CMV, and *P. jiroveci,* being successfully managed, EBV has emerged as a formidable obstacle to successful solid-organ transplantation in children.[29,61,63,66,100,127,233] The estimated overall risk for development of serious life-threatening EBV-associated illness is at least 4% and increases to 10% in children who experience a primary infection with EBV after undergoing renal transplantation.[61,112] Other risk factors for PTLD in children who have received solid-organ transplants include receipt of antilymphocyte therapy such as OKT3 for rejection, receipt of tacrolimus, sirolimus, or mycophenolate mofetil rather than cyclosporine for immunosuppression, and CMV or EBV donor/recipient (D^+/R^-) mismatch.[63,121,122]

Nonspecific viral syndromes and mononucleosis occur during the earlier posttransplant period, whereas lymphoma and leiomyoma are more likely to be a manifestation during the late posttransplant period.[31,66,83,100] Uncomplicated posttransplant mononucleosis is characterized by the self-limited illness of fever, pharyngitis, cervical adenopathy, and splenomegaly. The signs and symptoms of PTLD vary but often include persistent fever, weight loss, and generalized adenopathy.[112] The disease frequently is multisystemic and progressive, and involvement of the neck, chest, lungs, gastrointestinal tract, liver, spleen, eyes, and brain, as well as lesions, may be detected by computed tomography of the head, neck, chest, and abdomen.[4,5,195,228] The renal allograft also may be involved and show dysfunction. Lymphoma may be manifested as solid tumors in the renal allograft, lung, liver, spleen, brain, and soft tissues.[83,102] Smooth muscle tumors (leiomyoma) frequently are multicentric and multifocal; they often occur in lung, liver, and spleen but also may occur in unusual locations, including the brain and renal allograft.[29,100,111]

Laboratory diagnosis of posttransplant, EBV-associated disease is based on detection by PCR of EBV DNA in circulating lymphocytes.[5,54,75] Quantitative or semiquantitative PCR assays may show increasing or persistently high copies of EBV DNA in the circulating lymphocytes of patients who are at risk for developing PTLD.[5,99,212,223] If end-organ disease is observed, the diagnosis can be confirmed histopathologically by detection by PCR of EBV DNA in tissue or by in situ hybridization with an EBV-encoded RNA probe.[4,251]

The diseases associated with EBV also may be classified in the laboratory as polyclonal or monoclonal. Polyclonal illnesses seem to be more benign than are monoclonal diseases, which often are associated with chromosomal abnormalities and malignant transformation.[195] The virus cannot be cultivated by routine means; when studied by special culture techniques, EBV has been found frequently in the oropharyngeal secretions of seropositive transplant recipients and is not predictive of EBV-associated disease.[195,212] Similarly, serologic approaches to establishing the diagnosis of EBV infection after a transplant procedure also are nonspecific and difficult to interpret in most patients unless the recipient clearly has seroconverted during the posttransplant period.

Aggressive or intense treatment of uncomplicated EBV-associated viral syndrome or mononucleosis usually is unnecessary because these illnesses seem to be self-limited in most patients. Immunosuppression may be reduced, and acyclovir may be administered; the patient should be monitored carefully. If symptoms in the patient or EBV DNA levels in the blood persist or increase, PTLD should be suspected and the diagnosis should be confirmed.[245,252]

Treatment of established PTLD is challenging.[96] Mortality rates are high, and the best results seem to occur if the disease is diagnosed by quantitative PCR viral-load monitoring and serial imaging studies and treated aggressively.[251] Preemptive therapy instituted when viral surveillance monitoring detects an increase in EBV DNA in circulating lymphocytes before end-organ disease is evident also may be helpful in some patients.[4,54,154] Reduction in immunosuppression remains the most widely recommended strategy, but a variety of regimens have been studied as well.

Antiviral agents such as acyclovir and ganciclovir seem to reduce EBV replication early in the course of the disease process and may halt the progression of disease in some patients.[63,197,265] Antiviral agents are ineffective, however, against latent EBV or cells that have been transformed by the virus. Interferon-α, immunoglobulin, and anti–CD20 monoclonal antibody preparations such as rituximab have been used successfully in patients with established PTLD. Experimental protocols evaluating adoptive immunotherapy in transplant recipients are ongoing. In addition, some experts suggest that administration of intense anti-CMV therapy with ganciclovir and CMV hyperimmune globulin may improve chances of survival in certain patients with PTLD because CMV may serve as a cofactor in progression of disease caused by other members of the Herpesviridae.[1,20,66,200,236,250] Treatment of patients with lymphoma or leiomyoma includes a reduction in immunosuppression, chemotherapy, radiation therapy, and surgical resection of tumors.

Varicella zoster virus. VZV can cause primary (varicella, chickenpox) or reactivation (zoster, shingles) disease in a renal transplant recipient.[195,237] Infection with VZV can occur at any time but does so most often during the middle posttransplant period. Patients have fever and painful or pruritic vesicular skin lesions.[180] Hepatitis, encephalitis, acute or chronic recurrent cerebral vasculitis and vasculopathy, and pneumonia also may occur, even in the absence of skin lesions, especially in an immunocompromised host.[113] Varicella occurs more frequently in children, and zoster occurs more frequently in adolescent and adult transplant recipients.[44]

In contrast to other herpesviruses, VZV almost always is transmitted person to person or by aerosol in health care, family, and community settings; it rarely, if ever, has been linked to the transplanted allograft.[164,195] Before the advent of routine immunization and antiviral therapy, infection with VZV was a major cause of morbidity and mortality in children receiving solid-organ transplants.[44,77,219] Untreated primary varicella may continue for several weeks and result in visceral dissemination, pneumonitis, hepatic necrosis, encephalitis, vasculitis with stroke, disseminated intravascular coagulation, hemorrhagic skin lesions, and death.[77,197,227] Zoster in solid-organ transplant recipients may remain localized to a dermatome, but it often disseminates beyond the dermatomal distribution and produces widespread skin lesions and even visceral dissemination.

The diagnosis of VZV disease often is clinical, but it should be confirmed by isolation of VZV from fresh, vesicular skin lesions or detection of viral antigen by direct immunofluorescence assay on cells obtained by scraping the base of the skin lesion.[197] Tzanck smear may show multinucleated giant cells, suggesting a viral infection, but it cannot differentiate VZV from HSV. Other pathogens, especially HSV, may mimic VZV disease, so establishing an accurate viral diagnosis is important. VZV also may be detected by PCR-based DNA detection methods, which also may distinguish wild-type strains from the OKA vaccine strain of VZV; qualitative and quantitative VZV PCR tests may be performed by reference and research laboratories. Establishing a serologic diagnosis of active VZV infection is difficult. Routine serologic screening performed in the pretransplant period identifies patients who are seronegative and at risk for developing primary infection with VZV.

Treatment of established VZV disease should be instituted as early as possible during the course of the illness because survival is improved if treatment begins before the fifth day of illness.[77] Acyclovir is recommended for most renal transplant recipients experiencing either primary infection with varicella or zoster with dissemination; it is administered intravenously in high doses (500 mg/m^2 per dose every 8 hours if renal function is normal or adjusted for renal function as needed) for 5 to 10 days, or until new lesions have ceased to occur for 24 to 48 hours, old lesions have crusted, the fever has resolved, and disease has abated.[32,189,195,265] Uncomplicated zoster or very mild primary varicella may be treated with oral acyclovir, famciclovir, or valacyclovir, provided that the patient is monitored carefully for clinical response. Ganciclovir, foscarnet, or cidofovir also provide cross-cover protection for most VZV strains, if these antiviral agents are being administered for difficult CMV infections. If acyclovir-resistant varicella develops, then treatment with foscarnet or a combination of two or three antiviral agents may be necessary to control the infection.

Prevention of posttransplant VZV disease can be accomplished by several effective strategies, which should be discussed during the pretransplant evaluation. Transplant recipients who were seronegative for VZV during the pretransplant evaluation should receive varicella vaccine before undergoing transplantation, if possible.[84,131,275] Pretransplant varicella vaccination is safe, beneficial, and cost effective when administered to pediatric renal transplant candidates and in selected renal transplant recipients after a transplant procedure.[32,43,84,85,189]

Seronegative, unimmunized transplant recipients who are exposed to varicella or zoster during the posttransplant period should receive passive immunoprophylaxis with varicella zoster immunoglobulin (VariZig). Preemptive therapy with oral acyclovir also is recommended by some experts in this situation because varicella zoster immunoglobulin does not prevent, but only attenuates, the postexposure disease process. Finally, acyclovir, valacyclovir, ganciclovir, and valganciclovir administered prophylactically to transplant recipients who are seropositive for HSV or CMV also may provide protection against VZV disease.[143,195]

Human herpesviruses types 6, 7, and 8. HHV-6, HHV-7, and HHV-8 also infect renal transplant recipients by primary infection and by reactivation.[41,42,48,74,108,217,218,236] Infection with these viruses becomes evident during the middle posttransplant period, but their roles in specific disease processes are unclear.[197,230,246] HHV-6 and HHV-7 may act as cofactors in the progression of a disease, especially diseases caused by CMV and EBV.[74,129,180,191,250] HHV-8 is associated with Kaposi sarcoma after a transplant procedure in severely immunosuppressed adult renal transplant recipients, but to date it has not been appreciated as a major opportunistic pathogen in pediatric renal transplant recipients.[41,44,76,195,209,225] HHV-8 may be transmitted through the renal allograft or by blood product transfusion, or it can become reactivated in the recipient after transplant surgery.[209]

Polyomaviruses and Papillomaviruses

Polyomaviruses. Human polyomaviruses (JC, BK, and SV40) frequently infect children and are present in urine and stool.[258,259] They can be detected in the urine of 33% to 58% of renal transplant recipients and detected serologically in 56%, and they are found histopathologically and by PCR in blood, body fluids, and tissue in 8% to 13%.* Knowledge about the roles that these viruses play in the outcome of renal transplant patients is evolving.

The JC and BK polyomaviruses seem to have a significant impact on adult and pediatric renal transplant recipients.[6,24,86,153,170,181,183,210,221] BK virus has been implicated in various syndromes, including ureteral stenosis, hemorrhagic or chronic cystitis, interstitial nephritis with graft failure, allograft nephropathy (BK-associated nephropathy [BKAN]), and rejection, in renal transplant recipients.† Disease associated with these viruses most often occurs during the middle and late posttransplant periods. BK virus may be asymptomatic or cause increasing serum creatinine levels, cystitis, tubular necrosis, graft dysfunction, or allograft rejection.[192,207] Risk factors for BKAN seem to include BK serostatus at the time of transplant, greater immunosuppression with use of mycophenolate mofetil, and concurrent CMV infection.[72,88,89,107,146,253]

Ciprofloxacin prophylaxis in kidney transplant recipients has been shown in one recent study to reduce BK virus infection and BKAN 3 months posttransplant, but not at 1 year posttransplant.[270] BK virus historically was detected in urine by the presence of "decoy cells," which are cells containing intranuclear viral inclusions. Currently quantitative PCR assays that detect and quantify BK viral DNA are used for detection. BK viruria precedes BK viremia, which precedes BK nephropathy.[15,109] Patients with BK-associated nephropathy may have BK viral DNA detected in the urine, blood, or plasma, and renal biopsy specimens may show characteristic viral inclusions. Most recently quantitative PCR viral surveillance in blood or plasma has been shown in renal transplant recipients to be useful in predicting the development of BK nephropathy and in guiding preemptive antiviral and immunosuppressive strategies.

Pediatric kidney transplant recipients who have increasing BK viremia levels should be managed preemptively with carefully monitored reduction of immunosuppression to prevent development of more serious complications of BKAN and graft rejection.[205] This strategy usually results in reduction and then clearance of BK viremia and development of BK-specific cellular immunity coincident with BK virus clearance.[146] Treatment of established BKAN includes a reduction in immunosuppression. Cidofovir and fluoroquinolones have activity against BK virus, and both have been used to treat BK virus infection and treat severe disease caused by BKAN.[109,265] Intravenous immune globulin may also be of benefit; one report resulted in decrease of BK viremia and histologic resolution of BKAN.[8]

JC virus causes a rare syndrome called *progressive multifocal leukoencephalopathy.* It may be diagnosed by viral DNA detection using PCR-based assays available in reference and research laboratories or histopathologically by brain biopsy or autopsy examination. Successful treatment options for progressive multifocal leukoencephalopathy caused by JC virus are very limited, and most, if not all, patients die of progressive encephalopathy. An unusual case of JC virus encephalopathy transmitted from a donor kidney was successfully treated by removal of the donor organ.[22]

Papillomaviruses. Human papillomaviruses are common viruses that infect healthy children, adolescents, and adults. Adult renal transplant recipients are at increased risk for development of human papillomavirus–associated disease, such as cervical cancer and anogenital papillomas, whereas pediatric patients may develop numerous disfiguring cutaneous warts posttransplant, especially if they require severe immunosuppression.[186,195,211] Malignant transformation of cutaneous warts caused by high-risk types has been documented.[211] Treatment options are limited but include physical removal of papillomas with laser and cryotherapy and careful reduction of immunosuppression. In one case series report, careful transition of the immunosuppression regimen from tacrolimus-mycophenolate to tacrolimus-leflunomide resulted in resolution of cutaneous warts in four pediatric renal transplant recipients.[179] Human papillomavirus vaccines in patients with ESRD or renal transplant recipients are now recommended to be administered according to the standard immunization schedules.[162]

*References 6, 68, 72, 80, 81, 86, 88, 89, 107, 109, 111, 114, 146, 170, 181, 182, 183, 192, 194, 204, 205, 221, 253.

†References 24, 49, 59, 68, 80, 81, 111, 114, 182, 194, 204, 211, 221.

Adenoviruses

Adenoviruses may infect pediatric renal transplant recipients at any time, but they are most likely to cause significant disease during the middle posttransplant period. They continue to emerge as a significant pathogen in pediatrics, including transplant recipients. They do not seem to play as important a role in renal transplant outcome, however, as do other viruses, such as the herpesviruses, and they currently are not as prominent in renal transplant recipients as they are in other transplant recipients, such as recipients of liver, lung, bone marrow, or stem cell transplants.[94,159,187,195,197] Nonetheless infections with adenoviruses in pediatric renal transplant recipients, when they occur, can be serious and include hemorrhagic cystitis, diarrhea, allograft nephropathy, pneumonia, hepatitis, and disseminated disease with multisystemic involvement.[25,128,218,248,257,268,272]

The diagnosis is made by isolation or detection by PCR of the virus in respiratory secretions, stool, urine, blood, or tissue. Rapid diagnosis may be accomplished within 30 to 60 minutes, using a rapid immunochromatographic assay that detects adenovirus antigens in eye secretions, respiratory samples, urine, and stool. Viral DNA also may be detected by PCR or quantitative PCR available in reference or research laboratories, and characteristic changes may be seen by histopathology in tissue. Adenovirus serotyping by neutralization assays and genotyping by PCR sequence-based assays are available in reference laboratories.[94] Treatment of serious adenoviral disease primarily is supportive. Immunosuppression also may be reduced, when possible. Antiviral agents, such as ribavirin, ganciclovir, and cidofovir, have activity against adenoviruses. Clinical reports of use of cidofovir in traditional weekly dosing and intermittent renal sparing dosing is safe and well tolerated in pediatric transplant recipients with adenovirus disease.[21,40,67]

Human Erythrovirus (Parvovirus B19)

Human erythrovirus has been reported to cause acute and chronic infection, manifesting as chronic anemia, red blood cell aplasia, and pancytopenia in renal transplant recipients.[55,118,120,132,208,262,269] It also has been implicated in collapsing glomerulopathy and thrombotic microangiopathy in renal transplant recipients.[263] Unusual manifestations, such as hepatic necrosis or central nervous system infection with vasculitis, also have been reported.[19,23,137,138] Transmission most likely is person to person; however, some reports indicate that the virus may be transmitted by blood product transfusion or in the renal allograft.[18,19,136] More recent reports suggest that the role that this virus plays in the outcome of renal transplant recipients may be more important than previously recognized, but systemic studies in pediatric patients have not been done.[18]

The diagnosis of acute infection with human erythrovirus is supported by erythrovirus-specific IgG seroconversion; detection of erythrovirus-specific IgM antibodies in serum; or detection of viral DNA in plasma, blood, body fluids, bone marrow, or tissue. The virus is not cultivatable in clinical virology laboratories that use routine cell cultures, but laboratories using special erythroid precursor cell lines may be able to cultivate erythrovirus for research purposes. No specific antiviral therapy is available, but anecdotal experience and case reports support a beneficial role for intravenous immunoglobulin and carefully monitored reduction in immunosuppression as management strategies to resolve erythrovirus viremia and associated end-organ disease.[167]

West Nile Virus

WNV is a single-stranded RNA flavivirus is an important pathogen worldwide. It usually is transmitted by mosquitoes and causes a febrile illness, viral meningoencephalomyelitis, and acute flaccid paralysis in the normal host. Renal transplant recipients may become infected with WNV that is transmitted by the organ donor, by blood product transfusions, or naturally from mosquitoes.[55,118,120,132,208,262,269] Routine screening of solid-organ donors for WNV infection has been discussed but currently is not routinely performed.[118,177] Infection with WNV may manifest in the early posttransplant period if it is transmitted by the graft or blood products and, because of immunosuppression, produce severe febrile illnesses, seizures with status epilepticus, encephalitis, paralysis, and movement disorders. Death also may occur.[55] A high index of suspicion is required; if WNV is suspected, serum and cerebrospinal fluid should be sent for WNV-specific IgG and IgM antibody testing. The virus also may be isolated in special cell cultures and detected by reverse transcriptase PCR-based assays or through metagenomic deep sequencing.[269] Immunohistochemical staining may show WNV proteins in tissues from biopsy or autopsy examination. Outcome in renal transplant recipients with WNV disease improves with early establishment of the diagnosis and carefully managed reduction of immunosuppression.[208]

Zika Virus

Zika virus is another flavivirus that has emerged as an important global pathogen and that may potentially impact kidney transplantation. Zika virus causes a febrile illness with rash, conjunctivitis, headache, malaise, or muscle and joint pain. It may be transmitted from mosquitoes or through sexual transmission, by blood transfusions, or from mother to baby and cause congenital infection and congenital Zika syndrome.[173] The risk of Zika virus transmission through renal transplantation is unknown at this time, but the virus has been detected in the urine as well as the kidney and other organs of Zika-infected individuals.[93,184] Routine screening of donors or recipients for Zika virus infection is not currently recommended unless there is a recent history of travel or exposure or illness associated with Zika virus within 6 months of kidney transplantation. Pretransplant evaluation should include a careful travel history within 6 months to an area with active Zika virus transmission and a history for signs and symptoms associated with Zika virus infection in either the donor or the recipient. Since the risk of Zika virus transmission through renal transplantation is unknown at this time, Zika virus infection or exposure is not a contraindication to renal transplantation, but the risk of donor-derived infection should be balanced with the potential benefits of transplantation in each potential renal transplant recipient.[184]

Mycoplasma

Mycoplasma spp. commonly infect school-aged children. Children and adolescents who undergo renal transplantation also may experience respiratory tract infections with *M. pneumoniae* and *M. hominis.* The infection also may disseminate to extrapulmonary sites, causing hepatitis, septic arthritis, or perinephric fluid collections in pediatric renal transplant recipients.[126,157,239] *Mycoplasma* spp. may be detected using special biphasic culture media or PCR-based assays. Serologic diagnosis is difficult to accomplish owing to cross-reactivity of antigens producing the possibility of false-positive reactions in some patients. Antimicrobial therapy with macrolide antibiotics, along with carefully managed reduction of immunosuppression, may be beneficial in selected patients.[126,157]

Bacterial and Mycobacterial Diseases

Bacteria that commonly produce disease in renal transplant recipients during the middle posttransplant period include *L. monocytogenes,* which often causes sepsis or meningitis.[195,232] Routine bacterial illnesses that were not identified and properly treated during the pretransplant period also may emerge at this time and cause abscesses, sepsis syndrome, and death.

Mycobacterial disease caused by *M. tuberculosis* may occur at any time after transplantation, but it occurs most frequently during the middle posttransplant period.[141,144,195,206] *M. tuberculosis* causes disease in approximately 1% of renal transplant recipients in the developed continents, such as North America and Europe, and in 15% of renal transplant recipients in developing countries with a high prevalence of tuberculosis, such as India or Pakistan.[123,195,206,213,222,224] Tuberculosis may develop in renal transplant recipients as a result of primary and reactivation infection in almost any site, and transmission from the renal allograft and reactivation in the native kidney have occurred.[133,168,169,213] *M. tuberculosis* may cause various diseases, including pulmonary infiltrates, cavitary lesions, adenopathy, cutaneous lesions, bone and joint disease, liver or spleen granulomas, and meningitis. Fever frequently is noted, and miliary or disseminated disease may occur, especially in young children.

Because the TST is negative in most renal transplant recipients with active tuberculosis, the diagnosis is determined best by IGR assays, detection of acid-fast bacilli in smears from tissue or sputum, and isolation of *M. tuberculosis* in cultures of gastric aspirates, sputum, tracheal secretions, spinal fluid, or tissue.[144,195] The presence of granulomas in tissue also suggests the diagnosis of tuberculosis.

Treatment of tuberculosis in a renal transplant recipient usually includes isoniazid, rifampin, and pyrazinamide for 1 year, although shorter courses may be acceptable in some patients.[141,195] Other antituberculous drugs may be added to or substituted for this standard regimen, depending on the disease process, the susceptibility pattern of the organism, and potential drug interactions. Because many antituberculosis drugs are excreted by the kidney, doses may need to be adjusted in a renal transplant recipient. Because rifampin may interact with cyclosporine, levels of cyclosporine should be monitored closely to avoid rejection of the allograft.[185] If a history of tuberculosis exposure is elicited during the pretransplant evaluation, the transplant candidate should be evaluated for tuberculosis, including having a TST, IGR assay on blood, and chest radiograph.[168,169,206] All close contacts also should be investigated for evidence of having tuberculosis. Treatment is recommended if disease is discovered, and prophylaxis with isoniazid is indicated for most patients who have a recently positive result of a purified protein derivative (PPD) test on pretransplant evaluation.[141,195,197,224,274] A transplant recipient who receives an allograft from a donor with a history of tuberculosis or a positive TST or IGR assay also may be a candidate for prophylaxis with isoniazid after a transplant procedure.[141,195,197]

Atypical mycobacteria are ubiquitous nontuberculous mycobacteria that can infect and produce disease in renal transplant recipients. They can cause disease during the middle posttransplant period and so are included here. Their effects usually do not become evident, however, until many years after the patient has undergone transplantation, during the late posttransplant period.[53,169,198] Atypical mycobacteria that have been documented to cause disease in solid-organ transplant recipients include *M. kansasii, M. avium-intracellulare, M. fortuitum, M. xenopi, M. haemophilum, M. marinum, M. chelonae, M. abscessus, M. gastri, M. scrofulaceum,* and *M. thermoresistibile.*[123,195,197]

A high index of suspicion is necessary to detect these elusive pathogens. They should be considered as the cause of disease in patients with persistent cutaneous ulcers, abscesses, adenopathy, pulmonary nodules, chronic wound infections, or bone and joint disease after negative routine bacterial cultures have been obtained and the patient has failed to respond to standard antimicrobial therapy.[218] Disseminated, multisystemic disease also can occur. Environmental sources of atypical mycobacteria include contaminated dialysis equipment, soil, and contaminated water in aquariums and pools. The diagnosis is established by isolation of nontuberculous mycobacteria in fluid or tissue. Granulomas are not observed consistently in tissue, and acid-fast stains may be negative.[218] Atypical nontuberculous mycobacteria are difficult to treat, and treatment must be individualized to each patient. Strategies include reduction of immunosuppression and surgical débridement of localized disease. Antimicrobial therapy based on in vitro susceptibility testing of the isolate also should be administered, often for a prolonged period.

Nocardia

Nocardia asteroides is the most common *Nocardia* spp. causing illness in renal transplant recipients; however, other, more unusual *Nocardia* spp., including *N. transvalensis, N. brasiliensis, N. nova, N. otitidiscaviarum,* and *N. farcinica,* also have been shown to cause disease in solid-organ transplant recipients.[195,197,268] The most common manifestations of nocardial disease in transplant recipients are fever, cough, and pulmonary infiltrates.[268] Pleural effusion, pulmonary nodules, and cavitary lesions also may occur. Cutaneous infection, adenitis, arthritis, meningitis with brain abscesses, and infection of the renal allograft also may occur. *Nocardia* spp. can be seen on Gram and modified acid-fast stains of sputum, bronchoalveolar lavage fluid, abscess fluid, and tissue. They can be isolated on routine media but may take longer than conventional bacteria to grow. Prolonged treatment with sulfonamides, alone or in combination with trimethoprim, is recommended. Amikacin and other antimicrobial agents may be added in selected patients with severe disease, provided that renal function is monitored closely.[218] Trimethoprim-sulfamethoxazole prophylaxis for UTI and *P. jiroveci* also may be effective in preventing disease caused by *Nocardia.*

Fungal Diseases

Fungal infections occur infrequently in renal transplant recipients relative to other solid-organ transplant recipients.[12,195,197,218] This lower rate of infection probably is related to technical procedures performed at the time of transplantation and the lower level of immunosuppression required to maintain most renal allografts.[218] When they do occur, however, fungal infections often are serious and life threatening.[101,105,115] Fungal disease in a renal transplant recipient usually is manifested in one of two ways: (1) pulmonary or disseminated disease caused by one of the environmental mycoses, such as *H. capsulatum* or *C. immitis,* or (2) opportunistic infection with fungi that rarely cause disease in a normal host, such as *Candida* spp., *P. jiroveci, Aspergillus* spp., *Cryptococcus neoformans, Nocardia* spp., and others.[101,234]

Travel to endemic areas increases a transplant recipient's risk for development of histoplasmosis and coccidioidomycosis and may be identified during the pretransplant evaluation. Factors that increase a transplant recipient's risk for acquisition of opportunistic fungal disease include underlying conditions such as diabetes mellitus, repeated episodes of rejection, long-term administration of corticosteroids, prolonged use of antibiotics, and CMV infection. Similar to tuberculosis, invasive fungal disease can be a result of primary infection or reactivation infection with secondary dissemination.[218] *P. jiroveci,* currently classified as a fungus, may cause pneumonia in 10% of solid-organ transplant recipients, most often during the first 6 months after a transplant procedure.[9,195,197] It seems to occur more commonly in children than in adults and usually causes fever, dyspnea, tachypnea, hypoxemia, and a nonproductive cough.[69,195] Interstitial pulmonary infiltrates are typical findings, but almost any radiographic picture can be observed, and pneumothorax is common in severe disease. The diagnosis can be suspected clinically but is documented best by organisms being shown in lung biopsy specimens; bronchoalveolar lavage may provide the diagnosis in some patients.

Treatment with high-dose oral or intravenous trimethoprim-sulfamethoxazole for 14 to 21 days is used most often. Intravenous pentamidine may be administered to selected patients, but renal function should be monitored carefully.[218] Corticosteroids may be helpful in treating severe disease if given early in the course. Low-dose oral trimethoprim-sulfamethoxazole provides effective prophylaxis against *P. jiroveci* pneumonia and UTIs and usually is administered to renal transplant recipients for at least 6 months posttransplant.[82] Transplant recipients experiencing repeated episodes of rejection, allograft dysfunction, or CMV disease may require a longer period of prophylaxis.[195,197] Aerosolized pentamidine is an alternative prophylaxis strategy for some patients.[218]

Candida spp., especially *C. albicans,* are the opportunistic fungi most frequently isolated in renal transplant recipients.[195,197] Other *Candida* spp. isolated include *C. krusei, C. glabrata,* and *C. tropicalis,* and others. The newly recognized *C. haemulonii* and *C. auris,* potentially fatal, multidrug resistant species of *Candida* causing health care–associated bloodstream infections, have not yet been documented in pediatric renal transplant recipients but remain a potential risk for these patients.[36] Most fungal infections caused by *Candida* spp. occur during the first 2 months after transplant surgery, usually at the site of indwelling intravascular and urinary catheters.[218] Esophagitis, abscesses, and arthritis also can develop, and endocarditis with metastatic foci can occur if the fungemia persists. Other opportunistic fungi such as *Aspergillus* most often cause sinusitis and pulmonary disease, and, because of its angioinvasive nature, *Aspergillus* often disseminates and causes lesions in the liver, spleen, and brain.[195,197,234,235]

A thorough search for metastatic foci always should be undertaken when a primary focus of invasive fungal disease is documented. *C. neoformans* usually causes cutaneous lesions or abscesses and pneumonia with pleural effusion, but meningitis, arthritis, and pyelonephritis also can occur.[195,197,229] Exposure to soil or bird droppings provides an epidemiologic clue to the diagnosis. In addition, the Zygomycetes, including *Rhizopus, Mucor, Rhizomucor,* and *Absidia* spp., can cause disease in solid-organ transplant recipients.[234,235] They most often cause cutaneous, rhinocerebral, or pulmonary disease or brain abscesses in renal transplant patients. Cutaneous and soft tissue infections, wound infections, and gastrointestinal disease with perforation also have been described. The Zygomycetes, similar to *Aspergillus,* are angioinvasive and disseminate via the bloodstream to cause disease, which often is severe. A variety of unusual fungi, such as *Paecilomyces, Fusarium,* and *Bipolaris,* have been shown to cause cutaneous infection, usually at the site of indwelling catheters, and *Hansenula anomala* reportedly has caused UTI in a renal transplant recipient.[91]

The endemic dimorphic fungi include *H. capsulatum, C. immitis, B. dermatitidis,* and *Paracoccidioides brasiliensis.* Infection with these organisms can occur at any time after the patient has undergone transplantation but usually occurs during the intermediate posttransplant period.[249] These organisms usually are noted in renal transplant recipients who reside in endemic areas. Histoplasmosis is endemic in the central part of the United States and many foreign countries, and nosocomial outbreaks have occurred during hospital construction projects. Fever, chills, and cough are the usual initial signs. Skin lesions, hepatosplenomegaly, and meningitis also can occur. Pancytopenia often is present as well, and the organism frequently is found in the bone marrow of patients with disseminated disease. Coccidioidomycosis is endemic in the southwestern portion of the United States and northern Mexico. It usually is manifested as fever, cough, and pulmonary infiltrates, but extrapulmonary dissemination frequently occurs. Blastomycosis is endemic in the southern United States, along the Mississippi and Ohio River valleys, and in the Great Lakes area. It is a rare development after renal transplantation, but most often causes lung and skin lesions. Paracoccidioidomycosis rarely has been reported in renal transplant recipients.[244]

The diagnosis of invasive fungal disease is established best by isolating the fungus from sputum or tracheal aspirate, bone marrow, tissue, or fluid. Serum tests and bronchoalveolar lavage for galactomannan and 1-3-β-D-glucan levels support the diagnosis of invasive fungal disease, and DNA PCR tests on serum and bronchoalveolar lavage fluid also may now be performed to detect *Candida* spp. and other fungi.[12]

C. neoformans also may be isolated from urine. Fungal-specific serology and tests for cryptococcal antigen may support the diagnosis of cryptococcal infection.[244]

Fungal identification and susceptibility testing now can be performed in clinical and reference laboratories and should be used to guide therapy whenever possible. Amphotericin B usually is used to treat most invasive fungal disease in transplant recipients, and the deoxycholate, lipid complex, or liposomal forms can be used, provided that renal function is monitored closely.[142] Flucytosine may have additive or synergistic effects against many yeasts and fungi. The azole antifungal agents are not nephrotoxic and are used in renal transplant recipients whenever possible. Many *Candida* spp. are susceptible to fluconazole, although resistance is emerging in all *Candida* spp. and is present in a high percentage of *C. krusei* and *C. glabrata.* Itraconazole and voriconazole may be effective against other fungi, such as *Aspergillus.*[12] Voriconazole is the treatment of choice for most *Aspergillus* infections. Itraconazole should be used with caution because it has variable oral absorption and may interact with cyclosporine.[249] Caspofungin, an echinocandin, also has activity against most *Candida* spp. and a variety of opportunistic fungi, including some species of *Aspergillus.* The triazole posaconazole and the echinocandin micafungin have also been used successfully in pediatric renal transplant recipients with invasive fungal disease.

Surgical resection or drainage of abscesses, avascular cavities, or effusions may be required to treat some forms of invasive fungal disease of the lungs, liver, or spleen. Carefully monitored reduction in immunosuppression also may help the host recover from invasive fungal disease.

Parasitic Infections

The parasites most commonly encountered in renal transplant recipients during the intermediate posttransplant period are *T. gondii, S. stercoralis,* and *Trypanosoma cruzi.*[78,195] These infections occur most often in adults. Children also may be infected with routine parasites such as *Enterobius vermicularis, Ascaris, Giardia,* and others before a transplant operation. Other parasitic infections that may be found in renal transplant recipients include leishmaniasis, schistosomiasis, and malaria. Renal transplant recipients seem to be at much lower risk for acquisition of parasitic diseases than are other solid-organ transplant recipients.

Infection with *T. gondii* usually occurs as a result of reactivation of latent disease in the donor allograft or recipient.[149] It is encountered most frequently in heart transplant recipients, but any solid-organ recipient, including renal transplant patients, may be affected. Clinical manifestations of infection with *T. gondii* include focal meningoencephalitis, brain abscesses, pneumonia, myocarditis, pericarditis, hepatitis, and retinochoroiditis.[163,240,249,256] The diagnosis may be made by demonstration of the organism in tissue by histopathology, detection of DNA by PCR in body fluids or tissue, or serologically by detection of high titers of IgG and specific IgM antibody to *T. gondii.* Treatment with pyrimethamine, sulfadiazine, and folinic acid usually is recommended; however, some patients also may respond to clindamycin. Routine prophylaxis with trimethoprim-sulfamethoxazole for UTI and *P. jiroveci* infection may help prevent disease with *T. gondii.*

S. stercoralis is an important pathogen in adult transplant recipients, but it is rarely, if ever, a significant problem in pediatric patients. Because *S. stercoralis* can be maintained in the human intestinal tract for decades, it can disseminate and cause serious disease in transplant recipients who were infected before the procedure. A complete blood cell count for eosinophilia should be obtained, and stool and other specimens should be examined for rhabditiform larvae if the pretransplant evaluation reveals travel to endemic areas. Thiabendazole should be given before transplantation is performed if *S. stercoralis* infection has been documented or is suspected. *T. cruzi,* the cause of Chagas disease, rarely has been transmitted by renal transplantation.[78,139]

Infections Occurring During the Late Posttransplant Period

Infections occurring 6 months or more after the patient has undergone renal transplantation usually are less severe than infections experienced in the earlier periods, especially if the level of immunosuppressive therapy is low and the allograft is functioning well.[217] Constant vigilance for health care–associated and community-acquired viral and bacterial diseases and unusual infections should continue, however.

Chronic rejection or repeated episodes of acute rejection complicated by allograft dysfunction predispose the patient to development of more serious opportunistic infections, similar to infections encountered during the first 6 months after a transplant. UTIs that develop during this period, in contrast to UTIs in the early posttransplant period, usually are benign, especially if the patient is afebrile, and may be treated with conventional antimicrobial therapy in most instances if they do not seem to threaten the function of the allograft or the patient's survival. Patients also may experience community-acquired infections with respiratory viruses, such as influenza virus and respiratory syncytial virus, and with bacteria, especially *Streptococcus pneumoniae* (pneumococcus) or *S. aureus.* These common community-acquired bacterial pathogens may be resistant to usual β-lactam antibiotics.[241,254] In addition, patients vaccinated with 7-valent or 23-valent pneumococcal vaccines still may acquire invasive pneumococcal disease with emerging, nonvaccine serotypes, such as 19A and 3A. These serotypes often are also multidrug resistant. Opportunistic viral infections encountered during this period are zoster or, rarely, CMV retinitis.[172] The risk for developing PTLD and BKAN also persists during this late posttransplant period.

Renal transplant recipients may be chronically infected with HBV or HCV before a transplant is performed. Increased risk for mortality from fulminant hepatitis with hepatic failure may occur during the early pretransplant period, and chronic liver disease, cirrhosis, and liver failure may be seen 10 years or more after renal transplantation has been performed in hepatitis B surface antigen (HBsAg)–positive recipients.[273] All transplant recipients who are not immune to HBV should receive HBV vaccine before transplantation.[264] Most experts agree that renal allografts from HBsAg-positive donors should not be used, but the decision to perform renal transplantation in recipients who are HBsAg-positive is controversial and must be made on an individualized basis.

Renal transplant recipients who are infected with HCV before the transplant usually do well during the early posttransplant period, but long-term survival is poorer than in recipients who are not infected with HCV. Not only can chronic liver disease develop, but also membranoproliferative glomerulonephritis has been reported in renal transplant recipients infected with HCV.[33] Despite these risks, however, most experts do not consider infection with HCV a contraindication for renal transplantation in patients with ESRD.[201] Hepatitis G virus also has been detected in the serum of renal transplant recipients, and at least one association with membranous glomerulonephritis has been reported.[16,17] The role of HGV in clinical disease in renal transplant recipients is not established, however.

HIV may be transmitted by kidney transplantation despite routine screening of donors of blood and organs.[136,211] A transplant recipient also may become infected with HIV after undergoing transplantation.[195] Shortly after a patient has undergone transplantation, HIV infection may cause fever and a mononucleosis-like syndrome. Complications of acquired immunodeficiency syndrome may develop during the late transplant period. HIV-infected patients with ESRD are no longer excluded from receiving renal transplantation because recent studies have shown successful outcomes.[103,106,174,195]

NEW REFERENCES SINCE THE SEVENTH EDITION

22. Bialasiewicz S, Hart G, Oliver K, et al. A difficult decision: atypical JC polyomavirus encephalopathy in a kidney transplant recipient. *Transplantation.* 2016;101(6):1461-1467.
35. Caliskan B, Yazici H, Gulluoglu M, et al. Renal transplantation in a patient with 33aa. chronic granulomatous disease: case report. *Transplant Proc.* 2015;47(1):158.
36. Calvo B, Melo A, Perozo-Mena A, et al. First report of *Candida auris* in America: clinical and microbiological aspects of 18 episodes of candidemia. *J Infect.* 2016;73(4):369.
37. Cameron BM, Kennedy SE, Rawlinson WD, et al. The efficacy of valganciclovir for prevention of infections with cytomegalovirus and Epstein-Barr virus after kidney transplant in children. *Pediatr Transplant.* 2017;21(1).
47. Ciricillo J, Haslam D, Blum S, et al. Frequency and risks associated with *Clostridium difficile*-associated diarrhea after pediatric solid organ transplantation: a single-center retrospective review. *Transpl Infect Dis.* 2016;18(5):706.
93. Gourinat AC, O'Connor O, Calvez E, et al. Detection of Zika virus in urine. *Emerg Infect Dis.* 2015;21(1):84.
158. Michael M, Minard CG, Kale AS, et al. Outcomes of two-drug maintenance immunosuppression for pediatric renal transplantation:10 yr follow-up in a single center. *Pediatr Transplant.* 2016;20(1):49.
162. Miyairi I, Funaki T, Saltoh A. Immunization practices in solid organ transplant recipients. *Vaccine.* 2016;34(16):1958.
173. Musso D, Nhan T, Robin E, et al. Potential for Zika virus transmission through blood transfusion demonstrated during an outbreak in French Polynesia, November 2013–February 2014. *Euro Surveill.* 2014;19(14):62.
179. Nguyen L, McClellan RB, Chaudhuri A, et al. Conversion from tacrolimus/mycophenolic acid to tacrolimus/lefunomide to treat cutaneous warts in a series of four pediatric renal allograft recipients. *Transplantation.* 2012;94(5):450.
184. Nogueira M, Estofolate CF, Terzian AC, et al. Zika virus infection and solid organ transplantation: a new challenge. *Am J Transplant.* 2017;17(3):791-795.
215. Rocca S, Santilli V, Cotugno N, et al. Waning of vaccine-induced immunity to measles in kidney transplanted children. *Medicine (Baltimore).* 2016;95(37):e4738.
220. Saeed B. Pediatric renal transplantation. *Int J Organ Transplant Med.* 2012;3(2):62.
223. Sato T, Fjuieda M, Maeda A, et al. Monitoring of Epstein-Barr virus load and killer T cells in pediatric renal transplant recipients. *Clin Nephrol.* 2008;70(5):393.
226. Scotto G, Aucella F, Grandaliano G, et al. Hepatitis E in hemodialysis and kidney transplant patients in south-east Italy. *World J Gastroenterol.* 2015;21(11):3266.
243. Sue PK, Pisanic N, Heaney CD, et al. Hepatitis E virus infection among solid organ transplant recipients at a North American transplant center. *Open Forum Infect Dis.* 2016;3(1):ofw006.
261. Varghese PS. Pediatric kidney transplantation: a historical review. *Pediatr Res.* 2017;81(1-2):259-264.
269. Wilson MR, Zimmermann LL, Crawford ED, et al. Acute West Nile virus meningoencephalitis diagnosed via metagenomic deep sequencing of cerebrospinal fluid in a renal transplant patient. *Am J Transplant.* 2017;17(3):803-808.

The full reference list for this chapter is available at ExpertConsult.com.

Infections Related to Prosthetic or Artificial Devices

74

Tina Q. Tan • Leena B. Mithal

The development of biomaterials used in the manufacturing of temporary or permanent implantable prosthetic devices has been one of the greatest advances in modern medicine.[94,119,120] These devices have become an integral and important part of the current practice of medicine and have improved considerably the lives and health of countless patients. In the United States, the number and types of permanent prosthetic devices implanted to replace diseased or damaged body parts has increased substantially during the past several decades. An estimated 3 million or more people in the United States currently have some type of long-term biomedical implant.[108,434,511] Box 74.1 lists implantable prosthetic devices discussed in this chapter.

One of the major medical complications associated with the use of implantable prosthetic devices is infection, which may result in serious tissue destruction and dysfunction of the prosthetic device or in local and systemic consequences that may be life threatening. In most cases, these infections are very difficult to cure with antimicrobial agents alone, and removal of the device usually is required for resolution of the infection.

INTERACTION OF THE HOST WITH A PROSTHETIC DEVICE

The prosthetic devices currently in use are composed of a variety of biomaterials, including cobalt-chromium-molybdenum alloy, titanium alloy, and complex polymers such as polytetrafluoroethylene, silicone, and polyethylene, which in general are chosen for their inert, nonreactive, and nontoxic qualities. The interplay of both implant and host factors determines the risk for acquiring and the severity of infection. The human body has numerous well-developed defense mechanisms to protect it against possible invasion by various microorganisms. Such mechanisms include cellular and humoral immune systems, anatomic barriers, and an elaborate network of cells that phagocytize and destroy invading organisms. The presence of a foreign body may compromise one or more of these defenses and elicit a complex acute or chronic inflammatory response (or both) from the host. Many of these devices breach cutaneous and mucosal barriers, thereby creating a direct route by which bacteria and fungi may invade. In addition, implanted devices may alter the local immunity of the host directly or indirectly.[119,434,511,540]

Shortly after being implanted, hydrophobic polymeric materials such as polyethylene, Dacron, polydimethylsiloxane, and polyether urethanes become coated with a layer of host proteins such as plasma and interstitial fluid proteins (i.e., fibronectin, albumin, laminin, collagen, immunoglobulin G, fibrinogen) that bind to and are absorbed readily into the surface of the implant.[35,386,512] This protein layer (especially fibrinogen) has a major influence on the body's response to and the biocompatibility of the implant. The presence of fibrinogen attracts a large number of phagocytic cells (i.e., neutrophils, monocytes, and macrophages) to the implant; these cells interact with the implant surface and initiate an acute inflammatory response.[119,511] Some of these host proteins also serve as a receptor for various colonizing microorganisms. Collagen, laminin, and fibrinogen have been reported to play a role in adherence of bacteria,[545] and fibronectin has been found to be the major receptor for gram-positive cocci, especially *Staphylococcus aureus.*[418,523]

Chronic inflammatory responses, also known as *foreign body reactions,* are seen around many types of biomaterial implants and arise from interactions among the protein-coated surfaces of the implant and host tissues and adhering phagocytic cells such as macrophages and foreign body giant cells. These interactions may result in degradation and damage to the implant from the continuous generation of toxic catabolites and release of inflammatory mediators such as hydrolases, activated complement components, tumor necrosis factor (TNF), interleukins, prostaglandins, coagulation factors, and plasminogen activator by the phagocytic cells.[511,540,507]

INTERACTION OF MICROORGANISMS WITH A PROSTHETIC DEVICE

Once a prosthetic device is implanted, the surface of the device provides a potential area for adherence and multiplication of bacteria. Adherence is a complex process that involves electrostatic attachment of the bacteria to the surface of the implant, bacterial mechanisms that function specifically in attachment, and host-derived substances that coat the prosthetic device and serve as receptors for various bacteria. Bacteria arrive at the surface of the implant by many different routes; they may be inoculated at the time of implantation, the patient may have episodes of transient bacteremia, the device may be exposed by local trauma or infection, or the device may be implanted within an area in which the organism is part of the normal flora.[108,119]

Adherence of bacteria to the surface of an implant is influenced by numerous different factors, including the material used to make the device, the source of the device material (adherence is greater with synthetic material than with biomaterial), the surface of the device (i.e., irregular more than regular, textured more than smooth, hydrophobic more than hydrophilic), and the shape of the device.[108] Cell surface molecules or structures known as *adhesins* also play a role in adherence by attaching or binding an organism to specific receptors on implant surfaces; different bacteria use different adhesins to attach to and colonize medical implants. For example, *Staphylococcus epidermidis* uses proteinaceous autolysin and capsular polysaccharide intercellular adhesin for initial adherence to the implant surface and for adherence of bacteria to each other. These bacteria also produce a biofilm that increases cell-to-cell association and allows accumulation of bacteria.[442] *Streptococcus pyogenes* uses lipoteichoic acid as its adhesin, whereas *S. aureus* uses both lipoteichoic acid and host-tissue ligands (e.g., fibronectin, fibrinogen, and collagen) for adherence. Binding of *S. aureus* to host-tissue ligands is mediated by genetically defined microbial surface proteins known as *microbial surface components recognizing adhesive matrix molecules* (MSCRAMM).[109] *Escherichia coli* and other bacteria use fimbriae as an adhesin to mediate binding to receptors on the surfaces of target cells.

Bacteria also can protect themselves from host defenses by synthesizing and excreting numerous complex polysaccharides, known as *glycocalyces,* that function either as part of the bacterial capsule or as the slime layer. This slime layer is known to play a major role in keeping an organism attached to an implant surface by coalescing with the polysaccharides of other bacteria and with host products to produce a thick, adherent, and somewhat impenetrable biofilm.[541] The biofilm functions by trapping nutrients and protecting the organism from phagocytosis, antimicrobial agents, and competing microflora. It also plays a role in inhibiting the response to chemotactic stimuli, increases both *N*-formyl-methionyl-leucyl-phenylalanine (FMLP)-induced superoxide generation and release of specific granules, and impairs natural killer cell function while also altering the composition of T-lymphocyte cell subpopulations.[176,179,236,541] Therefore the biofilm aids bacteria in evading host cellular and humoral defense mechanisms and thereby allows the organism to colonize and infect an implanted device effectively.

Substantial progress has been made in our understanding of the pathogenesis, prevention, and treatment of foreign body infections; this increased knowledge has resulted in a dramatic decrease in the morbidity associated with these infections, as well as subsequent

BOX 74.1 Partial List of Implantable Devices Prone to Infection

Central nervous system shunts
Intracranial pressure monitors
Intrathecal pump infusion
Orthopedic prostheses (artificial hip, knee, and other joints; screws, pins, plates, and rods)
Intracardiac pacemakers and defibrillators
Left ventricular assist devices
Extracorporeal membrane oxygenation circuits
Ocular prostheses (artificial globes, intraocular lenses, ocular explants)
Cochlear implant devices
Tissue expander devices

improvement in the patient's quality of life. The following sections discuss specific device-related infections and the suggested treatment and management of these infections.

TISSUE EXPANDERS

The use of soft tissue expansion in reconstructive surgery was reported in the literature first in 1957, and since that time it has been used widely for the correction of multiple problems in plastic and reconstructive surgery in the adult and pediatric populations.[21,30] These expanders consist of an alloplastic prosthesis with a filling port that is implanted into a subcutaneous pocket. The expander is filled with saline through the filling port at various intervals to create adequate expansion of the skin. Subsequent improvements of this technique led to the development of osmotic tissue expanders. The Osmed osmotic tissue expander is made of an osmotically active hydrogel (vinyl pyrrolidone and methyl methacrylate) in a silicone construct. When implanted, water is drawn from the surrounding tissues into the device, which can spontaneously expand up to 10 times its original volume. In children, tissue expansion is used most commonly to provide coverage for skin defects caused by burns, trauma, hemangiomas, and other congenital deformities.[61,91,326,373,508,572]

The most common complication of tissue expansion is infection of the subcutaneous expander pocket, usually with skin organisms introduced during insertion of the expander.[393] Cellulitis of the overlying skin and hematogenous or lymphatic seeding of the expander pocket are seen as well but occur much less frequently.[21,154,165,221,318,326,365] In several pediatric case series, the infection rate ranged from 3.4% to 11%.[1,165,326] *S. aureus, S. epidermidis,* and group A streptococci are the microorganisms recovered most commonly from these infections.[165,221,321,326] Less commonly, nontypeable *Haemophilus influenzae,*[326] *Pseudomonas aeruginosa, E. coli,* and *Actinomyces* spp.[345] have been isolated from infections of expander pockets.[321]

In cases of infection of subcutaneous pockets, treatment consists of removal of the tissue expander, debridement and drainage of the subcutaneous pocket, and administration of intravenous antibiotic therapy tailored to the organism isolated. For cellulitis of the overlying skin of an expander pocket, treatment with intravenous antibiotics but without removal of the tissue expander has been shown to be successful.[21]

The most common empirical antimicrobial therapeutic regimen consists of a first-generation cephalosporin or an extended-spectrum, penicillinase-resistant penicillin. For all of the infections of prosthetic devices discussed in the chapter, empirical antistaphylococcal coverage should include agents effective against community strains of methicillin-resistant *S. aureus* (MRSA) if warranted by their frequency in the area.

Therapy is tailored once the organism has been identified and its antibiotic susceptibility has been determined.

COCHLEAR IMPLANTS

During the past several decades, cochlear implantation has emerged as one of the best methods of providing auditory rehabilitation for the profoundly deaf (congenital or acquired). The goal of this surgery in young children is to provide hearing that is adequate to facilitate the development of receptive and expressive language. The surgical technique involves the creation of a C-shaped flap in the postauricular and parietal-occipital scalp skin areas, elevation of the flap, implantation of a multichannel prosthesis, and insertion of an electrode array into the cochlea through openings drilled into the temporal bone.[97,102,312]

The most common infectious complications associated with these implants are cellulitis of the overlying skin flap,[305] acute mastoiditis,[143,429] meningitis, otitis media, and delayed cochlear implant infections leading to extrusion of the implant.* Rates of infection range from 0.3% to 0.5% for meningitis, 2% to 12% for cellulitis of the skin flap and delayed cochlear implant infections, and to 36% for otitis media. The reported cases of meningitis have occurred in association with leakage of cerebrospinal fluid (CSF) in persons with a malformed cochlea who undergo cochlear implantation, as a consequence of intracranial spread of a developing middle ear infection along the electrode pathway, or via pneumococcal bacteremia with hematogenous seeding of the cochlea—for example, at a site of tissue necrosis related to the electrode or positioner with contiguous spread to the CSF and meninges. In June 2002, the U.S. Food and Drug Administration (FDA) received numerous reports of bacterial meningitis in children with cochlear implants who were younger than 6 years when they received the implants. The most common causative organism identified was *Streptococcus pneumoniae,* followed by nontypeable and type b *H. influenzae.* Other less common organisms that have been reported include *S. pyogenes, Acinetobacter baumannii, E. coli,* and *Enterococcus* spp.[433] The incidence of pneumococcal meningitis in this group of patients was calculated to be 138.2 cases per 100,000 person-years—more than 30 times the incidence in the same-aged cohort in the general population. This increased incidence of meningitis was found to be associated strongly with the use of a cochlear implant with a positioner (a wedge-shaped insert that facilitates transmission of the electrical signal by pushing the electrode against the medial wall of the cochlea) in conjunction with the presence of radiographic evidence of a malformation of the inner ear and leakage of CSF. Cochlear implants with a positioner were voluntarily recalled in the United States in July 2002, although removal of existing implants containing a positioner was not recommended; use of appropriate vaccination against *S. pneumoniae* and type b *H. influenzae* was strongly recommended.[28,50,174,433] On February 24, 2010, a 13-valent pneumococcal conjugate vaccine (PCV13) was licensed by the FDA. This vaccine contains polysaccharides of the seven serotypes in PCV7 and polysaccharides from six additional serotypes. This vaccine replaces PCV7 for all scheduled doses of PCV7 in infants. A supplemental dose of PCV13 is recommended for children 14 months through 18 years of age with a cochlear implant.[2] Children with cochlear implants may have a higher risk for middle ear infections because of several factors, including the naturally high incidence of acute otitis media in this population, the presence of a foreign body in the area of the infection, and the potential for spread of the infection into the cochlea along the electrode pathway. In a study of 50 children who received cochlear implants between 1991 and 1995, researchers found that children prone to the development of otitis media before undergoing implantation were at higher risk for developing postimplantation acute otitis media but responded well to routine oral antimicrobial therapy. The overall prevalence and the severity of acute otitis media were not found to be increased in children with cochlear implants.[309]

In cases of cellulitis of the skin flap, intravenous antimicrobial therapy should include empirical broad-spectrum antimicrobial agents effective against community strains of MRSA, methicillin-susceptible strains of *S. aureus,* and group A streptococci. Empirical antimicrobial therapy for meningitis usually consists of vancomycin and a third-generation cephalosporin that is tailored to the organism isolated. An exception is for children with the onset of meningitis during the first 2 weeks after cochlear implantation; in these instances, causal bacteria may include a broader range of pathogens, including gram-negative bacilli and gram-positive bacteria. Selection of a combination of antimicrobial agents that provides broader-spectrum coverage against gram-negative

*References 47, 100, 101, 105, 111, 168, 189, 195, 204, 205, 215, 226, 228, 304, 341, 366, 384, 565.

bacilli should be chosen. For delayed development of cochlear implant infections, therapy consists of removal of the implant and administration of intravenous antibiotics.[434,440]

OCULAR PROSTHESES

The ocular prosthetic devices include artificial globes used primarily for cosmetic purposes, orbital implants, ocular explants, intraocular lenses, and contact lenses.

Orbital Implants

Orbital implants are made of hydroxyapatite or porous polyethylene and frequently are used in orbital reconstruction after enucleation or evisceration surgery. Infection of these implants is a rare event, with only a handful of cases reported in the literature.[6,167,214,240,247,139,584] Patients most commonly report anophthalmic socket pain or discomfort, pain with eye movement, and excessive conjunctival edema and irritation while wearing an artificial globe.[238] Papillary conjunctivitis of the socket with exudate and sometimes dehiscence of the overlying conjunctiva also may be seen.[166,357] Infection may develop months to years after placement of the implant, and severity ranges from cellulitis to the development of an abscess around the implant itself, with implant extrusion. In a retrospective clinical case series of 103 patients who underwent hydroxyapatite implant insertion at one institution, patients who had a freestanding polycarbonate peg placed to enhance the motility of their ocular prostheses had a significantly higher rate of infection than those patients with nonpegged hydroxyapatite implants, at 42.9% versus 19.5%.[140]

Radiographic studies that can aid in the detection of these types of infection include technetium 99m–labeled leukocyte scintigraphy, which is most useful in detecting early low-grade graft infection,[237] and computed tomography (CT) and magnetic resonance imaging (MRI), which are useful later in the course of the infection to detect the presence of abscesses and structural tissue changes. Gram-positive cocci, primarily *S. aureus,* and coagulase-negative staphylococci are the organisms associated most commonly with these infections; however, *H. influenzae, S. pneumoniae,* α-hemolytic streptococci, *Capnocytophaga, Pseudomonas,* and *Aspergillus fumigatus* have been cultured as well.[92,433,441,468,497,577,585] To cure the infection effectively, treatment involves both removal of the implant and institution of topical and parenteral antibiotic therapy directed against the organism isolated. Empirical therapy directed against gram-positive organisms may be started initially until the results of culture and sensitivity testing are available. This should include antimicrobial agents effective against community strains of MRSA. In addition, other common empirical regimens include a first- or second-generation cephalosporin or an extended-spectrum, penicillinase-resistant penicillin.

Intraocular Lenses

Insertion of polymethyl methacrylate (PMMA) intraocular lenses at the time of removal of a cataract is the standard surgical therapy for this disorder. Even though the rate of postoperative infection of intraoperative lenses is low (0.10–0.30%), the infection usually is serious and results in endophthalmitis and permanent loss of vision.[240,270] The predisposing factor for infection is bacterial adhesion to intraocular lenses during insertion. After adhesion is accomplished, the bacteria replicate, congregate, and form multiple layers of microcolonies that represent a biofilm in which the bacteria are embedded in a layer of slime. The major pathogens associated with this infection are *S. aureus* and *S. epidermidis,* which account for 90% of all isolates, although α-hemolytic *Streptococcus* spp. especially *Streptococcus pneumoniae,*[419] gram-negative bacilli, *Pseudomonas,* fungi,[364] *Chlamydia trachomatis, Nocardia* spp., and rapidly growing mycobacteria are isolated on occasion.[12,126,270,330,383,396,467,586] Intraocular lens–associated endophthalmitis is a serious infection that is difficult to diagnose and treat.[37,423,510,527,567] In a few cases, use of topical and systemic antibiotics alone has been successful in eradicating the infection, but in most cases surgical debridement and systemic antibiotics are required for cure. Empirical therapy for these infections consists of an extended-spectrum, penicillinase-resistant penicillin, a second-generation cephalosporin, or, in some instances, clindamycin or vancomycin. In cases of fungal endophthalmitis, treatment with the later-generation azoles alone and in combination with an echinocandin has been shown to have clinical success.[126] In rapidly growing mycobacterial endophthalmitis combinations of topical and intravenous antibiotics to which the organism is susceptible have been used for treatment.[330]

Contact Lenses

Primarily three different types of contact lenses are available. Hard lenses are made of PMMA, a substance that is impermeable to water and gas. This type of lens is designed to be worn only during waking hours because it limits oxygen flow to the cornea to that present in tears. Gas-permeable hard lenses are composed of silicone, cellulose acetate butyrate, or PMMA-silicone copolymers; they allow gas but not fluid to pass through the lens. Hydrophilic or soft lenses are made of a cross-linked hydrogel polymer or copolymer and consist of 38% to 85% water by weight; these lenses are permeable to both gas and water and allow the user to wear them continuously. However, for all these types of lenses, infection may result in damage to the corneal epithelium.

The two main infections that occur in association with contact lenses are conjunctivitis and keratitis.[81,257] The causative bacteria seen most commonly with these infections are *S. aureus,* streptococci, *Pseudomonas* spp. (found in improperly stored cleansing solutions), and fungi (including *Candida* spp., *Alternaria, Paecilomyces, Fusarium, Curvularia,* and other filamentous fungi, and *Acremonium*). Improper cleaning of soft or hydrophilic lenses may cause them to become a source of infection when bacteria penetrate the lens matrix. Risk factors for fungal keratitis include use of contaminated contact lens solution, trauma, contact lens wear, ocular surface disease, systemic diseases affecting the immune system, diabetes, use of systemic steroids, and recent chemotherapy.[9,83,535,588] Fungal keratitis frequently is a severe disease in which diagnosis may be difficult, response to medical therapy is generally slow, and the clinical outcome may be poor. Corneal perforation is 5 to 6 times more likely with fungal keratitis than in bacterial keratitis.[581] In a retrospective multicenter case series of 733 cases of fungal keratitis that looked at the epidemiology and microbiologic characteristics of fungal keratitis at tertiary eye care centers in the United States, it was found that filamentous fungi were more commonly found as the cause of keratitis among refractive contact lens wearers whereas yeasts, especially *Candida* spp., were the most common causative organisms in patients with ocular surface disease and ocular trauma.[249,587] Treatment of keratitis usually consists of removal of the lens and application of topical antibiotics or antifungals. The most commonly used topical antifungal regimen is a combination of natamycin 5% and amphotericin B 0.15%. Twenty-five percent of patients also may require systemic antifungal therapy in addition to the topical therapy. In fungal keratitis, 16% to 26% of patients require surgical intervention with therapeutic keratoplasty in addition to medical therapy.[227,249] To prevent the development of infections associated with contact lenses, users should adhere strictly to the manufacturer's suggested guidelines for wearing and cleaning the lenses.

A rare and often devastating infection associated with the use of contact lenses is infection with the fresh-water protozoan *Acanthamoeba.*[98,201,357,500] This organism contaminates the lens when sterility of the cleansing solutions is not maintained; it has been associated with users who prepare their own solutions and use of contaminated contact lens disinfection solution.[110,544,590] *Acanthamoeba* is very difficult to eradicate because it is not susceptible to standard antiparasitic agents, and it produces a chronic keratitis that can be complicated by corneal perforation and loss of the eye. Corneal transplantation may be necessary in many cases to restore vision.[201,500] In a study by Kaiserman and colleagues to assess the prognostic factors influencing visual prognosis and length of treatment after acanthamoeba keratitis, infection acquired by swimming or related to contact lenses, having neuritis and pseudodendrites, the absence of an epithelial defect, having been treated with chlorhexidine, and not having received steroids were factors that were associated with better final best spectacle-corrected visual acuity (BCVA); having an epithelial defect on presentation and having been treated with topical steroid were associated with worse BCVA.[239]

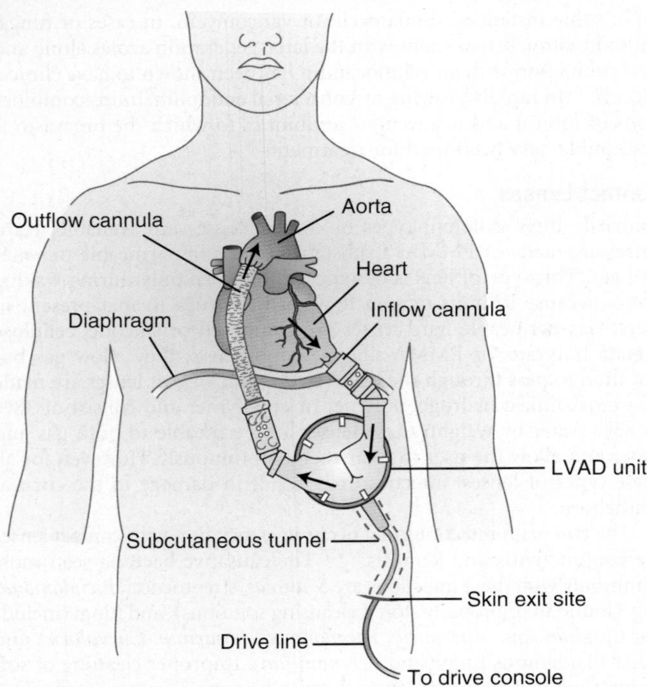

FIG. 74.1 Left ventricular assist device (LVAD). (Modified from Fisher SA, Trenholme GM, Costanzo MR, Piccione W. Infectious complications in left ventricular assist device recipients. *Clin Infect Dis.* 1997;24:18–23.)

LEFT VENTRICULAR ASSIST DEVICES

The development plus use of mechanical circulatory assist devices has grown very rapidly in the past several decades, especially with the shortage of available donor hearts. Such devices have improved considerably the hemodynamic status and quality of life of patients with heart failure who are awaiting cardiac transplantation. Fig. 74.1 shows a left ventricular assist device (LVAD), a pneumatically driven pump located outside the heart that draws blood from an inflow cannula in the left ventricular apex and ejects the blood through an outlet into the ascending aorta. Within the pump are several sections of Dacron graft material and two trileaflet porcine valves in the inflow and outflow positions to ensure that blood flow is unidirectional. The pump is encased in titanium and implanted via an extended median sternotomy into the left rectus sheath. A percutaneous driveline connects to an exterior power pack for venting or for pneumatic actuation and exits the body after passing through a subcutaneous tunnel, in the left lower quadrant. The interior surface of the pump is textured to prevent the formation of thrombi and encourage the deposition of a biologic pseudointimal lining. Most LVADs are surgically implanted through a median sternotomy, with pump placement primarily in the intraabdominal or preperitoneal space. Ventricular assist device designs primarily fall into two major categories: pulsatile and continuous flow devices. Pulsatile devices are first-generation devices that were designed to mimic nature by providing pulsatile circulation; they have many moving parts, including a diaphragm to hold and eject blood, valves to maintain directionality, and an air vent and conduit for cooling of the working parts. These requirements have limited the durability and size of these devices. Because of the multiple moving parts, these devices begin to wear out within the first 2 years of use, and the large size necessitates placement in the preperitoneal space or intraperitoneal space. The second-generation continuous flow devices are smaller and have fewer moving parts. These devices primarily consist of inflow and outflow pumps and a rotor, with a smaller conduit to the power source that does not include an air vent. Since January 2010, 98% of LVADs implanted are of continuous flow design.[259] Once the device is implanted, in most cases it cannot be removed without performing concurrent cardiac transplantation.[197,248,334,336,381]

Infection of an LVAD can involve any portion of the LVAD, including the surgical site, driveline, pocket, and pump. Infections occur most commonly within the first 3 months of device implantation, with the risk for severe infection and sepsis peaking at 1 month. The cumulative risk for device infection increases the longer the device remains in place; the incidence of infection significantly decreases after 3 months.[20,76,209,211,245,319,370] Based on data from the Interagency Registry for Mechanical Circulatory Support (INTERMACS), overall infection rates were 17.5 infections per 100 patient-months during the first 12 months after implantation.[260,480,498] The rates of infection have been shown to vary among generations of device, with 28.9 infections per 100 months in the pulsatile devices ($n = 406$) and 11.8 infections per 100 months in the continuous flow devices ($n = 548$) ($P < .0001$). It was also found that infection accounted for 16% of deaths associated with LVAD implantation.[209,259,451,457]

The approach taken by many centers for infection of an LVAD includes both preventive and interventional steps that are instituted before, during, and after implantation. Preventive strategies are focused on prevention of infections related primarily to the driveline and device pocket through the use of clean implantation techniques and limited traffic in the operating room in which the procedure is being performed. Antibiotic prophylaxis usually is given for 48 hours near the time of implantation of the LVAD and may include intravenous trimethoprim-sulfamethoxazole, rifampin, and fluconazole, along with the application of mupirocin ointment to the nares. Additional preventive measures include soaking the surfaces of the LVAD in vancomycin and gentamicin for 30 minutes before placing it, irrigating the device pocket with povidone-iodine (Betadine), and meticulously placing the subcutaneous tunnel in the appropriate position. Postoperative care with sterile and semisterile dressing changes around the driveline is emphasized.[24,146,153,209,335,336,400,505,569]

Despite the preventive measures taken, infection, thromboembolism, and hemorrhage at the time of implantation remain the most common complications associated with the use of mechanical circulatory support devices. Of these complications, infection has the most significant impact on morbidity and mortality.[158] Predisposing factors for development of device-related infections in these patients include a variety of host, device, and operative characteristics. Device-related risk factors are correlated with increased size and surface area of the device, turbulence of flow, contact of blood with the prosthetic surfaces, device-related pockets and cavities, transcutaneous drivelines, and power cables.[365,382] Operative and environmental risk factors include extent of surgery necessary for implantation hemorrhage, reoperation, frequent occurrence of multiple organ dysfunction or failure, duration of mechanical circulatory support, duration of hospitalization and intensive care unit stay, use of indwelling lines and catheters, parenteral nutrition, operative technique, and time.[299,417] The incidence of infection in patients on LVAD support for longer than 60 days is reported to be two times higher than that in patients with an LVAD in place for less than 30 days; initial episodes of infection after 90 days are rare.[363,408,476] With regard to patient-related risk factors, the severity of heart failure symptoms and presence of poor health and comorbid conditions, including diabetes, hyperglycemia, obesity, alcohol use, and renal disease, has been associated with increased risk for infection.[49,172,355,430,476] In addition, some evidence indicates that implantation of an LVAD itself may lead to defects in cellular immunity secondary to an aberrant state of T-cell activation that predisposes LVAD recipients to the development of candidal and other systemic infections.[19,170,225,258,408] The incidence of infection after implantation of an LVAD is reported to range between 13% and 80%, with most studies documenting an infection rate of 30% to 50%.[16,146,210,416,479,560] Most series report that the device pocket and drivelines are the device-related sites that account for most of the infections. Placement of the LVAD in the abdominal cavity instead of the preperitoneal area has been shown to decrease the chance for development of infection.[363]

Driveline infections are thought to result from a lack of integration of tissue around the driveline that allows the driveline to move and irritate surrounding tissues, which can result in an infection in the exit site and, in some cases, bacteremia. Such infections generally are defined by pain, erythema, warmth, drainage, or purulent discharge at the driveline exit site in the presence of a positive culture.[293] Bacteremia developing after implantation of a pump and infections of the pump itself are additional reported complications.[24,335] In a study of 205 patients who underwent placement of LVADs at the Cleveland Clinic, positive blood cultures were noted in 52%, infections of the driveline site occurred in 22%, and infections of the pump pocket developed in 9.2%.[248] Sun and colleagues[505] reported their experience with 95 patients who underwent insertion of an LVAD. Twenty-six (27%) of these patients experienced device-related infections involving the driveline, device pocket, or blood-contacting surfaces; 15 (57.7%) of the 26 had infections of the driveline site. Persistent bacteremia and progression of infection of the device pocket and driveline site can lead to the serious infection of LVAD endocarditis, which mimics prosthetic valve endocarditis, is very difficult to treat, and is associated with a high mortality rate. LVAD endocarditis is defined as positive cultures of the LVAD surface in conjunction with clinical signs and symptoms of infection during LVAD support. Manifestations of this condition are varied and range from persistent fever and bacteremia or fungemia to cerebral thromboembolism, LVAD inlet obstruction with hemorrhage, or LVAD outflow graft rupture.[24] In a report by Weyland and associates[569] of 27 patients who underwent insertion of LVADs, infections of the driveline developed in 8 (30%) of the 27 recipients, and LVAD endocarditis, defined as positive cultures from the pump chamber, was found in 12 (44%) of the patients; 8 (67%) of the 12 died of endocarditis.

Despite a high potential for the development of serious morbidity after placement of an LVAD, studies have shown that the presence of an infection after insertion of an LVAD does not seem to have very much influence on eventual cardiac transplantation and posttransplant outcome. A study by Argenziano found that infection subsequently developed in 29 (48%) of 60 patients who underwent insertion of an LVAD.[24] The most frequent sites of infection were the blood (27%), LVAD driveline (13%), LVAD surface (13%), and central venous catheter (10%); these sites thus represented 63% of all infections. The overall mortality rate, the rate of successful cardiac transplantation, and the rate of infection after transplantation were not influenced by the presence of infection during LVAD support.[24] In another study, Sinha and colleagues[479] reviewed their experience with 86 patients who received LVADs; device-related infections developed in six patients, five (83%) of whom had infections of the pocket. This study also found that the presence of infection during LVAD support did not influence successful cardiac transplantation or patient survival after transplantation. Over a 6-year period, Schulman and colleagues[458] reviewed their experience with 149 patients who received LVADs as a bridge to heart transplantation and sought to determine the impact of device-related infections on posttransplant survival and posttransplant infection. Of the 149 patients, 110 were successfully bridged to cardiac transplantation. Pretransplant device-related infections (e.g., pocket infections, wound infections, and postimplant bacteremia) had no negative effect on bridging to transplantation. However, patients with pretransplant sepsis were less often successfully bridged to cardiac transplantation. The presence of a pretransplant device-related infection was found to have no effect on posttransplant 1-year survival rates, although it was associated with an increased rate of posttransplant infection, especially if the patient had a driveline infection during LVAD support. Specifically having a driveline infection during LVAD support predisposed for having an infection in the former LVAD pocket or driveline site after cardiac transplantation, but did not predispose to having sternal wound infections, bacteremia, or sepsis in the posttransplant period. Diagnosing an infection early, determining the location and the extent of the infection, and assessing therapeutic efficacy can be a challenge in patients with LVADs. Anatomic imaging modalities such as CT and MRI may have limited value because of the presence of metallic CT artifacts and contraindications to using MRI. New imaging modalities, such as radiolabeled leukocyte single-photon emission computed tomography (SPECT/CT), are being studied to assess the accuracy of these modalities in revealing both anatomic location and extent of infection in patients with an LVAD. Preliminary results of leukocyte SPECT/CT have shown it to be very accurate in diagnosing an LVAD-related infection.[72,294,300]

Microbiology of Left Ventricular Assist Device Infections

Numerous organisms have been isolated from LVAD infections. In most series, *S. aureus* (including methicillin-resistant strains), *S. epidermidis* and other coagulase-negative staphylococci, and *Enterococcus* spp. are the organisms most commonly isolated from these infections, usually within the first 4 weeks after implantation. Other organisms such as *Enterobacter* spp., *P. aeruginosa, Serratia marcescens, Klebsiella* spp., *Stenotrophomonas maltophilia, Citrobacter koseri,* other gram-negative organisms, and polymicrobial organisms were seen more commonly later in the clinical course.* Fungal infections (e.g., *Candida albicans, Candida parapsilosis, Aspergillus* spp., and *Mucor* spp.) have been reported or observed as well and were responsible for approximately 16% of the infections.[33,116,121,210,333,389,471] However, colonization with fungi occurs in 35% to 39% of patients with LVADs.[170] Investigators suggested that treatment with broad-spectrum antibiotics (common in these patients) rendered them more susceptible to the development of fungal infection. When a fungal LVAD infection is suspected, signs of thrush, cutaneous rashes, esophagitis, retinal changes, peripheral embolization, and unexplained decrease in LVAD output should be investigated. The presence of yeast on Gram stain of the fluid surrounding the device and ultrasound showing increasing amounts of fluid around the device can be used to help confirm the diagnosis.[170]

Management of these infections, especially LVAD endocarditis, presents a major challenge, given that the device usually cannot be removed unless simultaneous heart transplantation is performed; moreover if transplantation is accomplished, multiple issues regarding the immunosuppressed condition of the patient are raised. In most cases, management involves a prolonged course (i.e., usually 4 to 6 weeks) of aggressive antimicrobial or antifungal therapy (or both) appropriate for the organism or organisms isolated, with meticulous attention given to skin care around the driveline exit site; debridement, drainage, surgical revision, and irrigation with povidone-iodine of infected wound sites; or, in certain instances, replacement of the LVAD unit or cardiac transplantation before completing antibiotic therapy if a donor heart becomes available and all blood culture results are negative.[146,210,335]

EXTRACORPOREAL MEMBRANE OXYGENATION CIRCUITS

Extracorporeal membrane oxygenation (ECMO) is a life support device used most commonly for treating severe cardiac and pulmonary failure in neonates and children. Patients undergoing repair for congenital cardiac lesions may require ECMO support (>1%). In addition a growing number of children are receiving ECMO support for acute decompensation from myocarditis; cardiomyopathy; post-cardiac arrest; acute respiratory distress syndrome; severe bacterial, viral, or aspiration pneumonia; and sepsis with hypotension thought to be due to cardiac output failure.[316,347,422,517] Specific indications for neonates include meconium aspiration syndrome, congenital diaphragmatic hernia, persistent pulmonary hypertension, and others.[521] Although the overall survival rate of children managed by ECMO has improved in recent years, it still is approximately 50% to 80%, and is lower in adults.[38,422,521,562,574] Multiple cardiac and noncardiac factors are associated with increased morbidity and mortality rates. Patients with a single ventricle or residual cardiac defect after surgery have a less favorable ECMO outcome.[52,107,266] Renal dysfunction, especially requiring hemodialysis, multiple organ system failure, initiation of ECMO in the operating room, blood product transfusion, mediastinal bleeding, ECMO circuit problems, and duration of ECMO for longer than 10 days also were predictors of increased risk for mortality.[3,266,356] The infection rate for patients on ECMO ranges from 6% to more than 40%, with a relatively recent report of 10.2% in about 40,000 patients in the Extracorporeal Life Support Organization registry.[555] Recent reports suggested a higher infection rate in older patients with culture-proven infections, at 6.1% to 10.1% in neonatal patients, 14% to 23% in pediatric patients, and 20.5% to 30.6% in adults.[51,460,574] The rate of development of sepsis in neonates while on

*References 24, 121, 146, 173, 210, 333, 335, 479, 522, 569.

ECMO in one study was 4.2% and was associated with higher complications and mortality.[348] Multiple risk factors for acquiring infection while on ECMO were identified, including indwelling vascular or urinary catheters,[356] duration of ECMO bypass (>10 days),[220,501] procedures before or during ECMO,[377] ECMO complications,[68] and changes in the humoral and cellular immunity.[539] Patients with infections usually will need longer bypass support[377] and will have a delay in post-ECMO lung recovery and increased mortality.[51,272,356] In one study, mediastinitis occurred in 11% of adults, with cardiac surgery noted to be a risk factor for this infection.[517]

Earlier reports suggested that gram-positive cocci (e.g., *S. aureus* and coagulase-negative staphylococci) are the most common etiologic agents and are still frequent pathogens.[501] However, gram-negative bacteria (both lactose fermenting and non–lactose fermenting[220]) and fungi[199] are becoming more commonly reported. *Candida* spp. were found to be frequently isolated pathogens in children and adults.[51,409,506] The distribution of these pathogens is similar to their distribution in other patients with infections treated in the intensive care unit.[199] The signs and symptoms of infection often are subtle and nonspecific. Fever develops in only half of these patients. The value of tachycardia and elevated cardiac output also is limited because these patients frequently are tachycardic, with increased cardiac output caused by a systemic inflammatory response (e.g., complement; cytokines such as TNF, interleukin-1 [IL-1], and IL-6; and acute phase reactants such as C-reactive protein and procalcitonin), which is characteristic of cardiopulmonary bypass procedures.[71,352,409,501,506] For the same reason, leukocytosis (unless developing acutely) and an elevated erythrocyte sedimentation rate (ESR) should be interpreted with caution. In addition, physical examination and radiologic tests may be difficult to interpret.[71] Consequently a high index of suspicion with careful evaluation of potential infection source (e.g., surgical wound and insertion site of catheter) and surveillance of blood and urine cultures is needed to identify these infections.

Most patients undergoing ECMO are treated with multiple broad-spectrum antibiotics. This practice probably is one of the reasons for the increased incidence of multidrug-resistant, gram-positive (e.g., *Enterococcus*) and gram-negative bacteria, as well as fungal (e.g., *Candida*) infections. In addition, many of these patients will be colonized with these same bacteria. Therefore if a deep bronchial suction or urine culture (performed routinely) becomes positive but without supporting evidence of infection (e.g., increased white blood cell [WBC] count, fever), serious effort to distinguish between colonization and infection should be made before initiating an unnecessary change in antimicrobial therapy. If a decision to treat is made, appropriate coverage for both gram-positive and gram-negative organisms should be chosen. If blood, urine, and bronchial cultures remain negative and the patient's condition is not improving or the culture becomes positive for a fungus, antifungal therapy should be added.

Most ECMO centers administer antibiotic prophylaxis; however, the optimal spectrum and duration of this practice are unknown. Some studies suggested that use of prophylaxis (for 24 hours before the ECMO is started) was effective in reducing infections[69,501]; others found no correlation between antibiotic prophylaxis and reduction in infection rate.[220] Of interest, despite advances in critical care for ECMO patients (including antibiotic prophylaxis), no significant decrease has occurred in infection rate during the past two decades.[68] The lack of specific guidelines and evidence from randomized trials evaluating different durations and spectrums of antibiotic contribute to the confusion and controversy in this area.[244] If prophylaxis is considered, antifungal prophylaxis (e.g., fluconazole) should be added because it was shown to decrease the incidence of fungal infections, which are increasing.[161]

PERMANENT CARDIAC PACEMAKER AND IMPLANTABLE CARDIOVERTER-DEFIBRILLATOR INFECTIONS

Permanent Cardiac Pacemaker Infections

Cardiac pacemakers have been widely used since the 1980s and the American Heart Association (AHA) has recently expanded the indications for their use.[134] Two types of permanent pacemaker generators are in use; those with transvenous electrodes and those with epicardial electrodes. Both types are implanted in either the chest or the abdominal wall; pacemakers with epicardial electrodes are the ones more commonly used in the pediatric population. Studies are currently being conducted on the next generation of pacemakers, which are miniaturized, fully self-contained leadless devices that are nonsurgically implanted in the right ventricle with the use of a catheter.[432]

Infection is one of the most common medical complications of implantation of permanent pacemakers, with reported rates ranging from 0.2% to 5.8% and a high mortality rate.[74,90,557] An estimated 25% of cardiac pacemaker–associated infections develop within 1 to 2 months of placement of the device, but delays of up to 12 months may occur before diagnosis is established. Several studies suggested that the relative rate of infection associated with permanent pacemakers has increased despite improved surgical techniques and better design of the devices themselves,[74,538,557] but a recent study demonstrated a fairly constant rate of infection over the course of 20 years.[235] Studies have shown that infections of permanent cardiac pacemakers seem to occur more commonly in patients with both local and systemic underlying medical problems, especially diabetes mellitus or an underlying renal insufficiency, or in those who are undergoing treatment with corticosteroids, anticoagulants, or other types of immunosuppressive therapy.[53,412,484,557] Other well-characterized independent risk factors include surgery related to any part of the pacemaker (especially replacement of a battery or upgrade of the pacemaker),[80,191,200,235,278,369] the presence of a hematoma after implantation,[75,369,483] temporary transvenous pacing,[200] and epicardial leads.[483] Multiple (two or more) pacemaker insertions and physician inexperience with insertion also represent significant risks for development of infection.[191,369] The presence of a central venous line also increases the risk for systemic infection.[80] Multivariable analysis of the largest reported pediatric pacemaker infections identified only presence of Down syndrome and manipulations of the pacing system during revisions as risk factors.[99]

Infections of permanent cardiac pacemakers are subdivided into groups depending on the specific site of involvement and whether they are early infections (<1 to 2 months after implantation) or late infections (>2 months after implantation). The groups are (1) local inflammation, infection, and the formation of an abscess in the generator pocket or subcutaneous portion of the lead, or in both sites; (2) secondary infection involving either the generator or the electrodes (including pacemaker endocarditis)[75,129]; (3) fever plus associated bacteremia, with or without concomitant infective endocarditis, in a patient without any apparent focus of infection[129]; and (4) mediastinitis, pericarditis, bronchopleural cutaneous fistulas, and mixed infections.[129]

The generator pocket and the subcutaneous portions of the leads (i.e., transvenous and epicardial) are the most common sites of infection. Infections of the pocket often are difficult to diagnose and may develop at any time after implantation; however, most tend to develop early and frequently are the result of contamination by skin flora at the time of the procedure.[353] Late infection usually occurs as a consequence of erosion of the device through the subcutaneous tissue and skin. The infection may remain localized to the pocket or may spread to the adjacent electrodes and lead to the development of bacteremia. Infection of transvenous pacemaker leads may occur in as many as 17% of patients who receive permanent pacemakers. These infections often are not apparent initially but have been associated with significant morbidity and mortality.[183] Infection generally develops along the subcutaneous portion of the leads and, if unrecognized, may progress centrally and result in sustained bacteremia, endocarditis, or both. Infections of the leads tend to occur later than infections of the pocket, with the median time of occurrence being 7 to 8 months after implantation of the pacemaker. Endocarditis as a complication of unrecognized infected transvenous leads can develop years (2 to 3 years) after placement of the pacemaker. Infections of permanent epicardial leads generally occur as a complication of infections of the generator pocket, skin erosion, or direct contamination at the time of placement. However, in contrast to infections of the transvenous leads, infections of the epicardial leads usually result in only local symptoms; rarely they may lead to more severe disseminated disease such as pericarditis, mediastinitis, bronchopleural cutaneous fistulas, bacteremia, or sepsis.

Microbiology

Staphylococci (*S. aureus* and coagulase-negative staphylococci) are the most common causes of pacemaker-related infections, accounting for more than 85% of such infections; however, a wide variety of organisms have been isolated.[75,80,328,369,483,486,549] An increasing number of the isolated staphylococci are methicillin resistant. Other gram-positive organisms such as viridans streptococci, other streptococci, enterococci, *Listeria,* and *Corynebacteria* have been isolated as well, but each causes fewer than 1% of cases. Gram-negative organisms such as *E. coli, Proteus, Enterobacter cloacae, P. aeruginosa, Klebsiella, S. marcescens,* and *Sphingomonas paucimobilis*[469] are isolated from 5% to 20% of device-related infections. In addition, *Candida, Aspergillus, Pseudallescheria, Trichosporon* spp.,[425] and other fungi have been isolated rarely, as well as *Mycobacterium* spp.; however, infections with these organisms generally are associated with poor clinical outcomes.*

Clinical and Laboratory Findings

Diagnosing a pacemaker-associated infection can be difficult because of its nonspecific symptomatology, and months may elapse after the onset of symptoms before the diagnosis is established. Symptoms may be confined to a local area or may be more widespread, with the development of bacteremia or other systemic effects. Rarely the only sign of infection is persistent pain at the pocket site.[265] Fever (84–100%) and chills (75–84%) are considered the most common systemic symptoms and are indicators of local infection, especially if they occur after the second postoperative day in association with other signs; however, they may be the only clinical manifestation in more than a third of patients.[75,264,354,375,573] Early infections are more likely to be accompanied by both local and systemic clinical findings and are manifested more commonly as infections of the generator pocket, bacteremia, or septicemia[75,311,597]; late infections, on the other hand, typically cause vague symptoms that evolve over the course of time and usually are lead-related infections and endocarditis.[278,549]

Infections of the generator pocket typically cause local swelling (21%), erythema (34%), pain (32%), drainage (through an incompletely healed incision or fistulous tract) over or adjacent to the generator pocket (25%), and warmth (11.5%).[90] Sterile breakdown of the pacemaker pocket develops in an estimated 5% of patients with permanent pacemakers, and skin or soft tissue erosion over the electrodes occurs in an additional 2% to 4%. Because these complications are associated with a high risk for the subsequent development of infections, the presence of any erosion is considered a potential indicator of device-related infection, especially if the erosion occurs more than 24 months after placement of the pacemaker, at which time the infection rate may be as high as 80%.[48,182] Pacemaker-related endocarditis is a relatively rare complication that occurs in 0.05% to 0.5% of cases after implantation of a pacemaker. Such endocarditis is associated with a mortality rate as high as 34% in some series.[75,157,264] It tends to be a late complication; only 27% to 36% of patients are seen within 6 to 12 weeks after the last procedure at the pacemaker implant site, with symptoms developing in most patients a mean of 25 months after the last procedure at the implant site. The diagnosis of pacemaker-related endocarditis is difficult to establish, and usually a delay occurs in making the diagnosis, with a mean interval of 5 to 8 months after the onset of symptoms.[75,264] Pulmonary symptoms are found in 20% to 45% of patients with pacemaker-related infections and may consist of bronchitis, lung abscess, pneumonia, or pulmonary embolism; these symptoms are seen more commonly in late-onset infection and in patients with intravenous lead–related infection.[75,264]

A variety of laboratory and imaging studies may be performed to aid in establishing the diagnosis of a pacemaker-related infection. A recent update from the AHA suggested two sets of cultures from blood, generator pocket site, and lead tips when infection is suspected.[32] A prospective study that looked at patients with pocket infections of cardiovascular implantable electronic devices found that sonication of generators and leads that were surgically removed was more sensitive than swab cultures or blood cultures alone in detecting bacteria in these types of infections.[436] An elevated ESR is found in 82% to 97% of patients, and peripheral leukocytosis is seen in 50% to 66%. The presence of a collection of fluid around the device as seen on ultrasound is suggestive of device-related infection. Gallium scanning may be performed in an attempt to determine the nature of the fluid (i.e., inflammatory vs. infectious). Transesophageal echocardiography (TEE) can be helpful in identifying endocarditis (especially when blood culture results are negative). TEE has emerged as a major tool in diagnosis; studies have shown that this test was able to demonstrate vegetations and other lesions on the electrodes, ventricular endocardium, and tricuspid valve in 90% to 96% of patients with pacemaker-related infections.[75,264,549] Only the combination of negative TEE and ECHO should be used to rule out endocarditis.[486]

*References 11, 75, 86, 89, 246, 277, 283, 320, 486, 549, 573.

Management and Treatment of Infection

Appropriate therapy for pacemaker-related infections is tailored to the specific clinical situation and depends on several factors: (1) whether the infection is limited to the generator pocket or subcutaneous electrodes, without bacteremia; (2) whether bacteremic pacemaker-related endocarditis is present with or without involvement of the subcutaneous electrodes; and (3) what organism is involved.

If the infection is limited to the generator pocket or subcutaneous electrodes, optimal treatment consists of both medical and surgical intervention in which all of the parts of the infected device are removed. Studies have shown that failure to remove completely all portions of the infected device results not only in failure to cure the infection but also in higher mortality rates.[32,75,556] In addition, infection relapse is higher.[90,324,484] The patient is given parenteral antimicrobial therapy, and an exchange of the pacing system with total removal of the infected device and simultaneous insertion of a new pacemaker at a different site is performed surgically. The infected subcutaneous pocket is drained, debrided, and packed open, and local wound care is instituted. Initial antibiotic therapy should provide coverage for both staphylococci and gram-negative bacteria; therapy is tailored once the organism is identified and its antibiotic susceptibility is known. Initial regimens include vancomycin plus an aminoglycoside. Oxacillin or nafcillin plus an aminoglycoside may be used if MRSA is rare in the community. In certain instances, a new pacemaker cannot be placed at the time of removal of the infected device; in such situations, a period of temporary transvenous pacing is instituted until a new pacemaker can be implanted. For local pocket infections, antimicrobial therapy targeted at the causative organism should be administered for 10 to 14 days.

The consensus approach to the management of pacemaker-related endocarditis and bacteremia involves removal of both the generator unit and the electrodes in conjunction with prolonged administration of parenteral antibiotic therapy designed to treat endocarditis (usual duration, 4 weeks).[32,484] In cases of MRSA, duration of treatment should be extended to 6 weeks.[301] A longer duration may be considered in patients with other sites of infection (e.g., osteomyelitis or septic thrombophlebitis). Vancomycin should be the initial antimicrobial treatment of choice before the etiologic agent is identified because the majority of infections are due to staphylococci species. More specific antibiotic regimens can be used when the pathogen is identified and in vitro susceptibility is available. Mortality rates may be as high as 50% for patients in whom total removal of the pacemaker unit is not performed.[75,264,399] Percutaneous removal of electrodes that have lead-associated vegetations smaller than 20 mm is acceptable,[32,145] but extraction of the electrodes with vegetations larger than 20 mm may be difficult and risky to perform, and surgical removal by cardiotomy may be necessary.[32] In patients who require a pacemaker, temporary transvenous pacing may be implemented until a new permanent pacemaker can be placed. Sterility of blood cultures should be ensured before a new pacemaker generator and electrode are placed.

Infection of Implantable Cardioverter-Defibrillators

The first implantable cardioverter-defibrillator (ICD) was placed in 1980, and, during the past several decades, the device has become a successful therapeutic modality for treatment of patients (both adults and children) with life-threatening ventricular arrhythmias. Older devices required surgical placement of a pulse generator, extrapericardial or epicardial defibrillation patches, and a transvenous rate-sensing electrode. More recent systems use transvenous approaches for placement of leads and a subcutaneous or submuscular pulse generator or newer methods of complete subcutaneous ICDs, including subcutaneous leads.[58,250,403,494,568,575]

Infection is the most serious complication of placement of an ICD.[75,280] Infection rate ranges associated with placement of ICDs were previously from 1% to 7%.[495,526] However, infection rates have decreased substantially with the advent of transvenous non–thoracotomy-placed systems, with rates ranging from 0.2% to 1.8%[344] and 3.1 per 1000 patient years.[169] Subcutaneous ICDs appear to have lower rates of infection, particularly endocarditis.[403] Results from some studies still suggest that ICDs are associated with a greater risk of infection than are permanent pacemakers.[557] Cost associated with hospital admission, length of stay, and mortality are substantially increased in patients with infection in contrast to those without it.[482,485,538] Several risk factors that have been identified as increasing the likelihood for development of infection include steroid use, diabetes, heart failure, renal failure, malignancy, chronic obstructive pulmonary disease, skin disorders, anticoagulant drug use, preprocedural fever, and previous device infection.[53,268] Previous generator replacement, abdominal implantation, postoperative hematoma, procedural duration, and surgeon experience also were reported as contributing to increased risk for infection.[53,289,537] Abnormal renal function is the most consistently identified risk factor for mortality. Mortality is high, ranging from 24.5% to 29%,[29,178,181] and is higher for patients with infective endocarditis or bloodstream infection compared to generator pocket infection only.[550]

Most ICD-related infections are clinically apparent within 3 to 6 months after placement, with infections of the generator pocket, subcutaneous patch wound site, epicardial patches, or bacteremia and endocarditis being the most common manifestations. Some infections can be indolent, and only a high index of suspicion will initiate an investigation. An increased WBC count and ESR, anemia, and microscopic hematuria are the most common laboratory findings. As with pacemaker infections, TEE is an effective test to exclude endocarditis because transthoracic echocardiography is helpful in only half of the cases.[151] Infection of the generator pocket or subcutaneous patch wound site usually causes local findings of pain, erythema, and collection and drainage of fluid. Occasionally these patients also may be bacteremic or hypotensive. In contrast, infection of the epicardial patches generally results in more systemic symptoms, bacteremia, or pericarditis.[379] At least two blood cultures should be obtained to rule out bacteremia. Cultures of the generator pocket and lead tips after removal of the device are essential for identifying the pathogen. Sonication of the extracted device increases the yield of positive cultures.[327]

Microbiology

Gram-positive bacteria, primarily coagulase-negative streptococci and *S. aureus* are the major pathogens seen with ICD-related infections and account for 68% to 93% of cases.*

However, a broad spectrum of other gram-positive, gram-negative, and fungal organisms, including *Enterococcus* spp., *P. aeruginosa, Corynebacterium,* streptococci, *E. coli, Klebsiella, Bacteroides fragilis, Propionibacterium acnes,* atypical mycobacteria, and *Candida* spp., have been isolated from ICD-related infections. Fungal infection is uncommon, reported in fewer than 2% of patients. Reported rates of polymicrobial infection range from 2% to 24.5%, and many patients with clinical infection are found to have negative cultures (12–49%).

Management

The same approach previously described for pacemaker infection should be applied to ICD infection. To eliminate ICD-related infections effectively, optimal management involves a combination of medical and surgical interventions, especially if the patient is bacteremic or has systemic findings or if the causative organism is *S. aureus*. Several studies have suggested that conservative management (i.e., antibiotic therapy without removal of the hardware) may be sufficient, but others have identified medical therapy as a risk factor for death. A medical management approach should be tried only in cases with superficial or incisional infection and in rare occasions when only the generator pocket is infected or in patients whose condition prevents removal of the entire device. In these cases, the treatment should consist of administration of parenteral antibiotics, wound care, and removal of only the generator portion of the device, with implantation of another generator at a different site.[379,533] The optimal management of any other ICD-related infection is parenteral antibiotics and complete removal of the entire ICD system, followed by reimplantation (after the infection is eradicated) at another site.[90,280,448,576] Although there are no clinical trial data to define the optimal duration of antimicrobial therapy, at least 2 weeks should be considered after hardware removal, and, if blood cultures continue to be positive 24 hours after removal of the ICD, a longer period (e.g., 4 weeks) should be considered. For infections limited to the pocket site, 7 to 10 days of appropriate antibiotics may be sufficient, with an oral agent being a reasonable option if there is only superficial or incisional involvement.[32]

*References 29, 57, 113, 178, 224, 232, 280, 379, 448, 495, 513, 552, 554.

PROSTHETIC JOINT AND ORTHOPEDIC IMPLANT INFECTIONS

The implantation of prosthetic joints along with the use of other implantable orthopedic devices (e.g., pins, screws, plates, rods, external fixators, or Ilizarov apparatus) has improved quality of life greatly and restored function to patients suffering from debilitating bone and joint disease, tumor, or injury. Based on conservative estimates, millions of people worldwide have some form of prosthetic joint or other implantable orthopedic device. Of the possible complications associated with implantation, infection is the second most common cause of prosthetic joint failure.[18] It occurs in 0.6% to 2.4% of total joint replacement[128] and results in postoperative prosthesis failure, chronic pain, immobility, and, in some cases, loss of the affected limb or, in the worst-case scenario, loss of life.[5,44,124,500] The health care cost in the United States for treating a single infection of a prosthetic joint is estimated to be more than $280 million per year nationwide.[196] The number of prosthetic joint infections is increasing.[276]

Prosthetic joints and implantable orthopedic devices may become infected by two major mechanisms: (1) the prosthetic device may be contaminated by microorganisms at the time of implantation, either as a result of airborne contamination in the operating room or by direct inoculation at the time of surgery; or (2) the prosthetic device may become infected as a result of hematogenous seeding from bacteremia or by direct contiguous spread from an infection adjacent to the prosthesis. Of infections of prosthetic joints, 20% to 40% arise by hematogenous seeding, with the remainder occurring as a result of airborne or direct inoculation.[4,297,298] Infections may remain asymptomatic for years before symptoms become apparent, and usually a long delay occurs between onset of the infection and the appearance of symptoms and confirmation of the diagnosis. The overall rate of infection of prosthetic joints has been shown to be highest in the first 6 months postoperatively, with a steady decline occurring after this time. The incidence rate for infection of total hip and total knee arthroplasties during the first 2 years postoperatively is reported to be 5.9 infections per 1000 joint-years; in contrast, during postoperative years 2 to 10, it is 2.3 infections per 1000 joint-years.[499] The risk for acquiring infection and the incidence of infection depend on the anatomic location of the implanted orthopedic device or prosthetic joint, with the hips having the highest risk, followed in descending order by the knees, elbows, shoulders, wrists, and ankles.[93,424,502] For implantable orthopedic devices, rates of infection range from 2% to 30%.[317,547]

Risk Factors

Numerous factors have been identified as increasing a patient's risk for developing infection of a prosthetic joint or orthopedic implant, including rheumatoid arthritis, diabetes mellitus, obesity, poor nutritional status, use of steroids, immunocompromised status, psoriasis, hemophilia, sickle-cell hemoglobinopathy, solid-organ transplant, dialysis-dependent renal failure, joint dislocation, and extremes of age.[44,114,190,387,574] In addition, procedure-related factors such as previous surgery at the site of the prosthesis or implant, extended operation time (>2.5 hours), postoperative bleeding, and hematoma also increase the risk for acquiring an infection.[114,391,583] The relative risk for the development of prosthesis-related infections in patients with poor healing and wound complications increases from 13- to 20-fold after total knee replacement and from 22- to 52-fold after total hip replacement.[583] In addition, bacteremia from any source increases the risk for prosthesis infection.[596] For example, prosthesis-related infection developed in 34% of patients with *S. aureus* bacteremia who were followed prospectively.[361]

The implanted metal prosthetic device and the PMMA cement that binds the prosthetic device to adjacent bone also predispose the joint space and bone to infectious processes, given that both are foreign bodies. In vitro studies have shown that the unpolymerized form of PMMA cement predisposes to infection by inhibiting phagocytic, lymphocytic, and complement function; the risk for acquiring infection seems to be enhanced further once the cement has polymerized in the body.[404,405] Cementless prostheses have been designed in an attempt to overcome the problem of infection associated with the PMMA cement. For certain orthopedic implants, the integrity of the skin is compromised chronically, thus providing ready access to organisms from the external environment.

Microbiology

Although any microorganism can cause prosthetic joint infections, more than half of the infections are caused by *S. aureus* or coagulase-negative staphylococci.[114,596] Other gram-positive bacteria (e.g., β-hemolytic streptococci, viridans streptococci, and enterococci) cause 20% to 25% of infections. Antibiotic resistance in these organisms is increasing, and multiple strains of staphylococci may be present in a single prosthetic joint infection.[229,317,449,547,578] Less commonly, aerobic gram-negative bacilli, including *E. coli, Proteus mirabilis, Klebsiella* spp., *Salmonella* spp., *S. marcescens*, other Enterobacteriaceae, and *P. aeruginosa*, may cause infection. In addition, 4% to 10% of infections are caused by anaerobic organisms such as peptostreptococci and *Bacteroides* spp.; polymicrobial infections occur in approximately 10% of cases, with *S. aureus* and anaerobes the most frequently found.[323] Infections with fungi, particularly *Candida, Aspergillus,* and *Penicillium* spp., or with mycobacteria (i.e., *Mycobacterium tuberculosis, Mycobacterium avium* complex [MAC], and other rapidly growing mycobacteria) also have been described.[31,43,321,531] Rarely a wide spectrum of other organisms, including *Corynebacterium, Propionibacterium, Bacillus* spp., and *Mycoplasma hominis,* have been reported to cause infection. Zoonotic bacteria such as *Brucella* spp., *Yersinia* spp., and *Pasteurella* spp. rarely can cause infection and should be considered in the correct epidemiologic setting.[321] Approximately 10% of infections are culture negative.

Certain clinical situations may predispose a patient to particular organisms as the cause of infection. Pyogenic skin infections commonly result in staphylococcal and streptococcal infections of prosthetic joints, whereas infections of the teeth and gums are frequent causes of viridans streptococcal and anaerobic infections in prostheses. Genitourinary and gastrointestinal tract procedures or infections frequently are associated with enterococcal and gram-negative bacillary infections of prostheses. The increased use of TNF-α blockers in patients with joint prosthesis predisposes them to infections with unusual pathogens (e.g., fungi or mycobacteria).

Clinical Manifestations

The clinical findings and severity of symptoms seen with infections of prosthetic joints are highly variable and determined primarily by three factors: (1) the route of infection—the hematogenous route versus direct inoculation; (2) the virulence of the infecting pathogen—*S. aureus* and, to a lesser extent, β-hemolytic streptococci and gram-negative bacilli seem to be particularly virulent pathogens capable of producing a fulminant clinical picture, whereas infection with organisms such as coagulase-negative streptococci is associated with a more chronic, indolent course; and (3) the nature of the tissue in which the microorganism proliferates—hematomas, seromas, ischemic wounds, and the tissues of diabetic patients and those receiving steroids all enhance the ability of the bacteria to proliferate and spread, thereby promoting the development of a more deep-seated fulminant infection.

The most common initial symptom is joint pain, which occurs in 95% of cases. Such pain can range from an acute fulminant illness with erythema, severe joint pain, swelling (38%), high fever (43%), and systemic symptoms to a chronic, slowly increasing pain in the joint without typical signs of inflammation that may be associated with the formation of a cutaneous draining sinus (32%) but no systemic symptoms.[114,596] The presence of constant joint pain is more indicative of infection than is the presence of pain occurring only with movement or weight-bearing, which is more common in aseptic and mechanical complications.

For implantable orthopedic devices, the most common initial symptom of infection is erythema, swelling, pain, or drainage from the area around and adjacent to the implant. Local symptoms also may be associated with fever, especially if the device is extensive or deep seated.

Diagnostic Studies

Laboratory screening tests commonly used to diagnose infection of a prosthetic joint or implanted orthopedic device such as peripheral WBC count, C-reactive protein (CRP), and ESR are neither specific nor sensitive (sensitivity, 60–96%; specificity, 55–92%).[114,492] Of these tests, CRP seems to be the better test. These test results may be normal, especially in patients with chronic, slowly progressing infection. Several biomarkers (e.g., procalcitonin, TNF, and IL-6[45,466]) have been suggested as diagnostic tests. Molecular techniques such as polymerase chain reaction (PCR), fluorescence in situ hybridization (FISH), and immunofluorescent microscopy were reported to have a sensitivity of 63% to 100% in detecting bacteria in prosthetic joint infections[202,325] but were not studied widely.[13,338]

The principal radiologic studies used for detection of an infected prosthetic joint include plain radiographs, arthrograms or sinograms, and radioisotope scans (indium and technetium diphosphate). Abnormalities that may be suggestive of infection and can be seen on plain radiographs include radiolucency at the bone-cement interface, motion and changes in position of the prosthetic components, evidence of osteomyelitis, cement fractures, and periosteal reaction. Intraarticular injection of dye (arthrogram or sinogram—in the presence of a sinus tract) may demonstrate abnormal communication between the joint space and the bone–cement interface. These radiographic abnormalities are present in approximately 50% of infected prostheses.[104,314] Nuclear scans with indium-111–labeled WBC or technetium-labeled sulfur colloid (^{99m}Tc) may be used to detect periprosthetic inflammation. Scanning techniques have a sensitivity of 80% to 86% and a specificity of 94% to 100%.[385,515] Of note, increased uptake can be seen around uninfected prostheses within the first 6 to 12 months after implantation. Therefore positive findings after this time are abnormal and reflect inflammation (which could be due to a variety of causes) but not specifically infection.[127,206,243,380] Of interest, ^{99m}Tc-labeled ciprofloxacin (which probably binds to live bacteria at the infection site) was shown to be 94% sensitive and 83% specific for diagnosis of chronic infection.[489] Use of this technique allowed 11 of 12 infections of prosthetic joints to be identified, whereas ^{99m}Tc-WBC scintigraphy was positive in only seven patients.[491] Combining antigranulocyte antibody (^{99m}Tc sulesomab) and ^{99m}Tc collodial rhenium sulfide (nanocolloids) was shown to be an acceptable alternative.[490] Positron emission tomography with fludeoxyglucose F-18 (18 FP-FDG PET) was also evaluated as a diagnostic technique.[114,279,504] CT and MRI are not used routinely in the evaluation of patients with suspected infection of a prosthetic implant because of the large amount of imaging artifact created by prosthetic devices.[62,351]

Aspiration of joint fluid for culture and culture of tissue obtained intraoperatively are the optimal ways to establish a specific diagnosis of infection of a prosthetic joint. Unfortunately the yield is only 50% to 90%. To optimize the yield, antibiotics should be stopped 2 to 3 days before aspiration or operative cultures are taken.[596] Although joint fluid findings indicative of an infectious process are a high leukocyte count (consisting mainly of polymorphonuclear leukocytes [PMNs]), a high protein content, and a low glucose concentration, these changes are not specific for bacterial infection and are present in only some patients. Using a cutoff value of 1700 WBC/μL with at least 65% PMN cells gave excellent results.[524] The fluid obtained should be cultured for a variety of organisms; Gram stain is positive in a third of cases, and a causative pathogen can be identified in only two-thirds of patients.[399,493] Intraoperative cultures should include, if possible, any purulent discharge, devitalized bone, and tissue from the bone–cement interface. Vortexing, bath sonication, or both of the explanted prosthesis may increase the yield.[394] Histopathologic examination of this tissue usually reveals an infiltration of PMNs consistent with an acute inflammatory reaction but not specific for infection.[184,525] More rapid, specific, and sensitive tests (e.g., FISH, PCR, immunofluorescent microscopy) are needed to differentiate between noninfectious inflammation and bacterial infection and identify the pathogen in patients already receiving antibiotic or infected with fastidious pathogens.

Treatment

Successful treatment of an infected prosthetic joint involves extensive surgical debridement of all devitalized bone and tissue, removal of the prosthesis and all associated cement, and prolonged parenteral antibiotic therapy.[36,95] For optimal results, the debridement should be performed within 1 to 3 weeks.[114,285,322] Microbiologic cure has been found to correlate well with the extent of debridement and the completeness of removal of all residual methylmethacrylate cement. Historically attempts at simple surgical debridement without removal of the prosthetic device in conjunction with parenteral antibiotic therapy had variable success, with relapse rates being as high as 88% by 2 to 4 years after therapy.[147,454,576] High failure rate was reported in *S. aureus* infections,[64,551] but in patients with a short duration of prosthetic joint infection caused by penicillin-susceptible streptococci, debridement and antibiotic therapy alone appear to be sufficient, with a low risk for relapse.[271,343]

Two protocols have been used for the treatment of these infections. A two-stage surgical procedure with prolonged parenteral antibiotic therapy has been shown to be one of the most successful treatment regimens with the best functional results. The first stage involves complete removal of the prosthesis and cement followed by a 6-week regimen of antibiotic therapy empirically chosen to cover the most likely organism and then tailored once the organism has been identified and its antibiotic susceptibility is known. The second stage involves reimplantation of a new prosthetic device at the end of the antibiotic course. Success rates with this procedure range from 87% to 100%.[144,292] An alternative method of therapy involves a one-stage exchange operation in which the infected prosthetic device and cement are removed, all devitalized tissue and bone are debrided, and a new prosthesis is reimplanted immediately, followed by 6 weeks of parenteral antibiotic therapy. Antibiotic-impregnated (i.e., tobramycin or gentamicin) methylmethacrylate cement is used in these situations, and success rates of more than 75% were reported.[78,131,132,190,397,428,536,596] This procedure is appropriate only for patients with infections caused by less virulent microorganisms because of the high failure rates seen when a more virulent organism such as *S. aureus* or a gram-negative bacillus is the cause of the infection. The Ilizarov method allows simultaneous treatment of infection, bone and joint deformities, bone loss, and shortening of the limb. This device includes proximal and distal circular external rings with wires passing through the bone and soft tissue from one side of the limb to the other. Although this method is used more often for the treatment of bone nonunion or bone loss with or without infection, David and colleagues[112] used this technique successfully to treat 12 patients who failed total knee arthroplasty because of infection. Wound infection and chronic osteomyelitis caused by infection of the wire tract occur infrequently and should be treated by debridement of the infected soft tissue and curettage of the infected bone.

The two-stage prosthetic removal-reimplantation procedure coupled with the incorporation of antibiotic-impregnated cement during reinsertion of the implant, in combination with a 6-week antibiotic regimen, is the mainstay of therapy for infections of prosthetic joints. Selection of antibiotics should take into account the recent increase in methicillin resistance among staphylococci for the following reasons: MRSA infections of the prosthetic joint result in a higher incidence of treatment failure than do infections with methicillin-susceptible *S. aureus*, and the former result in longer durations of hospitalization and a low survival rate free of treatment failure.[445] Thus vancomycin (with or without rifampin) should be the initial drug of choice for gram-positive bacteria until the susceptibility of the infecting organism is known.[491] In chronic and hematogenous infections (in which gram-negative bacteria are more common) carbapenems, aminoglycosides, or fluoroquinolones should be considered in addition to vancomycin until the microbiology results are available. Reports of treatment failures (even with vancomycin susceptibility within the treatment range [i.e., 2 to 4/μg per mL])[219,516] suggest that other antibiotics (e.g., trimethoprim-sulfamethoxazole or linezolid) should be considered. Several reports have shown that linezolid is a reasonable alternative that results in control of the infection.[346,546]

For infected implanted orthopedic devices, the success of therapy is based on total removal of the device together with parenteral antibiotic therapy. In cases in which the foreign body cannot be removed, extended parenteral antibiotic therapy should be instituted and continued until the device can be removed. The duration of therapy varies with the severity of the infection and ranges from several weeks to several years.

Prevention

Like other surgical procedures, prevention efforts should be focused on reducing the ability of the pathogen to reach the surgical site.[16] Patients should be screened for *S. aureus* colonization, and efforts should be made to decolonize those found to be carriers. The success of intranasal mupirocin or bathing with chlorhexidine in reducing the rate of surgical site infections suggests that such measures should be considered for patients receiving prosthetic joint or other implantable orthopedic devices.[55,401]

The use of prophylactic antibiotics for dental procedures in patients with an orthopedic device is controversial. Although no evidence supports such prophylaxis,[46] the American Academy of Orthopedic Surgery recommended it for all patients with joint implants.[14] The practice of using antimicrobial-loaded bone cements for prophylaxis is also controversial. Retrospective studies found it to be effective, but prospective studies found no extra benefit compared to systemic antibiotic prophylaxis. Animal models looking at the use of new biodegradable materials to replace antibiotic impregnated poly(methylmethacrylate) bone cement have shown promise in reducing the number of follow-up surgeries, enhancing antimicrobial efficacy, and regenerating bone in an infected defect.[223]

CEREBROSPINAL FLUID SHUNTS

Infection is a major cause of morbidity in children who undergo CSF shunting procedures.[252,273,477] Such procedures are performed to divert CSF in symptomatic hydrocephalic patients and are used commonly in patients with anatomic abnormalities (e.g., meningomyelocele and Chiari malformations), in premature newborns with intraventricular hemorrhage or intracranial infections (e.g., congenital cytomegalovirus, congenital toxoplasmosis, and bacterial meningitis), and in patients with central nervous system (CNS) tumors or head trauma. Usually the proximal end of the shunt is placed in the frontal or fourth ventricle and the distal end is inserted into the peritoneal cavity (i.e., ventriculoperitoneal shunt). Other compartments such as the right atrium (i.e., ventriculoatrial shunt), the pleural cavity, or the gallbladder can be used to place the distal end. CSF shunts are prone to complications, with a 10-year failure rate greater than 50%.[122] The most common complication is mechanical (such as obstruction or overdrainage), followed by shunt-related infection. The incidence of shunt-related infection varies considerably, from 0.3% to 26%, with more recent studies reporting a range of 8% to 12%.[23,70,103,136,188,252,273,286,477] These infections increase morbidity rates and, in some cases, significantly affect patient outcomes. In addition, the increased morbidity caused additional expenses and resulted in higher costs to the health care system.[532] Understanding some of the factors that contribute to the development of these infections has helped reduce their incidence.[141,564]

Epidemiology

Almost two-thirds of shunt-related infections occur within 1 month after placement of the shunt, and 90% of infections are manifested within 6 months.[187,269,339,459] The incidence of shunt-related infections is significantly higher in infants in the first 6 months of life than in older children or adults.[133,282,414,553] The infection rate is even higher in newborns with intraventricular hemorrhage who undergo shunting in the first week of life[15] and in premature infants.[273,340] Reasons for the increased incidence of shunt-related infection in very young patients are multifactorial. Several mechanisms that have been suggested include delayed wound healing, higher skin density of bacteria that are more resistant to antibiotics and more adherent to the shunt, longer duration of hospitalization, surgical technique, and increased exposure to antibiotics just before the shunt placement.

No significant difference in infection rate is seen in patients with ventriculoperitoneal or ventriculoatrial shunts,[376,473] but a lower infection rate was noted in those with lumboperitoneal or cholecystic shunts. An increased risk for development of infection was reported for shunts placed immediately after removal of a previously infected shunt, probably because of incomplete eradication of bacteria.[137,255] Several other factors, including the underlying cause of the hydrocephalus,[133] the surgeon's experience,[96,251] previous shunt infection,[336] the duration of surgery, the number of people in the operating room, perioperative factors (e.g., prophylactic antibiotics, skin preparation, and shaveless operation),[216] operative time, open surgery to insert the abdominal catheter versus direct puncture of the abdominal wall with a trocar, postoperative CSF leakage, and others,[273,477] have been reported to be associated with an increased incidence of shunt-related infection. Although a trend toward more shunt-related infections has been reported with these factors, it has not been demonstrated consistently. Malignant lesions and trauma as etiologies may have lower rates of infection.[478] A few studies suggest that tapping the shunt may result in an infection, with an incidence ranging from negligible to greater than 30% in premature infants with shunts tapped multiple times.[70] Reinfection rate was estimated to be around 25%.[252,274,528] Multiple factors were suggested as contributing to reinfection, including treatment duration of the first infection, age younger than 6 months, nonsurgical management, intraventricular hemorrhage (IVH) of prematurity, intracranial cysts, or aqueductal stenosis.[340,477,528] The median time to reinfection (i.e., second episode) ranged from 65 to 90 days.[274,528] Almost 60% of children with second infection developed a third reinfection, and 47% of them developed a fourth infection.[529] The median time to the second infection was 65 days, for the third infection 477 days, and for the fourth infection 2137 days.[528]

Etiology

Staphylococcal species are the most common cause of shunt-related infection, with coagulase-negative staphylococci (e.g., *Staphylococcus epidermidis, S. capitis, S. hominis,* and *S. lugdunensis*)[130] being isolated in 25% to 70% of cases (Table 74.1).[130,265,282,473] *S. aureus,* the second most common gram-positive bacterium, is responsible for 10% to 40% of cases. Streptococci (e.g., viridans, group B or C, *S. pyogenes, S. pneumoniae,* enterococci) are identified less commonly (3–7%). Other gram-positive bacteria such as *Propionibacterium*[282,518] and *Corynebacterium* (diphtheroids)[25,180] are isolated as well. The seemingly increased incidence of shunt-related infections caused by these two groups of bacteria probably is the result of poor culture technique (e.g., failure to use anaerobic culture media, less than 5 to 7 days' incubation period), misinterpretation of culture results (e.g., culture contamination) leading to underreporting, or both.

Gram-negative bacteria (e.g., *E. coli, Klebsiella* spp., and *Proteus* spp.) together are the cause of 5% to 25% of shunt-related infections.[496] *Pseudomonas* spp. and *Acinetobacter* spp. are reported as well, but less frequently. Many other etiologic agents, including fungi[86] (e.g., *Candida,*[34,163] *Histoplasma,*[461] *Cryptococcus,*[222] *Torulopsis*[563]), *Pasteurella multocida,*[284] *Neisseria* spp.,[217,503] *Serratia marcescens,*[67] *Listeria monocytogenes,*[290] nontuberculous mycobacteria,[82] and others, have been reported less commonly as causing shunt-related infections. With the increase in the number of patients who are immunocompromised or have significant risk factors for infection (e.g., neutropenia, chronic intravenous catheters, prolonged administration of broad-spectrum antibiotics, and hyperalimentation), the incidence of these rare infections may increase. Bacteria that traditionally cause meningitis, such as *Streptococcus pyogenes* (group A strep),[392] *H. influenzae,*[472,553] *S. pneumoniae,*[376,473,556] and *Neisseria meningitidis,*[287] have been reported as causing shunt-related infections. Whether these cases were isolated shunt-related infections or extensions of meningitis into the ventricular system (i.e., ventriculitis) is not clear. Therefore if such bacteria are isolated from a suspected shunt and the patient has a communicating hydrocephalus, lumbar puncture should be performed to rule out meningitis. Of interest, most children with

TABLE 74.1 Pathogens Causing Cerebrospinal Fluid Shunt Infection

Pathogens	Incidence (%)
Gram-Positive Bacteria	
Staphylococcus, coagulase-negative (e.g., *S. epidermidis, S. capitis, S. hominis, S. warneri, S. lugdunensis, S. haemolyticus*)	25–70
Staphylococcus aureus	10–40
Streptococci (e.g., *Streptococcus pyogenes*, group B or C streptococci, *Enterococcus, S. pneumoniae*)	3–7
Propionibacterium spp.	Rare
Corynebacterium spp.	1–2
Gram-Negative Bacteria	
Escherichia coli	5–25
Klebsiella spp.	5–10
Proteus spp.	2–6
Pseudomonas spp.	2–4
Acinetobacter spp.	1–3
Other gram-negative bacteria (e.g., *Neisseria* spp., *Haemophilus influenzae, Pasteurella*)	<1
Fungi	
Candida spp.	<1
Histoplasma	<1
Cryptococcus	<1
Torulopsis	<1

H. influenzae or *S. pneumoniae* infections recovered with antibiotic therapy alone and without shunt removal.[472]

Pathogenesis

Several observations suggest that most CNS shunt–related infections are caused by inoculation of the organism during surgery or bacterial colonization during the early phase of wound healing.[519] Contamination of the device by ward personnel during manipulation also was suggested.[405,561] These observations include the facts that common skin flora (e.g., coagulase-negative staphylococci and *S. aureus*) are the pathogens most frequently encountered, most of the infections occur within the first few weeks after surgery, and irrigation of the system is a risk factor for the development of infection. Another common mechanism (occurring with gram-negative bacterial infections) is retrograde progression of bacteria from the gastrointestinal tract (i.e., bowel perforation)[212,439] or from the urinary tract (in the case of a ventriculoureteral shunt).[160] Other mechanisms by which shunts become infected include (1) hematogenous infection in which a distant site of infection produces bacteremia leading to a shunt infection, although rare, and (2) wound or skin infection (e.g., cellulitis or decubitus ulcer) with direct extension from the infection site to the shunt.

The predominant role of coagulase-negative staphylococci and *S. aureus* in CNS shunt–related infection is the result of their being the major constituents of normal cutaneous flora, especially in young children,[295,465] and their having the ability to adhere directly to the shunt (e.g., *S. epidermidis*) or to host proteins covering the shunt (e.g., *S. aureus*). In addition, coagulase-negative staphylococci (and some *S. aureus* strains) produce large amounts of extracellular slime (i.e., biofilm).[66] More than 60% of staphylococci isolated from infected shunts produce biofilm.[117,138,185,592] The biofilm of *S. epidermidis* is a mixture of teichoic acid and protein. Production of biofilm also was reported in corynebacterial infection, which may explain the increasing importance of this organism in CNS shunt–related infections.[39] Biofilm facilitates attachment of these organisms to the surface of the shunt and protects the bacteria from the host immune defenses. Once the organisms are attached to the shunt material, they are extremely difficult to remove except by complete replacement of the shunt. In addition, penetration of antibiotic into the biofilm is variable, and the biofilm antagonizes the antimicrobial activity of some antibiotics, such as vancomycin.[123,142] Moreover infections caused by nonadherent organisms were significantly more likely to be cured by antibiotics alone (without removal of the shunt) than were infections caused by adherent organisms. Similarly Diaz-Mitoma and colleagues[117] found that both obstruction of ventriculoperitoneal shunts and failure to cure the infection with antibiotics alone occurred more frequently when infectious episodes were caused by biofilm-producing coagulase-negative staphylococci. Therefore complete removal of the shunt should be considered in patients with coagulase-negative staphylococci or *S. aureus* infection.

The immature humoral immune system of young infants is not likely to explain the increased incidence of shunt-related infections in patients younger than 6 months because these infants mount antistaphylococcal antibody responses that are comparable to those of older children.[415] Although levels of immunoglobulins and complement proteins are lower in this young group, levels of these proteins normally are very low in the CSF of older individuals (CSF levels of IgG and IgA are between 0.25% and 0.5% of those in serum). In addition, the types of bacteria causing CNS shunt–related infections are not associated commonly with humoral immunodeficiency states, thus suggesting that humoral protection is less important in CNS shunt–related infections. Little is known about the possible role of reduced tissue immunity in these infections.

The foreign body nature of the shunt apparatus plays an important role in the local host defense defect.[59] Electron-microscopic findings demonstrate irregularities in catheters, allowing microorganisms to be buried in the catheter. Other mechanisms that may contribute to shunt-related infections include (1) abnormal CSF flow (i.e., not being absorbed by the venous sinuses, thought to be important for prevention of infection in the CNS) and (2) interruption of the blood–brain barrier by the shunt catheter, with the creation of a direct tract between the subcutaneous tissues and the ventricles resulting in significant compromise in host defenses.[561]

Clinical Manifestations

The initial signs and symptoms of most patients with shunt-related infections are nonspecific and include mild to moderate fever, malaise, irritability, nausea, vomiting, vague abdominal pain, and headache. With such nonspecific findings, the physician must be careful to differentiate between a potential shunt-related infection and an intercurrent viral or bacterial infection of the upper respiratory, urinary, or gastrointestinal tract. Examination of the CSF (from a shunt tap) may be helpful. Only a minority of patients have the classic signs and symptoms of CNS inflammation, such as a stiff neck, bulging fontanelle, change in mental status, cranial nerve palsy, or papilledema. In some patients the shunt tract may be infected, with evidence of cellulitis, dehiscence, or both of the surgical wounds. Tenderness, edema, or erythema along the tract itself may be the only sign. Patients with known seizures frequently develop seizures with shunt malfunction (inducing in cases of infection).[261]

The type of shunt affects the nature of the infection. For example, ventriculoperitoneal shunt–related infections may cause symptoms and signs confined to the abdominal cavity, such as abdominal pain, tenderness (with or without guarding), intestinal obstruction,[435] or spontaneous bacterial peritonitis.[162,350] Rarely a distal shunt-related infection will be manifested as frank ascites as a result of CSF malabsorption.[275] A relatively common complication of ventriculoperitoneal shunts is an inflammatory peritoneal exudate that may lead to CSF loculation and the subsequent formation of a peritoneal pseudocyst.[17,437] These pseudocysts often are palpable and can be visualized by ultrasonography or CT. Bacteria are isolated in a third of cases, suggesting that infection may play a role in the pathogenesis of pseudocysts. In most cases, however, a high index of suspicion is required because the initial abdominal symptoms occur with no other signs of shunt malfunction.

A unique complication of patients with ventriculoatrial shunts is the development of immune complex disease such as shunt nephritis (a form of acute glomerulonephritis), arthritis, or rash.[447] In most of these cases, the infecting organism is *S. epidermidis,* but other bacteria such as *Corynebacterium* can cause this complication.[56] In the case of shunt nephritis, the patient has fever, edema, malaise, hepatosplenomegaly, hypocomplementemia, anemia, azotemia, hematuria, and proteinuria.[106] Pathologic findings consist of mesangial hypercellularity and granular deposits of immunoglobulins and complement along the glomerular membrane. Rarely arthritis may be the initial symptom.[288]

Diagnosis

Although shunt-related infections are not common, the nonspecific signs and symptoms and the insidious onset in many cases render establishing a diagnosis difficult. Therefore in any patient with a CNS shunt and fever without an obvious source, a shunt-related infection should be considered, especially in the case of persistent symptoms. A higher index of suspicion for shunt-related infection is needed in young patients with new fever within 3 to 6 months after shunt placement. The only definitive diagnostic test is direct staining and culture of CSF. Tapping the shunt or sampling fluid in direct contact with the shunt should be performed if no signs or symptoms of increased intracranial pressure are noted. CNS imaging (CT or MRI) is recommended before the tap is done if such symptoms exist. The shunt tap should be performed with careful sterile technique by a practitioner familiar with the technique and underlying hardware.

When percutaneous needle shunt aspiration is performed, the area around the shunt valve or reservoir should be sterilized and butterfly needle inserted. Measurement of opening pressure can help diagnose a distal malfunction (increased pressure) or proximal shunt obstruction (less than expected pressure). Gentle aspiration of CSF sometimes is performed if no fluid returns spontaneously. If only a few drops of CSF can be obtained, the more important tests, Gram stain and culture, should be performed first.

CSF should be tested for glucose concentration, differential cell count, Gram stain, and culture. Protein concentration is requested often but is of very limited help in evaluating the presence or absence of an infection because high protein levels are found in many patients with shunt malfunction and no infection. In contrast, normal protein levels have been reported in many patients with shunt-related infections. A low glucose level suggests an infection, although this is not sensitive for shunt-related infection. Typically CSF pleocytosis with a predominance of PMNs is indicative of a shunt-related infection. A count of 100 cells/μL or more is highly suggestive of infection.[281,291,337] According to one study, a CSF WBC count greater than 100 cells/μL with more than 10% PMN cells in febrile patients is 82% sensitive and 99% specific for shunt infection, with a positive predictive value of 93%.[337] In contrast, the negative predictive value is 95% for a sample with less than 10% PMNs. A recent review suggests that infection with gram-negative bacteria resulted in a higher initial and peak WBC count, with a greater percentage of PMNs than gram-positive bacteria.[156] In some cases the finding of a positive CSF culture is interpreted as a shunt-related infection despite a normal WBC count (<10 WBCs/mm^3) and the absence of clinical symptoms, when the positive culture probably represents colonization or contamination. Other cells, such as mononuclear cells[269,497] or eosinophils[337,571] can also predominate during an infection. If eosinophilia is the predominant cellular response, an allergy to the shunt (e.g., silicone[234]) or the materials used for sterilization (e.g., ethylene oxide[411]) or use of an antibiotic-impregnated catheter[529] or intraventricular administration of antibiotics (e.g., gentamicin[349] and vancomycin[177]) should be considered. It is important to note that eosinophilia (without these causes, including infection) is relatively common (but transient) in children with a CNS shunt.[155,194]

Interpretation of the WBC count should be done cautiously if the red blood cell count is high because the increased number of WBCs can be the result of blood spilling into the CSF or be part of the inflammatory response to the presence of blood (i.e., chemical ventriculitis).[406] A negative Gram stain result does not exclude an infection, and one should wait for the results of culture. Ventricular fluid always should be cultured anaerobically as well as aerobically. Although most bacteria causing shunt-related infections grow within 48 to 78 hours, cultures should be held for 7 days (if still negative) for fastidious organisms such as *Propionibacterium.*[27] The possibility of contamination or colonization of the shunt without infection should be considered when the culture is positive but other CSF parameters are normal. If such a scenario occurs and bacteria are growing only from one sample (e.g., a shunt tap) and not from subsequent CSF cultures, a shorter course of therapy may be sufficient.

Blood cultures, a peripheral complete blood count (CBC), and ultrasound of the abdomen (for ventriculoperitoneal shunts) are of limited value. For example, although 90% of patients with ventriculoatrial shunt–related infection will have a positive blood culture, fewer than 10% of patients with other shunt-related infections will have a positive culture. In more than a third of patients with shunt-related infections, no elevation in the peripheral WBC count was found. Some investigators suggest that blood CRP levels may be helpful in establishing the diagnosis of shunt-related infection when other concurrent infections (e.g., sinusitis, pneumonia) were excluded.[281,456] The triad of fever, abnormal CSF WBC count, and greater than 5% eosinophilia is highly predictive of a shunt-related infection.[337]

Treatment

A variety of medical and surgical approaches to treatment of an infected shunt have been suggested.[570] Regimens include (1) the use of antibiotics (systemically, with or without intraventricular administration) without removal of the shunt hardware; (2) removal of the infected shunt followed by immediate insertion of a new shunt and the administration of antibiotics[366]; (3) removal of the infected shunt and insertion of an extraventricular device (EVD) to monitor the patient's response to the accompanying antibiotic therapy, with a new shunt inserted only when the ventricular system is sterilized; (4) removal of the infected shunt followed by a stereotactic third ventriculostomy and administration of antibiotics; and (5) externalization of only the distal (e.g., peritoneal) catheter, along with the administration antibiotics.

The use of antibiotics alone without surgery was justified by the need to maintain CSF drainage and avoid costly operations and lengthy duration of hospital stay. The low success rate of this approach (33%) and the higher mortality rate associated with it suggest that it should not be used (Table 74.2). Of interest, the failure rate was much higher with infections caused by biofilm-producing organisms than with infections caused by bacteria that do not produce biofilm.[117] Only in shunted patients with purulent meningitis caused by *S. pneumoniae, N. meningitidis,* or *H. influenzae* did the administration of systemic antibiotics alone without removal of the shunt seem to be an effective option.[287,381]

Combining immediate replacement of the infected shunt with a new shunt and antibiotic therapy has a higher rate of success (70%; see Table 74.2) than does the use of antibiotics alone. Nonetheless it is less effective than removal of the infected shunt accompanied by insertion of an EVD and administration of antibiotic therapy (88% success rate; see Table 74.2). A decision analysis of 17 studies reached the same conclusion and suggested that "this treatment option has the highest cure rate and the lowest failure and mortality rates."[455] In addition, lack of the ability to monitor when the ventricular fluid is sterilized results in a longer period of systemic antibiotic therapy (e.g., 4 to 8 weeks) and may lead to an increase in iatrogenic infections and cost.

For infection that involves only the distal part of the shunt (e.g., pseudocyst, appendicitis,[395] erythema or swelling along the shunt tract, or surgical wound infection), externalization of only the distal end of the shunt along with the administration of antibiotic therapy is recommended by some neurosurgeons. Potential advantages of this technique include (1) diversion of CSF from an infected area to avoid ascending infection, (2) maintenance of CSF flow to prevent increased intracranial pressure (ICP), (3) the ability to perform frequent CSF sampling, and (4) the capability of monitoring therapy. The disadvantage is that early infection or colonization of the proximal portion of the shunt may be obscured by the antibiotic treatment and become active after discontinuation of therapy and reinsertion of the distal part. In patients with *P. acne*–related distal shunt infection, catheter removal without (or very short) antibiotic treatment is sufficient.[27]

Internal shunting by a third ventriculostomy with avoidance of a prosthetic device during the infected CSF shunt removal was investigated as another option to reduce reinfection. Although this procedure was shown to be effective in managing patients with refractory shunt-related infections who have a noncommunicating hydrocephalus, patent subarachnoid space, and adequate CSF absorption, the prevention of reinfection was marginal.[149,332,368,470,473] Yet it seems that the reinserted ventriculoperitoneal shunts after a third ventriculostomy have a better longevity than those inserted without this procedure.[470] Shunt independence for extended periods was documented in patients without

TABLE 74.2 Shunt Infection Cure Rates in Relation to the Therapeutic Approach

Study	Antibiotics Alone[a]	Antibiotics and Immediate Replacement With New Shunt	Antibiotics, Removal of Shunt, and Insertion of EVD
Schoenbaum[453]	5/30[b]		25/26
Nelson[367]	10/13		46/46
Salmon[446]		5/10	
Sells[464]	1/8	1/6	9/9
James[231]	3/10		9/10
Venes[543]		6/9	3/3
James[230]	4/11	11/13	21/22
Wald[559]	15/20		
Mates[329]	7/8		
Shurtleff[474]	2/27	6/20	19/19
Morrice[358]	4/14	19/23	14/18
Frame[152]	8/11	21/27	
Forward[149]	8/15	2/2	13/13
Luthardt[310]	1/17		
O'Brien[374]	11/11	15/19	9/9
Walters[561]	13/92	11/21	44/71
Swayne[509]			19/20
Ronan[438]	3/4	4/7	21/22
Stamos[496]			23/23
Younger[592]	4/11	42/46	
Total (success rate)	**99/302 (32.8%)**	**143/203 (70.4%)**	**275/311 (88.4%)**

Values are given as number cured/number treated.
[a]With and without intraventricular antibiotics.
EVD, Extraventricular device.

myelomeningocele. The success rate is lower in those with myelomeningocele or hemorrhage or after meningitis.[135]

The most effective treatment of shunt-related infections is to remove the entire infected shunt and insert an EVD to control ICP and monitor the infection. After antibiotic therapy has been successful, a new shunt is placed. With this approach, treatment success is very high (see Table 74.2), with more rapid clearance of the infection and a shorter duration of therapy.

The choice of intravenous antibiotic depends on local patterns of antimicrobial susceptibility and the ability of the antibiotic to penetrate the blood-brain barrier. With the notable rate of methicillin-resistant staphylococci, vancomycin should be used as initial therapy while awaiting bacteriologic identification and the results of antibiotic sensitivity testing. Effort should be made to discontinue vancomycin promptly following proof that organism is sensitive to the semisynthetic penicillins. In addition, despite in vitro data that bacteria are highly sensitive to first-generation cephalosporins (e.g., cephalothin, cefazolin), they should not be used due to poor penetration of the blood-brain barrier. Linezolid has been used successfully in cases of shunt infection.[54,79,372,548,589] This drug has a good CSF penetration, with concentrations above the minimal inhibitory concentration (MIC) of most gram-positive bacteria, including MRSA.[40,591] The limited data available suggest that linezolid should be considered cautiously when vancomycin fails or cannot be given. Rifampin should be considered as one of the drugs in the combination for gram-positive bacteria for three reasons. First, most staphylococci are still sensitive to this antibiotic and their MIC is significantly lower than that of other antistaphylococcal drugs. Unfortunately the use of rifampin alone may be followed rapidly by rifampin-resistant variants. Second, rifampin penetrates CSF well and easily achieves a greater than 10-fold level over the MIC of most staphylococci. Third, rifampin has demonstrated good bactericidal activity even when staphylococci were embedded in biofilm. In contrast, staphylococcal biofilm inhibits the antimicrobial activity of vancomycin.[142]

To achieve more consistent and efficient eradication of bacteria, the CSF drug level should be at least 10 times higher than the MIC of the pathogen. Therefore the dosage of antibiotic or antibiotics and the dosing interval should be maximized (i.e., "meningeal schedule"). If the selected antibiotic does not clear the infection within 2 to 3 days and no improvement occurs in CSF biochemical and WBC parameters (i.e., seemingly inadequate control of the infection), measurement of the bactericidal titer of ventricular fluid should be considered. To determine bactericidal titer, 1 mL of CSF (if CSF production is >5/mL/h) at the expected peak antibiotic level (i.e., 2 to 3 hours after the antibiotic is given parenterally) is diluted serially with culture media to produce dilutions of 1:2, 1:4, 1:8, and 1:16. To these dilutions, an equal amount of medium with 10^5 colony forming units/mL of the offending bacteria is added (the final CSF dilution is 1:4, 1:8, 1:16, and 1:32). After 24 hours of incubation, the tubes are observed for turbidity, which reflects the growth of bacteria. If no turbidity is seen in the 1:8 and 1:16 or higher dilution tubes, the CSF level of the antibiotic probably is sufficient, and continued growth of bacteria from CSF may be caused by colonization of the EVD or contamination. On the other hand, if turbidity is noted in the tube with less than a 1:8 dilution (i.e., a 1:4 dilution), the CSF level of antibiotic may not be sufficient to combat the infection and the addition of another antibiotic or change to a different antibiotic is warranted.

Selection of the initial antibiotic before culture results are known can be based on the patient's clinical and CSF findings. The initial diagnostic step after empiric antibiotic therapy is evaluation of the CSF Gram stain. If the Gram stain result is positive for gram-positive bacteria (e.g., *Staphylococcus* or *Streptococcus*), the drug of choice is vancomycin. If the Gram stain shows gram-negative bacteria, the drug of choice is cefotaxime (or ceftriaxone) or, in cases of suspected pseudomonas or multidrug-resistant infection, meropenem. Treatment with an aminoglycoside is acceptable, but the outcome seems to be less favorable because of poorer penetration into CSF.[386] If the Gram stain result is negative, other CSF parameters (e.g., WBC count and glucose) should be examined. If either is abnormal and the patient is not severely sick, vancomycin alone may be considered because the chance of having a gram-negative infection is low.[496]

In contrast, if the patient is more ill, coverage for gram-negative bacteria should be added (e.g., cefotaxime or ceftriaxone). In nontoxic patients with normal CSF parameters and no distal symptoms (e.g., peritonitis or wound or tract infection), antibiotic therapy can be withheld until the results of culture are known. On the other hand, if distal signs or symptoms exist, therapy is tailored according to the site. In patients with skin involvement, vancomycin is the drug of choice, whereas in febrile patients with abdominal symptoms, the combination of cefotaxime (or ceftriaxone) and metronidazole (to cover anaerobic bacteria) is preferred. An alternative for gram-negative plus anaerobic coverage in a seriously ill patient with history of broad spectrum antibiotic exposure or multidrug-resistant organism is meropenem.

Direct instillation of antibiotics into the ventricular system to increase their levels is suggested by some experts.[595] Such treatment may be considered in patients with persistently positive cultures despite intravenous therapy or multidrug-resistant organisms requiring specific antibiotics with inadequate CSF penetration. Several studies have reported promising results using combination of intravenous and intraventricular therapy.[132,303,512] Unfortunately the suggested doses for intraventricular treatment have been determined empirically on only a small number of patients, and their pharmacokinetics and pharmacodynamics have not been studied well. This therapy is not without risk, especially when the recommended doses often are much higher than those found to cause neurotoxicity.[262,481,566] Pleocytosis and eosinophilia also have occurred in patients receiving intraventricular vancomycin[307] or gentamicin.[349] In addition, preservative-containing preparations should be checked for appropriateness for intraventricular instillation. Limited pharmacokinetic data suggest that clearance of the instilled intraventricular antibiotic is sufficiently slow to allow once-daily administration. If possible, the EVD should be closed for 30 to 60 minutes after the drug is administered. If the EVD cannot be closed and the amount of CSF drainage exceeds 7 to 10 mL/h, the frequency of intraventricular antibiotic instillation should be increased to twice daily.

Antibiotics commonly recommended for intravenous and intraventricular use according to the etiologic agent are shown in Table 74.3, although antibiotic choice should be based on antimicrobial susceptibility results of the isolated pathogen. A small study in adults showed that administration of vancomycin 10 mg intraventricularly once daily was safe and achieved levels greater than 5 μg/mL (the recommended CSF trough level needed to achieve cure) for up to 21 hours.[407] Because of the potential toxicity of the empirically recommended intraventricular antibiotic doses and the unpredictability of CSF levels, irrigation of the ventricular system with a known concentration of an antibiotic solution is preferred when systemic antibiotics fail to eradicate the bacteria. To achieve irrigation, two EVDs must be inserted to produce a continuous flow of solution. The concentration of antibiotic in the solution should be equal to the highest safe plasma level when the drug is given intravenously. For example, for treating gram-negative bacteria sensitive to amikacin, amikacin at a dose of 30 to 40 mg/L of saline solution (producing a concentration of 30–40 μg/mL) is recommended. Gentamicin 10 to 12 mg/L (using a special intrathecal preparation) is an acceptable alternative when the gentamicin MIC for the bacteria is less than 1 μg/mL. The antibiotic solution is administered through one EVD at a rate of 10 mL/h, and the second EVD is left open to drain the fluid and to remove debris and pus from the ventricles.

When antibiotic therapy is completed, abnormal CSF findings such as low glucose or mildly elevated protein or cell counts should not delay reshunting. The duration of treatment is empirical and depends on the etiologic agent, the CSF parameters at initial evaluation, and the time to sterilization. In our institution, we found the following schedule to be successful: If CSF parameters are *normal* but culture yields coagulase-negative staphylococci from only the operating room (i.e., the initial sample), therapy should be given for only 3 to 4 days. If subsequent cultures also are positive, therapy should continue until negative cultures have been obtained for 7 days. If CSF parameters are *abnormal* in the operating room and culture is positive *only* from that specimen, therapy should continue for 7 days. If subsequent samples show abnormal CSF findings and positive cultures, therapy should be extended until negative cultures have been obtained for 10 days. This protocol was adopted by the Infectious Diseases Society of America guidelines for the management of CSF shunt infections.[530]

TABLE 74.3 Recommended Intravenous and Intraventricular Antibiotic Therapy for Shunt Infection According to Etiologic Agent

Etiologic Agent	Antibiotic	IV Dose (mg/kg/day) and Frequency	Intraventricular Dose (mg/day, 1 Dose)
Bacteria			
Staphylococcus aureus or coagulase-negative staphylococci			
Methicillin sensitive	Oxacillin[a,b]	200 (q8h)	NA
	or		
	Nafcillin[a,b]	200 (q8h)	50–75
Methicillin resistant	Vancomycin[b]	60 (q8h)	5–20
	or		
	Linezolid	30 (q8h)	
Streptococcal species	Penicillin[a]	200,000/U (q6h)	NA
	or		
	Ampicillin[a]	400 (q6h)	10–25
Diphtheroids	Ceftriaxone	100 (q12h)	
Enterococcus faecalis	Ampicillin[a]	Doses as above	
	or		
	Penicillin[a]		NA
	plus		
	Aminoglycoside[c]		
Anaerobic bacteria	Metronidazole	22.5–30 (q8h)	NA
Escherichia coli, Klebsiella, Proteus, Enterobacter	Cefotaxime	200–300 (q6h)	NA
	or		
	Ceftriaxone	100 (q12h)	NA
	or		
	Amikacin[§]	22.5 (q8h)	5–30
	or		
	Tobramycin[d]	7.5 (q8h)	5–20
	or		
	Gentamicin[d]	7.5 (q8h)	1–8
	or		
	Meropenem	120 (q8h)	
Pseudomonas spp.	Ceftazidime	200 (q8h)	NA
	or		
	Aminoglycoside		
	plus		
	Broad-spectrum penicillin		
	or		
	Carbapenem		
Fungi			
Candida spp.	Amphotericin B[e]	1 (q24h)	0.1–0.5
	AmBisome	5 (q24h)	

NA, Not available.
[a]In patients allergic to penicillin, use vancomycin.
[b]If cerebrospinal fluid levels are not sufficient and the bacteria are sensitive to rifampin, add rifampin, 20 mg/kg per day divided every 12 hours.
[c]See doses (for the specific aminoglycoside) for treatment of *E. coli* below.
[d]The addition of a broad-spectrum penicillin (e.g., piperacillin or ticarcillin, 300 to 400 mg/kg per day divided every 6 hours) may add to the bactericidal activity.
[e]If ventricular fluid remains positive after 5 to 7 days of therapy with amphotericin, add flucytosine (150 mg/kg per day divided every 6 hours).

A longer duration of antibiotic therapy is recommended with other bacteria (e.g., *S. aureus*, gram-negative bacteria). If culture is positive *only* on samples from the *operating room* and CSF findings are normal, treatment should be given until negative cultures have been obtained for 7 days. In all other situations, therapy should continue until negative cultures have been achieved for 10 days. Reshunting should take place immediately at the end of treatment. No benefit is found in observing the patient for a time without antibiotics for relapse of the infection.[564]

Complications

Shunt-related infections are associated with increased morbidity and mortality rates.[481] Patients with shunt-related infection have an increase in shunt-related operations, which contributes to the increased morbidity and cost. Even when the initial infection is treated successfully, secondary infection (or contamination) of the EVD occurs in 5% to 10% of cases. To minimize the risk for development of a secondary infection, a sterile closed-drainage system should be maintained. Only trained personnel should be allowed to drain CSF samples from the system, and injection into the system should be avoided. Continuous external drainage of CSF also causes loss of electrolytes and fluid. Therefore assessment of serum electrolytes is recommended, and, if significant, the total daily amount of drained CSF should be replaced. Recurrent shunt-related infection after completion of treatment is common, with two-thirds of such infections being caused by the same organism.[252] Unusual complications of ventricular shunt infections include brain abscess and subdural empyema.[136,558]

Prognosis

Complete removal of the shunt system results in better prognosis.[477] Long-term morbidity occurring after a shunt-related infection includes seizures, psychomotor retardation, and cognitive deficiency. The intelligence quotient (IQ) scores of children with myelomeningocele who had a shunt-related infection were found to be significantly lower (mean IQ, 72) than the scores of children with shunts but no infection (mean IQ, 95).[342] A trend was observed in which younger children with shunt-related infections had a lower IQ than older children with shunt-related infections, especially if the infection was caused by gram-negative bacteria. In addition, shunt-related infection adversely affected school performance.[553] With appropriate combined medical and surgical therapy, the mortality rate from shunt-related infection is low, but any episode of shunt-related infection appears to increase the probability of a subsequent episode.

Prevention

Standardized care protocols have been shown to reduce infections.[213,253,410,489] Preventive measures to reduce the incidence of shunt-related infection include attention to preoperative and intraoperative technique and the prophylactic use of antibiotics. Bactericidal shampoos (e.g., chlorhexidine) should be used to reduce the bacterial density of the scalp before surgery is performed. Shaving the scalp seems to be a risk factor, and thus shaveless surgery should be considered.[216] During the operation, only essential personnel should be present, and the skin should be cleaned with a fat solvent, followed by iodine solutions that reduce the number of bacteria[87] or bacteria's ability to adhere to the shunt (bacitracin).[176] Careful attention should be paid to surgical technique, with contact between the shunt and the skin avoided. A detailed preoperative protocol developed by the Hydrocephalus Clinical Research Network (HCRN) has reduced the infection rate from 8.8% to 5.7%.[253] Other investigators were able to reduce the infection rate by using measures similar to those suggested by the HCRN.[88] A single-center study showed that infection rate was reduced from 21% to 4.3% when impregnated sutures were used,[478] and other studies suggest that use of an antibiotic-impregnated shunt system significantly reduces the incidence of shunt infections in contrast to the use of a standard shunt.[175,362,390,396,462,463,593] However, no significant reduction in the overall shunt-related infection rate was observed in other studies.[193,242] In addition, the antibiotic-impregnated catheter may increase the rate of bacteria resistant to its antibiotic components.[115] Large, prospective, randomized studies are needed to evaluate the real contribution of an antibiotic-impregnated shunt to the reduction in infection rate.

Multiple studies have examined the effect of prophylactic antibiotics for the shunt insertion procedure on reducing the infection rate.[65,263,282,420,426,427] A recent meta-analysis and systematic review of nine studies, with seven being randomized controlled trials, found the infection rate in the prophylactic antibiotics group to be 5.9% compared with 10.7% in the control group.[263] A previous meta-analysis of 17 trials found a statistically significant benefit for either systemic antibiotic prophylaxis (15 studies) or antibiotic-impregnated catheters (two studies) in reducing the incidence of shunt-related infections, and some experts suggested adding intraventricular antibiotic administration (e.g., gentamicin or vancomycin) during the procedure.[421,426] The choice of antibiotics should be based on the local antibiotic sensitivity pattern of the pathogens commonly causing shunt-related infections in that area, although cefazolin is generally recommended, with vancomycin or clindamycin recommended in cases of β-lactam allergy and vancomycin preferred by some due to the frequency of coagulase-negative staphylococcus in these infections. Although many experts recommend giving the first dose 30 to 60 minutes before skin incision, prophylaxis should be considered to start 8 to 12 hours before surgery to allow higher levels of drug to accumulate in skin tissue than would do so if treatment were given just before the operation. The duration of prophylaxis should not exceed 24 to 36 hours. Further studies are needed to identify factors important in the development of shunt-related infections so that better techniques can be developed to further reduce or even eliminate this devastating complication of CNS shunting.

INTRACRANIAL PRESSURE MONITORS

Monitoring of ICP has become an important part of the evaluation, treatment, and management of children with a variety of intracranial pathologic processes,[308] including congenital anomalies (e.g., cranial or craniofacial dysostosis), metabolic diseases, trauma, intraventricular or subarachnoid hemorrhage, intracranial infections (e.g., meningitis, encephalitis), and other ischemic or hypoxic insults.[388] Several studies have demonstrated the therapeutic and prognostic benefit of monitoring ICP in children with high ICP[150,233,296,520]; nonetheless this procedure is not without complications such as hematoma, bleeding, leakage of CSF, and infection. Infections for which monitoring of ICP is used include ventriculitis, meningitis, brain abscess, subdural empyema, skin infection, and cranial bone infections.[264,307,580]

Several methods are available for monitoring ICP. Intraventricular placement of a catheter with the distal end connected to a pressure transducer is the method used most frequently because of its accuracy and ease of calibration. This procedure also allows drainage of CSF for biochemical or dynamic testing. Disadvantages of ventriculostomy are penetration of the meninges and brain, technical difficulties if the ventricles are small, and greater risk for the development of infection. Other methods used to monitor ICP include a subdural bolt or catheter (only the meninges are penetrated, but the brain remains intact), an epidural transducer (the dura remains intact), and a continuous intraparenchymal monitor (i.e., a fiberoptic cable is inserted through the dura into the brain parenchyma, not intraventricularly). Although both the epidural transducer and the intraparenchymal monitor have fewer complications (e.g., infection) than the intraventricular devices, they are prone to inaccuracy, which limits their use. Selection of the appropriate ICP-monitoring method depends on the patient's condition and the risk associated with the procedure.[315]

Epidemiology

Assessing the true infection rate of ICP monitoring devices is very difficult, mainly because the methods used to define infection (i.e., inclusion and exclusion criteria), the indication for ICP placement, and antibiotic use vary widely among reported studies. The incidence of infection ranged from less than 1% to 45%, with an average infection rate of 9.5%.[256,306,579] A much higher rate of infection was reported in patients who had devices that penetrated the meninges[208] than in those who had parenchymal monitors.[416]

Multiple factors were suggested as increasing the risk for development of ICP device–related infection including intraventricular or subarachnoid hemorrhage, open head trauma, perforation of the dura, CSF leak, neurosurgical procedure, pressure greater than 20 mm Hg, and frequent manipulations of device.[198] Patients with intracerebral hemorrhage usually do not have a higher risk for acquiring infection than those without such hemorrhage. In contrast, if the bleeding is intraventricular, the incidence of infection increases. The rate of infection also is higher in patients with open head trauma than in those with closed head trauma or intracranial malignancy.[218] Neurosurgical operations contributed significantly to the risk for acquiring infection,[250,397] and the same was noted if ICP was greater than 20 mm Hg.

Interruption of the monitoring system's integrity (e.g., CSF leak, number of times that the system was open, malfunction, and irrigation) was identified by several investigators as increasing patient risk for acquiring infection.[85,203,313] The effect of the duration of monitoring on the risk for infection is controversial, especially in patients with ventriculostomy catheters. Although several studies found a correlation between the length of time that the monitoring device was in place and the infection rate,[256,306] some investigators found no relationship with the duration of monitoring.[579] The different conclusions probably were the result of differences in the populations studied, the types of devices used to measure ICP, the definitions of infection, and analyses of the data. A critical review of the literature evaluating 23 major studies found a correlation between the duration of ICP monitoring and the rate of infections.[306]

The need to replace the device at a certain time has been challenged. Analysis of the outcome in 584 patients (receiving 712 ventriculostomy catheters) who had 61 infections showed a steady increase in the daily incidence of infection that peaked at day 10 with an average time to onset of infection 6.8 days.[208] These data suggest that the majority of infections occurred early after the ICP insertion and therefore that ICP monitoring devices should be removed as quickly as possible, but, if prolonged monitoring is required, catheter exchange is not indicated.

Etiology

In general, the microorganisms that cause infections related to ICP monitoring devices are the same as those causing CNS shunt–related infections (see Table 74.1). The major difference is that gram-negative bacteria are isolated more often in ICP monitor–related infection than in CNS shunt–related infections.[302,313,450] The more common bacteria include *Enterobacter* spp., *Klebsiella* spp., *S. marcescens*, and *Acinetobacter* spp. These bacteria are found in water and cause widespread colonization of hospitalized patients. Colonization of the respiratory tract is an especially common occurrence in patients in the intensive care unit and in those with serious underlying disease. Thus these organisms are occurring increasingly frequently in ICP monitor–related infections. Few infections are caused by *Corynebacterium, Propionibacterium,* and fungi.[186,452]

Clinical Manifestations

ICP monitor–related infections often occur in patients with an altered sensorium; therefore the signs and symptoms of meningeal irritation usually are not present. The clinical diagnosis is complicated further by the fact that these patients frequently are critically ill, and their signs and symptoms are caused by the underlying condition and are not a result of the ICP monitor–related infection. In addition, they may be receiving multiple antibiotics for other sources of infection (e.g., pneumonia, bacteremia, or urinary tract infection), both nosocomial and nonnosocomial. Although fever is the most frequent indication of infection, the presence of infections or inflammatory processes at other body sites causes the predictive value of fever to be low. Therefore providing close follow-up, having a high index of suspicion, and obtaining frequent cultures of CSF when available (e.g., ventriculostomy device) are recommended.

Diagnosis

The predictive value of the peripheral WBC count and differential count are very low, and the diagnostic specificity of the CSF parameters is questionable.[407,450] CSF biochemistry (i.e., protein and glucose) has a very low predictive value. Although a low glucose level may be of help in establishing the diagnosis, a normal level does not exclude the possibility of an infection. Calculation of the ratio of leukocytes to erythrocytes in CSF versus their ratio in peripheral blood was suggested as a potential diagnostic tool for early infection, but it was not validated in a subsequent study.[407,450] Most patients with ICP monitor–related infection will have an increased CSF WBC count with a predominance of PMNs, but in cases with low growth of bacteria, no elevation in CSF WBC counts ($<10/mm^3$) was reported. Most of these cases were caused by coagulation-negative staphylococci. In such cases, if no other indicators of infection (e.g., clinical symptoms or low glucose) are present, the possibility that the positive cultures represent colonization or contamination should be considered before treatment is initiated.

Treatment and Prophylaxis

Only a few control trials have evaluated treatment strategies for ICP infection; therefore the same principles used for the management of CNS shunt–related infections can be applied to infections associated with ICP monitoring devices. The use of antibiotics alone without removal of the device may be adequate for the treatment of infections associated with devices placed in the subdural or epidural space unless an abscess or empyema has formed. In the case of ventriculostomy, the infected device should be removed and appropriate antibiotic therapy instituted. Because gram-negative bacteria may also cause ICP device–related infections, initial antibiotic therapy should include both vancomycin and cefotaxime or ceftazidime if the Gram stain is negative. When the etiologic agent is identified, the specific antibiotic or antibiotics can be chosen from those listed in Table 74.3. The optimal treatment for fungal infections is unknown. Clinical experience with amphotericin B suggests that it is effective despite the fact that it achieves low levels in the CSF. Because fluconazole and voriconazole are known to achieve the best CSF levels, they should be considered as the first drugs of choice.[254] The duration of therapy depends on the etiologic agent and the CSF parameters. In patients with positive CSF culture but minimal CSF pleocytosis, if the CSF culture becomes negative immediately after removal of the catheter, therapy should be given for only 3 or 4 days because the cultures before removal of the catheter reflect colonization and not infection. If subsequent cultures are positive, therapy should continue for 10 days of negative cultures.

Although removal of the ICP monitor (if >5 days) and reinsertion at an alternative site was recommended as a prophylactic approach to reduce the infection rate, this practice is controversial, and several studies showed that routine changes of the ICP monitor did not reduce the risk for development of infection.[306,582]

Many physicians use prophylactic antibiotics for the duration of ICP monitoring in the hope of preventing infection. Unfortunately those studies that have evaluated the utility of antimicrobial agents in preventing such infections reported contradictory results.[431] A decreased rate of ICP monitor infection was reported in patients who received prophylaxis for the duration of the ICP monitoring, but these patients had an increase in MRSA and *Candida* infections.[413] Yet other studies showed no benefit of either preprocedural only prophylactic antibiotics or combined with prolonged antibiotic therapy (until the device was removed).[10,77] In addition, broad-spectrum antibiotic prophylaxis was associated with a shift to resistant gram-negative pathogens.[331] Observational studies suggested that use of antibiotic-coated devices significantly reduced infection rates,[361] and the same results were seen in a longitudinal study comparing infection rates in patients with and without antibiotic-coated catheter.[192] In contrast, a retrospective analysis of patients who developed ventriculitis after placement of either antibiotic-coated EVD or non–antibiotic-impregnated EVD found no major advantage for the impregnated device.[487] A recent systematic review of all studies evaluating systemic prophylactic antibiotic throughout the duration of the external ventricular drainage or placement of antibiotic-coated devices concluded that there is probably some benefit to using either of them.[488] The varying quality of the reviewed studies (most nonrandomized) suggests that cautious interpretation and further research is needed to confirm these findings. In the meantime, antibiotic-impregnated catheters (with or without systemic antibiotics) should be considered for prophylaxis.

INTRATHECAL PUMP INFUSION DEVICES

The intrathecal pump infusion system currently is used to infuse morphine to treat refractory pain,[378] deliver baclofen (a γ-aminobutyric acid agonist), or treat spasticity of spinal or cerebral origin.[8,26,399] In addition, patients with generalized dystonia also benefited from intrathecal baclofen.[7] Several pump systems are used. The simpler systems consist of an externalized catheter system similar to the Hickman catheter[123] or a subcutaneous reservoir system similar to an intravascular implanted port. The more sophisticated systems include a programmable pump that usually is implanted in an abdominal subcutaneous pocket and connected via a subcutaneous catheter to the subarachnoid space.[41] An optional sideport in some of these implanted pumps allows aspiration of CSF from the subarachnoid space.

Complications of the intrathecal pump system are relatively rare events[171,542] and include CSF leakage, intracatheter mechanical complications,[514] pump malfunctions resulting in baclofen withdrawal or overdosage, skin necrosis[159,514] and infection. Complications (especially wound complications such as CSF fistula, dehiscence, granuloma formation, and infection) occur more frequently in children than in adults.[10,148,542] Overdose that may result in coma, respiratory depression, apnea, cardiac conduction abnormalities, hypotension or hypertension, and abnormalities of the pupils was reported as well.[402] Intrathecal baclofen can induce both recurrent and new-onset seizures.[26,267] In addition, acute withdrawal syndrome was reported when treatment was stopped.[475] Infectious complications included suppuration at the exit site,[73,125,207] along the subcutaneous catheter (tunnel infection),[41,73,125,207] and around the pump,[41,73,84] or more severe deep-seated and organ space infections.

Epidemiology

The infection rate of intrathecal pump infusion devices ranges from 1.2% to 12%,[22,60,148] although a recent study reported a rate as high as 21.8%.[164] A more accurate description of the incidence would be the infection rate per 1000 catheter-days, which ranged from 0 to 2.5. The incidence of infections can be reduced by using perioperative antibiotic prophylaxis.[60,360,443]

Infections occurring less than 30 days from operative procedure were more likely to involve the skin and soft tissues, whereas those occurring more than 30 days post procedure were more likely to be deep incisional or organ space infections. Factors associated with infection are duration of procedure (>100 minutes)[73] and spasticity associated with underlying traumatic brain injury or genetic disorder being the indication for device implantation.[118] Multiple other factors, such as patient age, immune deficiency, other concurrent infections, previous intrathecal catheter, number of pump refills, intraspinal anesthetics, surgeon experience with the procedure, and operative complications (e.g., operative loss of blood), were not associated significantly with an increased risk for the acquisition of infection.[73] Very thin or malnourished patients may be prone to poor healing or skin breakdown, although a recent study did not find being underweight to be a risk factor for infection. This study also did not find a difference between subfascial versus subcutaneous pump implantation, whereas other studies have noted decreased infection in subfascial pump implantation.[118,359] One study reported an increased infection frequency in children with a percutaneous endoscopic gastrostomy (PEG) tube or urinary or fecal incontinence.[148] Pump replacement has also been reported as a risk factor for infection following the second operation.[359]

Etiology

The most common bacteria causing intrathecal device–related infection are from the skin flora. Coagulase-negative staphylococci and *S. aureus* lead the list, but *Streptococcus mitis,*[73,371] *Streptococcus* group A or G,[73] *Corynebacterium striatum,*[73] *Enterococcus faecalis,*[156] and polymicrobial infections are observed as well.[42,118] In addition, several studies have reported gram-negative bacteria as the cause of the pump-related infection. Such bacteria include *P. aeruginosa,*[73,156] *Pseudomonas paucimobilis,*[399] *E. coli,*[125] and *Klebsiella pneumoniae.*[398] A rare case of *C. albicans,*[125] *Mycobacterium* spp.,[125] and *Acinetobacter baumanii*[534] also has been reported. A rare case of baclofen vial contamination with the fungus *Wangiella* that caused infection was reported as well.[340,399]

Clinical Manifestations

Clinical findings depend on the site of the infection. Patients with more severe infections (i.e., epidural abscess or meningitis) may have symptoms of these infections (e.g., fever, irritability, headache, nerve root pain, or meningeal signs). In some patients, pain experienced during the injection may be the clue, but in many patients, a high level of awareness for possible infection is important because they will have nonspecific signs and symptoms.

Exit-site and superficial catheter-related infections usually cause local inflammation (e.g., swelling, redness), tenderness, and drainage. The more serious deep-tract (tunnel) infections are more difficult to assess. Visible inflammation along the tract or a soft fluctuant fluid collection around it may be the only clue. Fever is not always present.

Diagnosis

Performing a complete physical and neurologic examination may be helpful. A routine CBC is relatively unhelpful because leukocytosis is not always present, and screening with ESR or C-reactive protein may help identify inflammation in cases of deep-seated infection. MRI may be useful for diagnosing an epidural abscess and evaluating its extent. The only definitive diagnostic tests are Gram stain and culture of exudate or drainage from the exit site (if available), an aspirate of the fluid collection along the catheter tract if tunnel infection is suspected, or CSF for suspected meningitis. Irrigation of the epidural space with 1 or 2 mL of saline after removal of the pump filter (which should be sent for culture) may help in diagnosing an epidural abscess or empyema. Blood culture may be positive in cases of organ space infections, but is unlikely to be helpful in infections involving skin and soft tissue structures.

Treatment and Prophylaxis

If infection has occurred only at the exit site and the superficial catheter tract, local drainage with aggressive cleansing (i.e., topical antibiotics and antiseptics) but without removal of the catheter was suggested.[125] Unfortunately more severe or persistent infections occurred (e.g., deep-tunnel and epidural abscess) in some of these patients[73] (in the recent study by Dickey and colleagues, 71% of pump salvage attempts did not resolve and resulted in subsequent pump explantation).[118] In addition, failure of "catheter-sparing" treatment also was reported.[207] Therefore removal of the catheter should be considered even for mild infections if they do not respond promptly to therapy. In patients with pocket, epidural, and meningeal infections, the intrathecal pump system should be removed as soon as possible and systemic antibiotic therapy initiated (for selection of drugs and doses, see Table 74.3). The duration varies, and there are no trials to suggest a specific regimen, although superficial infections generally receive 7 to 14 days of therapy, whereas deeper infections may receive more than 4 weeks of therapy. With the increasing rate of multidrug-resistant staphylococci and the low CSF levels of vancomycin (only 20–30% of serum levels), linezolid may be considered as an alternative. Linezolid has good CSF penetration (60–70% of the serum level)[591] and has been shown effective in treating severe CNS infections,[444] including intrathecal infusion pump infection.[241] In the few reports that suggest successful treatment of severe pump infections (including meningitis) without removal of the pump system,[63,157,447,542,594] the pathogen was frequently considered to be of low virulence (e.g., coagulase-negative staphylococci) or colonization, which may be the reason for the success. In most of these cases, however, instillation of antibiotics into the reservoir with cautious flushing of the catheter or repetitive local application of antibiotic-impregnated fleece[398] was combined with systemic antibiotics. The main reason for the intrathecal administration of antibiotics is to increase the level of drug in the CSF. Before antibiotics are added to the baclofen infusion, their compatibility with baclofen should be verified or tested (vancomycin is compatible and can be used safely according to Zed and associates[594]).

No guidelines exist on how to treat severe infections of intrathecal pump systems, but, in most cases, removal of the pump system while systemic antibiotics are given and then reimplantation appear to be the treatment of choice. In rare cases in which removal of the pump will be detrimental to the patient, a trial of intrathecal administration of antibiotics may be justified, with close observation to ensure that the patient's condition is not deteriorating.

Although many physicians use perioperative (or longer) antibiotics for prophylaxis, their efficacy in preventing infection has not been proved. Therefore prophylactic antibiotics should not be administered for prolonged period (>24 hours) after the operation.

NEW REFERENCES SINCE THE SEVENTH EDITION

3. Aharon AS, Drinkwater DC Jr, Churchwell KB, et al. Extracorporeal membrane oxygenation in children after repair of congenital cardiac lesions. *Ann Thorac Surg*. 2001;72(6):2095-2102.
20. Ann HW, Ahn JY, Jeon YD, et al. Incidence of and risk factors for infectious complications in patients with cardiac device implantation. *Int J Infect Dis*. 2015;36:9-14.
29. Athan E, Chu VH, Tattevin P, et al. Clinical characteristics and outcome of infective endocarditis involving implantable cardiac devices. *JAMA*. 2012;307:1727-1735.
57. Bongiorni MG, Tascini C, Tagliaferri E, et al. Microbiology of cardiac implantable electronic device infections. *Europace*. 2012;14:1334-1339.
58. Bordachar P, Marquié C, Pospiech T, et al. Subcutaneous implantable cardioverter defibrillators in children, young adults and patients with congenital heart disease. *Int J Cardiol*. 2016;203:251-258.
65. Bratzler DW, Dellinger EP, Olsen KM, et al. Clinical practice guidelines for antimicrobial prophylaxis in surgery. *Am J Health Syst Pharm*. 2013;70(3):195-283.
113. Deharo JC, Quatre A, Mancini J, et al. Long-term outcomes following infection of cardiac implantable electronic devices: a prospective matched cohort study. *Heart*. 2012;98:724-731.
118. Dickey MP, Rice M, Kinnett DG, et al. Infectious complications of intrathecal baclofen pump devices in a pediatric population. *Pediatr Infect Dis J*. 2013;32(7):715-722.
143. Fawawi F, Cardona I, Akinpelu OV, et al. Acute mastoiditis in children with cochlear implants: is explanation required? *Otolaryngol Head Neck Surg*. 2014;151(3):394-398.
164. Ghosh D, Mainali G, Khera J, et al. Complications of intrathecal baclofen pumps in children: experience from a tertiary care center. *Pediatr Neurosurg*. 2013;49(3):138-144.

169. Gold MR, Peters RW, Johnson JW, et al. Complications associated with pectoral cardioverter-defibrillator implantation: comparison of subcutaneous and submuscular approaches. *J Am Coll Cardiol.* 1996;28:1278-1282.
178. Grammes JA, Schulze CM, Al-Bataineh M, et al. Percutaneous pacemaker and implantable cardioverter-defibrillator lead extraction in 100 patients with intracardiac vegetations defined by transesophageal echocardiogram. *J Am Coll Cardiol.* 2010;55:886-894.
181. Greenspon AJ, Prutkin JM, Sohail MR, et al. Timing of the most recent device procedure influences the clinical outcome of lead-associated endocarditis results of the MEDIC (Multicenter Electrophysiologic Device Infection Cohort). *J Am Coll Cardiol.* 2012;59:681-687.
223. Inzana JA, Schwarz EM, Kates SL, et al. Biomaterials approaches to treating implant-associated osteomyelitis. *Biomaterials.* 2016;81:58-71.
224. Ipek EG, Guray U, Demirkan B, et al. Infections of implantable cardiac rhythm devices: predisposing factors and outcome. *Acta Cardiol.* 2012;67:303-310.
230. James HE, Walsh JW, Wilson HD, et al. The management of cerebrospinal fluid shunt infections: a clinical experience. *Acta Neurochir (Wien).* 1981;59(3-4):157-166.
232. Jan E, Camou F, Texier-Maugein J, et al. Microbiologic characteristics and in vitro susceptibility to antimicrobials in a large population of patients with cardiovascular implantable electronic device infection. *J Cardiovasc Electrophysiol.* 2012;23:375-381.
257. Kim MJ, Yu F, Aldave AJ. Microbial keratitis after Boston type I keratoprosthesis implantation. *Ophthalmology.* 2013;120:2209-2216.
263. Klimo P Jr, Van Poppel M, Thompson CJ, et al. Pediatric hydrocephalus: systematic review and Evidence-Based Guidelines Task Force. *J Neurosurg Pediatr.* 2014;14(suppl 1):44-52.
268. Konstantinos A, Polyzos KA, Konstantelias AA, et al. Pacing and resynchronization therapy: risk factors for cardiac implantable electronic device infection: a systematic review and meta-analysis. *Europace.* 2015;17:767-777.
271. Kuiper JWP, Willink RT, Moojen DJF, et al. Treatment of acute periprosthetic infections with prosthesis retention: review of current concepts. *World J Orthop.* 2014;5(5):667-676.
286. Lee JK, Seok JY, Lee JH, et al. Incidence and risk factors of ventriculoperitoneal shunt infections in children: a study of 333 consecutive shunts in 6 years. *J Korean Med Sci.* 2012;27(12):1563-1568.
293. Leuck AM. Left ventricular assist device driveline infections: recent advances and future goals. *J Thorac Dis.* 2015;7(12):2151-2157.
294. Levy DT, Minamoto GY, Da Silva R, et al. Role of gallium SPECT-CT in the diagnosis of left ventricular assist device infections. *ASAIO J.* 2015;61(1):e5-e10.
305. Low WK, Rangabashyam M, Wang F. Management of major post-cochlear implant wound infections. *Eur Arch Otorhinolaryngol.* 2014;271:2409-2413.
316. MacLaren G, Butt W, Best D, et al. Extracorporeal membrane oxygenation for refractory septic shock in children: one institution's experience. *Pediatr Crit Care Med.* 2007;8(5):447-451.
319. Maniar S, Kondareddy S, Topkara VK. Left ventricular assist device-related infections: past, present and future. *Expert Rev Med Devices.* 2011;8(5):627-634.
347. Meyer DM, Jessen ME. Results of extracorporeal membrane oxygenation in children with sepsis. *Ann Thorac Surg.* 1997;63(3):756-761.
348. Meyer DM, Jessen ME, Eberhart RC. Neonatal extracorporeal membrane oxygenation complicated by sepsis. Extracorporeal Life Support Organization. *Ann Thorac Surg.* 1995;59(4):975-980.
359. Motta F, Antonello CE. Analysis of complications in 430 consecutive pediatric patients treated with intrathecal baclofen therapy: 14-year experience. *J Neurosurg Pediatr.* 2014;13(3):301-306.
364. Myint T, Dykhuizen MJ, McDonald CH, et al. Post operative fungal endopthalmitis due to *Geotrichum candidum*. *Med Mycol Case Rep.* 2015;10:4-6.
370. Nienaber JJC, Kusne S, Riaz T, et al. Clinical manifestations and management of left ventricular assists device-associated infections. *Clin Infect Dis.* 2013;57(10):1438-1448.
392. Patel C, Chaudhuri NR, Gaur S. Group A streptococcus ventriculoperitoneal shunt infection in a child. *Pediatr Infect Dis J.* 2012;31(6):660.
393. Patel PA, Elhadi HM, Kitzmiller WJ, et al. Tissue expander complications in the pediatric burn patient: a 10 year follow up. *Ann Plast Surg.* 2014;72(2):150-154.
403. Pettit SJ, McLean A, Colquhoun I, et al. Clinical experience of subcutaneous and transvenous implantable cardioverter defibrillators in children and teenagers. *Pacing Clin Electrophysiol.* 2013;36(12):1532-1538.
409. Pieri M, Greco T, De Bonis M, et al. Diagnosis of infection in patients undergoing extracorporeal membrane oxygenation: a case-control study. *J Thorac Cardiovasc Surg.* 2012;143(6):1411-1416.
412. Polyzos KA, Konstantelias AA, Falagas ME. Risk factors for cardiac implantable electronic device infection: a systemic review and meta-analysis. *Europace.* 2015;17:767-777.
419. Rachitskaya AV, Moysidis SN, Miller D, et al. Streptococcal endophthalmitis in pediatric keratoprosthesis. *Ophthalmology.* 2013;120(7):1506-1507.
420. Ragel BT, Browd SR, Schmidt RH. Surgical shunt infection: significant reduction when using intraventricular and systemic antibiotic agents. *J Neurosurg.* 2006;105(2):242.
422. Rajagopal SK, Almond CS, Laussen PC, et al. Extracorporeal membrane oxygenation for the support of infants, children, and young adults with acute myocarditis: a review of the Extracorporeal Life Support Organization Registry. *Crit Care Med.* 2010;38(2):382-387.
425. Rath PC, Purohit BV, Agrawal B, et al. Pacemaker lead endocarditis due to *Trichosporon* species. *J Assoc Physicians India.* 2015;63(4):66-68.
429. Raveh E, Ulanovski D, Attias J, et al. Acute mastoiditis in children with a cochlear implant. *Int J Pediatr Otorhinolaryngol.* 2016;81:80-83.
432. Reddy VY, Exner DV, Cantillon DJ, et al. Percutaneous implantation of an entirely intracardiac leadless pacemaker. *N Engl J Med.* 2015;373(12):1125-1135.
436. Rohacek M, Erne P, Kobza R, et al. Infection of cardiovascular implantable electronic devices: detection with sonication, swab cultures, and blood cultures. *PACE.* 2015;38:247-253.
460. Schutze GE, Heulitt MJ. Infections during extracorporeal life support. *J Pediatr Surg.* 1995;30(6):809-812.
469. Shi X, Liu R. *Sphingomonas paucimobilis* causing pacemaker pocket infection in a pediatric patient with a hemangioma. *Am J Infect Control.* 2016;44(5): 617-618.
485. Sohail MR, Uslan DZ, Khan AH, et al. Risk factor analysis of permanent pacemaker infection. *Clin Infect Dis.* 2007;45:166-173.
513. Tarakji KG, Chan EJ, Cantillon DJ, et al. Cardiac implantable electronic device infections: presentation, management, and patient outcomes. *Heart Rhythm.* 2010;7:1043-1047.
517. Thiagarajan RR, Laussen PC, Rycus PT, et al. Extracorporeal membrane oxygenation to aid cardiopulmonary resuscitation in infants and children. *Circulation.* 2007;116:1693-1700.
521. Toomasian JM, Snedecor SM, Cornell RG, et al. National experience with extracorporeal membrane oxygenation for newborn respiratory failure. *ASAIO Trans.* 1988;34:140-147.
530. Tunkel AR, Hartman BJ, Kaplan SL, et al. Practice guidelines for the management of bacterial meningitis. *Clin Infect Dis.* 2004;39(9):1267-1284.
550. Viganego F, O'Donoghue S, Eldadah Z, et al. Effect of early diagnosis and treatment with percutaneous lead extraction on survival in patients with cardiac device infections. *Am J Cardiol.* 2012;109:1466-1471.
554. Viola GM, Awan LL, Darouiche RO. Nonstaphylococcal infections of cardiac implantable electronic devices. *Circulation.* 2010;121:2085-2091.
555. Vogel AM, Lew DF, Kao LS, et al. Defining risk for infectious complications on extracorporeal life support. *J Pediatr Surg.* 2011;46(12):2260-2264.
568. Weiss R, Knight BP, Gold MR, et al. Safety and efficacy of a totally subcutaneous implantable-cardioverter defibrillator. *Circulation.* 2013;128(9): 944-953.
579. Winfield JA, Rosenthal P, Kanter RK, et al. Duration of intracranial pressure monitoring does not predict daily risk of infectious complications. *Neurosurgery.* 1993;33(3):424-430.
593. Zabramski JM, Whiting D, Darouiche RO, et al. Efficacy of antimicrobial-impregnated external ventricular drain catheters: a prospective, randomized, controlled trial. *J Neurosurg.* 2003;98(4):725.

The full reference list for this chapter is available at ExpertConsult.com.

75 Infections Related to Craniofacial Surgical Procedures

Marc A. Mazade • Gail J. Harrison

Craniofacial surgeons are operating more frequently in recent years in the management of traumatic injury, neoplasia, and syndromic and nonsyndromic craniofacial dysostosis, owing in part to the earthquakes in Haiti and Chile in 2010 that contributed to the need for craniofacial reconstructive procedures.[21] The incidence of associated craniofacial surgical infections was 14.7% in one study and 8.1% in another, but it varies greatly and may range from 3% to 45%, depending on the number of procedures undertaken during a single anesthesia, surgical duration, and the structures involved.[10,12] A review published in 2005 demonstrated a rate of 3.2 infections per 100 craniofacial surgical procedures and found that surgical duration longer than 7 hours, closure of skin under tension, use of bovine pericardium, and the presence of more than four surgeons in the operating suite were common risks for development of infection.[31] Determining when an infection has occurred is difficult. The overall facial appearance of the child may be so altered by the surgical intervention and postoperative swelling that even parents may not recognize that infection has occurred. Diagnostic needle aspiration may be helpful. Because infections tend to be caused by bacteria that reside in the sites through which incisions and osteotomies are performed, the main pathogens are skin, paranasal sinus, and oropharyngeal flora. Each additional site that is surgically violated increases the risk for development of an infection. Infections include cellulitis and dehiscence of the wound, infection of subgaleal fluid, osteomyelitis, focal soft tissue abscesses, epidural abscesses, and septicemia.[10,30,31] Exposure of harvested bone and use of metal plates, special cements, distraction pin systems, and wires render infection treatment decisions difficult, so follow-up plays a greater role in management of related infections than in management of simple surgical site infections. Routes of antibiotic administration and duration of antibiotic therapy are poorly established. Most procedures have required extensive preoperative planning, and what is done may not be so easily undone. The infectious diseases consultant must be prepared to engage in an ongoing dialogue with the surgeon and the patient's family, determining what can be removed and at what cost, providing objective feedback about the success of the treatment to that point, and declaring, when needed, that a failure of medical therapy has occurred. Stating dogmatically that all devitalized bone and foreign material must be removed will, in all likelihood, cause the surgeon to delay requesting consultation when infectious diseases services are again needed.

PROCEDURES AND INFECTIONS

Some children require palatal reconstruction, others need distraction osteogenesis by mandibular distraction pin device systems for mandibular hypoplasia.[17] Some require advancement of large portions of the face. One less commonly performed procedure to correct midfacial retrusion is the frontofacial monobloc advancement.[23] This procedure involves detachment and advancement of the entire facial bony mask and commonly requires a large frontal craniotomy, the bone from which may be shaped to complete the repair or used as needed to form a suitable foundation to which the advanced monobloc can be secured. Osteotomies are performed along the lower portion of the frontal bone and posteriorly along the roof of the orbits, along the lateral and medial inferior walls of the orbits, and through the zygomatic arches, with subsequent pterygomaxillary disjunction. A frontoethmoidal osteotomy divides the posterior portion of the nasal septum to free the monobloc so that it can be advanced and secured in place by wiring it anteriorly to a slightly fore-tilted strip of frontal bone and stabilizing it laterally with wired-in strips of calvarial bone grafts to bridge gaps in the zygomatic arches. Bone blocks in the pterygomaxillary area help to hold the maxillary portion forward. The temporary dead space created in the anterior cranial fossa is problematic in some patients.[29] This procedure is associated with an inherent risk for developing meningitis, which is associated less frequently with the extracranial procedures described later, although meningitis still may occur.[27] An alternative procedure that seeks to avoid entering sinus cavities and the cranium is the subcranial Le Fort III osteotomy.[13,23] Exposure is provided through a coronal incision with distraction of the soft tissues of the forehead. Osteotomies free part of the medial, lateral, and inferior walls of the orbit and the nasal bridge, and the remainder of the midface bloc is freed by pterygopalatine disjunction and osteotomies of the zygomatic arch and posterior nasal septum. Thus only the midface bloc is brought forward, and interposition grafts, hydroxyapatite, microplates, and wires secure the bloc in the advanced position. As in the frontofacial advancement, split calvarial bone grafts bridge the space in the zygomatic arches. A Le Fort I osteotomy is an isolated maxillary advancement procedure that might additionally be used to change the position of the upper teeth.[13,16,23]

Some cases of Treacher Collins syndrome require the integral (simultaneous midfacial and mandibular osteotomies).[23] In this complicated procedure requiring a tracheostomy, the midface osteotomies exclude the temporal, lateral walls of the orbits from the advanced bloc. In addition, osteotomies shaped like a C or inverted V through the mandibular rami with placement of the interposition bone grafts and wiring provide advancement of the mandible. Split calvarial bone grafts subsequently reestablish the zygomatic arches.

Reconstructive materials include bone autograft and solvent-treated allograft, titanium plates and mesh,[8] and alloplasts such as polymethyl methacrylate and hydroxyapatite cements, some of which readily accept bone ingrowth and wires. New materials are in development. In an effort to limit postoperative infection, antibiotics such as tobramycin may be mixed into hydroxyapatite cements, which are released into the surrounding field within the first 24 hours of placement.[20]

In many instances, infection permeates the entire operative field.[12] Donor bone graft sites may be involved in some instances. Bacteria may infect the wound or soft tissue area, may spread by contiguous extension through cortical bone during long periods of contact, or may extend through osteotomies that have disrupted the integrity of the periosteum and cortical bone barriers. Additionally surgical alteration of the local blood supply to the cranial bones through disruption of medullary channels and removal of the adherent periosteum, as well as the presence of hardware required to secure the bony structures in their new locations, can render infection difficult to treat. Repeated or prolonged hospitalizations for previous surgical procedures may predispose to subsequent postoperative infection with multidrug-resistant bacteria. Attempts to reduce the incidence of infection have made the use of parenteral prophylactic perioperative antibiotic regimens for 2 to 5 days commonplace.

The development of meningitis is a concern with many craniofacial procedures; however, the dura provides a significant barrier to infection when painstaking neurosurgical technique is applied during repair. The presence of a cerebrospinal fluid leak is a predisposing factor, and meningitis may be manifested years after the procedure in the case of a leak.[27] No cases of meningitis were identified from a combined report of complications after 567 procedures spanning 6.5 years at Medical City Dallas Hospital and at the Division of Plastic Surgery at the University of Pennsylvania in Philadelphia, primarily for cranial vault remodeling.[11] Similarly, meningitis was not identified from an earlier report of 170 transcranial operations spanning 10 years at the South Australian Cranio-Facial Unit in which 53 accidental dural tears occurred and 32 planned dural openings were performed.[9] Nonetheless meningitis has been documented to occur in association with a frontal abscess with osteomyelitis, subgaleal fluid infection, contamination of cerebrospinal fluid drains, and monobloc advancement.[12,27]

As with many procedures, longer operative times result in more infections. Staging of surgeries for complicated problems has helped manage the risk for infection. The Australian group mentioned above documented an average operative time of 10.5 hours for patients in whom a postoperative infection developed, which was 2.5 hours longer than operations on patients in whom an infection did not develop.[9] Longer and more complicated monobloc advancement procedures have been associated with infection rates as high as 45%,[12] whereas anterior cranial vault remodeling may be associated with infection rates as low as 2.5%.[11] The dura encountered during primary craniofacial procedures is manipulated more easily and has better vascularization than does the scarred dura encountered in more complicated and laborious secondary procedures, which are associated with higher rates of infection.[10,11] Additionally craniofacial postoperative infections develop in infants far less frequently than in adults.[9,11] Of the common procedures, infection remains a relatively rare complication of the less complicated Le Fort I maxillary osteotomy. In a large review of outcomes of 1000 such procedures, only 1.1% developed abscess or related infection.[14] Infections complicating distraction osteogenesis have been reported to occur in 9.5% of cases; however, osteomyelitis or deep infection requiring removal of instrumentation is less common, occurring in 0.5% to 0.9% of cases.[17]

As experience in craniofacial surgery has grown, the reduction in the frequency of infection has been attributed to shortened operative time, attempts to avoid entrance into the contaminated sinus cavities (an easier task in young children, in whom the sinuses often are still poorly developed), and mucosal repair at the end of surgery.[27] The mean time to diagnosis of infection is approximately 10 days.[12]

MICROBIOLOGY

Procedures that do not violate the mouth or paranasal sinuses, if infected, are usually infected by skin flora. Organisms causing these infections include flora of the skin such as *Candida albicans, Staphylococcus aureus* (both methicillin-susceptible and methicillin-resistant strains), *Staphylococcus epidermidis,* and other coagulase-negative staphylococci, group A β-hemolytic streptococci, and *Propionibacterium acnes.*[19] Resident flora of the oropharynx such as *Bacteroides* spp., *Corynebacterium* spp., and various α-hemolytic streptococci including *Streptococcus pneumoniae, enterococci, Morganella morganii, Eikenella corrodens, Haemophilus influenzae,* and *H. parainfluenzae* can be causative, especially in procedures that invade the sinus cavities. In addition, gram-negative organisms, such as *Pseudomonas aeruginosa, Escherichia coli, Klebsiella* spp., and *Acinetobacter calcoaceticus* may be involved.[6,11,31] Infections are often polymicrobial and may involve bacteria that are resistant or multidrug-resistant to antibiotics.[19] The frequency of infection with *Candida* spp. is also high and may rival the frequency of infection with more common bacteria.[11,29,31]

PREOPERATIVE PREPARATION, INTRAOPERATIVE IRRIGATION, AND PERIOPERATIVE ANTIBIOTIC THERAPY

Because wounds created during craniofacial surgery fall between the clean-contaminated category and the contaminated category,[6,7] screening for and treating dental caries, periodontal disease, and acute sinusitis is prudent before embarking on procedures involving intraoral incisions and trans-sinus osteotomies.[28] Vaccination of undervaccinated or unvaccinated children with pneumococcal vaccines during the planning process may be wise.[26] Some surgeons make use of intraoperative antibiotic-containing irrigants to help reduce the incidence of infection. These irrigants may be flushed over the intact cranium after subperiosteal exposure and again before skin closure. Other surgeons prefer to use a solution of one part povidone-iodine to four parts saline for intraoperative irrigation.[28] No strong evidence supports any one approach over another for reducing infection.[12]

Continuation of antibiotics beyond the intraoperative period is similar to the approach used in treatment of an open fracture and not very much like antibiotic prophylaxis in the traditional sense. The choice and duration of perioperative antibiotics vary among surgical centers and their surgical teams. Antibiotic regimens may include vancomycin, penicillin, ampicillin-sulbactam, a cephalosporin, clindamycin, or any two of these drugs in combination.[6,7,11,12,14] Erythromycin or other macrolides or vancomycin are used in penicillin-allergic patients in some centers.[1]

The optimal duration of perioperative antibiotic therapy is not clear, but duration at most centers ranges from 1 to 5 days. Higher infection rates occurred in some centers that tried restricting antibiotics to intraoperative use only.[1] Reports from one orthognathic surgical center showed a 10-fold reduction in infection rates with a 5-day antibiotic regimen in comparison with a single-day regimen.[2] However, recent studies have shown no difference in rates of infection when 1-day versus 5-day or longer durations for perioperative antibiotic prophylaxis was used for most procedures.[18,19] Longer durations of treatment with postoperative antibiotics may be needed for patients with more heavily contaminated wounds, however, including sinusitis or retained contaminated foreign materials.[6] Some advocates of a shorter duration of treatment with perioperative antibiotics suggested that longer administration of perioperative antibiotics contributes to infection with gram-negative organisms or may result in infection with more resistant gram-negative bacilli such as *P. aeruginosa* or other pathogens such as *C. albicans.*[8–12]

EVALUATION

Signs of postoperative craniofacial surgical infection include fever, warmth, tenderness, and erythema and rapid recurrence of swelling.[5] However, fever is a normal physiologic response to craniofacial surgery, occurring up to 5 days postoperatively.[10,23] Periorbital swelling may persist for some time and vary with sleeping position. Violaceous discoloration and bruising of the overlying skin are common. Distraction pins may dislodge as the integrity of the bone is compromised by infection.[26]

Purulent or seropurulent wound drainage may indicate underlying soft tissue and possibly bone infection. Wound drainage, pooling, and lack of wound healing at one location should prompt exploration for undiscovered infection elsewhere.[5] Laboratory abnormalities may be subtle. Leukocytosis may be present. The erythrocyte sedimentation rate has been shown to peak approximately 5 days after major orthopedic surgery and to decline slowly and irregularly for a period of 3 to 9 weeks, but it provides little diagnostic value initially.[3,15,25] C-reactive protein (CRP) levels peak within 2 to 3 days but usually normalize within 3 weeks.[3,15,22,25] Because an abrupt increase in CRP may be indicative of infection, some orthopedic centers monitor CRP levels to assist in early detection of infection after elective procedures such as total joint replacement and spinal surgery.[15,25] There may be value in following the CRP level in craniofacial patients postoperatively.

Needle aspiration of underlying fluid collections is the best primary means of diagnosing infection, especially if significant residual postoperative swelling has rendered clinical assessment of a particular area difficult. Diagnostic imaging such as computed tomography with contrast enhancement or magnetic resonance imaging may identify occult fluid collections, but diagnosing bone infection, especially in the flat bones of the cranium, is difficult with these modalities. Surgical exploration of suspected areas of infection remains the most helpful method to provide diagnostic information regarding infection.

TREATMENT

Management of infections complicating craniofacial procedures is primarily surgical. Open debridement, inspection and scraping of devitalized and contiguous bone, and copious pressurized saline irrigation may be curative. Removal of all hardware, while desirable, is often impractical. Successful treatment of these infections has been reported in some surgical centers in which the initial bony debridement was limited to areas of visibly apparent osteitis.[11] The value of adding antibiotics to the irrigant is questionable. Some physicians argue that irrigation with povidone-iodine may devitalize tissues that participate in the healing process and should not be used, whereas other physicians avoid using povidone-iodine irrigation because of concern about systemic iodine absorption.[11]

Placement of several drains prevents accumulation of sequestered focal soft tissue fluid collections. Resolution of drainage and subsequent wound healing can be a sign of cure. Continuous subgaleal flow-through irrigation with saline at a rate of 15 to 30 mL/h (with or without antibiotic additives) is an adjunctive measure instituted by some surgeons.[11]

In infections acquired during cranioplasty, some patient groups may fare well with attempted preservation of a bone flap with minor surgical debridement and systemic antibiotic therapy. Within a small group of five patients who had undergone craniotomy without a history of previous craniotomy, radiation therapy, or skull base surgery, operative debridement accompanied by culture and susceptibility data–driven systemic antibiotic therapy was successful in treating infection with a mean of 35 ± 20 months of follow-up. Several other patients required second-look operations with more debridement, but they did not require removal of the bone flap and were cured. In the same study, the two other subjects had undergone more extensive craniofacial surgery and had recurrent infection requiring removal of the bone flap at 2 months after presentation in one patient and at 29 months in the other; this finding bears out the concern that contamination of the bone flap can result in persistent, long-standing infection.[4]

For infections that complicate procedures not involving the oropharynx or sinus cavities, an antistaphylococcal antibiotic such as vancomycin, cefazolin, nafcillin, or clindamycin may be an appropriate empirical antibiotic choice pending the results of intraoperative drainage and debridement cultures. A third-generation cephalosporin with or without an aminoglycoside may be considered if the risk for developing an infection with a nosocomial gram-negative pathogen is high because of prolonged hospitalization or persistent tracheal colonization with gram-negative bacilli such as *Pseudomonas*[8,9] or if infection of the central nervous system is suspected or threatens. Infections complicating procedures involving the oropharynx or sinuses often are caused by organisms resistant to the perioperative antibiotic chosen.[6] Thus it may be reasonable to consider antibiotic therapy with clindamycin or metronidazole when a cephalosporin has been used or treatment with a second- or third-generation cephalosporin or ampicillin-sulbactam when clindamycin has been used prophylactically. Since *C. albicans* and other *Candida* spp. contribute significantly to these infections, initial treatment with fluconazole or other antifungal agents, depending on culture identification and susceptibility patterns, is also recommended, especially if *Candida* is isolated.[18,19] The duration of antibiotic therapy must be individualized to each case based on the organism and site of infection. A period of 6 weeks of antibiotic therapy has been suggested for patients with craniofacial surgical infections, especially those suspected of having osteomyelitis.[24] Long-term oral antibiotic suppression may be appropriate for patients who live long distances from the craniofacial surgery center who cannot be observed closely.

NEW REFERENCES SINCE THE SEVENTH EDITION

8. Dai J, Shen G, Yuan H, et al. Titanium mesh shaping and fixation for the treatment of comminuted mandibular fractures. *J Oral Maxillofac Surg*. 2016;74(2): 337-342.
18. Mottini M, Wolf R, Soong PL, et al. The role of postoperative antibiotics in facial fractures: comparing the efficacy of a 1 day versus prolonged regimen. *J Trauma Acute Care Surg*. 2014;76(3):720-733.
19. Orzechowska-Wylegala B, Wylegala A, Bulinski M, et al. Antibiotic therapies in maxillofacial surgery in the context of prophylaxis. *Biom Res Inst*. 2015;2015: 819086.

The full reference list for this chapter is available at ExpertConsult.com.

76 Infections in Burn Patients

Janak A. Patel • Gregory J. Berry • Natalie M. Williams-Bouyer

According to the American Burn Association, approximately 486,000 persons were treated for burns in 2011 in the United States; of these, approximately 40,000 were hospitalized and approximately 3240 died of the burn injury.[4] Most of the deaths were related to residential fires, and about 75% of the deaths occurred before arrival at the hospital. For those who are hospitalized, mortality rate peaks 20 days after hospital admission.[82] Improvement in the rate of burn-associated mortality is a direct result of advancement in burn care, comprising developments in fluid resuscitation, wound care, early excision and grafting, nutritional support, infection control, and antimicrobial therapy. The mortality rates and lengths of stay of children with burn injury have been reduced greatly in the past several decades. In the 1960s, the likelihood of survival was only 50% for pediatric patients with burns covering 35% to 44% of the total body surface area (TBSA), and few children with burns covering more than 45% of TBSA survived. The average length of stay was 103 days. In 2011, the LA_{50} (lethal burn size for 50% of patients) for children younger than 16 years exceeded 90% of TBSA.[4] The overall mortality rate for children is less than 1%, which is much lower than that of adults, who have mortality rates in the range of 2% to 26%.[4] At the Shriners Hospital for Children–Galveston, sepsis was found to be the leading cause of death and accounted for 47% of deaths.[154]

BURN WOUND

Burn Wound Depth

Burn wounds are categorized by their depth (Fig. 76.1).[51] Accurate assessment of the depth of burn wounds is important in planning the early definitive care of an individual patient. However, the majority of burn wounds are evaluated by clinical examination only. In this respect, laser Doppler imaging is an important advance in noninvasive techniques for predicting burn wound depth.[78]

Superficial-thickness burns consist of epidermal damage only. These wounds are painful and erythematous as a result of local vasodilation. They heal spontaneously, usually without forming scars, within 7 days.

Partial-thickness burns involve superficial portions of the dermis. These wounds are painful and often result in formation of blisters. Healing occurs through epithelial migration from the wound edges, hair follicles, and sebaceous glands. Relatively little scarring occurs, and reepithelialization occurs within 2 weeks. Deep partial-thickness burns are much more serious. The majority of the dermis is destroyed, leaving the bases of the epidermal appendages spared. The nerve endings also are destroyed, rendering the wound insensate. Blisters usually are not present, owing to the thicker formation of eschar. These wounds are

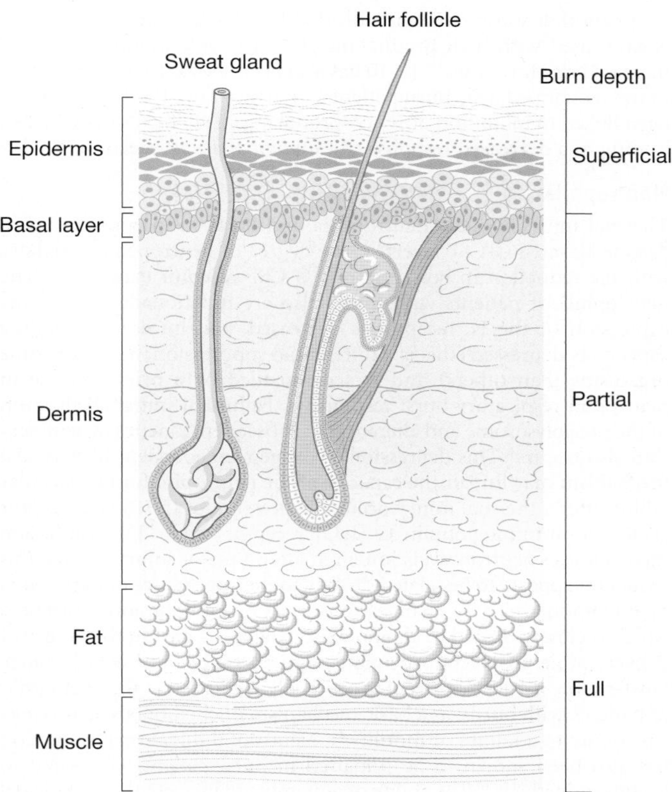

FIG. 76.1 Burn wound depth. (From Greenhalgh D. Wound healing. In: Herndon DN, editor. *Total burn care.* Philadelphia: WB Saunders; 2007: 579.)

treated as full-thickness injuries. Reepithelialization is tenuous and slow. The protracted inflammatory phase often results in excessive deposition of collagen and extensive scarring.

Full-thickness burns involve the entire epidermis, dermis, and the deeper subcutaneous tissues. Healing occurs by contraction and reepithelialization from the edges of the wound. These wounds are insensate and without blistering. Infants and young children have a much thinner dermal layer to their skin resulting in increased propensity for deeper burn injury. Treatment requires excision and skin grafting.

Full-thickness burns can extend into the deep tissue, which includes muscle, bone, and viscera. Treatment is debridement and possible amputation. Closure of these wounds may vary from primary closure after amputation to skin grafting and possibly flap reconstruction.

Cytologic Findings

The effects of extreme heat on the skin lead to cellular and subcellular impairment. The determining factors of how severe a burn will be are the temperature, the length of exposure, and the actual burning agent. Moritz and Henrique showed that the skin is able to withstand temperatures up to 40°C (104°F) for relatively long periods of time before an injury becomes apparent.[105] Increase in temperature leads to cell membrane dysfunction as ion channels are disrupted, resulting in sodium and water intake. As temperatures exceed 45°C (113°F), protein denaturation supersedes the cell's reparative capabilities, and oxygen radicals are liberated. Plasma membrane necrosis has been observed in cells exposed to 45°C for 1 hour. Other cytologic findings in thermal injury include the redistribution of solid and fluid components of the cell nuclei. Imbibition of fluid results in nuclear swelling, rupture of membranes, and pyknosis. As denaturation proceeds, vital cellular metabolic processes are injured. If enzyme activity is decreased to less than 50% of its normal level, cell death occurs. In lesser degrees of enzyme impairment, cell recovery may be possible.

Local Tissue Changes

Local burn injury is classically described by Jackson in three concentric zones. As temperature increases, protein denaturation results in coagulation.[65] The protein architecture is destroyed and new aberrant macromolecules are formed. The central area of a burn wound is that which is in direct contact with the source of heat. Cell necrosis is complete and is called the *zone of coagulation.* Cellular recovery is impossible, and the severity of injury decreases from the surface to the deeper levels. This zone is called the *burn eschar.* At the peripheral margins of the zone of coagulation, a less injured zone is present. The cells in this *zone of stasis* show direct injury from the heat, but the damage is not lethal. However, blood flow becomes progressively impaired to this area. Ischemia to the already compromised cells may lead to necrosis and conversion to dead eschar. Circulatory impairment occurs via adherence of neutrophils to the vessel wall, deposition of fibrin, formation of platelet microthrombus, vasoconstriction, and endothelial swelling. Heat-compromised erythrocytes lose their ability to deform, and their passage through microvessels is impeded. The circulatory embarrassment may be delayed for up to 24 hours, and the ischemia may progress for up to 48 hours after the burn has occurred. If stasis conditions are minimal, the injury may be halted and cell recovery may occur within 1 week. However, this tissue is fragile and further insults such as infection, hypovolemia, pressure, and overresuscitation can lead to further necrosis. Finally, the *zone of hyperemia* lies peripheral to the zone of stasis. This zone sustains minimal injury and often recovers within 7 to 10 days. Notable vasodilation is caused by potent vasoactive mediators secondary to the inflammatory response. Complete recovery is expected in this zone, barring further trauma or infection.

Burn Inflammation

Many of the just mentioned processes are either part of or result from the inflammatory process. Cellular infiltration, initiated by local inflammatory mediators such as prostanoids and leukotrienes, as well as proinflammatory cytokines from the burn wound, begins with the arrival of neutrophils at 4 to 5 days after the burn, followed by macrophages.[133] The neutrophils further mediate damage by releasing oxygen free radicals.[44] Reestablishment of blood flow in the zone of stasis is yet another setting in which oxygen free radicals are produced, leading to further injury. This phenomenon of ischemia-reperfusion injury occurs as oxygen is restored to the tissues.[72] Inflammation becomes prominent at 7 to 10 days. Consequently blood flow is maximal at this stage, creating a troublesome and hazardous setting for surgical excision of the eschar. Along with local inflammatory responses, several systemic responses occur with burns of more than 15% of the TBSA.

Inhalation Injury

Burn victims, especially those trapped in enclosed areas, injure the respiratory tract on inhalation of toxic gases from surrounding burning materials. An actual thermal airway injury is quite rare. The upper airway is rather effective in cooling and warming inspired air. Also, air has a very low heat capacity. To cause a direct injury to the airway, the flames must come into direct contact with them. Injury to the oropharynx after inhalation of toxic gases resembles thermal injury elsewhere in the body.[1] Protein denaturation, release of inflammatory mediators, and increased cellular and microvascular permeability all occur, leading to airway edema and consequent obstruction of the airway.

The chemical injury from inhalation of toxic gases can damage the tracheobronchial tree. First, separation of ciliated epithelial cells from the basement membrane occurs.[12] Next, the circulation of blood to the lung, as well as to the bronchial tree, is increased owing to vasodilation. Shortly thereafter, edema is evident. The inflammatory phase is followed by an exudative phase.[61] Furthermore the protein component of this fluid is composed of lung lymph and induces bronchoconstriction. As postburn time increases, fibrin casts are formed from the exudates, resulting in obstruction of the airway. As the epithelium sloughs and formation of fibrin casts increases, susceptibility to infection also increases. Pneumonia leading to sepsis and death are well-known sequelae at this stage. Finally formation of pseudomembranes proceeds and then squamous metaplasia follows.[118] Healing may take weeks to initiate, and permanent damage to the airway (e.g., stenosis and formation of tracheal granulomas) may occur.

INFLAMMATORY AND IMMUNE RESPONSES IN BURNS

Intact human skin is vital for preservation of the host's protection against infection. A combination of impaired local and systemic host defenses and loss of the skin barrier are major factors responsible for the increased susceptibility to infections in patients with burns. The major elements initially contributing to the inflammatory response that occurs after burns are incurred include the plasma proteins, mast cells, tissue macrophages, and systemically recruited neutrophils and monocytes.

Alterations in the host defenses include induction of local and systemic cytokine synthesis, decreased immunoglobulin levels, changes in the concentration and activity of both the classical and alternative complement pathways, reduced levels of circulating plasma fibronectin, depressed serum opsonic activity, and impairment of the macrophages, lymphocytes, neutrophils, and the reticuloendothelial system. However, many mechanisms of immune alterations remain unknown; for example, an association of the volume of blood transfusions with increased mortality rates and infectious episodes in patients with major burns was observed in two reports.[69,118] The immunologic status of the burn patient has a measurable impact on survival, death, and major morbidity.

The Cytokine Response

After burn injury occurs, numerous cytokines are induced rapidly. Many cytokines correlate with the severity of the burn injury and the prognosis. Studies at Shriners Hospital for Children–Galveston have shown a specific pattern of systemic cytokine responses in children with thermal injury. Compared with unburned healthy children, children with burns covering more than 40% of TBSA had significant increases in serum levels of 15 cytokines and immunoregulatory molecules during the first week after incurring the thermal injury: interleukin-1β (IL-1β), IL-2, IL-4, IL-5, IL-6, IL-7, IL-8, IL-10, IL-12p70, IL-13, IL-17, interferon-γ (IFN-γ), monocyte chemoattractant protein-1 (MCP-1), macrophage inflammatory protein-1α (MIP-1α), and granulocyte colony-stimulating factor (G-CSF).[39,82] The amount of granulocyte-macrophage colony-stimulating factor (GM-CSF) was significantly increased during the second week after burn occurred. Within 5 weeks, the serum concentrations of most cytokines decreased, approaching normal levels. In another study of children, serum IL-6, IL-8, IL-10, IL-12p70, IL-13, IFN-γ, tumor necrosis factor-α (TNF-α), MIP-1β, MCP-1, G-CSF, and GM-CSF values were significantly increased in large burns.[38,82] In general, there is a clear increase in these cytokines when the affected TBSA is greater than 60% when compared with burns affecting a lesser TBSA.[82]

A recent multicenter study specifically looked at the predictive value of IL-8 for sepsis and infection following burn injury. This study enrolled 468 pediatric burn patients with burns of greater than 30% TBSA and used IL-8 levels to stratify patients into IL-8 low and high groups. These patients were monitored for IL-8 levels for the first 60 days after injury. Based on the results, IL-8 may be a useful biomarker in pediatric burn patients for monitoring multiorgan failure, infections, sepsis, and mortality.[83] Another study also reported that pediatric patients with multiorgan failure had significant increases in serum IL-6, MCP-1, and TNF-α, but these were not predictive of outcome.[84] TNF-α may be the most important cytokine during acute inflammatory injury of burns because it induces production of C-reactive protein (CRP) and IL-6; migration of and phagocytosis by neutrophils and macrophages; hormone regulatory processes, particularly hypothalamic thermoregulation; and insulin hypersensitivity.

In children with inhalation injury, the serum cytokine studies at enrollment showed significant reduction in level of IL-7 and elevation of IL-12p70 compared with children without inhalation injury.[38] However, 5 to 7 days later, the levels were comparable. Host genetic factors also may affect the cytokine response in patients with burns. For example, single nucleotide polymorphisms for TNF-α (−308G), Toll-like receptor 4 (+896G), IL-6 (−174C), and CD14 (−159C) were significantly associated with an increased risk for severe sepsis after burns.[8]

In another study, children with IL-10 (−1082GG) genotype, which is associated with high production of IL-10, were found to have an increased risk for sepsis.[119] IL-10 has also been shown to be upregulated in the sera of pediatric burn patients.[46] Furthermore IL-10 has recently been linked to inhibition of IL-17–producing CD4$^+$ T cells (T_H17 cells), leading to a decreased response to *Candida albicans* infection.[64]

Neutrophils

Thermal injury induces neutropenia and myeloid maturation arrest despite elevated G-CSF levels.[135] The degree of neutropenia correlates with the reduction in bone marrow G-CSF receptor expression. The neutrophils of patients with burns also are functionally altered: the expression of the Fc receptor is decreased, and intracellular killing capacity is depressed (this is a differential suppression, more for some organisms than others) and is accompanied by a brief increase in neutrophil respiratory burst response.[107] Failure of initial alkalization of the phagolysosome and alteration of subsequent kinetics of acidification also occur.[16] This depression of oxygen-independent bactericidal mechanism may impair the capacity of the neutrophil for intracellular killing after a thermal injury occurs. Expression of CD16 (Fc receptor [FcR], Fc immunoglobulin G [IgG] receptor) and CD11 (adhesion molecule) on neutrophils is impaired after a major injury occurs; this reduction appears to be related directly to the appearance of bacteremia or pneumonia.[6] These changes in expression of adhesion molecules, which is closely related to chemotaxis, may play a part in the failure of delivery of neutrophils in adequate numbers to the local site of a burn. Furthermore a defect is present in actin polymerization in the neutrophils of patients with burns; as a basic mechanism of chemotaxis, it also may contribute to a failure of motility.[147] Neutrophil directional migration has also been shown to be impaired in burn patients compared to healthy individuals.[20] The ability of glutamine to increase the bactericidal function of neutrophils against *Staphylococcus aureus* has also been reported in neutrophils isolated from pediatric burn patients.[113]

Generation of leukotrienes from the neutrophils of severely burned patients also is impaired and appears to be based on the availability, or lack of availability, of the metabolizable substrate-free arachidonic acid.[77] Because leukotriene B also is a potent neutrophil chemotactic agent, this impairment may further contribute to the failure of neutrophil function.

Complements

The fluid of the burn blister shows much lower opsonic activity for bacteria such as *Pseudomonas aeruginosa* than the patient's own serum.[115] A mild impairment of production of C3 and release by macrophages of burn patients in vitro also occurs. Systemically both the classical and the alternative pathways are depleted, but the alternative pathway is more profoundly perturbed. After the development of bacteremia, additional complement activation and depletion occur.[145]

Macrophages

Suppression of the ability of the reticuloendothelial system to take up particulate material was among the original observations of burn immunology made in the 1960s. More recent reports, however, have described the demonstration of a differentially increased uptake of colloid in alveolar macrophages compared with other organs, perhaps indicating alveolar macrophage activation. Macrophages and monocytes appear to be activated in a fashion similar to that of lymphocytes after thermal injury occurs. Activation of macrophages, as measured by the serum neopterin level, is increased after thermal injury occurs.[7] This activation is confirmed by increased expression of the monocyte cell surface antigens C3b and iC3b.[103] At the same time, expression of human leukocyte antigen-DR (HLA-DR), HLA-DQ, and HLA-DP by monocytes is reduced, and these class II antigens are obligatory for many cell-mediated immunologic processes, thereby implying that a possible loss of function of monocytes occurs after thermal injury.[48] Production of C3 by macrophages is suppressed in patients with burns, but the synthetic ability for key cytokines such as IL-6 is increased.[159]

Peripheral blood monocytes are superstimulated to produce large amounts of IL-1, leading to exhaustion of the function on monocytes.[92] Reduced production of IL-1 by monocytes was found in patients with complicated organ injury, multiorgan failure, and systemic infection. Peripheral blood monocytes from severely burned patients also fail to produce MIP-1α, which has been shown to play an important role in recruitment and activation of various immune cells during infection.[79] Blood monocytes of patients with burns produce significantly more IL-10 at 7 to 10 days after burn injury, which correlates significantly with subsequent septic events.[74]

T Lymphocytes and Cell-Mediated Immunity

Early studies of T cells in patients with burns showed a variety of changes: impairment in mitogenic and antigenic responsiveness of lymphocytes, suppression of graft-versus-host reactivity related to the size of the burn, suppression of delayed cutaneous sensitivity tests, and diminution in both numbers of peripheral lymphocytes and concentration of thoracic duct lymphocytes. Whether the failure of T-cell functions is due to an intracellular defect related to thermal injury, the result of "overuse," or indirectly the result of downregulation by the cytokine cascade or other products of the inflammatory reaction remains controversial. A study has shown that severe burn injury could result in activation and maturation of regulatory T cells leading to immunosuppression.[63] The elevation of levels of cytokines produced by regulatory T cells and the activation markers on the surface of these cells correlate with burn size and are higher in those with sepsis than those without. However, among septic patients, the regulatory T-cell parameters in the survival group were markedly lower than those with fatal outcome, suggesting that persistence of a pronounced immunoparalysis induced by regulatory T cells after severe sepsis is associated with poor outcome after burns.

IL-17–producing $CD4^+$ T cells (T_H17 cells) have been shown to have an important role in protection from *Candida albicans* infection. A recent study looking at the ability of burn patients to generate T_H17 cells in response to *C. albicans* showed that their generation was impaired in pediatric and adult burn patients, presumably due to T_H17-inhibiting IL-10 produced as a result of burn injury. Since burn patients are quite susceptible to *C. albicans* infection, lack of T_H17 T-cell generation may be one mechanism by which infection occurs.[64]

Analysis of peripheral blood T cells supports the theory that, rather than an absolute reduction in CD4 and an increase in CD8 cells, a redistribution of lymphocyte traffic may occur.[116] Suppression in the numbers of the total population of lymphocytes is the only consistent overall change. Furthermore not only does lymphocyte traffic between stores of central lymphocytes and the peripheral blood occur after a thermal injury, but the responsiveness of these populations of lymphocytes also varies according to the site; for example, splenic lymphocytes of experimentally burned animals remain most profoundly depressed in response to antigenic stimulation compared with the peripheral blood and other organs.[30] In addition, in peripheral blood, the appearance of "activation" antigens on CD4 and CD8 cells (HLA-DR, IL-2 receptor [IL-2R], and transferrin receptor) is depressed significantly as early as 1 day after burn injury occurs.[96]

Addition of recombinant IL-2 does not appear to reverse the suppression of the appearance of surface markers such as IL-2R in burn patients, although it does not improve the response of natural killer (NK) cells to stimulation.[42] In experimental preparations, at least some of the observed T-cell suppression can be alleviated by early removal of the burn wound, thereby creating one further argument for promptly closing the burn wound.[54]

B Lymphocytes and Humoral Immunity

The function of B cells after the occurrence of a thermal injury is less well documented than is that of macrophages or T cells. The expression of this major histocompatibility complex is impaired and therefore some diminution of B-cell function can be expected as a result of diminished recognition of antigenic presentation.[111] Under the influence of stress-induced corticosteroids, the number of circulating B cells is relatively increased compared with T cells in peripheral blood.[71] Spontaneous cytokine (IL-4 and IL-2)-induced expression of the activation antigen CD23 is reduced significantly during the second to fifth week after burn injury occurs.[130]

If the products of B-cell activation, namely, the immunoglobulins, are measured in vivo, the results are somewhat difficult to interpret because of the increased catabolism of protein and the leakage through the burn wound. Briefly, marked diminution of serum IgG concentration (total and all subclasses) is present; these levels return to normal between 10 and 14 days after the burn injury has occurred. Extremely low levels of IgG on admission (300–400 mg/dL) are predictors of a poor prognosis. One study looking at immunoglobulin levels in pediatric burn patients found that the greatest drops were seen in IgG1 and IgG2 subclasses.[136] Levels of IgM and IgA appear to be relatively unaffected.

Overall the defective production of immunoglobulin after a thermal injury occurs appears to be a factor of macrophage/lymphocyte interaction rather than a failure of intrinsic activity by B cells.[37]

BURN WOUND MICROBIOLOGY

A working knowledge of the common flora of burn wounds is essential to appropriately tailor therapy. Pathogens peculiar to thermal injuries are basically no different from the normal flora of the environment. Table 76.1 shows the types of microorganisms found in various body tissues and secretions as either normal flora or as pathogens. However, the organisms causing infections change over the course of burn wound treatment. Gram-positive organisms prevail in the early postburn period and then are replaced by gram-negative bacteria and fungi.[35] Many of these organisms produce biofilms in burn wounds. The biofilms consist of organisms surrounded by a matrix consisting of various proteins, polymers, complex carbohydrates, and water. Biofilms are associated with development of antibiotic resistance because antibiotics do not penetrate through the matrix in sufficient concentration. Biofilm formation also inhibits effective local immune response as well as wound healing. Using electron microscopy, Kennedy and colleagues showed that in both ulcerated and escharotomy sites, evidence of biofilm was seen as early as 7 days after injury.[75] Formation of biofilm is best prevented by early excision and coverage of the wound with topical antimicrobial agents.

The organisms that predominate as causative agents of burn wound infection in any burn treatment facility change over time. For example, at Shriners Hospital for Children–Galveston, from 1989 to 1999, only 42% of children died of sepsis due to multidrug-resistant (MDR) organisms; in 25% of these children, *Pseudomonas* was the responsible organism. From 1999 to 2009, 86% of patients died of sepsis due to MDR organisms, and, in 64% of these children, again the cause was *Pseudomonas* infection. In this latter period, *Acinetobacter* also emerged as a major pathogen of death due to sepsis while the role of *Klebsiella* declined. In more recent years, there has been a further shift in the pathogens, described in the following sections.

Gram-Positive Bacteria

The gram-positive predominance is consistent with the normal inhabitants of the skin before the thermal injury. *Staphylococcus* spp., *Micrococcus* spp., *Streptococcus* spp., *Pediococcus* spp., and *Enterococcus* spp. are gram-positive cocci commonly encountered in burn wounds. Erol and colleagues demonstrated that coagulase-negative *Staphylococcus* and *S. aureus* were the most prevalent isolates in admission cultures, followed by diphtheroids.[35] These organisms can be life threatening as invasive infections or simply be locally colonized. The distribution of gram-positive bacteria at Shriners Hospital for Children–Galveston, which receives pediatric burn patients from all over the world, is shown in Table 76.2. In 2011, the gram-positive cocci accounted for 55% of bacterial isolates; however, by 2015, this rate had dropped to 46%. In this latter year, staphylococci were more prevalent (61%) than enterococci (29%). Interestingly the rates of methicillin-resistant *S. aureus* (MRSA) and methicillin-sensitive *S. aureus* (MSSA) isolates were equal in 2011, but, by 2015, the MRSA rates had dropped by two-thirds. This recent downward shift in MRSA rates is in keeping with the overall pattern observed in the United States.

Because of such resistance patterns, Cook stresses the importance of microbial surveillance and epidemiologic studies.[25] This approach is thought to reduce the prevalence of MRSA, yet it may be inadequate for eradicating or preventing outbreaks. Minimizing transmission and infection is emphasized. However, Reardon and associates suggest that this process is time-consuming and requires extensive resources for

TABLE 76.1 Tissue Association of Microorganisms Most Commonly Found in Burn Wound Infection

Organism	Soft Tissue Skin	Upper Respiratory Tract	Lower Respiratory Tract	Endocardial	Gastrointestinal	Urogenital	Bone and Joint
Staphylococcus aureus	NF, P	P, NF	P	P	P	NF, P	P
Staphylococcus epidermidis	NF, P	NF, P	P	P	P	NF, P	P
Other staphylococci	NF	NF, P	P	P	NF, P	NF, P	P
Streptococcus pyogenes	P, NF	P, NF	P	P	P	P	P
Other streptococci	NF	NF	P	P	NF	NF, P	P
Enterococcus spp.	P	P	P	P	NF, P	NF, P	P
Escherichia coli	NF, P	NF, P	P	P	NF, P	NF, P	P
Klebsiella pneumoniae	NF, P	NF, P	P	P	NF, P	NF, P	P
Enterobacter cloacae	NF, P	NF, P	P	P	NF, P	NF, P	P
Enterobacter aerogenes	NF, P	NF, P	P	P	NF, P	NF, P	P
Proteus spp.	NF, P	P	P	P	NF, P	NF, P	P
Serratia marcescens	NF, P	–	P	P	P	P	P
Other enterics	NF, P	NF, P	P	P	NF, P	P	P
Pseudomonas aeruginosa	P	NF, P	P	P	NF, P	P	P
Acinetobacter spp.	NF	NF	P	–	NF	NF	P
Candida albicans	NF	NF	P	P	NF	P, NF	P

NF, Normal flora; *P*, pathogens; –, normally not found, but these organisms should not be ignored when encountered.
Modified from Heggers J. Microbiology for surgeons. In: Kerstein MD, ed. *Management of Surgical Infections.* Mt. Kisco, NY: Futura Publishing; 1980: 27–55.

little gain.[122] Colonization with MSSA and MRSA in 86 patients was studied and found to have no significant changes on length of stay, number of operations, or mortality between these two organisms. However, the presence of either type of *S. aureus* significantly increased the number of surgical procedures performed and the lengths of stay. Many burn units report frequent colonization of burn patients with toxic shock toxin (TSS-1)–producing strains of staphylococci; however, their presence does not correlate well with increased morbidity or mortality rates.[24]

In the past, group A β-hemolytic streptococcus frequently was the cause of epidemics in burn units, but it seldom is encountered today because of the frequent empirical use of antibiotics for manipulations of burn wounds. Other β-hemolytic streptococci belonging to groups B, C, E, F, and G can be encountered as well.[90] Significant infection-control vigilance still is necessary because occasional clusters of outbreaks of group A streptococcal infection continue to be reported.[51,125] Fortunately group A streptococcus remains uniformly sensitive to penicillins, hence prophylaxis and treatment are easily accomplished.

Although enterococcal infections (*Enterococcus faecalis* and *E. faecium*) account for only 22% of burn wound infections caused by gram-positive bacteria (see Table 76.2), a significant cause for concern is the emergence of vancomycin-resistant *Enterococcus* (VRE) in burn units.[86,88] Although additional morbidity associated with VRE itself is not clear, when it occurs as a polymicrobial bacteremia, a mortality rate as high as 20% has been noted.[88]

Other gram-positive bacilli include the aerobic *Corynebacterium* spp. and *Listeria* spp., as well as the spore-forming *Bacillus* spp. (aerobe) and *Clostridium* spp. (anaerobe). *Bacillus* spp. and *Clostridium* spp. are associated with burn wounds that have come in contact with contaminated soil. In avascular muscle injuries (e.g., electrical injuries or crush injuries combined with burns), the risk for developing tetanus (from infection with *Clostridium tetani*) is high and has led to the practice of using tetanus immunoprophylaxis and booster vaccines.[87,132]

Gram-Negative Bacteria

The presence of the gram-negative bacteria in burn wounds is due in part to translocation of the bacteria from the gastrointestinal tract of the patients.[9] In a study of children with burns at Shriners Hospital for Children–Galveston, patients with large wounds (>50% TBSA) were found to have significantly higher colonization with their fecal gram-negative bacteria than were those with smaller wounds.[40] *P. aeruginosa* bacteremia is predicted by isolation of *P. aeruginosa* from another site (wound, urine, or sputum), and the prior nonblood isolates of *P. aeruginosa* can correctly predict the antimicrobial sensitivity pattern in 75% of patients.[95] At Shriners Hospital for Children–Galveston, gram-negative bacteria accounted for 54% of the total bacterial isolates of wounds in 2015 (see Table 76.2). Indeed, the rates increased from 2011 when it accounted for 48% of total isolates. A significant proportion of these bacteria produce extended spectrum β-lactamase (ESBL) enzyme. *Escherichia coli* and *Klebsiella pneumoniae* are the predominant ESBL-producing bacteria. Bennett and coworkers have shown that infections caused by ESBL-producing *K. pneumoniae* are predictive of death when occurring in older persons.[15]

Although the carbohydrate-fermenting Enterobacteriaceae account for 64% of the gram-negative isolates as a whole, *P. aeruginosa* and other nonfermenters are also important in burn patients. Other important gram-negative bacteria include the Enterobacteriaceae such as *E. coli, Enterobacter cloacae, K. pneumoniae,* and *Serratia marcescens.* Enterobacteriaceae also are encountered as a cause of nosocomial pneumonia in patients with inhalation injury who are on ventilators, and they are a cause of urinary tract infection in patients with indwelling urinary catheters. *Acinetobacter*, an increasingly more common cause of gram-negative infections, has been found more frequently in burn patients with glucose intolerance or preexisting diabetes mellitus[41] and in patients with more severe burns and comorbidities.[3]

Even without invasive infections, gram-negative bacteria have been implicated in systemic inflammatory diseases, including shock and disseminated intravascular coagulation, secondary to the circulation of bacterial endotoxin from the gut and the burn wound.[81,93] Often gut decontamination is instituted to reduce the incidence of endotoxin-mediated disease.

Fungi

Until the advent of topical antimicrobial agents and systemic antibiotics, fungal infections were not common developments in patients with burns. The burn wound is the site most commonly infected, although fungemia and dissemination to the respiratory tract in patients on ventilators and to the urinary tract in patients with indwelling catheters are encountered frequently. *Candida* spp. are the most common fungal colonizers of the wound; however, fewer than 20% of patients develop widespread candidiasis. Overall the rate of candidemia in the burn patient population is 3% to 5%, and burn wound invasion has a

TABLE 76.2 Bacteria Isolated From 156 Inpatient Acute Care Pediatric Burn Patients Admitted to Shriners Hospital for Children–Galveston (January 2015–December 2015)

	No. (%) of Isolates
Gram-Positive Organisms	
Coagulase-negative *Staphylococcus*	131 (37.9)
Enterococcus faecalis	63 (18.2)
Methicillin-sensitive *Staphylococcus aureus*	55 (15.9)
Enterococcus faecium	36 (10.4)
Other gram-positive organisms[a]	36 (10.4)
Methicillin-resistant *Staphylococcus aureus*	25 (7.2)
Total gram-positive isolates	**346**
Gram-Negative Organisms	
Enterobacteriaceae (Enterics)	
Klebsiella pneumoniae	45 (11.1)
Escherichia coli	34 (8.4)
Enterobacter cloacae	34 (8.4)
Proteus mirabilis	25 (6.2)
Escherichia coli (ESBL)	24 (5.9)
Other *Enterobacteriaceae*[b]	19 (4.7)
Klebsiella pneumoniae (ESBL)	19 (4.7)
Klebsiella spp.	16 (4.0)
Serratia marcescens	15 (3.7)
Enterobacter spp.	11 (2.7)
Morganella morganii	11 (2.7)
Non-Enterobacteriaceae	
Pseudomonas aeruginosa	60 (14.7)
Acinetobacter species	53 (13.1)
Stenotrophomonas maltophia	23 (5.7)
Other non-*Enterobacteriaceae*[c]	16 (4.0)
Total gram-negative isolates	**405**
Total bacterial isolates	**751**
Gram-positive organisms	**46.1%**
Gram-negative organisms	**53.9%**

[a]Includes other *Enterococcus* spp. ($n = 28$); *Streptococcus* spp. ($n = 7$); *Leuconostoc* spp. ($n = 1$).
[b]Includes *Citrobacter* spp. ($n = 9$); other *Proteus* spp. ($n = 2$); *Providencia* spp. ($n = 8$).
[c]Includes *Aeromonas hydrophila* ($n = 6$); *Alcaligenes* spp. ($n = 7$); *Burkholderia cepacia* ($n = 3$).

comparable rate. A study of children with burn injury at Shriners Hospital for Children–Galveston showed that those developing candidemia did so during the first week after the burn and 7 days after excision of burn eschar.[29] One hypothesis is that massive burns with immunosuppression are further suppressed by repeated surgical intervention, anesthesia, and perioperative use of broad-spectrum antibiotics, further predisposing these patients to early development of *Candida* septicemia. In one study, the attributable mortality rate with candidemia was 15%.[104] With early recognition of invasion of burn wounds by routine biopsies, wound swabs, and early amphotericin therapy, the mortality rate has been reduced to less than 10% compared with 60% to 90% reported in earlier series.[131]

Unlike *Candida,* true fungal infections caused by *Aspergillus, Penicillium, Rhizopus, Mucor, Rhizomucor, Fusarium,* and *Curvularia* occur early in the hospital course, specifically in those exposed to the spores on the ground or in water at the time the injury occurred. Once colonized, broad nonbranching hyphae extend into subcutaneous tissue and stimulate an inflammatory response. Vascular invasion occurs frequently and often is accompanied by thrombosis and avascular necrosis, which is clinically observed as rapidly advancing dark discolorations of the wound margin. Systemic dissemination occurs with invasion of the vasculature.

Viruses

Linnemann and MacMillan performed a retrospective survey of serum for viral antibodies in pediatric burn patients; 22% had fourfold increases in antibodies to cytomegalovirus (CMV), 8% had increases to herpes simplex virus (HSV) and to Epstein-Barr virus, and 5% had increases in antibodies to varicella zoster virus (VZV).[91] None of the patients had evidence of adenovirus or hepatitis B virus infection. On the basis of these observations, a prospective study of viral infections using both serologic and viral culture techniques was performed. This study showed that CMV infection developed in 33% of the children, HSV infection occurred in 25%, and adenovirus infection was noted in 17%. CMV infections developed in all of the most severely burned children, and both primary and reactivation infections were observed. Most primary CMV infections that develop during treatment for burns are likely to occur from transfusion of blood products. CMV infection typically occurs approximately 1 month after the burn occurs and clinically presents as fever of unknown origin with lymphocytosis; however, it rarely alters the patient's clinical course.[28] Kealey and colleagues[73] have shown that 56% of burn patients who initially were seropositive for CMV had a fourfold or greater rise in CMV antibodies as evidence of CMV reactivation. These patients tended to be younger, to have a larger burn area, and to have a longer hospital stay. No patient who experienced CMV infection, whether primary or reactivated, had serious complications attributable to CMV. On the basis of these observations, despite the availability of anti-CMV agents such as ganciclovir and valganciclovir, treatment of CMV infection remains controversial.[123]

Since the screening of blood began, hepatitis C virus (HCV) has been an important risk factor. Coursaget and colleagues screened 45 burn patients for anti-HCV antibodies at the time of burn injury and at more than 6 months after the burn.[26] HCV infection was detected in 18% of these patients as a consequence of the numerous transfusions of blood or blood derivatives used during the postburn treatment. Five patients displayed evidence of anti-C100, anti-C33c, and anticore antibodies together; two patients had only anti-C100 and anti-C33c antibodies, and the last patient showed only anticore antibodies. Chronic hepatitis was observed in 83% of HCV infections. Kinetics of appearance of anti-HCV antibodies varied among patients. Anticore antibodies generally are the first to be detected at high levels; however, in at least one case, they were detected only 2.5 months after C100 and C33c antibodies were detected. The incidence of HCV using polymerase chain reaction (PCR) assay to detect the viral genome has not been evaluated in burn patients. Nonetheless the current procedures used at blood banks have decreased the transmission of HCV by blood products.

Another transfusion-related agent is human immunodeficiency virus (HIV), which has become extremely rare as a result of the screening of donors that began in 1987 in the United States. However, significant risk existed prior to that period. A retrospective review of children with burn injury at Shriners Hospital for Children–Galveston who had received blood or blood products between 1978 and 1985 identified 52 patients at risk for developing HIV infection.[127] More than 50% of the identified population had received three or more units of blood or blood products during their acute hospital stay. A total of 214 patients (36.8%) were tested for HIV seroconversions: five tested HIV positive by enzyme-linked immunosorbent assay (ELISA) and four were confirmed by Western blot, yielding a 1.9% incidence. The four confirmed patients received two to nine total-body blood volume turnovers during their postburn period in the hospital. HIV may affect the outcome of burn wound injury. A study of Malawian children showed that with burns affecting 11% to 30% of the body surface area, HIV-positive children had a mortality rate approximately twice that of HIV-negative children.[66]

HSV is of significant concern in burn units because it is a dermatopathologic virus. A review of the literature suggests that patients younger than 10 years were at greater risk for acquiring an HSV infection when the size of the burn wound was greater than 15% TBSA.[55] However, the role of HSV in the healing of wounds is unclear. Bourdarias and associates showed that, in 11 patients with burns, local areas of active epidermal regeneration were affected most often.[17] Acyclovir therapy was not used, and the duration of hospitalization was normal when compared with that of other children. Nonetheless HSV in lungs may worsen morbidity. Byers and coworkers showed that the relative risk for developing HSV infection was higher for patients with acute respiratory distress syndrome but not for those with pneumonia.[21] Disseminated HSV infection also can be fatal.[21]

Another dermatopathologic virus is VZV. Mini-epidemics of VZV have occurred within pediatric burn units.[153] With the routine VZV vaccination of young children (at 1 year of age) in the United States, outbreaks of varicella in burn units are now uncommon. The characteristic fluid-filled lesions appear in partial-thickness burns that are healed or healing, as well as in uninjured epithelium and mucous membranes. The vesicles are much more destructive in the injured than uninjured skin and may present as hemorrhagic, oozing pock marks that are prone to development of secondary infection and subsequent scarring. Neovascularized skin grafts may be lost; therefore further grafting procedures should be delayed until the lesions are quiescent.

The morbidity due to respiratory virus infections, particularly in those with inhalation injury, has not been studied well. We tested more than 100 pediatric burn patients for respiratory syncytial virus (RSV) during the winter seasons of 1995 and 1996. Only six patients were found to be positive for RSV, with one death (1% mortality rate).

Parasites

Parasitic infestation also is seen, especially in children from the developing world. Because we see many patients who originate from Mexico, where such infestation is endemic, parasitemia has been found to complicate burn injuries. Parasites that are asymptomatic in sites such as the intestinal tract and the respiratory tract can become symptomatic as a result of the stress of a burn injury. At the Shriners Hospital for Children–Galveston, we have described three cases of *Ascaris* pneumonitis that exacerbated smoke-induced lung injury.[56] In 2006, the parasites isolated most frequently were *Giardia lamblia* and *Blastocystis hominis.*

CLINICAL MANIFESTATIONS

Local Signs

An open burn wound is a favorable target for bacterial colonization. The progression from simple eschar colonization to the invasive process is favored by a series of factors related to the patient, such as extension and depth of the burn, age, presence of previous disease, and local conditions of the wound; to the microorganism, such as density, motility, toxins, and antimicrobial resistance; to iatrogenic causes such as prosthetic devices; and to the nosocomial spread of bacteria. It is essential to recognize the early signs of infection of a local burn wound by examining the wound at least once a day.

The local signs of burn wound infection include black or dark brown focal areas of discoloration, conversion of partial-thickness injury to full-thickness necrosis, hemorrhagic discoloration of subcutaneous tissue, enhanced sloughing of burned tissue or eschar, and purplish discoloration or edema of skin around the margins of the wound. Presence of *Pseudomonas* infection can lead to ecthyma gangrenosa and green pigmentation of subcutaneous fat. In fungal infection, centrifugal advance of subcutaneous edema with central ischemic necrosis and hemorrhagic saponification of subcutaneous fat in fungal infection can be seen. In viral infection, vesicular lesions in healing or healed partial-thickness burns and crusted serrated margins of partial-thickness burns may be observed.

Systemic Signs

Progression from local to systemic invasion can occur rapidly, which correlates with the size of the burn wound, the extent of environmental contamination, and the surgical procedures. Early recognition of systemic invasion is critical to avoid high rates of mortality. Many of the signs of sepsis resemble complications of the burn itself; for example, fevers, tachycardia, shock, and elevated or depressed neutrophil count can occur in burn patients with or without infection. However, certain patterns of clinical signs and symptoms may help identify systemic bacterial invasion (Table 76.3).[43]

TABLE 76.3 Signs and Symptoms of Progression From Local Invasion to Systemic Illness

Gram-Negative Sepsis	Gram-Positive Sepsis
Burn wound biopsy >10^5 organisms/g tissue and/or histologic tissue invasion	Same
Rapid onset; well to ill in 8 to 12 hours	Gradual
Temperature of 37–39°C (98.6–102.2°F); can be normal, followed by hypothermia (34–35°C [93.2–95°F]), plus decrease in WBC	Temperature >40°C
WBC may be elevated	WBC 20–50 × 10^3, hematocrit decrease
Ileus	Same
Decreased blood pressure and urinary output	Same
Wounds develop focal gangrene, satellite lesions away from burn wound	Macerated wounds, ropy and tenacious exudate
Mental obtundation	Anorexic and irrational

Five or more signs or symptoms are definitive diagnostic parameters.
Modified from Gallagher JJ, Williams-Bouyer N, Villarreal C, et al. Treatment of infections in burns. In: Herndon DN, ed. *Total Burn Care.* Philadelphia: WB Saunders; 2007:143.
WBC, White blood cell count.

Biomarkers of Infection and Sepsis

A rise in CRP serum levels has been found useful in predicting systemic infection, although increases in the first 2 days after the burn or the day after surgery may occur without infection.[110] A recent large-scale study in pediatric burn patients showed that CRP cannot be used to predict infection or sepsis.[68] Another important biomarker is serum procalcitonin. Its relatively early rise within 4 hours of response to infection or trauma, with a long plateau of up to 24 hours, makes this marker very valuable in early assessment of sepsis. Egea-Guerrero and coworkers showed that procalcitonin levels could predict infection while CRP could not.[33] Furthermore Yang and coworkers showed that procalcitonin levels could predict severity of sepsis as well as mortality.[157] While the serum procalcitonin test is still not yet available widely, many medical centers are increasingly offering this test for routine clinical use. Studies of elevated levels of certain cytokines may also be useful biomarkers of infection, but they largely remain a research tool.

Complications of Infection

Other than the primary infection of the burned skin, several types of infectious complications in burn patients have been recognized. Bacteremia is a frequent complication.

Burn wound manipulations are responsible for development of bacteremias in approximately 50% of cases, but routine instrumentation and intravascular catheter devices also can cause bacteremia.[14,53] The risk for developing bacteremia also correlates with the TBSA affected by burns; Sasaki and associates showed that those patients with a positive blood culture had an average TBSA injury of 47%, whereas those with a 26% injury had negative blood cultures.[128] Bloodstream infection has been associated with longer duration of hospitalization and mechanical ventilation but not with mortality.[19] Toxic shock syndrome (TSS) caused by TSS toxin–producing strains of *S. aureus* has been identified in acutely burned children. Childs and coworkers found that 13% of children developed a toxic shock–like illness; however, its effect on overall burn mortality was not clear.[24]

Subacute bacterial endocarditis is a risk associated with persistent bacteremia of any cause, including repeated instrumentation, surgical intervention, and placement of central venous catheters.[13,22] *S. aureus* and gram-negative bacilli are the most frequent causes. In most cases, the antemortem diagnosis rarely is suspected in children with burn injury.[2,13] In addition to causing local valvular damage, infected vegetations may dislodge septic emboli. Suppurative thrombophlebitis occurs at the site of the insertion of the catheter. It may occur in as many as 5% of patients with burns covering 20% TBSA.[137]

Suppurative chondritis occurs in patients with full-thickness burn of the ear.[101] Because of the auricle's relatively low level of blood supply, chondritis frequently follows the progression of tissue ischemia, usually 3 to 5 weeks after burn injury occurs.[102] *P. aeruginosa* and *S. aureus* are the most common pathogens. However, with use of mafenide acetate as a topical agent, the incidence of suppurative chondritis has decreased significantly.

Suppurative sinusitis is seen in patients with long-term nasotracheal intubation. In one study, 8% of patients with burns who had nasotracheal intubation for more than 7 days developed sinusitis.[18] Pneumonia may occur with or without inhalation injury, although those with inhalation injury have a substantially higher risk.[134] Bronchopneumonia is the most common type of pulmonary infection, usually occurring in the second week of burn injury. Predisposing factors are size of the burn wound (hematogenous spread), aspiration, presence of tracheostomy or nasotracheal tube (nosocomial spread from burn wound), existence of inhalation injury, and disturbances of fluid and electrolyte balances. Causative organisms include gram-positive bacteria, especially *S. aureus;* gram-negative organisms such as *P. aeruginosa, E. coli,* and *K. pneumoniae;* and viruses, including HSV and CMV. Currently most infection-related deaths in burn patients are caused by pneumonia or bloodstream infections, rather than wound infection.[134] Fatal viral pneumonia due to CMV and HSV has been described as well.[27]

Urinary tract infection occurs in association with prolonged and often unnecessary catherization.[129] Osteomyelitis can occur when bones are exposed by the burn or by open fracture accompanying the burn; from extension of infection from a septic joint, introduction of organisms along traction pins, and internal fracture fixation devices; or by bacteremia. However, clinically significant osteomyelitis in burn patients is rare.[36] Septic arthritis occurs when a joint is exposed by a burn or by removal of burn eschar.[36] The joints most frequently exposed are the knee, the elbow, the proximal interphalangeal joints of the hand, and the metacarpophalangeal joints on the dorsal surfaces of the hand. The incidence of septic arthritis is obscured by its frequent association with signs and symptoms of severe burns that rarely are separable. Rarely in burns, a joint may become infected from adjacent metaphysical osteomyelitis. In children, most joints can be salvaged. Adult joints are less resilient.

Central nervous system infections in burn patients include meningitis, microabscesses, and septic infarcts. In one review, *Candida* spp., *S. aureus,* and *P. aeruginosa* caused almost 80% of infections, occurring most frequently in patients with extensive burns with wound infection or endocarditis.[155]

MICROBIOLOGIC INVESTIGATIONS

The three major approaches to determine burn wound infection are (1) quantitative burn wound cultures, (2) histologic assessment of bacterial invasion, and (3) bronchoalveolar lavage (BAL).

Quantitative Burn Wound Cultures by Biopsy

Teplitz demonstrated that quantitative bacterial counts of burn wound cultures correlated with histologic specimens showing invasion or colonization.[142] Burn wound infection (often referred to as "burn wound sepsis" in surgical literature) is suspected when proliferating microorganisms exceed 10^5 per gram of tissue and when invasion of subjacent unburned tissue has occurred (Fig. 76.2). The presence of microorganisms within the necrotic eschar cannot be considered evidence of burn wound infection. Furthermore although a bacterial count of 10^5 per gram of tissue is likely to indicate bacterial invasion, this is not invariably true. Only histologic sections can indicate the level of infection. Therefore burn wound cultures always should be accompanied by histologic sections from the same area.[120,121]

At the time that surgery is performed, the potentially infected tissues should be excised with a punch biopsy (Fig. 76.3) and divided into equal aliquots.[58] One aliquot should be placed into saline and delivered to the microbiology section for quantitative assessment. These biopsy samples are weighed aseptically and homogenized in a sterile tube in 3 mL of sterile saline. Known dilutions of the homogenate then are plated using precalibrated loops (10 μL) onto blood agar, colistin-neomycin agar, MacConkey agar, and Sabouraud agar for identification in initial dilutions of 0.1 mL with a 1-mL sterile pipette. After 24 hours, the number of colonies are counted and the quantitative wound culture is calculated according to the following formula:

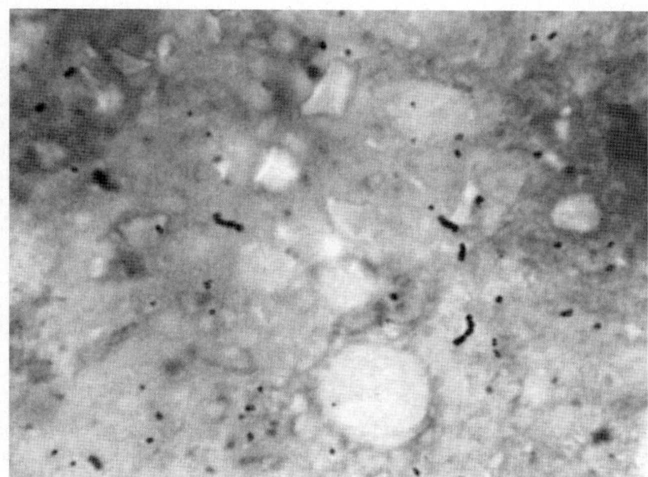

FIG. 76.2 Photomicrograph of a homogenized biopsy specimen stained with Gram stain. Gram-positive cocci are seen (cultures grew group A streptococcus at greater than 10^5 colony-forming units/gram tissue). (From Hunsicker L, Heggers JP, Patel JA. Infections in burn patients. In: Patrick CC, ed. *Clinical Management of Infections in Immunocompromised Infants and Children.* 2nd ed. Philadelphia: Lippincott Williams & Wilkins; 2001:338.)

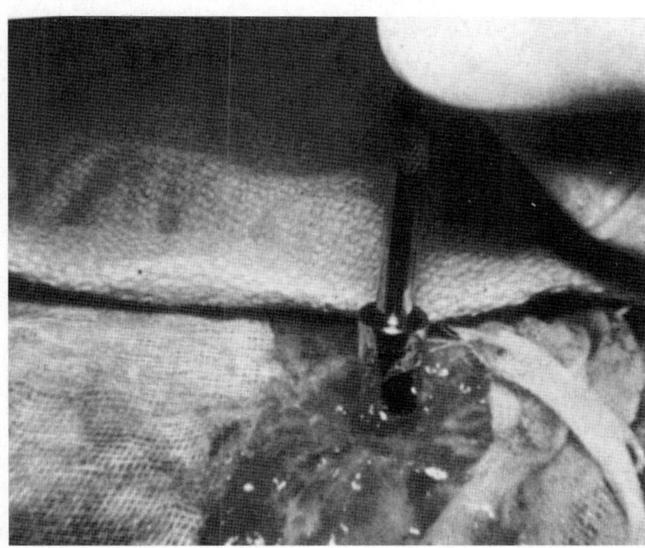

FIG. 76.3 Use of a 6-mm punch for collecting a skin biopsy specimen for tissue histology and quantitative culture. (From Hunsicker L, Heggers JP, Patel JA. Infections in burn patients. In: Patrick CC, ed. *Clinical Management of Infections in Immunocompromised Infants and Children.* 2nd ed. Philadelphia: Lippincott Williams & Wilkins; 2001:339.)

$$\text{Colony-forming unit} \times \text{g of Tissue} \times \text{Number of colonies}$$
$$\times \text{Volume} \times \text{Dilution weight of biopsy in grams}$$

Despite the dependence on quantitative tissue cultures, reliability of this procedure has been questioned because of the high degree of variability in quantitative counts. Woolfrey and colleagues found that when biopsy samples were divided and cultured separately, only 38% of paired quantitative results agreed within the same $\log_{10}$ unit, whereas 44% differed by 2 $\log_{10}$ units or more.[156]

Histologic Procedures

Standard histologic procedures, as well as cryostat examination, are necessary.[121] The tissues should be examined for morphologic changes and for the presence of pathogens. Many bacterial and fungal pathogens can be identified by staining with Gram stain and Gomori methenamine silver stain (Fig. 76.4). More specialized stains may be necessary to identify other fastidious bacteria and fungi. Tzanck stain can be used to identify inclusion bodies suggestive of invasion of HSV or VZV. Viral-specific antibodies also can be used to detect these viruses by immunohistochemistry. The microbial status of the burn wound (i.e., colonization or invasion), as assessed by histologic examination of a biopsy specimen, can be graded on the basis of the density and depth of penetration of microorganisms (Box 76.1).[121]

Bronchoalveolar Lavage

BAL fluid needs to be collected by personnel experienced in the evaluation of patients with inhalation injury who are at risk for developing airway edema and obstruction. Ventilator-associated pneumonia can be diagnosed if 10^4 or more organisms per milliliter are cultured. In a study reported by Wahl and colleagues, BAL eliminated the unnecessary antibiotic treatment of 21% of patients.[148] In winter months, BAL fluids also can be processed for prevalent respiratory viruses such as respiratory syncytial virus (RSV), influenza A and B viruses, and adenoviruses by rapid antigenic detection by immunoassays that are within the capability of most laboratories. Other respiratory viruses, as well as herpesviruses such as HSV and CMV in the respiratory tract, may be detected by viral culture or molecular diagnostics performed by a specialized virology laboratory or reference laboratory.

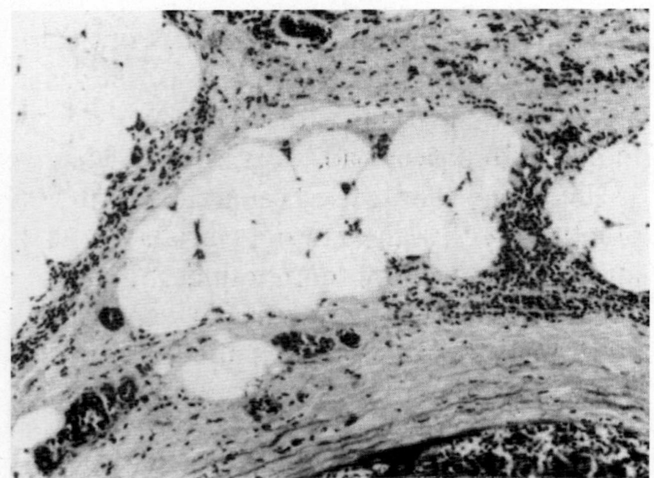

FIG. 76.4 Photomicrograph of a cross-section of tissue stained with hematoxylin and eosin showing invasion of *Pseudomonas aeruginosa*. (From Hunsicker L, Heggers JP, Patel JA. Infections in burn patients. In: Patrick CC, ed. *Clinical Management of Infections in Immunocompromised Infants and Children.* 2nd ed. Philadelphia: Lippincott Williams & Wilkins; 2001:338.)

BOX 76.1 Staging of Microbial Status of the Burn Wound by Biopsy Histology

Stage I: Colonization

A. Superficial: Microorganisms present only on burn wound surface
B. Penetrating: Variable depth of microbial penetration of eschar
C. Proliferating: Variable level of microbial proliferation at nonviable-viable tissue interphase (subeschar space)

Stage II: Invasion

A. Microinvasion: Microorganisms present in viable tissue immediately subjacent to subeschar space
B. Deep invasion: Penetration of microorganisms to variable depth and expanse within viable subcutaneous tissue
C. Microvascular involvement: Microorganisms within small blood vessels and lymphatics (thrombosis of vessels common)

Modified from Pruitt BA, Foley FD. The use of biopsies in burn patient care. *Surgery.* 1973;73:887–97.

Local and Systemic Viral Infection

Viral culture or molecular testing using qualitative or quantitative PCR of the wound surface obtained by swab or by tissue obtained by biopsy will detect the presence of HSV or VZV. Disseminated viral infection with HSV, VZV, CMV, and other viruses may be evaluated by sending whole blood or plasma for specific viral DNA detection and quantification by PCR.

PREVENTION AND TREATMENT OF INFECTION

Care of the wound is the mainstay of burn therapy. The goal is to minimize infection and facilitate healing of the burn wound. Wound care addresses both partial- and full-thickness burn injuries until all wounds are closed.

Wound Dressing

The superficial epidermal layer provides a barrier to microorganisms while the deeper lipid epidermal layer provides protection against loss of water vapor. In full-thickness burns, the eschar may extend beyond the skin into the subcutaneous fat and muscle. Closure of the wound cannot occur until the eschar is removed. Bacterial proteases lead to eschar pseudoseparation and are slowed with antiseptic therapies. Then the eschar is allowed to fragment and slough, with resultant decreased size. This process is called *wound contraction.* This eschar can also be excised and skin grafted. Full-thickness skin grafts have the least contraction rates. Deep dermal wounds allowed to heal spontaneously lead to hypertrophic scarring. Compression garments are used to prevent and treat hypertrophic scarring.

When approaching burn wound care, a plan must first be decided. Outer burn dressings provide comfort, metabolic enhancement, and protection. First, superficial burns are exquisitely sensitive to air currents, as are deeper burns after some healing. Also, dressings provide splinting and drainage containment. Next, occlusive dressings help eliminate shivering, cold stress, and evaporative heat loss. In open, granulating wounds, loss of water vapor is maximal. Finally, the protective component deals with the control of topical organisms. Supplies consist of large 9 × 9 inch burn gauze, Kerlix wraps, Ace wraps, and topical antimicrobial agents. Gentle cleansing of the wound and daily debridement also are important. Buttock burn wounds should be examined carefully and frequently for the presence of deep stool staining, an ominous predictor of burn wound sepsis and death.[124] Such wounds should be emergently excised.

Topical Antimicrobial Agents

Topical antimicrobial agents are used extensively in burn patients. Most patients with stage I and stage II A and B wounds (see Box 76.1) can be treated with topical or subeschar antimicrobial agents alone.

Silver Sulfadiazine (Silvadene, SSD, Thermazene, Flamazine, Burnazine)

Silver sulfadiazine is a 1% water-soluble cream combining sulfadiazine with silver (Ag^+). The Ag^+ ion binds with the DNA of an organism and consequently releases the sulfonamide that interferes with the intermediary metabolic pathway of the microbe. It is most effective against *P. aeruginosa,* the gram-negative enteric bacteria, and *C. albicans. S. aureus* and some strains of *Klebsiella* spp. have been less effectively controlled.[43] Caution is advised with use of sulfadiazine products because cases of *P. aeruginosa* resistance to sulfadiazine have been reported.[57] When compared with collagenase ointment, topical silver sulfadiazine has been shown to be associated with lower rates of wound infection.[117] Antimicrobial effectiveness has been observed to last for up to 24 hours. More frequent changes are required if a creamy exudate forms on the wound. The benefits of this topical agent are its ease of use and its ability to reduce pain. It has some tissue-penetrating ability, but it is limited to the epidermis.

Silver sulfadiazine can be used separately or in combination with other antibacterial agents or enzymatic escharotomy compounds. It can be combined with nystatin, which enhances the antifungal activity of this agent. By itself, silver sulfadiazine has been shown to retard wound healing; however, in conjunction with nystatin or aloe vera, the wound-retardant effect is reversed. When topical silver sulfadiazine was compared with the more expensive collagenase ointment for treatment of partial thickness burns in children, there was no significant difference in clinical course, outcome, or need for skin grafting.[117]

Cerium Nitrate–Silver Sulfadiazine (Flammacerium)

The lanthanide salt cerium nitrate has been added to silver sulfadiazine since the 1970s and has been shown to have increased bacteriostatic effect in large burn wounds. The antimicrobial spectrum is similar to that of silver nitrate. Methemoglobinemia has been seen only rarely, and no associated electrolyte disturbances occur. Only minimal cerium absorption has been noted in patients with large burns treated for weeks. No complications were noted. Its use is somewhat limited because it is not commercially available in the United States. It is, however, available in several western European countries. Koller and Orsag studied the effects of cerium sulfadiazine in 20 burn patients and found it to be safe and effective in the treatment of deep, extensive burn wounds.[80]

Silver Nitrate

Silver nitrate is available as a 0.5% solution that does not injure the regenerating epithelium in the wound and provides bacteriostatic effect against *S. aureus, E. coli,* and *P. aeruginosa.*[43] Silver nitrate is most effective when the wound is cleansed carefully of all emollients and other debris. Multilayered coarse mesh dressings should be placed over the wound and saturated with the silver nitrate solution. Like silver sulfadiazine, silver nitrate has limited penetration because the Ag^+ ion is bound rapidly to the body's natural anions such as Cl^-. Because it is hypotonic, it can cause osmolar dilution, resulting in hyponatremia and hypochloremia. Serum electrolyte levels should be monitored very carefully.

Notable detriments to the use of silver nitrate include its high expense and light sensitivity. Furthermore it also requires special handling because if it is allowed to dry or if it is covered with an impervious dressing hyperpyrexia could occur. *Klebsiella, Providencia,* and other Enterobacteriaceae are not as susceptible to it as are other bacteria. *E. cloacae* and other nitrate-positive bacteria can cause methemoglobinemia by converting nitrite to nitrate.

Mafenide Acetate (Sulfamylon)

Mafenide acetate is available both in a 10% water-soluble cream or a 5% solution and has more substantial bacteriologic data to support its efficacy than do any of the other topical antimicrobial agents.[85,99] It has been shown to be effective against a broad range of microorganisms, especially against all strains of *P. aeruginosa* and *Clostridium* spp.[128] After a wound has been cleansed of debris, mafenide acetate is "buttered" onto the wound. The treated burn surface is left exposed for maximal antimicrobial potency. The cream is applied a minimum of twice a day and can be reapplied as needed. The 5% solution is applied every 8 hours.

Additionally mafenide acetate has the ability to permeate burn eschar and thereby reduce the risk for bacterial colonization of a deep burn wound, and it is especially effective after the dead tissue is removed from the granulating bed. Unfortunately several detrimental aspects are associated with the use of mafenide acetate. Protracted use with the low environmental pH favors the growth of *C. albicans.* Mafenide acetate is converted to p-sulfamoyl benzoic acid by monamine oxidase, which is a carbonic anhydrase inhibitor; it subsequently causes metabolic acidosis in the patient. It also is painful when applied to superficial, partial-thickness burns with intact free nerve endings, and its requirement to remain uncovered for antimicrobial activity may be considered a disadvantage when a dressing is required.

Membrane Dressings

Acticoat and Aquacel are silver-coated dressings that have a broad antibacterial activity. Compared with silver nitrate or silver sulfadiazine use, Acticoat and Aquacel have been found easier to apply, were associated with less pain on removal, and have faster rates of reepithelialization.[23,143] In one clinical study, Acticoat was found to have better antibacterial activity than silver sulfadiazine.[76] Acticoat is also better than hydrogel (Solosite) and paraffin-embedded woven cotton fabric (Jelonet) in protection against wound colonization/infection.[149] Mepitel is another gridlike, silicone-coated, nylon dressing used in treatment of partial-thickness burn wounds. Gotschall and associates found this product to decrease the pain experienced during dressing change, the time needed for the wound to heal, and the overall duration of the hospital stay as compared with silver sulfadiazine.[49] This study did not find any difference in the incidence of infections between Mepitel and silver sulfadiazine treatments.

Topical Antibiotics

Several topical antibiotics have been tried in the management of burn infections. The use of these agents is highly discouraged in a burn unit because of rapid emergence of resistance:

1. *Gentamicin sulfate:* Available as a 0.1% water-soluble cream, this antibiotic is chemically similar to the other aminoglycosides, such as kanamycin and neomycin. It has a broad spectrum of antimicrobial activity. It is used for its activity against *P. aeruginosa;* however, its topical use is highly limited because of the high level of gentamicin resistance in burn units.
2. *Bacitracin/polymyxin:* This antibiotic combination has little or no effect on localized infections of burn wounds.
3. *Nitrofurantoin:* This agent is used topically as adjunctive therapy in patients with second- and third-degree burns. With good eschar penetration, it can be used in the treatment of invasive burn wound infections with sensitive agents. The drug presents some advantages for the ambulatory patient. Tissue granulation begins sooner and crusts separate more rapidly.
4. *Mupirocin (Bactroban):* Studies at Shriners Hospital for Children–Galveston have shown mupirocin to be superior to silver sulfadiazine in treating MSSA or MRSA infection.[138] Although mupirocin is weaker against gram-negative bacteria, it is also comparable to silver sulfadiazine and mafenide acetate against *P. aeruginosa, E. coli,* and *K. pneumoniae.* However, caution is advised for routine use of mupirocin in management of burn wound infection because it has been shown to lead to rapid development of resistance when it is used repeatedly.

Nystatin (Mycostatin, Nilstat)

Studies have shown that combining nystatin and silver sulfadiazine or nitrofurantoin results in effective prevention of local and systemic *Candida* infections, as well as burn wound sepsis.[59] However, in combination therapy with silver sulfadiazine and nystatin, mafenide acetate actually loses its antimicrobial activity. Therefore, use of nystatin with mafenide acetate is discouraged. Concentrated nystatin powder has also been studied for its effects on angioinvasive fungi (e.g., *Fusarium, Aspergillus*) refractory to systemic amphotericin B and serial excisions, including amputations.[11] A concentrated form of nystatin (6 million units/g) was used as dry aerosol every 6 hours with wet-to-dry dressings laid on top. Within 14 days, eradication of invasive fungal infections was noted in all four of the children studied. Also, all areas previously autografted underneath the nystatin powder healed well.

Sodium Hypochlorite (0.025% Heggers Solution)

Currently the most effective topical antibacterial agent for cleansing a wound is sodium hypochlorite (NaClO). It transcends the topical antimicrobial effects and tissue toxicity of such products as povidone-iodine, acetic acid, and hydrogen peroxide. The efficacy of NaClO has been determined to be at a concentration of 0.025%, which is bactericidal, is nontoxic to fibroblasts, and does not inhibit wound healing provided buffers are used.[60] It is a broad-spectrum antiseptic and is bactericidal for *P. aeruginosa, S. aureus* (MRSA and MSSA), enterococci, and other gram-negative and gram-positive organisms.[128]

Povidone-Iodine (Betadine)

The active antimicrobial component in this compound is the iodine. It has a broad spectrum of antibacterial and antifungal activities. However, there are disadvantages that limit its use in a burn center. It is painful when applied and is inactivated by wound exudates. Renal dysfunction and acidosis have been noted in association with systemic absorption when applied to open wounds.

Chlorhexidine

Chlorhexidine when combined with 0.5% silver nitrate has efficacy similar to that of silver sulfadiazine.[89] Some variants of this product have broader antimicrobial activities, but pain experienced by patients on application has limited its use. Unlike the sulfonamides, plasma-mediated resistance has not occurred.

Citric Acid

In a study from India,[109] citric acid was formulated into a 3% gel and was compared with silver sulfadiazine. Citric acid gel application was better in wound healing. However, large-scale studies are lacking.

Subeschar Antibiotics

Moncrief has described the technique of subeschar antibiotic infusion.[102] It is used for microbial invasion into unburned tissue when topical therapies have not been effective or in cases in which treatment has been delayed. The most common drugs used are tobramycin, gentamicin, and kanamycin. However, development of antimicrobial resistance is likely to be substantial, so subeschar infusion of antibiotics should be used infrequently. The antibiotic solution is administered via multiple needle infusions by subcutaneous lysis. The results of this technique are more rapid separation of eschar. The fluid infusion limit is 2000 mL (adult dose) and should be accounted for in a patient's fluid requirements. The infusion fluid should consist of 0.25 to 0.45 normal saline to avoid salt overload. Use of lactated Ringer solution should be avoided because some of the drugs are incompatible with calcium. Erythromycin has been studied but is too painful to use. Colistin, novobiocin, and cephaloridine have been used but found to be ineffective.

Systemic Antiinfective Agents

Drug pharmacokinetics are significantly altered in the burn patient and show significant interpatient and intrapatient variation.[152] Dolton and coworkers showed that vancomycin clearance is significantly higher in burn patients, but there is no significant difference in the volume of distribution.[32] Doh and associates also showed that meropenem clearance and volume of distribution were higher.[31] These studies suggest that higher dosing of vancomycin and meropenem may be needed in burn patients. Despite these studies, however, a review of the currently available literature shows that for many drugs there is a paucity of information to support current dosage recommendations, specifically in children of various age groups. In addition, many reports are based on small numbers of patients, and, even in larger studies, no standardization of the study population exists with regard to the important variables known to affect drug handling. For the subpopulation of burn patients who eliminate drugs extremely rapidly, a concern exists over the adequacy of antibiotic dosing. Researchers have suggested that antibiotic serum concentrations be measured, when available, in every patient to ascertain whether a significant problem exists with dosing.

Whereas stage I and stage II A and B wounds (see Box 76.1) can be treated with topical or subeschar antimicrobials alone, stage II C wounds require the immediate institution of systemic antiinfective agents. Systemic agents also are indicated for the treatment of various systemic infectious complications (see earlier discussion). Detailed information on selection of the appropriate systemic antimicrobial agents for specific bacterial, fungal, and viral pathogens is available elsewhere in this text. Nonetheless the following general principles can help guide the use of antimicrobial therapy:

1. Each antimicrobial agent must be selected for its specificity for the microbe present.
2. Such decisions should be made on appropriately collected culture and susceptibility data.
3. Colonizing flora should be distinguished from those responsible for inflammation and invasion.
4. The time, dosage, route of administration, and duration of treatment should be in accordance with what is required to make the organism nonpathogenic.
5. The need for broad-spectrum antibiotics should be balanced with the risk for promoting fungal infections.

Probiotics

Since burn injury results in exposure to MDR organisms in the hospital setting and the additional pressure of broad-spectrum antibiotics significantly alters the microbiome of the host, attempts have been made to reintroduce protective bacteria through the use of probiotics. No specific recommendations exist for the routine use of probiotics in the burn setting because there is concern for the potential for bacterial translocation and infection by the probiotic bacteria. Nonetheless some studies show encouraging results. Tahir and coworkers studied 64 Pakistani children with burns up to 50% TBSA; compared with controls, after treatment with an oral combination formulation of *Lactobacillus acidophilus, L. delbrueckii, Bifidobacterium*, and *Streptococcus thermophiles*, the loss of skin graft and mortality rates were modestly lower.[141] In a study of a small number of children, Mayes and coworkers showed that use of *Lactobacillus rhamnosus* was associated with a modest trend toward reduced antifungal use, diarrhea episodes, requirement for excision or graft procedure, and wound healing period.[97] Additional studies of a larger number children are needed.

Treatment of Multidrug-Resistant, Gram-Negative Bacteria

This issue deserves specific mention because it most severely affects burn units. As noted in the earlier review of burn wound microbiology, in many centers, MDR and extensively drug resistant (XDR) bacteria, particularly *P. aeruginosa* strains and *Acinetobacter* spp., are identified frequently. For ESBL strains, the drug choice is a carbapenem. Newer agents effective against ESBL bacteria include combinations of a cephalosporin with β-lactamase inhibitors; examples include ceftolozane/tazobactam and ceftazidime/avibactam.

For carbapenemase-producing bacteria, colistin and polymyxin B often remain the only effective antimicrobial agents. Goverman and coworkers have summarized their experience in 14 children treated with intravenous colistin: a favorable response was obtained in 79%, and the overall mortality rate was 14%.[50] Both colistin and polymyxin B are associated with significant elevation in serum creatinine value or with renal failure in 15% to 25% of recipients. Neurotoxicity in children is an infrequent occurrence. Intravenous and/or aerosol polymyxin B, doxycycline, and ampicillin/sulbactam (the active component is thought to be sulbactam) have been tried in XDR *Acinetobacter* infections as well.[112] Fosfomycin is also effective against carbapenemase-producing bacteria, but *Acinetobacter* spp is intrinsically resistant to it. Other studies have demonstrated in vitro susceptibility of XDR *Acinetobacter* to various synergistic combinations of antimicrobial agents, including carbapenems, colistin, rifampin, tigecycline, and ampicillin-sulbactam.[47,62,158] A significant challenge in managing children with these antibiotics is that their dosage is often unknown because their pharmacokinetics have not been studied across different pediatric age groups, and most have no regulatory approval for pediatric use.

Treatment of Viral Infections

If HSV or VZV infection of the wound surface, lungs, or disseminated viral infection with viremia is present, then systemic antiviral treatment with acyclovir is indicated. Pneumonitis and systemic infection with significant viremia with CMV should be treated with ganciclovir. If viral resistance to first-line antiviral agents occurs, then foscarnet or cidofovir may be administered. Respiratory tract infection, including pneumonia associated with influenza A or B virus may be treated with oseltamivir, which can be orally administered if the patient is able to absorb enterally administered medications.

Antibiotic Prophylaxis

Prophylactic use of antibiotics remains a highly controversial topic. Penicillin prophylaxis is used commonly in many burn centers during outbreaks of group A streptococcal infections.[52,125] Prophylactic antibiotics also are used before surgical manipulation or instrumentation because the risk for developing bacteremia is as high as 50%. The choice of perioperative antibiotics depends on the knowledge of existing microorganisms, which are present not only on injured skin but also in the wound that is ready for surgery. Nonetheless carefully controlled studies are necessary to identify the value of prophylactic antibiotics.

In a placebo-controlled study of cefazolin use in children with burn injury, researchers found that in children with burns of less than 35% TBSA, cefazolin was not necessary, and in those with burns of 35% or more, it was not effective.[126] In a retrospective review study, antibiotic prophylaxis was not associated with any reduction in the rate of wound infection; instead the duration of hospitalization was found to be longer.[34] A recent meta-analysis of studies of prophylactic antibiotics found that most of the studies were weak.[5] The most important finding was that staphylococcal infection rates declined with prophylaxis but resistance to prophylactic antibiotics increased. In a study by Mulgrew and coworkers, prophylactic antibiotic was found to have no effect on the occurrence of TSS in children.[106] Tagami and coworkers used a nationwide database of hospitalized burned children in Japan; use of antibiotic prophylaxis was associated with improved 28-day in-hospital mortality in mechanically ventilated patients but not in those who were not mechanically ventilated.[140] In another study, routine intranasal mupirocin use at admission was not associated with reduction of burn wound colonization.[67]

Wound Excision and Grafting

Studies have shown that early excision of wounds leads to significantly decreased rates of bacterial colonization and wound infection.[10] In a meta-analysis of six trials, it was found that early excision of burns is beneficial in reducing mortality (in patients without inhalational injury) and length of hospital stay. The only drawback is the greater volume of blood loss.[114]

Gut Support and Decontamination

The gut microflora have been implicated in the development of multiorgan failure when the gut barrier fails. Hence one theory is that early enteral feeding of the gut, which promotes function of the gut barrier, is important for preventing multiorgan failure. A decontaminated gut with nonabsorbable, broad-spectrum antibiotics might diminish the impact of failure of the gastrointestinal barrier. Although the suggestion has been made that the rate of pneumonia may be decreased by such maneuvers, no apparent impact on mortality rates has been noted.[94] Overall, convincing human data on the beneficial effect of enteral feeding and decontamination of the gut on sepsis and multiorgan failure are lacking.

Immunomodulators

In view of the intricate relationship between altered immune defenses in burn patients and increased susceptibility to infections, various types of immunotherapies have been tried. In an Italian study, treatment with intravenous pooled immunoglobulin (IVIG) was found to have a beneficial effect on septic phenomena and recovery.[100] However, in two U.S. studies, no change in rates of infection or mortality was shown. Overall the beneficial role of IVIG as prophylaxis or treatment remains unproved.[108,150] In a German study, prophylaxis with intravenous anti-*Pseudomonas* immunoglobulin did not appear to be beneficial to burn patients in general; however, it was shown to be effective in burn patients with inhalation injury.[139] In a South African study, prophylaxis with high-titer anti-lipopolysaccharide immunoglobulin G reduced the incidence of burn wound infection but did not affect mortality.[70] Benefits of plasmapheresis or fresh frozen plasma infusion have not been proved.

INFECTION CONTROL

Hospital-acquired infections in burn patients are common occurrences. In pediatric burn patients, wound infections, ventilator-related pulmonary infections, central-line bacteremias, and catheter-associated urinary tract infections are the most common nosocomial infections.[129,151] The rates of infections may be lower than those seen in adults, but urinary tract infections occur more frequently in children.[129] In a German study of children with burns, the overall infection rate was 59.7 nosocomial infections per 1000 inpatient days, and the device-associated infection rates per 1000 device days were 55.2 for pneumonia, 8.9 for primary bloodstream infections, and 41.7 for urinary tract infections.[45] The incident density of burn wound infections was 18.5 per 1000 inpatient days, which was associated with the percentage of TBSA of the burn wound. On the other hand, the rate of device-associated infections was not associated with the percentage of TBSA.

Surveillance of infection in a burn patient is performed to implement prompt treatment on the basis of surveillance cultures and antimicrobial sensitivities at the earliest sign of invasion. Such surveillance requires cultures of sputum, urine, and wounds about three times weekly; however, the need for such cultures and the frequency of monitoring remain controversial. Additional infection control measures involve surveillance of spread of pathogens among burn patients in a burn unit. In dealing with the burn wound, strict infectious disease precautions must be maintained to prevent contamination and worsening infection in these already immunocompromised patients.

In the past, poor hand-washing and shared hydrotherapy tubs were the source of many infections, some of which were life threatening. Strict enforcement of hand-washing and use of gowns, gloves, and masks have led to decreased rates of patient contamination. Also, disposable hydrotherapy tub liners are used to eliminated the risk for patient-to-patient transmission of infections.[144] In addition, isolation of burn patients in a single room compared with placing them in an open ward has dramatically affected infection rates. McManus and associates studied this measure in 2519 patients and found significantly lower incidence and mortality rates associated with gram-negative bacteremia in the isolated patients.[98] Also those patients in an open ward who had bacterial isolates showed significantly more antimicrobial resistance compared with patients in isolation.

Additional infection control measures include the daily use of germicidal solutions to clean all hardware, such as intravenous poles and pumps, monitoring equipment, bedside tables, and beds in patients' rooms. On discharge of the patient, everything in the room, including floors, walls, ceilings, and mattresses, must be cleaned with germicidal solutions. Air filters should be monitored repeatedly for fungal and bacterial growth.

Lai and colleagues studied the effects of strict isolation of patients with vancomycin-resistant enterococci, the use of vancomycin, and the cost-to-benefit analysis of barrier precautions.[86] The study showed that pharyngeal swabs were poor for surveillance but that rectal swabs were more useful. Also guidelines for use of vancomycin were adhered to by 85% of the staff. The overall cost for these implementations, including the barrier supplies and cleaning protocols, was $11,000. Nonetheless vancomycin-resistant enterococci were not eradicated. On the other hand, van Rijn and colleagues[146] have shown that isolation in a quarantine unit was highly effective in preventing outbreaks of MDR bacteria.

NEW REFERENCES SINCE THE SEVENTH EDITION

4. American Burn Association Fact Sheet. Available at http://www.ameriburn.org/resources_factsheet.php.
20. Butler KL, Ambravaneswaran V, Agrawal N, et al. Burn injury reduces neutrophil directional migration speed in microfluidic devices. *PLoS ONE*. 2010;5:e11921.
33. Egea-Guerrero JJ, Martínez-Fernández C, Rodríguez-Rodríguez A, et al. The utility of C-reactive protein and procalcitonin for sepsis diagnosis in critically burned patients: a preliminary study. *Plast Surg (Oakv)*. 2015;23:239-243.
46. Gauglitz GG, Herndon DN, Kulp GA, et al. Abnormal insulin sensitivity persists up to three years in pediatric patients post-burn. *J Clin Endocrinol Metab*. 2009;94:1656-1664.
64. Inatsu A, Kogiso M, Jeschke MG, et al. Lack of Th17 cell generation in patients with severe burn injuries. *J Immunol*. 2011;187:2155-2161.
67. Jaspers ME, Breederveld RS, Tuinebreijer WE, et al. The evaluation of nasal mupirocin to prevent *Staphylococcus aureus* burn wound colonization in routine clinical practice. *Burns*. 2014;40:1570-1574.
68. Jeschke MG, Finnerty CC, Kulp GA, et al. Can we use C-reactive protein levels to predict severe infection or sepsis in severely burned patients? *Int J Burns Trauma*. 2013;3:137-143.
79. Kobayashi M, Takahashi H, Sanford AP, et al. An increase in the susceptibility of burned patients to infectious complications due to impaired production of macrophage inflammatory protein 1 alpha. *J Immunol*. 2002;169:4460-4466.

84. Kraft R, Herndon DN, Finnerty CC, et al. Occurrence of multiorgan dysfunction in pediatric burn patients: incidence and clinical outcome. *Ann Surg*. 2014;259:381-387.
83. Kraft R, Herndon DN, Finnerty CC, et al. Predictive value of IL-8 for sepsis and severe infections after burn injury: a clinical study. *Shock*. 2015;43:222-227.
97. Mayes T, Gottschlich MM, James LE, et al. Clinical safety and efficacy of probiotic administration following burn injury. *J Burn Care Res*. 2015;36:92-99.
106. Mulgrew S, Khoo A, Cartwright R, et al. Morbidity in pediatric burns, toxic shock syndrome, and antibiotic prophylaxis: a retrospective comparative study. *Ann Plast Surg*. 2014;72:34-37.
113. Ogle CK, Ogle JD, Mao JX, et al. Effect of glutamine on phagocytosis and bacterial killing by normal and pediatric burn patient neutrophils. *J Parenter Enteral Nutr*. 1994;18:128-133.
136. Sobouti B, Fallah S, Ghavami Y, et al. Serum immunoglobulin levels in pediatric burn patients. *Burns*. 2013;39:473-476.
140. Tagami T, Matsui H, Fushimi K, et al. Prophylactic antibiotics may improve outcome in patients with severe burns requiring mechanical ventilation: propensity score analysis of a Japanese nationwide database. *Clin Infect Dis*. 2016;62:60-66.
141. Tahir SM, Makhdoom A, Awan S, et al. Role of probiotics in the management of burns patients. *World J Med Sci*. 2014;3:417-421.
157. Yang XJ, Jin J, Xu H, et al. Prognostic significance of serum procalcitonin in patients with extremely severe burn and sepsis. *Zhonghua Shao Shang Za Zhi (Chinese)*. 2016;32:147-151.

The full reference list for this chapter is available at ExpertConsult.com.

77 Kawasaki Disease

Stanford T. Shulman • Anne H. Rowley

Kawasaki disease (KD) is a multisystem acute febrile vasculitic syndrome of presumably infectious origin that affects predominantly infants and young children. The diagnosis is based on characteristic clinical features (Box 77.1). Serious complications include coronary arteritis, coronary artery aneurysms and stenoses, coronary thrombosis leading to myocardial infarction, and, very rarely, rupture of a coronary aneurysm. KD has become the leading cause of acquired heart disease in children in most developed countries, including the United States and Japan.[307,308] It has been reported in children of all racial groups and from all continents. Although the etiology of KD remains unknown and a specific diagnostic test is lacking, establishing a timely diagnosis is very important because administration of intravenous immunoglobulin (IVIG) and aspirin before the 10th day of illness generally has a dramatic effect on the clinical manifestations and markedly reduces the likelihood of development of coronary abnormalities (see the later sections on treatment).[87,196-199,267,311]

Synonyms for KD include *Kawasaki syndrome* and *mucocutaneous lymph node syndrome* (MCLS, MLNS, or MCLNS). The disease also has been referred to as *lymphomucocutaneous syndrome.* An earlier term used in autopsy reports was *infantile periarteritis nodosa* (IPAN), which is pathologically indistinguishable from fatal KD. The International Classification of Diseases (ICD-9) designates the condition as both KD and mucocutaneous lymph node syndrome (acute) (febrile) (infantile) under rubric 446.1 and ICD-10 under M30.3. Before 1983, the National Library of Medicine listed KD publications under various subject headings, particularly "Lymphatic Diseases." Since 1984, publications have been listed under "Mucocutaneous Lymph Node Syndrome," a name that has been replaced by KD.

HISTORY

The illness now bearing his name was first recognized as a clinical entity in 1961 by Dr. Tomisaku Kawasaki, who subsequently became chairman of the Department of Pediatrics at Tokyo's Japan Red Cross Medical Center. Between 1961 and 1967, Kawasaki identified 50 infants and young children who manifested a distinctive constellation of signs that included prolonged high fever, unilateral cervical lymphadenopathy, bilateral conjunctival injection, a polymorphous erythematous rash, changes of the mucosa of the lips and oral cavity, and edema and erythema of the extremities, with subsequent desquamation of the finger and toes. Although the syndrome was distinctive, its signs were nonspecific. Laboratory tests ruled out other disorders. A series of the first seven cases was presented by Kawasaki at the 61st Chiba General Meeting of the Japan Pediatric Society in 1962.[133] Convinced that he was observing a distinct clinical syndrome, Kawasaki published a report of his experience with 50 cases of "febrile oculo-oro-cutaneo-acrodesquamatous syndrome with or without acute nonsuppurative cervical lymphadenitis" in 1967.[134,135,137] Other Japanese physicians quickly recognized the syndrome after Kawasaki's report, although considerable discussion ensued about whether it was a distinct entity or an illness related to Stevens-Johnson syndrome.[136]

Cardiac involvement in this illness was suspected first in 1968, when Yamamoto and Kimura reported an infant with KD who had transient tachycardia with a gallop rhythm, cardiomegaly, and minor electrocardiographic (ECG) abnormalities.[339] In 1970, Kawasaki obtained funding to establish the Research Committee of Mucocutaneous Lymph Node Syndrome, sponsored by the Japanese Ministry of Health and Welfare, which was organized with Dr. Fumio Kosaki as chair.[137] In the first national survey of this committee, four autopsied and six nonautopsied cases of children who had died of coronary artery complications after apparent KD were identified.[147] These children were predominantly younger than 2 years of age and had died suddenly within 30 days of onset of disease, with evidence of coronary aneurysms and acute thrombosis. The first biennial Japanese national epidemiologic survey was conducted by this committee in 1970 under the leadership of Dr. I. Shigematsu and was published in 1972.[264] By this time, it had become well established that some patients who recovered apparently uneventfully from this acute illness were at risk for sudden cardiac death, with findings of acute myocardial infarction secondary to thrombosis within coronary arteries damaged by a severe vasculitic process.[147]

In 1971, physicians at the University of Hawaii who were unaware of the Japanese experience began to recognize patients with an unusual Reiter syndrome–like illness. When information about KD was published in the English-language literature,[137] the illness in Hawaii was recognized clearly as KD. Information exchanged between Japanese and U.S. investigators led to the 1974 publication of English-language articles by both groups[137,172,173] and triggered worldwide recognition of cases. In the early 1970s, death from myocardial infarction was reported to occur in approximately 2% of cases of KD; more recent data reflect much lower mortality rates of less than 0.02%.[105,188,327,345] Four deaths were recorded in Japan among 26,691 patients in 2011 to 2012 (0.015%). Four deaths occurred among 23,349 KD patients in Taiwan from 2000 to 2010 (0.017%).[163] With the availability of echocardiography in the late 1970s, researchers determined that 20% to 25% of patients developed evidence of coronary artery abnormalities.[123]

In the decades before Kawasaki recognized the clinical features of the illness, many individual reports of fatal coronary arteritis in children (usually labeled IPAN) were published in the non-Japanese pediatric and pathology literature.[48,72,182,218,232,237] Clinical details of these cases generally are highly suggestive of KD, and the pathologic features of IPAN are indistinguishable from those of KD, as demonstrated conclusively by Landing and Larson in 1977.[152] Almost 100 years before Kawasaki's description was published, Samuel Gee of St. Bartholomew's Hospital in London in 1871 reported the case of a 7-year-old boy who at death ("following scarlatinal dropsy") had three coronary aneurysms, each filled with a fresh clot; histologic examination of that patient's cardiac tissue is compatible with inactive KD with extensive coronary luminal myofibroblastic proliferation.[90,274,271] Shibuya and colleagues retrospectively identified cases of illnesses compatible with KD that occurred in Japan up to two decades before Kawasaki's description was published.[263] Likely, patients with KD in previous decades were misdiagnosed as having measles, scarlet fever, rubella, or other once common conditions, and reductions in the numbers of cases of those illnesses helped to facilitate recognition of KD.[136]

Kawasaki's clinical description of the syndrome has remained the foundation of diagnosis and the basis of the clinical and epidemiologic case definitions in use today (see Box 77.1). In 2017, the American Heart Association Committee on Rheumatic Fever, Bacterial Endocarditis, and Kawasaki Disease published updated guidelines for the management of patients with incomplete (or atypical) KD (see later discussion).[171a,199,]

EPIDEMIOLOGY

Sources of Epidemiologic Data

In the absence of a confirmatory diagnostic test, the epidemiologic case definitions of KD are relatively strict and exclude from surveillance

BOX 77.1 Diagnostic Criteria for Classic or Typical Kawasaki Disease

Fever for at least 5 days[a] *plus* four of the following features:

- Bilateral conjunctival injection
- Polymorphous exanthem
- Changes in the lips and oral cavity (erythema, cracking of lips; oropharyngeal erythema; strawberry tongue)
- Peripheral extremity changes (erythema and swelling of hands and feet; later periungual desquamation, Beau lines)
- Cervical lymphadenopathy (≥1.5 cm in diameter)

Exclusion of other diseases with similar features

The finding of fever plus three criteria in the presence of coronary abnormalities qualifies.
[a]In the presence of classic features, experienced clinicians may be able to establish the diagnosis before the fifth day of illness.

data other exanthematous conditions that could dilute "true" cases and thus could obscure secular trends. However, the original epidemiologic case definitions were not intended for clinical application, a very important point since effective treatment became available. Thus, less strict application of clinical case criteria is appropriate for management of patients. Clinicians must be aware that children often present with clinical illnesses that do not completely fulfill the diagnostic criteria for KD but who are nonetheless at risk for developing coronary artery sequelae and therefore warrant therapy. These patients generally are considered to have *incomplete* or *atypical* KD.[22,86,199,251] Incomplete presentations of KD are particularly common occurrences in young infants in whom clinical signs often are subtle or fleeting but who are at the highest risk for development of coronary artery abnormalities.[35,242] In the United States, the Centers for Disease Control and Prevention (CDC) case definition usually is used for epidemiologic purposes and the American Heart Association published an algorithm to aid in the diagnosis of incomplete (atypical) KD.[171a,199] The current Japanese diagnostic guidelines were revised in 2014 and also reflect the importance of incomplete cases.[117]

Incidence Rates

The incidence of KD varies throughout the world and reflects primarily the racial composition of various countries. Rates in Japan have climbed steadily, with an annual rate of 243.1 per 100,000 children younger than 5 years of age in 2011 and 264.8 in 2012 (22nd national survey).[166] The highest reported rate in Korea was 134 per 100,000 children younger than 5 years old in 2009–11.[140] Taiwan has the third highest reported rate, 82.8 per 100,000 children less than 5 years old.[163] In countries with predominantly non-Asian populations, the rate is 15 to 20 per 100,000 children younger than 5 years.[107]

Gender

In virtually all population-based studies in many countries, the ratio of male to female patients with KD approximates 1.5 : 1.[166,327,347] In addition, serious and fatal complications also are significantly more common findings among male patients with KD compared with female patients.[190,346] Examination of fatal Japanese cases indicated almost three times as many Kawasaki-related fatalities among males compared with females, with a higher ratio in infancy.[190,327] The basis for the preponderance of KD in males and for the even greater predominance of serious coronary artery disease in males with KD remains unclear. Of interest is that a male predominance is observed in many infectious diseases.

Race or Ethnic Background

The first cases of KD were recognized in Japanese children and in Hawaiian children of predominantly Japanese ethnicity, and subsequent data consistently support higher rates in those of Asian background. Annual incidence rates in Japan have climbed steadily to 264.8 cases per 100,000 children younger than 5 years of age in 2012,[166] from 102.6 in 1995 and 184.6 in 2005 to 2006,[187] and they are the highest in the world, approached only by rates for Japanese-American children in Hawaii (210.5 per 100,000 of children younger than 5 years).[108] More than 13,917 cases of KD were reported in Japan in 2012, with local clusters rather than nationwide epidemics, as were seen in 1979, 1982, and 1985–86.[166] In epidemic years in Japan, the annual age-specific incidence rates reached or exceeded 200 per 100,000 children younger than 5 years.[341] Incidence rates in white children in many communities are much lower, most often approximating 10 to 20 per 100,000 children younger than 5 years.[55,107,269] Surveys in countries with almost exclusively white populations often yield rates of 5 to 10 cases per 100,000 children younger than 5 years.[23,26,40,103,224,278] In Washington state, ethnic group–specific incidence rates per 100,000 children younger than 5 years were estimated to be 33.3 for Asian Americans, 23.4 for blacks, and 12.7 for whites.[55] In Hawaii, with its complex racial-ethnic makeup, the overall annual incidence is about 45 per 100,000 children younger than 5 years.[108] The yearly incidence for Japanese children in Hawaii approaches 200 cases per 100,000 children, and for whites it is 35 per 100,000, with intermediate rates for those of native Hawaiian and Chinese, Filipino, and other Asian ancestry.[107] Prospective Kawasaki disease surveillance in Germany in 2011–12 corrected for underreporting yielded an incidence of 7.2 per 100,000 children younger than 5 years.[115] Extrapolation of data from surveys of U.S. hospitals with large children's services led to estimates of approximately 2500 cases per year in the United States from 1984 to 1993,[307,308] with more recent estimates as high as 5000 cases annually.[29] A study of KD in the United States identified approximately 4200 hospitalizations in the year 2000, with highest rates among Asian and Pacific Islanders, lowest rates in whites, and intermediate rates in blacks and Hispanics.[107]

Age

KD occurs almost exclusively in children. In the United States and Japan, adult cases are quite rare, although some reports of adults diagnosed by accepted diagnostic criteria have been published.[157] Many of these adult patients have been infected with human immunodeficiency virus (HIV).[10,36,39,71,95,119,175,226,231,261] Most of the early reported adult cases, however, probably actually represented toxic shock syndrome or drug hypersensitivity reactions. Perhaps the best-documented adult case (confirmed by Dr. Kawasaki) was that of a 31-year-old Japanese man who later developed bilateral coronary artery aneurysms.[288] Because the signs and symptoms are nonspecific, adults suspected to have KD should be evaluated carefully for infectious, toxic, and other possible causes of illness.

The distribution of KD by age in childhood is highly characteristic. The disease occurs most frequently in young children: 50% are younger than 2 years, 80% are younger than 5 years, and cases seldom occur in those older than 12 years.[107,282,345] In 2009–10, 0.7% of Japanese patients with KD were 10 years old or older.[327] Infants in the first 3 to 5 months of life have a relatively low incidence of KD, but the incidence rises rapidly from that point.[327] In the United States, the peak age is about 10 months, whereas more recent data from Japan identified 25% as younger than 1 year, 88% as younger than 5 years, and the peak age incidence as 9 to 11 months of age.[166] In Hawaii, 29% of cases are in infants younger than 1 year, and 85% of patients are younger than 5 years.[107] The age-incidence curve may be helpful in elucidating risk factors for developing KD. Such a pattern is compatible with highly transmissible infectious agents, particularly respiratory agents, and suggests possible transplacental immunity. The features of 28 patients with KD who were aged 8 years and older at the time of diagnosis at Children's Memorial Hospital in Chicago have been reported.[282] Delays in establishing the diagnosis and in providing treatment were common occurrences and were at least partially related to the prominence of arthritic and gastrointestinal symptoms in this population. We recently cared for a 30-year-old man with classic KD.

Earlier Japanese mortality data suggested that fatality rates are approximately three times higher in children younger than 1 year at the time of onset of disease, compared with older children, and that fatalities occur predominantly in the first several months after onset of KD.[344] Male patients account for a disproportionate number of deaths in infants and older children.[105,186,327,344] Long-term mortality rates in a large Japanese KD cohort study were increased over background rates, particularly during and shortly after the acute stage of illness.[188,190]

A Taiwanese series of 25 infants who developed KD at 3 months or younger included 19 males and 6 females. Only 6 infants met KD diagnostic criteria, with the other 19 classified as incomplete. Coronary artery involvement was noted in 80%, although only one infant had persistent abnormalities at 1-year follow-up.[45]

Recurrent Kawasaki Disease

A recurrence of KD is defined generally as a new episode of illness meeting clinical criteria for KD that begins at least 3 months after the initial episode and after inflammatory markers such as the erythrocyte sedimentation rate (ESR) or serum C-reactive protein (CRP) level have normalized. The frequency of recurrences after first cases of KD in Japan was estimated to be approximately 1.9% during a 3-year follow-up period, with approximately 0.07% of patients experiencing a third episode.[187] This corresponds to a rate of 5.21 per 1000 person-years for one or more recurrences.[187] With longer follow-up, recurrence rates in Japan may approach 3%.[346] Data from the United States suggest a recurrence rate of 1% to 2%.[17] Recurrences occur most frequently within the first 2 years after the initial episode, especially in male patients and in children who have their initial episode before reaching their second birthday.[187] The frequency of recurrences in Chicago appears to be approximately 1%, occurring more often in Asian children, and recurrences were documented in about 2% of Hawaiian cases from 1996 to 2000,[108] a finding likely reflecting a racial difference. In the CDC's passive KD surveillance data, 97 of 5557 (1.7%) patients from 1984 to 2008 had recurrent KD, including 3.5% among Asian/Pacific Islander patients.[165] The true recurrence rate will be determined only when a specific diagnostic test becomes available for KD and thus minimizes recognition bias.

Family Cases

Simultaneous or sequential cases of KD in siblings, twins, or other family contacts also have been reported, particularly during outbreaks in Japan.[81,111,169,347] Japanese epidemiologists have documented secondary sibling cases in approximately 1% of cases, a rate that is approximately 10 times greater than that in the general child population.[81] However, such figures are difficult to interpret because they may be influenced by recognition and reporting biases. In the 2011–12 Japanese survey data, 1.5% of KD cases had one or more infected siblings, and 0.89% had at least one parent with history of KD.[166] Sibling cases are reported to occur more frequently in twins than in nontwins. Only three sibling pairs were recognized in more than 2100 Chicago patients, and none was reported in 400 children in Los Angeles.[168] A report from two US medical centers noted 18 families with multiple affected KD patients, including nine families with two affected siblings and nine with KD in two generations or in multiple affected members.[59]

Epidemics and Outbreaks

Japanese investigators noted large nationwide outbreaks of KD in 1979, 1982, and 1985 to 1986, with wavelike spread occurring from one prefecture to the next, suggesting an infectious origin.[189,340,342] The 1982 Japanese epidemic started simultaneously in four areas and spread outward from each region, similar to the way that epidemic influenza spreads in Europe and America.[189,340] In the 1985–86 Japanese epidemic, investigators identified epidemic "waves" that spread outward from an initial focus in the Tokyo metropolitan area and extended simultaneously northward and southward to involve most of the country within approximately 4 months.[189,340,342] A similar but less distinctive pattern of interprefectural progression in waves was noted in the 1982 Japanese epidemic. Within the northern Tohoku District, for example, KD spread from prefecture to prefecture over a period of approximately 7 months.[340] Korean epidemics were detected 7 and 15 months after the Japanese epidemics of 1979 and 1985–86, respectively.[156,340] More localized outbreaks also have been observed. In the United States and elsewhere, community-wide outbreaks were documented beginning in 1977.[18,56,317] Investigation of outbreaks provides opportunities to study potential risk and etiologic factors. Clustering of cases within families, schools, or neighborhoods is quite unusual, even during large-scale epidemics. Japanese investigators have associated epidemics with a significantly increased likelihood of second cases occurring in families, fatalities, and recurrent cases, but the implications of these findings are uncertain. It is striking that, since 1986, no further nationwide Japanese outbreaks have been identified, suggesting that the epidemiology of KD may have changed.[260,348] However, it is important to recognize that the current endemic rate of KD in Japan exceeds that of the largest previous endemic.

Geography

KD has been diagnosed throughout the United States and Japan and in virtually all developed and many developing countries on all continents, including temperate and tropical zones.[26,40,73,164,227,257,258,316] No striking rural–urban differences have been noted. Elevation, longitude, and latitude have not been implicated. Travel histories of patients are unremarkable, although an anecdotal report of a 7-month-old infant in Australia documented KD onset 17 days after leaving Japan during that country's 1982 epidemic,[278] and we diagnosed KD in infant in Chicago about 2 weeks after moving from Japan.

Seasonality

In Japan, KD occurs year round but is most prevalent in the winter, with peaks usually occurring in December or January, with a lower peak in June, and the lowest number of cases in October.[30,328,343,346] In Korea, peaks were observed in summer and winter[222]; in Taiwan, peaks occur in summer, with a nadir from November to January[110]; in Beijing and Shanghai, peaks occur in spring and summer[64], and in spring in Sichuan and Hong Kong.[159,200] In the United States and other temperate areas, the number of cases peak in the winter and early spring and is lowest in late summer; nonetheless, cases occur throughout the year.[17,19,42,107,168,233] No clear seasonality has been seen in Hawaii.[108] Winter predominance has been observed in at least some Southern Hemisphere countries.[32] That sporadic cases are recognized year round is somewhat different from the pattern usually observed with highly transmissible respiratory viral diseases, incidences of which peak sharply in the winter and spring (e.g., measles, rubella, influenza), and virtually disappear in summer.

Communicability

Although little direct evidence exists that KD is transmissible from person to person, considerable circumstantial evidence supports an infectious origin. Secondary or co-primary cases in families occur but are not common. Several outbreak investigations found a higher rate of antecedent respiratory tract illness in patients with KD compared with matched controls.[18,300] This finding is of particular interest in view of the finding that immunoglobulin A (IgA) plasma cells infiltrate the proximal respiratory tract and that viral-like inclusion bodies are observed in bronchial epithelial cells in fatal cases of KD, and it strongly supports a respiratory mode of spread of an inciting agent (see later discussion).[246,255] Japanese family data suggest that sibling cases cluster either on the same day as the index case or 7 days later.[81] Because these results are based on questionnaire data, however, the possibility of ascertainment bias is great; thus determining the degree to which Japanese familial cases represent co-primary or secondary cases is difficult.

Other Risk Factors

In addition to demographic risk factors for KD, specific exposures that could be related to an etiologic agent have been linked to the disorder by older epidemiologic investigations. History of more frequent recent antecedent respiratory illnesses in cases compared with controls was documented in the early 1980s.[18] Because many viral agents are prevalent in the winter and spring when KD is most prevalent, some "background" isolation of various viruses from patients and from matched controls is expected.

Other past reported KD associations include exposure to recent carpet cleaning or shampooing, exposure to house dust mites, and residence near bodies of water; very few recent reports support these associations. The association of KD with exposure to recently cleaned or shampooed carpets was observed in some reports[21,75,96,109,120,209,223,233,234] but not in others.[52,160,179,233,240,241,309] The significance of a possible association with shampoo is unclear because it is absent entirely in many well-studied outbreaks and because carpets are relatively uncommon in Japan.[52,179]

In a small number of outbreaks, investigators from the CDC found that patients with KD lived closer to bodies of water compared with control patients.[234,235] However, other studies, including one in Washington state, did not find living in proximity to water to be a risk factor.[55]

ETIOLOGY

The origin of KD remains unknown. However, clinical and epidemiologic features strongly suggest that the disease has an infectious cause. A self-limited, usually nonrecurring illness manifested by fever, rash, enanthem, conjunctival injection, swollen and red hands and feet, and cervical adenitis fits well with an infectious cause. The epidemiologic features noted earlier, including the striking age distribution, winter-spring seasonality in most areas, occurrence of community outbreaks with wavelike geographic spread, and apparent epidemic cycles, resemble those of a transmissible disease of childhood. The laboratory features, including leukocytosis with a "left shift," elevated acute-phase reactants, mildly elevated liver transaminases, and pyuria also suggest infection. The medium-size muscular arteritis of KD may result from infection of arterial walls by the causative agent(s) with a subsequent immune response or an immune attack on presently unknown host molecules as a consequence of infection with the agent(s).

A very attractive hypothesis is that KD is caused by a ubiquitous infectious agent that produces clinically apparent disease only in selected, genetically predisposed individuals, with particular predilection for Asians. Its rarity in the first few months of life and in older children and adults suggests an agent to which virtually all adults are immune and from which very young infants are protected to some degree by passive maternal antibody. Consistent with this hypothesis is the paucity of evidence of person-to-person spread of KD, because most infections are likely asymptomatic, and only very few of those infected likely develop clinical features of KD. This would be analogous to acute poliomyelitis, the relatively uncommon complication of poliovirus infection that occurs in only approximately 1 in 200 of those infected. However, efforts to identify an infectious agent of KD using conventional bacterial and viral culture and serologic methods, as well as inoculation of primates, mice, and guinea pigs, have failed to yield an infectious cause, and a long list of known infectious agents proposed as the cause has been disproved.[18,56,244] This includes *Leptospira* spp., retrovirus, TSST-1–producing *Staphylococcus aureus,* and coronavirus NL-63.[62,244] An oligoclonal, antigen-driven immune response has been well-documented[44,244,245,247]; whether a superantigen response also occurs in some children with KD is unclear[349] and will likely require identification of the causative agent to be determined.

The immune transcriptional profile of coronary arteritis in KD has features of an antiviral immune response such as activated cytotoxic T lymphocyte and type I interferon-induced gene upregulation.[256] Ultrastructural, immunofluorescence, and RNA evidence support the hypothesis of a presently unidentified "new" virus as the cause that enters through the respiratory tract and is carried by macrophages to the coronary arteries.[244,245,248,250] Another hypothesis is that the agent of KD, possibly a fungal toxin, may be carried via the wind as an aerosol.[238,239]

While some investigators suggest that KD can be triggered by any of a large number of diverse infectious agents in a genetically predisposed host,[289] recurrence of KD is quite uncommon, and KD children appear to experience subsequent infections without developing KD again. This theory also fails to explain epidemics and the wavelike geographic spread of illness during outbreaks.

Identification of the etiologic agent(s) of KD is an extremely important research goal because diagnostic test development, development of improved and specific therapies, and prevention are critical to improved patient care and outcomes but will likely only be achieved after the etiology is determined.

Genetic Susceptibility

The higher rates of KD in those of Japanese and, to a lesser degree, Korean and Taiwanese backgrounds indicate a genetic basis rather than environmental factors, as supported by increased rates among third- and fourth-generation immigrants from Japan to Hawaii.[108] The increased incidence of KD among siblings and parents of patients also supports a genetic predisposition.[329,344] The genetic basis is complex, and no single human leukocyte antigen (HLA) or MHC class II gene is common to most patients with KD. Immunoglobulin allotypic markers were studied as possible genetic markers for KD, and differences between patients and race-matched controls were found in Japanese and whites, supporting a complex genetic basis for susceptibility to KD.[270] Transmission disequilibrium studies involving children with KD and their parents demonstrated evidence of several functional single nucleotide polymorphisms in the calcineurin-NFAT pathway, the transforming growth factor-β (TGF-β) signaling pathway, and genes encoding Fcγ receptors. These studies show that single nucleotide polymorphisms (SNPs) within the inositol triphosphate kinase-3 *(ITPKC)* gene on chromosome 19 and in *CASP3* on chromosome 4 confer increased risk in Japanese, Taiwanese, and white children.[34,149,213,214]

Genome-wide association studies (GWAS) to define KD susceptibility risk loci have accelerated identification of additional loci on chromosome 8 and other chromosomes.[27,215,335] Davila and colleagues, also in a GWAS, identified a polymorphism in *FCGR2A* on chromosome 1 related to immune activation as a KD risk marker.[54] Other analyses have identified SNPs in *ITPKC* and *CASP3* that are associated with increased risk of IVIG unresponsive and coronary aneurysms.[216] Several additional loci have been identified in the Taiwanese population.[335] The picture is emerging that there are more than 6 to 10 genetic susceptibility markers for KD, each of which is associated with some increased risk for KD compared with controls. Onouchi et al. recently reported an SNP in the ORA/1gene in the Ca^{2+}/NFAT pathway that is associated with KD in Japanese and that is present with 20 times higher frequency in Japanese compared to European populations.[212] This is an area of intense research activity.

PATHOLOGY AND PATHOGENESIS

Relationship With Infantile Periarteritis Nodosa

When the first Japanese survey of KD in 1970 yielded reports of 10 deaths, the pathologic diagnosis was thought to be IPAN.[116,138,147] Japanese and Western investigators quickly recognized the pathologic similarities between fatal KD and IPAN, long known to have an unusual predilection for the coronary arteries.[1,15,16,302–305] In the most definitive study, Landing and Larson[152,155] showed clearly that IPAN and fatal KD were indistinguishable pathologically. Published case reports of autopsies of children with IPAN frequently contain clinical histories that include many or all features of acute KD and the development of severe vasculitis affecting primarily the coronary arteries.[237] The failure of some reported patients with IPAN to meet KD case criteria applied retrospectively is likely related to documentation bias and to the young age of many of the patients. Young infants with KD are less likely to have a classic presentation than are older children (see later discussion). When pathologic and clinical criteria are combined, the two diseases appear indistinguishable. Adult-type periarteritis nodosa was described first in 1866 by Kussmaul and Maier,[151] and it differs from IPAN primarily by the presence of hypertension and involvement of small and medium muscular arteries, especially in the lung, kidney, and intestines.[84,152,304,305] An early recorded case of possible IPAN dates from 1899.[148] In 1959, Munro-Faure[182] very clearly delineated a syndrome of infantile necrotizing arteritis with coronary artery involvement, fever, rash, conjunctival and pharyngeal infection, and cervical adenitis, distinct from classic periarteritis nodosa. Roberts and Fetterman[237] and others expanded on these observations to define a distinct clinicopathologic syndrome of IPAN shortly before Kawasaki recognized the clinical syndrome.[134,135]

Coronary artery aneurysms were described as early as the early 20th century, with a male to female ratio of roughly 3 : 1, including a male preponderance in childhood cases. Childhood death from multiple coronary artery aneurysms was known to occur at least as early as 1871, as reported by Samuel Gee.[90] The cardiac specimen from Gee's case, formalin fixed for more than 120 years in the pathology museum at St. Bartholomew's Hospital, London, recently was sectioned and examined histologically. The coronary arteries showed the characteristic histologic findings of inactive KD and IPAN.[274,272] Whether these early cases with childhood coronary artery aneurysms truly represented early examples of KD is not certain; details of the clinical histories usually were scant.[90,232]

What is clear, however, is that most of these cases greatly resemble (and very likely do, in fact, represent) KD.[48,72,90,182,232] From the features of many such early case reports, a reasonably accurate picture of KD as recognized today emerges. It is highly likely that in the decades before the introduction of the measles vaccine in the 1960s, cases of KD were misdiagnosed as measles, scarlet fever, drug hypersensitivity, or other common conditions. In fact, an autopsy study of pediatric vasculitis cases in Japan indicates that many pediatric vasculitis fatalities prior to 1977 had clinical and pathologic features that in retrospect were consistent with KD.[300] This study also demonstrated a marked decrease in all pediatric vasculitis fatalities in Japan following the advent of IVIG therapy in the late 1980s, suggesting that the majority of pediatric vasculitis fatalities in Japan prior to this time were actually the result of Kawasaki disease[300]

Pathologic Features of Kawasaki Disease

Cardiac death in KD generally occurs in the subacute or convalescent stages of illness but also can occur earlier.[186,189] KD results in medium-sized muscular arteritis, with a marked predilection for the coronary arteries.[5,6,85,152,299,304,305] Small arterioles, larger arteries, capillaries, and veins also are affected to a lesser extent.[6,84] In more than 80% of fatal cases in the acute stage, the immediate cause of death is acute thrombosis of inflamed coronary arteries, with resultant myocardial infarction. Less commonly, death can occur from acute coronary rupture, usually within a few weeks of the onset of illness, and rarely early deaths can result from pancarditis with inflammation of the atrioventricular conduction system and fatal arrhythmia or intractable congestive heart failure. Deaths that occur months to years after the acute episode of KD often are secondary to coronary stenosis, from luminal myofibroblastic proliferation (see below) and/or thromboses, resulting in myocardial ischemia. In some patients with coronary artery abnormalities (virtually always in those who also have quite severe coronary disease), aneurysms of other major medium-sized arteries, including the brachial, renal, and iliac arteries, also may be present. Although phlebitis may be found, vascular inflammation more typically and more severely affects medium-sized muscular arteries in their extraparenchymal portions. In the acute stage of KD, systemic inflammatory changes also are evident in many other organs, including myocardium, pericardium, cardiac valves, meninges, lung, lymph nodes, pancreas, spleen, joints, and liver.[7,84,178]

An extensive study of arterial tissues from 32 patients who died and 8 who received heart transplants shed new light on the pathologic features of severely affected KD patients.[217] Three characteristic vasculopathic processes were identified by light and transmission electron microscopy: (1) acute self-limited necrotizing arteritis (NA), (2) subacute/chronic (SA/C) vasculitis, and (3) luminal myofibroblastic proliferation (LMP). NA is a neutrophilic process that starts at the endothelial lining of vessels only in the first 2 weeks of illness, progressively destroying the vessel wall and causing development of saccular aneurysms, which can thrombose or rupture. In its most severe form, NA can result in necrosis of arteries to such an extent that only a thin layer of adventitia remains. These "giant aneurysms" can rupture but more commonly acquire multiple layers of thrombi which organize and can become recanalized and calcify.[5,192,217,260,295] SA/C vasculitis, consisting of lymphocytes, eosinophils, and plasma cells, with fewer macrophages, begins within the first 2 weeks of illness in the adventitia/perivascular tissue and damages the vessel wall during its progression toward the lumen. SA/C can lead to fusiform and saccular aneurysms that can thrombose, and it is associated with transition of medial and adventitial smooth muscle cells into smooth muscle cell–derived myofibroblasts which, with their matrix products, result in stenosing luminal lesions (SA/C-LMP). LMP can also occur in some areas without apparent local SA/C vasculitis.[217] NA is the only self-limiting of these three processes, is responsible for the earliest morbidity and mortality, and is consistent with acute viral infection. SA/C vasculitis can begin early but can persist for months or even years, whereas LMP can cause progressive arterial stenosis. Stenosis of the coronary arteries months to years after onset can result from LMP and/or thrombi.[217] The mechanism of persistent SA/C arteritis and LMP in a subset of KD children is unknown. Ongoing expression of vascular endothelial growth factor (VEGF) within smooth muscle cells,[296] TGF-β in myofibroblasts,[265] and matrix metalloproteinases in inflammatory and other cells[89] have been proposed to be involved.

Significant atrioventricular conduction system lesions have been identified in 5 of 10 autopsy specimens, with a strong correlation found between ECG findings, especially PQ-segment prolongation, and acute inflammation of the atrioventricular conduction system.[82,83] Severe acute changes were most pronounced at 21 to 31 days after onset. In a unique study of right ventricular endomyocardial biopsy specimens in 201 patients with uncomplicated acute KD, some degree of myocarditis and cellular infiltration ranging from very mild (subclinical) to quite severe myocardial inflammation was noted in all of the patients studied.[351,352]

Neutrophils infiltrate the arterial wall at sites of NA; NA appears limited to the first 2 weeks after fever onset.[217] In SA/C arteritis, which begins in the first 2 weeks after fever onset but can persist for months to years in a subset of KD children, lymphocytes (particularly $CD8^+$ lymphocytes[25]), plasma cells (particularly IgA plasma cells[253,255]), and eosinophils[217,312] predominate, while fewer macrophages[300,310] are also present. The transcriptome of KD SA/C arteritis demonstrates upregulation of genes associated with cytotoxic T-lymphocyte activation, antigen presentation, immunoglobulin production, and type I interferon response, features suggesting an antiviral immune response.[256] Both $CD8^+$ T lymphocytes[44] and IgA plasma cells have been demonstrated to be oligoclonal (i.e., they appear to be responding in an antigen-driven process).

Although arteritis is the most important pathologic feature of KD and results in the only known long-term sequelae of KD, the illness is associated with multisystem inflammation, and multiple organs and tissues are involved in the acute inflammatory process, including the digestive system (e.g., enteritis, hepatitis, cholangitis, pancreatitis), respiratory system (e.g., bronchitis, pulmonary nodules, segmental interstitial pneumonia), urinary system (focal interstitial nephritis, cystitis, prostatitis), nervous system (e.g., choriomeningitis), and hematopoietic system (e.g., lymphadenitis, splenitis), as well as the cardiovascular system (e.g., myocarditis, pericarditis).[7] IgA plasma cells have been observed in peribronchial, pancreatic, and renal tissues[255] and macrophages in pancreatic acini and islets.[178] Lymph node findings are nondiagnostic and can show severe lymphadenitis with necrosis.[94,302]

At present, it is not known what factors predispose children with KD to develop coronary artery stenosis from LMP. This complication can occur in children with persisting aneurysms, but can also result in critical stenosis in patients with aneurysms that appear to have "resolved" by echocardiography or angiography. In this latter circumstance, arterial luminal diameter initially returns to a more normal range as LMP fills the lumen, but the lumen subsequently narrows with progressive LMP, and coronary artery blood flow is impaired. Close follow-up of all children with KD with persisting or "resolved" aneurysms is strongly encouraged, according to the recommendations of the American Heart Association Committee on Rheumatic Fever, Endocarditis, and Kawasaki Disease.[171a,199]

CLINICAL MANIFESTATIONS

Clinical Phases of Illness

The clinical course of KD can be divided into acute, subacute, and late or convalescent phases. The *acute* febrile phase begins with fever, rash, conjunctival injection, "strawberry" tongue, red swollen lips, edema and erythema of the hands and feet, cervical lymphadenitis, and sometimes aseptic meningitis and mild hepatic dysfunction. Young children often are quite irritable. Evidence of myocarditis, rarely including congestive heart failure or arrhythmias, may develop during this time. Pericardial effusion, mitral regurgitation, and/or depressed myocardial function may be detected by echocardiogram. Without IVIG and aspirin treatment, the acute phase generally lasts 8 to 30 days (mean, 11 days).

After defervescence, the physical findings rapidly disappear, but, during this *subacute* phase, the child may remain irritable and anorectic, with decreased activity. Some conjunctival injection may persist. Arthritis or arthralgia, mainly of larger joints, may develop in the subacute phase. Desquamation of fingers and toes, typically beginning in the periungual region, and thrombocytosis are very common manifestations during this period. The subacute phase persists until the child has returned to his or her normal state of health at 6 weeks after the onset of fever, with normalization of inflammatory markers. The time of greatest risk for sudden death occurring from acute coronary artery thrombosis in patients with coronary lesions is during the subacute phase and the early convalescent phase. The *convalescent* phase begins when all clinical signs and symptoms have disappeared and inflammatory markers are normal, usually at 6 to 8 weeks after onset.

In its complete form, KD is a distinctive clinical entity with a fairly predictable course.[50,199] The principal clinical diagnostic criteria are presented in Box 77.1. A diagnosis of typical or classic KD, according to these accepted clinical criteria, is made in patients with fever and at least four of the five classic clinical criteria and with exclusion of other illnesses that mimic KD. Each of the five clinical features is present in 80% to 90% of patients with typical cases, except cervical lymphadenopathy, which is present in approximately 50% of patients. However, children who do not fulfill the classic criteria for diagnosis of KD, in fact, may have the illness and are at risk for developing complications, particularly coronary artery disease (see later discussion section on incomplete or atypical KD).[199,251] KD should be considered in the differential diagnosis of infants and children with fever for at least 5 days associated with two or more of the five classic features: (1) generalized polymorphous erythematous rash, (2) conjunctival injection, (3) characteristic changes of the lips and mouth, (4) bilateral redness and swelling of the hands and feet, and (5) unilateral nonfluctuant cervical lymph node enlargement greater than 1.5 cm.[199] All features are not necessarily present at the same time. The most commonly encountered diseases to be excluded are febrile exanthems, presumably viral, including measles; acute streptococcal and staphylococcal infections; and drug hypersensitivity reactions. Japanese diagnostic guidelines for KD are similar to the U.S. guidelines with rare exception: they consider fever and the other five major features to be six equal criteria and require at least five of those six criteria for diagnosis.[13] Thus a rare child could have no fever but all five other criteria and be considered a typical case by the Japanese criteria. The Japanese criteria also accept a course of fever lasting less than 5 days if it is shortened by early IVIG treatment.[13]

Several scoring systems using clinical and laboratory features have been developed, primarily in Japan.[11,102,191] The initial goal of these systems was to identify those patients with KD at highest risk for development of coronary abnormalities and who, therefore, would benefit most from receiving IVIG therapy, as well as those at low risk for coronary changes who could be spared IVIG treatment. This practice has decreased in Japan because no such scoring system appears sufficiently sensitive and specific to enable selective therapy (i.e., to allow nontreatment of patients predicted to be at low risk for development of coronary abnormalities). More recent scoring systems have focused on identifying patients at high risk for IVIG treatment failure and coronary abnormalities who may benefit from more aggressive primary therapy.[144,145] Patients who are at greatest risk are as follows: those younger than 1 year; male patients; those with prolonged or recurrent fever; and those with anemia, hypoalbuminemia, hyponatremia, and thrombocytopenia. The Kobayashi and other scoring systems are not effective in predicting treatment failure in multiracial populations as seen in the United States.[144,277] All patients diagnosed with KD within the first 10 days after onset of disease and those diagnosed later who are still manifesting significant inflammation should be treated with IVIG and aspirin.[199]

In KD, fever typically is high spiking and remittent, with peak temperatures generally exceeding 39°C (102.2°F) and in many cases exceeding 40°C (104°F). Unless treatment is initiated with IVIG and aspirin, fever persists for a mean of 11 days,[106] but it may continue for 3 to 4 weeks and rarely longer. In patients whose disease is treated with 80 to 100 mg/kg per day of aspirin and a single 2 g/kg dose of IVIG, fever generally resolves within 1 to 2 days.[197,198]

Bilateral painless vascular injection of the bulbar conjunctivae, clearly more severe than injection of the palpebral conjunctivae and often sparing the limbic region around the cornea, generally is seen in the first week of illness, usually beginning shortly after onset of fever. It generally is not associated with exudate, conjunctival edema, or corneal ulceration, thus distinguishing the eye findings of KD from purulent conjunctivitis and from Stevens-Johnson syndrome. Mild acute iridocyclitis or anterior uveitis, which may be noted by slit lamp examination, resolves rapidly and only rarely is associated with photophobia or eye pain.[28,91,154,210,279] Less common ocular findings include superficial punctate keratitis, vitreous opacities, vitreous and chorioretinal inflammation, lateral rectus palsy, and papilledema and other optic disk changes.[8,76,114,336]

Changes of the mouth and lips consist of the following: (1) erythema, dryness, fissuring, peeling, cracking, and bleeding of the lips; (2) a strawberry tongue indistinguishable from that associated with streptococcal scarlet fever, with erythema and prominent papillae; and (3) diffuse erythema of the oropharyngeal mucosae. Oral ulcerations, pharyngeal exudates, and Koplik spots are rarely if ever found in KD and when present help to exclude the diagnosis.

Changes in the extremities are among the most distinctive features of KD. The hands and feet become indurated and swollen with stretched, shiny skin, sometimes with painful induration. The palms and soles become erythematous, often with an abrupt change to normal skin at the wrist and ankle. Infants and young children frequently refuse to hold objects or to bear weight. In the subacute phase, a distinctive pattern of periungual desquamation of fingers and toes may occur from 2 weeks to 2 months after onset of KD in 50% to 70% of affected patients. Beau lines, which are transverse grooves across the nails, may appear at the nail base 1 to 2 months after a case of acute KD and grow out over several months. Peripheral gangrene is a rare complication (see later discussion).

The erythematous rash associated with KD may take many forms. Most common is a nonspecific, diffuse, maculopapular, primarily truncal erythematous rash. Occasionally diffuse scarlatiniform erythroderma, urticaria, or an erythema multiforme–like rash with target lesions develops. Vesicles and bullae are not seen, although very fine pustules occur rarely. Perineal erythema and then desquamation are quite common manifestations in diapered as well as toilet-trained children in the acute stage of illness. Although rashes in KD tend to be most prominent on the trunk, with perineal accentuation they frequently also involve the face and extremities.

Cervical lymphadenopathy is the least common of the five principal diagnostic criteria, but it sometimes is the dominant clinical feature along with fever.[281] It usually is unilateral and confined to the anterior cervical triangle. To fulfill diagnostic criteria, the enlarged node or mass of nodes exceeds 1.5 cm, is not fluctuant, usually is not associated with erythema of the overlying skin, and is not tender or only moderately tender. Lymphadenopathy generally is benign and transient. Clinicians should be aware that children with suspected acute bacterial cervical adenitis that is unresponsive to antibiotic therapy may have KD. Because other features of KD often are present but overlooked, KD should be considered in such febrile children without an alternate diagnosis.[281] The ultrasound appearance of lymph nodes in KD has been described to be similar to that of acute Epstein-Barr virus infection and distinct from bacterial adenitis.[306] The absence of changes suggesting suppuration on imaging (e.g., ultrasonography or computed tomography [CT]) of such lesions should strengthen the suspicion of possible KD in this setting. Impressive cervical adenopathy in patients with KD generally resolves remarkably promptly after administration of appropriate therapy.

The associated features of KD reflect its multisystemic nature (Box 77.2). Sterile pyuria as a manifestation of urethritis, occasionally with meatitis, is found in approximately half of patients. Arthritis appearing during the first week of illness can be polyarticular or oligoarticular, including the small interphalangeal joints as well as large weight-bearing joints, with a reported prevalence of approximately 7.5%.[97] Arthrocentesis during this early phase yields purulent-appearing fluid, with a mean white blood cell count of 125,000 to 300,000/mm^3, normal glucose levels, and negative Gram stain and bacterial cultures. Arthritis developing after the 10th day of illness has a predilection for large weight-bearing joints, especially the knees and ankles, with a somewhat lower synovial fluid white blood cell count.[106] Gastrointestinal complaints occur in approximately one-third of patients, especially in older patients; these complaints may be severe, even leading to laparotomy, and they include nausea, abdominal pain, and some diarrhea. These findings may be related to a hydropic gallbladder, pancreatitis, or appendicular vasculitis.[12,353] Obstructive jaundice and acute hydrops

BOX 77.2 Associated Noncardiac Features of Kawasaki Disease

Musculoskeletal System
Arthritis or arthralgia

Central Nervous System
Aseptic meningitis
Facial nerve palsy
Marked irritability
Sensorineural hearing loss

Gastrointestinal System
Hydrops of gallbladder
Abdominal pain, diarrhea
Hepatic dysfunction, obstructive jaundice
Pancreatitis

Genitourinary System
Urethritis, meatitis

Respiratory System
Perihilar infiltrates or pulmonary nodules
Preceding respiratory illness

Other
Erythema and induration of bacille Calmette-Guérin vaccine site
Anterior uveitis (mild)
Desquamating groin rash
Flare of atopic dermatitis or psoriasis
Peripheral gangrene (young infants)

of the gallbladder are not uncommon findings, whereas mild to moderate elevations of serum aminotransferases occur in almost half of patients. Central nervous system involvement including aseptic meningitis occurs in almost half of patients.[57] Transient unilateral lower motor neuron facial nerve palsy occurs rarely,[228] as does sensorineural hearing loss.[143] Characteristic marked irritability is very common, especially in young infants. Reactivation of inflammation at the site of a previous bacillus Calmette-Guérin (BCG) vaccination coincident with acute KD is a common finding in Japan, where BCG is used widely,[276] and Terp and associates observed a child in whom both a BCG site and a purified protein derivative (PPD) test site reactivated with acute KD.[313] Some patients experience a flare of atopic dermatitis or psoriasis during or after experiencing acute KD.[24,68] Various pulmonary manifestations of KD, including isolated pulmonary nodules,[80] pleural effusions, acute respiratory distress syndrome,[221] and pulmonary infiltrates,[330] all of which are interesting in view of the increased numbers of IgA plasma cells found in respiratory tract tissue,[253,255] have been observed.

By far the most important associated feature of KD is *cardiac involvement.* Cardiac manifestations can be prominent in acute KD and are the major cause of long-term morbidity and mortality. In addition to the coronary artery abnormalities that develop in 20% to 25% of untreated children, pericardial effusion and myocarditis with congestive heart failure, tachycardia, gallop rhythm, nonspecific changes on the ECG, or arrhythmia may occur.[123,126,128,199] An imperfect correlation exists between clinically apparent cardiac involvement and echocardiographic evidence of coronary abnormalities, although in the pre-IVIG era, echocardiographic evidence of mitral regurgitation, impaired left ventricular function, or pericardial effusion in the acute stage was shown to be predictive of subsequent coronary abnormalities.[92] Echocardiographic evidence of perivascular brightness of coronary arteries was suggested as a criterion for early diagnosis of KD, but subsequent reports did not confirm the reliability of this finding as a useful sign of incomplete KD.[350] Acute KD may involve pericardium, myocardium, endocardium, coronary arteries, and cardiac valves. Clinical and auscultatory features may include a hyperdynamic precordium, tachycardia out of proportion for the child's age and temperature, a gallop rhythm, and a flow murmur. Some infants may manifest very low cardiac output, and ECG changes (ST-segment and T-wave changes, prolonged PR interval, and arrhythmias) may be present.

A relatively recently recognized unusual presentation of acute KD is hypotension or shock.[63,122,161] Approximately 5% of patients may require admission to an intensive care unit for suspected septic shock or toxic shock but are ultimately recognized to have features of KD. In the few small series of cases, females and older patients have predominated, laboratory studies reveal more dramatically elevated markers of inflammation, and patients were more refractory to therapy compared with control subjects with KD. Hyponatremia was reported recently in a group of these patients, suggesting a possible association with the syndrome of inappropriate secretion of antidiuretic hormone.[275]

INCOMPLETE OR ATYPICAL KAWASAKI DISEASE

A substantial subset of children have illnesses that do not completely fulfill diagnostic criteria for KD but that include at least 5 days of fever and one, two, or three features of the disease. Incomplete or atypical KD (*incomplete* is the preferred term) is associated with a substantial risk for development of coronary artery aneurysms,[22,86,158,199,251] but it can be very difficult to diagnose. Incomplete KD occurs most frequently in young infants, who unfortunately are at greatest risk for developing coronary disease with KD,[242,251] and fatalities have occurred. The laboratory profile of incomplete cases is similar to that of classic cases, and laboratory results can increase or decrease the likelihood of the presence of KD in a particular patient.[199] Echocardiographic findings in the acute stage, including coronary ectasia, decreased myocardial contractility, pericardial effusion, and mild mitral regurgitation, can support the diagnosis of KD. Individual manifestations of KD in young infants tend to be more subtle than those in older children and can be fleeting.[242] KD should be considered in the differential diagnosis of prolonged fever in infants because patients are described in whom such fevers are virtually the sole manifestation of KD.

A committee of the American Heart Association developed a valuable algorithm to assist in the evaluation of patients with suspected incomplete KD (Fig. 77.1), with emphasis placed on clinical assessment and measurement of acute-phase reactants (CRP, ESR) in patients with 5 or more days of fever and two or three features of KD or in infants with 7 days or more of fever without other explanation.[171a,199] In addition to elevated ESR (≥40 mm/h) and/or CRP (≥3.0 mg/dL), a set of six supplementary laboratory criteria that can be useful in this regard include albumin, 3.0 g/dL or less; anemia for age; increased alanine aminotransferase; platelets after day 7 of more than 450,000/mm^3; white blood cell count of 15,000/mm^3 or more; and 10 or more white blood cells per high-power field in the urine sample.[199,171a] Hyponatremia is also useful in this regard. Echocardiographic features that support a KD diagnosis are Z score of left anterior descending (LAD) or right coronary artery (RCA) of 2.5 or greater, coronary aneurysm observed or three or more other suggestive features, including decreased LV function, mitral regurgitation, pericardial effusion, or LAD or RCA Z score of 2 to 2.5.

Retrospective diagnosis of KD often is based on finding coronary abnormalities on an echocardiogram, although the clinician's goal is to identify patients with incomplete KD before coronary changes have occurred. The existence of these patients again emphasizes the need to identify the etiologic agent of KD so that a diagnostic test can be developed. When possible, patients with illnesses suggesting incomplete KD should be referred to physicians with considerable experience in making the diagnosis.

LABORATORY FINDINGS

A specific diagnostic test for KD is not available and awaits discovery of the etiologic agent of the illness (Box 77.3). The laboratory features of KD, although quite nonspecific, are nonetheless characteristic of the illness. Leukocytosis, especially with neutrophilia, is typical in the acute stage, with a predominance of immature and mature granulocytes.

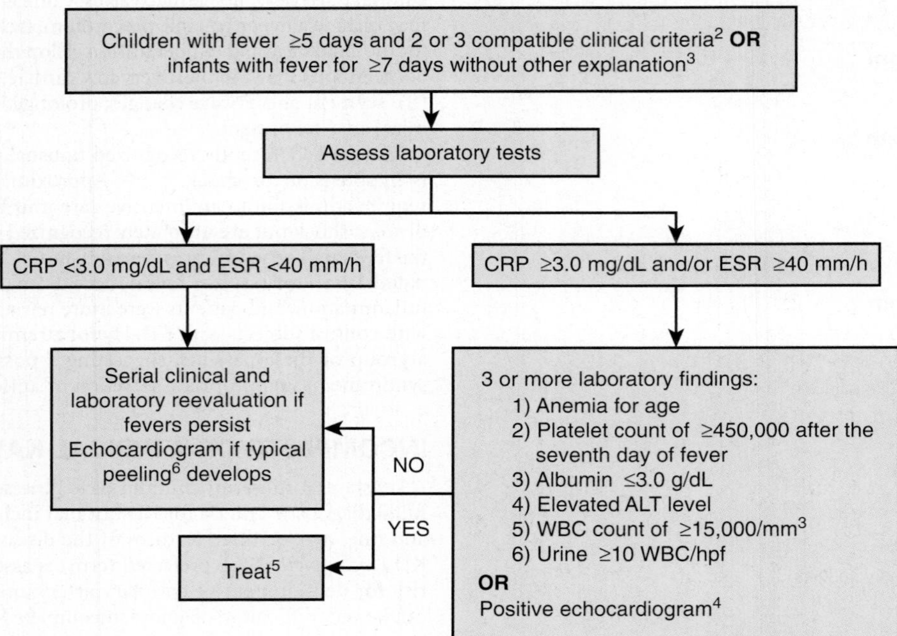

FIG. 77.1 Evaluation of suspected incomplete Kawasaki disease (KD). *1.* In the absence of a gold standard for diagnosis, this algorithm cannot be evidence based but rather represents the informed opinion of an expert committee. Consultation with an expert should be sought any time assistance is needed. *2.* Characteristics suggesting that another diagnosis should be considered include exudative conjunctivitis, exudative pharyngitis, ulcerative intraoral lesions, bullous or vesicular rash, generalized adenopathy, or splenomegaly. *3.* Infants age ≤6 months are the most likely to develop prolonged fever without other clinical criteria for KD; these infants are at particularly high risk of developing coronary artery abnormalities. *4.* Echocardiography is considered positive for purposes of this algorithm if any of three conditions are met: Z score of left anterior descending coronary artery or right coronary artery >2.5; coronary artery aneurysm is observed; or ≥3 other suggestive features exist, including decreased left ventricular function, mitral regurgitation, pericardial effusion or Z scores in left anterior descending coronary artery or right coronary artery of 2 to 2.5. *5.* If the echocardiogram is positive, treatment should be given within 10 days of fever onset or after the tenth day of fever in the presence of clinical and laboratory signs (C-reactive protein [CRP], erythrocyte sedimentation rate [ESR]) of ongoing inflammation. *6.* Typical peeling begins under the nail beds of fingers and toes. *ALT,* Alanine aminotransferase; *hpf,* high-power field; *WBC,* white blood cells. (From McCrindle BW, Rowley AH, Newburger JW, et al. Diagnosis, treatment, and long-term management of Kawasaki disease: a scientific statement for health professionals from the American Heart Association. *Circulation.* 2017;135(17):e927–e999.)

White blood cell counts in excess of 30,000/mm^3 occur rarely, and those in excess of 15,000/mm^3 occur in approximately 50% of patients. Leukopenia is unusual. Toxic granulations and Döhle bodies occasionally are seen on peripheral blood smear.[20] Anemia may develop, usually with normocytic red blood cell indices, particularly in patients with more prolonged duration of active inflammation. Severe hemolytic anemia requiring transfusions occurs but is unusual and usually is related to IVIG therapy.[47,268] Curiously Kawasaki's first patient in 1961 (and only rare subsequent patients) manifested Coombs-positive hemolytic anemia.[134,268]

Elevation of acute-phase reactants such as ESR, CRP, and α_1-antitrypsin is nearly universal in KD. CRP values rise and fall much more quickly than do ESR values. Additionally, IVIG therapy per se leads to elevation of the ESR (but not CRP) for several weeks, and thus ESR is not useful in assessing the degree of inflammatory activity in IVIG-treated patients; CRP or other acute-phase reactants clearly are superior for this purpose.[9,199]

A very characteristic feature of the subacute phase of illness is thrombocytosis, with platelet counts ranging from 500,000 to more than 1.5 million/mm^3. Thrombocytosis rarely is present in the first week of illness, usually appears in the second week, and peaks in the third week, with a gradual return to normal by 4 to 8 weeks after onset in uncomplicated cases. The mean peak platelet count is approximately 700,000/mm^3. In one study, infants younger than 1 year with fever without a source who had platelet counts greater than 800,000/mm^3 were 17 times more likely to be diagnosed with KD ultimately than were infants with platelet counts lower than 800,000/mm^3.[203] No difference exists in chromium-65–labeled autologous platelet survival between cases and controls, and little correlation exists between thrombocytosis and increased platelet aggregation. The latter has been detected in patients with KD from a few days until a year after onset.[131,337] The rare patients with thrombocytopenia in the acute stage of KD, most often young patients, are at increased risk for development of coronary artery disease and myocardial infarction.[204,205] The mechanism of thrombocytopenia appears to be low-grade consumptive coagulopathy.[205]

Plasma lipids are markedly perturbed in acute KD, with depression of plasma cholesterol, high-density lipoprotein (HDL) cholesterol, and apolipoprotein A-I (apoA-I).[37,194,259] Similar changes are observed in other conditions associated with an acute-phase response.[37] Marked appearance of serum amyloid A (SAA) protein in plasma, associated with HDL3-like lipoprotein particles, is seen acutely.[37] Cabana and colleagues[37] also showed that total cholesterol, HDL cholesterol, apoA-I, and triglyceride levels normalize over the course of several weeks and that SAA disappears from plasma. The core composition of HDL normalizes

BOX 77.3 Laboratory Features of Kawasaki Disease

Leukocytosis with neutrophilia
Elevated erythrocyte sedimentation rate
Elevated C-reactive protein (and other acute-phase reactants)
Anemia
Thrombocytosis after week 1
Sterile pyuria
Hypoalbuminemia
Hyponatremia
Elevated serum levels of aminotransferases and γ-glutamyltransferase
Plasma lipid abnormalities
Cerebrospinal fluid pleocytosis
Synovial fluid pleocytosis

more slowly than do plasma HDL cholesterol and apoA-I levels, a finding suggesting that KD has a profound effect on the lipoprotein profile acutely and a more subtle sustained effect on HDL composition.

Mild to moderate elevations in serum aminotransferase levels are present in as many as 40% of patients, and mild hyperbilirubinemia occurs in approximately 10%.[33] Plasma γ-glutamyl transpeptidase levels are elevated in most patients.[314] Hypoalbuminemia and hyponatremia are associated with more prolonged and more severe disease.[102,153,275,332] Urinalysis reveals intermittent mild to moderate sterile pyuria in approximately one-third of patients, although suprapubic urine generally does not show pyuria, a finding suggesting urethritis.[58,172] In those children who undergo lumbar puncture, evidence of aseptic meningitis, with a predominance of mononuclear cells, normal glucose, and normal to mildly elevated protein levels, is a common finding.[57]

Laboratory tests, even though nonspecific, can provide diagnostic support in patients with clinical features that are suggestive but not diagnostic, of KD[199] and may aid in prediction of nonresponder patients, at least in Japan.[144] A moderately to markedly elevated CRP (>3.0 mg/dL) or ESR (>40 mm/h), almost universal in KD, is an uncommon finding in most viral exanthems and hypersensitivity reactions. Platelet counts higher than 450,000 mm^3 usually are present in patients with KD after the seventh day of illness. In cases of incomplete KD associated with coronary abnormalities, thrombocytosis and elevated ESR/CRP are very common events in the acute stage. Clinical experience suggests that KD is unlikely if platelet counts and a full panel of acute-phase inflammatory reactants (e.g., ESR, CRP) are normal after the seventh day of illness.

Immunologic Findings

In the first 1 to 2 weeks of KD illness, marked peripheral blood neutrophilia is observed,[199] which coincides with the neutrophilic necrotizing arteritis that can occur in KD children who develop coronary arteritis.[217] Transcriptome studies of the peripheral blood in acute KD reveal neutrophil activation.[229,230] This prominent neutrophilic innate immune response is accompanied by secretion of many proinflammatory cytokines and chemokines[67,77] and abates as fever resolves, either spontaneously or in response to IVIG therapy. This response resembles that observed during many different infectious diseases associated with systemic inflammation and therefore has not been useful in establishing a specific KD diagnostic test. Nevertheless the presence of peripheral blood neutrophilia and elevated acute-phase reactants is so characteristic of KD that the absence of these findings argues against the diagnosis.

At 2 to 3 weeks after the onset of fever, elevation of all the immunoglobulins is observed in the peripheral blood,[162] suggesting an acquired B-lymphocyte immune response. Beginning in the first 2 weeks of illness, subacute/chronic arteritis can be observed in medium-sized muscular arteries, especially the coronary arteries, characterized by infiltration of lymphocytes, eosinophils, plasma cells, and macrophages.[217] This process may occur in adjacent or nonadjacent regions of the arteries affected by necrotizing arteritis or in different arteries.[217] This infiltrate is consistent with an acquired T- and B-lymphocytes immune response that appears to be oligoclonal or antigen driven.[44,247,252] CD8 T cells are prominent in the coronary artery infiltrate,[25] and plasma cells in this infiltrate and in other inflamed KD tissues produce predominately IgA antibodies in the first month after fever onset,[250,253] with IgM and IgG plasma cells present in lower numbers.[253] In a subset of children with KD, subacute/chronic arteritis can persist for months to years.[217] It does not appear that autoantibodies are more prevalent in KD sera than in febrile childhood control sera.[74,193] Circulating immune complexes can be detected in some KD patients but do not appear related to the development of coronary artery disease.[74]

The arterial immune transcriptome of KD subacute/chronic arteritis is notable for activated cytotoxic T lymphocyte and type I interferon-induced gene upregulation, suggestive of an antiviral response, with no apparent dysregulation of the TNF-α gene family.[254,256]

The stimulus resulting in these immunologic findings is likely to be a presently unidentified infectious agent(s). Whether the causative agent results solely in an antigen-driven immune response[244] or can result in a superantigen response in some KD children[170,349] is unclear and will likely require identification of the causative agent to be clarified.

The clinical response to IVIG treatment in KD patients generally is dramatic and rapid, and the majority of patients markedly improve during or immediately following completion of the infusion.[197,198] The mechanism of action of IVIG in KD is unknown. Potential mechanisms include modulation of cytokine production, suppression of endothelial cell activation, or modification of T- and B-lymphocyte response or function.[31] However, the very striking clinical response of KD patients to IVIG is unique and makes the theory of potential neutralization of a KD-specific agent or toxin or other product of the causative agent an appealing one.

In children with KD who do not develop cardiovascular sequelae, immune system function normalizes following resolution of the clinical signs, and inflammatory markers such as the CRP shortly after fever subsides. Although some investigators propose that many infectious agents may result in KD in genetically predisposed children,[290] KD recurrence is actually quite uncommon,[199] and KD children appear to have normal responses to future infections without developing KD recurrences.

MANAGEMENT

Treatment During the Acute Stage

Initial Therapy

Patients diagnosed with KD should be admitted to hospital, undergo a baseline echocardiogram, and receive IVIG 2 g/kg over the course of 10 to 12 hours, with high-dose aspirin at 80 to 100 mg/kg per day in four divided doses as soon as practical (Box 77.4).[50,199,273] When administered by the 10th illness day (onset of fever defines first day) this regimen is highly effective in reducing the risk for development of coronary abnormalities.[197] Because few data exist regarding management of patients treated later than the 10th illness day, the goal is to treat by illness day 10 whenever possible. Patients who are diagnosed after the 10th illness day and who are still febrile and/or with elevated inflammatory markers may benefit from therapy, but the ability to prevent coronary changes is less certain. IVIG and aspirin have been shown to prevent the development of giant coronary aneurysms[46,249] and to have direct benefits on cardiac function.[195] The mechanism of action of IVIG in KD remains unknown.[266] The single high-dose schedule is superior to the earlier regimen of 400 mg/kg/day IVIG for 4 days with high-dose aspirin with respect to rapidity of defervescence and normalization of acute-phase reactants, as well as in preventing development of coronary artery abnormalities.[197-199,208] The large single-dose infusion generally is well tolerated, even in patients with decreased myocardial function.[195] Patients should generally remain hospitalized until they have been afebrile for at least 24 hours, to ensure that they are available for retreatment if necessary.

Whether treatment with IVIG and aspirin earlier than the fifth illness day leads to better or worse outcomes remains unclear. Some reports indicate fewer coronary abnormalities in those treated before the fifth[322] or sixth[354] day of illness. Others report that those treated before day 5

BOX 77.4 Treatment of Kawasaki Disease

Acute and Subacute Stages

- IVIG 2 g/kg infusion over 10–12 hours *plus* aspirin 80–100 mg/kg per day in four divided doses (until patient is afebrile at least 3–4 days; some recommend until 14th illness day); then 3–5 mg/kg once daily for 6–8 weeks.
- IVIG may be repeated if fever persists or recurs together with at least one classic sign of disease and/or elevated C-reactive protein level (see text and Box 77.5 for other alternative "rescue therapies").
- For patients thought to be at particularly high risk for development of coronary complications, an adjunctive course of corticosteroid may be considered, although the optimal dosing and duration are unclear.

Convalescent Stage

- No coronary abnormalities: no therapy
- Transient coronary abnormalities: aspirin 3–5 mg/kg once daily at least until resolution of coronary abnormalities
- Persistent small to medium coronary aneurysms: aspirin 3–5 mg/kg once daily
- Giant or multiple small coronary aneurysms: aspirin 3–5 mg/kg once daily, with or without clopidogrel 1 mg/kg/day, with warfarin or low-molecular-weight heparin for most patients
- Coronary obstruction: thrombolytic therapy, surgical or interventional procedures

IVIG, Intravenous immunoglobulin.

were more likely to require additional therapy and/or have significantly worse coronary outcomes.[69,76,188] A more recent study concludes that the observed higher risk for cardiac complications in those treated on illness days 1 to 4 are due to underlying greater initial disease severity enabling earlier diagnosis and that KD patients should be treated as early as possible.[1a]

Single infusions of IVIG at doses of less than 2 g/kg have not been demonstrated to be as effective as 2 g/kg.[14,70] Terai's comprehensive meta-analysis of all Japanese and North American IVIG treatment trials showed that the coronary artery outcome is correlated directly with the *total* dose per kilogram of IVIG, with 2 g/kg superior to 1.6 g/kg, which is superior to 1.2 and 1.0 g/kg; the initial dose of aspirin did not appear to influence coronary outcome.[311] Another study confirmed this finding.[66]

Patients diagnosed after the 10th illness day who are still febrile and/or who manifest other signs of active disease may benefit from IVIG and aspirin therapy because this treatment may result in prompt clinical improvement, with subsidence of fever and other signs of inflammation. Little evidence supports that this approach results in lower rates of development of coronary abnormalities, however. Patients beyond the 10th to 12th illness day who have become afebrile and have resolved their clinical features of KD without therapy are unlikely to benefit from IVIG. Such children should be treated instead with low doses of aspirin, 3 to 5 mg/kg once daily, and should be evaluated carefully by serial echocardiograms. In patients who have already developed coronary aneurysms and whose acute manifestations of illness and elevated inflammatory markers have resolved, there is no convincing evidence of a beneficial effect of IVIG.

Various preparations of IVIG differ in manufacturing processes and therefore in composition (e.g., the proportion of IgG monomers and the presence of proteins other than IgG). Although adverse reaction rates differ among products, clinical efficacy does not seem to differ.[243] An exception is a report that showed IVIG prepared with β-propiolactone, which can affect the biologic activity of the Fc portion of IgG, to be less effective in KD.[321] Immunization with live virus vaccines such as for measles and varicella should be deferred for 9 to 11 months after administration of high-dose IVIG because of impaired immune responses.

The aspirin dosage for acute KD that is most thoroughly studied in the United States is 80 to 100 mg/kg per day in four divided doses. We generally recommend that this be maintained long enough to ensure that the patient has been afebrile for at least 3 to 4 days and then reduced to a daily dose of 3 to 5 mg/kg for antiplatelet activity. Others often lower the aspirin dose earlier. The lower dose should be continued until 6 to 8 weeks after onset of illness in those who have not developed coronary abnormalities.[199] Patients who develop coronary abnormalities should continue to take low-dose aspirin. High-dose aspirin is used for its antiinflammatory activity, whereas the much lower dose inhibits platelet aggregation. Japanese clinicians generally use an intermediate antiinflammatory dose of 30 to 50 mg/kg per day because of perceived higher rates of untoward effects in Japan.[13,150] Impaired absorption and bioavailability and enhanced salicylate clearance is present in acute KD.[146] Serum salicylate levels should be monitored only if symptoms of vomiting, hyperpnea, tinnitus, lethargy, or striking liver function abnormalities develop in children receiving aspirin.

A study that randomized U.S. patients to receive salicylates at 80 to 100 mg/kg per day or at 3 to 5 mg/kg per day for initial therapy (each regimen with 2 g/kg of IVIG) concluded that there was no difference in coronary outcome, but a more prompt clinical antiinflammatory benefit was noted in the high-dose aspirin group.[174] In the absence of IVIG, aspirin therapy does not decrease the frequency of coronary abnormalities.[66] Reye syndrome has been reported rarely in children taking high-dose aspirin for KD, but there are few data to suggest that low-dose aspirin poses this risk.[298]

Adjunctive Primary Therapy

The potential value of adding corticosteroid therapy to IVIG or aspirin for primary therapy has been addressed in several trials.[145,196,207,236] For example, Jibiki and colleagues compared 3 days of intravenous dexamethasone 0.3 mg/kg per day plus heparin and IVIG, with subsequent low-dose aspirin, to IVIG plus higher dose aspirin and found more prompt decreases in fever and inflammatory markers in the dexamethasone-treated group but no difference in rates of coronary abnormalities.[118] Okada and associates showed in high-risk patients that the addition of intravenous prednisolone (one pulse dose of 30 mg/kg) to IVIG and aspirin followed by a long taper of oral prednisolone was associated with shorter duration of fever, lower coronary abnormality rates, fewer treatment failures, and more a quicker fall in CRP and circulating interleukin-2 (IL-2), IL-6, IL-8, and IL-10 levels.[211] Inoue and colleagues[112] compared 88 patients treated with IVIG and aspirin to 90 patients who received in addition intravenous prednisolone 2 mg/kg per day in three divided doses until afebrile and then orally until the CRP value normalized, with a subsequent taper over the course of 15 days, for a median of 23 days of corticosteroids.[112] The results indicated fewer coronary abnormalities, shorter durations of fever, more rapid decline in CRP level, and fewer initial treatment failures in the steroid recipients. Caution must be exercised in the interpretation of the findings of these Japanese trials because the IVIG regimens and aspirin doses usually differ from those used in the United States, and echocardiograms were not interpreted by investigators blinded to the treatment group. A well-designed US trial in this regard showed little if any direct benefit of the addition of a single dose of intravenous methylprednisolone 30 mg/kg to the current IVIG and aspirin regimen, with the possible exception of the subset of patients who failed to respond to standard therapy and who required retreatment of the disease.[196]

Several attempts have been made in Japan to develop scoring systems to predict at the time of initial presentation those patients who are at increased risk for failure to respond to standard therapy[69,144] and/or to develop coronary lesions after therapy.[180] In a retrospective analysis of 193 patients, Mori and colleagues found that elevated white blood cell and neutrophil counts and CRP levels after IVIG treatment predicted increased risk for subsequent development of coronary lesions.[180] Egami and associates compared 279 patients who responded to initial standard treatment to 41 patients who were treatment resistant.[69] With their scoring system giving one point each for month younger than 6 months, treatment before 4 days of illness, platelet count 300,000/mm^3 or less, and CRP of 8 mg/dL or higher and two points for an alanine aminotransferase level of 80 IU/L or higher, a total score of three points or higher identified the IVIG-resistant group with 78% sensitivity and 76% specificity.[69] A similar predictive scoring system for IVIG unresponsiveness was developed by Kobayashi and colleagues,[144] who gave two points each for initial treatment on illness day 1 to 4, serum sodium level of less than 133 mmol/L, aspartate aminotransferase value of 100 IU/L or higher, and neutrophils of 80% or greater and two points each for CRP of 10 mg/dL or higher, platelet count up to 300,000/mm^3, and age 12 months or younger. This yielded 86% sensitivity and 67% to 68% specificity for patients with four or more points. The Kobayashi score was used to select patients at high risk for treatment failure in a randomized corticosteroid trial, as discussed earlier.[145]

A more recent Japanese multicenter, randomized, open-label, blinded end points trial (the RAISE study) assessed the benefit of adjunctive primary steroid therapy for KD patients considered at high risk to be refractory to initial therapy.[145] Using the Kobayashi score[144] to identify patients at high risk for nonresponse to IVIG and aspirin, high-risk subjects were randomized to IVIG and aspirin (30 mg/kg per day until afebrile, then 3–5 mg/kg) or to IVIG, aspirin, and intravenous prednisolone 2 mg/kg per day for 5 days, converting to oral dosage once free of fever and then a 15-day corticosteroid taper beginning when the CRP level normalized. Significantly fewer recipients of corticosteroids developed coronary changes (3% vs. 13% at 4 weeks), and coronary z-scores were significantly lower in corticosteroid recipients. In another recent Japanese study,[207] Ogata and colleagues evaluated corticosteroids with IVIG and aspirin 30 to 50 mg/kg per day in those patients with disease predicted to be refractory. Subjects were randomized to IVIG and aspirin alone or with a single 30 mg/kg dose of intravenously administered methylprednisolone and heparin from 2 hours before to 24 hours after the corticosteroid was given. Corticosteroid recipients had more rapid defervescence and decline in CRP levels with somewhat lower mean coronary z-scores ($z \geq 2.5$ in 9% of corticosteroid group, 38.5% in the noncorticosteroid group; $P = .04$), with transient adverse events only in the corticosteroid group.

It can be concluded that the addition of steroid to standard IVIG/ASA regimen in high-risk patients reduces the coronary abnormality rate and IVIG failure.

Unfortunately the Japanese scoring systems to identify high-risk patients are insensitive in ethnically diverse populations as seen in North America,[277,318] and it is thus difficult to know how to target adjunctive therapy outside Japan.

A well-designed trial evaluated Infliximab (Remicade), a monoclonal anti–TNF-α antibody, as adjunctive primary therapy.[320] The results showed safety but no significant benefit regarding IVIG resistance rates or rates of coronary artery abnormalities. Addition of infliximab for primary therapy with IVIG in not recommended.

Rescue Therapy for IVIG Treatment Failures

Most patients with acute KD respond promptly to treatment with IVIG and aspirin, with defervescence and subsidence of inflammatory manifestations occurring within 36 to 48 hours.[197,199,267] A subgroup of 10% to 20%, however, fails to show significant clinical response; these patients remain febrile 36 to 48 hours after receiving IVIG or they manifest only transient improvement, with recurrent fever and clinical evidence of inflammatory signs and elevated CRP levels. These patients need additional antiinflammatory therapy, and specific guidelines or controlled treatment trials do not exist (Box 77.5). Of course, when treating apparently treatment-refractory patients, it is also prudent to reconfirm the initial diagnosis of KD.

In these patients, administration of a second dose of 2 g/kg of IVIG generally is effective in suppressing disease activity.[80,104,199,273] In a retrospective study of 179 patients with KD, 89% responded to the first dose of IVIG and 67% of the nonresponders responded to a second IVIG dose; thus, only 3% to 4% of all patients failed to respond after a second dose of IVIG.[101] Some recommend a course (usually 3 days) of intravenous pulse methylprednisolone at 30 mg/kg per day instead of a second dose of IVIG.[334] We generally prefer to reserve pulse corticosteroid therapy for the patient with highly refractory acute disease who has failed to respond to at least two 2 g/kg doses of IVIG because most patients respond well to a second IVIG dose.[101,131,177] No adequately powered randomized comparison between repeat IVIG dosing and corticosteroids for refractory patients has been performed. In a few particularly treatment-refractory patients, we have employed a slow oral corticosteroid taper over the course of weeks to several months once inflammatory activity appeared to have been controlled.

BOX 77.5 Rescue Therapy for Patients Not Responding to Standard Therapy

Persistent or recurrent fever and/or elevated serum CRP levels 36–48 hours after primary therapy:

- Repeat 2 g/kg IVIG
- Failure of two doses of IVIG: therapeutic options
    - Third dose of IVIG (2 g/kg) with or without tapering course of prednisone starting at 2 mg/kg[145]
    - IV methylprednisolone (usually 30 mg/kg daily in three doses) with or without subsequent oral steroid, tapered over 1–3 weeks
    - Infliximab (5 mg/kg) single dose
    - Cyclosporin (4–8 mg/kg daily for 14–21 days), usually IV, with monitoring of serum levels and dosing adjustments
    - Methotrexate orally (10 mg/m^2) × 1–2 doses

CRP, C-reactive protein; *IV*, intravenous; *IVIG*, intravenous immunoglobulin.

Infliximab has been reported in a nonrandomized open-label experience to be effective in most patients with acute KD who are refractory to standard therapy.[280] Even more limited published experience exists regarding other therapies for IVIG-refractory KD. Cyclophosphamide with or without methotrexate has been used in a very small number of patients, as has plasmapheresis or plasma exchange.[331] Cyclosporine has been reported to be promising in this regard,[291] as has single-dose methotrexate.[139] Cyclosporine has been used for several weeks and requires assessment of blood levels and dosage adjustments.[319]

Sequelae

The major (and virtually the only) sequelae of KD are cardiovascular, particularly coronary artery abnormalities. Therefore appropriate cardiac imaging is critical for the evaluation of patients suspected to have acute KD and for their subsequent follow-up. Echocardiography has been considered the ideal imaging modality because it is noninvasive and has high sensitivity and specificity for detection of abnormalities of the proximal left main, left anterior descending, circumflex, and right coronary arteries.[199] This procedure should be performed under the supervision of an echocardiographer experienced with evaluating children, and internal arterial diameters should be measured and compared with normal standards for body surface area, expressed as z-scores.[60,167,199] The American Heart Association classifies coronary aneurysms as small (<5 mm), medium (5–8 mm), or giant (>8 mm); and de Zorzi and colleagues[60] and, more recently, Manlhiot and coworkers[167] showed that adjusting coronary dimensions for body surface area may identify more accurately those patients with enlarged coronary arteries. By z-scores, dilation is defined as a z of 2 to less than 2.5; a small aneurysm is defined as a z of 2.5 or more to less than 5; a medium aneurysm as a z of 5 or more to less than 10; and large or giant aneurysm as a z of 10 or greater or an absolute dimension of 8 mm or larger. Giant coronary aneurysms are associated with worse prognosis, and these patients require particularly close follow-up.[46,199] The sensitivity and specificity of echocardiography to identify coronary thrombi and coronary stenosis are uncertain, and visualization of coronary vessels is more difficult as body size increases. Therefore angiography, magnetic resonance angiography (MRA),[99,301] and ultrafast CT angiography (CTA)[38,225] have been useful for selected patients with KD.[199,262] Patients with significant coronary abnormalities are at risk for thrombotic events and are managed with antiplatelet agents and sometimes anticoagulants.[117,199]

Management Beyond the Acute Stage

Patients with KD should be re-evaluated within 2 weeks after hospital discharge and again 6 to 8 weeks after onset of illness because echocardiography at these time points is most likely to detect coronary artery aneurysms should they develop. If a baseline study and these two follow-up echocardiograms fail to detect evidence of coronary abnormality, performing further echocardiograms probably is unnecessary,[326] although a 6- to 12-month follow-up echocardiogram is performed at many centers.[51,199] Low-dose aspirin therapy (3–5 mg/kg per day) can be discontinued after the 6- to 8-week follow-up echocardiogram unless evidence of coronary abnormalities is present. To reduce the theoretical (and extremely low) risk for Reye syndrome in patients receiving low-dose aspirin, clopidogrel 1 mg/kg per day can be substituted for aspirin for a brief time in patients who develop varicella or influenza. Clopidogrel also can be used in the rare patient who is allergic to or intolerant of aspirin.

COMPLICATIONS

Myocardial Infarction

Myocardial infarction is the most common cause of death in KD (Box 77.6). In a classic cooperative Japanese study of 195 cases, the first myocardial infarction usually occurred in the first year after onset of disease and was fatal in 22% and asymptomatic in 37% of these patients. Major symptoms were shock, vomiting, and abdominal pain, with chest pain complaints only in children older than 4 years of age. Of those patients who survived a first infarct, 16% had a second myocardial infarct.[125,127] Patients with giant (>8 mm or z-score >10) coronary aneurysms are at greatest risk for having infarcts, particularly related to thrombi and/or to stenotic areas adjacent to a giant aneurysm. Most fatal infarctions are the result of obstruction of the left main coronary artery or both the right coronary and left anterior descending coronary arteries; survivors are most likely to have isolated right coronary involvement. Approximately half the survivors of acute myocardial infarction had one or more complications, including ventricular dysfunction, mitral regurgitation, and arrhythmias. Parents of all children with KD with significant coronary abnormalities should be instructed to seek emergency medical care if chest pain, dyspnea, lethargy, or syncope develops. Prompt fibrinolytic therapy should be attempted at a tertiary care center if acute coronary thrombosis is diagnosed.[124,199] The degree of reversibility of coronary thrombosis in children with KD may be somewhat less than that in adults with atherosclerotic disease. Late cardiac sequelae of KD may not manifest until adulthood.[130] A more recent Japanese study by Tsuda et al. assessed long-term outcomes of 60 KD patients who had a myocardial infarct between 1976 and 2007, with median follow-up of 16 years.[323] The 30-year survival rate was 63% (95% CI, 45–78%) and the 25-year ventricular tachycardia-free survival rate was 29% (CI, 15–46%).[323] Development of ventricular tachycardia was related to degree of nonviable myocardium.[323]

BOX 77.6 Cardiac Abnormalities in Kawasaki Disease

Acute Stage
- Pericardial effusion
- Decreased myocardial function
- Mitral regurgitation
- Enlargement (ectasia) of coronary arteries
- Arrhythmia (rare)

Subacute Stage
- Coronary aneurysms, irregularity, ectasia
- Significant mitral or aortic regurgitation, or both (rare)
- Coronary aneurysm rupture (very rare)
- Myocardial infarction (rare)

Convalescent Stage
- Persistent coronary aneurysms
- Regressed coronary aneurysms (residual fibrosis)
- Coronary artery stenosis
- Coronary aneurysm rupture (very rare)
- Myocardial infarction (rare)

Other Cardiovascular Complications

Other cardiac complications include myocardial fibrosis, valvulitis, and coronary rupture. Some researchers have suggested that valvular disease occurs in as many as 1% of patients with KD; most of these cases result in significant mitral regurgitation.[2,142] Patients with well-documented aortic regurgitation also have been observed. At least one patient with KD developed severe aortic and mitral regurgitation that necessitated double valve replacement.[93] In an autopsy study, coronary rupture was a rare finding but was noted more often among older children who died of KD within the first months after disease onset, whereas myocardial infarction was seen more often in younger fatal cases.[217]

Peripheral artery aneurysms develop in fewer than 1% of patients with KD, virtually always in those who also have significant coronary abnormalities.[132,294] These abnormalities generally involve medium-sized muscular arteries, such as subclavian, brachial, axillary, iliac, or femoral arteries and occasionally the hepatic or renal arteries or the abdominal aorta.

Peripheral Gangrene

A rare but very serious complication in the acute febrile stage of KD is severe peripheral ischemia and dry gangrene of distal extremities.[315] Virtually all such patients have been young infants up to approximately 7 months of age with giant coronary aneurysms, and some have developed peripheral (especially axillary or iliac) arterial aneurysms as well. This complication is virtually unknown in Japan[136] and has been reported primarily in non-Asian children in North America.[65,315] Possible pathogenic mechanisms of peripheral gangrene include the following: severe arteritis of digital or other small peripheral arteries; arteriospasm of peripheral arteries, perhaps in association with severe vasculitis; thrombosis of inflamed or spastic arteries as a result of stasis and damaged endothelium; thrombosis of a more proximal aneurysm (especially axillary) with embolism distally; rarely, cardiogenic shock; and, most likely, a combination of these factors.[291,309] This process has led to amputations in a small number of infants. Therapy has been empirical, primarily because the precise mechanisms of disease are unclear, and has included aggressive use of antiinflammatory agents; prostaglandin infusion; and antiplatelet, anticoagulant, and vasodilation therapies.[65,315,333]

Nonvascular Complications

As many as 5% to 10% of patients with KD develop painful arthritis or arthralgia in the acute stage of disease, often in the ankles or other lower extremity joints that can persist for several weeks, and they may benefit from treatment with a nonsteroidal antiinflammatory agent. Earlier-onset arthritis (≤10 days of illness) tends to be polyarticular, whereas later-onset arthritis involves primarily larger weight-bearing joints. We have used naproxen, usually 10 to 15 mg/kg per day divided into two or three doses, for several weeks with considerable success. However, if an NSAID is used, the antiplatelet effect of aspirin is decreased, and an alternative antiplatelet agent (such as clopidogrel) should be given to patients at high risk of thrombosis.

Abdominal pain and diarrhea in the early acute stage usually respond to intravenous hydration and supportive care. Acalculous distention (hydrops) of the gallbladder manifests clinically as right upper quadrant tenderness or a mass with or without obstructive jaundice and can be confirmed by ultrasonography.[199,284] Performing a cholecystectomy is not necessary. Hepatic involvement appears to be entirely self-limited and has not been associated with chronic liver disease.

Rare patients with KD develop hemophagocytic syndrome, also known as *macrophage activation syndrome,* as a complication.[49,181,220] This syndrome manifests as persistent fever associated with cytopenias, hepatosplenomegaly, hepatic dysfunction, often hyperferritinemia, elevated serum lactate dehydrogenase, hypofibrinogenemia, and hypertriglyceridemia. Therapy with high doses of prednisone or other immune modifiers is indicated for this rare but serious complication.

Rare events that occur in association with KD include sensorineural hearing loss,[143] transient unilateral facial nerve palsy,[88,228] and pneumonitis or pulmonary nodules.[79] We have cared for two older children who had sufficient abdominal findings to warrant appendectomy before establishing the diagnosis of KD. Consultation with a center that treats large numbers of patients with KD should be sought by the physician faced with patients with rare or serious complications.

LONG-TERM FOLLOW-UP AND PROGNOSIS

KD normally is an acute and self-limited illness. However, cardiac abnormalities that develop when the disease is active may be progressive, and prognosis clearly is related to the coronary artery status.[117] Twenty to 25% of patients not treated with IVIG develop coronary abnormalities that are detectable by two-dimensional echocardiography or angiography. The risk for development of coronary aneurysms is reduced to 2% to 3% overall when IVIG is given in the first 10 days of illness.[197,198] However, the rates for coronary abnormalities for young infants are somewhat higher, even with timely IVIG therapy. The risk for significant coronary events such as thrombosis, stenosis, myocardial ischemia, myocardial infarction, and even sudden death is correlated with higher coronary z-scores for many years after onset of illness and into adulthood.[127,171,199]

Children without apparent cardiac sequelae during the first month after onset of KD appear to return to their previous states of health without cardiac signs or symptoms. However, some reports suggest the possibility of generalized vascular endothelial dysfunction in patients with KD even in those who never had coronary abnormalities. These dysfunctions include altered lipid metabolism,[37] increased brachial-radial artery mean pulse wave velocity,[43] lower myocardial flow reserve,[185] and abnormal endothelium-dependent brachial artery reactivity,[61,176,201,338] but the data are not consistent and additional studies are needed.

Apparent "regression" of small and medium aneurysms as seen on an echocardiogram is a common occurrence. Overall, approximately half of all children with coronary aneurysms at 4 to 8 weeks after onset demonstrate normal luminal size by 1 to 2 years on angiography or echocardiography.[125,128] The likelihood that an aneurysm will appear to regress by echocardiography or angiography is higher with smaller aneurysms, age younger than 1 year at the onset of KD, fusiform rather than saccular morphology, and involvement of a more distal coronary segment.[4,297] "Regression" of the internal diameter of the vessel to normal may occur by luminal smooth muscle cell–derived myofibroblastic proliferation and/or by thrombus organization and recanalization.[85,217,260,273] Intravascular ultrasound studies have been interpreted to suggest that thickened intima and media sometimes with calcifications are present in areas of apparently regressed coronary aneurysms.[100,286] However, direct correlation of intravascular ultrasound findings and histology has not been performed. A recent histologic study of 41 heart specimens demonstrated that calcification was found only in areas of organized thrombus not in vascular media or intima.[217] Regressed aneurysmal segments are histologically abnormal and have abnormal functional responses with decreased vascular reactivity to exercise or pharmacologic agents such as isosorbide dinitrate or acetylcholine,[61,110,260] with the potential to progress to stenosis.[129,293,295]

Functional abnormalities of coronary vessel endothelium relaxation years after the onset of KD have been reported[61,110,176] and warrant further investigation. Newer imaging methods have demonstrated coronary vascular wall changes sometimes even in patients with no history of abnormalities in the acute phase. The meaning of these findings in patients thought to have escaped coronary abnormalities with acute KD and their long-term significance are uncertain.

Patients with giant coronary aneurysms are at the greatest risk for the development of significant stenosis with resultant myocardial ischemia.[117,132,199,283] The risk for significant stenosis, usually developing at the inlet or outlet of a moderate to large coronary aneurysm, shows a steady rise over 15 to 20 years of observation.[121,132,283,293] These markedly abnormal vessels are subject to luminal fibroblastic proliferation, calcification, and thrombosis, which may lead to myocardial ischemia or infarction. An analysis of 76 subjects with giant aneurysms from one Japanese center with median follow-up of 19 years showed 95%, 88%, and 88% 10-, 20-, and 30-year survival rates, respectively. Catheter and surgical coronary interventions resulted in 28%, 43%, and 59% cumulative coronary intervention rates at 5-, 15-, and 25-year follow-up, respectively.[283]

In 10- to 20-year follow-up studies of patients with KD, the arteries most likely to develop stenosis are the right main and left anterior descending coronary arteries.[121,132,283] A limited number of studies of young adults with ischemic heart disease and history of diagnosed KD or a compatible clinical illness have been performed.[53,130] A survey of Japanese adult cardiologists identified 130 adult patients with coronary aneurysms detected by angiography to evaluate myocardial infarction or ischemia.[130] Twenty-one of these patients (mean age, 34 years; range, 20–63 years) had a history compatible with KD in childhood. These patients had severe coronary disease with myocardial infarction, angina pectoris, mitral regurgitation, arrhythmias, congestive heart failure, and need for coronary bypass grafting. This study indicates that the coronary artery sequelae of KD likely are significant causes of ischemic heart disease in young adults. Daniels and coworkers evaluated 261 adults younger than 40 years who underwent angiography for suspected myocardial ischemia and found 16 with coronary aneurysms, 13 of whom had definite or presumed KD as the cause.[53] It is unknown whether patients with KD are at increased risk for developing premature or accelerated atherosclerosis, but there are no data to support this.

Long-Term Management

The risk for coronary artery thrombosis or stenosis that may result in myocardial ischemia and infarction remains the most important long-term clinical problem in the subset of patients with KD who develop significant coronary abnormalities (see Box 77.6). Patients classified as having medium (6–8 mm, or z ≥5 to <10), and large and giant (≥8 mm, z ≥10) aneurysms are at substantial risk for development of stenosis years after the acute illness, compared with patients with small aneurysms (z <5) or no aneurysmal changes.[4,121,125,128,132,294,325] Patients with giant aneurysms are at the highest risk for thrombosis.[199] Manlhiot and colleagues[167] documented that the previous American Heart Association classification scheme noted earlier underestimated the severity of coronary abnormalities and showed the following optimal definitions: small aneurysm, z-score of 2.5 to less than 5.0; medium aneurysm, z-score greater than or equal to 5.0 to less than 10.0; and large and giant aneurysm, z-score greater than or equal to 10.0. Echocardiography and electrocardiography often are not sufficiently sensitive to detect stenotic lesions. Various stress tests for detection of reversible myocardial ischemia, including nuclear perfusion scans with exercise, exercise echocardiography, and stress echocardiography with agents such as dobutamine, dipyridamole, or adenosine, have been used in children to detect stenosis.[199,206,219] Newer techniques, including stress magnetic resonance imaging (stress MRI), MRA, CTA, and position emission tomography (PET) are being utilized.[38,99,225,301] Coronary arteriography has been the most definitive method to determine the degree of stenosis and the adequacy of collateral circulation but is invasive. Intravascular ultrasonography is an effective method to evaluate vascular wall morphology in selected patients during angiography.[287,292] All patients with evidence of myocardial ischemia or infarction should be studied by angiography to determine the need for intervention.[199] Most experts agree that patients with moderate to severe coronary artery aneurysms, a single large aneurysm, or multiple aneurysms should have their coronary anatomy defined by angiography or MRA or CTA at least once after the acute stage of illness (after the inflammatory process has subsided) to define fully the extent of involvement and to identify potential sites of thrombotic or stenotic complications.[199] Aneurysms can also occur in noncoronary arteries, especially the subclavian, brachial, axillary, iliac, and femoral arteries, and occasionally in the abdominal aorta and renal arteries[294] (almost always in patients with coronary abnormalities).

Because KD patients with past or present aneurysms variably have evidence of chronic inflammation and reduced HDL-cholesterol levels, some have suggested that HMG CoA-reductase inhibitors (statins) may be beneficial. In addition to their LDL-cholesterol lowering effect, statins have potentially beneficial pleiotropic effects on inflammation, oxidative stress, endothelial function, platelet aggregation, fibrinolysis, and coagulation. Small short-term studies in KD patients with aneurysms showed improved endothelial function and lower hs-CRP levels. Safety studies have not identified an effect on growth. Empiric low-dose statin may be considered in KD patients with past or current aneurysms.[202]

Patients who have had KD are risk stratified into five levels based on their relative risk of myocardial ischemia and coronary z-scores for long-term management by the American Heart Association, as outlined here.[199] The American Heart Association recommendations should be consulted for more details[171a].

Patients With No Evidence of Coronary Artery Abnormalities at Any Time (Risk Level I)

Patients who have never manifested coronary artery abnormalities (z always <2) have no need for aspirin or other antiplatelet medication beyond 6 to 8 weeks after onset of illness or for restriction of physical activities in the convalescent stage. Only routine pediatric follow-up beyond 1 year, with routine cardiovascular risk assessment, is indicated.

Patients With Dilation (z ≥2 but <2.5, or >1 Decrease in z During Follow-up; Risk Level II)

Patients with transient coronary artery abnormalities that resolve by 6 to 8 weeks should be treated with aspirin 3 to 5 mg/kg per day until resolution of abnormalities. No restrictions are indicated after 6 to 8 weeks, angiography is not indicated, and risk assessment and counseling are recommended at 2- to 5-year intervals.[285]

Patients With Small (≥ 2.5 to <5) Coronary Aneurysm in One or More Coronary Arteries (Risk Level III)

Patients with small coronary artery aneurysms should be maintained on daily low-dose aspirin (3 to 5 mg/kg) at least until apparent regression is documented with annual echocardiographic follow-up.[285] No restriction on physical activity is indicated, and assessment for inducible myocardial ischemia should occur every 2 to 5 years depending on presence of symptoms of ischemia or ventricular dysfunction.

Patients With Medium Aneurysms (z-score ≥5 to <10, with Luminal Dimension <8 mm; Risk Level IV)

Long-term antiplatelet therapy with low dose aspirin 3 to 5 mg/kg once daily or clopidogrel 1 mg/kg per day up to adult dose of 75 mg is indicated for these children and should be continued indefinitely. Anticoagulant therapy with warfarin or daily subcutaneous low-molecular-weight heparin is not usually warranted. All such patients should be under the care of a physician with experience in managing patients with KD, usually a pediatric cardiologist. Cardiac evaluation with an echocardiogram and an ECG should be performed approximately every 1 to 2 years depending on persistence or return to normal luminal diameter, with stress testing performed every 1 to 4 years. Angiography may be considered 6 to 12 months after the patient has recovered from the acute stage of disease to define the coronary anatomy, and it should be repeated whenever symptoms or stress tests suggest the presence of myocardial ischemia. Physical activity should be regulated if receiving more than a single antiplatelet agent, and competitive sports should be based on periodic stress testing.

Patients With Large and Giant Coronary Artery Aneurysms (z-score ≥10 or ≥8 mm) and/or Obstructive Lesions (Risk Level V)

These patients should receive low-dose aspirin and/or clopidogrel as well as anticoagulation with either warfarin or low-molecular-weight heparin, and they require very close cardiac care with periodic stress testing to guide participation in physical activity. Patients with obstructive lesions or signs of myocardial ischemia must be evaluated urgently for possible intervention. Balloon angioplasty, rotablator angioplasty, coronary artery bypass grafting, stent placement, and even cardiac transplantation all have been employed for patients with KD who have particularly serious coronary artery disease.[3,41,98,113,183,324] Arterial bypass grafts are superior to venous grafts in these patients.[141] Balloon angioplasty procedures have been associated with high rates of recurrent stenosis in patients with KD and coronary stenosis.[3] Management details for this group of patients are beyond the scope of this chapter.

NEW REFERENCES SINCE THE SEVENTH EDITION

1a. Abrams JY, Belay ED, Uehara R, et al. Cardiac complications, earlier treatment, and initial disease severity in Kawasaki disease. *J Pediatr.* 2017;In press.

25. Brown TJ, Crawford SE, Cornwell ML, et al. CD8 T lymphocytes and macrophages infiltrate coronary artery aneurysms in acute Kawasaki disease. *J Infect Dis.* 2001;184:940-945.

31. Burns JC, Franco A. The immunomodulatory effects of intravenous immunoglobulin therapy in Kawasaki disease. *Exp Rev Clin Immunol.* 2015;11(7):819-825.

32. Burns JC, Herzog L, Fabri O, et al. Seasonality of Kawasaki disease. *PLoS ONE.* 2013;8:e74529.

42. Checkley W, Guzman-Cottrill J, Epstein L, et al. Short-term weather variability in Chicago and hospitalizations for Kawasaki disease. *Epidemiol.* 2009;20:194-201.

44. Choi IH, Chwae YJ, Shim WT, et al. Clonal expansion of CD8+ T cells in Kawasaki Disease. *J Immunol.* 1997;159:481-486.

56. Dean AG, Melish ME, Hicks R, et al. An epidemic of Kawasaki syndrome in Hawaii. *J Pediatr.* 1982;100(4):552-557.

63. Dominguez S, Friedman K, Seewald R, et al. Kawasaki disease in pediatric intensive care unit. *Pediatrics.* 2008;122:e786-e790.

74. Falcini F, Trapini S, Turchini S, et al. Immunological findings in Kawasaki disease: an evaluation in a cohort of Italian children. *Clin Exp Rheumatol.* 1997;15(6):685-689.

77. Feng S, Yadav SK, Gao F, et al. Plasma levels of monokine induced by interferon gamma/chemokine (C-X-X motif) ligand 9, thymus and activation-regulated chemokine/chemokine (C-C motif) ligand 17 in children with Kawasaki disease. *BMC Pediatr.* 2015;15:109.

115. Jakob A, Whelan J, Kordecki M, et al. Kawasaki disease in Germany. *Ped Inf Dis J.* 2016;35:129-134.

117. JCS Joint Working Group. Guidelines for diagnosis and management of cardiovascular sequelae in Kawasaki disease. *Circ J.* 2014;78:2521-2562.

140. Kim GB, Han JW, Park YW, et al. Epidemiologic features of Kawasaki disease in South Korea. *Ped Infect Dis J.* 2014;33:24-27.

149. Kuo HC, et al. CASP3 gene single nucleoside polymorphism and Kawasaki disease in Taiwanese children. *J Hum Genet.* 2011;56:161-165.

162. Lin CY, Hwang B. Serial immunologic studies in patients with mucocutaneous lymph node syndrome (Kawasaki disease). *Ann Allergy.* 1987;59(4):291-297.

163. Lin MC, Lai MS, Jan SL, et al. Epidemiologic features of Kawasaki disease in acute stages in Taiwan, 1997–2010. *J Chin Med Assn.* 2015;7:121-126.

161. Lin Y-J, Cheng M-C, Lo M-H, et al. Early differentiation of Kawasaki disease shock syndrome and toxic shock syndrome in a pediatric intensive care unit. *Ped Inf Dis J.* 2015;34:1163-1167.

165. Maddox RA, Holman RC, Uehara R, et al. Recurrent Kawasaki disease: U.S.A. and Japan. *Pediatr Int.* 2015;57:1116-1120.

166. Makino N, Nakamura Y, Yashiro M, et al. Descriptive epidemiology of Kawasaki disease in Japan: 2011–2012. *Epidemiol.* 2015;25:239-245.

171a. McCrindle BW, Rowley AH, Newburger JW, et al. Diagnosis, treatment, and long-term management of Kawasaki disease. *Circulation.* 2017;135:e927-e999.

193. Nash MC, Shah V, Reader JA, et al. Anti-neutrophil cytoplasmic antibodies and anti-endothelial cell antibodies are not increased in Kawasaki disease. *Br J Rheumatol.* 1995;34(9):882-887.

202. Niedra E, Chahal N, Manlhiot C, et al. Atorvastatin safety in Kawasaki disease patients with coronary artery aneurysms. *Pediatr Cardiol.* 2014;35:89-92.

212. Onouchi Y, Fukazawa R, Yamamura K, et al. Variations in ORAI1 gene associated with Kawasaki disease. *PLoS ONE.* 2016;11(1):e0145486.

216. Onouchi Y, et al. ITPKC and CASP3 polymorphisms and risk for IVIG unresponsiveness and coronary lesions. *Pharmacogenomics J.* 2013;13:152-159.

229. Popper S, Shimizu C, Shike H, et al. Gene-expression patterns reveal underlying biological processes in Kawasaki disease. *Genome Biol.* 2007;8(12):R261.

230. Popper SJ, Watson VE, Shimizu C, et al. Gene transcript abundance profiles distinguish Kawasaki from adenovirus infection. *J Infect Dis.* 2009;200(4):657-666.

239. Rodo X, Curcoll R, Robinson M, et al. Tropospheric winds from northeastern China carry the etiologic agent of Kawasaki disease from its source to Japan. *Proc Natl Acad Sci USA.* 2014;111(22):7952-7957.

244. Rowley AH, Baker SC, Orenstein JM, et al. Searching for the cause of Kawasaki disease—cytoplasmic inclusion bodies provide new insight. *Nat Rev Microbiol.* 2008;6:394-401.

252. Rowley AH, Shulman ST, Garcia FL, et al. Cloning the arterial IgA antibody response during acute Kawasaki disease. *J Immunol.* 2005;175:8386-8391.

256. Rowley AH, Wylie KM, Kim KY, et al. The transcriptional profile of coronary arteritis in Kawasaki disease. *BMC Genomics.* 2015;16:1076.

265. Shimizu C, Oharaseki T, Takahashi K, et al. The role of TGF-beta and myofibroblasts in the arteritis of Kawasaki disease. *Hum Pathol.* 2013;44:189-198.

274. Shulman ST, Rowley AH, Orenstein J. Histologic assessment of a case of likely Kawasaki disease in 1870 London. Abstract 110. 11th International Kawasaki Disease Symposium; February 2015; Honolulu.

273. Shulman ST, Rowley AH. Kawasaki disease: insights into pathogenesis and approaches to treatment. *Nat Rev Rheum.* 2015;11:475-482.

280. Sonada K, Mori M, Hokosaki T, et al. Infliximab plus plasma exchange rescue therapy in Kawasaki disease. *J Pediatr.* 2014;164:1128-1132.

289. Sundel RP. Kawasaki disease. *Rheum Dis Clin North Am.* 2015;41:63-73.

300. Takahashi K, Oharaseki T, Yokouchi Y, et al. A half century of autopsy results—incidence of pediatric vasculitis syndromes, especially Kawasaki disease. *Circ J.* 2012;76:964-970.
310. Terai M, Kohno Y, Namba M, et al. Class II HLA expression on coronary endothelium in Kawasaki Disease. *Human Path.* 1990;21:231-234.
320. Tremoulet AH, et al. Infliximab for intensification of primary therapy for Kawaski disease. *Lancet.* 2014;383:1731-1738.
319. Tremoulet AH, et al. Calcineurin inhibitor treatment of IVIG resistant Kawasaki disease. *J Pediatr.* 2012;161:506.e1-512.e1.
349. Yeung RS. Kawasaki disease: update on pathogenesis. *Curr Opin Rheumatol.* 2010;22:551-560.

The full reference list for this chapter is available at ExpertConsult.com

Chronic Fatigue Syndrome (Systemic Exertion Intolerance Disease) 78

Leonard R. Krilov

All cases are unique and very similar to others.
T.S. Eliot, *The Cocktail Party,* 1949.

Chronic fatigue syndrome (CFS) is an illness complex characterized by a prolonged (>6 months) period of constant or intermittent debilitating fatigue in association with multiple, often nonspecific, symptoms that may include new-onset headaches, decreased ability to concentrate, recurrent complaints of sore throat and tender cervical or axillary lymphadenitis, reports of low-grade fever, diffuse muscle or joint pain, postexertional increase in fatigue, and unrefreshing sleep. To date, no specific cause for this syndrome has been identified, and, despite similar arrays of signs and symptoms, patients with CFS likely represent a heterogeneous population. Still, evaluation of groups of patients with this symptom complex has provided information about pathophysiologic changes occurring in patients with CFS, and potentially beneficial, although not curative, approaches to therapy for affected individuals have been developed.

In an attempt to provide a degree of uniformity as a basis for research into the evaluation of such patients, the US Centers for Disease Control and Prevention (CDC) developed a definition of CFS in 1988.[51] These criteria were revised in 1994, with physical signs removed from the definition because they appeared to be unreliably documented in studies and the required number of symptoms for the diagnosis of CFS decreased from 8 of a list of 11 to 4 of 8 components (Box 78.1).[42] These changes, being less restrictive, may serve to increase the sensitivity of the diagnosis, but they also decrease the specificity. However these criteria are purely speculative in the absence of any gold standard or definitive diagnostic test for CFS. These 1994 criteria also suggest subdivisions of patients with CFS for research purposes and provide guidelines for nonresearch clinicians as well. Other international groups have generated similar definitions of CFS for evaluating this condition.[16,71,101]

The primary manifestations of CFS are severe fatigue of more than 6 months' duration that limits activity to less than 50% of premorbid function and the association of multiple other symptoms, as outlined in the case definitions of CFS.[42,51,71,101] These symptoms include new or more intense headaches, decreased ability to focus or concentrate, recurrent sore throats, a sensation of tender cervical or axillary lymph nodes, low-grade temperature elevations, myalgias and arthralgias, postexertional fatigue lasting longer than 24 hours, and sleep disturbances (hypersomnia or insomnia). The severity and persistence of these findings vary among individual patients with CFS. In addition, although not included in the case definitions, many patients report dizziness, especially with changes in position, feeling hot when others are cold or vice versa, chronic costochondritis, and a Raynaud-like phenomenon.

In 2015, the Institute of Medicine (IOM) recommended renaming the syndrome systemic exertion intolerance disease (SEID) in an effort to emphasize that any exertion (physical, cognitive, or emotional) can lead to adverse effects in these patients. This definition requires that patients have:

1. A substantial reduction or impairment in the ability to engage in premorbid levels of activities persisting for more than 6 months and be associated with new-onset fatigue that is not alleviated by rest.
2. Postexertional fatigue.
3. Unrefreshing sleep.

Additionally this definition includes the presence of cognitive impairment and/or orthostatic intolerance.[21,53]

HISTORICAL OVERVIEW

In all likelihood, CFS is not a new illness. Numerous conditions with features comparable to those of CFS have appeared in the medical literature during the past several centuries.[115] Many of these descriptions attempted to associate an illness characterized by prolonged debilitating fatigue and numerous other symptoms with an infectious agent. They have included chronic brucellosis,[108] chronic enteroviral syndrome,[23,29,46] chronic candidiasis,[94] myalgic encephalomyelitis,[2] chronic mononucleosis (Epstein-Barr virus [EBV] infection),[4,54,120,121] human herpesvirus–6 infection,[11,129] human herpesvirus–7 infection,[34] chronic Lyme disease,[109] parvovirus B19 infection,[60] and a new retroviral infection.[31] Noninfectious conditions described with similarities to CFS include total-allergy syndrome, hypoglycemia, neurasthenia, Iceland disease, Royal Free disease, and fibromyalgia rheumatica.[64] In addition to clinical similarity to CFS, all these conditions, at least at the time they were described, lacked a diagnostic test to confirm a definitive causative agent and, in their acute form, manifested as fatigue in association with multiple other complaints.

A review of the experience in the mid-1980s associated groups of patients with CFS-like illness with patients with chronic EBV infection.[4,54,120] These reports described elevated and aberrant patterns of EBV antibody responses in individuals with prolonged fatigue and multiple symptoms consistent with CFS. Acute infectious mononucleosis also often manifests as fatigue, fever, malaise, sore throat, lymphadenitis, and multiple systemic complaints, although typically in a more pronounced manner. Subsequent studies, however, revealed that the elevation or pattern of EBV antibody responses in such patients was not consistently different from findings in others who resolved symptoms of acute EBV infection.[79] Additionally shedding of EBV in secretions was not increased in these individuals, and no association was found between viral shedding and severity of symptoms.[122] Furthermore no response to the antiviral drug acyclovir occurred in a group of such patients in a placebo-controlled, double-blind crossover study in terms of improvement of clinical symptoms.[117] After these observations were made, the name *chronic fatigue syndrome* was chosen to define this illness,[51] at least until a specific cause or marker for this illness is identified.

Cameron and colleagues reported on a cohort of patients with prolonged fatigue after having infectious mononucleosis. No difference in EBV load was demonstrated in eight patients with 6 months or more of disabling symptoms after the diagnosis of infectious mononucleosis was established, and again there was a lack of correlation between persistent symptoms and viremia or altered host responses to EBV.[14]

BOX 78.1 Centers for Disease Control and Prevention 1994 Workshop Case Definition of Chronic Fatigue Syndrome

1. Fatigue (persistent or relapsing) that has new or definite onset, is of greater than 6 months' duration, and leads to a substantial (>50%) reduction in level of activity

   plus

2. At least four of the following:
   - Impaired memory or concentration
   - Sore throat
   - Tender lymph nodes: cervical or axillary
   - Myalgias
   - Arthralgias (multiple joints, without swelling or erythema)
   - New onset (or in severity) of headaches
   - Unrefreshing sleep (hypersomnia or insomnia)
   - Postexertional fatigue lasting more than 24 hours

   and

3. The absence of another diagnosis for the individual's signs and symptoms

Modified from Fukuda K, Straus SE, Hickie I, et al. The chronic fatigue syndrome: a comprehensive approach to its definition and study. *Ann Intern Med.* 1994;121:953–9.

TABLE 78.1 Symptoms Reported by 58 Children and Adolescents Evaluated for Chronic Fatigue Syndrome (1989–94)

Symptom	No. Patients	%
Fatigue	58	100
Headache	43	74
Sore throat	34	59
Abdominal pain	28	48
Fever	21	36
Impaired cognition	19	33
Myalgia	18	31
Diarrhea	17	29
Adenopathy	17	29
Anorexia	16	28
Nausea/vomiting	15	26
Congestion	13	22
Dizziness	10	17
Arthralgia	10	17
Otitis	6	10
Cough	6	10
Rash	5	9
Sweats	5	9
Chills	4	7
Depression	4	7

From Krilov LR, Fisher M, Friedman SB, et al. Course and outcome of chronic fatigue in children and adolescents. *Pediatrics.* 1998;102:360–6.

Despite the lack of association of ongoing EBV infection with CFS, Katz and colleagues observed that infectious mononucleosis may be an antecedent risk factor for CFS in adolescents.[59]

Recently increased detection of nucleic acid of a xenotropic murine leukemia virus (XMRV), a newly discovered retrovirus, was reported in two different series of CFS patients.[73,74] Subsequent studies failed to confirm these observations, including two reports that utilized samples from the same patients reported in the two positive studies just cited.[5,50,104,124] Contamination of the assays in the positive studies may have been responsible for the positive results, and both of those studies were subsequently retracted.[3,48,103]

EPIDEMIOLOGY

The definitions of CFS allow for attempts to characterize the prevalence and demographic features of this condition. Still, given the vagaries of the symptom complex, possible variations in application of the diagnosis by different health care providers, and the potential differences within groups of people to seek medical attention for this condition, data reported on these issues may not be a complete representation of the epidemiology of this condition. CFS has been reported in all age groups, including children as young as 5 years of age, and in all ethnic, racial, and socioeconomic groups, but most CFS cases have been reported to occur in middle- to upper-class white women with a median age of 35 to 40 years.[63] Based on a study of physician-diagnosed patients from four cities using the 1988 case definition of CFS,[1] the CDC estimates a minimum prevalence rate of CFS of 2 to 10 cases per 100,000 or higher in adults aged 18 years and older in the United States.[12,76,91] A population-based descriptive epidemiologic study conducted by the CDC in Kansas estimated the prevalence of CFS to be 235 per 100,000 persons and a 1-year incidence to be 180 per 100,000 persons.[95] Studies from outside the United States have reported similar or higher prevalence rates of CFS in adults.[35,71]

Although the CDC definition does not include age criteria for the diagnosis of CFS, the prevalence of CFS in the pediatric age range has not been studied well. Some researchers have suggested that the diagnosis of CFS should not be used in children to avoid potential delay in making an alternative medical or psychological diagnosis.[90] However many referral centers have reported groups of pediatric patients, primarily adolescents, with features and a clinical course similar to those reported in adults.[6,17,36,66,77,106] Furthermore in these studies, missed or alternative diagnoses were not found, despite years of follow-up. Rimes and colleagues reported prevalence rates of CFS in an adolescent population similar to those reported in adults.[96] The CDC estimates that between 0.2% and 2.3% of children or adolescents meet the diagnostic criteria for CFS, with the condition more prevalent in adolescents than younger children.[19] Collin and colleagues similarly estimated a prevalence of CFS at 1.86% in a population-based study of 16-year-olds, as reported by their parents.[24] In these pediatric studies, a predominance of female patients with a median age of 14 years at the time of diagnosis was noted. Additionally these patients were from predominantly middle- to upper-class families, and, as discussed later, their signs and symptoms at presentation (Table 78.1) and their course of illness were similar to those reported in adults with CFS. CDC studies suggest that the prevalence of CFS in adolescents approaches that reported in adults, but cases in children younger than 12 years of age occur much less often.[42] One suggestion is that a shorter duration of symptoms (3 to 4 months vs. 6 months) may be appropriate for establishing the diagnosis of CFS in pediatric patients.[42,55] Multiple family members with CFS may be seen as well, but, to date, evidence that CFS is contagious does not exist. Most often in this setting it is mothers of adolescents with CFS who exhibit similar symptoms.[126]

ETIOLOGY AND PATHOGENESIS

Infection

As noted previously, an infectious origin of CFS has not been demonstrated, and a single microorganism as the cause of CFS is unlikely. However an acute infection appears possibly to play a role in precipitating CFS because most (as many as two-thirds) patients with CFS relate a sudden onset of their symptoms to an acute infection, most often infectious mononucleosis. Lyme disease[75,109] and an influenza-like illness[52] also have been reported in association with the onset of CFS.

Immunologic Dysfunction

A role for immunologic dysfunction in CFS has been suggested based on numerous studies demonstrating abnormalities in lymphocyte function or cytokine production.[13,62,69,80,116,119,123] However these findings have not been reproducible in different groups of patients with CFS. Some evidence suggests that nonspecific elevation of antibody titers and an increase in allergic symptoms occur in patients with CFS.[118] However these findings are mild, and similar immunologic changes may be seen in other conditions, including depression. Individuals with CFS may report an increased frequency and duration of infections compared with their pre-CFS state, but they tend to be mostly routine viral illnesses. Neither unusual nor opportunistic infection nor increased risk for developing malignant disease has been observed in these individuals. Intravenous immunoglobulin infusions have not demonstrated long-term clinical benefit when they are administered to patients with CFS and may cause significant adverse reactions.[72,89,114]

Genetic Components

A number of recent studies of gene expression from peripheral blood samples have identified potential gene patterns associated with neuroendocrine function, stress reactions, and immune responses that may be associated with CFS.[49,61] Further definition of such genes may help further establish a biologic basis for development of CFS and eventually lead to diagnostic tests for CFS and targeted approaches to therapy.

Some studies have focused on potential genetic markers of CFS using DNA microarray technology.[110] An analysis of cytokine gene polymorphisms in 80 Italian patients with a diagnosis of CFS assessed using the 1994 CDC definition reported significant difference in tumor necrosis factor and interferon-γ phenotypes compared with controls. The authors hypothesized a potential altered immunologic or inflammatory response based on these differences as potentially contributing to the pathogenesis of CFS.[10,15,39] An analysis of prolonged postinfectious fatigue in patients who had had mononucleosis identified certain genes involved in immune responses, and hormonal and neurologic pathways that were altered in a subset of patients with mononucleosis were associated with the development of prolonged fatigue.[14,45,107] If reproducible gene expression markers are confirmed, they could potentially be used as diagnostic tools for CFS.

CLINICAL MANIFESTATIONS

Neurologic Factors

Many patients with CFS report cognitive impairment manifest as a decreased ability to concentrate and focus, difficulty in processing information, and trouble with word recall. Complaints of headache (new onset or altered pattern) and other neurologic symptoms, such as paresthesias and dysequilibrium, also are reported commonly by patients with CFS.

Despite these complaints, physical examination does not reveal abnormal neurologic signs. Formal neuropsychometric testing also may not reveal objective abnormalities to the extent reported by the patient. Whether this discrepancy reflects a problem with testing methods or altered perception on the part of the individual is uncertain at this time.[11,85]

Magnetic resonance imaging (MRI) has been reported to show an increase in cerebral white matter abnormalities in patients with CFS.[11,84,99] Similarly, in many studies, single photon emission computed tomography (SPECT) has demonstrated changes in perfusion in certain areas of the brain in patients with CFS.[27,38,100] In other studies, however, abnormalities specific to CFS have not been observed consistently, and methodological concerns have been raised regarding the interpretation of abnormal findings cited previously.[25,47] An abnormality at the base of the fourth ventricle detected on focal computed tomography (CT) of the base of the brain and responding to neurosurgical intervention was reported in a group of patients with CFS,[44] but this defect is not seen on routine CT or MRI and requires confirmation by other researchers before determining its significance for these patients. At present, imaging of the central nervous system is not indicated routinely in the evaluation of a patient with CFS.

Endocrinologic Factors

Subtle defects in the hypothalamic-pituitary-adrenal axis have been described in cohorts of patients with CFS. These abnormalities include decreased free urinary cortisol levels and exaggerated adrenal responsiveness to corticotropin infusion.[33] These changes are quantitatively minor, and mean values are still within normal for age and sex, thus rendering these values unreliable as a diagnostic test for CFS. Similar changes have been described in patients with fibromyalgia and posttraumatic stress disorder.

Cardiovascular Factors

In 1995, investigators at Johns Hopkins Hospital in Baltimore described a cohort of seven adolescents with chronic fatigue and autonomic dysfunction as assessed by tilt-table testing.[98] Furthermore these patients reported improvement or resolution of symptoms, including fatigue, with treatment of their orthostatic intolerance. Further studies from this group demonstrated some component of orthostatic hypotension in 92% of patients with CFS.[9] Studies in groups of adults, in contrast, showed tilt-table test abnormalities in only 25% to 40% of patients.[40,105] Whether this finding reflects true age-related differences in this phenomenon in patients with CFS is uncertain, given potential methodological differences in the performance of the tests.

The pattern of orthostatic intolerance among adolescents with CFS was characterized further by Stewart and colleagues and is consistent with the postural orthostatic tachycardia syndrome (POTS).[111–113] Symptoms of POTS may develop after an acute infectious illness or with severe deconditioning and include fatigue, lightheadedness, impaired cognition, inappropriate sweating, headache, palpitations, nausea, vomiting, and tremulousness. These authors suggest that CFS may be an extreme expression of POTS in at least some cases.

The importance of these cardiovascular findings in CFS remains unsettled. Subjective components may contribute to defining a tilt-table test as abnormal because these studies are not performed blinded. Some healthy individuals also may experience hypotension during these tests. Further studies defining the effect of treatment of POTS on the course of CFS should help to answer this question. In this context, evaluation of, and therapy for, orthostatic changes, especially if dizziness is a significant component of the patient's complaints, may be indicated.[137]

Sleep Physiology

Sleep disturbances have been described in selected groups of patients with CFS, and some of these conditions may be amenable to therapy.[68,93] However no single pattern of sleep abnormality has been reported for these patients, and, in our experience, the pattern of hypersomnia or insomnia tends to improve as the patient recovers.[125]

Psychological Factors

Psychological factors have been considered in the origin and perpetuation of CFS. Adults with CFS have demonstrated a higher frequency of depression and other psychiatric disorders before the onset of their CFS compared with age-matched controls.[1,67] Certainly many of the symptoms reported in CFS also are reported commonly in depression. They may include sleep disturbances, loss of energy, difficulty in concentrating, changes in appetite, and musculoskeletal complaints. Studies in children and adolescents with CFS also have shown significant psychological features, especially depression and somatization, compared with both healthy controls and those with other chronic illnesses (e.g., juvenile idiopathic arthritis, cancer, cystic fibrosis).[17,18,55,87,132] Still, certain features of CFS argue against its being solely a variant of depression. Individuals with CFS do not have the mood-related symptoms reported in patients with clinical depression. These mood-related symptoms include negative affect, anhedonia, low self-esteem, and suicidal ideation. Furthermore patients with CFS and their families have a firm belief that an infectious, immunologic, or other medical cause for their symptoms exists, and the patients desire a return to normal activities.

In considering the possible link between depression or psychological stress and CFS, several possible relationships may exist. Preexisting depression or stress may create a psychological vulnerability that allows for the development of CFS in combination with any of numerous other factors discussed previously. Studies have demonstrated a role for psychological factors predicting the response to mononucleosis and influenza.[52,57] Similar factors may be involved in the development of CFS. Alternatively depression may be a physiologic consequence of the central nervous system changes that occur in those who develop CFS, just as decreased concentration and memory occur as part of the syndrome.[55,132] Furthermore reactive depression may occur in these patients in response to the inability to participate in their usual activities and to absence from school and separation from friends. Finally CFS may be, at least in some cases, a manifestation of separation anxiety or school phobia in which secondary gain, as a conversion reaction, is playing a major role. Certainly, at least a subset of adolescents and children with CFS in our experience does not appear eager to return to school or activities, and secondary gain may play a role in the perpetuation of their illness.[52]

Coplan and colleagues recently described a group of patients with an anxiety disorder and a number of somatic comorbidities including joint laxity, pain syndromes (e.g., irritable bowel syndrome, fibromyalgia, chronic headaches), autoimmune and allergic disorders (e.g., hypothyroidism, asthma, allergic rhinitis with pharyngitis), and mood disorders (e.g., bipolar, major depression) that they termed anxiety-laxity-pain-immune-mood (ALPIM) syndrome.[26] These features share many similarities with CFS and emphasize the potential overlap of psychiatric and somatic complaints in such individuals.

In summary, each of these potential links among depression, anxiety, or stress and CFS likely plays a role, with the relative contribution of each feature varying for different people. This suggestion is consistent with the overall hypothesis that many different factors appear to contribute to the development and perpetuation of CFS. The relative contribution of these different features may vary from individual to individual and even for the same patient over the course of the illness. The assessment and management of the patient with CFS should attempt to consider these issues and their relative importance for that individual.

DIAGNOSIS AND DIFFERENTIAL DIAGNOSIS

The diagnosis of CFS is one of exclusion and requires a comprehensive history. In the pediatric population, this information is obtained best from the patient and parents. Additionally we request that families bring prior medical records, test results, and pertinent school records to facilitate a complete evaluation. This process may be lengthy because the details are complicated, of long standing, and often a source of debate between the patient and parents. The history should focus on the onset of illness, the duration and severity of symptoms, prior evaluations (often multiple) as well as medical history before the illness, family history, academic performance, and social history. The physical examination of the individual with suspected CFS almost always is essentially normal despite the multitude of symptoms. Findings of mild pharyngeal erythema and cervical adenopathy commonly are reported. However finding fever, weight loss, significant adenopathy, or organomegaly should alert the clinician to the possibility of an alternative diagnosis.

DeMeirleir and colleagues reported increased detection of a 37-kDa, 2-5A-synthetase binding protein in peripheral blood mononuclear cells from patients with CFS compared with healthy controls.[32] These binding proteins are related to the ribonuclease L antiviral pathway of these cells. This finding requires further confirmation before it can be considered a potential diagnostic test for CFS. At present, no specific tests for diagnosing CFS exist, and laboratory testing is aimed primarily at eliminating other possible diagnoses. Most patients have undergone multiple laboratory tests before a diagnosis of CFS has been considered, but these tests may be repeated or completed as part of the initial CFS evaluation. Additionally, interpreting previously performed tests may be part of the initial patient assessment. Screening studies may include a complete blood cell count with differential and platelets, erythrocyte sedimentation rate, hepatic and renal function studies, urinalysis, and thyroid function tests. Additional tests that may be indicated based on history and physical examination may include toxicology screening, human immunodeficiency virus serology, antinuclear antibody, rheumatoid factor, tuberculin skin test, and cortisol level. Serologic evaluations for EBV, Lyme disease, and group A streptococcal infection may be requested based on history and physical infection. In most instances, these tests are not indicated; however they often are obtained before CFS is suspected, and they need to be appropriately reviewed or repeated as part of the initial evaluation for CFS. Screening radiographic studies may include a chest radiograph or imaging of the paranasal sinuses based on the patient's symptoms.

Elimination of every possible disorder that may cause a patient to experience prolonged fatigue is impossible, but, when guided by history, physical examination, and laboratory screening tests as outlined previously, the clinician can make a reliable diagnosis of CFS. Follow-up for periods of 4 to 13 years for pediatric patients diagnosed with CFS have not identified cases of missed or alternative diagnoses for their complaints.[7,66] In general, the longer the duration and the greater the number of symptoms, the less the need for extensive laboratory evaluations to suggest the diagnosis of CFS. Conversely alternative diagnoses should be considered if a single symptom dominates the clinical presentation or if physical examination or laboratory tests reveal significant abnormalities.

Psychosocial assessment is indicated for all children and adolescents presenting for CFS evaluation. The extent of such evaluation may be limited to assessment by primary care personnel or may include collaboration with a social worker, psychologist, or psychiatrist based on the individual's needs and the comfort level of the examiner. Cardiopulmonary and neurologic evaluations may be used in some cases, both to consider possible alternative diagnoses and to assist in assessing factors that may be contributing to the symptoms of CFS.

MANAGEMENT

One of the essential qualities of the clinician is interest in humanity, for the secret of care of the patient is in caring for the patient.

Dr. Francis Peabody, 1926

Management of patients with CFS is aimed at providing a combination of supportive treatment and emotional support (Box 78.2).[41] This process can be initiated during the initial evaluation, with a discussion of the diagnostic criteria for CFS and a review of the results of previously obtained laboratory tests. The relationship between physical and psychological symptoms can be explained, and the patient and family can be reassured that symptoms are real, even if the symptoms have psychiatric components. Additionally the patient and family can be advised that most children and adolescents with CFS do well over time[7,36,65,66] and have a better long-term outlook than that described for adults with CFS.[56,136] Furthermore emphasizing the frequent ups and downs in symptoms that generally characterize the course of CFS is important in assisting the patient and family to develop coping skills. This assistance

BOX 78.2 Approach to Management of Chronic Fatigue Syndrome in Children and Adolescents

- Evaluation and explanation of the diagnosis, including overview of multifactorial components
- Reassurance that symptoms are real
- Anticipatory guidance regarding secondary problems, up-and-down course of syndrome, secondary gain
- Coping skills: lifestyle modification, decreased stress, and realistic expectations and schedule
- Cognitive behavioral approaches: gradual increases in activity, an exercise program, attention to sleep patterns, attention to nutrition
- Psychological support for individual and family
- Educational issues: return to classes, home tutors, neuropsychiatric testing as indicated
- Relationship issues: friends and family
- Follow-up plan: monitoring of physical symptoms and psychological issues, ongoing guidance and reassurance (follow-up visits every 4–6 weeks)
- Minimize shopping for a doctor, unnecessary testing, family strain, and unconventional, unproven, or experimental therapies

Modified from Krilov LR, Fisher M. Chronic fatigue syndrome in children and adolescents. *Contemp Pediatr.* 2002;19:61–8.

may include guidance on how to modify lifestyle most appropriately and how to set realistic schedules and goals. Studies from the United Kingdom suggest that formal cognitive behavioral therapy[30,92,102,135] or graded exercise programs, or both, may be beneficial for patients with CFS.[20,43,70,131,134]

Consistent with this approach, results from a series of interviews with children diagnosed with CFS reported by Parslow and colleagues suggest that supportive schools, families, and friends as well as development of coping skills to manage activities could help ameliorate symptoms.[86]

Although, as noted earlier, the prognosis for children and adolescents with CFS is generally favorable, Roberts and colleagues suggest a possible increase in rate of suicide in 2147 cases of CFS followed at a CFS referral center over a 7-year period.[97]

Many other therapies have been advocated by different groups for patients with CFS. These treatments may include supplements, such as essential fatty acids,[130] magnesium,[28] liver extract injections,[58] and vitamin and nutritional supplements,[78] as well as pharmacologic treatments, such as corticosteroids,[22,81,88] reduced nicotinamide adenine dinucleotide,[128] antidepressants,[83,127] and growth hormone.[82] A recent brief observation report suggested that methylphenidate may be beneficial in relieving fatigue and improving concentration in some patients with CFS.[8] Homeopathic therapies, osteopathy, and massage therapy[37] also have been reported to be beneficial in the management of CFS. Most of these approaches have not been studied adequately to allow definitive comment on their potential benefit for a given patient. Still, the clinician should be aware of them to help guide patients who are likely to hear about them from other patients or outside sources, including the Internet.[44,133,135]

PROGNOSIS AND FUTURE DIRECTIONS

CFS likely affects heterogeneous groups of patients, and a single cause or definitive treatment modality most likely will not be uncovered. Nonetheless studying groups of such patients yields helpful information on the pathophysiology of this condition, and useful steps to address and alleviate symptoms for patients have been reported. In recognition of the significance of this entity, the CDC launched an awareness campaign, including the development of an Internet site for health care professionals and the public (http://www.cdc.gov/cfs/). In addition, long-term follow-up data demonstrating improvement over the course of time, especially in children and adolescents, without emergence of significant other conditions, are encouraging for patients, families, and clinicians caring for such individuals.

NEW REFERENCES SINCE THE SEVENTH EDITION

19. Centers for Disease Control and Prevention. Chronic fatigue syndrome (CFS) in children and adolescents. Available at: http://www.cdc.gov/cfs/pediatric/index.html.
21. Clayton EW. Beyond myalgic encephalomyelitis/chronic fatigue syndrome: an IOM report on redefining an illness. *JAMA*. 2015;313(11):1101-1102.
24. Collin SM, Norris T, Nuevo R, et al. Chronic fatigue syndrome at age 16 years. *Pediatrics*. 2016;137(2):e20153434.
26. Coplan J, Singh D, Gopinath S, et al. A novel anxiety and affective spectrum disorder of mind and body-the ALPIM (Anxiety-Laxity-Pain-Immune-Mood) syndrome: a preliminary report. *J Neuropsychiatr Clin Neurosci*. 2015;27(2):93-103.
53. Institute of Medicine. Beyond myalgic encephalomyelitis/chronic fatigue syndrome: redefining an illness. 2015. Available at: http://www.iom.edu/mecfs.
70. Larun L, Brurberg KG, Odgaard-Jensen J, et al. Exercise therapy for chronic fatigue syndrome. *Cochrane Database Syst Rev*. 2016;(6):CD003200.
86. Parslow R, Patel A, Beasant L, et al. What matters to children with CFS/ME? A conceptual model as the first stage in developing a PROM. *Arch Dis Child*. 2015;100(12):1141-1147.
97. Roberts E, Wessely S, Chalder T, et al. Mortality of people with chronic fatigue syndrome: a retrospective cohort study in England and Wales from the South London and Maudsley NHS Foundation Trust Biomedical Research Centre (SLaM BRC) Clinical Record Interactive Search (CRIS) Register. *Lancet*. 2016;387(10028):1638-1643.
126. van de Putte EM, van Doornen LJ, Engelbert RH, et al. Mirrored symptoms in mother and child with chronic fatigue syndrome. *Pediatrics*. 2006;117(6):2074-2079.

The full reference list for this chapter is available at ExpertConsult.com.

PART

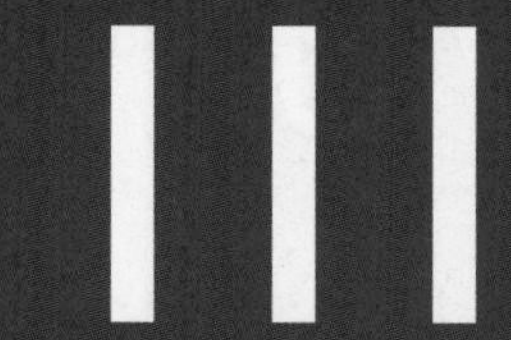

Infections With Specific Microorganisms

79 Nomenclature for Aerobic and Anaerobic Bacteria

David A. Bruckner

Table 79.1 represents an update of the current nomenclature, taxonomy, and classification of various microbial agents and is based on the organism's phenotypic and genotypic characteristics. Organisms included in this chapter are those that have been associated with pathologic processes or are medically significant. The current names are either officially recognized or proposed for recognition and currently used in the literature. Some organisms have been characterized but have never been cultured.

Taxonomic ranks for naming bacterial organisms include kingdom, division, class, order, family, genus, species, and subspecies. All of these ranks have official standing in nomenclature. Each taxonomic name should be represented by a nomenclature type. The species is represented by a type strain that is deposited in recognized culture collections.[3] Nomenclature priorities for bacteriologic names date back to May 1753. Because of difficulties in searching the literature and limited available information on described species, approved lists of bacterial names were published in the *International Journal of Systematic Bacteriology* in 1980. Names not included on those lists have lost all standing in nomenclature status.

Bacterial classification had relied on phenotypic information using physical characteristics and biochemical reactions; however these were poor parameters for establishing genetic relatedness. Multivariate analysis has played a large role in classification since the 1950s. DNA hybridization, rRNA-DNA hybridization, gene sequence analysis, and multilocus sequence analysis have played a major role in determining classifications. A prime example of this is reclassification of some species from the genus *Pseudomonas* to *Burkholderia* to *Ralstonia* (*R. pikettii*) or *Pseudomonas maltophilia* to *Xanthomonas maltophilia* to *Stenotrophomonas maltophilia.* Some changes are necessary due to a lack of criteria to define a genus or classification that was based on a single or limited number of isolates.

The *International Code of Nomenclature of Bacteria*[5] includes rules on how to name bacteria and use the name. Comprehensive taxonomic information for bacteriologic classification is found in *Bergey's Manual of Systematic Bacteriology,*[1,2,4,6,7] volumes 1 through 5. Names are validated only when they are included in the validation lists regularly published by the *International Journal of Systematic and Evolutionary Microbiology.*[3,5] An overview of validly published names can be viewed at http://www.bacterio.cict.fr or http://www.dsmz.de/bacterial-diversity/prokaryotic-nomenclature-up-to-date.

TABLE 79.1 Current Bacterial Nomenclature, Taxonomy, and Classification

Current Name	Synonym
I. Aerobic Gram-Positive Cocci	
Characteristics: Aerotolerant anaerobes that can occur singly or in pairs, tetrads, chains, or clusters; they can be catalase positive or catalase negative. Organisms positive for coagulase or clumping factor include *Staphylococcus aureus, Staphylococcus intermedius, Staphylococcus lugdunensis,* and *Staphylococcus schleiferi* subspecies *coagulans*	
Catalase-Positive Organisms	
Alloiococcus otitidis	*Alloiococcus otitis*
Auritidibacter ignavus	
Dermacoccus nishinomiyaensis	
Kocuria carniphila	
Kocuria kristinae	*Micrococcus kristinae*
Kocuria rhizophila	
Kocuria rosea	*Micrococcus roseus*
Kocuria varians	*Micrococcus varians*
Kytococcus schroeteri	
Kytococcus sedentarius	*Micrococcus sedentarius*
Micrococcus luteus	
Micrococcus lylae	
Rothia mucilaginosa	
Staphylococcus arlettae	
Staphylococcus aureus subspecies *anaerobius*	
Staphylococcus aureus subspecies *aureus*	
Staphylococcus auricularis	
Staphylococcus capitis subspecies *capitis*	
Staphylococcus capitis subspecies *ureolyticus*	
Staphylococcus caprae	
Staphylococcus carnosus subspecies *carnosus*	
Staphylococcus carnosus subspecies *utilis*	
Staphylococcus cohnii subspecies *cohnii*	
Staphylococcus cohnii subspecies *urealyticus*	
Staphylococcus condimenti	
Staphylococcus epidermidis	*Staphylococcus albus*
Staphylococcus felis	
Staphylococcus gallinarum	
Staphylococcus haemolyticus	
Staphylococcus hominis subspecies *hominis*	
Staphylococcus hominis subspecies *novobiosepticus*	
Staphylococcus hyicus	
Staphylococcus intermedius	
Staphylococcus kloosii	
Staphylococcus lentus	*Staphylococcus sciuri* subspecies *lentus*
Staphylococcus lugdunensis	
Staphylococcus massiliensis	
Staphylococcus nepalensis	
Staphylococcus pasteuri	
Staphylococcus pettenkoferi	
Staphylococcus pseudintermedius	
Staphylococcus saccharolyticus	*Peptococcus saccharolyticus*
Staphylococcus saprophyticus subspecies *bovis*	*Micrococcus* subgroup 3
Staphylococcus saprophyticus subspecies *saprophyticus*	*Staphylococcus saprophyticus* subspecies *saprophyticus*
Staphylococcus schleiferi subspecies *coagulans*	
Staphylococcus schleiferi subspecies *schleiferi*	
Staphylococcus sciuri subspecies *carnaticus*	
Staphylococcus sciuri subspecies *rodentium*	
Staphylococcus sciuri subspecies *sciuri*	
Staphylococcus simiae	
Staphylococcus simulans	
Staphylococcus succinus subspecies *casei*	
Staphylococcus succinus subspecies *succinus*	
Staphylococcus warneri	
Staphylococcus xylosus	
Catalase-Negative Organisms	
Abiotrophia defectiva	*Streptococcus defectivus* Nutritionally variant streptococci
Aerococcus christensenii	
Aerococcus sanguinicola	*Aerococcus sanguicola*
Aerococcus urinae	
Aerococcus urinaehominis	
Aerococcus viridans	
Dolosicoccus paucivorans	
Dolosigranulum pigrum	
Enterococcus avium	*Streptococcus avium* Group D *Enterococcus*
Enterococcus caccae	
Enterococcus casseliflavus	*Enterococcus flavescens* *Streptococcus casseliflavus*
Enterococcus cecorum	*Streptococcus cecorum*
Enterococcus dispar	
Enterococcus durans	*Streptococcus durans* Group D *Enterococcus*
Enterococcus faecalis	*Streptococcus faecalis* Group D *Enterococcus*
Enterococcus faecium	*Streptococcus faecium* Group D *Enterococcus*
Enterococcus gallinarum	*Streptococcus gallinarum*
Enterococcus gilvus	
Enterococcus hawaiiensis	
Enterococcus hirae	
Enterococcus italicus	*Enterococcus saccharominimus*
Enterococcus malodoratus	
Enterococcus mundtii	
Enterococcus pallens	
Enterococcus pseudoavium	
Enterococcus raffinosus	
Enterococcus sanguinicola	
Enterococcus thailandicus	
Facklamia hominis	
Facklamia ignava	
Facklamia languida	

Continued

TABLE 79.1 Current Bacterial Nomenclature, Taxonomy, and Classification—cont'd

Current Name	Synonym
Facklamia sourekii	
Gemella bergeri	*Gemella bergeriae*
Gemella haemolysans	*Neisseria haemolysans*
Gemella morbillorum	*Streptococcus morbillorum* *Peptostreptococcus morbillorum*
Gemella sanguinis	
Globicatella sanguinis	Salt-tolerant viridans streptococci
Granulicatella adiacens	*Abiotrophia adiacens* *Streptococcus adiacens* Nutritionally variant streptococci
Granulicatella elegans	*Abiotrophia elegans* Nutritionally variant streptococci
Granulicatella para-adiacens	
Helcococcus kunzii	
Helcococcus sueciensis	
Ignavigranum ruoffiae	
Lactococcus garvieae	*Streptococcus garvieae* Lancefield group N
Lactococcus lactis	
Leuconostoc citreum	
Leuconostoc lactis	
Leuconostoc mesenteroides	
Leuconostoc pseudomesenteroides	
Pediococcus acidilactici	
Pediococcus pentosaceus	
Streptococcus acidominimus	
Streptococcus anginosis group	Viridans streptococci
Streptococcus anginosus	
Streptococcus constellatus subspecies *constellatus*	
Streptococcus constellatus subspecies *pharyngis*	
Streptococcus constellatus subspecies *viborgensis*	
Streptococcus intermedius	
Streptococcus bovis group	Group D streptococci
Streptococcus alactolyticus	
Streptococcus bovis	
Streptococcus equinus	
Streptococcus gallolyticus subspecies *gallolyticus*	
Streptococcus gallolyticus subspecies *macedonicus*	
Streptococcus gallolyticus subspecies *pasteurianus*	
Streptococcus infantarius subspecies *coli*	
Streptococcus infantarius subspecies *infantarius*	
Streptococcus hongkongensis	
***Streptococcus mitis* group**	Viridans streptococci
Streptococcus australis	
Streptococcus cristatus	
Streptococcus gordonii	
Streptococcus infantis	
Streptococcus massiliensis	
Streptococcus mitis	
Streptococcus oralis	
Streptococcus oligfermentans	
Streptococcus orisratti	
Streptococcus parasanguinis	
Streptococcus peroris	
Streptococcus pneumonia	
Streptococcus pseudopneumoniae	
Streptococcus sanguinis	
Streptococcus sinensis	
***Streptococcus mutans* group**	*Viridans streptococci*
Streptococcus criceti	
Streptococcus downei	
Streptococcus mutans	
Streptococcus ratti	
Streptococcus sobrinus	
***Streptococcus pyogenes* group**	
Streptococcus agalactiae	
Streptococcus canis	
Streptococcus dysgalactiae subspecies *equisimilis*	
Streptococcus equi subspecies *zooepidermidis*	
Streptococcus iniae	
Streptococcus porcinus	
Streptococcus pyogenes	
***Streptococcus salivarius* group**	Viridans streptococci
Streptococcus salivarius	
Streptococcus thermophiles	
Streptococcus vestibularis	
Streptococcus suis	
Tetragenococcus halophilus	*Pediococcus halophilus*
Tetragenococcus solitarius	*Enterococcus solitarius*
Vagococcus fluvialis	
Weissella paramesenteroides	*Leuconostoc paramesenteroides*
II. Anaerobic Gram-Positive Cocci	
Characteristics: Occur singly or in pairs, chains, or clumps	
Anaerococcus hydrogenalis	*Peptostreptococcus hydrogenalis*
Anaerococcus lactolyticus	*Peptostreptococcus lactolyticus*
Anaerococcus murdochii	
Anaerococcus octavius	*Peptostreptococcus octavius*
Anaerococcus prevotii	*Peptostreptococcus prevotii*
Anaerococcus tetradius	*Peptostreptococcus tetradius*
Anaerococcus vaginalis	
Anaerosphaera aminiphila	
Atopobium parvulum	
Blautica coccoides	*Clostridium coccoides*
Blautica productus	*Peptostreptococcus productus* *Ruminococcus productus*
Blautica wexlerae	
Fingoldia magna	*Peptococcus magnus*
Murdochiella asaccharolytica	
Parvimonas micra	*Peptostreptococcus micros* *Micromonas micros*
Peptococcus niger	*Micrococcus niger*
Peptoniphilus asaccharolyticus	*Peptostreptococcus asaccharolyticus*
Peptoniphilus coxii	
Peptoniphilus duerdenii	
Peptoniphilus gorbachii	
Peptoniphilus harei	*Peptostreptococcus harei*
Peptoniphilus indolicus	
Peptoniphilus ivorii	*Peptostreptococcus ivorii*
Peptoniphilus koeoeneniae	
Peptoniphilus lacrimalis	*Peptostreptococcus lacrimalis*
Peptoniphilus olsenii	
Peptostreptococcus anaerobius	
Peptostreptococcus indolicus	*Peptococcus indolicus*
Peptostreptococcus magna	*Peptococcus magnus* *Peptococcus variabilis*
Peptostreptococcus massiliae	
Peptostreptococcus stomatis	
Peptostreptococcus trisimilis	
Ruminococcus gauvreauii	*Streptococcus hansenii*
Slackia heliotrinireducens corrig	*Peptostreptococcus heliotrinireducens*

TABLE 79.1 Current Bacterial Nomenclature, Taxonomy, and Classification—cont'd

Current Name	Synonym
III. Aerobic Gram-Negative Cocci	
Characteristics: Occur singly or in pairs or clumps; catalase and oxidase positive	
Lautropia mirabilis	*Sarcina mirabilis*
Neisseria bacilliformis	
Neisseria canis	
Neisseria cinerea	*Micrococcus cinereus* *Neisseria pharyngis*
Neisseria elongata subspecies *elongata*	*Neisseria elongata*
Neisseria elongata subspecies *glycolytica*	*Neisseria elongata*
Neisseria elongata subspecies *nitroreducens*	*Neisseria elongate* CDC group M-6
Neisseria flavescens	
Neisseria gonorrhoeae	
Neisseria lactamica	*Neisseria lactamicus*
Neisseria meningitidis	
Neisseria mucosa	
Neisseria polysaccharea	
Neisseria shayeganii	
Neisseria sicca	
Neisseria subflava biovar *flava*	*Neisseria subflava*
Neisseria subflava biovar *perflava*	*Neisseria subflava*
Neisseria subflava biovar *subflava*	*Neisseria subflava*
Neisseria wadsworthii	
Neisseria weaveri	Moraxella sp. M-5 CDC group M-5
IV. Anaerobic Gram-Negative Cocci	
Characteristics: Occur in pairs or clumps	
Acidaminococcus fermentans	
Acidaminococcus intestini	
Anaeroglobus geminatus	
Megasphaera elsdenii	*Peptostreptococcus elsdenii*
Megasphaera micronuciformis	
Negativivicoccus spp.	
Veillonella alcalescens	
Veillonella atypica	
Veillonella denticariosi	
Veillonella dispar	
Veillonella montpellierensis	
Veillonella parvula	
V. Aerobic Gram-Positive Bacilli	
Characteristics: Rodlike; catalase negative or catalase positive; some are acid-fast stain–positive, and some have branching. Only *Bacillus, Brevibacillus,* and *Brevibacterium* spp. produce spores	
Actinomadura chibensis	
Actinomadura cremea	
Actinomadura dassonvillei	
Actinomadura latina	
Actinomadura madurae	
Actinomadura nitritigenes	
Actinomadura pelletieri	
Actinomadura spuuti	
Arcanobacterium bernardiae	*Actinomyces bernardiae* CDC coryneform group 2
Arcanobacterium haemolyticum	*Corynebacterium haemolyticum*
Arcanobacterium pyogenes	*Actinomyces pyogenes* *Corynebacterium pyogenes*
Arthrobacter albus	
Arthrobacter cumminsii	

Current Name	Synonym
Arthrobacter oxydans	
Bacillus anthracis	
Bacillus cereus	
Bacillus circulans	
Bacillus coagulans	
Bacillus cytotoxicus	
Bacillus firmus	
Bacillus idriensis	
Bacillus infantis	
Bacillus lentus	
Bacillus licheniformis	
Bacillus megaterium	
Bacillus mycoides	
Bacillus pumilus	
Bacillus sphaericus	
Bacillus subtilis	
Bacillus thuringiensis	
Brevibacillus agri	*Bacillus agri*
Brevibacillus brevis	*Bacillus brevis*
Brevibacillus centrosporus	
Brevibacillus laterosporus	*Bacillus laterosporus*
Brevibacillus parabrevis	CDC coryneform groups B-1 and B-3
Brevibacterium casei	
Brevibacterium luteolum	
Brevibacterium mcbrellneri	
Brevibacterium sanguinis	
Cellulomonas denverensis	CDC coryneform group A-3
Cellulomonas hominis	
Cellulosimicrobium cellulans	*Cellulomonas cellulans* *Oerskovia xanthineolytica* CDC coryneform groups A-1 and A-2
Cellulosimicrobium funkei	
Corynebacterium accolens	
Corynebacterium afermentans subspecies *afermentans*	CDC coryneform group ANF-1
Corynebacterium afermentans subspecies *lipophilum*	CDC coryneform group ANF-1
Corynebacterium amycolatum	*Corynebacterium xerosis* *Corynebacterium minutissimum* *Corynebacterium striatum* CDC coryneform groups F-2 and I-2
Corynebacterium aquaticum	
Corynebacterium appendicis	
Corynebacterium argentoratense	
Corynebacterium atypicum	
Corynebacterium aurimucosum	CDC fermentive coryneform group 4
Corynebacterium auris	*Corynebacterium nigricans* CDC coryneform group ANF-1
Corynebacterium bovis	
Corynebacterium canis	
Corynebacterium confusum	
Corynebacterium coyleae	
Corynebacterium diphtheriae	
Corynebacterium durum	
Corynebacterium falsenii	
Corynebacterium freiburgense	
Corynebacteriun freneyi	
Corynebacterium glucuronolyticum	
Corynebacterium hansenii	
Corynebacterium imitans	

Continued

TABLE 79.1 **Current Bacterial Nomenclature, Taxonomy, and Classification—cont'd**

Current Name	Synonym
Corynebacterium jeikeium	*Corynebacterium* group JK CDC coryneform group JK
Corynebacterium kroppenstedtii	
Corynebacterium lipophiloflavum	
Corynebacterium macginleyi	CDC coryneform group G-1
Corynebacterium massiliense	
Corynebacterium matruchotii	*Bacterionema matruchotii*
Corynebacterium minutissimum	
Corynebacterium mucifaciens	
Corynebacterium nigricans	
Corynebacterium pilbarense	
Corynebacterium propinquum	CDC coryneform group ANF-3
Corynebacterium pseudodiphtheriticum	*Corynebacterium hofmannii*
Corynebacterium pseudogenitalium	
Corynebacterium pseudotuberculosis	
Corynebacterium resistens	
Corynebacterium riegelii	
Corynebacterium sanguinis	
Corynebacterium simulans	
Corynebacterium singulare	
Corynebacterium stationis	
Corynebacterium striatum	
Corynebacterium sundsvallense	*Corynebacterium thomssenii* *Rothia dentocariosa*
Corynebacterium thomssenii	
Corynebacterium timonense	
Corynebacterium tuberculostearicum	
Corynebacterium tuscania	
Corynebacterium ulcerans	
Corynebacterium urealyticum	*Corynebacterium* group D2 CDC coryneform group D2
Corynebacterium ureicelerivorans	
Corynebacterium xerosis	
Curtobacterium spp.	
Dermabacter hominis	CDC fermentative coryneform groups 3 and 5
Dermatophilus congolensis	*Actinomyces congolensis*
Dietzia maris	
Dietzia schimaea	
Erysipelothrix rhusiopathiae	*Erysipelothrix insidiosa*
Exiguobacterium acetylicum	*Brevibacterium acetylicum*
Exiguobacterium aurantiacum	*Brevibacterium aurantiacum*
Gardnerella vaginalis	*Haemophilus vaginalis* *Corynebacterium vaginalis*
Geobacillus stearothermophilus	
Gordonia bronchialis	*Rhodococcus bronchialis*
Gordonia effuse	
Gordonia otitidis	
Gordonia polyisoprenivorans	
Gordonia rubropertincta	*Rhodococcus rubiopertincta*
Gordonia sputi	*Rhodococcus sputi* *Rhodococcus chubuensis*
Gordonia terrae	*Rhodococcus terrae*
Listeria ivanovii subspecies *ivanovii*	*Listeria monocytogenes* serovar 5
Listeria monocytogenes	
Microbacterium foliorum	
Microbacterium oxydans	
Mycobacterium africanum	
Mycobacterium arosiense	
Mycobacterium arupense	
Mycobacterium asiaticum	
Mycobacterium avium subspecies *avium*	
Mycobacterium avium subspecies *hominissuis*	
Mycobacterium avium subspecies *paratuberculosis*	
Mycobacterium bacteremicum	
Mycobacterium boenickei	
Mycobacterium bohemicum	
Mycobacterium botniense	
Mycobacterium bouchedurhonense	
Mycobacterium bovis	
Mycobacterium branderi	
Mycobacterium brumae	
Mycobacterium canariassense	
Mycobacterium canettii	
Mycobacterium caprae	
Mycobacterium celatum	
***Mycobacterium chelonae/abscessus* group**	
Mycobacterium abscessus subspecies *abscessus*	
Mycobacterium abscessus subspecies *bolletii*	
Mycobacterium abscessus subspecies *massiliense*	
Mycobacterium chelonae	
Mycobacterium immunogenum	
Mycobacterium salmoniphilum	
Mycobacterium chimaera	
Mycobacterium colombiense	
Mycobacterium conspicuum	
Mycobacterium cookii	
Mycobacterium cosmeticum	
Mycobacterium doricum	
Mycobacterium elephantis	
Mycobacterium engbackii	
Mycobacterium europaeum	
Mycobacterium farcinogenes	
Mycobacterium florentinum	
***Mycobacterium fortuitum* group**	
Mycobacterium boenickei	
Mycobacterium brisbanense	
Mycobacterium fortuitum	
Mycobacterium houstonense	
Mycobacterium neworleansense	
Mycobacterium peregrimum	
Mycobacterium porcinum	
Mycobacterium senegalense	
Mycobacterium septicum	
Mycobacterium setense	
Mycobacterium fragae	
Mycobacterium gastri	
Mycobacterium genavense	
Mycobacterium gordonae	*Mycobacterium aquae*
Mycobacterium haemophilum	
Mycobacterium heckeshornense	
Mycobacterium heidelbergense	
Mycobacterium heraklionense	
Mycobacterium hiberniae	
Mycobacterium interjectum	

TABLE 79.1 Current Bacterial Nomenclature, Taxonomy, and Classification—cont'd

Current Name	Synonym
Mycobacterium intermedium	
Mycobacterium intracellulare	
Mycobacterium iranicum	
Mycobacterium kansasii	
Mycobacterium kubicae	
Mycobacterium kyorinrnse	
Mycobacterium lentiflavum	
Mycobacterium leprae	
Mycobacterium lepraemurium	
Mycobacterium llatzerense	
Mycobacterium longobardum	
***Mycobacterium mageritense/ wolinskyi* group**	
Mycobacterium mageritense	
Mycobacterium wolinskyi	
Mycobacterium malmoense	
Mycobacterium mantenii	*Mycobacterium balnei*
Mycobacterium marseillense	
Mycobacterium marinum	
Mycobacterium microti	
Mycobacterium monacense	
Mycobacterium monteofiorense	
***Mycobacterium mucogenicum* group**	
Mycobacterium aubagnense	
Mycobacterium mucogenicum	
Mycobacterium phocaicum	
Mycobacterium moriokaense	
Mycobacterium nebraskense	
Mycobacterium neoaurum	
Mycobacterium neworleansene	
Mycobacterium nonchromogenicum	
Mycobacterium noviomagense	
Mycobacterium novocastrense	
Mycobacterium palustre	
Mycobacterium paraffinicum	
Mycobacterium paragordonae	
Mycobacterium parakereense	
Mycobacterium parascrofulaceum	
Mycobacterium paraseoulense	
Mycobacterium parmense	
Mycobacterium pseudoshottsii	
Mycobacterium pulveris	
Mycobacterium riyadhense	
Mycobacterium saskatchewanense	
Mycobacterium scrofulaceum	
Mycobacterium senuense	
Mycobacterium seoulense	
Mycobacterium sherrisii	
Mycobacterium shimoidei	
Mycobacterium shinjukuense	
Mycobacterium simiae	*Mycobacterium habana*
Mycobacterium smegmatis group	
Mycobacterium goodi	
Mycobacterium smegmatis	
Mycobacterium stomatepiae	
Mycobacterium szulgai	
Mycobacterium terrae	
Mycobacterium timonense	
Mycobacterium triplex	
Mycobacterium triviale	
Mycobacterium tuberculosis	
Mycobacterium tusciae	
Mycobacterium ulcerans	*Mycobacterium buruli*
Mycobacterium vulneris	
Mycobacterium xenopi	
Mycobacterium youngonense	
Nocardia abscessus	
Nocardia africana	
Nocardia anaemiae	
Nocardia aobensis	
Nocardia araoensis	
Nocardia arthritidis	
Nocardia asiatica	
Nocardia asteroides type IV	
Nocardia beijingensis	
Nocardia blacklockiae	
Nocardia brasiliensis	
Nocardia brevicatena	*Micropolyspora brevicatena*
Nocardia carnea	
Nocardia concava	
Nocardia corynebacteroides	
Nocardia cyriacigeorgica	*Nocardia cyriacigeorgici*
Nocardia elegans	
Nocardia exalbida	
Nocardia farcinica	
Nocardia higoensis	
Nocardia ignorata	
Nocardia inohanensis	
Nocardia kruczakiae	
Nocardia mexicana	
Nocardia neocaledoniensis	
Nocardia nigatensis	
Nocardia ninae	
Nocardia niwae	
Nocardia nova	
Nocardia otitidiscaviarum	*Nocardia caviae*
Nocardia paucivorans	
Nocardia pneumoniae	
Nocardia pseudobrasiliensis	
Nocardia puris	
Nocardia shimofusensis	
Nocardia sienata	*Nocardia senatus*
Nocardia takadensii	
Nocardia terpenica	
Nocardia thailandica	
Nocardia transvalensis	
Nocardia vermiculata	
Nocardia veterana	
Nocardia vinacea	
Nocardia wallacei	
Nocardia yamanashiensis	
Nocardiopsis dassonvillei	*Actionmadura dassonvillei* *Nocardia dassonvillei*
Paenibacillus alvei	*Bacillus alvei*
Paenibacillus konsidensis	
Paenibacillus macerans	*Bacillus mascerans*
Paenibacillus polymyxa	*Bacillus polymyxa*
Paenibacillus popiliae	
Paenibacillus sanguinis	
Paenibacillus timonensis	

Continued

TABLE 79.1 Current Bacterial Nomenclature, Taxonomy, and Classification—cont'd

Current Name	Synonym
Prescottella equi	*Rhodococcus equi* *Corynebacterium equi*
Rothia aeria	
Rothia dentocariosa	*Nocardia dentocariosus*
Rothia mucilaginosa	*Stomatococcus mucilaginosus*
Streptomyces albus	
Streptomyces bikiniensis	
Streptomyces somaliensis	
Streptomyces thermovulgaris	
Tropheryma whipplei	*Tropheryma whippelii*
Tsukamurella inchonensis	
Tsukamurella paurometabola	*Gordona aurantiaca*
Tsukamurella pulmonis	
Tsukamurella stranjordii	
Tsukamurella tyrosinosolvens	
Turicella otitidis	*Rhodococcus aurantiacus*
Williamsia deligens	
Williamsia muralis	
VI. Anaerobic Gram-Positive Bacilli (Non–Spore-Forming)	
Characteristics: May be long-branching bacilli or pleomorphic coccobacilli	
Actinobaculum massiliae	
Actinobaculum schaalii	
Actinobaculum urinale	
Actinomyces cardiffensis	
Actinomyces dentalis	
Actinomyces europaeus	
Actinomyces funkei	
Actinomyces georgiae	*Actinomyces* D08
Actinomyces gerencseriae	*Actinomyces israelii* serotype II
Actinomyces graevenitzii	
Actinomyces hongkongensis	
Actinomyces israelii	
Actinomyces johnsonii	
Actinomyces massiliensis	
Actinomyces meyeri	
Actinomyces naeslundii	
Actinomyces nasicola	
Actinomyces neuii subspecies *anitratus*	
Actinomyces neuii subspecies *neuii*	CDC coryneform group 1
Actinomyces odontolyticus	
Actinomyces oricola	
Actinomyces radicidentis	
Actinomyces radingae	CDC coryneform group E; APL1
Actinomyces timonensis	
Actinomyces turicensis	CDC coryneform group E; APL10
Actinomyces urogenitalis	
Actinomyces viscosus	
Anaerofustis stercorihominis	
Atopobium fossor	*Eubacterium fossor*
Atopobium minutum	*Lactobacillus minutus*
Atopobium parvulum	*Streptococcus parvulus* *Peptostreptococcus parvulus*
Atopobium rimae	*Lactobacillus rimae*
Atopobium vaginae	
Bifidobacterium adolescentis	
Bifidobacterium breve	
Bifidobacterium dentium	*Bifidobacterium appendicitis*
Bifidobacterium infantis	*Bifidobacterium infantis*
Bifidobacterium longum	*Bifidobacterium longum*
Bifidobacterium scardovii	
Bifidobacterium suis	
Collinsella aerofaciens	*Eubacterium aerofaciens*
Collinsella intestinalis	
Collinsella stercoralis	
Cryptobacterium curtum	
Dorea formicigenerans	*Eubacterium formicigenerans*
Dorea longicatena	
Eggerthella hongkongensis	
Eggerthella lenta	*Eubacterium lentum*
Eggerthella sinensis	
Eggerthia catenaformis	*Lactobacillus catenaformis*
Eubacterium brachy	
Eubacterium contortum	
Eubacterium infirmum	
Eubacterium limosum	
Eubacterium minutum	*Eubacterium tardum*
Eubacterium moniliforme	
Eubacterium nitritogenes	
Eubacterium nodatum	
Eubacterium rectale	
Eubacterium saphenum	
Eubacterium sulci	*Fusobacterium sulci*
Eubacterium tenue	
Eubacterium ventriosum	
Eubacterium yurii subspecies *margaretiae*	
Eubacterium yurii subspecies *yurii*	
Holdemania filiformis	*Eubacterium* S14
Kandleria vitulinus	*Lactobacillus vitulinus*
Lachnoanaerobaculum saburreum	*Eubacterium saburreum*
Lactobacillus acidophilus	
Lactobacillus casei	
Lactobacillus colehominis	
Lactobacillus confusus	
Lactobacillus crispatus	
Lactobacillus fermentum	
Lactobacillus gasseri	
Lactobacillus iners	
Lactobacillus jensenii	
Lactobacillus johnsonii	
Lactobacillus plantarum	
Lactobacillus rhamnosus	*Lactobacillus* GG
Lactobacillus salivarius	
Lactobacillus ultunensis	
Mobiluncus curtisii	
Mobiluncus mulieris	*Falcivibrio grandis*
Mogibacterium timidum	
Mogibacterium vescum	
Olsenella profusa	
Olsenella uli	*Lactobacillus uli*
Parascardovia denticolens	*Bifidobacterium denticolens*
Propionibacterium acidifaciens	
Propionibacterium acnes	
Propionibacterium avidum	
Propionibacterium granulosum	
Propionibacterium propionicum	*Propionibacterium propionicum* *Arachnia propionica* *Actinomyces propionicus*
Pseudoramibacter alactolyticus	*Eubacterium alactolyticum*

TABLE 79.1 **Current Bacterial Nomenclature, Taxonomy, and Classification—cont'd**

Current Name	Synonym
Scardovia inopinata	*Bifidobacterium inopinatum* *Bifidobacterium dentium*
Scardovia wiggsiae	
Shuttleworthia satelles	
Slackia exigua	*Eubacterium exigaum*
Slackia heliotrinireducens	
Solobacterium moorei	
Varibaculum cambriense	
VII. Anaerobic Gram-Positive Bacilli (Spore-Forming)	
Characteristics: Broad, short bacilli with blunt ends. Most organisms readily produce spores, except *Clostridium perfringens* and *Tissierella praeacuta*	
Clostridium argentinense	*Clostridium botulinum* group G *Clostridium subterminale* *Clostridium hastiforme*
Clostridium baratii	*Clostridium barati* *Clostridium paraperfringens* *Clostridium perenne*
Clostridium bifermentans	
Clostridium bolteae	
Clostridium botulinum	*Clostridium putrificum*
Clostridium butyricum	*Clostridium pseudotetanicum*
Clostridium cadaveris	
Clostridium carnis	
Clostridium celerecrescens	
Clostridium chauvoei	
Clostridium clostridioforme	*Clostridium clostridioforme*
Clostridium coccides	
Clostridium cocleatum	
Clostridium difficile	*Clostridium difficilis*
Clostridium disporicum	
Clostridium fallax	*Clostridium pseudofallax*
Clostridium ghonii	*Clostridium ghoni*
Clostridium glycolicum	
Clostridium hastiforme	
Clostridium hathewayi	
Clostridium histolyticum	
Clostridium indolis	
Clostridium innocuum	
Clostridium intestinale	
Clostridium leptum	
Clostridium limosum	CDC group P-1
Clostridium neonatale	
Clostridium novyi	
Clostridium orbiscindens	
Clostridium paraputrificum	
Clostridium perfringens	*Clostridium welchii* *Welchia perfringens*
Clostridium putrificum	
Clostridium ramosum	*Eubacterium filamentosum* *Ramibacterium ramosum* *Actinomyces ramosus* *Eubacterium ramosum*
Clostridium septicum	
Clostridium sordellii	
Clostridium sphenoides	
Clostridium spiroforme	
Clostridium sporogenes	Nontoxigenic *Clostridium botulinum*
Clostridium subterminale	
Clostridium symbiosum	*Fusobacterium symbiosum* *Fusobacterium biacutus* *Bacteroides symbiosus*
Clostridium tertium	
Clostridium tetani	
Filifactor alocis	*Fusobacterium alocis*
Filifactor villosus	*Clostridium villosum*
Tissierella praeacuta	*Bacteroides praeacutus* *Clostridium hastiforme*
VIII. Aerobic Gram-Negative Bacilli: Enterobacteriaceae	
Characteristics: Ferment sugars; are oxidase-negative; most reduce nitrate to nitrite. Diagnostic laboratories may report *Salmonella* serovars by name (e.g., *Salmonella typhi* or *Salmonella* serovar *Typhi*)	
Buttiauxella gaviniae	
Buttiauxella noackiae	CDC enteric group 59
Cedecea davisae	CDC enteric group 15
Cedecea lapagei	
Cedecea neteri	
Citrobacter amalonaticus	*Levinea amalonatica*
Citrobacter braakii	*Citrobacter freundii*
Citrobacter farmeri	*Citrobacter amalonaticus* biogroup 1
Citrobacter freundii	*Colobactrum freundii*
Citrobacter gillenii	*Citrobacter genomospecies* 10 *Citrobacter freundii*
Citrobacter koseri	*Citrobacter diversus* *Levinea malonatica*
Citrobacter murliniae	*Citrobacter genomospecies* 11 *Citrobacter freundii*
Citrobacter rodentium	*Citrobacter genomospecies* 9 *Citrobacter freundii*
Citrobacter sedlakii	*Citrobacter genomospecies* 8 *Citrobacter freundii*
Citrobacter werkmanii	*Citrobacter genomospecies* 7 *Citrobacter freundii*
Citrobacter youngae	*Citrobacter genomospecies* 5 *Citrobacter freundii*
Cronobacter condimenti	*Enterobacter sakazakii*
Cronobacter dublinensis	*Enterobacter sakazakii*
Cronobacter malonaticus	*Enterobacter sakazakii*
Cronobacter muytjensii	*Enterobacter sakazakii*
Cronobacter sakazakii	*Enterobacter sakazakii*
Cronobacter turicensis	*Enterobacter sakazakii*
Cronobacter universalis	
Edwardsiella tarda	
Enterobacter aerogenes	*Aerobacter aerogenes*
Enterobacter agglomerans group	
Enterobacter amnigenus	
Enterobacter asburiae	CDC enteric group 17
Enterobacter cancerogenus	*Enterobacter cancerogenus* *Erwinia cancerogena* CDC enteric group 19
Enterobacter cloacae subspecies *cloacae*	
Enterobacter hormaechei subspecies *hormaechei*	
Enterobacter hormaechei subspecies *oharae*	
Enterobacter hormaechei subspecies *steigerwaltii*	
Enterobacter kobei	
Enterobacter ludwisii	
Erwinia persicinus	
Escherichia albertii	
Escherichia coli	

Continued

TABLE 79.1 Current Bacterial Nomenclature, Taxonomy, and Classification—cont'd

Current Name	Synonym
Escherichia fergusonii	CDC enteric group 10
Escherichia hermannii	CDC enteric group 11
Escherichia vulneris	CDC enteric group 1
Ewingella americana	CDC enteric group 40
Franconibacter heleviticus	
Franconibacter pulveris	
Hafnia alvei	*Enterobacter hafniae*
Klebsiella granulomatis	*Calymmatobacterium granulomatis*
Klebsiella oxytoca	
Klebsiella ozaenae	*Klebsiella ozaenae*
Klebsiella pneumoniae subspecies *pneumoniae*	*Klebsiella pneumoniae*
Klebsiella rhinoscleromatis	
Klebsiella variicola	
Kluyvera ascorbata	CDC enteric group 8
Kluyvera cryocrescens	
Kluyvera georgiana	CDC enteric group 36/37 *Kluyvera* spp. group 3
Leclercia adecarboxylata	*Escherichia adecarboxylata* CDC enteric group 41
Leminorella grimontii	CDC enteric group 57
Leminorella richardii	
Moellerella wisconsensis	CDC enteric group 46
Morganella morganii subspecies *morganii*	*Proteus morganii*
Morganella morganii subspecies *sibonii*	*Proteus morganii*
Morganella psychrotolerans	
Pantoea agglomerans	*Enterobacter agglomerans*
Pantoea brenneri	
Pantoea conspicua	
Pantoea eucrina	
Pantoea septica	
Photorhabdus asymbiotica subspecies *asymbiotica*	
Photorhabdus asymbiotica subspecies *australis*	
Photorhabdus luminescens	
Photorhabdus temperata	
Pluralibacter gergoviae	*Enterobacter gergoviae*
Proteus hauseri	*Proteus vulgaris* biogroup 3
Proteus mirabilis	
Proteus penneri	*Proteus vulgaris* biogroup 1
Proteus vulgaris	*Proteus vulgaris* biogroup 2
Providencia alcalifaciens	*Proteus inconstans*
Providencia heimbachae	
Providencia rettgeri	*Proteus rettgeri*
Providencia rustigianii	*Providencia alcalifaciens* biogroup 3
Providencia stuartii	*Proteus inconstans*
Rahnella aquatilis	
Raoultella ornithinolytica	*Klebsiella ornithinolytica*
Raoultella planticola	*Klebsiella planticola*
Raoultella terrigena	*Klebsiella terrigena*
Salmonella bongori	*Salmonella* subspecies V
Salmonella enterica subspecies *arizonae*	*Salmonella choleraesuis* subspecies *arizonae* *Salmonella* subspecies IIIa
Salmonella enterica subspecies *diarizonae*	*Salmonella choleraesuis* subspecies *diarizonae* *Salmonella* subspecies IIIb
Salmonella enterica subspecies *enterica*	*Salmonella choleraesuis* subspecies *choleraesuis* *Salmonella* subspecies I
Salmonella enterica subspecies *houtenae*	*Salmonella choleraesuis* subspecies *houtenae* *Salmonella* subspecies IV
Salmonella enterica subspecies *indica*	*Salmonella choleraesuis* subspecies *indica* *Salmonella* subspecies VI
Salmonella enterica subspecies *salamae*	*Salmonella choleraesuis* subspecies *salamae* *Salmonella* subspecies II
Serratia ficaria	
Serratia fonticola	
Serratia grimesii	
Serratia liquefaciens	*Serratia liquefaciens* *Enterobacter liquefaciens*
Serratia marcescens subspecies *marcescens*	
Serratia marcescens subspecies *sakuensis*	
Serratia odorifera	
Serratia plymuthica	
Serratia rubidaea	
Shigella boydii	*Shigella* biogroup C
Shigella dysenteriae	*Shigella* biogroup A
Shigella flexneri	*Shigella* biogroup B
Shigella sonnei	*Shigella* biogroup D
Schimuellia blattae	*Escherichia blattae*
Tatumella ptyseos	CDC group EF-9
Yersinia aldovae	
Yersinia aleksiciae	
Yersinia bercovieri	
Yersinia enterocolitica	*Yersinia enterocolitica* biogroup 3b *Pasteurella enterocolitica*
Yersinia entomophaga	
Yersinia frederiksenii	
Yersinia intermedia	
Yersinia kristensenii	
Yersinia massiliensis	
Yersinia mollaretii	*Yersinia enterocolitica* biogroup 3a
Yersinia nurmii	
Yersinia pekkanenii	
Yersinia pestis	*Pasteurella pestis*
Yersinia pseudotuberculosis	*Pasteurella pseudotuberculosis*
Yersinia rohdei	
Yersinia ruckeri	
Yersinia similis	
Yokenella regensburgei	*Koserella trabulsii* CDC enteric group 45
IX. Aerobic Gram-Negative Bacilli: Nonenterobacteriaceae; Fermentative	
Characteristics: Ferment sugars; are oxidase positive	
Aeromonas bestiarum	
Aeromonas caviae	
Aeromonas eucrenophilas	
Aeromonas hydrophila	*Pseudomonas hydrophila*
Aeromonas jandaei	
Aeromonas media	
Aeromonas salmonicida	

TABLE 79.1 **Current Bacterial Nomenclature, Taxonomy, and Classification—cont'd**

Current Name	Synonym
Aeromonas schubertii	
Aeromonas trota	
Aeromonas veronii	
Chromobacterium violaceum	*Bacillus violaceus*
Grimontia hollisae	*Vibrio hollisae*
Pasteurella aerogenes	
Pasteurella bettyae	CDC group HB-5
Pasteurella canis	*Pasteurella multocida* biotype 6
Pasteurella dagmatis	*Pasteurella* new sp 1 *Pasteurella* "gas"
Pasteurella multocida subspecies *gallicida*	
Pasteurella multocida subspecies *multocida*	
Pasteurella multocida subspecies *septica*	*Pasteurella septica*
Pasteurella pneumotropica	
Pasteurella stomatis	
Photobacterium damselae	*Vibrio damsel* CDC group EF5
Plesiomonas shigelloides	*Aeromonas shigelloides*
Vibrio alginolyticus	*Vibrio parahaemolyticus* biotype 2
Vibrio cholerae	*Vibrio comma*
Vibrio cincinnatiensis	
Vibrio fluvialis	CDC group EF-6
Vibrio furnissii	*Vibrio fluvialis* biogroup 2
Vibrio harveyi	
Vibrio metschnikovii	CDC enteric group 16 *Vibrio cholerae* biovar *proteus*
Vibrio mimicus	*Vibrio cholerae* sucrose negative
Vibrio parahaemolyticus	
Vibrio vulnificus	CDC group EF-3 *Beneckea vulnifica*
X. Aerobic Gram-Negative Bacilli: Nonenterobacteriaceae; Nonfermentative	
Characteristics: May or may not oxidize sugars; are catalase positive; are oxidase variable	
Achromobacter denitrificans	*Alcaligenes denitrificans* *Alcaligenes xylosoxidans* subspecies *denitrificans*
Achromobacter insolitus	
Achromobacter piechaudii	*Alcaligenes piechaudii*
Achromobacter spanius	
Achromobacter xylosoxidans	*Alcaligenes xylosoxidans* *Alcaligenes xylosoxidans* subspecies *xylosoxidans* *Alcaligenes denitrificans* subspecies *xylosoxidans* *Achromobacter xylosoxidans* CDC groups IIIa and IIIb
Acidovorax delafieldii	*Pseudomonas delafieldii*
Acidovorax facilis	*Pseudomonas facilis*
Acidovorax temperans	*Pseudomonas temperans*
Acidovorax wautersii	
Acinetobacter baumannii	*Acinetobacter anitratus*
Acinetobacter beijerinckii	
Acinetobacter bereziniae	
Acinetobacter boissieri	
Acinetobacter calcoaceticus	*Acinetobacter anitratus* *Acinetobacter calcoaceticus* subspecies *calcoaceticus*
Acinetobacter guillouiae	
Acinetobacter gyllenbergii	
Acinetobacter haemolyticus	*Acinetobacter anitratus*
Acinetobacter johnsonii	
Acinetobacter junii	*Acinetobacter anitratus* *Acinetobacter grimontii*
Acinetobacter lwoffii	*Acinetobacter calcoaceticus* subspecies *lwoffi*
Acinetobacter nectaris	
Acinetobacter nosocomialis	*Acinetobacter* genomic species 13TU
Acinetobacter parvus	
Acinetobacter pittii	*Acinetobacter* genomic species 3
Acinetobacter radioresisens	
Acinetobacter schindleri	
Acinetobacter soli	
Acinetobacter ursingii	
Advenella incenata	
Agrobacterium tumefaciens	CDC group Vd-3
Alcaligenes faecalis subspecies *faecalis*	*Alcaligenes odorans* *Pseudomonas odorans* CDC group VI
Asaia bogorensis	
Asia lannensis	
Azospirillum brasilense	*Roseomonas fauriae*
Balneatrix alpica	
Bergeyella zoohelcum	*Weeksella zoohelcum* CDC group IIj
Brevundimonas diminuta	*Pseudomonas diminuta* CDC group Ia
Brevundimonas vancanneytii	
Brevundimonas vesicularis	*Pseudomonas vesicularis* *Corynebacterium vesiculare*
Burkholderia ambifaria	
Burkholderia anthina	
Burkholderia arboris	
Burkholderia cenocepacia	
Burkholderia cepacia	*Pseudomonas cepacia* *Pseudomonas multivorans* *Pseudomonas kingae* CDC group EO-1
Burkholderia contaminians	
Burkholderia diffusa	
Burkholderia dolosa	
Burkholderia gladioli	*Pseudomonas gladioli* *Pseudomonas marginata*
Burkholderia lata	
Burkholderia latens	
Burkholderia mallei	*Pseudomonas mallei* *Actinobacillus mallei*
Burkholderia metallica	
Burkholderia multivorans	*Burkholderia cepacia* genomovar II
Burkholderia oklahomensis	
Burkholderia pseudomallei	*Pseudomonas pseudomallei*
Burkholderia pseudomultivorans	
Burkholderia pyrrocinia	
Burkholderia seminalis	
Burkholderia stabilis	*Burkholderia cepacia* genomovar IV
Burkholderia thailandensis	
Burkholderia ubonensis	*Burkholderia cepacia* genomovar V
Burkholderia vietnamiensis	

Continued

TABLE 79.1 Current Bacterial Nomenclature, Taxonomy, and Classification—cont'd

Current Name	Synonym
Chryseobacterium anthropi	
Chryseobacterium caeni	
Chryseobacterium gleum	*Flavobacterium gleum*
Chryseobacterium hominis	
Chryseobacterium indologenes	*Flavobacterium indologenes* CDC group Iib
Chryseobacterium massiliae	
Chryseobacterium treverense	
Comamonas aquatica	
Comamonas kerstersii	CDC group EF-19
Comamonas terrigena	
Comamonas testosteroni	*Pseudomonas testosteroni*
Delftia acidovorans	*Comamonas acidovorans* *Pseudomonas acidovorans*
Elizabethkingia meningoseptica	*Chryseobacterium meningosepticum* *Flavobacterium meningosepticum* CDC group Iia
Elizabethkingia miricola	*Chryseobacterium miricola*
Empedobacter brevis	*Flavobacterium breve*
Granulibacter bethesdensis	
Inquilinus limosus	
Kerstersia gyiorum	
Laribacter hongkongensis	
Leptotrichia hongkongensis	
Massilia oculi	
Massilia timonae	
Methylobacterium mesophilicum	
Methylobacterium zatmanii	
Moraxella catarrhalis	*Branhamella catarrhalis* *Neisseria catarrhalis*
Moraxella lacunata	*Moraxella liquefaciens*
Moraxella lincolnii	
Moraxella nonliquefaciens	
Moraxella osloensis	
Myroides odoratimimus	
Myroides odoratus	*Chryseobacterium odoratum* *Flavobacterium odoratum* CDC group M-4f
Ochrobactrum anthropi	*Achromobacter* spp. biotypes 1 and 2 CDC groups Vd-1, Vd-2
Ochrobactrumhaematophilum	
Ochrobactrum intermedium	
Ochrobactrum pseudogrignonense	
Ochrobactrum pseudointermedium	
Oligella ureolytica	CDC group Ive
Oligella urethralis	*Moraxella urethralis* CDC group M-4
Pandoraea apista	
Pandoraea norimbergensis	
Pandoraea pnomenusa	
Pandoraea pulmonicola	
Pandoraea sputorum	
Paracoccus yeei	*Paracoccus yeeii* CDC group EO-2
Photorhabdus asymbiotica	*Xenorhabdus luminescens*
Pseudomonas aeruginosa	*Pseudomonas pyocyanea* *Bacterium aeruginosum*
Pseudomonas alcaligenes	
Pseudomonas fluorescens	
Pseudomonas luteola	*Chryseomonas luteola* CDC group Ve-1
Pseudomonas mendocina	CDC group Vb-2
Pseudomonas monteilii	
Pseudomonas mosselii	
Pseudomonas oryzihabitans	*Flavimonas oryzihabitans* CDC group Ve-2
Pseudomonas pseudoalcaligenes	*Pseudomonas alcaligenes* biotype B
Pseudomonas putida	
Pseudomonas stutzeri	CDC group Vb-1
Pseudomonas veronii	
Psychrobacter faecalis	*Micrococcus cryophilus*
Psychrobacter phenylpyruvicus	*Moraxella phenylpyruvicus* CDC group M-2
Psychrobacter pulmonis	
Psychrobacter sanguinis	
Ralstonia insidiosa	
Ralstonia mannitolilytica	
Ralstonia pickettii	*Burkholderia pickettii* *Pseudomonas pickettii* CDC groups Va-1, Va-2, Va-3 *Pseudomonas thomasii*
Rhizobium radiobacter	*Agrobacterium radiobacter*
Roseomonas cervicalis	CDC "pink coccoid" group
Roseomonas genomospecies 4	CDC "pink coccoid" group
Roseomonas genomospecies 5	CDC "pink coccoid" group
Roseomonas gilardii subspecies *gilardii*	
Roseomonas gilardii subspecies *rosea*	
Roseomonas mucosa	
Shewanella algae	
Shewanella putrefaciens	*Alteromonas putrefaciens* *Pseudomonas putrefaciens* CDC groups Ib-1, Ib-2
Sphingobacterium mizutaii	*Flavobacterium mizutaii*
Sphingobacterium multivorum	*Flavobacterium multivorum* CDC group IIk-2
Sphingobacterium spiritivorum	*Flavobacterium spiritivorum* *Sphingobacterium versatilis* CDC group IIk-3
Sphingomonas parapaucimobilis	
Sphingomonas paucimobilis	*Pseudomonas paucimobilis* CDC group IIk-1
Stenotrophomonas maltophilia	*Xanthomonas maltophilia* *Pseudomonas maltophilia* *Stenotrophomonas africana*
Wautersiella falsenii	
Weeksella virosa	*Flavobacterium genital* CDC group Iif
Wohlfahrtimonas chitiniclastica	
XI. Anaerobic Gram-Negative Bacilli	
Characteristics: May appear as rods with rounded ends, curved rods, coccobacilli, or slender, spindle-shaped rods with tapered ends. *Dialister* and *Johnsonella* belong to the Clostridium subphylum	
Alistipes finegoldii	
Alistipes indistinctus	
Alistipes obesi	
Alistipes onderdonkii	
Alistipes senegalensis	
Alistipes shahii	
Alistipes timonensis	
Alloprevotella rava	
Alloprevotella tannerae	*Prevotella tannerae*

TABLE 79.1 Current Bacterial Nomenclature, Taxonomy, and Classification—cont'd

Current Name	Synonym	Current Name	Synonym
Anaerobiospirillum succiniciproducens		*Fusobacterium canifelinum*	
Anaerobiospirillum thomasii		*Fusobacterium gonidiaformans*	
Anaerostipes cocae		*Fusobacterium mortiferum*	
Anaerostipes hadrus		*Fusobacterium naviforme*	
Bacteroides caccae		*Fusobacterium necrogenes*	
Bacteroides capillosus		*Fusobacterium necrophorum* subspecies *animalis*	
Bacteroides cellulosilyticus		*Fusobacterium necrophorum* subspecies *funduliforme*	
Bacteroides clarus		*Fusobacterium necrophorum* subspecies *fusiforme*	
Bacteroides corrocola		*Fusobacterium necrophorum* subspecies *necrophorum*	
Bacteroides coprophilus		*Fusobacterium necrophorum* subspecies *nucleatum*	
Bacteroides distasonis		*Fusobacterium necrophorum* subspecies *polymorphum*	
Bacteroides dorei		*Fusobacterium necrophorum* subspecies *vincentii*	
Bacteroides eggerthii		*Fusobacterium nucleatum*	
Bacteroides faecis		*Fusobacterium perfoetens*	
Bacteroides finegoldii		*Fusobacterium periodonticum*	
Bacteroides fluxus		*Fusobacterium russii*	
Bacteroides forsythus		*Fusobacterium simiae*	
Bacteroides fragilis		*Fusobacterium ulcerans*	
Bacteroides fragilis group	True Bacteroides	*Fusobacterium varium*	*Fusobacterium pseudonecrophorum*
Bacteroides intestinalis	*Bacteroides putredinis* *Alistipes putredinis* *Bacteroides furcosus*	*Johnsonella ignava*	
Bacteroides massiliensis		*Jonquetella anthropi*	
Bacteroides merdae		*Leptotrichia amnionii*	
Bacteroides nordii		*Leptotrichia buccalis*	
Bacteroides oleiciplenus		*Leptotrichia goodfellowii*	
Bacteroides ovatus		*Leptotrichia hofstadii*	
Bacteroides plebeius		*Leptotrichia hongkongensis*	
Bacteroides pyogenes	*Bacteroides tectus* *Bacteroides tectum*	*Leptotrichia shahii*	
Bacteroides salyersae	*Baceroides suis*	*Leptotrichia trevisanii*	
Bacteroides splanchnicus		*Leptotrichia wadei*	
Bacteroides stercoris		*Meganonas funiformis*	
Bacteroides tectum		*Odoribacter laneus*	
Bacteroides thetaiotaomicron	*Bacteroides corrodens*	*Odoribacter splanchnicus*	*Bacteroides splanchnicus*
Bacteroides uniformis		*Parabacteroides distasonis*	*Bacteroides distasonis*
Bacteroides ureolyticus		*Parabacteroides goldsteinii*	*Bacteroides goldsteinii*
Bacteroides vulgatus		*Parabacteroides gordonii*	
Bacteroides xylanisolvens		*Parabacteroides johnsonii*	*Bacteroides merdae*
Barnesiella intestinihominis		*Parabacteroides merdae*	
Bilophila wadsworthia		*Paraprevotella clara*	
Butyrivibrio fibrisolvens		*Paraprevotella xylaniphila*	
Catonella morbi		*Parasutterella excrementihominis*	
Centipeda periodontii		*Parasutterella secunda*	
Cetobacterium somerae		*Phascolarctobacterium succinatutens*	
Christensenella minuta		*Phocaeicola abscessus*	
Coprobacter fastidiosus		*Porphyromonas asaccharolytica*	*Bacteroides asaccharolyticus* *Bacteroides melaninogenicus* subspecies *asaccharolyticus*
Desulfomicrobium orale		*Porphyromonas bennonis*	
Desulfovibrio desulfuricans		*Porphyromonas cangingivalis*	
Desulfovibrio fairfieldensis		*Porphyromonas canoris*	
Desulfovibrio intestinalis		*Porphyromonas cansulci*	
Desulfovibrio vulgaris		*Porphyromonas catoniae*	*Oribaculum catoniae*
Dialister invisus		*Porphyromonas endodontalis*	*Bacteroides endodontalis*
Desulfovibrio piger		*Porphyromonas gingivalis*	*Bacteroides gingivalis*
Desulfovibrio vulgaris			
Dialister invisus			
Dialister microaerophilus			
Dialister pneumosintes	*Bacteroides pneumosintes*		
Dialister propionicifaciens			
Fretibacterium fastidiosum			

Continued

TABLE 79.1 Current Bacterial Nomenclature, Taxonomy, and Classification—cont'd

Current Name	Synonym
Porphyromonas macacae	*Bacteroides macacae*
Porphyromonas somerae	
Porphyromonas uenonis	
Prevotella annii	
Prevotella aurantiaca	
Prevotella baroniae	
Prevotella bergensis	
Prevotella bivia	*Bacteroides bivius*
Prevotella buccae	*Bacteroides buccae* *Bacteroides ruminicola* subspecies *brevis* *Bacteroides capillus* *Bacteroides pentosaceus*
Prevotella buccalis	*Bacteroides buccalis*
Prevotella copri	
Prevotella corporis	*Bacteroides corporis*
Prevotella dentalis	*Mitsuokella dentalis* *Hallella seregens*
Prevotella denticola	*Bacteroides denticola*
Prevotella disiens	*Bacteroides disiens*
Prevotella enoeca	
Prevotella fusca	*Bacteroides heparinolyticus*
Prevotella heparinolytica	
Prevotella histicola	
Prevotella intermedia	*Bacteroides intermedius* *Bacteroides melaninogenicus* subspecies *intermedius*
Prevotella jejuni	
Prevotella loescheii	*Bacteroides loescheii*
Prevotella maculosa	
Prevotella marshii	
Prevotella massiliensis	
Prevotella melaninogenica	*Bacteroides melaninogenicus* *Bacteroides melaninogenicus* subspecies *melaninogenicus*
Prevotella micans	*Prevotella intermedia*
Prevotella multiformis	
Prevotella multisaccharivorax	
Prevotella nanceiensis	
Prevotella nigrescens	
Prevotella oralis	*Bacteroides oralis*
Prevotella oris	*Bacteroides oris* *Bacteroides ruminicola* subspecies *brevis*
Prevotella pallens	
Prevotella pleuritidis	
Prevotella ruminicola	
Prevotella saccharolytica	
Prevotella salivae	
Prevotella scopos	
Prevotella shahii	
Prevotella stercorea	
Prevotella timonensis	
Prevotella veroralis	*Bacteroides veroralis*
Prevotella zoogleoformans	*Bacteroides zoogleoformans*
Pseudoflavonifacter capillosus	
Pyramidobacter piscolens	
Selenomonas artemidis	
Selenomonas dianae	
Selenomonas flueggei	
Selenomonas infelix	
Selenomonas noxia	
Selenomonas sputigena	
Sneathia amnii	
Sneathia sanguinegens	*Leptotrichia sanguinegens*
Succinatimonus hippei	
Sutterella parvirubra	
Sutterella wadsworthensis	
Tannerella forsythia	*Bacteroides forsythus* *Tannerella forsythensis*
XII. Aerobic Gram-Negative Fastidious Coccobacilli	
Characteristics: Small, curved or straight gram-negative bacilli or coccobacilli; may require carbon dioxide and enriched media or special conditions for adequate growth	
Actinobacillus equuii	
Actinobacillus hominis	
Actinobacillus suis	
Actinobacillus ureae	*Pasteurella ureae*
Aggregatibacter actinomycetemcomitans	*Actinobacillus actinomycetemcomitans* CDC groups HB-3, HB-4
Aggregatibacter aphrophilus	*Haemophilus aphrophilus* *Haemophilus paraphrophilus* CDC group HB-2
Aggregatibacter paraphrophilus	*Haemophilus paraphrophilus*
Aggregatibacter segnis	*Haemophilus segnis*
Anaplasma phagocytophilum	*Ehrlichia egui* *Ehrlichia phagocytophila* HGE agent
Bartonella alsatica	
Bartonella bacilliformis	
Bartonella clarridgeiae	
Bartonella elizabethae	*Rochalimaea elizabethae*
Bartonella grahamii	
Bartonella henselae	*Rochalimaea henselae*
Bartonella koehlerae	
Bartonella quintana	*Rochalimaea quintana*
Bartonella rochalimae	
Bartonella vinsonii subspecies *arupensis*	*Rochalimaea vinsonii*
Bartonella vinsonii subspecies *berkhoffii*	
Bartonella tamiae	
Bordetella avium	CDC group IVa
Bordetella bronchiseptica	
Bordetella hinzii	
Bordetella holmesii	CDC group NO-2
Bordetella parapertussis	
Bordetella pertussis	
Bordetella petrii	
Bordetella trematum	
Brucella abortus	
Brucella canis	
Brucella melitensis	
Brucella suis	
Campylobacter concisus	CDC group EF-22
Campylobacter curvus	*Wolinella curva*
Campylobacter fetus subspecies *fetus*	*Vibrio fetus*
Campylobacter gracilis	*Bacteroides gracilis*
Campylobacter hominis	
Campylobacter jejuni subspecies *doylei*	

TABLE 79.1 Current Bacterial Nomenclature, Taxonomy, and Classification—cont'd

Current Name	Synonym
Campylobacter jejuni subspecies *jejuni*	
Campylobacter peloridis	
Campylobacter rectus	*Wolinella recta*
Campylobacter showae	
Campylobacter sputorum subspecies *sputorum*	
Campylobacter upsaliensis	
Campylobacterr ureolyticus	
Capnocytophaga canimorsus	CDC group DF-2
Capnocytophaga cynodegmi	CDC group DF-2
Capnocytophaga gingivalis	CDC group DF-1
Capnocytophaga granulosa	
Capnocytophaga haemolytica	
Capnocytophaga ochracea	CDC group DF-1
Capnocytophaga sputigena	CDC group DF-1
Cardiobacterium hominis	CDC group IId
Cardiobacterium valvarum	
Chlamydia pneumoniae	Taiwan acute respiratory agent (TWAR) *Chlamydophila pneumoniae*
Chlamydia psittaci	*Chlamydophila psittaci*
Chlamydia trachomatis	*Chlamydophila trachomatis*
Chromobacterium violaceum	
Coxiella burnetii	
Dysgonomonas capnocytophagoides	CDC group DF-3
Dysgonomonas gadei	
Dysgonomonas hofstadii	
Dysgonomonas mossii	
Ehrlichia chaffeensis	Human monocytic ehrlichiosis
Ehrlichia ewingii	
Ehrlichia muris	
Eikenella corrodens	
Francisella novicida	
Francisella philomiragia	CDC group HB-1
Francisella tularensis subspecies *mediaasiatica*	*Yersinia philomiragia*
Francisella tularensis subspecies *holarctica*	
Francisella tularensis subspecies *tularensis*	*Francisella tularensis* type A *Pasteurella tularensis* *Bacterium tularense*
Haemophilus aegyptis	
Haemophilus ducreyi	
Haemophilus haemolyticus	
Haemophilus influenzae	
Haemophilus parahaemolyticus	
Haemophilus parainfluenzae	
Haemophilus sputorum	
Haemophilus pittmaniae	
Helicobacter canadensis	
Helicobacter cinaedi	*Campylobacter cinaedi*
Helicobacter hepaticus	
Helicobacter pylori	*Campylobacter pylori*
Helicobacter suis	
Kingella denitrificans	CDC group TM-1
Kingella kingae	*Moraxella kingae* *Moraxella kingii*
Kingella oralis	
Kingella potus	
Legionella anisa	
Legionella birminghamensis	
Legionella bozemanii	*Fluoribacter bozemanae*
Legionella cardica	
Legionella cincinnatiensis	
Legionella dumoffii	*Fluoribacter dumoffii*
Legionella feeleii	
Legionella gormanii	
Legionella hackeliae	
Legionella jordanis	
Legionella lansingensis	
Legionella londiniensis	
Legionella longbeachae	
Legionella lytica	
Legionella maceachernii	
Legionella micdadei	*Tatlockia micdadei*
Legionella nagasakiensis	
Legionella oakridgensis	
Legionella parisiensis	
Legionella pneumophila	
Legionella rubrilucens	
Legionella sainthelensi	
Legionella steelei	
Legionella tucsonensis	
Legionella wadsworthii	
Neorickettsia sennetsu	*Ehrlichia sennetsu*
Orientia chuto	
Orientia tsutsugamushi	*Rickettsia tsutsugamushi*
Rickettsia aeschlimannii	
Rickettsia africae	
Rickettsia akari	
Rickettsia australis	
Rickettsia conorii	
Rickettsia felis	
Rickettsia heilongjiangensis	
Rickettsia honei	
Rickettsia japonica	
Rickettsia parkeri	
Rickettsia prowazekii	
Rickettsia rickettsii	
Rickettsia sibirica	
Rickettsia slovaca	
Rickettsia typhi	
Streptobacillus moniliformis	*Haverhillia multiformis*
Suttonella indologenes	*Kingella indologenes*
XIII. Mycoplasma (Pleuropneumonia-Like Organisms)	
Characteristics: Small, highly pleomorphic organisms that are difficult to observe with routine stains; require complex medium for growth	
Acholeplasma laidlawii	
Mycoplasma amphoriforme	
Mycoplasma buccale	
Mycoplasma faucium	
Mycoplasma fermentans	*Mycoplasma incognitus*
Mycoplasma genitalium	
Mycoplasma hominis	
Mycoplasma lipophilum	
Mycoplasma orale	
Mycoplasma penetrans	
Mycoplasma pirum	
Mycoplasma pneumoniae	
Mycoplasma primatum	

Continued

TABLE 79.1 **Current Bacterial Nomenclature, Taxonomy, and Classification—cont'd**

Current Name	Synonym	Current Name	Synonym
Mycoplasma salivarium		*Leptospira fainei*	
Mycoplasma spermatophilum		*Leptospira inadai*	
Ureaplasma parvum		*Leptospira interrogans*	
Ureaplasma urealyticum	T-mycoplasma	*Leptospira kirschneri*	
XIV. Treponemataceae (Spiral Organisms)		*Leptospira kmetyi*	
Characteristics: Filamentous, spiral organisms that may or may not stain with usual laboratory stains; require complex media or animal host for growth		*Leptospira licerasiae*	
		Leptospira noguchii	
Borrelia afzelii		*Leptospira santarosai*	
Borrelia anserine		*Leptospira weilii*	
Borellia bavariensis		*Treponema amylovorum*	
Borrelia burgdorferi		*Treponema carateum*	
Borrelia crocidurae		*Treponema denticola*	
Borrelia duttoni		*Treponema lecithinolyticum*	
Borrelia garinii		*Treponema maltophilum*	
Borrelia hermsii		*Treponema medium*	
Borrelia lonestari		*Treponema pallidum* subspecies *endemicum*	*Treponema pallidum*
Borrelia lusitaniae			
Borrelia miyamotoi		*Treponema pallidum* subspecies *pallidum*	*Treponema pallidum*
Borrelia parkeri			
Borrelia recurrentis		*Treponema pallidum* subspecies *pertenue*	*Treponema pertenue*
Borrelia spielmanii	*Borrelia spielmani*		
Borrelia turicatae		*Treponema parvum*	
Borrelia valaisiana		*Treponema pectinovorum*	
Brachyspira aalborgi		*Treponema phagedenis*	
Brachyspira pilosicoli	*Serpulina pilosicoli*	*Treponema putidum*	
Leptospira alexandria		*Treponema refringens*	
Leptospira alstonii		*Treponema socranskii*	
Leptospira borgpetersenii		*Treponema vincentii*	
Leptospira broomii			

CDC, Centers for Disease Control and Prevention.

NEW REFERENCES SINCE THE SEVENTH EDITION

1. Brenner DJ, Kreig NR, Staley JT, Garrity GM, eds. *Bergey's Manual of Systematic Bacteriology*. Vol. 2. 2nd ed. New York: Springer; 2005.
2. Garrity GM, Boone DR, Castenholz RW, eds. *Bergey's Manual of Systematic Bacteriology*. Vol. 1. 2nd ed. New York: Springer; 2001.
4. Kreig NR, Ludwig W, Whitman WB, et al, eds. *Bergey's Manual of Systematic Bacteriology*. Vol. 4. 2nd ed. New York: Springer; 2010.
6. Vos P, Garrity G, Jones D, et al, eds. *Bergey's Manual of Systematic Bacteriology*. Vol. 3. 2nd ed. New York: Springer; 2009.
7. Whitman WB, Goodfellow M, Kampfer P, et al, eds. *Bergey's Manual of Systematic Bacteriology*. Vol. 5. 2nd ed. New York: Springer; 2012.

The full reference list for this chapter is available at ExpertConsult.com.

SUBSECTION I Gram-Positive Cocci

80 *Staphylococcus aureus* Infections (Coagulase-Positive Staphylococci)

Sheldon L. Kaplan • Kristina G. Hulten • Edward O. Mason Jr

Staphylococcus aureus is a gram-positive coccus that occurs in pairs, chains, and grapelike clusters (Fig. 80.1). *S. aureus* is ubiquitous in nature and can be pathogenic for humans and animals. Staphylococci are nonmotile, are aerobic or facultative anaerobic, and are readily cultivated on routine laboratory media. These organisms are part of the normal human flora. *S. aureus* is responsible for an impressive variety of diseases ranging from minor skin and soft tissue infections to major life-threatening and fatal infections such as bacteremia, endocarditis, pericarditis, pneumonia, empyema, osteomyelitis, myositis, and septic arthritis. The focus of this chapter is on epidemiology, virulence factors, pathogenesis, diagnosis, and treatment of infections caused by *S. aureus*. The reader is referred to the many chapters in this textbook that address the specific infections noted.

On blood agar, *S. aureus* forms round, convex, shiny opaque colonies 1 to 4 mm in diameter, often with a zone of clear β-hemolysis

(Fig. 80.2) surrounding the colony. Pigment production is variable, with strains exhibiting a yellow or golden pigment on primary isolation; yellow pigment is actually an *S. aureus* virulence factor.[195] *S. aureus* secretes free coagulase, and this is the basis for the most definitive and most accepted method for identification of pathogenic staphylococci associated with human and animal infection. Free coagulase reacts with coagulase activator in plasma and converts fibrinogen to fibrin with the formation of a fibrin clot. Coagulase also can be evaluated by testing for bound coagulase or clumping factor in a rapid slide test (Fig. 80.3). Clumping factor bound to the organism acts directly on fibrinogen and converts it to fibrin; it is detected by visible clumping or agglutination when a suspension is incubated with plasma. The bound coagulase test is used commonly in clinical laboratories and is more rapid than the tube coagulase test. However, the slide test for clumping factor may be falsely negative in 10% to 15% of cases. Thus a negative slide coagulase test with an isolate that is highly suggestive of being *S. aureus* should be confirmed with a tube coagulase test for free coagulase.[178,262] A limited number of biochemical reactions can differentiate *S. aureus* from other staphylococci (Table 80.1). Commercially available molecular techniques can rapidly detect *S. aureus* from blood cultures with gram-positive cocci in clusters. By including gene targets both for an *S. aureus*–specific gene and a sequence near the insertion site of the staphylococcal cassette chromosome *mec* element (SCC*mec*) in the assay, it is possible to detect *S. aureus* and distinguish methicillin-susceptible (MSSA) isolates from methicillin-resistant (MRSA) isolates simultaneously. The rapid detection of *S. aureus* and methicillin susceptibility using these molecular tests impacts patient care by allowing more timely modification of treatment to the most appropriate antibiotic.[100,298]

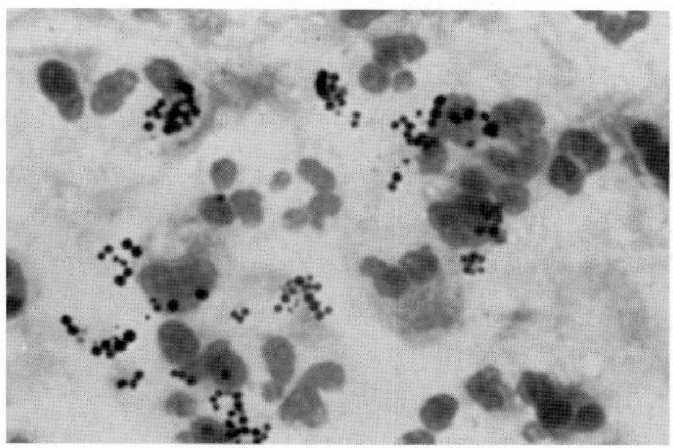

FIG. 80.1 Staphylococci in pus. The organisms tend to form clusters, are round, and stain purple with Gram stain (positive), similar to bunches of grapes.

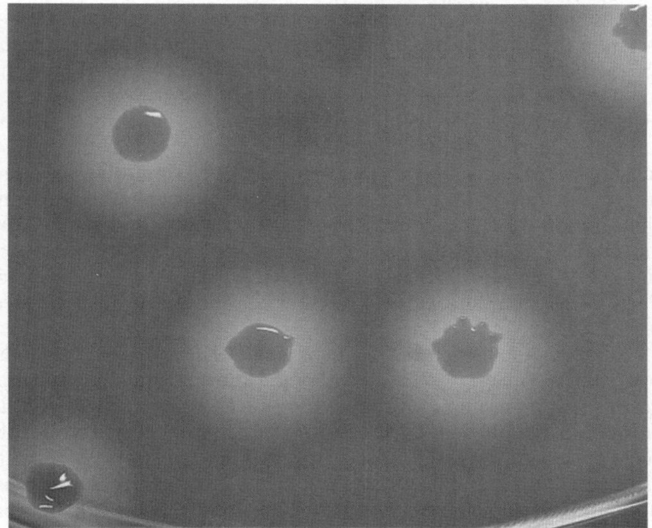

FIG. 80.2 Typical hemolysis produced by *Staphylococcus aureus* on sheep blood agar.

STRUCTURE

Capsule

Capsule production often is considered a virulence factor and frequently is used by bacteria to hinder phagocytosis by the host.[240] Karakawa and colleagues described a scheme of eight *S. aureus* capsular types in 1982.[164] Subsequently, Sompolinsky and associates described three more serotypes, bringing the total number to 11.[295] Most *S. aureus* organisms are encapsulated to a varying degree (Fig. 80.4). Two serotypes (1 and 2) produce mucoid colonies on agar media but are rare among clinical isolates.[295] Serotypes 5 and 8 account for about 75% of strains recovered from infections in humans, including children.[65,274,307] In practice, strains that do not belong to serotypes 1, 2, 5, or 8 are referred to as *nontypeable*.[136] The role of capsule polysaccharide in virulence comes primarily from studies of CP5 and CP8 and is not completely clear. These studies show that inhibition of phagocytosis by capsule can result in persistence on surfaces but modulates adherence to endothelial surfaces.[240] A protein conjugate vaccine composed of CP5 and CP8

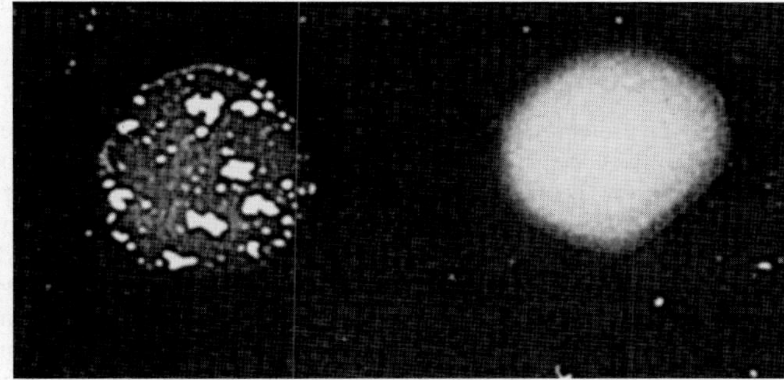

FIG. 80.3 Bound (slide) coagulase test. A suspension of organisms is mixed with plasma. Immediate clumping (reaction on the *left*) indicates both the presence of bound coagulase and the fact that the organism is coagulase positive.

TABLE 80.1 Identification of Staphylococci

Characteristics	*S. aureus*	*S. epidermidis*	*S. saprophyticus*
Coagulase	+	–	–
Acid aerobically from:			
Sucrose	+	+	+
Trehalose	+	–	+
Mannitol	+	–	+
Phosphatase	+	+	–
Novobiocin	Sensitive	Sensitive	Resistant

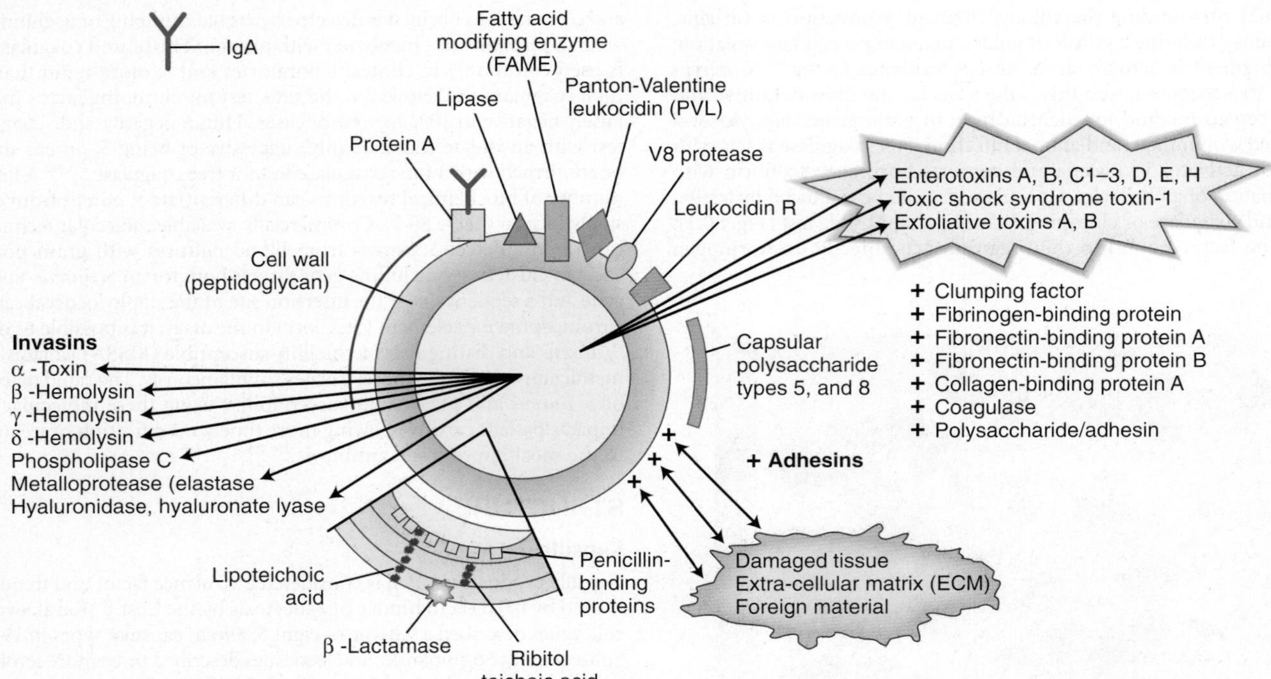

FIG. 80.4 Structure of *Staphylococcus aureus*. *TSST-1*, toxic shock syndrome toxin type 1. (From Daum RS, Spellberg B. Progress toward a *Staphylococcus aureus* vaccine. *Clin Infect Dis*. 2012;54[4]:560–567.)

conjugated to nontoxic recombinant *Pseudomonas aeruginosa* exotoxin A (StaphVax) initially appeared promising in prevention of *S. aureus* bacteremia in hemodialysis patients.[288] However, in a larger study this vaccine was not found to be efficacious.[287] Combinations including capsular polysaccharides in addition to other pathogenicity or virulence factors may prove more successful.[239] The major clone of MRSA associated with community-onset infections, USA300, as well as USA300 MSSA isolates and USA500 isolates do not express a capsular polysaccharide due to mutations in the cap5 locus, casting doubt on the contribution of the capsule to virulence of the organism.[33,307]

Protein A

Staphylococcal protein A, a major component of the cell wall of coagulase-positive staphylococci, has been found to bind to the Fc portion of immunoglobulin (Ig) G (IgG). This binding is nonimmune. It differs from specific antigen-antibody reactions in that the reaction is nonspecific, although both precipitation and agglutination are observed. Protein A binds the IgG of many mammalian species. This property has rendered protein A a major reagent in many immune assays. Protein A has also been found to bind to platelets through the platelet gC1qr, a 33-kDa cell protein,[237] as well as to von Willebrand factor,[127] both of which may be important in the pathogenesis of endovascular infections caused by *S. aureus*. Protein A plays a central role in the pathogenesis of staphylococcal pneumonia in that TNFR1, a receptor for tumor necrosis factor-α, is also receptor for protein A, and thus protein A is a principal staphylococcal proinflammatory factor in the lung.[109,249] The complex interactions of protein A, as well as other virulence factors, and the host in the pathogenesis of *S. aureus* pneumonia was reviewed by Parker and Prince.[249] Protein A also may play a role in modulating the duration of nasal carriage by influencing innate host defenses.[54] The gene encoding for protein A, *spa*, contains a polymorphic repeat region, which is the target for *spa* typing, a molecular method frequently used to characterize *S. aureus*.[126]

Extracellular Products

S. aureus elaborates a wide variety of extracellular toxins, many of which have potent biologic effects in the isolated state on intact animals, tissues, cells, and membranes. These toxins generally are thought to be responsible for the virulence of *S. aureus*, and the role of several of these products in staphylococcal infections has been proved definitively in humans. The important staphylococcal extracellular products include α-, β-, γ- and δ-hemolysins, coagulases, leukocidin, hyaluronidase, staphylokinase, bacteriocins, the epidermolytic toxins, toxic shock syndrome toxin type 1 (TSST-1), and the enterotoxins. In recent years a group of cytolytic peptides, the phenol-soluble modulins (PSM), have gained attention for their moderate cytolytic capacity, although the precise function of these molecules remains unclear.[172] PSM contribute to biofilm formation and are produced most highly by isolates recovered from skin and soft tissue infections, supporting the hypothesis that PSM play an important role in the pathogenesis of skin and soft tissue infections.[245,264] The pore-forming toxins include α hemolysin, γ hemolysin, Panton-Valentine leukocidin (PVL), LukED, and LukAB (also referred to as LukGH).[76,325]

S. aureus mobile genetic elements include pathogenicity islands, plasmids, and phages.[210] Almost half of the known toxins and virulence genes in *S. aureus* are found in pathogenicity islands. These genetic clusters, commonly of 15 to 20 kb, also contain genetic elements such as integrases and transposases. A high genetic instability is associated with many of these islands, and mosaic structures are common findings. A growing number of pathogenicity islands (νSa) have been described.[87,103,190,191,192,210,343] Although polymorphisms in gene content occur, studies have shown genetic conservation within specific lineages of *S. aureus*. All sequenced strains of *S. aureus* contain the genomic islands νSaα, νSaβ, and νSaγ.[70,103,137,122]

Hemolysins and Leukocidins

Encoded by *hla*, α hemolysin is produced by most *S. aureus* isolates and is a classic pore-forming bacterial toxin. The purified toxin has impressive hemolytic, dermonecrotic, and lethal properties. The protein interacts with and damages a variety of cell membranes, releases hemoglobin from erythrocytes of various mammalian and avian species, and is cytotoxic to a number of cell lines in tissue culture. It lyses rabbit and human platelets and disrupts lysosomes. It causes contraction in skeletal and vascular smooth muscle, with the latter action perhaps explaining its property of causing localized dermal necrosis. In a rat model, α toxin damaged the air–blood barrier in vivo during *S. aureus* pneumonia.[216] The α toxin forms pores in the membranes of endothelial cells, leading to vasoconstriction and increasing vascular permeability, and also has effects that lead to apoptosis of a number of different cells.[72] Damage from the α toxin to endothelial cells is mediated via its binding to the receptor for A-disintegrin and metalloprotease 10 (ADAM10).[256] This toxin also is an important activator of caspase 1/calpain signaling, which leads to pyroptosis, a form of inflammatory death, of human keratinocytes in vitro, which may allow *S. aureus* to penetrate across the skin to cause infection.[297]

Injection of α toxin is lethal to mammals and reptiles, with death occurring within 2 to 5 minutes. Anti–α toxin can be demonstrated in normal individuals,[55] and antibody to α hemolysin was protective in a mouse model of *S. aureus* pneumonia.[266] α Hemolysin also appeared to be a key factor in mortality associated with a rabbit model of MRSA osteomyelitis.[59] However, because the level of anti–α hemolysin is high in approximately 70% of patients with staphylococcal osteomyelitis and the antibody is also present in children with acute osteomyelitis at the time of admission to hospital, there is doubt regarding a protective role, at least in patients with osteomyelitis.[37,310]

The other hemolytic toxins, γ, β, and δ hemolysin, also possess hemolytic and cytotoxic activities. Highly cytotoxic, γ hemolysin lyses human neutrophils, and β toxin produces lethal and dermonecrotic effects. Eighty to 100% of adults possess antibody to β hemolysin. LukAB/GH has a reduced cytolytic action on neutrophils compared with γ hemolysin and PVL.[76] Children with invasive *S. aureus* infections develop high-titer neutralizing antibody to LukAB, but the role of LukAB in pathogenesis of infection or of antibody to LukAB for protection is unclear.[316] The biologic role of LukED remains unknown, although a variant of this molecule was highly toxic against human neutrophils.[232]

Despite evidence that these toxins are produced during infection, their roles in production of the typical staphylococcal tissue lesion remain unclear.[24,72] Although toxins likely play important roles in the establishment of infection by interacting with each other and with other biologically active staphylococcal products, the exact mechanisms have not been proved; human infection is not prevented by antitoxin antibody, and virulent staphylococci that lack one or more of these toxins are encountered.[293]

An in vitro study showed that α toxin was present in culture supernatants at seven- to ninefold greater concentrations in the USA300 strain compared with the USA400 strain when grown at midexponential and stationary phases of growth.[41] Further studies on how the strain-specific expression of virulence factors during the establishment and course of infection influence the pathology and host response are warranted.

Even though certain hemolysins are toxic to various leukocytes, PVL is the only known extracellular toxin that attacks the leukocyte exclusively.[248] It consists of two protein components, LukS-PV and LukF-PV, encoded by the genes *lukS-PV* and *lukF-PV* carried on a bacteriophage.

LukS-PV and LukF-PV assemble to form octameric β-barrel pores in polymorphonuclear leukocytes and macrophages.[32] Leukocidin injected into rabbits causes a striking fall in levels of circulating and bone marrow leukocytes, followed by marked granulocytosis; these changes occur without death of the rabbits. Leukocidin interacts with the membrane phospholipid and causes depolarization, increased permeability, and cell death. Local secretion of leukocidin might appear to confer an advantage to the staphylococcus by killing leukocytes and thereby preventing phagocytosis and intracellular killing. Levels of antileukocidin rise rapidly in the course of infection,[106,150] and some evidence indicates that infants and mothers with high levels of antileukocidin antibody are less likely to contract staphylococcal disease in high-risk epidemiologic situations.[20] In one study, a history of furunculosis suggesting a skin infection caused by PVL-producing *S. aureus* isolates was associated with a decrease in complications and mortality for patients with *S. aureus* PVL-associated necrotizing pneumonia.[268] Brown and colleagues noted that children who had invasive staphylococcal infections such as osteomyelitis or pneumonia had higher antibody concentrations to PVL at the time of admission to the hospital than children with skin and soft tissue infections, suggesting that PVL antibodies were not protective against invasive *S. aureus* infections.[37] Similarly, high levels of PVL antibody were not found to prevent initial or recurrent skin community-acquired MRSA (CA-MRSA) infections.[130]

In early studies, only a fraction of *S. aureus* isolates recovered from humans carried the PVL genes.[257] Interest in PVL greatly increased after reports that *S. aureus* isolates carrying PVL genes were associated with severe furunculosis[60] and particularly necrotizing pneumonia in children and adolescents that frequently was fatal.[105,189] Furthermore the independent emergence worldwide of CA-MRSA clones that generally carry the PVL genes led to further studies of the role of PVL in the pathogenesis of *S. aureus* infections.[322] PVL has been of particular interest in association with the USA300 CA-MRSA clone.[227,229] Using polymerase chain reaction (PCR) the PVL genes have been increasingly detected (*pvl*$^+$) in CA-MSSA strains in the United States as well.[38,140] In children with invasive *S. aureus* osteomyelitis, the presence of the PVL genes was associated with greater local and systemic inflammation, longer extent of fever, greater frequency of positive blood cultures, and more frequent complications such as the development of chronic osteomyelitis or venous thrombosis.[30,73,212] Pulmonary manifestations were also more frequently observed among children with invasive *S. aureus* infections caused by *pvl*$^+$ isolates[111]; *pvl*$^+$ strains were isolated almost exclusively among a group of children with staphylococcal pneumonia in one study.[42] In adults with staphylococcal pneumonia, *pvl*$^+$ isolates were associated with increased rates of mortality in one study but were not found to a significant factor in a larger study of hospital-acquired or ventilator-associated pneumonia.[203,252] In a multicenter international study, *pvl*$^+$ did not predict outcome of *S. aureus* skin and soft tissue infections in adults.[317] Thus the presence of PVL genes may be a marker for isolates capable of causing more severe disease in some populations of patients but not in others.[82]

The role of PVL in the pathogenesis of infection in experimental models also remains controversial. The contribution of PVL to severity of *S. aureus* infections has been examined in mice using isogenic *pvl*$^+$ or *pvl*$^-$ isolates. One study found no difference in lethality for sepsis or abscess volume in a skin abscess model,[328] as well as no difference in the destruction of human neutrophils by the isogenic strains. The investigators concluded that PVL was not a major virulence determinant of CA-MRSA. The other study found *pvl*$^+$ isolates caused much greater lung inflammation and necrosis in a mouse acute pneumonia model.[176] PVL was detected in the infected lung tissues. These investigators also discovered that staphylococcal protein A is more highly expressed in *pvl*$^+$ strains and postulated that PVL coupled with increased staphylococcal protein A could result in greater tissue inflammation than what is found with *pvl*$^-$ strains. A clear role for PVL has been shown in the pathogenesis of necrotizing pneumonia and necrotizing skin infections in a rabbit model.[69,193] In a rabbit model of osteomyelitis using an isogenic PVL genes negative derivative of a USA300 CA-MRSA isolate (LAC), PVL appeared to play a role in the persistence and extension of infection.[58] The discrepancy in these studies may be explained by use of different *S. aureus* isolates as well as different models of infection, especially the differential activity of PVL on neutrophils from humans or rabbits compared with murine or simian cells.[201]

Although the exact role of PVL in *S. aureus* infections has not been fully established, treatment measures directed against PVL have been proposed. These measures include the preferred use of protein-inhibiting antibiotics rather than or in addition to bactericidal antibiotics to decrease PVL production,[75,301] as well as adjunctive administration of intravenous immunoglobulin (IVIG) preparations containing PVL antibody.[102] However, currently there is no evidence that neutralizing PVL or decreasing PVL production affects outcomes.

Enzymes

Staphylococci express a variety of enzymes, including hyaluronidase, nuclease, proteases, lipase, catalase, lysozyme, and lactate dehydrogenase, that might play a role in the spread of infection in local tissues or the establishment of a nidus of infection.

Other biologically active extracellular products, as yet unidentified, undoubtedly are produced by the staphylococcus. The potency and number of these weapons in the armamentarium of the coagulase-positive staphylococcus, in contrast to the small number of extracellular products associated with the much less virulent coagulase-negative staphylococcus, suggest that the synergistic action of these toxins and enzymes may explain the superior ability of coagulase-positive staphylococci to establish infection and cause tissue necrosis. Several extracellular toxins have been proved to have specific roles in staphylococcal infection or disease: the epidermolytic toxins, TSST-1, and the enterotoxins.

Epidermolytic Toxins

Two biochemically and immunologically distinct exotoxins, epidermolytic toxins A and B (epidermolysins, exfoliatins), can separate adjacent cell layers within the epidermis and cause the various skin manifestations of the staphylococcal scalded skin syndrome (SSSS). These low-molecular-weight (~24,000 Da) protein exotoxins act extracellularly and specifically affect the upper epidermis by cleaving desmoglein-1, an important structural skin protein.[11,79] are now known.[11] Exfoliative toxin D has not been associated SSSS and only occasionally with bullous impetigo but was more commonly found among isolates derived from furuncles and abscesses.[286,342]

Toxic Shock Syndrome Toxin Type 1

TSST-1 was discovered independently in 1981 by two research groups. It was documented to be an excellent marker for staphylococci associated with vaginal toxic shock syndrome (TSS), in which it correctly identified more than 90% of strains in blinded testing. In experimental animal models, purified TSST-1 can induce the major physiologic changes of TSS: fever, mucous membrane suffusion, renal impairment, hepatic damage, hypocalcemia, lymphocytopenia, and hypotension. TSST-1 can be detected in blood, pus, urine, and tissues during human and experimental model TSS. USA300, the major CA-MRSA clone in the United States, typically does not carry the gene encoding TSST-1.[229] TSS and the role of TSST-1 as a super-antigen are discussed in Chapter 64.

Enterotoxins

More than 20 different staphylococcal enterotoxins (SEA to SE*l*V) have been identified, most of which cause emesis in primates.[72,129] The toxins are heat stable and resist boiling. Therefore once sufficient toxin has formed within food, even heating or boiling will not inactivate the toxin. Foods involved in outbreaks of food poisoning frequently have been inoculated by a lesion on the hand of a food handler in situations in which the food is then held at temperatures that allow bacterial growth (between 25°C and 60°C) for some time before the food is served. Foods implicated in particular are ham, salads with starch and mayonnaise, salami, poultry, cream sauces, pastries, and dairy products. The mode of action of enterotoxins is not well understood in part because of the lack of a convenient animal model.[207] Intravenous injection of purified enterotoxins in laboratory animals causes hypotension, cardiovascular collapse, and death. The significance of these properties of enterotoxins in naturally occurring human infections is unknown, although they may be linked to clinical syndromes, including TSS. Enterotoxin A often is elaborated with TSST-1 in menstrual-associated TSS, but it also has been identified without TSST-1 in patients with septicemia in whom TSS does not develop. Staphylococcal enterotoxin B, most often isolated in phage group V organisms, is associated with local infections and pneumonia.[211] USA300 strains typically do not contain the genes encoding most enterotoxins but frequently contain molecular variants of enterotoxins K and Q.[68] In contrast, other successful MRSA clones isolated from either the hospital or community setting carry several of the enterotoxin genes. For example, *seg, sei, sem, sen,* and *seo* were detected from isolates from USA100, USA200, and USA1100 isolates in one study.[68]

Staphylococcus aureus Microbial Surface Components Recognizing Adhesive Matrix Molecules

Bacterial adherence to host tissues is mediated by a number of bacterial surface components or adhesins that recognize and bind to host extracellular matrix and cell surface molecules.[149] The subfamily of adhesins that bind to the extracellular matrix are known as microbial surface components recognizing adhesive matrix molecules (MSCRAMMs). For *S. aureus,* important MSCRAMMs are protein A, fibronectin-binding proteins (A and B), clumping factors A and B (fibrinogen-binding proteins), and collagen-binding protein (Cna).[91] Many other less well-characterized adhesins also have been identified from the *S. aureus* genome.[273] The MSCRAMMs are linked to bacterial wall peptidoglycan after sortase cleavage of the LPXTG (LeuProXThrGly) motif that is a conserved C-terminal cell wall sorting signal among the adhesins.[49] Fibronectin-binding proteins play a role in *S. aureus* invasion into endothelial cells.[30,149] Collagen adhesin protein may contribute to the pathogenesis of *S. aureus* musculoskeletal infections,[78,246] although there are conflicting animal studies as well as clinical studies in this area.[151,278] USA300 CA-MRSA isolates do not carry the Cna gene, *cna,* yet osteomyelitis and septic arthritis are common CA-MRSA invasive infections in children.[43,212]

Clumping factor A has been the target for protective immunity in the prevention of *S. aureus* infections, and this approach has been successful in experimental models.[326] The safety and pharmacokinetics of an IVIG preparation enriched for antibody to clumping factor A were established in low-birth-weight infants; however, a large randomized trial did not document efficacy in prevention of staphylococcal infections in this population.[28] A monoclonal antibody (tefibazumab [Aurexis]) directed against clumping factor A has undergone preliminary evaluation as adjunctive therapy for *S. aureus* bacteremia in adults, but further development of the product has not occurred.[333]

Regulation

Bacterial pathogenesis is reliant on cell population, density-dependent gene expression. This quorum sensing acts to adjust the production of accessory genes (e.g., virulence genes), depending on the needs of the cell. Studies have shown that in low-density populations, when the bacterial cells are multiplying, accessory genes are either turned off or expressed at a low level to the advantage of other genes, such as genes involved in cell wall formation. In high-density bacterial populations, expression of the accessory genes is increased. The accessory gene regulator, *agr,* is genus specific, and the effector molecule is a regulatory RNA molecule, RNAIII. Many staphylococcal toxins and virulence factors are under the regulation of *agr,* and *agr* dysfunction is associated with reduced clearance of MRSA infection by vancomycin.[2,15,36,95,228] The staphylococcal accessory regulator, sar*A*, also functions as a global regulator in *S. aureus.* The *sar* locus produces three overlapping transcriptional units (*sarB, sarC,* and *sarA*), and the effector peptide, SarA, is a DNA-binding protein that functions as a transcriptional regulator. Both RNAIII and SarA have been shown to influence *S. aureus* virulence in animal models of infection. In addition to *agr* and *sar*A, several other factors have been described that affect accessory gene regulation.[27] Thus the complex network of regulatory operons that act on each other and/or directly on specific genes is not completely understood.

Staphylococcal Small Colony Variants

Small colony variants of *S. aureus* are isolates with atypical colony morphology, decreased hemolysis and pigmentation, decreased growth rate, and unusual biochemical characteristics that result in difficulty isolating and identifying these organisms.[324] Small colony variants also have been implicated in persistent and recurrent *S. aureus* infections, including osteomyelitis,[260] brain abscesses, and pulmonary infections in patients with cystic fibrosis.[156,284] Small colony variants can persist intracellularly, are often more resistant to antibiotics than the parent strain and antibiotics that penetrate into cells (e.g., rifampin), and do not activate innate host systems to the same degree as wild-type phenotypes, which helps to explain their successful intracellular persistence.[261,318] In one model of chronic osteomyelitis, some antibiotics induced small colony variants and only rifampicin was effective at reducing bacterial loads.[319]

Staphylococcal Cassette Chromosome *mec*

The staphylococcal cassette chromosome mec (SCC*mec*) is a region spanning between 20 and 70 kb located approximately 30 kb downstream of the chromosomal origin of replication. SCC*mec* contains the *mec*A gene encoding a penicillin-binding protein (PBP2a or 2′) with poor affinity to β-lactam antibiotics, allowing essential functions of cell wall formation to proceed in the presence of β-lactam antibiotics. The *mec*A gene is regulated by *mecR1* and *mec*I where activated *mec*R1 (signal transducer) inactivates *mec*I (repressor) through site-specific proteolytic cleavage, thereby initiating production of PBP2′. In vitro studies have suggested that the β-lactamase regulators *bla*R1 and *bla*I may also be effective regulators of *mec*A.[219]

The SCC*mec* classification systems are based on several genetic elements including the class of *mec* and the *ccr* genes, which are recombination genes involved in the mobility of the genetic cassette. Other elements that may be present are IS431, IS1272, Tn554, pUB110, and pT181. SCC*mec* types II and III also contain other antibiotic resistance genes such as *tet* (tetracycline resistance). All strains contain a J(unk) region of variable size and composition. Several schemes for SCC*mec* typing have been published.[170,242,243] Historically nosocomial MRSA isolates contained the SCC*mec* types I to III, and when community isolates were first described, three new types—IV, V, and VI—were introduced. Two more SCC*mec* types have been described, tentatively named VII and VIII. The smaller size (<30 kb) of SCC*mec* IV to VI is thought to explain an increased mobility between strains. Because the community strains have been brought into the health care setting, SCC*mec* typing cannot be used to predict whether an infection is health care or community related.[110,128,285]

TYPING METHODS

Staphylococcal strains were historically characterized by bacteriophage typing (World Health Organization method).[21] *S. aureus* isolates are susceptible to lysis when exposed to bacteriophages. Bacteriophage typing has been used primarily as an epidemiologic tool for identifying related strains in epidemics. Staphylococci of phage group 80/81 were widespread during the pandemic of staphylococcal disease in the late 1950s. At present, a wide variety of phage types are involved in staphylococcal disease.[272]

In the 1990s pulsed-field gel electrophoresis (PFGE) became the gold standard for strain typing utilized by both reference and research laboratories.[311] The method is reliable and reproducible, and the use of digital imaging and band analysis has enhanced the quality of interstrain and interlaboratory comparisons. The Centers for Disease Control and Prevention (CDC) used the PFGE method to define and interrelate *S. aureus* clones and designated 11 staphylococcal clones circulating in the United States as USA100 to USA1100.[215]

Multilocus sequence typing (MLST) is a nucleotide sequence-based method adapted from multilocus enzyme electrophoresis (MLEE). In MLST typing the alleles at each locus of seven housekeeping genes (*arc*C, *aro*E, *glp*F, *gmk*, *pta*, *tpi*, and *yqi*L) are determined through PCR amplification, nucleotide sequencing, and submission of sequence data via computer website to the MLST database (http://pubmlst.org/saureus).[80] In this database, strains can be compared with strains submitted by other investigators, and within-laboratory comparisons with control strains thus have become obsolete.

spa typing is a single-locus sequence method, based on the polymorphic X or the short sequence repeat (SSR) region of the protein A gene.[290] *spa* typing has some advantages over PFGE in terms of speed, interpretation, and exportability, the main limitation being the single-locus–based design.[121] Less commonly used methods include repetitive-element PCR (rep-PCR), restriction fragment length polymorphism (RFLP), and toxin typing. Reductions in the overall cost and advancements of techniques has led to an increased application of whole genome sequencing (WGS) in both clinical and research settings, enabling more detailed comparisons between isolates compared to previous methods.[182,202]

Staphylococcus aureus Clones in the Hospital and in the Community

Of the methods mentioned earlier, MLST has been especially useful in dividing *S. aureus* strains into lineages (or clonal clusters). Frequently these clones are described by their sequence type followed by the SCC*mec* type (e.g., ST8-IV). Most human *S. aureus* strains belong to 1 of 10 independent lineages. Five major clonal clusters (CC) that have been described to contain a majority of the human MRSA strains are CC5, CC8, CC22, CC30, and CC45. Of these, MRSA clones within the CC5 and CC8 clusters have been recognized as the main causes of hospital outbreaks worldwide.[53] Examples of widespread hospital MRSA clones are EMRSA15-ST22, EMRSA16 (ST36-II), the Archaic (ST250-I or 247-I), the Pediatric (ST5-IV), and the Brazilian (ST239-III) clones.[108]

Although a few hospital MRSA clones have circulated around the world, genetically distinct community clones have been reported from different geographic areas. Commonly these strains contain the smaller SCC*mec* elements, type IV or V.[271] Why these different clones emerged in parallel at this point in time is unknown.

In the United States, the currently most common community MRSA clone is USA300-ST8. USA400-ST1, originally described as MRSA strain MW2, which caused four pediatric deaths in Minnesota and North Dakota, was commonly observed in the Midwestern states in the early 2000s.[12] USA300 is the most frequently reported strain causing community-acquired disease in both pediatric and adult settings in the United States.[65] Like many other epidemic strains, it has been associated with a spectrum of disease presentations ranging from simple skin and soft tissue infections[157,162] to severe sepsis syndrome,[6,112] sometimes with fatal outcome. USA300 is a highly virulent strain that has been distributed over the continent and has become the most prevalent cause of community-acquired and community-onset health care–associated infections in less than a decade in the United States as well as in many other countries on different continents.[138,229,238] It has also become the most common source of hospital-acquired *S. aureus* infection in many hospitals, where it has acquired one or more antibiotic resistance markers.[66,110,139,285]

MLST typing has enabled the ancestry of many of these clones to be traced phylogenetically. For example, phage type 80/81 (ST30-MSSA) was epidemic in the 1960s and is the likely ancestor to the widely circulated Southwest Pacific clone ST30-MRSA-IV, which has been successful both as a colonizer and as a cause of diseases ranging from skin and soft tissue infections to invasive manifestations.[272] Similarly the USA300 (ST8-MRSA-IV) clone is postulated to have descended from an archaic ST8-MSSA.[81]

GENOMES

The list of current or completed *S. aureus* genome sequencing projects, submitted to the National Institutes of Health (NIH) genomes database (www.ncbi.nlm.nih.gov), contains more than 100 isolates and is continuously increasing. The sequenced genomes include CA-MRSA clones from the United States (e.g., MW2,[16] FPR3757,[70] and TCH 1516[133]). Among hospital-associated MRSA strains, genomes of the first reported MRSA clones, *S. aureus* COL,[103] as well as EMRSA-16,[152] N315, and Mu50,[175] are available. In addition, methicillin-susceptible isolates such as strains 476[137] and NCTC 8325[104] have been well defined.

Genome sizes range from 2.7 to 3.1 Mb, and the structures of the chromosomes are conserved. The core genome (the part of the genome that is the same in all strains) represents approximately 75% of the genome.[190] The biologic function remains unknown for at least a third of the predicted proteins. In the future the knowledge gained from these ongoing sequencing projects and analyses of the resulting large datasets will provide a deeper insight into the genetic differences of *S. aureus* strains and may give clues into the strain-specific causes of disease versus colonization, suggest candidate genes for potential vaccine or drug targets, or provide information into the acquisition of antibiotic resistance or virulence factors. For example, a comparative genome project of vancomycin-resistant strains provided proof that the vancomycin-resistant isolates reported to date in the United States all represented new acquisition of transposon Tn1546 from *Enterococcus* spp. and also identified a change in a gene important for uptake of foreign DNA, which may have facilitated the genetic exchange.[171] In another study using whole-genome sequencing, absence of patient-to-patient spread of sterile-site infection within the hospital was demonstrated.[202]

EPIDEMIOLOGY

S. aureus isolates are responsible for both sporadic infections and epidemics of varying extent ranging from the intrafamily outbreaks of staphylococcal disease commonly encountered to large and often prolonged hospital-associated outbreaks, such as those emanating from a neonatal nursery or a surgical service. Epidemic spread of staphylococci of phage type 80/81 was so widespread worldwide in the period encompassing the mid-1950s through the early 1960s that it constituted a pandemic. Researchers have suggested that a few "epidemiologically virulent" strains, such as 80/81, are particularly capable of spreading widely and causing disease. Robinson and colleagues[272] concluded that descendants of 80/81 have acquired methicillin resistance to emerge as a CA-MRSA clone, closely related to the Southwest Pacific ST30 clone. Because we are largely ignorant of the factors responsible for pandemic spread, we cannot prevent or predict recurrence.

Staphylococci may be transmitted by multiple routes, including contact with infected persons, contact with asymptomatic carriers, airborne spread, and contact with contaminated objects. Of these mechanisms, contact with a person who has a staphylococcal lesion appears to be particularly important in the spread of staphylococci. Persons with open draining lesions disseminate organisms into their environment and to others via direct contact. In a hospital, staphylococci may be spread from an infected patient to another on the hands of caretakers, such as physicians or nurses. Hospital personnel with mild or unapparent lesions, such as sties, furuncles, or paronychia, may themselves spread organisms. In family and small community outbreaks, multiple secondary cases can occur and frequently can be traced to an individual with a draining lesion. Secondary cases tend to appear for months after the initiating case within these small epidemiologic units.[299] Staphylococci also may be spread by asymptomatic carriers who have staphylococci in one or more body sites, including the nose, skin, hair, nails, axillae, and perineum.

At any one time, up to 30% of individuals are colonized in their anterior nose with *S. aureus*.[168] The rate of nasal carriage of MRSA appears to have increased. Nasal carriage of MRSA was 0.8% in 2001[236] and 9% in 2004[57] for children seen in an emergency center in Nashville, Tennessee. For children admitted to a hospital in Corpus Christi, Texas, in 2005, the rate of MRSA colonization was 22%.[8] In 2004 to 2005, an average of 2.6% (range, 0% to 9%) of children in 11 different practices in the St. Louis metropolitan area was colonized with MRSA in the nose.[97] Why nasal colonization of children by CA-MRSA has increased over the past decade is unclear but is likely related to unique properties of the major CA-MRSA clone USA300.[70] Actually for children with skin and soft tissue infections, CA-MRSA colonization of the groin is more commonly detected than is nasal carriage.[99,161]

Detailed studies have been performed to delineate factors regulating the carrier state and its establishment and perpetuation, as well as factors responsible for dispersion of organisms from carriers. Asymptomatic carriers may be a source of disease for themselves and others. For example, a wound infection appears to be more likely to develop in a hospitalized patient who becomes a carrier than in a noncarrier.[334] Much attention has been devoted to detecting and attempting to treat nasal carriers of staphylococci; however, studies of nursery outbreaks have indicated that nasal carriage is not as important as is hand transmission in the dispersal of staphylococci.[337] Transmission by hand contact can be minimized by effective hand washing.[107] The problem of hair carriage of staphylococci in operating room personnel has been minimized by using improved head coverings.

Staphylococci are widespread in the environment and can be cultured from clothing, carpets, toiletries (e.g., hairbrushes, razors), pets, and virtually all environmental surfaces, especially in the bathroom.[230] Airborne dissemination of organisms is possible, particularly in operating rooms with poor ventilation and heavy traffic; improved methods of ventilating operating rooms may have reduced the sepsis or colonization rate. Environmental staphylococci may serve as an important reservoir, but direct human-to-human transfer probably is a much more important means of transmission in epidemic situations than is airborne spread or contact with contaminated objects. This means of transmission is particularly true for spread of CA-MRSA among athletes.[166] Furthermore USA300 appears to be especially able to spread among household members, in part related to increased contamination of environmental surfaces.[225,320] Molecular methods of typing offer adjunctive information useful in characterizing strains involved in outbreaks.[71,80]

Few studies have reported the incidence of *S. aureus* infections in children. Over a 12-month period in 2004–05 in San Francisco, Liu et al.[196] reported the annual incidence of community-onset disease per 100,000 was 227 for children younger than 5 years, 100 for children 5 to 14 years old, and 284 for individuals 15 to 24 years old. The incidence of hospitalization per 100,000 for children with staphylococcal infections in California for the years 1985–2009 varied between 26 for children 6 to 9 years old and 83 for children 1 to 2 years of age.[118] The incidence of MRSA infections per 1000 patient-visits at Children's National Medical Center in Washington, DC, increased significantly from 0.93 in 2004 to a peak of 5.34 in 2007 but then decreased 5% per year through 2010.[296] The CDC Active Bacterial Core Surveillance study found the incidence of invasive CA-MRSA infection per 100,000 children increased from 1.1 in 2005 to 1.7 in 2010.[143] In Canada from 2000 to 2006, the incidence of *S. aureus* bacteremia in children younger than 19 years was 6.5 per 100,000; 52% of these patients had a significant underlying disease and 56% had the onset of infection in the community.[323] Since these studies are based on culture results, and many skin and soft tissue infections especially are not cultured, undoubtedly the overall incidence of *S. aureus* infections in children is underestimated.

The neonatal nursery has been an area of particular concern in the transmission of *S. aureus*. During the pandemic of strain 80/81 disease, outbreaks of serious neonatal disease were commonplace, high colonization rates were found in infants on discharge from the nursery, and the subsequent incidence of disease in some outbreaks was as high as 50% to 70%. Skin disease and infant and maternal mastitis usually appear within 1 to 4 weeks after discharge. Staphylococcal pneumonia, far more common during that period than at present, may not be seen for months after delivery, even though the infecting strain was acquired in a hospital. During the experience with strain 80/81 disease, a particularly high staphylococcal attack rate was seen in the families of colonized infants. The same epidemiology has been noted for the USA300 CA-MRSA clone that has been associated with staphylococcal infections in otherwise healthy newborns up through 30 days of life.[89] One study reported that 20% of infants with an *S. aureus* infection had a mother with a concomitant (proved or presumed) infection.[89] In a study of infants up to 30 days of age with community-onset *S. aureus* infections, the infecting strain in the neonate was the same as a nasal *S. aureus* strain recovered from the mother in eight of 34 (24%) mother-neonate pairs.[88] This suggests that maternal nasal colonization is not the sole source of *S. aureus* isolates causing infection in their otherwise healthy full-term neonate. In other studies, *S. aureus* colonization of infants was more likely to be related to horizontal than vertical transmission from the mother.[148]

Various control measures were used successfully to terminate individual outbreaks during the 1980s. Measures to protect the infant from colonization and subsequent development of disease by establishing a barrier at the site of initial colonization included hexachlorophene bathing, application of antibiotic ointment to the umbilicus and circumcision site, and application of an antiseptic dye to the umbilicus. Another approach, deliberate colonization of the umbilicus with an interfering "avirulent" strain, was successful in controlling several epidemics but itself has caused skin disease and, in one case, fatal septicemia.[289] Hexachlorophene bathing became a widespread practice during the period in which nosocomial staphylococcal infections were declining.[107,254] After approximately a decade of using hexachlorophene, researchers recognized that cutaneous absorption of hexachlorophene could result in potentially toxic hexachlorophene blood levels in infants, particularly premature ones, subjected to repeated daily baths over time. Brainstem abnormalities associated with the use of hexachlorophene were demonstrated in premature infants. For these reasons, controls were placed on the sale of hexachlorophene, and its routine use was discouraged in 1973. In one neonatal nursery outbreak of MRSA, the use of 0.3% triclosan (Bacti-Stat) was associated with cessation of an outbreak.[344]

Patterns of crowding of infants and understaffing contribute to outbreaks. Active clinical and bacteriologic surveillance and cohorting of infants may be effective in reducing outbreaks.[18,120] However, mandated active surveillance for MRSA nasal carriage during 5 years among neonates in the NICU did not appear to alter serial point prevalence of MRSA nasal colonization (4.2%) in 10 Chicago NICUs.[204]

S. aureus bacteremia related to intravenous catheters and *S. aureus* infections of prosthetic devices are common.[44,208,209] In particular, methicillin-resistant staphylococci are responsible for widespread nosocomial outbreaks of disease in hospitals.[31,39,56,62,83,167,281,304,332]

HOST DEFENSES

S. aureus is ubiquitous in the environment, and approximately 30% of the population are carriers. A major defense against staphylococcal infection is intact skin. Minor wounds frequently become colonized and infected and serve as portals to deeper, more significant staphylococcal infection. In some cases, the integumentary infection may be of major importance; in others, minor skin punctures may serve to introduce infection to distant internal sites. Burns, varicella virus and cutaneous herpesvirus infections, insect bites, minor lacerations or abrasions, primary skin diseases (e.g., atopic eczema), epidermolysis bullosa, and surgical wounds are important portals of entry for staphylococci. A deficiency in peptides (defensins and cathelicidins) important for innate immunity of skin against *S. aureus* has been shown in skin specimens from patients with atopic dermatitis and likely contributes to the increased susceptibility of the skin to *S. aureus* infections in these patients.[169,244] In hospitalized patients, intravenous needles and catheters may be sources of staphylococcal infection.[208,209]

Foreign bodies reduce local resistance to staphylococcal engraftment and are important in the pathogenesis and perpetuation of infection. Noteworthy foreign bodies are cerebrospinal fluid shunts, prosthetic cardiac valves, nonabsorbable sutures, vascular prostheses (including arteriovenous shunts for hemodialysis), orthopedic prostheses, nails, and wires. In neonates, the umbilicus and circumcision sites, which may be colonized within the first few hours of life and from which both local and distant infections may be established, are important portals of entry.

Viral respiratory diseases such as measles and influenza[119,255] predispose to development of pulmonary infection, again predominantly by damaging the integrity of the barrier at the portal of entry. In an animal model, differences in the ability of *S. aureus* strains to cause secondary bacterial pneumonia after influenza can be demonstrated.[142] Disruption of the respiratory epithelium and impairment of ciliary motion and other local defenses may allow secondary staphylococcal invasion. In a CDC study of complications of hospitalized children with influenza, *S. aureus* was the most commonly identified bacteria causing coinfections.[67]

Once the integumental barrier has been breached, the polymorphonuclear leukocyte appears to be the most important line of defense. Successful phagocytosis involves chemotaxis, opsonization, and intracellular killing. The incidence of difficulty with staphylococcal infection is highest in patients with defects in this area of host defense.[90,340] Granulocytopenia of any origin predisposes to the development of infection, particularly with the host's endogenous bacteria, including staphylococci.[17] Krishna and Miller have extensively reviewed the innate and adaptive immune response of the skin to *S. aureus* infections.[173]

Once the staphylococcus and the leukocyte are close to one another, opsonization of the bacterium must proceed for phagocytosis to occur. Two systems for opsonization of staphylococci have been described. Serum from normal adults has good opsonic activity when unheated but is generally inactive after heating at 56°C for 1 hour. The heat lability of normal opsonin and the observation of normal or only slightly decreased opsonic activity in unheated sera from patients with agammaglobulinemia[338] indicate that the major opsonin is complement. A few sera, generally from patients convalescing from serious staphylococcal disease, contain heat-stable opsonins, presumably antibody directed at the staphylococcal cell wall components.[179] Therefore either complement or antibody can provide opsonins for staphylococci; specific antibody is helpful but not required. The clinical correlate to these observations may be found in patients with defective defenses; patients with agammaglobulinemia and defective antibody generally have more severe problems with organisms other than staphylococci, whereas patients with deficiencies in complement components have been reported to have repeated and severe staphylococcal infections.[4,9,10,92,226,251]

Once the bacterium has been ingested, intracellular killing proceeds normally. Coagulase-positive staphylococci can survive within polymorphonuclear leukocytes for a considerably longer period than can coagulase-negative organisms.[222] Prolonged intracellular survival may be an important virulence factor separating coagulase-negative from coagulase-positive strains and may provide a mechanism whereby surviving organisms may be carried to distant body sites to establish metastatic foci of infection. A number of *S. aureus* exotoxins outlined earlier, such as PVL, contribute to the ability of *S. aureus* to evade human neutrophils. In addition, many *S. aureus* genes are regulated upward or downward after exposure to human neutrophils and there are differences in gene expression among various strains in response to human innate host response that might account for differences in the ability of the isolate to cause infection.[327]

Patients with chronic granulomatous disease of childhood have an inborn error in intraleukocytic killing of catalase-positive bacteria and fungi. These patients have an early onset of recurrent purulent infections of the skin, subcutaneous tissue, lungs, and reticuloendothelial organs, particularly the liver, that often are caused by *S. aureus.*[265] Staphylococcal infections are also characteristics of hyper-IgE syndrome and leukocyte adhesion deficiency syndromes. Neutrophil disorders are discussed in detail in Chapter 2.

In contrast to the primacy of polymorphonuclear defense against staphylococci, evidence for an important role of specific humoral and cellular immunity in host defense against staphylococci is either lacking or contradictory. Specific antibody is not required for opsonization of unencapsulated strains of staphylococci. The opsonic activity of serum from patients recovering from staphylococcal endocarditis or other serious disease is greater than that of otherwise normal persons.[179,335] Despite the presence of humoral antibodies to cell wall teichoic acids and to various toxins and enzymes, which are found regularly in those convalescing from serious staphylococcal infection, the patient remains susceptible to recurrence of infection with the same strain of staphylococci. Staphylococcal infections generally occur and progress in the presence of some degree of humoral immunity. Specific antibody to one or more staphylococcal components or products does not protect against infection.

Clinical evidence from patients with deficient cell-mediated immunity (combined immunodeficiency, thymic aplasia, Nezelof syndrome) suggests that staphylococcal infections are not among the most important pathogens in these patients. However, in an animal model, interleukin-17 production by local T cells is important for host defense against *S. aureus* cutaneous infections.[52]

Present evidence therefore suggests that intact local skin and mucous membrane barriers are the most important defense against the establishment of staphylococcal infection. Once infection is established, an intact polymorphonuclear response is essential for containment of the infection and clearance of the organisms.

Genomic studies are leading to a greater understanding of the host response to *S. aureus* and may lead to novel treatment or prevention modalities. Using microarray techniques to describe the host immune transcriptional profile in children with primarily invasive *S. aureus* infections, Banchereau and colleagues[19] found an overexpression of innate immunity and hematopoiesis genes and an underexpression of genes associated with adaptive immunity. Differences in gene expression were seen between children with musculoskeletal infections and those with pneumonia. Of interest, patients with osteoarticular infections displayed overexpression of transcripts linked to coagulation of blood that might relate to the venous thromboses that may occur with *S. aureus* osteomyelitis.[113]

PATHOGENESIS

Staphylococci cause disease by two mechanisms: direct invasion of tissues with liberation of toxins, which may have effects at sites distant from the focus of infection, and colonization. The hallmark of a staphylococcal lesion is the abscess. Local tissue destruction at the site of inoculation is followed rapidly by hyperemia and a vigorous inflammatory response marked by the accumulation of large numbers of polymorphonuclear leukocytes. Tissue necrosis in the center of the lesion occurs next. At the site of intensive hyperemia surrounding the lesion, a fibrin wall is formed. Liquefaction necrosis occurs centrally; the mature lesion consists of a fibrin wall surrounded by inflamed tissues enclosing a central core of pus consisting of organisms and leukocytes. Live bacteria may persist within these lesions for a considerable period of time. As pus accumulates, it may drain toward the skin surface or into adjacent tissues, where it forms sinus tracts and secondary abscesses. In the presence of an intact host inflammatory response, this type of reaction may be seen in diverse areas, including the skin and subcutaneous tissues, lymph nodes, joints, kidney, liver, parotid glands, muscles, lungs, and long bones.

In addition to local extension, *S. aureus* may disseminate hematogenously from this focus of infection, even from abscesses that are trivial in size. Hematogenous dissemination may result in infection of bones, joints, and heart valves. Given the ubiquitous nature of staphylococci, skin and wounds, which are the usual ports of entry, appear to be remarkably resistant to infection. This natural resistance is affected dramatically by the presence of foreign bodies within the wound, such as sutures and bits of soil or gravel. Natural resistance also is affected by the tissue compromise that occurs after ecchymosis or hemorrhage and by vascular insufficiency. Poor personal hygiene likewise predisposes to development of staphylococcal skin infection. Moist, macerated skin is invaded more easily and thus contributes to the increased frequency of staphylococcal skin infection in intertriginous areas and in tropical climates.

Toxigenic staphylococcal disease includes staphylococcal scalded skin syndrome, TSS, and staphylococcal food poisoning. Toxin can be elaborated from *S. aureus* isolates that are colonizing sites without a specific site of infection but leading to TSS. The major manifestations of these diseases are caused by the effects of specific toxins. Clinical manifestations of infections caused by *S. aureus* in children are discussed in multiple chapters, and the reader is referred to the specific infection of interest.

DIAGNOSIS

The diagnosis of significant staphylococcal infections should be pursued with vigor. Collections of pus, whether superficial or deep, should be aspirated or drained surgically for diagnostic and therapeutic purposes. Gram stain and culture should be performed. An aggressive approach to the diagnosis of osteomyelitis by bone aspiration and bone biopsy or surgical drainage provides an etiologic security that is helpful during the prolonged treatment phase that necessarily follows. When infection is associated with a foreign body, such as a central catheter or ventriculoperitoneal shunt, removal and culture of the foreign body help in determining the etiology and removal is almost always required for successful resolution of infection.

When possible, at least two blood cultures should be obtained before starting therapy for all serious infections. One need not wait for fever spikes or delay therapy to obtain specimens. Blood cultures frequently are negative in serious staphylococcal infection, a fact that demonstrates the need for performing other cultures. Blood cultures are positive in most cases of staphylococcal endocarditis, approximately half the cases of osteomyelitis and septic arthritis, and less than half the cases of pneumonia and deep tissue abscesses. PCR may detect evidence of *S. aureus* in normally sterile body fluids such as pleural fluid.[26] A number of molecular tests are available to rapidly identify MRSA once isolated (or growing in blood culture bottles) in the microbiology laboratory as well as to detect MRSA colonization in patients at the time of hospital admission.[321]

Measurement of nonspecific indicators of inflammation (e.g., erythrocyte sedimentation rate and C-reactive protein), although of limited value in diagnosis, can be helpful in monitoring the clinical course of infection and response to intervention. Accurate, sensitive serologic methods for making a diagnosis of serious staphylococcal infection are not available.

Enterotoxins can be identified by a variety of methods. Immunoassay is used routinely but may lack the sensitivity required to detect levels seen in staphylococcal food poisoning. DNA oligonucleotide probes are highly sensitive, but their clinical utility is limited by the identification of nonexpressed genes.[241]

TREATMENT

Successful treatment of staphylococcal infection depends on adequate drainage of collections of pus and the rational use of antibiotic therapy. Strategies for clinical management of MRSA infections, including those in children, are outlined in guidelines published by the Infectious Diseases Society of America.[194] Staphylococcal infections have a particular tendency to persist and recur; for these reasons, prolonged antibiotic therapy usually is required for all but minor infections. Surgical drainage is extremely important and, in some patients with minor superficial abscesses, may be all that is required.[51,77] In one study an abscess less than 5 cm in diameter was associated with successful outcome after incision and drainage regardless of whether the antibiotic administered was active against the isolated pathogen, which was CA-MRSA.[184] In other studies the size of the abscess was not associated with outcome.[51] But for some infections, a period of antibiotic therapy after surgical drainage better ensures that the infection has been contained. In an adult study, antibiotics active against CA-MRSA were associated with significantly greater cures than agents not active against CA-MRSA in patients who had undergone incision and drainage of skin and soft tissue infections.[276] Failure to provide surgical drainage is an important reason for persistence or recurrence of organisms. Antibiotics cannot be expected to penetrate into the avascular center of abscess cavities. When abscess cavities are undrained or when antibiotic therapy is discontinued before an area is sterilized, live bacteria may persist and disseminate to cause later recurrence at that site or distant sites. After incision and drainage, adjunctive antibiotics are recommended for patients with underlying conditions or with immunosuppression; multiple sites of infection; rapidly progressive lesions or lesions associated with cellulitis; abscesses located on the face, hand, or perineum; young children (<1 to 2 years old); or those patients whose condition has not improved with incision and drainage alone.[194]

For moderate to severe staphylococcal infection, the patient should be hospitalized initially for intravenous therapy. This strategy ensures peak antibiotic levels, which may allow greater penetration into relatively avascular areas. Once the patient is afebrile, has a negative blood culture, and there is definite evidence of clinical improvement, therapy can be completed with home administration of antibiotics or with oral agents, as deemed appropriate by the treating physicians.

Antibiotics for *Staphylococcus aureus* Infections

Since the mid 1960s, the vast majority of *S. aureus* isolates from most sections of North America and Europe have been penicillinase producers and, therefore, penicillin resistant. When *S. aureus* is likely to be the cause of infection, the most appropriate agents to administer for empirical treatment of infections with onset in the community in normal children are based on the relative frequency of CA-MRSA isolates in the particular community. In areas where CA-MRSA isolates are not a concern, treatment with a penicillinase-resistant penicillin or cephalosporin should be initiated before isolation of bacteria and susceptibility testing (Table 80.2). Methicillin-resistant organisms cannot be treated adequately with β-lactam antibiotics, including cephalosporins except for ceftaroline and ceftobiprole. In some locations, methicillin resistance is widespread in community isolates and thus alternative agents (see later discussion) are indicated for empirical treatment. When a penicillin-resistant organism that is susceptible to oxacillin is isolated (MSSA), the semisynthetic penicillinase-resistant penicillins or cefazolin are the drugs of choice.[187,267] Oxacillin, nafcillin and cefazolin are available for parenteral use. Dicloxacillin and cephalexin are the preferred oral agents.

If clinical response appears to be slow, nothing is to be gained by switching to another antibiotic within the same category; instead, microbiologic data should be reviewed and the dose of antibiotic rechecked to be certain it is correct, the patient is reassessed to be certain all sites requiring drainage have been addressed, and compliance with therapy is assured, especially if the antibiotics have been administered orally.

The cephalosporin antibiotics are active against penicillinase-producing staphylococci and cause less irritation of veins with intravenous infusion than do penicillinase-resistant penicillins. A potential disadvantage lies in their broader spectrum of activity, which may promote superinfection with cephalosporin-resistant, gram-negative organisms in a debilitated patient with serious staphylococcal disease. Cephalosporins have been advocated widely for use in patients allergic to penicillin, but because of considerable cross-reactivity, they should be used

TABLE 80.2 **Therapy for Staphylococcal Infections in Infants and Children (Excluding Neonates)**

	Oral (Mild to Moderate Infection)		Parenteral (Moderate to Severe Infection)	
Drug	***Children <40 kg***	***Children >40 kg and Adults***	***Children <40 kg***	***Children >40 kg and Adults***
Penicillins				
Oxacillin			150–200 mg/kg/24 h in 4–6 doses q4–6h IV	4–8 g/24 h in 4–6 doses q4–6h IV
Nafcillin			150–200 mg/kg/24 h in 4–6 doses q4–6h IV	4–8 g/24 h in 4–6 doses q4–6h IV
Cloxacillin	50–100 mg/kg/24 h in 4 doses	2–4 g/24 h in 4 doses		
Dicloxacillin	25–75 mg/kg/24 h in 4 doses	1–2 g/24 h in 4 doses		
Cephalosporins				
Cefazolin (Ancef, Kefzol)			75–100 mg/kg/24 h in 3 doses q8h	4–6 g/24 h in 3 doses
Cephalexin (Keflex)	25–100 mg/kg/24 h in 4 doses	1–4 g/24 h in 4 doses		
Cefadroxil (Duricef, Ultracef)	30 mg/kg/24 h in 2 doses	1–2 g/24 h in 2 doses		
Other Agents				
Erythromycin	35–50 mg/kg/24 h in 4 doses	1–2 g/24 h in 4 doses		
Clindamycin	25–40 mg/kg/24 h in 3 doses	600–1200 mg/24 h in 3–4 doses	30–40 mg/kg/24 h q6–8h IV	600–3000 mg/24 h q6–8h IV
Vancomycin			40–60 mg/kg/24 h q6h drip over 1 h or by continuous IV drip	1–2 g/24 h q6h over 1 h or by continuous IV drip
Linezolid	10 mg/kg/dose q8h[a]	10 mg/kg/dose q12h[b]	10 mg/kg/dose q8h[a]	10 mg/kg/dose q12h[b]
Doxycycline	2–4 mg/kg/24 h 1or 2 doses >7 years of age	100–200 mg/24 h		
Trimethoprim–sulfamethoxazole	8–12 mg/kg/24 h of TMP in 2 doses	160 mg of TMP q12h		

Refer to the 2015 Red Book for anti-staphylococcal antibiotic dosing for the neonate.
[a]Dose for children <12 y.
[b]Dose for children ≥12 y, not to exceed 600 mg/dose.
IV, intravenously; *TMP,* trimethoprim.
Modified from American Academy of Pediatrics. Table 4.2: Antibacterial drugs for neonates. In Kimberlin DW, Brady MT, Jackson MA, Long SS, eds. *Red Book: 2015 Report of the Committee on Infectious Diseases.* 30th edition. Elk Grove Village, IL: American Academy of Pediatrics; 2015:882–883.

extremely cautiously, if at all, in patients with a clear history of serious penicillin allergy or anaphylaxis. Among this group of antibiotics, cefazolin is the agent of choice for parenteral use.[253] It is well tolerated and can be administered every 8 hours intravenously. Serum concentrations of cefazolin are higher, and effective tissue levels appear to be easier to attain. Cefazolin also is associated with less bone marrow suppression than nafcillin or oxacillin. The efficacy of the second- and third-generation cephalosporins against *S. aureus* is reduced. Therefore, these drugs, especially cefotaxime, ceftriaxone, and cefuroxime, should be given in addition to specific antistaphylococcal agents if *S. aureus* is strongly suspected. Clindamycin and trimethoprim-sulfamethoxazole are alternative agents for patients who are seriously allergic to or intolerant of β-lactam antibiotics.[14,84,163] Clindamycin is an important option for treating invasive *S. aureus* infections but should only be considered if or when blood cultures are negative and endovascular infection, such as infective endocarditis, is not a concern because clindamycin is a bacteriostatic agent. In one study using a large insurance database for assessing outcome of large numbers of children with skin and skin structure infections (not *S. aureus*–specific infections), trimethoprim-sulfamethoxazole and cephalexin were more likely than clindamycin to be associated with treatment failures and recurrences.[299] However, in a large randomized trial, clindamycin and trimethoprim-sulfamethoxazole were found equivalent in the treatment of uncomplicated skin infections including cellulitis and abscesses (>5 cm in adults but smaller for children); abscesses were surgically incised and drained.[224] Almost 30% of the patients enrolled in this study were less than 18 years old and 19% were less than 9 years old.

The β-lactam resistance of MRSA is caused by the production of a novel penicillin-binding protein (PBP) designated PBP-2′, which, unlike the intrinsic set of PBPs (PBP-1 to PBP-4) of *S. aureus*, has remarkably reduced binding affinities to β-lactam antibiotics. Despite the presence of otherwise inhibitory concentrations of β-lactam antibiotics, MRSA can continue to synthesize cell walls solely through the uninhibited activity of PBP-2′ op 2α.[165,214] PBP-2′ is encoded by the *mec*A gene, which is carried by a unique mobile genetic element integrated into the *S. aureus* chromosome designated SCC*mec*.[134]

Some cases of MRSA actually may be caused by infection with *S. aureus* that lacks the *mec*A gene responsible for true methicillin resistance. The mechanism of resistance in these cases may be hyperproduction of β-lactamase.[154] Frequently in these cases, methicillin resistance is borderline, with minimal inhibitory concentrations (MICs) of 8 µg/mL or less. The clinical significance of these isolates is unknown.

Management of Methicillin-Resistant *Staphylococcus aureus*

MRSA first was described within 1 year of the introduction of penicillinase-resistant penicillins.[146] Initial reports of infection appeared in England in the early 1960s and subsequently were followed by reports from other European countries.[177,302] In the United States, only sporadic cases were observed initially[167,177] and not until 1968 was the first nosocomial outbreak described.[22] Since then, the prevalence of MRSA in the hospital setting has increased steadily. In a survey of US hospitals performed in 1989, 97% reported the presence of MRSA.[31] The SCOPE prospective surveillance project conducted between 1995 and 2001 identified more than 3400 episodes of nosocomial bacteremias in children. *S. aureus* accounted for 9% of isolates.[339] The proportion of *S. aureus* isolates that were MRSA increased from 10% in 1995 to 29% in 2001. Risk factors associated with infection or colonization with MRSA include recent or prolonged hospitalization, exposure to antibiotics, and stay in an intensive care unit.[197] Nosocomially acquired MRSA appears to be fully virulent, with in vitro characteristics similar to those of methicillin-susceptible staphylococci, and equivalent virulence in studies of experimental infection in mice. Clinical studies confirm comparable mortality rates.[132,315] These strains characteristically are multiresistant and usually show no, little, or decreased susceptibility to the standard cephalosporins, aminoglycosides, erythromycin, clindamycin, and tetracyclines.[5,331]

Epidemic outbreaks of nosocomially acquired MRSA are not uncommon. In these outbreaks, nasopharyngeal colonization with MRSA often occurs before infection. A high rate of nasal and hand carriage has been observed in health care workers associated with units that have MRSA outbreaks.[233] The usual approach to outbreaks has been to emphasize hand washing between examining and caring for patients. Strict isolation in a private room generally is advocated.[234] Single-room isolation may be impractical in neonatal and some pediatric intensive care units, where isolation facilities are in short supply and a single MRSA-colonized patient may occupy a room for months. Strict adherence to universal precautions (body substance isolation) with all moist body fluids and strict hand washing between seeing patients appear to be rational alternatives to "strict isolation."[205] Intranasal application of mupirocin ointment has been found to be capable of eliminating nasal and hand carriage of both colonized patients and hospital staff.[270] Interventions to control outbreaks of MRSA in intensive care or other units are multifaceted, and the reader is referred to major guidelines for recommendations.[234,292]

Occasional cases of MRSA infection apparently acquired in the community were observed sporadically in the 1970s. However, these infections were from patients who were chronically ill, and many gave a history of nursing home residence, recent admission to acute or chronic health care facilities, previous receipt of antibiotics, or intravenous drug abuse.[185,218,280,306] Hence, in these cases, infections usually were traceable to the hospital setting. By contrast, since the 1980s, cases of true CA-MRSA infection in patients without identified risk factors have appeared in the literature. The first reports in children arose from small MRSA outbreak investigations.[123] Subsequently Rathore and Kline described three patients with deep-seated infections caused by MRSA acquired in the community.[269] In the 1990s, reports of CA-MRSA in patients without known risk factors continued to appear sporadically in the literature. However, most of the infections described occurred in adults.[115,180,231] Four pediatric deaths in Minnesota and North Dakota in the period 1997 to 1999 demonstrated the potential for severe disease from CA-MRSA infections.[12] The landmark study describing the changing epidemiology of CA-MRSA in children was published in 1998.[131] Herold and colleagues performed a retrospective review of medical records and compared the frequency of *S. aureus* isolation in hospitalized children during two time periods: between 1988 and 1990 and between 1993 and 1995. The prevalence of CA-MRSA in children without identified risk factors was 25.9 times higher in 1993 to 1995 than in 1988 to 1990.[131] After the publication of this article, several reports of CA-MRSA in children without risk factors from different parts of the United States and many regions of the world have appeared.[40,50,155,162,263,283,345] This explosive increase in reporting that occurred in just a few years suggests that clones of CA-MRSA have unique properties that allow rapid spread once they are introduced into the community.[158]

All reports of the clinical characteristics of CA-MRSA infection in children without risk factors document a predominance of superficial infections, including subcutaneous abscesses and cellulitis.[65,162] However, a large proportion of children with abscesses require admission to the hospital for incision and drainage under anesthesia.[162] Recurrent skin infections are also very common.[7,29] Invasive disease with CA-MRSA, including severe, life-threatening infection, osteomyelitis, septic arthritis, and pneumonia, accounted for about 5% of cases in children seeking care in an emergency center of a large children's hospital in Houston.[111,112,162] As previously noted, the CDC ABC surveillance study noted an increasing incidence of invasive community-associated MRSA infections over the years 2005 to 2010 in children in the United States.[143] In another study using nationwide administrative data, the incidence of MRSA-coded osteoarticular infections increased from 0.02 per 1000 admissions in 1997 to 0.36 per 1000 admissions in 2012.[303]

Unlike hospital-acquired MRSA, CA-MRSA isolates usually are susceptible to most non–β-lactam antibiotics, including clindamycin, gentamicin, trimethoprim-sulfamethoxazole, and doxycycline or minocycline, in addition to vancomycin, daptomycin, and linezolid.[157] Erythromycin susceptibility is somewhat more variable, with the proportion of susceptible isolates varying from 29% to 80% in various studies.[116,131,141,235] Macrolide (erythromycin, azithromycin, clarithromycin)-resistant strains remain susceptible to clindamycin if the macrolide resistance is caused by an efflux pump (MEF). Clindamycin, lincosamide, and streptogramin B resistance can be constitutive (MLS_B) or inducible ($iMLS_B$). Both mechanisms can be detected with molecular methods and can also be detected reliably in the routine laboratory by the "D test" (Fig. 80.5).[85] The D test detects the presence of inducible MLS_B resistance by the disk approximation method. Clindamycin- and erythromycin-impregnated disks are set 15 to 20 mm apart over Mueller-Hinton agar containing a standard inoculum of bacteria. After a 24-hour incubation period, if the zone of inhibition around the clindamycin disk is flattened or blunted ("D shaped") on the side facing the erythromycin disk, the isolate is classified as having an inducible MLS_B resistance phenotype.[181] Alternative approaches include a single-well microdilution test containing both clindamycin and erythromycin and automated methods.[144]

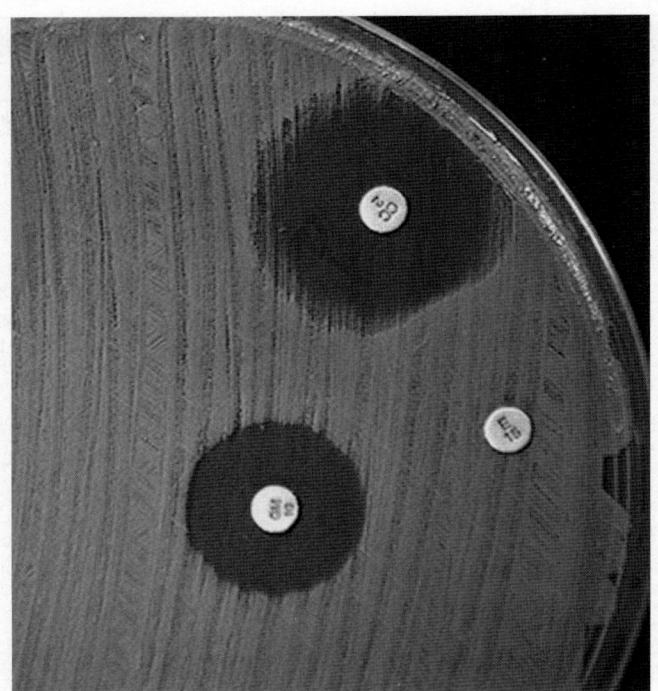

FIG. 80.5 D test.

Inducible macrolide-lincosamide-streptogramin B (MLS_B) resistance consists of modification of the target rRNA of *S. aureus* mediated by the presence of the resistance-conferring *erm* (erythromycin resistance methylase) gene, which encodes a 23S rRNA methylase.[145,181] In vitro and in vivo evidence indicates that, in the presence of erythromycin resistance, *S. aureus* could become resistant to clindamycin during therapy with this antibiotic.[74,217,247,330] Although 14-membered ring macrolides such as erythromycin are the most potent inducers, lincosamides such as clindamycin also can act as weaker inducers.[181] This ability may have clinical relevance in the setting of infections for which the bacteria are not eliminated quickly and may be exposed to subinhibitory concentrations of clindamycin for any amount of time. Examples include therapy for undrained deep-seated abscesses or treatment of osteoarticular infections. In patients infected with a strain having the inducible MLS_B resistance genotype and expressing the erythromycin-resistant, clindamycin-susceptible phenotype, cases of clindamycin therapeutic failure have been reported.[96,186,291] Vancomycin is the drug of choice for serious MRSA infections. There is no evidence that addition of an aminoglycoside or rifampin to vancomycin is beneficial for treatment of infections that do not involve prosthetic material.[250] Linezolid, an oxazolidinone antibiotic, has demonstrated significant activity against

MRSA, vancomycin-resistant enterococci, and penicillin-resistant *Streptococcus pneumoniae.* Linezolid is an important option for treatment of MRSA infections due to clindamycin-resistant isolates and may be a drug of choice for treating MRSA pneumonia.[160,341] It is available in both oral and intravenous formulations. Quinupristin-dalfopristin is an intravenous streptogramin antibiotic combination that has been found to be effective in the treatment of MRSA and vancomycin-resistant *Enterococcus faecium* infections in patients intolerant of or failing previous therapy. The frequent development of phlebitis with parenteral administration through a peripheral vein mandates the use of central venous access whenever possible. Both linezolid and quinupristin-dalfopristin are expensive, so their use should be restricted to situations for which other alternatives are not feasible. Quinupristin-dalfopristin has only been studied in children in compassionate use trials, and the development of other agents has limited its use in pediatrics.[200] Daptomycin has rapidly bactericidal activity in vitro against MRSA and is an effective agent for treating MRSA infections, including bacteremia and right-sided endocarditis in adults.[34,94] Pharmacokinetic studies in infants and older children indicate a larger dose per kilogram is required to obtain the same drug exposure in adults that resulted in effective treatment of MRSA infections.[1,35] The safety and efficacy of daptomycin for treating *S. aureus* infections in children are being studied but to date appears to be safe and effective in the treatment of serious gram-positive infections in children.[308] Ceftaroline is a fifth-generation cephalosporin that is approved for treatment of MRSA skin and soft tissue infections in adults, and studies are being conducted to determine the pharmacokinetics, safety, and efficacy of this agent in children.[282] Case reports suggest that daptomycin or ceftaroline provides a safe and effective option for the treatment of invasive MRSA infections in children.[25,336]

For severe infections caused by MRSA, the antibiotic of choice is vancomycin. In areas where CA-MRSA has been isolated from children without identified risk factors, severe, life-threatening infections suspected to be caused by *S. aureus* should be treated empirically with both nafcillin and vancomycin because nafcillin is a more active antibiotic than is vancomycin for the treatment of methicillin-susceptible isolates.[114] Antibiotic therapy can be adjusted subsequently after antibiotic susceptibility testing results are available. Clindamycin and linezolid are options for therapy depending on the susceptibility of the isolate, the desired route of administration, and the absence of endovascular involvement. Daptomycin is approved for serious *S. aureus* infections including bacteremia in adults but is not yet approved for children.[13,94] Tigecycline is another agent most useful for polymicrobial infections including MRSA in adults but has not been studied in children.[300] The role of parenteral trimethoprim-sulfamethoxazole in treating invasive MRSA infections is unclear owing to the paucity of reports.[223]

For mild to moderate skin and soft tissue infections caused by CA-MRSA, empirical treatment may include other antibiotics such as clindamycin or trimethoprim-sulfamethoxazole. Doxycycline and minocycline are options for children older than 8 years.[275] If more than 90% or so of community *S. aureus* isolates are susceptible to clindamycin, clindamycin can be used for empirical treatment of moderately invasive infections, such as in children with osteomyelitis or pneumonia and empyema who do not require intensive care and in whom bacteremia is not thought to be likely. This approach is not recommended when the clindamycin rate exceeds 10% of the CA-MRSA and CA-MSSA isolates combined.[64] Vancomycin or linezolid would be considerations in such circumstances.[160] Once an organism is isolated, therapy is modified based on susceptibility patterns. For moderate MSSA infections, nafcillin, oxacillin, and cefazolin are the preferred parenteral agents, and dicloxacillin and cephalexin are the preferred oral agents.

The origin of CA-MRSA is not known. The absence of health care exposure in patients harboring the bacterium, the unique antibiotic susceptibility characteristics of these isolates, and distinctive pulsed-field electrophoresis patterns that are different from the patterns of hospital-acquired MRSA isolates for a given institution suggest that the origin may be the community and that these isolates were not merely transferred from the hospital setting.[3,117] The unique combination of the gene complex and the much smaller SCC*mec* size than identified in the SCC*mec* of hospital-acquired MRSA also suggests a different origin.[206] Whether the origin is the hospital or the community, the changing epidemiology of MRSA is remarkably similar to the emergence of penicillin-resistant *S. aureus* that occurred in the 1940s and 1950s.[47] Finally the increasing rate of isolation of MRSA will mandate the use of alternative antibiotics, which in turn may promote the development of additional resistance to other antibiotic classes, the one of most concern being resistance to glycopeptide antibiotics such as vancomycin. Although vancomycin is the antibiotic of choice for severe MRSA infection, its use must remain monitored and controlled because clinical isolates with decreased susceptibility to this antibiotic—vancomycin- or glycopeptide-intermediate *S. aureus* (VISA or GISA)—have been reported.[294]

In June 2002, the first documented infection by vancomycin-resistant *S. aureus* in the United States was reported.[45] The isolate, obtained from a catheter exit site of a 40-year-old diabetic patient undergoing chronic dialysis, had high MICs for vancomycin (1024 μg/mL) and oxacillin (>16 μg/mL) but was susceptible to chloramphenicol, linezolid, minocycline, quinupristin-dalfopristin, and trimethoprim-sulfamethoxazole.[45,48] Since then, 14 total isolates have been reported from Michigan, Pennsylvania, Delaware, and New York.[46,188,313,314,329] All of the vancomycin-resistant *S. aureus* strains are resistant to the glycopeptides by virtue of the *van*A gene found in the enterococci. VISA strains (MIC of 4 or 8 μg/mL) do not harbor the *van*A gene and are intermediately resistant to vancomycin because of a thickened cell wall containing vancomycin-binding dipeptides.[61,124,135] Vancomycin (and other glycopeptides)-intermediate resistance is not detected by disk diffusion techniques and may not be consistently detected by automated systems.[312] In response to Clinical and Laboratory Standards Institute (CLSI) guidelines, microbiology laboratories have lowered the breakpoints for vancomycin susceptibility to 2 μg/mL or less, for intermediate resistance to 4 to 8 μg/mL, and for resistance to 16 μg/mL or more. In actuality, very few *S. aureus* have MICs greater than 4 μg/mL.[313]

Several studies in adults have reported worse outcomes for vancomycin treatment of MRSA infections, especially bacteremia or ventilator-associated pneumonia, when isolates have a vancomycin MIC greater than 1.0 μg/mL.[125,198,279] The relative increase in vancomycin MIC has been referred to as "vancomycin creep," but the MIC values are dependent on the method used to determine the MIC.[153] MIC results generally are higher using the E-test, but outcome of treatment may correlate better with E-test results compared with other methods.[174] As a result, dosing vancomycin such that the trough concentration remains between 15 and 20 μg/mL to achieve optimal drug exposure is recommended by experts for adults with serious MRSA infection.[194,277] However, "vancomycin creep" does not appear to be a problem in MRSA isolates recovered from children, and higher vancomycin troughs are associated with nephrotoxicity, and thus the need to target vancomycin trough levels at 15 to 20 μg/mL is unclear in children.[101,147,199,213,346] In fact, McNeil et al. found that over the years 2003 to 2013, vancomycin MICs for *S. aureus* isolates recovered from children with health care–associated bacteremia at Texas Children's Hospital had shifted to fewer isolates with MIC of 2 μg/mL or more over the study years.[221] This group also reported that the outcomes of patients whose vancomycin troughs were greater than 15 μg/mL compared to those with troughs of less than 15 μg/mL were similar. However, those with higher troughs had more nephrotoxicity. Furthermore doses of vancomycin much higher than the conventional dose (60 mg/kg per day) are often required in children to achieve this trough target. One approach would be to target this trough value for treatment of serious infections in selected patients when initiating vancomycin but to reduce the dose to 60 mg/kg per day once the patient has clearly improved clinically and blood cultures are negative. Daptomycin and ceftaroline will likely become primary option for treating serious invasive infections in children caused by MRSA strains with reduced susceptibility to vancomycin after the optimal doses and safety profiles of these agents have been established in children.

PREVENTION

Staphylococcal infections are so common that virtually everyone has had at least some minor encounters. Skin infections occur more commonly in tropical climates or during warm, humid weather in temperate areas and are likely to arise in moist areas of the body such as the axillae, perineal region, and skin creases. High standards of personal hygiene, careful cleaning, and adequate protection of abrasions and minor lacerations reduce the likelihood of a skin infection developing.[309] Early attention to minor infection in these small wounds with careful cleaning and antibiotic ointment may help prevent more serious or invasive infection. Even minor cutaneous infections can precede the development of more serious staphylococcal infections such as osteomyelitis, pneumonia, and endocarditis.

Person-to-person spread from an overt lesion is a major route for dissemination of infection within families, in hospitals, and in schools. A person with an infected, purulent wound should receive prompt treatment and be excused from school and from such occupations as hospital worker or food handler while the infection is open or draining. At home, special precautions should be taken in care and dressing of the wound. Disposable gauze pads should be used to wash and dry it, and towels and washcloths should not be shared with other members of the family. For children with recurrent infections or for families with multiple family members with infection, in addition to routine hygienic measures, Fritz and associates[98] found that a 5-day regimen of twice-daily intranasal mupirocin and daily chlorhexidine body washes for everyone in the household reduced the frequency of subsequent skin and soft tissue infections in the child as well as other household members. The Infectious Diseases Society of America guidelines also include mupirocin along with chlorhexidine as part of a strategy to decolonize patients with recurrent skin and soft tissue infections.[194] Resistance to mupirocin or chlorhexidine is likely to increase as these agents are used more frequently in the community for prevention programs.[183,220] Thus monitoring for resistance to mupirocin and chlorhexidine among *S. aureus* isolates should be more routinely performed. Dilute bleach kills *S. aureus* in vitro very quickly and has been used by dermatologists for years as part of a strategy to prevent staphylococcal skin infections.[86,159] We have found that, along with education regarding routine hygienic measures, having the patients take a bath for 15 minutes twice a week in water to which bleach (1 teaspoon/gallon of bath water) has been added may be somewhat helpful.[161]

To date no vaccine targeting polysaccharide, adhesion proteins, or other components of *S. aureus* has been successfully developed for the prevention of *S. aureus* infections.[63,93,258,259] One trial using immune globulin enriched for antibody to clumping factor A failed at preventing staphylococcal infections in low-birth-weight infants,[28] and a monoclonal antibody directed against clumping factor A was investigated preliminarily in adults with *S. aureus* bacteremia.[333] A polyclonal IgG preparation containing high levels of antibody to *S. aureus* capsular polysaccharides 5 and 8 has been developed by collecting plasma from healthy donors immunized with StaphVAX.[23] The pharmacokinetics and safety of this product in very-low-birth-weight infants were established in a phase 2 trial, but further development of this antibody preparation is questionable. The safety and pharmacokinetics of human chimeric monoclonal antibody directed against the lipoteichoic acid, an integral component of the cell wall of gram-positive organisms, including *S. aureus,* has been evaluated in a phase 2 study in very-low-birth-weight-infants.[28] This antibody (pagibaximab) also did not appear to be efficacious in preventing invasive *S. aureus* infections in very-low-birth-weight infants.

Perhaps taking advantage of the *S. aureus* genome with a reverse vaccinology approach will lead to a safe and efficacious vaccine.[305] But, until such time, simple measures such as frequent hand washing, attention to skin breaks, and avoiding contact of obviously infected skin lesions are the approaches for preventing common *S. aureus* infections.

NEW REFERENCES SINCE THE SEVENTH EDITION

7. Al-Zubeidi D, Burnham CA, Hogan PG, et al. Molecular epidemiology of recurrent cutaneous methicillin-resistant *Staphylococcus aureus* infections in children. *J Pediatric Infect Dis Soc.* 2014;3(3):261-264.
25. Billups KL, Stultz JS. Successful Daptomycin use in a pediatric patient with acute, bilateral osteomyelitis caused by methicillin-resistant *Staphylococcus aureus. J Pediatr Pharmacol Ther.* 2015;20(5):397-402.
26. Blaschke AJ, Heyrend C, Byington CL, et al. Molecular analysis improves pathogen identification and epidemiologic study of pediatric parapneumonic empyema. *Pediatr Infect Dis J.* 2011;30(4):289-294.
29. Bocchini CE, Mason EO, Hulten KG, et al. Recurrent community-associated *Staphylococcus aureus* infections in children presenting to Texas Children's Hospital in Houston, Texas. *Pediatr Infect Dis J.* 2013;32(11):1189-1193.
33. Boyle-Vavra S, Li X, Alam MT, et al. USA300 and USA500 clonal lineages of *Staphylococcus aureus* do not produce a capsular polysaccharide due to conserved mutations in the cap5 locus. *MBio.* 2015;6(2).
35. Bradley JS, Benziger D, Bokesch P, et al. Single-dose pharmacokinetics of daptomycin in pediatric patients 3–24 months of age. *Pediatr Infect Dis J.* 2014;33(9):936-939.
54. Cole AL, Muthukrishnan G, Chong C, et al. Host innate inflammatory factors and staphylococcal protein A influence the duration of human *Staphylococcus aureus* nasal carriage. *Mucosal Immunol.* 2016;9(6):1537-1548.
59. Cremieux AC, Saleh-Mghir A, Danel C, et al. alpha-Hemolysin, not Panton-Valentine leukocidin, impacts rabbit mortality from severe sepsis with methicillin-resistant *Staphylococcus aureus* osteomyelitis. *J Infect Dis.* 2014;209(11):1773-1780.
67. Dawood FS, Chaves SS, Perez A, et al. Complications and associated bacterial coinfections among children hospitalized with seasonal or pandemic influenza, United States, 2003–2010. *J Infect Dis.* 2014;209(5):686-694.
93. Fowler VG, Allen KB, Moreira ED, et al. Effect of an investigational vaccine for preventing *Staphylococcus aureus* infections after cardiothoracic surgery: a randomized trial. *JAMA.* 2013;309(13):1368-1378.
118. Gutierrez K, Halpern MS, Sarnquist C, et al. Staphylococcal infections in children, California, USA, 1985–2009. *Emerg Infect Dis.* 2013;19(1):10-20.
122. Hallin M, De Mendonca R, Denis O, et al. Diversity of accessory genome of human and livestock-associated ST398 methicillin resistant *Staphylococcus aureus* strains. *Infect Genet Evol.* 2011;11(2):290-299.
126. Harmsen D, Claus H, Witte W, et al. Typing of methicillin-resistant *Staphylococcus aureus* in a university hospital setting by using novel software for spa repeat determination and database management. *J Clin Microbiol.* 2003;41(12):5442-5448.
143. Iwamoto M, Mu Y, Lynfield R, et al. Trends in invasive methicillin-resistant *Staphylococcus aureus* infections. *Pediatrics.* 2013;132(4):e817-e824.
144. Jenkins SG, Schuetz AN. Current concepts in laboratory testing to guide antimicrobial therapy. *Mayo Clin Proc.* 2012;87(3):290-308.
162. Kaplan SL, Forbes A, Hammerman WA, et al. Randomized trial of "bleach baths" plus routine hygienic measures vs. routine hygienic measures alone for prevention of recurrent infections. *Clin Infect Dis.* 2014;58(5):679-682.
183. Lee GC, Long SW, Musser JM, et al. Comparative whole genome sequencing of community-associated methicillin-resistant *Staphylococcus aureus* sequence type 8 from primary care clinics in a Texas community. *Pharmacotherapy.* 2015;35(2):220-228.
187. Li J, Echevarria KL, Hughes DW, et al. Comparison of cefazolin versus oxacillin for treatment of complicated bacteremia caused by methicillin-susceptible *Staphylococcus aureus. Antimicrob Agents Chemother.* 2014;58(9):5117-5124.
188. Limbago BM, Kallen AJ, Zhu W, et al. Report of the 13th vancomycin-resistant *Staphylococcus aureus* isolate from the United States. *J Clin Microbiol.* 2014;52(3):998-1002.
195. Liu C, Graber CJ, Karr M, et al. A population-based study of the incidence and molecular epidemiology of methicillin-resistant *Staphylococcus aureus* disease in San Francisco, 2004–2005. *Clin Infect Dis.* 2008;46(11):1637-1646.
202. Long SW, Beres SB, Olsen RJ, et al. Absence of patient-to-patient intrahospital transmission of *Staphylococcus aureus* as determined by whole-genome sequencing. *MBio.* 2014;5(5):e01692-14.
204. Lyles RD, Trick WE, Hayden MK, et al. Regional epidemiology of methicillin-resistant *Staphylococcus aureus* among critically ill children in a state with mandated active surveillance. *J Pediatric Infect Dis Soc.* 2016;5(4):409-416.
210. Malachowa N, DeLeo FR. Mobile genetic elements of *Staphylococcus aureus. Cell Mol Life Sci.* 2010;67(18):3057-3071.
221. McNeil JC, Kok EY, Forbes A, et al. Healthcare-associated *Staphylococcus aureus* bacteremia in children: evidence for reverse vancomycin creep and impact of vancomycin trough values on outcome. *Pediatr Infect Dis J.* 2016;35(3):263-268.
225. Miller LG, Daum RS, Creech CB, et al. Clindamycin versus trimethoprim-sulfamethoxazole for uncomplicated skin infections. *N Engl J Med.* 2015;372(12):1093-1103.
230. Morelli JJ, Hogan PG, Sullivan ML, et al. Antimicrobial susceptibility profiles of *Staphylococcus aureus* isolates recovered from humans, environmental surfaces, and companion animals in households of children with community-onset methicillin-resistant *S. aureus* infections. *Antimicrob Agents Chemother.* 2015;59(10):6634-6637.
239. Nissen M, Marshall H, Richmond P, et al. A randomized phase I study of the safety and immunogenicity of three ascending dose levels of a 3-antigen *Staphylococcus aureus* vaccine (SA3Ag) in healthy adults. *Vaccine.* 2015;33(15):1846-1854.
245. Otto M. Phenol-soluble modulins. *Int J Med Microbiol.* 2014;304(2):164-169.
259. Proctor RA. Recent developments for *Staphylococcus aureus* vaccines: clinical and basic science challenges. *Eur Cell Mater.* 2015;30:315-326.
264. Qi R, Joo HS, Sharma-Kuinkel B, et al. Increased in vitro phenol-soluble modulin production is associated with soft tissue infection source in clinical isolates of methicillin-resistant *Staphylococcus aureus. J Infect.* 2016;72(3):302-308.
267. Rao SN, Rhodes NJ, Lee BJ, et al. Treatment outcomes with cefazolin versus oxacillin for deep-seated methicillin-susceptible *Staphylococcus aureus* bloodstream infections. *Antimicrob Agents Chemother.* 2015;59(9):5232-5238.

296. Song X, Cogen J, Singh N. Incidence of methicillin-resistant *Staphylococcus aureus* infection in a children's hospital in the Washington metropolitan area of the United States, 2003 - 2010. *Emerg Microbes Infect.* 2013;2(10):e69.
298. Spencer DH, Sellenriek P, Burnham CA. Validation and implementation of the GeneXpert MRSA/SA blood culture assay in a pediatric setting. *Am J Clin Pathol.* 2011;136(5):690-694.
303. Stockmann C, Ampofo K, Pavia AT, et al. National trends in the incidence, outcomes and charges of pediatric osteoarticular infections, 1997–2012. *Pediatr Infect Dis J.* 2015;34(6):672-674.
308. Syriopoulou V, Dailiana Z, Dmitriy N, et al. Clinical experience with daptomycin for the treatment of gram-positive infections in children and adolescents. *Pediatr Infect Dis J.* 2016;35(5):511-516.
316. Thomsen IP, Dumont AL, James DB, et al. Children with invasive *Staphylococcus aureus* disease exhibit a potently neutralizing antibody response to the cytotoxin LukAB. *Infect Immun.* 2014;82(3):1234-1242.
319. Tuchscherr L, Kreis CA, Hoerr V, et al. *Staphylococcus aureus* develops increased resistance to antibiotics by forming dynamic small colony variants during chronic osteomyelitis. *J Antimicrob Chemother.* 2016;71(2):438-448.
323. Vanderkooi OG, Gregson DB, Kellner JD, et al. *Staphylococcus aureus* bloodstream infections in children: A population-based assessment. *Paediatr Child Health.* 2011;16(5):276-280.
329. Walters MS, Eggers P, Albrecht V, et al. Notes from the field: vancomycin-resistant *Staphylococcus aureus*-Delaware, 2015. *MMWR Morb Mortal Wkly Rep.* 2015;64:1056.
335. Williams AW, Newman PM, Ocheltree S, et al. Ceftaroline fosamil use in 2 pediatric patients with invasive methicillin-resistant *Staphylococcus aureus* infections. *J Pediatr Pharmacol Ther.* 2015;20(6):476-480.

The full reference list for this chapter is available at ExpertConsult.com.

Coagulase-Negative Staphylococcal Infections 81

David Y. Hyun

Coagulase-negative staphylococci are some of the most common pathogens of healthcare-associated infections. Neonates, immunocompromised patients, and patients with indwelling medical devices are at higher risk for acquiring coagulase-negative staphylococcal infections.[180,199,227,276] Coagulase-negative staphylococci are the most frequently isolated organisms in the microbiology laboratory, in part owing to their commensal nature with human skin and mucosal membranes. Diagnostic challenges remain despite advances in molecular epidemiologic tools, owing to the difficulty of accurately differentiating true infections from contaminated clinical samples. Effective therapy can be difficult to achieve because of the high prevalence of resistance to multiple antibiotics. The discussion presented here is focused on the microbiology, epidemiology, pathogenesis, clinical manifestations, diagnoses, and treatment of infections caused by these ubiquitous organisms.

HISTORICAL BACKGROUND

Frederick Julius Rosenbach is credited with identifying *Staphylococcus epidermidis* in 1884, which at the time he named *S. albus* to denote the white colonies and to differentiate it from *S. aureus,* which was observed to have yellow colonies. The *S. albus* term was subsequently used as the descriptive terminology for all coagulase-negative staphylococci until the 1960s when coagulase-negative staphylococci began gaining recognition as significant infectious pathogens in certain patient populations. They were identified as etiologic agents of infections in neonates with sepsis and in adult patients with atrioventricular shunts and peritoneal catheters.[33,35,149,243] As a result, efforts to further differentiate and delineate species of coagulase-negative staphylococci led to the new nomenclature of *S. epidermidis* as well as to the identification and recognition of *S. saprophyticus* as a pathogen of the urinary tract. Descriptions and identifications of other species followed. Today there are more than 40 known species of coagulase-negative staphylococci.

MICROBIOLOGY

Staphylococci are gram-positive, nonmotile, non–spore forming, and catalase-positive bacteria. They are members of the family Micrococcaceae along with *Micrococcus, Planococcus,* and *Stomatococcus.* Members of the genus *Staphylococcus* have a low DNA G + C content (30 to 39 mol%), whereas members of the genus *Micrococcus* have a G + C content within the range of 66 to 75 mol%.[135] Staphylococci grow in irregular clusters, which are often described to resemble grapes when viewed microscopically. The cell wall is composed primarily of peptidoglycan with teichoic acid and an assortment of interspersed proteins, many of which are exposed on the surface and interact with host cells.[201] The teichoic acid has a glycerol backbone, in contrast to the ribitol of *S. aureus.*[188] Staphylococci are further divided by their ability to produce coagulase, the enzyme responsible for coagulation of rabbit plasma. *S. aureus* and *S. hyicus-intermedius* group constitute the coagulase-positive species. Most clinical laboratories utilize an alternative agglutination method that targets antigens specific to *S. aureus* to differentiate it from coagulase-negative staphylococci.[113] Fermentation of mannitol is another feature of *S. aureus* that differentiates it from most coagulase-negative staphylococci.

Species identification for coagulase-negative staphylococci requires assessment of a combination of features, including colony morphology, oxygen requirements, novobiocin resistance, aerobic acid production from carbohydrates, and selected liability to enzymatic activities.[133,136] Resistance to novobiocin is observed in several species including *S. saprophyticus.*[208] Commercial kits utilizing rapid biochemical reactions are available to identify species of coagulase-negative staphylococci. Although these kits have varying degrees of confidence and accuracy depending on the species, most systems can reliably identify species frequently associated with human disease, such as *S. epidermidis, S. haemolyticus,* and *S. saprophyticus.*[211] *S. lugdunensis,* which has recently emerged as a significant pathogen in humans, can be differentiated from other coagulase-negative staphylococci by a negative tube coagulase test, a positive pyrrolidonyl arylamidase (PYR) reaction, and positive ornithine decarboxylase activity.[76]

Matrix-assisted laser desorption ionization-time of flight (MALDI-TOF) uses mass spectroscopy for bacterial identification from clinical samples and has been demonstrated to be a rapid and accurate diagnostic tool for coagulase negative staphylococci.[9,65,155] By reducing the time to identification and speciation for coagulase negative staphylococci, MALDI-TOF can assist clinicians in making timely antibiotic treatment decisions.[181]

EPIDEMIOLOGY

Coagulase-negative staphylococci are primarily isolated from human skin and mucosal membranes (Table 81.1). The number of commensal coagulase-negative staphylococci on skin can vary from 10 to 10^6 colony-forming units per square centimeter depending on the anatomic location, with some species demonstrating a predilection for colonizing specific body sites.[134] Colonization can begin as early as the neonatal period. Two studies addressed the colonization of *S. epidermidis* in

TABLE 81.1 Coagulase-Negative Staphylococci Commensal to Human Skin and Mucosal Membranes

Species	Anatomic Site	Pathogenic Potential
S. epidermidis	Nares, axillae, skin	Common
S. saprophyticus	Occasionally skin	Common
S. haemolyticus	Skin of head, arms, and legs	Uncommon
S. hominis	Axillae, skin of head, arms, and legs	Uncommon
S. lugdunensis	Widely distributed on body	Uncommon
S. simulans	Occasionally skin	Uncommon
S. cohnii	Occasionally skin	Uncommon
S. warneri	Occasionally skin	Uncommon
S. saccharolyticus	Rarely skin	Rare
S. caprae	Occasionally skin	Rare
S. capitis	Skin of head, face, ears, and arms	Rare
S. auricularis	Ears	Rare
S. schleiferi	Skin	Rare
S. xylosus	Occasionally skin	Rare

Modified from Pfaller MA, Herwaldt LA. Laboratory, clinical, and epidemiological aspects of coagulase-negative staphylococci. *Clin Microbiol Rev.* 1988;1:281–99.

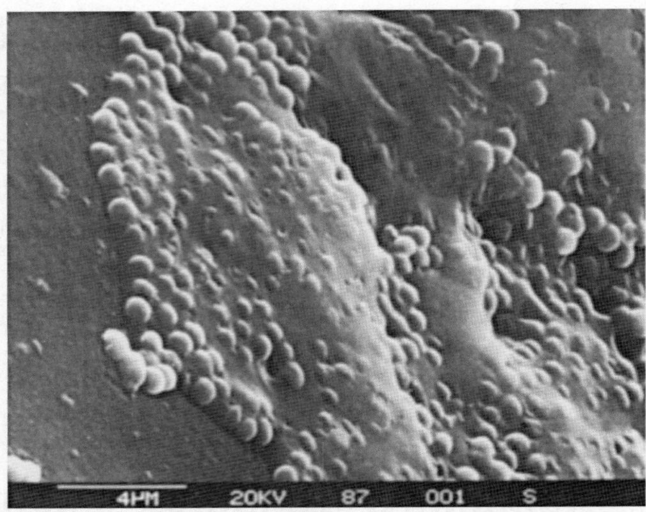

FIG. 81.1 Scanning electron microscopy of slime-producing coagulase-negative staphylococci. (From Peters G, Locci R, Pulverer G. Adherence and growth of coagulase-negative staphylococci on surfaces of intravenous catheters. *J Infect Dis.* 1982;146:479–482.)

TABLE 81.2 Methods of Epidemiologic Analysis of Coagulase-Negative Staphylococci

Conventional	Molecular
Biotyping[105,195]	Multilocus enzyme electrophoresis[187,264,276,293]
Colony morphology[135]	Plasmid analysis[8,135,193,194,239,240,261,281]
Antibiotic susceptibility[98,102,135,148,165,174]	Chromosomal analysis[23,85,116]
Serology[1,204,290]	Polymerase chain reaction amplification[135]
Polypeptide analysis[32,36,48,64,264]	
Biofilm production[44,51]	
Phage typing[43,54,196,195,254,259]	
Mass spectrometry[78]	

low-birth-weight neonates,[50,99] with both reports describing rapid colonization where 75% of neonates were colonized by 2 weeks of age. Although most infants acquire coagulase-negative staphylococci from environmental sources, including hospital personnel, a few are colonized by vertical transmission.[25,98,202]

Staphylococcus epidermidis continues to be the predominant species identified among commensal and clinical isolates.[284] Most coagulase-negative staphylococci cause nosocomial infections frequently associated with indwelling prosthetic devices such as central venous catheters. As a result, the increase in use of these medical devices has led to a proportional increase in the rates of infections.[227] *S. saprophyticus* and *S. lugdunensis* are notable exceptions that have been associated with community-acquired urinary tract infections and native-valve endocarditis, respectively.[13,147]

Epidemiologic typing methods are used in coagulase-negative staphylococcal infections when investigating a common-source outbreak or repeated infections within an individual (Table 81.2).[187,211,276] Older phenotypic typing tools such as antibiotic susceptibility pattern analysis, biochemical reactivity, slime production detection, and serologic typing lacked the power to differentiate closely related strains and were hampered by poor sensitivities and specificities.[255,284] In contrast, molecular genotyping methods have demonstrated higher discriminatory power with pulse-field gel electrophoresis (PFGE) becoming the method of choice when investigating patterns of transmission and sources of outbreaks.[29,145,175,263,276] Random amplification of polymorphic DNA (RAPD) by polymerase chain reaction (PCR) also has been successful in identifying clonal outbreaks and transmissions. Although it is less discriminatory than PFGE, RAPD is less costly and time consuming.[26,218] Multilocus sequence typing (MLST) can be used to delineate clonal relationships between strains and has been used to identify predominant clones from a group of clinical isolates.[159,292]

PATHOGENESIS

Risk factors for coagulase-negative staphylococcal infection are associated with nosocomial interventions that modify or bypass the host defense and immune mechanisms. They include immunosuppression,[72,127] prior antibiotic therapies,[128,245] and breakdown of mucocutaneous barriers, which is most commonly seen with the presence of prosthetic devices such as central venous catheters, cerebrospinal fluid (CSF) shunts, and peritoneal dialysis catheters.[14,21,67,152]

Biofilms (Fig. 81.1) are major virulence factors for coagulase-negative staphylococci especially in infections associated with prosthetic devices.[5,43,45,57–59,63,159,266,274] They are agglomerates of bacteria embedded in extracellular material and provide a mechanism of evasion against host defense and antibiotic activities.[68,89,120,140,247,248,275,279,280] They act as mechanical barriers to most immune cells, interfere with phagocytic activity, and limit antibiotic diffusion. Biofilm formation occurs in steps, with initial attachment followed by accumulation and detachment.

The initial attachment of *S. epidermidis* to polystyrene and other surfaces[160,159] is primarily mediated by several microbial surface components recognizing adhesive matrix molecules (MSCRAMMs).[109,114,228,265,279] MSCRAMMs facilitate binding to specific human matrix proteins, including fibrinogen, fibronectin, vitronectin, and collagen. Nonspecific electrostatic and hydrophobic interactions[106,111,267] and teichoic acids[114] also play roles in adhesion. Initial adhesion is followed by intercellular aggregation and accumulation of biofilms mediated by production of polysaccharide intercellular adhesion (PIA),[108,229] which acts as the primary component for the extracellular matrix of *S. epidermidis.* In addition to its role in biofilm formation, PIA also acts as a hemaglutinin[159,226] and provides protection against phagocytosis and killing by human polymorphonuclear leukocytes.[249,280] The *ica* operon encodes enzymes necessary for PIA production.[108]

In numerous epidemiologic studies, the presence of the *ica* operon has been associated more frequently with *S. epidermidis* strains isolated from hospitalized patients with prosthetic device infections than with community strains isolated from healthy individuals. Eighty-one to 89% of isolates from hospitalized patients have been reported to carry the *ica* operon. In contrast, only 6% to 38% of community-acquired isolates were found to carry the *ica* operon.[77,138,268] However, utilizing *ica* operon detection to differentiate between invasive and commensal strains of *S. epidermidis* has proven to be unreliable. Investigations of clinical strains obtained from patients in neonatal intensive care units, bone marrow transplant units, and oncology units have shown that although both invasive and commensal strains demonstrated high carriage rates of the *ica* operon, no significant difference was found between the two groups.[30,55,205,222] Higher proportions of invasive strains demonstrated biofilm production in quantitative assays compared with commensal strains.[30,222] Most of the commensal strains were biofilm-negative despite possessing the *ica* operon, a finding suggesting that regulation of gene expression plays a large role in virulence. Clinical strains of *S. epidermidis* producing biofilms independently of PIA have also been described.[137,222,221]

Unlike *S. aureus*, which is capable of producing various cytolytic and superantigenic toxins, *S. epidermidis* produces very few toxins.[278] More recently, phenol-soluble modulins (PSMs) have been identified and characterized as a family of peptides produced by *S. epidermidis* with cytolytic and proinflammatory capacities.[41,170] *Delta* toxin is part of the PSM complex and is an enteropathogenic toxin encoded by the *hld* component of the regulatory system agr that has been linked to necrotizing enterocolitis in infants.[241] *S. epidermidis* also produces antibacterial peptides called *lantibiotics* that may play a role in bacterial interference on skin and mucous membranes and in the creation of an ecologic niche for *S. epidermidis*.[142] Numerous extracellular enzymes are also produced by coagulase-negative staphylococci; an extracellular metalloprotease with elastase activity; a cysteine protease that degrades human secretory immunoglobulin A, immunoglobulin M, serum albumin, fibrinogen, and fibronectin; and an extracellular serine protease involved in epidermin processing.[107,278,282] Two lipases have been postulated to facilitate skin colonization.[107,278]

S. saprophyticus can cause urinary tract infections in the absence of indwelling catheters.[142] Several virulence factors have been described to explain its pathogenic potential to adhere and persistently grow in the urinary tract. A surface-exposed protein with hemagglutinin and adhesive properties[84] and a surface fibrillar protein,[83] designated *ssp*, are associated with attachment to urinary tract epithelium. Urease production also has been associated with invasiveness of this organism by causing damage to bladder tissues.[81,82] The whole genome of *S. saprophyticus* has been sequenced and compared with *S. aureus* and *S. epidermidis*.[142] Analysis revealed a single, unique cell wall–anchored protein with properties of hemagglutination and adherence to human bladder cells. A high population of ionic transport systems capable of providing osmotolerance in the highly variant ionic environment of urine also was demonstrated.

S. lugdunensis has emerged as a significant pathogen associated with more severe and aggressive forms of endocarditis compared to other coagulase-negative staphylococcal species. This may be explained by the ability of *S. lugdunensis* to directly bind to von Willebrand factor, thus facilitating adhesion to vessel walls and cardiac valves while allowing the organism to withstand shear forces.[154]

CLINICAL MANIFESTATIONS

Coagulase-negative staphylococci have been implicated in a variety of clinical infections, which are mostly nosocomial in immunocompetent and immunocompromised patients (Box 81.1).[133,199,230] Because of the commensal nature of these organisms, separating true infections from contaminated culture results continues to be a challenge. This is further complicated by the variability among clinical studies when defining the criteria for clinically significant cultures.[61] Repeated isolation of the same phenotypic or genotypic strains of coagulase-negative staphylococci can facilitate interpretation. Quantitative cultures can also add value in the diagnosis of catheter-associated bacteremia by demonstrating a five- to tenfold increase in the number of colony-forming units in cultures obtained from a catheter compared with cultures from a peripheral blood vessel. The Committee on Infectious Diseases of the American Academy of Pediatrics suggested the following considerations to distinguish pathogenic coagulase-negative staphylococci from contaminants: (1) two or more positive blood cultures from different collection sites, (2) a positive culture from blood and another usually sterile site with identical antimicrobial susceptibility patterns, (3) growth in continuously monitored blood culture system within 15 hours of incubation, (4) clinical findings of infection, (5) an intravascular catheter that has been in place for 3 days or more, and (6) similar or identical genotypes among all isolates.[4]

BOX 81.1 Clinically Significant Coagulase-Negative Staphylococcal Infections

Bacteremia:
- Neonates
- Patients with leukemia and lymphoma
- Bone marrow transplant recipients

Infections in patients with medical devices:
- Intravascular catheters
- Cerebrospinal fluid shunts
- Peritoneal dialysis catheter
- Prosthetic valves

Other infections:
- Prosthetic joints
- Vascular grafts and prostheses
- Hemodialysis catheter
- Pacemaker
- Scalp electrodes

Native valve endocarditis

Urinary tract infections

Miscellaneous infections:
- Endophthalmitis
- Postoperative wound infections
- Osteomyelitis
- Toxic shock syndrome

Modified from Patrick CC. Coagulase-negative staphylococci: pathogens with increasing clinical significance. *J Pediatr*. 1990;116:497–507.

Clinical presentation markedly differs from that of *S. aureus* infection. In general, infections caused by coagulase-negative staphylococci are more indolent and can have a subacute or even chronic course. They occur mostly as health care–associated bacteremia and infections of prosthetic medical devices.

Bacteremia

Coagulase-negative staphylococci, particularly *S. epidermidis*, are the most common pathogens in nosocomial bloodstream infections and have become the major nosocomial pathogens in most studies.[61,220] A large surveillance study between 1995 and 2001 among 49 hospitals in the United States showed that coagulase-negative staphylococci were identified in 43% of nosocomial bacteremias in pediatric patients.[285] In another single center study, analysis of 4405 episodes of bloodstream infections from a children's hospital during 2002 to 2012 demonstrated that coagulase-negative staphylococci were identified in 49% of these cases.[146] Among oncologic immunocompromised pediatric patients, coagulase-negative staphylococci accounted for up to 35% of all positive blood culture isolates.[2,12,144] A significant majority of all coagulase-negative bacteremia occurs with the use of indwelling vascular catheters.

Neonatal Bacteremia

Coagulase-negative staphylococci are the most frequent cause of late-onset septicemia and bloodstream infections among premature infants.[18,73,90,100,97,186,200] These infections are found predominantly in premature infants with a gestational age of less than 34 weeks and those with low birth weights,[90,104,118,200] owing to their higher likelihood of prolonged use of a central catheter and parenteral nutrition and their immature immune system, including quantitative and qualitative neutrophil deficiencies.[37,244,285] The presence of indwelling peripheral or umbilical catheters has been implicated in approximately half of neonatal coagulase-negative staphylococcal bacteremias.[18,97,185,195] The salient features from six large studies are listed in Table 81.3.[73,97,123,124,178,200]

TABLE 81.3 Clinical Characteristics of Coagulase-Negative Staphylococcal Bacteremia in Neonates

Characteristics	Munson et al., 1982[178] (*n* = 27)	Fleer et al., 1983[73] (*n* = 30)	Hall et al., 1987[97] (*n* = 29)	Patrick et al., 1989[200] (*n* = 32)	Kacica et al., 1994[123] (*n* = 47)	Kallman et al., 1997[124] (*n* = 27)
Patient						
Mean birth weight (g)	1130	1564	1607	1172	1259	NR
Gestational age (wk)	28.9	32.1	31	28.6	29	<30
Central lines (%)	85	NR	34	19	NR	NR
TPN (%)	78	77	NR	91	81	NR
Clinical						
Apnea or bradycardia (%)	>50	100	62	78	NR	NR
Temperature instability (%)	<50	70	7	22	NR	NR
Tachycardia (%)	>50	100	NR	6	NR	NR
Mortality (%)	0	0	0	0	NR	7.4
Laboratory						
Biofilm production (%)	NR	NR	79	54	65	NR
Antibiotic susceptibility	100% S to cephalothin	100% S to cephalothin	83% S to methicillin; 100% S to vancomycin	100% S to vancomycin	48% S to oxacillin; 100% S to vancomycin	86% S to methicillin[a] 55% S to methicillin[b]

NR, Not reported; *S*, susceptible; *TPN*, total parenteral nutrition.
[a]1981–86.
[b]1987–94.

Clinical findings of coagulase-negative staphylococcal bacteremia are mostly indolent and subtle and include bradycardia, apnea, and temperature instability (see Table 81.3). The frequency of fulminant late-onset sepsis caused by coagulase-negative staphylococcal bacteremia is very low (1%).[126] Mortality rates associated with coagulase-negative staphylococcal infections in neonates are much lower compared with those with other pathogens.[161,258] However, neonates with prolonged and persistent bacteremia have higher mortality rates that are comparable to those of other pathogens.[39,118] In addition, polymicrobial bloodstream infections that include coagulase-negative staphylococci as one of the pathogens are likely to have higher mortality rates.[192]

Laboratory studies need to be interpreted within clinical contexts and risk factors consistent with coagulase-negative staphylococcal bacteremia.[104,112,166,182] Leukocytosis may not be present, and there have been conflicting findings in regard to the utility of biofilm detection as a marker for infection.[97,200] Use of quantitative blood cultures correlated with clinical criteria may have a role in identifying the true pathogen.[257] The Centers for Disease Control and Prevention (CDC) defines laboratory-confirmed bloodstream infections for common skin contaminants including coagulase-negative staphylococci in patients 1 year or younger as (1) at least one finding of fever, hypothermia, apnea, or bradycardia; (2) signs, symptoms, and laboratory findings not consistent with infection at another site; and (3) isolation of an organism from two or more blood cultures drawn on separate occasions.[112]

Persistence of coagulase-negative staphylococcal bacteremia despite administration of adequate antibiotic therapy has been described in neonates.[60,131,200] Mean duration of persistent bacteremia is 10 to 14 days. This persistence was observed in patients with and without central venous catheters and in patients with normal findings on cardiac echocardiography. Neonates with persistent bacteremia had a significantly higher incidence of severe thrombocytopenia requiring platelet transfusions than did those with nonpersistent bacteremia.[60,131]

Rarely coagulase-negative staphylococcal meningitis in the absence of intraventricular devices has been reported in low-birth-weight neonates with normal CSF white blood cell counts.[95] CSF examination may be considered in neonates with coagulase-negative staphylococcal bacteremia because abnormal CSF findings or a positive CSF culture may influence the duration of therapy. Coagulase-negative staphylococci also have been implicated as etiologic agents of necrotizing enterocolitis,[94,241] although one report showed no association.[225]

Bacteremia in Immunocompromised Patients

Immunocompromised patients with leukemia or lymphoma are at risk for coagulase-negative staphylococcal bacteremia (Table 81.4).[2,12,79,144,212,213,246] In several reports, coagulase-negative staphylococci were the isolates most commonly causing bacteremia in pediatric patients with cancer and accounted for 35% to 50% of all initial isolates.[2,12,144,203] One-third of these patients did not have central venous catheters at the time of their bacteremia.[79] Risk factors for this patient population include indwelling catheters, malnutrition, and myelosuppression, especially neutropenia after chemotherapy. In addition to catheter-associated bloodstream infections, translocation of pathogens through inflamed mucosal surfaces secondary to chemotherapy, including the gastrointestinal tract, is a prominent mechanism of bacteremia. One study utilizing molecular epidemiologic tools, including RAPD and PFGE analysis of clinical isolates obtained from adult neutropenic oncology patients, showed that skin flora was the likely source for 75% of coagulase-negative staphylococcal catheter-associated infections.[187]

Coagulase-negative staphylococci have become the primary pathogens for bacteremia among hematopoietic stem cell transplant recipients.[34,173] These episodes occur most often during periods of agranulocytosis before marrow engraftment,[34] and they can be fatal.[20] Most bacteremic episodes are due to use of central venous catheters and broad-spectrum antibiotics. Coagulase-negative staphylococci is also a frequent pathogen for bloodstream infections in solid organ transplant recipients.[22]

Significant morbidity from coagulase-negative staphylococcal bacteremia can be attributed to the organism's acquisition of multiple antibiotic resistance that requires the use of antimicrobial agents with a higher risk for toxicity, such as vancomycin or linezolid.[79,127,144,157,158,214,238] Mortality rates have varied from 0% to 11%.[79,144]

Indwelling Medical Devices

Intravascular Catheter-Related Infections

Coagulase-negative staphylococci are the most common pathogens for catheter-related infections.[75,172,287] Risk for infections varies among the different types of catheters. Short-term central venous catheters (CVCs),

TABLE 81.4 Clinical Characteristics of Coagulase-Negative Staphylococcal Bacteremia in Pediatric Patients With Cancer

Characteristics	Friedman et al., 1984[79] (*n* = 150)	Langley and Gold, 1988[144] (*n* = 100)	Aledo et al., 1998[2] (*n* = 140)	Auletta et al., 1999[12] (*n* = 102)
Coagulase-negative staphylococci among total bacteremias (%)	12.7	35	31.4	35
Patients with central venous catheters (%)	32	53	95	95
Mortality rate (%)	10.5	38	<5	19
Patient isolates susceptible to:				
Methicillin (%)	17	38	NR	NR
Vancomycin (%)	100	100	NR	NR

NR, Not reported.

defined as those in place for fewer than 14 days, account for the majority of catheter-related infections. Peripherally inserted central catheters (PICCs) carry similar risks of infection to those of short-term CVCs when used in intensive care units.[172] However, the frequency of catheter-related infections for PICCs used for outpatient parenteral therapies appears to be significantly lower.[151,272] Long-term CVCs that are surgically implanted with a tunneled portion and a Dacron cuff just inside the skin exit site[32,110] also have lower infection rates at 0.14 per 100 catheter-days,[113] with the catheter hub being the major source of infection.[216] Finally totally implanted vascular devices with subcutaneous ports or reservoirs carry the lowest infection risk, with rates of 0 to 0.04 per 100 catheter-days.[113,224] Infections at the catheter insertion sites also can lead to bacteremia or septic thrombophlebitis, with further complications caused by metastatic spread.[215] Overall infectious complications involving central venous catheters have a variable reported frequency of 2.7% to 47%,[21,86,103,156,176,253,277] with coagulase-negative staphylococci identified as the pathogens in approximately half of these cases. The wide range of frequency is attributed to the intended use of the catheters, types of catheters, frequency of catheter access, characteristics of patients, and use of preventive strategies.[172]

As with other coagulase-negative staphylococcal infections, *S. epidermidis* is the predominant species associated with catheter-related infections, accounting for approximately 70% of cases.[21,103] This likely correlates to the high prevalence of the organisms colonizing the human skin.[134] Other implicated coagulase-negative staphylococcal species include *S. haemolyticus*, *S. warneri*, and *S. hominis*.[103]

Establishing accurate diagnoses of catheter-related coagulase-negative staphylococcal infections remains a challenge owing to the difficulty of differentiating true infections from contaminated specimens and depends on the patient's clinical status and the isolation of identical strains from repeated cultures. In addition, it is important to distinguish catheter-related bacteremia from secondary bacteremia caused by infections at other sites. The use of quantitative blood cultures has shown that catheter-related bacteremia has a 5- to 10-fold difference in bacterial concentration in blood cultures drawn from the catheter when compared with the concentration in peripheral cultures.[74,219] When a catheter is removed because of a suspected catheter-related infection, a semiquantitative culture of the distal 5 cm of the catheter is recommended.[172] This can be accomplished by rolling the distal portion of the catheter on an agar plate. Growth of more than 15 colony-forming units is indicative of catheter colonization.[162]

Duration of antimicrobial therapy for uncomplicated coagulase-negative staphylococcal catheter-related infections depends on whether the catheter is removed or retained.[172] When the catheter is no longer needed, it should be removed and the patient should be given 5 to 7 days of antimicrobial therapy. If the catheter is retained, the duration of antimicrobial therapy should be 10 to 14 days and accompanied by antibiotic lock therapy. Therapy with retention of a catheter carries a higher risk for recurrence.[217] Complicated catheter-related infections, including those with tunnel infections, port abscesses, septic thrombosis, endocarditis, and osteomyelitis, are indications for catheter removal. *S. lugdunensis* infections should be treated more conservatively in a manner similar to *S. aureus* infections owing to the higher virulence of this organism compared with other coagulase-negative staphylococci.

Central Nervous System Shunts

Coagulase-negative staphylococci are the predominant pathogens for infections of central nervous system shunts that are used to relieve hydrocephalus by diverting CSF.[130] They account for 60% to 75% of all bacterial causes of shunt infections.[130,183,250] Ventriculoperitoneal shunts that divert CSF into the peritoneal cavity have primarily been used since the 1960s because of their lower rate of mechanical complications.[130,179,189] Ventriculoatrial shunts that divert CSF into the right atrium are used infrequently because of higher complication rates.[189] However, the incidences of infection involving both ventriculoperitoneal and the ventriculoatrial shunts are comparable.[130,189,250] Infection rates are higher in neonates.

Shunt infections can begin at the insertion site by contamination of the catheter from the patient's skin flora[250] or during subsequent revisions. Short-term infection rates are reported to be 13%, and 10-year infection rates are 27%.[223] Seventy percent of ventriculoperitoneal shunt infections occur within the first 2 months after placement.[183]

CSF examination can be helpful in patients with signs and symptoms consistent with a shunt infection. Gram stain of ventricular fluid is often negative, but culture is sensitive. Subtle changes are noted in CSF and ventricular fluid cell counts or cytochemical findings.[289] Patients with ventriculoatrial shunts often have signs and symptoms compatible with septicemia. In patients with ventriculoperitoneal shunts, an intraabdominal cyst may develop at the distal end of the catheter. Dysfunctions of the shunt secondary to development of infections often lead to signs and symptoms consistent with increased intracranial pressure. Standard therapy for ventriculoperitoneal shunt infections has been removal of the shunt system and administration of systemic antibiotics.[250,289,291]

Peritoneal Dialysis Catheters

S. epidermidis is the bacterial pathogen most commonly isolated in peritoneal dialysis catheter infections,[93,209] accounting for up to 50% of infections.[209] These include catheter exit site infections as well as peritonitis.[209] The prevalence of peritonitis in patients undergoing continuous ambulatory peritoneal dialysis is approximately 60%. Signs of peritonitis include fever, abdominal pain, and cloudy peritoneal dialysis fluid. Removal of the catheter usually is not necessary for successful therapy but may be required in refractory cases or when the catheter malfunctions. Antibiotics can be administered systemically as well as intraperitoneally through the dialysis fluid.[70]

Prosthetic Valves

Coagulase-negative staphylococci are frequent pathogens causing prosthetic valve endocarditis, accounting for approximately 17% of cases.[52,283] This is in contrast to native valve endocarditis for which coagulase-negative staphylococci are rarely isolated. Although many cases of coagulase-negative staphylococcal prosthetic valve endocarditis occur within 60 days of device implantation,[150] they can also occur as late as 1 year after surgery, with inoculation of the organism at the time of surgery followed by abscess formation of the valvular ring being the likely mechanism.[29] Signs and symptoms can vary, but fever is the most common finding. Typical findings of endocarditis caused by other pathogens such as peripheral emboli can be mostly absent in coagulase-negative staphylococcal endocarditis, owing to the organism's indolent nature. Anemia is the abnormality identified most often by laboratory testing. Evaluation should include multiple blood cultures and echocardiography. The antimicrobial regimen for prosthetic valve endocarditis caused by coagulase-negative staphylococci usually involves vancomycin and rifampin for a minimum of 6 weeks along with gentamicin for the first 2 weeks because the majority of organisms are methicillin resistant.[15] Surgery may be indicated when infection is complicated by perivalvular or myocardial abscesses.

Other Indwelling Medical Devices

Coagulase-negative staphylococci are involved in an expanded spectrum of infections involving indwelling medical devices.[57,91] They include infections of prosthetic joints,[71,125] vascular grafts,[16,62] hemodialysis shunts,[197,242,243] and pacemaker pockets.[42,117,163,207] Additionally osteomyelitis secondary to *S. epidermidis* has been reported to occur after hemodialysis and in neonates after the use of a monitoring scalp electrode.[190]

Native Valve Endocarditis

Approximately 7% of cases of native valve endocarditis are caused by coagulase-negative staphylococci, and *S. epidermidis* is the most frequently isolated species.[46] These infections usually are subacute and arise from transient bacteremia. Pathogenesis is thought to involve seeding of a previously damaged valve or endocarditis that had not been previously identified.[6,19]

S. lugdunensis can cause acute, severe, and destructive endocarditis similar to *S. aureus* endocarditis,[270] with most favorable outcomes occurring in patients who undergo valve replacement.[53] Most patients with *S. lugdunensis* endocarditis have been older than 50 years. Mortality rates are higher compared with infections by other species.[13] Native aortic or mitral valves are involved most frequently.[269] The perineum appears to have a high colonization rate of *S. lugdunensis.*[121]

Surgical Site Infections

Coagulase-negative staphylococci are the second most common cause of postoperative surgical site infections after *S. aureus*, according to National Nosocomial Infections Surveillance Report survey data.[38] Most infections are likely caused by the patient's own endogenous skin flora, but outbreaks originating from operating room personnel have been reported.[29] Outbreaks of *S. epidermidis* surgical site infections, such as mediastinitis and endocarditis, among patients who have undergone cardiac valve replacements also have been reported.[28,218]

Urinary Tract Infections

S. saprophyticus is the most common coagulase-negative staphylococcal species that causes infections in both the upper and the lower urinary tracts.[147] These infections occur predominantly in young, healthy, sexually active women,[122,147,166] during late summer and fall, with a pattern similar to that of sexually transmitted diseases.[81] Recent sexual intercourse, outdoor swimming, and occupational meat processing have been identified as risk factors.[81] *S. epidermidis* and other coagulase-negative staphylococci rarely cause urinary tract infections, but they have been noted to produce disease in older adults with urinary tract complications.[96,153,184] Pyelonephritis caused by *S. epidermidis* have been described in healthy children.[100,168]

Miscellaneous Infections

Endophthalmitis secondary to *S. epidermidis* has been reported in patients undergoing ocular surgery or trauma.[17,31,210] One center reported coagulase-negative staphylococci as being the most common organisms isolated from patients with culture-positive endophthalmitis over a 20-year period, accounting for 38% of the cases.[40] Postoperative mediastinitis that develops after median sternotomy for open heart surgery can be caused by *S. epidermidis.*[27,66,92] Primary osteomyelitis secondary to coagulase-negative staphylococci is a rare occurrence in healthy children.[191] *S. caprae*[251] and *S. lugdunensis*[236] have been linked to bone and joint infections. Coagulase-negative staphylococci also have been implicated as a possible cause of toxic shock syndrome.[49] Rare cases of skin and soft tissue infections caused by *S. lugeunensis* have also been reported.[143,171]

TREATMENT

Vancomycin is the drug of choice for most coagulase-negative staphylococcal infections, owing to the high prevalence of methicillin resistance especially among nosocomial strains.[3,232,252] When susceptibility data are not available, vancomycin should be used for empirical therapy. If the coagulase-negative *Staphylococcus* is known to be susceptible to methicillin, oxacillin or nafcillin is the preferred therapeutic agent.[211,233]

Most coagulase-negative staphylococci, particularly *S. epidermidis* and *S. haemolyticus,* are resistant to multiple antibiotics, including methicillin.[7,9,43,56,69,88,101,245,256,275] Cross-resistance exists between penicillinase-resistant penicillins and cephalosporins. Therefore methicillin-resistant coagulase-negative staphylococci should be considered as cephalosporin resistant even if routine susceptibility testing indicates susceptibility to cephalosporins.[93,119,148,232] Methicillin-resistant coagulase-negative staphylococci are often resistant to other antibiotics, such as clindamycin, erythromycin, and gentamicin.[7] The *mecA* gene is responsible for methicillin resistance because it encodes a penicillin-binding protein (PBP2a) that interferes with the binding of β-lactams to the bacterial cell wall.[107,115] The same mechanism accounts for methicillin resistance in *S. aureus*. Consistent detection of methicillin resistance for coagulase-negative staphylococci can be a challenging process in the clinical laboratory owing to heterogeneous expression of the *mecA* phenotype in minimal inhibitory concentration or disk diffusion testing with only a minority of the bacterial population expressing the resistant phenotype.[7,115,232,288] To facilitate more reliable detection, the Clinical and Laboratory Standards Institute revised specific breakpoints for coagulase-negative staphylococci in 2007 (Table 81.5).[47] In addition, to enhance phenotypic expression of methicillin resistance, the use of lower incubation temperatures of 30°C to 35°C for prolonged periods and of increased sodium chloride content in culture medium is recommended.[164,169,231] Molecular detection of the *mecA* gene is an accurate method to predict methicillin resistance.[115]

Coagulase-negative staphylococci were the first organisms in which glycopeptide resistance was recognized.[245] A prolonged course of vancomycin is a well-recognized risk factor for the emergence of strains with decreased susceptibility to glycopeptides.[24,288] Although they are uncommon occurrences, infections caused by these strains have been described and may become more common. Decreased susceptibility occurs more frequently to teicoplanin than to vancomycin.[10,141,286] The minimal inhibitory concentrations of teicoplanin usually fall over a wide range, whereas vancomycin minimal inhibitory concentrations tend to remain more stable over a narrower range within the limits of susceptibility.[24] Intermediate resistance to vancomycin in coagulase-negative staphylococci has been rarely described.[237,245,273] Thickened cell walls, as seen by electron microscopy and altered cell metabolism that affects vancomycin binding, may be associated with glycopeptide resistance mechanisms.[107]

TABLE 81.5 Breakpoints for Antibiotic Susceptibility for Coagulase-Negative Staphylococci

	Oxacillin Susceptible	Oxacillin Intermediate	Oxacillin Resistant
MIC			
CoNS	≤0.25 µg/mL		≥0.5 µg/mL
S. aureus	≤2 µg/mL		≥4 µg/mL
Zone Size			
CoNS	≥18 mm	No intermediate zone	≤17 mm
S. aureus	≥13 mm	11–12 mm	≤10 mm

CoNS, Coagulase-negative staphylococci; *MIC,* minimal inhibitory concentration.
Data from Clinical and Laboratory Standards Institute. *Performance testing for antimicrobial susceptibility testing, 17th informational supplement M100-S17.* Wayne, PA: 2007.

Gentamicin and rifampin are active against coagulase-negative staphylococci, but rapid emergence of resistance has limited their use as single-drug regimens.[43,167,233] These two antibiotics have been shown to be synergistic with vancomycin against methicillin-resistant, coagulase-negative staphylococci.[157] Additionally rifampin has been used in neonates with persistent bacteremia to eradicate the organisms.[260,271] Combination therapies utilizing gentamicin or rifampin are frequently used for prosthetic device infections including endocarditis and CSF shunt infections.

Quinupristin-dalfopristin,[11] linezolid,[230] daptomycin,[87,139,235] ceftaroline,[234] and tigecycline[80,139] have all demonstrated significant in vitro activities against coagulase-negative staphylococci and may have a role in the treatment of multidrug-resistant strains. However, there is a paucity of clinical efficacy data for these therapies, and many lack pediatric pharmacokinetic data to guide appropriate dosing. Linezolid resistance in coagulase-negative staphylococci has been described and linked to increased utilization.[129,177]

PREVENTION

Preventing the development of coagulase-negative staphylococcal infection is difficult because of the ubiquitous and commensal nature of these organisms. A 3-year molecular analysis of coagulase-negative staphylococcal nosocomial infections in a neonatal intensive care unit showed that many of the infections were caused by clonal dissemination and potentially were preventable by hand washing, thus reducing the transmission rate from staff to patient or from patient to patient.[276]

Developing catheters that are both inert and resistant to bacterial colonization adherence has been only marginally successful.[132,198,206] The technique of impregnating the surface of catheters with antibiotics or disinfectants appears promising.[262] Prophylactic antibiotics are administered routinely for surgical procedures involving placement of a prosthetic device or material. However, the antimicrobial of choice to prevent infections caused by coagulase-negative staphylococci varies among institutions.[3] Vancomycin often is recommended for placement of a CSF shunt or prosthetic valve.

Infection control policies such as standardizing or "bundling" procedures for aseptic intravascular catheter placement and care is the single most important factor in preventing catheter-associated infections. Standard precautions should be used for methicillin-resistant, coagulase-negative staphylococci. For vancomycin-intermediate, coagulase-negative staphylococci, contact transmission precautions for multidrug-resistant organisms should be used.[4]

CONCLUSION

Coagulase-negative staphylococci, particularly *S. epidermidis,* are a major source of nosocomial infection in a variety of clinical situations. Most infections occur in patients who have indwelling medical devices. Epidemiologic studies have been limited by the commensal nature of the organisms, but newer molecular tools may help investigators to gain further insight and to differentiate true infections from contaminants. Therapy can be complex because of the usual presence of an indwelling medical device and the multiple antimicrobial resistances of the organisms.

NEW REFERENCES SINCE THE SEVENTH EDITION

9. Argemi X, Riegel P, Lavigne T, et al. Implementation of matrix-assisted laser desorption ionization-time of flight mass spectrometry in routine clinical laboratories improves identification of coagulase-negative staphylococci and reveals the pathogenic role of *Staphylococcus lugdunensis*. *J Clin Microbiol.* 2015;53:2030-2036.
22. Berenger BM, Doucette K, Smith SW. Epidemiology and risk factors for nosocomial bloodstream infections in solid organ transplants over a 10-year period. *Transpl Infect Dis.* 2016;18(2):183-190.
65. Dupont C, Sivadon-Tardy V, Bilie E, et al. Identification of clinical coagulase-negative staphylococci, isolated in microbiology laboratories by matrix-assisted laser desorption ionization-time of flight mass spectrometry and two automated systems. *Clin Microbiol Infect.* 2010;16:998-1004.
87. Gonzales-Ruiz A, Gargalianos-Kakolyris P, Timerman A, et al. Daptomycin in the clinical setting: 8-year experience with gram-positive bacterial infections from the EU-CORE(SM) registry. *Adv Ther.* 2015;32:496-509.
143. Lacour M, Posfay-Barbe KM, La Sacala GC. *Staphylococcus lugdunensis* abscesses complicating molluscum contagiosum in two children. *Pediatr Dermatol.* 2015;32:289-291.
146. Larru B, Gong W, Vendetti N, et al. Bloodstream infections in hospitalized children: epidemiology and antimicrobial susceptibilities. *Pediatr Infect Dis J.* 2016;35:507-510.
154. Liesenborghs L, Peetermans M, Claes J, et al. Shear-resistant binding to von Willebrand factor allows *Staphylococcus lugdunensis* to adhere to the cardiac valves and initiate endocarditis. *J Infect Dis.* 2016;213:1148-1156.
155. Loonen AJ, Jansz AR, Bergland JN, et al. Comparative study using phenotypic, genotypic, and proteomics methods for identification of coagulase-negative staphylococci. *J Clin Microbiol.* 2012;50:1437-1439.
171. Mehmood M, Khasawneh FA. *Staphylococcus lugdunensis* gluteal abscess in a patient with end stage renal disease on hemodialysis. *Clin Pract.* 2015;5:706.
181. Nagel JL, Huang AM, Kunapuli A, et al. Impact of antimicrobial stewardship intervention on coagulase-negative *Staphylococcus* blood cultures in conjunction with rapid diagnostic testing. *J Clin Microbiol.* 2014;52:2849-2854.
192. Pammi M, Zhong D, Johnson Y, et al. Polymicrobial bloodstream infections in the neonatal intensive care unit are associated with increased mortality: a case-control study. *BMC Infect Dis.* 2014;14:390.
234. Sader HS, Farrell DJ, Flamm RK, et al. Antimicrobial activity of ceftaroline and comparator agents when tested against numerous species of coagulase-negative *Staphylococcus* causing infection in US hospitals. *Diagn Microbiol Infect Dis.* 2016;85(1):80-84.

The full reference list for this chapter is available at ExpertConsult.com.

Group A, Group C, and Group G β-Hemolytic Streptococcal Infections

82

Linette Sande • Anthony R. Flores

Streptococcus pyogenes is the only organism within the group A β-hemolytic streptococci (GAS). GAS are among the most common pathogens that infect children and adolescents and are capable of causing a wide range of infections, including relatively benign pharyngitis and life-threatening invasive infections. Despite their uniform susceptibility to penicillin, GAS remain significant clinical and public health problems in this age group. Worldwide it is estimated that GAS are responsible for more than 500,000 deaths, the majority of which occur in underdeveloped countries.[26] GAS is unique among pyogenic streptococci in its ability to produce postinfectious sequelae such as acute rheumatic fever and acute poststreptococcal glomerular nephritis (APSGN). Infections caused by GAS were brought to the forefront in the United States in the late 1990s with a resurgence of acute rheumatic fever[96,158] and the appearance of serotype M1 and M3 strains causing severe morbidity and mortality.[10,151]

ORGANISM

GAS are gram-positive cocci, generally less than 2 μm, and tend to grow in chains in liquid media. GAS produce clear zones of hemolysis (β) on blood agar, differentiating them from streptococci producing partial (α) and nonhemolytic (γ) streptococci. Hemolysis is best observed when GAS are grown on agar containing 5% sheep blood. Some strains of GAS may appear to produce only partial hemolysis on blood agar plates. However, clear hemolysis can more easily be observed when grown anaerobically or by making a short cut or stab into the agar at the time of inoculation.[76] GAS are rarely nonhemolytic.[73,75] They can be differentiated from other β-hemolytic streptococci by their group-specific polysaccharide in the cell wall, the basis for latex agglutination and enzyme immunoassays, or by inhibition of growth by bacitracin.

GAS are frequently categorized or typed based on serologically distinct surface proteins, the M proteins, or by sequencing the gene encoding the M protein, *emm*.[42,43,76,87] The M protein is a major virulence factor of GAS. Acquired immunity to GAS is based, at least in part, on specific opsonic antibodies targeted against the M protein.[86] N-terminal sequence variation in the gene encoding the M protein has led to the description of more than 200 different *emm*-types,[14] and many more are being added to a curated database publicly available through the Centers for Disease Control and Prevention (CDC).[30] Certain GAS M serotypes have been associated with specific diseases and can be classified as skin or pharyngitis "specialists"; however, some M serotypes have the capacity to cause both types of infection.[16]

The GAS cell is complex and contains many antigenic substances. Freshly isolated clinical strains are typically covered with a hyaluronic acid capsule that is structurally similar to that found in mammals, including humans, and thus is nonimmunogenic.[19,50,79] The GAS capsule gives colonies a mucoid appearance. Recently some GAS serotypes (e.g., M4 and M22) have been shown to lack the genes necessary for hyaluronic acid biosynthesis.[48] Additionally a rise in the frequency of serotype M89 GAS has been linked to the absence of hyaluronic acid biosynthesis genes.[155,164] The M protein is a major constituent of the cell surface, and proteins similar to M protein have been identified. Genes encoding M and M-like proteins (e.g., *enn* and *mrp*) are part of an *emm* gene superfamily. Also found on the cell surface, protruding through the hyaluronic acid capsule, are fimbriae composed of lipoteichoic acid[13] that are frequently associated with M protein.[46] The surface proteins T and R and serum opacity factor are proteins of interest in part because of classification schemes based on each. The T protein is part of the GAS pilus structure,[98] and T-agglutination patterns are generally associated with specific M serotypes.[74] In strains that produce serum opacity factor, the serologically specific serum opacity factor proteins are closely correlated with a particular M serotype.[15]

The GAS cell surface contains a polysaccharide polymer of rhamnose with side chains of N-acetyl-glucosamine. The carbohydrate is found in sufficient quantities for antibody detection and forms the basis for group specificity originally described by Lancefield.[86] It has recently been recognized that the side chains of N-acetyl-glucosamine play a functional role in GAS pathogenesis.[156] Rigidity of the cell is provided by peptidoglycan consisting of alternating residues of N-acetyl-muramic acid and N-acetyl-glucosamine linked by a peptide bond. Lysozyme produced on mucosal surfaces and by phagocytic cells hydrolyzes the carbohydrate backbone, leading to lysis of the cell and release of bacterial fragments. Detection of the bacterial fragments by host pattern recognition receptors leads to initiation of the host immune response to infection. Some streptococci are able to modify their peptidoglycan, leading to lysozyme resistance,[38] and alter the host immune response. Whether GAS has this capability is unknown.

The innermost layer of the cell wall consists of the cell membrane composed of lipoprotein or lipid–protein complexes. Wall-less forms of streptococci, termed *L forms,* are osmotically fragile and lack the outermost constituents of the GAS cell wall. GAS L forms are of interest because of their resistance to penicillin[54] and their potential role in persistence.[95]

In addition to cell surface components, GAS produces many extracellular products. Among these are two distinct hemolysins: streptolysin O and streptolysin S. Streptolysin O, designated so because of its oxygen lability, is toxic to erythrocytes and many other cell types, including phagocytes. Streptolysin O is produced by almost all GAS strains, is antigenic, and measurement of anti–streptolysin O (ASO) antibodies is used as an indicator of GAS infection. Streptolysin S is stable in the presence of oxygen, heat labile, and not antigenic. Hemolysis on the surface of blood agar is the result of streptolysin S; streptolysin O results in hemolysis in the subsurface or in anaerobic conditions.

Several extracellular proteins allow the spread of GAS through tissue. Deoxyribonucleases (DNAses A, B, C, and D) break down extracellular DNA and are believed to facilitate escape from neutrophil extracellular traps consisting in large part of DNA.[23] Spread through connective tissue is achieved through the action of hyaluronidases that enzymatically degrade hyaluronic acid, a major component of connective tissue. GAS streptokinase dissolves clots through conversion of plasminogen to plasmin. GAS produces a C5a peptidase that specifically cleaves C5a, inhibiting phagocyte recruitment. Originally thought to be a GAS superantigen, streptococcal pyrogenic exotoxin B (SpeB) is a potent protease critical in the pathogenesis of severe invasive disease.[27]

The streptococcal pyrogenic exotoxins (Spe) constitute a family of bacterial superantigens believed to be associated with streptococcal toxic shock syndrome (TSS) and the pathogenesis of severe infections. SpeA and SpeC are bacteriophage-encoded and are associated with scarlet fever (i.e., scarlatinal toxins). Outbreaks of streptococcal TSS in the United States have been associated with strains producing SpeA.[33] Development of streptococcal TSS is multifactorial, and susceptibility may be associated with specific human leukocyte antigen haplotypes.[81]

TRANSMISSION AND EPIDEMIOLOGY

GAS are found almost exclusively in humans and rarely occur in other species.[87] Distinct and significant differences exist in the epidemiology and transmission of GAS based on the site of infection.[118,161]

Streptococcal pharyngitis is one of the most common infections of childhood. Whereas GAS cause the majority of infections, strains of other serogroups, including groups C and G, may instead be involved. GAS pharyngitis occurs primarily in children aged 5 to 15 years, with the peak incidence occurring during the first school years. Severe epidemics may occur in conditions of overcrowding, including daycare centers,[1] residential facilities,[117] and military barracks.[162] The effect of crowding may explain, at least in part, the seasonal occurrence in temperate and cold climates. Contaminated foods (e.g., milk and egg salad) may result in outbreaks of GAS pharyngitis.[70,92] Fomite contamination and airborne routes are unlikely to play any role in the spread of GAS pharyngitis.[29]

The mechanism of spread is facilitated by close personal contact. Early studies demonstrated that large droplets or direct transfer of respiratory secretions containing large amounts of infectious bacteria is required.[66,67] Experimental nonhuman primate studies[159] have elucidated the mechanisms of interpersonal GAS spread. The infection cycle consists of colonization, acute infection, and asymptomatic carrier phases of infection. During acute infection, GAS are present in large amounts in both the anterior nares and throat.[67] Although the acute symptomatic phase lasts only a few days, left untreated, the organism can persist for weeks in the absence of symptoms. During the asymptomatic carrier phase, bacterial burden decreases in the anterior nares and persists at lower numbers in the throat. Early studies also demonstrated that GAS in the asymptomatic carrier phase possess less hyaluronic acid capsule[127] and M protein.[124] The end result is that asymptomatic carriers are less likely to transmit the organism to close contacts than are those acutely infected. Antibiotic therapy rapidly reduces the bacterial burden and in most cases eradicates GAS from the throat. Thus, most patients are considerably less contagious within 24 hours of initiation of antibiotic therapy, reducing the risk for spread to contacts.[139]

The epidemiology and transmission of GAS skin infections is markedly different compared to throat infections. Prevalence of GAS skin infections appears to be influenced most by climate and level of hygiene. In contrast to throat infections, the peak age of incidence in impetigo and pyoderma is in children 2 to 5 years of age (i.e., preschool aged). GAS skin infections occur more frequently in hot or tropical climates[25] and, in temperate climates, infections are more common during the summer months.[45] Infection causing impetigo and pyoderma appears to be facilitated by disruption of the skin by trauma, insect bites, or preexisting skin disorders (e.g., eczema). The role of fomites and environmental contamination in the spread of GAS skin infections remains undefined.

Prospective studies on the transmission of streptococcal impetigo demonstrated that GAS initially colonize unbroken skin.[45] GAS skin colonization preceded development of impetiginous lesions by an average of 10 days.

Measures to prevent spread of GAS infections vary in their effectiveness. Spread of throat or skin infection within a family often occurs before the index case is identified and isolated or treated. In epidemic situations, especially situations involving cases of rheumatic fever or acute nephritis, a culture survey with treatment of all individuals with positive cultures (mass prophylaxis) may be indicated.[152] Reduction of crowding, especially in sleeping quarters, seems to be an effective long-term method of minimizing the incidence of transmission of streptococcal sore throat among some groups.

In families in which persistence or recurrence of streptococcal infection is a problem, simultaneous throat culture and culture of skin lesions of all members and treatment of all who have positive results have been successful in eradicating the organism. Control of environmental contamination would be expected to have little or no influence on the spread of GAS respiratory infections, although it possibly has an effect in controlling skin or wound infections. It also is suggested that family toothbrushes may have a role in the intrafamilial transmission of GAS. More recent guidelines have suggested, however, that performing cultures of all family members in instances in which invasive GAS infections occur is not always necessary. Because of reported instances in which secondary cases have occurred, this guideline remains controversial.[29,121,152]

PATHOGENESIS

Despite the numerous studies focusing on the pathogenesis of GAS infections, we understand little of mechanisms that give GAS predilection for certain body sites or why certain M serotypes are more frequently found in pharyngitis and yet others in skin infections. Infection begins with successful colonization of skin or pharyngeal epithelial surfaces. Initial interaction of GAS with epithelial surfaces is mediated by fimbriae and pili, believed to overcome the negative electrostatic forces between bacterial and host cell surfaces. More specific binding occurs through pili, M protein, hyaluronic acid capsule, and numerous fibronectin binding proteins. The complement of fibronectin binding proteins identified in GAS include proteins F1 (Prtf1) and F2 (Prtf2), SfbI, SfbII, FBP54, and others.[107]

Steps in initial colonization also require successful competition between resident flora on either the skin or pharyngeal epithelium. α-Hemolytic or viridans streptococci may interfere with throat colonization, and GAS elaborates bacteriocin-like substances that may facilitate competition.[107] Colonization of skin surfaces appears to be enhanced by physical removal of local bacterial flora.[4]

Several GAS virulence determinants participate in tissue invasion. Immune evasion is facilitated by expression of the antiphagocytic hyaluronic acid capsule, M protein, and IdeS (also known as Mac, which cleaves immunoglobulin [Ig]G bound to GAS); breakdown of neutrophil extracellular traps and host tissues by DNAses, hyaluronidases, and the cysteine protease SpeB; breakdown of chemoattractants by *S. pyogenes* cell envelope protease (SpyCEP) (cleaves IL-8), C5a peptidase (cleaves C5a); and others, including streptococcal inhibitor of complement (SIC), streptolysin O, and streptokinase. Together these virulence factors subvert immune defenses and facilitate spread through tissues.

Recently researchers have shed light on the in vivo molecular events that lead to invasive GAS infections. Many of the GAS virulence factors required for invasive infection are normally repressed by the CovRS two-component regulatory system. During invasive infection of serotype M1, mutations in the genes encoding the CovRS proteins result in de-repression (i.e., increased expression) of virulence factors, leading to more severe disease.[41,143] Extensive whole-genome sequencing studies of serotype M3[130] and M1[105] GAS isolates from human pharyngitis and invasive infections demonstrated that mutations in *covS* occur at a significantly higher frequency in isolates from invasive disease in contrast to pharyngitis. Moreover examination of paired superficial and invasive isolates from the same patient suggest that *covRS* mutation may facilitate the breaching of epithelial barriers leading to dissemination and invasive disease.[49,55]

We understand little of the mechanisms leading to early host defense against GAS infection. Although specific antibody targeted against the M protein promotes phagocytosis, it usually does not develop until 6 to 8 weeks after initial infection.[40] Rather than act during initial infection, type-specific antibody against the M protein more likely prevents reinfection by the same serologic type. Thus, in the early stages of infection, protection via phagocytosis by monocytes and polymorphonuclear leukocytes appears to be the primary mechanism of defense.

The rash and other toxic manifestations of scarlet fever have been attributed to the development of hypersensitivity to the pyrogenic toxins.[18] Toxic manifestations that have been noted in GAS TSS also may result from a direct influence of the pyrogenic exotoxins on lymphokines, such as tumor necrosis factor.[142] Hypersensitivity to other streptococcal products also may contribute to the manifestations of streptococcal disease.

Theories abound about the pathogenetic mechanism leading to the development of the nonsuppurative complications of streptococcal infections, acute rheumatic fever, and acute glomerulonephritis. Most of these hypotheses invoke immunologic processes in one way or another.[71,157] A major impediment toward clarifying the pathogenetic mechanism responsible for the development of nonsuppurative sequelae has been the lack of an appropriate animal model for study.

CLINICAL MANIFESTATIONS

Pharyngitis or tonsillitis caused by GAS has a brief incubation period of 12 hours to 4 days. Acute illness is characterized by abrupt onset of sore throat, malaise, fever, and headache. Children may present with nausea, vomiting, and abdominal pain. Severity can vary greatly from subclinical to a toxic appearance. Common physical findings include fever, erythema, edema, and lymphoid hyperplasia of the posterior pharynx, enlarged, hyperemic tonsils, exudate on the pharyngeal and tonsillar surfaces, and enlarged, tender lymph nodes at the mandibular angle.

Clinical manifestations generally subside spontaneously in 3 to 5 days in the absence of suppurative complications (e.g., otitis media, sinusitis, and peritonsillar abscess). Prompt antibiotic therapy (e.g., penicillin) shortens the period of fever, toxicity, and infectivity.[84,106,119] After acute streptococcal infection of the upper respiratory tract, the average latent period for glomerulonephritis is 10 days and the latent period for acute rheumatic fever is 18 days.[161]

Localized pharyngeal infection is less common in younger children, especially infants. An infantile form of streptococcal infection, streptococcal childhood fever, may be more prolonged, with persistent low-grade fever, generalized lymphadenopathy, and persistent serous nasal discharge. The term *streptococcosis* more correctly indicates the changing clinical picture with age analogous to that of tuberculosis.[116]

Infection with strains that elaborate streptococcal pyrogenic exotoxins may manifest as scarlet fever. Most commonly scarlet fever is associated with pharyngeal infection; however, it may also follow infection of wounds or puerperal sepsis. The characteristic rash is erythematous and finely punctate, with centrifugal spread beginning on the upper chest or trunk. The rash usually appears on the second day of illness, blanches with pressure, and spreads to cover the entire body within several hours to days. Lines of deeper red may be noted in the skinfolds of the neck, axillae, elbows, groin, and knees (Pastia's lines). The tongue may take on a strawberry appearance and become swollen and red. The skin may take on a sandpaper texture because of the occlusion of sweat glands, a particularly useful feature for diagnosis in dark-skinned people. Severe forms may be associated with local and hematogenous spread of the organism (i.e., septic scarlet fever) or toxemia (i.e., toxic scarlet fever). Rarely, scarlet fever may be complicated by arthritis, jaundice, and hydrops of the gallbladder. Severe manifestations are less frequent with the use of antibiotics.

Impetigo caused by GAS develops days or weeks after colonization on normal skin with an average latent period of 10 days.[45] The infection is usually painless in contrast to pharyngitis. Vesicles with minimal surrounding erythema rapidly develop into pustules and then into a thick, honey-colored crust that may persist for days or weeks. GAS impetigo does not involve the dermis, and depigmentation may be seen on healing but does not scar.

Strains of GAS that cause skin infections differ from those associated with tonsillitis and pharyngitis. The serologic types associated with skin infection tend to be higher-numbered M-types because of their more recent discovery. A small number of serotypes are capable of causing both pharyngitis and skin infections.[16]

APSGN may develop after cutaneous infection by a nephritogenic strain. Whereas rheumatic fever has not been proved to develop after skin infections with GAS, a clear association exists between GAS skin infections and rheumatic heart disease especially in Pacific populations.[109] The latent period for APSGN after skin infection is longer, 3 weeks on average, than is seen after pharyngitis (10 days).[77]

Erysipelas is a superficial streptococcal infection of the skin and sometimes adjacent mucous membranes. Three features distinguish erysipelas clinically from other forms of skin infection: (1) lesions are raised above the level of the surrounding skin, (2) a clear line of demarcation distinguishes infected from uninfected areas, and (3) lesions are a brilliant salmon-red color. Erysipelas is more common in infants and young children and most often involves the face. Lesions may be associated with wounds, an area of dermatosis (e.g., eczema), or the umbilical stump of a newborn. The cutaneous inflammation of erysipelas is often accompanied by systemic manifestations of toxicity observed in other forms of streptococcal infection.

If nothing else, GAS is notable for its ability to cause a wide range of infections. In addition to those already mentioned, suppurative complications of upper respiratory tract infection include otitis media, retropharyngeal or peritonsillar abscess, sinusitis, mastoiditis, pneumonia, and empyema. GAS are frequently isolated in cultures from peritonsillar abscesses[144] and likely act in concert with anaerobic bacteria to produce this entity.[21] Classically acute puerperal sepsis has been associated with GAS. Infection of the skin and subcutaneous tissues (streptococcal cellulitis) may complicate burns, wounds, surgical incisions, or seemingly mild trauma. More severe infections of the deeper subcutaneous tissues and fascia with rapid spread and necrosis (necrotizing fasciitis or streptococcal gangrene) also are associated with GAS. These bacteria are a common cause of perianal cellulitis and vaginitis in children.[7,80] Subpectoral abscesses and empyemas may develop as complications of streptococcal infections of the thumb and index finger as a result of the lymphatic drainage of that part of the hand.[7] Septic complications of varicella, including varicella gangrenosa,[24,138] osteomyelitis (especially in infants),[64] hand and foot syndrome,[65] blistering distal dactylitis,[69] necrotizing fasciitis, and TSS, are associated with β-hemolytic streptococci.

STREPTOCOCCAL UPPER RESPIRATORY TRACT CARRIER STATE

In addition to causing a wide range of diseases, asymptomatic carriage of GAS is a common occurrence among children and adolescents. Depending on the population studied, rates of GAS carriage range from 5% to 15% among children,[129] a rate greatly exceeding that of any disease caused by GAS. Very early studies demonstrated that pharyngeal carriers of GAS are less dangerous to others because they harbor fewer organisms and rarely spread the organism to close contacts.[66,67] However, multiple epidemiologic studies have shown that close contacts may harbor virulent organisms in the absence of symptoms.[34,99] Thus carriage represents a diagnostic and therapeutic dilemma for the clinician. The epidemiologic and immunologic reasons for the establishment and continuation of the carrier state are an active area of investigation.

A combination of host and bacterial factors are believed to contribute to the GAS carrier state. As opposed to true infection, in which an individual has the presence of the organism and evidence for an immunologic response, GAS carriers may harbor the organism for long periods in the absence of a host immune response.[76] Few studies have examined the bacterial or host factors that lead to persistent colonization by GAS. Bacterial studies suggest that GAS are able to internalize into epithelial cells and that internalization is associated with the presence of certain fibronectin-binding proteins.[12,104] Because penicillin does not effectively penetrate the epithelial cell, intriguingly, some have suggested that internalization of GAS into pharyngeal epithelial cells contributes to persistence despite antibiotic therapy.[78]

TREATMENT

GAS remain universally susceptible to penicillin in vitro. Oral penicillin V and intramuscular benzathine penicillin are the drugs of choice for the treatment of GAS, except in patients with a penicillin allergy.[58] The advantages of penicillin include a narrow spectrum of activity, proven efficacy, and low cost.[58]

Initial studies on the efficacy of penicillin for the primary prevention of acute rheumatic fever were conducted with military recruits in the 1950s.[39,161,162] Initial studies involved the use of injectable penicillin suspended in either sesame oil or peanut oil, and they showed therapeutic penicillin concentrations in serum for 9 to 10 days.[161] Later studies found an equal bacterial eradication rate of 10 days with either oral penicillin G or injectable benzathine penicillin.[162] Oral penicillin remains the first-line therapy because benzathine penicillin G is associated with pain and increased risk of allergic reactions.[112] However, in certain situations in which adherence to regimen or follow-up is not possible, intramuscular benzathine penicillin is preferred.

The regimen that has been established is 10 days of penicillin V treatment or a single dose of benzathine penicillin to prevent acute rheumatic fever.[17,58] The most recent guidelines by the Infectious Diseases Society of America (IDSA) for the prevention of rheumatic fever and treatment of acute streptococcal pharyngitis[133] recommend a dose of penicillin V for most children of 250 mg twice a day, and the dose usually recommended for adolescents and adults is 500 mg two or three times per day (see Table 82.1).[133] Penicillin V is preferred to penicillin G because it is more resistant to gastric acid. Although penicillin V is the recommended drug, many physicians prescribe amoxicillin because of its improved taste. An oral time-released formulation of amoxicillin was approved by the US Food and Drug Administration (FDA) for once daily therapy for patients 12 years of age and older.[133]

For patients with a penicillin allergy, a 10-day oral course of a narrow spectrum cephalosporin (e.g., cefadroxil or cephalexin) is recommended. Some studies have shown that 10 days of an oral cephalosporin is superior to a 10 day-course of oral penicillin.[63,115] Other studies suggest that treatment with 5 days of an oral broad-spectrum cephalosporin is comparable to treatment with 10 days of oral penicillin in the eradication of GAS tonsillopharyngitis.[58,114] However, at present, these shorter regimens have not been approved by the FDA. In the past, erythromycin was the drug of choice for penicillin-allergic patients, but it has been replaced by newer medications since they have lower rates of gastrointestinal side effects and easier administration regimens.[31,53,133] In patients with an immediate hypersensitivity (anaphylactic type) to penicillin, cephalosporins should be avoided, and macrolides (erythromycin or clarithromycin), azithromycin (an azalide), or clindamycin (a lincosamide) should be used. Recommended doses are shown in Table 82.1.

Macrolide resistance has been documented in many countries and remains an ongoing concern for the treatment of GAS infections.[53,90] Although erythromycin-resistant organisms were found in the 1950s, it was not until the 1970s that clinically significant macrolide resistance was noted.[53] Resistance to macrolides occurs by one of two mechanisms: an active efflux pump (M phenotype) related to enzymes encoded for by *mef* genes or ribosomal target site modification by methylation (*erm* genes), which causes coresistance to macrolide, lincosamide, and streptogramin (MLS) antibiotics (MLS phenotype).[90] Countries such as Japan, Finland, Italy, and the United States have reported treatment failures due to macrolide resistance.[53] A study in Finland[128] reported a decrease in the use of macrolide antibiotics from 2.40 defined daily doses per 1000 inhabitants per day in 1991 to 1.38 in 1992, after national recommendations were made to reduce the number of macrolides prescribed for respiratory and skin infections. This resulted in a decrease in macrolide resistance from 16.5% in 1992 to 8.6% in 1996.[128] Although the rate of resistance in the United States is relatively low compared with much of the rest of the world, a recent U.S. multicenter surveillance study[64] found an overall adjusted rate of macrolide resistance in GAS

TABLE 82.1 Antibiotic Regimens Recommended for Group A Streptococcal Pharyngitis

Drug, Route	Dose or Dosage	Duration or Quantity	Recommendation Strength, Quality[a]
Individuals Without Penicillin Allergy			
Penicillin V, oral	Children: 250 mg twice daily or 3 times daily; adolescents and adults: 250 mg 4 times daily or 500 mg twice daily	10 days	Strong, high
Amoxicillin, oral	50 mg/kg once daily (max = 1 g); alternate: 25 mg/kg (max = 500 mg) twice daily	10 days	Strong, high
Benzathine penicillin G, intramuscular	<27 kg: 600,000 U ≥27 kg: 1,200,000 U	1 dose	Strong, high
Individuals With Penicillin Allergy			
Cephalexin,[b] oral	20 mg/kg/dose twice daily (max = 500 mg/dose)	10 days	Strong, high
Cefadroxil,[b] oral	30 mg/kg once daily (max = 1 g)	10 days	Strong, high
Clindamycin, oral	7 mg/kg/dose 3 times daily (max = 300 mg/dose)	10 days	Strong, moderate
Azithromycin,[c] oral	12 mg/kg once daily (max = 500 mg)	5 days	Strong, moderate
Clarithromycin,[c] oral	7.5 mg/kg/dose twice daily (max = 250 mg/dose)	10 days	Strong, moderate

[a]Information is based on Grading of Recommendations Assessment, Development, and Evaluation criteria.
[b]Avoid in individuals with immediate-type hypersensitivity to penicillin.
[c]Resistance of group A *Streptococcus* to these agents is well known and varies geographically and temporally.
For other acceptable alternatives, see text. The following are not acceptable: sulfonamides, trimethoprim, tetracyclines, and fluoroquinolones.
From Shulman ST, Bisno AL, Clegg HW, et al. Clinical practice guideline for the diagnosis and management of group A streptococcal pharyngitis: 2012 update by the Infectious Diseases Society of America. *Clin Infect Dis.* 2012;55(10):e86–102.

of 5.2%. This represents a near twofold increase from rates reported in the United States in the 1990s. In recent years, macrolide resistance rates in the U.S. have ranged between 5% and 8%.[5] To avoid further increases in macrolide resistance that may result in treatment failures and acute rheumatic fever, some experts recommend that macrolide antibiotics be reserved for the treatment of GAS infections in patients with anaphylactic-type penicillin allergy.[90]

Certain broad-spectrum antibiotics should not be used against GAS. There is high prevalence of resistance to tetracycline and therefore it should not be used. Sulfonamides and trimethoprim-sulfamethoxazole should be avoided because they do not eradicate GAS from the pharynx. Ciprofloxacin has limited activity against GAS and therefore should not be used. Newer fluoroquinolones such as levofloxacin and moxifloxacin have shown in vitro activity against GAS, but should not be used because they are expensive and provide an excessive broad-spectrum activity.[36,57,58,133]

Even though penicillin remains the drug of choice in the treatment of GAS, penicillin treatment failures of 20% to 40% or higher have been reported.[113] It has been documented more often after oral penicillin than after benzathine penicillin.[44] Possible explanations for penicillin treatment failures include lack of compliance, penicillin tolerance, and carrier state.[58,113] Other considerations that have been proposed include copathogens in the pharynx[62,113,115,137] and antibiotic suppression of immunity.[20,58,163] Some authors have suggested that certain β-lactamase–producing organisms such as *Staphylococcus aureus*, *Haemophilus influenzae*, *Moraxella catarrhalis*, and anaerobes may be present in the pharynx during a GAS infection and inactivate penicillin. They argue that this may be one of the reasons for the superiority of β-lactamase stable antibiotics in cases of penicillin failures.[114] Studies from the 1940s and 1950s documented that antibiotics given shortly after onset of symptoms (within 24 to 48 hours) could suppress the immune response to the infection.[20,163] Other studies did not show a difference whether treatment was started early or delayed for 48 hours.[59] Penicillin therapy is effective in preventing rheumatic fever when started within 9 days after the onset of illness.[28,58,133] Delaying therapy for 24 to 48 hours until culture results are known does not increase the risk of rheumatic fever.[58,133] However, therapy should not be delayed in patients who appear toxic or are severely ill.

At present, recommendations in the management of GAS pharyngitis in children include obtaining a streptococcal rapid antigen detection test, with initiation of treatment when positive. Negative rapid antigen detection tests should be backed by a throat culture. Follow-up cultures in patients treated for GAS are no longer routinely recommended and should only be performed in those who remain symptomatic, have recurrence of symptoms, or have a history of rheumatic fever.[17,58,133] Children with recurrence of GAS pharyngitis symptoms after completing a 10-day course of a recommended oral antimicrobial agent can be retreated with the same antimicrobial agent, given an alternative oral drug, or given an intramuscular dose of penicillin G benzathine, especially if noncompliance is suspected. Alternative drugs include a narrow-spectrum cephalosporin, amoxicillin-clavulanate, clindamycin, a macrolide, azalide, or penicillin plus rifampin.[5,58,133]

Individuals found to have a positive rapid antigen detection test or throat culture without clinical evidence of infection or rise in antistreptococcal titers are considered chronic streptococcal carriers and do not need to be treated with antibiotics. However, because it may be difficult to distinguish a carrier state from true GAS infection when a viral upper respiratory infection develops in a carrier, appropriate antibiotics should be prescribed to any patient with acute pharyngitis and evidence of GAS from a positive rapid antigen detection test or throat culture.[5,58,133]

Although guidelines from the American Heart Association and from the IDSA exist for the treatment of GAS tonsillopharyngitis, no official guidelines exist for the treatment of streptococcal impetigo. For patients with a few lesions, topical therapy with mupirocin or retapamulin ointment may be useful for limiting person-to-person spread and for eradicating localized disease.[2] In more severe cases with multiple lesions or with nonbullous impetigo in multiple family members, child care groups, or athletic teams, impetigo should be treated with systemic antimicrobials.[5] Oral or parenteral penicillin may be used in the same doses as those for streptococcal infections. Regimens with first-generation cephalosporins or macrolides should be used for penicillin-allergic patients. With the increase in skin and soft tissue infections due to methicillin-resistant *Staphylococcus aureus* (MRSA), obtaining appropriate cultures and treating with antibiotics to cover this possible pathogen must also be considered.

Although treatment with penicillin has been shown to prevent the development of rheumatic fever, no definitive evidence exists that antimicrobial therapy after treatment of streptococcal skin infections prevents acute poststreptococcal glomerulonephritis.[2]

Otitis media and cervical adenitis due to GAS can be treated with the same regimens used for the treatment of streptococcal pharyngitis. Systemic parenteral antimicrobial therapy is indicated for severe infections, such as septicemia, pneumonia, endocarditis, meningitis, arthritis, osteomyelitis, erysipelas, necrotizing fasciitis, neonatal omphalitis, and streptococcal TSS. Treatment often is prolonged (2 to 6 weeks).[5] In the case of TSS and necrotizing fasciitis, clindamycin is also recommended because it is a protein-synthesis inhibitor and can neutralize bacterial toxins. Drainage of any lesions is warranted. Intravenous immunoglobulin (IVIG) can be considered as adjunctive therapy for GAS-related TSS or necrotizing fasciitis if the patient is severely ill.[5]

PREVENTION

Treatment of GAS pharyngitis with antimicrobials aims to prevent rheumatic fever through primary prevention. Prevention of recurrence of rheumatic fever (secondary prevention) requires continuous antimicrobial prophylaxis (see Chapter 29). A meta-analysis of 10 trials on primary prevention of rheumatic fever, which were carried out in the United States during 1950 to 1961, revealed that, although the methodology of the studies was poor, administration of antibiotics in patients with GAS infection reduced the risk of acute rheumatic fever by nearly 70%.[122] A subgroup analysis showed that the risk reduction was 80% when treated with intramuscular penicillin.[122]

Although the incidence of acute rheumatic fever has decreased in the developing world for the past 50 years, outbreaks in the community and the military continue to occur, and acute rheumatic fever remains a major cause of morbidity and mortality in the developing world.[35] Current strategies for disease prevention include infection-control measures such as isolation, appropriate hygiene measures for postpartum and postsurgical patients, and establishing nationwide surveillance systems.[35] During episodes of epidemic GAS infections, mass prophylaxis with penicillin, particularly intramuscular benzathine penicillin G, has been shown to be effective.

Children in the outpatient setting being treated for a GAS infection may return to daycare or school after 24 hours of treatment. For hospitalized children, droplet precautions are recommended for GAS pharyngitis or pneumonia until 24 hours after initiation of appropriate antimicrobial therapy. In the case of burns with secondary GAS infection and extensive or draining cutaneous infections that cannot be covered by dressings, patients should remain in contact precautions for at least 24 hours after the start of appropriate therapy.[2] Asymptomatic household contacts do not require diagnostic evaluation or chemoprophylaxis, unless exposure occurs during outbreaks or the contacts are at higher risk for developing sequelae of infection.[6]

In certain cases of GAS pharyngitis refractory to treatment, tonsillectomy has been performed, but at present, there are insufficient data to recommend routine tonsillectomy as part of the management of GAS pharyngeal infections.

Despite the use of antimicrobials, the persistence of acute rheumatic fever and its associated morbidity and mortality, especially in the developing world, has led to intensive research in vaccine development against GAS. However, despite more than 70 years of research, a commercial vaccine is still not available.[35] One of the main concerns for development of vaccines based on the M protein was the possibility of causing autoantibodies that could cross-react with heart, skeletal muscle, brain, and glomerular basement membrane tissues.[31,35] However, multivalent M protein–based strategies are at the forefront of GAS vaccine development. A 26-valent vaccine has been developed and shown to be both safe and immunogenic in healthy adults.[82,94] Such a vaccine would include 86% of the serotypes causing GAS pharyngitis, which could prevent 49% to 63% of invasive GAS infections among children and 43% to 50% among elderly individuals, with similar decreases in the number of deaths.[108] However, because of the geographic and temporal differences in M-types between countries, this vaccine may not be as effective in other countries, such as Japan, Ethiopia, or New Zealand.[35,125] More recently, a 30-valent vaccine has been developed, and early studies suggest that the vaccine may have broader coverage than originally anticipated.[37] Other components of GAS have been under investigation as potential candidates in the development of a vaccine. These include carbohydrate antigens, adhesins, C5a peptidase, and the GAS pilus.[31] Mucosal vaccines to GAS are also under investigation because mouse studies have found induction of specific IgA production during intranasal administration of vaccine, along with IgG production in serum.[31] Further research is needed in GAS vaccine development, with a goal of vaccines that may be useful globally.

PEDIATRIC AUTOIMMUNE NEUROPSYCHIATRIC DISORDERS ASSOCIATED WITH STREPTOCOCCAL INFECTIONS

Pediatric autoimmune neuropsychiatric disorders associated with streptococcal (PANDAS) infection is an autoimmune condition with obsessive-compulsive disorder (OCD) or tic disorder manifestations associated with GAS. Initially it was described as pediatric infection-triggered autoimmune neuropsychiatric disorders (PITANDS) by Allen, Leonard, and Swedo[3] in a four-patient case series and later coined as PANDAS by Swedo and associates[148] in a larger study involving 50 patients that established the diagnostic criteria, which include the following:

1. Presence of OCD and/or a tic disorder meeting lifetime *Diagnostic and Statistical Manual of Mental Disorders*, Fourth Edition (DSM-IV) diagnostic criteria
2. Age at onset between 3 years of age and the beginning of puberty
3. Clinical course characterized by the abrupt onset of symptoms or by dramatic symptom exacerbations
4. Temporal association with GAS infection, diagnosed by positive throat culture and/or elevated anti-GAS antibody titers
5. Association with neurologic abnormalities such as choreiform movements or tics

This proposed disorder is currently a hypothesis, and it remains a controversial topic. Several authors believe this disorder is a separate entity and recommend treatment and prophylaxis. Others argue that it is only a hypothesis and that further evidence with double-blinded studies is needed before recommending treatment and prevention for children given a diagnosis of PANDAS.

Proposed Pathogenesis

The hypothesis for PANDAS involves several factors, including pathologic strains of group A streptococcal bacteria, host susceptibility (e.g., genetics, development, or other), and abnormal immune response.[150] A pathogenesis model has been proposed to describe the disorder (Fig. 82.1).[145] Ongoing research is being conducted to understand the pathologic mechanisms involved in the PANDAS subgroup.

As part of the diagnostic criteria, temporal association with GAS infection and neuropsychiatric exacerbation is very important. It is essential to distinguish exacerbations of PANDAS due to GAS infection from the waxing and waning course seen in Tourette disorder and some cases of childhood-onset OCD.[145]

According to Swedo,[145] host susceptibility is thought to result from genetic, developmental, and immunologic factors. Children in the PANDAS subgroup may have similar genetic susceptibility for post-streptococcal sequelae as children with Sydenham chorea. Development also seems to play a role in the pathogenesis of PANDAS because the peak age of onset of symptoms is 6 to 7 years and prepubertal onset is characteristic. PANDAS is described as an autoimmune process, and many think that there are antineuronal cross-reactive antibodies similar to the autoantibodies found in Sydenham chorea.[145] These antibodies

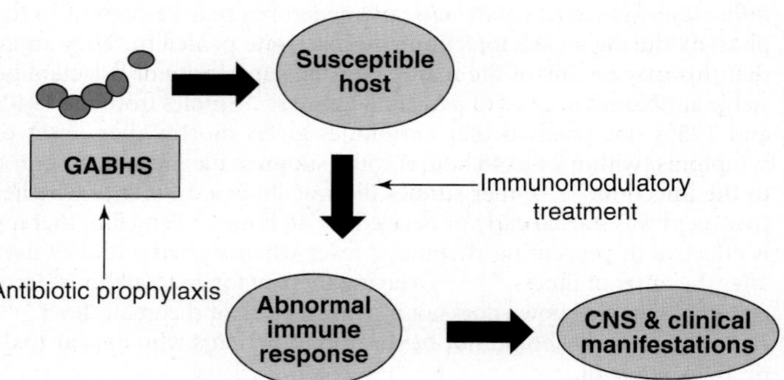

FIG. 82.1 Model of pathogenesis for pediatric autoimmune neuropsychiatric disorder associated with streptococcal infections. *CNS,* Central nervous system; *GABHS,* group A β-hemolytic *Streptococcus.* (From Swedo SE: Pediatric autoimmune neuropsychiatric disorders associated with streptococcal infections [PANDAS]. *Mol Psychiatry.* 2002;7:S24.)

are meant to react against group A *Streptococcus* epitopes, but, in the case of PANDAS, they cross-react with cells in the basal ganglia.[61] Studies using magnetic resonance imaging volumetric scans have shown bilateral enlargements of the caudate, putamen, and globus pallidus among patients in the PANDAS subgroup.[60,61]

Diagnosis

The diagnostic criteria defined by Swedo and colleagues during the description of the first 50 cases of PANDAS aimed to define a homogeneous subgroup of patients with OCD and tic disorders who had dramatic acute exacerbations usually following a GAS infection.[148,150] However, in the initial cohort, other psychiatric comorbidities were also found frequently, particularly attention-deficit/hyperactivity disorder (ADHD), affective disorders, and anxiety disorders. More recently other authors proposed the criteria be expanded to include related disorders such as ADHD[111] and anorexia.[141] In terms of the age at onset criterion, the authors based this on historical data showing that rheumatic fever and other poststreptococcal sequelae are rare before the age of 3 years and after the age of 12 years. Protective serum antibodies against streptococcal infections were found in 98% of healthy 12-year-old controls in a study by Fischetti.[47] OCD related to PANDAS usually can be distinguished from other forms of OCD because children in the PANDAS subgroup typically have a sudden onset of symptoms, reaching a peak in 24 to 48 hours, whereas in non-PANDAS OCD there is a more gradual onset of obsessions and compulsions. The authors also proposed that exacerbations of neuropsychiatric symptoms begin within 7 to 14 days after an infection with GAS and usually occur simultaneously.[150] However, since streptococcal infections are so common during childhood, for a child to fit this diagnostic criterion there should be prospective evaluation and documentation of at least two episodes of neuropsychiatric symptoms that correlate with streptococcal infections, as well as documentation of evidence of negative throat cultures or antibody titers when the patient goes into remission of neuropsychiatric symptoms. The last diagnostic criterion involves the presence of neurologic abnormalities during periods of symptom exacerbation. Choreiform movements seen in PANDAS patients are small, jerky movements that occur in an irregular and arrhythmic pattern in different muscles,[148] described as fine piano-playing movements of the fingers. Patients with a diagnosis of rheumatic fever, including chorea, should be excluded from the PANDAS subgroup.[148]

Children considered to have possible PANDAS syndrome who have symptoms suggestive of streptococcal infection should undergo evaluation for GAS infection. Rapid streptococcal antigen tests should be obtained, as well as a throat culture if the antigen test was negative. In patients with a negative throat culture, ASO and anti-DNase B titers could be obtained if the onset of PANDAS was at least 4 to 6 weeks prior. With acute exacerbations of tics or OCD symptoms, patients should be reevaluated for an acute infection due to GAS.[146]

A diagnostic marker present in children with rheumatic fever, D8/17, has been postulated to also identify children with PANDAS,[149] but its use in diagnosis of PANDAS remains controversial.[131]

Treatment

All patients who have an acute GAS infection should receive appropriate antibiotic therapy, usually with penicillin, because it remains the drug of choice. Treatment of the streptococcal infection has been noted by some authors to improve or cure the neuropsychiatric symptoms of PANDAS. A small prospective study of 12 patients showed resolution of symptoms of new-onset OCD, anxiety, and tics within an average of 14 days after starting treatment with an antibiotic (either penicillin, amoxicillin, amoxicillin/clavulanate, or a cephalosporin).[103] Every recurrent episode of PANDAS was associated with a GAS infection, and all patients with recurrences showed improvement after treatment with antibiotics.[103] However, this was a small study and not a double-blinded, randomized controlled trial.

Children with a significant tic disorder or OCD should receive appropriate psychiatric medications as necessary. Cognitive behavioral therapy also may be beneficial in the treatment of OCD. These treatments are commonly used in tics and OCD not related to PANDAS and have also been used for treatment of neuropsychiatric symptoms in patients given a diagnosis of PANDAS.[85]

Immunomodulators have been used in therapeutic trials based on the proposed model of immunologic dysfunction. One study reported benefits in patients fulfilling criteria for PANDAS in the group treated with plasma exchange as well as in the group treated with IVIG.[110] This study, however, was limited by small sample size, highly selective recruitment, and limited comparisons with controls. In addition, nearly two-thirds of patients receiving active treatment experienced adverse effects.[110] A small case series of 12 patients with severe PANDAS who had failed prior antibiotic and psychiatric therapies showed good response to IVIG given at 1.5 g/kg.[83] All patients had significant improvement or complete resolution of their symptoms after months or years of their last IVIG dose.[83]

Therapeutic plasma apheresis (TPA) has been recommended for patients with severe PANDAS who do not respond to other treatment modalities. A case series of 40 patients with PANDAS describes the use of TPA for patients who were severely ill with violent behavior or who were a danger to themselves or others, severe restrictions of food and/or fluid intake, or minimal or no response to oral steroids or IVIG.[88] All patients showed some benefit from TPA, with 65% showing a decrease in symptoms at 6 months and 78% at long-term evaluation. The procedure was well-tolerated with minimal adverse effects (bleeding at site of central line insertion in two patients). The authors recommend that IVIG and TPA should be reserved for patients who remain severely symptomatic after less-invasive therapies or if they exhibit life-threatening suicidality, aggressive behaviors, or severe restrictions of food and/or fluid intake.[88]

Experts of the PANDAS Physicians Network (PPN) recommend a multidisciplinary approach for the treatment of patients with PANDAS that should include a combination of antibiotic prophylaxis, targeted symptom treatments, and immunomodulatory therapy. The website www.pandasppn.org provides the clinical guidelines and therapeutic approach recommendations from expert clinicians across the United States.[83]

Prevention

The pathogenesis of PANDAS has been proposed to be an autoimmune process similar to rheumatic fever and Sydenham chorea.[145] Penicillin is recommended to prevent recurrences of the latter two conditions. Few clinical trials have been performed to determine whether antibiotic prophylaxis to prevent GAS infection can help reduce the neuropsychiatric morbidity seen in PANDAS and prevent future exacerbations. In a placebo-controlled, double-blinded crossover study involving 37 children with PANDAS published in 1999, penicillin failed to prevent streptococcal infections and there were no differences in the severity of OCD and tics between the two phases.[56] A double-blinded, randomized, controlled trial of 23 children published in 2005 compared penicillin (as "active placebo") and azithromycin in the prevention of GAS infection and exacerbation of PANDAS. Both penicillin and azithromycin prophylaxis were found to be effective in the prevention of recurrent GAS infections and decreased the neuropsychiatric symptom exacerbations in the PANDAS subgroup.[140] Of note, limitations of this study are a small sample size and lack of inactive placebo group.

Arguments Against PANDAS

Considerable controversy still exists surrounding the topic of PANDAS.[93,136] Many argue that sufficient evidence is lacking to support PANDAS as a diagnostic entity.[132] For instance, a prospective longitudinal study comparing PANDAS and non-PANDAS cases of Tourette syndrome and OCD did not show a temporal relation between exacerbation of neuropsychiatric symptoms and a GAS infection in the PANDAS group (a few exacerbations of symptoms were associated with a GAS infection in the control group).[89] An argument has even been proposed that the initial cases with choreiform movements could represent missed cases of chorea.[85] The authors in a study showing failure of immune markers to correlate with clinical exacerbations in PANDAS question the autoimmune pathogenesis of the disorder.[134] Similar concerns were raised by a study that failed to show differences in serum autoantibodies between PANDAS and Tourette syndrome (controls).[100]

Further research is needed to establish PANDAS as a clinical entity, to further describe the pathogenesis of the disease, to demonstrate disease in animal models, and to determine its appropriate treatment and prevention in randomized, double-blinded, placebo-controlled trials.

From PANDAS to PANS

Because the concept of PANDAS has generated much controversy and conflict regarding the scientific evidence to support this hypothesis, many researchers and clinicians have recently proposed to eliminate the diagnosis of PANDAS in favor of a broader diagnostic category.[135] To address the controversy surrounding PANDAS, experts met at the National Institutes of Health (NIH) in 2010, and modifications to the PANDAS criteria were made to broaden the spectrum of acute-onset OCD and related neuropsychiatric disorders. It was decided that the new syndrome should not exclude cases with postpubertal onset.[147] The term pediatric acute-onset neuropsychiatric syndrome (PANS) was accepted because it would extend the age to at least 18 years (and 21 years by some definitions).[147] The three PANS criteria, as defined by Swedo and colleagues,[147] are:

1. Abrupt, dramatic onset of OCD or severely restricted food intake
2. Concurrent presence of additional neuropsychiatric symptoms (with similarly severe and acute onset) from at least two of the following seven categories:
   a. Anxiety
   b. Emotional lability and/or depression
   c. Irritability, aggression, and/or severely oppositional behaviors
   d. Behavioral (developmental) regression (Fig. 82.2)
   e. Deterioration in school performance
   f. Sensory or motor abnormalities
   g. Somatic signs and symptoms, including sleep disturbances, enuresis, or urinary frequency
3. Symptoms are not better explained by a known neurologic or medical disorder, such as Sydenham chorea, systemic lupus erythematosus, Tourette disorder, or others

In 2013, a diverse group of clinicians and researchers met at Stanford University for the First PANS Consensus Conference. At this meeting, a consensus statement proposed recommendations for the diagnostic evaluation of patients presenting with PANS.[32]

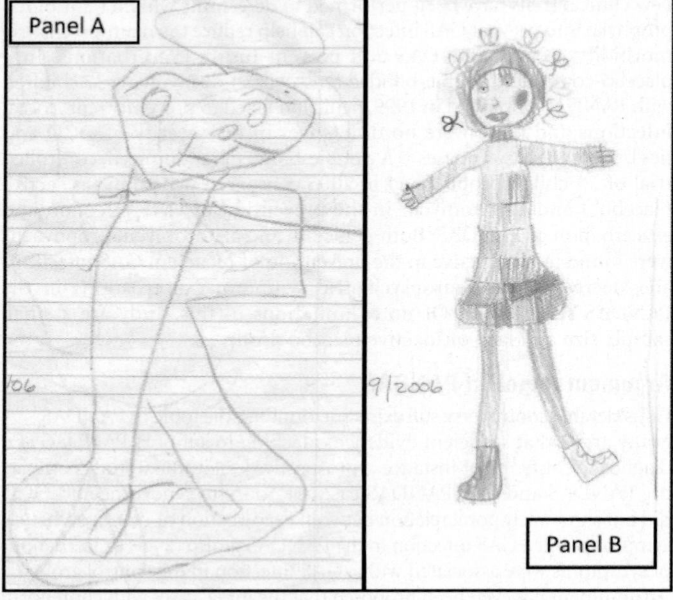

FIG. 82.2 Behavioral regression during a symptomatic episode. (A) Drawing produced during an acute exacerbation of obsessive-compulsive disorder and other symptoms of pediatric autoimmune neuropsychiatric disorder associated with streptococcal infections, which appears quite messy and immature. (B) Age-appropriate picture drawn after treatment with intravenous immunoglobulin and symptomatic improvement. (From Swedo SE, Leckman JF, Rose NR. Research Subgroup to Clinical Syndrome: modifying the PANDAS criteria to describe PANS (pediatric acute-onset neuropsychiatric syndrome). *Pediatr Therapeut.* 2012;2[2]:1–8.)

Most PANS cases are suspected to have a postinfectious etiology, although no organism other than GAS has been consistently associated with the onset of PANS.[32,51] The most common preceding infection is an upper respiratory infection (e.g., sinusitis, pharyngitis). Organisms most commonly mentioned as suspected etiologies for PANS include *Mycoplasma pneumoniae*, influenza virus, Epstein Barr virus, *Borrelia burgdorferi* (Lyme disease), herpes simplex virus, and varicella zoster virus.[32,147]

It is important to note that PANS is a "diagnosis of exclusion" and other medical diseases should be ruled out first. Many children can be extremely ill, with extreme compulsions, motor and phonic tics, behavioral regression, and extreme anxiety or aggression. In certain cases, the patients may have visual or auditory hallucinations, and it is important to exclude other diagnoses such as schizophrenia, bipolar disorder, and lupus cerebritis. Laboratory tests recommended for all patients meeting PANS criteria include complete blood cell count with manual differential, erythrocyte sedimentation rate, C-reactive protein, urinalysis with urine culture for those with pyuria, throat culture, ASO titer, and anti-DNAse B.[32]

Immunodeficiency workup should also be obtained if there is a history of recurrent infections, infection with an atypical organism, first-degree family member with history of overwhelming and/or fatal infection, or if the patient will receive IVIG therapy. Initial workup should include lymphocyte subsets, quantitative immunoglobulins, and vaccine responses (such as *Streptococcus pneumoniae* and tetanus antibody titers). If workup is abnormal, the patient should be referred to an immunologist. Brain magnetic resonance imaging should be obtained if other conditions are suspected (such as limbic encephalitis, CNS vasculitis) or if the patient has psychosis, altered mental status, or gait abnormalities. Electroencephalogram and lumbar puncture should also be considered in these cases.[32]

A study carried out at the University of South Florida involving 43 patients between the ages of 4 and 14 years who met criteria for PANS describes three symptom clusters.[102] The first cluster showed core characteristic PANS symptoms (emotional lability, anxiety, sleep disturbances, deterioration in school, and behavioral regression), the second showed classic streptococcal-related symptoms (ADHD, urinary symptoms, handwriting deterioration, sensory problems, and simple tics), and the third involved cytokine-driven/physiologic symptoms (food restriction, mydriasis, gastrointestinal problems, fatigue, depressive symptoms, psychosis, and complex tics).[102]

Some patients fit all criteria for PANDAS, but since testing for GAS infection may have been done after the window of opportunity to detect GAS passed, these patients end up being classified under PANS.[51,52] The role of inflammation in the etiology of PANS should be further investigated because there are cases of patients with PANS and overlap with other inflammatory diseases such as autoimmune encephalitis, immunodeficiency, sinusitis, inflammatory pain conditions, or food intolerance. These patients can respond to treatment modalities aimed at controlling the infectious or inflammatory condition, such as antibiotics, immunosuppression, IVIG, or removal of inflammatory foods.[52]

At the Stanford PANS clinic, 47 youth presenting with PANS symptoms were evaluated.[51] Those with acute onset usually had first-degree family members with autoimmune/inflammatory diseases and psychiatric disorders. GAS was the most common infection identified at onset (21%) and during relapses (74%).[51] Prospective studies are needed to investigate the connections between infections and psychiatric disorders, as well as the connections among infections, autoimmune diseases, and immune dysfunction.[51]

Food restriction in PANS has been associated with contamination fears, as well as with fears of vomiting or choking. Clues to distinguish disordered eating of PANS from other eating disorders include acuity of onset, male prevalence, and young age at presentation.[153] The management for children with PANS presenting with food restriction is different from the presentation for anorexia nervosa or avoidant/restrictive food intake disorder because children with PANS usually respond to treatment with antibiotics or immunomodulatory therapies.[153]

Recommendations for treatment of PANS cases are based on therapies that have been used for patients with PANDAS. Antibiotics used for treatment of PANS include amoxicillin, amoxicillin/clavulanic acid, cephalosporins, and azithromycin. A small randomized trial of cefdinir versus placebo for the treatment of recent-onset OCD and/or tics in PANS patients found small improvement in the OCD and tics symptoms in the cefdinir group, but these findings were not statistically significant.[101]

Just as in the cases for PANDAS who do not respond to other treatment modalities, patients with PANS refractory to other therapies could be considered for treatment with IVIG or TPA.[52]

GROUP C AND GROUP G STREPTOCOCCAL INFECTIONS

Organisms

The β-hemolytic streptococci include *Streptococcus pyogenes* (GAS), *Streptococcus agalactiae* (group B *Streptococcus*), and groups C, F, and G *Streptococcus*, based on the β-hemolysis they produce on blood agar plates. In addition, *Streptococcus anginosus* group organisms (*S. anginosus*, *S. constellatus*, and *S. intermedius*) may have variable hemolysis, and approximately one-third have group A, C, F, or G antigens.[6] Depending on their colony size, strains with either the group C or group G Lancefield carbohydrate antigens can be divided into small or large colony-forming strains. The small colony–forming strains (<0.5 mm in diameter) belong to the *S. anginosus* group, which are considered part of the viridans group streptococci. Large colony–forming strains (>0.5 mm) are considered true group C or group G streptococci (GCS and GGS, respectively).[22]

Lancefield group carbohydrate antigen and hemolytic reaction have been classically used for the identification of streptococci. However, streptococcal taxonomy has been significantly revised recently because there can be overlap between species. Currently three species of groups C and G have been described that are pathogenic in humans: *S. dysgalactiae*, *S. equi subsp. zooepidemicus*, and *S. canis*.[22]

GCS are catalase-negative, aerobic, facultatively anaerobic, coprophilic organisms. They are usually β-hemolytic, although all types of hemolysis have been seen with GCS. The group C antigenic determinant in their cell wall is rhamnose-*N*-acetylgalactosamine. Four species that possess this antigenic determinant were defined based on their ability to ferment various carbohydrates (*S. equisimilis*, *S. zooepidemicus*, *S. equi*, and *S. dysgalactiae*). Revision of the taxonomy after new research based on genetic studies (such as 16S RNA analysis) has shown that there are actually two GCS species, S. *dysgalactiae* and *S. equi*, each with two subspecies.

GGS typically show β-hemolysis on blood agar plates. They are facultative anaerobes. The group G antigenic determinant in their cell wall is L-rhamnose. The majority of GGS infections in humans are due to *S. dysgalactiae* subsp. *equisimilis*, but a few infections with *S. canis* have been reported.

Some of the same virulent factors found in GAS have been shown to be present in GCS and GGS, such as M protein, streptolysin, hyaluronidase, and C5a peptidase.[68,72,91,126] The most likely explanation for the overlap in these virulence factors is the horizontal transfer of genes between species.[120,154] The gene involved is the M-protein gene, which confers resistance to phagocytosis. The proposed mechanism is prevention of complete opsonization of the *Streptococcus* by interfering with the activation of the alternate complement pathway on the bacterial surface.[120]

Epidemiology

GCS and GGS in humans may colonize the skin, oropharynx, gastrointestinal tract, and vagina.[6] In addition, GCS have been cultured from the umbilicus of asymptomatic newborns and from routine puerperal vaginal samples. Classically these streptococcal groups have been thought to be a rare cause of infection in humans. They are common causes of animal infections, and many humans infected with these streptococci report animal contact. GCS and GGS have been known to cause foodborne outbreaks of pharyngitis.[6]

The classification and nomenclature of GCS and GGS has changed significantly, however, and clinical specimens are rarely identified to the species level by clinical laboratories, making it difficult to know the true burden of these infections. The first population-based study of the epidemiology and burden of invasive disease due to non–group A or B β-hemolytic streptococci (NABS) in the United States over a 2-year period was published in 2009.[22] According to this study, the majority of patients (87%) with invasive disease had underlying comorbid conditions, as has been previously reported.[68,91] Cardiovascular disease (44%), diabetes mellitus (42%), obesity (30%), and chronic skin disease (30%) were the most common underlying disorders among patients with *S. dysgalactiae* subsp. *equisimilis* bacteremia.[22,120] *S. dysgalactiae subsp. equisimilis* was the most common organism (80%) among patients with invasive disease. The case-fatality rate in bacteremia due to this species is as high as 15% to 18%.[120] However, the data for individuals younger than 20 years (6% of the patients) were different. Only 23% of the younger patients had underlying conditions, with asthma as the most common comorbidity. Isolates from pediatric patients were most often group F (40%), followed by group G (36%) and group C (24%). One very important finding of this study is that the burden of NABS infection in the United States during the study period was similar to that caused by invasive GAS infection: 3.2 cases per 100,000 population and 2.89 cases per 100,000, respectively.[22] A 6-month surveillance study published in Argentina in 2005 reported similar findings that most of the GCS and GGS *S. dysgalactiae subsp. equisimilis* infections occurred in adults and that diabetes was frequently seen as an underlying condition.[91]

Clinical Manifestations

GCS and GGS may cause invasive disease in infants, older children, and adults. The principal clinical manifestations of these organisms are upper and lower respiratory tract infections, septicemia, pneumonitis, skin and soft tissue infections, septic arthritis, osteomyelitis, meningitis with a parameningeal focus, brain abscess, puerperal and neonatal sepsis, peritonitis, and endocarditis.[6,8,160]

Pharyngitis caused by GCS and GGS has symptoms similar to those seen with GAS pharyngitis. GCS are a relatively common cause of acute pharyngitis among college students and among adults presenting to the emergency department.[57,133] Between 1% and 18% of asymptomatic pharyngeal carriers of GCS may be found in temperate climates, with higher percentages in the tropics. Similarly between 1% and 23% of asymptomatic pharyngeal carriers of GGS may occur in temperate climates. In addition, foodborne episodes of pharyngitis have been documented due to GCS and GGS.[6] These epidemic outbreaks may occur after consumption of contaminated products, such as unpasteurized cow's milk.

There are some studies that report an association with pharyngitis and acute poststreptococcal glomerulonephritis, and an association with acute rheumatic fever with isolation of *S. dysgalactiae* subsp. *equisimilis* from the upper respiratory tract.[120] Rare neonatal infections due to GGS and GCS have been reported, with symptoms similar to early-onset GBS sepsis.

GCS and GGS have been reported as a rare cause of skin and soft tissue infections. A report reviewing all cases of septic arthritis due to β-hemolytic streptococci at Stanford University Medical Center in California from 1985 through 1996 found that 40% of cases were due to GAS, 30% due to GBS, and 30% due to GGS. No cases due to GCS were reported during that time. Presence of infected prosthetic implants was found in the majority of patients with septic arthritis caused by GGS.[126] Rare cases of deep soft tissue infection resulting from GGS, such as necrotizing fasciitis, localized pyomyositis, and even myositis with subsequent fatal streptococcal TSS (STSS) have been reported in the literature.[160]

STSS typically has been associated with GAS, but recent case reports have shown cases resulting from GCS and GGS infection. Most of the cases have been due to *S. dysgalactiae subsp. equisimilis*, but a study from Japan reported the first case of STSS due to *S. equi subsp. zooepidemicus*.[68] Because most clinical isolates of GCS and GGS are β-hemolytic and some isolates are susceptible to bacitracin, some GCS and GGS may have been misidentified as GAS if Lancefield serologic testing was not performed.[68] Therefore the true rates of these diseases may be underestimated. For the accurate identification of GCS and GGS (such as *S. dysgalactiae* subspecies), molecular diagnostic tests, such as 16s rRNA sequencing, should be performed.[154] Patients with GAS-related STSS usually are previously healthy, whereas patients with infections due to GCS and GGS, including STSS, usually have underlying conditions such as diabetes mellitus, cardiopulmonary disease, malignancy, collagen disease, liver failure, or renal failure.[68]

Although rare, some cases of bacterial endocarditis may be caused by GCS and GGS infections. The mortality rates for these infections are high, reported as 41% for GCS and 35% for GGS, although the overall mortality rate of infective endocarditis by β-hemolytic streptococci was much lower (12.9%) in a questionnaire study by Baddour and the IDSA's Emerging Infections Network (EIN) members.[11]

S. anginosus is typically isolated from blood cultures, whereas *S. intermedius* tends to be associated with brain abscesses and *S. constellatus* with intraabdominal abscesses, soft tissue infections, or respiratory tract abscesses.[9] Children with *S. intermedius* brain abscess have been found to have certain predisposing factors, such as congenital heart disease (most common), sinusitis, otitis media, or dental caries. Infections at other sites caused by *S. intermedius*, such as liver abscess, lung abscess, or bronchiectasis, can also lead to brain abscess.[97]

Treatment

Penicillin remains the treatment of choice for GCS and GGS infections.[8,123] Penicillin-tolerant strains have been reported in laboratory findings, but the clinical significance is not known.[8,123] For most GCS and GGS infections, treatment with penicillin G alone is adequate. Other antimicrobial regimens that have been shown to work in vitro include penicillin with gentamicin, other β-lactam agents such as cephalosporins, vancomycin, and vancomycin with rifampin.[6] Resistance to macrolides, tetracycline, and chloramphenicol has been reported in the literature.[22,68,91] A few isolates of GCS and GGS *S. dysgalactiae subsp equisimilis* have shown high-level resistance to aminoglycosides.[22,91]

Guidelines for the treatment of endocarditis due to GCS and GGS have not been established because these infections are infrequent. Usually high-dose penicillin G is recommended for 4 to 6 weeks. Some experts recommend the addition of gentamicin to penicillin for at least the first 2 weeks of therapy.[11]

Patients may be treated with clindamycin in addition to penicillin in certain cases such as severe cellulitis, necrotizing fasciitis, or STSS, similar to patients with *S. pyogenes* severe infections. For meningitis, similar to endocarditis therapy, an aminoglycoside can be added in addition to penicillin.[120] For the treatment of a brain abscess (e.g., for *S. intermedius*) a combination of cefotaxime and metronidazole has been recommended.[97] IVIG in STSS may be considered, but there are not enough data to support its use at this time.

NEW REFERENCES SINCE THE SEVENTH EDITION

5. American Academy of Pediatrics. Group A streptococcal infections. In: Kimberlin D, Brady M, Jackson M, Long S, eds. *Red Book: 2015 Report of the Committee on Infectious Diseases*. 30th ed. Elk Grove Village, IL: American Academy of Pediatrics; 2015:732-744.
6. American Academy of Pediatrics. Non-group A or B streptococcal and enterococcal infections. In: Kimberlin D, Brady M, Jackson M, Long S, eds. *Red Book: 2015 Report of the Committee on Infectious Diseases*. 30th ed. Elk Grove Village, IL: American Academy of Pediatrics; 2015:750-753.
9. Asam D, Spellerberg B. Molecular pathogenicity of *Streptococcus* anginosus. *Mol Oral Microbiol*. 2014;29(4):145-155.
30. Centers for Disease Control and Prevention. *Streptococcus progenies emm* sequence database. 2016. Available at: http://www2a.cdc.gov/ncidod/biotech/strepblast.asp.
32. Chang K, Frankovich J, Cooperstock M, et al. Clinical evaluation of youth with pediatric acute-onset neuropsychiatric syndrome (PANS): recommendations from the 2013 PANS Consensus Conference. *J Child Adolesc Psychopharmacol*. 2015;25(1):3-13.
37. Dale JB, Penfound TA, Chiang EY, et al. New 30-valent M protein-based vaccine evokes cross-opsonic antibodies against non-vaccine serotypes of group A streptococci. *Vaccine*. 2011;29(46):8175-8178.
47. Fischetti VA. The *Streptococcus* and the host. Present and future challenges. *Adv Exp Med Biol*. 1997;418:15-20.
48. Flores AR, Jewell BE, Fittipaldi N, et al. Human disease isolates of serotype M4 and M22 group A *Streptococcus* lack genes required for hyaluronic acid capsule biosynthesis. *MBio*. 2012;3(6):e00413-2.
49. Flores AR, Sahasrabhojane P, Saldaña M, et al. Molecular characterization of an invasive phenotype of group A *Streptococcus* arising during human infection using whole genome sequencing of multiple isolates from the same patient. *J Infect Dis*. 2014;209(10):1520-1523.
51. Frankovich J, Thienemann M, Pearlstein J, et al. Multidisciplinary clinic dedicated to treating youth with pediatric acute-onset neuropsychiatric syndrome: presenting characteristics of the first 47 consecutive patients. *J Child Adolesc Psychopharmacol*. 2015;25(1):38-47.
52. Frankovich J, Thienemann M, Rana S, et al. Five youth with pediatric acute-onset neuropsychiatric syndrome of differing etiologies. *J Child Adolesc Psychopharmacol*. 2015;25(1):31-37.
55. Garcia AF, Abe LM, Erdem G, et al. An insert in the *covS* gene distinguishes a pharyngeal and a blood isolate of *Streptococcus progenies* found in the same individual. *Microbiology*. 2010;156(Pt 10):3085-3095.
82. Kotloff KL, Corretti M, Palmer K, et al. Safety and immunogenicity of a recombinant multivalent group A streptococcal vaccine in healthy adults: phase 1 trial. *JAMA*. 2004;292(6):709-715.
83. Kovacevic M, Grant P, Swedo SE. Use of intravenous immunoglobulin in the treatment of twelve youths with pediatric autoimmune neuropsychiatric disorders associated with streptococcal infections. *J Child Adolesc Psychopharmacol*. 2015;25(1):65-69.
88. Latimer ME, L'Etoile N, Seidlitz J, et al. Therapeutic plasma apheresis as a treatment for 35 severely ill children and adolescents with pediatric autoimmune neuropsychiatric disorders associated with streptococcal infections. *J Child Adolesc Psychopharmacol*. 2015;25(1):70-75.
94. McNeil SA, Halperin SA, Langley JM, et al. Safety and immunogenicity of 26-valent group A *Streptococcus* vaccine in healthy adult volunteers. *Clin Infect Dis*. 2005;41(8):1114-1122.
97. Mishra AK, Fournier PE. The role of *Streptococcus* intermedius in brain abscess. *Eur J Clin Microbiol Infect Dis*. 2013;32(4):477-483.
102. Murphy TK, Parker-Athill EC, Lewin AB, et al. Cefdinir for recent-onset pediatric neuropsychiatric disorders: a pilot randomized trial. *J Child Adolesc Psychopharmacol*. 2015;25(1):57-64.
103. Murphy TK, Patel PD, McGuire JF, et al. Characterization of the pediatric acute-onset neuropsychiatric syndrome phenotype. *J Child Adolesc Psychopharmacol*. 2015;25(1):14-25.
105. Nasser W, Beres SB, Olsen RJ, et al. Evolutionary pathway to increased virulence and epidemic group A *Streptococcus* disease derived from 3,615 genome sequences. *Proc Natl Acad Sci USA*. 2014;111(17):E1768-E1776.
120. Rantala S. *Streptococcus dysgalactiae* subsp. *equisimilis* bacteremia: an emerging infection. *Eur J Clin Microbiol Infect Dis*. 2014;33(8):1303-1310.
133. Shulman ST, Bisno AL, Clegg HW, et al. Clinical practice guideline for the diagnosis and management of group A streptococcal pharyngitis: 2012 update by the Infectious Diseases Society of America. *Clin Infect Dis*. 2012;55(10):e86-e102.
152. Torres RS, Santos TZ, Torres RA, et al. Management of contacts of patients with severe invasive group A streptococcal infection. *J Pediatric Infect Dis Soc*. 2016;5(1):47-52.
153. Toufexis MD, Hommer R, Gerardi DM, et al. Disordered eating and food restrictions in children with PANDAS/PANS. *J Child Adolesc Psychopharmacol*. 2015;25(1):48-56.
154. Tsai CT, Chi CY, Ho CM, et al. Correlation of virulence genes to clinical manifestations and outcome in patients with *Streptococcus dysgalactiae* subspecies *equisimilis* bacteremia. *J Microbiol Immunol Infect*. 2014;47(6):462-468.
155. Turner CE, Abbott J, Lamagni T, et al. Emergence of a new highly successful acapsular group A *Streptococcus* clade of genotype *emm89* in the United Kingdom. *MBio*. 2015;6(4):e00622.
156. van Sorge NM, Cole JN, Kuipers K, et al. The classical lancefield antigen of group A *Streptococcus* is a virulence determinant with implications for vaccine design. *Cell Host Microbe*. 2014;15(6):729-740.
164. Zhu L, Olsen RJ, Nasser W, et al. Trading capsule for increased cytotoxin production: contribution to virulence of a newly emerged clade of *emm89 Streptococcus progenies*. *MBio*. 2015;6(5):e01378-15.

The full reference list for this chapter is available at ExpertConsult.com.

83 Group B Streptococcal Infections

Pia S. Pannaraj • Carol J. Baker

HISTORY

Group B *Streptococcus*, or *Streptococcus agalactiae*, was isolated first by Nocard in 1887[266] and for decades was recognized as a cause of bovine mastitis[255] but not human infection. Serologic techniques for differentiating β-hemolytic streptococci were developed by Lancefield,[201] who also described isolation of group B streptococci (GBS) from parturient women in 1935.[203] In that same year, Congdon[88] included one fatal puerperal case of GBS sepsis and pneumonia in a report of streptococcal infections associated with childbirth. The significance of this organism as a human pathogen was reported first by Fry[136] in 1938, who described three cases of fatal puerperal sepsis. GBS infections continued to be reported sporadically until the 1960s, when maternal and neonatal infections increasingly were ascribed to this pathogen.[70,116,170] In the 1970s, GBS emerged as the predominant organism causing bacteremia and meningitis in neonates and young infants.[13,26,134,173,275] The incidence of infant infection remained stable, with reported attack rates ranging from 0.2 to 5.4 per 1000 live births, until the late 1990s, when maternal intrapartum chemoprophylaxis gained wide acceptance and incidence rates fell.[78,114,319] Invasive infection also occurs beyond the first 89 days of life in pregnant women, nonpregnant adults with underlying medical conditions, and elderly persons.[108,120,268]

MICROBIOLOGY

Isolation and Identification

GBS are facultative gram-positive diplococci that grow on a variety of bacteriologic media. Colonies are 3 to 4 mm in diameter, grayish white, flat, and somewhat mucoid. Colonies are surrounded by a narrow zone of β-hemolysis that for some strains is detectable only when the colony is lifted from the agar. Nonhemolytic strains account for 3% to 4% of isolates and can cause human disease.[13,309] Definitive identification of GBS relies on detection of the group B-specific antigen, a carbohydrate cell wall antigen common to all strains. The standard method, as described by Lancefield,[201] requires acid treatment of the bacteria to solubilize the carbohydrate group B antigen, followed by capillary precipitation with hyperimmune rabbit serum. Several newer methods using hyperimmune antisera have been developed, but latex agglutination is used widely because of the commercial availability of test kits, the ease of performing the assay, and the specificity of the results when organisms in pure culture are tested.[331] Other laboratory methods for presumptive identification include testing for resistance to bacitracin or trimethoprim-sulfamethoxazole, hydrolysis of sodium hippurate broth, failure to hydrolyze bile esculin, production of orange pigment when cultured under certain conditions, and CAMP testing. CAMP is an acronym of the names of the authors (Christie, Atkinson, Munch, Peterson) who first described the production of CAMP factor by GBS in the presence of the β-toxin of *Staphylococcus aureus* that results in synergistic hemolysis on sheep blood agar.[87] Chromogenic agars that undergo color change in the presence of β-hemolytic colonies can facilitate detection of β-hemolytic strains but will miss the majority of nonhemolytic strains (~4% of isolates).[345,361] In addition, recently developed rapid techniques for identifying GBS from enrichment broth include DNA probes and nucleic acid amplification tests (NAAT), such as polymerase chain reaction (PCR).[361]

Serologic Classification and Antigenic Structure

GBS possess two carbohydrate cell wall antigens, the group B–specific antigen and type-specific capsular polysaccharide. GBS are classified into serotypes based on type-specific capsular polysaccharides. Nine such polysaccharides are characterized and recognized: Ia, Ib, and II through VIII. The type-specific polysaccharides of GBS are repeating units of five to seven monosaccharides (glucose, galactose, glucosamine, and *N*-acetylneuraminic acid). All the characterized polysaccharides include an *N*-acetylneuraminic acid (sialic acid) residue, which is important in the pathogenesis of type III human infection and perhaps other types.[33,326,372] Despite structural relatedness, antibody directed against the capsular polysaccharide of one type does not provide cross-protection against other capsular polysaccharide types.[202,363,374] A few strains isolated from patients with systemic infection contain type-specific capsular polysaccharide genes by genotypic methods but express low levels of capsule or have modified capsular structures that do not react with hyperimmune sera or monoclonal antibodies to the characterized capsular polysaccharides.[297] These strains are called *nontypeable*.

Further differentiation of type Ia strains was based on the presence or absence of a protein antigen known as C, which led to the nomenclature of Ia and Ia/c serotypes. The C protein also is present in many other serotypes except type III strains. Two components make up the C protein: α (trypsin-resistant) found in 70% of non–type III capsular polysaccharide isolates and β (trypsin-sensitive) found in approximately 20% of isolates.[128,181,234] GBS express additional surface proteins including α-like repetitive proteins (Alp), also referred to as R proteins. R1 and R4 (shown to have an identical gene sequence to Rib) are the major R proteins found on clinical isolates.[127]

Pili, an essential virulence factor in many gram-negative pathogens, were discovered in GBS in 2005[208] and play a role in attachment and invasion of host cells[232] and resistance to macrophage phagocytosis.[180] Ongoing analyses of the GBS genome sequenced from multiple pathogenic strains will provide further insights into its antigenic structure, genes contributing to its virulence, and targets for treatment and prevention.[143,249,349,348]

Extracellular Products

Several bacterial products are elaborated by GBS. Type-specific capsular polysaccharide is released from cells, and the amount elaborated has been correlated with virulence.[196,383] These soluble polysaccharides inhibit opsonophagocytic killing in vitro, thereby providing a mechanism for the documented increase in virulence.[211] Most strains possess C5a-ase, an enzyme of the serine esterase class that inactivates complement component C5a.[168] Because C5a is a potent chemoattractant for neutrophils, this enzyme helps the bacteria to evade the host immune system by hindering the accumulation of neutrophils at the site of infection. The β-hemolysin elaborated by GBS was characterized in 1980; its role in virulence has been explored through the creation of nonhemolytic and hyperhemolytic mutants.[238,368] Expression of β-hemolysin correlated with tissue damage in an in vivo arthritis model,[293] activation of neutrophil signaling pathways in brain endothelium leading to development of meningitis,[104] induced neuronal damage,[303] increased virulence in pulmonary infection in rats and rabbits,[162,265] and directly impaired cardiomyocyte viability and function.[163] Other bacterial products of GBS, including CAMP factor,[164,189] lipoteichoic acid,[161,262,263] pigment,[223,344] hippuricase,[131] hyaluronidase,[247] and nucleases,[129] have been described, but the contributions of these substances to pathogenesis have not been elucidated.

Antimicrobial Susceptibility

To date, human isolates of GBS have remained uniformly susceptible to penicillin G. However, approximately 10-fold greater concentrations are required for inhibition and killing of GBS than for group A streptococci. Isolates with increasing minimum inhibitory concentration (MIC) to penicillin have been reported, but the significance of this finding is unclear.[91,324] GBS also are susceptible to other β-lactam agents, cephalosporins, carbapenems, and vancomycin. However, the first two cases of invasive infection with vancomycin-resistant GBS conferred by insertion of *vanG* elements were described in adults in 2014.[273,336] The prevalence of resistance to the macrolide-lincosamides (erythromycin, clindamycin, clarithromycin) is increasing since the 1970s from 3.4% to 7.4% of isolates and now up to 48% for erythromycin and 30% for clindamycin.[57,79,96,307] Resistance is related to the presence of *ermTR*, *ermB*, or *mefA* genes.[96] Macrolide resistance is highest in type V strains.[217] Furthermore inducible clindamycin resistance can occur in some strains that appear susceptible in broth susceptibility tests; therefore D-zone testing is important to identify these strains.[307] Ninety-five percent of strains are resistant to tetracycline, and resistance to bacitracin, nalidixic acid, trimethoprim-sulfamethoxazole, and metronidazole is uniform.[284] Low-level gentamicin resistance is typical, but when gentamicin is combined with either penicillin G or ampicillin, synergistic killing of GBS occurs in vitro and in vivo.[314,315,341]

As many as 5% to 17% of GBS isolates have been reported to be tolerant to penicillin.[49,192] Expression of tolerance requires laboratory conditions that promote a greater than 16-fold discrepancy between MICs and minimal bactericidal concentrations. Tolerant strains are characterized in vitro by delayed penicillin killing, similar rates of killing by penicillin whether growth is exponential or stationary, an additive rather than a synergistic response to the combination of penicillin and gentamicin, and deficient autolysis. The clinical significance, if any, of these laboratory-induced properties remains unknown.[193,194,329]

EPIDEMIOLOGY

Maternal Colonization

Asymptomatic colonization occurs at vaginal, rectal, urethral, and pharyngeal sites in up to one-third of healthy young women.[54,252] Much effort has been exerted trying to define groups of women at enhanced risk for colonization with GBS. Factors found to be associated with vaginal acquisition include African-American ethnicity, obesity, multiple sex partners, frequent sexual intercourse, male-to-female oral sex, tampon use, and infrequent hand washing.[54,197,236,252] Women younger than 20 years of age have higher prevalence of colonization.[14,31] Several studies have found significantly higher colonization rates among African-Americans,[73,167,252] whereas others found higher rates in Hispanics.[301] Asians have the lowest colonization rates.[73,252]

Maternal vaginal or rectal colonization rates during pregnancy vary from 18% to 35% in reported studies.[21,24,60,99,107,246,283,301] These rates relate to the body sites sampled, microbiologic techniques employed, and the period of gestation in which the cultures are performed. Specimens from the distal portion of the vagina yield GBS more frequently than do specimens from the proximal vagina or cervix.[228] Concomitant sampling of the rectal site results in a 10% to 15% increase in detection over culturing the vaginal site alone.[21,99] Several investigators have suggested the gastrointestinal tract as the principal reservoir for this organism, and sometimes the rectal site is the only one that yields GBS.[21,99,171,283] The urinary tract is an important site of infection (asymptomatic bacteriuria) because it is a surrogate for a high density or "heavy" (>10^5 colony-forming units per milliliter) genital inoculum and a marker of increased risk for development of early-onset sepsis in neonates.[228,379] Bacteriuria mandates therapy during pregnancy.[361]

The manner in which swab specimens from the vagina and rectum are processed also is important in accurately assessing colonization.[76,361] Anogenital culture swabs collected by patients themselves are as accurate as those performed by physicians.[17,292,351] Swabs can be placed in transport media at environmental temperatures for as long as 96 hours.[361] Specimens then should be placed in a selective antibiotic-containing enrichment broth medium, rather than on solid media, because solid media fail to detect as many as 50% of GBS carriers.[28,30] The addition of antibiotics to the broth limits the growth of competing flora, especially gram-negative enteric organisms, and enhances detection.[24,28,30,242] Todd-Hewitt broth with gentamicin and nalidixic acid (selective broth medium)[28] or with colistin and nalidixic acid (Lim broth)[216] is recommended for detection of GBS colonization.[361] After overnight incubation, the broth is subcultured onto a 5% sheep blood agar plate and is processed conventionally.

Ninety-two percent of culture-positive women are identified if lower vaginal and rectal cultures are obtained at a single visit with correct laboratory detection methods.[107] The proximity to delivery affects the accuracy of predicting colonization at delivery. Cultures obtained at 35 and 37 weeks' gestation predict colonization at delivery with 87% sensitivity and 96% specificity.[60,283,382]

Infant Colonization

Colonization and infection in the neonate are associated significantly with the presence of GBS in the maternal genital or gastrointestinal tract at delivery. Vertical transmission from colonized mothers to their infants occurs in 41% to 72% of cases (mean, ~50%).[7,15,24,62,106,167,246,385] Only 1% to 12% (mean, ~5%) of colonized infants are born to noncolonized mothers.[15,24,105,246,385] Acquisition is presumed to occur either by the ascending route through ruptured membranes or from contact with the organism in the genital tract during parturition. Heavy maternal inocula in the genital tract (>10^5 colony-forming units per milliliter) greatly increase the rates of vertical transmission to neonates and rates of heavy infant colonization.[10,15,61,171,183] Other factors associated with increased colonization rates in infants include prolonged rupture of membranes (>12 to 18 hours) and vaginal delivery.[15,167] Maternal intrapartum antibiotic therapy substantially diminishes the vertical transmission of GBS.[7,61,62,167,360,386] The body sites in neonates most likely to yield GBS are the rectum and throat, a finding reflecting replication of organisms at the respiratory or gastrointestinal tract sites after the ingestion of infected amniotic fluid or genital secretions.[167]

Horizontal transmission from nosocomial and community sources has been described.[1,106,138,267] Infant-to-infant or colonized staff member–to-infant spread may occur through hands of hospital personnel, but epidemics are rare.[106,267] The rate of community acquisition, presumably by an oral-fecal route, appears to be low, but this has not been investigated thoroughly.[138,235] Breast milk also has been proposed as a mode of transmission for late-onset infection; most reported cases involved a mother with postpartum mastitis. However, the role of breast milk in infants with late-onset disease, if any, is incompletely understood.[47,51,199,304]

Incidence of Disease

Before the widespread use of maternal intrapartum chemoprophylaxis to prevent early-onset disease, reported attack rates for GBS disease in infants ranged from 1.8 to 4.0 per 1000 live births.[268,369,388] Early-onset disease (onset within the first 6 days of life) accounted for approximately 80% of cases.[319] Late-onset disease (onset from 7 through 89 days of life) rates ranged from 0.3 to 1.8 per 1000 live births.[100,275] With the 2002 guidelines for universal screening of pregnant women at 35 to 37 weeks' gestation and administration of intrapartum chemoprophylaxis to carriers, the incidence of early-onset disease has decreased to approximately 0.25 cases per 1000 live births, a finding representing a decline of nearly 85% from 1990.[80,361] However, the incidence of late-onset disease remains unchanged at approximately 0.25 to 0.3 per 1000 live births.[80,185,361] Approximately 30% of cases of early-onset disease and up to 55% of those of late-onset and late, late-onset disease now occur in preterm infants.[219,317,322] Late, late-onset GBS disease occurs in infants older than 3 months of age and accounts for 7% to 13% of childhood GBS infections.[174,319,381] Affected infants typically were born before 34 weeks' gestation or have an underlying immunodeficiency or concomitant infection with human immunodeficiency virus (HIV).[80,97,174,381] Case fatality rates for all infants with GBS disease have dropped from 46% in the 1970s to 3% to 6% in recent years.[179,286,361]

GBS infection also is a common finding in pregnant women, with clinical manifestations that include urinary tract infection (usually asymptomatic bacteriuria but also cystitis or pyelonephritis), intraamniotic infection (i.e., chorioamnionitis), postpartum endometritis (often with bacteremia), and puerperal sepsis.[274,322,387] Occasionally meningitis, septic thrombophlebitis, and other serious complications occur.[387] Attack rates of 0.12 per 1000 deliveries have been reported, and 28% of maternal cases are associated with pregnancy loss or birth of an infant with early-onset GBS disease.[274,387] Nonpregnant women and men account for 68% of invasive GBS disease in adults.[120] These patients typically are more than 65 years old or have underlying medical conditions, especially diabetes mellitus, but also malignancy (e.g., breast cancer), HIV infection, liver disease, stroke and other neurologic disorders, decubitus ulcers, and neurogenic bladder.[108,120,177,268,355]

Risk Factors for Infant Disease

Vertical transmission is a prerequisite for the development of invasive, early-onset infection.[24,244,275] Evidence suggests that at least 50% of late-onset infections also occur after vertical transmission or from spread within the household.[100] The degree of colonization or inoculum also increases the likelihood of infant disease; heavily colonized mothers are more likely to have infants with invasive infection, and heavily colonized infants are more likely to have either early- or late-onset disease.[60,100,183,215] Other maternal factors associated with the development of early-onset disease include delivery before 37 weeks' gestation, premature rupture of membranes at any gestation (rupture of membranes more than one hour before onset of labor) or rupture of membranes more than 18 hours before delivery at any gestation, and intrapartum fever.[13,59,60,100,134,158,275] Women colonized with GBS also have a higher incidence of premature rupture of membranes and preterm labor, a finding suggesting a possible causal relationship between GBS and events leading to preterm birth.[6,243,248,301] Other maternal factors associated with an increased attack rate of early-onset infection are African-American ethnicity, age younger than 20 years, history of previous fetal loss, history of urinary tract infection with GBS during the current pregnancy, and primiparity.[321,322] Late-onset disease also is associated with young maternal age and African-American ethnicity.[322] Siblings of infected infants who are the product of a multiple pregnancy (e.g., twins, triplets) have enhanced risk for development of early- and late-onset GBS disease.[112,276]

Capsular Polysaccharide Types Causing Disease

Reports from the 1970s indicated that the GBS capsular polysaccharide types colonizing pregnant women and neonates were divided fairly evenly among types I, II, and III.[25,374,375] The current distribution of capsule polysaccharide types in invasive disease from multiple North American studies[93,153,218,370,387] is shown in Fig. 83.1. Serotypes Ia, followed by III, are the most common cause of early-onset infection, whereas serotype III is the most common cause of late-onset infection. In Europe, type III predominates in both early- and late-onset disease.[133,352,370] Serotype III is implicated in 80% to 93% of meningitis cases, either as a focus of early-onset disease or as a manifestation of late-onset infection.[25,26,375] Capsular polysaccharide type V emerged in the 1990s.[55,73,167,305] Type V causes both early- and late-onset infant disease and is the type most commonly isolated from adults with invasive disease.[55,305] In Japan, types VI and VIII are the most common isolates from pregnant women.[200] Recent studies from the Middle East, Africa, Europe, and North America suggest type IV may be an emerging pathogen.[98,130,132,346] The least common serotypes causing human disease are types Ib, VI, VII, and VIII.

PATHOGENESIS

For pediatricians, GBS disease predominantly afflicts neonates, a predilection that results from a unique combination of maternal, bacterial, and host factors. Fig. 83.2 shows a simplified flow chart of GBS transmission. First, an organism carried by an asymptomatically colonized mother is transmitted vertically to her neonate. Evidence suggests that this transmission may occur in utero shortly before birth or during

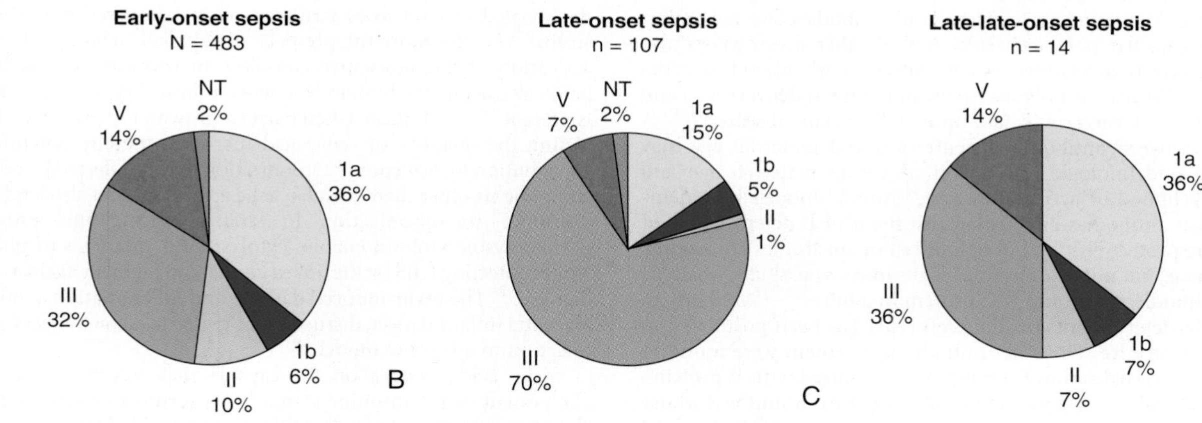

FIG. 83.1 Serotype distribution of invasive group B streptococcal strains causing (A) early-onset, (B) late-onset, and (C) late, late-onset disease in infants.[55,93,153,218,387] *NT*, Nontypeable.

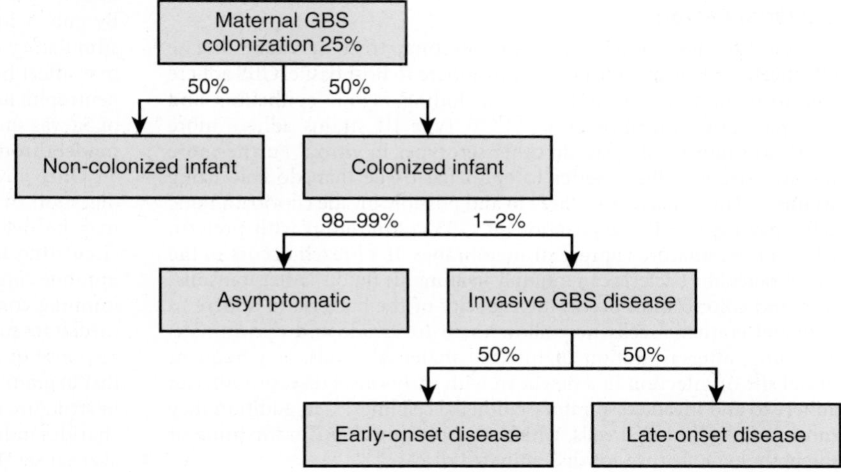

FIG. 83.2 Flow chart of vertical transmission and disease manifestation of group B streptococcal (GBS) disease in the era of intrapartum chemoprophylaxis.

parturition. This continuum in time of acquisition is reflected in the time of onset of symptoms; infected neonates often are ill at or within 12 hours of birth (up to 90% of cases), whereas others may not have evidence of disease for 48 hours or more.[26,322] The organism successfully colonizes approximately 50% of all infants born to GBS carriers, yet disease develops in only 1% to 2% of these infants.[13,320] A breach in the delicate interplay of maternal, infant, and bacterial factors allows the organism to invade. Once invasion occurs, a combination of host defenses and therapeutic interventions may halt the progression of disease, or the infant's defenses may fail and the disease may progress and result in tissue damage or death.

Maternal Factors

The bacterial inoculum in the maternal genital tract determines the likelihood that the organism will be transmitted vertically. Infants born to heavily colonized women are more likely to be colonized themselves and are more likely to have early-onset disease.[10,15,60,100,171,183] Infants delivered before 37 weeks of gestation have an increased risk for development of early-onset disease. Heavy maternal colonization may induce preterm delivery,[122,244,248,300,302] and disease is more likely to develop in the infant in this setting of high bacterial inoculum and immunologic immaturity. Invasive disease also has been reported in term neonates delivered by elective cesarean section with intact membranes, but this is a rare event.[13,95,116,190,274]

In addition to bacterial inoculum, another critical maternal factor is the concentration of serum antibody to the capsular type-specific polysaccharide of the colonizing strain of GBS at delivery. Antibodies to the capsular polysaccharide are protective against the homologous serotype in the mouse model of lethal infection; antibody to the group B polysaccharide is not.[204] Baker and associates[29,34] determined that invasive disease with type III GBS occurred primarily in infants born to women with low serum concentrations of antibodies directed against the type III capsular polysaccharide. Several other investigators also reported a correlation between low concentrations of antibody to types Ia, Ib, II, and III capsular polysaccharide in maternal delivery sera and the occurrence of early- and late-onset GBS infant disease.[145,147] A correlation between antibody concentration and maternal age may explain the epidemiologic association of young maternal age and increased likelihood of neonatal disease.[13] Animal models have demonstrated that antibodies directed against the α or β determinants of C protein are protective,[204,253] but definitive human studies are lacking. Invasive disease, but not colonization, elicits immunoglobulin M (IgM) and IgG antibodies to α- and β-C protein in adults.[269,270] Antibody to other protein determinants in some serotypes has been postulated to be partially protective. Titers of antibody to R protein were found to be higher in maternal serum from mothers colonized with R protein–bearing strains whose infants were healthy than from mothers whose infants were ill; such antibodies were protective in a mouse model against type II, but not type III strains.[220,221] Presence of maternal antibody to Rib also was associated with protection in neonates against Rib-expressing GBS strains.[207]

Bacterial Factors

To colonize the genital and gastrointestinal tract or cause disease effectively, organisms must be able to adhere to host tissue. GBS adhere well to many types of epithelium, including vaginal epithelium and chorioamniotic membranes.[137,227,332,343] Type III strains adhere more avidly to vaginal cells than do other serotypes in vitro.[58] Furthermore invasive strains adhere better to epithelial tissue than do colonizing strains.[159] This capacity to adhere to and possibly invade chorioamniotic cells may explain the association of GBS colonization with preterm labor and premature rupture of membranes. If a breach occurs in the membranes, the bacteria can multiply in amniotic fluid.[160] After transmission and colonization occur, the capacity of the bacteria to adhere to neonatal epithelial cells may allow them to invade and disseminate. The lung, after aspiration of infected maternal fluids, is a frequent initial site of infection in a newborn with early-onset disease. GBS can adhere to and invade respiratory epithelial cell lines.[311] In addition they can invade endothelial cells, which may be a mechanism for some of the pathologic features of disseminated disease.[141]

Several different factors may confer adherence properties of GBS including bacterial cell wall component lipoteichoic acid[263] or surface proteins.[69,343] Studies suggest that translocation across epithelial barriers is mediated by α-C protein binding to host cell surface glycosaminoglycan.[42,82] Several proteins with potential roles in adherence and invasion were identified by detecting upregulation during cell invasion using proteomics and include an undefined surface antigen, penicillin-binding protein 2b, glyceraldehydes-3-phosphate dehydrogenase, and an iron-binding protein.[182] Mouse antisera to these five proteins inhibited binding of GBS to cervical epithelial cells. Translocation also may occur by a paracellular route.[285,335] Fibrinogen-binding proteins and laminin-binding proteins also contribute to attachment and translocation.[205] Adherence to and invasion of the brain microvascular endothelial cells (BMEC) of the blood–brain barrier has been associated with proper anchoring of lipoteichoic acid,[103] β-hemolysin/cytolysin-induced cytolysis,[104] fibrinogen-binding protein FbsA,[347] and pilus proteins.[232] GBS also may attach, invade, and induce a proinflammatory response in human astrocytes that encircle the BMEC and contribute to neonatal meningitis.[339]

A well-defined virulence structure of GBS is the capsular polysaccharide. Mouse virulent strains are able to synthesize greater amounts of surface-bound capsular polysaccharide than avirulent strains.[196,383] An unencapsulated mutant, created by inserting a transposon into the gene regulating capsule expression, has significantly less virulence in neonatal rats than does the wild type III strain.[312] As with other encapsulated organisms, the capsule is thought to confer virulence primarily by interfering with opsonophagocytosis.[211] In vitro, the capsule of type III GBS has been shown to prevent the deposition of C3,[240] and the presence of the terminal sialic acid residue on the repeating unit of this polysaccharide is crucial to this interference.[113] Removal of sialic acid residues from the polysaccharide leads to diminished virulence, and a desialylated mutant loses virulence when compared with the parent strain.[373] Furthermore the presence of this sialic acid moiety prevents activation of the alternative complement pathway, the predominant pathway used by the human host when minimal type-specific antibody is present.[113] In addition, when bacteria grow in the presence of human serum, the quantity of sialic acid increases, thereby potentiating its contribution to virulence.[288] Opsonization may be affected by cell surface components other than capsular sialic acid. C protein also lends relative resistance to opsonization to strains bearing the antigen.[181,279] β-Hemolysin/cytolysin enables cytolysis and apoptosis of phagocytes while protecting GBS by the linked carotenoid pigment against oxidative damage.[223] The toxin-induced damage and inflammation contribute to placental inflammation, disruption of maternal–fetal barriers, and fetal infection in a murine model.[299]

Sialic acid residues on the capsule may interfere with another component of the immune system. In a serum-free system, the desialylated mutant of type III GBS elicited much larger quantities of leukotriene B_4 from macrophages than did the parent strain.[310] Leukotriene B_4 is a potent neutrophil chemoattractant, so this effect may result in diminished influx of effector cells. Similarly, C5a-ase may disable C5a, another host product capable of eliciting neutrophil influx. By enhancing phagocytosis and killing of GBS, C5a also has direct stimulatory effects on neutrophils.[342] Bacterial elaboration of C5a-ase may affect both the accumulation of neutrophils and the efficiency of neutrophil function. A novel peptide derived from the C-terminal region of 5a was shown to mediate clearance of GBS colonization in a murine model through direct bacterial killing.[75]

Once invasive infection is established, ongoing replication and digestion of bacteria can instigate host inflammatory responses that may be deleterious.[205] Neonates recovering from GBS disease have circulating immune complexes for a prolonged period of time, and immune complexes can contribute to end-organ damage.[356] Additionally immune complexes containing GBS components elicit inflammatory mediators such as leukotriene B_4 and interleukin-6 (IL-6). The cytokine response to gram-positive pathogens is not delineated as clearly as is that to gram-negative bacteria, partly because of the greater heterogeneity in structure of the latter.[56] Both group B and type III capsular polysaccharides induce the release of IL-6 from monocytes[335]; group B antigen also causes the release of tumor necrosis factor-α (TNF-α).[358] As with other gram-positive pathogens, the cell walls of GBS contain peptidoglycan and lipoteichoic acid. Peptidoglycans from other gram-positive organisms elicit a variety of proinflammatory cytokines such as TNF-α, IL-1, IL-6, and granulocyte colony-stimulating factor.[101,166,308] Lipoteichoic acid also induces the release of IL-1β, IL-6, and TNF-α.[50,191] GBS cell wall components likewise exert similar effects. Elaboration of these cytokines has been implicated in the clinical and hemodynamic effects of sepsis.[56,371] Specifically blockade of IL-1 activity by administration of an IL-1 receptor antagonist in a piglet model of GBS sepsis ameliorated systemic hypotension and prolonged survival.[359]

Infant Host Factors

Neonates have several domains of immune dysfunction that affect their ability to mount a sufficient defense against GBS. Neutrophils are the primary effector cell in host defense against extracellular bacterial pathogens, and neutrophils from neonates have many functional abnormalities.[212] The generation of chemotactic activity in neonatal serum in response to GBS is diminished, as is the release of chemotactic factors by neonatal monocytes.[11,12,20] Thus the diminished ability of neutrophils to migrate is amplified by a diminished level of chemotactic stimulation. Phagocytosis and bacterial killing also are impaired when opsonic activity is poor, as is the usual pattern in neonates with sepsis.[212] The neutrophil storage pools of neonates rapidly become depleted during invasive infection, thereby leading to profound neutropenia,[86] an ominous prognostic indicator.[278] These defects in neonatal neutrophils are even more pronounced in infants born prematurely.[212]

Cells of the monocyte/macrophage lineage also may play a role in host defense against GBS, especially in the lungs, where the alveolar macrophage is the first effector cell to encounter pathogens. Defects in the functions of these cells have been described in neonates, especially preterm infants.[90] Cord blood monocytes have impaired phagocytosis and killing of GBS.[239] In animal models, oxidative metabolism, bacterial uptake, and migration to the site of infection by neonatal macrophages are diminished in response to GBS.[241,323,325]

Humoral immunity is compromised in neonates. Both the alternative and classic complement pathways are affected, and preterm neonates are impaired more severely than are term neonates.[94,110] Both pathways are important in the opsonization of GBS.[114] The concentration of type-specific antibody passively acquired from the mother is an important protective factor. Because passive transfer of IgG increases dramatically during the final 8 weeks of pregnancy, premature neonates are again at a disadvantage because they may not receive sufficient amounts of type-specific IgG if they are born before protective levels are transferred.[85]

The pattern of production of cytokines by neonatal immune cells frequently is altered when compared with that of adults. For example, in response to GBS, the level of TNF-α and IL-6 released by neonatal monocytes is increased relative to adults,[357,358] but levels of IL-8 and leukotriene B_4 are decreased.[310,316] IL-12 and interferon-γ are associated with improved outcome in an animal model of GBS infection, but lower quantities of these mediators are released by neonatal mononuclear cells.[188,233] Impairment in the innate recognition systems including Toll-like receptors (TLR) and nucleotide-binding oligomerization domain (NOD)-like receptors may lead to reduced cytokine production and pathogen clearance.[89,313] Monocytes from newborns show lower TLR-mediated cytokine production compared to adults.[90,313] Cytokine networks are important both in the manifestations of sepsis and in the stimulation of an appropriate immune response, so alterations in expression of cytokines may affect the neonate's response to this pathogen both clinically and immunologically.

CLINICAL MANIFESTATIONS

Early-Onset Disease

GBS remains the leading cause of neonatal sepsis since the 1970s, and it accounts for 40% to 50% of early-onset sepsis cases.[40,53,114,175] The bimodal distribution of GBS infections corresponding to age of neonates and young infants was described first in 1973 and now is divided into two types, termed *early-* and *late-onset disease*.[26,134] The syndromes of early- and late-onset disease differ in epidemiologic characteristics, pathogenesis, clinical findings, and prognosis. Their major clinical features are detailed in Table 83.1. Early-onset disease is defined as onset of infection in the first 6 days of life, but most neonates (61% to 95%) become ill within the first 24 hours (median, 1 hour).[59,66,158,322] Premature infants often are ill at birth or within 6 hours of birth and account for 17% to 32% of neonates with early-onset GBS disease.[22,294,319,322] In very-low-birth-weight infants, GBS has dropped to the second most common cause of early-onset sepsis, after *Escherichia coli,* since the implementation of intrapartum antibiotic chemoprophylaxis.[338]

Early-onset disease often occurs in the setting of maternal complications, including labor before 37 weeks' gestation, prolonged rupture of membranes for more than 12 to 18 hours, intrapartum fever greater than 100.4°F, chorioamnionitis, and early postpartum febrile morbidity.[45,59,60,100,158,369] In one study, neonates born to a mother with one or more of these risk factors were 12.5 times more likely to develop early-onset GBS disease compared with those born to a mother with no risk factors.[59] A substantial number of term infants can develop GBS disease without definable maternal risk factors except vaginal/rectal colonization.[114] In other studies, 65% to 76% of mothers of neonates with early-onset disease had deliveries complicated by at least one of the foregoing identifiable risk factor or was known to be a GBS carrier.[158,294]

The three most frequent clinical manifestations are bacteremia without a focus, pneumonia, and meningitis.[13,369,381] The presentation for each may range from shock and respiratory failure at delivery to a healthy infant who has infection detected during evaluation because of maternal risk factors known to increase the risk for development of invasive infection.[294,369] Respiratory distress, including apnea, grunting respirations, tachypnea, and cyanosis, is the most common initial manifestation in all forms of early-onset GBS disease.[22,26,134,362,381] Other signs include lethargy, poor feeding, abdominal distention, pallor, jaundice, tachycardia, and hypotension. Fever usually is present in term neonates, but preterm infants often are normothermic or hypothermic.[369] Administration of intrapartum antibiotic prophylaxis to the mother does not alter the findings in infants, in whom early-onset disease develops despite administration of intrapartum chemoprophylaxis; most still become clinically ill in the first 24 hours of life.[40,66]

TABLE 83.1 Features of Group B Streptococcal Disease in Infants

Feature	Early-Onset Disease	Late-Onset Disease	Late, Late-Onset Disease
Age at onset[59,66,322]	≤6 days; mean, 8 h; median, 1 h	7–89 days; mean, 36 days; median, 27 days	≥90 days
Infants affected[369,322,77,151]	Premature neonates, births after maternal obstetric complications	Term and preterm infants equal	Premature neonates <32 wk gestation, immunodeficiency
Clinical findings[114,210]	Acute respiratory distress, apnea, and hypotension common	Fever, irritability, nonspecific signs, occasionally fulminant	Fever, irritability, nonspecific signs
Manifestations[13,134,369,381,23,109,185]	Bacteremia (40–55%), pneumonia (30–45%), meningitis (6–15%)	Bacteremia without a focus (55–67%), meningitis (20–35%), osteoarthritis (~5%), cellulitis/adenitis (~2%)	Bacteremia without a focus, focal infections as in late-onset disease
Case-fatality rate[78,319,322,369,381,185]	5–15%	2–6%	<5%

Bacteremia without a focus is present in 27% to 87% of neonates with early-onset disease.[322,369,381] Signs of septicemia, such as respiratory distress and poor perfusion, often are present, especially in neonates born at less than 37 weeks' gestation.[369] Bacteremia in healthy-appearing term infants also may develop, and in one series it occurred in 22% of cases.[173,369,381] These infants probably remained healthy because of early evaluation and institution of empirical antimicrobial therapy.[369] Most often, bacteremic infants are mildly ill and have fever and nonspecific signs that should prompt bacteriologic evaluation. Bacteremia also frequently accompanies pneumonia and meningitis.

Radiographic findings of pulmonary involvement include infiltrates suggestive of congenital pneumonia, small pleural effusions, a pattern similar to that of hyaline membrane disease or respiratory distress syndrome, and increased vascular markings as seen in transient tachypnea of the newborn; radiographs also may appear normal despite abnormal pulmonary signs.[214,224,362] In preterm neonates, the findings frequently are identical to those of respiratory distress syndrome, and at autopsy, hyaline membranes containing bacteria and minimal inflammatory infiltrates have been described.[2,362]

Meningitis is documented in 6% to 15% of neonates with early-onset disease (Fig. 83.3).[320,369,377] As a rule, no meningeal signs are present thus underscoring the need to evaluate all neonates with presumed early-onset disease for the possibility of meningeal involvement.[369,377] Early in the course, the cerebrospinal fluid (CSF) white blood cell count may be normal despite isolation of GBS.[13] Again respiratory distress is the most frequent clinical finding.[26,210,369,] Seizures rarely are the initial feature but do occur in as many as 50% of affected neonates early in the course of therapy; often these seizures are focal and subtle.[26] Postmortem evaluation of infants who die of early-onset GBS meningitis reveals hemorrhage, prominent basilar involvement, and abundant bacteria with relatively sparse inflammation.[134]

Late-Onset Disease

Late-onset disease is defined as infection in infants 7 to 90 days of age, and historically it primarily affected term infants with an unremarkable maternal history and early neonatal course.[26,100,185] However, one case series suggested that late-onset infection develops in a larger proportion of infants born quite prematurely (<34 weeks' gestation).[219] Bacteremia without a focus and meningitis are the two most common manifestations of late-onset disease.[134,280,381] Osteoarticular infections and cellulitis are additional clinical foci.[23,109,381] Whereas early-onset disease most frequently occurs acutely with apnea and hypotension, late-onset disease often is manifested by fever, irritability, and other nonspecific signs.[114] More fulminant, rapidly progressive cases do occur, however.[26]

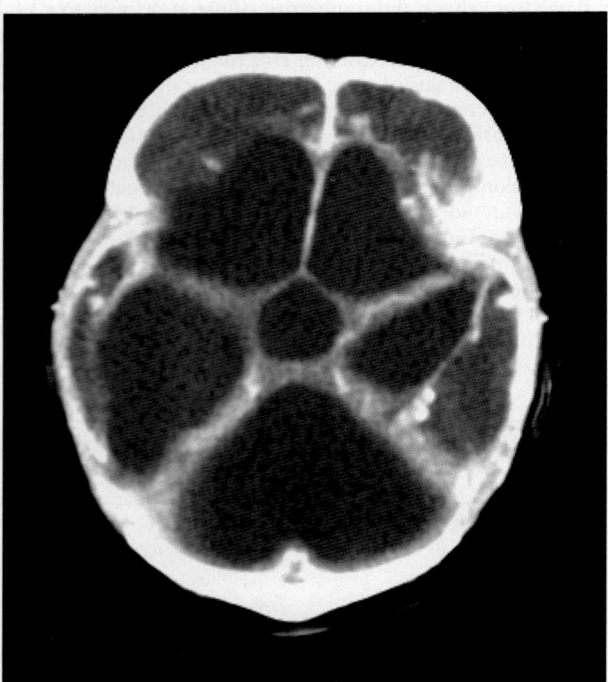

FIG. 83.3 Head computed tomographic scan at 6 weeks of age from a term infant with early-onset group B streptococcal meningitis shows significant loss of normal brain matter.

Meningitis is a frequent complication, occurring in 26% to 40% of late-onset disease cases.[26,185,369,381] GBS accounted for 86% of infant cases under 2 months of age with meningitis in a recent multistate epidemiologic study.[350] Late-onset meningitis most typically manifests with fever and lethargy, although respiratory distress, coma, and shock also may occur.[26] Classic signs of meningitis, such as a bulging fontanelle and nuchal rigidity, occur more commonly in neonates with late-onset than early-onset meningitis. Subdural effusions develop in as many as 20% of cases, but subdural empyema is a rare occurrence.[13,26,276] Infants who die of late-onset meningitis have purulent leptomeningitis at postmortem examination.[134]

Late, Late-Onset Disease

Contemporary studies show an increasing incidence of GBS infection in infants older than 3 months of age, defined as late, late-onset disease.[174,210,319,381] These infections tend to occur in infants who were born extremely prematurely and whose corrected postmenstrual age is less than 3 months.[174,319,381] Late, late-onset disease also occurs, albeit infrequently, in children co-infected with HIV and those with immunodeficiencies,[97,174,381] a finding supporting the recommendation that immunodeficiency be considered in any child infected beyond the usual period of risk.[97] The clinical manifestations in these older infants are similar to those in patients with typical late-onset infection; bacteremia without a focus and meningitis are the most common clinical features.[97,174] Endocarditis and central venous catheter infection also have been noted.[174]

Septic Arthritis and Osteomyelitis

Osteoarthritis occurs in approximately 5% of infants with late-onset infection but appears to be diminishing since implementation of maternal intrapartum prophylaxis.[381] Among neonates and young infants with osteomyelitis, GBS have been identified as the causal agent in 7% to 38% of cases.[109,378] The osteoarticular disease usually is more indolent than is the osteomyelitis caused by other etiologic agents in young infants. Diagnosis usually is established after a mean of 9 days of clinical signs at a mean age of 31 days.[109,114] Decreased motion of the involved extremity, typically the arm, and pain with manipulation are common signs. Warmth and redness are uncommon findings but have been described.[109] Systemic signs and symptoms, including fever, are unusual manifestations.[109,248]

GBS has a predilection for the proximal humerus.[109] The femur is the second most commonly affected bone. Involvement of more than one bone is an unusual finding.[109] However, involvement of the adjacent joint is described.[250] Blood cultures infrequently are positive, unlike neonatal osteomyelitis caused by other etiologic agents. A lytic lesion often is seen on radiographs at first evaluation (Fig. 83.4). This observation suggests that lytic lesions may be a late phenomenon that develops after seeding of the metaphysis during an episode of asymptomatic, early-onset bacteremia several weeks before presentation.[114]

The mean age at diagnosis in infants who have septic arthritis without osteomyelitis is 20 days. The clinical picture typically is acute, with a mean of 2 days of abnormal findings before diagnosis is established. The lower extremities are involved most often, with the hip joint predominating. Infants typically present with local joint signs in the absence of systemic symptoms.[250]

Cellulitis/Adenitis

In one case series, 2% of late-onset GBS infections were associated with cellulitis/adenitis syndrome.[381] Diagnosis is made at a mean age of 5 weeks, with a preponderance of cases in male patients.[23] Typical presentation includes fever, irritability, poor feeding, and swelling of the affected soft tissue area. Enlarged adjacent lymph nodes become palpable within a few days. The most frequent sites of cellulitis are the face and neck,[23,155,277] with enlarged lymph nodes in the submandibular area. Ipsilateral otitis media was noted in four of five infants with facial or

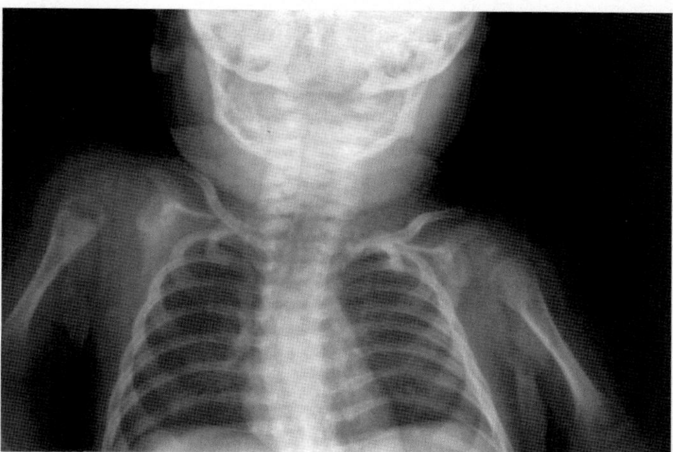

FIG. 83.4 Radiograph of the right arm of a 26-day-old infant with a 2-day history of diminished movement of that extremity. A well-defined, lytic lesion is present in the proximal end of the humerus. Necrotic material from this area was debrided surgically and grew group B streptococci on culture. (Courtesy Morven S. Edwards, MD.)

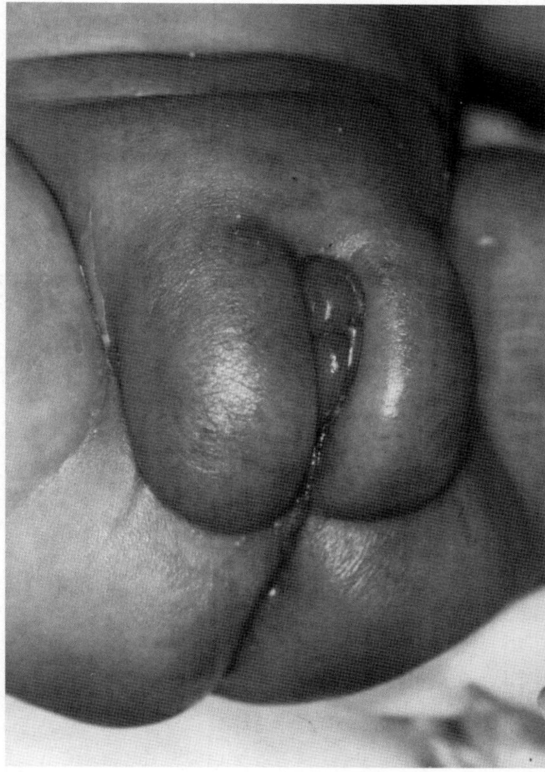

FIG. 83.5 This 3-month-old female infant born after 28 weeks' gestation had fever, lethargy, swelling of the external genitalia, and erythema that extended to the lower part of the abdomen and the thigh. Blood culture grew type Ib/c group B streptococci. (Courtesy Morven S. Edwards, MD.)

submandibular cellulitis in one case series.[23] Less commonly affected areas reported include the genital or inguinal region (Fig. 83.5), the hand, and the prepatellar bursa.[23,63,376] Aspiration of the affected area of cellulitis often yields GBS, and concomitant bacteremia almost always is present.

Other Manifestations

Nearly every organ has been reported to be a site of GBS infection in young infants. Table 83.2 lists these reported unusual manifestations of early- and late-onset disease.

Recurrent Infections

Second (and rarely third) episodes of GBS infection occur in approximately 1% to 2% of cases after early- and late-onset infection.[148] In a case series from Houston, the mean age at recurrence was 44 days, and the mean duration between the first course of therapy and recurrence was 19 days.[148] Molecular epidemiologic techniques have indicated that most, but not all, of these recurrent infections are caused by the strain implicated in the first episode; this finding suggests that persistent mucosal colonization after treatment of the first episode is followed by invasion of the bloodstream.[261] Contaminated breast milk also has been implicated as a source of recurrent infection, but this topic is controversial.[199] No specific risk factors are evident in these infants, but most of them are born prematurely.[148]

DIAGNOSIS AND DIFFERENTIAL DIAGNOSIS

Laboratory Studies

The diagnosis of GBS infection is confirmed by isolation of this pathogen from a normally sterile body site including blood, CSF, pleural fluid, bone aspirate, joint fluid, or soft tissue. Cultures of the skin, umbilicus, or mucous membranes do not have clinical significance. Tracheal aspirate cultures that grow GBS indicate neonatal colonization but do not prove pulmonary invasion (pneumonia). Rather isolation of the organism from blood (or in rare circumstances, lung tissue or the pleural space) is required.

Meningitis in early-onset disease is clinically indistinguishable from bacteremia without a focus, and 10% to 38% of neonates with meningitis have negative blood culture results,[377] so lumbar puncture is necessary to determine the presence or absence of meningeal involvement. Lumbar punctures also are indicated in patients with a focal site of GBS infection because each results from bacteremia. For example, GBS grew from CSF cultures in 24% of infants with cellulitis/adenitis who underwent lumbar puncture.[5] One study found that if selected criteria were used instead of routine lumbar punctures, the diagnosis of bacterial meningitis would have been missed or delayed in 17% of infants.[377]

CSF has had detectable group B antigen in 72% to 89% of neonates with meningitis; serum is much less likely to be positive. The only specimens that should be considered for antigen testing are blood and CSF; urine specimens should not be tested because they are unreliable. Antigen testing should not be used as a substitute for bacterial culture. Their proper use should be limited to the setting of symptomatic infants in whom rapid diagnosis may alter therapy or allow proper tailoring of antibiotic choice: for example, a sick neonate with CSF pleocytosis and previous antibiotic administration. These tests are never useful in infants who appear healthy.

A limited study of real-time PCR to detect DNA in blood of eight neonates with culture-proven GBS sepsis showed positive corresponding results.[184,187] However, larger prospective studies are required to evaluate sensitivity and specificity.

The white blood cell count of a neonate with proven GBS sepsis may be normal or demonstrate leukopenia, neutropenia, or leukocytosis.[237,278,362] Manroe and associates[237] found the ratio of absolute immature neutrophils to absolute total neutrophils (I:T index) to be the most reliable index for distinguishing respiratory distress caused by GBS infection from that with a noninfectious origin. Most infected neonates had an elevation greater than 0.20 (91% vs. 4% of uninfected infants). Other markers of inflammation such as C-reactive protein may also rise with acute infection and decrease in response to therapy.[287,291]

Differential Diagnosis

The signs and symptoms of early-onset GBS disease are clinically indistinguishable from neonatal sepsis caused by other bacterial pathogens such as *E. coli*. The timing is somewhat different, with GBS disease appearing in the first day and *E. coli* with onset on the second or third day of life.[179] The prominence of respiratory signs in early-onset disease may lead to confusion with noninfectious causes of respiratory distress such as transient tachypnea of the newborn, persistent fetal circulation, and respiratory distress syndrome.[2,22,278,362] Clinical features that suggest GBS infection include a history of prolonged rupture of membranes,

TABLE 83.2 **Unusual Clinical Manifestations of Group B Streptococcal Disease in Infants and Children**

Site and Manifestation	References	Site and Manifestation	References
Brain		Tracheitis	274
Abscess	329	Pleural empyema	173, 333
Cerebritis	195	**Skin and Soft Tissue**	
Chronic meningitis	334	Breast abscess	264, 305
Diabetes insipidus	229	Bursitis	65
Eosinophilic meningitis	256	Cellulitis/adenitis	23, 155, 173, 206, 277, 376
Subdural empyema	124	Dactylitis	135
Ventriculitis	257	Fasciitis	144, 296
Eye		Impetigo neonatorum	46, 198, 225
Conjunctivitis	16, 134, 289	Purpura fulminans	176, 226
Endophthalmitis	149, 209	Omphalitis	48, 178, 381
Ear and Sinus		Rhabdomyolysis	354
Ethmoiditis	173	Scalp abscess	121, 151
Otitis media/mastoiditis	23, 118, 327	**Abdomen**	
Cardiovascular/Hematologic		Adrenal abscess	19, 74, 365
Asymptomatic bacteremia	282, 173, 298	Delayed-onset diaphragmatic hernia	18, 41, 290, 340
Endocarditis	8, 43, 172, 267, 367	Gallbladder distention	281
Myocarditis	44	Peritonitis	72, 81
Mycotic aneurysm	3	**Urinary Tract**	
Pericarditis	152	Renal abscess	365, 380
Respiratory Tract		Urinary tract infection	337, 381
Epiglottitis	384		
Supraglottitis	222		

Modified from Edwards MS, Nizet V, Baker CJ. Group B streptococcal infections. In Wilson CB, Nizet V, Maldonado YA, Remington JS, Klein JO, eds. *Infectious Diseases of the Fetus and Newborn Infant*, 8th edition. Philadelphia: Elsevier; 2016:411–56.

TABLE 83.3 **Treatment of Group B Streptococcal Infections in Infants**

Focus of Infection	Antibiotic	Daily Dose	Duration
Suspected meningitis (initial empirical therapy)	Ampicillin *plus* gentamicin	300–400 mg/kg 4–7.5 mg/kg	Until cerebrospinal fluid is sterile
Suspected sepsis[a] (initial empirical therapy)	Ampicillin *plus* gentamicin	150–200 mg/kg	Until bloodstream is sterile
Meningitis	Penicillin G	450,000–500,000 U/kg	14 days minimum[b]
Bacteremia	Penicillin G	200,000 U/kg	10 days
Arthritis	Penicillin G	200,000–300,000 U/kg	2–3 wk
Osteomyelitis	Penicillin G	200,000–300,000 U/kg	3–4 wk
Endocarditis	Penicillin G	400,000 U/kg	4 wk[c]

[a]Assumes that lumbar puncture has been performed and the cerebrospinal fluid has no abnormalities.
[b]Should be extended to 21 days or longer if ventriculitis, cerebritis, subdural empyema, or other suppurative complications occur.
[c]In combination with low-dose gentamicin for the first 14 days.

apnea, shock in the first 24 hours of life, a 1-minute Apgar score of 5 or less, and rapid progression of pulmonary disease.[2,22,362]

The differential diagnosis of late-onset disease depends on the focus of infection. Meningitis in infants of this age also is caused rarely by *Streptococcus pneumoniae*, *Neisseria meningitidis*, *Listeria monocytogenes*, *Haemophilus influenzae* (type b and nontypeable), and more commonly with viruses.[350] The findings of osteomyelitis may be subtle; refusal to move the arm may be ascribed to neuromuscular disease or Erb palsy.[109] Careful physical examination usually reveals tenderness over the involved area, and radiographs generally show a lytic defect in the metaphyses.[109] If the organism is isolated from a bone aspirate, the diagnosis is definitive. Finally, as seen in Table 83.2, many unusual manifestations of GBS infection have been described, so this organism should be included in the differential diagnosis of any focal infection occurring in the age group at risk.

TREATMENT

Empirical Treatment

The antimicrobial regimens recommended for the treatment of GBS infection in infants are summarized in Table 83.3. Penicillin G remains the drug of choice because susceptibility is uniform. In the usual circumstance, however, antimicrobial therapy for GBS infection is initiated before culture results are known. Initial empirical therapy for early-onset disease includes ampicillin and gentamicin for the treatment of neonatal pathogens in addition to GBS. Irrespective of gestational age, neonates with suspected meningitis and those whose clinical condition will not permit lumbar puncture should receive high doses of ampicillin (300 mg/kg per day) plus gentamicin.[13] This combination is more effective than is either ampicillin or penicillin G alone in killing most GBS strains in vitro[314] and in vivo.[341] For suspected late-onset disease, the usual initial therapy includes intravenous ampicillin in combination with cefotaxime or ceftriaxone.[9] If an infant is receiving empirical vancomycin therapy and GBS meningitis has not been excluded, penicillin G or ampicillin should be added to the regimen because vancomycin is inhibitory rather than bactericidal in vitro, and CSF concentrations may not exceed the MIC if a high inoculum of GBS is present.[114]

Specific Treatment

Once GBS have been identified in cultures of blood, CSF, or other normally sterile body sites and blood and CSF cultures are shown to be sterile, penicillin G alone should be used to complete therapy. Recommendations concerning the optimal dose and duration have varied, but they should be dictated by the focus and severity of the infection (see Table 83.3). Several issues should be considered when selecting the appropriate dose: (1) the usual minimal bactericidal concentration of penicillin for GBS ranges from 0.04 to 0.8 μg/mL,[192] (2) only 10% of penicillin serum levels reach the CSF, (3) the inoculum of GBS in the CSF of infants with meningitis may reach 10^7 to 10^8 colony-forming units per milliliter,[123] and (4) high doses of penicillin G and ampicillin are safe in neonates.[114] To ensure rapid bacterial killing, especially in infants with meningitis, relatively high doses of penicillin are recommended for both early- and late-onset infections.

The infant with meningitis should undergo a second lumbar puncture 24 to 48 hours into therapy to document CSF sterility.[114] Infants with continued positive CSF cultures may have very high inoculum, ventriculitis with obstruction, severe infection with cerebritis and vasculitis, subdural empyema, or septic thrombophlebitis, or they may be receiving an insufficient dose of antibiotics; in this circumstance, appropriate studies should be initiated to determine which of these conditions is present. When CSF sterility is verified, penicillin G alone is given for a minimum of 14 days.[9] Longer treatment is indicated if the course is severe, the infant has ventriculitis, or CSF sterilization is delayed. Another lumbar puncture to evaluate CSF cell count and protein should be considered at the anticipated completion of therapy. Findings of polymorphonuclear cells greater than 30% or protein higher than 200 mg/dL may warrant further diagnostic evaluation and longer duration of therapy.[114] In addition, a contrast-enhanced neuroimaging study should be performed near completion of therapy in complicated cases, including infants who have prolonged fever (>5 days), cerebritis, abscess(es), subdural empyema, or venous thrombosis(es). Such complications often correlate with neurologic abnormalities that lead to a poor prognosis for complete central nervous system recovery.[115,364]

Infants with bacteremia without a focus should receive intravenous therapy for a total of 10 days.[9] A shorter duration has not been documented to be efficacious, and relapses, although rare, have been reported in these circumstances.[67,366] Patients with septic arthritis, osteomyelitis, or endocarditis should be treated for the durations summarized in Table 83.3. Oral therapy has no place in the management of infants with invasive GBS disease.[9,114] Alternative agents such as the third-generation cephalosporins are active against GBS in vitro.[125,217] The clinical efficacy of these agents is unknown, however, and these drugs are not recommended in most circumstances.

Supportive Treatment

The importance of prompt, vigorous, and careful supportive therapy in the successful treatment of infant GBS infections cannot be overemphasized. Neonates with early-onset disease accompanied by pneumonia should be suspected of having early respiratory failure, and ventilatory support should be initiated before the onset of apnea, septic shock, or frank respiratory failure occurs. Persistent metabolic acidosis and delayed capillary refill should prompt treatment for shock. All patients with signs of impending respiratory or circulatory failure or meningitis should be treated in an intensive care unit. When present, hypoxemia, severe anemia, and acidosis should be corrected, and seizures should be controlled with anticonvulsants. In addition, fluid and electrolyte status should be monitored meticulously. Surfactant should be used as per nursery protocol; improved gas exchange is seen in infected premature neonates who receive surfactant, although the response is slower than in patients with respiratory distress syndrome.[165] Finally, if an infant has persistent pulmonary hypertension or if conventional ventilatory therapy has failed, extracorporeal membrane oxygenation may be considered, if available.

Adjunctive Treatment

Adjunctive treatment of life-threatening GBS disease is aimed at correcting poor host defenses. Such treatments previously studied include intravenous human immunoglobulin, monoclonal antibodies to GBS polysaccharide antigen, leukocyte transfusion, and growth factors such as granulocyte colony-stimulating factor and granulocyte-monocyte colony-stimulating factor for neutropenia.[71,84,142] The efficacy of these agents has not been established, and, although they may be used occasionally, they should be considered experimental.

Recurrent Infections

In the few infants who experience a recurrence, suppurative foci, HIV infection, or humoral immune deficiency should be excluded or treated. Immunoglobulin levels should be determined to exclude humoral immune deficiency. Although it may be too early to document humoral immune deficiency unequivocally, total IgG usually is significantly lower than would be expected for age in weeks.[148] Susceptibility testing of isolates from the first and recurrent episodes should be determined, if possible, to ensure in vitro susceptibility to penicillin. If the reason for the recurrence remains unknown, persistent mucous membrane colonization with GBS is the likely source.[261] β-lactam antibiotics, even when administered by the parenteral route, do not eradicate GBS colonization reliably.[272] Some studies have shown the benefit of rifampin (20 mg/kg per day) to eradicate mucosal GBS colonization when given orally during the last 4 days of parenteral therapy.[148,254] However, a more recent study showed failure of rifampin to reliably eradicate GBS colonization in infants.[126]

PROGNOSIS

The outcome of GBS disease is related to the severity and site of infection at initial evaluation. Improved outcomes after early-onset infection have resulted from greater awareness among pediatricians and improved obstetric management. Improvements in obstetrics include the use of intrapartum antibiotic prophylaxis in women at risk for delivering an infant with early-onset GBS infection. However, the mortality rate remains substantial at 2% to 8%, especially in neonates born at less than 37 weeks' gestation, in whom the mortality rate often exceeds 20%.[78,320]

Little information is available on the long-term prognosis of survivors of GBS sepsis without meningitis. In infants with septic shock, the development of periventricular leukomalacia has been reported and associated with neurodevelopmental sequelae.[119] However, the frequency of this association is not known.

For infants with early- or late-onset meningitis, 20% to 30% will have permanent severe neurologic impairment such as cortical blindness, bilateral sensorineural hearing loss, cerebral palsy, motor deficits, or significantly delayed development and learning.[115,154,210,364] Another 25% will have mild to moderate impairment characterized by hydrocephalus requiring ventriculoperitoneal shunt, loss of a digit, seizure disorder controlled by medication, or mildly delayed development and learning. Despite advances in intensive care, a current assessment of term and near-term infants diagnosed with GBS meningitis followed up at 3 to 9 years of age shows that rates of neurologic impairment remain unchanged.[210,213] Only 51% demonstrate normal age-appropriate development. Features at admission associated with death after hospital discharge or severe impairment include lethargy, respiratory distress, coma or semicoma, bulging fontanel, hypotension requiring pressor support, leukopenia, CSF protein levels greater than 300 mg/dL, CSF glucose lower than 20 mg/dL, and neutropenia.[39,115,210,213,278] Features at hospital discharge associated with late death or severe impairment include failed hearing screen, abnormal neurologic examination, and abnormal brain imaging at the end of therapy.

To date, the prognosis for infants with osteoarticular or soft tissue infections with GBS has been excellent.[23,109] However, omission of early surgical intervention for infections that involve either the hip or shoulder joints can result in epiphyseal injury.

PREVENTION

The continuing magnitude and severity of GBS disease and its attendant mortality and morbidity have led to investigations aimed at its prevention. Several general approaches have been proposed: maternal prophylaxis to decrease transmission, infant prophylaxis to decrease colonization, and immunoprophylaxis to increase protection against disease.

Intrapartum Antibiotic Prophylaxis

Maternal Prophylaxis

Epidemiologic studies during the 1980s showed that women with GBS colonization during pregnancy had greater than 25 times likelihood of delivering infants with early-onset disease compared with women with negative prenatal cultures.[360,361] The idea of giving antibiotic therapy to the mother to prevent vertical transmission to her fetus was suggested first by Franciosi and colleagues.[134] The first strategy to be evaluated was antenatal treatment of GBS maternal carriers with oral or intramuscular penicillin. This method temporarily suppresses colonization density but does not eradicate colonization or interrupt vertical transmission of GBS to neonates.[139,150,295]

The next strategy, maternal intrapartum chemoprophylaxis, has been demonstrated to be efficacious in the prevention of vertical transmission of GBS from colonized mothers to their neonates, the development of early-onset disease, and maternal febrile morbidity. Infants are less frequently colonized with GBS if they are born to mothers treated with ampicillin during labor than to mothers not given antibiotics.[60,61,386] Several controlled trials involving thousands of deliveries indicated that intrapartum penicillin G or ampicillin given intravenously to GBS carriers during labor prevents early-onset disease in neonates.[62,244,353] Early-onset infection occurred in 0% to 1.1% of infants whose mothers received intrapartum ampicillin compared with 5% to 9% of infants of mothers in the groups not receiving prophylaxis. A large trial involving more than 50,000 live births in Australia showed similar results.[140]

In 1996, guidelines supported by the Centers for Disease Control and Prevention (CDC), the American College of Obstetricians and Gynecologists, and the American Academy of Pediatrics recommended a risk-based approach or culture-based approach.[361] The risk-based approach was based on the presence of one of more of the following: premature labor at less than 37 weeks' gestation, prolonged rupture of membranes (>18 hours), GBS bacteriuria, intrapartum fever (≥100.4°F [38°C]), or delivery of a previous infant with GBS infection. The culture-based approach required intrapartum chemoprophylaxis for all women with positive vaginal and rectal cultures routinely obtained at 35 to 37 weeks' gestation regardless of risk factors. Use of these methods to define women who were candidates for intrapartum chemoprophylaxis led to an approximately 70% decline in the incidence of early-onset GBS disease.[319,361]

In 2002, a population-based study compared the two approaches and found the culture-based approach to be 50% more effective than the risk-based approach in preventing early-onset GBS disease.[318] Sixty-two percent of infants with early-onset disease were born to mothers who were without identifiable risk factors. Therefore revised guidelines published by the CDC in 2002 recommended universal vaginal and rectal screening cultures of all pregnant women between 35 and 37 weeks of gestation, with intrapartum chemoprophylaxis for all women identified as GBS carriers.[317] The risk-based approach was to be reserved for any women in labor whose colonization status is unknown. Following release of these guidelines, active population surveillance showed that 85% of women were being actively screened, resulting in a 27% further decline in incidence of early-onset infection.[360] However, the retrospective cohort study also revealed missed opportunities for screening and chemoprophylaxis for women with unknown colonization status, especially those at risk for preterm delivery. Unpublished data from the CDC showed that antibiotic prophylaxis was 78% effective in preventing early-onset infection in preterm infants.[361] Thus revised intrapartum chemoprophylaxis guidelines with specific algorithms for women with preterm labor or premature rupture of membranes were released in 2010.[361] If a woman with unknown colonization status is admitted with signs and symptoms of preterm labor or premature rupture of membranes, a vaginal-rectal swab should be obtained for culture, and intrapartum chemoprophylaxis should be started and continued until delivery. If amniotic membranes are intact, prophylaxis should be discontinued if it is determined that the woman is not in true labor. Women with premature rupture of membranes who are not in labor should continue antibiotics per standard of care if receiving to prolong latency or continue antibiotics for 48 hours if receiving for GBS prophylaxis.

Colonization or bacteriuria during a previous pregnancy is not an indication for intrapartum chemoprophylaxis. Intrapartum chemoprophylaxis also is not indicated for cesarean section performed before onset of labor for a woman with intact amniotic membranes, regardless of GBS colonization status or gestational age. Women with GBS isolated from urine at a concentration of 10^4 cfu/mL or greater during the current pregnancy should receive intrapartum chemoprophylaxis because these women usually are heavily colonized. Women who previously gave birth to an infant with invasive GBS disease always should receive chemoprophylaxis. Table 83.4 shows the indications and nonindications for intrapartum chemoprophylaxis according to the current guidelines released in 2010.[361]

Optimal culture techniques are discussed earlier in the chapter. Many rapid tests are being studied because they offer the advantage of detecting colonization status in women who present for preterm labor or who have not had prenatal care. These tests include latex agglutination, optical immunoassay, DNA hybridization, enzyme immunoassay, Islam starch medium tests, and PCR.[169] With the exception of PCR, all tests showed poor sensitivity or specificity compared with the standard culture method and are not sufficiently accurate to replace routine culture in decision-making concerning intrapartum antibiotic prophylaxis. A multicenter

TABLE 83.4 Indications and Nonindications for Maternal Intrapartum Prophylaxis to Prevent Early-Onset Group B Streptococcal (GBS) Infection

Intrapartum GBS Prophylaxis Indicated	Intrapartum GBS Prophylaxis Not Indicated
Previous infant with invasive GBS disease	Colonization with GBS during a previous pregnancy
GBS bacteriuria during any trimester of current pregnancy[a]	GBS bacteriuria during previous pregnancy
Positive GBS vaginal-rectal screening culture within preceding 5 weeks[a]	Negative vaginal-rectal screening culture, regardless of intrapartum risk factors
Unknown GBS status at onset of labor and any of the following: • Delivery at <37 weeks' gestation • Prolong rupture of membranes for ≥18 hours • Intrapartum temperature ≥100.4°F (38°C)[b] • Intrapartum nucleic acid amplification test (NAAT) positive for GBS[c]	Cesarean delivery performed before onset of labor on a woman with intact amniotic membranes, regardless of GBS colonization status or gestational age

[a]Intrapartum chemoprophylaxis is not indicated in this circumstance if a cesarean delivery is performed before onset of labor on a woman with intact membranes.
[b]If amnionitis is suspected, broad-spectrum antibiotic therapy that includes an agent active against GBS should replace GBS prophylaxis.
[c]GBS NAAT are optional and may not be available in all settings (see text). If intrapartum NAAT is negative for GBS but any other above intrapartum risk factor is present, then intrapartum GBS prophylaxis is indicated.
Modified from Centers for Disease Control and Prevention. Prevention of perinatal group B streptococcal disease: Revised guidelines from CDC, 2010. *MMWR Morb Mortal Wkly Rep.* 2010;59:1–32.

study evaluated a real-time PCR assay that gave results in 40 minutes.[92] Compared with intrapartum culture, the PCR assay had a sensitivity of 94% to 98% and a specificity of 96% to 99%.[92,117] Nucleic acid amplification tests (NAAT) such as commercially available PCR assays, are an option for intrapartum testing for women who have unknown colonization status at labor onset.[361] However, NAAT should not replace antenatal culture or risk-based assessment of women with unknown colonization status. NAAT must be performed on samples placed in selective enrichment broths for adequate sensitivity of the assay, thereby lengthening the turnaround time and making it less useful in the real-world setting at this time.

Maternal chemoprophylaxis begins at hospital admission for delivery or at rupture of membranes and consists of intravenous penicillin G (initial dose, 5 million units; subsequent doses, 2.5 to 3 million units every 4 hours until delivery).[318,361] Although penicillin is preferred because of its narrow spectrum of activity, ampicillin (initial dose, 2 g; subsequent doses, 1 g every 4 hours) can be given as an alternative. For women who are allergic to penicillin, intrapartum chemoprophylaxis must take into account increasing resistance rates to clindamycin and erythromycin.[57,96] Women at low risk of developing anaphylaxis should be given cefazolin (initial dose, 2 g; subsequent doses, 1 g every 8 hours). Women at high risk of developing anaphylaxis should have susceptibility testing performed on their isolates obtained during screening at 35 to 37 weeks of gestation. Susceptibility testing should include checking for inducible clindamycin resistance. If the isolate is susceptible, clindamycin (900 mg every 8 hours) can be used. Erythromycin is not an acceptable alternative.[361] If susceptibility testing is not available, the results are not known, or the isolate is resistant to clindamycin, vancomycin (1 g every 12 hours) can be given as the alternative. The efficacy of vancomycin is not known.

Since the widespread adoption of chemoprophylaxis, the incidence of early-onset disease has plummeted but remains stable since 2010.[319,360,361] Racial disparities in early-onset disease have declined significantly,[319] but higher incidence of early-onset infection in black infants compared to non-black infants remains a problem. Opportunities to prevent early-onset disease still are missed, however, because of laboratory practices,[76] hospital or procedural errors in communication of the screening results, failure to administer intrapartum chemoprophylaxis to a mother known to be colonized, or failure to recognize preterm delivery in mothers with unknown colonization status as an indication for prophylaxis.[294,360] The incidence of late-onset disease remains unaffected by intrapartum chemoprophylaxis.[185,361]

Management of an infant born to a mother given intrapartum prophylaxis depends on the clinical findings at birth, antibiotic regimen, and the timing of doses administered to the mother (Fig. 83.6). Amniotic fluid levels of penicillin that will kill GBS are not achieved until at least 3 hours after administration of the first dose.[64] If the infant of any gestational age appears healthy and has a mother who received at least one dose of intrapartum chemoprophylaxis with intravenous penicillin, ampicillin, or cefazolin at least 4 hours before delivery, neither diagnostic evaluation nor empirical antimicrobial therapy is required.[361] However, to ensure their ongoing stability, such infants should be observed in the hospital for at least 48 hours unless they meet all criteria for early discharge. Keeping the infant hospitalized through day of life 2 has been challenging because the associated expense affects the cost-to-benefit ratio of intrapartum prophylaxis.[258] However, an analysis of all live births in the state of Florida for 1992 through 1994 demonstrated a 115% increase in the rate of readmission for GBS infection in infants discharged on day 1 of life; this finding supports the recommendation to observe infants for 48 hours.[146]

Neonates with signs of sepsis are evaluated and treated empirically for sepsis. Healthy-appearing neonates who either are born at least 37 weeks' gestation to a mother with an indication for chemoprophylaxis but received inadequate intrapartum chemoprophylaxis should be observed at least 48 hours. An infant born at less than 37 weeks' gestation or following prolonged duration of membrane rupture for greater or equal to 18 hours to a mother with inadequate chemoprophylaxis should undergo limited laboratory evaluation (complete blood count and blood culture) and observation in the hospital for 48 hours without therapy. Adequate intrapartum chemoprophylaxis is defined as at least 4 hours

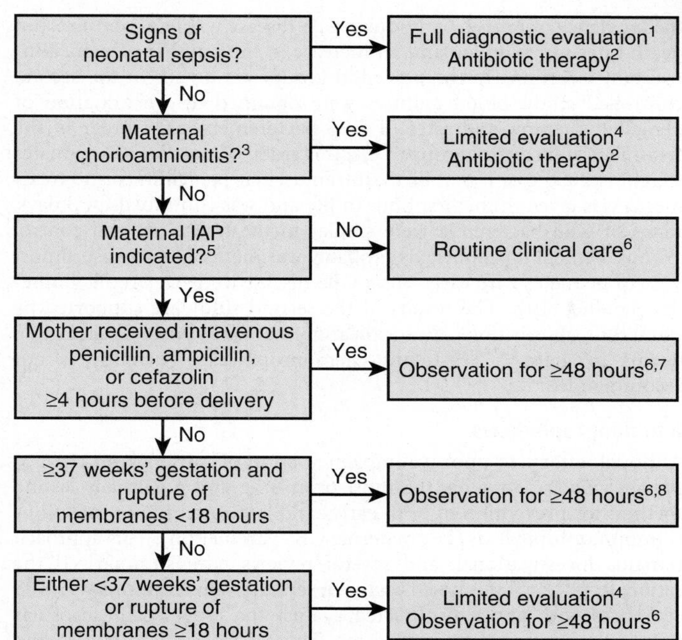

FIG. 83.6 Empirical management of a newborn for secondary prevention of early-onset group B streptococcal infection. *1,* Includes complete blood cell count (CBC) and differential, blood culture, and chest radiograph if respiratory abnormalities are present. When signs of sepsis are present, a lumbar puncture, if feasible, should be performed. *2,* Antibiotic therapy should be directed toward common causes of neonatal sepsis, including ampicillin for group B *Streptococcus* and coverage for *Escherichia coli* and other gram-negative pathogens, and should take into account local resistance patterns. *3,* Consultation with obstetric providers is important to determine the level of clinical suspicion for chorioamnionitis. Chorioamnionitis is diagnosed clinically, and some of the signs are nonspecific. *4,* Includes complete CBC and differential and blood culture. *5,* See Table 83.4 for indications for maternal intrapartum prophylaxis. *6,* If signs of sepsis develop, a full diagnostic evaluation should be conducted and antibiotic therapy initiated. *7,* A healthy-appearing infant who was ≥37 weeks' gestation at delivery and whose mother received ≥4 hours of appropriate intrapartum antibiotic prophylaxis *(IAP)* before delivery may be discharged home after 24 hours if other discharge criteria have been met, a person able to comply fully with instructions for home observation will be present, and access to medical care is readily available. If any one of these conditions is not met, the infant should be observed in the hospital for at least 48 hours and until criteria for discharge are achieved. *8,* Some experts recommend a CBC with differential at 6 to 12 hours. (Modified from Centers for Disease Control and Prevention. Prevention of perinatal group B streptococcal disease: revised guidelines from CDC, 2010. *MMWR Morb Mortal Wkly Rep.* 2010;59:1–32.)

of IV penicillin, ampicillin or cefazolin. All other agents are considered inadequate.[361] If the subsequent clinical course or the laboratory results suggest infection, full diagnostic evaluation and therapy is initiated.

Concern that widespread use of intrapartum ampicillin use will result in a greater incidence of ampicillin-resistant neonatal infection has been supported by some case series.[52,187,251] Development of penicillin- or ampicillin-resistant GBS has not been seen.[83] In most studies, incidence rates of *E. coli* and other gram-negative pathogens have remained stable.[4,187,251,306] The rate of ampicillin-resistant *E. coli* infections is increasing in preterm infants. However, rates of ampicillin resistance in term neonates before and after widespread intrapartum chemoprophylaxis are the same.

Infant Chemoprophylaxis

The two controlled trials evaluating neonatal prophylaxis reached contradictory conclusions.[295,328] In the first trial, more than 16,000 newborns received either intramuscular penicillin G or topical tetracycline (prophylaxis for gonococcal ophthalmia neonatorum) within an hour of birth during alternating weeks.[328] In penicillin-treated newborns, the incidence of proven early-onset GBS disease was less common, but death rates were similar, and an increase in the number of penicillin-resistant infections in the penicillin group was noted. In the second controlled study, blood cultures were obtained before initiation of penicillin therapy, and rates of GBS bacteremia were similar in the treatment and control groups.[295] In this study of nearly 1200 neonates weighing 2000 g or less at birth, intramuscular penicillin (or no treatment) was given in the first hour of life and was continued for 3 days. Rates of GBS bacteremia were similar in the treatment and control groups. Penicillin prophylaxis probably was ineffective because almost 90% of neonates with early-onset GBS disease were bacteremic immediately after birth. The results of the second study are supported by numerous observations, thus indicating that early-onset disease often begins in utero.[61,275,321] Infant chemoprophylaxis currently is not recommended.[361]

Immunoprophylaxis

Although efforts to improve implementation of intrapartum chemoprophylaxis are ongoing, the most promising and potentially lasting method for prevention of both early- and late-onset infant infections is immunoprophylaxis (i.e., maternal GBS vaccination). This approach remains investigational, and several reviews have summarized the rationale.[32,111,157,230] It is based on the observation that immunity to GBS correlates with antibody directed against the type-specific capsular polysaccharides of these organisms. These IgG class antibodies and complement promote opsonization, phagocytosis, and bacterial killing of GBS and protect animals against lethal challenge.[271,372] Thus provision of protective levels of type-specific immunity to the infant could be achieved through active immunization of the mother. A study immunizing women with a III capsular polysaccharide-tetanus toxoid conjugate reported a 95% immune response, with persistence of opsonophagocytic antibodies at 2 months of age in 100% of infants born to maternal responders.[38] Other studies immunizing nonpregnant adults with purified capsular polysaccharide-tetanus toxoid conjugate vaccines showed the safety and immunogenicity of these vaccines.[35–37] A recent phase 2, randomized, observer-blind, multicenter study of a trivalent CPS conjugate vaccine at 24 to 35 weeks' gestation resulted in placental antibody transfer ratios of 66% to 79%.[102] Infant antibody concentrations remained at 22% to 25% of birth levels for at least 3 months after birth. Clinical trials are planned with multivalent CPS conjugate vaccines with CRM197 as the carrier protein and a protein vaccine made from the N-terminal domains of the Rib and α-C surface proteins of GBS.[157]

Availability of the complete genome sequences for GBS has led to the discovery of many potential surface proteins and secreted proteins that can be expressed in recombinant form and used for production of antibodies.[231,349] A set of proteins shared by the disease-causing serotypes theoretically can be used in combination to create a vaccine capable of providing protection against multiple serotypes. GBS pili with at least one of the pilus islands present in all sequenced GBS genomes may be included in a future vaccine.[68,180]

Because most pregnant women in the United States (estimated at 85–90%) have nonprotective levels of these antibodies in their sera at delivery, active immunization of women of childbearing age before or during pregnancy would optimize the strategy to induce high maternal antibody levels. Human studies have demonstrated efficient antibody transfer to the neonate, as discussed earlier.[38,102] Transfer of high levels of maternal antibody would provide protection of the neonates from early- and late-onset GBS disease.[27,186] In addition, immunization also would offer protection for the mother against preterm deliveries and fetal loss caused by GBS infection. Finally vaccination of elderly or nonpregnant adults with defined medical conditions could reduce the disease burden significantly. Because immunoprophylaxis most likely is the most cost-effective and beneficial prevention strategy for GBS disease,[156,259,330] it should be promoted by physicians, public health officials, parents, pharmaceutical manufacturers, and legislators.

NEW REFERENCES SINCE THE SEVENTH EDITION

27. Baker CJ, Carey VJ, Rench MA, et al. Maternal antibody at delivery protects neonates from early onset group B streptococcal disease. *J Infect Dis*. 2014;209(5):781-788.
47. Berardi A, Rossi C, Creti R, et al. Group B streptococcal colonization in 160 mother-baby pairs: a prospective cohort study. *J Pediatr*. 2013;163(4):1099-1104, e1091.
75. Cavaco CK, Patras KA, Zlamal JE, et al. A novel C5a-derived immunobiotic peptide reduces *Streptococcus agalactiae* colonization through targeted bacterial killing. *Antimicrob Agents Chemother*. 2013;57(11):5492-5499.
76. Centers for Disease Control and Prevention. Active Bacterial Core Surveillance (ABCs) report, Emerging Infections Program Network, group B Streptococcus, provisional-2014. 2014. Available at: http://www.cdc.gov/abcs/reports-findings/survreports/gbs14.html.
77. Centers for Disease Control and Prevention. Antimicrobial susceptibilities among group B *Streptococcus* isolates (GBS)–active bacterial core surveillance, 2010. 2012. Available at: http://www.cdc.gov/abcs/reports-findings/survreports/gbs10-suscept.html.
91. Dahesh S, Hensler ME, Van Sorge NM, et al. Point mutation in the group B streptococcal pbp2x gene conferring decreased susceptibility to beta-lactam antibiotics. *Antimicrob Agents Chemother*. 2008;52(8):2915-2918.
102. Donders GG, Halperin SA, Devlieger R, et al. Maternal immunization with an investigational trivalent group B streptococcal vaccine: a randomized controlled trial. *Obstet Gynecol*. 2016;127(2):213-221.
111. Edwards MS, Gonik B. Preventing the broad spectrum of perinatal morbidity and mortality through group B streptococcal vaccination. *Vaccine*. 2013;31(suppl 4):D66-D71.
114. Edwards MS, Nizet V, Baker CJ. Group B streptococcal infections. In: Wilson CB, Nizet V, Maldonado YA, Remington JS, Klein JO, eds. *Infectious Diseases of the Fetus and Newborn*. 8th ed. Philadelphia: Elsevier; 2016:411-456.
130. Ferrieri P, Lynfield R, Creti R, et al. Serotype IV and invasive group B *Streptococcus* disease in neonates, Minnesota, USA, 2000–2010. *Emerg Infect Dis*. 2013;19(4):551-558.
132. Florindo C, Damiao V, Silvestre I, et al. Epidemiological surveillance of colonising group B *Streptococcus* epidemiology in the Lisbon and Tagus Valley regions, Portugal (2005 to 2012): emergence of a new epidemic type IV/clonal complex 17 clone. *Euro Surveill*. 2014;19(23).
156. Heath PT. Status of vaccine research and development of vaccines for GBS. *Vaccine*. 2016;34(26):2876-2879.
197. Kleweis SM, Cahill AG, Odibo AO, et al. Maternal obesity and rectovaginal group B *Streptococcus* colonization at term. *Infect Dis Obstet Gynecol*. 2015;2015:586767.
205. Landwehr-Kenzel S, Henneke P. Interaction of *Streptococcus* agalactiae and cellular innate immunity in colonization and disease. *Front Immunol*. 2014;5:519.
213. Libster R, Edwards KM, Levent F, et al. Long-term outcomes of group B streptococcal meningitis. *Pediatrics*. 2012;130(1):e8-e15.
231. Madhi SA, Dangor Z, Heath PT, et al. Considerations for a phase-III trial to evaluate a group B *Streptococcus* polysaccharide-protein conjugate vaccine in pregnant women for the prevention of early- and late-onset invasive disease in young-infants. *Vaccine*. 2013;31(suppl 4):D52-D57.
273. Park C, Nichols M, Schrag SJ. Two cases of invasive vancomycin-resistant group B *Streptococcus* infection. *N Engl J Med*. 2014;370(9):885-886.
299. Randis TM, Gelber SE, Hooven TA, et al. Group B *Streptococcus* β-hemolysin/cytolysin breaches maternal-fetal barriers to cause preterm birth and intrauterine fetal demise in vivo. *J Infect Dis*. 2014;210(2):265-273.
324. Seki T, Kimura K, Reid ME, et al. High isolation rate of MDR group B streptococci with reduced penicillin susceptibility in Japan. *J Antimicrob Chemother*. 2015;70(10):2725-2728.
336. Srinivasan V, Metcalf BJ, Knipe KM, et al. vanG element insertions within a conserved chromosomal site conferring vancomycin resistance to *Streptococcus agalactiae* and *Streptococcus anginosus*. *MBio*. 2014;5(4):e01386-14.
339. Stoner TD, Weston TA, Trejo J, et al. Group B streptococcal infection and activation of human astrocytes. *PLoS ONE*. 2015;10(6):e0128431.
346. Teatero S, Athey TB, Van Caeseele P, et al. Emergence of serotype IV group B *Streptococcus* adult invasive disease in Manitoba and Saskatchewan, Canada, is driven by clonal sequence type 459 strains. *J Clin Microbiol*. 2015;53(9):2919-2926.

The full reference list for this chapter is available at ExpertConsult.com.

Enterococcal and Viridans Streptococcal Infections 84

84A ■ Enterococcal Infections

J. Chase McNeil

ENTEROCOCCAL INFECTIONS

The enterococci are gram-positive ovoid bacteria that are related closely to the streptococci but are phylogenetically distinct and make up the genus *Enterococcus*. These organisms are found in normal bowel flora of humans and many animals and commonly are isolated from environmental sources. Enterococci generally are considered to be of low virulence but have been known to cause human infection since 1899 (reviewed by Murray[206]). Although these ubiquitous bacteria are important causes of both nosocomial and community-acquired infection in adults* and children,† the role of *Enterococcus* spp. as a pathogen (or co-pathogen) in certain clinical settings, particularly intraabdominal and pelvic infections, often remains unclear.

Enterococci are intrinsically resistant to many antimicrobial agents (including the cephalosporins, oxacillin, clindamycin, and aminoglycosides). Since the emergence of high-level aminoglycoside resistance in *Enterococcus* spp. more than 40 years ago,[193] increasing percentages of these organisms have acquired clinically significant resistance to β-lactam antibiotics, vancomycin and other glycopeptides, and aminoglycosides. Vancomycin-resistant enterococcal (VRE) infections, especially those caused by vancomycin-resistant *Enterococcus faecium* (VREF), are of particular concern because VREF isolates frequently are resistant to other bactericidal antimicrobial agents.[5,205,207,259] The dramatic increase in nosocomial VRE infections[4,78,204,219] has resulted in failure of antimicrobial therapy[156] and has inspired comparisons with the preantibiotic period[6] and even speculation about a "postantimicrobial era."[56] Fortunately new classes of antimicrobials active against most VRE isolates have become available recently, but pediatric experience with these agents is limited, and enterococci resistant to these agents already have been detected (see later discussion). Concern about the continued nosocomial spread of VRE isolates and the documented transfer of vancomycin resistance determinants to *Staphylococcus aureus*[36,38,291,303] led to the development of stringent hospital infection control guidelines designed to interrupt the spread of vancomycin-resistant organisms.[214] Although the impact of VRE infections in children has been less dramatic, many pediatric centers report infections caused by these organisms.‡

MICROBIOLOGY

The genus *Enterococcus* consists of gram-positive cocci that are catalase-negative and occur singly, in pairs, and in short chains. Morphologically enterococci are indistinguishable from streptococci and traditionally were classified as members of the genus *Streptococcus*. Sherman's early classification scheme[269] divided the streptococci into four groups: pyogenic, viridans, lactic, and enterococcal. By the Lancefield criteria, enterococci were classified as group D streptococci, along with the "nonenterococcal" *Streptococcus bovis* group. However, genetic evidence has indicated that the enterococci are sufficiently different from the streptococci to merit establishment of a separate genus.[84]

Fig. 84A.1 is a scheme for the differentiation of enterococci from other gram-positive cocci. Catalase-negative gram-positive cocci that have been isolated from human sources include the streptococci, the enterococci, *Lactococcus* spp., *Leuconostoc* spp., *Pediococcus* spp., and *Gemella* spp. Most enterococci produce no (γ) or partial (α) hemolysis on blood agar; differentiation between enterococci and certain α-hemolytic or nonhemolytic streptococci and other nonstreptococcal gram-positive cocci may require a series of biochemical tests.[82,84] Clinical laboratories may identify an organism presumptively on a primary isolation plate as an enterococcus based on colony morphology, Gram stain, and the pyrrolidonyl arylamidase (PYR) test. Most enterococci produce PYR, as do *Streptococcus pyogenes* and nutritionally variant streptococci *(Abiotrophia)*, but not other streptococci. The PYR test is particularly useful for differentiating enterococci from group D streptococci and *Leuconostoc* spp. (see Fig. 84A.1). *S. pyogenes* and *Abiotrophia* spp. are distinguished easily from enterococci by colony morphology, hemolysis, and special growth requirements.

Enterococci are able to hydrolyze esculin in the presence of 40% bile salts; of the true streptococci, only group D streptococci (*S. bovis* group) and approximately 5% to 10% of viridans streptococci share this characteristic.[84] Enterococci are facultatively anaerobic and grow under harsh conditions that inhibit the growth of streptococci; growth in 6.5% sodium chloride at 45°C (113°F) is a useful confirmatory test. Enterococci produce leucine aminopeptidase, as do streptococci, lactococci, pediococci, and some *Gemella* strains. The presence of group D streptococcal antigen is of limited value because the *S. bovis* group, most pediococci, and half of the clinical *Leuconostoc* spp. isolates share this antigen.[84]

Occasional clinical isolates of *Leuconostoc* spp., *Pediococcus* spp., and *Lactococcus* spp. may be difficult to distinguish from the enterococci. Some strains of *Leuconostoc* spp. and *Pediococcus* spp. may grow in 6.5% NaCl at 45°C, but they are PYR negative. Lactococci are PYR-positive, and some isolates will grow in 6.5% NaCl; however, most lactococci fail to grow (or grow very slowly) at 45°C. Consequently definitive confirmation of an organism as an enterococcus may require complete identification to the species level. Molecular techniques allow rapid, reliable identification and speciation of enterococci[62,72,76] but usually are available only in the research setting.

The genus *Enterococcus* now includes at least 14 "typical" species and three additional "atypical" species (the latter are PYR negative and grow very slowly in the presence of 6.5% NaCl) (Box 84A.1). However, most human clinical isolates are either *Enterococcus faecalis* (50–90%) or *E. faecium* (5–37%), although clusters of human infection caused by *E. raffinosus*,[45] *E. casseliflavus*,[212] *E. avium*,[226] and *E. durans*[263] and occasional human infections attributable to *E. gallinarum*, *E. mundtii*, and *E. flavescens* have been reported.[83] Even though *E. faecalis* and *E. faecium* continue to account for most clinical isolates, the percentage of *E. faecium* isolates has been increasing, and relatively more "other" (i.e., non-*faecalis* and non-*faecium*) enterococci are being identified by clinical laboratories.[139,141,170]

Speciation of enterococci has been useful primarily for epidemiologic purposes, but distinction between the more antibiotic-susceptible *E. faecalis* and the more antibiotic-resistant (see later discussion) *E. faecium* may be helpful in selecting optimal therapy for endocarditis and other

*References 37, 78, 92, 110, 116, 117, 130, 171, 194, 195, 205-207, 218, 227, 239.

†References 9, 17, 18, 26–28, 40, 50, 75, 77, 88, 90, 114, 115, 131, 146, 153, 164, 168, 177, 188, 197, 210, 217, 219, 234, 236, 241, 245, 261, 262, 267, 268, 276, 283, 316.

‡References 26, 40, 43–50, 73–75, 88, 90, 91, 99, 114, 116, 119, 131, 153, 164, 168, 189, 197, 210, 217, 234, 235, 245, 283, 316.

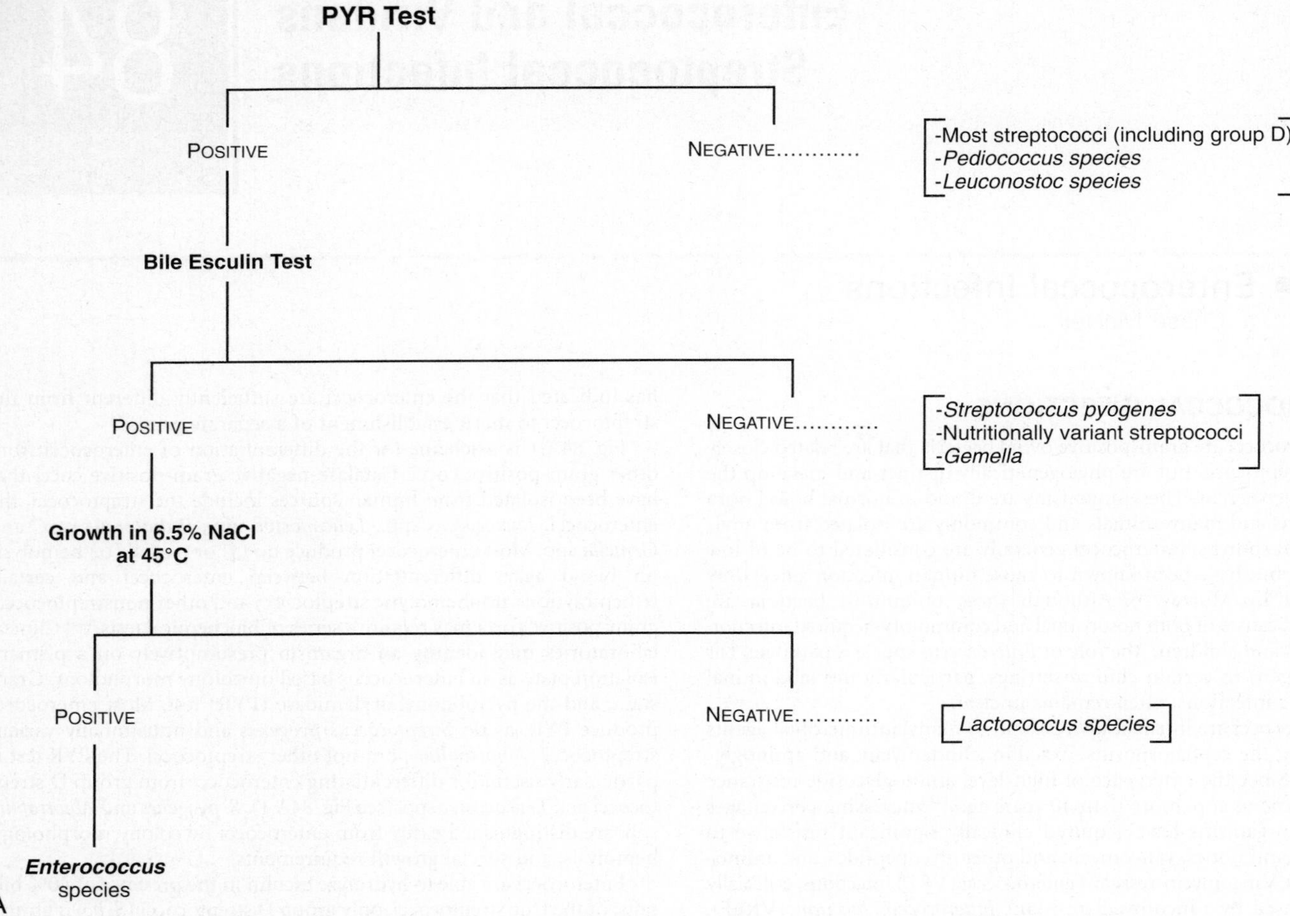

FIG. 84A.1 Differentiation of enterococci from other gram-positive cocci. *PYR*, Pyrrolidonyl.

BOX 84A.1 *Enterococcus* Species

Typical Enterococci (PYR⁺)

E. faecalis
E. faecium
E. avium
E. casseliflavus
E. durans
E. raffinosus
E. gallinarum
E. malodoratus
E. hirae
E. mundtii
E. pseudoavium
E. dispar
E. flavescens
E. sulfureus

Atypical Enterococci (PYR⁻)

E. cecorum
E. columbae
E. saccharolyticus

PYR, Pyrrolidonyl arylamidase.

serious enterococcal infections. A panel of biologic tests can differentiate these two common enterococcal species readily.[84,147,206] Most *E. faecalis* isolates (unlike those of *E. faecium*) grow in the presence of 0.04% tellurite, reduce tetrazolium to formazan, and produce acid from sorbitol and glycerol.

A variety of molecular techniques are available to assist in the identification of enterococci and determination of the relatedness of enterococcal isolates.[51,52,71,76,198,308] These molecular techniques have been particularly valuable in investigations of possible nosocomial transmission of multiresistant enterococci.[51,52,72,76,84,198,222,252,308]

EPIDEMIOLOGY

Enterococci are normal flora of the gastrointestinal tract of most humans and have been found in as many as 97% of fecal samples from adults in Europe, Asia, and North America.[206] Approximately half of newborn infants become colonized with enterococci by the time they are 1 week of age.[215] Enterococci are isolated less commonly (<20% of specimens) from other sites, including the vagina, oral cavity, and skin. These organisms also are common inhabitants of the bowel flora of many animals and frequently are present in soil, water, and food. Enterococci are hardy organisms and may persist for long periods on environmental surfaces, thereby contributing to potential nosocomial spread of these bacteria.

Human infection caused by enterococci was reported before the beginning of the 20th century, but the initial reports included patients with infections that seldom are associated with enterococci today: enteritis, meningitis, and appendicitis.[206] The ubiquitous presence of enterococci in fecal samples led to the mistaken impression that these organisms cause enteritis and food poisoning. Enterococci are isolated commonly as part of mixed flora in intraabdominal and pelvic infections, but the contribution of these organisms to the pathogenesis of such infections remains unclear.[102,213] However, enterococci were identified as pathogens causing urinary tract infection and endocarditis as early as 1906,[5] with later confirmation by many studies. Subsequently, enterococci have been documented to cause invasive infection in neonates,[9,71,98,115,151,234] patients with malignancies,[106,107,153,197,217,268] recipients of bone marrow and solid organ transplants,[15,88,91,145,149,189,225,257] burn victims,[158] patients with indwelling catheters,[15,63,195,204,206,219] and other immunosuppressed or debilitated patients.[39,168,173,185,189,227,242]

In general, enterococcal infections occur less frequently in children (outside the neonatal period) than in adults, and enterococci are less common causes of pediatric (vs. adult) urinary tract infection[312] and endocarditis.[279] There are relatively fewer series of pediatric enterococcal infection published than those in adults.[22,25,30,51,63,90,106,114,177,246] Much of the published experience with enterococcal infection in children focuses on the neonatal period,[59,71,98,115,173,238] and some evidence suggests that late-onset (but not early-onset) neonatal enterococcal infection may be increasing in frequency.[51,71] In one recent series, *E. faecalis* was the third most common organism to cause late-onset sepsis in neonates.[21]

Enterococci are important nosocomial agents, and they rank as either the second or third most common hospital-acquired pathogens in this country.[5,37,78,142,202,244,258,314,315] Evidence of nosocomial spread of enterococci is relatively recent. Initially, all enterococci isolated from hospitalized patients were thought to have originated from the patient's endogenous bowel flora. However, the emergence of multiantibiotic-resistant enterococci prompted the performance of careful epidemiologic studies that documented the nosocomial spread of these organisms.[5,37,78,142,202,244,258,314,315] Many groups have reported that VRE and other enterococcal isolates may persist for long periods in the environment and may be spread either by direct patient-to-patient contact via the hands of colonized health care personnel[238] or from contaminated beds or other hospital material or contaminated patient equipment, including thermometers.[5,26,146,164,195]

The growing problem of nosocomial infection by VRE organisms is multifactorial; the diversity of isolates found in many hospitals indicates that resistant organisms may be introduced via multiple sources.[50,76,98,198,204,244,269] Consequently outbreaks of VRE infection in institutions may be caused by single or multiple clones, although the first recognized outbreak of VRE infection or colonization in a hospital usually is associated with a single clone.[40,99]

Distinguishing risk factors for VRE colonization from those for invasive disease caused by these organisms has often not been possible, and certain factors probably increase the risk for both colonization and development of infection caused by VRE organisms. Major risk factors for VRE colonization or the development of infection, or for both, appear to be the severity of the underlying illness or immunosuppression; the proximity to patients colonized with VRE organisms (e.g., admission to an intensive care unit [ICU] or a transplant unit); receipt of a bone marrow or solid organ (especially liver) transplant; increasing length of hospital stay; recent cardiothoracic or abdominal surgery; the presence of indwelling central venous or urinary catheters; and previous treatment with vancomycin, broad-spectrum antibiotics (particularly those lacking appreciable antienterococcal activity, such as the third-generation cephalosporins), or agents with broad antianaerobic activity.[17,18,52,109,238,242,244,246,276,315] Among neonates specifically, VRE colonization has been especially associated with the use of broad-spectrum antibiotics.[129] Patients infected with human immunodeficiency virus (HIV) also appear to be at higher risk for the development of VRE bacteremia.[15] Factors contributing to nosocomial spread of these organisms probably differ from those responsible for the gradual overall increase in resistant strains.[242]

Since the first report of a vancomycin-resistant isolate in 1988,[160] infection and colonization with VRE bacteria in the United States have been observed primarily in the ICUs of large teaching hospitals.[37,205,207] For example, data reported to the National Nosocomial Infection Surveillance (NNIS) system of the Centers for Disease Control and Prevention (CDC) from January 1989 through March 1993 revealed no vancomycin resistance in hospitals with fewer than 200 beds, a resistance rate of 1.8% in hospitals with 200 to 500 beds, and a rate of 3.6% in hospitals with more than 500 beds.[37] A 1995 report from the multicenter *Enterococcus* Study Group analyzed 1936 isolates collected from 97 laboratories in 47 states during the last quarter of 1992 and generally confirmed the findings of the NNIS survey.[139] However, VRE infections are not limited to ICUs. A 1999 report from the Surveillance and Control of Pathogens of Epidemiologic Importance (SCOPE) group's ongoing surveillance of nosocomial bloodstream infections in 49 US hospitals revealed no overall differences in rates of vancomycin resistance in enterococci isolated from patients located in critical care versus hospital ward settings.[78] In a multicenter surveillance study in Canada, a dramatic increase was seen in the incidence of VRE bacteremia increasing from less than 0.01 per 1000 hospital admissions in 2006 to more than 0.08 per 1000 in 2009.[181] In this study much of this shift was associated with the emergence of new sequence types of VRE. Fortunately VRE infections have occurred much less frequently in children than in adults, and overall rates of vancomycin resistance in enterococci isolated from children's hospitals remain very low. That being said, many pediatric centers, however, have reported VRE infections.[22,25,58,71,98,151,173,183,238,273] In a large survey of European bloodstream isolates, a similar proportion of *E. faecium* isolates from children were resistant to vancomycin as was seen among isolates from adults.[16]

In the United States, VRE isolates generally have not been detected in environmental sources or in patients who have not had exposure to hospitals,[205,206] with rare exceptions.[40] VRE was only isolated from one of 1,813 stool specimens in healthy children in the community setting.[113] However, the ecology of VRE organisms in Europe differs: they have been detected in the feces of nonhospitalized patients and healthy volunteers in several European studies, with rates of VRE colonization as high as 28% in adults living in some parts of Belgium.[205,206] The more widespread occurrence of VRE strains in Europe probably was related to the use of oral glycopeptides such as avoparcin in animal feed and the oral administration of bacterial preparations (possibly contaminated with resistant enterococci) to humans and animals for therapeutic purposes.[203,205,206]

Initial reports of VRE organisms in the United States were clustered in the northeast region, particularly New York, Maryland, and Pennsylvania,[37] and geographic differences in rates of VRE colonization and infection persist. However, subsequent reports indicate that VRE strains are found in most parts of the United States[138,170] and that rates of vancomycin resistance among enterococci isolated from patients in this country generally are higher than those found in isolates from Canada, Western Europe, or Latin America.[137,140,170] The reasons for these geographic differences remain unclear, but the high rates of resistance in the United States may be related to the increased use of vancomycin in this country during the past 3 decades.[150]

Interestingly, new evidence has emerged regarding the origin of drug-resistant *E. faecium*. Using whole genome sequencing, Lebreton et al. were able to demonstrate that a dominant multidrug resistant strain of *E. faecium* evolved from a population that included animal strains and not from human commensal strains. This diversion from animal strains occurred approximately 75 years ago at the time of the widespread introduction of antibiotics.[159] Other investigators have noted similar antibiotic resistance determinants in processed meat products and human clinical isolates despite genomic diversity between these sources, suggesting horizontal transfer of antibiotic resistance from animal to human strains of enterococci.[208]

PATHOGENESIS AND VIRULENCE

Enterococci are organisms of low virulence, and their ubiquitous presence in the human gastrointestinal tract probably has contributed to both the spurious association of these organisms with some illnesses (e.g., enteritis) and the failure to recognize other situations in which enterococci are true pathogens (e.g., immunosuppressed and debilitated patients and neonates). When contrasted with organisms such as *S. pyogenes* and *S. aureus*, enterococci are much less virulent in animal models of infection,[133,194] but they are capable of causing disease at a higher inoculum.

Enterococci rarely cause primary cellulitis or abscesses, although these organisms are isolated frequently as components of polymicrobial wound infections and intraabdominal and pelvic infections. The contribution of enterococci to the pathogenesis of these polymicrobial infections remains uncertain.[102,213] In animal models, synergy between enterococci and a variety of other organisms (particularly anaerobes) can be demonstrated, but enterococci injected alone have little propensity to cause either peritonitis or subcutaneous infection.[133,134,206,221] Many clinical trials have concluded that provision of antienterococcal therapy generally is not necessary to effect a cure of human intraabdominal and pelvic infections, even though *Enterococcus* frequently (14–33% of cases) is isolated from primary peritoneal cultures.[102]

Enterococci are an important cause of urinary tract infections in adults (particularly in elderly men, patients with structural abnormalities of the urinary tract, and those with indwelling urinary catheters), but they are associated less frequently with urinary tract infections in children.[9,312] Enterococci also are important but less frequent (than in adults) causes of bacterial endocarditis in children.[186,280]

Adherence of bacteria to tissue is a necessary first step in the pathogenesis of both urinary tract infection and endocarditis, and evidence suggests that pathogenic enterococci produce factors that mediate adherence to urinary epithelial cells and endocardial tissue.[133,134] Enterococcal adhesins include an enterococcal surface protein known as aggregation substance[47,154] and surface carbohydrates. Lipoteichoic acid, an important adhesin for *S. pyogenes,* does not appear to mediate adherence of enterococci,[275] but it may trigger the host inflammatory response to these organisms.[287] The innate immune response to enterococci is poorly understood, although one report has implicated the intracellular sensor nod2 in mediating the host inflammatory response to these organisms.[148] Recent studies have implicated an enterococcal surface protein, Esp, in biofilm formation by *E. faecalis*.[34,290] Enterococcal secreted antigen A (SagA) as well as extracellular DNA appear to be critical components of biofilm formation among clade A1 *E. faecium*, the dominant hospital-acquired strain.[223] In addition, many virulent *E. faecalis* isolates express a cytolysin in the presence of target cells.[55,60]

Nosocomial enterococcal bacteremia in adults frequently is associated with urinary tract and wound infections, but catheter-related bacteremia is of increasing importance. Enterococcal bacteremia without a source occurs relatively more commonly in children,[25,242] although Bonadio[22] reported that many children with enterococcal bacteremia had an identifiable focus of infection. Enterococcal bacteremia occurs more frequently in patients with severe underlying disease and may be life threatening. However, the precise contribution of enterococcal bacteremia to morbidity and mortality in the severely ill remains unclear in individual patients. Adult ICU patients with enterococcal bacteremia have a very high mortality rate,[104] and some early studies suggested that isolation of *Enterococcus* from blood merely served to identify a very high-risk group of patients.[206] In several studies, clearance of VRE organisms from blood was not associated with a reduced mortality rate in this high-risk population. In other studies, spontaneous resolution of VRE bacteremia has been reported, thus suggesting that transient VRE bacteremia or pseudobacteremia (or both) may occur.[297] However, a series of subsequent studies clearly associated vancomycin resistance with an increased risk for mortality in certain patients and has demonstrated that effective antienterococcal therapy reduces the overall mortality rate in patients with VRE bacteremia.[69,70,77,123,205,227] Taken together, these findings indicate that at least a subset of high-risk patients with VRE bacteremia are at risk for the development of significant morbidity and mortality directly related to the infection.

CLINICAL MANIFESTATIONS

Enterococcal infections generally occur less frequently in children than in adults, but *Enterococcus* is a relatively frequent cause of neonatal infections.[71] The types of infections caused by enterococci in children are similar to those in adults,[22,25,63,114,242] although enterococcal bacteremia may be associated with fewer sequelae in children.[63] In children, as well as in adults, enterococci have become increasingly important nosocomial pathogens.* They are important causes of endocarditis, urinary tract infection, and bacteremia (particularly catheter-related bacteremia) in pediatric patients, and these organisms commonly are isolated as components of polymicrobial wound, intraabdominal, and pelvic infections in children.[22,25,195,206] Meningitis[283] and septic arthritis[235] are rare manifestations of enterococcal infection. Enterococci are also important causes of peritonitis in children being treated with peritoneal dialysis.[283] Respiratory tract infections caused by enterococci are rarely recognized, although many neonates with enterococcal infection have pulmonary symptoms.[71]

Urinary Tract Infection

Urinary tract infections are the most common enterococcal infections in adults,[5,195] and enterococci are important urinary pathogens in children.[8,64,177] Most enterococcal urinary tract infections occur in elderly men after they have undergone urinary catheterization, instrumentation, or both.[86,200] Enterococci are infrequent causes of cystitis and pyelonephritis in otherwise healthy children, infants, and neonates[8,312] and are infrequent causes of urinary tract infection in young women.[206] Notably, however, some centers are reporting an increasing incidence of both community-acquired and nosocomial urinary tract infection caused by enterococci.[86] Cantey et al.[33] reported that *E. faecalis* was the second most common cause of urinary tract infection in otherwise healthy febrile infants younger than 60 days in Dallas, Texas, accounting for 16 of 171 cases (9.4%). Investigators from Israel found that enterococci were responsible for 5.6% of community-acquired urinary tract infections.[177]

Most enterococcal urinary tract infections in children[8,64,166] and adults[86,94] are nosocomial. Risk factors for the development of urinary tract infection by *Enterococcus* include indwelling urinary catheters, instrumentation of the urinary tract, structural abnormalities of the urinary tract, and previous broad-spectrum antimicrobial therapy.[200,206] The increasing problem of nosocomial enterococcal urinary tract infection[86] is compounded by the growing problem of multiantibiotic-resistant enterococci.[37] While the emergence of multidrug resistance is certainly concerning, a multicenter survey of antimicrobial susceptibility among pediatric uropathogens in the United States revealed that 99% of *E. faecalis* were susceptible to amoxicillin,[288] although this study was biased toward community-acquired isolates.

The genitourinary tract reportedly is the most common entry site leading to enterococcal bacteremia in adults,[104,155] but it is implicated much less frequently in the cause of enterococcal bacteremia in children.[22,25,63] Christie and colleagues[51] reported that urosepsis was the cause of 12% of episodes of nosocomial enterococcal bacteremia in one children's hospital, but Das and Gray[63] failed to detect any cases of urosepsis in 75 consecutive cases of enterococcal bacteremia in another pediatric hospital during a 3-year period. Other complications of enterococcal urinary tract infection in adults include prostatitis and perinephric abscess.[195]

Endocarditis

Enterococcal endocarditis was reported first in 1906,[4] and these organisms are important causes of native-valve and prosthetic-valve endocarditis in children and adults.[2,4,186,240] Either normal or previously damaged valves may be involved. Enterococci cause approximately 5% to 20% of cases of native-valve endocarditis in adults (excluding cases in intravenous drug users),[186] approximately 6% to 7% of prosthetic-valve endocarditis,[186,293] and approximately 5% to 10% of endocarditis in intravenous drug users.[206] Enterococcal endocarditis in intravenous drug users generally involves the aortic or mitral valves, unlike staphylococcal endocarditis in this setting, which usually involves the tricuspid valve.[206] As with other enterococcal infections, *E. faecalis* causes most cases of endocarditis.

Enterococcal endocarditis primarily is a disease of older men, and the genitourinary tract is the most commonly identified source of the initial bacteremia. Enterococci are relatively less frequent causes of endocarditis in children—less than 5% of cases in most series.[135,136,278,279,289,317] Typically enterococcal endocarditis occurs after a subacute course that is clinically indistinguishable from that caused by streptococci.[186] Although the enterococcus is a common neonatal pathogen,[71] reports of neonatal enterococcal endocarditis are extremely rare.[289] The prognosis of enterococcal prosthetic-valve endocarditis is somewhat better than that of native-valve endocarditis caused by these organisms.[2,240] Aortic-valve involvement is associated with increased rates of morbidity and mortality.[186] Endocarditis rarely complicates nosocomial enterococcal bacteremia.[175,206,227] Consequently VRE-associated endocarditis is a rare development, although cases have been reported even in neonates.[14,281]

Bacteremia

Enterococcal bacteremia often represents a conundrum. Bacteremia in severely ill hospitalized patients, particularly that caused by VRE organisms, is associated with considerable morbidity and mortality. However, only a portion of that morbidity and mortality can be attributed directly to enterococcal bacteremia per se. Nosocomial enterococcal bacteremia frequently occurs as a component of polymicrobial bacteremia, with

*References 25, 37, 51, 75, 90, 91, 114, 153, 183, 194, 217, 244, 315.

21% to 45% of bloodstream isolates of *Enterococcus* being accompanied by one or more other pathogens.[63,175,227,271] As many as half of cases of catheter-related enterococcal bacteremia are polymicrobial.[183,227] Pammi et al. found that *Enterococcus* spp. were more common as a contributor to polymicrobial bacteremia (14.9%) than monomicrobial bacteremia (6.9%) in neonates.[224] Many,[112,175] but not all,[122,183] series of patients with enterococcal bacteremia have reported increased mortality rates in patients with polymicrobial bacteremia (including *Enterococcus*) versus isolated enterococcal bacteremia. Mortality in adults with nosocomial enterococcal bacteremia has ranged from 23% to 46%,[175,176,227] but patients at risk for the acquisition of nosocomial enterococcal bacteremia are severely ill and have a poor prognosis independent of the bacteremic event. However, hospital-acquired enterococcal infections can be life-threatening,[76,206,227,232] and specific therapy does appear to reduce the overall mortality rate.[77,123,227] Furthermore a meta-analysis concluded that vancomycin resistance is independently correlated with increased mortality in patients with enterococcal bloodstream infections.[69,70] Nonetheless many episodes of enterococcal bacteremia in high-risk patients apparently resolve in the absence of specific therapy.[123,297] The mortality rate associated with enterococcal bacteremia in children has been lower than that reported in adults in most studies but has ranged from 7.5%[63] to 12% with some series as high as 20%[22] to 26%,[51] depending on the population studied.

In adults, many cases of enterococcal bacteremia are associated with a primary focus, most commonly a urinary tract infection.[67,106] In contrast, few children with enterococcal bacteremia have urosepsis, and most episodes of enterococcal bacteremia in children have not been associated with any identifiable focus.[25,242] However, Christie and coworkers[51] identified a primary focus in 21 of 57 children (37%) with nosocomial enterococcal bacteremia, including seven patients with urosepsis and six with peritonitis. Many children with enterococcal bacteremia do have underlying disease involving the gastrointestinal or respiratory tract.[22,25] Central venous catheter–related enterococcal bacteremia is a significant problem in both children[22,25,51,63,71,227] and adults.[103,227] In earlier series, infections of vascular catheters were reported to account for only 2% to 14% of cases of enterococcal bacteremia,[104] but subsequent reports have implicated intravascular devices in as many as 22% to 28% of these episodes in adults and children.[63,227] Nosocomial transmission appears to be a factor in the development of VRE bacteremia in children and, in at least one study, played a larger role than individual patient exposure to vancomycin.[65]

Most episodes of enterococcal bacteremia do not lead to endocarditis,[175,206,227] and endocarditis is particularly uncommon in the setting of nosocomial enterococcal bacteremia. Maki and Agger[175] identified only one case of endocarditis in 118 episodes of hospital-acquired enterococcal bacteremia, whereas endocarditis was diagnosed in 12 of 35 patients with community-acquired enterococcal bacteremia.

Intraabdominal Infections

Most of the published information about the role of *Enterococcus* in intraabdominal and pelvic infections comes from series of adult patients. Enterococci commonly are isolated as components of polymicrobial infections involving the abdomen or pelvis,[102] and animal models suggest that these organisms can play a synergistic role in the pathogenesis of such infections.[133] However, evidence that the addition of specific antienterococcal therapy improves the outcome of human intraabdominal and pelvic infections, even when enterococci are isolated from peritoneal cultures, is not compelling.[102]

Children with enterococcal bacteremia frequently have underlying conditions related to the gastrointestinal tract.[22,25,51] Bonadio[22] reported five cases of enterococcal bacteremia in previously healthy infants with gastroenteritis, six cases associated with bowel obstruction, and one case associated with acute appendicitis without perforation. Boulanger and coworkers[25] identified underlying conditions affecting the gastrointestinal system in eight of 32 pediatric patients, but they were unable to specifically implicate any of these conditions as the source of the bacteremia. Das and Gray[63] detected underlying chronic gastrointestinal pathology (short-gut syndrome, congenital anomalies of the gastrointestinal tract, ulcerative colitis, chronic liver disease) in fully a third (25 of 75) of pediatric patients with enterococcal bacteremia.

Meningitis

Enterococci are rare causes of bacterial meningitis in adults and children. Stevenson and colleagues[282] found only four cases of enterococcal meningitis among 493 episodes (0.8%) of bacterial meningitis in adults, and they identified an additional 90 cases in a literature search of the interval from 1966 to 1992. These authors reviewed 16 published cases of enterococcal meningitis in children: 11 of these 16 pediatric cases were complications of central nervous system (CNS) trauma or surgery, but four children (three of the four were neonates) had primary meningitis.[282] Enterococci are uncommon but well-recognized causes of infection involving cerebrospinal fluid (CSF) shunts and related devices.[131,152,209,261,316] Meningitis rarely complicates nosocomial bacteremia in adults,[175,227] but it has been reported more frequently in children (particularly neonates) with bacteremia. For example, meningitis developed in 7% (four of 57) of episodes of nosocomial enterococcal bacteremia in children in Cincinnati[51] and in 15% (four of 26) of premature neonates with late-onset enterococcal sepsis in Houston.[71]

Stevenson and associates[282] found that most adults with enterococcal meningitis were immunocompromised (most were receiving steroids) or had a history of CNS, surgery, or both. Enterococcal meningitis has been reported in an adult patient with HIV infection who had completed a course of steroids for presumed *Pneumocystis* pneumonia.[229] Although many children with enterococcal meningitis do have a history of CNS trauma or surgery or are premature infants, most do not have other identifiable predisposing conditions or a history of immunosuppressive therapy. As with the majority of enterococcal infections, most isolates from CSF are *E. faecalis,* but meningitis and ventriculoperitoneal shunt infections caused by *E. faecium* also have been reported in children and adults.[209,211,230]

Neonatal Infections

Enterococci are important neonatal pathogens,* and the published experience with neonatal enterococcal infections constitutes much of the pediatric experience with these organisms. Although several large series of neonatal sepsis included few cases of enterococcal infection,[151] many centers have reported that *Enterococcus* is a relatively frequent cause of neonatal bacteremia. Siegel and McCracken[273] found that enterococci were second only to group B streptococci as causes of neonatal sepsis at Parkland Hospital in Dallas from 1974 to 1977, with an incidence rate of approximately one case per 1000 live births. Gladstone and colleagues[98] reported that *Enterococcus* caused 18 of 270 (6.7%) episodes of neonatal sepsis at Yale–New Haven Hospital during the period 1979 to 1988, which ranked fourth in incidence behind group B streptococci (64 cases; 23.7%), *E. coli* (46 cases; 17.0%), and coagulase-negative staphylococci (36 cases; 13.3%). During the 1990s, reports from Houston,[71] Cincinnati,[51] and New York City[183] documented sharp increases in the rate of late-onset neonatal infection with enterococci in both hospitalized high-risk premature neonates and infants[71,183] and otherwise healthy term newborns with "community-acquired" infection.[71] By contrast, a study of otherwise healthy term infants aged 1 week to 3 months cared for in the Kaiser Permanente Health System revealed that *E. faecalis* accounted for one of 92 culture confirmed cases of bacteremia from 2005 to 2009.[111]

Enterococci cause both early-onset (<7 days of age) and late-onset (>7 days of age) neonatal sepsis. Early-onset disease is indistinguishable from that caused by other neonatal pathogens, but it tends to be less severe.[71] Dobson and Baker[71] identified 56 neonates with enterococcal sepsis during a 10-year period at Jefferson Davis Hospital in Houston; 18 of 56 (32%) had early-onset sepsis, 26 of 56 (46%) had late-onset sepsis, and 12 of 56 (21%) had sepsis associated with necrotizing enterocolitis (2 early onset, 10 late onset). In this study, 25 of 26 (96%) infants with late-onset enterococcal sepsis were premature infants. Christie and colleagues[51] identified 83 cases of enterococcal bacteremia between 1986 and 1992 at Children's Hospital of Cincinnati; 58 of the 83 episodes occurred in neonates. Most cases (57 of 83; 68.7%) were

*References 7, 9, 39, 40, 44, 59, 77, 85, 98, 110, 115, 116, 146, 162, 173, 195, 199, 203, 206, 207, 214, 234, 243, 243, 246.

nosocomial, but many (26 of 83; 31.3%) were community acquired. Young infants (<3 months of age) accounted for almost all (24 of 26; 92.3%) of the community-acquired episodes and for many (34 of 57; 59.6%) of the nosocomial infections. Bonadio[22] and Boulanger and colleagues[25] also reported community-acquired enterococcal bacteremia in young infants.

McNeeley and associates[183] identified 138 episodes of enterococcal bacteremia in a New York City neonatal ICU during a 20-year period and reviewed 100 of the episodes in detail. These authors noted a sharp increase in the rate of enterococcal bacteremia during the second decade (1984–94) of this study and found that most cases occurred in older infants; during this decade, the mean age at onset was 44.7 days (vs. 16.1 days during the first decade of the study), and 65% (51 of 78) of the episodes occurred after the infants reached 30 days of age. Most of the infections occurred in neonates with indwelling central venous catheters (77%), and more than half of the patients had evidence of gastrointestinal disease (necrotizing enterocolitis in 33% and abdominal distention in an additional 21%). The overall mortality rate in this study was 28%, although many of the deaths were not attributed to the enterococcal infection. Most (64%) of the episodes of enterococcal bacteremia in this series were polymicrobial.[183] In a recent 10-year survey by Bizarro et al., *E. faecalis* accounted for 13% of 368 episodes of late-onset neonatal sepsis.[21] Enterococci are an uncommon but known cause of neonatal meningitis; in a recent study from the United Kingdom of 256 episodes of meningitis among infants younger than 90 days, a single case was attributed to *E. faecalis*.[128] By contrast, in a study from Dallas, Texas, two of 21 meningitis cases in febrile infants younger than 60 days were caused by *E. faecalis*.[33]

Nosocomial outbreaks of enterococcal infection, including VRE infection, have been reported in several neonatal units in the United States.[51,59,173,234,238] Indwelling central venous catheters, necrotizing enterocolitis, and intraabdominal surgery are important predisposing factors for the development of nosocomial enterococcal bacteremia in neonates, whereas the genitourinary tract is implicated much less frequently as a source.[51,183] Colonization with VRE in the NICU at Parkland Hospital in Dallas, Texas, was associated with a strain that was considered endemic among adult nonobstetric inpatients at their institution, underscoring the potential for transfer of drug-resistant pathogens from one hospital unit to another.[234]

Enterococcal bacteremia in neonates and young infants has been associated with diarrhea and respiratory disease,[22,71] although a causative role for *Enterococcus* in the pathogenesis of gastroenteritis or pneumonia remains undefined. Enterococci rarely cause urinary tract infections in neonates,[22,51,71,183] but nosocomial and community-acquired cases have been reported. Enterococci have been noted to cause a variety of other neonatal infections, including focal skin and soft tissue infections such as scalp abscess,[71] omphalitis,[71] and conjunctivitis.[301]

Most enterococcal infections in neonates are caused by *E. faecalis,* but outbreaks of infection with *E. faecium* have been reported.[59] In the series from Cincinnati consisting largely of neonates, 82% of enterococcal isolates were *E. faecalis* and 14% were *E. faecium*.[20] McNeeley and colleagues[183] reported the isolation of *E. faecalis* from 94/100 patients and *E. faecium* from 15 of 100 patients in their series (both organisms were isolated from nine of the patients). Six of the *E. faecium* isolates were resistant to vancomycin, and all six patients with VRE bacteremia died, although only one death appeared to be related directly to the VRE infection.

Septic Arthritis

Enterococci rarely have been reported to cause septic arthritis, but they can infect native or prosthetic joints. Raymond and colleagues[235] reported a case of enterococcal septic arthritis involving a prosthetic hip and reviewed an additional 18 cases from the literature. Of these 19 episodes, 11 involved prosthetic joints (two hips, nine knees), and eight involved native joints; only one of the eight individuals with native-joint arthritis had an underlying abnormality of the joint. In seven of the 19 episodes, *Enterococcus* was isolated from synovial fluid, along with a second organism (three with coagulase-negative staphylococci, one with group B streptococci, one with *Pseudomonas,* one with *Streptococcus,* and one with *Kingella kingae*). Only one pediatric case was identified: a 21-month-old girl with septic arthritis of the wrist whose joint aspirate grew *Enterococcus* spp. and *K. kingae*.[272] Other musculoskeletal infections such as osteomyelitis and pyomyositis secondary to enterococci have been reported; however, these are also quite rare.[248,302]

DIAGNOSIS

Enterococcal infections usually are diagnosed by isolation of *Enterococcus* from a culture of blood or another normally sterile site. As discussed earlier, enterococci are ubiquitous inhabitants of the human gastrointestinal tract, and isolation of these organisms from stool or surface cultures is not evidence of invasive infection. Although enterococci are uncommon blood culture contaminants, transient bacteremia, pseudobacteremia, or both may be caused by these organisms.[123,297]

More problematic is the interpretation of a positive culture for enterococcus as a component of polymicrobial infections, particularly intraabdominal and pelvic infections. In this setting, the role of the enterococcus in pathogenesis is unclear, and therapeutic regimens that do not include antienterococcal agents usually suffice to effect a clinical cure.[102] However, rare cases of breakthrough enterococcal bacteremia have been reported with these regimens, and one study found a decreased rate of abdominal surgical wound infections when antienterococcal coverage was provided in a prophylactic regimen.[306]

ANTIMICROBIAL SUSCEPTIBILITY AND RESISTANCE

The increasing importance of *Enterococcus* as a human pathogen, especially in the nosocomial setting,[37,78,141,183,194,206,244,314,315] is of particular concern because of the concomitant development of antimicrobial resistance by these organisms. Furthermore antibiotic resistance probably has played a critical role in allowing the organism to persist and eventually cause disease in high-risk patients despite its relatively low virulence.

Some enterococci have acquired high-level resistance to all three classes of antimicrobial agents that traditionally have been used to treat life-threatening enterococcal infections—β-lactams, aminoglycosides, and glycopeptides. This acquired resistance has occurred in the context of intrinsic (usually lower level) resistance of enterococci to many antibiotics, and physicians have been confronted with the possibility that invasive disease caused by these organisms might not respond to any available antibiotics. Some enterococci also have acquired resistance to recently developed agents (e.g., linezolid, daptomycin) that are active against most antibiotic-resistant gram-positive cocci (see later discussion). The molecular basis of enterococcal resistance to commonly used antimicrobials is summarized in Table 84A.1.

Intrinsic Resistance

β-Lactam Antibiotics

Relative resistance to β-lactam antibiotics is an intrinsic characteristic of enterococci that occurs even in human populations without previous exposure to antibiotics[190]; such resistance is due to the lower affinity of enterococcal (vs. streptococcal) penicillin-binding proteins, especially PBP-5.[195,309] In general, the minimal inhibitory concentration (MIC) of penicillin for most *E. faecalis* isolates (2 to 8 μg/mL) is at least 10 to 100 times higher than that of most streptococci, and *E. faecium* is even more resistant (MIC of 8 to 32 μg/mL or higher).[206] Ampicillin is the most active of the β-lactam antibiotics against enterococci, with average MIC values approximately twofold lower than those for penicillin.[190,195,206] Nafcillin generally is less active than penicillin, and methicillin is much less active (MIC >50 μg/mL for *E. faecalis*), as is ticarcillin. Importantly enterococci exposed to β-lactam antibiotics rapidly become tolerant of the killing effects of these agents.[195,206] Along with intrinsic resistance to these agents, tolerance limits the utility of β-lactam monotherapy for the treatment of endocarditis or other severe enterococcal infections.

Imipenem has some activity against *E. faecalis* but is much less active against *E. faecium*.[195,206] None of the cephalosporins currently approved for use in pediatrics has clinically useful activity against the enterococci, and frequent use of broad-spectrum cephalosporins and imipenem has been identified as a risk factor for the acquisition of nosocomial enterococcal infection.

TABLE 84A.1 Summary of *Enterococcus* spp. Mechanisms of Resistance to Commonly Used Antimicrobials

Antimicrobial	Intrinsic or Acquired Resistance	Acquired Genes/ Gene Products, Method of Acquisition	Mechanism	Comments
β-lactams	Intrinsic		Decreased affinity of PBP5 for β-lactams. Alterations in PBP5 may confer high-level ampicillin resistance in *E. faecium.* Rarely can possess a plasmid-mediated β-lactamase.	Ampicillin has lower MICs for *Enterococcus* spp. than any other β-lactam.
Aminoglycosides	Intrinsic		All enterococci exhibit relative resistance to aminoglycosides (lack of bactericidal activity) because of diminished intracellular uptake of these drugs. *E. faecium* produce an acetyltransferase that confers complete resistance to some aminoglycosides (tobramycin, kanamycin, etc.).	Increased bacterial uptake of aminoglycosides in the presence of a cell wall active antibiotic has been described.
High-level aminoglycoside resistance (HLAR)	Acquired	AAC(6′)-Ie/APH (2′)-Ia APH (2′)-Ic aadA/ANT(3′) (specific to streptomycin)	High-level gentamicin resistance through acquisition of a dual function enzyme with a combination of acetyltransferase and phosphotransferase. Streptomycin resistance acquired through acquisition of an adenyltransferase.	HLAR eliminates synergism with cell wall active antibiotics (β-lactams and glycopeptides).
Glycopeptides	Acquired	*vanA, vanB*	Alteration of peptidoglycan pentapeptide crosslink from d-Ala-d-Ala to d-Ala-d-Lac or d-Ala-d-Ser.	VanA phenotype associated with resistance to vancomycin and teicoplanin, more commonly seen in *E. faecium.* VanB phenotype associated with resistance to vancomycin but not teicoplanin, more commonly seen in *E. faecalis.* Other van phenotypes are very uncommon in human clinical isolates.
Oxazolidinones (linezolid)	Acquired	Multiple copy mutations in genes for 23s rRNA L3 or L4 ribosomal protein mutations *cfr* methyltransferase	Altered drug target	
Daptomycin	Acquired	Mutations within LiaFSR system which helps regulate cell membrane homeostasis	Unclear mechanism but likely involves alterations in phospholipid metabolism.	Lipopeptide resistance remains rare with >99% isolates susceptible
Streptogramins (Quinupristin-Dalfopristin)	Intrinsic (*E. faecalis*) Acquired (*E. faecium*)	*E. faecalis* (intrinsic): *lsa* encoding a presumptive efflux pump	Possible efflux of drug in *E. faecalis.*	All *E. faecalis* are intrinsically resistant but is a rare finding among *E. faecium.*
		E. faecium (acquired): VatD and VatE acetyltransferases, VgbA, VgbB	Modification of drug in *E. faecium.*	

Aminoglycosides

Enterococci are intrinsically resistant to all aminoglycosides because of diminished uptake of these drugs. For most *E. faecalis* isolates, the MIC for gentamicin or tobramycin ranges from 8 to 64 μg/mL and for streptomycin ranges from 12 to 250 μg/mL.[185,228,294] Moellering and Weinberg[192] and Zimmerman and colleagues[320] first demonstrated that the addition of a cell wall–active antibiotic results in dramatically increased aminoglycoside uptake by enterococci and that combinations of β-lactam and aminoglycoside antibiotics can lead to synergistic killing of these organisms. All *E. faecium* strains exhibit higher MICs than does *E. faecalis* to certain aminoglycosides, including tobramycin, netilmicin, kanamycin, and sisomicin, and these aminoglycosides do not exhibit synergy with β-lactam antibiotics against *E. faecium.*[49,206]

Other Antibiotics

Under carefully standardized laboratory conditions, enterococci are inhibited by the combination of trimethoprim and sulfamethoxazole (TMP-SMX). However, *Enterococcus* isolates should be considered resistant to TMP-SMX because these organisms are capable of using exogenous folinic acid to evade the antimicrobial action of TMP-SMX.[319] TMP-SMX fails to eradicate enterococci in animal models of infection,[43,109] and breakthrough enterococcal bacteremia has occurred in patients being treated with TMP-SMX for enterococcal urinary tract infection.[101] Enterococci also are intrinsically resistant to clindamycin, a drug with excellent activity against many other gram-positive cocci. Most enterococci have a clindamycin MIC of 12.5 to 100 μg/mL.[206] As with low-level β-lactam resistance, clindamycin resistance is found in enterococcal isolates from human populations with no previous antibiotic exposure.[190]

Acquired Resistance

Enterococci have acquired resistance to antibiotics by the acquisition of both narrow and broad host range plasmids and via the exchange of conjugative transposons.[206] Resistance mediated by broad host range plasmids is of particular concern because glycopeptide resistance encoded by broad host range plasmids has been transferred to staphylococci in vitro[216] and in vivo.[36,38,292,305]

High-Level Resistance to Aminoglycosides

Intrinsic resistance of enterococci to aminoglycosides is caused by poor drug uptake by these organisms and can be overcome effectively both in vitro and in vivo by the addition of cell wall–active antibiotics. In contrast, high-level resistance to aminoglycosides is mediated either by the acquisition of plasmids encoding aminoglycoside-modifying enzymes (affecting all aminoglycosides via several different enzymes) or by ribosomal mutations (streptomycin only). High-level aminoglycoside resistance is of great clinical importance because it eliminates synergism between the affected aminoglycoside or aminoglycosides and β-lactam or glycopeptide antibiotics.[49,206,228] All *E. faecium* strains produce a chromosomally encoded aminoglycoside acetyltransferase that eliminates synergistic killing between cell wall–active antibiotics and certain aminoglycosides (including tobramycin, kanamycin, netilmicin, and sisomicin),[49] but it does not result in high-level resistance to these compounds. Consequently these particular aminoglycosides should not be used to treat infections caused by *E. faecium*.

Enterococci with high-level resistance (MIC usually ≥2000 μg/mL) to streptomycin, kanamycin, and several other aminoglycosides (excluding gentamicin) were identified more than 40 years ago[193] and were widely prevalent in the United States by the mid-1970s.[32] High-level resistance to streptomycin occurs via two mechanisms, ribosomal mutation or enzymatic modification by 6′-adenylyltransferase. Initial reports of high-level resistance to kanamycin were associated with the production of 3′-phosphotransferase.[49,206]

Horodniceanu and colleagues[125] first reported high-level resistance to gentamicin in *E. faecalis* in 1979, and this resistance was shown later to be mediated by a fusion enzyme containing both 6′-acetyltransferase and 2″-phosphotransferase activity. Expression of this fusion enzyme conferred resistance to all clinically useful aminoglycosides except streptomycin.[161,162] Enterococci expressing this fusion protein usually have gentamicin MICs that are 2000 μg/mL or higher. Thus, enterococci expressing this fusion enzyme and the 6′-adenylyltransferase mediating streptomycin resistance (or chromosomally mediated streptomycin resistance) are highly resistant to all available aminoglycosides and generally fail to be killed synergistically by any combination of β-lactam antibiotics and aminoglycosides. Strains of *E. faecalis* resistant to both streptomycin and gentamicin (and thus to all aminoglycosides) were detected first in Houston, Bangkok, and Santiago in 1983.[185,206] Subsequently strains of *E. faecalis, E. faecium,* and other enterococci resistant to gentamicin, streptomycin, or both (or all) aminoglycosides have become increasingly prevalent[103,137,138,140,170,228] (see Table 84A.2). Although high-level resistance to both streptomycin and gentamicin was described first in *E. faecalis,* it now is at least as common in *E. faecium.*[139]

Enterococci resistant to all aminoglycosides frequently have been isolated from clinical specimens for the past 2 decades. Jones and colleagues and the *Enterococcus* Study Group[138] found that fully 20% of 1936 enterococcal isolates from late 1992 (from 97 participating laboratories in 47 states) exhibited high-level resistance to both gentamicin and streptomycin. Low and associates and the SENTRY Antimicrobial Resistance Surveillance Program[170] reported similar rates of high-level resistance to both gentamicin and streptomycin from 1997 to 1999 (see Table 84A.2). Almost a third (32.8%) of enterococci collected by the SENTRY group from 1997 to 2005 were highly resistant to gentamicin.[140] Many medical centers in the United States now report that most enterococcal isolates exhibit high-level resistance to all aminoglycosides.[207]

Several new aminoglycoside-resistant genes were identified in enterococci during the late 1990s.[49] Some enterococci produce three or more enzymes. Strains expressing some of the recently described resistant genes may fail to exhibit synergy between gentamicin and β-lactams despite MICs below those usually associated with high-level resistance. For example, the *aph (2″)-Ic* gene[48] found in clinical isolates of both *E. faecalis* and *E. faecium* results in gentamicin MICs of approximately 256 to 384 μg/mL, lower than the standard screening cutoff for high-level resistance to gentamicin (500 μg/mL). Nonetheless these organisms are resistant to ampicillin-gentamicin synergism and would not be detected by standard screening methods.

High-Level Resistance to β-Lactams and Production of β-Lactamase

The mechanisms of resistance to penicillin, ampicillin, and other β-lactam antibiotics differ among enterococcal species. High-level β-lactam resistance (ampicillin MIC ≥16 μg/mL) of *E. faecium*[27,108,180] and some other non-*faecalis* enterococcal strains[27] is now common and is mediated by additional alterations in penicillin-binding proteins (PBPs), particularly PBP-5.[89,108,241] Thus high-level resistance to ampicillin and other β-lactams in *E. faecium* (and other non-*faecalis* strains) represents an exaggerated form of intrinsic β-lactam resistance. *E. faecalis* isolates also are intrinsically resistant to β-lactams (though less so than *E. faecium*), but little change has occurred in the level of this resistance in recent years. However, some strains of *E. faecalis*[139,203,202] and *E. faecium*[58] have acquired clinically significant resistance to ampicillin and penicillin via the plasmid-mediated, constitutive production of a β-lactamase enzyme identical to that of *S. aureus.*[321] β-Lactamase–producing strains of *E. faecalis* and *E. faecium* will not be detected by routine susceptibility testing because of a pronounced inoculum effect. Therefore enzymatic methods such as the nitrocefin test must be used to screen for β-lactamase–producing strains.[147,203] Fortunately such strains remain very uncommon.[5,195]

Glycopeptide Resistance

Enterococci resistant to vancomycin were identified first in 1988[158,298] and rapidly have become a major nosocomial problem. Data collected by the CDC NNIS revealed a dramatic increase in the rate of vancomycin resistance in nosocomial isolates of *Enterococcus* during the interval 1989 to 1993.[37] The NNIS survey documented a 26-fold increase in vancomycin resistance among all nosocomial isolates (from 0.3% of enterococcal isolates in 1989 to 7.9% in 1993) and a 34-fold increase in vancomycin resistance among isolates obtained from adult patients in ICUs (from 0.4% of isolates in 1989 to 13.6% in 1993). Rates of vancomycin resistance in enterococci continued to increase during the next decade (Table 84A.2). The NNIS reported that fully 25% of enterococci associated with nosocomial infections in adult patients in ICUs in the United States were resistant to vancomycin in 1999 and 2000; by 2003 to 2004, approximately 30% of the enterococcal isolates from these patients were vancomycin resistant. (See CDC website: http://www.cdc.gov/ncidod/dhqp/pdf/ar/ICU_RESTrend1995-2004.pdf.) Isolates of *E. faecium* are particularly likely to be vancomycin resistant. Jones and colleagues[140] in the SENTRY Antimicrobial Resistance Surveillance Program reported that 69.4% of 1512 US bloodstream isolates of *E. faecium* collected between 1997 and 2005 were resistant to vancomycin. Similarly Wisplinghoff and colleagues[314] in the SCOPE surveillance study found that 60% of US bloodstream isolates of *E. faecium* collected between 1995 and 2002 were resistant to vancomycin, whereas only 3% of *E. faecalis* bloodstream isolates were vancomycin resistant.

Enterococci were the second most common organisms associated with pediatric bloodstream infections in both the 1992 to 1997 NNIS database[246] and the pediatric component of the 1995 to 2001 SCOPE survey.[314] However, VRE organisms were detected much less frequently in these pediatric patients: only 11% of *E. faecium* and 1% of *E. faecalis* bloodstream isolates (of 357 total enterococcal isolates) obtained from pediatric patients in the SCOPE study were vancomycin resistant.[314] This finding is important because vancomycin-resistant isolates, particularly those of *E. faecium,* also may exhibit high-level resistance to both β-lactam antibiotics and aminoglycosides, thus rendering treatment of these infections extremely challenging.*

Vancomycin resistance among enterococci is phenotypically and genotypically heterogeneous[7,99,204,207] and may or may not be associated with resistance to other glycopeptides, including teicoplanin. Five major phenotypes of vancomycin resistance (VanA, VanB, VanC, VanD, and VanE) have been well characterized in *Enterococcus* spp. The VanA and VanB phenotypes are most common, and both are transferable. The VanA phenotype is characterized by high-level resistance to vancomycin and teicoplanin, whereas strains with the VanB phenotype exhibit variable

*References 26, 94, 116, 142, 164, 197-199, 242, 243, 246, 267, 268.

TABLE 84A.2 Antimicrobial Resistance Patterns of Enterococci (United States)

	Gordon et al.[103] (7/1988–4/1989)			Jones et al.[139] (Enterococcus Study Group) (10/1992–12/1992)			Edmond et al.[78] (4/1995–4/1998) (Bloodstream Isolates)			Low et al.[170] (SENTRY Antimicrobial Surveillance Program) (1997–99)	Jones et al.[140] (SENTRY Antimicrobial Resistance Surveillance) (1997–2005)	Sader et al.[250] (Daptomycin Surveillance Study of Nosocomial Isolates, 2007–08)		
Agents	*E. faecalis* (*N* = 632) (%)	*E. faecium* (*N* = 58) (%)	*Total* (*N* = 705) (%)	*E. faecalis* (*N* = 1428) (%)	*E. faecium* (*N* = 306) (%)	*Total* (*N* = 1936) (%)	*E. faecalis* (*N* = 598) (%)	*E. faecium* (*N* = 303) (%)	*Total* (*N* = 1354) (%)	*Total enterococcal isolates* (*N* = 2303) (%)	*E. faecium* (*N* = 1512) (%)	*E. faecalis* (*N* = 1401) (%)	*E. faecium* (*N* = 843) (%)	*Total (N = 2307)*
Ampicillin resistance (MIC ≥16 μg/mL)	0[a]	41[b]	4	0.6–0.7[c]	58.7–59.3	12	2.7	81.1	NA	24	89	0	93.5	34.6
Streptomycin high-level resistance (MIC >2000 μg/mL)	14	33	16	31.5	55.7	36	NA	NA	NA	40	NA	24.4	41.8	30.6
Gentamicin high-level resistance (MIC >500 μg/mL)	11	2	10	26.0	30.8	27	NA	NA	NA	31	32.8	29.5	19.7	25.2
Vancomycin resistance (MIC >4 μg/mL)	0.3	0	0.3	2.0	21.9	5.6	3.2	50.5	17.7	17	69.4	5.6	75.9	31

[a]However, 11/632 (1.7%) *E. faecalis* isolates were β-lactamase producers.
[b]No β-lactamase–producing strains were identified.
[c]Only two β-lactamase–producing isolates were identified.

levels of resistance to vancomycin but not teicoplanin.[7,99,206,207] The VanC phenotype is limited to *E. gallinarum* and *E. casseliflavus* and is associated with constitutive, low-level, chromosomally mediated (nontransferable) resistance to vancomycin but not teicoplanin.[99,206,207,242] VanD and VanE phenotypes occur uncommonly and are not transferable.

High-level resistance to both vancomycin and teicoplanin (the VanA phenotype) is found primarily in strains of *E. faecium,* whereas most vancomycin-resistant strains of *E. faecalis* express the VanB phenotype and remain susceptible to teicoplanin. Jones and associates and the *Enterococcus* Study Group found that 10 of 11 (91%) vancomycin-resistant strains of *E. faecalis* remained susceptible to teicoplanin (VanB phenotype), whereas 49 of 62 (79%) vancomycin-resistant strains of *E. faecium* were resistant to teicoplanin (VanA phenotype).[139]

The biochemical mechanisms responsible for the major vancomycin-resistant phenotypes are the subject of intense study. [99,205] Glycopeptides prevent cross-linkage of peptidoglycan through binding to the terminal d-Alanine (Ala)-D-Ala residues on the N-acetylmuramic acid component of the cell wall. This in turn interferes with the formation of a glycine pentapeptide that links individual peptidoglycan chains. Vancomycin resistance in enterococci is mediated through alteration of d-Ala-d-Ala to D-Ala-D-lactate (Lac) or D-Ala-D-Serine (Ser). Both VanA and VanB phenotypes are mediated by homologous enzymes that catalyze the formation of an altered, vancomycin-resistant D-Ala-D-Lac peptide that is incorporated into cell wall peptidoglycan for which vancomycin has diminished affinity.[7,207,242] The *vanA* and *vanB* gene clusters share functional similarities but are regulated quite differently.[99,207] VanA resistance is transferable by either a transposon or conjugative plasmids. VanB resistance often is encoded by chromosomal DNA but may be transferred by at least two different transposons.[99,207] Vancomycin induces the production of enzymes encoded by both the *vanA* and *vanB* gene clusters, whereas teicoplanin induces VanA but not VanB enzymes.[99]

Resistance to Other Antibiotics

Recently licensed antimicrobials active against most antibiotic-resistant, gram-positive cocci (including VRE organisms) include linezolid and daptomycin. The minocycline derivative tigecycline also is active against most enterococci but has not been well studied for the treatment of these infections. Finally, another agent, the streptogramin quinupristin-dalfopristin, is active against *E. faecium* but not *E. faecalis* isolates and, because of this limitation and its considerable toxicity, it has little utility in pediatrics.

The oxazolidinones are a novel class of synthetic protein synthesis inhibitors that act to inhibit the formation of ribosomal initiation complexes in bacteria.[53] Linezolid, the first oxazolidinone antimicrobial approved for human use, is active against both *E. faecalis* and *E. faecium,* including most VRE isolates. Initial studies demonstrated virtually uniform activity of this agent against clinical isolates of enterococci,[24,81,219] with 100% of 180 strains (representing multiple resistance profiles) inhibited by linezolid concentrations of 1 to 4 μg/mL in one study.[81] Furthermore initial in vitro studies suggested that the development of resistance would occur very rarely.[53,141,322] However, resistance to linezolid has been reported in several patients receiving prolonged courses of therapy with this drug [4,100,178,187,264] and in some patients who have not previously received the agent,[23] and it has been associated with clinical failures.[5,100] Resistance to linezolid is conferred by single nucleotide changes in varying numbers of copies of the bacterial genes encoding 23S ribosomal RNA.[187] Resistance increases in strains containing multiple copies of these mutations.[177,187] In addition, mutations within the L3 and L4 ribosomal proteins can confer resistance to oxazolidinones in enterococci and staphylococci.[41] A gene encoding a methylase known as *cfr* confers resistance to phenicols, oxazolidinones, pleuromutilins, macrolides, and streptogramins. *cfr* was first observed in staphylococci but was ultimately recognized to occur, albeit rarely, among enterococci of human origin.[68] Another gene with 75% peptide identity to *cfr* has recently been recognized in linezolid-resistant *E. faecium* isolates from New Orleans and has been termed *cfr*(B).[66] Recent work has identified a novel gene in both *E. faecalis* and *E. faecium* of animal origin, *optrA,* encoding a membrane transporter that confers resistance to both oxazolidinones and phenicols; the presence of these gene in enterococci of human origin remains quite rare, however.[304] Although some centers have reported increasing rates of linezolid resistance in VRE isolates[187] and nosocomial spread of linezolid-resistant VRE strains,[121] overall rates of linezolid resistance in enterococci remain low. For example, only 0.9% of 1512 US bloodstream isolates of *E. faecium* collected from 1997 to 2005 by the SENTRY group were resistant to linezolid,[140] and only 0.75% of 934 enterococcal isolates studied in 2010 as part of the LEADER surveillance program were resistant to linezolid.[87]

Daptomycin is a novel cyclic lipopeptide antimicrobial that exhibits rapid, concentration-dependent bactericidal activity against gram-positive pathogens, including methicillin-resistant *Staphylococcus aureus* (MRSA) and VRE strains.[35,280] Daptomycin has a novel method of action in which binding to bacterial membranes and triggering of rapid depolarization of membrane potential lead to inhibition of protein and nucleic acid synthesis.[94] Daptomycin was found to have potent activity against a panel of VRE isolates from the United States and Europe—all 75 VRE isolates tested (i.e., 55 *E. faecium* and 20 *E. faecalis*) were susceptible to this agent.[253] Daptomycin also was reported to be active against a collection of VRE strains resistant to linezolid or quinupristin-dalfopristin.[3] However, daptomycin resistance has developed during therapy with this agent,[167,201,249] although resistance rates remain very low. Sader and colleagues[251] studied 4312 *E. faecalis* isolates (195 VRE) and 2462 *E. faecium* isolates (1867 VRE) collected between 2005 and 2010; 99.98% of the *E. faecalis* isolates and 99.68% of the *E. faecium* isolates were susceptible to daptomycin. The mechanisms responsible for daptomycin resistance are poorly understood but are believed to involve genes associated with phospholipid metabolism and bacterial cell membrane integrity, specifically *liaR,* which appears to be involved in cardiolipin distribution[237,295]

Streptogramins are protein synthesis inhibitor antibiotics and are natural combinations of two chemically unrelated molecules, streptogramin A and B.[172] Quinupristin-dalfopristin is a streptogramin agent that is active against *E. faecium* (including most strains of VREF) but lacks activity against *E. faecalis* at clinically achievable concentrations.[57] An early study found that more than 95% of 875 initial patient isolates of VREF were susceptible to quinupristin-dalfopristin,[80] but both emergence of resistance to this agent[191,253] and superinfection with *E. faecalis* and other organisms[46,313] have been reported during therapy with this drug. In the United States, overall rates of enterococcal resistance to quinupristin-dalfopristin remain low, in the range of 1% to 2% in most areas.[122]

Testing for Antimicrobial Resistance in Enterococci

All enterococci isolated from cultures of blood, CSF, or other normally sterile sites (with the possible exception of urine) should be tested for resistance to β-lactam antibiotics (i.e., ampicillin, penicillin, or both, including a test for β-lactamase production), vancomycin, and high levels of aminoglycosides (streptomycin and gentamicin)[84,235,242] by using the methodology and interpretative guidelines published by the Clinical and Laboratory Standards Institute (CLSI).[54] For multiantibiotic-resistant isolates, testing for susceptibility to alternative agents, including linezolid and daptomycin, should be performed.

Testing of enterococci for ampicillin (or penicillin) resistance must involve determination of the MIC of these agents and a test for β-lactamase production.[54] Jones and colleagues[138] and the *Enterococcus* Study Group compared three techniques that are used commonly to determine the ampicillin MIC of enterococcal isolates—disk diffusion, broth microdilution, and E-test strips—and found excellent agreement among the three methods. Enterococcal isolates with an ampicillin or penicillin MIC of 16 μg/mL or greater are considered resistant to these agents.[54] β-Lactamase–producing enterococci cannot be detected by these methods but are identified routinely by performance of the chromogenic nitrocefin assay.[286]

High-level resistance to gentamicin and streptomycin usually may be detected by either agar dilution (high-level resistance to gentamicin, MIC >500 μg/mL; high-level resistance to streptomycin, MIC >2000 μg/mL) or broth microdilution (high-level resistance to gentamicin, MIC >500 μg/mL; high-level resistance to streptomycin,

MIC >1000 μg/mL).[54,284,286] These isolates also may be identified by disk diffusion with the use of high-content aminoglycoside disks (120-μg gentamicin disk, 300-μg streptomycin disks, ≥10-mm zone = susceptible)[284] or high-range E-test strips.[138,256] However, the recent identification of novel genes encoding gentamicin resistance in both *E. faecalis* and *E. faecium* has raised concern about continued use of the 500-μg/mL cutoff for detection of high-level resistance to gentamicin.[49] These enterococcal isolates are not killed synergistically by combinations of ampicillin or penicillin and gentamicin, even though gentamicin MICs are 256 to 384 μg/mL. If these isolates become more widely prevalent, modification of the standard screening procedures for high-level aminoglycoside resistance may be required.

Commercially available automated antimicrobial susceptibility testing methods may fail to detect vancomycin resistance in enterococci, particularly the VanB phenotype of moderate resistance,[291] although newer versions of these systems appear to be much more reliable.[96,299] Routine disk diffusion testing is more dependable but requires an extended incubation time and the use of transmitted light for examination of zone size to be highly accurate.[285,291] Agar dilution screening using brain-heart infusion agar supplemented with 6 μg/mL vancomycin reliably identifies VRE strains,[54,286,307] as does the standard broth microdilution method.[139,291] E-test glycopeptide strips are a useful alternative to the more cumbersome broth dilution methodology.

THERAPY FOR ENTEROCOCCAL INFECTIONS

Before the emergence of VRE infection as a major nosocomial problem in high-risk patients, the optimal management of serious enterococcal infections (especially endocarditis) was well established. Successful treatment of enterococcal endocarditis required the administration of combination therapy consisting of a cell wall–active agent (usually ampicillin) and an aminoglycoside (gentamicin or streptomycin). Combination therapy also was recommended for other potentially life-threatening enterococcal infections (e.g., sepsis or meningitis) based on the extensive experience with endocarditis. Other enterococcal infections, including urinary tract infections, responded well to monotherapy with a variety of antimicrobials.

In contrast, the optimal therapy for many infections caused by VRE strains remains uncertain. Both linezolid and daptomycin have now been used extensively for the treatment of VRE infections in adults. However, only one of these antibiotics (linezolid) has been approved for use in children, and enterococci resistant to these new agents already have been detected.[187,201]

Treatment of Infections Caused by Antibiotic-Susceptible Enterococci

Any discussion of the treatment of serious enterococcal infection must begin with a review of the large experience in the treatment of enterococcal endocarditis. The difficulty of treating enterococcal endocarditis has been apparent since early reports showed that penicillin alone failed to cure as many as two-thirds of patients with enterococcal endocarditis but was highly effective in the treatment of streptococcal endocarditis.[206] The early failures of penicillin therapy stimulated studies of the in vitro and in vivo effects of β-lactam antibiotics on enterococci. These studies led to the discovery that enterococci were "tolerant" of the killing effects of cell wall–active agents and provided evidence that bactericidal therapy was required to cure bacterial endocarditis reliably.

For more than 65 years, standard therapy for enterococcal endocarditis has included an aminoglycoside plus a cell wall–active agent. Hunter[127] first reported clinical evidence of synergism between penicillin and streptomycin in the treatment of enterococcal endocarditis in 1947, and this synergism subsequently was confirmed for combinations of penicillin or ampicillin and streptomycin or gentamicin, both in vitro and in vivo.[206] Moellering and Weinberg[192] first demonstrated that synergy between β-lactams and aminoglycosides was a consequence of increased aminoglycoside uptake by enterococci exposed to cell wall–active agents. Glycopeptides and aminoglycosides also exhibit in vitro and in vivo synergy against "susceptible" (not expressing high-level resistance) strains of enterococci.[124,195]

The preferred therapy for endocarditis caused by "susceptible" strains of enterococci in both adults[5,20,186,195,240,310] and children[62,279] consists of combination therapy with parenteral ampicillin (or penicillin G) plus parenteral gentamicin (or streptomycin) for a minimal duration of 4 to 6 weeks.[11] Patients with severe penicillin allergy should be treated with vancomycin plus gentamicin or streptomycin. Selected adult patients with a short duration of symptoms and an uncomplicated course may be treated with 4-week regimens[310]; most other patients, including those with mitral valve involvement, a longer duration of symptoms (especially those with symptoms for >3 months), or prosthetic valve endocarditis, probably should receive 6-week courses of therapy.[186,310] Interestingly, several reports indicate that the prognosis of enterococcal prosthetic valve endocarditis is better than that of native valve disease, perhaps because of the generally shorter duration of symptoms before the diagnosis is made.[186,240] Many patients with prosthetic valve endocarditis caused by enterococci can be cured without surgery. Rice and colleagues[240] reported a 69% cure rate with medical therapy in patients with enterococcal endocarditis involving prosthetic valves.

The general consensus, based on experience with enterococcal endocarditis, is that other life-threatening enterococcal infections, including meningitis and septicemia, should be treated with bactericidal regimens.[194,206,282] The duration of therapy for uncommon enterococcal infections such as meningitis must be individualized, although 2- to 3-week courses of antibiotics have been reported to cure enterococcal meningitis.[282] The optimal treatment of enterococcal bacteremia, particularly that occurring in the nosocomial setting, remains controversial. A recent retrospective study compared the outcomes of children with *E. faecalis* bacteremia without endocarditis treated with ampicillin plus synergistic gentamicin (1 mg/kg per day) with those treated with ampicillin monotherapy.[128] While only 313 patients total were included in this study, the difference in duration of bacteremia between these two groups was only 0.4 days and there was no difference in the frequency of relapse of infection. There was, however, a higher rate of acute kidney injury in the combination therapy group (18.4% vs. 9.3%). While this study has limitations, given the modest improvements in duration of bacteremia and risk of renal toxicity, it does call into question the need for combination therapy in patients without endocarditis.

The prognosis for patients with enterococcal bacteremia varies widely and often is related more closely to the underlying disease than to the enterococcal infection. In adults, single-drug regimens generally are successful in the treatment of enterococcal bacteremia, thus indicating that bactericidal therapy is not required in all cases.[194,206]

Considerable clinical experience supports the routine use of single-drug therapy for uncomplicated enterococcal urinary tract infection and for soft tissue infection caused by enterococci. Urinary tract infections by susceptible strains of enterococci generally respond promptly to ampicillin, penicillin, nitrofurantoin, or vancomycin.[194,195,200,206]

Treatment of Infections Caused by Antibiotic-Resistant Enterococci (Including Vancomycin-Resistant Enterococci)

Unfortunately the emergence of enterococci with clinically significant resistance to aminoglycosides, β-lactams, and glycopeptides has greatly complicated the management of endocarditis and other serious infections caused by these organisms. This discussion focuses on the management of endocarditis caused by drug-resistant enterococci because the need to provide bactericidal therapy has been well established in this setting. The general principles probably apply to the management of other life-threatening enterococcal infections (see earlier discussion).

Endocarditis caused by enterococci with high-level resistance to either streptomycin or gentamicin may be treated by substituting the other aminoglycoside in a combination regimen, but isolation of strains with high-level resistance to both aminoglycosides means that no available aminoglycoside will provide synergistic killing in concert with cell wall–active agents.[186,206,311] Based on animal studies, some experts recommend prolonged treatment (≥8 to 12 weeks) with high-dose intravenous ampicillin given by continuous infusion in this situation (if the isolate is susceptible).[79,195] Surgical excision of infected valves may be required in such patients.[240] Studies in adults have shown that patients with endocarditis due to *E. faecalis* with high-level aminoglycoside resistance can be treated with a combination of ampicillin and ceftriaxone[97]; furthermore in vitro synergism is exhibited by such a combination. National guidelines now endorse the use of "double β-lactam therapy" with ampicillin plus ceftriaxone for patients with endocarditis due to enterococci with resistance to aminoglycosides but susceptibility to ampicillin.[11]

Endocarditis and other serious infections caused by enterococci resistant to β-lactam antibiotics also are increasing in frequency.[108] Endocarditis caused by enterococci (usually *E. faecium*) highly resistant to β-lactams may be treated with vancomycin plus an aminoglycoside (if the strain is susceptible to vancomycin). Endocarditis caused by β-lactamase–producing strains of *E. faecalis* (or, rarely, *E. faecium*) would be expected to respond to ampicillin-sulbactam because this combination is highly effective in animal models[79]; the most recent American Heart Association (AHA) guidelines however, endorse the use of a combination of vancomycin plus an aminoglycoside in this circumstance however.[11] Higher-dose or continuous-infusion ampicillin may be effective in the treatment of endocarditis caused by some strains of enterococci that are "resistant" to ampicillin by current guidelines (MIC ≥16 μg/mL) because sustained plasma concentrations in excess of 100 μg/mL may be achieved with these regimens.[207] However, even high-dose ampicillin therapy probably will fail to cure endocarditis caused by enterococci with ampicillin MICs greater than 64 μg/mL.[29,99]

Enterococci resistant to vancomycin may remain susceptible to teicoplanin (VanB phenotype). Teicoplanin with or without the addition of an aminoglycoside has been used successfully in the treatment of serious enterococcal infections caused by susceptible isolates,[260] including some cases of endocarditis[232,260] and meningitis.[169] However, teicoplanin is not available in the United States, treatment of endocarditis with this agent has been associated with both treatment failure and relapse,[232,260] and high-level teicoplanin resistance may develop even without exposure to the drug.[118] Endocarditis caused by VanB strains of enterococci should be treated with high-dose ampicillin plus gentamicin or streptomycin if resistance to these agents is not present.

Similarly, endocarditis caused by enterococci highly resistant to both vancomycin and teicoplanin (VanA phenotype) but susceptible to β-lactams should be treated with ampicillin plus an aminoglycoside (if high-level resistance to aminoglycosides is not present). Unfortunately the VanA phenotype is associated primarily with strains of *E. faecium*, which increasingly are resistant to β-lactams.[89,108,138] Endocarditis caused by enterococci highly resistant to both glycopeptides and β-lactams is especially difficult to treat. Combinations of ampicillin and vancomycin are not bactericidal against these isolates but may[270] or may not[39] provide additive or synergistic inhibition in vitro. If high-level resistance to aminoglycosides is not present, triple-combination therapy with a β-lactam, a glycopeptide, and an aminoglycoside may achieve bactericidal activity; such combinations are reported to be highly effective in animal models of endocarditis caused by ampicillin- and vancomycin-resistant *E. faecium*.[34] For endocarditis caused by enterococci exhibiting high-level resistance to both gentamicin and streptomycin along with resistance to β-lactams and glycopeptides, AHA guidelines endorse the use of daptomycin or linezolid (see later discussion).

Newer Options for Treatment of Vancomycin-Resistant Enterococcal Infections

Four newer antimicrobials with activity against most VRE strains have been licensed: linezolid, daptomycin, tigecycline, and quinupristin-dalfopristin. Of these drugs, only linezolid has been approved for use in children.

Linezolid, the first oxazolidinone antibiotic, was approved by the US Food and Drug Administration (FDA) in April 2000 for the treatment of selected infections caused by antibiotic-resistant, gram-positive bacteria in adults, including those caused by VRE strains (*E. faecium* or *E. faecalis*). In December 2002, the FDA approved this agent for treatment of pediatric patients with pneumonia, skin and skin structure infections, and VREF infections. Linezolid is available in both parenteral and oral formulations (with comparable bioavailability). Linezolid is active against many antibiotic-resistant, gram-positive pathogens, including MRSA, penicillin-resistant *S. pneumoniae*, and vancomycin-resistant isolates of both *E. faecium* and *E. faecalis*.[24,53,80,87,219] This agent is bacteriostatic against most susceptible organisms, including the enterococci, but it does exhibit bactericidal activity against some strains of pneumococci. Initial studies demonstrated virtually uniform activity of linezolid against clinical isolates of enterococci.[24,79,220]

Linezolid has been reported to effect both bacteriologic and clinical cure in patients with life-threatening VRE infections, including endocarditis,[10,19,45,280] bacteremia,[45,184,220] and meningitis,[266,316,318] although clinical experience with this agent in the treatment of endocarditis or meningitis remains limited. Linezolid therapy has been reported to cure several patients with VRE endocarditis,[10,19,44,281] including 10 of 22 patients in one study[19] and all of 3 patients who received at least 6 weeks of the drug in another report.[281] These results are encouraging, but enthusiasm for the use of linezolid to treat serious VRE infection must be tempered by its generally bacteriostatic activity and the potential for increasing resistance to this agent. Some experts suggest caution in using linezolid for treatment of VRE endocarditis because of reported therapeutic failures, toxicity, and potential for emergence of resistance.[5,245] Pediatric experience with linezolid is not as extensive as that in the adult literature, but the drug was demonstrated to be well tolerated and as effective as vancomycin in the treatment of children with serious gram-positive infections in a large multicenter trial.[143]

Linezolid generally has been tolerated well in both adults and children.[52,93,255] Longer courses of linezolid therapy have been associated with more serious adverse effects, including optic neuropathy that usually is reversible and peripheral neuropathy that may be irreversible.[132,247] Enterococcal resistance to linezolid remains very uncommon[87] but has been associated with clinical failures in both adults and children. A new oxazolidinone, tedizolid, has been approved by the FDA for treating skin and soft tissue infection in adults. In vitro studies have demonstrated that tedizolid remains active against enterococci with elevated MICs to linezolid and may be an additional therapeutic option in adolescents with linezolid nonsusceptible enterococci.[13,42]

Daptomycin is a novel cyclic lipopeptide antimicrobial that exhibits rapid, concentration-dependent bactericidal activity against enterococci, including VRE strains.[35,280] It was approved by the FDA in September 2003 for the treatment of adult patients with complicated skin and soft tissue infections caused by gram-positive bacteria, including staphylococci, streptococci, and vancomycin-susceptible strains of *E. faecalis*. Daptomycin is available in an intravenous formulation. It is not approved for use in children, and pediatric experience with the drug is limited. Daptomycin should not be used for the treatment of pneumonia because it is inactivated by pulmonary surfactant.[274]

Considerable published experience exists now with daptomycin therapy (alone and in combination with other agents) in adult patients with VRE bloodstream infections, although pediatric data remain limited. Half (11 of 22) of the adult patients with VRE bacteremia or endocarditis treated with daptomycin summarized in three early reports were cured.[157,231,265] Subsequently anecdotal reports have been published documenting successful treatment of VRE bacteremia or endocarditis with daptomycin alone or in combination with other agents.[5] Higher doses of daptomycin (e.g., 8 mg/kg per day in adults) may be more effective for the treatment of bacteremia caused by VRE (and other bacteria). A number of retrospective comparisons have failed to identify significant differences in the outcomes of VRE bacteremia treated with daptomycin or linezolid.[61,296] At least one meta-analysis, however, has shown a small but statistically significant increase in mortality among adults with VRE bacteremia treated with daptomycin compared to those treated with linezolid.[12] The published pediatric experience is limited, and clinical trials in children are under way. Based on pharmacokinetic studies, children may require higher doses of daptomycin (8 to 10 mg/kg in children 2 to 6 years old) to achieve comparable serum levels to adults with 4 to 6 mg/kg dosing.[1]

Daptomycin resistance remains uncommon among enterococci[251] but may develop during therapy. Patients being treated with daptomycin should be monitored for the development of muscle toxicity by serial measurement of serum creatine kinase concentrations and screening for muscle pain or weakness.

The streptogramin antibiotic quinupristin-dalfopristin[172] was approved by the FDA in September 1999 for the treatment of adults with infections caused by VREF. This agent is not approved for the treatment of *E. faecalis* infections, nor for pediatric use.

Quinupristin-dalfopristin has been reported to effect clinical cures of several serious infections caused by multiresistant *E. faecium,* including ventriculoperitoneal shunt infections in two patients,[209,296] an infected aortic graft in one patient,[254] and VREF peritonitis in a series of adults.[174] Clinical response to quinupristin-dalfopristin has been reported in approximately 74% to 80% of patients with VREF bacteremia.[95,105,163,165,179,191,301,313] The lack of a consistent bactericidal effect may limit the utility of this agent in the treatment of endocarditis and other life-threatening infections. Quinupristin-dalfopristin therapy generally has been tolerated fairly well in both adults and children, although a high rate of venous phlebitis in recipients has led to a recommendation that the agent be administered through a central venous catheter. Myalgias and arthralgias are other commonly reported side effects of this agent. The potential utility of quinupristin-dalfopristin for the treatment of pediatric patients is limited by its venous toxicity, its lack of a consistent bactericidal effect against VREF, and its lack of clinically useful activity against *E. faecalis.*[57]

Tigecycline is a novel glycylcycline antibiotic derived from minocycline. It is FDA approved in adults for treatment of complicated skin and soft tissue infections and abdominal infections caused by susceptible bacteria, including vancomycin-susceptible *E. faecalis.* It is active in vitro against both vancomycin-susceptible and vancomycin-resistant *E. faecalis* and *E. faecium,* but the clinical experience with this agent for treatment of VRE infections is limited and mostly consists of case reports involving combination antimicrobial therapy.[5,31] Pediatric experience is even more limited.[131]

Several other promising new antibiotics with in vitro activity against VRE isolates are being studied in clinical trials, including the lipoglycopeptides oritavancin and telavancin,[188] as well as new members of the oxazolidinone and streptogramin classes of antibiotics.

PREVENTION OF ENTEROCOCCAL INFECTIONS

The explosive increase in nosocomial infections caused by vancomycin-resistant and multiantibiotic-resistant enterococci[37,77] has rendered prevention of enterococcal infections, particularly those caused by VRE strains, a public health priority in the United States.[40,99,207,236,267] In 1995, the Hospital Infection Control Practices Advisory Committee (HICPAC) recommended a series of overlapping strategies designed to prevent the development of serious VRE infections.[236] These strategies remain useful today and are designed to simultaneously reduce vancomycin resistance in enterococci and prevent nosocomial infections caused by these organisms. Implementation of such strategies has been reported to reduce or eliminate the transmission of VRE organisms in health care facilities.[222] However, overall rates of nosocomial infection by VRE continued to increase in the United States from 1995 to 2004, perhaps because the HICPAC guidelines were followed inconsistently.[40] (See the CDC website http://www.cdc.gov/ncidod/dhqp/pdf/ar/ICU_RESTrend 1995-2004.pdf.)

Reversing the Trend Toward Vancomycin and Multiple-Antibiotic Resistance in Enterococci

The use of vancomycin[236,267] and treatment with broad-spectrum antibiotics, including the third-generation cephalosporins and carbapenems, [77,107,182,199,205,213,243] are risk factors for colonization and the development of infection with VRE strains. Consequently the HICPAC and CDC recommend that all hospitals, even those at which VRE organisms have not been isolated, should (1) develop a comprehensive antimicrobial utilization plan, (2) oversee surgical prophylaxis, and (3) develop institution-specific guidelines for the proper use of vancomycin.[236] These strategies are echoed in the recommendations for development of antimicrobial stewardship programs that have been made jointly by the Society for Healthcare Epidemiology of America, the Infectious Diseases Society of America (IDSA), and the Pediatric Infectious Diseases Society.[277]

Efforts to eliminate unnecessary use of vancomycin are of critical importance[236,267] but may be inadequate unless the use of other classes of antimicrobials is reduced as well (see later discussion). In 1995, HICPAC provided recommendations regarding the acceptable and appropriate use of vancomycin (Box 84A.2), as well as recommendations regarding situations in which vancomycin use should be discouraged[236] (Box 84A.3). These recommendations remain useful, but the emergence of community-acquired MRSA infections[120,126,144] has resulted in increased empirical and definitive use of vancomycin for an HICPAC-approved indication: "treatment of serious infections caused by β-lactam–resistant, gram-positive microorganisms."[236]

In addition, efforts should be undertaken to reduce the unnecessary use of broad-spectrum antibiotics and certain agents with potent

BOX 84A.2 Situations in Which Vancomycin Use Is Appropriate or Acceptable

Treatment

- Treatment of serious infections caused by β-lactam–resistant, gram-positive microorganisms
- Treatment of gram-positive infections in patients with serious allergies to β-lactams
- Treatment of antibiotic-associated colitis only when it fails to respond to metronidazole or is severe and potentially life threatening

Prophylaxis

- Endocarditis prophylaxis after certain procedures in high-risk patients according to the American Heart Association guidelines
- Prophylaxis for major surgical procedures involving implantation of prosthetic materials or devices (single-dose prophylaxis usually is adequate)

Modified from Recommendations for preventing the spread of vancomycin resistance: Recommendations of the Hospital Infection Control Practices Advisory Committee (HICPAC). *MMWR Recomm Rep.* 1995;44(RR-12):1–13.

BOX 84A.3 Situations in Which Vancomycin Use Should Be Discouraged

Treatment

- Empiric therapy for febrile neutropenic patients (unless there is presumptive evidence of an infection caused by gram-positive organisms, such as a Hickman catheter exit-site infection, and the local prevalence of methicillin-resistant *Staphylococcus aureus* strains is substantial)
- Treatment of an isolated, single blood culture positive for coagulase-negative *Staphylococcus*
- Treatment (chosen for dosing convenience) of infections caused by β-lactam–susceptible, gram-positive microorganisms in patients with renal failure
- Continued empirical use of presumed infection in patients whose cultures are negative for β-lactam–resistant gram-positive microorganisms
- Primary treatment of antibiotic-associated diarrhea
- Eradication of methicillin-resistant *S. aureus* colonization

Prophylaxis

- Routine surgical prophylaxis except in patients with life-threatening allergy to β-lactams
- Systemic or local prophylaxis for infection of indwelling intravascular catheters
- Routine prophylaxis for infants with very low birth weight
- Routine prophylaxis for dialysis patients
- Use of vancomycin solution for topical application or irrigation
- Selective decontamination of the gastrointestinal tract

Modified from Recommendations for preventing the spread of vancomycin resistance: Recommendations of the Hospital Infection Control Practices Advisory Committee (HICPAC). *MMWR Recomm Rep.* 1995;44(RR-12):1–13.

antianaerobic activity, particularly in settings with high rates of nosocomial infection (such as ICUs). These efforts are necessary because many studies indicate that nonglycopeptide antibiotics also exert selective pressure for VRE strains and that limitation of the use of vancomycin alone has only a modest effect on reducing VRE colonization and infection.[243] Exposure to agents with broad-spectrum activity (but lacking antienterococcal activity), such as the extended-spectrum cephalosporins, appears to predispose to colonization with VRE organisms,[74,243] whereas exposure to antimicrobials with potent antianaerobic activity (even if they are also active against enterococci) may promote high-density, prolonged VRE colonization (by eliminating gut anaerobes that may interfere with colonization by VRE strains).[73,233,243]

Preventing and Controlling the Spread of Nosocomial Infection by Vancomycin-Resistant Enterococci

The increasing prevalence of *Enterococcus* in nosocomial infections is related to the intrinsic and acquired antimicrobial resistance of these organisms, but the factors leading to increased antibiotic resistance in enterococci are not identical to those that predispose to enterococcal colonization, infection, or both. Enterococcal infections are concentrated increasingly in debilitated and immunocompromised patients, including those with malignancies, recipients of bone marrow and solid organ transplants, burn victims, premature neonates, and critically ill patients with indwelling intravascular catheters. Consequently special attention should be paid to potential outbreaks of VRE infection in hospital wards caring for these high-risk patients.[40]

Efforts to prevent the spread of VRE colonization, infection, or both probably will be more successful if the VRE isolates are confined to a few patients in a single area of the hospital. Widespread colonization with VRE strains may precede identification of infections by these organisms. Therefore all hospitals should implement active VRE surveillance and formulate a multidisciplinary plan to prevent nosocomial spread of VRE strains if such organisms are identified. In hospitals that have not isolated VRE strains, periodic antimicrobial susceptibility testing should be performed on enterococcal isolates from all sources, particularly from high-risk patient populations such as those in intensive care or transplant units. If VRE organisms are identified, a comprehensive plan to prevent nosocomial spread of these bacteria should be instituted immediately. The HICPAC guidelines summarized the essential elements of such a plan.[236] Hospital infection control staff and clinical staff must be notified promptly when VRE strains are isolated from a clinical sample, and isolation precautions should be implemented immediately to prevent patient-to-patient transmission of VRE organisms. These precautions include gown and glove isolation, vigorous hand washing, dedicated use of noncritical patient items such as thermometers and stethoscopes, and prompt surveillance of any possibly exposed patients for VRE colonization. Additional measures may be necessary in hospitals with endemic or continued VRE transmission despite implementation of the aforementioned measures.[236] Ostrowsky and colleagues[222] reported that an active infection control program that included surveillance cultures and prompt isolation of infected patients successfully reduced the spread of VRE strains in health care facilities throughout the Siouxland region of Iowa, Nebraska, and South Dakota.

Once VRE organisms become endemic in a hospital unit, achieving complete eradication is very difficult. The duration of VRE colonization in individual patients may be weeks or months,[40,197] although spontaneous resolution of colonization occurs frequently.[40,196] Attempts to eradicate colonization in individual patients generally have been unsuccessful.[40,196] Consequently the measures recommended by HICPAC and others are directed at preventing the initial establishment of VRE strains in hospitals. Implementation of these policies will require the involvement of hospital pharmacy and therapeutics committees, quality assurance programs, and medical staff. Ongoing monitoring of the efficacy of these programs is necessary.

NEW REFERENCES SINCE THE SEVENTH EDITION

2. Alminrante B, Tornos M, Gurgui M, et al. Prognosis of enterococcal endocarditis. *Rev Infect Dis*. 1991;13:1248-1249.
11. Baddour LM, Wilson WR, Bayer AS, et al. Infective endocarditis in adults: diagnosis, antimicrobial therapy and management of complications: A scientific statement for healthcare professional from the American Heart Association. *Circulation*. 2015;132:1435-1486.
12. Balli EP, Venetis CA, Miyakis S. Systematic review and meta-analysis of linezolid versus daptomycin for treatment of vancomycin-resistant enterococcal bacteremia. *Antimicrob Agents Chemother*. 2014;58:734-739.
13. Barber KE, Smith JR, Raut A, Rybak MJ. Evaluation of tedizolid against *Staphylococcus aureus* and enterococci with reduced susceptibility to vancomycin, daptomycin or linezolid. *J Antimicrob Chemother*. 2015;epub.
14. Beneri CA, Nicolau DP, Seiden HS, Rubin HG. Successful treatment of a neonate with persistent vancomycin-resistant enterococcal bacteremia with a daptomycin-containing regimen. *Infect Drug Resis*. 2008;1:9-11.
16. Bielicki JA, Lundin R, Sharland M, et al. Antibiotic resistance prevalence in routine bloodstream isolates from children's hospitals varies substantially from adult surveillance data in Europe. *Pediatr Infect Dis J*. 2015;34:734-741.
21. Bizzarro MJ, Shabanova V, Baltimore RS, et al. Neonatal sepsis 2004-2013: the rise and fall of coagulase negative staphylococci. *J Pediatr*. 2015;166:1193-1199.
33. Cantey JB, Lopez-Medina E, Nguyen S, Doern C, Garcia C. Empiric antibiotics for serious bacterial infection in young infants: opportunities for stewardship. *Pediatr Emerg Care*. 2015;31:568-571.
41. Chen H, Wu W, Ni M, et al. Linezolid-resistant clinical isolates of enterococci and *Staphylococcus cohnii* from a multicenter study in China: molecular epidemiology and resistance mechanisms. *Int J Antimicrob Agents*. 2013;42:317-321.
42. Chen KG, Huang YT, Liao CH, Sheng WH, Hsueh PR. In vitro activities of tedizolid and linezolid against gram-positive cocci associated with acute bacterial skin and and skin structure infections and pneumonia. *Antimicrob Agents Chemother*. 2015;59:6262-6265.
65. DePentima MC, Chan S, Briody C, et al. Driving forces of vancomycin-resistant *E. faecium* and *E. faecalis* bloodstream infections in children. *Antimicrob Resis Infect Control*. 2014;3:29.
66. Deshpande LM, Ashcraft DS, Kahn HP, et al. Detection of a new cfr-like gene, cfr(B), in *Enterococcus faecium* isolates recovered from human specimens in the United States as part of the SENTRY antimicrobial surveillance program. *Antimicrob Agents Chemother*. 2015;59:6256-6261.
68. Diaz L, Kiratisin P, Mendes RE, et al. Transferable plasmid-mediated resistance to linezolid due to cfr in a human clinical isolate of *Enterococcus faecalis*. *Antimicrob Agents Chemother*. 2012;56:3917-3922.
97. Gavalda J, Len O, Munoz P, et al. Brief communication: treatment of *Enterococcus faecalis* endocarditis with ampicillin plus ceftriaxone. *Ann Intern Med*. 2007;146:575-579.
111. Greenhow TL, Hung YY, Herz AM. Changing epidemiology of bacteremia in infants aged 1 week to 3 months. *Pediatrics*. 2012;129:e590-e596.
113. Gurnee EA, Ndao IM, McGhee JE, et al. Fecal carriage of methicillin-resistant *Staphylococcus aureus* and vancomycin-resistant *Enterococcus* in healthy children. *Antimicrob Agents Chemother*. 2014;58:1261-1262.
128. Ibrahim SL, Zhang L, Brady TM, et al. Low-dose gentamicin for uncomplicated Enterococcus faecalis bacteremia may be nephrotoxic in children. *Clin Infect Dis*. 2015;61:1119-1124.
129. Iosifidis E, Evdoridou I, Agakidou E, et al. Vancomycin-resistant *Enterococcus* outbreak in a neonatal intensive care unit: epidemiology, molecular analysis and risk factors. *Am J Infect Control*. 2013;41:857-861.
159. Lebreton F, van Schaik W, McGuire AM, et al. Emergence of epidemic multidrug-resistant *Enterococcus faecium* from animal and commensal strains. *MBio*. 2013;20:4.
181. McCracken M, Wong A, Mitchell R, et al. Molecular epidemiology of vancomycin-resistant enterococcal bacteremia: results from the Canadian Nosocomial Infection Surveillance Program, 1999-2009. *J Antimicrob Chemother*. 2013;68:1505-1509.
208. Musarrat J, Zhanel GG, Sparling R, Holley RA. Horizontal transfer of antibiotic resistance from Enterococcus faecium of fermented meat origin to clinical isolates of *E. faecalis* and *E. faecium*. *Int J Food Microbiol*. 2015;199:78-85.
223. Paganella F, deBeen M, Braat JC, et al. Distinct SagA from hospital associated clade A1 *Enterococcus faecium* strains contributes to biofilm formation. *Appl Environ Microbiol*. 2015;81:6873-6882.
224. Pammi M, Zhong D, Johnson Y, Revell P, Versalovic J. Polymicrobial bloodstream infections in the neonatal intensive care unit are associated with increased mortality: a case-control study. *BMC Infect Dis*. 2014;14:390.
237. Reyes J, Panesso D, Tran TT, et al. A *liaR* deletion restores susceptibility to daptomycin and antimicrobial peptides in multidrug-resistant *Enterococcus faecalis*. *J Infect Dis*. 2015;211:1317-1325.
248. Rusconi R, Bergamaschi S, Cazzavillan A, Carnelli V. Clivus osteomyelitis secondary to *Enterococcus faecium* infection in a 6-year-old girl. *Int J Pediatr Otorhinolaryngol*. 2005;69:1265-1268.
250. Sader HS, Jones RN. Antimicrobial susceptibility of gram-positive bacteria isolated from US medical centers: results of the daptomycin surveillance program (2007-2008). *Diag Microbiol Infect Dis*. 2009;65:158-162.
288. Tamma PD, Sklansky DJ, Palazzi DL, Swami SK, Milstone AM. Antibiotic susceptibility of common pediatric uropathogens in the United States. *Clin Infect Dis*. 2014;59:750-752.

295. Tran TT, Panesso D, Gao H, et al. Whole-genome analysis of a daptomycin-susceptible *Enterococcus faecium* strain and its daptomycin-resistant variant arising during therapy. *Antimicrob Agents Chemother.* 2013;57:261-268.
302. Viani RM, Bromberg K, Bradley JS. Obturator internus muscle abscess in children: report of seven cases and review. *Clin Infect Dis.* 1999;28:117-122.
304. Wang Y, Lv Y, Cai J, et al. A novel gene, *optrA*, that confers transferable resistance to oxazolidinones and phenicols and its presence in *Enterococcus faecalis* and *Enterococcus faecium* of human and animal origin. *J Antimicrob Chemother.* 2015;70:2182-2190.

The full reference list for this chapter is available at ExpertConsult.com.

84B ■ Viridans Streptococcal Infections

J. Chase McNeil

VIRIDANS STREPTOCOCCAL INFECTIONS

The group of *Streptococcus* species characterized as viridans, α-hemolytic, or oral streptococci is ubiquitously present on the human oral mucosa. These organisms are important pathogens in children and adults alike; they cause infections ranging from caries and bacterial endocarditis in immunocompetent hosts to fatal sepsis in neutropenic persons.

None of the terms applied to this group is entirely satisfactory. Not all members of the α-hemolytic streptococci are α-hemolytic, some being γ-hemolytic (nonhemolytic) or even β-hemolytic. Furthermore *Streptococcus pneumoniae,* which is α-hemolytic, is not considered a member of the viridans group. The term "viridans streptococci" is likewise inadequate, because "viridans," derived from the Latin *viridis* (green), refers to the sheen caused by partial hemolysis around α-hemolytic colonies on sheep blood agar. The term "oral streptococci" circumvents the dilemma of outliers in the hemolytic classification schema; however, viridans streptococci are found in sites other than the oral cavity, and nonviridans streptococcal species are frequently present in the oral cavity. In accordance with the American Society for Microbiology's most recent guidance,[273] the term "viridans streptococci" is used here for this diverse group of bacteria, with the understanding that member organisms are typically but not invariably α-hemolytic. We further note that viridans refers not to a species of streptococci but rather to a group of species, notwithstanding erroneous references to *Streptococcus viridans.*[297]

Streptococci have been reclassified on the basis of molecular and genetic studies[66,273]; however, this reclassification may cause clinical confusion for the short term. For example, certain small-colony β-hemolytic streptococci, including some in Lancefield group A, are now considered to be viridans streptococci. The hope is that classification based on molecular similarities will eventually lead to a clearer understanding of the infectious diseases associated with these organisms. One should recognize, however, that the current knowledge of viridans streptococcal infections is based predominantly on studies of the α-hemolytic members of the viridans group.

MICROBIOLOGY

Streptococci are gram-positive, catalase-negative bacteria that are spherical or ovoid and less than 2 μm in diameter. They are facultatively anaerobic and nonmotile and do not produce spores or gas. Some strains require an atmosphere enriched with carbon dioxide (5%). The enterococci (distinguished by their ability to grow in 6.5% sodium chloride) and lactococci (formerly Lancefield group N streptococci) were previously classified as streptococci but have now been assigned to separate genera.

Fig. 84B.1 is a classification schema for the clinically important streptococcal species. Hemolysis of blood agar remains a key tool for classifying streptococci. Strains that are β-hemolytic are further characterized according to colony size and Lancefield group (a serologic

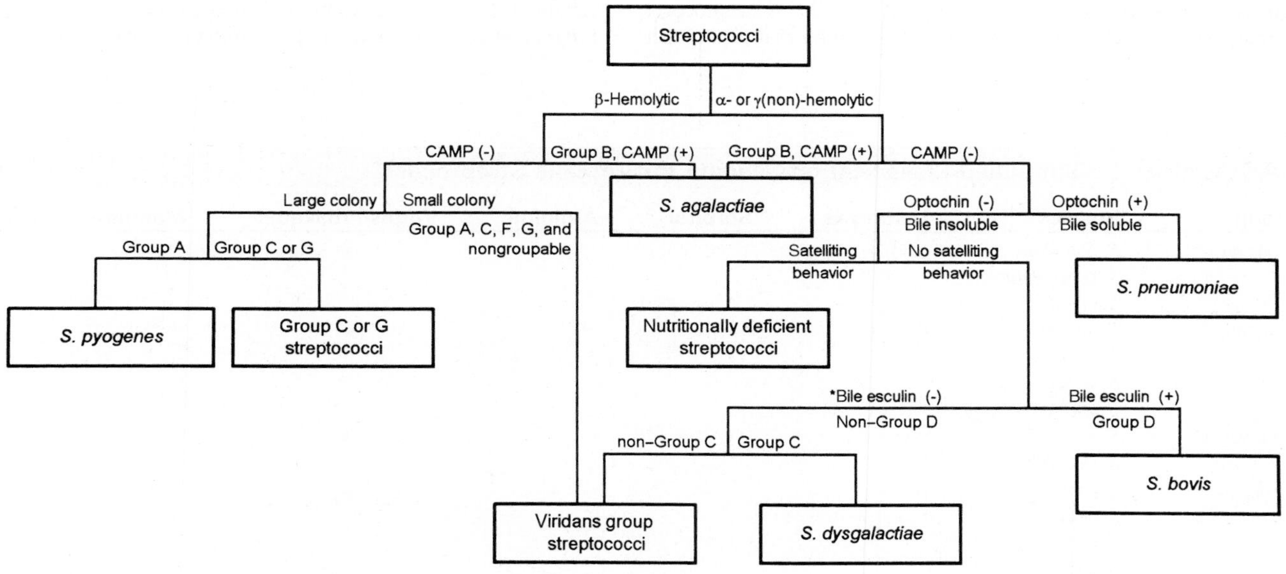

FIG. 84B.1 Schema for the identification of clinically important streptococcal species. Viridans group species are, in general, those remaining after identification of other streptococcal species. *CAMP,* Christie, Atkins, and Munch-Peterson test.

classification system based on cell wall carbohydrate). Group B *Streptococcus agalactiae* strains can typically be identified by β-hemolysis and a positive Christie, Atkins, and Munch-Peterson (CAMP) test result[273]; however, some strains of *S. agalactiae* that are α- or γ-hemolytic also produce a positive CAMP test result.

Large-colony, β-hemolytic, group A streptococci make up the species *Streptococcus pyogenes.* Most other large-colony, β-hemolytic streptococci are group C or G streptococci, and they are occasionally pathogenic. Among the α- or γ-hemolytic streptococci, *S. agalactiae* (group B streptococci) and *S. pneumoniae* are generally identified by positive CAMP and Optochin test results, respectively. Bile solubility confirms an Optochin-susceptible isolate as *S. pneumoniae*; however, some *Streptococcus mitis* isolates (as determined by genetic sequencing) yield similar results.[178]

Nutritionally deficient streptococci are identified by their requirement for the presence of a second bacterial species (*Staphylococcus aureus* is typically used in testing) to maintain growth on agar. These streptococci will generally grow in blood culture media in the absence of reduced nicotinamide adenine dinucleotide produced by a second bacterial species and may demonstrate some growth on agar in the absence of other bacteria. Nutritionally deficient streptococci were once classified as viridans streptococci, but more recent studies have assigned these organisms to a new genus: *Abiotrophia adjacens* and *Abiotrophia defectiva.*[164] With the exception of *Enterococcus* spp., streptococci that are α- or γ-hemolytic, possess Lancefield group D antigen, and are bile esculin positive may be tentatively identified as *Streptococcus bovis.* This species was once considered a viridans streptococcus but is now classified separately.

Strains of one species of group C streptococci, *Streptococcus dysgalactiae,* are α- or γ-hemolytic. These strains must also be distinguished from the viridans group. A species once included in the viridans group, *Streptococcus morbillorum,* was reclassified as *Gemella morbillorum.*[167]

The *S. anginosus* group, sometimes referred to as the *S. milleri* group, includes *S. anginosus, S. constellatus,* and *S. intermedius.* These can be either β-hemolytic or nonhemolytic, often have small colonies, and may belong to any number of different Lancefield groups (A, C, G, F, or un-typeable). The *S. anginosus* group can be distinguished from other β-hemolytic streptococci based on a positive Voges-Proskauer reaction.[104] These organisms are often grouped together with viridans streptococci (and will be discussed briefly later); however, they truly have a different taxonomic classification.

The remaining streptococcal organisms may tentatively be identified as viridans group streptococci. Thus, in practice, viridans streptococci continue to be characterized by the absence of features that distinguish other major streptococcal pathogens. Viridans streptococci have no characteristics that can be used to definitively confirm their identity in the standard microbiology laboratory.

Classification of species within the viridans streptococci group has also been challenging. Several schemata have been developed over the years, including those of Carlsson,[48] Coleman and Williams,[62] Facklam,[103] Ruoff and Kunz,[271,272] and Coykendall.[66] However, each of these schemata lacks reliable markers for member species, and clinical isolates are inconsistently classified as a result. Consequently efforts to characterize the clinical features of infections according to individual viridans streptococcal species have been largely unsuccessful. Molecular and polymerase chain reaction (PCR)–based taxonomies have been used to classify viridans streptococci,[5,66,232,270,359] but these techniques are generally unavailable in the clinical laboratory. Given the current flux in the taxonomy of these organisms, the American Society for Microbiology has advocated a simplified, practical approach to classifying viridans streptococci (Table 84B.1).[273] The biochemical tests available in many clinical microbiology laboratories can be used to assign clinical isolates to one of the five groups to which the 14 clinically important viridans streptococcal species belong. Rapid molecular nucleotide sequence analysis and PCR–based tests are available for tentative identification of individual viridans streptococcal species.[110,121,239,272,323] However, precise identification of species currently has clinical significance only as an epidemiologic tool.

EPIDEMIOLOGY

Viridans streptococci are the predominant oral microflora of humans; they are also commonly found in other areas of the upper respiratory tract, throughout the gastrointestinal tract, and in the female genital tract. Viridans streptococci are occasionally identified as skin flora.

Viridans streptococci begin colonizing neonates shortly after birth. By 1 month of age, virtually all infants are colonized with at least one species of viridans streptococci.[236] The mix of colonizing species varies with human ontogeny. For example, *Streptococcus mutans,* a species implicated in the development of caries, is rarely found in predentate children but is commonly present after the eruption of teeth.[50,90,321] The ecology of other viridans streptococcal species also appears to be affected by the eruption of teeth.[51,90,299,321] In addition to these temporal factors in the colonization of infants and children, individual viridans streptococcal species preferentially colonize certain anatomic areas of the oral cavity and pharynx. For example, *Streptococcus sanguis* is the predominant isolate of the buccal mucosa but is rarely found on the dorsum of the tongue, where *S. mitis* is the predominant species.[114] Diet may also

TABLE 84B.1 Simplified Classification Schema for Viridans Streptococci

Group	Species	Hemolysis	Sorbitol	Arginine	Voges-Proskauer	Mannitol	Esculin
S. anginosus[a]	*S. anginosus*	α, β, γ	–	+	+	±	±
	S. constellatus					–	
	S. intermedius					±	
S. mutans	*S. mutans*	β, γ, α	+	–	+	+	+
	S. sobrinus						
	S. rattus						
	S. cricetus						
S. salivarius	*S. salivarius*	γ, α	–	–	+	–	+
	S. vestibularis						
S. sanguis	*S. sanguis*	α	–	+	–	–	+
	S. gordonii						+
	S. parasanguis						±
	S. crista						–
S. mitis	*S. mitis*[b]	α	–	–	–	–	–

[a]Previously referred to as *S. milleri* group.
[b]Previously included *S. mitis, S. sanguis II,* and *S. oralis.*
Data from Coykendall AL. Classification and identification of the viridans streptococci. *Clin Microbiol Rev.* 1989;2:315–28; and Ruoff KL. *Streptococcus.* In: Murray PR, Baron EJ, Pfaller MA, et al, eds. *Manual of Clinical Microbiology.* 6th ed. Washington, DC: American Society for Microbiology; 1995:299–307.

affect viridans streptococcal ecology. For example, the low oral pH that can result from consumption of sugar-containing beverages and other carbohydrates favors colonization with caries-producing *S. mutans.*[129,318]

Little is known about the transmission of viridans streptococci in general, but studies have shown that *S. mutans* is commonly transmitted within families, especially from mother to child, and among young school children.[4,47,82,136,274] Toothbrushes may be an important vehicle of transmission of viridans streptococci in children.[193] A normal dishwasher cycle eliminates *S. mutans* from toothbrushes.[22] The hands of hospital personnel, especially those with skin disorders such as eczema, may also be a vehicle for transmission.[59] In addition, paper dental records have been suggested as a vehicle for the transmission of viridans streptococci.[68]

Viridans streptococci play an important role in the ecology of the oral flora by protecting against potentially more invasive pathogens via colonization resistance.[21,119] This mechanism was demonstrated by a double-blind study in which patients who had completed antibiotic therapy for group A streptococcal pharyngitis were treated with either a preparation containing four species of viridans streptococci or a placebo. None of the 17 patients in the treated group experienced recurrence of group A streptococcal pharyngitis, whereas pharyngitis recurred in 7 (37%) of the 19 patients in the placebo group.[263] A second double-blind, placebo-controlled multicenter trial by the same group confirmed these findings.[264] Viridans streptococci may also contribute to colonization resistance to pathogens such as methicillin-resistant *S. aureus* in the infant oral cavity[337]; nontypeable *Haemophilus influenzae*, *S. pneumoniae*, and *Moraxella catarrhalis* at the eustachian tube orifice[320]; and *Neisseria gonorrhoeae* in the female genital tract.[203] In addition to competing for mucosal adherence sites, viridans streptococci produce hydrogen peroxide and bacteriocins that inhibit certain competing bacteria; this mechanism may also contribute to colonization resistance.[69,71,338,343] Conversion of the hydrogen peroxide to ozone in the oral cavity may play a role in colonization resistance to other bacterial species and to *Candida* species.[336]

PATHOGENESIS

Viridans streptococci are typically low-virulence organisms; when they do cause infection, it is usually nonpyogenic with the exception of infections caused by the *Streptococcus anginosus (milleri)* subgroup. They are implicated most often in localized infections of the sinuses and oral cavity, including the teeth, after the tissues are directly invaded by colonizing organisms. Caries is a dental disease that develops during a period of years, often in association with *S. mutans* infection interacting with other oral flora.[171] Patients with cystic fibrosis may be particularly susceptible to caries because of a decreased buffering capacity.[49] Viridans streptococci are associated with a variety of gingival diseases, possibly including gingival hyperplasia accompanying chronic phenytoin administration. In an experimental animal model, phenytoin-induced gingival hyperplasia was more advanced in rats infected with *Streptococcus sobrinus* than in uninfected control animals.[220] On occasion, viridans streptococci, usually organisms of the *S. anginosus* subgroup, cause pyogenic infections, including abscesses in the brain, lung, and abdomen. An intriguing preliminary study suggested that viridans streptococcal–related dental disease is associated with the subsequent development of coronary artery disease.[185] Viridans streptococci are among the microorganisms isolated from atherosclerotic plaque, although their role in the pathogenesis of atherosclerosis is unknown.[57] Typically viridans streptococci cause life-threatening infection only when the oral mucosa is disrupted and the host's mechanisms of microbial clearance are compromised by conditions such as neutropenia or cardiac valve disease.

It is the preponderance of viridans streptococci in the oral flora, rather than their virulence, that accounts for their predominance in infections originating in the mouth. In a study of 36 children who underwent extraction of normal or abscessed teeth, 11 (30%) had postextraction positive blood cultures, and viridans streptococci were exclusively isolated in all 11.[306] Bacteremia occurred more commonly after removal of diseased teeth (37%), but it also occurred after removal of normal teeth (23%). In a small study, children with dental caries had a higher burden of *S. mutans* in the saliva than those children without caries, suggesting that the relative proportion of oral species play a role in dental pathology.[224]

Another study of 58 children who underwent dental extraction included 26 who received penicillin, amoxicillin, or erythromycin prophylaxis because of a risk of endocarditis.[65] Bacteremia was detected in only 9 (35%) of the 26 children who received prophylaxis and in 20 (63%) of 32 children who did not ($P < .05$). In this study, viridans streptococci accounted for 37% of the blood isolates, strict anaerobes accounted for 26.5%, and a variety of organisms accounted for the remainder. The number of colony-forming units per milliliter of blood ranged from 2 to 12. Even within a single colony-forming unit, more than one bacterial species was sometimes identified after subculture.

In a study from Spain, bacteremia was detected in 96%, 64%, and 20% of patients 30 seconds, 15 minutes, and 1 hour after dental extractions, respectively.[330] This study indicates that bacteremia after dental procedures may not be as transient as was generally believed.

A study of 30 subjects with chronic periodontitis and 30 subjects with periodontal health showed that 40% and 41% had bacteremia during dental flossing; viridans streptococci were the most common isolate in both groups.[67] Roughly half of positive subjects remained positive 10 minutes after flossing.

Although these two studies differed in the diversity of organisms isolated, both indicated that viridans streptococci are the organisms most likely to invade the blood after trauma to the oral cavity. Viridans streptococcal bacteremia also occurs commonly during orthodontic banding[102] and esophageal stricture dilation, also reflecting the predominance of these organisms in the oral and salivary flora.[365]

The ability of viridans streptococci to bind to oral mucosa, dental surfaces, and dental plaque by interaction with specific microbial and host "receptors" accounts for the preferential colonization of the oral cavity by these organisms.[341] This interaction also helps explain the localization of the various viridans streptococcal species to distinct anatomic sites as well as the involvement of ontologic factors in colonization. The precise nature of bacterial adherence to the oral mucosa is not defined but appears to involve streptococcal lipoteichoic acid.[146] Through release of modulin protein I/II, viridans streptococci induce the expression of adhesion molecules such as E-selectin and intercellular (ICAM-1) and vascular cell (VCAM-1) adhesion molecules on endothelial cells, promote transendothelial migration of neutrophils in vitro, and induce cytokine release in epithelial (interleukin-6 [IL-6]) and endothelial (IL-6 and IL-8) cells.[345,346] Orthodontic appliances favor the proliferation of *S. mutans.*[332] The host's immune status also may be an important determinant of adherence and subsequent invasion. For example immunocompetent persons produce secretory IgA to *S. mutans,*[13] and these antibodies are capable of preventing caries in a rodent model.[212] Viridans streptococci within the biofilm present in dental plaque are at least 500 times more resistant to antibiotic treatment than is predicted on the basis of their susceptibility in culture medium; this finding suggests that antibiotic treatment cannot eradicate viridans streptococci from dental plaque, even temporarily.[173]

At the University of Texas M. D. Anderson Cancer Center in Houston, the incidence of viridans streptococcal bacteremia increased extraordinarily between 1972 and 1989, from one to 47 cases per 10,000 admissions.[93] A risk factor analysis indicated that patients were significantly predisposed to the development of bacteremia by prophylactic administration of TMP-SMX or a fluoroquinolone, profound neutropenia, or the administration of antacids or histamine type 2 receptor antagonists.[93] Presumably, administration of the implicated antibiotics and antacids favored the overgrowth of viridans streptococci and their proliferation throughout the gastrointestinal tract, which in turn would favor viridans streptococcal bacteremia in an immunocompromised host, especially a neutropenic host whose mucosal barrier was disrupted by cytotoxic chemotherapy. Notably although administration of cytosine arabinoside (cytarabine, Ara-C) was identified as a major risk factor for viridans streptococcal sepsis in many other studies,34·35·45·84·152·198·209·257 it did not emerge as a risk factor in this study. In a recent Canadian study, a higher cumulative dose of cytarabine was associated with viridans streptococcal bacteremia in children with acute myelogenous leukemia, although this was not associated with streptococcal septic shock per se.[181]

The ability to adhere to damaged cardiac valves and vegetations is a key factor in the pathogenesis of viridans streptococcal endocarditis. Strains of viridans streptococci carried by healthy children adhered less well to buccal and endocardial cells than did strains isolated from children with viridans streptococcal endocarditis.[283,284] Lipoteichoic acid is thought to help mediate adhesion of viridans streptococci to endocardium, and the effectiveness of penicillin prophylaxis may reflect its reduction of lipoteichoic acid on the bacterial cell surface.[187]

The ability of antibiotics to alter the surface properties of bacteria, even those resistant to the bactericidal action of the drug, may be an important determinant of the effectiveness of prophylactic antibiotics.[187,295] In the host, fibronectin is an important determinant of viridans streptococcal binding to damaged endothelium. Although viridans streptococci do not bind to soluble fibronectin, a reactive fibronectin binding domain becomes available when the fibronectin molecule is immobilized, as in endocarditis.[186] Mutant viridans streptococci that were unable to bind to fibronectin were shown to be significantly less virulent in an animal model of endocarditis.[186]

The ability of viridans streptococci to induce platelet aggregation also may be a factor in the pathogenesis of endocarditis.[111,194] In viridans streptococci–challenged, anticoagulated rabbits, only microscopic vegetations developed despite fulminant sepsis, indicating inability to limit the infection. In contrast, viridans streptococci–challenged, nonanticoagulated animals tended to have large vegetations and a subacute course.[149] These findings are concordant with those of a separate study showing that the density of bacteria within vegetations was greater in viridans streptococci–challenged thrombocytopenic rabbits than in nonthrombocytopenic control animals; these results suggest that platelets limit progression of the disease.[314] Surprisingly neutropenia appears to have little effect on susceptibility to endocarditis in animal models, although it impedes containment of the infection.[207,208]

In neutropenic cancer patients and those who have undergone bone marrow transplantation, viridans streptococci cause septic shock and adult respiratory distress syndrome (ARDS). Viridans streptococci also induce nephritis in experimental models.[6,325] Little is known about the mechanisms involved in the pathogenesis of these conditions. Viridans streptococci produce no endotoxin, and no specific exotoxins have been identified. Nonetheless products of these organisms can activate complement[218] and induce production of tumor necrosis factor-α (TNF-α) and TNF-β, IL-1, IL-2, IL-6, IL-8, interferon-γ, and nitric oxide.[23,98,138,202,230,301,303,317] Strains isolated from patients with sepsis were found to induce TNF-β and IL-8 production more potently than colonizing strains isolated from healthy subjects.[304] A study of two neutropenic patients with fatal viridans streptococcal sepsis showed high blood levels of IL-6, especially late in the course of infection, whereas levels of IL-1 and TNF-α were unremarkable.[96] Viridans streptococcal lipoteichoic acid induces production of cytokines and nitric oxide in vitro,[98,218] but the clinical significance of these observations is not known. Unlike blood-borne group A streptococci isolated from patients with septic shock, viridans streptococci isolated from the blood of pediatric cancer patients with septic shock do not express superantigens in vitro.[228] Thus intravenous immune globulin, which has been suggested as an adjuvant therapy for group A streptococcal shock, may not be effective in cases of viridans streptococcal sepsis.

CLINICAL MANIFESTATIONS

The viridans streptococcal species are diverse, and consequently the infections they cause show a variety of clinical manifestations. Typically the viridans streptococci cause nonpyogenic infections such as bacteremia and endocarditis, whereas the *S. anginosus* group tends to cause invasive pyogenic infections, including bone infections, brain abscesses, appendicitis, and pulmonary and abdominal abscesses.[221]

Sepsis in Immunocompromised Hosts

For obscure reasons, the relative incidence of gram-positive bacterial infections, especially viridans streptococcal infections, has increased in immunocompromised hosts during the past 2 or 3 decades. Viridans streptococci were first identified as an important cause of sepsis in neutropenic patients with cancer in 1978, when 29 episodes were reported in adults and children at the National Cancer Institute[243] and six episodes were reported in children at the M.D. Anderson Cancer Center.[145] The significance of blood isolates of viridans streptococci in the setting of cancer had previously not been generally appreciated. The fact that no deaths occurred in the original National Cancer Institute series or in a subsequent series from that institute[268] suggested that viridans streptococci produce a benign bacteremia similar to that caused by coagulase-negative staphylococci. In contrast, three of the six children at M. D. Anderson died. Several other centers in Europe and North America have reported fulminant, sometimes fatal viridans streptococcal sepsis in patients with cancer and in patients who have received transplants.* Overall, the reported death rate associated with viridans streptococcal sepsis has ranged from 0% to 50%; most centers report mortality rates of approximately 10%. In some centers, viridans streptococci are the most common cause of fatal and nonfatal sepsis.[26,34,128,135] The incidence of viridans streptococcal sepsis appears to be higher in children than in adults.[201,310] In a study from St. Jude's Children's Research Hospital from 1983 to 2008, viridans streptococci accounted for 63 of 702 (8.9%) bloodstream isolates from children with cancer.[204] In a recent Italian study of both adults and adolescents who underwent hematopoietic stem cell transplantation, viridans streptococci accounted for 8% of bloodstream infection posttransplant with an 8% 30-day mortality.[214]

The oral cavity is the most common portal of entry in immunocompromised hosts. Catheter-related viridans streptococcal bacteremia is unusual as determined by quantitative culture of simultaneous peripheral and catheter blood specimens. However, because administration of antacid is a risk factor,[93] the lower gastrointestinal tract is likely to be a portal of entry in some patients taking antacids and potentially in other circumstances. Several factors predispose patients to viridans streptococcal sepsis. Profound neutropenia is clearly a predisposing factor,[34,93] although viridans streptococcal bacteremia occasionally develops in cancer patients with absolute neutrophil counts greater than 1000/mm^3. Mucositis, especially oral mucositis, is a well-recognized risk factor.[34,35,93,128,198,209] Cytarabine appears to incur a risk even greater than that caused by its induction of clinically apparent mucositis,[34,35,45,84,97,152,198,209,257] although this greater risk has not been observed in at least one study.[122] Chemotherapy does markedly alter the oral flora, with 25 species identified only after chemotherapy in one study.[222] The use of prophylactic TMP-SMX or quinolones is also an important risk factor.[34,35,60,93,108,128,238] The observation that administration of acyclovir may decrease the incidence of viridans streptococcal bacteremia in transplant patients suggests that herpes simplex virus infection may be a risk factor as well.[258] Allogeneic bone marrow transplantation has also been associated with increased risk of viridans streptococcal sepsis, which increases the mortality rate by a factor of 4.[198] Development of viridans streptococcal sepsis has also been observed to be associated with menstruation.[93]

The hallmark clinical feature of viridans streptococcal sepsis in an immunocompromised host is fever that typically is high, coincides with neutropenia and mucositis, and frequently lasts for several days after viable organisms are cleared from the blood. Most patients recover uneventfully. However, fulminant septic shock may occur. Shock may appear early, although it is often delayed for 2 or 3 days after the onset of sepsis, and it occurs despite prompt sterilization of blood by effective antibiotics.[310] ARDS frequently occurs in severe cases, usually 2 or 3 days after the initial bacteremia.[12,93,322] Focal complications, including pneumonia, encephalopathy,[280] and meningitis, are uncommon. Rash and palmar desquamation may be present but are not common.[93] For unexplained reasons, the incidence of aspergillosis is increased after viridans streptococcal sepsis in children with cancer.[229]

Several studies have implicated *S. mitis* as a more pathogenic species of viridans streptococci that has a greater likelihood of causing shock and ARDS in patients with cancer,[12,35,61,88,137,205,310,322] but other studies have found no clear relationship between clinical features and species.[93] *S. mitis* is the closest known relative of *S. pneumoniae,* and the two species share numerous pathogenicity genes.[75] Investigators at M. D. Anderson Cancer Center used multilocus sequence analysis to classify

*References.12, 15, 26, 34, 35, 45, 61, 63, 93, 128, 131, 140, 151, 174, 198, 201, 238, 255, 257, 294, 302, 310, 349.

viridans streptococci into species and investigate associations with severity of illness. *S. mitis/oralis* species were more often associated with a severe bacteremia phenotype even when correcting for the presence of neutropenia.[293] *S. mitis* isolated from cancer patients with sepsis has also been found to be more antibiotic resistant than other species of viridans streptococci isolated from the same patient population.[137]

Neonatal Sepsis, Meningitis, and Other Infections

Viridans streptococci are normal inhabitants of the female genital tract and are a common cause of chorioamnionitis and subsequent abortion.[10] They are also a frequent cause of neonatal sepsis and meningitis.[2,30,40,115,182,219,352] Viridans streptococci do not ordinarily colonize the skin of newborns and should not entirely be dismissed as contaminants when they are isolated from normally sterile sites.[2] At some newborn centers, the incidence of bacteremia and meningitis caused by viridans streptococci has approached or exceeded that caused by group B streptococci, although viridans streptococcal infections tend to be less severe.[40,219] *Streptococcus oralis* (*S. mitis*) caused more than half of the cases in one study.[352] The portal of entry of the organism is generally unknown in this setting, but a fetal scalp electrode was implicated in one case.[116] Unusual manifestations in newborns include pharyngitis and epiglottitis,[37] endocarditis,[206] and conjunctivitis.[170] Viridans streptococci also account for 6% to 12% of community-acquired bacteremias, with a higher prevalence in children than in adults.[319]

Endocarditis

Viridans streptococci are a common cause of endocarditis at all ages because of the organism's ability to adhere to diseased endocardium and its frequent implication in bacteremia after dental procedures and routine mouth care. A study at a teaching hospital in Finland found that, starting in 1995, *S. aureus* overtook viridans streptococci as a cause of endocarditis.[139] A review of published series by Elder and Baltimore showed a shift in the microbiologic etiologies of endocarditis in children from viridans streptococci to *S. aureus* predominance in the modern era of surgical repair of congenital heart disease.[91] However, a study in Minnesota found no significant change in the etiology of endocarditis between 1970 and 2000; viridans streptococci remained the most common cause.[329] A study in Israel noted that *Candida albicans* was the most common cause of hospital-associated endocarditis in children, whereas viridans streptococcus was the most common cause of community-acquired endocarditis in children.[195] Viridans streptococci tend to cause subacute endocarditis; blood cultures may be only intermittently positive. *S. sanguis* and *S. mitis* are the species most commonly identified.[85,253,259,315,354] Complications of viridans streptococcal endocarditis include septic pulmonary emboli, congestive heart failure, pericarditis, myocardial abscess, meningitis, osteomyelitis, and glomerulonephritis.[172,253] Shock and ARDS occur in immunocompromised patients but uncommonly in immunocompetent patients with endocarditis.

Pneumonia

Pulmonary infiltrates frequently complicate viridans streptococcal sepsis in neutropenic hosts. In most cases, these infiltrates represent ARDS and not primary pneumonia. However, several cases of primary viridans streptococcal pneumonia have been reported in previously healthy persons.[118,127,196,223,249,279] In some cases, the diagnosis was supported by multiple viridans streptococcus isolates from blood in the absence of endocarditis. The incidence of viridans streptococcal pneumonia may be significantly underestimated because tracheal isolates of viridans streptococci are usually discounted as contaminants, which they may not be in all cases.[265] In children with *S. milleri* group pleuropulmonary infections, computed tomography often shows complex pleural effusion and lung abscesses, which may require drainage for optimal treatment.[177] Viridans streptococci are increasingly recognized as contributing to pulmonary infections in children with cystic fibrosis (CF), a population with a higher prevalence of antibiotic resistance among viridans streptococcal isolates.[130,233,298] The presence of certain viridans streptococci may augment the virulence of an epidemic strain of *Pseudomonas aeruginosa* among CF patients in an airway biofilm model.[355] Given the increasing incidence of viridans streptococcal infection and the escalating prevalence of antibiotic resistance among these organisms, clinicians should consider viridans streptococci as potential causes of pneumonia when they are isolated in the absence of other pathogens.

Osteomyelitis and Septic Arthritis

Viridans streptococci are unusual causes of osteomyelitis and septic arthritis. Extension of an oral infection into the mandible or maxilla is the most common cause of viridans streptococcal osteomyelitis,[235] but several cases of vertebral osteomyelitis caused by these organisms have been described.[3,44,74,269,339,350] Infection of the long bones[227,256] and septic arthritis[17] occur infrequently.

Caries

Although caries was recognized as an infectious disease in 1890 by workers trained in Robert Koch's laboratory, its infectious nature is still not accepted universally.[9,14,89] Evidence that *S. mutans* is the main cause of caries in children and adults alike is substantial,[9,14,38,290,324,335,342] but other viridans streptococci, *Lactobacillus* spp., and *Actinomyces* spp. also have cariogenic potential among the more than 700 species found in the indigenous microflora.[162,251,290,342] *S. mutans,* which colonizes the oral cavity only after the eruption of teeth, has a predilection for the dental surfaces, metabolizes sucrose, and produces a strong acid that weakens the mineral matrix of teeth, allowing the organisms to penetrate the dental structure.[52,290] Fluoridation of the water supply has been credited with strengthening tooth enamel, thereby fostering resistance to the harsh acids produced by *S. mutans.*[290] Fluoride exerts potent antibacterial activity against *S. mutans,* particularly at low pH.[52,344] Thus fluoridation of water supplies may represent, albeit in a unique form, the most widespread and successful use of antibacterial prophylaxis. Topical treatments also provide protection against the cariogenicity of *S. mutans* and in some circumstances depend on the antibacterial action of fluoride.[144,328,340,363] Short courses of oral antibiotics can substantially reduce colonization with *S. mutans* and may be an important adjunct to the treatment of caries.[309] Specially designed culture systems are available to detect and measure the concentration of *S. mutans* in plaque to monitor the effects of therapy.[38,351] Because the development of cavities typically requires a few years of infection, there is ample opportunity to interrupt the pathogenesis of this disease.[9] Meticulous attention to teeth brushing and dental hygiene can reduce the burden of *S. mutans* in the oropharynx of preschool-aged children in one randomized clinical trial, but the effect was short lived.[184] A study in Germany showed that a special long-term program begun during pregnancy and continued through the teenage years increased caries-free dentitions from 57% in the control group to 90% in the treatment group.[210]

Abscesses and Other Infections

Suppurative infections produced by viridans streptococci are typically caused by the *S. anginosus* (formerly *S. milleri*) group: *S. anginosus, S. constellatus,* and *S. intermedius.* Like *S. aureus,* members of this group resist killing by polymorphonuclear leukocytes and stimulate less chemotaxis than other viridans streptococci do.[348] *S. anginosus* is particularly prevalent in odontogenic abscesses, subdural empyemas, and epidural abscesses.[134,300] Because *S. anginosus* inhabits the upper respiratory tract and the gastrointestinal tract and is relatively invasive, this organism causes sinusitis; otitis media; meningitis; and abdominal, splenic, and perianal abscesses. It is also often identified in brain abscesses, sometimes in association with tongue piercing.* *S. anginosus* group organisms may infect the brain through a hematogenous route that originates in the oral cavity or intestinal tract or by direct invasion through the upper respiratory tract. In a recent series from Paris of children with sinogenic intracranial infections, the *S. anginosus* group were the most commonly isolated pathogens.[120] Furthermore *S. anginosus* is associated with more frequent need for neurosurgical intervention and long-term neurologic deficits.[77] Molecular analysis indicates that some cases of culture-negative intracranial abscess are caused by the *S. anginosus* group.[240] Similarly these organisms may be emerging pathogens in orbital cellulitis/abscesses in children, being the most common cause in a study from the University of Colorado.[286] Sepsis is uncommon with these purulent infections in non-neutropenic patients, usually occurring in association with an intraabdominal source.[190,276]

*References 29, 64, 95, 141, 176, 213, 217, 221, 276, 311.

Other unusual infections caused by viridans streptococci include a large outbreak of *S. mitis* pharyngitis accompanied in 50% of cases by a toxic shock–like syndrome.[189] Meningitis resulting from both hematogenous and direct spread has been observed in healthy adults.[188] Iatrogenic meningitis due to contamination by oral viridans streptococci may complicate lumbar puncture or other central nervous system procedures.[100,282,360] Lung abscesses caused by viridans streptococci may result from the aspiration of saliva.[158,249] Empyema and mediastinitis are other reported thoracic infections associated with viridans streptococci.[24,158] Myositis complicated by rhabdomyolysis in children with leukemia has been reported.[277] Viridans streptococci also are found occasionally in liver abscesses,[20,112,123] peritonitis,[28] appendicitis,[244] and endophthalmitis.[55] In solid organ transplantation patients, viridans streptococci are a common cause of cholangitis.[312]

DIAGNOSIS

Infections caused by viridans streptococci cannot be distinguished clinically from those caused by other gram-positive and gram-negative bacteria. Collection of adequate culture specimens is essential for diagnosis. Viridans streptococcal infections are typically diagnosed by culture of blood or other normally sterile tissues. The organisms may be present in low concentration. A volume of 30 mL of blood has been suggested as the optimal volume for culture in an adult-sized patient.[289] The addition of agents that neutralize the antibacterial effects of fresh blood, such as sodium polyanethol sulfonate, significantly improves the yield of blood cultures.[288] Chemotherapeutic agents may interfere with detection of viridans streptococci in blood.[237] Viridans streptococci have been reported to cross-react with *S. pneumoniae* omnisera, potentially causing false-positive results.[148]

ANTIBIOTIC SUSCEPTIBILITY

Viridans streptococci were once considered universally penicillin susceptible. Today, however, penicillin-resistant and penicillin-tolerant viridans streptococci are identified worldwide as causes of sepsis, endocarditis, meningitis, and other infections, including conjunctivitis of the newborn, making knowledge of specific antimicrobial susceptibility more important.* Penicillin resistance occurs commonly, particularly in patients receiving long-term penicillin therapy,[8,32,234,307,313] although even short courses of antibiotics may predispose patients to colonization with resistant viridans streptococci.[101,124,216] Monthly injections of penicillin do not appear to increase penicillin resistance in oral viridans streptococci.[31] In a study of more than 732 viridans groups streptococci bloodstream isolates from the M. D. Anderson Cancer Center, more than 50% were nonsusceptible to penicillin, and nonsusceptibility to third- and fourth-generation cephalosporins and meropenem was seen almost exclusively when the penicillin MIC was 2 μg/mL or greater. In a multivariate analysis, β-lactam nonsusceptibility was independently associated with nosocomial onset of infection, use of a β-lactam antibiotic as prophylaxis, and receipt of a β-lactam in the previous 30 days.[292] Antibiotic resistance is found more commonly in viridans streptococci isolated from children compared with adults, perhaps reflecting greater use of antibiotics in children.[80] Infection with penicillin-resistant viridans streptococci is associated with a higher risk for mortality than is infection with penicillin-susceptible strains.[79,305] All species of viridans streptococci may develop antibiotic resistance, although *S. mutans* rarely exhibits resistance.[157] Investigators from Seoul examined 1448 clinical isolates of viridans streptococci for antimicrobial resistance. The proportion of isolates nonsusceptible to penicillin is 40.2% of *S. sanguinis*, 60.3% of *S. mitis*, and 78.9% of *S. salivarius*.[58] By contrast, only 6.2% of the members of the *S. anginosus* group were penicillin-nonsusceptible.

Resistance to a variety of antibiotic classes has developed during the past 2 decades,[247] although resistance is still uncommon in community residents who have not had recent antibiotic treatment.[361] Resistance to cephalosporins is widespread; the general pattern of susceptibility is that cefotaxime and ceftriaxone are usually more active than cefepime and cefuroxime, which are both more active than ceftazidime and cephalexin.[81,197,241,356] Previous cephalosporin therapy is a risk factor for cephalosporin resistance, an observation particularly relevant to patients with cancer.[42,165] Resistance to fluoroquinolones, especially ciprofloxacin and ofloxacin, is common.[54,72,78,11,281,359]

Levofloxacin has greater activity against viridans streptococci than the older fluoroquinolones do, and the newer agents garenoxacin, gatifloxacin, and moxifloxacin have enhanced activity against most gram-positive pathogens, including viridans streptococci.[260,261,262,300] However, resistance develops rapidly when patients receive prophylactic quinolones, including levofloxacin and moxifloxacin.[248,326] At the Mayo Clinic in Rochester, Minnesota, 6 (16%) of 37 transplant patients receiving levofloxacin prophylaxis developed viridans streptococcal sepsis (3 experienced shock); blood isolates were resistant to levofloxacin and to gatifloxacin and moxifloxacin.[254] Resistance was associated with mutations in the quinolone resistance–determining region of GyrA or ParC. In the M. D. Anderson study, more than 70% of isolates were fluoroquinolone nonsusceptible.[292] Resistance of viridans streptococci to aminoglycosides,[163] tetracycline,[72,81,359] TMP-SMX,[72,78,81,359] clindamycin,[78,333,359] erythromycin,[39,72,78,352,353,359] other macrolide antibiotics,[7] and vancomycin[296] has also been reported. Meropenem resistance of viridans streptococci appears to increase in children with cancer who receive multiple courses of empirical therapy.[1] Isolates of *S. anginosus* have been identified with resistance to vancomycin mediated through a vanG element closely related to that seen in *E. faecalis* [308]; thankfully, however, such isolates remain extraordinarily rare.

The penicillin resistance of viridans streptococci appears to involve chromosomally mediated alterations in the organisms' penicillin-binding proteins.[252,364] Initially researchers suspected that genes conferring penicillin resistance had been acquired from *S. pneumoniae*.[87] Subsequent studies, however, indicated that penicillin resistance may have evolved first in *S. mitis* and that *S. pneumoniae* might have acquired genes mediating penicillin resistance from this and other closely related viridans streptococcal species,[53,86,246] although a recent study favors the other pathway.[153] Quinolone resistance determinants are also transmitted efficiently between viridans streptococci and *S. pneumoniae*,[156] and the *mef*(E) gene, which confers resistance to macrolides, is readily transmitted from viridans streptococci to *S. pyogenes*.[160]

The clinical impact of the development of penicillin resistance among viridans streptococci has been far reaching. The emergence of penicillin-resistant viridans streptococci may in fact be encouraging the development of vancomycin-resistant enterococci because of the increased use of vancomycin to prevent and treat viridans streptococcal infection in patients with cancer.

Overall vancomycin is the antibiotic most reliably active against viridans streptococci. Teicoplanin also has been used successfully to treat viridans streptococcal endocarditis.[357] Daptomycin, dalbavancin, quinupristin/dalfopristin, tigecycline, and linezolid are active in vitro against most clinical isolates of viridans streptococci,[107,159,168,215,275] although breakthrough septic shock due to resistant *S. anginosus* has been reported during daptomycin therapy,[231] and 43% of viridans streptococci were resistant to quinupristin/dalfopristin in a study from Finland.[183]

TREATMENT

Empirical antibiotic therapy for viridans streptococci should be based on the pattern of antibiotic susceptibility among recent local clinical isolates. Antimicrobial susceptibility testing of viridans streptococcal isolates is necessary. Limited data indicate that antibiotic susceptibility testing performed with the E-test is well correlated with agar dilution susceptibility testing.[266] Although vancomycin-resistant clinical isolates are rarely identified at present, inclusion of vancomycin in susceptibility testing is advisable. For infections other than endocarditis and meningitis, single-antibiotic therapy is usually preferred. However, in neutropenic patients with cancer, restricting antibiotic therapy to drugs active against gram-positive bacteria may increase the risk for gram-negative bacterial infections.[242] Some investigators have advocated reserving vancomycin for neutropenic patients with shock or ARDS,[333] whereas others have advocated inclusion of vancomycin in initial empirical therapy for patients with fever and neutropenia.[94,294] The IDSA guidelines for the

*References 36, 41, 92, 106, 126, 147, 170, 180, 245, 252, 334.

management of fever and neutropenia in patients with cancer recommends only including vancomycin empirically in patients with specific risk factors for gram-positive infections including cellulitis, severe mucositis, hemodynamic instability, pneumonia, or suspected catheter-related bloodstream infection.[117] Viridans streptococcal sepsis may occur in neutropenic patients despite ongoing antibiotic therapy with β-lactam agents to which the organisms are susceptible in vitro[294]; however, this phenomenon has not been observed during vancomycin therapy, thus supporting the use of this antibiotic for viridans streptococcal sepsis in neutropenic patients. In addition, various methods to measure the susceptibility of viridans streptococcus to various antibiotics commonly yield discrepant results.[191]

Combination therapy is often advocated for treatment of viridans streptococcal endocarditis[33,113,200,347] and may be considered for treatment of meningitis, especially when the pathogen is penicillin tolerant.[99] A combination of either penicillins and aminoglycosides or of vancomycin and aminoglycosides is used most commonly. Penicillin and vancomycin are thought to increase the uptake of aminoglycosides, thereby providing synergistic bactericidal activity.[362] However, a meta-analysis of five clinical trials failed to identify any overall improvement in the outcome of patients with endocarditis who were treated with β-lactam and aminoglycoside combination therapy versus β-lactam monotherapy.[105] The 2015 AHA guidelines for the management of endocarditis[16] recommend 4 weeks of intravenous penicillin G or ceftriaxone for native valve endocarditis secondary to viridans streptococci susceptible to penicillin (MIC ≤0.12 μg/mL). An alternative to this regimen in patients with good renal function and uncomplicated endocarditis is a 2-week course of penicillin or ceftriaxone both, along with gentamicin. This recommendation is based on data showing similar outcomes in select patients treated with monotherapy for 4 weeks compared to combination therapy for 2 weeks.[287] For prosthetic valve endocarditis secondary to penicillin-susceptible viridans streptococci, 6 weeks of penicillin or ceftriaxone are recommended with the optional addition gentamicin for the first 2 weeks. In the case of prosthetic valve endocarditis from penicillin-resistant streptococci, the combination of a β-lactam and gentamicin are recommended for 6 weeks. Vancomycin monotherapy has been successfully used to treat patients with penicillin-resistant viridans streptococcal endocarditis[150,169]; monotherapy with linezolid[226] or ceftriaxone[169,291] has also been used successfully.

Frequent dosing of antibiotics is generally recommended. However, because viridans streptococci exposed to combinations of penicillin or cephalosporin plus aminoglycoside appear to be susceptible to a postantibiotic effect,[46,166,175] longer dosing intervals may be satisfactory, although data are currently insufficient to support a recommendation. The duration of therapy for viridans streptococcal infections other than endocarditis has not been studied but can generally be guided by site-specific practice and individual clinical response.

In the treatment of endocarditis, penetration of antibiotics into the fibrin vegetation may be markedly impeded. Viridans streptococci produce an exopolysaccharide composed predominantly of dextran, which may limit penetration. Experimental studies indicate that the extent of exopolysaccharide production by viridans streptococcal strains affects the success rate of antimicrobial therapy.[250] Administration of dextranase to animals with experimental viridans streptococcal endocarditis enhances antibiotic efficacy, consistent with this observation.[211] In the future, such adjuvant therapies designed to reduce the size or density of valvular vegetations may offer promise for patients with endocarditis who are not helped by conventional antibiotic therapy.

Another setting in which adjuvant therapy may be considered is viridans streptococcal sepsis in neutropenic patients who have received cytarabine chemotherapy. One uncontrolled trial suggested that the early addition of high doses of corticosteroids to the antimicrobial therapeutic regimen may reduce the incidence of associated ARDS and death.[83] However, data are insufficient to recommend this approach routinely.

PREVENTION

Attempts to prevent viridans streptococcal infection have focused on three distinct settings: prevention of caries, prevention of endocarditis, and prevention of sepsis in neutropenic patients with cancer. Efforts have been successful in the first two settings. However, the emergence of penicillin-resistant viridans streptococci and concern about the future emergence of vancomycin resistance highlight the need for new approaches to prevent infection with these ubiquitous organisms. In developing such methods, investigators should keep in mind that the resistance to colonization provided by viridans streptococci can protect the host from more virulent pathogens (see Epidemiology).

The incidence of caries in the United States has been sharply reduced by fluoridation of water supplies, inclusion of fluoride in toothpaste, and modification of diet (e.g., use of sugar substitutes). Fluoride acts as an antibacterial agent that also strengthens the resistance of teeth to invasion by bacteria. The use of dental varnishes, gels, and rinses that contain fluoride or other antibacterial agents such as chlorhexidine or vancomycin may be beneficial in selected cases.[109,161,199,225] *Streptococcus salivarius*, a relatively nonpathogenic organism that produces potent bacteriocins, has been proposed for study as a probiotic.[278] There is evidence for and against the use of xylitol gum to reduce the levels of *S. mutans* in the oral cavity.[143,285]

The AHA has led a successful effort to prevent endocarditis by the administration of systemic antibiotic prophylaxis to patients with known endocardial defects who are undergoing dental procedures.[70] These efforts are aimed especially at preventing viridans streptococcal endocarditis, and penicillin is the antibiotic most commonly used. The mechanism or mechanisms by which antibiotic prophylaxis prevents endocarditis are not completely understood. In animals, endocarditis can be prevented by administration of bacteriostatic antibiotics and by maintenance of serum levels of bactericidal antibiotics that are well below the minimum inhibitory concentration for the colonizing viridans streptococci.[125] Vancomycin has been observed to prevent development of vancomycin-tolerant *S. sanguis* endocarditis in experimentally challenged animals without reducing the incidence or level of bacteremia; thus antibiotics may prevent endocarditis by reducing bacterial adherence to endocardium.[25] This hypothesis is supported by a study in which 21% of children receiving antibiotic prophylaxis developed bacteremia, in some cases with antibiotic-resistant organisms, but endocarditis rarely occurred.[142] However, studies in animals have indicated that the probability of preventing endocarditis is related to the antibiotic susceptibility of the challenging streptococcal strains.[142] A study from Sydney found that 11 of 30 patients undergoing dental scaling developed viridans streptococcal bacteremia after mouth rinsing for 2 minutes with normal saline, whereas none of 30 patients developed viridans streptococcal bacteremia after rinsing with 7.5% povidone-iodine.[56] A similar study of patients undergoing dental extraction showed a decreased duration of bacteremia if chlorhexidine mouthwashes were used prior to extraction.[18] These studies provide promising alternatives for prophylaxis, given the increasing resistance to antibiotics found in oral flora.

Prophylaxis should be carefully targeted[331] and administered immediately before dental procedures. An increase in the number of blood-borne antibiotic-resistant viridans streptococci can be detected within 6 hours of antibiotic treatment and persists for 9 days or longer.[179] Experimental studies of the prevention of endocarditis by antibiotic administration *after* challenge with bacterial inocula have yielded inconsistent results,[27,155,192] and the clinical utility of this approach is unknown. Topical treatment with vancomycin or chlorhexidine has been advocated as an adjuvant in preventing endocarditis, but its efficacy is unproved.[316,358] In 2007, the AHA revised its guidelines on the criteria for antibiotic prophylaxis to prevent endocarditis making the criteria more restrictive in an effort to curb unnecessary antibiotic administration. Notably, this has not been associated with a rise in endocarditis cases, suggesting that indeed many more patients were being previously prescribed prophylaxis than was necessary.[76]

In recent years, viridans streptococcal infections have presented a major problem in neutropenic patients with cancer and in patients who have received bone marrow transplants. Because penicillin-resistant viridans streptococci are widespread, some cancer centers include vancomycin in the initial empirical antibiotic regimen for febrile neutropenic patients.[294] In addition, despite concern about promoting vancomycin resistance, bone marrow transplant physicians are administering intravenous vancomycin prophylactically to high-risk patients in an effort to prevent viridans streptococcal sepsis; results of an observational cohort study support this practice.[154]

Uncontrolled trials of oral vancomycin paste[19] and vancomycin mouthwash[43] in children receiving cytotoxic chemotherapy suggested their efficacy in preventing viridans streptococcal infection. However, an increase in colonization and infection with vancomycin-resistant enterococci is a predictable consequence of increased vancomycin use. Therefore the CDC has recommended that empirical vancomycin therapy be avoided when it is feasible and encouraged investigators to explore alternatives to the empirical or prophylactic use of vancomycin.

In a comparative trial, penicillin prophylaxis was superior to TMP-SMX prophylaxis in preventing viridans streptococcal infections in patients with cancer, despite extensive colonization with penicillin-resistant streptococci.[133] In other studies, oral prophylaxis with penicillin or roxithromycin (a macrolide antibiotic) also appeared to reduce the incidence of viridans streptococcal infection in patients with cancer in comparison to historical controls.[73,267,305] In contrast, prophylactic ampicillin did not reduce the incidence of viridans streptococcal sepsis in patients receiving autologous bone marrow transplants, and the incidence of penicillin resistance increased.[32] Other penicillin prophylaxis trials have also observed increased penicillin resistance.[32] The CDC does not recommend the routine use of penicillin prophylaxis in patients receiving bone marrow transplants.[132]

Levofloxacin prophylaxis is currently commonly used to prevent bacterial infections in adults with cancer, but there is concern that viridans streptococci rapidly develop quinolone resistance.[327] Among 45 children with acute myeloid leukemia cared for at Children's Hospital Los Angeles, ciprofloxacin prophylaxis was associated with a decline in bacteremia episodes from gram-negative bacteria but a subsequent increase in bacteremia due to gram-positive agents, largely viridans streptococci.[108] Innovative prophylactic methods and carefully designed clinical trials are needed to identify effective prophylactic measures, especially for patients at high risk, such as children undergoing chemotherapy for acute myeloid leukemia.

NEW REFERENCES SINCE THE SEVENTH EDITION

16. Baddour LM, Wilson WR, Bayer AS, et al. Infective endocarditis in adults: diagnosis, antimicrobial therapy and management of complications: A scientific statement for healthcare professional from the American Heart Association. *Circulation.* 2015;132:1435-1486.
18. Barbosa M, Prada-Lopez I, Alvarez M, et al. Post-tooth extraction bacteraemia: a randomized clinical trial on the efficacy of chlorhexidine prophylaxis. *PLoS ONE.* 2015;10:e0124249.
58. Chun S, Huh HJ, Lee NY. Species-specific difference in antimicrobial susceptibility among viridans group streptococci. *Ann Lab Med.* 2015;35:205-211.
76. DeSimone DC, Tleyiah IM, Correa de Sa DD, et al. Incidence of infective endocarditis due to viridans group streptococci before and after the 2007 American Heart Association's prevention guidelines: an extended evaluation of the Olmsted County, Minnesota, population and nationwide inpatient sample. *Mayo Clin Proc.* 2015;90:874-881.
77. Deutschmann MW, Livingstone D, Cho JJ, et al. The significance of *Streptococcus anginosus* group in intracranial complications of pediatric rhinosinusitis. *JAMA Otolaryngol Head Neck Surg.* 2013;139:157-160.
91. Elder RW, Baltimore RS. The changing epidemiology of pediatric endocarditis. *Infect Dis Clin North Am.* 2015;29:513-524.
103. Facklam R. What happened to the streptococci: overview of taxonomic and nomenclature changes. *Clin Microbiol Rev.* 2002;15:613-630.
108. Felsenstein S, Orgel E, Rushing T, et al. Clinical and microbiologic outcomes of quinolone prophylaxis in children with acute myeloid leukemia. *Pediatr Infect Dis J.* 2015;34:e78-e84.
117. Freifeld AG, Bow EJ, Sepkowitz KA, et al. Clinical practice guideline for the use of antimicrobial agents in neutropenic patients with cancer: 2010 update by the Infectious Diseases Society of America. *Clin Infect Dis.* 2011;52:e56-e93.
120. Garin A, Thierry B, Leboulanger N, et al. Pediatric sinogenic epidural and subdural empyema: the role of endoscopic sinus surgery. *Int J Pediatr Otorhinolaryngol.* 2015;79:1752-1760.
181. Lewis V, Yanofsky R, Mitchell D, et al. Predictors and outcomes of viridans group streptococcal infections in pediatric acute myeloid leukemia: from the Canadian infection in AML research group. *Pediatr Infect Dis J.* 2014;33:126-129.
184. Liu M, Ge L, Zheng S, et al. Short-term effect of mechanical plaque control on salivary mutans streptococci in preschool children. *Oral Health Prev Dent.* 2014;12:219-224.
204. McCullers JA, Williams BF, Wu S, et al. Healthcare-associated infections at a children's cancer hospital, 1983–2008. *J Ped Infect Dis Soc.* 2012;1:26-34.
214. Mikulska M, Del Bono V, Bruzzi P, et al. Mortality after bloodstream infections in allogeneic hematopoietic stem cell transplant (HSCT) recipients. *Infection.* 2012;40:271-278.
224. Neves AB, Lobo LA, Pinto KC, et al. Comparison between clinical aspects and salivary microbial profile of children with and without early childhood caries: a preliminary study. *J Clin Pediatr Dent.* 2015;39:209-214.
286. Seltz LB, Smith J, Durairaj VD, et al. Microbiology and antibiotic management of orbital cellulitis. *Pediatrics.* 2011;127:e566-e572.
287. Sexton DJ, Tenenbaum MJ, Wilson WR, et al. Ceftriaxone once daily for four weeks compared with ceftriaxone plus gentamicin once daily for two weeks for treatment of endocarditis due to penicillin-susceptible streptococci. Endocarditis treatment consortium group. *Clin Infect Dis.* 1998;27:1470-1474.
292. Shelburne SA III, Laskey RE, Sahasrabjojane P, et al. Development and validation of a clinical model to predict the presence of β-lactam resistance in viridans group streptococci causing bacteremia in neutropenic cancer patients. *Clin Infect Dis.* 2014;59:223-230.
293. Shelburne SA, Sahasrabhojane P, Saldana M, et al. *Streptococcus mitis* strains causing severe clinical disease in cancer patients. *Emerg Infect Dis.* 2014;20:762-771.
308. Srinivasan V, Metcalf BJ, Knipe KM, et al. vanG element insertions with a conserved chromosomal site conferring vancomycin resistance to *Streptococcus agalactiae* and *Streptococcus anginosus. MBio.* 2014;5:e01386-14.
355. Whiley RA, Fleming EV, Makhija R, et al. Environment and colonization sequence are key parameters driving cooperation and competition between *Pseudomonas aeruginosa* cystic fibrosis strains and oral commensal strains. *PLoS ONE.* 2015;10:e0115513.

The full reference list for this chapter is available at ExpertConsult.com.

85 Pneumococcal Infections

Stephen I. Pelton • Michael R. Jacobs

RELEVANCE OF PNEUMOCOCCAL DISEASE TO CHILD HEALTH

The pneumococcus (*Streptococcus pneumoniae*) continues to be a leading cause of morbidity and mortality in persons of all ages. Its impact on child health is demonstrated by Elliott and Beeson's conclusion that it is one of the five pathogens that account for nearly half of infection-related deaths among children less than 5 years of age (Fig. 85.1)[154] Pneumococcal infections include serious diseases such as meningitis, bacteremia, and bacteremic pneumonia, as well as milder but more common illnesses, such as community-acquired pneumonia (CAP), sinusitis, and otitis media. The causative agent, *Streptococcus pneumoniae*, is found in the nasopharynx of 30% of children in high-income countries and as many as 80% of children in low-income countries.* The

*References 6, 18, 106, 119, 122, 160, 167, 191, 217, 332, 369, 380, 617.

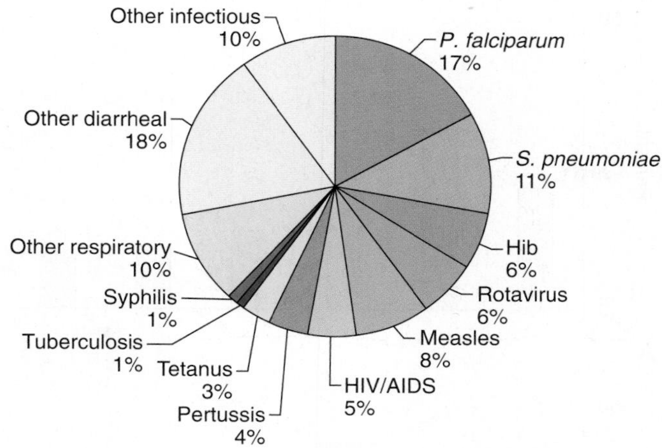

FIG. 85.1 Pathogen-specific infection-related mortality among children <5 years. Among deaths from respiratory infection, 41% were attributed to *Streptococcus pneumoniae*. (From Elliott SR, Beeson JG. Estimating the burden of global mortality in children aged <5 years by pathogen-specific causes. *Clin Infect Dis.* 2008;46:1794–5.)

pneumococcus is transmitted mainly through respiratory droplets among children and to adult contacts and was estimated to cause nearly 500,000 global deaths annually among children less than 5 years of age in 2008 by the World Health Organization.[577] Many children experience some form of pneumococcal infection (e.g., otitis media or pneumonia), but sepsis or meningitis occur in few. The continued incidence and severity of pneumococcal disease, coupled with significant case-fatality rates despite antimicrobial therapy and the increasing prevalence of strains of pneumococci resistant to antimicrobial agents, serve to underscore the necessity for ongoing surveillance and expanded research into treatment and prevention of pneumococcal infections.

Pasteur and Sternberg, working independently in 1880 and 1881, discovered the pneumococcus. Pasteur called the organism *microbe septicémique de la salive*, and Sternberg called it *Micrococcus pasteri*. Each researcher recovered pneumococci from rabbits injected with human saliva. Friedlander demonstrated pneumococci in tissue from humans with pneumonia in 1882 and, in the following year, found them in most cases of acute pneumonia. Friedlander described both the characteristic capsule and colonial morphologic features of pneumococci and, in 1884, recovered pneumococci from the blood of patients with pneumonia for the first time. During the next few years, pneumococci were found in virtually all types of infection, including meningitis and otitis media. By 1890, researchers had established the pneumococcus as the most common cause of acute pneumonia, at which point the term *pneumococcus* emerged. In addition, the pneumococcus became recognized as a principal cause of meningitis and other serious infections. In 1926, the pneumococcus was called *Diplococcus pneumoniae* because it usually appears in pairs. In 1974, it was renamed *Streptococcus pneumoniae* because it forms long chains when grown in liquid medium.

Early researchers immunized animals with cell-free filtrates of pneumococci, demonstrated that serum from immune animals could protect against experimental pneumococcal infection, deduced the role of immunity in promoting phagocytosis, and noted agglutination of pneumococci by serum from immune animals. In 1897, Pane treated humans suffering from pneumonia with serum from such animals. By 1900, researchers had laid the foundation for immunotherapy for pneumococcal pneumonia, the only effective treatment until the advent of chemotherapy. Investigators noted that agglutination of pneumococci appeared to depend on the strain isolated. In 1910, Neufeld and Haendel classified pneumococci into several discrete serotypes on the basis of the appearance of capsular swelling (the Quellung reaction). Only strains exposed to homologous serum showed capsular swelling. Their work made possible all subsequent epidemiologic investigations of pneumococcal infection, immunotherapy with type-specific serum, and the development of vaccines. The original classification of pneumococci was limited to types I, II, III, and IV (others). Currently, 94 serotypes have been identified and certain serotypes have proved to be more virulent than others. Virulence depends, to some extent, on the species of animal infected.

The use of antisera for the treatment of pneumococcal pneumonia proved strikingly effective when type-specific sera were administered. As early as 1913, Cole and associates showed that treatment with antisera lowered fatality rates from 25% to 30% to 10.5%. In addition to allergic reactions, difficulties associated with this treatment included the necessity of identifying the causative serotype, the need for the earliest possible administration of antisera, and the availability of antisera to only types I, II, and III. White[594] compared the efficacy of early antisera therapy and found that 403 of 1614 (25.0%) patients that did not receive any therapy died, while 32 of 377 (8.5%) who received therapy within 3 days of onset died and 24 of 127 (18.9%) who received therapy 4 or more days after onset died. Therapy with antisera had no beneficial effect on pneumococcal infections such as meningitis and endocarditis. Despite these drawbacks, the use of antisera soon became widespread. The advent of chemotherapy—first sulfa compounds, then penicillin—was followed by a precipitous decline in the use of antisera. Antimicrobial agents killed or inhibited pneumococci, regardless of serotype, and cured patients with previously incurable localized infections.[594] Coincident with research resulting in the use of antisera came research into the efficacy of pneumococcal vaccines. Proof of efficacy lagged, and indisputable evidence of protection induced by vaccination was not available until 1945. The ability of pneumococci to cause epidemic pneumococcal pneumonia in young men crowded into army camps or gold mines allowed large-scale trials to be performed. Highlights of the development of effective vaccines include the trial of Wright and associates[605] in South Africa beginning in 1911. Using a vaccine made with whole killed pneumococci, this trial produced inconclusive results. Many trials followed, with some showing trends toward protection. In 1923, Heidelberger and Avery[237] published their classic article in which they stated that protective antibodies were reactive with surface capsular polysaccharides. In 1930, Francis and Tillett[178] showed capsular polysaccharides to be immunogenic for humans. Ekwurzel and colleagues[153] used a vaccine containing such polysaccharides during 1933 to 1937 and showed it to be effective. Smillie and associates used a preparation of serotype 1 polysaccharide to abort a hospital epidemic of pneumonia at State Hospital in Worcester, Massachusetts.[517]

Although many of these studies suggested that specific pneumococcal polysaccharide antigens could confer protection against severe pneumococcal infection, not until 1945, in a trial performed on US Army and Air Force recruits, were they finally proved by MacLeod and associates to do so.[356] This trial showed vaccination to be strikingly effective in preventing pneumococcal pneumonia caused by serotypes contained in the vaccine but not in preventing disease caused by other serotypes, thus showing serotype-specific protection.

Regrettably, interest in vaccination waned rapidly with the general availability of penicillin, and manufacturers voluntarily withdrew their vaccines from the market. This unfortunate attitude persisted for the next 2 decades until the inability of chemotherapy to prevent many deaths from pneumococcal disease was recognized.[33] The rapid development and spread of antibiotic resistance among many clinically important strains further emphasized that prevention could be more effective than treatment for pneumococcal disease. A few farsighted individuals continued to maintain surveillance of the serotypes causing human disease, and their work allowed the reintroduction of pneumococcal vaccines. The current status of vaccines is discussed later in this chapter. Interested readers should consult both White's *The Biology of Pneumococcus* and Heffron's *Pneumonia, with Special Reference to Pneumococcus Lobar Pneumonia*, as well as a comprehensive review by Watson and colleagues, for a complete account of the long and fascinating history of this organism.[594,236,586]

EPIDEMIOLOGY

The incidence of pneumococcal disease is highest in children less than 2 years old and adults greater than 65 years of age and varies substantially by country, by individual health status, and by season. Prior to

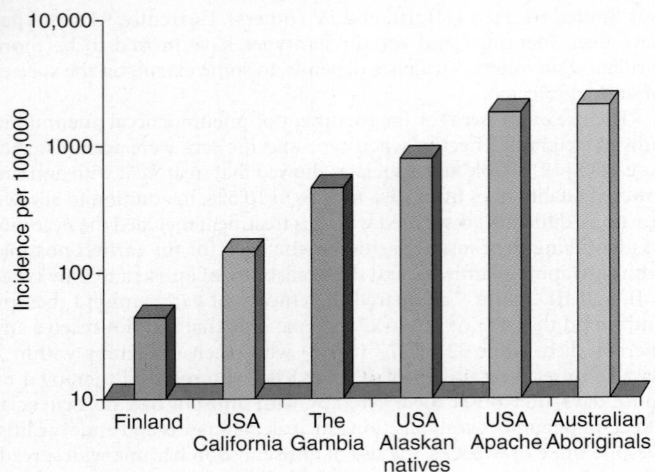

FIG. 85.2 Incidence of invasive pneumococcal disease in children <2 years old in The Gambia and in various high- and low-risk populations. (From Greenwood B. The epidemiology of pneumococcal infection in children in the developing world. *Philos Trans R Soc Lond B Biol Sci.* 1999;354:777–85.)

introduction of pneumococcal conjugate vaccines for universal administration in young children, the highest rates were observed in infants, with a rapid decrease in incidence after 5 years of age. Greenwood reported that the incidence of invasive pneumococcal disease (IPD) in children under 2 years of age varies 10-fold—from less than 100 cases per 100,000 in Finland to more than 1000 per 100,000 in Australian Aboriginal children (Fig. 85.2).[214] In part, the variability reflects the increased risk among children with sickle cell disease or HIV, indigenous populations such as Native Americans, Inuit or Aboriginee children, and malnourished children. However, as IPD impacts primarily healthy children, the susceptibility of high-risk groups contributes only slightly to the large geographical differences in incidence. Specific populations can have rates of IPD that are as much as 100-fold greater than age-matched healthy children residing within the same country. The incidence of IPD is also correlated with standard of living, with children in high-income countries having less disease than in low-income countries or less privileged populations. The incidence of IPD in children younger than 5 to 6 years in western Europe (e.g., Finland, the United Kingdom, Germany, Switzerland, Denmark, and Spain) was lower than 25 cases per 100,000 population per year in various studies; in Chile, Australia, and New Zealand, it was 25 to 60 per 100,000; and during the same period in the United States, the range was approximately 65 to 75 cases per 100,000.[232] The rates of IPD in US children appear to be atypical, with higher rates reported than in comparable high-income nations, although rates of pneumococcal meningitis appear more similar across countries.[232,359] The difference in US incidence rates is most likely a reflection of the higher use of blood cultures in nontoxic febrile infants and toddlers in the United States than elsewhere.

Despite the increasing proportion of invasive pneumococcal disease among children with comorbid illness, the majority of cases occur in healthy infants and toddlers. Such children represent an immunologically naïve population susceptible to bloodstream invasion or direct invasion of the lower respiratory tract. Differences in the proportion of disease by age also vary globally. In The Gambia and comparable countries, a larger proportion of disease occurs in children less than 5 months of age compared with representative populations of US children (Fig. 85.3). Similarly, in many countries, colonization is more prevalent and begins earlier, usually in the first months of life, compared with industrialized countries.[5]

As virtually all children carry pneumococci belonging to several serotypes during their childhood, a focus on the epidemiology of carriage is warranted. In a study conducted in the United States, the prevalence of nasopharyngeal carriage in preschool children was 38% to 60% versus 29% to 35% and 9% to 25% in elementary school and junior high

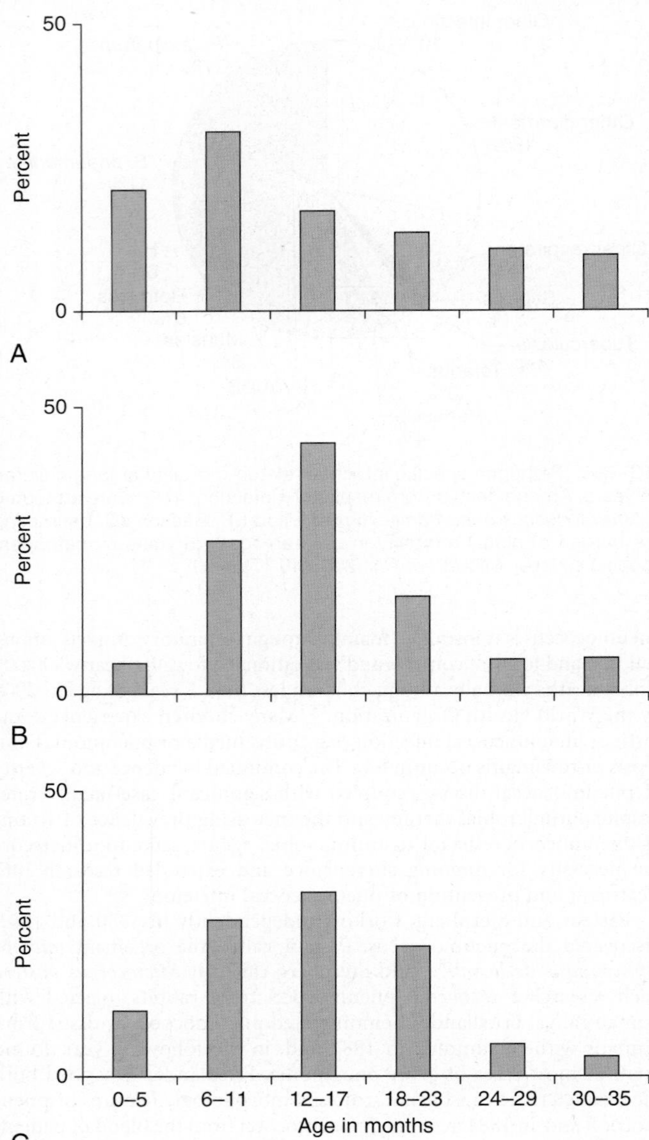

FIG. 85.3 Age distribution of invasive pneumococcal disease in (A) young children in The Gambia and (B) high-risk and (C) low-risk communities in the United States. (From Greenwood B. The epidemiology of pneumococcal infection in children in the developing world. *Philos Trans R Soc Lond B Biol Sci.* 1999;354:777–85.)

school students, respectively.[239] The prevalence in adults with no children at home was 6%. In studies in closed populations, such as kibbutzim in Israel or a poor and crowded community in southern Israel, the same differences between children and adults were noted.[68,117] Contact with young carriers increases the carriage rates in older children and adults. In the United States, adults with no children living in the household had a carriage rate of 6%, whereas the carriage rate increased to 29% when children were present at home. Similarly, primary school–aged children who have siblings younger than 2 years old carried *S. pneumoniae* more often than did those without young siblings.[353] In a study in Costa Rica, cultures in mother-child dyads showed an increased prevalence of carriage in infancy: from 6% at 1 month of age to 39% at 12 months of age. At the same time, carriage in mothers increased from 0% to 9.8%, thus supporting our understanding that pneumococci are transmitted from infants to adults—in this case, mothers.[372] In a Swedish study, the observed average duration of carriage was longer in children who had family carriers of the same serotype and, therefore, was suggestive of ongoing recirculation in the family.[152]

Acquisition of *S. pneumoniae* may occur during the very first days of life. In infants aged 2 months, the prevalence of carriage ranges from less than 15% in most high-income countries to greater than 60% in low-income countries.[18] Colonization peaks during the second and third year of life in high-income countries.[122,213,238] The relationship of age to carriage is not understood, but it depends, at least in part, on the development of specific anticapsular antibodies.[211,212] In toddlers vaccinated with a pneumococcal conjugate vaccine, nasopharyngeal acquisition of new *S. pneumoniae* vaccine serotypes was inversely related to serum levels of specific antipolysaccharide IgG antibodies.[115] In another study, the presence of both circulating IgG and secretory immunoglobulin A (IgA) antibodies to the surface pneumococcal protein PsaA was associated with a lower prevalence of nasopharyngeal pneumococcal carriage.[455,511] A 2004 study showed that mucosal anticapsular IgA developed in response to colonization in preschool-aged children, regardless of vaccination status.[66] This phenomenon has been hypothesized to contribute to the falling carriage rates observed with increasing age.[618] Potentially, maturation of innate immunity may also contribute to the declining prevalence of colonization with increasing age; however, a specific role or mechanism has not been established.

Crowding is an important factor that facilitates the spread of *S. pneumoniae*. Therefore, it is not surprising that in high-income countries the nasopharyngeal carriage rate and spread are highest in infants and toddlers attending daycare centers, with levels exceeding 90% in some studies, followed by those living with one or more siblings at home.[18,122,448,568] In addition, the viral infections that are very prevalent in infants and toddlers attending daycare centers enhance colonization of the nasopharynx with *S. pneumoniae*.[213,351,568] The combination of young age and increased incidence of respiratory viral infections renders daycare centers an important site for transmission of *S. pneumoniae* from child to child and subsequently child to parent or child to younger sibling.

The duration of carriage depends on age and serotype and may be related to additional factors, such as antibiotic treatment, immune status of the child, and unknown factors. Carriage lasts longer in infants and young toddlers than in older children and adults.[116,152,211] Infants are colonized for an average of 30 days; however, carriage can persist for as long as 12 months in some.[150] In a study in the United States in adults, individual serotypes usually persisted for 2 to 4 weeks.

The relative risk for a specific serotype to colonize the nasopharynx of a child and its ability to cause respiratory or invasive infection appears to vary by serotype but not geographic location. Some serotypes—such as 6A, 6B, 9V, 14, 18C, 19A, 19F, and 23F—are among the most frequent colonizers in infants and young children in most parts of the world and thus often are considered "pediatric" serotypes.[70,117] These serotypes are acquired frequently by infants and young children and often are carried for prolonged periods. After children reach the age of 2 years, carriage of these "pediatric" serotypes declines. Although pneumococcal carriage decreases overall with age, the proportion of "nonpediatric" serotypes increases with age. This phenomenon is demonstrated in Fig. 85.4.

In contrast to the "pediatric" serotypes, serotypes such as 1, 5, 7F, and 12 are carried infrequently and are eliminated from the nasopharynx rapidly. However, these serotypes are able to cause disease and even clusters or epidemics.[70,117] The different distribution of serotypes among colonized children, children with invasive infections, and adults with pneumonia is depicted in Fig. 85.5.[498]

Although most colonization occurs without the development of disease, prospective, longitudinal studies have suggested that most systemic infections develop soon after colonization with a new pneumococcal serotype.[160,209,211] Some carriers are protected from invasive disease by the presence of circulating antibodies. However, such antibodies do not always protect against invasion of contiguous sites. Other investigators have shown that a substantial number of pneumococcal otitis media cases occur at any time following nasopharyngeal colonization.[534]

The emergence of resistance to more than one antibiotic class has become a serious problem.[266] In 1993, approximately a fifth of the pneumococcal strains in Iceland were penicillin nonsusceptible and 80% were multidrug resistant. When the risk for carriage of penicillin-resistant *S. pneumoniae* was investigated, a clear association was found not only with use of β-lactam drugs but also with the use of

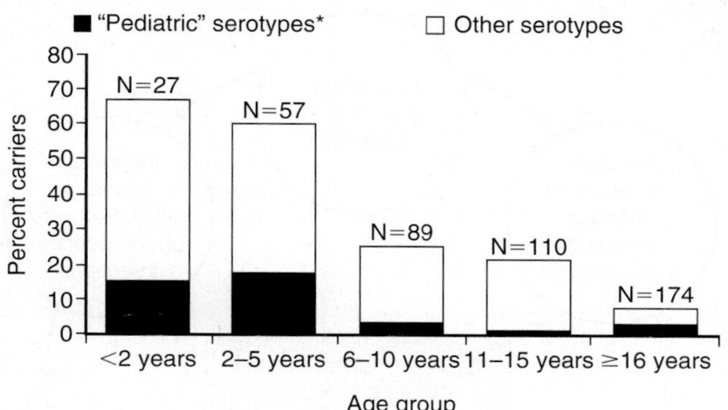

FIG. 85.4 Nasopharyngeal carriage of *Streptococcus pneumoniae* in closed community living in crowded conditions in Southern Israel. *Pediatric serotypes 6A, 6B, 9V, 14, 18C, 19A, 19F, and 23F. (Modified from Dagan R, Gradstein S, Belmaker I, et al. An outbreak of *Streptococcus pneumoniae* serotype 1 in a closed community in southern Israel. *Clin Infect Dis*. 2000;30:319–21.)

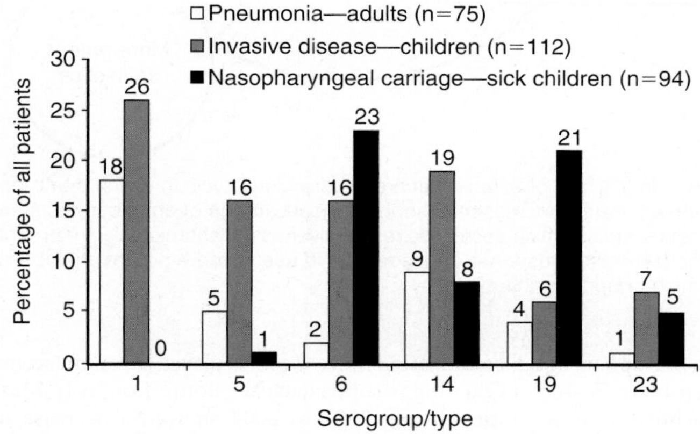

FIG. 85.5 Distribution of selected serogroups/serotypes in *Streptococcus pneumoniae* isolates from adults with pneumonia, children with invasive pneumococcal disease, and nasopharyngeal specimens from sick children in Kenya. (Modified from Scott JAG, Hall AJ, Hannington A, et al. Serotype distribution and prevalence of resistance to benzylpenicillin in three representative populations of *Streptococcus pneumoniae* isolates from the coast of Kenya. *Clin Infect Dis*. 1998;27:1442–50.)

trimethoprim-sulfamethoxazole and erythromycin.[23] Following treatment of acute otitis media (AOM), carriage of trimethoprim-sulfamethoxazole–resistant *S. pneumoniae* was found in 23% of patients by day 6 and in 33% by day 40. Additionally, non–penicillin-susceptible *S. pneumoniae* was carried at these times by 26% and 43% of children, respectively. This remarkable promotion of colonization with penicillin-resistant strains by trimethoprim-sulfamethoxazole treatment occurred because many strains were resistant to both penicillin and trimethoprim-sulfamethoxazole.

The dramatic change in nasopharyngeal flora after initiation of antibiotic therapy has two important consequences. Antibiotic treatment not only can increase nasopharyngeal carriage of antibiotic-resistant *S. pneumoniae* but also can result in subsequent infection of the middle ear with that resistant strain within a few days.[119] Second, the increased prevalence of antibiotic-resistant *S. pneumoniae* in the nasopharynx leads to enhanced transmission within extended families and daycare centers.[122,191,238,448,474,609] The widespread use of antibiotics is likely to be responsible for the increase in antibiotic-resistant *S. pneumoniae*, especially in crowded populations such as daycare centers, thus creating a vicious cycle that is difficult, if not impossible, to overcome (Fig. 85.6).[569]

Since the use of pneumococcal conjugate vaccine has become widespread in the United States, the serotypes found most commonly

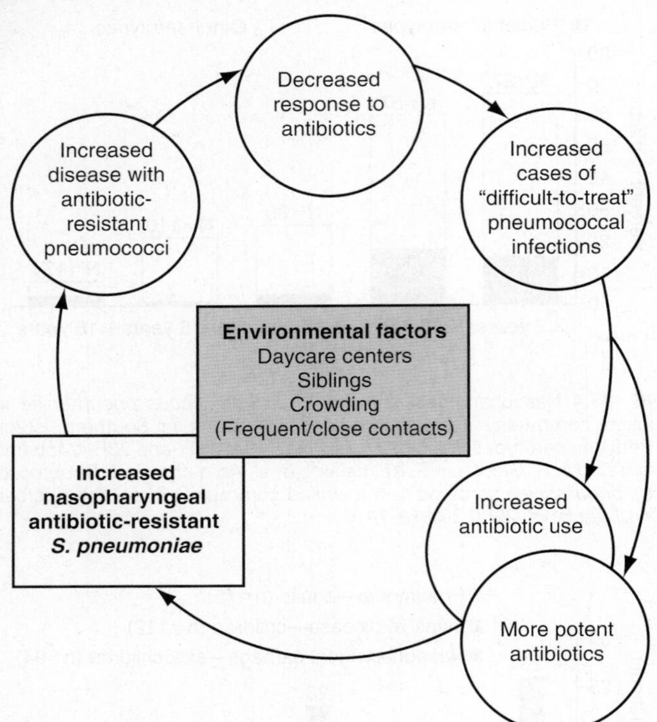

FIG. 85.6 Chain of events that creates a vicious cycle in which treatment with antibiotics increases nasopharyngeal carriage of antibiotic-resistant pneumococci, which decreases responsiveness to antimicrobial treatment. The decreased responsiveness results in use of more potent antibiotics, which continues the cycle.

in nasopharyngeal colonization have been replaced by nonvaccine serotypes. A study evaluating nasopharyngeal colonization in 16 Massachusetts communities during 2001 to 2004 showed a decrease in serotypes found in the 7-valent pneumococcal conjugate vaccine (PCV-7) from 36% to 14% along with an increase in non–PCV-7 serotypes from 34% to 55%.[257] Another study showed that 25% of children colonized with pneumococci carried antibiotic-resistant, nonvaccine serotypes, including serotypes 19A and 35B, rarely detected before introduction of the pneumococcal conjugate vaccine. Further changes in the distribution of pneumococcal serotypes—specifically types 19A, 7F, and 6A—subsequent to the implementation of universal vaccination of children less than 5 years of age with the 13-valent pneumococcal conjugate vaccine (PCV13) has been observed.[354] Both a reduction in overall carriage of the unique PCV13 serotypes and specific declines in serotypes 19A and 7F have been significant. The rapid decline in colonization with PCV13 led to a decline in prevalence of antibiotic resistance among pneumococcal isolates recovered from the nasopharynx.[293] However, replacement pneumococcal strains (serotypes 6D, 15A, 15C, 16F, 23A, and 35B) have begun to acquire macrolide and/or β-lactam resistance.[558] Pneumococcal serotype diversity among adults has been shown to be influenced by pediatric pneumococcal vaccination uptake.[207] Analysis of differences in serotype proportions and incidence of adult IPD matching the 23-valent pneumococcal polysaccharide vaccine (PPSV23) and 13-valent conjugate vaccine showed that the median differential between the 23 and 13 serotypes increased from 16.3% to 24.4% ($P < .003$). This difference can be used to guide national recommendations for vaccine use in various populations.

Risk Factors for Pneumococcal Infection

Demographic Features

Age. Young age is a major risk factor for pneumococcal infection because of immunologic immaturity and the absence of acquired immunity. The relationship between age and the development of protective immunity to pneumococcal infection was published in 1932 by Sutliff and Finland.[532] Maternal antibody, passively transferred to the fetus, protects against invasive infection in the first few months of life. These antibodies decay over the first few months and the incidence of invasive pneumococcal disease increases, peaking between 12 and 18 months of age, presumably as specific immunity is acquired following exposure. Following the introduction of pneumococcal conjugate vaccine (PCV), the peak incidence in children is now between 6 and 12 months of age.[612] This age distribution reflects the ongoing susceptibility of young infants to nonvaccine serotypes due to naïvete of the infant immune system despite acquisition of protective antibody to vaccine serotypes following immunization.[362,381,596] IPD in developing countries occurs earlier in life. It is hypothesized that this is related to earlier and more intense exposure to pneumococci in such children.[6]

Gender

In most studies of pneumococcal disease, there is a greater proportion of males than females. Yildirim reported that the proportion of male cases was significantly higher (58.5% vs. 41.5%; $P = .01$), but gender-specific incidence rates were not significantly different.*

Race/Ethnicity

Prior to the introduction of PCV, the incidence of pneumococcal bacteremia and meningitis in Alaskan Native children younger than 5 years ranges from 598 cases per 100,000 population in those 6 to 11 months of age to 56 cases per 100,000 population in those 36 to 47 months of age, which is approximately four times the incidence in similarly aged non–Alaskan Native/non–Native American children.[130] The highest incidence for any ethnic group in the United States is found in Navajo and Apache populations living on reservations in the southwestern United States. The incidence in children aged 1 to 2 years in these populations ranged from 557 to 2396 per 100,000.[109,417] Among children younger than 5 years, the incidence of invasive pneumococcal disease in African American children in the United States was two to three times higher than that in white children of the same age.[53,75,229,469] In a case-control study of risk factors for the development of invasive disease in young children, the association of race with disease risk was not statistically significant in an analysis that controlled for socioeconomic status.[340] However, other studies have reported persistence of increased risk even when controlling for income.[75,94,168,229,240] Whether environmental differences (e.g., poverty, use of wood burning stoves, crowding) completely explain the increased incidence in some populations in comparison to others in the United States or whether genetic differences are also contributory remains unclear. Universal immunization with PCV in children less than 5 years of age has resulted in a reduction in the incidence of invasive pneumococcal disease in Native Americans, African Americans, and other high-risk populations but has not completely eliminated differences in rates of disease, likely reflecting increased susceptibility to nonvaccine serotypes.[587]

In other geographic regions, differences among populations also can be observed, again being higher in populations that live in less privileged conditions. Such observations raise the question of the importance of genetic versus environmental risk factors. In southern Israel, the incidence of pneumococcal invasive infection during the first year of life in Bedouin infants (a population with a lifestyle, birth rate, and general disease incidence similar to that of low-income countries) was fourfold higher than in Jewish infants (a population with standards of living comparable to the middle/low social class in the high-income countries).[180]

In New Zealand, when Maoris, Pacific Islanders, and others were compared, incidence rates of invasive pneumococcal disease in the first year of life per 100,000 population were 153, 276, and 52, respectively. These rates in children younger than 5 years were 67, 117, and 36 per 100,000, respectively.[575]

Seasonality

Pneumococcal infection occurs in a seasonal pattern with increased cases of invasive infections, pneumonia, and otitis media between September/October and April/May in the Northern Hemisphere, with the opposite picture in the Southern Hemisphere. Peak incidence often

*References 72, 147, 233, 376, 407, 425, 466, 506, 545, 612.

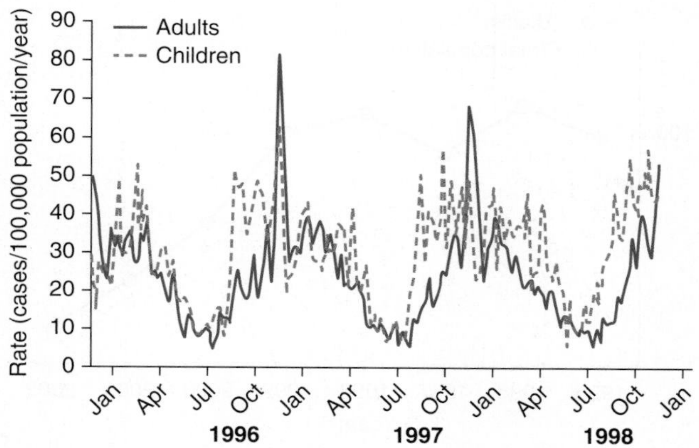

FIG. 85.7 Weekly rates of invasive pneumococcal disease in children (*dotted line:* birth to 17 years) and adults (*solid line:* >18 years) in the United States, 1996–98. (From Dowell SF, Whitney CG, Wright C, et al. Seasonal patterns of invasive pneumococcal disease. *Emerg Infect Dis.* 2003;9:573–9.)

occurs from December through February (Fig. 85.7).[146] The same seasonal variation in nasopharyngeal carriage of pneumococci is also observed with lowest rates in the summer months.[213,351] This pattern is likely related to the seasonal variations in viral respiratory infections, which play an important role in increasing pneumococcal carriage and subsequent infection and in attendance at school and daycare centers. However, other factors are likely to be important. In one study, adults had higher incidence of pneumococcal disease following school holidays and presumably increased contact with children.[583] In Israel, the Jewish and Bedouin populations in southern Israel demonstrate distinct and different seasonal patterns. The Jewish population appears similar to traditional Western populations with distinct seasonal variation. The Bedouin live in crowded and less hygienic conditions, with a high birth rate and a disease pattern similar to that in low-income countries, without a clear pattern of seasonality.[342] Recently, a subtle difference in the seasonal difference between bacteremia and pneumonia has been described in which bacteremic and nonbacteremic pneumonia peaked in winter (in Israel) while IPD peaked in the fall. The authors suggest these differences may imply differences in pathogenesis.[52]

Lack of Breastfeeding

Breastfeeding may be protective against pneumococcal infection. The reduction in colonization and decreased attachment to pharyngeal cells is thought to be mediated through several components of the immune system, including secretory IgA, lactoferrin, and lysozyme. Some studies have suggested that breastfeeding protects against otitis media,[19] but others have failed to show this effect.[48] Studies in the United States demonstrated a protective effect of breastfeeding against invasive pneumococcal infection in children in the general population[48] and in Alaskan Natives.[190] However, in Finland, no protective effect was observed.[538]

Crowding

Crowding contributes to many factors that increase the risk for acquiring pneumococcal infection, including viral infections, poor hygiene, and potentially increased person-to-person transmission of *S. pneumoniae.* Attendance at daycare centers was the most important risk factor for acquiring invasive pneumococcal infection in children and infants in several studies.* In a population-based, case-control study, adults aged 18 to 64 years who lived in households that included children attending daycare were at greater risk of acquiring invasive pneumococcal infection.[412] In high income countries, attendance at daycare centers is also the most important risk factor for AOM, including pneumococcal otitis.[406,478]

*References 65, 200, 337, 408,448, 451, 458, 474, 478, 535, 572.

Immunocompromising Conditions

Congenital and Acquired Absence of Spleen or Splenic Function

The spleen is critical for the clearance of pneumococci from the bloodstream.[531,584] Children in whom the spleen is absent or dysfunctional are at risk for the development of overwhelming pneumococcal infection (see clinical syndrome, sepsis, and purpura). In children with absence or dysfunction of the spleen, the mortality rate is multifold higher. Schutze and colleagues reported 27% mortality from prospective surveillance of eight US children's hospitals in children with splenic dysfunction.[496] Splenic dysfunction is also regarded as explaining the increased incidence and severity of pneumococcal bacteremia in sickle-cell disease and other sickle hemoglobinopathies (e.g., hemoglobin sickle-cell disease or S-β-thalassemia).[432,496,615] Children with hemoglobin sickle-cell disease, thalassemia, and other hemaglobinopathies demonstrate a higher incidence of IPD compared to healthy children, albeit lower than in persons with sickle-cell disease.[327,554] Other factors that contribute to the high incidence and poor outcome for pneumococcal infection in persons with sickle-cell disease include low levels of circulating antibodies and complement deficiency.[432,599] Penicillin prophylaxis is effective in reducing the risk of pneumococcal disease in children with absent or abnormal splenic function; however, the rate of disease remains increased compared to healthy children. PCV has been demonstrated to be immunogenic and effective in reducing disease due to vaccine serotypes in children with hemoglobinopathies (Fig. 85.8).[8,223,570] However, increased rates of disease due to serotypes not contained in the current vaccines are observed.[8,170,223,429,570,601,615]

Defective Antibody Formation

Reduced antibody formation is associated with increased risk of pneumococcal infection. Congenital agammaglobulinemia, acquired common variable hypogammaglobulinemia, and defective antibody production associated with diseases such as malignancies and human immunodeficiency virus (HIV) infection are associated with increased risk of pneumococcal disease.[113,560] In the era preceding the introduction of highly active antiretroviral treatment, HIV-infected children had a 100-fold to 1000-fold increase in incidence compared to healthy children.[16,55,162,179,360,388] In one study, the incidence of invasive pneumococcal disease was 6.1 cases per 100 patient-years in HIV-infected children through the age of 7 years.[367] Despite the introduction of highly active antiretroviral treatment, HIV-infected African children remain a high-risk group for IPD and pneumococcal pneumonia.[411]

Neutropenia and Neutrophil Dysfunction

The risk of pneumococcal disease is not uniform across all neutrophil abnormalities. Primary and secondary neutropenia, such as cyclic neutropenia, drug-induced neutropenia, and aplastic anemia, are associated with an increased incidence of severe pneumococcal infection. However, the incidence is not increased in other granulocyte dysfunction syndromes, such as leukocyte adhesion deficiency syndromes.[15,183]

Genetic Variation in Mannose-Binding Lectin

Approximately 5% of the population in Europe and North America and an even larger population in many developing countries are homozygous for mannose-binding lectin (MBL) codon variants. These subjects have a greater than 2.5-fold increased risk for the acquisition of pneumococcal infection than do those who do not have this variant or are only heterozygous for this variant.

Immunocompetent Conditions

Studies of IPD since the introduction of PCV in 2000 have identified that an increasing proportion of cases occur in children with comorbid conditions. Children over the age of 5 years with IPD were threefold more likely to have a comorbid condition compared to those less than 5 years old. Specific conditions identified by the Committee on Infectious Diseases of the American Academy of Pediatrics include children with chronic lung and heart disease, diabetes mellitus, cerebrospinal fluid leak, chronic renal failure and nephrotic syndrome (at least in part due to hypogammaglobulinemia), and cochlear implants are at increased risk for pneumococcal disease (Table 85.1). Children with asthma and

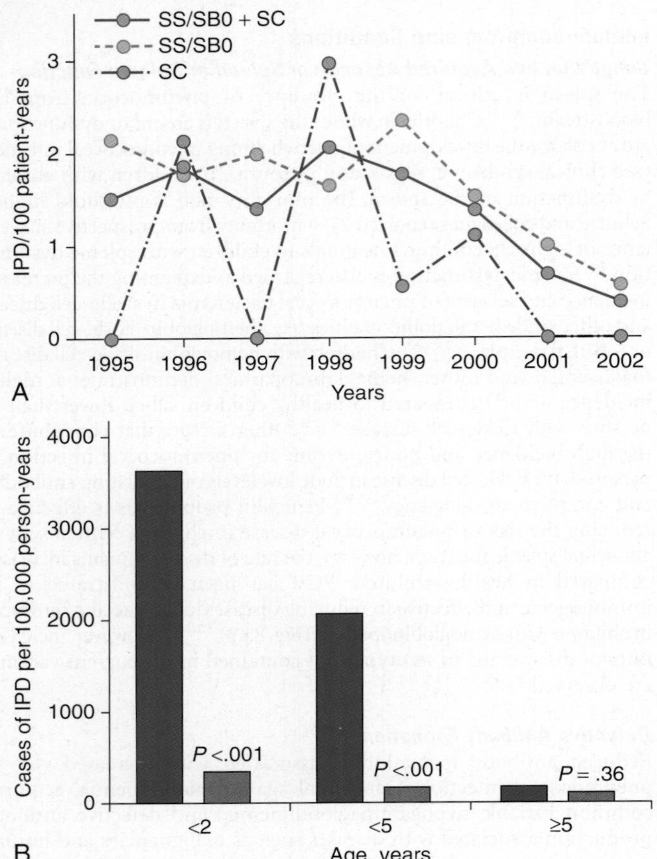

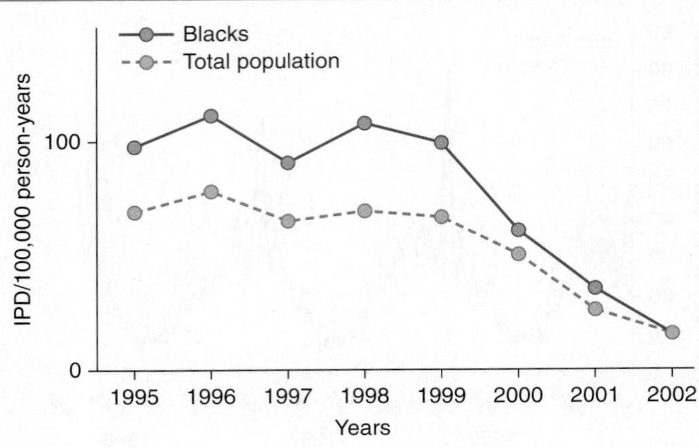

FIG. 85.8 (A) Rates of invasive pneumococcal disease (IPD) in children ≤10 years with sickle-cell disease and in the general population. *Left*, IPD rates in children with sickle cell disease. *Right*, IPD rates in the general population of children. Surveillance data are from the Georgia Emerging Infections Program.[7] (B) Comparison of rates of IPD (cases per 100,000 person-years) in children with sickle-cell disease enrolled in Tennessee Medicaid 1995–99 with 2001–04. (From Halasa NB, Shankar SM, Talbot TR, et al. Incidence of invasive pneumococcal disease among individuals with sickle cell disease before and after the introduction of the pneumococcal conjugate vaccine. *Clin Infect Dis*. 2007;44:1428–33.)

TABLE 85.1 Underlying Medical Conditions That Are Indications for Pneumococcal Immunization Among Children, by Risk Group[13]

Risk Group	Condition
Immunocompetent children	Chronic heart disease[a] Chronic lung disease[b] Diabetes mellitus Cerebrospinal fluid leaks Cochlear implant
Children with functional or anatomic asplenia	Sickle cell disease and other hemoglobinopathies Chronic or acquired asplenia, or splenic dysfunction
Children with immunocompromising conditions	HIV infection Chronic renal failure and nephrotic syndrome Diseases associated with treatment with immunosuppressive drugs or radiation therapy, including malignant neoplasms, leukemias, lymphomas, and Hodgkin disease; or solid organ transplantation Congenital immunodeficiency[c]

Modified from American Academy of Pediatrics. Pneumococcal Infections. Red Book: 2012 Report of the Committee on Infectious Diseases. In: Pickering LK, editor. Elk Grove Village, IL: American Academy of Pediatrics; 2012. pp. 571–582.

[a]Particularly cyanotic congenital heart disease and cardiac failure.

[b]Including asthma if treated with prolonged high-dose oral corticosteroids.

[c]Includes B- (humoral) or T-lymphocyte deficiency; complement deficiencies, particularly C_1, C_2, C_3, and C_4 deficiency; and phagocytic disorders (excluding chronic granulomatous disease).

neurologic conditions, including seizure disorders and muscular dystrophies, are also at increased risk. The risk is further increased in children with two or more comorbidities. In addition to increased incidence, children with such comorbid illnesses have poorer outcomes following IPD or pneumococcal pneumonia. Yildirim reported 2.5-fold greater rates of hospitalization and 3.7-fold higher case-fatality ratios for children with comorbid conditions.[611]

Pneumococcal Serotype

A characteristic of most disease-causing strains of *S. pneumoniae* is the presence of a polysaccharide capsule. The capsular polysaccharides are composed of repeating units of oligosaccharides, for most of which the exact chemical structure is known. To date, 94 distinct capsular types have been described, several very recently (Table 85.2). Understanding serotype distribution and characteristics is important for several reasons. First, a selected number of serotypes are responsible for the majority of disease. However, the serotypes vary somewhat by geography. For example, prior to the introduction of PCV, 7 serotypes (4, 6B, 9V, 14, 18C, 19F, and 23F) accounted for 80% of cases of IPD in North American children (Fig. 85.9A). Globally, a larger number of serotypes—including serotypes 1, 3, and 5—must be included to account for a similar 80% of IPD cases (Fig. 85.9B).[282] A significant positive association between disease and serotype has been demonstrated in children younger than 36 months, with serotypes 1, 5, and 12F associated with IPD, serotypes 1, 3, 5, 12F, 19A, and 19F with AOM, and serotype 3 with necrotizing pneumonia and nontypeable strains with conjunctivitis. A significant negative association with IPD was demonstrated for nontypeable *S. pneumoniae*. Understanding the distribution of serotypes causing serious pneumococcal disease is relevant to developing vaccine strategies for prevention and estimating the impact of a vaccine that provides coverage for a limited number of serotypes. Serotype distribution also

TABLE 85.2 **Capsular Serotypes of *Streptococcus pneumoniae*, Now 94, Includes 25 Individual Serotypes and 21 Serogroups Containing 69 Serotypes**

Serotypes (*n* = 25)	Serogroups (*n* = 21)
1	6A, 6B, 6C, 6D, 6E
2	7A, 7B, 7C, 7F
3	9A, 9L, 9N, 9V
4	10A, 10B, 10C, 10F
5	11A, 11B, 11C, 11D, 11E, 11F
8	12A, 12B, 12F
13	15A, 15B, 15C, 15F
14	16A, 16F
20	17A, 17F
21	18A, 18B, 18C, 18F
27	19A, 19B, 19C, 19F
29	22A, 22F
31	23A, 23B, 23F
34	24A, 24B, 24F
36	25A, 25F
37	28A, 28F
38	32A, 32F
39	33A, 33B, 33C, 33D, 33F
40	35A, 35B, 35C, 35F
42	41A, 41F
43	47A, 47F
44	
45	
46	
48	

varies over time, as experience with serotype 1 disease in Europe demonstrated.

The serotype distribution of nasopharyngeal carriage and invasive and other pneumococcal diseases varies, as not all pneumococci have the same relative risk of progressing from carriage to disease. Invasive capacity, the term describing the relative risk of disease occurring following a colonizing event, appears to be an intrinsic property of pneumococcal strains, predominantly determined by the capsular polysaccharide. The invasive capacity for common serotypes has been computed by several investigators. Large differences among serotypes (>10-fold) have been reported and, in general, estimates of relative risk have been similar across studies. Dagan and colleagues were able to demonstrate that capacities to cause IPD and AOM were not comparable and that differences among serotypes were blunted for AOM compared to IPD (Fig. 85.10). Following the introduction of PCV7, investigators in many countries reported increases in both carriage and disease due to serotype 19A. In part, the increase in carriage resulted from intrinsic characteristics of specific clones of serotype 19A, permitting them to out-compete other serotypes; multidrug resistance, which allowed its persistence as a result of selective pressure from antimicrobial usage in the community; and the lack of significant cross-protection by antibodies generated in response to 19F capsular polysaccharide. It was initially hypothesized that including the capsular polysaccharide from serotype 19F in the vaccine would elicit cross-protective antibody against serotype 19A. The hypothesis was that antigenically related serotypes (those within serogroups)—for example, serotype 9A—would elicit cross-protective antibody against serotypes 9L, 9N, and 9V. However, although antibody to the 19A capsule increased following immunization with 19F as measured by enzyme-linked immunosorbent assay (ELISA), it was not sufficiently functional to prevent carriage or disease due to 19A following immunization with PCV7. Proof of cross-protection currently exists for antibody elicited by the 6B capsular polysaccharide, which demonstrates protection against disease and carriage due to serotype 6A, as well as for 6A, which elicits protection against 6C strains.[108] For serotype 23F, an increase in carriage of the cross-reacting serotypes 23A and 23B has been observed following immunization with PCV containing 23F capsular polysaccharide. Insufficient data is available to understand whether capsular polysaccharides elicit cross-protection for other serotypes of the same serogroup. The extent of cross-reactivity between types within the respective serogroups may differ—for example, serotypes 6A and 6B have identical chemical composition except for one of the bonds between two sugars and are extensively cross-reactive, while types 19F and 19A are clearly less cross-reactive. Poolman suggested that the process of protein conjugation of the 19F polysaccharide during conjugation with CRM altered its structure such that antibody elicited was not functional against serotype 19A strains and that by using alternative strategies, such as employed for PCV10, greater functional activity against serotype 19A can be achieved.[446] Another important reason for understanding serotype differences relates to clinical disease. Different serotypes may cause specific clinical syndromes. For example, serotype 3 is associated with necrotizing pneumonia, while serotype 1 is associated with empyema and "epidemic disease," specifically in central Africa. Serotype 1 epidemiology also differs in that it causes disease across a broader age spectrum than the usual serotypes, which are primarily found in infants.[42,189,566] High mortalities have been associated with specific serotypes as well.[444,564,589] Serotype is also linked to antimicrobial susceptibility. Prior to introduction of PCV7, the majority of antibiotic-resistant pneumococci were associated with five serotypes: 6B, 9V, 14, 19F, and 23F.

Other attributes beyond capsular polysaccharide also impact on clinical syndromes. Differences between strains of serotype 1 in Europe and Africa have been described. In Africa, disease due to serotype 1 is often meningitis and the strain is wild type with regard to the pneumolysin produced, whereas in Europe the clinical syndromes are bactermia and pneumonia and the strain has a mutant pneumolysin, unable to produce hemolysis.[383,589]

Evidence is clear that introduction of PCV13 has again impacted serotype distributions in the nasopharynx and in pneumococcal disease syndromes. Epidemiologic studies highlight differences in carriage by geographic locations that have major relevance as to whether replacement disease is more or less observed. For example, in France, serotypes with high invasiveness—such as 24F, 22F, 33F, and 15A—are more prevalent in carriage (than prior to PCV13 introduction) and appear to be increasing in invasive pneumococcal disease cases as well, suggesting that replacement disease will remain a challenge but likely vary by geography.[567] Additional changes in serotypes recently reported include the following. A multidrug-resistant invasive serotype 8 has emerged in Spain that is resistant to erythromycin, clindamycin, tetracycline, and quinolones, likely originating from the multidrug-resistant Sweden 15A-ST63 clone.[24] Multidrug-resistant putative serotype 6E isolates belonging to clonal complex 90 have been described from 11 Asian countries.[38,39] A high prevalence of genotype 6E (putative serotype 6E) has been reported among noninvasive/colonization isolates of *Streptococcus pneumoniae* in northern Japan.[294] Serotype 11E has been described and differentiated from serotype 11A strains.[87]

PATHOGENESIS

To cause disease, pneumococci, like other extracellular bacterial pathogens, must adhere to mammalian cells, replicate in situ, escape phagocytosis, and damage tissue by causing inflammation or producing substances that directly damage cells and, in some cases, invade the bloodstream.[399] The vast array of virulence mechanisms available to pneumococci are countered by numerous host defense mechanisms, although some host responses facilitate infection. Even though colonization with a pneumococcal strain can progress to disease, it usually does not occur, and the development of anticapsular type-specific antibodies occurs within 30 days in older children and adults.[210,211,401,402] If organisms find their way into the eustachian tubes, sinuses, or bronchi, clearance mechanisms—chiefly, ciliary action—lead to their rapid removal. After the development of humoral immunity, colonization with a strain may persist for 1 to 12 months, during which time disease may occur in contiguous sites, but the host is protected from invasive disease by

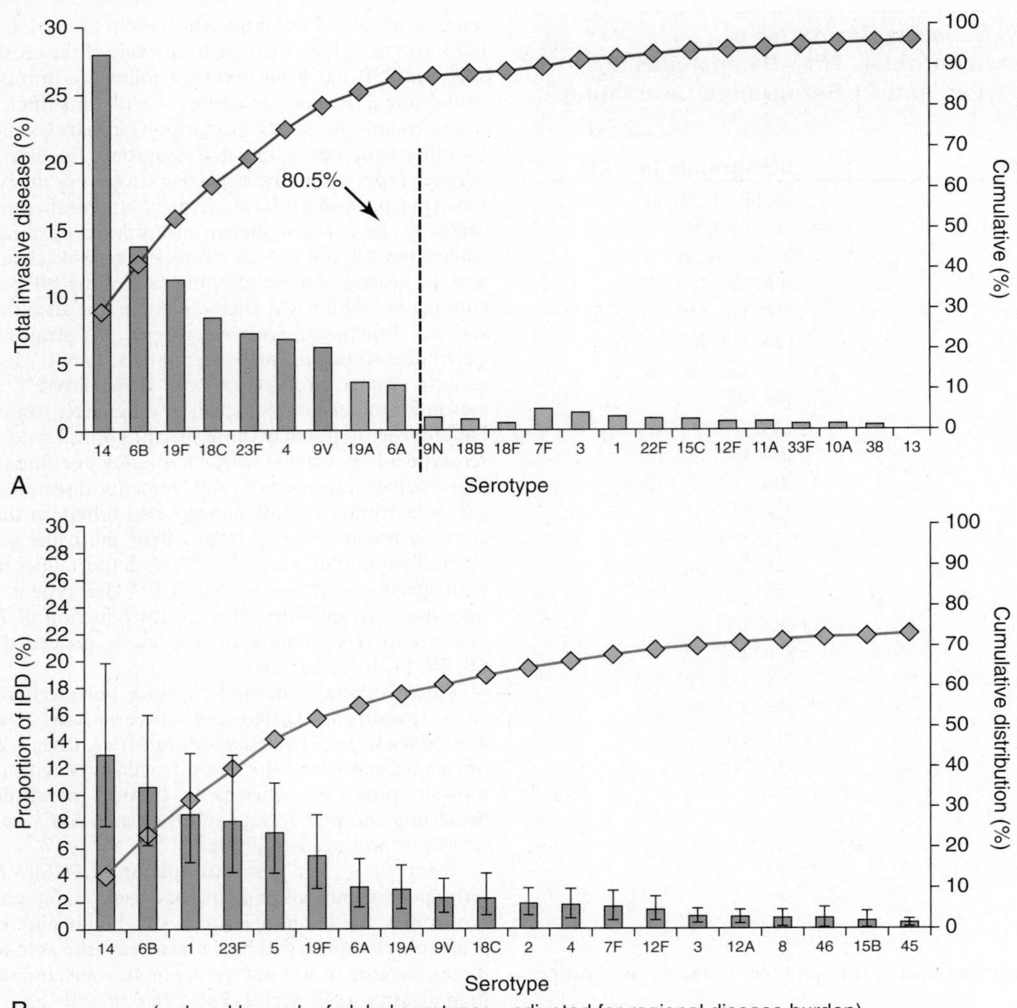

FIG. 85.9 (A) Pneumococcal serotypes causing invasive disease in North American young children prior to PCV7. (B) Proportion of invasive pneumococcal disease (IPD) in young children due to the most common serotypes globally. Error bars indicate 95% confidence interval; cumulative line indicates proportion of IPD due to the 21 serotypes detailed. (A, From Hausdorff WP, Bryant J, Kloek C, et al. The contribution of specific pneumococcal serogroups to different disease manifestations: implications for conjugate vaccine formulation and use, part II. *Clin Infect Dis.* 2000;30:122–40. B, From Johnson HL, Deloria-Knoll M, Levine OS, et al. Systematic evaluation of serotypes causing invasive pneumococcal disease among children under five: the pneumococcal global serotype project. *PLoS Med.* 2010;7:e1000348.)

circulating type-specific anticapsular IgG. Loss of colonization with a strain is followed, after a variable colonization-free interval, by colonization with a different serotype. Because 94 antigenically distinct serotypes exist, this cycle of colonization accompanied by the development of humoral immunity occurs many times.

Progression of colonization to disease usually requires the combination of two events: first, acquisition of a serotype to which the host is not immune; and, second, a concurrent respiratory viral infection, chronic damage to respiratory epithelium (e.g., smoking or exposure to smoke or occupational exposure), allergy, or other conditions that result in the development of disease rather than just colonization.[399] Many of these concurrent conditions initiate cytokine activation of the respiratory epithelium, which facilitates increased adhesion of pneumococci to respiratory epithelial cells and invasion of these cells.[341] Mechanisms by which cytokine activation facilitate pneumococcal adhesion include expression of platelet-activating factor and polymeric immunoglobulin receptor (pIgR). This combination of factors leads to a higher density of colonizing organisms and enables pneumococci to cause infection—including pneumonia, acute exacerbations of chronic bronchitis, sinusitis, otitis media, and mastoiditis—in contiguous respiratory tract sites. Adherence of *S. pneumoniae* to host cells involves an array of surface adhesin molecules, such as CbpA, PspA, PspC, Hyl, Ply, PsaA, and both neuraminidases (see section on virulence factors to follow). These proteins are involved in interactions with the host complement system (PspA), degradation of hyaluronan of the extracellular matrix (Hyl), lysis of cholesterol-containing membranes (pneumolysin), and binding of metals (divalent cations) such as Mn^{2+} or Zn^{2+} (PsaA), followed by their transport inside the cytoplasm of pneumococci. Additionally, transepithelial and transendothelial transport of organisms into the bloodstream results in bacteremia; subsequent transport across other epithelial cells leads to infection of noncontiguous sites such as the leptomeninges, peritoneum, and joint spaces. Such infection occurs in nonimmune hosts by virtue of the fact that pneumococci are able to escape ingestion and killing by host phagocytic cells in the absence of type-specific antibody because the capsule inhibits phagocytosis. *S. pneumoniae* produces few toxins and largely causes disease by its capacity to replicate in host tissues and generate an intense inflammatory response. Cell wall teichoic acid and peptidoglycan stimulate the production of cytokines (interleukin-1 [IL-1], IL-6, IL-8, and tumor necrosis factor [TNF]) and activate complement by the alternative pathway. The polysaccharide capsule also activates the alternative complement pathway in vitro. Such activation is associated with the release of C5a, a potent

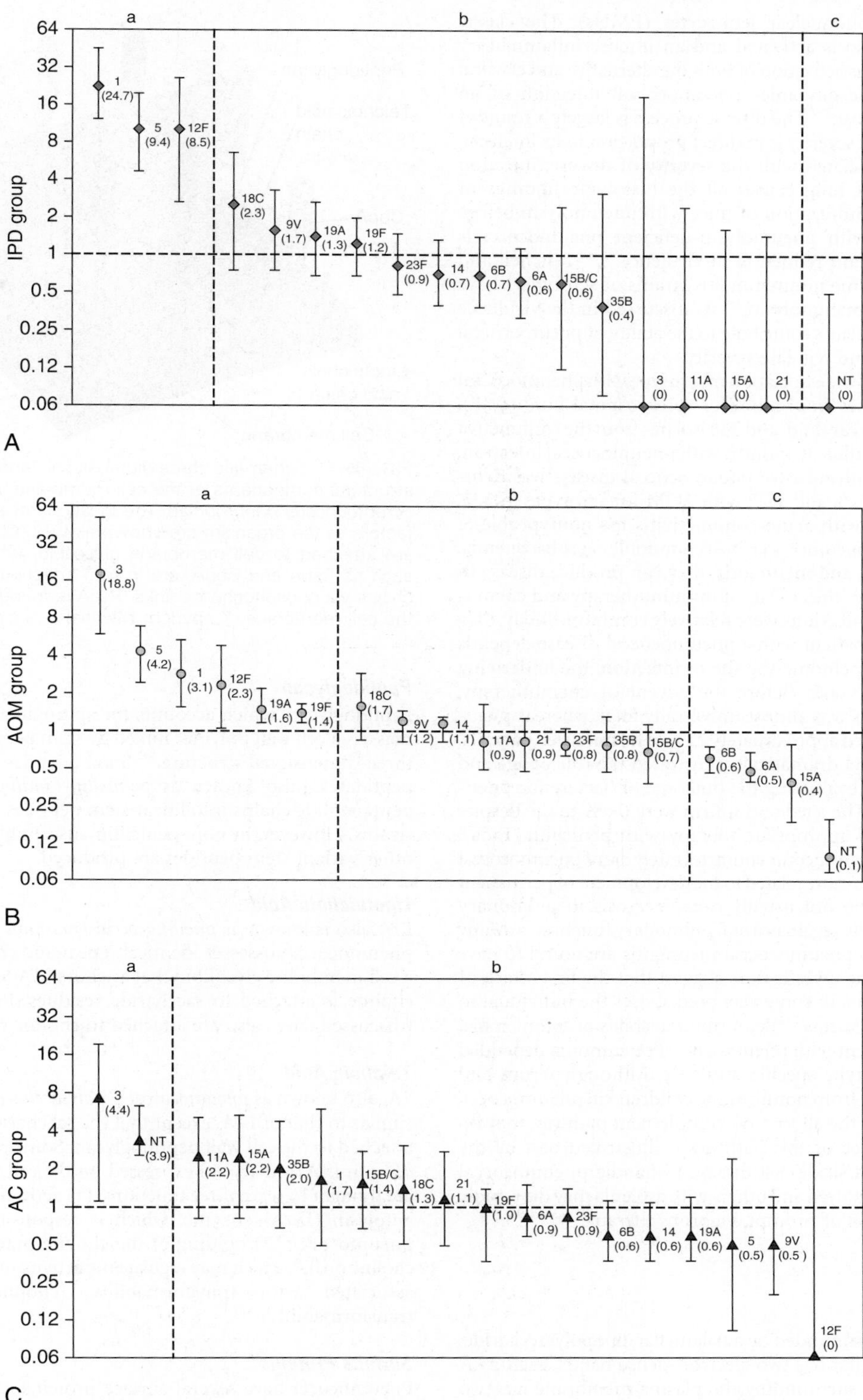

FIG. 85.10 Site-specific odds ratio for different *S. pneumoniae* serotypes for invasive pneumococcal disease (IPD), acute otitis media (AOM), and acute conjunctivitis (AC). (A) Serotypes with significant positive associations. (B) Serotypes with no significant positive or negative associations. (C) Serotypes with a significant negative association. *NT,* Nontypeable. Odds ratios are shown in parentheses. (From Shouval DS, Greenberg D, Givon-Lavi N, et al. Site-specific disease potential of individual *Streptococcus pneumoniae* serotypes in pediatric invasive disease, acute otitis media, and acute conjunctivitis. *Pediatr Infect Dis J.* 2006;25:602-7.)

attractant for polymorphonuclear leukocytes (PMNs). The classic complement pathway also is activated and an intense inflammatory response fueled by vigorous activation of both the alternative and classical complement pathways accompanies pneumococcal infection of an immunologically naïve host.[399] The disease process is largely a result of this inflammation, and its severity is in direct proportion to its intensity. Pneumolysin also is associated with the severity of disease: injection of pneumolysin into rat lung causes all the histologic findings of pneumonia, whereas immunization of mice with pneumolysin before infection or challenge with pneumolysin-deficient pneumococci is associated with a significant reduction in virulence.[41,166] Mitchell and Mitchell reported that some nonmeningitis strains of serotype 1 have a mutant nonhemolytic pneumolysin.[384] As discussed in the virulence section, numerous other factors contribute to the ability of pneumococcal strains to cause disease and regulate severity.

A 2006 study evaluated the association of serotype with pneumococcal disease among 189 isolates from blood or cerebrospinal fluid (CSF), 3200 isolates from middle ear fluid, and 348 isolates from the conjunctiva of children aged younger than 36 months with pneumococcal infection. A positive association with invasive pneumococcal disease was demonstrated for serotypes 1, 5, and 12F; with AOM for serotypes 1, 3, 5, 12F, 19A, and 19F; and with acute conjunctivitis for nontypeable *S. pneumoniae*.[506] Although pneumococci most commonly cause bacteremia, otitis media, pneumonia, and meningitis, they can produce disease in virtually any organ. Before the advent of immunotherapy and chemotherapy, such "unusual" infections were relatively common. Today, they are less so. Survival of a patient with a pneumococcal disease depends on numerous variables, including the site of infection, the underlying disease, and the patient's age. Before the advent of chemotherapy, pneumococcal meningitis was almost universally fatal, whereas pneumococcal pneumonia killed approximately 25% of hospitalized patients. Austrian and Gold in 1964 dramatically illustrated the role of age and underlying disease when evaluating the outcome of bacteremic pneumococcal pneumonia.[33] The aged and infirm were likely to die despite receiving immediate and appropriate therapy with penicillin. Today, healthy children living in high-income countries rarely die of pneumococcal disease; thus, the concern is more related to the development of permanent sequelae. Pneumococci do not usually cause necrosis in pulmonary tissue, and survivors rapidly regain normal pulmonary function.[277] Many children recovering from pneumococcal meningitis are found to have neurologic sequelae. Some investigators suggest that the first attack of pneumococcal otitis media in some way predisposes the individual to subsequent attacks of otitis media.[252] Before the availability of antimicrobial agents, recovery of a patient with pneumococcal pneumonia depended on the development of type-specific antibody. Although serum and white blood cells (WBCs) from nonimmune children kill pneumococci, probably by activation of the alternative complement pathway, they do so slowly. The importance of this pathway is illustrated best by the inability of children with sickle-cell disease to handle pneumococcal infection.[139,284,433] These children and others with asplenia may die rapidly despite the administration of prompt, vigorous therapy.[286,304,499]

MICROBIOLOGY

Structure

Pneumococcal cells are surrounded by a trilamellar, lipopolysaccharide, cytoplasmic membrane that has two electron-dense bands, each 25 Å to 30 Å wide. A cell wall surrounding the plasma membrane has two bands—an inner 30- to 40-Å-wide band and an outer 60- to 80-Å-wide band. Numerous bridges connect the cell wall and the plasma membrane. The polysaccharide capsule covers the cell wall in encapsulated strains and is seen as a wider, less structured band.[551] A schematic representation of the major structural components and selected cell wall components is shown in Fig. 85.11.

Cell Wall Structure

The predominant structural components of the pneumococcal cell wall are peptidoglycan, teichoic acid (TA), lipoteichoic acid (LTA), and several choline-bound proteins. Choline is a lipid that is an essential growth factor for *S. pneumoniae*.

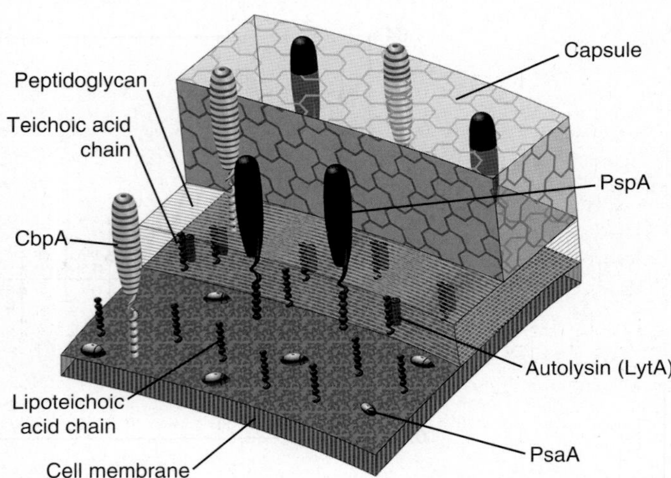

FIG. 85.11 Schematic three-dimensional representation of the major structural components of the cell membrane, cell wall, and capsule of *Streptococcus pneumoniae*. The locations of selected major virulence factors of the organism are shown as well. Chains of lipoteichoic acid are attached to cell membrane glycolipid, whereas surface proteins, such as PspA and CbpA, are in turn attached to the lipoteichoic acid chains via phosphocholine links. PsaA is found on the outer surface of the cell membrane. (Copyright Michael R. Jacobs.)

Peptidoglycan

Peptidoglycan, which accounts for approximately half of the cell wall mass, is a cell wall polymer linked by stem peptides to form a complex, three-dimensional structure.[502] Stem peptides are formed when transpeptidases (also known as *penicillin-binding proteins* [PBPs]) link pentapeptide chains into linear stem peptides in penicillin-susceptible strains. However, in non–penicillin-susceptible strains, branched and other variant stem peptides are produced.

Lipoteichoic Acid

LTA also is known as *pneumococcal Forssman (F) antigen*. The LTA of pneumococci possesses identical repeat and chain structures linked to a cell membrane glycolipid that anchors LTA to the cell.[172,173] Phosphocholine is attached to saccharide residues. PspA and other proteins (discussed later) also are attached to choline residues on LTA.

Teichoic Acid

TA, also known as *pneumococcal C polysaccharide*, has a chain structure similar to that of LTA, except that the saccharide differs. TA chains are attached to the cell wall peptidoglycan. Some phosphocholine residues of both LTA and TA are expressed on the cell wall surface, where they are thought to serve three functions: (1) activation of the pneumococcal autolysin (LytA) enzyme, which is responsible for the autolysis of pneumococci; (2) binding of the choline-binding domain of LytA to choline on TA, which may regulate the activity of LytA; and (3) a function associated with transformability (choline-deficient cells lack transformability).[510]

Surface Proteins

Pneumococci have several surface proteins, the five most important being *pneumococcal surface protein A* (PspA), *pneumococcal surface adhesin A* (PsaA), *choline-binding protein A* (CbpA), *hyaluronate lyase* (Hyl), and *pilin protein* (RrgB).

PspA is a cell wall protein with a molecular size of 67 kd to 99 kd that is bound to TA and LTA by phosphocholine links.[278] This protein extends through the cell wall and capsule to the surface of the organism.[613] PspA exists in various antigenic forms, and epitopes within one PspA molecule can recombine into different types.[77] However, PspA variants usually are sufficiently cross-reactive that immunization with one PspA serotype elicits immunity to other PspA serotypes.

PsaA is a 37-kd surface protein thought to be anchored to the cell membrane and associated with magnesium and zinc transport.[140] It appears to be a lipoprotein and is common to virtually all *S. pneumoniae* isolates.[457] Considerable variation in the amino acid sequences of PsaA from different strains has been detected.[431] The relationship of this protein to other cell wall components has not been determined.[541]

CbpA is a protein similar to PspA and has a mass of 75 kd. It is an adhesin involved in the adherence of pneumococci to cytokine-activated human cells.[476] Several other choline-binding proteins also have been identified.

Hyl is a hyaluronidase that results in breakdown of the hyaluronan and chondroitin sulfate present in the extracellular matrix of human tissues.[476]

Pilin protein (RrgB) is present on the surface of virulent pneumococci in the form of a pilus shaft, which is a long, thin proteinaceous filament extending from the cell wall that aids bacterial colonization in the nasopharynx through epithelial cell binding.[430] It has a large adhesive pilin at the tip, a polymeric shaft, and a smaller cell wall anchor, and is comprised of four immunoglobulin-like domains. Isopeptide bond formation in the N-terminal domains, which provides the covalent linkage to the next pilin subunit in the shaft, appears to take place only upon assembly of the pili.

Capsule

The capsule of pneumococci consists of polysaccharides that vary in the make-up of monosaccharides, the sequence of monosaccharides in polysaccharides, the linkage of monosaccharides to each other, and the presence of nonsaccharide components.[167] Currently, 94 serotypes consisting of 25 individual serotypes and 69 serotypes grouped into 21 serogroups are known (see the upcoming section, microbiology, and Table 85.2). Each serotype has a specific capsular structure, and serotypes within a serogroup often have the same oligosaccharide sequences linked differently. The capsular structure of many serotypes has been determined.[369]

Several epidemic clones have different serotypes, and extensive genetic changes involving the replacement of entire cassettes of genes related to capsule production are required for capsular switching to take place.[6]

Changes in serotype distribution are the result of both serotype replacement and capsular switching. The role of capsular switching and the extent of vaccine-induced selective pressures on this are not clear. Analysis of serotype and multilocus sequence typing data and whole-genome sequence data for a subset of 426 pneumococci dated from 1937 through 2007 showed that 36 independent capsular switch events had occurred during this time period.[607] Two events took place no later than 1960, and the imported DNA included the capsular locus and the nearby penicillin-binding protein genes pbp2x and pbp1a. Capsular switching has therefore been a regular occurrence among pneumococcal populations throughout the past 7 decades. Recombination of large DNA fragments (>30 kb), sometimes including the capsular locus and penicillin-binding protein genes, predated both vaccine introduction and widespread antibiotic use and has likely been an intrinsic feature throughout the history of pneumococcal evolution. These recombination events, including the capsular locus and penicillin-binding protein genes, help explain the evolution of penicillin resistance in pneumococci.

Genome

The complete pneumococcal genome has been mapped. The genome has been estimated to be 2.0 to 2.1 megabases in size, approximately half that of *Escherichia coli*.[44,143] The locations of more than 100 genes, including 20 tRNA synthetase and 20 ribosomal protein genes, have been mapped. Genes involved in cell wall synthesis also have been identified. *S. pneumoniae* is a naturally transformable bacterium, which means that it is able to take up single-stranded DNA from its environment and incorporate this exogenous DNA into its genome. This process is known as *transformational recombination*.[393,523] Recombination is a powerful means of genome evolution and provides a great degree of genome flexibility to this organism. Transformation occurs only at high cell densities (10^5–10^8 colony-forming units/mL), and a peptide pheromone quorum-sensing signal called *activator* or *competence factor* is required.[453] This factor also is called *competence-stimulating peptide*.[526] The genes associated with capsule synthesis have been characterized for several serotypes as well. The complete nucleotide sequence of many of these genes of several *S. pneumoniae* serotypes has been determined.[27,185,390,586]

While next-generation sequencing has revolutionized bacterial genomics, major barriers still exist to its implementation for routine microbiological use in public health and clinical microbiology laboratories.[481] These limitations include the inherent complexity and high frequency of data analyses on very large sets of DNA sequence data, the ability to ensure data integrity, the need for quick and accurate results, and the lack of a user-friendly interface.

Virulence Factors

Animal models of pneumococcal infection have provided considerable insight into the pathogenesis of disease and the association of virulence factors with disease. However, the pneumococcus is primarily a human pathogen, and the host defenses of animal models can vary significantly from those in humans. For example, pneumococci adhere to human but not to rabbit pIgR.[50,619] Additionally, virulence in mice varies considerably with the strain of pneumococcus: pneumococci belonging to serogroups 6, 14, 19, and 23 rarely are virulent in mice, whereas serotypes 1, 2, and 3 usually are virulent.[76,619] Virulence also may vary according to the mouse strain.[1,31,35,319,462,548]

Some serotypes can be virulent to one species of animal but not to others. An example is serotype 19F, which rarely is virulent in mice[35] but is highly virulent in guinea pigs.[31] In addition, penicillin resistance appears to be linked to decreased virulence by virtue of the fact that virulence of isogenic mutants of a virulent, penicillin-susceptible strain was reduced significantly when transformed into a penicillin-resistant strain with an abnormal *pbp2x* gene.[462] Therefore, many animal models of pneumococcal virulence may not be representative of virulence in humans or representative of all pneumococcal serotypes or antimicrobial-resistant strains.

Although the polysaccharide capsule has been recognized as the major determinant of virulence, relatively little is known about the molecular basis of the pathogenesis of pneumococcal disease. A library of 1786 pneumococcal mutants created by insertion-duplication mutagenesis was analyzed for their ability to survive and replicate in murine models of pneumonia and bacteremia.[328] A total of 186 mutant strains exhibited attenuated virulence; 56 of these strains were genetically characterized, and genomic DNA inserts were sequenced and subjected to database searches. Most of the insertions were in probable operons, but no pathogenicity islands were found. Forty-two novel virulence loci were identified. Five strains showed mutations in genes involved in gene regulation, cation transport, or stress tolerance; the virulence of these strains was shown to be highly attenuated in a murine respiratory tract infection model. Additional experiments also suggest that induction of competence for genetic transformation has a role in virulence.[328] This approach has revealed several previously unrecognized genes required for virulence.

A similar genomic approach was used to look for genes coding for surface-localized proteins that could be targets for protective humoral immunity. By exploiting the whole genome sequence of *S. pneumoniae*, researchers found 130 open-reading frames encoding proteins with secretion motifs or similarity to predicted virulence factors.[591] Mice were immunized with 108 of these proteins; 6 conferred protection against disseminated pneumococcal infection. Each of the six protective antigens showed broad strain distribution and immunogenicity in human infections. Some of these proteins have been identified as LytB, LytC, and a cell wall–anchored serine protease. Another genomic-based study used a genomic expression library of *S. pneumoniae* screened with convalescent-phase serum for immunoreactive proteins.[623] Six known and 17 unknown pneumococcal proteins were detected. Five of the known proteins, including PspA and SpsA (CbpA), were surface-located virulence factors; eight of the unknown proteins were putative membrane proteins. Use of these genomic approaches for the identification of novel microbial targets to elicit a protective immune response has been validated. These new antigens may play roles in the development of improved vaccines against *S. pneumoniae*.

Capsule

The capsule is the major determinant of virulence in pneumococci. It prevents phagocytosis by PMNs and macrophages, thereby allowing unrestricted extracellular multiplication of the organism. Because the pneumococcus has 94 antigenically distinct serotypes, production of anticapsular antibody in response to one serotype provides protection against only that serotype or serogroup, whereas nonencapsulated strains are considerably less virulent.[399] The importance of the capsule as a virulence factor is emphasized by the fact that protection from pneumococcal infection can be achieved by capsular-specific antibodies. Despite the large number of additional virulence factors (described in the following), the capsule remains the single most important determinant of virulence in avoiding host defenses after the epithelial barriers have been breached. Other virulence factors are important in breaching host defenses, such as epithelial barriers.

Neuraminidases

Neuraminidases are enzymes that cleave terminal sialic acid residues from glycolipids, glycoproteins, and oligosaccharides on eukaryotic cell surfaces; such cleavage may unmask cell surface receptors for pneumococcal adhesins.[431] The neuraminidase NanA has been implicated in the ability of *S. pneumoniae* to colonize and persist in the nasopharynx and middle ear.[552] A second neuraminidase, NanB, has much weaker activity than NanA does but exhibits optimal activity at pH 5, whereas NanA is most active at pH 7.[431]

Pneumolysin

Pneumolysin, also known as hemolytic pneumolysin (PLYh), is a 53-kd cytoplasmic protein produced by all pneumococci. It is essential for the initial binding to membrane cholesterol and the interaction leading to subsequent membrane damage.[36]

Functions of pneumolysin include the following:

1. Pore formation in host epithelial cell membranes: Pneumolysin binds to cholesterol in host epithelial cell membranes, where oligomers of pneumolysin molecules assemble to form 35- to 45-nm pores in the cell membrane, which results in lysis of the targeted cell. Pneumolysin is, therefore, cytotoxic to epithelial cells. It also slows ciliary beating of bronchial epithelial cells and disrupts the tight junctions between epithelial cells. In addition, pneumolysin disrupts alveolar epithelial cells and the alveolar-capillary boundary, thereby facilitating entry of pneumococci into the bloodstream and through the blood–brain barrier.[195,624]
2. Effects on phagocytic and immune cell function: Pneumolysin attracts neutrophils in the early phases of disease and lymphocytes at a later stage.
3. Direct activation of the complement system: Expression of pneumolysin by pneumococci reduces serum complement levels and serum opsonic activity.[10]
4. Promotion of nitric oxide (NO) production by macrophages: NO is produced by an inducible NO synthase during inflammation as an essential element of antimicrobial defense, but it also can contribute to host-induced tissue damage.[74]

Some serotypes, such as 1 and 8, express an ahemolytic pneumolysin, PLYa, in place of PLYh.[299] These serotypes are associated with low colonization rates but high rates of invasive disease. Mice colonized with PLYa-expressing strains had significantly higher colonization densities than those colonized with hemolytic pneumolysin (PLYh)–expressing strains, irrespective of capsular background. PLYa-expressing strains induced diminished innate (dendritic cell cytokines, costimulatory receptor, and apoptotic) and adaptive ($CD4^+$ T-cell proliferative and memory interleukin 17A) responses. Replacement of PLYh with PLYa can therefore change colonization and virulence properties of serotypes.

Surface-Located Choline-Binding Proteins

The virulence of members of the choline-binding protein (Cbp) family and two cell wall hydrolases, LytB and LytC, has been characterized.[205] Cbp-, LytB-, and LytC-deficient mutants show significantly reduced colonization of the nasopharynx. The following proteins of the Cbp family and their virulence mechanisms have been described:

1. *PspA* is a serologically variable protein that has undergone extensive recombination.[247] It is thought to exert its virulence function in systemic infection by interfering with deposition of the complement component C3b onto pneumococci or by blocking recruitment of the alternative pathway, thereby reducing the effectiveness of complement receptor–mediated pathways of clearance.[556] PspA has been shown to bind to lactoferrin, an iron-sequestering glycoprotein found in mucosal secretions, when the level of free extracellular iron is not sufficient for the growth of pneumococci. This binding is thought to overcome the iron limitation at mucosal surfaces and might represent a potential virulence mechanism for colonization of mucosal surfaces.[226]
2. CbpA, or SpsA, is a surface protein adhesin that acts as a bridging element between pneumococci and host-cell glycoconjugates on cytokine-activated host cells.[227] This process is thought to be associated with change from nasopharyngeal colonization to invasion of epithelial and endothelial cells.[476] One mechanism by which this process occurs, wherein CbpA binds to the pIgR of human epithelial cells, has been described.[620] The pneumococcus co-opts the IgA transcytosis machinery and gains entry into and across airway epithelial cells. This process is a novel example of a pathogen co-opting the transcytosis machinery to promote translocation across a mucosal barrier.[288]
3. PsaA is a surface protein that also is associated with virulence via adhesion to epithelial cells.
4. Pneumococcal histidine-containing protein A (PhpA) is a 20-kd protein with putative proteolytic activity against the human complement component C3. PhpA is a potential candidate for use as a vaccine against systemic pneumococcal disease and otitis media.[619]
5. The pneumococcal histidine triad (Pht) proteins PhtA, PhtB, PhtD, and PhtE constitute a novel family of homologous surface proteins associated with virulence; they are also potential vaccine candidates.[9] Although antibodies targeting PhtA, PhtB, or PhtD are protective, the function of these proteins remains unknown. The number of histidine and tyrosine residues in these proteins suggests that they may be involved in metal or nucleoside binding.
6. Hic, a member of the pneumococcal surface protein C (PspC) family, is associated with resistance of serotype 3 strains to opsonophagocytosis due to recruitment of the complement inhibitor factor H by Hic.[314] Hic also interacts with vitronectin, a fluid-phase regulator involved in hemostasis, angiogenesis, the terminal complement cascade and a component of the extracellular matrix. This interaction of Hic with vitronectin and factor H may contribute to colonization and invasive disease caused by serotype 3 pneumococci.

Phase Variation

Phase variation in the colonial opacity of *S. pneumoniae* has been implicated as a factor in bacterial adherence, colonization, and invasion.[590] On clear media, colonies can appear as opaque or translucent when viewed under magnification with oblique transmitted light. All strains of *S. pneumoniae* are thought to be capable of phase variation. Opaque colonies are less likely to autolyze, contain less TA but more PspA in their cell walls, and colonize the nasopharynx poorly in animal models but are more virulent when inoculated into sterile sites. Conversely, translucent colonies are more likely to autolyze, contain more TA but less PspA in their cell walls, and colonize the nasopharynx well but are less virulent when inoculated into sterile sites. Translucent colonies become umbilicated as a result of autolysis, whereas opaque colonies remain dome shaped.

Phosphorylcholine Esterase

This enzyme has activity that removes phosphorylcholine residues from cell wall TA and LTA.[574]

Inactivation of the gene encoding for the enzyme in pneumococcal strains caused a change in colony morphology from translucent (colonizing) to opaque (virulent) and a striking increase in virulence in the intraperitoneal mouse model. Phosphorylcholine esterase therefore appears to be a regulatory element involved in the interaction of *S. pneumoniae* with its host.

Pneumococcal Autolysin

Pneumococcal autolysin (LytA) is a 36-kd cell wall protein attached to choline residues on TA and LTA. It is associated with unlinking of cell wall glycan from stem peptides during cell remodeling and division.

Autolysin initially was considered to be a significant virulence factor, but more recent work has shown that it plays only a minor role and that immunization with autolysin does not provide protection.[431]

Cell Wall Stem Peptides

The peptidoglycan of gram-positive bacteria triggers the release of cytokines from peripheral blood mononuclear cells.[364] However, 100 to 1000 times more gram-positive peptidoglycan than gram-negative lipopolysaccharide endotoxin is required to release the same amount of cytokine. Simple stem peptides were 10-fold less active than was undigested peptidoglycan in stimulating TNF. In contrast, complex branched peptides such as tripeptides were at least 100-fold more potent than was the native material. These complex branched peptides represented 2% or less of the total material, but their activity in stimulating TNF was almost equal to that of endotoxin.

Iron Transport

The availability of iron is a major requirement for the growth and survival of many organisms, including *S. pneumoniae.* Two *S. pneumoniae* genetic loci, *pit1* and *pit2,* which encode homologues of ABC iron transporters, are required for uptake of iron by this organism.[80] Virulence in mouse models of pulmonary and systemic infection is attenuated moderately with a *pit2*-disrupted strain and attenuated strongly with a *pit1/pit2*-disrupted strain.

IgA Protease

IgA proteases belong to a family of proteins used by a diverse group of bacteria, including *S. pneumoniae,* for colonization and invasion. IgA1 protease allows bacteria to cleave human IgA1 in the hinge region. The exact role of these enzymes in bacterial pathogenesis is not understood completely, but they are important in bacterial colonization of mucosal membranes in the presence of secretory IgA antibodies by causing local IgA deficiency.[300] The IgA protease genes of *S. pneumoniae* and *Streptococcus mitis* show extensive polymorphism, which results in enzymes with considerable antigenic diversity.[447]

Phosphoglucomutase

Phosphoglucomutase is an enzyme that is necessary in one of the early steps in capsular polysaccharide synthesis. *S. pneumoniae* mutants lacking this enzyme do not produce a capsule and are avirulent in immunocompetent but not in immunosuppressed mice.[228] Other metabolic pathways also are thought to be affected by this enzyme.

Free Oxygen Radicals

Release of free oxygen radicals has been implicated in the pathogenesis of otitis media by *S. pneumoniae.* Antibiotic killing of bacteria leads to the release of further free oxygen radicals, which results in tissue damage despite the administration of appropriate antibiotic therapy.[539] Reactive oxygen intermediates also mediate brain injury in bacterial meningitis.[30,352]

Nicotinamide Adenine Dinucleotide Plus Hydrogen Oxidase

Reduced nicotinamide adenine dinucleotide plus hydrogen (NADH) oxidase has been shown to be a virulence factor necessary for *S. pneumoniae* infection. The basis of NADH oxidase as a virulence factor is the conversion of O_2 to H_2O. If O_2 is not reduced fully, it can form superoxide anion (O_2^-) and hydrogen peroxide (H_2O_2), both of which can be toxic to cells.[614]

Pyruvate Oxidase

Pyruvate oxidase decarboxylates pyruvate to acetyl phosphate plus H_2O_2 and CO_2 and appears to be associated with regulation of the multiple adhesive properties of pneumococci.[522] A pneumococcal mutant lacking the gene encoding pyruvate kinase showed a greater than 70% loss of the ability to attach to all cell types.

Plasminogen Binding and Penetration of the Basement Membrane

Binding of plasminogen plus penetration of the basement membrane is thought to be an essential step in the pathogenesis of bacterial meningitis.[149] Most strains adhere to reconstituted basement membrane, as well as to its purified laminin and collagen IV components, and to bound plasminogen. Penetration of the basement membrane was achieved within 3 to 4 hours in the presence of plasminogen; without plasminogen, no penetration occurred.

Hyaluronidase

Virtually all pneumococcal strains produce the enzyme hyaluronidase, a 107-kd protein. Models used to simulate human meningitis generally involve the direct intracerebral route of infection. However, intranasal inoculation would provide a more realistic model; this was achieved by intranasal administration of *S. pneumoniae* with hyaluronidase. This model induced meningitis in 50% of inoculated mice; meningitis did not develop in any of the mice inoculated without hyaluronidase. Hyaluronidase was found to facilitate pneumococcal invasion of the bloodstream after colonization of the upper respiratory tract. This murine model mimics important features of human disease, which allows the model to be used to study issues related to the pathogenesis and treatment of pneumococcal meningitis.[622]

Peptidoglycan N-Acetylglucosamine Deacetylase A

The glucosamine and muramic acid residues of the pneumococcal cell wall traditionally are regarded as being *N*-acetylated. However, more than 80% of the glucosamine and 10% of the muramic acid residues have been shown to be deacetylated, thereby explaining the resistance of peptidoglycan to the hydrolytic action of lysozyme, a muramidase that cleaves the glycan backbone.[573] A gene that encodes for peptidoglycan *N*-acetylglucosamine deacetylase A has been identified. This gene may contribute to pneumococcal virulence by providing protection against host lysozyme, which is known to accumulate in high concentrations at sites of infection.

Phages

Whereas transformation is recognized as occurring in pneumococci, another mechanism of DNA transfer in pneumococci is transduction of DNA carried by bacteriophages (lysogeny). A high proportion (76% of 791 isolates) of clinical isolates of pneumococci were found to carry multiple copies of LytA, thus indicating the widespread occurrence of lysogeny in pneumococci.[454] The LytA hybridization pattern of a strain has been found to be stable during extensive serial culturing; it is specific for the clonal type of the strain and can be used as a molecular epidemiologic marker. In addition, phage DNA integrated into the pneumococcal genome acts as an integrase to facilitate the introduction of foreign genes into the pneumococcal chromosome.[196]

Tolerance

The ability of *S. pneumoniae* to escape lysis and killing by vancomycin and penicillin, a property termed *tolerance,* has been described.[242] Among 116 clinical isolates of pneumococci, 3% and 8% were tolerant to vancomycin and penicillin, respectively. Tolerance may contribute to treatment failure, particularly in meningitis, in which bactericidal activity is critical for eradication. A vancomycin- and cephalosporin-tolerant strain of *S. pneumoniae,* the Tupelo strain, has been isolated from the CSF of a patient in whom recrudescence of meningitis developed despite treatment with vancomycin and a third-generation cephalosporin.[373] The defect leading to tolerance in this strain involves the control pathway for triggering of autolysis via a mutated CiaH histidine kinase.[394] A frameshift mutation in the *lytA* gene encoding the main pneumococcal autolysin was associated with vancomycin tolerance in another strain.[394]

Respiratory Viral Infections

The role of respiratory viral infection in predisposing the host to secondary bacterial infection—including pneumonia, empyema, and lung abscess—is well recognized.[341] The lungs of immunocompetent mice infected with influenza A virus on day 1 and *S. pneumoniae* on day 8 demonstrate greater *S. pneumoniae* colony counts, more extensive neutrophil infiltration, and higher lung levels of IL-1β and TNF-α after exposure to *S. pneumoniae* than do the lungs of control mice not preinfected with influenza virus.[341] Influenza A virus facilitates *S. pneumoniae* transmission and disease, with secondary bacterial pneumonia representing an important cause of excess mortality during both influenza epidemics and pandemics.[11,138] This lethal synergism between influenza virus and *S. pneumoniae* was first suggested by studies performed on samples collected during autopsy from victims of the 1918 influenza pandemic and was confirmed by data collected during the 2009 A/H1N1v influenza pandemic.

Glycerophosphodiester Phosphodiesterase (GlpQ)

This enzyme is produced by the lung epithelium and metabolizes glycerophosphorylcholine to produce free choline, which is transformed into phosphorylcholine, which is present on the surfaces of many respiratory pathogens.[100] *S. pneumoniae* has two orthologs of glpQ genes: glpQ is widespread in pneumococci, whereas glpQ2, which is similar to glpQ in *Haemophilus influenzae* and *Mycoplasma pneumoniae*, is present only in *S. pneumoniae* serotype 3, 6B, 19A, and 19F strains. The presence of glpQ2 in serotype 19A enhances surface phosphorylcholine expression and contributes to the severity of pneumonia by promoting adherence and host cell cytotoxicity.

Regulatory System 11

This is a two-component regulatory system, TCS11, consisting of the sensor kinase, hk11, and its cognate response regulator, rr11. Regulatory system 11 is associated with biofilm formation and is postulated to be associated with airway colonization.[104] This regulatory system is upregulated by exposure to cigarette smoke, which would thereby enhance colonization.

ftsY

ftsY is a gene coding for a central component of the signal recognition particle (SRP) pathway that is responsible for delivering membrane and secretory proteins to their proper cellular destination.[473] Deletion of this pathway is lethal to many bacterial species but is tolerated in streptococci, although these strains have decreased virulence. Such strains are therefore attractive live vaccine candidates, as they colonize but do not cause invasive disease. In a mouse model, a live vaccine candidate with deletion of *ftsY* induced serotype-independent protection against otitis media, sinusitis, pneumonia, and invasive pneumococcal disease. This protection was maintained in animals coinfected with influenza virus but was lost if mice were depleted of $CD4^+$ T cells.

spxB Mutations

Large-colony variants of serotype 1 strains are associated with higher numbers of viable faster-growing bacteria that produce no or little hydrogen peroxide.[533] These variants contain mutations in the *spxB* gene and have been shown to be considerably more virulent in mice and less susceptible to early host clearance than wild-type strains after intravenous infection but impaired in colonization. Additionally, *spxB* mutants were less efficiently phagocytosed by macrophages. These *spxB* mutants are hypervirulant in both mice and patients and are resistant to early macrophage-mediated clearance.

Diagnostic Microbiology

S. pneumoniae is a gram-positive coccus that replicates in pairs and chains in liquid medium. The shape of the individual organism is a lanceolate coccus, usually in pairs, with the long axis forming a straight line. Elongated or pointed forms are commonly found.

Isolation

Pneumococci are cultured readily on blood and chocolate agar media, as well as in suitable liquid culture media for isolation from blood. Isolates are facultative anaerobes, and most strains require atmospheric enrichment with 5% to 10% CO_2 for primary isolation[32]; occasional strains are strict anaerobes. Strains can be adapted for growth without CO_2 supplementation by repeated subculture. Detection of nasopharyngeal carriage of pneumococci is a problem because of the presence of other flora; the use of antimicrobial-containing media, such as blood agar supplemented with gentamicin (5 μg/mL), has led to improvements in isolation of pneumococci, particularly resistant strains.[434,451] However, the sensitivity of current in vitro methods is poor in comparison to the sensitivity of mouse inoculation, although not all serotypes are virulent in mice.[246,312]

Identification

Pneumococci usually are identified readily by standard features such as colonial morphology, alpha-hemolysis, negative catalase reaction, optochin susceptibility, bile solubility, and specific reactions with antisera to capsular polysaccharides.[264] *S. pneumoniae* produces an autolytic intracellular enzyme, LytA, that causes the organism to autolyze rapidly when grown on artificial media. Bile salts and optochin accelerate this natural autolytic process by combining with the pneumococcal cell and activating its autolysin. Strains with atypical features—such as rounded rather than flat or concentrically ringed colonies, optochin resistance, or lack of capsules—do occur and can result in misidentification of such strains as viridans streptococci. Atypical strains are more likely to be encountered from normal flora sites and with penicillin-resistant strains. Molecular methods for identification of pneumococci include PCR detection of *ply* and *psaA* genes, multilocus sequence typing, 16S rRNA gene sequencing, and pyrosequencing. The presence of *psaA* is useful in distinguishing between atypical pneumococci and other streptococcal species.[264]

Strains with optochin zones greater than 14 mm can be identified presumptively as pneumococci, strains with 7- to 14-mm zones require confirmation by bile solubility, and strains with no zone usually are not *S. pneumoniae*. However, incubation in carbon dioxide has been recognized for a long time as decreasing the size of the zone around optochin disks, and incubation in room air generally results in an increase in zone size if the strain is a pneumococcus or a decrease if the strain is a member of the viridans group of streptococci.[452] Optochin-resistant variants of pneumococci can occur and usually are seen as a subpopulation within the zone of inhibition of an optochin disk, and optochin-resistant mutants can be selected by passage of strains in the presence of optochin.[398] Strains with equivocal optochin zones or atypical colonial morphology can be tested for bile solubility either directly by placing a drop of bile salt solution (10% sodium deoxycholate) onto colonies and observing for lysis of the colonies or by suspension of organisms in a bile salt solution with a bile salt–free control. Care must be taken in the tube bile solubility test to avoid obtaining false-positive results, which can be caused by the organism suspension being too light or by organisms being suspended in broth rather than saline.[264]

Matrix-assisted laser desorption ionization-time of flight mass spectrometry fingerprinting systems are increasingly being used for bacterial identification in the routine diagnostic microbiology laboratory but may not adequately differentiate pneumococci from species within the *Streptococcus mitis* group, which includes *S. pneumoniae*. A comparative analysis of matrix-assisted laser desorption ionization-time of flight spectra of several species from the *S. mitis* group suggests that it is possible to distinguish different species of the *S. mitis* group by close analysis of their mass peak profiles.[592]

Identification of the capsular polysaccharide serotype or serogroup also is useful in characterizing strains and confirming the identity of problem strains. Such identification is performed by the capsular swelling technique, in which equal volumes of an organism suspension—0.3% methylene blue dye solution and antiserum—are mixed on a glass slide, covered with a coverslip, and read at ×1000 magnification by phase-contrast microscopy. Alternatively, organism suspensions can be dried on slides and antiserum and methylene blue dye solution mixed on a coverslip, which then is placed on the slide. The polysaccharide capsule of the pneumococcal organism binds with type-specific antiserum and organisms can be seen to clump or agglutinate. The resulting change in the refractive index of antibody-coated capsule causes the capsule to appear swollen. Currently, antisera to each serotype or serogroup and factoring antisera to subtype serogroups are available from Statens Serum Institut, Copenhagen, Denmark.[241] The numbering system for pneumococcal serotypes is shown in Table 85.2.

Currently, 94 serotypes have been identified and are divided into 25 individual serotypes and 21 serogroups in the Danish classification, which now is used universally. Most serotypes have one antigenic determinant, whereas serogroups have one or more antigenic determinants common to the group and one or more determinants unique to each serotype. Serotypes within a serogroup usually are identified by the serogroup number, followed by a letter indicating the serotype to which a strain belongs. Except for serogroups 6 and 9, the letters are F for the first subtype, followed by A, B, and so on. Each serogroup contains 2 to 6 related types; the 21 serogroups currently include over 67 individual subtypes. Serotype numbers 26 and 30 are not in use. Serotype 2, an extremely uncommon pneumococcal serotype, was detected as the leading pneumococcal serotype (20% of 221 cases) in childhood meningitis in Bangladesh.[484] These serotype 2 strains had three closely related pulsed field gel electrophoresis types.

Omniserum containing antibodies to all serotypes is available and can be used to confirm the identity of isolates as pneumococci. Because many serotypes or serogroups are included in this reagent, reactions may not always be optimal and usually are stronger in pool or monovalent reagents. Nine antiserum pools classified from A to I, each containing four to seven serotypes or serogroups, also are available and can be used to identify strains in a group of serotypes before individual serotype or serogroup reagents are tested. Other methods of capsular typing can be used—such as latex agglutination, coagglutination, and capillary precipitation—but these methods are not available commercially.

The ability of a polymerase chain reaction (PCR) method to identify the capsular serotype of pneumococci has been developed on the basis of polymorphisms in two genes common to the different capsule loci.[331] PCR holds promise as a noncultural method for determining serotype, and multiple methods have been developed. An example is a high throughput nanofluidic real-time PCR-based assay using 29 primer pairs to cover 50 serotypes. This assay is able to differentially quantify 29 pneumococcus groups for 45 test samples in a single run and can be used for large-scale epidemiologic studies.[136]

Detection of Clonality

In addition to phenotypic features, such as serotype and antimicrobial resistance markers, various DNA fingerprint methods for epidemiologic typing of *S. pneumoniae* have been applied. The currently recognized reference method is multilocus sequence typing, in which 450 bp fragments of seven housekeeping loci are determined. The combination of alleles at these seven loci provides a sequence type, and the relatedness between isolates is obtained by constructing a dendrogram from the matrix of pairwise differences between sequence types.[156,148,363] Other typing methods include ribotyping, BOX fingerprinting with the BOX repetitive sequence of *S. pneumoniae* used as a DNA probe, PCR fingerprinting with a primer homologous to the enterobacterial repetitive intergenic consensus sequence, pulsed-field gel electrophoresis of large DNA fragments digested by restriction enzymes, and detection of polymorphic DNA sequences for a Multiple-Locus Variable-Number Tandem-Repeat Analysis.[243,374]

Diagnosis of Pneumococcal Disease

Definitive diagnosis of pneumococcal infection is based on recovery of pneumococci from the site of infection or documentation of pneumococcal bacteremia, whereas presumptive diagnosis is based on detection of pneumococcal cellular components, such as capsular polysaccharide, or on species-specific DNA and RNA sequences from the site of infection or from remote sites, such as urine.[264] Definitive diagnosis is confounded in many instances by the need for invasive procedures to obtain specimens (e.g., from the middle ear space) and by nasopharyngeal carriage of pneumococci when sputum is cultured. Pneumococci almost invariably are isolated from CSF in pneumococcal meningitis, even in patients receiving oral antibiotics.[477]

However, establishing the diagnosis of pneumococcal pneumonia is more challenging because sputum rarely is available from children and direct lung puncture is performed very infrequently. Detection of pneumococcal bacteremia to confirm the diagnosis of pneumococcal pneumonia or other localized infection is valuable, but it does not occur frequently and the actual prevalence of bacteremic pneumococcal pneumonia in children is not known,[547] although a study suggests that the prevalence is approximately 17% (11/64).[378] Therefore, pediatricians must use other methods to diagnose pneumococcal pneumonia. Signs and symptoms significantly associated with bacteremic pneumococcal pneumonia in children include high temperature (>38.9°C [>102°F]), leukocytosis (>15,000/mm^3), and lobar or segmental consolidation.[547] However, the frequency with which these findings are associated with nonbacteremic pneumococcal pneumonia is not known.

With the widespread deployment of pneumococcal vaccine, occult bacteremia caused by *S. pneumoniae* occurs less commonly. The likelihood that a positive blood culture will be a false-positive result is increased if the WBC count is less than 15,000/mm^3, the time for the blood culture to become positive exceeds 24 hours, or the Gram stain result is suggestive of a contaminant.[491]

Direct examination of Gram-stained smears of clinically appropriate material remains the fastest diagnostic method and can be augmented if necessary by direct demonstration of capsular swelling of organisms in the presence of anticapsular antisera. The availability of antigen-detection systems that can be used in urine, serum, CSF, and other specimens, such as capsular antigen detection by counterimmunoelectrophoresis and latex agglutination with polyvalent pneumococcal reagent, generally has not improved patient management because of the low sensitivity and specificity of these methods and the fact that they usually are positive only when a Gram stain also is positive. The concentration of pneumococcal capsular antigen in saliva was evaluated by latex agglutination in a study consisting of children with CAP and healthy controls. None of the children with pneumonia in this study had a positive blood culture, and pneumococcal capsular antigen was detected in the saliva of 27% of children with pneumonia versus 17% of controls. More cases (20%) than controls (2%) had a pneumococcal capsular antigen titer of 10 or greater ($P < .01$). Quantitative measurement of pneumococcal capsular antigen in saliva may be valuable in helping to make an etiologic diagnosis in children with pneumonia, but its sensitivity is poor and it is confounded by false-positive results caused by pneumococcal carriage.[175]

A rapid (15-minute) immunochromatographic membrane test to detect pneumococcal polysaccharide capsular antigen in urine samples (Binax NOW) has been developed and was evaluated in the diagnosis of bacteremic and nonbacteremic pneumococcal pneumonia. Urine samples were studied in 51 patients with bacteremic and nonbacteremic pneumonia caused by *S. pneumoniae*. The pneumonia was diagnosed by blood culture and pneumococcal polysaccharide capsular antigen was detected by counterimmunoelectrophoresis in urine samples. Pneumococcal antigen was detected in urine by the immunochromatographic membrane test in 41 of 51 patients with pneumococcal pneumonia (80.4%), including 23 of 28 bacteremic cases (82.1%) and 18 of 23 nonbacteremic cases (78.3%). Antigen also was detected in seven of 16 patients with a diagnosis of presumptive pneumococcal pneumonia (43.7%) and in one of the 16 patients with pneumonia but in whom no pathogen was identified. The specificity of the immunochromatographic membrane test was 97.2%, but its sensitivity was only approximately 80%, thus limiting its value.[175] Furthermore, the usefulness of this test is questionable because the antigen was detected in the urine in 30 of 138 (22%) healthy children with nasopharyngeal carriage of *S. pneumoniae* versus only 3 of 71 (4%) noncarriers ($P < .001$).[225] Thus, the test was shown to be often positive in healthy pneumococcal carriers.

One study found that immunochromatographic testing for *S. pneumoniae* in CSF was both 100% sensitive and specific. The simplicity of the test and the longevity of the CSF antigen even after treatment suggest potential utility of this method in identifying *S. pneumoniae* meningitis in resource-poor countries with widespread prehospital antimicrobial use.[485] Another study showed immunochromatographic testing to be more sensitive than culture in detecting *S. pneumoniae* as the causative agent in thoracic empyema.[442]

Newer molecular-based methods for establishing the diagnosis of pneumococcal disease include the use of DNA probes to detect pneumolysin, autolysin, and PsaA protein. However, considerable practical problems must be overcome before these methods will be applicable clinically.[125] Examples include a commercial method involving real-time PCR for simultaneous detection of *N. meningitidis*, *H. influenzae*, and *S. pneumoniae* in patients suspected of having meningitis and septicemia. This method is based on detection of the pneumolysin gene for *S. pneumoniae* and uses a single-tube, 5′-nuclease multiplex PCR assay on samples of CSF, plasma, serum, and whole blood. Amplified products are monitored with sequence-specific, fluorescent dye–labeled probes. The sensitivity of using clinical samples (CSF, serum, plasma, and whole blood) from culture-confirmed cases of *S. pneumoniae* infection was 91.8%. The multiplex assay also was used to test a large number of culture-negative samples, which resulted in the detection of numerous cases of meningococcal, *H. influenzae*, and pneumococcal disease that had not been detected by culture.[536] However, whether these results are true positives or false positives is not known and, in another study, although the sensitivity of PCR amplification of the pneumolysin gene in the serum and CSF of infants and children with culture-proven pneumococcal bacteremia and meningitis was 100%, the specificity was poor, with 17% of healthy controls having positive results.[125] The prevalence of false-positive reactions was highest (33%) in 2-year-old children, the age group with the highest rate of nasopharyngeal carriage of pneumococci. Therefore, although PCR of serum and CSF is a sensitive test for the detection of *S. pneumoniae* in these sites, its high rate of positivity in healthy controls as a result of nasopharyngeal carriage limits its utility in detecting systemic pneumococcal infection.[125]

Another rapid PCR method involving the use of a set of primers that amplify 273 base pairs of the autolysin gene has been developed to identify *S. pneumoniae*. In addition, three sets of primers were designed to amplify a 240–base pair fragment of the PBP-2B gene (*pbp2b*) of penicillin-susceptible *S. pneumoniae* and two common *pbp2b* mutations present in penicillin-resistant *S. pneumoniae* in order to simultaneously identify the penicillin susceptibility of strains. The autolysin gene was identified in all 1062 clinical isolates of *S. pneumoniae* evaluated. In addition, 98.9% of 621 penicillin-susceptible isolates were shown to have DNA fragments amplified by the penicillin-susceptible primers, whereas 72.1% of 441 penicillin-resistant isolates were detected by the penicillin-resistant *S. pneumoniae* primers.[557] A gene probe for the gene encoding the PsaA protein also has been developed on the basis of PCR assay. PsaA was confirmed to be present in representative strains of all 90 known (at that time) serotypes of *S. pneumoniae*. The specificity of the assay was verified by the lack of signal from analysis of heterologous bacterial species ($n = 30$) and genera ($n = 14$), including viridans group streptococci. The potential of the assay for clinical application was shown by its ability to detect pneumococci in culture-positive nasopharyngeal specimens.[391]

While a wide variety of molecular methods have been developed for the diagnosis of pneumococcal disease, use of these methods to rapidly detect *S. pneumoniae* remains problematic, with assays such as those targeting the pneumolysin gene cross-reacting with other streptococcal species, while assays that target the autolysin and *psaA* genes appear to be more specific.[4,90,368,420,528,608,40,303,493] The significance and clinical implications of *S. pneumoniae* DNA detected in clinical samples is therefore difficult to determine.[61] The diagnosis of pneumococcal CAP has been improved by use of real-time PCR in blood and World Health Organization–validated serotype-specific serology.[133] A study using these methods to diagnose CAP in children hospitalized for CAP in Belgium after implementation of PCV7 increased the diagnosis of a pneumococcal etiology from 12% to 74%, with nonvaccine-serotypes accounting for the majority of cases.

Susceptibility Testing

Susceptibility testing of pneumococci has been well standardized, and testing can be performed by determination of the minimal inhibitory concentration (MIC) and, for selected agents, by disk diffusion.[356] MICs can be performed by macrodilution or microdilution in cation-supplemented Mueller-Hinton broth enhanced with 5% whole defibrinated sheep or horse blood or 5% percent lysed and centrifuged horse blood.[103] If sulfonamides are tested, only the latter supplement should be used to avoid the presence of sulfonamide antagonists. MICs also can be determined by dilution in Mueller-Hinton agar supplemented as just described. Many systems based on frozen or dried microdilution trays are available commercially and used extensively for surveillance testing.[265] As with any system, commercial microdilution panels should be validated and used with appropriate quality controls. Another method for determination of MICs, the E-test (bioMerieux), is much simpler to use than are the other methods for MIC determination. Evaluation of the E-test has shown that this method generally is reliable, although problems are encountered with some agents because acidification of the medium occurs during incubation of the plates in CO_2, which is required to ensure the growth of clinical isolates. Agents particularly affected are macrolides and some quinolones.

Disk diffusion also has been standardized well for testing pneumococci against selected agents. Distinction between susceptible and resistant strains is accomplished readily by using the current Clinical and Laboratory Standards Institute method involving macrolides, tetracycline, chloramphenicol, trimethoprim-sulfamethoxazole, and clindamycin.[103,264] For testing penicillin and other β-lactams, disk diffusion is used best as a screening method with 1-μg oxacillin disks that have a susceptible cutoff zone of 20 mm or larger. Strains with zones of 20 mm or larger are fully susceptible to penicillin and other β-lactams. However, strains with zones that are less than 20 mm need to have MICs of penicillin and other appropriate β-lactams determined. Penicillin-susceptible strains with MICs of 0.06 μg/mL usually screen out with resistant strains.

Although interpretative categories for clarifying the significance of MIC values are available, many limitations to the currently available Clinical and Laboratory Standards Institute pneumococcal breakpoints exist, particularly for agents that can be administered in multiple-dosing regimens and by multiple routes of administration and that are used for infections in different body sites. Breakpoints for parenteral β-lactam agents generally are based on the use of agents in meningitis, whereas those of oral β-lactam agents are based on nonmeningeal infections, such as otitis media.[103,264] Nonmeningeal breakpoints for some parenteral β-lactam agents were introduced in 2002, which to some extent will avoid the use of non–β-lactam agents for serious nonmeningeal pneumococcal infections. These breakpoint changes classify strains previously interpreted as intermediate in sensitivity to penicillin G, cefotaxime, and ceftriaxone as susceptible if the agents are administered parenterally to treat pneumonia and other nonmeningeal infections. Pharmacokinetic and pharmacodynamic parameters have been shown to correlate with clinical outcome and offer a more rational approach to predicting antimicrobial efficacy and determining clinically relevant susceptibility breakpoints.[111,120,268,271]

The activity of antimicrobial agents against penicillin-susceptible, penicillin-intermediate, and penicillin-resistant pneumococci, based on the original penicillin breakpoints (susceptible, ≤0.06 μg/mL; intermediate, 0.12–1 μg/mL; resistant, ≥2 μg/mL), are shown in Table 85.3.[267] There is considerable variation in antimicrobial susceptibility between pneumococcal serotypes, and the in vitro activity of selected antimicrobial agents against a collection of 891 pneumococci collected in 2008 from 22 centers in the United States is shown in Table 85.4 for all isolates and for the 11 predominating serotypes.[269] All serotype 7F isolates were susceptible to all agents tested, as were greater than 95% of serotype 3 isolates. In contrast, many isolates of serotypes 19A, 6C, and 19F were multidrug resistant. Serotypes and antimicrobial susceptibility of pneumococci isolated from blood or lower respiratory tract specimens from hospitalized patients in the United States (all age groups) during 2011 to 2012 ($n = 1190$) were compared with those from a similar study performed in 2008 ($n = 694$).[377] Percentages of PCV7 types were 6.3% and 4.9% in 2008 and 2011 to 2012, respectively, and the most common PCV7 serotypes (19F and 6B) comprised only 3.7% and 4.0% of all isolates from both periods, respectively. PCV13 serotypes represented 42.9% of isolates in 2008 and 30.1% in the second period. Non-PCV13 serogroups/serotypes 23A, 15B/15C, 7C, 8, and 31 increased. Penicillin nonsusceptibility rates (using parenteral nonmeningitis breakpoint of ≥4 μg/mL) were 9.6% and 38.9%, respectively.

Antibiotic Resistance

Resistance to Β-Lactam Drugs

Widespread resistance to β-lactam and other drug classes has evolved in the most common pathogens, including *S. pneumoniae*. Although pneumococci are naturally transformable organisms, β-lactamase production never has been described in this organism. Instead, a much more complex resistance mechanism has evolved in *S. pneumoniae* that is mediated by sophisticated restructuring of the targets of the β-lactams, the PBPs, and by other newly described mechanisms.[222] The PBP targets in penicillin-resistant strains of *S. pneumoniae* are modified, low-binding affinity versions of the native PBPs. PBP targets may be modified by mutation or by transformation and homologous recombination with DNA from the PBP genes of viridans streptococci. The level of resistance

TABLE 85.3 Activity of Antimicrobial Agents Against Penicillin-Susceptible, Penicillin-Intermediate, and Penicillin-Resistant Pneumococci, Based on the Original Penicillin Breakpoints[a]

			MIC$_{90}$ (µ/mL)		
Agent Class	**Antimicrobial Agent**	**Breakpoints (≤S/I/≥R) µg/mL**	**Penicillin Susceptible**	**Penicillin Intermediate**	**Penicillin Resistant**
Penicillins	Penicillin G (meningitis)	0.06/–/0.12	0.015–0.06	0.5–1	2–4
	Penicillin G (nonmeningitis)	2/4/8	0.015–0.06	0.5–1	2–4
	Amoxicillin	2/4/8	0.015–0.03	0.12–1	2
	Amoxicillin/clavulanate	2/4/8[b]	0.015–0.05	0.12–1	2
	Ampicillin	NA	0.015–0.06	0.5–2	2–4
	Ticarcillin	NA	1–2	64	64–128
	Piperacillin	NA	≤0.06	1–2	4–8
Oral cephalosporins	Cefdinir	0.5/1/2	0.06–0.125	1–4	8
	Cefpodoxime	0.5/1/2	0.06–0.25	1–4	4
	Cefuroxime axetil	1/2/4	0.03–0.125	1–4	4–8
	Cefaclor	1/2/4	0.5–2	8–16	16≥32
	Cefixime	NA	0.25–1	8–32	>32
	Cefprozil	2/4/8	0.25–1	4–8	>32
Parenteral cephalosporins	Cefuroxime sodium	0.5/1/2	0.03–0.125	1–4	4–8
	Ceftriaxone (nonmeningitis)	1/2/4	0.01–0.06	0.5–1	1–2
	Ceftriaxone (meningitis)	0.5/1/2	0.01–0.06	0.5–1	1–2
	Cefotaxime (nonmeningitis)	1/2/4	0.01–0.12	0.25–0.5	1–4
	Cefotaxime (meningitis)	0.5/1/2	0.01–0.12	0.25–0.5	1–4
	Cefepime (nonmeningitis)	1/2/4	0.06–0.12	0.5–1	1–2
	Cefepime (meningitis)	0.5/1/2	0.06–0.12	0.5–1	1–2
	Ceftazidime	NA	0.25–0.5	16–32	>32
	Ceftaroline	0.25/–/–	0.015	0.06	0.25
Penems	Imipenem	0.12/0.25–0.5/1	≤0.008–0.015	0.12–0.25	0.25
	Meropenem	0.25/0.5/1	0.015–0.03	0.5	1
	Ertapenem	1/2/4	0.03	0.5	1
	Doripenem	NA	≤0.015	0.25	1
Macrolides, lincosamides, azalides, ketolides, streptogramins	Erythromycin	0.25/0.5/1	0.06–0.12	16≥64	>64
	Azithromycin	0.5/1/2	0.12–0.25	16≥64	>64
	Clarithromycin	0.25/0.5/1	0.03–0.06	8≥64	>64
	Clindamycin	0.25/0.5/1	0.03	0.12	>64
	Telithromycin	1/2/4	0.03	0.25	0.25
	Quinupristin/dalfopristin	1/2/4	0.5–1	0.5–1	0.5–1
Fluoroquinolones	Levofloxacin	2/4/8	2	2	2
	Moxifloxacin	1/2/4	0.25	0.25	0.25
Other agents	Tetracycline	2/4/8	≤2	>32	>32
	Doxycycline	0.25/–/0.5	0.12	8	8
	Vancomycin	1/–/–	0.12–0.5	0.12–0.5	0.12–0.5
	Rifampin	1/2/4	≤0.12	≤0.12	≤0.12
	Trimethoprim-sulfamethoxazole	0.5/–/1[c]	>4	>4	>4

Modified from Jacobs MR. Antimicrobial-resistant *Streptococcus pneumoniae*: trends and management. *Expert Rev Anti Infect Ther.* 2008;6(5):619–35.

[a]Susceptible, ≤0.06 µg/mL; intermediate, 0.12–1 µg/mL; resistant, ≥2 µg/mL). Values are shown as MIC values or ranges in µg/mL that inhibit 90% or more of isolates (MIC$_{90}$).

[b]Amoxicillin component.

[c]Trimethoprim component.

MIC, Minimum inhibitory concentration; *NA,* not available.

is determined by how many and to what extent targets are modified.[93] Restructuring of PBPs is mediated by stepwise alterations in PBPs. The high-molecular-weight PBPs—types 1A, 2X, and 2B—that usually are detected in *S. pneumoniae* are involved in transpeptidase activity and play an important role in resistance.[222] Alterations in PBP-2B are associated with low-level resistance to penicillin, and alterations in PBP-2X mediate low-level resistance to cephalosporins. The additional alterations in PBP-1A raise penicillin MICs to 1 µg/mL or greater and cefotaxime MICs to 0.5 µg/mL or greater. Genomic comparison between *S. pneumoniae* and commensal *S. mitis* and *S. oralis* strains has documented the mosaic nature of PBPs among these species, with pneumococci acquiring their altered PBP genes from *S. mitis* and *S. oralis*.[221] Many other mosaic gene clusters not associated with penicillin resistance also have been found.[187] The capacity to produce branched cell wall stem peptides encoded by altered *murM* and *murN* genes, as well as altered PBPs, is required for expression of penicillin resistance in *S. pneumoniae*.[169] The *fibA* and *fibB* genes, which are homologous to the *Staphylococcus aureus femA/B* genes required for expression of methicillin resistance in this organism, encode proteins involved in the formation of interpeptide bridges and also are required for expression of PBP-mediated penicillin resistance.[588] Other mechanisms of β-lactam resistance have been described in laboratory mutants and in a clone of Hungarian pneumococcal strains with notably high levels of β-lactam resistance (penicillin MIC, 16 µg/mL; cefotaxime MIC, 4 µg/mL).[222,519]

Resistance to Non–B-Lactam Drugs

The molecular and genetic mechanisms of resistance to macrolides, chloramphenicol, tetracycline, fluoroquinolones, and trimethoprim-sulfamethoxazole in *S. pneumoniae* also have been determined. Resistance genes for several agents are carried on a transposon, Tn1545.[110] It confers

TABLE 85.4 In Vitro Activity of Selected Antimicrobial Agents Against 891 Pneumococci Collected in 2008 From 22 Centers in the United States for All Isolates and for the 11 Predominating Serotypes

	PERCENT SUSCEPTIBILITY OF ISOLATES BY SEROTYPE (NO. OF ISOLATES)											
Agent (CLSI Breakpoint for Susceptibility [μg/mL])	**All (891)**	**19A (189)**	**3 (82)**	**35B (59)**	**7F (52)**	**11A (49)**	**6C (43)**	**15A (38)**	**22F (35)**	**23A (33)**	**23B (33)**	**19F (29)**
Penicillin G (≤2)	86.2	46.6	100	98.3	100	100	100	100	100	100	100	37.9
Ceftriaxone (≤1)	90.7	65.6	100	98.3	100	98.0	100	100	100	100	97.0	65.5
Imipenem (≤0.12)	76.2	40.2	100	15.3	100	95.9	90.7	100	100	100	100	20.7
Penicillin V (≤0.06)	58.6	13.8	98.8	10.2	100	95.9	37.2	10.5	100	36.4	84.8	20.7
Amoxicillin/clavulanate (≤2)	83.1	45.0	100	62.7	100	98.0	100	100	100	100	100	37.9
Cefuroxime (≤1)	70.1	36.1	100	9.6	100	95.2	47.5	91.4	100	96.4	96.8	20.7
Erythromycin (≤0.25)	61.6	26.5	95.1	64.4	100	75.5	41.9	5.3	88.6	78.8	75.8	17.2
Clindamycin (≤0.25)	79.2	43.4	96.3	100	100	95.9	97.7	10.5	100	81.8	100	31.0
Levofloxacin (≤2)	99.4	100	100	98.3	100	100	100	100	100	100	97.0	96.6
Moxifloxacin (≤1)	99.6	100	100	100	100	100	100	100	100	100	97.0	96.6
Vancomycin (≤1)	100	100	100	100	100	100	100	100	100	100	100	100
SXT (≤0.5)	66.2	16.9	97.6	100	100	87.8	34.9	55.3	97.1	90.9	84.8	17.2
Linezolid (≤2)	100	100	100	100	100	100	100	100	100	100	100	100

Modified from Jacobs MR, Good CE, Windau AR, et al. Activity of ceftaroline against recent emerging serotypes of *Streptococcus pneumoniae* in the United States. *Antimicrob Agents Chemother*. 2010;54(6):2716-9.
CLSI, Clinical and Laboratory Standards Institute; *SXT*, trimethoprim-sulfamethoxazole.

resistance to three antimicrobial classes—kanamycin (*aphA-3*), macrolide-lincosamide-streptogramin B–type antibiotics (*ermB*), and tetracycline (*tetM*). This transposon has been conjugated and transposed to the chromosome of *Enterococcus faecalis*, oral streptococci, and *Listeria monocytogenes*. The properties of this transposon account for the sudden emergence, rapid dissemination, and stabilization of resistance to multiple antibiotics in *S. pneumoniae* in the absence of plasmids.

Resistance mechanisms include the production of chloramphenicol acetyltransferase, an enzyme capable of catalyzing the conversion of chloramphenicol to nonfunctional derivatives. Chloramphenicol acetyltransferase is encoded by a chloramphenicol acetyltransferase (*cat*) gene identical to the *cat* gene from the *S. aureus* plasmid pC194. Tetracycline resistance occurs through ribosomal protection encoded by the genes *tetM* and *tetO*. The tetM and tetO proteins are thought to cause tetracycline to be released from the ribosome. Resistance to fluoroquinolones primarily involves mutations in the DNA gyrase gene *gyrA* and in the topoisomerase IV genes *parC* and *parE*, as well as an efflux mechanism that affects some fluoroquinolones. Resistance to trimethoprim is mediated through a single amino acid substitution in the chromosomal dihydrofolate reductase gene of *S. pneumoniae*, which is thought to disrupt the bond with trimethoprim without affecting the action of dihydrofolate reductase. Sulfonamide resistance appears to result from repetitions of one or two amino acids in the chromosomal dihydropteroate synthase.[597]

Two major mechanisms have been described for resistance to erythromycin. Co-resistance to macrolides, clindamycin, and streptogramin B–type antibiotics is a result of modification of the ribosome through methylation of an adenine residue in domain V of the 23S rRNA. Methylation is encoded by a methylase gene, *ermB* (previously called *ermAM*). Resistance to 14- and 15-membered macrolides (erythromycin, azithromycin, and clarithromycin) but not to 16-membered macrolides (roxithromycin, josamycin, and spiramycin), ketolides, or clindamycin is a result of efflux of the antibiotic from the cell; such resistance is encoded by the gene *mefE* in *S. pneumoniae* and appears to be emerging rapidly as the predominant mechanism of resistance to erythromycin in many countries.[187] Other macrolide resistance mechanisms that have been described include mutations in position 2059 of the 23S rRNA and in genes encoding ribosomal protein L4.[537]

Vancomycin Tolerance

Although vancomycin resistance has not been described in pneumococci, antibiotic tolerance, or the ability of bacteria to survive but not grow in the presence of antibiotics, has been described. It has been shown to be caused by loss of function of the VncS histidine kinase of a two-component gene expression sensor-regulator system in *S. pneumoniae* that produces tolerance to vancomycin and other classes of antibiotics.[409]

Evolution of Antibiotic Resistance

Pneumococci initially were susceptible to many antimicrobial agents, but they became resistant with varying degrees of rapidity to many of these agents. The earliest example was the development of resistance to optochin (ethylhydrocupreine) when this agent was used experimentally in mice in the early part of the 20th century. With the introduction of sulfonamides in 1939, pneumococci similarly exhibited an ability to acquire resistance in experimental infections in mice, as well as in a human case of meningitis.[310] Sulfonamide resistance was identified sporadically thereafter, and a trimethoprim-sulfamethoxazole–resistant strain was recognized first in 1972. Trimethoprim-sulfamethoxazole resistance subsequently has become widespread in virtually all serotypes throughout the world, including developing countries, and resistance to this agent is greater than that to any other antimicrobial class worldwide.[245] Tetracycline resistance emerged in the 1960s and chloramphenicol resistance in 1970. However, little attention was paid to the development of resistance in this species until 1977, when isolates resistant to several antimicrobial classes—including penicillins, chloramphenicol, tetracyclines, macrolides, clindamycin, and trimethoprim-sulfamethoxazole—were detected in South Africa.[22,270]

Subsequently, multiresistant clones of pneumococci have spread throughout many regions of the world. Noteworthy is that multiresistant clones are confined mostly to serotype 14 and serogroups 6, 9, 19, and 23.[131] Whereas resistance to penicillins occurs in a stepwise fashion and in many cases can be overcome by using β-lactams with appropriate pharmacokinetics, resistance to other drug classes usually is absolute, and distinct populations of strains are found to be susceptible and resistant to agents such as macrolides, clindamycin, tetracyclines, trimethoprim-sulfamethoxazole, and chloramphenicol. Unlike enterococci, resistance to vancomycin has not developed in pneumococci yet, although vancomycin-tolerant strains have been detected.[46,242]

Cross-resistance among *S. pneumoniae* to macrolides and other classes of antibiotics usually increases with increasing MICs to penicillin[268] (Fig. 85.12). Whereas only 6% of penicillin-susceptible pneumococci are resistant to macrolides and 14% to trimethoprim-sulfamethoxazole, approximately half of the penicillin-intermediate isolates were resistant to these agents. In the case of penicillin-resistant strains, three-quarters were resistant to macrolides, 90% to trimethoprim-sulfamethoxazole,

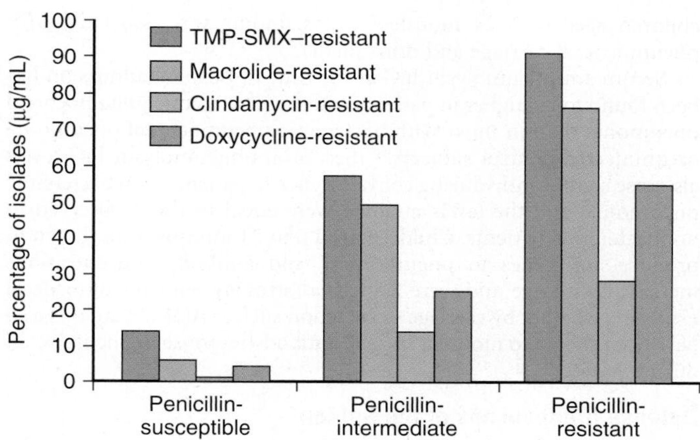

FIG. 85.12 Pneumococci often are resistant to several drug classes, and cross-resistance to macrolides and other classes of antibiotics increases as minimal inhibitory concentrations of penicillin increase. TMP-SMX, trimethoprim-sulfamethoxazole. (From Jacobs MR. Antimicrobial-resistant *Streptococcus pneumoniae:* trends and management. *Expert Rev Anti Infect Ther.* 2008;6:619–35.)

and 28% to clindamycin. However, this pattern is not the case in all countries, and at least one multiresistant clone resistant to chloramphenicol, tetracycline, erythromycin, clindamycin, and trimethoprim-sulfamethoxazole has remained susceptible to penicillin.[135,536]

Strains of *S. pneumoniae* were exquisitely susceptible to penicillin (MICs of 0.01 to 0.03 µg/mL) when this agent initially was used clinically in the 1940s and 1950s, and this MIC range is referred to as the baseline activity of penicillin against "wild-type" *S. pneumoniae.*[264] Evolution of resistance to this class of agents was noted first when a few strains of *S. pneumoniae* were isolated in the 1960s in Australia and New Guinea. These strains had decreased susceptibility to penicillin, with MICs of 0.1 to 0.25 µg/mL, approximately 10-fold higher than the MICs of baseline strains. Strains with penicillin MICs of 2 to 4 µg/mL, approximately 100-fold higher than baseline strains, were isolated in South Africa in 1977; subsequently, strains with even higher MICs (16 µg/mL, approximately 1000-fold higher than baseline strains) were described in Hungary.[519] Pneumococci conventionally are classified as penicillin-susceptible if the MICs are 0.06 µg/mL or less, intermediate if the MICs are 0.12 to 1.0 µg/mL, and resistant if the MICs are 2.0 µg/mL or greater. This classification is useful mainly in characterizing strains as fully susceptible to β-lactams if susceptible or as having decreased susceptibility if intermediate or resistant. Strains with such decreased susceptibility are better referred to as β-lactam drug-challenged because the mechanism of resistance can be overcome if the pharmacokinetics of the β-lactam drug used in serum or at the site of infection exceeds the MIC for 40% to 50% of the dosing interval.[112] Similar variations in MIC ranges are seen with all β-lactams, although MIC ranges for many β-lactams are much higher than that for penicillin itself. Agents such as ampicillin, amoxicillin, cefotaxime, and ceftriaxone have MIC ranges similar to that of penicillin, whereas agents such as cefazolin, cefaclor, cefprozil, ceftazidime, and cefixime have much higher MIC ranges. For example, the baseline activity of cefaclor against *S. pneumoniae* is 0.5 to 1 µg/mL, which is a concentration approximately 20- to 30-fold higher than that required for penicillin to inhibit the most susceptible strains. Changes in susceptibility that occur over the course of time were illustrated in a study of recent versus archived otitis media strains. In this study, the MIC_{90} for cefaclor against archived isolates was 1 µg/mL, whereas the MIC_{90} against recent isolates was greater than 64 µg/mL.[266] A few agents, such as imipenem and meropenem, have slightly lower MIC ranges than those of penicillin. The proportion of pneumococci that are penicillin susceptible, intermediate, and resistant vary considerably throughout the world.

Resistance to macrolides in strains of *S. pneumoniae* was noted first in 1964 and was detected sporadically in the United States until it became widespread in the latter half of the 1990s.[245,259,310] The baseline activity of macrolides (0.03 µg/mL) and MIC distributions (1000-fold concentration range, 0.03 to >32 µg/mL) against *S. pneumoniae* are somewhat similar to those of penicillin. The MIC distribution of macrolides is trimodal, with strains being exquisitely susceptible (erythromycin MIC ≤0.03 µg/mL) or highly resistant (erythromycin MIC ≥32 µg/mL) or demonstrating low-level resistance (MICs of 1–16 µg/mL).[163] These distributions closely correlate with macrolide ribosomal methylase and efflux resistance mechanisms. The prevalence of macrolide resistance and reports of clinical failure resulting from strains with efflux and ribosomal methylase resistance mechanisms continue to increase. Some authors, however, have argued that isolates with efflux-mediated resistance could be susceptible to the high intracellular concentrations that these agents achieve in phagocytic cells and in epithelial lining fluid of the alveoli.[14] However, no clinical or animal data support these arguments for extracellular pathogens such as *S. pneumoniae,* whereas considerable clinical and animal data support the use of current breakpoints.[43,111,112,385] The rising incidence of macrolide-resistant pneumococci was directly proportional to the increasing use of macrolides in various communities and age groups.[184,259,440]

Strains with multiple antibiotic resistance have greater selective advantages than do strains resistant to just one antibiotic because the opportunity for positive selection is increased as the number of drug classes to which isolates are resistant increases.[311] Exposure to different classes of antibiotics allows more opportunity for selective advantage to a multiple antibiotic–resistant organism than to a monoresistant strain, which must wait to encounter the one antibiotic to which it is resistant and is likely to be killed by agents of other antibiotic classes. Thus, the increasing prevalence of antibiotic-resistant pneumococci is associated with the increasing prevalence of multidrug-resistant strains. Therefore, one is not surprised that the use of one class of antibiotics (mainly macrolides and trimethoprim-sulfamethoxazole) can be associated with an increase in resistance to other classes of antibiotics (mainly β-lactam drugs).[3,23,202,440] Many authorities now think that antibiotic agents such as the newer macrolides (e.g., clarithromycin and azithromycin) and trimethoprim-sulfamethoxazole are stronger promoters of antibiotic resistance among *S. pneumoniae* strains than are the β-lactam drugs.[23,202,440] Researchers also have suggested that among the β-lactam drugs, cephalosporins are stronger promoters of resistance in *S. pneumoniae* than are the aminopenicillins.[184,488] Although many strains are resistant to tetracyclines and macrolides, they are susceptible to the new tetracycline derivatives, the glycylcyclines, as well as to streptogramins, ketolides, glycopeptides, oxazolidinones, and rifampin. Many strains are resistant to trimethoprim-sulfamethoxazole worldwide, with more than 40% being resistant in the United States. Fluoroquinolones with antipneumococcal activity (e.g., gatifloxacin, levofloxacin, moxifloxacin) are active against most strains of *S. pneumoniae.* However, in several countries where fluoroquinolones have been prescribed widely, clinically relevant levels of resistance have been described.[95,245] No doubt, antibiotic resistance will continue to evolve and challenge us.

HOST DEFENSES

Although anticapsular antibody is the most prominent protective mechanism against pneumococcal infection, many host responses to infection occur and many other factors are associated with protection against disease.[399] Pneumococcal infection and disease have been modeled in several animal species. Most are models of sepsis arising from intravenous or intraperitoneal inoculation of bacteria, and only a few were designed to study disease arising from intranasal infection. Chinchillas provide the only animal model of middle ear pneumococcal infection in which the disease can be produced by very small inocula injected into the middle ear or intranasally. This model, developed at the University of Minnesota in 1975, has been used to study pneumococcal pathogenesis at a mucosal site, the immunogenicity and efficacy of pneumococcal capsular polysaccharide vaccine antigens, and the kinetics and efficacy of antimicrobial drugs.[193]

Anticapsular Serum IgG Antibody

IgG to the capsular polysaccharide of *S. pneumoniae* is thought to provide the greatest degree of protection against systemic pneumococcal disease and limited protection against colonization. The reference method for measurement of antibody is the opsonophagocytosis assay, which involves serial dilutions of serum, viable pneumococci, complement, and viable PMNs incubated together for 1 hour.[472] An infant mouse assay system for assessment of protective concentrations of human serum pneumococcal anticapsular antibodies correlated well with opsonophagocytic titer but not with naturally occurring IgG antibody concentrations or IgG produced in response to nonconjugated polysaccharide vaccines, as determined by ELISA.[283,404] However, the ELISA method of serotype-specific antibody assay with absorption of cross-reacting antibody to cell wall polysaccharides does correlate well with protection after vaccination with conjugated vaccine, and it is the method used most commonly to predict serotype-specific immunity.[21,561,562]

The development of a phagocytosis assay based on flow cytometry has not overcome the limitations of the ELISA method and is inferior to the opsonophagocytosis method.[276] Investigation of polymorphisms in the variable region of IgG that affect protective function has indicated that the capsular polysaccharide antibody repertoire in adults is derived from memory B-cell populations that have switched class and undergone extensive hypermutation.[355] Functionally disparate anticapsular polysaccharide antibodies can arise within individuals both by activation of independent clones and by intraclonal somatic mutation, which illustrates the complexity of assaying and interpreting serum capsular polysaccharide antibody levels.

Anticapsular IgA Antibody

The role of IgA in the control of invasive mucosal pathogens such as *S. pneumoniae* is understood poorly. Human pneumococcal capsular polysaccharide–specific IgA initiates dose-dependent killing of *S. pneumoniae* in the presence of complement and phagocytes. The majority of specific IgA in serum is of the polymeric form, and the efficiency of killing initiated by this polymeric form exceeds that of monomeric IgA–initiated killing. In the absence of complement, specific IgA induces minimal bacterial adherence, uptake, and killing. Killing of *S. pneumoniae* by resting phagocytes with immune IgA requires complement, predominantly via the C2-independent alternative pathway, which, in turn, requires factor B but not calcium. Pneumococcal capsule–specific IgA may have distinct roles in effecting the clearance of pneumococci in the presence or absence of inflammation, and the polymeric form may control pneumococcal infections locally and after the pathogen's entry into the bloodstream by several mechanisms.[274]

Phagocytosis and Leukocyte IgG Receptors

IgG-mediated phagocytosis by PMNs is the main defense against *S. pneumoniae*. Two leukocyte IgG receptors, FcγRIIa and FcγRIIIb, are expressed constitutively on PMNs. Blocking experiments have shown that FcγRIIa is crucial for opsonophagocytosis of serum-opsonized *S. pneumoniae*. In adults, serum-induced phagocytic activity depends mainly on antipneumococcal IgG2 antibodies.[471] However, in infants and young children, the main response to pneumococcal conjugate vaccines occurs in the IgG1 subclass.[21,571] Investigators have suggested that IgG1 subclass antibodies are at least as highly functional as IgG2.[158] Recruitment and function of neutrophils also are important host defenses. In a pneumococcal infection model in immunocompetent and immunodeficient mice intranasally infected with *S. pneumoniae* type 2, immunocompetent BALB/c mice were resistant and immunodeficient CBA/Ca mice were susceptible to infection. BALB/c mice recruited significantly more neutrophils in the lungs, and inflammatory lesions were visible much earlier than in CBA/Ca mice.[197]

Antibodies to Surface Proteins and Pneumolysin

PspA, PsaA, and pneumolysin are common to virtually all pneumococcal isolates. The development of antibodies to PspA, PsaA, and pneumolysin as a result of pneumococcal infection and carriage in young children was determined by measurement of serum antibodies to these proteins by ELISA in children at ages 6, 12, 18, and 24 months and in their mothers. All age groups were shown to produce antibodies to the three proteins, which increased with age and were associated strongly with pneumococcal exposure as a result of carriage or AOM.[456] IgA to PspA, PsaA, and pneumolysin has been detected by ELISA in the saliva of children aged 6 to 24 months.[511] This finding was associated with pneumococcal carriage and otitis media.

Serum antipneumolysin IgG at the time of hospital admission has been found to be higher in patients with nonbacteremic pneumococcal pneumonia than in those with bacteremic pneumococcal pneumonia or uninfected control subjects.[403] Serum antipneumolysin IgG levels also rose significantly during convalescence in patients with bacteremic pneumonia, and the levels attained were equal to those observed in nonbacteremic patients. Children aged 6 to 24 months were shown to produce antibodies to pneumolysin, and antibody concentrations increased with age and were associated strongly with pneumococcal exposure, whether by carriage or infection such as AOM.[456] Infants also have been shown to mount a specific antibody response to pneumolysin during AOM.[457]

Defense Mechanisms of the Spleen

The spleen is the principal organ that clears pneumococci from the bloodstream.[399,326] Opsonized particles are removed from the circulation by the liver, but with decreasing opsonization, the spleen increasingly assumes the role of clearance. The slow passage of blood through the spleen and the prolonged contact time with reticuloendothelial cells in the cords of Billroth and the splenic sinuses allow time for the removal of nonopsonized particles. Overwhelming pneumococcal infection occurs in children and adults whose spleens have been removed or do not function normally. Pneumococcal disease progresses so rapidly in such individuals that pneumonia is not detectable clinically or by chest radiographs, although it is seen at autopsy. The increase in the incidence of pneumococcal bacteremia and meningitis in children with sickle-cell disease is due largely to splenic dysfunction. Splenectomy also results in a marked, sustained elevation in risk of severe infection due to *S. pneumoniae* in HIV patients.[445]

Vitamin A

The association of nasopharyngeal colonization with *S. pneumoniae* and vitamin A supplementation in infants in an area with endemic vitamin A deficiency in southern India showed that neonatal vitamin A supplementation delayed the age at which colonization occurs. Therefore, it may play a role in lowering morbidity rates associated with pneumococcal disease.[107]

C-Reactive Protein

C-reactive protein (CRP) is a normal constituent of human serum that is synthesized by hepatocytes and induced by proinflammatory cytokines. The function of this acute-phase reactant includes activation of complement and enhancement of opsonophagocytosis. CRP binds to phosphorylcholine, a constituent of eukaryotic membranes that also is found on the cell surface of the major bacterial pathogens of the human respiratory tract, including *S. pneumoniae* and *H. influenzae*. CRP is present in inflamed (0.17–42 μg/mL) and uninflamed (<0.05–0.88 μg/mL) secretions from the human respiratory tract in sufficient quantities to have an antimicrobial effect. In addition, the CRP gene was expressed in human respiratory epithelial cell cultures. The complement-dependent bactericidal activity of normal nasal airway surface fluid and sputum was abolished when the secretions were pretreated to remove CRP. Human respiratory epithelial cells are capable of expressing CRP, which may contribute to bacterial clearance in the human respiratory tract.[206]

Platelet-Activating Factor Receptors of Airway Epithelial Cells

Adherence of pneumococci to cultured human tracheal epithelial cells increased after exposure to acid and decreased after exposure to a specific inhibitor of the receptor for platelet-activating factor.[261] Exposure to acid thus may stimulate the adherence of *S. pneumoniae* to airway epithelial cells via increases in platelet-activating factor receptors. The clinical significance of these findings is not clear.

Cytokines

Polymorphonuclear granulocytes, which provide a major defense against *S. pneumoniae* infection, are attracted to and activated by various cytokines, including IL-1β, IL-6, TNF-α, IL-8, IL-10, IL-12, interferon-γ, and granulocyte-macrophage colony-stimulating factor.[28] The inflammatory response in bacterial meningitis also is mediated by TNF-α and IL-1, which are produced in the subarachnoid space by cells such as leukocytes, astrocytes, and microglia.[424] Inoculation of pneumococcal cell wall components directly into the CSF of rabbits also results in the induction of an inflammatory response with pleocytosis and increased levels of CSF TNF-α and IL-1.[208] Both TNF-α and IL-1β increase mucosal adhesion of pneumococci to tracheal epithelium in a chinchilla trachea whole-organ perfusion model.[553] Induction of type I interferon response in the lung has been postulated to be a key factor in early progression of invasive disease. In a mouse model, a serotype 1 strain infection progressed beyond the lung during development of IPD.[258] The pneumococcal virulence factor associated with this type I interferon induction has not been described.

L-Ascorbic Acid (Vitamin C)

Degradation of the connective tissue component hyaluronic acid by the hyaluronate lyase produced by *S. pneumoniae* is inhibited competitively by L-ascorbic acid (vitamin C).[343] One L-ascorbic acid molecule was found to bind to the active site of the enzyme. The high concentration of L-ascorbic acid in human tissues probably provides a low level of natural resistance to pneumococcal invasion by this mechanism.

Leukotrienes

Leukotrienes are produced by macrophages and are considered important for antibacterial defense in the lung. Leukotrienes comprise a group of highly potent lipid mediators synthesized by the enzyme 5-lipoxygenase. Multidrug-resistance protein 1 (mrp1) is a transmembrane protein responsible for the cellular extrusion of leukotrienes from macrophages. In a mouse pneumonia model, mrp1-deficient mice display diminished growth of pneumococci in the lungs and low mortality by a mechanism that involves increased release of leukotriene B_4.[495] Pneumococci also induce the production of leukotrienes in the middle ear, which has been related to up-regulation of two genes that govern the lipoxygenase pathway.[348]

Human Alveolar Macrophage Binding and Phagolysosomes

Human alveolar macrophages are the major resident phagocytic cells of the lung. After contact with macrophages, bacteria enter phagosomes, which gradually acquire the characteristics of terminal phagolysosomes, with incorporation of lysosome-associated membrane protein. Opsonization with serum containing immunoglobulin resulted in significantly greater binding of pneumococci to macrophages than did opsonization with immunoglobulin-depleted serum.[203] Binding, intracellular localization, and killing of pneumococci by macrophages all are increased significantly by opsonization with serum containing immunoglobulin, complement, or both.

Intracellular Killing

Once pneumococci undergo phagocytosis by "professional" phagocytes (leukocytes and macrophages), they are killed.[399] However, researchers have shown that pneumococci can enter and survive inside A549 cells, a human lung alveolar carcinoma (type II pneumocyte) cell line.[540] Not all clinical *S. pneumoniae* isolates were capable of penetrating these cells, and the presence of a polysaccharide capsule also reduced their capacity to penetrate A549 cells significantly. The intracellular activity of various antibiotics against pneumococci in A549 cells showed that, in the presence of antibiotics for 18 hours, more than 98% of the A549 cells were viable and less than 3% of the pneumococci that initially were phagocytosed could be detected intracellularly after exposure to peak serum concentrations of penicillin G, azithromycin, moxifloxacin, trovafloxacin, rifampin, and telithromycin.[366]

In the absence of antibiotics, pneumococci were phagocytosed efficiently but then paradoxically went on to kill all the A549 cells within 18 hours. The clinical significance of these findings is unknown.

Complement

The second component of complement (C2) is an important factor associated with host defense against encapsulated organisms. Homozygous deficiency of C2 is the deficiency of complement most commonly inherited. Although C2 deficiency can be asymptomatic, patients usually have either autoimmune disease or recurrent pyogenic infection caused by encapsulated bacteria such as *S. pneumoniae*, *H. influenzae* type b (Hib), and *Neisseria meningitidis*. An association between C2 deficiency and IgG subclass deficiency also has been described.[29] *S. pneumoniae* challenge of mice deficient in the third component of complement (C3) results in a 2000-fold increase in organism load in the bloodstream in comparison to controls.[102] Binding of pneumococcal CbpA to epithelially produced C3 results in adhesion of pneumococci to type II pulmonary epithelial cells. CbpA-deficient pneumococcal mutants and lysates therefore fail to bind C3 and demonstrate a moderate decrease in adhesion to type II pulmonary epithelial cells, thus confirming the interaction of CbpA and C3 in adhesion.[518]

Polymeric Immunoglobulin Receptor

pIgR plays a crucial role in mucosal immunity against microbial infection by transporting polymeric immunoglobulins such as IgA across the mucosal epithelium. Polymeric IgA consists of two IgA molecules joined by a small polypeptide J chain. The J chain shows high affinity for the glycoprotein pIgRs of epithelial cells, which are responsible for externalization of polymeric IgA across cell membranes.[280] However, pIgR also can act as a "Trojan horse" and participate in the pathogenesis of invasive pneumococcal disease as pIgR binds to a major pneumococcal adhesin, CbpA.[620] Expression of pIgR in human nasopharyngeal cells greatly enhances pneumococcal adherence and invasion; this effect is abolished either by insertional knockout of CbpA in pneumococci or by antibodies against either pIgR or CbpA.

Basic Fibroblast Growth Factor

Basic fibroblast growth factor is a neurotrophic factor in the central nervous system that is expressed at high levels in response to seizure or stroke. It also occurs in pneumococcal meningitis, as shown in experimental bacterial meningitis in mice and in children with bacterial meningitis.[256] Patients with meningitis in whom major sequelae or death occurred had much higher levels of CSF basic fibroblast growth factor than did those who survived. In patients with bacterial meningitis who survived, basic fibroblast growth factor decreased significantly in CSF after 24 to 50 hours of administration of antibiotic therapy. However, its biologic role in the pathogenesis of bacterial meningitis is not known.

Granulocyte Colony-Stimulating Factor

In a limited study of 22 nonneutropenic adult patients with pneumococcal meningitis, granulocyte colony-stimulating factor (G-CSF), in addition to cefotaxime and dexamethasone, was administered subcutaneously for 6 days. All patients survived, and in only one patient did a complication develop (bilateral hearing deficit). Improvement of inflammation indices in CSF was rapid.[132] However, controlled clinical trials are needed. In a rabbit meningitis model, G-CSF increased the percentage of granulocytes in blood but not in CSF and increased CSF TNF-α and IL-1β concentrations.[492] However, G-CSF did not reduce the density of apoptotic neurons in the dentate gyrus of the hippocampus. A second study in a rabbit meningitis model used longer pretreatment with G-CSF and showed more positive results.[423] G-CSF pretreatment attenuated meningeal inflammation and enhanced systemic killing of bacteria. Pretreatment with recombinant human G-CSF in a murine model of pneumococcal pneumonia resulted in improved survival with low, but not high, bacterial inocula. Therefore, the benefits of using G-CSF are limited, as pneumococci already have recruited large numbers of neutrophils in the lungs by this time.[128]

Intracellular Signaling Pathways

Pneumococcal cell walls activate multiple intracellular signaling pathways in microglial brain cells, with induction of an outwardly rectifying K^+ channel; suppression of the constitutively expressed inwardly rectifying K^+ current; and release of TNF-α, IL-6, IL-12, and other inflammatory mediators.[449] The presence of serum strongly facilitated these effects. The mechanisms involved in microglial activation by pneumococcal cell walls were different from those activated by gram-negative lipopolysaccharide.

Lactoferrin

Human lactoferrin is an iron-binding glycoprotein that is particularly prominent in exocrine secretions and leukocytes and also is found in serum, especially during inflammation. It is able to sequester iron from microbes and has immunomodulatory functions, including inhibition of both activation of complement and production of cytokines. Binding of human lactoferrin to the surface of *S. pneumoniae* depends entirely on PspA.[220] Prevention of the binding of lactoferrin to pneumococcal PspA could be an important host defense mechanism.

Mannose-Binding Lectin

MBL is a key mediator of innate host immunity that activates the complement pathway and directly opsonizes some infectious pathogens. Mutations in three codons in the MBL gene have been identified, and individuals homozygous for a mutant genotype have very little or no serum MBL. In a study conducted in the United Kingdom of 229 patients in whom *S. pneumoniae* was isolated from sterile sites, 28 (12%) were homozygous for MBL codon variants versus only 18 of 353 (5%) controls (odds ratio, 2.59; 95% confidence interval, 1.39–4.83).[479]

Ficolin-2

Serotype 11E has been described among isolates previously typed as 11A.[73] Serotype 11A pneumococci express capsule beta-galactose-6-O-acetylation mediated by the capsule synthesis gene *wcjE*, while serotype 11E strains contain loss-of-function mutations in *wcjE* and completely lack expression of beta-galactose-6-O-acetylation.[86] Serotype 11E is rarely carried, but is a common invasive strain, suggesting that it survives better during invasion. This has been postulated to be associated with the innate host factor ficolin-2, an initiator of the lectin complement pathway leading to complement-dependent opsonophagocytosis. Low ficolin-2 binding to serotype 11A has been postulated to account for the low invasive potential of this serotype 11A.[73]

CLINICAL SYNDROMES

The pneumococcus causes disease over the entire age spectrum from early-onset neonatal sepsis to pneumonia, IPD, and meningitis in geriatric patients. It is found frequently in the nasopharynx of children younger than 5 years, yet only a small fraction of colonized children develop either invasive disease syndromes or respiratory tract infection. New data from both animal and human studies suggest that colonization is associated with a mild inflammatory response within the nasopharynx that, in general, resolves spontaneously.[287,604] In those children in whom the pneumococcus evades host defenses, it has the potential to cause local respiratory tract illnesses such as AOM, acute sinusitis, and nonbacteremic pneumonia or to enter the bloodstream and result in a spectrum of clinical syndromes, including bacteremia, sepsis, meningitis, or focal infections such as septic arthritis, osteomyelitis, endocarditis, soft tissue infection, or peritonitis. Infection may also spread directly to the central nervous system from the nasopharynx in children with cochlear implants and in children with basal skull fracture and CSF leak. Peritonitis is also reported, most often in children with nephrotic syndrome. Colonization of the genital tract in women is also reported and may be the source for early-onset sepsis in vulnerable newborns or spread through the fallopian tubes to the peritoneal cavity.

The clinical signs and symptoms of patients with pneumococcal infection can be nonspecific, reflective of the bacteremia/sepsis syndrome, or specific to the organ system involved. In general, bacteremia presents with high fever and temperatures that can exceed 40°C.[37] Pneumococcal pneumonia most often will present with fever, cough and tachypnea, and possibly chest pain when consolidation is also present.

Bacteremia and "Occult" Bacteremia

Unsuspected or "occult" bacteremia in children 3 to 36 months of age presenting with fever without evidence of toxicity or focal infection has been reported in up to 4% of febrile infants and toddlers in the era prior to the introduction of pneumococcal conjugate vaccines. Where clinical practice includes performance of blood cultures on febrile children with mild or moderate toxicity, bacteremia has been identified from emergency or walk-in clinics as well as office practice settings.[75] In the United States, *S. pneumoniae* represented ~ 60% of pathogens identified in children well enough to be discharged home while *H. influenzae* type b (Hib) was identified in up to 25% of cases. This distribution was dramatically altered with the introduction of Hib conjugate vaccines, increasing the proportion of bacteremic cases from which *S. pneumoniae* was isolated from blood culture to 80% to 90%.[12,307,602] Age less than 24 months and temperature greater than 39°C were the demographic and clinical features initially described that characterized the majority of children with "occult" pneumococcal bacteremia in US studies. Clinically, the risk of bacteremia increases with increasing temperature being greatest, with temperature greater than 40°C. Subtle clinical differences in alertness, color, quality of cry, hydration and responsiveness have been described in bacteremic children compared to otherwise similar febrile children.[371,602,372] Laboratory studies reveal that elevated WBC counts above 15,000 per mm^3, absolute neutrophil counts above 5,000 per mm^3, or elevated erythrocyte sedimentation rate or procalcitonin[17] are associated with increased risk of pneumococcal bacteremia, but each has a poor predictive value. These tests are best used as negative predictors, as a WBC count below 10,000 per mm^3, normal absolute neutrophil count, or a normal erythrocyte sedimentation rate have negative predictive values that are near 99%.

The clinical significance of "occult" bacteremia in untreated children has been of considerable interest and debate, as some have argued "occult" bactermia is the prologue to serious pneumococcal disease and others that it is primarily a self-resolving syndrome of less significance. Observational studies demonstrate spontaneous clearance in approximately one-third of cases and persistent signs or symptoms of illness in as many as two-thirds.[307]

Persistent bacteremia, even in those with persistent clinical illness, is not common even in the absence of antimicrobial therapy. However, the development of focal, presumed pneumococcal infection is not uncommon (Table 85.5). Temperature greater than 39°C at follow-up best correlates with the presence of persistent bacteremia or a new focus of infection. Persistent bacteremia and new focal infections were associated with higher temperature (mean, 38.8°C vs. 37.7°C), greater elevation in WBC count (18,900/mm^3 vs. 14,900/mm^3), age younger than 20 months, and no antibiotic treatment being prescribed during the initial visit.[37] Complications such as meningitis, pneumonia, cellulitis, periorbital cellulitis, and AOM are the most common focal infections reported at follow-up. Children in whom a lumbar puncture was performed at the initial presentation with fever without a focus, at the time of pneumococcal bacteremia as reflected by a positive culture of blood, have been reported to have a fivefold greater risk of having CSF pleocytosis and meningitis at follow-up.[602]

The role of antibiotics in initial management of the febrile child at risk of bacteremia for the prevention of serious focal complications is controversial. Bachur and Harper reported higher rates of persistent

TABLE 85.5 Outcome in Children With Pneumococcal Bacteremia Initially Managed at Home

Outcome	Number (%) of Children
Antimicrobial therapy at first visit	46 (47)
Improved at second visit	37 (79)
Not improved at second visit	9 (20)
Persistent bacteremia at second visit	2 (4)
Meningitis at second visit	2 (4)
No antimicrobial therapy at first visit	51 (53)
Improved at second visit	16 (31)
Not improved at second visit	35 (69)
Persistent bacteremia at second visit	13 (25)
Meningitis at second visit	2 (4)
TOTAL	97

From Teele DW, Marshall R, Klein JO. Unsuspected bacteremia in young children: a common and important problem. *Pediatr Clin North Am.* 1979;26(4):773-84.

clinical illness, persistent bacteremia, and focal infection in those not treated at the visit during which the blood culture was drawn compared to children receiving oral or parenteral therapy at the initial visit.[37] They also identified that only 1 of 8 patients with meningitis at follow-up returned prior to notification of a positive blood culture, suggesting that the practice of blood culture at initial visit enhances the early identification of at-risk children prior to clinical progression of disease, at least in some children. Whether this syndrome is unique to the United States or industrialized countries or is universal, including developing countries, is unclear largely because of differences in clinical practices in performing blood cultures in ambulant febrile children. The syndrome of "pneumococcal bacteremia without a focus" represented 61% to 70% of IPD in the United States in the pre-PCV era.[615]

Comparable to reports from the United States, bacteremia without a focus, defined as a positive blood culture with no obvious focus after clinical and laboratory evaluation, was identified in 179 (70.5%) cases at a Canadian hospital in Alberta.[329] Of those cases, 40% admitted to the hospital and 89% of those not admitted to the hospital did not have a focus of infection. Of the cases, 29% had focal infection; 8% percent had meningitis, almost 10% had pneumonia, 5.5% had periorbital cellulitis, and 6% had other clinical syndromes. Few cases were identified in the first 90 days of life, with the majority occurring in children between 3 and 36 months. Comorbid illness, primarily cardiac, respiratory, and neurologic conditions, was present in 21.6% of hospitalized children compared to 3.8% of those managed as an outpatient. The overall mortality rate was low at 0.7%. In other industrialized countries, primarily Europe, a low proportion of IPD is characterized as bacteremia without a focus (18–20%). In developing countries, the proportion is even lower (~ 1%).[330,418,503]

Reports from cities such as Bangkok suggest that the "benign" nature of bacteremia without a focus is not a universal observation. In a hospital-based study in Bangkok, IPD without a focus was associated with 23% mortality rate, which was especially high in children with comorbid conditions.[513] These reports suggest that the syndrome IPD without a focus is different in severity and associated complications in Thailand compared to that described in the United States and Canada, with a large proportion of cases developing pneumonia or meningitis and high death rates during the initial few days of hospitalization. Earlier age of onset, nutritional status, comorbid conditions, or genetic factors may result in a different syndrome with more rapid progression of pneumococcal bacteremia and reduced likelihood of spontaneous clearance than the slower progression and relatively high rate of spontaneous resolution described in US children. Yildirim reported that during the years 2007 through 2009, bacteremia without any focus was the most common clinical presentation among children younger than 24 months (46.9% of all cases), whereas the majority of the cases in children older than 24 months presented as bacteremic pneumonia (45.9%).[612]

Pneumococcal Sepsis With Purpura

Sepsis, characterized by hypotension and even purpura that mimics meningococcemia, is also reported with pneumococcemia (Fig. 85.13). It has been observed most often in children with sickle-cell anemia and in asplenic children, although it has also been reported in children with immunodeficiency as well on rare occasions in otherwise healthy children. Unlike meningococci, pneumococci do not produce an endotoxin. However, pneumococcal autolysin has been proposed as a potential mechanism. This glycan-teichoic acid fragment released from the bacterial cell wall has produced purpura when injected into monkeys and mice.[97,234]

Acute hemorrhagic edema in association with pneumococcal sepsis has also been described, possibly suggesting a vasculitic mechanism.[392]

Pneumococcal Meningitis

S. pneumoniae has become the most common bacterial cause of bacterial meningitis in most countries following the introduction of *H. influenzae* type b conjugate vaccines, as well as the falling incidence of meningococcal disease in North and South America and Europe, in part as a result of meningococcal C conjugate vaccine programs. Although meningitis is a less common presentation of IPD in children compared with bacteremia, sepsis, and pneumonia, the case-fatality rates are high (6–54%) and neurologic morbidity is frequent in survivors (0–50%).[214,435]

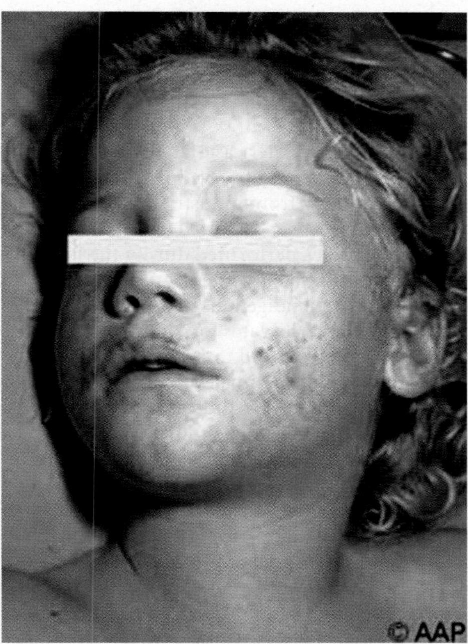

FIG. 85.13 *Streptococcus pneumoniae* sepsis with purpura fulminans in a child who had undergone splenectomy for refractory idiopathic thrombocytopenic purpura. (From American Academy of Pediatrics. Pneumococcal infections. In: Pickering LK, ed. *Red Book: 2012 Report of the Committee on Infectious Diseases.* Elk Grove Village, IL: American Academy of Pediatrics; 2012:571–82.)

Examination of CSF for the presence of bacteria by microscopy and culture yield a bacterial etiology in more than 70% of children that have not as yet received antimicrobial therapy.[214] Antigen-detection assays, such as latex agglutination and now PCR assays, enhance the identification of bacterial pathogen and are of most value in those children who received antimicrobial treatment before performance of the lumbar puncture.[298] PCR assays can also effectively identify pneumococcal serotypes in CSF samples, especially when patients have already been started on antibiotics.[92]

Prolonged fever, lasting more than 10 days, or recurrence of fever after initial defeverescence is reported in pneumococcal meningitis.[67] Most often, an alternative diagnosis of a nosocomial infection is found in children with recurrent fever. Diagnoses such as viral infection, phlebitis, urinary tract infection (especially in children requiring catheterization) or drug fever are common. Occasionally, complications of pneumococcal infection–such as subdural effusion, complicated pneumonia with effusion, endocarditis, or pericarditis—may be the source.[129] Relapse of the meningitis has been reported rarely as the cause for prolonged or secondary fever.[129] The outcome and long-term complications of pneumococcal meningitis include severe hearing loss, seizures, learning or mental difficulties, or paralysis.[25] Patients with pneumococcal meningitis have a higher mortality rate and are at greater risk for the development of neurologic sequelae than are patients with *N. meningitidis* or Hib infection.[289,407] The mortality rate varies from 6.3% to 20%, with the highest mortality in the youngest children.[494] A peripheral WBC count of less than 5000/mm^3 at initial evaluation was recognized as a poor prognostic factor. A high mortality rate and a trend toward a higher mortality rate also was noted if the CSF WBC count was less than 1000/mm^3.[3,315] A similarly poor outcome can be predicted in patients with pneumococcal meningitis when low CSF glucose concentrations (<1.11 mmol/L)[177] or high CSF protein concentrations (>250 mg/dL) are present.[315] A multicenter US study reported a 7.7% mortality rate, with 25% of children suffering neurologic morbidities and 32% with moderate or severe hearing loss.[25]

Children who have cochlear implants are more than 30 times more likely than healthy children to acquire pneumococcal meningitis, presumably from direct extension from the nasopharynx or middle ear. Implants with positioners were associated with a greater risk than those without. The risk period for development of pneumococcal meningitis appears to extend for 24 months after implantation.[56,460] Delayed sterilization of CSF cultures after antimicrobial treatment also has been associated with a poorer outcome.[333]

Higher incidence rates, greater case-fatality rates, and more frequent neurologic sequelae have been observed in children from developing countries compared to those from industrialized countries. Case-fatality rates in excess of 50% have been reported from some African and Asian countries, including studies performed during the late 1990s and early 2000s.[88,418,427,470,486] The case-fatality rates from pneumococcal meningitis in developing countries and indigenous native populations in fact exceed the overall annual incidence rates of pneumococcal meningitis in industrialized countries by 15-fold to 100-fold.[524] The in-hospital case-fatality rates provide a minimal estimate as to the true mortality associated with pneumococcal meningitis, as indicated by studies with follow-up beyond the hospitalization period. A study in The Gambia showed that 23% of hospital survivors subsequently died in the community, mainly related to neurologic sequelae resulting from the meningitis.[260] Late clinical presentation of cases to the hospital as well as delays in diagnosing meningitis—for example, 22% initial erroneous misdiagnosis of pneumococcal meningitis as malaria in Malawi[387]—may contribute to this high mortality. The review by Peltola reported that mortality rates for pneumococcal meningitis (45%) were greater than for *H. influenzae* (29%) or *N. meningitidis* (8%).[435] A meta-analysis on mortality due to bacterial meningitis in developed countries also found higher mortality rates associated with pneumococcal meningitis (15.3% vs. 3.8% for *H. influenzae* type b and 7.5% for *N. meningitidis*).[47]

Pneumonia

Defining pneumococcal pneumonia in children remains a challenge, as a specific pathogen cannot be documented in most cases unless bacteremia or empyema occur. Vaccine probe studies have helped to redefine the spectrum of clinical pneumonia associated with *S. pneumoniae* and extended the clinical description beyond lobar pneumonia. Lobar pneumonia remains the classical pulmonary disease resulting from pneumococcal infections. High fever exceeding 40°C, general fatigue, a productive cough, and dyspnea are the prototypic presenting signs and symptoms. In older children, chest pain is often associated with a lobar infiltrate. Fever and cough are nearly universal, occuring in 90% and 70%, respectively. Severe abdominal pain is often a presenting symptom in left lower lobe disease; chest pain occurs in 10% to 50% of patients[542] and meningeal signs may be present with apical infiltrates, especially in young children. Comparison of pneumococcal pneumonia with respiratory syncytial virus demonstrates significant overlap in presentation. Children with pneumococcal pneumonia less often have tachypnea but more often high WBC counts (mean of 20,800/mm^3 in pneumococcal pneumonia) and high CRP level (mean of 137 mg/L). Alveolar infiltrates are observed more frequently, but not exclusively, in pneumococcal pneumonia.[285] Children with bacteremic pneumococcal pneumonia appeared more ill than children with nonbacteremic pneumococcal pneumonia. Lobar infiltrates on chest radiographs were present in the majority of bacteremic cases. Pleural effusion is common and occurs in up to 40% of patients; however, only 10% have substantial fluid accumulation and 2% develop empyema.[345] Patients with pleural fluid secondary to pneumonia have the usual signs and symptoms, with chest pain, abdominal pain, egophony, and/or dullness on percussion. A pleural friction rub, abdominal pain, and dullness on percussion may also be present. Persistent fever, lasting as long as 3 weeks, can be associated with even relatively small effusions.[542] Several studies have reported *S.pneumoniae* as the most common cause of empyema in children.[85] It was most commonly reported in children between 3 and 5 years of age. Serotypes 1, 19A, and 3 were the most common pneumococcal serotypes identified in children with empyema.[84]

Establishing the diagnosis of a specific pathogen in children with pneumonia remains challenging. Blood culture is positive in no more than 10% of patients with pneumococcal pneumonia.[585] Children with bacteremic pneumococcal pneumonia usually have a high temperature and leukocytosis on admission, with peripheral WBC counts exceeding 15,000/mm^3, similar to those without bacteremia.[550] Based on vaccine probe studies, Madhi et al. reported that procalcitonin and CRP were equally useful in children infected and not infected with HIV to improve the specificity of the pneumococcal pneumonia efficacy endpoint in the vaccine trial among children with radiologically confirmed pneumonia.[358]

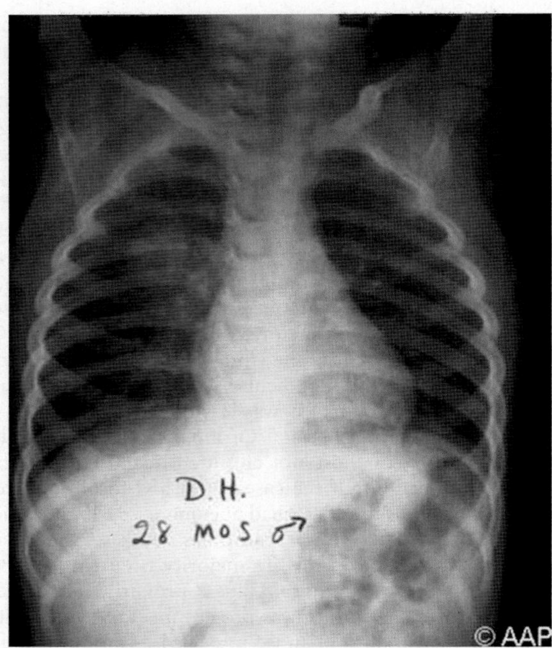

FIG. 85.14 Segmental (round) pneumococcal pneumonia in 28-month-old child. (From American Academy of Pediatrics. Pneumococcal infections. In: Pickering LK, ed. *Red Book: 2012 Report of the Committee on Infectious Diseases*. Elk Grove Village, IL: American Academy of Pediatrics; 2012:571–82.)

No strict radiologic definition of pneumococcal pneumonia in children is accepted broadly. At one end is the typical appearance of severe lobar consolidation (Fig. 85.14), which is recognized as associated with bacterial pneumonia.[603] At the other end are the mild interstitial and perihilar changes that are often associated with viral infections or asthma and that may be part of the spectrum of normal appearances for children in developing countries. In studies performing lung aspiration in cases of radiologically proven lobar infiltrates, the proportion of patients in whom *S. pneumoniae* was detected was high.[161,576,581] *S. pneumoniae* was the predominant bacterial pathogen in most studies of childen with lobar infiltrates (Table 85.6).[359] The role of the pneumococcus in children with lobar infiltrates is further supported by the observed 63% reduction in pneumonia with alveolar infiltrates in children vaccinated with a PCV-7 compared to children receiving placebo.[60]

While the role of the pneumococcus in children with lobar consolidation is known, its role in cases with other radiologic findings is not as well defined. Studies demonstrating a reduction in hospitalizations associated with viral pneumonia in children immunized with PCV suggests a role for the pneumococcus in disease manifesting as interstitial and perihilar infiltrates, as least in countries such as South Africa. A study found that the incidence of human metapneumovirus lower respiratory tract infection was reduced by 45% and the incidence of clinical pneumonia was reduced by 55% percent in non–HIV-infected children who had received three doses of conjugate pneumococcal vaccine. In fully vaccinated HIV-infected children, the incidence of human metapneumovirus–associated lower respiratory tract infection was reduced by 53% and that of clinical pneumonia by 65%.[357]

In the preantibiotic era, the natural course of pneumococcal pneumonia consisted of 7 to 9 days of a stationary phase of symptoms followed by worsening of the systemic signs ("precrisis") and high mortality. Today, the mortality rate in industrialized countries is extremely low—less than 1%—even in cases of bacteremic pneumonia and long-term complications are uncommon.[291] However, hemolytic uremic

TABLE 85.6 **Etiology of Pneumonia Based on Lung Aspirate Studies**[357]

Continent	Age	No.	% Culture Positive	INFECTIOUS AGENT, N (%)				
				S. pneumoniae	*H. influenzae*	*S. aureus*	*E. coli*	Other
Europe	6 wk–11 y	255	66	40 (32)	21 (17)	13 (5)	0.5 (0)	13 (10)
North America	2 mo–15 y	240	34	77 (26)	5 (2)	12 (4)	2 (0.1)	15 (5)
South America	1 mo–14 y	885	44	22 (10)	14 (6)	44 (19)	3 (1)	22 (9)
Africa	1 mo–12 y	949	66	25 (17)	17 (12)	29 (20)	4 (3)	44 (31)
Asia	11d–14 y	674	51	10 (2)	9 (5)	45 (24)	4 (2)	29 (15)
Oceania	1 mo–10 y	101	58	57 (34)	71 (42)	1 (1)	0 (0)	39 (23)

Modified from Madhi S, Pelton SI. Epidemiology, diagnosis and treatment of serious pneumococcal infections in children from pneumococcal vaccines. In: George R. Siber, Keith P. Klugman, P. Helena Makela, eds. *The Impact of Conjugate Vaccine.* Washington, DC: ASM Press; 2008:95–108.

syndrome in association with pneumococcal pneumonia and bacteremia is being reported with increasing frequency. Thirty-seven cases occurring between 1997 and 2009 in North America were reported from the Emerging Infection Network.[45] In general, the patients were severely ill, presented with pneumonia and bacteremia, and half of the patients required mechanical ventilation and chest tube placement or video-assisted thoracoscopic surgery. Ninety-two percent of cases were associated with PCV13 serotypes, with serotype 19A recovered from half of the children. Twenty cases have been reported from Taiwan.[334]

Otitis Media

Between 25% to 60% of cases of AOM are attributable to the pneumococcus. The bacteriologic outcome of *S. pneumoniae* AOM is less favorable than is the outcome of AOM caused by other organisms when untreated or treated inappropriately.[308,400,421] The pathogenesis is thought to reflect recently acquired colonization in combination with viral respiratory tract infections in most cases.[308,400] Some studies have suggested that pneumococcal AOM is more severe than that caused by other pathogens; however, the overlap in signs and symptoms prevents clinical criteria alone from accurately predicting the etiologic pathogen. Observations from 1970 support that pneumococcal AOM is accompanied more frequently by greater pain and higher fever than was AOM caused by other pathogens, is more purulent as characterized by higher middle ear fluid WBC counts, and that the tympanic membrane is more erythematous.[78,251] Subsequent studies have reported that when *S. pneumoniae* is recovered from the nasopharynx at the time that AOM is present, there are greater abnormalities in the tympanic membrane, as reflected in higher severity score and greater likelihood of persistent symptoms on day five, persistence of tympanic membrane abnormalities on day 28, and recurrence before day 28.[160] Spontaneous remission of the infection occurs less commonly in patients with pneumococcal AOM than in those with other pathogens.[250] Tympanic membrane perforation is also more commonly observed with pneumococcal otitis.

Mastoiditis

Acute mastoiditis is the most common suppurative complication of AOM.[114] *S. pneumoniae* is the most common cause of acute mastoiditis in children and accounts for 25% to 46% of all culture-proven cases.[198,248] Increased cases of mastoiditis due to multidrug-resistant *S. pneumoniae* have been reported following the introduction of PCV7 in the United States.[422] Studies of the incidence of mastoiditis suggest a higher rate of disease in countries in which observation is the first-line approach to children with otitis media; however, the risk still remains remarkably small in such countries.[565]

Sinusitis

Studies suggest that 5% to 10% of all upper respiratory tract infections are complicated by bacterial sinusitis when defined as either acute, febrile illness with facial swelling (usually localized to the eye), initial improvement in upper respiratory tract infection signs and symptoms, and then recurrence of signs and symptoms or persistence of rhinorrhea, low-grade fever, facial swelling without improvement beyond 10 days.[579] *S. pneumoniae* is the pathogen most commonly isolated from patients with sinusitis, and it causes 35% to 42% of all bacterial cases.[580]

Conjunctivitis

Purulent bacterial conjunctivitis due to *S. pneumoniae* is well described, with nonencapsulated strains most often involved. Clinically, bilateral, purulent discharge is the most common clinical presentation and often distinguishes it from viral disease.[62,194,578,591] When conjunctivitis is present with AOM, the so-called "conjunctivitis-otitis" syndrome, *H. influenzae* is the most common pathogen.[64]

A study in Minnesota[551] evaluated children with conjunctivitis in two cities. A total of 49% of positive cultures were *S. pneumoniae*. All isolates were nontypeable. Pulsed-field gel electrophoresis identified three clonal groups, with 84% of the isolates belonging to one clonal group. Multilocus sequence typing revealed that isolates had the same multilocus sequence type as that of isolates from a 2002 pneumococcal disease outbreak at a New England college. It has been suggested that certain pneumococcal strains have a predilection for causing conjunctivitis.[83] These reports suggest that pneumococcal conjunctivitis can be highly contagious in school settings.

Bone and Joint Infections

Septic arthritis caused by *S. pneumoniae* is a relatively rare condition that accounts for 2.2% to 9.7% of all cases.[219,482] Its main initial clinical features are single or multiple swollen, warm, and painful joints. The joints most commonly involved are the knee and the ankle.[262] In one study, the mean duration of symptoms before hospitalization was 2 days, and patients were hospitalized for an average of 11 days. The mean peripheral WBC count was 20,600/mm^3, the erythrocyte sedimentation rate usually was greater than 90 mm/h, and the CRP concentration generally was higher than 100 mg/L. *S. pneumoniae* can be isolated from synovial fluid or blood in most patients.[482] The outcome is favorable in the majority of cases unless underlying diseases or sepsis occurs concomitantly.[262]

Soft Tissue Infections

S. pneumoniae has become an uncommonly recognized etiologic agent of soft tissue infections but can cause serious infections. Most commonly, facial cellulitis has been described in otherwise healthy children in conjunction with recovery of *S. pneumoniae* from either local or systemic cultures.[141] Periorbital infection can be a complication of sinus disease and can uncommonly spread to the orbit, resulting in orbital cellulitis or abscess manifested as proptosis and ophthalmoplegia.[504] Most patients with such complications are younger than 3 years of age and previously were healthy. Fever and peripheral WBC counts higher than 15,000/mm^3 can be observed in most patients, and blood cultures frequently are positive. Overall, response to therapy generally is good, and patients usually recover.[199] In patients with connective tissue diseases, such as systemic lupus erythematosus and HIV infection, or undergoing corticosteroid treatment, pneumococcal cellulitis has been reported and may be severe.

Peritonitis

Primary peritonitis, in which the pathogen travels from the blood or via the lymphatic system to the peritoneal cavity, is an uncommon condition that accounts for only 17% of all cases of peritonitis. *S. pneumoniae* is the major pathogen in primary peritonitis, responsible for 38% of all cases.[204] Primary pneumococcal peritonitis should be considered in the differential diagnosis of children with an acute abdominal syndrome,[181] particularly in children with nephrotic syndrome, immunocompromised status, or sickle-cell disease.[204] Colonization of the perineum and subsequent spread via the fallopian tube to the peritoneal cavity has been suggested as the pathogenesis of primary pneumococcal peritonitis and is consistent with the observation that 87% of cases occur in females.[501,514] Most of the patients are between 4 and 10 years of age.[501] Symptoms include diffuse abdominal pain, fever, vomiting, and diarrhea. Abdominal tenderness can be maximal in the right lower quadrant, which can lead to confusing it with acute appendicitis. In some cases, *S. pneumoniae* can be isolated as the only cause of peritonitis secondary to appendicitis. Cultures should include blood, peritoneal fluid, and a vaginal swab. Some patients need laparotomy or laparoscopy to exclude other pathologies, such as appendicitis or a tubo-ovarian abscess.[514] Morbidity and mortality rates can be high when the period without treatment exceeds 1 week, but in most cases, the outcome is favorable when treated adequately.[501]

Endocarditis

S. pneumoniae endocarditis is most often reported to involve the aortic and mitral valves. The syndrome of pneumococcal meningitis, pneumonia, and endocarditis was previously more common. It was initially described by Osler but is also known as Austrian syndrome. This triad is now uncommon and *S. pneumoniae* currently accounts for less than 3% of cases of bacterial endocarditis.[263,396,543] This triad is rarely present in children. In children, mitral valve involvement has been described most frequently. A history of congenital heart disease is often present. Medical therapy alone has a high mortality rate that was improved in a group of patients receiving combined medical and surgical interventions.[98]

Pericarditis

In the preantibiotic era, pneumococcal pericarditis was a relatively frequent complication of lobar pneumococcal pneumonia and the most common pathogen in purulent pericarditis in children. After the introduction of antibiotics, the pneumococcus declined as a cause of pericarditis, decreasing from 51% to 9% of cases and occurring mainly in adults. Currently, infections of the pericardium are rare in children and often are related to underlying medical conditions, such as immunodeficiency.[436]

Infection in Immunocompromised Hosts

Patients with functional asplenia, including those with hemoglobinopathies, are at high risk for invasive pneumococcal disease. In 19 asplenic patients with invasive pneumococcal infection, the clinical findings included fever (86%), shock (27%), petechiae or purpura (27%), disseminated intravascular coagulopathy (18%), and respiratory distress (18%). Clinical illness included bacteremia alone (52%), meningitis (26%), bacteremia with otitis/sinusitis (13%), and bacteremia with pneumonia (9%). The mortality rate was 32%.[496]

HIV-infected children with pneumonia usually have the typical symptoms of fever, shortness of breath, and productive cough associated with pleuritic pain. The chest radiograph shows unilobar or multilobar infiltrates, and peripheral WBC counts often are elevated. A comparison between HIV-infected and non–HIV-infected children with CAP showed no significant differences between groups with regard to the duration of hospitalization and mortality rates.[361] In contrast, when only patients infected with isolates belonging to the traditional "pediatric serotypes" (see the sections on epidemiology and prevention) were compared, a higher rate of pneumonia with or without concurrent meningitis in the HIV-infected group was observed. Recurrence of pneumococcal infection within 6 months from the initial episode is also common in patients infected with HIV, particularly children.[188] Most HIV-infected patients recover without significant sequelae, and the clinical course of their systemic infection does not appear to be markedly different from that in healthy children.[275]

Patients with immunodeficiency disorders consisting of antibody and complement deficiencies are at high risk for acquisition of invasive and recurrent pneumococcal infection.[275] Children with nephrotic syndrome have a particularly increased risk for the development of pneumococcal peritonitis, mainly during relapse of their renal disease.[165] Children with sickle-cell disease are prone to the development of overwhelming *S. pneumoniae* bacteremia and sepsis; in children younger than 3 years of age, the incidence of bacteremia is 6.1 events per 100 patient-years, and the case-fatality rate is 24% for *S. pneumoniae* sepsis.[616]

S. pneumoniae is an important pathogen in patients undergoing bone marrow transplantation (BMT) or peripheral blood stem cell transplantation with two patterns of disease recognized. Early onset is observed in both allogeneic and autologous BMT and peripheral blood stem cell transplantation patients within the first 35 days. Later-onset disease occurs after 100 days and is more frequent in allogeneic compared to autologous BMT and is the most common bacterial infection in such patients. Functional hyposplenism secondary to irradiation, chronic graft versus host disease, and decreased IgG2 antibody contribute to the risk of invasive pneumococcal disease and the poor outcome. Case-fatality rates approximate 20%.[322] Chronic graft versus host disease is associated with long-term risk for pneumococcal infections in recipients of BMTs.[155,322]

Solid-organ transplant patients are at increased risk of pneumococcal disease. The risk varies with the nature of the transplant. However, recipients have a lifelong increase in risk due to the immunosuppressive therapy required for transplant survival and recurrent disease is common. Of 42 children who had undergone BMT or solid-organ transplantation and became infected with *S. pneumoniae*, 8 (19%) had recurrent pneumococcal infections.[497] Solid-organ recipients were more likely to have recurrent invasive disease than were recipients of BMTs. Death occurred in 2 of 42 recipients (5%). Cardiac transplant patients have an incidence of 39 cases of invasive pneumococcal infection per 1000 patients per year,[527] the highest risk of which occurs in African American heart transplant recipients who undergo transplantation because of idiopathic dilated cardiomyopathy.

TREATMENT

The pneumococcus is the causative bacterial agent in many respiratory and invasive infections, many of which are often treated empirically. Empiric and pathogen-directed treatment guidelines are available for the major disease syndromes associated with pneumococcal infection. In the absence of rapid methods for diagnosis of disease and identification of drug-resistant strains, empiric treatment will continue to be the rule in clinical practice.

Dosing regimens and susceptibility of β-lactam and non-β-lactam antimicrobial agents used to treat pneumococcal infections are shown in Tables 85.7 and 85.8, respectively.[267] Dosing regimens are shown as total recommended daily dose and number of doses per day and should be used in conjunction with local prescribing information. Susceptibility data reflect overall findings from US and international studies; local susceptibility data should be taken into consideration as susceptibility patterns may vary considerably.

Pneumonia

Guidelines for the management of infants and children older than 3 months of age with presumed bacterial CAP have been published by the Pediatric Infectious Diseases Society and the Infectious Diseases Society of America.[71] Children with mild disease severity should be considered for outpatient treatment with antibiotics; amoxicillin should be used as first-line therapy for previously healthy, appropriately immunized infants and preschool children with mild to moderate CAP. In children allergic to amoxicillin, second- or third-generation cephalosporins, oral levofloxacin, or oral linezolid may be appropriate. For children who do not have clinical, laboratory, or radiographic evidence that distinguishes bacterial from atypical pneumonia, a macrolide can be added to the β-lactam antibiotic, especially in school-aged children and adolescents. Hospitalization is required for any child requiring

TABLE 85.7 **Dosing Regimens and Susceptibility of β-Lactam Antimicrobial Agents Used to Treat Pneumococcal Infections**

Antimicrobial Agent	TOTAL DAILY DOSE (NO. OF DOSES/DAY) Adolescents	Infants and Children	Susceptible Breakpoint (μg/mL)[a]	% Susceptibility
Parenteral Agents—Meningitis				
Penicillin G	24 million units (6–8)	300,000–400,000 units/kg (4–6)	≤0.06	63.5
Ampicillin	12 g (6)	300 mg/kg (4)	Penicillin ≤0.06	68.3
Ceftriaxone	4 g (1–2)	100 mg/kg (1–2)	≤0.5	82.2–86.2
Cefotaxime	8–12 g (4–6)	225–300 mg/kg (4–6)	≤0.5	87.4
Cefepime	6 g (3)	150 mg/kg (3)	≤0.5	85.3
Meropenem	6 g (3)	120 mg/kg (3)	≤0.25	78.1–93.9
Parenteral Agents—Nonmeningeal Infections				
Penicillin G (regular dose)	12 million units (6)	250,000–400,000 units/kg (4–6)	≤2[b]	92.6
Penicillin G (high dose)	18–24 million units (6)	400,000 units/kg (4–6)	≤4	99.7[c]
Ampicillin	4–8 g (4)	50–100 mg/kg (4)	Penicillin ≤2	92.6
Ceftriaxone	1-2 g (1)	50–75 mg/kg (1-2)	≤1	95.2
Cefotaxime	3 g (3)	75–100 mg/kg (3–4)	≤1	95.1–96.5
Cefuroxime sodium	2.25 g (3)	50–100 mg/kg (3–4)	≤0.5	75.3
Cefepime	2 g (2)	100 mg/kg (2)	≤1	96.5
Ceftaroline	1.2 g (2)	NA	≤0.25	100
Meropenem	1.5–3 g (3)	60–120 mg/kg (3)	≤0.25	78.1–93.9
Imipenem	1–2 g (3–4)	60 mg/kg (4)	≤0.12	92.4–96.3
Ertapenem	1 g (1)	30 mg/kg (2)	≤1	93.2–93.3
Oral Agents				
Penicillin V	1–2 g (3–4)	25–50 mg/kg (3-4)	≤0.06[b]	63.5
Amoxicillin (regular dose)	1.5 g (2–3)	45 mg/kg (2–3)	≤2	84–92.2
Amoxicillin/clavulanate (regular dose)	1.5 g/250 mg (2–3)	45/6.4 mg/kg (2–3)	≤2	84–93.6
Amoxicillin (high dose)	6 (3)	90 mg/kg (2–3)	≤4	86–92.2
Amoxicillin/clavulanate (high dose and extended release)	4 g/250 mg extended release (2)	90/6.4 mg/kg (2–3)	≤4	86–93.6
Cefaclor	750–1,500 mg (3)	20–40 mg/kg (3)	≤0.5	60.2
Cefuroxime axetil	500–1,000 mg (2)	20–30 mg/kg (2)	≤1	68–78.2
Cefixime	400 mg (1–2)	8 kg/kg (1–2)	≤1	68.3
Cefprozil	500–1,000 mg (2)	15–30 mg/kg (2)	≤1	79.7
Cefdinir	600 mg (1–2)	14 mg/kg (1–2)	≤0.5	68–76.8

Modified from Jacobs MR. Antimicrobial-resistant *Streptococcus pneumoniae*: trends and management. *Expert Rev Anti Infect Ther.* 2008;6(5):619-35.

Dosing regimens are shown as total recommended daily dose and number of doses per day and should be used in conjunction with local prescribing information. Susceptibility data reflect overall findings from US and international studies, and local susceptibility data should be taken into consideration, as susceptibility patterns may vary considerably.

[a]Susceptibility breakpoint for agent shown unless specified otherwise.

[b]Nonmeningeal isolates susceptible to penicillin G at this breakpoint can be considered susceptible to parenteral ampicillin, cefepime, cefotaxime, and ceftriaxone. Nonmeningeal isolates susceptible to ≤0.06 μg/mL of penicillin G can be also considered susceptible to these parenteral agents as well as to parenteral ertapenem, imipenem, and meropenem and to oral ampicillin, amoxicillin, amoxicillin/clavulanate, cefaclor, cefdinir, cefditoren, cefprozil, cefuroxime, and cefpodoxime.

[c]Includes penicillin G susceptible (92.6%) and intermediate (7.1%) isolates based on new, nonmeningeal, parenteral penicillin G susceptibility breakpoints.

NA, Not available.

intravenous therapy, hydration, or respiratory support. For inpatient treatment of children fully immunized with conjugate pneumococcal and *H. influenzae* type b vaccines, parenteral ampicillin, penicillin G, ceftriaxone, or cefotaxime are recommended, with the addition of clindamycin or vancomycin if community-acquired methicillin-resistant *S. aureus* is suspected. Except for ampicillin and penicillin G, the same agents are recommended for children who are not fully immunized. If atypical pneumonia cannot be excluded from the differential diagnosis, addition of azithromycin is recommended, with doxycycline and levofloxacin alternatives for older children. Other agents approved for treatment of pneumococcal pneumonia in adults include linezolid, tigecycline, and ceftaroline, a cephalosporin with anti–methicillin-resistant *S. aureus* activity.[279] Recently, the US Food and Drug Administration added a black box warning for quinolones (levofloxacin included) that such antibiotics may cause potentially permanent damage to muscles, tendons, joints, nerves, and the central nervous system and should not be used in patients with "minor" infections.[176] While bacterial pneumonia is not included in the Food and Drug Administration categorization of minor infections and the linkage between permanent damage and quinolones is primarily associative, caution should be used in prescribing levofloxacin in children for cases of pneumonia in which the likelihood of bacterial disease is small.

Sinusitis

While fewer than 2% of cases of acute viral rhinitis are complicated by acute bacterial rhinosinusitis, patients with symptoms lasting more than a week or increasing in severity after 5 to 7 days can be indicative of bacterial superinfection requiring treatment with antimicrobial agents. Detailed recommendations for treatment of acute bacterial sinusitis are found in Chapter 14.

Acute Otitis Media

AOM is the most commonly treated bacterial infection in children. Current guidelines for treatment are discussed in details in Chapter 16.

TABLE 85.8 Dosing Regimens And Susceptibility of Antimicrobial Agents Other Than β-Lactams Used to Treat Pneumococcal Infections

Antimicrobial Agent	TOTAL DAILY DOSE (NUMBER OF DOSES PER DAY)		Susceptible Breakpoint (μg/mL)[a]	Percent Susceptibility
	Adolescents	Infants and Children		
Parenteral Agents—Meningitis				
Vancomycin	30–60 mg/kg (3–4)	60 mg/kg (4)	≤1	100
Rifampin	600 mg (1)	20 mg (1–2)	≤1	99.9
Chloramphenicol	4–6 g (4)	75–100 mg/kg (4)	≤4	88.1
Parenteral Agents—Nonmeningeal Infections				
Vancomycin	2 g (2–4)	40–45 mg/kg (3–4)	≤1	100
Oral Agents				
Doxycycline	200 mg day 1, then 100 mg (1)	NR	≤0.25	71.3
Co-trimoxazole	320/1600 mg (2)	8/40 mg/kg (2)	≤0.5/9.5	56–69.0
Oral and Parenteral Agents				
Levofloxacin	500–750 (1)	NR	≤2	99.2
Gemifloxacin	320 (1)	NR	≤0.25	99.9
Moxifloxacin	400 (1)	NR	≤1	99.6
Erythromycin	1–2 g (4)	30–50 mg/kg (4)	≤0.25	70.9
Clarithromycin	500–750 mg (1–2)	15 mg/kg (2)	≤0.25	71.1
Azithromycin	500 mg day 1, then 250–500 mg (1)	10 mg/kg day 1, then 5–10 mg/kg (1)	≤0.12	55–65.5
Clindamycin	600–1200 mg (4)	16–40 mg/kg (4)	≤0.25	66.7
Linezolid	1200 mg (2)	30 mg/kg (3)	≤2	100

Modified from Jacobs MR. Antimicrobial-resistant *Streptococcus pneumoniae*: trends and management. *Expert Rev Anti Infect Ther.* 2008;6(5):619-35.
Dosing regimens are shown as total recommended daily dose and number of doses per day and should be used in conjunction with local prescribing information. Susceptibility data reflect overall findings from US and international studies; local susceptibility data should be taken into consideration as susceptibility patterns may vary considerably.
[a]Susceptibility breakpoint for agent shown unless specified otherwise.
NR, Not recommended for use in infants and children.

Bacteremia

S. pneumoniae is a common cause of bacteremia in children, frequently associated with pneumonia, and treatment guidelines follow recommendations for treatment of pneumonia.[99,267]

Meningitis

After PCV7 introduction, an estimated 3330 pneumococcal meningitis hospitalizations and 394 deaths were prevented in persons of all ages during 2001 to 2004 in the United States, and pneumococcal meningitis is now more common in adults than in children.[555] The Infectious Diseases Society of America has published practice guidelines for the management of bacterial meningitis.[224] Detailed treatment strategies are discussed in Chapter 31.

PREVENTION

Nonimmunologic Strategies

This category includes interventions that aim at (1) reducing risk factors predisposing to the development of pneumococcal infection, (2) providing antimicrobial prophylaxis to abort or prevent pneumococcal colonization or disease, and (3) modifying anatomic abnormalities that predispose to the development of pneumococcal infection.[309]

A factor that is important not only for pneumococcal infection but also for many other serious bacterial infections is the need to improve general health and nutrition worldwide, particularly in low-income countries. Many risk factors for the acquisition of pneumococcal infection that can be alleviated include poor living conditions, overcrowding, poor hygiene, malnutrition, and a high prevalence of viral infections, particularly respiratory viruses, measles, and HIV. In high-income countries, carriage of pneumococci, especially antibiotic-resistant strains that result in sporadic infections and outbreaks, is related to daycare attendance and is proportional to the number of children per group.[96,105,120,122,340,458,538] Therefore, reducing the number of children per group in daycare centers and developing alternative forms of childcare may reduce the rate of pneumococcal morbidity.

The importance of passive smoking (namely, being in close contact with smokers in the same household) has been highlighted as a risk factor for the development of pneumococcal disease.[412] Thus, efforts to prevent smoking in the home may have an important role in the prevention of pneumococcal infection. Breastfeeding may protect against some infections related to *S. pneumoniae*, such as otitis media.[19,81,147,475,559] Therefore, breastfeeding should be encouraged, especially in families in which otitis media occurs commonly, although the precise role of prolonged breastfeeding in protecting against pneumococcal infection has not been established.

Antimicrobial chemoprophylaxis is used predominantly for two indications: prevention of recurrent AOM and prevention of pneumococcal sepsis in children with anatomic or functional asplenia. Data now exist to support the common practice of prescribing regular doses of penicillin for children with asplenia or sickle-cell disease.[186]

The potential benefits of otitis media chemoprophylaxis have been weighed against the ability of chemoprophylaxis to alter the nasopharyngeal flora, foster colonization with resistant organisms, and thereby compromise the long-term efficacy of the prophylactic drug and contribute to the propagation of resistant organisms throughout the community. As a result, the practice of otitis media chemoprophylaxis has been reduced greatly. In one study, prophylaxis with amoxicillin induced a dramatic increase in the carriage of penicillin-resistant *S. pneumoniae* and increased carriage of other resistant pathogens.[79] The fear of increasing resistance led the Committee on Infectious Diseases of the American Academy of Pediatrics to issue a warning against the widespread use of otitis media prophylaxis and to state that "Antimicrobial prophylaxis should be reserved for control of recurrent acute otitis media, defined by 3 or more distinct and well-documented episodes during a period of 6 months or 4 or more episodes during a period of 12 months." Surgical otitis media prophylaxis by insertion of tympanostomy tubes or adenoidectomy (with or without tonsillectomy) has been recommended for otitis-prone children[307] (see Chapter 16).

Immunoprophylaxis

Unconjugated Capsular Polysaccharide Vaccines

It is well established that both passive immunization by administration of specific antibodies and active immunization with polysaccharides can provide protection against many pneumococcal infections.

Passively administered serotype-specific antibodies can protect animals and humans against diseases caused by pneumococci, with administration of antisera associated with improved clinical outcome, including reduced mortality, in humans.[89] Human immunoglobulins can prevent experimental pneumococcal bacteremia in mice[101,480] and otitis media in chinchillas.[507] The finding of low cord blood IgG antibodies, mainly of the IgG1 subset, is predictive of early-onset AOM in infancy.[49,349,487] In several clinical studies, bacterial polysaccharide immune globulin obtained by immunizing healthy adults with a 14-valent pneumococcal vaccine (in addition to group C meningococcal and Hib polysaccharide vaccines) decreased the prevalence of AOM[509] and invasive infection[509] in children.

Immunization with pneumococcal polysaccharide antigens, mainly in adults, has been studied for a long time. First, hexavalent polysaccharide vaccines were introduced in the late 1940s, followed by 14-valent vaccines in the late 1970s and 23-valent vaccines in the early 1980s. The last, produced by several manufacturers, contains 25 μg of purified, nonconjugated polysaccharide antigens per dose for serotypes 1, 2, 3, 4, 5, 6B, 7F, 8, 9N, 9V, 10A, 11A, 12F, 14, 15B, 17F, 18C, 19A, 19F, 20, 22F, 23F, and 33F. These 23 serotypes accounted for approximately 90% of the serotypes responsible for invasive pneumococcal infection in all age groups in both developed and developing countries.[230,231,467,520] The 23-valent polysaccharide vaccines are tolerated well by healthy children for primary[335,500] or repeated immunization.[69] However, the presence of preexisting antibodies was associated with an increased incidence of adverse events at the site of injection.[63,317,415]

Generally speaking, these bacterial polysaccharide-based vaccines are poorly immunogenic in infants and toddlers for important disease-causing serotypes, which is to be expected because bacterial capsular polysaccharides induce antibody production primarily by T-cell–independent mechanisms that still are not fully developed in this age group.[463] Polysaccharide-specific IgG concentrations are relatively high in very young infants because they are acquired transplacentally and consist mainly of IgG1. Nasopharyngeal colonization with various serotypes of *S. pneumoniae* results in the natural production of serotype-specific antibodies.[82,235,549,600] The immune response to pneumococcal polysaccharides is serotype dependent, and some serotypes commonly associated with disease are especially poor immunogens until children reach the age of approximately 5 years.[145] Serotypes 6A, 6B, 12, 19A, 19F, and 23F are examples of this phenomenon.[121,145,316,335,338,521,549,600] The IgG subclasses that are produced after exposure to polysaccharide antigens of other bacterial species are mainly IgG2 and IgG4.[346] A second dose of polysaccharide vaccine does not provide a booster effect and even may result in a reduced immune response when compared with the response after the first dose, which may suggest antigenic tolerance.[63,413,570] Children with many underlying conditions that predispose to the development of pneumococcal infection often respond more poorly to pneumococcal polysaccharide vaccines than do otherwise normal children. Published studies of children with recurrent respiratory tract infections all have demonstrated this phenomenon.*

In addition to a relatively poor systemic immune response, the polysaccharide vaccines have been shown to induce only minimal mucosal immune responses. Serotype-specific antibodies to pneumococcal serotypes 6A, 14, 18C, and 23F were measured in the sera and middle ear effusions of 14 children who had received a 14-valent pneumococcal capsular polysaccharide vaccine and in controls.[316] Serotype-specific antibody concentrations in middle ear effusions correlated with serum concentrations and generally were higher in pneumococcal vaccine recipients than in control vaccine recipients. IgM class antibodies frequently were seen only in the serum samples, thus suggesting that antibodies diffuse into the middle ear space rather than being synthesized in situ in response to the vaccine. This finding refutes previous theories that local production of antibodies occurs in the middle ear after vaccination.[318,515,516]

Limited data exist regarding the efficacy of polysaccharide pneumococcal vaccines in preventing disease in infants and children. A large study conducted in Papua New Guinea on more than 7000 children showed a reduction in mortality rates from acute lower respiratory tract disease.[336,465,464] In this study, the effect was dramatic: a 59% reduction in mortality rates in all children vaccinated (5 months to 5 years of age) and a 50% reduction in children vaccinated before they reached 2 years of age. However, the vaccine did not protect against nonfatal disease. In the United States, researchers have suggested that the polysaccharide vaccines would be 62% effective in preventing invasive pneumococcal disease caused by vaccine serotypes in children aged 2 to 5 years.[170]

The effectiveness of polysaccharide pneumococcal vaccines in preventing otitis media is not clear. Several studies have shown some reduction in the incidence of otitis media in vaccinated children.[144,253,292,365,544] No effect of the use of polysaccharide pneumococcal vaccine on pneumococcal nasopharyngeal carriage could be demonstrated.[117,121] These studies on T-cell–independent polysaccharide pneumococcal vaccines clearly show that their benefit in children is at best limited to the minority of serotypes that are immunogenic in this age group.

Recent meta-analyses have examined the effect of PPV23 on invasive pneumococcal disease and pneumococcal pneumonia in adults.[137,320] One concluded that PPV23 provided significant protection against IPD (~50% efficacy) in adults greater than 50 years of age with lower efficacy against CAP (4–17%), dependent on study design. The second reported that PPV23 provided weak protection against all-cause pneumonia in immunocompetent adults and, although a trend toward protection against pneumococcal pneumonia was present, it was not statistically significant.

Conjugated Capsular Polysaccharide Vaccines

The conjugation of pneumococcal polysaccharides to protein alters the immune response by recruiting T-cells that both amplify the B-cell response and create memory B-cells in contrast to the T-cell–independent nature of the immune response that occurs after the administration of bacterial polysaccharides[34,150,296,468,508,525] (Fig. 85.15). These polysaccharide-protein antigens elicit protective antibody in infants and prime the immune system for future boosting with reexposure to the polysaccharide either alone or conjugated. Antibodies elicited by polysaccharide–protein conjugates demonstrate improved functional capacity (determined by avidity and opsonization assays), persist, and result in a booster response with reexposure.[158] The concept of conjugation technology, highly successful with capsular polysaccharide from *H. influenzae* type b, was modified to permit development of vaccines with multiple polysaccharide while maintaining immunogenicity for each individual polysaccharide.

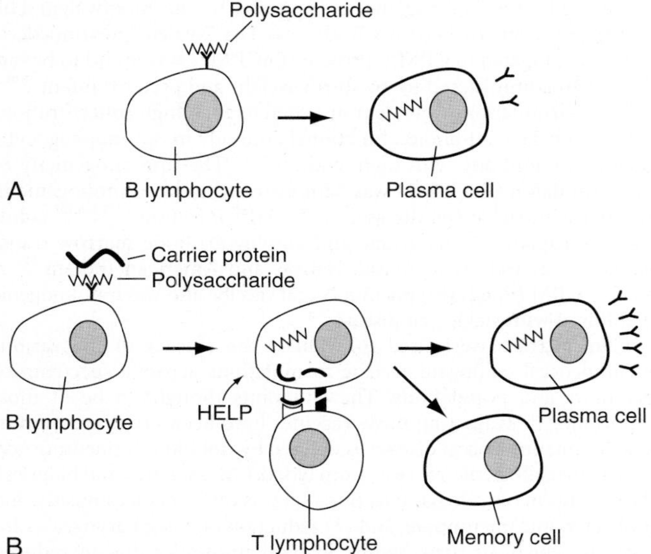

FIG. 85.15 (A) T-cell–independent and (B) T-cell–dependent antibody responses to polysaccharide or polysaccharide-protein conjugate antigens. (From Eskola J, Anttila M. Pneumococcal conjugate vaccines. *Pediatr Infect Dis J.* 1999;18:543–51.)

*References 2, 26, 57, 157, 182, 192, 244, 323, 437, 459, 461, 483, 489, 490, 523, 570.

TABLE 85.9 Pneumococcal Conjugate Vaccines Licensed in at Least One Country or Being Tested in Clinical Trials

Vaccine	Valency	Pneumococcal Polysaccharides	Carrier Protein	Current Status	Manufacturer
PnOMPC7	7-valent	4, 6B, 9V, 14, 18C, 19F, 23F	Meningococcal outer-membrane protein complex	Research formulation only	Merck Research Laboratories
PnCRM7	7-valent	4, 6B, 9V, 14, 18C, 19F, 23F	CRM_{197} protein	Licensed	Pfizer
PnCRM9	9-valent	1, 4, 5, 6B, 9V, 14, 18C, 19F, 23F	CRM_{197} protein	Research formulation only	Pfizer
PHiD-CV	10-valent	1,4,5,6B,7F,9V,14,18C 19F,23F		Licensed	GlaxoSmithKline
PncT/D	11-valent	1, 3, 4, 5, 6B, 7F, 9V, 14, 18C, 19F, 23F	A mixture of tetanus and diphtheria toxoids	Not in commercial development	Aventis Pasteur
Pn-PD	11-valent	1, 3, 4, 5, 6B, 7F, 9V, 14, 18C, 19F, 23F	*Haemophilus influenzae*—protein D	Prototype for PHiD-CV; not in commercial development	GlaxoSmithKline
PnCRM13	13-valent	1, 3, 4, 5, 6A, 6B, 7F, 9V, 14, 18C, 19A, 19F, 23F	CRM_{197} protein	Licensed	Pfizer
PCV 15	15-valent	1, 3, 4, 5, 6A, 6B, 7F, 9V, 14, 18C,19A, 19F, 22F, 23F, 33F	CRM_{197} protein	In clinical trials	Merck

Currently, vaccines with 7 to 13 different conjugated pneumococcal polysaccharide antigens are licensed and next-generation vaccines with even greater numbers of polysacchardies are in clinical trials.[324]

Table 85.9 shows pneumococcal conjugate vaccines that are licensed in at least one country, are being tested in phase III efficacy studies, or are in advanced phase II (safety and immunology) stages. The selection of serotypes for inclusion in the various formulations is based on serotype epidemiology discussed earlier. These conjugate vaccines were developed primarily targeting serotypes responsible for invasive pneumococcal disease, including meningitis, bacteremic pneumonia, and empyema.

The primary target population for polysaccharide conjugate vaccines is infants and toddlers, as disease incidence is highest, global mortality substantial, and polysaccharide vaccines demonstrated to be poorly immunogenic and of limited value at this age. Pneumococcal conjugate vaccines are immunogenic, safe, and well tolerated, with vaccine reactions primarily being pain, redness, and swelling at the injection site. The incidence of fever and irritability was somewhat higher than reported in studies with Hib conjugate vaccines or hepatitis B vaccines, perhaps because the pneumococcal vaccines represent 7 to 13 separate monovalent vaccines administered together as opposed to the monovalent Hib conjugate vaccine or hepatitis B vaccine. The 7-valent pneumococcal vaccine conjugated to CRM_{197} protein (PnCRM7) was found to be safe even when administered to low-birth-weight and preterm infants.[505]

PCV formulations were demonstrated to elicit high concentrations of IgG1 subclass antibodies, functional antibody in opsonophagocytic assays, and antibody with high avidity.[158,164] The immunogenicity of one formulaton (PnCRM7) was demonstrated to be immunogenic in children with sickle-cell disease,[410,415,570] HIV infection,[6,305,306,405] solid-organ transplants,[347] allogeneic and autologous bone marrow transplants,[20,155] as well as in Alaska Natives and American Indians.[379] A 9-valent CRM (PnCRM9) pneumococcal vaccine also was immunogenic in children with sickle-cell disease.[201]

Clinical trials were used to evaluate the efficacy of the various pneumococcal conjugate vaccine formulations across a spectrum of endpoints and populations. The endpoints thought to be of most importance in evaluating these vaccines have been (1) prevention of invasive pneumococcal disease as defined by isolation of pneumococci from a normally sterile site (e.g., from blood, CSF, aspirates, and biopsies); (2) prevention of mucosal infections such as otitis media, sinusitis, and nonbacteremic pneumonia; and (3) reduction of nasopharyngeal colonization, which, in turn, results in herd immunity due to reduced transmission of organisms.

Three efficacy studies of conjugate vaccines with the endpoint of a reduction in the number of invasive infections were completed by mid-2002, two with PnCRM7 and one with the PnCRM9 vaccine. The first study was a prospective double-blind study of 37,868 healthy infants in northern California to whom either the PnCRM7 vaccine or a control vaccine was administered at 2, 4, 6, and 12 to 15 months of age.[59] The vaccine was 97.4% efficacious (95% confidence interval [CI], 82.7–99.9%) against invasive disease caused by the 7 serotypes included in the vaccine in fully vaccinated infants and 93.9% efficacious (95% CI, 79.6–98.5%) in partially vaccinated infants. No evidence of an increase in invasive disease caused by serotypes that were not included in the vaccine was detected; thus, the overall effect was a reduction in total invasive pneumococcal disease by 89.1% (95% CI, 73.7–95.8%). This trial led to US licensure of the vaccine in February 2000, with subsequent licensure in many other countries. Additional analysis has shown that the vaccine was as effective in the subset of low-birth-weight and premature infants as it was in the full study cohort.[505] Secondary analyses demonstrated reductions in all-cause pneumonia and AOM.

A second large-scale efficacy study with the PnCRM7 vaccine was conducted among American Navajo and White Mountain Apache children in the United States using a cluster randomization strategy in which communities rather than individuals are randomized. This population has rates of invasive pneumococcal infection that are approximately five times those of the general US population.[414] In this double-blind, community-randomized study, infants and young children aged 2 months to 2 years received the PnCRM7 vaccine or a control vaccine. A total of 8292 infants from 43 communities were enrolled; of these, 8091 lived in 38 communities that were randomized to the pneumococcal or the control vaccine. During the study period, two cases of invasive pneumococcal infection caused by the serotypes included in the vaccine occurred in the vaccine group versus eight in the control group. After controlling for community randomization, the primary efficacy of the vaccine was 76.8% (95% CI, 9.4–95.1%) and the intent-to-treat efficacy was 86.4% (95% CI, 11–96.1%).

A third efficacy study was conducted with the PnCRM9 vaccine among black infants in South Africa. In this double-blind, randomized, placebo-controlled study, PnCRM9 was administered to children at the ages of 6, 10, and 14 weeks according to the World Health Organization's Expanded Programme on Immunization. The infants were monitored until they reached 2 years of age. The intent-to-treat analysis showed a reduction of 82.5% (95% CI, 39.0–96.7%) in the number of invasive infections caused by the serotypes included in the vaccine for children not infected with HIV and a reduction of 65.4% (95% CI, 23.8–85.7%) in antiretroviral-naïve children infected with HIV.[313]

Once licensed in the United States (February 2000), universal immunization for children less than 2 years of age and selected immunization for high-risk children was implemented in the United States. The Committee on Infectious Diseases of the American Academy of Pediatrics recommended routine administration as a four-dose series for infants at ages 2, 4, 6, and 12 to 15 months (known at the 3+1 schedule); catch-up immunization was recommended for all children up to 23 months of age. Infants of very low birthweight could be immunized when they reached a chronologic age of 6 to 8 weeks, regardless of their calculated gestational age. The PCV-7 vaccine also was recommended for all children younger than 60 months of age at high risk of acquiring invasive pneumococcal infection, including patients with sickle-cell disease, asplenia, HIV/acquired immunodeficiency syndrome, diabetes, cancer, liver disorders, lung diseases, and cardiac diseases. For some high-risk children, administraton of PPV23 was recommended for supplemental protection.

The incidence of invasive pneumococcal disease decreased sharply in infants and toddlers following the widespread use of PCV7 in US children.[58,254,595] Effectiveness studies demonstrated a rapid decline in IPD due to vaccine serotypes in children less than 5 years of age (Fig. 85.16) within 2 years of vaccine introduction, with a further gradual decline that persisted through 2010, when a second-generation pneumococcal conjugate vaccine was introduced (PCV13).[441,612] Rates of bacteremia without a focus, meningitis, and bacteremic pneumonia all declined. By 2006 to 2007, PCV7 serotypes accounted for only 2% of IPD cases in children compared to 83% prior to 2000. By 2009, nasopharyngeal PCV7 serotypes comprised only 2% of pneumococcal isolates carried in the nasopharynx of children less than 6 years of age[606] (Fig. 85.17). Despite the decline in carriage of PCV7 serotypes, overall pneumococcal carriage did not change as a result of increases in carriage of nonvaccine serotypes, particularly serotypes 19A, 15A, 15B, 15C, 6C, 23A, 23B, and 35B. These changes in serotype distribution resulted in reduced transmission of PCV7 serotypes and a decline in IPD due to vaccine serotypes in all age groups, including infants less than 90 days of age and too young to be protected directly, as well as adults.[444] In fact, Simonsen noted that 90% of the reduction in pneumococcal disease mortality occurred though herd immunity among adults 18 years and older (Table 85.10).[512] Consistent with the observed differences in virulence between pneumococcal serotypes as discussed earlier, the current belief is that the lower capacity to produce disease following colonization with nonvaccine serotypes provides the explanation for the fall in invasive disease and pneumonia without a change in overall colonization. However, some of the non-PCV7 serotypes that emerged, specifically 19A and 7F, were associated with modest increases in invasive disease syndromes as well as pneumonia and otitis media both in children and adults. By 2007, the incidence of IPD due to serotype 19A had increased from 2.6 cases per 100,000 to 11.1 per 100,000 in children less than 5 years of age and represented nearly 40% of all IPD in this age group (Fig. 85.18).[612]

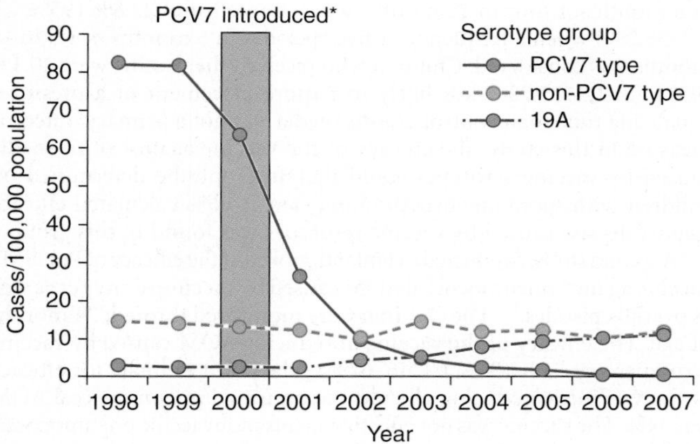

FIG. 85.16 Changes in invasive pneumococcal disease in US children <5 years by serotype groupings. PCV7 serotypes include 4, 6B, 9V, 14, 18C, 19F, and 23F. (From Pilishvili T, Lexau C, Farley MM, et al. Active Bacterial Core Surveillance/Emerging Infections Program. Sustained reductions in invasive pneumococcal disease in the era of conjugate vaccine. *J Infect Dis.* 2010;201:32–41.)

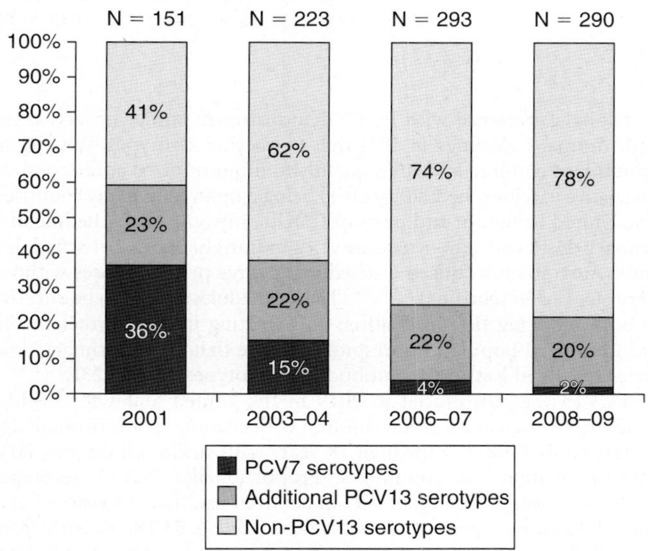

FIG. 85.17 Percent of pneumococcal isolates within each sampling period by vaccine serotype grouping. PCV7 serotypes are 4, 6B, 9V, 14, 19C, 19F, and 23F. Additional 13 valent serotypes are 1, 3, 5, 6A, 7F, and 19A. Non-PCV13 serotypes are all other serotypes. (From Wroe PC, Lee GM, Finkelstein JA, et al. Pneumococcal carriage and antibiotic resistance in young children before 13-valent conjugate vaccine. *Pediatr Infect Dis J.* 2012;31:249–54.)

TABLE 85.10 Estimated PCV7 Reductions In Mortality During Hospitalizations for Invasive Pneumococcal Disease, Pneumococcal Pneumonia, and All-Cause Pneumonia: 1999–2000 Through 2004–05

Age Group	Estimated IPD Reduction	95% CI	Estimated Pneumococcal Pneumonia (ICD9 481) Reduction	95% CI	Estimated All-Cause Pneumonia Reduction	95% CI
<2	212	81–275	34	−66 to 67	548	425–646
2–4	46	12–62	26	−3 to 38	191	136–235
5–17	103	65–130	13	−14 to 29	350	252–431
18–39	810	674–922	1088	888–1245	2495	2220–2754
40–64	1045	709–1349	2304	1990–2596	8513	7674–9312
≥65	4007	3246–4693	10,895	9772–11,934	71,556	61,644–81,013
Total[a]	6222	4788–7431	14,360	12,568–15,908	83,653	72,351–94,391

Modified from Simonsen L, Taylor RJ, Young-Xu Y, et al. Impact of pneumococcal conjugate vaccination of infants on pneumonia and influenza hospitalization and mortality in all age groups in the United States. *MBio.* 2011;2(1):e00309–00310.

[a]Number of deaths prevented.

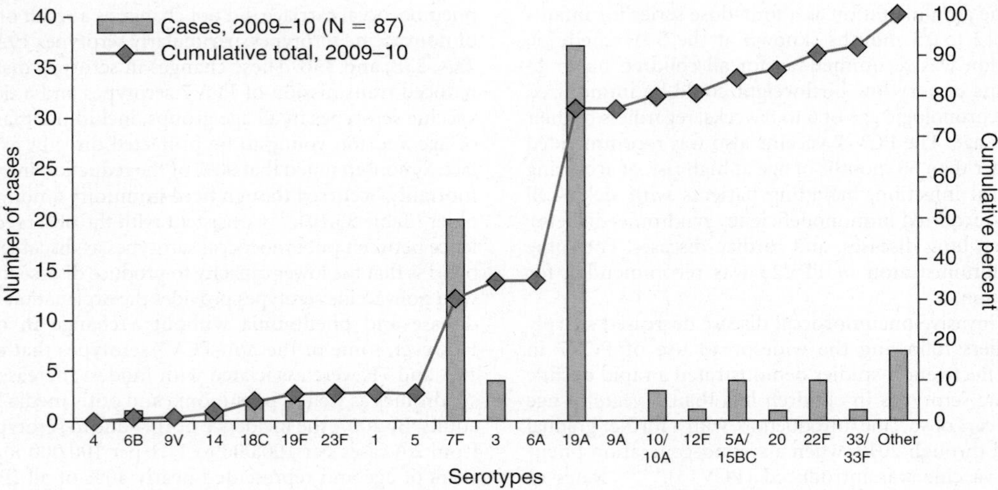

FIG. 85.18 Serotypes causing invasive pneumococcal disease in children <18 years in Massachusetts between October 31, 2009, and September 1, 2010. (From Yildirim I, Stevenson A, Hsu KK, et al. Evolving picture of invasive pneumococcal disease in Massachusetts children: a comparison of disease in 2007–2009 with earlier periods. *Pediatr Infect Dis J.* 2012;31:1016–21.)

Global experience with PCV7 demonstrated similar observations, with dramatic declines in IPD due to vaccine serotypes, initially in immunized children and subsequently in unimmunized adults, despite alternative vaccine schedules (to 3+1) being employed in many countries. The United Kingdom and parts of Canada introduced a schedule of 2 primary doses with a booster dose at 12 months of age (a 2+1 schedule), while Australia introduced a schedule of three primary doses without a booster (a 3+0 schedule).[134,281,382] These schedules proved to be effective in both reducing IPD in children and creating indirect protection in unimmunized populations despite evidence that a two–primary dose series results in less serum antibody for serotypes 6B and 23F.[295,350]

PCV13 was introduced in 2010 in the United States for healthy children through age 5 years, children with chronic illness through age 6 years, and children 6 through 18 years with sickle-cell disease, HIV, and other high-risk conditions. Proportionally, PCV13 serotypes comprised nearly 75% of all IPD in children less than 18 years of age, with 19A disease representing nearly 40% (see Fig. 85.18). Reports from multiple US surveillance programs[290,389,610] demonstrate further declines in IPD in children under 5 years of age and a decline in disease due to serotype 19A.

Current surveillance data from the Centers for Disease Control and Prevention report that as of 2015, IPD in children less than 5 years of age had declined from 100 per 100,000 in 1998 to 9 per 100,000 in 2015 primarily due to a decline in vaccine serotypes, with little evidence of replacement (Fig. 85.19).[91] The United Kingdom introduced PCV13 early in 2010 and has also reported a decline IPD due to PCV13 unique serotypes.[381] Similar declines in IPD in children have been reported from both high- and low-income countries following introduction of PCV13 or PCV10.[142,249,563]

Although not licensed in the United States, PCV10 was also demonstrated to be efficacious against IPD using a population-based strategy, cluster randomized design in Finland. The reduction in vaccine-type IPD was 92% (95% CI, 86–95%) in children less than 2 years of age, with an overall reduction in IPD of 80%. A nonsignificant increase in nonvaccine type IPD was observed. The study demonstrated a substantial decrease in IPD rates among vaccine-eligible children and a smaller and temporally delayed reduction among older, unvaccinated children, confirming the presence of indirect protection.[281]

Although invasive infections are the most dramatic part of the pneumococcal disease spectrum, respiratory infections such as otitis media are far more frequent.[344] Efficacy studies have shown protection against AOM due to vaccine serotypes in children immunized with pneumococcal conjugate vaccines. In one study, PnCRM7 vaccine reduced the number of clinically diagnosed otitis media episodes by 7% (95% CI, 4.1–7.9%).[171] The effectiveness of the PnCRM7 vaccine against frequent otitis media was 9.3% (95% CI, 3.0–15.1%) when three episodes in 6 months or four in 12 months were counted, and 22.8% (95% CI, 6.7–36.2%) when a frequency of five episodes in 6 months or six in 12 months was considered. Children who received the vaccine were 20.1% (95% CI, 1.5–35.2%) less likely to require placement of a pressure-equalizing tube than controls. Otitis media was not a primary outcome measure in this study; the efficacy of the vaccine against otitis media caused by vaccine serotypes could therefore only be determined on children with spontaneously draining ears. A 66% calculated efficacy against disease caused by vaccine serotypes was found in this group.

A second study, conducted in Finland, looked at the efficacy of PnCRM7 vaccine against pneumococcal AOM caused by vaccine serotypes as well as overall episodes.[159] The children were monitored through 24 months of age. The efficacy of the vaccine in reducing AOM caused by vaccine serotypes was 57% (95% CI, 46–67%). The point estimate for efficacy of the vaccine in reducing all culture-confirmed pneumococcal AOM was 34%. The vaccine was not effective against nonvaccine pneumococcal serotypes, except against serotype 6A. The overall high protection provided against the serotypes included in the vaccine was offset partially by an increase in the number of episodes of otitis media caused by other serotypes of pneumococci and other pathogens. The overall reduction in the number of episodes of AOM of any cause in the pneumococcal vaccine group was 6%. Although this difference did not reach statistical significance, it was similar to the 7% reduction in AOM observed in the California study.[59] In addition, similar to the California study, by the time children reached the age of 4 to 5 years, tympanostomy tube placement was reduced 39% compared to controls.[426]

A third study was conducted by the same Finnish group in parallel with the study just described, with a different 7-valent vaccine (serotypes 4, 6B, 9V, 14, 18C, 19F, and 23F conjugated to the meningococcal outer-membrane protein complex [OMPC]—PnOMPC7).[301] This vaccine was administered in 4 doses at 2, 4, 6, and 12 months of age. At 12 months of age, approximately 22% of the PnOMPC7 conjugate vaccine recipients received a nonconjugate 23-valent polysaccharide vaccine as a booster, while the others received a fourth dose of PnOMPC7. The efficacy of the vaccine in reducing the number of cases of otitis media caused by the serotypes included in the vaccine was 56%, with 25% for reduction of any pneumococcal AOM. However, there was no overall reduction in the number of episodes of otitis media, with nonvaccine serotype pneumococci and other pathogens producing replacement disease.

A fourth study, using an 11-valent PCV (the prototype for PCV10), conjugated to outer membrane protein D of nontypeable *H. influenzae*,

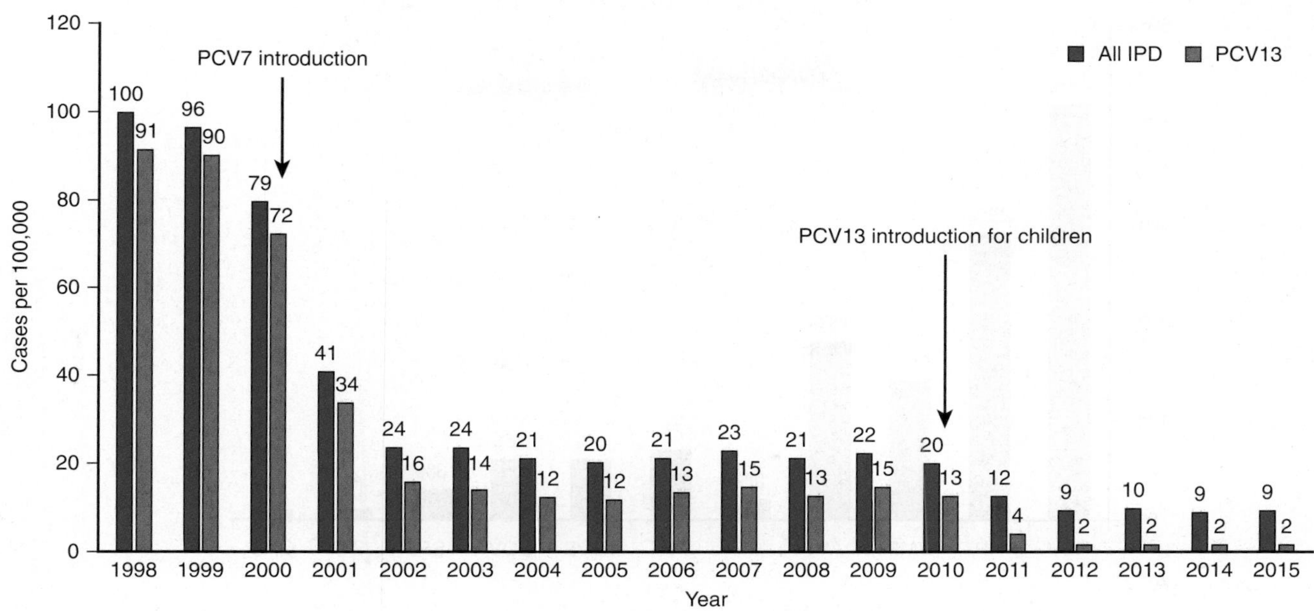

FIG. 85.19 Changes in the incidence of invasive pneumococcal disease (IPD) among children <5 years from 1998 through 2015 in the United States. Rates of IPD expressed as cases per 100,000 population are shown on the *y*-axis, and calendar year of surveillance on the *x*-axis. Blue bars represent overall IPD incidence, while the orange bars represent IPD incidence caused by serotypes included in the 13-valent pneumococcal conjugate vaccine (PCV13). PCV13 serotype: 1, 3, 4, 5, 6A, 6B, 7F, 9V, 14, 18C, 19A, 19F, and 23F. (From Active Bacterial Core surveillance data. Available at http://www.cdc.gov/pneumococcal/surveillance.html.)

demonstrated a similar magnitude of protection against vaccine serotype AOM despite a markedly different study design.[450] As the 11-valent PCV was conjugated to protein D from nontypeable *H. influenzae*, a 35% reduction in AOM episodes due to this pathogen was also reported, with an overall reduction in all episodes of AOM of approximately 33%. Further studies confirming the efficacy of PCV10, in which some serotypes are conjugated to protein D, are pending completion.

Since licensure and universal immunization of children younger than 2 years with PCV7, several studies have shown that the reduction in AOM exceeds that reported in clinical trials.[216,443,582,621] Several hypotheses have been proposed to explain the observation. First, that with widespread immunization and dramatic reduction in nasopharyngeal carriage of vaccine serotypes, effectiveness against vaccine serotypes will increase to nearly 100%. Second, prevention of early episodes of pneumococcal AOM will change the natural history of AOM in children, reducing subsequent episodes.[174] Pneumococcal AOM is now primarily caused by nonvaccine serotypes.[529,530]

Postmarketing studies from Israel demonstrated both direct protection following PCV13 against vaccine type pneumococcal otitis media and indirect protection reducing disease in children less than 4 months of age. In addition, Dagan and colleagues have proposed that prevention of early otitis media, and specifically early pneumococcal otitis media, had downstream benefits resulting in declines in the incidence of complex otitis media.[51,124] Consistent with this hypothesis, tympanostomy tube insertion has declined following introduction of PCV13 in US children.[124]

Reports of AOM and mastoiditis unresponsive to antimicrobial therapy requiring drainage and systemic antimicrobial therapy due to multidrug resistant serotype 19A increased prior to the introduction of PCV13.[422,439] Antibiotic susceptibility and serotype distribution of pneumococcal isolates from children with AOM in France changed significantly after the introduction of the PCV-7 (2003) and PCV-13 (2010) vaccines.[297] Resistance rates in 2001 and 2011were 76.9% and 57.3% for penicillin, 43.0% and 29.8% for amoxicillin, and 28.6% and 13.0% for cefotaxime, respectively. After PCV-7 implementation, vaccine serotypes were markedly reduced, from 63.0% in 2001 to 13.2% in 2011, while the incidence of the additional six serotypes included in PCV-13, particularly serotype 19A, increased during this period. Following introduction of PCV13, studies from Israel and Rochester, New York documented the decline in disease due to vaccine serotypes, specifically 19A.[438]

As most cases of pneumococcal pneumonia are nonbacteremic, the role of *S. pneumoniae* can best be demonstrated indirectly in vaccine probe studies by determining the proportion of disease reduction following vaccine implementation. In the northern California PnCRM7 vaccine study, 3711 clinically diagnosed episodes of pneumonia were identified by the age of 3.5 years.[60] The efficacy of the vaccine in reducing the incidence of clinical pneumonia was 6.0%. For children in whom a chest radiograph was obtained, an 8.9% reduction was observed; for those with a positive chest radiograph (defined as parenchymal infiltrates, consolidation, or effusion), a 22.7% (95% CI, 8.7–34.5%) decline in disease occurred. As the reduction in pneumonia was a secondary endpoint, the precision of the decline has some limitations. However, the findings suggest that more cases of clinically and radiologically proven pneumonia in children are caused by *S. pneumoniae* than previously suspected, with the reduction in disease extending beyond the "classic" lobar pneumonia pattern associated with *S. pneumoniae* to cases with non–lobar infiltrates. Comparable observations from South Africa documented a 22.1% reduction in children not infected with HIV immunized with PCV9.[313] Recent studies highlight the challenge of measuring the burden of pneumococcal pneumonia. Jain identified a pathogen in 1802 of the 2222 children (81%): one or more viruses in 1472 (66%), one or more bacteria in 175 (8%), and both bacterial and viral pathogens in 155 (7%). *S. pneumoniae* was identified in 4% of cases.[273] Yet, in contrast, Griffin reported that annual pneumonia hospitalization rates declined in Tennessee children younger than 2 years old from 14.5 to 4.1 per 1,000 from pre-PCV years to PCV13 years (72%).[215] A 27% decline following introduction of PCV13 compared to the PCV7 era suggests that the role of the pneumococcus in hospitalized pediatric pneumonia is much larger than can be ascertained by traditional diagnostic approaches (Fig. 85.20).[272]

Additional supportive evidence that *S. pneumoniae* has an important role in a broader spectrum of respiratory infections can be derived from a study in southern Israel involving toddlers aged 12 to 35 months who attended daycare centers.[126] In this study, a 15% reduction in non–otitis media upper respiratory tract infection was reported. Episodes

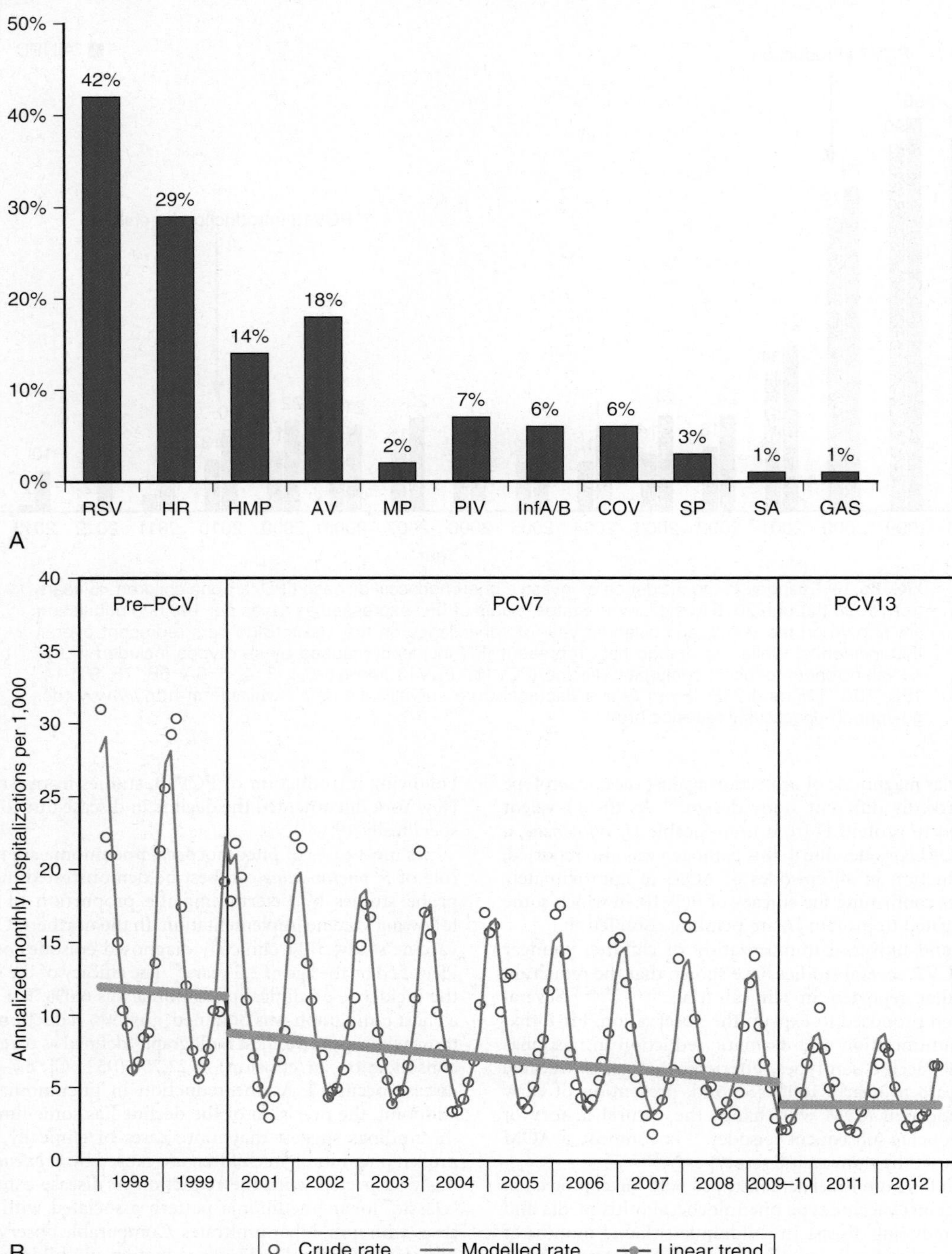

FIG. 85.20 The paradox of pneumococcal pneumonia. (A) Pathogens detected in 980 cases of hospitalized pneumonia in children <2 years. *AV,* Adenovirus; *COV,* coronavirus; *GAS,* Group A *Streptococcus; HMP,* human metapneumovirus; *HR,* human rhinovirus; *MP,* mycoplasma pneumonia; *PIV,* parainfluenza virus 1-3; *Inf A/B,* influenza A or B; *RSV,* respiratory syncytial virus; *SA, Staphylococcus aureus*; *SP, Streptococcus* pneumonia. (B) Monthly all-cause pneumonia hospitalizations in children <2 years. Pneumonia hospitalization rates decreased 27%, from 5.6 to 4.1 per 1000, after the switch from PCV7 to 13-valent pneumococcal conjugate vaccine in 2010. (A, Data from Jain S, Williams DJ, Arnold SR, et al. Community-acquired pneumonia requiring hospitalization among U.S. children. *N Engl J Med.* 2015;372(9):835-845. B, Modified from Griffin MR, Mitchel E, Moore MR, et al. Declines in pneumonia hospitalizations of children aged <2 years associated with the use of pneumococcal conjugate vaccines — Tennessee, 1998–2012. *MMWR Morb Mortal Wkly Rep.* 2014;63[44]:995-998.)

of lower respiratory tract disease—including bronchiolitis, cough, and pneumonia—were reduced. A reduction of 10% in the number of days that antibiotics were given for upper respiratory tract infections was achieved, as was a reduction of 47% for lower respiratory tract problems in the pneumococcal vaccine group.

Person-to-person spread is the major route of transmisson for *S. pneumoniae*. The nonconjugate pneumococcal polysaccharide vaccines do not have a significant effect on carriage of *S. pneumoniae* in children and adults.[121,356] In contrast, the conjugate vaccines have a significant effect on carriage that expands its public health value. Table 85.11 shows

TABLE 85.11 **Studies on the Effect of Conjugate Pneumococcal Vaccine on Carriage of *Streptococcus pneumoniae* and Antibiotic-Resistant *S. pneumoniae***

Author	Conjugate Vaccine (Valence)	Site	Age (mo) at Vaccination	Reduction in Serotypes Included in the Vaccine	Reduction in Resistant Pneumococci	Increase in Nonvaccine Serotypes
Dagan[122]	PnOMPC7	Israel	12–18	Yes	Yes	No
Dagan[123]	PnT, PnD (4-valent)	Israel	2, 4, 6	Yes	Yes	±
Obaro[419]	PnCRM5	The Gambia	2, 3, 4	Yes	ND	Yes
Kristinsson[321]	PnT, PnD (8-valent)	Iceland	3, 4, 6	Yes	ND	Yes
Mbelle[370]	PnCRM9	South Africa	1.5, 2.5, 3.5	Yes	Yes	Yes
Edwards[151]	PnCRM9	US	2, 4, 6, 12	Yes	ND	Yes
Dagan[127]	PnT/D (11-valent)	Israel	2, 4, 6, 12	Yes	Yes	No
Dagan[118,116]	PnCRM9	Israel	12–35	Yes	Yes	Yes
O'Brien[416]	PnCRM7	US (Native American)	2, 4, 6, 12–15	Yes	ND	Yes
Kilpi[302]	PnCRM7	Finland	2, 4, 6, 12	Yes	ND	ND

ND, Not done; *PnCRM,* Pneumococcal vaccine conjugated to CRM_{197} protein (PnCRM5, 5-valent; PnCRM7, 7-valent; PnCRM9, 9-valent); *PnD,* pneumococcal vaccine conjugated to diphtheria toxoid; *PnOMPC,* 7-valent pneumococcal vaccine conjugated to the outer-membrane complex of *Neisseria meningitidis* B; *PnT,* pneumococcal vaccine conjugated to tetanus toxoid; *PnT/D,* pneumococcal vaccine conjugated to a mixture of tetanus and diphtheria toxoid.

selected studies conducted and published documenting the effect of pneumococcal vaccines on carriage of *S. pneumoniae.* Despite variations in the nature of the conjugate vaccines, populations, and the ages at which the vaccines were administered, a significant reduction in carriage of the serotypes included in the vaccine was observed in all studies. In most studies, serotype replacement was observed as the overall pneumococcal colonization remained relatively constant despite the decline in prevalence of vaccine serotypes.

Changes in nasopharyngeal colonization are important because they reduce exposure of unimmunized children and adults to these potential pathogens. This reduction has been demonstrated in studies of toddlers attending daycare centers who were vaccinated with a PnCRM9 vaccine or a control vaccine.[116] In this study, the younger siblings of immunized and control children, who stayed home, were monitored. A marked reduction in the incidence of vaccine-type pneumococcal carriage was seen in the young siblings of those who were vaccinated with the PnCRM9 vaccine when compared with siblings of the controls. In a second study, Navajo and White Mountain Apache children younger than 2 years old were randomized according to their community of residence to receive either PnCRM7 or meningococcus C conjugate vaccine.[380] A reduction in carriage of vaccine-associated serotypes was found both in infants who lived with a PnCRM7-vaccinated sibling and in those who did not have direct contact with a PnCRM7-vaccinated child but lived in a vaccine community, demonstrating the indirect protective effect of pneumococcal vaccination on those in the household. Because most antibiotic-resistant *S. pneumoniae* strains belong to a limited number of serotypes that are included in the conjugate pneumococcal vaccines or are related to these serotypes (see the section on epidemiology and microbiology), conjugate vaccines reduce disease, carriage, and spread of antibiotic-resistant *S. pneumoniae* and have an impact on the use of antibiotics. In all vaccine studies that evaluated the effect of conjugate vaccines on nasopharyngeal carriage of antibiotic-resistant *S. pneumoniae,* a reduction in carriage of such strains was observed[116,121,123,127,370] (see Table 85.11). However, this reduction is both limited in time, as resistance had increased among the nonvaccine serotypes that replaced vaccine serotypes in carriage, and differs by geographic location depending on the serotypes most prevalent in a specific community.

Although invasive infections are the most dramatic part of the pneumococcal disease spectrum, respiratory infections such as otitis media and sinusitis occur far more frequently.[344] In a study investigating current estimates of pneumococcal disease burden, clinical outcome, and vaccine efficacy, researchers estimated that for each annual US birth cohort, routine use of a 7-valent vaccine could prevent 12,000 cases of pneumococcal bacteremia and meningitis, 53,000 cases of pneumococcal pneumonia, and more than1 million clinical cases of otitis media per year.[344] Pneumonia has a greater impact globally than does otitis media or even invasive infections because of its high mortality rate in children in the developing world.[54,218,339] Thus, the protection conferred by the conjugate pneumococcal vaccines with regard to reduction in the number of episodes of otitis media, pneumonia, and other mucosal infections have an even greater public health impact on the burden of disease than on prevention of invasive infections.

Pneumococcal disease remains a burden on children throughout the globe. In young babies and children, the elderly, and those with serious comorbidities, the disease can be deadly. Progress in prevention, both in the development of effective vaccines and in implementation of vaccine delivery programs in developing countries, has exceeded expectations, resulting in decreased incidence of and mortality from invasive pneumococcal disease, including meningitis and both bacteremic and nonbacteremic pneumonia.[395] The virtual elimination of nasopharyngeal colonization with vaccine serotypes enhances their public health value by reducing transmission of vaccine serotypes from children to adults, thereby reducing overall rates of pneumococcal disease. Vaccine failure is uncommon; Park et al. reported only 155 vaccine serotype infections identified by US surveillance systems with only 25 in fully vaccinated children, suggesting that the combination of direct and indirect effects protects infants as well as children with chronic illness from vaccine serotype disease.[428] These findings demonstrate the major reduction in the burden of vaccine serotype pneumococcal disease in children associated with use of conjugate vaccines.

Nevertheless, potential challenges to the successful scenario observed to date are found in the distribution of disease due to nonvaccine serotypes. The US surveillance program reported a doubling of the proportion of children with comorbidities and IPD, which increased from 3% in 1998–1999 to 7% in 2007. In Massachusetts, a report noted that 16% of children with IPD have comorbidities that proportionally increased with age. Among the 155 cases of vaccine failure referred to earlier, a disproportionate proportion were reported to have comorbidities (37%).[428] Ladhani also reported that comorbidities were present in 17.7% of UK children with IPD caused by PCV7 serotypes.[325] Case-fatality rates also reflected great vulnerability of children with comorbidities, with mortality from pneumococcal disease (4.4% overall) higher for meningitis (11.0%) and for children with comorbidities (9.1%).

The most common comorbidities associated with pneumococcal disease reported include malignancies and immunocompromised conditions.[255] Children with asthma, diabetes, and neurologic disorders such as seizures and muscular dystrophies have increased relative risk for IPD compared to age-matched healthy controls.[593] Although the risk is modest with a single comorbidity, it escalates in children with two or more. Certainly, the high incidence of HIV and sickle-cell disease in developing countries in Africa are likely to result in these children being at high risk for nonvaccine serotype disease. Children with malnutrition, tuberculosis, or exposed to secondhand smoke may also have higher risks for disease due to nonvaccine serotypes that erode vaccine success that requires ongoing surveillance and analysis.

CONCLUSIONS

Pneumococcal disease, most notably invasive disease and pneumonia, has decreased considerably, specifically in children in industrialized countries over the past decade, in association with the introduction of protein-conjugated polysaccharide vaccines as part of national childhood vaccination schedules. The decline in disease has been larger in unimmunized adults than in immunized children as a result of herd protection created by the reduction in carriage and transmission of vaccine serotypes. Decreases in antimicrobial-resistant vaccine serotypes also has resulted.

However, in developing countries, acute respiratory infections in general and pneumonia in particular remain the leading causes of morbidity and mortality.[375] The mortality rate from respiratory infections in developing countries is estimated to be 10- to 30-fold higher than that in developed countries.[397,598] Otitis media, although often not perceived as a severe problem in developing countries, may progress to chronic suppurative otitis media and acquired hearing loss in children.[7] Global Alliance for Vaccines and Immunization programs have been critical in reducing the time line for introduction of pneumococcal conjugate vaccine into developing countries.

These advances have been limited by replacement of nasopharyngeal colonization by vaccine serotypes with nonvaccine and frequently antimicrobial-resistant serotypes, resulting in some erosion of vaccine effectiveness as a result of disease with nonvaccine serotypes in IPD and pneumonia as well as other respiratory pathogens in otitis media. These limitations, in turn, have been countered by the introduction of "second-generation" vaccines containing additional serotypes. These next-generation pneumococcal conjugate vaccines resulted in further declines in pneumococcal disease specifically due to the additional serotypes. However, as there are currently 94 recognized serotypes, replacement disease due to nonvaccine serotypes continues to be observed with variable incidence depending on the serotypes present. Evolution of additional serotypes in this genetically promiscuous organism is likely to continue. Development of alternative, broadly conserved vaccine targets that elicit protection against all pneumococcal strains would be very beneficial in the long term, yet currently identification of such potential vaccine antigens remains elusive.[386]

NEW REFERENCES SINCE THE SEVENTH EDITION

24. Ardanuy C, de la Campa AG, Garcia E, et al. Spread of *Streptococcus pneumoniae* serotype 8-ST63 multidrug-resistant recombinant Clone, Spain. *Emerg Infect Dis.* 2014;20(11):1848-1856.
38. Baek JY, Park IH, So TM, et al. Prevalence and characteristics of *Streptococcus pneumoniae* "putative serotype 6E" isolates from Asian countries. *Diagn Microbiol Infect Dis.* 2014;80(4):334-337.
39. Baek JY, Park IH, Song JH, et al. Prevalence of isolates of *Streptococcus pneumoniae* putative serotype 6E in South Korea. *J Clin Microbiol.* 2014;52(6):2096-2099.
51. Ben-Shimol S, Greenberg D, Givon-Lavi N, et al. Impact of PCV7/PCV13 introduction on invasive pneumococcal disease (IPD) in young children: comparison between meningitis and non-meningitis IPD. *Vaccine.* 2016;34(38):4543-4550.
52. Ben-Shimol S, Greenberg D, Hazan G, et al. Seasonality of both bacteremic and nonbacteremic pneumonia coincides with viral lower respiratory tract infections in early childhood, in contrast to nonpneumonia invasive pneumococcal disease, in the pre-pneumococcal conjugate vaccine era. *Clin Infect Dis.* 2015;60(9):1384-1387.
73. Brady AM, Calix JJ, Yu J, et al. Low invasiveness of pneumococcal serotype 11A is linked to ficolin-2 recognition of O-acetylated capsule epitopes and lectin complement pathway activation. *J Infect Dis.* 2014;210(7):1155-1165.
86. Calix JJ, Brady AM, Du VY, et al. Spectrum of pneumococcal serotype 11A variants results from incomplete loss of capsule O-acetylation. *J Clin Microbiol.* 2014;52(3):758-765.
87. Camilli R, Spencer BL, Moschioni M, et al. Identification of *Streptococcus pneumoniae* serotype 11E, serovariant 11Av and mixed populations by high-resolution magic angle spinning nuclear magnetic resonance (HR-MAS NMR) spectroscopy and flow cytometric serotyping assay (FCSA). *PLoS ONE.* 2014;9(6):e100722.
91. Centers for Disease Control and Prevention. Invasive pneumococcal disease among children <5 years old from 1998 through 2015 in the United States. 2016. www.cdc.gov/pneumococcal/surveillance.html.
100. Chuang YP, Peng ZR, Tseng SF, et al. Impact of the glpQ2 gene on virulence in a *Streptococcus pneumoniae* serotype 19A sequence type 320 strain. *Infect Immun.* 2015;83(2):682-692.
108. Cooper D, Yu X, Sidhu M, et al. The 13-valent pneumococcal conjugate vaccine (PCV13) elicits cross-functional opsonophagocytic killing responses in humans to *Streptococcus pneumoniae serotypes* 6C and 7A. *Vaccine.* 2011;29(41):7207-7211.
124. Dagan R, Pelton S, Bakaletz L, et al. Prevention of early episodes of otitis media by pneumococcal vaccines might reduce progression to complex disease. *Lancet Infect Dis.* 2016;16(4):480-492.
133. De Schutter I, Vergison A, Tuerlinckx D, et al. Pneumococcal aetiology and serotype distribution in paediatric community-acquired pneumonia. *PLoS ONE.* 2014;9(2):e89013.
136. Dhoubhadel BG, Yasunami M, Yoshida LM, et al. A novel high-throughput method for molecular serotyping and serotype-specific quantification of *Streptococcus pneumoniae* using a nanofluidic real-time PCR system. *J Med Microbiol.* 2014;63(Pt 4):528-539.
137. Diao WQ, Shen N, Yu PX, et al. Efficacy of 23-valent pneumococcal polysaccharide vaccine in preventing community-acquired pneumonia among immunocompetent adults: a systematic review and meta-analysis of randomized trials. *Vaccine.* 2016;34(13):1496-1503.
140. Dintilhac A, Alloing G, Granadel C, et al. Competence and virulence of *Streptococcus pneumoniae*: Adc and PsaA mutants exhibit a requirement for Zn and Mn resulting from inactivation of putative ABC metal permeases. *Mol Microbiol.* 1997;25(4):727-739.
142. Domingues CM, Verani JR, Montenegro Renoiner EI, et al. Effectiveness of ten-valent pneumococcal conjugate vaccine against invasive pneumococcal disease in Brazil: a matched case-control study. *Lancet Respir Med.* 2014;2(6):464-471.
176. Food and Drug Administration. Risks May Outweigh Benefits for Antibiotics Levaquin, Cipro. https://www.drugwatch.com/2016/05/16/fda-black-box-warning-for-levaquin-cipro-antibiotic-risk/.
207. Grabenstein JD, Weber DJ. Pneumococcal serotype diversity among adults in various countries, influenced by pediatric pneumococcal vaccination uptake. *Clin Infect Dis.* 2014;58(6):854-864.
215. Griffin MR, Mitchel E, Moore MR, et al. Declines in pneumonia hospitalizations of children aged <2 years associated with the use of pneumococcal conjugate vaccines—Tennessee, 1998-2012. *MMWR Morb Mortal Wkly Rep.* 2014;63(44):995-998.
249. Hortal M, Estevan M, Laurani H, et al. Hospitalized children with pneumonia in Uruguay: pre and post introduction of 7 and 13-valent pneumococcal conjugated vaccines into the National Immunization Program. *Vaccine.* 2012;30(33):4934-4938.
258. Hughes CE, Harvey RM, Plumptre CD, et al. Development of primary invasive pneumococcal disease caused by serotype 1 pneumococci is driven by early increased type I interferon response in the lung. *Infect Immun.* 2014;82(9):3919-3926.
272. Jain S, Self WH, Wunderink RG, et al. Community-acquired pneumonia requiring hospitalization among U.S. adults. *N Engl J Med.* 2015;373(5):415-427.
273. Jain S, Williams DJ, Arnold SR, et al. Community-acquired pneumonia requiring hospitalization among U.S. children. *N Engl J Med.* 2015;372(9):835-845.
293. Kaur R, Casey JR, Pichichero ME. Emerging *Streptococcus pneumoniae* strains colonizing the nasopharynx in children after 13-valent pneumococcal conjugate vaccination in comparison to the 7-valent era, 2006-2015. *Pediatr Infect Dis J.* 2016;35(8):901-906.
294. Kawaguchiya M, Urushibara N, Kobayashi N. High prevalence of genotype 6E (putative serotype 6E) among noninvasive/colonization isolates of *Streptococcus pneumoniae* in northern Japan. *Microb Drug Resist.* 2015;21(2):209-214.
297. Kempf M, Varon E, Lepoutre A, et al. Decline in antibiotic resistance and changes in the serotype distribution of *Streptococcus pneumoniae* isolates from children with acute otitis media; a 2001-2011 survey by the French Pneumococcal Network. *Clin Microbiol Infect.* 2015;21(1):35-42.
299. Khan MN, Coleman JR, Vernatter J, et al. An ahemolytic pneumolysin of *Streptococcus pneumoniae* manipulates human innate and CD4(+) T-cell responses and reduces resistance to colonization in mice in a serotype-independent manner. *J Infect Dis.* 2014;210(10):1658-1669.
314. Kohler S, Hallstrom T, Singh B, et al. Binding of vitronectin and Factor H to Hic contributes to immune evasion of *Streptococcus pneumoniae* serotype 3. *Thromb Haemost.* 2015;113(1):125-142.
320. Kraicer-Melamed H, O'Donnell S, Quach C. The effectiveness of pneumococcal polysaccharide vaccine 23 (PPV23) in the general population of 50 years of age and older: a systematic review and meta-analysis. *Vaccine.* 2016;34(13):1540-1550.
324. Musey L. Safety, Tolerability, and Immunogenicity of 15-Valent Pneumococcal Conjugate Vaccine (PCV15) in Healthy Adults. 2013. Poster 658. Presented at IDSA, San Diego, CA.
377. Mendes RE, Costello AJ, Jacobs MR, et al. Serotype distribution and antimicrobial susceptibility of USA *Streptococcus pneumoniae* isolates collected prior to and post introduction of 13-valent pneumococcal conjugate vaccine. *Diagn Microbiol Infect Dis.* 2014;80(1):19-25.
383. Mitchell AM, Mitchell TJ. *Streptococcus pneumoniae*: virulence factors and variation. *Clin Microbiol Infect.* 2010;16(5):411-418.

399. Musher DM. *Streptococcus pneumoniae*. In: Mandell GL, Bennett JE, Dolin R, eds. *Principles and Practice of Infectious Disease*. 5th ed. Philadelphia: Churchill Livingstone; 2000:2218-2246.
446. Poolman J, Frasch C, Nurkka A, et al. Impact of the conjugation method on the immunogenicity of *Streptococcus pneumoniae* serotype 19F polysaccharide in conjugate vaccines. *Clin Vaccine Immunol*. 2011;18(2):327-336.
473. Rosch JW, Iverson AR, Humann J, et al. A live-attenuated pneumococcal vaccine elicits CD4+ T-cell dependent class switching and provides serotype independent protection against acute otitis media. *EMBO Mol Med*. 2014;6(1):141-154.
481. Rusu LI, Wyres KL, Reumann M, et al. A platform for leveraging next generation sequencing for routine microbiology and public health use. *Health Inf Sci Syst*. 2015;3(suppl 1 HISA Big Data in Biomedicine and Healthcare 2013 Con):S7.
533. Syk A, Norman M, Fernebro J, et al. Emergence of hypervirulent mutants resistant to early clearance during systemic serotype 1 pneumococcal infection in mice and humans. *J Infect Dis*. 2014;210(1):4-13.
563. van der Linden M, Weiss S, Falkenhorst G, et al. Four years of universal pneumococcal conjugate infant vaccination in Germany: impact on incidence of invasive pneumococcal disease and serotype distribution in children. *Vaccine*. 2012;30(40):5880-5885.
567. Varon E, Cohen R, Bechet S, et al. Invasive disease potential of pneumococci before and after the 13-valent pneumococcal conjugate vaccine implementation in children. *Vaccine*. 2015;33(46):6178-6185.
577. WHO Publication. Pneumococcal vaccines WHO position paper—2012—recommendations. *Vaccine*. 2012;30(32):4717-4718.
587. Weatherholtz R, Millar EV, Moulton LH, et al. Invasive pneumococcal disease a decade after pneumococcal conjugate vaccine use in an American Indian population at high risk for disease. *Clin Infect Dis*. 2010;50(9):1238-1246.
607. Wyres KL, Lambertsen LM, Croucher NJ, et al. Pneumococcal capsular switching: a historical perspective. *J Infect Dis*. 2013;207(3):439-449.

The full reference list for this chapter is available at ExpertConsult.com.

Miscellaneous Gram-Positive Cocci 86

Randall G. Fisher

The focus of this chapter is on relatively uncommon gram-positive cocci that are of importance because of their unusual antimicrobial sensitivities and increasing recognition as pathogens in hospitalized patients. The reader is referred to a review of these organisms for more details.[22]

LEUCONOSTOC SPECIES

Bacteriology

Leuconostoc spp. are facultatively anaerobic, gram-positive cocci that usually appear in pairs or chains. They are catalase negative, Vogues-Proskauer positive, and leucine aminopeptidase positive. In addition, colonies often are α-hemolytic on blood agar and also may react with group D streptococcal antiserum. These properties are shared by viridans streptococci, with which *Leuconostoc* spp. often are confused.[24] They also may resemble enterococci, except that they are pyrrolidone carboxylyl peptidase negative. Differences include the production of gas from glucose and high-level vancomycin resistance. *Leuconostoc* spp. have been divided into three subclusters[20]; members of the first of these (the *L. mesenteroides* subcluster) are the only ones of human clinical importance. The most common pathogens are *L. mesenteroides, L. lactis, L. citreum, L. paramesenteroides,* and *L. pseudomesenteroides.*

Epidemiology

Leuconostoc spp. are found commonly on plants, especially sugar cane and leafy vegetables. They also are present in dairy products and wine.[67] They are used in the food industry as starter cultures in food production.[42,81] Dextransucrase derived from *L. meserentoides* is used to make gentio-oligosaccharides, which are prebiotics that have a lower degree of digestibility than inulin; these compounds are also toxic to human colon carcinoma cells in vitro.[47] Studies using culture methods have suggested that, although they occasionally are recovered from vaginal swabs in healthy individuals[71] and from mucosal surfaces in some hospitalized individuals,[34] *Leuconostoc* spp. are not part of the normal human flora.[4] Case reports of pediatric infection began to appear in the 1980s.[15,35,65,88]

Pathophysiology

Leuconostoc spp. rarely are pathogenic. Underlying disease states or compromised immune system, gastrointestinal tract disease (especially short-gut syndrome), previous or current antibiotic therapy, venous or gastrointestinal tract access devices, recent invasive procedures, and infancy are thought to be risk factors.[19,21,34,67] In patients with short-gut syndrome, the presence of central venous catheters and disrupted bowel mucosa are likely the most important risks.[25] Frequently, the organisms are isolated as part of a polymicrobial infection after a patient has been treated with vancomycin.[22] Of the first 21 cases reported in the English literature, 12 were in children, 10 of which occurred in patients younger than 1 year. Documented portals of entry include central lines,[4,35] peritoneal dialysis and urinary catheters,[9] and gastrostomy tubes.[40] A case of nosocomial meningitis apparently caused by frequent lumbar puncture after intracranial hemorrhage has been reported.[36] Contaminated enteral formula also has been implicated.[10,40,62] One outbreak involving 42 patients in Spain was traced to contaminated total parenteral nutrition solution.[5] Occasional sporadic cases without a known risk factor have been described, including one in a mildly premature baby who had not undergone instrumentation.[15,34,56]

Clinical Manifestations

Bacteremia, heralded by fever and usually leukocytosis, is by far the most common clinical manifestation of *Leuconostoc* infection. Gastrointestinal disturbances, especially diarrhea, are common manifestations.[4] Infants are prone to emesis. *Leuconostoc* bacteremia, in association with cough and chest radiographic findings consistent with pneumonia, was reported in a child with acquired immunodeficiency syndrome (AIDS).[67] *L. citreum* has been isolated from the lung tissue of a 33-year-old patient with AIDS who also had *Pneumocystis jiroveci* pneumonia.[28] Small necrotic cavities scattered through both lungs were associated with gram-positive cocci in tissue. Patients with associated dental infections,[88] peritonitis,[29] osteomyelitis,[58] and meningitis[15,26] also have been described. Meningitis has been reported in an otherwise healthy 16-year-old patient and in a neonate with fatal infection despite high cerebrospinal fluid (CSF) bactericidal antibiotic titers.[15,26] A nosocomial cluster of five cases of urinary tract infection caused by *L. pseudomesenteroides* (strictly a species of a new genus, *Weissella*)[14] has been reported,[9] as has a cluster of three cases of *Leuconostoc* septicemia in critically ill postsurgical patients.[74] In a series of 20 cases from Taiwan, 19 of the 20 had health care–associated bacteremia. Eleven of the 20 had an underlying malignancy, and the same number had been hospitalized for 30 days or more at the time the diagnosis was made.[49]

Diagnosis

Cultures usually are positive within 24 to 48 hours. Identification of vancomycin-resistant *Streptococcus* should raise the suspicion of

Leuconostoc infection and prompt additional biochemical studies,[67] including gas production in MRS broth, failure to hydrolyze arginine, and delayed esculin hydrolysis. Accurate identification to the species level may require molecular techniques.[17]

Treatment

Treatment with relatively high doses of penicillin or ampicillin frequently is successful in eradicating infection. Many species produce biofilms[51]; when possible, access devices should be removed. Leuconostocs are most sensitive to the primitive β-lactam antibiotics, especially penicillin and ampicillin, although penicillin tolerance is a common finding.[40,84] They also frequently are sensitive to erythromycin, cephalothin, and the aminoglycosides. Leuconostocs are variably resistant to clindamycin and trimethoprim-sulfamethoxazole. Resistance increases with later generations of cephalosporins.[34,84] Leuconostocs are intrinsically vancomycin resistant because their pentapeptide cell wall precursors end in D-Ala-lactate rather than the usual D-Ala-alanine.[33] Vancomycin cannot bind the lactate. This mode of resistance is the same as that possessed by vancomycin-resistant enterococci. However, whereas resistance in enterococci is plasmid derived and transferable, in *Leuconostoc* spp. it is chromosomally mediated, constitutional, and not transferable.

PEDIOCOCCUS SPECIES

Bacteriology

Pediococci also are intrinsically vancomycin resistant, facultatively anaerobic gram-positive cocci. They appear most characteristically in tetrads on Gram staining, although they may appear in pairs or clusters.[31] The genus name *Pediococcus* is derived from the Greek word *pedium,* which means "plane." This name, therefore, suggests that this is a genus of cocci that grow in a single plane. It is a misnomer, however, because pediococci are the only lactic acid bacteria that divide in two planes.[27] They are catalase and oxidase negative. They do not reduce nitrates, and no gas is produced in MRS broth.[79] They are pyrrolidone carboxylyl peptidase negative.[22] Most isolates react with Lancefield group D streptococcal antibodies.[79] They are leucine aminopeptidase positive, which distinguishes them from *Leuconostoc* spp.[23] They produce white, opaque, nonhemolytic colonies on sheep's blood agar. A new broth medium, a combination of 90% Iso-Sensitest broth and 10% MRS broth and called LAB susceptibility test medium, has been found to provide optimal support of growth and to yield the most accurate minimal inhibitory concentration values.[46]

Pediococci produce powerful bacteriocins, which are substances that kill other bacteria. The bacteriocins of pediococci are active against other gram-positive organisms in particular[13] but also are active against *Clostridium botulinum* spores,[63] some gram-negative organisms,[80] and *Listeria monocytogenes.* This has led to investigation of *P. pentosaceus* as a vaginal probiotic. Reports have suggested that some species of *Pediococcus* have antifungal activity[55]; however, this activity in other studies has been found to be present only at low pH and has been attributed to acetic acid in the medium.[8]

Pediococcus acidilactici inhibits growth of *H. pylori* in vitro and provides benefit in a mouse model of *H. pylori* gastric ulcer disease.[43] Several species of *Pediococcus* have the characteristics of a good probiotic; they adhere to Caco-2 cells, possess desirable enzyme activities, and survive in feces for up to 2 weeks in human volunteers.[2,50]

Epidemiology

Like leuconostocs and other lactic acid bacteria, pediococci are found on plants, in dairy products, and in alcohol-containing beverages, where certain species are associated with spoilage.[85] They also are used in the formation of silage[42] and as starter cultures for some meat products. They are not thought to be part of the normal flora. They have been isolated from saliva and stool on rare occasion.[72] Although formerly thought to be nonpathogenic, they now are considered rare opportunistic pathogens with minimal virulence.

Pathophysiology

Pediococci rarely are pathogenic. Many cases of blood isolates are found in patients without symptoms of infection or in polymicrobial cultures in which the significance of the isolate could not be assessed adequately.[57] One patient with a clinical picture of septic shock in whom the only organism recovered was *P. pentosaceus* has been reported.[16] Risk factors for bacteremia, with or without symptoms, appear to be the extremes of age, recent abdominal surgery or tube feeding, broad-spectrum antimicrobial therapy, and the presence of severe underlying disease states.[57] However, because the overall number of reported cases is small, the relative risks of these factors are uncertain.

Clinical Manifestations and Diagnosis

Most patients either are asymptomatic or have fever as the only symptom. Six of the first 12 reported cases of *Pediococcus* bacteremia had concomitant pneumonia. Fifty-six percent of adult patients either were receiving tube feeding or had undergone abdominal surgery within 30 days of isolation of the organism.[57] The three reported pediatric cases occurred in infants, and all had underlying gastrointestinal tract anomalies. A 16-day-old infant with congenital jejunoileal atresia had undergone surgical repair just 8 days before being evaluated.[57] Her acute illness was characterized by emesis and a 200-g weight loss. She was afebrile when initially examined. The second patient was a 64-day-old infant with gastroschisis who had undergone two abdominal surgical procedures.[1] His fever reached 38.6°C (101.5°F), and his peripheral white blood cell count was 38,000/mm^3 with a significant left shift. The third patient was a 3-month-old female infant who had undergone surgical repair of gastroschisis on the first day of life.[3] Lethargy, direct hyperbilirubinemia, and a CSF pleocytosis were noted. Blood cultures grew *Pediococcus* spp., and the CSF (obtained after initiation of antibiotics) was sterile. The patient responded to a 21-day course of ampicillin and gentamicin. An adult case of infective endocarditis in a man who had a history of bowel transplantation for short-gut syndrome[41] and a case of persistent bacteremia in a patient with metastatic adenocarcinoma of the gallbladder have been reported[82]; both responded rapidly to therapy with daptomycin.

Pediococci are isolated frequently in localized infections, especially from abdominal sites, but they are virtually always part of a polymicrobial process. The relative importance of pediococci in these sites is difficult to assess. A case of *Pediococcus* bacteremic pneumonia was reported in a previously healthy pregnant woman.[73] Among 31 cases of *Pediococcus* infection submitted to the U.S. Centers for Disease Control and Prevention laboratory, 17 were from blood culture isolates (including two reported cases of endocarditis) and four were associated with urinary tract infections. Other sources included catheter tips, wounds, peritoneal fluid, CSF, lung, and bone.[22]

Diagnosis of infection with pediococci is established by identifying catalase-negative, vancomycin-resistant, gram-positive cocci in the characteristic tetrads. Many pediococci are misidentified initially as *Streptococcus equinus, S. constellatus,* or group D streptococcus, not *Enterococcus.* Reported cases of pediococcal infection may therefore represent only a fraction of the total number of infections.

Treatment

Pediococci generally are susceptible to penicillin, ampicillin, imipenem, clindamycin, and first- and second-generation cephalosporins. Although both imipenem and penicillin are highly active against pediococci, they do not appear to be bactericidal. Pediococci are moderately resistant to the quinolones, tetracycline,[85] and trimethoprim-sulfamethoxazole.[70] Pediococci, like leuconostocs, are intrinsically resistant to vancomycin. Resistance is not plasmid mediated, nor can it be transferred to other bacteria.[85] Sensitivity to ticarcillin and cefotaxime, when measured by agar dilution, is poor despite large zones of inhibition on disk susceptibility testing.[85] Occasionally inducible resistance to erythromycin is found, although most isolates remain sensitive. Aminoglycoside sensitivity is variable. Daptomycin appears to be active.

AEROCOCCUS SPECIES

Bacteriology

The genus *Aerococcus* contains at least five species, but only three, *A. viridans, A. sanguinicola,* and *A. urinae,* have known clinical significance. In earlier papers, *A. urinae* was referred to as *Aerococcus*-like organism.[12]

Aerococci are catalase-negative, nonmotile, gram-positive cocci that appear preferentially in tetrads but sometimes in pairs or clusters. These relatively slow-growing organisms produce small, well-delineated, translucent, α-hemolytic colonies on blood agar.[11] They also are weakly bile esculin positive and pyrrolidone carboxylyl peptidase negative. They ferment mannose and mannitol.[68] Like enterococci, most aerococci will grow in 6.5% salt.[48]

Epidemiology

Aerococci are distributed throughout the world and are contaminants of air and dust.[37] They also have been found on meat, on raw vegetables, and in small numbers on human skin.[7] In hospitals, aerococci have been cultured from all areas, including operating suites and delivery rooms.[44] They also are found in saltwater, where they cause a fatal disease in lobsters.[64]

Disease in humans is an uncommon event, and the organism usually is recovered from the bloodstream of patients with infective endocarditis. Most patients are elderly, but infection of infants and neonates also has been reported.[61,64] A rapidly fatal bacteremia has been described in patients with profound neutropenia.[45] Aerococci are agents of urinary tract infection in elderly and institutionalized persons[78]; these organisms can also cause pediatric urinary tract infections and even pyelonephritis, usually in the setting of obstructive uropathy.[52,59]

Pathophysiology

In most circumstances, aerococci are saprophytic. The exact conditions that favor the development of infection have not been elucidated clearly. Some cases of *A. urinae* infection have occurred after genitourinary tract surgery. One case of septic arthritis developed after an elective abortion.[86] Septic arthritis of the hip developed in a paraplegic man; infection started in the urinary tract.[30] Immunocompromised patients are at higher risk, but infection in otherwise well persons has been described.[68] One report of meningitis in neonates found adherence of aerococci to inflammatory cells and suggested a role of as-yet-undefined adhesion factors.[61] Work in laboratory animals also has shown that a protease isolated from *A. viridans* cleaves the hemagglutinin of influenza virus and potentiates both viral replication and disease in mice.[75] In vitro experiments show that the organism forms biofilms and causes platelet aggregation, features that explain why endocarditis is a common manifestation.[77]

Clinical Manifestations

Most cases of *A. viridans* bacteremia have been found in association with signs and symptoms of subacute infective endocarditis. Severe disease requiring valve replacement surgery has been described, but not in pediatric patients.[6] In one series of four cases of *A. viridans* infective endocarditis, two of the patients required surgical intervention.[69] *A. urinae* causes urinary tract infection with dysuria and frequency, usually in the absence of fever.[11] There have been several reports of foul-smelling urine in otherwise healthy children being caused by colonization of the urinary tract with *A. urinae*. Trimethylaminuria was suspected, but the odor went away with treatment.[18,53] *Aerococcus* infection in childhood is an uncommon occurrence. One case of bacteremia in a 1-month-old infant has been reported.[64] The patient had a 2-day history of loose stools, irritability, and drowsiness and on physical examination was noted to have mottled skin, circumoral cyanosis, and agitation. CSF and urine studies were normal, but blood cultures exhibited pure growth of *A. viridans*. No predisposing factors were identified.

Nathavitharana and associates[61] reported three cases of meningitis caused by *A. viridans*. They occurred in a 7-month-old female infant with jerking movements of the extremities, irritability, and a bulging fontanelle; a 5-month-old female infant with fever, decreased appetite, and generalized convulsions; and a 24-month-old girl whose illness was manifested as fever, vomiting, and the neurologic signs of truncal ataxia, flaccidity, and hypoactive deep tendon reflexes. All three patients had elevated CSF white blood cell counts with 55% to 93% segmented forms. Remarkably all these patients had a history of prolonged illness (1 week to 2 months) before being evaluated, in contrast to patients with other causes of bacterial meningitis. No risk factors for infection were identified in any of these patients, who were thought to have normal immune function.

Swanson and colleagues[83] reported a case of penicillin-resistant *A. viridans* bacteremia in an 11-month-old girl receiving prophylactic penicillin for sickle-cell disease. The patient responded clinically to a 10-day course of therapy with cephalosporins.

Bone and joint infections and wound or other localized infections are exceedingly rare occurrences and not distinguishable from similar syndromes caused by more common organisms. However, there are a number of case reports of spondylodiscitis in patients with *A. urinae* bacteremia or infective endocarditis.[60,87]

Diagnosis

Careful observation of both appearance on Gram stain and growth in culture is key to establishing the diagnosis of aerococcal infection. On Gram stain, aerococci resemble staphylococci. On blood agar, they resemble viridans group streptococci. One series revealed that 1% of 719 cultures called streptococci actually were aerococci[66]; another study reclassified 3% of 168 cultures.[7] In one study of 24 α-hemolytic, nonenterococcal bacterial isolates from urine, standard identification methods were compared with 16S rRNA sequencing and special biochemical profiling. Thirteen of the isolates were aerococci; all were identified correctly by sequencing, but typical procedures failed to differentiate them from nonaerococcal isolates. The ability to grow the organisms at 45°C improved the discrimination of standard testing.[32] In their propensity toward tetrad formation, they mimic pediococci. However, all aerococci are vancomycin sensitive. In their bile esculin hydrolysis and growth in 6.5% salt, they resemble enterococci; unlike enterococci, however, aerococci are pyrrolidone carboxylyl peptidase negative and do not form chains. Molecular modalities such as matrix-assisted laser desorption/ionization time of flight (MALDI-TOF) are able to identify pediococci to the species level.[76]

Treatment

Broth microdilution susceptibility testing of 128 isolates of *A. urinae* showed that they were all susceptible to penicillin, amoxicillin, cefotaxime, ceftriaxone, doxycycline, tetracycline, linezolid, meropenem, and vancomycin. A substantial portion had clindamycin and erythromycin minimum inhibitory concentrations (MICs) of greater than 0.25 μg/mL; 16% had levofloxacin MICs of greater than 2 μg/mL.[39] Reports of nonsusceptibility to penicillin or resistance to ceftriaxone have appeared but are the exception.[54] One report of an isolate resistant to vancomycin has been published.[89] They usually are intermediately susceptible or resistant to sulfonamides and aminoglycosides.[7,37] Susceptibility testing for trimethoprim-sulfamethoxazole appears to be affected by the medium used in the testing.[38] One report suggests that *A. viridans* and *A. urinae* have distinct antibiograms[48]; that is, *A. urinae* is more sensitive to penicillin and resistant to sulfonamides, whereas *A. viridans* is more resistant to penicillin and sensitive to the sulfonamides.[7] Individual case reports do not confirm these in vitro observations, and no large clinical trials of antimicrobial susceptibility have been conducted.

Acknowledgments

I thank Dr. William Gruber and Dr. Thomas Boyce for their invaluable assistance with earlier versions of this chapter.

NEW REFERENCES SINCE THE SEVENTH EDITION

2. Balgir PP, Kaur B, Kaur T, et al. In vitro and in vivo survival and colonic adhesion of Pediococcus acidilactici MTCC5101 in human gut. *Biomed Res Int*. 2013;583850.
17. Deng Y, Zhang Z, Xie Y, et al. A mixed infection of *Leuconostoc lactis* and vancomycin-resistant *Enterococcus* in a liver transplant recipient. *J Med Microbiol*. 2012;61:1621-1624.
18. deVries TW, Brandenburg AH. Foul smelling urine in a 7-year-old boy caused by *Aerococcus urinae*. *Pediatr Infect Dis J*. 2012;31:1316-1317.
30. Goetz LL, Powell DJ, Castillo TA, et al. Hip abscess due to *Aerococcus urinae* in a man with paraplegia: case report. *Spinal Cord*. 2013;51:929-930.
39. Humphries RM, Hindler JA. In vitro antimicrobial susceptibility of *Aerococcus urinae*. *J Clin Microbiol*. 2014;52:2177-2180.
43. Kaur B, Garg N, Sachdev A, et al. Effect of the oral intake of probiotic *Pediococcus* acidilacticiBA28 on *Helicobacter pylori* causing peptic ulcer in C57BL/6 mice models. *Appl Biochem Biotechnol*. 2014;172:973-983.

47. Kothari D, Goyal A. Gentio-oligosaccharides from *Leuconostoc mesenteroides* NRRL B-1426 dextransucrase as prebiotics and as a supplement for functional foods with anti-cancer properties. *Food Funct*. 2015;6:604-611.
49. Lee KW, Park JY, Sa HD, et al. Probiotic properties of *Pediococcus* strains isolated from jeotgals, salted and fermented Korean seafood. *Anaerobe*. 2014;28:199-206.
53. Lenherr N, Berndt A, Ritz N, et al. *Aerococcus urinae*: a possible reason for malodorous urine in otherwise healthy children. *Eur J Pediatr*. 2014;173:1115-1117.
54. Lupo A, Guilarte YN, Droz S, et al. In vitro activity of clinically implemented beta-lactams against *Aerococcus urinae*: presence of non-susceptible isolates in Switzerland. *New Microbiol*. 2014;37:563-566.
56. Martinez-Pajares JD, Diaz-Morales O, Acosta-Gonzalez F, et al. Sepsis by *Leuconostoc* spp. in a healthy infant. *Arch Argent Pediatr*. 2012;110:332-334.
76. Senneby E, Nilson B, Petersson AC, et al. Matrix-assisted laser desorption ionization-time of flight mass spectrometry is a sensitive and specific method for identification of aerococci. *J Clin Microbiol*. 2013;51:1303-1304.
89. Zhou WQ, Niu DM, Zhang ZZ, et al. Vancomycin resistance due to VanA in an *Aerococcus viridans* isolate. *Indian J Med Microbiol*. 2014;32:462-465.

The full reference list for this chapter is available at ExpertConsult.com.

SUBSECTION II Gram-Negative Cocci

87 *Moraxella catarrhalis*

Barbara W. Stechenberg

Once thought to be an unimportant commensal organism in the human respiratory tract, *Moraxella catarrhalis* now is recognized as an important pathogen in respiratory tract diseases, particularly otitis, sinusitis, and lower tract disease. The initial paper by Ghon and Pfeiffer[24] published in 1902 described gram-negative cocci in sputum referred to as *Micrococcus catarrhalis*. Since then, the organism has undergone several changes in nomenclature, first to *Neisseria catarrhalis* because of its resemblance to other *Neisseria* organisms. In 1970, in recognition of the contributions of Sarah Branham, the name was changed to *Branhamella catarrhalis*.[11] More recently, that this organism should be a member of the genus *Moraxella* has become clear; thus the name was changed to *M. catarrhalis*. With the transition in nomenclature, the past 2 decades have seen a parallel rebirth of this organism as a mucosal pathogen.

MICROBIOLOGY

M. catarrhalis is a gram-negative diplococcus that is morphologically indistinguishable from *Neisseria*. It has a tendency to resist decolorizing.[1] The organism is kidney shaped, with the flat sides abutting each other. The size varies, but it may be larger than meningococcus or gonococcus. However, the resemblance on sputum Gram stain or conjunctival smear to gonococcus can be striking and clinically confusing.

The organism grows well on blood or chocolate agar and forms small, opaque, grayish colonies that are circular and nonhemolytic. They have poor adhesion to the agar surface, on which they act like hockey pucks when pushed over the surface of the agar plate.[17] The use of selective media such as modified Thayer-Martin or TV broth (Müeller-Hinton broth supplemented with trimethoprim and vancomycin) increases the likelihood of recovering *M. catarrhalis* from the complex flora of the mucosal surfaces.

Isolates of *M. catarrhalis* cannot use maltose, glucose, lactose, or sucrose as carbohydrate sources. *M. catarrhalis* is oxidase-positive and produces deoxyribonuclease. Valuable differentiating tests are hydrolysis of DNA and tributyrin. Several rapid tests such as butyrate hydrolysis, Tween 80 hydrolysis, and selective DNase agar have been described.[51,56] Fatty-acid analysis also has been used to identify atypical strains.

The surface of *M. catarrhalis* is composed of outer-membrane proteins, lipo-oligosaccharide, and pili. The organism does not appear to have a capsule, and the role of the pili is not defined well. By using a technique involving the collection of outer membrane vesicles, which are released into the culture medium, and then examining by sodium dodecyl sulfate–polyacrylamide gel electrophoresis (SDS-PAGE), Bartos and Murphy[6] identified eight proteins designated outer membrane proteins A through H. The outer membrane protein patterns of strains from diverse geographic and clinical sources were strikingly homogeneous.

Preliminary studies of the lipo-oligosaccharide of *M. catarrhalis* show that it is more antigenically conserved than those of other gram-negative bacteria.[40] One study suggests that the lipo-oligosaccharide is not an adhesin, but its surface charge plays a critical role in the initial stage of attachment to human epithelial cells.[2] Several adhesins have been identified and may be potential candidates for a vaccine.[40]

Restriction endonuclease analysis has been used as an epidemiologic tool to distinguish strains of *M. catarrhalis*. Patterson and associates[43] used the technique to evaluate a nosocomial outbreak and demonstrate the lack of association of other strains. Dickinson and coworkers[16] used a similar technique to study isolates from children with otitis media.

PATHOGENESIS

The ability of *M. catarrhalis* to produce disease, particularly in sequestered areas such as the ear and lung, indicates that this organism possesses virulence mechanisms that allow it not only to grow in these anatomic sites but also to produce pathologic effects. However, a subset of strains of *M. catarrhalis* associated with selected virulence traits resulting in complement inactivation suggests that some strains are more virulent than others.[9,55]

A body of literature concerning the immune response to *M. catarrhalis* and the antigenic composition of this organism has accumulated.[12,13,35] Goldblatt and associates[25] demonstrated that children younger than 4 years possess immunoglobulin (Ig) G1 and IgG2 that recognize an 82-kDa outer membrane protein exclusively but that older children mount an IgG3 response to a broad range of outer membrane proteins. Faden and colleagues[22] developed a technique to measure opsonic antibody with the use of outer membrane, antigen-coated beads. Convalescent sera opsonized homologous, antigen-coated beads significantly more often than did acute sera.

Unhanand and coworkers[53] used a murine model to study pulmonary clearance of *M. catarrhalis* from infected lungs. They investigated 10 strains and found marked variability in clearance rates and recruitment of phagocytic cells. With this model, Maciver and associates[37] actively immunized animals with the outer membrane vesicles of *M. catarrhalis* and passively immunized animals with rabbit antiserum raised against these vesicles. Both experiments resulted in enhanced pulmonary clearance of both homologous and heterologous strains. The same model has been used to evaluate the role of a large, antigenically conserved protein of *M. catarrhalis* in pulmonary clearance, as well as the role of outer membrane protein B in defense mechanisms of the lung.[31] The contribution of these proteins, as well as lipo-oligosaccharide, in host defense continues to unfold.

Initially thought to be an exclusively extracellular pathogen, *M. catarrhalis* invades multiple cell types. It is present intracellularly in human pharyngeal tissue, where it is a potential reservoir for persistent colonization.[30] The organism forms biofilms, which may contribute to its role in chronic otitis with effusion.[28,29] Colonization of healthy children is characterized by genotypic heterogeneity, virulence gene diversity, and co-colonization with *Haemophilus influenzae*.[57]

EPIDEMIOLOGY

M. catarrhalis is a normal inhabitant of the upper respiratory tract and is recovered exclusively from humans. The rate of colonization is highest in the early years and then declines steadily to less than 5% in adult life.[54] Prevalence studies report that as many as 50% of children are colonized with *M. catarrhalis*.[33,38] Faden and associates[21] monitored a large cohort of children from birth to 2 years of age. Sixty-six percent became colonized by the time they reached 1 year of age, and 77.5% did so by 2 years of age. The frequency of nasopharyngeal colonization was higher during visits for otitis media than during well-child visits. Otitis-prone children were colonized by 6 months of age. Restriction endonuclease analysis showed marked heterogeneity, with children acquiring and eliminating many different strains over time.[21,43]

Numerous studies have documented the increased prevalence of *M. catarrhalis* as a pathogen in otitis media, either alone or as a copathogen.[33,44] Shurin and colleagues[49] noted that isolation of *M. catarrhalis* from middle ear exudates increased from 6.4% between 1979 and 1980 to 26.5% between 1980 and 1982. A similar increase in *M. catarrhalis* as a pathogen in sinusitis has been reported.[58] In the pneumococcal conjugate vaccine (PCV7) era, a significantly higher proportion of PCV7-immunized children exhibit nasopharyngeal colonization with *M. catarrhalis*.[45]

Once colonization of the oropharynx occurs, colonization of the tracheobronchial tree may follow, but usually only if other risk factors are operative. In adults, such risk factors include previous cardiorespiratory disease, smoking, use of corticosteroids, use of immunosuppressive agents, malignancy, and intercurrent viral illnesses.[27,56] In children, many cases of pneumonia are associated with a preceding viral illness, prematurity, underlying lung disease, IgG deficiency, or other risk factors.

Nosocomial transmission has been well documented by DNA restriction endonuclease analysis.[14,43] In pediatric intensive care units, endotracheal intubation and frequent suctioning have been identified as risk factors for the development of pneumonia and bacterial tracheitis.[14,20]

Other interesting associations need to be investigated further. Seddon and associates[48] noted that colonization with *M. catarrhalis* occurred more commonly in asthmatic than in normal children. Whether the organism might be a trigger or pathogen in these children remains to be seen. Gottfarb and Brauner[26] found a high carriage rate of *M. catarrhalis* in children with severe persistent cough.

Infection with *M. catarrhalis* exhibits seasonality in both adults and children.[27,49] Infection is much more likely to occur in the winter and spring months.

CLINICAL MANIFESTATIONS AND DIAGNOSIS

Otitis media caused by *M. catarrhalis* is indistinguishable clinically from otitis caused by other pathogens, such as *Streptococcus pneumoniae* and *Haemophilus influenzae*. *M. catarrhalis* may be isolated as a single agent or in combination with other organisms. There is some suggestion that otitis caused by this organism may be associated with less fever; a lower likelihood of a red, bulging membrane or perforation; and a lower C-reactive protein level.[40] Mastoiditis is not commonly seen with *M. catarrhalis*.

Because tympanocentesis usually is not performed in routine cases, the exact cause of an episode of acute otitis media generally is not known. One study found that *Moraxella* was an unusual organism as a single agent in children in whom acute otitis media had been treated recently.[29] Nonetheless, in a study of persistent otitis, Pichichero and Pichichero[44] demonstrated *Moraxella* in 7% of specimens. The spontaneous resolution rate of *M. catarrhalis* may be high,[4] and this fact should be considered when therapy is planned.

The clinical manifestations of acute sinusitis caused by *M. catarrhalis* are similar to those of other organisms; therefore selection of antibiotics should be made with consideration of this organism as a potential pathogen.

Lower respiratory tract disease caused by *M. catarrhalis* may have a broad clinical spectrum; however, because sputum samples often are not available in children, many cases documented in the literature have been severe. Berg and Bartley[7] described five premature infants, all younger than 6 months of age, in whom precipitous clinical deterioration developed after 2 to 4 days of a prodrome consisting of cough, tachypnea, and intercostal retractions. They all required assisted ventilation, which is common in young infants with severe pneumonia.[7,14,19] Some cases of *M. catarrhalis* pneumonia have been associated with bacteremia.

Underlying conditions such as leukemia, acquired immunodeficiency syndrome, and trauma have been reported to predispose a patient to the development of infection with *M. catarrhalis*.[38,59] An association with Ig deficiency has been demonstrated in some patients with disease caused by this organism.[12] In adults, *M. catarrhalis* pneumonia occurs more commonly in patients with human immunodeficiency virus infection, malignancy, or chronic lung problems.[25,56] The role of this organism in less severe manifestations probably is limited.[34]

Bacterial tracheitis caused by *M. catarrhalis* has been reported in both immunocompromised hosts and those with normal immune systems.[20]

M. catarrhalis also has been responsible for a wide variety of other infections. Urethritis caused by this organism can be mistaken for infection with *Neisseria gonorrhoeae*.[50] Several cases of conjunctivitis have been reported; when present in the newborn period, *M. catarrhalis* can mimic the ophthalmia neonatorum of *N. gonorrhoeae*.[52] The relationship of neonatal infections to maternal vaginal carriage of *Moraxella* has not been established.[42]

More severe infections with *M. catarrhalis* include meningitis and bacteremia, so this organism should be considered in appropriate circumstances, especially in immunocompromised children.

Children with *M. catarrhalis* bacteremia may have many different manifestations. Some patients have petechial or purpuric rashes, thus rendering the clinical picture indistinguishable from that of meningococcemia. Others have been neutropenic and have required mechanical ventilation.[8] Baron and Shapiro[5] reported two cases of unsuspected bacteremia in children with nonspecific symptoms. Their manifestations were similar to those of children with occult pneumococcal bacteremia. An immunocompetent child with *M. catarrhalis* bacteremia and preseptal cellulitis has been reported.[47]

Meningitis can occur from hematogenous spread of *M. catarrhalis* from the nasopharynx or as a consequence of ventriculoperitoneal shunt placement or surgery. Rarely suppurative arthritis has been seen in children and adults.[32,39] Endocarditis is a rare occurrence, as is peritonitis.

TREATMENT

In the past, *M. catarrhalis* was susceptible to all β-lactam antibiotics. In the late 1970s, however, β-lactamase–producing strains of *M. catarrhalis* were isolated in Europe. In the United States, a parallel increase in the frequency of isolation of β-lactamase–producing *M. catarrhalis* has been noted, so it is not unusual for a laboratory to report that more than 90% of strains are β-lactamase producers.

The β-lactamases BRO-1, BRO-2, and BRO-3 are of chromosomal origin. BRO-1 is the most common β-lactamase in North American strains.[15] Because of the high prevalence of β-lactamase–producing strains, many laboratories choose not to do any such testing. The β-lactamase inhibitors clavulanic acid, sulbactam, and tazobactam are active against the enzymes produced by *Moraxella*. Most β-lactamase–positive isolates will respond to achievable concentrations of β-lactam/β-lactamase inhibitor antimicrobial combinations, cephalosporins, and cephamycins.[18,23]

Among the oral cephalosporins active against β-lactamase–positive strains of *Moraxella*, the minimal inhibitory concentration increases two- to fourfold in the presence of the β-lactamase BRO-1 but not the β-lactamase BRO-2; cefixime is more active than are the older cephalosporins.[41] Resistance to tetracycline (by the nontransferable tetB determinant) and erythromycin has been reported, but such resistance is a rare finding.[10,46]

In vitro, *M. catarrhalis* usually is susceptible to ampicillin-sulbactam, amoxicillin-clavulanate, erythromycin, azithromycin, clarithromycin, trimethoprim-sulfamethoxazole, tetracyclines, chloramphenicol, fluoroquinolones (e.g., ciprofloxacin), aminoglycosides, and second- or third-generation cephalosporins, such as cefuroxime, cefprozil, cefpodoxime, cefixime, cefdinir, and loracarbef.[36] Levofloxacin also exhibits good activity against *M. catarrhalis*.[3] The *Moraxella* organism is resistant to clindamycin, vancomycin, and oxacillin.

PREVENTION

Prevention of nosocomial *M. catarrhalis* infection depends on sound practices of infection control, especially with regard to pulmonary toilet. Prevention of other infections with this organism has not been attempted. Development of a vaccine has been hampered by a lack of an animal model.

The full reference list for this chapter is available at ExpertConsult.com.

88 Meningococcal Disease

Lucila Marquez

Epidemic meningococcal meningitis was first described by Gaspard Vieusseux in Geneva in the spring of 1805. In a monograph entitled "The Disease Which Raged During the Spring of 1805," he wrote:

> *It commences suddenly with prostration of strength, often extreme: the face is distorted, the pulse feeble. There appears a violent pain in the head, especially over the forehead; then there comes pain of the heart or vomiting of greenish material, stiffness of the spine, and in infants, convulsions. In cases which were fatal, loss of consciousness occurred. The course of the disease is very rapid, termination by death or by cure. In most of the patients who died in 24 hours or a little after, the body is covered with purple spots at the moment of death or very little time afterward.*[230]

Today, *Neisseria meningitidis* continues to be a cause of endemic and epidemic disease. In the United States since 2012, approximately 550 cases of invasive meningococcal disease are reported each year, and 95% to 97% of these cases are sporadic.[46] Although cases in the United States are at a historic low, epidemics in developed and developing countries continue, and it is estimated that at least 1.2 million cases of invasive meningococcal disease occur annually, with an associated 135,000 deaths.[118]

The reader is referred to the excellent reviews of meningococcal disease that have been published recently.[54,90,106]

MICROBIOLOGY

The *Neisseria* genus was named for Dr. Albert Neisser, who described the organism of gonorrhea in 1879. The genus *Neisseria* contains two species important in human disease, *N. gonorrhoeae* and *N. meningitidis*. In addition, several species are part of the normal flora of humans and animals. *N. sicca, N. lactamica, N. subflava, N. flavescens, N. mucosa, N. cinerea, N. polysaccharea*, and *N. elongata* are human commensals; they only occasionally cause human disease.[147]

N. meningitidis is a gram-negative coccus, usually less than 1 µm in diameter. It classically occurs in pairs, with adjacent sides flattened, resembling kidney beans. Occasionally the organism divides in two planes at right angles to one another, which results in the formation of tetrads. The organisms are nonmotile, are aerobic (but facultatively anaerobic), produce catalase and oxidase, and may be encapsulated. *N. meningitidis* oxidizes glucose and maltose to acid. This distinguishes it from *N. gonorrhoeae,* which oxidizes only glucose. However, certain rare strains of *N. meningitidis* have been reported that fail to produce acid from either glucose or maltose. Fresh isolates have complex nutritional requirements, growing best on chocolate or blood agar. Incubation in a humidified 10% carbon dioxide environment is not essential, but enhances growth. Morphologically the colonies are bluish-gray in appearance and will produce β-hemolysis after 48 to 72 hours of incubation on 5% horse blood agar.[32]

N. meningitidis can be transformed by DNA originating in other *Neisseria* spp. Thus when a *Neisseria* spp. cohabiting the nasopharynx with *N. meningitidis* dies and releases its DNA, the coresident meningococcus can take up the DNA and incorporate it into its genome. Although this sequence of events is very rare, if the new DNA confers a selective advantage to the recipient meningococcus, the trait encoded by the incoming DNA may be retained in future progeny. This is the mechanism by which sulfonamide and penicillin G resistance have arisen in *N. meningitidis*.[147] Many commensal *Neisseria* spp., which inhabit the nasopharynx, are relatively resistant to penicillin G. DNA fragments from these commensal strains, encoding penicillin resistance, can be detected in penicillin-resistant *N. meningitidis*.[201] Transformation of new DNA into *N. meningitidis* also can introduce genes that modify the structure of the bacterium. Serotyping of groups A, B, and C meningococci has provided valuable macroepidemiologic information.[87] It is clear that as a population develops immunity to one capsular polysaccharide, the organism is capable of acquiring DNA encoding for an alternative capsule. Serogroup B to C and C to B switching has been reported.[210,217,231] Additionally the serogroup W strain responsible for the Hajj pilgrim outbreak in 2000 was genetically associated with serogroup C strains.[54] In the United States, vaccination is not felt to be the driving force for capsular switching because serogroup B incidence declined even in the absence of vaccination against this serogroup, and more switching from serogroup B to C was observed in an epidemiologic study that compared pre- and postmeningococcal conjugate vaccine (MenACWY) periods.[54,233] Horizontal gene transfer appears to occur from commensal *Neisseria* to *N. meningitidis*, offering products that aid the bacterium in surviving in the host or are involved in housekeeping functions.[143] This phenomenon is probably responsible for the occasional report of commensal *Neisseria* causing meningitis.[14]

In addition to the transformation route for varying the antigenic phenotype, meningococci also may exhibit phase variation, which allows for variance of the number of surface antigens. It has been estimated that there are at least 65 genes in *N. meningitidis* subject to phase variation including *por*A, which is an immunogenic outer membrane protein with more than 600 variants.[80,224] Capsule synthesis may be switched on and off by this mechanism.

Like other gram-negative bacteria, the outer and inner cell membranes of *Neisseria* are phospholipid bilayers. These membranes sandwich a layer of peptidoglycan. Lipooligosaccharide, which is similar to the lipopolysaccharide seen in gram-negative enteric bacteria, is associated with the outer leaflet of the outer cell membrane. Outer membrane proteins that function as porins are an integral part of the outer membrane. Some of these outer membrane proteins are opacity proteins and facilitate adherence and invasion.[162] Beyond the outer membrane, meningococci possess a polysaccharide capsule that protects them from phagocytosis.

Meningococci also have pili, which seem to be important in some phases of adherence to host cells, colonization, and invasion. The genes that code for pili can be turned on and off, so that the organism at times may not express pili. A recent study reported that posttranslational modification of the type IV pili by phosphoglycerol altered the pili structure and destabilized the pili bundles, resulting in reduced bacterial aggregation on the mucosal surface, which allowed the organism to better cross epithelial monolayers to produce systemic invasion.[49] Antigenic variation of pili by a cassette mechanism allows the bacterium to escape the host's immune system.[99] In addition, both outer membrane proteins and lipooligosaccharide display antigenic variation by phase variation.

For epidemiologic purposes, meningococci are divided into serogroups, serotypes, and subtypes. Differences in capsular polysaccharides, outer membrane proteins, and lipooligosaccharides constitute the basis for these classifications. The capsular polysaccharides are antigenic and the basis for serogroup designation. Twelve serogroups currently are recognized: A, B, C, H, I, K, L, X, Y, Z, W-135, and 29E.[240] Serogroup D has been reclassified as a serogroup C variant.[90] Serogroups A, B, C, W-135, X, and Y are the most common causes of invasive disease worldwide. Furthermore, more than 90% of meningococcal disease is caused by serogroups A, B, C, and Y.

Serotyping of organisms is based on antigenic differences in outer membrane proteins termed *porins.* Porins are protein channels in the outer membrane that permit nutrients and certain antibiotics to diffuse into the periplasmic space. A single locus encodes porin B, but two mutually exclusive alleles have antigenic differences. All meningococci have either antigenic class 2 or class 3 porin B. These differences permit serotyping. Subtypes are differentiated based on antigenic differences in porin A. This highly variable antigen is called a class 1 outer membrane protein. Multiple serotypes and subtypes have been identified. Antigenic specificity is achieved by the generation of monoclonal antibodies to the major protein (primarily class 2 or 3), lipooligosaccharide, and class 1 protein. The designation B:2a:P1.1:L3,7 indicates that the serogroup B strain is an "a" subtype of class 2 proteins, is a "1" of class 1 protein, and possesses two lipooligosaccharide antigens: 3 and 7.[93]

Type 2 protein antigen is isolated from more than 50% of cases in the United States and Canada and is an antigenic determinant in serogroup B and C strains. These protein antigens not only are important as epidemiologic markers but also can induce protective bactericidal antibodies.[86]

EPIDEMIOLOGY

Epidemiology in the United States

Invasive infections caused by *N. meningitidis* are reportable through the National Notifiable Surveillance System in the United States. The number of cases reported to the Centers for Disease Control and Prevention (CDC) between 2011 and 2014 were 845, 551, 556, and 564, for each year, respectively.[43–46] The recent numbers reflect the lowest number of cases ever reported in the United States. In adolescents, the rate of meningococcal disease due to serogroups C, W, and Y dropped by 80% between 2004 and 2005 and 2012 and 2013 following introduction of quadrivalent meningococcal conjugate vaccine.[54]

The Active Bacterial Core surveillance (ABCs) system in the United States tracks invasive disease caused by encapsulated organisms in selected counties of 10 states geographically dispersed throughout the country. This reporting system covers a population of 43 million people. In 2014, the overall incidence of invasive meningococcal disease for the United States was estimated to be 0.14 per 100,000 population.[46] Of cases reported through the ABCs system, 46% were meningitis, with a fatality rate of 6.9%; and 25% of cases were bacteremia, with a fatality of 20%. The case rate of invasive disease was similar between blacks and whites, 0.16 per 100,000 population and 0.15 per 100,000, respectively. The serogroup distribution was 26% serogroup B, 36% serogroup C, 9% serogroup Y, and 28% other serogroups. These data exclude cases from Oregon due to hyperendemic rates in the state after a prolonged outbreak of serogroup B disease.[46]

Certain serogroups are predominant causes of invasive disease depending on the age of the afflicted individuals. In the United States, serogroup B is responsible for 65% of infant disease. In contrast, disease in unvaccinated adolescents is principally due to serogroups C and Y, and disease in the elderly is due to serogroup Y.[54] Disease caused by serogroup W-135 is infrequent and, like disease in serogroup Y, has been associated with meningococcal pneumonia.[199,234] The incidence of serogroup C and serogroup Y disease has increased in the United States over the past few years, associated with antigenic shifts involving outer membrane protein genes.[107] Outbreaks in the United States are typically due to serogroup C, although there have been a few notable outbreaks of serogroup B disease in recent years (see Outbreaks section).[90] Meningococcal disease in the United States peaks during the months of November through March.[199] The highest attack rate is seen in February, and the lowest attack rate occurs in September.

The risk for meningococcal disease is inversely related to age, with the highest rates of disease occurring in children younger than 1 year.[47] Between 2006 and 2012, the estimated annual incidence of meningococcal disease in infants was 3.30 cases per 100,000 infants.[145] However, in epidemics an age shift occurs, with older children, adolescents, and young adults more often affected.[39] A progressive increase in the development of protective antibodies against meningococci occurs between the ages of 2 and 12 years. In general, the development of bactericidal antibodies to meningococci increases in children at a rate of about 5% per year.[93] Neonates usually are protected if the mother has antimeningococcal antibody by passive in utero immunoglobulin (Ig) G transfer.

International Epidemiology

Reduction in invasive serogroup C disease has been observed in several European countries, including the United Kingdom and Italy, after introduction of a conjugate serogroup C vaccine in the 1990s and 2000s.[90,151,208] Overall in Europe, serogroup B is now responsible for the majority of cases of invasive disease, accounting for an estimated 60% to 72% of cases.[90] In the United Kingdom, it was estimated that serogroup B caused 85% of cases of meningococcal disease prior to the introduction of MenB vaccine.[151] Other changes include an increase in disease due to serogroup Y observed in Northern European countries.[90]

As was the case in Europe, Australia has also experienced a reduction in the number of cases due to serogroup C resulting from vaccination efforts.[90] Serogroup B now accounts for nearly three-quarters of invasive disease cases in the continent.[171]

In contrast, New Zealand has controlled an epidemic of serogroup B disease that began in 1996. At the peak of the epidemic in the early 2000s, the average incidence was 9.7 cases per 100,000 individuals. A tailor-made MenB vaccine that was introduced in 2004 subsequently controlled the epidemic. By 2013, the incidence of invasive disease due to serogroup B in New Zealand was down to 0.67 cases per 100,000 individuals.[208]

In developing countries, the incidence rate of invasive meningococcal disease is many times higher than in the United States (10 to 25 per 100,000 inhabitants per year).[97] Historically, the highest rate of meningococcal disease was found in a multicountry belt across sub-Saharan Africa, termed the *meningitis belt,* that had long been afflicted with endemic and epidemic serogroup A disease. Epidemics occurred in the meningitis belt each year, affecting thousands of individuals, typically during the dry season and decreasing once the rainy season started.[177,184] Every 7 to 12 years, explosive outbreaks of disease occurred, causing extensive morbidity and mortality. The World Health Organization defines a meningococcal epidemic as more than 100 cases per 100,000 inhabitants per year, but in African epidemics the incidence could reach as high as 1000 per 100,000 inhabitants per year.[118] Spread of clonal strains of serogroup A meningococcus may be a factor in Africa's unusually high rate of epidemic disease. Clonal strains can migrate transcontinentally and cause epidemics, such as the clonal serogroup A meningococcus, electrophoretic type III-1 (ET III-1) that caused epidemics in China, Nepal, Saudi Arabia, Chad, and Kenya in the 1980s.[156,158,177]

The epidemiology of meningococcal disease in Africa has been greatly impacted by the introduction of a conjugate meningococcal A vaccine (MenAfriVac) in 2010.[90] In 2009, the year prior to MenAfriVac introduction, 14 African countries implemented enhanced surveillance during the epidemic season and reported 88,199 suspected cases, including 5352 deaths, the largest number since a 1996 epidemic. However, the epidemiology has vastly changed since 2010. Mass vaccination campaigns have led to a dramatic drop in the incidence of meningococcal disease cases.[171] Burkina Faso is one exemplary country were disease incidence fell by 99.8% after 94% vaccine coverage was achieved.[54] Similarly dramatic changes have occurred in Chad after mass vaccination.[88]

Since the introduction of MenAfriVac, serogroup W has emerged as the predominant cause of meningococcal disease in the meningitis belt.[171] Additionally in Africa the incidence of disease due to serogroup X has been increasing, even prior to the introduction of MenAfriVac.[90] MenX was responsible for more than half of the fatalities from meningococcal meningitis in Burkina Faso in 2010.[185,243] As there is no licensed vaccine for serogroup X, this poses a real threat to disease control in this region of the world.

International outbreaks of *N. meningitidis* infections occurred in 1987 and 2000 and were associated with Muslims making the annual pilgrimage to Mecca. The disease spread to persons of all nationalities represented, some of whom returned home before becoming ill.[158,181] In some cases, close contacts of travelers were infected. Several cases in US citizens were attributed to the outbreaks. The 1987 outbreak was linked to serogroup A, and the 2000 outbreak was due to serogroup W-135.[8,158,181] Saudi Arabia now requires meningococcal vaccine for travelers entering the country to participate in the annual pilgrimage to Mecca.[129] Quadrivalent meningococcal vaccines should be used for travel to these areas given the need to protect against serogroups A and W.[4]

Serogroup W has emerged in other regions, including the southern cone of South America. In Argentina and Chile, serogroup W was responsible for 0% to 2% of cases of invasive disease in 2000, but by 2010 accounted for 50% to 55% of invasive cases.[208] In Chile in 2012, serogroup W replaced serogroup B as the predominant cause of invasive meningococcal disease.[134] Similarly, England experienced the emergence of serogroup W, which led to incorporation of the quadrivalent conjugate vaccine for adolescents in the national program.[134]

COLONIZATION AND CARRIAGE

The epidemiology of meningococcal disease was defined elegantly in a series of observations in New Jersey military recruits. An inverse correlation was noted between the age-related incidence of meningococcal disease in the United States and the prevalence of serum bactericidal activity against three pathogenic strains of *N. meningitidis*.[93,94] Investigators prospectively studied all incoming recruits to Fort Dix and demonstrated that recruits who lacked bactericidal activity to case strains had a 38% attack rate if they were exposed and acquired a pathogenic meningococcus strain.[93] Usually nasopharyngeal carriage was an immunizing process. Carriage induced the formation of protective antibodies against homologous strains but also produced cross-reacting antibodies to heterologous strains of pathogenic meningococci. Antibody production typically was seen within 2 weeks of acquisition of carriage.[93,94]

In addition to nasopharyngeal carriage, other processes may contribute to meningococcal antibody formation. Certain strains of cross-reacting bacteria, such as *Escherichia coli* and *Bacillus*, produce capsular polysaccharides that immunologically are identical to the capsules of meningococci serogroups A, B, and C. This is a potential immunizing source against invasive meningococcal disease in the general population.[93,123,229]

Nasopharyngeal carriage of *N. meningitidis* is lowest in infants and children and highest in adolescents and young adults. Overall, 1 in 10 individuals in industrialized countries carry *N. meningitidis*, but the range varies from about 2% in young children to as high as 25% to 32% in adolescents and young adults.[54] One study determined that 2.4% of asymptomatic infants and children had a positive nasopharyngeal culture for *N. meningitidis* during a nonepidemic period.[150] A study of 1500 Norwegians found the carriage rate in persons 20 to 24 years of age was 32.7% and in individuals beyond 25 years of age was 10%.[38] Other investigators have shown that approximately 20% of children harbor meningococcal species in their nasopharynx, but the majority of these isolates are atypical, nontypeable strains, which ferment lactose in addition to glucose and maltose.[93,94]

Nasopharyngeal meningococcal carriage in household contacts of persons with documented meningococcal disease is about 10%.[153,169,191] Several studies demonstrated that the carriage rate increases if infants or children are in the home.[124,169] In one outbreak of serogroup C meningococcal disease, the carriage rates were 37.8% in households with a case in an infant, 17.5% in households with a case in a child, and 6.9% in households with disease in an adult.[123]

Nasopharyngeal carriage is common after household contact with an index case, and colonization can persist for weeks to months. Without chemoprophylaxis, up to 35% of contacts become colonized by the eighth week. The median duration of carriage is 9 months.[150] However, in nearly 40% of individuals, it may exceed 16 months.[96] An association between smoking and increased rate of meningococcal carriage has been demonstrated.[209,215]

RISK FACTORS FOR INVASIVE DISEASE

The factors responsible for converting nasopharyngeal colonization to invasive disease have not been firmly established. Many people who subsequently develop invasive disease are colonized shortly before the illness begins, usually within 2 weeks of colonization.[35] Likely these individuals lack bactericidal antibody and do not develop protective antibody after acquisition of the pathogenic strain. Some sequence types, such as ST-11, have the propensity to cause invasive disease, whereas others are more likely to be associated with asymptomatic carriage.[35,90] Other risk factors associated with invasive disease include young age, crowding (e.g., military barracks and college dormitories),[9,31,40] lower socioeconomic class,[198] concurrent upper respiratory tract infections,[157,245] intimate kissing with multiple partners,[221] specific immune deficiencies (i.e., properdin or terminal complement),[81] functional or anatomic asplenia,[85] and active or passive smoking, presumably due to its effects on mucosal immunity.[83,90,209] Passive smoke has been implicated to increase the risk for meningococcal disease in children younger than 5 years by 7.5 times that of the general population.

Speculation as to the role of other upper respiratory tract pathogens in meningococcal disease prompted several observations. It was noted that the peak incidence of meningococcal infection mirrors the peaks of agents such as influenza and *Mycoplasma*. Several studies have shown an association between colonization or infection with respiratory tract viruses or *Mycoplasma* and the increased risk for development of meningococcal disease.[36,113,157,204] Simultaneous outbreaks of meningococcal and influenza or echovirus infections have been documented.[112,141,245] In addition, one study suggested that the incidence of meningococcal disease and the resultant morbidity and mortality increased in the 5 weeks after influenza-like syndromes.[157] It has been postulated that viral pathogens may temporarily affect the immune response and facilitate meningococcal disease. It is also possible that disruption of the normal respiratory epithelium occurs with viral infection, and this increases the likelihood that colonizing meningococci might become invasive.[157] Preceding viral respiratory tract disease is not a prerequisite for the establishment of meningococcal carriage or disease. However, its occurrence may increase the risk for invasive meningococcal disease.

A variety of host genetic factors also may influence susceptibility to invasive meningococcal disease, including deficiencies of components of the immune system (complement, properdin, and immunoglobulins) and single nucleotide polymorphisms (SNPs).[90] Individuals with complement component deficiencies (C3, properdin, Factor D, Factor H, or C5-C9) have up to a 10,000-fold increased risk for meningococcal disease.[55,81] This usually is an inherited defect, and a history of other members of the family with meningococcal disease or repeated meningococcal infections may exist. Complement factor H is a complement-related protein, and certain polymorphisms in the complement factor H gene have been associated with an increased susceptibility to meningococcal disease.[63,103] Acquired complement deficiencies associated with diseases such as systemic lupus erythematosus, nephrotic syndrome, and chronic liver disease also are associated with increased risk for meningococcal disease.[137] A Russian study found the incidence of complement deficiency in first episodes of meningococcal disease to be about 1%.[179] In Italy, the prevalence of complement deficiency in patients with meningococcal meningitis was 17%.[61] The decision of whom to screen for complement deficiency should be partly based on the prevalence of meningococcal disease in a given country. In countries where the incidence of meningococcal disease is high, complement deficiency is less likely to be found. In countries such as the United States, where the incidence is relatively low, complement screening should be considered because it has implications for family members who can be tested, immunized, and educated regarding their increased risk for meningococcal disease.

The chance of finding a complement or alternative pathway (properdin) deficiency substantially increases in patients with recurrent meningococcal disease or with uncommon serogroups. The prevalence of complement or properdin deficiency in a patient with infection by an unusual serogroup was found to range from 31% to 50%.[82,165] Therefore screening all individuals with unusual serogroups is reasonable. CH_{50} is a generally available test and will screen for combined activity of C1 to C9. If complement deficiency is found, the individual should receive meningococcal vaccines as recommended for high-risk individuals. In addition, family members should be screened for complement deficiency and should be educated about the disease.

Some investigators demonstrated that although persons with complement deficiency are more at risk for meningococcal disease, the disease they get often is mild. Meningococcal infection activates the complement system, and lipooligosaccharide present in the bacterium's outer membrane is probably responsible for the activation. In fatal cases, intense activation has continued until the time of death.[29] The case-fatality rate in complement-deficient individuals is about 3%.[200] It is thought that complement-deficient individuals are unable to maintain the high-level complement pathway activation and therefore have less severe disease.

Properdin deficiency, which impairs activation of the alternative complement pathway, is X-linked and has been associated with fulminant meningococcal disease.[67,82] The case-fatality rate in one kindred was 75%.[22] Screening of individuals with exceptionally fulminant disease or individuals who have a family history of meningococcal infections should be considered. AP_{50} will screen for properdin deficiency in the alternative complement pathway.

SNPs can influence progression to or protection from meningococcal disease. Variants in mannose-binding lectin (MBL), Toll-like receptors (TLR) 2 and 4, and nucleotide oligomerization domain (NOD) 2 have all been associated with progression to meningococcal disease.[90] MBL is a pattern recognition receptor and a component of the innate immune system. Patients with meningococcal disease during childhood have a significantly increased incidence of structural mutations in the genes coding for MBL, leading to deficient MBL function in contrast to that in healthy age-matched controls.[78] Similarly human TLR4 mutations are associated with susceptibility to invasive meningococcal disease in infancy.[77] In one study, a TLR4 SNP was associated with mortality, skin grafting, and limb loss.[90] In contrast, SNPs of TLR9 have been shown to be protective of invasive meningococcal infections.[90]

PATHOLOGY AND PATHOGENESIS

The mechanisms by which meningococci invade humans are only partially understood. We do know that encapsulated, typeable meningococci are virulent, whereas nonencapsulated strains are relatively nonpathogenic. The presence of a polysaccharide capsule enhances invasiveness by resisting opsonization and subsequent phagocytosis. Even among encapsulated strains, differences in virulence between case and carrier strains of *N. meningitidis* have been demonstrated in an animal model.[111]

The human nasopharynx is the only natural reservoir of *N. meningitidis*.[212] Once pathogenic meningococci have colonized the respiratory tract of susceptible persons, either the organisms become invasive or the individual develops antibody to the organism, conferring immunity. Meningococci adhere to nonciliated, columnar epithelial cells in the nasopharynx via pili. Binding induces endocytosis of the organism into the epithelial cell, and the bacteria may penetrate the epithelial barrier via phagocytotic vacuoles.[211] If antibody is insufficient and invasion occurs, the individual may become bacteremic. Occasionally unsuspected meningococcal bacteremia has been detected on blood culture and spontaneously cleared on a follow-up culture without antibiotics.[215] However, in most cases, this does not occur and the individual becomes progressively sicker. Bacteria in the blood may seed the meninges and cause meningitis.

Meningococci are gram-negative organisms, and lipooligosaccharide is a major component of the bacterial cell membrane. Meningococci release blebs from their surfaces that contain an outer membrane laden with lipooligosaccharide. Lipooligosaccharide is a potent endotoxin and concentrations of it correlate with severity of disease.[27–29] Lipooligosaccharide induces release of a host of inflammatory and antiinflammatory mediators whose concentrations are also correlated with severity of disease: tumor necrosis factor-α (TNF-α), γ-interferon, interleukin-1 (IL-1), IL-6, IL-8, IL-10, and IL-1 receptor antagonist.[91,138,225,226,236] TNF-α downregulates thrombomodulin expression on endothelial cells, leading to decreased activity of proteins S and C.[56,163] Like TNF-α, many of the mediators directly or indirectly contribute to the formation of a procoagulant state, which results in the formation of microthrombi that are characteristically found in the skin, digits, extremities, and organs. The disseminated intravascular coagulation commonly seen in meningococcemia is believed to be a consequence of activation of the coagulation system by endotoxin.[195] Experimental animal work suggests a synergistic effect of meningococcal endotoxin and materials egested from leukocytes containing meningococci in the initiation of disseminated intravascular coagulation.[69]

Cytokines play an important role in the development of shock frequently seen in meningococcemia. Cytokine release causes neutrophil activation and upregulation of adhesion molecules that may promote endothelial damage and capillary leak.[75] Vasodilation also may occur secondary to increased production of nitric oxide by endothelial cells.[155] Compensatory vasoconstriction of splanchnic, skin, and renal vessels may subsequently not suffice to maintain adequate blood pressure. Endotoxin-related or cytokine-mediated cardiac dysfunction also may contribute to development of heart failure and hypotension.[172] Profound capillary leak in the pulmonary bed may lead to the development of acute respiratory distress syndrome (ARDS). The pathologic purpuric lesions seen in fulminant meningococcal disease are similar to those that the generalized Shwartzman reaction induces in rabbits by endotoxin. Pathologically these lesions show evidence of microthrombi in the small dermal vessels, endothelial damage, and hemorrhage. Inflammatory vasculitis is mediated by upregulation of endothelial adhesion molecules, neutrophil activation, and effects of cytokines and bacterial endotoxin.[11,60,110] Circulating concentrations of endotoxin in patients with meningococcemia may be 50 to 100 times that of other gram-negative infections.[180] In addition, meningococcal endotoxin is more potent than endotoxin from enteric bacilli.[64]

A pathologic study of 200 fatal meningococcal infections illustrates the ability of the meningococcus to affect virtually any organ, either directly or indirectly.[105] Approximately 40% of patients in this study had both meningococcemia and meningitis. Except for adults with meningitis, the average survival time for all cases was 72 hours or less. The major organ systems involved at autopsy in these 200 cases were heart, central nervous system (CNS), skin, mucous and serous membranes, and adrenals. Myocarditis occurred in 78% of cases. Cutaneous hemorrhages occurred in 69% of the fatal infections and ranged from isolated petechiae to diffuse purpura. Acute meningitis was noted at autopsy in 68%, with brain abscesses noted in two patients. In almost half of the cases with acute meningococcemia, *N. meningitidis* was isolated from otherwise normal cerebrospinal fluid (CSF). Adrenal hemorrhage and necrosis were found in 48% of autopsy cases. Diffuse adrenal hemorrhage occurred in approximately 50% of adult cases and in more than 80% of pediatric cases. Focal areas of inflammation and petechial hemorrhage were seen in many other tissues, including the synovium, skeletal muscle, and the tracheobronchial tree. An association was seen between the pathologic findings and the infecting serogroup of *N. meningitidis*. Serogroup A infections most frequently were associated with encephalitis; serogroups B and C infections were associated with necrotizing myocarditis.

CLINICAL MANIFESTATIONS AND DIFFERENTIAL DIAGNOSIS

The spectrum of disease caused by *N. meningitidis* ranges from asymptomatic transient bacteremia, which clears spontaneously, to fulminant sepsis resulting in death only a few hours from symptom onset.[215] In 2006, Kaplan and colleagues (the US Multicenter Meningococcal Surveillance Study Group)[122] reviewed 159 episodes of invasive meningococcal disease seen at 10 children's hospitals in the United States between January 2001 and March 2005. Meningitis was the most common manifestation of disease seen in 70% of cases. In this study, 27% of children had bacteremia alone and 4.4% had fulminant disease. Hypotension was present in 10% and thrombocytopenia in 6% on admission. The overall mortality rate was 8% and was significantly greater in children older than 10 years compared to those younger than 11 years ($P < .01$).

Meningococcemia and Meningitis

Serious or invasive disease usually presents in one of two ways: meningococcemia or meningitis (either with or without meningococcemia). It is important to consider other etiologies in the differential diagnosis of meningococcemia (Box 88.1).

The signs and symptoms of meningococcemia are variable. Early on, evidence of an upper respiratory tract infection may be seen, including coryza, pharyngitis, tonsillitis, and laryngitis. Patients generally are febrile, with complaints of headache, lethargy, and vomiting. Severe myalgias with muscle tenderness and joint pain also may be the presenting symptom.[114] The typical patient with meningococcemia has a short history of upper respiratory tract symptoms, fever, and a hemorrhagic rash. The patient often develops signs of severe circulatory collapse. It is not unusual for purpura and shock to develop within hours of the first onset of symptoms.

The skin manifestations of meningococcemia range from diffuse mottling to extensive purpuric lesions (Figs. 88.1 and 88.2). Unfortunately some variation exists in the type of rash seen. Petechiae or purpura are present in 50% to 60% of patients.[124,242] In a multicenter study of invasive disease in children, 55% of patients had petechiae and 38% had purpura.[122] Maculopapular rash alone is reported in 10% to 13% of patients.[152,242] This makes differentiation from a viral exanthem particularly difficult. A pink macular rash resembling early varicella is another variant sometimes seen in children with meningococcemia; these lesions often are tender. They may occur in crops, as do the petechiae, and are seen most frequently on the trunk and extremities.[71,109] Furthermore 20% to 30% of children may have no rash at presentation.[242]

The finding of petechiae or purpura in a febrile child should increase the index of suspicion for meningococcemia or other serious disease (e.g., infectious, neoplastic, immunologic). Acral distribution of a rash is particularly worrisome for meningococcemia or another infectious vasculitic process. In two studies involving more than 200 patients with fever and petechiae (not purpura), 8.0% to 20.2% had invasive bacterial disease.[228,242] Seven to 10% of the total group had infections

BOX 88.1 Differential Diagnosis Meningococcemia

Infectious

- Rocky Mountain spotted fever
- Ehrlichiosis
- Streptococcal *pneumoniae* sepsis
- *Haemophilus influenzae* type b sepsis
- Group A streptococcus sepsis
- *Staphylococcus aureus* sepsis
- Other bacterial sepsis with disseminated intravascular coagulation (i.e., enteric gram-negative organisms)
- Infective endocarditis
- Gonococcemia
- Rat bite fever
- Typhus
- Secondary syphilis

Noninfectious

- Henoch-Schönlein purpura
- Acute hemorrhagic edema of infancy
- Idiopathic thrombocytopenic purpura
- Collagen vascular disease
- Neoplastic processes

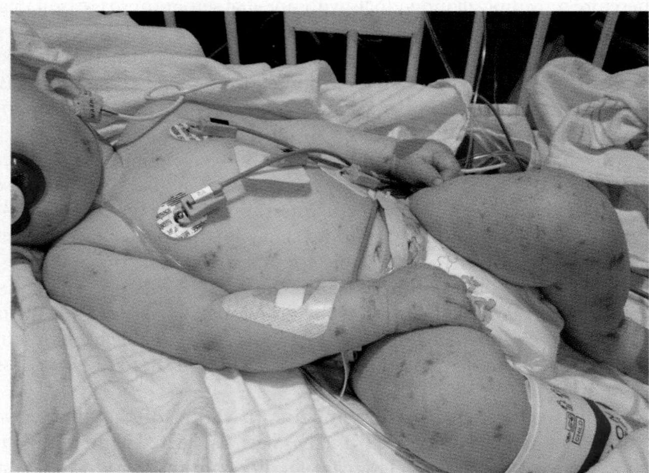

FIG. 88.1 Purpuric lesions are seen on the trunk and extremities of a young child with meningococcemia.

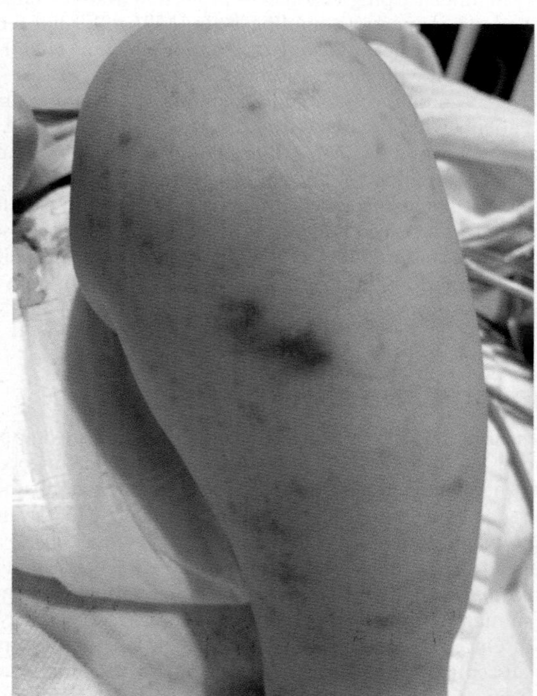

FIG. 88.2 Close-up of leg lesions in the child shown in Fig. 88.1.

caused by *N. meningitidis*. Therefore it seems reasonable to obtain blood cultures on most febrile patients with petechiae. Lumbar puncture should be performed if clinically indicated or if the blood culture ultimately is positive. Antibiotic therapy should include coverage for meningococcus.

Wong and colleagues[242] reviewed 100 cases of meningococcal infections in children seen at their institution between 1985 and 1988. Fifty-five percent of patients had meningitis. Leukopenia (white blood cell count <5000/mm^3) was present in 21%, and thrombocytopenia was noted in 14%. Eleven percent of those with culture-positive meningitis had no CSF abnormalities on chemistries or examination. Other laboratory abnormalities seen in patients with sepsis or shock include abnormal coagulation panels (disseminated intravascular coagulation), acidosis, and abnormal liver function studies.

Purpura is noted in 16% to 24% of patients.[182,242] When purpura is extensive and accompanied by shock, it is referred to as *purpura fulminans*. Acquired protein S and C deficiencies have been described in some patients with purpura fulminans.[182,183] One study showed a mortality rate of 50% in patients who developed purpura. Progressive purpura was accompanied by declining protein C levels, and the level of protein C was related inversely to the clinical severity of disease.[182]

Patients with meningitis often are febrile, with headache, vomiting, irritability, stiff neck, and sometimes seizures. A history of lethargy may be present, or the patient may be obtunded. In neonates, physical findings of meningismus, such as Kernig and Brudzinski signs, often are absent. The anterior fontanelle, if open, may be full and tense.

Hyponatremia is seen in some patients with meningitis. Inappropriate secretion of antidiuretic hormone is the mechanism. In a study of 43 children with meningococcal meningitis, 7% developed syndrome of inappropriate secretion of antidiuretic hormone.[76]

The most common neurologic complications of meningitis are cerebral edema, cranial nerve palsies (especially hearing loss), subdural effusions or empyemas, cortical vein thrombosis, cerebral infarctions, and hydrocephalus (see section on Prognosis, Morbidity, and Mortality).

Cerebral edema and cranial nerve palsies may be seen at presentation or develop shortly thereafter. Sixth- or third-nerve palsies are suggestive of increased intracranial pressure and impending herniation, respectively. The development of either of these signs indicates an urgent intracranial process. Auditory testing should be performed on all patients with meningitis after recovery.

Subdural effusions or empyemas should be considered in patients with fever persisting after 8 days of therapy, vomiting, or development of signs of increased intracranial pressure after the initial few days of treatment. Drainage is recommended only if the effusions are infected (empyemas) or are large enough to produce either focal neurologic signs or increased intracranial pressure.[170]

Vascular thrombosis and cerebral infarction can be due to arterial or venous thrombosis. Venous thrombosis is more common and generally is not seen before the second week. Hemorrhagic infarction of the brain may occur then. Cerebral infarction also may be seen in patients without arterial or venous thrombosis who are in shock with prolonged hypotension and cerebral ischemia. Cerebral infarction in these individuals is an early event.

Hydrocephalus occurs most frequently in young children and those with delayed diagnosis or severe disease. It tends to present 3 to 4 weeks after the onset of illness. Inflammation, with collagen deposition and proliferation of fibroblasts in the meninges, produces an obstruction to the flow of CSF. Progressive increase in head circumference should alert the clinicians to the possibility of hydrocephalus.[170] Imaging (i.e., computed tomography or magnetic resonance imaging) studies are diagnostic.

Neonatal meningococcemia and meningitis are uncommon but have been reported. In one report, a 2-week-old infant died after a brief febrile illness with both CSF and blood cultures positive for meningococcus. Maternal endocervical colonization was documented. In addition, the mother's pharyngeal culture grew *N. meningitidis*.[120] If endocervical colonization by *N. meningitidis* is found prenatally, treatment with antibiotics should be considered in an attempt to eradicate colonization before delivery or intrapartum antibiotics should be given. Ceftriaxone would seem to be a reasonable choice. Rifampin and ciprofloxacin are not advocated for use during pregnancy.

Chronic Meningococcemia

Chronic meningococcemia, first described in 1902, is defined as meningococcal septicemia without meningeal symptoms in which fever has persisted for at least a week before any antibiotic therapy.[73,168] Benoit[17] reviewed 148 cases of chronic meningococcemia in the United States in 1963 in patients ranging in age from 3 months to 62 years. The major symptoms included fever and chills (present in 100% of patients), skin rash (93.2%), arthralgias (70.3%), and headache (61.5%). The patients generally were not in a toxic state and were in good health before becoming infected. The mean duration of illness before diagnosis was 6 to 8 weeks (range, 1 to 40 weeks). Symptoms tended to be intermittent; the rash often appeared in association with fever and then disappeared over the next several days. Bacteremia also was intermittent in some patients. In the Benoit study, on average, five blood cultures were obtained before meningococci were isolated. However, after a blood culture yielded the organism, most subsequent cultures were positive. In children, some investigators report that it is common to isolate the organism in the first blood culture.[139] Arthralgias also tended to be intermittent in nature.

In Benoit's series,[17] almost 40% of the patients with chronic meningococcemia developed localizing complications. The meninges were the most common site of localization; meningitis developed in 15.5% of patients. Other localized infections included carditis, nephritis, epididymitis, conjunctivitis, iritis, and retinitis. In only one instance was an organism recovered from a joint. The average duration of meningococcemia in those patients with complications was 10.2 weeks, in contrast to 4 to 8 weeks in patients without any localization.

The diagnosis is established by identifying the organism in blood cultures. Antibiotic therapy results in prompt defervescence and dramatic recovery.

The pathophysiologic mechanisms permitting chronic meningococcemia remain unclear. No evidence suggests that the organisms are less virulent than other meningococci; thus, a defect in host immunity has been suggested. A hypersensitivity basis for this disease has been postulated, and it is theorized that the skin changes and arthritis may be secondary to antigen-antibody complexes.[169] In contrast to acute meningococcemia, bacteria are almost never found by biopsy or culture of skin lesions. The histologic findings of the skin lesions are distinct from those seen in skin lesions of patients with acute meningococcemia.[17,105,169]

Meningococcal Pneumonia

Meningococcal pneumonia occurs in conjunction with meningococcemia or meningitis in 8% to 15% of cases.[128] However, meningococcus also can play a role as a primary respiratory pathogen.

Primary meningococcal pneumonia, once considered a rare disease, now is recognized as the most common form of meningococcal disease in certain military recruit populations and has been reported to cause 4.5% of all bacterial pneumonias in a general hospital population.[128,142]

Patients with preceding viral pneumonias are at risk for meningococcal pneumonia; more than 100 cases of meningococcal pneumonia occurred during the influenza pandemic of 1918 and 1919. In addition to disease among military recruits, nosocomial acquisition of meningococcal pneumonia in hospitalized patients has been reported.[53]

The diagnosis of meningococcal pneumonia is difficult because isolation of the organism from the sputum does not distinguish a meningococcal carrier from an individual with meningococcal pneumonia. In addition, routine sputum cultures do not include media selective for meningococcus. Blood cultures are positive in only 15% of individuals.[128]

Koppes and associates[128] reported on 68 cases of meningococcal pneumonia; diagnostic criteria included a compatible clinical syndrome and isolation of *N. meningitidis* from pleural fluid or blood.[128] All 68 meningococcal pneumonia cases were serogroup Y; during the same period, 10 cases of meningococcemia and 6 cases of meningitis were caused by serogroup Y. The high ratio of pneumonia to meningitis in this study suggests that serogroup Y organisms may be more likely to cause pneumonia than other serogroups, which has been substantiated by other investigators.[186,198] Pneumonia caused by serogroup B or C meningococci has been reported, usually in association with meningococcemia or meningitis.[241]

Primary meningococcal pneumonia usually is associated with a gradual onset of symptoms. Rales and fever are found in most patients, and 80% have pharyngitis. The radiograph often shows involvement of lower lobes with patchy alveolar infiltrates. More than one lobe is involved in 40% of cases. Twenty-five percent have pleural effusions. Petechiae, purpura, or shock were not present in any of the patients with pneumonia reported by Koppes and colleagues.[128]

The pathogenesis of this disease is thought to be pulmonary infection via droplet inhalation. The epidemiologic importance of meningococcal pneumonia was emphasized in a report from the CDC discussing nosocomial transmission of serogroup Y *N. meningitidis* in oncology patients.[53] The index case had meningococcal pneumonia. One other patient in an adjacent room developed meningococcal bacteremia; in three additional patients, serogroup Y *N. meningitidis* was isolated from nasopharyngeal cultures. Airborne dissemination seemed to be the mode of transmission. Respiratory isolation for a patient with suspected meningococcal pneumonia is indicated.

Penicillin therapy of penicillin-sensitive meningococcal pneumonia results in a prompt clinical response. Of the patients reported by Koppes and colleagues,[128] 93% were afebrile after 3 days of therapy. Third-generation cephalosporins, such as ceftriaxone, may be the current drugs of choice pending definitive identification.

Other Meningococcal Syndromes

Conjunctivitis

Primary meningococcal conjunctivitis is indistinguishable clinically from acute bacterial conjunctivitis caused by other organisms. Usually it presents in children as the acute onset of unilateral purulent conjunctivitis.[15] It has been reported in individuals from 2 days of age to adulthood.[8] Gram stain of the purulent material typically shows gram-negative diplococci that may sometimes be confused with gonococcal organisms. Barquet and colleagues[16] showed that 44% of the isolates were serogroup B meningococci.

The complications of primary meningococcal conjunctivitis reported by Barquet and colleagues[16] included sepsis or meningitis in approximately 18% of patients. The symptoms of systemic meningococcal disease occurred 3 to 96 hours after the onset of the conjunctivitis (mean, 41 hours). Patients treated only with topical therapy at the time of conjunctivitis were 19 times more likely to develop systemic disease than were patients treated with systemic therapy ($P = .001$). Ocular complications occurred in 15.5% of patients and included corneal ulcers (10.7%), keratitis, hemorrhage, and iritis.

Pharyngitis

The diagnosis of meningococcal pharyngitis is difficult because, like group A β-hemolytic streptococci, the isolation of meningococcus from the pharynx does not establish that this organism is the etiologic agent. In fact, most individuals who harbor meningococci in their nasopharynges are asymptomatic carriers. However, Banks[13] noted overt nasopharyngitis in one third of patients with meningococcal sepsis or meningitis. Pizzi,[178] describing a severe epidemic of meningococcal meningitis, noted that individuals with sore throats often had a pure culture of meningococci.[180] Olcen and associates[169] cultured family members of 21 consecutive cases of meningococcal disease and found that 61% of family members with sore throat or other upper respiratory tract symptoms were meningococcal carriers, in contrast to 14% of asymptomatic family members.[169]

On occasion, culture samples are obtained in individuals in the community with symptomatic pharyngitis, and the laboratory reports growth of *N. meningitidis*. If the patient is febrile but otherwise appears well, we recommend a blood culture and intramuscular or intravenous ceftriaxone. If the blood culture result is negative, the patient should be treated with an antibiotic. If the patient is afebrile and asymptomatic at the time the culture results are obtained, we recommend eradication of the organism using one of the antibiotics recommended for chemoprophylaxis (see discussion of chemoprophylaxis).

Arthritis

Meningococcal arthritis occurs primarily in adults. The overall incidence, as a complication of bacteremia, is approximately 2% to 14%.[98,242] Meningococcal arthritis has two forms. The first is seen within the first few days of treatment and is characterized by severe arthralgias and few objective signs of joint inflammation. It is suggested that the pathogenesis of this arthritis is an inflammatory response to viable organisms that have seeded the synovium during the initial bacteremia. The second, more common form appears to be an immune complex phenomenon. It usually is noted 3 to 7 days after the recognition of meningococcemia, often at a time when the patient appears to be improving from the meningitis or sepsis. The knee, wrist, elbow, and ankle joints are involved most commonly.[98]

In both forms, the arthritis usually is monoarticular or oligoarticular with an effusion, with minimal pain, erythema, and limitation of motion. It is very unusual to culture organisms from the effusion; joint fluid culture yields meningococci in fewer than 10% of cases. The exception to this is a child with suppurative arthritis on initial presentation. In one study, 8% of patients with meningococcal infections had arthritis; 75% had positive culture results when cultures were obtained before receiving antibiotics.[241,242]

Synovial fluid leukocyte counts vary widely, but counts greater than 100,000/mm^3 have been reported.[176] The appearance of arthritis often is accompanied by a rise in temperature; in 7 of 47 patients with arthritis, a characteristic skin lesion appeared at the same time.[99] These lesions began as skin hyperpigmentation but progressed to vesiculation and ulceration; biopsies showed vasculitis. Additional evidence of concurrent vasculitis is suggested by reports of patients developing episcleritis and mild proteinuria simultaneously with arthritis.[99]

On histologic examination, the synovium is infiltrated with mononuclear cells that contain IgM, C3, and meningococcal antigen.[97] This strongly suggests an immune complex–mediated disease. No specific therapy is indicated, and the arthritis resolves spontaneously. Controversy exists regarding the role of intermittent closed drainage of the joint space.[23] Permanent joint deformity is uncommon in this disease, occurring in approximately 10% of cases.[203] Edwards and Baker[74] reported immune-mediated complications of meningococcal disease in 10% of the 86 children followed prospectively. More than 83% were serogroup B, although late-onset arthritis and vasculitis also have been reported with disease due to serogroups A and C.

Permanent joint damage is unusual, occurring in about 1.5% of patients with arthritis. Potential sequelae include ankylosis, decreased range of motion, and bone necrosis.[137]

Pericarditis and Myocarditis

Pericarditis as a complication of meningococcal disease occurs in 3% to 5% of cases, although one series reported a 19% incidence in 32 patients with meningococcal meningitis.[72,159] It generally occurs in patients with meningococcemia but has been reported as an isolated event without septicemia or meningitis.[108]

Pericarditis is presumed to be a late complication of meningococcal disease because clinical symptoms such as fever, dyspnea, or substernal chest pain (or even cardiac tamponade) usually do not appear until the fourth to the seventh day of illness. However, several investigators have noted early evidence of pericarditis based on electrocardiographic or radiographic data of patients examined at the time of hospital admission.

Because most symptomatic pericardial effusions develop late in the course of the illness, are serous, and are sterile, the pathophysiologic mechanism is presumed to be an immune complex reaction. Uncontrolled studies report the successful use of steroids in the treatment of this complication. However, one report documents pericarditis and the development of tamponade in a patient receiving steroids.[173] Although an immune complex phenomenon is the most likely scenario, *N. meningitidis* may cause as many as 20% of cases of purulent pericarditis.[35]

The clinical course of meningococcal pericarditis usually is benign, but pericardial compression requiring pericardiocentesis occurs.[175] Early relapses also have been reported, but these were self-limited. The development of constrictive pericarditis requiring pericardectomy has been reported.[173,205,235]

Myocarditis was noted at autopsy in 78% of patients with fatal meningococcal disease.[105] Myocarditis was noted most often in adults but was more severe when it occurred in children. Rosenblatt and colleagues[196] noted myocarditis at autopsy in 10 of 12 children with fatal meningococcal infection. On pathologic examination, these cases showed collections of inflammatory cells in the myocardial interstitium and focal extravasation of erythrocytes with acute vasculitis. Abscesses and endocarditis were not seen. Inflammation occasionally may involve the atrioventricular node and has been reported as a cause of sudden death in a patient recovering from meningococcal meningitis.[193]

Miscellaneous Meningococcal Infections

Several unusual syndromes have been reported, including primary meningococcal pericarditis,[228] mesenteric adenitis,[133] peritonitis,[133] and genitourinary infections.[79]

PROGNOSIS, MORBIDITY, AND MORTALITY

Various scoring systems have been devised in an attempt to predict prognosis in patients with meningococcal disease. Most prognostic scoring systems and clinical reviews agree that purpura fulminans and shock uniformly are poor prognostic signs. These scoring systems were reviewed in an article by Kirsch and colleagues.[127]

The Glasgow Meningococcal Septicaemia Prognostic Score (GMSPS) is a validated scoring system developed to clinically assess patients and facilitate admission of the most severely ill children to intensive care units.[206,218] This scoring system, which evaluates seven key items (hypotension, difference in skin-core temperature, coma, acute deterioration, absence of meningismus, progressive purpura, and base deficit) has been used by many to define entry criteria into clinical trials.

In a review of 100 cases of meningococcal disease at the Los Angeles Children's Hospital, five features were identified that correlated with poor prognosis: shock or seizures on presentation, hypothermia, total white blood cell count less than 5000/mm,[118] platelet count less than 100,000/mm^3, and development of purpura fulminans. The overall mortality in this series was 10%.[242]

Long-term complications can occur in 20% to nearly 60% of patients.[151] Survivors of meningitis can be left with neurologic and hearing impairment. In an Australian study, any neurologic impairment occurred in 8.5% of cases with CNS infection.[151] Neurologic sequelae are much more common in patients with meningitis, but complications such as cerebral infarction also can be seen in children with meningococcemia and shock.[169] In studies of adults with meningococcal meningitis, cognitive impairment was identified in 28% of patients, hearing impairment in 8% of patients, and cranial nerve palsies in 3% of patients.[35] In a United States multicenter study conducted from 2001 to 2005, hearing loss occurred in 12.5% of children with meningitis.[122]

Sequelae of meningococcemia are disfiguring and debilitating. In one study, skin necrosis occurred in 9.4% of children, and 2.4% required skin grafts.[122] In this study, 1% of children underwent amputations; one child lost all four limbs. However, limb amputation has been reported in as many as 20% of survivors, although incidence is likely influenced by geography.[90] Other consequences include renal failure.[90]

The overall mortality of invasive meningococcal disease in the United States is 7% to 19%.[122,166,197,213] Individuals with only meningitis have a lower case-fatality rate than those with bacteremia or an isolate from another source (2% vs. 12%).[197] Presumably this is a function of the virulence of the organism, ability of the immune system to contain the infection, or both. Case-fatality rates also differ by serogroup and are higher in W-135 disease (21%) than in serogroup C (14%), Y (9%), or B (6%).[197]

Evidence suggests a genetic component exists in host cytokine production that may be associated with severity of disease. Westendorp and associates[237] reported that families with low TNF production or high IL-10 production are at increased risk for fatal outcomes with meningococcal disease. Variants of proinflammatory host genes (TNF-α, IL-1) might be linked to severity of disease. Read and colleagues found that homozygosis of certain alleles at the IL-1 locus increased risk for death in individuals with meningococcal disease and suggested that IL-1 genotype may be associated with fatal outcomes.[190]

DIAGNOSIS

The gold standard for diagnosis is based on recovering the organism from blood, CSF, or skin lesions. Blood culture alone is positive in about 50% of patients who have not received antibiotics.[242] Rapid diagnosis can be made by Gram stain of CSF in patients with meningitis, which reveals characteristic gram-negative diplococci in approximately 90% of samples obtained before starting antibiotics.[35] However, caution should be exercised in relying solely on the Gram stain to determine the initial antibiotic regimen. Overdecolorized gram-positive cocci of *Streptococcus pneumoniae* on occasion have been confused with meningococci on Gram stain. Thus broad-spectrum antibiotic therapy should be initiated pending identification of the organism by culture.

In patients who have skin lesions, a rapid presumptive diagnosis of meningococcemia often can be made by needle aspiration and Gram stain of a skin lesion, which reveals gram-negative diplococci in 50% to 80% of patients with acute meningococcal infections.[35,227] Culturing the obtained aspirate increases the yield further. Skin lesion gram stain and culture may be useful in individuals pretreated with antibiotics as they have been shown to be positive up to 45 hours and 13 hours, respectively, after administration of antibiotics.[35] Correlation of the Gram stain with the clinical presentation is important because disseminated gonococcal infections also may present with skin lesions that yield gram-negative diplococci on Gram stain.

Latex agglutination has been used to detect circulating antigen in serum, CSF, and urine of patients with meningococcal disease.[238] Latex agglutinin tests using serum and urine are not recommended. Cross-reactions with certain *E. coli* K1 (cause of neonatal meningitis) or *Bacillus* strains may occur.

Polymerase chain reaction (PCR) may be very helpful in the diagnosis of patients who have partially treated meningococcemia or meningitis. Confirmation of the diagnosis impacts patient management, follow-up, and prompt institution of chemoprophylaxis to contacts. Once antibiotics have been given, the chances that a blood culture will be positive decreases to less than 5%.[37] CSF culture can be negative as early as 15 minutes after antibiotics and is expected to be negative when obtained 2 or more hours afterwards.[35] One study showed the sensitivity and specificity of PCR for *N. meningitidis* to be 91% in cerebrospinal fluid specimens. Treatment with antibiotics before the test did not decrease the test's sensitivity or specificity.[164] One report from the United Kingdom describes use of a multiplex PCR assay for the simultaneous detection of *N. meningitidis, H. influenzae,* and *S. pneumoniae* from clinical samples of CSF and whole blood. Corless and colleagues[58] found that the sensitivities for detection of the three organisms ranged from 88.4% to 91.8%, with 100% specificity. A 2012 article from China and Australia reported development of a multiplex PCR assay for detection of 12 meningococcal serogroups.[246] Commercially available assays such as this would greatly facilitate etiologic diagnosis in children with sepsis or meningitis. Currently meningococcal PCR is in use in the United Kingdom but is not routinely available in the United States. Investigators in the United Kingdom have utilized quantitative PCR of CSF in patients with culture-proved meningococcal disease. In their experience, the sensitivity of CSF PCR was 89% for detection of *N. meningitidis*. In addition, they noted that patients with serogroup B infection had extremely high quantities of bacteria within the CSF regardless of the peripheral blood bacterial quantitation.[62]

TREATMENT

The first antibiotics used for meningococcal infections were the sulfonamides, and their use lowered the death rate to 5% to 10%.[100] With the emergence of sulfa-resistant strains, penicillin was added to the regimen and is still recommended for susceptible meningococcal infections. In the late 1980s, reports began to appear of meningococci relatively resistant to penicillin. The mechanism of resistance is reduced binding affinity of penicillin-binding proteins, though resistance is not entirely explained by mutations in PBP2.[104] Relatively resistant strains have been reported in the United States, Canada, Europe, South Africa, Romania, and Croatia.[25,116,174,216,245]

In a United States multicenter descriptive study of invasive disease in children conducted between 2001 and 2005, only one penicillin-intermediate isolate was identified, and no penicillin-resistant isolates were found.[122] Later, in a United States study by Harcourt and colleagues, susceptibility testing was performed on isolates collected through the ABCs system and found that, overall, 10.3% of isolates in 2004, 2008, 2010, and 2011 were penicillin-intermediate.[104] The overall trend in the United States is concerning given that only 3% of isolates in 1997 were penicillin-intermediate compared to 16.7% in 2010.[104] Yet the clinical significance of intermediate resistance to penicillin is unknown, and the proportion of penicillin-intermediate isolates in fatal cases in the United States was low.[54,104]

In the study that tested ABC system isolates, 3 of 466 isolates tested between 2004 and 2010 were penicillin-resistant.[104] There were no resistant isolates in 2011. The three penicillin-resistant isolates were serogroup Y, which was also the serogroup most likely to have intermediate resistance to penicillin. Isolates that are absolutely resistant to penicillin (minimum inhibitory concentration >1.0 µg/mL) have also been documented from Spain and the United Kingdom.[174,216] These European strains had acquired a gonococcal plasmid encoding for the production of a β-lactamase.[216] Ceftriaxone-nonsusceptible strains have been reported from India.[149]

In 2009, ciprofloxacin-resistant isolates were identified from four unrelated patients with invasive meningococcal disease in three U.S. states. Three of the cases were infected with serogroup B meningococcus and one with serogroup Y meningococcus. Genetic studies suggested that the Y strain acquired resistance by a point mutation. However, the B strains may have acquired resistance through horizontal gene transfer from *N. lactamica,* a commensal organism carried in the nasopharynx.[244] Resistance to rifampin has also been reported but is sporadic.[104]

Prompt institution of antibiotic therapy in suspected meningococcal infections may be life saving. Children who present with fever and purpura should be considered to have meningococcemia until proved otherwise while recognizing that other pathogens or disease processes may present with fever and purpura. A purpura fulminans–like presentation also has rarely been described in infections due to *Staphylococcus aureus,*[131] group A streptococcus,[70] group B streptococcus, and overt sepsis with other organisms causing disseminated intravascular coagulation. Antibiotics should be administered as soon as possible. A systematic review of the effectiveness of antibiotics given before admission concluded that "the data are consistent with benefit when a substantial proportion of cases are treated."[101] If possible, blood cultures should be drawn before antibiotic administration, but specimen collection should not delay administration of antibiotics. A lumbar puncture can be performed in stable patients, but the procedure should not delay antibiotic administration. CSF obtained after antibiotic therapy may be sterile, but pleocytosis should be apparent and other diagnostic modalities such as PCR can be considered. Patients who are unstable or have significant coagulopathy should have the lumbar puncture deferred. Shortly after administration of bactericidal antibiotics, some patients have marked clinical deterioration, including hypotension and sometimes death. Rapid liberation of endotoxin (and resultant stimulation of cytokine release) from lysing organisms may be the cause of this phenomenon.[153]

The clinical presentation of *N. meningitidis* meningitis may be similar to that of meningitis caused by *S. pneumoniae* or *H. influenzae.* Empirical antibiotic therapy should therefore take into consideration the most likely pathogens. In children older than 1 month of age with meningitis, vancomycin and ceftriaxone is an appropriate regimen until a definitive diagnosis is made. Similarly, empirical therapy for children younger than 1 month of age includes ampicillin, with consideration given to the addition of vancomycin.[199]

The 2015 American Academy of Pediatrics Red Book states that, for cases in the United States, treatment can be narrowed to penicillin once *Neisseria meningitidis* is identified. However, continuation of ceftriaxone is recommended for travelers from areas where penicillin resistance has been reported, including Spain, Italy, and parts of Africa.[6] Some experts recommend susceptibility testing before narrowing to penicillin, and the previously described study that documented penicillin resistance in the United States supports the need to ascertain penicillin susceptibility prior to narrowing from empirical therapy. In the United States, large microbiology laboratories should be able to perform susceptibility testing. Susceptibility testing should especially be considered in circumstances in which resistance is clinically or epidemiologically suspected.

For penicillin-susceptible meningococcemia or meningitis, intravenous penicillin G 300,000 U/kg per day (maximum 12 million U/day) given in divided doses every 4 to 6 hours for 7 days, is effective. Third-generation cephalosporins, such as ceftriaxone 100 mg/kg per day intravenously in two divided doses, also are effective. The recommended treatment for patients with anaphylactic reactions to penicillin is chloramphenicol. Meropenem is a treatment option for those with severe allergies, although there is a small proportion of penicillin-allergic patients who may cross-react with the carbapenems.[5]

In confirmed cases of meningococcal disease, comparisons of penicillin G with ceftriaxone have shown ceftriaxone to be as efficacious. Necrotic skin lesions were seen more commonly in the penicillin group, but otherwise complication and mortality rates were equivalent.[222] Meningococcal disease has been treated successfully with ceftriaxone intravenously in both the 80 to 100 mg/kg per day in one daily dose and 100 mg/kg per day in two divided doses regimens.[222]

With all cases of meningococcal disease, eradicating colonization of the index case is important (see discussion of chemoprophylaxis). One dose of ceftriaxone effectively eradicates nasal carriage.

Steroid administration in patients with septic shock and meningococcemia is controversial, but several studies have reported adrenal insufficiency (or partial adrenal insufficiency) in 10.3% to 16.9% of severely ill children with meningococcemia.[24,65,66,192] For patients with Waterhouse-Friderichsen syndrome, treatment with steroids is indicated. However, treatment of meningococcal meningitis with steroids has been debated in the literature for years. Steroid proponents point to the *Haemophilus influenzae* type b meningitis and *Streptococcus pneumoniae* studies, in which treatment with steroids decreases hearing loss and may reduce neurologic sequelae. They postulate that steroids, through antiinflammatory effects, may decrease polymorphonuclear neutrophils, macrophages, and cytokines in the CNS and thus decrease CNS immune-mediated damage and hearing loss. Steroid opponents say that no conclusive studies show steroids to be of benefit in meningococcal meningitis and that risks include gastrointestinal ulceration, decreased penetration of antibiotics into the CNS (because of decreased meningeal inflammation), and steroid psychosis. If steroids are used, it seems prudent to use them early (preferably close to the time the first dose of antibiotic is administered). However, antibiotics should never be withheld waiting for steroids to be given.

Experimental and Adjunctive Therapies

Many adjunctive and experimental therapies have been tried, including antiendotoxin therapies and protein C concentrate infusions. Two antiendotoxin therapies have been evaluated in clinical trials: HA-1A and recombinant bactericidal/permeability increasing protein (rBPI). HA-1A, a human monoclonal antibody to endotoxin, was evaluated in a randomized, double-blind, placebo-controlled trial in 269 children with severe meningococcemia that was published in 1999. Although the 28-day mortality rate in the treatment group was 18% in contrast to 28% in the placebo group, this was not statistically significant ($P = .11$).[68] BPI is a naturally occurring protein in neutrophil azurophilic granules that binds to and neutralizes the effects of endotoxin. A randomized, double-blind, placebo-controlled trial that was published in 2000 studied rBPI in 393 children with presumed meningococcal disease. There was no difference in mortality rates (7.4% rBPI vs. 9.9% placebo). There was a trend in reduction of amputations in the treatment group that approached statistical significance ($P = .067$).[140]

The efficacy of recombinant human activated protein C in sepsis has been studied extensively. In a large randomized, placebo-controlled trial of 1690 adult patients with severe sepsis, known as the PROWESS study, a reduction in mortality was demonstrated, but the treatment group had an increased risk for bleeding.[18,21] A large study, published in 2007, compared activated protein C to placebo in children with severe sepsis.[161] The study was terminated by the Data and Safety Monitoring Board because of a low likelihood of improved outcome in the treatment group. Subsequently a follow-up large trial in adults, the PROWESS-SHOCK study, was published in 2012 and found no mortality benefit. Ultimately these findings led to removal of the drug from the market.[35,189]

Additional supportive measures such as prophylactic low-dose heparin are used by some clinicians.[239] Many investigators have studied the effect of heparin on survival and disseminated intravascular coagulation in patients with meningococcemia, and no consistent beneficial effect on these parameters has been noted. Serious side effects directly attributed to heparin therapy have been reported rarely.[89] The difficulty in adjusting the dose in small infants may lead to heparin intoxication. A retrospective chart review of 24 patients with purpura fulminans showed less necrosis of the digits and extremities in patients treated with heparin, but the results were not statistically significant.[134] A randomized, placebo-controlled trial evaluated the use of continuous heparin in patients with sepsis and found no benefit on 28-day mortality or length of stay.[119]

Other experimental therapies have been attempted in patients with fulminant meningococcemia. Anecdotal reports or small case series describe use of tissue plasminogen activator,[2,160] antithrombin III infusion,[52] topical nitroglycerin,[115,154] plasmapheresis,[50] and extracorporeal membrane oxygenation (ECMO).[136] Continuous caudal block has been used to restore lower extremity perfusion.[219] Insufficient evidence exists to say that any of these therapies have a significant impact on outcomes in meningococcal disease. Larger, multicenter studies are needed to evaluate efficacy.

TABLE 88.1 Chemoprophylaxis Regimens for Eradication of *Neisseria Meningitidis*

Drug	Age	Dose/Duration
Rifampin[a]	Children <1 mo	5 mg/kg/dose PO twice daily for 2 days (4 doses)
	Children ≥1 mo	10 mg/kg/dose (maximum dose 600 mg) PO twice daily for 2 days (4 doses)
	Adults	600 mg dose PO twice daily for 2 days (4 doses)
Ceftriaxone	Children <15 y	125 mg IM, single dose
	Children ≥15 y and adults	250 mg IM, single dose
Ciprofloxacin[b]	Children	Not recommended
	Adults	500 mg PO, single dose
Azithromycin[c]	Children	10 mg/kg PO (maximum dose 500 mg), single dose
	Adults	500 mg PO, single dose

IM, Intramuscularly; *PO,* orally.

[a]Rifampin is not recommended for pregnant women (teratogenicity in laboratory animals). The reliability of oral contraceptives may be affected by rifampin therapy; therefore alternative contraceptive measures should be used during and for the month after rifampin administration.

[b]Ciprofloxacin is not recommended in children, pregnant women, or lactating women. Ciprofloxacin can be used in children if there is no acceptable alternative.

[c]Azithromycin is *not* routinely recommended and is not listed in the US Centers for Disease Control recommendations for prophylaxis.

CONTROL AND PREVENTION

Chemoprophylaxis

The mode of transmission of *N. meningitidis* is direct contact with respiratory droplets or secretions. The ability of it to spread from person to person and cause epidemic disease has been recognized since the 1800s. Chemoprophylaxis is recommended for individuals with close contact to cases with invasive disease if the contact occurred in the 7 days preceding onset of illness in the case. Candidates for prophylaxis include household members, child-care center contacts, and persons with direct exposure to oral secretions.[55] The secondary attack rate in households with an index case is approximately 1000 times the attack rate in the general population.[7,209] Household crowding and young age are factors that increase the secondary attack rate. For close contacts, chemoprophylaxis is recommended regardless of immunization status.[5] Additionally airline passengers who had direct contact with respiratory secretions or who were seated directly next to an index case during a flight lasting 8 hours or longer should receive chemoprophylaxis.[5]

Several epidemiologic studies suggest that casual acquaintances (e.g., school-aged classmates) are not at increased risk, although some authors report secondary cases in this population.[117,121] Therefore casual acquaintances are not candidates for chemoprophylaxis. Additionally contact with individuals who have *N. meningitidis* isolated from nonsterile sites, such as respiratory secretions, would not qualify for chemoprophylaxis.[55] Mass prophylaxis is not recommended to control large outbreaks; instead vaccine is used in this setting.[55]

The period of communicability of the index patient is not well established. Most public health authorities recommend that persons in contact with the patient up to 7 days before onset of illness be considered for prophylaxis. Prophylaxis should be instituted as soon as possible, ideally within 24 hours, after identification of the index case.[55] It is not necessary to wait for laboratory confirmation of a case if the clinical picture is most consistent with meningococcal infection. Nasopharyngeal cultures are not recommended as they can delay therapy.[55] Secondary cases originally were defined as occurring more than 24 hours but less than 31 days after onset in the index case.[42] Approximately 70% of secondary cases will occur in the first 7 days after presentation of the index case.[42]

In the hospital setting, other preventative measures should be pursued. Droplet precautions should be continued for 24 hours after initiation of appropriate antibiotics in the hospitalized patient. The index patient should receive chemoprophylaxis before discharge unless he or she has been treated with ceftriaxone. A single dose of ceftriaxone is sufficient to eradicate nasopharyngeal colonization.[5] Abramson and Spika[1] reported that four of 14 (29%) patients with meningococcal infection treated with intravenous penicillin had positive culture results from the respiratory tract 1 week after completion of therapy. The original drug used for chemoprophylaxis was sulfadiazine. However, a large percentage of strains now are resistant to sulfa. Table 88.1 lists four antibiotics that are highly effective in eradicating meningococcus from the nasopharynx. Rifampin is generally the drug of choice for chemoprophylaxis of children. It is generally well tolerated but has side effects, including orange urine and sweat, orange staining of contact lenses, and stimulation of liver microsomal enzymes leading to reduction in levels of other concurrent medications (e.g., oral contraceptives, anticoagulants, digoxin, and phenytoin). Development of resistant strains has been reported rarely.[57] Rifampin, ciprofloxacin, and ceftriaxone have been evaluated in a randomized, comparative study.[59] All three drugs are highly effective, eradicating carriage in 90% to 95% of individuals.[54] Ceftriaxone is the drug of choice for a pregnant contact and also should be considered for children because a single intramuscular injection may result in greater compliance than four doses of rifampin. A single oral dose of ciprofloxacin is highly effective in eradicating carriage of meningococcus, but it is less desirable in individuals younger than 18 years because fluoroquinolones tend to be reserved to select circumstances in children. In addition, a 2009 article reported four cases of invasive meningococcal disease in the United States with isolates resistant to ciprofloxacin, although this remains rare.[55,244]

Although not recommended as a first-line agent, azithromycin was studied in a randomized, controlled trial comparing 500 mg of azithromycin orally once to rifampin 600 mg orally twice daily for 2 days. Carriage was eradicated in 56 of 60 (93%) colonized adults treated with azithromycin compared to eradication in 95% of the 59 colonized adults treated with rifampin.[92] Azithromycin is a consideration in areas where ciprofloxacin resistance has been detected.[42]

As mentioned in the next section, secondary disease can also be prevented by immunization of contacts, which is the preferred intervention for large outbreaks.[42] The single most important element of chemoprophylaxis is education regarding the need for immediate medical attention if contacts develop signs or symptoms of a febrile illness. No prophylactic strategy is 100% effective, and ill contacts should be medically evaluated with a high suspicion for meningococcal disease.

Outbreaks

A meningococcal outbreak is defined as three or more confirmed or probable primary cases within a three month period.[42] Between 1994 and 2002, there were 69 outbreaks of meningococcal disease in the United States.[171] Of these, 43 were due to serogroup C.[90] Outbreak-associated cases represented less than 2% of total cases of invasive disease, but they were associated with a higher case fatality rate than sporadic cases (21% vs. 11%; odds ratio, 3.3; 95% confidence interval [CI], 2.0–5.5).[30]

Meningococcal vaccines, described in detail later, are crucial in control of large meningococcal outbreaks. Internationally meningococcal vaccines have been used to control epidemics for several decades.[171] Reasons to not use chemoprophylaxis in large outbreaks include cost, concern for emergence of drug resistance, and difficulty in assuring simultaneous administration of drug in many individuals.[42] Vaccination for a population at risk (within an institution or a geographic setting) should be considered when the primary attack rate is more than 10 cases per 100,000 persons.[42,55] Usually vaccine candidates are those younger than 30 years within the population at risk in a community outbreak or all persons at risk in an organization-based outbreak.[55] The outbreak serogroup dictates the candidate vaccine.

Outbreaks in the past few decades have been defined geographically, while others have affected individuals with common risk factors. For example, in the mid-1990s an outbreak of serogroup B disease occurred in Oregon that resulted in a peak incidence of 4.5 cases per 100,000 individuals.[171] Although the rate in Oregon has since decreased, meningococcal disease continues to be hyperendemic in the state. Other examples include outbreaks in illicit drug users and men who have sex with men in New York.[130]

There were seven serogroup B college outbreaks between 2009 and 2015 that resulted in 41 cases and 3 deaths.[146] In 2013, two unrelated outbreaks in college campuses (Princeton and University of California-Santa Barbara) due to serogroup B were contained with use of MenB-4C vaccine, which is now licensed by the US Food and Drug Administration (FDA) but was dispensed at the time under an Investigational New Drug designation.[54] At Princeton, 95% of students received at least one dose of vaccine starting in December 2013, and no further cases were identified after introduction of the vaccine.[171] Additionally MenB-FHbp vaccine was used in a 2015 University of Oregon outbreak.[171]

Meningococcal Vaccines

Primary prevention of meningococcal disease is essential for several reasons. The presentation may be fulminant, with no opportunity for antibiotics to influence the course of the disease. Antibiotic-resistant strains now are recognized, and chemoprophylaxis of contacts is a cumbersome and often ineffective public health measure. Mass immunization offers the opportunity to prevent both endemic and epidemic disease worldwide.

Three types of vaccines, meningococcal polysaccharide vaccine (MSPV4), meningococcal conjugate vaccine (MCV), and recombinant meningococcal B vaccines are currently licensed in many countries around the world for prevention of meningococcal disease. There is no licensed vaccine for serogroup X.[90] Although more costly, meningococcal conjugate vaccines are superior to polysaccharide vaccines in several ways. Children younger than 2 years do not produce high levels of antibody in response to pure polysaccharide antigens. Polysaccharide antigens do not induce T-cell–dependent immunity with memory cell production. Polysaccharide vaccines have little effect on nasopharyngeal carriage.[151] Last, repeated boosting with MSPV4 has resulted in a blunting of antibody response, termed *hyporesponsiveness*.[26,144] In contrast, licensed conjugate vaccines have been shown to be immunogenic when used in an appropriate series with boosters, even in infants.[167] Conjugate vaccines produce stimulation of both T-cell and B-cell–dependent immunity and have been shown to decrease nasopharyngeal carriage.[42] For these reasons, although meningococcal polysaccharide vaccines are licensed and available in many countries, meningococcal conjugate vaccines have significant advantages.

Previously MenB vaccine development had been problematic because group B capsular polysaccharide is poorly immunogenic due its similarities to human fetal neural cell adhesion molecule. Additionally similarities to neural tissue raised concerns for induction of autoimmunity. In a few countries, including New Zealand, Norway, and Cuba, serogroup B vaccines had been developed utilizing outer membrane vesicle (OMV) in order to control epidemics. However, OMV vaccines are limited in that they are only serosubtype specific. Researchers would later capitalize on the New Zealand vaccine and create MenB-4C by adding three protein antigens (factor H-binding protein [fHbp], neisserial adhesion A [NadA], and neisserial heparin-binding antigen [NHBA]) to the New Zealand outbreak vaccine. MenB-FHbp (Trumenba) contains fHbp from the two subfamilies of this outer membrane protein providing broad serogroup B coverage.[151]

MenB-4C and MenB-FHbp have been shown to be immunogenic, and MenB-4C has been shown to have a modest impact on carriage, although efficacy is difficult to demonstrate due to rarity of meningococcal disease.[151] A large multicountry European study examined the immunogenicity and reactogenicity of MenB-4C in 1885 infants. The vaccine was highly immunogenic against two of the three meningococcal strains tested. For the third strain, 79% of infants developed sufficient antibody response that would be considered protective. Injection site pain and fever were relatively common after vaccination.[95] A study in more than 1600 Chilean adolescents showed that a two-dose series of MenB-4C performed better than a single dose in terms of good immunogenicity that lasted at least 6 months.[202]

Because MenB vaccines contain antigens among non-B meningococci, MenB vaccines have the potential to provide cross-protection against other capsular groups, as supported by in vitro studies.[135,151] However, the duration of long-term protection with these vaccines is not known.[208]

Meningococcal Vaccines in the United States

Meningococcal polysaccharide vaccine. Meningococcal polysaccharide vaccine (MPSV4, Menomune) is a capsular polysaccharide vaccine that targets serogroups A, C, Y, and W-135 and is licensed for use in individuals older than 2 years of age who are at increased risk for meningococcal disease. This vaccine was licensed in 1981 and was the only meningococcal vaccine widely available in the United States until the licensing of meningococcal conjugate vaccines. Conjugate vaccines are generally preferred over meningococcal polysaccharide vaccines in people for whom conjugate vaccines are licensed due to inferior efficacy of polysaccharide vaccines, as previously described.[151] Additionally, although MSPV4 is the only vaccine licensed in persons older than 55 years, off-label use of conjugate vaccine is recommended in persons older than 55 years if ongoing risk in the future is anticipated. MSPV4 is given subcutaneously as a single dose.

Meningococcal conjugate vaccines. Three meningococcal conjugate vaccines are currently licensed in the United States: MenACWY-D (Menactra), MenACWY-CRM (Menveo), and HibMenCY-TT (MenHibrix). Quadrivalent vaccines were first licensed in the United States in 2005.[54] MenACWY-D and MenACWY-CRM are quadrivalent vaccines that couple polysaccharide capsular antigens (i.e., serogroups A, C, Y, and W-135) to a protein carrier. In MenACWY-D, the protein carrier is diphtheria toxoid and in MenACWY-CRM, the protein carrier is CRM_{197} (mutant diphtheria toxin). MenHibrix is a combination *H. influenza* type b and bivalent meningococcal conjugate vaccine (i.e., serogroups C and Y) licensed in the United States for young children aged 6 weeks to 18 months.

MenACWY-D, MenACWY-CRM, and HibMenCY-TT vaccines have been found to be safe and immunogenic in infants, children, adolescents, and adults.[12,20,85,102,125,167,175,223] Efficacy was inferred by the demonstration of development of serum bactericidal antibodies to each of the meningococcal antigens the vaccines contain at a level that was noninferior to the response generated by polysaccharide vaccines.[20,214]

Close monitoring for potential adverse events initially suggested a possible association between MenACWY-D (Menactra) and Guillain-Barré syndrome based on case reports through the Vaccine Adverse Event Reporting System (VAERS) shortly after the licensure of MenACWY-D.[10] Subsequently the results of two large observational studies (collectively representing 2 million doses of vaccine) found no risk for Guillain-Barré associated with meningococcal conjugate vaccine.[1] Language about Guillain-Barré was removed from the meningococcal vaccine information statement.

Meningococcal conjugate vaccines are administered intramuscularly (as opposed to MPSV4, which is administered subcutaneously). Soon after licensure of meningococcal conjugate vaccines, numerous cases of misadministration of MenACWY-D (Menactra) were reported. The CDC studied 100 such cases and found that misadministration of MenACWY-D by the subcutaneous route still resulted in a protective immune response. While this route of administration is not recommended, persons who received the vaccine by this route do not need to be revaccinated.[41]

The duration of protection of quadrivalent meningococcal vaccination was originally thought likely to persist for 10 years. This was part of the rationale to incorporate meningococcal conjugate vaccine into the United States preadolescent vaccine platform. It was presumed that by vaccinating 11- to 12-year-old children, antibody levels would be sufficient for protection through the early college years, when there is increased risk for meningococcal disease. Subsequent studies showed significant decline in meningococcal antibody (vaccine serogroups) in adolescents 3 to 5 years after vaccination. Additionally a limited number of cases of meningococcal C or Y disease were reported to the CDC in previously vaccinated teenagers. The average time between vaccination and meningococcal disease was 3.25 years.[232] In 2010, as a result of concerns that adolescents may not be protected against invasive meningococcal disease for more than 5 years, the CDC's Advisory Committee on Immunization Practices (ACIP) recommended a booster dose of quadrivalent meningococcal vaccine be administered at age 16 years (Table 88.2).[54]

Meningococcal conjugate vaccines are currently licensed in the United States for persons as young as 6 weeks through 55 years. MenACWY-CRM is licensed in persons age 2 months through 55 years; MenACWY-D is licensed in persons 9 months through 55 years; HibMenCY-TT is licensed in infants and children 6 weeks through 18 months of age. As in adolescents, waning antibody has been detected 3 to 5 years after primary immunization and is the basis for the current recommendations for boosters if an ongoing risk factor exists for meningococcal disease.[54]

In the United States, the incidence of invasive meningococcal infections is highest in infants. Surveillance data from 2006 to 2012 suggest that vaccination to protect infants from meningococcal serogroups B, C, and Y by 4 months of age would prevent 63% of infections in infants.[145] However, because there would be a large subset of infants who would remain vulnerable to infection prior to being able to receive the two or three doses of necessary vaccine, alternate vaccination strategies could include maternal vaccination and the reduction of colonization in adolescents who serve as a reservoir of infection.[145]

Recombinant MenB vaccines. There are two licensed recombinant serogroup B vaccines, MenB-FHbp (Trumenba) and MenB-4C (Bexsero). In 2014, MenB-FHbp (Trumenba) became the first serogroup B vaccine licensed in the United States. This was followed shortly by MenB-4C (Bexsero) in 2015.[84] MenB vaccines in the United States are licensed for individuals 10 to 25 years of age.[54] Currently MenB vaccines are recommended for high-risk individuals and can be considered for routine vaccination in adolescents.

US recommendations for use of meningococcal vaccines. Tables 88.2 to 88.6 summarize the ACIP recommendations for the use of vaccines to prevent meningococcal disease.[4,55,113,126,194] Quadrivalent meningococcal vaccine is recommended for all US children (who have no contraindication) at the 11- to 12-year-old preadolescent visit, with a booster dose at age 16 years. The booster is recommended because vaccine efficacy wanes by up to 60% 2 to 5 years after vaccination.[54] Teenagers who receive their primary dose of quadrivalent meningococcal conjugate vaccine at 13 to 15 years should receive a booster at 16 to 18 years. If the primary dose of meningococcal conjugate vaccine is given on or after the 16th birthday, no booster is recommended. In the 2016 vaccine schedule, meningococcal B vaccine is offered as a consideration for any adolescent 16 to 23 years of age.[6,194] Meningococcal vaccines are also recommended in other scenarios including (1) underlying condition that predisposes to developing invasive meningococcal infection (complement component deficiencies and persons with functional or anatomic asplenia), (2) travel or residence in regions with endemic disease, (3) in the setting of outbreaks, and (4) for microbiologists who routinely work with *Neisseria meningitidis*. Recommendations for vaccines in these groups are listed in Tables 88.3 to 88.6. Of note, when vaccinating for travel to the meningitis belt or the Hajj it is necessary to administer quadrivalent meningococcal vaccine in order to immunize against MenA.[54]

Meningococcal Vaccines Outside the United States

Meningococcal A vaccine. The story of development and delivery of a conjugate serogroup A meningococcal vaccine to Africa is an inspirational public health achievement. In 2001, a partnership was developed between the World Health Organization (WHO) and the Program for Appropriate Technology in Health (PATH) around the Meningitis Vaccine Project. This project was funded by the Bill and Melinda Gates Foundation, and its goal was to develop and introduce an affordable meningococcal conjugate serogroup A vaccine in Africa. The vaccine was developed with help from additional agencies at a cost of $0.40 per dose. Two

TABLE 88.2 Recommendations for Adolescent Meningococcal Vaccination

Targeted Serogroup	Age	Primary Series	Booster Recommendations
A, C, W, Y	Age 11–18 y (preferably at age 11 or 12 y), routinely	Give one dose[a] of MCV4[b]	Booster at age 16 y if primary dose given at age 12 y or younger Booster at 16–18 y if primary dose given at 13–15 y[c] No booster if primary dose given at ≥16 y
	Age 19–21 y, first-year college students living in residence halls	Give one dose[a] of MCV4 if person has not received a dose on or after 16th birthday	No booster, unless other risk factors
B[d]	Age 16–23 y (preferred 16–18 y)	Give two doses of MenB-4C (Bexsero), 1 mo apart *or* Give three doses of MenB-FHbp (Trumenba) at 0, 2, and 6 mo, or give 2 doses at 0 and 6 mo	No booster

[a]If the person is HIV-positive, give a two-dose primary series, 8 weeks apart.
[b]*MCV4,* Menveo or Menactra.
[c]The minimum interval between doses of MCV4 is 8 weeks.
[d]Vaccination against serogroup B is not routinely recommended but can be considered.
Data from references 6, 126, 194.

TABLE 88.3 Recommendations for Meningococcal Vaccination in Individuals With Underlying Conditions (Persistent Complement Component Deficiencies[a] or Persons With Functional or Anatomic Asplenia)

Targeted Serogroup	Age of First Meningococcal Vaccination	Primary Series	Booster Recommendations
A, C, W, Y	Age 2–6 mo	Give four doses of MenACWY-CRM (Menveo) at 2, 4, 6, and 12 mo	See booster for age 2–55 y
	Age 7–23 mo	Give two doses of MenACWY-CRM (Menveo) (if age 7–23 mo)[c] or MenACWY-D (Menactra) (if age 9–23 mo with complement deficiency ONLY)[d], 12 wk apart	See booster for age 2–55 y
	Age 2–55 y	Give two doses of MCV4,[b,d] 8 wk apart	If primary series at: 2 mo–6 y: booster 3 y after primary series, then every 5 y thereafter ≥7 y: Booster every 5 y
	Age ≥56 y	Give two doses of MCV4,[b,e] 8 wk apart	Boost every 5 y with MCV4
C, Y	Age 2–11 mo	Give four doses of Hib-MenCY (MenHibrix) at ages 2, 4, 6, and 12–15 mo	No booster for Hib-MenCY (MenHibrix)
	Age 12–18 mo	Give two doses Hib-MenCY (MenHibrix), 8 wk apart	No booster for Hib-MenCY (MenHibrix)
B	Age ≥10 y[f]	Give two doses of MenB-4C (Bexsero), 1 mo apart *or* Give three doses of MenB-FHbp (Trumenba) at 0, 2, and 6 mo	No booster for MenB

[a]Persistent complement component deficiencies include C3, C5-C9, properdin, factor H, and factor D.
[b]*MCV4,* Menveo or Menactra.
[c]MenACWY-CRM (Menveo) second dose should be after first birthday.
[d]Children with functional or anatomic asplenia should complete a series of PCV13 vaccine before vaccination with MCV4; if MenACWY-D (Menactra) is to be given, begin at age 2 years and administer meningococcal vaccination at least 4 weeks after the fourth dose of pneumococcal conjugate vaccine to avoid possible interference with immune response to the pneumococcal vaccine series.
[e]MCV4 is preferred for those 56 years of age or older who have previously received MCV4 or for whom multiple doses are anticipated, as would be the case for someone with an underlying condition. MPSV4 is recommended for those ≥56 years who have not previously received MCV4 and for whom only one dose is anticipated.
[f]Approved for those aged 10–25 years but recommended for ≥10 years.
Data from references 55, 126, 194.

TABLE 88.4 Recommendations for Meningococcal Vaccinations for Travel (Travelers to or Persons Residing in Countries Where Meningococcal Disease Is Endemic or Hyperendemic)

Targeted Serogroup	Age of First Meningococcal Vaccination	Primary Series	Booster Recommendations
A, C, W, Y	Age 2–6 mo	Give four doses[a] of MenACWY-CRM (Menveo) at 2, 4, 6, and 12 mo	
	Age 7–23 mo	Give two doses[a,c] of MenACWY-CRM (Menveo) (if age 7–23 mo) or MenACWY-D (Menactra) (if age 9–23 mo), 12 wk apart	See booster for age 2–55 y
	Age 2–55 y	Give one dose of MCV4[b]	If risk continues and primary series at: 2 mo–6 y: booster 3 y after primary series, then every 5 y thereafter ≥7 y: booster every 5 y
	Age ≥56 y	Give one dose of MCV4 or MPSV4 (Menomune)[d]	If risk continues: boost every 5 y with MCV4
B	All ages	Not recommended	

[a]Completion of the entire series is preferred before travel.
[b]*MCV4,* Menveo or Menactra.
[c]If a child aged 7–23 months will enter endemic area in less than 3 months, give doses as soon as 2 months apart.
[d]MCV4 is preferred for those aged ≥56 years who have previously received MCV4 or for whom multiple doses are anticipated. MPSV4 is recommended for those aged ≥56 years who have not previously received MCV4 and for whom only one dose is anticipated.
Data from references 4, 126, 194.

studies (one in children 12 to 23 months of age and one in persons 2 to 29 years of age) showed the vaccine to be more immunogenic than and with a similar safety profile to the polysaccharide serogroup A vaccine.[207] Burkina Faso became the first country to conduct a nationwide rollout of the meningococcal conjugate serogroup A vaccine (MenAfriVac) nationwide. More than 11 million people aged 1 to 29 years were immunized in a 10-day period in December 2010. During the subsequent 2011 winter dry season only 2665 suspected meningococcal cases were reported (80% reduction over prior years). From the suspect cases, 1437 specimens were cultured (or submitted for PCR), and only four isolates were identified to be serogroup A—all from unvaccinated individuals.[51] Carriage studies done before and after vaccine implementation in Burkina Faso show a decrease in oropharyngeal carriage. Before vaccine implementation, examination of 20,326 oropharyngeal cultures yielded a carriage rate of 0.4%. Fifteen thousand oropharyngeal samples obtained after the MenAfriVac implementation program revealed none of the samples was positive for serogroup A *N. meningitidis.*[48,132] More than 55 million Africans have now been vaccinated in at least six countries. Large-scale institution of this vaccine has dramatically decreased the incidence of serogroup A meningococcal disease.[171]

Meningococcal B vaccines. Tailor-made Men-B vaccines using serogroup B outer membrane proteins were developed for outbreaks that began in the 1970s in Norway and Cuba and in the 1990s in New Zealand.[171] In addition to the United States, MenB-4C (Bexsero) is licensed in Europe and Australia.[3,135] In the United Kingdom, MenB-4C has been offered as part of the routine vaccination program since September 2015.[135]

Meningococcal C vaccines. Meningococcal C conjugate vaccination in the United Kingdom has been effective[187,220] and has produced herd immunity (67% disease reduction in unvaccinated 1- to 17-year-olds)[188] and a 66% reduction in adolescent nasopharyngeal carriage. A meningococcal serogroup C conjugate vaccine program was begun in the United Kingdom in 1999 with a 2-, 3-, 4-month primary series schedule for infants. Children 1 to 18 years of age received a single dose of meningococcal serogroup C conjugate vaccine (MCCV). In 2002, MCCV was offered to all individuals up to age 25 years. Later studies from the United Kingdom showed rapid waning of immunity in vaccinated infants (vaccinated at 2, 3, and 4 months). Despite high vaccine efficacy during the first year after immunization, vaccine efficacy fell significantly at 1 year or more after vaccination.[34] As of 2013, the vaccine schedule was changed to a single infant vaccine at 4 months, with two boosters at 12 months and 14 years of age, respectively.[3]

The United Kingdom's meningococcal conjugate serogroup C program has been highly effective in producing a dramatic and sustained reduction in serogroup C disease. The overall incidence rate of serogroup C disease has fallen by 98.7% in England and Wales, and no evidence exists for serogroup replacement.[33,148]

Several other countries also incorporated meningococcal C conjugate vaccines into their immunization programs because of circulating clonal serogroup C strains. Canada's staggered serogroup C vaccine implementation program allowed for a comparison of the meningococcal disease incidence in provinces with and without vaccine implementation; provinces with vaccine implementation showed substantial reduction in meningococcal C disease, and no serogroup replacement was seen.[19]

TABLE 88.5 Recommendations for Meningococcal Vaccinations for Outbreaks (Persons in a Defined Risk Group During an Institutional or Community Outbreak[a])

Targeted Serogroup	Age of First Meningococcal Vaccination	Vaccine
A, C, W, Y	Age 2–6 mo	Give 4 doses of MenACWY-CRM (Menveo) at 2, 4, 6, and 12 mo
	Age 7–23 mo	Give 2 doses of MenACWY-CRM (Menveo) (if age 7–23 mo)[c] or MenACWY-D (Menactra) (if age 9–23 mo), 12 wk apart
	Age 2–55 y	Give 1 dose of MCV4[b]
	Age ≥56 y	Give 1 dose of MCV4[b] or MPSV4 (Menomune)[d]
C, Y	Age 2–11 mo	Give 4 doses of Hib-MenCY (MenHibrix) at ages 2, 4, 6, and 12–15 mo
	Age 12–18 mo	Give 2 doses Hib-MenCY (MenHibrix), 8 wk apart
B	Age ≥10 y	Give 2 doses of MenB-4C (Bexsero), 1 mo apart *or* Give 3 doses of MenB-FHbp (Trumenba) at 0, 2, and 6 mo

[a]Seek advice of local public health authorities to determine if vaccination is recommended.
[b]*MCV4,* Menveo or Menactra.
[c]MenACWY-CRM (Menveo) second dose should be after first birthday.
[d]MCV4 is preferred for those aged ≥56 years who have previously received MCV4 or for whom multiple doses are anticipated. MPSV4 is recommended for those aged ≥56 years who have not previously received MCV4 and for whom only one dose is anticipated.
Data from references 126, 194.

Future for Meningococcal Vaccines

A deeper understanding of the pathophysiologic mechanism of meningococcal disease and the bacterial structures critical for antigenicity and immunogenicity in humans is needed. A safe and effective vaccine that could induce protection against all encapsulated meningococci in all age groups is the ultimate goal.

Acknowledgments

I acknowledge Marsha S. Anderson, Mary P. Glodé, and Arnold L. Smith, who were the previous authors of this chapter.

TABLE 88.6 Recommendations for Meningococcal Vaccinations for Microbiologists (Microbiologists Routinely Working With *Neisseria Meningitides)*

Targeted Serogroup	Age	Primary Series	Booster Recommendations
A, C, W, Y	Age 19–55 y	Give 1 dose of MCV4[a]	If risk continues, boost every 5 y with MCV4
	Age ≥56 y	Give 1 dose of MCV4 or MPSV4 (Menomune)[b]	If risk continues, boost every 5 y with MCV4
B	Age ≥19 y	Give 2 doses of MenB-4C (Bexsero), 1 mo apart *or* Give 3 doses of MenB-FHbp (Trumenba) at 0, 2, and 6 mo	No booster

[a]*MCV4,* Menveo or Menactra.
[b]MCV4 is preferred for those aged ≥56 years who have previously received MCV4 or for whom multiple doses are anticipated. MPSV4 is recommended for those aged ≥56 years who have not previously received MCV4 and for whom only 1 dose is anticipated.
Data from references 126 and 194.

NEW REFERENCES SINCE THE SEVENTH EDITION

3. Ali A, Jafri RZ, Messonnier N, et al. Global practices of meningococcal vaccine use and impact on invasive disease. *Pathog Glob Health*. 2014;108(1):11-20.
4. American Academy of Pediatrics Committee on Infectious Diseases. Recommended childhood and adolescent immunization schedule: United States, 2016. *Pediatrics*. 2016;137(3):e20154531.
5. American Academy of Pediatrics Committee on Infectious Diseases. Updated recommendations on the use of meningococcal vaccines. *Pediatrics*. 2014;134(2):400-403.
6. American Academy of Pediatrics. Meningococcal infections. In: Kimberlin DW, Brady MT, Jackson MA, Long SS, eds. *Red Book:2015 Report of the Committee on Infectious Diseases*. Elk Grove Village, IL: American Academy of Pediatrics; 2015:547-558.
35. Campsall PA, Laupland KB, Niven DJ. Severe meningococcal infection: a review of epidemiology, diagnosis, and management. *Crit Care Clin*. 2013;29(3):393-409.
39. Centers for Disease Control and Prevention. Active bacterial core surveillance report, Emerging Infections Program Network, *Neisseria meningitidis*, 2011. Available at: http://www.cdc.gov/abcs/reports-findings/survreports/mening14.pdf.
40. Centers for Disease Control and Prevention. Active bacterial core surveillance report, Emerging Infections Program Network, *Neisseria meningitidis*, 2012. Available at: http://www.cdc.gov/abcs/reports-findings/survreports/mening13.pdf.
41. Centers for Disease Control and Prevention. Active bacterial core surveillance report, Emerging Infections Program Network, *Neisseria meningitidis*, 2013. Available at: http://www.cdc.gov/abcs/reports-findings/survreports/mening12.pdf.
42. Centers for Disease Control and Prevention. Active bacterial core surveillance report, Emerging Infections Program Network, *Neisseria meningitidis*, 2014. Available at: http://www.cdc.gov/abcs/reports-findings/survreports/mening11.pdf.
46. Centers for Disease Control and Prevention. Meningococcal disease. In: Roush S, Baldy L, eds. *Manual for the Surveillance of Vaccine-Preventable Diseases*. Atlanta, GA: Centers for Disease Control and Prevention; 2011:1-11.
54. Cohn A, MacNeil J. The changing epidemiology of meningococcal disease. *Infect Dis Clin North Am*. 2015;29(4):667-677.
55. Cohn AC, MacNeil JR, Clark TA, et al. Prevention and control of meningococcal disease: recommendations of the Advisory Committee on Immunization Practices (ACIP). *MMWR Recomm Rep*. 2013;62(RR-2):1-28.
84. Folaranmi T, Rubin L, Martin SW, et al. Use of serogroup B meningococcal vaccines in persons aged ≥10 years at increased risk for serogroup B meningococcal disease: recommendations of the Advisory Committee on Immunization Practices, 2015. *MMWR Morb Mortal Wkly Rep*. 2015;64(22):608-612.
88. Gamougam K, Daugla DM, Toralta J, et al. Continuing effectiveness of serogroup A meningococcal conjugate vaccine, Chad, 2013. *Emerg Infect Dis*. 2015;21(1):115-118.
90. Gianchecchi E, Torelli A, Piccini G, et al. *Neisseria meningitidis* infection: Who, when and where? *Expert Rev Anti Infect Ther*. 2015;13(10):1249-1263.
104. Harcourt BH, Anderson RD, Wu HM, et al. Population-based surveillance of *Neisseria meningitidis* antimicrobial resistance in the United States. *Open Forum Infect Dis*. 2015;2(3):ofv117.
118. Jafri RZ, Ali A, Messonnier NE, et al. Global epidemiology of invasive meningococcal disease. *Popul Health Metr*. 2013;11(1):17.
119. Jaimes F, De La Rosa G, Morales C, et al. Unfractioned heparin for treatment of sepsis: a randomized clinical trial (The HETRASE Study). *Crit Care Med*. 2009;37:1185-1196.
126. Kim DK, Bridges CB, Harriman KH. Advisory Committee on Immunization Practices (ACIP), ACIP Adult Immunization Work Group. Advisory Committee on Immunization Practices recommended immunization schedule for adults aged 19 years or older—United States, 2016. *MMWR*. 2016;65(4):88-90.
130. Kratz MM, Weiss D, Ridpath A, et al. Community-based outbreak of *Neisseria meningitidis* serogroup C infection in men who have sex with men, New York City, New York, USA, 2010–2013. *Emerg Infect Dis*. 2015;21(8):1379-1386.
135. Ladhani S, Giuliani M, Biolchi A, et al. Effectiveness of meningococcal B vaccine against endemic hypervirulent *Neisseria meningitidis* W strain, England. *Emerg Infect Dis*. 2016;22(2):309-311.
145. MacNeil J, Rubin L, Folaranmi T, et al. Use of serogroup B meningococcal vaccines in persons adolescents and young adults: recommendations of the Advisory Committee on Immunization Practices, 2015. *MMWR*. 2015;64(41):1171-1176.
146. MacNeil JR, Bennett N, Farley MM, et al. Epidemiology of infant meningococcal disease in the United States, 2006–2012. *Pediatrics*. 2015;135(2):e305-e311.
151. Marshall H, Wang B, Wesselingh S, et al. Control of invasive meningococcal disease: Is it achievable? *Int J Evid Based Healthc*. 2016;14(1):3-14.
171. Oviedo-Orta E, Ahmed S, Rappuoil R, et al. Prevention and control of meningococcal outbreaks: the emerging role of serogroup B meningococcal vaccines. *Vaccine*. 2015;33:3628-3635.
189. Ranieri VM, Thompson BT, Barie PS, et al. Drotrecogin alfa (activated) in adults with septic shock. *N Engl J Med*. 2012;366:2055-2064.
194. Robinson CL. Advisory Committee on Immunization Practices (ACIP), ACIP Child/Adolescent Immunization Work Group. Advisory Committee on Immunization Practices recommended immunization schedules for persons aged 0 through 18 years—United States, 2016. *MMWR*. 2016;65(4):86-87.
208. Sridhar S, Greenwood B, Head C, et al. Global incidence of serogroup B invasive meningococcal disease: a systematic review. *Lancet Infect Dis*. 2015;15(11):1334-1346.
233. Wang X, Shutt KA, Vuong JT, et al. Changes in the population structure of invasive *Neisseria meningitidis* in the United States after quadrivalent meningococcal conjugate vaccine licensure. *J Infect Dis*. 2015;211(12):1887-1894.

The full reference list for this chapter is available at ExpertConsult.com.

89 Gonococcal Infections

Charles R. Woods Jr

Gonorrhea, the foremost manifestation of human disease caused by *Neisseria gonorrhoeae* (the gonococcus), is one of the oldest known human diseases. Gonorrhea has been known as "the clap" since the late 1300s. This term may have derived from the Les Clapier district of Paris, where prostitutes were housed during the Middle Ages.[131,182]

The description by Neisser of *N. gonorrhoeae* in stained smears of urethral and other exudates in 1879 and culture of the organism by Leistikow and Löffler in 1882 provided the foundation for modern understanding of the clinical spectrum of gonococcal diseases. The advent of safe and effective antimicrobial agents, first sulfonamides in 1936 and then penicillin in 1943, was the next major advance in combating gonorrhea.[182,131] Modern knowledge of the molecular pathogenesis of *N. gonorrhoeae* infection began in 1963 with the observation by Kellogg and colleagues[186] that gonococcal strains with differences in colony morphology also varied in virulence. Further understanding of the clinical aspects of the disease was facilitated by development of the Thayer-Martin medium in 1964.[322]

N. gonorrhoeae remains a major international public health problem because of reproductive sequelae of infection (e.g., infertility), the ever-growing resistance to antimicrobial agents, and disproportionate case burdens in public clinics.[54,62,184,209,210,265] Efforts to develop an effective vaccine are ongoing.[50,345] Additional information on gonococcal infections is provided in Chapter 42.

EPIDEMIOLOGY

Gonococcal infections remain second in incidence only to *Chlamydia* infections among reportable diseases in the United States.[55,62] The United States reached a historic nadir of 98.1 cases per 100,000 population in 2009, but rates have subsequently increased to 110.7 in 2014.[62] Regions with higher rates of adult disease have higher numbers of pediatric cases,[99,122] a finding that reflects the adult origin of virtually all pediatric cases. (For the most current national data for the United States, see the

Gonococcal Isolate Surveillance Project [GISP] website: http://www.cdc.gov/std/gisp/default.htm.)

An estimated 820,000 new cases of gonococcal infection occur annually in the United States.[343] At least half of the cases are thought to go undiagnosed or unreported. In 2014 in the United States, 350,062 cases were reported.[62] US national trends in reported rates are shown in Fig. 89.1. Rates of gonorrhea are based primarily on detection of symptomatic infection. Asymptomatic chronic infection in adults is well documented and may account for 5% of cases.[166] Such infections can be transmitted. Some untreated cases will resolve over time. Data also indicate that asymptomatic infection occurs in children, including prepubertal children.[3,115,153,166] Gonococcal infections rarely are fatal (approximately four deaths per year in the United States), with death being caused by gonococcal sepsis.[55,210]

Gonorrhea rates remain highest among adolescents and young adults (Fig. 89.2). In 2014, rates of reported cases were 430.5 of 100,000 and 221.1 among adolescent females and males 15 to 19 years of age, respectively, and 533.7 and 485.6 among females and males 20 to 24 years of age, respectively.[62] Rates among African Americans were 10.6 times higher than among whites, which represents a decline from 18.7 in 2010.[60,62] Low socioeconomic status, early onset of sexual activity, unmarried marital status, and past gonococcal infections are risk factors for acquiring gonococcal infection, as are prostitution and illicit drug use.[15,37] Limited access to health care also may contribute to increased prevalence of disease in impoverished populations.[57] The prevalence of gonococcal infection in adolescents attending private clinics probably is lower than that in those seeking care in publicly funded settings.[21] For women, the use of hormonal contraceptives may increase the risk for acquiring infection, whereas the use of spermicides or diaphragms appears to be at least partially protective.[206,207]

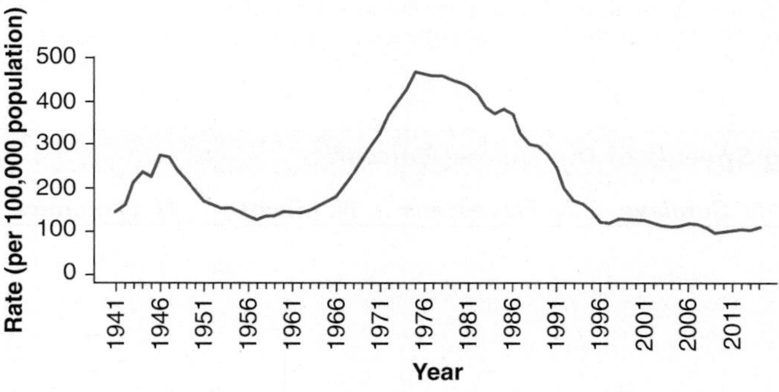

FIG. 89.1 Rates of gonorrhea in the United States, 1941–2014. After steady decline from 1975 through 1997, overall gonorrhea rates have plateaued, reaching a historic nadir of 98.1 cases per 100,000 population in 2009. The rate in 2014 was 110.7. Gonorrhea is substantially underdiagnosed and underreported. (From Centers for Disease Control and Prevention: http://www.cdc.gov/std/stats14/figures/12.htm. For the most currently available data, see http://www.cdc.gov/std/gisp/default.htm.)

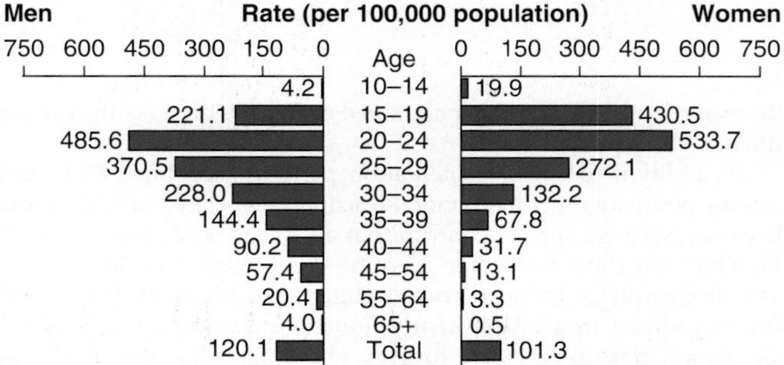

FIG. 89.2 Rates of gonorrhea by age and sex: United States, 2014. This pattern has been the same for decades. Rates in males may be underreported compared to females. (From Centers for Disease Control and Prevention: http://www.cdc.gov/std/stats14/figures/17.htm. For the most currently available data, see http://www.cdc.gov/std/gisp/default.htm.)

Among persons seeking care in clinics participating in the STD Surveillance Network, rates of gonococcal infection among men who have sex with men (MSM) are higher than those among men who have sex only with women (MSW) and among women, especially among adolescent MSM 19 years of age or younger.[62]

The southeastern United States continues to have rates of gonorrhea higher than those of other regions of the country. In 2014, rates in the South, Midwest, West, and North were 131.4, 106.6, 101.1, and 84.7 cases per 100,000 population, respectively.[62] About 50% of reported cases occurred in only 70 counties or independent cities in the United States in 2014 (Fig. 89.3). Humans are the only reservoir of *N. gonorrhoeae*. Exudate and secretions from infected mucosal surfaces allow transmission to occur during the intimate contact of sexual acts, parturition, and, rarely, household exposure. The incubation period usually is 2 to 7 days. No evidence of airborne transmission of gonococci exists; contact with viable microbes is required for transmission. Gonococci survive on surfaces outside the human body for only short periods (probably minutes). Although organisms can be cultured from environmental sources (e.g., toilet seats) for up to 3 hours after artificial inoculation in large numbers, viable gonococci have not been recovered from random samplings in public restrooms.[125]

Nonsexual transmission of *N. gonorrhoeae* to the genitalia, rectum, or oropharynx of children rarely occurs and never should be presumed without extensive investigation of the social setting of the infected child.[236] Childhood infection potentially could be acquired when a child cosleeps in the same bed with an infected family member,[125] and sharing of bath towels and other similar objects has been suspected as the cause of epidemics in prepubescent girls living together.[305] Although persistence of apparently perinatally acquired gonococcal infection for up to 1 year of age has been reported, and fomite or maternal nonsexual transmission to young infants is plausible,[33] these possibilities should not be generalized beyond infancy. Gonococcal conjunctivitis can be acquired nonvenereally.[197]

The risk for males acquiring urethral infection after a single episode of vaginal intercourse with infected females is estimated to be 20%. With four exposures, the risk increases to 60% to 80%. The prevalence of infection in females named as sexual contacts of males with gonococcal urethritis has been reported to be 50% to 90%.[159,163]

MICROBIOLOGY

Neisseria spp. are aerobic, gram-negative, nonmotile, non–spore-forming cocci that occur in pairs (diplococci), with adjacent sides flattened. They have the typical gram-negative microbial outer membrane overlying a thin peptidoglycan layer and cytoplasmic membrane. The species lacks a true polysaccharide capsule but produces a surface polyphosphate that provides a hydrophilic, negatively charged surface.[242] In Gram stains of clinical specimens, the microbes frequently are observed within phagocytes.[300]

Gonococci are able to use glucose, lactate, and pyruvate as carbon sources but cannot use other carbohydrates, which is the basis for the carbohydrate utilization tests for speciation of *Neisseria* (Table 89.1). Catalase and cytochrome oxidase are produced by the gonococcus, as in most *Neisseria* spp., but gonococci do not produce appreciable amounts of superoxide dismutase. Growth is optimal in a 5% carbon dioxide atmosphere at 35°C to 37°C (95°F–98.6°F) and a pH of 6.5 to 7.5. Gonococci do not survive below pH 6.0, grow poorly below 30°C (86°F), and do not survive above 40°C (104°F).

Neisseria spp. require enriched media, including free iron, to support their growth. Multiple colony types are evident when a single isolate is grown on clear agar. Small convex glistening colonies are piliated, whereas larger, flatter colonies are nonpiliated. In vitro passage usually results in loss of pili. Under low-power microscopy, some colonies appear opaque or granular and others are transparent. The former represent colonies in which most cells express one or more opacity-associated proteins (Opa), whereas in the latter colonies, most cells do not express these proteins.[36,40,186,307,317,318,333]

Culture and Speciation From Clinical Specimens

The organisms are cultured best on chocolate blood agar in an atmosphere enriched by carbon dioxide. If the clinical specimen has been obtained

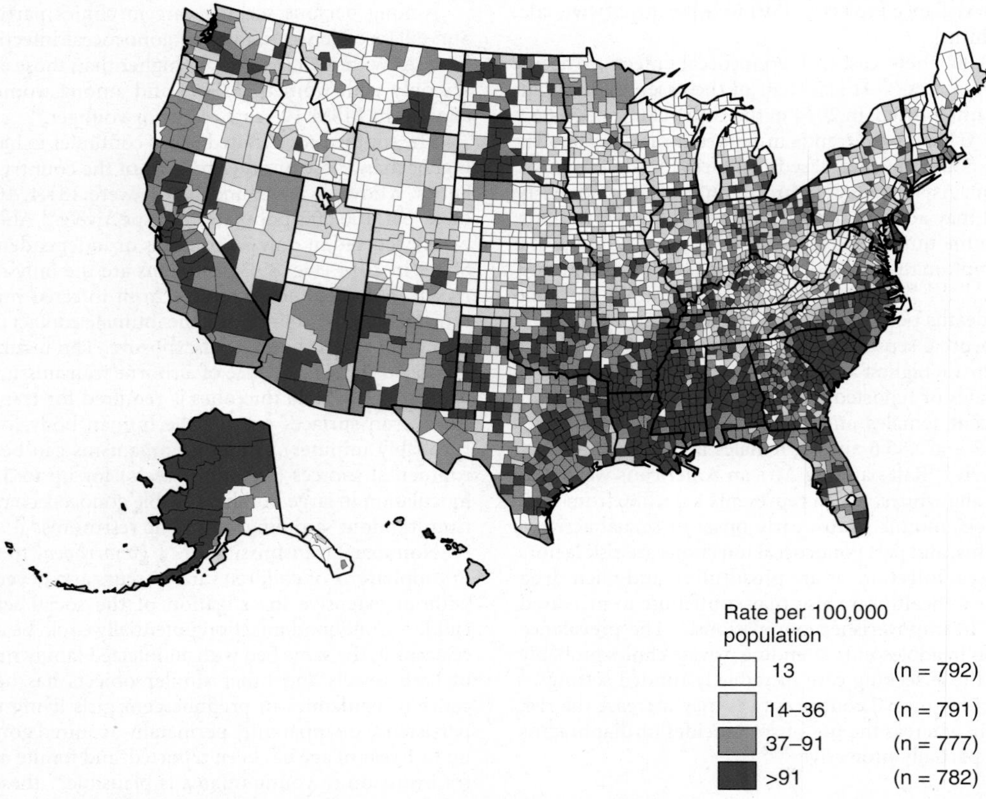

FIG. 89.3 Rates of gonorrhea by county in the United States, 2014. (From Centers for Disease Control and Prevention: http://www.cdc.gov/std/stats14/figures/16.htm. For the most currently available data, see http://www.cdc.gov/std/gisp/default.htm.)

TABLE 89.1 Biochemical Characteristics Differentiating Species of the Genus *Neisseria*

	N. Gonorrhoeae	*N. Meningitidis*	*N. Sicca*	*N. Subflava*	*N. Flavescens*	*N. Mucosa*	*N. Lactamica*
Acid from:							
Glucose	+	+	+	+	−	+	+
Maltose	−	+	+	+	−	+	−
Sucrose	−	−	+	±	−	+	−
Lactose	−	−	−	−	−	−	+
Polysaccharide produced from 5% sucrose	0	0	+	±	+	+	0
Reduction of:							
Nitrate	−	−	−	−	−	+	−
Nitrite	−	±	+	+	+	+	+
Pigment	−	−	±	+	+	+	−
Extra CO_2 for growth	+	+	−	−	−	−	−

from a highly contaminated site (e.g., rectum or cervix), a selective medium containing nystatin, vancomycin, trimethoprim, and colistin (e.g., modified Thayer-Martin medium) to suppress contaminating flora allows the growth of most *Neisseria* spp. A few strains of gonococci are inhibited by vancomycin.[36,223] Chocolate agar without antimicrobial agents is preferred if the culture is taken from a usually sterile area such as blood, cerebrospinal fluid (CSF), synovial fluid, or a skin lesion. Gonococcal colonies usually are evident on agar plates within 24 to 48 hours after inoculation. Frequent propagation is necessary to maintain isolates because viability is lost rapidly after 48 hours of growth.

Because gonococci cannot tolerate drying, clinical specimens must be plated as soon as possible onto appropriate media. Transport bottles that contain medium and a carbon dioxide–enriched atmosphere should be used if definitive processing of the specimen must be delayed. Transport bottles should be maintained upright to preserve the carbon dioxide atmosphere.

In addition to sugar fermentation patterns (see Table 89.1) and oxidase positivity, other biochemical reactions can be used to differentiate between *Neisseria* spp. or confirm that an isolate is *N. gonorrhoeae*.[343] Enzyme substrate tests that identify the presence or absence of 1-hydroxyprolylaminopeptidase, γ-glutamyl aminotransferase, and β-galactosidase are available as an adjunctive means of confirmation.[86] Gonococci possess only the former. These reactions alone will not distinguish *N. gonorrhoeae* from several commensal *Neisseria* spp. Antigen-detection–based tests, including fluorescent antibody staining, also have been used to confirm the identity of an isolate as *N. gonorrhoeae*.[185] Tests based on detection of gonococcal nucleic acid sequences, which are being used increasingly for diagnostic purposes, can be used to confirm the identity of gonococcal isolates from cultures. Additional information about laboratory methods that should be used to distinguish *N. gonorrhoeae* from other *Neisseria* species is available at http://www.cdc.gov/std/gonorrhea/lab/ident.htm.[63]

Matrix-assisted laser desorption/ionization time-of-flight mass spectrometry (MALDI-TOF MS) can be used to identify *N. gonorrhoeae* in clinical specimens.[287] As databases of MALDI-TOF MS patterns of various neisserial species are expanded, misidentification of species within this genus by this method should decrease.

Genetic Characteristics

Gonococci have a circular chromosome consisting of 2219 kilobases (kb), which is about half the size of the *Escherichia coli* genome.[97] The gonococcal genome has approximately 2250 predicted open-reading frames.[34] The entire genomes of *N. gonorrhoeae* strains FA1090, NCCP11945, and ST1407 have been sequenced. A macrorestriction map with the positions of many genetic markers has been available since 1991.[71,154,251] More than 1300 open-reading frame sequences have been validated.[34] *N. gonorrhoeae* are polyploid, with two to five genome equivalents present in each cell. These copies are ultimately haploid in that strains cannot be made to carry two different alleles at the same locus.[276]

RNA expression analyses of cervicovaginal lavage specimens collected from women recently exposed to infected male partners compared to the same isolates after growth in chemically defined medium showed that 140 genes had increased expression and 165 genes had decreased expression during natural infection.[211] A large portion of the genes with increased expression are related to regulatory functions and iron scavenging.

Piliated gonococcal cells (the natural in vivo state) are competent for genetic transformation by exogenous DNA at all stages of growth.[24] Only homologous DNA is taken into the cell.[103] Gonococci are highly autolytic and release DNA in a biologically active form. Thus different strains are able to exchange genetic material readily. Such exchange can lead to further genetic and phenotypic diversity, which helps maintain the species in its human hosts and facilitates transfer of chromosomal antibiotic resistance genes.[285]

A 36-kb conjugal plasmid is present in many gonococci. It efficiently mobilizes its own transfer and other non–self-mobilizable plasmids (e.g., the 4.5- and 7.5-kb penicillinase plasmids), but not chromosomal genes.[238,248,272] Extrachromosomal, nonplasmid DNA circles recently have been identified in wild-type gonococcal isolates. They may play a role in gene recombination, amplification of chromosomal genes, and transformation.[17] Gonococci possess multiple restriction endonucleases and their corresponding DNA methylases.[316] The species is relatively nonmutagenic and lacks photoreactivation and error-prone repair systems.[46]

Strain Typing

The ability to differentiate one strain from another allows investigation of the epidemiology of transmission of gonorrhea across populations and assessment of virulence factors. Numerous methods have been applied to gonococci.

Auxotyping classifies strains according to their ability to grow or not grow in the absence of 11 specific compounds, including amino acids (e.g., arginine and proline), purines, pyrimidines (e.g., hypoxanthine and uracil), and other nutrients (e.g., thiamine). Approximately 20 auxotype phenotypes are recognized. A single auxotype can represent many genotypes.[295] The auxotype of greatest importance is designated arginine, hypoxanthine, and uracil negative (AHU^-). Such strains are unable to grow in the absence of these compounds. AHU^- strains typically are more resistant to killing by normal human serum, are more likely to cause asymptomatic infections in males, and are found more frequently in patients with disseminated infection.[107,187] AHU^- strains often are susceptible to vancomycin.[223]

A serologic technique based on antigenic heterogeneity of the porin protein contained in the outer membrane of the gonococcus is able to divide strains into two immunochemically distinct serogroups, PorA and PorB, with various serovars within each.[9,162,174,188,282,283] This method is no longer used for epidemiologic evaluations.

Multiple genotyping methods have been applied to *N. gonorrhoeae*.[204] Simple restriction endonuclease methods[113,256] have been supplanted by polymerase chain reaction (PCR)-based methods and pulsed-field gel electrophoresis (PFGE). *N. gonorrhoeae* multiantigen sequence typing (NG-MAST) is based on internal variation of two highly polymorphic loci and has been used for cluster identification, tracing sexual contacts, and investigating treatment failures.[324] These methods appear most useful for local microepidemiologic purposes.

Multilocus sequence typing is the primary typing method used now for macroepidemiologic analyses such as monitoring global spread of clones or clonal complexes with particular virulence traits or antimicrobial resistance patterns. At least two seven-loci–based schemes have been developed.[324] Whole-genome sequencing has been applied to a set of 169 isolates and grouped these into 12 clades.[95] This method may supplant all others as its associated costs decrease over time. The high ratio of recombination to mutation events, estimated at 2.2 in a recent study,[112] may make comparison on clonality over longer periods of time more difficult.

PATHOGENESIS

A continuously expanding body of literature is devoted to the pathogenesis of *N. gonorrhoeae*.[79,85,106,114,156,203,260] *N. gonorrhoeae* is well adapted to its human host and is able to co-opt components of the innate immune system for its survival. Species specificity is demonstrated by greater adherence of gonococci to human cells than to nonhuman cells. Close interactions of *N. gonorrhoeae* with mucosal cells, erythrocytes, spermatozoa, and polymorphonuclear cells are well described.

Gonococci are able to survive in the urethra in the face of hydrodynamic forces that tend to wash other microbes away and persist there despite close proximity and even attachment to the hordes of neutrophils that respond to their presence. These observations indicate an ability to adhere to mucosal epithelia and evade the host acute innate immune response. Individuals also can have repeated infections by the same gonococcal strain, suggesting that the organism can thwart establishment of local adaptive immune responses. The tissue damage that occurs in the fallopian tubes during salpingitis implies that one or more directly toxic moieties or factors can trigger a deleterious host response.[116,305]

In the male human model of experimental infection, gonococci are recovered in urine at low levels for about 2 hours after urethral inoculation. The microbes then disappear from the urine for variable periods before becoming shed in increasing numbers. The bacteriuria persists until signs and symptoms of dysuria and urethritis appear after an incubation period of 1 to 6 days after inoculation. Severity of symptoms does not correlate with the shed microbial burden. Pyuria and detectable urinary concentrations of interleukin-6 (IL-6) and IL-8 usually appear within 24 hours after inoculation. Phenotypic variation of gonococcal surface determinants is seen during the course of experimental infection.[156]

This human model and multiple in vitro molecular studies involving cell lines and fallopian tube organ cultures have provided many insights into the molecular pathogenesis of gonococcal infection.[72,152,213,214,266]

Invasion of Mucosal Epithelial Cells

In addition to the ability to resist killing by neutrophils, gonococci are able to persist in human hosts via their ability to invade epithelial cells. The initial steps of intracellular invasion involve attachment of microbes to epithelial cell surfaces through synergistic effects of pili, Opa proteins, and porin proteins.[18,85,137] Gonococci also exploit the production of complement factors, including C3, by cervical epithelial cells. In females, especially during the luteal phase and menses, C3 is secreted into the extracellular milieu, where it is activated to C3b. The gonococcal surface binds C3b and cleaves it to iC3b (inactive), which then serves as a ligand for the complement receptor 3 molecules on host cells that facilitates microbial attachment independently of pili and Opa proteins.[106]

After adhering to host epithelial cells, some microbes are internalized by endocytosis triggered by interaction of gonococcal phospholipase D with host cell Akt (protein kinase B).[106] The vast majority of invading gonococci are ingested and killed by neutrophils. Gonococci are susceptible to the oxidative burst products of phagocytes, as well as to nonoxidative products such as cathepsin G.[49,293] Those that survive

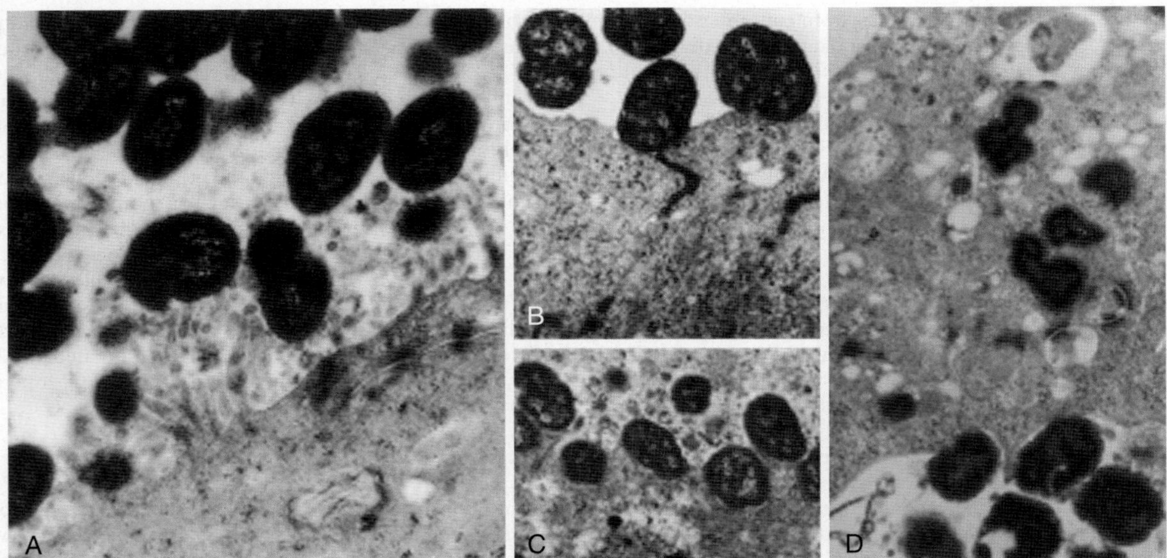

FIG. 89.4 Electron micrographs of *Neisseria gonorrhoeae* (strain MS11) interactions with polarized T84 human epithelial cell monolayers. At early stages of infection, the microbes adhere to the apical plasma membrane as microcolonies. (A) Adherent bacteria are surrounded by a matrix of microvilli. (B–C) Bacteria subsequently disperse from the microcolony and adhere as a monolayer in which bacterial and host-cell membranes are tightly apposed. (C) The region of contact between the bacteria and the host-cell membrane enlarges, with subsequent internalization of the microbes. (D) Bacteria then traverse the host cell and exit via the basolateral membrane. (From Merz AJ, So M. Interactions of pathogenic *Neisseriae* with epithelial cell membranes. *Annu Rev Cell Dev Biol.* 2000;16:423-457.)

intracellularly may replicate inside the phagosomes and ultimately exit the basal (but not lateral) surface of the cell via exocytosis[214,219,234] (Fig. 89.4). Adjacent nonepithelial cells are sloughed, probably because of the toxicity of LOS and peptidoglycans.[135] Mucosal cell damage and submucosal invasion are followed by an influx of neutrophils along with the formation of submucosal microabscesses and exudation of purulent material into the lumen of the infected organ.[341]

Adherence of gonococci to mucosal epithelial cells causes activation of nuclear factor-κB (NFκB) and activator protein 1, which in turn leads to upregulation and release of multiple cytokines and chemokines, including macrophage colony-stimulating factor, tumor necrosis factor-α (TNF-α), tumor growth factor-β (TGF-β), monocyte chemoattractant protein 1, IL-1β, IL-6, and IL-8.[235,259]

N. gonorrhoeae can form biofilms during cervical infection. Membrane blebs that contain DNA elements and outer membrane structures are key components of these biofilms. A gonococcal thermonuclease is involved in remodeling of biofilm matrix. Cells in the biofilm activate gene sets involved in anaerobic respiration.[114]

Resistance to Phagocytosis and Intracellular Killing

Subsets of infecting gonococci are able to resist extracellular killing by neutrophils through mechanisms that are increasingly understood. The microbes also resist phagocytosis via blocking deposition of opsonic antibodies and complement components on their own surfaces and by antigenic variation of their surface structures to evade any preexisting humoral immune responses. Antibody binding is inhibited by sialylation of surface lipo-oligosaccharide (LOS). Gonococci thwart the effects of complement via binding of the complement cascade inhibitor complement factor H to porin proteins and LOS.[85]

N. gonorrhoeae have multiple mechanisms by which they resist oxidative and nonoxidative killing after phagocytosis by neutrophils. The species produces catalase, cytochrome *c* peroxidase, superoxide dismutase, and a metalloproteinase that detoxify superoxide compounds produced in phagolysosomes. Gonococci also have repair systems for oxidatively damaged DNA. Nonoxidative antibacterial factors such as lysozyme, elastase, cathepsin G, defensins, and cathelicidins can be counteracted by gonococcal efflux pump systems, metalloproteinase, and other protein and regulatory systems.[85]

Neutrophil extracellular traps (NETs) form from chromatin and neutrophil granule components as neutrophils undergo programmed cell death in association with the oxidative burst in response to bacterial infection. Gonococci elicit NETs but may be able to degrade these with expression of the thermonuclease and also are able to suppress the oxidative burst process.[142,178]

Specific Virulence Factors

Specific *N. gonorrhoeae* virulence factors include (1) pili, (2) opacity proteins, (3) porin protein, (4) the ability to survive in low iron environments, (5) immunoglobulin (Ig)A protease, (6) LOS, (7) cell wall peptidoglycan, (8) reduction modifiable protein (Rmp), and (9) a type IV secretion system. Many other gonococcal gene products and molecular systems have been identified, and a more detailed and complex understanding of virulence at the molecular level is steadily forthcoming.

Pili

Gonococci are piliated predominantly in vivo and express type IV pili. Pili cover essentially the entire surface of the cell and are arranged in individual fibrils or fibrillar aggregates. Pili consist primarily of polymers of an 18-kd subunit now denoted as PilE. A single pilus is approximately 6 nm in diameter and up to several microns in length.[219] Each may contain thousands of PilE subunits.[42] The PilC protein is present in lower numbers in the pilus but appears to be the key pilus adhesin. PilC interacts with CD46 molecules, which are present on most human cells and serve as receptors for C3b, C4b, measles, and other viruses. PilC-CD46 attachment appears to be a key step in the initiation of microbial adherence to host cells.[44,181,190,277,279]

Binding of pili to a host-cell membrane induces at least two responses in the host cell: release of Ca^{2+} from intracellular stores[180] and cytoskeletal rearrangements with the formation of cortical plaques that represent an accumulation of actin, ezrin, and other phosphotyrosine-containing proteins.[217,263] The latter results in elongation of the microvilli that embrace the microbe. Formation of plaque appears to be induced by retraction of the attached pilus, and retraction depends on another pilus protein designated PilT.[220]

Gonococcal pili undergo both phase variation (switching from piliated to nonpiliated states) and high-frequency antigenic variation.[43] These variations occur during natural infection and in vitro passage.[289] Pili have a common N-terminal domain, semivariable domains in the midportion, and two hypervariable regions in the carboxyl-terminal of the pilin protein subunit.[306] Relatively invariant regions occur between the variable domains. The pilin protein consists of 159 to 160 amino acids. The chromosome contains either one or two complete pilin genes. The expressed gene contains an intact promoter region, a ribosome binding site, and a seven–amino acid signal sequence in addition to the pilin sequence. Scattered around the chromosome are six to eight loci that contain varying portions of the pilin sequence without the promoter region or the 5′ end of the structural gene. Some loci may contain many incomplete pilin sequences arranged head to tail that differ slightly from one another. Movement of these sequences into the active expression site through nonreciprocal combination events results in antigenic variation of the pilus protein. If recombination leads to a faulty pilin subunit product that cannot be processed into a mature pilus, the progeny of that organism become nonpiliated (phase variation). Subsequent recombination events can allow reversion back to the piliated phase.[145,221,222,239,288,306,319]

In addition to promoting adhesion to epithelial cells, pili also provide a twitching motility, are involved in DNA transformation, and may play a role in resistance to ingestion by phagocytic cells.[228] The presence of pili, perhaps mediated through their promotion of adhesion, affects the activation of $CD4^+$ T-lymphocytes and the production of IL-10. This property may help gonococci diminish the T-cell response to their presence.[253]

Opacity-Associated Proteins

Opa proteins also influence adherence of the gonococcus to host cells. The isolation of particular Opa protein phenotypes from different anatomic sites or at different times during the menstrual cycle has suggested that these proteins contribute to the ability of the organism to succeed in a given niche. Opa proteins (formerly designated protein II) are a set of as many as 12 related proteins that are variably present in gonococcal outer membranes. Opa proteins are 24 to 28 kDa in size and confer increased opacity to colonies of organisms by promoting adherence of the organisms to one another. A given strain has the capacity to make at least 10 different Opa proteins but appears to express no more than five at the same time. Some cells express no Opa proteins. Like pili, Opa proteins undergo both antigenic and phase variation. Both types of variations can occur within a single colony, so sector variations in opacity can be seen.[27,305,317,318]

Each *opa* gene is present as a complete gene with its own promoter and is transcribed at all times. Phase variation in expression occurs at the translational level. Each gene has a varying number of pentameric CTCTT repeat units adjacent to the ATG start codon. When the number of repeats is divisible by three, the transcribed mRNA is translationally in frame and the Opa protein is expressed. The number of pentameric repeats is subject to high-frequency variation. Antigenic variation results from recombination between the two hypervariable regions in each of the *opa* genes.[75,308–320]

Two classes of host-cell receptors for Opa proteins have been identified. Heparan sulfate–proteoglycan (HSPG) receptors are present on epithelial cells and interact with one particular Opa protein variant (Opa_{50}). HSPG binding can stimulate the lipid hydrolysis enzymes phosphatidylcholine-specific phospholipase C and acid sphingomyelinase and thereby lead to clathrin-independent endocytosis. HSPG-Opa binding also can lead to interactions with serum factors such as vitronectin and fibronectin, which then mediate endocytosis via host-cell integrin receptors. The CD66 family is present on epithelial cells and neutrophils, recognizes many different Opa proteins, and mediates nonopsonic phagocytosis, a process distinct from antibody- and complement-mediated phagocytosis.[92,91,134,193,218,219,330]

Porin Protein

Formerly designated protein I, porin protein is the most common gonococcal outer-membrane protein. Porin is 34 to 36 kDa, is exposed on the surface, exists as a trimer in the membrane, and is physically proximate to LOS and Rmp.[28,155] The trimer forms an anion-specific pore in the bacterial membrane that allows small water-soluble molecules to enter the cell.[344] The *por* locus has two alleles that encode chemically and immunologically distinct classes of porin protein—PorA and PorB—that are similar to porin proteins in other gram-negative bacteria. A given strain expresses only PorA or PorB, and many antigenic variants of both exist (thereby forming the basis for serotyping).[48,188]

The porin trimer appears to translocate into the host-cell membrane and is able to disrupt neutrophil degranulation, the oxidative burst, and phagosome maturation,[146,205,227] in addition to induction of apoptosis in epithelial cells and neutrophils in vitro.[231] Exposure to gonococcal porin protein induces the typical structural and biochemical changes seen in apoptotic cells.[230] Porin translocation permits rapid influx of Ca^{2+} into the host cell from the external environment.[231] Porin proteins also may play a role in endocytosis mediated by the binding of HSPG and Opa protein[18] and in downregulation of complement by binding with C4b-binding protein.[258]

Iron Metabolism

Iron is an essential nutrient for *N. gonorrhoeae,* and, in host tissues, iron is sequestered in hemin compounds as ferritin or is bound to lactoferrin or transferrin. The species does not produce any siderophores but relies on an iron-repressible system that scavenges iron from transferrin, lactoferrin, and hemoglobin. This system comprises numerous proteins, some of which serve as receptors for the aforementioned iron-bearing ligands.[25,69,80,335] Other components include a TonB-dependent transporter and an associated lipoprotein that are expressed ubiquitously by gonococci, have limited antigenic variability, and are important for growth in vivo.[79] These proteins thus have potential as vaccine targets.

Immunoglobulin A Protease

All gonococci (and meningococci, but not nonpathogenic *Neisseria* spp.) make a protease that cleaves both serum and secretory IgA1 (but not IgA2) at the hinge region with the release of Fab and Fc fragments. This protease may help the organism evade host IgA at the mucosal surface, especially early in secondary infections, when preexisting antibodies may be present. However, mutant strains without the IgA protease have limited ability to grow inside epithelial cells. The protease appears to cleave a host-cell intracellular protein (LAMP1) involved in phagosome compartmentalization.[199] IgA1 protease is not required for gonococci to cause experimental urethritis,[173] thus suggesting that its intraphagosome function may be more important in pathogenesis.

Lipo-Oligosaccharide

Gonococci express LOS complexes of 3 to 7 kDa on their cell surface. LOS consists of a lipid A moiety and a core polysaccharide comprising ketodeoxyoctanoic acid, heptose, glucose, galactose, glucosamine, galactosamine, or any combination of these constituents.[139] The lack of a long polymeric sugar attached to the core distinguishes LOS from the lipopolysaccharides of other gram-negative bacteria. The core sugar antigens of LOS are subject to intrastrain and interstrain variation, and a single strain may express as many as six variants of LOS.[94,138] Numerous genes are involved in LOS synthesis; these genes undergo high-frequency phase variation similar to *opa* genes.[133] LOS terminal sugars mimic the structure of certain human glycosphingolipids.[139]

Gonococci with predominately short LOS molecules appear to be more sensitive to killing by human serum but also more able to invade eukaryotic cells. Strains with longer LOS are more serum-resistant but noninvasive.[331] Longer LOS moieties are sialylated readily with host neuraminic acid by a bacterial sialyltransferase that appears to shield both LOS and porin molecules from antibody binding, thus providing protection from complement-mediated killing in serum.[32,336]

LOS from serum-sensitive strains is able to activate the classic complement pathway and may do so in the absence of antibody.[292] LOS induces the production of cytokines (i.e., TNF-α, IL-1β, IL-6, and IL-8) by urethral epithelial cells[148] and can mediate host defensin-enhanced adherence to epithelial cells.[132]

Cell Wall Peptidoglycan and Lytic Transglycosylases

Gonococci shed membrane fragments with peptidoglycan into their environment during exponential growth. Peptidoglycan monomers have numerous biologic properties, including activation of complement and modulation of mononuclear cell proliferation. These fragments also damage fallopian tube mucosa in organ culture, thus suggesting a pathogenic role for the compounds in invasive disease.[135,214] Production of peptidoglycan monomers is a by-product of lytic transglycosylases that act during cell growth and division. At least five such enzymes are encoded by *N. gonorrhoeae*. These also may facilitate gene transfers as part of type IV secretion.[65]

Reduction Modifiable Protein

Rmp (formerly designated protein III) is an antigenically conserved, 30- to 31-kDa protein that is present in all pathogenic *Neisseria*. Rmp is located proximate to LOS and porin in the outer membrane. Antibodies that bind to Rmp epitopes block the bactericidal effect of the complement-fixing IgM antibodies that recognize LOS. Women with preexisting anti-Rmp antibodies appear to be more susceptible to the development of infection than do those without such antibodies.[268,269,305]

Ribosomal Protein L12

Ribosomal protein L12 mimics the structure of human chorionic gonadotropin, the natural ligand for lutropin receptors. It is able to bind to lutropin receptors in the upper female genital tract, which may facilitate ascending infection in females.[104,309]

Type IV Secretion System

About 80% of *N. gonorrhoeae* strains encode a horizontally acquired 57-kb genetic island that encodes a type IV secretion system (T4SS). A T4SS is a multiprotein complex that functions as a conjugation system. In gonococci the T4SS secretes single-stranded chromosomal DNA into the extracellular environment. T4SS expression may enhance microbial survival inside human cells in addition to its role in genetic recombination and natural transformation among gonococcal strains.[260]

Characteristics of Strains Causing Disseminated Disease

The increased virulence of some strains is suggested by observations such as a microepidemic of gonorrhea involving one asymptomatic infected male and eight female contacts.[149] Seven of the women were infected symptomatically, and four experienced disseminated infection. Overall many infections are asymptomatic and dissemination is relatively rare.

Strains of *N. gonorrhoeae* obtained from adult patients with disseminated disease usually are less susceptible to the bactericidal activity of sera.[38,73,266,267,294] These strains have an atypical growth pattern on agar[224] that reflects the absence of Opa protein expression, which suggests that the genetic variation capacity described earlier allows adaptation to different niches and probably helps organisms elude the host response.[22] Unlike most gonococcal strains, many invasive strains (designated AHU$^-$) require arginine, uracil, and hypoxanthine for growth.[186] A high degree of sensitivity to penicillin also has been characteristic of most strains from patients with disseminated disease.[340] Many also are susceptible to vancomycin, which may prevent detection in selective media. These strains should be detected in the usual media used for blood culture.

Host Response

The adult response to local and systemic infection with *N. gonorrhoeae* has been investigated extensively, but no such studies have been performed on infected children. Gonococcal infections usually are characterized by intense inflammation that involves neutrophilic and mononuclear granulocytes. The vast majority of gonococcal cells ingested by neutrophils are killed.[49] Gonococci are susceptible to the oxidative products produced by neutrophils but also can be killed efficiently by nonoxidative products such as cathepsin G.[293]

An intact complement system is essential for successful eradication of the organism. Properdin-mediated recruitment of C4b-binding protein facilitates antibody-mediated complement-dependent killing of gonococci that resist destruction via the classic complement pathway.[141] Persons with inherited or acquired complement deficiencies may be predisposed to contracting disseminated gonococcal infection, as is the case with meningococcal infection. Approximately 13% of patients with disseminated disease have complement deficiencies.[109,242]

Adherence of gonococci in vitro induces the activation of NFκB and activator protein 1, which leads to upregulation of messenger RNA (mRNA) and release of numerous cytokines and chemokines: macrophage colony-stimulating factor, TNF-α, TNF-β, monocyte chemoattractant protein 1, IL-1β, IL-6, and IL-8.[235] Intraurethral challenge leads to increased levels of IL-8, IL-6, and TNF-α in urine before the onset of symptoms and in plasma at the onset of symptoms.[259]

Multiple episodes of gonorrhea may occur in a single individual in a short period and may be caused by the same strain. The antigenic diversity and ease of altering the antigenicity of both pili and opacity proteins undoubtedly contribute to the insufficiency of the host response in preventing reinfection. Noninvasive mucosal infections elicit production of low-affinity, broadly reactive IgM antibody by IgD$^+$, CD27$^+$ B cells in a T-cell–independent manner that may partially explain the limited humoral response to typical infections.[304] In a mouse model of vaginal infection, gonococci induce T_H17 inflammatory responses, which drive neutrophil influx. T_H1- and T_H2-adaptive specific antibody responses are suppressed by increased production of TGF-β plus enhanced development of T-regulatory cells. TGF-β production is mediated by interaction of Opa proteins with carcinoembryonic antigen related–cellular adhesion (CEACAM) molecules on human cells.[203]

Circulating humoral antibody to the infecting strain is present in most persons who have prolonged mucosal colonization with *N. gonorrhoeae*.[183] Women who develop pelvic inflammatory disease (PID) usually produce bactericidal antibody during the infection. IgA- and IgG-blocking antibodies against some gonococcal antigens appear to block killing of the bacteria mediated by otherwise bactericidal IgG and IgM antibodies.[266] Serum antibody responses are greater in patients with invasive disease (e.g., bacteremia or salpingitis).

Secretory IgA antibody is present in the urethral exudate of men with gonorrhea and in the genital secretions of women with gonorrhea.[243] The development of local IgA antibody occurs more rapidly and is more transient than development of the serum bactericidal response. Microbial IgA1 protease is not required for infection but may play a role in reinfection.

A cellular immune response to gonococcal antigens in patients with uncomplicated gonorrhea has been demonstrated in vitro.[196] The significance of this response in controlling or preventing infection is unknown.

PERINATAL GONOCOCCAL INFECTIONS

Since the 1970s, health clinics have encouraged the routine screening of sexually active women for gonorrhea, especially during pregnancy. Adolescent girls have a higher prevalence of gonorrhea than do older women of child-bearing age. This probably translates into higher rates of gonorrhea in pregnant adolescents. Rates of gonococcal infection in neonates reflect the frequency of infection in pregnant women. Recognition of gonorrhea early in pregnancy identifies a population at risk who should be monitored sequentially for reinfection throughout pregnancy.[175]

The spectrum of infection with *N. gonorrhoeae* appears to be similar in pregnant and nonpregnant women. Most are asymptomatic. Pharyngeal infection seems to occur more commonly during pregnancy, perhaps reflecting altered sexual practices. One study reported that 39% of patients with *N. gonorrhoeae* at any site had concurrent involvement of the pharynx and that 30% had pharyngeal infection as the sole manifestation.[78] In adolescent girls, pregnancy and menstruation are associated with disseminated disease.[158]

Gonorrheal infection puts both the mother and infant at risk for the development of other forms of gonococcal disease. Pregnant women, including those of adolescent age, have an increased risk for the development of gonococcal septic arthritis, and most such cases occur during the third trimester or in the immediate postpartum period.[39,158]

Gonococcal PID and acute salpingitis may complicate the pregnancy of an infected woman.[123] When these complications occur during the first trimester there is a high rate of fetal loss. Untreated gonorrhea late in pregnancy can lead to postpartum fever in the mother.[170]

Hazards to the fetus posed by maternal gonorrhea include septic abortion, perinatal death, prematurity, perinatal distress, and premature

TABLE 89.2 Pregnancy Complications and Outcomes of Mothers Who Were Infected With *Neisseria Gonorrhoeae* at Delivery

Pregnancy Complications and Outcomes	Charles et al[66] (*N* = 14)[a] (%)	Sarrel and Pruett[284] (*N* = 37) (%)	Israel et al[170] (*N* = 39) (%)	Amstey and Steadman[6] (*N* = 222)[a] (%)	Edwards et al[105] (*N* = 19)[a] (%)	Handsfield and Holmes[149] (*N* = 12)[a] (%)
Normal or term infant	—	13 (35)	30 (77)	142 (64)	7 (37)	—
Aborted	—	13 (35)	1 (2)	24 (11)	—	—
Perinatal death	—	3 (8)	1 (2)	15 (7)	2 (11)	—
Premature	—	6 (16)	5 (13)	49 (22)	8 (42)	8 (67)
Perinatal distress	—	—	2 (5)	—	2 (11)	—
Premature rupture of membranes	6 (43)	8 (22)	—	52 (23)	12 (63)	9 (75)

[a]Data were provided in which the outcomes of pregnancies of mothers not infected with *N. gonorrhoeae* were shown to be significantly more favorable.

rupture of membranes. Prolonged rupture of membranes, premature delivery, chorioamnionitis, funisitis, and a clinical diagnosis of sepsis occur frequently in infants with *N. gonorrhoeae* detected in the gastric aspirate during delivery.[6,105,108,148,273] Table 89.2 tabulates the proportions in six studies of infants born to infected mothers who experienced these problems.

Gonococcal Ophthalmia Neonatorum

Epidemiology

The increased risk for ophthalmia neonatorum among infants born to women with vaginal discharge has been recognized for centuries. Recommendations for flushing the eyes of a newborn commonly were given before the 20th century.[216] In the late 1800s, Neisser helped establish the relationship between the gonococcus and neonatal ophthalmia.

By 1881, Dr. Carl Sigmund Franz Credé recognized that asymptomatic disease in the mother was a potential source of infection.[84] Gonorrhea was highly prevalent in Europe; gonococcal ophthalmia neonatorum (GON) was occurring in approximately 10% of newborns in major cities. The infection was the cause of a large proportion of admissions to schools for the blind.[16] Credé described the technique of instillation of 2% silver nitrate into the infant's conjunctival sac, which remains one method recommended for preventive procedures today.

By 1930, most states in the United States required that all newborns receive silver nitrate prophylaxis (i.e., the Credé procedure). GON decreased as a cause of admission to schools for the blind in the United States, from an average of 24% from 1906 to 1911 to 0.5% from 1951 to 1955.

The worldwide decline in adult gonorrhea in the 1950s probably contributed to the decreased recognition of disease in newborns during that period. The incidence of GON rose in the 1960s and 1970s along with the increased incidence of gonorrhea in the general population and was very high in some developing nations.[193] In Los Angeles, the rate rose from nine per 100,000 live births in 1957 to 1958 to 56 per 100,000 live births in 1962 to 1963. In a New York hospital between 1970 and 1973, a rate of 145 per 100,000 births was reported; in a hospital in North Carolina during 1969 and 1970, a rate of 265 per 100,000 live births was proved by culture.[303] In the late 1970s and 1980s, GON again subsided in developed countries but has remained a problem in underdeveloped nations.

Factors associated with higher rates of GON include lower socioeconomic class of the mother and longer duration of rupture of membranes before delivery.[10] An increased incidence of GON in infants of unwed mothers and mothers who have not had prenatal care also may exist.[299] Previous treatment of gonorrhea during pregnancy also is associated with an increased incidence of GON.[175] The incidence of prematurity in infants with GON often is reported to be higher. Premature rupture of membranes appears to increase the risk for GON.

Prevention

In the United States, prophylaxis for GON is recommended for all infants immediately after birth and is required by law in most states.[327] Prophylaxis regimens using a 1% solution of silver nitrate, 1% tetracycline ointment, or 0.5% erythromycin ophthalmic ointment are equally effective. In the United States, erythromycin 0.5% ophthalmic ointment is the only one of these agents available for prophylaxis of GON. Single-dose units are preferred over multidose tubes. One unit should be instilled into the eyes of every neonate as soon as possible after delivery. Instillation may be delayed for as long as 1 hour to facilitate parent-infant bonding.

The efficacies of tetracycline and erythromycin preparations in the prevention of tetracycline-resistant *N. gonorrhoeae* ophthalmia are unknown.[244] Both probably are effective because of the high concentration of drug in these preparations.

Silver Nitrate and Gonococcal Ophthalmia Neonatorum

Numerous studies have compared the efficacy of silver nitrate and no prophylaxis or prophylaxis with another agent in the prevention of GON.[67,226,274] Such studies consistently showed lower rates of GON in treated versus untreated infants. Decreased frequency of blindness from GON in the population during the past half century, even during periods of increased rates of gonorrhea in women of child-bearing age, further supports the benefits of silver nitrate prophylaxis.

In a randomized trial of Kenyan infants born to mothers with gonorrhea reported in 1988, rates of GON were 42% in the control group, 7% in the group treated with 1% silver nitrate (83% reduction), and 3% in the group treated with 1% tetracycline (93% reduction). The two treatment arms were not statistically different.[195] In a randomized trial in the United States involving infants born to women without gonococcal infection, infants treated with 1% silver nitrate had a 39% lower rate (statistically significant) of conjunctivitis of any type in the first 2 months of life than did infants who received no prophylaxis. Infants treated with 0.5% erythromycin ointment in this trial had a 31% reduction in contrast to control infants, but this result was not statistically significant.[19]

The major advantages of the use of silver nitrate for prophylaxis are the lack of allergic potential, the absence of development of bacterial resistance to the compound, and very low cost. Two outbreaks of erythromycin-resistant staphylococcal conjunctivitis in newborn nurseries have been associated with the use of erythromycin eye ointment as ocular prophylaxis, but the outbreaks remitted when silver nitrate was substituted. Disadvantages include the occurrence of conjunctival irritation with associated development of exudate in many neonates. Failure of silver nitrate prophylaxis (as well as other agents for prevention of GON) does occur. Improper administration of silver nitrate such that the solution does not reach the conjunctival sac, irrigation performed too quickly after instillation, and inadvertent omission of prophylaxis can lead to apparent failure. When gonococcal infection of the eye has become established before birth, silver nitrate is not expected to prevent further progression. The increased risk for GON associated with premature rupture of membranes is due to exposure to and establishment of infection before actual delivery. In some cases of premature rupture of membranes, clinically apparent GON can be present at the time of birth.

Despite these problems, the use of 1% silver nitrate remains a widely accepted, carefully evaluated, and safe form of GON prophylaxis. The occasional failure of silver nitrate prophylaxis emphasizes that it is preferable to prevent GON through identification and treatment of pregnant women.

Clinical Features

The newborn eye is subject to colonization with numerous bacterial organisms that cause infections that usually are clinically mild, nonprogressive, and characterized by conjunctival discharge. The bacteria most commonly associated with conjunctival discharge are *Haemophilus influenzae, Streptococcus pneumoniae, Staphylococcus aureus, Neisseria cinerea, Klebsiella pneumoniae,* enterococci, and *C. trachomatis.*[100,192] Viral causes include herpes simplex virus and adenoviruses. In contrast, infection of the eye of a newborn with *N. gonorrhoeae* results in disease of a severity that, despite frequently being mild, can be rapidly destructive and lead to scarring and blindness. The chemical conjunctivitis that can result from silver nitrate prophylaxis typically starts within 6 to 24 hours after administration and disappears within 24 to 48 hours.

Colonization during delivery is followed by an incubation period of 2 to 5 days and usually less than 3 days, but cases occasionally may be recognized for 2 to 3 weeks after delivery.[121] A discharge typically develops that initially is watery but usually becomes thick and mucopurulent within a short time and may contain blood (Fig. 89.5). The disease generally is bilateral. Early findings include prominent edema of the conjunctivae and lids, followed by edema and later ulceration of the cornea or spread to wider areas in severe cases. Rapid arrest of the disease is essential because the degree of corneal involvement determines whether vision will be preserved. Some cases are self-limited and have benign outcomes, and occasional cases of asymptomatic GON have been discovered during routine screening.[255] Perforation of the globe and panophthalmitis can result from extensive local disease. The conjunctivae may serve as a portal of entry for gonococcal septicemia, arthritis, or other manifestations of invasive disease, but such events seldom occur.

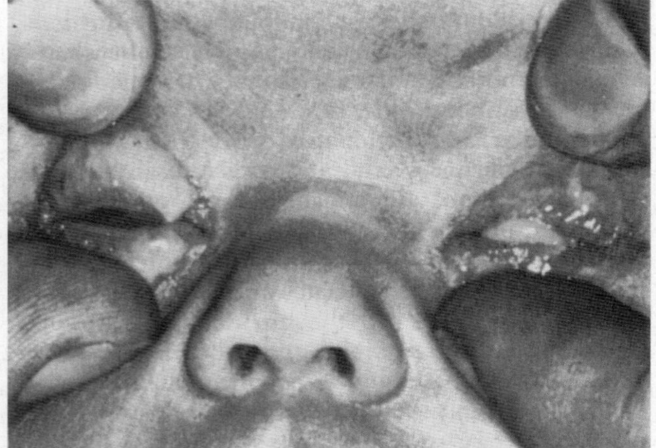

FIG. 89.5 Gonococcal ophthalmia neonatorum. The usual clinical finding is bilateral conjunctivitis that becomes progressively purulent if untreated. (From Gutman LT. Gonococcal infections. *Semin Pediatr Infect Dis.* 2005;16:4.)

A presumptive diagnosis may be made by demonstrating typical gram-negative diplococci by Gram stain of conjunctival exudate. Because other organisms also may cause exudative infection of the conjunctivae, laboratory confirmation of the diagnosis of GON depends on culture results of *N. gonorrhoeae.*

Invasive disease rarely occurs in association with GON, but neonates with clinical evidence suggestive of GON should be evaluated for disseminated disease. The evaluation should include a thorough physical examination, especially of the joints. Exudate from the eyes or other sites of apparent local infection should be sent for Gram stain and culture on appropriate media.

Current recommendations in the United States are to obtain cultures of blood, eye discharge, and other potential sites of infection, including CSF.[343] The absolute necessity of obtaining CSF for analysis and culture in otherwise well-appearing neonates is not certain but likely prudent. Neonates with GON generally should be hospitalized as part of initial management.

Testing for *C. trachomatis* infection of the conjunctiva also should be performed.

Gonococcal Scalp Abscess and Other Local Infections

Gonococcal infections of scalp wounds occur especially after fetal monitoring electrodes have been used on infants born to infected mothers.[88] The lesions may produce extensive local inflammatory disease and necrosis and can be a focus for disseminated infection. A scalp wound in a neonate should be cultured for gonococci, as well as other likely pathogens, which include *Staphylococcus* spp., group B streptococci, *H. influenzae,* and gram-negative enteric flora. Herpes simplex also may be present in areas of injury to the scalp of newborns. Overall approximately one in 200 births that are monitored with fetal scalp electrodes are complicated by infection at the monitoring site.[254]

Neonatal gonococcal vulvovaginitis, proctitis, rhinitis, funisitis, and urethritis have been described but are rare.[144] Gonococcal colonization of the oropharynx, gastric fluid, or both occurs relatively frequently in perinatally exposed infants, however. Pharyngeal colonization is present in as many as 35% of neonates who have GON.[119] A summary of selected studies on the incidence of neonatal gonococcal colonization and disease in exposed infants is presented in Table 89.3.

Infants with localized gonococcal infection other than GON should have cultures obtained of blood, CSF, and the site of infection, if feasible. They should be hospitalized pending the availability of culture results.

Systemic Disease in the Neonate

Disseminated disease occurs in 1% or fewer of infants who are perinatally exposed to gonococcal infection[12] (see Table 89.3). Septic arthritis is the most common form of disseminated gonococcal infection in neonates. Gonococcal arthritis of the newborn was described extensively between 1900 and 1930,[76,77,334] and recent case reports suggest that the disease remains similar. Clinical findings usually become evident when the infant is 1 to 4 weeks old. Although a few infants with gonococcal arthritis will have evidence of GON or other sites of mucosal or skin infection at the time of onset of arthritis, most do not. Concurrent gonococcal arthritis in both mother and newborn infant has been described.[136]

The signs and symptoms of gonococcal septic arthritis are similar to those of joint infection caused by other microbes in the neonatal

TABLE 89.3 Incidence of Neonatal Gonococcal Disease in Exposed Infants

Site of Neonatal Infection	Rate of Positive Cultures (%)	Population	References
Conjunctiva	0–10	Exposed infants who underwent silver nitrate ocular prophylaxis	4, 10, 105,193
	2–48	Exposed infants who had no ocular prophylaxis	119, 188, 274
Orogastric fluid	26–40	Infants of infected mothers	105, 148
Oropharynx	35	Infants with gonococcal ophthalmia	193
Disseminated disease as a proportion of all neonatal gonorrhea	0–1 (rare)	Reported series of neonatal gonococcal disease	105, 117, 119, 323, 332

period, including a predominance of polyarticular involvement. Infection most frequently involves the ankles, knees, wrists, and hands.[76] The hip may be infected with minimal signs other than pseudoparesis. Involvement of a joint may include suppurative arthritis, inflammatory disease of the periarticular structures, and tenosynovitis. Leukocytosis usually occurs, and most infants have a positive culture and compatible Gram stain results from the synovial fluid of the involved joint.[128]

Prompt drainage of septic hips, along with initiation of antimicrobial therapy, is necessary because of the risk for development of aseptic necrosis of the femoral head. Long-term dysfunction from gonococcal infection of other joints seldom occurs.[77,144,160,189]

Although gonococcal sepsis can develop in neonates with or without associated septic arthritis, the bacteremic phase of spread to the joints from the initial sites of infection generally is typically clinically silent. Premature infants seem to be more at risk for the development of sepsis with bacteremia than are term infants. Meningitis is an exceedingly rare manifestation of neonatal gonococcal infection.[31,144,148]

GONOCOCCAL DISEASE BEYOND THE NEONATAL PERIOD

Lower Genital Tract Infection in Prepubertal Girls

Gonococcal vaginitis or vulvovaginitis is the most common form of gonorrhea in prepubertal girls beyond the neonatal period. In contrast to that of postpubertal females, the anestrogenic vaginal mucosa of prepubertal girls creates an alkaline environment that is colonized and infected more readily with *N. gonorrhoeae*. Infection of the endocervix, urethra, paraurethral and Bartholin's glands, and upper genital tract occurs only rarely.

Gonococcal vaginitis in prepubertal girls almost always is symptomatic, with vulvar erythema and a profuse vaginal discharge (Fig. 89.6). The girl may complain of dysuria, urinary frequency, vulvar discomfort, or pain while walking.[232,294,296] Asymptomatic cases are uncommon.

Signs and symptoms should resolve promptly within a few days after treatment is initiated, but acute manifestations may persist for several weeks if the child is not treated. The natural course of disease is for the inflammation to subside and the discharge to become scant and seropurulent. Infection may resolve spontaneously but occasionally may persist until the girl reaches puberty.

Prepubertal vulvovaginitis can be caused by numerous irritative and infectious agents, including pinworms, foreign bodies, group A streptococci, *Neisseria meningitidis, Neisseria sicca,* and *Moraxella catarrhalis* (see Chapter 42). Vulvovaginitis can mimic urinary tract infection, and pyuria can be seen on urinalysis with gonococcal and other causes of vulvovaginitis.[120,202]

Although ascending infection seldom occurs in this age group, it may result in salpingitis or peritonitis. One study found that 10% of young girls with gonorrhea had signs compatible with peritonitis, including fever, diffuse abdominal pain, leukocytosis, and decreased bowel sounds.[45] Salpingitis and periappendicitis may cause findings similar to those of appendicitis.[11]

In children with gonorrheal infection of the genitourinary tract resulting from sexual abuse concomitant anorectal and tonsillopharyngeal colonization are common.[237]

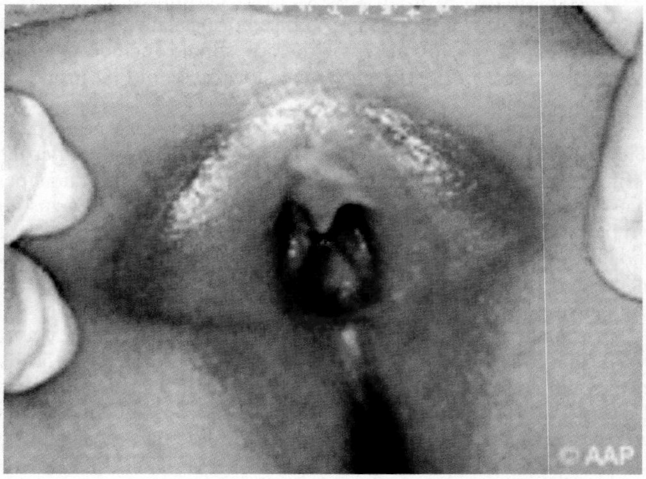

FIG. 89.6 Profuse, purulent vaginal discharge in an 18-month-old girl with gonococcal vulvovaginitis. Gonococcal infections in prepubertal children are almost always the result of sexual abuse. (From American Academy of Pediatrics 2012 Red Book Collection.)

Lower Genital Tract Infection in Postmenarchal Females

Gonococcal infections in adolescent girls are similar to those in adults. The endocervix is the primary site of urogenital infection, although the external genitalia, urethra, vulvar mucosa, and vestibular glands also may be infected. Symptoms of acute infection usually begin 3 to 5 days after exposure with the development of a profuse, purulent vaginal discharge. The vulvar tissues are inflamed, with resultant pruritus and a burning sensation. Urethritis often is present initially and can lead to dysuria with urinary frequency and urgency. Urethral discharge can be seen but is much less prominent than in males. A purulent discharge from the vestibular and paraurethral glands also may be noted.

The endocervical mucosa is edematous, inflamed, and often friable (Fig. 89.7). A profuse yellow-green discharge is present and detaches easily from the surface. The zone of endocervical ectopy that normally is present in as many as 50% of adolescents may appear bright red, does not bleed easily when touched with swabs, and should not be mistaken for cervicitis. Ectopy that appears swollen and friable suggests cervicitis. Nabothian inclusion cysts (transparent and grayish) also are normal findings.

Infection of Bartholin's (major vestibular) gland or paraurethral (Skene's) gland ducts may develop during acute gonorrhea. Bartholin's gland abscesses appear as large, circumscribed painful swellings of the dorsal aspect of the labium minus (Fig. 89.8). This occurs in about 5% of females with endocervical gonorrhea.[262] Paraurethral duct abscesses appear as small painful swellings in the urethrovaginal septum and may cause dysuria. Rupture into the urethra can create a urethral diverticulum. Bartholin's gland or paraurethral duct abscesses should be incised and drained.

If the gonococcal infection goes untreated, the acute symptoms generally subside in 8 to 10 weeks. In a cohort of 387 adolescents 14 to 17 years of age who were evaluated by weekly quantitative cultures, 16 developed acute infection. Microbial load did not correlate with genitourinary symptoms.[315]

Persisting acute symptoms are more likely to represent reinfection than chronic infection. Chronic urethritis, thickening of the vestibular glands and paraurethral ducts, and chronic cervicitis can occur. A

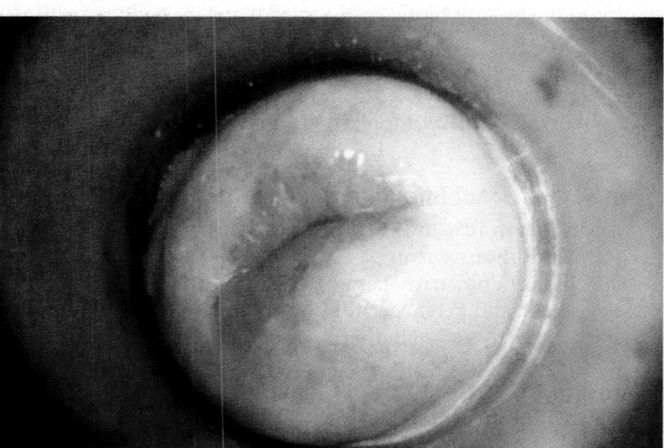

FIG. 89.7 Colposcopic view of cervix showing eroded ostium resulting from gonococcal infection. (From American Academy of Pediatrics 2012 Red Book Collection.)

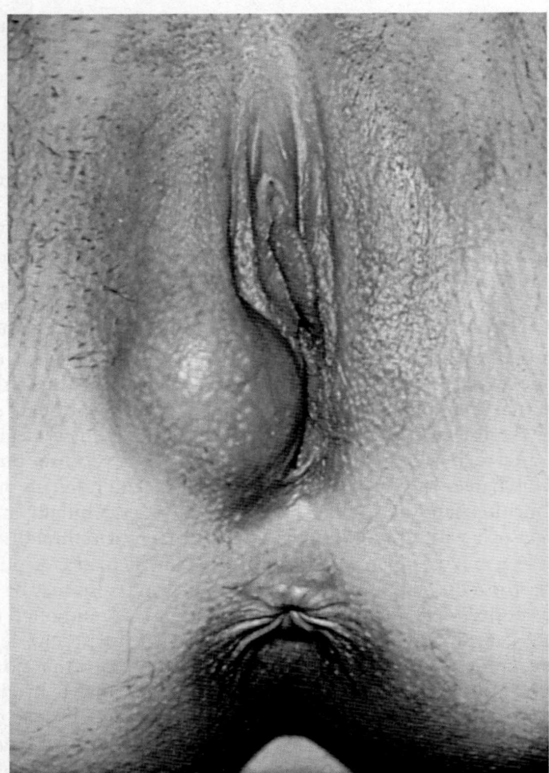

FIG. 89.8 Acute Bartholin's duct abscess.

secondary nonspecific vaginitis can develop as a result of irritation of the mucosa from persisting profuse endocervical discharge.

Mucopurulent cervicitis can be caused by *N. gonorrhoeae, C. trachomatis, Gardnerella vaginalis, Mycoplasma hominis, Ureaplasma urealyticum,* and group B streptococci. The overlap in clinical manifestations of infections caused by these microbes and the frequency of infection by two or more simultaneously preclude establishing the diagnosis by clinical findings alone.

Adolescents may be unaware of their infection, especially if they have a preexisting profuse discharge as a result of nonspecific vaginitis or trichomoniasis. Early recognition and treatment of lower genital tract gonococcal infection may prevent extension to and complications of upper genital tract infection. Therefore sexually active adolescent females should be examined for gonococcal infection as part of their routine health care.[153,280]

A review of reported complications in 1232 cases of gonococcal vaginitis in the pre-antibiotic era revealed that 35% had urethritis, 19% had proctitis, and 6% had peritonitis.[20]

Urinalysis may provide clues to gonococcal infection in some cases. In a cross-sectional study of 296 sexually active females 14 to 22 years of age, gonorrhea or trichomoniasis was present in 65% who had sterile pyuria.[164]

Upper Genital Tract Infection in Postmenarchal Females

PID will develop in 10% to 17% of females with endocervical gonococcal infection. Conditions encompassed by the term *pelvic inflammatory disease* include endometritis, parametritis, salpingitis, oophoritis, tubo-ovarian abscess, and pelvic peritonitis. PID can be caused by a variety of bacteria. Anaerobes, including *Bacteroides, Peptococcus,* and *Peptostreptococcus* spp., are the organisms usually recovered. *N. gonorrhoeae* is present in 25% to 50% of cases, similar to the proportion of cases from which *C. trachomatis* is recovered. Coliform organisms, *G. vaginalis, M. hominis, U. urealyticum,* and various streptococcal species also may be involved. PID develops when these organisms are able to ascend into the uterus, fallopian tubes, and beyond from the lower genital tract. Multiple species may be involved in a single episode. Gonococcal PID often occurs during or just after menses.[110,158] Identification of the specific microbial cause or causes of PID is complicated by the difficulty of obtaining fallopian tube specimens before initiating therapy.

Common findings in PID include an acute onset of lower abdominal pain with tenderness, fever, tenderness on lateral motion of the cervix, adnexal tenderness that generally is bilateral, and adnexal fullness. Vaginal discharge, urinary symptoms, and irregular vaginal bleeding also may be present. In moderate to severe cases, abdominal pain frequently is bilateral, exacerbated with movement, and continuous. Nausea, vomiting, marked abdominal tenderness, an abdomen that appears tense, and fever exceeding 39°C (102.2°F) may be present. Such patients often appear to be ill and may have tachycardia consistent with the height of fever.[291] Leukocytosis and elevated erythrocyte sedimentation rates are common findings. Alternatively, PID may be clinically silent or cause only mild pain without discernible tenderness, vaginal discharge, or leukocytosis. Such mild cases can go unrecognized by patients and physicians.

Establishing the diagnosis of PID may be difficult, and the differential diagnosis includes numerous other lower abdominal conditions, such as appendicitis, ectopic pregnancy, cholecystitis, mesenteric adenitis, pyelonephritis, and septic abortion. Sonography and pregnancy testing may be helpful in diagnostic decision making. No single symptom, sign, or laboratory finding is sensitive and specific for the diagnosis of PID. Combinations of findings can improve the sensitivity but do so at the expense of reduced specificity, and vice versa.

Initiation of empirical therapy for PID should be considered if the minimal criteria of lower abdominal tenderness, adnexal tenderness, and cervical motion tenderness all are present and no other cause for these findings is readily apparent. More elaborate evaluation may be needed in some cases because incorrect diagnosis and management might lead to unnecessary morbidity. Additional criteria that support the diagnosis of PID include an oral temperature higher than 38.3°C (101°F), an abnormal cervical or vaginal discharge, elevated erythrocyte sedimentation rate, increased C-reactive protein level, and laboratory documentation of cervical infection with *N. gonorrhoeae* or *C. trachomatis.* Some cases may require pursuit of definitive criteria for diagnosing PID, which include histopathologic evidence of endometritis on endometrial biopsy, transvaginal or abdominal ultrasonography or other imaging studies that show thickened fluid-filled fallopian tubes with or without free pelvic fluid or a tubo-ovarian abscess, and laparoscopic abnormalities consistent with PID.[171]

The outcome for fertility probably is improved with prompt and vigorous therapy. Hospitalization is recommended when the patient is pregnant, a surgical emergency (e.g., ectopic pregnancy or appendicitis) cannot be excluded, when compliance with or tolerance of an outpatient treatment regimen cannot be ensured (e.g., presence of nausea or vomiting), when the illness appears to be severe (e.g., presence of high fever, pelvic or tubo-ovarian abscess, overt peritonitis, or sepsis), or when the patient is immunocompromised or has failed to respond to outpatient therapy. All courses of therapy should include treatment that is appropriate for *C. trachomatis* and other causes of PID, in addition to *N. gonorrhoeae.*[343]

Complications of PID include tubo-ovarian abscess, perihepatitis (Fitz-Hugh-Curtis syndrome), future ectopic pregnancy, and infertility. Perihepatitis is characterized by right upper quadrant abdominal pain that may radiate to the shoulder. Nausea, fever, and other signs and symptoms of PID may be present as well. Leukocytosis occurs commonly, and liver enzymes are elevated in some cases. The differential diagnosis of perihepatitis includes pleuritis, cholelithiasis, subphrenic abscess, and perforated ulcers.[201]

An estimated 15% of women may become sterile after a single episode of PID and 50% after three infections. Because of scarring and fibrosis in the fallopian tube, patency is compromised and fertility is jeopardized.[51,110,111] PID in adolescents is particularly likely to result in infertility and ectopic pregnancy (Fig. 89.9), and PID is the single most common cause of infertility in young women.[41] Between 1970 and 1980, the rate of ectopic pregnancies per 1000 live births increased from 4.8 to 14.5, and between 1975 and 1981, the rate of hospitalization of females 15 to 19 years of age for salpingitis was four per 100,000.[332] These increases correlated with rising rates of gonococcal infection in the affected

TABLE 89.4 Prevalence of Gonorrhea and Other Sexually Transmitted Diseases in Clinics for Adolescents

Reference	Location	Total Clinic Population Studied	Gonorrhea (%)	*Chlamydia* Infection (%)	Other
Shafer et al., 1984[292]	California	366	15	4	*Trichomonas* infection
Golden et al., 1984[129]	New York	186	10	10	Syphilis, *Trichomonas* infection
Demetriou et al., 1984[96]	Oklahoma	839	14	—	
Mulcahy and Lacey, 1987[229]	Leeds, UK	210	14	16	*Trichomonas* infection
Jamson et al., 1995[172]	Colorado	632	7	—	Human papillomavirus infection
Giannini et al., 2010[124]	Ohio	16,039[a]	9	—	Human papillomavirus infection
		525[b]	16	—	

[a]Females age 14–21 years seen at a children's hospital adolescent clinic, 2003–07.
[b]Females age 14–21 years seen at a health department sexually transmitted infection clinic, 2006–07.

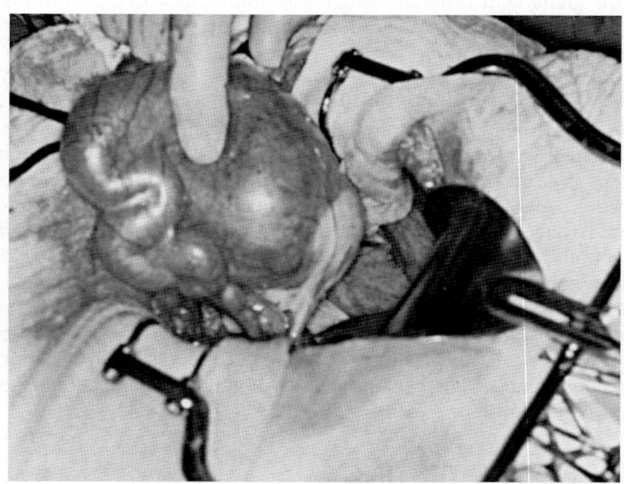

FIG. 89.9 Large hydrosalpinx resulting from gonococcal salpingitis in an adolescent female with repeated gonorrheal infections.

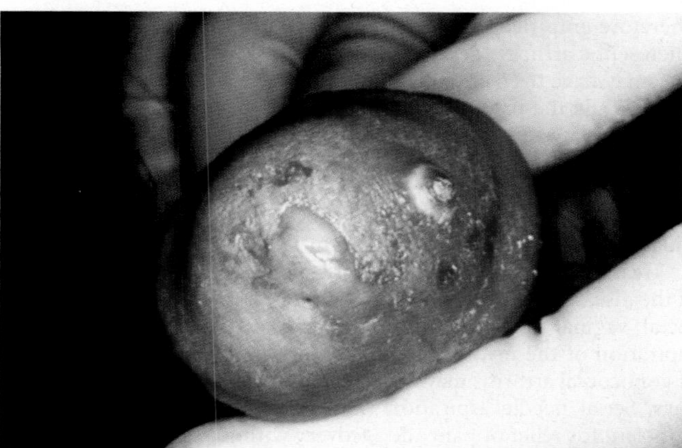

FIG. 89.10 Purulent male urethral discharge resulting from gonorrhea with an associated pyodermal lesion on the glans. (From American Academy of Pediatrics 2012 Red Book Collection.)

populations. Data from several studies of gonococcal disease in adolescents are presented in Table 89.4.

Risk factors for the development of PID include young age at the time of acquisition of gonococcal disease or other STIs, a history of previous PID, multiple sexual partners, and the use of an intrauterine device (IUD) for contraception. The immature cervix may be at particular risk for progression to upper tract disease.[298] Disseminated gonococcal infection may accompany asymptomatic infection of an IUD,[74] and the rate of acute PID in those who use IUDs may be increased.

Genital Tract Infection in Males

Gonococcal urethritis in prepubertal boys is a less frequent event than vaginitis in girls because of gender differences in rates of sexual abuse. As in girls with gonorrheal infection of the genitourinary tract, concomitant anorectal and tonsillopharyngeal colonization is a frequent finding.[237]

Urethritis is the primary manifestation of gonococcal infection in males of all ages beyond the neonatal period (Fig. 89.10). Even in young boys, the disease usually is symptomatic and resembles gonococcal urethritis in men.[83,122] Dysuria, purulent discharge, or both develop 2 to 7 days after exposure. Patients generally are afebrile. Purulence typically is greater than with nongonococcal urethritis, but symptoms often are mild enough that patients (or their parents) may delay seeking medical care for weeks. Associated inguinal adenopathy occurs rarely.

At least 5% of cases of gonococcal urethritis in males are asymptomatic, and asymptomatic infection can occur at all ages. Asymptomatic pyuria is a manifestation with which the pediatrician should be familiar.[89] It may be the only finding in some cases and should raise suspicion of gonococcal or chlamydial infection in boys who may have been sexually abused or in sexually active adolescent males.

Males with asymptomatic infection are a major reservoir for transmission to their sexual partners. Untreated male urethral infection may persist for as long as 6 months.

Complications of gonococcal infection in males now occur much less frequently than in the pre-antibiotic era. Epididymitis is the most common complication. Unilateral swelling, pain, and erythema in the posterior aspect of the scrotum are the usual features. Fever may occur. If untreated, the infection may progress to involve the ipsilateral testis. Hydrocele may result from secretion of fluid into the potential space of the tunica vaginalis. Epididymitis can lead to testicular infarction, abscess, infertility, prostatitis, paraurethral abscesses, and penile lymphangitis, but these local complications are rare findings. Perihepatitis in males has been described but occurs extremely infrequently.[191]

Disseminated Disease

Dissemination requires invasion of the bloodstream from local infection of the mucous membranes of the genital tract, rectum, pharynx, or conjunctiva. Bacteremia then can lead to infection of other sites. The risk for dissemination in children after mucosal infection appears to be higher than the 1% to 3% rate in adults. Dissemination in adults seems to be more common with asymptomatic infections, many of which are caused by AHU$^-$ gonococcal strains.[185] The frequency of deficits in the complement system associated with disseminated disease in children is unknown.

As in neonates, gonococcal arthritis is the most common form of disseminated disease in older children, adolescents, and adults. The ankles, knees, wrists, and hands are involved most frequently. The clinical findings are not distinct from those of other microbial causes of septic arthritis. Polyarticular involvement occurs less frequently than in neonates.[81] Gram stain and synovial fluid cultures often are negative.

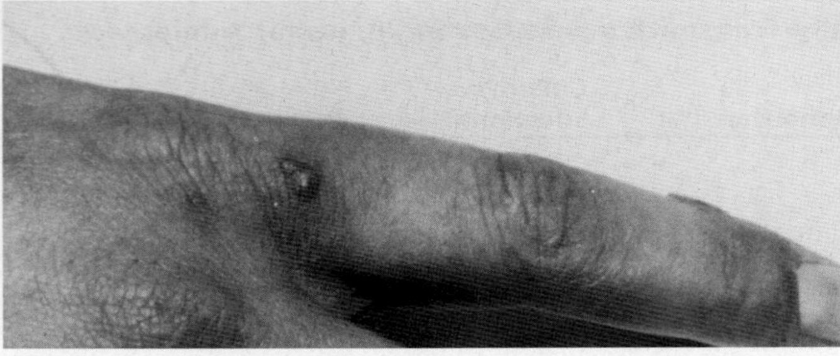

FIG. 89.11 Skin lesion typical of the arthritis-dermatitis syndrome of disseminated gonococcal infection: necrotic pustule with an erythematous halo overlying proximal phalanx of index finger. (Courtesy Daniel P. Krowchuk, MD.)

Therefore empirical coverage for *N. gonorrhoeae* must be considered when septic arthritis develops in a sexually active adolescent or a child who may have been sexually abused.

Typically the patient has a single most severely affected joint, and associated myositis and tenosynovitis may be prominent findings. Gonococcal arthritis in older children and adolescents resembles that in adults and may be accompanied by cutaneous lesions (Fig. 89.11).[4] Osteomyelitis rarely occurs but has been reported in all age groups, usually in association with septic arthritis.[8]

Treatment of gonococcal arthritis depends on prompt recognition of the disease. Cultures of all mucous membranes (i.e., nasopharyngeal, rectal, vaginal or endocervical, and conjunctival), blood culture, and aspiration of the involved joint should be performed. The local signs of gonococcal arthritis may not respond to antibiotic therapy for several days. Serial needle aspiration rather than open drainage usually is sufficient for relief of pain and recovery without sequelae (the hip may be an exception).

Gonococcemia is clinically silent generally but can cause a syndrome of migratory polyarthralgia, fever, and rash that precedes the onset of arthritis by several days to a week. The symptomatic course normally is only mild to moderate in severity. Blood cultures often are negative by the time care is sought. Gonococcemia-related symptoms may resolve after several days, even without treatment. Rare cases can resemble meningococcemia with purpura and fulminant sepsis with disseminated intravascular coagulopathy. These cases sometimes can be fatal.[248]

The skin lesions associated with gonococcemia usually are pustules on an erythematous base (see Fig. 89.11), but petechiae, papules, and hemorrhagic bullae can develop. Skin lesions in conjunction with septic arthritis also has been referred to as the arthritis-dermatitis syndrome. The lesions usually arise on the extremities and are fewer than 20 in number. Low-grade fever is most common, but high fever with shaking chills may occur. Tenosynovitis is present in a fourth of these patients. Leukocytosis, pyuria, and elevated liver enzyme test results may be seen. The resultant septic joints generally become clinically apparent during the second week after the onset of disseminated infection.

Anorectal Gonorrhea

Gonococcal anorectal infection (proctitis) frequently is asymptomatic but can be associated with pruritus, tenesmus, purulent discharge, or rectal bleeding. Rectal infection can occur as a result of rectal intercourse or inoculation from vaginal secretions. Approximately 40% of females with genital gonococcal infection have positive anorectal cultures. Rectal infection is an unusual finding in males who have not engaged in rectal intercourse.[308]

Pharyngeal Gonorrhea

Pharyngeal gonococcal infection in all age groups beyond the neonatal period is acquired by orogenital contact. Pharyngeal gonorrhea may be asymptomatic, without evidence of inflammation, or may cause an exudative tonsillopharyngitis that can mimic group A streptococcal or viral infection. Cervical adenopathy may be present in some cases. In sexually abused children, the pharynx may be the only site of infection. It may be the sole culture-positive site in some cases of disseminated gonococcal infection, and pharyngeal infection possibly is a factor predisposing to dissemination. Pharyngeal infection usually resolves spontaneously within 10 to 12 weeks but should be treated when recognized.[1,41,64,82,140,237,245,297,337,341] In a recent study of 14- to 21-year-old females hospitalized in a children's hospital or seeking care in a public health clinic, pharyngeal gonorrhea prevalence among adolescents was 3.5% and 6.8%, respectively.[124]

Conjunctivitis Beyond Infancy

Gonococcal ophthalmia occasionally is seen in children and adults. Direct inoculation of the eye can occur as a result of transmission of fomites from infected persons. Clinical findings typically include a profuse purulent discharge, chemosis, eyelid edema, keratitis, and fever. The initial ocular discharge may be watery before turning purulent. The acute phase may mimic orbital cellulitis. Untreated infection, as with neonates, can lead to corneal opacification, ulceration, and rupture of the globe with resultant visual loss. Some cases may be minimally symptomatic, with a low-grade inflammatory response followed by spontaneous resolution.[197,202,255]

Other Forms of Gonococcal Disease

Gonococcal meningitis is a rare condition that may occur with or without associated signs of gonococcemia or septic arthritis. Pyomyositis of the biceps and soft tissue abscesses remote from the genital area have been reported. A gonococcal abscess arising in an area of blunt trauma to a hand has been described in an adolescent with associated endocervical infection.[130] An abdominal wall abscess resulting from *N. gonorrhoeae* infection in a 22-month-old male child without other foci of infection has been described.[101] Ventriculoperitoneal shunt–associated infection, endocarditis, and myocarditis caused by *N. gonorrhoeae* have been reported in adults and can be expected to occur occasionally in children and adolescents.[158] These manifestations of gonococcal infection seldom are seen in children.

DIAGNOSTIC TESTING

Isolation of *N. gonorrhoeae* in culture remains important for diagnosing gonococcal infection, but nonculture, DNA-based tests have become widely used in recent years. Serologic tests based on complement fixation, latex agglutination, enzyme-linked immunosorbent assays, and other techniques have been developed, but the sensitivity of these methods is only about 70%. These methods are limited now to studies of immune response and pathogenesis.[157,161,281]

The Centers for Disease Control and Prevention (CDC) also has defined three levels of diagnosis based on clinical and laboratory findings. They are more stringent than the case definitions used for public health surveillance. A *suggestive diagnosis* is defined by presence of mucopurulent endocervical or urethral exudate and sexual exposure to a person with gonococcal infection. A *presumptive diagnosis* requires two of three criteria: (1) typical gram-negative *intracellular* diplococci on Gram stain of urethral exudate from males or endocervical secretions; (2) growth of apparent *N. gonorrhoeae* from such specimens on culture medium, defined as typical colonial morphology, positive oxidase reaction, and typical gram-negative morphology; and (3) detection of *N. gonorrhoeae* by a nonculture laboratory test. A *definitive diagnosis* requires (1) isolation of *N. gonorrhoeae* from clinical specimens by culture, as in the second criterion for a presumptive diagnosis, and (2) confirmation of identity by biochemical, enzymatic, serologic, or nucleic acid testing.[59]

A diagnosis of *N. gonorrhoeae* infection at any site should prompt evaluation for the presence of other common STIs, if not already done (see Chapter 42).[272]

Culture

In adults, culture of clinical specimens is 80% to 95% sensitive when promptly inoculated and incubated. Cultures of adult male urethral specimens, blood, and other normally sterile body sites tend to have sensitivities in the higher range.[161] Because false-positive cultures with appropriate laboratory confirmation are not thought to occur, specificity and positive predictive values are 100%. Culture in adolescents and children probably has sensitivity similar to that of adults.

TABLE 89.5 Treatment of Gonococcal Infections in the Neonatal Period

Disease Category	Treatment Regimen	Comments
Infants born to mothers with gonococcal infection *or* Gonococcal ophthalmia neonatorum (GON) or other focal sites of infection (i.e., rectum, pharynx, vagina, urethra)	Ceftriaxone 25–50 mg/kg IV or IM, not to exceed 125 mg (single dose)[a,b,c]	Infants with GON should receive eye irrigation with saline solution immediately on recognition and at frequent intervals subsequently until the discharge is eliminated
Disseminated gonococcal infection (septic arthritis, sepsis, meningitis) or scalp abscess	Ceftriaxone 25–50 mg/kg IV or IM once daily for 7 days (10–14 days for meningitis) *or* Cefotaxime 25 mg/kg IV or IM every 12 h for 7 days (10–14 days for meningitis)	Cefotaxime is preferred for infants with hyperbilirubinemia who require more than a single dose of therapy If meningitis is present, higher or more frequent doses in the recommended ranges may be needed

IM, Intramuscularly; *IV,* intravenously.
[a]If ceftriaxone is unavailable or contraindicated, cefotaxime, 100 mg/kg IV or IM (single dose) is an alternative.
[b]Topical agents alone are inadequate and unnecessary when recommended systemic antibiotics are given.
[c]For GON, some experts prefer to continue parenteral therapy with one of these agents until blood (with or without cerebrospinal fluid) cultures have been negative for 48 to 72 hours.
Data from Workowski KA, Bolan GA. Sexually Transmitted Diseases Treatment Guidelines, 2015. *MMWR Recomm Rep.* 2015;64:1–137. For potential updates to these recommendations, see http://www.cdc.gov/std/gonorrhea/treatment.htm.

The use of selective media such as modified Thayer-Martin is required for culture of endocervical, rectal, and pharyngeal specimens to suppress contaminating flora. Selective or nonselective media (chocolate agar) can be used with equal sensitivity for male urethral cultures. Plating of specimens on both types of media may improve the sensitivity, but the incremental yield is small and probably not cost-effective for routine practice.[29,87,263]

Gonococcal colonies become evident on agar plates within 24 to 48 hours after inoculation. Isolates are considered presumptively positive if Gram stain shows gram-negative diplococci and colonies are oxidase-positive. Further testing that demonstrates the gonococcal phenotypic pattern of acid production from selected carbohydrates or a positive result by a nucleic acid method, or both is required for confirmation as *N. gonorrhoeae* (Table 89.5).[63]

Gonococci do not tolerate drying, so clinical specimens must be plated onto appropriate media as soon as possible. Transport bottles containing medium and a carbon dioxide–enriched atmosphere should be used if definitive specimen processing will be delayed. Transport bottles should be maintained upright during inoculation to preserve the carbon dioxide atmosphere.

Adolescents

Endocervical and vaginal swab specimens are preferred for culture in females at risk for or with clinical suspected gonococcal infection.

Culture of the rectum and pharynx in females can be considered optional except when evaluating for sexual abuse.[29,177] However, in a recent study, addition of pharyngeal culture allowed detection of an additional 11% to 26% of cases versus cervical culture alone among 14- to 21-year-old females.[124]

In males, sites to be cultured depend on the sexual practices and the anatomic sites exposed. Among MSM, rectal and pharyngeal infections occur with frequencies similar to that of gonococcal urethritis.[35,161,215,225]

Prepubertal Children

Cultures remain of paramount importance in evaluation of prepubertal children with clinically suspected gonococcal infection or who are being screened for STIs that may have been acquired during potential sexual abuse. Culture is preferred for diagnosis of genital tract and rectal, oropharyngeal, and other extragenital sites of infection in children (see Medicolegal section). Vaginal specimens are adequate for diagnosis in prepubertal girls, for whom obtaining endocervical specimens is unnecessary. Urethral specimens are required in boys. Gram stains are considered inadequate for diagnosis or exclusion of gonococcal infection. Nucleic acid amplification tests (NAATs) can be used for rapid diagnosis on vaginal and urine specimens from girls, but there are insufficient data for their use in boys.[343]

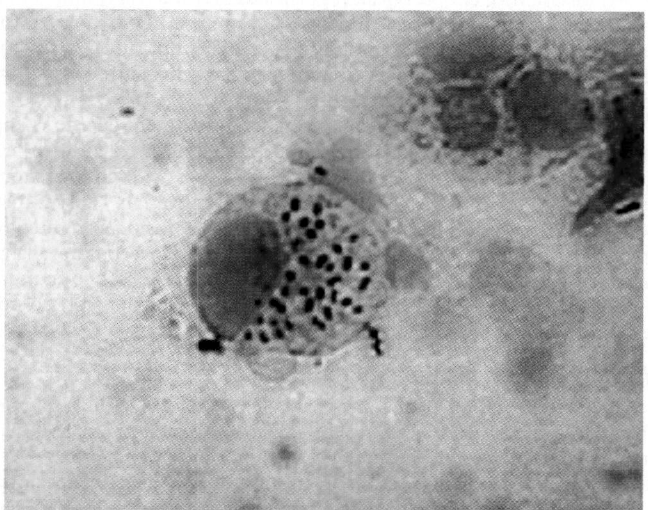

FIG. 89.12 Gram stain of gonorrheal exudate showing multiple intracellular diplococci. In male urethral specimens, this is considered diagnostic of gonococcal infection. In children and adolescent females, confirmation by culture or nucleic acid–based tests is needed. (From American Academy of Pediatrics 2012 Red Book Collection.)

Gram-Stained Smears

In symptomatic males, a Gram stain of a urethral specimen that demonstrates polymorphonuclear leukocytes with intracellular gram-negative diplococci can be considered diagnostic of infection with *N. gonorrhoeae* (Fig. 89.12). Gram stain in this population has greater than 99% specificity and greater than 95% sensitivity.[343] Negative Gram stain results are not sufficient to exclude the diagnosis of gonorrhea. Although nonpathogenic *Neisseria* spp. and *N. meningitidis* are morphologically indistinguishable from gonococci, the former rarely are cell-associated.

Gram stains of endocervical, pharyngeal, and rectal specimens are not recommended because of lower sensitivity in detection of infection at these sites. The specificity of a negative Gram stain appears to be at least 95% for specimens from the endocervix and rectum.[161,275,343]

Gram stains of eye exudates, joint fluid, and pustular fluid should be performed because the presence of gram-negative diplococci may help guide initial therapeutic interventions pending culture results.

Nonculture Diagnostics

Nonculture diagnostic tests are widely used for rapid diagnosis of gonococcal (and chlamydial) infection. Many offer the advantage of using urine samples rather than the more invasive swabs and also allow *C. trachomatis* to be evaluated with the same specimen. Numerous gonococcal antigen-detection tests were developed but have been supplanted largely by NAATs. Nucleic acid hybridization tests (NAHTs) also are available. NAHTs are based on a single-stranded DNA probe complementary to gonococcal ribosomal RNA (rRNA). Sensitivities are about 95% (less than culture), with a specificity of 99%.[147,161,198,247]

NAATs use standard PCR-based assays, transcription-mediated amplification, or strand-displacement assays (SDA). These are more sensitive than culture. False-positive reactions with PCR- or SDA-based NAATs can occur as a result of the carry-over contamination that occurs during processing or because of occasional cross reactions with commensal *Neisseria* spp. that may be present in some clinical specimens. Specificities are generally greater than 98%. False-negative results can occur as a result of target sequence differences (or absence) in some gonococcal clones. NAATs can be used to evaluate first-void urine specimens, which facilitates screening for gonococcal infection in lieu of more invasive genital tract specimens.[70,301,328,329,338] NAATs can detect the presence of nonviable gonococcal microbes thereby possibly reducing the need for the stringent transport conditions often required for culture. Currently available NAATs are multiplex tests that also can detect *C. trachomatis.*

NAATs are approved by the US Food and Drug Administration (FDA) for use with endocervical, vaginal, and urethral (male only) swab specimens and with urine specimens. They are not FDA approved for rectal, oropharyngeal, or conjunctival specimens but can be used for tests of these sites when clinical laboratories have met CLIA regulatory requirements for off-label procedures.[343]

Results of NAATs are adequate for making treatment decisions and public health case identifications. Culture remains the definitive test for medicolegal purposes, although use of NAATs with confirmatory testing with a second NAAT based on an alternative DNA target may be acceptable for forensic use on urine samples from girls but not boys.[26,290] In addition, because of ever-increasing resistance to the available antimicrobial agents, monitoring of gonococcal susceptibility by culture is necessary at the local level, at the very least in patients who do not respond to apparently adequate therapy.[338,343]

Medicolegal Issues Related to Diagnostic Tests

N. meningitidis and other members of the Neisseriaceae family are morphologically and often biochemically similar to *N. gonorrhoeae* and may be isolated from sites such as the vagina, blood, and nasopharynx.[98,102,339] Accurate identification of *Neisseria* organisms from any pediatric specimen is essential because misidentification of nongonococcal species as *N. gonorrhoeae* may lead to very serious social consequences for children and their families by precipitating concern regarding sexual abuse. A recent report of two cases of meningitis in young children initially misidentified as having *N. gonorrhoeae* but subsequently confirmed as having *N. meningitidis* illustrates that this may be an ongoing issue.[310] Nonculture methods consistently identify more clinical specimens as positive than do standard cultures.[329] Determining whether such results indicate greater sensitivity, increased false positivity, or a combination of both has been difficult.

Because of this potential for obtaining false-positive results with NAATs, culture has been considered the medicolegal standard for children who require evaluation for suspected sexual victimization, including prepubertal girls with obvious vaginal discharge. Sequential testing using nonculture tests followed by culture if the former is positive has been proposed as a more sensitive approach than culture alone.[246] A recent multicenter study using NAATs on urine specimens and using a second NAAT based on an alternative DNA target or species-specific *N. gonorrhoeae* PCR to confirm positive results found no false-positive results.[26] The NAAT-based approach increased the number of confirmed gonococcal infections among 485 girls who were suspected victims of sexual assault from 12, based on culture alone, to 16. This approach is now considered an alternative to culture alone on vaginal and urine specimens in girls. Culture remains preferred for urethral specimens from boys and for extragenital specimens from all children.[343]

Proper Collection of Clinical Specimens

Urethral exudate from males may be obtained by passing small swabs or bacteriologic loops 2 to 4 cm into the urethra.[150] Endocervical specimens from postpubertal females are obtained by speculum examination with swabs inserted 1 to 2 cm into the external os after the cervix has been cleansed of external exudate and vaginal secretions.[271] The swab should be rotated one full revolution and withdrawn. Self-obtained vaginal swabs also provide adequate specimens for nonculture methods.[302] This technique has been studied in adolescents. Vaginal specimens collected with tampons also can be used with nonculture methods.[320]

In prepubertal girls, cultures can be obtained from the vaginal introitus by gently swabbing the hymenal opening. Deeper insertion is not necessary. Swabs of exudates emanating from the urethral meatus or vaginal orifice also are sufficient for culture.

In persons with symptomatic anorectal infection, rectal specimens should be obtained by anoscopic means, which increases the sensitivity. In asymptomatic persons, rectal specimens can be procured by blindly inserting a swab 2 to 3 cm into the anal canal and applying lateral pressure to avoid entering any fecal mass. Swabs that are grossly contaminated with fecal matter should be discarded.[90,342]

The posterior pharynx, tonsillar areas, and faucial pillars should be swabbed to obtain adequate specimens for the diagnosis of pharyngeal infection.[161]

When urine specimens can be used for nonculture methods, the first 15 to 30 mL of voided urine should be collected.[208,233] Collection of urine should be delayed at least 1 hour after the most recent void to maximize sensitivity.

ANTIMICROBIAL RESISTANCE AMONG GONOCOCCI

Gonococcal strains have been able to acquire resistance to antibiotics since the first agents were introduced. In 1986, the CDC initiated the Gonococcal Isolate Surveillance Program (GISP) to monitor the antimicrobial sensitivities of *N. gonorrhoeae* in STI clinics in 21 cities in the United States.[53] This system consisted of 29 sites in 2010.[60]

Sulfanilamide became available in 1936, but widespread resistance to sulfanilamide occurred by 1944.[250] As successive agents have become available, multidrug-resistant strains are being seen with increasing frequency in many parts of the world. Ongoing analysis of gonococcal isolates for antibiotic susceptibility to the available antimicrobial agents remains essential for maintaining effective empirical therapeutic regimens.

In the 1940s, virtually all gonococcal isolates were highly susceptible to penicillin. Despite a gradual increase in the mean minimal inhibitory concentration (MIC) to penicillin from the mid-1950s through the mid-1970s, almost all strains had penicillin MICs of less than 0.5 μg/mL. This low-level resistance is mediated by alterations at a genetic locus called *penA* that result in modification of its product, penicillin-binding protein 2. Two other loci designated *mtr,* which encode an efflux pump that reduces concentrations of multiple antibiotics, and *penB,* which is an allele of *por,* the gene of the porin protein, also mediate low-level resistance to penicillins. *penB* encodes a porin with a mutation that decreases permeability to hydrophilic antibiotics.[126]

In 1976, strains of *N. gonorrhoeae* were discovered that had acquired plasmid-conferring resistance to penicillin through the production of penicillinase (a TEM-1 β-lactamase). These strains were found in many parts of the Far East and in London, and in the former they constituted approximately 30% of the isolates in some cities. The strains caused the expected spectrum of clinical disease, and treatment with penicillin was not effective. Penicillinase-producing gonococci contain one of two closely related 5.3- or 7.2-kb plasmids (Pc^r) that carry a Tn2 transposon system. This plasmid appears to have been acquired from *Haemophilus ducreyi.*[7,23,47,68,252] In 1983, an outbreak of chromosomally mediated, penicillin-resistant (MICs of 2 to 4 μg/mL), non–penicillinase-producing gonococci was reported from North Carolina.[116] Such strains were seen subsequently in other areas of the country.

Resistance to tetracycline antibiotics emerged in the 1980s and subsequently increased. Three chromosomal loci designated *mtr, penB,* and *tet* mediate low-level resistance. High-level resistance to tetracycline is conferred by *tetM,* which resides on a 38-kb plasmid (Tc^r) that is a derivative of the 36-kb conjugal plasmid. *tetM* produces a cytoplasmic protein that protects ribosomes from tetracycline. Tc^r gonococci can transfer this plasmid, as well as Pc^r, efficiently to other gonococcal strains.[231,311]

Spectinomycin resistance was described first in 1987 in US military personnel in Korea. This agent had been introduced as the drug of choice there in 1981 because of high rates of penicillin resistance. Treatment failures actually began to occur in 1983. Resistance is chromosomally mediated and results in alteration of the ribosomal target site of the drug.[30,47] The widespread use of spectinomycin was associated with a decline in the rate of penicillin resistance.[30] All gonococcal strains tested in the United States since 1994 have been susceptible to streptomycin.[62]

Ciprofloxacin and other fluoroquinolone antibiotics became widely available for the treatment of gonococcal infection in the 1980s. Low-level resistance to fluoroquinolones is associated with mutations in the DNA gyrase gene *gyrA*, and high-level resistance has been linked to mutations in the topoisomerase gene *parC*.[169] Resistance to these agents has been noted since the early 1990s in areas of Southeast Asia.[118] In April 2007, the CDC no longer recommended the use of fluoroquinolones for the treatment of gonococcal infections in the United States[58] as prevalence of resistances to ciprofloxacin increased to 14.8% among GISP isolates. In 2014, 19.2% of GISP isolates were resistant.[62]

In 1989, 13% of the *N. gonorrhoeae* isolates evaluated were resistant to penicillin, tetracycline, or both.[54] In 1999, such strains accounted for 28% of all isolates.[56] Overall in 2014, 37% of isolates evaluated by GISP were resistant to penicillin, tetracycline, ciprofloxacin, or some combination of these antibiotics.[62] The distribution of azithromycin MICs among gonococcal isolates has shifted upward in the last decade. The proportion of GISP strains with reduced susceptibility (MICs ≥2.0 μg/mL) has risen from 0.3% in 2011[61] to 2.5% in 2014.[62] Rifampin resistance is also high in some areas of the world.[240]

During the past few years cefixime MICs have crept upward in the United States and other countries, along with reports of treatment failures with the recommended 400 mg oral dose of this agent.[61,209,325] MICs of 0.5 μg/mL or higher are considered to have decreased susceptibility to cefixime. The mechanism of this reduced susceptibility is chromosomally mediated and multifactorial. Mutations in the *penA* encode alterations in penicillin binding protein (PBP) 2 that confer reduced affinity for penicillins. Mutations in the promotor *mtrR* and *porB1b (penB)* result in increased efflux capacity and decreased permeability of the cell membrane, respectively, which decrease concentrations of these agents in the periplasm. High-level resistance can result from a mutation of *ponB* that encodes an altered PBP 1.[200]

Nationally in the United States in 2011, 1.5% of GISP isolates had cefixime MICs of 0.25 μg/mL or higher, a threshold used by GISP for monitoring emerging resistance to cephalosporins (Fig. 89.13). In the Western United States, 3.2% of isolates had MICs at or above 0.25 μg/mL. These observations prompted removal of cefixime from recommended options for empirical treatment of uncomplicated gonococcal infections in the United States in August 2012. In 2014, 0.8% of GISP isolates had MICs at or above 0.25 μg/mL.

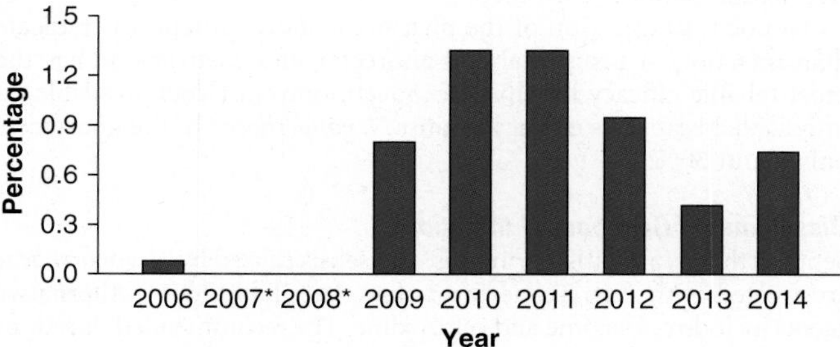

FIG. 89.13 Percentage of *Neisseria gonorrhoeae* isolates with elevated cefixime minimum inhibitory concentrations (MICs) (≥0.25 μg/mL), Gonococcal Isolate Surveillance Project (GISP), 2006–14. The rise in MIC since 2006 is the result of alterations in the microbial penicillin-binding proteins. Cefixime susceptibility was not tested by GISP during 2007 and 2008. (From Centers for Disease Control and Prevention: http://www.cdc.gov/std/stats14/figures/27.htm. For the most currently available data, see http://www.cdc.gov/std/gisp/default.htm.)

Ceftriaxone MICs have increased minimally overall to date, with MICs at or above 0.125 μg/mL fluctuating between 0.1 and 0.4% among GISP isolates in recent years.[62] A few isolates with MICs of 0.5 to 2 μg/mL have been reported.[61,62,325]

These ongoing events raise concerns about potential emergence of near "pan-resistant" gonococcal strains.

TREATMENT

Because of ever-changing gonococcal susceptibility patterns and variations in susceptibility in different international regions, practitioners must remain alert for modifications of treatment guidelines for their respective geographic locations. Based on the current patterns of antimicrobial resistance in prevalent *N. gonorrhoeae* strains in the United States, the third-generation cephalosporin ceftriaxone is the only remaining agent routinely recommended as initial therapy in children and adults as of August 2012.[61] Dual therapy with azithromycin also may enhance treatment efficacy for gonococcal infections, especially against pharyngeal gonococcal infections in combination with oral cephalosporins. Azithromycin is thus now preferred over doxycycline for treatment of potential concomitant *C. trachomatis* infection.[343]

The recommendations for treatment of childhood gonorrhea in the United States discussed in this section and listed in Tables 89.5 and 89.6 are based primarily on 2015 guidelines from the CDC.[343] CDC guidelines are based on the stringent clinical efficacy criterion of an expected 95% efficacy with lower bound of 95% confidence interval of 90%.[238] Up-to-date information on treatment regimens for gonorrhea and other STIs can be obtained from the CDC website http://www.cdc.gov/std/treatment.

Treatment of Infants Born to Mothers With Gonococcal Infection

Infants born to mothers with untreated gonorrhea are at high risk for acquiring infection; consequently, even without overt signs of infection, such infants should be treated with a single injection of ceftriaxone (see Table 89.5). Ceftriaxone should be given cautiously to hyperbilirubinemic infants, especially premature ones. A single dose of cefotaxime 100 mg/kg intravenously or intramuscularly is an acceptable alternative. Topical prophylaxis for neonatal ophthalmia is not adequate therapy for documented infections of the eye or other sites.[343]

Treatment of Neonates With Gonococcal Infection

Neonates with suspected gonococcal infection of any site, including GON, should be admitted to the hospital for parenteral antibiotics and any needed supportive care. Many but not all experts recommend that CSF studies be performed even in afebrile, otherwise well-appearing infants whose only clinical manifestation is apparent GON.

The presence of typical gram-negative diplococci in Gram-stained specimens is sufficient justification to begin treatment of GON or gonococcal infection in other sites. The absence of gram-negative diplococci in Gram-stained specimens is not sufficient to abrogate presumptive treatment of GON in a neonate with conjunctival exudate.

Tests for concomitant *C. trachomatis* infection, HIV infection, and congenital syphilis should be performed in infants with gonococcal infection at any site. The mother and her partner(s) should be evaluated for gonococcal infection (and other STIs) and treated according to the recommendations for gonococcal infection in adolescents and adults.

Infants with GON can be treated with a single dose of ceftriaxone 25 to 50 mg/kg intravenously or intramuscularly, not to exceed 125 mg (see Table 89.5). This regimen also may be used for infants with other sites of nondisseminated gonococcal infection, including the rectum, pharynx, vagina, and urethra. A single dose of cefotaxime 100 mg/kg given intravenously or intramuscularly is an alternative treatment of GON. Some experts prefer to continue parenteral therapy with one of these agents until blood cultures (with or without CSF cultures) have been negative for 48 to 72 hours. Infants with GON also should receive eye irrigation with saline solution immediately on recognition and at frequent intervals until the discharge is eliminated. Topical antimicrobial agents alone are inadequate and unnecessary when the recommended systemic antibiotics are given.[59,120,194]

TABLE 89.6 Recommended Treatment of Gonococcal Infections in Children and Adolescents Beyond the Neonatal Period

	Prepubertal Children <45/kg	Patients Age ≥8 Years, ≥45/kg
Uncomplicated Gonococcal Infections[a,b]		
Vulvovaginitis, endocervicitis, urethritis, proctitis, or pharyngitis	Ceftriaxone 25–50 mg/kg IV or IM in a single dose, not to exceed 125 mg	Ceftriaxone 250 mg IM in a single dose
Conjunctivitis[c]	Ceftriaxone 50 mg/kg (maximum, 1 g) IM in a single dose	Ceftriaxone 1/g IM in a single dose
Disseminated or Complicated Gonococcal Infections[a,b]		
Septic arthritis, sepsis, or arthritis-dermatitis syndrome[d287]	Ceftriaxone 50 mg/kg/day (maximum, 1 g/day) IV or IM once daily for 7 days[e,f]	Ceftriaxone, 1/g IV or IM once daily for 7 days[e,f]
Meningitis or endocarditis[g286]	Ceftriaxone 50 mg/kg/day (maximum, 2 g/day) IV or IM given twice daily; for meningitis, duration is 10–14 days; for endocarditis, duration is at least 28 days	Ceftriaxone 1–2/g IV every 12 to 24 h; for meningitis, duration is 10–14 days; for endocarditis, duration is at least 28 days
Epididymitis		Ceftriaxone, 250/mg IM in a single dose[95]
Treatment for presumed coinfection with *C. trachomatis*	Erythromycin base or ethylsuccinate 50 mg/kg/day (maximum 2 g/day) PO in 4 divided doses for 14 days *or* Azithromycin 20 mg/kg (maximum 1 g) PO in a single dose[j]	Azithromycin 1/g PO in a single dose is preferred[290] *or* Doxycycline[i] 100/mg PO twice daily for 7 days[h]

See text for discussion of alternative treatment options, including those for patients with allergies to the recommended regimens above.
IM, Intramuscularly; *IV,* intravenously; *PO,* orally.
[a]Therapy for potential (presumptive) coinfection with *Chlamydia trachomatis* also is recommended. See bottom row of Table.
[b]Azithromycin provides potential dual therapy for gonococcal strains with reduced susceptibility to cephalosporins, in addition to its role in treatment of chlamydial infection. Prevalence of tetracycline resistance is high among Gonococcal Isolate Surveillance Project isolates, particularly among those with elevated minimum inhibitory concentrations to cefixime.
[c]Eyes should be lavaged with saline initially and at regular intervals until secretions no longer continue to accumulate.
[d]Hospitalization for arthritis-dermatitis syndrome should be considered for children based on clinical severity, including those (1) who are unlikely to receive the prescribed treatment because of personal or parent/guardian failure to adhere to the regimen or (2) whose infection has not responded to prior outpatient therapy.
[e]Some experts advise a 10- to 14-day course of therapy for gonococcal sepsis or septic arthritis.
[f]For older children and adolescents, parenteral therapy can be discontinued 24 to 48 h after improvement occurs and the 7-day course completed with an appropriate oral antimicrobial agent, based on antimicrobial susceptibility results.
[g]Children or adolescents with gonococcal meningitis or endocarditis should be hospitalized initially.
[h]Add doxycycline 100 mg PO twice daily for 10 days for coverage of chlamydia; for males at risk for epididymitis due to enteric organisms (e.g., those who practice insertive anal sex), add levofloxacin 500 mg PO once a day for 10 days *or* ofloxacin 300 mg PO twice a day for 10 days.
[i]Children who weigh 45 kg or more but are < 8 years generally should not be prescribed doxycycline for treatment of STIs due to concerns about dental staining.
[j]Data are limited regarding efficacy of azithromycin for treatment of chlamydia in young children, but the single dose and favorable side-effect profile make this agent a reasonable choice.
Data from Workowski KA, Bolan GA. Sexually Transmitted Diseases Treatment Guidelines, 2015. *MMWR Recomm Rep.* 2015;64:1–137; and American Academy of Pediatrics: Gonococcal infections. In: Kimberlin DK, ed. *2015 Red Book: Report of the Committee on Infectious Diseases.* 30th ed. Elk Grove Village, IL: American Academy of Pediatrics; 2015:356–67. For potential updates to these recommendations, see http://www.cdc.gov/std/gonorrhea/treatment.htm.

Simultaneous infection with *C. trachomatis* should be considered a potential explanation for neonates who do not respond satisfactorily to the recommended treatment.

Disseminated Gonococcal Infection or Scalp Abscess

The recommended therapy for gonococcal arthritis, scalp abscess, and sepsis is ceftriaxone 25 to 50 mg/kg intravenously or intramuscularly given once per day for 7 days. Cefotaxime is an alternative and is preferred for infants with hyperbilirubinemia. For gonococcal meningitis, treatment should be continued for 10 to 14 days, with consideration of the use of higher daily doses of these agents (see Table 89.5).[343]

Treatment of Gonococcal Infections Beyond the Neonatal Period

Treatment recommendations for children and adolescents with uncomplicated and complicated gonococcal infection, including PID, are outlined in Table 89.6. Children who weigh 45 kg or more may be treated with dosage regimens as defined for adults. All treatment regimens include agents active against *C. trachomatis* in addition to *N. gonorrhoeae.* Choice of chlamydial regimen also is impacted by age, where routine use of doxycycline is generally avoided for STI treatment in those younger than 8 years.

The recommended regimens generally have not been studied in populations of prepubertal children with either uncomplicated or complicated gonococcal infection, but these regimens are likely to be highly effective in most cases, as they are for older adolescents and adults. As a general rule, children treated with ceftriaxone do not require follow-up cultures, but if treatment regimens other than ceftriaxone are used, follow-up cultures may be indicated.[343]

Uncomplicated Gonococcal Infections

Ceftriaxone is the preferred agent for treatment of uncomplicated gonococcal vulvovaginitis, endocervicitis, urethritis, proctitis, pharyngitis, and conjunctivitis beyond the neonatal period (see Table 89.6). Higher dosage is recommended for conjunctival infection. Oral cefixime is no longer recommended as routine therapy since it does not provide bactericidal concentrations as high or sustained as ceftriaxone. Cefixime still may be considered as an alternative agent for a few more years (MICs are expected to continue to climb over time); use of other previously recommended oral cephalosporins, such as cefpodoxime or cefuroxime, should be avoided.[343]

Gonococcal infection of the pharynx is more difficult to eradicate than infection of urogenital and anorectal sites. Ceftriaxone has the most reliable efficacy for this site. Spectinomycin (when available) is unreliable because its efficacy against *N. gonorrhoeae* in the pharynx is only about 50%.[343]

Disseminated Gonococcal Infection

Septic arthritis, arthritis-dermatitis, and sepsis caused by *N. gonorrhoeae* are treated with ceftriaxone for 7 days (see Table 89.6). Alternative agents include cefotaxime and ceftizoxime. The recommended durations of ceftriaxone therapy for meningitis and endocarditis are 10 to 14 days and at least 28 days, respectively. These treatment durations have not been systematically studied.[343]

Pelvic Inflammatory Disease

PID is presumed to be polymicrobial, including anaerobes, in addition to *N. gonorrhoeae.* Combination antimicrobial regimens are required. Hospitalization is warranted for adolescents who are pregnant; have

TABLE 89.7 Recommended Treatment of Pelvic Inflammatory Disease

Recommended Parenteral Regimens	Recommended Intramuscular Plus Oral Regimens
Option 1[a,b]	**IM/PO Options**
Cefotetan 2 g IV every 12 h	One of
or	Ceftriaxone 250 mg IM in a single dose
Cefoxitin 2 g IV every 6 h	*or*
plus	Cefoxitin 2 g IM in a single dose with Probenecid, 1 g PO concurrently as a single dose
Doxycycline[c] 100 mg PO or IV every 12 h	*or*
Option 2[a,b]	Another parenteral third-generation cephalosporin (e.g., cefotaxime, ceftizoxime)
Clindamycin 900 mg IV every 8 h	*plus*
plus	Doxycycline 100 mg PO twice a day for 14 days
Gentamicin loading dose IV or IM (2 mg/kg) followed by 1.5 mg/kg every 8 h (single daily dosing of 3 to 5 mg/kg can be substituted)	*with or without*[d]
	Metronidazole 500 mg PO twice a day for 14 days

[a]Ampicillin-sulbactam 3 g IV every 6 h plus doxycycline 100 mg orally or IV every 12 h is an alternative option for initial parenteral therapy that provides needed broad-spectrum coverage with a modicum of clinical trial data demonstrating efficacy.
[b]Adolescents with PID usually can be transitioned from the parenteral regimen to oral therapy for completion of the course within 24 to 48 h. Those with tubo-ovarian abscess should be observed for at least 24 h in an inpatient setting.
[c]Doxycycline should be administered PO when possible due to pain associated with its IV infusion.
[d]None of the recommended parenteral third-generation cephalosporins provides adequate anaerobic coverage. Metronidazole should be added unless or until it is known that extended anaerobic coverage is not needed for a particular episode of acute PID.
Data from Workowski KA, Bolan GA. Sexually Transmitted Diseases Treatment Guidelines, 2015. *MMWR Recomm Rep.* 2015;64:1–137. For potential updates to these recommendations, see http://www.cdc.gov/std/gonorrhea/treatment.htm.

potential surgical emergencies other than PID, including tubo-ovarian abscess; have not responded to an oral regimen already prescribed for the episode; are unable to follow or tolerate an oral regimen; or have severe illness, nausea and vomiting, or high fever.

Two parenteral regimens are recommended for those requiring hospitalization (Table 89.7 for dosages): (1) *either* cefotetan *or* cefoxitin intravenously combined with doxycycline orally or intravenously; or (2) clindamycin intravenously plus gentamicin, using a loading dose intravenously or intramuscularly followed by maintenance doses. Single daily dosing of gentamicin also can be used. Parenteral therapy can be discontinued 24 to 48 hours after clinical improvement. Oral doxycycline or clindamycin should then be continued to complete a total of 14 days of therapy. Clindamycin is preferred for course completion when tubo-ovarian abscess is present to provide more effective anaerobic coverage.[343]

Outpatient regimens recommended for adolescents who are not severely ill, as discussed earlier, and appear able to tolerate oral agents also are listed in Table 89.7. These include a cephalosporin, generally single intramuscular doses of ceftriaxone or cefoxitin (with addition of an oral dose of probencid with the latter), in combination with 14-day oral courses of doxycycline plus metronidazole. Metronidazole provides anaerobic coverage and treatment for often associated bacterial vaginosis. Other parenteral third-generation cephalosporins (e.g., cefotaxime or ceftizoxime) may be substituted for ceftriaxone or cefoxitin in these regimens. Other regimens may become recommended over time when supported by data from more clinical trials.[343]

Quinolone-based oral regimens are no longer recommended for routine use because of prevalence of gonococcal resistance to these agents. However, if a cephalosporin-based regimen is not feasible, a fluoroquinolone plus metronidazole may be used (both for 14 days) if a culture for *N. gonorrhoeae* showing susceptibility to quinolones is documented. Levofloxacin 500 mg, moxifloxacin 400 mg, or ofloxacin 400 mg, each orally once daily, are the agents of choice.[343]

Substantial clinical improvement is expected within 72 hours after initiation of therapy. Those failing oral regimens should be hospitalized and switched to parenteral regimens. Diagnostic testing (i.e., imaging or laparoscopy) should be considered in such cases.

Severe Allergies to Cephalosporins

Selection of alternative antibiotic therapies for persons with a history of a reaction to a cephalosporin must be guided by the severity of the reaction and the availability of suitable alternative regimens. Desensitization can be considered but may be impractical. There are no data for specific alternative regimens for treatment of gonococcal infections in children with apparent severe IgE-mediated penicillin or cephalosporin allergy or other adverse reactions such as Stevens-Johnson syndrome. In adults, currently suggested options for treatment of uncomplicated infection in such persons are *either* a single dose of oral gemifloxacin (320 mg) *or* a single intramuscular dose of gentamicin (240 mg) *plus* a single oral dose azithromycin (2 g). Spectinomycin can be considered for urogenital or anorectal infection is available.[343] Agents such as fluoroquinolones or doxycycline may be used if the isolate is known to be susceptible.

Infection With Human Immunodeficiency Virus

Children and adolescents infected with HIV who acquire a gonococcal infection should receive the same treatment as persons without HIV infection.

Concurrent Syphilis Infection

A single dose of ceftriaxone is not adequate for treating syphilis. Longer courses of therapy are required with penicillin-based regimens (see Chapter 144).

Pregnancy

Quinolone and tetracycline agents should be avoided during pregnancy. Those unable to take one of the recommended cephalosporin regimens can be treated with the 2-g dosage of azithromycin. Spectinomycin would be appropriate if available.

Presumptive Treatment of *Chlamydia Trachomatis* Coinfection

Persons with gonococcal infection, including children, are at high risk for acquiring concurrent chlamydial infection.[241] Coinfection may occur in more than 50% of teens with gonorrhea.[179] In adolescents, treatment of gonococcal cervicitis with drug regimens that are effective against gonococci but not *Chlamydia* has been associated with a high incidence of residual salpingitis in females and urethritis in males because of persisting *C. trachomatis*.[249,261,264,291]

Therefore treatment recommendations for gonococcal infections beyond the neonatal period include agents active against both organisms (see Table 89.7). Neonates with gonococcal infections also should be evaluated for *C. trachomatis* coinfection as dual vertical transmission can occur. Penicillin, amoxicillin, ceftriaxone, or spectinomycin alone will fail to eradicate *C. trachomatis*. Trimethoprim-sulfamethoxazole, tetracycline, doxycycline, azithromycin, and erythromycin are effective in vitro and in many clinical forms of chlamydial disease.

Follow-Up

The recommended ceftriaxone regimens have such high cure rates that routine testing for cure is not recommended. As with adults, children or adolescents who receive treatment regimens other than ceftriaxone should have test of cure by culture or NAAT 14 days after treatment.[343] If a NAAT is performed and is positive, culture should be obtained prior to initiation of a second treatment regimen to provide antimicrobial susceptibility data and assess for the possibility of infection by a different microbe. Reinfection is generally more likely than treatment failure, though ongoing surveillance for the latter due to antimicrobial resistance is a critical public health function.

Adolescents treated for gonorrhea and remaining sexually active, regardless of whether they believe their partner(s) have been treated, should be retested at 3 months for potential reinfection or whenever they next present for health care. Partners who have had sexual contact within the previous 60 days with an adolescent diagnosed with gonococcal infection should be evaluated and treated.[343]

GONOCOCCAL INFECTION AND SEXUAL ABUSE OF CHILDREN

When gonococcal infection or any other STI is identified in a prepubertal child or in adolescents who are not sexually active within their peer groups, sexual abuse must be considered to have occurred unless proved otherwise. Nonsexual transmission never should be assumed without extensive investigation of the social setting of an infected child and even then rarely.[236,343] Isolation of *N. gonorrhoeae* in cultures from children should be reported to local public health authorities and also to child protective services to ensure that the child is not exposed to further abuse. Sexual abuse has been reported in approximately 10% of all self-reporting populations of girls during childhood in numerous studies, and rates in boys are about 3%.[13,278] Approximately 1% of children appear to experience serious forms of sexual abuse yearly.[5]

STIs occur in 3% to 20% of sexually abused children, with gonococcal infections found in about 3% to 15%.[93,127,166,168,167,228,270,296,332,337] The absence of STDs does not rule out sexual abuse when other findings suggest that it has occurred. The prevalence and clinical manifestations of gonococcal infection in sexually abused children are determined by the prevalence of infection in the adults who constitute the population with whom the child resides, the age of the child, and the type and frequency of sexual contact.[246] As a result of improved control of gonorrhea in the 1980s, fewer pediatric cases have been recognized in the United States in recent years. Nonetheless girls who are exposed to an infected male appear to have a high rate of acquired disease. In an outbreak in an orphanage, 53 of 95 abused girls were found to have contracted infection.[2]

Among prepubertal girls who develop vaginal discharge after being sexually abused, gonococcal infection is the etiology in 9% to 24%.[127,166,294,296] Although most cases of gonorrhea in prepubertal children are associated with vaginal discharge, infection without evident discharge can occur.[127] The oropharynx also is a common site of gonococcal infection associated with sexual abuse of children and may be the only site of infection in children forced to perform orogenital sexual acts with an infected abuser. Pharyngeal infection may be asymptomatic. When STIs result from sexual abuse, these may be the only evidence that such abuse has occurred.[165]

Children with suspected gonococcal infection (or suspected to have suffered sexual abuse) should undergo a thorough physical examination by someone familiar with the medicolegal and clinical aspects of sexually abused children. Genital, rectal, and pharyngeal cultures should be obtained. Vaginal cultures are satisfactory in prepubertal girls. Endocervical cultures should be obtained only after puberty. Blood culture should be performed if disseminated disease is a consideration. Other sites (e.g., conjunctivae and joint fluid) should be cultured if clinically indicated. Cultures should be handled in a manner that will ensure legal acceptance if needed. When gonococcal isolates are available from both the sexual abuse victim and the alleged assailant, comparison of DNA fingerprints by methods such as PFGE may provide supporting evidence.[286]

NAATs occasionally may be used as an alternative to culture for forensic purposes for vaginal and urine specimens in girls, but not for these specimens from boys or extragenital specimens in boys or girls.[246,290]

Children who are being evaluated for sexual abuse should be evaluated for other STIs, including chlamydial disease, syphilis, hepatitis B, and HIV infection. Girls also should be evaluated for evidence of *Trichomonas vaginalis* and bacterial vaginosis by wet mount of vaginal swabs.[59,143,280] As a general rule, children undergoing evaluation for STIs should not have initiation of treatment until all appropriate diagnostic specimens have been obtained.[343]

Repeat physical examination and specimen collection may be warranted 2 weeks after initial evaluation, especially when the suspected abuse event was very recent. Repeat examination and serologic testing for syphilis, hepatitis B, and HIV should be provided at 6 weeks and 3 months after the last suspected sexual exposure.[343] A single evaluation may be sufficient if suspected abuse occurred over an extended period and a substantial amount of time has elapsed since occurrence of the last suspected episode. This is determined on a case-by-case basis.[59]

PREVENTION AND CONTROL OF GONOCOCCAL INFECTIONS

The US Preventive Services Task Force and the CDC both recommend that all sexually active women aged 24 years or younger at high risk of gonorrhea and chlamydia infection be screened with a NAAT that can detect these microbes.[321,343] Risk factors to be assessed include new or multiple sex partners, inconsistent condom use in persons not in a monogamous relationship, prior or concurrent STIs, and exchanging sex for money.[321] The CDC also recommends such testing annually for males who have sex with other males.[343]

All gonococcal infections must be reported to public health officials. Effort should be made to evaluate, counsel, and treat all sexual partners who were exposed to the index case within 60 days before the onset of symptoms or diagnosis in the index case. If a patient's last sexual intercourse occurred more than 60 days before the onset of symptoms, the most recent sexual partner of the patient should be evaluated and treated. Patients should be instructed to avoid engaging in sexual activity until therapy is completed and any symptoms have resolved. Cases in prepubertal children must be investigated to identify the source of infection (and potential perpetrator of abuse).[343]

Condoms provide a high degree of protection against the acquisition and transmission of genital gonococcal infection.[176,326] Other barrier contraceptive measures and topical spermicidal and bactericidal agents likewise can reduce the likelihood of acquiring gonococcal (and chlamydial) infection.[14,52,212,314] Postexposure prophylactic antibiotics also reduce the risk for infection developing but are unlikely to be cost-effective.[151]

When patients, including infants with ophthalmia neonatorum, with gonococcal infection are hospitalized, standard precautions are recommended.

Prevention of Neonatal Infection

Pregnant adolescents are at higher risk for contracting gonococcal infection than are older women. Pregnant women should have an endocervical culture for *N. gonorrhoeae* as part of their initial prenatal care visit. A second culture late in the third trimester should be performed for those at high risk for exposure during pregnancy.

Infants born to mothers known to have active gonococcal infection are at risk for acquiring local and disseminated infection from colonization during birth. Such infants should be treated as listed in Table 89.5. Standard preventive measures for GON were described earlier.

Vaccine Development

Research into the development of vaccines for gonococcal infection is ongoing. Although natural infection induces antibody responses directed primarily against pili, Opa, porin protein, and LOS, these antibodies do not protect against reinfection even with the same strain. Serologic correlates of immunity remain elusive, making vaccine development more difficult. A killed whole-cell vaccine studied in the 1970s induced antibody responses and was well tolerated but not protective. A purified pilin vaccine was studied in high-risk military personnel and also was not protective.[345]

Molecular analysis of gonococcal transferrin binding proteins may have potential as vaccine antigens because of their exposure on the microbial surface. These proteins are expressed in all strains, have highly conserved gene sequences, and lack antigenic and phase variation. Natural infection, however, generates little systemic or local antibody response to transferrin binding proteins.[50,257] Recent structure–function analysis of the transferrin receptor system may be an important step toward identifying an approach to immunogenic epitopes or novel therapeutic small-molecule inhibitors of this gonococcal system.[50]

As with meningococcal serogroup B strains, use of combinations of recombinant antigens, potentially delivered in different formats, may be necessary. The continued emergence of antimicrobial resistance in *N. gonorrhoeae* makes vaccine development increasingly urgent.

NEW REFERENCES SINCE THE SEVENTH EDITION

50. Cash DR, Noinaj N, Buchanan SK, et al. Beyond the crystal structure: insight into the function and vaccine potential of TbpA expressed by *Neisseria gonorrhoeae*. *Infect Immun.* 2015;83(11):4438-4449.
62. Centers for Disease Control and Prevention. *Sexually transmitted disease surveillance 2014.* Atlanta, GA: U.S. Department of Health and Human Services; 2015.
63. Centers for Disease Control and Prevention. Identification of N. gonorrhoeae and related species. Available at: http://www.cdc.gov/std/Gonorrhea/lab/ident.htm.
95. Demczuk W, Lynch T, Martin I, et al. Whole-genome phylogenomic heterogeneity of Neisseria gonorrhoeae isolates with decreased cephalosporin susceptibility collected in Canada between 1989 and 2013 [abstract]. *J Clin Microbiol.* 2014;53(1):191-200.
112. Ezewudo MN, Joseph SJ, Castillo-Ramirez S, et al. Population structure of *Neisseria gonorrhoeae* based on whole genome data and its relationship with antibiotic resistance. *Peer J.* 2015;3:5.
142. Gunderson CW, Seifert HS, et al. *Neisseria gonorrhoeae* elicits extracellular traps in primary neutrophil culture while suppressing the oxidative burst. *MBio.* 2015;6(1):e02452-14.
178. Juneau RA, Stevens JS, Apicella MA, et al. A thermonuclease of *Neisseria gonorrhoeae* enhances bacterial escape from killing by neutrophil extracellular traps. *J Infect Dis.* 2015;212(2):316-324.
200. Lindberg R, Fredlund H, Nicholas R, et al. *Neisseria gonorrhoeae* isolates with reduced susceptibility to cefixime and ceftriaxone: association with genetic polymorphisms in penA, mtrR, porB1b, and ponA. *Antimicrob Agents Chemother.* 2007;51(6):2117-2122.
211. McClure R, Nudel K, Massari P, et al. The gonococcal transcriptome during infection of the lower genital tract in women [abstract]. *PLoS ONE.* 2015; 10(8).
276. Rotman E, Seifert HS. The genetics of *Neisseria* species. *Annu Rev Genet.* 2014;48(1):407-411.
286. Sathirareuangchai S, Phuangphung P, Leelaporn A, et al. The usefulness of *Neisseria gonorrhoeae* strain typing by pulse-field gel electrophoresis (PFGE) and DNA detection as the forensic evidence in child sexual abuse cases: a case series. *In J Legal Med.* 2014;129(1):153-157.
287. Schweitzer VA, Dam AP, Hananta IP, et al. Identification of *Neisseria gonorrhoeae* by the Bruker biotyper matrix-assisted laser desorption ionization–time of flight mass spectrometry system is improved by a database extension. *J Clin Microbiol.* 2016;54(4):1130-1132.
290. Sena AC, Hsu KK, Kellogg N, et al. Sexual assault and sexually transmitted infections in adults, adolescents, and children. *CID.* 2015;61(suppl 8):S856-S864.
321. Tanksley A, Cifu AS. Screening for gonorrhea, chlamydia, and hepatitis B. *JAMA.* 2016;315(12):1278-1279.
343. Workowski KA, Bolan GA. Sexually transmitted diseases treatment guidelines, 2015. *MMWR Recomm Rep.* 2015;64:1-137.

The full reference list for this chapter is available at ExpertConsult.com.

SUBSECTION III Gram-Positive Bacilli

Diphtheria 90

Barbara W. Stechenberg

Diphtheria is an acute infectious disease caused by *Corynebacterium diphtheriae* or, less commonly, *C. ulcerans. C. pseudotuberculosis,* which primarily causes infections in sheep and goats, is not discussed here because it only rarely causes a diphtheria-like disease in humans. Infection by toxigenic strains of *C. diphtheriae* causes disease that is mediated by the production of an extracellular protein. Nontoxigenic strains also can cause disease, but it is usually less severe.

Before the discovery of antitoxin at the turn of the 20th century, the "strangling angel of children," as diphtheria once was called, was a significant cause of mortality in children and adults.[108] Apparent reference to diphtheria can be traced to the 5th century BC in the works of Hippocrates, *Epidemics III,* case 7.[79] In 1821, it was recognized as a specific entity by Brettoneau, who suggested that the disease was caused by a germ and that it could be transmitted from person to person. Brettoneau coined the origin of the modern term *diphtheria* from the Greek root *diphtheria,* which means "skin" or "hide."[50] In 1883 the causative agent was identified by Klebs in stained smears from diphtheritic membranes; in 1884, Löffler grew the organism on artificial media and showed that in guinea pigs it caused a fatal infection closely resembling human disease.

The toxin was purified in 1889 by Roux and Yersin, who found that toxin alone could cause the disease. Shortly thereafter, Behring and Kitasato discovered antitoxins when they immunized animals with toxins rather than bacteria. The use of antitoxin to treat children with diphtheria at the turn of the 20th century resulted in one of the largest decreases in mortality rates by a therapeutic intervention. In Germany alone, an estimated 45,000 lives were saved each year.[62]

ETIOLOGY

Corynebacteria (Klebs-Löffler bacilli) are irregularly staining, gram-positive, nonmotile, nonsporulating, pleomorphic bacilli.[54] The club-shaped appearance of the bacillus is not a true morphologic feature, but results from attempting to grow the bacillus on media that are nutritionally inadequate (Löffler media). The organism can be recovered most readily on media containing selective inhibitors that retard the growth of other microorganisms; a sheep blood agar–based medium containing fosfomycin (for selectivity) and Tindale medium (tellurite medium with cystine) are ideal.[43,44] *C. diphtheriae* and *C. ulcerans* grow on supplement-free blood agar, chocolate agar, and other standard media.[43]

Colonies of *C. diphtheriae* (with the exception of the lipophilic, gray *C. intermedius*) and *C. ulcerans* appear grayish white on Löffler medium. On tellurite medium, three diphtheria colony types can be distinguished: *mitis, gravis,* and *intermedius. Mitis* colonies are smooth, black, and convex; they do not ferment starch or glycogen and are hemolytic. *Gravis* colonies are gray, radially striate, and semirough; they ferment starch and glycogen and usually are not hemolytic. *Intermedius* colonies are small and smooth and have a black center; they do not ferment starch or glycogen and are not hemolytic. *C. ulcerans* colonies resemble *gravis* on Tindale medium but differ in that they are hemolytic. Similar to *gravis,* they ferment starch and glycogen. All diphtheria biotypes and *C. ulcerans* are characterized by cystinase activity and absence of pyrazinamidase activity. *C. ulcerans* may be distinguished from *C. diphtheriae* by its urease activity and ability to liquefy gelatin. Biotype *belfanti,* which does not occur in a toxigenic form, may be distinguished from the three potentially toxigenic diphtheria biotypes by its inability to reduce nitrate on Tindale medium and from *C. ulcerans* by its lack of production of urease.[43] Ribotyping and pulsed-field gel electrophoresis, both of which involve restriction digestion of genomic bacterial DNA, followed by gel electrophoresis and Southern blotting, permit more specific typing within each diphtheria biotype and aid in the epidemiologic study of outbreaks.[41,95]

C. diphtheriae biotypes *intermedius, gravis,* and *mitis* and *C. ulcerans* all have been observed in a toxigenic form. *Intermedius* was the biotype isolated most commonly in the United States between 1971 and 1981. Of the strains isolated, *intermedius* was found to be toxigenic more often than *mitis* or *gravis.*[36] In the United Kingdom between 1993 and 1998, and similarly in other parts of Europe, the biovar *gravis* has represented most nontoxigenic isolates, followed by *mitis* and *belfanti.*[45] Of the four nontoxigenic isolates obtained during a surveillance study of a U.S. Northern Plains Native American Community in 1996, two were of biotype *mitis* and two were *gravis.*[59] According to a UK diphtheria reference laboratory, between 1993 and 1998, the toxigenic isolates originating from Asia, Africa, and the Middle East were reported to be of the biotype *mitis* or *gravis,* with the exception of one *intermedius* isolate.[44] Golaz and associates[59] reported similar findings when they surveyed the different biotypes in South Dakota. A significant overall increase in the proportion of nontoxigenic isolates has been observed in Europe and Australia in recent years.[58] The reason for this increase is unclear, but one hypothesis is that increased immunity to toxigenic strains secondary to immunization has altered this epidemiology.

The complete genome sequence of *C. diphtheriae* biotype *gravis* has been elucidated.[33] The genome is approximately 2.48 Mb with a G+C content of 53% and has approximately 2320 predicted coding sequences. Metabolic analysis of the genome has revealed that *C. diphtheriae* has a complete set of enzymes for glycolysis, gluconeogenesis, pentose-phosphate pathways, anaerobic and aerobic respiration, amino acid biosynthesis, and purine nucleotide biosynthetic pathway. Most of the enzymes for the tricarboxylic acid cycle are present, with the exception of an enzyme succinyl coenzyme A (CoA) synthetase that catalyzes the conversion of succinate to succinyl CoA. An alternative enzyme present in *C. diphtheriae* may fulfill this conversion, however. The pyrimidine pathway in *C. diphtheriae* lacks an enzyme that interferes with the production of cytidine; the pathway to the biosynthesis of thymidine is complete. The genome has revealed 13 regions that are unique to *C. diphtheriae* and may serve as pathogenicity islands.[33]

No functional or significant differences have been detected in the exotoxins elaborated by the three strains of *C. diphtheriae* or by *C. ulcerans.* Only strains that are lysogenic for β-prophage or a closely related phage carrying the gene for toxin production produce diphtheria toxin. One or more *tox* gene sequences may exist in the bacterial genome, and the most highly toxigenic strains contain three or more copies.[82] Phage multiplication is not a prerequisite for the production of toxin. The capacity to synthesize toxin depends on genetic and nutritional factors. Toxin-producing cells apparently are cells in which spontaneous induction of the prophage to the phage occurs.[53] The most important factor controlling the yield of toxin is the concentration of inorganic iron in the culture medium.[39] Growth of *C. diphtheriae* in iron-deficient media prolongs the duration of induction lysis and is associated with a high yield of toxin. High concentrations of iron inhibit the production of toxin. Production of toxin also can be increased by the use of ultraviolet radiation. Conversion to a toxigenic strain occurs in nature, as has been shown by restriction enzyme studies of carriers of toxigenic and nontoxigenic strains in Manchester, England.

The ability of a strain of *C. diphtheriae* to elaborate diphtheria toxin can be shown by using several methods. In vivo studies involving necrosis of tissue in guinea pigs has been replaced by the widely used Elek[46] or modified Elek test.[49] Enzyme immunoassay[48] and polymerase chain reaction (PCR)[94] have been used to detect toxigenicity.

Diphtheria toxin is lethal to humans in an amount of approximately 130 μg/kg body weight. Cytoplasmic internalization of 1 molecule of toxin has been shown to cause cell death.[11] Toxigenic and nontoxigenic strains of *C. diphtheriae* can cause disease, but only strains that produce toxin cause disease with symptoms of myocarditis and neuritis.

EPIDEMIOLOGY

Asymptomatic human carriers serve as the reservoir for *C. diphtheriae.* Infection by *C. diphtheriae* is acquired by contact with either a carrier or an individual with active disease. The bacteria may be transmitted via droplets during coughing, sneezing, or talking. Rarely transmission of *C. diphtheriae* occurs from skin lesions or fomites. Some reports suggest that skin carriers of *C. diphtheriae* are more infectious than nose or throat carriers and that skin carriers may serve as potential reservoirs for the initiation of epidemic spread.[12,68] In areas in which skin infections are endemic, levels of natural immunization may be high.[20] This phenomenon is illustrated particularly well in a survey of tetanus and diphtheria immunity in a rural Kenyan community, where age was not found to be predictive of immunity, and no correlation was found between levels of antibody for tetanus and diphtheria.[77]

Person-to-person transmission of *C. ulcerans* is not known to occur, although *C. ulcerans* was isolated from the siblings of two patients reported in the United Kingdom between 1995 and 1997.[17] Cases of respiratory diphtheria caused by *C. diphtheriae* and *C. ulcerans* have been documented in association with contaminated unpasteurized milk taken from cows with infected teats.[18,60,104] *C. diphtheriae* has been isolated from horses, dogs, and other domestic animals. *C. ulcerans* has been reported to infect ground squirrels in the United States, but transmission to humans has not been reported.[67,93] *C. ulcerans* is a commensal in animals and has been isolated in a wide range of wild and domestic animals.[105]

According to World Health Organization (WHO) reports, diphtheria is distributed worldwide and remains endemic in many developing areas of the world, including Asia, Africa, South America, and the Mediterranean regions.[19] Worldwide, diphtheria epidemics have occurred in a cyclic manner since the 16th century. In 2014, 7321 cases of diphtheria were reported to the WHO, although many others were likely unreported.

In the United States, the incidence and mortality rates from diphtheria in the 1920s were 140 to 150 cases/100,000, with 13,000 to 15,000 deaths each year. The number of cases gradually declined to 15 cases/100,000 population in 1945 with the extensive use of diphtheria toxoid vaccine. From 1970 through 1979, the average number of cases of diphtheria reported annually in the United States was 196.[8] From 1980 to 2004, only 57 cases of diphtheria were reported in the United States. Approximately 75% of the cases were in patients older than 15 years who were unimmunized or inadequately immunized.[8] Only two cases of diphtheria have been reported in the United States between 2004 and 2015. Maintenance of immunity in adults requires a booster vaccination every 10 years. The Centers for Disease Control and Prevention (CDC) estimated in the mid-1990s that fewer than 50% of adults in the United States had received their 10-year boosters and that 40% to 50% of adults were susceptible to diphtheria.[52,96] In addition, the toxoid vaccine does not provide protection against nontoxigenic strains.

The incidence peaks during the cooler autumn, winter, and spring months. Several epidemics, primarily in the southern United States, have occurred in late summer and fall and corresponded to a high prevalence of *C. diphtheriae* skin infections. Between the years 1971 and 1981, the incidence of diphtheria was highest in the western United States. A 100-fold greater incidence of diphtheria occurs in Native Americans than in the general population.[36] This difference may be attributable to socioeconomic factors more than to race. In 1996, a surveillance study was conducted in a Northern Plains Native American community after *C. diphtheriae* was isolated from the skin of a resident of the community. The woman was a chronic alcoholic admitted to the hospital for detoxification and treatment of severe necrotizing leg ulcers, from which a toxigenic *mitis* biotype was isolated. In the following 4 months, 11 positive cultures were obtained from the community, including four positive throat swabs from asymptomatic household contacts of the index cases. Ribotyping indicated that the isolates were related closely to each other genetically and to strains obtained from past cases from the same area; they were different from organisms obtained from other parts of the United States and from the former Soviet Union, where an ongoing epidemic was occurring at the time.[25,59] A similar study was conducted in a Koorie (Aborigine) community in Victoria, Australia, in 1994, after three cases of nontoxigenic *C. diphtheriae* endocarditis were diagnosed in the community. After screening 359 asymptomatic (with the exception of four people who had chronic skin ulcers swabbed) contacts of the index cases, 12 produced positive cultures for nontoxigenic *C. diphtheriae*. Of them, five were of the same biovar *gravis* clone as the three index cases.[69] Evidence that diphtheria is diagnosed more frequently in chronic alcoholics and the indigent than in the general population is significant. In a 1993 to 1994 outbreak in St. Petersburg, Russia, 69% of a total of 42 deaths occurred in individuals classified as chronic alcoholics.[98] Between 1972 and 1982, three outbreaks occurred in the indigent alcoholic population living in Seattle's Skid Road.[66] Cutaneous infections accounted for 86% of the 1100 total cases. The first outbreak was caused by a single toxigenic *intermedius* biotype clone, whereas the other two involved nontoxigenic *mitis* and *gravis* strains. The incidence was highest in winter and spring.

A major epidemic began in 1990 in the new independent states of the former Soviet Union and spread throughout the area. Between 1990 and 1997, approximately 150,000 cases of diphtheria were reported, with approximately 4000 fatalities.[65,95] The epidemic was attributed to decreasing immunization rates and immunity in adults and children and to movement of large numbers of people during the collapse of the former Soviet Union.[23,106] Apparently multiple foci of infection existed across the continent. Most of the epidemic isolates from Ukraine and Russia were biotype *gravis,* but further molecular characterization of the *tox* genes from these areas revealed distinct epidemic strains in each location.[70] A mass immunization program was initiated in Russia in 1993, with a resultant 10% decrease in the number of new cases reported between 1994 and 1995 (vs. two- to threefold increases in the number of cases each year for the preceding 3 years).[57] The WHO also held training workshops and assembled laboratory kits to assist in establishing the proper diagnosis of diphtheria. Because cases also began to appear in Europe with increasing frequency during this period, the European Working Group on Diphtheria (ELWGD) and reference laboratories were assembled to assist in an effort to increase routine screening for diphtheria. The ELWGD since has expanded and currently includes 20 participating countries, including representatives in Western and Eastern Europe, the United States, Australia, and Southeast Asia.[45] Surveillance from Europe from 2000 to 2009 has documented a decrease in incidence of more than 95% across the region, with the Russian Federation and Latvia accounting for 83% of the cases. In Western Europe, toxigenic *C. ulcerans* has increasingly been identified, often in association with contact with companion animals.[107] More recently there have been documented cases, particularly of cutaneous diphtheria, in refugees and asylum seekers in Europe.

PATHOGENESIS AND PATHOLOGY

Diphtheria is initiated by entry of *C. diphtheriae* into the nose or mouth, where the bacilli remain localized on the mucosal surfaces of the upper respiratory tract. Occasionally the ocular or genital mucous membranes serve as the site of localization. The bacilli are unable to invade intact skin but may infect preexisting skin lesions. After a 2- to 4-day period of incubation, lysogenized strains may elaborate toxin.

Diphtheria toxin is secreted as a single polypeptide of 535 amino acids with a molecular weight of 58,342 Da.[70] The toxin is composed of two subunits: a large B subunit that is involved in receptor binding and an A subunit that is the enzymatically active portion of the toxin. The toxin initially is absorbed onto the target cell membrane by binding a receptor on the cell surface and then undergoes receptor-mediated endocytosis. When it is in the endolysosomal complex, it undergoes a conformational change with subsequent release of the A subunit into the cytoplasm. The A subunit transfers an adenosine diphosphate (ADP)-ribosyl group from nicotinamide adenine dinucleotide (NAD) to elongation factor 2. This ADP-ribosylation inactivates elongation factor 2 and inhibits protein synthesis in the cell. Cholera and pertussis toxins also mediate target protein ribosylation by this mechanism. In addition to the inhibition of cellular protein synthesis, an independent mechanism of cytolysis has been described. In the presence of calcium and magnesium, diphtheria toxin has a nuclease-like activity that causes DNA fragmentation that results in cytolysis.[34,35,70,78]

Marked toxin-mediated tissue necrosis occurs in the vicinity of *C. diphtheriae* colonization and induces a robust local inflammatory response. The inflammatory response coupled with the necrotic tissue produces a patchy exudate that initially can be removed. As the infection progresses, the increased production of toxin causes a centrifugal widening of the area of infection, and eventually a fibrinous exudate develops. A tough adherent membrane results from coagulation of the exudate. The color of the pseudomembrane initially is white but, over the course of time, becomes dirty gray. Late in the course of the infection, green or black spots appear on the membrane, representing areas of necrosis. Histologic analysis of the pseudomembrane differs based on the site of formation and maturation of the membrane. Analysis of the pharyngeal pseudomembrane shows fibrin; inflammatory cells, primarily composed of neutrophils, red blood cells, and colonies of organisms; and superficial epithelial cells.

With severe infections, significant vascular congestion, interstitial edema, fibrin exudate, and intense neutrophilic infiltration develop.[64] Profuse bleeding can occur when the membrane is torn off. The edematous tissue and the diphtheritic membrane may encroach on the airway. The membrane sloughs spontaneously during the recovery period, although sloughing can occur during the acute phase of the illness, leading to aspiration. Occasionally secondary bacterial infection (classically caused by *Streptococcus pyogenes*) develops. Respiratory embarrassment or suffocation may occur, with involvement of the larynx or tracheobronchial tree. Bronchopneumonia may develop if the exudate enters the small airways and alveoli. Infection of these sites is an uncommon occurrence, however. Infections of the esophagus and stomach, with pseudomembranous lesions indistinguishable from lesions found in the respiratory tract, have been reported.[72]

Toxin produced at the site of infection is distributed throughout the body by the bloodstream and the lymphatics. This distribution occurs most readily when the pharynx and tonsils are covered by a diphtheritic membrane. Any organ or tissue can be damaged as a result of diphtheria toxin, but lesions of the heart, nervous system, and kidneys are particularly prominent. Clinical manifestations appear after a variable latent period of 10 to 14 days for myocarditis and 3 to 7 weeks for manifestations in the nervous system, such as peripheral neuritis. In a study of 102 patients who died of diphtheria caused by *C. diphtheriae,* the hearts appeared dilated, flabby, and pale, with a characteristic "streaky" appearance in the myocardium. The most prominent pathologic findings are necrosis and hyaline degeneration of the myocardium. The myocardium also appears edematous and is infiltrated with mononuclear cells with eosinophilic cytoplasm. In a significant proportion of cases, fatty accumulation in muscle fibers and the conducting system may be observed.[89] Burch and associates[21] showed mitochondrial damage with depletion of glycogen and accumulation of lipid droplets in the damaged myofibrils. Toxin may be observed within the myocardial cells with fluorescent antibody staining.[64] If the patient survives, muscle regeneration and interstitial fibrosis can be seen.

Peripheral neuropathy occurs secondary to *C. diphtheriae* infections. Histologic studies have shown that affected nerves have significant degeneration of myelin sheaths and axons. Toxic neuritis with fatty degeneration of paranodal myelin can be noted early in the disease course; segmental demyelination occurs later.[9] Axonal damage is secondary to the application of external pressure from the swollen Schwann cell cytoplasm and myelin.[81]

C. diphtheriae infections also can lead to necrosis and hyaline degeneration of the liver, which can lead to hypoglycemia. Adrenal hemorrhage and acute tubular necrosis of the kidney have been known to occur secondary to *C. diphtheriae* infections.[64]

CLINICAL MANIFESTATIONS

The signs and symptoms of diphtheria depend on the site of infection, the immunization status of the host, and whether toxin has been distributed to the systemic circulation. The incubation period is 1 to 6 days (range, 1 to 10 days). Diphtheria can be classified clinically on the basis of the anatomic location of the initial infection and the diphtheritic membrane (nasal, pharyngeal/tonsillar, laryngeal or laryngotracheal, skin, and others) involved. More than one anatomic site may be involved simultaneously.

Nasal diphtheria initially resembles a common cold and is characterized by mild rhinorrhea and a paucity of systemic symptoms. Gradually the nasal discharge becomes serosanguineous and then mucopurulent. A foul odor may be noticed, and careful inspection reveals a white membrane on the nasal septum. In severe cases, the infection may excoriate the nares and upper lip. Nasal diphtheria is a mild form of the disease because absorption of toxin usually is slow from this site. Frequently delays in establishing an accurate diagnosis of nasal diphtheria occur because of the lack of systemic symptoms. The nasal form of the disease occurs most often in infants.

Pharyngeal and tonsillar diphtheria begin insidiously with anorexia, malaise, low-grade fever, and pharyngitis. Within 1 or 2 days, a membrane appears. The extent of membrane formation correlates with the immune status of the host; in some partially immune individuals, a membrane may not develop. The white or gray adherent membrane may cover the tonsils and pharyngeal walls and extend on to the uvula and soft palate or down on to the larynx and trachea. Attempts to remove the membrane are followed by bleeding. Cervical lymphadenitis varies. In some cases, it is associated with edema of the soft tissues of the neck and may be so severe that it gives the appearance of a "bull neck." In a 1970 epidemic, "erasure" edema of the neck was noted in patients with pharyngeal diphtheria.[85] Patients with erasure edema did not have a classic bull neck appearance, but the edema was characterized by obliteration of the sternocleidomastoid muscle border, the mandible, and the median border of the clavicle. The edema was brawny, pitting, warm to the touch, and tender to palpation. Erasure edema was noted in 29% of immunized patients and 30% of nonimmunized or inadequately immunized patients. It occurred most commonly in children older than 6 years and generally was associated with infection by the *gravis* or *intermedius* strain of *C. diphtheriae.*

The course of pharyngeal diphtheria depends on the degree of elaboration of the toxin and the extent of the membrane. In severe cases, respiratory and circulatory collapse may occur. The pulse rate is increased disproportionately to body temperature, which generally remains normal or slightly elevated. The palate may be paralyzed. This paralysis may be unilateral or bilateral and associated with difficulty swallowing and nasal regurgitation of swallowed fluids.[42] Stupor, coma, and death may occur within 7 to 10 days. In less severe cases, recovery may be slow and may be complicated by the development of myocarditis or neuritis. In mild cases, the membrane sloughs off in 7 to 10 days, and recovery is uneventful.

Laryngeal diphtheria generally reflects a downward extension of the membrane from the pharynx. Rarely laryngeal diphtheria is primary and does not reflect an extension of disease from the pharynx. In these cases, toxicity and signs of toxemia generally are less prominent. Two cases of isolated diphtheritic tracheitis have been reported in the literature.[13,103] The clinical findings of laryngeal diphtheria are indistinguishable from those of other types of infectious croup. Noisy breathing, progressive stridor, hoarseness, and a dry, barking cough may be noted. Suprasternal, subcostal, and supraclavicular retractions reflect severe laryngeal obstruction, which may be fatal unless alleviated. Occasionally in a mild case, an acute and fatal obstruction may occur because of a partially detached piece of membrane that occludes the airway. In severe cases of laryngeal diphtheria, the membrane may extend downward and invade the entire tracheobronchial tree.

Cutaneous disease, in contrast to pharyngeal disease, is more common in warmer climates and often is caused by nontoxigenic strains. In some countries with tropical and subtropical climates, such as Uganda, Tanzania, Sri Lanka, and Samoa, *C. diphtheriae* has been isolated from 60% of skin lesions in children.[74] Cutaneous diphtheria is more contagious than respiratory diphtheria. Cutaneous diphtheria may be an important source of person-to-person transmission of diphtheritic organisms and outbreaks in indigenous populations in which overcrowding and poor hygiene are important risk factors.[12,20,68] The skin lesions begin as vesicles or pustules that progress to typical ulcers with sharply defined borders, membranous bases, and surrounding erythema and edema. They may be covered with a dark pseudomembrane. The lesions occur most commonly on the legs, feet, and hands. For the first 1 to 2 weeks, the lesions are painful. Spontaneous healing generally takes 6 to 12 weeks, but lesions have been reported to persist for 1 year.[68]

Conjunctival, aural, and vulvovaginal diphtheria also may occur. Conjunctival lesions usually are limited to the palpebral conjunctiva, which appears red, edematous, and membranous. Rarely conjunctival lesions have been associated with corneal erosion.[99] Diphtheria infections of the ear are characterized by the development of otitis externa with a persistent purulent and frequently foul-smelling discharge.

Clinical presentations other than typical diphtheria have been associated with isolation of the organism from patients with meningitis, endocarditis, osteomyelitis, and hepatitis. In most cases, these infections have occurred in patients with underlying problems, such as structural or valvular heart disease or intravenous drug use, or in individuals from poor socioeconomic backgrounds.[40,104]

Several cases of septic arthritis caused by nontoxigenic *C. diphtheriae* have been described.[1,63,104] Afghani and Stutman[1] reported the case of a 27-month-old child who had septic arthritis of the hip and skin lesions on the lower extremities. In this case, the skin lesions were presumed to be the portal of entry for nontoxigenic *C. diphtheriae.* Although the child had received four doses of diphtheria and tetanus toxoids and pertussis vaccines, immunization with toxoid does not provide protection against nontoxigenic strains of *C. diphtheriae.* In this case, the organism was sensitive to penicillin, cefuroxime, cephalothin, and clindamycin but was resistant to oxacillin, an antistaphylococcal antibiotic often used for the treatment of septic arthritis when the causative organism cannot be identified. A similar case was described in an immunocompetent, fully vaccinated 2-year-old child who had skin lesions from which *C. diphtheriae* was isolated. The skin lesions also were assumed to be the portal of entry for the organism because pan-sensitive *C. diphtheriae* were isolated from the skin and the articular aspirate.[63]

Within a 12-month period, in New South Wales, Australia, four cases of septic arthritis complicating endocarditis caused by the nontoxigenic *gravis* variety of *C. diphtheriae* were reported. In addition, the same strain caused three cases of endocarditis without the development of septic arthritis. Demographic distribution of these seven cases included a 12-year-old boy who died, five patients who were in their 20s, and a patient who was 49 years old. Three of the patients had underlying cardiac abnormalities, and one had a history of intravenous drug use.[104] This same clone of nontoxigenic *C. diphtheriae* was isolated from three patients in Koorie, an aborigine community in Victoria, Australia, who had endocarditis, and five asymptomatic contacts.[69] Two of the three patients with endocarditis were members of the same family, and one of them had a history of alcohol abuse. The third patient had a septic sternoclavicular joint, in addition to endocarditis, with isolation of the same organism. Nontoxigenic *C. diphtheriae* sepsis can lead to splenic and hepatic abscesses, as reported in a patient with chronic lymphocytic leukemia in British Columbia, Canada.[71]

Complications secondary to elaborated diphtheria toxin may affect any system, but myocarditis and involvement of the nervous system are most characteristic. Myocarditis may occur after mild and severe cases of diphtheria. Generally it develops in patients in whom administration of antitoxin is delayed. Myocarditis most commonly appears in the second week of the disease, but it can appear as early as the first or as late as the sixth week of illness. Tachycardia, a muffled S_1, murmurs, and arrhythmias such as atrioventricular dissociation indicate myocardial involvement. Echocardiography may show left ventricular dysfunction.[3,61,80] Although some cases may result in cardiac failure, most myocardial complications are temporary.

Neurologic complications appear after a variable latent period. Approximately 75% of all patients with severe diphtheria develop neuropathies. The incidence of neurologic sequelae has been shown to correlate with the severity of respiratory symptoms; 20% of all patients with respiratory problems develop polyneuritis. Neurologic complications from diphtheria infections predominantly are bilateral, are motor rather than sensory, and usually resolve completely. Paralysis of the soft palate is the most common occurrence and generally appears in the third week. It is manifested by a nasal quality in the voice, nasal regurgitation, and difficulty swallowing. Ocular paralysis usually occurs around the fifth week of illness and is characterized by blurring of vision and difficulty with accommodation. Internal strabismus also may be noted. Paralysis of the diaphragm, peripheral neuropathy involving the limbs, and loss of deep tendon reflexes likewise are reported as complications of diphtheria. When they occur, along with an elevated cerebrospinal fluid protein, the syndrome is clinically indistinguishable from Guillain-Barré syndrome.

Rarely, 2 or 3 weeks after the onset of illness, involvement of the vasomotor centers results in hypotension and cardiac failure. Gastritis, hepatitis, nephritis, and hemolytic-uremic syndrome also have been reported as complications of diphtheria.[102]

Information on the effects, if any, of diphtheria on the fetus during pregnancy is sparse. El Seed and associates[47] reported a case of pharyngeal diphtheria in a pregnant woman that occurred during the first trimester of pregnancy. Apart from vaginal bleeding, no complications of pregnancy were noted. Severe diphtheritic toxemia in the mother was characterized by quadriparesis, from which she fully recovered. A physically normal female infant was delivered at term. In this single case, severe diphtheritic toxemia during pregnancy was not associated with any teratogenic effect in the fetus and did not impair intrauterine fetal growth.

DIAGNOSIS

The diagnosis of diphtheria should be based on clinical findings because any delay in initiating therapy poses a serious risk to the patient. Isolation of the organism is used to confirm the clinical diagnosis. Material obtained from beneath the membrane, where organisms are concentrated most highly, or a portion of the membrane itself should be obtained for culture.[5,33]

C. diphtheriae is relatively resistant to drying. The use of a nonnutritive, moisture-reducing transport medium helps prevent the overgrowth of other microorganisms. The laboratory should be notified about the possibility of diphtheria so that appropriate culture media are inoculated. A Löffler slant, a tellurite plate, and a blood agar plate should be inoculated. Tellurite-containing media inhibit the growth of normal oral flora, allowing *C. diphtheriae* to grow into characteristic black colonies. Other corynebacteria, staphylococci, and yeast also can reduce tellurite and grow into black colonies.[38] Although examination of direct smears of colonies or diphtheritic lesions remains an important supplement to clinical examination, it often is inaccurate. Screening the colonies from the tellurite plate for catalase, urea, nitrate, pyrazinamidase, and cystinase is important. Most biotypes of *C. diphtheriae* are catalase positive, urease negative, nitrate positive (except biotype *belfanti*), pyrazinamidase negative, and cystinase positive.[43]

All diphtheria bacilli that are recovered should be tested for toxigenicity. In 1949, the Elek immunoprecipitation assay replaced in vivo testing for toxigenicity using guinea pigs or rabbits.[46] The Elek test is based on gel diffusion and immunoprecipitation of toxin from organisms inoculated onto agar adjacent to an antitoxin-containing well. A strain that is positive for toxin is indicated by the formation of a precipitin band between the toxin and antitoxin.[44,46] The Elek test takes 48 hours to yield results on the toxigenic nature of a *C. diphtheriae* strain. A modified Elek test that consists of placement of an antitoxin-impregnated disk onto an agar plate surrounded by inoculates of clinical specimen and positive control has been described. In contrast to the conventional Elek test, the modified test has the advantage of using "spot" inoculations of numerous colonies directly from the primary plate. In addition, the modified Elek test has fewer false-positive and false-negative results and yields results more rapidly (16 to 24 hours).[43]

A rapid enzyme immunoassay is another test for detection of diphtheria toxin. This method uses equine polyclonal antibody to capture the diphtheria toxin and an alkaline phosphatase–labeled monoclonal antibody to detect fragment A of the toxin. It is a rapid test that takes 3 hours and has a limit of detection of 100 pg/mL.[48]

Rapid testing for diphtheria toxin by PCR specific for the A or B portion of the toxin gene, *tox*, is sensitive and has produced positive results in specimens stored for 12 months before performing the assay.[7,74,75,91,92,94] The absence of the *tox* gene by PCR excludes the diagnosis of diphtheria. PCR may give false-positive results, however, because it does not differentiate between partial or nonfunctional *tox* genes and functional *tox* gene products. An increasing number of cases of nontoxigenic diphtheria that are positive for the *tox* gene by PCR have been reported from Ukraine and Russia.[58,83]

The immune status of patients can be determined by toxin neutralization in Vero cells.[88] This method is used frequently, although it is difficult to standardize and relies heavily on individual interpretation of results. Enzyme-linked immunosorbent assay is a more rapid and quite sensitive method, but it detects some nonspecific antibodies; when antitoxin levels are in the low range, the assay may generate falsely elevated results.[86] Finally a delayed fluorescence immune assay method was developed by Aggerbeck and colleagues[2] in 1996 and has been reported to have good sensitivity, specificity, and reproducibility.[16] Levels of diphtheria antitoxin of 0.01 IU/mL or greater generally are accepted as protective. A skin-testing method, the Schick test, also has been used to assess immunity.

The Schick test was used previously to determine the immune status of the patient. It is not helpful in establishing an early diagnosis because it cannot be read for several days, and currently it is not widely used. In the Schick test, a measured amount of purified diphtheria toxin (0.1 mL) is injected subcutaneously. A hypersensitivity reaction indicates an inadequate presence of antitoxin. A toxoid control also is injected, in the opposite arm, to help distinguish between a reaction to toxin and a reaction to other antigens in the toxin preparation.

Other laboratory studies are of little diagnostic value. The white blood cell count may be normal or elevated. Rarely anemia develops as a result of rapid hemolysis of red blood cells. Examination of cerebrospinal fluid may reveal a minimal elevation of protein and, rarely, a mild pleocytosis in patients with diphtheritic neuritis. Hypoglycemia, glucosuria, or both may occur and reflect hepatic toxicity. An elevation in blood urea nitrogen may develop in patients with acute tubular necrosis. An electrocardiogram should be obtained and may reveal ST-segment and T-wave changes or arrhythmias indicative of myocarditis.

Differential Diagnosis

Mild forms of nasal diphtheria in a partially immunized host may resemble the common cold. When the nasal discharge is more serosanguineous or purulent, nasal diphtheria must be distinguished from a foreign body in the nose, sinusitis, adenoiditis, or the snuffles of congenital syphilis. Careful examination of the nose with a nasal speculum, sinus radiographs, and appropriate serologic tests for syphilis are helpful in excluding these disorders.

Tonsillar or pharyngeal diphtheria must be differentiated from streptococcal pharyngitis. Generally streptococcal pharyngitis is associated with more severe pain on swallowing, higher temperature, and a nonadherent membrane limited to the tonsils. In some patients, pharyngeal diphtheria and streptococcal pharyngitis coexist.

Tonsillar and pharyngeal diphtheria also must be differentiated from infectious mononucleosis (lymphadenopathy and splenomegaly are common findings, atypical lymphocytes are generally present, and heterophile antibody may be present), nonbacterial membranous tonsillitis (white blood cell count generally is low, throat cultures reveal normal flora, and the course is unaffected by antibiotics), primary herpetic tonsillitis (presence of gingivitis, stomatitis, and discrete lesions of the tongue and palate may be helpful), Vincent angina (may be indistinguishable), and thrush (constitutional symptoms are absent, and lesions are present on the buccal mucosa and tongue). Tonsillar and pharyngeal diphtheria also must be differentiated from blood dyscrasias such as agranulocytosis and leukemia (complete blood count and bone marrow study are helpful); post-tonsillectomy faucial membranes (membranes are stationary and do not spread); and oropharyngeal involvement by toxoplasmosis, *Arcanobacterium,* cytomegalovirus, tularemia, and salmonellosis (associated signs and symptoms and appropriate cultures and serologic tests may be diagnostic).[55]

Laryngeal diphtheria must be differentiated from spasmodic or nonspasmodic croup; acute epiglottitis; laryngotracheobronchitis; bacterial tracheitis (particularly staphylococcal); aspirated foreign bodies;

peripharyngeal and retropharyngeal abscesses; and laryngeal papillomas, hemangiomas, or lymphangiomas. A careful history, followed by careful visualization in the hospital under controlled conditions, aids in making a correct diagnosis.

PREVENTION

Diphtheria is prevented on a community-wide basis most effectively by active immunization. Diphtheria toxoid is available in combination with tetanus toxoid as pediatric DT or adult Td and in combination with acellular pertussis as DTaP and Tdap. Combination regimens with DTaP and inactivated poliovirus and hepatitis B (Pediatrix) and inactivated poliovirus and *Haemophilus influenzae* type B (Pentacel) are also available. Pediatric formulations of diphtheria toxoid vaccines contain three to four times more diphtheria toxoid but the same tetanus toxoid in contrast to the adult formulations. Children younger than 7 years should be given the pediatric formulations of vaccine, whereas children older than 7 years should receive the adult Td. Two forms of Tdap are available: Boostrix, which is approved for children beginning at age 10 through 65 years or older, and Adacel, which is approved for individuals 11 to 64 years old.[22,26–29]

Primary immunization is carried out conveniently and effectively by giving diphtheria and tetanus toxoids and pertussis vaccine, DTaP, at 2, 4, and 6 months of age, with booster doses given at 15 to 18 months and again when the child is 4 to 6 years of age. Booster doses with the adult type of diphtheria and tetanus toxoids adsorbed (Td) should be given at 10-year intervals to all immunized individuals. Current recommendations are to give Tdap as the first booster dose in patients who are 11 to 12 years old and to anyone older who has not received a dose of Tdap.[30] Td and Tdap contain 2 to 2.5 flocculation units (Lf) diphtheria toxoid per dose in contrast to 7 to 25 Lf in the pediatric diphtheria, tetanus toxoid, and pertussis vaccine preparations (DTaP and DT). Primary immunization of children older than 7 years may be performed with Td. Two doses are given intramuscularly at least 4 weeks apart, with a booster dose provided 1 year later. Children and adults who are severely immunocompromised or undergoing long-term hemodialysis should use the standard immunization schedule, although response may be suboptimal.[51,56,76]

Most local and systemic reactions to the diphtheria and tetanus toxoids and whole cell pertussis vaccine (DTP), including fever, were related to the pertussis component.[10,37] Administration of tetanus and diphtheria toxoids is not followed by the high incidence of reactions associated with the use of pediatric DTP vaccines. At least one study showed that 7.5 Lf toxoid can be given safely to adults without a higher risk for reactions occurring.[14] Primary immunization against diphtheria for infants with progressive neurologic disorders and completion of the primary immunization series in patients who had experienced an untoward reaction to an earlier DTP vaccine injection may be performed with diphtheria and tetanus toxoids rather than diphtheria and tetanus toxoids and pertussis vaccine.[4]

A report of 97 preterm infants who received diphtheria and tetanus toxoids and acellular pertussis vaccine (DTaP) (94 of these infants also received *H. influenzae* type B vaccine) showed that most infants tolerated the vaccination without side effects, although a subgroup of infants with very low birth weight (mean, 873 g) had either a recurrence or an increase in the number of apneic and bradycardic episodes in the 48 hours after receiving vaccination. The apneic and bradycardic episodes were present before immunization in every case.[100]

Booster doses of tetanus and diphtheria toxoids should be given at 10-year intervals to all immunized individuals. The CDC Advisory Committee on Immunization Practices now recommends that all adults aged 19 years and older who have not received a dose of Tdap should receive a single dose.[31,84] A recent update recommends a dose of Tdap during every pregnancy.[32] As mentioned earlier, levels of diphtheria antitoxin of 0.01 IU/mL or greater generally are accepted as protective.

Diphtheria immunization is not always followed by complete protection.[78] Immunization is directed against the phage-mediated toxin, not against infection. Fully immunized individuals may be carriers or may have disease caused by nontoxigenic strains. An investigation conducted during an epidemic in Texas showed no statistical difference in the risk for diphtheria infection developing in individuals with full, lapsed, inadequate, or no previous diphtheria immunization; however, a 30-fold increased risk for development of symptomatic diphtheria in individuals with no immunization and an 11.5-fold increase in individuals with inadequate immunization were noted.[87]

The most important health problem in the United States today is inadequate immunization of the population. Immunization rates in adults are poorer than those in infants and children because of failure to maintain adequate immunity through appropriate booster immunization. A 70% to 80% immunization level is thought to be required to prevent epidemic spread.[36]

Prevention of diphtheria also depends on management of the contacts of known cases of diphtheria and carriers of the organism and on isolation of patients to minimize the spread of disease. Individuals at risk for contracting the disease from the index case include those who have had close respiratory or physical contact or prolonged close proximity with the infected individual, including members of the index case's household.[17] Specifically, family members who share body towels and cups or eating utensils, share a bed or a bedroom with more than two people, or take a bath less than once per week have a significantly greater risk for contracting the disease from the infected patient. A history of eczema in the contact also has been associated with a significantly increased risk for contracting diphtheria from the index case.[97] The patient is infectious until diphtheria bacilli no longer can be cultured from the site of infection. Two or three consecutive negative cultures at least 24 hours apart are required, and antibiotic therapy must be complete for 24 hours before the patient is released from isolation. If obtaining cultures is impossible, isolation may be ended after the completion of 14 days of appropriate antibiotic treatment.[6]

Cultures should be taken from the nose and throat of all close contacts, who should be kept under surveillance for 7 days (surveillance as an outpatient is acceptable).[5] Regardless of their immunization status, contacts should be treated with a single intramuscular dose of benzathine penicillin G 600,000 U for individuals weighing less than 30 kg and 1.2 million U for individuals weighing more than 30 kg or a 7-day course of erythromycin 40 to 50 mg/kg per day (maximum 2 g/day) divided into four doses.[5] The immune status of each contact should be determined; individuals for whom immune status is inadequate, including individuals who have had the primary series but more than 5 years has elapsed since they received their last booster dose, should receive an injection of diphtheria toxoid. In addition, patients with diphtheria should be immunized during convalescence because infection may not confer immunity.[6]

Asymptomatic carriers who previously were not immunized against diphtheria should have cultures taken, receive diphtheria toxoid and penicillin or erythromycin (as described earlier), and be seen daily by a physician. Asymptomatic contacts who are found to carry a toxigenic strain should be subjected to the same isolation and treatment measures as the index case.[6] If daily surveillance is impossible, benzathine penicillin is preferred over erythromycin for treatment because failure to adhere to an oral drug regimen is a concern. If a contact is experiencing symptoms when seen, treatment of diphtheria is indicated. It is important to initiate prophylactic therapy in contacts who have not been immunized before the results of culture are received. Management of carriers is described in the next section. Contacts whose occupations involve close contact with unimmunized children or food handling (especially milk) should refrain from working until cultures are confirmed to be negative.[6]

TREATMENT

Treatment of diphtheria is predicated on neutralization of free toxin and eradication of *C. diphtheriae* or *C. ulcerans* with antibiotics. Disease caused by *C. ulcerans* should be treated in the same manner as disease caused by *C. diphtheriae*.[3,24] The decision to administer equine antitoxin should be based on the site and size of the membrane, the degree of toxicity, and the duration of illness and should be made clinically as soon as possible.[15]

Antitoxin can neutralize circulating toxin or toxin that is absorbed onto cells, but is ineffective when cells have been penetrated. Early treatment is essential to limit tissue damage. An adequate dose of antitoxin must be administered intravenously as early as possible to neutralize all free toxins. A single dose is used to avoid the risk for developing sensitization from repeated doses of horse serum. Tests for sensitivity to horse serum must be performed before antitoxin is administered. Antitoxin and its indications for use as well as instructions for sensitivity testing and administration are available through the CDC (Emergency Operations Center, 770-488-7100; www.cdc.gov/diphtheria/dat.html).[5] The antitoxin dosage is empirical. Pharyngeal or laryngeal disease of 48 hours' duration or less should be treated with 20,000 to 40,000 U, nasopharyngeal disease with 40,000 to 60,000 U, and severe pharyngeal or laryngeal diphtheria with 80,000 to 120,000 U of antitoxin. The last dose also should be given to patients with mixed clinical symptoms and to patients with brawny edema or disease of longer than 48 hours' duration. The value of antitoxin in the treatment of cutaneous disease is debated, but some experts recommend 20,000 to 40,000 U because toxic effects have been reported.[5] The use of intravenous immunoglobulin (IgIV) for therapy of respiratory or cutaneous diphtheria has not been approved or evaluated for efficacy. A human monoclonal antibody to replace equine diphtheria antitoxin is under development and holds promise as a potential therapeutic agent.[101]

Although antibiotics are not a substitute for treatment with antitoxin, they should be given when diphtheria is suspected clinically. Penicillin and erythromycin are still effective against most strains of *C. diphtheriae*. Penicillin and erythromycin also are effective in eradicating group A hemolytic streptococci, which may complicate 30% of cases of diphtheria. Treatment consists of a 14-day course of penicillin or erythromycin. Penicillin may be given as aqueous penicillin G 100,000 to 150,000 U/kg per day in four divided doses intravenously or as procaine penicillin 25,000 to 50,000 U/kg per day (maximum of 1.2 million U) in two divided doses intramuscularly. Patients who are sensitive to penicillin should be given erythromycin in a daily dosage of 40 to 50 mg/kg (maximum of 2 g/day) in four divided doses for 14 days. When the patient is able to tolerate oral medications, erythromycin or penicillin V may be used in place of the intravenous antibiotics.[5]

Follow-up cultures should be obtained at least 2 weeks after antibiotic therapy is completed; if they are positive, erythromycin should be given for an additional 10 days.[5] Some resistance to erythromycin has been observed, but it is uncommon, and its epidemiologic significance is unknown.[5,6] Penicillin is recommended as first-line treatment in Vietnam, based on sensitivity data.[73] Amoxicillin, rifampin, and clindamycin provided in appropriate dosages also may be effective. Lincomycin and tetracycline have proved to be less effective, and cephalexin, oxacillin, and colistin have been shown to be ineffective against *C. diphtheriae*. The endpoint of therapy is two or three consecutive negative cultures at least 24 hours apart. In addition to receiving antibiotic therapy, patients with diphtheria should be immunized during convalescence because infection may not confer immunity.[5]

The carrier state has been treated effectively with a single intramuscular dose of benzathine penicillin G 600,000 U for children weighing less than 30 kg or 1.2 million U for individuals weighing 30 kg or greater or oral erythromycin 40 to 50 mg/kg per day for children and 1 g/day for adults for 7 to 10 days.[5] Carriers should have repeat pharyngeal cultures performed a minimum of 2 weeks after antibiotic therapy is complete; if the repeat cultures are positive, carriers should receive an additional course of antibiotics.

Treatment of deep infections caused by nontoxigenic *C. diphtheriae* can be accomplished with a wide variety of susceptible agents. Endocarditis with these organisms treated with either a β-lactam alone or in combination with an aminoglycoside has been associated with favorable outcomes.[90]

Supportive Treatment

Bed rest is extremely important and should be required for 2 to 3 weeks. Serial electrocardiograms should be obtained two or three times each week for 4 to 6 weeks to detect myocarditis as early as possible. Absolute bed rest must be enforced if myocarditis is detected, because sudden death has been precipitated by excessive activity. A patient with myocarditis may receive digitalization if congestive heart failure develops. Digitalization for arrhythmias caused by diphtheria may be contraindicated, however. In severe disease, prednisone 1 to 1.5 mg/kg per day for 2 weeks has been shown to lessen the incidence of myocarditis.

Hydration should be maintained, and a high-calorie liquid or soft diet should be provided. Secretions should be suctioned as needed to prevent aspiration. Palatal and pharyngeal paralysis increases the risk for aspiration occurring, so gavage via a nasogastric tube is indicated in these patients.

The quality of the voice and the gag reflex should be checked regularly for assessment of progression of the disease. Laryngeal diphtheria may require relief of obstruction with a tracheostomy. This procedure should be performed before the patient has become exhausted.

Adequate immunity does not develop in at least half of patients who recover from diphtheria, and they remain subject to reinfection. Immunization is indicated after the patient recovers.

PROGNOSIS

Many factors affect the prognosis in cases of diphtheria, the most important being the immunization status of the host. Morbidity and mortality rates are increased significantly in patients who are unimmunized or inadequately immunized. The rapidity with which medical care is sought and the diagnosis of diphtheria is suggested has a great impact on outcome. If specific treatment is provided on the first day of disease, the mortality rate may be reduced to less than 1 percent; delay in providing treatment until day 4 may be associated with a 20-fold increase in the mortality rate.

The virulence of the infecting organism and the location of infection are important prognostic factors. Infection with a nontoxigenic *C. diphtheriae* strain may cause disease but does not lead to myocarditis, neuritis, and other toxin-related phenomena. Toxigenic disease may vary from mild to severe. In cases of mild diphtheria, membrane sloughing and full recovery generally occur within 7 days. Disease caused by toxigenic *gravis* strains tends to be more severe and carries a poorer prognosis. Although diphtheria may affect the skin, nasopharynx, and other mucous membranes, involvement of the larynx heralds a more complicated course. Laryngeal diphtheria increases the risk for development of airway obstruction and promotes systemic absorption of the toxin. These patients require close monitoring of respiratory function and for involvement of other organ systems. Laryngeal diphtheria is more likely to be fatal in infants.

Few laboratory parameters indicate the severity of diphtheria. The development of amegakaryocytic thrombocytopenia and leukocytosis with counts of greater than 25,000 cells/mm^3 has been associated with a poor outcome.

The prognosis in a patient with diphtheria remains guarded until recovery is complete. At any time during the course of the illness, complications such as laryngeal obstruction, shock, and ventricular fibrillation may occur suddenly and unexpectedly. In patients with myocardial involvement, permanent damage to the heart, specifically fibrosis, may occur and lead to later complications. In addition, potentially severe neurologic manifestations, such as phrenic nerve paralysis, may appear late in the course of the disease.

Persistence of *C. diphtheriae* may be noted in the nasopharynx of 5% to 10% of convalescing patients. Recovery from diphtheria is followed by immunity that is demonstrable for at least 1 year after illness in 50% of patients. Second attacks are rare; nonetheless, immunization should be performed after the patient recovers.

Before the use of antitoxin and the availability of antibiotics, the mortality rate from diphtheria was 30% to 50%. Death was most common in children younger than 4 years old and was the result of suffocation. At present, the worldwide mortality rate is 5% to 10%, with no clear association with age.

NEW REFERENCES SINCE THE SEVENTH EDITION

5. American Academy of Pediatrics. Diphtheria. In: Kimberlin DW, Brady MT, Jackson MA, et al, eds. *Red Book: Report of the Committee on Infectious Diseases.*

30th ed. Elk Grove Village, IL: American Academy of Pediatrics; 2015:60-63, 325–9.
32. Centers for Disease Control and Prevention. Updated recommendation for the use of tetanus toxoid, reduced diphtheria toxoid and acellular pertussis vaccine (Tdap) in pregnant women – Advisory Committee on Immunization Practices (ACIP), 2012. *MMWR Morb Mortal Wkly Rep*. 2013;62:131-135.
101. Sevigny LM, Booth BJ, Rowley KJ, et al. Identification of a human monoclonal antibody to replace equine diphtheria antitoxin for the treatment of diphtheria intoxication. *Infect Immun*. 2013;81:3992-4000.

The full reference list for this chapter is available at ExpertConsult.com.

ADDITIONAL READING

Barksdale L. Corynebacterium diphtheriae and its relatives. *Bacteriol Rev*. 1970;34:378-422.
Pappenheimer AM Jr. Diphtheria toxin. In: Ajl SJ, Kadis S, Montie TC, eds. *Microbial Toxins*. Vol. 11B. New York: Academic Press; 1973.
Wood WB Jr. *From Miasmas to Molecules*. New York: Columbia University Press; 1961.
Zamiri I. Corynebacterium. In: Collee VG, Fraser AG, Marmion BP, Simmons A, eds. *Mackie and McCartney Practical Medical Microbiology*. 14th ed. New York: Churchill Livingstone; 1996:299-307.

91 Anthrax

Morven S. Edwards

Anthrax, also known as charbon, woolsorter's disease, and ragpicker's disease, is a toxigenic disease of herbivores for which humans are an incidental host. The term *anthrax*, derived from the Greek *anthrakos*, or "coal," refers to the black eschar characteristic of cutaneous anthrax. The three clinical manifestations of anthrax are cutaneous, which accounts for 95% of infections in the United States; inhalation; and gastrointestinal. Each can occur in children,[38] and all can be complicated by meningitis.

HISTORICAL ASPECTS

Anthrax has been recognized since antiquity. The earliest reference to a disease thought to be anthrax is a description in Exodus of the plague that caused the death of all of the Egyptians' cattle. Hippocrates described carbuncles that are thought to represent the cutaneous form of anthrax. An account of anthrax in animals is detailed in the third of the Roman poet Virgil's four *Georgics*.[35] In the early 17th century, an anthrax pandemic referred to as "Black Bane" caused 60,000 human deaths in Europe. By the 18th century, several excellent descriptions of the clinical disease in humans had been published.

Bacillus anthracis has a unique niche in infectious diseases. The organism, seen microscopically by Delafond in 1838, was isolated and cultivated in 1877 by Koch, who showed its proliferation in vivo, establishing a model for the causation of infectious disease. In 1881, both Pasteur and Greenfield[40] showed that a live-attenuated anthrax bacillus vaccine provided protection against subsequent challenge in animals, demonstrating the efficacy of immunization to prevent an infectious disease. In the late 1800s, anthrax was proved to be the cause of inhalation anthrax, contracted by factory workers handling anthrax-contaminated animal hides.

During World War I, *B. anthracis* was manufactured as an agent for biologic warfare. Because anthrax transmitted by inhalation is usually fatal and *B. anthracis* spores are stable in the environment, anthrax continues to be a focus of biologic warfare research programs. The accidental release of anthrax spores from a military research facility in Sverdlovsk in the former Soviet Union in 1979 resulted in at least 68 inhalation anthrax deaths.[31]

The first confirmed outbreak associated with intentional anthrax release in the United States occurred in October 2001.[23] Anthrax spores were disseminated by mail, resulting in five deaths from inhalation and 22 total cases of cutaneous and inhalation anthrax. Envelopes containing anthrax spores were sent through the US Postal Service to offices of newspaper and broadcast media and US senators. The spores were "weaponized," or finely milled, and treated with chemicals to prevent clumping so they dispersed when the envelopes were opened and leaked from sealed envelopes as they passed through mail-sorting machines. A single anthrax strain was implicated. Outbreak-related expenditures exceeded billions of dollars and revealed the potential impact of a bioterrorism event.[7,13] It is estimated that the aerosolized release of 100 kg of anthrax spores upwind of Washington, DC, could result in 130,000 to 3 million deaths.

A distinct form of anthrax, injectional anthrax, emerged in drug users in Europe in 2009 and has been attributed to contaminated heroin.[1]

BACTERIOLOGY

B. anthracis is an aerobic, nonmotile, spore-forming rod in the family Bacillaceae. Optimal growth occurs at 36°C in nonselective media. Colonies are gray-white, rough, and flat and can have comma-shaped projections caused by the outgrowth of chains of bacilli from the edges of the colony, giving it a "Medusa head" appearance. Individual colonies are 4 to 5 mm in diameter with a ground-glass appearance and exhibit tenacity or a "beaten egg white" appearance when lifted with an inoculating loop. The capsule, a γ-linked poly-D-glutamic acid, can be produced in blood or by culture in carbon dioxide. Gram stain reveals large, square-ended, gram-positive rods singly or in short chains without a visible capsule. The equatorial or paracentral spores are invisible in smears fixed promptly after collection. After 24 to 48 hours of aerobic incubation, strands of rods are arranged in "boxcar" or "bamboo" fashion and sporulation occurs. Small numbers of bacteria are pathogenic for mice, guinea pigs, and rabbits, and death usually occurs 2 to 5 days after inoculation. Genotyping methods are available to determine molecular relatedness of clinical isolates and their geographic origin.[30]

EPIDEMIOLOGY AND TRANSMISSION

Domestic herbivores—cattle, sheep, horses, goats, and swine—are the most important agricultural sources of anthrax, but all domestic and many wild animals can serve as hosts. Animals are infected by ingestion of spores from infected pastures. Spores germinate in vivo, and death, associated with massive septicemia, usually occurs in 1 or 2 days. Anthrax is endemic in areas where an animal–soil–animal cycle is established because the spores can survive indefinitely in a dry environment. Uncultivated soil with a pH greater than 6.0 and ambient temperature greater than 15.5°C provides an environment favorable for persistence of spores.

An estimated 20,000 to 100,000 human cases of anthrax occur yearly.[36] Regions of high endemicity include Central and South America, southern and eastern Europe, Asia, Africa, the Caribbean, and the Middle East. The number of human cases probably correlates with the enzootic status of the disease in livestock in these countries. Familial clustering can occur in association with exposure to diseased animals. Children who live in endemic areas can contract cutaneous anthrax from direct animal contact.[32] Cases of illness were identified in four states and in Washington, DC, during the 2001 bioterrorism-related outbreak.

The incidence of human anthrax in the United States has decreased markedly since the early 1900s, when more than 100 cases were reported annually. Cutaneous infections are reported sporadically. Cases often are associated with exposure to contaminated animal products in commercial preparations, but exposure to indigenous animal anthrax does occur.[39] Two members of a farmer's family ate hamburgers made from an anthrax-infected steer in Minnesota in 2000. The family members received antibiotic prophylaxis and anthrax vaccine and remained well.[14]

Direct contact with contaminated animal meat or carcasses or with contaminated animal products, such as hides, hair, wool, bone meal, and animal feed, are sources of transmission of anthrax spores to humans. Children of industrial workers have acquired infection, presumably from contact with their parents' contaminated clothing. Processed products, such as shaving brushes and saddle blankets, have been implicated as sources of infection. Use of contaminated goat hides from West Africa caused cutaneous anthrax in a drum maker in Connecticut and, through his work clothing or objects from his shed, led to cutaneous anthrax in his 8-year-old child.[16] Cutaneous anthrax is transmitted by deposition of spores or bacilli into abrasions or cuts in the skin. Blood-sucking insects, including mosquitoes and stable flies, can be vectors.[41]

The mode of acquisition may be difficult to determine in children; in one child with cutaneous anthrax, the only potential exposure was proximity to a bone meal factory that he walked past on his way to school.[27] Tying the umbilicus with a dirty thread was the presumed portal of entry for a neonate with *B. anthracis* sepsis.[32] Rubbing with contaminated fingers or deposition by an insect vector can lead to cutaneous involvement of the eyelids.[43] Discharge from cutaneous lesions theoretically is infectious, but person-to-person transmission has not been confirmed. Skin-to-skin contact through his mother's exposure at her workplace was proposed as the route of transmission to an infant in the US bioterrorism-related outbreak.[20] Maternal anthrax has been associated with preterm delivery.[24]

Inhalation anthrax results from inhalation of spores. The estimated infectious dose in humans is 8000 to 50,000 spores. Cases of inhalational anthrax in the United States have occurred in a weaver whose imported yarn was contaminated and a drum maker whose imported hand-dried animal hide was contaminated with *B. anthracis*.[9,15] In some patients no specific source is identified, as with a man who acquired inhalation anthrax while vacationing through states in which animal anthrax is sporadic or enzootic.[21] Eleven adults acquired inhalational anthrax during the 2001 bioterrorism outbreak of anthrax in the United States. Gastrointestinal anthrax usually is caused by ingestion of contaminated meat but has occurred after exposure to a contaminated animal-hide drum.[17,25] Neonates can contract anthrax meningitis if a mother is bacteremic at the time of delivery.

PATHOGENESIS AND PATHOLOGY

Anthrax toxicity results from the capsule and from the activity of three polypeptides—protective antigen, edema factor, and lethal factor—that combine to form two exotoxins: lethal toxin and edema toxin. Protective antigen is integral to the action of both toxins. Toxin entry into cells is initiated when protective antigen binds to membrane receptors of susceptible cells. Two related proteins, tumor endothelial marker 8 and capillary morphogenesis protein 2, function as receptors. Cleaved protective antigen oligomerizes and a heptamer of protective antigen provides binding sites for edema factor or lethal factor. The complex is endocytosed as edema toxin or lethal toxin.

Edema factor is a calmodulin-dependent adenylate cyclase that increases intracellular cyclic adenosine monophosphate levels and is responsible for the massive edema that occurs in cutaneous anthrax.[28] Lethal factor is a metalloproteinase that cleaves mitogen-activated protein kinase-kinases so that they are unable to activate their downstream substrates, the mitogen-activated kinases.[19] Lethal factor stimulates production of tumor necrosis factor-α and interleukin-1β. The capsule of *B. anthracis* contributes to virulence by inhibiting phagocytosis.[23,42]

Cutaneous infection is initiated when anthrax spores are ingested at the site of entry by macrophages and germination occurs in skin tissues. Production of toxin results in local edema. Regional lymphangitis and lymphadenopathy can occur.[18] Interstitial edema, lymphatic dilation, and thrombosis and necrosis of blood vessels are characteristic microscopic features of cutaneous anthrax lesions. Erythrocytes extravasate freely into interstitial fluid. Few neutrophils or other inflammatory cells are present unless a lesion is infected secondarily. Hemorrhagic lymphadenitis involving regional lymph nodes occurs in all forms of anthrax.

In inhalation anthrax, spores entering alveoli are ingested by alveolar macrophages and dendritic cells and carried to mediastinal lymph nodes, where they germinate. Inhalation anthrax is not pneumonia, although primary focal hemorrhagic necrotizing pneumonia can occur at the pulmonary portal of entry.[2] Massive hemorrhagic mediastinal lymphadenitis can block lymphatic drainage routes and can be causally related to the pulmonary edema, respiratory distress, and systemic disease observed clinically.

Gastrointestinal anthrax results from ingestion of spores or vegetative bacilli in contaminated meat. The primary sites of infection are the epithelium of the stomach or bowel wall.[8] Edema and necrotic ulcers of the mucosa of the gastrointestinal tract, especially the ileum or cecum, are characteristic findings. Dissemination to the CNS can occur by hematogenous or lymphatic routes from any site of primary involvement. Hemorrhage involving the meninges and intense arteritis are uniform findings in patients who die of anthrax meningitis.

Injectional anthrax results from direct injection or "skin popping" among persons who become infected by injecting heroin. At least 70 confirmed cases have been attributed to contaminated heroin distributed throughout Europe.[1]

CLINICAL MANIFESTATIONS

Cutaneous Anthrax

The lesions of cutaneous anthrax occur mainly on exposed areas of the body.[3] In one report, the distribution in young children was 52% of lesions on the head and neck, 28% on the trunk, and 20% on the extremities, whereas in older children the distribution was 70% on the head and neck, 16% on the trunk, and 14% on the extremities.[22] Spores are introduced through abraded or injured skin. Children can have one or several lesions, and they are associated with regional adenitis.[29] After an incubation period of 2 to 5 days, a small, nontender, but often pruritic, papule develops at the site of inoculation. The lesion progresses within 36 hours to a serous or serosanguineous vesicle with surrounding nonpitting edema. Satellite vesicles, sometimes referred to as a "pearly wreath,"[43] can be seen occasionally.

The lesion undergoes central necrosis, and a 1- to 3-cm black eschar with well-defined margins forms 1 week to 10 days after onset of illness (Fig. 91.1).[34] The term *malignant edema* is used to describe severe lesions, particularly those involving the head and neck, which can be associated with systemic toxicity and occlusion of the airway. Small children can appear acutely ill with a temperature of 39° to 40°C (102.2° to 104°F) and leukocytosis with counts of 20,000 to 30,000 cells/mm^3.[20,27] Bacteremia is uncommon. The edema usually resolves within 2 to 3 days, but separation of the eschar can take several weeks, and healing occurs with variable central scarring.

Inhalation Anthrax

Inhalation anthrax is a biphasic illness. Symptoms in the initial stage—malaise, low-grade fever, myalgia, and nonproductive cough—are nonspecific and resemble an upper respiratory tract illness. Adults who have inhalational anthrax more often present with tachycardia, high hematocrit, and low albumin and sodium levels and less often with myalgias, headache, and nasal symptoms than do adults who have influenza-like illnesses.[26] After several days of illness, dyspnea and hypoxemia initiate onset of the second stage, which usually terminates fatally within 24 hours. Chest radiographs can show a widened mediastinum with smooth borders and evidence of hemorrhagic mediastinitis and large, often bloody pleural effusion. Pulmonary infiltrates usually are the result of superimposed bacterial infection. In the more recent cases from the United States, computed tomography of the chest showed the characteristic findings of hemorrhagic mediastinal and hilar lymph nodes and mediastinal edema and pleural effusions.[7]

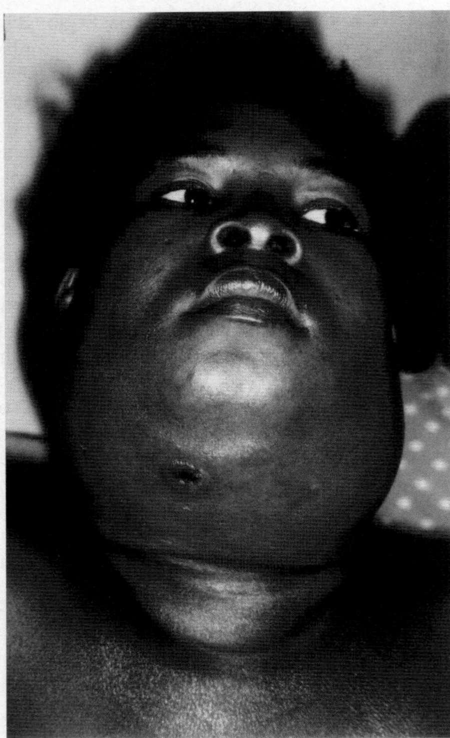

FIG. 91.1 Cutaneous anthrax with associated massive submental edema. The lesion is located at the site of a small, initially trivial laceration that served as the portal of entry for the anthrax endospores. The patient received ampicillin and recovered completely. (Courtesy M. Thomas Casey, MD.)

Gastrointestinal Anthrax

Gastrointestinal anthrax can manifest as oropharyngeal or intestinal disease.[12] Each has an incubation period of 2 to 5 days after the ingestion of contaminated meat. The oropharyngeal form results in an oral or esophageal ulcer.[8,23] Presenting features include fever, severe sore throat, neck swelling caused by edema and enlargement of the cervical lymph nodes, dysphagia, and respiratory difficulty. Lesions on the tonsils or posterior oropharynx progress over 1 to 2 weeks from edema to a pseudomembrane-covered ulcer. Oropharyngeal anthrax, although uncommon, has a more favorable prognosis than intestinal anthrax.

Initial features of intestinal anthrax are fever, nausea, anorexia, vomiting, and diffuse abdominal pain that progresses rapidly to severe abdominal pain with rebound tenderness. Vomiting of blood-tinged or coffee ground–like material and melena are common and are caused by ulceration of the intestinal mucosa.[8,23] Pain decreases, and massive ascites develops within 24 to 48 hours. Abdominal radiographs show edematous loops of bowel and decreased air. If the abdomen is explored, findings include enlarged, erythematous mesenteric lymph nodes and straw-colored to purulent ascitic fluid in which organisms are readily visible.[4] Death usually occurs in association with significant blood loss, electrolyte imbalance, and shock. If the patient survives, the edema and melena subside in 10 to 14 days.

Injection Anthrax

Direct injection has resulted in a distinct clinical presentation. Extensive painless edema occurs at the injection site. There is a notable absence of the eschar typical of cutaneous anthrax. Extensive tissue involvement can necessitate surgical debridement. Biphasic illness, with initial recovery followed by deterioration with systemic findings occurs in some patients.[1]

Meningitis

Most reports of anthrax meningitis are associated with cutaneous disease, likely owing to the higher frequency of cutaneous disease. Anthrax can disseminate to the meninges from any site of primary involvement. In the 2001 bioterrorism event, one adult with inhalation anthrax presented with meningitis, and several others had features suggestive of CNS involvement.[33] In one group of 70 patients with anthrax meningitis who ranged from younger than 1 to 71 years of age, no primary focus was evident in 12%.

Anthrax meningitis is characterized by a fulminant, rapidly progressive course. Initial symptoms include intense headache, nausea and vomiting, myalgia, chills, dizziness, and, occasionally, a petechial rash. Meningismus is usually present, but not invariably, because of the acuity of the course. Progressive neurologic deterioration with delirium, convulsions, and coma can occur in hours or over the course of 2 to 4 days. Overall survival is approximately 5%, but survival without sequelae has been reported in children.[33,37,38]

Examination of cerebrospinal fluid (CSF) reveals gross or microscopic hemorrhage, leukocytosis consisting predominantly of neutrophils, elevated protein, and depressed glucose. Gram-positive rods are easily visible on smears of CSF. Peripheral leukocytosis is common, and the white blood cell count can be 60,000 to 80,000 cells/mm^3. Blood cultures yield the organism in 70%, and CSF cultures are positive in virtually 100% of patients. Neuroimaging findings are notable for multiple hemorrhages in the ventricles, subarachnoid space, and deep gray matter.[33]

DIAGNOSIS AND DIFFERENTIAL DIAGNOSIS

B. anthracis can be visualized by direct smear and cultured from tissue biopsy specimens or discharge from cutaneous lesions and from pleural fluid, blood, and CSF in systemic infections. Gram-positive bacilli seen on a peripheral smear, in vesicular fluid or CSF are an important finding, and polychrome methylene blue-stained smears showing blue staining bacilli with a capsule visualized in red (McFadyean reaction) provide a presumptive identification. The commercially available QuickELISA Anthrax-PA Kit can be used as a screening test.[5] Traditional microbiologic methods can provide presumptive identification from cultures. Definitive identification can be obtained through the Laboratory Response Network in each state by methods that include detection of antigen by polymerase chain reaction (PCR), an enzyme immunoassay to detect IgG to protective antigen in paired sera, a matrix-assisted laser desorption/ionization time-of-flight (MALDI-TOF) mass spectrometry assay measuring lethal factor activity in serum samples, and tissue immunochemistry. Specimens suitable for PCR include blood, CSF, pleural fluid, vesicular fluid or eschar material, and tissue biopsy specimens.

The lesion of cutaneous anthrax must be differentiated from ecthyma gangrenosum and from ulcerative skin lesions with regional lymphadenopathy, including rat-bite fever, ulceroglandular tularemia, plague, glanders, scrub typhus, rickettsialpox, cowpox, and orf. Staphylococcal lymphangitis can be distinguished by the discharge of purulent material and by the inflammatory response observed microscopically. Noninfectious causes of eschars include arachnoid bites and vasculitides.[23] The first stage of inhalational anthrax and the clinical features of the intestinal form are nonspecific, so a history of exposure is crucial to establishing the diagnosis. Mediastinal widening of inhalational anthrax can cause confusion with that seen in acute bacterial mediastinitis and in fibrous mediastinitis caused by *Histoplasma capsulatum*.[18] Gastrointestinal anthrax must be differentiated from other causes of acute abdominal illness and, if bleeding is present, from duodenal ulcer, typhoid, and intestinal tularemia. Injectional anthrax must be differentiated from other causes of soft tissue infection; the degree of edema, excessive bleeding at time of surgery, and lack of a clear demarcation between affected and healthy tissue are suggestive of injectional anthrax.[1] Anthrax meningitis must be differentiated from subarachnoid hemorrhage.

TREATMENT

First-line agents for treatment of naturally occurring uncomplicated cutaneous anthrax include ciprofloxacin or an equivalent fluoroquinolone, or doxycycline. Clindamycin is an alternative, as are penicillins if the isolate is shown susceptible. Treatment for 7 to 10 days is adequate. Treatment of bioterrorism-associated cutaneous disease should be initiated with ciprofloxacin (30 mg/kg per day orally divided every 12 hours, not to exceed 1000 mg every 24 hours), or doxycycline (100 mg orally 2 times/day for children 8 years of age or older; or 4 mg/kg per day divided every 12 hours, for children younger than 8 years of age with a maximum of 200 mg per day), until susceptibility data are available. The antimicrobial regimen should continue for 60 days to provide postexposure prophylaxis (PEP) and is administered in conjunction with vaccine.[5]

The initial regimen for treatment of all forms of systemic anthrax including cutaneous anthrax with systemic signs should include intravenously administered ciprofloxacin as the primary component of a multidrug regimen (30 mg/kg per day, intravenously, divided every 8 hours, not to exceed 400 mg per dose) until results of susceptibility testing are known. Levofloxacin and moxifloxacin are considered equivalent alternatives to ciprofloxacin. At least two additional antimicrobial agents with CNS penetration, one a bactericidal and the other a protein synthesis-inhibiting agent, should be administered in conjunction with ciprofloxacin until meningitis is excluded. Meropenem is recommended as the second bactericidal agent, with imipenem/cilastatin or doripenem as alternatives; if the strain is known to be susceptible, penicillin G or ampicillin are equivalent alternatives. Linezolid is the suggested protein synthesis inhibiting agent.

If meningitis has been excluded, treatment can consist of two antimicrobials, including a bactericidal and a protein synthesis-inhibiting agent. Clindamycin is preferred as the latter agent, with linezolid, doxycycline, and rifampin as acceptable alternatives. Ciprofloxacin is the preferred bactericidal agent, with meropenem, levofloxacin, imipenem/cilastatin, and vancomycin as alternatives. If susceptible, penicillin G or ampicillin are equivalent alternatives. Therapy should continue for at least 14 days; intravenous can be changed to oral treatment to complete the course as symptoms permit. For bioterrorism-associated anthrax, treatment should be continued for at least 60 days to provide PEP.

For anthrax with evidence of systemic disease, administration of anthrax immune globulin (Anthracil) or raxibacumab (ABthrax), a humanized monoclonal antibody, should be considered in consultation with the Centers for Disease Control and Prevention (CDC). Anthrax immune globulin can be accessed under a CDC-sponsored investigative new drug (IND) protocol. Raxibacumab is approved by the US Food and Drug Administration.[5] Supportive therapy includes attention to details of fluid and electrolyte balance, endotracheal intubation if indicated to maintain a patent airway, and local care for cutaneous lesions. Systemic corticosteroids can reduce the severity of infections in patients with massive edema or meningitis.[38]

PROGNOSIS

Before penicillin was introduced, cutaneous anthrax was fatal in approximately 20% of patients. With effective treatment, the mortality rate is less than 1%. Cutaneous anthrax of the eyelid may be complicated by ectropion of the upper lid and corneal scarring with blindness.[43] Immunity probably is lifelong in most patients. Although second attacks of cutaneous anthrax have been recorded, they have not been confirmed serologically and usually are mild.[22] Fatality rates are high for systemic anthrax and range from 50% to 100% for gastrointestinal anthrax to virtually 100% for inhalation anthrax, but children who have survived these infections have no apparent sequelae.

PREVENTION AND CONTROL

The only human anthrax vaccine licensed in the United States is anthrax vaccine adsorbed (AVA), marketed as BioThrax, which is prepared from cell-free filtrates of microaerophilic cultures of a toxigenic, nonencapsulated strain of *B. anthracis* V770-NP1-R. Each 0.5-mL dose contains proteins including the protective antigen and contains no dead or live bacteria. The vaccine is licensed for use in persons 18 to 65 years of age at high risk for exposure. Preexposure vaccination is recommended for persons at risk for repeated exposure to anthrax spores, including some laboratory personnel, persons involved in environmental investigations or remediation efforts, military personnel, and some emergency responders. The preexposure vaccination schedule consists of five intramuscular doses administered at day 0; 4 weeks; and 6, 12, and 18 months, followed by an annual booster to maintain immunity.

The CDC updated its recommendations for exposure to anthrax through bioterrorism and the American Academy of Pediatrics published a pediatric anthrax management document in 2014.[10,11] In the event of a bioterrorism threat, updates will be posted on the CDC anthrax website (https://www.cdc.gov/anthrax/bioterrorism/index.html). Public health authorities will provide a 10-day course of antimicrobial prophylaxis to those likely exposed and will determine those who should continue PEP to complete a 60-day course. Ciprofloxacin (30 mg/kg per day orally divided every 12 hours, not to exceed 1000 mg every 24 hours) and doxycycline (100 mg orally 2 times/day for children 8 years of age or older; or 4 mg/kg per day divided every 12 hours, for children younger than 8 years of age with a maximum of 200 mg per day) are equivalent first-line agents for children; levofloxacin or clindamycin are second-line agents for PEP. If susceptible (minimal inhibitory concentration less than or equal to 0.125 μg/mL), use of amoxicillin (80 mg/kg per day divided into 3 doses with a maximum of 500 mg/dose) may be advised by public health authorities. AVA is not licensed for use in children but will be made available in a bioterrorism event as an investigational vaccine. The process required for use of AVA will be accessible at the CDC website (www.cdc.gov/anthrax) as well as through the American Academy of Pediatrics and the FDA.[10,11] All exposed children older than 6 weeks of age should receive 3 doses of AVA at 0, 2, and 4 weeks by the subcutaneous route in addition to 60 days of PEP. Infants younger than 6 weeks of age at the time of exposure should begin vaccine when they reach 6 weeks of age.

Worldwide, anthrax is controlled through livestock immunization programs. Procedures to prevent the spread of anthrax in animals include disposal of contaminated carcasses by burning and annual vaccination of livestock in known enzootic areas. Novel approaches to the treatment of anthrax are under investigation and include nonantimicrobial drugs with activity against anthrax toxin components and evaluation of agents that inhibit binding or assembly of toxins.[6] Suspected or proven cases of anthrax should be reported to public health officials. Hospitalized patients should be kept under isolation until the lesions are bacteriologically sterile. Contaminated dressings and clothing must be burned or sterilized, and the patient's room must be disinfected to destroy spores.

NEW REFERENCES SINCE THE SEVENTH EDITION

1. Abbara A, Brooks T, Taylor GP, et al. Lessons for control of heroin-associated anthrax in Europe from 2009–2010 outbreak case studies, London, UK. *Emerg Infect Dis.* 2014;20:1115-1122.
5. American Academy of Pediatrics. Anthrax. In: Kimberlin DW, Brady MT, Jackson MA, Long SS, eds. *Red book: 2015 Report of the Committee on Infectious Diseases.* 30th ed. Elk Grove Village, IL: American Academy of Pediatrics; 2015:234-240.
9. Bradley JS, Peacock G, Krug SE, et al. Pediatric anthrax clinical management: executive summary. *Pediatrics.* 2014;133:940-942.
10. Bradley JS, Peacock G, Krug SE, et al. Pediatric anthrax clinical management. *Pediatrics.* 2014;133:e1411-e1436.
21. Griffith J, Blaney D, Shadomy S, et al. Investigation of inhalation anthrax case, United States. *Emerg Infect Dis.* 2014;20:280-283.

The full reference list for this chapter is available at ExpertConsult.com.

92 *Bacillus cereus* and Other Bacillus Species

Sarah M. Labuda • Richard A. Oberhelman

Bacillus cereus is an environmental gram-positive rod that can give rise to two distinct forms of foodborne diseases, the emetic and the diarrheal syndromes, and occasionally to localized and systemic disease.[57,91] *B. cereus* pathogenicity has been recognized since the early 1950s, with clarification of the taxonomy of the genus *Bacillus*. Multiple early reports of food poisoning and other infections, including gastroenteritis, bacteremia-septicemia, cellulitis, ear and eye infections, endocarditis, and urinary tract infections, which were attributed to *Bacillus subtilis* or to other *Bacillus* spp., probably were caused by *B. cereus*.[145]

The diarrheal syndrome was recognized first by Hauge[65] in 1955 after four clinically similar outbreaks in Norway occurred. This common form of disease was related to a great variety of foods, such as meat and vegetable soup, poultry, pudding, sauce, pasta, cake, and milk. In 1974, Mortimer and McCann[111] described a vomiting syndrome associated with the consumption of fried rice in Chinese restaurants. Despite widespread recognition in Europe, *B. cereus* outbreaks have been reported infrequently in the United States. The first documented outbreak in the United States occurred in 1970.[108]

BACTERIOLOGY

Members of the genus *Bacillus* are aerobic or facultative anaerobic, gram-positive or gram-variable, spore-forming rods. They are distributed widely in the environment because of the high resistance of their endospores to extreme conditions, including heat, cold, desiccation, salinity, and radiation.[46,132]

Bacillus cereus belongs to the group of gram-positive rods that produce central or terminal ellipsoid or cylindrical spores that do not distend the sporangia.[151] Studies of DNA-DNA hybridization and 16S and 23S ribosomal RNA (rRNA) sequencing and enzyme electrophoretic patterns have shown a close relationship among *B. cereus, Bacillus anthracis, Bacillus mycoides, Bacillus pseudomycoides, Bacillus weihenstephanensis,* and *Bacillus thuringiensis;* these organisms are so closely related that they all may be considered variants of *B. cereus* and are labeled the *B. cereus* group, or *B. cereus sensu lato*. Based on the high variability in guanine and cytosine content (32% to 69%), the debate ensues regarding the classification of *Bacillus* spp.[151] Whole-genome sequencing has shown large amounts of gene transfer between members of the *B. cereus sensu lato,* complicating identification.[20,99] Pathogenic strains of *B. cereus* are shown to have pathogenic plasmids shared with *B. anthracis* and other species, leading to confusion in clinical and laboratory identification.[20,99] Differentiating, particularly between *B. cereus* and the insect pathogen *B. thuringiensis,* sometimes is difficult in the diagnostic laboratory, and overlap occurs among clinical syndromes reported.[64,80] Polymerase chain reaction (PCR) technology, including multiplex-PCR capable of distinguishing members of *Bacillus cereus sensu lato*, pulse field gel electrophoresis, and genomic sequencing, as well as detection of specific emetic and diarrheagenic toxins, have been used for identifying species.[22,115,93]

B. cereus sensu stricto (i.e., the species *B. cereus* only) is a flagellated, motile, gram-positive rod, typically 1 to 1.2 μm in diameter by 3 to 5 μm in length. The organism sporulates freely on many media under well-aerated conditions, but vegetative cells also can grow anaerobically. It is able to metabolize glucose, fructose, and sucrose, but not pentose and other sugar alcohols. It produces acid from glucose, but not from arabinose, xylose, or mannitol. Starch hydrolysis and catalase production are similar to those of the other members of the genus. The presence of lipid globules or protoplasts is a characteristic that it shares with *Bacillus megaterium*.[92] Colonies on blood agar are large, flat, granular, and slightly green tinged. *B. cereus* is differentiated from *B. anthracis* by motility, hemolysis, lack of lysis by γ phage, penicillin resistance, and absence of a capsule in *B. cereus*.[46] Identifying morphologic differentiation with nonmotile *B. cereus* strains and *B. anthracis* strains that are occasionally weakly hemolytic may be difficult.

Growth and multiplication of vegetative cells occur in a temperature range of 10°C to 50°C (50°F to 122°F), with an optimum of 28°C to 35°C (82.4°F to 95°F). Variations in toxin levels found in certain foods also can be related to pH levels, sugar content, the presence of other lactic acid bacteria, and aeration.[138,139] Some strains responsible for milk spoilage can grow at temperatures of 5°C (41°F),[92,132] but few strains are able to produce toxin at temperatures less than 7°C (44.6°F).[132] Ribosomal DNA characterization and genotyping based on the major cold shock protein homologue cspA have defined the species, *Bacillus weihenstephanensis,* which can grow at 4°C to 7°C (39.2°F to 44.6°F) but not at 43°C (109.4°F).[96] These strains form a subgroup of *B. cereus* organisms described as psychrotolerant or psychrotropic, meaning they are able to grow at temperatures of 7°C (44.6°F) and less.[95,126,140] Spore formation allows some *B. cereus* strains to survive pasteurization and heating, as well as transit of the acidic conditions of the human gastrointestinal tract to cause diarrheal disease.[95,28,29] A crystalline cell surface protein layer or "S-layer" has been described as a determinant of cell hydrophobicity. S-layer–producing cells are hydrophilic and able to bind to human matrix proteins, and presence of the S-layer in some *B. cereus* strains is associated with resistance to phagocytosis and increased radiation resistance against γ irradiation.[91]

Serologic differentiation of *Bacillus* spp. is hampered by cross-reactive antigens and autoagglutination of spores caused by hydrophobic surface properties. Serologic typing based on the flagellar (H) antigen can be used during an outbreak to distinguish among strains and to determine the similarity of isolates obtained from humans with the strains isolated from suspect foods.[46] The serotype scheme is based on H antisera raised against prototype strains. In addition to serology, biochemical typing, plasmid analysis, and phage typing have proved useful epidemiologically.[2,92,114,136,155] A *B. cereus*-specific, repetitive, extragenic, palindromic sequence-based PCR analysis (Bc-Rep-PCR) appears to be a promising newer technique.[120,129] Pulsed-field gel electrophoresis (PFGE) has been less successful in differentiating among *B. cereus* group species.[166] Developments in genomics, proteomics, and metabolomics have increased ability to distinguish species in *B. cereus sensu lato* for research purposes, but have yet to be used commonly in clinical practice.[77]

Diagnosis of the less common extraintestinal infection is made by isolation from normally sterile sites (blood or tissue) after overnight incubation on nutrient or blood agar; clinical specimens from normally nonsterile sites (feces, vomitus) and food or environmental samples require selective techniques. Polymyxin B is used as a selective agent, and the lecithinase reaction of the organism on egg yolk and its inability to catabolize mannitol permit presumptive identification to be made with a variety of media: mannitol–egg yolk–polymyxin B, Kim and Goepfert medium, and polymyxin B–pyruvate–egg yolk–mannitol with bromothymol blue or bromocresol purple.[46]

EPIDEMIOLOGY

Bacillus cereus in the spore and vegetative form is a ubiquitous organism found in soil, water, vegetation, and food products, especially cereals, dairy products, dried foods, spices, meat products, and vegetables.[92] The emetic syndrome typically is associated with cooked rice, usually fried, from Chinese restaurants.[88,111] Saving portions of boiled rice at room temperature overnight until required for frying previously was a common practice. Refrigerating boiled rice makes the grains stick together, which is less convenient for frying. The spores of *B. cereus* survive cooking and are capable of germination and outgrowth.[58,60] The optimal temperature for growth in boiled rice is 30°C to 37°C (86°F to 98.6°F), although growth does occur during storage at 15°C to 43°C (59°F to 109.4°F).[58] Most samples of uncooked rice contain multiple serotypes of *B. cereus,* and little difference occurs in the growth rate of the various serotypes in boiled rice at 22°C (71.6°F).[118] In laboratory conditions, using high pressure along with high temperatures for treating cooked rice has been shown to reduce survival of spores, perhaps indicating a method for reduction of clinical disease from contaminated rice dishes.[36]

Starchy dried foods other than rice, such as cereals, frequently are contaminated.[19] Tortillas can be contaminated with the water used in preparation and from the hands of producers.[26] Specific foods incriminated in outbreaks in the United States include Chinese food (accounting for 50% of reported outbreaks between 1973 and 1987), followed by Mexican food, beef, fruits, and vegetables. Other foods implicated, particularly in the enterotoxin syndrome, include beef stew, turkey loaf, barbecued pork, macaroni and cheese, potatoes, spaghetti and other pastas, dairy and dried milk products, and seafoods.[40,56,70,72,82,91,100]

In a study of 96 milk and milk product samples collected from retail shops in Nairobi, Kenya, 57% of samples were contaminated with *B. cereus* and 81% of the bacterial isolates (38 of 47) produced nonhemolytic enterotoxins, including 6 of 43 pasteurized milk products (43%).[117] Infant complimentary foods tested in urban and rural Bangladesh found high levels of diarrheagenic bacteria present, including 6% to 8% of all samples showing growth of *B. cereus.*[78] In Korea, survey of 687 powdered infant formulas and ready-to-eat-foods from markets found 347 isolates of *B. cereus,* with 95% harboring at least one toxin gene.[73] A study of donor breast milk in Spain found that *B. cereus* were the only bacteria to survive the pasteurization process, though they were not genetically virulent strains.[39] However, a cluster of two cases of severe *B. cereus* enterocolitis in very-low-birthweight preterm neonates in France found pooled donor breast milk to be the likely source.[41]

Among the factors thought to contribute to outbreaks, the most frequent were inadequate cold-holding temperatures, preparing foods a half-day or more before serving, contaminated equipment, and storage in a contaminated environment.[10,27] Outbreaks of *B. cereus* have been recognized widely in Europe but less often in the United States and Asia. In the Netherlands, *B. cereus* reportedly was the cause of 22.4% of foodborne disease outbreaks of known bacterial cause. Similarly, in Finland, it accounted for 11.9% of outbreaks. In most places, *B. cereus* is incriminated in 0.9% to 7% of outbreaks of food-related disease and 0.7% to 3% of cases.[92] In Korea, for 36,745 cases of food poisoning referred to the Korea Center for Disease and Prevention between 2007 and 2008, only 129, or 0.35% of cases, were stool culture positive for *B. cereus,* despite concerns that the rate might be higher in a culture with a very rice-dependent diet.[116] In the United States, between 1998 and 2002, *B. cereus* was identified as the cause of 37 of 6647 (0.6%) foodborne outbreaks reported to the Centers for Disease Control and Prevention (CDC), with a total of 571 cases and no deaths recorded.[103] The location of the outbreak is known for 24 of these outbreaks, and most of these (15 of 24 [62.5%]) occurred in commercial food outlets, such as restaurants, delicatessens, or workplace cafeterias. In outbreaks for which the implicated source was known, cereal products were the most common vehicle.[103] From 1998 to 2008, the CDC reported 56 confirmed and 179 suspected foodborne outbreaks of *B. cereus* with a total of 2050 cases resulting in 0 deaths. Fifty percent of confirmed outbreaks involved rice dishes as the implicated source, and 67% of confirmed outbreaks were associated with foods prepared in a restaurant or deli.[17] The susceptibility of children to this pathogen is evident from the report of an outbreak involving two daycare centers[88] and other reports that included neonates, children, and adolescents.[42,49,67,81,113,119,131,146,161] Only a small fraction of outbreaks are reported to the CDC; small outbreaks of mild, brief illness are less likely to be reported. It is thought that 10^5 to 10^8 organisms per gram need to be ingested to cause the emetic syndrome and 10^5 to 10^7 cells or spores (total dose) ingested to cause the enterotoxin syndrome.[61]

For infections not related to food, groups at risk include neonates,[49,119,133] immunocompromised hosts,[4,30,48,60,67,81,87,136,143] patients with recent eye surgery or trauma, intravenous drug users,[33,146] and patients with intravascular devices or artificial prostheses.[6,8,48,49,136,137] *B. cereus* has been known to contaminate a variety of unusual environmental niches, including alcohol prep pads,[45] steam-dried towels,[44] hospital linens during a period of hospital construction,[5] and unopened boxes of nonsterile nitrile gloves.[84] Studies in three populations in South Africa and London, including school-aged children, found the organism in 18% to 43% of fecal samples.[150] The organism can be part of the normal intestinal flora. *B. cereus* does not persist in the intestine after ingestion and so is not spread by the fecal-oral route.[55]

PATHOGENESIS

Bacillus cereus produces an enormous range of extracellular metabolites, including peptides with antibiotic properties (biocerin, cerein, thiocillins), β-lactamases, hydrolases, nuclease, urease, and proteases.[145] Two groups of toxins, known as diarrheal enterotoxins and emetic toxins, are responsible for the clinical syndromes of food poisoning.[106,148] There is great variability of toxicity and clinical spectrum of illness among *B. cereus* isolates.[86] Some strains may be able to produce both toxins based on the evidence that culture filtrates derived from strains isolated from emetic poisoning occasionally are able to produce a positive rabbit ileal loop assay.[132]

Biologic activities of diarrheal enterotoxins can be shown in multiple different assay systems. Three enterotoxins, nonhemolytic enterotoxin (Nhe), hemolysin BL (Hbl), and cytotoxin K (CytK), are produced and regulated by multifactorial, complex processes.[83] Purification plus isolation of multiple toxic fractions with some, but not all, of these activities has caused confusion.[46,144] Evaluation of the toxic activity of whole-cell suspension, cell-free culture filtrates, and the purified enterotoxin complex classically has included the rabbit ileal loop fluid accumulation assay, vascular permeability in rabbit skin, dermonecrosis and intestinal necrosis, mouse lethality, cytotoxicity, and hemolysis.[15,24,98,141,147,152] Hemolytic *B. cereus* enterotoxin has been characterized as a complex termed *hemolysin BL,* composed of a binding component B (35 kDa) and two lytic components, L1 and L2 (36 kDa and 45 kDa, respectively)[11]; all three are needed for fluid accumulation in the rabbit ileal loop.[13] Other *B. cereus* enterotoxins, a nonhemolytic enterotoxin and cytotoxin K, also have been described.[21,91,102] These toxins also damage lung epithelial cells in cases of *B. anthracis*-like pneumonia, with varying levels of cytotoxicity depending on the level of aeration.[89]

The emetic toxin cereulide, encoded in a megaplasmid and produced by a large enzyme complex known as the Ces-non-ribosomal cereulide peptide synthetase, is well characterized.[51] It is a heat-stable (126°C [258.8°F] for 90 minutes), ring-shaped peptide with a molecular weight of 1.2 kDa[107]; it is stable between pH 2.0 and 11.0 and is protease-resistant. Cereulide variants with differing cytotoxicity have been found among different isolates of *B. cereus,* likely contributing to the spectrum of clinical illness possible with the emetic syndrome.[105] In contrast to the diarrheal toxins, it is preformed in foods, so the presence of living organisms at the time of ingestion is not necessary to cause symptoms.[57,145] Rice culture filtrates derived from emetic syndrome-associated strains cause cytoplasmic vacuolation and swollen mitochondria in Hep-2 cells, characteristics suggestive of uncoupling of oxidative phosphorylation.[127] Emetic activity occurs through the serotonin 5-HT_3 receptor and stimulation of the vagus afferent nerve.[1]

Among the multiple other substances with relevant activity, two groups are associated with local infection.[147,149] Cereolysin, or hemolysin I, is a thiol-activated cytolysin. Phospholipase C–like or lecithinase-like substances, including a sphingomyelinase and two hydrolases with preference for phosphatidylcholine and phosphatidylinositol, also exist. These enzymes induce the release of lysosomal enzymes from neutrophils that probably are involved in tissue damage, especially in wound and ocular infections.[46,163]

CLINICAL MANIFESTATIONS

Food Poisoning

Diarrheal Syndrome

The enterotoxins preformed in food or produced in vivo in the intestine after the ingestion of bacilli cause profuse, watery, nonbloody diarrhea accompanied by abdominal pain and cramps, nausea, and, occasionally, vomiting or low-grade fever.[4,40,56,82,92,101,135] The typical incubation period is 8 to 16 hours, and the clinical characteristics resemble the food poisoning of *Clostridium perfringens*. The interval between ingestion and the onset of symptoms reflects the time required for production of toxin in the gut. The symptoms resolve within approximately 12 to 24 hours but occasionally can last 2 days to 2 weeks.[56] The diarrhea (three to ten bowel movements per day) rarely leads to dehydration in healthy individuals. The most prevalent flagellar H serotypes are 1, 2, 6, 8, 10, 12, and 19. Serotyping is available at research laboratories.[19,40,100,150]

Emetic Syndrome

The usual illness is characterized by a rapid onset (within 1 to 5 hours after the ingestion of contaminated food) of nausea, vomiting, and malaise, occasionally followed by diarrhea hours later.[111] Infrequently, the diarrhea is reported to last several days.[157] The short incubation reflects the ingestion of preformed emetic toxin.

Extraintestinal Infections

Eye Infection

Keratitis, conjunctivitis, endophthalmitis, and panophthalmitis can be produced by *B. cereus*. Endophthalmitis that develops after the occurrence of penetrating wounds is caused by this organism in 27% to 46% of cases.[37,154] A history of soil contamination or the presence of a metal foreign body should raise clinical suspicion. Less frequently, corneal ulcers and surgical procedures are predisposing factors.[66,154,9,123] Exogenous endophthalmitis usually progresses rapidly, with deterioration of vision occurring in less than 48 hours. Severe pain is accompanied by chemosis, periorbital swelling, proptosis, and pus in the anterior chamber. The classic lesion is a corneal ring abscess, similar to that produced by *Pseudomonas* and *Proteus* spp. Endogenous cases may have subretinal exudation, retinal hemorrhage, and perivasculitis. Associated systemic symptoms are not unusual manifestations.[33] CT imaging may show posterior dislocation of the lens, hyperdense vitreous humor, and increased density of retroorbital soft tissue.[94] The outcome is poor, with almost half of patients left with visual acuity no better than simple light perception.[154] Clinical severity was shown to be associated with *vrr* genotype in a series of 24 cases of *B. cereus* endophthalmitis in China.[71] Many patients require enucleation. Endogenous ophthalmitis is associated with the use of illicit intravenous drugs or transfusion of contaminated blood products and subsequent bacteremic seeding of one eye.[33,136,143,154]

The pathogenesis of *B. cereus* on ocular tissue has been linked to the lecithinase activity of phospholipase C. A toxin fraction, hemolysin BL, which is formed by three separate components, produces similar destruction of retinal tissue in vitro and in animal experiments.[12] Its relationship with the diarrheal enterotoxin is unclear.[15]

Wound and Soft Tissue Infections

Wound infections of variable severity related to trauma, burns, or postsurgical complications occasionally are reported.[149,146,147,161] Because *Bacillus* is a common environmental contaminant, proof of the relevance of a *B. cereus* isolate is clearer if the organism is obtained from deep tissue in heavy pure growth. Severe infections in individuals involved in motor vehicle accidents can be complicated by necrotizing fasciitis and require extensive debridement.[161] Superficial, benignly infected wounds are common findings in the tropics.[47] Immunosuppressed patients may contract a severe gas gangrene-like infection with myonecrosis similar to disease caused by *Clostridium* spp.,[107,125] requiring amputation,[63] or a less severe primary cutaneous infection manifested by vesicles, pustules, or cellulitis.[67]

Skeletal Infections

Cases of chronic osteomyelitis occur rarely and result from accidental or surgical trauma. Radical debridement and antibiotic treatment are required.[136] Because *B. cereus* can be found as a copathogen with other, more frequent pathogenic bacteria, resolution of symptoms is delayed until eradication of the organism.[134] Acute osteomyelitis may occur in drug users.[136,143]

Bacteremia and Septicemia

Bacteremia occurs with indwelling catheters and other foreign bodies, contaminated intravenous drugs (e.g., heroin), and blood products, particularly platelets.[23,48,164,75,158] Immunosuppression and impaired neutrophil killing, such as occur in individuals with neutropenia secondary to malignancy or chemotherapy and in neonates with immaturity of the immune system, are major contributors to morbidity in systemic *B. cereus* infection.[6,24,68,74,76,119,122,153] Disseminated intravascular coagulation, multiorgan failure, and a fulminant course may occur in neonates and compromised hosts. Intestinal perforation with abdominal infection in neonates also has been described.[59] Outbreaks of sepsis in newborn nurseries have been linked to contaminated ventilation balloon devices.[156] Endocarditis is an infrequent complication of bacteremia that usually occurs in intravenous drug users or individuals with a long-term intravascular device.[112,136,143] Vegetations can form over mechanical prosthetic valves or pacemaker wires, requiring their replacement.[136,137] Morbidity and mortality rates are high in patients with valvular heart disease. Fatal serosanguineous pericarditis in a patient undergoing hemodialysis has been reported.[52]

Pneumonia

Primary pulmonary disease rarely has been recorded. Underlying predisposing conditions include leukemia, alcohol abuse, chronic hepatitis, and steroid use.[16,48,74,136] Multiorgan disease in premature neonates with necrotizing pneumonia usually is fatal.[85] Outbreaks of *B. cereus* pneumonia in neonates have been linked to contaminated ventilators.[62] Blood culture is positive in 75% of cases, followed by pleural fluid and sputum culture in 40% to 60%.[16] The pleural space may become contaminated with *B. cereus* by mishandling of the thoracic drainage system in patients with other causes of pleuritis.[79]

A dramatic pulmonary syndrome similar to that of inhalational anthrax has been seen in adults (all metal workers) with *B. cereus* infection. The organisms in these cases possessed some *B. anthracis* toxin genes while being clearly phenotypically *B. cereus*.[3,69,70]

Infection of the Central Nervous System

Premature neonates are susceptible to meningeal seeding by dissemination of intravascular infection related to catheters.[119] As in patients with other serious infections, patients who are immunosuppressed are at higher risk.[74] The cerebrospinal fluid in *B. cereus* meningitis is purulent, with white blood cell counts of more than 1000/mm^3, a predominance of polymorphonuclear leukocytes, and moderate increments in protein content. Gram stain is positive in 70% of cases. Multiple brain abscesses may result from hematogenous spread in patients with leukemia.[74,81,121,35,159] Sequelae include hydrocephalus and brain damage. Often, these infections are fatal.

Intracranial shunts and penetrating surgical or traumatic cranial wounds expose the central nervous system to environmental *B. cereus*.[49,134] Spinal anesthesia[48] was associated with *Bacillus* infection in the past. Contamination in the operating room through the linen is a potential source.[7,8] These infections are typically more benign.

Liver Failure

Fulminant hepatitis and rhabdomyolysis have been associated with the emetic toxin. The toxin inhibits hepatic mitochondrial fatty acid oxidation. Liver changes include fatty infiltrates and midzonal necrosis.[104] This has been implicated in sudden death within hours of onset in cases of *B. cereus* emetic syndromes[43,105] and has been treated in at least one reported case with emergent liver transplant in a young child,[142] though in other cases the liver failure has been reversible.[128] Most reported cases are in children and adolescents.

Pseudoinfections

Pseudoepidemics with *B. cereus* are a challenge for the clinical microbiologist.[109] Because these spore formers are so hardy, they are common laboratory contaminants. *Bacillus* spp. isolated from a single clinical specimen usually should be considered a contaminant, although their pathogenic potential is well known.[34,48,76,122,136,143,147,149] Pseudoinfections have been associated with contaminated blood culture media, syringes, blood culture analyzers, and fiberoptic bronchoscopes.[34] Colonization of umbilical cord stumps and eye surfaces by contaminated linens may cause pseudo-outbreaks in nurseries.[162]

COMPLICATIONS

Death rarely ever results from the food-poisoning syndromes. Rapidly spreading wound infections may require amputation of extremities,[60] and ocular infections can lead to loss of vision with or without enucleation.[66,154,163] The risk for death in patients with septicemia, endocarditis, and meningitis, as well as fulminant liver failure, is related to the underlying condition and severity of the disease.[6,67,110,119,137]

DIAGNOSIS

The laboratory finding of *B. cereus* in a foodstuff without quantitative cultures and without epidemiologic data is insufficient to establish its role in an outbreak.[157] In practice, appropriate specimens often either are unavailable or are submitted long after the incident, rendering their microbiologic significance questionable. During analysis of foods not involved in foodborne illness, the bacteria may be found in counts of 10^1 to 10^6 organisms per gram.[18,19,26,58,118,138] Emerging advances in diagnostics including multiplex PCR for identification of toxin-encoding genes,[165] real-time PCR for detection of spores in contaminated foods,[50] transcriptionomics, and genomics[77,130] will allow for more rapid and specific identification and classification of strains of *B. cereus* found in incriminated foods, as well as from patient samples in outbreak investigations. Diagnosis of the diarrheal form of *B. cereus* food poisoning is supported by the isolation of 10^5 or more organisms per gram from epidemiologically incriminated food.[110] The levels of *B. cereus* found in the implicated foods usually are in the range of 5×10^5 to 9.5×10^8 colony-forming units per gram. With the exception of milk, the products rarely appear to be spoiled, despite the bacteria's high density. Isolation of more than 10^5 organisms per gram in feces during an acute attack provides supportive evidence for the presumed diagnosis and confirms the association if the same serotype is isolated from incriminated food.

The organisms that produce emetic toxin are present in concentrations of 1×10^3 to 5×10^{10} colony-forming units per gram. Reheating may decrease or eliminate the organisms and leave the toxin intact, but render isolation of the organism difficult to accomplish.[46,157] Accurate PCR assays for the presence of the emetic toxin-producing *B. cereus,* as well as liquid chromatography-tandem mass spectrometry for quantification of cereulide toxin, have been developed and can be performed on food samples.[53,90,124]

Commercial immunoassay kits (reversed passive latex agglutination test, enzyme-linked immunosorbent assay, and microslide immunodiffusion assay) are available for the detection of *B. cereus* diarrheal toxin. The kits may detect a variety of proteins, however.[12,14,38] Experimental techniques based on the detection of genes for phospholipase C and sphingomyelinase by PCR have been developed for the identification of *B. cereus* in food products.[107]

The relevance of clinical isolates in extraintestinal syndromes can be assessed by the degree of growth (heavy vs. scanty), the number of occasions that growth was obtained, the source of the material cultured, and predisposing or underlying conditions.[149] For suspected endophthalmitis, aqueous and vitreous samples should be obtained.[37]

TREATMENT

During a mild, self-limited attack of food poisoning, patients require only supportive therapy. Usually, oral fluid and electrolyte replacement is adequate (Table 92.1).[56]

No antibiotic therapy is required except in cases of nongastrointestinal infection. The production of three β-lactamases by most of the organisms renders penicillin derivatives, including third-generation cephalosporins, ineffective against *B. cereus.* Most strains are susceptible to chloramphenicol, vancomycin, clindamycin, aminoglycosides, erythromycin, tetracycline, imipenem, and ciprofloxacin.[6,31,147,149,160] Definitive antibiotic therapy should be based on the antibiogram susceptibility, but initial empirical therapy with clindamycin or vancomycin, with or without an aminoglycoside, is appropriate, pending susceptibility data.[6,16,34,81,131,161] Ciprofloxacin has also been reported to be useful in the treatment of recurrent pneumonia and bacteremia[54] and may have advantages in the penetration of respiratory and eye secretions.[97] Immediate empirical coverage for *B. cereus* is indicated

TABLE 92.1 Management and Complications Associated With *Bacillus Cereus* Infections

Condition	Management	Complications
Food poisoning	Supportive measures; hydration	Usually none; liver failure and sudden death rarely reported
Ocular	Systemic, topical, intravitreal antibiotics: vancomycin and/or ciprofloxacin; surgical—early vitrectomy[31]	Severe decreased visual acuity, blindness, enucleation
Septicemia	Removal of IV device, foreign body; IV antibiotics (according to sensitivity): vancomycin	Localization of infection: endophthalmitis, endocarditis, meningitis; death
Pneumonia/pleuritis	IV antibiotics; drainage of pleural space; resection of necrotic tissue	Death
Meningitis	IV antibiotics; removal of infected intracranial shunts or cerebrospinal fluid reservoirs	Hydrocephalus, brain damage, death
Wound/subcutaneous infection	IV antibiotics; surgical debridement	Amputation, death

IV, Intravenous.

for endophthalmitis in groups at risk. Vancomycin and ciprofloxacin administered intravitreally are the best options.[25] In cases of penetrating trauma, early vitrectomy should be considered.[37,154]

Surgical debridement of necrotic tissue, drainage of closed-space infections, and prompt removal of foreign bodies and indwelling catheters are important aspects of successful therapy.[16,32,131] Some bacteremic patients may be cured by removal of the intravenous catheter only.[136]

PREVENTION AND CONTROL

Low-level contamination in food products is difficult to avoid, but proper food handling should diminish the proliferation of bacilli.[132] Practical precautions for handling cereals and rice include not preparing large quantities at a single time and maintaining the food at a hot temperature (>63°C [96.8°F]) or cooling it quickly. The food must not be stored under warm conditions, especially in the range of 15°C to 50°C (59°F to 122°F).[19,58]

NEW REFERENCES SINCE THE SEVENTH EDITION

5. Balm MN, Jureen R, Teo C, et al. Hot and steamy: outbreak of *Bacillus cereus* in Singapore associated with construction work and laundry practices. *J Hosp Infect.* 2012;81(4):224-230.
9. Basak SK, Deolekar SS, Mohanta A, et al. *Bacillus cereus* infection after Descemet stripping endothelial keratoplasty. *Cornea.* 2012;31(9):1068-1070.
17. Bennett SD, Walsh KA, Gould LH. Foodborne disease outbreaks caused by *Bacillus cereus, Clostridium perfringens,* and *Staphylococcus aureus*—United States, 1998-2008. *Clin Infect Dis.* 2013;57(3):425-433.
20. Böhm M, Huptas C, Krey VM, Scherer S. Massive horizontal gene transfer, strictly vertical inheritance and ancient duplications differentially shape the evolution of Bacillus cereus enterotoxin operons hbl, cytK and nhe. *BMC Evol Biol.* 2015;15(246):1-17.
28. Ceuppens S, Uyttendaele M, Drieskens K, et al. Survival of *Bacillus cereus* vegetative cells and spores during in vitro simulation of gastric passage. *J Food Prot.* 2012;75(4):690-694.
29. Ceuppens S, Van de Wiele T, Rajkovic A, et al. Impact of intestinal microbiota and gastrointestinal conditions on the in vitro survival and growth of *Bacillus cereus. Int J Food Microbiol.* 2012;155(3):241-246.
35. Dabscheck G, Silverman L. *Bacillus cereus* cerebral abscess during induction chemotherapy for childhood acute leukemia. *J Pediatr Hematol Oncol.* 2015;37(7):568-569.

36. Daryaei H, Balasubramaniam VM, Legan JD. Kinetics of *Bacillus cereus* spore inactivation in cooked rice by combined pressure-heat treatment. *J Food Prot.* 2013;76(4):616-623.
39. de Segura AG, Escuder D, Montilla A, et al. Heating-induced bacteriological and biochemical modifications in human donor milk after holder pasteurization. *J Pediatr Gastroenterol Nutr.* 2012;54(2):197-203.
41. Decousser JW, Ramarao N, Duport C, et al. *Bacillus cereus* and severe intestinal infections in preterm neonates: putative role of pooled breast milk. *Am J Infect Control.* 2013;41(10):918-921.
42. Delbrassinne L, Botteldoorn N, Andjelkovic M, et al. An emetic *Bacillus cereus* outbreak in a kindergarten: detection and quantification of critical levels of cereulide toxin. *Foodborne Pathog Dis.* 2015;12(1):84-87.
43. Dierick K, Van Coillie E, Swiecicka I, et al. Fatal family outbreak of *Bacillus cereus*-associated food poisoning. *J Clin Microbiol.* 2005;43(8):4277-4279.
50. Fischer C, Hu T, Jarck J, et al. Food Sensing: Aptamer-based trapping of *Bacillus cereus* spores with specific detection via real time PCR in milk. *J Agric Food Chem.* 2015;63:8050-8057.
51. Frenzel E, Marxen S, Stark TD, et al. Ces locus embedded proteins control the non-ribosomal synthesis of the cereulide toxin in emetic *Bacillus cereus* on multiple levels. *Front Microbiol.* 2015;6:1-14.
68. Hirabayashi K, Shiohara M, Suzuki T, et al. Critical illness polyneuropathy and myopathy caused by *Bacillus cereus* sepsis in acute lymphoblastic leukemia. *J Pediatr Hematol Oncol.* 2012;34(3):e110-e113.
71. Hong M, Wang Q, Tang Z, et al. Association of genotyping of *Bacillus cereus* with clinical features of post-traumatic endophthalmitis. *PLoS ONE.* 2016;17:1-10.
72. Hoornstra D, Andersson MA, Teplova VV, et al. Potato crop as a source of emetic *Bacillus cereus* and cereulide-induced mammalian cell toxicity. *Appl Environ Microbiol.* 2013;79(12):3534-3543.
73. Hwang JY, Park JH. Characteristics of enterotoxin distribution, hemolysis, lecithinase, and starch hydrolysis of *Bacillus cereus* isolated from infant formulas and ready-to-eat foods. *J Dairy Sci.* 2015;98(3):1652-1660.
75. Ikeda M, Yagihara Y, Tatsuno K, et al. Clinical characteristics and antimicrobial susceptibility of *Bacillus cereus* blood stream infections. *Ann Clin Microbiol Antimicrob.* 2015;14(43):1-7.
77. Iriyama N, Uchino Y, Matsumoto K, et al. The significance of genome-based diagnosis for the *Bacillus cereus* species. *Intern Med.* 2013;52(5):651.
78. Islam MA, Ahmed T, Faruque AS, et al. Microbiological quality of complementary foods and its association with diarrhoeal morbidity and nutritional status of Bangladeshi children. *Eur J Clin Nutr.* 2012;66(11):1242-1246.
83. Jessberger N, Dietrich R, Bock S, et al. *Bacillus cereus* enterotoxins act as major virulence factors and exhibit distinct cytotoxicity to different human cell lines. *Toxicon.* 2014;77:49-57.
86. Kamar R, Gohar M, Jehanno I, et al. Pathogenic potential of *Bacillus cereus* strains as revealed by phenotypic analysis. *J Clin Microbiol.* 2013;51(1):320-323.
87. Kelley JM, Onderdonk AB, Kao G. *Bacillus cereus* septicemia attributed to a matched unrelated bone marrow transplant. *Transfusion.* 2013;53(2):394-397.
89. Kilcullen K, Teunis A, Popova TG, Popov SG. Cytotoxic potential of *Bacillus cereus* strains ATCC 11778 and 14579 against human lung epithelial cells under microaerobic growth conditions. *Front Microbiol.* 2016;7:1-12.
93. Krawczyk AO, De Jong A, Eijlander RT, Berendsen EM, Holsappel S. Next-generation whole-genome sequencing of eight strains of *Bacillus cereus*, isolated from food. *Genome Announc.* 2015;3(6):e01480-15.
94. Lam KC. Endophthalmitis caused by *Bacillus cereus*: a devastating ophthalmological emergency. *Hong Kong Med J.* 2015;21(5):475.e1-475.e2.
99. Liu Y, Lai Q, Göker M, et al. Genomic insights into the taxonomic status of the *Bacillus cereus* group. *Sci Rep.* 2015;5(14082):1-11.
105. Marxen S, Stark TD, Frenzel E, et al. Chemodiversity of cereulide, the emetic toxin of *Bacillus cereus*. *Anal Bioanal Chem.* 2015;407(9):2439-2453.
112. Ngow HA, Wan Khairina WM. *Bacillus cereus* endocarditis in native aortic valve. *J Infect Chemother.* 2013;19(1):154-157.
113. Nicholls M, Purcell B, Willis C, et al. Investigation of an outbreak of vomiting in nurseries in South East England, May 2012. *Epidemiol Infect.* 2016;144:582-590.
115. Ogawa H, Fujikura D, Ohnuma M, et al. A novel multiplex PCR discriminates *Bacillus anthracis* and its genetically related strains from other *Bacillus cereus* group species. *PLoS ONE.* 2015;10(3):e0122004.
116. Oh SK, Chang H, Choi S, Ok G, Lee N. and Molecular characterization of emetic toxin–producing *Bacillus cereus* group isolates from human stools. *Foodborne Pathog Dis.* 2015;12(11):914-920.
121. Rhee C, Klompas M, Tamburini FB, et al. Epidemiologic investigation of a cluster of neuroinvasive *Bacillus cereus* infections in 5 patients with acute myelogenous leukemia. *Open Forum Infect Dis.* 2015;2(3):ofv096.
123. Rishi E, Rishi P, Sengupta S, et al. Acute postoperative *Bacillus cereus* endophthalmitis mimicking toxic anterior segment syndrome. *Ophthalmology.* 2013;120(1):181-185.
124. Ronning HT, Asp TN, Granum PE. Determination and quantification of the emetic toxin cereulide from *Bacillus cereus* in pasta, rice and cream with liquid chromatography-tandem mass spectrometry. *Food Addit Contam Part A Chem Anal Control Expo Risk Assess.* 2015;32(6):911-921.
125. Rosenbaum A, Papaliodis D, Alley M, et al. *Bacillus cereus* fasciitis: a unique pathogen and clinically challenging sequela of inoculation. *Am J Orthop (Belle Mead NJ).* 2013;42(1):37-39.
128. Saleh M, Al Nakib M, Doloy A, et al. *Bacillus cereus*, an unusual cause of fulminant liver failure: diagnosis may prevent liver transplantation. *J Med Microbiol.* 2012;61(Pt 5):743-745.
130. Savini V, Polilli E, Marrollo R, et al. About the *Bacillus cereus* Group. *Intern Med.* 2013;52(5):649.
133. Shimono N, Hayashi J, Matsumoto H, et al. Vigorous cleaning and adequate ventilation are necessary to control an outbreak in a neonatal intensive care unit. *J Infect Chemother.* 2012;18(3):303-307.
142. Tschiedel E, Rath PM, Steinmann J, et al. Lifesaving liver transplantation for multi-organ failure caused by *Bacillus cereus* food poisoning. *Pediatr Transplant.* 2015;19(1):E11-E14.
153. Uchino Y, Iriyama N, Matsumoto K, et al. A case series of *Bacillus cereus* septicemia in patients with hematological disease. *Intern Med.* 2012;51(19):2733-2738.
158. Veysseyre F, Fourcade C, Lavigne J, Sotto A. *Bacillus cereus* infection: 57 case patients and a literature review. *Med Mal Infect.* 2015;45(11-12):436-440.
165. Zhang Z, Feng L, Xu H, et al. Detection of viable enterotoxin-producing *Bacillus cereus* and analysis of toxigenicity from ready-to-eat foods and infant formula milk powder by multiplex PCR. *J Dairy Sci.* 2016;99:1047-1055.
159. Vodopivec I, Rinehart EM, Griffin GK, et al. A cluster of CNS infections due to *B. cereus* in the setting of acute myeloid leukemia: neuropathology in 5 patients. *J Neuropathol Exp Neurol.* 2015;74(10):1000-1011.

The full reference list for this chapter is available at ExpertConsult.com.

93 *Arcanobacterium haemolyticum*

Natascha Ching

Arcanobacterium haemolyticum is a pleomorphic gram-positive coryneform rod that causes pharyngitis and exanthem in children and young adults.[19,42,46,51]

HISTORY

This diphtheroid was first noted by MacLean and colleagues[46] in association with exudative pharyngitis in American servicemen in the South Pacific during World War II. The organism was originally named *Corynebacterium haemolyticum,* but was reclassified in 1986 as *A. haemolyticum* on the basis of phenetic, peptidoglycan, fatty acid, menaquinone, and DNA data.[17–19] The association between infection with *A. haemolyticum* and pharyngitis was observed repeatedly over the years, but a cause-and-effect relationship between the organism and illness has been established only relatively recently.[11,46,51]

ORGANISM

Microbiology[19,21,27,78,81]

A. haemolyticum is a gram-positive to gram-variable pleomorphic rod. Its laboratory characteristics are presented in Table 93.1. The organism

TABLE 93.1 Identification Characteristics of *Arcanobacterium haemolyticum*[a]

Test or Characteristic	Finding
Catalase	Negative
β-Hemolysis	Positive (a narrow zone of slight hemolysis after 48 hr on sheep blood)
Nitrate reduction	Negative
Pigment production	White or gray
Urease	Negative
Gelatin hydrolysis	Negative
Motility	Negative
Esculin hydrolysis	Negative
Carbohydrate use:	
Glucose	Positive
Maltose	Positive
Sucrose	Positive (requires rabbit serum for growth in peptone water)
Mannitol	Negative
Xylose	Negative

[a]Data from Collins MD, Cummins CS. Genus *Corynebacterium*. In: Sneath PHA, Main NS, Sharpe ME, et al, editors. Bergey's manual of systemic bacteriology. Vol. 2. Baltimore, MD: Williams & Wilkins; 1986:266-276.

grows best at 37°C (98.6°F) on a blood- or serum-enriched medium with the addition of 5% carbon dioxide. Alternatively, it grows well anaerobically. On rabbit or human blood agar, colonies are pinpoint (0.5 mm) at 24 hours; they increase to 1 to 1.5 mm after 48 hours. At this time, a unique black opaque dot is noted in the center of the colony, and this dot remains on the agar when the colony is scraped away.

At 24 hours, a 1-mm zone of hemolysis develops around colonies grown on human or rabbit blood agar. The hemolytic zone increases to 3 to 5 mm by 48 hours. Both growth and red cell hemolysis are minimal on horse and sheep blood agar. Because throat cultures usually are performed on sheep blood agar plates, the hemolytic activity of *A. haemolyticum* may be missed.

Colonies of *A. haemolyticum* can be of either the smooth or rough biotypes on horse blood agar.[13] These biotypes also differ in their hemolysis and biochemical properties. Smooth colonies predominate in wound infections and frequently use sucrose and trehalose, are β-hemolytic, and lack β-glucuronidase. Rough colonies are found almost exclusively in the respiratory tract and do not use sucrose and trehalose, are nonhemolytic, and are β-glucuronidase positive.

A. haemolyticum resembles *Actinomyces pyogenes* (formerly *Corynebacterium pyogenes*), a common cause of bovine mastitis and a rare cause of skin ulcers in children.[38] These organisms can be differentiated by several means. *A. pyogenes* is able to hydrolyze gelatin and to ferment xylose. In addition, *A. haemolyticum* has a positive reverse Christie, Atkins, and Munch-Petersen (CAMP) test in that it inhibits the β-hemolysis of *Staphylococcus aureus*, whereas *A. pyogenes* shows slight enhancement of β-hemolysis.[26] The poor growth of *A. haemolyticum* on tellurite medium and lack of catalase help to distinguish it from *Corynebacterium diphtheriae*, which also causes pharyngitis.[32,39,42]

Toxin Production

A. haemolyticum liberates three toxins: phospholipase D (PLD), a hemolysin, and neuraminidase.[19] PLD is a dermonecrotic toxin that, after intradermal inoculation in rabbits and guinea pigs, causes local hemorrhagic necrosis; injection of PLD also is lethal in rabbits.[61] The PLD gene of *A. haemolyticum* has a high degree of homology to that of *Corynebacterium pseudotuberculosis*.[20,49] PLD has been shown to be involved in the virulence of *C. pseudotuberculosis;* PLD mutants are less pathogenic in experimental infections in goats.[48] The PLD of *C. pseudotuberculosis* is similar biochemically and shares some biologic activity with the PLD that is found in brown recluse spider venom where it plays a role in the venom's toxicity.[6,42] *A. haemolyticum* carries a gene similar to the gene encoding the erythrogenic toxin of *Streptococcus pyogenes*.[19]

Antimicrobial Susceptibility

Almost all *A. haemolyticum* strains are highly susceptible to erythromycin (minimal inhibitory concentration <0.06 μg/mL). However, erythromycin is not bactericidal.[10,46,78] Carlson and colleagues[12] reported an *A. haemolyticum* isolate from a diabetic foot ulcer that was exceptionally resistant to macrolides, clindamycin, tetracycline, and ofloxacin. Waagner[78] noted that of 100 pharyngeal isolates, all were inhibited by concentrations of 0.25 μg/mL or less of penicillin G and by 1 μg/mL of penicillin V. However, tolerance to penicillin has been observed.[46,58] In one study, the minimal bactericidal concentration/minimal inhibitory concentration ratio varied from 1:1 to 1:8.[46] In addition to being susceptible to penicillin and erythromycin, *A. haemolyticum* also is susceptible to other β-lactams, clindamycin, chloramphenicol, azithromycin, vancomycin, ciprofloxacin, tetracyclines, and rifampin; most strains are resistant to sulfonamides and trimethoprim-sulfamethoxazole.[10,12,78]

Carlson[9] compared the E test and agar dilution methods for susceptibility testing of 12 antimicrobial agents in 70 *A. haemolyticum* isolates. E test and agar dilution method results for benzylpenicillin, clindamycin, erythromycin, imipenem, levofloxacin, rifampin, and vancomycin were in 100% agreement. Tetracycline, ciprofloxacin, and ofloxacin were in agreement between 97% and 99% of the time, but a lower percentage of agreement was found for cefotaxime and cefuroxime, at 93% and 84%, respectively. The author reinforces the concept that, because there are no universal standards for the organism in regard to susceptible, intermediate, or resistant categories, results should be interpreted with caution for clinical care. Almuzara and associates[1] also evaluated the susceptibility of 19 strains of *A. haemolyticum* according to National Committee for Clinical and Laboratory Standards (now the Clinical and Laboratory Standards Institute [CLSI]) interpretative standards for aerobic organisms. The majority of isolates were susceptible to penicillin, cephalosporins, clindamycin, ciprofloxacin, vancomycin, and macrolides (erythromycin and azithromycin). However, only 68% of isolates were found to be sensitive to tetracycline.

Recommendations for antimicrobial susceptibility testing of *Arcanobacterium* are provided in the CLSI document M45 entitled "Methods for Antimicrobial Dilution and Disk Susceptibility Testing of Infrequently Isolated or Fastidious Bacteria." Table 5 in this document is for *Corynebacterium* spp. and coryneforms and also applies to *Arcanobacterium* spp. The recommended MIC method for testing *Arcanobacterium* spp. uses broth microdilution with cation-adjusted Mueller-Hinton broth (CAMHB) supplemented with 2.5% to 5% lysed horse blood (CAMHB-LHB); there is currently no disk diffusion method recommended.[16] This method involves testing in cation-adjusted Mueller-Hinton broth supplemented with lysed horse blood (2.5% to 5% v/v). Some investigators have used agar dilution or E test satisfactorily.[9]

A vancomycin-resistant *A. haemolyticum* isolated from stool during an outbreak of vancomycin-resistant enterococci has been described. It contained the *vanA* gene primarily found in *Enterococcus faecium*.[62] Two other case reports have described organisms resistant to ciprofloxacin[76] and tetracycline.[41]

Miyamoto et al. reported seven elderly patients with skin and soft tissue infections with *A. haemolyticum* that were susceptible to minocycline, vancomycin, and β-lactam antibiotics, but resistant to gentamicin and levofloxacin.[53]

EPIDEMIOLOGY

Although similar organisms are common causes of infection in animals, humans appear to be the primary host of *A. haemolyticum*.[66,78] The organism is isolated primarily from throat specimens in patients with pharyngitis,[46,51,78] although it also may be a commensal of human skin.[45] It likewise may be a commensal in the throat but often is overlooked because laboratories frequently do not differentiate diphtheroids, which are considered "normal flora." In addition, because *A. haemolyticum* often is found in polymicrobial respiratory tract infections with classic respiratory pathogens, including *S. pyogenes*, it sometimes is missed when these more classic pathogens are identified.[42]

Although no definitive data are available, spread from person to person is assumed to be from the throat discharge of an infected person to the throat of a susceptible host. Transmission could occur directly or indirectly by fomites. Secondary cases in families indicate that spread is from person to person rather than from an environmental source.[24,51]

In an 8-year study, the organism was isolated from throat specimens in each year, with isolation rates varying from 0.2% to 0.7%.[51] The peak age for contracting illness caused by *A. haemolyticum* is during the second decade of life; in contrast, the peak age for developing pharyngitis caused by *S. pyogenes* is during the first decade of life.[24,46,51] In two studies, illnesses occurred more commonly in females than in males.[24,51] In a review of *A. haemolyticum* systemic and deep-seated infections, a preponderance of males over females was found in adolescents, with no risk factors for development of invasive disease.[71] No seasonal prevalence has been reported.

Screening throat cultures for pharyngotonsillitis in northern Israel was performed in 518 throat cultures in patients aged 1 to 90 years.[15] Only one culture was positive (0.2%) for *A. haemolyticum* in contrast to 26% recovery of group A *Streptococcus*. However, the one case was in a 9-year-old patient and only 58.7% of patients were 1 to 18 years old, the more common age of isolation for this organism.

PATHOGENESIS AND PATHOLOGY

Few data are available regarding pathogenesis and pathology. The dermonecrotic toxin probably plays a role in pharyngitis. Skin biopsy specimens taken from the exanthem in two patients both showed only a mild lymphohistiocytic perivascular infiltrate.[51] Cultures of both samples were negative, and no IgG, IgA, or IgM deposition was noted. These findings suggest that the rash may be toxin mediated, similar to the rash in group A streptococcal infections.

A. haemolyticum persists intracellularly,[59] which might account for failure of penicillin treatment in some cases.

In one study, five of 42 patients were found to have apparent dual infections with Epstein-Barr virus and *A. haemolyticum*.[46] The authors of this study suggested that immune suppression by the virus contributes to a more marked effect of the bacterial infection in the throat.

With regard to the immune response to *A. haemolyticum*, paired acute and convalescent sera showed the development of a humoral response to four distinct cell wall–associated proteins on Western blot analysis in seven of eight patients with culture-confirmed infection.[56]

CLINICAL MANIFESTATIONS

Pharyngitis

Pharyngitis is the most common finding in *A. haemolyticum* infection.* Signs and symptoms associated with pharyngitis are presented in Table 93.2. The illness is indistinguishable from that caused by group A streptococci; frequently it resembles Epstein-Barr virus infectious mononucleosis. Several patients with typical infectious mononucleosis had laboratory evidence of infection with both Epstein-Barr virus and *A. haemolyticum*.[29,30,46] Peritonsillar abscess caused by *A. haemolyticum* has been reported on several occasions.[4,39,43,52] The most common exanthem is scarlatiniform, which has an onset 1 to 4 days after the beginning of pharyngeal symptoms. The rash is most prominent on the extensor surfaces of the arms and legs (Fig. 93.1). Circumoral pallor, which is seen with group A streptococcal scarlet fever, does not seem to occur with *A. haemolyticum* infection. The rash may progress to involve the chest and back; it usually spares the palms, soles, and face, and it rarely involves the abdomen and buttocks.

The rash frequently is pruritic and may be urticarial. Erythema multiforme has been described.[3] Gaston and Zurowski[28] reported a 20-year-old man who had, in addition to pharyngitis, a rash involving mainly his hands and feet. His feet were swollen, and erythematous macules, petechiae, and vesicles were on the soles. His palms were tender, and 2- to 4-mm erythematous macular lesions that contained small central vesicles were present. Recently, Mehta[50] reported a 19-year-old woman who presented with pharyngitis and a pruritic rash on her arms and legs 4 days before evaluation. Physical examination revealed an erythematous, urticarial rash with large and small annular rings over

*References 3, 11, 24, 28, 30, 32, 36, 45, 46, 51, 55, 57, 67, 68, 70, 77, 78.

TABLE 93.2 Signs and Symptoms in Children, Adolescents, and Young Adults With *Arcanobacterium haemolyticum* Infection

	Frequency (%)
Symptoms	
Sore throat	100
Rash	40–70
Pruritus	50
Fever	40–75
Hoarseness	60
Cough (nonproductive)	40–60
Vomiting	30
Signs	
Pharyngitis or tonsillitis	100
Exudative	50–70
Palatal petechiae	30
Glossitis	25
Cervical lymphadenitis	40–75
Rash	40–70
Scarlatiniform	50
Urticarial	5
Maculopapular	25

Data from references 24, 33, 43, 48, 71.

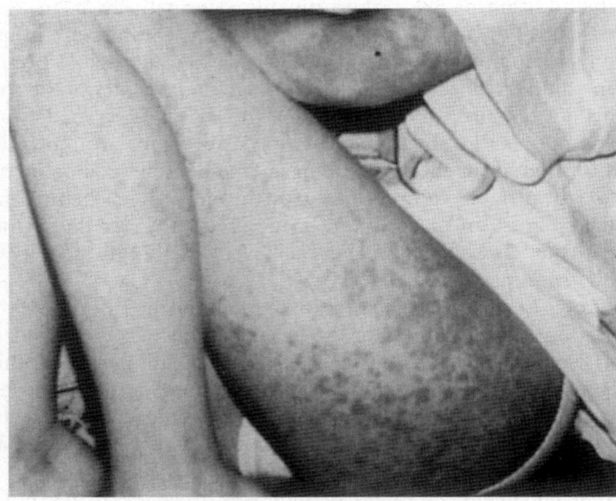

FIG. 93.1 An erythematous maculopapular discrete and confluent rash on the thigh and arm of a 16-year-old girl with pharyngitis and *Arcanobacterium haemolyticum* isolated from her throat. (From Mackenzie A, Fuite LA, Chan FTH, et al. Incidence and pathogenicity of *Arcanobacterium haemolyticum* during a 2-year study in Ottawa. *Clin Infect Dis.* 1995;21: 177–1781.)

the whole body with confluence on the upper thighs, and smaller lesions groups on distal dorsal parts of the hands and feet.

Carlson and associates[14] also reported a 19-year-old man who presented with a 2-day history of a pruritic exanthem on the upper back and chest that spread centrifugally. The patient had pharyngitis that worsened to exudative tonsillitis, and a throat culture was positive for *A. haemolyticum*. He also had swollen fingers and worsening erythematous maculopapular exanthem over his trunk and proximal extremities. Interestingly, Pastia's lines were observed on the third day. Two weeks after antimicrobial treatment and discharge, a mild late desquamation was noted on the palms and around fingernails.

The duration of the exanthem has not been described adequately in the literature. In one study, exanthem was noted to persist for longer than 2 days in 69% of patients.[48]

On occasion, *A. haemolyticum* infection has been manifested as a grayish-white pharyngeal pseudomembrane that has been confused with diphtheria.[3,32,35,39] *C. diphtheriae* and *A. haemolyticum* are diphtheroids that cannot be distinguished on Gram stain but can be differentiated by their biochemical properties.

Skin Infections

In the initial report of infections with *A. haemolyticum* in 1946, MacLean and associates[46] noted both pharyngitis in US servicemen and skin infections in the native populations of the South Pacific Islands. Cutaneous infections have been observed mainly in tropical countries.[78] The most common manifestations are ulcerative lesions that resemble ecthyma. Cellulitis, wound infections, and paronychia all have been noted.* In wound infections, mixed infections with *A. haemolyticum* and other organisms are common findings.

Tan and colleagues[74] report five cases of *A. haemolyticum* bacteremia associated with soft tissue infections in adults. These patients had a history of soft tissue infections; two elderly bedridden patients had decubitus ulcers, and three diabetic patients had foot ulcers with extensive involvement that required surgical debridement. Four patients also had *A. haemolyticum* isolated from the suspected soft tissue focus of infection. A 3-year retrospective review of clinical samples over the same period as the five reported cases revealed 25 isolates of *A. haemolyticum*. Isolates from wound infections or cellulitis were found in 96% of cases; 20% of those patients also had bacteremia. Cultures from nonsterile sites were often polymicrobial, but the authors report *A. haemolyticum* was usually the predominant isolate.

Malini and colleagues[47] report three individuals with soft tissue infections with mixed infections with *A. haemolyticum* and β-hemolytic streptococci group G in a patient with cellulitis, β-hemolytic streptococci group A in postoperative wound infection, and *Proteus vulgaris* in a diabetic patient with chronic osteomyelitis. Each of these patients responded to erythromycin alone or in combination with penicillin or ciprofloxacin therapy. *A. haemolyticum* may have a synergistic role in tissue damage in these mixed soft tissue infections.

Sinusitis/Orbital Cellulitis

Individual cases have been reported in healthy children and young adult patients diagnosed with sinusitis and complications of orbital cellulitis. The cases seem to have acute refractory orbital cellulitis, possibly preceded by pharyngitis, sinusitis, or history of rash. These cases have similar clinical histories with an aggressive clinical course requiring repeat surgical drainage and debridement.

Limjoco-Antonio and colleagues[41] report a 9-year-old girl with a swollen right eye after blunt trauma. She had ethmoid and maxillary sinusitis and orbital cellulitis, which required surgical drainage, debridement of subperiosteal abscess, and a second procedure with external ethmoidectomy and endoscopic sinus surgery. Cultures from the ethmoid sinus grew *A. haemolyticum*, and she was treated with ceftriaxone and clindamycin.

Stone and Harshbarger report a rare case of ethmoid sinusitis that progressed to orbital necrotizing fasciitis and osteomyelitis due to *A. haemolyticum* in a 16-year-old male.[73] He initially presented with concerns of periorbital cellulitis and sinusitis but progressed on intravenous vancomycin, clindamycin, and ampicillin-sulbactam. He had soft tissue swelling of the right orbit, forehead, and ethmoid sinusitis, with rapid progression of swelling leading to increased intraorbital pressure, diplopia, and a dilated pupil unresponsive to light and diminished visual acuity. Surgical exploration revealed necrotic fascia and periosteum of the orbit. Cultures were positive for *A. haemolyticum* and orbital osteomyelitis was noted on pathology. He required three debridement surgeries, delayed wound closure, and prolonged intravenous antibiotics.

Ramey and Burket report a 20-year-old male who presented with pharyngitis, fatigue, malaise, and rash, was diagnosed with EBV infection, and received a course of oral steroids.[63] After 4 days of steroids, the patient had fevers, headache, right periorbital swelling, decreased extraocular motility, and blurry vision. He was diagnosed with orbital cellulitis and started on ceftriaxone. CT scans revealed deep subperiosteal fluid collection; MRI revealed extraconal, optic nerve sheath enhancement and hyperintensities, complete bilateral maxillary and ethmoid opacification, and air fluid levels from both frontal sinuses. There was also pachymeningeal and leptomeningeal enhancement and subdural fluid collection. Despite sinus drainage and orbital exploration, he remained with orbital pain and proptosis with pupillary defect. Repeat imaging revealed reaccumulation of subperiosteal abscesses. This patient required multiple surgical procedures and drainage, in addition to prolonged antibiotics.

Burroughs and colleagues also present an 18-year-old man with pansinusitis, right orbital abscess, and rapid clinical deterioration, who had multiple abscess and sinus drainage procedures with sinus cultures positive for *A. haemolyticum* and orbital cultures positive for both *A. haemolyticum* and *Fusobacterium necrophorum*.[8]

The lessons from these cases alert clinicians that an early diagnosis requires high suspicion for this organism, and good communication with microbiology for appropriate measures to isolate this organism. Along with prolonged antimicrobial therapy, repeated debridement may be required for effective management.[8,26,29,41,63–65,73]

Other Manifestations

Isolated instances of septicemia, brain abscess, meningitis, meningoencephalitis, orbital cellulitis, endocarditis, osteomyelitis, septic arthritis, deep soft tissue infections, pleural empyema, cavitary pneumonia, pyothorax, Lemierre disease, and sinusitis have been attributed to *A. haemolyticum* infection.* Most of these serious infections occurred in adults and frequently were associated with underlying conditions such as diabetes, a malignancy, or intravenous drug use. In a 1998 review of systemic and deep-seated infections caused by *A. haemolyticum,* Skov and associates[71] identified two groups of patients. The first group was composed of middle-aged to elderly adults who were immunocompromised or had other known risk factors for development of serious infectious disease. The second group consisted of preteens to young adults with no known risk factors except for one individual receiving steroid treatment for Epstein-Barr virus infection. Therriault and colleagues[75] report a case of sepsis with *A. haemolyticum* bacteremia, cavitary pneumonia, and pyomyositis that resolved with combination therapy of penicillin and azithromycin in an 18-year-old man with only a past history of mild asthma. Cultures were positive for *A. haemolyticum* from blood, bronchoalveolar fluid, and surface and surgical cultures from a lower extremity abscess.

A pyothorax with multiloculated hydropneumothorax has been reported in a 19-year-old man in India with no history of pharyngitis.[60] Pure growth of *A. haemolyticum* was obtained from the thoracocentesis. Treatment consisted of a therapeutic thoracocentesis and continued chest tube drainage for 1 month. Ceftriaxone and metronidazole were given for a month, and the patient had clinical and radiologic resolution.

A brain abscess was documented in an 18-year-old man in Venezuela with history of multiple periodontal problems, with periodontitis, dental caries, and multiple tooth extractions.[76] The patient had headache, vomiting, and neurologic deficits in the left extremities. Computed tomography (CT) of the brain revealed a left-sided hypodense frontoparietal lesion with cystic, contrast ring enhancement, edema, and midline mass effect. With worsening neurologic status, a craniotomy was performed and aspiration of purulent material from the encapsulated mass revealed positive cultures with pure *A. haemolyticum* growth. Therapy consisted of ceftriaxone and metronidazole for 1 week and was switched after susceptibility testing to penicillin for 3 weeks.

Infective endocarditis caused by *A. haemolyticum* was reported in a 21-year-old woman with a history of congenital heart disease repaired as a child; she was on lifelong warfarin anticoagulation therapy.[83] This patient had fever, lethargy, and a swollen, painful left calf. A transthoracic echocardiogram raised concerns of vegetations on the mitral valve and ventricular septal defect patch. As a result of the occurrence of a grand mal seizure, a large right frontal parenchymal hematoma with smaller frontal abscesses was found on CT of the head. She required a frontal craniotomy for evacuation of the hematoma. Blood culture revealed *A. haemolyticum* in one of 12 sets, which was confirmed by 16S rRNA

*References 7, 23, 24, 37, 52, 54, 78, 82.

*References 2, 5, 8, 22, 26, 29–31, 33, 34, 40, 41, 44, 60, 63–65, 71, 73–75, 77–80, 83–85.

gene sequencing. Antimicrobial therapy consisted of ceftriaxone with addition of gentamicin, for 6 weeks total therapy. The initial therapy of vancomycin and metronidazole was given for only 2 weeks after identification of *A. haemolyticum.*

Fernandez-Suárez and colleagues[25] report that *A. haemolyticum* was associated with Lemierre's disease and septicemia in a 23-year-old man who presented with acute pharyngotonsillitis. The patient underwent cervical contrast-enhanced CT, which revealed complete thrombosis of the left internal jugular vein. Enoxaparin was initiated, with a transition to another anticoagulant (acenocoumarol) for 3 months as an outpatient. Antimicrobial therapy consisted initially of high-dose amoxicillin-clavulanate and metronidazole, but was changed to imipenem-cilastatin and metronidazole when right basal pneumonia was diagnosed, along with bilateral pleural effusions. The patient completed 7 days of intravenous antibiotics and was transitioned to clindamycin as an outpatient for 10 days. All three blood cultures were positive for *A. haemolyticum.*

Lemierre disease with coinfection of *A. haemolyticum* and *Fusobacterium necrophorum* bacteremia was reported by Younus and colleagues.[85] A 21-year-old man presented with fever, sore throat, tenderness along the border of his left sternocleidomastoid muscle, crackles, a blanching maculopapular rash, sepsis, and worsening pulmonary symptoms. The initial blood culture had *F. necrophorum,* and repeat blood cultures from day of admission had *A. haemolyticum* before antimicrobial therapy. CT of the chest revealed multiple nodular densities in the lungs, with evidence of central necrosis in one area. Therapy consisted of anticoagulation with heparin, initial antimicrobial therapy of gatifloxacin and metronidazole, which was switched to vancomycin and piperacillin-tazobactam for 2 weeks, followed by an oral course of amoxicillin-clavulanate for 3 months, but no surgical intervention was needed.

Sayyahfar et al. report a 2-year-old girl with a thyroid abscess who presented with fever without a source for 10 days but was eventually noted with a painful neck mass.[69] She had a CT scan that revealed a cystic lesion in the left thyroid lobe causing tracheal shift, compatible with abscess. This patient had surgical exploration and aspiration of the abscess after 2 days of antibiotics; cultures revealed *A. haemolyticum.* She was treated with clindamycin and ceftriaxone before surgery and transitioned to clindamycin to complete oral therapy.

DIFFERENTIAL DIAGNOSIS

Pharyngitis caused by *A. haemolyticum* must be differentiated from all other causes of pharyngitis (see Chapter 9). Of particular importance is distinguishing *A. haemolyticum* pharyngitis from *S. pyogenes* pharyngitis. Such differentiation can be achieved with certainty only by specific culture. In *A. haemolyticum* infection, the rapid group A streptococcal antigen tests will be negative, as will the usual group A streptococcal culture. These negative tests in specimens from adolescents should suggest strongly the possibility of *A. haemolyticum* pharyngitis.

When exanthem occurs, the confusion with illness caused by *S. pyogenes* is more pronounced. In many cases, the rash in patients infected with *A. haemolyticum* is scarlatiniform. However, the lack of typical circumoral pallor and a tendency for more discrete lesions in *A. haemolyticum* infection occasionally may help in making the clinical diagnosis.

Other common causes of pharyngitis and exanthem in adolescents and young adults are *Mycoplasma pneumoniae* and Epstein-Barr virus infections. As noted by Mackenzie and colleagues,[45] *A. haemolyticum* and Epstein-Barr virus coinfections are not uncommon occurrences. Concurrent *M. pneumoniae* pneumonia and *A. haemolyticum* empyema and bacteremia have been reported in a previously healthy 20-year-old man.[72]

Cutaneous infections, including subacute ulcerations, wound infections, cellulitis, and paronychia caused by *A. haemolyticum,* must be differentiated from those caused by other organisms, such as staphylococci and streptococci.

SPECIFIC DIAGNOSIS

A specific diagnosis is made by culturing *A. haemolyticum* from the pharynx, a skin lesion, or a sterile body site in invasive infections. Culturing is done best with rabbit or human blood agar and the addition of 5% carbon dioxide.[19,21,78,81] An important note is that horse or sheep blood agar, which generally is used for culture of *S. pyogenes,* is not satisfactory for the growth and identification of *A. haemolyticum.* Using biochemical identification systems, such as the API (RAPID) Coryne strip or the Biolog system, can help differentiate *A. haemolyticum* from other coryneform bacteria. The Biolog system can make the identification in 4 hours.[27]

TREATMENT

A. haemolyticum is highly susceptible to numerous antibiotics.[10,13,46,57,78] Although no specific treatment studies have been performed, the experience in several large studies suggests that both penicillin and erythromycin are effective.[10,36,46,51] Clinical failure with penicillin has been noted.[3,55,78] Therefore, erythromycin has been suggested for first-line therapy for certain indications, such as *A. haemolyticum* tonsillitis.[12] Carlson and coworkers[12] suggest using either a broad-spectrum β-lactam antibiotic, clindamycin, or macrolides for serious systemic *A. haemolyticum* infections, although these authors do acknowledge that macrolides do not provide anaerobic coverage. An alternative approach would be to use high-dose penicillin plus an aminoglycoside.[71,78]

PROGNOSIS

The prognosis in cases of *A. haemolyticum* pharyngitis is good, even in untreated patients. However, invasive disease can be fatal, and peritonsillar abscess or sinusitis with orbital cellulitis requires prompt surgical intervention and appropriate antimicrobial therapy.

NEW REFERENCES SINCE THE SEVENTH EDITION

8. Burroughs JR, Hsueh JB, Pelton RW. Re: "*Arcanobacterium hemolyticum* orbital cellulitis: a rare but aggressive disease". *Ophthal Plast Reconstr Surg.* 2013;29(4):332-333.
40. Lee S, Roh KH, Kim CK, et al. A case of necrotizing fasciitis due to *Streptococcus agalactiae, Arcanobacterium haemolyticum,* and *Finegoldia magna* in a dog-bitten patient with diabetes. *Korean J Lab Med.* 2008;28(3):191-195.
53. Miyamoto H, Suzuki T, Murakami S, et al. Bacteriological characteristics of *Arcanobacterium haemolyticum* isolated from seven patients with skin and soft-tissue infections. *J Med Microbiol.* 2015;64(Pt 4):369-374.
63. Ramey NA, Burkat CN. *Arcanobacterium hemolyticum* orbital cellulitis: a rare but aggressive disease. *Ophthal Plast Reconstr Surg.* 2013;29(3):e69-e72.
64. Ramey NA, Burkat CN. Re: Orbital necrotizing fasciitis and osteomyelitis caused by *Arcanobacterium haemolyticum:* a case report. *Ophthal Plast Reconstr Surg.* 2015;31(3):250.
65. Ramey NA, Burkat CN. Reply re: "*Arcanobacterium hemolyticum* orbital cellulitis: a rare but aggressive disease". *Ophthal Plast Reconstr Surg.* 2013;29(4):333.
69. Sayyahfar S, Nasiri SJ. First report of a thyroid abscess in the pediatric age group-caused by *Arcanobacterium haemolyticum. J Infect Chemother.* 2012;18(4):584-586.
73. Stone LA, Harshbarger RJ 3rd. Orbital necrotizing fasciitis and osteomyelitis caused by *Arcanobacterium haemolyticum:* a case report. *Ophthal Plast Reconstr Surg.* 2015;31(2):e31-e33.

The full reference list for this chapter is available at ExpertConsult.com.

Erysipelothrix rhusiopathiae

94

Randall G. Fisher

Erysipelothrix rhusiopathiae (insidiosa) was identified definitively first by Rosenbach[40] in 1884 as a cause of the cutaneous disease erysipeloid. Although most commonly associated with localized skin infection in humans, this organism has been associated with sepsis,[17,38,50] chronic skin eruption,[12,24] and endocarditis.[4,17,30,31,39,50]

BACTERIOLOGY

E. rhusiopathiae is a slender, pleomorphic, gram-positive, unencapsulated rod that produces 0.1-mm bluish colonies on blood agar. On Gram staining, the rods may appear singly, in short chains, or, rarely, in long branching filaments. Although they are gram positive, they decolorize readily, sometimes producing a spotted appearance. Some strains produce α-hemolysis in 48 to 72 hours. Gelatin inoculated by stab inconsistently forms a "test-tube brush" or "pipe cleaner" appearance diagnostic for this organism.[17] *Erysipelothrix* is differentiated from morphologically similar *Listeria monocytogenes* and diphtheroids by the absence of motility and catalase production and by the presence of hydrogen sulfide production in triple-sugar iron medium.[17,50]

EPIDEMIOLOGY

First isolated from mice in 1880 by Koch, *Erysipelothrix* is a common commensal of wild and domestic mammals, birds, and fish.[17,50] The organism also may lead a saprophytic existence in soil. First identified by Loeffler in 1882 as the causative agent of swine erysipelas, it remains an important epidemic cause of disease in these animals.[17] Sheep, rabbits, cattle, turkeys, and rats are subject to infection. *Erysipelothrix* has been recovered from wild moose and domestic emus.[7,18,28] *E. rhusiopathiae* survives salting and smoking procedures. Pieces of meat may contain the organism for 170 days after pickling, but exposure to moist heat for 15 minutes at 55°C kills most strains.[17,48] Fish handlers, meat processors, poultry workers, veterinarians, abattoir workers, and food handlers are at risk for exposure to *Erysipelothrix*.[33,35] Almost 90% of cases are linked to high-risk occupational exposures.[22] Isolates of the same serotype may show genetic diversity, thus serotyping may not be completely reliable as an epidemiologic tool for tracking outbreaks.[8]

PATHOPHYSIOLOGY

Human infection is largely accidental and results from contamination of skin abrasions during handling of infected material. Males are infected more commonly than females, perhaps because of an increased risk for exposure. The presence of an antiphagocytic capsule may be a virulence factor for *E. rhusiopathiae*.[43] In vitro study shows that encapsulated strains are poorly phagocytized by macrophages, unless immune serum is provided; ingested bacteria are able to replicate within the macrophage. Knock-out isolates that lack surface protective antigen A (SpaA) are 76-fold less virulent and are sensitive to the bactericidal activity of swine serum.[5] The ability to survive and replicate within macrophages probably is due to failure of the encapsulated strains to induce the oxidative burst;[42] full genomic sequencing shows that *E. rhusiopathiae* encodes for nine antioxidant factors and nine phospholipases that facilitate intracellular survival.[36] The disease usually is self-limited, most often involving the hands. Biopsy of skin lesions shows a marked inflammatory response. Difficulty establishing bacteriologic confirmation has been attributed to the organism's location in the deep part of the pars reticularis of the corium.[10]

CLINICAL MANIFESTATIONS

Human disease typically manifests as a mild, localized cutaneous eruption; a more severe, generalized cutaneous form; or a septicemia often associated with endocarditis. Localized cutaneous infection, the erysipeloid of Rosenbach,[40] is the most common manifestation of *Erysipelothrix* disease.[35] After a 1- to 4-day incubation period, an acute localized lesion appears at the site of an abrasion contaminated with *E. rhusiopathiae*-colonized material. Slowly progressive, purplish red, painful induration is typical. Absence of suppuration and involution without desquamation help to distinguish this lesion from streptococcal or staphylococcal infections. Occasionally, the skin may show sharply circumscribed bluish red lesions, which are similar to the cutaneous manifestations in swine.[17,50] Fever and other constitutional symptoms are uncommon manifestations, occurring in less than 10 % of cases, unless bacteremia supervenes.[12,35] Untreated infection usually is self-limited, with an average duration of 3 weeks.

Lymphangitis and adenitis occur in 10% of cases; in 20% of cases, progression of disease extends from lesions on the hand to the wrist and forearm.[25] In one case, a patient with type 2 diabetes was discovered at the time of surgery to have necrotizing fasciitis; *E. rhusiopathiae* was the predominant but not only organism isolated from surgical specimens.[44] A 7-week-old infant with localized *E. rhusiopathiae* infection of the knee without a known source of exposure has been reported,[27] and a 6-year-old girl with *Erysipelothrix* pyopneumothorax has been described.[37] Septic arthritis has been described in a healthy 18-year-old man in whom disease developed after he underwent arthroscopic knee surgery,[2] in association with infective endocarditis,[41] and in a patient with systemic lupus erythematosus and chronic monarthritis without associated systemic symptoms.[49] One case of septic arthritis of the hip in a 5-year-old boy without risk factors or obvious immune deficiency has been reported.[32]

Cutaneous eruptions may occur rarely in areas distant from the site of inoculation,[26] appearing as violaceous lesions with advancing pink borders. Bullous vesiculation has been described.[12] In 1921, Prausnitz[38] reported the first case of apparent septicemia in childhood, isolating the organism from the blood of a 10-year-old boy.

E. rhusiopathiae rarely is associated with the bite of a domestic dog or cat.[1] In one prospective study of infected domesticated animal bite wounds, two patients who had been bitten by a cat infected with *E. rhusiopathiae* were identified.[45] Cultures were carefully processed and were performed in reference laboratories. Cats are not natural hosts of the organism.

An uncommon but important complication of *Erysipelothrix* infection is endocarditis. Presumed or proven endocarditis accounts for 90% of serious *E. rhusiopathiae* infections.[16] Patients with congenital heart disease or heart valve damage secondary to acute rheumatic fever are at the greatest risk for development of endocarditis. However, previously normal heart valves can be infected.[17,30] Valvular and myocardial abscesses have been described.[34] In contrast to diphtheroid endocarditis, *E. rhusiopathiae* endocarditis usually does not involve prosthetic valves; and in contrast to *Bacillus* spp. endocarditis, it is not associated with intravenous drug abuse.[16] In a review of 1989 cases of endocarditis from 13 series,[4] *Erysipelothrix* was documented in two patients. *Erysipelothrix* endocarditis commonly involves the aortic or mitral valves or both. Overall mortality in reported cases is 38%, despite appropriate surgery and antibiotic therapy, which is considerably higher than that associated with other pathogens of endocarditis.[15] Many patients with endocarditis are treated empirically with vancomycin, a drug to which all *Erysipelothrix* isolates are constitutively resistant.[20] No history nor physical evidence of cutaneous lesions is found in 50% of cases of endocarditis, and history of exposure to contaminated material often is lacking. Although immunocompromised individuals[31] may be at increased risk, serious infection also occurs in otherwise normal hosts,[6,17,30] particularly in association with occupational exposure. Many case reports involve patients with diabetes mellitus and/or alcoholic hepatitis.

Multiple case reports of septic arthritis, usually involving prosthetic joints, have been published.[19,46,47] In rare cases, *E. rhusiopathiae* can cause pneumonia,[29] osteomyelitis,[9] spinal abscess,[3] or meningitis.[21] Meningitis may be acute[21] or chronic.[23]

DIAGNOSIS

For localized disease, diagnosis depends largely on clinical appearance of the lesion in association with an appropriate history of exposure. Attempts to culture the organism from material collected by swab or aspirate of a local lesion almost always are unsuccessful.[10,50] Biopsy specimens of affected skin cultured in broth generally yield the offending bacteria. Amplification and detection of *Erysipelothrix* DNA by polymerase chain reaction show promise in animal models of infection.[28] Other newer mechanisms for identification include matrix-assisted laser desorption ionization-time of flight (MALDI-TOF)[13] and loop-mediated isothermal amplification (LAMP) assays.[51] *Erysipelothrix* is isolated commonly from the blood of patients with septicemia or endocarditis and can be found in affected heart valves at autopsy or at the time of valve replacement.[12] Growth of the organism may be slow; cultures should be monitored for at least a week. A high index of suspicion is important for establishing the diagnosis of endocarditis. The organism has been misidentified as a viridans group streptococcus because of its pleomorphic coccoid appearance, α-hemolysis, and catalase-negative character. Abbreviated identification schema that do not include testing for hydrogen sulfide production sometimes lead to misidentification as *Lactobacillus* spp. or enterococci.[11]

TREATMENT

E. rhusiopathiae is exquisitely sensitive to penicillin. Most isolates also are sensitive to ceftriaxone.[14] Clindamycin or ciprofloxacin may be used for patients who are allergic to penicillin.[14] Localized disease usually can be treated with oral medication, but high parenteral doses occasionally are necessary, particularly for disseminated disease.[17] Treatment of endocarditis is similar to treatment of endocarditis caused by viridans streptococci. At least 12 million units of penicillin administered for 4 weeks has been curative in adult patients, but many cases have been treated for 6 weeks or longer. Concomitant administration of an aminoglycoside has been used in some cases. *Erysipelothrix* is resistant to vancomycin.[20] Prompt microbiologic differentiation of *E. rhusiopathiae* from other gram-positive organisms is important in guiding antimicrobial choice because vancomycin often is employed in empiric therapy of endocarditis. Risk of disease is minimized by protecting individuals exposed to potentially contaminated materials.

NEW REFERENCES SINCE THE SEVENTH EDITION

3. Andrychowski J, Jasielski P, Netczuk T, Czernicki Z. Empyema in spinal canal in thoracic region, abscesses in paravertebral space, spondylitis: in clinical course of zoonosis erysipelothrix rhusiopathiae. *Eur Spine J.* 2012;21(suppl 4):S557-S563.
5. Borrathybay E, Gong FJ, Zhang L. Nazierbieke W. Role of surface protective antigen A in the pathogenesis of Erysipelothrix rhusiopathiae strain C43065. *J Microbiol Biotechnol.* 2015;25:206-216.
9. Denes E, Camilleri Y, Fiorenza F, Martin C. First case of osteomyelitis due to Erysipelothrix rhusiopathiae: pubic osteomyelitis in a gored farmer. *Int J Infect Dis.* 2015;30:133-134.
13. Farfour E, Leto J, Barritault M, et al. Evaluation of the Andromas matrix-assisted laser desorption ionization-time of flight mass spectrometry system for identification of aerobically growing Gram-positive bacilli. *J Clin Microbiol.* 2012;50:2702-2707.
21. Joo EJ, Kang Ci, Kim WS, et al. Acute meningitis as an initial presentation of Erysipelothrix rhusiopathiae endocarditis. *J Infect Chemother.* 2011;17:703-705.
23. Kichloo AA, Hallac A, Mousavi B, Herkhan O. Nonspecific Erysipelothrix rhusiopathiae bacteremia in a patient with subclinical alcoholic liver disease. *Case Rep Infect dis.* 2013;474593.
30. Meric M, Ozcan SK. Erysipelothrix rhusiopathiae pneumonia in an immunocompetent patient. *J Med Microbiol.* 2012;61:450-451.
33. Mukhopadhyay C, Shah H, Vandana KE, Munim F, Vijayan S. A child with Erysipelothrix arthritis—beware of the little known. *Asian Pac J Trop Biomed.* 2012;2:503-504.
37. Ogawa Y, Ooka T, Shi F, et al. The genome of Erysipelothrix rhusiopathiae, the causative agent of swing erysipelas, reveals new insights into the evolution of firmicutes and the organism's intracellular adaptations. *J Bacteriol.* 2011;193:2959-2971.
52. Yamazaki Y, Oba E, Kashiwagi N, et al. Development of a loop-mediated isothermal amplification assay for rapid and simple detection of Erusipelothrix rhusiopathiae. *Lett Appl Microbiol.* 2014;58:362-369.

The full reference list for this chapter is available at ExpertConsult.com

95 Listeriosis

Sing Sing Way • Ghada N. Al-Rawahi • Tobias R. Kollmann

Listeria species are found widely in the environment in soil, water, and decaying vegetation.[4,46,124] Pathogenic *L. monocytogenes* was described first by Murray and associates in 1926 while investigating an epidemic of fatal infections in laboratory rabbits during pregnancy.[100] The first case of human *L. monocytogenes* infection was identified 3 years later,[102] with neonatal infection first recognized in 1936.[17] The first outbreak confirming transmission from animals to humans was reported in 1983.[125] *L. monocytogenes* is now recognized as a ubiquitous bacterium that colonizes the intestinal tract of virtually all mammalian species. It has specialized virulence features that make it an often lethal pathogen in a wide variety of susceptible hosts, including newborn infants, pregnant women, older adults, and other individuals with immunocompromising conditions.[14,27,80] The frequent occurrence of outbreaks underscores the necessity for the continued high level of attention afforded to this organism.[18]

ORGANISM

The genus is named after Sir Joseph Lister, the pioneer of antiseptic surgical techniques.[132] *Listeria* are facultative anaerobic, non–spore-forming, motile, small gram-positive bacilli that form whitish-gray colonies with narrow zones of β-hemolysis on nutrient agar. They are catalase positive, non–acid-fast and non–capsule-forming bacteria. Of the nineteen defined species within the *Listeria* genus,[37] the majority of clinical infections are caused by *L. monocytogenes*.[58,87] The few case reports on human infection caused by other species usually involve immunocompromised hosts.[121] In direct smears, *Listeria* may have a coccoid morphology and be confused with Gram positive cocci. However, the following features of *L. monocytogenes* may be used to distinguish it from other Gram-positive bacteria[131]:

1. All *Listeria* species exhibit tumbling motility at 25°C to 30°C, owing to the uniform distribution of flagella across the bacterial surface (peritrichous) flagella, with reduced motility at 37°C (98.6°F).[155]

2. *L. monocytogenes* grows with a narrow zone of β-hemolysis (nonhemolytic, non-invasive mutant strains exist but are rare[67]) and exhibits a rectangular area of increased hemolysis when streaked on blood agar in proximity to *Staphylococcus aureus* (Christie, Atkins, Munch-Peterson [CAMP] test).
3. *L. monocytogenes* ferments methyl-D-mannoside and L-rhamnose but not D-xylose.

Listeria tolerate low temperatures, high salt concentrations, and high pH, which allows survival and replication in soil, water, sewage, manure, animal feed, and refrigerated foods. Cold enrichment has been used to improve isolation from clinical samples.[11,45,58,130] In this regard, the ability of *Listeria* to survive and replicate even at refrigeration temperatures distinguishes it from most other food-borne bacterial pathogens. Paterson,[107] and Seeliger and Finger[133] performed extensive serologic characterization of *L. monocytogenes.* At least 17 serotypes have been identified on the basis of somatic and flagellar antigens, with 3 (1/2a, 1/2b, 4b) accounting for most clinical and food isolates.[92,109]

TRANSMISSION

The ability of *L. monocytogenes* to tolerate high salt concentrations and an alkaline environment allows it to survive for months in soil, water, animal feed, and refrigerated foods.[25] Contaminated food is the most common source of human *Listeria* infection.[20,54,78] Despite implementation of a "zero tolerance" policy for *L. monocytogenes* by the US Department of Agriculture in 1987, outbreaks involving various meat and dairy products, along with contaminated fruits and vegetables, remain common.[18] *L. monocytogenes* still is the most common cause of foodborne illness–related hospitalization and death in the United States.[20] Nonetheless, despite frequent foodborne outbreaks, most infections are sporadic and have no epidemiologic explanation.[149] These sporadic clinical cases could reflect invasive infection from intestinal colonization. Indeed, the rate of asymptomatic fecal carriage in healthy individuals is common, ranging from 2% to 10%[124] or higher.[66,80] However, fecal shedding of *L. monocytogenes* appears to be of short duration.[54] Although maternal colonization does not invariably lead to invasive illness, pregnancy-associated infection represents approximately 17% of all invasive cases.[61] About 20% of pregnancy-associated infection results in stillbirth or neonatal death.[61] Transmission of *L. monocytogenes* from mother to fetus can occur in utero by ingestion of infected amniotic fluid or transplacentally from the maternal circulation.[80] The factors contributing to cases of late-onset infection of the newborn (up to 2 months of age) are unknown.[12,69,111]

EPIDEMIOLOGY

Despite its ubiquitous presence and frequent sporadic outbreaks, *L. monocytogenes* is a relatively uncommon cause of infection in the general population (ranging from 0.1 to 10 per 1 million individuals).[14,27,44,120,140] Listeriosis has a nonuniform age distribution, with most cases occurring among newborn infants or older adults (Fig. 95.1). In these susceptible subpopulations, infection confers a disproportionately high mortality rate ranging from 20% to over 60%.[120] Invasive *L. monocytogenes* infection is also 20- to 100-fold more common among women during pregnancy compared with the general population.[51,61,80] As a result, perinatal attack rates during outbreaks are extremely high and can reach 1% to 2% of all deliveries.[12,111] Although preventative measures, monitoring, and voluntary recall of contaminated food products have reduced the incidence of perinatal listeriosis in recent decades,[80] risk for foodborne infection remains high, with increasing incidence in older adults.[12,94,120]

PATHOGENESIS AND PATHOLOGY

Listeria is a facultative intracellular organism. Infection with *L. monocytogenes* begins after oral ingestion of the bacteria. In adults, the infectious dose is estimated to be 10^4 to 10^6 organisms per gram of ingested food but may be as low as 10 organisms in immunocompromised hosts and patients who have diminished gastric acidity or injured intestinal barrier function.[124,126,12,123] *L. monocytogenes* infects intestinal M cells through phagocytosis and intestinal epithelial cells through actions of listerial surface proteins called internalin A (InlA).[43,84] InlA binds to host E-cadherin that is transiently exposed to the luminal surface of the intestinal villi during remodeling of epithelial junctions.[108] InlA also facilitates placental invasion since E-cadherin is expressed on syncytiotrophoblasts.[10,85] After intestinal epithelial cell invasion, *L. monocytogenes* translocates systemically to infect target tissues that include the liver, spleen, mesenteric lymph nodes, and other organs via the blood and lymph.[150] Binding of listerial internalin B (InlB) to the host hepatocyte growth factor receptor (also known as the tyrosine kinase receptor Met) and complement component C1q[8] permits efficient hepatocyte entry via endocytosis.[15,16,31,53,105] InlB may also have a role facilitating the transfer of *L. monocytogenes* across the blood-brain barrier.[53]

After cell entry, *L. monocytogenes* quickly escapes from endocytic vacuole and enters the cytosol of host cells. In the cytosolic compartment, the bacterium replicates and spreads to adjacent neighboring cells through intercellular protrusions, avoiding recognition and subsequent destruction

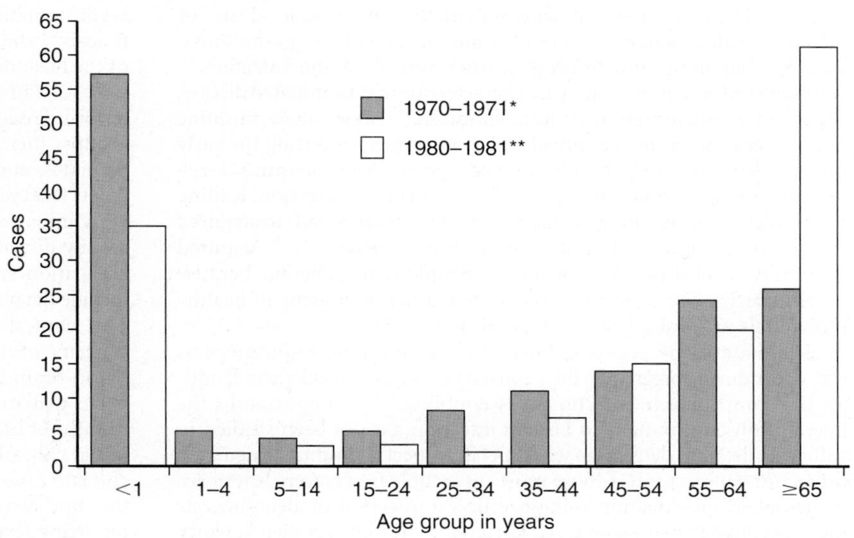

FIG. 95.1 Human listeriosis cases by age group for the United States, 1970–71 and 1980–81. (From Albritton WL, Cochi SL, Feeley JC. Overview of neonatal listeriosis. *Clin Invest Med.* 1984;7:311–314.)

by antibodies or neutrophils.[79] *L. monocytogenes* vacuolar escape is mediated by two virulence-associated bacterial proteins: listeriolysin O (LLO) and phospholipase C.[25] LLO is a pore-forming, cholesterol-dependent cytolysin.[7,70,127,151] Although LLO is absolutely required for vacuolar escape in murine cells, it appears dispensable in human cells, where phospholipases play unique and functionally redundant roles.[110] Once in the host cell cytoplasm, *L. monocytogenes* retains motility by active recruitment and polymerization of actin filaments into organized tails though the actin assembly-inducing protein ActA. Motile bacteria create membrane-bound protrusions into adjacent cells; within the newly infected cells, the membrane layers are then lysed by LLO and phospholipases, propagating the unique intracellular life cycle of this bacterium. Thus, key *L. monocytogenes* virulence determinants include efficient invasion and access to the cytoplasmic compartment of host cells, followed by rapid spread into adjacent cells, thereby avoiding intracellular degradation (autophagy) as well as extracellular host defense mechanisms (e.g., antibodies, complement, neutrophils).[97,143-145] In animal infection models, *L. monocytogenes* mutants lacking the molecules required for cytoplasmic entry from the endocytic vacuole (e.g., LLO or phospholipase C) or actin recruitment within the host cell cytoplasm (ActA) are highly attenuated.[151] Although ActA is one of the major virulence determinants of *L. monocytogenes,*[29] strains lacking ActA retain the ability to infect the placenta, although at a lower rate than wild-type strains.[83]

To counteract infection, a protective host response that aims to restrict bacterial invasion and survival is set into motion shortly after *L. monocytogenes* host cell adherence.[25,148] This has been best characterized after infection of mouse macrophage cells, where *L. monocytogenes* activates at least three unique host defense pathways[157]: (1) a MyD88-dependent pathway emanating from the cell surface and phagosome, leading to expression of cytokines and reactive oxygen species; (2) a STING/IRF3-dependent pathway emanating from the cytosol, leading to the expression of interferons and coregulated genes; and (3) an AIM2/caspase-1–dependent inflammasome pathway, resulting in proteolytic activation and secretion of interleukin (IL)-1 and IL-18 and pyroptotic cell death. *L. monocytogenes,* on the other hand, has developed elaborate mechanisms to counterbalance these host defense strategies.[28] The outcome of this molecular "tug of war" is likely dictated by the bacterial inoculum and activation properties of individual host cells.

Cytokines and chemoattactant chemokine proteins released by *L. monocytogenes* infected cells recruit neutrophils, which efficiently eliminate extracellular bacteria and dying infected cells.[75] Infected macrophage cells also produce the proinflammatory cytokine IL-12, which induces the synthesis of interferon-γ (IFN-γ) by natural killer cells and CD4 T helper-1 cells. IFN-γ in turn activates infected macrophages to become listericidal through the production of free oxygen and nitrogen radicals.[104,150] The recruitment of acute inflammatory cells to local sites of infection with *L. monocytogenes* in some cases results in granulomas, thereby containing and limiting further spread of the infection.[134] Although multiple granulomas are characteristic of disseminated disease, suppurative inflammation is more common.[74] These innate immune effector cascades limit the spread of *L. monocytogenes* during the early phase of infection. In the immune-competent host, adaptive T-cell immune responses peak about 1 week after primary infection, leading to complete clearance of infected cells; this process also leads to acquired resistance to subsequent infection (immune memory).[104] Acquired immunity is not dependent on clinical symptomatic infection, because T cells specific for *L. monocytogenes* are frequently present in healthy individuals without a history of listeriosis.[26,47,77,98,111,112]

There are many poorly defined shifts in immune responsiveness that occur during pregnancy, the neonatal period, and in elderly individuals that contribute to infectious susceptibility.[76,86,101] Importantly, the host response in humans to *Listeria* infection has not been studied in sufficient detail to determine what specific aspect of immune-mediated protection fails to protect those most susceptible from severe listeriosis. Nonetheless, investigation using preclinical infection models suggests that susceptibility to invasive *L. monocytogenes* infection during pregnancy is primarily conveyed by the selective expansion of immune suppressive regulatory CD4 T cells that are essential for maintaining maternal tolerance to genetically foreign paternal antigens expressed by the developing fetus.[35,64] Fetal wastage readily occurs with systemic maternal *L. monocytogenes* infection in animals. However, fetal wastage does not require *L. monocytogenes* invasion of the placental unit, but instead is driven by fractured maternal tolerance to immunologically foreign fetal antigens.[117,119] Disrupted fetal tolerance with ensuing inflammation at the maternal-fetal interface draws circulating pathogen into the placenta, bypassing innate host resistance properties of trophoblast cells and other cell types unique to this tissue.[115,158,159] These recent findings demonstrating a causative role for "unintentional" attack by maternal immune components in driving fetal wastage that occurs with prenatal infection also highlights the exciting possibility of protecting the developing fetus from injury using immune modulatory therapies.[21,118] In turn, naturally occurring strategies for reinforcing fetal tolerance, including immunological tolerance to noninherited maternal antigens, have recently been shown to protect against fetal injury and congenital transmission after *L. monocytogenes* prenatal infection.[72,73]

In animal models of neonatal infection, *L. monocytogenes* susceptibility is associated with blunted production of innate proinflammatory cytokines, and delayed activation of protective T cells.[12] Recently, active immunological suppression by erythroid precursor cells that express the transferrin receptor, CD71, has been shown to play a dominant role skewing neonatal T cell differentiation towards susceptibility of newborns to invasive infection by *L. monocytogenes* and other neonatal pathogens.[34,114] However, the physiological enrichment of erythoid precursor cells in early postnatal development that increase susceptibility to *L. monocytogenes* and other neonatal pathogens may play more essential roles in averting pathological inflammation during primary colonization with commensal microbes during the abrupt transition from the sterile in utero compartment that occurs with parturition.[34] Therefore, the susceptibility of neonates to invasive infection by *L. monocytogenes* and other neonatal pathogens likely reflects the need for active immunological suppression during this unique developmental window.

In older children and young adults, *L. monocytogenes* infection is rare; however, underlying diseases or medications that interfere with cell-mediated immunity are known to increase susceptibility.[12,24,30,60,111,135,148,157] On the other hand, neutropenia and disorders of the humoral immune system (complement or immunoglobulin) are not associated with excessive prevalence of listeriosis.[80] This suggests a central role of at least the innate and adaptive cell-mediated immune system in optimal defense against *L. monocytogenes* in the human host.

CLINICAL MANIFESTATIONS

The incubation period for listeriosis is variable, ranging from 6 hours to 10 days for gastroenteritis to 1 to 70 days for invasive disease.[89,103] Most infections with *L. monocytogenes* in the healthy host remain entirely asymptomatic.[12] Clinical infection with *L. monocytogenes* is called listeriosis[123] and exists in two forms depending on the immunologic status of the host: noninvasive gastrointestinal listeriosis and invasive listeriosis.[12,120,151] In immunocompetent children and adults, noninvasive listeriosis develops as a febrile gastroenteritis.[123,126] However, in vulnerable groups, including women during pregnancy, the developing fetus, neonates, and infants up to approximately 2 months of age,[88] older adults (>60 years of age), and immune-compromised children and adults with impaired cell-mediated immunity,[12,120] *L. monocytogenes* more readily disseminates from the gastrointestinal tract into the systemic circulation and from there to other tissues.[12] The main target tissues include the placenta, the central nervous system, liver, and spleen.[12,32,111,123] This clinical pattern of invasive listeriosis derives from the unique capacity of *L. monocytogenes* to cross the placental, intestinal, and blood-brain barriers.[84]

In pediatric listeriosis, most severe infections occur in the first 2 months of life. Similar to those of group B streptococcal infection, the initial clinical features of neonatal listeriosis can be divided into early and late-onset disease (Table 95.1). In 50% to 74% of early-onset cases, the mother reports a history of an "influenza-like illness," with 65% reporting fever, 21% backache (which may be mistaken for a urinary tract infection), 10% headache, 7% vomiting and diarrhea, and 4% muscle pains or sore throat. Importantly, despite this range of clinical symptoms, approximately one-third of infected pregnant women remain

TABLE 95.1 Clinical and Laboratory Findings of Early-Onset and Late-Onset Neonatal Listeriosis

Feature	Early Onset[80,65,1,3,39]	Late Onset[2,40,71,80,128]
Median (range) age (days)	1 (birth to 6)	14 (7–35)
Male (%)	60	67
Preterm (%)	65	20
Mortality rate (%, range)	38 (22–63)	3 (0–10)
Respiratory involvement (%)	38–50	10
Meningitis (%)	24	67–93
Blood isolate (%)	81–88	17–95
Maternal perinatal illness (%)	50–74	0

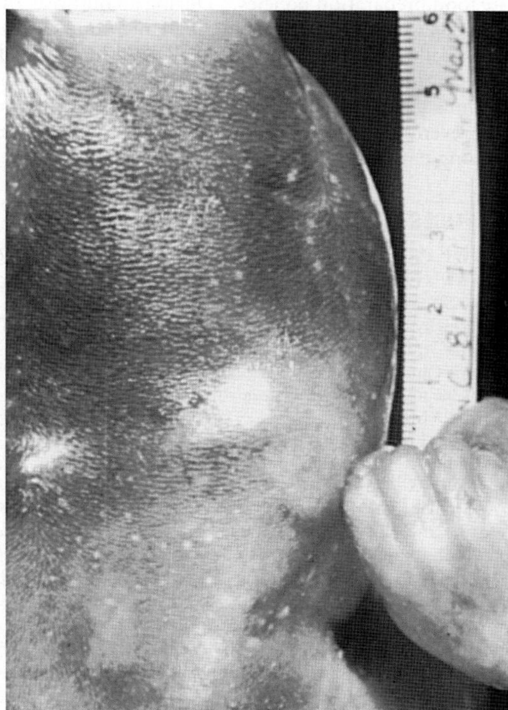

FIG. 95.2 Typical pustular rash on the abdomen of a stillborn infant with listeriosis. Note the small pale granuloma measuring 1 to 3 mm and the dark erythema surrounding these lesions.

entirely asymptomatic.[80] Spontaneous abortion occurs in 10% to 20% of clinically symptomatic listeriosis cases during pregnancy, with another approximately 50% delivering preterm, and 11% ending in intrauterine fetal demise.[80] Thirty-four percent of infected pregnancies demonstrate fetal distress, and 75% display meconium-stained amniotic fluid; microabscesses are frequently histologically evident in infected placentas.[80]

Early-onset neonatal listeriosis has a high mortality rate (20–60%); even in those who survive, a significant number (12.7%) develop long-term neurologic sequelae.[12,80] At birth, respiratory distress, apnea, lethargy, and fever are common manifestations; diarrhea, conjunctivitis, and myocarditis also have been described.[12] The respiratory symptoms may mimic symptoms of respiratory distress syndrome. Patchy bronchopneumonic infiltrates, probably caused by aspiration of infected amniotic fluid, may be seen on chest radiographs.[12] Occasionally, discrete roseolar or pustular lesions on the skin and pharynx occur that on histology appear as microabscesses and macroabscesses and contain culturable *L. monocytogenes;* this rash has been termed *granulomatosis infantisepticum* (Fig. 95.2).

The late-onset form of neonatal listeriosis is less common than the early-onset form and usually affects term infants, who appear healthy until the onset of meningitis or, less commonly, septicemia and colitis 1 to 8 weeks after birth.[40,59,71,81] Clinical manifestations of late-onset meningitis are often subtle and include fever, irritability, lethargy, and poor feeding.[71,129] Cerebrospinal fluid findings vary; although pleocytosis usually is significant, not all infections have a polymorphonuclear cell predominance. The maternal history in these cases usually is negative, suggesting postnatal, possibly even nosocomial, exposure in affected infants.[130]

Although the incidence of listeriosis in immunocompromised children is higher, the clinical features are similar to those of non-immunosuppressed patients and include most commonly meningitis or septicemia. Rare clinical manifestations of *L. monocytogenes* infection include rhombencephalitis, brain abscess, arthritis, osteomyelitis, endocarditis, endophthalmitis, liver abscess, and peritonitis.[90,129,130,135]

DIAGNOSIS

Appropriate specimens for staining and culture vary with the clinical syndrome, but the organism can be readily cultured from blood, cerebrospinal fluid, amniotic fluid, and genital secretions. Examination of gram-stained material (ear, meconium, and placenta) from neonates is recommended in suspected, early-onset sepsis.[83] Pathologic specimens (e.g., biopsy material, placental or fetal tissue) may reveal the characteristic Gram-stain morphology and pathologic features, such as microabscesses and granulomas. Selective and differential culture media, such as lecithin and levofloxacin (LL) medium, CHROMagar *Listeria*, PALCAM (polymyxin B–acriflavine–lithium chloride–ceftazidime–esculin–mannitol agar) or modified Oxford agar, may be helpful for isolation of *Listeria* from nonsterile sites such as stool or vaginal secretions.[91,106,109] Laboratories undertaking primary isolation must be aware of the similarities between *L. monocytogenes* and frequently disregarded "commensals."[92]

After 48 hours of incubation at 37°C on 5% sheep blood agar, typical colonies are whitish/gray with a narrow zone of β-hemolysis. Traditionally, identification is based on morphology; tumbling motility; β-hemolysis; positive catalase, esculin, and CAMP tests; and carbohydrate-use pattern. Commercial kits are available for the rapid identification of *Listeria* from culture. These kits include DNA probes, latex agglutination, and enzyme immunoassay methods. Despite extensive attempts to develop serologic techniques for the diagnosis of listeriosis, none has proved satisfactory and few centers attempt serodiagnosis. More recently, matrix-assisted laser desorption ionization-time of flight mass spectrometry (MALDI-TOF MS) has become a valuable tool for the rapid identification, and possibly typing, of *Listeria* species.[6,62]

Histologic diagnosis from pathologic material should be attempted if the organism is not cultured. Specific fluorescent antibody staining,[22] nucleic acid hybridization,[139] and polymerase chain reaction[5,63] have all been used for detection of *Listeria.* The application of molecular detection to food safety programs has been growing rapidly, with clinical applications of molecular *Listeria* detection lagging somewhat behind with regard to the limited commercial options available. However, several centers have reported the development of sensitive and specific molecular assays for detection of *L. monocytogenes* in cerebrospinal fluid. For cases of suspected meningitis with prior antibiotic treatment, broad-range 16s rDNA polymerase chain reaction is becoming widely used in North America and can be key in establishing the diagnosis.[13,82]

TREATMENT

Intravenous ampicillin and an aminoglycoside, typically gentamicin, remain the treatment of choice for invasive *L. monocytogenes* infections. Ampicillin may be used alone in immunocompetent patients with less severe infections or once clinical response has occurred. *L. monocytogenes* shows tolerance to some antibiotics in vitro,[36,93] but antibiotic resistance in clinical *Listeria* isolates remains low (although surveillance of food and dairy products has shown an increase in resistance to multiple antibiotics including ampicillin).[55,137,154] Ampicillin plus gentamicin has demonstrable synergy on most *Listeria* strains both in vitro and in animal models[33,96,146]; however, human clinical trial data for dual treatment are lacking. Antibiotics commonly recommended for treatment—including ampicillin—are bacteriostatic at concentrations usually achieved in blood.[36,48,49,147,152]

For penicillin-allergic patients, trimethoprim-sulfamethoxazole has been used successfully.[54,138] This is supported by in vivo data with and without the addition of rifampin.[41,56,57,96,122] In an in vivo model of *L. monocytogenes* encephalitis, the combinations ampicillin/gentamicin and trimethoprim-sulfamethoxazole/rifampin were highly active against intracerebral bacteria.[9] Trimethoprim-sulfamethoxazole cannot be recommended for use in perinatal infections because of the concern of bilirubin toxicity developing with sulfonamides.[41]

For patients with both penicillin and sulfa allergies, vancomycin has been used successfully, albeit with much less accumulated clinical experience than ampicillin-based regimens.[113] One group has reported a case of bacteremia with vancomycin-resistant *L. grayi,* the first such documented invasive infection with this species.[121] More recently, cases of invasive *Listeria* infections treated successfully with linezolid have been published; this oxazolidinone antimicrobial exhibits bactericidal activity against *Listeria.*[96,99]

L. monocytogenes is intrinsically resistant to cephalosporin antibiotics.[36] Acquired resistance to clindamycin, tetracyclines, quinolones macrolides and daptomycin has been reported, although clinical experience with these agents is very limited.[95,136,156] Antagonism also seems to occur between certain antibiotic combinations (erythromycin and penicillins, erythromycin and aminoglycosides, penicillin and chloramphenicol, and penicillin and tetracycline).[36,48]

Duration of therapy depends on the clinical syndrome, the presence of underlying disease, and the response to treatment. For most invasive infections without meningitis, 10 to 14 days of therapy is usually sufficient. When meningitis is present, many experts recommend 2 to 3 weeks of therapy. Longer courses may be necessary for patients with endocarditis, rhombencephalitis, and severe complicated infections. When treating central nervous system infections, diagnostic imaging of the brain near the end of anticipated therapy may be used to evaluate the possibility of parenchymal involvement and determine the need for an extended duration of therapy.

Listeria gastroenteritis in otherwise healthy individuals is generally a self-limited illness, and no data exist with regard to the efficacy of antimicrobial therapy. In high-risk individuals such as pregnant women and immunocompromised patients, who have either symptomatic illness or who are known to have ingested a contaminated food, it may be prudent to administer treatment or prophylaxis with a course of oral amoxicillin or trimethoprim-sulfamethoxazole.[103]

PROGNOSIS

Maternal listeriosis may result in abortion, stillbirth, or early neonatal death.[80] Although the relative risk for fetal death is difficult to estimate, spontaneous abortion rates of 10% to 20% and stillborn rates of 11% have been noted.[80] Fetal distress and/or meconium staining of amnionic fluid is estimated to occur in 75% of perinatal cases.[80] Convincing evidence that *L. monocytogenes* is associated with repeated abortions is lacking.[52]

Among cases of early-onset sepsis, the mortality rate in North America is approximately 40% (see Table 95.1).[1,39] Most survivors appear normal at short-term follow up.[38,39,142] Sequelae are related to the associated complications of prematurity, pneumonia, and sepsis; hydrocephalus and cerebral palsy also have been reported.[38,68] Early treatment of maternal disease affects fetal and neonatal outcome favorably.[39,68]

Late-onset *Listeria* meningitis has a mortality rate of less than 10%. The outcome after *Listeria* meningitis may be more favorable than the outcome associated with other types of bacterial meningitis.[71,153] Major sequelae are hydrocephalus and mental retardation. Beyond the neonatal period, the outcome of listeriosis depends on the nature of any underlying disease and the availability of intensive medical care. Among adults with no underlying malignancy, the long-term outcome of *Listeria* meningitis is excellent.[116]

PREVENTION

The sporadic nature of the disease in North America emphasized the need for collaborative investigation and reporting of infections by physicians and veterinarians to public health authorities.[11,45] In the early 1990s, listeriosis became a notifiable disease in the United States and Canada.[109,141] Since then, the important role of food in the transmission of sporadic cases has been firmly established.[130,141] Inspection of food production facilities and dissemination of educational materials may have contributed to a general reduction of outbreaks of listeriosis since then as well.[5,42,50,141] Strict adherence to regulations for pasteurization of raw milk is important to inactivate the organism.[19] Contamination of food can occur during the preparation and processing of pasteurized milk products and ready-to-eat meat or poultry products. The source of an outbreak is sometimes found by tracking strains of *L. monocytogenes* isolated from a patient's food to the retail sources. Recommendations for individuals at high risk, such as pregnant women and immunocompromised patients, include avoiding soft cheeses and delicatessen meats, and avoiding reheating leftover foods or ready-to-eat foods (e.g., hot dogs).[109] Despite this, many hospitals have failed to implement appropriate food preparation policies.[23] During an outbreak of *Listeria,* prompt investigation and treatment of pregnant women with a febrile "influenza-like" illness have been advocated.[11,68] Although treatment of symptomatic mothers may prevent perinatal listeriosis, there is no evidence to show that treatment of colonized infants can either eradicate carriage or prevent infection. Standard precautions are recommended when managing patients with listeriosis.

NEW REFERENCES SINCE THE SEVENTH EDITION

2. Albritton WL, Cochi SL, Feeley JC. Overview of neonatal listeriosis. *Clin Invest Med.* [Review]. 1984;7(4):311-314.
6. Barbuddhe SB, Maier T, Schwarz G, et al. Rapid identification and typing of listeria species by matrix-assisted laser desorption ionization-time of flight mass spectrometry. *Appl Environ Microbiol.* 2008;74(17):5402-5407.
18. CDC. Listeria Outbreaks. Atlanta, GA: Centers for Disease Control and Prevention; 2016. Available from: http://www.cdc.gov/listeria/outbreaks/. Updated March 17, 2016; Cited 23 March 2016.
21. Chaturvedi V, Ertelt JM, Jiang TT, et al. CXCR3 blockade protects against Listeria monocytogenes infection-induced fetal wastage. *J Clin Invest.* 2015;125(4):1713-1725.
26. Darji A, Mohamed W, Domann E, Chakraborty T. Induction of immune responses by attenuated isogenic mutant strains of Listeria monocytogenes. *Vaccine.* 2003;21(suppl 2):S102-S109.
34. Elahi S, Ertelt JM, Kinder JM, et al. Immunosuppressive CD71+ erythroid cells compromise neonatal host defence against infection. *Nature.* 2013;504(7478):158-162.
35. Ertelt JM, Rowe JH, Mysz MA, et al. Foxp3+ regulatory T cells impede the priming of protective CD8+ T cells. *J Immunol.* 2011;187(5):2569-2577.
37. Euzeby JP. List of Prokaryotic names with Standing in Nomenclature. bacterio.net. Available at http://www.bacterio.net/listeria.html.
62. Jadhav S, Gulati V, Fox EM, et al. Rapid identification and source-tracking of *Listeria monocytogenes* using MALDI-TOF mass spectrometry. *Int J Food Microbiol.* 2015;202:1-9.
64. Jiang TT, Chaturvedi V, Ertelt JM, et al. Regulatory T cells: new keys for further unlocking the enigma of fetal tolerance and pregnancy complications. *J Immunol.* 2014;192(11):4949-4956.
67. Kathariou S, Pine L, George V, Carlone GM, Holloway BP. Nonhemolytic Listeria monocytogenes mutants that are also noninvasive for mammalian cells in culture: evidence for coordinate regulation of virulence. *Infect Immun.* 1990;58(12):3988-3995.
72. Kinder JM, Jiang TT, Ertelt JM, et al. Cross-Generational Reproductive Fitness Enforced by Microchimeric Maternal Cells. *Cell.* 2015;162(3):505-515.
73. Kinder JM, Jiang TT, Ertelt JM, et al. Tolerance to noninherited maternal antigens, reproductive microchimerism and regulatory T cell memory: 60 years after 'Evidence for actively acquired tolerance to Rh antigens'. *Chimerism.* 2015; 30:1-13.
88. Lewis DB, Larsen A, Wilson CB. Reduced interferon-gamma mRNA levels in human neonates. Evidence for an intrinsic T cell deficiency independent of other genes involved in T cell activation. *J Exp Med.* 1986;163(4):1018-1023.
89. Linnan MJ, Mascola L, Lou XD, et al. Epidemic listeriosis associated with Mexican-style cheese. *N Engl J Med.* 1988;319(13):823-828.
95. Moreno LZ, Paixao R, Gobbi DD, et al. Characterization of antibiotic resistance in Listeria spp. isolated from slaughterhouse environments, pork and human infections. *J Infect Dev Ctries.* 2014;8(4):416-423.
101. Corbett N, Ho KC, Cai B, et al. Ontogeny of toll-like receptor mediated cytokine responses of human blood mononuclear cells. *Plos One.* 2010;5(11):e15041.
106. Park SH, Chang PS, Ryu S, Kang DH. Development of a novel selective and differential medium for the isolation of Listeria monocytogenes. *Appl Environ Microbiol.* 2014;80(3):1020-1025.

114. Rincon MR, Oppenheimer K, Bonney EA. Selective accumulation of Th2-skewing immature erythroid cells in developing neonatal mouse spleen. *Int J Biol Sci.* 2012;8(5):719-730.
115. Robbins JR, Skrzypczynska KM, Zeldovich VB, Kapidzic M, Bakardjiev AI. Placental syncytiotrophoblast constitutes a major barrier to vertical transmission of Listeria monocytogenes. *PLoS Pathog.* 2010;6(1):e1000732.
117. Rowe JH, Ertelt JM, Xin L, Way SS. Listeria monocytogenes cytoplasmic entry induces fetal wastage by disrupting maternal Foxp3+ regulatory T cell-sustained fetal tolerance. *PLoS Pathog.* 2012;8(8):e1002873.
118. Rowe JH, Ertelt JM, Xin L, Way SS. Pregnancy imprints regulatory memory that sustains anergy to fetal antigen. *Nature.* 2012;490(7418):102-106.
119. Rowe JH, Ertelt JM, Xin L, Way SS. Regulatory T cells and the immune pathogenesis of prenatal infection. *Reproduction.* 2013;146(6):R191-R203.
128. Schuchat A. Listeriosis and pregnancy: food for thought. *Obstet Gynecol Surv.* [Editorial]. 1997;52(12):721-722.
132. Seeliger HP. Listeriosis–history and actual developments. *Infection.* 1988;16(suppl 2):S80-S84.
136. Spanjaard L, Vandenbroucke-Grauls CM. Activity of daptomycin against Listeria monocytogenes isolates from cerebrospinal fluid. *Antimicrob Agents Chemother.* 2008;52(5):1850-1851.
155. Way SS, Thompson LJ, Lopes JE, et al. Characterization of flagellin expression and its role in Listeria monocytogenes infection and immunity. *Cell Microbiol.* 2004;6(3):235-242.
156. Wieczorek K, Dmowska K, Osek J. Characterization and antimicrobial resistance of Listeria monocytogenes isolated from retail beef meat in Poland. *Foodborne Pathog Dis.* 2012;9(8):681-685.
158. Zeldovich VB, Clausen CH, Bradford E, et al. Placental syncytium forms a biophysical barrier against pathogen invasion. *PLoS Pathog.* 2013;9(12): e1003821.
159. Zeldovich VB, Robbins JR, Kapidzic M, Lauer P, Bakardjiev AI. Invasive extravillous trophoblasts restrict intracellular growth and spread of Listeria monocytogenes. *PLoS Pathog.* 2011;7(3):e1002005.

The full reference list for this chapter is available at ExpertConsult.com.

Tuberculosis 96

Andrea T. Cruz • Jeffrey R. Starke

Tuberculosis still ranks as one of the three most important infectious diseases in the world in terms of morbidity and mortality. The disease is recognizable in skeletons from the Stone Age and in mummified corpses from the Egyptian Old Kingdom. Tuberculosis became more widespread in western Europe after the plague years of the Middle Ages, and the epidemic worsened during the era of urbanization and industrialization in the 18th and 19th centuries.[172] With improving socioeconomic conditions, the mortality rate fell to 200 per 100,000 around 1900, and to 26 per 100,000 by 1950, even before the advent of effective chemotherapy. Stress in all its forms—famine, war, rationing, long working hours, child labor, population displacement, crowded living, and working conditions—favors the spread of tuberculosis in humans, whereas years of peace and plenty favor its rapid decline.[171,508] Improving socioeconomic conditions in the United States resulted in a decline in TB mortality during the early 20th century. The decrease in the Western world in the incidence of tuberculosis was accentuated by the discovery, development, and widespread use of antituberculosis drugs beginning in the late 1940s.

Another important factor leading to the decline of tuberculosis in Western countries was the recognition in the 1920s of the importance of bovine tuberculosis and its successful eradication as a public health problem in the United States by gradual slaughter of infected cattle and almost universal pasteurization of milk.[216] Although *Mycobacterium bovis* disease now accounts for a small fraction (1% to 2%) of all tuberculosis in the United States,[246] it has been implicated in 5% to 10% of cases in children along border regions of the United States.[139,202]

STAGES: EXPOSURE, INFECTION, AND DISEASE

The pathophysiologic process of tuberculosis is complicated, and the delay between acquisition of infection and manifestation of disease renders certain pathophysiologic events less distinct.[11] There are three major stages of tuberculosis: exposure, infection, and disease.[612]

Exposure implies that the child has had significant recent contact with another person who has infectious pulmonary tuberculosis. The contact investigation—examination of individuals close to a person suspected of having tuberculosis by performing a test of infection (tuberculin skin test [TST] or interferon-γ release assay [IGRA]), chest radiograph, and physical examination—is the most important activity in a community to prevent cases of tuberculosis in children.[14,52,255] The most frequent setting for exposure of a child is the household, but it can occur in a school, daycare center, or other closed setting.[148,247] In this stage, the test of infection is negative, the chest radiograph is normal, and the child lacks signs or symptoms of disease. Some exposed children may have inhaled droplet nuclei infected with *M. tuberculosis* and have early infection, but the clinician cannot know it because delayed hypersensitivity to tuberculin—a positive TST response—takes up to 3 months to develop. Children younger than 5 years old or immunocompromised children of any age who are in the exposure stage should be treated to prevent the rapid development of disseminated or meningeal tuberculosis, which can occur before the test of infection becomes positive.[179,363,452,487,629]

Infection occurs when the individual inhales droplet nuclei containing *M. tuberculosis*, which becomes established intracellularly within the lung and associated lymphoid tissue. The hallmark of tuberculosis infection is a reactive TST or a positive interferon gamma release assay (IGRA). In this stage, the child has no signs or symptoms and the chest radiograph is either normal or reveals only granuloma or calcifications in the lung parenchyma, regional lymph nodes, or both. In industrialized countries, virtually all children with tuberculosis infection should receive treatment to prevent the development of disease.

Disease occurs when signs or symptoms or radiographic manifestations caused by *M. tuberculosis* become apparent. The word *tuberculosis* refers to disease. Not all infected individuals have the same risk for contracting disease. An immunocompetent adult with untreated tuberculosis infection has a 5% to 10% lifetime risk for development of disease; half the risk exists in the first 2 to 3 years after infection occurs. Adults with tuberculosis infection who then become infected with human immunodeficiency virus (HIV) have a 5% to 10% annual risk for development of tuberculosis disease.[561] Historical studies have shown that often serious, life-threatening forms of the disease will develop within a year in as many as 40% of immunocompetent infants with untreated tuberculosis infection.[385]

EPIDEMIOLOGY

Incidence and Prevalence

Between 20% and 45% of the world's population (approximately 2 billion people) are infected with *M. tuberculosis*, and more than 90% of new cases occur in the developing world. The World Health Organization (WHO) estimates that 9.6 million incident cases, 12 million prevalent cases, and 1.5 million deaths from tuberculosis occur annually worldwide.[714] Twelve percent of all persons with tuberculosis are HIV coinfected, but this percentage is as high as 40% in sub-Saharan Africa. True rates of HIV and tuberculosis coinfection are unclear, because many nations do not screen all newly diagnosed tuberculosis patients for HIV.

According to the WHO, in 1997, only 32% of the world's population lived in areas where effective tuberculosis control programs were fully operational[448]; this situation has not improved in the subsequent two decades. Poor tuberculosis control selects for drug-resistant isolates. Multidrug-resistant tuberculosis (MDR-TB), in which the isolate is resistant to at least isoniazid and rifampin, and extensively drug-resistant tuberculosis (XDR-TB),[569] with resistance to isoniazid, rifampin, non-streptomycin injectable drugs, and fluoroquinolones, have become important problems in many areas of the world.[178] MDR-TB was not described until 1990[87] but has spread widely. In adults, drug resistance in *M. tuberculosis* often is secondary, with the resistance emerging during therapy because treatment is inadequate or interrupted.[199] In children, drug resistance usually is primary in that the child is infected with a strain that already has become resistant.[451,542,544,644] Rates of drug resistance in children tend to mirror those in adults in the same population[618,619] and may be higher in developing countries because of difficulty in completing therapy and an inadequate supply of child-friendly medication formulations. Three percent of new and 20% of retreatment tuberculosis cases globally (300,000 estimated MDR-TB cases in 2014)[714] are MDR-TB; 54% of MDR-TB cases occur in India, China, and the Russian Federation.[714] The true rates of drug-resistant tuberculosis are unclear. Limitations to accurate estimates include variation in laboratory capacity and reporting, and selection of particular patients for drug susceptibility testing (e.g., patients who are failing standard therapy). Additionally, not all patients have culture-confirmed tuberculosis. Finally, the manner in which rates are reported is important. Although incident cases are a better marker of spread of strains in the community, prevalence rates provide a better reflection of the chronicity of MDR-TB and XDR-TB.

Estimates for children are less accurate for many reasons. In developing countries where the burden of disease is greatest, the only available diagnostic test often is an acid-fast smear of sputum, the result of which rarely is positive from infants and children with pulmonary tuberculosis. This leads to underestimation of the pediatric tuberculosis disease burden. Up to 11% of deaths from adolescence to early adulthood are attributable to tuberculosis and HIV infection/AIDS in high-prevalence areas.[483] In areas with both accurate reporting and high rates of tuberculosis, it is thought that children younger than 15 years of age comprise 15% to 20% of the disease burden.[389] This figure varies widely among countries: although only 6% of all cases in the United States occur in children,[98] children are reported to account for 1.4% (Nigeria) to 17% (Swaziland) of cases in sub-Saharan African nations.[715] Some of this variation is real but some likely is due to underreporting and underdiagnosis.

More recent mathematical models have provided more accurate estimates for the 22 high-burden countries (HBCs). In these HBCs, it was estimated that over 15 million children had household contact to a person with infectious tuberculosis, resulting in 7.5 million cases of infection and 650,000 cases of disease annually. The authors estimated that only 35% of all pediatric TB cases were reported.[154] A different group of investigators evaluated the global burden of MDR-TB in children, estimating almost 1 million cases of disease, of which almost 32,000 were MDR-TB.[283] Using similar modeling approaches, in 2015 WHO increased its annual estimates of childhood tuberculosis to 1 million cases and 140,000 deaths annually.[714] In addition, it has been estimated that 9.7 million children had been orphaned as of 2009 after at least one of their parents died of tuberculosis.

The situation in the United States is markedly different. Declining incidence preceded the advent of effective TB treatment and likely reflected improved health status for the American populace. The United States became a low-incidence nation (incidence rate <20/100,000) in the late 1960s. Between 1985 and 1992 in the United States, the total tuberculosis case numbers rose 20%.[91] During that same time, the number of pediatric tuberculosis cases rose 40%.[284,668] Most experts cite four probable causes for the increases: (1) the co-epidemic of HIV infection; (2) the increasing rates of tuberculosis in foreign-born individuals in the United States[73]; (3) the increased transmission among adults in congregate settings, including jails and prisons, nursing homes, homeless shelters, HIV treatment facilities, hospitals, and, rarely, schools[36,39,54,409]; and (4) a decline in the public health infrastructure in many areas of the country.[67,117,509,613] After several years of intense and expensive effort were expended, the number of tuberculosis cases in the United States declined again.[438]

In 2015, a total of 9563 incident tuberculosis cases (three cases per 100,000 population) were reported in the United States.[98] Six percent of cases occurred in HIV-coinfected persons. MDR-TB is uncommon in the U.S., accounting for 1.3% of all isolates, with 90% occurring in foreign-born persons. Tuberculosis remains concentrated in certain high-risk groups[92] (Box 96.1) and regions in the United States (Fig. 96.1). Four states—California, Florida, New York, and Texas—accounted for one-half of all U.S. tuberculosis cases in 2015.[98] These states are characterized by high numbers of immigrants and ethnic and

BOX 96.1 High-Risk Groups for Tuberculosis Infection and Disease

Groups at High Risk for Exposure or Infection

Close contacts of person with tuberculosis
Foreign-born persons from high-risk countries (Asia, Africa, Latin America, Russia, Eastern Europe)
Residents and employees of high-risk congregate settings (correctional institutions, nursing homes, homeless shelters, hospitals serving high-risk populations, drug treatment centers)
Medically underserved, low-income populations
High-risk racial or ethnic minority populations
Injection drug users
Children exposed to adults in high-risk categories

Groups at Higher Risk for Disease Once Infected

Immunosuppressed patients, including those HIV infected
Recent tuberculosis infection (within past 2 years)
Persons with certain medical conditions (diabetes mellitus, silicosis, cancer, end-stage renal disease, gastrectomy, body weight ≤90% of ideal)
Injection drug users
History of inadequately treated tuberculosis
Children age ≤4 years, especially infants

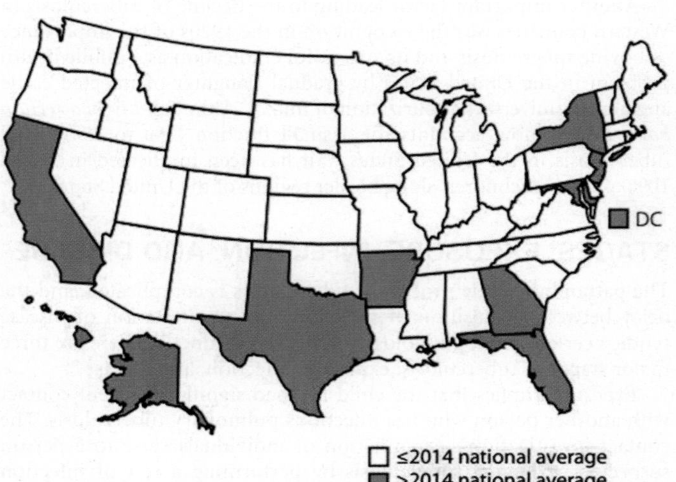

FIG. 96.1 Tuberculosis case rates (cases per 100,000) by state, 2014. (From Centers for Disease Control and Prevention. Tuberculosis trends—United States, 2014. *MMWR* 2015;64:265-9.)

minority group members. In 2015, when compared with U.S-born non-Hispanic whites, tuberculosis rates among U.S.-born Hispanics, non-Hispanic blacks, and Asians were 2.8, 5.7, and 2.8 times greater, respectively.[98]

Sixty-seven percent of all U.S. TB cases occur in foreign-born persons; over half of cases are from persons born in Mexico, the Philippines, Vietnam, India, and China. This trend reflects several themes: declining rates of TB in U.S.-born persons; failure to screen and/or treat adult immigrants for infection; high prevalence of TB infection and disease in these nations; and limited access to care after arrival in the United States. During the immigration process, adults are screened for tuberculosis disease with a chest radiograph, but testing to detect tuberculosis infection is not required. In 2009, the United States began requiring tests of infection for children 2 to 14 years old prior to immigration but not treatment for a positive test.[96] Before this, children emigrating to the United States were entirely unscreened for TB. Tuberculosis is endemic in most developing countries, and between 30% and 50% of recent immigrants to the United States have tuberculosis infection before entry into the country.[113,639] Foreign-born adopted children also are at risk for having tuberculosis infection and disease.[198,334,526] People who enter the United States without documentation may be unable or afraid to seek medical treatment, even when they are ill. Studies have shown that in most immigrants in whom tuberculosis develops, it does so within 5 years of immigration, thus indicating that many cases could be prevented if appropriate screening and treatment programs were conducted.

Other important risk factors for tuberculosis in adults include lower socioeconomic status, migrant work, HIV infection, drug use, homelessness, travel to high-prevalence countries, history of incarceration, and occupations with exposure to high-risk populations (Box 96.1). Children from high-risk population groups or children who have contact with adults in these groups may be at increased risk for tuberculosis infection.[361] Age has an important influence on tuberculosis case rates.[442] During 2014, 6% of cases in the United States occurred in children younger than 15 years, 11% in persons 15 to 24 years old, 33% in persons 25 to 44 years old, 31% in persons 45 to 64 years old, and 20% in persons older than 64 years.[98] The highest case rates among children are in those younger than 3 years. Children aged 5 to 14 years, the so-called favored age, have a consistently lower case rate than that of any other segment of the population.[384,442] In early childhood, the incidence is not significantly different in girls and boys, although higher rates of disease are generally experienced by adolescent girls than adolescent boys.[62]

An estimated 4% to 6% of the U.S. population, or approximately 13 million people, are infected with *M. tuberculosis*.[252] The percentage of infected people varies widely by racial and ethnic groups and socioeconomic status. Foreign-born persons residing in the United States have a prevalence of infection of 19%. Among African-Americans the prevalence is 7%; Mexican-Americans, 9%; and persons living in poverty, 6%.[41] This group of infected persons represents a large reservoir from which cases of tuberculosis disease will emerge in the future if these individuals are not treated.[7]

The HIV epidemic has had a profound effect on the epidemiology of tuberculosis in children by two mechanisms[537]: (1) most important in the United States, HIV-infected adults with tuberculosis may transmit *M. tuberculosis* to children in their environment and tuberculosis disease will develop in some of them[315]; and (2) important in many developing countries, children with HIV infection are at increased risk for progressing from asymptomatic tuberculosis infection to disease.[265,366] Several studies have demonstrated increased rates of childhood tuberculosis associated with increased rates of disease among HIV-infected adults in the community.[232,288] Tuberculosis probably is underdiagnosed in HIV-infected children, especially in the developing world, because of the similarity of its clinical manifestations with other opportunistic pulmonary diseases and the difficulty of confirming the diagnosis with the skin test or culture. All children with suspected tuberculosis disease should have HIV serotesting because the two infections are linked epidemiologically and many experts prolong treatment in HIV-infected children with tuberculosis.[226,545,701]

Children comprise a small fraction of tuberculosis cases in the United States, in part because of low rates of coinfection with HIV, an older

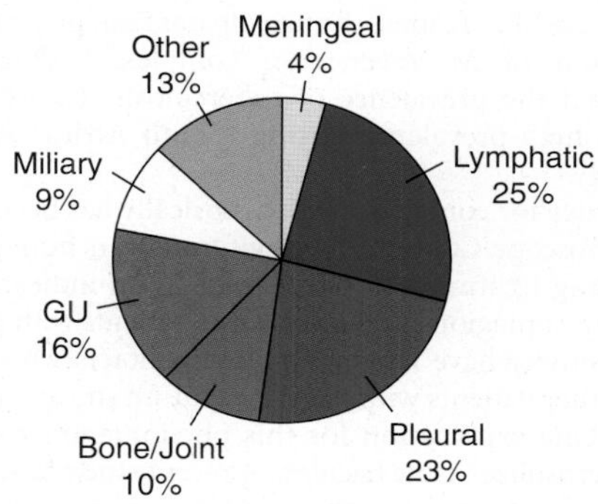

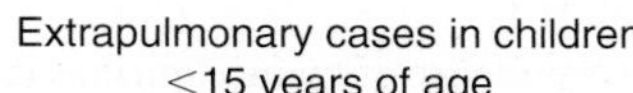

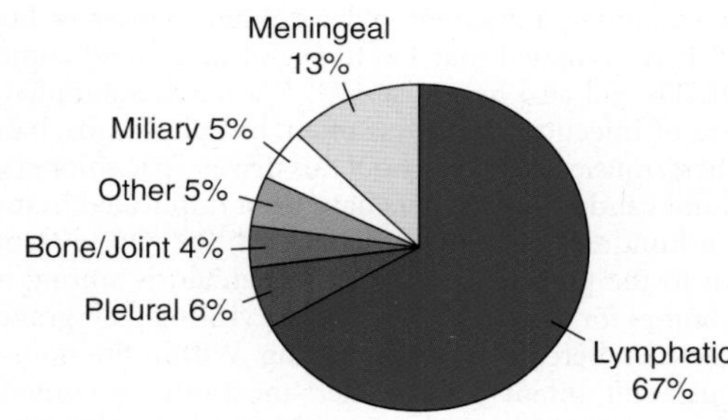

FIG. 96.2 Extrapulmonary disease by site in adults and children in the United States. (From the Centers for Disease Control and Prevention.)

population structure than many developing nations, and far less recent transmission. The site of manifestation of tuberculosis disease differs between adults and children. Although pulmonary disease is most common for all ages, extrapulmonary tuberculosis occurs more often in children.[442] In general, 25% of pediatric cases are extrapulmonary, with 75% being pulmonary. In 1985, before widespread HIV infection occurred, 85% of adults had pulmonary disease and 15% had extrapulmonary disease. With the spread of HIV infection, these numbers have shifted; and in recent years, the Centers for Disease Control (CDC) reported that 79% of all new cases, including those in adults and children, were pulmonary and 21% were extrapulmonary. Comparison of the site of extrapulmonary disease in children and adults in 1985, before the AIDS epidemic, shows some important differences. First, approximately 70% of extrapulmonary tuberculosis in children involved the lymph nodes, as opposed to 25% in adults (Fig. 96.2). Second, tuberculous meningitis accounted for 13% of extrapulmonary disease in children versus 4% in adults. Genitourinary involvement occurred in 16% of adults, but it was a rare finding in children. Although the proportion of extrapulmonary cases in adults has increased as a result of the HIV-AIDS epidemic, extrapulmonary disease still occurs more commonly in children.

TRANSMISSION

Transmission of tuberculosis is from one human to another, usually through infected droplets of mucus that become airborne when an individual coughs, sneezes, or laughs.[108] The droplets dry and become droplet nuclei, which may remain suspended in air for hours. Only particles less than 10 μm in diameter are small enough to reach the alveoli.[538] Transmission sometimes occurs by direct contact with infected discharges (sputum, saliva, urine, or drainage from an open sinus or abscess); it occasionally occurs by means of heavily contaminated fomites, such as gastric lavage tubes, bronchoscopes, or syringes prepared by someone with positive sputum.[244] Rare cases of tuberculosis transmitted by a lung or kidney transplant have been reported.[93,437] Dogs, pigs, goats, and camelids (camels, llamas, alpacas) can play a role in interspecies transmission of *M. tuberculosis* complex.[496] One necropsy study showed that the prevalence of tuberculosis disease and infection in dogs in a high-prevalence setting (South Africa) was 1% and 50%, respectively.[481]

The proxy for contagiousness historically has been acid-fast sputum smear microscopy. Conversion of sputum smears from positive to negative after starting treatment has been used as an indication that a patient is no longer contagious. However, some patients with prolonged sputum smear positivity have few or no close contacts who become infected, whereas other patients with negative sputum smears have many infected contacts. One explanation for this phenomenon may be that not all patients aerosolize viable bacteria. A recent study found that the density of cough-generated aerosols correlated more with TST and IGRA positivity in contacts than the degree of sputum smear positivity. Even among sputum smear-positive adults, only 30% produced cough-generated aerosols.[289]

The collective experience of many clinicians is that children usually are infected by an adult or adolescent in the immediate household, most often a parent, grandparent, older sibling, boarder, or household employee.[38] It is estimated that 1% to 5% of household contacts of a person with TB will also have disease.[719] Casual extrafamilial contact is the source of infection much less often, but physicians, babysitters, schoolteachers, music teachers, school bus drivers, parishioners, nurses, gardeners, and candy store keepers have been implicated in individual cases and in hundreds of mini-epidemics.[23,60,174,340,348,695] Attention has been drawn to the prevalence of active tuberculosis among residents of nursing homes for the elderly.[268] Children visiting their grandparents have contracted tuberculosis in this setting. Within the household of an infectious adult, infants and toddlers most often become infected. Adults with pulmonary disease who are receiving regular, appropriate chemotherapy probably rarely infect children; much more dangerous are those with chronic tuberculous disease that is unrecognized, inadequately treated, or in relapse because of the development of resistance. Modeling studies suggest that increasing case detection by 25% can result in an almost 50% reduction in TB mortality and an almost 30% reduction in TB incidence.[719]

Wallgren[688] was the first to point out that children with tuberculosis rarely infect other children. Many children with the disease have tuberculin-negative siblings and parents. Children with tuberculosis often have been cared for by their families or in hospitals and institutions without infecting their contacts.[126,436] When transmission of *M. tuberculosis* has been documented in children's hospitals, it almost invariably has come from an adult with undiagnosed pulmonary tuberculosis.[24,294,295,425,697] Adults accompanying a child with suspected tuberculosis disease should be screened as soon as possible for pulmonary tuberculosis.[63,95,112,126,296,297,436,608] In tuberculous children, tubercle bacilli in endobronchial secretions are relatively sparse and cough is not characteristic of endothoracic tuberculosis or miliary disease. When young children cough, they lack the tussive force of adults. Specimens collected by bronchoalveolar lavage or early-morning gastric aspiration from children with clinically suspected tuberculosis seldom have acid-fast bacilli seen on smears. Only approximately 40% eventually will grow *M. tuberculosis* by culture.[597] Young infants with congenital tuberculosis or advanced, postnatally acquired pulmonary disease are more likely to have smear- or culture-positive specimens (80%) than older children.[541,669] Therefore, specimens and secretions from infants, children with cavitary lesions, and intubated patients should be handled as potentially infectious.[95,397] Most preadolescent children with tuberculosis, however, are not contagious and do not require isolation. Tuberculosis in adolescents may be more typical of adult-type reactivation disease, including the presence of cavitary lesions with smear- and culture-positive sputum. Children or adolescents who have symptomatic pulmonary tuberculosis with features of adult-type tuberculosis should be treated as potentially contagious until mycobacterial smears and cultures are negative.[77,133]

Children, nonetheless, play an extremely important role in the transmission of tuberculosis, not so much because they are likely to contaminate their immediate environment, but rather because they may harbor a partially healed infection that lies dormant, only to be reactivated as infectious pulmonary tuberculosis many years later under the social, emotional, and physiologic stresses arising during adolescence, pregnancy, or old age. Thus, children infected with *M. tuberculosis* constitute a long-lasting reservoir of tuberculosis in the population. From an epidemiologic perspective, the diagnosis of tuberculosis disease in a child is a marker of recent transmission in the community, owing to the short incubation periods seen for childhood tuberculosis.

The risk for infection developing in child contacts of adults receiving antituberculosis chemotherapy often is a matter of practical concern. Several studies reveal that most contacts are infected by the index case before the diagnosis is made and treatment is initiated. Although it is not possible to carry out a definitive clinical study, evidence indicates that patients receiving effective chemotherapy rarely transmit *M. tuberculosis.* Nonetheless, it seems prudent to avoid exposure of children to adults with positive sputum smears or positive cultures and to assume that adults positive by smear or culture remain infectious for at least several weeks after the start of therapy.

MYCOBACTERIOLOGY

The genus *Mycobacterium,* closely related by its cell wall antigens to the genera *Corynebacterium* and *Nocardia,* is classified in the order Actinomycetales and the family Mycobacteriaceae. Several species are termed *M. tuberculosis* complex (MTBC): *M. tuberculosis, M. africanum, M. bovis, M. canetti,* and *M. microti.* Phylogenetic analysis indicates an origin for MTBC approximately 40,000 years ago, coinciding with expansion of humans out of Eastern Africa.[706]

Mycobacteria are nonmotile, non–spore-forming, pleomorphic, weakly gram-positive rods measuring 1 to 5 μm long and typically slender and slightly "bent." Some appear beaded, and some are clumped. The cell wall constituents of mycobacteria determine their most striking biologic properties. The cell walls contain 20% to 60% lipids by dry weight, largely bound to proteins and carbohydrates. These organisms are more resistant than are most others to light, alkali, acid, and the bactericidal action of antibodies. Their growth is slow, with a generation time of 14 to 24 hours, perhaps because of the slow metabolic exchange through the waxy "capsule." Their hydrophobic properties render them difficult to study.

Acid-fastness, that is, the capacity to form stable mycolate complexes with certain aryl methane dyes (specifically, carbolfuchsin, crystal violet, auramine, and rhodamine, which then are not removed readily even by rinsing with 95% ethanol plus hydrochloric acid), is the hallmark of mycobacteria. The cells appear red when stained with fuchsin (as with the Ziehl-Neelsen or Kinyoun stains), appear purple with crystal violet, or exhibit yellow-green fluorescence under ultraviolet light (when stained with auramine and rhodamine, as in Truant stain). Truant stain, in experienced hands, is considered the best stain for specimens expected to contain small numbers of organisms. Fluorescent staining can decrease staining time by 50% and increase sensitivity capacity in high-volume laboratories in developing countries when compared with Ziehl-Neelsen staining.[341] One study of LED fluorescence microscopy in adults showed that fluorescence microscopy was more sensitive but less specific than Ziehl-Neelsen staining, in part because in the fluorescence microscopy artifacts can fluoresce, leading to false-positive results.[130]

Identification of mycobacteria depends on their staining properties and on their biochemical and metabolic characteristics. Mycobacteria are obligate aerobes. On the whole, their growth requirements are simple. *M. tuberculosis* can grow in "classic" media, whose essential ingredients are egg yolk and glycerin (Löwenstein-Jensen, Petragnani, Dorset). These media often include a dye, such as malachite green, to inhibit contaminants or potatoes and charcoal, which probably neutralize growth inhibitors. They also can grow in synthetic media, frequently with an admixture of asparagine, glutamate, or amino acid mixtures (Middlebrook 7H9, Tween-albumin). Once grown, they can be replated on media also containing antituberculosis drugs to determine drug susceptibility patterns. Isolation on solid media often takes 3 to 6 weeks, followed by another 2 to 4 weeks for drug susceptibility results. Improvements in laboratory methods have permitted more rapid culture, identification, and drug susceptibility testing of mycobacteria, such as by an automatic radiometric method known as the BACTEC method, in which a decontaminated, concentrated specimen is inoculated into a bottle of medium containing carbon 14-labeled palmitic acid as the substrate.[577] As mycobacteria metabolize the carbon 14-labeled palmitic acid, carbon dioxide 14 accumulates in the head space of the bottle, where radioactivity can be measured. Unfortunately, cross-contamination of bottles has been reported and has resulted in false-positive culture results.[173] The addition of appropriate dilutions of antituberculosis drugs permits an evaluation of drug susceptibility to be made. The time for identification and drug susceptibility testing can be reduced to 1 to 3 weeks, depending on the size of the inoculum.

Restriction fragment length polymorphism (RFLP) analysis and whole-genome analysis of mycobacterial DNA have become powerful tools for determining strain relatedness in both outbreaks and routine epidemiology of tuberculosis in a community, allowing for social network analysis.[9,206,582,710]

RESISTANCE AND IMMUNITY

Natural resistance to tuberculosis infection varies greatly among animal species; humans, guinea pigs, and rabbits are highly susceptible. Multiple single nucleotide polymorphisms (SNPs) have been associated with disease susceptibility in a number of racial and ethnic groups: *CCL2-2518G* in Asians and Latinos,[194] *IRGM*[312] and interleukin-12B in African-Americans, and *P2X7* and Toll-like receptor 2 and 8 mutations in Turkish children.[134,135,645] However, few mutations, apart from *SLC11A1*,[345] have been identified that appear to increase susceptibility across racial and ethnic groups. Many of these mutations are in genes influencing macrophage-mediated destruction of the bacillus.[312,645] Other risk factors for the development of TB disease include young age,[442,540,669] poorly controlled diabetes mellitus,[696] and wild-type measles and perhaps influenza.[40,238,730] Unfortunately, natural resistance is ill defined and poorly understood.

Cell-mediated immunity is regarded as most important in host defense against *M. tuberculosis*.[164,344] The T cell–mediated immune response involves a variety of cell subsets that are involved in numerous functions, including protection, delayed hypersensitivity, cytolysis, and establishment of memory immunity.[468] The functions also involve an array of cytokines, several of which direct cells of the monocyte-macrophage axis to contain and destroy the invading bacilli.[15,635] An emerging concept is that much of the clinical response to the presence of *M. tuberculosis* is determined by the balance of the cellular cytokine response,[164] which to some degree is under genetic influence.[468] In general, T-helper 1 (Th1) responses are more beneficial to the host than are Th2 responses, in part owing to the former's role in activating macrophages in granulomas.[164] Unfortunately, infants and young children have increased propensity to develop Th2 responses to mycobacterial immunogens.[344] Although different strains of *M. tuberculosis* can evoke different host immune responses, there is no apparent association between the genotype and the phenotype expressed in children with disease.[391]

More details about the immune response to *M. tuberculosis* are emerging as new immunotherapies are developed. During the past decade, several monoclonal antibodies directed against tumor necrosis factor-α have been used to manage inflammatory bowel disease and rheumatologic disorders. Unfortunately, use of these agents, particularly infliximab, has been associated with up to a 25-fold increased risk for tuberculosis disease.[596] All immunocompromised patients, including those who will undergo any form of immunotherapy, should be evaluated carefully for tuberculosis infection or disease.

PATHOGENESIS

Portal of Entry

The tubercle bacillus usually is inhaled. The observations of Riley[517] suggest that a single tubercle bacillus can initiate infection. Ghon, Kuedlich, and their associates (Table 96.1) reported that the primary focus found in 2114 autopsies on children was the lung in 96% of cases. Especially significant is that their study was done at a time when bovine tuberculosis, which might have produced many primary gastrointestinal foci, was much more common than it is today. Ingestion probably accounts for a small percentage of primary pulmonary foci and for some gastrointestinal foci, particularly in infants who have consumed milk containing bovine tubercle bacilli. *M. tuberculosis* has also been transmitted by organ transplantation.[93] Contamination of marijuana bongs has been associated both with clusters of pulmonary tuberculosis[435] and uvulitis.[224] Contamination of a superficial skin or mucous membrane lesion, such as an abrasion of the sole of the foot or the elbow, insect bite, ritual circumcision, or infection of the vulva, may lead to infection. Infection by inoculation with a sputum-contaminated syringe has been reported in more recent years.[244] True congenital infection, although rare, may be a result of either lymphohematogenous spread in the mother during pregnancy or smoldering endometritis.[671]

TABLE 96.1 Portal of Entry of Tubercle Bacilli

Respiratory (%)		Nonrespiratory (%)	
Lung	95.93[a]	Bowel	1.14
Tonsils	0.09	Skin	0.14
Nose	0.09	Eye	0.05
Middle ear	0.09	Parotid	0.05
Total[b]	*96.20*	*Total*	*1.38*

[a]Of 2114 autopsies on children.
[b]Undetermined, 2.4%.
Data from Ghon A, Kuedlich H. Die Eintrittspforten der Infektion. In: Engel S, Pirquet C, editors. *Handbuch der Kindertuberkulose*. Stuttgart: Georg Thieme; 1930.

Incubation Period

The incubation period from the time that the tubercle bacillus enters the body until cutaneous sensitivity develops has been found to be 3 weeks to 3 months.[385] With both bacille Calmette-Guérin (BCG) and experimental infections, the incubation period is shorter and the clinical manifestations are more severe when the inoculum is large; clinical experience suggests that the same is true in humans. Debré, for example, noted long ago that tuberculosis acquired by an infant from its mother was likely to be much more severe than was an infection acquired from a visitor to the home.[144]

"Timetable" of Tuberculosis

Wallgren's tremendous experience with tuberculous children in institutions permitted him to recognize and describe the usual early course and timing of the initial infection and each of its best-known complications.[691] His timetable concept is an extremely useful one for clinicians because it permits a realistic prognosis, an understanding of what complications to look for and when, and a more productive approach to finding the infectious source case (Fig. 96.3).[385] Half of the lifetime risk of progression to disease occurs within 2 years of infection.[57]

The relationship between the anatomic site of tuberculosis and the median age at onset in children is shown in Table 96.2. Symptomatic, massive lymphohematogenous spread (i.e., miliary or acute meningeal tuberculosis) is seen in only 0.5% to 3% of infected children. When it does occur, the usual onset is 2 to 6 months after initial infection. Endobronchial tuberculosis, possibly with segmental pulmonary lesions, develops slightly later on average. The metastatic lesions of bones and joints, which can be expected in 5% of untreated infected children, usually do not appear until approximately 1 year after infection occurs, at the earliest. Renal lesions come later still, 5 to 25 years after initial infection. The interval between the acquisition of initial infection and the appearance of chronic pulmonary tuberculosis is extremely variable but can be months to decades, depending mainly on the age of the child at the time of infection. The interval is likely to be short in adolescents but much longer in infants.

In summary, the first 5 years after initial acquisition of tuberculosis infection in childhood, especially the first year, is when complications usually occur. Later in life, during times of stress, a previously silent or arrested lesion may reactivate and become dangerous to the patient as well as highly infectious to others.

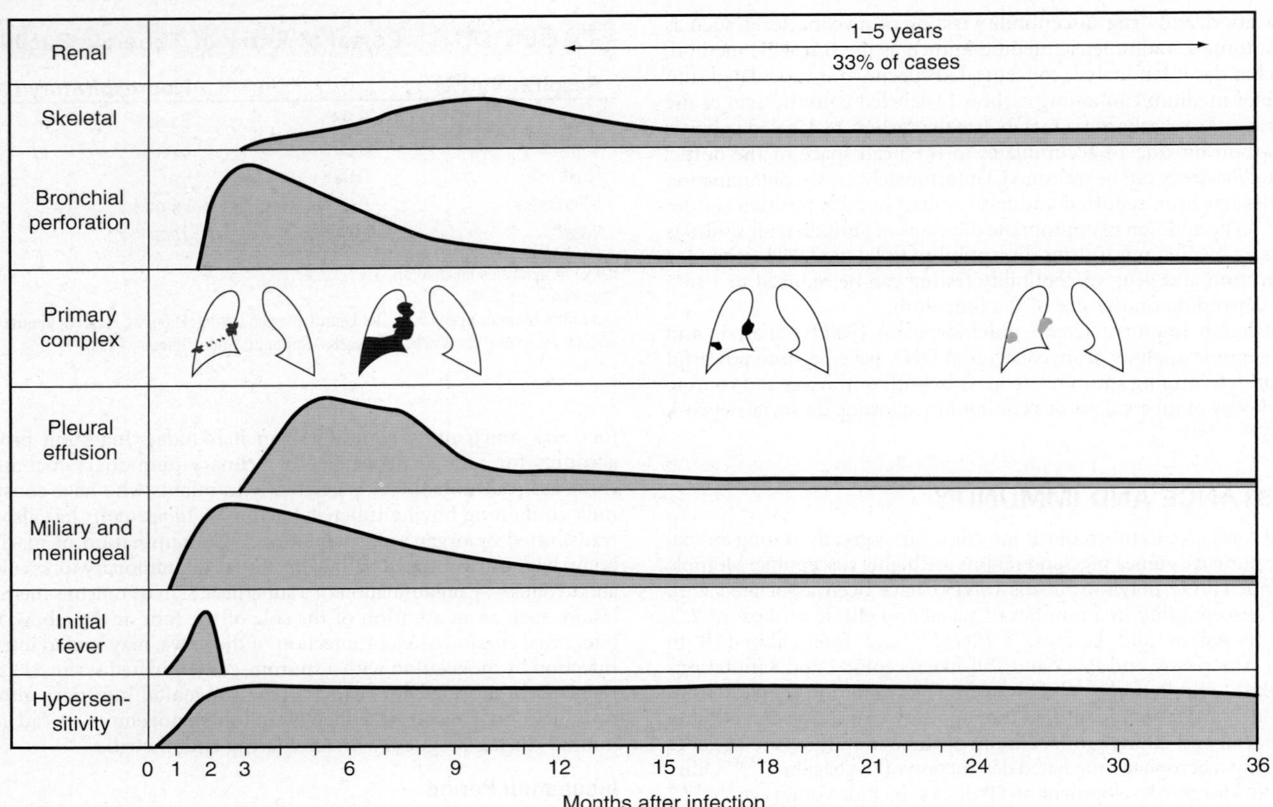

FIG. 96.3. Timetable of tuberculosis.

TABLE 96.2 Median Age of Children[a] With Tuberculosis by Predominant Site of Involvement, United States, 1988

Site	No. of Cases (%)	Median Age (y)
Pulmonary	1213 (77.5)	6
Lymphatic	209 (13.3)	5
Pleural	49 (3.1)	16
Meningeal	29 (1.9)	2
Bone or joint	19 (1.2)	8
Other	15 (1.0)	12
Miliary	14 (0.9)	1
Genitourinary	13 (0.8)	16
Peritoneal	4 (0.3)	13
Not stated	1 (0.1)	—
Total	*1566 (100.0)*	*6*

[a]<20 years.

CLINICAL FORMS OF TUBERCULOSIS IN CHILDREN

Endothoracic Asymptomatic Tuberculosis Infection

Asymptomatic (or latent) infection can be defined as tuberculin hypersensitivity and a positive tuberculin test result without striking clinical or radiographic manifestations. Computed tomography (CT)—which is not recommended in the routine evaluation for pulmonary TB in children—may reveal enlarged lymph nodes in the chest, even though the plain radiograph is normal.[17,146] On occasion, low-grade fever is found at the onset, usually by chance. If the child has been in recent contact with a person who has contagious tuberculosis and the TST result is positive, disease should be ruled out immediately with a chest radiograph and a thorough physical examination. The lifetime risk of progression from infection to disease is lowest for elementary school-aged children (<5%), intermediate for adolescents and preschool-aged children (10–20%), and highest for infants (40–50%).[485]

A clinician making a diagnosis of tuberculosis infection in a child must assume that the patient might be in the earliest stage of infection and at risk for the development of symptomatic disease in the near future.[385] A careful history and investigation of contacts should be undertaken immediately for determination, if possible, of the date of exposure. Chemotherapy must be started, and the patient closely monitored not only to detect any toxic effect of chemotherapy and to monitor adherence with treatment, but also to be sure that disease does not develop.

Endothoracic Primary Complex and Its Complications

The primary complex, described by Ghon,[209] includes three elements: the primary focus, lymphangitis, and regional lymphadenitis. This complex holds true for every primary infection, regardless of the portal of entry. Ghon noted that at least 70% of primary pulmonary foci are subpleural. Thus, pleurisy is almost a regular feature of the primary complex. Evolution of the primary pulmonary focus begins with an acute inflammatory reaction around tubercle bacilli inhaled into an alveolus, with the localized alveolar consolidation varying from the size of a pea to the size of a walnut. Macrophages appear within hours in the inflammatory exudate and change into clusters of epithelioid cells to form tubercles. In turn, these tubercles may resolve and disappear, or central caseation consisting of incomplete cell autolysis may develop. The caseous lesion contains large numbers of multiplying tubercle bacilli that spread rapidly from the primary focus through the regional lymphatic vessels to the regional lymph nodes, with areas of inflammation being set up along the way that later may caseate and calcify.[497] The primary pulmonary focus (Table 96.3) can be located in any part of the lung. The thought that the primary focus has a predilection for the lower fields of the lung probably arises from the fact that the lung is pyramid shaped, with more basilar than apical lung tissue. Seventy to

TABLE 96.3 Location of Primary Pulmonary Focus

Location	No. of Patients (%)
Right upper lobe	138 (27)
Right middle lobe	40 (7)
Right lower lobe	107 (20)
Left upper lobe	122 (24)
Left lower lobe	104 (20)
Total	*511 (98)*

Data from Ghon A, Kuedlich H. Die Eintrittspforten der Infektion. In: Engel S, Pirquet C, editors. *Handbuch der Kindertuberkulose.* Stuttgart: Georg Thieme; 1930.

TABLE 96.4 Lymphatic Drainage of the Lung

Right upper lobe	→	Right paratracheal chain
Right middle lobe	→	Right and left paratracheal nodes
Right lower lobe	→	Subcarinal nodes
Left upper lobe	→	Left paratracheal nodes
Left lower lobe	→	Left paratracheal nodes
Lingula	→	Subcarinal nodes
Subcarinal nodes	→	Right paratracheal nodes

Based on data of Rouviere, cited in Courtice FC, Simmonds WJ. Physiological significance of lymph drainage of the serous cavities and lungs. *Physiol Rev.* 1954;34:419–42.

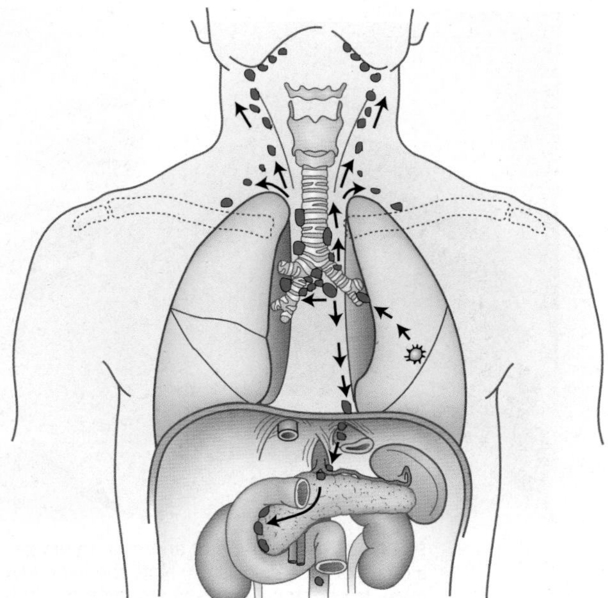

FIG. 96.4. Composite image illustrating wide lymphogenic spread of tuberculosis infection from a primary pulmonary focus in the base of the left upper lobe. The infection extends cephalad to the submandibular nodes in the head and caudad as far as the pancreatic nodes in the abdomen. (From Caffey J. *Pediatric x-ray diagnosis.* 7th ed. Chicago: Year Book; 1978.)

85% of primary infections are initiated by one focus.[636] Multiple lung foci can result, although rarely, from the ingestion and inhalation of tubercle bacilli. This pattern of disease was shown clearly in the results of pathologic studies of the 71 infants who died in the Lübeck disaster of the 1930s, an incident in which 251 neonates mistakenly had been given live tubercle bacilli by mouth instead of BCG vaccine. Fifteen of the neonates were found to have primary lung lesions at autopsy, and all 251 had primary intestinal lesions.

Although the lymphadenitis cannot be detected clinically and rarely is apparent even on radiographs, the hallmark of initial tuberculosis infection is the relatively large size and importance of the adenitis as opposed to the relatively insignificant size of the initial focus in the lung, skin, or elsewhere. The development of tuberculin hypersensitivity within 3 to 12 weeks after initial acquisition of infection enhances the cellular reaction throughout the primary complex, but with a particularly prominent effect on the primary focus and the regional lymph nodes. At this time, the infection may spread along nearby lymphatic chains to involve more distant nodes. The lymphatic drainage of the lungs is outlined in Table 96.4; it occurs predominantly from left to right. It is not surprising, therefore, that the nodes in the right upper paratracheal area appear to be the ones most often affected. Many primary lesions are subpleural, and the lymphatic drainage of the apical pleura is to the cervical nodes. Moreover, the paratracheal chains have communications with both the deep cervical nodes and the abdominal nodes, as shown in Fig. 96.4. Calcification of regional lymph nodes is a late finding, usually seen after at least 2 to 6 months.

Extrinsic bronchial obstruction can result from enlargement of peribronchial lymph nodes.[351,554,604] Clinically, bronchial obstruction can result in one of three outcomes: sudden death from asphyxiation (very rare),[331] hyperaeration, or atelectasis. At the end of the incubation period, as tuberculin sensitivity develops, the hilar lymph nodes enlarge greatly and, in many cases, caseous foci appear within them. Acid-fast studies of smears and sections have confirmed that this caseum has few tubercle bacilli. As the nodes enlarge, they frequently impinge on the neighboring regional bronchus and compress it and cause diffuse inflammation of its wall, even to the point of obstructing the lumen.[351,554,604] Other mechanisms of obstruction include damage to the bronchial cartilage leading to gradual (or, rarely, abrupt) perforation of the bronchus and the formation of plugs of semiliquid toothpaste-like caseum that partially or completely occludes the bronchus. In some cases, endobronchial granulomatous tissue forms around the stoma of the fistula and obstructs the lumen.

Obstructive hyperaeration (also called *obstructive emphysema*) can involve a lobar segment, a lobe, or even an entire lung. Hyperaeration is most common in children younger than 2 years old. Physical examination can demonstrate wheezing that is not relieved by beta agonists. Radiographs, best taken on expiration, show hyperaeration, which usually is not accompanied by mediastinal displacement, probably because of fixation by the tuberculous mediastinal nodes (Fig. 96.5). Aspiration of a foreign body always must be considered in the differential diagnosis. The obstruction ultimately resolves by itself; however, corticosteroids may be added to the chemotherapeutic regimen to hasten recovery.[443,444,659] Surgical removal of the obstructing nodes has been successful but rarely is performed.[142]

The third possible result of bronchial obstruction is the appearance of a segmental lesion (termed *collapse-consolidation lesion*) that is fan-shaped on a radiograph, representing mainly atelectasis and almost always involving the very segment occupied by the primary pulmonary focus[328,383,427] (Fig. 96.6). Actually, the radiographic opacity results from a combination of several elements: the primary pulmonary focus, the caseous material from an eroded bronchus, the inflammatory response elicited by the caseum, and atelectasis. In some instances, acute secondary infection plays a role. Children with secondary bacterial pneumonia often initially have high fever, cough, and rales; the signs and symptoms respond to conventional antibiotics, but the chest radiographic findings usually do not clear because of the underlying tuberculosis. The younger the child, the more frequently collapse-consolidation lesions occur (Table 96.5). The segmental lesion is likely to form during the first 3 to 6 months after acquisition of infection (50 of 65 in Payne's series[485]) and multiple segmental lesions can occur simultaneously. Sometimes, segmental lesions and obstructive hyperaeration occur simultaneously. The physical signs and symptoms of segmental lesions—cough, rales, localized wheezing, egophony—are surprisingly meager but are seen more frequently in infants because of the smaller size of their airways.

Although segmental lesions and hyperaeration are the most common findings produced by enlarging thoracic lymph nodes, others occur. Enlarged paratracheal nodes may cause stridor and respiratory distress.[382] Subcarinal nodes may impinge on the esophagus, causing difficulty

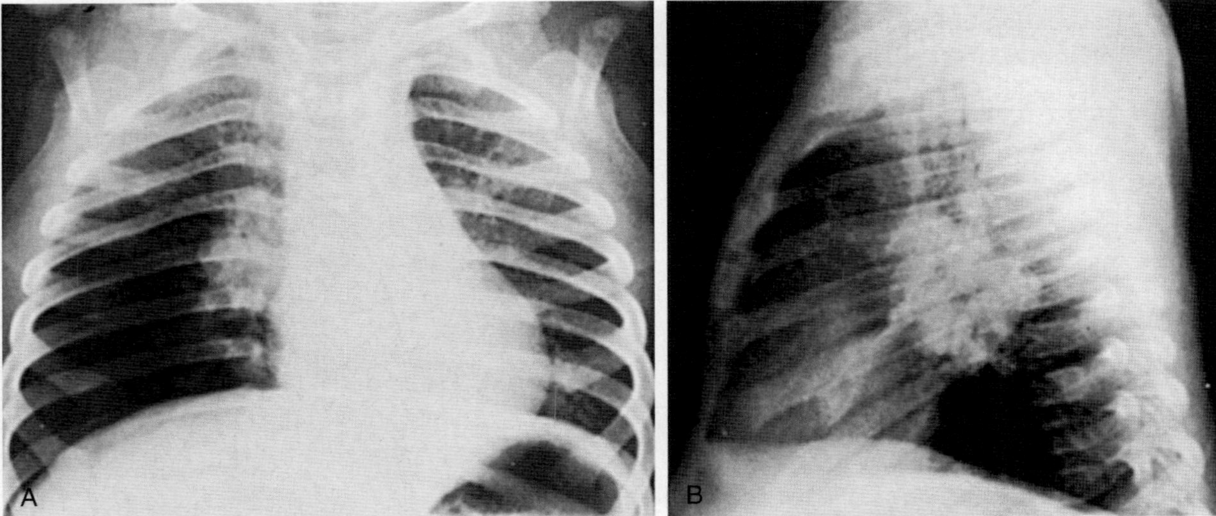

FIG. 96.5. Radiograph of an 8-month-old girl with obstructive hyperaeration of the right lower lobe as a result of tuberculosis. (A) Note the hyperlucent right lower lobe and shift of the heart and mediastinum away from the ball-valve obstruction to the left. (B) Note the large hilar lymph nodes compressing the right lower lobe bronchi. Tuberculosis should be considered in patients with hyperaeration of unknown cause.

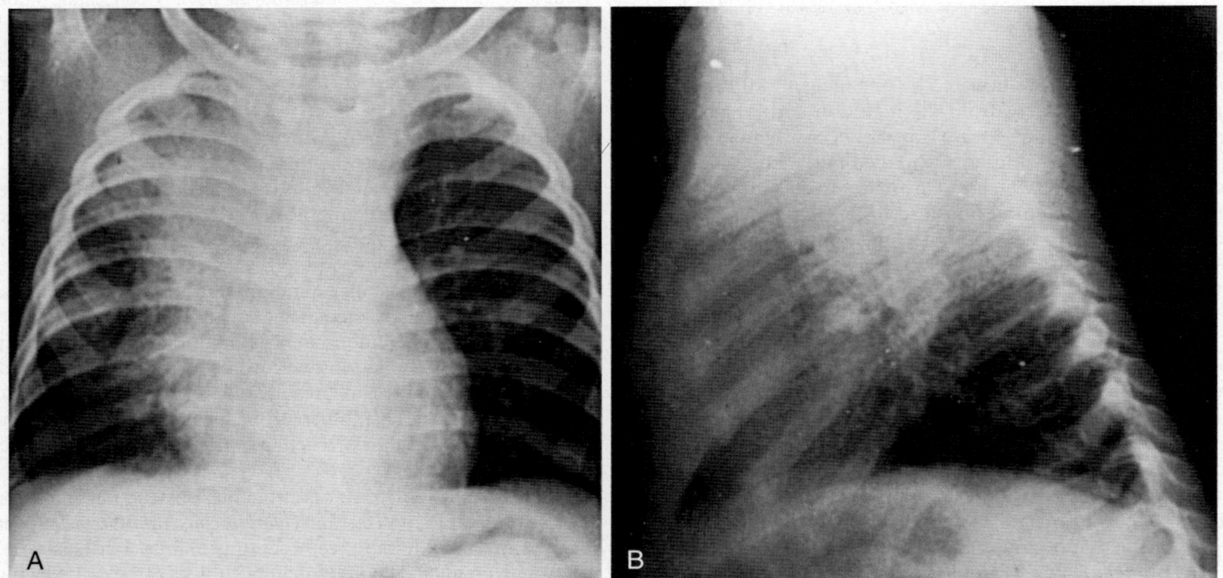

FIG. 96.6. (A) Posteroanterior and (B) lateral radiographs of an 8-month-old boy with primary tuberculosis. (A) shows collapse-consolidation of the right upper lobe, hilar and paratracheal adenopathy, and pleural reaction. Note the narrowed right bronchi.

TABLE 96.5 Percentage of Tuberculin Converters and Age at Which Segmental Lesions Develop

Age at Infection (y)	CONVERTERS WITH SEGMENTAL LESIONS Number (%)	No. of Total Converters
Birth–1	77 (43)	180
1–5	35 (24)	147
6–10	31 (25)	121
11–15	16 (16)	97
Total	*159 (29)*	*545*

Based on Payne M, cited in Miller FJW, Seale RME, Taylor MD. *Tuberculosis in children.* Boston: Little, Brown; 1963.

swallowing, or erode into the esophagus, producing a bronchoesophageal fistula. Enlarged lymph nodes may compress the subclavian vein and produce edema of the hand and arm, or they may erode major blood vessels, including the aorta. They also may rupture into the mediastinum and point in the left or more often the right supraclavicular fossa. Compression of the left recurrent laryngeal nerve has been reported. Compression of the left phrenic nerve leads to paralysis of the left leaf of the diaphragm in an estimated 0.1% to 0.3% of tuberculous children. Rupture into the pericardial sac is described later.

The late results of bronchial obstruction include the following possibilities: complete reexpansion of the lung and resolution of the radiographic findings; disappearance of the segmental lesion, with residual calcification of the primary focus or the regional lymph nodes; or scarring and progressive contraction of the lobe or segment, usually associated with bronchiectasis.[351,385] Permanent anatomic sequelae result

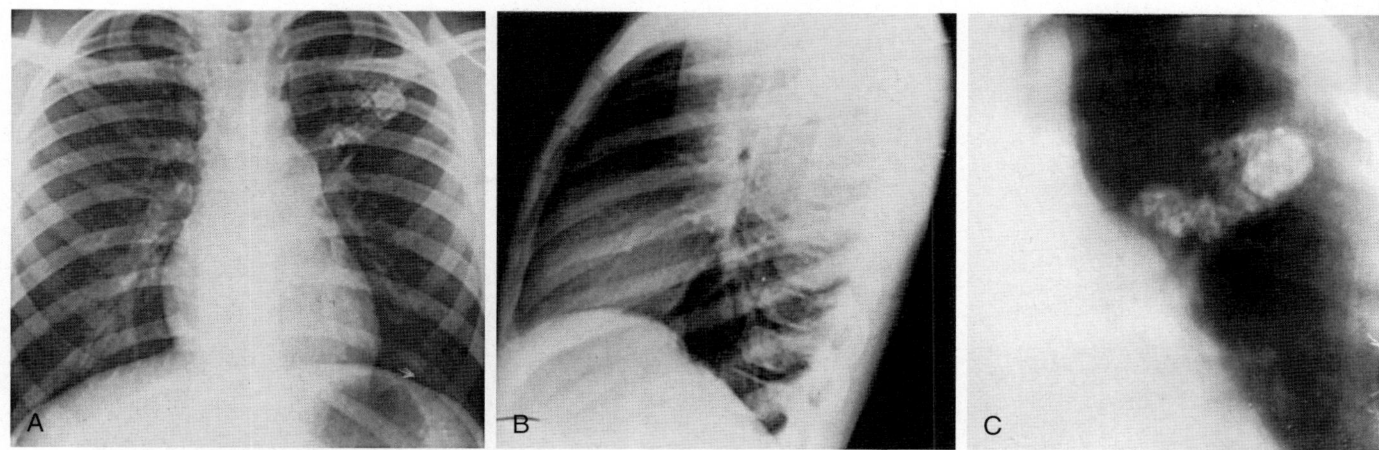

FIG. 96.7. (A) Posteroanterior and (B) lateral radiographs of a 7-year-old boy with a calcified left upper lobe, primary complex. (C) Tomogram showing the fine granular calcific pattern.

from segmental lesions in approximately 60% of all cases, even though the abnormality usually is not apparent on plain radiographs. Fortunately, most of these abnormalities are asymptomatic in the upper lobes. However, secondary infection may occur in the middle and lower lobes and cause the middle lobe syndrome.[66] On occasion, the chronic vascularity that accompanies bronchiectasis leads to poor oxygen saturation during exercise and to restricted body growth. In addition, bronchogenic carcinoma may arise years later in the old scarred lesions remaining in the bronchus.

Calcification of the primary complex (Fig. 96.7), when it appears, always results from caseation. Calcification of caseous lesions occurs much more readily in children than in adults, probably because children's calcium and phosphorus plasma levels are higher. Payne,[485] in a study of calcification in 299 English children, reported calcification visible on the chest radiographs of one child within 6 months of infection, 13% within 12 months, 35% within 18 months, 55% within 24 months, 84% within 3 years, and 100% within 4 years.

Calcification may persist without much change, or it may start resorbing within 5 years and eventually disappear completely. Calcification, if it is visible at all on radiographs, most often involves the regional lymph nodes.[61] Sometimes, however, the primary pulmonary focus or the entire primary complex, including the lymphangitis, calcifies (Fig. 96.8). Currently, extensive calcification occurs uncommonly in the Western world, probably because tuberculous lesions treated early with isoniazid rarely caseate and caseation is a prerequisite for calcification.

Pleural Effusion

Pleural effusion (Fig. 96.9) can be localized or generalized and unilateral or bilateral.[349] Most children will have concomitant pulmonary parenchymal disease and/or intrathoracic lymphadenopathy.[127] All tuberculous serous effusions probably originate in the discharge of bacilli into the cavity from an adjacent lesion—in the case of the pleura, from a subpleural pulmonary focus or from subpleural caseous lymph nodes. The breakthrough may be small and the pleuritis localized and asymptomatic, or it may occur in the form of a generalized effusion, usually 3 to 6 months after infection occurs (see Fig. 96.11). In 75% of Wallgren's cases,[689] later calcification of the pulmonary focus or regional lymph nodes proved the effusion to be on the same side as the original primary focus. Seemingly without logical explanation are the following clinical observations: tuberculous pleural effusion is a rare occurrence in children younger than 2 years and an uncommon one in children younger than 5 years (perhaps because sensitivity to tuberculin is lower in the very young); occurs more frequently in boys than in girls; almost never is associated with a segmental lesion; and rarely is associated with miliary tuberculosis.

The onset of pleurisy usually is abrupt and resembles bacterial pneumonia, with fever, chest pain, shortness of breath, and, on physical examination, dullness to percussion and diminished breath sounds. Fever may be high and, in untreated cases, last for several weeks. On occasion, differentiation of an effusion from an extensive pneumonic lesion is difficult; lateral decubitus radiographic views are helpful in confirming the presence of pleural fluid.

Thoracentesis is the essential diagnostic procedure. The puncture should be made in the area shown on the radiograph to have the greatest accumulation of fluid. No more than 30 mL of pleural fluid should be withdrawn; otherwise, the protein loss from this usually protein-rich fluid may be considerable. The fluid generally is greenish yellow, occasionally tinged with blood, with a specific gravity of 1.012 to 1.022, a high protein content, and often a low glucose level (<30 mg/dL), and it has several hundred white cells/mm^3 with a predominance of neutrophils (early in disease) or lymphocytes, depending on the age of the effusion. Polymerase chain reaction (PCR), adenosine deaminase levels of greater than or equal to 38 IU/L, and absolute lymphocyte count of greater than or equal to 275 cells/mm^3 in pleural fluid had a sensitivity and specificity of 74% and 88%, 81% and 75%, and 90% and 83%, respectively, in one study of children with tuberculous effusions.[416] Acid-fast smears almost always are negative, and pleural fluid cultures are positive in less than 30% of cases. Pleural biopsy is a useful diagnostic procedure because both the finding of typical tubercles on histologic study and culture of the tissue are much more likely to establish the diagnosis than is culture of pleural fluid.[343]

The prognosis for children with tuberculous effusions always has been relatively good compared with that for other overt forms of tuberculosis, even in the days before chemotherapy.[353] Clinical improvement occurs well before radiographic resolution of disease; the majority of children have radiographic abnormalities at the completion of therapy.[127] Permanent impairment of pulmonary function is a surprisingly uncommon event after pleural effusion.[197] The development of scoliosis is a remote possibility.

Progressive Pulmonary Tuberculosis

In this serious complication of the primary complex, the primary pulmonary focus, instead of resolving or calcifying, enlarges steadily and develops a large caseous center. This center then liquefies and empties into an adjacent bronchus to create a "primary cavity"[643,673] (Fig. 96.10); the liquefaction is associated with particularly large numbers of tubercle bacilli. The tubercle bacilli further disseminate to other parts of the lobe and to the entire lung, where other foci of infection form. On rare occasion, an enlarging primary focus ruptures into the pleural cavity and creates a pneumothorax, bronchopleural fistula, or caseous pyopneumothorax or ruptures into the pericardial sac or the mediastinum.

A progressive lesion often is accompanied by more severe fever, cough, malaise, and weight loss, as well as classic signs of cavitation, such as egophony.[223,541] Before chemotherapy was available, the inability

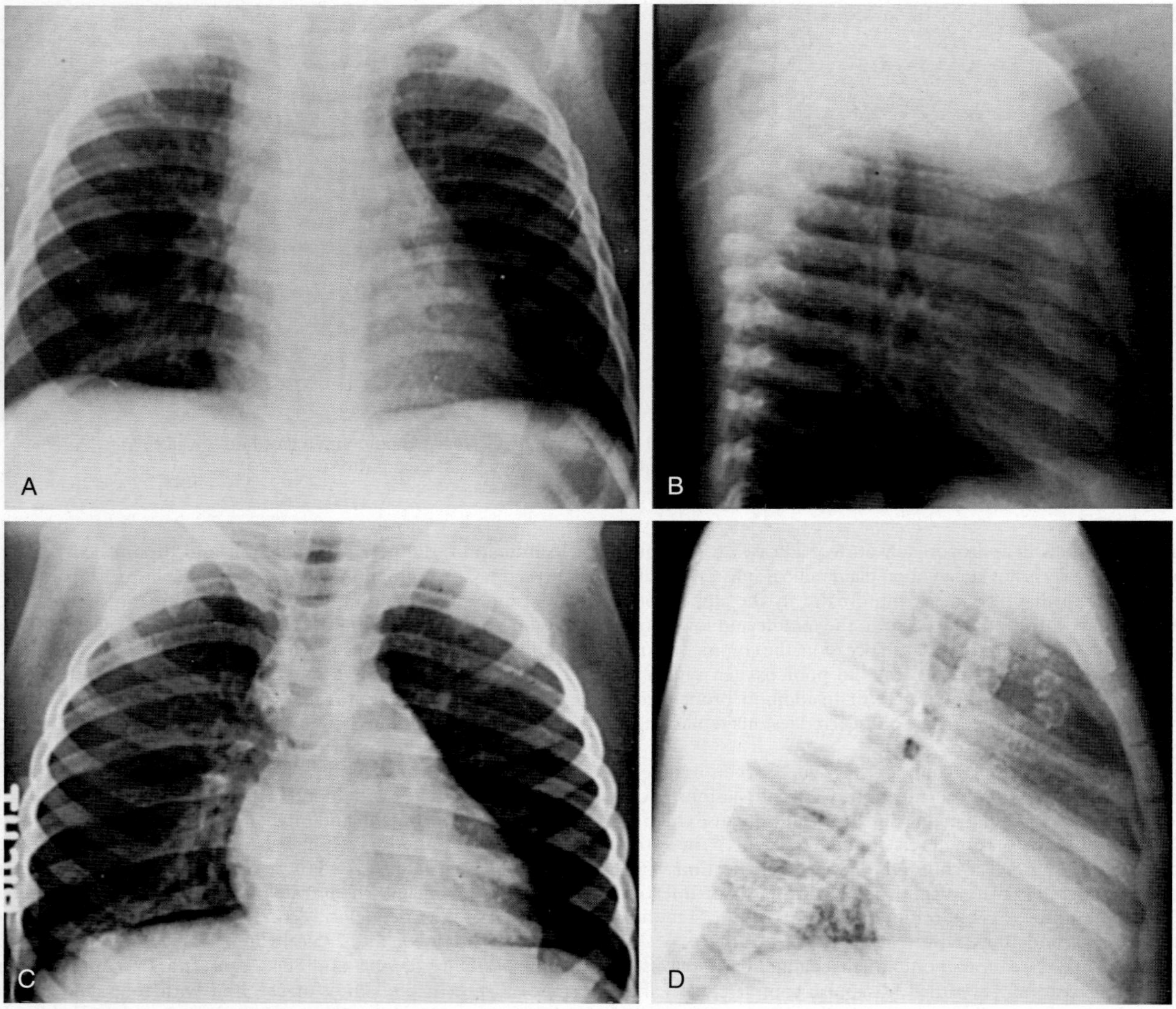

FIG. 96.8. (A–B) Radiographs of a 7-month-old girl with mild fullness of the right upper mediastinum and a hazy infiltrate in the right lower lobe. The result of a skin test for tuberculosis was positive. She was treated for tuberculosis and clinically improved. (C) The same patient 3.5 years later has a calcified primary complex in the right upper and lower lobes over the diaphragm. (D) The anterior location of the upper lobe complex is seen clearly on the lateral chest radiograph.

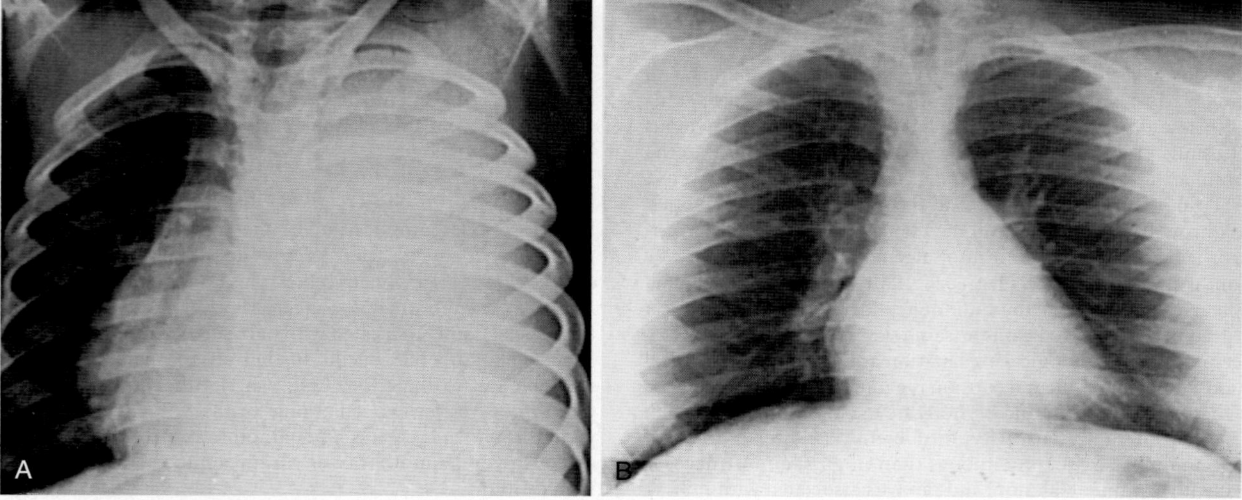

FIG. 96.9. (A) Posteroanterior chest radiograph of a 5-year-old boy with massive left pleural effusion caused by tuberculosis. (B) Normal radiograph 6 years later from the same patient who had no physical complaint.

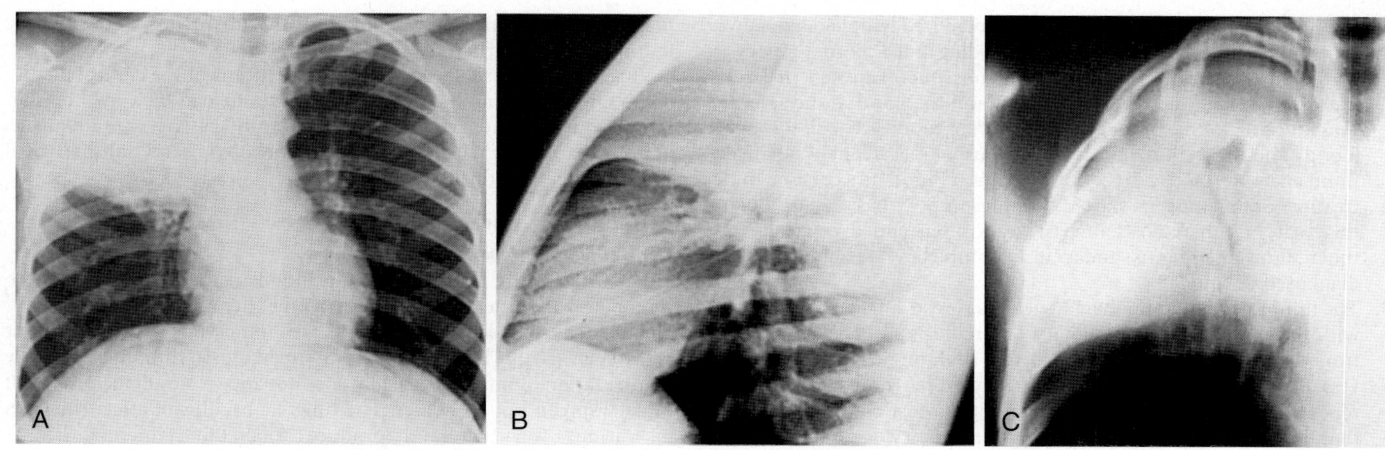

FIG. 96.10 Tuberculosis in a 9-year-old boy with an expanding right upper lobe consolidation. (A) Posteroanterior and (B) lateral chest radiographs. (C) Tomogram showing an air bronchogram and a cystic cavitary lesion.

to contain the primary focus was associated with a grave outlook; 25% to 65% of affected patients died. Now, with appropriate treatment, the prognosis is good.

Distinguishing between progressive pulmonary tuberculosis and a simple tuberculous focus with a superimposed acute bacterial pneumonia caused by *Staphylococcus, Klebsiella,* or anaerobes may be difficult. Antimicrobial agents effective against these pathogens may be indicated, in addition to appropriate antituberculosis drugs. Sometimes, especially during convalescence from pulmonary parenchymal lesions, bullous lesions appear and persist for several months. They seem to be associated, in children as in adults, either with "tears" in damaged alveolar walls or with the emptying of caseum out of cavities.[398]

Chronic Pulmonary Tuberculosis

Chronic pulmonary tuberculosis, sometimes referred to as adult or reactivation tuberculosis, is the type of disease seen in pulmonary tissue sensitized and immunized by an earlier tuberculosis infection. Endogenous reinfection is the usual event.[615] However, reinfection with a different strain of *M. tuberculosis* has been documented and may be more common in areas where tuberculosis is prevalent.[583]

Careful long-term studies of children have revealed a continuum of involvement in many cases: first the primary focus, followed within a few years in some patients by infraclavicular small round foci in the lung apices that often were calcified (Assmann foci, Simon foci) and thought to result from hematogenous spread at the time of initial infection. Later, these foci disappear spontaneously or remain visible as tiny calcifications or as larger "round foci," which may, if untreated, progress to the typical lesions of chronic pulmonary tuberculosis.

Even before antituberculosis drugs were discovered, chronic pulmonary tuberculosis was a rare occurrence in children (e.g., 6–7% in the series of Lincoln and colleagues[350] of closely monitored patients at Bellevue Hospital). It appears more frequently in children in the lower socioeconomic strata of society and more frequently in girls than in boys. Chronic pulmonary tuberculosis is much more frequent in children who acquire their initial infection after reaching 7 years of age and particularly if they become infected close to the onset of puberty. Cough, fever of unknown origin, chest pain, hemoptysis, and supraclavicular adenitis are the most common clinical manifestations. Essential diagnostic procedures are the tuberculin skin test and appropriate chest radiographs, often including lordotic views (with cephalic angulation). An intense search for tubercle bacilli must be made in sputum, gastric washings, and, if necessary, secretions obtained by bronchoscopy.

Myocardial and Pericardial Tuberculosis

Tubercles often are found in the heart in miliary tuberculosis. Although it is exceedingly rare, myocardial caseation has been described that is usually secondary to direct spread from mediastinal glands and accompanied by paroxysmal tachycardia or arrhythmias.[690]

Tuberculous pericarditis, although more common than symptomatic tuberculous myocarditis, occurred in only 0.4% of 2500 children monitored by Lincoln and Sewell[353] at Bellevue Hospital, and in 4% of 200 children in Boyd's series.[59] TB accounts for approximately 70% of all pericarditis cases in sub-Saharan Africa.[270] In most cases, tuberculous pericarditis probably arises by direct invasion or by lymphatic drainage from caseous lymph nodes in the subcarinal area or from nodes close to the ductus arteriosus, with resulting exudation of hemorrhagic fluid and the development of granulation tissue on both the parietal and visceral surfaces of the pericardium. Pericardial fluid may be serofibrinous or hemorrhagic; tubercle bacilli rarely are found on smears.[263] Sometimes, extensive fibrosis leads to obliteration of the pericardial sac, with the development, usually years later, of constrictive pericarditis.

The initial symptoms generally are nonspecific: low-grade fever, poor appetite, failure to gain weight, and, rarely, chest pain. On examination, a pericardial friction rub may be heard, or if a large effusion already is present, distant heart sounds, tachycardia, and a narrow pulse pressure may suggest the diagnosis. The diagnosis then is confirmed by radiography, echocardiography, electrocardiography (widespread ST-segment elevation or PR depression; dampened voltages in the presence of a large pericardial effusion), tuberculin skin test, and aspiration of fluid for culture. Culture yield is higher for pericardial tissue than for pericardial fluid. In one study, IGRAs were more sensitive than pericardial adenosine deaminase levels and Xpert MTB/RIF for the diagnosis of tuberculous pericarditis.[477] Before the advent of chemotherapy, approximately half the patients succumbed. Now, with appropriate drugs and corticosteroids to diminish the size of the effusion[630] and also occasional partial pericardiectomy, the outlook is excellent.

Lymphohematogenous Spread

Tubercle bacilli from the lymphadenitis of the primary complex are disseminated during the incubation period in all cases of tuberculosis infection. The results of liver biopsy of young asymptomatic tuberculin converters (indicating recent infection) show that the liver always is involved.[111] Tubercle bacilli can reach deep, distant organs through the bloodstream or lymphatic channels. Autopsies on individuals who have died soon after development of initial infection show that bacilli often are deposited in the liver, spleen, skin, and apical pulmonary tissue.

The clinical picture produced by lymphohematogenous spread probably is determined by host susceptibility at the time of spread and by the quantity of tubercle bacilli released.[571,674] Three clinical forms can be recognized:

1. The lymphohematogenous spread may be occult, in which case it usually remains so, or it may be occult initially with metastatic, extrapulmonary lesions appearing months or years later (e.g., renal tuberculosis).[514]
2. So-called protracted hematogenous tuberculosis, rarely seen today, is characterized by high, spiking fever, marked leukocytosis,

hepatomegaly and splenomegaly, and generalized lymphadenopathy, sometimes with evidence of metastatic seeding in the choroid, kidneys, and skin. Calcifications may appear subsequently, often in large numbers, in the pulmonary apices (Simon foci) and in the spleen, thus attesting to the earlier dissemination of tubercle bacilli through blood. The tuberculin skin test result usually is strongly positive. Bone marrow biopsy may confirm the clinical impression, but treatment often must be started on a presumptive basis.[522] Although this type of tuberculosis in past years often ended tragically in tuberculous meningitis, today it is completely treatable if it is diagnosed in time.

3. The third form of lymphohematogenous spread, analogous to sepsis with pyogenic bacteria, is miliary tuberculosis.[571] It usually arises from discharge of a caseous focus, often a lymph node, into a blood vessel such as a pulmonary vein; it may be self-propagating, with repeated discharge arising at various sites. Most common during the first 2 to 6 months after infection in infancy, it can arise even in adults who have apparently well-healed, calcified lesions.[310,553]

Miliary disease provides a striking illustration of the difference in susceptibility of tissue to tubercle bacilli; tubercles tend to be larger and more numerous in the lung, spleen, liver, and bone marrow than in the heart, pancreas, and brain. The number of fixed intravascular phagocytes, as well as the relative tortuosity of the smaller blood vessels themselves, must play an important role in determining tissue susceptibility. In acute caseating miliary tuberculosis, the lesions are likely to be numerous and sometimes almost coalescent.

The clinical picture of miliary tuberculosis varies greatly, probably depending on the number of bacilli in the bloodstream. Sometimes, the patient is afebrile and appears to be well, and the condition is diagnosed by chance during contact investigation of another individual with infectious tuberculosis. The onset can be insidious, often occurring after the patient has had another precipitating infection. In rare cases, the onset is abrupt. Drowsiness, loss of weight and appetite, persistent fever, weakness, rapid breathing with a rustling sound on auscultation of the lungs, occasionally cyanosis, and almost always a palpable spleen are the clinical manifestations that lead the clinician to obtain a chest radiograph.

Usually within no more than 3 weeks after the onset of symptoms, tubercles can be seen evenly distributed throughout both lung fields[465]; in the early stages, they often are detected best on a lateral view of the retrocardiac space (Fig. 96.11). The incidence of choroidal tubercles varies greatly; it has been reported variously as 13% and 87%. Recurrent pneumothorax (including tension pneumothoraces), subcutaneous emphysema, pneumomediastinum, and pleural effusion are well-recognized complications of miliary tuberculosis. Cutaneous lesions, including painful nodules, papulonecrotic tuberculids, and purpuric lesions, may appear in crops.[304]

The diagnosis usually is established by means of the clinical picture and a chest radiograph. Sometimes it is confirmed by a liver or skin biopsy; by culture of *M. tuberculosis* from the gastric aspirate, urine, or bone marrow[111,236]; or by fiberoptic bronchoscopy and transbronchial biopsy.[69] Treatment usually is successful.

Extrathoracic Spread

Central Nervous System Tuberculosis

Tubercle bacilli are distributed by the bloodstream into all parts of the central nervous system (CNS) during lymphohematogenous spread.[352,607] Surprisingly, they do not multiply as well in nervous tissue as in other areas such as the lung. Thus, CNS tuberculosis, although an early manifestation of infection, usually does not appear simultaneously with miliary spread but days later. The tubercle bacilli can affect the CNS in various ways[667,685] and produce tuberculous meningitis,[267,633] serous meningitis,[347,667] tuberculoma,[660,667] or tuberculous brain abscess, or it can affect mainly the spinal cord and cause spinal tuberculous leptomeningitis.[456]

Tuberculous meningitis arises from caseous foci[515] that discharge tubercle bacilli directly into the subarachnoid space. The thick, gelatinous exudate lies in the meshes of the pia–arachnoid in the brain, where it infiltrates the walls of meningeal arteries and veins and produces inflammation, caseation, and obstruction; the exudate can extend along small vessels into the cortex, where it causes occlusion and produces infarcts. This same exudate interferes with normal flow of cerebrospinal fluid (CSF) in and out of the ventricular system and with CSF absorption. The predilection of the exudate for the base of the brain accounts for the frequent involvement of the third, sixth, and seventh nerves and the optic chiasm. The combination of vascular lesions producing infarcts,[342] interference with CSF flow resulting in hydrocephalus, and direct cranial nerve involvement, especially of the eye, causes the devastating damage that all too often results from tuberculous meningitis.[20]

Tuberculous meningitis has been estimated to develop in one of every 300 untreated infections.[279] Virtually never seen in infants younger than 4 months, it occurs most frequently in children younger than 6 years, usually appears within 2 to 6 months after initial infection, and accompanies miliary tuberculosis in approximately 50% of cases. Tuberculosis should be suspected as the cause of meningitis that is accompanied by cranial nerve involvement, hydrocephalus, or evidence of inflammation at the base of the brain.[672]

The onset of tuberculous meningitis usually is gradual and occurs during a period of approximately 3 weeks. On occasion, the onset is abrupt and marked by a convulsion. A convenient approach is for the

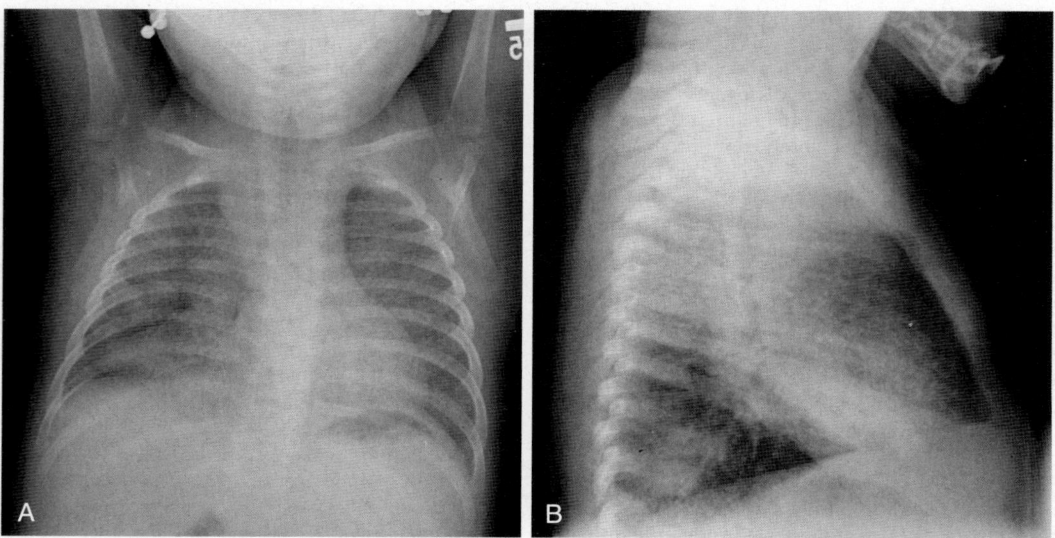

FIG. 96.11. Miliary tuberculosis in an infant. The numerous tubercles can be seen on both the (A) posteroanterior and (B) lateral views.

clinician to divide the course into three stages. The first stage is characterized by personality change, irritability, anorexia, listlessness, and some fever. After 1 or 2 weeks, the disease passes into the second stage, when signs of increased intracranial pressure and cerebral damage appear: drowsiness, stiff neck, cranial nerve palsies, inequality of the pupils, vomiting, absence of the abdominal reflexes, and convulsions that may be tonic or clonic and focal or generalized. The third stage is characterized by coma, irregular pulse and respirations, and rising fever. Papilledema occasionally is noted.

Aids in establishing the diagnosis are a history of contact with an adult who has tuberculosis (however, the family history of tuberculosis often is "negative" because the incubation period of meningitis is short and the contagious adult has not been discovered yet)[155]; a tuberculin skin test (positive result in only 50% of cases); positive tuberculin skin test results in siblings; a chest radiograph, which often reveals pulmonary disease; and changes in, and the characteristic findings from, CSF. However, the ventricular CSF may be relatively normal because it is obtained proximal to the site of inflammation. The lumbar CSF usually is clear and under substantially increased pressure. It will contain 50 to 500 white blood cells/mm^3, with polymorphonuclear leukocytes predominant early and lymphocytes predominant later. The CSF glucose level may be at the lower limits of normal if the patient is examined early in the second stage, and it falls by 5 mg or so each day; by the third stage, hypoglycorrhachia is profound. The protein content may be normal at the time of the first lumbar puncture, but it rises steadily to very high concentrations. Tubercle bacilli are scarce. Only 30% to 50% of cases of tuberculous meningitis in children can be confirmed by culture of CSF; CSF acid-fast smear positivity is seen in fewer than 10% of cases. Gastric washings should be cultured, not only to confirm the diagnosis in retrospect but also to permit drug susceptibility testing of the organisms.[723]

CT or magnetic resonance imaging (MRI)[18,20,225,461,707] is recommended for the evaluation of all patients with tuberculous meningitis. Both permit recognition and follow-up of tuberculomas,[666,703] infarction or vasculitis, and hydrocephalus that might require shunting.[20,131,285,624] Involvement of the basal ganglia often is a diagnostic clue for the presence of tuberculosis.[18] High levels of antidiuretic hormone (the syndrome of "inappropriate" antidiuretic hormone secretion [SIADH]) may cause hypotonic expansion of the extracellular fluid. Hyponatremia is a nonspecific finding seen with various causes of vasculitis. Salt wasting in the urine occurs in rare cases. Because intense vomiting and dehydration usually accompany tuberculous meningitis, the electrolyte disturbances usually include severe hypochloremia.

A good prognosis depends on immediate initiation of treatment without awaiting epidemiologic and bacteriologic confirmation of the diagnosis.[264,528] Before chemotherapy was used, every case of true tuberculous meningitis was fatal within 3 to 4 weeks, whereas today appropriate treatment during the first stage allows survival in nearly every case, although the patient's intelligence may never return to its previous level. Unfortunately, the nonspecific signs and symptoms of stage 1 TB meningitis mean that few children are diagnosed at this early stage. When treatment is initiated during the second stage, treatment results in survival in 75% or more of patients. If patients are obtunded or comatose when treatment is begun, they rarely recover unscathed. Very young age and the occurrence of convulsions generally are poor prognostic factors.[528,550] Hydrocephalus, usually of the communicating type, occurs frequently (38% in one series) and is largely responsible for poor outcomes. Relieving the hydrocephalus surgically appears to improve the sensorium, vision, and neurologic deficits. Studies support the early use of ventriculoperitoneal shunting in patients severely ill at the time of admission.[329,475] Some neurosurgeons may prefer to place an external ventricular drain initially if there is concern that the high CSF protein levels could result in shunt malfunction. Infarcts caused by vasculitis also can leave catastrophic residua. The presence of drug-resistant tuberculous meningitis greatly worsens the prognosis,[474] as does coinfection with HIV.[687] The role of corticosteroids in the treatment of intracranial tuberculosis is discussed later in this chapter.

The long-term sequelae of tuberculous meningitis are numerous and include blindness, deafness, intracranial calcification, diabetes insipidus, syndrome of inappropriate antidiuretic hormone secretion, obesity, paraplegia, and mental retardation.[550] A recent meta-analysis found that the mortality rate for TB meningitis was 19% and that the probability of neurologically intact survival was only 37%.[107]

Serous tuberculous meningitis is an uncommon occurrence (13% of 500 cases in the experience of Udani and associates[667]). Apparently, it develops when a tuberculous focus close to the subarachnoid space causes a lymphocytic reaction in the subarachnoid space without the actual presence of tubercle bacilli.[728] Isolated tuberculoma is manifested clinically as a brain tumor.[26,141,156] As many as 30% of mass-occupying CNS lesions are tuberculomas, depending on the incidence of tuberculosis in the particular population under study (e.g., in India). Tuberculomas occur most often in children younger than 10 years old and often are located at the base of the brain around the cerebellum.[686] In contrast, tuberculomas in adults more often are supratentorial. Headache, convulsions, fever, and other symptoms and signs usually associated with brain abscess or tumor also characterize tuberculoma. Only careful evaluation, including inquiry about exposure to tuberculosis, a TST, chest radiography, and a CT, will permit these cases to be recognized in time to begin appropriate chemotherapy before neurosurgical intervention is needed. The widespread use of neuroimaging has revealed that small, multiple tuberculomas are a frequent feature of tuberculous meningitis in infants and young children.[18,20] A phenomenon recognized fairly recently is a symptomatic intracranial tuberculoma appearing and enlarging during treatment of meningeal, miliary, and even pulmonary tuberculosis.[6,339,507,572,649] This phenomenon appears to be mediated immunologically; it usually responds to corticosteroids and does not necessitate a change in antituberculosis chemotherapy. In addition, some small children with severe pulmonary or disseminated tuberculosis have one or several tuberculomas but normal findings on CSF evaluation.[155,280] CT or MRI of the head should be performed whenever neurologic signs or symptoms accompany tuberculosis.

Tuberculous brain abscess is a rarely reported form of CNS tuberculosis that tends to occur at an older age than tuberculoma does.[323,702] On pathologic examination, the lesion lacks the giant cell and granulomatous reaction associated with tuberculoma. Focal neurologic signs occur commonly. CT and MRI, if used routinely in cases of tuberculous meningitis, may permit this type of abscess, which requires surgical intervention as well as chemotherapy, to be recognized more frequently. Intramedullary tuberculoma of the spinal cord is exceedingly rare. It can be manifested as recurrent abdominal pain.

Spinal tuberculous leptomeningitis occurs more often in older children and adults than in infants; in the series of 500 cases studied by Udani and coworkers,[667] only 2% fell into this last age group. Protein levels in the CSF are elevated substantially, and sometimes partial or total block may be noted on myelography. Exudate may completely surround the spinal cord.

Cutaneous Tuberculosis

The manifestations of cutaneous tuberculosis can be classified in children according to a modification of the earlier classifications designed for adults[324]: (1) lesions produced by inoculation from an exogenous source[493] or after inoculation with BCG vaccine; (2) lesions resulting from hematogenous dissemination[304]; (3) lesions arising from an endogenous source; and (4) erythema nodosum.

Skin lesions associated with the primary complex may be caused by direct inoculation of tubercle bacilli into a traumatized area, such as a lesion on the sole of a child's bare foot, a mosquito bite on the face, an abraded elbow, or the foreskin at the time of ritual circumcision.[478,560] The initial skin focus usually is a small, painless nodule, sometimes with tiny satellite lesions that soon turn into indolent ulcers without surrounding inflammation. The most striking feature is painless regional lymphadenitis, which often is what convinces the patient to see a physician. Fever and systemic reactions generally are minimal; low-grade pyogenic infection and cat-scratch fever (*Bartonella* infection) always must be considered in the differential diagnosis. A strongly positive TST result usually is obtained. Needle aspiration and culture may differentiate disease caused by *M. tuberculosis* from that caused by nontuberculous mycobacteria.

Scrofuloderma indicates tuberculosis of the skin overlying a caseous lymph node (most often in the cervical area) that has ruptured to the outside and left either a shallow ulcer or a deep sinus, sometimes surrounded by a cluster of nodules. Today, it is a rare occurrence because the diagnosis generally is made before the node ruptures. Administration of chemotherapy often forestalls the need for surgical excision. Needle aspiration of fluctuant nodes can help with decompression and may decrease the risk of sinus tract formation.

Manifestations that result from hematogenous dissemination are papulonecrotic tuberculids and tuberculosis verrucosa cutis. Papulonecrotic tuberculids[580] are miliary tubercles in the skin that usually appear as tiny papules with "apple jelly" centers, most often on the trunk, thighs, and face. They frequently are similar to papular urticaria or early varicella lesions, or they may be confused with the skin lesions of Letterer-Siwe disease. Skin biopsy provides a reliable diagnosis. Lupus vulgaris is a rare form of chronic, indolent tuberculosis, usually on the face, that often seems to evolve from tuberculids, very rarely at the site of BCG inoculation.

Tuberculosis verrucosa cutis is a condition characterized by large (several centimeters in diameter) papulonecrotic tuberculids. The lesions usually appear on the arms, legs, or buttocks, suggesting that trauma may play some part in their causation. Fungal infection is the main consideration in the differential diagnosis.

Erythema nodosum formerly was a common manifestation of hypersensitivity to tuberculin. It occurs mostly in teenage girls. Usually beginning with fever and systemic toxicity manifesting soon after initial infection develops, erythema nodosum is characterized by large, deep, painful, indurated nodules on the shins and sometimes on the thighs, elbows, and forearms. The nodules gradually change from light pink to a bruise-like color. Erythema nodosum is not specific for tuberculosis but also occurs with streptococcal and meningococcal infections, histoplasmosis, coccidioidomycosis, sarcoidosis, drug sensitivity reactions, and perhaps cat-scratch disease. Tuberculin hypersensitivity is pronounced in children with tuberculosis underlying erythema nodosum, and tuberculin skin testing should be performed with caution. These patients may or may not have associated tuberculous lesions, but some clinicians hold that these patients have a greater chance of suffering complications. Skin biopsy reveals only nonspecific changes regardless of cause and, therefore, is useless in establishing the diagnosis. Both fever and nodules clear within 2 or 3 weeks.

Skeletal Tuberculosis

Bone and joint tuberculosis can be expected in 1% to 5% of children whose initial infection with tubercle bacilli is untreated. Usually, the tubercle bacilli are disseminated to skeletal structures during lymphohematogenous spread of the initial infection.[33] The disease becomes symptomatic during the first 1 to 3 years after infection. Each of the most frequently involved bones and joints has a characteristic "incubation period" (e.g., 1 month for dactylitis but about 30 months for tuberculosis of the hip). In very young children, blood flow through growing bone is intense; consequently, they suffer from skeletal tuberculosis more often than older children do. The lesion usually starts as an area of endarteritis in the metaphysis of the long bone, where the blood supply is particularly abundant; lesions can be single or multiple.[504,570] Bone infection can be initiated by two other mechanisms, particularly in the vertebrae: (1) direct extension through the lymphatics from a caseous paravertebral lymph node[70] and (2) direct local hematogenous or lymphatic extension from a neighboring bone. As bone is destroyed progressively by pressure necrosis and formation of a cold abscess, a nearby joint may become involved.[505,670,687]

The bones most often affected are the vertebrae.[464] In one study of 1074 patients with the disease, 41% had vertebral involvement, 8% each had hip or knee involvement, and 5% had elbow involvement.[664] Non–weight-bearing bones, such as the skull, clavicle, and mandible, rarely are involved.[235,239] Often a history of trauma is present and may play some part in activation of an underlying lesion or may serve simply to draw attention to the process.

Tuberculous spondylitis, or tuberculosis of the vertebrae, frequently affects the thoracic vertebrae, particularly the 12th one.[246] In one series of 64 cases of spinal tuberculosis in children, thoracic lesions were most common (38%), followed by lumbar involvement (29%); in 20%, both the thoracic and lumbar spine were involved. Cervical involvement is rare.[258] Usually, two vertebrae are involved, but sometimes 3, 4, or even as many as 11 (usually contiguous, but at times with "skips") are affected. The body of the vertebra is affected far more often than the spinous processes or the arch.

The progression of tuberculous spondylitis, as seen on radiographs, is from slight narrowing of the disk space with only minimal disk involvement and slight collapse and "wedging" of the vertebral body to marked narrowing of the disk space with collapse, wedging of the bodies, and resulting angulation of the spine (gibbus), and to extensive destruction of the bodies with severe kyphosis (Pott disease).

Paravertebral abscess (Pott abscess), retropharyngeal abscess, psoas abscess, and neurologic lesions are serious complications seen in 10% to 30% of cases of spondylitis. Neurologic complications most often arise from cervical and lumbar vertebral lesions and consist of various degrees of neuroplegia, paraplegia, or even quadriplegia. The complications are caused by inflammation of the spinal cord secondary to a neighboring cold abscess, by caseum or granuloma in the extradural space, or by spinal vessel thrombosis.

The signs and symptoms of spondylitis include pain that is worse at night, low-grade fever, and a peculiar position (e.g., torticollis with cervical lesions) or gait. Findings on physical examination may include marked "guarding" because of dorsal muscle spasm, pain when the back is "pounded," a gibbus deformity (e.g., acute angle thoracolumbar kyphosis), or reflex changes (including clonus).[399] On occasion, the presence of referred chest pain leads to discovery of a paravertebral abscess on the chest radiograph. With chemotherapy and, when necessary, surgery, the outlook for both eventual clinical healing and neural recovery is in the range of 80% to 90%, although patients may not gain their full expected height.

Tuberculosis of the knee can be divided into several clinical types[245]: isolated effusion (with little restriction of motion); synovial thickening and fibrosis of the synovial membrane without bone erosion (with considerable restriction of motion); or synovial disease and a bone focus but an intact joint space.[627] Some degree of pain, stiffness, and limping, usually intermittent in milder cases, first calls attention to the problem.

Tuberculosis of the hip, in some series of patients more common than tuberculosis of the knee, should be considered in the differential diagnosis of the child with an antalgic gait or refusal to weight bear. Isolated involvement of the acetabulum or femoral head without intraarticular disease has a good prognosis.

Tuberculous dactylitis (spina ventosa)[231] is the most common form of skeletal tuberculosis in infants. Endarteritis is followed by swelling (often painless), and cystic bone lesions are seen on radiographs. A cold abscess may form and drain spontaneously. The prognosis for recovery without deformity is surprisingly good and was so even before chemotherapy was available.

Tuberculous arthritis is rare in children. Usually monoarticular, it involves primarily the weight-bearing joints; upper extremity involvement is rare. Bacterial cultures and histologic examination of the synovium establish the diagnosis.[687] Poncet disease is a form of rheumatic joint disease associated with tuberculosis characterized by nondestructive, transient, migratory polyarthritis. Poncet disease is exceedingly rare in children.[136] The diagnosis of skeletal tuberculosis should be considered immediately in any child with known TB infection in whom a bone or joint lesion develops and in any child with a persistent, otherwise unexplained bone or joint lesions.[682] The differential diagnosis must include low-grade infections caused by *Staphylococcus, Haemophilus influenzae, Salmonella,* and *Brucella;* fungal infections; rheumatoid arthritis; malignancy; eosinophilic granuloma, particularly with skull or pelvic lesions; and osteochondrosis resulting from aseptic necrosis of bone, particularly Legg-Calvé-Perthes disease and tuberculosis of the hip.

Children with bone and joint tuberculosis usually react strongly to tuberculin. Chest radiographs are abnormal in up to 50% of children with TB skeletal disease. Although the number of tubercle bacilli in an active bone lesion is much lower than in a lung lesion, the organisms almost invariably can be recovered on culture, and a great effort to do so should be made by means of aspiration or open biopsy.[222]

Treatment of skeletal tuberculosis includes both chemotherapeutic and orthopedic interventions, with the chemotherapeutic interventions by far the more important.[502] Orthopedic procedures can be used for several purposes: establishment of the diagnosis, evacuation of caseum and necrotic bone, immobilization of a joint, and reconstruction or strengthening of damaged bone. Since the advent of chemotherapy, any indicated surgical procedure can be performed without fear of subsequent development of sinus formation. However, the trend has been toward reliance on drug therapy with increasingly conservative surgical management. Controlled trials of treatment undertaken in different parts of the world (Southeast Asia) by the Medical Research Council Working Party on Tuberculosis of the Spine and others have demonstrated the remarkable effectiveness of ambulatory treatment with different regimens of chemotherapy in children and adults,[271,403–405] including short-course chemotherapy.[229]

Tuberculosis of the Superficial Lymph Nodes (Scrofula)

Striking enlargement of the superficial regional lymph nodes is an integral component of the primary tuberculous complex. The tonsillar and submandibular nodes are involved most often and probably represent extension from the paratracheal lymph nodes (and not from a primary lesion in the tonsil, as once was thought); occasionally, these nodes are involved when the primary lesion occurs in the mucous membranes of the mouth, a rare event. Enlarged supraclavicular nodes may accompany a primary pulmonary lesion in the upper lung fields.[555] Enlarged axillary and epitrochlear nodes can result from a primary skin lesion of the elbow or hand, often a small, insignificant-looking area that has, however, been present for some time. Preauricular adenitis suggests a focus on the scalp or forehead or in the lacrimal sac, sometimes attributed to an insect bite. With inguinal adenitis, careful examination of the sole of the foot may reveal a small ulcer, often at the base of the toes.

When the superficial lymph nodes are involved early in the course of infection—the normal event—the enlargement usually is painless and the node or nodes are rubbery and discrete.[390] Low-grade fever generally is present, sometimes unnoticed by the parents. On occasion, acute respiratory tract infections seem to precipitate or to aggravate superficial tuberculous lymphadenitis and the patient has high fever, some local pain, and perilymphadenitis. Rarely, the patient is seen first with a fluctuant mass and the overlying skin is shiny and erythematous.[138,600]

The diagnosis usually is not obvious, so it is wise in all cases of chronic superficial cervical and supraclavicular lymphadenitis to perform a throat culture, radiography of the chest, and a TST. If the node is fluctuant, it should be aspirated and cultured for mycobacteria, as well as for pyogenic bacteria.[332] In preauricular, axillary, and inguinal adenitis, a possible primary skin lesion should be sought diligently. If a lesion is found, a biopsy should be performed, in addition to a tuberculin skin test, chest radiography, and a careful history. In one study conducted in a tuberculous hyperendemic region in children with chronic (greater than 4 week duration) lymphadenopathy whose nodes were at least 2 × 2 cm and were unresponsive to antibiotic therapy, tuberculosis lymphadenitis was diagnosed in over 90% and sensitivity was excellent.[390] In areas with lower incidences of tuberculosis, this scoring system cannot be used.

In addition to pyogenic infection, the following need to be considered as possible causes: cat-scratch disease, tularemia, malignant tumors, sarcoid, and nontuberculous mycobacterial (NTM) infections.[32,327] If the adenitis is caused by infection with *M. tuberculosis,* the TST induration usually is greater than 15 mm, whereas most NTM produce a less intense reaction. IGRAs can also help distinguish *M. tuberculosis* from most NTM species (a notable exception is *M. kansasii*). The key to distinguishing tuberculosis from infection by another mycobacterium generally is epidemiologic—has the child been exposed to tuberculosis?

Because infection with pyogenic bacteria often enhances mycobacterial adenitis, frequently a wise approach is to institute therapy with a conventional antibacterial agent while awaiting the results of the TST, chest radiography, and cultures. If the adenitis persists and evidence of mycobacterial infection is elicited, antituberculosis drug therapy should be initiated and surgical excision seriously considered.[327,554] Surgical excision currently is the treatment of choice for adenitis caused by mycobacteria other than *M. tuberculosis.* In the case of lymphadenitis caused by *M. tuberculosis,* the response to antituberculosis drugs is likely to be good. On the other hand, the adenitis is more likely to extend down into the mediastinum and to be difficult to remove. Under these circumstances, surgical excision probably is unwise, whereas a few weeks of corticosteroid and antituberculosis therapy may be effective.[282,327]

Superficial tuberculous lymphadenitis sometimes occurs early in the course of lymphohematogenous spread, in which case it often is manifested as generalized lymphadenopathy with associated fever, malaise, and weight loss. The TST result almost always is positive in immunocompetent patients, and the TST should be included in the investigation of every patient with generalized lymphadenopathy.

Finally, tuberculous adenitis, either localized or generalized, can occur in adolescents or young adults who were infected months or even years earlier, whose infection has been quiescent, and in whom the appearance of lymphadenitis heralds reactivation of the tuberculosis infection.[326]

Ocular Tuberculosis

Ocular tuberculosis is an uncommon finding in children. When it does occur, the conjunctiva and the cornea are the areas most often involved.[153]

The conjunctiva can serve as the initial portal of entry for tubercle bacilli, especially after trauma. Unilateral lacrimation and reddening may lead to the discovery of yellowish gray nodules, usually on the palpebral conjunctiva. Preauricular adenitis appears early; the submandibular and cervical nodes also may enlarge. A TST and biopsy of the lymph node with culture can be performed to confirm the diagnosis.

Phlyctenular conjunctivitis probably is one of the hypersensitivity phenomena of childhood tuberculosis. Tubercle bacilli have, on rare occasion, been isolated from the small, grayish, jelly-like nodules usually clustered on the limbus and surrounded by dilated conjunctival vessels. Pain and photophobia are intense, and the lesions may recur in crops for weeks and affect one or both eyes. In the differential diagnosis, foreign body, herpes simplex virus conjunctivitis, vernal conjunctivitis, and trachoma should be considered. Tuberculin sensitivity is likely to be pronounced, and 1 tuberculin unit of purified protein derivative (PPD) should be used in the initial tuberculin skin test. Fortunately, hydrocortisone drops are effective in controlling both a strong local reaction to the diagnostic tuberculin test and the discomfort from the underlying disease. The prognosis for complete recovery is excellent, provided the phlyctenules do not ulcerate and leave corneal scars. Systemic chemotherapy should be started immediately after the diagnostic procedures are completed. The data for systemic corticosteroids are heterogeneous, but many experts would consider a 4- to 6-week course of systemic corticosteroids for ocular manifestations of tuberculosis.

Although tuberculosis of the ciliary body and iris has been reported rarely in children, tubercles of the choroid often have been found in patients with miliary tuberculosis (up to 70% of patients in some series) and occasionally in children with a seemingly uncomplicated infection.[428,462] Frequently multiple, the tubercles heal slowly with deposition of retinal pigment; residual scarring apparently can be prevented with corticosteroid therapy. Tuberculous uveitis and tuberculosis manifested as an orbital mass are rare clinical entities.[573]

Tuberculosis of the Middle Ear

Tuberculosis of the middle ear is a relatively rare manifestation of the disease.[187,365,367,434,534] It occurs as a primary focus in the area of the Eustachian tube (because of reflux up the tube) in neonates who have aspirated infected amniotic fluid, or in older infants who have ingested tuberculous material. It can occur as a metastatic lesion in older children who have a primary focus elsewhere. If it is a primary focus, regional lymphadenitis involves the preauricular lymph node or the anterior cervical chain and facial paralysis occurs frequently. The primary focus always is unilateral. Chronic painless otorrhea is a common occurrence and may become foul smelling because of bacterial contamination with enteric organisms. Direct intracranial extension is rare, but contiguous involvement of the mastoid can be seen. Older patients may complain of tinnitus and "funny noises." The eardrum often is damaged extensively. A large central perforation or several perforations are characteristic findings. MRI is superior to CT in visualizing abscesses and bony destruction, and for monitoring response to therapy radiographically.[430]

A TST, biopsy, and careful cultures for tubercle bacilli are essential. Once greatly feared for the almost inevitable loss of hearing and the frequent occurrence of tuberculous meningitis, tuberculous otitis media now heals well with appropriate chemotherapy.[434]

Gastrointestinal and Abdominal Tuberculosis

Tuberculosis of the mouth occurred more commonly in the days of bovine tuberculosis than it does today; at that time, scrofula often represented a primary complex in the mouth or tonsils, with associated submandibular or cervical lymphadenitis.[414] A primary focus in the mouth generally consists of a painless ulcer or mass of granulation tissue around a tooth socket or in the gingivolabial sulcus, with enlarged submental or submandibular nodes. Primary tuberculosis of the tonsils begins as a painless swelling of one tonsil, sometimes with an ulcer or yellowish node and, of course, enlargement of the regional lymph nodes. If tubercles found on histologic examination of a tonsil removed at tonsillectomy are unaccompanied by lymphadenitis, the lesion is considered a metastatic rather than a primary lesion. Tuberculosis of the esophagus occurs rarely, if ever, in children; sometimes, dysphagia is produced by a mass of mediastinal nodes, which may rupture into the lumen and later heal, possibly leaving an esophageal diverticulum.

Abdominal tuberculosis may occur after the ingestion of tubercle bacilli or as a part of generalized lymphohematogenous spread, but tuberculous enteritis always has been uncommon.[19,46,525,637,640] When tubercle bacilli penetrate the gut wall, they usually do so through the Peyer patches or the appendix, where they give rise to local ulcers followed by mesenteric lymphadenitis and sometimes peritonitis.[19] On occasion, especially in older children, tuberculous enteritis accompanies extensive pulmonary cavitation. Symptoms and signs include vague abdominal pain, intussusception, blood in the stool, and sinus formation after a seemingly routine appendectomy.

The spleen is seeded during the initial lymphohematogenous spread. Only rarely are the tubercles numerous and large enough to undergo caseation and to calcify.[316] The reticuloendothelial system of the liver is involved also. Symptoms rarely are manifested except in miliary tuberculosis, in which the liver may be enlarged markedly, or in congenital tuberculosis, in which both the liver and spleen usually are enlarged.[371]

Mesenteric lymphadenitis can arise as part of an intraabdominal primary complex or by extension from tuberculous thoracic or pelvic lymph nodes; often asymptomatic, it may be discovered later when calcified. It can cause ascites and dilation of the superficial abdominal veins, but the symptom most frequently attributed to mesenteric lymphadenitis is colicky abdominal pain after exercise, probably because adhesions are stretched.

Tuberculous peritonitis can be a result of direct extension from a primary intestinal focus, adjacent mesenteric lymph nodes, or tuberculous salpingitis.[104,152,208] It may be "plastic" or accompanied by a serous effusion. On palpation, a mass of lymph nodes often can be felt and the abdomen may have a characteristic "doughy" feeling. Paracentesis should be performed with care because the intestine may be immobilized by adhesions. Even with a large effusion, absorption usually occurs within a month. Malignant disease must, of course, be considered strongly in the differential diagnosis, and it may be necessary to obtain a biopsy specimen even if the tuberculin skin test result is positive. Laparoscopy frequently is useful, as is fine-needle aspiration[359] and ultrasonography.[293] CT is more sensitive than ultrasound. CT findings may include lymphadenopathy (often with central necrosis and rim enhancement), solid masses, and multisegment symmetrical intestinal mural thickening.[727] CT is less helpful for ascites, as it does not detect septations well.[677] The ascitic fluid–blood glucose ratio of the aspirated peritoneal fluid can be helpful in differentiating tuberculous peritonitis from ascites of other causes.[703]

Renal Tuberculosis

Renal tuberculosis is a late and uncommon complication of pulmonary disease; it rarely occurs less than 4 or 5 years after primary infection and is therefore likely to be diagnosed during adolescence.[182,587] However, tubercle bacilli can be recovered from the urine in many cases of miliary tuberculosis and some cases of pulmonary tuberculosis in young children. Hematogenous dissemination can give rise to tubercles in the glomeruli, with resultant caseating and sloughing but tiny lesions, which then discharge tubercle bacilli into the tubules. An encapsulated caseous mass occasionally develops in the zone between the renal pyramid and cortex; it may calcify in situ or discharge into the pelvis of the kidney and form a cavity analogous to a pulmonary cavity. Infection can be unilateral or bilateral and can spread downward to involve the bladder. Frequently, dysuria, hematuria, and "sterile" pyuria are the initial findings in the urine; they may occur grossly but often not until late in the course of a disease that causes strikingly few symptoms. CT findings can include renal parenchymal cavities, hydronephrosis, ureteral strictures, and thickening of the renal pelvis or ureter.[532] Appropriate examination and culture of single early-morning urine specimens rarely fail to reveal tubercle bacilli. Intensive chemotherapy renders surgical intervention a rare necessity.[587] Urine from patients with renal tuberculosis is highly infectious, and such children should be isolated until their urine is sterile.

Dialysis- and Renal Transplant–Associated Tuberculosis

Infections are a common cause of morbidity and mortality in patients with end-stage renal disease. The frequency of extrapulmonary disease is higher in dialysis recipients, and one recent study of adults receiving dialysis in the United Kingdom found that one-fourth of patients had drug-resistant isolates.[469] Depressed cellular immunity, as manifested by cutaneous anergy, delayed homograft rejection, and depressed lymphocyte count, has been demonstrated in uremic patients, whereas cell-mediated immunity appears to recover in stable patients treated by long-term hemodialysis. Thus, it is not surprising that tuberculosis occurs more frequently in patients maintained on dialysis than in the general population and that when it does become active, it does so before or early in the course of dialysis. Extrapulmonary involvement (mediastinal, meningeal, pleural, osseous, and renal) and miliary tuberculosis appear relatively frequently in this group. In these patients, fever of unknown origin should lead to suspicion of active tuberculosis.[15] Tuberculosis also can originate in the transplanted organ.[437,681]

Genital Tuberculosis

Tuberculosis of the genital tract is an uncommon finding in both sexes before puberty.[587] It usually arises as a metastatic lesion during lymphohematogenous spread and occasionally by direct extension from an adjacent lesion of bone, gut, or the urinary tract. Genital tuberculosis is a particular hazard for adolescent girls with tuberculosis infection. Frequently, other forms of tuberculosis associated with initial infection, such as a pleural effusion, also are present. Acute or chronic salpingitis is the most common manifestation (seen in over 90% of cases). This results in nodular thickening and a "corkscrew" appearance of the fallopian tubes, and, ultimately, tubular obstruction. Endometritis is seen in 50% of cases and is characterized by intrauterine adhesions. Ovarian involvement (in 20–30%) may include perioophoritis (from direct spread from the fallopian tubes) and tuboovarian masses. Cervical involvement is seen in 5% to 20% of cases; cervical stenosis is the most common finding, and this results in infertility in one-half of cases.[547,567] With tubal involvement, peritoneal tuberculosis occurs frequently.

Lower abdominal pain and amenorrhea usually prompt the patient to seek medical care. A lower abdominal mass, free peritoneal fluid, and constitutional symptoms may or may not be present. Chemotherapy is effective, but infertility remains a potential sequela of the disease.

Tuberculosis of the external genitalia has been seen as a manifestation of child abuse.

Genital tuberculosis can occur in males as primary tuberculosis of the penis after ritual circumcision; many such instances were reported in the past.[248,478] Massive inguinal lymphadenopathy in a circumcised infant should arouse suspicion of a possible tuberculous etiology. Epididymitis or epididymoorchitis can occur in early childhood.[217] These disorders are characterized by nodular, painless swelling of the scrotum, and a dragging pain in the groin and have a gradual onset rather than the acute onset that results after trauma, torsion of the testis, mumps orchitis, or epididymitis associated with bacterial infection.

Inoculation Tuberculosis

More than 200 cases of syringe-transmitted tuberculosis have been described in the world literature.[244] It has become more common since the widespread use of injectable penicillin and routine childhood immunization and usually has been a result of contamination of the syringe or the solution by an individual with infectious sputum. If the recipient has not been infected previously, the lesion in the muscle or subcutaneous tissue will be the primary focus and the regional lymph nodes will enlarge, caseate, and, under favorable circumstances, calcify. However, at least 10 infants thus infected have died as a result of generalized tuberculosis, and in others bone tuberculosis has developed. If the recipient already is tuberculin positive, a tuberculous abscess will form without regional lymphadenitis. In this case, an injection abscess must be differentiated from a deep tuberculous abscess arising in the stage of hematogenous dissemination.

Perinatal Tuberculosis (Congenital and Postnatal)

Transmission of *M. tuberculosis* from mother to infant through the placenta or amniotic fluid has been reported in approximately 300 patients.[76] Infection of the placenta has been demonstrated, and tubercle bacilli have been grown from the tissues of stillborn infants and from living infants within a few days of birth. Perinatal tuberculosis can be acquired by the infant through one of several routes:

1. Transplacental spread through the umbilical vein from a mother with primary hematogenous tuberculosis occurring during pregnancy (i.e., true congenital tuberculosis). The liver is enlarged, enlarged lymph nodes may be present at the porta hepatis, and evidence of widespread miliary disease may be seen in the infant (i.e., the infant may have a primary liver complex or primary lung complexes).
2. In utero aspiration of amniotic fluid infected from endometritis in the mother or from the placenta. This route of infection also constitutes true congenital tuberculosis. In both these situations, clinical onset of signs and symptoms is likely to be rapid (by 2 to 3 weeks of age) and to include failure to thrive, fever, respiratory distress, and hepatosplenomegaly.
3. Ingestion of infected amniotic fluid or secretions during delivery. This mechanism would seem to be less well documented than the first two routes, but it certainly is a possibility.
4. Inhalation of tubercle bacilli at or soon after birth from the mother, other relatives, or attendants with infectious pulmonary tuberculosis. This route is the most common mode of transmission to neonates.
5. Ingestion of infected breast milk or cow's milk.

One cannot always be sure of the type of infection in a particular neonate; only clear-cut evidence of a primary complex in the liver establishes a definite diagnosis of congenital tuberculosis. However, the presence of early forms of tuberculosis (e.g., pleural, miliary, or meningeal) in the mother during pregnancy or the puerperium also is strong evidence of true congenital tuberculosis in the infant.

The last two listed routes are really means of "postnatally" acquired tuberculosis and need, for epidemiologic purposes, to be distinguished from the first three routes. Neonates with these types of tuberculosis usually lack striking clinical features until they are 1 or 2 months of age.

The diagnosis of perinatal tuberculosis is likely to be difficult to establish and often delayed.[336] Disease in the mother often is overlooked; the mother may have pleural effusion, fever of unknown origin, cough, endometritis, and other symptoms without the tuberculous etiology being recognized. The early symptoms and signs in the neonate likewise are overlooked frequently and may be similar to those caused by other congenital infections. Once the diagnosis is suspected, treatment should be started immediately, and diagnostic procedures should be carried out rapidly and aggressively.

The clinical manifestations vary, probably depending on the size of the infecting dose of bacilli and the site and size of the caseous lesions.[400,445] In many of the reported cases, tuberculosis disease was discovered only at autopsy.[262] Symptoms usually appeared during the second week of life and included loss of appetite and failure to gain weight, fever, nasal or ear discharge, cough, bronchopneumonia, jaundice, hepatomegaly, and splenomegaly occurring later.[76] Wasting has been noted frequently and, in one case, clearly was shown to be caused by hypoadrenocorticism.[426]

Because the result of the tuberculin skin test very rarely is positive in infants, demonstration of tubercle bacilli in gastric washings, middle ear fluid, lymph node biopsy specimens, skin biopsy specimens, bone marrow aspirate, endotracheal aspirate, or lung biopsy specimens is essential.[226] Examination of the placenta for organisms or characteristic histopathologic changes can be extremely helpful and should be done when tuberculosis is diagnosed in the mother around the time of delivery. Successful treatment of congenital tuberculosis has been reported by several investigators, although clinical response may be very slow, and extensive calcification of the lungs, liver, spleen, and muscles may result.[298,302,445,590,603]

Tuberculosis in Adolescents

Tuberculosis in adolescents has become relatively more important as the incidence of infection in childhood has lessened.[143,380,586] Logically, it should be considered in two ways: first, tuberculosis acquired as an initial infection during the adolescent years and, second, tuberculosis infection acquired in early life and reactivated during adolescence.[384,447] In actual practice, separating the two often is difficult or impossible, and most clinical reports and studies do not do so.

Tuberculosis in adolescents may occur exactly as it does in young children, or a classic primary complex may progress rapidly to chronic pulmonary tuberculosis while the hilar lymph node involvement characteristic of childhood tuberculosis remains present. The Medical Research Council in 1963 published a report of 504 cases of tuberculosis in adolescents, including 316 cases of pulmonary tuberculosis, 44 cases of pleural effusion, 44 with hilar lymph node enlargement, 6 cases of miliary and 5 of meningeal tuberculosis, 13 with bone and joint disease, and 8 with genitourinary tuberculosis. In a series of cases of primary tuberculosis in adults, Stead[615] included 11 adolescents, 5 with simple primary tuberculosis, 5 with pleurisy and effusion, and 1 with progressive pulmonary tuberculosis.

From the extensive clinical experience of Lincoln and Sewell[353] and others, several observations emerge. Tuberculosis infection in early infancy rarely leads to pulmonary tuberculosis in adolescence, perhaps because it has several years in which to heal, whereas tuberculosis infection acquired after 7 years of age and, in particular, acquired after 10 years of age is likely to progress. When *M. tuberculosis* is acquired during adolescence, chronic pulmonary tuberculosis may develop within 1 to 3 years. Moreover, the risk for acquiring pulmonary tuberculosis is two to six times greater for adolescent girls than for adolescent boys. In both sexes, the adolescent growth spurt is the time of greatest risk. The work of Johnston[287] suggests that the depressant effect of puberty on calcium and nitrogen retention, at least in girls, may be correlated with the failure of tuberculosis infection to heal.

While clinical manifestations may overlap with those of younger children, psychosocial factors impacting adolescents are unique. The treating clinician must (without caregivers in the room) discuss use of illicit and prescription drugs and alcohol use, as well as recommending alternatives to oral contraceptives to the sexually active young woman who will be receiving rifamycin. As many adolescents with intrathoracic tuberculosis may be contagious, certain infection control considerations are present for these patients that are not found in younger children: respiratory isolation while in the community; missed school or work; and the attendant depression that often stems from this social isolation.

Tuberculosis and Pregnancy

In the era before chemotherapy, whether pregnancy and tuberculosis affected each other adversely was an ongoing controversy. Since the advent of chemotherapy, however, the prognosis has improved greatly.[196] The main problems now are serious unrecognized tuberculosis in a pregnant woman, sometimes with a fatal outcome, and serious unrecognized disease in her infant. Another problem is whether pregnancy influences the risk for progression of tuberculosis infection to disease; the data are conflicting. Tuberculin skin testing probably is valid during pregnancy; chest radiographs (with shielding) should be obtained for all tuberculin-positive pregnant patients. Therapy, when indicated, can safely include isoniazid (which crosses the placenta but apparently without ill effects), rifampin, and ethambutol. The safety of pyrazinamide in pregnancy has not been established, but a growing number of experts recommend it because anecdotal data have not shown it to be harmful to the mother or fetus. Streptomycin, because of fetal ototoxicity, is not recommended.[594] However, one study of seven pregnant women with multidrug-resistant tuberculosis showed no adverse effects on their neonates when mothers were treated with second-line drugs, including aminoglycosides.[169,574] Mothers receiving antituberculosis therapy can safely breast-feed; the drugs are found in milk at very low concentrations.[595]

Tuberculosis and Human Immunodeficiency Virus Infection

In adults infected with both HIV and *M. tuberculosis,* the rate of progression from asymptomatic infection to disease is increased greatly.[538] The clinical manifestations of tuberculosis in HIV-infected adults are typical when the $CD4^+$ cell count is higher than 500/mm^3. As the $CD4^+$ cell count falls, manifestations become "atypical." Extrapulmonary foci occur in as many as 60% of profoundly immunocompromised patients.[29] In up to one-fourth of children, intrathoracic and extrathoracic tuberculosis may occur simultaneously.[243] Pulmonary cavities are rare findings; lower lobe infiltrates or nodules often accompanied by thoracic adenopathy are common occurrences, especially if the patient's tuberculosis infection is recent. Focused assessment with sonography for HIV/TB (FASH) was developed to help diagnose pleural and pericardial effusions and extrathoracic TB in HIV-infected children and adults. FASH can demonstrate intraabdominal lymphadenopathy, splenic abscesses, and hepatic lesions.[237]

Many HIV-infected patients have a nonreactive tuberculin skin test. IGRAs have been poorly studied in this patient population, and studies have found poor correlation between IGRAs and TSTs and between IGRAs and TB risk factors.[520,521] Sputum is less likely to be produced or to contain visible acid-fast organisms on stained smears; more invasive procedures, such as bronchoscopy, often are required to isolate *M. tuberculosis* and to rule out other causes of opportunistic lung disease.[387] Malabsorption of antituberculosis drugs in HIV-infected patients can lead to prolonged symptoms and disease.[490]

When tuberculosis develops in HIV-infected children, the clinical features tend to be fairly typical of childhood tuberculosis in immunocompetent children, although the disease often progresses more rapidly and the clinical manifestations are more severe.[55,100,109,181,183,253,309,429,474,652] Many children have sizeable pulmonary radiographic findings with minimal respiratory signs or symptoms. An increased tendency for extrapulmonary disease may be noted. Nonspecific signs and symptoms,[692] overlap in symptomatology with other opportunistic infections, and higher rates of culture-positive patients with negative radiographs make the diagnosis challenging. Consequently, studies evaluating the utility of symptom-based scoring systems have shown discrepant results.[181,381,488] Establishing the diagnosis can be very difficult; a diligent search for an infectious adult in the child's environment may yield the best clues to the correct diagnosis.[314] Recurrent disease and relapse occur more frequently in HIV-infected children.[545] The prognosis generally is good if tuberculosis disease is not far advanced when the patient is diagnosed and appropriate antituberculosis drugs are available.[243]

Tuberculosis and Immune Reconstitution Inflammatory Syndrome

The introduction of highly active antiretroviral therapy (HAART) into regions where tuberculosis is prevalent has had a profound effect on the epidemiology and clinical expression of both diseases. One manifestation may be immune reconstitution inflammatory syndrome (IRIS). IRIS manifestations can include either worsening of tuberculosis symptoms while on effective therapy (paradoxical IRIS) or new-onset tuberculosis symptoms after initiation of HAART (unmasking IRIS).[408,610] Sometimes it is difficult to tell if a deterioration in the clinical course of a patient with an opportunistic infection who is started on HAART is due to IRIS, poor compliance with treatment for the opportunistic infection, or drug resistance.[333–335] Consensus case definitions were created in 2008 to help differentiate among these diagnostic possibilities. Paradoxical IRIS is defined for patients diagnosed with tuberculosis before starting HAART and who showed an initial response to antituberculous medication. Major criteria include new or enlarging lymph nodes or focal tissue involvement, central nervous system findings, serositis, or new or worsening radiographic findings. Minor criteria include new or worsening constitutional or respiratory symptoms or new or worsening abdominal pain accompanied by peritonitis, organomegaly, or intraabdominal lymphadenopathy. At least one major or two minor criteria are needed for diagnosis. Unmasking IRIS is defined in patients not receiving tuberculosis treatment when HAART is initiated who then develop tuberculosis with evidence of substantial inflammation (e.g., tuberculous lymphadenitis, pulmonary tuberculosis accompanied by respiratory failure).[408]

There continues to be a paucity of data on IRIS in HIV-infected children. One systematic review included 303 cases of TB-IRIS, 90% of which were unmasking IRIS, but noted few data on risk factors, immunopathogenesis, or treatment.[357] Factors suggesting IRIS are temporal association (within 4 months of starting HAART), unusual clinical manifestations, unexpected clinical course, exclusion of alternative explanations, evidence of preceding immune restoration (rise in CD4 lymphocyte count), and fall in HIV viral load. In adults, the risk for developing IRIS in patients with tuberculosis who are started on HAART is greatest if they have extrapulmonary tuberculosis, high initial HIV viral loads and low CD4 lymphocyte counts, and rapid response to HAART.[56,433] One metaanalysis showed that paradoxical IRIS developed in 16% percent of adults with tuberculosis.[433] Although the risk for IRIS is higher when HAART is initiated shortly after antituberculosis medications are begun, most reactions are mild and the survival benefit in patients receiving HAART outweighs the risk for IRIS.[50,291]

Published reports of IRIS in children have been rare,[290,441,467,500,693,720] although anecdotal evidence from pediatric acquired immune deficiency clinics in Africa suggest it is becoming common as HAART is introduced to more children with HIV infection. One study indicated that IRIS was seen in almost 40 percent of HIV-infected children and was more common in boys than girls and more common in children 5 to 12 years of age, and that unmasking IRIS comprised more than three fourths of cases.[467] Other studies have shown lower incidence of IRIS,[500,693] but the finding that IRIS is more common in children with disseminated disease and malnutrition has been documented in multiple studies.[467,693] IRIS in children has been associated with nontuberculous mycobacteria,[500] disseminated viral[500,693] or fungal infections,[467] bacterial pneumonia,[467] and previous BCG vaccination.[320,501,576] The finding that IRIS occurs in children with tuberculosis and HIV infection who receive HAART is not surprising. For decades, so-called paradoxical reactions have been described in HIV-uninfected children with tuberculosis after antituberculosis therapy is started. The most common manifestations are fever, cough, new skin lesions, enlarging lymph nodes in the thorax or neck, and appearance or enlargement of tuberculomas in the brain, with or without accompanying meningitis.[408,467] The risk for unmasking IRIS appears to be highest in the first 3 months after initiation of HAART.[27]

IRIS also can be seen in HIV-uninfected children. One study in HIV-uninfected children showed that unexpected deterioration while on therapy was seen in almost 15% of children, most commonly manifest as enlarging intrathoracic lymphadenopathy. In this cohort, IRIS was more common in children with multiple sites of disease and in children whose weight was in the lowest quartile.[650]

The best management of IRIS is unknown. As with paradoxical reactions that cause tissue damage or obstruction, corticosteroids may be beneficial to "quiet" the local immune response, although no randomized clinical trials have been reported. Less severe reactions may respond to nonsteroidal antiinflammatory drugs. The high frequency of IRIS associated with tuberculosis has led some experts to recommend delay of HAART until appropriate (for drug susceptibility pattern) antituberculosis chemotherapy has been given for at least 2 months.[346] No consensus on this approach has been reached, however, and data from children may indicate that they are more likely to die of complications of HIV than of tuberculosis when they are dually infected.[243]

DIAGNOSIS

In the developing world, the only way that children with tuberculosis disease are discovered is passively, when they have a profound illness that is consistent with a manifestation of tuberculosis. Having an ill adult contact is an obvious clue to establishment of the correct diagnosis. The only available laboratory test usually is an acid-fast smear of sputum, which the child rarely produces. In many regions, chest radiography is not available. To aid in establishing the diagnosis, a variety of scoring systems based on available tests, clinical signs and symptoms, and known exposures have been devised.[413,699] No single clinical scoring system has been validated. Sensitivities and specificities tend to be low, resulting in both overdiagnosis and underdiagnosis of tuberculosis. Sensitivity is quite low in HIV-infected children.[307,390,413] Finally, differing prevalences of tuberculosis can skew predictive values.

In industrial countries, children with tuberculosis usually are discovered in one of two ways.[167,311,540] Obviously, one way is to consider tuberculosis as the cause of a symptomatic illness.[529] Discovering an adult contact with infectious tuberculosis is an invaluable aid to establishing the diagnosis; the "yield" from a contact investigation usually is higher than that from cultures from the child.[37] Culture from the infectious adult case may yield the only drug susceptibility results for the child because cultures from children with tuberculosis frequently are negative. Children often are the first in the family to be diagnosed with tuberculosis, potentially owing to different thresholds for seeking medical attention for children and adults, and more rapid onset of severe manifestations in young children. A negative exposure history does not rule out tuberculosis in a child. The yield of contact investigations is higher for children than adults, owing to the former's more limited social network. Yield of contact investigations may be lower in foreign-born children, whose source cases may still reside in their country of origin.[568] The second way is to discover a child with pulmonary tuberculosis during the contact investigation of an adult with tuberculosis.[392,421,598,629,631] Typically, the affected child has few or no symptoms, but investigation reveals a positive tuberculin skin test result and an abnormal chest radiograph. In some areas of the United States, as many as 50% of children with pulmonary tuberculosis are discovered in this manner, before significant symptoms have begun.

The recent use of molecular epidemiology techniques has shown, however, occasional discordance between the isolate from the child and that from the presumed source, meaning that the real source of transmission to the child is undiscovered.[710,718] It is less common to find tuberculosis disease in a US-born child as the result of a community- or school-based tuberculin skin testing program, although foreign-born children with tuberculosis may be found in this manner.[168,487]

Tuberculin Sensitivity and the Skin Test

Sensitization to tuberculin is induced by infection with living tubercle bacilli. Specific tuberculin sensitivity to either *M. tuberculosis* or other mycobacteria can be transferred in humans by injection of lymphocytes from sensitized donors and also by injection of certain purified mycobacterial protein antigens. Sensitization to tuberculin as a result of infection with *M. tuberculosis* tends to persist undiminished for life.[180,230,256]

The time of appearance of sensitivity in animals after infection with *M. tuberculosis* has occurred depends on the number of tubercle bacilli in the infective dose and on the virulence (i.e., the rate of multiplication of the organisms), and such is also likely to be the case in humans.[30] For all practical purposes in humans, tuberculin reactivity seems to appear in 3 to 6 weeks, and occasionally as long as 3 months after initial infection. The size of the induration depends on the amount of tuberculoprotein injected and the availability of sensitized T lymphocytes in sufficient number. The size of the induration seems to depend on at least two additional factors: the local behavior of the skin (the disappearance time for wheals of normal saline solution, the so-called Aldrich-McClure test, is accelerated during fever, pregnancy, cachexia, and extreme malnutrition) and the number of actively multiplying tubercle bacilli in the body. That still other factors must be involved is clear because 10% to 20% of immunocompetent patients with proven tuberculosis are tuberculin negative during initial disease, with tuberculin sensitivity often regained during treatment.[495]

Falsely negative tuberculin skin tests can be seen in a number of circumstances. Temporary desensitization to tuberculin occurs most strikingly during wild-type measles and has been studied carefully. Full reactivity diminished during the incubation period and returned within approximately 1 month after appearance of the exanthem.[238] Influenza and administration of influenza and measles vaccines tend to depress sensitivity but rarely suppress it entirely.[319,730] Whether other viral diseases and vaccines regularly are less active in this regard and what the important factors may be are not known.[40] If a temporary desensitizing effect occurs in bacterial infections such as scarlet fever, it probably depends on factors such as hyperthermia and dehydration. Corticosteroids,[58,368,548] HIV infection,[376,506] adrenocorticotropic hormone,[533] nitrogen mustard,[694] and irradiation[137] diminish tuberculin reactivity, perhaps simply by inducing lymphopenia.[612]

False-positive results of tuberculin skin tests also are seen. That degrees of sensitivity to *M. tuberculosis* are induced by nontuberculous mycobacteria also is clear.[227] Previous receipt of BCG vaccine can cause increased reactivity to tuberculin, but the association is weaker than many clinicians suspect.[10,80,364,431,563] Less than 50% of infants given BCG vaccination have a reactive tuberculin skin test at 9 to 12 months of age, and the great majority will have a nonreactive skin test by the time they are 5 years of age. Older children and adults who receive BCG vaccination have a reactive skin test and keep it longer, but by 10 to 15 years after vaccination most individuals have lost tuberculin skin test reactivity.[119,411,536] However, a Chinese population-based cohort of persons 5 years old and older found significantly higher rates of TST positivity (15–42%) than IGRA positivity (13–20%).[204] This raised concerns that the prevalence of TB infection was being overestimated by the TST. Repeated administration of BCG vaccine can maintain tuberculin reactivity.[269] Repeated tuberculin skin tests in a person sensitized previously by BCG vaccination, infection with *M. tuberculosis,* or probably infection by an environmental mycobacterium may increase the reaction to subsequent tuberculin skin tests (called the booster phenomenon).[44,298,562,656]

The Mantoux test is the reference test. A graduated syringe and a 26- or 27-gauge needle are used to inject 0.1 mL of PPD into the most superficial layer of the epidermis of the forearm, which raises an immediate wheal (Fig. 96.12). Under optimal circumstances, the needle should not be withdrawn for a few seconds to minimize leakage. If there is leakage or if the injection was too deep and no wheal is noted, the skin test should be repeated at least 5 cm from the original site. The reference test uses a dose of 5 tuberculin units of PPD-S or 2 units of RT-23. The reading should be made at 48 to 72 hours, with the forearm slightly flexed. Any induration (not erythema) should be measured, preferably with calipers, and the diameter at right angles to the axis of administration recorded in millimeters. Any blistering or ulceration also should be noted. Use of the words "negative" and "positive" should be avoided because interpretation can change as more

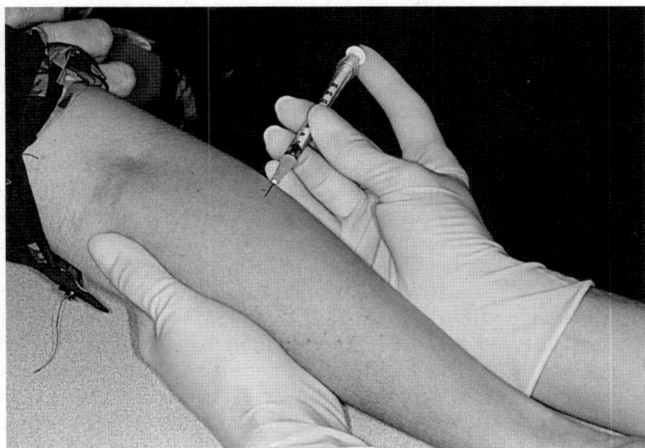

FIG. 96.12. A useful technique for performing a Mantoux tuberculin skin test on a child. The needle is applied perpendicular to the long axis of the arm to attain better control.

epidemiologic information becomes known. No study has demonstrated that parents or patients can read positive skin test results accurately, but that they may not correctly interpret or report positive results has been well documented.[106,106,220,254,470] Two studies have demonstrated that pediatric care providers tend to under-read Mantoux tuberculin skin tests.[72,276] Several studies have shown great variability in readings of Mantoux tests.[34,79,301,470] Such variability can be minimized only by ongoing training of both testers and readers and by concentrating the responsibility of testing and reading to a small number of trained individuals.

The importance of the tuberculin test cannot be overemphasized as the main criterion for diagnosis of tuberculosis infection in an individual child. Only rarely is the tuberculin test response negative in an infected child, usually as a result of anergy from overwhelming infection, from viral infection, from HIV infection, from the use of immunosuppressive drugs, or because of factors not yet understood.[621] Anergy in tuberculosis can be selective for tuberculin; results of "control" skin tests may be positive but the Mantoux test result negative in a child with tuberculosis disease.[614] The utility of candidal or tetanus controls is limited and they are not recommended. In lieu of controls, clinicians need to be cognizant of the decreased sensitivity of the test in young children and immunocompromised patients.

The Mantoux test has a sensitivity and specificity of only approximately 95% at 10 mm of induration.[260] When a test with these characteristics is applied to a population with a 90% prevalence of tuberculosis infection, the positive predictive value of the skin test is 99%, an excellent result. However, if the same test is applied to a population with only a 1% prevalence of infection, the positive predictive value drops to 15%; 85% of the "positive" results are false-positive findings created by biologic variability, nonspecific reactions, and infection with environmental mycobacteria. These false-positive results lead to unnecessary treatment, cost, and anxiety for the patient, family, and clinician. In short, the low sensitivity and specificity of the tuberculin skin test render the test undesirable for use in persons from low-prevalence groups. The trend in the United States is to reduce or to eliminate routine testing of low-risk children but to target children with specific risk factors for one-time or periodic tuberculosis skin testing.[12,90,422]

In lieu of mass screening using tuberculin skin tests, children should be screened by history. Several recently published studies have shown that a questionnaire can be used in the United States to identify children with significant risk factors for tuberculosis infection, who then can receive a tuberculin skin test.[201,361,471,527] Factors that consistently correlate with having a positive tuberculin skin test result include contact with a case of tuberculosis, other family members with a positive tuberculin skin test result, and foreign birth or extensive travel to a high-prevalence country.[551] The predictive value of these questions may be diminished in high-prevalence areas. Having a parent born in a high-incidence nation is a risk factor for a child having TB disease[705]; however, the association of parental foreign birth on TB infection is unclear.

The CDC and the American Academy of Pediatrics (AAP) have recommended varying the size of induration considered positive in various groups, according to their risk factors (Table 96.6). This is an attempt to increase sensitivity in children most likely to have rapid progression of asymptomatic tuberculosis infection to disease and to increase specificity in persons with no known risk factors for tuberculosis. In general in the United States, previous receipt of BCG vaccine should not influence interpretation of the initial tuberculin skin test of a child.[286]

Advances in interferon-γ release assays (IGRAs) in molecular biology and genomics have led to use of alternatives to the tuberculin skin test.[473,609] Two in vitro formats have been developed that measure interferon-γ release by sensitized lymphocytes after stimulation by *M. tuberculosis* antigens.[611] Both formats use proteins—early secreted antigen target 6, culture filtrate protein (CFP)-10—that are found on *M. tuberculosis* and only a few species of nontuberculous mycobacteria (*M. kansasii, M. marinum, M. szulgai,* and *M. flavescens*) but not on the bacilli BCG or the *M. avium* complex. The first test licensed in the United States was QuantiFERON-TB and includes an extra antigen (TB7.7). The test measures whole-blood interferon production. The second format licensed in the United States is the enzyme-linked immunospot (T-SPOT.TB), which measures the number of mononuclear cells that produce interferon.

TABLE 96.6 Amount of Induration in Reaction to a Mantoux Tuberculin Skin Test Considered Positive (Indicating Probable Infection With *Mycobacterium Tuberculosis*)

Reaction Size	Risk Factors
≥5 mm	Contact with infectious cases Abnormal chest radiograph HIV infection or other immunocompromise
≥10 mm	Birth or previous residence in a high-prevalence country Residence in long-term care or corrections facility Certain medical risk factors: diabetes mellitus, silicosis, renal disease Occupation in health care field, exposure to patients with tuberculosis Member of a local high-risk group Close contact with a high-risk adult (except health care workers) Age <4 y
≥15 mm	No risk factors

Both formats of IGRAs have been studied extensively in adults.[473] Sensitivity in HIV-uninfected adults with disease has ranged from 73% to 96%,[412,472] and reported specificities range from 86% to 99%.[150,564] In HIV-infected adults with disease, sensitivity and specificity have ranged from 30% to 92% and 52% to 76%, respectively.[105,412] One metaanalysis of IGRA performance in HIV-uninfected adults with infection demonstrated specificities ranging from 98% to 100%.[149] There is some evidence that the T-SPOT.TB is less affected by immunosuppression in HIV-infected adults than the QuantiFERON.[84,472]

In many clinical situations, these tests have a higher specificity than that of the TST, better correlation with surrogate measures of recent exposure to *M. tuberculosis* in low-incidence settings, and less cross-reactivity than does the TST because of previous BCG vaccination [Table 96.7]. Like the tuberculin skin test, interferon release assays cannot differentiate between tuberculosis infection and disease. Two clear advantages of the interferon release assays are the need for only one patient encounter (vs. two with the tuberculin skin test) and the lack of possible boosting of the result, because the patient is not exposed to any biologic material. It is unclear to what degree an IGRA can be boosted by a preceding tuberculin skin test. One metaanalysis reported substantial within-subject variation in IGRAs before and after tuberculin skin testing, but the frequency varied dramatically (16–80%).[676] Two more recent studies did not demonstrated boosting.[518,539] Although the potential risk for boosting can be avoided by obtaining the IGRA before or at the same time as placing the tuberculin skin test, prior receipt of a tuberculin skin test is not a contraindication to IGRA use.

There are fewer pediatric studies of IGRAs but several metaanalyses of the available studies have been performed.[369,375,634] Sensitivity in children with microbiologically confirmed or all children diagnosed with tuberculosis disease (clinically diagnosed disease and microbiologically confirmed) has ranged from 53% to 100% and from 53% to 94%, respectively. However, low sensitivity of the IGRAs in children with microbiologically confirmed disease may be due, in part, to the immunosuppression caused by the disease; these children also are more likely to have a negative tuberculin skin test. As with the tuberculin skin test, a negative IGRA result never rules out tuberculosis disease.[355,552]

The performance of IGRAs is limited in certain groups by an increased rates of indeterminate results, most often caused by failure of the positive control of the test. Immunocompromised children, including those with cancer[81,616] and HIV infection,[122,292,375] are more likely to have indeterminate test results,[234,377] as are children younger than 2 years of age.[292] Whereas some studies have shown no association between indeterminate results and age,[484] others have reported high rates of indeterminate test results in children younger than 4 or 5 years of age.[42,125] It appears that technical

TABLE 96.7 Suggested Uses of TST and IGRAs in Children

Preferred Test	Scenario
TST preferred	Children age <5 y[a]
IGRA preferred, TST acceptable	Children age ≥5 y who have received the BCG vaccine
	Children ≥5 y who are unlikely to return for TST reading
Both the TST and an IGRA should be considered	Initial and repeat IGRA results are indeterminate/invalid
	Initial test (TST or IGRA) is *negative and:* There is clinical suspicion of TB disease[b]; The child has a TB risk factor and is at high risk of progression and poor outcome (especially therapy with an immunomodulating biologic agent, such as a tumor necrosis factor-α antagonist)[b]
	Initial TST is *positive and:* Patient is ≥5 y and has a history of BCG vaccination; Additional evidence is needed to increase adherence with therapy

From Starke JR and the Committee on Infectious Diseases, American Academy of Pediatrics. Interferon-γ release assays for diagnosis of tuberculosis infection and disease in children. *Pediatrics.* 2014;134:e1763–e1773.

[a]Some experts will use an IGRA in children aged 2 to 4 y, especially if they have received a BCG vaccine but have no other significant risk factors. Most experts do not use IGRAs in children age <2 y because of the lack of data in this age group and the high risk of progression from infection to disease.

[b]Either the TST or the IGRA result being positive would be considered significant in these groups.

IGRA, Interferon-γ release assay; *TST,* tuberculin skin test.

factors such as inadequate shaking of the test tube contribute significantly to indeterminate results.[68,472] Helminthic infections have also been associated with indeterminate results,[654] a particular concern when screening international adoptees.[599]

Determining performance for children with tuberculosis infection is more challenging, because there is no reference standard. One proxy is degree of exposure to a documented source case. Sensitivity and specificity for infection have ranged from 90% to 92% and 91% to 95%, respectively.[369] Concordance between results from the tuberculin skin test and IGRAs vary widely. Although high concordance (>90%) has been reported from low-prevalence settings where BCG is not used, concordance decreases in BCG-immunized children.[42,125,369] IGRAs appear to correlate more closely than tuberculin skin tests for BCG-vaccinated children identified in contact investigations.[192,521] However, data are conflicting, and other studies have shown similar performance for the tuberculin skin test and IGRAs for the diagnosis of pediatric tuberculosis infection.[5] Some studies have demonstrated a decrease in the sensitivity of both the IGRAs and the tuberculin skin test with decreasing age and in HIV-infected children,[375] while other studies have demonstrated good performance in these two groups.[51,378]

The American Academy of Pediatrics (AAP) has suggested that IGRAs be used with caution in children younger than 5 years of age given the relative paucity of data for this age group.[97,611] The main reason for caution is that sensitivity is paramount for infants and toddlers who have a higher risk of progression to disease if they have untreated tuberculosis infection. However, many experts use the IGRAs in children down to 2 years of age. An optimal use for these assays—when one wants to maximize specificity—is in the BCG-immunized older child (≥5 years of age) who lacks tuberculosis risk factors aside from birth in a high-prevalence nation. Another use may be for a child whose family is reluctant to treat infection based on a tuberculin skin test result alone or when there may be difficulty having the child return for the reading of the tuberculin skin test. In children with suspected disease, or for children with a high risk of progression to disease (such as those about to undergo significant immune suppression with drug therapy), obtaining both a tuberculin skin test and one or both IGRAs provides maximum sensitivity. Because most studies have not shown a consistent, significant difference between the two IGRAs, the CDC and the AAP recommend that the assays may be used interchangeably.[97]

Given the brief period of time during which IGRAs have been used, some questions remain unanswered, including the dynamics of IGRAs—when they become positive after exposure to a person with tuberculosis disease, how long they remain positive, and the degree to which conversions and reversions occur on therapy. These questions may be best answered with longitudinal studies.

Diagnostic Mycobacteriology in Children

The demonstration of acid-fast bacilli in stained smears of sputum is presumptive evidence of pulmonary tuberculosis in most patients.[531] However, children have paucibacillary disease. Gastric washings, which often are used in lieu of sputum, can be contaminated with nonpathogenic oral acid-fast organisms. Tubercle bacilli in CSF, pleural fluid, lymph node aspirate, and urine are sparse; thus, only rarely are direct-stained smears for tubercle bacilli of any use in pediatric practice.[626] Cultures for tubercle bacilli are of great importance, not only to confirm the diagnosis but increasingly to permit testing for drug susceptibility. If culture and drug susceptibility data are available from the associated adult case and the child has classic features of tuberculosis (positive skin test result, consistent abnormal chest radiograph), obtaining cultures from the child adds little to management. In many low-incidence countries, a child usually will have contact with only one adult with potentially contagious TB. This is a poor assumption in hyperendemic areas, and cultures on the child should still be obtained. Similarly, cultures in the child should be attempted in children with suspected TB disease if the associated adult case has drug-resistant tuberculosis, as different drug susceptibility profiles would alter management substantially.

Painstaking collection of specimens is essential for diagnosis of children because fewer organisms usually are present than in adults.[575] Yield may be increased by obtaining multiple specimens from the same site, or by obtaining specimens from different locations (e.g., urine samples and gastric aspirates).[653] Gastric lavage should be performed in the very early morning, when the patient has had nothing to eat or drink for 8 hours and before the patient has a chance to wake up and start swallowing saliva, which could dilute the bronchial secretions that were brought up during the night and made their way into the stomach. The stomach contents should be aspirated first. No more than 50 to 75 mL of sterile distilled water (not saline) should be injected through the stomach tube and the aspirate added to the first collection. The gastric acidity (poorly tolerated by tubercle bacilli) should be neutralized immediately. Concentration and culture should be performed as soon as possible after collection. However, even with optimal, in-hospital collection of three early-morning gastric aspirate samples, *M. tuberculosis* can be isolated from only 30% to 40% of children and 70% of infants with pulmonary tuberculosis.[71,614,669] One review of 31 studies on gastric aspirate yield in children found that smear-positivity was seen in 1% to 21% and culture positivity rates of 7% to 75%, depending on the inclusion criteria for the study.[625] Higher rates of smear and culture positivity were seen in studies where children with longer symptom duration, positive TSTs, or specific radiographic findings were included.

Sputum induction is an alternative to gastric aspiration. Sputum induction is an outpatient procedure that can be performed in clinic settings[424] and requires the child to be fasting for only 3 hours. A nebulized treatment with a β agonist is given, followed by a nebulized treatment with hypertonic saline. The β agonist decreases the risk for bronchospasm occasionally seen with hypertonic saline. Saline increases the tussive force in children (even those who had no cough initially). As children begin to cough up secretions, the child's oropharynx is suctioned. One study from a high-prevalence nation showed that one specimen obtained via sputum induction had the same smear and culture yield as three gastric aspirates.[273,722] Sputum induction in HIV-infected and HIV-uninfected adults had the same diagnostic yield as specimens obtained via bronchoscopy.[121] In most studies, the yield of *M. tuberculosis* from bronchoscopy specimens has been lower than from properly obtained gastric aspirates.[1,99]

The string test is a less invasive approach to diagnosing childhood tuberculosis. This procedure, originally designed for enteric pathogens such as *Giardia* and *Helicobacter*, entails the child swallowing a gelatin capsule containing a coiled absorbent string. One end is taped to the cheek before the child swallows the pill. After 2 hours, the string is gently removed via the mouth and placed in sterile normal saline. While best studied in adult patients, one pediatric study found comparable smear (4–5%) and culture (9%) in for string test and sputum induction.[440] One obvious limitation is the need for a child to be able to swallow an intact pill, which has limited data collection predominantly to school-aged children.

CSF, pleural fluid, and synovial fluid (as much fluid as possible should be collected) usually are centrifuged, and the sediment is used for stained smear and culture. An overnight urine specimen should be obtained in the early morning and taken immediately to the laboratory for processing because the organisms tolerate the low pH of urine poorly. Lymph node aspirates and biopsy tissue can be inoculated directly into a fluid medium such as Middlebrook 7H9.

Staining and examination of smears as well as inoculation of special media, incubation in a carbon dioxide environment, strain differentiation based on many cultural characteristics, and drug susceptibility testing require equipment, skills, and experience beyond those available in the usual clinic or hospital laboratory.[242] Thus, most laboratories depend on regional or reference laboratories for procedures beyond their scope.

Traditional drug susceptibility testing ordinarily is performed for isoniazid, rifampin, ethambutol, and streptomycin. For many years, pyrazinamide susceptibilities were not routinely performed owing to testing complexities. This made the diagnosis of *Mycobacterium bovis* (which is inherently pyrazinamide resistant) challenging. Recently, laboratory advances have resulted in pyrazinamide susceptibility testing being more widely available. Drug susceptibilities are performed using one of two systems: agar proportions and growth in liquid media. For agar proportions, the organism is inoculated onto two plates: one with a specified concentration of an antibiotic and one that is drug free. The proportion of colonies on each plate is compared, and if there is more growth on the antibiotic plate, the isolate is considered resistant to that drug. For automated liquid media systems (e.g., BACTEC), the isolate is inoculated into vials with and without antibiotic. If the drug-containing vial grows faster than or at the same rate as the drug-free vial, then the isolate is considered resistant to that drug. Susceptibilities to other medications can be requested if the isolate is resistant to first-line medications.

Pyrosequencing, detecting pyrophosphate release during DNA synthesis, has been used to detect mutations associated with resistance to several first- and second-line medications. One advantage is the ability of pyrosequencing to detect mutations in multiple loci in several isolates in real time.[190]

Nucleic Acid Amplification

The main form of nucleic acid amplification studied in children with tuberculosis is PCR, which uses specific DNA sequences as markers for microorganisms.[379,423] Various PCR techniques, most using the mycobacterial insertion element IS6110 as the DNA marker for *M. tuberculosis* complex organisms,[12,85] have a sensitivity and specificity of more than 90% in comparison to sputum culture for detecting pulmonary tuberculosis in adults. Other advantages include the ability to detect even low organism burdens, a particular consideration in children with paucibacillary disease; rapidity of results and decreased time to initiation of therapy and patients lost to follow-up; ability to differentiate between *M. tuberculosis* and nontuberculous mycobacterial species; and potentially diminished biosafety requirements.[450] Disadvantages include diminished sensitivity in patients with smear-negative disease; expense of equipment; variation in test performance even among reference laboratories[454,704]; and concern for cross-contamination. One study in Peru found that cross-contamination was so common that PCR positivity was as likely to be seen in well controls as from suspected cases.[458]

Evaluation of PCR in childhood tuberculosis has been limited. Compared with a clinical diagnosis of pulmonary tuberculosis in children, the sensitivity of PCR has varied from 25% to 83% and specificity has varied from 80% to 100%.[423,457,482,549,589] PCR of stool had a sensitivity of 30% to 40% and a specificity of 100% in children with pulmonary tuberculosis,[709] offering a noninvasive diagnostic modality. PCR of gastric aspirates may be positive in a recently infected child even when the chest radiograph is normal, demonstrating the occasional arbitrariness of the distinction between tuberculosis infection and disease in children. PCR may have a useful but limited role in evaluating children for tuberculosis. A negative PCR analysis never eliminates tuberculosis as a diagnostic possibility, and a positive result does not confirm it. PCR may be particularly helpful in evaluating immunocompromised children with pulmonary disease, especially those with HIV infection, although published reports of its performance in such children are lacking. PCR also may aid in confirming the diagnosis of extrapulmonary tuberculosis, but only a few reports have been published.[214,374,415]

Xpert TB/RIF is a real-time PCR assay for *M. tuberculosis* that simultaneously detects rifampin resistance. Rifampin resistance is used as a proxy for MDR-TB, because rifampin monoresistance is uncommon.[166] Rifampin mutations, in contrast to isoniazid mutations, cluster on a small part of the mycobacterial genome and synonymous mutations are rare, facilitating molecular detection of drug resistance. This assay uses a self-contained cartridge system and is not as operator dependent as traditional PCR. A metaanalysis conducted in 2013 included over 2600 children. Specificity was excellent (98%); pooled sensitivity was only 66%, but this was still a higher sensitivity than smear microscopy (which has reported sensitivities of 30–40%).[449] Sensitivity was higher among smear-positive (95–96%) than smear-negative (55–62%) patients. This study found no difference in performance between HIV-infected and -uninfected children.[713] A metaanalysis from 2015 compared Xpert TB/RIF to culture; sensitivity of Xpert was 62% and specificity was 98%, which was 36% to 44% higher than the sensitivity for smear microscopy. Xpert's sensitivity in detection of rifamycin resistance was 86%.[147] Although cartridges for the Xpert system are expensive, the self-contained system offers advantages in rapid detection of MDR-TB and the prospect of increasing available diagnostics in settings that lack laboratory infrastructure. However, Xpert does not replace the need for obtaining mycobacterial cultures. Culture remains more sensitive than Xpert[147,210,713] and the need to identify additional drugs to which the isolate is susceptible is crucial for advancing patient care.

Line probe assays (e.g., GenoType MTBDR*plus* by Hain) detects mutations conferring resistance to rifamycins (*rpoB*) and low- and high-level resistance to isoniazid (*inhA* and *katG*, respectively). There are few pediatric data for line probe assays; in adults, specificity is excellent (>99%), but sensitivity varied from 57% to 100%.[356]

In the United States, samples can be sent to the CDC laboratory for molecular detection of drug resistance (MDDR). This PCR-based platform evaluates for mutations that commonly result in resistance to different drugs (e.g., *katG* and *inhA* mutations for isoniazid, *rpoB* mutations for rifamycins, *pncA* mutations for pyrazinamide, *embB* mutations for ethambutol, and *gyrA* mutations for fluoroquinolones). The average turnaround time is 2 days. Sensitivity is highest for *rpoB* and *katG* mutations, where most mutations conferring resistance are found on a specific part of the genome; specificity is excellent.[75]

TREATMENT

Management of Tuberculous Children

Treatment of cavitary tuberculosis in adults is one of the most scientifically accurate areas in all of medicine and one of the finest examples of international professional cooperation in all of history. The ability to quantify the extent of disease and the large numbers of cases of tuberculosis have allowed researchers to address specific questions about optimal drug regimens and doses, duration of therapy, and nonmedical management. Historically, treatment recommendations for children have been extrapolated from data in adults.[22,53,88,114,249,250,281,578,581] However, during the past 3 decades, a large number of treatment trials for children have been reported, which has led to dramatic changes in the therapeutic approach to childhood tuberculosis.

As recently as the early 1980s, the recommended treatment duration for children with tuberculosis disease was 12 to 18 months. Although these regimens are effective when they are used properly, actual failure rates are high because of poor adherence during the long period of treatment. Newer regimens often are called short-course chemotherapy because treatment durations as short as 6 months are routinely successful. However, the key to the new approach is not the short duration but the intensive initial therapy with three or more antituberculosis drugs.

Antituberculosis Drugs

Isoniazid is the mainstay of therapy for tuberculosis in children (Tables 96.8 and 96.9). Inexpensive, bactericidal, of low molecular weight and therefore readily diffusible to all tissues in the body,[159] and relatively nontoxic to children, isoniazid is one of the most nearly perfect drugs in the pediatrician's armamentarium. It can be administered orally, intramuscularly, or intravenously. When the drug is taken orally, high plasma, sputum, and CSF levels are reached within a few hours and persist for at least 6 to 8 hours.[330,463] Because of the slow multiplication of *M. tuberculosis,* the total daily dose can be given at one time. The usual level necessary to inhibit multiplication of tubercle bacilli is 0.02 to 0.05 µg/mL.

Human variation in the acetylation rate of isoniazid to an inactive compound is known to be determined genetically.[396] Rapid acetylation occurs more frequently in blacks and Asians than in whites. Although a simple method, specifically the use of a urine sample, now is available for classifying patients as slow or rapid inactivators of isoniazid, the normal way of coping with the problem in children has been to give a sufficiently large dose of isoniazid to ensure an adequate level even in rapid inactivators.[393,679]

The principal toxic effects of isoniazid are peripheral neuritis and hepatitis. Peripheral neuritis resulting from competitive inhibition of pyridoxine utilization is a rare event in North American children because both milk and meat are the main dietary sources of pyridoxine.[48] In some well-nourished children, serum pyridoxine concentrations are depressed by isoniazid but clinical signs are not apparent.[489] In the case of most children, therefore, the use of supplementary pyridoxine is not necessary. However, in teenagers whose diets may be inadequate, in children from ethnic groups with low milk and meat intake, in HIV-infected children, and in breast-fed infants, pyridoxine supplementation (25 to 50 mg/day) is important. Peripheral neuritis, when it does occur, usually is manifested by "pins and needles" sensations in the hands and feet.

The risk for development of hepatotoxicity from isoniazid, which is rare in children, increases in frequency with age.[35,83,318,358,439,459,503,601,617] Its cause is unclear.[322] Rapid acetylators are no more susceptible than are slow acetylators.[184,393] Simultaneous use of alcohol, phenytoin, piperazine, and

TABLE 96.8 Commonly Used Drugs for the Treatment of Tuberculosis Disease in Children

Drug	Dosage Forms	Daily Dose (mg/kg/day)	Twice-Weekly Dose (mg/kg/dose)	Thrice-Weekly Dose (mg/kg/dose)	Maximal Daily Dose
Ethambutol	Tablets: 100 mg, 400 mg	20–25	50	Not recommended for young children 1.5 g if 40–55 kg 2.5 g if 56–75 kg 3 g if >75 kg	2.5 g
Isoniazid[a]	Scored tablets: 100 mg, 300 mg Syrup[b]: 10 mg/mL	10–15[b]	20–30	15	Daily: 300 mg Twice weekly: 900 mg Thrice weekly: 900 mg
Pyrazinamide	Scored tablets: 500 mg	20–40	50 (max: 2 g) if <56 kg 3 g if 56–75 kg 4 g if >75 kg	Not recommended for young children 1.5 g if 40–55 kg 3 g if 56–75 kg 4 g if >75 kg	2 g
Rifampin[c]	Capsules: 150 mg, 300 mg Syrup: formulated in syrup from capsules	10–20	10–20	Not recommended for young children Adolescents: 10	Daily: 600 mg Twice weekly: 900 mg
Streptomycin	Vials: 1 g, 4 g	20–40	20–40		1 g

[a]When isoniazid is used in combination with rifampin, the incidence of hepatotoxicity increases if the isoniazid dose exceeds 10 mg/kg/day.
[b]Most experts advise against the use of isoniazid syrup because of instability and a high rate of gastrointestinal adverse reaction (diarrhea, cramps).
[c]Rifamate is a capsule containing 150 mg of isoniazid and 300 mg of rifampin. Two capsules provide the usual adult (>50 kg body weight) daily doses of each drug.

TABLE 96.9 Treatment of Drug-Resistant Tuberculosis in Children[a]

Drug	Dosage Forms	Daily Dosage (mg/kg/day)	Maximum Daily Dose
Amikacin	Vials: 500 mg, 1 g	15–30 (IM, IV)	1 g
Capreomycin	Vials: 1 g	15–30 (IM, IV)	1 g
Clofazimine	Capsules: 50 mg, 100 mg	50–100 mg/day	200 mg
Cycloserine	Capsules: 250 mg	10–20	1 g
Ethionamide	Tablets: 250 mg	15–20 given in 2 or 3 divided doses	1 g
Kanamycin	Vials: 75 mg/2 mL, 500 mg/2 mL, 1 g/3 mL	15–30 (IM, IV)	1 g
Levofloxacin	Tablets: 250 mg, 500 mg, 750 mg	Adults: 500–750 mg total/day Pediatric: 20–30 mg	1000 mg
Linezolid	Vials: 2 mg/mL Tablets: 600 mg Suspension: 20 mg/mL	10 (PO, IV)	600 mg
p-Aminosalicylic acid	Packets: 4 g	200–300 given in 2 to 4 divided doses	12 g

[a]There are no data to support intermittent dosing for second-line medications except for injectable agents.
IM, Intramuscularly; *INH,* isoniazid; *IV,* intravenously; *PO,* orally; *PZA,* pyrazinamide; *RIF,* rifampin; *STM,* streptomycin.

especially rifampin seems to increase the likelihood of hepatotoxicity.[83,325] Monitoring of aspartate aminotransferase and alanine aminotransferase activity sometimes reveals transient increases during treatment with isoniazid in up to 40% of children,[338] but the levels usually return spontaneously to normal without interruption of treatment.[476] Liver enzyme abnormalities in adolescents receiving isoniazid are common occurrences and usually disappear spontaneously, but severe hepatitis can occur.[362,591] The estimated incidence of hepatic failure in children on isoniazid monotherapy was 3.2 per 100,000,[716] jaundice was rare (0.06%), and transient elevations in hepatic transaminase levels were seen in 8%.[158] In children receiving isoniazid as part of multidrug therapy, rates of jaundice and elevated hepatic transaminase levels are higher, but still extremely low.[158]

The possible occurrence of hepatitis raises the question of routine monitoring of liver enzyme levels once a month in all children receiving isoniazid. The advantage of doing so has to be weighed not only against the expense but particularly against the difficulty of ensuring regular monthly visits if the patient and parents know that every clinic visit entails a venipuncture. Most experts prefer to substitute routine questions about appetite and well-being, determination of weight, and a check of the appearance of the sclera and the size of the liver.[72,487] Patients should be counseled to stop taking isoniazid and to contact the clinician immediately if significant nausea, vomiting, abdominal pain, or jaundice occurs during the use of isoniazid.

Allergic manifestations of isoniazid hypersensitivity are extraordinarily rare. Convulsions have been reported after doses of 100 mg/kg or more, as in suicide attempts.[401,453,479,566] The treatment for isoniazid overdose is intravenous pyridoxine.

The usual dosage in children is 10 to 15 mg/kg/day, to a maximum of 300 mg/day. Isoniazid is available in tablets of 100 and 300 mg. A syrup of isoniazid in sorbitol (10 mg/mL) also is available; however, it is unstable at 37°C and should be kept cool. Significant gastrointestinal intolerance (nausea, diarrhea) develops in many children while they are taking the isoniazid suspension. If tablets are used, they are crushed easily in a dessert spoon, to which then is added in the same spoon a vehicle such as applesauce, mashed banana, or another palatable medium. The crushed tablets must never be added to the nursing bottle or offered in milk or water because they will be ingested only partially. If isoniazid is given concurrently with rifampin, the dose should not exceed 10 mg/kg/day.[459] If the intramuscular form is used, for example, in a child with meningitis who is vomiting, the daily dose is the same as the daily oral dose but usually is divided and given every 8 to 12 hours. Isoniazid can interact with several other drugs, including acetaminophen, some antiepileptics (carbamazepine, phenytoin), and a few antituberculosis medications (INH increases the serum concentration of cycloserine and rifamycins and ethionamide can result in increased levels of INH). The dosage of each may need to be modified in a patient taking several drugs.[25]

RIF is a semisynthetic drug derived from *Streptomyces mediterranei*. Active against a wide variety of both intracellular and extracellular organisms, it is bactericidal and more effective against mycobacteria than is any other drug except isoniazid. Most clinical isolates are susceptible to 5 μg/mL or less. The drug is absorbed readily from the gastrointestinal tract in the fasting state; peak serum levels of 6 to 10 μg/mL are achieved within 2 hours, and the drug is distributed widely in body fluids and tissues, including CSF. Excretion is mainly through the biliary tract; however, effective levels are achieved in the kidneys and urine. In many patients receiving treatment with rifampin, tears, saliva, urine, and stool turn orange as the result of a harmless metabolite, but patients and parents always must be warned in advance. Drawbacks include the relatively high cost; the rare occurrence of explosive hypersensitivity reactions with hemolytic anemia (associated with intermittent rifampin therapy[211]); and the occasional occurrence of leukopenia or thrombocytopenia.[221] Cholestatic hepatitis can be seen, and rifampin should be suspected as the culprit in children with transaminitis associated with elevated conjugated bilirubin. Rifampin has a number of drug interactions, including inactivation of oral contraceptives. It decreases levels of protease inhibitors, thus limiting its use in HIV-coinfected children on antiretroviral therapy. Rifabutin is preferred in this circumstance. Finally, there is a "therapeutic orphan" clause in the United States for children younger than 5 years, which also means that no formulation is commercially available for young children. However, rifampin easily can be made into a suspension for use in children.

Rifampin should be used alone in treating tuberculosis infection with an isoniazid-resistant organism or for children who do not tolerate isoniazid. If isoniazid 20 mg/kg and RIF 15 to 20 mg/kg are used, the incidence of hepatotoxicity is appreciable. Therefore, when the two are used together, one would be wise to approximate the doses to isoniazid 10 mg/kg and RIF 15 to 20 mg/kg. Rifamate is a capsule containing both isoniazid (150 mg) and rifampin (300 mg). Two capsules supply the usual adult (more than 50 kg) daily dose of each drug. Rifamate may be appropriate for older children and adolescents.[4] Rifater contains isoniazid, rifampin, and pyrazinamide together in one pill in varying concentrations. Rifapentine is a new rifamycin with a very long half-life, allowing for weekly administration. It is now recommended in combination therapy with isoniazid for the treatment of tuberculosis infection for persons 12 years of age or above.[623] This regimen currently is recommended only under directly observed preventive therapy. Few pharmacokinetic data for rifapentine are available for young children. It appears that children require larger weight-normalized doses than adults.[52] Long-term efficacy data for children and adolescents are scant.

Pyrazinamide contributes to the killing of *M. tuberculosis*, particularly at a low pH, such as within macrophages.[530] The exact mechanism of action of this agent is a subject of controversy. Pyrazinamide has no effect on extracellular tubercle bacilli in vitro but clearly contributes to the killing of intracellular bacilli. Primary resistance is very rare, except that *Mycobacterium bovis* is intrinsically resistant. The drug diffuses readily into all areas, including CSF.[157,185] The usual adult daily dose is 30 to 40 mg/kg. The adult dose is tolerated well by children, results in high CSF concentrations, and clearly is effective in therapy trials for tuberculosis in children.[162,523,535,605] However, serum concentrations are lower in children than in adults taking a weight-equivalent dose.[218] Pyrazinamide appears to exert its maximal effect during the first 2 months of therapy. Hepatotoxicity can occur at high doses but rarely does at the usual dose. That said, pyrazinamide is the most common cause of drug-associated hepatitis in children receiving multidrug therapy for TB disease. Pyrazinamide routinely causes an increase in serum uric acid concentration by inhibiting its excretion through the kidneys. Toxic reactions in adults include flushing, cutaneous hypersensitivity, arthralgia, and overt gout; however, the considerable experience with this drug in children in Latin American countries, Hong Kong, and the United States has revealed few problems. It plays a major role in intensive, short-course treatment regimens.[212,605] Use of pyrazinamide for the first 2 months allows therapy to be shortened from 9 to 6 months for most nonskeletal, nonmeningeal forms of tuberculosis. While pyrazinamide has few drug interactions, it can increase the levels of cyclosporine and rifamycins.

Ethambutol has been used for many years as a companion drug for isoniazid in adults. The usual oral dose is 20 mg/kg per day.[160] At this dose, the drug primarily is bacteriostatic, its major role being to prevent the emergence of resistance to other drugs. However, at doses of 25 mg/kg per day or 50 mg/kg given twice a week, ethambutol has some bactericidal action.[123,203] Unfortunately, at these higher doses, optic neuritis or red-green color blindness has occurred in some adults. Regular visual field and color chart testing should detect these reversible effects early. The incidence of ophthalmologic toxicity in children is extremely low (0.05%), if it occurs at all, in part because children metabolize the drug faster than adults.[160] It is used frequently and safely in children, including in preverbal children in whom visual acuity evaluation is not possible, with life-threatening forms of tuberculosis or who are at risk for drug-resistant tuberculosis. However, it diffuses poorly into CSF.[157] In the United States, it is used with isoniazid, rifampin, and pyrazinamide as first-line therapy for children with suspected tuberculosis when drug-susceptibility results are not yet known. Ethambutol has few drug interactions.

Ethionamide is an effective and well-tolerated drug in children at a dose of 15 to 20 mg/kg/day divided into two or three doses given after meals. Children rarely complain about its sulfurous taste, which is repulsive to adults. Related to isoniazid, it likewise diffuses readily into CSF.[161,163,261] Ethionamide is used in cases of drug-resistant tuberculosis and tuberculous meningitis, where it can replace ethambutol in the regimen. Unfortunately, no convenient pediatric dosage form is available. Use of ethionamide may be limited by its most common side effect—vomiting. Ethionamide can increase serum concentrations of isoniazid and cycloserine. Ethionamide resistance is common in children with isoniazid resistance.[546]

Second-line medications are used when patients have drug-resistant strains of *M. tuberculosis* or when they are intolerant of first-line mediations. Second-line medications are notable for more frequent or severe adverse effects, fewer pediatric pharmacokinetic data, and fewer available child-friendly formulations than first-line drugs. Drug susceptibility testing for some second-line agents (cycloserine, linezolid, clofazimine) is less well validated than for first-line medications, and correlation between in vitro susceptibility and clinical response is less evident.

Streptomycin is used in conjunction with isoniazid and rifampin in life-threatening forms of tuberculosis. It is bactericidal and tolerated well in children in the usual dose of 20 to 40 mg/kg/day intramuscularly up to 1 g. Usually, streptomycin can be discontinued within 1 to 3 months if clinical improvement is definite, whereas the other two or three drugs are continued by mouth. Use of streptomycin and other injectable drugs (amikacin, capreomycin, kanamycin) is limited by the dose-dependent incidence of ototoxicity and nephrotoxicity. An isolate may be resistant to some injectable agents and remain susceptible to others. Streptomycin is rarely used in the United States, where less toxic alternative injectables are available.

p-Aminosalicylic acid formerly was part of the standard treatment of tuberculosis. However, it is a purely bacteriostatic drug that has been superseded by more powerful drugs (e.g., rifampin, pyrazinamide). It is used only for the treatment of drug-resistant tuberculosis. Cycloserine, linezolid, and clofazimine are other drugs sometimes used in patients with MDR-TB.[558] Cycloserine diffuses well into tissues and CSF,[157] but its use may be limited by neuropsychiatric side effects (including depression, suicidality, psychosis, aggression, tremors, paresthesias),[655] which are more common in adults. Toxicity is more common when serum levels exceed 30 µg/mL. Linezolid demonstrates modest early bactericidal activity but little extended early bactericidal activity[151]; its use may be limited by optic neuritis, peripheral neuropathy, and bone marrow suppression. Despite these adverse effects, it has been widely used in the treatment of patients with MDR-TB and XDR-TB. Almost 90% of adults experience sputum conversion after receipt of linezolid-containing regimens.[725] There are few published data regarding linezolid use in children with drug-resistant tuberculosis. Clofazimine has antiinflammatory properties, and there is little documented resistance. Addition of clofazimine to an optimized background regimen resulted in more rapid cavity closure and sputum culture conversion, as well as increased cure in a cohort of patients with MDR-TB in China.[641] Clofazimine's use may be limited by pink or brownish-black skin pigment changes.[110]

Several of the fluoroquinolones, especially levofloxacin and moxifloxacin, have significant antituberculosis activity,[303,420] but they are not used routinely in children with drug-susceptible tuberculosis because of the possible destruction of growing cartilage seen in animal models. However, the dire consequences of drug-resistant tuberculosis lead many experts to use them successfully and with little apparent toxicity in children with MDR-TB disease.[559] These drugs are bactericidal and diffuse into tissues and CSF well.[157] Children require higher milligram per kilogram dosing to achieve the same serum levels observed in adults.[205] If an isolate is resistant to one fluoroquinolone, resistance to other fluoroquinolones is common.

Microbiologic Basis for Treatment

Laboratory observations of *M. tuberculosis* and the results of clinical therapy trials have led to a hypothesis concerning the actions of various drugs and drug combinations.[176,221,417,418] The tubercle bacillus can be killed only during replication, which occurs in organisms that are active metabolically. In one model, bacilli in a host exist in different populations. They are active metabolically and replicate freely where oxygen tension is high and the pH is neutral or alkaline. Environmental conditions for growth are best within cavities, and such conditions can lead to a large bacterial population. Adults with reactivation-type pulmonary tuberculosis usually have all three populations of tubercle bacilli. Children with pulmonary tuberculosis, and patients of all ages with only extrapulmonary tuberculosis, are infected with a much smaller number of tubercle bacilli because the cavitary population is not present.

Naturally occurring drug-resistant mutant organisms occur within large populations of tubercle bacilli even before chemotherapy is started. All known genetic loci for drug resistance in *M. tuberculosis* are located on the chromosome; no plasmid-mediated resistance is known. The rate of resistance within populations of organisms is related to the rate of mutations at these loci.[407,638,646,724,726] Although a large population of bacilli as a whole may be considered drug susceptible, a subpopulation of drug-resistant organisms occurs at a fairly predictable rate. The mean frequency of these drug-resistant mutants is about 10^{-6} but varies among drugs: streptomycin, 10^{-5}; isoniazid, 10^{-6}; and rifampin, 10^{-7}.[138] A cavity containing 10^{9} tubercle bacilli has thousands of single drug–resistant mutant organisms, whereas a closed caseous lesion contains few if any resistant mutants.

The two microbiologic properties of population size and drug resistance mutation explain why single antituberculosis drugs cannot cure cavitary tuberculosis. In the mid 1940s, streptomycin alone was given to adults with cavitary pulmonary tuberculosis.[402] Within 3 months, 80% of patients had significant numbers of streptomycin-resistant organisms. This phenomenon has been observed for every antituberculosis drug developed subsequently. However, the natural occurrence of resistance to one drug is independent of resistance to any other drug because the resistance loci are not linked. The chance of having even one organism "naturally" resistant to two drugs is on the order of 10^{-11} to 10^{-13}. Populations of this size in patients are extremely rare, and mutants naturally resistant to two drugs are nonexistent.

The population size of tubercle bacilli within a patient determines the appropriate therapy. For patients with large bacterial populations (tuberculosis disease), many single drug–resistant mutants are present and at least two antituberculosis drugs must be used.[140] Conversely, for patients with tuberculosis infection but no disease, the bacterial population is small (10^{3} to 10^{4} organisms), drug-resistant mutants are rare findings, and a single drug can be used.

Some antituberculosis drugs, such as isoniazid, rifampin, streptomycin, and fluoroquinolones, are bactericidal against *M. tuberculosis.* Other drugs, including ethionamide, *p*-aminosalicylic acid, and low-dose ethambutol, are bacteriostatic. The earliest treatment regimens for tuberculosis combined the killing action of a bactericidal drug with a bacteriostatic drug that would suppress replication of drug-resistant mutant organisms. A small number of organisms survived despite administration of chemotherapy, and 18 to 24 months of treatment was necessary to permit host defenses to eliminate persisting organisms. Despite the prolonged treatment period, relapse rates were 5% to 15%, mostly a result of poor adherence.

The availability of rifampin and the rediscovery of pyrazinamide in the early 1970s effected radical change in antituberculosis chemotherapy. These two drugs have the most potent sterilizing action, the ability to kill tubercle bacilli within lesions as quickly as possible. The addition of rifampin to isoniazid for the treatment of pulmonary tuberculosis leads to cure rates approaching 100% with only 9 months of treatment. The further addition of pyrazinamide shortens the necessary treatment duration to only 6 months.

In the international community, there has been a shift away from intermittent therapy, driven in part by concern about intermittent rifamycin use in HIV-infected adults selecting for rifamycin-resistant isolates. However, there is a wealth of operational experience with intermittent therapy in the United States for both adults and children. Duration of therapy may need to be extended in HIV-infected patients. One metaanalysis found that relapse and failure rates were higher in thrice-weekly compared with daily therapy and there was a trend toward higher relapse rates in patients who were treated for 6 months when compared with those treated for at least 8 months.[306]

Treatment of the Stages of Tuberculosis

Exposure

Children exposed to potentially infectious adults with pulmonary tuberculosis should begin treatment, usually with isoniazid only, if the child is younger than 5 years or has other risk factors for the rapid development of tuberculosis disease, such as immunocompromise.[629,711] Failure to do so may result in the development of severe tuberculosis disease even before the tuberculin skin test becomes reactive; the "incubation period" of disease may be shorter than that for the skin test. The child is treated for a minimum of 2 months after contact with the infectious case is broken (by physical separation or by effective treatment of the case). After 2 months, the tuberculin skin test is repeated. If the second test result is positive, infection is documented and isoniazid should be continued for a total duration of 9 months; if the second skin test result is negative, treatment can be discontinued. If the exposure was to a person with an isoniazid-resistant but rifampin-susceptible isolate, then rifampin is the recommended treatment for 4 months.

Two special circumstances of exposure deserve attention. A difficult situation arises when exposed children are anergic because of HIV infection. These children are particularly vulnerable to rapid progression of tuberculosis, and it will not be possible to determine whether infection has occurred. In general, these children should be treated as though they have tuberculosis infection.

The second situation is potential exposure of a neonate to a mother (or other adult) with a positive tuberculin skin test result or, rarely, a nursery worker with contagious tuberculosis.[346,620] Management is based on further evaluation of the mother:

1. *The mother has a normal chest radiograph:* no separation of the infant and mother is required. Although the mother should receive treatment for tuberculosis infection and other household members should be evaluated for tuberculosis infection or disease, the infant needs no further workup and no treatment is needed unless a case of disease is found.
2. *The mother has an abnormal chest radiograph:* the mother and child should be separated until the mother has been evaluated thoroughly. If the radiograph, history, physical examination, and analysis of sputum reveal no evidence of pulmonary tuberculosis in the mother, a reasonable assumption is that the infant is at low risk for acquiring infection. The radiographic abnormality is due to another cause or a quiescent focus of previous tuberculosis infection. However, if the mother remains untreated, contagious tuberculosis may develop later and the infant will be exposed. Both the mother and infant should receive appropriate follow-up care, but the infant does not need treatment. If the radiograph and clinical history are suggestive of pulmonary tuberculosis, the child and mother should remain separated until both have begun appropriate chemotherapy. The infant should be evaluated for congenital tuberculosis. The placenta should be examined. If the mother has no risk factors for drug-resistant tuberculosis, the infant should receive isoniazid and close follow-up care. The infant should have a tuberculin skin test at 3 or 4 months after the mother is judged to be contagious no longer; evaluation of the infant at this time follows the guidelines for other exposure of children. If the mother has tuberculosis caused by a multidrug-resistant isolate of *M. tuberculosis* or she has poor adherence to therapy, the child should remain separated from her until she is no longer contagious or the infant can be given BCG vaccine and be kept separated until the vaccine "takes" (marked by a reactive tuberculin skin test).

Infection

The recommendation for treatment of asymptomatic tuberculin-positive individuals is based on data from several well-controlled studies; it applies particularly to children and adolescents who are at high risk for the development of overt disease but at very low risk for development of the main toxic manifestation of isoniazid therapy, which is hepatitis.[165,195,446,459,593] The large, carefully controlled US Public Health Study of 1955, followed by others both in this country and abroad, demonstrated the favorable effect of 12 months of isoniazid on the incidence of complications as a result of both lymphohematogenous and pulmonary spread.[259] The younger the infected person, the greater the benefit.[120]

The American Thoracic Society and the CDC[13] recommend that isoniazid for treatment of tuberculosis infection be given to several high-risk groups (Box 96.2). The question arises regarding how long the protective effect can be expected to last. Comstock and associates,[118] in their final report on isoniazid prophylaxis in Alaska, demonstrated

BOX 96.2 Persons in Whom Isoniazid (or Other Regimens) Should Be Initiated to Prevent Progression to Tuberculosis

Household members and other close associates of potentially infectious tuberculosis cases

All contacts of any age with a Mantoux tuberculin skin test reading of 5 mm or greater and without a documented history of reaction in the past or with a positive interferon gamma release assay (IGRA) should be considered recently infected and receive therapy if they have not been previously treated

Newly infected people, regardless of age, who have had a tuberculin skin test or IGRA conversion within the past 2 years

People with HIV infection who have a reaction of 5 mm or greater to a Mantoux test

People of any age with tuberculosis infection in the past who received inadequate treatment

People of any age with a positive tuberculin skin test or positive IGRA and an abnormal but stable chest radiograph

People with significant tuberculin reactions or positive IGRAs who have special clinical situations, including silicosis, diabetes mellitus, prolonged corticosteroid therapy, immunosuppressive therapy, hematologic malignant disease, and end-stage renal disease

All children and adolescents with a "positive" tuberculin skin test reaction or interferon release assay result

the protective effect of 1 year of chemoprophylaxis to be at least 19 years. Hsu[257] described 2494 patients monitored for up to 30 years and showed that adequate drug prophylaxis prevented reactivation of tuberculosis infection during adolescence and into young adulthood. It seems reasonable to hope that the decreased risk for active tuberculosis after isoniazid prophylaxis may, in fact, be lifelong in individuals infected with isoniazid-susceptible tubercle bacilli. Optimal treatment of infection caused by isoniazid-resistant *M. tuberculosis* is unclear. Rifampin alone is recommended and widely used, although failures have been reported.[360]

The duration of isoniazid treatment initially was set arbitrarily at 12 months.[272] A large trial comparing regimens of daily isoniazid for 12, 24, and 52 weeks with placebo for their ability to prevent tuberculosis disease was conducted in eastern Europe with adults who had old fibrotic lesions caused by tuberculosis. Therapy for 1 year was most effective, especially if the patients were adherent to it. However, therapy for 24 weeks afforded a fairly high level of protection. A subsequent analysis concluded that the 24-week duration of preventive therapy was more cost effective for adults than was the 52-week duration.[592] Subsequently, many health departments have accepted 6 months of isoniazid preventive therapy as their standard regimen for adults. However, the cost-effectiveness analysis does not apply to children. A recent review of all published studies concluded that the effectiveness of isoniazid therapy increased up to 9 months' duration, but no additional benefit was achieved with a longer duration.[13]

AAP and CDC recommend three regimens[13] for tuberculosis infection: 9 months of isoniazid; 4 months of rifampin; and 12 once-weekly doses of isoniazid and rifapentine. These three and other regimens used for TB infection therapy caused by presumably susceptible strains are described in Table 96.10.[124] While 9 months of isoniazid is very efficacious, adherence is abysmal, with approximately 50% of children completing therapy.[128] A shorter duration of effective treatment for tuberculosis infection is highly desirable to improve compliance and effectiveness.[386] Short-course regimens (3–4 months) with isoniazid and rifampin have been used frequently in the United Kingdom,[188,602] but are not yet recommended in the United States. Four months of rifampin is the shortest regimen recommended for daily administration in the United States. In one study, children receiving rifampin were over 7 times more likely to complete therapy than children receiving 9 months of isoniazid.[129]

More recently, pediatric data (children ≥2 years) were published for 12 weekly doses of isoniazid combined with a long-acting rifamycin,

TABLE 96.10 **Available Regimens for the Treatment of Tuberculosis Infection**

Regimen	Formulations	Dose (mg/kg) [Maximum Dose (mg)]	Advantages/Disadvantages	Selection Scenario(s)
INH + RPT × 12 doses (3HP)	INH: as above Rifapentine: Tablets: 150 mg	*INH*: 15 (round to nearest 50 mg or 100 mg) [900] *RIF*[c]: 10–14 kg: 300 mg 14.1–25 kg: 450 mg 25.1–32 kg: 600 mg 32.1–49.9 kg: 750 mg ≥50 kg: 900 mg	Pro: adherence Con: availability; need for administration via DOT	Short-course therapy desirable; need to complete therapy urgently (e.g., because child will be traveling or completion is necessary before child is to receive immunosuppressive therapy)
RIF × 4 mo	Capsule: 150 mg, 300 mg	10–20 [600]	Pro: adherence; availability Con: cost; potential drug interactions	Short-course therapy is desirable and not a candidate for 3HP (e.g., age <2 y); infected child had contact with adult with INH-resistant TB
INH × 9 mo (CDC)	Tablets: 100, 300 mg Suspension: 10 mg/mL[a]	Daily: 10–15 [300] Biweekly[b]: 20–30 [900]	Pro: ~20% added benefit over INH × 6 mo; low cost Con: low (<50%) adherence	Medication interactions preclude use of RIF; intolerant of RIF; cannot afford RIF and not eligible to receive medication via local health department; infected child had contact with adult with RIF-resistant, INH-susceptible TB
INH × 6 mo (WHO)	As above	Daily: 10–15 [300] Biweekly[b]: 20–30 [900]	Pro: adherence >9 mo Con: slightly reduced benefit compared with 9-mo regimen (assuming both taken as indicated)	
INH + RIF × 3 mo (BTS)	As above	INH: 10–15 [300] RIF: 10–15 [600]	Pro: adherence Con: slightly increased risk of side effects compared to monotherapy	Short-course therapy desirable and 3HP unavailable or family reluctant to receive medication under DOT Use of this regimen likely to be low in the US given availability of 3HP
RIF + PZA × 2 mo	RIF: as above PZA: Tablets: 500 mg	Study in adults: RIF: 600 mg PZA: 15–20 mg/kg/day [2 g]	Pro: adherence Con: hepatotoxicity; now only recommended for patients initially suspected of having TB disease	Children initially started on therapy for TB disease and later suspected of having TB infection instead; if at least 2 mo of RIF/PZA have been completed, this comprises adequate TB infection therapy

[a]Many commercially available formulations of INH suspension are sorbitol based and cause profuse diarrhea; providers should limit use of INH suspension only to very young infants. INH tablets can be crushed and mixed with pureed food or a small volume of formula even for young babies.
[b]Intermittent dosing should only be used if the child is receiving DOT.
[c]Rifapentine dose is in mg, not mg/kg.
BTS, British Thoracic Society; *CDC,* Centers for Disease Control and Prevention; *DOT,* directly observed therapy; *INH,* isoniazid; *PZA,* pyrazinamide; *RIF,* rifampin; *RPT,* rifapentine; *TB,* tuberculosis; *WHO,* World Health Organization.

rifapentine (termed 3HP).[623,683] This regimen was as safe and at least as effective in preventing disease as 9 months of isoniazid, but had far higher completion rates. Use of this regimen has been limited by drug availability and by the need to administer medications under directly observed therapy. While in adults, influenza-like illness, myalgias (which peak in the second or third week of therapy and are responsive to nonsteroidal antiinflammatory drugs), and skin rashes are common,[622] these seem to be infrequently observed in children.

Isoniazid preventive therapy in HIV-infected patients has been best studied in adults.[394] The theoretical advantages of this therapy in settings with high tuberculosis prevalence are that persons may be exposed without knowledge of a specific source case; HIV-infected patients may be anergic to the tuberculin skin test (and have high rates of indeterminate IGRA results); and HIV-infected persons with tuberculosis infection are at high risk for rapidly progressing to tuberculosis disease. The potential disadvantages are the potential of selecting for isoniazid-resistant isolates, inadvertently treating patients for infection when they have disease, drug toxicity in a patient who may not have infection, and cost. Randomized trials have shown IPT to be effective in preventing tuberculosis disease-free survival in adults, irrespective of the use of HAART. Isoniazid preventive therapy in HIV-infected children is controversial. Two large randomized studies have evaluated its impact on survival and tuberculosis disease-free survival in HIV-infected African children. Whereas one study showed decreased all-cause mortality and decreased cases of tuberculosis disease,[721] a second study found no benefit.[370] Additional data are needed to determine what role isoniazid preventive therapy should have in national tuberculosis programs in settings with high prevalence of both HIV and tuberculosis.

Chemotherapy for Children

Clinical trials of antituberculosis drugs in children are difficult to perform, mostly because of the difficulty in obtaining positive cultures at diagnosis or relapse and the need for long-term follow-up.[605,606] Historically, recommendations for treating children with tuberculosis have been extrapolated from clinical trials of adults with pulmonary tuberculosis.[585] However, during the past 2 decades, a large number of clinical trials involving only children have been reported. In 1983, Abernathy and colleagues[2] reported successful treatment of 50 children with tuberculosis in Arkansas using isoniazid and rifampin daily for 1 month, then twice weekly for 8 months. The success rate virtually was 100%. Most pulmonary infiltrates cleared by the end of therapy, but hilar adenopathy usually was still present radiographically and then gradually cleared over 2 to 3 years. Patients with only hilar adenopathy can be treated successfully with isoniazid and rifampin for 6 months.[277,511] In children with cavitary lung disease or children with persistently positive sputum cultures after 2 months of effective therapy, therapy may be extended to 9 months to decrease relapse rates.[94]

Several major studies of 6-month therapy in children with at least three drugs in the initial phase have been reported.[8,47,266,321,636,642,662] The regimen used most commonly was 6 months of isoniazid and rifampin supplemented during the first 2 months with pyrazinamide. The overall success rate was greater than 98% and the incidence of clinically significant adverse reactions less than 2%. Use of streptomycin did not improve treatment outcomes. Use of twice-weekly medications (under directly observed therapy) during the continuation phase was as effective and safe as was daily administration. Three studies used twice-weekly therapy throughout the treatment regimen with excellent success.[321,642,678] The 6-month, three-drug regimen is successful, tolerated well, and less expensive.[627,663] It also effects a cure faster, so the likelihood of successful treatment is greater if the child becomes nonadherent later in therapy. Current CDC and ATS recommendations are to include ethambutol with isoniazid, rifampin, and pyrazinamide during the initial phase unless the child's source case is known to have an *M. tuberculosis* isolate susceptible to first-line medications.

The optimal duration of therapy and dosing interval for antituberculous medications in children coinfected with HIV is unclear. Relapse or failure in up to 12% of HIV-infected children treated for 6 months has been reported.[545] The optimal timing for initiation of HAART in children with tuberculosis disease is unclear, but extrapolation from adult data suggests a survival benefit from initiation within 2 to 8 weeks.[291,568] Selection of a HAART regimen may be complicated by the known interaction of rifampin with protease inhibitors. Although these interactions are decreased by using rifabutin, some nations have deferred protease inhibitors to second-line HAART because of these interactions. Further complicating care of the coinfected child is the risk for IRIS and that children on both HAART and antituberculous medications tend to tolerate both classes of medication more poorly than children receiving one or the other.[680]

Extrapulmonary Tuberculosis

Controlled treatment trials for various forms of extrapulmonary tuberculosis are rare. In most reports, extrapulmonary cases have been combined with pulmonary cases and often are not analyzed separately. Several of the 6-month, three-drug trials in children included extrapulmonary cases.[47,321] Most non–life-threatening forms of extrapulmonary tuberculosis respond well to a 9-month course of isoniazid and rifampin[175,177] or to a 6-month regimen including isoniazid, rifampin, and pyrazinamide.[275] One exception may be bone and joint tuberculosis, which may have a high failure rate when 6-month chemotherapy is used, especially if surgical intervention has not occurred.[175] Tuberculous meningitis usually is not included in trials of extrapulmonary tuberculosis therapy because of its serious nature and low incidence. Treatment with isoniazid and rifampin for 9 to 12 months generally is effective.[684] Data from Thailand showed that a 6-month regimen that included pyrazinamide for serious tuberculous meningitis led to fewer deaths and better outcomes than did longer regimens that did not contain pyrazinamide.[278] Most children are treated initially with four drugs (isoniazid, rifampin, pyrazinamide, and ethionamide or an injectable agent). Ethambutol crosses the blood-brain barrier very poorly,[157] making it a suboptimal choice for treating children with tuberculous meningitis. Treatment with pyrazinamide and the fourth drug is stopped after 2 months, and isoniazid and rifampin are continued for a total of 9 to 12 months.[161]

Drug-Resistant Tuberculosis in Children

The incidence of drug-resistant tuberculosis is increasing because of poor adherence by the patient, the availability of some antituberculosis drugs in noncontrolled over-the-counter formulations, and poor management by physicians.[49,199,200,372,455] In the United States, approximately 13% of *M. tuberculosis* isolates are resistant to at least one drug and 1.2% are MDR-TB[112]; rates of drug resistance are more than twice as high in foreign-born cases than in US-born persons with disease. Initial drug resistance rates of up to 80% have been noted in adults with pulmonary tuberculosis in some countries,[373] and rates of 20% to 30% are common findings. Resistance is most common to streptomycin and isoniazid and still is relatively rare to rifampin.[144,251,419,729] Rifampin monoresistance is unusual[166]; in the vast majority of cases, rifampin resistance is seen in conjunction with isoniazid resistance. Certain epidemiologic factors—disease in an Asian or Hispanic immigrant to the United States, homelessness in some communities, and history of previous antituberculosis therapy—correlate with drug resistance in adult patients.[16] Patterns of drug resistance in children tend to mirror those found in adult patients in the population.[86,543,565,619] Outbreaks of drug-resistant tuberculosis in children occurring at schools have been reported.[86,516] Individual cases also have been recognized. The key to determining drug resistance in childhood tuberculosis usually comes from the drug susceptibility results of the infectious adult contact case's isolate.

Therapy for drug-resistant tuberculosis is successful only when at least two bactericidal drugs are given to which the infecting strain of *M. tuberculosis* is susceptible.[74,480,542,647] If only one effective drug is given, secondary resistance will develop. Exact treatment regimens must be tailored to the specific pattern of drug resistance. The duration of therapy usually is extended to at least 9 to 12 months if either isoniazid or rifampin can be used and to at least 18 to 24 months if resistance to both drugs is present.[274] Children tend to tolerate second-line antituberculosis drugs well, and community-based treatment usually is successful.[170,432] This is reflected in the lower mortality rates seen in children than in adults with MDR-TB. One pediatric series of children with MDR-TB in South Africa demonstrated 25-fold and almost 40-fold increases in mortality for children with MDR-TB and HIV coinfection and extrapulmonary tuberculosis, respectively.[559] On occasion, surgical resection of a diseased lung or lobe is required.[276,717] One metaanalysis showed that estimated success rates for pulmonary resection in adults with MDR-TB were over 80%,[716] a substantial improvement over the 50% to 65% survival seen with medical therapy alone.[466]

Treatment of a child with MDR-TB or XDR-TB exposure or infection is controversial. The benefit of preventing progression to disease, especially in a child with ongoing exposure, must be balanced against the scant pharmacokinetic, safety, and efficacy data available for many second-line medications. The role of treating the exposed child with contact to an adult with MDR-TB is unclear. For infected children whose source case has MDR-TB, combination therapy with one or two drugs to which the isolate is susceptible may be considered; use of a 12-month course of fluoroquinolones in the regimen (either as monotherapy or as part of combination therapy) has been effective,[28,395] although longitudinal outcomes are unknown. Many children require treatment modification due to adverse events if more than one drug is given. Optimal treatment duration is unknown. At least 6 to 9 months of therapy should be attempted. An expert in tuberculosis always should be involved in the management of children with drug-resistant tuberculosis infection or disease.

Adherence and Directly Observed Therapy

Nonadherence with drug treatment by patients is a major problem in control of tuberculosis because of the long-term nature of its treatment.[410,632,675] As treatment regimens become shorter in duration, adherence assumes an even greater importance. Suspected cases of tuberculosis must be reported to the local health department so that it can perform the necessary contact investigations and assist both patients and health care providers in overcoming barriers to adherence. To comply, the patient and family must know what is expected of them through verbal and written instructions in the patient's preferred language. Missed appointments should be brought quickly to the attention of the responsible public health officials, who may be able to use incentives or enablers, behavior modification, or, rarely, confinement to ensure adherence. The success of twice-weekly therapy, especially after a period of daily administration of medications, allows directly observed therapy to be given by a health care professional in cases of proven or suspected nonadherence.[102,103,275,651] Most experts hold that twice-weekly medication should be administered only under the direct observation of a health care worker.[317,698] Direct observation means that a health care worker or other nonrelated third party (e.g., teacher, school nurse, social worker) is physically present while the patient ingests the medication. A substantial number of children and their families are nonadherent with therapy. One study of isoniazid preventive therapy after tuberculosis exposure showed that 33% took medications for at least 4 months and only 12% completed a 6-month course.[207] Adherence is inaccurately predicted by physicians. There are no documented differences in completion rates by child's age or duration of time the family has been in the United States.[498] In one study, the only factor associated with completion of tuberculosis infection therapy was health department-enabled medication administration.[128] In most communities in the United States and in an increasing number of other nations, directly observed therapy is the standard of care for all patients with tuberculosis disease.[90,189] However, when directly observed therapy cannot be used, structured behavior interactions can increase compliance with treatment.[82,642]

Summary of Treatment Recommendations

1. A regimen of isoniazid and rifampin for 6 months, supplemented with pyrazinamide during the first 2 months and ethambutol for 2 months or until the source case is known to be susceptible to all first-line agents, is standard therapy for children with suspected intrathoracic tuberculosis in the United States and Canada.
2. An alternative regimen is isoniazid and rifampin for 9 months. The disadvantages of this regimen include a longer duration, the potential for increased drug resistance during therapy, and less effectiveness if the patient absconds from treatment. This regimen should be used only if pyrazinamide cannot be tolerated.
3. After an initial 2 weeks to 2 months of daily drug administration, drugs can be given twice weekly under directly observed therapy with excellent effectiveness.[494] With patients for whom social or other restraints prevent reliable daily self-administration even during the initial phase of therapy, drugs can be given two or three times per week from the beginning under directly observed therapy.
4. In most cases, extrapulmonary tuberculosis can be treated with the same regimens as used for pulmonary tuberculosis, although data for tuberculous meningitis and bone or joint disease are relatively lacking. The duration of therapy is extended for tuberculous meningitis, osteoarticular tuberculosis, and children with substantial pulmonary disease after 6 months of therapy.[94,712]
5. Optimal therapy for tuberculosis in children with HIV infection has not been established.[628] Most HIV-infected adults with tuberculosis respond well to antituberculosis drugs but may require longer durations of treatment; higher failure and relapse rates were noted if rifamycins were used for only 6 months.[306] Immunosuppressed children with tuberculosis, including those with HIV infection, should be treated with at least three drugs initially, and treatment should be continued for a minimum of 9 months. Intermittent therapy is not recommended for HIV-infected children.[712] HIV testing is recommended for all infants and children with tuberculosis disease.
6. Tuberculosis disease occurring during pregnancy should be treated with a 9-month regimen of isoniazid and rifampin, supplemented during the initial phase with ethambutol (streptomycin should not be used). The use of pyrazinamide in pregnant patients is controversial although probably safe.

Corticosteroids

Corticosteroids have a place in the treatment of patients with tuberculosis. They should never be used except under cover of effective antituberculosis drugs. Corticosteroids would be expected to be beneficial in situations in which the host inflammatory reaction is contributing to tissue damage or is impairing function.

Corticosteroids often are a useful addition to antituberculosis drugs if suppression of inflammatory reaction is desired, such as in the following situations[584]:

1. In patients with tuberculous meningitis in whom increased intracranial pressure is present.[657] The major actions are to reduce vasculitis, inflammation, and, ultimately, intracranial pressure. Not only is reduction of pressure desirable, but lowering of the pressure also probably favors the circulation of chemotherapeutic drugs through the brain and meninges.[193] One metaanalysis demonstrated lower rates of mortality and long-term neurologic sequelae in patients with tuberculous meningitis treated with corticosteroids than in children and adults not treated with corticosteroids.[499]
2. In patients with acute pericardial effusion in whom tamponade is occurring. Relief of symptoms takes place within hours. Use of corticosteroids reduced symptoms and mortality but not echocardiographic resolution of the effusion in both HIV-infected[228] and HIV-uninfected[630] children and adults. There appears to be a reluctance to use corticosteroids in HIV-infected patients with tuberculous pericarditis,[708] but increased mortality has not occurred when corticosteroids are utilized in conjunction with antituberculosis chemotherapy.
3. In patients with pleural effusion associated with mediastinal shift and impending respiratory failure.[337] The long-term course probably is the same with or without corticosteroids, but symptomatic improvement usually is dramatic. One randomized trial of corticosteroid use for pleural tuberculosis in HIV-infected adults showed more rapid disease resolution, but increased rates of Kaposi sarcoma and no change in mortality, in corticosteroid recipients[186]; although both groups had similar CD4 cell counts and viral loads, no antiretroviral agents were provided, making it difficult to extrapolate the findings. Similar data are unavailable for children.
4. In patients with miliary tuberculosis if the inflammatory reaction is so severe that it produces alveolocapillary block with cyanosis.
5. In patients with enlarged mediastinal lymph nodes that are causing respiratory difficulty or a severe collapse-consolidation lesion, particularly in the middle or lower lobes, when bronchiectasis is likely to be a troublesome sequela.[444] Under either of these circumstances, a course of corticosteroids is warranted, with the realization that it will be more successful in an early infection because inflammation characterizes the first stages of tuberculosis. If caseation already is advanced, corticosteroids will be of little benefit.
6. In patients with IRIS whose reactions are either severe (e.g., airway compromise, brainstem herniation) or whose symptoms are refractory to therapy with nonsteroidal antiinflammatory medications.[408]

The dosage of corticosteroids should be in the antiinflammatory range, that is, prednisone 1 to 2 mg/kg per day for 4 to 6 weeks with gradual withdrawal. Some experts prefer dexamethasone, but no comparative trials have been published.

Activity

Activity need not be restricted in children with tuberculosis, except when a particular complication is inevitable (shortness of breath in pleural effusion, immobilization for a vertebral lesion).

Isolation

Isolation should be maintained for children with cavitary lesions, productive cough with acid-fast stain-positive sputum, draining sinuses, or renal tuberculosis until their secretions are negative on smear and preferably on culture. Young children are virtually noninfectious because they rarely cough and because their bronchial secretions contain few bacilli compared with those of adults with tuberculosis. Guidelines issued by the CDC state that most children with typical tuberculosis do not require isolation in the hospital.[95] Children with possible pulmonary tuberculosis should be treated as potentially infectious if they have a cavity or extensive upper lobe infiltrate, if they have a productive cough (especially if the sputum is acid-fast smear positive), or during high-risk procedures such as bronchoscopy. Although most children are not contagious with tuberculosis, the same cannot be said of their adult caregivers. Two studies in a relatively high-prevalence area of the United States showed that up to 17% of children admitted to the hospital for tuberculosis were accompanied by an adult with as yet undiagnosed tuberculosis.[126,436] Consideration should be given to screening caregivers of these children symptomatically or radiographically.

Follow-Up

Follow-up of children treated with antituberculosis drugs has become somewhat more streamlined in recent years. While receiving chemotherapy, the patient should be seen monthly, both to encourage regular intake of the prescribed drugs and to check, by a few simple questions (concerning appetite, well-being) and a few observations (weight gain; appearance of the skin and sclerae; palpation of the liver, spleen, and lymph nodes), that the disease is not spreading, and that toxic effects of the drugs are not appearing.[700] Repeated chest radiographs should be obtained 1 to 2 months after the onset of chemotherapy to ascertain the maximal extent of disease before chemotherapy takes effect; thereafter, radiographs rarely are necessary.[313] Radiographic worsening at this time may be an indication of IRIS, the presence of drug-resistant tuberculosis, and/or adherence difficulties. Therefore, it is important to obtain this radiograph before stopping four-drug therapy and starting isoniazid and rifampin. If the radiograph at 1 to 2 months has normalized, subsequent imaging is unnecessary unless the child's disease worsens clinically. If the radiograph at 1 to 2 months is abnormal, repeating imaging at the conclusion of therapy is helpful to reestablish a new radiographic baseline for the child. Chemotherapy has been so successful that follow-up beyond its termination is not necessary, except for children with serious disease, such as tuberculous meningitis, or those with extensive residual chest radiographic findings at the end of chemotherapy.

Case Reporting

Every case of definite or suspected tuberculosis, by United States law,[89] must be reported immediately by telephone to the health authority[213] to ensure prompt contact investigation.[255] Free antituberculosis drugs are available for diagnosed cases and for close contacts in almost every state of the United States and in many countries.

Prevention

Prevention of tuberculosis can be subdivided logically to consider the following circumstances:

1. Protection against exposure to the disease
2. Use of antituberculosis drugs in tuberculin-negative individuals at high risk for development of infection[556]
3. Immunization of tuberculin-negative individuals

Protection against exposure to disease is the ideal form of prevention.[388,406] It presupposes thorough preemployment and ongoing case-finding programs among all who come in contact with children, including daycare center and school personnel, Sunday school personnel, teachers, health care workers, babysitters, household servants, food handlers, beauticians, and barbers. Numerous epidemics, miniepidemics, and mass exposures in neonatal nurseries have been traced to such infected individuals.

Immunization

Immunization against tuberculosis theoretically would be a tremendous boon to humanity, but in practice it has been fraught with very great difficulty. The impossibility of standardizing vaccines in the early days,[45,219,648] differences in inoculation techniques and amount of bacteria inoculated, the lack of any clinically useful test reflecting the immune status of the individual, and the relatively slow course of the disease have handicapped epidemiologic studies. A number of new vaccines are in human clinical trials. These studies use surrogate markers of interferon, interleukin, and other cytokine responses as measures of vaccine take, because finding correlates of protection remains elusive.[233,557]

BCG was developed in 1908 using an attenuated strain of *M. bovis*. In 1921, it first was administered orally to neonates and since then has been given to more than 4 billion people. BCG vaccine attempts to replace the potentially dangerous primary infection with *M. tuberculosis* with an innocuous primary infection with the bacillus of Calmette and Guérin, thus activating host cell-mediated immunity with minimal chance of causing progressive disease so that an infection with *M. tuberculosis* will be of the "reinfection" type.[354]

Difficulties in evaluation the BCG vaccine include variation in strain and differences in inoculation techniques and doses used. For almost 60 years, several BCG strains of different potencies were in use. The WHO, through its International Reference Preparation for BCG vaccine and through quality control testing, has helped decrease the gross variations in BCG vaccine found until recent years. Vaccination techniques and dosages are variable. Intradermal injection is the most precise technique. Multiple-puncture techniques are popular because they are easy, but less effective than intradermal injection. Oral vaccination, the original method of administration, largely has been abandoned because of poor results. The actual dose of BCG at present usually is approximately 10^6 culturable particles. Because in animals large doses produce better resistance to challenge than small ones do, the largest convenient dose is used. However, in neonates, who have a higher incidence of untoward reactions, the customary approach is to halve the dose generally used in older infants and children to prevent local complications.

The usual local reaction to intradermal BCG vaccine is the development of a papule at the site of vaccination, and this papule reaches its maximal diameter (10 to 20 mm) in the sixth week. A small crust that may form on the papule detaches at about this time, with only a small ulcer remaining that may discharge a surprising amount of pus. Most ulcers are healed by the 10th week. A small scar is visible in over 80% of BCG-vaccinated individuals.[308,536] Enlargement of the regional (axillary) lymph nodes occurs regularly and is painless, sometimes ending in calcification. Formation of an abscess with breakdown is a rare event, but it occurs more often in infants.

Untoward reactions to BCG rarely have been a problem.[665] Fatalities caused by progressive disease have been reported in no more than 60 vaccine recipients (of an estimated 4+ billion), usually (but not always) children with well-documented immunodeficiency.[78,145,191,215,486,491] No return of the attenuated strain to virulence has ever been noted. In countries where BCG is used routinely for immunization of neonates, osteomyelitis has been diagnosed in some 5 per 100,000 neonates. It usually becomes manifested when the child is between 5 and 33 months of age, when a tender swelling is noted near a joint; bone destruction is well localized and responds to conservative treatment.[101] On the whole, BCG is one of the safest vaccines in use.

In many countries where BCG is given routinely, the incidence of HIV infection in adults and children is high.[64,524] Reports of local and systemic complications from BCG vaccine in HIV-infected people are increasing, but the true magnitude of the interaction is not yet known.[43,240,241,460,510] However, in more recent studies, the rate of adverse BCG reactions in HIV-infected children appears to be higher than thought previously.[240,241] In most cases, BCG complications occur shortly after vaccination, but in one man with AIDS, adenitis as a result of BCG occurred 30 years after inoculation.[513] Routine treatment of patients with previous BCG vaccination who subsequently become immunocompromised is not recommended, but the clinician should be aware of previous BCG vaccination if signs or symptoms of mycobacterial infection occur.

The efficacy of BCG vaccines in humans has been evaluated in several large, well-controlled studies (Table 96.11). Three of these trials showed excellent protection, two showed mediocre protection, and two showed

TABLE 96.11 Summary of Eight Large Controlled Trials of BCG Immunization Against Tuberculosis

Subjects	Investigators	Intake Period	Vaccine Laboratory	Duration of Observation (y)	% Protection from BCG
North America: American Indians	Stein and Aronson, 1953	1935–38	Phipps	9–11	80
Chicago: infants	Rosenthal et al., 1961	1937–48	Tice	12–23	75
Britain: schoolchildren	Medical Research Council, 1971	1950–52	Copenhagen	15	78
South India: rural population	Frimodt-Moller et al., 1964	1950–55	Madras	2.5–7	60/31[a]
Puerto Rico: children	Palmer et al., 1958	1949–51	New York State	5.5–7.5	31
Georgia, Alabama: population	Comstock and Palmer, 1966	1950	Tice	14	14
Georgia: schoolchildren	Comstock and Webster, 1969	1947	Tice	20	0
Brazil: schoolchildren[b]	Pereira et al., 2011	1996–98	Moreaux	9	25

Modified from Sutherland, quoted by Eickhoff TC. The current status of BCG immunization against tuberculosis. *Annu Rev Med.* 1977;28:411–23.

[a]Initial estimate of efficacy was 60%. Subsequently, when follow-up was extended to 9 to 14 y, the efficacy figure declined to 31%.

[b]BCG vaccine given for the first time to children age 7–14 y.

BCG, Bacillus Calmette-Guérin.

little or no effect of BCG. Explanations for these differences in outcomes among trials must be sought in the quality and characteristics of the BCG vaccine used in the particular trial, the possible immunizing effect (in Georgia and Alabama) of infections with other mycobacteria,[588] the possibly greater effectiveness of BCG vaccine in areas of high tuberculosis prevalence, and methodological variations among the trials.

The most recent large study of BCG effectiveness is the Chingleput study, started in 1968 near Madras, South India, an area where sensitization with nontuberculous mycobacteria is prevalent. People of all ages were vaccinated with one of two BCG vaccines or a placebo; only the incidence of adult-type pulmonary tuberculosis in the three groups was compared (i.e., not the forms usually found in children). During the ensuing years, no difference in incidence was noted among the three groups.[21] This disturbing result has been the subject of several WHO investigations because BCG is one of the vaccines recommended for all children in the Expanded Program of Immunization sponsored by the WHO itself.[512] Another study of neonatal vaccination with BCG in England reported very favorable results with BCG.[132] Most countries administer BCG to infants. In some nations, multiple doses of BCG are used. The few data that are available on revaccination show a modest efficacy (9%).[31,519] Revaccination with BCG is not recommended by the WHO. Higher effectiveness (up to 25% more effective than when BCG is given to neonates) is seen when BCG is given to school-aged children who never received BCG as infants.[492]

A group at the Harvard School of Public Health reviewed all published studies of BCG efficacy in a metaanalysis.[116] Most published trials were not analyzed because of serious flaws in their experimental design or reporting. Among all trials and case-control studies included, the average protection against tuberculosis disease by various BCG preparations was 50%. The protective levels were higher for disease in children, particularly for meningitis and tuberculosis-associated death.[115,661] However, ascertainment bias and lack of standardized case definitions render the results of these analyses very difficult to interpret. A more recent metaanalysis included 132 studies and indicated that there was evidence of measurable protection against intra- and extrathoracic TB for at least 10 years after vaccination.[3] The BCG vaccines prevent many cases of tuberculosis in children, but the effect is quite variable. Variation in effectiveness of BCG in pulmonary tuberculosis has been seen across a number of trials. It has been hypothesized that these differences may be due to differences in BCG strains, overattenuation of BCG strains, interference in immunologic response caused by nontuberculous mycobacteria, and polymorphisms seen in human populations.[305] That BCG vaccines are not an instrument of tuberculosis control also has become apparent because they do not prevent infection with *M. tuberculosis,* their protective effect is short lived, and vaccination of infants does little to prevent future cases of contagious tuberculosis among adults in a community.

The role of BCG vaccine in the United States today is very limited. The Advisory Committee on Immunization Practices of the US Public Health Service and the Advisory Council for the Elimination of Tuberculosis recommend BCG only for tuberculin-negative infants and children in the United States who (1) are at high risk for having intimate and prolonged exposure to persistently untreated or ineffectively treated adults with infectious pulmonary tuberculosis, cannot be removed from the source of infection, and cannot be prescribed long-term preventive therapy or (2) continuously are exposed to people with tuberculosis resistant to isoniazid and rifampin. A few experts, however, are more inclined toward the use of BCG in neonates who are at any risk for exposure to tuberculosis whatsoever.[299,300,579,658]

The BCG vaccine has been used in healthcare workers in settings with high MDR-TB incidence to decrease their risk for nosocomial infection.[65] The utility of this strategy is unclear, but in regions where healthcare workers, many of whom are HIV infected, are continually exposed to MDR-TB, BCG vaccination may be a sustainable strategy.

Contraindications to the use of BCG for prevention of tuberculosis include congenital immunodeficiency, known HIV infection (in the United States), leukemia, lymphoma, and generalized malignant disease, as well as treatment with corticosteroids, alkylating agents, antimetabolites, and radiation. The WHO recommends giving BCG to asymptomatic HIV-infected infants who reside in areas with high tuberculosis rates.

NEW REFERENCES SINCE THE SEVENTH EDITION

3. Abubakar I, Pimpin L, Ariti C, et al. Systematic review and meta-analysis of the current evidence on the duration of protection by bacillus Calmette-Guérin vaccination against tuberculosis. *Health Technol Assess.* 2013;17:1-372.
28. Bamrah S, Brostrom R, Dorina F, et al. Treatment for LTBI in contacts of MDR-TB patients, Federated States of Micronesia, 2009-2012. *Int J Tuberc Lung Dis.* 2014;18:912-918.
51. Blandinières A, de Lauzanne A, Guérin-El Khourouj V, et al. QuantiFERON to diagnose infection by Mycobacterium tuberculosis: performance in infants and older children. *J Infect.* 2013;67:391-398.
65. Brewer TF, Colditz GA. Bacille Calmette-Guérin vaccination for the prevention of tuberculosis in healthcare workers. *Clin Infect Dis.* 1995;20:136-142.
68. Bui DH, Cruz AT, Graviss EA. Indeterminate QuantiFERON-TB gold in-tube assay results in children: possible association with procedural specimen collection. *Pediatr Infect Dis J.* 2014;33:220-222.
75. Campbell PJ, Morlock GP, Sikes RD, et al. Molecular detection of mutations associated with first- and second-line drug resistance compared with conventional drug susceptibility testing of *Mycobacterium tuberculosis. Antimicrob Agents Chemother.* 2011;55:2032-2041.
81. Carvalho AC, Schumacher RF, Bigoni S, et al. Contact investigation based on serial interferon-gamma release assays (IGRA) in children from the hematology-oincology ward after exposure to a patient with pulmonary tuberculosis. *Infection.* 2013;41:827-831.
95. Centers for Disease Control and Prevention. Leveling of tuberculosis incidence – United States, 2013-2015. *MMWR Morb Mortal Wkly Rep.* 2016;65:273-278.
96. Centers for Disease Control and Prevention. CDC Immigration Requirements: technical instructions for tuberculosis screening and treatment; 2009. Available online at: http://www.cdc.gov/immigrantrefugeehealth/pdf/tuberculosis-ti-2009.pdf. Accessed 28 January 2015.
107. Chiang SS, Khan FA, Milstein MB, et al. Treatment outcomes of childhood tuberculous meningitis: a systematic review and meta-analysis. *Lancet Infect Dis.* 2014;14:947-957.
124. Cruz AT, Ahmed A, Mandalakas AM, Starke JR. Treatment of latent tuberculosis infection in children. *J Pediatric Infect Dis Soc.* 2013;2:248-258.
129. Cruz AT, Starke JR. Safety and completion of a 4-month course of rifampicin for latent tuberculosis infection in children. *Int J Tuberc Lung Dis.* 2014;18:1057-1061.
147. Detjen AK, DiNardo AR, Leyden J, et al. Xpert MTB/RIF assay for the diagnosis of pulmonary tuberculosis in children: a systematic review and meta-analysis. *Lancet Respir Med.* 2015;3:451-461.
154. Dodd PJ, Gardiner E, Coghlan R, Seddon JA. Burden of childhood tuberculosis in 22 high-burden countries: a mathematical modelling study. *Lancet Glob Health.* 2014;2:e453-e459.
202. Gallivan M, Shah N, Flood J. Epidemiology of human *Mycobacterium bovis* disease, California, USA, 2003-2011. *Emerg Infect Dis.* 2015;21:435-443.
204. Gao L, Lu W, Bai L, et al. Latent tuberculosis infection in rural China: baseline results of a population-based, multicentre, prospective cohort study. *Lancet Infect Dis.* 2015;15:310-319.
205. Garcia-Prats AJ, Draper HR, Thee S, et al. Pharmacokinetics and safety of ofloxacin in children with drug-resistant tuberculosis. *Antimicrob Agents Chemother.* 2015;59:6073-6079.
210. Giang DC, Duong TN, Ha DTM, et al. Prospective evaluation of GeneXpert for the diagnosis of HIV-negative pediatric TB cases. *BMC Infect Dis.* 2015;15:70.
237. Heller T, Goblirsch S, Bahlas S, et al. Diagnostic value of FASH ultrasound and chest X-ray in HIV co-infected patients with abdominal tuberculosis. *Int J Tuberc Lung Dis.* 2013;17:342-344.
270. Imazio M, Gaita F, LeWinter M. Evaluation and treatment of pericarditis: a systematic review. *JAMA.* 2015;314:1498-1506.
283. Jenkins HE, Tolman AW, Yuen CM, et al. Incidence of multidrug-resistant tuberculosis disease in children: systematic review and global estimates. *Lancet.* 2014;383:1572-1579.
289. Jones-Lopez EC, Namugga O, Mumbowa F, et al. Cough aerosols of Mycobacterium predict new infection: a household contact study. *Am J Respir Crit Care Med.* 2013;187:1007-1015.
338. Leeb S, Buxbaum C, Fischler B. Elevated transaminases are common in children on prophylactic treatment for tuberculosis. *Acta Paediatr.* 2015;104:479-484.
356. Ling DI, Zwerling AA, Pai M. GenoType MTBDR assays for the diagnosis of multidrug-resistant tuberculosis: a meta-analysis. *Eur Respir J.* 2008;32:1165-1174.
355. Ling DI, Nicol MP, Pai M, et al. Incremental value of T-SPOT.TB for diagnosis of active pulmonary tuberculosis in children in a high-burden setting: a multivariable analysis. *Thorax.* 2013;68:860-866.
357. Link-Gelles R, Moultrie H, Sawry S, et al. Tuberculosis immune reconstitution inflammatory syndrome in children initiating antiretroviral therapy for HIV infection: a systematic literature review. *Pediatr Infect Dis J.* 2014;33:499-503.
377. Mandalakas AM, Kirchner HL, Walzl G, et al. Optimizing the detection of recent tuberculosis infection in children in a high tuberculosis-HIV burden setting. *Am J Respir Crit Care Med.* 2015;191:820-830.

378. Mandalakas AM, van Wyk S, Kirchner HL, et al. Detecting tuberculosis infection in HIV-infected children: a study of diagnostic accuracy, confounding and interaction. *Pediatr Infect Dis J.* 2013;32:e111-e118.
395. Mase SR, Jereb JA, Gonzalez D, et al. Pharmacokinetics and dosing of levofloxacin in children treated for active or latent multidrug-resistant tuberculosis, Federated States of Micronesia and Republic of the Marshall Islands. *Pediatr Infect Dis J.* 2015 [e-published ahead of print December 10, 2015].
430. Moya PA, Malinvaud D, Mimoun M, et al. Tuberculous otomastoiditis: advantage of MRI in the treatment survey. *Rev Laryngol Otol Rhinol (Bord).* 2008;129:301-304.
440. Nansumba M, Kumbakumba E, Orikiriza P, et al. Detection yield and tolerability of string test for diagnosis of childhood intrathoracic tuberculosis. *Pediatr Infect Dis J.* 2016;35:146-151.
458. Oberhelman RA, Soto-Castellares G, Gilman RH, et al. A controlled study of tuberculosis diagnosis in HIV-infected and uninfected children in Peru. *PLoS ONE.* 2015;10:e0120915.
469. Ostermann M, Palchaudhuri P, Riding A, et al. Incidence of tuberculosis is high in chronic kidney disease patients in South East England and drug resistance is common. *Ren Fail.* 2016;38:256-261.
472. Pai M, Denkinger CM, Kik SV, et al. Gamma interferon release assays for detection of *Mycobacterium tuberculosis* infection. *Clin Microbiol Rev.* 2014;27:3-20.
477. Pandie S, Peter JG, Kerkbelker ZS, et al. Diagnostic accuracy of quantitative PCR (Xpert MTB/RIF) for tuberculous pericarditis compared to adenosine deaminase and unstimulated interferon-gamma in a high-burden setting. *BMC Med.* 2014;12:101.
496. Pesciaroli M, Alvarez J, Boniotti MB, et al. Tuberculosis in domestic animal species. *Res Vet Sci.* 2014;97(suppl):S78-S85.
521. Rose W, Kitai I, Kakkar F, et al. Quantiferon Gold-in-tube assay for TB screening in HIV infected children: influence of quantitative values. *BMC Infect Dis.* 2014;14:516.
522. Rose W, Read SE, Bitnun A, et al. Relating tuberculosis (TB) contact characteristics to QuantiFERON-TB-Gold and tuberculin skin test results in the Toronto pediatric TB clinic. *J Pediatric Infect Dis Soc.* 2015;4:96-103.
532. Sallami S, Ghariani R, Hichri A, et al. Imaging findings of urinary tuberculosis on computed tomography versus excretory urography: through 46 confirmed cases. *Tunis Med.* 2014;92:743-747.
552. Schopfer K, Rieder HL, Bodmer T, et al. The sensitivity of an interferon-γ release assay in microbiologically confirmed pediatric tuberculosis. *Eur J Pediatr.* 2014;173:331-336.
567. Shah HU, Sannanania B, Baheti AD, et al. Hysterosalpingography and ultrasonography findings of female genital tuberculosis. *Diagn Interv Radiol.* 2015;21:10-15.
599. Spicer KB, Turner J, Wang S-H, Koranyi K, Powell DA. Tuberculin skin testing and T.SPOT.*TB* in internationally adopted children. *Pediatr Infect Dis J.* 2015;34:599-603.
614. Starke JR; the Committee on Infectious Diseases, American Academy of Pediatrics. Interferon-γ release assays for diagnosis of tuberculosis infection and disease in children. *Pediatrics.* 2014;134:e1763-e1773.
622. Sterling TR, Moro RN, Borisov AS, et al. Flu-like and other systemic drug reactions among persons receiving weekly rifapentine plus isoniazid or daily isoniazid for treatment of latent tuberculosis infection in the PREVENT Tuberculosis Study. *Clin Infect Dis.* 2015;61:257-535.
625. Stockdale AJ, Duke T, Graham S, et al. Evidence behind the WHO guidelines: hospital care for children – what is the diagnostic accuracy of gastric aspiration for the diagnosis of tuberculosis in children? *J Trop Pediatr.* 2010;56:291-298.
634. Sun L, Xiao J, Miao Q, et al. Interferon gamma release assay in diagnosis of pediatric tuberculosis: a meta-analysis. *FEMS Immunol Med Microbiol.* 2011;63:165-173.
641. Tang S, Yao L, Hao X, et al. Clofazimine for the treatment of multidrug-resistant tuberculosis: prospective, multicenter, randomized controlled study in China. *Clin Infect Dis.* 2015;60:1361-1367.
653. Thomas TA, Heysell SK, Moodley P, et al. Intensified specimen collection to improve tuberculosis diagnosis in children from rural South Africa, an observational study. *BMC Infect Dis.* 2014;14:11.
683. Villarino ME, Scott NA, Weis SE, et al. Treatment for preventing tuberculosis in children and adolescents: a randomized clinical trial of a 3-month, 12-dose regimen of a combination of rifapentine and isoniazid. *JAMA Pediatr.* 2015;169:247-255.
705. Winston CA, Menzies HJ. Pediatric and adolescent tuberculosis in the United States, 2008-2010. *Pediatrics.* 2012;130:e1425-e1432.
711. World Health Organization. 2015 Global Tuberculosis Report. WHO Press; Geneva, Switzerland; 2015.
715. World Health Organization. Xpert MTB/RIF assay for the diagnosis of pulmonary and extrapulmonary TB in adults and children. Policy update. WHO Press; Geneva, Switzerland; 2013. Available online at: http://apps.who.int/iris/bitstream/10665/112472/1/9789241506335_eng.pdf?ua=1. Accessed 24 February 2016.
719. Yuen CM, Amanulla F, Dharmadhikari A, et al. Turning off the tap: stopping tuberculosis transmission through active case-finding and prompt effective treatment. *Lancet.* 2015;386:2334-2343.
724. Zhang X, Falagas ME, Vardakas KZ, et al. Systematic review and meta-analysis of the efficacy and safety of therapy with linezolid-containing regimens in the treatment of multidrug-resistant and extensively drug-resistant tuberculosis. *J Thorac Dis.* 2015;7:603-615.
727. Zhao J, Cui MY, Chan T, et al. Evaluation of intestinal tuberculosis by multi-slice computed tomography enterography. *BMC Infect Dis.* 2015;15:577.

The full reference list for this chapter is available at ExpertConsult.com.

97 Other Mycobacteria

W. Matthew Linam • Richard F. Jacobs

The definition of mycobacteria other than tubercle bacilli is quite confusing. Runyon[155] in his address to the International Conference on Atypical Mycobacteria probably defined them best: "Tubercle bacilli include *Mycobacterium tuberculosis, Mycobacterium bovis,* and *Mycobacterium africanum.* Together with *Mycobacterium microti* (not pathogenic for humans), these organisms constitute the tubercle bacillus complex." Any mycobacteria not listed in this group are considered to be in the "other" grouping. Mycobacteria other than those causing tuberculosis and leprosy were not recognized as causes of disease in humans until the 1950s.[189] The most common forms of the disease are chronic pulmonary disease resembling tuberculosis (occurring mainly in adults), cervical adenopathy in children, skin and soft tissue infection, and disseminated disease in immunocompromised individuals.[131] In the mid-1980s, the incidence of infections with nontuberculous mycobacteria (NTM) increased markedly, probably because of the increased number of immunocompromised patients (e.g., because of AIDS, hematopoietic cell transplant, and organ transplantation) and the significant improvement in microbiologic methods for cultivating these organisms.[215,218] With the continued proliferation of immunocompromised patients because of AIDS and new treatment modalities that induce an immunocompromised state (e.g., organ transplantation, new immunosuppressive drugs), NTM probably will continue to remain important pathogens.

EPIDEMIOLOGY

NTM are ubiquitous in nature. They are found in soil, water, animals, milk,[49] and food. Of importance in some hospital-acquired infections or infections in immunocompromised hosts is the presence of the organisms in common tap water.[18,67,118,181] Exposure to environments, especially soil, colonized by these organisms seems to be important for acquisition of disease in children. Organisms commonly found in soil include *Mycobacterium scrofulaceum, Mycobacterium flavescens, Mycobacterium avium* complex (MAC), *Mycobacterium gastri, Mycobacterium terrae, Mycobacterium fortuitum,* and *Mycobacterium chelonae.* Water is an important source for all of the previously named organisms and for *Mycobacterium kansasii, Mycobacterium marinum, Mycobacterium gordonae,* and *Mycobacterium xenopi.* In a multi-site study evaluating the presence of NTM in tap water, 78% of the water samples were positive for NTMs. The most frequently identified species were: *Mycobacterium mucogenicum* (52%), *M. avium* (30%), and *M. gordonae* (25%).[46] A recent outbreak of rapidly growing mycobacterium (*M. chelonae*) in pediatric hematopoietic cell transplant patients was linked with the hospital water supply.[86]

The estimated prevalence of NTM disease in the United States in the 1980s was 1.8 per 100,000 persons.[132] More recent studies suggest that the prevalence has increased. A population study from Oregon in 2005 to 2006 estimated the prevalence at 7.2 cases per 100,000 persons.[21] In a survey from the Centers for Disease Control and Prevention (CDC) from 1980, 35% of mycobacteria isolated in laboratories were nontuberculous.[61] MAC (*M. avium* and *Mycobacterium intracellulare*) accounted for 66% of the nontuberculous isolates, followed by *M. fortuitum* (19%), *M. kansasii* (9%), and *Mycobacterium scrofulaceum* (6%). Two studies from 2009 showed a similar distribution of nontuberculous isolates. The distribution in the Australian study was MAC (48.5%), *Mycobacterium abscessus* or *M. chelonae* (13.2%), *M. fortuitum* (11.8%), and *Mycobacterium ulcerans* (5.9%).[15] The distribution in a California study was MAC (47%), *M. abscessus* or *M. chelonae* (22%), and *M. fortuitum* (5%).[148] Some of the variation seen may be due to geographic differences.

Geography apparently has some bearing on the prevalence and type of these infections. MAC was seen most commonly along the coastal borders of the United States and in the states bordering Canada. The highest rates were seen in Hawaii (10.9 cases per 100,000 population), Connecticut (8.9 cases per 100,000 population), and Florida (8.4 cases per 100,000 population). High rates also were seen in Kansas and the desert Southwest, however, showing the widespread nature of this organism in causing disease. In contrast, *M. kansasii* was seen most commonly in the Midwest of the United States and almost never in the Southeast.[52] *M. marinum* frequently was isolated from coastal areas, whereas *M. xenopi* was scattered across the United States, with 50% of cases found in just three states (Connecticut, Wisconsin, and California). Internationally, incidence rates of NTM infections in children range from 0.84 per 100,000 (Australia) to 3.1 per 100,000 (Germany).[15,147] For all of the nontuberculous species, males and rural residents had a much higher incidence of infection.[161] Extrapolation of these rates to determine disease patterns is not without problems, however. The number of mycobacterial isolates could be skewed easily by the presence of multiple isolates from a single patient, or it may just represent colonization. Nonetheless, these rates can help predict which species of NTM are most likely to be encountered in a particular geographic region.

The site of isolation from the human source can be helpful in determining the type of mycobacteria that may be involved in the disease process. MAC is responsible for lymphadenitis, particularly in children. MAC also is responsible for pulmonary disease and disseminated disease to bones and occasionally to the meninges. *M. kansasii* is associated most commonly with infections of pulmonary origin and disseminated lesions in adults; rarely, it is associated with adenitis and skin granuloma in children. *M. scrofulaceum* also causes lymphadenitis in children, and *M. marinum* is responsible for skin granuloma and ulcers after exposure to certain salt water beaches, swimming pools, and tropical fish tanks. The rapidly growing mycobacteria, such as *M. fortuitum* and *M. chelonae*, often cause skin and soft tissue infection and, rarely, pulmonary and disseminated disease in adults and children. A notable exception is the rapidly growing mycobacterium *M. abscessus*, which is the third most common NTM species recovered from respiratory specimens.[66] Healthcare-associated NTM infections have been reported in patients with long-term vascular catheters, peritoneal dialysis catheters, and various surgical procedures. Rapidly growing mycobacteria are frequently implicated. The source is often contaminated tap water.

A familial immune defect predisposing to disseminated NTM infection in childhood has been reported.[107] Interleukin (IL)-12 and interferon (IFN)-γ play an important role in the control of mycobacterial infections, primarily through upregulation of tumor necrosis factor (TNF)-α. Defects in either the synthesis or signaling pathways of these cytokines have resulted in disseminated NTM infections.[48] In addition, patients receiving anti–TNF-α therapy may be at increased risk for NTM disease, especially if they are receiving additional immune suppressive medications.[212] In a recent study of patients receiving anti–TNF-α therapy, the rate of NTM was 74 per 100,000 person-years compared to the background rate of NTM infection of 4.1 per 100,000 person-years.[211]

MICROBIOLOGY

Runyon and Timpe[153,154,189] in their monumental work on NTM suggested a useful classification system based on three characteristics of the organisms: production of pigment, rate of growth, and colonial characteristics. The four groups are as follows: group I—photochromogens, which produce bright yellow to red pigment in the presence of light; group II—scotochromogens, which produce yellow to orange pigment in the dark; group III—nonphotochromogens, which are non–pigment producers; and group IV—rapid growers, which generally grow in less than 1 week. Kubica[99] published an updated version of Runyon's classification in 1978, and it was useful for many years. Subsequently, a more "simplified" classification based on the growth rates of the organisms alone was proposed.[215] More recently, reliable DNA sequencing, using the highly conserved *16S rRNA* gene, has allowed for rapid recognition of new species. A sequence difference of greater than 1% usually indicates a new species. Currently, at least 160 NTM species have been identified.[74,122,133,190]

The NTM still are differentiated by most clinical laboratories based on various morphologic, physiologic, and biochemical characteristics (Tables 97.1 and 97.2). The difficulty with identifying many of these organisms is their slow growth rates with standard techniques. Because antibiotic susceptibility varies for different species, it is important to identify organisms to the species level to ensure the appropriate therapy is chosen.[64] Results from identification and susceptibility testing are often delayed; therefore, this process should begin as soon as a NTM is cultivated and thought to be the responsible pathogen. In clinical medicine, serologic tests rarely are valuable for establishing a diagnosis in an individual patient. A study using humoral immunoglobulins against mycobacterial antigens failed to diagnose tuberculosis or nontuberculous adenitis in children.[194] Blood cultures for mycobacteria are best performed with the Isolator lysis-centrifugation system or the radiometric BACTEC 13A blood culture bottle.[2,93,92] Blood collected in ethylenediaminetetraacetic acid or coagulated blood is unacceptable. Body fluids such as cerebrospinal fluid, pleural fluid, and peritoneal fluid can be inoculated directly into BACTEC or Septi-Chek broth, particularly if only small volumes are available. To aid in detection and growth, cultures should include both solid and broth media, whenever possible. Gene probes became commercially available in the late 1980s. They involve DNA probes complementary to species-specific sequences of rRNA for the identification of *M. tuberculosis*, MAC, *M. gordonae*, and *M. kansasii*.[63]

Polymerase chain reaction (PCR) assay has been evaluated for the routine detection of *M. tuberculosis* in the clinical laboratory and compared with fluorochrome smear and culture. Multiplex, real-time PCRs also have been developed to aid in the rapid identification of NTM. In a study by Kim and colleagues,[96] a multiplex, real-time PCR was developed capable of identifying 23 mycobacterial species and was tested using 77 reference strains and 369 clinical isolates. The test correctly identified all 189 (100%) isolates of the *M. tuberculosis* and 169 (93.9%) of the NTM isolates. Another multiplex, real-time PCR test using 314 clinical isolates had a 95% to 99% sensitivity and 99% to 100% specificity for distinguishing *M. tuberculosis* complex, MAC, the *M. chelonae–M. abscessus* group, the *M. fortuitum* group, and *Mycobacterium mucogenicum*.[148] The PCR testing offered by commercial laboratories at present is not approved by the US Food and Drug Administration for in vitro diagnosis. With newer isolation techniques and new technology such as DNA probes, the ability to diagnose these infections and understanding of the pathogenesis of the infections that these organisms produce should improve, as should the ability to treat these infections.

MANIFESTATIONS OF NONTUBERCULOUS MYCOBACTERIAL INFECTION IN CHILDREN

Lymphadenitis

Lymphadenitis is the most common manifestation of NTM infection in children, but it also occurs rarely in adults.[43,103,110] All nodes in the

TABLE 97.1 Characteristics of Slow-Growing Pathogenic Mycobacteria

Organism	GROWTH PRESENT (°C) 25	37	45	Growth Rate (Days)	Niacin	Nitrate Reduction	Pigment Dark	Pigment Light	Growth in 5% NaCl
M. tuberculosis	−	+	−	12–28	+	+	−	−	−
M. bovis	−	+	−	21–40	−	−	−	−	−
Photochromogens, Runyon Group I									
M. kansasii	+	+	−	10–21	−	+	−	+	−
M. marinum	+	±	−	7–14	−	−	−	+	−
Scotochromogens, Runyon Group II									
M. scrofulaceum	+	+	−	10–28	−	−	+	+	−
M. szulgai	+	+	−	12–28	−	+	+	+	−
M. gordonae	+	+	−	10–28	−	−	+	+	−
Nonchromogens, Runyon Group III									
M. avium	+	+	+	10–21	−	−	−	−	−
M. intracellulare	+	+	−	10–21	−	−	−	−	−
M. ulcerans	−	−	−	28–60	−	−	−	−	?
M. xenopi	−	+	−	14–28	−	−	−	−	−

TABLE 97.2 Characteristics of Rapid Mycobacterial Growers

Runyon Group IV	Optimal Temperature (°C)	Growth Rate (Days)	Niacin	Nitrate Reduction	Growth in 5% NaCl
M. fortuitum	37	3–7	−	+	+
M. abscessus	37	3–7	−	−	+
M. chelonae	37	3–7	−	−	

cervical chain can be affected, but the nodes of the submandibular region seem to be most commonly involved.[45,116] The parotid gland also can be affected.[39] The differential diagnosis frequently centers on deciding whether a malignant process or a nonmalignant process is present. Nonmalignant processes to consider include mononucleosis, bacterial adenitis, cat-scratch disease, toxoplasmosis, tularemia, and *M. tuberculosis* infection.

Although most mycobacterial cases of lymphadenitis are caused by the nontuberculous organisms, the clinician also must consider *M. tuberculosis*.[35] No clinical features help the clinician discern between NTM infection and tuberculosis. The use of histopathology has been postulated to help differentiate between atypical and tuberculous infections.[138] In a retrospective study, the findings of ill-defined (nonpalisading) granulomas, predominantly sarcoid-like granulomas, or lack of significant caseation were seen more commonly with nontuberculous lymphadenitis. Additionally, nontuberculous infections had neutrophils predominantly in the center of the necrosis, whereas in tuberculous infections, neutrophils were scattered throughout the specimen.[138] A prospective study investigating these findings has not been published to date, and other authors have not noted similar patterns.[12]

In a Canadian study, the rate of NTM as a cause of lymphadenitis was 1.21 cases per 100,000 children, whereas the rate for tuberculosis was 0.3 cases per 100,000 children.[171] Investigators from San Diego as well as other areas from around the world have reported a marked increase in the number of infections in immunocompetent children.[59,139] In one study, the incidence increased from 1 case between 1987 and 1990 to 85 cases between 1991 and 1993.[102] A recent Canadian study compared the incidence of NTM cervicofacial adenitis in children from 1994 to 1998 (25.1 per 100,000 hospitalizations) and 1999 to 2004 (107.4 per 100,000 hospitalizations) and showed a statistically significant increase. In a large study compiled by Lincoln and Gilbert[109] involving 243 children, more than 50% were younger than 3 years of age and 80% were younger than 5 years. Contact with NTM sources such as soil and water may account for the frequency of cervical lymphadenitis in young children.[192]

Infections are caused mainly by MAC and *M. scrofulaceum*. A large prospective study spanning 32 years from 1958 to 1990 showed that MAC has become the predominant etiologic agent and has surpassed *M. scrofulaceum* from earlier in the study.[217] Current data estimate that 72% of NTM lymphadenitis cases are caused by *M. avium*.[137] A series of 190 patients from India showed, however, that 60% of the nontuberculous adenitis cases were caused by *M. scrofulaceum*, followed by 40% by *M. avium-intracellulare*.[88] This difference may be due in part to differences in water chlorination. Additional causes of NTM lymphadenitis in children include *Mycobacterium haemophilum*,[8,158] *Mycobacterium malmoense*,[191] *M. fortuitum*,[150] and recently described *Mycobacterium heidelbergense*.[70]

Most patients have no systemic symptoms and exhibit normal chest radiographs; other laboratory studies generally are not helpful. The mean duration of swelling is approximately 6 weeks. Affected lymph notes are often unilateral and nontender. Over time, NTM infections involving superficial lymph nodes may develop a violaceous discoloration of the overlying skin. Nodes may spontaneously rupture or develop draining sinus tracts.

Currently, no NTM skin test is commercially available in the United States. All patients with suspected NTM lymphadenitis should have a tuberculin skin test placed. Children with NTM lymphadenitis can have a variety of reactions to tuberculin skin tests, ranging from 0 mm to greater than 10 mm of induration. Needle aspiration of an affected node can be a valuable diagnostic tool. Cultures for bacterial and mycobacterial etiologies should be performed, with recovery rates in children with cervical lymphadenitis ranging from 60% to 88%.[10,16,80,91,221] The aspirate should be inoculated onto aerobic and anaerobic media and Sabouraud agar and mycobacterial media (Löwenstein-Jensen slants or Middlebrook media). Use of the BACTEC system can be helpful, especially in isolation of more fastidious species. Samra and colleagues[158] showed that the BACTEC radiometric system or MB Redox broth is superior to Löwenstein-Jensen media for isolation of *M. haemophilum*, and this may account for the increased identification of this organism. Mycobacteria can be isolated 12 to 17 days after inoculation.[177] PCR is being used with increasing frequency in the diagnosis in NTM lymphadenitis.[31,137] More recently, preoperative diagnosis of *M. avium* lymphadenitis was accomplished with the use of PCR of gastric aspirates in two children.[69]

The best treatment of lymphadenitis caused by NTM is complete excision of the involved lymph node.[117,198] Incision and drainage without excision results in a high rate of secondary drainage, and subsequent excision of the remaining tissue is required for cure.[5,157,164] Complete excision may not be possible when affected nodes are adjacent to large vessels or the facial nerve. In those situations, adjunctive antibiotic therapy may be necessary. The majority (59%) of clinicians manage NTM lymphadenitis by surgical excision followed by adjunctive antibiotics.[137] A randomized controlled trial involving 100 children with NTM cervicofacial lymphadenitis compared surgical excision to antibiotic therapy with clarithromycin and rifabutin.[111] Esthetic outcome was significantly better in the surgical group. Another small study showed successful nonsurgical management of deep cervical NTM lymphadenitis.[73]

Pulmonary Infections

Reviews from the late 1970s showed that pulmonary disease caused by NTM usually was caused by *M. kansasii* and MAC.[32,62,151] Historically, NTM pulmonary infections have occurred most commonly in men (ratios as high as 4 : 1), with most patients have underlying pulmonary disease such as chronic obstructive pulmonary disease (COPD). MAC infection most commonly occurred during the sixth decade, whereas *M. kansasii* infection occurred in individuals a decade younger. Two recent prevalence studies in the United States have shown that the epidemiology and clinical features have changed. An Oregon study estimated the 2-year prevalence of NTM pulmonary disease to be 8.6 cases/100,000 persons (20.4 per 100,000 for persons >50 years).[213] In a large multisite study, the age-adjusted annual prevalence was 5.4 cases per 100,000 persons.[140] Both studies show an increased prevalence of NTM pulmonary disease. This increase is most evident in women, especially those older than 60 years of age.[140] MAC was the most common isolate (80–87.5%), followed by *M. abscessus* or *chelonae* (6–12%).[140,213] The epidemiology of NTM pulmonary infections in Europe is similar, but the rate of infections is lower.[149] Other species causing NTM pulmonary disease include *Mycobacterium simiae, M. kansasii, M. fortuitum, M. mucogenicum, Mycobacterium szulgai,* and *M. xenopi.*[115,140,172,204] Underlying comorbidities such as COPD, bronchiectasis, and lung cancer were common, with bronchiectasis more common in women.[140,213] Most common imaging findings were nodules (59%), bronchiectasis (39.7%), and cavitary lesions (8.5%).[140] Rare case reports of mediastinal mass lesions in children caused by NTM have been published.[54] NTM pulmonary disease is uncommon in children and most frequently seen in children with cystic fibrosis.[38]

Patients with cystic fibrosis have been noted to have an increased incidence of infection with NTM with prevalence rates of 2% to 20%.[4,78,79,95,165] In a large multicenter prospective prevalence study of NTM in patients with cystic fibrosis from France, which included 1582 patients, the prevalence of patients with at least one positive NTM culture was 6.6%.[152] *M. abscessus* complex and MAC were the most common species responsible for both colonization and disease. Mycobacterial infections are seen more commonly in older patients with cystic fibrosis. The peak prevalence for *M. abscessus* was 11 to 15 years and 25 years for MAC.[152] Frequent intravenous antibiotic use is a possible risk factor for colonization with NTM.[190] *M. abscessus* has emerged as a clinically significant pathogen in patients with cystic fibrosis, especially patients on steroid therapy for allergic bronchopulmonary aspergillosis.[53,127,190] Persistent *M. abscessus* infection has been associated with lung function decline.[52] Despite antibiotic therapy, less than a third of patients with *M. abscessus* clear their infection.[142] Other organisms cultured from patients with cystic fibrosis include *Mycobacterium peregrinum, M. kansasii, M. fortuitum, M. chelonae,* and *M. xenopi.* Bacterial contamination, particularly with *Pseudomonas aeruginosa,* of the acid-fast bacilli cultures from patients with cystic fibrosis has been a major problem that has rendered isolation of mycobacteria more difficult.[174] Another confounding problem is the difficulty in differentiating infection from colonization in these patients.[95]

The American Thoracic Society recommends radiographic changes (i.e., nodules, cavitary opacities, or multifocal bronchiectasis), isolation of multiple colonies of the same species, and the absence of other potential pathogens as criteria for the diagnosis of pathogenic infection with NTM.[3] Discernment is even more difficult in the setting of the chronic lung disease seen in patients with cystic fibrosis. Kilby and associates[95] suggest that repeated isolation of NTM associated with pulmonary cavities or infiltrates that do not improve with aggressive standard antibacterial treatment could indicate active mycobacterial disease in patients with cystic fibrosis.

Treatment of NTM pulmonary disease recommended by the American Thoracic Society requires prolonged courses using multidrug regimens. Drugs are administered for 18 to 24 months, with a minimum of 12 months of culture negativity required while receiving therapy. Treatment of MAC pulmonary infections involves clarithromycin or azithromycin, ethambutol, and rifampin. In fibrocavitary or other severe disease, streptomycin or amikacin may be added.[64] Treatment success is variable. The median efficacy of macrolide-based regimens reported in a review of 12 clinical trials was 56% (range, 26–71%).[55] A case was reported of a 7-year-old boy with leukemia in whom pneumonia with *M. xenopi* developed and was treated successfully with 2 years of therapy that included ethambutol and clarithromycin.[106] *M. simiae,* which has been isolated in adults with underlying pulmonary abnormalities, is the most drug-resistant of all the NTM, with some isolates resistant to all drugs tested.[11,98]

Skin Infections

Mycobacterium marinum

M. marinum is photochromogenic and was identified as a pathogen in fish in 1926 by Aronson.[109] The natural reservoir for *M. marinum,* which requires a cool incubator (32°C [89.6°F]), is in fish and other cold-blooded animals. Skin lesions usually result from light trauma (abrasions) in swimming pools or other bodies of water when the surfaces of the pool are colonized by *M. marinum.*[41,124] Fish tanks also have been implicated and generally involve the upper limb or a finger.[9,185] Most cases occur in children aged 10 to 16 years old. The most common sites are the elbows, knees, and ankles. Cooler superficial portions of the body are affected most frequently. Other exposed body areas can be involved, depending on what part of the body has made contact with the water containing the mycobacterium (e.g., the nose in divers).[125] Lesions are usually solitary but may have a sporotrichoid pattern. Regional spread of lesions has been reported.[179]

The incubation period from exposure to formation of a small, indurated papule that ulcerates generally is 3 weeks. The lesion then crusts and forms a granuloma with a small crater. The lesions usually are painless and resolve in several months; occasionally, they can last longer. In contrast to other mycobacterial diseases, regional nodes are usually not involved. Infection with this organism usually is benign, but it frequently results in the conversion of a purified protein derivative stabilized with Tween (PPD-T) test to positive.[109] Generally, only a few organisms may be isolated in some granulomas.

M. marinum is usually susceptible to rifampin, ethambutol, clarithromycin, and trimethoprim-sulfamethoxazole and intermediately susceptible to doxycycline. Treatment regimens usually include two active agents. Treatment of *M. marinum* has been successful with rifampin and ethambutol,[196,214] Other studies have shown success with a combination of clarithromycin and rifampin.[9] The duration of therapy, according to the literature, varies from several weeks to 18 months. Generally, response to therapy is rapid, and treatment should be continued for 4 to 6 weeks after clinical resolution.[47]

Mycobacterium ulcerans

Infections caused by *Mycobacterium ulcerans* result in chronic necrotizing cutaneous ulcers known as Buruli ulcers. *M. ulcerans* and Buruli ulcer are covered in greater detail in Chapter 98. In 1948, MacCullum[114] reported the first cases of disease caused by *M. ulcerans.* Most cases have occurred in remote, tropical, or subtropical areas of the world, including parts of Africa and Australia.[113,146] Cases also have been reported in Mexico.[109] Most patients harboring this organism are in otherwise good health without underlying immunodeficiency.[33] Scraping of the skin by thorns or pieces of wood or insect bites have been implicated as possible routes of inoculation in many of the cases. The natural reservoir for *M. ulcerans* is unknown. One report suggests the spines of a tall prickly grass known as *Echinochloa pyramidalis* as a reservoir.[180]

An Australian study found evidence that mosquitoes may play a role in the transmission of *M. ulcerans*.[104] The lesions caused by *M. ulcerans* occur mainly on the cooler superficial portions of the body. The organism is fastidious, with growth requiring 6 to 12 weeks and seen only between 25°C and 33°C (77°F–91.4°F).

The incubation period is approximately 3 weeks. Disease forms include: papules, nodules, plaques, edema, and ulcers. Lesions often begin as nodules or plaques and can progress to ulcers. Ulcers can become large with significant tissue destruction. Occasionally, disease spreads to bone resulting in osteomyelitis. Complications can result when the infection extends into adjacent tissues and organs resulting in tissue destruction. Disseminated infection in an immunocompetent child, along with the development of multifocal osteomyelitis, has been described.[80] Healing frequently results in scarring and fibrosis, which in the setting of large or deep ulcers can result in functional limitations and deformities. Treatment for Buruli ulcers includes antibiotics and surgery. Surgery is typically reserved for removal of necrotic tissue, coverage of skin/tissue defects and restoration of function. Recommended antibiotic regimens include rifampin in combination with an aminoglycoside or clarithromycin and is usually administered for at least 8 weeks.

Other Mycobacteria in Skin Disease

A study of archived skin biopsy specimens using PCR for NTM identified additional NTM skin infections.[195] *M. haemophilum* was the most common organism identified. *M. haemophilum* has produced painful subcutaneous nodules in immunocompromised patients, particularly patients with renal transplants.[42,216] *M. chelonae* has been found to be a cause of disseminated cutaneous infection.[200] Steroid use is the predisposing factor for infection with this organism. *M. fortuitum-chelonae* complex has been responsible for superficial skin abscesses in children.[14] *M. fortuitum* was implicated as the cause of cutaneous lesions in a child involved in a motor scooter accident, with the subsequent development of lesions at the site of knee lacerations; regional adenopathy of the inguinal nodes also developed.[169] A recent outbreak of cutaneous hand and foot infections in 29 children caused by *M. abscessus* was linked to a school swimming pool.[173] *M. avium* has been isolated from an eyelid abscess.[163] Contaminated pedicure footbaths have been implicated in outbreaks of NTM skin infections, including a recent outbreak from *Mycobacterium bolletii* and *Mycobacterium massiliense*.[207] NTM skin infections also have occurred at insulin injection sites, acupuncture sites, and filler injection sites, with many of these caused by rapidly growing mycobacteria.[105,178] Treatment of cutaneous disease caused by these organisms is difficult at best. Four- or five-drug therapy has been tried, but with poor results.

Other Sites of Infection

Although infections involving lymph nodes, lungs, and skin are the most frequent sites of infection, NTM infections have been reported from nearly every organ system. Carpal tunnel syndrome in adults has been reported as being caused by *M. szulgai*, an uncommon scotochromogenic mycobacterium.[183] In a review of 21 cases of *M. szulgai*, pulmonary disease was most common, with disseminated disease more common in immune-suppressed patients.[197] Effective treatment included debridement, ethambutol, and rifampin. Other infections in humans include choroiditis,[34] panniculitis,[159] parotitis,[29] genitourinary tract infection,[17,188] and synovitis.[184] Ear infections with NTM also have been reported, as has mastoiditis.[56,130,182] Importantly, infection of Broviac catheters in pediatric patients with leukemia and hemodialysis and peritoneal dialysis catheters has been described.[24,28,106,166,193] In all cases, removal of the catheter was required for resolution of the infection. NTM are a rare cause of ventriculoperitoneal shunt infections including infections in children.[20,187] *M. fortuitum* is the most common species identified. Patients frequently present with subacute meningitis. Catheter removal is imperative.

Acquired Immunodeficiency Syndrome and Nontuberculous Mycobacteria

Before the availability of combination antiretroviral therapy (cART), NTM infections, most commonly MAC, were the second most common opportunistic infections in children in the United States with human immunodeficiency virus (HIV) infection. The incidence rate in the pre-cART era was 1.3 to 1.8 episodes per 100 person-years.[60,129] Approximately 6% of adults and 4% of children with AIDS reported to the CDC had disseminated MAC infection as the AIDS-defining disease.[22] Autopsy studies show that MAC infection is present in 20% to 50% of adult HIV-infected patients.[145,206,209] In a retrospective study from 1990 to 1996 in New York City, 26% of children had evidence of MAC infection at the time of their deaths.[89] MAC infection was thought to be the cause of death in 13% of the 54 children with HIV infection, and the mean age at death was 7.8 years. More than 70% of children with MAC and AIDS had evidence of disseminated disease. Almost all had $CD4^+$ counts less than 100 cells/mm^3. Since the availability of cART, incidence of MAC has decreased to 0.14 to 0.2 episodes per 100 person-years.[60,129]

In the CDC study, MAC was the NTM most commonly isolated in HIV patients. In adult studies, *M. kansasii* and *M. scrofulaceum* have been identified as causes of infection, but the incidence of infection is low.[44,83] In patients with HIV, *M. fortuitum* complex is the most frequently isolated rapidly growing mycobacteria and typically causes lymphadenitis and pulmonary disease.[143] *Mycobacterium genavense* has been shown to cause infection in children with HIV infection with the organism identified in stool and lymph node specimens.[128]

Clinical findings included failure to maintain growth curves, anorexia, persistent or recurrent fever, fatigue, and abdominal pain. MAC has been shown to infect the esophagus, stomach, and intestine of pediatric patients with AIDS.[90] Patients with extensive MAC infection of the small and large intestines have severe, persistent diarrhea. Respiratory symptoms are uncommon. Clinical findings may include hepatomegaly, splenomegaly, or lymphadenopathy. Bone marrow suppression also may occur. The median age at diagnosis was 46 months, with a median of 9 months elapsing between the onset of symptoms and positive cultures. When NTM infection was diagnosed in these patients, they survived less than 10 months. Blood cultures have 90% to 95% sensitivity in detecting disseminated MAC infection in adult patients with AIDS.[76] Infection is also confirmed by isolation of MAC from a normally sterile body site such as lymph node or bone marrow. Isolates should be tested for susceptibility to azithromycin and clarithromycin.

For treatment of MAC infection in HIV-infected children, combination therapy is recommended.[170] Clarithromycin or azithromycin and ethambutol should be included. Clarithromycin/ethambutol has been shown to be more effective than azithromycin/ethambutol in one randomized trial.[202] Rifabutin can be added as a third drug, but its use is controversial. The decision to start rifabutin should balance the degree of immune suppression and the extent of infection with the effect increased cytochrome P450 has other medications. Lack of clinical response after 8 to 12 weeks of treatment suggests treatment failure. Repeating susceptibility testing and initiating a new combination regimen based on the results are recommended. Additional antibiotics to consider include rifabutin, amikacin, and quinolones. The use of granulocyte colony-stimulating factor as an adjunct to antimicrobial therapy for disseminated MAC infection has been reported,[134] but additional data are needed to determine the usefulness of this agent. Immune reconstitution inflammatory syndrome has been reported in adults and children with MAC infection receiving cART.[37,167]

Secondary prophylaxis is recommended for all children with a history of disseminated MAC infection. Clarithromycin is recommended in combination with ethambutol, with or without rifabutin. In most situations, secondary prophylaxis is lifelong. Guidelines are available for discontinuing prophylaxis in children who have completed appropriate therapy, are without evidence of ongoing infection, are stable on cART, and have sustained recovery of their $CD4^+$ cells above the threshold for initiating primary prophylaxis.[170]

The US Public Health Service and the Infectious Disease Society of America have published guidelines for the prevention of opportunistic infections, including disseminated MAC.[170] These guidelines incorporate age-specific $CD4^+$ counts at which primary prophylaxis should be used: children 6 years of age or older, fewer than 50 cells/mm^3; children 2 to 6 years old, fewer than 75 cells/mm^3; children 1 to 2 years old, fewer than 500 cells/mm^3; and children younger than 1 year, fewer than 750 cells/mm^3. Before initiating prophylaxis, patients should be evaluated for disseminated MAC infection by obtaining a blood culture for MAC. The use of clarithromycin or azithromycin for primary prophylaxis is recommended for adults and children with advanced immunosuppression. In HIV-infected children older than 2 years of age, primary prophylaxis may be discontinued once they are stable on cART (>6 months) with sustained immunologic response for over 3 months (children age ≥6 years, >100 cells/mm^3; children age 2–6 years, >200 cells/mm^3). Rifabutin can be used as an alternative agent; although poor efficacy and side effects limit its utility.[170,175] Combination therapy for prophylaxis is not recommended.

The emergence of resistance is a concern with the MAC prophylactic regimens in patients with AIDS. In some trials, 9% of adults receiving azithromycin prophylaxis and 5% of adults receiving clarithromycin prophylaxis had breakthrough MAC bacteremia. Of these cases, 11% and 58% of the azithromycin and clarithromycin, respectively, breakthrough isolates were macrolide-resistant.[6,75]

ORGANISMS SEEN IN CHILDREN

Specific organisms and treatment guidelines are discussed in the following sections. Table 97.3 provides a quick guide to some of the more commonly used antimycobacterial agents.

Mycobacterium avium-intracellulare Complex

MAC consists of *M. avium* and *M. intracellulare. M. avium* was recognized in 1890 as the causative agent of disease in chickens.[216] *M. intracellulare* was designated in 1967 and at the time was difficult to distinguish routinely from *M. avium,* thus the name *M. avium-intracellulare.* Today, with the use of DNA probes, most seroagglutination types have been discerned between the two groups. *M. avium* is the most common NTM causing disease in humans, but isolates from environmental sources are more likely to be *M. intracellulare.* Both organisms can be found in birds, soil, dust, and fresh or salt water. Infections caused by MAC strains isolated from adult patients with AIDS could be identified as either serotype 4 or 8, in contrast to patients without AIDS, in whom no predominant serotype has been identified.[94,219] Nearly all isolates of MAC from patients with AIDS have been identified as *M. avium;* in patients without AIDS, the rate of *M. avium* is approximately 55%, and the rate of *M. intracellulare* is 32% to 40%.[68,219]

In a study of 56 isolates from pediatric patients involving sequence analysis of the ribosomal internal transcribed spacer, Hazra and colleagues[77] showed that the closely related Mav-B and Mav-A sequevars caused most disease. Patients from geographically diverse areas of the United States (i.e., Boston, Miami, and Los Angeles) had isolates with closely related patterns. The finding of related strains causing disease in epidemiologically unrelated patients is most consistent with two hypotheses: a similar subset of *M. avium* strains is more virulent and more likely to cause disease in humans, or pathogenic strains are more prevalent in the environment.

These organisms are slow-growing, obligate aerobes that require 2 to 6 weeks for colony formation on solid media. MAC infection is diagnosed most commonly by culture of blood, bone marrow, or tissue. These organisms grow on routine bacterial media, but growth is achieved best on selective mycobacterial media, such as Löwenstein-Jensen medium or Middlebrook 7K10 and 7K11 agar. Colonies usually are smooth but may be rough and can be transparent or opaque. Nucleic acid hybridization probes using target sequences of ribosomal RNA are available commercially for rapid identification of clinical isolates.[108,126]

In children, lymphadenitis is the most common manifestation of MAC. Please refer to the section on lymphadenitis for more information. In non-immunocompromised adults, lung disease has been the major manifestation of MAC infection. Most investigators thought that MAC infection occurred mainly in patients with deficient immunity or underlying lung disease; however, later reports seemed to indicate that normal adult hosts are at risk for development of infection with MAC and that rates are increasing.[87,141] The incidence of NTM lung disease in postmenopausal women has increased over the last 20 years, especially

TABLE 97.3 Antimycobacterial Agents

Drug	Dosage	Form
Amikacin (A)	15–30 mg/kg/day divided 3 times daily	IV or IM
Azithromycin (Z)	500 mg bid (adults/adolescents); 10–12 mg/kg/day (children)	PO
Cefoxitin (X)	80–160 mg/kg/day divided 4 to 6 times daily	IV or IM
Ciprofloxacin (C)	20–30 mg/kg/day divided 2 times daily (adults only in United States)	PO or IV
Clarithromycin (CL)	15–30 mg/kg/day divided 2 times daily	PO
Clofazimine (CLO)	1–2 mg/kg/day	PO
Doxycycline (D)	2–4 mg/kg/day divided 2 times daily (>8 yr old)	PO, IV
Ethambutol (ETB)	15 mg/kg/day	PO
Ethionamide (ETH)	15–20 mg/kg/day divided 2 times daily	PO
Imipenem (IMP)	60–100 mg/kg/day divided 4 times daily	IV
Isoniazid (I)	5 mg/kg/day	PO
Pyrazinamide (PZA)	15–30 mg/kg/day	PO
Rifabutin (RIB)	5–10 mg/kg/day; maximum 300 mg/day	PO
Rifampin (RIF)	10–20 mg/kg/day once or divided 2 times daily	PO or IV
Streptomycin (S)	20–30 mg/kg/day	IM
	INFECTIONS	
Disseminated MAC: HIV infected: CL (or Z) + ETB (± RIB)		
MAC lung disease: CL (or Z) + ETB + RIF ± S or A (severe or cavitary disease)		
Mycobacterium abscessus: CL or Z + one or more of A, X, or IMP		
Mycobacterium chelonae: CL alone (skin disease), two or more of the following: CL, linezolid, IMP, or tobramycin (invasive disease)		
Mycobacterium fortuitum: two or more of the following: CL, C, A, X, IMP, or TMP-SMX		
Mycobacterium kansasii: RIF + ETB + I		
Mycobacterium marinum: ETB + RIF, or CL + RIF		

Data from references 64, 67, 83, 106, 107, 155, 194, 204, 216, 218.
HIV, Human immunodeficiency virus; *MAC, M. avium* complex; *TMP-SMX,* trimethoprim-sulfamethoxazole.

in slender women with scoliosis or pectus excavatum.[23] Case reports involving children are lacking in detail because they usually appear within discussions of adult patients.[144]

Pediatric case reports of disseminated disease caused by MAC have appeared in the literature. Children have had ulcerative lesions of the colon[40]; mesenteric disease with abscess formation[163]; hematogenous spread to the liver, spleen, kidneys, and adrenal cortex; lesions of the epididymis[176]; bone lesions[199]; and skin lesions. Disseminated osteomyelitis rarely is caused by NTM, but if it occurs, *M. intracellulare* most commonly is isolated.[30,97] Septic arthritis also has been reported in association with osteomyelitis.[58] Immunocompromised patients with disseminated MAC infection historically require multiple-drug therapy, including a combination of azithromycin or clarithromycin and ethambutol. Rifabutin is frequently added as a third agent.[64] Some reports indicate, however, that disseminated disease in HIV-infected patients may respond to only two agents, as mentioned earlier in the discussion of AIDS patients. The addition of other agents may be necessary because of the high incidence of resistant organisms. A preliminary report showed that IFN-γ might be effective when combined with conventional therapy in some patients who are refractory to standard chemotherapy alone.[82]

Bacterial peritonitis is a common occurrence in patients regularly undergoing ambulatory peritoneal dialysis for chronic renal failure. Reports of NTM causing peritonitis have been noted.[71,135,208] In cases involving NTM with foreign bodies, such as Tenckhoff catheters, the development of infected sinus tracts is frequent. Additionally, antituberculous drug regimens in these cases generally are unsuccessful. Although the mycobacteria were sensitive to the agents used, the patients continued to have sinus tract drainage without improvement, even after removal of the foreign body.

Mycobacterium scrofulaceum

M. scrofulaceum has many characteristics similar to those of *M. avium* and *M. intracellulare* and can be found in soil, water, and dairy products. This organism is associated most commonly with lymphadenitis in children 1 to 5 years old and rarely causes other manifestations in humans. Skin and bone lesions have been reported in two children chronically infected with *M. scrofulaceum* for 10 years.[50,205] Disseminated disease caused by *M. scrofulaceum* is rare, but was recently reported in a child with IFN-γ receptor 1 deficiency.[119] Few data are available on chemotherapeutic agents for treatment of infection with this organism. Based on susceptibility patterns, three or more drugs may be necessary for treatment of serious disease. Lymphadenitis can be cured with complete excision of the lymph node.

Mycobacterium kansasii

Of the photochromogens, *M. kansasii* is the one most commonly isolated in humans. It is also the second most commonly identified NTM causing disease in the United States. In contrast to *M. avium-intracellulare* and *M. scrofulaceum, M. kansasii* rarely is isolated in soil but has been cultured from water and milk.[26,27] Chronic pulmonary infection is the most common manifestation of this disease and is seen mainly in adults, particularly adults with AIDS. A survey from Israel of 56 adults with *M. kansasii* pulmonary infection showed that 64% occurred in men, 59% had underlying lung disease, and none was infected with HIV.[168] Pulmonary disease occurs infrequently in children. Some children have a course similar to that of adults, with underlying pulmonary disease caused by previous tuberculosis or chronic pulmonary disease.[13,123] The clinical presentation of *M. kansasii* lung disease is similar to that of *M. tuberculosis,* including cavitary infiltrates and more frequent involvement of the upper lobes, although bilateral disease, pleural effusions, and lymphadenopathy are less common.[168] In contrast, other children have acute symptoms of classic bacterial pneumonia with an abrupt onset of fever and sputum production and lung consolidation on physical examination and radiographs.[13,25]

In contrast to some other nontuberculous organisms, *M. kansasii* is sensitive to most of the antituberculous drugs, particularly rifampin. Most authorities recommend the use of three drugs, including rifampin, isoniazid, and ethambutol. The treatment course usually requires a minimum of 12 months of negative sputum cultures, with therapy for 24 months needed in some patients. A study of 18 patients showed that thrice-weekly clarithromycin, ethambutol, and rifampin were effective, with a mean follow-up of 46 months.[65] Patients with AIDS and *M. kansasii* infection have responded to this three-drug regimen, but the total duration of therapy is unknown at this time. In children with AIDS, the diagnosis of *M. kansasii* infection is rare, and the clinical response to therapy has been poor.[84] Cases have been reported in other immunocompromised children, including a 7-month-old boy with disseminated *M. kansasii* infection and numerous organisms found in his spleen at autopsy.[121] *M. kansasii* also has been reported to cause meningitis; the patients died despite the use of antimycobacterial therapy.[85,160] In another report, an 18-month-old previously healthy boy developed chronic septic arthritis of the ankle with adjacent osteomyelitis of the distal tibia[210] resulting in significant bone destruction.

Mycobacterium malmoense

Buchholz and coworkers[19] reviewed infections with *M. malmoense* in the United States from 1993 to 1995. Only 1 of 73 patients was younger than 10 years. This patient had cervical lymphadenitis and was cured with surgical excision alone. This organism, which frequently is overlooked on standard Löwenstein-Jensen egg medium, grows at 25°C to 37° C (77° to 98.6°F). The organism is slow-growing, and it may require 8 to 12 weeks for colonies to become visible on solid media. The BACTEC system was shown to be superior in isolating *M. malmoense* in one study of children with lymphadenitis.[81] Bone marrow involvement also was described in a patient with chronic granulocytic leukemia.[51] PCR may improve the identification of this organism. The study by Buchholz and colleagues[19] showed that prolonged combination therapy with isoniazid, rifampin, ethambutol, and pyrazinamide after surgical excision was effective in some cases.

RAPIDLY GROWING MYCOBACTERIA

NTM that form colonies on subculture within 7 or fewer days are referred to as *rapidly growing mycobacteria.* The *M. chelonae-abscessus* group consists of *M. chelonae, M. abscessus, M. bolletii, and M. massiliense.* The *M. fortuitum* complex consists of *M. fortuitum, M. peregrinum,* and biovariant 3.[101,72] Multilocus DNA sequencing may be needed to differentiate rapidly growing mycobacteria to the species level.[1,223] Patients typically have an underlying condition such as immune suppression or cystic fibrosis and may have a catheter or other implanted device. The most frequent manifestations of rapidly growing mycobacteria include pulmonary infections, bloodstream infections, skin and soft tissue infections, osteomyelitis, device-associated infections, and disseminated disease.[143,72]

M. abscessus, as stated earlier, is related closely to *M. chelonae* but should be designated as a separate species.[101] Manifestations of *M. abscessus* infection usually involve pulmonary, bloodstream, cutaneous, or occasionally disseminated disease.[66,201,72] *M. abscessus* is the most common rapidly growing mycobacteria isolate causing pulmonary disease.[66] Underlying conditions such as bronchiectasis, gastroesophageal disorders with chronic vomiting, and cystic fibrosis are frequently present. Multilobar nodular bronchiectatic disease is the most common presentation. Cutaneous disease is often related to surgery or trauma and manifests as purple nodules. Maxson and associates[120] reported a case of osteomyelitis caused by *M. abscessus.*

Wallace and associates[200] provided the largest series of patients with skin, soft tissue, and bone involvement with *M. chelonae,* which is the primary clinical manifestation. Steroid use seemed to be the factor associated most commonly with the development of disease. Adult renal transplant patients also have been described with skin and subcutaneous tissue involvement caused by *M. chelonae.*[36] *M. chelonae* has also been described as an etiologic agent for otitis media, probably from contamination of ear, nose, and throat instruments with colonized water sources.[112] Cases of keratitis caused by *M. chelonae* have been reported after laser in situ keratomileusis (LASIK).[57,220] Pulmonary disease is less common.[66] With the improved ability to distinguish *M. abscessus* and *M. chelonae,* many isolates that were once identified as *M. chelonae* may now be identified as *M. abscessus.*[72]

M. fortuitum complex is one of the most frequently isolated rapidly growing mycobacteria and causes a range of diseases, including pulmonary, wound, lymphadenitis, and catheter infections.[143,72] *M. fortuitum* and *M. chelonae* have been implicated in sternal wound infections and endocarditis and have occurred in outbreak-type settings.[100,156,186] Patients responded to surgical debridement and amikacin with cefoxitin. A case series from Hong Kong reported successful treatment of *M. fortuitum* sternotomy infections with the use of a single daily dose ofloxacin as monotherapy in three patients.[222] Pulmonary disease with findings similar to those in *M. abscessus* occur in patients with *M. fortuitum,* but primarily in patients with gastroesophageal disorders with chronic vomiting.[66]

Other rapidly growing mycobacteria include *M. mucogenicum,* which is commonly isolated in cancer patients. In this population, *M. mucogenicum* is the rapidly growing mycobacteria most frequently associated with bloodstream and catheter-associated infections.[72] An outbreak of *M. mucogenicum* catheter-associated bloodstream infections occurred in eight pediatric hematology and oncology patients.[166] Six of the patients were successfully treated with catheter removal alone. *Mycobacterium neoaurum* also has been associated with catheter-associated bloodstream infections in immune-suppressed patients, including children.[203] *Mycobacterium smegmatis,* which resembles *M. fortuitum,* is a rapidly growing mycobacterium responsible for skin and soft tissue infections.[201] A case of disseminated infection has been reported in a child with inherited IFN-γ receptor deficiency.[136] *M. massiliense,* which is a rapidly growing mycobacterium closely related to *M. abscessus,* was associated with an outbreak of intramuscular injection–associated soft tissue infections in adults and children.[95] *Mycobacterium septicum* is a recently described rapidly growing mycobacterial species associated with catheter-related bacteremia.[162] *Mycobacterium wolinskyi* is an uncommon cause of posttraumatic and postsurgical wound infections and osteomyelitis.[7] As our ability to detect and distinguish different mycobacterial species improves, the number of mycobacterial species implicated in human infection will likely continue to increase.

Treatment of rapidly growing mycobacteria usually requires combination therapy involving at least two agents. Because susceptibility differs across species, these bacteria should be identified to the species level and treatment based on susceptibility testing. In general, skin and soft tissue disease should be treated for at least 4 months and bone disease for at least 6 months. Surgery may be required for extensive disease. For infections involving implants, the foreign body should be removed. Pulmonary disease often is difficult to treat, but a goal of at least 12 months of negative sputum is reasonable.[64]

NEW REFERENCES SINCE THE SEVENTH EDITION

20. Cadena G, Wiedeman J, Boggan JE. Ventriculoperitoneal shunt infection with Mycobacterium fortuitum: a rare offending organism. *J Neurosurg Pediatr.* 2014;14:704-707.
21. Cassidy PM, Hedberg K, Saulson A, et al. Nontuberculous mycobacterial disease prevalence and risk factors: a changing epidemiology. *Clin Infect Dis.* 2009;49:e124-e129.
46. Donohue MJ, Mistry JH, Donohue JM, et al. Increased frequency of nontuberculous Mycobacteria detection at potable water taps within the United States. *Environ Sci Technol.* 2015;49:6127-6133.
74. Hatzenbuehler LA, Starke JR. Common presentations of nontuberculous mycobacterial infections. *Pediatr Infect Dis.* 2014;33:89-91.
86. Iroh Tam PY, Kline S, Wagner JE, et al. Rapidly growing mycobacteria among pediatric hematopoietic cell transplant patients traced to the hospital water supply. *Pediatr Infecti Dis.* 2014;33:1043-1046.
132. O'Brien RJ, Geiter LJ, Snider DE Jr. The epidemiology of nontuberculous mycobacterial diseases in the United States. Results from a national survey. *Am Rev Respir Dis.* 1987;135(5):1007-1014.
142. Qvist T, Gilljam M, Jonsson B, et al. Epidemiology of nontuberculous mycobacteria among patients with cystic fibrosis in Scandinavia. *J Cyst Fibros.* 2015;14(1):46-52.
149. Ringshausen FC, Apel RM, Bange FC, et al. Burden and trends of hospitalisations associated with pulmonary non-tuberculous mycobacterial infections in Germany, 2005-2011. *BMC Infect Dis.* 2013;13:231.
165. Seddon P, Fidler K, Raman S, et al. Prevalence of nontuberculous mycobacteria in cystic fibrosis clinics, United Kingdom, 2009. *Emerg Infect Dis.* 2013;19(7):1128-1130.
170. Siberry GK, Abzug MJ, Nachman S, et al. Guidelines for the prevention and treatment of opportunistic infections in HIV-exposed and HIV-infected children: recommendations from the National Institutes of Health, Centers for Disease Control and Prevention, the HIV Medicine Association of the Infectious Diseases Society of America, the Pediatric Infectious Diseases Society, and the American Academy of Pediatrics. *Pediatr Infect Dis J.* 2013;32(suppl 2):i-KK4.
173. Sinagra JL, Kanitz EE, Cerocchi C, et al. Mycobacterium abscessus hand-and-foot disease in children: rare or emerging disease? *Pediatr Dermatol.* 2014;31(3):292-297.
187. Talati NJ, Rouphael N, Kuppalli K, et al. Spectrum of CNS disease caused by rapidly growing mycobacteria. *Lancet Infect Dis.* 2008;8(6):390-398.
202. Ward TT, Rimland D, Kauffman C, et al. Randomized, open-label trial of azithromycin plus ethambutol vs. clarithromycin plus ethambutol as therapy for Mycobacterium avium complex bacteremia in patients with human immunodeficiency virus infection. Veterans Affairs HIV Research Consortium. *Clin Infect Dis.* 1998;27(5):1278-1285.
211. Winthrop KL, Baxter R, Liu L, et al. Mycobacterial diseases and antitumour necrosis factor therapy in USA. *Ann Rheum Dis.* 2013;72(1):37-42.

The full reference list for this chapter is available at ExpertConsult.com.

98 Leprosy and Buruli Ulcer: The Major Cutaneous Mycobacterioses

Andrea T. Cruz

Mycobacterial infections in humans date to at least the 10th millennium BCE, with evidence of tuberculosis in Neolithic skeletons from Heidelberg, Germany,[15] Egyptian mummies,[279] and from pre-Columbian Mesoamerica.[77] Evidence of lepromatous leprosy has been found in burials in India dating back to 2000 BCE, correlating with Vedic scriptural references to leprosy.[269] Although the origins of mycobacterial infections in humans are unknown, most authorities speculate that domestication of animals in the Neolithic era promoted the transmission of mutants of *Mycobacterium tuberculosis* from livestock to humans. The origins of leprosy and Buruli ulcer and their respective etiologic agents are understood less well but may involve interplay among nontuberculous mycobacteria, animals, and humans.[294] After tuberculosis, leprosy and Buruli ulcer are the second and third most common mycobacterial infections in humans. Leprosy and Buruli ulcer are the two most common cutaneous mycobacterioses.

Tuberculosis and other cutaneous mycobacterial infections are discussed in Chapters 96 and 97. This chapter is devoted to the two cutaneous mycobacterioses that are of greatest medical importance: leprosy and Buruli ulcer.

LEPROSY

Leprosy is a chronic infectious disease caused by *Mycobacterium leprae* that principally affects the cooler parts of the body, especially the skin, upper respiratory tract, testes, eyes, and superficial segments of peripheral nerves. The World Health Organization (WHO) reported that in 2013 there were 215,000 incident cases and 180,000 prevalent cases.[377] Many authorities consider that the total global prevalence of patients with active leprosy is much higher (1.5–2 million),[11] however, and are underreported because of the stigma associated with leprosy.[139] Several million more patients experience serious sequelae.[182]

In the Middle Ages, leprosy was common in Europe, reported in up to one quarter of skeletons in one ordinary (nonleprous colony) Danish village cemetery.[27] European emigration and the West African slave trade, rather than crossing from Asia via the Bering Strait, likely introduced leprosy to the New World. The Silk Road may have then spread leprosy from Europe to China.[221] At least two foci in the United States were established in the 19th century by specific immigrations: Asians brought leprosy to the Hawaiian Islands and started an epidemic in the highly susceptible Hawaiians[224] and Scandinavians introduced leprosy into the northern Midwest region of the United States.[191]

Patients with leprosy frequently experience severe stigmas. This has been noted in the Old Testament (Leviticus 13:4) and in 8th century BCE Chinese literature.[315] Similarly, the *Laws of Manu* (India, circa 1500 BCE) punished persons marrying into families with leprosy.[33] Although suicide was considered a sin under Hinduism, leprosy was an exception.[139] The stigma persists to the modern era. In 2009, the chairman of India's human rights commission recommended prosecuting leprosy patients if they had children.[37] Continuing efforts must be made to minimize the stigma peculiarly associated with leprosy. To help achieve this goal, the Fifth International Leprosy Congress in 1948 adopted a resolution to abandon the word *leper* for the leprosy patient.[179] Some physicians prefer Hansen disease as a synonym for leprosy.

Organism

M. leprae is a species in the order Actinomycetales and the family Mycobacteriaceae. This bacillus was seen first by Hansen in 1873 in Bergen, Norway, in lepromas from Norwegian patients, and this organism was the first reported bacterium causing chronic disease in humans.

M. leprae is an acid-fast bacillus 0.3 to 0.5 µm wide by 4 to 7 µm long. The acid-fastness of *M. leprae* is weaker than that of other mycobacteria. Viable *M. leprae* organisms stain solidly, but degenerating bacilli first stain irregularly, then become granular, and eventually lose acid-fastness completely. The persistence of bacillary carcasses can be verified by silver staining techniques.[350] Because *M. leprae* still cannot be cultivated, identification depends on criteria other than those used routinely for cultivable mycobacteria. Current criteria for *M. leprae* are the following: (1) it does not grow on routine laboratory media; (2) it infects the footpads of mice in a characteristic manner[180,309]; (3) acid-fastness is extractable with pyridine[53]; (4) the organism invades nerves of the host; (5) suspensions of dead bacilli produce a characteristic pattern of reactions when injected into the skin of patients (lepromin reaction) with the various clinical forms of leprosy; (6) it produces the species-specific antigen phenolic glycolipid-1 (PGL-1)[105]; and (7) it exhibits species-specific DNA sequences.[365]

Gene deletion and decay have markedly limited the metabolic activities of *M. leprae* and may contribute significantly to failure to cultivate the organism and to its long generation time in the mouse footpad (14 days).[29,86] Localization of infections to the cooler parts of the body,[26] selective growth in the footpads of immunologically intact mice and in the ears of hamsters, and the high susceptibility of the armadillo (central body temperature of 32°C to 35°C [89.6°F to 95°F]) to disseminated infections all suggest that the optimal temperature for growth of *M. leprae* is less than 37°C (98.6°F).[201]

Transmission

The modes of transmission of *M. leprae* in nature have not been fully established. The frequency in children of a single early lesion in skin that usually is covered by clothing argues against the development of such lesions at the site of contact with *M. leprae*.[18] For many years, skin-to-skin contact between the patient and healthy subjects was considered the most important means of transmission, and this concept cannot be abandoned readily.[178] Intact skin of heavily infected patients discharges a few *M. leprae,* but ulcers in the skin may be a source of numerous bacilli. In some studies, bacillary load was the only factor associated with leprosy spread to index case contacts.[284] Skin-to-skin contact and fomites containing *M. leprae* could be sources of infection, but this mode has been minimized in recent years in favor of the nasorespiratory route.[147]

Studies suggest that the respiratory passages could be an important source of infecting bacilli.[73] In one study, 80% of patients with multibacillary leprosy had *M. leprae* DNA in skin washings and 60% had nasal secretions testing positive for *M. leprae* by polymerase chain reaction (PCR). Household contacts were PCR-positive from skin and nasal secretion samples in 17% and 4% of instances, respectively.[147] *M. leprae* organisms ejected in nose blowing remain viable under ambient conditions for 1 week,[64] and disseminated leprosy develops in immunosuppressed mice after the inhalation of aerosol that contains *M. leprae.*[264] Breast tissue and milk from lepromatous patients contain *M. leprae,* and infants may acquire infection from this source.[248]

Placental transmission of leprosy has been a subject of conjecture for some time, but evidence is growing for a significant influence of leprosy on fetal development and for intrauterine fetal infection. In a study of 156 pregnant leprosy patients in Ethiopia, the placentas were small, and infants had lower birth weight, higher risk for intrauterine growth restriction, and higher infant mortality rates than infants of nonlepromatous mothers.[81] Immunoglobulin A (IgA) and IgM antibodies for *M. leprae* are present in the cord blood of 30% to 50% of infants delivered by mothers with lepromatous leprosy.[197] Evidence is strong for synthesis of fetal antibodies to *M. leprae*. Occasionally, *M. leprae* has been shown in placentas and cord blood and can be detected until 2 years of age.[137,198,336] Two young children with intrauterine exposure developed leprosy before 18 months of age.[80]

Leprosy in young infants may be a common occurrence in areas of high endemicity.[111] In a report combining cases from the literature and observations by experienced leprologists, a total of at least 49 infants with leprosy were identified.[31] In only half of these infants did the mother have a history of leprosy. The youngest infant was 2.5 months old at the time of diagnosis. The fact that many of the mothers never had clinical leprosy suggests that they had transient *M. leprae* bacteremia during gestation. Persistent bacteremia is a common finding in multibacillary disease[78,171] and is detectable in 15% of paucibacillary patients.[162]

The discoveries of a naturally acquired leprosy-like disease in recently captured wild armadillos in Louisiana,[332,355] chimpanzees,[76,114] and Old World monkeys[204,212] provide reason to consider that leprosy is a zoonosis.[337] Naturally acquired leprosy was found in 16% of nine-banded armadillos in the southeastern United States.[306] In all of these species, the histopathologic features resemble those in leprosy in humans, and the bacilli that cause the infection cannot be distinguished from *M. leprae.*[25,205,211] Leprosy has been transmitted successfully from the mangabey monkey to other mangabey, rhesus, and African green monkeys.[149,367] No cases of transmission of leprosy to humans from naturally infected mangabey monkeys or chimpanzees have been reported, but this potential exists.[114,203] Some authorities suggest that insects, including *Aedes aegypti* mosquitoes, may ingest *M. leprae* during a blood meal from lepromatous patients and harbor viable bacteria.[12] The natural transmission of leprosy by insects remains unproven, however.

Epidemiology

The highest incidence rates of leprosy are found in Southeast Asia (including India), which accounted for 72% of new leprosy cases in 2013. The Americas accounted for 15%, followed by Africa (10%), Western Pacific nations (2%), and Eastern Mediterranean countries (1.7%).[377] While prevalence has fallen substantially in recent years, this decrease is partially due to decreased treatment durations.[271] Based on limited whole-population surveys in endemic areas, the total number of active patients may exceed the number reported by the WHO by a significant margin. The stigma of the disease and inefficiency in health care delivery systems contribute to this disparity in statistics.[139]

Between 1994 and 2011, leprosy incidence rates declined from 0.52 to 0.43 per million in the United States; 2323 new cases were reported during this time period. Incidence rates were 14 to 23 times higher in foreign-born persons than in persons born in the United States.[239] Since 2000, an increased number of cases in immigrants from the Marshall Islands and Micronesia has been reported.[369] A few indigenous patients regularly come from Louisiana, Texas, other southeastern states, and Hawaii.[172] No instances of secondary transmission from imported cases within the United States have been reported; immigrants with leprosy present no known public health risk to the population of the United

States. The same situation probably is true for other nonendemic countries that receive many immigrants from endemic areas.

In 1871 and 1872, Hansen studied 69 Norwegian families in which several members had leprosy. The prevailing concept of that era was that leprosy was hereditary, but from data gathered on these families, Hansen showed that patients always had contact with another leprosy patient.[121] Hansen reasoned that the spread of leprosy depended on dissemination of this etiologic agent in a susceptible population. The leprosy epidemic in Nauru in the central Pacific area shows how rapidly leprosy can spread in a leprosy-naïve population.[115] Leprosy was introduced into this small island in 1912, and by 1924, one-third of the 2500 inhabitants had leprosy.

The prevailing concept has been that an individual becomes infected only after experiencing repeated exposure. This concept now is doubted, and a single exposure may be sufficient in optimal conditions. One report describes leprosy transmission occurring after a single exposure from a patient to a surgeon who practiced in a leprosy nonendemic area.[1] Other reports describe inoculation leprosy after injury with a broken glass bangle[110] and after tattooing.[314] In any patient-contact situation, the number of viable *M. leprae* being shed by the patient and the degree of susceptibility of the contact both may vary. Lymphocyte transformation studies show that occupational contacts of leprosy patients in Ethiopia have the highest rate of sensitization (58%) to *M. leprae,* followed closely by household contacts (47%). Noncontacts living in endemic areas have a lower rate of sensitization, but approximately 29% of the population still is sensitized.[112]

Factors facilitating spread of leprosy include multibacillary (versus paucibacillary disease), the nutritional status of a population, and living conditions. The percentage of patients with multibacillary disease (lepromatous leprosy) varies by ethnicity. Multibacillary disease is seen in up to 50% of Asians and only 5% to 10% of Africans. Social factors, such as low educational level, bathing weekly in open water bodies, low frequency of bed linen changes,[164] and food shortages[94,115,280,316] were associated with leprosy transmission. Nonetheless, convincing evidence that the prevalence of leprosy is unusually high in chronically malnourished populations is lacking, in part because of the collinearity between malnutrition and other markers of socioeconomic deprivation.

Improvements in housing and other living conditions may play a role in the declining prevalence of leprosy. No other factor satisfactorily explains the virtual disappearance of leprosy from northern Europe after the Middle Ages and from Scandinavia in the 20th century, long before any effective chemotherapy was available. If the disease is predominantly airborne, the construction of dwellings that provide less confined sleeping quarters in this era could have contributed to reduced incidence rates in these regions. Consistent with this concept is the inadequate housing that prevails in all geographic areas in which leprosy is common today. Another explanation for declining leprosy cases in Europe after the 15th century was that the rudimentary infection control and isolation of lepromatous patients may have had an impact.[307]

The presumed increased susceptibility of children is difficult to establish and may depend more on exposure to contagious patients and genetic predisposition than on other factors. In most populations studied, only 5% to 10% of individuals are susceptible to leprosy. The proportion of children among all detected patients is 20% to 30%.[106,241] Lara,[174] in a study of 2000 Filipino children who lived in a leprosarium in the prechemotherapy era, noted that leprosy developed in 470 (23%). In 75%, the lesions healed spontaneously; active, persistent disease developed in approximately 6% of heavily exposed children. In adults, leprosy occurs more commonly in men than in women (2:1 to 3:1). In children, the sex ratio is approximately 1:1.

Genetic factors likely influence the susceptibility of some individuals to leprosy and the form of disease that develops.[95,99,100,311] Several polymorphisms have been associated with leprosy susceptibility. These include a mannose gene, interleukin (IL)-10, and tumor necrosis factor (TNF) receptor mutations.[286,308] TNF promoter mutations are particularly associated with development of lepromatous or multibacillary leprosy.[276] Other mutations identified include those on chromosome 6 near the Parkinson disease gene *PARK2* and *PACRG* genes,[213,214] vitamin D receptor gene,[99] interferon (IFN)-γ receptor-1 gene promoter (*IFNGR1*) polymorphisms,[344] and the nucleotide-binding oligomerization domain-containing protein 2 (NOD2)-mediated signaling pathway, which helps mediate innate immune responses.[382] Certain human leukocyte antigens (*HLA-DR*) seem to be associated with specific forms of leprosy. *HLA-DR2* and *HLA-DR3* alleles are associated with tuberculoid disease, and *HLA-DQ1* is associated with lepromatous disease.[55] HLA-DR antigens may influence the presentation of antigens of *M. leprae* to T cells and may affect the immune response to leprosy.[245]

Toll-like receptors (TLRs), molecules present on the surface of innate or native immune cells, mediate cytokine production on encountering a foreign invader, including mycobacteria, and ultimately may influence the pattern of specific immunity.[193,275] Lepromatous leprosy occurs more commonly in patients with a mutation in the TLR-2, associated with altered production of IL-10 and IL-12, underscoring the role early cytokine responses against *M. leprae* may play.[152–154] Another SNP, this one in the TLR-1 transmembrane domain, was associated with diminished nuclear factor-κB (NFκ-B) activity and found to have reduced cytokine responses to *M. leprae*.[215,368] In African patients, polymorphisms in the *NRAMP1* gene, a gene also associated with cellular immunity to *M. tuberculosis,* are associated with lepromatous leprosy,[196] as shown in the Mitsuda reaction.[6,260]

Pathogenesis and Pathology

M. leprae causes disease by its ability to survive and multiply in macrophages (Fig. 98.1).[294] If macrophages of the host digest the bacilli early, disease is undetectable or the patient has only minimal lesions. If the macrophages are totally incapable of destroying the organisms, widely disseminated lepromatous leprosy follows. Survival of *M. leprae* in macrophages depends on the immune response of the patient; knowledge of immunity to *M. leprae* is necessary for understanding the mechanism of pathologic changes in leprosy.

Immunity

The immunopathogenesis of leprosy can be understood by examining the polar nature of the condition, whereby tuberculoid disease is characterized by one or several well-demarcated lesions, borderline disease manifests with a modest number of medium-sized lesions, and lepromatous disease manifests with widespread poorly demarcated lesions (Table 98.1). Each type is associated with a different immunologic profile, especially within the lesions.

The ability of an individual to resist *M. leprae* is assessed readily by the induration provoked by an intradermal injection of a suspension of killed *M. leprae* prepared from lepromatous tissue from armadillos.[206] The reagent is known as *lepromin,* and the response is known as the *lepromin reaction.*[217] This reaction has two components: an early response at 48 hours (Fernandez reaction) and a late response at 3 to 4 weeks

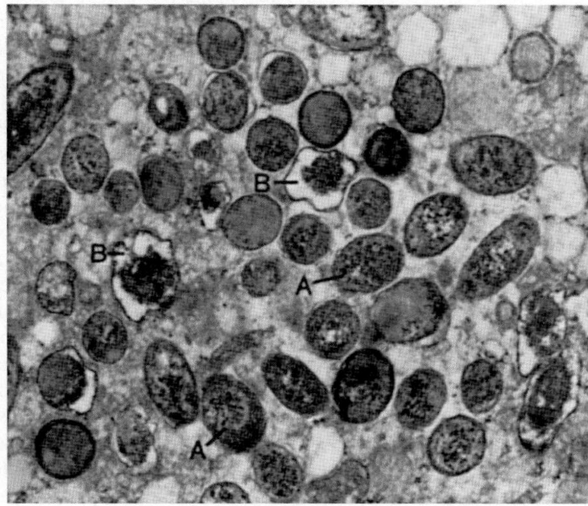

FIG. 98.1 Electron micrograph of a portion of a globus of *M. leprae* within a histiocyte in a leproma in the skin. Cross sections of (A) well-preserved and (B) degenerated bacilli are presented (×45,000). (Courtesy Dr. S.C. Chang.)

TABLE 98.1 Criteria for Classification of Leprosy

Group	Clinical Features	Histologic Features	Lepromin Reaction (Mitsuda)	Bacillary Density
Tuberculoid	Single or few anesthetic macules or plaques Borders well defined Peripheral nerve involvement common	Epithelioid-lymphocyte granulomas, with or without giant cells, in skin and nerves No subepidermal clear zone Bacilli in nerves, but rare	Strongly positive	Rare
Borderline tuberculoid	Lesions similar to those of tuberculoid, but more numerous Borders of lesions less distinct Satellite lesions sometimes present around larger lesions Peripheral nerve involvement common	Granulomas similar to those in tuberculoid Nerves are infiltrated Bacilli frequently found in nerves	Positive	Scanty
Borderline	More lesions than in borderline tuberculoid Borders more vague Satellite lesions often seen Peripheral nerve involvement common	Epithelioid cells and histiocytic infiltrations focalized by lymphocytes Nerves show increased cellularity Bacilli readily found in nerves	Negative or weakly positive	Moderate
Borderline lepromatous	Lesions are numerous and similar to those of borderline Some nerve damage	Histiocytic infiltrations show a tendency to evolve toward epithelioid cells and foamy cells Lymphocytes present Nerves have less cellular infiltration Bacilli plentiful in nerves	Negative	Heavy
Lepromatous	Multiple, nonanesthetic, macular or papular, symmetrically distributed lesions No neural lesions until late Late complications of madarosis, leonine facies, testicular damage	Foamy histiocytes containing large numbers of bacilli Few or no lymphocytes Subepidermal clear zone Numerous bacilli in nerves and perineurium without significant intraneural cellular infiltration	Negative	Very heavy
Indeterminate	Vaguely defined hypopigmented or erythematous macule	Often indistinguishable from mild nonspecific dermatitis Lymphocytes and histiocytes around skin appendages and nerves	Weakly positive or negative	Negative or scanty

(Mitsuda reaction). The Mitsuda reaction is the most consistent and is used by clinicians as an aid in classifying the clinical forms of leprosy.

Mitsuda reactions are strongly positive (>5 mm in diameter) in tuberculoid patients, weak or negative (0 to 2 mm) in lepromatous patients, and intermediate (3 to 5 mm) in patients with borderline disease. The reactions are a direct measure of delayed hypersensitivity or cell-mediated immunity to *M. leprae* antigens; lepromatous patients are anergic to *M. leprae*, akin to anergy to the tuberculin skin test (TST) seen in children with tuberculous meningitis or miliary tuberculosis. Also similar to the TST, the lepromin reaction has no value in establishing the diagnosis because a high percentage of any population is Mitsuda positive. One study evaluated the Mitsuda response in Indian children residing in leprosy-endemic regions. Percent positivity was higher in low-endemic regions than high-endemic areas (93% and 88%, respectively), indicating that the Mitsuda response is independent of *M. leprae* exposure.[303] Nonspecific factors participate in host defense against *M. leprae*. Complement promotes phagocytosis of leprosy bacilli.[290] Although the precise mechanisms of specific immunity remain elusive, abundant experimental evidence indicates that in a lepromatous leprosy (multibacillary) patient, cell-mediated immunity to *M. leprae* is markedly suppressed.[35] The degree of suppression is gradually less pronounced in clinical forms of disease that are progressively nearer tuberculoid (paucibacillary) leprosy.[356] Patients with multibacillary forms of leprosy are found to have decreases in the total numbers of circulating T lymphocytes,[84] despite normal T-cell subsets,[261] or decreased lymphocyte function.[228] $CD4^+$ T lymphocytes predominate in paucibacillary disease and produce IFN-γ,[285,380] whereas $CD8^+$ lymphocytes predominate for multibacillary disease and produce IL-4.[285] This immunologic dichotomy between tuberculoid and lepromatous lesions is consistent with the paradigm that robust cell-mediated immunity limits disease progression and that humoral immunity has little or no effect.

Macrophages of lepromatous patients are thought to have the capacity to kill, digest, and clear *M. leprae* if they are activated.[130] Patients with lepromatous leprosy fail to produce IL-2, but IL-2 restores the proliferation of lymphocytes in response to specific antigens.[123] Defective IFN-γ is produced by lymphocytes from lepromatous patients on stimulation by *M. leprae* antigens.[238] IL-2–bearing lymphocytes are reduced markedly in lepromatous infiltrations in tissues.[219] These combine to result in macrophages not being activated. The injection of IFN-γ or recombinant IL-2 into the skin of lepromatous patients causes a local influx of $CD4^+$ T cells along with the formation of epithelioid and giant cells and a reduction in bacillary load.[156,346] Therapy with IL-2 or IFN-γ induces the secretion of TNF-α; however, the activity of this toxic molecule may be inhibited by thalidomide or pentoxifylline.[155,328] TNF-α is associated with macrophage infiltration of peripheral nerves in reversal reactions.[165] Whether the increasing use of TNF-α antagonists would be associated with the development of leprosy from latent infections or perhaps be useful in the management of leprosy reactions remains unclear.[88,295]

Immunoglobulin production (i.e., IgG, IgA, and IgM) usually is elevated only slightly in tuberculoid patients but is elevated markedly in lepromatous patients, consistent with the predominant T_H1 versus T_H2 responses.[36] The total number of B lymphocytes is increased in the blood of lepromatous patients, as is the circulating antibody to mycobacterial antigens.[234]

Histopathology

Biopsy specimens from well-defined lesions of leprosy should be taken from the active border (not the center of the lesion) and fixed in buffered 10% formalin or other suitable fixative. The Fite-Faraco staining method conventionally is used because the Ziehl-Neelsen (ZN) stain does not show *M. leprae* optimally in tissue sections. However, Fite-Faraco staining is time-consuming, can result in observer fatigue (particularly in paucibacillary cases), and has sensitivities of 45% to 60%. In contrast, ZN stains[265] and rhodamine-auramine fluorescent stains[235] have sensitivities of 50% and 70%, respectively. Combining Fite-Faraco staining with PCR can provide more rapid diagnoses than other modalities used in isolation.[265] A histopathologic diagnosis of leprosy must not be made unless the evidence is convincing. In nonendemic regions, providing additional history to the pathologist can allow for clinicopathologic correlation.[273]

Indeterminate leprosy. Indeterminate leprosy (Fig. 98.2) is characterized by mild chronic inflammation (Fig. 98.3). If leprosy is suspected, all nerves in the dermis and subcutaneous tissue in numerous sections of the biopsy specimen must be searched for acid-fast bacilli, even if no inflammatory changes within the nerves are present. Sometimes acid-fast bacilli are more common in the arrector pili muscles or subepidermal zone,[267] but are rarely seen in normal-appearing skin.[32] Angiogenesis is not common in indeterminate leprosy skin lesions, in contrast to other forms.[21] A histopathologic diagnosis requires demonstration of acid-fast bacilli. PCR is less sensitive in paucibacillary forms, such as indeterminate leprosy, when compared to multibacillary forms. However, given the diagnostic difficulties for indeterminate leprosy, PCR can greatly augment diagnostic yield compared to slit-skin smears for acid-fast organisms.[13]

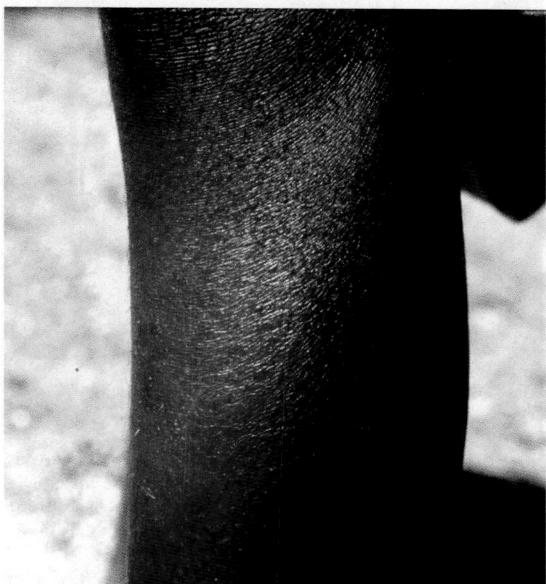

FIG. 98.2 Hypopigmented macule of indeterminate leprosy on the anterior surface of the leg of an Indian girl.

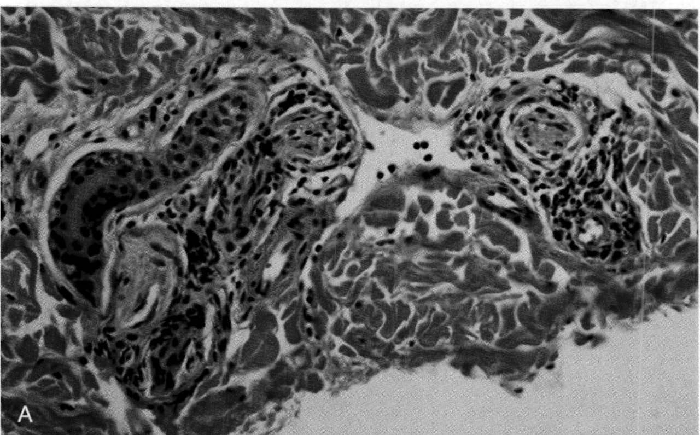

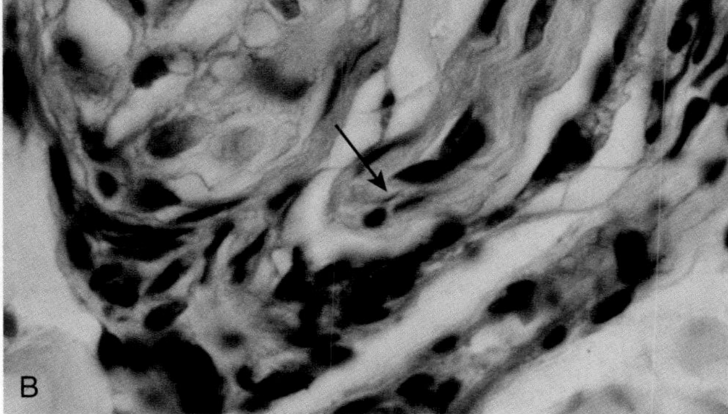

FIG. 98.3 (A) Indeterminate leprosy showing only mild infiltrations along neurovascular channels in the deep dermis (hematoxylin and eosin stain). (B) Only a single acid-fast bacillus was found in one deep dermal nerve (*arrow*) after a search of multiple sections (Fite-Faraco stain).

Tuberculoid leprosy. Tuberculoid leprosy (Fig. 98.4) is characterized by granulomata in the dermis, epidermis, and subcutaneous tissues (Fig. 98.5A). Damage to nerves is a distinctive feature; in advanced lesions, all cutaneous nerves may be damaged beyond recognition (see Fig. 98.5B). This nerve damage is best visualized by S-100 immunostaining, which reveals a neural pattern of Schwann cells. Bacilli rarely are found, and often many sections must be searched to locate a single bacillus. The bacilli usually are within remnants of dermal nerves but sometimes are located just beneath the epidermis. When major nerve trunks are involved, they contain typical tuberculoid infiltrates that eventually may replace the entire nerve. Occasionally, caseous "abscesses" are present in large nerves; these are rare in children.

Borderline leprosy. Borderline leprosy represents a broad spectrum of clinical (Fig. 98.6) and histopathologic variations (see Table 98.1). In the borderline-tuberculoid variety, nerves usually are damaged less and are identifiable more readily than in tuberculoid leprosy. *M. leprae* often remain rare but are seen more readily than in tuberculoid leprosy in nerves (Fig. 98.7) or in the subdermal zone. Acid-fast bacilli can be seen in arrector pili muscle in normal-appearing skin in 17% to 25% of cases of borderline leprosy.[32] Some histopathologists do not recognize borderline leprosy as an entity because there is usually a suggestion that the lesion is on either the borderline-tuberculoid or the borderline-lepromatous side of the spectrum of the disease.[146] Borderline-lepromatous lesions are characterized by granulomas, easily identified nerves with perineurium infiltration, and readily visualized bacilli.

Lepromatous leprosy. Prelepromatous lesions show only a mild proliferation of macrophages around vessels, nerves, and appendages. Acid-fast bacilli are few and often difficult to show. As the disease progresses, the bacilli-laden macrophage (Virchow cell or lepra cell) becomes the predominant inflammatory cell (Fig. 98.8). In early lesions, they tend to accumulate around vessels, nerves, and appendages, but they eventually may replace the entire dermis (Fig. 98.9A). As the macrophages age, they become vacuolated (foamy), largely from their lipid content. In developing lesions, the intracellular bacilli are arranged in small bundles (see Fig. 98.9B); in advanced lesions, dense masses of bacilli termed *globi* may replace nearly the entire cytoplasm of the

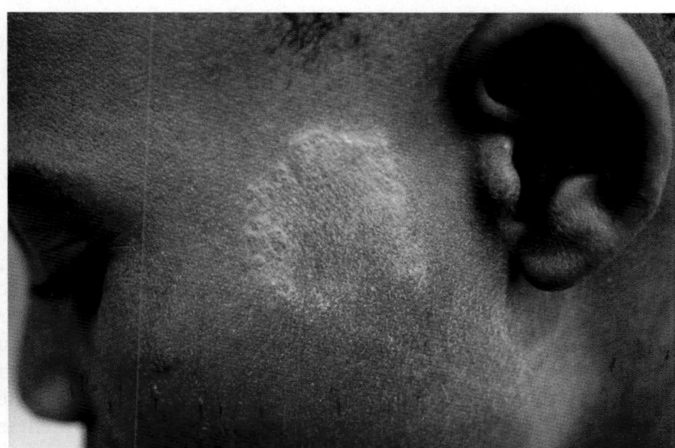

FIG. 98.4 Tuberculoid leprosy in a 12-year-old Congolese boy. This was the only lesion; it has a well-defined papulated border with central healing.

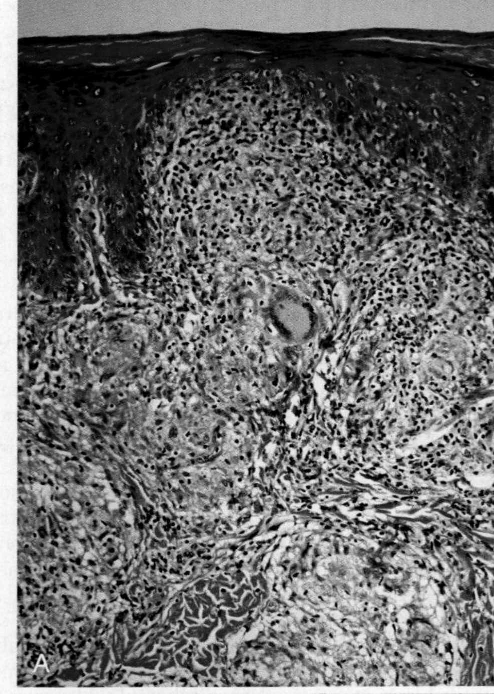

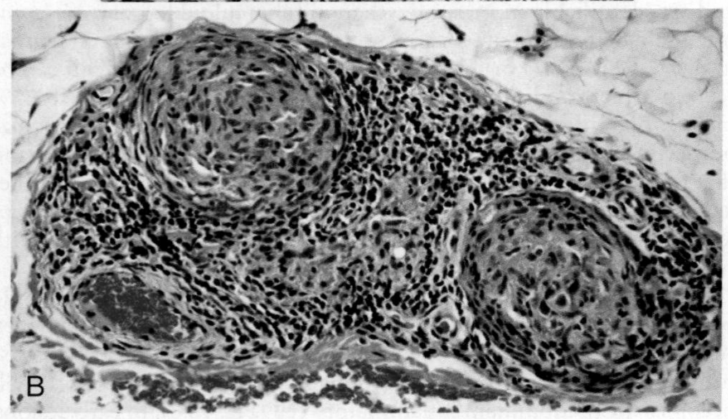

FIG. 98.5 (A) Tuberculoid leprosy with a dense granulomatous infiltration that invades the epidermis. Granulomata contain epithelioid cells, Langhans giant cells, and lymphocytes (hematoxylin and eosin stain). (B) High magnification of a nerve bundle in the subcutaneous tissue of section in (A). Granulomata have nearly completely destroyed the nerves. Remnants of nerves contained rare acid-fast bacilli (hematoxylin and eosin stain).

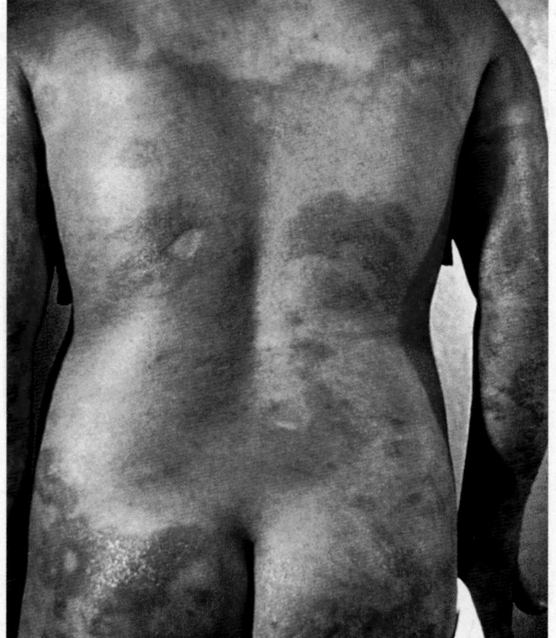

FIG. 98.6 Borderline lepromatous leprosy in a Filipino. There are many plaques, some with well-defined borders and others vaguely defined. The erythematous plaques indicate that the patient is undergoing an upgrading reversal reaction (type 1).

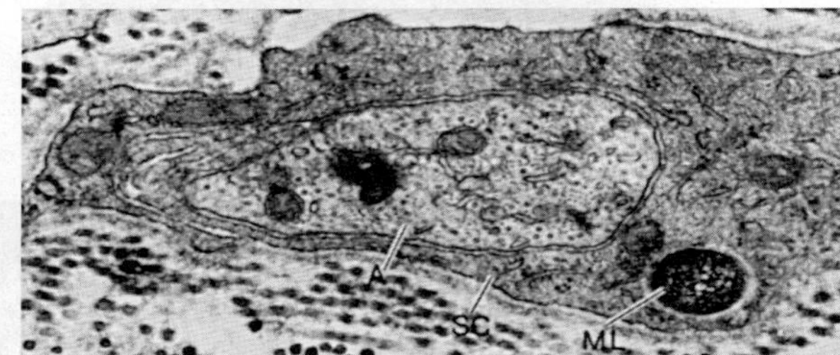

FIG. 98.7 Electron micrograph of a portion of a damaged dermal nerve in borderline leprosy. A nonmyelinated axon *(A)* is surrounded by a Schwann cell (*SC*) that contains a single *M. leprae* bacillus *(ML)* (×60,000). (Courtesy Dr. S.C. Chang.)

macrophage. Many bacilli are found in the dermal nerves and frequently in endothelial cells, walls of blood vessels, arrector pili muscles, and epithelial cells of hair follicles.[226] In one case series, acid-fast bacilli were found in arrector pili muscle in normal-appearing skin in more than 50% of patients with lepromatous leprosy,[32] with implications for both disease extent and recurrence risk. Lymphocytes are scant. Large nerve trunks may show typical lepromatous infiltrations.

Occasionally, in patients with lepromatous leprosy, elevated firm nodules form in the skin, especially in relapsing disease. Because of the characteristic histologic pattern of these lesions, in which the spindle-shaped histiocytes resemble fibrocytes, this form is called *histoid leprosy*.[297,351] Lepromatous leprosy is disseminated widely, and lepromatous infiltrations frequently are found in the upper respiratory tract, as far down as the larynx, and in the eyes and testes. In adults, the testes sometimes are densely infiltrated, with subsequent development of sterility and gynecomastia, but these complications are rare findings in children. Lymph nodes often are infiltrated by bacilli-laden macrophages, especially in the medulla and paracortical areas.

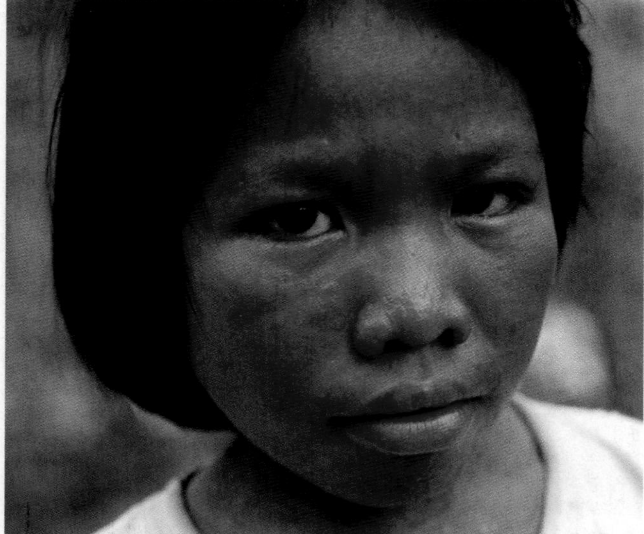

FIG. 98.8 Advanced lepromatous leprosy in an adolescent Filipino. Skin of most of the face, especially the alae nasi, is diffusely thickened. Eyebrows are thinned.

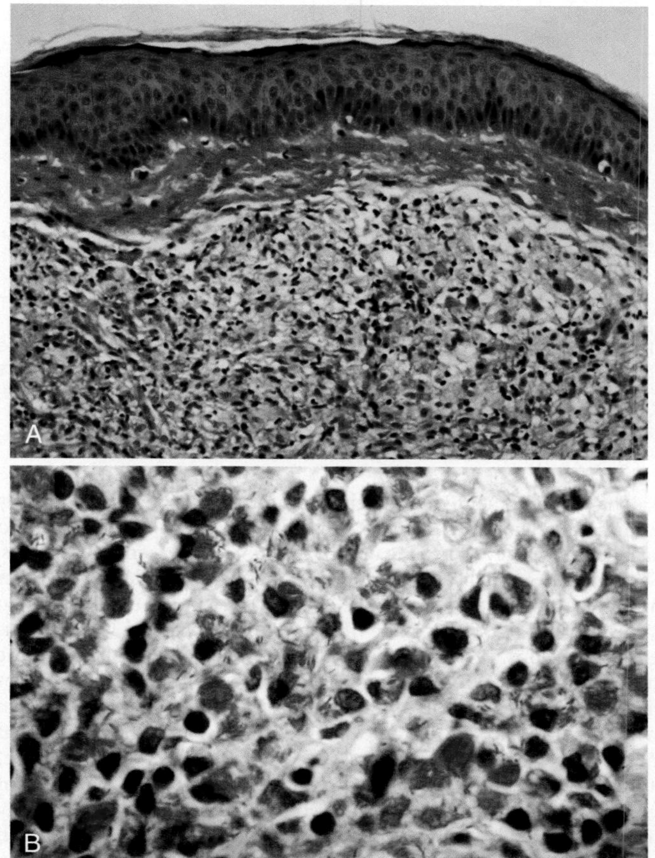

FIG. 98.9 (A) Advanced lepromatous leprosy showing replacement of dermis by foamy histiocytes and very few lymphocytes. Note thin subepidermal clear zone (hematoxylin and eosin stain). (B) Higher magnification of same biopsy specimen showing clumps of *M. leprae* (globi) in histiocytes in a leproma in the skin (Fite-Faraco stain).

Clinical Manifestations

The incubation period varies (usually 2 to 5 years), and no prodromal manifestations are well established. Some experienced clinicians working in areas of high prevalence recognize early signs of nerve involvement (i.e., localized paresthesia, itching, or numbness) before any visible lesions develop. Paucibacillary leprosy is defined as having one to five skin lesions, and includes all smear-negative cases. Multibacillary leprosy includes more than five skin lesions and includes all smear-positive cases. The extreme forms of leprosy include tuberculoid (paucibacillary disease) and lepromatous (multibacillary) leprosy, with other forms falling between these extremes. Differentiation of paucibacillary from multibacillary disease is important for selection of the number of empirical medications started, duration of therapy, and risk for relapse and sequelae.

After the incubation period, various lesions appear. The nature of the lesions depends on the immune response of the patient to *M. leprae*. So far, no variations in strain have been found to explain the leprosy phenotype.[363,364] Most clinicians today follow the classification scheme outlined by Ridley and Jopling (see Table 98.1).[268] This classification system is based on clinical features, histopathologic findings, bacterial load, and reaction to the Mitsuda test. On one extreme is tuberculoid leprosy, characterized by a robust cell-mediated immune response and paucibacillary disease. On the other extreme is lepromatous leprosy, a multibacillary form characterized by more of a humoral immune response. Classification is important because it aids in establishing the prognosis and treatment program for the patient. The distribution of leprosy types varies geographically. In Latin America, lepromatous leprosy was the most common,[342] whereas borderline leprosy was more common in India.[240]

Virtually all patients with leprosy have peripheral neuropathy if cutaneous sensory changes are included, and approximately 25% have significant deformity. In experimental studies, the pathogenesis of peripheral neuritis in leprosy involves bacillation of the endothelial cells of epineural and perineural blood vessels and lymphatics.[293,294,296]

Ocular complications in leprosy are well known, especially in lepromatous leprosy. These lesions can include corneal scarring; conjunctivitis; and eyelash abnormalities, including ectropion (eversion of lid margin from globe), lagophthalmos (inability to close eyelids completely), madarosis (loss of eyelashes), and trichiasis (eyelashes growing back toward globe).[56,60,61,85,128] All patients with leprosy should be evaluated by an ophthalmologist at diagnosis and periodically thereafter, especially during any reactional episodes. Reactional episodes can involve ocular hypotension, punctate keratitis, and uveitis.[63]

Indeterminate Leprosy

An indeterminate lesion is the first manifestation of leprosy in most patients and may heal spontaneously, remain unchanged for months or years, or gradually progress toward tuberculoid or lepromatous disease. Patients with indeterminate leprosy have a single or a few macules in the skin (see Fig. 98.2). The macule is defined poorly and is mildly hypopigmented in deeper pigmented skin and slightly erythematous in lighter skin. Skin texture, presence of body hair over the lesion, sensation, and sweating within early macules are normal or only slightly altered. Peripheral nerves are normal, and skin smears from lesions rarely contain bacilli. The definitive diagnosis can be made only by finding acid-fast bacilli in histopathologic sections.

Tuberculoid Leprosy

Tuberculoid leprosy is the paucibacillary extreme of leprosy. Patients with tuberculoid leprosy have a single or several asymmetrically distributed hypopigmented skin lesions (see Fig. 98.4). Tuberculoid lesions arise de novo or evolve from indeterminate macules. The lesion may be macular or infiltrated, but the borders always are sharply demarcated, usually elevated from the surrounding normal skin, and frequently are finely papulated. Lesions range in size from less than 1 cm to large enough to cover entire regions, such as the thigh or buttock. Many tuberculoid lesions heal spontaneously. In large, active lesions, the centers often are healed and repigmented, although somewhat atrophic. The lesions often are hairless, hypohidrotic, and anesthetic. Sensation is lost in a specific order: first is loss of thermal sensation, then tactile, and loss of pain sensation is seen in more advanced disease. On the face, because of its rich innervation, the detection of hypoesthesia in early lesions requires discriminating tests. Conversely, clinicians may mistakenly diagnose leprosy in areas of the body that normally are hypoesthetic (e.g., over the elbows or knees). Despite hypoesthesia, deep pain on percussion of lesions over bone in tuberculoid leprosy, termed the *tap sign,* has been described, with a sensitivity of 67% and specificity of 100%.[169]

Involvement of peripheral nerves commonly occurs in tuberculoid leprosy (Fig. 98.10), and cutaneous nerves often can be palpated adjacent to or within lesions. The regional nerve trunks most commonly enlarged are the ulnar from the olecranon groove to midarm, lateral popliteal just distal to the head of the fibula, and posterior tibial in the medial aspect of the ankle. Enlarged or tender nerves anywhere should alert the clinician to the possibility of leprosy. Any readily palpable cutaneous nerve probably is enlarged, but evaluating the size of nerve trunks requires experience because of the wide range in normal size. Slit-skin smears are usually negative for acid-fast organisms.

Borderline Leprosy

Borderline leprosy, sometimes called *dimorphous* or *intermediate leprosy,* has features of the lepromatous and tuberculoid forms and represents a continuous spectrum of disease ranging from near-tuberculoid to near-lepromatous. It is an unstable form of leprosy and may evolve gradually toward tuberculous leprosy by undergoing reversal reactions or be downgraded toward lepromatous leprosy. Table 98.1 describes the three major subgroups of borderline leprosy: borderline-tuberculoid, borderline, and borderline-lepromatous.

In borderline-tuberculoid leprosy, the number of lesions (>10) usually is greater than in tuberculoid leprosy, and the borders of each lesion,

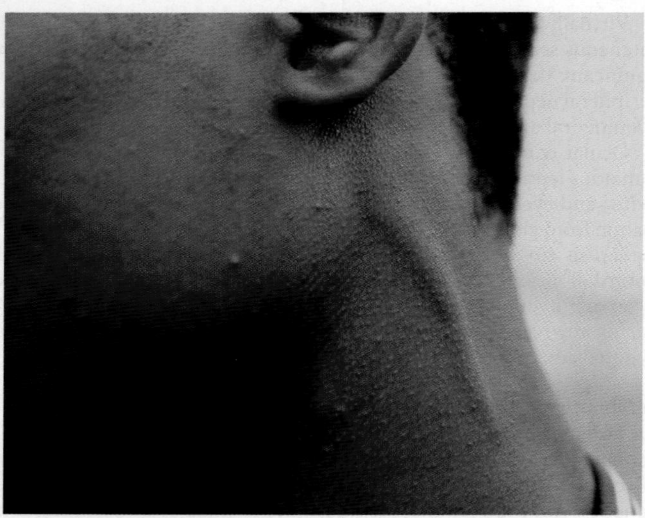

FIG. 98.10 Enlargement of the great auricular nerve in an adolescent Congolese boy. A large macule of tuberculoid leprosy over the angle of the mandible is now nearly inactive and barely visible.

macule, or plaque are defined less sharply than in tuberculoid leprosy. Ulceration of cutaneous lesions may occur. Small satellite lesions may develop around larger macules or plaques or extend as finger-like projections from larger lesions. Acid-fast smears are variably positive.

Borderline leprosy is characterized by hypochromic plaques that are well defined and have apparent central sparing of the skin. Skin findings may include papules, plaques, macules, or nodules and the lesions are sometimes described as having a "Swiss cheese" appearance.[329] Acid-fast smears often are strongly positive.

Borderline-lepromatous leprosy often manifests with widespread nodular infiltrations or plaques of varying size (see Fig. 98.6). The lesions are hypochromic and symmetrically distributed. Over time, the lesion borders become irregular as normal skin is invaded. Nontender peripheral nerve involvement is common. Acid-fast smears are strongly positive.

Damage to nerves and the resulting deformity develop early and often are widespread. Most patients who are disabled due to neuropathy are within the borderline spectrum of leprosy. It is often these neuropathic changes (e.g., sensory changes that lead to damaged hands or feet or a muscular weakness such as footdrop) that bring the patient to medical attention. Severe damage to nerves occurs infrequently in young children, but can be disastrous. Prevention of this complication is an important goal of leprosy detection programs and of treatment in every patient with leprosy.

Lepromatous Leprosy

Lepromatous leprosy is the classic multibacillary disease extreme. Here, peripheral blood smears can be positive for acid-fast bacilli (up to 80% in one study),[78] and the disease disseminates widely, often before striking cutaneous manifestations develop. In its earliest form, lepromatous leprosy manifests as "juvenile leprosy," a clinical entity delineated from observations of large numbers of children in homes for children of patients with leprosy in India.[225] This form, also called *prelepromatous leprosy,* is difficult to detect and frequently goes unrecognized until a more advanced stage develops. Skin texture may be altered slightly, but the vague macules with indistinct borders are detected only under appropriate lighting, preferably daylight. No changes in sensation or sweating occur in the macules, and frequently acid-fast bacilli are not detectable in skin smears. Histopathologic sections may reveal a few bacilli to confirm the diagnosis; however, if leprosy is suspected, the patient should be monitored until an explanation for the mild skin changes is found. If leprosy is present and not detected and treated, advanced forms of lepromatous leprosy develop in many of these patients (Fig. 98.11).

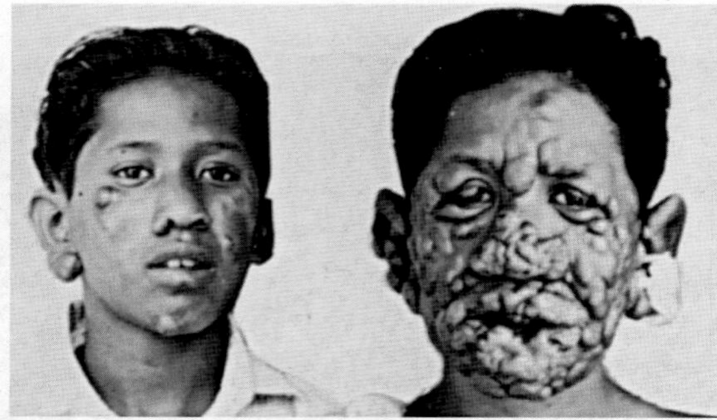

FIG. 98.11 Progression of lepromatous leprosy in a Hawaiian boy. The photograph at *left* was taken in 1931, when the patient was 13 years old; the photograph at *right* was taken 2 years later. No effective chemotherapy was available in that era.

The hypopigmented or slightly erythematous macules of early lepromatous leprosy, similar to those of juvenile leprosy, are missed easily because they are vague and have slight, if any, sensory changes. These macules usually are small but gradually may coalesce and cover large areas of skin, even nearly the entire body. Clinical diagnosis often is missed, and over the course of a few years, advanced lepromatous leprosy develops. If skin smears or biopsy specimens are taken in the macular stage, diagnosis is virtually ensured. If the disease is not diagnosed and treated in the macular stage, infiltration of the skin increases gradually and nodules may develop. The skin is infiltrated most heavily in the cooler portions of the body, notably the ears (pinnae) and face. By this time, nerves usually are enlarged, with early signs of sensory loss in the hands and feet. Eyebrows are thinned and eventually lost, beginning at the lateral edges. Loss of eyelashes (madarosis) often is seen. These well-known advanced changes of lepromatous leprosy are not common findings in young children.

Involvement outside the integument is common in patients with lepromatous leprosy. This includes involvement of the upper respiratory tract, characterized by mucopurulent nasal drainage and epistaxis due to involvement of the palate, larynx, and nasal bones. Destruction of eyelashes and eyebrows can result in corneal trauma, including ulceration, perforation, and infection. Iritis, uveitis, and glaucoma are late findings. Dissemination to the reticuloendothelial system, adrenals, and testes can be seen during hematogenous spread. Acid-fast smears are strongly positive.[329]

Histoid leprosy, one variant of multibacillary leprosy, often is classified with lepromatous leprosy. Here, firm, dome-shaped nodular or papular lesions show constriction around the base. They are more commonly found in the axial skeleton.[297] This form of leprosy is more common among patients whose isolates are resistant to dapsone.[351]

Patients of Latin American ancestry, especially patients from Mexico and Costa Rica, may contract the highly anergic diffuse form of lepromatous leprosy called *Lucio-Latapi leprosy*. The disease may be so diffuse that it is not recognized until sensory changes appear in the hands and feet, and the eyebrows and other body hair begin to disappear. The skin appears shiny and moist, resulting in a healthy appearance to the skin that led this condition to be called *lepra bonita* (pretty leprosy). In advanced forms of Lucio leprosy, a necrotizing panvasculitis in the skin is present, with the production of dermal infarcts and irregular ulcers (Lucio phenomenon).[175,262] Lucio leprosy has been reported in children 7 years old.[289]

Neuritic Leprosy

Neurotic leprosy, a relatively rare form of the disease, manifests as motor or sensory impairment in one or multiple nerves in the absence of cutaneous changes. Symptoms include anesthesia, paresis, and wasting of muscles in the affected area. Nerve trunks frequently are painful, enlarged, and tender. Leprosy must be suspected in patients with any peripheral neuritis that has these features. Chronic neuropathy and nerve enlargement often persist for years after the patient has completed chemotherapy for leprosy.[127] Large leprotic nerve abscesses are rare occurrences but are exquisitely painful and may require surgical intervention for drainage.[300] Most clinicians prefer to treat such lesions with corticosteroids. From a classification standpoint, patients with one to two nerves are deemed to have paucibacillary disease and those with more than two nerves involved are considered to have multibacillary disease. The diagnosis is difficult and may require PCR, as acid-fast smears usually are negative.

Leprosy and Acquired Immunodeficiency Syndrome

Given the history of acquired immunodeficiency syndrome (AIDS) altering the epidemiology and undermining control efforts for the other mycobacterial species with human-to-human transmission, *M. tuberculosis,* concern exists that a similar phenomenon might be seen with *M. leprae.*[335] The degree to which HIV impacts leprosy incidence is unclear. Some studies in sub-Saharan Africa have shown that HIV seroprevalence was two to five times higher in leprosy patients than controls.[28,194] Perhaps the positivity of some of these patients with leprosy can be explained by cross-reactivity between antibodies to HIV-1 and the lipoarabinomannan of *M. leprae.*[160]

However, most studies have shown that HIV seroprevalence among leprosy patients is no higher than the general population and that clinical manifestations are similar in coinfected patients and patients with leprosy alone.[143,163,170,222,299,335] Other prospective studies show that HIV infection may not be a risk factor for acquisition of leprosy in some populations.[163,299] However, HIV-infected patients seem to be more at risk for leprosy complications than HIV-seronegative patients. The incidence of reversal reactions (type 1, described later) and neuritis is increased in multibacillary patients coinfected with HIV.[38] These reactions, similar to immune reconstitution inflammatory syndrome (IRIS), have been described for both forms of IRIS.[335] Paradoxical IRIS, in which worsening of leprosy lesions is seen while on both appropriate leprosy and antiretroviral therapy, has been described with borderline leprosy; reactions often are local, not systemic.[16] Unmasking IRIS, in which leprosy symptoms develop anew in a person on antiretroviral therapy, has been described in a patient with borderline tuberculoid leprosy.[177]

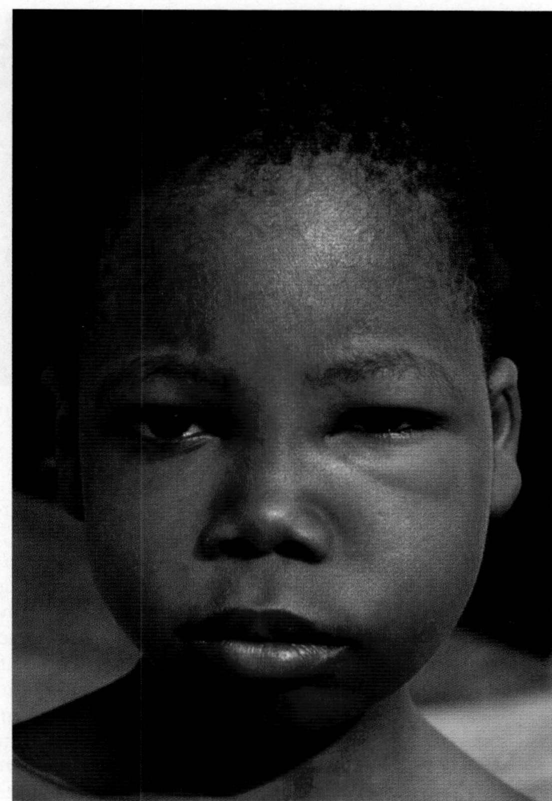

FIG. 98.12 Reversal reaction (type 1) in an 8-year-old Congolese boy with borderline-tuberculoid leprosy. The left side of his face is swollen and displays mild palsy from facial nerve damage. The patient responded rapidly to oral steroid therapy.

Reactions

The course of leprosy, treated or untreated, often is interrupted by acute episodes known as reactions, which fall into two general categories: reversal reactions (or type 1) and erythema nodosum leprosum (or type 2).[72]

Reversal Reactions

Reversal reactions complicate borderline leprosy and represent delayed hypersensitivity reactions, with an upgrading of cell-mediated immunity toward tuberculoid leprosy. Lesions become erythematous and edematous, and neuritis is common (Fig. 98.12). Risk factors for reversal reactions include being lepromin positive and having PGL-1 IgM antibodies.[270] Proliferation of sensitized T lymphocytes initiates reversal reactions and amplifies the inflammatory response by releasing lymphokines and activating macrophages.[274] Effective chemotherapy for paucibacillary and multibacillary patients may activate cell-mediated immunity and provoke clinical or subclinical reversal reactions (similar to IRIS). In severe reactions, necrosis may occur, almost always in nerves. Increased levels of TNF-α may partially explain this necrosis.[23] Cyclooxygenase-2 (COX-2) levels are elevated in nerves and blood vessels during reversal reactions, a finding that explains why nonsteroidal antiinflammatory drugs, including selective COX-2 inhibitors, often improve the condition.[249] Patients experiencing such reactions must be observed closely so that sensory loss and deformities are minimized.

Differentiating reversal reactions from relapsing lesions frequently is difficult and requires careful correlation of clinical and histopathologic findings. This correlation is becoming increasingly important in endemic areas, where shorter term chemotherapeutic regimens of fixed duration are used.[101,200] The following criteria for differentiating relapses and reversal reactions are suggested: a relapse involves an increased number of lesions; positive skin smears for acid-fast bacilli (for patients with a borderline area of leprosy and borderline-lepromatous leprosy); tissue reaction inconsistent with a reversal reaction; and a favorable response to chemotherapy. A reversal reaction involves an exacerbation of existing lesions; skin smears negative for acid-fast bacilli; tissue reaction consistent with a reversal reaction; and a rapid response to antiinflammatory drugs.

Erythema Nodosum Leprosum

Formerly, erythema nodosum leprosum (ENL) developed in approximately 50% of lepromatous leprosy patients after they had undergone a few months of chemotherapy; however, with the addition of clofazimine to the standard therapeutic regimen, the frequency is much lower.[91] One systematic review found that ENL developed in 1.2% of all leprosy cases, but was higher in patients with multibacillary disease (including 15% of patients with lepromatous leprosy).[349] Tender erythematous subcutaneous nodules develop rapidly (Fig. 98.13) and may ulcerate; the nodules often are accompanied by fever, synovitis, and iridocyclitis.[252] Erythema nodosum leprosum resembles the Arthus reaction and is thought to result from immune complex formation.[107] Erythema nodosum leprosum is associated with serum TNF-α elevation[23,288] and intralesional increases in helper T lymphocytes.[218]

A neutrophilic vasculitis is the hallmark of the tissue reaction. Demonstration of serum amyloid A and C-reactive protein may aid in establishing the diagnosis in patients without neutrophilic infiltration.[133] Glomerulonephritis sometimes complicates this condition; secondary amyloidosis is a late sequela of repeated reactions and may be a consequence of the neutrophilic leukocytosis.[190] More recent studies indicate that renal involvement is less severe and more reversible in the modern era, likely due to the use of multidrug therapy and more effective treatment of reversal reactions.[253] Occasional patients may have mixed reversal (upgrading) reactions and erythema nodosum leprosum. These patients usually have leprosy in the borderline-lepromatous area of the spectrum.

Diagnosis and Differential Diagnosis

The cardinal signs of leprosy are hypoesthetic lesions of the skin, enlarged peripheral nerve or nerves, and acid-fast bacilli in skin smears. In the

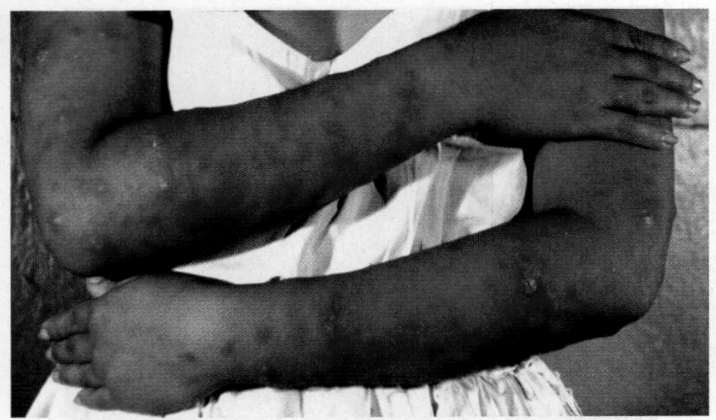

FIG. 98.13 Erythema nodosum leprosum in a adolescent Filipino girl with lepromatous leprosy.

absence of another clear explanation, any one of these signs strongly suggests leprosy.

An experienced observer can establish a clinical diagnosis in most patients, except those with early leprosy, with a high degree of accuracy. Because leprosy is considered one of the "great imitators,"[354] however, histopathologic evaluation is strongly recommended to supplement and confirm the clinical diagnosis. Patients with leprosy may be found in almost any geographic area, an awareness of which would minimize missed and delayed diagnoses, especially in areas of low prevalence. In the United States, the usual delay in establishing the diagnosis after the patient's first visit to a physician for symptoms related to leprosy is approximately 1.5 to 2 years. This delay often significantly worsens the prognosis.

History is important. Contact with patients with leprosy or residence in an endemic area raises suspicion of leprosy in a patient with a chronic lesion of the skin. Sensory loss or unexplained damage to hands or feet suggests damage to nerve trunks. Sometimes, a footdrop or clawhand brings the patient to a physician. Occasionally, patients with lepromatous leprosy consult an otolaryngologist first because of a chronic stuffy nose.

Clinicians must evaluate sensory changes in a lesion using the precautions already mentioned. The modalities usually tested are light touch with the use of a few fibers of cotton or calibrated nylon threads and heat and cold discrimination with the use of warm and cold water in test tubes. Much patience and repeated testing often are necessary in evaluating young children. Spontaneous sweating can be observed directly, or induced sweating can be evaluated. Hair may be completely preserved in early lesions but lost in advanced lesions. The main nerve trunks must be palpated for tenderness and enlargement. Skin in the area of discrete lesions also must be palpated gently to detect enlargement of cutaneous nerves. Globally, leprosy is the most common cause of peripheral neuropathy and must be considered in any patient with peripheral neuropathy.[281]

The histamine test can assist in the diagnosis of indeterminate leprosy in light-skinned patients. This test consists of applying one drop of histamine (1/1000 dilution) within and around hypochromic lesions. The test is positive if, after 1 to 2 minutes, a triphasic (response of Lewis) is observed. This response consists of a line of erythema followed by a wheal and flare response. This triphasic response is *not* seen with leprosy, but is seen for other causes of hypochromic skin.[329]

Obtaining and examining smears for acid-fast bacilli is an important diagnostic procedure and should be controlled carefully by experienced laboratories. Briefly, smears are made from the edge of discrete macules or plaques, nodules, ear lobes, and nasal mucosa. Fine needle aspirate has a sensitivity over 90%.[195] Slit-skin smears are made by squeezing and holding a fold of skin between the thumb and forefinger to avoid getting blood in the smear and by making a short, shallow slit in the skin with a razor blade or scalpel. The instrument is turned at a right angle to the slit, and the edges of the incision are scraped. The cells and fluid thus obtained are spread on a slide, heat fixed, and stained by the Ziehl-Neelsen method.[345] Evaluation of smears should not be done by researchers unfamiliar with their interpretation. An occasional acid-fast bacillus may be a harmless contaminant in the staining reagents. DNA probes specific for *M. leprae* are available and are useful in identifying leprosy bacilli in tissue or nasal secretions.[73,365]

The lepromin reaction is useless for the diagnosis of leprosy.[34] Currently available skin tests with soluble *M. leprae* antigens are unreliable.[120] Enzyme-linked immunosorbent assays and gelatin particle agglutination tests for antibodies to the PGL-1 of *M. leprae* are available.[45,113,138] Although specificity for *M. leprae* is high, these tests are insensitive (50%) for patients with paucibacillary leprosy. Other serologic tests for antibodies to *M. leprae*-specific epitopes on protein moieties of the bacillus are being evaluated.[247] PGL-1 antigen is detectable in the serum and urine of most multibacillary patients.[242,381] PGL-1 antibodies also have been used for early leprosy diagnosis in household contacts.[17]

Interferon gamma release assays (IGRAs) evaluating *M. leprae*-specific cell-mediated immunity have more recently been developed.[244] The optimal combination of antigens remains unclear, and these assays likely will not distinguish among healthy endemic controls and patients.

Reliance on DNA probes and PCR technology may prove useful in establishing the diagnosis of leprosy in tissue sections, skin smears, and nasal smears.[73,327,363,365] Whole-blood PCR is more sensitive for patients with multibacillary than paucibacillary disease (95% versus 70%), and can also be positive in asymptomatic household contacts.[362] Because these methods can detect a single leprosy bacillus, interpreting results, particularly in highly endemic areas, is difficult. Careful clinicopathologic correlation is essential when basing a diagnosis on DNA findings.[338] Multiplex PCR has also been piloted to detect early cases of leprosy in community-based contact tracing, and was more sensitive than acid-fast bacillus smear examination.[14] One pediatric study showed that, whereas slit-skin acid-fast bacillus smears were positive in only 20% of cases, PCR was positive in almost 90% of children with borderline and lepromatous leprosy and 72% of leprosy cases overall.[151] Specimens for PCR amplification should be preserved in 70% ethyl alcohol.[44,96,116]

Historically, mouse footpad (MFP) assays have been used to screen for *M. leprae* drug resistance; however, the MFP assay is time-consuming (often requiring more than 6 months before result availability). Molecular targets for drug resistance have been identified. Resistance to rifampin (similar to *M. tuberculosis*) is associated with the *rpoB* gene, fluoroquinolone resistance with the *gyrA* gene, and dapsone resistance is associated with the *folP1* gene.[231] In one study, sensitivity was higher for PCR than for MFP.[298] A newer modality, which uses reverse hybridization DNA strips, is now commercially available. This assay, the GenoType Leprae DR, evaluates for mutations in *rpoB, gyrA,* and *folP*. In one study conducted in 120 strains, concordance with PCR and MFP assays was 100%[39]

The differential diagnosis of leprosy in children is an extensive subject and can be discussed only briefly here. Superficial mycoses and postinflammatory changes commonly are confused with early leprosy. Changes in pigmentation may be caused by scars, birthmarks, and actinic dermatitis. In areas where dermal filariasis is endemic, vague macules in a black-skinned patient may appear identical to the early macules of leprosy.[30,192,202] Among the many infiltrated lesions of the skin that can resemble leprosy are leishmaniasis, lymphoma, granuloma annulare, granuloma multiforme (Mkar disease), lupus erythematosus, psoriasis, pityriasis alba, rosea, and versicolor, sarcoidosis, seborrheic dermatitis, vitiligo, and neurofibromatosis. Histoid leprosy especially mimics other diseases—von Recklinghausen lesions, molluscum, erythema nodosum, subcutaneous rheumatoid nodules, and nodular syphilis.[297,329] Peripheral neuropathies that may simulate leprosy are those seen in Morvan syndrome, syringomyelia, lead intoxication, diabetes mellitus, primary amyloidosis of nerves, and familial hypertrophic neuropathy. Pure neuritic leprosy is in the differential diagnosis of hypertrophic neuropathies, such as those caused by amyloidosis and chronic relapsing polyneuritis, and progressive hypertrophic interstitial lepromatous leprosy frequently gives false-positive reactions for syphilis.

Prognosis

Without chemotherapy, the prognosis in all patients except those with limited and self-healing disease potentially is poor. Patients with borderline or advanced tuberculoid leprosy frequently become mutilated because of neuropathy. Borderline patients can decline toward lepromatous leprosy. In patients with lepromatous leprosy, the disease is progressive and can cause death from laryngeal obstruction. Secondary amyloidosis is a frequent late sequela. Blindness may result from repeated episodes of iridocyclitis or ocular desiccation and/or keratitis from eyelash anomalies. Nerve damage as identified by electrophysiologic tests may be more widespread than realized on clinical examination. In one series of adults with multibacillary leprosy, before treatment, 92% of patients had abnormal nerve conduction studies, with sensory nerves being more involved than motor nerves (52% vs. 37%), and almost two-thirds of patients had involvement of five or more sensory or motor nerves or both.[40] General debility and deformity eventually prevent gainful employment in many patients. Additionally, the stigma associated with the disease may have pervasive effects on the lives of affected children and adults.

If therapy is started early, the prognosis usually is excellent, and deformity and mutilation are prevented. Even after receiving successful chemotherapy, however, some patients continue to experience significant neuritis and loss of peripheral nerve function. Sometimes this "silent neuropathy" goes unnoticed by the patient and the physician.[65,359] Appropriate early attention to anesthetic hands and feet and restoration of function by reconstructive surgery can prevent most mutilation.

The lepromin test is a valuable prognostic tool because it measures the cell-mediated immunity potential of the host to acquisition of infection by *M. leprae*.[145] Patients with early macular lesions who are lepromin negative have a poorer prognosis than patients who are lepromin positive if treatment cannot be administered. Histopathologic evaluation made before instituting chemotherapy is important for determining the prognosis and, if available, should not be neglected.

Treatment

When a diagnosis of leprosy is established, chemotherapy must be initiated and appropriate measures must be instituted for preventing or correcting deformity in patients with neurotropic changes.[47,103,173] The three chemotherapeutic agents most commonly used are dapsone, clofazimine, and rifampin.[223] Although the WHO recommends only clinical findings for assessment of the therapeutic response in field programs, clinicians may wish to use additional evaluations. The effectiveness of chemotherapy is assessed readily in patients with lepromatous or near-lepromatous leprosy by the staining quality of *M. leprae* in skin smears. The response to chemotherapy in patients with tuberculoid leprosy and most borderline patients is determined by the clinical response and by histopathologic evaluation. Viability of *M. leprae* in tissues is assessed in unusual cases in the mouse footpad.

Combined chemotherapy is being accepted increasingly for all forms of active leprosy. Although experimental data are limited,[310] multidrug therapy has replaced monotherapy (Table 98.2).[74,379] Monotherapy with any chemotherapeutic agent is not advised for concern for selection of resistant isolates. As previously discussed, conventional methodologies for leprosy drug susceptibility are cumbersome, leading to increased emphasis on detection of resistance using molecular modalities. This has also resulted in increased surveillance capabilities. During 2010, sentinel surveillance data from nine nations (Brazil, China, Colombia, India, Myanmar, Pakistan, the Philippines, Vietnam, and Yemen) evaluated drug resistance in patients with relapsed multibacillary leprosy. Of 88 samples tested for drug resistance, 9 were dapsone resistant, 1 was rifampin resistant, and none was fluoroquinolone resistant. No isolate was found to be multidrug resistant.[376] More recent reports from China have found that, among 85 isolates, 1.5%, 8.8%, and 25.9% had mutations associated with resistance to clofazimine, rifampin, and ofloxacin, respectively, and 3.5% of isolates were multidrug resistant.[181]

Dapsone

Dapsone, a bacteriostatic sulfone antimetabolite for *M. leprae*, was the first chemotherapeutic agent found to be effective; it was first used in 1941 in Carville, Louisiana.[90] The drug usually is given orally at 1 to 2 mg/kg per day as a single daily dose. The adult dose is 100 mg daily,

TABLE 98.2 Suggested Dosing Regimens for Leprosy From the World Health Organization[378,379] and National Hansen's Disease Program[233]

Leprosy Classification	Drug	DOSE[D] Age <10 y	Age 10–14 y	Age ≥15 y	Duration
Paucibacillary[a]	Dapsone	1–2 mg/kg/day	1–2 mg/kg/day	100 mg daily	WHO: 6 months
	Rifampin	10–20 mg/kg/day	10–20 mg/kg/day	600 mg daily (NHDP) 600 mg monthly (WHO)	NHDP: 12 months
Multibacillary[b]	Dapsone	1–2 mg/kg/day	1–2 mg/kg/day	100 mg daily	WHO: 12 months
	Rifampin	10 mg/kg/day	10 mg/kg/day	600 mg monthly (WHO) 600 mg daily (NHDP)	NHDP: 24 months
	Clofazimine[c]	50 mg biweekly + 100 mg monthly (WHO) 1 mg/kg/day (NHDP)	50 mg every other day + 150 mg monthly (WHO) 1 mg/kg/day (NHDP)	50 mg daily (NHDP, WHO) ± 300 mg load monthly (WHO)	
	Minocycline (second line for dapsone or clofazimine)	25 mg monthly if <15 kg; 50 mg monthly if 15–30 kg (WHO) ND (NHDP)	50 mg monthly (WHO) ND (NHDP)	100 mg monthly (WHO) 100 mg daily (NHDP)	Extend multidrug therapy to 2 years[347]
	Ethionamide (second line for clofazimine)	50–75 mg daily if <15 kg, 150–175 mg daily if 15–30 kg (WHO) ND (NHDP)	275–375 mg daily (WHO) ND (NHDP)	275–375 mg daily	
	Ofloxacin (second line for clofazimine or rifampin)	100 mg monthly if <15 kg, 200 mg monthly if 15–30 kg (WHO) Not recommended (NHDP)	200 mg monthly (WHO) Not recommended (NHDP)	400 mg monthly (WHO) 400 mg daily (NHDP)	

Because the National Hansen's Disease Program may change its recommendation for patient management, clinicians in the United States are advised to seek consultation prior to treating any patient with leprosy (800-642-2477, 225-756-3709; Mtemplet@hrsa.gov; www.bphc.hrsa.gov/nhdp/).

[a]Tuberculoid leprosy, borderline-tuberculoid, and indeterminate.

[b]Lepromatous, borderline, and borderline-lepromatous.

[c]Higher doses may be used for patients with erythema nodosum leprosum.

[d]Pediatric dosing should never exceed adult maximum. Approximate pediatric dosing,[150] as a percentage of adult dosing, can be estimated as 25% for children <15 kg, 50% if 15–30 kg, 75% if 30–45 kg, and 100% if >45 kg.

ND, No dosing information available; *NHDP,* National Hansen's Disease Program; *WHO,* World Health Organization.

and in the United States, dapsone is available as 25- and 100-mg tablets. The effect of dapsone on the bacilli is slow; 3 to 6 months of treatment is necessary to render bacilli from patients with lepromatous leprosy noninfectious for the mouse footpad. Sulfone-resistant strains of *M. leprae* are being detected with increasing frequency[359,360,376]; monotherapy with dapsone is not recommended. Dapsone usually is well tolerated but may provoke one or more of the following signs or symptoms: fever, exfoliative dermatitis, generalized lymphadenopathy, hepatosplenomegaly, or psychosis. Laboratory findings may include leukocytosis, hemolytic anemia, eosinophilia, or elevated bilirubin and serum transaminases.[3] Children should be screened for glucose-6-phosphate dehydrogenase (G6PD) deficiency before initiation of therapy.

Rifampin

Rifampin is a bactericidal antibiotic inhibiting bacterial DNA-dependent RNA polymerase. A single large dose can render a highly positive lepromatous patient noninfectious within 1 week. Available formulations include capsules (150 and 300 mg) and a parenteral formulation. The dose for persons 15 years of age and older is 600 mg, with pediatric doses of approximately 10 mg/kg given as a single daily dose. Optimal doses for children with leprosy have not been reported. Adult doses range from 300 to 600 mg daily.[370] Many side effects (e.g., hepatotoxicity, myalgias, thrombocytopenia) and drug-drug interactions with rifampin have been described, and the relevant literature must be consulted.[35] Rifampin-resistant leprosy has been reported.[140,366] Rifampin is not felt to interact with dapsone or clofazimine.

Clofazimine

Clofazimine (Lamprene) is a bacteriostatic riminophenazine dye that has anti–*M. leprae* and antiinflammatory activities, of particular utility for patients with erythema nodosum leprosum reactions, and is part of multidrug therapy for multibacillary leprosy (in conjunction with dapsone and rifampin).[91] The mechanism of action may involve enhancement of oxygen-dependent killing of *M. leprae* and binding to bacterial DNA. Clofazimine is available in 50- and 100-mg capsules, but is not commercially available in the United States (the National Hansen's Disease Program [NHDP] can facilitate US practitioners obtaining the medication). The WHO recommends clofazimine for patients with multibacillary leprosy.[379] The lower dosages are used for maintenance therapy when a good clinical response has been achieved, and the higher dosages (up to 100–300 mg daily in two or three divided doses) may be needed to control erythema nodosum leprosum; these regimens have not been well studied in children. The major adverse reactions to clofazimine are hyperpigmentation of skin and enteritis. Enteritis is experienced only at the higher dosages generally used for erythema nodosum leprosum. The pink to black hyperpigmentation is most prominent on exposed body parts, usually begins within 1 to 4 weeks of therapy initiation, subsides with the clinical improvement in leprosy, and resolves within a year of drug withdrawal. Pigmentary staining of the cornea and lacrimal fluid have been reported, but infrequently affects visual acuity. Ichthyosis can also be seen, especially in dry climates. This can be reduced by application of skin moisturizers and decreasing exposure to bright sunlight. Although two instances of clofazimine-resistant *M. leprae* infection have been reported, the validity of these observations is uncertain.[157,357] Cross-resistance between clofazimine and dapsone or rifampin has not been reported. For some time, clofazimine has been considered safe in pregnancy, but one report described three neonatal deaths in 15 observed pregnancies.[92] Whether the drug was associated with the deaths was not established.

Fluoroquinolone Therapy

The last decade has seen use of fluoroquinolones, primarily ofloxacin, for leprosy after nonhuman animal studies and early clinical studies in humans demonstrated that this class of drugs was more effective against *M. leprae* than dapsone and clofazimine. One Brazilian trial[59] of patients with multibacillary leprosy found that short-course treatment with short-course rifampin-ofloxacin therapy had higher failure rates than the recommended WHO regimen (below) and that addition of 1 month of daily ofloxacin to the 12-month WHO regimen did not increase efficacy. However, a study of a 4-week course of ofloxacin and rifampin for paucibacillary disease[10] found that short-course therapy was efficacious and few patients had relapses when compared to standard multidrug therapy. As such, the role of fluoroquinolones in the treatment of leprosy remains unclear. In addition, the optimal dose of fluoroquinolones in children is unclear, as children often require a higher milligram per kilogram dose than adults to achieve similar serum concentrations.

Multidrug Therapy

Because of the existence of drug-resistant *M. leprae,* combined drug regimens are mandatory for the treatment of all forms of leprosy.[87,310,358,359]

Combined drug therapy minimizes development of drug-resistant strains of *M. leprae* and may eliminate some "persisting" organisms. Persisting *M. leprae* are viable bacilli that can be isolated in small numbers from patients who are clinically responding well to therapy. These persisting *M. leprae* bacilli are sensitive to the drug in question when tested in the mouse footpad and may account for relapses when treatment is discontinued. Persisting *M. leprae* organisms have been detected after 5 years of therapy with rifampin, 6 years of clofazimine therapy, and 22 years of dapsone therapy.

In 1982, a WHO study group recommended the multidrug therapy (MDT) regimens that are described hereafter.[371] The MDT regimens were designed primarily for field programs, and they use pulsed supervised monthly rather than daily rifampin.[20] MDT is well tolerated, and compliance in large-scale control programs has been satisfactory. The efficacy of MDT has been promising.[42,359] In two surveys involving approximately 112,000 patients with multibacillary disease monitored for 9 years after receiving therapy, the cumulative risk for relapse was 0.77%. Anecdotal descriptions of certain groups of highly bacilliferous patients with relapse rates of 20% and recurrences developing 5 years or more after therapy have been reported.[142] These and other results suggest that therapeutic regimens for multibacillary patients should be given for longer than 2 years. In most reports, relapse rates in paucibacillary patients exceed those in multibacillary patients. The potential for relapse after receiving MDT regimens must await long-term, large-scale follow-up results.[141,319] Factors associated with relapse include having declining IgG antibodies against PGL-1, requiring treatment for reactions, and having lepromatous leprosy.[83,119] Peripheral neuropathy sometimes persists after completion of these therapeutic regimens.[4,127]

The trend since 2001 has been to reduce the duration of treatment and change the therapeutic regimens—even to the extreme of a single-dose regimen composed of rifampin, ofloxacin, and minocycline (ROM) for single-lesion therapy. One meta-analysis concluded that single-dose ROM was less effective than multidrug therapy for paucibacillary leprosy.[301] Many of these innovations are interwoven into the WHO Elimination of Leprosy Program and have provoked critical concern by some authorities.[97,182,229,317] The NHDP recommends daily therapy,[233] as opposed to the intermittent dosing recommendations for rifampin recommended by the WHO for resource-limited settings. Both WHO- and NHDP-recommended regimens are listed in Table 98.2. Laboratory monitoring should include baseline complete blood count, transaminases, bilirubin, blood urea nitrogen, creatinine, and calcium and then repeated every 3 months.

Other Drugs Under Investigation

Recent years have seen escalating use of fluoroquinolones, macrolides, tetracyclines, and ethionamide for patients intolerant of standard regimens.[108,109,117,144] Knowledge of the *M. leprae* genome will potentially lead to targeted drug development after computational genomic analysis. For example, one study identified several genes mapping to peptidoglycan cell wall biosynthesis; these *Mur* genes have no homolog to human genes, decreasing the risk for cross-reactivity of agents.[304]

Treatment of Reactions

Patients experiencing a reaction should be observed daily in the early stages and hospitalized if the symptoms are severe. Formerly, specific therapy was stopped or the dosage reduced during reactions, but these measures are no longer recommended.[371] Damage to eyes and neurotropic changes may ensue rapidly without immediate attention. Nerve tenderness and function must be assessed frequently during reactions. Acute inflammation of isolated lesions without damage to nerves is likely to be of little consequence except for cosmetic considerations, but the patient should be monitored closely. It is difficult for clinicians to identify children who may be at increased risk for a leprosy reaction. One retrospective cross-sectional study identified laboratory factors associated with increased risk of reactions. These included PCR positivity, anti–PGL-1 ELISA, leukocytosis, thrombocytopenia, and elevated lactate dehydrogenase.[7]

Reversal (type 1) reaction. Patients with painful, tender nerves must receive immediate care, usually in the hospital. Analgesics are given, and the affected area is rested. Large daily doses of corticosteroids are started and tapered to a minimal effective dose until the reaction subsides. Conversion to alternate-day steroid regimens may be attempted when long-term treatment is necessary. One randomized, double-blind trial compared methylprednisolone with placebo in conjunction with oral corticosteroids for adults with type 1 reactions; persons treated with methylprednisolone were less likely to have nerve damage and recurrent type 1 reactions.[353] However, one meta-analysis indicated that, although corticosteroids may be useful for treating acute nerve damage, long-term benefit may not be seen.[40,341] A 12-week course of topical tacrolimus was used in one case of steroid-refractory type 1 reaction in a child with borderline lepromatous leprosy, with resolution of all skin lesions.[282] Some clinicians use clofazimine for chronic reversal reactions, but it is not recommended for the initial treatment of reactions with acute neuritis. For reactions, clofazimine probably is consistently efficacious only for erythema nodosum leprosum (ENL).[136]

Erythema nodosum leprosum (type 2) reaction. Mild erythema nodosum leprosum (ENL) is treated with analgesics; more severe disease is treated with corticosteroids, thalidomide, clofazimine, or other drugs.[348] Pediatric doses of thalidomide in ENL have not been established, but the initial adult dose is 100 mg four times daily followed by a minimal effective dose, usually 100 mg daily. In the United States, thalidomide is available for ENL under the Celgene REMS Program (http://www.celgeneriskmanagement.com). The teratogenic action of thalidomide demands that appropriate measures be taken in the treatment of fertile women. For the rare patient who does not respond to thalidomide or in fertile women, corticosteroids or clofazimine is used. Corticosteroids, if used, are administered in the usual dosage schedules (1 to 2 mg/kg daily), beginning with large doses and tapering to a minimal effective level. The total duration of corticosteroid therapy is unclear; one study found that patients treated for 5 months were less likely to have recurrence than those treated for only 3 months.[352] One systemic review indicated that clofazimine was superior to thalidomide or corticosteroids, but analysis was hindered by variation in the quality of studies in the pooled data.[340] Clofazimine is effective in most patients with erythema nodosum leprosum and does not have the disadvantages of thalidomide or corticosteroids. The antiinflammatory action of clofazimine is not manifested until after 4 to 6 weeks of continuous use. The dosage must be adjusted to the minimal effective level, and high doses are recommended by the WHO for erythema nodosum leprosum reactions.[379] A few studies suggest that pentoxifylline or pentoxifylline plus clofazimine is effective.[236,328,361] While clofazimine provides sustained improvement, it acts slowly; in contrast, pentoxifylline is more effective in reducing initial severity.[277] However, one randomized double-blind clinical trial comparing thalidomide (300 mg) to pentoxifylline (1.2 g) administered daily for 1 month found that thalidomide was more effective in treating ENL. Nonetheless treatment with pentoxifylline seemed to help with limb edema and constitutional symptoms.[283] One case report described the successful treatment of a chronic erythema nodosum leprosum reaction with a 6-week course and slow taper of the TNF inhibitor etanercept.[259] A recent case series demonstrated that 80% of adults with ENL who had failed corticosteroids responded to minocycline (100 mg/day for up to 3 months). The potential mechanism of action is that minocycline has immunomodulatory, antiinflammatory, and neuroprotective effects.[232]

Iridocyclitis requires emergency measures. Local corticosteroids must be added to systemic antiinflammatory regimens. Ophthalmologic consultation should be obtained.

Prevention

Precise recommendations for the prevention of leprosy in individuals have not been formulated. Control programs today are based on the general principles that (1) the number of contagious patients is reduced by chemotherapy and (2) the surveillance of contacts detects early leprosy. To accomplish these goals, appropriate education of the public and medical personnel and population surveys in areas of higher prevalence must be implemented. In endemic areas, improved housing probably is a highly important preventive measure by reducing close contact of patients with healthy individuals. In health care settings, infection control precautions include hand hygiene for all patients with lepromatous leprosy. Standard precautions are indicated for the hospitalized patient. Leprosy is a reportable disease in the United States.

Chemoprophylaxis

Chemoprophylaxis for close contacts was first attempted with dapsone, showing efficacy rates ranging from 34% to 99%,[319] but was not recommended for large populations[65] given concerns that long-term use would select for dapsone-resistant isolates.[370] More recently, rifampin has been evaluated for chemoprophylaxis. One study on leprosy hyperendemic Indonesian islands used rifampin every 3.5 months, showing protective efficacy of 75% to 90%.[9] A cluster randomized trial in Bangladesh showed that single-dose rifampin had protective efficacy of 57% within 2 years of administration.[220] Single-dose rifampin chemoprophylaxis is both culturally acceptable[93] and cost-effective, particularly in social contacts and neighbors of cases.[135] However, concern exists that single-dose rifampin chemoprophylaxis may select for rifampin-resistant *M. leprae* isolates.

Vaccination, Immunoprophylaxis, and Immunotherapy

Vaccines composed of heat-killed whole *M. leprae* (from experimentally infected armadillos) have been found to be safe and to induce delayed-type hypersensitivity to *M. leprae* in a high percentage of lepromin-negative individuals. Several other vaccines based on cultivable mycobacteria (*Mycobacterium vaccae, Mycobacterium w,* and the Indian Cancer Research Centre bacillus) induce similar responses.[22,158,322] Vaccine progress has been thwarted by the need for extended follow-up observations[24] and concern that vaccines containing only *M. leprae* would not be protective given that infection-induced immunity is infrequently observed for leprosy. Consequently, combined vaccines of killed *M. leprae* and live bacillus Calmette-Guérin (BCG) have been studied. Such vaccines convert lepromin-negative contacts of patients with leprosy to positive reactors and upgrade patients with lepromatous leprosy toward the tuberculoid region of the disease spectrum.[52,207]

BCG immunization alone had a protective effect of 26% in one meta-analysis; this analysis also found that age at immunization did not affect efficacy and that receipt of a second dose of BCG vaccine was more protective for leprosy than receipt of a single BCG dose.[302] Subsequent studies have had variable results.[371] Combining BCG with killed *M. leprae* did not protect against leprosy.[54,159] BCG vaccination was combined with single-dose rifampin for close contacts of leprosy patients in Bangladesh, showing a protective effect of 80%.[292] The WHO does not recommend BCG vaccination for the prevention of leprosy.[19]

Leprosy vaccines as adjuvant to multidrug therapy also have been attempted in multibacillary leprosy patients. *Mycobacterium w* vaccine given in 3-month intervals (up to eight doses) was associated with improvement in clinical scores and decline in bacteriologic indices for up to 2 to 3 years, but no impact was seen on clinical relapse or incidence of neuropathy after this interval. Rates of type 1 reactions were more common in the vaccine group in contrast to a placebo group receiving multidrug therapy alone.[305]

Elimination

In 1991, the World Health Assembly defined leprosy elimination as a prevalence of fewer than 1 case/10,000 persons. By this definition, only three nations with populations over 1 million have yet to attain this goal: Brazil, Nepal, and Timor-Leste (East Timor).[37] However, pockets of high endemicity exist in several countries: Angola, Brazil, the Central African Republic, the Democratic Republic of the Congo, India, Madagascar, Mozambique, Nepal, and Tanzania. The prospect of truly eliminating leprosy is poor due to several factors. First, a zoonotic focus[203,332] can lead to continued introduction into human populations. Second, vaccination development efforts have been hindered by poor correlates of immunity. Third, surveillance for new cases can be hindered by the stigma attached to the disease. This can lead to either failure to seek medical attention or seeking medical attention in alternative medical settings, where reporting of cases may not occur.[139] One study modeled the impact of various interventions on leprosy incidence rates. Variables included passive versus active case detection, multidrug therapy, contact tracing, BCG vaccination of infants, early diagnosis of subclinical infection, and chemoprophylaxis. A multifaceted approach including BCG vaccine coverage, contact tracing, early diagnosis, and chemoprophylaxis of household contacts seemed to reduce leprosy incidence rates most substantially.[98] However, these strategies would require an infrastructure and investment that fall outside the health budgets of many developing nations. Given the lack of tools to diagnose subclinical infection, long treatment duration, and continued uncertainty regarding aspects of patterns of exposure, modes of transmission, persistence of leprosy in treated cases, and early host response, many experts believe that control, rather than eradication, should be the goal.[318]

BURULI ULCER

Mycobacterium ulcerans causes indolent, necrotizing cutaneous ulcers that are known classically as *Buruli ulcers*.[183,339] Other names for these lesions include Bairnsdale or Searles ulcer in Australia, and Kumusi ulcer in Papua New Guinea. Today, researchers recognize that many infections with *M. ulcerans* are not manifested as ulcers and that *M. ulcerans* infection is a technically more appropriate name for the disease. The WHO has recognized Buruli ulcer as a reemerging infectious disease in western Africa with an important public health impact.[374]

Organism

The organism was first isolated in 1948.[184] *M. ulcerans* is strongly acid-fast, with an optimal growth temperature of 30°C to 33°C (86°F–91.4°F) on routine mycobacteriologic media such as Löwenstein-Jensen medium. Unlike *M. marinum, M. ulcerans* is slow growing, nonphotochromogenic, microaerophilic, and heat sensitive.[208,246]

Comparative genomic analysis indicates that *M. ulcerans* arose from *M. marinum,* with which it shares 98% genomic homology.[71] *M. ulcerans* is the only mycobacterial pathogen of humans known to elaborate a necrotizing, immunosuppressive exotoxin, mycolactone.[62,263,313] The mycolactone mechanism of action is unclear, but evidence exists for the toxin triggering apoptosis[122,354] and decreasing satellite cell proliferation.[131] Variations in the 3′ end of the 16S rRNA gene sequence are related to geographic origin and are used to divide the organism into African, American, Asian, and Australian strains.[256]

Transmission and Epidemiology

Endemic foci of *M. ulcerans* infections usually appear in rural settings near permanent wetlands in warm countries, especially in terrain subject to seasonal flooding. Reports of patients with Buruli ulcers have come from at least 33 countries, principally in the tropics.[375] A few patients live in nontropical climates, such as China,[89] Japan,[333] and southern Australia.[343] Today, the largest numbers of reported patients live in West Africa (Cameroon, Côte d'Ivoire, the Democratic Republic of the Congo, and Ghana report the most cases).[339] In these countries, the disease is reemerging rapidly, with an estimated total annual incidence exceeding 2200 patients from 12 of the 33 nations. Other countries in which the disease is known to be endemic include Angola, Equatorial Guinea, French Guiana, Gabon, Indonesia, Malaysia, Papua New Guinea, Peru, Suriname, and Uganda.[66,129,200,250] In the Western Hemisphere, cases have been reported primarily in French Guyana, but also in Brazil, Mexico, Peru, and Suriname.[375]

Observers attribute this reemergence to environmental factors such as deforestation, artificial topographic alterations (e.g., dams and irrigation systems),[69,185] increasing populations engaged in basic manual agriculture in wetlands, and possibly climactic changes.[210] These manmade environmental modifications may lead to changes in water temperature or turbidity, potentially protecting *M. ulcerans* biofilms.[199] In North America, two cases of Buruli ulcer were reported in 2005 in central Mexico, the nearest location to the United States to date.[48] Individuals of all ages are affected, but the highest frequencies are in children 15 years of age or younger—approximately 50% to 75% of all cases.[189] A second peak occurs in the seventh to eighth decade of life, suggesting that latent infection can reactivate with age.[67] The sexes are affected equally, and a racial predilection is unknown.[67] Seasonal variations in incidence occur in some foci.[125,266] Approximately 80% of the lesions are on the limbs, with the highest frequencies involving the lower extremities.

Although the ultimate source of *M. ulcerans* remains obscure, the organism has been discovered in aquatic insects, such as water bugs, firefly larvae, and beetles, and obtained from stagnant water in endemic areas of West Africa, as well as newly dammed areas in Cameroon.[185,188,255] In some cases, the organisms were found only in the salivary glands of aquatic insects, supporting the notion that insect bites may play a role in transmitting *M. ulcerans*.[186,187] Adult mosquitoes trapped outside Victoria, Australia also had detectable *M. ulcerans* DNA. *Aedes* spp. were most likely to have DNA identified, followed by *Anopheles* spp.; lowest detection was seen in *Culex* spp.[176] This may explain the observation that having daily contact with a natural water source was a risk factor for Buruli ulcer disease according to one study in Benin,[320] and that lower rates of Buruli ulcer were seen in higher altitude villages in Benin.[321] Wading into rivers was a risk factor for Buruli ulcer in one study, which also found that the most common lesions occurred on uncovered extremities[258]; both also suggest transmission from biting aquatic insects. A group from Melbourne, Australia, evaluated both environmental sources and nonhuman animal (koala, opossums, small rodent) feces for *M. ulcerans* DNA.[82,104,216] *M. ulcerans* DNA was not detected in fecal samples from Buruli ulcer patients, suggesting that the human gastrointestinal tract is not likely to be a significant reservoir.[287]

Buruli ulcer rarely, if ever, is contagious. The distribution of patients, even in highly endemic foci, is random, suggesting that each patient is exposed to environmental sources, such as swamps where villagers work their gardens and obtain water for domestic use and especially where children play. The mode or modes of transmission to humans have not yet been delineated completely; however, the most plausible route is by trauma at sites of skin recently contaminated by *M. ulcerans*.[79,209] Many patients give a history of specific antecedent penetrating trauma at the site of their initial lesion, which may include wounds from a gunshot or land mine, thrown stones, hypodermic injection, or even a human bite (Fig. 98.14).[70] The organism may be spread by aerosol from the surface of ponds or be carried by fomites or insects to skin surfaces.

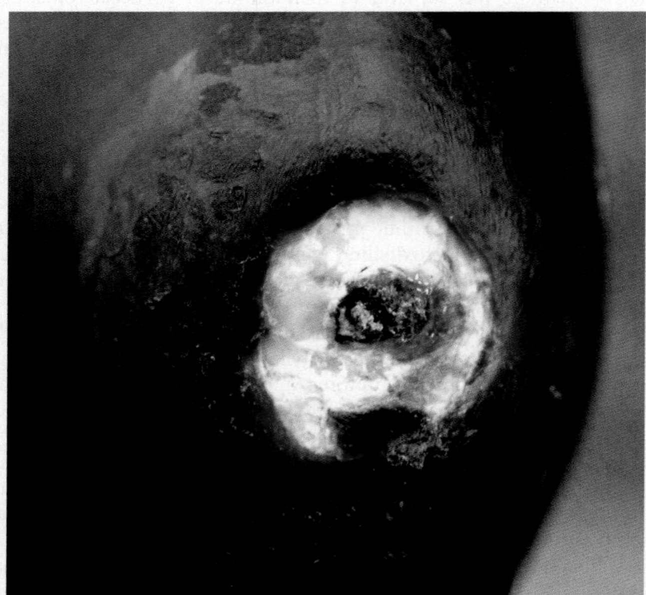

FIG. 98.14 A major Buruli ulcer in the deltoid area of a 12-year-old Angolan boy. This pristine ulcer developed 3 months after a documented hypodermic anticholera vaccine injection at this site. Typical Buruli ulcer features are represented—undermining of borders, necrotic base, and induration of the adjacent skin.

Insects may introduce *M. ulcerans* into the skin, but this means of transmission has not been proved. Although proposed by some authorities, transmission by nasorespiratory passage with a subsequent bacteremia seems to be unlikely.

Pathogenesis and Pathology

Three properties determine the pathologic features of early *M. ulcerans* infection: optimal growth at 30°C to 33°C (86°F–91.4°F), slow growth rate, and elaboration of the toxin mycolactone.[313] The temperature requirement tends to favor the development of lesions in the skin (versus deeper tissues). The slow growth rate results in slowly progressive lesions. Mycolactone destroys tissues and suppresses immune responses. The spectrum of clinical and histopathologic forms of infection suggests that some patients have innate resistance, or resistance develops soon after infection is acquired, whereas others acquire resistance later or, occasionally, never.

Many of the differences in pathogenicity between *M. ulcerans* and *M. marinum* may be explained by the presence of mycolactone in the former species. Mycolactone has broad-spectrum cytotoxic activity for a variety of cell types. It can cause apoptosis, vasculitis, and thromboses. Mycolactone is also thought to inhibit TNF-γ and IL-2 production and augment IL-10 production.[2,58,168] These activities partly explain the immunologic unresponsiveness and reduced inflammatory reaction at the site of the lesion. One study in Benin found that the rate of hemoglobinopathies was almost seven times higher in Buruli ulcer osteomyelitis patients than the general population, suggesting these disorders facilitate the growth of the organism in bony matrices.[230]

Based on the current understanding of the natural history of *M. ulcerans* infection, pathogenesis may proceed as follows: after inoculation of the etiologic agent deep into the skin or subcutaneous tissue, a latent phase occurs during which the mycobacterium proliferates slightly, probably initially intracellularly,[243] and begins to elaborate small amounts of toxin that causes necrosis, especially of fatty tissue. During this necrotic phase, no significant cellular response occurs.[49,75]

In some patients, at this stage, a subcutaneous nodule begins to develop, with clusters of *M. ulcerans* in the center surrounded by a zone of necrosis. In highly resistant patients, this lesion may self-heal, perhaps without ulceration, or form a small, sharply delineated ulcer. In others, the skin is undermined by the necrosis and eventually breaks down into larger ulcers with widely undermined skin. In the least resistant individuals, a nodule never develops and the necrosis spreads rapidly and widely to cover large body surface areas, but ulceration, if it occurs at all, is a late event.

Eventually, the necrotic stage ceases in most patients, either because the toxin is neutralized or because production is interrupted. At this time, a granulomatous stage begins to develop, followed by healing and scarring. Some of the variability in clinical presentation and progression of the disease may be related to heterogeneity in the *M. ulcerans* genome and in the plasmid that encodes the production of mycolactone.[227,325,326]

Histopathologic findings are characterized by extensive coagulation necrosis of the soft tissues (Fig. 98.15)[118] masses of acid-fast bacilli, marked edema, and extensive vasculitis. Fat cells enlarge and die, with only their cellular ghost outlines remaining (Fig. 98.16). The dermis and surrounding tissue seldom contain acid-fast bacilli. Lesions sometimes provoke a reactive (contiguous) osteitis that leads to necrosis of cortical bone and osteomyelitis. Metastatic lesions may develop in the skin and bone from bacteremia and produce skin lesions distant from the original lesion and frequently focal or multifocal osteomyelitis. Regional lymph nodes may show massive necrosis and contain large numbers of acid-fast bacilli. Visceral organs are not known to be involved, but no necropsies of patients who died of disseminated disease have been reported.[331]

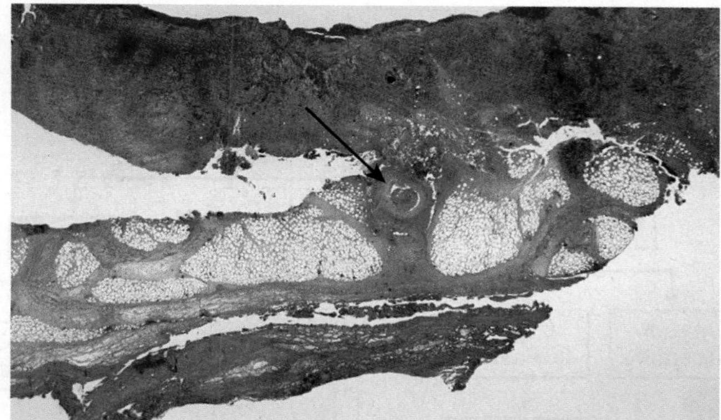

FIG. 98.15 Histopathologic section of the undermined edge of a major Buruli ulcer. Note the coagulation necrosis of the entire panniculus and fascia, and vasculitis with thrombosis of a blood vessel *(arrow)* (hematoxylin and eosin stain).

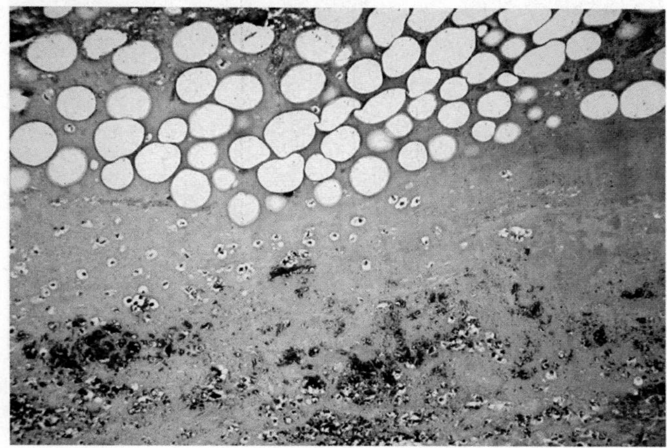

FIG. 98.16 High magnification of the necrotic panniculus of a Buruli ulcer showing dead fat cell "ghosts," coagulation necrosis, and masses of acid-fast bacilli (Ziehl-Neelsen stain).

Clinical Manifestations

Incubation and Forms of Lesions

In one study of specific trauma related to lesions, the incubation period ranged from 2 weeks to 3 years, with a mean of 3 months.[209] The following are the various forms of lesions of *M. ulcerans* infection according to WHO designations.[376] Fig. 98.17 presents a proposed classification of the clinical forms of *M. ulcerans* disease and their possible interrelationships. The WHO also designates three categories of lesions. Category I consists of single lesions less than 5 cm in diameter; these may heal completely with medical therapy. Category II consists of a single lesion 5 to 15 cm in diameter; only some heal completely with medical therapy. Category III lesions encompass large (>15 cm diameter) lesions, lesions in multiple locations, osteomyelitis, or lesions in critical sites (e.g., ocular, genitalia, or breast). These lesions usually require combined medical and surgical therapy.[378,375]

Papule. The papular stage has been described only in patients from Australia. These papules are painless, elevated, and measure up to 1 cm in diameter.

Nodule. Nodules are primarily subcutaneous and firm, measure approximately 2 cm in diameter, and are painless, although they are often pruritic. The overlying skin may be discolored. Although usually mobile, they can become attached both to the skin and to deeper tissues.[334] This stage is the initial one in most Africans, and in the Kikongo language, the disease is called *mputa matadi* because the nodule is a "rock-hard lesion." Unlike ulcerative forms, acid-fast bacilli are aggregated in the center of nodules.[334] Patients with nodular lesions have fewer functional limitations than other forms of Buruli ulcer disease.[291]

Plaque. Plaques are firm, elevated, painless, well-defined lesions more than 2 cm in the largest dimension. Their borders are irregular. This stage often is the one in which physicians initially see the patient, but the lesion may or may not arise from a nodule. The skin over the lesion is reddened or discolored. These lesions may ulcerate in the late stages.

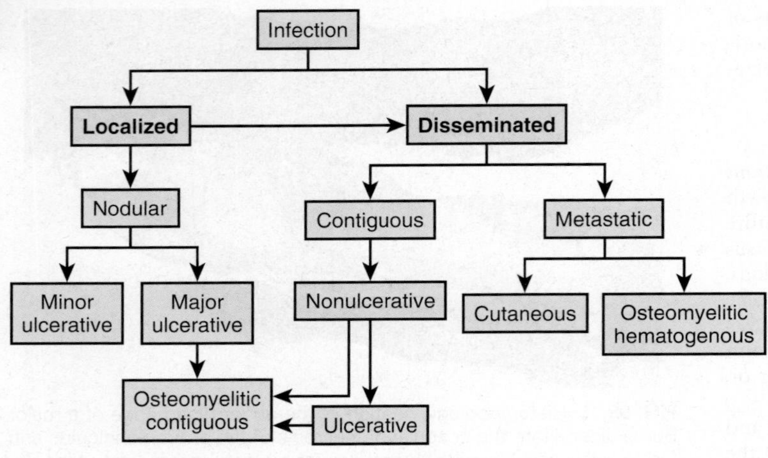

FIG. 98.17 Proposed classification of clinical forms of *M. ulcerans* infections, indicating possible progression of lesions after the initial cutaneous infection. Without treatment, lesions may self-heal at any stage or advance according to the schema.

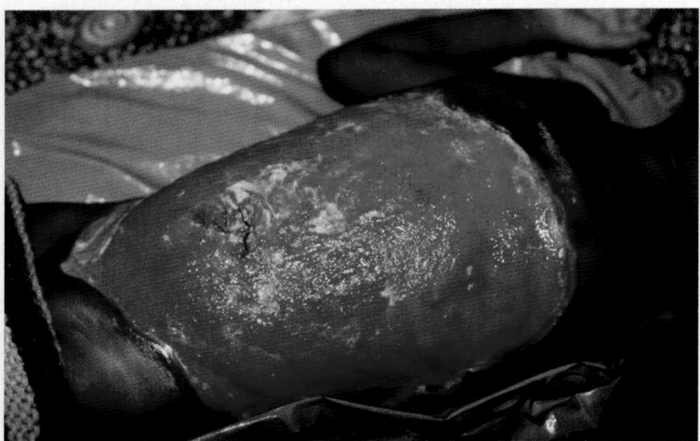

FIG. 98.18 Edematous form of *M. ulcerans* infection in a 6-year-old Ghanaian girl after surgery to remove all necrotic tissue. There was never any ulceration. Note ablation of breast tissue.

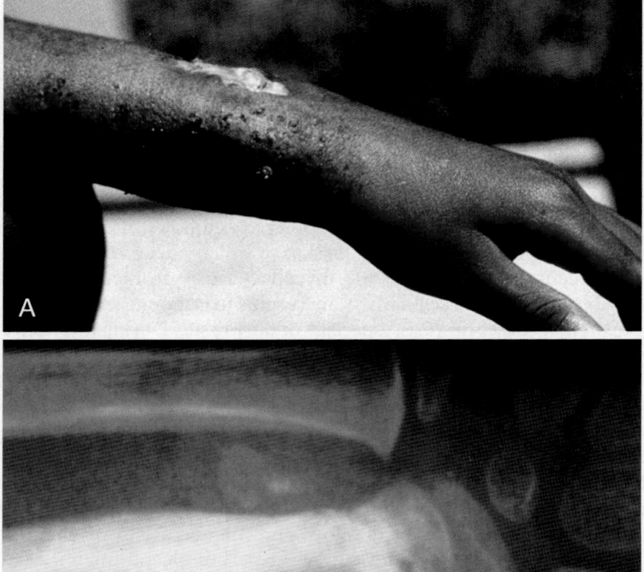

FIG. 98.19 (A) *M. ulcerans* infection in a young Congolese boy. Note swelling and ulcer on dorsum of forearm. (B) Radiograph of forearm shows reactive osteitis, necrosis of cortex of distal end of the radius, and early sequestration with osteomyelitis.

These lesions are more likely to relapse after surgical therapy than ulcerative forms.[167]

Edematous form. Most edematous lesions do not begin in the nodular stage but spread directly from the initial nidus of infection. Spread often is rapid and wide and covers entire limbs or major portions of the trunk (Fig. 98.18). This type of lesion is characterized by diffuse nonpitting swelling and vague margins. Lesions are firm and frequently painful, with changes in color and scaling on the skin surface. These lesions, along with plaques, are more likely to relapse after surgical therapy than ulcerative forms.[167]

Ulcerative forms. When fully developed, pristine ulcers have undermined edges surrounded by a zone of induration and often desquamation of the epidermis (see Fig. 98.14). In the base of the ulcerated area, a whitish necrotic slough and sometimes eschar develop. An oily exudate frequently oozes from the dependent area. Old ulcers tend to begin healing in the uppermost part while activity continues in the dependent portion. Collections of fluid in this area probably continue to support the growth of *M. ulcerans,* which sustains progression of the lesion.

The ulcerative forms are divided into major and minor ulcers. Both forms tend to self-heal. A major ulcer is large and chronic and can form a contiguous osteomyelitis. Minor ulcers are small (1 to 2 cm in diameter), are sharply delineated, and heal early. Both ulcerative forms begin as subcutaneous nodules.

Bone Involvement

Contiguous osteomyelitis. Reactive osteitis occasionally develops beneath destroyed overlying skin and soft tissue, particularly with major ulcers. Bone becomes devitalized and necrotic, with the development of sequestra (Fig. 98.19).

Metastatic osteomyelitis. *M. ulcerans*–specific osteomyelitis develops in approximately 10% of all patients, underscoring that Buruli ulcer should always be considered a potentially systemic disease.[257] Most likely, metastatic osteomyelitis is a result of lymphohematogenous spread of *M. ulcerans* from a distant, earlier cutaneous lesion (Fig. 98.20). The overlying skin ordinarily is intact, but swelling and inflammation occur over the site of bone involvement. If the condition goes untreated, a draining fistula usually develops. Osteomyelitis often requires amputation (Fig. 98.21).

Complications. Infection may traverse the deep fascia and damage tendons, nerves, joints, genitalia, and periorbital tissues, requiring subsequent enucleation of the eye. Healing leads to fibrosis and scarring, causing functional limitations.[323] The scar may form keloids and often causes major contraction deformities, especially in lesions that cross joints (Fig. 98.22). Squamous cell carcinoma may develop in healed

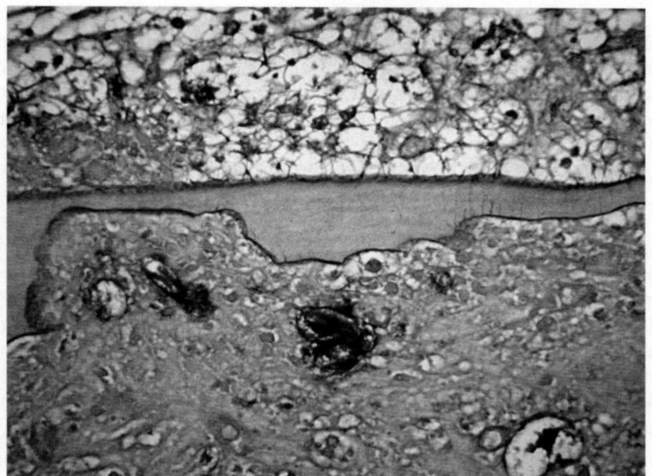

FIG. 98.20 Ziehl-Neelsen–stained section shows metastatic osteomyelitis of the tibia in a 6-year-old boy in Benin. This lesion developed after *M. ulcerans* infection of the contralateral leg. Note necrosis of marrow, erosion of a trabecula, and many clusters of acid-fast bacilli.

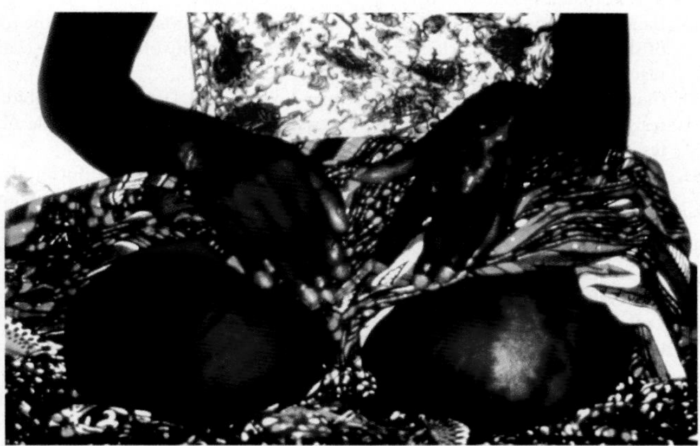

FIG. 98.21 This 13-year-old girl in Benin initially had a cutaneous lesion of Buruli ulcer. Subsequently, metastatic spread to bones of the lower extremities occurred, resulting in bilateral high-thigh amputations. Note also the spread to bones of both wrists and left hand.

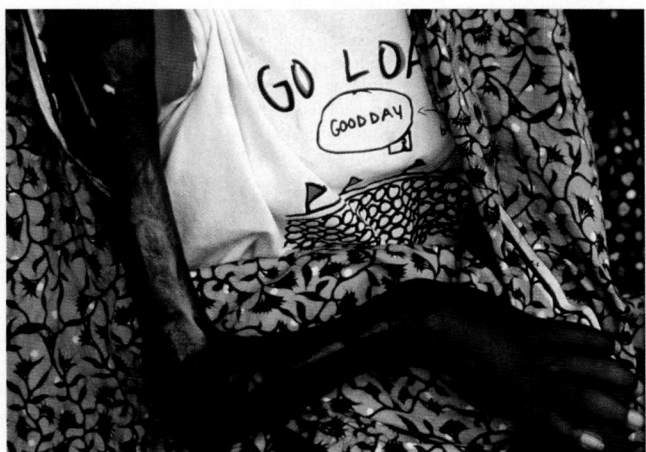

FIG. 98.22 Ghanaian adolescent girl with healed *M. ulcerans* infection that extended from the wrist to the shoulder. The scarring resulted in contraction deformities of the wrist and elbow and disuse atrophy of the entire extremity. Appropriate physiotherapy would have minimized these sequelae.

lesions, especially nonpigmented lesions.[161] Skin grafting and physiotherapy prevent most of these complications. Most disease-related deaths result from septicemia, gas gangrene, or tetanus.

Human Immunodeficiency Virus and Buruli Ulcer

Studies indicate that HIV infection increases the risk of Buruli ulcer by sevenfold to eightfold,[46,148] including a fivefold increase in HIV-infected children. HIV infection was also associated with more severe forms of Buruli ulcer: larger lesions and slower time to healing. Rapidly spreading *M. ulcerans* osteomyelitis has developed in several patients with AIDS.[166,284] Chronic diarrhea in an HIV-infected adult has also been attributed to *M. ulcerans*.[132]

Diagnosis and Differential Diagnosis

To an experienced observer, an accurate clinical diagnosis often can be made with ease.[372,373] In the ulcerated forms, a Ziehl-Neelsen stain of exudate from the ulcer edge obtained with a cotton swab reveals clusters of extracellular acid-fast bacilli. Punch biopsies and fine-needle aspiration also have been used to obtain samples from nonulcerative lesions.[378] Smears have an estimated sensitivity of 40%.[375] The same material, obtained by swab after decontamination, may be used for culture on Löwenstein-Jensen or other suitable mycobacterial media. The incubation temperature must be 30°C to 33°C (86°F–91.4°F). If culture cannot be performed locally, transport media may be inoculated with material from the cotton swab and maintained at 4°C (39.2°F) while in transport to a specialized laboratory. The transport medium is composed of Middlebrook 7H9 broth supplemented with polymyxin B, amphotericin B, nalidixic acid, trimethoprim, azlocillin, and 0.5% agar. Cultures often require at least 6 to 8 weeks to grow and have a sensitivity of 20% to 60%, in part because of the fastidious temperature requirements of the organism.[375] PCR is available and increasing in popularity and convenience.[312,324] PCR sensitivity is high (approximately 98%).[375] Tissue for histopathologic analysis should be obtained from the edge of the ulcer and must include all levels, including the fascia. Fixation in 4% buffered formalin is adequate. Histopathology has a sensitivity of 90% in experienced hands.[375] Mycolactone can be found in peripheral blood and ulcer exudates (including exudates obtained at the conclusion of therapy) by high-performance liquid chromatography. Reduction in mycolactone is a proxy for response to therapy in nonhuman animal models.[51] This modality may be more specific than smear microscopy, faster than culture, and more simple than PCR, making mycolactone an interesting target for diagnostic testing.

Some of the differential diagnostic possibilities are as follows:

Papules: Insect bites, verruca vulgaris, pityriasis, granuloma annulare
Nodules: Lipoma, sebaceous cyst, onchocerciasis, furuncle
Plaques: Leprosy, mycosis, necrobiosis, psoriasis
Edema: Bacterial cellulitis, actinomycosis, elephantiasis, pyomyositis
Ulcers: Tropical phagedenic ulcer, noma, stasis ulcer, leishmaniasis

Prognosis

Without treatment, Buruli ulcer often leads to deforming depressed scars, contraction deformities, or amputation. Delays in diagnosis are statistically related to the kind of Buruli ulcer disease. In one study, diagnosis for patients with nonulcerative forms was 32 days, 60 days for those with ulcerative manifestations, and 1 year for those with bony lesions.[41] One study found that almost 60% of patients had functional limitations a median of 4 years after completing therapy. Functional limitations and risk factors for stopping work or school were collinear and included lesion over a joint or on hands or feet, female sex, older age, and presence of a persistent wound.[323] The stigma of the deformities and the socioeconomic burden of the disease often are marked.[8] With early appropriate treatment, including excision and grafting, the prognosis usually is excellent. Metastatic lesions and local recurrences occur frequently enough, however, to warrant vigilant follow-up.[5] Paradoxical worsening of lesions while on appropriate antibiotic therapy has been noted, similar to immune reconstitution inflammatory syndromes seen for other mycobacterial infections. These are thought to be due to mycobacterial antigens and inflammatory cytokines released from clinically unrecognized bacterial foci.[278]

Treatment

Treatment options for Buruli ulcer include antibiotics and surgical intervention, the latter commonly used for category III lesions. In the preantibiotic era, wide local excision was commonly used.[334] The WHO now recommends surgery as an adjunct to medical therapy, particularly to remove necrotic tissue, cover skin defects, and correct deformities resulting in functional limitations.[378]

The WHO recommends an 8-week course of rifampin 10 mg/kg (maximum 600 mg) daily and either streptomycin or amikacin 15 mg/kg (maximum 1 g) daily as first-line therapy for all forms of active disease.[378,379] Intramuscular administration of aminoglycosides in children may be limited by the small muscle mass in many children. Macrolide therapy (clarithromycin, 7.5 mg/kg, maximum 1 g/day divided into two daily doses) has been substituted for aminoglycoside therapy during pregnancy. Monitoring for side effects is essential. For streptomycin, treatment should be stopped if hearing impairment or vertigo with nystagmus develops. For rifampin, treatment should be stopped if hepatitis, jaundice, or acute renal failure occurs, side effects that generally are associated with intermittent therapy of more than 10 mg/kg. One randomized trial in Ghana for patients with ulcers less than 10 cm in diameter compared the WHO-recommended regimen to streptomycin and rifampin for 4 weeks, followed by rifampin and clarithromycin for 4 weeks; they found no difference in response to therapy acutely or at 1-year follow-up.[237] An entirely oral regimen of 8 weeks of rifampin and clarithromycin was evaluated in a pilot study of 30 Beninese patients with lesions less than 10 cm in diameter. The treatment was well tolerated, and all patients had healed by 12 months without disease recurrence.[43] One Australian study combined with rifampin with either ciprofloxacin or clarithromycin; this entirely oral regimen was well tolerated with low rates of recurrence and relapse.[102] The extent to which these studies would apply to patients with more invasive or multifocal disease is unclear.

If surgical intervention is chosen, to minimize the danger of development of *M. ulcerans* bacteremia, many surgeons prescribe clarithromycin and rifampin 1 to 2 weeks before performing surgery and have the patients continue antibiotic therapy for several weeks after surgery. Although reasonable, this antibiotic complement to surgery is not of proven efficacy. In preulcerative Buruli disease, bacilli may extend well beyond the apparent border of the lesion, and having positive margins may increase the risk of recurrence.[126] As such, margins of at least 2.5 cm are recommended,[334] and the need for postoperative medical management in these cases is unclear.

Plaques and edematous forms are excised widely down to the fascia, or through the fascia if it is necrotic. Muscle usually is not damaged, but if so, the excision is extended into muscle. The lateral extent of excision often is difficult to determine. By careful palpation, the physician can establish an approximate limit of the disease. Exploratory incisions and blunt dissection may help determine the limit of induration and necrosis. Use of real-time PCR for determining the extent of disease is being evaluated.[272]

Very small ulcers can be excised and closed primarily, as for nodules. Large ulcers are excised widely. The required extent of surgery may be determined by exploratory lateral excision and blunt dissection. Split-skin autografting of surgical defects usually is performed after a bed of granulation tissue has formed. Postoperative care, including physiotherapy, should be designed to prevent contractures.

Bone lesions should be referred to specialists. Heat therapy without surgical excision has been successful for appropriate lesions, but must be applied assiduously, with all necessary controls.[208] Recurrences after surgical treatment are frequent, but rates are not well established.[68]

Prevention

In an endemic tropical rural setting where children usually are scantily attired, prevention of contamination of the skin from environmental sources is virtually impossible. Wearing long trousers seems to prevent development of infection.[189] Protected water supplies in villages would reduce exposure; however, such protective measures usually are futile in rural areas of developing countries. Standard precautions are indicated for the hospitalized patient. Buruli ulcer disease is not a reportable disease in the United States.

Vaccination with BCG has a moderate (40% to 50%) protective effect against *M. ulcerans* infections for 6 to 12 months,[134] although effect wanes with time and has been variable in both human and animal studies.[50,251] One form of Buruli ulcer disease for which BCG appears to have a sustained protective effect for children and adults is for the disseminated osteomyelitic form.[254] The role of repeated BCG immunization to increase immunity[159,254,302,330] to *M. ulcerans* infection is unclear. Using a recombinant BCG vaccine encoding an *M. ulcerans* mycolyl transferase, has been effective in murine models.[124] One *M. ulcerans*–specific vaccine target would be mycolactone, but this polyketide is poorly immunogenic, and antimycolactone antibodies are not detected in either cases or controls.[50] Mycobacterial heat shock protein (HSP) 45 is very immunogenic and protective in mouse models, but homology to a human HSP increases risk for autoimmune reactions.[57] In the absence of an effective vaccine, control strategies have focused on early detection and treatment, combined with physiotherapy to reduce scarring and functional limitations.[375]

NEW REFERENCES SINCE THE SEVENTH EDITION

7. Antunes DE, Araujo S, Ferreira GP, et al. Identification of clinical, epidemiological, and laboratory risk factors for leprosy reactions during and after multidrug therapy. *Mem Inst Oswaldo Cruz.* 2013;108:901-908.
10. Balagon MF, Cellona RV, Abalos RM. The efficacy of a four-week, ofloxacin-containing regimen compared with standard WHO-MDT in PB leprosy. *Lepr Rev.* 2010;81:27-33.
13. Banerjee S, Biswas N, Kanti Das N, et al. Diagnosing leprosy: revisiting the role of slit-skin smear with critical analysis of the applicability of polymerase chain reaction in diagnosis. *Int J Dermatol.* 2011;50:1522-1527.
39. Cambau E, Chauffour-Nevejans A, Tejmar-Kolar L, et al. Detection of antibiotic resistance in leprosy using GenoType LepraeDR, a novel ready-to-use molecular test. *PLoS Negl Trop Dis.* 2012;6:e1739.
41. Capela C, Sopoh GE, Houezo JG, et al. Clinical epidemiology of Buruli ulcer from Benin (2005-2013): effect of time-delay to diagnosis on clinical forms and severe phenotypes. *PLoS Negl Trop Dis.* 2015;9:e0004005.
46. Christinet V, Comte E, Ciaffi L, et al. Impact of human immunodeficiency virus on the severity of Buruli ulcer disease: results of a retrospective study in Cameroon. *Open Forum Infect Dis.* 2014;1:ofu021.
51. Converse PJ, Xing Y, Kim KH, et al. Accelerated detection of mycolactone production and response to antibiotic treatment in a mouse model of *Mycobacterium ulcerans* disease. *PLoS Negl Trop Dis.* 2014;8:e2618.
59. Cunha Mda G, Virmond M, Schettini AP, et al. OFLOXACIN multicenter trial in MB leprosy FUAM-Manaus and ILSL-Bauru, Brazil. *Lepr Rev.* 2012;83:261-268.
102. Friedman ND, Athan E, Hughes AJ, et al. *Mycobacterium ulcerans* disease: experience with primary oral therapy in an Australian cohort. *PLoS Negl Trop Dis.* 2013;7:e2315.
119. Guerrero-Guerrero MI, Muvdi-Arenas S, Leon-Franco CI. Relapses in multibacillary leprosy patients: a retrospective cohort of 11 years in Colombia. *Lepr Rev.* 2012;83:247-260.
124. Hart BE, Hale LP, Lee S. Recombinant BCG expressing *Mycobacterium ulcerans* Ag85A imparts enhanced protection against experimental Buruli ulcer. *PLoS Negl Trop Dis.* 2015;9:e0004046.
126. Herbinger KH, Brieske D, Nitschke J, et al. Excision of pre-ulcerative forms of Buruli ulcer disease: a curative treatment? *Infection.* 2009;37:20-25.
181. Liu D, Zhang Q, Sun Y, et al. Drug resistance in *Mycobacterium leprae* from patients with leprosy in China. *Clin Exp Dermatol.* 2015;40:908-911.
232. Narang T, Sawatkar GU, Kumaran MS, et al. Minocycline for recurrent and/or chronic erythema nodosum leprosum. *JAMA Dermatol.* 2015;151:1026-1028.
239. Nolen L, Haberling D, Scollard D, et al. Incidence of Hansen's disease – United States, 1994-2011. *MMWR Morb Mortal Wkly Rep.* 2014;63:969-972.
244. Olveira RM, Hungria EM, de Araujo Freitas A, et al. Synergistic antigen combinations for the development of interferon gamma release assays for paucibacillary leprosy. *Eur J Clin Microbiol Infect Dis.* 2014;33:1415-1424.
251. Phillips RO, Phanzu DM, Beissner M, et al. Effectiveness of routine BCG vaccination on Buruli ulcer disease: a case-control study in the Democratic Republic of the Congo, Ghana, and Togo. *PLoS Negl Trop Dis.* 2015;9:e3457.
253. Polito MG, Moreira SR, Nishida SK, et al. It is time to review concepts on renal involvement in leprosy: pre- and post-treatment evaluation of 189 patients. *Ren Fail.* 2015;37:1171-1174.
265. Reja AH, Biswas N, Biswas S, et al. Fite-Faraco staining in combination with multiplex polymerase chain reaction: a new approach to leprosy diagnosis. *Indian J Dermatol Venereol Leprol.* 2013;79:693-700.
276. Roy K, Sil A, Das NK, et al. Effectiveness and safety of clofazimine and pentoxifylline in type 2 lepra reaction: a double-blind, randomized, controlled study. *Int J Dermatol.* 2015;54:1325-1332.

283. Sales AM, de Matos HJ, Nery JA, et al. Double-blind study of the efficacy of pentoxifylline vs thalidomide for the treatment of type II reaction in leprosy. *Braz J Med Biol Res*. 2007;40:243-248.
306. Sharma R, Singh P, Loughry WJ, et al. Zoonotic leprosy in the southeastern United States. *Emerg Infect Dis*. 2015;21:2127-2134.
328. Talhari C, Talhari S, Oliveira Penna G. Clinical aspects of leprosy. *Clin Dermatol*. 2015;33:26-37.
349. Voorend CG, Post EB. A systematic review on the epidemiological data of erythema nodosum leprosum, a type 2 leprosy reacation. *PLoS Negl Trop Dis*. 2013;7:e2440.
352. Walker SL, Lockwood DN. Leprosy type 1 (reversal) reactions and their management. *Lepr Rev*. 2008;79:372-386.
362. Wen Y, Xing Y, Yuan LC, et al. Whole-blood nested-PCR amplification of *M. leprae*-specific DNA for early diagnosis of leprosy. *Am J Trop Med Hyg*. 2013;88:918-922.
378. World Health Organization. Global leprosy update, 2013: reducing disease burden. *Weekly Epidemiol Record*. 2014;36:389-400.

The full reference list for this chapter is available at ExpertConsult.com.

99 Nocardia

Nada Harik • Richard F. Jacobs

Nocardia spp. are obligate aerobic bacilli that exist throughout the world as soil and dust saprotrophs. They are also found in salt and fresh water and rotting vegetable matter. These organisms are non–spore-forming, thin, branching, gram-positive, partially acid-fast, filamentous bacteria. Humans become infected with *Nocardia* by two primary routes: inhalation of contaminated airborne dust particles or traumatic implantation of the bacterium into subcutaneous tissue. Pulmonary disease is the form of nocardiosis recognized most commonly in the United States.[5] The pulmonary event may be subclinical or transient, or it may provoke an acute or chronic process mimicking staphylococcal or fungal pneumonia, tuberculosis, or carcinoma. Hematogenous dissemination may occur, especially in immunocompromised hosts. The central nervous system (CNS) is the most common site of dissemination, with involvement manifested most often as a brain abscess. Cutaneous nocardiosis may be acute, subacute, or chronic (mycetoma). This form of disease is seen predominantly in immunocompetent hosts, with *Nocardia brasiliensis* being the agent identified most frequently.[50]

In 1888, Nocard, a veterinarian, noted an aerobic actinomycete in bovine farcy, a chronic wasting disease in cattle characterized by pulmonary abscesses and draining cutaneous sinus tracts. H.L. Eppinger first described human disease in 1890. The earliest pediatric case was documented in 1895 in a boy with pulmonary and subcutaneous infection.[8]

ORGANISM

Nocardia spp. are included among the aerobic actinomycetes. They are gram-positive bacteria that are filamentous and branched and grow more slowly than other aerobic and facultatively anaerobic bacteria. They commonly produce a fungus-like mycelium that fragments or breaks up into rod-shaped and short coccoid forms. *Nocardia* spp. grow slowly on a variety of simple media (e.g., blood agar and brain-heart infusion agar); addition of carbon dioxide (10%) promotes more rapid growth. The organisms are inhibited by antibiotics and antifungal agents, so media containing such agents do not support the growth of *Nocardia*. Because of their growth on commonly used fungal media (e.g., Sabouraud dextrose agar) and on some mycobacterial media (e.g., Löwenstein-Jensen medium), many *Nocardia* samples may be misdirected to the mycology or mycobacteriology section of clinical laboratories for identification.

Nocardia spp. grow best at temperatures of 25°C to 45°C (77°F–113°F); growth at higher temperatures may be used for differentiation. In pure culture, small, chalky white, heaped, wrinkled, or verrucous colonies appear in 3 to 5 days. Mature colonies usually are light orange and have a velvety appearance caused by the production of rudimentary aerial mycelia. They have the odor of a musty basement or freshly turned soil. Detection of colonies from clinical specimens, such as respiratory secretions, may require 2 to 4 weeks. In mixed culture, rapidly growing bacteria may obscure small *Nocardia* colonies. Use of modified Thayer-Martin medium may enhance recovery.

Gram stain of a portion of a colony shows delicate, branching filaments no more than 1 µm in diameter. The filaments may fragment and produce bacillary or coccoid forms. Many *Nocardia* spp. are partially acid-fast (i.e., in contrast to *Mycobacterium* spp., they retain fuchsin less tenaciously). A modified Ziehl-Neelsen or Kinyoun stain that decolorizes with 1% sulfuric acid instead of the more active acid alcohol is best for showing beaded acid-fast *Nocardia* in clinical specimens. Acid-fastness is characteristic of *Nocardia* in tissue or primary colony isolates but is lost quickly on subculture; not all pathogenic strains of *Nocardia* are acid-fast.[9] *N. asteroides* often survives the *N*-acetylcysteine digestion procedure (without sodium hydroxide) performed on sputum or bronchial washings; however, some positive sputum specimens may be rendered falsely negative.[58] Cultures of sputum and bronchial washings for isolation of *Nocardia* should be performed before and after the digestion procedure. Grocott's methenamine silver histochemical stain (GMS) can be used to detect *Nocardia* spp. in tissue specimens.

In the past, microscopic and colonial morphology, biochemical tests, chemotaxonomic methods, or antimicrobial susceptibility patterns were used to speciate *Nocardia*. 16S rRNA gene sequencing, multilocus sequence analysis, and polymerase chain reaction (PCR) restriction fragment length polymorphism (RFLP) analysis are the current methods most frequently used for speciation; use of these molecular techniques has resulted in changes in the nomenclature of *Nocardia* spp.[14] Analyzing *Nocardia* spp. with molecular techniques has demonstrated that many species were previously misidentified using conventional techniques.[52] Utilizing matrix-assisted laser desorption ionization-time of flight mass spectrometry (MALDI-TOF) with custom databases for the identification of *Nocardia* spp. is promising.[16,90]

More than 30 species of *Nocardia* of human clinical significance have been identified.[14] Formerly, the term *Nocardia asteroides* complex was used to account for the heterogeneity in antimicrobial resistance patterns seen among *N. asteroides.* Detailed molecular analyses and susceptibility testing have established clearly that *N. asteroides* complex represented many different *Nocardia* spp.[14] Various previously under recognized *Nocardia* spp. have recently been reported to cause infection in humans.[25,33,63] However, the most medically important species of *Nocardia* remain: *N. asteroides, Nocardia abscessus, Nocardia brasiliensis, Nocardia farcinica, Nocardia brevicatena/paucivorans* complex, *Nocardia nova* complex, *Nocardia otitidiscaviarum* complex, *Nocardia pseudobrasiliensis,* and *Nocardia transvalensis* complex.

EPIDEMIOLOGY, TRANSMISSION, AND PATHOGENESIS

Nocardia spp. can occasionally contaminate skin or colonize the upper respiratory tract.[30,66,78] Bronchial obstruction and/or decreased bronchociliary clearance predisposes to colonization.[66] The importance of *Nocardia* spp isolated in the sputum of individuals with cystic fibrosis remains uncertain.[65,70] The presence of signs and symptoms that correlate with nocardiosis can help ascertain the clinical significance of a positive *Nocardia* culture.

Most infections occur in the lungs, via inhalation.[5] The second most common site of infection is the CNS.[5] Although nocardiosis occurs in immunocompetent individuals, approximately 70% of patients are immunosuppressed by medications or underlying disease.[5] The typical patient has compromised cellular immunity (secondary to steroids, organ transplantation, hematopoietic stem cell transplant, cytotoxic chemotherapy, chronic granulomatous disease, chronic alcoholism, diabetes mellitus, or human immunodeficiency virus [HIV] infection). Nocardiosis also is seen more commonly in patients with a history of surgery or trauma.[55] The risk of acquiring infection is increased in patients with chronic pulmonary disease and in any patient who is receiving long-term corticosteroid treatment. Person-to-person communicability has not been a problem. Historically the incidence of nocardiosis in the United States has been estimated to be approximately 500 to 1000 new cases per year.[5,6] However, this number most likely is an underrepresentation, given the marked increase in the number of immunocompromised individuals. In addition, nocardial infections can be difficult to recognize, resulting in underestimation of the true incidence of nocardiosis. Presumed nosocomial nocardiosis has been reported.

Nocardiosis has been diagnosed in individuals of all ages (4 weeks to 83 years of age). Except in cases of cutaneous nocardiosis, almost all patients have one or more severe underlying diseases (e.g., lupus erythematosus, asthma, glomerulonephritis, ulcerative colitis, bronchiectasis, tuberculosis, rheumatoid arthritis, diabetes mellitus, or sarcoidosis) and/or are immunocompromised. Patients with lymphoreticular neoplasms and transplant recipients seem to be particularly at risk. The incidence of nocardiosis varies among transplant recipients with lung transplant recipients having the highest incidence.[48] In a literature review of nocardiosis in transplant recipients, the median time to infection was 7.5 months after hematopoietic stem cell transplantation and 21 months after solid organ transplantation.[48] Anti-tumor necrosis factor therapy (with infliximab, etanercept, and adalimumab) has been associated with the development of nocardial infection.[1,2,83,88] This catalase-positive organism is one of the five main pathogens seen in children with chronic granulomatous disease and can cause severe infection.[36] Although *Nocardia* is not a surveillance organism for acquired immunodeficiency syndrome (AIDS), patients with HIV may contract nocardiosis.[37] In a review of all cases ($n = 25$) of nocardiosis at an urban adult teaching hospital from 1999 to 2004, 76% of patients with nocardiosis also were infected with HIV; all had CD4 counts less than 100 cells/mm^3.[17]

Cutaneous nocardiosis usually is an infection of immunocompetent hosts. *N. brasiliensis* is isolated from approximately 80% of cases of primary cutaneous or subcutaneous nocardiosis.[68] Traumatic implantation of *Nocardia* into deep subcutaneous tissue may result in an indolent condition termed *actinomycotic mycetoma* (to distinguish it from the eumycotic mycetomas caused by true fungi).[61] Mycetoma is a chronic, progressive infection that can extend to underlying bone. Actinomycotic mycetomas usually involve the lower extremities or hands and typically are caused by *Actinomadura* spp., non–acid-fast aerobic actinomycetes, or *Streptomyces* spp. Actinomycotic mycetomas caused by *Nocardia* frequently involve the chest and back. Mycetomas, the cause of which may be *N. brasiliensis,* have been described in Mexican and South American field workers. *N. brasiliensis* also has been documented as an opportunistic pathogen prevalent in Florida, with a predilection for diabetics.[73]

In addition to the classic mycetoma, traumatic introduction of *Nocardia* spp. from soil may result in wound infections that occur after a more acute or subacute course. The organism can be introduced into the skin by tick[49] and other insect bites[27,59] or by a cat scratch[28,67] and result in cellulitis, pustules, or pyoderma; these conditions occasionally disseminate in immunocompromised individuals.[39,40] Posttraumatic endophthalmitis,[29] necrotizing fasciitis,[51] and poststernotomy mediastinitis[79,91] have been described.

N. farcinica is a medically important pathogen.[71,87] In a series of 200 cases of *Nocardia* infection reported by Wallace and associates,[87] the isolates designated *N. farcinica* were from patients with severe illness, 56% of whom had disseminated infections. *N. farcinica* isolates were characterized by increased resistance to antimicrobials, specifically third-generation cephalosporins. Evidence from mouse models indicates that *N. farcinica* seems to be more virulent than are other *Nocardia* spp.[24] Because the various species of *Nocardia* seem to have different pathogenicities, determination of the infecting species of *Nocardia* is important.

In a retrospective review of cases of pediatric nocardiosis admitted to Arkansas Children's Hospital, five children with nocardiosis were identified from more than 100,000 admissions in a 10-year period. Four of the five patients had received a transplant within the previous year. Three of these patients had pulmonary disease caused by *N. asteroides,* and one transplant recipient had skin involvement with *N. brasiliensis* at a central venous line site. One immunocompetent 5-year-old boy contracted CNS infection caused by *N. asteroides* 2 months after incurring a penetrating brain injury.[34]

The immune response to *Nocardia* is multifaceted.[5] Neutrophils are mobilized to the site of infection and are the predominant cell type found in lesions. Neutrophils only inhibit the organisms, however, and limit the spread of infection until an adequate cell-mediated immune response develops or effective antimicrobial agents are administered. Immune T cells are vital in clearing *Nocardia* from the lung and preventing dissemination; many predisposing conditions for nocardiosis involve inadequate cell-mediated immunity. Activated macrophages induce cytotoxic T cells effective against *N. asteroides. Nocardia* may survive inside neutrophils and macrophages by inhibiting phagosome-lysosome fusion and production of catalase and superoxide dismutase, which inactivate the myeloperoxidase system. *Nocardia* organisms exhibit a differential ability to evade phagosome-lysosome fusion that depends on their state of growth, possibly related to specific cell wall mycolic acids detected only in log-phase cells.[7] Differential cell wall characteristics also may influence the ability of *Nocardia* organisms to exhibit specific organ tropism (e.g., the brain).[10] Antibody may play a role in host defense through enhancement of macrophage activities. Although antecedent conditions of nocardiosis frequently involve dysfunctional cellular immunity, other important preconditions include neutrophil disorders (chronic granulomatous disease) and immunoglobulin disorders.

PATHOLOGY

The lesions of nocardiosis are suppurative, whether in the lung or in subcutaneous tissue, and they involve primarily proliferation of neutrophils rather than formation of granulomas. Pulmonary nocardiosis in immunocompetent patients often resembles pulmonary actinomycosis in that it results in a chronic localized pneumonia that often abuts the pleura.[35] Indolent progressive fibrosis resembling fibronodular tuberculosis may occur. Pulmonary nocardiosis is more aggressive in immunocompromised patients and is manifested as multifocal necrotizing pneumonia with confluent abscess formation. *Nocardia* spp. tend to invade the pleura and chest wall, with tissue planes disregarded in the process. Little evidence of encapsulation is characteristic of all organs invaded and probably accounts for the ready dissemination of organisms from the initial pulmonary focus.

Nocardia spp. appear as delicate, beaded, branching filaments in tissue stained with Gram stain or modified acid-fast stain (Fig. 99.1). *Nocardia* spp. are invisible in hematoxylin and eosin preparations and in sections stained with periodic acid–Schiff for fungi. GMS preparations sometimes detect tissue organisms; overstaining with silver enhances visualization.

CLINICAL MANIFESTATIONS

The most common manifestation of nocardiosis (>40% of all cases) in the United States is pulmonary disease in a patient with underlying immunosuppression.[22,62,66] Infection may remain localized to the lung or may disseminate hematogenously to the CNS and skin and, more rarely, to almost any organ in the body. In high-risk patients, the diagnosis should be suspected when CNS manifestations, particularly signs of a brain mass, abscess, or soft tissue swelling, develop in conjunction with a current or recent subacute or chronic pulmonary infection. Although sulfonamides are the most effective drugs for treatment of nocardiosis, invasive infections have been described in immunocompromised individuals receiving oral trimethoprim-sulfamethoxazole (TMP-SMX) as prophylaxis for *Pneumocystis jirovecii* pneumonia[19,86] and in patients with chronic granulomatous disease receiving TMP-SMX prophylaxis.[74]

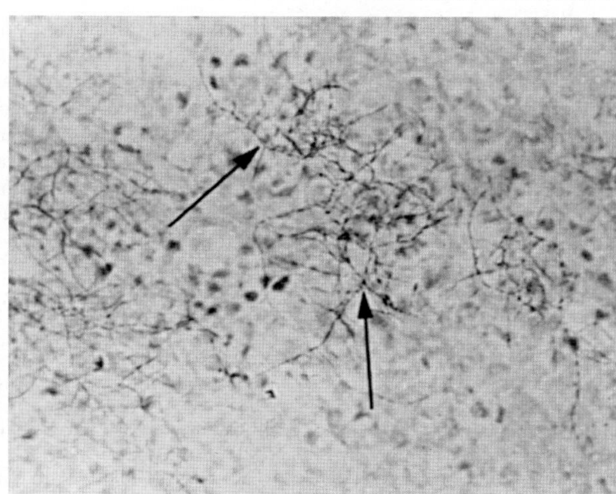

FIG. 99.1 Appearance of *Nocardia asteroides* and *Nocardia brasiliensis* *(arrows)* in a properly decolorized acid-fast smear. Organisms appear as fragmented bacilli with stain concentrated in a beaded fashion along portions of the filaments (×160).

Clinical manifestations of pulmonary nocardiosis are not specific and include anorexia, weight loss, productive cough, pleural pain, dyspnea, and, occasionally, hemoptysis.[22] Therefore, diagnosis of pulmonary nocardiosis is often delayed. In a recent study from China of adults with pulmonary nocardiosis, the median time to diagnosis was 25 days.[18] Untreated pulmonary nocardiosis usually runs a chronic course, similar to that of tuberculosis, but it also may clear spontaneously and obscure the source of subsequent metastatic infection. The diverse clinical and radiographic manifestations, including acute bronchopneumonia, lobar pneumonia or necrotizing pneumonia with single or multiple abscesses, and pleural empyema, may mimic more common pulmonary infections, such as mycobacterial, staphylococcal, and fungal pneumonia. For example, common computed tomography (CT) findings of pulmonary nocardiosis include solitary or more often multiple lung nodules and lung consolidation with or without cavitation that are nonspecific.[41] Pleural involvement (i.e., thickening or effusion) and chest wall extension are seen less commonly on CT.[41] Normal hosts or patients with only slightly impaired host defenses may have only mild respiratory tract symptoms of several months' duration.[26]

The CNS is the most common secondary site of infection, and such infection occurs in approximately one-third of patients.[5] Most experts recommend performing routine cranial CT for patients with pulmonary nocardiosis even when they are asymptomatic because of the frequency of involvement of the CNS. Brain abscesses are the most common manifestation; meningitis is reported less frequently.[4,12,19] In a literature review of 84 cases of CNS nocardiosis from 2000 to 2012, the most common signs and symptoms of infection were: focal neurologic abnormalities (51%), headache (45%), fever (40%), altered mental status (36%), seizures (28%), visual changes (21%), and nausea/vomiting (21%).[4]

Traumatic inoculation may result in localized disease manifested as cellulitis, mycetoma, subcutaneous abscess, or a lymphocutaneous syndrome in which one or more cutaneous nodules are associated with regional adenopathy or suppurative lymphadenitis.[47] Lymphocutaneous nocardiosis is clinically indistinguishable from sporotrichosis. Over a 5-year period, 31 cases of localized cutaneous nocardiosis with *N. brasiliensis* were identified in immunocompetent children in South Texas.[28] *Nocardia* spp. may cause cervicofacial disease and cervical adenitis in children.[46] Cutaneous nocardiosis can be mistaken for tularemia, mycobacterial infection, sporotrichosis, or superficial cellulitis due to *S.pyogenes* or *S.aureus*.

Other reported clinical manifestations of nocardiosis include tracheitis, peritonitis, iliopsoas abscess, hematogenous endophthalmitis, keratitis, endocarditis, mediastinitis, necrotizing faciitis, septic arthritis, ventriculitis and choroid plexitis, sinusitis/orbital cellulitis, and osteomyelitis.[22,42,45,51,56,75]

Bacteremic nocardiosis is reported rarely and usually is associated with endovascular foreign bodies in patients receiving long-term steroid therapy.[44] Catheter-associated *Nocardia* bacteremia also has been reported in a child with acute lymphoblastic leukemia (ALL) on maintenance chemotherapy.[89] In a report of six cases of central venous catheter–related *Nocardia* bacteremia, four cases were in children 18 years or younger.[27] All six patients received antibiotic therapy; the catheter was retained in three of the six. Relapse occurred in one of the three patients in whom the catheter was not removed.[27]

DIAGNOSIS

The diagnosis of nocardiosis is established in one-third of cases by sputum analysis and culture. Humoral methods used to diagnose nocardiosis generally lack specificity because of the high degree of serologic cross reactivity that occurs among *Nocardia* spp. and between *Mycobacterium* and *Streptomyces* spp.[11] The decreased sensitivity for detection of an antibody response in immunocompromised individuals is also likely a limitation of serologic testing. It is important to notify the laboratory when nocardial infection is suspected so that steps can be taken to optimize its recognition and recovery. Although *Nocardia* colonies usually are evident by 3 to 5 days after culture, prolonged incubation may be necessary.

Bronchoalveolar lavage or lung biopsy may be required to establish the diagnosis. Although these procedures are invasive, given the overlap in symptoms with other infectious and neoplastic processes and potential for rapid progression of disease, bronchoalveolar lavage or lung biopsy should be considered early in immunodeficient patients to establish a definitive diagnosis. The demonstration of tissue invasion confirms active infection.

Tentative species identification of most *Nocardia* can be made by biochemical methods, chemotaxonomic methods, or antimicrobial susceptibility patterns. However, only *N. brasiliensis, N. farcinica,* and *N. pseudobrasiliensis* can be identified reliably by these methods.[14] Molecular confirmation (e.g., DNA probes, PCR and PCR-RFLP molecular analyses, DNA sequencing, pyrosequencing, and ribotyping) of species identification is the method of choice. Molecular testing by hsp 65 PCR and 16S restriction enzyme analysis identifies more than 90% of currently recognized clinical species.[14] PCR assays for identifying *Nocardia* spp. are not commercially available. Accurate identification of *Nocardia* spp. by MALDI-TOF with custom databases has been reported.[16,90]

TREATMENT AND PROGNOSIS

Sulfonamides have been the best-studied drugs for the treatment of nocardiosis.[69,74,85] In the United States, TMP-SMX, the only intravenous sulfonamide formulation available, has been the agent of choice for treatment of nocardiosis. TMP-SMX has been used successfully at doses of 15 mg/kg per day of TMP and 75 mg/kg per day of SMX, either parenterally or orally.[74,82,84] Few cases have been reported of failure of TMP-SMX therapy for the treatment of nocardiosis.[3,31,60,76] TMP-SMX resistance among *Nocardia* spp. has been documented. However, a study of sulfonamide resistance in isolates of *Nocardia* spp. from six major laboratories across the United States from 2005 and 2011 showed only 2% resistance to TMP-SMX or sulfamethoxazole.[13] *N. farcinica* and *N. otitidiscaviarum* isolates are reported to have higher rates of resistance to TMP-SMX.[38,80,81] However, in a recent study of 22 *N. farcinica* clinical isolates, 100% were susceptible to TMP-SMX (94% were resistant to ceftriaxone).[43] The 2011 Clinical and Laboratory Standards Institute document on susceptibility testing of mycobacteria and other aerobic actinomycetes recommends that all clinically significant isolates of *Nocardia* spp. be tested for susceptibility to multiple antimicrobial agents.[20] No published prospective clinical trials have correlated in vitro susceptibilities with clinical outcome for nocardiosis. Susceptibility testing is the best available guide for selecting appropriate combination therapy and alternative therapies if sulfonamides fail or cannot be given because of patient intolerance or allergy.

No prospective randomized trials have established the optimal antimicrobial therapy for nocardiosis. Recommended antimicrobial therapy regimens are based on efficacy in animal models of nocardiosis, in vitro susceptibility and synergy testing, and retrospective clinical reviews and clinical case reports.[14]

TMP-SMX as a single agent usually is sufficient for patients with cutaneous nocardiosis. Many infectious disease specialists administer empiric combination drug therapy, consisting of TMP-SMX, amikacin, and a carbapenem or third-generation cephalosporin, for patients with severe disease, CNS nocardiosis, disseminated nocardiosis, and for immunosuppressed patients because of documented treatment failure and mortality associated with sulfonamide monotherapy in those settings.[53,58,76] Currently, no *Nocardia* spp. are resistant to amikacin and a β-lactam in vitro; the use of both (plus TMP-SMX) ensures that all clinical isolates would be susceptible to at least one other drug.[14] Antimicrobial therapy can be narrowed to two agents when results of in vitro susceptibility testing become available. Since antimicrobial resistance patterns vary by species, clinical isolates identified initially as *Nocardia* should be speciated further using molecular techniques. Children allergic to sulfonamides can be treated with amikacin and a carbapenem or third-generation cephalosporin.

The oxazolidinone linezolid is the first antimicrobial shown to be active in vitro against all clinically important *Nocardia* spp.[15] Linezolid, which is available for oral administration, has been used successfully to treat 11 patients with nocardiosis.[37,57] In one study, linezolid-associated hematologic toxicity was seen in three of six patients.[57] Peripheral neuropathy has also been observed in individuals with nocardiosis treated with linezolid.[38] Myelosuppression occurs more commonly in individuals receiving linezolid for longer than 2 weeks. Therefore, the use of linezolid for nocardial infection is limited by the prolonged treatment required for nocardiosis.

Clinical experience with minocycline, the tetracycline with best in vitro activity against *Nocardia*, has been encouraging. Amoxicillin-clavulanic acid has been effective in treating infections with *N. brasiliensis*, commonly a β-lactamase producer.[84] However, a case of acquired resistance to β-lactamase inhibitor antibiotics has been reported.[77] Other species with susceptibility to amoxicillin-clavulanic acid include *N. abscessus* and *N. farcinica*, whereas isolates of the *N. nova* complex are ampicillin susceptible or intermediate but resistant to amoxicillin-clavulanic acid.[14] Susceptibility of some *Nocardia* spp. to fluoroquinolones has been reported. In an in vitro study, gatifloxacin and moxifloxacin generally were more active than was ciprofloxacin against isolates of *Nocardia*, especially against isolates of *N. farcinica* and *N. brasiliensis*.[14] A patient with disseminated *N. farcinica* nocardiosis initially treated with aspiration, TMP-SMX, and imipenem had recurrence of brain lesions after a change to monotherapy with moxifloxacin despite in vitro susceptibility to moxifloxacin.[23] Recently, a benzothiazinone (PBTZ169) was shown to have significant in vivo activity against *N.brasiliensis* in a murine model of cutaneous nocardiosis.[32]

Clinical improvement typically is seen within 7 to 10 days after initiation of appropriate therapy.[55] Patients with unchanged or worsening symptoms after receiving 2 weeks of therapy should be reassessed thoroughly. Intravenous antibiotic therapy may be changed to an oral regimen after at least 3 to 6 weeks if clinical improvement is noted. The variable and chronic course of nocardiosis precludes determining precise therapeutic end points. Metastatic lesions can appear during or after an otherwise effective course of sulfonamide therapy with maintenance of the recommended 100- to 150-μg/mL level in serum or plasma. Because the tendency for relapse or the late appearance of metastatic disease is a concern, therapy often is continued for many months. Patients with mycetomas may require 6 to 12 months of therapy; localized cutaneous nocardiosis usually is treated for 3 to 6 months. Therapy for 6 to 12 months is suggested for patients with serious infection. Therapy for 12 months is indicated for patients with CNS nocardiosis and for immunocompromised patients.[50] Immunosuppressive medications should be reduced, if possible, during treatment for nocardiosis. Patients with CNS disease should be monitored with serial neuroimaging studies. Patients with AIDS probably should be treated with suppressive therapy indefinitely.

Surgical drainage of abscesses is important because metastatic abscesses can appear in the face of adequate therapy until surgical drainage is achieved.[30] Select brain abscesses may respond to antimicrobial treatment without surgery.[54]

Historically, the overall mortality rate for nocardiosis is 25% to 40%[64,66] with higher rates having been reported in immunocompromised hosts with disseminated nocardiosis.[6] Factors associated with increased mortality rates in one patient series were treatment with corticosteroids or antineoplastic agents, underlying Cushing disease, disseminated disease involving two or more noncontiguous organs or the CNS, and the presence of symptoms for less than 3 weeks before initial evaluation.[64] However, recent studies in immunocompromised patients with nocardiosis have reported mortality rates of 0% to 20%.[21,43,72]

NEW REFERENCES SINCE THE SEVENTH EDITION

1. Abreu C, Rocha-Pereira N, Sarmento A, et al. Nocardia infections among immunomodulated inflammatory bowel disease patients: a review. *World J Gastroenterol*. 2015;21:6491-6498.
2. Ali T, Chakraburrtty A, Mahmood S, et al. Risk of nocardial infections with anti-tumor necrosis factor therapy. *Am J Med Sci*. 2013;346:166-168.
4. Anagnostou T, Arvanitis M, Kourkoumpetis TK, et al. Nocardiosis of the central nervous system. *Medicine (Baltimore)*. 2014;93:19-32.
16. Buckwalter SP, Olson SL, Connelly BJ, et al. Evaluation of Matrix-Assisted Laser Desorption Ionization-Time of Flight Mass Spectrometry for Identification of Mycobacterium species, Nocardia species, and Other Aerobic Actinomycetes. *J Clin Microbiol*. 2016;54:376-384.
18. Chen J, Zhou H, Xu P, et al. Clinical and radiographic characteristics of pulmonary nocardiosis: Clues to earlier diagnosis. *PLoS ONE*. 2014;9:e90724.
21. Coussement J, Lebeaux D, van Delden C, et al. Nocardia infection in solid organ transplant recipients: a multicenter European case-control study. *Clin Infect Dis*. 2016;63:338-345.
25. Ercibengoa Arana M, Marimon Ortiz de Zarate JM. First report of Nocardia fusca isolated in humans. *BMJ Case Rep*. 2015;Jun 2:2015.
32. Gonzalez-Martinez NA, Lozano-Garza HG, Castro-Garza J, et al. In vivo activity of the benzothiazinones PBTZ169 and BTZ043 against Nocardia brasiliensis. *PLoS Negl Trop Dis*. 2015;9:e0004022.
33. Hagerman A, Rodriguez-Nava V, Boiron P, et al. Imipenem-resistant Nocardia cyriacigeorgica infection in a child with chronic granulomatous disease. *J Clin Microbiol*. 2011;49:1185-1187.
42. Kapur N, Adib N, Grimwood K. Nocardia brasiliensis infection mimicking juvenile idiopathic arthritis in a 4-year-old girl. *Pediatrics*. 2013;132:e1424-e1427.
43. Kim YK, Sung H, Jung J, et al. Impact of immune status on the clinical characteristics and treatment outcomes of nocardiosis. *Diagn Microbiol Infect Dis*. 2016;85: 482-487.
48. Lebeaux D, Morelon E, Suarez F, et al. Nocardiosis in transplant recipients. *Eur J Clin Microbiol Infect Dis*. 2014;33:689-702.
51. Lin Y-C, Huang Z-Y, Wang C-H. First case report of Nocardia brasiliensis infection causing necrotizing faciitis in an immunocompetent patient. *J Microbiol Immunol Infect*. 2016;49:824-825.
52. Liu WL, Lai CC, Ko WC, et al. Clinical and microbiological characteristics of infections caused by various Nocardia species in Taiwan: a multicenter study from 1998 to 2010. *Eur J Clin Microbiol Infect Dis*. 2011;30:1341-1347.
61. Pai S, Pai K, Sharma S. Cutaneous nocardiosis: an underdiagnosed pathogenic infection. *BMJ Case Rep*. 2015. www.ncbi.nlm.nih.gov/pmc/articles/PMC4369048/.
63. Plau C, Kerjouan M, Le Mouel M, et al. First case of disseminated infection with Nocardia cerradoensis in a Human. *J Clin Microbiol*. 2015;53:1034-1037.
65. Rodriguez-Nava V, Durupt S, Chyderiotis S, et al. A French multicentric study and review of pulmonary Nocardia spp. in cystic fibrosis patients. *Med Microbiol Immunol*. 2015;204:493-504.
70. Schoen L, Santoro JD, Milla C, et al. Pulmonary nocardiosis in an immunocompetent patient with cystic fibrosis. *Case Rep Pulmonol*. 2015;2015:984171.
72. Shrestha S, Kanellis J, Korman T, et al. Different faces of Nocardia infection in renal transplant recipients. *Nephrology*. 2016;21:254-260.
75. Sorichetti B, Westerberg B, Tan R, et al. Nocardia asteroids sinusitis in a pediatric patient: case report with 20 year follow-up and review of the literature. *Int J Pediatr Otorhinolaryngol*. 2015;79:1152-1154.
80. Torres OH, Domingo P, Pericas R, et al. Infection caused by Nocardia farcinica: case report and review. *Eur J Clin Microbiol Infect Dis*. 2000;19:205-212.
81. Uhde KB, Pathak S, McCullum I Jr, et al. Antimicrobial-resistant nocardia isolates, United States, 1995-2004. *Clin Infect Dis*. 2010;51(12):1445.
83. Verma R, Walia R, Sondike SB, et al. Pulmonary nocardiosis in an adolescent patient with Crohn's disease treated with infliximab: a serious complication of TNF-alpha blokers. *W V Med J*. 2015;111:36-39.
90. Xiao M, Pang L, Chen SC, et al. Accurate Identification of Common Pathogenic Nocardia Species: Evaluation of a Multilocus Sequence Analysis Platform and Matrix-Assisted Laser Desorption Ionization-Time of Flight Mass Spectrometry. *PLoS ONE*. 2016;11:e0147487.

The full reference list for this chapter is available at ExpertConsult.com.

Corynebacterium and Rhodococcus

100

Randall G. Fisher

CORYNEBACTERIUM

The genus *Corynebacterium* comprises a wide number of organisms possessing little pathogenic potential, with some notable exceptions. The most infamous member of this genus, *C. diphtheriae* (see Chapter 90), is a cause of a potentially lethal pharyngeal infection with systemic manifestations. *Corynebacterium jeikeium* (formerly *Corynebacterium* group JK) can be a major nosocomial agent of bacteremia and endocarditis; other species commonly are associated with infections in animals and rarely cause invasive infection in humans.[85,125] For an exhaustive consideration of coryneform bacteria, the reader is referred to the review by Funke and colleagues.[51]

Bacteriology

Corynebacterium spp. derive their name from their clublike shape. Because of their resemblance to *C. diphtheriae,* they are included in the heterogeneous group of diphtheroids. Snapping division produces the angular and palisade arrangement of cells responsible for their characteristic gram-positive, "Chinese letters" microscopic appearance.[27] Organisms are facultatively anaerobic or aerobic and do not produce spores. They are nonmotile and catalase positive and contain mycolic acid in their cell walls. Clinically relevant species include *C. diphtheriae, C. jeikeium, C. pseudotuberculosis, C. xerosis, C. amycolatum, C. pseudodiphtheriticum, C. minutissimum, C. striatum, C. ulcerans,* and *C. urealyticum.* Species can be differentiated according to biochemical tests and fermentation of sugars.[27,51,121]

Epidemiology

Corynebacterium spp. can be part of the normal skin and upper respiratory tract flora and commonly colonize hospitalized patients. Nosocomial acquisition of *C. jeikeium* has been characterized most completely. Thirty-five percent of hospitalized patients may be colonized with *C. jeikeium,* and the organism may be isolated at the time of admission.[53] The skin, groin, and rectum are common sites of recovery of organisms. Wounds and suppurative sites quickly become colonized.[53] Longer duration of hospitalization, receipt of broad-spectrum antimicrobial agents, and impaired skin integrity are risk factors for invasive infection. Hospital personnel caring for oncology patients have higher rates of hand colonization with pathogenic *Corynebacterium* spp. than do nurses caring for dermatology patients.[67] Transmission from patient to patient in the hospital environment can occur, and selective antibiotic pressure has been shown to augment colonization with *Corynebacterium* spp.[83,99,167] Outbreaks of bacteremic infection have been reported in hematology wards,[116,141] and DNA restriction fragment analysis and hybridization techniques have been used to document spread.[83,113]

It has been shown by whole genome sequencing that *C. jeikeium* actually comprises four different genomospecies, two of which can be differentiated from the other two by conventional microbiologic methods. Clinical isolates generally do not match the type strains.[127]

Pathophysiology

C. jeikeium and *C. urealyticum* are lipophilic, which may account for their ability to proliferate on skin that has a higher lipid content; organisms have been isolated from sebum-filled eccrine gland biopsy specimens in an adolescent with malignancy.[72] Breach of the integrity of the skin is an important risk factor for acquisition of local infection and bacteremia with *Corynebacterium.* Intravascular catheters increase the risk for infection.[119] Certain isolates of *C. pseudotuberculosis* and *C. ulcerans* can express diphtheria-like toxins,[165] which may confer virulence.

Some *Corynebacterium* spp., notably *C. jeikeium* and *C. urealyticum,* commonly show resistance to penicillins, cephalosporins, aminoglycosides, erythromycin, and tetracycline.[38,53,85,99,106,121,139] Strains with a significant DNA relationship to the *C. jeikeium*–type strain show penicillin resistance.[120] Resistant organisms have been noted to have significantly thickened cell walls compared with susceptible strains, but the functional importance of this feature is unknown.[16]

Clinical Manifestations

Systemic infections with *Corynebacterium* spp. generally are not clinically distinguishable from serious infections caused by other pathogens. Immunocompromised patients are at the highest risk for developing disease caused by *Corynebacterium,*[63,124] but infections also have been described in neonates and immunocompromised older children.[14,38,76] Risk factors include male gender, neutropenia, broad-spectrum antibiotic exposure, and prolonged hospital stay.[116,141] Catalase production may be responsible for the rare infection with non-JK *Corynebacterium* spp. in children with chronic granulomatous disease.[76] *Corynebacterium* spp. are responsible for approximately 9% of early-onset and 4% of late-onset prosthetic valve endocarditis.[164]

C. jeikeium is a pathogen of particular concern. In 1976, this agent first was described as a cause of serious infection in four patients, including an 11-year-old boy with a ventriculoatrial shunt.[63] The other three patients had hematologic malignancies and were neutropenic at the time of infection. Immunocompromised patients, particularly patients with leukemia, are vulnerable to bacteremia. These high-risk subjects may show a local inflammatory lesion at the site of infection or a disseminated, hemorrhagic, or necrotic papular exanthem.[109] Subcutaneous nodules also may be seen. *C. jeikeium* has been recovered from disseminated lesions in a 14-year-old boy with leukemia.[72] A literature review of 83 neutropenic patients (nearly all adults) with *C. jeikeium* sepsis found the following risk factors for development of infection: presence of a central venous catheter, being male, profound and prolonged neutropenia, and exposure to multiple antibiotics. Skin lesions were reported in 48% of patients, and pulmonary infiltrates were found in 36% of patients. The overall case-fatality rate was 34%, but it was reduced to 5% in patients with recovery from neutropenia.[154]

Infections with *C. jeikeium* also have been reported after trauma, ventriculoperitoneal shunting procedures,[3,78] orthopedic procedures,[26] bone marrow aspiration,[38] and central venous catheter placement.[38] *C. jeikeium* now is recognized to be one of the most common causes of prosthetic valve endocarditis in adults.[106] Cutaneous findings of bacteremia so commonly observed in patients with cancer generally are absent in patients with endocarditis.[33] In a series of 38 patients with *C. jeikeium* endocarditis, 74% of patients had prosthetic valves. The mortality rate was 33% and was not altered by valve replacement surgery.[104] According to a newer study, cases of endocarditis caused by *C. jeikeium* are more likely to require valve replacement than are those caused by other *Corynebacterium* spp.[12] Exit-site infections in patients on continuous ambulatory peritoneal dialysis also may be caused by *Corynebacterium* spp.; in the largest series published to date, *C. striatum* caused almost twice as many of these infections as did *C. jeikeium.* Most infections are manageable without removal of the dialysis catheter.[130] A case of malignant otitis externa that led to osteomyelitis of several skull bones and an epidural abscess which grew *C. jeikeium* along with *C. xerosis* and *Enterococcus faecalis* has been reported.[86]

Although primarily a pathogen in farm animals, *C. pseudotuberculosis* can cause localized suppurative granulomatous lymphadenitis in humans[85,103]; almost all cases are associated with animal contact, particularly sheep and goats.[54] Presentation and histology may mimic the much more common cat-scratch disease, and Gram stain and culture are required to differentiate the two entities.[85] Most cases have been reported from Australia.[111] The complete genome of an isolate taken from a 12-year-old girl with suppurative lymphadenitis has been sequenced.[152]

C. xerosis has been reported as a rare cause of endocarditis, arthritis, and ventriculoperitoneal shunt infection.[7,17] Most individuals with endocarditis have a prosthetic heart valve.[42,89] In one case an implantable cardioversion device became infected with the organism.[93] *C. xerosis* also can be a cause of eye infections in patients with superficial corneal foreign bodies; in one study of 101 patients, *C. xerosis* caused three of 15 culture-positive cases.[90] It also is an extremely rare cause of post-LASIK (laser-assisted in-situ keratomileusis) infectious keratitis.[37] Using chemical testing and molecular genetic investigation, Funke and colleagues[50] showed that many isolates tentatively identified as *C. xerosis* are actually *C. amycolatum. C. amycolatum* is much more likely to be multidrug-resistant than *C. xerosis.*[51] *C. amycolatum* is a comparatively common cause of bacteremia in children with cancer; of 12 cases of corynebacterial bacteremia reported from St. Jude Children's Research Hospital, three were caused by this species. In contrast to reports in adults, corynebacterial bacteremia in children usually started in the outpatient setting, happened in patients who were nonneutropenic, occurred relatively late in the course of cancer therapy, and had a relatively benign outcome.[1] In adults with cancer, *C. amycolatum* was often recovered from the upper urinary or lower respiratory tracts or found in surgical wounds or as an infection of ulcerating tumors.[96] It is generally seen in adults with solid tumors rather than hematologic malignancy.[96] A case of fatal sepsis in a premature neonate caused by *C. amycolatum* has been reported.[14]

C. pseudodiphtheriticum, a commensal of the oropharynx, can cause pneumonia, bronchitis, or tracheitis.[2,28,31] Lung disease usually occurs in the context of underlying cardiopulmonary pathology or immunocompromise.[61] Onset typically is acute, but fever may be noticeably absent.[91] One cystic fibrosis center in France reported that 10 children had exacerbations that appeared to be related to respiratory tract infection with *C. pseudodiphtheriticum;* matrix-assisted laser desorption ionization time-of-flight (MALDI-TOF) mass spectrometry was used to identify the isolates.[15] At least 18 cases of *C. pseudodiphtheriticum* endocarditis, including three infections in children with congenital heart disease, have been reported.[105] Infection of allograft material is a common finding; native heart valves may be involved but usually in the context of preexisting lesions or intravenous drug abuse. In adults, endocarditis due to *C. pseudodiphtheriticum* has a predilection for men who have had a previous prosthetic valve replacement; infection with toxigenic strains appears to have a higher mortality rate.[12] Three cases of exudative pharyngitis with a pseudomembrane mimicking diphtheria, including one in a 4-year-old girl from Arkansas, have been reported to be caused by *C. pseudodiphtheriticum.*[71] In one case, a surface swab from a draining wound after arthroscopy was reported to harbor "normal skin flora" but joint fluid grew the same organism, which was finally identified as *C. pseudodiphtheriticum.* Treatment resulted in resolution of symptoms of septic arthritis.[77] Patients who are immunocompromised and have corneal epithelial defects can get severe eye infections with this organism.[84] Rarely, ulcerative skin lesions have been described due to *C. pseudodiphtheriticum.*[22]

C. minutissimum traditionally has been regarded as the cause of the mild cutaneous disease erythrasma, which is characterized by scaly, pruritic red-brown patches, usually occurring in the axilla, groin, or between the toes. Although *C. minutissimum* may play a role, erythrasma probably is a polymicrobial process.[51] It may also be a secondary infection in patients with intertrigo.[74] *C. minutissimum* is recognized as a rare nosocomial infectious complication of malignancy and dialysis and has been implicated in a case of pyelonephritis in an 8-month-old infant with posterior urethral valves.[30] An adult who developed native-valve endocarditis caused by *C. minutissimum* has been reported.[6] Bacteremia and meningitis due to this organism has been described in a patient with sickle-cell disease with an intravenously implanted right subclavian port.[32]

C. striatum has been recovered from purulent sputum of hospitalized patients and from infected central venous catheter sites.[132,160] It also is a cause of exit-site infections in patients on long-term ambulatory peritoneal dialysis.[130] It has been reported as a cause of fatal pulmonary infection and endocarditis.[83,95,125] *C. striatum* was responsible for a nosocomial outbreak among 14 patients over a 12-month period in a surgical intensive care unit. Endotracheal intubation for longer than 24 hours was the only risk factor found to predispose to infection.[19] A second intensive care unit outbreak was reported from Italy; in this series, one of the patients was a 16-year-old admitted for severe trauma that resulted in having a sepsis-like picture and three blood cultures positive for *C. striatum.* Despite therapy with teicoplanin and meropenem, the patient died.[69] *C. striatum* also has been reported as a cause of meningitis and ventriculoperitoneal shunt infections.[68,161] Several cases of septic arthritis have been reported.[45, 131,156]

C. ulcerans derives its name from its association with ulcerative pharyngitis. Although it is more commonly a pathogen of nonhuman primates,[110] infection can occur in humans after contact with an animal or consumption of contaminated raw milk.[11,34] Toxigenic strains of *C. ulcerans* can produce a syndrome indistinguishable from that caused by toxigenic *C. diphtheriae.*[23,149] The toxin has a different DNA and amino acid sequence from that of *C. diphtheriae,*[136] and is apparently carried by a different prophage.[134] In the United Kingdom, domestic *C. ulcerans* is now a more common cause of diphtheria than *C. diphtheriae.*[159] Cases in the United States are decidedly rare; the case of an 80-year-old man in Idaho reported in 2010 was the first case in 5 years.[24] Skin lesions that exactly mimic cutaneous diphtheria, caused by diphtheria toxin–secreting strains of *C. ulcerans,* also have been reported.[158]

C. urealyticum (formerly *Corynebacterium* group D2) is a cause of alkaline-encrusted cystitis and pyelitis, primarily in the elderly.[44,139] A case series of four children with encrusted cystitis and pyelitis has been published. The mean age was 9 years (range, 4–13 years). Treatment was with prolonged antibiotics and endoscopic debulking. Cure was effected in three of the four patients; the other patient was a renal transplant recipient who lost the graft.[102] A prospective study of renal transplant recipients suggested that it is likely an underdiagnosed cause of obstructive uropathy in this group of patients; risk factors for infection were receipt of antibiotics in the previous month, nephrostomy, and skin colonization with the organism.[88] Routine urine culture may miss the organism; it may grow with prolonged incubation of sheep's blood agar.[135] It is associated less commonly with infection at other sites and with bacteremia.[138] An 8-year-old boy with chemotherapy-induced neutropenia and a necrotic soft tissue infection of the scrotum caused by *C. urealyticum* has been reported.[126] Cure of bacteremia in a patient with obstruction due to prostate cancer was not effected until his percutaneous nephrostomy tube was removed.[25]

Diagnosis

Diagnosis of *Corynebacterium* infection is based on isolation of the organism from clinical material. This organism commonly is accompanied by other pathogens. Similar to *Mycobacterium* and *Nocardia* spp., *Corynebacterium* organisms have mycolic acids in their cell wall. The chains are shorter, however, and the organisms are not acid fast. *Corynebacterium* spp. may be difficult to distinguish from some *Rhodococcus* spp.[27] Colonies of *C. jeikeium* may show a metallic sheen when grown on agar.[63] Growth of *C. jeikeium* is enhanced by the addition of lipids to the medium. Most *Corynebacterium* spp. can be differentiated quickly from each other by sugar fermentation, hydrolysis of urea, and reduction of nitrate.[148] Selective media containing kanamycin or trimethoprim-sulfamethoxazole have been useful in the recovery of multidrug-resistant strains of *Corynebacterium.*[62] The API Coryne system version 2.0 correctly identified 162 of 178 (91%) isolates in one study.[5] Polymerase chain reaction testing and MALDI-TOF spectrometry are quite accurate for specific identification at the species level, and are increasingly being used. Erythrasma usually is diagnosed by the typical coral red fluorescence under Wood lamp examination.

Treatment

Empirical therapy for infection must account for the frequency of infection with *C. jeikeium,* which often is multiresistant to antibiotics but is susceptible to vancomycin.[51] In some series of immunocompromised patients, this organism is the most common *Corynebacterium* spp. encountered.[140,163] Vancomycin is recommended for empirical therapy for suspected *Corynebacterium* infection until susceptibilities are known.

Treatment can be changed to a penicillin or cephalosporin, if appropriate. In vitro, *C. jeikeium* is sensitive to linezolid,[56] and most strains also are sensitive to quinupristin-dalfopristin[128] and daptomycin.[55] Treatment with daptomycin, however, has been associated with development of resistance in *C. striatum* strains during therapy.[98,162] This phenomenon has also been replicated in vitro.[98] In one worrisome case, a man who had received two long courses of daptomycin for MRSA infection developed native valve endocarditis with a strain of *C. striatum* that was heteroresistant to daptomycin.[151] A majority of strains is also sensitive to tigecycline, but experience with the antibiotic in childhood is sparse.[46] Linezolid is bacteriostatic against all species of *Corynebacterium,* and in vitro its activity is slower against *C. jeikeium* than it is against *C. striatum* and *C. amycolatum.*[56]

Two-drug therapy generally is recommended for treatment of *Corynebacterium* endocarditis; for gentamicin-susceptible strains, penicillin-gentamicin combinations have been shown to be synergistic, regardless of whether the strains are susceptible to penicillin.[106] Rarely, resistance to vancomycin is encountered. A woman with prosthetic valve endocarditis caused by a vancomycin-resistant *Corynebacterium* spp. was treated successfully with imipenem and ciprofloxacin.[10] Removal of infectious sources, such as central nervous system shunts and central venous catheters, may be required for cure. Scrupulous attention given to skin hygiene may reduce colonization of hospital personnel and the incidence of patient-to-patient transmission of pathogenic strains.[40,116] Management of toxigenic *C. ulcerans* infection is identical to that for infection caused by toxigenic *C. diphtheriae,* including the use of antitoxin.[149] Erythrasma usually responds to treatment with a macrolide.

RHODOCOCCUS

The genus *Rhodococcus* contains at least 15 species, of which *Rhodococcus equi* is the most clinically relevant to humans. Infections with other species are rare. Suppurative keratitis caused by *Rhodococcus ruber* after penetrating trauma has been described.[80] One case of bacteremia with *R. globerulus* was reported in a stem-cell transplant patient.[117] *R. equi* derives its name from its role as a cause of pyogranulomatous pneumonia in young horses.[114] It has assumed a prominent role as a cause of human pulmonary disease in immunocompromised patients, particularly in patients with acquired immunodeficiency syndrome (AIDS).[43,64,132] For a comprehensive discussion of this organism, the reader is referred to the review by Cornish and Washington.[29]

Bacteriology

R. equi is a catalase-positive, urease-positive, oxidase-negative, gram-positive rod. The organism assumes a more coccoid morphology in solid media and a more bacillary form in liquid media. Its cell wall contains mycolic acid, rendering it acid fast when grown on Lowenstein-Jensen media and stained with Kinyoun stain.[57]

Epidemiology

R. equi is a soil organism, and its growth is enriched by the manure of herbivores. Despite the common occurrence of this pathogen as a cause of veterinary infections, exposure to animals apparently is not necessary for human infection to occur[114]; most reported human patients have not had farm or animal exposure.[64] Hospital outbreaks of infection associated with patient-to-patient transmission have not been reported. In a retrospective analysis of 24 cases of *R. equi* infection, however, six patients had shared a hospital room with a patient with *R. equi* pneumonia, raising the possibility of nosocomial transmission.[8] Most patients diagnosed with *Rhodococcus* infection are immunocompromised; AIDS is the most common underlying diagnosis, but infection also has been reported in transplant patients[9] and rarely in patients believed to be immunocompetent.[153] In one case, infective endocarditis with severe complications including subarachnoid hemorrhage and subdural hematoma was reported in a patient with a normal immune workup.[97] On the other hand, a chronic, nonhealing ulcerative lesion caused by *R. equi* in a man believed to be immunocompetent led to a diagnostic workup that proved the cause to be a CD8 deficit.[36]

Chemotherapeutic agents such as fludarabine, which causes prolonged CD4 lymphocytopenia, can predispose to *R. equi* infection.[52] Receipt of high-dose corticosteroids[122] and alemtuzumab (an anti-CD52 monoclonal antibody) have also been reported as antecedents of infection.[101]

Pathophysiology

The prominence of pulmonary infection suggests that the respiratory tract is a common portal of entry. After gaining access to the lower respiratory tract, organisms are taken up by alveolar macrophages; Mac-1 macrophage receptors and complement are required for binding.[65] The organism replicates within a modified phenotypic vacuole; pathogenicity is dependent upon a plasmid that prevents phagosome-lysosome fusion.[155] The appearance of pyogranulomatous lesions is consistent with the role of *R. equi* as an intracellular parasite containing mycolic acid, a possible virulence factor in the cell wall.[58,115] Surface 15- and 17-kDa antigens expressed by an 85-kb plasmid seem to confer virulence in mice and foals,[143] and virulent strains seem to have an increased capacity for intracellular survival in macrophages.[66]

Most *R. equi* isolates from patients with AIDS express either the 15- to 17-kDa antigens or a 20-kDa antigen that seems to confer intermediate virulence. Most isolates from patients without AIDS express none of these antigens, however.[144] Other factors may play a role in promoting *Rhodococcus* disease in humans.[145] Death of parasitized macrophages may release enzymes, which contribute further to tissue damage. In vitro, infected respiratory epithelial cells upregulate the production of IL-6 and IL-8.[118] $CD4^+$ lymphocytes are essential for pulmonary clearance of *R. equi* in a mouse model,[75] which may help to explain the high risk for infection associated with cellular immunodeficiency.

Clinical Manifestations

Infection typically manifests as a subacute pneumonia developing over several weeks. Symptoms such as cough and fever are common, but progression of disease may be silent. Although most infections currently occur in patients with AIDS, malignancy and transplantation[166] also pose risks. Pulmonary infection in children with leukemia has been described.[4,100] Infection may be accompanied by other pathogens, particularly in patients with AIDS.

Pulmonary infection often is pleura based and associated with cavitation.[64] Empyema may occur as a complication. Computed tomography most frequently reveals pneumonia with cavitation, but other patterns, including ground-glass opacities, peribronchial nodules, and centrilobular nodules, may be seen.[92] Lung tissue showing malakoplakia, an unusual-appearing granulomatous inflammation with aggregates of histiocytes that contain concentrically layered basophilic inclusions, should raise suspicion of the presence of *R. equi* infection.[21,59,129]

Extrapulmonary disease is seen at diagnosis in 7% of patients with pneumonia.[157] Manifestations of infection include otitis/mastoiditis,[4,70,87] abscesses,[47] osteomyelitis,[18,48,108] meningitis,[35,133] pericarditis,[82] lymphadenitis,[82] and endophthalmitis.[41] The organism has been grown from a biopsy of a granulomatous skin lesion in an immunocompetent 7-year-old girl.[94] *R. equi* also has been reported as a cause of peritonitis in patients receiving long-term peritoneal dialysis.[20,146] A case report of ventriculitis in a premature infant with a ventriculoperitoneal shunt has been reported.[142]

Diagnosis

Diagnosis relies on isolation of *Rhodococcus* from clinical material. Although sputum specimens may be positive, bronchoalveolar lavage or lung biopsy may be required. Blood cultures may be positive in half or more of patients with AIDS and with focal pneumonic disease.[150] The physician should be alert to the possible coexistence of *R. equi* with other pathogens. In the laboratory, confusing this organism with *Corynebacterium,* acid-fast organisms, and other gram-positive coccobacilli has been shown to delay establishment of the diagnosis.[39] Positive findings on Gram stain and Kinyoun stain should be interpreted in the context of clinical information.[132] Organisms appear salmon-pink when grown on blood agar and orange on Lowenstein-Jensen medium.[13] Differentiating from acid-fast bacteria on smear sometimes can be difficult. Combined use of a siderophore detection medium, ethylene glycol degradation, and β-galactosidase activity may help differentiate

Rhodococcus from *Nocardia* and rapid-growing mycobacteria.[49] DNA restriction fragment analysis and ribotyping show promise in aiding the identification and tracking of *Rhodococcus* spp.[81] An *R. equi*–specific polymerase chain reaction assay has been used to confirm infection in some cases in which identification was difficult.[1]

Differentiation of *R. equi* from other species of the genus *Rhodococcus* can be difficult and may frequently be incorrect; 16S rRNA genome sequencing analysis sometimes identifies a different species of *Rhodococcus* from specimens originally signed out as *R. equi.*[60] Also, organisms of the genus *Dietzia* are often misidentified as *R. equi.*[79] In one study, only 7 of 15 clinical specimens originally called *R. equi* by the microbiology laboratory were actually *Rhodococcus* isolates; the 8 others were all members of the genus *Dietzia.*[112]

Treatment

Clinical isolates commonly are resistant to penicillins and cephalosporins. Even if susceptible in vitro, β-lactam antibiotics should be avoided because of rapid development of resistance.[73] Erythromycin, clarithromycin, azithromycin, clindamycin, rifampin, aminoglycosides, vancomycin, fluoroquinolones, and imipenem are active against *R. equi.*[107] Moxifloxacin is more active in vitro than is either ciprofloxacin or levofloxacin.[123] Synergy has been shown with various combinations of these agents. Including rifampin or azithromycin in a two-drug combination has been recommended because of penetrance of macrophages.[13,137] Combinations of antibiotics that included vancomycin were found to be most effective in clearing infection in a mouse model.[107] The combination of levofloxacin or ciprofloxacin and azithromycin is sometimes successfully employed. Cure rates in adults with lung infection are approximately 60% when antibiotic therapy alone is employed but may reach 75% when combined with surgical resection of infected pulmonary tissue.[64] Surgery has not been shown to increase survival rates, however.[8]

Pediatric patients generally have fared better than adults, but most reported cases in children have been in non-AIDS patients.[13] Relapse is a common occurrence, but the optimal duration of therapy to prevent relapse is unknown. For patients with AIDS, some authors recommend a minimum of 2 months of therapy followed by long-term suppressive therapy.[73] Relapse has been reported to occur at extrapulmonary sites in 13% of immunocompromised patients,[157] often without reappearance of pulmonary disease. Treatment of *R. equi* peritonitis in patients receiving peritoneal dialysis has been reported to be successful with intraperitoneal imipenem or vancomycin for 14 days.[20,147] Removal of the peritoneal dialysis catheter may be required for cure.

NEW REFERENCES SINCE THE SEVENTH EDITION

45. Feced Olmos CM, Alegre Sancho JJ, Ivorra Cortex J, Roman Ivorra JA. Septic arthritis of the shoulder due to Corynebacterium striatum. *Reumatol Clin.* 2013;9:383.
74. Kalra MG, Higgins KE, Kinney BS. Intertrigo and secondary skin infections. *Am Fam Physician.* 2014;89:569-573.
86. Liu XL, Peng H, Mo TT, Liang Y. Malignant otitis externa in a healthy non-diabetic patient. *Eur Arch Otorhinolaryngol.* 2016;273(8):2261-2265.
98. McElvania TeKippe E, Thomas BS, Ewald GA, Lawrence SJ, Burnham CA. Rapid emergence of daptomycin resistance in clinical isolates of Corynebacterium striatum…a cautionary tale. *Eur J Clin Microbiol Infect Dis.* 2014;33:2199-2205.
117. Ramanan P, Deziel PJ, Razonable RR. Rhodococcus globerulus bacteremia in an allogeneic hematopoietic stem cell transplant recipient: report of the first transplant case and review of the literature. *Transpl Infect Dis.* 2014;16:484-489.
118. Remuzzo-Martinez S, Pilares-Ortega L, Alvarez-Rodriguez L, et al. Induction of proinflammatory cytokines in human lung epithelial cells during Rhodococcus equi infection. *J Med Microbiol.* 2013;62:1144-1152.
127. Salipante SJ, Sengupta DJ, Cummings LA, et al. Whole genome sequencing indicates Corynebacterium jeikeium comprises 4 separate genomospecies and identifies a dominant genomospecies among clinical isolates. *Int J Med Microbiol.* 2014;304:1001-1010.
134. Sekizuka T, Yamamoto A, Komiya T, et al. Corynebacterium ulcerans 0102 carries the gene encoding diphtheria toxin on a prophage different from the C. diphtheriae NCTC 13129 prophage. *BMC Microbiol.* 2012;12:72.
136. Sing A, Berger A, Schneider-Brachert W, Holzmann T, Reischl U. Rapid detection and molecular differentiation of toxigenic Corynebacterium diphtheriae and Corynebacterium ulcerans stains by Lightcycler PCR. *J Clin Microbiol.* 2011;49:2485-2489.
151. Tran TT, Jaijakul S, Lewis CT, et al. Native valve endocarditis caused by Corynebacterium striatum with heterogeneous high-level daptomycin resistance: collateral damage from daptomycin therapy? *Antimicrob Agents Chemother.* 2012;56:3461-3464.
155. Vasquez-Boland JA, Giguere S, Hapeshi A, et al. Rhodococcus equi: the many facets of a pathogenic actinomycete. *Vet Microbiol.* 2013;167:9-33.
156. Verma R, Kravitz GR, Westblade LF, et al. Septic arthritis of a native knee joint due to Corynebacterium striatum. *J Clin Microbiol.* 2014;52:1786-1788.
162. Werth BJ, Hahn WO, Butler-Wu SM, Rakita RM. Emergence of high-level daptomycin resistance in Corynebacterium striatum in two patients with left ventricular assist device infections. *Microb Drug Resist.* 2016;22:233-237.

The full reference list for this chapter is available at ExpertConsult.com.

SUBSECTION IV Gram-Negative Bacilli

101 *Citrobacter*

Lawrence A. Ross • Randall G. Fisher

Citrobacter, a genus of enteric gram-negative rods closely related to *Salmonella,* has been increasingly associated with human disease. Although *Citrobacter* strains usually are not considered normal inhabitants of the intestinal tract of humans and animals,[69,119] a study using 16S rDNA polymerase chain reaction (PCR) showed that normal newborns are colonized with these organisms by day 6 of life.[79] The impact of perinatal factors, such as Caesarean section, upon intestinal colonization with *Enterobactereaciae,* including *Citrobacter species,* is of growing interest.[105] *Citrobacter* species are associated with a broad spectrum of clinical diseases, including urinary tract infections,[9,31,50,61,64,69] osteomyelitis,[64] diarrhea,[25,38,122] and invasive disease in the immunocompromised host.[46,50,64,69] Further, *Citrobacter* species are identified as emerging nosocomial pathogens,[5] including potential acquisition from contaminated transfusion products.[44,26] As detailed in a review by Doran,[23] *Citrobacter* commonly is associated with sepsis, meningitis, and brain abscess in neonates.

BACTERIOLOGY

In 1931, Werkman and Gillen[119] proposed the generic term *Citrobacter* for citrate-positive coli-aerogenes intermediates isolated from stool. This genus now includes 11 species, of which the most commonly identified are *Citrobacter freundii, Citrobacter koseri* (formerly *Citrobacter diversus*), and *Citrobacter farmeri* (formerly *Citrobacter amalonaticus*).[10] Additional species are likely to be identified using advanced analytic methodology.[18] *Citrobacter rodentium* induces inflammatory colitis in laboratory animals that is similar to that induced by pathogenic strains of *Escherichea coli.* Such research models have been useful for delineation of the pathogenesis of microbial-mediated colonic inflammation.[20] *Citrobacter* are straight, facultatively anaerobic bacilli possessing peritrichous flagellae that confer motility. In addition to using citrate, these organisms hydrolyze urea and ferment glucose, with production of gas.[102] They grow on ordinary media as gray, opaque, round colonies that produce a strong, fetid odor. In contrast to *Salmonella, Citrobacter* grows in the presence of potassium cyanide. Indole-negative strains that produce hydrogen sulfide are classified as *C. freundii*. Indole-positive, hydrogen sulfide–negative strains are differentiated by their ability to ferment malonate; *C. koseri* ferments malonate, whereas *C. farmeri* does not.[3] Antigenic schemata have been developed to classify the O somatic antigens of *Citrobacter*[33,37,122]; these antigens show cross reactivity with O antigens of other *Enterobacteriaceae*.

EPIDEMIOLOGY

Meningitis caused by *Citrobacter* was reported first in 1960, with two cases of *C. freundii*.[42] In the decade from 1970 to 1979, 69 cases of *Citrobacter* meningitis were reported,[34] and 4% of neonatal meningitis cases reported in the First Neonatal Meningitis Cooperative Study Group were caused by *Citrobacter*.[74] *C. koseri* is the species usually isolated with meningitis; central nervous system infection caused by *C. freundii* occurs less commonly.[23,34,92] Most cases in the United States are reported from southern states; biotype d or serotypes O2 and O1[34] are the most common isolates of *C. koseri* encountered.

Most cases of neonatal meningitis caused by this organism have been sporadic. The source of sporadic cases usually is unknown, but nine cases clearly have been documented to be vertically transmitted from mother to infant.[23] In addition, several well-documented nosocomial outbreaks of infection have been reported.[27,31,33,63,80,91,122] The source usually is the gastrointestinal tract or hands of nursery staff. One cluster was associated with contaminated formula.[112] When *Citrobacter* is introduced into the neonatal nursery, colonization may exceed 79%.[33] Parry and associates[80] described a nursery outbreak in which 11 of 128 infants were colonized with *C. koseri* over an observation period of 3 months; two of the colonized infants developed meningitis. Additional colonization of neonates seemed to be eliminated by removal of a nurse with persistent hand carriage of the organism.

In another outbreak,[122] introduction of *C. koseri* into the nursery was linked to an infant admitted with meningitis. Thirty-one percent of infants in the nursery subsequent to the index case were found to be colonized with *C. koseri* of the same serotype and biotype. A second infant from this study developed meningitis with the organism during the observation period. Umbilical colonization of infants in this cluster was more common than was rectal colonization, but rectal colonization was more persistent, lasting 4 months. Two nurses were found to have hand colonization with the organism, and the reintroduction of these bacteria into the nursery was linked to a pregnant nurse who had perineal cultures at delivery yielding the epidemic strain. She was implicated in the colonization of her own infant and three other neonates. Corresponding culture data from a reference hospital revealed an overall neonatal colonization rate with *Citrobacter* of 1% to 10% over a 5-year period, with no invasive disease. Of interest, a research study performed in very-low-birth-weight infants administered human recombinant lactoferrin developed altered fecal microbiomes, including increased colonization with *Citrobacter*; the relevance of this observation is unclear.[100]

Although *Citrobacter* has been isolated increasingly from debilitated adult patients,[120,97] particularly as a urinary tract,[50,64,69,89] soft tissue,[24,64,69] and bone[69] pathogen, *Citrobacter* infection in children is unusual after the first 2 months of life. One case of meningitis was reported in a teenager who lacked apparent risk factors or immunodeficiency.[87] In older children, *Citrobacter* spp. are more likely to cause opportunistic infections in immunocompromised hosts, including a recent association of *C. freundii* infections in patients with heterotaxy syndrome.[15] *Citrobacter* are established etiologic agents of urinary tract infections in pediatric patients; one study showed *Citrobacter* spp. to be responsible for 37 (1.4%) urinary tract infections in children over a 3-year period.[29] One-quarter of infections were nosocomially acquired, and one-third occurred in children with urinary tract abnormalities. A more recent study from Kosovo of 299 children with urinary tract infections found that *Citrobacter* spp. caused 5.4% of cases, making it the fourth most common cause.[104]

PATHOPHYSIOLOGY

Citrobacter infrequently colonizes the intestinal tract and perineum of humans.[50] Vertical transmission of strains shown to be identical by DNA typing shows that the newborn can acquire colonization at the time of passage through the birth canal of a colonized mother.[43,78] Onset of disease beyond the first week of life is related commonly to colonization of the infant in the nursery. As with other types of gram-negative neonatal meningitis, central nervous system infection results from bacteremia in a colonized infant, leading to seeding of the meninges.

The basis for the particular invasiveness of *Citrobacter* in the neonate and its propensity to cause multiple brain abscesses are largely unexplained. *Citrobacter* spp. possess the ability to invade, transcytose, and multiply within human brain microvascular endothelial cells in vitro.[6] Additionally, in the neonatal rat model, after being taken up into macrophages, *C. koseri* is able to survive phagolysosomal fusion and replicate therein.[113] Many strains of *C. koseri* seem to be able to produce brain pathologic processes in the mouse, but the degree of damage seems to be related to virulence of the strain and the age of the mouse.[57,103] Differences in strains, related to the presence of an outer-membrane protein with a molecular weight of 32,000 kDa, have been associated with differences in brain histopathology in one infant rat model of *C. koseri* meningitis.[56] Strains isolated from cerebrospinal fluid of infants with meningitis more commonly possess this outer-membrane protein than do strains isolated from other body sites.[57] In the mouse model, early proinflammatory mediator release was dependent on MyDD88 (a signaling adapter of Toll-like receptor 4 [TL4]). MyDD88 knockout mice had enhanced mortality and elevated bacterial burdens versus wild-type mice.[65] In vitro, microglial cells respond with inflammation via TL4 and MyDD88.[66]

In an immunocompromised patient, broad use of antimicrobial agents may produce selective pressure, leading to increased colonization with *Citrobacter*. Increased bacterial density combined with a blunted immune response may result in invasive disease. Some strains of *C. freundii* produce Shiga toxins (verotoxins) nearly identical to those produced by enterohemorrhagic strains of *Escherichia coli*.[98] At least one outbreak of gastroenteritis and the hemolytic-uremic syndrome caused by Shiga toxin–producing *C. freundii* has been reported.[115] Investigation of pathogenesis and molecular correlates of colitis in murine models using *C. rodentium* have clarified the basis for intestinal defense and response to infection.[95]

Citrobacter spp. contain type 3 fimbriae, which are vital to the production of biofilms.[77] The formation of biofilms in *Citrobacter* isolates is important in the pathogenesis of catheter-associated urinary tract infections.[77]

CLINICAL MANIFESTATIONS

Citrobacter, similar to other neonatal pathogens, can cause early-onset and late-onset infection. In a review of 74 cases of neonatal meningitis caused by these bacteria, the mean age of onset reported for early disease was 7 days; 85% of patients were included in this group.[34] Fifteen percent of cases occurred after 3 weeks of age. Twenty-three (31%) of 74 patients were younger than 36 weeks of gestational age at birth, suggesting that preterm infants are at increased risk for acquisition of *Citrobacter* infection. Prematurity is even more common (71%) in cases that are proved to be vertically acquired.[23]

Clinical signs and symptoms are typical of neonatal sepsis. Fever, lethargy, poor feeding, vomiting, irritability, bulging fontanelle, seizures, and jaundice are common presenting features. Umbilical infection and surgical manipulation of colonized umbilical stumps occasionally have preceded development of bacteremia and meningitis.[80] The white blood cell count may show leukocytosis or leukopenia. Cerebrospinal fluid findings are consistent with those of most types of neonatal bacterial meningitis and usually show polymorphonuclear cell elevation, elevated protein, and depressed glucose; gram-negative rods may be seen on smear. Although growing the organism in culture normally is not difficult, in one reported case standard cultures were negative, but the organism was recovered by direct inoculation of cerebrospinal fluid into a BACTEC blood culture bottle.[19] Of *Citrobacter* meningitis cases in which the results of blood cultures are reported, 80% document concurrent bacteremia.[23]

Citrobacter is a particularly devastating cause of neonatal meningitis. The most common *Citrobacter* spp. causing neonatal meningitis is *C. koseri,* which accounts for more than 80% of the cases.[23] Central nervous system infection with this organism produces multiple brain abscesses with unusually high frequency.[34,40,51,57,62] In the extensive reviews by Graham and Band[34] and by Doran,[23] three-quarters of *Citrobacter* meningitis cases resulted in intracerebral abscesses. By comparison, the incidence of abscess formation in non-*Citrobacter* gram-negative meningitis is reported to be as low as 10%.[34] The case-fatality rate for *Citrobacter* meningitis is approximately 30%, and at least three-quarters of surviving infants have neurologic sequelae, such as mental retardation, hemiparesis, seizures, and developmental delay.[23]

The presence of brain abscess seems to contribute substantially to morbidity and mortality[21,33,34]; however, a favorable outcome may be observed.[1] For unknown reasons, neonates with vertically acquired *Citrobacter* meningitis seem to be less likely to develop intracerebral abscesses.[23] At least four cases in which diffuse pneumocephalus developed in association with *Citrobacter* meningitis have been reported; in one, gas was noted to accumulate within the brain and in the anterior chamber of the eye, a condition known as *pneumatosis oculi.*[2,85,99] Rarely, *Citrobacter* infection in the neonatal period may lead to focal infection not involving the central nervous system. A case of septic arthritis and osteomyelitis of the shoulder in a 3-week-old infant has been reported.[45]

In adults, *Citrobacter* is isolated most commonly from the urinary tract.[50,64,69,89] In earlier studies, 5% to 12% of bacterial isolates from urinary tract infections in adult patients were *Citrobacter.*[25,121] More recently, in a health maintenance organization, *Citrobacter* spp. accounted for only 0.8% of 4342 isolates from women with acute uncomplicated cystitis.[39] *Citrobacter* spp. are a similarly uncommon cause of urinary tract infection in children.[29] Sputum is the second most common clinical specimen to yield *Citrobacter* in adults[50]; lung abscess,[30] pneumonia,[64,69] bronchitis,[46] and septic arthritis[64] have been reported. *Citrobacter* is an occasional cause of bacteremia in hospitalized patients, accounting for approximately 0.5% of blood culture isolates.[83,101] In one series, all 45 patients had at least one underlying disease, with malignancies (particularly intraabdominal tumors) and hepatobiliary stones being the most frequent coexisting conditions.[101] Polymicrobial bacteremia occurred in one-third of patients. Bacteremia with *Citrobacter* has been observed in a recipient of haematopoietic stem cell transplantation with fever and neutropenia.[117] In a series of six bacteremic patients who had *Citrobacter* species other than *freundii* or *koseri,* five of the six had associated intraabdominal infection; cancer and cirrhosis were the most common underlying diseases.[60]

A broad spectrum of organ-specific infections caused by *Citrobacter* have been reported; these include liver abscess,[58] infective endocarditis,[90] spinal epidural abscess,[59] folliculitis,[88] and sinus disease complicated by orbital extension.[68]

Gastrointestinal disease occasionally has been attributed to *Citrobacter*, but frequent isolation of this agent from normal stools often renders this diagnosis equivocal. This genus was implicated first in an outbreak of mild gastroenteritis by Barnes and Cherry[8] in 1946, and an outbreak of watery diarrhea in a Virginia infant care unit included two infants in whom isolates of enterotoxin-liberating *Citrobacter* were obtained from the stool.[38] Some studies have found higher incidences of *Citrobacter* isolation from the stool of patients with enterocolitis syndrome than from stools of control patients.[122] Shiga-toxin (verotoxin)-producing *C. freundii* isolated from organically grown parsley was associated with an outbreak of diarrhea and hemolytic-uremic syndrome in a daycare setting.[115] *C. freundii* has been found as a cause of appendicitis in a healthy adult,[64] peritonitis in adults with liver disease or pancreatitis,[64] neutropenic colitis after chemotherapy for breast cancer,[17] and meningitis in adults as a complication of neurosurgery.[111] A case of Meleney gangrene occurring after cesarean section delivery has been reported.[110]

A patient with diabetes developed necrotizing fasciitis caused by *C. freundii* associated with injury from a fish fin.[16] Bone and soft tissue infections occur[11,35,106]; 3% of *Citrobacter* pathogens were isolated from joint or bone in one adult series.[64] One 53-year-old man developed infection 3 weeks after total hip arthroplasty, a condition normally expected to be caused by *S. aureus.*[52] Eye infections, including keratitis,[32] traumatic endophthalmitis,[12,94] and endogenous endophthalmitis[14] have been reported. *Citrobacter* has been identified as a pathogen in patients with dacryocystitis.[4] A case of *C. freundii* pharyngitis complicated by retropharyngeal abscess and mediastinitis was cured by minimally invasive surgery and intravenous antibiotics.[114]

DIAGNOSIS

Biochemical characteristics of *C. koseri* include lack of hydrogen sulfide production on triple-sugar iron agar, negative Voges-Proskauer reaction, use of citrate, motility, production of indole, decarboxylation of ornithine but not lysine, and production of acid from adonitol.[3] Identification of this organism as a pathogen in a nursery setting should heighten suspicion of its possible role in subsequent neonatal infections. *C. freundii* is indole negative and hydrogen sulfide positive, which differentiates it from *C. koseri. C. farmeri* differs from *C. koseri* because of the former's inability to ferment malonate. *C. freundii* and *C. farmeri* account for a significant portion of disease caused by *Citrobacter* in immunocompromised individuals and should be suspected particularly in this group of patients.[46] In some cases, *C. freundii* can be misidentified as *Cronobacter* spp. by commercial systems.[28]

Infants with invasive *Citrobacter* disease present in a similar fashion to infants with sepsis and meningitis of other causes. Such infants should undergo a thorough evaluation, including blood and urine culture and cerebrospinal fluid studies. Emerging laboratory methods have facilitated more rapid identification of gram-negative isolates, as well as identifying the presence of antimicrobial-resistance factors.[107] Brain imaging studies should be obtained and when indicated, sequentially followed when the diagnosis of meningitis is established. Magnetic resonance imaging (MRI) is the most sensitive diagnostic tool for early identification of cerebritis and early abscess formation; however, computed tomography is the most common imaging evaluation performed. Ultrasound often is more feasible for an unstable neonate and may be nearly as sensitive in detecting abscesses.[62,75,123] Serial imaging studies should be done because abscesses may develop during the first few weeks of illness. In cases in which the cerebrospinal fluid cultures are negative because of prior antimicrobial therapy, surgical aspiration of abscesses sometimes enables identification of the organism.

TREATMENT

As with other species of *Enterobacteriaciae,* effective antimicrobial therapy for *Citrobacter* is challenged by the continuing worldwide emergence of a broad array of β-lactamases, including metallo-β-lactamases (MBL).[53] Many different types of β-lactamases, including a novel TEM-type (TEM-134),[81] the class A β-lactamase CKO,[82] and a VIM-1 metallo-β-lactamase, have been described in various isolates of *Citrobacter.*[118] Most *C. koseri* organisms are resistant to ampicillin (97% in one series)[64] and susceptible to aminoglycosides and third-generation cephalosporins.[23] A 4-year experience with neonatal septicemia caused by *C. koseri* has been described, however, in which all of 13 isolates were resistant to gentamicin but susceptible to third-generation cephalosporins.[27] The resistance patterns of *C. freundii* were reported in a national surveillance study of nosocomial bloodstream infections.[83] Of the 23 *C. freundii* isolates tested, resistance to piperacillin, piperacillin/tazobactam, ceftriaxone, and ceftazidime was a common (39% to 48%) finding. Isolates generally were susceptible to the aminoglycosides and ciprofloxacin (91% to 96%), and all *C. freundii* tested were susceptible to cefepime and imipenem.

The growing challenge of antimicrobial resistance amongst *Citrobacter* sp. is exemplified by a study performed in a tertiary care facility in India of bacterial isolates identified from 2010 to 2013.[86] Of 221 *Citrobacter* isolates, 179 (81%) were found to have diminished susceptibility to carbapenems. These resistant isolates were capable of elaborating extended-spectrum-β-lactamases as well as MBLtransferable on plasmids. Additional reports have confirmed the presence of *Klebsiella pneumoniae*

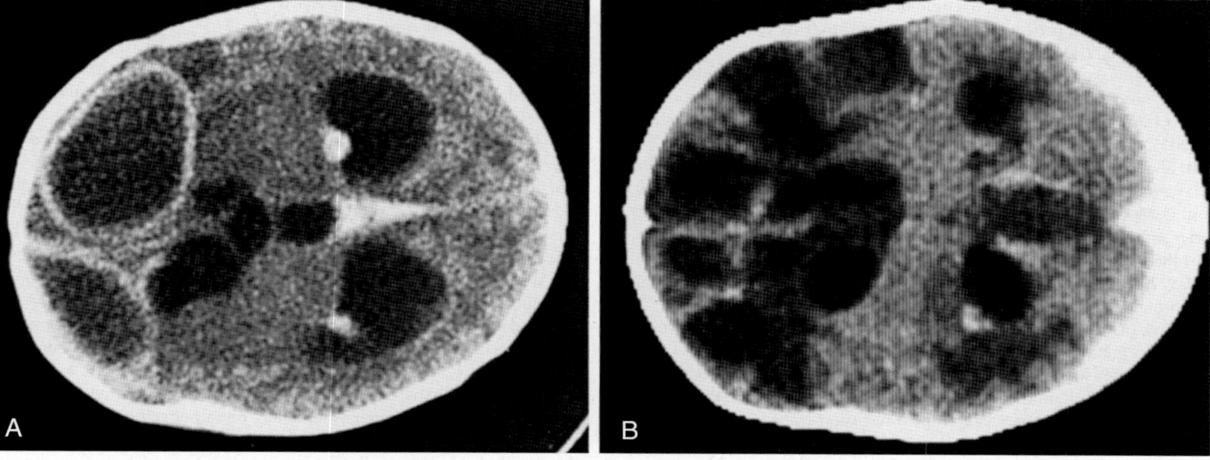

FIG. 101.1 Computed tomography scans showing progressive abscess formation and encephalomalacia in an infant (A) at 3 weeks of age and (B) 6 weeks of age, despite bacteriologic cure of *Citrobacter* meningitis.

carbapenemase-2 (KPC-2) from *Citrobacter* isolates.[13,71] Some *Citrobacter* isolates contain chromosomally mediated group I β-lactamases. These bacteria possess a gene that, when triggered by exposure to cephalosporins or by spontaneous mutation, produces a cephalosporinase capable of inactivating cephalosporins.[47] Clinically, it manifests as treatment failure and emergence of drug resistance to various cephalosporins despite initial susceptibility.[70] In one study, the presence of group I β-lactamases was much more common with *C. freundii* (9 of 22 isolates) than with *C. koseri* (0 of 7 isolates).[47] Resistance was associated with previous receipt of an extended-spectrum β-lactam antibiotic. Reliable estimates of the percentage of *Citrobacter* strains that contain the chromosomal resistance gene are difficult to obtain because most studies lump *Citrobacter, Enterobacter,* and *Serratia* isolates together. In one Korean study, of 152 *Enterobacter/Citrobacter/Serratia* isolates, 45 (30%) were derepressed Amp C mutants.[79] In an in vitro study, Amp C production was inducible in eight of nine clinical isolates of *C. freundii* and in one of three isolates of *C. koseri*. Amp C synthesis was stably derepressed in 1/9 *C. freundii* isolates.[24] In contrast, an investigation from Johns Hopkins University Hospital of isolates collected in 2010 detected Amp C β-lactamases in only 1% of *Citrobacter* spp.[1,109] Cefepime seems to be less likely to induce production of these β-lactamases and more resistant to hydrolysis by them,[96,109] although a highly cefepime-resistant strain has been described.[7] Of 3030 ceftazidime-resistant Enterobacteriaceae in a US study, 99% retained susceptibility to imipenem and 96.7% of ceftazidime-resistant *Citrobacter* isolates were susceptible to cefepime.[84] Quinolone resistance via *qnr* genes has also been found in *C. koseri*[49]; in one study from Korea, 29% of *C. freundii* isolates were quinolone resistant. Most of these had *qnrB* genes.[48] Extensively resistant isolates are more likely to be susceptible to colistin[67] and polymyxin B[124] than to tigecycline; however there is a paucity of experience in the use of these antimicrobials for treatment of *Citrobacter* infections.

Treatment of *Citrobacter* meningitis often requires a multidisciplinary effort involving the neurosurgeon and the pediatrician. Although cerebral abscesses usually are aspirated or drained surgically, some patients are treated with antibiotics alone, and neither approach is clearly shown to be superior. When abscesses are inaccessible or small and not progressive, conservative management may be considered.[23] Ventriculostomy and craniectomy with open drainage of abscesses have been required in some children to effect bacteriologic cure, and placement of a shunt for hydrocephalus often is required.

Generally, antimicrobial therapy for gram-negative neonatal meningitis has proved disappointing (see Chapter 66).[72,73] While no evidence supports one combination of antimicrobials over another in the treatment of *Citrobacter* meningitis, initial therapy usually combines a third- or fourth-generation cephalosporin or carbapenem (usually meropenem) with an aminoglycoside.[23] Careful evaluation of pharmacodynamic and pharmacologic data has led to a recent recommendation to consider meropenem as the preferred antimicrobial for therapy of *C.koseri* infections.[22] Chloramphenicol,[21,33,41] imipenem-cilastatin,[25,41] and trimethoprim-sulfamethoxazole[36] also have been used successfully.

Poor meningeal penetration of aminoglycosides in addition to the presence of intracranial abscesses render antibiotic therapy for *Citrobacter* meningitis especially difficult. The ability of this organism to persist in the brain is shown by its recovery 4 years after neonatal infection.[25] Cranial computed tomography usually is used for evaluation of complications such as hydrocephalus and multicystic encephalomalacia (Fig. 101.1). Administration of antibiotics intrathecally or directly into abscess cavities has been tried but has not been shown convincingly to be beneficial.[36,37,40,55,63,76,93,108,116] In a randomized controlled trial, intraventricular administration of gentamicin in the treatment of neonates with gram-negative meningitis was associated with a poorer outcome.[74]

Neonates with gram-negative meningitis should undergo repeat lumbar puncture approximately 72 hours after beginning therapy to document sterilization of cerebrospinal fluid. Duration of therapy with intravenous antibiotics generally is a minimum of 21 days for gram-negative neonatal meningitis. For cases complicated by intracranial abscesses, prolonged therapy (usually 4 to 6 weeks after sterilization of cerebrospinal fluid) is indicated.[23,54]

Scrupulous attention to preventive infection control practices has been recommended to stem nursery outbreaks.[33,80,122] These prophylactic measures include care of skin and the umbilical cord, elimination of crowding with isolation of infected infants and carriers, and good hand washing practices. Exclusion of colonized personnel and temporary closing of the nursery have been followed by a reduction in neonatal *C. koseri* colonization. Although cohorting of colonized infants is a reasonable practice, multiple sources of introduction of *Citrobacter* may limit the efficacy of this approach in some outbreaks.[31]

Treatment of *Citrobacter* infection beyond the neonatal period requires choice of an appropriate antimicrobial, with drainage of abscesses and débridement of wounds. Therapy should be guided by antimicrobial susceptibility testing. Outcome depends largely on the preceding debility of the host and location of the infection. Significant mortality is associated with immunocompromised patients with septicemia or pulmonary disease.[46,50,64,69,101]

Acknowledgments

We thank Dr. William Gruber and Dr. Thomas Boyce for their invaluable assistance with earlier versions of this chapter.

NEW REFERENCES SINCE THE SEVENTH EDITION

1. Algubaisi S, Buhrer C, Ulrich-Wilhelm T, Spors B. Favorable outcome in cerebral abscesses by *Citrobacteer koseri* in a newborn infant. *IDCases*. 2015;2:22-24.

4. Assefa Y, Moger F, Endris M, et al. Bacteriologic profile and drug susceptibility patterns in dacryocystitis patients attending Gondar University Teaching Hospital, Northwest Ethiopia. *BMC Ophthalmol.* 2015;15:34.
5. Avinash G, Sreenivasulu RP, Jithendhara K, et al. Significance of Citrobacter as an emerging nosocomial pathogen with special reference to its antibiotic susceptibility pattern in a tertiary care hospital Nellore, AP India. *Int J Curr Microbiol App Sci.* 2015;4:841-847.
15. Chiu SM, Shao PL, Wang JK, et al. Severe bacterial infections in patients with heterotaxy syndrome. *J Pediatr.* 2014;164:99-104.
18. Clermont D, Motreff L, Passet V, et al. Multilocus sequence analysis of the genus *Citrobacter* and description of *Citrobacter pasteurii sp.nov. Int J Syst Evol Microbiol.* 2015;65:1486-1490.
20. Collins JW, Keeney KM, Crepin VF, et al. *Citrobacter rodentium*: infection, inflammation and the microbiota. *Nat Rev Microbiol.* 2014;12:612-623.
22. Deveci A, Caban AY. Optimum management of *Citrobacter koseri* infection. *Expert Rev Anti Infect Ther.* 2014;12:1137-1142.
26. Fernandes C, Oliveira MC, Jorge MT. A case report of *Citrobacter koseri* bacteremia after transfusion of contaminated red cells. *Transfus Med.* 2012;22:450-451.
44. Hauser L, Menasie S, Bonacorsi S, et al. Fatal transfusion-transmitted *Citrobacter koseri. Transfusion.* 2016;56(6):1311-1313.
53. Kazmierzak KM, Rabine S, Hackel M, et al. Multiyear, multinational survey of the incidence and global distribution of Metallo-beta-lactamase-producing *Enterobacteriaceae* and *P. aeruginosa. Antimicrob Agents Chemother.* 2015;60:1067-1078.
58. Kumar P, Ghosh S, Deepak R, Gadpayle AG. Multidrug resistant Citrobacter: an unusual cause of liver abscess. *BMJ Case Rep.* 2013;2013.
59. Kumar A, Jain P, Singh P, Diuthane R, Badole CM. *Citrobacter koseri* spinal epidural abscess: a rare occurrence. *J Indian Med Assoc.* 2013;111:67-68.
68. Lovato A, De Filippes C. Acute rhinosinusitis and intraorbital abscess caused by *Citrobacter koseri* infection. *Epidemiol Infect.* 2016;144(12):2670-2671.
86. Praharaj AK, Khajuria A, Kumar M, Grover N. Phenotypic detection and molecular characterization of beta-lactamase genes among *Citrobacter species* in a tertiary care hospital. *Avicanna J Med.* 2016;6:17-27.
88. Raia DD, Barbareschi M, Veraldi S. *Citrobacter koseri* folliculitis of the face. *Infection.* 2015;43:595-597.
89. Ranjan KD, Ranjan N. *Citrobacter*: an emerging health care associated urinary pathogen. *Urol Ann.* 2013;5:313-314.
90. Raval J, Nagaraja V, Poojara L, et al. *Citrobacter koseri* native valve endocarditis: a case report and review of the literature. *J Indian Coll Cardiol.* 2014;4:246-248.
92. Rodrigues J, Rocha D, Santos F, Joao A. Neonatal Citrobacter *koseri* meningitis: report of 4 cases. *Case Rep Pediatr.* 2014;2014:195204.
94. Roy R, Pradeepkumar P, Malathi J, et al. Endophthalmitis caused by *Citrobacter species*: a case series. *Can J Ophthalmol.* 2013;48:216-217.
95. Ryz NR, Lochner A, Bhullar K, et al. Dietary vitamin D3 deficiency alters intestinal mucosal defense and increases susceptibility to *Citrobacter rodentium*-induced colitis. *Am J Physiol Gastrointest Liver Physiol.* 2015;309(9):G730-G742.
97. Samonis G, Karageorgopoulos DE, Kofteridis DP, et al. *Citrobacter* infections in a general hospital: characteristics and outcomes. *Eur J Clin Microbiol Infect Dis.* 2009;28:61-68.
99. Shenoi AN, Shane AL, Fostenberry JD, et al. Spontaneous pneumocephalus in vertically acquired, late-onset neonatal *Citrobacter* meningitis. *J Pediatr.* 2013;163:1791.
100. Sherman MP, Sherman J, Arcinue R, Niklas V. Randomized control trial of human recombinant lactoferrin: a substudy reveals effects on the fecal microbiome of very low birth weight infants. *J Pediatr.* 2016;173S:S37-S42.
105. Stokholm J, Thorsen J, Chaives BL, et al. Caesarian section changes neonatal gut colonization. *J Allergy Clin Immunol.* 2016;138(3):881-889.
107. Sullivan KV, Debarger B, Roundtree SS, et al. Pediatric multicenter evaluation of the Verigene gram-negative blood culture test for rapid detection of inpatient bacteremia involving gram-negative organisms, extended-spectrum beta-lactamases and carbapenemases. *J Clin Microbiol.* 2014;52:2416-2421.
109. Tamma PD, Girdwood SC, Goparel R, et al. The use of cefepime for treating AmpC beta-lactamase-producing *Enterobacteriaceae. Clin Infect Dis.* 2013;57:781-788.
117. Wang L, Wang F, Fan X, et al. Prevalence of resistant gram-negative bacilli in bloodstream infections in febrile neutropenia patients undergoing Hematopoietic Stem Cell Transplantation: a single center retrospective cohort study. *Medicine (Baltimore).* 2015;94:e1931.

The full reference list for this chapter is available at ExpertConsult.com.

102 Enterobacter

Laura A. Sass • Randall G. Fisher

Enterobacter is a genus of Enterobacteriaceae that is an increasingly frequent cause of health care–associated pediatric infection. *Enterobacter* can cause infection of postsurgical wounds, meningitis, and infection of the gastrointestinal, urinary, and respiratory tracts. Development of resistance to antibiotics commonly used for treatment of infection is an increasingly common challenge. For a more detailed overview of *Enterobacter* spp., the reader is referred to the review by Sanders and Sanders.[187]

BACTERIOLOGY

Enterobacter spp. are named for their enteric recovery as gram-negative bacteria.[181] They commonly are found in soil, water, and sewage. More reports are appearing of resistant species found in the community, often in hospital wastewater.[213,227] *Enterobacter* spp. also cause botanical disease. These organisms are facultatively anaerobic and motile by peritrichous flagella, with the exception of *E. asburiae*. Most species yield positive results on malonate, citrate, sucrose fermentation, and Voges-Proskauer tests. *Cronobacter sakazakii* (formerly known as *E. sakazakii*) is distinguishable from the other species by its yellow-pigmented colonies.[94] There are now at least seven species included in the *Cronobacter* genus, with *C. sakazakii* remaining the predominant human pathogen.[59,215] Taxonomic studies have led to several classifications of species contained in this genus. With the reclassification of *E. agglomerans* as *Pantoea agglomerans* (see Chapter 114), *E. cloacae, E. hormaechei,* and *E. aerogenes* are the most common species recovered from clinical material.[8,18,34,37,53,66,96,139,221,223]

Additional species in the *Enterobacter* genus rarely recovered from human infections include, *E. asburiae, E. cancerogenus* (formerly *E. taylorae*), *E. kobei*,[111] *E. cloacae* subsp. *dissolvens, E. massiliensis*,[116] *E. bugandensis*,[49] and *E. hormaechei*.[1,39,70,88,105,137,138,151,181,226] *E. ludwigii* is another new species isolated from clinical specimens that is closely related to the *E. cloacae* complex.[89] Numerous former *Enterobacter* species have been reclassified into new genera including *E. cowanii* as *Kosakonia cowanii, E. intermedius* as *Kluyvera intermedia* (formerly *Kluyvera cochleae*),[162] *E. amnigenus* and *E. nimipressuralis* as *Lelliottia amnigenus* and *L. nimipressuralis*, as well as *E. gergoviae* as *Pluralibacter gergoviae*.[24,154]

EPIDEMIOLOGY

Enterobacter is encountered most commonly as a hospital-acquired pathogen in patients with chronic illness.[8,18,37,53,96,221,223,231] A surveillance study at 50 American medical centers showed *Enterobacter* as the eighth most common cause of health care–associated bloodstream infections, accounting for 230 of 4725 (5%) isolates.[169] Of these, 71% were *E. cloacae*, 23% were *E. aerogenes*, and 6% were other species of *Enterobacter*. *Enterobacter* infections are particularly common in intensive care units (ICUs).[141] A report from the Centers for Disease Control and Prevention (CDC) describing the epidemiology of health care–associated infections in 61 pediatric ICUs in the United States revealed that *Enterobacter* spp. were isolated with increasing frequency from patients with pneumonia and were the most common gram-negative isolates from bloodstream infections.[96] The frequency of *Enterobacter* spp. increased from 7% to

12% of reported pathogens over a 6-year period. *Enterobacter* spp. also accounted for 6% of health care–associated blood stream infections in a prospective collection of surveillance data from an Australian public hospital system[194] and were found to cause 22% of the neonatal gram-negative infections from neonatal ICUs (NICUs) in the UK.[104] *Enterobacter* spp. also were found to be second only to *Pseudomonas aeruginosa* in prevalence in health care–associated sinusitis.[182]

In other CDC surveys focusing on data from the National Healthcare Safety Network (NHSN), *Enterobacter* was one of the five pathogens most commonly encountered in ICUs and accounted for 5.0% to 8.6% of reported health care–associated infections.[85,96] In one large academic hospital, the relative proportion of *Enterobacter* spp. in health care–associated infections had decreased as a result of an increase in gram-positive and anaerobic infections.[101] During a 10-year period in six Brazilian NICUs, gram-negative pathogens accounted for more than half of all bloodstream infections, with *Enterobacter* spp. representing 2%.[41] In Canada, similar results were found in a nationwide surveillance program, with *E. cloacae* found in 2.2% of all health care–associated infections, including blood, wound, and urine sources.[238] Multiple outbreaks caused by *Enterobacter* have been described in neonatal ICUs.[71,86,186] *E. cloacae* has been found in some NICUs as the predominant pathogen, representing almost 40% of bloodstream isolates,[130] in addition to being responsible for outbreaks of sepsis.[44] In some series, one-third of *Enterobacter* bacteremias were polymicrobial, which represents a greater prevalence than that of bacteremia caused by other gram-negative organisms.[21,66]

The most frequently cited risk factor for *Enterobacter* infection is the recent receipt of antibiotics, particularly third-generation cephalosporins.[4,7,8,17,26,66,97,218] Other risk factors include prolonged hospital stay (especially in an ICU), presence of serious underlying illness (e.g., burns, malignancy, and diabetes); prematurity in a neonate; immunosuppression; organ transplantation; and the presence of a foreign device.* Vertical spread of *Enterobacter* from mother to infant may occur at the time of birth,[64] but infant colonization is usually from an environmental source. A surveillance program in an NICU that screens for *E. cloacae* colonization determined that only 8.8% of colonized infants were the result of mother-to-child transmission.[71] Environmental sources implicated in outbreaks of infection have included intravenous fluids,[9,28,31,131,134,204,216,220,222] chronic hand dermatitis of a care provider,[12] contaminated infant formula,[10,15,30,38,150] blood gas machines,[2,115] contaminated transesophageal echocardiography probes,[99] cardioplegia ice,[25] therapeutic bed mattresses and mattress covers,[209] and rectal thermometers.[208]

Ribotyping, pulsed-field electrophoresis, and restriction-fragment polymorphism analysis of DNA from clinical isolates have been useful in discriminating possible sources of contamination and patient-to-patient transfer of individual strains.† Integrons, discrete mobile units of DNA that can confer antibiotic resistance, have been reported in *Enterobacter* spp. and are more common findings in infections acquired in a health care setting.[43] Molecular diagnostic testing has proved useful in outbreak situations, especially in tracking antibiotic-resistant strains caused by plasmid acquisition of extended-spectrum β-lactamases (ESBL).[69] Most cases are not outbreak-associated, and endogenous origin of infection is a more common means of acquisition than is the patient's environment.[169] This factor explains why recent antimicrobial use by the patient is such a strong predictor of infection.

PATHOPHYSIOLOGY

Newborns often are colonized by *Enterobacter* spp. in the gastrointestinal tract soon after birth,[14,160] and acquisition of hospital strains, including ESBL-producing strains, in immunocompromised newborns is common.[7,14,58,65,92,211] *Enterobacter* spp. may contaminate the compromised respiratory tract. The oropharynx commonly is colonized by *Enterobacter* by the time the infant is 1 month of age; colonization rates generally are lower in breast-fed infants.[11] Newborns with gastrointestinal abnormalities requiring prolonged parenteral nutrition have higher rates of colonization with *Enterobacter* and a higher incidence of sepsis.[170,171] Other risk factors for increased *Enterobacter* colonization in neonates include prematurity and prior antibiotic use.[164] Enteric organisms are recovered less frequently from the oropharynx of healthy older children and adults, but increased colonization, including increased risk for third-generation cephalosporin-resistant strains, especially with prior cephalosporin treatment of at least 3 days, is noted during illness.[225]

The ability of *Enterobacter* spp. to develop inducible resistance to penicillins and cephalosporins increases their pathogenic potential. All *Enterobacter* spp. possess an inducible chromosomally encoded class C (Bush group I) β-lactamase type cephalosporinase (*ampC*), which usually is produced in small amounts, conferring resistance to both first- and third-generation cephalosporins.[187] An inducible plasmid-encoded *ampC* (gene bla_{ACT-1}) also has been described and can be present in *Enterobacter* spp. and other Enterobacteriaceae.[184] Both enzymes have a high affinity for third-generation cephalosporins but a low maximum hydrolysis rate.[137] Consequently β-lactamase mediates resistance to these antibiotics only when it is produced in large quantities or large numbers of plasmids are present.[123,180]

Resistance emerges after a mutation occurs in the *ampD* gene, which normally prevents high-level expression of β-lactamase.[95,98] Such mutants are considered "stably derepressed" and may be induced by exposure to β-lactam antibiotics, especially ampicillin and cephalosporins. Mutations in the *ampR* gene produce similar effects.[114] The addition of a β-lactamase inhibitor (e.g., clavulanic acid) does not increase the activity of β-lactam antibiotics against *Enterobacter* spp.; rather, it may decrease the activity against the organism by inducing the class C β-lactamase, as can the presence of *ampR* mutants.[98,114,212]

Emergence of resistance can occur during therapy for an isolate that initially is shown to be susceptible.[84,187] Resistance can be detected 24 hours after initiation of therapy or may be delayed 2 to 3 weeks.[36] Reports of resistant strains of *Enterobacter* that produce plasmid-mediated, ESBL began to be published in 1993 and have persisted over time.[90,132,172] Various ESBL genes, including genes from the TEM, SHV, and CTX-M families, have been found.[29,69,159,198,237] This variation can complicate choosing antimicrobial agents because discerning the source of the β-lactam resistance in the clinical microbiology laboratory often is difficult without performing specific testing, such as the double-disk diffusion method. Newer rapid methods of identification, such as rapid biochemical tests for ESBL and carbapenemase producers, polymerase chain reaction (PCR) technology, and mass spectroscopy are becoming more prevalent in the clinical microbiology laboratory, replacing the traditional double-disk diffusion methodology.[56] A survey of 11 clinical laboratories in Germany to determine ESBL prevalence found that 40% of *E. cloacae* complex organisms were resistant to extended-spectrum cephalosporins, and only 6% carried ESBL genes.[90] This finding is in contrast to other reports with prevalences of 36% in some Asia-Pacific regions.[13] There continues to be wide variability in the prevalence of multidrug resistance throughout the world.

The global spread of carbapenemase-producing Enterobacteriaceae (CRE) has affected *Enterobacter* spp. as well as other members of the class. Infections with these multidrug-resistant organisms have been reported worldwide. Class A carbapenemases are plasmid-mediated, effectively hydrolyze carbapenems, and are partially inhibited by clavulanic acid, with one of the most common being *Klebsiella pneumoniae* carbapenemases (KPC).[149] KPC-mediated resistance in *Enterobacter* spp. has been reported.[125,190] Class B metallo-β-lactamases (MBLs) are Verona integron–encoded metallo-β-lactamase (VIM), New Delhi metallo-β-lactamase–1 (NDM-1), and *IMP* (imipenem resistance gene). VIM producers can be endemic to a certain region, but have been reported globally in outbreaks and sporadic infections.[79,83,155] These enzymes hydrolyze all β-lactam antibiotics, including carbapenems, but do not hydrolyze monobactams such as aztreonam. NDM-1 producers have also been reported worldwide and are likely endemic in India. These genes are not associated with a single clone and have varied resistance to carbapenems. Of concern is the likelihood of other antibiotic resistance genes to be included on the bla_{NDM-1} gene, including ESBL, aminoglycoside, macrolide, and rifampin resistance.[27,149] The CDC had three reports of NDM-1 isolates in 2010, one of which was *E. cloacae*. All patients had recent medical care in India as their risk factor.[33] Class D OXA-β-lactamases have also been reported in *Enterobacter* species. They

*References 3, 43, 62, 86, 93, 128, 186, 187, 200, 214, 239.
†References 16, 25, 30, 37, 38, 76, 81, 82, 118, 168, 187, 191, 210.

are serine-carbapenemases along with oxacillinases and are generally plasmid-mediated, conferring broad-spectrum resistance to cephalosporins due to point mutations in the enzyme itself.[57,61] The prevalence of CRE is increasing in the United States, especially in the adult population. A seven-region survey of the United States for CRE found an incidence of 2.93 per 100,000 population, with regional differences. Most of the cases were isolated from urine and were associated with prior hospitalizations, indwelling devices, or residence in long-term chronic care facilities.[78] The Surveillance Network-USA database reviewed antimicrobial susceptibilities of Enterobacteriaceae from 1999 to 2012, finding that 0.08% were CRE. The CRE infection rate increases were highest for *Enterobacter* spp., blood culture isolates, and isolates originating from an ICU setting. This is still a low overall rate, but it did increase 3% to 5% over the course of 12 years.[126]

In one study, gram-negative fecal aerobic flora were eradicated completely after 24 hours of ceftriaxone therapy, only to be replaced within 10 days (mean, 6.7 days) of therapy by *P. aeruginosa, Enterobacter,* and *Citrobacter* resistant to all β-lactam antibiotics.[77] Although uncommon, the combination of reduced outer-membrane permeability and high-level β-lactamase production renders some clinical isolates of *E.* resistant to carbapenems (imipenem, meropenem, and ertapenem) and fourth-generation cephalosporins (cefepime).[19,47,50,120,122,137,166,199,206]

Other than the presence of endotoxin, factors responsible for the virulence of *Enterobacter* spp. are not well defined but may include cytotoxins, type III secretion systems, altered pili, and efflux pumps.[103,113,119,156,158,167] In vitro, it is possible to transfer and express an *Escherichia coli* enterotoxigenic plasmid in *Enterobacter,* implying the potential for transfer of virulence factors to *Enterobacter* spp. from other species.[236] Shiga toxin–producing *E. cloacae* has been isolated from the stool of a 5-month-old girl with hemolytic-uremic syndrome.[161] Shiga-toxin producing *E. coli* OR:H9 also was isolated from the child's stool, rendering the cause of the child's symptoms unclear. Similar to other organisms associated with central venous catheter infections, *Enterobacter* spp. may adhere irreversibly to catheter material, promoting colonization and infection via biofilm formation.[108,106,165] Certain ribotypes have been encountered more commonly as community or blood stream isolates, indicating the presence of as yet undefined factors affecting virulence.[224] The propensity of *C. sakazakii* to produce neonatal meningitis complicated by abscesses and cerebral infarction is unexplained.[15,38,158,230] Proposed mechanisms have included brain capillary and intestinal endothelial cell invasion, persistence in human macrophages, biofilm formation, and a possible role for outer membrane protein A (OmpA).[42,108,143,144,202,203]

CLINICAL MANIFESTATIONS

Infection caused by *Enterobacter* commonly is indistinguishable from illness caused by other enteric pathogens. Sources of infection include central venous catheters and the urinary and biliary tracts.[8,10,66,87,96,127] *Enterobacter* commonly colonizes the respiratory tract secretions of intubated patients, and it is implicated increasingly as a cause of ventilator-associated pneumonia.[96,182,189] It can also be a cause of severe community-acquired pneumonia, generally in patients with serious comorbidities. This type of pneumonia strongly resembles health care–associated pneumonia, and patients may appear septic. Empirical antibiotic therapy may be very difficult because of unpredictable resistance patterns.[23] It also is one of the most common causes of pneumonia after lung transplantation[129] and can be found as part of the oral flora in patients with strokes.[75] Neonatal infection warrants special mention because of the prominence of *Cronobacter sakazakii* as a cause of devastating meningitis.

Similar to *Citrobacter koseri* (see Chapter 101), *C. sakazakii* causes neonatal meningitis complicated by cerebral abscesses or infarctions.[15,32,38,51,102,230,232] Poor feeding, irritability, jaundice, a full anterior fontanelle, and fever or hypothermia are presenting features shared with other gram-negative causes of bacterial meningitis. The mortality rate has been reported to range from 33% to 80%, and almost all survivors experience severe neurologic complications, including quadriplegia, developmental impedance, and impaired sight and hearing.[51,230] This severe morbidity is consistent with the development of multiple cystic lesions of the brain in 50% of surviving neonates. Serial computed tomography (CT) scans commonly reveal evolution of lesions most consistent with initial cerebral infarction, rather than primary abscess formation.[67,117,230] Subsequent cystic lesions may be purulent abscesses, from which the organism can be cultured; alternatively, they sometimes represent sterile fluid collections.[27] Meningitis tended to develop in infants of greater gestational age and birth weight than in infants with only bacteremia, but they tended to be younger in chronologic age.[22]

Enterobacter also may be associated with necrotizing enterocolitis in the newborn, which became more apparent during the outbreaks of *C. sakazakii* associated with contaminated powdered infant formula.[117,207] *Enterobacter* spp. were the third most common isolate recovered from peritoneal fluid in a series of patients with necrotizing enterocolitis.[117,146]

In older immunocompromised children, bacteremia complicated by sepsis is a significant risk. Central venous catheterization and gastrointestinal tract pathologic processes seem to pose greater risks for development of bacteremia than infection of the urinary tract.[8,37,66,127] Bacteremia is accompanied by shock in almost one-third of patients, but disseminated intravascular coagulation occurs in fewer than 5%.[17,21,66] Seeding of metastatic foci is uncommon. Overall case-fatality rates with bacteremia vary but usually are approximately 30%.[187] Predictors of poor prognosis include age younger than 18 months, inadequacy of antimicrobial chemotherapy, infection with extended-spectrum cephalosporin-resistant isolates, septic shock, type of underlying disease, presence of pulmonary infection, thrombocytopenia, unknown primary site of infection, and requirement for intensive care.[17,21,34,46,66,100,133] Absence of fever during the course of infection may be a particularly ominous sign; four of five afebrile subjects died in one series.[17] One study found that the use of an aminoglycoside as part of the empirical antibiotic management was a factor contributing to survival of *Enterobacter* or *Citrobacter* bacteremia.[46]

Some *Enterobacter* spp. recovered from children with diarrhea have been reported to produce enterotoxin,[35] although a causative role in enteritis has not been established. Other presentations of *Enterobacter* infection include endophthalmitis,[110,140,142] endometritis,[73] wound infections,[66] diskitis,[175,196] endocarditis,[205] and osteomyelitis.[40,52,109,197] *Enterobacter* also has caused syndromes classically associated with other agents, such as gas gangrene,[60] childhood purpura fulminans,[80] ecthyma gangrenosum,[176] and necrotizing fasciitis.[112]

DIAGNOSIS

Diagnosis of infection caused by *Enterobacter* relies primarily on isolation of the organism in culture from clinical material. Motility, production of ornithine decarboxylase, and the absence of deoxyribonuclease help distinguish the genus from *Klebsiella* and *Serratia.* The presence of yellow-pigmented colonies can help identify *C. sakazakii.* Patterns of sugar fermentation and production of decarboxylase also distinguish the species. Molecular techniques that are becoming available for rapid identification of bacteria include PCR single-strand conformation polymorphism analysis using 16S ribosomal DNA. This technique allows the potential identification of pathogens to be made from a wide range of clinical specimens with low numbers of bacteria.[228,234] Matrix-assisted laser desorption ionization time of flight mass spectrometry (MALDI-TOF) and real-time PCR for rapid nonculture detection of *Enterobacter* and other clinical isolates are becoming more common in the clinical setting.[135,163,183] In light of the increase of *C. sakazakii* invasive disease after ingestion of contaminated powdered infant formula, several techniques have been introduced for the rapid identification of this pathogen clinically and in foodstuffs. The use of a specific PCR amplification of the outer membrane protein A gene *(ompA)* is being investigated,[145] as is reverse-transcriptase[124] and the use of selective media.[5,48,107] DNA microarray technology is also being investigated for use.[219] Ribotyping is a highly discriminatory and reproducible method for the typing of *E. cloacae,* the most common cause of infection.[68] Other useful molecular techniques include restriction endonuclease analysis of chromosomal DNA, pulsed-field gel electrophoresis, random amplification of polymorphic DNA, and amplification of short interspersed repetitive sequences.[187] Most often, molecular typing methods are used in concert with biotyping, serotyping, or bacteriocin typing.

TREATMENT

Treatment of *Enterobacter* infection is made problematic by inducible resistance to cephalosporins and intrinsic resistance to aminopenicillins, cefazolin, and cefoxitin.[20] The recognition that *Enterobacter* spp. may carry ESBL plasmids in addition to expressing chromosomal *ampC* β-lactamases can be problematic using automated ESBL detection systems. The use of the double-disk synergy method for ESBL detection can indicate the presence of plasmid-mediated resistance but is challenging because high production of *ampC* can mask the inhibition of ESBL by clavulanic acid.[229] New selective media for the identification of ESBL-producing isolates are available but still may have problems with high *ampC* producers.[177,179] Identification of carbapenemase-producing isolates is more difficult, although there are increased commercial applications becoming available such as rapid biochemical tests for both ESBL and carbapenamase producers.[56,173,174] The Clinical and Laboratory Standards Institute (CLSI) lowered carbapenem breakpoints in the United States in 2010 to allow for better identification, and these were also lowered in Europe in 2013 by the European Committee on Antimicrobial Susceptibility Testing (EUCAST). They are not perfect, and the use of molecular confirmation for ESBL carriage is suggested.[147] The modified Hodge test has potential, but, like the double-disk synergy method for ESBL detection, it is manual and can be time-consuming while still lacking in specificity and sensitivity (e.g., allows detection of high-level *ampC* producers, but has weak detection of NDM-1 producers). Molecular techniques, mostly PCR, are now the standard for detection.[149] It is important to know the local antibiotic resistance patterns to determine the risk for multidrug resistance. Therapeutic options in this setting can include the use of older medications, including fosfomycin and colistin, in addition to newer antibiotics such as tigecycline and doripenem.[72]

Antibiotic resistance may be present at the time of initial isolation or may develop during therapy.[37,84] This problem is compounded by the common observation of resistance to extended-spectrum penicillins and, to a lesser extent, aminoglycosides.[6] The risks for development of resistance to cephalosporins, piperacillin, and aminoglycosides have been reported to be higher at a tertiary care center than at a primary care hospital.[55] Previous administration of third-generation cephalosporins increases the risk for having multiresistant *Enterobacter* isolates in an initial positive blood culture.[8,36,148] Hospitalized newborns quickly may acquire multiresistant strains, even though they themselves have not been treated with cephalosporins.[14] Isolation of multiresistant *Enterobacter* spp. in blood culture is associated with a higher case-fatality rate in contrast to mortality after isolation of a more sensitive strain.[36,192] A recent study from the United Kingdom noted that increased mortality from gram-negative infections, including *Enterobacter* spp., was associated with increasing gentamicin minimum inhibitory concentration (MIC), even for isolates deemed susceptible.[104] Although less common, resistance to imipenem has been reported.[54,120,201] Cefepime, a fourth-generation cephalosporin, generally maintains activity against *Enterobacter* spp. that possess the class C β-lactamase,[188] although MICs may be higher.[137]

Emergence of cefepime resistance during therapy has been described in a liver transplant recipient with a hepatic abscess caused by *E. aerogenes*.[122] The accompanying editorial warns about the risk for failure using cefepime in patients who have high-density infections (e.g., poorly drained liver abscess) caused by ceftazidime-resistant strains of *Enterobacter*.[137] The presence of an SHV-type ESBL has been associated with cefepime resistance, highlighting the need to identify those strains.[196] Vigilant antibiotic stewardship may aid in decreasing resistance. One institution restricted the use of cefepime and compared the 2 years before with the 2 years after the policy, demonstrating an improvement in ciprofloxacin susceptibility in their *Enterobacter* clinical isolates.[152]

In a nationwide survey of nosocomial bloodstream infections, rates of *Enterobacter* resistance to third-generation cephalosporins (ceftazidime, ceftriaxone) and broad-spectrum semisynthetic penicillins (piperacillin) with or without a β-lactamase inhibitor (tazobactam) was high, ranging from 35% to 50%.[169] Cefepime and imipenem inhibited 97% to 100% of isolates. Susceptibility to aminoglycosides and fluoroquinolones ranged from 92% to 98%, and 85% to 96% of isolates were susceptible to trimethoprim-sulfamethoxazole. Fluoroquinolone resistance is now being reported and likely is plasmid-mediated.[157,235] Plasmid-mediated quinolone resistance can be more common in ESBL-producing isolates as well, so caution should be used.[195] Because resistance patterns may vary based on geographic location, local susceptibility data should be used to guide initial therapy.

Some investigators recommend initial combination therapy that includes an aminoglycoside plus either cefepime or a carbapenem (imipenem or meropenem), until results of susceptibility testing are available. Third-generation cephalosporins should be used with caution, even when initial susceptibility results seem favorable. When strains are resistant to gentamicin and tobramycin, amikacin may be a suitable alternative. Good responses to therapy and return of gentamicin susceptibility of hospital *Enterobacter* strains have occurred after routine substitution of amikacin for gentamicin.[178,193] Trimethoprim-sulfamethoxazole alone (or combined with an aminoglycoside) and quinolones seem to be good alternatives for the treatment of *Enterobacter* infections, including meningitis.[8,45,74,138,232] Fluoroquinolones have been reported to be effective in bone and joint infections, in combination with cefepime.[121] Tigecycline has been used for the treatment of multidrug-resistant strains, although reports of resistance are emerging.[91,217,233] Colistin has also been used, but it is hampered by its side-effect profile. As newer antimicrobial agents become available, more testing will be required to determine their effectiveness. Ceftazidime-avibactam, a combination drug with a novel non–β-lactam/β-lactamase inhibitor that inhibits class A, class C, and some class D enzymes, may have some promise in treating these difficult infections.[185]

Enterobacter meningitis creates special concerns. As is common with other forms of neonatal enteric meningitis, even susceptible organisms often persist in cerebrospinal fluid for 5 days or longer.[102] Monotherapy with a cell wall–active agent seems to be less effective than combination therapy with an aminoglycoside. Trimethoprim-sulfamethoxazole also has been used successfully.[63,232] Intrathecal administration of antibiotics does not seem to be beneficial in infants,[136] but it has been used with some success in adults.[153] The physician should anticipate the potential development of cerebral abscesses, infarctions, and cysts in newborns with *C. sakazakii* infection. Serial CT scans should be considered, and a neurosurgeon should be sought for drainage of abscesses and management of fluid accumulation.

NEW REFERENCES SINCE THE SEVENTH EDITION

24. Brady C, Cleenwerck I, et al. Taxonomic evaluation of the genus Enterobacter based on multilocus sequence analysis (MLSA): proposal to reclassify. *Syst Appl Microbiol*. 2013;36(5):309-319.
49. Doijad S, Imirzaligoglu C, et al. Enterobacter bugandensis sp. nov., from a neonatal unit in Tanzania. *Int J Syst Evol Microbiol*. 2015. Epub ahead of print.
56. Endimiani A, Jacobs MR. The changing role of the clinical microbiology laboratory in defining resistance in gram-negatives. *Infect Dis Clin North Am*. 2016;30: 323-345.
57. Evans BA, Amyes SGB. OXA β-lactamases. *Clin Microbiol Rev*. 2014;7:241-263.
59. Farmer JJ. My 40-year history with *Cronobacter/Enterobacter sakazakii*: lessons learned, myths debunked, and recommendations. *Front Pediatr*. 2015;3:84.
61. Fernandez J, Montero I, et al. Dissemination of multiresistant *Enterobacter cloacae* isolates producing OXA-48 and CTX-M-15 in a Spanish hospital. *Int J Antimicrob Agents*. 2015;46(4):469-474.
78. Guh AY, Bulens SN, et al. Epidemiology of carbapenem-resistant Enterobacteriaceae in 7 US communities, 2012–2013. *JAMA*. 2015;314(14):1479-1487.
91. Huang LF, Lee CT, et al. A snapshot of co-resistance to carbapenems and tigecycline in clinical isolates of *Enterobacter cloacae*. *Microb Drug Resist*. 2017;23(1):1-7.
92. Huerta-Garcia GC, Miranda-Novales G, et al. Intestinal colonization by extended-spectrum beta-lactamase producing Enterobacteriaceae in infants. *Rev Invest Clin*. 2015;67(5):313-317.
93. Ivady B, Kenesei E, et al. Factors influencing antimicrobial resistance and outcome of Gram-negative bloodstream infections in children. *Infection*. 2016;44(3):309-321.
104. Kent A, Kortsalioudaki C, et al. Neonatal gram-negative infections, antibiotic susceptibility and clinical outcome: an observational study. *Arch Dis Child Fetal Neonatal Ed*. 2016;Epub ahead of print.
116. Lagier JC, El Karkouri K, et al. Non contiguous-finished genome sequence and description of *Enterobacter massiliensis* sp. nov. *Stand Genomic Sci*. 2013;7:399-412.

126. Logan LK, Renschler JP, et al. Carbapenem-resistant Enterobacteriaceae in children, United States, 1999–2012. *Emerg Infect Dis.* 2015;21(11):2014-2021.
139. Mezzatesta ML, Gona F, Stefani S. *Enterobacter cloacae* complex: clinical impact and emerging antibiotic resistance. *Future Microbiol.* 2012;7(7):887-902.
147. Morrissey I, Bouchillon SK, et al. Evaluation of the Clinical and Laboratory Standards Institute phenotypic confirmatory test to detect the presence of extended-spectrum β-lactamases from 4005 *Escherichia coli, Klebsiella oxytoca, Klebsiella pneumoniae* and *Proteus mirabilis* isolates. *J Med Microbiol.* 2014;63:556-561.
154. Oren A, Garrity GM. List of new names and new combinations previously effectively, but not validly, published. *Int J Syst Evol Microbiol.* 2013;63:3931-3934.
173. Poirel L, Fernandez J, Nordmann P. Comparison of three biochemical tests for rapid detection of extended-spectrum-β-lactamase-producing Enterobacteriaceae. *J Clin Microbiol.* 2016;54(2):423-427.
174. Poirel L, Nordmann P. Rapid carbaNP test for rapid detection of carbapenemase producers. *J Clin Microbiol.* 2015;53(9):3003-3008.
185. Sader HS, Castanheira M, et al. Ceftazidime-avibactam activity against gram negative organisms isolated from intra-abdominal infections in United States hospitals, 2012–2014. *Surg Infect (Larchmt).* 2016;17(4):473-478.
194. Si D, Runnegar N, et al. Characterising health care-associated bloodstream infections in public hospitals in Queensland, 2008–2012. *Med J Aust.* 2016; 204(7):276.
200. Tebano G, Geneve C, et al. Epidemiology and risk factors of multidrug-resistant bacteria in respiratory samples after lung transplantation. *Transpl Infect Dis.* 2016;18(1):22-30.
213. Vaz-Moreira I, Varela AR, et al. Multidrug resistance in quinolone-resistant gram-negative bacteria isolated from hospital effluent and the municipal wastewater treatment plant. *Microb Drug Resist.* 2016;22(2):155-163.
215. Vojkovska H, Karpiskova R, et al. Characterization of *Cronobacter* spp. isolated from food of plant origin and environmental samples collected from farms and from supermarkets in the Czech Republic. *Int J Food Microbiol.* 2016;217: 130-136.
227. White L, Hopkins KL, et al. Carbapenemase-producing Enterobacteriaceae in hospital wastewater: a reservoir that may be unrelated to clinical isolates. *J Hosp Infect.* 2016;93(2):145-151.

The full reference list for this chapter is available at ExpertConsult.com.

103 Extraintestinal Pathogenic *Escherichia coli*

Patrick C. Seed

Escherichia coli are ubiquitous among terrestrial mammals, including humans, occupying approximately 0.1% of the microbes in the human enteric tract.[25] *E. coli* is a common commensal with normal homeostatic functions within intestinal-associated microbial communities. However, some subtypes are virulent and produce infectious diseases.[57,66] Genetic mutations and the loss and gain of genetic material through genetic rearrangements, transposons, phages, and plasmids have produced *E. coli* lineages with a wide capacity to occupy different host niches and yield different clinical syndromes.[66] Animal and human subtypes are closely related and in many cases are the same, differentiated based only on the hosts from which they were isolated. The pathotypes of *E. coli* have specific associated virulence factors and genetic islands.

E. coli is the common cause of a wide range of bacterial infections within and outside of the intestinal tract, including traveler's diarrhea, dysentery, cholecystitis, cholangitis, urinary tract infection (UTI), bacteremia, neonatal meningitis, and pneumonia (Table 103.1). The pathogenic *E. coli* may be divided into two major categories: extraintestinal pathogenic *E. coli* (ExPEC) and diarrheagenic *E. coli.* ExPEC is the focus of this chapter.

E. coli are facultative anaerobic gram-negative bacilli in the Enterobacteriaceae family.[40] Common physiologic and biochemical features include fermentation of lactose (~90% of isolates), indole production, and lysine decarboxylase activity.[73] Many isolates are motile, with peritrichous flagella constituting one of 56 flagellar antigen (H) serotypes.[71] In addition, there are 171 somatic antigens (O). The most common O subtypes have been reported as O1, O2, O4, O6, O7, O8, O18, O25, O68, and O75.[13,35,103,128]

EPIDEMIOLOGY

E. coli produces three major types of extraintestinal invasive diseases in children: (1) UTIs, (2) bacteremia and sepsis, and (3) meningitis. Lower incidence infections produced by ExPEC include pneumonia, osteomyelitis, and endocarditis. Antibiotic resistance in ExPEC has undergone a shift in the past decade and has important implications in the treatment of ExPEC-related infections. In particular, ExPEC sequence type 131 (ST131), a pandemic community-associated strain, is frequently multidrug resistant (three or more antibiotic classes).[104]

Urinary Tract Infection

E. coli is the leading cause of culture-proven UTI in children, producing more than 80% of community-acquired UTI, regardless of the presence of vesicoureteral reflux.[45] Other etiologies in pediatric community-acquired UTI include *Klebsiella pneumoniae, Proteus mirabilis, Enterococcus* spp., and, primarily in female adolescents, *Staphylococcus saprophyticus. E. coli* is also the leading cause of hospital-acquired UTI among children. Unlike in adult patients, in whom *E. coli* may account for more than 50% of nosocomial UTIs, *E. coli* produces approximately 30% of nosocomial UTIs in children.[69,75] Organisms such as *Candida* spp., *Klebsiella* spp., and *Pseudomonas aeruginosa* collectively assume a greater proportion of pediatric nosocomial UTIs.

In general, the prevalence of UTI is 7% among infants with febrile illness, of which, as noted earlier, *E. coli* is by far the most likely cause.[113] Among female infants, 7.5% with febrile illnesses have a UTI. Of male infants, the prevalence differs greatly based on whether the infant is circumcised. Among uncircumcised male infants, the prevalence of UTI is 20.1%, in contrast to a prevalence of 2.4% among those who are circumcised. Circumcision status does not alter the high proportion of UTIs associated with *E. coli.* Black infants have a lower prevalence of UTI, at approximately 4.7%, in contrast to white children, at 8%. The prevalence of UTI drops significantly after age 1 year, but increases during adolescence such that the pooled prevalence among children younger than 19 years of age is 7.8%.[113] Factors increasing the risk for UTI include vesicoureteral reflux, bladder dyssynergia, other urinary tract anomalies, sexual intercourse, spermicide use, pregnancy, and diabetes mellitus (Table 103.2).

Fever without localizing signs is a major cause of presentation for medical care among infants younger than 90 days of age. Recent studies indicate that in the era of vaccinations for *Haemophilus influenza* type b and *Streptococcus pneumoniae, E. coli* UTI is the leading cause of fever without localizing signs.[129,130] UTI was responsible for 76% of all episodes, and bacteremia and meningitis were 19% and 3%, respectively. Of the UTIs, *E. coli* was the causative agent in 96% of the cases.

Some female children experience colonization of the bladder without urinary symptoms, termed asymptomatic bacteriuria (ASB). *E. coli* is also the most common cause of ASB. In U.S. female school children at 5 to 6 years of age, the incidence of ASB was observed to be 1.9% to 2.2%, whereas only 0.2% of age-matched boys had ASB.[20,110] The cumulative prevalence of ASB between the ages of 6 and 12 years is reported to be 4.6%. No ethnic or socioeconomic risk factors have been associated with ASB. In addition to sex, risk factors include diabetes and sickle-cell disease.[17,102]

TABLE 103.1 Major *Escherichia coli* Classifications

Main Group	Subgroup	Associated Diseases
Intestinal pathogenic *E. coli* (IPEC)	Enterohemorrhagic *E. coli* (EHEC)	Afebrile, bloody colitis
	Enteropathogenic *E. coli* (EPEC)	Watery diarrhea
	Enterotoxigenic *E. coli* (ETEC)	Watery diarrhea
	Enteroaggregative *E. coli* (EAEC)	Chronic, persistent diarrhea
	Enteroinvasive *E. coli* (EIEC)	Watery diarrhea or dysentery
Extraintestinal pathogenic *E. coli* (ExPEC)	Uropathogenic *E. coli* (UPEC)	Urinary tract infection, urosepsis
	Neonatal meningitis *E. coli* (NMEC)	Meningitis
	Sepsis-causing *E. coli* (SEPEC)	Bacteremia, sepsis
Animal-associated pathogenic *E. coli* (AAPEC) reservoir groups	Avian pathogenic *E. coli* (APEC)	Bird sepsis, chronic respiratory disease, swollen head syndrome
	Mammary pathogenic *E. coli* (MPEC)	Bovine mastitis
	Endometrial pathogenic *E. coli* (EnPEC)	Bovine endometriosis

TABLE 103.2 Risk Factors for Extraintestinal Pathogenic *Escherichia coli* Urinary Tract Infection in Children

Factor	Type	Mechanism	References
Female gender	Physical-anatomic	Shorter urethra and closer proximity to the rectum increases access of uropathogens to the urinary tract	135
Vesicoureteral reflux	Physical-anatomic	Reflux of urine through the ureteral valves moves contaminated urine from the bladder to the kidneys	7, 11, 114
Bladder dyssynergia	Physical-anatomic	Incoordination of voiding; failure to clear microbes	117
Urinary tract anomalies	Physical-anatomic	Urinary stasis; failure to clear microbes	7
Catheterization	Physical-anatomic	Introduction of organisms into urinary tract; persistence of less virulent organisms	70, 109, 123
Sexual intercourse	Behavioral	Introduction of periurethral organisms into urinary tract	26, 87
Spermicide use	Behavioral	Inhibition of vaginal lactobacilli with outgrowth of *E. coli*	46
Diaphragm use	Behavioral	Spring-rim–mediated minor bladder trauma; co-use of spermicidal gels	46
Diabetes mellitus	Immune	Glucosuria; neutrophil functional impairment	32, 89, 94

Bacteremia and Sepsis

E. coli may produce bacteremia or sepsis. Pediatric *E. coli* bacteremia and sepsis occur mostly in young infants and special groups of children such as patients with chemotherapy-induced immunodeficiency, central venous catheters, urinary tract anomalies, and human immunodeficiency virus.[16,105] Patients in the neonatal and pediatric intensive care units have a heightened risk for bloodstream *E. coli* infections, as do patients with obstructive urinary tract disease and UTI, leading to urosepsis.

Among infants, *E. coli* bloodstream infections are most common in the first month of life, with decreasing numbers of cases in the second to third months of life. Among neonates, *E. coli* has been associated with approximately 18% of early-onset sepsis and a similar percentage of late-onset sepsis, placing it as the second or third most common etiology in this age group.[126] In preterm infants, the infection rate for *E. coli* was more than 10%, with a contemporary study demonstrating a rate of 29%.[9,120] Prematurity, low birth weight, prolonged labor, prolonged rupture of membranes, intrapartum maternal fever, and maternal antibiotics may increase the risk for complicated, high morbidity or mortality infections.[124] Neonatal early-onset group B streptococcal disease has decreased significantly with the use of intrapartum ampicillin for women at risk because of known colonization, prolonged rupture of membranes, or maternal fever. However, more than 50% of *E. coli* organisms are resistant to ampicillin such that prophylaxis has not had a positive impact on early-onset *E. coli* infection. Retrospective data suggest that ampicillin-resistant *E. coli* may be responsible for more fulminant and higher mortality disease among premature infants,[1,9,53] although this remains controversial and in need of further study.[112]

Meningitis

In the pediatric population, *E. coli* meningitis occurs almost exclusively among young infants and highly immunocompromised children. It is the leading cause of meningitis among preterm infants and equal to group B streptococcus.[19,119] *E. coli* meningitis frequently results in intensive care, severe neurologic impairment, and high mortality, at 34%, 21%, and 14%, respectively.[48,49] Twenty-eight percent of infants have a concurrent UTI and are older than 6 days of life.[48] Concurrent bacteremia is present in up to 81% of infants.

Peritonitis

Peritonitis in children is most typically a complication of appendicitis. Intestinal perforation is an infrequent cause in children. Overall it is a rare entity in children, in contrast to adults. *E. coli* accounts for more than 50% of bacterial peritonitis in children, with 60% of the infections being polymicrobial.[23]

Pneumonia, Endocarditis, and Osteomyelitis

E. coli is an infrequent cause of infections of the lungs, heart, and bones. Pneumonia may arise from oropharyngeal or hematogenous sources and endocarditis through hematogenous spread after translocation of bacteria from the intestinal tract or following urosepsis. Osteomyelitis is most frequently hematogenous after intestinal translocation or urosepsis but also may occur after traumatic injuries and direct inoculation into areas proximal to bone.

PATHOGENESIS

ExPEC produces a wide variety of invasive infections outside of the gastrointestinal tract, including those of the urinary tract, bloodstream, and central nervous system (CNS). ExPEC is a normal commensal organism in the enteric and genital tracts, and colonization alone does not have any measurable consequence to individuals harboring these strains. ExPEC colonizes through oral-fecal transmission where food may be contaminated, through cross-transmission between humans, or, as more recently described, through transmission between domesticated animals such as cats and dogs.[52] Sexual transmission of ExPEC also has been shown to occur, with male partners appearing to transmit

ExPEC bearing virulence gene characteristics typical of those producing UTIs to their female partners.[27] The relative frequency of acquisition of ExPEC by oral-fecal and sexual routes is not clear at present.

ExPEC infections occur after bacteria invade sterile sites such as the urinary tract or the bloodstream from commensal reservoirs such as the enteric tract and vagina. When the immune system is unable to limit the spread of bacteria, invasive infections such as UTI, bacteremia, meningitis, and, more rarely, pneumonia or osteomyelitis may occur.

Urinary Tract Infection

ExPEC is the leading cause of UTI,[28] and UTI may precede more invasive infections of the bloodstream, bones, heart, and CNS. ExPEC colonizing the periurethral area may be introduced into the urethra and ascend through the urinary tract. The infection may involve only the urethra (urethritis), but most commonly involves the bladder, resulting in cystitis. More advanced infections may ascend through the ureters to the kidneys, resulting in pyelitis, pyelonephritis, or pyelonephrosis. Anatomic variation or defects, such as voiding dysfunction and vesicoureteral reflux, increase the risk for lower tract and upper tract UTI.[31]

Infrequently ExPEC UTI may occur through hematogenous spread in which bloodstream organisms infect the kidneys and are subsequently isolated from the urine in a descending infection. This may occur during bacteremia after organisms have translocated from the enteric tract. Perinephric abscesses may be the sole consequence of hematogenous infection of the urinary tract.

The specific host and bacterial factors that favor transition from the external genital region into the urethra remain poorly understood in the prepubescent, non–sexually active child. After the initiation of sexual activity, UTI rates increase.[28] Spermicides and intercourse are both associated with an increased risk for UTI in women, primarily through promotion of ExPEC in the vagina and mechanical introduction of bacteria into the female urethra, respectively. The size of the inoculum necessary to start an infection in humans is not well understood and is likely overestimated in animal models.

Many of the molecular events during ExPEC cystitis have been elucidated through animal and human studies (Fig. 103.1). ExPEC produces numerous virulence factors that persist in the urinary tract (Table 103.3). Once in the urinary bladder, ExPEC adheres to the bladder epithelium to initiate an infection. Attachment is essential because micturition is a potent host defense to flush the bacteria out of the organ.[131] Type 1 pili, fibrous extensions from the bacteria with adhesive tips, have been established as a major *E. coli* factor promoting adherence to the bladder epithelium. On attachment of ExPEC to the apical surface of the bladder epithelium via type 1 pili, ExPEC can invade into bladder epithelial cells through a variety of routes, including lipid rafts and caveolin, clathrin-coated pits, and fusiform vesicles.[8,24,59] Within the epithelium, ExPEC may persist long term in late endosomes[82,83] or escape into the cytosol of the epithelial cell and form intracellular bacterial communities (IBCs), biofilm-like structures with bacteria enmeshed in type 1 pili, aggregative antigens, and polysaccharide capsules.[3,4] From the IBC state, bacteria may amass and escape as long filaments, only to bind to more bladder epithelial cells and reinvade naïve epithelium.[54,55]

ExPEC isolates from children with pyelonephritis are more likely to produce P pili, hemolysin, and cytotoxic necrotizing factor (CNF-1) and be serum resistant than cystitis strains or commensal isolates.[21,49] In the kidneys, ExPEC uses P pili and type 1 pili to adhere to the renal tubule epithelium and persist in the kidney.[68,77] Local toxin production, including hemolysin, CNF-1, and Sat, damage the epithelium and may permit bacterial penetration and translocation across the border into the adjacent capillary system.[76,116] The toxins also may inhibit infiltrating granulocytes and limit their capacity to contain the infection.[18]

In response to acute infection of the bladder, the lipopolysaccharide-recognition receptor Toll-like receptor 4 (TLR4) is triggered by ExPEC, initiating a signal cascade that results in proinflammatory events, including the expression of cytokines interleukin (IL-6), IL-8, and granulocyte-macrophage colony-forming unit (GM-CSF).[41,118] Neutrophils and macrophages are recruited into the bladder to assist in clearing the infection.[65,133] The superficial bladder epithelium is also shed in the process of exfoliation, resulting in elimination of attached and invasive

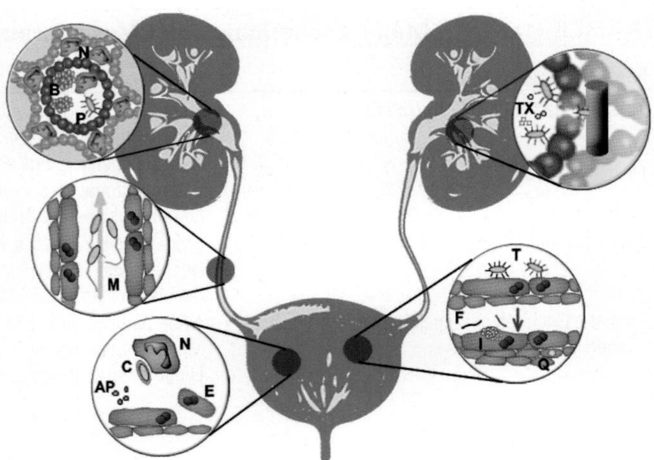

FIG. 103.1 Pathogenesis of extraintestinal pathogenic *E. coli* (ExPEC) urinary tract infection. ExPEC produces lower and upper tract infection. In the bladder, *E. coli* adheres to the bladder epithelium by using adherence factors such as type 1 pili *(T, lower right circle)*. ExPEC can invade the epithelium, replicate, and reemerge as filamentous bacteria *(F)*. Infection of the bladder results in a strong inflammatory response *(lower left circle)* involving production of antimicrobial peptides *(AP)*, neutrophil infiltration *(N)*, and exfoliation, or sloughing, of the epithelium *(E)*. ExPEC produces a capsule *(C)* to protect against the innate immune response. ExPEC can migrate up the ureters *(middle left circle)* against urinary flow using flagella *(M)*. In the kidneys, ExPEC produces P pili *(P)* and other adhesive factors to bind to the renal epithelium, where biofilms *(B)* may be formed. An inflammatory response includes neutrophils *(N)* and other factors such as complement and antimicrobial peptides. From the kidney tubules, ExPEC may also produce toxins *(TX; upper right circle)*, damaging the local epithelial and endothelial borders to invade capillaries and disseminate in the bloodstream, producing bacteremia.

intracellular ExPEC. Microscopy of urine from young women with acute cystitis revealed leukocytes and exfoliated bladder epithelial cells, including filamentous ExPEC and cells harboring IBC.[107] In animal studies, the clearance of ExPEC is incomplete even with the application of antibiotics, resulting in chronic latent intravesical infection, predicted to be a reservoir for some recurrent infections.[83,111]

The determinants that balance acute inflammatory infections and ASB are not fully known. ASB and cystitis isolates have reduced virulence gene numbers relative to strains causing pyelonephritis.[10,122] Despite similar known virulence gene content in cystitis strains of ExPEC, a prototypic ASB isolate of *E. coli* has been previously shown to have reduced virulence factor gene expression in contrast to cystitis isolates, and ASB isolates may outcompete cystitis strains for growth in urine.[106] The host response to bacteria within the urinary tract is likely to be important to the development of ASB. Children with reduced TLR4 expression have been shown to have an increased risk for ASB.[100]

Bacteremia

ExPEC are frequent causes of bacteremia secondary to translocation from the intestinal tract into the bloodstream. This frequently occurs in patients with loss of intestinal epithelial barrier integrity or compromised immunity. ExPEC produces protective factors that favor survival in serum, including polysaccharide capsules known to inhibit complement deposition, opsonization, and phagocytosis by granulocytes.[12,47,108] Toxins such as hemolysin A and CNF-1 have roles in inhibiting phagocyte function,[18,99] thus limiting ExPEC clearance. ExPEC also responds to the bloodstream environment by downregulating factors that may stimulate immunity or promote phagocytosis such as the adhesive factor type 1 pili.

Critical metabolic pathways are necessary for successful dissemination of ExPEC in bloodstream infections. Sialic acid usage and iron acquisition have been previously shown to be essential for ExPEC survival during disseminated infection.[115]

TABLE 103.3 **Representative Extraintestinal *Escherichia coli* Virulence Factors**

Functional Category	Virulence Factor	Role	References
Adhesin	Type 1 pili *(fim)*	Adherence to urinary tract epithelium, particularly in bladder; lectin-recognizing mannosylated glycoproteins	50, 51, 60
	P pili *(pap/prf)*	Adherence to urinary tract epithelium, particularly in bladder; lectin-recognizing glycolipids	68, 74, 101, 125
	S pili *(sfa/foc)*	Bind to α-sialyl-2,3-β-galactoside found in urinary tract and central nervous system	131
	Auf pili	Expression in urinary tract but unknown function	15
	Dr adhesins	Examples include Dr and Afa I-IV; binding to decay-activating factor	33, 91
	TosA	Repeats-in-toxin (RTX) protein; adherence to renal tubular cells	127
	UpaB	Autotransporter-type adhesion; binding to extracellular matrix proteins	2
	Tsh	Serine protease-type autotransporters; associated with pyelonephritis strains	42
Invasin	IbeA	Invasion of the brain endothelium	52, 74
	OmpA	Outer membrane protein A	88
Toxins	HlyA	α-Hemolysin	79
	Cyclomodulins	Examples include cytolethal distending toxin (CDT-1) and cytotoxic necrotizing factor 1 (CNF-1)	22
	Sat	Serine autotransporter	37
Protectins	Groups II and III polysaccharide capsules	K1, K2, and K5 capsules, among others	3, 5
	OmpT	Outer membrane protease T	121
	Curli	Amyloid-like extracellular fibers	56
Iron acquisition	IreA	Siderophore receptor	30
	Iro	Salmochelin	30
	Iuc	Aerobactin	30
	SitA	Periplasmic iron binding protein	30
	Ybt	Yersiniabactin	30
Immune regulators	TcpC	Immunomodulator	74
	SisA/B	Inflammation suppressors	72
Other	DsdA	D-Serine deaminase	39
	Flagella	Motility	67, 132
	Cellulose	Biofilm formation	90

Meningitis

ExPEC disseminates from mucosal surfaces through the bloodstream to the CNS. Neonatal animal models have suggested that ExPEC disseminates to the CNS within macrophages and that dissemination depends on nitric oxide production.[78] The burden of organisms during bacteremia correlates with the likelihood of developing meningitis in both infant and adult animal models.[63] At the blood-brain barrier (BBB), ExPEC transverses the brain microvascular endothelial cells by first binding and invading the cells through actin rearrangement and transcellular traversal of the barrier.[63] Type 1 pili and OmpA (Table 103.4) are key adhesive factors mediating the initial interaction between *E. coli* and the vasculature via gp96 and CD48, respectively.[62,97] The *E. coli* factor IbeA has been shown to enhance brain microvascular endothelial cell invasion.[29,98] K1 polysaccharide encapsulation, common among ExPEC causing neonatal meningitis, prevents late endosome–lysosomal fusion and thus killing of intracellular *E. coli,* whereas lack of encapsulation results in bacteria proceeding through early to late endosomes and lysosomal fusion with eventual degradation of the bacteria-containing vacuoles.[64] The consequence of brain endothelial cell invasion by *E. coli* is cytokine release such as the proinflammatory factor IL-8, brain endothelial cell apoptosis, BBB dysfunction, and increased permeability, ultimately leading to encephalopathy.[63]

TABLE 103.4 **Susceptibility to Antibiotic-Class Representative Agents Commonly Used in the Treatment of Urinary Tract Infection and Invasive *Escherichia coli* Infections**

Antibiotic[a]	Resistance (95% CI)	Reference
Ampicillin/amoxicillin	53.4% (46–60.8%)	14
Amoxicillin-sulbactam	8.2% (7.9–9.6%)	14
Trimethoprim-sulfamethoxazole	23.6% (13.9–32.3%)	14
Nitrofurantoin	1.3% (0.8–1.7%)	14
Ciprofloxacin[c]	2.1% (0.8–4.4%)	14
Levofloxacin[c]	9%	Unpublished[b]
Ceftriaxone	5%	Unpublished[b]
Gentamicin	8%	Unpublished[b]
Tobramycin	6%	Unpublished[b]
Amikacin	0%	Unpublished[b]
Meropenem	0.5%	Unpublished[b]

[a]Oral agents are listed first.
[b]Data are representative of the Research Triangle Region in North Carolina.
[c]US Food and Drug Administration–approved for complicated *E. coli* urinary tract infections.

CLINICAL PRESENTATION

Urinary Tract Infection

Acute UTI with *E. coli* is associated with dysuria, urinary frequency, urgency, and often cloudy or odorous urine. Cystitis typically has low-grade fever or no elevation in temperature and may include anterior abdominal or pelvic pain or pressure. In contrast, *E. coli* pyelonephritis includes flank or lower back pain, and high fever, often higher than 38.9°C (102°F). Pyelonephritis may also include chills, sweats, rigors, nausea, vomiting, and headache. In patients with perinephric abscesses or intrarenal necrosis, the patient may have pleuritic chest pain from irritation of the diaphragm, and a flank mass may be palpable on physical examination. Bacteremia and urosepsis may develop secondary to pyelonephritis, especially among patients with diabetes, urinary tract abnormalities, urinary obstruction, or pregnancy. Pyelonephritis with and without urosepsis must be differentiated from intraabdominal processes, including appendicitis, psoas abscess, ruptured ovarian cyst, and ectopic pregnancy.

E. coli UTIs are not easily distinguished symptomatically from the syndromes caused by other organisms, including *S. saprophyticus* in the female adolescent, *K. pneumoniae, P. mirabilis,* or group B streptococcus.

Bacteremia and Sepsis

Bacteremia by *E. coli* is not readily distinguished in signs and symptoms from bloodstream infections produced by other gram-negative bacteria. Children may have fever, fatigue, lethargy, or irritability. Nausea and vomiting may accompany bloodstream infections. Some children may have a diffuse erythematous rash and, in the case of sepsis, generalized edema. Tachycardia may occur in the presence and absence of fever. Urine output may be diminished accompanying renal failure in cases of severe infection.

Meningitis

Neonates with *E. coli* meningitis present with general nonspecific features, including fever, vomiting, irritability, and failure to thrive. In advanced circumstances, neurologic signs, including apnea, seizures, decreased muscular tone, and ocular or limb palsies, may be present. Jaundice may accompany the presentation. In the infant older than 3 months, nuchal rigidity and a tense fontanelle may be part of the presentation. Acute *E. coli* meningitis in the older child is accompanied by headache, nausea, vomiting, lethargy, confusion, and fever. Neurologic features such as seizure or focal symptoms may accompany *E. coli* meningitis. The clinical presentation of *E. coli* meningitis overlaps with other etiologies of meningitis. Acute *E. coli* meningitis must be differentiated from other processes, including seizure disorder, brain abscess, aneurysm, sepsis, and, in the case of the neonate, tetanus.

E. coli meningitis is a rare complication of neurosurgical procedures. The clinical presentation may not be different from that of acute meningitis in the nonsurgical patient. However, infectious meningitis must be differentiated from other infectious and noninfectious complications of surgery.

Intraabdominal Infection

E. coli produces cholecystitis and cholangitis associated with right upper quadrant pain, fever, and jaundice. In advanced cases, bacteremia and sepsis may complicate the infections. Both infections are associated with high fever, typically above 38.9°C (102°F). Cholangitis is accompanied by chills and sometimes hepatic abscess. Children with *E. coli* cholecystitis or cholangitis develop right upper quadrant pain, fever, and jaundice. In severe cases, hypotension and confusion also develop. Cholecystitis manifests with fever (>38.9°C [102°F]). Cholangitis manifests with fever (>38.9°C [102°F]), shaking chills, and right upper quadrant pain and can be complicated by hepatic abscess. Other infectious etiologies may bear resemblance to *E. coli* intraabdominal infection, including *Klebsiella* spp., enterococcus, and, with appropriate exposure histories, amoebic abscess or *Echinococcosis* spp.

E. coli also may cause intraabdominal abscesses with and without peritonitis. Abscess alone may be associated with low-grade fever and nonspecific abdominal pain, as well as occasional malaise and anorexia. Peritonitis is associated with higher fever and rebound pain. In severe cases, septic shock may accompany peritonitis. Patients with *E. coli* intraabdominal abscesses may have low-grade fever, but the spectrum of clinical presentations ranges from nonspecific abdominal examination findings to frank septic shock. Peritonitis manifests as localized pain with rebound and fever. Abdominal abscess with E. coli are often polymicrobial with anaerobes, gram-negative bacilli, and enterococci.

Pneumonia

Children with *E. coli* pneumonia typically present with a febrile illness, shortness of breath, tachypnea, increased respiratory secretions, and rales and crackles with auscultation. *E. coli* pneumonia may be ventilator-associated and bacteremia-associated. *E. coli* is a rare cause of community-acquired pneumonia in a child with otherwise normal immune defenses. *E. coli* pneumonia is difficult to distinguish clinically from other bacterial pneumonia.

DIAGNOSIS

General

The definitive diagnosis of ExPEC infection is isolation of the organism from a sterile site such as urine, blood, or cerebrospinal fluid (CSF). Isolation from sputum or wounds is also indicated in some circumstances, such as pneumonia and abdominal infections, respectively. In these circumstances, recovery of the bacterium must be regarded in the context of the patient's clinical presentation to determine if the isolation of the organism is compatible with infection or represents colonization.

E. coli is readily isolated from a wide variety of clinical samples at 37°C (98.6°F) and aerobic conditions.[40] Nonselective and selective media, including MacConkey agar, will isolate *E. coli.* Approximately 90% of isolates are lactose fermenting, and approximately 99% produce indole, making this an optimal biochemical test for the identification of *E. coli.*[85] *E. coli* does not typically produce pigments, but many isolates are β-hemolytic, although a significant percentage from sites such as the urinary tract may not display β-hemolysis on blood agar.

Urinary Tract Infection

For suspicion of UTI, a urine dipstick test may be performed to rapidly determine if the patient has pyuria or bacteriuria based on the detection of leukocyte esterase and nitrites, respectively. Definitive diagnosis is based on urine culture results. The specimen should be collected from a midstream clean void in children old enough to provide such a sample or by straight sterile catheterization in younger children. A contaminated specimen and asymptomatic colonization must be differentiated from infection based on clinical symptoms and signs, as well as the urinalysis consistent with inflammation. In cases of infection, pyuria usually is present. In urinalysis, leukocyte esterase and nitrite each have a sensitivity of 0.88 and a false-positive rate of 0.05. Bacteria identified by Gram stain on noncentrifuged samples have a sensitivity of 0.93 and false-positive rate of 0.05. White blood cells alone have poor sensitivity and increased false-positive rate.[34]

Routine screening of the urine for cure after antibiotic therapy and screening for asymptomatic colonization are not recommended because screening produces a large number of false-positive results and does not alter rates of renal scarring.[58,61]

Imaging studies may be indicated in some patients to assist in making a diagnosis of *E. coli* infection, determining the necessity for an interventional procedure, or assessing the prognosis. For UTI, renal ultrasonography, computed tomography (CT), or dimethylsuccinic acid scans may be indicated to evaluate the kidneys and look for any other source of abscess, stones, or obstruction. Vesicoureterogram may be indicated for the diagnosis of vesicoureteral reflux, which may predispose a patient to pyelonephritis.

Other Infections

Recovery of the organism in contaminated sites, such as sputum and wounds, must be analyzed in the context of the patient's clinical state to determine if it represents colonization or infection. Recovery from sterile sites, such as the CSF, should be considered diagnostic of infection.

Lumbar puncture and a CSF culture for *E. coli* will establish the diagnosis of acute *E. coli* meningitis. Before culture data are available, CSF parameters alone will not be specific for *E. coli* infection. Elevated protein, depressed glucose, and the presence of leukocytes with a neutrophilic predominance may be present. Before culture information is available, Gram stain may reveal gram-negative bacilli without being solely indicative of *E. coli.* Justification for a lumbar puncture and analysis must be made based on indications for possible CNS infection, including a positive blood culture, altered behavior, and abnormal neurologic signs, such as seizures.

Patients with pneumonia should have blood cultures and sputum Gram stain and culture performed. The results of a Gram stain of the sputum help differentiate a good specimen (i.e., many polymorphonuclear [PMN] leukocytes and few squamous epithelial cells) from a bad specimen (i.e., few PMN leukocytes and many squamous epithelial cells). Culture should be obtained before antibiotic therapy is initiated.

Additional studies may be indicated for non-UTI ExPEC infections. In pneumonia, chest radiography or CT is indicated. In cholecystitis and cholangitis, ultrasonography or CT of the right upper quadrant is indicated. For suspicion of intraabdominal abscess, abdominal and pelvic ultrasound or CT may be indicated.

TREATMENT

General

Therapy for ExPEC infections depends on the site and severity of infection. The choice of antibiotics must be determined on the basis of local regional antibiotic susceptibilities, site to which the antibiotic is to be delivered, and appropriateness and tolerance of oral or parenteral agents.

Urinary Tract Infection

Determination of therapy for UTI is first contingent on the appropriateness of oral therapy or intravenous antibiotics. Most community-acquired UTIs may be treated with oral therapy, assuming that antibiotic resistance that would preclude therapy with an available oral agent is not suspected, the child is able to tolerate oral therapy (e.g., not vomiting), and the child does not have underlying urinary tract anomalies or other comorbidities such as diabetes mellitus, renal transplantation, systemic lupus erythematosus, or other conditions. Infants with UTI in the first month of life should be given parenteral antibiotics at the start of their treatment because of the challenge of differentiating lower and upper tract infections, the high prevalence of concomitant bacteremia (~10%), and concurrent urinary tract pathology, including posterior urethral valves, obstructed duplex systems, and high-grade vesicoureteric reflux with serious metabolic disturbance, such as hyperkalemia and hypernatremia. Furthermore past trials have excluded young infants, leaving no specific data to further guide management of UTI in this group.

The duration of therapy for cystitis should be 5 to 7 days, although pediatric-specific data regarding sufficient minimum duration of therapy are not available. Caution must be taken because it may be difficult in the young child to differentiate lower and upper urinary tract involvement, especially given that fever is a typical presenting symptom suggesting upper tract involvement. Typical therapy entails oral trimethoprim-sulfamethoxazole (TMP-SMX), trimethoprim alone, cephalexin, amoxicillin-clavulanate, or nitrofurantoin. The fluoroquinolone ciprofloxacin is not approved for use in children except for complicated *E. coli* UTI.

Prior research has indicated that oral therapy for pyelonephritis using the cephalosporins cefixime and ceftibuten or amoxicillin-clavulanate is effective in treating acute infections and does not result in a significant increase in renal scarring in contrast to initial parenteral therapy.[44,81,86] Pyelonephritis should be treated for a longer duration of 10 to 14 days. In children who are not candidates for initial oral therapy, 2 to 3 days of parenteral therapy should be provided until the child is able to tolerate an oral agent. However, no difference in renal scarring was identified in children receiving initial parenteral therapy before oral therapy in contrast to children receiving oral therapy for the entire course.[86] Longer initial intravenous therapy (8 days vs. 3 days) also was not shown to decrease renal scarring.[12] The combined duration of parenteral and oral therapy should then be the same as for children receiving only oral therapy.

E. coli UTI complicated by perinephric or intrarenal abscess may require surgical drainage and longer therapy. Ultrasound evaluation may be indicated before discontinuation of therapy.

Antibiotic prophylaxis has been used to prevent recurrent UTI for the primary purpose of reducing the risk of renal scarring and long-term renal insufficiency. The role of prophylactic antibiotics for the prevention of UTI has changed in recent years as more studies indicate they do not provide significant protection from recurrent infections and in particular renal scarring[30,80,92,95] and demonstrate that prophylactic antibiotics, particularly β-lactams like amoxicillin and cephalosporins, may result in subsequent infections with resistant organisms.[36,84] Even the most recent data from the largest randomized controlled study yet of children with VUR demonstrated no reduction in renal scarring attributable to daily prophylaxis (8.2% vs. 8.4%, with and without prophylaxis).[43] Prophylaxis did reduce recurrent UTI (14.8% vs. 27.4%, with and without prophylaxis) with a number needed to treat of 8 and 2 years of therapy, although an increase in antibiotic-resistant organisms was noted in a number of children. Exceptions may be for children with high-grade vesicoureteral reflux grades IV and V awaiting surgical interventions, for whom the benefits of daily antibiotic prophylaxis to prevent recurrent UTI and renal scarring may outweigh the risks that include cost and the emergence of multidrug-resistant organisms. TMP-SMX or nitrofurantoin may be considered in these circumstances.

Other Infections

The treatment of invasive infections for *E. coli* should entail parenteral antibiotics of the appropriate spectrum, accounting for local resistance patterns and, in the case of empirical coverage, for other possible etiologic agents. Two antimicrobials with independent mechanisms of action such as a β-lactam and an aminoglycoside should be considered in patients at risk for multidrug-resistant *E. coli* infections. Past hospitalization and antibiotic exposure are among the risk factors for multidrug resistance.

The treatment of *E. coli* bloodstream infections is generally 10 to 14 days. Serious consideration should be given to the removal of central venous catheters in the presence of a high degree of suspicion that the catheter may be involved or responsible for the infection, although mixed data exist for the necessity of catheter removal.[6,16,38,93] *E. coli* meningitis should be treated for a minimum of 21 days or 14 days after obtaining a negative CSF culture, whichever is longer.[96] Parenteral therapy is indicated for both bloodstream infection and meningitis. Treatment of *E. coli* meningitis should include an agent with known penetration of the BBB, for example, an advanced cephalosporin such as cefotaxime or a carbapenem such as meropenem, as well as an aminoglycoside, until full antibiotic susceptibilities are available.

Antibiotic Susceptibility

Specific antibiotic susceptibility data for pediatric *E. coli* isolates in North America are severely lacking. However, the antibiotic resistance of *E. coli* causing invasive infections among the population as a whole, particularly UTI, has undergone major shifts over the past decade. Previously *E. coli* was widely susceptible to a range of antibiotics, but, in the past decade, resistance has increased in prevalence (see Table 103.4). Susceptibilities of *E. coli* to cephalexin and cefixime, often employed in treating pediatric *E. coli* infections in the outpatient setting, are notably unavailable. Antibiotic resistance to ampicillin, amoxicillin, and TMP-SMX is now broadly distributed. Neonates delivered to mothers treated with ampicillin for the prevention of group B streptococcus infection have an increased risk for ampicillin-resistant *E. coli* early-onset sepsis.[9] Furthermore multidrug resistance is common. Of the *E. coli* resistant to TMP-SMX, they are twice as likely to be resistant to ampicillin and 33 times more likely to be resistant to the fluoroquinolones and nitrofurantoin.[134]

Risk factors associated with infection with extended-spectrum β-lactamase (ESBL)-producing *E. coli* include underlying illness and hospitalization in the previous 3 months.[126]

OUTCOMES

General

Outcomes of *E. coli* infections depend on the degree of invasiveness and status of the host immunologic defenses.

Urinary Tract Infection

Cystitis has the lowest morbidity, mostly incurred in terms of socioeconomic costs and emergence of antibiotic resistance. In contrast, pyelonephritis and other renal infections require more extended antibiotic therapy, incurring more cost and lost time from school and work. Furthermore renal infections may result in progressive renal scarring with the concern for loss of renal function and early renal insufficiency. In some circumstances, particularly in young children, children with anatomic variations of the urinary tract and those with diabetes, UTI may precede bloodstream infections.

Other Infections

The mortality rate for early-onset and late-onset sepsis in neonates has been previously shown to be approximately 15% and 9%, respectively.[52]

In infants with very low birth weight (<1500 g) the odds ratio of death with early-onset and late-onset sepsis was 1.45 and 1.30, respectively, with *E. coli* contributing to this degree of risk.[46] Among older children with central venous catheter–related *E. coli* bloodstream infections, the mortality rate is approximately 7% despite appropriate antibiotic therapy, with parenteral nutrition and mechanical ventilation being predictors for poor outcome.[16]

In a 25-year retrospective study of neonates with meningitis in a tertiary medical center, of which *E. coli* was one of the top three pathogens, approximately 14% died and 40% had significant morbidity, including seizures and hearing loss.[72]

NEW REFERENCES SINCE THE SEVENTH EDITION

14. Bryce A, Hay AD, Lane IF, et al. Global prevalence of antibiotic resistance in paediatric urinary tract infections caused by *Escherichia coli* and association with routine use of antibiotics in primary care: systematic review and meta-analysis. *BMJ*. 2016;352:i939.
43. Hoberman A, Greenfield SP, Mattoo TK, et al. Antimicrobial prophylaxis for children with vesicoureteral reflux. *N Engl J Med*. 2014;370(25):2367-2376.
52. Johnson JR, Clabots C, Kuskowski MA. Multiple-host sharing, long-term persistence, and virulence of *Escherichia coli* clones from human and animal household members. *J Clin Microbiol*. 2008;46(12):4078-4082.
104. Rogers BA, Sidjabat HE, Paterson DL. *Escherichia coli* O25b-ST131: a pandemic, multiresistant, community-associated strain. *J Antimicrob Chemother*. 2011;66(1):1-14.
120. Stoll BJ, Hansen NI, Bell EF, et al. Neonatal outcomes of extremely preterm infants from the NICHD Neonatal Research Network. *Pediatrics*. 2010;126(3): 443-456.
132. Wright KJ, Seed PC, Hultgren SJ. Uropathogenic *Escherichia coli* flagella aid in efficient urinary tract colonization. *Infect Immun*. 2005;73(11):7657-7668.

The full reference list for this chapter is available at ExpertConsult.com.

104 Diarrhea-Causing and Dysentery-Causing *Escherichia coli*

Jorge J. Velarde • James P. Nataro

Escherichia coli has been long recognized as the most common facultative anaerobe in the human gastrointestinal tract. Virtually all *Homo sapiens* (and most other mammals) harbor this bacterium. Yet within the *E. coli* biomass lurk highly evolved pathogenic subtypes that have adapted themselves to a new niche—human pathogenicity. These pathotypes may prefer the gastrointestinal tract, the genitourinary tract, or disseminated sites (including the meninges)—the last almost exclusively in neonates. This chapter focuses on *E. coli* associated with enteric infections.

The first implication of *E. coli* with diarrhea occurred more than 75 years ago, when Adam[3] postulated the existence of a group of "dyspepsia" *E. coli* responsible for neonatal and infantile diarrhea. In the 1940s, Bray reported that many, but not all, *E. coli* from severe infant diarrhea cases in summer agglutinated with antiserum prepared from a diarrheal isolate, whereas *E. coli* organisms from other sources did not.[13] The isolate used by Bray to develop the antiserum was later serotyped by the Kauffman scheme as O111:B4, one of the now classic serogroups of enteropathogenic *E. coli* (EPEC) (Table 104.1). Although this initial description was made possible by serologic fingerprinting, the advent of molecular biology rapidly produced a plethora of reports describing the several discrete *E. coli* pathotypes.

CAUSATIVE ORGANISMS

Six distinct diarrheogenic pathotypes are recognized currently on the basis of clinical, biochemical, and molecular or genetic criteria (Table 104.2) as follows:

1. Enterotoxigenic *E. coli* (ETEC), a major cause of traveler's diarrhea and infant diarrhea in developing countries, elaborates the heat-stable enterotoxin, the heat-labile enterotoxin, or both and causes infection of the small intestine.
2. EPEC, the original pathotype defined by Bray,[13] causes infant diarrhea in less-developed countries. The bacteria induce a characteristic attaching and effacing lesion in the small intestine. Classic EPEC requires the chromosomally encoded locus of enterocyte effacement (LEE) and a high-molecular-weight virulence plasmid termed EPEC adherence factor (EAF) plasmid.
3. Enterohemorrhagic *E. coli* (EHEC) causes outbreaks of hemorrhagic colitis and hemolytic-uremic syndrome (HUS) in temperate climates. The essential virulence factor is the Shiga toxin, which circulates through the bloodstream and acts by inhibition of protein synthesis in the target cell.
4. Enteroinvasive *E. coli* (EIEC) is an unusual cause of diarrhea and dysentery. It is similar to *Shigella* epidemiologically and pathogenetically and shares similar virulence genes.
5. Enteroaggregative *E. coli* (EAEC) causes diarrhea in individuals of all ages in industrialized and less-developed countries and in travelers. The organism adheres to the intestinal mucosa and secretes several enterotoxins and cytotoxins.[142]
6. Diffusely adherent *E. coli* (DAEC) is a highly heterogeneous pathotype; its association with diarrhea is controversial. The epidemiologic scenario for this organism has not been well elucidated.

TRANSMISSION AND EPIDEMIOLOGY

Diarrheogenic *E. coli* strains are worldwide in distribution. The route of infection is fecal-oral, predominantly via contaminated food and water, although person-to-person transmission may occur with EHEC and possibly EPEC in infants.[175] As discussed subsequently, environmental contamination by EHEC is an emerging problem in industrialized countries, whereas ETEC continues to be ubiquitous worldwide. Table 104.3 lists the age-specific predilections of the various *E. coli* pathogens.

Enterotoxigenic *Escherichia coli*

The infectious dose for ETEC is approximately 10^8 bacteria.[69] The incubation period is 14 to 50 hours.[171] Transmission typically occurs via contamination of food and water,[232] and person-to-person transmission is thought to be uncommon due to its high infectious dose. In developing countries, contamination of food and water sources occurs commonly.[208] ETEC has been detected in the United States in numerous food samples, including cheese, hamburger, sausage, and seafood.[116,159,232] A domestic US outbreak of diarrhea at Crater Lake National Park in Oregon was traced to ETEC organisms in the water supply.[226] Additional outbreaks in developed countries have been described.[47,76,152,199] Because large numbers of organisms are required for experimental infection, transmission probably would require multiplication of the inoculum within the vehicle, which probably contributes to the well-documented propensity of ETEC infection to occur in warm months.[208]

ETEC is a major cause of diarrhea in infants and children in the developing world.[92,208] The incidence typically increases during the first 6 months of life and decreases after 2 years. ETEC has been estimated to cause approximately 20% of diarrheal episodes in the developing world,[208] although this percentage varies substantially by location. A

TABLE 104.1 Serotypes Characteristic of the Diarrheogenic Pathotypes of *Escherichia coli*

Enteropathogenic	Enterotoxigenic	Enteroinvasive	Enterohemorrhagic	Enteroaggregative
O44:H34	O6:H–, 12, 16, 40	O28:H–	O26:H11	Nontypeable
O55:H6, 7, 32	O8:H–, 42	O29:H–	O77:H18	Rough
O86:H2, 34	O25:H–, 42	O32:H–	O103:H2	O3:H2
O111:H2, 7, 12	O27:H7	O42:H–	O104:H21	O6:H1
O114:H2	O29:H21	O89:H–	O111:H8	O11:H16
O119:H6	O63:H–, 12	O112:H–	O113:H21	O15:H21
O124:H?	O78:H11, 12	O121:H–	O128:H2	O44:H18
O125:H21	O117:H4	O124:H–	O145:H–	O92:H23
O127:H4, 6, 21	O125:H30	O136:H–	O157:H–, 7	O111:H21
O128:H2, H21	O126:H10, 27	O144:H–	O178:H19	O126:H2, 27, H–
O142:H6, 34	O127:H2	O152:H–		O104:H4
O158:H23	O128:H8, 35			
	O143:H–			
	O146:H39			
	O148:H28			
	O153:H45			
	O159:H4, 21			

TABLE 104.2 Relationship of *Escherichia coli* Virulence Genes to Clinical Patterns of Diarrhea

Pathogen Group	VIRULENCE GENES										Clinical Disease
	EAF	A/E	LA	AA	LT/ST	CFA	Afa/Dr/F1845	Invasion Factors	Stx	ShET-2	
ETEC	–	–	–	–	+	+	–	–	–	–	Watery
EPEC	+	+	+	–	–	–	–	–	–	–	Watery
EHEC	–	+	–	–	–	–	–	–	+	–	Bloody (hemorrhagic colitis)
EIEC	–	–	–	–	–	–	–	+	–	+	Bloody (dysentery)
EAEC	–	–	–	+	+[a]	–	–	–	–	–	Watery (persistent)
DAEC	–	–	–	–	–	–	+	+	–	–	Watery

[a]Enteroaggregative stable toxin (EAST) is a member of the ST family.

AA, autoaggregative attaching pattern; *A/E*, attaching and effacing changes; *CFA*, colonization factor antigens; *Afa/Dr/F1845*, DAEC adherence factors; invasion factors, chromosomal and plasmid factors mediating cell invasion; *EAEC*, enteroaggregative *E. coli; EAF*, EPEC adherence factor; *EHEC*, enterohemorrhagic *E. coli; EIEC*, enteroinvasive *E. coli; EPEC*, enteropathogenic *E. coli; ETEC*, enterotoxigenic *E. coli; LA*, localized adherence pattern; *LT/ST*, heat-labile and heat-stable toxins; *ShET-2*, plasmid-encoded Shigella enterotoxin-2, highly homologous to the plasmid-encoded EIEC toxin; *Stx*, Shiga family cytotoxins.

TABLE 104.3 Age-Related Patterns of *Escherichia coli* Diarrhea

Pathogen Classification	Age at Highest Risk	CHARACTERISTICS OF DIARRHEA		
		Bloody	Watery	Inflammatory
EAEC	<6 mo	–	+++	–
EPEC	<1 y	–	+++	–
ETEC	<2 y	–	+++	–
EIEC	>2 y	++	+	+++
EHEC	2-10 y	+++	+	–
DAEC	>1 y	–	+++	–

DAEC, Diffusely adherent *E. coli; EAEC*, enteroaggregative *E. coli; EHEC*, enterohemorrhagic *E. coli; EIEC*, enteroinvasive *E. coli; EPEC*, enteropathogenic *E. coli; ETEC*, enterotoxigenic *E. coli.*

study in rural Egypt found that ETEC accounted for 66% of all first episodes of diarrhea, with an incidence of 1.7 episodes per child-year during the first 6 months of life and 2.3 during the second 6 months.[211] In Tehran, researchers found that ETEC could be isolated from 15.5% of patients younger than 5 years old with diarrhea.[236] The prevalence was 18% in Bangladesh,[207] 33% to 37.5% in Mexico,[56,75] and 20.5% among children with diarrhea in Nicaragua.[288] A study in Hanoi found, however, that only 2.2% of diarrheal episodes could be attributed to ETEC.[182] Prevalence was 9.2% in a study in the Brazilian northeast,[185] and the frequency in Mongolia[240] was similarly low. A large multicenter case-control study of moderate-to-severe diarrhea among children under 5 years of age at seven sites in sub-Saharan Africa and south Asia implicated ETEC consistently among the top five etiologic pathogens.[135] In this study, STh-producing strains accounted for the large majority of attributable cases.

ETEC disease is primarily a childhood problem, with the incidence decreasing after the child reaches 5 years of age.[207,208] After infection with a particular ETEC strain, the host is resistant to disease but still may excrete the organism asymptomatically, a characteristic that contributes to the environmental burden.[175,266] Adults still may be susceptible to ETEC diarrhea.[92,208] In a study of elderly individuals in Dhaka, Bangladesh, researchers found that 13% of adults older than 60 years with diarrhea were noted to have ETEC.[77] Although the incidence of ETEC diarrhea decreases after age 5 years, the incidence seems to increase again in patients older than 15 years, and 25% of ETEC infections are seen in adults.[207,208]

ETEC is the most common cause of traveler's diarrhea, typically accounting for approximately 30% to 40% of cases, except in southeast Asia where it has been found to account for approximately 7% of cases.[2,120,243,248] Illness is acquired by ingestion of contaminated food or water. The diarrhea is acute and watery and typically resolves spontaneously without severe limitation of activities.[2]

ETEC organisms are extremely diverse, and children in endemic areas experience multiple infections. The basis of immunity, which increases with repeated exposure, is unknown.[266] Strains producing heat-stable enterotoxin cause more severe disease than strains producing only heat-labile enterotoxin, and the former is not immunogenic. Colonization of the small intestinal mucosa is mediated by surface fimbriae termed *colonization factor antigens*, which are immunogenic and may elicit some element of protective immunity.[212] Despite the existence of more than 25 known colonization factor antigens (or CFAs), a few are overrepresented among clinical isolates;[184,231,249,288] in a study from Bangladesh for instance, seven colonization factor antigens constituted more than 75% of the colonization factor antigens isolated.[207] In an analysis of multiple studies, Wolf [296] suggested that most ETEC express colonization factor antigens I, II (CS1, CS2, CS3), or IV (CS4, CS5, CS6). A recent study looking at more than 360 ETEC isolates from around the world also suggested that there are multiple lineages with CFA and associated toxin profiles that appear to be stable over time.[291] Of note, in some epidemiologic studies, more than 50% of strains do not express known colonization factor antigens.[249,250] This may be second to the presence of colonization factor antigens that are as yet unrecognized.[170] ETEC is predominantly an infection of warm weather months in endemic areas, coincident with conditions promoting bacterial replication in the environment. Some sites report that a second peak occurs after the rainy season.[207,208]

Enteropathogenic *Escherichia coli*

Neter and associates[181] first coined the term EPEC to denote a group of *E. coli* serotypes associated with dramatic and highly lethal nursery outbreaks of diarrhea in the United States and the United Kingdom (see Table 104.1). We now recognize that these serotype antigens serve as surrogate markers for a package of chromosomal and plasmid-borne virulence genes, which together orchestrate enteric pathogenesis.[137,179,299] The epidemiology of EPEC has changed since its original description was provided. Gone are the lethal outbreaks formerly reported in industrialized countries, to be replaced by sporadic endemic disease in resource-poor countries. The infection retains its dramatic predilection for infants and children younger than 24 months, is rarely seen in older children and adults, and is not a cause of traveler's diarrhea.[55,56,93,135,281] The basis of this age-dependent incidence is unknown.

Globally, EPEC is among the most common causes of infant diarrhea.[55,56,93,188,189,221] EPEC has a propensity to cause persistent infection and wasting, suggesting that its burden may comprise more than simple dehydration. Breast-feeding offers some protection against EPEC because of the presence of immune factors and oligosaccharides that inhibit adherence of EPEC to epithelial cells.[58] In industrialized countries such as the United States, EPEC generally is no longer considered to be a cause of endemic diarrhea, although EPEC may be present in infants immigrating from or visiting resource-poor settings. Rare indigenous cases may occur.[95] In an outpatient setting in the United States, two of 147 cases of nondysenteric acute diarrhea were caused by EPEC.[38] In 166 Swiss children admitted to hospitals with diarrhea, 13 (7.8%) had EPEC isolated from stool cultures.[74]

As noted previously, EPEC strains of the classic serotypes (also known as typical EPEC) require the chromosomal locus of enterocyte effacement (LEE) and the EPEC adherence factor plasmid (encoding the bundle-forming pilus, or BFP) to cause diarrhea. Controversy exists over whether so-called atypical EPEC (which are positive for the locus of enterocyte effacement and negative for BFP) are a cause of diarrhea.[172] Several studies and outbreak descriptions suggest there is a relationship.[4,52,220,300] Other studies, however, have failed to identify atypical EPEC as a cause of diarrhea.[135,177] Recent molecular epidemiologic studies have suggested that atypical EPEC may require a chromosomally encoded adhesion factor termed Efa1,[5,189] which may substitute for the EPEC plasmid-encoded BFP.

Enterohemorrhagic *Escherichia coli*

Since its discovery in 1977, EHEC has emerged as an important and increasingly common human pathogen. Although most occurrences of disease are sporadic and not all occurrences are related to ground beef,[276] EHEC is notably carried asymptomatically in cattle and other ruminants, from whence it can be transmitted widely. The organisms may be excreted by cattle herds, and large outbreaks of human infection have been associated with the ingestion of undercooked hamburger and other foods contaminated directly and indirectly by cattle manure. Careful prospective epidemiologic surveillance in Minnesota revealed an increase in the incidence of EHEC from 0.5 to 2 per 100,000 children younger than 18 years old during the period 1979 to 1988,[155] similar to the incidence of EHEC determined in the state of Washington in the late 1980s: 2.1 per 100,000. Recent data from the CDC FoodNet surveillance network in 2012 indicated current incidence rates in the United States of 1.11 cases of O157 STEC and 1.16 cases of non-O157 STEC per 100,000 population.[45] In a multicenter study of mild acute diarrhea in outpatients in the United States, five (3.4%) of 147 cases were caused by EHEC,[38] a frequency similar to that in Swiss children hospitalized for community-acquired diarrhea.[74] Very young children are not commonly infected; rather, infection occurs most commonly and severely in children 2 to 10 years old or in the elderly.

Ground beef is identified as the most common source of EHEC infection. Several outbreaks have been associated with fast-food consumption.[210] In meat-processing plants where bulk ground beef is prepared for the fast-food industry, meat from one contaminated carcass can contaminate and distribute the organisms to a huge number of beef patties. Several other food sources of transmission that have been documented include other beef; produce, including spinach and lettuce; milk; water; and processed foods, including unpasteurized apple cider, mayonnaise, and dry fermented sausage. Person-to-person, cattle-to-person, and waterborne outbreaks have been described. Person-to-person spread as sequelae of point-source epidemics is common.[247] Many unusual modes of transmission linked with cattle have occurred and include poorly washed apples dropped in cow pastures and used to make cider, surface water supplies in proximity to areas where cattle graze, spread of aerosolized particles at agricultural fairs, and transmission by contact at petting zoos. Contaminated swimming holes have been implicated in several outbreaks.

A multistate outbreak of O157:H7 EHEC infections associated with the consumption of fresh bagged spinach occurred in the United States in 2006, affecting 26 states and resulting in 205 confirmed illnesses, 103 hospitalizations, 31 cases of hemolytic-uremic syndrome, and three deaths.[15,39] This outbreak exemplifies the widespread effect of a foodborne outbreak caused by the mass production and distribution of produce.

Hemolytic-uremic syndrome is a not infrequent sequelae of EHEC-associated infection. A review of O157:H7 outbreaks (defined as two or more cases) reported to the Centers for Disease Control and Prevention in the United States from 1982 to 2002 found 350 outbreaks representing 8598 cases, 1493 (17%) hospitalizations, 354 (4%) cases of hemolytic-uremic syndrome, and 40 (0.5%) deaths.[210] During a large outbreak of *E. coli* O157:H7 infection associated with fast-food restaurant hamburgers on the West Coast of the United States in 1993, of the 732 affected individuals identified, 195 were admitted to the hospital, hemolytic-uremic syndrome developed in 55 (7.5%), and four died.[95] Investigation of this outbreak showed that small numbers of bacteria (in the range of a few hundred) constituted an infectious dose. Among 93 cases of O157:H7 infection reported in Washington State in 1987, hemolytic-uremic syndrome or thrombotic thrombocytopenic purpura developed in 11 (12%), for an approximate incidence of 0.23 per 100,000.[196]

The highest incidence of hemolytic-uremic syndrome occurs in children younger than 5 years, in whom the age-specific incidence ranged from 2.6 to 5.8 per 100,000 in Minnesota,[155] Washington,[196] and Oregon.[224] More recently, improvements in animal processing and public health interventions including detection and investigation of outbreaks has lead to a U.S. national decrease in the incidence of hemolytic-uremic syndrome to less than one case per 100,000.[43] The incidence of hemolytic-uremic syndrome in Argentina was reported in 2002 as 12.2 per 100,000 children younger than 5 years, which is among the highest reported incidence of hemolytic-uremic syndrome in the world.[148,219]

In the United Kingdom and the United States, hemolytic-uremic syndrome is associated predominantly with Stx2-producing *E. coli* O157:H7[155,197]; however, this finding may represent more facile detection of this serotype. In addition, the incidence of non-O157:H7 infections in the United States is increasing (serotypes associated with EHEC infection are presented in Table 104.1).[35,122,295] In Argentina, non-O157:H7, Stx2-producing strains are commonly isolated.[148,219] Similarly, in Australia, other serotypes, especially O111, have been associated with major outbreaks and a significant number of hemolytic-uremic syndrome cases.[41] Many of these serotypes have been implicated in sporadic and outbreak disease in the United States[33] (e.g., an outbreak caused by O104:H21 acquired from contaminated milk[42]).

Non-O157:H7 EHEC infections have increased in prevalence in the United States and are now known to account for 20% to 50% of all EHEC infections.[45,122] Although some non-O157 strains are not pathogenic, others have been shown to cause disease as severe as that caused by O157:H7 strains, suggesting that a clinical suspicion for EHEC should be maintained even when testing for O157:H7 is negative.[122] Non-O157, Stx-producing *E. coli* infection was made a reportable disease in the United States in 2000.[35]

In 2011, a large, international outbreak of hemorrhagic colitis and hemolytic-uremic syndrome occurred due to a Shiga toxin *E. coli* of serotype O104:H4.[117] The outbreak originated in Germany, and was traced to the consumption of contaminated fenugreek sprouts, most likely coming from Egypt. More than 4000 infections were identified among 16 countries, resulting in more than 50 deaths.[44] Interestingly, the implicated pathogen was an enteroaggregative *E. coli* strain which had become lysogenized with the Shiga toxin-encoding phage. Such strains had previously been identified, and may become an emerging threat.[117]

Hemolytic-uremic syndrome occurs seasonally in the United States and Canada (most common during the summer months), although no specific seasonal risk factor or factors for infection with Shiga toxin-producing *E. coli* are known. Other epidemiologic data suggest that poor children are at lower risk for the development of hemolytic-uremic syndrome, perhaps because they already have immunity to EHEC or Shiga toxins through early contact with the organisms in their environment.[50]

Enteroinvasive *Escherichia coli*

EIEC is closely related to *Shigella* microbiologically and pathogenetically. The pathotype typically is found in areas with a high burden of *Shigella*. The infectious dose may be higher than that of *Shigella*, and person-to-person transmission seldom is reported. Foodborne outbreaks occur sporadically.[94,154] The first description of EIEC as a pathotype occurred in 1971, when bloody diarrhea was traced to the consumption of French Camembert cheese contaminated with *E. coli* O124.[154] Small outbreaks or sporadic cases involving a limited number of serotypes have been reported from numerous countries, including the United States, France, Japan, and Brazil.[154,190,259,282,285] The prevalence varies by region. In a rural community in Ecuador up to 20.5% of diarrheal cases were due to EIEC[230]; in Tunisia 11.3% of children with diarrhea had EIEC.[10] Prospective studies in Thailand using DNA probes for EIEC pathogenicity genes indicated that 6% of cases of dysentery may be caused by EIEC strains.[70] Studies in Nicaragua, South India, Vietnam, Gabon, Tanzania, Denmark, and multiple sites in Africa including Kenya, Ghana, and Nigeria, demonstrated low to nondetectable rates of EIEC.[108,169,191,192,209,216,237] The epidemiology of the cases is complicated by the fact that in contrast to the initial descriptions of EIEC-associated disease, most EIEC infections probably are neither dysenteric nor characterized by bloody diarrhea but instead manifest as watery diarrhea with low-grade fever, similar to that caused by viral agents and ETEC.

Infection with 10^8 bacteria has been shown to be necessary for experimental dysentery in human volunteers,[69] a dose substantially higher than that for *Shigella* spp. ($<10^4$ organisms). In a foodborne outbreak caused by a nontypeable EIEC, secondary person-to-person transmission was not reported.[259]

Enteroaggregative *Escherichia coli*

EAEC was implicated first as a cause of diarrheal disease in studies of children in Chile, Mexico, and India.[26,27,57,176] The pathogenicity of at least some EAEC strains has been established by several observations. First, volunteer studies by Nataro and associates[174] revealed that some EAEC could elicit diarrhea in healthy subjects, whereas other strains may not be pathogenic. Second, EAEC strains have been implicated in outbreaks of diarrhea, the largest of which involved nearly 2700 schoolchildren in Japan.[102,115,301] A metaanalysis performed by Huang and colleagues[112] of more than 20 years of studies revealed convincingly that EAEC is a cause of diarrhea in infants; adults, especially those with human immunodeficiency virus (HIV) and acquired immunodeficiency syndrome (AIDS) in developing countries; children in industrialized countries; and adult travelers to less-developed areas. In addition, a study from the United States by Nataro and colleagues[177] suggested that EAEC was the most frequent bacterial cause of diarrhea among all ages in Baltimore, Maryland, and New Haven, Connecticut.

A persisting controversy surrounding EAEC epidemiology and pathogenesis is the definition of the pathotype. The metaanalysis described earlier implicated EAEC, as defined by the characteristic stacked-brick adherence pattern to epithelial cells in culture.[112] A study of infant diarrhea in Cincinnati suggested, however, that only strains hybridizing with an EAEC gene probe (see later) were truly associated with clinical diarrhea.[52] A full understanding of what constitutes a truly pathogenic EAEC strain is unavailable.

Diffusely Adherent *Escherichia coli*

The association between DAEC and diarrhea remains controversial. When DAEC was given to adult volunteers, it failed to convincingly elicit symptoms.[272] Additionally, this strain has been found in both healthy individuals and patients with diarrhea.[191,246] An age-related association may exist in children older than 12 to 18 months.[124,175,193,242,264] Of note, the commonly used *daaC* probe has been found to cross-react with some strains of EAEC, which may have led to overestimation of DAEC in some studies.[258] Finally, DuPont and colleagues[163] suggest that DAEC may also play a role in traveler's diarrhea cases previously identified as pathogen negative.

CLINICAL MANIFESTATIONS

Diarrhea-causing *E. coli* may be responsible for a variety of clinical syndromes because virtually all known mechanisms of diarrhea, including secretory toxins, cytotoxic toxins, invasion, and pathogenic adherence, are manifested by the various *E. coli* pathotypes. The clinical manifestations are largely a function of the complement of virulence genes (see Table 104.2), and identification of the essential pathogenicity genes provides the definitive diagnostic maneuver. As with other pathogens, invasive *E. coli* strains (i.e., EIEC) produce inflammatory diarrhea with fever, abdominal pain, nausea, vomiting, and leukocytes and blood in the stool. Noninvasive, cytotoxin-producing EHEC strains cause a frankly bloody diarrhea associated with leukocytosis but without fecal leukocytes or fever. Producers of heat-labile or heat-stable enterotoxins (i.e., ETEC) elicit brisk, watery diarrhea with the potential for significant dehydration.

Enterotoxigenic *Escherichia coli*

ETEC causes watery, nonmucoid, nonbloody diarrhea in infants, older children, and adults, and it is a common cause of traveler's diarrhea.[208] The onset of diarrhea is abrupt, with an incubation period of 14 to 50 hours.[171] The frequency of stools varies from a few to more than 10 per day, and a striking absence of leukocytes is noted when the diarrheal stool is examined by light microscopy. Young affected children may vomit and commonly are febrile (38°C to 40°C), although adults typically are afebrile. ETEC disease cannot be distinguished clinically from most other causes of acute nonspecific watery diarrhea. The illness usually is self-limited to 3 to 5 days but occasionally lasts more than 1 week. Severely dehydrating illness that resembles clinical cholera can occur but is uncommon.

Variability in the clinical picture may be due to age differences and preexisting immunity, but it also may be attributed to differences in the infecting inoculum. DuPont and colleagues[69] produced mild diarrhea (three watery stools per day for 2 to 3 days) when 10^8 bacteria were fed to adult volunteers, whereas 10^{11} organisms caused more pronounced diarrhea (more than five stools per day for 4 to 5 days), with mucus but no blood observed in some subjects. Many subjects also had abdominal cramping, but no tenesmus was present, and all remained afebrile. This clinical picture is typical of traveler's diarrhea in adults.[165]

ETEC diarrhea can result in severe dehydration necessitating aggressive fluid therapy.

Enteropathogenic *Escherichia coli*

EPEC diarrhea typically is copious and watery, without blood or fecal leukocytes.[143] Patients may have low-grade fever. In a Swiss study conducted with modern diagnostic methods, the mean age of 13 hospitalized children with EPEC diarrhea was 1.4 years (range, 0.5 to 3 years).[74] Fever was low-grade, and vomiting occurred in 69%. Volume depletion was considered moderate in five children and severe in two. Although nursery outbreaks no longer occur commonly, severe illness still can develop in infants infected with EPEC,[119] with high mortality rates ranging from 25% to 70%.[63] The cause of death of patients in nursery outbreaks is not well documented. Investigations using an experimental EPEC infection model in adult volunteers (who are not naturally susceptible) revealed that watery diarrhea occurred 3 to 16 hours after inoculation and generally lasted less than 2 days. Diarrhea occasionally was copious and in some cases was associated with abdominal cramps, nausea, vomiting, malaise, and fever.[65] This clinical picture is consistent with disease caused by outbreaks of EPEC in adults.

EPEC also has been implicated in chronic diarrhea in the United States and elsewhere, with serious nutritional consequences that may require total parenteral nutrition and hospital stays of 120 days.[227] In prospective studies of EPEC diarrhea in young infants in Brazil[93] and Ethiopia,[280] fever, vomiting, and dehydration all were observed commonly. The clinical significance of chronic diarrhea may be increased by the underlying malnutrition of infants in resource-poor countries. In many settings, especially where effective oral rehydration programs are in place, chronic diarrhea and associated malnutrition are now more important causes of diarrheal deaths than are acute diarrhea and dehydration.[31]

In the course of the classic, severe nursery outbreaks caused by typical EPEC strains, the first signs and symptoms were mild and nonspecific, but they commonly were followed by vomiting and diarrhea of increasing severity. Stools contained neither mucus nor blood, and the volume fluctuated over a period of weeks. Plain abdominal radiographs revealed only nonspecific dilation of small bowel loops, although severe ileus not attributable to hypokalemia developed in many patients. Infected infants lost as much as 15% of body weight, leading to profound electrolyte disturbances and severe dehydration along with central nervous system manifestations, such as irritability, hypertonicity, seizures, and coma. Circulatory collapse occurred despite adequate replacement of fluids and achievement of electrolyte balance. In an epidemic in Virginia, Belnap and O'Donnell[22] described fatal infections caused by *E. coli* O111:B4 occurring after 3 weeks of illness and associated with renal failure, coma, and signs of disseminated intravascular coagulation, but blood cultures typically remained negative. The fatality rate was age dependent; although the overall mortality rate was 16%, the rate in neonates was 40%. Recent epidemiologic studies suggest that typical EPEC may be common causes of diarrhea in parts of Africa with high HIV/AIDS burden.[203] The etiologic link between HIV and EPEC is not clear.

The clinical description of atypical EPEC, when thought to be responsible for an outbreak, is similar to the presentation of typical EPEC.[4] Patients present with vomiting, diarrhea, and abdominal pain. They can also present with low-grade fever. Typically, no macroscopic blood is present but the stool can be hemoccult positive and fecal leukocytes have been described in a minority of patients. Atypical EPEC has also been associated with prolonged diarrhea greater than 14 days.[4,183]

Enterohemorrhagic *Escherichia coli*

In 1971, a distinctive clinical diarrheal syndrome was recognized that was characterized by afebrile bloody diarrhea in addition to cramping and colonic inflammatory changes, usually right-sided.[217] In 1983, this illness was associated with an otherwise rare *E. coli* serotype, O157:H7, and a characteristic syndrome, hemorrhagic colitis, was defined.[218] O157:H7 subsequently was recognized as the most virulent prototype of a Shiga toxin-producing pathotype designated EHEC. EHEC now has been shown to cause a wide spectrum of diseases that may be confined to the gastrointestinal tract or, in a sizable proportion (typically 5–10%), can become systemic.[21,276] After an incubation period of 3 to 4 days (range, 1–8 days), the local gastrointestinal illness usually begins with nonbloody diarrhea that can progress to bloody diarrhea after 1 or 2 days. Hemorrhagic colitis occurs in 50% to 90% of O157:H7 infections.[196,276]

Further progression may occur over the course of the next day or two and result in the passage of frank blood, the pathognomonic clinical feature of hemorrhagic colitis. Associated manifestations include vomiting in approximately 50% of patients and abdominal pain. Fever may occur but typically is low grade. This clinical picture may be confused with other conditions, such as appendicitis, intussusception, inflammatory bowel disease, ischemic colitis, and diverticulitis. The difficulty in establishing the diagnosis can lead to inappropriate drug therapy or even surgery.[96,113]

A serious complication of hemorrhagic colitis is the development of hemolytic-uremic syndrome.[96] Hemolytic-uremic syndrome is characterized by the triad of acute renal failure, thrombocytopenia, and hemolytic anemia and develops in approximately 10% to 20% of infected children younger than 10 years.[175] It is the most common cause of acquired renal failure in the United States.[283,284] The acute mortality rate is approximately 55%, and renal failure is expected to develop eventually in many more patients during the next several decades. After renal failure, cerebrovascular accident and colonic perforation are the most common serious sequelae. Thrombotic thrombocytopenic purpura and hemolytic-uremic syndrome have some overlapping clinical and pathologic features, but thrombotic thrombocytopenic purpura is increasingly regarded as a separate clinical entity that is not associated with an antecedent EHEC infection[275]; the separation is supported by its separate pathophysiology (see later discussion).

A prospective study in Canada identified *E. coli* O157:H7 in 15% of 125 patients with grossly bloody diarrhea over a 6-month period.[198] The age range was 15 months to 73 years; however, almost half of the patients were younger than 10 years old. The illness was similar to that described earlier, with a mean duration of 7.8 days, but it was significantly longer in children (9.1 ± 2 days) than in adults (6.6 ± 1.1 days). Sigmoidoscopy findings were abnormal in seven of eight adults examined, with hyperemic mucosa in six and superficial ulcerations in one. Biopsy samples showed mild mucosal inflammation in four of five patients. In another study, the findings on colonoscopy in 10 patients with hemorrhagic colitis caused by *E. coli* O157:H7 included severe inflammation (predominantly right sided), marked edema, easy hemorrhage, and the frequent appearance of longitudinal ulcer-like lesions.[253]

Because local and systemic manifestations in EHEC infection are caused, at least partially, by Shiga toxins, the presence of these same toxins in the intestinal lumen in patients with non-O157:H7 infection puts them at risk for development of hemorrhagic colitis and hemolytic uremic syndrome. Available longitudinal data suggest that O157:H7 infection results in more bloody diarrhea, hospitalization, and hemolytic-uremic syndrome than non-O157:H7 EHEC infection.[101,105]

Enteroinvasive *Escherichia coli*

Naturally acquired EIEC infection causes a mild to moderately severe dysentery syndrome consisting of fever, malaise, diarrhea, tenesmus, and abdominal cramping.[69,285] Watery diarrhea usually occurs at the onset of the illness and progresses to mucoid diarrhea with streaks of blood or microscopic hematochezia but rarely to the classic small-volume, grossly bloody, dysenteric stool seen with *Shigella* infection. Of 229 cases reported in one study, grossly bloody stool occurred in only four.[154] In two of these patients, sigmoidoscopy revealed superficial ulcerations in one and hyperemia alone in the second patient. As in *Shigella* infection, the stool reveals abundant polymorphonuclear cells, compatible with the inflammatory, invasive nature of the organism. Vomiting and dehydration can occur; the latter generally is mild. Fever of 38°C to 39.5°C (100.4°F to 103.1°F) is a typical symptom that occurs early in association with malaise, myalgia, and headache and lasts for 2 to 3 days. In most instances, the diarrhea ceases in 1 week or less, but in some patients, it may continue for 2 weeks or more.

In adult volunteers with experimentally induced EIEC disease, febrile illness developed approximately 11 hours (range 8 to 24 hours) after the inoculum was ingested.[69] Chills, myalgia, headache, and profuse diarrhea or abdominal cramps and tenesmus rapidly followed. In two of 13 subjects, this picture was associated with systemic toxicity and transient hypotension consistent with bacteremia, even though blood cultures were negative for all patients. Clinical dysentery with bloody stools occurred in several subjects, and reddened, friable mucosa with multiple bleeding points was seen by sigmoidoscopy. Clinical illness was controlled quickly with parenteral ampicillin therapy.

Enteroaggregative *Escherichia coli*

Descriptions of EAEC clinical features are derived from outbreak investigations, volunteer studies, and studies of traveler's diarrhea.[112] Most EAEC infections are accompanied by watery diarrhea, which may progress to persistent diarrhea that lasts 14 days or longer.[27,175,176] Bloody diarrhea is observed in a subset of patients.[57] An EAEC strain was implicated in a school lunch outbreak in Tajimi City, Japan, in 1993.[115] Of 6636 children who ate the school lunch at 16 schools, 2697 (rate of attack 40.6%) reported gastrointestinal symptoms. Major symptoms were abdominal pain (73.6%), nausea (51.1%), and diarrhea (39.9%). The incubation period for the onset of gastrointestinal illness was 40 to 50 hours on average. Duration of symptoms was not reported. A nursery outbreak in Serbia involved 19 normal infants.[51] All experienced watery diarrhea, which persisted beyond 2 weeks in three patients. A report of 17 pediatric patients with illness caused by EAEC of serotype O126:H27 in Israel suggested that patients typically manifested diarrhea (in all), vomiting (in eight), and fever (in 12, ≤40°C [104°F]).[251] In this report, one 6-week-old infant developed diarrhea persisting for 40 days. Studies in travelers suggest that EAEC disease may be mildly inflammatory, although fever and fecal leukocytes are present in a few patients.[112] Inflammation due to EAEC may be associated with growth faltering among children in developing countries even in the absence of frank diarrhea.[265]

The particularly severe epidemic linked to an O104:H4 Stx-producing EAEC strain[214] differed from O157:H7 induced disease in several ways. Sequelae were more severe in adults than children, and overall the frequency of hemolytic-uremic syndrome and death was unusually high. Diarrhea in patients infected with O104:H4 was similar to that described in patients infected with O157:H7, suggesting that presentation of Stx at the site of infection does not require a set of virulence factors unique to EHEC strains.

Diffusely Adherent *Escherichia coli*

The association between DAEC and diarrhea remains controversial. Typically in cases in which a relationship is thought to exist, it causes a watery diarrhea that can be prolonged.[175]

PATHOGENESIS

Enterotoxigenic *Escherichia coli*

ETEC was identified first as a porcine pathogen,[100,256] which elicited fluid secretion when injected into ligated ileal loops.[100] Two secretogenic activities were characterized; one could be inactivated by heating, and the other could not, and the activities could be found both in the same strain or independently. These activities now have been assigned to two well-characterized enterotoxins, heat-stable and heat-labile enterotoxins. The heat-labile enterotoxin is genetically, structurally, and mechanistically similar to cholera toxin produced by *Vibrio cholerae* O1 strains.[91,175] The heat-stable enterotoxin is actually two distinct toxins: STa (including closely related STI peptides STI-a and STI-b) is associated with human disease, whereas STb is associated with disease only in animals.[82,175]

The essential pathogenic strategy for ETEC involves colonization of the proximal small intestine, followed by release of one or both of the enterotoxins. Colonization of the intestinal epithelium (Fig. 104.1) is likely initially mediated by the ETEC flagella aided by the tip adhesin, EtpA.[228,229] The organism also secretes mucinases to facilitate access to epithelial cells.[84,83,136,151] Colonization then becomes dependent on proteinaceous, hair-like bacterial surface appendages termed *fimbriae* (or *pili*), of which greater than 25 antigenic types are known to exist.[170,296] As noted above, these adherence factors are termed *colonization factor antigens* or *coli surface antigens* (Fig. 104.2).[88]

Human STa is a small, nonimmunogenic molecule that is translated as a 72-amino acid polypeptide.[260] The first 19 amino acids serve as a signal sequence for secretion into the periplasmic space; a further cleavage event occurs after secretion, which results in the final 18- (ST-Ia) to 19- (ST-Ib) amino acid active peptide.[82,175,213] The sequence of the mature heat-stable enterotoxin has six cysteine residues that form stabilizing disulfide bonds, contributing to the high stability of the toxin to heat and proteases.[302] The heat-stable enterotoxin receptor on the apical surface of the intestinal epithelial cells is guanylyl cyclase C. This receptor is a large transmembrane protein with an extracellular ligand-binding domain and intracellular catalytic domain; binding to guanylyl cyclase C results in its activation, which is responsible for an increase in cellular cyclic guanosine monophosphate (cGMP).[244] cGMP is an intracellular signaling molecule that induces activation of apical chloride channels and inhibition of absorptive mechanisms, contributing to a secretory diarrhea.[81,97,166] The heat-stable enterotoxin exploits an endogenous signaling pathway, the natural agonist of which is the peptide guanylin, a natural controller of electrolyte homeostasis.[59]

The heat-labile family of toxins includes LT-I, which has significant homology in structure and function with cholera toxin, and LT-II, which

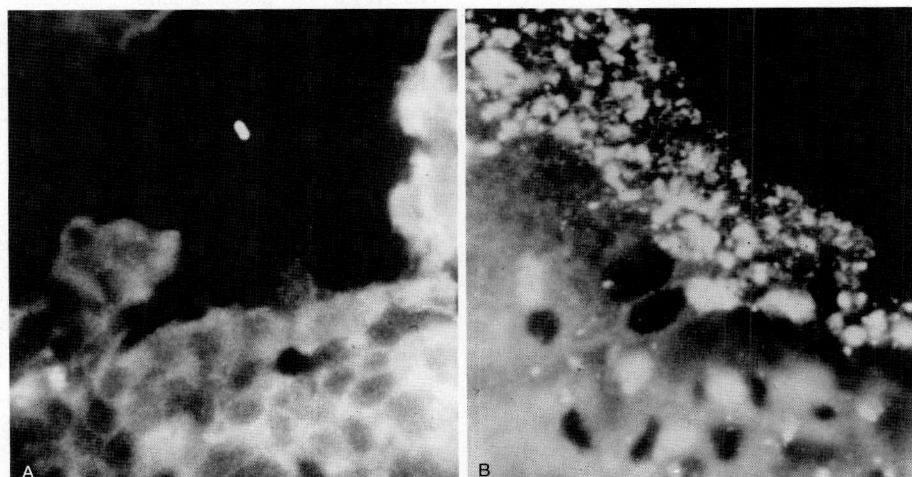

FIG. 104.1 (A) Laboratory-passaged avirulent *Escherichia coli* H10407 in infant rabbit intestine. No adherent colonizing bacteria are seen. (B) Fresh virulent H10407 organisms at the same time interval in infant rabbit intestine are closely adherent to the brush border (indirect immunofluorescent stained section, ×1000). (Courtesy Drs. Dolores and Doyle Evans, Department of Microbiology, Baylor College of Medicine.)

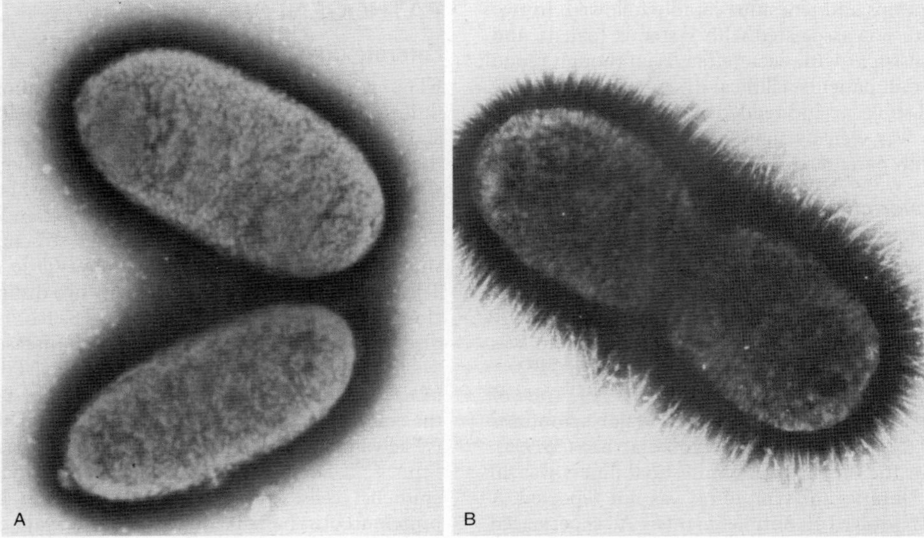

FIG. 104.2 (A) Electron micrograph of negatively stained cells of avirulent plasmid-cured *Escherichia coli* H10407. Note the bald appearance of the outer surface of the organism. (B) Similar view of virulent fresh *E. coli* H10407. Note the hairy surface of the organism as a result of colonization factor antigen I (×20,000). (Courtesy Drs. Dolores and Doyle Evans, Department of Microbiology, Baylor College of Medicine.)

does not seem to cause human or animal disease.[175] LT-I shares 80% identity with cholera toxin and similarly has an A_1-B_5 stoichiometry.[90,164,175,255,268] The 28-kd A subunit is the catalytically active moiety, whereas the 11-kd B subunit pentamer mediates cell binding and entry. Heat-labile enterotoxin interacts with G_{M1} gangliosides on the surface of the epithelial cells.[82,141,175] The A subunit is composed of two domains, termed A1 and A2, which are bound via a disulfide bond. A1 has adenosine diphosphate–ribosyl transferase activity, which targets the cellular guanosine triphosphate binding protein $G_{s\alpha}$, a regulator of cellular cyclic adenosine monophosphate (cAMP) levels. Ribosylation of $G_{s\alpha}$ leads to constitutive activation of adenylate cyclase, which greatly increases cAMP levels.[82,245] Increased cAMP leads to increased phosphorylation of chloride channels, especially the Cystic Fibrosis Transmembrane Conductance Regulator (CFTR), by protein kinase A, and increased chloride secretion, which also may contribute to secretory diarrhea.[82,245] The heat-labile enterotoxin additionally seems to promote *E. coli* adherence to epithelial cells, a function which is dependent on ADP-ribosylation, although the mechanism remains unclear.[121]

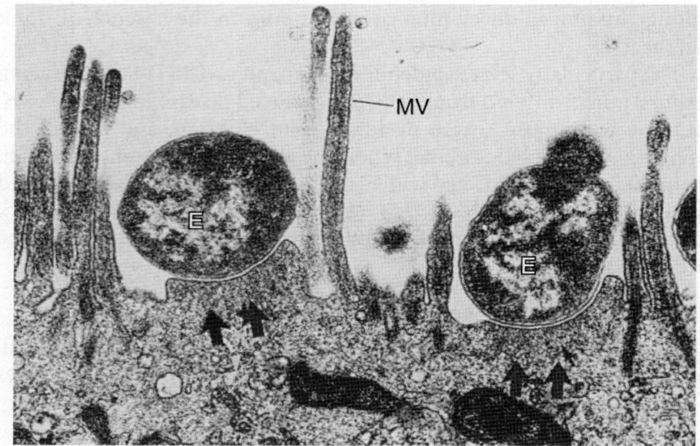

FIG. 104.3 High-power electron micrograph of intestinal epithelium infected by typical enteropathogenic *Escherichia coli* strains *(E),* with occasional intact microvilli *(MV)* and pedestal formation *(double arrows).* This figure shows not only the structural alterations and loss of the brush border but also the close apposition of the organisms to the epithelial cells. (Courtesy Ralph A. Gianella, Department of Medicine, University of Cincinnati School of Medicine.)

Enteropathogenic *Escherichia coli*

EPEC pathogenesis is complex and only partly understood. In contrast to ETEC, it possesses no potent secretogenic toxin but rather induces changes to the enterocyte signal transduction environment, which transforms the enterocyte from an absorptive cell to a secretory cell. EPEC pathogenesis has been described as a multistep process. The first step comprises attachment to the small bowel mucosa, an event mediated by the EPEC adherence factor plasmid-encoded, bundle-forming pilus. The bundle-forming pilus is a complex surface fimbrial structure, expressed by classical or typical EPEC, that may undergo contraction, not only tethering the bacteria to the cell but also pulling itself close to the cell's apical membrane.[133] Atypical EPEC are missing the bundle-forming pilus and must rely on other adhesion factors.[189] Approach of the bacteria is followed by induction of a characteristic lesion, termed *attaching and effacing.* Under electron microscopy, the normal microvillus architecture is dissolved, and the bacterium adheres tightly (<20 mm distance) to the now protruding cell membrane (Fig. 104.3). This deceptively simple phenotype is mediated and accompanied by a dizzying array of invisible changes to the cell's internal environment.[63]

Cellular changes are induced largely by a platoon of protein toxins that the bacterium injects directly into the cytoplasm of the target host cell. This injection process is mediated by a complex bacterial organelle termed an *injectisome,* also known as a *type III secretion system.* The first toxin injected is referred to as the *translocated intimin receptor* (Tir). Tir inserts itself into the apical plasma membrane, where it serves as the receptor for the bacterial outer membrane adhesion protein, *intimin.* As its name suggests, intimin mediates very close attachment of the bacterium to the cell and contributes to the resulting cytoskeletal damage.[46]

The net effect of Tir, intimin, and other injected toxins is dissolution of the microfilament and microtubule networks, phosphorylation of membrane ion transporters, and disruption of tight junctions at the cell's periphery.[137,179,299] Diarrhea apparently is caused by a combination of ion transport and paracellular leakage.[293] Release of proinflammatory cytokines may complete the pathogenic cascade. The relative contributions of each of these events to EPEC disease are unknown.[46]

EPEC adhere to HEp-2 epithelial cells in a characteristic localized pattern, which has been suggested as a diagnostic assay (Fig. 104.4).[63]

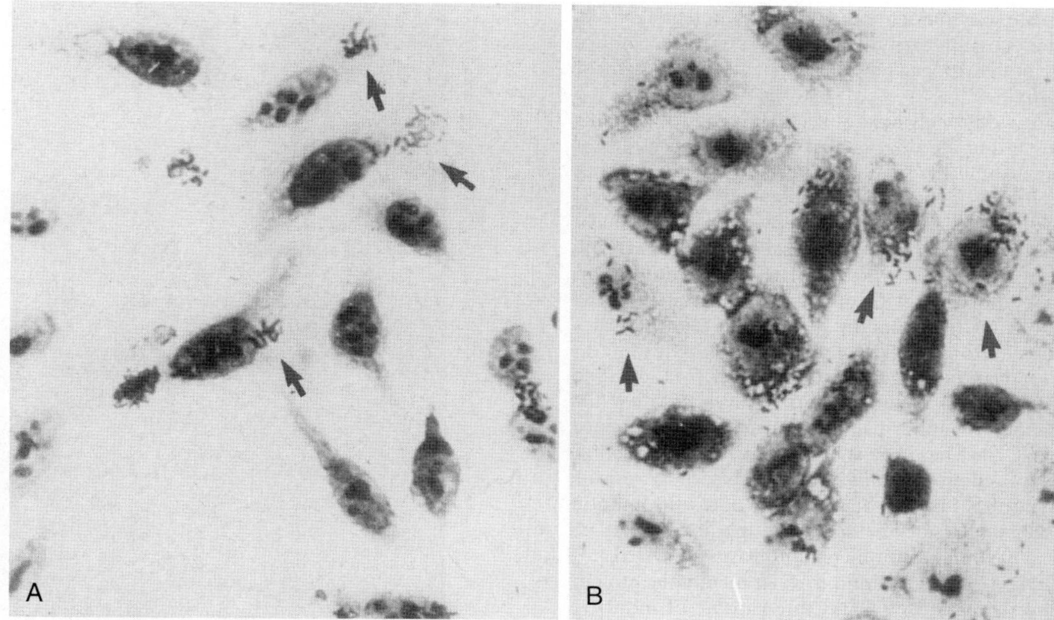

FIG. 104.4 Patterns of adherence of *Escherichia coli* to HEp-2 cells in tissue culture. Typical enteropathogenic *E. coli* associates with HEp-2 cells in the pattern shown in (A) termed localized adherence (LA). *Arrows* point to cells where growing microcolonies of bacteria are attached to focal areas of the cell membrane. Other *E. coli* organisms isolated from patients with diarrhea adhere over the entire HEp-2 cell membrane, as shown in the cells identified with *arrows* in (B). This pattern of interaction is termed diffuse adherence (DA). Although the LA phenotype has been associated definitively with the capacity to induce diarrhea in experimental models, evidence of virulence in DA strains remains controversial.

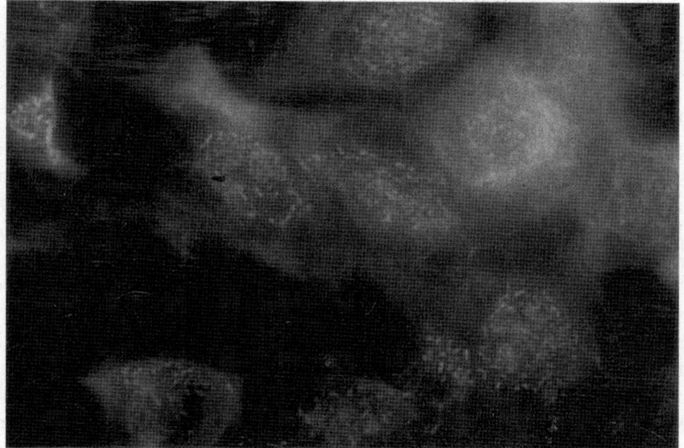

FIG. 104.5 Some *Escherichia coli* strains have the capacity to attach to the eukaryotic cell membrane and induce polymerization of actin beneath the membrane. This property may be shown by the fluorescent actin staining test, in which polymerized F-actin is detected by a fluorescein-tagged mushroom toxin specific for this form of actin. In this figure, the bacteria are attached to HEp-2 cells, and the induced actin polymerization revealed by the fluorescent reagent highlights the organisms, which are seen as bright rods on the infected cells.

Also, EPEC causes actin polymerization of target cells at sites of attachment, a virulence property readily detected in tissue culture (e.g., HEp-2 cells) by a fluorescent actin-staining test (Fig. 104.5).[132] As discussed subsequently, these phenotypic assays, although useful for pathogenesis studies, have largely been replaced by molecular diagnostic tests.

Enterohemorrhagic *Escherichia coli*

The cardinal pathogenic feature of the EHEC pathotype is the production of Shiga toxin, accompanied by a cohort of accessory virulence factors. As with EPEC, these factors are encoded by the bacterial chromosome and a high-molecular-weight virulence plasmid. Shiga toxin is encoded on a lysogenic phage, which is capable of infecting some non-EHEC *E. coli* strains. The full package of virulence genes has been well characterized in serotype O157:H7; studies which characterize locally obtained EHEC strains suggest that non-O157 pathogens are a heterogeneous group and tend to share some, but not all, of the virulence traits, accounting for their reduced virulence and frequency.[19,125,153] Shiga toxins were discovered by Konowalchuk and associates,[134] who reported finding Vero cell toxic activity in culture filtrates of certain strains of *E. coli* isolated from patients with diarrhea (Shiga toxin occasionally has been referred to by the archaic synonym *Vero toxin*).

Shiga toxins constitute a family of protein toxins that share identical enzymatic action and target cell binding specificity. Shiga toxins are subdivided into two families, Stx1 and Stx2, each consisting of the major Stx type and variants (i.e., Stx1c, Stx1d, Stx2c, Stx2c2, $Stx2d_{EH250}$, $Stx2d_{activatable}$, Stx2e, and Stx2f).[29] Stx2 and Stx2c have been associated with severe disease, including hemorrhagic colitis and hemolytic-uremic syndrome.[87,197] $Stx2d_{activatable}$ can be activated by mouse and human intestinal mucus and is associated with a severe clinical phenotype.[29] The greater pathogenicity of Stx2 may be due to greater accessibility of the active site on the Stx2 structure.[85] The *stx1* gene differs from the *Shigella stx* gene by three nucleotide changes, which result in a single conservative amino acid substitution in the A subunit: threonine to serine.[109]

Shiga toxins have the same structure and mechanism of action. They have an A_1-B_5 stoichiometry, comprising a single enzymatically active A subunit and a pentamer of B subunits responsible for toxin binding. The B subunits bind to globotrioacyl ceramide (Gb_3) and related glycolipids on host cells, including epithelial enterocytes, vascular endothelial cells, smooth muscle cells, renal endothelial cells, and erythrocytes.[66,139] The catalytic A subunit cleaves the *N*-glycosidic bond in a specific adenosine of the 28S rRNA in the 60S ribosomal subunit.[71] This single cleavage event results in irreversible cessation of protein synthesis and ultimately leads to cell death via multiple signal transduction pathways.[53] Intestinal villus cells are susceptible to the action of Shiga toxin, which includes reduced absorption of sodium. Data suggest that Shiga toxin induces local inflammatory cytokine production, with potential effects on epithelial cell and mucosal integrity. This host response may induce a vicious cycle because both hydrogen peroxide and neutrophils augment production of Shiga toxin.[292]

Epidemiologic evidence strongly links Shiga toxin-producing strains to hemorrhagic colitis and to the associated systemic complications of hemolytic-uremic syndrome.[95,127,218] The mechanisms underlying hemolytic-uremic syndrome are becoming clearer. Shiga toxin-induced disease appears to be due to the effects of toxin on vascular endothelial cells, possibly in concert with bacterial lipopolysaccharide. These activate secretion of a variety of cytokines, which initiate events resulting in endothelial cell injury and platelet thrombi, and subsequently, the characteristic thrombotic microangiopathy.[50,128,187] Shiga toxin activates complement and binds Factor H, a complement regulator, leading to excess complement activation and deposition.[54,194] Other possible pathophysiologic derangements include abnormal levels of von Willebrand factor, but whether this abnormality is a cause or a consequence of disease is unknown.[167] Stx1 has been shown to decrease production of prostacyclins; however, the role of this event in the pathogenesis of hemolytic-uremic syndrome is uncertain.[128] Of note, thrombotic thrombocytopenic purpura results from autoantibodies against or mutations in the von Willebrand factor metalloprotease ADAMTS13.[275]

Similar to EPEC, EHEC express the intimin outer membrane protein and a type III secretion apparatus.[175] EHEC are capable of inducing complex cytoskeletal alterations similar to those caused by EPEC infection, although certain subtle differences are observed. EHEC infects the human colon, whereas EPEC is an infection of the small bowel. The genes encoding intimin, Tir, the type III secretion system, and secreted proteins reside on a 35-kb pathogenicity island called the locus of enterocyte effacement, which may be more crucial for EPEC than for EHEC for virulence.[66] A 60-Md plasmid, pO157, which contains genes encoding an enterohemolysin, is commonly found in O157:H7 strains, but its role in production of disease is unclear.[175] Subtilase cytotoxin (SubAB), a novel cytotoxin with an A_1-B_5 stoichiometry, is associated with hemolytic-uremic syndrome in diverse EHEC strains in Australia and the United States.[130,202] SubAB is heat-stable, more toxic to Vero cells than Shiga toxin, and lethal when injected in mice.[130,202] Cytotoxicity is the result of direct cleavage of an endoplasmic reticulum chaperone protein, BiP.[201]

Enteroinvasive *Escherichia coli*

In 1967, Trabulsi and coworkers[282] in Brazil and Sakazaki and associates[235] in Japan described the isolation of certain *E. coli* serotypes from patients with a disease resembling bacillary dysentery, but with cultures negative for *Shigella*. These isolates possessed a critical virulence hallmark associated with *Shigella*—the ability to invade intestinal and other epithelial cells (Fig. 104.6).[187] They have been referred to as EIEC, and a limited number of serotypes, distinct from the EPEC O groups, but often cross-reactive with *Shigella* O antigens, have been found to possess this property (see Table 104.1). The genetic and molecular basis of invasion by *Shigella* was well defined in the 1990s, and the same plasmid and chromosomal genes encoding invasion properties and mechanisms seem to be present in EIEC as well.[111,144,200,238]

The invasive process for EIEC is thought to be the same as that for *Shigella* spp. It involves four main steps: (1) initial entry into cells, (2) intracellular multiplication, (3) intracellular and intercellular spread, and (4) host-cell killing. The process is complex and involves multiple genes on the invasion plasmid and the chromosome.[1,12,287] Intracellular *Shigella* and likely EIEC are able to escape autophagy/xenophagy.[12] They additionally take advantage of the immune response to promote an invasive phenotype.[287] EIEC produces toxins reported to be structurally distinct from the Stx of *Shigella dysenteriae* type 1 and the Shiga toxins 1 and 2 of EHEC.[78] Nonetheless, studies suggest that EIEC toxins possess many properties in common with the Shiga toxin family of toxins, including the ability to cause fluid secretion in animal models.[78] EIEC may contain a plasmid-borne gene that encodes a 63-kd protein called *ShET2* (*Shigella* enterotoxin 2); a mutation in this gene substantially decreases the enterotoxic activity of the parent strain.[178] The virulence of EIEC is notably less severe than *Shigella*. Several groups have noted that the expression of virulence genes by EIEC using in vitro models of infection is diminished as compared to *Shigella*.[261,263] However, the differences leading to less severe disease in vivo are still not clear.

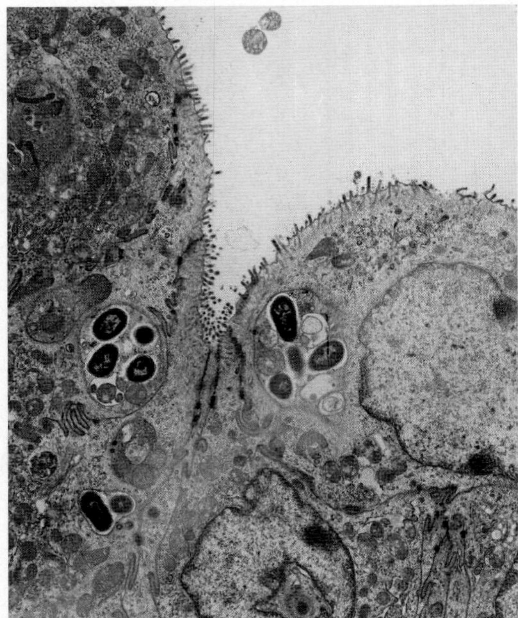

FIG. 104.6 Electron micrograph of enteroinvasive *Escherichia coli* infection of intestinal mucosa. The intracellular location of the bacteria clearly is seen within membrane-bound vesicles in two adjacent infected cells. The pathogenesis of enteroinvasive *E. coli* infection involves the invasion of intestinal cells and local cell-to-cell spread, as shown here, by a mechanism identical to that of *Shigella* spp. (Courtesy Saul Tzipori, DVM, Department of Comparative Medicine, Tufts University School of Veterinary Medicine.)

Enteroaggregative *Escherichia coli*

The pathogenesis of EAEC includes adherence to the intestinal epithelium as a thick biofilm, accompanied by mucus hypersecretion, intestinal damage, and induction of an inflammatory response. Most of these phenotypes seem to be mediated by a set of bacterial cytotoxins and enterotoxins.[103]

Adherence and colonization of the intestinal epithelium are mediated by pili called *aggregative adherence fimbriae,* of which several allelic variants exist. EAEC may colonize the large and small intestines.[107] All known aggregative adherence fimbriae variants are encoded on high-molecular-weight virulence plasmids collectively termed *pAA*. Also encoded on pAA is a transcriptional activator of the fimbrial genes, *AggR*. AggR is emerging as a global regulator of virulence functions in EAEC[67]; also under AggR control is a gene encoding a surface protein nicknamed *dispersin*. In the absence of dispersin, the aggregative adherence fimbriae adhesins collapse onto the surface of the bacterium.[305] Several cryptic genes, including a large chromosomal locus, also are under AggR control. One recently discovered gene product, termed Aar, acts to check AggR-mediated activation, resulting in finely tuned gene regulation.[239]

Damage to the intestinal mucosa has been linked to the presence of a secreted enterotoxin named plasmid-encoded toxin (*Pet*).[73] Pet is a protease that is internalized by target epithelial cells, where it cleaves cytoskeletal proteins, including spectrin. The net effect of these cleavage events is induction of fluid, secretion of electrolytes, and, ultimately, exfoliation of cells from the mucosal surface.[106]

EAEC strains also harbor a homologue of the ETEC heat-stable toxin, enteroaggregative heat-stable enterotoxin,[241] and a chromosomally encoded toxin called *Shigella* enterotoxin 1.[79] Inflammation by EAEC has been linked to the expression of the bacterial flagellum, although studies in polarized epithelial monolayers suggest that additional factors under control of AggR also are required.[103]

Diffusely Adherent *Escherichia coli*

As their name implies, DAEC are categorized by their adherence pattern on Hep-2 cells. Their pathogenesis is not well delineated. They characteristically contain nonfimbrial adhesins referred to as Afa/Dr adhesins (Afa/Dr DAEC). Along with a fimbrial adhesin, F1845 found in prototypical strain C1845 and a majority of DAEC strains, these adhesins bind to human decay-accelerating factor and, depending on the subtype of DAEC, carcinoembryonic antigen related molecules.[124,140,246] Binding then leads to invasion by a zipper-like mechanism[123] and a resulting inflammatory response.[17,23,24,40,246] Few virulence factors have been elucidated for DAEC. However, Sat, a member of the autotransporter family of toxins, has been found in DAEC strains thought to be diarrheagenic, causes lesions, triggers autophagy in vitro in epithelial cells, and causes intestinal damage in an animal model.[99,145,274]

DIAGNOSIS AND DIFFERENTIAL DIAGNOSIS

Diarrheogenic *E. coli* can be identified best by detecting their defining virulence genes. Many molecular tests are described for this purpose. The FDA has recently approved multiplex platforms for use in the diagnosis of enteric pathogens, including PCR-based techniques to identify multiple *E. coli* pathotypes (EPEC, ETEC, STEC, EIEC, EAEC) from patient samples.[36,304] However, these are not yet widely utilized. For most pathotypes, consultation with an expert, such as the senior author or the *E. coli* reference laboratories at the CDC, is recommended. Detection of *E. coli* generally is indicated for severe and persistent diarrhea lacking any other diagnosis (particularly in returning travelers) or in the setting of diarrheal outbreaks of unknown cause. With the exception of EHEC, most infections caused by diarrheogenic pathotypes are self-limiting.

Because of the potential of EHEC to cause serious sequelae, establishing a specific diagnosis is of clinical and epidemiologic importance. The earlier in the course of illness that a stool specimen is obtained, the more likely that *E. coli* O157:H7 will be recovered[277]; recovery more than 7 days after onset of diarrhea is unusual. The laboratory can use sorbitol-MacConkey agar to screen colonies for lack of sorbitol fermentation or substrates such as 4-methylumbelliferyl-β-D-glucuronide (MUG) for the production of γ-glucuronidase; *E. coli* O157:H7 is almost uniquely sorbitol negative and glucuronidase negative. These techniques have limited sensitivity, with the sensitivity of sorbitol-MacConkey agar reported as 50% to 60%.[129] Some sorbitol-fermenting O157:H7 isolates and many other sorbitol-fermenting, non-O157 EHEC capable of causing severe illness and hemolytic-uremic syndrome would be missed by sorbitol-MacConkey agar.

Detecting *Shiga* toxin in stool specimens, either directly or after overnight broth enrichment, currently is the most sensitive method for identifying EHEC after the first 7 days of illness.[129] These tests, immunoassays and PCR assays that identify shiga toxin 1 or 2 or *stx* genes, are more sensitive than culture techniques and are not dependent on serotype.[25,80,173] Despite the detection of Shiga toxin by these rapid assays, isolation of the organism, usually performed at reference laboratories, remains crucial for serotyping and other epidemiologic purposes. Serotype-specific commercial antigen immunoassays also are available.[173]

Diagnosis of ETEC traditionally would require identifying the heat-labile enterotoxin or heat-stable enterotoxin genes in an isolate or, after isolation and growth in vitro, by DNA probes or by detecting their products using enzyme-linked immunosorbent assay (ELISA). Multiplex PCR assays for detection of toxins and colonization factor antigens have been developed and are rapid, sensitive, and used with increasing frequency.[61,223] PCR techniques are additionally available that allow virulence factors to be detected directly from stool or environmental sources without the need for performing culture.[37,149] A retrospective diagnosis can be made by detecting an increase in antitoxin antibody, especially for the heat-labile enterotoxin. ELISA for colonization factor antigens of ETEC also could be useful.

EPEC can be detected reliably by DNA probes for the 60-Md EPEC adherence factor plasmid or by adherence to cells in culture. The ability of *E. coli* to adhere to HEp-2 cells in culture in distinct morphologies led to the description of EPEC, EAEC, and DAEC as different pathotypes (see Fig. 104.3). After a 3-hour incubation of bacteria with cells, EPEC adheres to the cell in tight microcolonies, called the *localized adherence* pattern. Although it remains sensitive and specific for EPEC, this method has been replaced by molecular detection methods to detect the locus of enterocyte effacement island (via the intimin-encoding gene *eae*) and the EPEC adherence factor plasmid (often via detection of the BFP-encoding genes).[64]

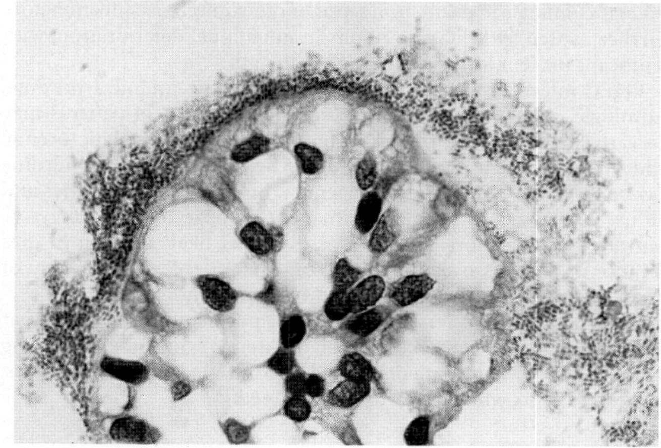

FIG. 104.7 Enteroaggregative *Escherichia coli* (EAEC) infection of the gnotobiotic pig intestine. This photomicrograph shows the characteristic "stacked brick" appearance of the aggregative organisms over the surface of the intestinal epithelium in vivo in the same manner described for EAEC adherence to HEp-2 cells in tissue culture. (Courtesy Saul Tzipori, DVM, Department of Comparative Medicine, Tufts University School of Veterinary Medicine.)

EAEC can be detected by the presence of the aggregative adherence pattern in the Hep-2 adherence assay (Fig. 104.7). DNA probes and PCR are available to detect the AggR regulon, and these tests are likely to provide more specific detection of EAEC pathogens.[52]

EIEC is detected best using molecular techniques that are specific for detection of pathogenesis-related genes. Several multiplex PCR assays that allow the user to screen for multiple *E. coli* pathotypes simultaneously have been described.[16,146,205] Additionally, it is possible to differentiate between *Shigella* spp. and EIEC using these techniques,[204] which can be introduced readily into any molecular biology laboratory and produce excellent results.

DAEC can be detected by a diffuse adherence pattern on Hep-2 cells.[191,246] A probe, commonly used in epidemiologic studies, which targets *daaC*, part of the F1845 operon, has recently been shown to cross-react with some strains of EAEC.[246,258] PCR methods are available for detection from stool.[163,246]

PROGNOSIS

EPEC, EAEC, and ETEC do not cause systemic infections or complications except those resulting from dehydration or the consequences of nutritional depletion. The prognosis is related directly to the availability and adequacy of fluid therapy. When this need is dealt with correctly in an otherwise healthy and well-nourished patient, the principal complication is the rare instance of monosaccharide intolerance. In infants or young children in developing countries with protein-energy malnutrition, however, chronic diarrhea and progressive worsening of nutritional status frequently are observed, sometimes resulting in mortality. When food is withheld from either well-nourished or poorly nourished children, hypoglycemia may occur and produce seizures, coma, or death. Rarely, loss of water in excess of salt causes hypertonic dehydration, with serum sodium concentrations greater than 160 mEq/L, a situation that may cause seizures, coma, and death.

As noted earlier, EAEC has been associated with persistent diarrhea lasting longer than 14 days in young infants and children. Persistent diarrhea leads to nutritional deterioration, may be difficult to control, and may culminate in death from sepsis or other infections. Inflammatory diarrhea caused by EIEC also results in nutritional deterioration, with significant protein losses occurring via the gut.

EHEC infections can be followed by hemolytic-uremic syndrome, neurologic, and intestinal complications. Ten percent of patients may die early in the course of the systemic phase of hemolytic-uremic syndrome. Although the renal failure of hemolytic-uremic syndrome may be reversible with good management of fluid and electrolytes and the use of dialysis as needed, permanent damage to the kidneys is, contrary to earlier more optimistic assessments, likely to occur in 25% or more of patients over the course of 1 or 2 decades, and many of them require permanent dialysis or transplantation in the future.[89] Symptoms of chronic renal disease may appear more than one year after the initial presentation of hemolytic-uremic syndrome, suggesting that follow-up of these patients should be continued for at least 5 years, even for patients who appear to be recovered.[225]

TREATMENT

In all age groups, the principal treatment of the intestinal manifestations of *E. coli* enteric infection is replacement of fluids and electrolytes; with maintenance of fluid balance, the disease is self-limited to 1 week or less in most patients and lasts no more than 2 weeks in nearly all patients. The earlier that fluid replacement therapy is begun, the better the prognosis, particularly considering that clinical signs of dehydration do not develop until a 5% loss of body weight occurs, and that sustained loss of more than 10% of body weight is incompatible with survival.

When shock is present (usually with altered consciousness and an absent or thready pulse) or oral rehydration is unsuccessful because of persistent vomiting, patients must be rehydrated by intravenous infusion of an isotonic electrolyte solution, such as lactated Ringer solution or normal saline. Alternatively, several prerequisites must be ensured for oral therapy: (1) the patient must not be in shock; (2) the patient must be fully conscious; (3) the patient must be able to drink (vomiting, particularly common in children, is not an absolute contraindication because frequent small oral feedings usually are largely retained; when the metabolic abnormality begins to reverse toward normal, vomiting ceases); (4) bowel sounds must be present; and (5) renal function must be normal. Current recommendations for oral rehydration in the United States and Europe suggest the use of hypotonic fluid containing 60 to 75 mEq of sodium per liter (along with potassium and carbohydrates). In the developing world, where cholera is a common occurrence, the World Health Organization recommends that a solution containing 75 mEq of sodium be used for all cases of diarrhea.[9,294] Monitoring for electrolyte imbalances may be required. Rice-based solutions for oral rehydration currently are favored in many diarrheal centers because of their reduced osmotic load.[131] Additionally, zinc supplementation may be of benefit in reducing the duration of acute diarrhea and preventing further episodes.[28,131,267]

A prospective cohort study comparing *E. coli* O157:H7 hemolytic-uremic syndrome patients who developed oligoanuric renal failure requiring dialysis with patients with nonoligoanuric renal failure found that the patients who required dialysis had received less intravascular volume expansion and sodium than the patients who did not require dialysis, suggesting that intravascular volume expansion with isotonic fluid was protective for oligoanuric renal failure when given early in the course of O157 infection.[8] The authors advocate hospitalizing all children with suspected EHEC infection for volume expansion with isotonic fluids and close monitoring.

Although rehydration therapy is the cornerstone of management, antibiotic therapy should be considered in some cases. In most *E. coli*–associated diarrheal illnesses, the disease is mild and of short duration, and no specific antimicrobial therapy is required. Studies to address this issue have found antibiotics to be beneficial in some circumstances. In traveler's diarrhea secondary to ETEC, antibiotic therapy can shorten the duration of illness and decrease its severity.[14,72] Prophylactic antibiotic therapy probably carries more risk than benefit, however, and generally is not recommended unless a significant reason exists for the traveler to require prophylaxis. Because of increasing rates of resistance to trimethoprim-sulfamethoxazole (TMP-SMX), it is no longer recommended for treatment or prophylaxis.[68] For moderate to severe traveler's diarrhea (both ETEC and EAEC), rifaximin, ciprofloxacin, and azithromycin for 1 to 3 days have been shown to have some efficacy. Rifaximin is not absorbed from the gastrointestinal tract which provides a more favorable side effect profile. However, if symptoms occur, such as high fever (39.4°C [102.9°F]) or grossly bloody stools, suggesting a more invasive pathogen, azithromycin is recommended instead (10 mg/kg per day for 3 days in children >6 months).[61,68] Fluoroquinolones (ciprofloxacin) are considered to have a potential undesirable side effect profile in children although 1 to 3 days as recommended for traveler's diarrhea would likely be safe. Of note, resistance to fluoroquinolones does continue to increase which warrants continued monitoring and judicious use.[162] Children in developing countries with ETEC diarrhea also may benefit from receiving antibiotic therapy.[168,186]

EIEC infection theoretically would benefit even more from antibiotic therapy, given its pathogenic similarity to shigellosis and the known benefits of the early use of antibiotics. No controlled studies have validated this benefit for EIEC, however. In experimentally induced disease, DuPont and colleagues[69] reported that parenteral ampicillin produced a bacteriologic cure and rapid clinical response with defervescence and improvement of diarrhea in adults. They have also used ampicillin in the pediatric population for severe dysentery caused by EIEC.[262] TMP-SMX and ampicillin are the current drugs of choice, although resistance has been reported.[6]

Immunocompromised hosts, especially children with AIDS, may require prolonged antibiotic therapy for protracted or recrudescent diarrhea, even when it is caused by bacteria that normally produce only self-limited disease. Malnourished children and children with other serious underlying illness also fit this category. In these patients, systemic invasion may develop along with associated complications, including shock and renal failure. In addition, prolonged carrier states are common findings, with frequent relapses requiring long-term antibiotic therapy for suppression of relapse.

Epidemic EPEC infection, especially in newborns, seems to be affected favorably by antibiotic therapy.[180] The potential for this pathogen to cause prolonged disease and a history of high rates of mortality in neonates suggest the need for antibiotic trials in this age group. Based on limited data, either TMP-SMX or oral nonabsorbable antibiotics, such as gentamicin or colistin, usually are recommended, although antibiotic resistance is common and may alter the choice of antibiotics based on local susceptibility patterns.[18,289]

Antibiotic treatment of EHEC is not recommended. Antibiotics in clinical use do not improve the course or prevent sequelae, and they may exacerbate the illness by promoting production and release of Shiga toxin.[11,30,48] In vitro data suggest that subinhibitory concentrations of TMP-SMX and other antibiotics may increase expression of Shiga toxin.[18,126,156] The most rigorous prospective study to address this question found that the cohort who received antibiotics had a higher incidence of hemolytic-uremic syndrome (of 25 patients who received antibiotics, nine developed hemolytic-uremic syndrome) than the cohort who did not (of 234 patients who did not receive antibiotics, 27 developed hemolytic-uremic syndrome; $P < .001$).[297,298] Other studies have found no association.[196,234]

Notably, no studies have used a randomized placebo-controlled design, so the association may reflect selection bias because both the use of antibiotics and systemic complications are associated with more severe disease. A metaanalysis[234] did not show a higher risk of hemolytic-uremic syndrome associated with antibiotics; however, this metaanalysis has been criticized because it included a study in which all of the patients received antibiotics[114] and because comparisons were made among different antibiotics, which may not induce similar sequelae.

Eculizumab, a monoclonal C5 antibody that targets terminal complement complex formation, has been shown in a small case series (n = 3) to be effective in improving refractory severe hemolytic-uremic syndrome.[138] Further follow-up of hundreds of patients in Germany who had Shiga toxin-positive EAEC during a 2011 continental outbreak suggests possible benefit.[62,195]

Antimotility agents such as loperamide generally are not needed and should be used cautiously if prescribed, with great attention paid to dosage, especially in very young patients.[279] Dysentery is a contraindication to the use of antimotility agents, which may be a risk factor for the development of ileus and abdominal distention.[3] The prolonged use of antimotility agents is reported to be associated with more serious systemic complications of EHEC infection and is not recommended.[48,49]

In most instances of *E. coli* diarrhea, the clinician is left to make therapeutic decisions without knowing the etiologic agent responsible. For reasons already outlined, routine diagnostic microbiology laboratories cannot distinguish pathogenic from nonpathogenic *E. coli,* with the exception of classic EPEC serotypes and Shiga toxin producing *E. coli* including O157:H7 EHEC. Clinical decisions regarding the administration of antibiotic therapy are made on purely clinical grounds with criteria such as the history, duration, and severity of the illness; the age and immunologic competence of the patient; and the nature of the diarrheal stool (e.g., watery, inflammatory, bloody, or dysenteric). Empiric antimicrobial therapy is more justifiable for immunocompromised hosts, for patients with prolonged or severe illness or a history of relevant risk factors (e.g., specific food ingestion, travel, exposure to known contacts), and for cases of inflammatory or dysenteric illness.

Research on alternative treatments of EHEC and prevention of hemolytic-uremic syndrome is ongoing. A synthetic verotoxin receptor, SYNSORB Pk, was not shown to prevent death, dialysis, or serious extrarenal events in a trial of 145 children with EHEC-induced hemolytic-uremic syndrome.[286] Although antibodies against *E. coli* O157 intimin were protective for colonization and disease in a pig model,[60] plasmapheresis and intravenous immunoglobulin have not been shown to ameliorate hemolytic-uremic syndrome in humans.[222,290] Investigation of monoclonal antibodies directed against Shiga toxin are under way.[161,286] The complete genome sequence of *E. coli* O157:H7 is now known and may lead to greater understanding of the pathogenesis of hemorrhagic colitis and hemolytic-uremic syndrome and perhaps innovative approaches to treatment and prevention.[104]

PREVENTION

Epidemic nursery outbreaks of diarrhea in newborns can be controlled by the application of classical principles of preventive medicine. Prompt diagnosis and treatment and scrupulous attention given to details of hand washing and environmental sanitation to eliminate person-to-person transmission are still effective, whereas prophylactic antimicrobials have no role. Outbreaks in neonatal nurseries can be contained by epidemiologic control measures such as cohorting; by screening staff for carriage; and, if necessary, by closing the unit until it is decontaminated. In contrast, preventing sporadic cases of *E. coli* diarrhea is difficult. In communities with obvious deficits in water supply and feces disposal, correction of these problems would lead to a diminished incidence of diarrheal diseases in general.

For traveler's diarrhea, avoidance of contaminated sources such as tap water, unpeeled fresh fruits, and large quantities of ice can be effective in prevention. Several studies additionally indicate that prophylactic antibiotics can protect adult travelers, at least for a limited time.[98] The risk of selection of resistant organisms and drug side effects limits the use of antibiotic prophylaxis to short-term travelers with business or diplomatic missions that would be hindered significantly by an episode of diarrhea. Fluoroquinolones, azithromycin, and rifaximin have been evaluated for prophylaxis and presumptive treatment, and all are efficacious.[254] Some evidence has been presented for the moderate efficacy of bismuth compounds, such as bismuth subsalicylate, for the prevention of ETEC diarrhea in adults. The concern for bismuth toxicity with prolonged use in young children would render it a problematic solution for pediatric *E. coli* diarrhea and its prevention.[68,215]

ETEC vaccine development has been propelled by the observation that ETEC infection confers some protection from reinfection with the same strain,[266] also evident in the decreasing rates of infection in children older than 5 years.[208] The challenge is that more than 25 colonization factor antigens have been identified, and strain serotypes vary tremendously across the world.[92] As noted previously, however, it also is known that certain serotypes and colonization factor antigens are most common (i.e., colonization factor antigens I, II, and IV) and tend to co-segregate with certain virulence factor combinations.[88,92,291,296] This factor would limit the antigenic variability needed in an effective vaccine. Many isolates of ETEC expressing only the heat-labile enterotoxin do not express known colonization factors and would be unaffected by a colonization factor antigen–based vaccine. Although no ETEC vaccine currently is licensed and available, several approaches have been attempted. Dukoral, a vaccine licensed in Europe and Canada for prevention of cholera, has been demonstrated to have some short-term efficacy against ETEC-associated traveler's diarrhea and may be useful to for travelers to high-risk areas.[118] Among the ETEC vaccines furthest in development is one that began as a combination of recombinant cholera toxin B (as a surrogate for the LTB toxin subunit) with strains of formalin-killed ETEC expressing the most prevalent colonization factor antigens in developing countries (rCTB-CF ETEC).[269] This vaccine was found to prevent 77% of nonmild ETEC diarrhea in travelers to developing countries.[208,233,269] In a study of Egyptian children, however, it was not efficacious in preventing disease.[32,208] Reformulation of this vaccine (ETVAX) now includes increased content of CF antigen as well as a new adjuvant (dmLT, an attenuated form of LT) and has shown promise in clinical trials.[34,110,150,269]

Other avenues of vaccine development that have been pursued include live, attenuated ETEC vaccines[34,158] and subunit vaccines. The heat-stable enterotoxin does not create a significant immune response; however, the heat-labile enterotoxin is a known adjuvant similar to cholera toxin and has been conjugated to the heat-stable enterotoxin.[32,92,147,303] Concerns for human use of this construct come, however, from the homology of heat-stable enterotoxin to guanylin, which is produced endogenously.[32,59,278] Live, attenuated *Shigella* vaccine vectors also are being studied in an attempt to elicit a mucosal immune response. Researchers have studied new methods of delivering antigens to the mucosa, including encapsulation in microspheres, delivery in recombinant foods,[271,270,273] and a transcutaneous heat-labile enterotoxin patch vaccine, which was shown to elicit an antibody response but not protect against symptomatic infection.[20,86,157] Finally, new vaccine candidates are being identified, such as novel virulence factors including the EtpA adhesin, EatA and YghJ, secreted metalloproteases, and EaeH, an ETEC surface protein. Many of these virulence factors are conserved in a majority of ETEC strains.[34,84,136,228,229,252] Although no vaccine is yet licensed in the United States, work continues to advance in this field in an attempt to decrease the incidence and severity of morbidity from dysentery in the developing world and from traveler's diarrhea.

Vaccine development for other diarrheogenic *E. coli* strains lags behind that for ETEC. Because EHEC-induced hemolytic-uremic syndrome is a rare disease, vaccine development for humans is limited. However, one group is pursuing vaccination as part of the primary infant series because young age is a risk factor for the development of hemolytic-uremic syndrome. An O157:H7 O-specific polysaccharide conjugated to recombinant exotoxin A of *Pseudomonas aeruginosa* (O157-rEPA) vaccine was shown to be safe and immunogenic in children in a phase 2 study.[7,160] Vaccine development for cattle, the major reservoir, is ongoing[257] and has now yielded two available cattle vaccines.[160] A vaccine composed of type III secreted proteins resulted in decreased shedding of *E. coli* O157:H7 in contrast to controls, although prevalence of shedding increased over the study period. Repeat vaccination of cattle may serve as a mode to decrease human exposure to EHEC.[206]

NEW REFERENCES SINCE THE SEVENTH EDITION

4. Afset JE, Bergh K, Bevanger L. High prevalence of atypical enteropathogenic *Escherichia coli* (EPEC) in Norwegian children with diarrhoea. *J Med Microbiol.* 2003;52(Pt 11):1015-1019.
11. Alam NH, Yunus M, Faruque AS, et al. Symptomatic hyponatremia during treatment of dehydrating diarrheal disease with reduced osmolarity oral rehydration solution. *JAMA.* 2006;296(5):567-573.
20. Behrens RH, Cramer JP, Jelinek T, et al. Efficacy and safety of a patch vaccine containing heat-labile toxin from *Escherichia coli* against travellers' diarrhoea: a phase 3, randomised, double-blind, placebo-controlled field trial in travellers from Europe to Mexico and Guatemala. *Lancet Infect Dis.* 2014;14(3):197-204.
34. Bourgeois AL, Wierzba TF, Walker RI. Status of vaccine research and development for enterotoxigenic *Escherichia coli. Vaccine.* 2016;34(26):2880-2886.
36. Buss SN, Leber A, Chapin K, et al. Multicenter evaluation of the BioFire FilmArray gastrointestinal panel for etiologic diagnosis of infectious gastroenteritis. *J Clin Microbiol.* 2015;53(3):915-925.

41. CDC Centers for Disease Control and Prevention. Foodborne Diseases Active Surveillance Network (FoodNet): FoodNet Surveillance Report for 2012 (Final Report). Atlanta, GA: US Department of Health and Human Services, CDC; 2014.
45. CDC Centers for Disease Control and Prevention. Outbreak of *Escherichia coli* O104:H4 infections associated with sprout consumption—Europe and North America, May-July 2011. *MMWR Morb Mortal Wkly Rep*. 2013;62(50):1029-1031.
47. Cho SH, Kim J, Oh KH, et al. Outbreak of enterotoxigenic *Escherichia coli* O169 enteritis in schoolchildren associated with consumption of kimchi, Republic of Korea, 2012. *Epidemiol Infect*. 2014;142(3):616-623.
54. Conway EM. HUS and the case for complement. *Blood*. 2015;126(18):2085-2090.
62. Delmas Y, Vendrely B, Clouzeau B, et al. Outbreak of *Escherichia coli* O104:H4 haemolytic uraemic syndrome in France: outcome with eculizumab. *Nephrol Dial Transplant*. 2014;29(3):565-572.
76. Ethelberg S, Lisby M, Bottiger B, et al. Outbreaks of gastroenteritis linked to lettuce, Denmark, January 2010. *Euro Surveill*. 2010;15(6).
80. Feng P, Weagant S, Jinneman K. Bacteriological Analytical Manual, Chapter 4A, Diarrheagenic *E. coli*. Available at: http://www.fda.gov/food/foodscienceresearch/laboratorymethods/ucm070080.htm.
82. Fleckenstein J, Sheikh A, Qadri F. Novel antigens for enterotoxigenic *Escherichia coli* vaccines. *Expert Rev Vaccines*. 2014;13(5):631-639.
84. Fleckenstein JM, Munson GM, Rasko D. Enterotoxigenic *Escherichia coli*: Orchestrated host engagement. *Gut Microbes*. 2013;4(5):392-396.
110. Holmgren J, Bourgeois L, Carlin N, et al. Development and preclinical evaluation of safety and immunogenicity of an oral ETEC vaccine containing inactivated *E. coli* bacteria overexpressing colonization factors CFA/I, CS3, CS5 and CS6 combined with a hybrid LT/CT B subunit antigen, administered alone and together with dmLT adjuvant. *Vaccine*. 2013;31(20):2457-2464.
117. Jandhyala DM, Vanguri V, Boll EJ, et al. Shiga toxin-producing *Escherichia coli* O104:H4: an emerging pathogen with enhanced virulence. *Infect Dis Clin North Am*. 2013;27(3):631-649.
135. Kotloff KL, Nataro JP, Blackwelder WC, et al. Burden and aetiology of diarrhoeal disease in infants and young children in developing countries (the Global Enteric Multicenter Study, GEMS): a prospective, case-control study. *Lancet*. 2013;382(9888):209-222.
136. Kumar P, Luo Q, Vickers TJ, et al. EatA, an immunogenic protective antigen of enterotoxigenic *Escherichia coli*, degrades intestinal mucin. *Infect Immun*. 2014;82(2):500-508.
137. Lai Y, Rosenshine I, Leong JM, et al. Intimate host attachment: enteropathogenic and enterohaemorrhagic *Escherichia coli*. *Cell Microbiol*. 2013;15(11):1796-1808.
150. Lundgren A, Bourgeois L, Carlin N, et al. Safety and immunogenicity of an improved oral inactivated multivalent enterotoxigenic *Escherichia coli* (ETEC) vaccine administered alone and together with dmLT adjuvant in a double-blind, randomized, placebo-controlled Phase I study. *Vaccine*. 2014;32(52):7077-7084.
151. Luo Q, Kumar P, Vickers TJ, et al. Enterotoxigenic *Escherichia coli* secretes a highly conserved mucin-degrading metalloprotease to effectively engage intestinal epithelial cells. *Infect Immun*. 2014;82(2):509-521.
152. MacDonald E, Moller KE, Wester AL, et al. An outbreak of enterotoxigenic *Escherichia coli* (ETEC) infection in Norway, 2012: a reminder to consider uncommon pathogens in outbreaks involving imported products. *Epidemiol Infect*. 2015;143(3):486-493.
161. Melton-Celsa AR, O'Brien AD. New Therapeutic developments against Shiga toxin-producing *Escherichia coli*. *Microbiol Spectr*. 2014;2(5).
179. Navarro-Garcia F, Serapio-Palacios A, Ugalde-Silva P, et al. Actin cytoskeleton manipulation by effector proteins secreted by diarrheagenic *Escherichia coli* pathotypes. *Biomed Res Int*. 2013;2013:374395.
182. Nguyen RN, Taylor LS, Tauschek M, et al. Atypical enteropathogenic *Escherichia coli* infection and prolonged diarrhea in children. *Emerg Infect Dis*. 2006;12(4):597-603.
199. Pakalniskiene J, Falkenhorst G, Lisby M, et al. A foodborne outbreak of enterotoxigenic *E. coli* and *Salmonella anatum* infection after a high-school dinner in Denmark, November 2006. *Epidemiol Infect*. 2009;137(3):396-401.
203. Pavlinac PB, John-Stewart GC, Naulikha JM, et al. High-risk enteric pathogens associated with HIV infection and HIV exposure in Kenyan children with acute diarrhoea. *AIDS*. 2014;28(15):2287-2296.
215. Rendi-Wagner P, Kollaritsch H. Drug prophylaxis for travelers' diarrhea. *Clin Infect Dis*. 2002;34(5):628-633.
219. Rivas M, Miliwebsky E, Chinen I, et al. Characterization and epidemiologic subtyping of Shiga toxin-producing *Escherichia coli* strains isolated from hemolytic uremic syndrome and diarrhea cases in Argentina. *Foodborne Pathog Dis*. 2006;3(1):88-96.
220. Robins-Browne RM, Bordun AM, Tauschek M, et al. *Escherichia coli* and community-acquired gastroenteritis, Melbourne, Australia. *Emerg Infect Dis*. 2004;10(10):1797-1805.
239. Santiago AE, Ruiz-Perez F, Jo NY, et al. A large family of antivirulence regulators modulates the effects of transcriptional activators in gram-negative pathogenic bacteria. *PLoS Pathog*. 2014;10(5):e1004153.
265. Steiner TS, Lima AA, Nataro JP, et al. Enteroaggregative *Escherichia coli* produce intestinal inflammation and growth impairment and cause interleukin-8 release from intestinal epithelial cells. *J Infect Dis*. 1998;177(1):88-96.
278. Taxt AM, Diaz Y, Bacle A, et al. Characterization of immunological cross-reactivity between enterotoxigenic *Escherichia coli* heat-stable toxin and human guanylin and uroguanylin. *Infect Immun*. 2014;82(7):2913-2922.
291. von Mentzer A, Connor TR, Wieler LH, et al. Identification of enterotoxigenic *Escherichia coli* (ETEC) clades with long-term global distribution. *Nat Genet*. 2014;46(12):1321-1326.
294. WHO World Health Organization. Oral Rehydration Salts. Production of the new ORS. Geneva, Switzerland: World Health Organization, UNICEF; 2006.
299. Wong Fok Lung T, Pearson JS, Schuelein R, et al. The cell death response to enteropathogenic *Escherichia coli* infection. *Cell Microbiol*. 2014;16(12):1736-1745.
304. Zhang H, Morrison S, Tang YW. Multiplex polymerase chain reaction tests for detection of pathogens associated with gastroenteritis. *Clin Lab Med*. 2015;35(2):461-486.

The full reference list for this chapter is available at ExpertConsult.com.

105 *Klebsiella*

Debra J. Lugo • Randall G. Fisher

Klebsiella is a genus of Enterobacteriaceae, a frequent cause of nosocomial pediatric infection. Classically described by Friedländer[48] as a cause of pneumonia, *Klebsiella* can cause infections of the urinary tract, lung, and central venous catheters in high-risk newborns and immunocompromised older children.[21]

BACTERIOLOGY

Klebsiella organisms were named for Edwin Klebs, the noted German bacteriologist.[108] Distinguishing features of *Klebsiella* spp. include the absence of motility and the presence of a polysaccharide capsule that gives rise to large mucoid colonies on solid media. However there was one recent report of a *K. pneumoniae* clinical isolate that demonstrated a swim-like motility by electron microscopy and staining revealing polar flagella.[23] The organisms are oxidase-negative and citrate-positive; they ferment inositol and hydrolyze urea but do not produce ornithine decarboxylase or hydrogen sulfide. Acetoin and 2,3-butanediol predominate over acidic end products during sugar fermentation (positive result on the Voges-Proskauer test). Four species of *Klebsiella* commonly are agreed on by microbiologists: *K. pneumoniae* (the most common human pathogen), *K. oxytoca* (a less common human pathogen), *K. terrigena*, and *Raoultella planticola*. Previously *R. planticola* was recovered almost exclusively from soil and aquatic environments; reports now suggest that this organism may be a relatively common neonatal pathogen in some parts of the world.[116,147] *R. planticola* isolates with increased drug resistance have been reported worldwide. A 4-year retrospective study of 42 isolates listed the bloodstream as the most common site of *Raoultella* infection, with indwelling catheters and intensive care unit

(ICU) stays as risk factors.[37] *R. planticola* may express virulence factors similar to those of *K. pneumoniae*.[117] Recently the frequency of reports of *R. planticola* infection has increased likely due to increased identification. Organisms are defined serologically by their capsular polysaccharide (K antigens) and lipopolysaccharide (O antigens). Significant cross-reactivity exists between the capsule of some pneumococci (e.g., 19F) and *Klebsiella*.[88] The reader is referred to a review by Podschun and Ullman[119] for a detailed description of *Klebsiella* spp.

EPIDEMIOLOGY

Friedländer[48] proposed that *K. pneumoniae* was the most common cause of community-acquired pneumonia, an observation that was refuted by Fraenkel's[46] observations on pneumococcal pneumonia. *K. pneumoniae* accounts for fewer than 10% of hospitalized cases of pneumonia in adults.[24] *Klebsiella* spp. were historically thought to cause serious infection in immunocompromised hosts, but recent hypervirulent strains have caused increased infections in immunocompetent patients.[110] *Klebsiella* spp. are in greatest evidence as opportunistic nosocomial pathogens of the urinary tract, respiratory tract, biliary tract, and bloodstream. In one survey of the Centers for Disease Control and Prevention (CDC), the infection rate of nosocomial *K. pneumoniae* was 16.7 infections per 10,000 patients discharged.[69] Hand carriage generally is regarded as the most common mode of transmission.[52] Environmental sources of *Klebsiella* spp. include contaminated blood pressure monitoring equipment,[125] ventilator traps,[52] dialysate,[82] ultrasound coupling gel,[50] dextrose solution,[86] and hand disinfectant.[128] The emergence of plasmid-mediated, β-lactamase resistance can be responsible for the rapid spread of resistant organisms to susceptible patients in ICUs.[13,15] Outbreaks may be complex; patient-to-patient transmission of epidemic strains containing different plasmids may be interspersed with sporadic, nonepidemic *Klebsiella* infections.[15]

Klebsiella spp. are second only to *Escherichia coli* as causes of sepsis,[51] with the highest rates of infection being reported from larger hospitals affiliated with medical schools. Strains expressing extended-spectrum β-lactamases (ESBL) may become endemic and may present a complex and diverse pattern of production of enzymes with resistance to β-lactamase inhibitors.[40,45] Although broad-spectrum resistance to β-lactams and carbapenems[92] has been described, previous longitudinal studies have shown that the frequency of ESBLs in *K. pneumoniae* isolates is decreasing.[131] Hypervirulent strains and multidrug-resistant isolates have evolved separately but are both contributing to increased morbidity. The dissemination of resistance is due to mobile elements that may also transfer increased virulence.[60] In 2012, 4% of acute care hospitals reported at least one carbapenem-resistant enterobacteriaceae (CRE) hospital-acquired infection, an increase from 1% in 2001. Carbapenem resistance is increasing, but most CRE infections are still health care associated.[26]

Klebsiella spp. commonly are highlighted as pathogens of debilitated adults and alcoholics,[76] but by 1985, nearly 50% of reported outbreaks of *Klebsiella* were in neonatal ICUs.[69] Outbreaks in newborns continue to occur frequently worldwide.[2,10,31,39,62,114,127] Most outbreaks in newborns have been associated with *K. pneumoniae* infection, but scattered outbreaks of *K. oxytoca* infection in nurseries also have been reported.[9,146] A high percentage of infants in ICUs may become colonized with hospital strains of *Klebsiella*.[58] In one longitudinal study in which weekly rectal swabs were cultured, 80 of 368 (22%) neonates in an ICU harbored ESBL-producing *Klebsiella* spp.[18] Infecting organisms have been isolated from care providers and from mothers of colonized infants.[31] One report described an outbreak among newborns associated with infestation of a neonatal unit by cockroaches colonized with infecting *Klebsiella* strains.[32] *Klebsiella* may spread from newborn units to adult units; interhospital and international spread of resistant strains has been described.[30,39,135] In a newer report, 31 neonates became colonized, 10 were infected, and five died from a neonatal ICU (NICU) outbreak in Maryland. Understaffing of an overcrowded NICU was thought to be important in the genesis of the outbreak.[145] In another NICU outbreak, the use of proton pump inhibitors and prior receipt of third-generation cephalosporins were identified as the principal risk factors for colonization and infection with an ESBL-producing strain.[55] Outbreak control usually depends on cohorting, careful hand washing, and intensive cleaning. However *K. pneumoniae* isolates that are extremely antibiotic resistant also may be more resistant to chlorhexidine; cleaning with this agent in such cases may provide a selective advantage to the resistant strain.[105]

CRE outbreaks have increased over the past 2 decades, and plasmid-encoded carbapenem hydrolyzing enzymes have the potential for rapid dissemination. *K. pneumoniae* carbapenemases (KPC) are responsible for most carbapenem resistance in the United States. A CDC report from 2013 examined the resistance of enterobacteriaceae isolates in the United States and found that it was increasing and that most infections with CRE were associated with health care exposure.[26] New Delhi metallo-β-lactamase (NDM)–producing CRE isolates were shown to be increasing in the United States.[27] OXA-48 was first identified in Turkey in 2001, but was retrospectively identified in isolates in the United States from 2009 and 2012,[93] and OXA-48-like carbapenemases were increasingly identified in the United States from 2010 to 2015.[93] In 2012, the spread of the bla (OXA 48) gene was linked to a single self-transferable plasmid that did not carry any additional resistance genes and only demonstrated decreased susceptibility to carbapenems, not broad-spectrum cephalosporins.[120] OXA-48–like carbapenemase-producing enterobacteriaceae hydrolyze penicillins and carbapenems and differ by one to five amino acids from the OXA-48-like genes associated with a plasmid.[120] These variants can combine variability and demonstrate high levels of resistance to carbapenems. Verona integron encoded metallo β-lactamase–producing Enterobacteriaceae were identified in a NICU and in an adult ICU outbreak in Kentucky in 2015, with isolates from six different patients. However, most of these were *Enterobacter*, with one *E. coli*, one *Raoultella*, and one *K. pneumoniae*.[148]

Ribotyping, pulsed-field gel electrophoresis, and DNA amplification techniques have proved valuable in characterizing *Klebsiella* strains associated with outbreaks.[90,137,138] Whole-genome sequencing was compared with pulsed-field gel electrophoresis in one outbreak study. Neither could definitively determine relatedness, but whole-genome sequencing identified an additional plasmid.[149] Experimental techniques include multiplex real-time polymerase chain reaction, which can identify carbapenem-resistant *K. pneumoniae* strains in 2 hours.[144] The modified Hodge test is used in resource-limited settings and works quite well at identifying organisms that produce carbapenemases.[5] Different ribotypes that share plasmids conferring antibiotic resistance can be responsible for pediatric infections in a particular institution.[15] Strains expressing ESBL may become endemic and may present a complex and diverse pattern of production of enzymes with resistance to β-lactamase inhibitors.[40,45] Active surveillance, carrier cohorting, and increased barrier protection resulted in a decrease in the frequency of KPC-producing *K. pneumoniae* in one Greek hospital.[121]

PATHOPHYSIOLOGY

Pneumonias caused by *Klebsiella* most commonly arise from colonization of the upper respiratory tract, followed by aspiration of organisms to the lower respiratory tract. Some degree of gram-negative oropharyngeal colonization is a normal finding in newborns. The oropharynx of nearly one-third of healthy newborns is colonized by gram-negative rods, including *Klebsiella*, by the time infants reach 1 month of age; colonization rates generally are lower in breast-fed infants.[12] Antibiotic pressure in high-risk newborns and older children has been observed to promote overgrowth of *Klebsiella*.[14,134] Enteric organisms are recovered less frequently from the oropharynx of healthy older children and adults; oral colonization with gram-negative rods is increased during illness,[73] after postoperative viral infections,[72,124] and in debilitated adults.[94] Increased adherence of gram-negative rods to oropharyngeal cells contributes to increased colonization.[72] Elastase made by polymorphonuclear cells contributes to such colonization by reducing the fibronectin coating of sugar receptors.[35] The capsule plays an initial role in interactions of epithelial cells but is not required for an adhesin interaction with the cell surface.[43] Adherence properties may be affected by plasmid content[38] and may be transferred between *E. coli* and *K. pneumoniae*.[68]

In animal models of sepsis, capsular polysaccharide (K antigens) is a virulence factor; monoclonal antibodies to the K antigens reduce the severity of illness in mice.[87] In a mouse model of urinary tract infection (UTI), the K antigens seemed to be more important in infection than the lipopolysaccharide (O antigens), and clinical strains deficient in lipopolysaccharide retained virulence by resistance of capsule to complement.[4,22] In one series of adult patients, capsular type K2 frequently was associated with asymptomatic bacteriuria and cystitis, but not pyelonephritis; the presence of type 1 fimbriae bore a closer relationship to upper UTI.[118] In a retrospective study, patients bacteremic with hyperviscous strains were more likely to develop invasive localized disease, such as liver abscess, meningitis, pleural empyema, or endophthalmitis.[89] Patients bacteremic with the hypermucoviscous phenotype are more likely to come to the hospital from the community and less likely to have underlying disease states, suggesting increased virulence.[77] Liver abscess is almost always caused by hypermucoviscous organisms[44]; surprisingly, disruption of the genes that produce this phenotype did not affect serum sensitivity in vitro and did not alter abscess formation in a mouse model.[83] In another study, the lipopolysaccharide O1 was found to be important; O1 serotypes had higher serum resistance and mutation of the O1 gene greatly reduced the virulence of the organism in a mouse model.[66] Neutrophils play an important role in clearance of *Klebsiella,* and phagocytosis is augmented by leukotrienes.[95]

CLINICAL MANIFESTATIONS

Klebsiella infection shows little clinical distinction from diseases produced by other enteric pathogens. The organism generally is less common than group B streptococcus or *E. coli* as a cause of early-onset or late-onset infection in newborns.[53,98] Investigators from Spain,[62] however, reported one 7-year interval in which *K. pneumoniae* was the most common cause of bacteremia in newborns. In Yemen, gram-negative rods accounted for almost all of 90 cases of neonatal sepsis; *E. coli* outnumbered *K. pneumoniae* by only one case.[3] Risk factors for neonatal *Klebsiella* infection include prematurity, presence of indwelling catheters, previous antibiotic treatment, and parenteral nutrition.[127] Infection in newborns is characterized by typical features of pneumonia, sepsis, and meningitis.[98] In one unusual case, *K. pneumoniae* bacteremia manifested on day 4 of life as a morbilliform maculopapular exanthem, more severe on the face. The infant was afebrile, but the mother had had fever in the peripartum period, and the amniotic fluid had been meconium stained.[25] There was also one reported case of confirmed ophthalmia neonatorum in a healthy newborn, and urgent treatment was recommended.[85]

Although hepatic abscesses have been associated principally with adults with poorly controlled diabetes mellitus, one case report described a 32-week-gestation neonate with *K. pneumoniae* sepsis who developed a liver abscess large enough to be noted on physical examination as an abdominal "lump."[139] In adults, hepatic abscess occasionally is complicated by endophthalmitis or central nervous system infection, with devastating outcomes. A study from Taiwan found that infection with genotype K1 was the only significant risk factor for these complications.[42] This series also revealed that eight of 19 (42%) of the complicated K1 strain infections occurred in patients without identifiable underlying medical disease.[42] Other investigators have emphasized that serotype K2 also can be virulent in patients with liver abscess.[49] Careful study of the pathophysiology and epidemiology of complicated *K. pneumoniae* liver abscesses is ongoing, and the picture is likely to continue to be clarified.

Klebsiella spp. have been isolated commonly from blood and peritoneal fluid in outbreaks of necrotizing enterocolitis.[54,102] Less common manifestations in infants include toxic epidermal necrolysis,[59,113] conjunctivitis,[84] parotitis,[29] retropharyngeal abscess,[33] subdural hematoma,[107] psoas abscess,[6] and renal abscess.[143]

Klebsiella is an unusual cause of infection in an otherwise healthy older child. The classic Friedländer pneumonia that occurs in debilitated adults[48] is rare in children. The identification of pulmonary infection should suggest the possibility of underlying immunodeficiency or significant malnutrition, if not suspected previously.[67,74] If pneumonia caused by *Klebsiella* does occur, progression to lung abscesses should be anticipated.

Lung abscesses may develop within days to weeks after *Klebsiella* infection. Formation of abscesses occurs more frequently during *Klebsiella* pulmonary infection than during any other community-acquired infection.[24] A rare but devastating outcome is massive pulmonary gangrene—the rapid total destruction of part of the lung presumed to be due to vascular compromise. This complication is heralded by radiographs that show small cavities that later coalesce into a large cavity with an intracavitary mass of necrotic lung.[104,109] Some researchers speculate that *Klebsiella* lung infection is accompanied by coincident anaerobic infection that contributes to or is primarily responsible for the pathologic process.[24]

Catheterization of the urinary tract can be associated with urinary tract *Klebsiella* infection, but bacteremia is an uncommon complication in an immunocompetent child.[36,91] Asymptomatic bacteriuria is also frequently encountered. In one retrospective study, a carbapenem-resistant *Klebsiella* strain was isolated on a urine culture in an asymptomatic patient. This did not lead to increased risk of UTI or other *Klebsiella* infections.[123] Approximately 10% of nosocomial UTIs observed in infants after surgery are caused by *Klebsiella*.[36] Focal renal infection progressing to renal abscess has been described.[81] *K. pneumoniae* bacteremia has been associated with lesions of the gastrointestinal tract, presence of an indwelling central venous catheter, and neutropenia. Patients with short-bowel syndrome seem to be at greater risk than are patients with inflammatory bowel disease or malignancy for development of catheter-associated *Klebsiella* or *Enterobacter* bacteremia. *K. pneumoniae* was a constituent of polymicrobial bacteremia in 15 such patients (26%).[17] Mortality rates have ranged from 5% to 20%, with higher death rates occurring in children infected with an aminoglycoside-resistant strain.[16,69] Pneumonia, shock, and disseminated intravascular coagulation are poor prognostic factors in children with underlying malignancy. Rare clinical presentations include multifocal osteomyelitis[80] and endophthalmitis.[96] Pediatric recipients of solid organ transplants may have high rates of acquisition of drug-resistant *Klebsiella*.[126] *Klebsiella* spp. have been described as a frequent pathogen in children and adults with sickle-cell disease in West Africa.[1]

Of four patients who received organ transplants from people who had been infected with KPC-producing *K. pneumoniae,* one developed invasive infection despite tigecycline prophylaxis.[8] *K. pneumoniae* was the most common cause of bloodstream infection in children undergoing liver transplantation in Korea, accounting for 22% of all infections.[129] In New York City, *K. pneumoniae* was the second most common etiology of infection among adult liver transplant recipients. The mortality rate was 71% among those who contracted KPC-positive strains; the odds ratio for death was 4.9 for those with the KPC-producing isolates.[78]

Of six patients with clinical and colonoscopic findings suggestive of antibiotic-associated hemorrhagic colitis (pseudomembranous enterocolitis) but negative evaluation for *Clostridium difficile,* five had stool cultures positive for *K. oxytoca*.[65] All five patients had been receiving penicillin therapy. *K. oxytoca* was cultured from only 1.6% of 385 healthy controls. Additionally the disease could be reproduced in a rat model when rats were inoculated with *K. oxytoca* and administered amoxicillin-clavulanate, but disease was not seen if rats were not given the injection and the antibiotic treatment.[65]

DIAGNOSIS

Klebsiella spp. characteristically grow as large mucoid colonies on MacConkey agar. Citrate-containing media can be used to facilitate isolation of *Klebsiella* strains because these organisms can use citrate as a sole carbon source.[108] Serotyping with specific antisera usually is determined by countercurrent immunoelectrophoresis or a Quellung test.[11] In situ hybridization techniques have been used to identify *Klebsiella* in phagocytes from blood specimens,[97] and restriction-enzyme analysis and ribotyping of clinical isolates have been used to characterize nosocomial spread of antibiotic-resistant strains.[15,56,57] Conventional, commonly used microbiologic methods may misidentify some *Klebsiella* spp., particularly *R. planticola* and *K. terrigena*.[103] Rarely blood cultures have required longer than 72 hours of incubation for radiometric detection of *Klebsiella*.[99]

TREATMENT

Empirical antimicrobial therapy should be guided by an understanding of antimicrobial susceptibilities of *Klebsiella* in the hospital. Therapy with a cephalosporin plus an aminoglycoside (rather than a cephalosporin alone) has been associated with a more favorable outcome in patients with cancer who are infected with susceptible strains.[16] Antimicrobial therapy of *Klebsiella* spp. is made problematic, however, by the resistance to penicillins and cephalosporins conferred by ESBLs.[13,15,19,61] *Klebsiella* with ESBL are widely distributed, and regional differences in susceptibility occur.[75] As described earlier, carbapenems have also become ineffective in cases of CRE; plasmid-encoded carbapenemases pose a major public health concern. Outer membrane protein changes and porin deficiencies of some strains can augment resistance to third-generation cephalosporins.[7,130] Some investigators have reported significant correlation between production of ESBL and resistance to ciprofloxacin.[112,136] Plasmid-mediated resistance to aminoglycosides also is common.[9,31,51,106] Endocarditis isolates that developed resistance to piperacillin-tazobactam and to ciprofloxacin during therapy have been reported.[150]

In cases of CRE, aminoglycosides may be a possible treatment if strains are susceptible and no cell wall active agent is available. Aminoglycosides were associated with a 70% 30-day survival rate in bacteremia cases.[141] Prediction of response to aminoglycosides depends on presence of both KPC and ESBL in *Klebsiella*. Resistance to gentamicin and tobramycin was as high as 100% for isolates that were both KPC and ESBL positive. These isolates were more likely to contain aminoglycoside-modifying enzymes.[56,57] Aminoglycoside monotherapy is more likely to be successful when infection is limited to the urinary tract. There may be a role for plazomicin in some cases.

Effective treatment of multidrug-resistant isolates sometimes requires creativity or use of antibiotics no longer commonly employed. In one case report, a 15-year-old girl developed bacteremia with a meropenem-intermediate strain; bacteremia persisted despite thrice-daily administration of meropenem combined with gentamicin, to which the isolate was sensitive. Clearance was achieved eventually with meropenem administered as a continuous infusion.[41] In another case, bacteremia and peritonitis developed in a patient on continuous ambulatory peritoneal dialysis; infection persisted despite removal of the catheter and treatment with meropenem and amikacin (to which the isolate was intermediately resistant). Cure required a switch to intravenous polymyxin B.[111] Treatment of carbapenem-resistant strains is even more difficult. In vitro, the combination of doripenem and colistin produced bactericidal activity in 75% and synergy against 50% of colistin-resistant KPC-positive strains.[70] Treatment failures in carbapenem-colistin combination therapies are much more likely if isolates show resistance in vitro, with colistin having a minimum inhibitory concentration (MIC) of more than 2 and doripenem a MIC of more than 8 in KPC-producing strains. This resistance may also depend on the absence of other porin mutations.[142] In gentamicin-susceptible, KPC-2–producing isolates with minor ompK36 mutations, doripenem-colistin was inferior to gentamicin alone or combinations of doripenem-colistin and gentamicin. This suggests that genotyping and susceptibility testing may be necessary to select an effective treatment regimen.[28] In an animal model, isolates that were carbapenem-resistant because of OXA-48 were more sensitive to ceftazidime than to piperacillin-tazobactam, imipenem, ertapenem, or cefotaxime.[101] New approaches to the treatment of so-called pan-resistant strains include the novel β-lactamase inhibitor MK-7655[64] (Relebactam) and an antibacterial "designer peptide" called Api88, which binds a chaperone protein and rescues mice from lethal challenge.[34] Ceftazidime-avibactam has been shown to be potent against organisms that are resistant to most other antibiotics, including KPC-producing strains.[133,140] Ceftazidime is a β-lactam, and avibactam is a novel non–β-lactam/β-lactamase inhibitor. It is recommended for use in combination with other agents due to risk of multiple mechanisms of resistance, unless susceptibility testing can be performed.

Antibiotic pressure is important in increasing the risk for development of resistant isolates.[122] In some nursery outbreaks, switching from gentamicin to amikacin has been associated with return of the susceptibility of *Klebsiella* isolates to gentamicin.[9,63] Imipenem or the combination of piperacillin and tazobactam may show good antimicrobial activity against multiply-resistant organisms.[71,115,122] The combination of β-lactamase and porin deficiency has been associated with resistance to imipenem,[20] and hyperproduction of some β-lactamases can limit the effectiveness of β-lactam/β-lactamase inhibitor combinations.[47] Experience with ciprofloxacin in young children is limited because of observations of irreversible cartilage injury in juvenile laboratory animals after administration of this quinolone. Successful treatment of a multidrug-resistant *K. pneumoniae* has been reported in a preterm infant, however, without observable short-term adverse effects.[79] Avoidance of excessive antibiotics is also important due to rapid development of resistance, and, for carbapenem-resistant *K. pneumoniae* limited to the urinary tract, doxycycline monotherapy may be effective.[123] Strict adherence to infection control policies that promote restricted antibiotic use, cohorting, and hand washing may help to prevent the spread of resistant *Klebsiella* strains.[9,31,58,100,132]

Acknowledgments

We thank Dr. William Gruber and Dr. Thomas Boyce for their invaluable assistance with earlier versions of this chapter.

NEW REFERENCES SINCE THE SEVENTH EDITION

23. Carabarin Lima A, Leon-Izurieta L, Rocha Gracia RD, et al. First evidence of polar flagella in a *Klebsiella pneumoniae* isolated from a patient with neonatal sepsis. *J Med Microbiol.* 2016;65(8):729-737.
26. Centers for Disease Control and Prevention. Vital signs: carbapenem-resistant Enterobacteriaceae. *MMWR.* 2013;62(9):165-170.
27. Centers for Disease Control and Prevention. Notes from the field: New Delhi metallo-beta-lactamase-producing *Escherichia coli* associated with endoscopic retrograde cholangiopancreatography–Illinois, 2013. *MMWR.* 2014;62(51-52):1051.
28. Clancy CJ, Hao B, Shields RK, et al. Doripenem, gentamicin, and colistin, alone and in combinations, against gentamicin-susceptible, KPC-producing *Klebsiella pneumoniae* strains with various ompK36 genotypes. *Antimicrob Agents Chemother.* 2014;58(6):3521-3525.
37. Demiray T, Koroglu M, Ozbek A, et al. A rare cause of infection, *Raoultella planticola:* emerging threat and new reservoir for carbapenem resistance. *Infection.* 2016;44(6):713-717.
57. Haidar G, Alkroud A, Cheng S, et al. Association between presence of aminoglycoside modifying enzymes and in vitro activity of gentamicin, tobramycin, amikacin and plazomicin against KPC and ESBL-producing *Enterobacter* spp. *Antimicrob Agents Chemother.* 2016;60(9):5208-5214.
60. Hennequin C, Robin F. Correlation between antimicrobial resistance and virulence in *Klebsiella pneumoniae. Eur J Clin Microbiol Infect Dis.* 2016;35(3):333-341.
85. Kumar JB, Silverstein E, Wallace DK. *Klebsiella* pneumonia: an unusual cause of ophthalmia neonatorum in a healthy newborn. *J AAPOS.* 2015;19(6):564-566.
93. Lyman M, Walters M, Lonsway D, et al. Notes from the field: carbapenem-resistant Enterobacteriaceae producing OXA-48-like carbapenemases—United States, 2010–2015. *MMWR.* 2015;64(47):1315-1316.
110. Paczosa MK, Mecsas J. *Klebsiella pneumoniae*: going on the offense with a strong defense. *Microbiol Mol Biol Rev.* 2016;80(3):629-661.
120. Poirel L, Potron A, Nordmann P. OXA-48-like carbapenemases: the phantom menace. *J Antimicrob Chemother.* 2012;67(7):1597-1606.
123. Qureshi ZA, Syed A, Clarke LG, et al. Epidemiology and clinical outcomes of patients with carbapenem-resistant *Klebsiella pneumoniae* bacteriuria. *Antimicrob Agents Chemother.* 2014;58(6):3100-3104.
133. Sader HS, Castanheira M, Flamm RK, et al. Antimicrobial activity of ceftazidime-avibactam against gram-negative organisms collected from U.S. medical centers in 2012. *Antimicrob Agents Chemother.* 2014;58(3):1684-1692.
140. Shields RK, Clancy CJ, Hao B, et al. Effects of *Klebsiella pneumoniae* carbapenemase subtypes, extended-spectrum beta-lactamases, and porin mutations on the in vitro activity of ceftazidime-avibactam against carbapenem-resistant *K. pneumoniae. Antimicrob Agents Chemother.* 2015;59(9):5793-5797.
141. Shields RK, Clancy CJ, Press EG, et al. Aminoglycosides for treatment of bacteremia due to carbapenem-resistant *Klebsiella pneumoniae. Antimicrob Agents Chemother.* 2016;60(5):3187-3192.
142. Shields RK, Nguyen MH, Potoski BA, et al. Doripenem MICs and ompK36 porin genotypes of sequence type 258, KPC-producing *Klebsiella pneumoniae* may predict responses to carbapenem-colistin combination therapy among patients with bacteremia. *Antimicrob Agents Chemother.* 2015;59(3):1797-1801.
148. Yaffee AQ, Roser L, Daniels K, et al. Notes from the field: verona integron-encoded metallo-beta-lactamase-producing carbapenem-resistant Enterobacteriaceae in a neonatal and adult intensive care unit—Kentucky, 2015. *MMWR.* 2016; 65(7):190.
149. Yang S, Hemarajata P, Hindler J, et al. Investigation of a suspected nosocomial transmission of blaKPC3-mediated carbapenem-resistant *Klebsiella pneumoniae* by whole genome sequencing. *Diagn Microbiol Infect Dis.* 2016;84(4):337-342.

The full reference list for this chapter is available at ExpertConsult.com.

106 Morganella morganii

Leidy J. Tovar Padua • Randall G. Fisher

Similar to *Proteus* and *Providencia* spp., *Morganella morganii* has emerged as an important nosocomial pathogen, most often associated with urinary tract or wound infections. Although most descriptions of infection are in adults, infections in children do occur.

HISTORY

In 1905, Castellani isolated and described a bacterium that caused typhoid-like fever. He later called this isolate and two other identical strains *Bacterium columbense.* In 1906, Morgan described a nonlactose fermenting organism associated with summer infantile diarrhea occurring in Germany, Philippines, and the United States. This organism was known as Morgan's bacillus until Winslow and colleagues named it "*Bacillus morganii*" in 1919. Two decades later, Rauss demonstrated that *B. morganii* had similar spreading phenomenon exhibited by *Proteus* species and renamed this bacterium "*Proteus morganii.*" Fulton proposed a new genus called *Morganella* after discovering that *B. columbense* and *P. morganii* were the same species in 1943. However, *B. columbense* was reclassified as *Escherichia coli* leaving *M. morganii* solitary within its genus. As a result, *M. morganii* was relegated to the genus *Proteus.* Finally, the organism was elevated to genus rank in 1978 after molecular phylogenetic analysis revealed genetic differences from *Proteus,* with which it is otherwise biologically similar.[40]

BACTERIOLOGY

M. morganii (formerly *Proteus morganii*) is a motile gram-negative bacillus commonly found in the feces of humans, other mammals, and reptiles.[43] Most strains do not ferment lactose. *M. morganii, Proteus* spp., and *Providencia* spp. are distinguished from other Enterobacteriaceae by their ability to deaminate phenylalanine and lysine. Similar to *Proteus* and *Providencia* spp., *M. morganii* produces urease, but this enzyme is unrelated genetically and serologically to urease produced by the other two genera.[24,43] In contrast to *Proteus* spp., neither *Providencia* spp. nor *M. morganii* shows swarming activity on 1.5% agar[43]; *M. morganii* is ornithine positive, whereas *Providencia* spp. are ornithine negative. *M. morganii* organisms do not hydrolyze gelatin and do not produce hydrogen sulfide. For a detailed discussion of taxonomy and characterization of *M. morganii,* the reader is referred to the review by O'Hara and colleagues.[40]

EPIDEMIOLOGY

Similar to *Proteus* and *Providencia* spp., *M. morganii* organisms commonly are found in soil, sewage, and manure. Similar to *Proteus mirabilis, M. morganii* often invades urinary bladder catheters and surgical wounds; patients in adult inpatient surgical units have the greatest risk for colonization and infection.[1] Institutionalized elderly patients also are infected frequently with these organisms. Urinary tract colonization with *M. morganii* accompanying groin skin colonization in elderly individuals may account for the greater frequency of urinary tract infections in this population.[18] *M. morganii* accounted for nearly 10% of 145 consecutive complicated, multidrug-resistant urinary tract infections in one study.[13] *E. coli* and *P. mirabilis* account for most urinary tract infections in children, but *M. morganii* has been implicated in some cases of cystitis and pyelonephritis. In contrast to well-described nursery epidemics of *P. mirabilis* infection,[3,8] no *M. morganii* neonatal outbreaks have been described, and infections of the central nervous system are rare in newborns.[16,35,57] A fatal case of early-onset sepsis in which both the mother's lochia and the neonate's blood were culture positive has been reported; the baby died at 17 days of age despite appropriate antimicrobial therapy.[41] Ribotyping is a sensitive method for molecular characterization of isolates that may aid in analyzing outbreaks.[45]

PATHOPHYSIOLOGY

Factors that predispose the urinary tract to invasion by *P. mirabilis* and *Providencia* spp. also may favor *M. morganii* colonization and infection. These organisms all split urea, forming ammonium hydroxide and increasing local pH, which results in toxicity to renal cells and potentiation of urolithiasis.[6,37] The ability of *P. mirabilis* to regenerate more rapidly in urine with faster generation of alkaline pH compared with *M. morganii* may provide a selective advantage for the former organism in establishing itself as a urinary tract pathogen.[52]

CLINICAL MANIFESTATIONS

Urinary tract infection with *M. morganii* often is associated with an elevated urinary pH. Urolithiasis can occur, although perhaps less frequently than during *P. mirabilis* infection.[4] *M. morganii* has been recovered from less than 10% of adult bacteremic episodes, but mortality rates have exceeded 20%.[1] Approximately three fourths of all cases of adult *M. morganii* bacteremia are hospital associated.[27] In a series of 132 patients with bacteremia from Proteeae, preexisting biliary or hepatic disease (especially the presence of biliary drainage catheters) was associated with *Morganella* bacteremia.[27] In a series of 73 patients with *Morganella* bacteremia in Taiwan, 92% had at least one underlying disease, the most common of which was solid tumor. The only independent risk factor for mortality was inappropriate antibiotic treatment.[31] Other reported complications identified in immunocompromised or instrument-fitted patients include meningitis,[21,33] pericarditis,[38] arthritis,[26,50] osteomyelitis,[29] empyema,[22] spontaneous bacterial peritonitis,[22] peritoneal dialysis-related peritonitis,[28,55] intratesticular abscess,[59] prostatitis,[32] otitis media,[19] and skin infection.[2] Many cases of postoperative *M. morganii* endophthalmitis and panophthalmitis have been reported, as have rare cases of endogenous endophthalmitis, all in adults.[12,56,58,60]

M. morganii has been recovered alone or in combination with other organisms from surgical wounds[13] and soft tissue abscesses in children.[7,14] A 12-year-old with *M. morganii* meningoencephalitis secondary to chronic otitis, whose immune system was apparently normal, has been reported.[39] Septic arthritis with *M. morganii* was described in an otherwise healthy 23-month-old.[49] Another rare manifestation of *M. morganii* infection was pericarditis, seen in a child with X-linked agammaglobulinemia.[10] A 3-year-old boy developed hemorrhagic bullae and necrotizing fasciitis after being scratched by a chicken; cultures grew both *M. morganii* and enterococci.[30] Meningitis and brain abscess have been described.[35,42,57] Approximately 13 cases of neonatal sepsis with *M. morganii* have been reported in the literature.[9,35,36] Mortality rates exceed 30% in this age group. Lower gestational age and smaller birth weight were associated with higher morbidity and mortality.[9] In four cases of early-onset neonatal sepsis with *M. morganii*, premature rupture of membranes and maternal receipt of antepartum amoxicillin were documented.[5,9,17]

DIAGNOSIS

M. morganii produces a reddish brown pigment when cultured on nutrient media supplemented with 5% tryptophan.[43] Production of urease and deamination of tryptophan help to distinguish this bacterium from other organisms. In contrast to the closely related *Proteus* and

Providencia spp., *M. morganii* generally ferments only glucose and mannose and does not produce a red color on lysine iron agar.[43] *M. morganii* may be missed or mistaken for other organisms in the common circumstance of polymicrobial infection in a catheterized patient. In one series, *M. morganii* was among the most common bacteriuric species in patients on long-term catheterization but commonly was missed by reference laboratories.[15] Automated systems provide rapid and reliable genus and species-level identification for *Morganella spp.*[47] The clinical laboratory should be directed to look for this organism, particularly in circumstances of nosocomial urinary tract infection and sepsis.

TREATMENT

Effective treatment of local infections or septicemia relies on appropriate choice of an antibiotic, often including an aminoglycoside, combined with removal of invasive devices, surgical debridement, and drainage of abscesses, as necessary. Antimicrobial susceptibility can vary widely among *M. morganii* and the related *Proteus* and *Providencia* strains, emphasizing the importance of species identification and susceptibility testing.[25,44] Complex combinations of aminoglycoside resistance that differ by hospital and geographic region can occur.[34] Most isolates are intrinsically resistant to ampicillin and first- and second-generation cephalosporins. Some carry a chromosomal broad-spectrum AmpC β-lactamase that can be stably derepressed on treatment with third-generation cephalosporins, similar to *Enterobacter* spp., although it appears that this problem arises much less frequently among *Morganella* isolates.[11] Most urinary tract infections respond to treatment with third-generation cephalosporins. Failure to clear bacteriuria should alert the physician to the possibility of urolithiasis or structural abnormality[4]; stone removal or surgical correction of anatomic defects often is required for cure. The approach to the treatment of sepsis or serious infection of sites other than the urinary tract should be considered carefully in light of local susceptibility patterns, keeping in mind that isolates with AmpC β-lactamases may seem to be sensitive to cephalosporins on initial testing but develop resistance during therapy. Treatment failure, with prolonged culture-positive ventriculitis, has been described in an infant with *M. morganii* meningitis after initial therapy that included cefotaxime led to stable derepression of an AmpC β-lactamase, showing the potentially devastating clinical relevance of this phenomenon.[53] Data from the SENTRY Antimicrobial Surveillance Program has shown reduced susceptibility to imipenem for *M. morganii* in the United States.[46] Carbapenemases (including IMP-1, VIM-1, NDM-1, and OXA-48) and plasmid-mediated quinolone resistance gene qnrS1 activity have been reported among *M. morganii*.[20,23,48,51] Addition of avibactam enhances the activities of aztreonam, ceftaroline, and ceftazidime against resistant Enterobacteriaceae.[54]

Acknowledgments

We thank Dr. William Gruber and Dr. Thomas Boyce for their invaluable assistance with earlier versions of this chapter.

NEW REFERENCES SINCE THE SEVENTH EDITION

9. Chang HY, Wang SM, Chiu NC, et al. Neonatal *Morganella morganii* sepsis: a case report and review of the literature. *Pediatr Int*. 2011;53(1):121-123.
14. D V, Jv S, Mk Y, et al. *Morganella morganii* causing abscess over the anterior chest wall- a case report. *J Clin Diagn Res*. 2014;8(9):DD03.
20. Hammoudi D, Ayoub Moubareck C, Aires J, et al. Countrywide spread of OXA-48 carbapenemase in Lebanon: surveillance and genetic characterization of carbapenem-non-susceptible Enterobacteriaceae in 10 hospitals over a one-year period. *Int J Infect Dis*. 2014;29:139-144.
23. Jamal WY, Albert MJ, Khodakhast F, et al. Emergence of new sequence type OXA-48 carbapenemase-producing enterobacteriaceae in Kuwait. *Microb Drug Resist*. 2015;21(3):329-334.
28. Kimura Y, Ito A, Miyamoto K, et al. *Morganella morganii* Peritonitis associated with continuous ambulatory peritoneal dialysis (CAPD) after colonoscopy. *Intern Med*. 2016;55(2):165-168.
29. Koyuncu S, Ozan F. *Morganella morganii* osteomyelitis complicated by secondary septic knee arthritis: a case report. *Acta Orthop Traumatol Turc*. 2012;46(6):464-467.
32. Li X, Chen J. Septic shock induced by bacterial prostatitis with *Morganella morganii* subsp. *morganii* in a posttransplantation patient. *Case Rep Transplant*. 2015;2015:850532.
35. Milligan KL, Barenkamp SJ. Neonatal meningitis due to *Morganella morganii*. *Clin Pediatr (Phila)*. 2013;52(5):462-464.
36. Murphy K, Ryan C, Dempsey EM, et al. Neonatal sulfhemoglobinemia and hemolytic anemia associated with intestinal *Morganella morganii*. *Pediatrics*. 2015;136(6):e1641-e1645.
38. Nakao T, Yoshida M, Kanashima H, et al. *Morganella morganii* pericarditis in a patient with multiple myeloma. *Case Rep Hematol*. 2013;2013:452730.
42. Patil AB, Nadagir SD, Lakshminarayana S, et al. *Morganella morganii*, subspecies *morganii*, biogroup A: an unusual causative pathogen of brain abscess. *J Neurosci Rural Pract*. 2012;3(3):370-372.
46. Rennie RP, Jones RN. Effects of breakpoint changes on carbapenem susceptibility rates of Enterobacteriaceae: results from the SENTRY Antimicrobial Surveillance Program, United States, 2008 to 2012. *Can J Infect Dis Med Microbiol*. 2014;25(5):285-287.
47. Richter SS, Sercia L, Branda JA, et al. Identification of Enterobacteriaceae by matrix-assisted laser desorption/ionization time-of-flight mass spectrometry using the VITEK MS system. *Eur J Clin Microbiol Infect Dis*. 2013;32(12):1571-1578.
48. Rozales FP, Ribeiro VB, Magagnin CM, et al. Emergence of NDM-1-producing Enterobacteriaceae in Porto Alegre, Brazil. *Int J Infect Dis*. 2014;25:79-81.
49. Sanz Santaufemia FJ, Suarez Rueda C, Garcia Talavera ME, et al. *Morganella morganii:* an unusual bacterium in joint effusions]. *An Pediatr (Barc)*. 2012;76(5):298-299.
51. Seija V, Medina Presentado JC, Bado I, et al. Sepsis caused by New Delhi metallo-beta-lactamase (blaNDM-1) and qnrD-producing *Morganella morganii*, treated successfully with fosfomycin and meropenem: case report and literature review. *Int J Infect Dis*. 2015;30:20-26.
54. Testa R, Canton R, Giani T, et al. In vitro activity of ceftazidime, ceftaroline and aztreonam alone and in combination with avibactam against European gram-negative and gram-positive clinical isolates. *Int J Antimicrob Agents*. 2015;45(6):641-646.
55. Tsai MT, Yeh JT, Yang WC, et al. CAPD-related peritonitis caused by *Morganella morganii*. *Perit Dial Int*. 2013;33(1):104-105.
59. Zaid UB, Bagga HS, Reese AC, et al. Intratesticular abscess in a solitary testicle: the case for testicle sparing management. *Case Rep Med*. 2013;2013:184064.

The full reference list for this chapter is available at ExpertConsult.com.

Proteus 107

Randall G. Fisher

BACTERIOLOGY

Proteus spp. are motile, gram-negative bacilli that do not ferment lactose and are distinguished from other Enterobacteriaceae by their ability to deaminate phenylalanine and lysine. Rapid and abundant production of urease further differentiates *Proteus* spp. from *Providencia* spp.[37] *Proteus vulgaris* and *Proteus mirabilis* tend to form a thin, spreading growth (swarm) on the surface of moist agar media, often overgrowing other bacterial isolates. They also produce hydrogen sulfide and liquefy gelatin. *P. mirabilis* is distinguished from other *Proteus* spp. (e.g., *P. vulgaris*) by its inability to produce indole from tryptophan. Most indole-negative clinical *Proteus* isolates are classified by laboratories as *P. mirabilis;* however, in one study, eight of 61 were found to be *P.*

penneri when extensive biochemical testing was performed.[35] Disparate DNA content and anomalous biochemical and serologic reactions have caused *Proteus morganii* to be renamed *Morganella morganii* (see Chapter 106),[37] and both terms for this organism appear in the clinical literature. For detailed discussion of taxonomy and characterization of *Proteus* spp., the reader is referred to the review by O'Hara and colleagues.[49]

EPIDEMIOLOGY

Proteus spp. commonly are found in soil, sewage, and manure. Although they are normal inhabitants of the colon and perineum, their numbers can be increased in individuals receiving antibiotic therapy.[33]

First reported by Buisine and Henninot in 1949,[13] neonatal meningitis caused by *P. mirabilis* accounts for approximately 4% of all neonatal meningitis cases.[45] Outbreaks in nurseries have been attributed to contaminated equipment and human carriers. Vertical transmission from mother to infant has been confirmed by DNA fingerprinting and ribotyping methods.[10] In Becker's series[7] of *P. mirabilis* neonatal meningitis, all affected infants came from the same nursery and all were exposed to mist from an apparatus that yielded *P. mirabilis.* The importance of hand carriage was well documented by Burke and associates[14]; neonatal umbilical colonization and invasive disease were linked to a single nurse from whom *P. mirabilis* was cultured from her hands, rectum, and vagina. Ribotyping is a sensitive method for molecular characterization of isolates and may aid in analyzing outbreaks.[53]

Proteus infection after the first few months of life most commonly involves the urinary tract. Although *Escherichia coli* accounts for most urinary tract infections in children, *Proteus* spp. commonly are implicated in reported series of cystitis and pyelonephritis[9,24,34,50,73]; in a large pediatric series, they were the third most common cause of urinary tract infection, after *E. coli* and *Klebsiella pneumoniae.*[11] *P. mirabilis* is the most common species of *Proteus* isolated: it has been cultured more frequently from the urethra of uncircumcised than of circumcised male infants and replaced *E. coli* as the most prevalent pathogen in one consecutive series of male patients presenting with initial urinary tract infection.[34,74]

Urinary tract infection with *Proteus* spp. is one of the most common presenting signs of urolithiasis in children,[20] and *P. mirabilis* supplants *E. coli* as the major urinary tract pathogen in children prone to renal stone formation.[9] Diagnosis of greater than 50% of pediatric urolithiasis cases is based on preceding urinary tract infection, and *Proteus* is responsible for 65% of these infections.[9] Isolation of this organism as a pathogen on urine culture should alert the physician to the possible presence of a urinary tract stone.

PATHOPHYSIOLOGY

Most cases of central nervous system infection caused by *Proteus* spp. occur in neonates and are thought to arise by bacteremic spread of the organism to the brain or meninges. Contiguous spread to the brain from localized infections is reported occasionally.[44,62] As is the case with *Citrobacter* meningitis, a propensity for formation of abscesses of the central nervous system remains unexplained. Rabbit models of *P. mirabilis* meningitis have shown that in vivo concentrations of gentamicin necessary to produce bacterial killing are 10 to 30 times higher than the concentrations predicted from in vitro susceptibility testing.[69] Reduced aminoglycoside effect may be secondary to depressed cerebrospinal fluid pH associated with *P. mirabilis* infection.[69] Whatever the mechanism, lack of effective antimicrobial activity in the ventricles accounts partly for the persistence of organisms at these sites.

Crystallization of urinary catheters and stents leads to obstruction of outflow of urine. Urease produced by *Proteus* infection causes calcium phosphate and magnesium phosphate to precipitate and accumulate in the catheter lumen.[68] This process is less likely to occur when the urine is dilute and acidic.[68] In vitro, increasing the concentration of magnesium, calcium, and phosphate strongly intensifies crystallization, although decreasing their concentrations below physiologic levels has no effect on crystal formation.[70] Mannose-resistant/*Proteus*-like fimbriae (often shortened to MR/P fimbriae) are important in the formation of biofilms on catheter material[57] and also, apparently, in attachment and cytotoxicity.[59] *Proteus* isolates obtained from catheter-associated urinary tract infection have increased swarming motility and form biofilms more readily than *Proteus* isolates from stool of healthy volunteers.[28] Methods of preventing crystallization of catheters include coating them with agarose[67] and impregnating them with chlorhexidine and triclosan.[23]

Numerous factors may predispose the urinary tract to invasion by *Proteus* spp. *Proteus* spp. split urea, forming ammonium hydroxide and increasing local pH, which results in toxicity to renal cells and potentiation of urolithiasis.[12,47] The ability of *P. mirabilis* to regenerate more rapidly in urine with faster generation of alkaline pH when compared with *M. morganii* may provide a selective advantage for the former organism in establishing itself as a urinary tract pathogen.[61] Biochemically complex struvite ($MgNH_4PO_4$) stones provide a refuge for *Proteus* organisms and form a barrier to effective antimicrobial therapy.[9] Formation of struvite stones is a major cause of urinary bacterial persistence in women without azotemia,[66] and a similar case probably can be made for pediatric patients with urolithiasis. *P. mirabilis* ureases showed lower affinities for substrate but hydrolyzed urea 6 to 25 times faster than enzymes from other species, which may explain the frequent association of this species with formation of stones.[30]

Organisms have been shown to be taken up by human renal epithelium, by an actin-independent mechanism.[16] Pili may enhance the virulence of *Proteus* in pyelonephritis by increasing adherence of organisms to the renal pelvis.[57,63] Flagella have been implicated in the spread of this organism in the urinary tract[40]; the ability to invade host uroepithelial cells is coupled closely with the ability of *P. mirabilis* to differentiate into hyperflagellated, filamentous swarm cells capable of rapid spread on the surface of moist agar media.[4] The role of fimbriae as a factor predisposing to ascending infection is less clear.[6,43] Swarming behavior might inherently assist ascending colonization of the urinary tract, as shown in a mouse model of infection.[5] A putative gene regulator for swarming behavior (RsbA) may act to identify environmental conditions that favor swarming.[8] The reader is referred to the review by Rozalski and colleagues[58] for a more in-depth review of *Proteus* virulence factors.

A growing body of literature suggests that adult rheumatoid arthritis may be triggered by infection of the urinary tract with *Proteus* spp. In one study, increased levels of total and class-specific immumoglobulin G antibodies directed at three *Proteus* peptides were found in patients with rheumatoid arthritis but not in control subjects.[56] Patients with active disease had measurable IgM, and a positive correlation was found between antibody indices and inflammatory markers.[56] This association is still speculative and is being investigated; at this time, no suggestion has been made that juvenile idiopathic arthritis is related in any way to *Proteus* infection.

CLINICAL MANIFESTATIONS

P. mirabilis can produce a broad spectrum of symptoms associated with neonatal infection. Most patients have typical symptoms of early-onset neonatal sepsis, including nonspecific lethargy, fever, and poor feeding; manifestations of sepsis may include septic arthritis and osteomyelitis. In a few patients the disease presents after the first week of life. Meningitis may occur with either early-onset or late-onset disease. Brain abscesses associated with subtle clinical abnormalities rarely develop for weeks to months before presentation.[14] *Proteus* brain abscesses are associated with a high degree of mortality, frequent complications, and increased risks of neurologic deficits in survivors.[18,31,39,64] Hydrocephalus is a particularly frequent complication and should be anticipated. Destruction of the brain may progress to porencephaly or compartmentalization of ventricles and often requires surgical intervention.[31] Computed tomography is useful, especially in diagnosing and following progression of cerebral complications.[64]

Urinary tract infection with these bacteria involves predominantly younger patients and often is associated with elevated urinary pH; clinical findings and urine abnormalities often are less striking than in patients with *E. coli* urinary tract infections.[34] Thirty percent of patients may show recurrent infection during the 12 months after receiving initial treatment.[34] Indwelling urinary catheters increase the risk for *Proteus* colonization and infection. Long-term indwelling urinary catheters or stents may become blocked by encrustations of aggregated struvite crystals; prolonged colonization with urease-producing *P. mirabilis* is associated with this complication.[38] *P. mirabilis* is the most common pathogen associated with xanthogranulomatous pyelonephritis,[3] which can mimic Wilms tumor and usually is not seen in childhood except in malnourished patients.

Proteus spp. often are implicated as agents of septicemia in adult patients and account for approximately 8% of gram-negative bacteremias in this group.[21,36] In 60% of *Proteus* bacteremic episodes in adults, the urinary tract has been determined to be the source[21]; no anatomic source is identified in 20% of cases of *Proteus* bacteremia. *P. mirabilis* and *P. vulgaris* are the species responsible for most cases of *Proteus* bacteremia. The overall incidence of gram-negative enteric bacteremia in pediatric patients is lower than that of adults; 5% of such cases are caused by *Proteus* spp.[21] As in adults, the genitourinary tract is the source identified most frequently.[21] Predictors of bacteremia in adults with *Proteus* urinary tract infection are community acquisition, hydronephrosis, bandemia greater than 10%, a C-reactive protein value greater than 10 mg/dL, and hypothermia or hyperthermia at diagnosis.[15] Mortality rates average less than 40% and strongly depend on the severity of underlying disease in the host.[21,36]

Osteomyelitis,[32,52,69] pneumonia,[21,36,54] mastoiditis,[44] and wound infections[36] also occur. Rarely, native-valve endocarditis has been caused by *P. mirabilis*.[17] Severe multifocal osteomyelitis requiring bilateral above-knee amputation for cure has been reported in a patient with human immunodeficiency virus infection despite a reasonably good $CD4^+$ cell count.[51] *Proteus* spp. have been isolated commonly from chronic suppurative otitis media on several different continents.[25,72] Reports that *Proteus* spp. are major pathogens of otogenic brain abscess in pediatric and adult patients support this association.[26,55] Pediatric osteomyelitis secondary to contiguous infection of traumatized soft tissue often is polymicrobial, and *Proteus* spp. have been implicated as co-pathogens in at least 10% of such cases.[52] Sickle cell anemia is a risk factor.[2,32]

DIAGNOSIS

Proteus is suspected readily because of its ability to swarm on the surface of moist agar. A selective medium developed for the isolation of *Proteus* organisms relies on the ability of all members to produce a dark brown pigment in medium containing DL-tryptophan.[27] Production of urease, lack of indole production from tryptophan, and a positive result with ornithine decarboxylase testing distinguish *P. mirabilis* from *Providencia* spp. and other *Proteus* spp.[37]

TREATMENT

Treatment of meningitis caused by *Proteus* spp. should conform to standard regimens recommended for gram-negative meningitis. *P. mirabilis* usually is sensitive to ampicillin, however, and this drug alone or combined with an aminoglycoside often is suitable therapy when the identity and susceptibilities of the infecting organism are known.[60] A third-generation cephalosporin often is an alternative, but resistant extended-spectrum β-lactamase–producing strains and β-lactamase inhibitor–resistant strains have been described in pediatric patients.[19,40] Consecutive lumbar punctures should be performed for *Proteus* meningitis until cerebrospinal fluid cultures are sterile. A minimum of 2 weeks of antibiotic therapy is recommended after bacteriologic cure has been achieved. Ventricular aspiration or drainage of abscesses may be required to direct therapy, based on persistence of organisms at these sites. Open drainage of abscesses often is necessary, but resolution of abscess formation with the use of antibiotic therapy alone has been reported.[65] Intraventricular antibiotics are not of proven benefit in terms of mortality or morbidity but have been used to clear ventricular colonization. A 15-year-old boy with *Proteus* mastoiditis and meningitis was treated successfully with intravenous trimethoprim-sulfamethoxazole.[44]

Effective treatment of local infections or septicemia relies on appropriate choice of antibiotics, often including an aminoglycoside, combined with surgical debridement and drainage of abscesses as necessary. Many experts recommended "double coverage"—a cell wall-active agent plus an aminoglycoside—especially when the infection is severe or is caused by an indole-positive strain. In a large, three-continent longitudinal survey, approximately 5% of *P. mirabilis* strains exhibited phenotypic extended-spectrum β-lactamase resistance patterns.[22] In France, 59% of 1008 urinary *P. mirabilis* isolates were resistant to amoxicillin, 48% were resistant to piperacillin, 34% were resistant to amoxicillin-clavulanate, and 2.8% were resistant to piperacillin-tazobactam.[41] One third of isolates were resistant to trimethoprim-sulfamethoxazole.[41] In Japan, extended-spectrum β-lactamase production in *P. mirabilis* went up from 7% in 2000 to 12.9% in 2009.[48] Over a 10-year period in Taiwan, susceptibility to cefotaxime decreased from 93% to 82%; to ceftazidime from 100% to 95%; to ciprofloxacin from 80% to 54%; about 8% were extended-spectrum β-lacatamase producers.[71] A report from China details the combination of carbapenem resistance and quinolone resistance in 19 isolates; all of them had the *Klebsiella pneumoniae* carbapenemase-2 gene.[29] Complex combinations of aminoglycoside resistance that differ by hospital and geographic region can occur.[46] In one study, amikacin retained better activity than did other aminoglycosides.[41] In France, 65% of all colistin-resistant gram-negative isolates were *Proteus* species.[1] Most *P. mirabilis* urinary tract infections respond to ampicillin, but some organisms have been shown to acquire a plasmid-mediated β-lactamase.[42] Failure to clear bacteria should alert the physician to the possibility of urolithiasis or structural abnormality; removal of stones or surgical correction of anatomic defects often is required for cure.

NEW REFERENCES SINCE THE SEVENTH EDITION

1. Abat C, Desboves G, Olaitan AO, et al. Increasing burden of urinary tract infections due to intrinsic colistin-resistant bacteria in hospitals in Marseille, France. *Int J Antimicrob Agents*. 2015;45:144-150.
59. Scavone P, Villar S, Umpierrez A, Zunino P. Role of *Proteus mirabilis* MR/P fimbriae and flagella in adhesion, cytotoxicity and genotoxicity induction in T24 and Vero cells. *Pathog Dis*. 2015;73.
70. Torzewska A, Rozalski A. Various intensity of *Proteus mirabilis*-induced crystallization resulting from changes in the mineral composition of urine. *Acta Biochim Pol*. 2015;62:127-132.
71. Wang JT, Chen PC, Chang SC, et al. Antimicrobial susceptibilities of *Proteus mirabilis*: a longitudinal nationwide study from the Taiwan surveillance of antimicrobial resistance (TSAR) program. *BMC Infect Dis*. 2014;14:486.

The full reference list for this chapter is available at ExpertConsult.com.

108 Providencia

Randall G. Fisher

The genus *Providencia* comprises pathogens most commonly associated with urinary tract infection. *Providencia* spp. are encountered most often as pathogens in hospitals or long-term care facilities and can be responsible for outbreaks of multidrug-resistant infection.[44]

BACTERIOLOGY

Providencia spp. (named after the city of Providence, Rhode Island) are motile gram-negative bacilli that do not ferment lactose and are distinguished from other Enterobacteriaceae by their ability to deaminate phenylalanine and lysine.[9,33] The genus distinguishes "urease-negative" organisms, *P. rettgeri, P. stuartii, P. alcalifaciens, P. rustigianii,* and *P. heimbachae,* from the otherwise biochemically similar "urease-positive" *Proteus* spp.[16,33] Urease is produced by most strains of *P. rettgeri* and by 15% or less of *P. stuartii* strains.[28] *Providencia* spp. also differ from other Proteeae in their ability to produce acid from inositol. Strains are differentiated further by reactivity with straight-chain hydroxy alcohols.[33] For a detailed discussion of taxonomy and characterization of *Providencia* spp., the reader is referred to the review by O'Hara and colleagues.[29]

EPIDEMIOLOGY

Providencia organisms are recovered uncommonly from stool in healthy humans, but they frequently colonize indwelling or condom urinary catheters, particularly in patients receiving antibiotic therapy.[5,6,11,17,44,45] In a Japanese study of patients with traveler's diarrhea, *Providencia* spp. were recovered, using a new selective medium, from 23 of 130 specimens tested.[46] *P. alcalifaciens* has also been associated with a foodborne outbreak of gastrointestinal disease with seven primary and four secondary cases.[36] A study of retail meats in Thailand found *Providencia* strains in 68% of chicken, 68% of pork, and 72% of beef sampled; *P. alcalifaciens* was the most common organism identified.[37] *Providencia* spp. have been recognized as pathogens for more than 50 years[8]; *P. rettgeri* and *P. stuartii* are the most common species implicated in urinary tract infection.[11,13,14,25,45] Multiple biotypes of *P. stuartii* have been identified in hospital outbreaks, indicating the probability of multiple sources of colonization.[1] Ribotyping is a sensitive method for molecular characterization of isolates that may aid in analysis of outbreaks.[35]

PATHOPHYSIOLOGY

P. stuartii does not seem to have greater access to the urinary tract compared with other bacteria; in patients with long-term catheters, the incidence of bacteriuria caused by this organism is equivalent to that caused by other uropathogens.[44] Rather, *P. stuartii* manifests an extraordinary ability to persist within the catheterized urinary tract.[45] Bacteriuria may take weeks to months to clear. A mannose-resistant, *Klebsiella*-like hemagglutinin may play an important role in the persistence and adherence of *P. stuartii* to urinary tract catheters.[27]

Despite the similarities between *P. mirabilis* (the major pathogen responsible for urolithiasis in children)[4] and urease-producing *Providencia* spp., the latter organisms rarely are associated with formation of stones. *P. stuartii* occasionally produces urease with a higher affinity for substrate, but *P. mirabilis* ureases hydrolyze urea 6 to 25 times faster.[15] Restriction-enzyme analysis of genes coding for the respective enzymes shows significant divergence.[15] These differences may explain the more frequent association of *P. mirabilis* with formation of stones.

Some strains of *P. alcalifaciens* have been isolated more commonly in children with diarrhea, and enteropathogenicity has been shown in HEp-2 cells and a rabbit model.[1,2] In vitro, *P. alcalifaciens* prefers basolateral to apical entry into Caco-2 cells; they are taken up by endocytosis and appear to require an invasion.[24] Ex vivo *P. alcalifaciens* strains show the ability to translocate and to resist complement-mediated lysis.[43] In children with diarrhea, *P. alcalifaciens* often is associated with other enteric pathogens, so its role in pathogenesis remains unclear.[3]

CLINICAL MANIFESTATIONS

Although *Escherichia coli* and *Proteus* spp. account for most urinary tract infections in children, *Providencia* spp. have been reported as a cause of infection in children with spinal injury and long-term urinary tract catheterization.[18,25] Most infections have been described, however, in elderly patients or adults with spinal injury who require long-term urinary tract catheterization.[44] Clinical findings are typical of those associated with urinary tract infection. Bacteremia is uncommon but devastating.[19] In a study of 132 cases of bacteremia caused by members of the tribe Proteeae, only eight were caused by *Providencia* spp., but four of those patients died of the infection.[19] A single case of endocarditis and a case of relapsing pericarditis both caused by *P. stuartii* have been reported.[20,39] In a newer case series of *Providencia* bacteremia, 11 of 14 cases were nosocomial, nine were polymicrobial, and the mortality rate was 29%; patients were a median age of 64.5 years, and cerebrovascular/neurologic disorders were the most common underlying illnesses.[6]

Eye infections caused by *P. rettgeri,* including conjunctivitis, dacryocystitis, keratitis, and endophthalmitis, have been reported. These infections generally occurred in patients with compromise in ocular surface or in immunity.[31]

Providencia spp. have been implicated in the so-called purple urine bag syndrome, in which an enzyme from the organism causes 3-indoxyl sulfate to be formed, which discolors the urine blue or blue-violet. This syndrome usually occurs in patients with indwelling cystotomy or nephrostomy tubes.[21,42] Xanthogranulomatous pyelonephritis with a nephrocutaneous fistula has also been reported.[22]

Although central nervous system infection with *Providencia* spp. is extremely rare, meningitis occurred after a neurosurgical procedure in a patient in Turkey[40] and a left frontal lobe cystic mass was reported that was originally thought to be a tumor but proved to be a brain abscess caused by *P. stuartii.*[29]

DIAGNOSIS

Infection with *Providencia* spp. should be suspected when indole-positive, urease-negative, gram-negative rods, which oxidatively deaminate tryptophan, are isolated in culture. Because patients with long-term catheterization may be colonized with multiple organisms, *Providencia* spp. frequently are overlooked or misidentified.[8] Clinical laboratories should be encouraged to identify all bacterial colonies in patients with long-term catheterization in whom infection is suspected. Identification is particularly important because of the marked differences in susceptibility of uropathogens.[34]

TREATMENT

Empirical therapy should be guided by antimicrobial susceptibility testing of the patient's isolate and knowledge of susceptibilities of previously identified *Providencia* within the care facility. Removal of urinary tract catheters speeds eradication of these pathogens. Strains of *P. stuartii* and *P. rettgeri* commonly are resistant to many antibiotics. In a longitudinal Italian study of 223 *P. stuartii* isolates, 116 (52%) were extended-spectrum β-lactamase positive.[41] The rate of extended-spectrum β-lactamase–positive isolates increased from 31% in 1999 to 62% in

2002.[33] Since the 1970s, multidrug resistance has emerged[32,38]; many strains are resistant to sulfonamides, trimethoprim, nitrofurantoin, nalidixic acid, penicillins, cephalosporins, and aminoglycosides; some singular strains are resistant to most antibiotics in common use.[34] Imipenem-resistant strains have now been described.[38] One case report describes an isolate that carried *blaPER-1, blaVIM-2,* and *armA* (a 16S methylase gene that confers resistance to aminoglycosides).[23] Much of the observed resistance seems to be plasmid based[12]; quinolones and aztreonam have shown some promise in the treatment of such cases.[7,10] One isolate in Israel was found to be carrying 27 different antibiotic resistance genes, most of them located on mobile genetic elements.[30] Complex combinations of aminoglycoside resistance that differ by hospital and geographic region can occur.[26] Organisms that are resistant to gentamicin and tobramycin may remain susceptible to amikacin.

Acknowledgments

I thank Dr. William Gruber and Dr. Thomas Boyce for their invaluable assistance with earlier versions of this chapter.

NEW REFERENCES SINCE THE SEVENTH EDITION

6. Choi HK, Kim YK, Kim HY, Park JE, Uh Y. Clinical and microbiological features of *Providencia* bacteremia: experience at a tertiary care hospital. *Korean J Intern Med.* 2015;30:219-225.
30. Olaitan AO, Diene SM, Assous MV, Rolain JM. Genomic plasticity of multidrug-resistant NDM-1 positive clinical isolate of *Providencia rettgeri. Genome Biol Evol.* 2016;8(3):723-728.
36. Shah MM, Odoyo E, Larson PS, et al. First report of a foodborne *Providencia alcalifaciens* outbreak in Kenya. *Am J Trop Med Hyg.* 2015;93:497-500.
37. Shima A, Henenoya A, Somosornsuk W, et al. Prevalence of *Providencia* strains among patients with diarrhea and retail meats in Thailand. *Jpn J Infect Dis.* 2016;69(4):323-325.

The full reference list for this chapter is available at ExpertConsult.com.

109 Shigella

Theresa J. Ochoa • Margaret Kosek

HISTORICAL BACKGROUND

The term *dysentery* classically has been used to describe the frequent, painful passage of stools containing blood and mucus. The syndrome has been recognized since the time of Hippocrates. The differentiation of dysentery into bacillary and amebic forms followed the recognition by Shiga in 1898 that one form of dysentery was associated with a bacterium in the stools of affected individuals; their sera also were found to agglutinate the bacillus. In recognition of Shiga's achievement, the genus was eventually named after him. *Shigella flexneri* was first described in 1900, and only 14 years later shigellae became the main diarrheal agent in World War I.[30]

The most important subsequent advance has been the recognition of the molecular basis of *Shigella* virulence. In the 1960s, researchers showed that shigellae invade the corneal epithelium of guinea pigs and cause keratoconjunctivitis (Sereny test). Subsequently, Formal and colleagues[96] showed that *Shigella flexneri* invades the intestinal epithelium. Since 1980, Sansonetti and colleagues[256–258] and other investigators[261] have identified multiple plasmid and chromosomal virulence genes.

BACTERIOLOGY

Shigellae are small, nonencapsulated gram-negative rods that are members of the Enterobacteriaceae. Shigellae do not ferment lactose, or do so slowly, and are nonmotile (they lack the H [flagellar] antigen). They lack urease and do not produce hydrogen sulfide on triple sugar iron media or gas during metabolism of carbohydrate.[88] The somatic antigen (or O antigen) side chains that determine serotype and serogroup are attached as multiple repeating units to the lipid A core and core oligosaccharides shared with other members of Enterobacteriaceae. Envelope or K antigens that are heat labile also have been described, although their clinical relevance is uncertain. *Shigella* and *Escherichia coli* are closely related. Enteroinvasive *E.coli* (EIEC) strains have remarkable phenotypic and genotypic similarity with *Shigella* species and are difficult to differentiate. The sequencing of multiple housekeeping genes indicates that *Shigella* has risen on several different occasions from several independent ancestors by acquisition of the transferable forms of ancestral virulence plasmids within the group of nonpathogenic *E. coli.*[285]

Serogroup Classification

The genus *Shigella* has four species or subgroups (A, B, C, and D) and 43 serotypes.[65] Subgroups A, B, C, and D have historically been treated as species: subgroup A is referred to as *S. dysenteriae*; subgroup B as *S. flexneri*; subgroup C as *S. boydii*; and subgroup D as *S. sonnei*. Subgroups and serotypes are differentiated from each other by their biochemical characteristics and antigenic properties. *Shigella dysenteriae* (subgroup A), mannitol nonfermenters, includes 15 serotypes having O antigens that do not cross react immunologically. *Shigella sonnei* (subgroup D), ornithine decarboxylase–positive, slow lactose fermenters, share the same lipopolysaccharide (1 serotype). *Shigella* strains that ferment mannitol (in contrast to *S. dysenteriae*) but do not decarboxylate ornithine or ferment lactose (in contrast to *S. sonnei*) are classified as serogroups B and C. Of these, the strains that express lipopolysaccharides that are related to each other immunologically are group B *(Shigella flexneri)*, whereas the strains whose O antigens are unrelated to each other or to other shigellae are group C *(Shigella boydii)*. *S. flexneri* has eight serotypes; serotypes 1 through 5 are subdivided into 11 subserotypes. Although the numbering scheme for group C (*S. boydii*) serotypes extends to serotype 20, there are only 19 serotypes because *S. boydii* 13 is now reclassified as *Escherichia albertii*, and has been removed from the scheme[122] (Table 109.1).

EPIDEMIOLOGY

Based on the findings of the Child Health Epidemiology Reference Group (CHERG) of the World Health Organization (WHO), it is estimated that globally 89 million community cases and 37 million outpatient cases of shigellosis occur annually in children younger than age 5 years.[157] Most of these cases occur in developing countries. In 1999, a review of the literature for 1966 through 1997 suggested that around 1.1 million persons die annually of shigellosis, including around 880,000 in Asia.[149] A review of the literature from 1990 through 2009 indicates that around 125 million shigellosis cases occur annually in Asia, of which, 14,000 are fatal.[31] A systematic review of global causes of diarrheal disease mortality in children of articles published between 1990 and 2011, estimated 28,000 deaths due to shigellosis in children under 5 years in the world.[156] This estimate is much lower than a previous

TABLE 109.1 Classification of *Shigella* Subgroups

Serogroup	Species	Number of Serotypes
A	*dysenteriae*	15
B	*flexneri*	8[a]
C	*boydii*	19[b]
D	*sonnei*	1

[a]Group B serotypes 1–5 are subdivided into 11 groups.
[b]Although the numbering scheme for group C serotypes extends to serotype 20, there are only 19 serotypes.

estimate of approximately 600,000 deaths due to shigellosis published by Kotloff et al. in 1999[149]; and is compatible with the Asian estimate of 14,000.[31] The lower estimates of deaths are associated with markedly reduced case-fatality rates rather than fewer cases.

Generally, *Shigella* spp. are associated with 5% to 10% of all diarrhea cases and 30% of dysentery cases, although estimates based on PCR-based diagnostics are higher.[205] Dysentery associated with *Shigella* spp is often severe and with longer duration.[231] Although epidemic *Shigella* dysentery is the most dramatic manifestation of *Shigella* infections in developing countries, most infections are caused by endemic shigellosis. Despite the fact that severe dehydration usually is not seen in shigellosis, shigellosis is disproportionately represented in severe and fatal cases of diarrhea, particularly in children younger than 5 years old. The incidence of *Shigella* is increased by undernutrition, particularly wasting,[146] and *Shigella* is one of the enteric infections that has shown to be most strongly correlated with linear growth deficits following infection.[44,161] *Shigella* is a common cause of prolonged and persistent episodes of diarrhea, and the dominant cause of the clinical dysentery syndrome in populations living in poverty or exposed to conditions where hygiene and water quality are suboptimal. Therefore, the empirical management of dysentery should always include an antibiotic that has been demonstrated to have low levels of resistance as defined by the best available regional data on antimicrobial resistance.

According to surveillance reports of the Centers for Disease Control and Prevention, 10,000 to 15,000 cases of shigellosis have been documented each year during the past 30 years in the United States,[63] and it is currently estimated that nearly 500,000 cases occur annually in the United States, one fourth of which are domestically acquired; with 40 annual deaths.[66,262] *Shigella* is the third most important Foodborne Diseases Active Surveillance Network pathogen in 10 sentinel states in the United States, with a population-based incidence of 5.7 per 100,000 population. The groups with the highest incidence are children younger than 5 years, black race, and Hispanic ethnicity.[66] However, incidence rates have decreased significantly in 2014 when compared with rates documented in 1996 and 1998 (46% decrease).[64,66] Around 10% to 18% of persons with culture-confirmed *Shigella* infection in the United States are hospitalized.[209]

Because shigellae are spread through a fecal-oral route, they are especially prevalent where hygiene is poor. The organisms can be cultured from around toilets in homes where shigellae have caused disease. Shigellae are transmitted easily from person to person because the inoculum size required to cause disease is only 10 organisms in the case of *S. dysenteriae* serotype 1[85] and a few hundred organisms in the cases of *S. sonnei* and *S. flexneri*.[83] Hand washing and wearing gloves are mandatory procedures for individuals caring for patients with bacillary dysentery. Patients who lack the acid barrier provided by a normally functioning stomach because of prior gastrectomy or use of antacids are at increased risk for acquiring infection.

Epidemics usually are associated with exposure to contaminated water or food, although as might be predicted from the inoculum size, outbreaks related to swimming also occur.[177] Houseflies can be mechanical vectors of shigellosis, particularly where the fly population is large. A study in Bangladesh demonstrated that housefly population density correlates with shigellosis among children.[89] *Shigella* infection shows seasonal variation. In North America, few cases occur in the winter, whereas in tropical regions, the peak is during the rainy season. Shigellae are worldwide and thrive where susceptible individuals are grouped together (including institutions for retarded or mentally ill individuals, prisoner-of-war camps, Indian reservations, the military, daycare centers, and the developing world).[138,229,275] The devastating impact of *S. dysenteriae* type 1 epidemics in vulnerable concentrated populations is still notable as can be seen in refugee camps in Goma and Tanzania in the 1990s where attack rates ranged from 6.3% to 39.1% and case-fatality rates were estimated to be as high as 9% at some camps.[101,137]

The species of *Shigella* causing most infections varies according to region. In developed countries, *S. sonnei* is the most common species, followed by *S. flexneri* (approximately 86% *S. sonnei* and 12% *S. flexneri*); however, in the developing world, this pattern is reversed, with *S. flexneri* being more common than *S. sonnei* (66% vs. 24%).[66,143,175] In recent years, *S. sonnei*, which has historically been more commonly isolated in developed countries, is undergoing an expansion across industrializing regions in Asia, Latin America, and the Middle East. *Plesiomonas shigelloides* is hypothesized to protect populations with poor water supplies against *S. sonnei*. Improving the quality of drinking water supplies would, therefore, result in a reductionin *P. shigelloides* exposure and a subsequent reduction in environmental immunization against *S. sonnei*. This phenomenon would explain why *S. sonnei* is more common in industrialized countries.[280]

S. dysenteriae serotype 1 occurs primarily in Africa, India, and Bangladesh. *S. boydii* is found primarily on the Indian subcontinent.[205] However, *Shigella* has shown temporal procession in serogroup dominance. Recently, epidemiologic transition has favored the emergence of *S. sonnei* as the dominant serogroup in some countries (i.e., Israel, Argentina, Vietnam), although the reason for this is not clear.[145] A large molecular epidemiology investigation in China has provided convincing evidence for numerous serotype switching events, as well as changing antibiotic resistance, of an emergent sequence type that has replaced *S. flexneri* 2a as the dominant serotype.[295]

Based on a study in South Africa, systemic shigellosis is associated with HIV-infected patients, primarily in older girls and women, potentially due to the burden of caring for sick children in the home. Death rates are higher in HIV-infected versus uninfected individuals.[136]

Humans and other primates can be infected with shigellae, and an age-related risk for acquiring symptomatic shigellosis exists. In contrast to *Salmonella* spp., which causes disease most frequently in the first few months of life, shigellae infrequently cause illness in the first 6 months of life. The peak incidence occurs in children between 1 and 4 years of age, with fewer cases occurring in children aged 5 to 9 years old. Adults are at lower risk.

PATHOGENESIS

Invasiveness and Toxin Production

Shigella invades the colonic epithelium where it elicits an intense inflammation leading to tissular destruction. The main steps of colonic infection by *Shigella* are adhesion, invasion, intracellular replication, and cell-to-cell spread. The ability to invade mammalian cells is the most important virulence trait of *Shigella* spp.[2,14,99,154,166,201,213,263] Uptake by M cells overlying Peyer patches with ingestion by macrophages under the M cells induces production of cytokines and recruitment of polymorphonuclear leukocytes (Fig. 109.1). Apoptosis is induced in macrophages after ingestion of shigellae; these events are accompanied by release of interleukin (IL)-1, IL-1β, and IL-18, which triggers other inflammatory events.[259,302,304] *Shigella* induces a controlled inflammatory response which includes release of both inflammatory (IL6, IL8, IL1β, TNFα and β) and anti-inflammatory cytokines (IL10, TGFβ).[181] Polymorphonuclear leukocytes enter the gut lumen by moving between epithelial cells. *Shigella* enters the intestinal epithelium via the basolateral surface of polarized enterocytes by delivering several effectors that subvert cell signaling pathways, which then direct bacterial internalization by the epithelial cells.[14] After penetration of intestinal epithelial cells, shigellae are located in vacuoles derived from the cytoplasmic membrane of the mucosal cells. The bacteria lyse these vacuoles, move intracellularly, multiply, kill the epithelial cells, and infect adjacent cells.[57,189] Cell death is followed by formation of ulcerations and microabscesses in the colon.

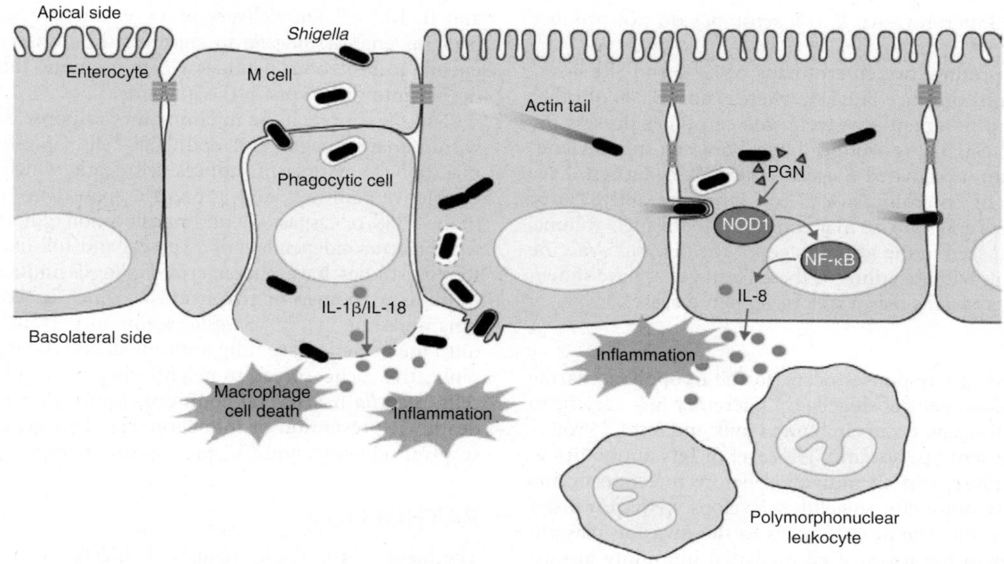

FIG. 109.1 Cellular pathogenesis of *Shigella* spp. *Shigella* passes the epithelial cells barrier by transcytosis through M cells and encounters resident macrophages. The bacteria evade degradation in macrophages by inducing an apoptosis-like cell death, which is accompanied by proinflammatory signaling. Free bacteria invade the epithelial cells from the basolateral side, move into the cytoplasm by vectorial actin polymerization, and spread to adjacent cells. Proinflammatory signaling by macrophages and epithelial cells further activates the innate immune response and attracts polymorphonuclear leukocytes. (From Ashida H, Ogawa M, Kim M, et al. *Shigella* deploy multiple countermeasures against host innate immune responses. *Curr Opin Microbiol.* 2011;14:16–23.)

In contrast to *Salmonella* infection, *Shigella* infection rarely spreads beyond the lamina propria, so bacteremia and metastatic infections are uncommon.

The genetic basis of virulence has been studied extensively.[215,219] Invasiveness is the result primarily of genes on a large virulence plasmid (200 kb), containing a mosaic of around 100 genes and insertion sequences.[109,110,115,226–228,261,263] These genes encode a molecular apparatus called a type III secretion system (T3SS) that is capable of injecting bacterial proteins through bacterial and host membranes into host cells (translocation) or the extracellular milieu (secretion) to influence host biochemistry and cell physiology directly.[219] More than 50 effector proteins of the T3SS have been identified and their virulence function and phenotype described.[15,214,263] Recent structural and functional studies suggest that two different sets of effectors are involved in inducing actin cytoskeleton reorganization to promote entry of bacteria into epithelial cells and in modulating cell signaling pathways to dampen innate immune responses induced on infection, respectively. Effectors involved in entry are produced independently of the T3TSS activity, whereas effectors involved in controlling the cell responses are produced on activation of the T3SS.[220] The invasive plasmid antigen (ipa) region includes genes for four polypeptides needed for invasion: *ipaA, ipaB, ipaC,* and *ipaD.* The proteins produced by these loci are recognized by the humoral immune system. IpaB function depends on the face of invasion; plays a role as a T3SS needle tip protein, as a pore-forming translocator protein, and as an effector protein.[230] The product of the *ipaB* locus is essential for induction of apoptosis in macrophages.[302,303] The IpaH protein family has E3 ubiquitin ligase activity.[245] *Shigella* modulates macrophage cell death by activating nucleotide-binding oligomerization domain–like receptor (NLR) inflammasome to secure its own dissemination via IpaH7.8. This allows bacteria to escape from macrophages and spread to neighboring cells.[277] The mxi-spa region of the virulence plasmid is necessary for orientation of the ipa-encoded proteins into the outer membrane of the bacteria. The *virG* gene encodes a protein that causes intracellular and intercellular spread of shigellae after invasion of epithelial cells. The *virF* gene regulates a locus *(virB)* that is responsible for positive regulation of the ipa genes.[249]

Chromosomal loci regulate expression of the virulence plasmid.[218] The keratoconjunctivitis provocation *(kcpA)* gene is a positive regulator of the *virG* virulence plasmid gene that determines ability to spread within and between cells. Lipopolysaccharides play a role in resistance to nonspecific host defense mechanisms that are encountered during invasion of tissue. The *Shigella* lipopolysaccharides induce the trafficking of Toll-like receptor 4, the dominant mediator of the innate immune response.[58] Smooth colonies express the complete complex of lipopolysaccharide O side chains required for full virulence—the ability to invade epithelial cells, to multiply within them, and to resist phagocytosis.[103,216] Rough colonial variants that lack complete lipopolysaccharides do not penetrate epithelial cells efficiently and are avirulent.

Some strains of *Shigella* spp. produce toxins that injure mammalian cells. A chromosomal locus in *S. dysenteriae* serotype 1 encodes a protein synthesis-inhibiting exotoxin (Shiga toxin, Stx) that is a major virulence factor in this serotype (and in the enterohemorrhagic *E. coli* serotypes that have the same or closely related genes).[34,268] In addition to being potent protein synthesis inhibitors, Stxs are also multifunctional proteins capable of activating multiple cell stress signaling pathways, which may result in apoptosis, autophagy, or activation of the innate immune response.[160] This toxin is composed of a single copy of an A subunit (32,000 Da) that is linked to five copies of B subunits (7790 Da).[211] The B subunits bind to a glycolipid cell receptor, globotriaosylceramide, followed by internalization. The A subunit cleaves an adenine residue from the eukaryotic 28S ribosomal subunit. The resulting block in elongation factor 1-dependent binding of aminoacyl tRNA to the ribosome causes cell death through inhibition of protein synthesis.[211] Shiga toxin previously was considered to be a neurotoxin because its administration to mice or rabbits caused paralysis and death[51,62,119]; it now is thought to target primarily the vascular endothelium. It causes fluid accumulation in rabbit ileal loops[91,139] that probably is related to reduced fluid uptake by damaged villus cells.

The severity of *S. dysenteriae* serotype 1 infection relative to other *Shigella* serotypes is thought to be caused by production of Shiga toxin. Enterohemorrhagic *E. coli* serotypes, such as *E. coli* O157:H7, produce an identical (Shiga toxin 1) or similar (Shiga toxin 2) toxin and, similar to *S. dysenteriae* serotype 1, cause bloody diarrhea and hemolytic-uremic syndrome. Recently, stx producing *S. sonnei* has been described to produce more severe disease than is typical of non-stx producing infections, and 71% of 56 cases reported in California derived from Mexico had clinical dysentery.[155] Enteroinvasive *E. coli* serotypes do not produce these toxins.[72]

Shigella spp. also produce two enterotoxins, ShET-1 and ShET-2.[286] All *S. flexneri* 2a strains produce ShET-1, whereas only 3.3% of other *Shigella* serotypes and no enteroinvasive *E. coli* serotypes possess the gene for this toxin.[206] ShET-2 is produced by all *Shigella* spp.[286] Genes of an additional toxin, designated *Shigella* enterotoxin, or Sen, have been found in 75% of enteroinvasive *E. coli* serotypes and 83% of *Shigella* strains.[200] These enterotoxins may contribute to the high-volume, watery diarrhea often seen in the initial stages of the disease.[25] Vaccine studies using a mutant with deletions of these toxin genes have shown that one or both enterotoxins play a role in human disease.[148]

Immune Response

Serum IgG, IgM, and IgA responses occur to the lipopolysaccharide and invasion plasmid antigens of shigellae.[210] Secretory IgA, specific to both of these sets of antigens, occurs in human milk and feces.[73] Protection is thought to be serotype specific. The level of IgG antibodies to lipopolysaccharides present in an individual before infection occurs determines whether symptomatic shigellosis develops.[77] No clear proof currently exists about the role of antibodies to the invasion plasmid virulence proteins or to the toxins. Cell-mediated immunity against shigellae also may play a role in resolution of infection. Production of αβ T cells and natural killer cells mediates interferon-γ production that may be essential to defense from *Shigella.*[159,292] Antibody-dependent cellular cytotoxicity against shigellae has been shown.

During infection, shigellae use several effectors to direct various cellular signaling pathways and to modify the innate immune activation of the host.[215,225] *Shigella* release bacterial components (lipopolysaccharide, LPS, and peptidoglycan -PGN) and T3SS components.[16,17,15,191] These are recognized as pathogen-associated molecular patterns (PAMPs) and danger-associated molecular patterns (DAMPs) by recognition receptors, such as toll-like receptors (TLRs), nucleotide-binding oligomerization domain-like receptors (NLRs), AIM2-like receptors (ALRs), and RIG-like receptors; and trigger host immune response against bacterial infection. Upon recognition, a subset of NLRs (NLRP1, NLRP3, and NLRC4) and ALRs (AIM2) form inflammasomes, which are multi-protein signaling complexes composed of NLR/ALR, the adaptor protein ASC, and inflammatory caspase, such as caspase-1 (canonical inflammasomes) and caspase-11 (non-canonical inflammasomes). Inflammasome activation results in release of pro-inflammatory cytokines (IL-1β and IL18) and induction of pyroptosis.[135] In addition, the remnants of the host cell membrane that result from the disruption of the phagocytic vacuolar membrane may also stimulate inflammatory responses.[84] As *Shigella* cells multiply within macrophages, the T3SS effector IpaB assembles an ion channel within cell membrane to allow for potassium influx, which is recognized by the NLRC4-inflammasome and triggers pyroptosis.[265]

All this causes activation of the nuclear factor κB and other terminal kinase pathways, with IL-8 appearing as a major chemokine, mediating the inflammatory burst that is dominated by massive infiltration of the mucosa by polymorphonuclear leukocytes.[225] The levels of cytokines tumor necrosis factor-α, IL-1β, IL-1RA, IL-6, IL-8, and granulocyte-macrophage colony-stimulating factor in stool correlate with the severity of shigellosis. In contrast to other cytokines, interferon-γ and its receptor[239] are depressed early and increase during recovery. Fecal concentrations of tumor necrosis factor-α, IL-1β, IL-1RA, IL-6, IL-8, and granulocyte-macrophage colony-stimulating factor are significantly higher in patients with *S. dysenteriae* serotype 1 than in patients with *S. flexneri* infection.[241] Elevated tumor necrosis factor-α and IL-6 levels in stool and serum have been associated with complications during infection with *S. dysenteriae* serotype 1.[80] Infiltration of polymorphonuclear leukocytes and lymphocytes into the intestine is controlled by these cytokines. Epithelial cell production of IL-8 and a low ratio of IL-1RA to IL-1 are responsible for the severe inflammation.[13,255] T lymphocytes with suppressor-cytotoxic and helper-inducer phenotypes are recruited into the epithelium and lamina propria during infection with *Shigella,* related partly to the induction of HLA-DR expression in the rectal mucosa.[240] Peripheral blood lymphocytes of infected individuals respond to *Shigella* antigens in vitro with production of interferon-γ and IL-10.[215,254] The delivery of as yet uncharacterized T3SS-secreted proteins enables *Shigella* to suppress the transcription of genes that encode antimicrobial peptides, which promotes the advance of bacteria deeper into the crypts in the intestine.[271]

Shigella spp. elicits an inflammatory response during multiplication within macrophages and epithelial cells. *Shigella* multiplication in macrophage cytoplasm induces cell death, which is achieved by two distinctive pathways: activation of caspase-1 by IpaB, MxiI, or MxiH of the T3SS, or caspase-11, and translocation of lipid A from the cytosol, which occurs independent of caspase-1 and Toll-like receptor 4 activities. Recent studies have characterized *Shigella*-induced macrophage cell death as pyroptosis or pyronecrosis, which is accompanied by severe inflammation.[16,15,108,241] *Shigella* seems to prevent epithelial cell death until the bacteria have fully multiplied, because it prefers these cells as replicative niche, spread to neighboring cells, and evasion of immune cells. *Shigella* has several countermeasures that inhibit epithelial cell death: (i) prevention of mitochondrial damage, (ii) activation of cell survival signaling, and (iii) prevention of caspase activation.[15]

PATHOLOGY

The main morphologic changes of shigellosis (superficial ulcerations, focal hemorrhages, mucosal edema, erythema, and friability) occur in the colon where the organisms invade.[125,269] The rectosigmoid and distal segments of the colon typically are involved more severely than is the proximal colon. The epithelial cell damage may cause development of a pseudomembrane composed of thick, fibropurulent exudate tightly adherent to the necrotic ulcerated colonic mucosa. Pseudopolyposis also has been reported.[53] On microscopic examination, damage to epithelial cells, ulcerations, goblet cell depletion, and intense polymorphonuclear and mononuclear infiltration with crypt abscesses are seen. Rectal mucosa shows increased numbers of $CD8^+$ and $\gamma\delta^+$ T cells.[124] Vessels in the lamina propria are congested or thrombosed. Perforation of the colon usually does not occur as part of the colitis.[29] Evidence of inflammation and proinflammatory cytokines persists for at least 1 month after clinical resolution.[238] Histologic changes generally are more severe and persistent[105] with *S. dysenteriae* than with *S. flexneri.*[10]

CLINICAL MANIFESTATIONS

The incubation period ranges from 12 hours to a few days (if a low number of organisms are ingested). Onset of high fever, toxicity, and crampy abdominal pain is sudden and typically precedes the onset of diarrhea. During the first 48 hours, high-volume watery diarrhea may occur (small bowel phase of disease); subsequently, low-volume, bloody, and mucous diarrhea develops in association with urgency and tenesmus (large bowel or "dysenteric" disease). In some cases, the watery diarrhea persists for several days without subsequent development of dysentery. *Shigella* is the predominant cause of dysentery in the world, and the appropriate management of dysentery is directed primarily at the appropriate antimicrobial coverage as described by regional surveillance.

Physical examination shows fever, signs of toxicity, tenderness over the lower abdominal quadrants, and hyperactive bowel sounds. Signs of dehydration may be present. Rectal examination reveals severe tenderness. Rectal prolapse may be present, particularly when diarrhea is associated with malnutrition.

The course without therapy typically lasts 5 to 7days. Although it is true that many enteric infections exacerbate undernutrition, initiating a "viscous cycle" of diarrhea and undernutrition, *Shigella* infections are particularly likely to do so. *Shigella* incidence is increased in underweight children.[146] *Shigella* causes a severe protein-losing enteropathy[45] (which is lessened by early appropriate antibiotic therapy)[41] and wasting of large amounts of vitamin A and zinc.[61,193] Shigellosis is associated with prolonged and persistent illness and linear growth shortfalls in children.[44] Groups at risk for severe disease include young children, the elderly, and malnourished children (Box 109.1).

Children infected with *S. dysenteriae* type 1, when compared to children infected with other species, are more likely to have severe gastrointestinal manifestations: grossly bloody stools (78% vs. 33%),

BOX 109.1 Risk Factors for Severe Disease

Infants and adults >50 y
Children who are not breastfed
Children recovering from measles
Patients with HIV
Malnourished children and adults
Any patient who develops dehydration, unconsciousness, hypothermia or hyperthermia, or has a history of convulsion with first seen

BOX 109.2 Complications of Shigellosis

Abdominal
Persistent diarrhea
Postdysenteric irritable bowel syndrome
Ileus, toxic megacolon, intestinal perforation
Protein-losing enteropathy, malnutrition
Surgical complications: intestinal perforation and obstruction, appendicitis, intraabdominal abscesses

Neurologic
Seizures
Headache, lethargy, disorientation, hallucinations
Coma
Severe toxin encephalopathy or ekiri syndrome

Bacteremia
In malnourished children, young infants, and HIV-AIDS patients

Hemolytic-Uremic Syndrome
Only with *Shigella dysenteriae* serotype 1

Urogenital
Vulvovaginitis, urinary tract infections

Other
Conjunctivitis, keratitis, corneal ulcers
Reactive arthritis
Reiter syndrome
Hepatitis
Myocarditis

more stools in the 24 hours before admission (median 25 vs. 11), rectal prolapse (52% vs. 15%), and extraintestinal manifestations: leukemoid reaction (22% vs. 2%), hemolytic-uremic syndrome (8% vs. 1%), severe hyponatremia (58% vs. 26%) and neurologic abnormalities (24% vs. 16%).[143]

The need for surgical intervention in shigellosis is rare but is associated with significant morbidity and mortality. In a series of 57 children with complications of shigellosis requiring surgical intervention,[192] intestinal obstruction (53%), appendicitis (28%), and colonic perforation (17%) were the most common occurrences (Box 109.2).

Although the organism usually is excreted for only a few days or weeks (range, 1 to 30 days), carriage of the organism has been described.[75,167] Asymptomatic or mildly symptomatic infection of infants and toddlers living in an endemic area occurs commonly and is usually transient, lasting no more than a few days.[106]

Extraintestinal Manifestations and Complications

Multiple extraintestinal complications have been described with *Shigella* infection (see Box 109.2). Seizures have been reported in 10% to 45% of hospitalized children with culture-proven shigellosis.[23,27,33,81,94] In outpatient settings, the frequency of seizures is very low. Children who develop neurologic complaints may have lethargy, severe headache, disorientation, hallucinations, or self-limited convulsions lasting less than 15 minutes.[21,24,27,197] Seizures are most likely to occur in very young patients, patients with a high peak body temperature, and patients with a family history of convulsive disorders.[23,150] Seizures can be focal, although typically, they are generalized.

When symptoms related to the nervous system occur, they are likely to appear early in the illness, even preceding development of diarrhea. Death rarely has been described[118]; most children recover completely with no residual neurologic deficits.[24] In contrast, in Bangladesh, where seizures in shigellosis typically are associated with factors known to alter consciousness (e.g., hypoglycemia, hyponatremia, fever), mortality rates are high.[142] Children with *Shigella* encephalopathy have significantly higher case-fatality rates than children with shigellosis without encephalopathy.[68] The pathogenesis of neurologic signs and symptoms during episodes of shigellosis is unclear. Hypoglycemia and electrolyte abnormalities are found in a few patients.[24] Direct invasion of the central nervous system during *Shigella* bacteremia is very rare.[293] Simple febrile seizures might explain convulsions in a few children with dysentery, but some children who have seizures during episodes of shigellosis do not experience seizures during other febrile infections and are outside the age range usually associated with febrile seizures.[24] Shiga toxin formerly was thought to cause the neurologic symptoms because it was considered to be a neurotoxin; however, data now clearly show that Shiga toxin is not responsible.[22] In an animal model of *Shigella*-related seizures, corticotropin-releasing hormone, a stress neurohormone, was associated with increased susceptibility to seizures after exposure to *S. dysenteriae*.[298] Studies from the same group have demonstrated that proinflammatory mediators are involved in *Shigella*-related seizures[297]; however, these researchers found that prostaglandins, which are host mediators induced during the inflammatory process, are not involved in the enhanced seizure response after exposure to *Shigella*.[299]

Severe toxic encephalopathy has been described. This syndrome (ekiri), as originally described in Japan, was characterized by dysentery with hyperpyrexia, convulsions, sensory disturbances, and rapid progression to death.[250] The children died of cerebral edema early in the course of disease (6 to 48 hours after onset). Mild hyponatremia has been a common finding.[102] Children with ekiri did not have sepsis, disseminated intravascular coagulation, hemolytic-uremic syndrome, or severe dehydration. This toxic encephalopathy is rare. Whether this syndrome is part of a continuum of central nervous system dysfunctions with seizures and other encephalopathic symptoms or has a completely different pathogenesis is unclear.

Hemolytic-uremic syndrome (microangiopathic hemolytic anemia, thrombocytopenia, and acute renal failure) or isolated hemolysis has been reported, mainly after infections with *S. dysenteriae* serotype 1 and rarely after infection with *S. flexneri*.[236] Vascular endothelial cell damage by Shiga toxin is considered to be the initial event, although endotoxin absorbed from the gut also may play a role.[147]

Ileus that progresses to toxic megacolon with distended loops and eventual intestinal perforation occurs.[28] It is seen mainly with *S. dysenteriae* serotype 1 infection.

Septicemia in shigellosis is a rare occurrence except in human immunodeficiency virus (HIV)-infected patients, malnourished children, young infants, and children with *S. dysenteriae* serotype 1 infections.[112,136,186,264] The mortality rate is at least twice as high in dysentery-associated sepsis as in shigellosis uncomplicated by bacteremia. The serogroup-related mortality risk in cases of *Shigella* bacteremia has been reported to be 85% for infection with *S. dysenteriae,* 43% for infection with *S. flexneri,* and 25% for infection with *S. sonnei;* bacteremia rarely is reported with *S. boydii* infection.[182] In Bangladesh, *Shigella* bacteremia was found in 4% of patients.[276] When bacteremia occurs with dysentery, it is as likely to be caused by other enteric bacteria as by the *Shigella* itself. The occurrence of *Klebsiella, E. coli,* and other enteric pathogens in blood cultures of children with shigellosis presumably reflects loss of the barrier function during severe colitis.[202] *Shigella* bacteremia may be complicated by disseminated intravascular coagulation and multiorgan failure. Bronchopneumonia may develop in septicemic children,[5] but its pathogenesis is unclear. Children who die of shigellosis often have pneumonia at autopsy.[53] HIV-infected patients with systemic shigellosis are more likely to die than patients not infected with HIV.[136]

Other extraintestinal infections rarely are caused by *Shigella* spp. Vaginitis with a bloody discharge (sometimes lasting for months in the absence of specific therapy) may occur, usually without concurrent or recent diarrhea.[78,199] *Shigella* cystitis, not always associated with diarrhea, has been described, usually in girls.[33] Conjunctivitis, keratitis, corneal ulcers, and iritis are other uncommon manifestations of shigellosis that usually are assumed to occur after autoinoculation.[33,281] Hepatitis with mildly abnormal liver function test results has been described.[274] Myocarditis manifested clinically by hypotension despite fluid replacement, arrhythmia, heart block, or low voltage on electrocardiography and pathologically by interstitial lymphocytic infiltrates and focal necrosis has been described.[247]

Postinfectious complications of shigellosis include reactive arthritis and postinfectious irritable bowel syndrome. Reactive arthritis may develop after infections with enteric pathogens such as *Shigella, Campylobacter, Salmonella,* or *Yersinia.*[59] However, the lack of a clear case definition precludes assessing the real disease burden of postinfectious arthritis. In general, reactive arthritis after shigellosis occurs especially in adults who are HLA-B27 positive; is uncommon in children[55]; and is unlikely to be associated with *Shigella* vaccines in developing countries.[98] Postdysenteric irritable bowel syndrome occurs in some patients after recovery.[291] In a recent case-control study of children in Italy, 43% of children with prior *Shigella* infections were found to have symptoms of postinfectious irritable bowel syndrome versus 11% of controls.[260] However, in a study conducted in the Netherlands the prevalence of postinfectious irritable bowel syndrome after *Campylobacter, Salmonella,* or *Shigella* infections was 9%.[107]

Shigellosis in the Neonatal Period

Bacillary dysentery is rare in neonates.[34,86,92,111,158] More than half of the reported neonatal cases occurred during the first 3 days of life, which is consistent with fecal-oral transmission during delivery,[104,204] usually from a symptomatic mother. Although a neonate with shigellosis usually has only low-grade fever with diarrhea of variable severity,[6,152,195] septicemia[164,248] and chronic diarrhea are more common than in older children. Intestinal perforation has been reported in neonatal shigellosis.[273] Diarrhea more often is nonbloody in infants; fever also occurs less commonly than in older children.[121] Data on age-related mortality caused by shigellosis in developing countries suggest that the mortality rate of the neonate is more than twice that of older children.

Shigellosis in Acquired Immunodeficiency Syndrome

In patients with acquired immunodeficiency syndrome (AIDS), shigellosis not only is more common and more severe but also is associated more often with bacteremia.[35,120,136] In contrast to the usual short, self-limited course of shigellosis, *Shigella* infection in patients with AIDS may be chronic and relapsing, despite appropriate antibiotic treatment.[153,267]

LABORATORY FINDINGS

The fecal leukocyte examination is helpful in evaluating a patient with fever and watery diarrhea and in monitoring the response to antimicrobial therapy. Direct microscopic examination of fecal mucus stained with methylene blue reveals sheets of polymorphonuclear leukocytes in patients with colitis, including most patients with shigellosis.[114] The blood leukocyte count in patients with shigellosis often is normal, although leukopenia or leukocytosis may occur.[19] The differential of the blood leukocyte count typically shows an increased percentage of band forms. Approximately one-third of children with shigellosis have more bands than segmented neutrophils in their peripheral blood smear. A leukemoid reaction, with a peripheral leukocyte count greater than 50,000/mm^3, has been reported, mainly with infections caused by *S. dysenteriae* serotype 1.[54] A leukemoid reaction has been reported in 10% of patients infected with the Shiga bacillus. When examination of cerebrospinal fluid is performed in children with neurologic symptoms, normal results usually are obtained, although some patients have a mild lymphocytic pleocytosis. Likewise, when electroencephalography is performed, the results usually are normal.[24]

DIAGNOSIS

Bacillary dysentery usually is suspected in children who present with bloody diarrhea, high fever, tenesmus, and generalized toxicity. However, approximately half of children do not develop bloody diarrhea during the course of their disease. This fact is especially relevant in developed countries, where most infections are caused by *S. sonnei.* The presence of only watery diarrhea does not exclude the possibility of shigellosis, especially in an ill patient with high fever.

Isolation Techniques

Proof of the diagnosis of suspected bacillary dysentery often is problematic and no licensed rapid diagnostic tests currently exist for shigellosis. Definite diagnosis of *Shigella* infection routinely depends on isolation of the organism from stool specimens or rectal swabs. The bacteria may not survive in fecal specimens during transit, however, and special selective media are necessary for isolation. Recovery of shigellae is easier early in the course of the disease than later because the number of viable organisms in stools decreases significantly during late stages of the disease. Even in adult volunteer studies, when appropriate stool cultures were obtained daily, cultures failed to isolate shigellae in approximately 20% of volunteers who had ingested the organism and developed diarrhea.

Several measures increase the likelihood of isolating *Shigella.* Specimens should be processed without delay. Pre-enrichment broth does not significantly impact isolation rates, and the main determinant of success in isolating *Shigella* is rapid processing time (time between voiding and storage in an appropriate transport medium) and minimal time to primary plating. If a specimen cannot be processed immediately, a transport medium, preferably Cary-Blair, should be used. More than one stool culture or rectal swab should be obtained and inoculated promptly onto at least two different culture media, and rapid plating onto primary media is rewarded by increased rates of isolation. Specimens should be plated lightly onto MacConkey, xylose-lysine-deoxycholate, or Hektoen enteric agar, whereas heavier plating is necessary for the more inhibitory *Shigella-Salmonella* medium.[196,279] After overnight incubation at 37°C, suspect colonies are transferred to triple sugar iron and lysine iron agar slants and incubated again overnight. Slants showing characteristic reactions of alkaline red slants, acid butt, and production of gas are tested biochemically for presumptive identification and then serologically for definitive identification.

Other Diagnostic Methods

Because presumptive identification of *Shigella* takes at least 48 hours and definite identification takes approximately 72 hours, attempts to develop rapid diagnostic methods are being made, especially because the early institution of treatment is important in shigellosis. PCR can detect as few as 10 colony-forming units of *S. flexneri* in stool specimens, whereas the sensitivities of DNA probe hybridization (with no amplification, often which are serotype specific) and standard biochemical methods are 10^3 and 10^6 colony-forming units, respectively and is the current gold standard diagnostic test in the research setting. Most PCR diagnostics rely on the detection of the *ipaH* gene, a multicopy element that is found on the chromosome and on the invasion plasmid of shigellae, has been developed and found to be more sensitive than the probes that were used previously, and is conserved across serogroups.[288] Molecular-based diagnoses have revealed that the sensitivity of culture is quite low, and now have an important role in attributing an increased burden of moderate and severe diarrhea to shigellosis.[173] Recently in a subset of specimens from the Global Enterics Multisite Study (GEMS), the fraction of attributable disease in moderate to severe diarrhea was 9.6% based on culture, and 17.6% based on a detection threshold of 1.4 × 104 ipaH copies.[173] The development of a broadly reactive point of care diagnostic test is a priority to improve care in settings where most cases of shigellosis occurs.

Serologic studies are not helpful in establishing the diagnosis of shigellosis in individual patients; humoral antibodies develop after clinical recovery. Serologic studies may be helpful, however, in epidemiologic studies to define the level of endemicity of shigellosis.

DIFFERENTIAL DIAGNOSIS

Colitis of any etiology manifesting as acute-onset bloody diarrhea with fever and abdominal cramps can mimic shigellosis. Etiologic agents to be considered include *Campylobacter* spp., *Salmonella* spp., *Clostridium difficile, Yersinia enterocolitica, Vibrio parahaemolyticus,* enteroinvasive *E. coli,* enterohemorrhagic *E. coli* (e.g., serotype O157:H7), and *Entamoeba histolytica.* The initial presentation of inflammatory bowel disease can mimic shigellosis.

An etiologic diagnosis of acute colitis syndrome on the basis of clinical presentation is difficult to make, although some data suggest a specific causative agent. In developed countries, *Campylobacter* is the most common cause of acute infectious colitis. Shigellosis should be suspected when evidence exists of person-to-person spread and when convulsions or other neurologic symptoms develop. A history of previous antibiotic treatment suggests diarrhea related to *C. difficile,* and previous consumption of seafood suggests *V. parahaemolyticus. Yersinia* infections are found mainly in the cooler regions of Europe and North America; the disease may mimic acute appendicitis because of the right lower quadrant pain associated with mesenteric lymphadenitis.

Enterohemorrhagic *E. coli* (EHEC) or Shiga toxin producing *E. coli* (STEC) infection often causes bloody diarrhea with little or no fever, in contrast to shigellosis, in which high fever is typical. Negative stool cultures for the mentioned bacterial pathogens may suggest infection by enteroinvasive *E. coli.* Amebiasis causes a colitis similar to the colitis caused by *Shigella,*[270] although it is of slower onset, with a lower degree of fever; the findings on fecal leukocyte examination are negative. The involvement of the colon with amebiasis is less diffuse than in shigellosis; areas of normal mucosa are found between ulcerations.

A prolonged course with negative cultures, especially with ancillary PCR-based diagnostics targeting the ipaH antigen, should raise concern about the possible presence of either ulcerative colitis or Crohn disease. When watery diarrhea is present, the list of possible etiologic agents is even longer, although many agents that cause watery diarrhea are associated with little or no fever and are not often confused with shigellosis. The diagnosis usually cannot be made by clinical presentation alone and requires laboratory confirmation.

TREATMENT

Fluid Administration

Dehydration is less a problem with shigellosis than with rotavirus or toxigenic *E. coli* infection. Some children with shigellosis, particularly young infants, have dehydration during the course of the disease. The high-volume watery diarrhea seen early in the course of the disease may cause excess losses of fluids and electrolytes; likewise, in patients with severe colitis, systemic toxicity and vomiting may cause anorexia that interferes with fluid intake.

Assessment of the hydration status of the patient on admission is mandatory, with early institution of appropriate fluid and electrolyte therapy needed. Low osmolarity oral rehydration (total osmolarity 245 mOsm/L, 75 mEq sodium, 20 mEq potassium, 10 mmol/L citrate, 75 mmol/L glucose), an improved choice especially in undernourished children, should be administered when available. Oral rehydration with commercially available solutions (e.g., Pedialyte) also is acceptable, and continued feeding is to be encouraged whenever possible. Administration of intravenous fluid therapy is necessary in children who are comatose, have an ileus, or are in shock. Early (12 to 24 hours after oral fluids are begun) breast-feeding and age-appropriate feeding in these children is a priority, especially in undernourished patients. Children with severe disease, seizures, and/or obtundation should have glucose and serum sodium levels monitored because hyponatremia and hypoglycemia are treatable complications seen in severe disease and possibilities to consider in severe cases or in patients who decompensate while receiving appropriate antibiotic therapy.

Antibiotic Therapy

Children who have dysentery and fever should be treated empirically with antimicrobial agents. WHO guidelines suggest that dysentery should be treated with antibiotics, the choice being decided by the antimicrobial susceptibility pattern of locally circulating *Shigella* strains (WHO/CDR/95.3). If after 2 days of therapy, the patient's condition improves, a full course of therapy for 5 days should be given. If the patient does not improve, the antibiotic should be changed. If after the second antibiotic the patient does not show signs of improvement, the diagnosis must be reviewed, and stool microscopy, culture, and susceptibility testing should be performed where available.[205]

Appropriate antimicrobial therapy for shigellosis shortens the duration of fever and diarrhea, reduces the risk for developing complications,[14] and shortens fecal carriage, thus attenuating transmission. Therapy should be stopped or changed on the basis of culture results (e.g., another pathogen or a resistant *Shigella* strain is isolated) and clinical response.

The choice of antimicrobial agent is complicated by the increasing frequency of antibiotic resistance.[90,93,145,253] Organisms resistant to ampicillin, trimethoprim-sulfamethoxazole, tetracycline, and chloramphenicol have been reported from the Middle East,[2,7,12,25,91,113,130,296] Africa,[2,46,60,133,185,201] South America,[170,200,207,234] Europe,[34,67,127,131,151,169,180,289] Eurasia,[29,217,300] Asia,[3,8,43,140,169,171,173,178] and the South Pacific. Currently, none of these agents should be used for empirical therapy; they should be used only if the organism has been shown to be susceptible.[18]

Strains exhibiting resistance to one or several antimicrobials also are found commonly in some parts of the United States. Among 4021 *Shigella* strains evaluated by the National Antimicrobial Resistance Monitoring System between 2004 and 2013, 95.9% were resistant to one or more antimicrobial agents and 61% were resistant to two or more agents. Fifty three percent of strains were resistant to ampicillin and 43.5% to trimethoprim-sulfamethoxazole. Resistance to current first line antibiotics in the same series was 3.7% for azithromycin (data from 2011–13 only), 1.0% for ciprofloxacin, 3.0% for nalidixic acid, and 0.5% for ceftriaxone, so despite reports of clusters of cases with decreased sensitivity to azithromycin and ciprofloxacin in the United States, the best available evidence supports their continued use.[48,49,116,266]

Multiresistant *Shigella* spp. are particularly likely to emerge in individuals who are exposed to multiple antibiotics[278] (e.g., patients with AIDS) and individuals who recently have traveled to areas with known resistance (particularly India and Vietnam).[79,144] Likewise, children in daycare centers are at risk for acquiring resistant organisms because the frequent use of antibiotics for otitis media may favor selection and emergence of resistant enteric organisms and because crowded living conditions and poor hygiene facilitate transmission.[50]

Shigella has a long history of the rapid development of antimicrobial resistance. Generally, shigellae are susceptible in vitro to azithromycin, ceftriaxone, cefotaxime, cefixime, nalidixic acid, and quinolones. However, the rapid disseminations of resistance to these antibiotics is being reported in several regions, most notably Southeast Asia. Nalidixic acid-resistant *Shigella* has rapidly developed principally in Asia in particular, although it has also been well documented in Africa.[70,105] Resistance to ciprofloxacin is increasingly common in India and in travelers returning from India.[49,190,272] These fluoroquinolone-resistant strains have mutations in *gyrA* and *parC* and have developed efflux pumps.[223] Similarly, azithromycin resistance is being increasingly reported. Resistance to ceftriaxone[179,290] and extended spectrum beta lactamase producing (ESBL) made up 8.7% of isolates in a recent series.[47,287]

In vitro susceptibility does not always predict clinical efficacy or superiority of one drug over another, however. The first-generation and second-generation cephalosporins are active in vitro but have been ineffective in clinical trials. Clinical studies have shown some drugs to be clearly superior to others when susceptibility data have suggested that either might work well.

Prevalent serotypes and resistance patterns can vary from year to year in a given locale. Typically, rates of resistance are related to the severity of disease caused by a given serotype. The more likely an organism is to cause severe disease, the more likely that resistant strains will emerge. *S. dysenteriae* serotype 1 is more likely to be multiply resistant than *S. flexneri; S. flexneri* is more likely to be resistant than *S. sonnei.* In Africa[46,133] and Asia,[37,39,71,178,198] *Shigella dysenteriae* resistance to nalidixic acid and ciprofloxacin has been reported. Nalidixic acid-resistant *S. flexneri* also have been recognized occasionally.[70] Local resistance patterns,

TABLE 109.2 **Antibiotic Treatment of Shigellosis in Children**

Antibiotic	Dosage[a]	Comments
Azithromycin	12 mg/kg/day once daily PO on day 1, followed by 6 mg/kg/day once daily on days 2–5 (maximum 500 mg/day)	Although published data in children are limited, its use is recommended by many experts Evidence of emerging resistance
Nalidixic acid	55 mg/kg/day PO divided every 6 h (maximum 2 g/day)	Not available in the United States; contraindicated in infants <3 mo Rates of resistance are rapidly increasing in Southeast Asia
Ciprofloxacin	15–30 mg/kg/day PO divided every 12 h (maximum 1.5 g/day)	Rates of resistance are increasing in Southeast Asia
Ceftriaxone	50 mg/kg/day IM or IV (maximum 2 g/day)	Current drug of choice for empirical therapy for severe dysentery in children ESBL strains are now well documented, particularly in India
Pivmecillinam	80 mg/kg/day divided 4 times a day	Limited geographic availability
Meropenem	120 mg/kg/day IV divided 3 times a day	Option for severe disease in patients with drug-resistant or suspected drug-resistant strains (from Southeast Asia)
Cefixime	8 mg/kg/day PO divided every 12–24 h (maximum 400 mg/day)	Not recommended as therapy in adults

[a]Recommended duration of antibiotic therapy for shigellosis usually is 5 days.
IV, Intravenously; *PO*, orally.

history of travel to an area of frequent resistance,[278] and severity of illness should determine antimicrobial selection.

Given the frequent occurrence of resistant organisms, optimal empirical therapy in children with dysentery should include azithromycin, a third-generation cephalosporin, nalidixic acid, or ciprofloxacin (Table 109.2).[18,36,87,126,162,205,227] Although less well studied, ampicillin-sulbactam and pivmecillinam also have been shown to be effective in children. In children, oral cefixime seems to be superior to ampicillin-sulbactam.[117] Adults do not respond well to usual doses of cefixime.[252]

In the absence of local susceptibility data, the WHO recommendations should be followed.[282,294] First-line therapy is ciprofloxacin (in all age groups, including children), and second-line therapy is pivmecillinam (where available), ceftriaxone, or azithromycin. Azithromycin has the advantage of additionally being appropriate for use for campylobacteriosis, the second most common cause of dysentery. The use of quinolones in children has been controversial. An oral fluoroquinolone (ciprofloxacin, norfloxacin) seems to be optimal for adults.[20,36,42,117,163,183,233] A considerable body of evidence from the long-term use of these drugs in children with cystic fibrosis has been accumulated, as has evidence from short-term use to treat typhoid fever and dysentery in children[162]; no evidence of bone or joint toxicity or growth impairment has been found, except for transient musculoskeletal events (arthralgia) in some children.[1,246] Nalidixic acid does not cause arthropathy or limit growth when it is used for a short time.[208]

Data for children suggest that norfloxacin at a dose of 10 to 15 mg/kg per day or ciprofloxacin at a dose of 10 mg/kg every 12 hours (maximum, 500 mg/dose) for 5 days is effective therapy.[102,163,176,251] In adults, short-course therapy (1 or 2 days) with ciprofloxacin has been effective for treatment of infections caused by *Shigella* spp. other than *S. dysenteriae*, for which a 10-dose, 5-day regimen is superior.[40] Pediatric data suggest that even for *S. dysenteriae* serotype 1 a short course of ciprofloxacin 15 mg/kg per dose every 12 hours for 3 days is as effective as a 5-day course.[301]

Because the patterns of antibiotic resistance of shigellae change, susceptibility testing should be performed on all clinical isolates if facilities are available, and the treatment should be changed accordingly. The recommended duration of antibiotic therapy for shigellosis usually is 5 days. Studies in adults and children have shown, however, that short-course treatment is nearly as effective as multiple doses in terms of symptomatic improvement,[100,183] although eradication of the organism from stools is less likely to occur with a single-dose regimen.[128] Because a major goal of antibiotic therapy is to reduce person-to-person transmission, multiple doses are preferred.

After initiation of therapy, a resistant organism can be suspected in the event of persistence of fever, grossly bloody stools, or unchanged frequency of stools by day 3 of therapy.[123] Persistent presence of numerous fecal leukocytes (>50 per high-power field) and erythrocytes (>5 per high-power field) at day 5 also suggests resistance. These findings are important because morbidity and mortality rates are higher when the organism is not susceptible to the initial drug of choice.[129] Protein-losing enteropathy is a more likely occurrence with resistant *Shigella* spp. if an inadequate agent has been used.[41]

Adjunctive Therapy

As with other forms of infectious colitis, antimotility agents should be avoided. Antimotility drugs, such as diphenoxylate (Lomotil), prolong the duration of fever, diarrhea, and excretion of the organism.[82] It has been speculated that intestinal motility and the constant fluid flow are important host defense factors for clearing of the organism and recovery from the infection.

Nutritional therapy is a key in undernourished children living in poverty, where the burden of global *Shigella* infections is focused. A high-protein, high-calorie diet during convalescence is important, and children should receive at least one additional meal a day until pre-illness weight is achieved. Nutritional therapy based on green bananas, a food rich in amylase-resistant starches, has been shown to be more efficacious than diet therapy with rice- or yogurt-based therapies in different trials in Bangladesh and Venezuela.[9,235] Because this is an affordable staple in many regions where shigellosis is endemic, its adjunctive use should be considered. Zinc should be given to all children at 20 mg/day (dosed as elemental zinc with sulfate and gluconate preparations being equally efficacious) for 10 to 14 days in children older than the age of 6 months; younger children should receive 10 mg/day for the same duration.

PROGNOSIS

Most patients recover eventually with or without specific antimicrobial therapy, although illness may be prolonged and severe if it is not treated with appropriate antibiotics.[52] The mortality rate in developed countries is less than 1%, and life-threatening complications are rare events. With appropriate antibiotic therapy, defervescence usually occurs within 24 hours and the diarrhea decreases dramatically in 1 to 2 days. If left untreated, the disease usually lasts 1 week or more. In developing countries, childhood shigellosis is associated with significant morbidity and mortality (10% to 30%),[38] particularly if it is caused by *S. dysenteriae* serotype 1. Children with malnutrition are particularly likely to have a complicated course.[69] Shigellosis in malnourished children often causes a vicious cycle of further impaired nutrition, and repeated infections may be associated with impaired growth. Young infants and severely undernourished children are more likely to have bacteremia, which markedly increases mortality rates.[212]

PREVENTION

In developed countries where person-to-person transmission of shigellae is the major mode of infection, personal hygiene measures are most important.[141] Special attention to hygiene should be given in daycare centers, which sometimes play a central role in community-wide outbreaks of shigellosis.[194] The close contact among children too young to control their excretions renders this setting ideal for fecal-oral spread of the organism. Children attending daycare centers frequently transmit infection to their families. Washing hands after defecating and before eating or preparing meals is important and helpful in preventing spread.[141] Daycare personnel who prepare food should avoid performing diaper-changing duties. Sick children should be excluded from the daycare center or cohorted, and mothers should be educated regarding the possibility of being infected by their children and the use of the necessary precautions. Proper cooking of potentially infected food, appropriate refrigeration, and exclusion of individuals with diarrhea from handling food are important precautions. Education of staff members in proper hygiene is essential to infection control.[228]

Patients with diarrhea in institutional and hospital settings should be isolated for prevention of outbreaks. Aggressive investigation and early initiation of appropriate antibiotic therapy in cases of bacillary dysentery are important measures in reducing excretion of virulent shigellae and stopping spread of the disease. Use of antibiotics for prophylaxis is not recommended.

In developing countries, a safe water supply and appropriate sanitation systems are important measures for reducing the risk for shigellosis. Chlorination of drinking water is important. Water stored in vessels that permit hand dipping has been defined as a risk factor.[284] Food prepared by street vendors also has been recognized as a risk factor. Prolonged breast-feeding is the best practical strategy for prevention of shigellosis (and most other enteric infections) in infants in most of the developing world.[4,74,187] Educational efforts to promote breast-feeding in these areas are key to children's survival. Human milk contains specific secretory IgA antibodies against *Shigella* lipopolysaccharides and virulence plasmid-coded antigens.[73] Lactoferrin and other nonspecific (nonantibody) factors in human milk, the effect of human milk on the type of intestinal flora, and the supply of an uncontaminated food source all may contribute to the protective effect of breast-feeding against diarrheal disease.

Natural clinical *Shigella* infection confers approximately 75% protection against illness on subsequent exposure to the homologous *Shigella* serotype and in some instances against heterologous serotypes. Antibodies (serum or mucosal) directed against the lipopolysaccharide O-antigen appear to play a major role in protection. The first line of defense, however, occurs at the mucosa.[221] Serotype-specific (lipopolysaccharide-based) vaccines have been produced.[95,96] Although early studies showed that immunization by the parenteral route with killed vaccines was ineffective, interest in this approach continues.[26,76,165] Several oral, live organism-based *Shigella* vaccines have been studied. Avirulent mutants of *S. flexneri* that lack the ability to invade the intestinal mucosa are safe and effective in monkeys. Multiple doses of large numbers of organisms were required to protect humans, however. Attenuated vaccines prepared from streptomycin-dependent mutant strains were effective but unstable.[188] Genetically attenuated *S. flexneri* strains conferred protection but caused diarrhea when fed to some volunteers. Prototype-attenuated *S. flexneri* strains CVD 1208[148] and WRSS[134] have provided encouraging results in early clinical trials. Two nonliving vaccine approaches include the oral administration of proteosomes[97] and of inactivated *Shigella* bacteria.

A recent trial of a new set of O-specific polysaccharide conjugate vaccines in Israeli children has demonstrated immunogenicity; however, there was no significant level of protection for the *S. sonnei* conjugate in children 1 to 2 years old, the age when *Shigella* infections peak in most endemic regions. Additionally, the incidence rates at the study site did not allow for estimates of the efficacy of the *S. flexneri* conjugate.[222] New studies are being conducted using improved techniques for enhancing immunogenicity of the polysaccharide unit and using synthetic conjugates.[226,244] Other new candidate vaccines are being evaluated, including the use of the major outer membrane proteins (OmpA) of *S. flexneri* 2a[232]; outer membrane vesicles (OMVs) from *S. flexneri*[56]; invasin-complex-based vaccines (Invaplex) from *S. flexneri* 2a containing lipopolysaccharides[243,283]; type III secretion system (TTSS) IpaB and IpaD proteins, which are more likely to be cross protective[184]; and second-generation *virG (iscA) S. sonnei* live attenuated candidate vaccines.[32,237]

No effective, licensed vaccine against shigellosis is available.[132,145,165,168,172,221,224] Whatever prototype *Shigella* vaccines prove to be well tolerated, immunogenic, and protective, the final formulation will have to confer protection against multiple epidemiologically important serotypes to have a meaningful impact on the burden of shigellosis. Inclusion of multiple cross reactive *S. flexneri* serotypes to control the majority of the burden of endemic shigellosis in developing countries is the priority. The additional availability of a vaccine against *S. dysenteriae* 1 has the potential to severe and most lethal epidemics, but the relative decline of *S. dysenteriae* infections seen over the last 20 years is notable in most settings. *S. sonnei* is responsible for 5% to 15% of shigellosis in developing countries and is an important cause of traveler's shigellosis and of shigellosis in diarrhea in daycare centers in industrialized countries.[165] Given that there is only one serotype, that there is evidence that the relative burden of disease is increasing, and the recently noted presence of stx producing *S. sonnei*, the inclusion of *S. sonnei* appears to be increasingly advantageous. Clearly the rapid and progressive emergence of antimicrobial resistance that now includes all oral therapies available in the developing world argues strongly for increased investment in *Shigella* vaccines.

NEW REFERENCES SINCE THE SEVENTH EDITION

16. Ashida H, Kim M, Sasakawa C. Manipulation of the host cell death pathway by *Shigella*. *Cell Microbiol.* 2014;16:1757-1766.
17. Ashida H, Mimuro H, Sasakawa C. *Shigella* manipulates host immune responses by delivering effector proteins with specific roles. *Front Immunol.* 2015;6:219.
30. Baker KS, Mather AE, McGregor H, et al. The extant World War 1 dysentery bacillus NCTC1: a genomic analysis. *Lancet.* 2014;384:1691-1697.
48. Bowen A, Eikmeier D, Talley P, et al. Notes from the Field: Outbreaks of *Shigella sonnei* infection with decreased susceptibility to azithromycin among men who have sex with men: Chicago and metropolitan Minneapolis-St. Paul, 2014. *MMWR Morb Mortal Wkly Rep.* 2015;64:597-598.
49. Bowen A, Hurd J, Hoover C, et al. Importation and domestic transmission of *Shigella sonnei* resistant to ciprofloxacin–United States, May 2014-February 2015. *MMWR Morb Mortal Wkly Rep.* 2015;64:318-320.
57. Carayol N, Tran Van Nhieu G. Tips and tricks about *Shigella* invasion of epithelial cells. *Curr Opin Microbiol.* 2013;16:1-6.
65. Centers for Disease Control and Prevention (CDC). *National Shigella Surveillance Overview.* Atlanta, Georgia: US Department of Health and Human Services, CDC; 2011.
66. Centers for Disease Control and Prevention (CDC). *Foodborne Diseases Active Surveillance Network (FoodNet): FoodNet Surveillance Report for 2014 (Final Report).* Atlanta, Georgia: U.S. Department of Health and Human Services, CDC; 2014.
79. De Lappe N, O'Connor J, Garvey P, McKeown P, Cormican M. Ciprofloxacin-resistant *Shigella sonnei* associated with travel to India. *Emerg Infect Dis.* 2015;21:894-896.
88. Farag TH, Faruque AS, Wu Y, et al. Housefly population density correlates with shigellosis among children in Mirzapur, Bangladesh: a time series analysis. *PLoS Negl Trop Dis.* 2013;7:e2280.
105. Guerrero L, Calva JJ, Morrow AL, et al. Asymptomatic *Shigella* infections in a cohort of Mexican children younger than two years of age. *Pediatr Infect Dis J.* 1994;13:597-602.
107. Hagar JA, Miao EA. Detection of cytosolic bacteria by inflammatory caspases. *Curr Opin Microbiol.* 2014;17:61-66.
115. Heiman KE, Karlsson M, Grass J, et al. Notes from the field: *Shigella* with decreased susceptibility to azithromycin among men who have sex with men: United States, 2002-2013. *MMWR Morb Mortal Wkly Rep.* 2014;63:132-133.
121. Hyma KE, Lacher DW, Nelson AM, et al. Evolutionary genetics of a new pathogenic *Escherichia* species: *Escherichia albertii* and related *Shigella boydii* strains. *J Bacteriol.* 2005;187:619-628.
134. Kayagaki N, Wong M, Stowe I, et al. Noncanonical inflammasome activation by intracellular LPS independent of TLR4. *Science.* 2013;341:1246-1249.
142. Khan WA, Griffiths JK, Bennish ML. Gastrointestinal and extra-intestinal manifestations of childhood shigellosis in a region where all four species of *Shigella* are endemic. *PLoS ONE.* 2013;8:e64097.
143. Kim JS, Kim JJ, Kim SJ, et al. Outbreak of ciprofloxacin-resistant *Shigella sonnei* associated with travel to Vietnam, Republic of Korea. *Emerg Infect Dis.* 2015;21:1247-1250.
154. Lamba K, Nelson JA, Kimura AC, et al. Shiga toxin 1-producing *Shigella sonnei* Infections, California, United States, 2014-2015. *Emerg Infect Dis.* 2016;22:679-686.
155. Lanata CF, Fischer-Walker CL, Olascoaga AC, et al. Global causes of diarrheal disease mortality in children <5 years of age: a systematic review. Sestak K, ed. *PLoS ONE.* 2013;8:e72788.

160. Lee MS, Koo S, Jeong DG, et al. Shiga toxins as multi-functional proteins: induction of host cellular stress responses, role in pathogenesis and therapeutic applications. *Toxins (Basel)*. 2016;8:77.
161. Lee G, Paredes Olortegui M, Peñataro Yori P, et al. Effects of *Shigella-, Campylobacter-* and ETEC-associated diarrhea on childhood growth. *Pediatr Infect Dis J*. 2014;33:1004-1009.
172. Lindsay B, Ochieng JB, Ikumapayi UN, et al. Quantitative PCR for detection of *Shigella* improves ascertainment of *Shigella* burden in children with moderate-to-severe diarrhea in low-income countries. *J Clin Microbiol*. 2013;51:1740-1746.
175. Livio S, Strockbine NA, Panchalingam S, et al. *Shigella* isolates from the Global Enteric Multicenter Study Inform Vaccine Development. *Clin Infect Dis*. 2014;59:933-941.
181. Marteyn B, Gazi A, Sansonetti P. *Shigella*: a model of virulence regulation in vivo. *Gut Microbes*. 2012;3:104-120.
188. Mellouk N, Weiner A, Aulner N, et al. *Shigella* subverts the host recycling compartment to rupture its vacuole. *Cell Host Microbe*. 2014;16:517-530.
208. Nygren BL, Schilling KA, Blanton EM, et al. Foodborne outbreaks of shigellosis in the USA, 1998–2008. *Epidemiol Infect*. 2013;141:233-241.
229. Picking WL, Picking WD. The many faces of IpaB. *Front Cell Infect Microbiol*. 2016;6:12.
231. Platts-Mills J, Babji S, Bodhidatta L, et al. Pathogen-specific burdens of community diarrhoea in developing countries: a multisite birth cohort study (MAL-ED). *Lancet Glob Health*. 2015;3:e564-e575.
241. Rayamajhi M, Zak DE, Chavarria-Smith J, et al. Cutting edge: mouse NAIP1 detects the type III secretion system needle protein. *J Immunol*. 2013;191:3986-3989.
264. Senerovic L, Tsunoda SP, Goosmann C, et al. Spontaneous formation of IpaB ion channels in host cell membranes reveals how *Shigella* induces pyroptosis in macrophages. *Cell Death Dis*. 2012;3:e384.
277. Suzuki S, Mimuro H, Kim M, et al. Shigella IpaH7.8 E3 ubiquitin ligase targets glomulin and activates inflammasomes to demolish macrophages. *Proc Natl Acad Sci USA*. 2014;111:E4254-E4263.
280. Thompson CN, Duy PT, Baker S. The rising dominance of *Shigella sonnei*: an intercontinental shift in the etiology of bacillary dysentery. *PLoS Negl Trop Dis*. 2015;9:e0003708.
285. Ud-Din A, Wahid S. Relationship among *Shigella* spp. and enteroinvasive *Escherichia coli* (EIEC) and their differentiation. *Braz J Microbiol*. 2014;45:1131-1138.
287. Varghese SR, Aggarwal A. Extended spectrum beta-lactamase production in *Shigella* isolates: a matter of concern. *Indian J Med Microbiol*. 2011;29:76-78.

The full reference list for this chapter is available at ExpertConsult.com.

110 Serratia

Randall G. Fisher

Similar to other members of the Enterobacteriaceae, the genus *Serratia* contains species increasingly associated with opportunistic infection in the compromised host. One of the oldest bacterial organisms to be named,[124] *Serratia marcescens* is the chief species associated with disease in humans and has been associated with infection of the urinary tract, the respiratory tract, local wounds, and central venous catheters. Illness may be complicated by bacteremia and meningitis. Treatment of infection may be made exceptionally difficult because these organisms frequently are resistant to penicillins, cephalosporins, and aminoglycosides.

BACTERIOLOGY

S. marcescens can produce a red pigment resembling blood on contaminated foodstuffs. In the 6th century, the "miraculous" appearance of blood on food provoked superstition and scientific investigation. Troops were goaded into battle, and religious beliefs gained support because of the fortuitous growth of the saprophyte in bread.[124] In vitro, the red pigment produced by these strains (called "prodigiosin") is toxic to cancer cells but not to nonmalignant cell lines.[34] In addition, prodigiosin has activity against the mitochondria of *Trypanosoma cruzi*,[45] is larvicidal against *Aedes aegypti*,[95] and, together with serratolomide, is broadly antimicrobial, presumably allowing *S. marcescens* to compete with other microorganisms for limited nutients.[115]

In 1819, *S. marcescens* was named by Bizio, who correctly interpreted the discoloration of cornmeal to be due to a living organism.[79] The genus name honors the Italian physicist Serrafino Serrati, who Bizio thought had been slighted in favor of Robert Fulton as inventor of the steamboat; the species name *marcescens* was drawn from the Latin word meaning "to decay."

We now recognize the genus *Serratia* as comprising organisms that are straight, motile, catalase-positive, gram-negative rods. On solid agar, colonies are opaque; iridescent; and white, pink, or red. Organisms appear positive with the Voges-Proskauer test.[54] The genus may be distinguished from other Enterobacteriaceae by its use of caprylate or L-fucose as a sole carbon source and its hydrolysis of gelatin.[54,119] Clinically relevant strains include *S. marcescens, S. liquefaciens, S. odorifera, S. ficara,* and *S. plymuthica*.[19,42] For a detailed review of the properties of *S. marcescens,* the reader is referred to the review by Hejazi and Falkiner.[55]

EPIDEMIOLOGY

S. marcescens was thought to be nonpathogenic in earlier times and was used as a biologic marker of transmission in 1906. In that year, N.H. Gordon, commissioned to study the atmospheric hygiene of the British House of Commons, gargled a liquid culture of *S. marcescens* and then quoted Shakespeare to an audience of agar plates in the otherwise empty House of Commons chamber.[49,124] The organism subsequently was recovered from the plates, documenting the possibility of aerosol transmission of bacteria (Gordon reported no ill effects). The importance of *S. marcescens* as a biologic marker for hand-to-hand bacterial transmission, ascension of bacteria in the urinary tract in catheterized patients, and bacteremia after dental extraction is reviewed in detail by Yu.[124] Most remarkably, in investigations in 1950 and 1952 to judge the threat of biologic warfare to the United States, the US Navy released *S. marcescens* into the Pacific, where it became aerosolized and drifted 80 miles inland.[13] Although an epidemic of *S. marcescens* infection in a San Francisco hospital coincided with this event, subsequent serotype and biotype analyses cast doubt on any relationship to the U.S. Navy experiments.[39] Rather the early San Francisco hospital experience heralded the increased frequency of nosocomial infections that would be observed in subsequent years.[124]

In some studies, *S. marcescens* is the organism most frequently isolated from contact lens solutions and contact lens cases.[96,126] Ex vivo mouse cornea studies show that the organism adheres to injured but not to intact corneas.[96] It is a cause of postoperative and posttraumatic endophthalmitis, with generally dire visual outcomes.[113] All commercial multipurpose disinfectant solutions are active against the type strain but vary in their activity against actual clinical isolates. Polyquaternium-1–based solutions fared the worst in their activity against circulating strains.[58]

Sporadic nosocomial outbreaks of infection were reported first in the 1950s and 1960s.[75,97,122] Early outbreaks in a pediatric ward and neonatal nursery were attributed to contaminated intravenous solution and caps of bottles containing saline used to moisten umbilical cords.[75] As reviewed by Yu,[124] environmental sources before 1979 included disinfectants, water from ultrasonic nebulizers, respirators, arterial pressure monitors, and fiberoptic bronchoscopes. Environmental sources since have included suction traps,[84] intraaortic pressure transducers,[10,120] contaminated handwashing brushes,[5] illicit intravenous drug paraphernalia,[30] contaminated urologic instruments,[37] colonized disinfectants or soaps,[38,70,77] contaminated infant parenteral nutrition fluid,[43] contaminated whole blood or blood products,[48,98] and inadequately sterilized breast milk pumps.[51] In one report, a woman elected to discontinue breastfeeding when the breast pump tubing turned bright pink and was culture positive for *S. marcescens.*[40]

Hand-to-hand transmission seems to be the primary mechanism of nosocomial spread. In one dramatic outbreak, spread of an organism with the same serotype, phage type, and antimicrobial sensitivity pattern was documented among four geographically separated teaching hospitals in the same region[103]; spread likely was due to passive carriage of *S. marcescens* on the hands of rotating personnel. By 1979, it was apparent that nosocomial increase in *S. marcescens* infection was becoming a worldwide concern.[19]

Outbreaks in neonatal units and pediatric wards have been widespread, persistent, and associated with high morbidity and mortality rates.[5,16,84,114] At the peak of one epidemic of invasive *S. marcescens* disease in a neonatal nursery, more than 90% of infants were colonized with the epidemic strain.[36] Increased rates of colonization have been associated with nearly 10-fold increases in rates of *S. marcescens* bacteremia and meningitis.[127] In a case-control study, neonates with *S. marcescens* bloodstream infection were at least three times more likely to have associated meningitis than were neonates whose blood cultures grew *Escherichia coli.*[14] Outbreaks of multidrug-resistant strains have been especially troublesome in surgical subspecialty wards, and an outbreak has been reported in a bone marrow transplant unit.[20,63] In the United States a multistate outbreak of *Serratia* infections was caused by contaminated prefilled saline and heparin syringes.[24]

Biotyping may be successful in characterizing isolates, which can be traced in the hospital environment.[53,111] Ribotyping or identification of a unique biochemical characteristic has proved useful for showing cross-contamination across hematology, gastroenterology, and neonatology units in a pediatric hospital.[12,44] Use of typing methods may be particularly important because drug-resistant and drug-susceptible isolates of *Serratia* organisms may co-circulate.[28] Banding differences from pulsed-field gel electrophoresis of DNA digests are restricted in number from outbreak strains; increases in banding pattern may reflect genetic drift over time.[7] Such DNA techniques have aided decisions regarding cohorting and closure of neonatal units and have been used to show cross-contamination of wards.[57,82] DNA amplification techniques offer promise for characterizing isolates in future outbreaks and defining antimicrobial susceptibility.[56,70,106]

PATHOPHYSIOLOGY

Pathologic findings of sepsis are similar to the findings of other gram-negative enteric bacilli. Postmortem examination of the lungs of patients with radiologic findings of *S. marcescens* pneumonia reveals a focal necrotizing pneumonia in most cases and hemorrhagic manifestations in some.[9]

Several properties may enhance virulence of *Serratia* organisms in human infection. The 56-kDa protease of *S. marcescens* seems to possess properties of a virulence factor. It enhances vascular permeability through activation of the Hageman factor–kallikrein–kinin pathway in vivo.[73] The protease also has the capacity to degrade host proteins important in humoral immune response, such as immunoglobulins and fibronectin,[83] and inactivates the chemotactic effect of C5a.[90] *Serratia* hemolysin indirectly may increase vascular permeability, local edema, and granulocyte accumulation.[64] Clinical strains seem to possess increased adherence properties compared with environmental isolates.[8] Compared with some enteric organisms, *Serratia* organisms adhere better to epithelial cells of the bladder, which may facilitate development of urinary tract infection.[32] Protease activity correlates with cytotoxicity in an in vitro model of eye infection; clinically strains from patients with keratitis have more protease activity than do those from patients with conjunctivitis.[109] Outer membrane vesicles (OMVs) are formed by *S. marcescens* in response to stress; OMVs likely play a role in virulence because it appears they function in toxin delivery.[76]

Cell-mediated immunity and humoral immunity may be important in protection from *Serratia* infection and illness. In a murine model of immunization against *S. marcescens,* only the transfer of antiserum and spleen cells from vaccinated mice increased bacterial clearance from the liver and survival after infection developed.[67] In nonphagocytic cells in vitro, *S. marcescens* can survive and even proliferate within autophage-like vacuoles by delaying or preventing fusion with lysosomes.[41]

Resistance of *S. marcescens* to aminoglycosides generally is plasmid mediated. Resistance to aminoglycosides may be conferred by one of several genes producing acetylating, phosphorylating, or adenylating enzymes.[1,2,20,59,80] Risk for acquiring infection with aminoglycoside resistance increases with exposure to these agents.[50,125] In some patients, repeated hospitalizations have shown greater importance, however, than aminoglycoside use as a risk factor for developing infection with resistant strains.[6] High levels of resistance to penicillins and cephalosporins are mediated by one or more plasmids. Cephalosporin resistance also may be derived chromosomally (see also Chapter 102).[28,46,78,93] Chromosomally mediated β-lactam resistance may be inducible in the presence of high levels of penicillin or cephalosporins, particularly when plasmid-derived β-lactamase is blocked by clavulanic acid.[21]

A group of researchers found and cloned a multidrug efflux pump of the major facilitator superfamily from *S. marcescens.*[108] Transposable plasmid elements may seem partly responsible for the rapid spread of multidrug resistance.[99,100,105] In one survey, 2.6% of *S. marcescens* isolates were deemed "multidrug resistant," defined as resistant to three or more classes of antimicrobial agents.[35] Plasmids conferring multidrug resistance are transferable from *S. marcescens* to *Klebsiella* spp. and may be responsible for sequential nosocomial outbreaks of different genera sharing common drug-resistance patterns.[118] A report from Spain suggested probable in vivo transmission between *E. coli* and *S. marcescens* of a plasmid containing both β-lactamase and quinolone resistance genes.[72] Carbapenem-resistant isolates have also been found.[112]

CLINICAL MANIFESTATIONS

First described in a patient with bronchiectasis as a cause of "blood-tinged" sputum colored by the organism,[123] *S. marcescens* commonly is associated with urinary tract, respiratory tract, central venous catheter, and bacteremic infections.[2] Other species, including *S. liquefaciens, S. ficara, S. odorifera,* and *S. plymuthica,* are less common causes of disease.[14,25,33,42,107]

Chromogenic *S. marcescens* was responsible for the historically interesting and reportedly benign "red diaper syndrome," which persisted for 7 months in the infant of a genetics professor.[121] In at least one series, the organism has been identified as one of the top five causes of neonatal sepsis[52] and now is recognized as a major pathogen of compromised newborns. Disease in neonatal intensive care units is associated commonly with high rates of underlying respiratory illness.[87] Other preexisting risk factors include necrotizing enterocolitis, surgical procedures, intravenous catheters, prolonged intubation, and cardiac disease.[14] Clinical illness shares features in common with other neonatal enteric pathogens; apnea, hypotension, and respiratory distress are seen frequently. Pneumonia with empyema has been reported.[62] Meningitis occurs as a complication in 24% of cases of neonatal bacteremia,[14] and antibiotic resistance may emerge during therapy for bacteremia or localized infection.[22] Significant brain injury caused by ventriculitis, brain abscesses, or porencephalic cysts is observed in most infants with meningitis.[22,68]

In older children and adults, *Serratia* spp. are isolated most frequently from the urinary tract.[2,103] Instrumentation, catheterization, and clustering of susceptible individuals are important risk factors.[6,23,59,101,104] By the 1970s, increased frequencies of serious infection, such as endocarditis, were noted in intravenous drug abusers.[30] In some series of respiratory and urinary tract infections, *S. marcescens* was observed to be associated more commonly with the complication of bacteremia than was any other enteric pathogen.[61,66] As is true of other causes of gram-negative sepsis, *Serratia* sepsis characterized by shock, pneumonia, or hemorrhage confers a substantially poorer prognosis.[15,17,102] The risk for these complications in cancer patients was observed by Saito and associates[102] to be lower, however, than their previous experience with other pathogens, such as *E. coli* and *Pseudomonas aeruginosa.* When predictive factors of mortality were sought in 385 subjects with nosocomial bacteremia, *S. marcescens* was not an independent predictor of death.[81] Other infections caused by *Serratia* include soft tissue infections, abscesses, endophthalmitis (including a case occurring after septicemia in an infant),[3,4] osteomyelitis and arthritis,[117] spinal epidural abscess, ventriculoperitoneal shunt infection,[27] and peritonitis in dialysis patients.[29] A severe case of epiglottitis including fasciitis, myositis, and bacteremia was seen in a 58-year-old woman; prior cases were all in immunecompromised patients.[86] In one report, sternal osteomyelitis recurred 15 years after apparent successful treatment.[94] Necrotizing soft tissue infection with *Serratia* has been reported in a patient with rheumatoid arthritis who was on steroids, tacrolimus, and tocilizumab.[74]

DIAGNOSIS

The diagnosis of *Serratia* infection relies primarily on isolation of organisms from clinical material. Nonspecific laboratory tests occasionally may be misleading. *Serratia* meningitis in a neonate may be accompanied by a normal cerebrospinal fluid white blood cell count or only a modest cerebrospinal fluid pleocytosis.[22] Although *S. marcescens* is famous historically because of its chromogenic potential, most strains are nonpigmented. Hydrolysis of gelatin distinguishes *S. marcescens* from *Klebsiella* and *Enterobacter* in the clinical microbiology laboratory. The presence of ornithine decarboxylase and fermentation of sorbitol but not arabinose helps to differentiate further *S. marcescens* from other *Serratia* spp.[54] Biotyping,[53] DNA and RNA detection techniques,[70] and antimicrobial susceptibilities[111] can be used to characterize strains.

TREATMENT

Empirical decisions about antibiotic treatment of *Serratia* infection should rely on knowledge of hospital flora. Therapy should be tailored when susceptibilities are known. In newborns, meningitis and its complications should be suspected and interventions should be guided by imaging of the central nervous system. Imaging techniques may be useful in guiding needle aspiration of abscesses.[89] Recommended antibiotic therapy for neonatal meningitis is a cephalosporin and an aminoglycoside for susceptible strains. Mortality rates remain high (>45%) even with appropriate antibiotic management.[22]

In older children and adults, reported response rates for bacteremic infection have been 75% for patients who received appropriate antibiotics, 22% for patients who received inappropriate antibiotics, and 29% for patients who received no antibiotics.[102] Patients who continue to have positive blood culture results while receiving appropriate antibiotic therapy have a poor prognosis. In the review by Saito and associates[102] of 118 patients with *Serratia* bacteremia, patients who received only an aminoglycoside had the poorest response rate among those who received appropriate therapy; patients who received a cephalosporin, alone or in combination, fared better. *Serratia* organisms generally have proved susceptible to third-generation cephalosporins in surveys of hospitals from North America.[60] The physician needs to be wary, however, of potential resistance to cephalosporins and penicillins owing to the production of extended-spectrum β-lactamases; this resistance may arise during therapy. In an illustrative case, cefotaxime therapy failed to clear the spinal fluid in a child with a shunt infection; by day 17 of therapy, the cefotaxime MIC had risen from less than 1 μg/mL to more than 16 μg/mL. Intermittent meropenem therapy also failed, but the patient was cured when meropenem was given by continuous infusion.[27] An extended-spectrum, metallo-β-lactamase that mediates resistance to imipenem has been described,[92] but it is uncommon. Physicians should strongly consider empirical use of a carbapenem in combination with an aminoglycoside in critically ill patients.[88] A worldwide surveillance study from 2004 to 2009 suggested that more than 90% of *Serratia* strains were susceptible to meropenem, imipenem, and tigecycline.[11] However, outbreaks due to meropenem-resistant clones have also been described.[116]

Amikacin historically has been effective in the treatment of gentamicin-resistant strains.[31,69] In 1985, amikacin was recommended as a first-line antibiotic for treatment of pediatric nosocomial infection when *Serratia* spp. or other enteric agents with resistance potential were suspected.[110] Since the 1980s, however, outbreaks of *S. marcescens* infections caused by amikacin-resistant strains have been reported.[91] Quinolones have been used successfully for treatment of organisms resistant to other agents,[47] but resistance to these drugs also has been identified.[65] Many multiresistant strains remain susceptible to tigecycline.[71,85]

Cohorting and attempts to remove environmental sources of infection have been successful in ending epidemics but typically require several months.[26] Rarely neonatal intensive care units have been closed to admissions to halt epidemics.[18,84]

NEW REFERENCES SINCE THE SEVENTH EDITION

27. Cies JJ, Moore WS 2nd, Calaman S, et al. Pharmacokinetics of continuous-infusion meropenem for the treatment of Serratia marcescens ventriculitis in a pediatric patient. *Pharmacotherapy*. 2015;35:332-336.
71. Margate E, Magalhaes V, Fehlberg LC, et al. KPC-producing Serratia marcescens in a home-care patient from Recife, Brazil. *Rev Inst Med Trop Sao Paulo*. 2015;57:359-360.
74. Matsuo H, Kosaka K, Iwata K, et al. Necrotizing soft tissue infection caused by Serratia marcescens in a patient treated with tocilizumab. *Kansenshogaku Zasshi*. 2015;89:53-55.
85. Morfin-Otero R, Noriega ER, Dowzicky MJ. Antimicrobial susceptibility trends among gram-positive and –negative clinical isolates collected between 2005 and 2012 in Mexico: results from the Tigecycline Evaluation and Surveillance Trial. *Ann Clin Microbiol Antimicrob*. 2015;14:53.
109. Shanks RM, Stella NA, Hunt KM, et al. *Infect Immun*. 2015;83:2907-2916.
112. Silva KE, Cayo R, Carvalhaes CG, et al. Coproduction of KPC-2 and IMP-10 in carbapenem-resistant Serratia marcescens isolates from an outbreak in a Brazilian teaching hospital. *J Clin Microbiol*. 2015;53:2324-2328.
113. Sridhar J, Kuriyan AE, Flynn HW Jr, et al. Endophthalmitis caused by Serratia marcescens: clinical features, antibiotic susceptibilities, and treatment outcomes. *Retina*. 2015;35:1095-1100.
115. Stella NA, Lahr RM, Brothers RM, et al. Serratia marcescens cyclic AMP receptor protein controls transcription of EepR, a novel regulator of antimicrobial secondary metabolites. *J Bacteriol*. 2015;197:2468-2478.

The full reference list for this chapter is available at ExpertConsult.com.

111 *Salmonella*

Theresa J. Ochoa • Javier Santisteban-Ponce

Salmonellosis is a foodborne disease of global public health importance. *Salmonella* infections most often cause gastroenteritis, but can also cause invasive infections. Based on the clinical disease and pathogenesis, *Salmonella* organisms are classified as nontyphoidal *Salmonella* (NTS) and *Salmonella* associated with typhoid fever or enteric fever (*Salmonella enterica* ser. Typhi). NTS causes asymptomatic infection or carriage, gastroenteritis, bacteremia, or metastatic focal infections.

MICROBIOLOGY

Salmonellae are motile (owing to peritrichous flagella), nonencapsulated, gram-negative bacilli and facultative anaerobes of the Enterobacteriaceae family. *Salmonella* serotype is defined by the serogroup, the flagellar (H), and the virulence (Vi) antigens. H antigens can be either phase 1 (nonspecific) or phase 2 (specific). The Vi antigen, a heat-labile polysaccharide found on *S.* ser. Typhi, *S.* ser. Dublin, and *S.* ser. Paratyphi C may block agglutination caused by antibodies to O antigen. Serotyping is important for defining outbreaks, although it is most useful when an unusual type is associated with disease. When a common serotype is associated with an outbreak (e.g., *S.* ser. Typhimurium), biochemical phenotype, antibiogram, plasmid characterization, bacteriophage typing, outer-membrane protein analysis, pulsed-field gel electrophoresis, and randomly amplified polymorphic DNA may help determine whether a single-strain, common-source outbreak is in progress.

Based in host adaptability, Salmonellae are divided into three groups. Group 1 encompasses *Salmonella* highly adapted to humans and primates, group 2 identifies highly specific animal-adapted *Salmonella,* and group 3 includes those serovars not host adapted but capable of infecting both humans and a wide range of animals and consisting mainly of *Salmonella* ser. Typhimurium and *S.* ser. Enteritidis.[7] Blood agar or chocolate agar supports their growth when they are present as the sole organisms in blood, cerebrospinal fluid (CSF), or joint fluid. For specimens containing mixed flora (e.g., stool), selective media such as *Salmonella-Shigella* (SS) agar or bismuth sulfate agar must be used.

TAXONOMY AND NOMENCLATURE

The genus *Salmonella* is divided into two species, *enterica* and *bongori.* The species *S. enterica* is further subdivided into six subspecies that are designated by taxonomic names: *enterica, salamae, arizonae, diarizonae, houtenae* and *indica*; these are sometimes abbreviated by Roman numerals. For example, *S. enterica* subsp. *enterica* is subspecies I.[67]

Serotyping is used to differentiate isolates of *Salmonella* beyond the subspecies level. *Salmonella* serotypes are designated based on the immunoreactivity of two cell surface structures, the O and H antigens. A substantial amount of diversity exists in these two antigens, resulting in the designation of more than 2500 serotypes; about 60% belong to subspecies I. In the United States, 99% of reported human *Salmonella* isolates belong to subspecies I.[67] All *Salmonella* serotypes can be designated by a formula; subspecies I serotypes are also given a name (e.g., Typhimurium, Enteritidis, Typhi).

The complete, formal designation of a *Salmonella* serotype is its genus-species or genus-species-subspecies name, followed by "serotype" and the serotype name or formula. Some scientific journals require the formal designation of serotypes; others allow the use of an abbreviation. For example *Salmonella enterica* subsp. *enterica* serotype Typhimurium, is shortened to *Salmonella* serotype (ser.) Typhimurium or *Salmonella* Typhimurium. However, there is no international standard for abbreviating *Salmonella* serotypes.

In this chapter, we use the nomenclature of the Centers for Disease Control and Prevention (CDC) rather than either the complete name or the traditional clinical shorthand (Table 111.1). In hospital laboratories, *Salmonella* ser. Choleraesuis and *Salmonella* ser. Typhi are distinguished biochemically from other *Salmonella* spp. serogroup, based on O (somatic) antigen; organisms that are not *S.* ser. Typhi or *S.* ser. Choleraesuis are reported as *Salmonella* serogroup A, B, C1, D1, and so on. Common *Salmonella* spp. and their serogroups are shown in Table 111.2. Complete serotyping is performed only in public health laboratories.

TABLE 111.1 Examples of Current *Salmonella* Nomenclature

CDC Designation	Complete Name	Previous Designation
S. ser. Typhi	*S. enterica*[a] subsp. *enterica* ser. Typhi	*S. typhi*
S. ser. Enteritidis	*S. enterica* subsp. *enterica* ser. Enteritidis	*S. enteritidis*
S. IIIa 18:z_4,z_{23}:-	*S. enterica* subsp. *arizonae* ser. 18:z_4,z_{23}:-	*Arizona hinshawii* ser. 7a, 7b:1,2,5:
S. ser. Marina	*S. enterica* subsp. *houtenae* ser. Marina	*S. marina*

CDC, Centers for Disease Control and Prevention.
[a]*S. choleraesuis* and *S. enteritidis* also are designations commonly used for the species.

EPIDEMIOLOGY

Nontyphoidal *Salmonella*

Public Health Issues

In most of the world, the prevalence of *Salmonella* varies according to the water supply, waste disposal, food preparation practices, and climate. The incidence of NTS is 31 to 211 million gastroenteritis cases worldwide each year, causing 36,000 to 89,000 deaths globally and leading to the loss of 2 to 6 million of life-years.[171] Most of the deaths occurred in the African region.[171] Globally NTS is the worst foodborne hazard (2.5 to 6.3 million disability-adjusted-life-years).[171] In the United States the incidence of the disease has increased steadily despite good public health interventions, while NTS-related mortality declined over years.[99] A more than sixfold increase in reported NTS infection in the United States has occurred during the past 40 years,[391] with an estimated 1.2 million illnesses, 23,000 hospitalizations, and 450 deaths annually during 2000 to 2008.[69,341] This increase reflects industrial-scale food production and distribution,[66] misuse of antimicrobial agents (in humans and animals) that alter the competing gastrointestinal flora and induce multidrug-resistant strains of *Salmonella,*[381] and probably an increasing number of immunocompromised individuals in the population. Direct medical costs are estimated to be $365 million annually.[70]

Targeted interventions, including on-farm control measures, refrigeration, and education contributed to an important decrease in the incidence of *S.* ser. Enteritidis infections in the United States.[248] From 1996 to 2011, serotypes Typhimurium, Enteritidis, Newport, Heidelberg, and Javiana jointly were 63% of isolates.[51] While average incidence decreased for serotypes Typhimurium (16%) and Heidelberg (30%), increases in Newport (27%), Javiana (63%), Saintpaul (43%), and Mississippi (63%) were found from the second half of the time period.[51]

Globally 2.1 to 6.5 million cases per year are due to invasive NTS.[19] In some developing countries, mortality rates of bacteremic NTS infections in infants remain at 20% or higher over the years, leading to 415,000 to 1.3 million deaths annually.[19,155]

TABLE 111.2 *Salmonella* spp. Included in Major Serogroups

Serogroup[a]	Representative Serotypes
A	*S.* ser. Paratyphi A
B	*S.* ser. Paratyphi B
	S. ser. Saint-Paul
	S. ser. Agona
	S. ser. Derby
	S. ser. Typhimurium
	S. ser. Heidelberg
C1	*S.* ser. Paratyphi C
	S. ser. Choleraesuis
	S. ser. Montevideo
	S. ser. Infantis
C2	*S.* ser. *Newport*
C3	*S.* ser. Santiago
D1	*S.* ser. Typhi
	S. ser. Enteritidis
	S. ser. Dublin
D2	*S.* ser. Strasbourg
E1	*S.* ser. Anatum
E2	*S.* ser. Newington
E3	*S.* ser. Illinois

[a]Human infections with organisms in serogroups E4, F, G1, G2, H, and I and the O antigens not given serogroup designation (O17 through O67) are uncommon.

Significance of Animal Reservoirs and Other Food Sources

In contrast to *Shigella* spp., which infect only primates, nontyphoidal *Salmonella* spp. infect a variety of animals (including poultry, livestock, and pet reptiles and rodents).[1,27,34,68,130,158,178,255,362] Salmonella has been isolated from flies, mites, and other arthropods taken from animal farms; it is able to multiply inside some insects and is transmitted within insects and to birds, rodents, and livestock.[397] These arthropods, birds, and rodents could contribute to *Salmonella* transmission to wildlife.[176] Animals and animal products (including meat and dairy products),[299,320,415] water,[104,120,211,260] and infected humans[384] can be the source of infection. *Salmonella* is the leading cause of foodborne illness in the United States and the second most common cause of death from foodborne pathogens.[240] Spread of resistant organisms from food animals to humans has been shown.[270] *Salmonella* spp. have been isolated from 50% of poultry,[53] 16% of pork, 5% of beef, and 40% of frozen egg products in retail stores. Slicing food with contaminated tools and surfaces transfers *Salmonella* in progressively decreasing amounts per slice, resulting in higher bacterial contamination for the first sliced portions.[65] Undercooked eggs (e.g., in Caesar salad, egg-dipped bread, and homemade eggnog) may be contaminated by organisms on the shell surface or transovarially directly through the egg yolk. Grade A shell eggs have been implicated in more than 40% of more recent outbreaks.[240] Even in the absence of recognized outbreaks, undercooked eggs probably are important vehicles of infection.[162,173,401]

The impact of *Salmonella* outbreaks was shown when milk contaminated with *S.* ser. Typhimurium was distributed in Chicago, Illinois. Reports estimated that more than 150,000 people became ill, with more than 16,000 culture-confirmed cases, 2777 individuals hospitalized, and 14 fatalities.[37] Ice cream, cream cakes, and mayonnaise commonly have been incriminated as the source of infections. Fruits and vegetables are vehicles reported less frequently in outbreaks but better identified and reported in recent years as a result of molecular methods and country-wide database reporting.[40,135,175,236,245,315] From 2010 to 2014 the CDC's Foodborne Disease Outbreak Surveillance System reported 120 multistate foodborne disease outbreaks in the United States; *Salmonella* was the leading pathogen, responsible for 63 of these outbreaks.[94]

Of the 10 most frequent *Salmonella* serovars causing disease in humans, eight are included within the 10 serovars most frequently identified in at least one of the major food-animal species.[137] Some serotypes are associated with particular reservoirs. *S.* ser. Dublin is associated with dairy cattle and is frequently found in individuals who drink raw milk.[369] *S.* ser. Choleraesuis is associated with pigs.[77] *S.* ser. Typhimurium is associated with contact with pet rodents.[362] Infection with *S.* ser. Marina is associated with contact with pet iguanas.[363] *Salmonella* group F, *S.* ser. Typhimurium, *S.* ser. Muenchen, *S.* ser. Poona, and *S.* ser. Java infections have been traced to pet turtles.[219] Reptiles, including rattlesnakes, are important *S.* IIIa 18:z_4,z_{23}: *(Arizona hinshawii)* reservoirs and have been associated with almost all the 20 serovars isolated in animals in the United States during 2006.[177]

Humans as a Reservoir

After infection occurs, NTS are excreted in feces for a median of 5 weeks. Children younger than 5 years may excrete the organisms for 20 weeks after having an illness, but older children and adults usually excrete *Salmonella* for less than 8 weeks. Up to 5% of children younger than 5 years have been found to excrete NTS for 1 year after disease[59]; 2.2% to 2.7% of children in endemic settings have been found to excrete NTS.[192] *S.* ser. Typhi may be excreted chronically, particularly in the presence of gallbladder disease and sustained by biofilms for decades.[93,154,174,249] Food handlers who are excreting *Salmonella* spp. represent an important risk group. NTS infection index cases have been mapped to isolation of the same clones in 65% of children and adults living in the same household versus less than 2% of home rural environment samples.[205] NTS may be excreted for longer periods in feces of children with primary immunodeficiency.[293]

Bacterial Characteristics Favoring Survival

Salmonella spp. survive refrigeration and sometimes heating; they may remain viable at ambient or reduced temperatures for weeks, even in low-moisture foods.[308] Salmonellae may remain viable in foods after cooking for less than 12 minutes at less than 65°C (140°F). *Salmonella* spp. are killed by heating to 54.4°C (130°F) for 1 hour or 60°C (140°F) for 15 minutes. Food industry ingredients with low water activity and high fat content provide a marked thermal resistance to *Salmonella*, making it necessary to use higher heating temperatures and longer times.[308] Salmonellae survive for hours on the hands of slaughterhouse workers and in flour for nearly 1 year.[301] *S.* ser. Tennessee has been reported to remain viable for 2 to 8 days on glass, stainless steel, enameled surfaces, a rubber mattress, linen, and a rubber tabletop.[399] Small *Salmonella* inoculates (<100 colony-forming units [cfu]/g) are able to survive 30 to 40 days in vacuum dust.[172] Nosocomial infections have been related to contaminated medical equipment (e.g., endoscopes) and diagnostic or pharmacologic preparations, particularly those of animal origin (e.g., bile salts, pancreatic extracts, pepsin, and vitamins). *Salmonella*'s capability to form complex surface structures called biofilms in both host and nonhost environments is an important mechanism for survival and persistence.[64,216,249] Biofilm formation increases resistance of *Salmonella* to disinfectants and even to antibiotics, resulting in 2000-fold resistance to ciprofloxacin in vitro.[355]

Relationship of Age to Risk for Disease

The highest incidence rates occur in children younger than 5 years (69.5 infections per 100,000 children),[171] especially infants younger than 1 year, and in individuals older than 70 years. Among infants in the United States, the incidence of invasive salmonellosis (7.8 cases/100,000 inhabitants) is the highest within age groups.[392] Nursery outbreaks often can be traced to an infected mother,[28,222] with subsequent spread occurring through health care personnel.[340,400] The mother of the index case can be symptomatic[136,199,328] or asymptomatic,[400] recovering from recent infection,[283,346] or a chronic carrier.[337] Low-birth-weight infants seem to be at higher risk than full-term infants for acquiring *Salmonella* infection.[33,340,400] The source of infection occasionally is contaminated food, but more often it is fomites (e.g., delivery room resuscitators,[329] rectal thermometers,[191,256] suction devices,[209] water baths for heating formula,[201] soap dispensers,[266] scales,[6,35,400] tables,[400] air-conditioning filters,[400] and plumbing[262]). Outbreaks in nurseries often are extraordinarily difficult to stop. They have been reported to last months[222,290,400] to years.[136,262,366] Contamination sometimes can become so widespread that other areas of the hospital also experience cases.[251,345] These outbreaks occur far more commonly with *Salmonella* than with other bacterial enteropathogens. Such outbreaks sometimes are caused by multiresistant *Salmonella*.[222] Multidrug-resistant *Salmonella* has been isolated from cockroaches found in a neonatal intensive care unit in Africa.[375]

Seasonality

Salmonella infection occurs throughout the year with a predilection for warm months,[223] especially for some serotypes as Norwich, Javiana, Mississippi, and Newport,[51] whereas serotypes Senftenberg, Mbandaka, Anatum, and Derbyare are distributed throughout the seasons.[51,223]

Inoculum Size Required to Cause Disease

The estimated inoculum size required to cause symptomatic disease in healthy adult volunteers is 10^5 to 10^{10} organisms,[47] but the number of organisms required to cause symptoms in infants and children probably is much lower. In contrast, large inocula are not required for *Shigella* infection, which occurs in adult volunteers exposed to only 10 organisms. In some outbreaks, very small inocula of *Salmonella* seem to have caused disease. Pharmacologic suppression of gastric acid secretion increases the risk for disease caused by *Salmonella*.[36] Large inocula (e.g., 10^9 organisms) may cause severe symptoms, even in healthy children.[369] The incubation period usually is 6 to 72 hours but depends on inoculum size, bacterial virulence, and host immunocompetence. Communicability parallels the duration of fecal excretion. The probability of salmonellosis occurring is increased when a member of the household is infected. Infants especially may be susceptible to acquiring *Salmonella* infection directly or indirectly from ill family members. Infants also may acquire infection via exposure to raw meat while riding in a grocery cart or while having contact with infected pets.[198] In a retrospective review of 187 infants younger than 1 year with *Salmonella* gastroenteritis, 39%

had at least one family contact with diarrhea, and 71% of the contacts had stool cultures positive for *Salmonella*.[403] *Salmonella* spp. rarely have been isolated during studies of gastroenteritis in daycare centers, suggesting that larger inocula are required to cause illness in toddlers and older children.[80,231,304]

Antibiotic Selection Pressure

Since the mid-1960s, *Salmonella* spp. have become increasingly resistant to ampicillin, chloramphenicol, and trimethoprim-sulfamethoxazole (TMP-SMX). Multiresistant strains have included *S.* ser. Typhimurium, which is the most common serotype in Europe and the United States. Multidrug-resistant *S.* Typhimurium phage type DT104 (DT104) rapidly emerged globally in the 1990s and became the most prevalent phage type isolated from humans and animals in many countries. DT104 is typically resistant to ampicillin, chloramphenicol, streptomycin, TMP-SMX, and tetracycline, along with its capacity to acquire additional resistance to other clinically important antimicrobials, including fluoroquinolones.[152,227] Another important resistance trend among NTS isolates has been the development of resistance to fluoroquinolones, especially in Asia. The development of NTS isolates resistant to extended-spectrum cephalosporins, such as ceftriaxone, represents a substantial global public health concern.[98]

Antibiotic resistance usually is transferable between organisms through plasmids that carry genes encoding resistance factors. Some serotype-specific virulence plasmids form hybrid plasmids through recombination with resistance plasmids or acquire gene cassettes consisting of multiple resistance genes. Such evolutionary events provide a virulent strain with the advantage of survival in an unfavorable drug environment.[361] Patients who are infected with antibiotic-resistant strains are more likely to be hospitalized, to be very young, to be black, and to have been exposed recently to antibiotic agents.[224] Previous use of antimicrobial agents for treatment of other illnesses is a significant risk factor for acquiring multiresistant *Salmonella* infection.[242,319]

In the United States, 30.5% of NTS isolates from blood from 1996 to 2007 were found resistant to at least one antimicrobial tested.[96] The National Antimicrobial Resistance Monitoring System (NARMS) during the years 2009–2011 reported 3% ceftriaxone resistance and 3% ciprofloxacin resistance in NTS *Salmonella* strains.[71]

Perhaps the most important factor is the overuse and misuse of antibiotics in animals raised for food.[87,182,183,230,354] Subtherapeutic concentrations of antibiotics used to enhance growth and prevent infection in animals promote intestinal colonization by antibiotic-resistant bacteria, including *Salmonella;* these organisms may be found in feces and may contaminate instruments and meat at the time of slaughter.[64,135] Plasmid analysis and antibiotic susceptibility patterns have linked *Salmonella* outbreaks to specific farms and slaughterhouses.[182,183,270]

Salmonella Ser. Typhi

The CDC estimates that 22 million typhoid cases occur each year in the world, with an annual incidence varying from less than 10 to more than 1000 cases per 100,000 population.[336] The global mortality estimates from typhoid also have been revised downward from 600,000 to 200,000, on the basis of regional extrapolations.[95] Globally the major nondiarrheal causes of foodborne deaths were due to *Salmonella* Ser. Typhi (~52,000) in 2010.[171] *S.* ser. Typhi is the most common *Salmonella* isolate in many developing countries. Although the overall ratio of disease caused by *S.* ser. Typhi to disease caused by *S.* ser. Paratyphi is about 10 : 1, the proportion of *S. paratyphi* infections is increasing in some parts of the world,[42] sometimes paralleling *S.* ser. Typhi isolations.[97] The human immunodeficiency virus (HIV) and acquired immunodeficiency syndrome (AIDS) epidemic in Africa has been associated with a concomitant increase in community-acquired bacteremia caused by NTS.[41,157] In the United States, approximately 1700 total cases were reported (one case per 100,000) in 1955. In 1988, approximately 400 total cases were reported (0.018 case per 100,000). Approximately 28% of infections occurred in individuals 19 years old or younger. Frequently, the highest incidence is stated as occurring in individuals 5 to 12 years of age. More recent population-based studies from South Asia and India suggest, however, that the incidence is highest in children younger than 5 years, with higher rates of complications and hospitalization.[42,349]

In the United States, individuals traveling to developing countries are a high-risk group; 62% to 81% of infections are related to foreign travel, especially to Mexico, India, the Philippines, Pakistan, El Salvador, and Haiti. Of these areas, the Indian subcontinent has the highest incidence of typhoid among travelers.[4,65,264,333]

Reservoir

Humans are the reservoir for *S.* ser. Typhi; infection implies direct or indirect contact with an infected person. Animal products transmit *S.* ser. Typhi if they are contaminated by infected humans during processing. The most common mode of transmission is food or water contaminated by human feces. Waterborne typhoid fever epidemics are especially important. Congenital transmission can occur from a bacteremic mother to her fetus transplacentally[269,342] or at the time of delivery.[269]

Relevance of Inoculum Size to Disease

As with NTS, more than 10^5 organisms are required to cause clinical illness in adults.[185,186]

Antibiotic Resistance

The worldwide frequency of antibiotic-resistant *S.* ser. Typhi has been increasing since the 1960s.[351] Drug resistance in *Salmonella* Typhi (resistance or partial resistance to ciprofloxacin) has increased significantly from about 20% in 1999 to more than 70% in 2011.[70] Travel-associated infections are more likely to be antibiotic resistant. The CDC has reported some level of resistance (resistance or partial resistance) to ciprofloxacin in 67% of *Salmonella* Typhi tested (3-year average, 2009–11). The CDC has not yet seen resistance to ceftriaxone or azithromycin in the United States, but this has been reported in other parts of the world. Resistant infections are likely to cost more than susceptible infections because illness may last longer.[70] Extensive protracted outbreaks have been reported throughout Asia, the Middle East, and Central and South America. These outbreaks may have been related to widespread and inappropriate use of antimicrobial agents in these areas. After sporadic outbreaks of chloramphenicol-resistant typhoid between 1970 and 1985, many strains of *S.* ser. Typhi developed plasmid-mediated, multidrug resistance to the three primary antimicrobials used (i.e., ampicillin, chloramphenicol, and TMP-SMX).[327] This pattern of simultaneous resistance of *S.* ser. Typhi to formerly recommended first-line antimicrobials (i.e., ampicillin, chloramphenicol, and TMP-SMX) is defined as multidrug-resistant typhoid fever.[405] Chromosomally acquired quinolone resistance in *S.* ser. Typhi and *S.* ser. Paratyphi has been described more frequently in some parts of Asia and the rest of the world, possibly related to the widespread and indiscriminate use of quinolones.[316,348] With the advent of quinolone resistance, third-generation cephalosporins were used for treatment, followed initially by occasional reports of resistance.[416] Today *Salmonella* serovar Typhi isolates displaying resistance to extended-spectrum cephalosporins are described worldwide. For example, extended-spectrum β-lactamase (ESBL) enzymes of the SHV-12 and CTX-M types and an AmpC β-lactamase of the ACC-1 type have been reported among isolates from Germany, the Philippines, Bangladesh, and India.[98] Similarly there have been sporadic reports of azithromycin resistance.[195]

PATHOPHYSIOLOGY

The severity and outcome of *Salmonella* infections depend on the combination of the virulence of the infecting bacterial strain, the infectious dose, the route of infection, and the genetic makeup and immunologic status of the host.

Salmonella can (1) adhere to, invade, and multiply in intestinal epithelium; (2) produce cholera toxin–like enterotoxin that increases cyclic adenosine monophosphate levels within intestinal crypt cells, causing a net efflux of electrolytes and water into the intestinal lumen; (3) be taken up by M cells overlying Peyer's patches of the distal ileum and proximal colon; (4) survive in macrophages of Peyer's patches, mesenteric lymph nodes, and the extraintestinal reticuloendothelial system; and (5) survive in the bloodstream.[134,136,145] Specific genes encode virulence factors necessary for each step in these processes and for specific disease manifestations (Table 111.3).

TABLE 111.3 Putative Pathophysiologic Basis of Selected Clinical Features of Salmonellosis

Disease Manifestation	Mechanisms and Bacterial Genes
Bloody diarrhea	*sip* A-D–mediated invasion and interleukin-8–mediated inflammation
Watery diarrhea	*stn* enterotoxin (cholera-like toxin) *SopB*-mediated intestinal inflammation and fluid secretion Serotypes that induce transepithelial polymorphonuclear leukocyte migration (e.g., *S.* ser. Typhimurium) are more likely to cause diarrhea than are serotypes that do not (e.g., *S.* ser. Typhi)
Bacteremia	*viaB* (Vi synthesis) capsular antigen interferes with C3 binding (*S.* ser. Typhi, *S.* ser. Dublin, *S.* ser. Paratyphi C) *rck* resistance to serum complement (virulence plasmid encoded) *rfb* encodes lipopolysaccharide synthesis; lipopolysaccharide contributes to persistence of bacteremia
Relapses, prolonged fever, failure of certain antibiotics	Survival in macrophages (*sseABC, spiC, mgtCB,* cytotoxin and virulence plasmid genes *spvRABCD*)

Pathologic findings in *S.* ser. Typhi infection include hypertrophy and hyperplasia of the intestinal and mesenteric lymphoid tissues, liver, and spleen. In contrast, *S.* ser. Typhimurium and other nontyphoidal serotypes cause diffuse colitis, mucosal edema, and crypt abscesses as the major pathologic abnormalities.[53,103]

Some virulence genes are shared by all *Salmonella* strains, whereas others are serotype-specific. Differences in invasiveness of various serotypes exist. *S.* ser. Typhi, *S.* ser. Choleraesuis, *S.* ser. Heidelberg,[190,258] and *S.* ser. Dublin[369] are more likely to enter the blood and to seed distant sites. Virulence plasmids have been identified in *S.* ser. Typhi, *S.* ser. Typhimurium, and *S.* ser. Dublin.[29] The presence of virulence plasmids seems to be more common in blood isolates of *S.* ser. Typhimurium than in fecal isolates (76% vs. 42%).[128]

Nursery outbreaks of *Salmonella* have shown dramatically the variability in severity of illness related to strain or serotype. In nursery outbreaks of *S.* ser. Oranienburg[366] and *S.* ser. Newport,[222] grossly bloody stools were found in 76% to 90% of infected infants, with 10% to 11% febrile and only 9% to 11% asymptomatic. Watery, green, nonbloody diarrhea has been common with *S.* ser. Typhimurium,[2] *S.* ser. Virchow,[325] and *S.* ser. Nienstedten.[345] A high frequency of asymptomatic infections has been seen during nursery outbreaks with *S.* ser. Heidelberg (38% asymptomatic),[33] *S.* ser. Virchow (42% asymptomatic),[325] and *S.* ser. Tennessee (100% asymptomatic).[400]

Which genes are required for disease in humans versus animals remains unclear. *S.* ser. Typhimurium has genes that allow it to cause a nondiarrheal typhoidal illness in mice; in humans, it typically causes symptoms related primarily to intestinal involvement. An estimated more than 200 genes determine *S.* ser. Typhimurium virulence in mice. The clinical variability in host range and disease manifestations is due to the fact that *Salmonella* strains vary in their possession and expression of virulence genes.[248]

Salmonella has developed two complex virulence functions to actively interact with the host and modify host cell functions. These interactions are hallmarks of *Salmonella* pathogenesis: (1) *Salmonella* infects cells of the gastrointestinal epithelium and is thus able to invade nonphagocytic cells, and (2) *Salmonella* may survive and replicate inside the phagocytes. Of critical importance for these interactions are the *Salmonella* pathogenicity islands (SPI), in particular SPI-1 (invasion and penetration of the gastrointestinal epithelium) and SPI-2 (systemic spread and colonization of host organs) (Fig. 111.1).[169] Both SPIs encode a molecular apparatus termed type III secretion system (TTSS). This apparatus is structurally and functionally related to the flagella assembly systems and typically contains more than 20 different protein subunits located in the inner and outer membrane and in the periplasm and cytoplasm of the bacterial cells.[169] TTSSs are capable of injecting bacterial proteins through bacterial and host membranes into host cells (translocation) or the extracellular milieu (secretion) to influence host biochemistry and cell physiology directly.[85]

Genes relevant to the intestinal phase of illness are encoded primarily in SPI-1. The *invA-H* chromosomal genes are necessary for adherence to and invasion of intestinal mucosal cells[133]; most of the genes described so far seem to be involved in secretion or transport of virulence proteins.[160,383] Genes related to the *Shigella* invasion plasmid antigens *(ipaA-D)* have been described in *Salmonella* spp.[203,204]; these *Salmonella* genes *(sipA-D)* encode the proteins that interact with host cells to cause bacterial uptake and intracellular movement. The major TTSS effector proteins used to invade epithelial cells and induce inflammation in the *Salmonella typhimurium* mouse model are SipA, SopB, SopE, and SopE2.[202] Although initially characterized as an invasiveness island, SPI-1 has additional functions related to the activation of the innate immune pathway, including (1) induction of polymorphonuclear recruitment across the intestinal epithelium by the SPI-1 secreted effect SipA, (2) activation of nuclear factor-κB signaling by the concerted activity of SPI-1 translocated effectors, and (3) activation of caspase-1–mediated interleukin-1β (IL-β)/IL-18 activation and proinflammatory cell death by the SPI-1 translocator effector SipB.[85]

The role of host cells in the invasion process is complex. After *S.* ser. Typhimurium comes in contact with epithelial cells, activation of epidermal growth factor receptor occurs, which activates a kinase that turns on phospholipase A_2 so that arachidonic acid is generated. Arachidonic acid is converted to leukotriene D_4, which opens calcium channels and causes membrane ruffling, cytoskeletal changes, and uptake of bacteria.[133] Nonphagocytic cells, including epithelial cells, are adapted poorly for killing of internalized bacteria. Not only do *Salmonella* spp. survive in vacuoles within epithelial cells, but they also can replicate actively.[134] *S.* ser. Typhi survives better in human than in mouse macrophages, whereas *S.* ser. Typhimurium survives better in mouse macrophages.[38,58,343] *Salmonella* is capable of infecting a wide variety of cells, including dendritic cells, macrophages, hepatocytes, neutrophils, colonocytes, and other epithelial cells. In vitro, within minutes of contact with cells, *Salmonella* organisms are internalized and take up residence in a unique membrane-bound compartment distinct from a phagosome or lysosome, the *Salmonella*-containing vacuole.[156] Live neutrophils recruited during acute *Salmonella* colitis engulf pathogens in the gut lumen and may thus actively engage in shaping the environment of pathogens and commensals in the inflamed gut.[235]

SPI-2 is essential for intracellular parasitism and systemic virulence in murine typhoid and for evasion of phagocyte oxidase machinery of the host.[388] Intracellular replication occurs in a specialized membrane compartment, the *Salmonella*-containing vacuole, and depends on translocation of approximately 30 effector proteins via the SPI-2 TTSS into the host endomembrane system and cytoplasm.[129] SPI-2 has additional roles in inflammatory disease, such as induction of cyclooxygenase and modulation of host cytokine expression and signaling. In addition, SPI-2 function affects antimicrobial defense mechanisms of the host, intracellular transport processes, integrity and function of the cytoskeleton, and host cell death.[217] SPI-2 is crucial for early and complete induction of enterocolitis and systemic disease.[85]

Several pathogen-associated molecular patterns of pathophysiologic importance are presented by *Salmonella* during infection, principally lipopolysaccharides and flagellin. The activation of Toll-like receptor 4 (TLR4) in response to *Salmonella* lipopolysaccharides is essential for inducing host responses.[387] *Salmonella* flagellin is a potent inducer of host inflammation in polarized epithelial monolayers when delivered to the basolateral surface of the epithelium. When delivered there, *Salmonella* flagellin induces IL-8 secretion by stimulating basolateral

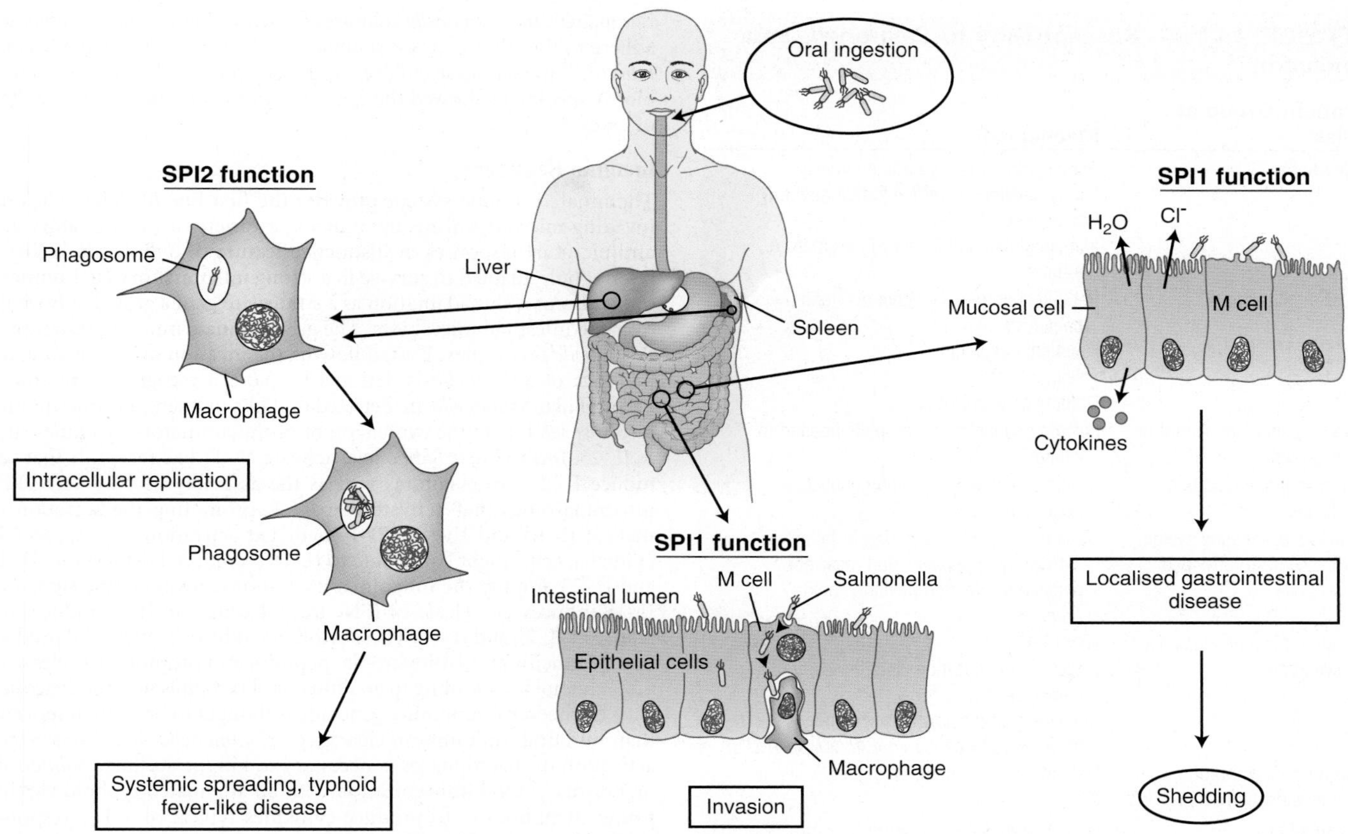

FIG. 111.1 Host-pathogen interactions during pathogenesis of *Salmonella* infection. SPI1 function is required for the initial stages of salmonellosis (i.e., the entry of *Salmonella* into nonphagocytic cells by triggering invasion and the penetration of the gastrointestinal epithelium). Furthermore, SPI1 function is required for the onset of diarrheal symptoms during localized gastrointestinal infections. The function of SPI2 is required for later stages of the infection (i.e., systemic spread and the colonization of host organs). The role of SPI2 for survival and replication in host phagocytes appears to be essential for this phase of pathogenesis. (From Hansen-Wester I, Hensel M. *Salmonella* pathogenicity islands encoding type III secretion systems. *Microbes Infect.* 2001;3:549–59.)

TLR5.[417] Flagellin stimulation of innate immune responses is crucial for intestinal inflammation but not for murine typhoid.[85]

The development of diarrhea depends on host and pathogen factors. An influx of polymorphonuclear leukocytes into the mucosa must occur for diarrhea to develop.[398] Neutropenic animals fail to develop fluid secretion when they are infected with *Salmonella*[398]; infiltration of leukocytes is thought to trigger production of prostaglandin because fluid secretion can be blocked by indomethacin.[146] A cholera toxin–like enterotoxin is made by approximately two-thirds of *Salmonella* strains, including *S.* ser. Typhimurium and *S.* ser. Typhi.[196]

For most NTS strains, infection does not extend beyond the lamina propria and the local lymphatics. In contrast, *S.* ser. Typhi, *S.* ser. Dublin, and *S.* ser. Choleraesuis rapidly invade the bloodstream, with little intestinal involvement. Some virulence genes confer a survival advantage to the organisms if they get into the extraintestinal milieu. Vi capsular antigen present in *S.* ser. Typhi, *S.* ser. Dublin, and *S.* ser. Paratyphi C interferes with C3 binding. Mutations in lipopolysaccharide genes decrease invasiveness of *S.* ser. Typhi and *S.* ser. Choleraesuis, but not of *S.* ser. Typhimurium.[134,277] *S.* ser. Dublin, *S.* ser. Typhimurium, and *S.* ser. Enteritidis have virulence genes that confer resistance to complement by preventing the formation and insertion of the C5b-9 membrane attack complex.

The mechanisms governing homeostasis and immune defense are of great importance for *Salmonella* infection. *Salmonella* uses multiple strategies to evade and modulate host innate and adaptive immune responses, to persist in the presence of a robust immune response.[273] Chronically infected hosts are often asymptomatic and transmit disease to naïve hosts via fecal shedding of bacteria, thereby serving as a critical reservoir for disease. The ability of *Salmonella* to persist depends on a balance between immune responses that lead to the clearance of the pathogen and avoidance of damage to host tissues.[330] In addition, the intestinal microbiota plays a critical role in controlling *Salmonella* infection, disease, and transmissibility.[273] However the molecular nature of the homeostatic interactions, the pathogen's ability to overcome colonization resistance, and the triggering of native and adaptive mucosal immune responses are still poorly understood.[201,202]

Host Factors

Multiple host defense strategies have evolved to deal with the bacteria virulence factors; host susceptibility often can be related directly to defects in these defense mechanisms (Table 111.4). The host tries to kill ingested organisms in the stomach, to inhibit their growth in the gut, to limit their spread beyond the intestine, and to clear them by immune mechanisms. At a pH of 2.0, most *Salmonella* spp. are killed rapidly.[144] When gastric pH is increased by oral administration of antacid, susceptibility increases.[143,185,186,319] A *Salmonella* inoculum ingested in water passes through the stomach more rapidly than when the same inoculum is ingested in food. Rapid transit through the small bowel decreases the contact time of organisms with the mucosa. Patients with decreased intestinal motility caused by medication or anatomic factors have increased severity and complications and may have a prolonged carrier state. Prior antimicrobial exposure increases the risk for incurring infection with antimicrobial-susceptible and antimicrobial-resistant strains of *Salmonella*.[300] The normal flora may compete for substrates, lower the local pH by production of short-chain fatty acids, and produce antibacterial substances such as colicins. Some patients with

TABLE 111.4 Susceptibility to *Salmonella* spp. Infection

Patient Group at Risk	Mechanism
Newborn	Achlorhydria, rapid gastric emptying Poorly developed cell-mediated immunity Complement deficiency Immunoglobulin deficiency in premature infants
Sickle-cell anemia	Reticuloendothelial system overload owing to hemolysis Functional asplenia Tissue infarcts Defective opsonization
Neutropenia (congenital or acquired)	Polymorphonuclear neutrophils needed for killing
Chronic granulomatous disease	Defective killing by polymorphonuclear neutrophils
Defects of immune system IL-12/interferon-γ axis	Defective signaling resulting in failure to activate macrophages and recurrent/ persistent infection by nontyphoid *Salmonella*
Acquired immunodeficiency syndrome	Low CD4 Effects of malnutrition on cell-mediated immunity Survival of organisms in macrophages (owing to *Salmonella* genes *PhoP/PhoQ, spvA-D, R*)
Organ transplantation, immunosuppression	Defective cell-mediated immunity
Gastrectomy	Loss of stomach acid barrier
Malaria	Reticuloendothelial overload during hemolysis Abnormal complement levels Abnormal macrophage function
Bartonellosis (verruga peruana)	Reticuloendothelial overload during hemolysis
Schistosomiasis	*Salmonella* sequestered in schistosomes protected from host defenses and antibiotics

gastroenteritis have progression or exacerbation of symptoms when antibiotics are given.[324]

Children with compromised immune systems are at increased risk for serious focal infections. *Salmonella* organisms are able to survive in macrophages but not in polymorphonuclear leukocytes. Patients with neutropenia (e.g., congenital or related to chemotherapy) or neutrophil dysfunction (e.g., chronic granulomatous disease) are at high risk for development of disseminated infection. Patients who have been bacteremic with a NTS strain are at increased risk for having a relapse if leukopenia is present.[141]

An increased risk for acquiring disease exists in settings in which reticuloendothelial function or cell-mediated immunity is impaired[282,353] or immature.[280] Hemolytic anemias are thought to cause reticuloendothelial overload. Children with sickle-cell anemia are at risk for developing bacteremia and osteomyelitis, and *Salmonella* spp. is 2 to 5 times more common than *Staphylococcus aureus* in these patients.[5,5,247,364,410] Within febrile children with sickle-cell anemia, *Salmonella* spp. was found in 3.1% of positive urine cultures.[254] Children with sickle-cell and S-Thal also sometimes develop osteomyelitis.[86] Patients with sickle-cell anemia have complement defects and defects in opsonization of *S.* ser. Typhimurium.[168] Newborns also have complement deficiencies that may explain the high frequency of *Salmonella* infection in newborns and the susceptibility of newborns to bacteremic complications seldom seen in normal hosts.

Malaria predisposes to salmonellosis by multiple mechanisms.[241] Schistosomiasis predisposes to development of *Salmonella* infections and prolonged bacteremia[319]; reticuloendothelial cell killing of *Salmonella* is impaired, and *Salmonella* colonizes the schistosomes. Pili on *Salmonella* adhere to the surface of *Schistosoma mansoni* and *Schistosoma haematobium*.[237] In Gabonese children with bacteremic NTS infection, rectal biopsy specimens showed the eggs of *Schistosoma intercalatum* in 90% of cases.[142]

Immune Response

The innate immune system provides the first line of defense against invading microorganisms by inducing a variety of inflammatory and antimicrobial responses. A distinctive feature of *Salmonella* is that it has not only adapted to survive in a strong inflammatory environment, but it also uses this adaptation as a strategy to gain a growth advantage over the intestinal microbiota. The gastric innate immune response to *Salmonella* is complex. First, following the invasion of the mucosa, the presence of *Salmonella* is detected by pattern recognition receptors. Extracellular *Salmonella* are detected by TLRs inducing a transcriptional response leading to the expression of proinflammatory cytokines such as IL-23. Intracellular *Salmonella* activate NOD-like receptors that can induce IL-23 expression, as well as the assembly of NLRC4/NLRP3 inflammasomes that activate caspase-1, promoting the secretion of mature IL-1β and IL-18. SPI-1–mediated activation of caspase-1 in epithelial cells might contribute to IL-18 secretion. Furthermore IL-18 and IL-23 amplify the inflammatory response by paracrine signaling. IL-18 induces the release of IFNc from T cells, and IL-23 induces the release of IL-22 and IL-17. These cytokines induce the increased production of mucins and antimicrobial peptides and promote the release of CXC chemokines, leading to an influx of neutrophils into the mucosa.[56]

Cell-mediated immunity generally is thought to be more important than humoral immunity in clearance of *Salmonella* organisms. T-cell activation of macrophages is necessary to kill intracellular *Salmonella* organisms.[244] Oral immunization with an attenuated typhoid vaccine primes lymphocytes to produce cytokines typical of a T_H1 response (high interferon [IFN-γ]/low IL-4) to the flagellar antigen.[367] Healthy individuals vaccinated with either oral or parenteral typhoid vaccines develop antibody-dependent cellular cytotoxicity mediated by IgA, IgG, or both.[100] Studies of serum and secretory antibodies to O and H antigens have not shown protection, however; relapses of typhoid fever have occurred despite high antibody titers. Immunity may be short lived. In a study of 14 individuals (17 to 28 years old) with acute typhoid fever, cell-mediated immunity persisted for 16 weeks; intestinal secretory IgA persisted for 48 weeks; and IgG, IgM, and anti-O and anti-H agglutinins persisted for 2 years, 16 weeks, 16 weeks, and 36 weeks, respectively.[339]

Cytokines play a crucial role in initiating and regulating the innate and adaptive immune response against *Salmonella*. These bacteria can trigger synthesis of cytokines and chemokines in epithelial cells, macrophages, and dendritic cells. The consequences of cytokine activation vary. Although IFN-γ, IL-12, tumor necrosis factor-α, IL-18, transforming growth factor-β, and CCL2 have protective functions during *Salmonella* infection, IL-4 and IL-10 interfere with host defenses.[117] The main immunologic mechanisms that control the course of *Salmonella* infection in mice are described in Fig. 111.2.[252]

Impaired cell-mediated immunity probably explains the high frequency of bacteremia with nontyphoidal *Salmonella* strains in children with HIV infection[332] and with malnutrition.[350] Defective cell-mediated immunity can be congenital or acquired (from tumors,[165] collagen vascular disease, organ transplantation,[119] chemotherapy, glucocorticosteroids).[313] Inherited deficiency in the IL-12/IL-23/IFN-γ pathway results in susceptibility to recurrent *Salmonella* and *Mycobacterium* infections.[109] Defects have been described in which patients have mutations in IL-12, IL-12 receptor, IL-23, IL-23 receptor, IFN-γ receptor, or signal transducer and activator of transcription (STAT). Complete and partial deficiency syndromes have been described.[15,21,200] Isolated persistent or recurrent nontyphoidal *Salmonella* infection without history of infectious episodes by other microorganisms has been reported in 15% of children with deficiency of the β-1 receptor for IL-12.[38]

Humoral immunity is less important.[49] Preterm neonates who are infected with *S.* ser. Typhimurium may have a lower risk for developing complications (e.g., intestinal perforation, meningitis, endophthalmitis, sepsis, and pyelitis) if they are given intravenous immunoglobulin plus

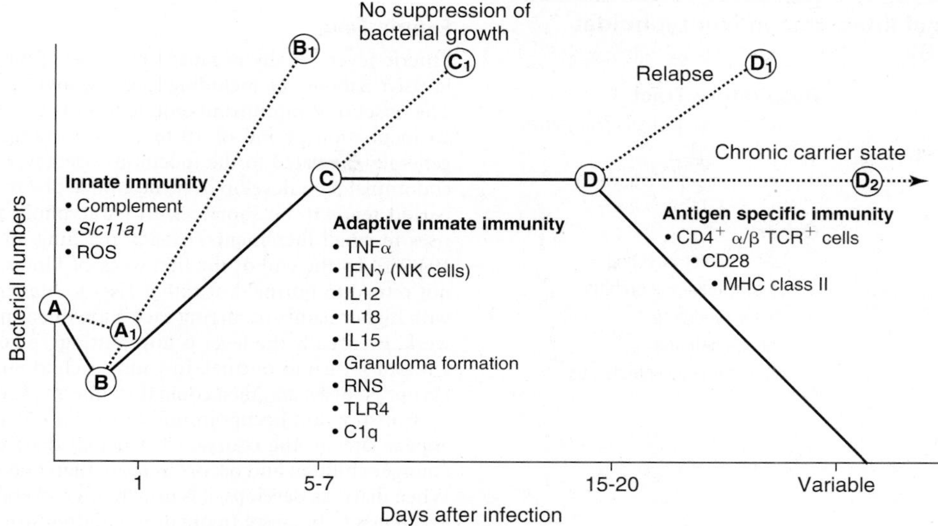

FIG. 111.2 Immunologic mechanisms that control the progression of a sublethal *Salmonella enterica* infection in the mouse model. The *solid line* shows the course of a sublethal infection in wild-type immunocompetent mice. The *dotted lines* show the course of the infection when immunologic mechanisms required at points *A→D* are absent. Lack of complement and/or reactive oxygen species (*ROS*) affects the early blood clearance and killing of the bacteria with a shift of the growth curve from *A→B* to *A→A1*. The *Slc11a1* gene and ROS influence the net growth rate, and their absence determines a shift of the curve from *B→C* to *B→B1*. Point *C* coincides with the onset of the adaptive innate immunity response. The lack of any of the immunologic factors that form part of adaptive innate immunity determines failure to suppress bacterial growth in the tissues *(C→D)* and the unrestrained progression of the infection process *(C→C1)*. Point *D* coincides with the intervention of antigen-specific immunity that is required to clear the infection and prevent relapse *(D→D1)* of the establishment of a chronic carrier state *(D→D2)*. (From Mastroeni P, Maskell D, editors. *Salmonella infections.* Cambridge, MA: Cambridge University Press; 2006:209).

cefoperazone than if given cefoperazone alone (16% vs. 82%); the mortality rate also is decreased (12% vs. 41%).[153]

CLINICAL MANIFESTATIONS

Salmonella spp. may cause acute or chronic asymptomatic infection. Symptomatic infections include acute gastroenteritis, bacteremia with or without local suppuration, and enteric fever.

Acute Asymptomatic Infection

Asymptomatic infections are identified by stool cultures obtained during prospective or epidemiologic investigations. Detections range from no signal by polymerase chain reaction (PCR) in 410 schoolchildren from rural Madagascar[140] to 74% positive stool cultures for NTS in Mexican infants.[92]

Acute Gastroenteritis

The most common clinical illness caused by *Salmonella* infection is gastroenteritis. Nausea, vomiting, and crampy abdominal pain begin 6 to 72 hours (median, 24 hours) after ingestion of contaminated food or water. The abdominal pain may be severe enough to suggest appendicitis. Diarrhea usually is moderate in volume and, depending on the serotype, may contain blood. Dysentery is more common in children from developed countries than in those from developing regions.[303] Headaches, malaise, myalgias, and fevers are common. These symptoms usually resolve in approximately 1 week without antibiotic therapy; symptoms may persist in very young patients and patients with underlying diseases. In neonates, loose, green, mucous stools or, less often, bloody diarrhea is seen; fever is common with *Salmonella* gastroenteritis during the first months of life.[190] Reactive arthritis develops rarely in children after having *Salmonella* gastroenteritis.[208]

Bacteremia With or Without Metastatic Focal Infection

Some *Salmonella* serotypes (e.g., *S.* ser. Typhi; *S.* ser. Choleraesuis; *S.* ser. Paratyphi A, B, and C; *S.* ser. Heidelberg; *S.* ser. Typhimurium; *S.* ser. Enteritidis; *S.* ser. Saint-Paul; *S.* ser. Newport; *S.* ser. Panama; and *S.* ser. Dublin) have a propensity to invade the bloodstream; others (e.g., *S.* ser. Tennessee and *S.* ser. Weltevreden)[405] rarely seem to cause bacteremia. *Salmonella* has been found as one cause of occult bacteremia in infants and children,[10,213] and, when not treated with appropriate parenteral antibiotics, 45% to 68% of infected children developed persistent *Salmonella* bacteremia.[218] *Salmonella* is also found within cases of clinically suspected community-acquired invasive bacterial disease in children from tropical regions.[18] Fever, chills, diaphoresis, myalgias, anorexia, and weight loss may last for days or weeks. Stool cultures may be negative. A child sometimes can have afebrile diarrhea and yet be bacteremic for several days.[206] Warm climate, previous gastrointestinal disease, and recent exposure to antibiotics are some reported risk factors for bacteremia in children.[170] Severe malnutrition, HIV infection, prolonged illness, and recent hospital admission are risk factors for nontyphoidal *Salmonella* bacteremia in developing countries.[54] The true frequency of bacteremia is unclear. Depending on the patient's age, geographic location, and nature of the study (prospective vs. retrospective), 2% to 45% of infections are bacteremic.[101,190,258,280,350,376,404,405,413] Bacteremia probably occurs more commonly in newborns (in some studies 30% to 50%) than in older children,[190] although this is debatable.[258] The true risk for bacteremia developing in the first year of life is likely to be 2% to 6%.[101,376]

Palpable purpura and leukocytoclastic vasculitis have been described with bacteremia and sepsis due to *Salmonella*.[12,90,132,418] In the preantibiotic era this was an ominous sign.[323] Recently, it has been described in patients affected by a defect in IL-$12_{\beta 1}$ receptor (IL-12/IFN-γ axis).[13,131,220,334] A high index of suspicion for defects in this axis is recommended because the usual panels for immunodeficiency are within normal in this group of conditions.[13,38,285,382]

Hemolytic anemia, especially sickle-cell anemia, is associated with a high risk for development of *Salmonella* bacteremia.[276] Persistent or recurrent bacteremia occurs in patients with AIDS, schistosomiasis, and intravascular focal infection.[276,284] Immunocompromised adults who become bacteremic with *Salmonella* are more likely to do so without

BOX 111.1 Focal Infections in Nontyphoidal Salmonellosis (NTS)

Brain
- Meningitis
- Brain abscess and empyema

Osteoarticular
- Arthritis
- Osteomyelitis
- Pyomyositis and psoas abscess
- Prosthetic osteoarthritis
- Subcutaneous abscess

Cardiovascular
- Endocarditis
- Pericarditis
- Mycotic aneurysm
- Myocardial abscess
- Septic thrombophlebitis

Respiratory Tract
- Retropharyngeal and pharyngeal abscess
- Pneumonia and empyema

Other
- Urinary tract infection
- Epididymitis and orchitis
- Reiter syndrome
- Endophthalmitis
- Suppurative lymphadenitis

having had preceding gastroenteritis and to have a high mortality rate.[167] Children more typically are relatively immunocompetent; most often, they develop bacteremia associated with diarrhea and have a much better prognosis.[226,258] In a large study in African children, NTS were the second most common cause of community-acquired bacteremia in all children and in HIV-positive patients.[41] The risk for development of focal infections during bacteremia is higher (36%) in children with underlying conditions than in previously healthy children (2.5%).[414]

Focal suppurative infections may occur almost anywhere (Box 111.1); the most common sites are bones (particularly in sickle-cell anemia)[267,318] and the central nervous system.[57,113,212,238,322,414] Meningitis has a high morbidity, with acute hydrocephalus, seizures, ventriculitis, abscesses, subdural empyema, and cerebral infarction.[411] Long-term neurologic sequelae include developmental delay, which could be severe; motor disabilities (i.e., cranial nerve palsy, hemiparesis, quadriparesis); chronic hydrocephalus; epilepsy; visual and auditory impairment; and athetosis.[87,292,411] Neurologic sequelae are particularly common in infants with delayed presentation, prolonged fever (>10 days) or seizures during hospitalization, and marked alteration of consciousness on admission.[188,292,411] Mortality rates from meningitis were 40% to 60% before the introduction of third-generation cephalosporins, fluoroquinolones, and carbapenems. With the use of these antibiotics, the mortality rate has decreased to almost 10% but still carries a high rate of sequelae.[292,411] Relapses even after prolonged therapy occur commonly (reflecting the intracellular localization of *Salmonella* and the difficulty of achieving adequate intracellular levels of antibiotics). Of NTS meningitis, 50% to 75% occur in the first 4 months of life.[86,292] The serotypes causing meningitis, including *S.* ser. Typhimurium, *S.* ser. Heidelberg, *S.* ser. Enteritidis, *S.* ser. Saint-Paul, *S.* ser. Havana, *S.* ser. Oranienburg, *S.* ser. Newport, and *S.* ser. Panama,[86,403] are commonly associated with bacteremia. In infants, complications include pneumonia,[33] osteomyelitis,[107,215,410] septic arthritis,[33,50,340] pericarditis,[9,48,166,257] pyelitis,[366] peritonitis,[2,389] otitis media,[2] mastitis,[279,344] cholecystitis,[164,221] endophthalmitis,[91] cutaneous abscesses,[32,233,311] phlebitis[233] and infected cephalohematoma.[107] In adults and occasionally in older children, femoral and distal aorta (mycotic aneurysms),[86,126] heart valves,[86] mediastinum,[126] scrotum,[379] testicles,[86] prostate,[338] vulva,[46] vagina,[46] ovaries,[86] and fallopian tubes[338] also may be infected.

Hemolytic-uremic syndrome associated with *S.* ser. Typhimurium[114,253] and *S.* ser. Typhi[31] has been reported. Because the cytotoxins produced by various *Salmonella* strains are distinct immunologically from Shiga toxin produced by *Shigella dysenteriae* 1 and the Shiga toxins produced by enterohemorrhagic *Escherichia coli*,[22] the association of hemolytic-uremic syndrome with salmonellosis may represent undiagnosed dual infection with toxin-producing organisms.

Enteric Fever

Enteric fever usually is caused by *S.* ser. Typhi and, less often, other invasive *Salmonella*, including *S.* ser. Paratyphi and *S.* ser. Choleraesuis. The onset of symptoms in enteric fever is usually insidious.[185,186] After an incubation period of 10 to 14 days (range, 6 to 21 days), which generally is related to the inoculum size, fever, malaise, anorexia, and abdominal pain develop over the course of 2 to 3 days. The incubation period tends to be shorter with paratyphoid fever. The temperature rises in small increments, usually reaching 40°C to 40.5°C (104°F to 104.9°F) by the end of the first week of illness. The temperature does not return to normal but rather rises to higher peaks each afternoon, with higher nadirs occurring each subsequent morning during the first week. Eventually the fever is unremitting; spikes in temperature occur without return to normal. In younger children, onset of fever is more abrupt on onset and then could turn intermittent or remain sustained.[121]

Constipation occurs in one-fourth of older children and tends to appear later in the course,[26,210] whereas diarrhea is more frequent in younger children and occurs in more than one-third of patients.[26,259,373] When diarrhea develops, it is usually after several days of febrile illness[209] and tends to be more frequent in children from nonendemic settings, where it can even lead to dehydration.[359] It is small in volume and of loose consistency, resembling a greenish pea soup; it contains erythrocytes but usually is not grossly bloody.[115,259,358] Fecal leukocytes are present in nearly all patients with diarrhea.[115] Diarrhea occurs more commonly with paratyphoid than with typhoid fever.[373] Vomiting is mild and not sustained.

A dull, continuous frontal headache begins during the first 2 days of fever and is easier to explore in adolescents.[210] Children commonly complain of headache and often are drowsy, irritable, or delirious.[106]

A relative bradycardia for the degree of fever can be found over the first week, but it is not a constant or specific finding.[102,368] Patients have a toxic facies; coated tongue; a musty, "damp hay–like" odor; and a tender, doughy abdomen with slight guarding. Occasionally a child may have a low-level cough. The skin is dry with little sweating. Meningismus may occur early in the illness.

During the second week, rose-colored spots measuring 2 to 4 mm may appear on the abdomen or chest and rarely on surrounding locations. They are blanching, erythematous, slightly raised lesions that last approximately 3 days. Rose spots occur in a few patients and are difficult to recognize in dark-skinned individuals. Infrequently, new crops of rose spots continue for 1 to 2 weeks.

A soft, tender spleen becomes palpable by the second week of illness. Respiratory symptoms may progress, and epistaxis occasionally may occur. If left untreated, enteric fever has a prolonged course, with continuous high temperatures of 39.5°C to 40.5°C (103.1°F to 104.9°F) for up to 4 weeks, followed by a gradual return to normal beginning during the third or fourth week. A rapid decrease in temperature late in illness suggests intestinal hemorrhage or perforation[45]; such a decline in temperature typically is followed by an increase a few hours later as peritonitis develops. Intestinal hemorrhage and intestinal perforation[147,45,61,61,] may occur in the second to fourth week in 1% to 3% of patients with typhoid fever.[26,61]

Complications occur in 10% to 15% of patients; mainly during the second or third week of illness. Many complications, of which gastrointestinal bleeding, intestinal perforation, and typhoid encephalopathy are the most important, have been described (Box 111.2).[228,291,295] Gastrointestinal bleeding is the most common, occurring in 5% to 10% of patients.[26,26] It results from erosion of a necrotic Peyer's patch through the wall of an enteric vessel. Suppurative lymphadenitis,[278] mesenteric lymphadenitis,[148,232] tonsillitis,[197,338] endocarditis,[111] and pancreatitis[20,250,412] rarely occur. Patients who have thalassemia or glucose-6-phosphate dehydrogenase deficiency may have hemolysis during typhoid fever.[373]

The relapse rate is 5% to 10%, even when appropriate therapy has been given.[8] Relapses typically occur 2 to 3 weeks after the resolution of fever and are milder than the initial illness. The *Salmonella* isolate from a patient in relapse usually has the same antibiotic susceptibility pattern as the isolate obtained from the patient during the original episode. Reinfection also may occur and can be distinguished from relapse by molecular typing.[394]

BOX 111.2 Complications of Typhoid Fever

Abdominal
- Gastrointestinal hemorrhage
- Intestinal perforation
- Hepatitis
- Cholecystitis
- Pancreatitis
- Neuropsychiatric
- Encephalopathy
- Delirium
- Psychosis
- Meningitis
- Impairment of coordination

Cardiovascular
- Asymptomatic electrocardiographic changes
- Myocarditis
- Infected prosthetic valve
- Shock
- Respiratory
- Bronchitis
- Pneumonia

Hematologic
- Anemia
- Disseminated intravascular coagulation

Other
- Focal abscess
- Suppurative lymphadenitis
- Mesenteric lymphadenitis
- Pharyngitis
- Tonsillitis
- Osteomyelitis
- Arthritis
- Parotiditis
- Orchitis
- Pyelonephritis
- Miscarriage
- Relapse
- Chronic carriage

In some geographic areas, such as Indonesia, where an exceptionally virulent *S.* ser. Typhi is endemic, toxemia, delirium, obtundation, coma, and shock sometimes occur.[228,186,185] Some serotypes in Indonesia (e.g., H1-j) seem to be less virulent than others, suggesting that properties of the flagellar antigen may be important to virulence.[161]

Typhoid fever varies in its clinical course. Variations on the classic theme include a completely afebrile course occurring in debilitated patients, a high spiking fever from the first day (particularly in children), a focal presentation (e.g., pneumonia and nephritis), and a severe course during relapses. Infants are said to be at higher risk for development of massive hepatomegaly, thrombocytopenia, and other complications.[312] The mortality rate is high in the neonatal period.[314] Children younger than 5 years may have a nonspecific illness that is not recognized clinically as typhoid[349]; infants and toddlers often have a febrile illness misinterpreted as a "viral syndrome." In children younger than 2 years, the fever may last for only 1 to 5 days, despite the presence of *S.* ser. Typhi or *S.* ser. Paratyphi in the blood; low-grade fever (temperature of 38.3°C–38.8°C [100.9°F–101.8°F]) and cough may be the only findings in such children.[127,127] Deaths are up to 6 times more frequent in children younger than 5 years compared to older children and adolescents.[26] The most important contributor to a poor outcome is probably a delay in instituting effective antibiotic treatment.[295]

Enteric fever from infection with multidrug resistant *Salmonella* ser. Typhi (MDRST) is found globally in 22% to 25% of children and is more frequently associated with the presence of fever, toxic appearance, hepatomegaly, splenomegaly, and abdominal tenderness and distention on admission in contrast to non-MDRST.[26,416] Children with MDRST also tend to present later in the course, with current or prior antibiotic treatment, and are more likely have complications such as dehydration, gastrointestinal bleeding, ileus, shock, myocarditis, and/or pneumonia.[26]

Typhoid and nontyphoidal *Salmonella* infections during pregnancy increase the risk for spontaneous abortion.[266,360] Spontaneous abortion or premature labor usually can be prevented by early treatment.[347] Transmission of *S.* ser. Typhi rarely occurs in utero.[75] Typically premature delivery occurs during the second to fourth week of untreated maternal typhoid fever.[159] In the preantibiotic era, 40% of women with typhoid delivered prematurely; the remainder carried to term, although only 17% of infants survived.[105] If infection occurs late in gestation and is treated appropriately, the infant may survive.

Asymptomatic Chronic Carrier State

Chronic carriers excrete *Salmonella* organisms in stools for longer than 1 year after having gastroenteritis-enterocolitis or enteric fever. Approximately 1% to 4% of patients who recover from enteric fever caused by *S.* ser. Typhi chronically excrete the organism[265]; fewer than 1% of patients with NTS excrete for a prolonged period.[59,72] Twenty-five percent of prolonged carriers have no history of typhoid.[295] Nontyphoidal infection is associated with excretion for a mean of 5 weeks, although children younger than 5 years,[59] female patients, elderly patients, and patients with biliary tract disease are more likely to become carriers. The biliary tract is infected in almost all chronic carriers of *S.* ser. Typhi. As many as 10^6 organisms per 1 g of feces may be excreted.[265]

Chronic excretion in such patients serves as the source of infection to their contacts. Chronic carriers represent an epidemiologically important reservoir of *S.* ser. Typhi; they often are the source of outbreaks of typhoid fever. In the United States, although typhoid fever generally is imported, 30% of infections result from exposure to previously diagnosed or newly diagnosed chronic carriers.[335]

Patients who have a history of *Schistosoma haematobium* or tuberculous infections of the urinary tract may develop chronic urinary carriage after a bout of typhoid fever.[122,321]

DIAGNOSIS

The symptoms in *Salmonella* gastroenteritis overlap sufficiently with symptoms seen in other diarrheal illnesses that laboratory studies generally are required to prove the diagnosis. Proctoscopy is rarely done; typical findings include mucosal edema, hyperemia, friability, and hemorrhages.[103] The fecal leukocyte examination is positive for polymorphonuclear leukocytes in 36% to 82% of nontyphoidal cases,[170] but this finding is nonspecific. Stool culture is preferable to swab culture, particularly for evaluation of long-term carriers. Overnight enrichment in selenite broth increases the yield from stool cultures. The optimal agar for isolation of the organism (SS, Hektoen enteric, MacConkey, xylose-lysine-deoxycholate, xylose-lysine-Tergitol 4, brilliant green, or modified semisolid Rappaport-Vassiliadis medium) is debated. Modified semisolid Rappaport-Vassiliadis medium has a high yield but cannot be used for isolating *S.* ser. Typhi or nonmotile strains and has lower specificity than SS agar.[331] Increasing the volume of stool sample improves the yield of *Salmonella* in cultures.[393]

Salmonella organisms usually can be isolated readily from blood by use of conventional media if the patient is bacteremic. In patients with extraintestinal focal nontyphoidal infection, specimens from the affected areas may have positive Gram stains and grow the organism.

Enteric fever should be suspected on the basis of the setting and clinical course. Laboratory abnormalities are common but nonspecific findings. Normocytic, normochromic anemia and leukopenia or neutropenia, perhaps caused by hemophagocytosis in the bone marrow, often are present.[246] Clotting abnormalities consistent with disseminated intravascular coagulation (e.g., thrombocytopenia, hypofibrinogenemia) may occur[60] but usually are transient and not associated with clinically significant bleeding. In enteric fever, electrolyte values usually are normal, but increases in alkaline phosphatase, serum lactate dehydrogenase, serum aspartate aminotransferase, and serum cholesterol occur frequently. Transient proteinuria sometimes occurs during the first week of enteric fever.

Cultures from multiple sites should be submitted for suspected enteric fever; culture of bone marrow has the highest yield,[179,181,380] particularly if the patient has had antibiotic pretreatment. During the first week of typhoid fever, approximately 90% of patients have positive blood and bone marrow cultures, but negative stool and urine cultures. During subsequent weeks, the yield of blood and bone marrow cultures decreases as the yield of stool and urine cultures increases. Culture of duodenal fluid obtained by string capsules can be as sensitive as culture of bone marrow aspirates.[25,181,380] Over the third week of enteric fever, bone marrow culture could remain positive despite negative blood cultures.[396] The ratio of nonviable to viable *Salmonella* bacteria in blood ranges from 1000 : 1 to 47,000 : 1.[30] The overall frequencies of positive cultures during the course of typhoid are found in blood (40–54%), urine

(7–10%), stool (~35%), bone marrow (80–90%), rose spots (~65%), and duodenal string test culture (58–85%).[149,181]

Blood volume is the most important factor for *Salmonella* isolation in blood cultures, and it is recommended that 10 to 15 mL be drawn per sample from infants, as in adults.[406] Because bacterial counts in blood are higher in children[393] and the volumes of drawn samples are worrisome both for personnel and caregivers, recommended blood volume for toddlers and infants is 2 to 4 mL.[406] The Widal test measures antibodies against the O and H antigens of *S.* ser. Typhi. Although many patients with enteric fever may have a fourfold increase in the titer of paired sera during the second week of illness, many false-negative and false-positive test results occur. Widal test titers could rise before clinical onset of disease, preventing the expected fourfold rise in titers of paired sera.[298] False-positive results in the Widal test can be caused by infection with other Enterobacteriaceae, malaria, dengue, nontyphoidal *Salmonella,* and other diseases and previous exposure to *Salmonella* antigens (including typhoid vaccines). Variability and poor standardization of commercial test antigens are identified causes for both false-positive and false-negative results.[289] Widal test titers may be more useful in children with typhoid who are living in a nonendemic area. Interpretation of Widal test results is aided by information about seropositivity in the population to which the patient belongs.[82,378] Some centers have found the Widal test helpful when it is used with locally determined cutoff points.[84,297] The Widal test could be used to diagnose typhoid fever, but only under unfavorable circumstances when no confirmatory microbiologic test result is available; this approach is not to be encouraged.[289] Various diagnostic kits, including serologic tests such as passive hemagglutination, passive bacterial agglutination, latex particle agglutination slide tests, counterimmunoelectrophoresis, radioimmunoassay, and enzyme-linked immunosorbent assay with use of monoclonal antibodies, have been developed.[193] These commercial assays (i.e., Typhidot, Typhidot-M, and Tubex) have not proved to be sufficiently robust in large-scale evaluations in community settings.[42] Molecular techniques used primarily in epidemiologic studies include DNA hybridization studies, phage typing, chromosome analysis, and plasmid analysis. Recent evaluation of blood culture, typhoid IgM flow assay, and *Salmonella* ser. Typhi/Paratyphi A real-time PCR in children with typhoid fever found typhoid IgM flow assay sensitivity near to that of blood culture (77.9% vs. 80%). However, given that no blood marrow culture was used for comparison, blood culture performance could be overestimated as well as the new IgM flow assay.[274] Of interest was the poor performance of real-time PCR sensitivity (37.8%).[274]

DIFFERENTIAL DIAGNOSIS

Salmonella gastroenteritis cannot be distinguished clinically from other infectious causes of acute diarrhea reliably, although history and epidemiology sometimes may suggest an etiologic agent. Bloody diarrhea with mucus can be caused by *Salmonella, Shigella,* enteroinvasive *E. coli,* enterohemorrhagic *E. coli, Campylobacter* spp., *Yersinia enterocolitica, Clostridium difficile, Trichuris trichiura,* and *Entamoeba histolytica.* Watery diarrhea may be caused by rotavirus or other viral enteropathogens or enterotoxin-producing bacterial pathogens. When abdominal pain and tenderness are severe, the differential diagnosis includes appendicitis, perforated viscus, and mesenteric adenitis.

Enteric fever can mimic other infections of the reticuloendothelial system,[43] including Epstein-Barr virus infection, disseminated histoplasmosis, and tuberculosis, among others (Box 111.3). Noninfectious illnesses with prolonged fever that sometimes can be confused with typhoid include juvenile rheumatoid arthritis and other collagen vascular diseases, Kawasaki syndrome, and lymphomas. An early diagnosis often is difficult to establish because the findings are nonspecific. Findings that are particularly helpful in discriminating typhoid fever from other prolonged febrile illnesses include severe cough and chest pain (more typical of lobar pneumonia), diarrhea with grossly obvious blood (more typical of dysentery), acute onset of chills (more typical of malaria), and marked lower abdominal pain early in the febrile illness (more typical of bacillary dysentery, *Y. enterocolitica* infection, and salpingitis). For patients in countries where typhoid is not endemic, a history of travel is crucial. In endemic developing countries, the widely variable false-positive and false-negative results of the Widal test complicate the differential diagnosis workup, favoring the misuse of antimicrobials.[298] *Salmonella* infections could be a cause of fever of unknown origin, especially in developing countries.[81]

BOX 111.3 Differential Diagnosis of Enteric Fever

Epstein-Barr infection	Tularemia
Dengue	Ehrlichiosis
Tuberculosis	Plague
Brucellosis	Typhus
Bartonella henselae	Malaria
Leptospirosis	Disseminated histoplasmosis

TREATMENT

For children with salmonellosis for whom antibiotic treatment is appropriate, the interpretation of antimicrobial susceptibility studies is important. Drugs such as aminoglycosides, polymyxins, tetracyclines, and first- and second-generation cephalosporins (e.g., cephalothin, cefazolin, cefuroxime, cefamandole) have a poor clinical track record despite apparent in vitro susceptibility. Table 111.5 shows the drugs that typically are useful in treatment of children with *Salmonella* infections. The emergence and dramatic increase of multidrug-resistant *Salmonella* strains represent an important challenge for empirical antibiotic management.

Gastroenteritis

As with all forms of gastroenteritis, fluid and electrolyte replacement and maintenance are the first objective of management. For most patients, oral rehydration is all that is necessary to treat *Salmonella* gastroenteritis. Generally *Salmonella* gastroenteritis should not be treated with antibiotics because these agents do not shorten the course of illness[21,23,78,79,207,243,281,302,335] but prolong excretion of *Salmonella.*[21,23,108,207,281,302] *Salmonella* serotypes typically have been grouped together for these treatment studies, however, as though they were all the same organism. Given the variability in expression of virulence genes, whether treatment may be useful for some serotypes that possess particular virulence traits remains an open question.

Exceptions to the generalization that *Salmonella* gastroenteritis should not be treated include children at high risk for developing complications, including children with underlying diseases or receiving therapies that impair host defenses. Examples of children who probably ought to be given antibiotics are infants 6 months or younger; children with AIDS or malignant diseases; those splenectomized; children with primary immunodeficiencies[38]; children with chronic hepatopathy; children with hemolytic anemias, particularly sickle-cell anemia; and malnourished children. Treatment of these patients is debatable; the data from neonates suggest that antibiotics make little difference in the course.[2,118,207,318,365] Because the risk for development of bacteremia is high, however, antibiotics likely will continue to be used in such settings. Bacteremia occurs in a small fraction of infections; therefore, proving the concept is impossible without conducting a massive placebo-controlled clinical trial. When treatment is given, probably 5 days or fewer of antibiotics is indicated, barring complications. Ciprofloxacin or a third-generation cephalosporin (i.e., ceftriaxone or cefotaxime) are recommended in preference to former suggestions in favor of ampicillin or amoxicillin.[55] Parenteral therapy with a third-generation cephalosporin or fluoroquinolone has been related to reductions in duration of fever and hospitalization in one retrospective study of children with more severe gastroenteritis.[377]

Extraintestinal Infections

Any child who appears to be sufficiently toxic that bacteremia is suspected also should be started on antibiotic treatment until blood cultures exclude the diagnosis. For children with bacteremic NTS and focal extraintestinal complications, a third-generation cephalosporin (e.g.,

TABLE 111.5 Antibiotics Commonly Used in the Treatment of *Salmonella* Infections

Drug	Dose	Comments
Ciprofloxacin	20–30 mg/kg/day in 2 doses PO or IV	First-line therapy[a]
Ceftriaxone	75–100 mg/kg/day in 1 or 2 doses IM or IV	First-line therapy
Cefotaxime	100–300 mg/kg/day in 3–4 doses IM or IV	First-line therapy
Cefixime	20–30 mg/kg/day in 1 or 2 doses PO	Alternative therapy
Azithromycin	10 mg/kg/day in 1 dose PO	Alternative therapy
Chloramphenicol	50–100 mg/kg/day in 4 doses PO	High frequency of resistance; use only for susceptible strains
Ampicillin	200–400 mg/kg/day in 4 doses PO, IM, or IV	High frequency of resistance; use only for susceptible strains
TMP-SMX	10 mg/kg/day TMP, 50 mg/kg/day SMX in 2 doses PO or IV	High frequency of resistance; use only for susceptible strains

[a]Not approved by the US Food and Drug Administration in children <18 years; current expert opinion agrees in recommending this agent as an effective therapy for regions with susceptible *Salmonella* strains and especially for severe infections.
TMP-SMX, Trimethoprim-sulfamethoxazole.

ceftriaxone, cefotaxime) or fluoroquinolone is an appropriate choice. If the patient seems to have a life-threatening infection, ampicillin and chloramphenicol should be used only if evidence exists that the pathogen is not resistant to ampicillin or chloramphenicol and that no meningitis or related involvement is suspected. Children at high risk for having recurrence of bacteremia (children with congenital or acquired immunodeficiencies, such as AIDS) may require a third-generation cephalosporin or a fluoroquinolone to achieve cure.[88,184] Combinations of fluoroquinolones, cephalosporins, and azithromycin are used in patients with severe disease who fail to respond promptly, or in the face of potential drug-resistant strains, or potentially to reduce the emergence of resistant strains during the course of treatment. However there are few studies of the in vitro interactions between antimicrobials for *Salmonella* isolates.[98] Frequent recurrences of life-threatening infection sometimes necessitate use of prolonged or life-long maintenance therapy with an oral agent, after controlling the episode with prolonged combined parenteral therapy guided by antibiogram results.[184]

Many presumed recurrent episodes of NTS in the same child are actually a persistent infection by the same clone in nearly 80% of cases[288] and merit evaluation in search of primary or acquired immune deficiencies. In some primary immunodeficiencies, even NTS could elicit fatal hemophagocytic lymphohistiocytosis.[39,357,371]

Meningitis should be treated with a third-generation cephalosporin because these agents have good penetration into the CSF; ampicillin and chloramphenicol use is associated with higher relapse rates and lower cure rates.[212,292] Meningitis must be treated for at least 4 to 6 weeks for children with apparent good response;[16] for complicated patients (ventriculitis, hydrocephalus, extensive damage) prolonged therapy of more than 12 weeks could be neccesary[411]; approximately three-fourths of patients who have relapses have been treated for 3 weeks or less.[86] *Salmonella* may persist for more than 3 weeks inside CSF mononuclear leukocytes despite negative CSF cultures.[79] Some authors suggest combined antimicrobial therapy with cefotaxime or ceftriaxone plus ciprofloxacin for meningitis.[74,163,184,292,309] Dexamethasone before or at the time of initiation of antimicrobials, aimed at reducing the severity of sequelae of bacterial meningitis in children, is recommended by extension to *Salmonella* meningitis by some authors[17,187,411] but available data are very limited and lead to no definitive conclusions.[271,272,386] Timely initiation of appropriate active bactericidal antimicrobials and severity of disease on arrival are important determinants of outcome, especially in developing countries.[112] Moderate to severe sequelae could affect more than half of infants after complete antimicrobial therapy for *Salmonella* meningitis.[411] Carbapenems such as imipenem and meropenem have been used with good results in a few cases of *Salmonella* meningitis,[73,292] but risk for seizures with imipenem therapy must be considered.[309] Regarding ceftriaxone effectiveness in contrast to ceftazidime and cefotaxime, data from case series suggest a better response to ceftriaxone, especially compared to ceftazidime.[225]

For other extraintestinal infections in children, the duration of antibiotic treatment usually is 10 to 14 days for bacteremia and 4 to 6 weeks for acute osteomyelitis. Collections of pus should be drained, and, for intracranial collections, the total duration of antimicrobial therapy should be extended to 4 to 6 weeks after drainage if this is feasible.[73] Nonaccessible collections in the central nervous system need more prolonged therapy and complicate outcomes. Schistosomiasis, when present, must be treated to achieve resolution of the coincident *Salmonella* infection.[284,321] If combined resistance to all first- and second-line drugs develops, the carbapenems (e.g., imipenem, meropenem, and ertapenem), and tigecycline could be potential alternatives.[98]

Typhoid Fever

The response to antibiotics is slow. Fever may persist for many days, even after bacteremia has resolved.[416] The emergence and spread of MDRST since 1989, defined as combined resistance to chloramphenicol, TMP-SMX, and ampicillin,[416] caused a shift in empirical therapy from once first-line drugs to a fluoroquinolone; a third-generation cephalosporin, such as ceftriaxone; or azithromycin in children (Table 111.6). MDRST is particularly common in the Indian subcontinent, Southeast Asia, and Africa, and resistance to ciprofloxacin is increasing.[83,327]

In the United States, MDRST has been less problematic than it is elsewhere, but resistance to ampicillin, chloramphenicol, and TMP-SMX has continuously increased since the 1990s.[4,239,333] Currently most *S.* ser. Typhi isolates are still sensitive to ceftriaxone and ciprofloxacin, although nalidixic acid–resistant isolates are common in travelers returning from the Indian subcontinent.[4,239] Such strains respond poorly to fluoroquinolones, with a 30-fold chance of requiring retreatment.[395] Recent reports from India found 98.9% resistance to nalidixic acid and 75% resistance to ciprofloxacin in *S.* ser. Paratyphi A from 264 blood culture isolates.[263,395] When the patient has a history of recent travel to or of contact with a traveler from an area with MDRST, the choice of empirical treatment should take this information into account. New minimum inhibitory concentration (MIC) breakpoints have been established for determination of *Salmonella* susceptibility, intermediate sensitivity, or resistance against ciprofloxacin.[189] As a result, MICs of 1 μg/mL or less but 0.06 μg/mL or greater are associated with delayed antimicrobial responses to ciprofloxacin or even to clinical failure.[189] Third-generation cephalosporins are effective against MDRST[123,193,212,261,275,294,352,374] and appropriate for children in such circumstances. Although older, small trials in adults suggested shorter courses could be comparable to longer courses of treatment, caution is warranted for decisions on treatment duration for children given the low quality of evidence and changing susceptibility patterns over time.[407] For MDRST in children, ceftriaxone given at 65 mg/kg per day was associated with relapses with short-course therapy (7 days) in contrast to 14 days of therapy.[44]

Current evidence supports ceftriaxone, cefotaxime, azithromycin, and fluoroquinolones as the most effective drugs for the treatment of typhoid fever.[16,55,407] Fluoroquinolone drugs have proved safe in all age groups, are rapidly effective, and are associated with lower rates of stool carriage than traditional first-line drugs. The three main issues regarding the use of fluoroquinolones are (1) the potential for toxic effects in children, (2) the cost, and (3) the potential emergence of resistance.[296]

TABLE 111.6 Recommended Antibiotic Treatment of Typhoid Fever

Susceptibility	Antibiotic	Days
Fully susceptible	Chloramphenicol *or*	14–21
	Amoxicillin *or*	14
	Trimethoprim-sulfamethoxazole *or*	14
	Third-generation cephalosporin (e.g., cefixime or ceftriaxone) *or*	7–10[a]
	Fluoroquinolone (e.g., ofloxacin or ciprofloxacin)	7–10[a]
Multidrug-resistant	Azithromycin	5–7
	Third-generation cephalosporin (e.g., cefixime or ceftriaxone) *or*	7–10[a]
	Fluoroquinolone (e.g., ofloxacin or ciprofloxacin)	7–10[a]
Quinolone-resistant	Azithromycin *or*	5–7[a]
	Third-generation cephalosporin (e.g., cefixime) *or*	7–10[a]
	Parenteral third-generation cephalosporin (e.g., ceftriaxone) *or*	7–10[a]

[a]For severe typhoid fever, consider 10–14 days of therapy.

In preclinical testing, the fluoroquinolones damaged the articular cartilage of young beagles. A considerable body of evidence exists supports the safety of fluoroquinolones in the long-term use of these drugs in children with cystic fibrosis and in short-term use to treat typhoid fever and dysentery in children. The availability of generic fluoroquinolones in many developing countries and its subsequent misuse has favored the emergence of fluoroquinolone resistance and marks the greatest limitation on their use.[295]

In the developed world, described concerns about the toxicity of fluoroquinolones in children have limited their use to situations of MDRST infections with confirmed resistance to all of the usual antibiotics but sensitive to a fluoroquinolone. If a fluoroquinolone is used, ciprofloxacin or ofloxacin is preferred because of better oral bioavailability. Ciprofloxacin 15 mg/kg per dose twice daily for 7 to 10 days in children causes defervescence in an average of 4.2 days, with infrequent relapses, even with MDRST.[11] Children with MDRST who have been treated with ciprofloxacin 10 mg/kg per day became afebrile in 3.3 days, and 94% achieved clinical cure, with no relapses or carriers detected on follow-up.[116] Ofloxacin is associated with more rapid defervescence and better cure rates than cefixime.[63] Very short courses of ofloxacin (2 or 3 days) may be followed by relapse.[286,390]

Fluoroquinolone treatment for typhoid fever produced lower relapses (relative risk [RR], 0.04–0.52) and length of hospital stay (−3.53 to −1.62 days) in contrast to chloramphenicol.[372] Clinical failure (RR, 0.01–0.54) and microbiologic failure (RR, 0.03–0.64) were reduced for fluoroquinolones in contrast to β-lactam antibiotics treatment.[372] Fluoroquinolones performed better than third-generation cephalosporins, leading to lower clinical failures and duration of hospital stay.[372]

Other agents have been described that occasionally may be useful. Furazolidone 7.5 mg/kg per day is nearly as effective as is chloramphenicol in strains susceptible to both drugs (86% vs. 90% cure).[86] Despite low serum levels, azithromycin seems to be equivalent to chloramphenicol or ciprofloxacin; the high intracellular concentration in macrophages (>100 times serum levels) of azithromycin presumably accounts for its efficacy.[62,150,151] When MDRST is resistant to nalidixic acid, azithromycin is more effective than ofloxacin, resulting in faster resolution of fever and very effective control of fecal carriage in contrast to ofloxacin and even to combined therapy of azithromycin with ofloxacin.[76,296]

A 5-day course of oral azithromycin 20 mg/kg per day (maximum 1000 mg/day) is as effective as intravenous ceftriaxone 75 mg/kg per day (maximum 2.5 g/day for 5 days).[139] Various non-antimicrobial measures should be considered as part of the management of *S.* ser. Typhi infections.

No good level of evidence exists to establish superiority of fluoroquinolones over first-line antibiotics for typhoid fever specifically in children, but fluoroquinolones are suggested at this time as first-line therapy. Because of the high level of resistance in some regions of the world, the World Health Organization (WHO) recommendations for second-line therapy options include third-generation cephalosporins and azithromycin.[407]

Dexamethasone, although potentially increasing the relapse rate,[89] is indicated for patients with severe typhoid fever with delirium, stupor, shock, or coma; the dose is 3 mg/kg initially and then eight doses of 1 mg/kg every 6 hours for 48 hours. This therapy reduces mortality rates from 35% to 55%, to 10%.[180,310] Parenteral fluoroquinolones are probably the antibiotic of choice for severe infections, but no randomized trials of such treatment have been performed.[116] Antipyretics were thought at one time to be dangerous in typhoid fever[110]; whether this concern is correct is doubtful on the basis of more recent experience.[287]

Intestinal hemorrhage or perforation during enteric fever generally is considered to be an indication for surgical intervention.[45,61,147,234] Resection of 10 cm of intestine proximal and distal to the perforation seems to improve outcome in contrast to other surgical approaches.[24] Antibiotic coverage should be broadened to include anaerobes and gram-negative enterics when perforation occurs.[45]

Chronic Carriers

Generally patients who are not food handlers probably should not be cultured or given special treatment after having a bout of gastroenteritis caused by a NTS strain. Carriers of *S.* ser. typhi should be decolonized to decrease the risk to close contacts. Carriers who have a normal gallbladder can be treated with oral ciprofloxacin or norfloxacin for 4 weeks; these drugs concentrate highly in bile.[16] If oral fluoroquinolone therapy is not tolerated, then high-dose intravenous ampicillin for 4 weeks could be indicated.[16] Other options are oral ampicillin or amoxicillin combined with probenecid for 6 weeks. Chronic carriers who cannot be decolonized are treated with cholecystectomy if cholelithiasis or cholecystitis is present; these patients should receive ampicillin intravenously for 7 to 10 days before and 30 days after cholecystectomy.

PREVENTION

Public Health Measures

Recognition of an increased frequency of human infections with an unusual serotype should be followed by an epidemiologic investigation aimed at detecting the source and vehicle. Intervention to stop such outbreaks then can be attempted. Judicious use of antibiotics in dairy and livestock animals,[182] careful food processing and storage, and proper preparation of foods are helpful in decreasing transmission of infection. Appropriate sewage disposal, assurance of a safe water supply, prevention of sale of pet turtles, inspection of cosmetics for contamination, and adequate cleaning of medical equipment are important public health strategies. Families with small children should be informed of the risks associated with pet reptiles and encouraged to avoid such unnecessary risks.

Personal Hygienic Measures

Person-to-person spread can be decreased by hand washing after defecating or changing diapers, frequent hand washing during preparation of foods that might be contaminated (e.g., meat), and excluding infected individuals from food-handling tasks.

Infection Control

Hospitalized children with *Salmonella* gastroenteritis should be isolated (enteric precautions) until stool cultures are negative. Children with extraintestinal infections should be isolated until stool studies exclude intestinal infection or colonization.

Nursery Outbreaks

Neonatal *Salmonella* infection outbreaks should be investigated to determine the source. Cultures of fomites sometimes reveal a removable focus. Neonates and staff members caring for them should be cohorted during outbreaks, with use of enteric precautions in dealing with infants who are excreting the organism. Surveillance cultures should be done on feces of not only sick infants but also well infants to cohort more appropriately. With current early postpartum discharge policies, reporting *Salmonella* infections in infants is important in detecting outbreaks. Isolation and cohorting can be effective in controlling such outbreaks.[317]

Breast-Feeding

In the developing world, breast-feeding is key in prevention because human milk contains secretory IgA and other factors that protect infants from *Salmonella* spp.[14,52,124,125,138,305,306] Case-control studies conducted in the United States and Australia also found breast-feeding to have a strong protective effect against sporadic *Salmonella* infections.[326,402] Pediatric health care providers and community education programs should encourage mothers to breast-feed.

Vaccination

Vaccination of children is indicated when the risk for development of typhoid fever is high (e.g., living with a chronic carrier or in an endemic area) but probably is underused.[356,370] Only 4% of U.S. travelers to endemic settings who acquired enteric fever were previously vaccinated.[356] An updated position paper from the WHO on typhoid vaccine policy recommendations is under development.[409] Two vaccines are extensively available: (1) an oral live attenuated Ty21a vaccine (Vivotif Berna) and (2) a parenteral purified Vi capsular polysaccharide vaccine (Typhim Vi).[214,307]

The Ty21a vaccine has been evaluated in liquid and capsule forms. Ty21a oral vaccine is well tolerated; abdominal pain, nausea, vomiting, and rashes occur rarely. The form licensed in the United States is an enteric-coated capsule preparation meant to be given in four separate doses on alternate days and taken 1 hour before meals. It is not recommended for children younger than 6 years. The four doses should be completed 1 week before potential exposure.[16] Revaccination with the entire four-dose series is recommended every 5 to 7 years in high-risk settings. Because the Ty21a oral vaccine is a live-attenuated *Salmonella*, it should not be used in immunocompromised hosts or in individuals taking antibiotics at the time of vaccination.[16,65,194] Mefloquine, chloroquine, and any combination of atovaquone/proguanil and pyrimethamine/sulfadoxine can be administered together with Ty21a vaccine only if given at doses for malaria prophylaxis.[194] Proguanil use other than prophylaxis must be delayed after 10 days from receipt of the fourth dose of Ty21a vaccine.[16] Other antimalarial drugs could be given 3 days after the last Ty21a vaccine dose.[194]

Several large field trials suggest that the Vi capsular vaccine as a single 25-μg dose (0.5 mL) has an efficacy of 55% and 75% in adults and children older than 5 years, respectively.[3,307] Although fever, malaise, local pain, and tenderness occur with this vaccine, it has two major advantages over the Ty21a oral vaccines. It does not require refrigeration, and only a single dose is required for protection; it is repeated every 3 years.[408] It may be used in children 2 years of age. Vaccination must occur at least 2 weeks before exposure.[16]

Two parenteral Vi vaccines conjugated with tetanus toxoid are licensed and produced in India (PedaTyph and Typbar-TCV).[268,385] The first dose of PedaTyph is advised for subjects older than 2 years of age, followed by a second dose at 4- to 8-week intervals, and then by a booster every 10 years.[229] Only the Typbar-TCV vaccine is recommended by the Indian Academy of Pediatrics (IAP), to be given as a first dose to infants 9 to 12 months old followed by a booster dose at 2 years of age. There should be at least a 4-week interval between Typbar-TCV and any MMR vaccine dose due to paucity of data regarding any possible interference between these vaccines.[385] The IAP has urged the Indian government to recommend universal typhoid immunization.[385] Several vaccine producers from Asia, Russia, and Cuba manufacture local-use parenteral polysaccharide Vi vaccines.[229] Typhoid vaccination is recommended additionally for curtailing typhoid fever outbreaks.[408]

PROGNOSIS

Salmonella gastroenteritis usually is a self-limited disease in the normal host, although chronic diarrhea sometimes develops after an acute episode. Extraintestinal focal infections with nontyphoidal *Salmonella* strains are difficult to cure, particularly if they involve the meninges or occur in compromised hosts. *Salmonella* spp. meningitis may relapse if the course of treatment is too short. Likewise, bacteremia and focal infection recur after treatment in severely compromised hosts, particularly patients with AIDS. Relapse after typhoid fever has long been recognized as a risk.

NEW REFERENCES SINCE THE SEVENTH EDITION

1. Aarestrup FM. The livestock reservoir for antimicrobial resistance: a personal view on changing patterns of risks, effects of interventions and the way forward. *Phil Trans R Soc Lond B Biol Sci.* 2015;370(1670):20140085.
9. Ailal F, Tazi A, Bustamante J, et al. Péricardite purulente et infiltration colique à Salmonella enteritidis compliquée d'invagination intestinale aiguë dans un cas de déficit en IL-12Rβ1. *Arch Pediatr.* 2014;21(12):1348-1352.
12. Alexander M, Bieva C, Butzler JP, et al. Chronic salmonella infection with hypergammaglobulinemic purpura and cryoglobulinemia in a five year old girl. *Acta Paediatr Belg.* 1978;31(4):245-249.
13. Al-Mayouf SM, Bahabri S, Majeed M. Cutaneous leukocytoclastic vasculitis associated with mycobacterial and *Salmonella* infection. *Clin Rheumatol.* 2007;26(9):1563-1564.
14. Al-Shehri SS, Knox CL, Liley HG, et al. Breastmilk-saliva interactions boost innate immunity by regulating the oral microbiome in early infancy. *PLoS ONE.* 2015;10(9):e0135047.
16. American Academy of Pediatrics. Salmonella infections. In: Kimberlin DW, Brady MT, Jackson MA, et al, eds. *Red Book: 2015 Report of the Committee on Infectious Diseases.* Elk Grove Village, IL: American Academy of Pediatrics; 2015:695-702.
19. Ao TT, Feasey NA, Gordon MA, et al. Global burden of invasive nontyphoidal salmonella disease, 2010. *Emerg Infect Dis.* 2015;21(6):941-949.
26. Azmatullah A, Qamar FN, Thaver D, et al. Systematic review of the global epidemiology, clinical and laboratory profile of enteric fever. *J Glob Health.* 2015;5(2):20407.
27. Baily JL, Foster G, Brown D, et al. Salmonella infection in grey seals (*Halichoerus grypus*), a marine mammal sentinel species: pathogenicity and molecular typing of *Salmonella* strains compared with human and livestock isolates. *Env Microbiol.* 2016;18(3):1078-1087.
32. Baliga S, Shenoy S, Saldanha DRM, et al. Scalp abscess due to *Salmonella typhimurium*. *Indian J Pathol Microbiol.* 2010;53(3):572-573.
34. Barbour EK, Ayyash DB, Alturkistni W, et al. Impact of sporadic reporting of poultry *Salmonella* serovars from selected developing countries. *J Infect Dev Ctries.* 2015;9(1):1-7.
39. Benz-Lemoine E, Bordigoni P, Schaack JC, et al. Histiocytose réactionnelle systémique avec hémophagocytose et troubles de l'hémostase associés à une granulomatose septique. *Arch Fr Pediatr.* 1983;40(3):179-182.
46. Black PH, Kunz LJ, Swartz MN. Salmonellosis—a review of some unusual aspects. *N Engl J Med.* 1960;262(16):811-817.
48. Bobylev D, Sarikouch S, Meschenmoser L, et al. Uncommon case of intrapericardial nontyphoidal Salmonella infection in a preterm baby presenting as a cardiac tumor. *Ann Thor Surg.* 2016;101(4):1577-1580.
49. Bonilla FA, Khan DA, Ballas ZK, et al. Practice parameter for the diagnosis and management of primary immunodeficiency. *J Allergy Clin Immunol.* 2015;136(5):1186-1205, e1-78.
50. Bono KT, Samora JB, Klingele KE. Septic arthritis in infants younger than 3 months: a retrospective review. *Orthopedics.* 2015;38(9):e787-e793.
51. Boore AL, Hoekstra RM, Iwamoto M, et al. *Salmonella enterica* infections in the United States and assessment of coefficients of variation: a novel approach to identify epidemiologic characteristics of individual serotypes, 1996–2011. *PLoS ONE.* 2015;10(12):e0145416.
55. British Medical Association, and Royal Pharmaceutical Society. *British National Formulary BNF 70: September 2015–March 2016.* 70th ed. London: BMJ Group; Pharmaceutical Press; 2015.
67. Centers for Disease Control and Prevention. *National Enteric Disease Surveillance: Salmonella Surveillance Overview.* Atlanta, GA: CDC; 2011.
68. Centers for Disease Control and Prevention. Turtles and other reptiles are risky pets. Available at: http://www.cdc.gov/media/matte/2012/09-turtles-salmonella.pdf.
69. Centers for Disease Control and Prevention. *An Atlas of Salmonella in the United States, 1968–2011.* Atlanta: CDC; 2013.
70. Centers for Disease Control and Prevention. *Antibiotic Resistance Threats in the United States, 2013.* Atlanta: CDC; 2013.
71. Centers for Disease Control and Prevention. *NARMS National Antimicrobial Resistance Monitoring System: Enteric Bacteria 2011 Human Isolates Report.* Atlanta: CDC; 2013.
90. Corcos A, Tabbane C, Roussel H. Un cas de septicémie à salmonella typhimurium avec purpura important et atteinte cardiaque chez une fillette de 9 ans. *Arch Fr Pediatr.* 1953;10(9):985-988.
94. Crowe SJ, Mahon BE, Vieira AR, et al. Vital signs: multistate foodborne outbreaks: United States, 2010–2014. *MMWR.* 2015;64(43):1221-1225.

98. Crump JA, Sjölund-Karlsson M, Gordon MA, et al. Epidemiology, clinical presentation, laboratory diagnosis, antimicrobial resistance, and antimicrobial management of invasive *Salmonella* infections. *Clin Microbiol Rev.* 2015;28(4):901-937.
104. Dekker DM, Krumkamp R, Sarpong N, et al. Drinking water from dug wells in rural Ghana—Salmonella contamination, environmental factors, and genotypes. *Int J Environ Res Public Health.* 2015;12(4):3535-3546.
120. Eleazar CI, Philip IP, Ogeneh BO. Dissemination of Salmonella bacilli through carriers and domestic water sources in Enugu urban/peri-urban of Nigeria. *Adv Microbiol.* 2015;5(4):278-284.
125. Fernández L, Langa S, Martín V, et al. The human milk microbiota: origin and potential roles in health and disease. *Pharmacol Res.* 2013;69(1):1-10.
126. Fernández Guerrero ML, Aguado JM, Arribas A, et al. The spectrum of cardiovascular infections due to Salmonella *enterica*. *Medicine (Baltimore).* 2004;83(2):123-138.
130. Figueiredo R, Henriques A, Sereno R, et al. Antimicrobial resistance and extended-spectrum beta-lactamases of *Salmonella enterica* serotypes isolated from livestock and processed food in Portugal: an update. *Foodborne Pathog Dis.* 2015;12(2):110-117.
131. Filiz S, Kocacik Uygun DF, Verhard EM, et al. Cutaneous leukocytoclastic vasculitis due to *Salmonella* enteritidis in a child with interleukin-12 receptor beta-1 deficiency. *Pediatr Dermatol.* 2014;31(2):236-240.
132. Fincher RE, Threadgill ST, Cranford MS, et al. Case report: salmonellosis complicated by leukocytoclastic vasculitis. *Am J Med Sci.* 1991;302(5):296-297.
140. Frickmann H, Schwarz NG, Rakotozandrindrainy R, et al. PCR for enteric pathogens in high-prevalence settings. What does a positive signal tell us? *Infect Dis (Lond).* 2015;47(7):491-498.
148. Gil-Fortuño M, Yagüe-Muñoz A, Tirado-Balaguer MD, et al. Aislamiento de Salmonella enterica serovar Typhi en una adenopatía mesentérica. *Rev Esp Quimioter.* 2013;26(2):162-163.
151. Girgis NI, Sultan Y, Hammad O, et al. Comparison of the efficacy, safety and cost of cefixime, ceftriaxone and aztreonam in the treatment of multidrug-resistant *Salmonella typhi* septicemia in children. *Pediatr Infect Dis J.* 1995;14(7):603-605.
154. Gonzalez-Escobedo G, Gunn JS. Gallbladder epithelium as a niche for chronic Salmonella carriage. *Infect Immun.* 2013;81(8):2920-2930.
158. Grant A, Hashem F, Parveen S. Salmonella and Campylobacter: antimicrobial resistance and bacteriophage control in poultry. *Food Microbiol.* 2016;53:104-109.
162. Gu W, Vieira AR, Hoekstra RM, et al. Use of random forest to estimate population attributable fractions from a case-control study of *Salmonella enterica* serotype Enteritidis infections. *Epidemiol Infect.* 2015;143(13):2786-2794.
171. Havelaar AH, Kirk MD, Torgerson PR, et al. World Health Organization Global estimates and regional comparisons of the burden of foodborne disease in 2010. *PLoS Med.* 2015;12(12):e1001923.
174. Herman HK, Hampshire KN, Khoshnam N, et al. Suppurative granulomatous cholecystitis in a pediatric chronic carrier with *Salmonella enterica* serotype Typhi: a case report and review of literature. *Fetal Pediatr Pathol.* 2016;35(2):129-132.
175. Herman KM, Hall AJ, Gould LH. Outbreaks attributed to fresh leafy vegetables, United States, 1973–2012. *Epidemiol Infect.* 2015;143(14):3011-3021.
177. Hoelzer K, Moreno Switt A, Wiedmann M. Animal contact as a source of human non-typhoidal salmonellosis. *Vet Res.* 2011;42(1):1-27.
178. Hoff GL, White FH. *Salmonella* in reptiles: isolation from free-ranging lizards (Reptilia, Lacertilia) in Florida. *J Herpetol.* 1977;11(2):123-129.
191. Im J, Nichols C, Bjerregaard-Andersen M, et al. Prevalence of *Salmonella* excretion in stool: a community survey in 2 sites, Guinea-Bissau and Senegal. *Clin Infect Dis.* 2016;62(suppl 1):S50-S55.
194. Jackson BR, Iqbal S, Mahon B. Updated recommendations for the use of typhoid vaccine—Advisory Committee on Immunization Practices, United States, 2015. *MMWR.* 2015;64(11):305-308.
195. Jain S, Das Chugh T. Antimicrobial resistance among blood culture isolates of Salmonella *enterica* in New Delhi. *J Infect Dev Ctries.* 2013;7(11):788-795.
208. Keithlin J, Sargeant JM, Thomas MK, et al. Systematic review and meta-analysis of the proportion of non-typhoidal *Salmonella* cases that develop chronic sequelae. *Epidemiol Infect.* 2015;143(7):1333-1351.
211. Kim S. *Salmonella* serovars from foodborne and waterborne diseases in Korea, 1998–2007: total isolates decreasing versus rare serovars emerging. *J Korean Med Sci.* 2010;25(12):1693-1699.
219. Kuroki T, Ito K, Ishihara T, et al. Turtle-associated *Salmonella* infections in Kanagawa, Japan. *Japan J Infect Dis.* 2015;68(4):333.
220. Kutukculer N, Genel F, Aksu G, et al. Cutaneous leukocytoclastic vasculitis in a child with interleukin-12 receptor beta-1 deficiency. *J Pediatr.* 2006;148(3):407-409.
221. Lai C-Y, Huang L-T, Ko S-F, et al. *Salmonella* gastroenteritis complicated with bacteremia and ruptured cholangitis in an infant with congenital choledochal cyst. *J Formos Med Assoc.* 2007;106(3 suppl):3.
227. Leekitcharoenphon P, Hendriksen RS, Le Hello S, et al. Global genomic epidemiology of *Salmonella enterica* serovar Typhimurium DT104. *Appl Environ Microbiol.* 2016;82(8):2516-2526.
232. Likitnukul S, Wongsawat J, Nunthapisud P. Appendicitis-like syndrome owing to mesenteric adenitis caused by *Salmonella typhi*. *Ann Trop Paediatr.* 2002;22(1):97-99.
233. Lin W-J, Wang C-C, Cheng S-N, et al. Hand abscess, phlebitis, and bacteremia due to *Salmonella enterica* serotype Augustenborg. *J Microbiol Immunol Infect.* 2006;39(6):519-522.
249. Marshall JM, Flechtner AD, La Perle KM, et al. Visualization of extracellular matrix components within sectioned *Salmonella* biofilms on the surface of human gallstones. *PLoS ONE.* 2014;9(2):e89243.
254. Mava Y, Bello M, Ambe JP, et al. Antimicrobial sensitivity pattern of organisms causing urinary tract infection in children with sickle cell anemia in Maiduguri, Nigeria. *Niger J Clin Pract.* 2012;15(4):420-423.
255. Mayor S. Over a quarter of *Salmonella* cases in English children are caused by pet reptiles, study finds. *BMJ.* 2014;349:g7796.
260. Melloul AA, Hassani L. Salmonella infection in children from the wastewater-spreading zone of Marrakesh city (Morocco). *J Appl Microbiol.* 1999;87(4):536-539.
263. Menezes G, Harish B, Khan M, et al. Antimicrobial resistance trends in blood culture positive *Salmonella* Paratyphi A isolates from Pondicherry, India. *Indian J Med Microbiol.* 2016;34(2):222.
268. Mohan VK, Varanasi V, Singh A, et al. Safety and immunogenicity of a vi polysaccharide–tetanus toxoid conjugate vaccine (typbar-TCV) in healthy infants, children, and adults in typhoid endemic areas: a multicenter, 2-cohort, open-label, double-blind, randomized controlled phase 3 study. *Clin Infect Dis.* 2015;61(3):393-402.
284. Neves J. Salmonelose septicêmica prolongada. In: Neves J, ed. *Doencas Infectuosas e Parasitárias em Pediatria.* Rio de Janeiro: Guanabara Kogan; 1981:477-486.
285. Newport MJ, Holland SM, Levin M, et al. Inherited disorders of the interleukin-12/23-interferon gamma axis. In: Ochs HD, Smith CIE, Puck J, eds. *Primary Immunodeficiency Diseases: A Molecular and Genetic Approach.* 2nd ed. New York: Oxford University Press; 2007:390-401.
299. Patrick ME, Mahon BE, Zansky SM, et al. Riding in shopping carts and exposure to raw meat and poultry products: prevalence of, and factors associated with, this risk factor for *Salmonella* and *Campylobacter* infection in children younger than 3 years. *J Food Prot.* 2010;73(6):1097-1100.
315. Regunath H, Saizer W. Sources and vehicles of foodborne infectious diseases. In: Khardori N, ed. *Food Microbiology: in Human Health and Disease.* Boca Raton, FL: CRC Press; 2016:67-90.
320. Roccato A, Uyttendaele M, Cibin V, et al. Survival of *Salmonella typhimurium* in poultry-based meat preparations during grilling, frying and baking. *Int J Food Microbiol.* 2015;197:1-8.
323. Rolleston HD, Molony JB. Purpura in infective diarrhoea. *Proc R Soc Med.* 1921;5:54-59.
334. Sanal O, Turul T, De Boer T, et al. Presentation of interleukin-12/-23 receptor β1 deficiency with various clinical symptoms of *Salmonella* infections. *J Clin Immunol.* 2006;26(1):1-6.
341. Scallan E, Hoekstra RM, Angulo FJ, et al. Foodborne illness acquired in the United States—major pathogens. *Emerg Infect Dis.* 2011;17(1):7-15.
344. Seah XFV, Ngeow JHA, Thoon KC, et al. Infant with invasive nontyphoidal salmonellosis and mastitis. *Glob Pediatr Health.* 2015;2.
356. Steinberg EB, Bishop R, Haber P, et al. Typhoid fever in travelers: who should be targeted for prevention? *Clin Infect Dis.* 2004;39(2):186-191.
357. Stéphan JL, Koné-Paut I, Galambrun C, et al. Reactive haemophagocytic syndrome in children with inflammatory disorders. A retrospective study of 24 patients. *Rheumatology (Oxford).* 2001;40(11):1285-1292.
363. Sylvester WRB, Amadi V, Pinckney R, et al. Prevalence, serovars and antimicrobial susceptibility of *Salmonella* spp. from wild and domestic green iguanas (Iguana iguana) in Grenada, West Indies. *Zoonoses Public Health.* 2014;61(6):436-441.
371. Tesi B, Sieni E, Neves C, et al. Hemophagocytic lymphohistiocytosis in 2 patients with underlying IFN-γ receptor deficiency. *J Allergy Clin Immunol.* 2015;135(6):1638-1641.
382. van de Vosse E, Hoeve MA, Ottenhoff THM. Human genetics of intracellular infectious diseases: molecular and cellular immunity against mycobacteria and salmonellae. *Lancet Infect Dis.* 2004;4(12):739-749.
384. Vanhoof R, Gillis P, Stévart O, et al. Transmission of multiple resistant *Salmonella* Concord from internationally adopted children to their adoptive families and social environment: proposition of guidelines. *Eur J Clin Microbiol Infect Dis.* 2012;31(4):491-497.
385. Vashishtha VM, Choudhury P, Kalra A, et al. Indian Academy of Pediatrics (IAP) recommended immunization schedule for children aged 0 through 18 years—India, 2014 and updates on immunization. *Indian Pediatr.* 2014;51(10):785-800.
389. Vidal E, Marzollo A, Betto M, et al. Automated peritoneal dialysis-related peritonitis due to *Salmonella enteritidis* in a pediatric patient. *Clin Exp Nephrol.* 2012;16(2):342-344.
401. Whiley H, Ross K. Salmonella and eggs: from production to plate. *Int J Environ Res Public Health.* 2015;12(3):2543-2556.
402. Williams S, Markey P, Harlock M, et al. Individual and household-level risk factors for sporadic salmonellosis in children. *J Infect.* 2016;76(1):36-44.

409. World Health Organization. SAGE Working Group on Typhoid Vaccines (established March 2016). Available at: http://www.who.int/immunization/policy/sage/sage_wg_typhoid_mar2016/en/.

415. Zaidi MB, McDermott PF, Fedorka-Cray P, et al. Nontyphoidal *Salmonella* from human clinical cases, asymptomatic children, and raw retail meats in Yucatan, Mexico. *Clin Infect Dis*. 2006;42(1):21-28.

418. Zucchini A, Manfredi R. Malattia di Schoenlein-Henoch in corso di infezione da salmonella: una nuova associazione? *Minerva Pediatr*. 1992;44(11):559-563.

The full reference list for this chapter is available at ExpertConsult.com.

Plague *(Yersinia pestis)* 112

Walter Dehority • Gary D. Overturf

HISTORY AND EPIDEMIOLOGY

Yersinia pestis has been responsible for the most devastating epidemics in human history. Plague was first mentioned in 1320 BCE in the Old Testament in I Samuel. The first of three pandemics was heralded by the Justinian plague in northern Africa and the Mediterranean (541–700).[55,73] The second pandemic occurred in Sicily in 1346. In the same year, plague appeared during the siege of Kaffa in the Crimea, thereafter spreading throughout most of Europe, where it became known as the "Black Death," having been introduced by accompanying rodent populations from China along Asian-European trade routes. One-third of the population of Europe died in its aftermath. Between the 14th and 20th centuries, plague occurred throughout Europe and Russia, with resultant frequent outbreaks.[48]

In 1894, Yersin and Kitasato, working independently, first described the plague bacillus while investigating plague spread from mainland China to Hong Kong,[54] and the role of rats and fleas in the spread of disease was defined.[67] In 1900, plague was introduced into San Francisco by rats aboard ships docking there and subsequently to ground squirrels and many other wild animals of the American Southwest.[45] In 1943, effective antibiotics against *Y. pestis* became available. Although antibiotics have been effective in the treatment and prophylaxis of plague, plasmid-borne antibiotic resistance is increasingly being noted.[22] The potential for aerosolized *Y. pestis* as a biologic weapon has led to renewed interest in the understanding and study of this organism.[32]

Plague is now a worldwide disease. The World Health Organization reported 38,359 human cases of plague from 1989 to 2003 with 2845 deaths.[75] Approximately 80% of the cases occurred in Africa, with endemic sites in east Africa and Madagascar; 15% were reported from Asia, including China, southeast Asia, and India; and 5% occurred in the Americas.[75] An African predominance continued into the first decade of the 21st century, with 97% of 21,725 cases reported originating from Africa, with the Congo and Madagascar reporting 82% of these cases.[6] Plague remains endemic in the American Southwest, with more than 80% of cases occurring in New Mexico, Arizona, and Colorado and approximately 10% in California.[11,14] Plague occurs in rodent populations of 17 contiguous states west of the 100th meridian.[19,20]

BACTERIOLOGY

Y. pestis is in the family *Enterobacteriaceae* and is one of 14 *Yersinia* spp. It is a small, pleomorphic, nonmotile, gram-negative bacillus and is closely related to one of the three pathogenic representatives of the genus, *Yersinia pseudotuberculosis*.[1,51,63,65] Wayson, Giemsa, and Gram stains of the bacillus take on bipolar or "safety pin" morphologic features.[18] *Y. pestis* grows on blood, chocolate, and MacConkey agars at temperatures ranging from 0°C to 40°C (32°F–104°F); the optimal temperature is 28°C (82.4°F). On first isolation at 35°C (95°F) on 5% blood agar, the colonies are pinpoint in size, growing to 1 to 2 mm after 2 days. They are nonhemolytic on 5% sheep blood agar.[65]

Depending on the clinical nature of the disease, blood cultures, sputum, or aspirates of enlarged nodes should be examined for typical bacilli. The isolated bacilli can be identified by the following criteria: *Y. pestis*, the sole *Yersinia* spp. that is nonmotile at 37°C and 22°C (98.6°F and 71.6°F), is the sole *Yersinia* spp. that is urease negative, but it may be positive in freshly isolated strains. The organism is positive for esculin, β-galactosidase, catalase, and methyl red. Oxidase, indole, and Voges-Proskauer reactions are negative. It ferments glucose, maltose, salicin, xylose, arabinose, dextrin, trehalose, and mannitol. It does not produce acid from lactose, sucrose, rhamnose, melibiose, ribitol, cellobiose, sorbose, or dulcitol. It does not use citrate, and it does not grow in potassium cyanide. *Y. pestis* is negative for lysine, ornithine decarboxylase, and arginine dihydrolase.[49,65]

Positive cultures show pinpoint colonies within 24 to 48 hours after inoculation. Many laboratories use fully automated or semiautomated identification systems that may not detect *Y. pestis*, often confusing *Y. pestis* and *Y. pseudotuberculosis* or *Y. enterocolitica* with plague bacillus. Nonautomated laboratories may require 6 days to identify the organism. Currently because of the concerns for the use of plague as a biological weapon, suspected isolates should be referred to public health or other reference laboratories for final identification to the species level; this complies with the select agent requirements of the Title II Enhanced Controls for Dangerous Biological Agents and Toxins Act.[32]

Several chromosomal-mediated virulence factors are responsible for the virulence of *Y. pestis*, including (1) an antiphagocytic capsular material known as fraction 1, (2) the endogenous purine synthesis that allows the organism to grow within macrophages, and (3) the ability to absorb iron from the medium.[24,49,62,73] Several plasmids have been implicated in the development of other virulence factors.[66,68,73] Several lines of evidence suggest proteins produced by *Y. pestis* may provide an immunomodulatory function, attenuating the human immune response to provide a more favorable environment for the organisms' survival.[50,66] A prolonged immune response to the F1 antigen is common in survivors of plague and has been documented to persist for at least 10 years.[39] A plasmid of 9-kb pairs contains the determinant of secretory protein that kills other bacterial strains. A plasmid of 72-kb pairs, which all pathogenic *Y. pestis* strains contain, confers the requirement for environmental calcium to be present for the organism to grow at 37°C (98.6°F). When grown under this condition, *Y. pestis* produces V and W antigens that are necessary for virulence.[24] An exotoxin and an endotoxin have been found to contribute to the lethal effects of plague as well.[65,71]

TRANSMISSION

Host

More than 200 mammalian species have been reported to be naturally infected with *Y. pestis*. Epidemics of plague usually are transmitted by fleas of infected domestic rats, which is more likely to occur in urban, rat-infested, and crowded dwellings. In the United States, plague is transmitted sporadically to humans after contact with an enzootic sylvatic focus.[34] Infected wild rodents perpetuate the plague bacillus in a given ecosystem by virtue of their ability to withstand an inoculum of *Y. pestis* many times greater than that necessary to cause disease in humans or domestic animals. After inoculation, wild rodents may become bacteremic and infect fleas that feed on them; these fleas transmit the plague bacillus to another rodent. Hibernating animals are especially resistant to clinical infection. Animals inoculated before going into hibernation may survive through the winter and not die until after they come out of their burrows, reintroducing the bacillus in the new season.[29] Carnivores are relatively resistant to infection but contribute to the spread of the organism by transporting infected fleas from one area to another.[34,67]

The role of domestic animals in bridging the gap between sylvatic plague and human infection has been studied extensively.[47,54,60] Cats and dogs are susceptible to natural and experimental plague.[60] Epizootics in cats have been observed in conjunction with plague epidemics in humans.[54] Experimentally infected cats develop severe systemic illness, with bacteremia and abscess formation at the site of inoculum. Between 1977 and 1998, 23 cases of feline-associated human plague in the United States were reported[25]; five cases were fatal; two of the patients had primary pneumonic plague, and one had septicemic plague. Many of these cases were misdiagnosed at presentation, leading to delays in treatment and, in some cases, fatalities. This diagnosis should be considered especially in the western states of Arizona, California, Colorado, and New Mexico. No seasonal variation in the occurrence of cat-associated illness was noted.[20,25] Ten other cases reported in the literature of feline transmission of plague to humans involved four veterinarians.[21] Dogs also are susceptible, but the disease is milder.[60] Dogs are less likely to transmit plague to humans, though this has been documented on five occasions in the literature.[58] Swine are resistant to plague disease, the only evidence of subclinical infection being the presence of antibodies to the fraction 1 antigen of *Y. pestis*. Domestic animals, by virtue of their intimate contact with wildlife and humans, may be responsible for some cases of human plague. This danger is accentuated by a dearth of symptoms in some animals.[47]

Vector

Plague is transmitted to humans by bite of an infected flea, the skinning and evisceration of infected animals,[35] or inhalation of infected droplets from a case of pneumonic plague.[42] Infrequent portals of entry include the conjunctiva[47] and the pharynx.[46,56] *Y. pestis* has been detected in both head and body lice recovered from patients with suspected plague in the Democratic Republic of the Congo, leading to speculation that transmission could occur through lice as well as flea vectors.[53]

The efficiency of fleas as vectors for human disease depends on the likelihood that an infected flea will feed on a person and that the flea will regurgitate bacilli into the victim's bloodstream in the process of feeding.[34] Flea species vary in both of these attributes. Wild rodent fleas are reluctant to feed on humans and do it only under duress (e.g., when the natural host dies). Fleas of domestic animals are more likely to bite humans. The Oriental rat flea, *Xenopsylla cheopis,* is the most efficient transmitter of plague because of its willingness to bite people and its propensity for regurgitating large numbers of bacilli in the process.[34] When the Oriental rat flea ingests infected blood, the actions of a coagulase produced by *Y. pestis* and a trypsin-like enzyme present in the flea's stomach result in the formation of an infected clot that blocks the flea's proventriculus. In obstructing the flea's intestinal tract, the clot allows further replication of bacteria. When the flea tries to feed again, it regurgitates large numbers of plague bacilli. The formation and dissolution of the fibrin clot are temperature dependent. At temperatures greater than 27°C (>80.6°F), a fibrinolytic enzyme is activated that dissolves the clot and allows the flea to dispose of plague bacilli. One postulation is that this temperature-dependent phenomenon is responsible for the observed cyclic nature of urban plague epidemics, which tend to subside with the advent of hot weather.[8] However *X. cheopis* fleas with a blockage in the proventriculus are inefficient transmitters of plague given the long (12- to 16-day) extrinsic incubation period before blockage and transmission occur, followed by the death of the flea after a relatively short infectious window. This model may not adequately explain the rapid spread of disease often seen in epidemics of plague. However *Oropsylla montana*, a primary vector of *Y. pestis* in North America, rarely becomes blocked after feeding and has a very short extrinsic incubation period (24–96 hours).[23] This flea is subsequently able to transmit *Y. pestis* in a murine model with 83% to 100% efficiency only 1 to 4 days after feeding, which may better explain the rapidity with which epidemics of plague may spread.[23] Fleas in which the intestinal tracts do not become blocked may also contribute to the endemicity of plague by harboring the organism and transmitting it in sublethal doses.[9] Sylvatic plague depends on the rodent flea as the vector. This flea, although not as efficient as the rat flea in transmitting the bacillus, may itself become a reservoir of *Y. pestis* by surviving for 12 to 15 months after the original host dies. In the new season, it reintroduces the plague bacillus into a new rodent population.[54] The observation that *Y. pestis* can survive in soil between epizootics suggests another possible mechanism of transmission of plague.[27]

EPIDEMIOLOGY

Recent studies have suggested that plague is an ancient disease of mammals; the bacterium emerged 1500 to 20,000 years ago as a clone that evolved from *Y. pseudotuberculosis* that first caused outbreaks in Africa.[1] Plague bacteria exist in enzootic cycles involving wild animals or domestic rats. In urban plague, the course of events usually is initiated by the introduction of plague from an enzootic focus into a susceptible rat population. With humans and rats living in proximity, an epizootic in rats may be followed by an epidemic in humans.[54] The epidemic may subside with the advent of hot, humid weather[8] or the obliteration of the rat population.[54] Such epidemics rarely occur today but have been described in Southern Vietnam[5,37] and more recently in India.[16] Between 1985 and 1999, 23 countries reported a total of 29,020 cases of plague to the World Health Organization, with an average mortality rate of 11%; major epidemics and outbreaks occurred in Tanzania (1991), Zaire (1992, 1993), Peru (1993, 1994), India (1994), and Madagascar (1995), with fatality rates ranging from 4.6% to 22.3%.[74]

In the United States, humans become infected most frequently by direct contact with a sylvatic reservoir of infection. Sporadic human cases usually result from working or hunting in a plague-infested area[34] or living near foci of infection as suburban spread encroaches on the natural habitats of rodents.[13] Although poor socioeconomic status has been associated with an increased incidence of plague, particularly in resource-limited settings, recent analyses from New Mexico suggest that this is changing in the United States. Prior to 1990, plague cases clustered in regions with poor housing conditions, older homes, and high proportions of the population living below the poverty line.[61] In the past two decades, plague is increasingly clustered in regions with newer homes, higher home values, and in areas of higher median income.[61] This is presumed secondary to migration of upper- to middle-class families to regions ecologically supportive of sylvatic plague. Hence epidemiological suspicion of plague should primarily be driven by local epidemiological data and ecological factors, not socioeconomic considerations.[61]

In recent years, domestic animals, especially cats, have been responsible for a significant proportion of human cases. Sylvatic plague epizootics occur in the summer, and most cases of rural plague occur between April and September. The rare occurrence of human plague in the winter usually is associated with hunting and direct exposure to infected animal tissues.[12,35] Many resurgences of plague occur after ecologic changes resulting in population increases in ground rodents such as prairie dogs, ground squirrels, mice, and rats in the American Southwest.[9]

The continental United States has a large enzootic focus that includes 130 counties in 15 western states. Surveillance for plague in rodents during the 1990s has identified infected animals farther east than ever before reported. The plague bacillus now has been isolated in wild rodents in eastern Montana, western Nebraska, western North Dakota, and eastern Texas.[13] A summary of all 1006 human cases of plague in the United States reported to the US Public Health Service (1900–81) or the Centers for Disease Control and Prevention (1981–2012) revealed plague cases in 18 states.[36] Overall the median age was 29 years, with 65% of patients male; 82% of cases were bubonic, 10% septicemic, 8% pneumonic, 1% pharyngeal, and two cases (<1%) were gastrointestinal.

Approximately half of all cases occurred prior to 1925 and were primarily clustered around port cities, with tremendous variation in yearly incidence. The median age of patients was 30, with 71% male and just over 30% of Asian descent. The last case of confirmed person-to-person spread of pneumonic plague was documented in 1924. Four percent of cases were reported from 1926 to 1964, with just over half of cases (52%) reported from California; no cases were reported in 17 of these years. The median age was 15 years during this time period, with 83% of patients male and 83% white. Forty-seven percent of all cases occurred from 1965 to 2012, with approximately 90% of reports originating from the Southwest (54% of which were from New Mexico). In contrast to the preceding era, at least one case was reported in every year during this time period. The median age of infected patients was 28 years, with 57% of patients male and 33% of Native American descent. Many patients were infected within 1 mile of their residence and almost all within their state of residence.[30] Seven of the 10 patients described in 1993 were exposed in their home sites, and one, a veterinarian, was exposed at work.[13]

Occasionally plague has been acquired by a traveler in an endemic area who then traveled during the incubation period to a plague-free region of the country. This set of circumstances demonstrates why all physicians need to be aware of the presenting symptoms and signs of plague and to obtain an accurate travel history.[38] Laboratory-acquired infection with *Y. pestis* in laboratory workers has also been described, including two fatal cases.[57]

PATHOGENESIS AND PATHOLOGY

The portal of entry of the plague bacillus determines, to some extent, the form of disease. The most common portal of entry is the skin when it is bitten by an infected flea. Broken skin may provide access for direct inoculation while infected animals are being handled. After overcoming the skin barrier, the organisms move through the lymphatics to the regional lymph nodes, where they elicit an inflammatory response. The infection may be localized at this site, with subsequent formation of antibody and recovery. This clinical form is known as *pestis minor*. The bacillus commonly is disseminated through the bloodstream. Distant organ involvement may include the liver, spleen, kidneys, lungs, and meninges. Disseminated intravascular coagulation is common in fatal cases. Coagulation defects, including thrombocytopenia and elevated fibrin split products[5] and fibrin deposits in the glomeruli[24,54] may be present. Bacteremia is not synonymous with severe disease and occurs commonly in mild cases.[54]

The major determinant of severity seems to be the presence of high levels of endotoxin. The toxin of *Y. pestis* has the biologic properties of a typical endotoxin. When injected into experimental animals, it can cause clinical symptoms, signs, and pathologic changes characteristic of endotoxic shock and death. The quantity of endotoxin necessary to kill is estimated to be comparable to that present in a lethal dose of live bacteria.[2,71] The murine toxin of *Y. pestis* has a direct inhibitory effect in vitro on the respiration of heart mitochondria of rats and mice, whereas it has little or no effect on the mitochondria of rabbits, chimpanzees, dogs, and monkeys. The differing sensitivities in vitro correlate with the susceptibilities in vivo of these species to *Y. pestis* infection.[59] Achieving high levels of toxin depends on the ability of the bacillus to replicate in the infected host. Although resistance to phagocytosis had been assumed to be related to virulence, experimental evidence has shown that virulent *Y. pestis* organisms are phagocytosed, but, in contrast to avirulent ones, are not killed. They continue to replicate freely in macrophages, allowing the accumulation of endotoxin.[33,59]

When the lung is the portal of entry, the disease usually is more fulminant. After being inhaled, bacilli replicate freely in the alveolar spaces. Severe pneumonia, endotoxemia, and septicemia ensue and, if untreated, cause death. In fatal cases, the thoracic lymph nodes have infarction, necrosis, and liquefaction with pus formation. Edema and inflammation of surrounding tissue are common.[54] The mucosa of the trachea and bronchi is covered by bloody, frothy exudate. Submucosal hemorrhages and areas of necrosis may surround the trachea. The pleural surfaces contain hemorrhagic lesions and fibrinous adhesions. Lung parenchyma may be consolidated or show signs of acute edema.[54] The predominant histologic feature is an alveolar exudate consisting of histiocytes and polymorphonuclear leukocytes.[24]

Other organs also are involved. The kidneys may appear grossly hemorrhagic and contain areas of necrosis. Microscopic examination reveals leukocytic infiltrates of congested veins and capillaries. Glomeruli with fibrin thrombi frequently are found in patients with disseminated intravascular coagulation.[24] Biopsy of purpuric skin lesions reveals subepithelial hemorrhages and fibrin deposit in capillaries. These changes are indistinguishable from changes seen in a generalized Shwartzman reaction.[5]

CLINICAL MANIFESTATIONS

The incubation period of *Y. pestis* generally is 3 to 4 days but ranges from a few hours to 10 days. The onset of illness usually is abrupt, beginning with fever, malaise, weakness, and headache.[54,55] Fever is high, frequently accompanied by shaking chills.[47] The appearance of a visible and palpable bubo may be preceded by pain and tenderness at that site.[55]

On physical examination, the patient is "toxic," apprehensive, and tachycardic. The skin inoculation site may not be evident or may be marked by an abscess. In bubonic plague, typical large, fixed, edematous, and exquisitely tender nodes are present at one anatomic site.[37] In decreasing order of frequency, the areas of nodal involvement are the groin (femoral and inguinal nodes), axilla, and neck.[54] Any lymph node may suppurate, sometimes presenting an atypical picture (e.g., if intraabdominal nodes are involved, an acute abdominal emergency may be suspected).[55] Septicemia as an initial presentation of *Y. pestis* infection is common.[30] Among 71 confirmed cases of plague in New Mexico from 1980 to 1984, 25% presented without adenopathy. All patients with septicemia presented with fever and chills, and most had tachycardia, tachypnea, and relative hypotension. Seventy-two percent had gastrointestinal symptoms. Plague pneumonia was twice as likely to occur among septicemic patients as among patients with bubonic plague. Septicemic patients were significantly older and more likely to die than were patients with a bubonic presentation. Although septicemic plague occurred more often in older patients, those younger than 30 years with a septicemic presentation were more likely to die.[30]

As a result of its nonspecific presentation, septicemic plague is difficult to diagnose early. Of 27 patients with plague admitted to Indian Medical Center in Gallup, New Mexico, between 1965 and 1989, five had a nonspecific febrile syndrome with upper respiratory tract symptoms and were prescribed penicillin; three of these five patients died. Another five patients had a nonspecific febrile syndrome associated with chills, myalgias, and anorexia. These patients were not treated initially with antibiotics, and three died.[21] The index of suspicion must be high because early diagnosis is imperative to avoid a high risk of mortality. Individuals who appear to have community-acquired, gram-negative sepsis who reside in or have a history of recent travel to endemic areas of plague must be evaluated for and treated with antibiotics effective against *Y. pestis*.[45]

Gastrointestinal symptoms often occur in patients with plague, especially patients with septicemic plague.[29] Between1980 and 1984, more than half of the 71 patients with plague in New Mexico had gastrointestinal symptoms. In bubonic cases with these symptoms, 39% of the time the symptoms preceded the appearance of the buboes.[29] Common symptoms are abdominal pain, nausea, vomiting, and diarrhea. These symptoms are believed to be a general response to gram-negative septicemia. Occasionally, hepatosplenomegaly and mesenteric or retroperitoneal lymphadenopathy have masqueraded as an acute abdomen.[31,38]

Neurologic manifestations caused by the effects of toxin on the brain are common. A patient with plague may have insomnia, delirium, stupor, weakness, staggering gait, vertigo, disorders of speech, and loss of memory.[44] *Y. pestis* meningitis is rare. Children younger than 15 years appear to be more susceptible, and septicemic patients are four times more likely to develop meningitis than are patients with bubonic plague.[44] It often manifests while the patient is well into a course of antibiotic therapy for bubonic or septicemic plague.[3] When intravascular coagulation supervenes, renal involvement may manifest as acute cortical or tubular necrosis. Hepatic involvement may be evidenced by mildly elevated liver enzymes.[54] Hantavirus pulmonary syndrome may mimic septicemic or pneumonic plague; both share a similar geographic distribution, and patients for whom this diagnosis is contemplated should be treated with antibiotics to cover the possibility of plague.[52]

Primary pneumonic plague has similar constitutional symptoms but follows a fulminant course with a more pronounced pulmonary component. Within 20 to 24 hours after the onset of the illness, tachypnea, dyspnea, and cough productive of bloody, mucopurulent sputum supervene. If early and effective treatment is not instituted, the patient usually dies.[54] In the preantibiotic era in the United States, 18% of pneumonic plague patients transmitted *Y. pestis* to at least one other person.[28] No confirmed secondary transmission of pneumonic plague has been reported since 1924.[36] A potential case of human-to-human spread of pneumonic plague was reported in Colorado in 2015, but proved difficult to confirm given that the patient had contact with both an infected dog and a patient with pneumonic plague.[58]

DIFFERENTIAL DIAGNOSIS

Because of the rare incidence of plague today, the diagnosis often is delayed or missed. Bubonic plague may be confused with other diseases affecting the skin and lymph nodes. The diagnosis of staphylococcal or streptococcal adenitis can be established easily by culture. Lymphogranuloma venereum is more indolent, has milder systemic symptoms, and is associated with anogenital ulcer. Syphilitic adenitis usually is nontender. With cat-scratch disease and *Pasteurella multocida* infections, the constitutional symptoms are few and the patient typically has a history of animal exposure. Tularemia has a more gradual onset.[54] In their later stages, the ulcerated skin lesions of plague may resemble anthrax.[37]

DIAGNOSIS

The most important factor in promptly establishing the diagnosis of plague is having a high index of suspicion. Suspicion should trigger immediate notification to the local or state health department. The state reference laboratory can arrange for rapid and confirmatory diagnostic tests. Bacterial staining of lymph node material by Giemsa, Wayson, or Wright stain may reveal typical bipolar plague organisms. In the septicemic form of the disease, similar bacterial staining of venous blood frequently permits visualization of the plague bacillus.[43] Although culture is a mainstay of diagnosis, *Y. pestis* isolates may be misidentified by automated bacterial identification systems as a variety of gram-negative organisms (often with a high probability), including *Acinetobacter spp.*, various species of *Pseudomonas*, and *Y. pseudotuberculosis*.[69] Hence clinical suspicion is essential when interpreting blood culture results from automated systems with gram-negative rods in patients with the possibility of plague.[69] *It is essential to inform the laboratory that plague is suspected.* Fluorescent antibody staining of direct smears and tissues may provide a rapid, presumptive diagnosis of plague.[32] More recent rapid tests, such as an enzyme-linked immunosorbent assay for the F1 antigen[17] or polymerase chain reaction for F1 antigen genes (*pla* and *caf1*), are now often available in public health laboratories.[6]

TREATMENT

Therapeutic decisions cannot await culture results. All patients suspected of having plague should receive prompt antimicrobial therapy after appropriate blood and tissue samples have been obtained for cultures, fluorescent antibody staining, and serologic testing.

The sulfonamides and streptomycin proved effective when they were first introduced in the 1940s. Resistant strains to one or the other of these antibiotics soon appeared.[7,56] Despite the paucity of published trials in humans on antibiotic effectiveness, other than streptomycin and tetracycline, the Working Group on Civilian Biodefense Consensus Statement[32] recommends gentamicin as an effective alternative to streptomycin for patients needing parenteral antibiotics. Gentamicin has been used frequently in recent years and has shown comparable outcomes to streptomycin in one case series.[4] In vitro and in vivo studies in mice corroborate its effectiveness against *Y. pestis* infections.[64,65]

For acutely ill patients thought to have plague infection, streptomycin or gentamicin are the drugs of choice. If available, streptomycin is given intramuscularly, 20 to 40 mg/kg per day in two divided doses up to a maximum of 1 g every 12 hours.[44] Gentamicin is administered intravenously or intramuscularly, 7.5 mg/kg per day to children and 3 to 5 mg/kg per day to adults in three divided doses. Although single daily doses of gentamicin are commonly recommended today and may be effective in infections due to *Y. pestis*, they have not been studied to date. During the first 36 to 72 hours after infection, *Y. pestis* invades host macrophages to evade innate immune responses. This intracellular state may result in an organism less susceptible to commonly used antibiotics than the extracellular form of *Y. pestis*. Indeed, minimum bactericidal concentrations (MBCs) for ciprofloxacin, chloramphenicol, gentamicin, and doxycycline are 2 to 4 times higher for intracellular than for extracellular forms of *Y. pestis*, whereas MBCs for streptomycin are unchanged.[72]

Antibiotic susceptibility testing should be done because *Y. pestis* with plasmid-mediated, multiple-antibiotic resistance has been described.[26] The antimicrobial efflux pump AcrAB-TolC mediates resistance to many antibiotics commonly used for the treatment of *Y. pestis*.[40] Though plasmid-mediated multidrug resistance has been documented in *Y. pestis*, a 2012 analysis of 392 isolates from humans, animals, and fleas collected from 17 different countries failed to document any resistance to gentamicin, streptomycin, tetracycline, doxycycline, ciprofloxacin, levofloxacin, chloramphenicol, or trimethoprim-sulfamethoxazole (TMP-SMX), indicating that such resistance may be uncommon.[70]

When plague meningitis develops, chloramphenicol, 50 to 100 mg/kg per day intravenously in four divided doses (maximum dose, 4.0 g/day), is the treatment of choice. Duration of therapy is determined by the length and severity of the illness. Treatment is continued for at least 7 days in patients with uncomplicated disease.[15] Patients older than 8 years who do not require hospitalization may receive tetracycline at a dose of 25 to 50 mg/kg per day every 6 hours up to a total daily dose of 1 g in children and 2 g in adults. When outpatient treatment is given, the patient should be observed closely for the first 3 days to ensure resolution of the disease.[15] In vitro data suggests that moxifloxacin at a dose of 400 mg/day may also be effective in the treatment of *Y. pestis* in adults.[41]

Sulfonamides may be used for prophylaxis in pediatric patients as an alternative to the tetracycline class of antibiotics, and, as noted under prevention, TMP-SMX is now currently recommended for prophylaxis in young children.[32] Doxycycline at a dose of 4 mg/kg per day (up to a maximum of 200 mg) divided into two doses may be substituted for tetracycline.

PROGNOSIS

An analysis of all 1006 cases of human plague reported in the United States from 1900 to 2012 revealed that, prior to the use of antimicrobial therapy, 66% of cases overall were fatal, with higher mortality rates for septicemic (89%) and pneumonic plague (93%).[36] In the antibiotic era, mortality overall decreased to 16%, with a significantly lower mortality rate among those patients who received at least one dose of an appropriate antibiotic compared with those who did not (9% vs. 52%). In the antimicrobial era, the mortality rate for pneumonic plague (36%) remained higher than for septicemic plague (27%) and bubonic plague (13%).[36]

With prompt specific antimicrobial therapy, the overall mortality rate for plague has decreased to 5%.[42] Complications during convalescence include polyarthritis, small lung abscesses, delayed suppuration of buboes,[37] and meningitis. *Staphylococcus aureus* and *Pseudomonas* spp. may superinfect involved lymph nodes.[55] Immunity usually ensues after clinical or asymptomatic infection occurs, but natural reinfection rarely has been observed.[55]

PREVENTION AND CONTROL

Institution of hygienic measures and eradication of rats from areas of human habitations have all but eliminated epidemics of urban plague. When epizootics occur in wild rodents, control measures must be directed against rodents and fleas. Vector control can be achieved by the use of insecticides in fields and housing areas. In plague-endemic areas, the public must be instructed to avoid burrows, not to handle sick or dead rodents, to de-flea household pets, and to eliminate trash near living areas.[10] Immune surveys of wild or domestic animals can be used as a surveillance tool to ascertain the presence of *Y. pestis* in the community because dogs, cats, and swine develop antibodies to the fraction 1 antigen of *Y. pestis*.[47,60]

Patients with plague should be isolated with respiratory precautions until they are bacteriologically sterile. Close contacts of patients with pneumonic plague should receive chemoprophylaxis with tetracycline at 25 to 50 mg/kg per day up to 2 g in adults and up to 1 g in children 8 years and older. Younger children should receive TMP-SMX at 8 mg/kg per day (trimethoprim component) in two equal doses orally.[32] The 6-day quarantine period for international travel for contacts of patients with plague does not guarantee the clearance of the bacillus from asymptomatic pharyngeal carriers.[7] Public and professional education in endemic zones is paramount for ensuring prompt reporting of human and animal cases.

Plague vaccines have been used since the late 19th century for individuals at high risk for occupational exposure. They are no longer being manufactured in the United States. Research in this area is continuing.[32,63]

NEW REFERENCES SINCE THE SEVENTH EDITION

6. Butler T. Review article: plague gives surprises in the first decade of the 21st century in the United States and worldwide. *Am J Trop Med Hyg*. 2013;89:788-793.
23. Eisen R, Bearden S, Wilder A, et al. Early-phase transmission of *Yersinia pestis* by unblocked fleas as a mechanism explaining rapidly spreading plague epizootics. *Proc Natl Acad Sci USA*. 2006;103:15380-15385.
28. Hinckley A, Biggerstaff B, Griffith K, et al. Transmission dynamics of primary pneumonic plague in the USA. *Epidemiol Infect*. 2012;140:554-560.
36. Kugeler K, Staples E, Hinckley A, et al. Epidemiology of human plague in the United States, 1900–2012. *Emerg Infect Dis*. 2015;21:16-23.
39. Li B, Du C, Zhou L, et al. Humoral and cellular immune response to *Yersinia pestis* infection in long-term recovered plague patients. *Clin Vaccine Immunol*. 2012;19:228-234.
40. Lister I, Raftery C, Mescas J, et al. *Yersinia pestis* acrAB-tolC in antibiotic resistance and virulence. *Antimicrob Agents Chemother*. 2012;56:1120-1124.
41. Louie A, Heine H, VanScoy B, et al. Use of an in vitro pharmacodynamics model to derive a moxifloxacin regimen that optimizes kill of *Yersinia pestis* and prevents emergence of resistance. *Antimicrob Agents Chemother*. 2011;55:822-830.
50. Osei-Owusu P, Condry D, Toosky M, et al. The N terminus of type III secretion needle protein YscF from *Yersinia pestis* functions to modulate innate immune responses. *Infect Immun*. 2015;83:1507-1523.
53. Piarroux R, Abedi A, Shako J, et al. Plague epidemics and lice, Democratic Republic of the Congo. *Emerg Infect Dis*. 2013;19:505-506.
57. Ritger K, Black S, Weaver K, et al. Fatal laboratory-acquired infection with an attenuated *Yersinia pestis* strain: Chicago, IL, 2009. *MMWR Morb Mortal Wkly Rep*. 2011;60:201-205.
58. Runfola J, House J, Miller L, et al. Outbreak of human pneumonic plague with dog-to-human and possible human-to-human transmission: Colorado, June-July 2014. *MMWR Morb Mortal Wkly Rep*. 2015;64:429-434.
61. Schotthoefer A, Eisen R, Kugeler K, et al. Changing socioeconomic indicators of human plague, New Mexico, USA. *Emerg Infect Dis*. 2012;18:1151-1155.
66. Spinner J, Camody A, Jarrett C, et al. Role of *Yersinia pestis* toxin complex family proteins in resistance to phagocytosis by polymorphonuclear leukocytes. *Infect Immun*. 2013;81:4041-4053.
69. Tourdjman M, Ibraheem M, Brett M, et al. Misidentification of *Yersinia pestis* by automated systems, resulting in delayed diagnoses of human plague infections: Oregon and New Mexico, 2010–2011. *Clin Infect Dis*. 2012;55:e58-e60.
70. Urich S, Chalcraft L, Schriefer M, et al. Lack of antimicrobial resistance in *Yersinia pestis* isolates from 17 countries in the Americas, Africa and Asia. *Antimicrob Agents Chemother*. 2012;56:555-559.
71. Wendte J, Ponnusamy D, Reiber D, et al. In vitro efficacy of antibiotics commonly used to treat human plague against intracellular *Yersinia pestis*. *Antimicrob Agents Chemother*. 2011;55:3752-3757.

The full reference list for this chapter is available at ExpertConsult.com.

Other *Yersinia* Species 113

Charles R. Woods Jr

Yersinia spp. are gram-negative, coccobacillary organisms that are primarily zoonotic. The genus is a member of the family Enterobacteriaceae and consists of at least 11 species, three of which clearly are human pathogens[73]: *Yersinia pestis, Y. pseudotuberculosis* (both formerly included in the genus *Pasteurella*), and *Y. enterocolitica*. *Y. pestis,* the causative agent of plague, is found in rodents and insect vectors and is discussed in Chapter 112.

Y. enterocolitica and *Y. pseudotuberculosis* are responsible for a variety of syndromes, some of which originally were called *pseudotuberculosis*. Infections caused by these primarily enteropathogenic *Yersinia* spp. now are collectively referred to as *yersiniosis,* which is the focus of this chapter. Molecular phylogenetic analysis suggests that *Y. pestis* evolved from *Y. pseudotuberculosis* 1500 to 20,000 years ago.[4] The genomes of representative strains of the three pathogenic *Yersinia* spp. have been sequenced.[210]

During the past 4 decades, *Y. enterocolitica* has been recognized as an important human pathogen worldwide and is a common cause of gastroenteritis in some pediatric populations of the industrialized world.[1,50,60,128] *Y. enterocolitica* also has drawn attention because of its immunologic or postinfectious manifestations, which include reactive arthritis and erythema nodosum.[50] *Y. pseudotuberculosis,* although widespread, is a much less common cause of human disease.[73] In Japan, it has been associated with clinical illness that sometimes has resembled Kawasaki disease.

HISTORICAL ASPECTS

In 1883, Malassez and Vignal[141] described a bacterium that produced a disease they named *pseudotuberculosis*. The first case of mesenteric adenitis, the most common syndrome produced by *Y. pseudotuberculosis,* was reported in 1913 by Saisawa.[186] In 1954, Knapp and Masshoff[116] first reported the clinical features of infection produced by this organism.

The existence of a species of *Yersinia* other than that causing pseudotuberculosis was suggested in 1933 by Gilbert,[66] who reported an unusual infection in animals. In 1964, it was named *Y. enterocolitica* by Frederiksen.[63]

The genus is named for A. J. Yersin, the French bacteriologist who first isolated the plague bacillus.[200] During the past 50 years, an extensive literature detailing the microbiology, pathology, epidemiology, molecular pathogenesis, and clinical features of disease caused by *Y. pseudotuberculosis* and *Y. enterocolitica* has accumulated.*

*References 13, 23, 25, 26, 48, 50, 58, 88, 89, 94, 100, 114–117, 128, 136, 148, 183, 197, 199, 203, 216, 229.

MICROBIOLOGY

Yersinia organisms are large (0.5 to 1 μm × 1 to 2 μm or larger), gram-negative, and ovoid or rod-shaped. *Y. enterocolitica* and *Y. pseudotuberculosis* are motile at 22° to 25°C (71.6°F–77°F) but not at 37°C (98.6°F). Similar to other members of Enterobacteriaceae, *Yersinia* organisms are facultative anaerobes and grow well on ordinary media. On Gram staining, *Y. pseudotuberculosis* appears as a large coccobacillus. Staining with methylene blue and carbol fuchsin discloses a bipolar (safety pin) morphology of most, but not all, strains. *Y. enterocolitica* is smaller and shows little, if any, bipolarity.[197,200]

Unless careful biochemical and physiologic studies are conducted, *Yersinia* organisms may be confused with coliforms, such as *Morganella, Proteus, Shigella, Salmonella,* and *Providencia* spp., or *Escherichia coli* or with *Y. pestis* or *Brucella,* and *Achromobacter* organisms. *Yersinia* organisms reduce nitrates and are oxidase negative, catalase positive, and andurease positive. *Yersinia* organisms usually do not ferment lactose but produce α-galactosidase. All strains of *Y. pseudotuberculosis* and most strains of *Y. enterocolitica* isolated in Europe are indole negative. Most strains of *Y. enterocolitica* found in the United States have been indole positive.[53,70,95,158,164,197,200]

Although these two species of *Yersinia* share many properties, they are distinguishable on the basis of several biochemical activities, antigenic structure, and sensitivity to various *Yersinia* phages.[185] *Y. enterocolitica* produces an acid slant and acid butt on triple sugar iron agar caused by fermentation of sucrose, whereas *Y. pseudotuberculosis* produces an alkaline slant and an acid butt. *Y. enterocolitica* elaborates ornithine decarboxylase and ferments sucrose and amygdalin. *Y. pseudotuberculosis* does none of these, but it ferments adonitol, which *Y. enterocolitica* does not.[95,200]

Commercially available tests used to identify Enterobacteriaceae in clinical laboratories may not contain the biochemical reactions needed to identify specific *Yersinia* spp. Traditional macroscale biochemical testing may be required to distinguish *Y. enterocolitica* and *Y. pseudotuberculosis* from nonpathogenic *Yersinia* spp.[80,132] On solid culture media, colonies of the pathogenic species typically are small, smooth, opaque colonies. The colonies of nonpathogenic species are larger and more translucent.[109] The emerging bacterial identification method, matrix-assisted laser desorption ionization–time of flight (MALDI-TOF) mass spectrometry, appears reliable for distinguishing *Yersinia* isolates at the species level.[201]

Genomes and Typing of *Yersinia* Strains

Biotyping and serotyping have been the predominant methods used to characterize strains of *Y. enterocolitica*. At least 54 to 60 serotypes of *Y. enterocolitica* exist on the basis of variability of somatic O antigens, but only 11 typically are associated with human disease.[23,25,60,73,213] Six biotypes of *Y. enterocolitica,* designated 1A, 1B, and 2 to 5, have been defined on the basis of phenotypic differences in 12 biochemical reactions.[25,35,212]

Biotypes 1A, 2, 3, 4, and 5, now designated as *Y. enterocolitica* subsp. *palearctica*, are considered generally low pathogenic.[191] Biotype 1B, now designated as *Y. enterocolitica* subsp. *enterocolitica,* is considered highly pathogenic. Further subspecies distinctions may be forthcoming.[192] The genomes of biotypes 1A, 1B, and 2 to 5 are about 4.9, 4.6, and 4.5 Mb, respectively.[177] Genomic size differences are primarily related to number and distribution of insertion sequences.

Only a few serotype:biotype combinations are regarded as human pathogens: O:8, O:4, O:13a,13b, O:18, O:20, and O:21 (biotype 1B); O:9 and O:5,27 (biotype 2); O:1,2,3 and O:5,27 (biotype 3); O:3 (biotype 4); and O:2,3 (biotype 5).[218] These pathogenic strains, which carry *Yersinia* virulence plasmids (pYV), generally have negative test results for pyrazinamidase activity, esculin hydrolysis, and salicin fermentation. Nonpathogenic strains, generally of biotype 1A, have positive test results for each of them.[44,51,107] Data suggest that some biotype 1A strains that lack pYV and other *Yersinia* virulence factors also may cause gastroenteritis.[72,191,193]

Strains of *Y. enterocolitica* can be typed genetically by multilocus sequence typing (MLST),[192] repetitive element-based (interrepeat) polymerase chain reaction (PCR), pulsed-field gel electrophoresis,[153] and ribotyping.[133] An MLST schemed derived from whole-genome sequence data has recently been described[79] and likely will become a standard for epidemiologic investigations.

The complete genomes of the Old World biotype 3/O:9 strain 105.5R(r), prototypical of isolates common in Europe and Japan, and New World biotype 1B/O:8 strain 8081, prototypical of isolates in China, have been compared. The type III secretion systems differ, and strain 8081 has lost ancestral clusters of genes that contribute to enteric survival and pathogenesis.[223] Other genomic studies have shown that low pathogenic *Y. enterocolitica* subsp. *palearctica* biotype 4/O:3, which causes sporadic human disease and commonly colonizes pigs worldwide, also possess a type III secretion system and other alternative virulence determinants in contrast to the high pathogenic *Y. enterocolitica* subsp. *enterocolitica* (biotype 2) strains associated with outbreaks of human disease in Northern Europe.[16]

At least 11 antigenic groups of *Y. pseudotuberculosis* exist on the basis of variation of somatic O antigens. They have been labeled 1a, 1b, 2a, 2b, 2c, 3, 4a, 4b, 5a, 5b, and 6.[76,99,140] Type 2 is related antigenically to *Salmonella* group B, and type 4 is related to *Salmonella* groups D and H.[71] Two clusters of *Y. pseudotuberculosis* have been described using MLST. Strains of one cluster are distributed worldwide and usually harbor pYV. The second cluster lacks pYV and is currently restricted to the Far East.[43]

EPIDEMIOLOGY

Although most of the early reports of yersiniosis caused by *Y. pseudotuberculosis* and *Y. enterocolitica* came from northern Europe, these microbes have been identified with increasing frequency in all parts of the world.[12] *Y. enterocolitica* infections are more common in the United States than *Y. pseudotuberculosis.* Between 1996 and 2007, 1355 cases of foodborne *Y. enterocolitica* infections were identified by FoodNet in contrast to only 18 cases of foodborne *Y. pseudotuberculosis.*[135] The median ages of infected persons were 6 years (0 to 94 years) and 47 years (16 to 86 years), respectively.

During 1996 to 2009, FoodNet data show that the rate of foodborne disease caused by *Y. enterocolitica* in the United States was stable at 0.5 per 100,000 population.[161] Rates have been highest in blacks, but declined from 3.9 to 0.4 per 100,000 during this time period. The rate in black children younger than 5 years declined from 41.5 to 3.9 per 100,000. The overall rate among blacks was lower than whites in 2013. Rates are highest in children younger than 10 years and adults 70 years and older. In 2013, the rates of *Y. enterocolitica* infection in children younger than 5 years and 5 to 9 years were 1.35 and 0.6 per 100,000 population. Cases were reported year-round with highest frequency in April followed by January and December.[36]

Yersinia enterocolitica

Y. enterocolitica is distributed worldwide but is isolated most frequently in cooler climates.[149] Whether such geographic differences reflect differences in reservoirs or culinary practices that may enhance the risk for acquisition of this organism or instead represent differences in surveillance for the disease and use of more sensitive culturing techniques in these areas is unclear.[50] Increased frequency of infections during fall and winter has been reported from Europe[189] and the United States,[1] but no seasonality is evident among outbreaks of disease in which more than three cases of *Y. enterocolitica* disease have been identified.[50]

Geographic differences in serotype distribution and frequency also exist. Sporadic infections caused by biotype 4/serotype O:3 and biotype 3/serotype O:9 strains are common in Europe,[9,92] but outbreaks rarely have occurred.[50] In North America, multiple serotypes have been responsible for sporadic disease,[18,24,35,69,189,195] but more recently serotype O:3 has become predominant.[35,54,128] Outbreaks have been caused by serotype O:8 in the United States and by serotypes O:5 in Canada.[50] Disease caused by serotype O:8 has been reported in Europe.[92] Biotype 2/serotype O:9 is predominant in China.[223]

The true incidence and prevalence of *Y. enterocolitica* infection are unknown.[50] The reported proportional frequency of isolation of *Y. enterocolitica* from stool cultures from patients with diarrhea has ranged

TABLE 113.1 Percentage of Stool Cultures Yielding *Yersinia enterocolitica*

Location	Years	Population	Total Cultures	Percentage *Y. enterocolitica*
Canada[142]	1977–78	Symptomatic children	6364	2.8
The Netherlands[93]	1982–84	Enteritis patients <40 y	827	2.9
Italy[147]	1981–85	Children with diarrhea	2500	1.4[a]
New Zealand[60]	1988–93	Patients with gastroenteritis	231,128	0.6
Detroit, MI[52]	May–November 1977	Children with diarrhea	1262	0
New York state[189]	1976–80	Survey of cultures from a state laboratory, six hospitals, and several daycare centers	2487	0.9[b]
US[c] (seven cities)[128]	November 1989–January 1990	All stool cultures submitted to seven hospitals	4841	0.8
St. Louis, MO[113]	1998–2001	Children presenting to an emergency department with diarrhea	1626	0.1

[a]Yearly percentages during the 5 years ranged from 0% to 4.4%.
[b]This increased to 4% of 3035 isolates when cultures from an outbreak and other screenings were included.
[c]Includes Detroit, MI.

from 0% to 3.2% in series from Europe, the United States, and New Zealand (Table 113.1).[52,60,92,128,142,147,189] Symptomatic infection occurs more commonly in children. Most series show a slight male predominance of approximately 1.3 : 1.[54,60,142,212] Animals and water sources are the primary environmental reservoirs for *Y. enterocolitica,* but the biotypes and serotypes of the strains found in them usually differ from those causing human disease.[35,50,189] Blood transfusions also may be a source of *Y. enterocolitica* infection.[37]

Animal Reservoirs

Y. enterocolitica strains have been isolated from a wide variety of mammals (dogs, pigs, sheep, rabbits, guinea pigs, cows, horses, chinchillas, and monkeys), frogs, fish, flies, fleas, snails, crabs, and oysters. Birds do not seem to be a major reservoir for *Y. enterocolitica,* although avian isolates have been reported.[50,95,136] The proportion of enteric illness attributable to animal contact in the United States in recent years is 1%.[78]

Pigs seem to be an important reservoir for the human pathogenic serotypes O:3 and O:9 in Europe and Japan and serotype O:3 in North America and South Africa.[50,128,171] The biochemical and phage typing profiles of isolates from pigs are similar to those of strains commonly responsible for human infections.[216] *Y. enterocolitica* has been isolated from the tongue, tonsils, and cecal contents of swine and from pork, ham, and butcher shop cutting boards.[50,70] Pig farmers in Finland were 3 times and 2.4 times as likely to have seropositivity to serotypes O:3 and O:9, respectively, than were berry farmers.[188]

Wild rodents captured in areas of Japan where human infections caused by *Y. enterocolitica* serotype O:8 had occurred were shown to harbor isolates of the same serotype.[46] Two distinct serotype O:8 strains, defined by restriction enzyme analysis of the virulence plasmids, were isolated from humans and rodents. This finding suggests that rodents are a potential source of sporadic human infection in Japan.

Apparent transmission to humans from dogs and cats also has been reported. A fecal–oral or oral–oral route has been postulated but not confirmed. Little evidence supports airborne or insect vector–borne transmission.[50]

Foods and Water

In countries with high numbers of cases of yersiniosis, ingestion of raw pork has been common. Infection with serotypes O:3 and O:9 was highly associated with ingestion of raw pork during the 2 weeks preceding the illness in a case-control study.[208] In Belgium, laboratory surveillance that began in 1967 showed yearly increases in cases through 1986. After a media campaign was launched to dissuade people from eating raw or undercooked pork or pork products and to educate consumers regarding good hygiene practices during food preparation, the number of isolations of *Y. enterocolitica* decreased from a high of 1469 in 1986 to 707 in 1996.[218] Eating raw minced pork or other foods prepared from raw pork products remains an ongoing risk factor for *Y. enterocolitica* infection for young children.[22,97,182] Preparation of chitterlings in the household was a risk factor for *Y. enterocolitica* infection in outbreaks among children in Michigan[1] and Illinois.[38]

Ingestion of contaminated water has led to sporadic cases and outbreaks.[50,57] Bean sprouts immersed in contaminated water and ingestion of tofu (bean curd) packed in untreated spring water led to outbreaks in Washington state in 1981 and 1982.[206] However serotypes commonly found in water samples rarely are isolated from humans with symptomatic disease.[35]

Contaminated milk has been implicated as the source of several large outbreaks of *Y. enterocolitica* infection.[5,19,50,213] Whipped cream and ice cream may harbor the organism. Contamination of milk products after pasteurization has been documented. *Y. enterocolitica* has been found in raw milk samples from cows and goats. Samples of beef, lamb, poultry, oysters, and a variety of vegetables also have been found to be contaminated with *Y. enterocolitica.*[32,50,70]

Serotypes O:3, O:4,33, O:5,27, O:7,8, O:8, O:10, O:13, and O:16 cause most human disease in North America but rarely are isolated in surveillance of water or food samples. Serotype O:8 strains have been cultured from cattle, milk, and water samples[158]; serotype O:4,33 strains have been isolated from pigs and cattle; and serotype O:4,32 strains have been found in cheese, ham, sausage, raw beef, and one pancake specimen.[35,189,213]

Outbreaks of *Y. enterocolitica* disease have involved communities, families (with interfamily spread), hospitals, and schools.[14,18,37,75,142,213,231] The sources of the organism have been various foods and animals, especially dogs, as noted earlier. Yersiniosis also resembles disease caused by *Salmonella* and *Shigella* organisms in many respects, including the environmental sources of the organisms, the clinical syndromes, and the occurrence of asymptomatic infection.

Incubation, Carriage, and Transmission in Humans

The incubation period of *Y. enterocolitica* enterocolitis ranges from 1 to 14 days, with a median of approximately 4 days.[35,50,128] The minimal infective dose of *Y. enterocolitica* is unknown. Ingestion of 3.5×10^9 organisms by a volunteer resulted in diarrhea in less than 1 day, but such large inocula are unlikely to be encountered clinically. The duration of excretion of the organism after development of infection in children ranges from 14 to 97 days (mean, 42 days).[142] The impact, if any, of antibiotic treatment on the duration of carriage is unknown.

Transmission to household members occurs uncommonly, even among young children, who are at higher risk for development of symptomatic disease.[19,142,206] Six percent of household contacts developed disease in one outbreak,[206] but several large outbreaks with no secondary household cases have been reported.[50]

Nosocomial transmissions have been documented. A young child who was hospitalized in Finland with acute gastroenteritis was the source case of infection in a housekeeping worker and four nurses who cared for her.[211] Person-to-person contact was considered the likely mode of transmission in a hospital outbreak that involved nine patients in Canada.[174]

Yersinia Enterocolitica *and Blood Transfusion–Related Sepsis*

In this era of screening for viral infections in blood donations, bacterial sepsis has become the most frequent infectious complication of blood transfusions in developed countries. Sporadic cases of *Y. enterocolitica* sepsis related to contamination of transfusions of red blood cells (RBCs) have been recognized since 1987 and have occurred in the United States, Europe, and Australia.[37,74] *Y. enterocolitica* is the most common cause of transfusion-related sepsis.[105] Rapid-onset septic shock, fever, chills, and atypical signs such as explosive diarrhea are common. Case fatality is about 50%.[45,74]

In many cases of transfusion-related sepsis, the contaminated RBC units had been stored for 25 days or more.[87] After experimental inoculation of small numbers of *Y. enterocolitica* into packed cells kept at 4°C (39.2°F), the organisms continue to replicate, reaching concentrations of 100 colony-forming units (CFU)/mL in 7 days and 10^6 CFU/mL in 21 days. This lag of 1 to 3 weeks in rapid growth is consistent with the increasing iron stores released from hemolyzing RBCs during storage. *Y. enterocolitica* multiplication is supported by glucose and adenine, which are part of RBC anticoagulant and additive solutions. Although growth is calcium-dependent during human infection at body temperatures, *Y. enterocolitica* can replicate in calcium-free media (e.g., RBCs anticoagulated via citrate chelation) at temperatures less than 30°C (86°F).[74] High levels of endotoxin can result from bacterial replication in RBC products and have been documented in samples from RBC units that led to transfusion-related sepsis.[45] Timely administration of effective antimicrobial agents appears to improve outcomes, suggesting a significant contribution from viable microbes.[74]

Prevention of Disease

During outbreaks, efforts should be made to identify environmental sources and vehicles of transmission.[50] A single environmental source can harbor multiple serotypes of *Y. enterocolitica*, such that resulting outbreaks may be polyclonal.[206] Enteric precautions should be used for hospitalized patients with diarrhea caused by *Y. enterocolitica* (as with other causes of gastroenteritis).[50] At the population level, decreased consumption of raw or undercooked pork products potentially can reduce the incidence of infection.[208,218]

Yersinia pseudotuberculosis

Y. pseudotuberculosis may infect individuals of all ages, but at least 75% of patients with clinically apparent disease are children younger than 15 years.[99,185] Infection in young infants has been reported.[99,225] Of 130 cases diagnosed in Great Britain from 1959 to 1970, boys were involved three times more frequently than girls.[136] Infections occur more commonly during the cold months of the year.[99,184] The seasonal winter peak of human infection produced by *Y. pseudotuberculosis* is similar to that seen in wild and domesticated animals.[114,115,185]

The attack rates for children living in rural and urban areas seem to be the same. *Y. pseudotuberculosis* occasionally has been recovered from healthy individuals. Exposure to the organism seems to be uncommon; antibody to *Y. pseudotuberculosis* was detected in only one of 2000 sera samples from individuals with no history of yersiniosis.[63,185]

Y. pseudotuberculosis is distributed worldwide in a large variety of animals and birds, but infection seldom occurs.[67] Guinea pigs, rodents, and rabbits are infected most often[136] and may experience a plaguelike illness.[67,95] Lesions in guinea pigs may be confused easily with lesions caused by *Y. pestis*. Rats and other rodents also may have plaguelike disease caused by *Y. pseudotuberculosis*. The microbe can be cultured from tongue, tonsils, intestines, and large organs of infected animals.[157]

Infection has been reported in various domestic animals (cattle, sheep, goats, cats, dogs, hamsters), commercially raised fur bearers (chinchillas, mink, coypu), and other wild or captive animals (rabbits, raccoons, foxes, deer, beavers, monkeys, puma, kangaroos). *Y. pseudotuberculosis* has been found in more than 50 species of birds,[82,108,136] and epizootics have occurred among turkeys, ducks, pigeons, and doves and in aviaries of canaries and finches. Strains obtained from animals and birds in the United States are predominantly of serotypes 1a, 1b, and 3.[136,185]

The incubation period for human disease ranges from 41 hours to 20 days.[99] In a food-associated outbreak in Finland, the median incubation period was 8 days (Fig. 113.1).[102] The organism can survive in fresh tap water for 46 days at room temperature and for 8 months at 4°C (39.2°F). It can survive at 4°C in meat for 145 days and in milk and bread for 2 to 3 weeks.[136]

A family outbreak of mesenteric adenitis caused by *Y. pseudotuberculosis* that involved four siblings aged 7 to 14 years has been reported.[173] A pet dog was shown to have increasing antibody titers at the time the children were ill.

Periodic outbreaks have been reported in Japan, northern Europe, and areas of the former Soviet Union. Sandwiches prepared by a single bakery were the primary risk factor for 67 cases that occurred in a 3-week period in Japan.[99] Drinking unchlorinated well water or mountain stream water has been the source of other outbreaks. Children were much more likely to have clinical disease than adults. More recent outbreaks in Finland have been associated with contaminated lettuce and grated carrots.[102]

PATHOLOGY

The diseases produced by *Y. enterocolitica* and *Y. pseudotuberculosis* are similar and share the histopathologic theme of involvement of the lymphoid tissues of the intestinal mucosa and mesentery.

Yersinia enterocolitica

Y. enterocolitica infection predominantly affects the gastrointestinal tract. The most severe clinical symptoms correlate with an acute terminal ileitis. The mucosal surface of the ileum and other involved sites may be inflamed diffusely. Ulcerations may occur throughout the gastrointestinal tract and may be small and superficial or extend to the muscularis propria. Mucosal and submucosal hyperplasia of Peyer's patches occurs with scattered microabscess formation.

Ulcers occur primarily over the sites of lymphoid tissue within the mucosa, which accounts for their more longitudinal appearance in the small intestine and an oval or punctate appearance in the stomach and colon. Ulcerations are characterized by necrosis of the epithelial layer. In the colon, the necrosis also may extend through the superficial third of the crypts. Large colonic ulcerations covered by pseudomembranes or mucoid debris are seen occasionally. Ulcerations may progress to perforation, with subsequent development of peritonitis or gastrointestinal hemorrhage in severe cases.[29,68,216,217]

The inflammatory response in the mucosa consists mainly of neutrophils and mononuclear cells. Lymphocytes and plasma cells also may be seen. Giant cells are not seen, although a granulomatous appearance can be imparted by the presence of plump epithelioid histiocytes. Numerous colonies of gram-negative bacteria often can be seen beneath the mucosal ulcerations and within the microabscesses that occur in the lymphoid tissues.[68,216,217]

The appendix usually appears normal on gross inspection, but small focal ulcerations frequently are present.[7] Large areas of necrosis are found occasionally, and acute, suppurative appendicitis has been reported.[29,104,142] Periappendicular inflammation may result from a true appendicitis or an adjacent terminal ileitis.[216]

Mesenteric adenitis, the hallmark of infection caused by *Y. pseudotuberculosis*, also is a common feature of enterocolitis caused by *Y. enterocolitica*. The lymph nodes usually show numerous large pyroninophilic cells and mitotic figures in the cortical area and marginal sinuses. Small collections of leukocytes in the germinal centers are seen in some cases and suggest formation of microabscesses. In severe cases, extensive areas of necrosis circumscribed by a neutrophilic infiltrate may be seen. The sinusoids can become filled with neutrophils and mononuclear cells. The germinal centers often appear reactive.

The histopathologic appearance of the mesenteric adenitis of infection caused by *Y. enterocolitica* can resemble the adenitides caused by cat-scratch disease *(Bartonella henselae)*, toxoplasmosis, infectious mononucleosis, and *Y. pseudotuberculosis*.[7,216,228] The necrotizing epithelioid granulomata that may be present in mesenteric adenitis caused by *Y.*

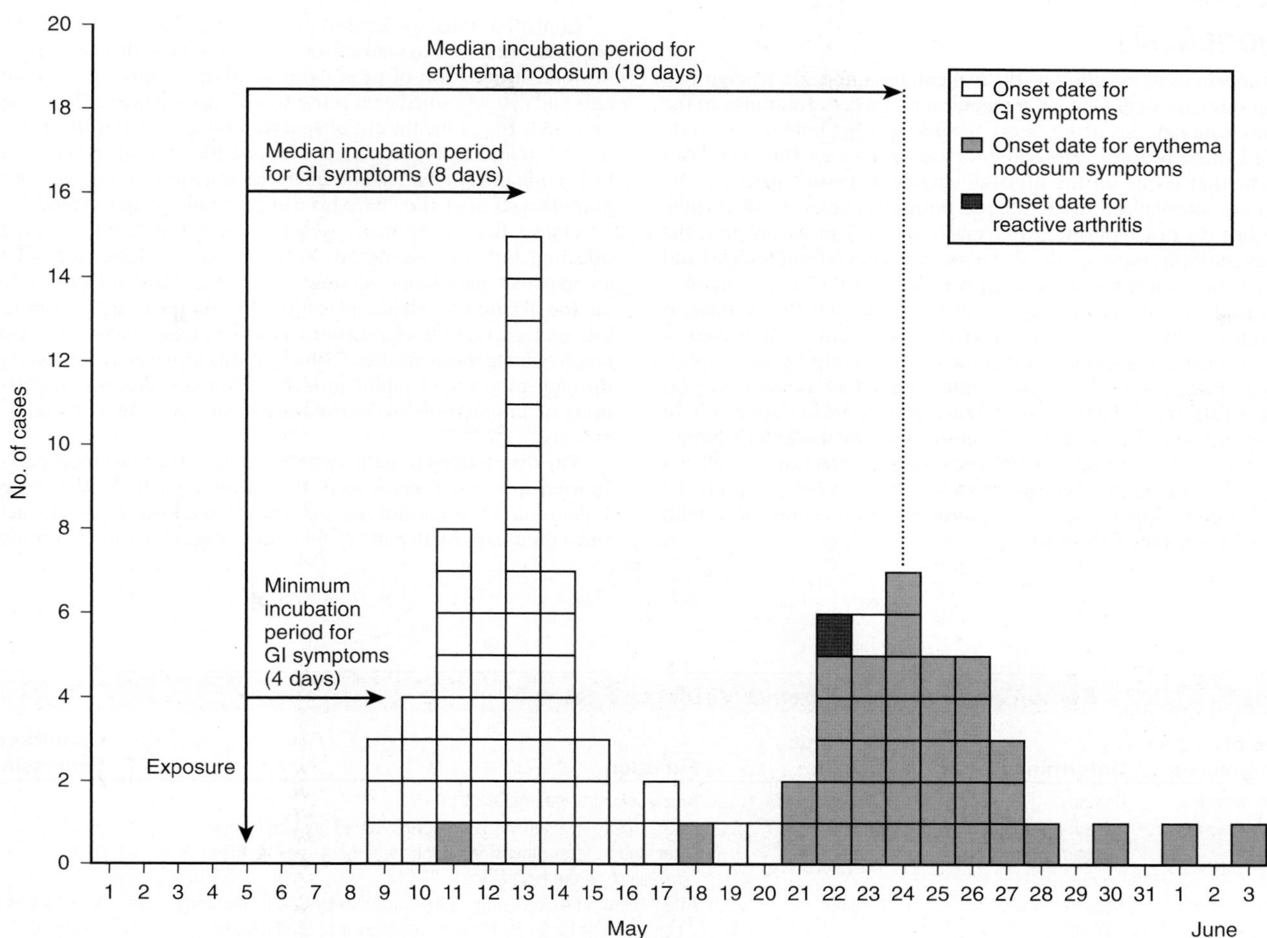

FIG. 113.1 Distribution of incubation periods for *Yersinia pseudotuberculosis* infection to onset of gastrointestinal (GI) symptoms and erythema nodosum after point source exposure to contaminated carrots. Of 72 case patients with a known date of onset, 51 had GI symptoms and 38 had erythema nodosum only; 28 had GI symptoms and erythema nodosum and appear twice in the graph. (From Jalava K, Hakkinen M, Valkonen M, et al. An outbreak of gastrointestinal illness and erythema nodosum from grated carrots contaminated with *Yersinia pseudotuberculosis*. *J Infect Dis.* 2006;194:1209–16.)

pseudotuberculosis have not been described in infection caused by *Y. enterocolitica*. A more recent study of six cases suggests that biotype 1B strains may be more likely to cause suppurative inflammation, whereas biotype 2 through 5 strains may be more likely to cause granulomatous infection.[125]

Yersinia pseudotuberculosis

Numerous reports collectively have described the pathology of infection caused by *Y. pseudotuberculosis*.[53,61,94,115,137,143,144,148,173,224] Grossly enlarged, soft, and inflamed mesenteric lymph nodes are the predominant finding on laparotomy. They frequently are located at the ileocecal angle. Punctate hemorrhages and small, yellow microabscesses may be present on the surfaces of the nodes at the height of infection. The appendix usually appears normal, but the terminal ileum and cecum occasionally appear inflamed. A necrotic purulent mass sometimes is seen in the mesentery.

Histopathologic findings in the mesenteric lymph nodes include enlarged follicles and small abscesses; hyperplasia of reticulum cells; necrosis of the nodes with infiltrates of neutrophilic leukocytes and plasma cells; and, in some instances, punctate hemorrhages. Scattered clusters of neutrophils may be seen within the sinusoids and germinal centers without formation of abscess or necrosis. Atypical mononuclear cells, some of which may be mitotic, may be present in the sinusoids. When necrosis is absent, large numbers of eosinophilic leukocytes occasionally are seen surrounding reticulogranulocytic infiltrates in the nodes. Giant cells can occur and may cause the histologic picture to be confused with that of tuberculosis.

The mesenteric adenitis produced by *Y. pseudotuberculosis* seems to progress through histopathologic stages akin to those of other pyogenic infections that can lead to formation of abscesses.[53,76] Reticulogranulocytic infiltration is followed by formation of an abscess, with subsequent organization and clearing of the abscess. The inflammatory process of *Y. pseudotuberculosis* seems to remain confined to the lymph nodes without rupture through the nodal capsule.

Focal mucosal ulcerations may be seen in the ileum, and are more likely to be found at the site of Peyer's patches. Aggregates of neutrophilic leukocytes similar to those in mesenteric nodes may be seen in germinal centers within mucosal lymphoid tissue. Fibrinoid material may be a prominent feature at these sites. Small areas of necrosis surrounded by reticulum cells and leukocytes also may be present in the submucosal follicles.[61,115,117,224] Ulcerated lymphoid follicles in the intestinal wall are connected to the regional lymph nodes by a lymphangitis. This anatomic situation is analogous to the primary complex of tuberculosis.

Despite a clinical picture of acute appendicitis as the presenting feature of infection by *Y. pseudotuberculosis*, the appendix typically is grossly and microscopically normal. Inflammatory changes, when present, usually are in the form of a periappendicitis. Phlegmonous appendicitis can result from infection caused by *Y. pseudotuberculosis* but is rare.[53,91]

PATHOGENESIS

The pathogenesis of infection by the two enteropathogenic *Yersinia* spp. has been studied extensively. After ingestion and successful transit to the small intestine have occurred, these *Yersinia* spp. are able to penetrate into the lamina propria primarily by passing through the cytoplasm of M cells that reside on the mucosal surface of Peyer's patches. The bacteria are internalized in membrane-bound vacuoles in which they survive but do not replicate. After reaching the lamina propria, the microbes multiply as extracellular microcolonies in lymph follicles and Peyer's patches, where they may reach densities of 10^9 CFU/g of tissue.[56]

Neutrophils and macrophages infiltrate these sites in response to the infection, ultimately creating microabscesses, but *Y. enterocolitica* is able to resist phagocytosis and intracellular killing by neutrophils and macrophages. *Yersinia* spp. also inhibit production of tumor necrosis factor-α (TNF-α) and interferon-γ (IFN-γ) and induce apoptosis in host macrophages. The microbes disseminate to the mesenteric lymph nodes, apparently through lymphatic vessels. Infection usually is contained at this point, although abscesses often develop within the nodes. Systemic spread occurs occasionally, more commonly with infection by serotype O:8 strains.

Control of infection caused by *Y. enterocolitica* is the result of T-cell responses that lead to restriction of bacterial growth in infected organs through stimulation of production of *Yersinia*-specific antibody by B cells and cytokine-mediated activation of macrophages. These responses ultimately overcome the antiphagocyte strategies of *Yersinia*. Production of TNF-α and IFN-γ seems to be an essential part of the host response to *Yersinia* infections. *Yersinia* microbes generally do not survive within granulocytes after they have been successfully phagocytosed.[46,48,49,162]

Only a few of the many serotypes of *Yersinia* spp. are capable of infecting humans. Numerous virulence factors have been identified among these "pathogenic" strains (Table 113.2). Most of them are encoded on the *Yersinia* virulence plasmid pYV. At least eight chromosomal loci that encode novel *Yersinia* virulence factors have been found by tagged mutagenesis studies.[66] Much of this knowledge has been gained through mouse and rabbit models of human infection and observations of interactions of *Yersinia* organisms with in vitro cell culture models.[28,46,90,138,169]

The distinctions in pathogenesis between the two enteropathogenic *Yersinia* spp. and *Y. pestis* seem to be caused partly by the presence in *Y. pestis* of (1) two additional plasmids that encode a plasmin activator and a mouse exotoxin and (2) a hemin storage locus on its chromosome.

TABLE 113.2 Known and Putative *Yersinia* Virulence Factors[a]

Stage of Pathogenesis	Determinant	Genomic Origin[b]	Function	Conditions of Expression
Gastric transit	Urease	Chromosome	Aids survival of gastric acidity	
Mucosal invasion	Invasin (inv)	Chromosome	Attachment, invasion via β_1 integrins; broad host/cell range	28°C
	Attachment invasion locus (AiL)	Chromosome	Attachment, lesser invasion factor; more host-specific than invasion; serum resistance	37°C
	Yersinia adhesin A (YadA)	Plasmid	Attachment, invasion; reduces opsonization by C3b by binding complement factor H; ? role in resistance to antibacterial polypeptides (e.g., bactericidal permeability-increasing protein)	37°C and *any* calcium concentration
Disruption of phagocyte function	Effector proteins (act on host cells)	Plasmid		37°C and low calcium concentration
	YopH		Tyrosine phosphorylase that prevents phagocytosis by macrophages by preventing assembly of focal adhesion structures of phagocytes	
	YopE		Phagocytosis resistance via induction of host cell actin filament rearrangements	
	YopJ/P		Cysteine protease/acetyltransferase that inhibits mitogen-activated protein kinase and nuclear factor κB signaling via interruption of posttranslational covalent additions of ubiquitin-like molecules to these enzymes; this prevents production of cytokines (tumor necrosis factor-α), inhibits the host immune response, and triggers apoptosis of macrophages.	
			Inhibits kinase phosphorylation via an acetyltransferase function	
	YpkA/YopO		Serine kinase, causes rounding up of cells, specific target unknown	
	YopT		Disruption of actin filaments	
	YopM		Role unclear	
			Inhibits thrombin-induced platelet activation in vitro but is delivered intracellularly during infection	
			Leads to depletion of natural killer cells and alters expression of IL-15 and IL-15 receptors	
	Membrane attachment, pore insertion into host cell	Plasmid		37°C and low calcium concentration
	YopB and YopD		Pore formation in host cell membrane to allow translocation of effector proteins into the host cell	
			Suppression of IL-8 secretion by epithelial cells	
	YopQ (YopK)		Controls translocation via modulating the size of the YopB, YopD pore in the host cell membrane	
	YopN		Involved in control of translocation, perhaps stabilizing contact between the bacterium and host cell membranes	

TABLE 113.2 Known and Putative *Yersinia* Virulence Factors—cont'd

Stage of Pathogenesis	Determinant	Genomic Origin[b]	Function	Conditions of Expression
	LcrV[e]		Assists extrusion of YopB and YopD to the host cell membrane Homologue of the *Y pestis* V antigen Antibodies against V antigen seem to be protective at the serotype level	
	Yop secretion apparatus (Ysc) (28 proteins in total; part of microbe)	Plasmid		37°C and low calcium concentration
	YscD, YscR, YscU, and LcrD/YscV		Form a complex that spans the inner bacterial membrane (gated pore/channel)	
	YscC secretin		Forms a pore in the outer bacterial membrane that may connect with the inner membrane pore	
	YscN		ATPase that energizes Yop transfer across the membranes	
	LcrQ (in *Y. pseudotuberculosis*), YscM1 and YscM2 (in *Y. enterocolitica*)		Negative *yop* gene regulators that, when secreted, decrease in concentration in the bacterium, allowing *yop* expression	
	Cytosolic chaperones (Syc) (6 proteins in total; within microbe)	Plasmid	Secretion/translocation pilots or antidegradation roles for effector proteins	37°C and low calcium concentration
Colonization of Peyer's patches and lymph nodes	*Yersinia* phospholipase A	Plasmid	Serum resistance, inhibition of phagocytosis	37°C and low calcium concentration
Iron metabolism	Yersiniabactin	Chromosome (high pathogenicity island)	Siderophore	37°C, iron starvation
Diarrhea	*Yersinia* heat-stable enterotoxin (Yst)	Chromosome	Fluid secretion in intestine Precise role in pathogenesis of disease in humans is unclear, but found in clinical isolates from children with diarrhea	28°C (in vitro)
Systemic invasion	O antigen	Chromosome	Component of lipopolysaccharide Complement/serum resistance	

IL, Interleukin; *Lcr,* low calcium response; *Yop, Yersinia* outer membrane protein (although not all such designated proteins reside in the outer membrane).
[a]The complete pathogenesis/virulence roles of several gene products encoded on the *Yersinia* virulence plasmid pVY and chromosomal sites have yet to be determined.
[b]Plasmid refers to the *Yersinia* virulence plasmid pYV.
Data from references 25, 47, 48, 71, 75, 111, 121, 129, 151, 152, 162, 180, 187, 193, 194, 232, 233.

These additional factors may enable *Y. pestis* to survive in and transmit between fleas and rodents. Such transmission does not occur with the enteropathogenic *Yersinia* spp.[180]

Bacterial Determinants of Mucosal Invasion

Two outer-membrane proteins encoded by chromosomal genes permit entry into various mammalian cell types in vitro and are likely to be responsible for the ability of *Yersinia* to invade into and through the intestinal mucosal epithelium. They have been named *invasin* and the *attachment invasin locus protein* (Ail). All isolates of *Y. enterocolitica* that are virulent in humans contain DNA sequences that encode for invasin and Ail. Nonpathogenic strains do not contain the genetic code for Ail, but most contain invasin genes that cannot be expressed because of chromosomal rearrangements. These proteins apparently are unique to the genus *Yersinia*.[100,146,166]

Invasin attaches to receptors in the β_1 integrin family and induces an actin-mediated endocytosis of the microbe. It binds to β_1-chain integrin receptors with approximately 100-fold higher affinity than do natural ligands, such as fibronectin. Such high-affinity binding triggers endocytosis-like internalization that involves clathrin.[49] Invasin is expressed maximally at ambient temperatures when the organism is in stationary phase. *Y. enterocolitica* microbes living in the environment probably exist in a stationary phase–like state and may be primed maximally for invasion of the host after ingestion. Invasin expression also can remain elevated at 37°C (98.6°F) when the pH is 5.5, and such conditions are encountered during passage through the intestinal tract. Ail is expressed maximally at 37°C, functions as an adhesin and an invasion factor, and plays a role in the resistance of *Y. enterocolitica* to the bactericidal activity of human serum.[100,101,166]

High levels of β_1-chain integrin receptors are found on the luminal surface of M cells, which are antigen-sampling epithelial cells found in highest numbers overlying Peyer's patches in the intestinal tract.[83] Flagellum-dependent motility seems to be required for invasin-mediated invasion of cells by *Y. enterocolitica*.[230]

The following determinants are primarily relevant to *Y. enterocolitica*, although *Y. pseudotuberculosis* shares many of these features.

Yersinia Adhesin A

Yersinia adhesin A (YadA) is a multifunctional virulence factor of *Y. enterocolitica*. YadA is approximately 50 kDa and probably forms tetrameric fibrillae on the microbial surface. Its gene resides on the pYV plasmid and is transcribed at 37°C independently of the calcium concentration. YadA binds to extracellular matrix proteins, such as collagen, and mediates adhesion to cells. It may play a role in translocation of Yop effector proteins into eukaryotic phagocytic cells. YadA also inhibits the terminal complement attack complex, reduces opsonization by C3b through binding of complement factor H, and contributes to the ability of *Y. enterocolitica* to resist killing by antimicrobial polypeptides of human granulocytes. YadA knockout mutants are far less virulent in mice than is the parent wild-type strain.[48,89,221]

Virulence Plasmid and Type III Secretion System

Pathogenic strains of *Y. enterocolitica* harbor a plasmid that consists of approximately 70 kb (denoted pYV) and encodes the low-calcium response system of *Yersinia* spp., which involves a complex response to environmental conditions of 37°C and calcium concentrations of less than 2.5 mM, both of which describe the intracellular compartment of mammalian cells.[48,194] Plasmid-encoded factors are required for survival and extracellular multiplication after reaching Peyer's patches. Plasmid-cured derivatives are ingested rapidly and killed by neutrophils in Peyer's patches, whereas wild-type strains are able to proliferate and spread through the lamina propria to adjacent villi. Plasmid-encoded factors are not required for *Y. enterocolitica* to penetrate the intestinal mucosa.[89]

In DNA cross-hybridization studies, the pYVs of *Y. enterocolitica* serogroups O:9, O:3, and O:5 show 90% nucleotide identity with one another, 75% identity with the pYV of serogroup O:8, and 55% identity with the pYV of *Y. pestis* and *Y. pseudotuberculosis*. Despite the nucleotide divergence among the pYVs of the three *Yersinia* spp., the overall structures and most of the genes are highly similar among them. The *Yersinia* low calcium response plasmids are nonconjugative.[48,194]

The *Y. enterocolitica* pYV contains approximately 70 genes, of which around 53 have protein products with known or putative functions (many of these are listed among the virulence factors in Table 113.2). pYV encodes *Yersinia* adhesin A and a system of six effector proteins that are delivered into host cells (primarily phagocytic granulocytes) through a complex mechanism of regulatory proteins, secretion chaperones, and proteins that act as secretion channels or pores in the bacterial and host cell membranes. This system, called a type III secretion system, denotes secretion of the bacterial proteins only in response to contact with a mammalian cell. The effector proteins and several others involving pore formation are designated Yops (*Yersinia* outer-membrane proteins), although most of them do not reside in the outer membrane. Similar type III secretion systems are found in other *Enterobacteriaceae*.[48,194]

The secretion system is composed partially of syringe-like organelles—called *Ysc injectisomes*—that develop when *Yersinia* organisms are incubated at mammalian body temperatures. These injectisomes are protein pumps that span the peptidoglycan layer and the two bacterial cell membranes, topped by a needle-like structure protruding outside the bacterium. Twenty-seven proteins are involved in the structure; 10 of them are located internally and form a structure similar to the basal body of a flagellum, which also includes an ATPase that functions as a proton pump. A homomultimeric ring-shaped structure extends through the outer membrane, with a central pore diameter of about 50 Å.[33]

As the injectisomes assemble, stocks of intracellular Yops are synthesized. Active transcription of *Yop* genes is limited to bacteria in close contact with eukaryotic cells. The secretion channel of the injectisome remains closed, with negative feedback mechanisms to prevent overproduction of Yops. On close contact with a phagocyte, the injectisome channels open, and secretion of effector Yops into the target cell begins.[33] This is accomplished through insertion of YopB and YopD into the host cell membrane, where these form a multimeric complex that serves as a pore for effector injection.[151]

After secretion into a phagocytic cell occurs, YopH, YopE, YopT, and YopO/YpkA disrupt its cytoskeletal dynamics, blocking phagocytosis (see Table 113.2). YopT is a cysteine protease that cleaves and inactivates Rho proteins, which are small membrane-associated GTPases that control the host cell actin cytoskeleton.[187] Other Yops inhibit production of TNF-α, interleukin-8 (IL-8), and other inflammatory chemokines and induce apoptosis of macrophages.[33]

A similar type III secretion system is present in *Y. pseudotuberculosis*, which is considered to be primarily an extracellular pathogen.[233] *Y. pseudotuberculosis* can survive within macrophages, and mouse studies suggest a small minority of invading microbes may reside intracellularly in multiple tissue sites. This system is able to transport Yops from phagosomes in macrophages into the cytosol and to inject Yops into mouse dendritic cells. YopJ inhibits dendritic cell–mediated T-cell responses via induction of apoptosis and reduction of surface molecule expression.[207]

Summary *of Yersinia* Pathogenesis

Pathogenic strains of *Y. enterocolitica* require calcium concentrations equivalent to those of serum and extracellular fluids in humans for growth at body temperature. Plasmid proteins are synthesized maximally; however at 37°C and under conditions of low calcium concentrations, such as those found intracellularly. These regulatory effects of environmental calcium concentrations permit free growth of *Yersinia* organisms during extracellular life and production of factors that inhibit phagocytosis by macrophages and neutrophils when *Yersinia* organisms pass through the intracellular compartment during mucosal invasion or come into contact with these granulocytes.[46,48,89]

A model of how pathogenic *Yersinia* organisms living in cold (≤28°C [≤82.4°F]) environmental reservoirs are able to establish infection in the mammalian host can be described at the molecular level (see Table 113.2). *Yersinia* microbes living in the environment express invasin, which renders them ready to attach and invade the intestinal mucosal M cells after ingestion. Expression of invasin continues at body temperature during gastric passage to the intestines. Survival of gastric acidity is assisted by a urease-producing system.

During intracellular passage through M cells in the small intestine, *pYV* genes are likely to be activated (conditions of low calcium, 37°C). YadA can be produced at body temperature and may assist in mucosal invasion. Transcytosis from the intestinal lumen to the lamina propria seems to occur by a clathrin-mediated process that probably is a normal function of the host cell, after internalization is triggered. Ail also is synthesized after ingestion occurs and probably promotes attachment to migrating cells in the lamina propria that may facilitate extracellular spread of the microbes to regional lymph nodes and perhaps the liver and spleen.

To survive this journey, *Yersinia* organisms must evade phagocytosis by macrophages and neutrophils. YadA can inhibit complement opsonization, reducing the likelihood that phagocytosis will occur. When contact between the microbe and a host granulocyte occurs, the previously activated type III secretion system (described earlier) encoded by the pYV plasmid comes into play. A contiguous pore is inserted into the granulocyte cell membrane (involving YopB, YopD, YopQ, YopN, and LcrV). Effector proteins (YopE, YopH, YopJ/P, YopO/A, YopM, and YopT) then are translocated into the granulocyte cytoplasm, disrupting its abilities to ingest the bacterium and produce cytokines and triggering apoptotic cell death (see Table 113.2). Although this system of virulence factors is robust enough to facilitate short-lived infection that often causes mild to moderate clinical symptoms, the microbes that do not succumb to the innate immune response ultimately are contained and then eliminated by the adaptive host response.

Y. pseudotuberculosis, which does not express Ail or invasin, is able to penetrate the intestinal epithelial barrier through a cascade of steps initiated via binding to Toll-like receptor 2 on monocytes. This involves caspase 1 and IL-1β production that ultimately leads to myosin light chain kinase activation in intestinal epithelial cells that disrupts tight junctions between them.[106]

Iron Metabolism and Virulence

Iron is an essential growth factor for most bacteria, many of which release siderophores (high-affinity chelators) that bind ferric iron and then are taken up again through receptors by the microbe. *Y. enterocolitica* serotype O:8 and other biotype 1B strains synthesize a chromosomally encoded siderophore, designated *yersiniabactin,* which sits on the outer membrane of the bacterium. The presence of this siderophore decreases the concentration of environmental iron required for optimal growth and probably accounts for the increased virulence observed for serotype O:8 strains.[50,89] The gene encoding yersiniabactin and the genes required for its biosynthesis, transport, and regulation compose the core of what is termed a *high-pathogenicity island* because of the high lethality for mice that its presence confers.[172]

Serotypes O:8, O:4, O:13, O:18, O:20, and O:21 (all biotype 1B and historically considered American strains) are highly lethal to mice after intraperitoneal injection and are able to evoke a keratoconjunctivitis after inoculation into the conjunctival sac of guinea pigs (the positive Sereny test result). Oral infection in mice predominantly produces the features of mesenteric adenitis and systemic infection, rather than simple gastroenteritis, which is characteristic of human infection by American strains. The European serotypes, O:3, O:9, and O:5,27, yield a negative Sereny test result and cause mild diarrhea but not death in mice. The

TABLE 113.3 Clinical Features of *Yersinia enterocolitica* Infection in Children

	Sweden,[18] 1967–73	Finland,[139] 1974–78	Canada,[54] 1972	Canada,[142] 1977–78	US,[128] 1989–90	US,[154] 1988–91	Combined Totals
No.	31	35	40	57	37[a]	48	248
Age ≤5 y	28	26	19	NS[b]	≥28	NS	≥101/142 (≥71%)
Fever (>38°C)	15	6	36	39	35	44	175/248 (71%)
Diarrhea	31	26	32	56	37	45	227/248 (92%)
Grossly bloody diarrhea	2	NS	7	NS	14	22	45/156 (29%)
Abdominal pain	4	6	20	31/48	NS	NS	61/154 (40%)
Vomiting	NS	12	12	22	18	23	87/217 (40%)
Rash[c]	NS	2	2	NS	NS	NS	4/75 (5%)
Appendectomy	0	0	4	1	0	0	5/200 (2%)
Serotype O:3	31	NS	34	57	34	NS	156/165 (94%)

NS, Not specified.
[a]All were black children; seven cities, 3-month period.
[b]More than half of these children were <2 years old.
[c]Maculopapular rash or urticaria.

European serotypes of *Y. enterocolitica* do not produce yersiniabactin but are able to use siderophores synthesized by other organisms.[46,89,146]

Deferoxamine, a *Streptomyces*-derived siderophore used clinically to treat iron overload states, can be used by *Y. enterocolitica* strains as a source of iron. The increased availability of ferric iron that exists in iron overload states—for example, hemochromatosis and diseases such as thalassemia, which require frequent red blood cell transfusions—also facilitates survival and growth of *Y. enterocolitica*. Iron overloading and deferoxamine are independent risk factors for development of systemic disease after intestinal infection with *Y. enterocolitica*.[50]

Enterotoxin Production

All enteropathogenic strains of *Y. enterocolitica* produce a heat-stable enterotoxin that closely resembles the heat-stable toxin of *E. coli*. Both enterotoxins induce increases in levels of cyclic guanosine monophosphate levels in intestinal epithelial cells. The *Y. enterocolitica* enterotoxin is not plasmid encoded, and its presence does not correlate with the expression of other virulence phenotypes.[67] Because the enterotoxin is not produced in vitro at temperatures exceeding 30°C (86°F), production in the gastrointestinal tract and a causative role in diarrhea were thought to be unlikely.[50] Observations in the young rabbit oral infection model have shown, however, that enterotoxin-negative mutants did not induce diarrhea and the wild-type strain did. Clinical biotype 1A isolates from children with diarrhea in India produce *Y. enterocolitica* stable toxin-b. These findings suggest that *Yersinia* enterotoxins may play a role in causing the diarrhea frequently associated with *Y. enterocolitica* infection in children.[89,164,193]

Gastric Acidity as a Protective Host Factor

Although *Y. enterocolitica* is able to grow under conditions at pH 5.0 to 9.0, optimal growth occurs at pH 7.0 to 8.0. Gastric acidity may play a protective role against some *Yersinia* inocula, although pathogenic *Yersinia* organisms produce a urease enzyme that facilitates survival. Therapeutic agents or clinical conditions that result in reduced gastric acidity may predispose patients to development of infection. *Y. enterocolitica* bacteremia has been reported after gastrectomy.[50,121]

CLINICAL MANIFESTATIONS

Clinical disease caused by *Y. enterocolitica* occurs far more frequently than that caused by *Y. pseudotuberculosis*.[60,131,130] Historically diarrheal illness has been considered the hallmark of *Y. enterocolitica* and the pseudoappendicular syndrome of mesenteric adenitis indicative of *Y. pseudotuberculosis*. Each species can cause enterocolitis and mesenteric adenitis, however. Various other clinical infections and postinfection syndromes also are caused by these microbes. In a series of patients presenting with acute abdominal pain suggestive of appendicitis, the incidence of serologic evidence of *Yersinia* infection has ranged from 7% to 31%.[15]

Yersinia enterocolitica

The clinical features of the disease caused by *Y. enterocolitica*, primarily an acute enteritis, have been described by many investigators.* The clinical manifestations depend partly on the age and physiologic condition of the host.[50,142,173] Enterocolitis is the most common presentation and occurs most often in young children. The pseudoappendicular syndrome, which results primarily from mesenteric adenitis and mimics acute appendicitis, occurs more commonly in older children and young adults.[19,50,93,104,159,179] Asymptomatic infection can occur, but the relative frequency in contrast to symptomatic disease is unknown. The predominant clinical features of *Y. enterocolitica* infection in children are summarized in Table 113.3. Disease manifestations may be strain-related in some cases. The so-called pathogenic strains of biotype 1B are more likely to cause fever, whereas those of so-called nonpathogenic strains of biotype 1A may cause more vomiting.[97]

Enterocolitis

Y. enterocolitica enterocolitis is characterized by diarrhea and abdominal pain. The diarrhea usually persists for 7 to 14 days.[128,142,216] A range of 1 to 46 days of diarrhea has been reported.[109] Ten percent of cases may persist for 30 days or more,[142] and chronic diarrhea persisting for several months has been described.[54]

During the first week of symptoms, patients commonly have three to 10 stools per day, with a gradual decrease in frequency thereafter. Stools typically are greenish, exhibit variable consistency (usually watery or mucoid), and are not remarkably malodorous. Gross blood is noted in approximately 25% to 50% of patients. Vomiting occurs in 40% of cases. Nausea is a common symptom. The abdominal pain can be colicky, diffuse, or localized to the right lower quadrant or epigastrium. Fever occurs commonly and usually is of low grade, but may exceed 40°C (104°F); it usually resolves within 1 week.[1,139]

Most cases are self-limited, but some children require hospitalization. Among 60 children hospitalized in Michigan between 1990 and 1997, the mean number of hospital days required was 4 (range, 1 to 17 days).[1]

Fecal leukocytes are present commonly but not universally. The peripheral white blood cell count may range from 5600/mm^3 to more than 30,000/mm^3. Most counts are greater than 15,000/mm^3. Band forms often exceed 15% of the total. Infants frequently exhibit an immature-to-total neutrophil ratio greater than 0.5.[1,128,139] An absolute monocytosis

*References 17, 40, 50, 54, 81, 120, 127, 128, 138, 139, 142, 174, 179, 212, 229.

may be seen in two thirds of patients.[123] Culture-negative cerebrospinal fluid pleocytosis can occur.[1]

Radiologic examination by upper gastrointestinal barium studies in 24 adult patients with severe diarrhea caused by *Y. enterocolitica* showed abnormalities of the terminal ileum in 21 cases.[217] Diffuse thickening of the mucosal folds was seen in 16 cases, and nodular filling defects were seen in 11. The radiographic appearance suggested the presence of one or more ulcerations of the terminal ileum in 11 patients. Dilation of the terminal ileum was noted in 12 patients, and extrinsic compression, presumably from enlarged lymph nodes, was present in four. In some instances, the findings suggested the terminal ileitis of Crohn disease. Follow-up studies performed 2 months after acute illness showed decreased but persistent thickening of mucosal folds in eight patients. Barium enema studies were done in 15 patients and showed no striking abnormalities other than mucosal ulcerations, which were seen best on air-contrast studies.[216]

Mesenteric lymphadenopathy can be seen on computed tomography scans.[215] Among 13 adults who had colonoscopy or sigmoidoscopy for severe diarrhea caused by *Y. enterocolitica,* abnormalities were seen in eight; the mucosa appeared diffusely swollen, erythematous, and friable in six individuals, and two had only small, 1- to 2-mm aphthoid ulcerations. Serial procedures showed macroscopic and microscopic healing of ulcers within 4 to 5 weeks.[217] Mucosal ulcers may develop in the ileum and aphthoid ulcerations may be seen throughout the colon (Fig. 113.2).[215]

Pseudoappendicitis-Mesenteric Adenitis

The syndrome of pseudoappendicitis, characterized in most cases by a normal appendix and an intense suppurative mesenteric adenitis, has attracted considerable attention since it was reported first in 1953.[143,144] The first recognized cases were caused by *Y. pseudotuberculosis,* but most cases reported in recent years have been caused by *Y. enterocolitica.*[30,103,127]

Fever, abdominal pain, right lower quadrant tenderness, and leukocytosis are the primary features of *Y. enterocolitica*–induced pseudoappendicular syndrome.[50,104] Some patients also have features of enterocolitis (i.e., nausea, vomiting, and diarrhea). The clinical presentation often is highly suggestive of acute appendicitis, such that laparotomy is required. Among a series of 581 patients in Scandinavia who underwent laparotomy for suspected appendicitis, 3.8% of cultures of stool or operative specimens yielded *Y. enterocolitica.*[159] Another 284 patients with similar symptoms were observed, and 5.6% of stool cultures from

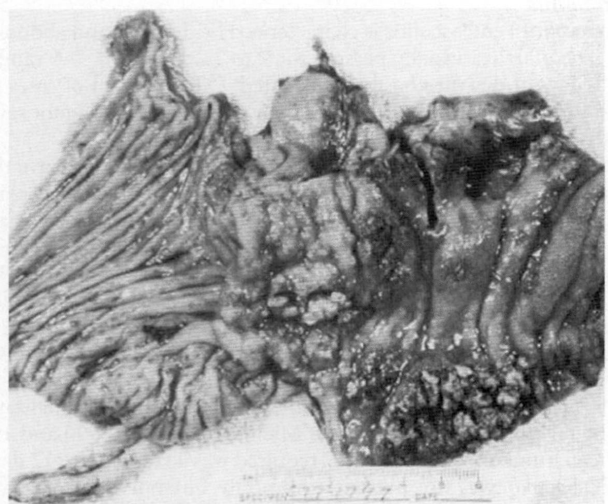

FIG. 113.2 Surgical specimen from a 12-year-old girl with 6 days of fever and abdominal pain localizing to the right lower quadrant. The proximal colon (*left*) shows evenly distributed apthoid ulcers and a normal appendix (*lower left*). The terminal ileum (*right*) shows ulcers of varying size with normal intervening mucosa. (From Gleason TH, Patterson SD. The pathology of *Yersinia enterocolitica* ileocolitis. *Am J Surg Pathol.* 1982;6:347–55.)

these cases yielded *Y. enterocolitica.* In a similar Scandinavian series of 205 patients who underwent appendectomy, 22 subsequently were diagnosed by serology as having *Y. enterocolitica* infection.[104] The findings on laparotomy usually are mesenteric lymphadenitis, terminal ileitis, and a normal or slightly inflamed appendix.[19,50,104,159]

A study of 40 cases of granulomatous appendicitis found evidence suggesting infection caused by *Y. enterocolitica* in four specimens, *Y. pseudotuberculosis* in four specimens, and both in two specimens by PCR analysis.[126] Two patients in the series subsequently were diagnosed as having Crohn disease, but causation cannot be inferred.

Asymptomatic Infection

In an unknown number of cases, infection by *Y. enterocolitica* is entirely asymptomatic. In a study of the distribution of antibodies to *Y. enterocolitica* in sera collected for various purposes in Ontario, Canada, from 4209 individuals who had no evidence of infection by this organism, specific antibody was present in 199 (serotype O:3 in 158 and serotype O:9 in 41).[212]

Other Presentations of Acute Infection

Bacteremia can occur[34,41,50,150] and may result in spread of infection to virtually any body site. Such events occur uncommonly and are seen more often in adults than in children. In children, bacteremia occurs more commonly in infants than in older children.[1] The risk for development of bacteremia during gastroenteritis in infants younger than 3 months may be 30%.[154] Bacteremias may be transient and asymptomatic or lead to septic shock and death. Septic cases tend to occur among patients with underlying illnesses and are associated with mortality rates of 34% to 50%.[50]

Y. enterocolitica may cause focal infections in many extraintestinal sites, even in the absence of detectable bacteremia. Pharyngitis has been reported and occurs primarily in adults. Cervical adenopathy may be associated with *Y. enterocolitica* pharyngitis, and gastrointestinal symptoms may be absent.[50] One adult with pharyngitis died of associated septic shock.[181] Conjunctivitis and panophthalmitis caused by *Y. enterocolitica* have been described. Parinaud oculoglandular syndrome,[42] inguinal adenopathy,[225] and suppurative lymphadenitis[214] have been reported, including a neonate with inguinal adenitis.[160]

Cellulitis, soft tissue abscesses, and wound infections also have been reported. Cellulitis may have associated vesiculobullous lesions. An erysipelas-like rash, maculopapular rash, and urticaria also have been described in association with infection caused by *Y. enterocolitica.*[17,30,50,77,189,206,226]

Pancreatitis, cholecystitis, diverticulitis, and intestinal perforation have been described.[131,170] Peritonitis also can occur but is extremely rare,[175] especially considering the frequency of mesenteric adenitis. Pneumatosis intestinalis has been reported in an infant.[1] Pneumonia, pleural empyema, lung abscess, hepatic and splenic abscesses, urinary tract infection, and renal abscess also have been reported.[50] Glomerulonephritis that usually is transient has been reported.[51,64] Cases of meningitis, osteomyelitis, septic arthritis, pyomyositis (including psoas muscle abscess), endocarditis, mycotic aneurysm, and intravenous catheter–related infection caused by *Y. enterocolitica* have been described.[11,31,50,90,198,200] Thrombocytopenia[69] and hemolytic anemia[118] have occurred in association with infection caused by *Y. enterocolitica.*

Underlying Conditions That Predispose to Bacteremia

Y. enterocolitica bacteremias that occur in patients beyond early infancy most often occur in patients with chronic illnesses or iron overload states. Thalassemias are such conditions that occur most commonly in children.[40,62,110] Among 144 Italian children with thalassemia who were receiving deferoxamine therapy and frequent blood transfusions, 14 developed infection caused by *Y. enterocolitica* during a 12-month period.[40] Septicemia occurred in five of the 14 and was preceded by enterocolitis or mesenteric adenitis in each case. All 14 recovered after receiving 2 weeks of therapy with intravenous trimethoprim-sulfamethoxazole. A similar proportion of children with thalassemias observed in two centers in Canada between 1979 and 1994 also developed invasive disease caused by *Y. enterocolitica.*[6] Bacteremia can be associated temporally with blood transfusions in such patients, suggesting that transfusions may be the source of infection or predispose to development of infection in some cases.[131]

Hemochromatosis, cirrhosis, and other liver diseases may facilitate development of *Y. enterocolitica* bacteremia, also on the basis of excess availability of serum iron. Deferoxamine therapy itself is a risk factor for development of sepsis caused by *Y. enterocolitica* because of the ability of the microbe to extract iron from this compound. Immunosuppressive therapies, diabetes mellitus, and malnutrition also may predispose to development of *Y. enterocolitica* bacteremia.[50]

Postinfectious Syndromes

A reactive arthritis may occur 1 to 14 (usually 4–10) days after the cessation of acute illness.[7,8,10,12,90,92,179,209,217,227] Most such events occur in adults, with a slight female predominance, but 8 of 74 cases in one series from Sweden were in children aged 11 to 20 years (five boys, three girls).[227] In a series from The Netherlands, 10% of children with yersiniosis, most of whom were 7 years of age or older, developed arthritis.[92] The knees, ankles, and wrists are affected most commonly, and in approximately 50% of cases, only one or two joints are involved. Hands, fingers, toes, shoulders, hips, and elbows also may be involved. Pain usually is severe, and the arthritis is additive and usually not migratory. The inflammatory process is self-limited and may persist for 2 months or longer in two-thirds of cases, with one-third persisting for 4 months or longer.

The erythrocyte sedimentation rate exceeds 60 mm/h in approximately 50% of cases. Joint effusions usually are inflammatory, but cell counts and differentials vary and occasionally mimic septic arthritis. Immune complexes have been found in joint fluid. Nonsteroidal antiinflammatory drugs and corticosteroids, intraarticularly and systemically administered, have been used for symptomatic relief for this process.[178]

Erythema nodosum also occurs as a postinfectious manifestation, more often in adults than in children. It can occur alone or in association with arthritis.[86] Tendinitis, myositis, myocarditis, urethritis, uveitis, and conjunctivitis also can occur in association with arthritis. Many but not all patients who develop these postinfectious reactions are human leukocyte antigen (HLA)-B27 positive.[1] Some patients manifest full Reiter syndrome.[92,119,184,196] Acute glomerulonephritis has been linked to infection with serotype O:3 strains in one series of adults.[64]

Yersinia antigens, but not intact bacteria, have been found in synovial tissue obtained several weeks to months after onset of reactive arthritis. *Y. enterocolitica* is able to survive within in vitro cultures of human synovial cells for 6 weeks, with resultant deposition of residual antigen aggregates within the cells.[98] Synovial fluid–derived T cells from patients with *Y. enterocolitica*–induced reactive arthritis have been shown to respond to several *Y. enterocolitica* antigens: heat shock protein 60, urease β subunit, ribosomal L2 protein, and a region of the plasmid-encoded tyrosine phosphatase YopH that is highly homologous to the catalytic domain of eukaryotic protein tyrosine phosphatases.[124,145,168]

Epitopes on *Yersinia*-produced proteins likely trigger cross-reactive immunologic recognition of host proteins that leads to chronic inflammation in susceptible individuals.[95] High levels of antibodies that react with 60-kDa recombinant *Yersinia* heat shock protein have been found in HLA-B27–positive individuals with acute anterior uveitis or pars planitis.[33]

Antibodies against *Y. enterocolitica* have been detected in patients with disorders of the thyroid, including Graves disease, thyroid adenoma, and Hashimoto thyroiditis.[190] A Danish twin study found no increased risk for thyroid antibodies after *Y. enterocolitica* infection, however.[84] These observations may reflect autoantibodies that cross react with *Yersinia* epitopes, rather than a causal link between yersiniosis and thyroid disease.[50,176]

Yersinia pseudotuberculosis

The pseudoappendicular syndrome that results from mesenteric adenitis is the primary disease produced by *Y. pseudotuberculosis*.* The chief complaint is abdominal pain, either diffuse or localized to the right lower quadrant. Fever (38°–40°C) (100.4°–104°F) almost always is present. Tenderness over the McBurney point usually is present. All of these symptoms are highly suggestive of acute appendicitis. Diarrhea may occur but often is absent. Mild leukocytosis occurs, but white blood cell counts usually are less than 20,000/mm^3. The clinical course almost always is benign, with recovery typically beginning approximately the fifth day of illness. On laparotomy, the appendix is normal in most cases but occasionally appears inflamed or suppurative. The mesenteric lymph nodes are enlarged and may appear necrotic.

Efforts have been made to distinguish the pseudoappendicular syndrome caused by *Y. pseudotuberculosis* from that caused by *Y. enterocolitica*.[26,70] *Y. pseudotuberculosis* adenitis is less likely to have associated enterocolitis and may have a shorter febrile course but no clear distinction can be made on clinical grounds alone.

A fulminant typhoidal or septicemic form of infection caused by *Y. pseudotuberculosis* can occur but seems to affect primarily older adults with debilitating conditions, such as diabetes or liver disease. This syndrome often is fatal.[115,184] Isolated cervical adenitis, liver abscess, and terminal ileitis have been described.[86,224] Subacute and recurrent disease can occur.[137] Erythema nodosum[184] and nonsuppurative arthritis[39] also have been reported in association with infection caused by *Y. pseudotuberculosis*. In an outbreak related to eating contaminated grated carrots in Finland in 2003, erythema nodosum was seen in numerous patients with gastrointestinal illness.[102] Median time from exposure to development of gastrointestinal symptoms was 8 days. Median time from exposure to development of erythema nodosum was 19 days (see Fig. 113.2). One patient developed reactive arthritis in a similar time frame.

Yersinia pseudotuberculosis *and Kawasaki Disease–Like Illness*

In Korea and Japan, *Y. pseudotuberculosis* strains have been responsible for a clinical syndrome that can mimic Kawasaki disease.[39] This manifestation of disease occurs primarily in outbreaks and has been described as scarlet fever–like.[163] A transient (2–3 days) erythematous maculopapular rash, strawberry tongue, conjunctivitis, and desquamation can occur, generally in association with gastrointestinal symptoms and fever. Erythema nodosum, lymphadenopathy, uveitis, and coronary aneurysms have occurred in some of these cases, as has acute interstitial nephritis, which can lead to transient renal failure.[3,122,163] Among a series of 33 patients (median age, 5 years) with such presentations, 20 had elevated antibody titers against *Y. pseudotuberculosis*–derived mitogen, which can function as a superantigen.[3] As in Kawasaki disease, Vβ3 T lymphocytes were increased in many of these patients in contrast to healthy control subjects.

DIFFERENTIAL DIAGNOSIS

The differential diagnosis of *Yersinia* enterocolitis includes viral and other bacterial causes of acute gastroenteritis. When the symptoms of mesenteric adenitis are predominant and severe, appendicitis and other causes of an acute abdomen must be considered. The acute terminal ileitis caused by *Yersinia* infections also can be similar to the gastrointestinal manifestations of Crohn disease, ulcerative colitis, cat scratch disease, anisakiasis, amebiasis, actinomycosis, typhoid fever, and lymphoma.[68,92,163,216,224] Cases of infection caused by *Y. enterocolitica* with concomitant recovery of *Salmonella* and *Campylobacter* spp. and rotavirus antigen in stool specimens have been observed.[1]

DIAGNOSIS

The most effective approach to the diagnosis of yersiniosis is isolation of the organism from the stool of patients with enteritis caused by *Y. enterocolitica* or from the infected mesenteric lymph nodes of patients infected by *Y. pseudotuberculosis*. *Y. enterocolitica* occasionally can be recovered from involved mesenteric lymph nodes or the distal ileum.[50] Cultures of feces from individuals with acute suppurative mesenteric adenitis usually fail to grow either organism.

Isolating *Yersinia* organisms from extraintestinal specimens such as lymph nodes and blood is not difficult because they grow on ordinary media (e.g., blood agar) and on several selective and differential media

*References 20, 53, 61, 70, 91, 96, 114, 115, 137, 163, 183, 184, 219, 224.

employed for enteric bacteria. Isolating from fecal specimens is more difficult, however, because *Yersinia* multiply more slowly than other enteric bacteria at 37°C (98.6°F) and have no characteristic colony morphology. Selective media have been developed, but many clinical laboratories culture stool specimens for *Yersinia* spp. only on request because of the costs of these media and the relatively low frequency of occurrences of these pathogens in the community.

Yersinia organisms grow well on MacConkey agar but are much smaller than are other enteric bacteria after standard incubation at 37°C. Cefsulodin-irgasan-novobiocin agar plates have been designed specifically for the isolation of *Yersinia* spp. from stool specimens. After being incubated for 48 hours, *Yersinia* colonies appear dark pink with translucent borders and occasionally are surrounded by a zone of precipitated bile. Cefsulodin-irgasan-novobiocin agar inhibits the growth of most other bacteria except for *Citrobacter* spp. (positive citrate reactions of which allow their distinction). If a dedicated medium for *Yersinia* isolation is not used, MacConkey agar can be examined after 24 hours at 35° to 37°C (95°F–98.6°F) for small colorless colonies that become much larger after an additional 24 hours of incubation at room temperature. Most *Y. enterocolitica* strains are lactose-negative.[73] *Yersinia* spp. grow faster at 37°C than at room temperature. Growth occurs readily at 22° to 28°C (71.6°F–82.4°F), however, and these lower temperatures are recommended for primary isolation.[73] Because of the ability of *Yersinia* spp. to grow at even colder temperatures, specimens can be inoculated into phosphate-buffered saline, refrigerated at 4° to 6°C (39.2°F–42.8°F), and subcultured periodically (up to 4 weeks) if the routine plates that were inoculated with the specimen remain negative. Such "cold enrichment" greatly enhances the isolation rate of *Yersinia* spp. and may be the most reliable method for isolating these organisms from fecal specimens. Many of the *Yersinia* isolates recovered by cold enrichment represent either *Y. enterocolitica* serotypes that usually are not associated with human disease or other *Yersinia* spp. that have roles in disease that remain unclear.

Pathologic or virulent *Yersinia* strains can be distinguished in most instances from nonpathogenic strains by three biochemical tests that are associated with absence of the virulence plasmid. The virulent strains lack pyrazinamidase activity, do not ferment salicin, and do not hydrolyze esculin. On Congo red–magnesium oxalate agar during incubation at 36°C (96.8°F), fresh pathologic isolates (but not those that have been subcultured serially) grow as small red colonies, showing the virulence plasmid-determined properties of Congo red dye uptake and calcium-dependent growth.[59]

Serology

Serology can be performed with microtiter techniques and is most reliable for serotypes O:3 and O:9 of *Y. enterocolitica*. Antibody to the infecting serotype usually is absent at the onset of disease. Peak titers usually are reached 3 to 4 weeks after onset of clinical illness and decrease during the next 3 to 5 months. Low postconvalescent titers may persist for months. Microhemagglutination, complement fixation, and enzyme immunoassays are available in a few commercial laboratories.[27,73,216]

Agglutinin titers of 1 : 128 or higher for *Y. enterocolitica* in previously normal healthy individuals suggest infection. Titers of 1 : 200 or greater were present within 3 weeks of onset of illness in 62 of 65 Canadian children who had infection with serotype O:3. Fourfold increases in titer rarely were seen. Negative or minimal titers (≤1 : 32) do not rule out yersiniosis in infants or immunosuppressed patients. Serologic responses occur more commonly and are of higher titer among patients with extraintestinal systemic infection. Prozone reactions may occur at dilutions of 1 : 32 or lower. Marked cross agglutination occurs between *Y. enterocolitica* serotype O:9 and *Brucella abortus, Morganella morganii,* and *Salmonella*.[27,142] Antibodies to *Y. pseudotuberculosis* often are detectable at the onset of clinical signs of infection and may be highest during the acute phase of illness.[91]

Molecular Techniques

PCR assays have been developed for *Y. enterocolitica* and *Y. pseudotuberculosis* with use of primers that allow assessment of 16S rRNA sequences and of specific plasmid-encoded and chromosome-encoded genes.[39,126,155,156,220,222] PCR techniques have been used to identify *Yersinia* organisms in blood, tissue, stool, water, and food samples.[85,125] *Y. enterocolitica* can be detected by several commercially available multiplex PCR panels marketed for detection of common bacterial, viral, and protozoan pathogens in stool specimens.[112]

TREATMENT

Most patients with yersiniosis do not require treatment because the disease usually is self-limited. Seriously ill patients generally have responded to treatment with chloramphenicol, gentamicin, or tetracyclines, but clinical success has not been uniform. Of these agents, tetracyclines have been the traditional agent of choice.[70,216] *Y. enterocolitica* isolates resistant to the tetracyclines have been reported in recent years, however. Two percent of a sample of *Y. enterocolitica* isolates from Canada in 1992 were resistant to tetracycline,[167] and 10% of a sample of *Y. enterocolitica* isolates from the Netherlands from 1982 to 1991 were resistant to doxycycline.[202]

More than 99% of 1060 isolates of *Y. enterocolitica* collected in Canada in 1972 to 1976, 1980, 1985, and 1990 were susceptible in vitro to piperacillin, cefotaxime, aztreonam, gentamicin, tobramycin, amikacin, trimethoprim-sulfamethoxazole, chloramphenicol, and ciprofloxacin. No evidence of decreasing susceptibility to any of these agents was found across the periods sampled. These results were mirrored by a study of 335 isolates obtained in the Netherlands from 1982 to 1991. All of these isolates were susceptible to ceftazidime, cefepime, imipenem, trimethoprim-sulfamethoxazole, ciprofloxacin, and ofloxacin. Aminoglycosides were effective against more than 99%, chloramphenicol was effective against 94%, and cefuroxime was effective against 90%. Seven multidrug-resistant isolates were present among the isolates from Canada, but none was found among the isolates from the Netherlands.[167,202]

Most *Y. enterocolitica* isolates, regardless of serotype, are resistant to ampicillin, ticarcillin, and first-generation cephalosporins. Most of them also are resistant to amoxicillin-clavulanic acid. This is likely due to expression of β-lactamase *BlaA* and/or *BlaB* genes, because most *Y. enterocolitica* strains harbor both.[21] Azithromycin was active in vitro against 50% of the 335 isolates in the Netherlands, but almost all isolates were resistant to erythromycin and clarithromycin.[167,202] Antimicrobial resistance of *Y. enterocolitica* strains in Europe does not appear to have increased in recent years.[21]

The decreasing effectiveness of tetracyclines in vitro raises the question of whether these agents should be the first choice for treatment of infection caused by *Y. enterocolitica*. A retrospective review of 43 cases (with patient ages ranging from 3 to 89 years) treated for *Y. enterocolitica* septicemia in France between 1985 and 1991 showed that third-generation cephalosporins were effective in 85% of cases in which they were used, although aminoglycosides or fluoroquinolones usually were administered concurrently.[65] Fluoroquinolones alone or in combination with other agents cured all 15 patients. Seven children with bacteremia and diarrhea in Michigan responded well to cefotaxime.[1]

In a double-blind, placebo-controlled trial of trimethoprim-sulfamethoxazole for treatment of children with gastroenteritis caused by *Y. enterocolitica,* the clinical course of illness was not shortened.[165] The children had been ill for a mean of 12 days before treatment was begun, however.

Systemic infections, extraintestinal focal infections, and enterocolitis in compromised hosts should be treated with antibiotics.[50] The in vitro susceptibilities and limited clinical data suggest that children with such infections should be treated with a third-generation cephalosporin, an aminoglycoside, or both. Trimethoprim-sulfamethoxazole also may be used.[40,92] Fluoroquinolones also probably would be effective. Cefotaxime and ceftriaxone were effective in treating bacteremia in a series of 12 children.[2]

Even fewer clinical and in vitro susceptibility data are available for *Y. pseudotuberculosis*. These infections probably can be managed identically to *Y. enterocolitica* infections. A recent analysis of 12 strains in Germany found no resistance to agents tested, including ampicillin.[21] All isolates of *Y. enterocolitica* and *Y. pseudotuberculosis* should be examined for susceptibility to a variety of antibacterial drugs.

VACCINES

There are no vaccines for *Yersinia* species at this time in the United States, although a live attenuated *Y. pestis* vaccine is available in some countries.[205] An attenuated *Y. pseudotuberculosis* strain (IP32953) transformed to express the *Y. pestis* F1 capsule conferred 100% protection in mice against a high challenge dose of *Y. pestis* after a single oral dose of the vaccine strain.[55]

OTHER *YERSINIA* SPECIES

Other "non-pestis" *Yersinia* spp. (*Y. frederiksenii, Y. intermedia, Y. kristensenii, Y. aldovae, Y. bercovieri, Y. mollaretii, Y. rohdei, Y. alecksiciae, Y. similiensis, Y. massiliensis,* and *Y. ruckeri*) occasionally have been isolated from clinical specimens, but their roles as human pathogens remain unclear.[73,189,191,203] These microbes also can be found in fresh-water sources, sewage, dogs, pigs, cattle, wild mammals, birds, reptiles, fish, and some foods, especially milk and meat products.

These organisms are similar biochemically to one another and have been termed atypical *Y. enterocolitica*.[50] None contains the *Yersinia* virulence plasmid pYV.[146] Some contain other large plasmids distinct from pYV, carriage of which may be associated with the ability to cause diarrhea in humans.[164,203] A heat-stable enterotoxin has been found in isolates of *Y. bercovieri*.[204] These *Yersinia* spp. can grow at 4°C (39.2°F) and on cefsulodin-irgasan-novobiocin agar and can multiply in refrigerated foods.

These species occasionally may cause diarrhea and other gastrointestinal symptoms, especially in immunocompromised hosts or individuals with gastric acid suppression.[134] Use of cold enrichment techniques may enhance recovery of these organisms. Their isolation from clinical specimens should not be disregarded or deemed causative of clinical disease without careful epidemiologic considerations.[73] Isolates of these species sometimes can be misidentified as *Y. enterocolitica* by commercial identification systems used in many clinical laboratories. Differences in colony morphology, pyrazinamide reactions (negative for *Y. enterocolitica*), and other biochemical tests can be used to distinguish them from *Y. enterocolitica*.[80,109]

NEW REFERENCES SINCE THE SEVENTH EDITION

36. Centers for Disease Control and Prevention. FoodNet 2013 Annual Report. Available at: http://www.cdc.gov/foodnet/reports/annual-reports-2013.html.
79. Hall M, Chattaway MA, Reuter S, et al. Use of whole-genus genome sequence data to develop a multilocus sequence typing tool that accurately identifies *Yersinia* isolates to the species and subspecies levels. *J Clin Microbiol.* 2015;53:35-42.
112. Khare R, Espy MJ, Cebelinski E, et al. Comparative evaluation of two commercial multiplex panels for detection of gastrointestinal pathogens by use of clinical stool specimens. *J Clin Microbiol.* 2014;52:3667-3673.
205. Sun W, Curtiss R. Rational considerations about development of live attenuated *Yersinia pestis* vaccines. *Curr Pharm Biotechnol.* 2013;14:878-886.

The full reference list for this chapter is available at ExpertConsult.com.

Miscellaneous Enterobacteriaceae 114

Randall G. Fisher

Three less commonly isolated organisms of the family Enterobacteriaceae are *Edwardsiella tarda, Hafnia alvei,* and *Pantoea agglomerans.* Each of these organisms, although uncommon, can cause significant disease in certain clinical circumstances.[75]

EDWARDSIELLA TARDA

Bacteriology

E. tarda is a non–lactose-fermenting, gram-negative bacillus that is indole positive and produces hydrogen sulfide. It ferments only glucose and maltose. The species name *tarda* reflects its biochemical inactivity. Most, if not all, *E. tarda* isolates have peritrichous flagellae (from one to about seven); a higher number of flagellae correlates with better motility and improved biofilm formation in vitro.[43] It usually is lysine positive and ornithine decarboxylase positive.[30] The organism resembles *Salmonella* biochemically and clinically.[49] *Salmonella* usually ferments mannitol, sorbitol, and rhamnose, however. The innate resistance of *Edwardsiella* to colistin also distinguishes it from *Salmonella*.[78] *E. tarda* grows well on usual differential media in the laboratory and produces smooth, glistening, semitranslucent colonies.

Epidemiology

E. tarda is an organism associated with freshwater and marine life and has been isolated from turtles, fish, pelicans, alligators, seals, and toads.[49] It also is found in snakes and lizards. Case reports of human disease have implicated ornamental fish,[107] pet turtles,[79] snakes,[91] and catfish[8,20,41] and injuries in fresh and brackish water.[98]

Patients with chronic liver disease, chronic ethanol abuse, corticosteroid therapy, and hemoglobinopathy particularly are prone to developing infection with *E. tarda*.[68] Any condition associated with iron overload also is a potential risk factor. Serious infections, including pyomyositis and bacteremia, can occur even in otherwise well individuals.[40,98] A single case of infected distal aortic arch aneurysm has been reported.[83]

Infection with *E. tarda* is global but occurs more commonly in tropical and subtropical climates, particularly Southeast Asia, Africa, and Latin America.[57] The elderly and the very young seem to be at increased risk for developing severe illness.[12] Asymptomatic carrier states have been documented as well,[85] but no true epidemic has been reported, and person-to-person transmission has not been established directly.[27]

Pathophysiology

Invasiveness of the organism in HeLa and HEp-2 cells,[88] siderophore production, the elaboration of a cell-associated hemolysin,[44] and resistance to complement-mediated lysis may contribute to virulence, although no clear associations have been made.[53] Hemolytic activity requires the presence of two genes, *ethA* and *ethB*. The *ethA* gene codes for the hemolysin, whereas the *ethB* gene codes for an activation/secretion protein, which is necessary for activation of the hemolysin. Transcription of the *ethB* gene is regulated by iron, which may explain the association between iron overload states and severe *E. tarda* infection.[44] Hemolysin activity seems to be necessary for cell entry and cytotoxicity.[101] *E. tarda* produces an iron-cofactored superoxide dismutase that inhibits macrophage-mediated innate immune responses.[18] *E. tarda* has both type III and type VI secretion systems; expression of these gene products is regulated by phosphorus and iron concentrations.[16]

Clinical Manifestations

Infections with *E. tarda* can be divided broadly into two types: intestinal and extraintestinal. Approximately 80% of infections are intestinal.[98] Gastrointestinal infection usually causes self-limited enteritis, with intermittent watery diarrhea and low-grade fever.[47] Nausea and vomiting usually are not seen. Occasionally enterocolitis or a dysentery-like illness is noted.[71] Because most laboratories do not culture stool specimens specifically for *Edwardsiella,* most cases are unrecognized.

Wound infection is the most common extraintestinal infection. Most of the wounds are caused by fish fins or snakes; wounds sustained in automobile accidents also have been implicated.[50] Cellulitis or abscesses may be produced. Coinfection with other organisms, particularly *Aeromonas hydrophila,* is common.[41,98] One case of necrotizing fasciitis and myonecrosis in an immunocompetent man has been reported. Cultures obtained at surgical debridement yielded a pure growth of *E. tarda.*[98] In one case, a puncture wound from a catfish led to a rapidly progressive, necrotizing soft tissue infection in a man with chronic active hepatitis C infection; after failing multiple debridements, he received a transhumeral amputation.[23]

Septicemia with *E. tarda* is a rare but serious infection that carries a mortality rate of approximately 45%. Most patients with septicemia have underlying conditions, such as liver disease, iron overload, diabetes mellitus, and immunosuppression. Septicemia occasionally follows a mild diarrheal illness.[20] Infants without other risk factors have been reported.[108] Septicemia manifests as high fever, shock, and, often, disseminated intravascular coagulation. Meningitis and multiple brain abscesses also have been reported.[84,95,102,110] Death sometimes occurs despite administration of appropriate antimicrobial therapy.

Other syndromes associated with *E. tarda* infection include an enteric fever–like illness,[20] multiple or solitary liver abscesses,[59,115] osteomyelitis,[91] septic arthritis,[8] cellulitis,[34] myonecrosis,[98] necrotizing fasciitis,[74] endocarditis,[80] uterine pyomyoma,[113] tubo-ovarian abscess,[89] and peritonitis.[20] A case of puerperal intrauterine infection in a woman without obvious risk factors has been reported; her infant was not affected.[76] In another case, neonatal sepsis resulted from maternal chorioamnionitis.[42] Patients with sickle-cell disorders may be predisposed to bony infection with *E. tarda,* as they are with *Salmonella.*[95,112] Reported cases all are in patients with sickle-cell hemoglobinopathy, rather than homozygous sickle-cell disease. Osteomyelitis has also been reported in X-linked chronic granulomatous disease.[55]

Diagnosis and Treatment

Diagnosis rests on identification of *E. tarda* in culture. The major pitfall is mistaking it for *Salmonella.*

E. tarda is sensitive in vitro to most antibiotics used routinely in the treatment of gram-negative infections, including β-lactams, cephalosporins, aminoglycosides, and fluoroquinolones.[19] It also is sensitive to chloramphenicol, trimethoprim-sulfamethoxazole, and tetracycline.[100] Resistance to polymyxin B, colistin, and, occasionally, penicillin has been shown.[19,20] The organism almost universally elaborates a β-lactamase, but no resistance to β-lactams other than penicillin[19] and oxacillin[100] has been reported.

Gastrointestinal disease usually does not require treatment. Severe disease, such as septicemia or meningitis, probably should be treated with the combination of a β-lactam and an aminoglycoside,[49] even though synergy has not been shown.

HAFNIA ALVEI

Bacteriology

H. alvei is a facultatively anaerobic, gram-negative bacillus, formerly referred to as *Enterobacter hafnia.*[96] This indole-negative, catalase-positive, and oxidase-negative organism is positive for lysine and ornithine decarboxylases. It is motile at lower temperatures but may be immotile at temperatures of 35°C (95°F) and greater. *H. alvei* ferments mannitol, maltose, and sucrose. It grows well on blood or MacConkey agar as a nonlactose fermenter, producing gray-white, slightly elevated, glistening colonies.[29] Historically *H. alvei* was thought to be the only species within the genus *Hafnia;* however, in 2010, members of DNA hybridization group 2 were reclassified as *H. paralvei* sp. nov.[45]

Epidemiology

H. alvei has been found in soil, dairy products, sewage, and the feces of humans and animals. Some question whether it exists as part of the endogenous microflora of the gut[92] or whether an asymptomatic "carrier" state exists. One study from Japan cultured *H. alvei* from 13% of healthy subjects[73]; other epidemiologic surveys have shown the incidence to be less than 2%.[94] Long regarded as a nonpathogen, *H. alvei* now has been associated clearly with enteritis and rarely has been isolated in pure culture from other sites, including blood, cerebrospinal fluid, peritoneal fluid, and urine. Infection seems to be opportunistic.

Pathophysiology

The pathophysiology of *H. alvei* has been investigated most thoroughly with regard to its production of gastrointestinal symptoms,[3] although whether *H. alvei* is actually a diarrheagenic pathogen remains controversial. Albert and associates[4] showed that although *H. alvei* elaborated neither enterotoxins nor a Shiga-like toxin and was not invasive in HeLa cell assays or by Sereny test, it did produce diarrhea in experimental animals whether given parenterally or by mouth. Sections of intestines from infected animals showed lesions indistinguishable from those caused by enteropathogenic *Escherichia coli.* "Diarrheagenic strains" of *H. alvei* also were thought to differ from other strains in that they possessed the *eaeA* gene.[47] Janda and colleagues[52] first presented data suggesting that diarrheagenic *H. alvei* isolates were actually either unusual biotypes of *E. coli* or a new species in the genus *Escherichia.* Subsequently the same group showed that organisms originally called *H. alvei* reported to produce attaching-effacing lesions and to possess the *eaeA* gene are actually a novel species, *Escherichia albertii.*[46] *H. alvei* does cause damage to intestinal epithelial cells but does not use the attaching-effacing mechanism, nor does it use the same mechanism as *E. coli* O157:H7.[28] Information about the pathophysiology of extraintestinal infection is sparse.[51]

Clinical Manifestations

Cases of diarrhea caused by *H. alvei* (possibly *E. albertii*) have been reported primarily in children.[3,4] Most patients with gastroenteritis secondary to *H. alvei/E. albertii* report six to 12 episodes of watery diarrhea per day, low-grade or no fever, and nausea with or without vomiting. Mucus sometimes is found in stools, but blood is not.[92,111] In most patients, symptoms last for a few days, but in some patients, symptoms persist for more than a week.[92] One patient with a reactive arthritis from *H. alvei/E. albertii* enteritis has been reported.[81] A unique case has been reported of an 11-year-old girl who had a 3-day history of red lesions on the forehead, neck, and trunk associated with abdominal pain, emesis, and decreased urinary output, with one bloody diarrheal stool the day before admission; she then developed hemolytic-uremic syndrome. Stool cultures repeatedly were negative for *E. coli* O157:H7 but positive for a toxigenic strain of *H. alvei* from two consecutive cultures.[22]

Traditionally extraintestinal *H. alvei* infections were thought to occur mostly in hospitalized patients and to be hospital acquired. In one large series, the organism was isolated from 80 samples collected from 61 patients; 57 (93%) patients had underlying illnesses, most commonly malignancies.[38] Nearly half of isolates were from the respiratory tract. Other sites included blood, skin, wounds, urine, and intraabdominal abscesses. In 60 (75%) samples, other organisms were cultured concomitantly. In a larger study from Canada, two-thirds of 138 isolates were of community onset, 112 (81%) were from the urinary tract, and 94 (68%) were from monomicrobial infections.[60] Older age and female gender were risk factors for development of infection.

One 20-day-old premature infant with necrotizing enterocolitis exhibited *H. alvei* in blood and stool.[36] Yeager and associates[114] reported four cases of pneumatosis intestinalis in patients after they had undergone bone marrow transplantation; in one of the four cases *H. alvei* was grown in pure culture from blood. An 8-year-old boy with acquired immunodeficiency syndrome (AIDS) developed recurrent episodes of *H. alvei* bacteremia.[21] Both episodes were associated with fever and diarrhea; the second episode also was associated with pneumonia and pleural effusion, the cause of which is unclear. A well-documented case of pneumonia in a 54-year-old woman with AIDS has been reported in which the pleural fluid grew a pure culture of *H. alvei.*[31] A patient with graft-versus-host disease developed *H. alvei* colonization with mild symptoms suggesting infection.[97] Pyelonephritis[64] and gangrenous cholecystitis[87] have been reported. A 39-day-old infant without obvious risk factors developed urosepsis.[63] A single case report of *H. paralvei* bacteremia, in an 85-year-old man, exists. His culture was also positive for an enterococcus.[86]

Wound abscess caused by *H. alvei* has been reported.[2] A 2-year-old liver transplant recipient developed hepatic abscess and bacteremia with *H. alvei* and *Enterococcus faecalis.*[9] One case of meningitis in a 1-year-old infant without known predisposing risk factors has been reported.[77] A case of a woman with rheumatoid arthritis who contracted endophthalmitis with *H. alvei* in mixed culture has been described; the woman used snake powder as a food seasoning.[15] Two case reports are described in the older literature of persistent bacteremia with this organism, alone and in mixed cultures. One of these patients was a previously well 13-year-old girl.[37]

Diagnosis and Treatment

Diagnosis is established by isolation of the organism from stools or from normally sterile body fluids. Gunthard and Pennekamp[38] reported the susceptibility results of 80 *H. alvei* isolates recovered from 61 patients over a 2.5-year period. All isolates tested were susceptible to ciprofloxacin. Isolates also were generally susceptible to tobramycin (99%), imipenem (99%), piperacillin (92%), trimethoprim-sulfamethoxazole (90%), ceftriaxone (88%), and ceftazidime (88%). Nearly all isolates were resistant to ampicillin and to amoxicillin-clavulanate.

H. alvei is constitutively cephalothin resistant.[111] One report describes an inducible β-lactamase that rendered the isolate ceftazidime resistant.[103] In a study of 17 isolates from a single institution in France, six were noted to have a high-level constitutive, inducible cephalosporinase production profile similar to that of *Enterobacter* spp.[59] In one study, the antimicrobial susceptibility of *H. alvei* was compared with that of *E. albertii,* the organism with which *H. alvei* is confused most frequently. *E. albertii* isolates were naturally susceptible to all β-lactams except for penicillin and oxacillin; they also were susceptible to azithromycin. In contrast, *H. alvei* strains were naturally resistant to tetracycline, amoxicillin, amoxicillin-clavulanate, ampicillin-sulbactam, azithromycin, and the narrow-spectrum cephalosporins.[100] Most are also resistant to colistin.[1]

Treatment probably is unnecessary for most cases of gastroenteritis. Treatment of invasive infection should be based on susceptibility testing. Empirical therapy with a third-generation cephalosporin and an aminoglycoside is reasonable pending susceptibility results.

PANTOEA AGGLOMERANS

First identified as a plant pathogen and named after Erwin Smith in 1917, the genus *Erwinia* has an extended domain as an infectious microbe, including production of disease in humans.[14,90,99] A member of this group of organisms, *Pantoea agglomerans (Enterobacter agglomerans, Erwinia herbicola)* has been established as a cause of conjunctivitis,[14] central nervous system infections,[14,96] urinary tract infections,[89,95] pneumonia,[5] and nosocomial infections secondary to contaminated intravenous fluids.[34,56] Other species in the genus *Pantoea* are extremely rare causes of infection, including *P. dispersa,*[39] *P. ananatis,*[69] and *P. calida.*[35]

Bacteriology

Species definition within *Erwinia* has been controversial and confusing. It has been suggested to rename the anaerogenic clinically relevant *Erwinia herbicola-lathryi* group *E. agglomerans* or *P. agglomerans.*[30,49,99] In clinical microbiology, both of the latter terms tend to be used interchangeably. This species consists of facultatively anaerobic, fermentative, hydrogen sulfide–negative, gram-negative rods; they do not possess oxidase, phenylalanine deaminase, proteinase, or arginine dehydrolase.[30] None decarboxylates ornithine.[49] They are motile, have peritrichous flagella, and produce a yellow pigment. Strains grow well at 37°C (98.6°F) on standard agar. When colonies are viewed microscopically after growth for 18 to 20 hours, characteristic biconvex spindle-shaped bodies and bacterial aggregates often can be seen.[14,96] Almost all strains isolated from clinical specimens and grown on agar slants show characteristic elongated, spheroidal aggregates,[98] termed *symplasmata* by Cruickshank,[24] who first described them. It is difficult to identify them to the species level without using molecular methods.[93]

Epidemiology

Microorganisms of the genus *Erwinia* long have been recognized as phytopathogens producing dry necrosis, wilts, and soft rots in plants; more recently they have been associated with disease in trout and leafhoppers.[90,99]

The first reports of *P. agglomerans* as a human pathogen appeared in the 1960s. Many infections are local skin/soft tissue infections or synovitis/septic arthritis cases from thorn injuries. Subsequently a nationwide outbreak of infection caused by this organism was traced to contaminated liners from caps of parenteral solution bottles.[66,67] The importance of this organism as a nosocomial cause of bacteremia is emphasized by the 17% mortality rate in patients receiving an infusion with the contaminated intravenous fluid.[66] A trend was noted for an increased mortality rate in infected individuals younger than 20 years. In neonatal intensive care units, the situation seems to be even more dire; in one study, the mortality rate for infants with blood cultures positive for *P. agglomerans* was 88% (seven of eight).[106] Lipid-based medications support rapid bacterial growth at room temperature and, in the absence of strict aseptic handling, have been implicated in more recent nosocomial *P. agglomerans* bloodstream infections.[11] An outbreak of eight cases of bacteremia occurring in a 3-week period was traced to an anticoagulant citrate-dextrose solution that was prepared in house.[13] *Pantoea* outbreaks also have been traced to contaminated blood products; prolonged storage of packed red blood cells at 4°C provides conditions that allow these organisms to grow and subsequently produce high concentrations of endotoxin.[7] Cotton used to filter heroin has been implicated as a source of infection ("cotton fever") in intravenous drug users.[32]

Outbreaks in pediatric hospitals and urgent care centers caused by contaminated intravenous solutions[72] or tubing[10] also have been described. At least one retrospective review of *Erwinia* organisms isolated from clinical specimens suggested a predisposition to infection in the pediatric age group[14]; however other studies have noted no preference based on season, sex, age, or residence in hospitals.[99] A large pseudo-outbreak traced to contamination of cotton pledgets also has been reported.[56]

Pathophysiology

The true incidence of clinical infection caused by *P. agglomerans* is difficult to ascertain because of the common association of this microbe with other organisms when obtained from clinical specimens. Nonetheless the accumulation of case reports in which this organism is isolated in pure culture from infected material leaves little doubt that *P. agglomerans* can be a human pathogen, apart from its role as a nosocomial contaminant. This organism has little inherent invasiveness. Evidence for animal pathogenicity of *Erwinia* strains isolated from plants and humans is limited[62]; 10^{15} washed organisms injected intraperitoneally into mice or guinea pigs do not cause symptoms, whereas inoculation of 10^{30} organisms leads to death within 36 hours.[24]

Most strains seem to act as saprophytes in humans,[109] but the organism has been isolated from purulent wounds of the extremities acquired through lacerations or thorn pricks. In one series of nine infected superficial wounds seen in an emergency department and not getting better more than 10 days later, *P. agglomerans* was responsible for all of them. Most failed antibiotic treatment for a month or more, leading to discovery of retained plant material; wounds healed within 2 to 3 days after said material was removed.[105] In one fascinating case, a 25-year-old man was found to have a mass in his right posterior thigh, thought to be a benign tumor. Biopsy specimens grew *P. agglomerans.* Upon further questioning, the man recalled a fall that had resulted in a thorn injury to the thigh some 4 years previously.[48] Thorn injuries also have led to septic arthritis and osteomyelitis.[25] A delay of 4 to 6 weeks often occurs between the injury and the bone or joint infection. In one case, an 8-year-old girl developed osteomyelitis due to *P. agglomerans* about a month after a closed fracture of the radius and ulna.[58] Most serious infections have occurred in individuals with a breach of host defenses (e.g., immunocompromised individuals or patients who received contaminated intravenous fluid).

Clinical Manifestations

P. agglomerans bacteremia often is associated with fever, shaking chills, and systemic toxicity characteristic of gram-negative sepsis. These symptoms frequently have been misinterpreted, however, in hospitalized patients who unknowingly were administered contaminated intravenous fluids.[67] Premature neonates with sepsis owing to *P. agglomerans* tend to have a rapidly progressive sepsis with prominent pulmonary involvement, including hemorrhage and acute respiratory distress syndrome. A case series of five premature infants with *P. agglomerans* bacteremia has been reported; all infants had a birth weight of less than 1500 g, and in all cases the onset of sepsis was after age 7 days. Lethargy, mottling, and bradycardia were common; patients had desaturations but no evidence of pulmonary disease. Thrombocytopenia developed in four of the five infants, with metabolic acidosis in two and jaundice in two.[6] In the largest pediatric series reported to date, 21 of 53 (about 40%) *P. agglomerans* isolates from normally sterile sites were grown from central venous lines; of these, two-thirds were polymicrobial.[25]

Eye and skin infections caused by *P. agglomerans* are particularly prominent. Bottone and Schneierson[14] included six cases of conjunctivitis, five of which occurred in infants, from whom this organism was isolated. Only two of the isolates were in pure culture, however, and a description of the clinical course of these children was not included in the report. *Erwinia* endophthalmitis has been associated with foreign-body penetration of the eye in a 14-year-old boy.[82]

Skin infection in association with a casted fracture has been described in an elderly patient,[109] and wound infections from which this organism was isolated have been described subsequently, most often in association with agricultural injury.[109] Four isolates were obtained in mixed cultures from skin lesions of children younger than 5 years, but their possible role in those infections was not confirmed.[14] In a recent series, 14 cases of abscesses required drainage; all 14 were polymicrobial.[25] *P. agglomerans* was the only organism isolated from six consecutive blood cultures in a 9-year-old boy with osteomyelitis.[70] A 13-year-old boy developed septic arthritis caused by *P. agglomerans* 1 month after sustaining a plant thorn injury to his knee.[26] A case of *P. agglomerans* spondylodiscitis has been reported.[90] In many cases of *P. agglomerans* osteomyelitis or septic arthritis, the patient is afebrile and blood cultures are negative. In addition, measures of inflammation and joint fluid findings may be largely unremarkable.[25] A high index of suspicion of *P. agglomerans* must be maintained when bone or joint infection follows plant thorn injury.

Primary lung disease caused by these bacteria is a rare occurrence; it has been reported in an adult with chronic bronchitis[6] and also in a heart-lung transplant recipient.[6] This organism is a very rare cause of meningitis. A contaminated incubator has been implicated in two cases of neonatal central nervous system infection,[104] and a cisternal tap revealed the presence of *P. agglomerans* in an unrelated case in a newborn whose clinical course was not described.[14] A 57-year-old man with tetralogy of Fallot and cyanosis had a brain abscess in which *P. agglomerans* organisms grew in pure culture.[110] Presenting manifestations included headaches, seizures, and left-sided weakness, which occurred over a 2-week period before admission. The patient recovered after undergoing drainage of the abscess and gentamicin therapy. A woman developed *P. calida* meningitis after surgical resection of a pituitary adenoma.[35] Several cases of peritonitis in patients on continuous ambulatory peritoneal dialysis have been reported[33,54,65]; in one case the infection was thought to be secondary to a rose thorn injury.[61]

Diagnosis

Difficulty in identifying this organism is common; in March 1972, as part of a quality control program, *P. agglomerans* was sent as an unknown organism to 250 US hospitals and was identified incorrectly 45% of the time.[67] Even when fully identified in isolates from human sources, *P. agglomerans* often is considered a contaminant or saprophyte. The organisms have been identified mistakenly as *Citrobacter, Escherichia coli, Flavobacterium,* and *Klebsiella.* In addition to routine microbiologic studies, identification of yellow-pigmented colonies and observation of the characteristic spindle-shaped bodies and symplasmata can aid in this differentiation.

MALDI-ToF and 16srRNA sequencing is reliable if species identification is required. Prognosis may not be much different, however, in patients said to have "*P. agglomerans*" bacteremia by conventional culture results, regardless of what genus and species is ultimately identified.[17]

Treatment

Most localized infections respond to treatment that includes an aminoglycoside. The presence of persistent localized infection with this organism should prompt a search for an organic foreign body, given the organism's tendency to live as a saprophyte or as a pathogen in vegetable material. In addition to appropriate antimicrobial therapy, treatment of bacteremia should include removal of any potentially contaminated intravenous access. The physician should be alert to the possibility of a common source of infection in nosocomial outbreaks.[67] In view of the rarity of bacteremia caused by *P. agglomerans,* single sporadic cases should be investigated, and clusters of two or more cases should lead to immediate inquiry into possible sources of contamination. In catheter-related infections, successful treatment did not always require catheter removal.[17] Formal surveillance programs have been the key to early recognition and abortion of epidemics.[67]

Acknowledgments

I thank Dr. William Gruber and Dr. Thomas Boyce for their invaluable assistance with earlier versions of this chapter.

NEW REFERENCES SINCE THE SEVENTH EDITION

1. Abbott SL, Moler S, Green N, et al. Clinical and laboratory diagnostic characteristics and cytotoxigenic potential of Hafnia alvei and Hafnia paralvei strains. *J Clin Microbiol.* 2011;49:3122-3126.
13. Boszczowski I, Nobrega de Lmeida Junior J, Peixoto de Miranda EJ, et al. Nosocomial outbreak of Pantoea agglomerans bacteraemia associated with contaminated anticoagulant citrate dextrose solution: new name, old bug? *J Hosp Infect.* 2012;80:255-258.
17. Cheng A, Liu CY, Tsai HY, et al. Bacteremia by Pantoea agglomerans at a medical center in Taiwan, 200–2010. *J Microbiol Immunol Infect.* 2013;46:187-194.
23. Crosby SN, Snoddy MC, Atkinson CT, et al. Upper extremity myonecrosis caused by Edwardsiella tarda resulting in transhumeral amputation: case report. *J Hand Surg Am.* 2013;38:129-132.
35. Fritz S, Cassir N, Noudel R, et al. Postsurgical Pantoea calida meningitis: a case report. *J Med Case Rep.* 2014;16:195.
39. Hagiya H, Otsuka F. Pantoea dispersa bacteremia caused by central line-associated bloodstream infection. *Braz J Infect Dis.* 2014;18:696-697.
40. Hara K, Ouchi H, Kitahara M, et al. [A case of fasciitis localized in the calf muscles associated with Edwardsiella sepsis.]. *Rinsho Shinkeigaku.* 2011;51:694-698.
43. He Y, Xu T, Han Y, et al. Phenotypic diversity of Edwardsiella tarda isolated from different origins. *Lett Appl Microbiol.* 2011;53:294-299.
48. Jain S, Bohra I, Mahajan R, et al. Pantoea agglomerans infection behaving like a tumor after plant thorn injury: an unusual presentation. *Indian J Pathol Microbiol.* 2012;55:386-388.
58. Labianca L, Montanaro A, Turturro F, et al. Osteomyelitis caused by Pantoea agglomerans in a closed fracture in a child. *Orthopedics.* 2013;36:3252-3256.
69. Manoharan G, Lalitha P, Jeganathan LP, et al. Pantoea ananatis as a cause of corneal infiltrate after rice husk injury. *J Clin Microbiol.* 2012;50:2163-2164.
83. Okada K, Yamanaka K, Sakamoto T. In situ total aortic arch replacement for infected distal aortic arch aneurysms with penetrating atherosclerotic ulcer. *J Thorac Cardiovasc Surg.* 2014;148:2096-2100.
93. Rezzonico F, Stockwell VO, Tonolla M, et al. Pantoea clinical isolates cannot be accurately assigned to species based on metabolic profiling. *Transpl Infect Dis.* 2012;14:220-221.
105. Vaiman M, Lazarovich T, Lotan G. Pantoea agglomerans as an indicator of a foreign body of plant origin in cases of wound infection. *J Wound Care.* 2013;22:184-185.

The full reference list for this chapter is available at ExpertConsult.com.

Aeromonas

115

Santhosh Nadipuram • James D. Cherry

Aeromonas spp. were recognized for their role in disease first by Sanarelli in 1891. His findings associated aeromonads with bacteremic "red leg" disease in frogs.[168] Studies by Hill and associates in 1954 linked the first human disease, acute fulminating metastatic myositis, with *Aeromonas* infection.[32] Generally *Aeromonas* spp. have been considered opportunistic pathogens for humans; however these organisms have been identified with increasing frequency as primary pathogens in normal individuals as well as in compromised hosts.

Aeromonas bacteria are ubiquitous. They are found as normal flora in nonfecal sewage and are isolated from tap water, canals, streams, and rivers. They also have been isolated from clinical and food samples. Aeromonads are pathogens for cold-blooded animals (fish, shellfish, amphibians, and reptiles) as well as commensal organisms of leeches.

EPIDEMIOLOGY

Ewing and associates[64] and other investigators have isolated *Aeromonas* from tap water and from the water or sediments of rivers, especially during periods when the water temperature was relatively warm.[99,126,175] Hazen and colleagues[85] recovered *A. hydrophila* from 135 of 147 natural water sources in 30 states of the United States and reported that its density was higher in flowing (lotic) than in calm (lentic) water systems and lower in freshwater than in saline systems; *Aeromonas* could not be recovered from waters in which the saline content approached that of seawater or from extremely polluted waters. Leclerc and Buttiaux[109] found *Aeromonas* in 30% of more than 9000 samples of drinking water in France. Drinking water sampling by the US Environmental Protection Agency (EPA) in 2011 revealed the presence of aeromonads in 42 of 293 (14.3%) samples of public water systems in the United States.[57] *Aeromonas* spp. also have been recovered from hospital water supplies.[126,149,150] Pin and colleagues[152] isolated these organisms from clinical and food samples, including poultry, shellfish, pork, and beef, where they thrived even at low temperatures.

Aeromonas organisms survive readily on surfaces such as bench tops and moistened paper towels. Slotnick[183] recovered *Aeromonas* organisms from a moistened paper towel that had been allowed to dry 24 hours after the application of the organisms. When the towel was placed in a humidified closed environment, the period was extended to 2 weeks.

A. hydrophila may be found in the mouths of fish, alligators, turtles, tadpoles, and frogs.[89] Importantly *Aeromonas hydrophila* is a commensal organism in the digestive tract of leeches, required for the digestion of blood. This was originally found in 1983 when the practice of using leeches to control venous congestion after surgery began to rise in prominence. This form of leech therapy has now expanded to the pediatric population, which has resulted in cases of *Aeromonas* skin and soft tissue "flap" infection (see Clinical Manifestations).[49,73,201] Studies done in Thailand and Turkey have found high percentages of *Aeromonas* in uncooked commercially sold seafood (27% of samples from Thailand, 94% of fish from Turkey).[202,206] Another investigation of fish and animal meats bought at markets in northern India revealed *Aeromonas* species in 38 of 332 (11%) food samples.[180] It also has been found in the feces of guinea pigs and laboratory mice.[55] Unusual sources of *Aeromonas* infection include contamination of home or hospital hemodialysis equipment,[94,158] tsunami-associated wound contamination,[88] and contamination of blood or blood products.[154,159] San Joaquin and colleagues[170] noted that *Aeromonas* organisms also have been found in ornamental aquaria belonging to patients with *Aeromonas*-associated gastroenteritis; however they found that isolates from the aquaria differed in susceptibility testing from the gastrointestinal isolates, so the aquaria probably were not the sources of infection. A multicenter study of more than 150 extraintestinal clinical isolates showed the presence of 22 isolates of *A. aquariorum,* a species once believed to be only virulent to ornamental aquaria.[67]

Aeromonas also have been isolated from a large proportion of ready-to-eat salads.[122] Of *Aeromonas* salad isolates, 35% were *A. hydrophila* or *A. sobria.* All isolates tested in this study had at least one marker of enteropathogenicity, including hemolysin and cytotoxin production. Nonetheless, few if any cases of diarrhea have been associated with ingestion of these salads in immunocompetent hosts.

In 1988, California made infection by *Aeromonas* a reportable condition, permitting the first population-based study of the epidemiology of infection caused by this organism. The overall incidence rate for *Aeromonas* isolation was 10.6 cases per 1 million population. The gastrointestinal tract was the most common site of infection (81% of cases), followed by wounds (9%). Five (2%) of 219 patients with *Aeromonas* infection died; all had serious underlying medical conditions.[103] Studies of traveler's diarrhea revealed the presence of *Aeromonas* spp. in eight of 56 (14%) stool samples in Thailand.[41] A retrospective review of diarrhea in neonates in Bangladesh showed the presence of *Aeromonas* spp. in 222 of 699 stool samples that were positive for bacteria (222 of 2511 overall), making it the second most common isolate after *Vibrio cholerae* in this cohort.[102] A study involving patients with diarrhea in Spain showed *Aeromonas* spp. in 32 of 800 (4%) diarrheal stools.[143] The bacteria isolated were found to be similar (by pulsed-field gel analysis) to isolates from drinking water isolates. Data from a study in southern Brazil using 680 stool samples from patients with diarrhea compared with 300 healthy controls showed that 2.6% of the diarrheal samples contained *Aeromonas,* whereas only 0.3% of the control samples contained this organism.[189] *A. hydrophila* has been placed on the EPA's contaminant candidate list of emerging pathogens in drinking water because it has the potential to grow in water distribution systems and to be resistant to chlorination.[23]

ETIOLOGIC AGENT

Aeromonas organisms are motile, asporogenic, gram-negative rods that contain a single polar flagellum. The organisms are oxidase positive and catalase positive and produce acid or gas during carbohydrate fermentation. They can grow at temperatures between 0°C and 41°C. Growth may occur within a pH range of 5.5 to 9. Lipase, gelatinase, DNase, and other exoenzymes are formed by these organisms.[63,174,198]

Aeromonads grow well on blood agar; most strains produce a large zone of β-hemolysis on this medium, although nonhemolytic strains exist. *Aeromonas* colonies on blood agar have a ground-glass appearance and a fruity odor.[200] Aeromonads also grow on MacConkey, eosin-methylene blue, *Salmonella-Shigella,* and triple-sugar iron media.

The sensitivity and specificity of various media for detection of *Aeromonas* spp. in fecal specimens have been evaluated.[7,136,164,197] Isolation is achieved readily on any of the following: Pril-xylose-ampicillin agar, xylose-sodium, deoxycholate citrate agar, alkaline peptonic water, inositol–brilliant green bile salts agar, trypticase soy broth with ampicillin, and dextrin-fuchsin-sulfite agar.[197] The colonies appear almost colorless on these media, with the exception of growth on dextrin-fuchsin-sulfite agar, on which they appear dark red.

Mishra and associates[130] evaluated five selective agars. Of these, sheep blood agar with 30 mg of ampicillin per liter (ASBA 30) permitted the greatest number of *Aeromonas* colonies to grow while also inhibiting the competing fecal flora. These researchers recommend that ASBA 30 be used with DNase-toluidine blue agar (DNTA) to detect the ampicillin-susceptible strains and the nonhemolytic strains. The combination of ASBA 30 and DNTA allowed 98% of all isolates to be detected.

Strains of motile *Aeromonas* isolates can be identified to species level by use of the following tests: production of nitrate reductase; fermentation of D-glucose and trehalose; failure to use mucate; and the inability to produce acid from D-arabitol, dulcitol, erythritol, and xylose.[1] More recently, the use of restriction fragment length polymorphism analysis of the 16s RNA, along with gene sequencing of common genes has contributed to the identification and speciation of *Aeromonas* isolates.[67,156] Detection of *Aeromonas* organisms by use of strain-specific fluorescent antibody has been described.[197] The technique is not satisfactory; only a small percentage of isolates react with prepared antisera, which suggests the presence of numerous serogroups. The use of a monoclonal antibody against *A. hydrophila* has been shown to overcome this problem however.[53] This monoclonal antibody could prove beneficial in the future as a screening tool. Additionally the study of selected housekeeping genes has been helpful in establishing phylogenetic relationships among members of the aeromonads.[186]

Aeromonas previously was considered a member of the Vibrionaceae, which included the genera *Vibrio* and *Plesiomonas.*[155] Molecular genetic techniques have identified that these three genera are not related evolutionarily, however, and aeromonads represent a family of their own.[48] Genome sequencing has further added to the growing knowledge of *Aeromonas* taxonomy and has also given great insight into the diversity of virulence factors, such as quorum sensing and biofilm formation.[16,36,37,39,47,132,191] *Aeromonas* have long been viewed as belonging to one of two major groups on the basis of their ability to grow at different temperatures. Mesophiles were strains that grew at 35°C to 37°C, and psychrophilic strains were more prevalent at lower temperatures (22°C–28°C). These two groups could be distinguished not only by optimal growth conditions but also by elaboration of pigmentation on tyrosine agar and production of indole. The mesophilic strains are motile, and the psychrophilic strains are nonmotile.

Twenty-two *Aeromonas* spp. have been recognized, and this number is expected to increase as new strains are isolated and identified.[1,146] Although the number of strains of psychrophilic *Aeromonas* spp. has remained stable, the number of various strains of mesophilic species isolated has increased. Several classification schemes within the genus are in use. The strains are classified based on biochemical assays or the use of genotyping techniques such as DNA-DNA hybridization and restriction fragment length polymorphism of the 16S rRNA, or both. Genetic techniques have been used to differentiate the genus into genomospecies or hybridization groups (HG), allowing more precise identification.[24]

Abbott and associates[1] classified *Aeromonas* based on the results of the Møeller decarboxylase and dihydrolase reactions. They also were able to place the strains they studied into complexes based on certain biochemical reactions. The *Aeromonas* strains that produced elastase, pectinase, and stapholysin were grouped into the *A. hydrophila* complex (*A. hydrophila, A. bestiarum,* and *A. salmonicida*). Similarly the *A. caviae* complex includes *A. caviae, A. media,* and *A. eucrenophil.* The *A. sobria* complex comprises *A. veronii* HG8, *A. jandaei, A. schubertii,* and *A. trota.*

In addition, other species, including *A. media* (similar to *A. salmonicida*),[8] *A. veronii,*[87] *A. schubertii,*[31,86] *A. jandaei,*[30] *A. trota,*[29] *A. allosaccharophila,*[120] *A. encheleia,*[62] *A. bestiarum,*[10] *A. popoffii,*[92] and *A. eucrenophila,*[174] have been described. A new species, *A. culicicola,* was isolated more recently.[151] Other isolates include *A. enteropelogenes* and *A. ichthiosmia,* which seem to be similar to previously identified species.[46] Of the species isolated currently, *A. hydrophila, A. caviae,* and *A. veronii* have been associated most often with human infections.[128]

Aeromonas is confused most frequently with Enterobacteriaceae. The oxidase test always should be performed to aid in differentiation; *Aeromonas* organisms generally are oxidase positive, whereas the Enterobacteriaceae are oxidase negative. McGrath and associates[124] described oxidase-variable strains of *A. hydrophila.* These strains are oxidase positive when grown on nonselective media but oxidase negative when grown on differential or gram-negative media. Organic acid end-products of lactose fermentation can inhibit the oxidase reaction. Paik[144] also has shown that a platinum wire loop should be used for oxidase testing; use of an iron-containing loop can cause false-positive oxidase results.

Although drug resistance is a rapidly emerging concern, *Aeromonas* has traditionally shown susceptibility to ceftriaxone (8 μg/mL), chloramphenicol (2–4 μg/mL), gentamicin (0.5–2 μg/mL), streptomycin (16 μg/mL), trimethoprim-sulfamethoxazole (<0.5–9.5 μg/mL), and imipenem and meropenem.[14,64,65,141,142,161,197] Reinhardt and George[162] determined that the most active on a weight basis were ciprofloxacin, enoxacin, and norfloxacin; nalidixic acid and trimethoprim-sulfamethoxazole also possessed good activity. Neither sulfamethoxazole nor trimethoprim alone was active. In addition, these investigators did not note appreciable differences in susceptibility among species or in susceptibility between fecal versus nonenteric isolates. In contrast, Motyl and colleagues[135] noted higher levels of resistance to various antibiotics among *A. hydrophila* strains compared with *A. sobria* or *A. caviae,* as judged by minimal inhibitory concentration. Susceptibility to cephalothin may serve as a useful criterion in the identification of *A. sobria.*[135,170] Resistance to fluoroquinolones has been shown to be based on chromosomal mutations of the *gyrA* and *parC* genes,[2,9,73] along with a plasmid containing a *qnrS* gene[11,12,84] and a separate plasmid with the aac(6′)-Ib-cr.[66]

Aeromonas organisms consistently are resistant to penicillin, ampicillin, carbenicillin, cephalothin, erythromycin, clindamycin, and vancomycin. Sawai and associates[173] showed that resistance to β-lactam antibiotics is caused by the production of a species-specific, chromosome-mediated β-lactamase. Two studies of *Aeromonas* spp. cultures examining for the presence of the *cphA* gene encoding for metallo-β-lactamase have been published. In Brazil, 87 *Aeromonas* isolates recovered from environmental sources showed a prevalence of the *cphA* gene in 97.6% of *A. hydrophilia* isolates and 100% of *A. jandaei* isolates. Likewise, 51 consecutive blood isolates of *Aeromonas* spp. were examined; it was found that, overall, *cphA* was present in 69% of these isolates. The rise of these resistant strains of *Aeromonas* spp. is very troubling.[14,61,118,203] Multidrug-resistant *Aeromonas* have been recovered both in the stool of children with gastroenteritis, as well as in environmental samples.[61,118,14,203] Tetracycline resistance was found in environmental and fish isolates of *Aeromonas* by Han and colleagues.[83] This resistance was conferred by several *tetA* through *tetE* genes; *tetE* was found on a plasmid. It is not R plasmid-mediated. In 1980, McNicol and coworkers[125] reported the recovery of *Aeromonas* isolates from the Chesapeake Bay that were resistant to tetracycline and polymyxin B. They also noted that 57% of isolates from Bangladesh had a multiple streptomycin-chloramphenicol-tetracycline resistance phenotype that correlated with the presence of a larger plasmid. Extended-spectrum β-lactamase (ESBL)-producing *Aeromonas* infections are also becoming more prevalent. A report from Taiwan highlighted the presence of ESBL-producing isolates from 4 of 156 patients with *Aeromonas* bloodstream infection. Resistance was encoded by bla(TEM), bla(CTX-M), and bla(SHV) genes, and conferred resistance to cefotaxime, ceftazidime, and cefepime.[204]

PATHOGENESIS

In addition to its pili, *A. hydrophila* produces numerous virulence factors, including extracellular toxins and enzymes that are involved in the pathogenesis of *A. hydrophila* infection. Some of the toxins elaborated by *A. hydrophila* include hemolysins, aerolysin, and enterotoxins.[18,72,156,160,176] Like many other gram-negative bacteria, *Aeromonas* spp. employ a type III secretion system to bind to host cells and deliver toxins.[2] *Aeromonas* spp. have also been found to produce quorum-sensing molecules which control the expression of many virulence determinants.[36,37,39,190,191]

α-Hemolysin is released from cells during a stationary growth phase. It has a molecular weight of 50[113,114] to 65[114] kDa and is stable at room temperature between pH 3.5 and 9.5. It is heat labile and is cytotoxic to HeLa cells and human embryonic lung fibroblasts.[196] When injected into rabbit skin, it causes dermonecrosis. Intraperitoneal injection of α-hemolysin is lethal for rabbits and mice.

β-Hemolysin has a molecular weight of 49 to 53 kDa and is released near the end of the logarithmic phase of growth of the *Aeromonas* organism. It is heat labile and resists destruction by trypsin and pronase.[114] It causes dermonecrosis of rabbit skin and is lethal for rabbits, rats, and mice. It is cytotoxic to HeLa cells and to human diploid lung fibroblasts.[194] It also has been shown to induce impairment in the intestinal epithelial barrier and to stimulate active chloride secretion in human colon cell monolayers, contributing to enteritis.[60]

α-Hemolysin and β-hemolysin may be significant virulence factors. Most clinical isolates are β-hemolytic, and hemolysis is a common feature of infection caused by *Aeromonas* spp. α-Hemolysin and β-hemolysin in high concentrations produce hemorrhagic enteritis in a rabbit ileal loop; however neither is clearly established as a virulence factor in diarrheal disease.[115] Antibodies to either hemolysin neutralize both toxins.

Aerolysin is a pore-forming toxin that shares some homology with β-hemolysin.[60] After inserting into its target cells, it disrupts ion gradients and membrane potentials, leading to cell lysis.[108] Caco-2 cells derived from human intestine have been shown to be very sensitive to the effects of aerolysin.[4]

In 1975, Sanyal and associates[171] showed that the enterotoxins from *A. hydrophila* were enterotoxigenic. Subsequently, enterotoxigenic *A. hydrophila* has been isolated from humans,[28,76-79,99,199] water sources,[18] fish, and pigs.[25,141] Sha and colleagues[177] have characterized three enterotoxins from *A. hydrophila.* The cytotoxic enterotoxin has hemolytic, cytotoxic, and enterotoxic activities and has a molecular weight of 52 kDa. It is a pore-forming toxin that has been shown to cause fluid secretion and tissue damage in mouse ileal loops.[108] The other two are cytotonic enterotoxins. One has a molecular weight of 44 kDa and is heat labile. The second has a predicted molecular weight of 71 kDa and is heat stable. These cytotonic enterotoxins cause elevation of cyclic adenosine monophosphate and prostaglandin levels in Chinese hamster ovary cells and fluid secretion in rabbit ileal loops.[177] All three enterotoxins have been implicated in *A. hydrophila*–induced gastroenteritis. *Aeromonas* spp. also produce proteinase A and B, endopeptidase, staphylolytic enzyme, fibrinolysin, and leukocidin.[113] The precise relationship of these toxins and enzymes to the pathogenesis of human infection is unclear.

Strains of *Aeromonas* produce proteases, DNase, lecithinase, and elastase.[5] These extracellular enzymes may have pathologic significance. *Aeromonas* strains that possess hemolytic and cytotoxic capabilities and that are characterized as HG1/BD-2 type strains have been related strongly to patients with diarrheal disease.[106] Human *Aeromonas* isolates have been found also to express Shiga toxins (much like Shiga toxin–producing *Escherichia coli*).[11]

Antihemolysin and agglutinating and precipitating antibodies to *A. hydrophila* have been detected in patients with systemic *Aeromonas* infections but not in patients with superficial infections. Increases in the antihemolysin titer to 1 : 1280 and in the agglutinin titer to 1 : 640 have been noted.[33]

Burke and colleagues[27] found that many strains associated with diarrhea were able to hemagglutinate cells from human, horse, rat, and guinea pig. Of these strains, 68% displayed fucose-resistant hemagglutination. The investigators suggested that these properties may contribute to virulence. The ability of *Aeromonas* spp. to create biofilm allowing for colony protection and quorum sensing has been demonstrated.[38,58]

Ketover and associates[100] showed that normal serum promotes phagocytosis and intracellular killing of *Aeromonas* organisms by normal white blood cells. In contrast, sera from two patients with fatal *Aeromonas* infections failed to do so. One patient had an increase in the serum opsonic antibody titer from less than 1 : 5 in the acute stage of disease to 1 : 5120 in the convalescent stage. These studies suggest that a specific opsonizing antibody that is present in normal serum and normal bactericidal activity of neutrophils are required to prevent invasive *A. hydrophila* infections.

The flexible type IV pili of *Aeromonas* are the predominant pili expressed on fecal isolates of diarrhea-associated species of *Aeromonas.* They represent a family of type IV pili that has been designated as bundle-forming pili (Bfp). Kirov and associates[104] have presented compelling evidence to support the concept that Bfp are important intestinal colonization factors. More recently, this group also showed that *Aeromonas* flagella are adhesins for human intestinal cells, playing a role in its enteropathogenicity.

Serogroup analysis may be helpful in establishing which *Aeromonas* isolates can cause human disease. Serogroups O:11, O:34, and O:16 predominate as causes of clinical infection.[93] Hadi and colleagues successfully isolated a 22-kb region of the *A. veronii* bv. *sobria* genome, demonstrating many functions of the Bfp subunits by mutations.[82]

Clear correlation between known virulence properties and enteropathogenicity in humans is lacking. This lack of a clear correlation has been attributed to the heterogeneity of *Aeromonas* spp., the great variety of *Aeromonas* virulence factors, and the loose association between virulence factors and the phenotype and genotype.[128] Consequently many researchers have proposed a multifactorial pathogenesis with the involvement of numerous cellular and extracellular virulence factors.[42]

CLINICAL MANIFESTATIONS

Aeromonas spp. have been implicated as a cause of septicemia, gastroenteritis, peritonitis, skin and wound infections, osteomyelitis, septic arthritis, ocular infections, myositis, urinary tract infections, pneumonia, meningitis, and hemolytic-uremic syndrome in children. Infections have been noted in normal and immunocompromised hosts.[17,22,68,147,148]

Sepsis caused by *Aeromonas* spp. has been reported in children.* Because *Aeromonas* infection is not a reportable disease, the total number of affected children is unknown. Although septicemia caused by *Aeromonas* spp. has occurred in normal children, most children affected have had a disorder known to impair the normal host response to infection or a disorder in which the intact skin as a barrier to infection has been destroyed. *Aeromonas* infection has been noted in children with leukemia (particularly those with neutropenia), aplastic anemia, cirrhosis, hemoglobinopathies, malnutrition, burns, and renal failure. Neonates are susceptible to sepsis when exposed to contaminated water. Chaudhari and Todd detailed neonatal sepsis, necrotizing enterocolitis, and death associated with *A. hydrophilia* in a 27-week-gestation neonate born in a toilet.[40]

The clinical manifestations of septicemia are similar to the manifestations noted in other gram-negative enteric bloodstream infections with high fever and shock. During the course of septicemia in some of these patients, ecthyma gangrenosum also has been noted. The reported case-fatality rate of 50% despite administration of antibiotic therapy presumably is related to the severity of the underlying disorders and not to an unusual virulence of the organism. The propensity for infection in the compromised host suggests that *Aeromonas* organisms are of low virulence for the human host. Bacteremia with *A. sobria, A. punctate, A. veronii, A. caviae,* and *A. schubertii* also has been described.[43,94,98,159,182]

Meningitis caused by *Aeromonas* spp. also has been reported in children.[69,70,205] In one reported review of 21 years' experience with gram-negative bacillary meningitis, *Aeromonas* spp. accounted for 2% of the cases.[196] The course was fulminant, and the patients died despite having received antibiotic therapy. All of these children could be considered immunocompromised as a result of sickle-cell anemia (a 23-month-old child) or age (neonates).

Gastrointestinal infections caused by *Aeromonas* spp. have been reported with greater frequency in pediatric patients. *A. hydrophila, A. sobria, A. caviae,* and *A. punctata* have been recovered from stool specimens of patients with gastroenteritis.[28,35,71,94,134] In 1961, Martinez-Silva and colleagues[121] described an epidemic of enteritis in a newborn nursery affecting nine infants (eight as neonates and one at 7 days old). *Aeromonas* spp. were found in the stools of six of these infants. One neonate, the only patient with a pure growth of *Aeromonas* in a stool specimen, died. In 1964, Rosner[166] reported severe gastroenteritis in a child with growth of *A. hydrophila* from four stool cultures. In 1991, one study reported 224 cases of *Aeromonas* gastroenteritis in Iowa from January to June.[157] Taneja and associates[192] described an outbreak of diarrhea caused by *Aeromonas* spp. on a hematology-oncology ward in a pediatric hospital during March/April 2001, where six of 18 children were infected. *Aeromonas* spp. were found to be the sole enteropathogen in five of the six children. Aeromonads have been detected worldwide as the sole pathogen causing diarrhea in 2% to 20% of affected children and in only up to 2% of children without diarrhea.[42,54,79,193]

In an attempt to assess the role of *Aeromonas* spp. in diarrheal disease, numerous investigators have evaluated the fecal carriage rate of the

*References 26, 45, 51, 80, 91, 100, 138, 147, 165, 172, 200, 205, 207.

organism.[81] Freij[70] described a study performed by other investigators who recovered *Aeromonas* from none of 300 adults and from 31 of 4426 (0.7%) children younger than 2 years. Pitarangsi and coworkers[153] reported carrier rates of 16% to 27% in various districts in Thailand and noted the same frequency of *A. hydrophila* in stools of Thais with and without diarrhea. In contrast, *A. hydrophila* was recovered from the stools of American Peace Corps volunteers more frequently when they had diarrhea than when their stool frequency was normal.[41] Only three *Aeromonas* isolates were reported from 1685 rectal swab cultures obtained from 1217 children hospitalized for gastroenteritis in Manitoba, Canada. Bhat and colleagues[19] recovered *Aeromonas* organisms from seven of 133 patients with acute diarrhea in a valley in India and found *Aeromonas* and *Plesiomonas shigelloides* in the well water commonly used by these individuals. Soltan Dallal and Moezardalan[187] isolated *Aeromonas* spp. from 14 of 310 Iranian children in a case-control study. A large, retrospective study on the island of Crete found the prevalence of *A. hydrophilia* to be 0.44% in submitted stool cultures from children over an 18-year period.[119]

Gracey and associates[77,78] described a prospective study in Australia of 1156 children with diarrhea and an equal number of age- and sex-matched control subjects. Enterotoxigenic *Aeromonas* organisms were isolated from 10.2% of children with diarrhea compared with 0.6% of healthy children. *Aeromonas* was the only potential pathogen recovered in 6.5% of children with diarrhea. Cases of *Aeromonas* infection peaked during the summer months. The mean duration of diarrhea was 15.3 days, and 33% of the children required hospitalization. These investigators described three clinical syndromes of *Aeromonas* gastroenteritis: (1) watery diarrhea, vomiting, and low-grade fever in 41%; (2) diarrhea with blood and mucus in 22%; and (3) prolonged diarrhea of more than 2 weeks' duration in 37%.

Many investigators[6,34,137,139,169] have attempted to describe gastrointestinal infections caused by *Aeromonas* spp. Gluskin and associates[74] performed a 15-year study of the rate of *Aeromonas* spp. in gastroenteritis in hospitalized children. A total of 146 strains of *Aeromonas* spp. were isolated from 32,810 fecal specimens from 13,820 hospitalized patients. These isolates constituted 4% of all pathogenic bacterial strains cultured. Most of the cases of diarrhea (94%) occurred in children younger than 3 years. The peak incidence occurred in infants aged 2 to 6 months. Bloody diarrhea occurred in 7% of children. Several investigators[6,169] have detected a larger number of cases of *Aeromonas*-associated diarrhea in the summer months than in other months, whereas Challapali and colleagues[34] found no seasonal patterns of *Aeromonas* isolation. The greatest number of cases occurred in children younger than 12 months to 3 years of age.

Symptoms included diarrhea, bloody stools, vomiting, abdominal cramps, mild dehydration, and fever. *Aeromonas*-associated diarrhea resembled other types of bacterial diarrhea, except that fecal leukocytes were absent in children with *Aeromonas*-associated diarrhea; in contrast, fecal leukocytes were found in 60% of children with other types of bacterial enteritis.[34] A cholera-like illness caused by enterotoxigenic *A. sobria* has been described.[35,107] Gastroenteritis caused by *A. sobria* and *A. hydrophila* tended to be acute, whereas diarrhea associated with *A. caviae* frequently was chronic, lasting 4 to 6 weeks in untreated patients.

San Joaquin and Pickett[169] described three patients with *A. caviae* diarrhea who originally presented with failure to thrive presumed to be secondary to formula intolerance. Diarrhea in these patients improved after administration of trimethoprim-sulfamethoxazole. Moyer[137] noted that although *A. caviae* is considered nonpathogenic, five pediatric patients with otitis media who were treated with penicillin or ampicillin subsequently developed diarrhea in which *A. caviae* was the only potential enteric pathogen. The prior therapy with antibiotics to which *Aeromonas* spp. are known to be resistant probably contributed to colonization of the gastrointestinal tract with *A. caviae* and subsequent development of diarrhea. These four patients also were treated successfully with trimethoprim-sulfamethoxazole.

Outbreaks of diarrhea associated with *Aeromonas* in daycare centers have been described.[54] *A. caviae, A. hydrophila,* and *A. sobria* were the strains recovered most commonly.

Complications of *Aeromonas* intestinal infection included gram-negative bacteremia, intussusception, internal hernia strangulation, hemolytic-uremic syndrome,[22,131,163] and failure to thrive. Peritonitis has been reported in a 5-year-old patient with a ruptured appendix.[91] No additional clinical information about this patient was provided. Peritoneal dialysis catheter–related peritonitis was described in one patient.[112] The patient was involved in gardening and had poor adherence to peritoneal dialysis protocol and hand washing guidelines.

A. hydrophila has been recovered from the skin or from wound infections of children.* Most of these patients have been normal hosts; three had leukemia. In 40% of these cases, *Aeromonas* organisms were not recovered from the lesion in pure culture. The lower extremity was involved in 75% of these cases. Exposure to water was noted in 40% of these cases; alligator bites, snake bites, stepping on glass, and burns were other presumed predisposing factors. Clinical manifestations included cellulitis, hemorrhagic blebs, and purulent diarrhea with fever and leukocytosis. Secondary bacteremia and osteomyelitis have been reported.[21,90] In a study of neonates with omphalitis in Karachi, Pakistan, 19 of 583 (3.2%) of purulent secretions from umbilical stumps yielded a positive culture with *Aeromonas* spp. The clinical implications of the presence of *Aeromonas* in these neonates was not discussed.[129]

Aeromonas organisms have been recovered from skin lesions that have been the result of tick bites. In each of the cases, a circumscribed area of purple discoloration has surrounded the bite, and nonpurulent drainage from the center of the lesion yielded the organism. These patients sought medical attention because the local lesion had persisted or had increased in size over the course of 1 to 2 weeks. *A. schubertii* also has been isolated from traumatic wound infections.[31]

Ecthyma gangrenosum caused by *A. hydrophila* has been described in several children with leukemia.[100,138,178] Ecthyma gangrenosum has been seen in several children with *Aeromonas* septicemia who have had malignant or hepatobiliary disease. Clark and Chenoweth[44] isolated *A. hydrophila* from an 18-month-old boy and a 2-year-old boy, both of whom had liver transplants for biliary atresia and subsequently developed cholangitis. In both instances, these were polymicrobial infections.

Current practice by plastic surgeons to use medicinal leeches to control venous congestion after reimplantation of limbs or closure of skin flaps has led to sepsis and skin and soft tissue infection with *Aeromonas* spp. in adults.[111] This practice is now becoming more prevalent in children, and practitioners should be aware that therapy with leeches requires antibiotic prophylaxis. Leeches can harbor *Aeromonas* spp. resistant to the prophylaxis of choice.

Lopez and associates[116] described an 8-year-old child with acute myelogenous leukemia with bacteremia and osteomyelitis; *Aeromonas* organisms grew from a bone aspirate of this patient. Blatz[21] reported finding osteomyelitis and *Aeromonas* bacteremia in a previously healthy 16-year-old patient; a bone aspirate was not attempted. Septic arthritis caused by *A. hydrophila* also has been described in a child with leukemia; the organism was recovered from the second metacarpophalangeal joint at autopsy.[51] Elwitigala and colleagues[59] also recovered *A. hydrophila* in a previously healthy 13-year-old girl who developed severe septic arthritis of the knee after injury sustained in a private freshwater lake. This infection frequently is rapidly progressive.

Aeromonas has been recovered from the conjunctiva of a previously healthy 7-year-old boy whose eye had been penetrated by a safety pin[185] and from the anterior chamber of an 8-year-old boy who developed endophthalmitis after receiving a corneal laceration from a fishhook.[45] *A. sobria* endophthalmitis has been described in a 14-year-old patient after a penetrating eye injury occurred in which a cormorant pecked the patient's eye.[110]

Although numerous cases of *Aeromonas* urinary tract infections have been reported in adults, only a few cases have been reported in children. McCracken and Barkley[123] reported the recovery of *A. hydrophila* in pure culture from the urine of a 5-month-old boy with diarrhea. Bartolomé and colleagues[15] described a case of urinary tract infection associated with diarrhea in a male neonate with bilateral ureterohydronephrosis and bladder involvement from posterior urethral valves. Ojeda-Vargas and associates[140] reported the case of an 18-year-old girl with severe pyelonephritis requiring admission to an intensive care unit: *A. hydrophila*

*References 15, 21, 52, 68, 91, 100, 123, 138, 148, 163, 178, 188, 197.

and *Pseudomonas* were isolated from her urine cultures. In a case series of seven patients with *Aeromonas* urinary tract infections in a hospital in Puducherry, India, one 4-year-old girl with chronic renal failure was found to grow *A. caviae* from a urine specimen.[117]

Myositis caused by *Aeromonas* also has been described in children. A 9-year-old girl and a 16-year-old boy required amputation of their legs as a result of *Aeromonas* myositis.[52,184] Another case of sepsis accompanied by myositis of the thigh was described by Papadakis and associates in a 36-month-old girl with acute lymphoblastic leukemia; this child recovered well with prompt antibiotic therapy and surgical debridement.[145] Necrosis of muscle was noted in both cases, and gas was seen on the radiographs before amputation in the 9-year-old girl. Fatal myofascial necrosis also has been reported in a patient with a history of aplastic anemia.[75] *A. hydrophila* also has been isolated from abscesses caused by snake bites.[95]

Pneumonia caused by *A. hydrophila* is a rare event in children. Kao and associates[97] reported that there have been a total of seven case reports in the literature so far, and four patients died of fulminant disease. Of the seven patients, four had accompanying medical conditions, including acute leukemia (two patients), cavernous hemangioma with thrombocytopenia (one patient), and nephrotic syndrome (one patient). One patient was the victim of a near-drowning, and two patients were previously healthy.[97,161,181] One of the previously healthy patients was described by Kao and associates[97] in their case report and literature review. The patient was a 5-year-old girl who presented with fulminant sepsis and pneumonia and quickly died. *A. hydrophila* was recovered from her blood, endotracheal aspirate, and postmortem pleural fluid. Neither a bone marrow aspirate nor an immunologic workup was performed, so whether she had an underlying malignancy or immunodeficiency that might have contributed to her rapid demise is unknown. *A. hydrophila* has been isolated from lung abscess at autopsy of a 16-year-old girl with *A. hydrophila* septicemia and leukemia.[51]

DIAGNOSIS AND DIFFERENTIAL DIAGNOSIS

Aeromonas should be considered a possible cause of infection in children with any of the disorders previously noted. In addition, *Aeromonas* infection should be considered in any child noted to be exposed to a contaminated water source (e.g., sewage, waste). It also always should be included as a possible cause of gastroenteritis, bacteremia, and skin infection in a compromised host. Generally *Aeromonas* organisms are recognized only when they grow from body fluids or tissues that normally are sterile. Also, as noted earlier, *Aeromonas* infection should be suspected in ill children after the use of medicinal leech therapy in surgery or subsequent to an alligator, snake, or shark bite.[3] The best methods for isolation of *Aeromonas* organisms have been described (see the section on Etiologic Agents).

A. hydrophila in food can be detected by an enzyme-linked immunosorbent assay and polymerase chain reaction.[20,127,195] These organisms also have been identified in environmental samples by use of 16S rDNA–targeted oligonucleotide primers.[56] Many sophisticated techniques, including rRNA sequencing, DNA-DNA reassociation techniques, and polymerase chain reaction, have been used to continue to identify and differentiate *Aeromonas* spp.[24,50,101,128]

TREATMENT AND PROGNOSIS

Penicillin-hydrolyzing β-lactamases have been detected in most strains of *Aeromonas,* rendering those strains resistant to ampicillin.[133] Piperacillin shows variable activity against *Aeromonas* spp., whereas ticarcillin-clavulanate generally is active. In vitro, *Aeromonas* organisms generally are susceptible to chloramphenicol, aminoglycosides, trimethoprim-sulfamethoxazole, aztreonam, quinolones, and the third-generation cephalosporins.[96,105,167] Great care must be taken to obtain minimal inhibitory concentrations on *Aeromonas* isolates, and carbapenems should be initiated when there is lack of clinical response because ESBL-producing organisms are known to occur both in the environment and in clinical isolates.[14] Likewise, rates of tetracycline, fluoroquinolone, and aminoglycoside resistance should be known before considering these agents.[2,12–14,84,179]

Initial empirical treatment with a third-generation cephalosporin is suggested. Following this, a drug to which the organism is sensitive should be provided (usually intravenously). The duration of administration depends on the site of infection and the clinical response to therapy. The occurrence of *Aeromonas* infections predominantly in compromised hosts accounts for the high case-fatality rate despite administration of an antibiotic agent to which the organism is susceptible.

NEW REFERENCES SINCE THE SEVENTH EDITION

3. Abrahamian FM, Goldstein EJ. Microbiology of animal bite wound infections. *Clin Microbiol Rev*. 2011;24(2):231-246.
7. Aguilera-Arreola MG, Portillo-Munoz MI, Rodriguez-Martinez C, et al. Usefulness of chromogenic CromoCen(R) AGN agar medium for the identification of the genus *Aeromonas*: assessment of faecal samples. *J Microbiol Methods*. 2012;90(2):100-104.
16. Beatson SA, das Gracas de Luna M, Bachmann NL, et al. Genome sequence of the emerging pathogen *Aeromonas caviae*. *J Bacteriol*. 2011;193(5):1286-1287.
36. Chan KG, Chin PS, Tee KK, et al. Draft genome sequence of Aeromonas caviae strain L12, a quorum-sensing strain isolated from a freshwater lake in Malaysia. *Genome Announc*. 2015;3(2).
39. Chan KG, Tan WS, Chang CY, et al. Genome sequence analysis reveals evidence of quorum-sensing genes present in *Aeromonas hydrophila* strain M062, isolated from freshwater. *Genome Announc*. 2015;3(2).
37. Chan XY, Chua KH, Puthucheary SD, et al. Draft genome sequence of an *Aeromonas* sp. strain 159 clinical isolate that shows quorum-sensing activity. *J Bacteriol*. 2012;194(22):6350.
47. Colston SM, Fullmer MS, Beka L, et al. Bioinformatic genome comparisons for taxonomic and phylogenetic assignments using *Aeromonas* as a test case. *MBio*. 2014;5(6):e02136.
49. Dabb RW, Malone JM, Leverett LC. The use of medicinal leeches in the salvage of flaps with venous congestion. *Ann Plast Surg*. 1992;29(3):250-256.
61. Esteve C, Alcaide E, Gimenez MJ. Multidrug-resistant (MDR) *Aeromonas* recovered from the metropolitan area of Valencia (Spain): diseases spectrum and prevalence in the environment. *Eur J Clin Microbiol Infect Dis*. 2015;34(1):137-145.
72. Ghenghesh KS, Ahmed SF, Cappuccinelli P, et al. Genospecies and virulence factors of Aeromonas species in different sources in a North African country. *Libyan J Med*. 2014;9:25497.
73. Giltner CL, Bobenchik AM, Uslan DZ, et al. Ciprofloxacin-resistant *Aeromonas hydrophila* cellulitis following leech therapy. *J Clin Microbiol*. 2013;51(4):1324-1326.
107. Kumar KJ, Kumar GS. Cholera-like illness due to *Aeromonas caviae*. *Indian Pediatr*. 2013;50(10):969-970.
118. Mansour AM, Abd Elkhalek R, Shaheen HI, et al. Burden of *Aeromonas hydrophila*-associated diarrhea among children younger than 2 years in rural Egyptian community. *J Infect Dev Ctries*. 2012;6(12):842-846.
132. Moriel B, Cruz LM, Dallagassa CB, et al. Draft genome sequence of Aeromonas caviae 8LM, isolated from stool culture of a child with diarrhea. *Genome Announc*. 2015;3(3).
156. Puthucheary SD, Puah SM, Chua KH. Molecular characterization of clinical isolates of *Aeromonas* species from Malaysia. *PLoS ONE*. 2012;7(2):e30205.
160. Rather MA, Willayat MM, Wani SA, et al. A multiplex PCR for detection of enterotoxin genes in *Aeromonas* species isolated from foods of animal origin and human diarrhoeal samples. *J Appl Microbiol*. 2014;117(6):1721-1729.
176. Senderovich Y, Ken-Dror S, Vainblat I, et al. A molecular study on the prevalence and virulence potential of *Aeromonas* spp. recovered from patients suffering from diarrhea in Israel. *PLoS ONE*. 2012;7(2):e30070.
190. Tan WS, Yin WF, Chan KG. Insights into the quorum-sensing activity in Aeromonas hydrophila strain M013 as revealed by whole-genome sequencing. *Genome Announc*. 2015;3(1).
191. Tan WS, Yin WF, Chang CY, et al. Whole-genome sequencing analysis of quorum-sensing *Aeromonas hydrophila* strain M023 from freshwater. *Genome Announc*. 2015;3(1).
201. Whitaker IS, Josty IC, Hawkins S, et al. Medicinal leeches and the microsurgeon: a four-year study, clinical series and risk benefit review. *Microsurgery*. 2011;31(4):281-287.
204. Wu CJ, Chuang YC, Lee MF, et al. Bacteremia due to extended-spectrum-beta-lactamase-producing Aeromonas spp. at a medical center in Southern Taiwan. *Antimicrob Agents Chemother*. 2011;55(12):5813-5818.

The full reference list for this chapter is available at ExpertConsult.com.

116 Pasteurella multocida

Deborah Lehman

In 1878, Kitt first isolated a bacterium of the *Pasteurella* group from wild hogs during an epidemic; 2 years later, Pasteur described the organism that causes fowl cholera. Since that time, the same organism has been implicated in rabbit septicemia, swine plague, hemorrhagic septicemia, and wildseuche (a fatal disease in deer). Hueppe applied the term *hemorrhagic septicemia* to this group of infectious diseases in lower animals because of the characteristic hemorrhagic areas seen scattered throughout the viscera. Original names for the causative organisms included *Pasteurella aviseptica, P. boviseptica, P. suiseptica,* and *P. lepiseptica,* but these organisms now are classified under the name *P. multocida,* a small, nonmotile, gram-negative rod.[57]

Although *P. multocida* was originally recognized as an animal pathogen, its role in human disease following animal exposure is now well established. Brugnatelli reported the first bacteriologically proven case in a human in 1913,[10] and Hundeshagen described the first systemic human infection in 1919.[35] Schipper[58] did an extensive review of the literature from 1930 through 1947, and reported only 40 cases of infection with *P. multocida.* Since then an increasing number of human infections with *P. multocida* have been reported,[61] and it has been recognized to be one of the primary pathogens implicated in wound infection and septicemia following bites from cats, dogs, and other mammals.[50,64]

THE ORGANISM

P. multocida generally appears as a short, ovoid, gram-negative rod; however, it also may appear as a coccobacillus with convex sides and rounded ends. The length ranges from 0.3 to 1.25 µm, and the diameter ranges from 0.15 to 0.25 µm. *P. multocida* may appear singly or in pairs, chains, or clusters. Healthy organisms stain easily with aniline dyes and are gram negative. They may show bipolar staining, especially when smears are made directly from animal tissue or fluids. The organism becomes increasingly pleomorphic on subculture and may resemble Enterobacteriaceae in broth. They do not grow on eosin–methylene blue, MacConkey, deoxycholate, or any other bile-containing agar. They are facultatively anaerobic and nonmotile. They do not require X or V factor for growth, an important differential point in distinguishing *Pasteurella* species from *Haemophilus influenzae.* Its unique susceptibility to penicillin also differentiates it from other small gram-negative rods such as *H. influenzae*, a property noted in 1947 by Schipper.[58]

Colonies are nonhemolytic and translucent, 1 to 2 mm in diameter, and generally, convex, and butyrous. Occasionally, they may be larger and mucoid or iridescent. Colonies on blood agar appear smaller, opaque, and grayish white. In broth culture, turbidity, often with flocculent sediment, is present.

Cultures tend to autoagglutinate in saline and have a peculiar musty odor. The organism is catalase positive and usually oxidase and indole positive. It usually ferments galactose, glucose, fructose, mannitol, mannose, and sucrose without production of gas. Some variability occurs in the fermentation of other sugars, and patterns of fermentation can be used to differentiate different strains of the organism.[19] Using fermentation reactions, Oberhofer[49] developed a biotyping system in which correlation of biotype, 61% A and B, was found for cat-bite isolates but not with dog-bite isolates. *Pasteurella* reduces nitrates but has negative urease, methyl red, and Voges-Proskauer reactions. The pathogenicity of the organism varies; most mucoid and smooth colony-forming strains produce a capsule and usually are highly pathogenic for mice and rabbits. The capsule is antiphagocytic allowing the organism to resist intracellular killing by neutrophils, and each of the five capsular types (A, B, C, D, E, and F) is generally restricted to a specific host.

Nielsen and Rosdahl[47] developed a bacteriophage typing system for typing toxigenic and nontoxigenic strains. DNA hybridization studies have led to a reclassification of the genus *Pasteurella. P. multocida* now includes three subspecies: *P. multocida* subsp. *multocida, P. multocida* subsp. *septica,* and *P. multocida* subsp. *gallicida.* Of 159 strains recovered from 46 infected humans, 95 were identified as *P. multocida* subsp. *multocida* and 21 were identified as *P. multocida* subsp. *septica;* the remainder were divided among multiple other species.[29] Other less common *Pasteurella* spp. include *P. canis, P. dagmatis,* and *P. stomatis.* The use of serology in conjunction with DNA fingerprinting can classify isolates for epidemiologic studies.[74]

Polymerase chain reaction (PCR) analysis using universal primers for 16S rRNA genes, genomics, and molecular techniques are now the primary methods for identification, characterization, and differentiation of *P. multocida* and other Pasteurelleae in research settings.[73]

Immunity to *P. multocida* can be demonstrated in many animals, and animal vaccines have been developed with known efficacy, especially in birds and cattle.[4] The precise mechanisms involved in the development of both vaccine immunity and, more importantly, natural immunity, are currently being elucidated. Antibodies to somatic and capsular antigenic determinants develop within 2 weeks of infection; with the capsular antibodies being longer lasting.[12] Woolcock and Collins[76] developed models in pathogen-free mice that may help uncover the mechanisms of immunologic protection. The efficacy of heat-killed vaccine is greatest when multiple doses are administered.

TRANSMISSION

Pasteurella is found in the oral flora of many different animals; 67% of cats may harbor this organism in their mouths or throats.[70] Smith[60] found that *P. multocida* could be recovered from the tonsils of 54% and from the nose of 10% of dogs. Schipper[58] grew *P. multocida* from 14% of wild rats trapped in the Baltimore area. Hansmann and Tully[28] showed that *P. multocida* can remain as a commensal for prolonged periods in the mouth of a cat. They described a patient who had been bitten on two occasions, 3 years apart, by the same healthy pet cat; each time, an abscess caused by *P. multocida* developed. *P. multocida* also has been isolated from panthers, komodo dragons, Tasmanian devils, buffalos, minks, pigs, and opossums.[2,11,33,42] *Pasteurella* infection is of particular concern following bites from large cats such as lions, tigers, and cougars.[73]

Although verifying the mode of transmission has been easiest when an infection has been related specifically to a pet or a farm animal, many cases of infection caused by *P. multocida* have been documented despite a negative history of animal exposure. Respiratory tract infection with this organism has been described in veterinarians, farmers, dairy workers, and individuals employed in locations where animal tissues are processed. A recent case series reported three life-threatening *P. multocida* respiratory tract infections associated with palliative pet care in the home.[45]

The possibility of a reservoir of infection in humans with resultant interhuman transmission has been considered. In a study of veterinary students, Smith[60] described two of 71 with positive throat cultures for the organism. *Pasteurella* was present in 1 student for a few days and in the other for the full 4 months of the study; both patients were asymptomatic. Several other cases of isolation of the organism from the human respiratory tract, many without associated symptoms or known animal contact, have been reported.

Interhuman spread by nasopharyngeal excretions, feces, and urine may occur and the organism has been recovered from these sites. The female genital tract is another potential source, especially for cases of septicemia and meningitis that occur during pregnancy and in the newborn period.

Investigators of an outbreak in a chronic disease hospital showed that *P. multocida* was potentially viable on a towel for 24 hours. Although the source in this outbreak was not established, this finding may have implications for spread in other situations, particularly for pet owners.[36]

EPIDEMIOLOGY

P. multocida has been isolated from humans in all areas of North America and Europe, with some reports coming from other areas. In the United States, it is not a reportable organism, so incidence and prevalence data are unavailable. Lee and Buhr[40] have cited a seasonal variation in the number of reported cases related to dog bites, with the highest incidence being in the fall and winter months, possibly related to increased nasal carriage in dogs during that period. Other investigators have found no seasonal differences.[18,44]

No difference in attack rate has been found between the sexes. The attack rate is higher in individuals of both sexes in very young (birth to 4 years old) and in older (>55 years old) individuals.

PATHOGENESIS AND PATHOLOGY

Animal Infection

In animals the organism is typically a colonizer, but it may invade via mucous membranes in animals under stress. Highly virulent strains can invade and cause septicemia, characterized by high fever, cardiac weakness, toxemia, and early death. Organisms can be cultured from the blood; autopsy findings from the affected animal may be minimal or include petechial hemorrhages on mucosal and serosal surfaces and in various organs. Animals can also develop pneumonia with a serofibrinous exudate in the interlobular septa of the lungs, a hemorrhagic gastroenteritis, and subacute and chronic infections such as otitis media.[72] The mechanisms by which these bacteria invade the mucosa and cause systemic disease continue to unfold. Key virulence factors are the capsule and lipopolysaccharide, with others still being identified.[29]

Human Infection

The most common infection for humans is the result of direct inoculation following an animal bite or scratch resulting in skin and soft tissue infection. Invasive disease, including septicemia and meningitis, as well as chronic pulmonary infection are described in humans. The pathology and pathogenesis are similar to those of other organisms, particularly other gram-negative organisms. Pulmonary infection is most common at the extremes of age as well as in immunocompromised individuals. Increasing numbers of invasive infections due to *Pasteurella multocida* have been reported in recipients of solid organ transplants.[13]

CLINICAL MANIFESTATIONS

In humans, three major types of infections occur.[71] In the most common type, local skin infection occurs after a cat bite or scratch, a dog bite, or, rarely, the bite of another animal. Many cases have also been associated with non-bite exposure, such as licking.[21] Local skin infection that follows an animal bite or scratch has a rapid onset of symptoms, a rapidly progressive acute cellulitis typically with in the first few hours of the incident, in contrast to infection caused by other organisms such as *Staphylococcus aureus*, where onset of symptoms is more typically delayed. The infection may be associated with generalized lymphatitis, local lymphadenitis, or both. A gray serous or sanguinopurulent discharge from the puncture sites may be noted at presentation, with surrounding soft tissue erythema and swelling. *Pasteurella* infection can also cause necrotizing fasciitis with similar pathophysiology to that caused by *Streptococcus pyogenes*. Puncture wounds can result in osteomyelitis or tenosynovitis if the injury is deep and penetrates these tissues. These deeper infections most often occur after bites from animals with sharp incisor teeth deposit the organism on or under the periosteum. These infections are most common following cat bites, but have been reported following puncture bites from other animals including dogs.

Signs of systemic toxicity, such as chills and fever, may be present and regional lymphadenopathy develops later. Less commonly, the infection may be lower grade and more indolent.[55] Patients typically have elevated leukocyte count with left shift and elevated inflammatory markers. Lee and Buhr[40] found *P. multocida* to be the most common infecting organism in a report of 69 dog bites that had been cultured; 20 of the bites became grossly infected, and *P. multocida* was isolated from 10. Of 30 wounds that were sutured, 14 (47%) were infected with *P. multocida*. Talan et al.[64] found that *Pasteurella* spp. were the most commonly isolated organisms isolated from 107 cat and dog bite infections. It was isolated from 50% of dog bites and 75% cat bites, with the majority of infections being polymicrobial for both types of bite. Other unusual localized infections include chronic skin ulcers, secondary infection of a gouty joint, and infection of a compound fracture site and an amputation site.[67]

The respiratory tract is the second most common location for *Pasteurella* infections, and, as with skin and soft tissue infections, *Pasteurella* is typically isolated along with other organisms in chronic pulmonary infections. Cases of bronchiectasis, pulmonary abscess, and empyema have been reported, usually in patients with underlying chronic pulmonary disease such as cystic fibrosis or bronchiectasis.[1,6,27,38]

Disseminated infection is the third major clinical manifestation of *Pasteurella* infection and these are commonly associated with antecedent animal exposure.[65] Many of these cases have associated meningitis, many of which were mistaken for *Haemophilus influenzae* or *Neisseria meningitidis* infection because of the morphologic similarities among these organisms. In a review of the subject in 1967, Controni and Jones[15] noted 14 confirmed cases of *Pasteurella* meningitis; 11 occurred in adults, and three occurred in children. Eight of the 14 patients had a history of accidental or surgical trauma. The mortality rate was 50%, but only five patients were treated with antibiotics. Evaluation of the cerebrospinal fluid showed white blood cell counts ranging from 580 to 5200/mm^3, all with a predominance of polymorphonuclear leukocytes. More recently, Green and coworkers[25] reviewed 29 cases of *P. multocida* meningitis in adults.

The first reported neonate with *Pasteurella* meningitis died at 88 hours of age.[7] The infant's mother had a fever in the postpartum period, but her pretreatment cultures were lost, so verification of the source was not possible.[15] Since then, a case of *Pasteurella* chorioamnionitis associated with premature delivery and neonatal sepsis and death within 1.5 hours of delivery has been reported,[63] as has a case of a fatal outcome for both mother and fetus after the mother sustained a cat bite at 37 weeks' gestation, resulting in overwhelming sepsis, death, and fetal demise.[54] Several young infants with septicemia and meningitis due to *Pasteurella* survived without apparent sequelae after treatment with penicillin or ampicillin and gentamicin. Pizey[52] reported infection in a 3-week-old infant with septic arthritis with no recognized animal contact. *P. multocida* infection may take a rapidly fatal course even in an older infant.[58,66] Clapp and associates[14] described two infants with invasive *Pasteurella* infection following nontraumatic facial licking by pets. In another report, in utero infection at 12 weeks' gestation was described, resulting in fetal death. In this case there was no known animal-related trauma, but the mother had both cats and dogs, and *Pasteurella* was isolated from gingival cultures of all animals in the home.[69] A neonate with meningitis and cervical spine osteomyelitis with full recovery has also been reported.[31,32] Other neonatal infections, primarily sepsis and meningitis, have been described with similar incidental exposure, usually licking by a pet. Bacteremia caused by *P. multocida* with concomitant meningitis due to echovirus 9 was described in a 22-day-old with good outcome.[3]

Guet-Revillet et al.[26] described 6 neonates with *P. multocida* meningitis in France over a 10-year period and reviewed an additional 42 cases reported worldwide in infants less than 1 year of age. The majority of these infections followed nontraumatic animal exposures; there was a high rate of neurologic complications (37.5%), and 6 (14%) of the infants died. Siahanidou et al.[59] reported horizontal household transmission from a dog to a grandmother to a neonate causing sepsis and meningitis. In this case, the mother of the infant tested negative for colonization or infection.

More unusual invasive infections have also been reported in children and adults. Larsen and Holden[39] described a 14-year-old girl with chronic otitis media for 2 years who developed a *P. multocida* cerebellar abscess. Nguefack et al.[46] described a case of a healthy 5-year-old boy with a large brain abscess caused by *P. multocida*, with the hypothesis that the infection was transmitted from a dog's saliva through an occult skull fracture A healthy man developed endocarditis with no known animal exposure,[9] and a case of epiglottitis caused by *P. multocida* has been reported in an adult.[37] A child developed Ludwig angina after non-bite exposure, and an adolescent boy with Kikuchi disease and *P. multocida* bacteremia has been described.[75] A 15-year-old boy with chronic lymphedema developed *P. multocida* bacteremic cellulitis of his penis and scrotum after local exposure to cat hair.[8] In a report of 136 cases of non–bite-related *P. multocida* infections, the respiratory tract was the most commonly reported site, followed by the abdomen and genitourinary tract. The organism has also been recovered from patients with appendicitis, and it has been cultured from the female reproductive tract, urine, and from a chronic sacral abscess.[5,34] Whether these cases were a result of ingestion of the organism or from hematogenous spread has not been determined. Raffi and colleagues[53] described three children with appendiceal peritonitis associated with *P. multocida.* The organism also has been isolated from infected peritoneal fluid in cases of peritoneal dialysis–associated peritonitis secondary to animal puncture of dialysis tubing[41,43] and from the conjunctival secretions in an immunocompromised man with acute conjunctivitis after ocular exposure to his dog's respiratory secretions.[16]

Giordano et al.[20] described the clinical features and outcomes of 44 cases of *P. multocida* infection with and without animal bite exposure. This report concluded that infections associated with non-bite exposure more frequently occurred in immunocompromised patients or in those with comorbidities. Non–bite-associated infections in these patients more frequently resulted in bacteremia, longer length of hospital stay, and higher mortality rate.

DIAGNOSIS AND TREATMENT

Diagnosis of *P. multocida* infection is made definitively by culture. *Pasteurella* may resemble several other organisms morphologically, which may lead to initial misidentification, but identification is not difficult for an experienced microbiologist. The organism does not require X and V factors for growth, distinguishing it from *H. influenzae.* Its production of indole differentiates it from the *Neisseria* group and its inability to grow on MacConkey agar or a bile salt medium distinguishes it from *Acinetobacter* spp. and the enteric organisms. Multiplex PCR allows laboratories to differentiate *P. multocida* strains on the basis of the organism's LPS genotype.[30]

The drug of choice for *P. multocida* infection is penicillin, to which the organism is exquisitely susceptible. This feature may be used to distinguish it from *H. influenzae* or the Enterobacteriaceae, organisms which are typically resistant to penicillin due to β-lactamase production. Rare strains of *P. multocida* that produce β-lactamase and are resistant to penicillins have been recovered.[56] The organism usually is sensitive to a wide variety of other antibiotics, including ampicillin, other broad-spectrum penicillins (e.g., piperacillin/tazobactam), amoxicillin/clavulanic acid,[22] tetracyclines, parenteral cephalosporins (particularly second- and third-generation agents and ceftaroline fosamil),[24,48] and chloramphenicol. Semisynthetic penicillins (e.g., nafcillin, dicloxacillin), erythromycin, some orally administered cephalosporins (cephalexin, cefaclor), and clindamycin (all antibiotics commonly used empirically for treatment of wound infections) have relatively low activity against *P. multocida*[61,17,23] and may lead to failure of initial therapy if used alone to treat or provide prophylaxis for wound infections due to animal bites. Azithromycin seems to have acceptable activity,[14] as does ciprofloxacin.[36] Trimethoprim-sulfamethoxazole is an acceptable alternative treatment, particularly for patients unable to take a β-lactam antibiotic,[57] but it will not provide adequate coverage for *Streptococcus pyogenes*, so must be used with in combination with another agent. Surgical drainage or debridement also may be necessary for areas of abscess or necrotic tissue. The duration of treatment depends on the primary disease process. Seven to 10 days generally is adequate for local infections, with longer courses indicated for meningitis and deeper infections, including those involving bones and joints.

PROGNOSIS AND PREVENTION

Proper cleansing and debridement of wounds caused by animal bites or scratches is important to prevent bacterial infection, including those caused by *P. multocida*. Lee and Buhr[40] found that suturing wounds caused by a dog bite was associated with a higher incidence of infection. Whether a wound is sutured often depends on the site and the potential cosmetic consequences of not suturing the wound. The use of prophylactic antibiotics following animal bites to prevent infection is guided by several factors. Most experts recommend their use for facial bites, those with delayed medical attention, for all cat bites and other deep puncture wounds, or for patients with immunocompromising conditions.[62]

Choice of antibiotic for prophylaxis following a bite should include coverage for *P. multocida* in addition to other common organisms implicated in skin and soft tissue infection. Typically amoxicillin-clavulanate is effective, and guidelines are available for other treatment options for patients with drug allergies.[62] Limiting contact with wild and domestic animals that may harbor the organism is probably the only definitive way to prevent infection. Teaching the proper handling of pets and keeping pets from licking infants and young children, as well as pregnant women, particularly on the face, may help.[51] No vaccine for human use is currently available.

Prognosis of infection with *P. multocida* depends on the particular site of infection, the extent of infection, and the immune status of the host. With appropriate and timely treatment, resolution usually occurs, but the healing process may be slow, particularly for local infections with extension to the bone or tendons.[18,68]

NEW REFERENCES SINCE THE SEVENTH EDITION

1. Abdelkarim A, et al. Empyema due to severe Pasteurella multocida treated with a quinolone: a case report. *Am J Ther.* 2014;21(6):e204-e206.
2. Abrahamian FM, Goldstein EJ. Microbiology of animal bite wound infections. *Clin Microbiol Rev.* 2011;24(2):231-246.
3. Aguado I, Calvo C, Wilhelmi I, et al. Sepsis and meningitis caused by *Pasteurella multocida* and echovirus 9 in a neonate. *Pediatr Infect Dis J.* 2014;33(12).
4. Ahmad TA, Rammah SS, Sheweita SA, Haroun M, El-Sayed LH. Development of immunization trials against *Pasteurella multocida. Vaccine.* 2013;32:909-917.
5. Arashima Y, Kumasaka K, Tsuchiya T, Kawano K, Yamazaki E. Current status of *Pasteurella multocida* infection in Japan. *Kansenshogaku Zasshi.* 1993;67:791-794.
6. Atin HL, et al. Pasteurella multocida empyema. Report of a case. *N Engl J Med.* 1957;256:979-981.
8. Blasiak RC, Morrell DS, Burkhart CN. *Pasteurella multocida* cellulitis in a 15-year-old male with chronic lymphedema. *J Am Acad Dermatol.* 2013;68(6):e183-e184.
9. Branch J, Kakutani T, Kuroda S, Shiba Y, Kitagawa I. *Pasteurella multocida* infective endocarditis: a possible link with primary upper respiratory tract infection. *Intern Med.* 2015;54(24):3225-3231.
10. Brugnatelli E. Batteriemia puerperale da bacillo del gruppo della "setticemia emorragica" (Pasteurelle). *Pensiero Med.* 1913;3:305-308.
13. Christenson ES, Ahmed HM, Durand CM. *Pasteurella multocida* infection in solid organ transplantation. *Lancet Infect Dis.* 2015;15:235-240.
16. Corchia A, Limelette A, Hubault B, et al. Rapidly evolving conjunctivitis due to *Pasteurella multocida,* occurring after direct inoculation with animal droplets in an immuno-compromised host. *BMC Ophthalmol.* 2015;15:21.
19. Hunt Gerardo S, Citron DM, Claros MC, Fernandez HT, Goldstein E. *Pasteurella multocida* subsp. *multocida* and *P. multocida* subsp. *septica* differentiation by PCR fingerprinting and alpha-glucosidase activity. *J Clin Microbiol.* 2001;2558-2564.
20. Giordano A, Dincman T, Clyburn BE, Steed LL, Rockey DC. Clinical features and outcomes of *Pasteurella multocida* infection. *Medicine (Baltimore).* 2015; 94(36):e1285.
24. Goldstein EJ, Citron DM, Merriam CV, Tyrrell KL. Ceftaroline versus isolates from animal bite wounds: comparative in vitro activities against 243 isolates, including 156 *Pasteurella* species isolates. *Antimicrob Agents Chemother.* 2012;56:6319-6323.
26. Guet-Revillet H, Levy C, Andriantahina I, et al. Paediatric epidemiology of *Pasteurella multocida* meningitis in France and review of the literature. *Eur J Clin Microbiol Infect Dis.* 2013;32:1111-1120.
27. Hamada M. Infective exacerbation of *Pasteurella multocida. Case Rep Infect Dis.* 2016;2016:2648349.
30. Harper M, John M, Turni C. Development of a rapid multiplex PCR assay to genotype *Pasteurella multocida* strains by use of the lipopolysaccharide outer core biosynthesis locus. *J Clin Microbiol.* 2015;53:477-485.
35. Hundeshagen K. Ein Bacillus aus der Gruppe der hamorrhagischen septikamie bei einem fall von influenza-pleuritis. *Med Klin.* 1919;15:1008-1010.

38. Kagihara JM, Brahmbhatt NM, Paladino J. A fatal *Pasteurella* empyema. *Lancet.* 2014;384:468.
42. López C, Sanchez-Rubio P, Betrán A, Terré R. *Pasteurella multocida* bacterial meningitis caused by contact with pigs. *Braz J Microbiol.* 2013;44(2):473-474.
46. Nguefack S, Moifo B, Chiabi A, et al. Pasteurella multocida meningitis with cerebral abscesses. *Arch Pediatr.* 2014;21(3):306-308.
50. Oehler RL, Velez AP, Mizrachi M, Lamarche J, Gompf S. Bite-related and septic syndromes caused by cats and dogs. *Lancet Infect Dis.* 2009;9:439-447.
51. Pickering LK. Exposure to nontraditional pets at home and to animals in public settings: risks to children. Committee on Infectious Diseases. *Pediatrics.* 2008;122(4):876-886.
54. Rasaiah B, Otero JG, Russell IJ, et al. *Pasteurella multocida* septicemia during pregnancy. *Can Med Assoc J.* 1986;135:1369-1371.
59. Siahanidou T, Gika G, Skiathitou AV, et al. *Pasteurella multocida* Infection in a neonate: evidence for a human-to-human horizontal transmission. *Pediatr Infect Dis J.* 2012;31(5):536-537.
62. Stevens DL, Bisno AL, Chambers HF, et al. Practice guidelines for the diagnosis and management of skin and soft tissue infections: 2014 update by the Infectious Diseases Society of America. *Clin Infect Dis.* 2014;59(2):147-159.
64. Talan DA, Citron DM, Abrahamian FM, Moran GJ, Goldstein EJ. Bacteriologic analysis of infected dog and cat bites. Emergency Medicine Animal Bite Infection Study Group. *N Engl J Med.* 1999;340:85-92.
65. Talley P, Snippes-Vagnone P, Smith K. Invasive Pasteurella multocida infections-report of five cases at a Minnesota hospital, 2014. *Zoonoses Public Health.* 2016;63(6):431-435.
72. Wilkie IW, Harper M, Boyce JD, Adler B. Pasteurella multocida: diseases and pathogenesis. *Curr Top Microbiol Immunol.* 2012;361:1-22.
73. Wilson BA. Pasteurella multocida: from zoonosis to cellular microbiology. *Clin Microbiol Rev.* 2013;26(3):631-655.

The full reference list for this chapter is available at ExpertConsult.com.

Cholera 117

Randy G. Mungwira • Matthew B. Laurens

Cholera is a toxin-mediated, secretory diarrheal illness caused by the bacteria *Vibrio cholerae.* Disease course varies from mild and self-limiting to severe and life-threatening. The most serious manifestation, *cholera gravis,* presents with rapid intravascular volume depletion and shock and can lead to death within 12 to 24 hours. The rapid progression to dehydration and explosive nature of outbreaks give reason for cholera to be one of the most feared public health threats. Cholera is also considered a disease of poverty because it disproportionately affects low-income countries.[115] Epidemic, endemic, and a mixture of the two forms occur. Epidemic cholera typically occurs in populations with little preexisting immunity and affects both children and adults. Endemic cholera tends to affect children with a higher incidence and severity because of lower levels of acquired immunity relative to adults.[31]

Cholera incidence has increased since 2000.[129] In 2014, 42 countries, mostly in sub-Saharan Africa and Asia, reported 190,549 cases, 2231 deaths, and a 1.2% case-fatality rate.[129,130] The United States reported seven cases in 2014, all imported.[129,130] Cholera disease burden is considered vastly underreported, and the actual number of cases is estimated at 2.9 million annually (range, 1.3–4 million), with 95,000 deaths (range, 21,000–143,000 deaths).[92] In recent times, outbreaks occurred in Tanzania, Malawi, Democratic Republic of Congo, the Republic of Congo, Cameroon, Chad, Niger, Iraq, Nigeria, Sudan, Somalia, Angola, Zimbabwe, and Haiti.[126,131,134] In 2011, Haiti reported more than 500,000 cholera cases and 7000 deaths shortly after the October 2010 outbreak,[78] caused by a *V. cholerae* O1 variant similar to epidemic isolates from Southern Asia and Africa.[49] The case-fatality rate during the Haitian outbreak began at 7%, one of the highest recorded in recent history, and then fell to 1.3%, just slightly above the generally accepted benchmark of 1%.[33] Many organizations advocate for an integrated and comprehensive approach to control and prevention of this relatively neglected global public health problem.

HISTORY

Cholera has long been indigenous to the Ganges River Valley in northern India; however, the modern history of cholera is described in seven discrete pandemics, all originating from Asia and all presumably caused by the O1 serogroup.[10] The first six pandemics, caused by the classic biotype, occurred between 1817 and 1923. The ongoing seventh pandemic began in Indonesia and South East Asia in 1961, and then spread throughout Asia and Africa. By 1991, it appeared in Peru and spread throughout Latin America. This most recent pandemic was caused by the El Tor biotype, which has almost completely replaced the classic biotype and is the longest and most widespread of all pandemics to date.[10] Several atypical El Tor variants containing phenotypic and genetic characteristics of the classic biotype have been identified, suggesting the emergence of hybrids.[103] In 1992, the first non-O1 serogroup isolated in association with an epidemic was reported.[102] This new O139 Bengal serogroup emerged in India and Bangladesh, raising concern for an eighth pandemic, but it has not spread beyond the region to date. A novel strain of disease causing nontoxigenic O139 serogroup has recently been reported in Bangladesh.[26]

The disastrous saga of cholera over the past 2 centuries helped shape public health as a discipline. Beginning in 1826, during the second cholera pandemic, many jurisdictions were induced to establish local sanitation and health boards, eventually evolving into the first organized public health apparatus. During the 1854 London cholera epidemic, investigations by Dr. John Snow demonstrated that disease transmission was associated with contaminated drinking water consumption from the city's infamous Broad Street pump; this episode is considered the first scientific public health investigation and gave rise to modern epidemiology.[39] In 1866, an epidemic in New York City led to the creation of the first Board of Health in the United States, and cholera became the first reportable disease.

The Italian scientist Fillipo Pacini identified the comma-shaped organism in 1854, but this discovery was overlooked until Robert Koch identified the cholera bacillus in 1883 during the fifth pandemic. Koch's cholera discoveries contributed to his pioneering work that began the field of Medical Microbiology.[39] The addition of glucose to enhance the absorption of sodium in oral rehydration therapy, the cornerstone of cholera treatment, has saved millions of lives and is heralded as one of the most important medical advancements of the 20th century.[39]

MICROBIOLOGY

V. cholerae is a curved gram-negative rod classified by biochemical tests and subdivided into serogroups based on the somatic O antigen. It belongs to the family Vibrionaceae of Proteobacteria, which differs from the related family Enterobacteriaceae in being oxidase-positive and motile with a single flagellum. Vibrios are fermentative and oxidative in metabolism. They have few nutritional requirements and can grow in glucose as the sole carbon and energy source. Most vibrios are marine organisms, and most grow best in 2% to 3% sodium chloride under aerobic conditions. Although neither the typical comma shape of *V.*

cholerae nor its motility is seen on Gram stain, both are apparent in wet mount even on fresh fecal samples. If motility stops after adding anti-*Vibrio* antiserum, this establishes a presumptive diagnosis of the homologous organism.

Numerous *Vibrio* spp. exist, most of which are nonpathogenic in humans. *V. cholerae* spp. includes more than 200 serogroups classified according to the antigenic characteristics of the lipopolysaccharide O antigen.[13] To date, only *V. cholerae* organisms carrying the somatic O antigens O1 and O139 are associated with epidemic disease. Some non–O1 *V. cholerae* serogroups cause sporadic diarrheal illness, which can be severe and sometimes invasive and inflammatory.

The O1 serogroup is divided further into two biotypes, classic and El Tor, based on biochemical properties and phage susceptibilities. The classic biotype traditionally causes a more severe disease, but the El Tor biotype may be better adapted to persist in the environment and establish epidemics. The classical biotype expresses genes conferring human virulence more than the El Tor biotype, which shows enhanced gene expression for biofilm formation, chemotaxis, and transport of amino acids, peptides, and iron.[13] Classic and El Tor biotypes are divided into three serotypes (i.e., Ogawa, Inaba, and Hikojima) based on their dominant heat-stable lipopolysaccharide somatic antigens. The O139 serogroup comprises several genetically diverse strains, including nontoxigenic variants, and is genetically related to the O1 El Tor biotype.[35] Media used to isolate cholera organisms in stool include thiosulfate citrate bile salts sucrose (TCBS) agar and tellurite taurocholate gelatin agar. The appearance of yellow ("popcorn") colonies on TCBS agar is considered highly suggestive of *V. cholerae*. The bacterium is confirmed further by its ability to grow in the presence (or absence) of salt and by serology.

PATHOGENESIS

The pathogenic paradigm of *V. cholerae* comprises small bowel mucosa colonization followed by release of one or more enterotoxins, the most potent of which is the oligomeric cholera toxin itself. *V. cholerae* attaches to the intestinal mucosa by virtue of proteinaceous hairlike fimbriae, the most important being the toxin-coregulated pilus.[102] These pili mediate microcolony formation of the intestinal epithelium. Colonization is facilitated by a protease that degrades mucin[110] and epithelial tight junction–associated proteins and a single flagellum, which accelerates approach to the intestinal mucosa in conjunction with chemotactic receptors and intracellular sensor molecules.[17]

V. cholerae organisms shed in an infected individual's stool act more virulently than strains acquired from an environmental source. Serial passage through multiple patients may augment virulence further, partly accounting for the violent epidemics occurring throughout history.[77] On intestinal passage, genes required for acquiring nutrients and motility are upregulated, whereas genes required for chemotaxis are downregulated. This increased virulence was confirmed in an animal model in which *V. cholerae* shed by mice has a 10-fold lower infectious dose than organisms grown in vitro.[77] Reduced chemotaxis prevents dispersion in environmental waters and increases bacterial clumping[18]; the resulting increased concentration of organisms also may contribute to the vigor of cholera outbreaks.

Cholera toxin is composed of five identical binding (B) subunits and one active (A) subunit. Similar in structure and function to the heat-labile toxin produced by enterotoxigenic *Escherichia coli*,[83] cholera toxin binds to the GM_1 ganglioside receptor on the intestinal epithelial cell surface. The A subunit is internalized into the cell, where it activates adenylate cyclase by ADP-ribosylation of the $G_{s\alpha}$ protein. This results in cyclic adenosine monophosphate upregulation, causing an increase in chloride secretion from the intestinal crypt cells via the cystic fibrosis transmembrane conductance regulator chloride channel and a decrease in sodium chloride absorption by the villous cells. In addition to this mechanism, cholera toxin may have effects on prostaglandins and the enteric nervous system that could contribute to the voluminous diarrhea characteristic of the disease.[64] Water follows electrolyte loss along the osmotic gradient into the intestinal lumen. The dramatic fluid and electrolyte loss rapidly leads to decreased intravascular volume and to the complications of hypovolemic shock and metabolic acidosis. Although cholera toxin is responsible for much of the pathogenicity associated with the organism, strains mutated in cholera toxin still elicit mild diarrhea.[64] Several other toxins have been identified, but their exact role in pathogenesis and immune modulation is not completely understood. These include the zonula occludens toxin, which increases small intestinal mucosa permeability through internal tight junction modulation, and the accessory cholera enterotoxin, an integral membrane protein thought to function as an ion-permeable pore.[23,36,122] The multifunctional cholera toxin protein is also a powerful immunomodulator and may have potential applications in immunotherapeutics and as a mucosal or possibly epicutaneous adjuvant.[14,90]

The genetics of *V. cholerae* provide insight into the organism's pathogenicity and spread. The genome of 4 million DNA base pairs comprises two circular chromosomes,[32,51] the larger of which contains genes for growth and pathogenicity, and the smaller contains metabolism and regulation elements. The genes required for virulence can propagate laterally and among different strains. Required for pathogenicity are the cholera toxin genetic element and the *Vibrio* pathogenicity island, which encodes toxin-coregulated pilus and the critical regulator ToxT, the primary direct transcriptional virulence gene activator. The pathogenicity island can be moved between strains by phage transduction and chitin-induced transformation. Toxigenic strains emerge through the acquisition of the bacteriophage CTXΦ, which harbors the *ctxAB* gene encoding cholera toxin.[76] The complex regulatory system controlling virulence gene expression includes the ToxT/ToxR regulator proteins, quorum sensing, and small RNA molecule, and differs among in vivo and in vitro life stages[16,53,76] and between clinical and environmental isolates.[80]

EPIDEMIOLOGY

Cholera is classically described as a waterborne illness, but it can also be transmitted via contaminated food. The incubation period depends on the inoculum, with lower inocula corresponding to a longer incubation period and decreased stool volumes.[64] Incubation generally is 1 to 3 days, with a range of several hours to 5 days. Symptoms usually last 2 to 3 days, and patients treated with antibiotics may be infectious for several days. Patients who are untreated remain infectious for 1 to 2 weeks. Although waterborne transmission is typical in developing countries of Asia and Africa, *V. cholerae* found in marine environments can be transmitted via undercooked shellfish.[30] The role of household animals in transmission is probably minimal.[107] Person-to-person transmission was previously considered rare due to the high infectious dose,[84] but a recent study in Bangladesh documented up to 5% risk of household transmission during an 11-day infectious period compared to a 5% to 9% risk of infection over a 30-day period due to community-based exposure.[111] This investigation also documented increased susceptibility of children younger than 5 years compared to adults (odds ratio, 1.5–1.7).

Seasonal patterns in endemic areas have long been recognized for cholera outbreaks, with a predilection for warmer months. Studies conducted during interepidemic periods suggest a complex interaction between humans and the environment. *V. cholerae* exists in saline aquatic environments in a viable but nonculturable state, mostly in the form of metabolically dormant biofilm associated with zooplankton.[55,116] This latent form originates from human stool, survives gastric acidity, and causes infection. When human cases begin to occur in a community, direct food and water contamination may occur, circumventing the need for the aquatic reservoir.[34] Seasonal epidemics are associated with other factors that affect the environmental reservoir, including changes in zooplankton blooms, chitin abundance, and rainfall. Several cholera prediction models have been developed based on these factors and may be critical in preventing epidemics.[2,60,61,75,97,98] Recent evidence from Bangladesh and Haiti suggests that increases in vibrio-infecting bacteriophages can facilitate *V. cholerae* genetic evolution, affecting virulence and human infection, factors that may contribute to outbreak cessation and also allow epidemic-free periods in cholera endemic regions.[108,109]

Host factors associated with susceptibility to *V. cholerae* include age, immunity, blood type, and reduced gastric acid production. Age groups commonly affected by cholera typically include young children because susceptibility depends on preexisting immunity. In endemic areas such as Bangladesh, cholera cases are concentrated in the 2- to 9-year-old age category, followed by women of childbearing age.[29,64] The increased susceptibility of children is further supported by a more recent prospective study in Kolkata, India, where cholera burden was greatest in children younger than 2 years, and cases were more likely where a household member had diarrhea.[47,112] Mucosal humoral immune responses in both children and adults to *V. cholerae* may be decreased with intestinal helminth coinfection.[47] Breastfeeding protects against disease in children colonized with *V. cholerae*.[29,41] Animal models suggest that offspring acquire passive immunity from vaccinated female mice.[93] Achlorhydric patients are at higher risk for acquiring infection because bacteria are more likely to survive the gastric environment and colonize the small intestine.[87] Observations of increased cholera severity among people with blood type O were confirmed through challenge and cohort studies,[46,70] presumably because of blood type O antigen binding to cholera toxin.[50] For reasons that are not completely understood, individuals with the Lewis blood group Le(a+b–) phenotype may also be at increased risk for symptomatic disease in contrast to those with Le(a–b+) and Le(a–b–).[7] Other host genetic factors likely also play a role, as evidenced by familial clustering of cases and gene association studies.[43,65,69,95]

CLINICAL MANIFESTATIONS

Most individuals infected with *V. cholerae* have only mild symptoms, indistinguishable from symptoms caused by other enteric infections. Individuals who develop disease urgently need fluid resuscitation and replacement of ongoing losses. Among all causes of infectious diarrhea, the stool volumes passed and the rapidity by which dehydration develops are greatest with cholera.[106] In severe disease, stool volume can exceed 250/mL per kg body weight in a 24-hour period.[81,94]

The most distinctive clinical feature of cholera is the painless passage of voluminous, watery stools. Termed "rice water stools" because of the watery, colorless diarrhea dotted with mucus, cholera stools may have a fishy smell or may be nearly odorless. Other common symptoms include abdominal cramping and vomiting. Abdominal cramping is probably due to increased abdominal secretions and resulting small bowel distention. Vomiting commonly occurs a few hours after diarrhea onset due to decreased gastric and intestinal motility, but it also occurs later in the course of the illness due to lactic acidosis.[19,48,86,105] Patients with clinical symptoms do not typically present with fever.[21,105]

Complications of cholera relate mostly to the massive intravascular volume and electrolyte loss. If cholera is not treated promptly, diarrhea and vomiting eventually lead to dehydration, which is most often isotonic. Patients with severe cholera may experience vascular collapse, shock, and death rates of 50%, starting within hours after diarrhea onset.[102] Related to the massive intravascular volume loss and hypoperfusion, bicarbonate losses in stool, and hyperphosphatemia, acidosis also may develop.[124,125] Compensatory tachypnea may be seen in patients with acidosis. In addition to bicarbonate losses in stool, potassium is also lost and may not be reflected in serum potassium levels; acidosis induces the intracellular potassium shift into the intravascular space in exchange for hydrogen ions, resulting in decreased total body potassium and potentially normal serum potassium values. As the acidosis is corrected, serum hypokalemia may result. In cases complicated by severe malnutrition, in which body potassium stores already are depleted, hypokalemia may be quite severe and manifest as paralytic ileus. This hypokalemia is rarely associated with severe cardiac arrhythmias, but it may manifest as changes on electrocardiogram.

After dehydration, hypoglycemia is the second most common cause of death in pediatric patients with cholera.[12] In one study, the mortality rate in pediatric patients with hypoglycemia caused by cholera was 15% in contrast to 1% mortality in patients with normoglycemia.[12] Although the precise mechanism of hypoglycemia is unknown, malnourished children who are acutely ill have lower glycogen stores and impaired gluconeogenesis. Special attention should be given to monitor patients with concomitant malnutrition and cholera for hypoglycemia.

Severe cholera is diagnosed in individuals who present with clinical signs and symptoms of severe dehydration (loss of ≥15% of total body water or loss of ~10% of body weight). Common signs of severe volume depletion include a combination of decreased skin turgor, depressed anterior fontanelle in infants, lack of tears and sunken eyes, dry mouth, anuria, tachycardia, decreased peripheral perfusion, and hypotension (Fig. 117.1). In some cases, mental status changes may be a sign of volume depletion, but more common are somnolence, restlessness, and lethargy.

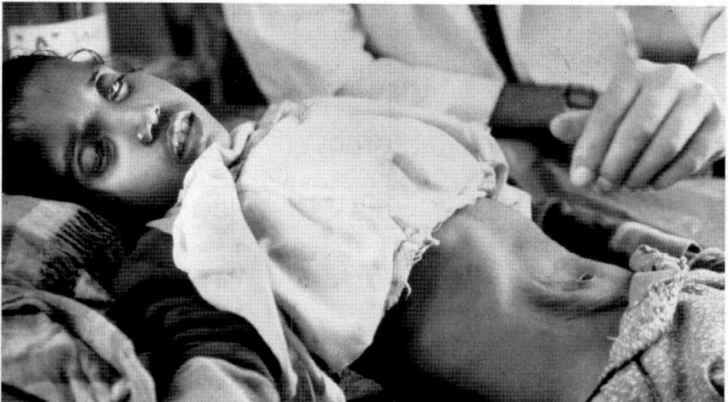

FIG. 117.1 An adolescent girl with severe dehydration from cholera. Characteristic features include obtundation, sunken eyes, and "tenting" of the abdominal skin and subcutaneous tissues after firmly pinching the abdomen.

LABORATORY FINDINGS AND DIAGNOSIS

Laboratory abnormalities in patients with cholera relate to the massive volume and electrolyte loss. The hypovolemic state can lead to hemoconcentration, causing increased hematocrit, serum specific gravity, serum protein, serum creatinine, and blood urea nitrogen.[124,125] Because of the sodium loss that accompanies water loss, serum sodium is either slightly low or normal.[64,94] As noted earlier, although potassium loss occurs in the stool, serum potassium may be normal, whereas total body potassium may be decreased. Acidosis caused by bicarbonate loss in stool and lactic acidosis can result in a serum bicarbonate concentration of less than 15 mmol/L.[124,125] Serum creatinine and blood urea nitrogen also are elevated as a result of a decreased glomerular filtration rate. The common abnormalities of sodium, potassium, bicarbonate, and glucose mandate early determination of serum glucose and electrolytes as a guide to therapy.

Although presumptive diagnosis is made on the basis of typical oxidase-positive colonies from stool samples that agglutinate with O1 or O139 antiserum, conventional culture methods remain the gold standard. The characteristically motile organisms can be visualized directly using darkfield microscopy,[11] but few laboratories except those in cholera-endemic regions are experienced with this technique. If cholera is suspected, special culture media, such as TCBS agar, should be used to culture the organism.

In epidemic settings or in areas of intense transmission, a rapid vibrio dipstick test may be used. This is a one-step immunochromatographic test developed by the Institut Pasteur for rapid detection of cholera O1 and O139 from stool samples. The method was tested in Madagascar, Bangladesh, and Mozambique, achieving 84% to 100% specificity and 94% to 100% sensitivity.[88,123] It is especially advantageous because it requires minimal technical skill, can be read in 10 minutes,[88] and detects cholera from rectal swabs.[15,123] Rapid diagnostic test specificity improves with alkaline peptone water enrichment of fecal samples.[38] Several other rapid diagnostic tools have been developed for field use including immunochromatographic lateral flow tests which can diagnose *V. cholerae* O1 serotype Ogawa within 5 minutes.[25] Confirmation of *V. cholerae* in stool also can be done using polymerase chain reaction amplification or oligoprobes.[54,79,121]

TREATMENT

The cornerstone of cholera management is fluid resuscitation. When fluid resuscitation is initiated, previous losses must be estimated based

TABLE 117.1 Electrolyte Concentration in Cholera Stool and in Fluids Used for Rehydration and Replacement of Stool Losses

	ELECTROLYTE CONCENTRATION (MMOL/L)				
	Na^+	Cl^-	K^+	HCO_3^-	Osmolality
Cholera Stool					
Adults	130	100	20	44	300[a]
Infants and children	100	90	33	30	300[a]
Hydration Solutions					
WHO oral rehydration	75	65	20	10[b]	170[c]
Intravenous					
Dhaka	133	98	13	48	273
Lactated Ringer's solution	130	109	4	28[d]	251
5:4:1[e]	129	97	11	44	281

WHO, World Health Organization.
[a]Osmolality includes unmeasured osmotically active molecules (primarily organic acids) in addition to electrolytes.
[b]As citrate.
[c]From electrolytes only; also contains 75 mmol/L of glucose.
[d]As lactate.
[e]Intravenous solution containing 5 g sodium chloride, 4 g sodium bicarbonate, and 1 g potassium chloride per liter.

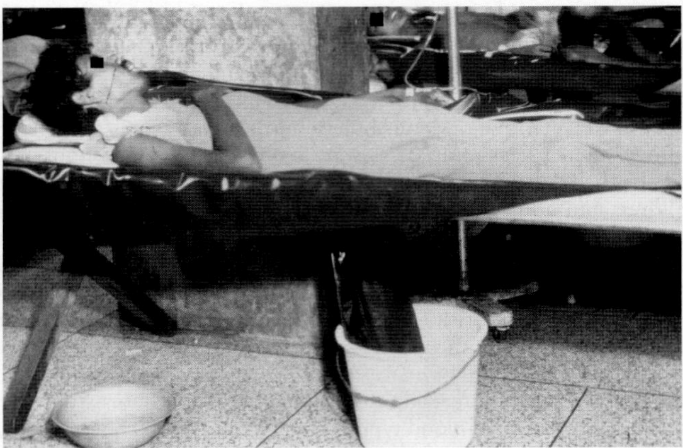

FIG. 117.2 A cholera cot is a simple folding cot covered with plastic that has a hole and bucket for collecting the stool output, as used for the care of cholera patients at the International Centre for Diarrhoeal Disease Research, Bangladesh. The bucket is calibrated, and the volume of stool (and replacement fluids required) can be calculated easily. The plastic sheet is cleaned daily and between patients.

on the degree of dehydration and replaced, and ongoing losses must be quantified and replenished. Replacement fluids in children with cholera should be similar to fluids that are lost, such as lactated Ringer solution (Table 117.1).[52,127] The ideal solution contains amounts of bicarbonate and potassium sufficient to replace what is lost in stool.

At the International Centre for Diarrhoeal Disease Research, Bangladesh, where thousands of cholera patients are treated annually, patients of all ages are seen with severe dehydration of rapid onset. Many arrive for treatment in hypovolemic shock. The extent of dehydration is determined, one or two intravenous catheters are inserted, and isotonic resuscitation solution is administered rapidly. The composition of the preferred solution at the Center (Dhaka solution) is listed in Table 117.1. The solution contains Na^+, Cl^-, K^+, and HCO_3^-, but no glucose. The complete estimated deficit is administered over the course of 4 hours, whereupon ongoing losses and maintenance fluids are provided. Serum glucose and electrolytes are determined rapidly, with glucose administration as needed based on these results. Because severely dehydrated patients characteristically are anuric, concern may exist over early potassium administration. The rapid onset of dehydration in cholera patients reduces this risk, however, and acute tubular necrosis is rarely seen.[94,125] A greater concern may be the rapid shift of potassium from the circulation on correction of acidosis. Patients treated in this manner respond dramatically. After the 4-hour resuscitation phase, most patients can begin to accept oral rehydration solution. Close attention to fluids and electrolytes is required for the duration of diarrhea.

Although oral and intravenous rehydration methods are acceptable in theory for cholera management, the severity of losses in severe cholera renders intravenous rehydration the mainstay for treatment initiation in these cases. Not only do intravenous fluids allow predictable and rapid intravascular fluid volume expansion to occur, they also ensure timely replacement of ongoing losses that may be challenging because of excessive purging.[91] As massive fluid volumes are lost in severe cholera, the volume deficit is frequently underestimated and rehydration therapy is often inadequate. Treatment of severe cases is best carried out by those with adequate training and experience in managing cholera. In cases where peripheral intravenous access is challenging, parenteral fluid resuscitation in severely dehydrated children can be achieved via scalp veins or via intraosseous access.[105] Mild cases can be managed with oral rehydration solution (see later discussion). Oral rehydration can also be administered via nasogastric tube in patients who are not able to drink or when IV access is problematic. Guidelines for the initial management of cholera in an outbreak setting have been published by the World Health Organization (WHO) Global Task Force on Cholera Control.[128]

Use of a "cholera cot" is extremely helpful in quantifying ongoing fluid loss and for patient comfort (Fig. 117.2) and can easily be set up in cholera treatment centers. It is constructed of a simple cot with a hole in the center through which a plastic sheet drains into a graduated bucket below via a funnel. This allows for accurate quantification of ongoing losses and permits the patient to remain horizontal, an important advantage if the patient is initially hypotensive. Attention given to tachycardia and signs of hypoperfusion in prostrate patients is essential.

The WHO-approved oral rehydration salts (see Table 117.1) are recommended for patients with no detectable dehydration or mild dehydration, provided that the patient can drink sufficient quantities to replace the deficit and keep pace with ongoing losses. Oral rehydration solution can also be used for patients with severe dehydration to replace ongoing losses after initial intravenous replacement therapy. For cholera, oral rehydration solution that is made with rice rather than with glucose is preferred because carbohydrate reduces the purging rate.[44,82,135] In resource-limited settings and remote areas, homemade oral rehydration salts can be prepared by dissolving half a small spoon of salt and six level small spoons of sugar in 1 L of clean water to initiate rehydration.[100] Food should be offered to patients as soon as they are able to eat, and breast-feeding in children should not be restricted. Supplementation with zinc reduces diarrhea duration and stool volume in children with cholera.[101] Effective oral rehydration solution use requires extra effort in pediatric patients. Parents need instruction to encourage and supervise oral rehydration solution intake by the child, including taking as much as 20 ml/kg body weight per hour.[20] Parents also need reassurance that oral rehydration is still effective despite occasional vomiting.

A short course of antibiotics should be given to children with clinically significant cholera. This approach reduces the amount of diarrhea, the duration of illness, and the infectious dose in stools.[42,102] Antibiotic therapy may also favorably affect transmission dynamics and hence have public health implications.[89] Because of high resistance rates in some areas, the organism should be isolated and tested for susceptibility using standard methods for gram-negative enteric bacteria. On average, patients not treated with antibiotics may continue to shed organisms for 5 or more days.[71]

Treatment options for cholera in pediatric patients are listed in Table 117.2. First-line therapies for *V. cholerae* in children include single-dose azithromycin or erythromycin for 3 days in younger children, and a single dose of doxycycline may be given to children older than 8 years. Tetracycline and doxycycline are generally not recommended

TABLE 117.2 Antimicrobial Therapy of Cholera[a]

Agent	Single Dose	Multiple Dose
Azithromycin	20 mg/kg; maximal dose 1 g	
Erythromycin	Not evaluated	50 mg/kg/day erythromycin divided into 4 doses for 3 days; maximal dose 2 g/day
Doxycycline	2–4 mg/kg; maximal dose 300 mg	
Tetracycline	Not evaluated	50 mg/kg/day divided into 4 doses for 3 days; maximal dose 2 g/day
Ciprofloxacin[b]	20 mg/kg; maximal dose 1 g	30 mg/kg/day divided into 2 doses for 3 days; maximal dose 1 g/day
Trimethoprim-sulfamethoxazole	Not evaluated	10 mg trimethoprim/50 mg sulfamethoxazole/kg/day divided into 2 doses for 5 days; maximal doses 320 mg trimethoprim and 1.6 g sulfamethoxazole daily
Ampicillin	Not evaluated	50 mg/kg/day divided into 4 doses for 3 days; maximal dose 2 g/day
Furazolidone	7 mg/kg; maximal dose 300 mg[c]	5 mg/kg/day divided into 4 doses for 3 days; maximal dose 400 mg/day

[a]Antimicrobial therapy is an adjunct to fluid therapy for cholera and is not an essential component. It reduces diarrhea volume and duration, however, by approximately 50%. The choice of antimicrobial agent is determined by the susceptibility pattern of local strains of *Vibrio cholerae* O1 or O139. Resistance to all agents has been reported and is common in some areas.
[b]The fluoroquinolones, such as ciprofloxacin, are only approved for use in children younger than 18 years in the United States for special indications because of concerns about arthropathy; multidose therapy has not been evaluated systematically in children, and recommendations are extrapolated from experience in adults.
[c]Single-dose therapy with these drugs has not been evaluated systematically in children, and recommendations are extrapolated from experience in adults.

in children younger than 8 years because of the risk for dental staining. In addition, ciprofloxacin is also effective against susceptible strains.[89] Trimethoprim-sulfamethoxazole has demonstrated efficacy in children,[62] although resistance may be present among O139 strains.[3] Both single-dose azithromycin 20 mg/kg and single dose ciprofloxacin 20 mg/kg achieved clinical success rates similar to a 12-dose course of erythromycin in children 15 years of age or younger, but ciprofloxacin was less effective in eradicating *V. cholerae* from the stool.[67,104] Recently, single-dose azithromycin showed superiority to single-dose ciprofloxacin in children.[66]

Multidrug-resistant *V. cholerae* strains have been isolated from both clinical and environmental settings, and the number of pathogenic strains resistant to one or more antibiotics is increasing.[68] Several different drug resistance mechanisms have been reported and include extended-spectrum β-lactamase production, enhanced multidrug efflux pump activity, plasmid-mediated quinolone and fluoroquinolone resistance, and chromosomal mutations.[9,40,45,117] The horizontal transfer of resistance determinants with mobile genetic elements such as integrons and the integrating conjugative elements assist in drug resistance dissemination.[40] SXT, first identified in a *V. cholerae* O139 strain from India, is an integrating conjugative element carrying a resistance gene for trimethoprim-sulfamethoxazole, streptomycin, and chloramphenicol.[40] Appropriate antibiotics, usually prescribed before obtaining sensitivity testing results, should be administered according to local resistance patterns and should be monitored for changes in sensitivity. Antibiotic prophylaxis is not indicated for health care workers providing care to cholera patients.[56]

PREVENTION

Because contaminated food and water are the main transmission routes of pathogenic *V. cholerae,* strategies to improve access to safe water sources and a clean food supply are the best methods for prevention. Proper sanitation methods also play a key role. During outbreaks, measures to increase awareness of cholera transmission and means to decrease spread should be communicated to the public. These measures include proper hand washing (especially after defecating), proper food preparation, and identifying ill individuals so they can be treated. Setting up an organized response amid explosive outbreaks is challenging in resource-limited settings, but a coordinated, multidisciplinary response can limit mortality and secondary transmission.[118]

Vaccination is another prevention method. Whole-cell, inactivated parenteral vaccines have been superseded by inactivated oral vaccines and are currently the only cholera vaccines commercially available and are used mostly as travel vaccines. The whole-cell plus B subunit vaccine (WC-rBS; Dukoral) consists of approximately 1×10^{33} inactivated whole cell classic and El Tor *V. cholerae* O1, serotypes Inaba and Ogawa with 1 mg of recombinant cholera toxin B subunit. The vaccine is WHO-prequalified and approved for children 24 months of age or older. It is supplied as 3 mL single-dose vials that require refrigeration, each provided with a sachet of sodium bicarbonate buffer prepared by dissolving the contents in 150 mL of water immediately before consumption. Two doses administered at least 15 days apart are recommended for adults and three doses for children younger than 5 years of age. A large field trial in Matlab, Bangladesh, showed 85% protective efficacy for 6 months after vaccination among women and children older than 2 years,[27] but protection was not sustained in children younger than 5 years of age.[28] In Beira, Mozambique, one or more doses of WC-rBS vaccine during a mass campaign protected nearly 80% of children and adults against culture-confirmed cholera in a setting where the human immunodeficiency virus seroprevalence rate is 20% to 30%.[72] All confirmed cases were due to an O1 El Tor Ogawa variant strain expressing the classic cholera toxin, indicating that the vaccine also provided protection against these newer cholera strains.[31] The WC-rBS vaccine also may provide herd immunity in endemic settings.[4]

Two closely related oral vaccines are also available (mORCVAX and Shanchol). These killed bivalent (O1 and O139) vaccines do not contain the B subunit, do not require an oral buffer, and appear safe and immunogenic in trials conducted in Vietnam, India, and Haiti,[5,22,58,74] including a study in HIV-seropositive Haitian women.[57] Protective efficacy after two doses was about 60% and remained near 50% for 3 to 5 years after vaccination.[113] The Vietnamese vaccine (mORCVAX) is licensed and used nationally. The Indian vaccine (Shanchol) is prequalified by the WHO and licensed for use in adults and children older than 1 year of age. Two doses are administered in a 2-week interval, with a booster dose recommended 2 years after primary vaccination.[31] Limited evidence suggests that oral cholera vaccination is safe in pregnancy.[73] During a cholera outbreak in Malawi's southern region in February 2015 affecting more than 160,000 people, the Malawi Ministry of Health initiated a mass vaccination campaign using Sanchol and targeting people aged 1 year and older, including pregnant women.[132,133] An ongoing interventional study in the same region aims to assess inactivated oral cholera vaccination safety in pregnancy.[37]

The live, attenuated cholera vaccine, CVD 103-HgR is genetically engineered from an O1 classic Inaba strain by *ctxA* subunit deletion and insertion of a marker mercury ion receptor gene into the chromosomal *hlyA* locus. Protection of 100% was seen against homologous strain in challenge studies of North American volunteers and lasts at least 6 months.[114] It was previously licensed in the 1990s, but subsequently did not demonstrate protection in children or adults living in an endemic area,[99] potentially as a result of both direct and indirect protection.[4] In an outbreak setting, however, a single dose provided 79% protection,[18] making CVD 103-HgR more cost effective than the registered two-dose inactivated OCV regimens in terms of cases averted and fatalities.[1,8,59,119] In 2015, the US Food and Drug Administration accepted a Biological License Application and granted priority review status for the CVD 103-HgR–based single dose OCV, Vaxchora, a step toward the first licensed single-dose OCV for US travelers.[59] Phase 3 clinical trials of Vaxchora in Australia and North America enrolled more than 3000 participants total and showed a 90.3% and 79.5% efficacy rate against wild-type cholera challenge at 10 and 90 days postvaccination, respectively. Age-dependent immunity seen with CVD 103-HgR and other OCV products may be due to *Helicobacter pylori* gastritis and subsequent gastric acid secretion.[85] Several other candidate oral cholera vaccines, mostly live, attenuated, are under development, including Peru-15, a genetically engineered strain derived from an O1 El Tor Inaba strain,[31] with safety and immunogenicity demonstrated in both healthy American[24] and Thai adults who are HIV seropositive.[96] Other live attenuated oral cholera vaccine under development include *V. cholerae* 638 and IEM 101/108 constructed from O1 El Tor Ogawa strain[63,120] and VA1.3/VA1.4 derived from a nontoxigenic O1 El Tor strain.[6]

Cholera vaccines should be used in conjunction with other prevention and control strategies in areas where the disease is endemic and considered in areas at risk for outbreaks.[129] The impact of reactive vaccination in response to outbreaks is less clear, although mathematical models predict a substantial benefit with prompt institution.[31]

NEW REFERENCES SINCE THE SEVENTH EDITION

1. Clinical Trials Organization. A phase 2 randomized, double-blinded study to compare in Malian adults the immunogenicity, clinical acceptability and excretion pattern following the ingestion of a single dose of PXVX0200 (CVD 103-HgR) live oral cholera vaccine containing either 108 colony forming units [Cfu] or 109 Cfu using Shanchol™ killed whole cell oral cholera vaccine as an immunological comparator. 2014: ClinicalTrials.org. Available at: https://clinicaltrials.gov/ct2/show/NCT02499172.
2. Akanda AS, Jutla AS, Gute DM, Evans T, Islam S. Reinforcing cholera intervention through prediction-aided prevention. *Bull WHO.* 2012;90(3):243-244.
6. Anita HJ, Biggelaar VD, Poolman JT. *Live-Attenuated and Inactivated Whole-Cell Bacterial Vaccines.* New York: Springer; 2015.
8. Azman AS, Luquero FJ, Ciglenecki I, et al. The impact of a one-dose versus two-dose oral cholera vaccine regimen in outbreak settings: a modeling study. *PLoS Med.* 2015;12(8):e1001867.
20. Centers for Disease Control and Prevention. Vibrio choreal infection: rehydration therapy. 2014. Available at: http://www.cdc.gov/cholera/treatment/rehydration-therapy.html.
21. Centers for Disease Control and Prevention. Non-O1 and non-O139 *Vibrio cholerae* infections. 2014. Available at: http://www.cdc.gov/cholera/non-01-0139-infections.html.
22. Charles RC, Hilaire IJ, Mayo-Smith LM, et al. Immunogenicity of a killed bivalent (O1 and O139) whole cell oral cholera vaccine, Shanchol, in Haiti. *PLoS Negl Trop Dis.* 2014;8(5):e2828.
24. Chen WH, Garza J, Choquette M, et al. Safety and immunogenicity of escalating dosages of a single oral administration of peru-15 pCTB, a candidate live, attenuated vaccine against enterotoxigenic *Escherichia coli* and *Vibrio cholerae. Clin Vacc Immunol.* 2015;22(1):129-135.
25. Chen W, Zhang J, Lu G, et al. Development of an immunochromatographic lateral flow device for rapid diagnosis of *Vibrio cholerae* O1 serotype Ogawa. *Clin Biochem.* 2014;47(6):448-454.
26. Chowdhury F, Mather AE, Begum YA, et al. *Vibrio cholerae* serogroup O139: isolation from cholera patients and asymptomatic household family members in Bangladesh between 2013 and 2014. *PLoS Negl Trop Dis.* 2015;9(11):e0004183.
29. Colombara DV, Cowgill KD, Faruque ASG. Risk factors for severe cholera among children under five in rural and urban Bangladesh, 2000–2008: a hospital-based surveillance study. *PLoS ONE.* 2013;8(1):e54395.
37. Follow-up of pregnant women after a mass vaccination of oral cholera vaccine (ShancholTM) in Nsanje Malawi. 2015. Available at: https://clinicaltrials.gov/ct2/show/NCT02499172.
38. George CM, Rashid MU, Sack DA, et al. Evaluation of enrichment method for the detection of Vibrio cholerae O1 using a rapid dipstick test in Bangladesh. *Trop Med Intl Health.* 2014;19(3):301-307.
49. Hasan NA, Choi SY, Eppinger M, et al. Genomic diversity of 2010 Haitian cholera outbreak strains. *Proc Natl Acad Sci USA.* 2012;109(29):E2010-E2017.
56. Infection Control for Cholera in Health Care Settings. 2014. Available at: http://www.cdc.gov/cholera/infection-control-hcp.html.
57. Ivers LC, Charles RC, Hilaire IJ, et al. Immunogenicity of the bivalent oral cholera vaccine Shanchol in Haitian adults with HIV infection. *J Infect Dis.* 2015;212(5):779-783.
58. Ivers LC, Hilaire IJ, Teng JE, et al. Effectiveness of reactive oral cholera vaccination in rural Haiti: a case-control study. *Lancet Global Health.* 2015;3(3):e162-e168.
59. Jackson SS, Chen WH. Evidence for CVD 103-HgR as an effective single-dose oral cholera vaccine. *Future Microbiol.* 2015;10(8):1271-1281.
61. Jutla A, Aldaach H, Billian H, et al. Satellite based assessment of hydroclimatic conditions related to cholera in Zimbabwe. *PLoS ONE.* 2015;10(9):e0137828.
63. Kanungo S, Sen B, Ramamurthy T, et al. Safety and immunogenicity of a live oral recombinant cholera vaccine VA1.4: a randomized, placebo controlled trial in healthy adults in a cholera endemic area in Kolkata, India. *PLoS ONE.* 2014;9(7):e99381.
65. Karlsson EK, Harris JB, Tabrizi S, et al. Natural selection in a Bangladeshi population from the cholera-endemic Ganges River Delta. *Sci Trans Med.* 2013;5(192):192ra186.
73. Lutgarde Lynen M, Sokkab An M, Olivier Koole M, et al. An algorithm to optimize viral load testing in HIV-positive patients with suspected first-line antiretroviral therapy failure in Cambodia. *J AIMS.* 2009;52(1):40-48.
75. Mari L, Bertuzzo E, Finger F, et al. On the predictive ability of mechanistic models for the Haitian cholera epidemic. *J R Soc Interface.* 2015;12:104.
85. Muhsen K, Lagos R, Reymann MK, et al. Age-dependent association among *Helicobacter pylori* infection, serum pepsinogen levels and immune response of children to live oral cholera vaccine CVD 103-HgR. *PLoS ONE.* 2014;9(1):e83999.
92. Phillips A, Shroufi A, Vojnov L, et al. Sustainable HIV treatment in Africa through viral-load-informed differentiated care. *Nature.* 2015;528(7580):S68-S76.
93. Price GA, McFann K, Holmes RK. Immunization with cholera toxin b subunit induces high-level protection in the suckling mouse model of cholera. *PLoS ONE.* 2013;8(2):e57269.
96. Ratanasuwan W, Kim YH, Sah BK, et al. Peru-15 (Choleragarde (R)), a live attenuated oral cholera vaccine, is safe and immunogenic in human immunodeficiency virus (HIV)-seropositive adults in Thailand. *Vaccine.* 2015;33(38):4820-4826.
100. Roberts T, Bygrave H, Fajardo E, Ford N. Challenges and opportunities for the implementation of virological testing in resource-limited settings. *J Intl AIDS Soc.* 2012;15(2):17324.
105. Handa S, King JW, Thaker VV, Windle ML, Schleiss MR. Cholera treatment and management. *Medscape.* 2014;Available at:: http://emedicine.medscape.com/article/962643-treatment#d11.
108. Seed KD, Bodi KL, Kropinski AM, et al. Evidence of a dominant lineage of *Vibrio cholerae*-specific lytic bacteriophages shed by cholera patients over a 10-year period in Dhaka, Bangladesh. *MBio.* 2011;2(1):e334-e310.
109. Seed KD, Yen M, Shapiro BJ, et al. Evolutionary consequences of intra-patient phage predation on microbial populations. *eLife.* 2014;3:e03497.
111. Sugimoto JD, Koepke AA, Kenah EE, et al. Household transmission of *Vibrio cholerae* in Bangladesh. *PLoS Negl Trop Dis.* 2014;8(11):e3314.
118. Ticona E, Kirwan DE, Soria J, Gilman RH. Implementation of a symptomatic approach leads to increased efficiency of a cholera treatment unit. *Am J Trop Med Hyg.* 2014;91(3):570-573.
119. Troeger C, Sack DA, Chao DL. Evaluation of targeted mass cholera vaccination strategies in Bangladesh: a demonstration of a new cost-effectiveness calculator. *Am J Trop Med Hyg.* 2014;91(6):1181-1189.
120. Uddin T, Aktar A, Xu P, et al. Immune responses to O-specific polysaccharide and lipopolysaccharide of *Vibrio cholerae* O1 Ogawa in adult Bangladeshi recipients of an oral killed cholera vaccine and comparison to responses in patients with cholera. *Am J Trop Med Hyg.* 2014;90(5):873-881.
130. World Health Organization. Weekly epidemiological record. 2014. Available at: http://www.who.int/wer/2015/wer9040.pdf?ua=1.
131. World Health Organization. WHO intensifies support to cholera outbreak in Malawi and Mozambique [press release]. Available at: www.afro.who.int/news/who-intensifies-support-cholera-outbreak-malawi-and-mozambique.
132. World Health Organization. Malawi completes round one of the oral cholera vaccination campaign in Nsanje District. 2015. Available at: http://www.afro.who.int/en/malawi/press-materials/item/7556-malawi-completes-round-one-of-the-oral-cholera-vaccination-campaign-in-nsanje-district.html.
133. World Health Organization. 84% of flood victims living in camps and people from surrounding villages immunized against cholera in Nsanje, Malawi. 2015. Available at: http://www.afro.who.int/en/malawi/press-materials/item/7665-84-of-flood-victims-living-in-camps-and-people-from-surrounding-villages-immunized-against-cholera-in-nsanje-malawi.html.
134. World Health Organization.Cholera – United Republic of Tanzania. 2015. Available at: http://www.who.int/csr/don/11-september-2015-cholera/en/.

The full reference list for this chapter is available at ExpertConsult.com.

Vibrio parahaemolyticus

118

Deborah Lehman

Vibrio parahaemolyticus is recognized worldwide as a cause of foodborne disease associated with consumption of seafood—in particular, crustaceans and mollusks—and occasionally as a cause of wound infections and sepsis in immunocompromised hosts. *V. parahaemolyticus* was first isolated in 1950 and was associated with a foodborne outbreak in Japan traced to dried sardines. In this outbreak, there were 272 infections and 20 deaths.[12] The organism was originally classified as *Pasteurella parahaemolyticus* due to its similarity to other gram-negative rods with bipolar staining. Five years later, the halophilic bacterium was isolated from a patient with food poisoning and was renamed *Pseudomonas enteritis*. Almost 10 years after the original outbreak, the organism was classified correctly in the genus *Vibrio*,[9] with the scientific name of *Vibrio parahaemolyticus*, and its distribution in coastal waters and estuaries of temperate climates around the world was recognized.[89] The regional differences in disease incidence are related to patterns of consumption of marine products and practices of food preparation. In Japan and Taiwan, where fish and shellfish are a major source of dietary protein and frequently consumed raw, *V. parahaemolyticus* accounts for 10% to 40% of foodborne outbreaks.[80,103] In the United States, the incidence is lower, but with increasing consumption of raw or partially cooked seafood, *V. parahaemolyticus* is recognized as the leading cause of seafood-associated gastroenteritis. The first confirmed foodborne outbreak in the United States occurred in Maryland in 1971 and was linked to the consumption of contaminated crabmeat.[26] Since then, sporadic outbreaks have been reported,[6,7,15,26,28,73,40,92] demonstrating the risk of infectious and toxic syndromes from marine products in the United States.[33] *Vibrio parahaemolyticus* can also cause wound infections, particularly in immunocompromised patients. An increase in such infections was reported in 2005 following Hurricane Katrina off the Gulf Coast of the United States; these infections were epidemiologically linked to exposure to brackish water in the hurricane areas.[17]

BACTERIOLOGY

V. parahaemolyticus is a gram-negative, non–spore-forming, curved rod with rounded ends that possess a polar flagellum.[65] On surfaces or in viscous environments, *V. parahaemolyticus* can differentiate into swarmer cells equipped with additional shorter lateral peritrichous flagella.[64] *V. parahaemolyticus* is a facultative anaerobe with respiratory and fermentative metabolisms. Similar to other *Vibrio* species, it is an oxidase-positive nonfermenter of lactose.[8] It is arginine dihydrolase negative and ornithine decarboxylase positive. The requirement of sodium and enhancement of growth in a specific range of concentration differentiate it from *Vibrio cholerae* and *Vibrio mimicus*. Optimal growth occurs in solutions containing 2% to 4% sodium; concentrations greater than 8% sodium inhibits growth.[101]

V. parahaemolyticus produces round, blue-green colonies on the widely used *Vibrio*-selective thiosulfate citrate bile salt sucrose (TCBS) agar. This medium inhibits most fecal flora by the presence of bile salts and a highly alkaline pH. Direct plating on TCBS agar may be used for feces and other clinical specimens, but food samples that are not heavily contaminated require enrichment either in alkaline peptone water supplemented with 3% sodium chloride or in a strongly selective medium, such as Glucose Salt Teepol Broth.[101] The optimal pH for growth is in the neutral range, but *V. parahaemolyticus* can survive in alkaline media. Optimal growth temperatures are between 35°C and 39°C (95°F–102.2°F).[109] Growth is rapid in conventional media and foodstuff, with generation times of only 8 minutes[50]; a significant number of organisms can be found after only a short period of inappropriate storage. Growth is inhibited at temperatures of 44°C (111.2°F) or greater and at temperatures less than 4°C (39.2°F). The degree of inactivation is greater with increased temperatures; a million-fold decline occurs in viable bacteria in shrimp homogenate kept for only 1 minute at 100°C (212°F).[99] In laboratory conditions with low temperature and nutrient supply, *V. parahaemolyticus* enters a viable but nonculturable state, during which the organism can no longer be cultured on routine growth media, but its viability can be confirmed using direct microscopic assays.[35,49,107]

The genome of *V. parahaemolyticus* consists of two circular chromosomes. Genes for a type III secretion system (TTSS) were identified in a pathogenicity island on chromosome 2.[59] Two types of nonredundant TTSS have been identified.[77] TTSS, also a central virulence factor in both salmonellae and shigellae, possesses needle-like structures that facilitate direct injections of bacterial proteins into a target host cell and confers pathogenicity of the inflammatory diarrhea seen in *V. parahaemolyticus* infections. The presence of TTSS in *V. parahaemolyticus* differentiates its pathogenicity from that of *V. cholerae*, which does not carry these genes.[59]

EPIDEMIOLOGY

In the United States, *V. parahaemolyticus* is found along the East, West, and Gulf Coasts, and an increasing number of outbreaks have been reported.[19,29,50] Water, sediments, suspended particulates, plankton, fish, and shellfish have all been shown to harbor the organism.[5,68] The organisms are present in highest numbers in water at temperatures between 17°C and 35°C (62.6°F–95°F) and containing 0.5% to 2.5% salinity.[48] Marked seasonal and geographic variations occur, with maximal mean concentrations occurring during late summer and spring along the Gulf Coast.[29] Outbreaks, predominantly between June and October, correlate with seasonal distribution of the organism.[4]

Finfish and all types of shellfish products—including oysters, clams, crabs, and shrimp—may be involved in the transmission of the infection.[48] The risk for acquiring infection is higher with molluscan shellfish due to their ability to concentrate the bacteria by filter feeding.[5,35,109] In oysters, the density of *V. parahaemolyticus* may be 100 times greater than that in the surrounding water.[29] The levels of contamination are generally low in freshly collected oysters, with the highest mean density of only 160 bacteria/g found in the United States.[29] In Japan, high counts (up to 10^3–10^4/g) have been reported in market shellfish.[22] The minimum infective dose is thought to be in the range of 10^5 to 10^7 organisms, based on volunteer feeding studies.[31] More recent outbreaks of illness caused by oysters that met bacteriologic safety standards have raised questions about the adequacy of current food storage recommendations.[27] Noningestion *Vibrio* infection has been demonstrated in the marine-estuarine environment, potentially placing swimmers at risk for infection.[87]

Between 1973 and 1987, shortly after the first outbreaks in the United States were reported, only 23 of 1869 foodborne disease outbreaks with known bacterial etiology reported to the Centers for Disease Control and Prevention (CDC) were caused by *V. parahaemolyticus*.[6] In 18 of these outbreaks, a shellfish was recognized as the food vehicle. No fatal cases were reported. Contributing factors included inadequate cooking (92%), improper holding temperature (75%), and food acquired from an unsafe source (75%).[6,7] Most affected individuals were adults, and no patterns of unusual susceptibility by age group or gender were noted. Unlike other bacterial and viral pathogens that cause gastroenteritis, secondary spread of *V. parahaemolyticus* does not occur between family members or other close contacts. Between 1988 and 1997, 345 sporadic cases were reported to the CDC. The majority of these infections (59%)

resulted in gastroenteritis and were related to ingesting raw oysters.[28] In the summer of 2006, outbreaks of *V. parahaemolyticus* associated with consumption of contaminated shellfish harvested from a common area were reported across the states of New York, Oregon, and Washington. Of these isolates, 78% tested had a subtype of O4:K12.[18]

Until more recently, *V. parahaemolyticus* infections were causally associated with multiple serotypes and occurred as sporadic cases or localized outbreaks.[70] In 1996, a sudden increase in infections was seen in India, and 50% to 80% of cases were attributed to a single serotype, O3:K6.[78] Shortly thereafter, O3:K6 strains were isolated from clinical samples from other countries in Asia.[71] In 1998, two outbreaks of gastroenteritis in the United States were associated with O3:K6.[16,28] By 2005, this pandemic clone was found in patients from Europe, South America, and Africa.[3,39,63] Other clones that genetically diverged from O3:K6, such as O4:K68 and O1:KUT, were first isolated in the Pacific Northwest in 1988 and were responsible for large outbreaks in the United States in 1997 and 2004.[25,66] Spread of these clones from the West Coast to the East Coast and to Europe traced to transport of seafood with improper storage.[40,62,73] In 1997, oceanic eastward dispersion of *Vibrio* from Asia to the Americas was attributed to El Niño, which occurred the previous fall.[60,62]

Although rates of *V. parahaemolyticus* stabilized during the late 2000s,[37] cases and outbreaks associated with these pandemic clones continue to be reported in high numbers globally.[79,102]

Vibriosis became a notifiable disease nationally in 2007. Prior to routine reporting, the CDC relied on two surveillance systems to monitor the incidence of vibriosis in the United States. The Centers for Disease Control's Vibrio Surveillance (COVIS) system, initiated in 1988, is a passive surveillance system that relies on laboratories to report positive tests. The FoodNet system, established in 1996, is an active surveillance system for 10 states reporting *Vibrio* infections in addition sto other foodborne enteric infections. Between 1996 and 2010, these surveillance systems demonstrated an increase in vibriosis overall, with the rise being driven primarily by an increase in *V. parahaemolyticus* infections reported by both systems (44.9%% and 54%, respectively).[72] FoodNet reporting from 2013 showed the highest incidence in *Vibrio* infections to date.[106] Although rates of *Vibrio* infections remain lower than those of *Salmonella* or *Campylobacter* infections, the overall incidence is increasing and may be related to rising surface seawater temperatures.[61,105] From 1996 to 2010, there were 3460 and 820 *V. parahaemolyticus* infections reported by the COVIS and FoodNet systems, respectively. Of these 4280 cases, 845 (20%) patients were hospitalized and there were 28 (0.65%) deaths.[72]

Given the specific culture media required for *Vibrio* isolation, and the limited access to more sophisticated diagnostic techniques, the number of infections reported to the CDC each year likely vastly underestimates the true number of infections. The CDC estimates that the number of *V. parahaemolyticus* infections approaches 4500 annually in the United States.[21]

PATHOGENESIS

The ability of certain strains of *V. parahaemolyticus* to produce β-hemolysis on Wagatsuma agar, known as the Kanagawa phenomenon (KP), was first epidemiologically associated with human pathogenicity.[67] KP is observed in the vast majority of strains from clinical specimens and in only rarely in strains from environmental sources.[31,50,97] Thermostable direct hemolysin (TDH) produces KP.[96] TDH has a molecular weight of 42,000 consisting of two subunits of 21,000[68] and, in contrast to other hemolysins produced by *V. parahaemolyticus*, is not inactivated by heating for 10 minutes at 100°C (212°F). TDH is a pore-forming toxin that causes hemolysis by binding to and disrupting erythrocyte membranes.[44] TDH also has been shown to have enterotoxic activities, such as causing accumulation of fluid in rabbit ileal loop assays, invading intestinal mucosa,[24,100] and increasing intracellular calcium concentrations that trigger secretion of chloride by intestinal cells.[86,94,95] TDH is cytotoxic, lethal to small experimental animals, and cardiotoxic.[111]

Certain KP-negative isolates from outbreaks have been shown to produce a TDH-related hemolysin (TRH).[46] Although TRH is heat labile, it shares similarities with TDH, such as hemolysis, production of fluid accumulation in the rabbit ileal loop model, and induction of chloride secretion in human colonic epithelial cells.[45,83] Likewise, some variants closely related to the original TDH by molecular analysis (Vp TDH/I and Vp TDH/II) have been isolated from KP-negative strains.[69] Both TDH and TRH are considered to be the major *V. parahaemolyticus* virulence factors, although the mechanism for enteric pathogenicity is not fully understood.

When the *tdh* and *trh* genes were cloned and sequenced, researchers realized that certain strains possess the genetic material but are phenotypically incomplete. Strains with a typical hemolysin-positive phenotype carried two chromosome gene copies, whereas *tdh* gene–positive strains with weakly positive or negative hemolysin phenotype possessed only a single chromosome gene copy.[75] Less than 50% percent of *trh* gene–positive strains produce TRH when examined by enzyme-linked immunosorbent assay.[91] Low-level expression of the *tdh* genes may be the reason for the KP-negative phenotype.[76] The expression of the *tdh* genes is controlled by the Vp-toxRS operon. The basal production of mRNA and the degree of transcriptional activation seem to be related to differences in the nucleotide sequences and strength of the promoter region.[76] Studies have also suggested that conditions that simulate the human intestine, 37°C to 42 °C and the presence of bile, upregulate *tdh* gene expression, explaining increased production in pathogenic strains compared to those isolated from the environment.[85,88]

Some studies, however, suggest additional virulence mechanisms and that the mere presence of the *tdh* or *trh* genes does not reliably correlate with virulence of a given strain.[100,109] Up to 10% of clinical isolates have been shown to be TDH or TRH toxin negative by polymerase chain reaction (PCR).[58] *V. parahaemolyticus* requires intestinal colonization factors to cause disease. A variety of pili and other potential virulence factors have been isolated, but their roles are still incompletely defined.[22] Adherence of *V. parahaemolyticus* to intestinal epithelial cells of rabbits[23] and human small intestine[38,108] seems to require binding to complex carbohydrates or hemagglutinins of the host. A multivalent adhesion molecule, MAM7, conserved in many other gram-negative intestinal pathogens, appears to be a key factor in the initial attachment of bacteria to intestinal cells and is constitutively expressed, allowing for rapid attachment with host cells. *V. parahaemolyticus* can also disrupt epithelial barrier function, regardless of TDH and TRH production.[58] Type 3 secretion systems 1 and 2 are organelles that span the bacterial inner and outer membranes and likely facilitate bacterial toxin delivery into the eukaryotic cell, resulting in cytotoxicity. Like the TDH and TRH system, the expression of these virulence factors is influenced by the presence of bile acids and higher temperatures.[12,112]

Additional virulence factors include a capsule and two different types of flagella with distinct functions for swimming and swarming. These factors likely aid the organism in the colonization and infection of the human host and enhance its survival in the environment.[56]

The occurrence of cases with grossly bloody stools[15,47] is suggestive of the organism's invasiveness and is consistent with the production of cytotoxin.[1] KP-positive and KP-negative strains from clinical specimens can invade and colonize the mucosal cells of the rabbit ileum, producing acute inflammation, degeneration, and erosion of the villi.[8] *Vibrio* infection is not isolated to the intestinal lumen; organisms can be cultured from tissue specimens of spleen, liver, and heart in experimental animals, indicating spread through the lymphatic or circulatory systems.[11]

CLINICAL MANIFESTATIONS

The spectrum of intestinal disease varies from mild gastroenteritis to dysenteric syndrome. The incubation period is typically 15 to 24 hours (range, 4–96 hours)[4,93]; this variability is likely related to the number of organisms ingested. Resolution of symptoms usually occurs after approximately 3 days[68] but varies from several hours to more than 10 days.[4,13] Diarrhea (96%) and abdominal pain (95%) are the most common and earliest symptoms, accompanied by nausea, vomiting, and headache in 40% to 70% of cases. Chills and moderate fever are less frequent (20%).[4,26] Diarrhea caused by *V. parahaemolyticus* is watery and explosive,[14] with patients having up to 15 stools during the first day. Shock caused by loss of intestinal fluid is unusual but has been reported.[29] Diarrheal stools may contain mucus, but grossly bloody stools are less common.[9,47,57] Small superficial ulcerations may be seen on sigmoidoscopy.[9] No difference in symptoms exists in cases caused by KP-negative strains.[44]

V. parahaemolyticus can also cause wound infections and septicemia. COVIS, initiated in 1988 in four Gulf Coast states, demonstrated that 18% to 34% of *V. parahaemolyticus* isolates were isolated from wound infections, and 3% to 5% were associated with septicemia.[27,57] In 2009, 11% of isolates from the United States were obtained from wounds and 2% of isolates from blood cultures.[20] Wound infection occurs after contamination of skin lacerations with seawater or after direct trauma with pieces of shellfish, fish hooks, or utensils contaminated with seawater.[10] Superficial infection can extend to deeper soft tissue and, in some cases, lead to fatal necrotizing fasciitis.[81] Septicemia is of most concern in immunocompromised patients, particularly patients with leukemia[31] and liver disease.[30,41] Bacteremia may develop after either wound infection[10,31] or ingestion of seafood.[41,84] Skin bullae,[41] intravascular hemolysis,[31] and disseminated intravascular coagulation[41] may also complicate wound and bacteremic infections.

COMPLICATIONS

An acute diarrhea episode may require medical attention but less frequently leads to hospitalization.[13,26,57,93] Children younger than 5 years of age are more likely to require hospitalization compared to older individuals.[98] Long-term sequelae from *V. parahaemolyticus* infection is unusual, although severe dehydration, shock,[47,82] and death (0.04% of cases in Japan) can occur.[8,101] Primary septicemia,[54,57,84] septicemia secondary to wound infection,[10,31,54] and septicemia secondary to gastroenteritis[41,54] have higher mortality rates, especially in immunosuppressed patients or in patients with liver disease.[10,34]

DIAGNOSIS

Epidemiologic data are the basis for the presumptive diagnosis. In a patient with compatible symptoms, a history of recent seafood consumption or exposure to warm seawater should suggest the diagnosis. Leukocytosis and fecal leukocytes may be found[9,47] but are nonspecific findings. A positive stool culture on selective media, such as TCBS agar, can confirm the clinical impression. Routine use of TCBS agar, however, is not cost-effective, even in coastal areas, unless an appropriate clinical setting is available.[10,57,65] The use of a transport medium, such as Cary-Blair (Thermo Fisher Scientific), is necessary if a delay in sample processing is expected. Isolation of more than 10^5 *V. parahaemolyticus* from epidemiologically implicated food supports the diagnosis and identifies the vehicle.[65] A correlation between the serotype found in the food and the clinical isolate is not always present because multiple strains can contaminate a single food.[4] Adding an enrichment broth to the processing increases the yield of isolation. The use of chromogenic (chromogenicCHROMagar *Vibrio* [CV] agar) agar has facilitated the identification and isolation of *V. parahaemolyticus* and has simplified laboratory differentiation of *V. parahaemolyticus* from other *Vibrio* species. Generally, culture methods are laborious, have low sensitivity, and are not able to distinguish pathogenic strains from nonpathogenic strains. More advanced diagnostic techniques, such as immunoassays and PCR, are preferable and becoming increasing available commercially.[43]

For testing blood specimens, use of routine culture media followed by selective media is appropriate.[41,84] Immunoassays (enzyme-linked immunosorbent assay, immunoprecipitation in agar medium, reversed passive latex agglutination) are available in research laboratories and commercially in Japan (KAP-RPLA, Denka Seiken; BT test, Nissui Pharmaceutical) to detect the TDH. Strains producing TRH may be detected by cross reactions.[110] DNA probe hybridization[74] and PCR with a sequence of a highly conserved DNA fragment[55] or targeting the *tdh* or *trh* genes can be used to detect low numbers of the organism in environmental and clinical specimens.[52,53] Loop-mediated isothermal amplification is a newer technique[56] that does not require thermal cycling and has been used to identify *tdh* and *trh* genes in addition to other genes encoding virulence factors in *V. parahaemolyticus.* Serologic methods (slide agglutination) can detect H antigens in lateral flagella.[90] Histologic findings from duodenal and rectal biopsy samples from patients infected with *V. parahaemolyticus* show a nonspecific acute inflammatory response, with epithelial degradation, polymorphonuclear neutrophil infiltration of villi and crypt cells, and hemorrhage.[83]

TREATMENT

For the management of gastroenteritis, supportive therapy with careful attention to fluid and electrolyte balance is indicated. Oral rehydration is usually appropriate, although intravenous fluids may be required if massive fluid losses and significant dehydration occurs.[9,47,82] Antibiotic treatment for most *V. parahaemolyticus* infections is unnecessary, as it is a self-limited disease. For protracted cases, tetracycline or a fluoroquinolone may be beneficial.[8,9,50]

For wound infections and septicemia, antibiotics are always indicated. Patients with septicemia should be treated with a third-generation cephalosporin plus doxycycline. Trimethoprim-sulfamethoxazole plus aminoglycoside is an alternative regimen for young children. Penicillins are ineffective because of the presence of β-lactamases in 50% of isolates.[36,51] Multidrug-resistant strains have been reported in fresh and frozen oysters as well as in water samples.[2] Few clinical strains have been shown to be resistant to trimethoprim-sulfamethoxazole, third-generation cephalosporins, aztreonam, imipenem, fluoroquinolones, and aminoglycosides.[10,31,36,41] Wound infections with necrotic tissue require surgical debridement.

PREVENTION AND CONTROL

Ensuring the lack of contamination of seafood is difficult, but avoiding food-handling errors decreases the risk for infection. A recommendation for an acceptable upper limit of 100 colony-forming units per gram of *V. parahaemolyticus* in raw shrimp was established by the International Commission on Microbiological Specification for Foods.[48] Heating seafood to 60°C (156.2°F) for 15 minutes[32] or boiling for 7 minutes[13] seems to be adequate to reduce the risk for infection; thorough cooking eliminates the organism.[99] When undercooked or raw seafood is consumed, adequate refrigeration prior to ingestion to preclude multiplication of organisms is important. Cooked seafood that comes in contact with contaminated water can also transmit infection; thus, attention to food service is critical to preventing infections. During the preparation of seafood, special attention should be paid to possible cross-contamination. Use of the same utensils, board surfaces, or containers for fresh and recently cooked seafood should be avoided.[82,99] Finally, raw seafood consumption should be discouraged, particularly for individuals at high risk for development of septicemia.[30,54,57] Governmental regulations established in 1999 in Japan guiding the collection, storage, and preparation of seafood resulted in significant declines in *V. parahaemolyticus* infections, specifically those due to pathogenic TDH producing serotype 03:K6[42] Investigation into new and novel methods to prevent seafood contamination with pathogenic *Vibrio* while preserving the taste of the food will be important to reduce future outbreaks and maintain the safety of seafood consumption.[104]

NEW REFERENCES SINCE THE SEVENTH EDITION

2. Albuquerque R, et al. Raw tropical oysters as vehicles for multidrug resistant *Vibrio parahaemolyticus. Rev Inst Med Trop Sao Paulo.* 2015;57:193-196.
12. Broberg CA, et al. *Vibrio parahaemolyticus* cell biology and pathogenicity determinants. *Microbes Infect.* 2011;13:992-1001.
21. Centers for Disease Control and Prevention (CDC). *Vibrio parahaemolyticus*; 2013a. Centers for Disease Control and Prevention, Atlanta. Available at http://www.cdc.gov/vibrio/vibriop.html.
17. Centers for Disease Control and Prevention. *Vibrio* Illnesses After Hurricane Katrina–Multiple States, August-September 2005. *MMWR Morb Mortal Wkly Rep.* 2005;54:928-931.
19. Centers for Disease Control and Prevention. *Vibrio parahaemolyticus* infections associated with consumption of raw shellfish—three states, 2006. *MMWR Morb Mortal Wkly Rep.* 2006;55:854-856.
40. Haendiges J, et al Pandemic *Vibrio parahaemolyticus*, Maryland, USA, 2012. Emerging Infectious Diseases. https://www.nc.cdc.gov/eid/article/20/4/13-0818_article.
42. Hara-Kudo Y, et al. Impact of seafood regulations for *Vibrio parahaemolyticus* infection and verification by analyses of seafood contamination and infection. *Epidemiol Infect.* 2014;142:2237-2247.

43. He P, et al. Multiplex real-time PCR assay for detection of pathogenic *Vibrio parahaemolyticus* strains. *Mol Cell Probes*. 2014;28:246-250.
56. Letchumanan V, et al. *Vibrio parahaemolyticus*: a review on the pathogenesis, prevalence, and advance molecular identification techniques. *Front Microbiol.* 2014;11:1-13.
61. Martinez-Urtaza J, et al. Climate anomalies and the increasing risk of *Vibrio parahaemolyticus* and *Vibrio vulnificus* illnesses. *Food Res Int*. 2010;43:1780-1790.
60. Martinez-Urtaza J, et al. Emergence of *Asiatic vibrio* diseases in South America in phase with El Niño. *Epidemiology*. 2008;19:829-837.
62. Martinez-Urtaza J, et al. Spread of Pacific Northwest *Vibrio parahaemolyticus* strain. *N Engl J Med*. 2013;369:1573-1754.
66. McLaughlin JB, et al. Outbreak of *Vibrio parahaemolyticus* gastroenteritis associated with Alaskan oysters. *New Engl J Med*. 2005;353:1463.
72. Newton A, et al. Increasing rates of vibriosis in the United States, 1996-2010: Review of surveillance data from 2 systems. *Clin Infect Dis*. 2012;54:S391-S395.
73. Newton A, et al. Increase in *Vibrio parahaemolyticus* infections associated with consumption of Atlantic Coast shellfist—2013. *MMWR*. 2014;63(15):335-336.
85. Raghunath P. Roles of thermostable direct hemolysin (TDH) and TDH-related hemolysin (TRH) in *Vibrio parahaemolyticus*. *Front Microbiol*. 2015;5:1-4.
87. Shaw KS, et al. Recreational swimmers' exposure to *Vibrio vulnificus* and *Vibrio parahaemolyticus* in the Chesapeake Bay, Maryland, USA. *Environ Int*. 2015;74:99-105.
88. Shimohata T, et al. Diarrhea induced by infection of *Vibrio parahaemolyticus*. *J Med Invest*. 2010;57:179-182.
89. Shinoda S. Sixty years from the discovery of *Vibrio parahaemolyticus* and some recollections. *Biocontrol Sci*. 2011;16:129-137.
92. Slayton RB, et al. Clam associated vibriosis, USA, 1988-2010. *Epidemiol Infect*. 2014;142:1083-1099.
104. Wang W, et al. Intervention strategies for reducing *Vibrio parahaemolyticus* in seafood: A review. *J Food Sci*. 2015;80:R10-R19.
105. Weis KE, et al. *Vibrio* illness in Florida, 1998-2007. *Epidemiol Infect*. 2011;139:591-598.
106. Wilken JA, et al. Incidence and trends of infection with pathogens transmitted commonly through food—Foodborne Diseases Active Surveillance Network, 10 U.S. Sites, 2006–2013. *MMWR. Morb Mortal Wkly Rep*. 2014;63:328-332.
112. Zhang L, et al. Virulence determinants for *Vibrio parahaemolyticus* infection. *Curr Opin Microbiol*. 2013;16:70-77.

The full reference list for this chapter is available at ExpertConsult.com.

119 *Vibrio vulnificus*

Randall G. Fisher

BACTERIOLOGY

Vibrio vulnificus is a small, curvilinear, gram-negative rod of the family Vibrionaceae.[7] This facultative anaerobe is oxidase positive and lysine positive, similar to other species of the genus *Vibrio*. Its major difference is that it ferments lactose, a feature that accounts for its original name, Lac + *Vibrio*. *V. vulnificus* is arginine negative and ornithine variable. This halophilic (salt-loving) organism grows in concentrations of sodium chloride of 1% to 8% and seems to grow best at approximately 3%.[39]

EPIDEMIOLOGY

V. vulnificus, similar to *Vibrio parahaemolyticus,* is a marine organism that is a common inhabitant of offshore waters, especially estuarial waters.[62] It has been isolated from sediment, plankton, water, finfish, crabs, and oysters.[70] Peak recovery occurs in the summer and early fall,[18] possibly because at higher water temperatures *V. vulnificus* is released and rises to surface waters. There, it attaches to plankton and shore fish and then is taken up and concentrated by filter-feeding mollusks and crustaceans.

V. vulnificus has been isolated from wild and commercial oysters throughout the world. It especially is prevalent in warm coastal waters. Reports about the survival of the organism in oysters stored at low temperatures are conflicting.[33] Nilsson and associates[60] revealed, however, that even if *V. vulnificus* is rendered nonculturable by storage at low temperatures, it can be "resuscitated" by allowing the oysters to warm up to room temperature. This cycle could be carried out twice without any reduction in bacterial count. Because of the ubiquity of the organism in the marine environment and its ability to thrive under even the most careful conditions of sanitation, storage, and transport,[17,37] ensuring that commercial shellfish do not contain viable *V. vulnificus* is very difficult.

So-called heat shock shucking, during which the internal meat temperature exceeds 50°C (122°F) for 1 to 4 minutes, reduces the *V. vulnificus* and total bacterial levels in oysters 10-fold to 10,000-fold compared with conventional processing.[23] A separate study confirms that low-temperature pasteurization, which brings oyster temperatures to 50°C for 10 to 15 minutes, reduces colony counts from greater than 100,000/g of oyster meat to undetectable levels.[2] Ice immersion for 3 hours is ineffective at reducing *V. vulnificus* and actually increases coliform counts in oysters.[61,65] High-pressure processing is a promising new approach to eliminating *V. vulnificus* from oysters; in preliminary studies, *V. vulnificus* could be reduced to undetectable levels by processing at 586 MPa with a 7-minute "come up" time.[40]

Disease in humans is initiated by contact with the organism. Contact occurs either through marine contamination of a wound or in the gastrointestinal tract after ingestion of the organism in raw shellfish, most commonly oysters.[7] The incidence of disease caused by *Vibrio* species, including *Vibrio vulnificus*, almost tripled (from approximately 0.09 to 0.3 per 100,000 population) in the United States from 1996 through 2010. *V. vulnificus*, not surprisingly, caused the most hospitalizations and death.[59]

PATHOPHYSIOLOGY

V. vulnificus causes three distinct diseases in humans: wound infection and gastrointestinal infection, which may be self-limited or progress to septicemia. Local infection occurs after a wound is exposed to contaminated seawater. Wound infections with *V. vulnificus* are marked by rapid spread, the formation of bullae, and necrosis of involved tissues.[7] Marked edema and vascular thromboses occur in experimental and natural infection. *V. vulnificus* elaborates a cytolysin,[21,22,39,43] a collagenase,[68] and a protease,[54] which enhance its rapid spread in tissues. The protease activates the plasma kallikrein-kinin system to produce bradykinin[53]; histamine also is released locally. These factors account for the intense inflammatory reaction seen in these lesions. One group of researchers constructed an isolate that lacked a flagellum and found that its ability to adhere to cells was decreased, as was its lethality in mice.[48] Another group found that three different TonB systems (these transport iron-bound substrates across the bacterial outer membrane) are required for flagellar biosynthesis.[20] Hemorrhagic complications may be due to the presence of a metalloprotease that interferes with blood homeostasis through prothrombin activation and fibrinolysis.[11]

In otherwise healthy individuals, a mild, self-limited gastrointestinal illness similar to that caused by *V. parahaemolyticus* has been described.[38] The most serious infection produced by *V. vulnificus* is primary septicemia, which occurs most commonly in patients with liver disease after they have ingested the organism in raw shellfish.[8,52,53] The organism contains an elastase called VvpE that mediates disruption of intestinal tight junctions, allowing access to the bloodstream.[46]

For patients with hepatic disease, the risk for acquiring septicemia is 40 to 80 times greater, and the case-fatality rate is 2.5 times higher than for otherwise healthy individuals.[25] *V. vulnificus,* similar to many other gram-negative organisms, requires iron for growth and grows better in an excess of iron.[78] It is able to extract iron from hemoglobin, even if it is complexed completely to haptoglobin.[78,82] Liver damage, excess iron, deferoxamine therapy, and hepcidin deficiency[3] have been shown to decrease the median lethal dose (LD_{50}) of *V. vulnificus* in experimental animals. Deferoxamine alone decreased the LD_{50} by four orders of magnitude.[9] Iron overload almost certainly underlies *V. vulnificus* septicemia in patients who require repeated transfusions and deferoxamine therapy for anemia.[32,80] Some evidence indicates that alcoholism, even in the absence of demonstrable liver disease, is a risk factor for developing sepsis.[63] Fatal septicemia has been reported in patients with other chronic diseases, such as diabetes mellitus and lymphomas.[64]

Virulence factors of the organism have been described.[79] Virulent strains are resistant to the bactericidal activity of human serum,[42] probably because of the presence of a polysaccharide capsule.[1] Poor uptake of virulent strains into phagocytes[71] and opaqueness of the colony on agar have been correlated with the presence of the capsule.[67,79] RTX toxin is a cytolysin that also may be important in protecting the organism from phagocytosis.[49] No difference has been shown in the lipopolysaccharides of virulent versus avirulent strains.[6] The production of recalcitrant shock in patients with septicemia is secondary to toxins, loss of vascular tone, capillary leak, and possibly negative inotropy, as in other forms of gram-negative sepsis.

CLINICAL MANIFESTATIONS

Patients commonly have wound infection or primary septicemia. Wound infection occurs after injury in seawater or after the contamination of a recently acquired wound with seawater. Often, the wound is caused by the shell of a crustacean or mollusk. Many patients with wound infections work in shellfish-related industries. Apparently, wound infection with *V. vulnificus* can develop from superficial wounds acquired within 24 hours of "uneventful" fish handling; the physiologic characteristics of human sweat may be conducive to the survival of the organism on the skin, allowing for later inoculation.[10] A worker at a fish hatchery who had other risk factors, including diabetes mellitus and fatty liver disease, developed necrotizing fasciitis from acupuncture therapy, again suggesting prolonged survival on the skin.[41] Cellulitis may develop and spread rapidly. Overlying skin often is covered with tense bullae. At debridement, the extent of necrosis may exceed presurgical expectations.[77] Primary wound infection may progress to systemic infection; for this reason, wound infection with *V. vulnificus* carries a mortality rate of 7% to 24%.[7,38] Findings associated with mortality in patients with necrotizing fasciitis include low white blood cell counts, low platelet counts, hypoalbuminemia, high immature neutrophil percentages, and hypotension at presentation.[74]

Patients with primary septicemia generally give a history of recent (i.e., 6 to 72 hours) consumption of raw seafood. Illness is marked by the rapid onset of fever, hypotension, and septic shock. Prodromal symptoms—such as malaise, chills, and fever—are common manifestations. Vomiting and diarrhea are seen in approximately 20% of patients.[8] Shock progresses quickly and is difficult to reverse. Secondary skin lesions develop in approximately half of patients[7] and may be bullous, petechial, or maculopapular. *V. vulnificus* frequently is isolated from cultures of secondary lesions, providing evidence of septicemic spread to those sites.[7] The mortality rate from primary septicemia has been reported to be 46% to 79%.[8,63] A poor outcome is portended by pH less than 7.35,[81] white blood cell count less than 10,000/μL, platelet count less than 100,000/μL, creatinine greater than 1.3 mg/dL, albumin less than 2.5 g/dL, increased prothrombin time, multiple skin lesions (implying septicemic spread), and delay in initial therapy.[45]

In addition to causing the described syndromes, *V. vulnificus* has been reported as a cause of corneal ulcer,[19] myositis,[34] adult epiglottitis,[50] osteomyelitis,[75] endocarditis,[73] peritonitis,[27] tubo-ovarian abscess,[51] and meningitis.[32,63] In one case, a patient had endogenous endophthalmitis without systemic symptoms that developed after ingestion of raw seafood.[31] A case of fatal septicemia has been described in which the presenting symptom was a compartment syndrome of the forearm.[29] A 9-year-old girl with thalassemia and iron overload had septic arthritis as the presenting feature of her septicemia.[44] Ninety percent of reported patients are 40 years old or older.[7,63] Childhood cases of septicemia have been associated with thalassemia major,[31] for which frequent transfusions and deferoxamine therapy are required. Wound infections in previously healthy children and adolescents have been reported. *V. vulnificus* also has been isolated from a premature infant's stool sample obtained on the infant's first day of life; the infant's mother worked as an oyster shucker.[5]

DIAGNOSIS

The diagnosis of *V. vulnificus* infection is made by isolating the organism from blood or tissue culture. It also may be recovered from stool specimens.[5,64] Agars designed specifically to aid in the growth and identification of *V. vulnificus* have been developed; cellobiose-colistin agar outperforms thiosulfate citrate bile salts sucrose agar for recovery of *V. vulnificus* from environmental samples.[26] From a practical standpoint, however, most hospital microbiology laboratories do not stock cellobiose-colistin agar. Of the commercially available media, *V. vulnificus* tends to grow best in thiosulfate citrate bile salts sucrose agar,[7] but it also may be recovered from ordinary blood agar plates[4,66] or MacConkey plates.[7]

A very sensitive nested polymerase chain reaction technique that is capable of detecting 1 pg of bacterial DNA and one colony-forming unit of *V. vulnificus* has been described; it was positive in 94% of clinical samples that grew the bacteria in culture and in 42% of culture-negative samples from patients with suspected *V. vulnificus* infection.[24,47] A multiplex polymerase chain reaction was developed that had 100% sensitivity and specificity for identification and differentiation of *V. cholerae*, *V. parahaemolyticus*, and *V. vulnificus* in validation tests with 488 strains.[57] An enzyme immunoassay also has been developed.[71]

The diagnosis of *V. vulnificus* wound infection or septicemia can be suspected on clinical grounds and appropriate therapy initiated while awaiting culture results. A history of ingestion of raw shellfish or contamination of a wound with either seawater or brackish inland waters[69] should be sought. *V. vulnificus* infection should be given high consideration in patients with hemosiderosis, anemia with transfusion therapy, liver disease, or other chronic diseases.

TREATMENT

For severe wound infections and necrotizing fasciitis, performing surgical therapy as rapidly as possible is paramount. In some cases, in which septic shock combined with multiorgan system dysfunction syndrome makes prolonged surgical procedures difficult or impossible, temporizing with rapid incision and drainage followed by full debridement 24 hours later may be a feasible approach.[28] However, in a large retrospective study, debridement within 12 hours of admission held the most favorable prognosis.[12] For primary septicemia, support of the patient's airway, along with aggressive pressor support and other adjunctive therapies for severe septic shock, is of primary concern. Secondarily, appropriate antibiotic treatment for *V. vulnificus* should be started as early as possible.[55]

In vitro, the organism is susceptible to many antibiotics, including ampicillin, third-generation cephalosporins, fluoroquinolones, tetracycline, chloramphenicol, and gentamicin.[7] Most of what we know about effective antimicrobial therapy for *V. vulnificus* sepsis comes from mouse studies and retrospective human case series. In the mouse model, ciprofloxacin is the single most effective agent, and the combination of ciprofloxacin plus cefotaxime tends to have the highest survival rate[30] despite the fact that cefotaxime by itself has virtually no salutary effect. In humans, similarly, mortality rates are highest when cephalosporins are used by themselves[16] despite good minimum inhibitory concentrations in the laboratory. Combination therapy with cefotaxime and minocycline or cefotaxime and ciprofloxacin looks far superior, with the latter combination being perhaps the best.

In the largest retrospective case series, outcomes were similar in those who received a fluoroquinolone with or without minocycline and those who received a third-generation cephalosporin plus minocycline. Mortality was 61% in those who were treated with a third-generation cephalosporin alone.[14] In vitro synergy studies show that the combination of ciprofloxacin and cefotaxime is synergistic for *V. vulnificus*,[36] and in a murine model, the newer fluoroquinolones (e.g., moxifloxacin) worked as well as combination therapy in preventing lethality in mice.[15] Given these data, combination therapy with ciprofloxacin and cefotaxime should be used without regard to the age of the patient.

In vitro, the addition of the iron chelator deferasirox to antimicrobial treatment (in this study, ciprofloxacin) resulted in synergistic antimicrobial activity.[58] One case has been reported of a patient iron-overloaded from hemochromatosis who survived after treatment with the combination of ciprofloxacin and deferasirox.[35]

The addition of modified Dakin solution (0.025% sodium hypochlorite) may have some utility in the treatment of skin and wound infections. An in vitro study of eight topical antibiotic preparations showed that *V. vulnificus* was most sensitive to modified Dakin solution.[52] Although no controlled trial has been performed, a series has been reported of 10 patients with culture-proved *V. vulnificus* wound infections treated with doxycycline and topical modified Dakin solution, none of whom experienced progression of infection or required surgical debridement.[76] Autologous platelet concentrate spray was used successfully as adjunctive wound therapy in a renal transplant patient.[72]

PREVENTION

Patients with severe anemia, liver disease, hemosiderosis, or other debilitating chronic diseases and patients on deferoxamine therapy should be advised against eating raw seafood of any kind. Awareness of the disease has been shown to be low in high-risk patients; physicians need to educate at-risk patients.[56] Patients with open wounds probably should avoid contact with seawater or brackish inland waters. In a mouse model, intramuscular VvpE (a recombinant metalloprotease/elastase antigen of *V. vulnificus*) elicits a good antibody response and confers protection against lethal challenge.[13]

NEW REFERENCES SINCE THE SEVENTH EDITION

3. Arezes J, Jung G, Gabayan V, et al. Hepcidin-induced hypoferremia is a critical host defense mechanism against the siderophilic bacterium *Vibrio vulnificus*. *Cell Host Microbe*. 2015;17:47-57.
12. Chao WN, Tsai CF, Chang HR, et al. Impact of timing of surgery on outcome of *Vibrio vulnificus*-related necrotizing fasciitis. *Am J Surg*. 2013;206:32-39.
14. Chen SC, Lee YT, Tsai SJ, et al. Antibiotic therapy for necrotizing fasciitis caused by *Vibrio vulnificus*: retrospective analysis of an 8 year period. *J Antimicrob Chemother*. 2012;67:488-493.
20. Duong-Nu TM, Jeong K, Hong SH, et al. All three TonB systems are required for *Vibrio vulnificus* CMCP6 tissue invasiveness by controlling flagellum expression. *Infect Immun*. 2015;2:254-265.
28. Hong GL, Dai XQ, Lu CH, et al. Temporizing surgical management improves outcome in patients with *Vibrio* necrotizing fasciitis complicated with septic shock on admission. *Burns*. 2014;40:446-454.
30. Jang HC, Choi SM, Kim HK, et al. In vivo efficacy of the combination of ciprofloxacin and cefotaxime against *Vibrio vulnificus* sepsis. *PLoS ONE*. 2014;9:3101118.
41. Kotton Y, Soboh S, Bisharat N. *Vibrio vulnificus* necrotizing fasciitis associated with acupuncture. *Infect Dis Rep*. 2015;29:5901.
46. Lee SJ, Jung YH, Ryu JM, et al. VvpE mediates the intestinal colonization of *Vibrio vulnificus* by the disruption of tight junctions. *Int J Med Microbiol*. 2016;306(1):10-19.
45. Lee YC, Hor L, Chiu HY, Lee JW, Shieh SJ. Prognostic factor of mortality and its clinical implications in patients with necrotizing fasciitis caused by *Vibrio vulnificus*. *Eur J Clin Microbiol Infect Dis*. 2014;33:1011-1018.
59. Newton A, Kendall M, Vugia DJ, Henao OL, Mahon BE. Increasing rates of vibriosis in the United States, 1996-2010: review of surveillance data from 2 systems. *Clin Infect Dis*. 2012;54(suppl 5):S391-S395.
81. Yun NR, Kim DM, Lee J, Han MA. pH level as a marker for predicting death among patients with *Vibrio vulnificus* infection, South Korea, 2000-2011. *Emerg Infect Dis*. 2015;21:259-264.

The full reference list for this chapter is available at ExpertConsult.com.

120 Miscellaneous Non-Enterobacteriaceae Fermentative Bacilli

Randall G. Fisher

Fermentative bacilli that are not of the family Enterobacteriaceae are discussed in this chapter. Specifically examined are *Chromobacterium violaceum, Plesiomonas shigelloides,* and *Pasteurella* organisms other than *Pasteurella multocida*.

CHROMOBACTERIUM VIOLACEUM

C. violaceum is a facultatively anaerobic, gram-negative rod that is a saprophyte of soil and water and is found especially in tropical and subtropical climates. It causes occasional illness in animals and, rarely, in humans. Infection with *C. violaceum,* when it does occur, is a serious disease with a high mortality rate.

Bacteriology

C. violaceum is a long, motile, gram-negative bacillus that appears singly or in pairs on Gram stain. It has a polar flagellum and one to four subpolar or lateral flagella that antigenically are distinct from the polar flagellum.[96] Most isolates produce an insoluble pigment, violacein. This pigment is intense and makes colonies appear dark purple to black, especially on blood agar. Violacein induces apoptotic death in certain cell types in vitro, including leukemia and lymphoma cells.[72] The therapeutic potential of violacein and structural analogs is being explored. Violacein also has antibacterial, antitrypanosomic, antimalarial,[65] and weak antiviral effects.[8] In a rat model, violacein displays immunomodulatory, analgesic, and antipyretic effects[11]; in addition, it protects against gastric ulcers[12] and is an effective treatment for diarrhea.[13] *C. violaceum* grows readily on standard agar (any medium that contains tryptophan supports growth). The colonies are low convex, violet, smooth, and not gelatinous. Colonies produce hydrogen cyanide; thus, a faint almond odor may be present.[96]

C. violaceum is catalase positive and oxidase positive, although the latter may be difficult to interpret because of the production of pigment. Growing the organism anaerobically inhibits pigment formation.[58] Pigment also may be lost on subculture[85] or as effective treatment is initiated. *C. violaceum* has a fermentative, not oxidative, attack on carbohydrates.

Epidemiology

C. violaceum commonly is found in soil and water of areas with tropical or subtropical weather patterns. It also has been recovered from soil as far north as New Jersey.[28] Ten of the first 12 cases reported in the United States occurred in Florida; the other two were in Louisiana. Subsequently, one case from New Jersey[79] and one from Ohio[98] have been reported, along with more from southeastern states. All but one case occurred during summer.[85] Patients tend to be young, with a median age of 14 years.[85]

Pathophysiology

Although *C. violaceum* is a common inhabitant of soil and water, human infection is rare. Disorders of neutrophil function are important risk factors. A disproportionately high number of *C. violaceum* infections have occurred in patients with chronic granulomatous disease[67] (CGD); in one case, *C. violaceum* septic shock with multiple skin, liver, and lung abscesses was the presenting feature of CGD.[88] *C. violaceum* infection in a child with another disorder of neutrophil function, polymorphonuclear leukocyte glucose-6-phosphate dehydrogenase deficiency, has been reported.[68] Organisms may show variable virulence, and differences in endotoxin activity, resistance to phagocytosis, and production of catalase and hydrogen peroxide have been observed between clinical and soil isolates.[76] An elastase activity, expressed through the entire life cycle and produced by a zinc metalloproteinase, may account for the propensity of *C. violaceum* to cause abscesses.[113] Because *C. violaceum* is a free-living organism that is exposed to diverse environmental conditions, it exploits a wide range of energy resources and is able to thrive in aerobic and anaerobic conditions.[27] It is equipped to be tolerant of harsh conditions, including acid and ultraviolet stress, temperature stress, heavy metal exposure, and antibiotic exposure.[50] The complete sequencing of its genome has allowed researchers to identify putative virulence genes that are likely involved in host cell adhesion, cell invasion, and cytolysis.[19] Cytotoxicity is caused by pore formation on host cell membranes; this is mediated by a type 3 secretion system product of pathogenicity island 1.[75] A *Serratia*-type hemolysin has also been described.[21] *C. violaceum* is able to produce an exopolysaccharide biofilm.[16]

The organism usually gains entrance to the body through cuts or abrasions that come in contact with contaminated soil or water. After entrance, a localized infection usually develops at or around the site of entry, which is commonly followed by dissemination of infection via the bloodstream to distant sites. Rapid debridement and appropriate antibiotic therapy may arrest the infection at the wound stage.[62] Two cases of systemic infection occurred in near-drowning victims. One case report describes fulminant infection and death in an immunocompetent host from *C. violaceum* sepsis that began as conjunctivitis after a fall that splattered mud into the patient's eye.[33] Another severe case with sepsis and multiorgan dysfunction began as a small prick injury to a finger.[10] Numerous microabscesses are found in multiple organs, especially liver, lung, and kidneys. Spread to bone, joints, and the central nervous system also has been described.

Clinical Manifestations

The pattern of illness in all reported patients is similar, with a contaminated inoculation site, localized disease, regional lymphadenopathy, and hematogenous spread to visceral organs. Progression of symptoms tends to be rapid after a variable incubation period.

Most patients have cutaneous lesions,[67] which are described as being nodular or pustular and sometimes with surrounding cellulitis.[104] They may progress to suppuration and drainage or to ulceration. Occasionally, classic ecthyma gangrenosum lesions have been described.[20] Regional lymphadenopathy is common; some of the nodes suppurate and require surgical drainage or removal.

Severe disease is heralded by high fever (39°C–41°C [102.2°F–105.8° F]), confusion or lethargy, abdominal pain, headaches, nausea and vomiting, and sometimes myalgias. Patients with systemic illness appear toxic. Hepatosplenomegaly develops frequently, and jaundice may be present. Progression from high fever and moderate toxicity to septic shock with disseminated intravascular coagulation and multisystem organ failure is precipitous.[10] After the liver, the lung is the most common site of dissemination of infection, and evidence of pneumonia often is found. Adult respiratory distress syndrome is rare.[63] Brain and liver abscesses have been noted.[77] The overall mortality rate is 65%.[67] Rarely, there may be recurrence, which can prove fatal.[58,85] A review of all 25 pediatric cases reported between 1971 and 2005 revealed, counterintuitively, that the case-fatality rate was 12 of 16 (75%) in patients without CGD and in none of 9 in patients with a known diagnosis of CGD.[94] One case in a patient with CGD who suffered three separate episodes of *C. violaceum* sepsis has been reported.[100]

A review of all cases reported between 1952 and 2009 (N = 106) found that all patients had fever. Sepsis developed in 82% of patients. Localized abscesses were found in about half of the patients, with the liver being the most common site. Relapse occurred in 6.6%, with a median interval of 135 days. Risk factors for mortality were young age at diagnosis, the presence of a localized abscess, a shorter clinical course, and inappropriate initial antimicrobial therapy.[110]

Diagnosis

Diagnosis is made by recovery of the organism from blood, lymph nodes, skin lesions, or abscesses. Gram-negative bacilli sometimes can be seen in smears or grown in culture[10] of material from skin lesions. Laboratory values reveal either very low or very high white blood cell counts with marked left shifts. Mild to moderate anemia is common. Serum levels of liver enzymes may be elevated, and evidence of early renal failure sometimes is present. The organism grows readily and is easy to identify if it produces the characteristic violet pigment. Nonpigmented forms exist in soil and have similar virulence in mice[95] but are recovered only rarely from clinical specimens.[98] Other cases may have been missed, however, because the nonpigmented forms often are misidentified as *Aeromonas hydrophila* or as pseudomonads.[95] Reports that *C. violaceum* infection causes a melioidosis-like illness were probably due to misidentification of *Burkholderia pseudomallei* by the API 20NE system.[51]

A clinical history of contamination of a wound with water or soil—especially in the southeastern United States or in Southeast Asia—with subsequent local infection, lymph node suppuration, and lack of response to conventional antibiotic therapy should arouse suspicion of *C. violaceum* infection. The clinician particularly should be aware of the possibility of *C. violaceum* infection in patients with CGD.

Treatment

C. violaceum is sensitive in vitro to chloramphenicol, gentamicin, fluorinated quinolones, tetracyclines, imipenem, trimethoprim-sulfamethoxazole, and semisynthetic penicillins. *C. violaceum* often is resistant to cephalosporins, penicillin, ampicillin, and the antistaphylococcal penicillins. All isolates are resistant to vancomycin and rifampin.[5] Some strains have been shown to elaborate a β-lactamase, which is chromosomal and inducible in vitro.[32] At least one case report gives in vivo evidence of inducible resistance to ceftazidime.[104] Laboratory evidence of susceptibility to erythromycin cannot be relied on. In vitro, the fluoroquinolones have the highest activity.[5] Clinical experience with the fluoroquinolones in *C. violaceum* infection is scarce; an impressive case of a 4-month-old infant with severe disseminated *C. violaceum* infection who survived after therapy with trimethoprim-sulfamethoxazole and ciprofloxacin has been reported.[77] The review of 25 cases mentioned earlier found that all survivors had been given one or a combination of the following agents: ciprofloxacin, trimethoprim-sulfamethoxazole, chloramphenicol, or imipenem.[94]

Because infection with *C. violaceum* is rare and often rapidly fatal, optimal antimicrobial therapy is unknown. Duration of therapy also is unknown, but because of late recurrences, some authors recommend 3 to 4 weeks of intravenous therapy followed by 1 month or more of oral trimethoprim-sulfamethoxazole.[85]

PLESIOMONAS SHIGELLOIDES

Plesiomonas shigelloides is the only species of the genus *Plesiomonas*. These organisms are facultatively anaerobic, motile, gram-negative rods that are common inhabitants of surface water and fish. They have been implicated in gastrointestinal infections and, rarely, have been recovered from extraintestinal sites.

Bacteriology

P. shigelloides is a member of the Vibrionaceae, although some authorities suggest that it is related more closely to Enterobacteriaceae.[66] The organisms are motile by means of a polar flagellum. They can produce lateral flagellae when grown in solid or semi-solid media.[74] They are lysine positive, ornithine positive, and arginine decarboxylase positive. They can be distinguished from Enterobacteriaceae by oxidase positivity. They also are catalase positive and indole positive. They grow well on MacConkey agar but not on thiosulfate citrate bile salts sucrose agar. Growth may be enhanced by the use of selective media, such as trypticase soy broth with ampicillin[86] and inositol brilliant green–bile salts agar. Growth is maximal at 40°C to 44°C and completely inhibited at 8°C. Usually within 24 hours, 1.0- to 1.5-mm grayish, shiny, opaque colonies with a slightly raised center and a smooth surface are visible. A few isolates of *P. shigelloides* share a common O antigen with *Shigella sonnei.*

Epidemiology

The organism is a ubiquitous freshwater inhabitant at temperatures greater than 8°C. It sometimes also is found in estuarial waters in temperate or tropical climates and can exist in seawater during the summer. It has been cultured from finfish, shellfish, pigs, birds, and dogs.[108] Although infection with *P. shigelloides* has been associated with ingestion of raw or improperly cooked fish (especially oysters), it is unknown what role, if any, other animals play in the ecology of the organism. Asymptomatic carriage of *P. shigelloides* is rare in developed countries[90] but may be 15% in some parts of China.[108]

Pathophysiology

Despite the ubiquity of the organism in nature, human infection is uncommon. Most often, infection is associated with gastroenteritis. Evidence for the role of *P. shigelloides* in the production of gastrointestinal symptoms is that it has been isolated much more frequently from patients with diarrhea than from healthy control subjects[48]; there have been some outbreaks, especially in Japan; it often is the only organism detected in the stools of patients with gastroenteritis[71]; and patients who have *P. shigelloides* growing from a stool culture recover more quickly with than without antibiotic therapy.[55] Acquisition of disease has been linked specifically to consumption of raw seafood or untreated water and to foreign travel, especially to Mexico.[45,70] A study in China found *P. shigelloides* in 2.9% of 3564 outpatients with diarrhea; it accounted for 7.3% of bacterial isolates.[23]

The mechanism by which the organism produces disease has been elusive. It is not enteroinvasive by laboratory tests, most investigators fail to find either a Shiga toxin or an enterotoxin,[1,45] no animal model of gastrointestinal disease has been found,[18] patients in the recovery phase do not show serologic evidence of infection, and inoculation of volunteers fails to produce illness.[45] In a suckling gnotobiotic piglet model in which the animals became septic, histology of the gastrointestinal tract showed neither destruction of cells nor invasion of tissues.[45] Neonatal BALB/c mice became chronically infected with *P. shigelloides,* however; histopathologic findings included some cases of necrosis of the mucosal surface of the ileum and colon.[107]

Some potential virulence factors (i.e., a cholera-like toxin, a weak cytolysin, serum resistance, and a large [>150-kDa] plasmid) have been described, but their exact roles in pathophysiology are uncertain; attempts to correlate these features with virulence have been fruitless.[1] Investigators have characterized a cytotoxin derived from *P. shigelloides* using strains from patients with a diarrheal illness. The cytotoxin is a complex of three lipopolysaccharide-binding proteins and lipopolysaccharide in a 6:5 ratio.[81] Cytotoxic activity was inhibited 80% in vitro by proteinase K or when incubated with anticholera toxin antibody. This cytotoxin produced a positive reaction in the suckling mouse assay, whereas the purified lipopolysaccharide exhibited almost no cytotoxicity.[81] The lipopolysaccharide downregulates complement and has been shown to be important in attachment, invasion, and biofilm formation.[14]

Transmission electron microscopy has provided investigators with the first definitive proof that *P. shigelloides* can adhere to and invade eukaryotic intestinal cells. Organisms attached to microvilli and plasma membranes of the cells; they also were seen within vacuoles in the cell cytoplasm, suggesting a phagocytotic entry mechanism.[102] In one in vitro system using Caco-2 cells, adherence occurred within 10 minutes and internalization occurred within 60 minutes. Cytotoxicity was due to the induction of apoptosis.[105] In vitro, cell-free and cell-associated hemolysis is demonstrable,[40] and low levels of elastase, proteinase, histidine decarboxylase, and moderate levels of triacylglycerol lipase activity have been found.[26] Culture filtrates are capable of inducing vacuolation of a variety of mammalian cells in vitro.[31]

P. shigelloides rarely, but more clearly, is a pathogen in extraintestinal sites. Osteomyelitis, endophthalmitis, cholecystitis, pseudoappendicitis, spontaneous peritonitis,[4] meningitis,[101] and septicemia have been reported sporadically.[18] Most patients with septicemia have been immunocompromised hosts, but the organism has been isolated from blood cultures in otherwise healthy individuals.[52,84] The mode of infection in extraintestinal sites is unclear, but most cases are thought to arise from the gastrointestinal tract. The case of a newborn with *P. shigelloides* meningitis, septicemia, and endophthalmitis who was born to a mother who reported severe diarrhea after eating raw oysters 2 weeks before delivery raises the possibility of transplacental transmission.[69]

Clinical Manifestations

Patients with *P. shigelloides* gastroenteritis complain of diarrhea, crampy abdominal pain, nausea and vomiting, headache, and fever. Symptoms usually begin 24 hours to 4 days after contact with the organism.[48] Diarrhea tends to be secretory, although some patients have symptoms more consistent with colitis.[55] Passage of blood, mucus, or both in the stools is a common manifestation, as is the presence of white blood cells by Wright stain.[48] Patients with *P. shigelloides* gastroenteritis tend to have disease that is more acute, associated with more severe abdominal pain, and of longer duration than patients with diseases caused by other enteropathogens.[55]

In one case-control study, 76% of patients were sick for more than 2 weeks and 32% were sick for more than a month.[55] In contrast, a large Japanese study of returning travelers suggested that for most patients, the symptoms abated within approximately 3 days.[93] In a series of 38 pediatric cases in Bangladesh, 84% had secretory diarrhea and 71% had associated emesis. Only three patients (8%) had fever, and only five (13%) had diarrhea for 14 days or longer.[60] In a separate report, one child developed migratory polyarthritis during an otherwise typical case of culture-proven gastrointestinal infection. All symptoms and signs of arthritis disappeared when the gastrointestinal infection was treated with antibiotics.[42]

Localized extraintestinal infections have been reported but are rare. Two cases of severe polymicrobial endophthalmitis resulting from fishhook trauma progressed to enucleation.[22] A rapidly progressive keratitis after corneal laceration has been reported.[61] Two cases of peritonitis associated with continuous ambulatory peritoneal dialysis were reported from Hong Kong. Both patients recovered after 10 days of therapy with intraperitoneal cefazolin and tobramycin.[109] There has been one report of spontaneous bacterial peritonitis.[83] In one odd case, a woman had pyosalpinx from *P. shigelloides* thought to have been acquired by swimming in contaminated water.[91] A cavitary pneumonia was found in a 78-year-old woman who underwent gastrectomy and esophagojejunostomy because of adenocarcinoma of the stomach. Biopsy showed granulomatous changes.[92] One patient developed a skin abscess after incurring trauma in fresh water.[46]

Septicemia, meningitis, or both usually occur in immunocompromised hosts. Severe, rapidly progressive sepsis complicated by disseminated intravascular coagulation, adult respiratory distress syndrome, renal insufficiency, hepatic dysfunction, adrenal hemorrhage, and splenic abscess has occurred in patients with hemoglobinopathies and absence of splenic function, including thalassemia intermedia and sickle-cell disease.[7,106] Unusual sites of infection sometimes are noted in immunocompromised individuals, such as epididymo-orchitis in a patient with human immunodeficiency virus infection.[112] Newborns constitute most of the reported cases of *P. shigelloides* meningitis, in whom the mortality rate is 80%.[1] Cerebrospinal fluid parameters may be normal, even when the culture is positive.[82] Septicemia also has a high mortality rate in adults, although otherwise well patients may recover with appropriate antimicrobial therapy.

Diagnosis

A clinical history of foreign travel or of ingestion of raw seafood or untreated water should raise suspicion of possible *P. shigelloides* infection, especially when the clinical illness matches the description just mentioned. Oxidase tests should be done on any predominant or solitary organisms to distinguish them from Enterobacteriaceae.[48] The organisms can be shown not to be aeromonads or pseudomonads by production of ornithine decarboxylase and fermentation of inositol. Selective medium can be used if the index of suspicion is high. A new indicator medium (UNISC agar) for the identification of *Aeromonas* and *Plesiomonas* has been developed; colonies turn yellow if xylose is fermented and turn blue if it is not.[89] Loop-mediated amplification assays[73] and polymerase chain reactions have also been developed; it is included in some commercial multiplex polymerase chain reactions that are increasingly available.

Treatment

Most strains of *P. shigelloides* produce a β-lactamase,[87] which seems to be specific for the penicillins. In one study, all isolates were resistant to ampicillin, ticarcillin, carbenicillin, and piperacillin.[37] *P. shigelloides* is universally susceptible to trimethoprim-sulfamethoxazole, the fluoroquinolones, most cephalosporins, carbapenems,[99] tetracycline,[99] and chloramphenicol. It is variably susceptible to the aminoglycosides and mostly resistant to erythromycin.[54]

P. shigelloides gastroenteritis resolves without therapy, but the illness may be prolonged. Treatment seems to shorten the course.[55] Extraintestinal infections carry a poor prognosis and should be treated aggressively. For meningitis, cephalosporins and carbapenems have good cerebrospinal fluid penetration and are effective therapy against most isolates.

OTHER PASTEURELLA ORGANISMS

The genus *Pasteurella* consists of a group of pleomorphic, gram-negative coccobacilli that are part of the normal flora of many animals. These organisms are frequent animal pathogens. *P. multocida* is a common human pathogen and is discussed in Chapter 116. The other species of the genus *Pasteurella* are rare but occasionally cause serious infection in humans.

Bacteriology

These organisms, similar to *P. multocida*, grow readily on most common laboratory media, including blood agar. Most of the species do not grow on MacConkey agar. They are non–spore forming, nonmotile, aerobic, and facultatively anaerobic. These glucose-fermenting organisms all are oxidase positive. Most are nitrate positive and catalase positive, and all except *Avibacterium gallinarum* (formerly *Pasteurella gallinarum*, discussed later) produce indole. They are small, coccoid or rod-shaped bacilli that may show prominent bipolar staining on Gram stain. Colonies are small, translucent, and gray and may be smooth or rough. A browning discoloration may develop around them, and they are nonhemolytic with a distinctive musty or "mushroom" odor.[25]

The taxonomy of these organisms is confusing and continues to be revised. *Pasteurella ureae* was moved to the genus *Actinobacillus*. *Pasteurella haemolytica* has been reclassified into the genus *Mannheimia*.[9] *Pasteurella dagmatis* is the name now given to what formerly was called *P.* new species, or *P.* "gas."[78] *Pasteurella gallinarum*, *Pasteurella avium*, and *Pasteurella volantium* have 96.8% sequence similarity and are phenotypically separate from other *Pasteurella* spp.; therefore, they have been moved into the genus *Avibacterium*.[17] Most experts agree that the genus *Pasteurella sensu stricto* should include *P. multocida*, *P. canis*, *P. stomatis*, and *P. dagmatis*.[56] *Pasteurella* spp. B has now been reclassified as *P. oralis* sp. nov.[24] Clinically recovered species other than *P. multocida* include *Actinobacillus ureae*, *Mannheimia haemolytica*, *Pasteurella pneumotropica*, *P. dagmatis*, *P. canis*, *Pasteurella aerogenes*, *Pasteurella bettyae*, *P.* "SP" group, *P. oralis*, and *P. stomatis*. *Pasteurella caballi* has caused wound infections after horse bites.[29] *Avibacterium gallinarum* is an extremely rare pathogen in humans.

Pathophysiology

Infection with *Pasteurella* spp. has been divided clinically into three types: (1) from animal bites, (2) from animal contact,[36] and (3) without known animal contact.[27] Infections from animal bites include cellulitis, abscesses, tenosynovitis, and bone and joint infection, but infection can become generalized, especially in patients who are immunocompromised. Infections caused by animal contact can be similar to infections described earlier and are caused by animals licking broken skin or wounds. Sometimes pulmonary infections occur, possibly related to aerosolization of organisms. In some cases, these organisms have been reported as respiratory flora in patients with pets, but at present no proof exists that such colonization is an antecedent of infection.[34] Cases without known animal contact history constitute 3% to 30% of all cases.[49,53]

Infection usually occurs when the organisms are inoculated into deeper tissues either on animal teeth that break the skin or in animal saliva that comes in contact with nonintact skin. Bite wound infections often are polymicrobial. Infection in cases without known animal contact is harder to explain but definitely happens.[57] Most cases of serious infection occur in patients with underlying diseases, such as diabetes mellitus, chronic alcoholism, and other types of liver disease.[80] Central nervous system infection with these organisms has occurred after head trauma or neurosurgery in 10 of 11 reported cases.[57] One intrauterine death of the fetus of a 20-year-old woman who worked at a pig farm has been attributed to *P. aerogenes*.[103] Case reports of unusual infections with rare species of *Pasteurella*, such as fatal sepsis and meningitis in a 4-day-old infant caused by *A. gallinarum*,[2] should be considered doubtful unless molecular identification methods have been used.[44]

Clinical Manifestations

Pasteurella infections produce pain, swelling, pus, and sometimes abscess formation at the site of inoculation, beginning within 24 to 36 hours. Clinically, these infections are indistinguishable from wound infections with *Staphylococcus aureus* or other gram-positive organisms. Gram stain may show the characteristic pleomorphic bacilli with bipolar staining. Growth on standard agar is rapid.

Patients with peritonitis,[4,80] meningitis,[57] osteomyelitis,[37] or infectious endocarditis[6] have symptoms typical of these diagnoses. Risk factors—such as household pet exposure, animal contact, animal bites, and comorbid conditions—should heighten suspicion of possible *Pasteurella* infection. One report describes a previously healthy 21-month-old girl who developed *P. canis* bacteremia after exposure to rabbit saliva.[111] Bacteremia due to *P. canis* has also been described in a cirrhotic patient whose leg wound was licked by a dog.[3] Children on continuous ambulatory peritoneal dialysis may rarely develop peritonitis with *Pasteurella* species.[41]

In one eastern European study of an outbreak in a child welfare agency, *P. canis* was cultured from the anterior fornix of several infants with refractory conjunctivitis.[15]

Diagnosis

Establishing the diagnosis of *Pasteurella* infection can be difficult, not because the organism is fastidious or slow growing but because it often is misidentified. Other organisms of the same family (i.e., *Actinobacillus* spp. and *Haemophilus* spp.) have similar biochemical profiles and can be misidentified by commonly used systems, such as API. Lester and associates[64] reported that of 30 species firmly identified as *Pasteurella* by biochemical means, only 3 were identified correctly by the API 20E system. *Actinobacillus* (*Haemophilus*) *aphrophilus* and *Actinobacillus actinomycetemcomitans* are sometimes misidentified as *Avibacterium gallinarum* by commercial systems.[35] Additionally, Hamilton-Miller[43] reported that four strains of *Haemophilus influenzae* and three strains of *Haemophilus parainfluenzae* were identified falsely as *Pasteurella* spp. by API and suggested that if the clinical history renders *Pasteurella* infection unlikely, then tests for X and V factor requirements should be performed (see Chapter 133). Clinical case reports corroborate these laboratory observations.[30,80,97] Notifying the bacteriology laboratory of suspicion of *Pasteurella* infection is helpful. These problems are being minimized by newer techniques, including matrix-assisted laser desorption ionization-time of flight.

Treatment

Penicillin has been considered the drug of choice for *Pasteurella* infection in the past and, despite some reports of penicillin resistance, still is effective against most strains. *Pasteurella* spp. also are susceptible to ampicillin, β-lactamase–inhibitor combination drugs, tetracycline, and chloramphenicol. Truncated but fully functional tetracycline resistance genes have been identified in isolates from animal sources.[59] The aminoglycosides, erythromycin, clindamycin, cefadroxil, and cefaclor are not recommended. Dicloxacillin and cephalexin have poor activity against *Pasteurella* spp. and should not be used as monotherapy for animal bite wounds.[38] In one study of bite wound infections, ertapenem was found to be active against all *Pasteurella* spp.[39] Of fluoroquinolones tested in vitro against 75 clinical isolates of *Pasteurella* spp., levofloxacin was the most active.[47]

Acknowledgments

I thank Dr. William Gruber and Dr. Thomas Boyce for their invaluable assistance with earlier versions of this chapter.

NEW REFERENCES SINCE THE SEVENTH EDITION

10. Ansari S, Paudel P, Gautam K, et al. *Chromobacterium violaceum* isolated from wound sepsis: a case study from Nepal. *Case Rep Infect Dis.* 2015;181946.
12. Antonisamy P, Kannan P, Aravinthan A, et al. Gastroprotective activity of violacein isolated from *Chromobacterium violaceum* on indomethacin-induced gastric lesions in rats: investigation of potential mechanisms of action. *Scientific World J.* 2014;616432.
14. Aquilini E, Merino S, Tomas JM. The *Plesiomonas shigelloides* sb(O1) gene cluster and the role of O1-antigen LPS in pathogenicity. *Microb Pathog.* 2013;63:1-7.
15. Balikoglu-Yilmaz M, Yilmaz T, Esen AB, Engin KN, Taskapili M. *Pasteurella canis* and *Granulicatella adiacens* conjunctivitis outbreak resistant to empirical treatment in a child welfare agency. *J Pediatr Ophthalmol Strabismus.* 2012;49:314-319.
23. Chen X, Chen Y, Yang Q, et al. *Plesiomonas shigelloides* infection in Southeast China. *PLoS ONE.* 2013;8:e77877.
41. Gundluru R, Bheemanathini P, Rafee Y. *Pasteurella canis* peritonitis in a child on peritoneal dialysis. *Pediatr Infect Dis J.* 2015;34:332.
61. Klatte JM, Dastjerdi MH, Clark K, et al. Hyperacute infectious keratitis with *Plesiomonas shigelloides* following traumatic corneal laceration. *Pediatr Infect Dis J.* 2012;31:1200-1201.
73. Meng S, Xu J, Xiong Y, Ye C. Rapid and sensitive detection of *Plesiomonas shigelloides* by loop-mediated isothermal amplification of the *hugA* gene. *PLoS ONE.* 2012;7:e41978.
74. Merino S, Aquilini E, Fulton KM, Twine SM, Tomas JM. The polar and lateral flagella from *Plesiomonas shigelloides* are glycosylated with legionaminic acid. *Front Microbiol.* 2015;6:649.
83. Patel S, Gandhi D, Mehta V, Bhatia K, Epelbaum O. Plesiomonas shigelloides: an extremely rare cause of spontaneous bacterial peritonitis. *Acta Gastroenterol Belg.* 2016;79:52-53.
88. Richard KR, Lovvorn JJ, Oliver SE, et al. *Chromobacterium violaceum* sepsis: rethinking conventional therapy to improve outcome. *Am J Case Rep.* 2015;19:740-744.

The full reference list for this chapter is available at ExpertConsult.com.

121 Acinetobacter

Armando G. Correa

First recognized as a human pathogen in 1908,[94] the ubiquitous organism *Acinetobacter* has emerged as a rather common cause of health care–associated infections in immunocompromised hosts.[8] Some of the confusion regarding this organism may be attributed to the many changes in nomenclature that the members of this genus have undergone over the years. Names used in the past to identify this genus include *Herellea, Bacterium, Mima, Achromobacter, Alcaligenes, Neisseria, Micrococcus, Diplococcus, Moraxella,* and *Cytophaga.* Treatment of infection caused by *Acinetobacter* is complicated by its widespread multidrug resistance and the difficulty encountered in eradicating the organism.

ORGANISM

The genus *Acinetobacter* is now classified in the Moraxellaceae, a recently proposed family that also includes the *Moraxella* and *Psychrobacter* genera.[65] *Acinetobacter* is a gram-negative bacterium that typically appears as a rod 0.9 to 1.6 μm in diameter and 1.5 to 2.5 μm in length, but it may become spherical in the stationary phase of growth. It frequently occurs in pairs or short chains. Many strains are encapsulated. The organism has a strictly aerobic respiratory metabolism and does not grow under anaerobic conditions. It does not form spores or exhibit swimming mobility. *Acinetobacter* grows well in all common complex media between 20°C and 30°C, with optimal growth occurring between 33°C and 35°C, and it has no growth factor requirements.

Convex, grayish white colonies 1.0 to 2.5 mm in diameter are typical findings. The colonies may appear mucoid if the strain is encapsulated. *Acinetobacter* is catalase positive and may be differentiated readily from other closely related genera by virtue of its negative reaction to oxidase.

Formerly, the genus *Acinetobacter* contained the single species *A. calcoaceticus* subdivided into two subspecies or biovars: *anitratus* and *lwoffii.*[42] However, in 1986, the taxonomy of the genus *Acinetobacter* was changed extensively on the basis of DNA hybridization studies,[13] and at least 46 genomic species have been proposed, of which 41 have been assigned species names, according to the list of prokaryotic names with standing nomenclature (www.bacterio.net, as of June 2016). At least 19 of these nomenspecies have been isolated from human specimens, including: *A. baumannii, A. calcoaceticus, A. haemolyticus, A. johnsonii, A. junii, A. lwoffii, A. radioresistens, A. parvus, A. schindleri,* and *A. ursingi.*[20,42,59,60] Several genospecies that have been isolated from human clinical samples and had been given the provisional designation of genomic species 3, 13TU, 10, and 11 have now been named as *A. pittii, A. nosocomialis, A. bereziniae,* and *A. guillouiae,* respectively.[59,60] *A. soli,* a species previously isolated only from soil, has recently been implicated in an outbreak in a neonatal care unit.[66] Newly named species that have recently been isolated for human samples include *A. beijerinckii, A. gyllenbergii, A. seifertii,* and *A. variabilis.* These species may be difficult to differentiate in the clinical laboratory on the basis of their growth characteristics and biochemical activity.[43,65] In light of their closely related phenotypic properties and antimicrobial resistance, four of these species, *A. baumannii, A. calcoaceticus, A. pittii* (formerly genomic species 3), and *A. nosocomialis* (formerly genomic species 13TU), are grouped under the term *A. baumannii-calcoaceticus* complex. Furthermore the three clinically relevant members of this complex (*A. baumannii, A. pittii,* and *A. nosocomialis*) cannot be separated by currently available commercial identification systems, prompting the use of the term *A. baumannii* group to accommodate these three species that share epidemiologic and clinical features.[42,65] Under the new classification, most

TABLE 121.1 Illustrative Nosocomial Clusters of Acinetobacter Infection in Pediatric Patients Over the Past 3 Decades

Country	Year	Type of Unit	Infected Children	Colonized Children	Presentation	Mortality (%)	Suspected Source
United Kingdom[58]	1981	NICU	4	0	Meningitis	0	None identified
United Kingdom[88]	1983	NICU	9	1	Pulmonary infection	22	Ambu bag
India[45]	1988	Oncology	8	NA	Meningitis	38	Intrathecal needle
Germany[80]	1988	NICU	3	41	Sepsis	100	Humidifier
Israel[71]	1988–1990	NICU	9	NA	Sepsis	44	None identified
India[56]	1995	NICU	79	NA	Sepsis	14	None identified
Bahamas[55]	1996	NICU	8	1	Sepsis	37	Air conditioner
South Africa[67]	1997	NICU	9	NA	Sepsis	22	Suction catheters
Taiwan[39]	2000	NICU	9	NA	Sepsis	0	HCW hands
US[87]	2004	NICU	4	3	Sepsis	57	Referring hospital
Brazil[66]	2005	NICU	5	NA	Sepsis	20	Intravenous fluids
Turkey[37]	2006–2007	NICU	64	NA	Sepsis	83	Multiple sources
South Korea[36]	2001–2011	PICU	13	7	Bacteremia (10), pneumonia (3)	85[a]	Sinks/water taps

HCW, Health care workers; *NA*, data not available; *NICU*, neonatal intensive care unit; *PICU*, pediatric intensive care unit.
[a]Outbreak was due to imipenem-resistant *A. baumannii.*

A. baumannii strains represent organisms that were classified formerly as biovar *anitratus,* whereas *A. junii* and *A. lwoffii* previously were listed under the biovar *lwoffii.*

EPIDEMIOLOGY

Acinetobacter strains are distributed widely in nature and can be found in soil, fresh water, and sewage.[10,33] *Acinetobacter* also can be isolated from many animals, fresh meats, poultry, contaminated milk, and frozen foods.[10,33] The organism can be part of the bacterial flora of the skin in healthy individuals,[10,15] and the skin frequently becomes a reservoir for *Acinetobacter* in hospitalized patients and the health care staff.[8,10] It occasionally forms part of the normal flora of the oral cavity and the upper respiratory, genital, and lower gastrointestinal tracts.[10,15] Colonization by *Acinetobacter* is particularly common in patients who have undergone a tracheostomy.[75] The organism frequently can be found in the hospital environment, particularly in moist areas, such as in humidifiers, water sinks, and ventilators.[10] In an outbreak of bacteremia due to *A. junii* among children in an pediatric oncology ward, faucet aerators were found to be reservoirs.[44] Nosocomial outbreaks have been linked to colonized medical equipment such as ventilator tubing and other respiratory equipment,[31] intravenous catheters,[10] hygroscopic bandages,[87] gloves,[64] and mattresses.[84]

The frequency of occurrence of health care–associated infections by *Acinetobacter* is not easy to assess because the pathogenic role of this organism often has been underestimated. However a national surveillance study conducted from 1974 to 1977 identified *Acinetobacter* as a pathogen in 0.76% of nosocomial infections.[72] The estimated rate of health care–associated infections caused by this organism was 3.11 per 10,000 patients discharged, and approximately 15% of 1372 reported episodes occurred in the pediatric age group.[72] By 1978, this rate increased by 14% and accounted for 1% of the bacterial isolates associated with healthcare-associated infections.[15] An unusual seasonal pattern was observed, with most infections occurring in late summer.[15,72] The cause of this increase is unknown. In a national prospective survey of US hospitals from 1995 through 2002, *Acinetobacter* spp. accounted for 1.3% of all health care–associated bloodstream infections and was associated with a crude mortality rate of 34%.[98] By 2003, the percentage almost doubled to 2.4% of nosocomial bloodstream infections from the same surveillance system.[26] When comparing data from 1986 to 2003, *Acinetobacter* spp. were the only gram-negative pathogens associated with a consistently increasing proportion of hospital-acquired pneumonias, as well as surgical site, urinary tract, and bloodstream infections.[26] Between 2006 and 2007, *A. baumannii* was the ninth most common pathogen associated with cases of health care–associated infections, accounting for nearly 3% of them.[35]

Data from SENTRY, an international surveillance program that monitors the frequency of occurrence and antimicrobial susceptibility of bacterial pathogens, revealed a significantly greater frequency of *Acinetobacter* infections in Latin America than in all other regions.[25] Data from another international surveillance consortium study of ICU infections from 2003 to 2008 revealed a striking increase in frequency of resistance to imipenem among *A. baumannii* when compared to that reported in a similar US system (46% vs. 29%).[76] A higher prevalence rate of *Acinetobacter* infections was noted in patients ranging in age from birth to 10 years.[25] In the pediatric age group, at least 20 outbreaks of invasive nosocomial infections due to *Acinetobacter* have been reported in the past three decades[37,38,87]; the vast majority of them were concentrated in neonatal ICUs (Table 121.1).[38,58,87]

More recently, *Acinetobacter* emerged as a particularly important pathogen in unusual situations such as earthquakes and war zones.[41] This prevalence was illustrated by reports of outbreaks of multidrug-resistant *Acinetobacter* infections associated with the US-Iraq conflict.[81]

PATHOGENESIS

Limited information is available regarding the pathogenesis of *Acinetobacter* infections. The lipopolysaccharide of *Acinetobacter,* a normal constituent of the outer membrane of gram-negative bacteria, is capable of eliciting multiple pathogenic host responses. Strains producing exopolysaccharide have been shown to be more pathogenic than are nonproducers.[41] Nonspecific adherence factors, such as fimbriae, also have been described in *Acinetobacter.*[41] The role of quorum sensing as a regulatory mechanism for autoinduction of multiple virulence factors in *Acinetobacter* is under investigation.[41]

In animal models, *Acinetobacter* can enhance the virulence of other bacteria in mixed infections, perhaps by slime-induced inhibition of neutrophils.[62] Researchers have speculated that the ability of this organism to grow in an acidic pH at lower temperatures may enhance its ability to invade devitalized tissue.[2] The organism also may survive in a dry environment for as long as a week.[16]

CLINICAL MANIFESTATIONS

Acinetobacter can cause suppurative infection of virtually any organ, and the clinical manifestations typically are similar to those seen with other bacterial infections because no unique features are suggestive of *Acinetobacter* infection. The clinical manifestations also may depend on the underlying immune status of compromised hosts. Infections caused by *Acinetobacter* are rare occurrences in normal children[21] and have mostly occurred in tropical areas.

Intracranial Infection

Most cases of *Acinetobacter* meningitis are the result of a penetrating injury or occur after a neurosurgical procedure, although sporadic cases of meningitis have been reported in the absence of these factors. A cluster of eight children in whom *Acinetobacter* meningitis developed after the administration of intrathecal methotrexate was reported.[44] All patients had fever, headache, nausea, and vomiting; and lumbar puncture revealed cerebrospinal fluid (CSF) pleocytosis.

The earlier literature contains several reports of *Acinetobacter* meningitis developing in apparently normal children.[18,19,34,91,95] CSF pleocytosis with a predominance of segmented forms occurred commonly.[19] Because as many as 30% of these patients had a petechial rash and gram-negative diplococci on CSF smears, the diagnosis of meningococcal meningitis was made erroneously in most of these cases, thereby leading to a delay in the institution of appropriate therapy and possibly contributing to a mortality rate as high as 27%.[19]

Siegman-Igra and associates,[86] in a review of 25 cases of *Acinetobacter* meningitis secondary to invasive procedures that included some children, found that fever, leukocytosis, and neck stiffness, along with other clinical signs of central nervous system (CNS) infection, were common features. The CSF in these patients showed pleocytosis with a predominance of polymorphonuclear leukocytes, elevated protein concentration, and a low glucose level. Most of the infections were associated with indwelling ventriculostomy tubes or a fistula into the CSF space. A case series from Pakistan[78] reported eight cases of *Acinetobacter* meningitis that occurred over the course of a 4-year period in children who had undergone neurosurgical procedures. Mortality in this series was 25%, and the use of intrathecal antibiotics was explored as an adjunctive therapy.[78]

Researchers have suggested that an inherited or acquired complement deficiency may be associated with meningitis caused by *Acinetobacter*[23] because it is seen with *Neisseria meningitidis* and other related species. Treatment of CNS infections caused by *Acinetobacter* requires a minimum of 3 weeks of parenteral antibiotics.

Bacteremia

Acinetobacter bacteremia may occur as an isolated event or may be secondary to a primary infected site, such as the respiratory tract, urinary tract, or a wound. Primary bacteremia appears to occur more commonly in immunocompromised neonates, and clinical manifestations can vary from an absence of clinical signs of infection to fulminant septic shock and disseminated intravascular coagulation.[46,80] Thrombocytopenia has been reported to be a prominent feature in these neonates.[39,61,71] Pneumonia has been seen more commonly in early-onset sepsis.[56] Predisposing factors include low birth weight,[77,80] previous antibiotic therapy,[71,77,80] and the presence of indwelling catheters.[39,55,77]

Acinetobacter bacteremia in children with malignant diseases also has been noted to occur rarely. Fuchs and colleagues[24] reported 29 episodes of sepsis caused by this organism over the course of a 12-year period in an oncology center. All these children were febrile and appeared ill at the time of diagnosis, and a high association of *Acinetobacter* sepsis with the presence of intravascular catheters was noted. Surprisingly no connection was found with the level of neutropenia.[24]

Community-acquired *Acinetobacter* bacteremia among infants less than 2 months of age has been reported in some developing countries.[30]

Respiratory Tract Infections

Because *Acinetobacter* may be a transient colonizer of the pharynx in 7% of healthy children[7] and adults[27] and this rate is increased in hospitalized patients, the relative importance of *Acinetobacter* in comparison with other potential pathogens isolated from sputum is difficult to ascertain. The tracheobronchitis and pneumonia attributed to *Acinetobacter* are mostly nosocomial infections associated with the presence of an endotracheal tube or tracheostomy.[27] Pneumonias frequently are multilobar and occasionally may lead to cavitary destruction or pleural empyema.[27]

Community-acquired pneumonia caused by *A. baumannii* has been reported to occur in adults in the Northern Territory of Australia and other tropical regions.[5] This entity generally is seen in patients with diminished host defenses caused by alcoholism, cigarette smoking, or underlying pulmonary disease and is characterized by the rapid onset of fever, dyspnea, pleuritic chest pain, and purulent sputum. The mortality rate has been as high as 53% to 64%,[5] although increased awareness and implementation of empiric antibiotic protocols that cover this organism has led to a dramatic reduction in mortality in these regions.[17] A case of necrotizing pneumonia due to *A. lwoffii* in a previously healthy toddler has been reported.[57]

Miscellaneous Infections

Urinary tract infections occur almost exclusively in patients with indwelling bladder catheters, usually are limited to the bladder, and generally are mild.[27] Burns, as well as traumatic and surgical wounds, frequently become colonized by *Acinetobacter* as a result of the ability of this organism to thrive on compromised tissue and foreign material.[27] Bacteremia may occur as a consequence of this colonization, which is often polymicrobial. *Acinetobacter* is a prominent cause of peritonitis in children undergoing peritoneal dialysis when gram-negative organisms are involved.[96]

Other rare infections caused by *Acinetobacter* that have been reported include suppurative otitis media,[73,91] cellulitis (frequently in association with trauma, a foreign body, or an animal bite),[27,73] synergistic necrotizing fasciitis,[4] native-valve and prosthetic-value endocarditis,[29] septic arthritis,[73] osteomyelitis,[91] and liver abscesses.[27] Ocular infections also have been documented.[53] A case of osteomyelitis occurring after a hamster bite in a child has been described.[54]

DIAGNOSIS

The diagnosis of *Acinetobacter* infection is made by culture of appropriate body fluids or tissue specimens. No serologic or antigen-detection tests are available. A selective medium containing MacConkey agar with cephaloridine has been used to culture skin specimens during investigation of outbreaks[88] because of its ability to inhibit most of the skin flora but not *Acinetobacter.*

Biotyping, phage typing, electrophoretic analysis of isoenzyme and cell wall proteins, plasmid analysis, polymerase chain reaction–based DNA fingerprinting, and restriction endonuclease digestion of DNA have been used for investigation of nosocomial outbreaks.[9,65] Antibiogram typing no longer is considered an effective method in the investigation of *Acinetobacter* epidemics because the susceptibility pattern may change rapidly within the same outbreak.[9,14]

TREATMENT

As with many other opportunistic gram-negative organisms, treatment of infections caused by *Acinetobacter* spp., particularly those of the *A. baumannii* group,[82,93] has become more complicated by the rapid increase in resistance to the antibiotics used commonly in hospitals. Selection of an antibiotic regimen should be based on in vitro susceptibility testing and ideally should include both a β-lactam antibiotic and an aminoglycoside, which may have synergistic activity[27] and prevent the emergence of resistance.[8]

Species of the *A. baumannii-calcoaceticus* complex have shown decreased susceptibility to ampicillin, broad-spectrum penicillins, cephalosporins, aminoglycosides, and ciprofloxacin.[25,82] Resistance to extended-spectrum cephalosporins may be the result of the presence of cephalosporinases (particularly the chromosomally encoded cephalosporinase AmpC),[12] other broad-spectrum β-lactamases, or changes in the outer-membrane porins and penicillin-binding proteins.[12,63] Resistance to aminoglycosides is mediated by aminoglycoside-modifying enzymes.[93] The carbapenems imipenem and meropenem appear to be the most active agents against *A. baumannii,*[86,93] but reports have found more than 10% of such strains to be resistant to these antibiotics in some areas,[25,52] and increasing numbers of nosocomial outbreaks of carbapenem-resistant *Acinetobacter* infections have been reported.[28,65,92,100] The incidence of carbapenem-resistant *Acinetobacter* strains has been particularly high in Latin America, Africa, Europe, and the Asian Pacific rim region.[11,25,51] Resistance to the carbapenems has been associated with the presence of serine and metallo-β-lactamases (carbapenemases). Of particular concern are the numerous carbapenem-hydrolyzing OXA enzymes that have emerged in *A. baumannii.*[12] Caution should be exercised when using imipenem in high doses in children for the treatment of meningitis (i.e., 100 mg/kg per day) because of an unusually high rate of seizures.[99] Thus, meropenem is recommended for this indication. Doripenem, a newer carbapenem antibiotic, has more potent in vitro activity against *Acinetobacter* species compared with other carbapenems,[22] but its safety and effectiveness in pediatric patients have not been established. On the other hand, ertapenem has poor in vitro activity against *Acinetobacter*[49] and should not be used for the treatment of these infections. Combinations of a β-lactam antibiotic with a β-lactamase inhibitor, such as ampicillin-sulbactam, piperacillin-tazobactam, or ticarcillin-clavulanate, have been used for infections caused by carbapenem-resistant strains.[92,100]

The fluoroquinolones, in particular ciprofloxacin, have been used successfully to treat infections caused by multidrug-resistant *Acinetobacter* in children[56,67] and adults. Although ciprofloxacin has been approved for the treatment of complicated urinary tract infections in children and levofloxacin for postexposure treatment of inhalation anthrax in the pediatric age group, the other systemic fluoroquinolones are not approved for use in children younger than 16 years because of the theoretic concern for damage to growth cartilage. Of the quinolones, gatifloxacin exhibits the best in vitro activity against *A. baumannii,* followed by levofloxacin and trovafloxacin.[32] Although 76% to 86% of sporadic isolates of *A. baumannii* are susceptible to the fluoroquinolones, only 32% to 55% of outbreak-related strains remain susceptible to this antibiotic class.[32] Topoisomerase mutations in both *gyrA* and *parC* have been identified in quinolone-resistant *A. baumannii.*[12]

In some cases, the polymyxin drugs polymyxin B and colistin are the only therapeutic options for the treatment of multidrug-resistant *Acinetobacter* infection.[28,48,85] Unfortunately with the increase in the use of colistin to treat these infections, the emergence of colistin-resistant *A. baumannii* has surged, particularly among patients who had previously received colistin for treatment of carbapenem-resistant, colistin-susceptible *A. baumannii.*[70] Efflux pumps capable of conferring resistance to multiple antibiotic classes have been identified in *Acinetobacter* spp.[12,51,74]

Tigecycline is the first member of the glycylcycline antimicrobial class to gain approval in the United States. Because this agent demonstrates in vitro activity against multidrug-resistant strains of *A. baumannii,* its potential use as an alternative therapy for severe infections caused by this organism is being investigated.[74] However an increase in all-cause mortality observed in a meta-analysis of clinical trials in tigecycline-treated patients has prompted a warning to reserve its use to situations where alternative treatments are not available.[68] Data regarding the use of this agent in pediatric patients are lacking, and it should not be used in children unless no alternative agents are available.[40] In such circumstances, the suggested tigecycline dose for children 8 to 11 years is 1.2 mg/kg every 12 hours (maximum of 50 mg every 12 hours), and those 12 to 17 years should receive 50 mg every 12 hours.[69,89] The development of resistance to tigecycline among clinical isolates of *Acinetobacter* has been documented and appears to be increasing in some regions.[3,51]

Recently two novel combinations of a cephalosporin with a β-lactamase inhibitor, ceftalozane/tazobactam and ceftazidime/avibactam, gained approval in the United States for the treatment of complicated gram-negative infections in adults.[89] Although the former has shown good in vitro activity against *A. baumannii,*[89] there is no clinical data on its efficacy in the treatment of infections due to this organism. On the other hand, the addition of avibactam to ceftazidime does not appear to enhance activity against *A. baumannii* despite having action against carbapenemases.[47,89] Safety and efficacy of these drug combinations in the pediatric population have not been established.

Lack of suitable options and efficacy data has made the treatment of multidrug-resistant *A. baumannii* infections a difficult task.[89] Based on limited in vitro and animal models data, it appears that combinations of antibiotics may be superior than single-agent regimens against carbapenem-resistant *A. baumannii,*[65,89] such as polymyxin plus rifampicin, colistin plus tigecycline, or two- or three-drug combinations with carbapenem plus rifampicin and/or sulbactam.[65,89]

Imipenem, meropenem, amikacin, ciprofloxacin, ceftazidime, and ceftriaxone have exhibited good in vitro activity against isolates identified as species other than the *A. baumannii-calcoaceticus* complex.[82] In addition to antimicrobial therapy, prompt drainage of focal suppurative sites and removal of infected indwelling catheters are essential. Intraventricular administration of amikacin, polymyxin B, or colistin has been used in the treatment of CNS infections caused by this organism.[78,97] Similarly the use of adjunctive aerosolized therapy with colistin or tobramycin has been explored in adults with pulmonary infections.[6]

PROGNOSIS

Because *Acinetobacter* strains often are resistant to the antibiotics used commonly, prompt recognition of the specific cause and institution of effective antibiotic therapy are critical to achieving a successful outcome. The reported mortality rate in a series of pediatric patients ranged from 0% to more than 50% (see Table 121.1), and the outcome appeared to correlate more closely with the underlying condition than with other factors such as polymicrobial bacteremia.[90] In a series of 58 infections caused by this organism that occurred over the course of a 2-year period from 1973 through 1974 at the Massachusetts General Hospital in Boston, the mortality rate was 23%.[27] A 1999 prospective study in the Slovak Republic revealed that the case-fatality rate for 157 episodes of *A. baumannii* bacteremia was significantly higher in adults than in children (34% vs. 12%).[46] A recent systematic review that included a total of 469 children from 51 outbreaks and case series of invasive *Acinetobacter* infections revealed an attributable mortality of 14.5%.[38]

The nosocomial acquisition of multidrug-resistant *A. baumannii* group has been associated with high mortality rates and prolonged hospitalization in adult patients in ICUs,[50,79] in contrast to the more benign clinical outcome usually seen with other species of *Acinetobacter.*[83] Mortality rates as high as 85% have been reported in outbreaks of imipenem-resistant *A. baumannii* infection among pediatric patients.[36]

PREVENTION

Nosocomial acquisition of *Acinetobacter* by high-risk compromised hosts can be prevented by placing emphasis on the control measures routinely used for endemic infections, such as careful hand washing by personnel, limitation of the frequency and duration of use of devices, proper isolation of colonized and infected patients, application of strict techniques for invasive procedures, restricted use of antibiotics, and implementation of antibiotic stewardship programs.[16,50,51,87]

NEW REFERENCES SINCE THE SEVENTH EDITION

17. Davis JS, McMillan M, Swaminathan A, et al. A 16-year prospective study of community-onset bacteremic *Acinetobacter* pneumonia: low mortality with appropriate initial empirical antibiotic protocols. *Chest.* 2014;146:1038-1045.
30. Hamer DH, Darmstadt GL, Carlin JB, et al. Etiology of bacteremia in young infants in six countries. *Pediatr Infect Dis J.* 2015;34:e1-e8.
35. Hidron AI, Edwards JR, Patel J, et al. Antimicrobial-resistant pathogens associated with healthcare-associated infections: annual summary of data reported to the National Healthcare Safety Network at the Centers for Disease Control and Prevention, 2006–2007. *Infect Control Hosp Epidemiol.* 2008;29:996-1011.
36. Hong KB, Oh HS, Song JS, et al. Investigation and control of an outbreak of imipenem-resistant *Acinetobacter baumannii* infection in a pediatric intensive care unit. *Pediatr Infect Dis J.* 2012;31:685-690.
40. Iosifidis E, Violaki A, Michalopoulou E, et al. Use of tigecycline in pediatric patients with infections predominantly due to extensively drug-resistant gram-negative bacteria. *J Pediatr Infect Dis Soc.* 2017;6(2):123-128.
42. Jung J, Park W. Acinetobacter species as model microorganisms in environmental microbiology: current state and perspectives. *Appl Microbiol Biotechnol.* 2015;99:2533-2548.
44. Kappstein I, Grundmann H, Hauer T, Niemeyer C. Aerators as a reservoir of *Acinetobacter junii*: an outbreak of bacteraemia in paediatric oncology patients. *J Hosp Infect.* 2000;44:27-30.
47. Lagancé-Wiens P, Walkty A, Karlowsky JA. Ceftazidime-avibactam: an evidence-based review of its pharmacology and potential use in the treatment of gram-negative bacterial infections. *Core Evid.* 2014;9:13-25.

65. Peleg AY, Seifert H, Paterson DL. *Acinetobacter baumannii*: emergence of a successful pathogen. *Clin Microbiol Rev*. 2008;21:538-582.
68. Prasad P, Sun J, Danner RL, Natanson C. Excess deaths associated with tigecycline after approval based on noninferiority trials. *Clin Infect Dis*. 2012;54:1699-1709.
69. Purdey J, Jouve S, Yan JL, et al. Pharmacokinetics and safety profile of tigecycline in children aged 8 to 11 years with selected serious infections: a multicenter, open-label, ascending-dose study. *Clin Ther*. 2012;34:496-507.
70. Qureshi ZA, Hittle LE, O'Hara JA, et al. Colistin-resistant *Acinetobacter baumanii*: beyond carbapenem resistance. *Clin Infect Dis*. 2015;60:1295-1303.
76. Rosenthal VD, Maki DG, Jamulitrat S, et al. International Nosocomial Infection Control Consortium (INICC) report, data summary for 2003–2008, issued June 2009. *Am J Infect Control*. 2010;38:95-104.e2.
85. Siddiqui NU, Qamar FN, Jurair H, Haque A. Multi-drug resistant gram-negative infections and use of intravenous polymyxin B in critically ill children of developing country: retrospective cohort study. *BCM Infect Dis*. 2014;14:626.
89. Taneja N, Kaur H. Insights into newer antimicrobial agents against gram-negative bacteria. *Microbiology Insights*. 2016;9:9-19.

The full reference list for this chapter is available at ExpertConsult.com.

122 Achromobacter (Alcaligenes)

Randall G. Fisher

Organisms of the genus *Achromobacter* are gram-negative bacilli that live in aqueous environments. Originally considered commensals, they increasingly are recognized as important, although rare, hospital pathogens. *Achromobacter* can be especially problematic in immunocompromised patients and in neonates, in whom infection can be life-threatening. These organisms have been isolated from such diverse clinical specimens as sputum, urine, feces, blood, cerebrospinal fluid, cornea, and peritoneal and pleural fluids.

BACTERIOLOGY

Achromobacter spp. are gram-negative, motile, indole-negative, obligate aerobes that are oxidase and catalase positive. They are considered to be nonfermenters because of their extremely limited action on carbohydrates. Most ferment xylose, and some ferment glucose. All reduce nitrate to nitrite. They are urease, lysine, and ornithine negative. They grow well on both blood and MacConkey agar and produce colonies that are smooth and glistening and have a distinct edge. *Achromobacter* spp. alkalinize organic salts and amides, a property that led to the name *Alcaligenes*, which means *alkali producing*. *Alcaligenes faecalis* has a distinct, sweet odor that has been described as resembling that of green apples.[32]

Bacteriologically, these bacilli may be confused with other nonfermenting gram-negative organisms, especially *Pseudomonas* spp. Morphologically, however, they can be distinguished easily from pseudomonads by the presence of peritrichous flagella: *Pseudomonas* spp. have polar flagella.[27]

The taxonomy of these organisms is confusing and undergoes frequent changes. They were classified as *Achromobacter* spp., then reclassified as *Alcaligenes,* and have been reassigned the name *Achromobacter*. The genera *Achromobacter* and *Alcaligenes* are closely related and comprise many species, but clinically important ones are as follows: (1) *Achromobacter xylosoxidans,* which has two subspecies: *xylosoxidans* and *dentrificans,* the former of which is the most common cause of clinically recognizable infection; (2) *A. faecalis,* which is a less common pathogen but has a distinct antimicrobial susceptibility pattern[6]; (3) *Achromobacter piechaudii,* which has been isolated from clinical specimens[49] but is of doubtful significance, and (4) *A. dentrificans*, which is a rare pathogen.[57] In the discussion that follows, the abbreviation *A. xylosoxidans* refers to *Achromobacter xylosoxidans* subspecies *xylosoxidans.*

EPIDEMIOLOGY

Like *Pseudomonas* spp., *Achromobacter* are water organisms and prefer aqueous environments and moist soil. They do not survive long on porous surfaces or fomites or if they become desiccated.[55] They also may be part of the normal flora of the ear and of the gastrointestinal and respiratory tracts of some people. These organisms establish a niche within the hospital environment and have been recovered from ventilators, humidifiers, "sterile" saline, intravenous fluids, and irrigation and dialysis solutions. *Achromobacter* spp. also have been recovered from infant formula,[20] children's soap bubbles,[42] well water,[62] and swimming pools.[29] Organisms also survive many disinfectants and have been cultured from chlorhexidine,[59] 1% eosin,[7] and alcohol- or quaternary amine–containing compounds.[55,59] Shigeta and associates[59] reported an outbreak of *A. xylosoxidans* ventriculitis secondary to contaminated chlorhexidine used on a surgical ward. Foley and colleagues[23] reported an outbreak accompanied by deaths in a neonatal intensive care unit (NICU) secondary to contamination of saline used as an eyewash. Boukadida and coworkers[7] reported a neonatal death caused by meningitis contracted by dissemination after treatment of a diaper rash with 1% eosin. An outbreak of 37 cases (with two fatalities) that was caused by bacterial contamination of deionized water in a hemodialysis system was described by Reverdy and associates.[50] Surgical wound infection also has occurred in which infection was suspected to be secondary to contaminated irrigation fluids used in surgery.[71] One outbreak of four cases in a hemodialysis unit was linked to an atomizer of 2.5% chlorhexidine used to disinfect the skin.[65] Three kinds of pseudo-outbreaks have been described: in one, seven patients in a pediatric hospital were infected with *A. xylosoxidans,* but restriction fragment-length polymorphism analysis proved they all were genetically unrelated[5]; in another, *A. xylosoxidans* was isolated from three different clinical specimens but was later proved to be a contaminant of the saline used in their processing[26]; in a third, blood cultures were positive when drawn on the night shift because the nurses were cleaning the top of the blood culture bottles with a contaminated disinfectant.[61]

Studies have documented that *A. xylosoxidans* colonization of patients with cystic fibrosis (CF) is on the rise. In one large study, *A. xylosoxidans* was isolated from the sputum culture of 52 of 595 patients (8.7%).[8] In other studies, isolates of *A. xylosoxidans* at a single CF center were not genetically related, a finding implying no common source of infection and little or no patient-to-patient spread within the center.[18,70] However colonization of multiple patients with identical strains also is well documented.[53] Colonization rates as high as 17.6% have been reported; many of these patients were shown to be chronically colonized.[34] Molecular methods prove that other species of *Achromobacter* are also colonizers in CF patients, including *A. ruhlandii*, *A. insuavis*, and *A. dolens*.[11] In one study, all less common *Achromobacter* species were misidentified as *A. xylosoxidans* by matrix-assisted laser desorption/ionization-time of flight (MALDI-TOF).[52] Other investigators have reported 75% concordance between MALDI-TOF and 16SrDNA sequencing, however.[30] Most investigators report no significant changes in forced expiratory volume in 1 second (FEV_1) or growth parameters in *A. xylosoxidans*–colonized patients,[34] and the presence of pan-resistant

A. xylosoxidans had no influence on survival after lung transplantation.[38] Environmental cultures at one CF center were positive for *A. xylosoxidans* only 0.8% of the time, whereas 22.8% of such cultures were positive for *Pseudomonas aeruginosa*.[22]

PATHOPHYSIOLOGY

Achromobacter spp. are weakly virulent bacteria. Medical care commonly provides the conduit through which organisms are introduced into their host by way of indwelling catheters, endotracheal tubes, and so forth. The bacteria may take advantage of a weakened immune system and disseminate, causing sepsis, meningitis, and death. Preterm or term infants who are small for gestational age are at particular risk for acquiring such severe *Achromobacter* infections.[23] Although most neonatal infections are considered to be nosocomial, vertical transmission from mother to baby may occur.[27] An increased incidence of infection has been reported for patients with neoplasms[35] and those receiving long-term steroid therapy.[31] Sporadic cases of *Achromobacter* infection in patients with idiopathic immunoglobulin (Ig)M deficiency,[19] Waldenström macroglobulinemia,[64] granulomatosis with polyangiitis (Wegener granulomatosis),[48] and systemic lupus erythematosus have been reported.[54] My colleagues and I have seen one boy with hyper-IgM syndrome in whom 14 separate episodes of *Achromobacter* bacteremia occurred; an exhaustive environmental search for a source was fruitless. The source was eventually proved to be deep infection of a cervical lymph node, and the episodes ceased when the node was removed.[72] *Achromobacter* infections occur in patients with acquired immunodeficiency syndrome (AIDS),[10,25] but whether this syndrome is an independent risk factor for infection is unclear.

In one study, patients with CF and colonized with *A. xylosoxidans* tended to be older (mean age, 20 years) and at baseline had worse lung function than did uncolonized controls; however, over the course of the study, the rate of decline of lung function did not differ between cases and controls.[13] In a second similar case-control study, lung function decline and growth parameters generally were not affected by colonization; however a subset of patients had rapidly increasing antibody titers against *A. xylosoxidans*, and this group did experience more accelerated decline.[53]

In unusual circumstances, patients with neither overt underlying disease nor obvious immune deficiency will develop infection with *Achromobacter* spp. Most of these cases involve penetrating trauma. One case of corneal infection complicating epidemic keratoconjunctivitis in a normal host has been described.[44] Eye infections, including conjunctivitis and keratitis, also have occurred in patients who wear contact lenses; the organism was also recovered from contact lens cases and solutions.[33,39] Post-LASIK *A. xylosoxidans* keratitis can be misdiagnosed as recurrent corneal erosion owing to a lack of signs suggesting acute inflammation.[51] In some cases, post-LASIK infection may require corneal transplantation.[37]

CLINICAL MANIFESTATIONS

Signs of sepsis or meningitis caused by *A. xylosoxidans* in the newborn are difficult to differentiate from other causes of bacterial sepsis. However some babies may develop a distinctive rash in association with this infection, in which 1- to 2-cm, sharply demarcated red patches appear, especially in the head and neck region. This rash was noted in 29 of 33 newborns with *A. xylosoxidans* infection reported by Doxiadis and associates in 1960[16] and was seen again in a case reported in 1993.[7] *A. xylosoxidans* sepsis and meningitis tend to manifest later in life than do infections with the usual vertically acquired pathogens and may have a more insidious onset.[40] In some cases, cerebrospinal fluid profiles may resemble those usually associated with viral meningitis, with white blood cell counts in the hundreds, and with monocytic predominance.[56] Neonatal *Achromobacter* sepsis or meningitis has an extremely poor prognosis; one series noted a mortality rate that approached 75%, and 36% of survivors had severe neurologic deficits.[23] The incidence of intracranial hemorrhage also was high.

Three large series of bloodstream infections with *A. xylosoxidans* all revealed a similar story; most cases are nosocomial, most patients have an underlying malignant disease, many are neutropenic or receiving high-dose steroids, and many have indwelling vascular catheters.[2,24,58] Polymicrobial bacteremia was not rare in these series. Mortality rates ranged from 15%[24] to 48%.[58] Risk factors for mortality were age older than 65 years at diagnosis, neutropenia, nosocomial acquisition, and polymicrobial bacteremia. An earlier review of reported cases revealed that the case-fatality rate was lowest in patients with catheter-associated bacteremia and highest (65%) in those with pneumonia, meningitis, or endocarditis.[17]

An outbreak of urinary tract infection was traced to ultrasound gel used in transrectal ultrasound-guided prostate biopsies.[45] Urinary tract infections are generally seen in elderly patients with underlying malignancies or urologic abnormalities.[66] A large NICU outbreak in Brazil involved 22 neonates over the course of 6 months. Features of illness were abdominal distention, thrombocytopenia, and neutropenia. The mortality rate was almost 14%. The source of the outbreak was never determined, and the outbreak ceased only after the NICU was physically moved.[67]

One child developed osteomyelitis caused by *A. xylosoxidans* after stepping on a nail through old sneakers (a clinical situation classically associated with *Pseudomonas* infection)[28,29]; another developed *Achromobacter* infection as a consequence of a gunshot wound.[12] In the setting of a patient with an artificial heart valve, *A. xylosoxidans* endocarditis has been described.[46] In another case, endocarditis was associated with an abandoned pacemaker lead.[1] A case series of liver abscesses included three patients from whom *A. xylosoxidans* was isolated, all of whom shared a clinical pattern—history of cholecystectomy, "coral-like" multilobulated appearance on computed tomography, and epithelioid granulomas at the periphery of the abscesses.[3] *A. xylosoxidans* infection in older patients usually is not suspected on clinical grounds but rather in the context of a common-source outbreak or because of microbiologic clues. *A. faecalis* infection is less common and usually is part of a polymicrobial process.

A review of *Achromobacter* pulmonary infections found that the majority of cases presented as pneumonia, usually in people with malignancy.[63] Two patients suffering from a pertussis-like illness were found to be infected with *A. xylosoxidans* strains carrying the *ptxA* gene.[47]

DIAGNOSIS AND TREATMENT

Generally the diagnosis of *Achromobacter* infections rests on recovery of the organism from clinical samples, although newer methods sometimes have been employed. In one case of culture-negative endophthalmitis, fluid obtained from the anterior chamber was subjected to polymerase chain reaction (PCR) using a 16S rDNA primer set, finding a 214 base pair sequence from *A. xylosoxidans*.[69] These organisms often are mistaken for pseudomonads, and the clinician should suspect *A. xylosoxidans* when the laboratory reports an organism as a *Pseudomonas* spp. that is resistant to all aminoglycosides.[55] Key differentiation features include the antibiogram and the morphology of the organism, with its distinctive peritrichous flagella. The organism can be identified in the sputum of CF patients using a PCR for the *bla* (OXA-114-like) gene, which is constitutive in *A. xylosoxidans*.[68] MALDI-TOF also has been used to identify nonfermenting gram-negative rods in CF sputum with great accuracy, correctly identifying 549/559 strains.[15]

Achromobacter spp. typically are resistant to a large number of antibiotics, including ampicillin, aztreonam, aminoglycosides, first- and second-generation cephalosporins, tetracyclines, and rifampin. They variably are resistant to chloramphenicol, fluoroquinolones, macrolides, ureidopenicillins, and β-lactamase combination drugs.[6] *Achromobacter* spp. have been shown to produce β-lactamases, some of which are chromosomal, constitutive, and inducible[14] and some of which are on plasmids.[36] Some isolates overproduce β-lactamase,[14] which stoichiometrically can render β-lactamase inhibitors useless. In addition, their porins are small, thus rendering antibiotic entry difficult. More recently, a multidrug efflux pump of the RND-type has been described.[4] Although there is no antibiotic to which all isolates have been shown to be sensitive,[46] most are sensitive in vitro to trimethoprim-sulfamethoxazole, piperacillin-tazobactam, imipenem, ceftazidime, and cefoperazone.

Carbapenem-resistant strains also have been discovered. These strains produced VIM-2, OXA-30, and a chromosomal AmpC β-lactamase.[60] One isolate harbored both a chromosomal and a plasmid-mediated carbapenemase.[9] Two case reports describe treatment failures of ceftazidime[41] and piperacillin[14] in clinical isolates that were sensitive at the time of isolation but developed resistance during the course of therapy. In one case of a 14-year-old girl with *A. xylosoxidans* meningitis secondary to a baclofen pump infection, standard treatment with 30-minute infusions of meropenem every 8 hours led to apparent success but with recurrence despite removal of the pump; treatment was successful when a 4-hour infusion was substituted, maintaining the serum level above the minimum inhibitory concentration (MIC) of the organism for at least 75% of the dosing interval.[43]

Because resistance patterns vary across isolates, the combination of a third-generation cephalosporin, piperacillin (or piperacillin-tazobactam), or meropenem with trimethoprim-sulfamethoxazole is reasonable empirical therapy for suspected *Achromobacter* infection, pending susceptibility results. In general, in vitro susceptibilities seem to correlate well with in vivo results,[35] but the risk for inducible resistance to β-lactam antibiotics should be acknowledged. One report described synergy in microbial killing with an aminoglycoside, even though the isolate was resistant to the same aminoglycoside when it was tested alone.[10] This phenomenon was confirmed by two-disk Kirby-Bauer approximation methods using 11 clinical blood culture isolates; all were resistant to gentamicin, but 10 of 11 were inhibited synergistically when gentamicin was added to ticarcillin-clavulanate, and nine of 11 displayed synergy when gentamicin was added to piperacillin or ceftazidime.[17]

Removal of infected catheters may speed recovery, although some patients have been treated successfully through indwelling lines.[10] Because of a high recurrence rate, experts in the care of patients with renal failure treated with continuous ambulatory peritoneal dialysis recommend removal of peritoneal catheters in patients who develop peritonitis with *A. xylosoxidans.*[21]

NEW REFERENCES SINCE THE SEVENTH EDITION

9. Chen Z, Fang H, Wang L, et al. IMP-1 encoded by a novel Tn402-like class 1 integron in clinical *Achromobacter xylosoxidans*, China. *Sci Rep.* 2014;27:7212.
11. Coward A, Kenna DT, Perry C, et al. Use of nrdA gene sequence clustering to estimate the prevalence of different *Achromobacter* species among cystic fibrosis patients in the UK. *J Cyst Fibros.* 2015;15(4):479-485.
30. Homem deMello deSouza HA, Dalla-Costa LM, Vicenzi FJ, et al. MALDI-ToF: a useful tool for laboratory identification of uncommon glucose non-fermenting gram-negative bacteria associated with cystic fibrosis. *J Med Microbiol.* 2014;63:1148-1153.
38. Lobo LJ, Tulu Z, Aris RM, Noone PG. Pan-resistant *Achromobacter xylosoxidans* and *Stenotrophomonas maltophilia* infection in cystic fibrosis does not reduce survival after lung transplantation. *Transplantation.* 2015;99:2196-2202.
43. Nichols KR, Knoderer CA, Jackson NG, Manaloor JJ, Christenson JC. Success with extended-infusion meropenem after recurrence of baclofen pump-related *Achromobacter xylosoxidans* meningitis in an adolescent. *J Pharm Pract.* 2015;28:430-433.
47. Orellana-Peralta F, Jacinto M, Pons MJ, et al. Characterization of two *Achromobacter xylosoxidans* isolates from patients with pertussis-like symptoms. *Asian Pac J Trop Med.* 2015;8:464-467.
48. Patel PK, vonKeudell A, Moroder P, et al. Recurrent septic arthritis due to *Achromobacter xylosoxidans* in a patient with granulomatosis with polyangiitis. *Open Forum Infect Dis.* 2015;2(4):ofv145.
51. Riaz KM, Feder RS, Srivastava A, Rosin J, Rasti S. *Achromobacter xylosoxidans* keratitis masquerading as recurrent erosion after LASIK. *J Refract Surg.* 2013;29:788-790.
52. Rodrigues ER, Ferreira AG, Leao RS, et al. Characterization of *Achromobacter* species in cystic fibrosis patients: comparison of blaOXA-114 PCR amplification, MLST, and MALDI-ToF-MS. *J Clin Microbiol.* 2015;53:3894-3896.
57. Sgrelli A, Mencacci A, Fiorio M, et al. *Achromobacter dentrificans* renal abscess. *New Microbiol.* 2012;35:245-247.
63. Swenson CE, Sadikot RT. *Achromobacter* respiratory infections. *Ann Am Thorac Soc.* 2015;12:252-258.
67. Turel O, Kavuncuoglu S, Hosaf E, et al. Bacteremia due to *Achromobacter xylosoxidans* in neonates: clinical features and outcome. *Braz J Infect Dis.* 2013;17:450-454.

The full reference list for this chapter is available at ExpertConsult.com.

123 *Eikenella corrodens*

Jeffrey M. Bender • Randall G. Fisher

Eikenella corrodens is a facultatively anaerobic, fastidious gram-negative rod that is part of the normal flora of the mouth and the gastrointestinal and genitourinary tracts. Long regarded as a commensal, its pathogenicity no longer is in doubt. It frequently is a pathogen of periodontitis in both adults and children and is a common isolate from wounds that have been contaminated by oral secretions. It also has been recovered from pleuropulmonary infections, central nervous system infections, orbital cellulitis, peritonsillar abscesses, abdominal infections, osteomyelitis, and bloodstream infections, including endocarditis.

BACTERIOLOGY

In 1948, Hendriksen described the organism and called it the "corroding bacillus" because it pitted the agar.[20] It was characterized more fully in 1958 by Eiken, who named it *Bacteroides corrodens.*[12] In 1972, Jackson and Goodman separated two species of corroding bacteria; the strict anaerobe kept the name *B. corrodens* (now called *B. ureolyticus*), and the facultative anaerobe was classified as *Eikenella.*[21] It is a small, straight, nonmotile gram-negative rod that occasionally is coccobacillary. It is oxidase positive and catalase negative. Most strains are positive for lysine and ornithine decarboxylase. The organism is nonfermentative, reduces nitrate to nitrite, and is negative for urease and indole. *E. corrodens* cell surface components vary from isolate to isolate; these differences probably relate to virulence.[6]

E. corrodens will grow either aerobically or anaerobically, but its growth is not rapid. Growth can be enhanced by 3% to 10% carbon dioxide. It grows on blood or chocolate agar but poorly or not at all on MacConkey agar. Selective medium, which contains clindamycin, may increase the yield. Colonies are small and grayish. They look slightly yellow when they are old. Although *E. corrodens* is nonhemolytic, a faint green appearance may be seen on blood agar. Approximately 50% will produce the characteristic pitting. They release an odor that resembles that of bleach or hypochlorite.[21]

E. corrodens is a member of the so-called HACEK family of organisms, which have the following in common: slow growth, a requirement for carbon dioxide, and a predilection for infecting heart valves. The other members of the family are *Aggregatibacter*[35] (formerly *Haemophilus*) *aphrophilus, Aggregatibacter* (formerly *Actinobacillus*) *actinomycetemcomitans, Cardiobacterium hominis,* and *Kingella kingae.*

EPIDEMIOLOGY

Infection with *E. corrodens* occurs when mucosal or skin barriers are disrupted and the organism gains access to deeper tissues. Puncture of the skin with forks[37] or toothpicks[43] may result in deep-seated infections.

One case of vertebral osteomyelitis that occurred after a woman accidentally inoculated the organism into the paravertebral space by penetration of a fish bone through the posterior pharynx has been reported.[32] In a similar case, a fish bone stuck in the throat for 2 months eventually led to a spinal epidural abscess.[25] Infection commonly occurs after clenched-fist injury as a result of fistfighting.[16] Hand infections in children are more likely to be secondary to digital biting or sucking.[18] Intravenous drug abusers are at risk for injection site and soft tissue abscesses,[17] bacteremia, and endocarditis.[10,36] Elderly persons and patients with advanced carcinomas are the other high-risk groups. However children are at particularly high risk for serious *E. corrodens* infections.[42] Thyroid abscesses[7,51] and purulent thyroiditis[41] all have been reported in children. In one review, more than 20% of *E. corrodens* pleuropulmonary infections occurred in children younger than 14 years.[27] A separate review demonstrated more than 50% of abdominal *E. corrodens* infections were reported in patients younger than 25 years.[9] *E. corrodens* orbital cellulitis,[19] empyema,[48] peritonsillar abscess,[28] paronychia,[1] and osteomyelitis[39,45] have been observed in children. A review of 54 cases of *E. corrodens* infection in children and adolescents revealed that 41% of pediatric infections occurred in the head and neck. The most common single site was the thyroid gland.[37]

PATHOPHYSIOLOGY

E. corrodens infections often are polymicrobial and may include other anaerobes or gram-negative rods.[49] However *E. corrodens* is accompanied most frequently by recovery of α-hemolytic streptococci. In most reports, the streptococci were not speciated further, but Jacobs and associates made a case for the *Streptococcus anginosus* group because of similarities between the two organisms (i.e., both are found in the mouth and gastrointestinal tract, both produce local suppurative infection, and both thrive in carbon dioxide–rich, oxygen-poor environments).[23] Brooks and colleagues also reported synergy of the two organisms in a rabbit model of skin infection.[4] In vitro studies of *E. corrodens* co-cultivated with members of the *S. anginosus* group showed that a significant degree of coaggregation occurs. In addition, exponential growth of *Streptococcus constellatus* and *Streptococcus intermedius* occurs 6 hours into incubation when these species are grown in the presence of *E. corrodens*; in its absence, exponential growth does not occur until 25 hours after inoculation.[53]

The possible role of *E. corrodens* in periodontitis has not been delineated precisely. However, soluble products of *E. corrodens* induce gene expression and protein production of vascular endothelial growth factor and cause phosphorylation of mitogen-activated protein kinase in vitro, a process that leads to increased production of interleukin-8 and adhesion molecules.[54] This cascade of inflammatory responses could promote chronic periodontitis.

E. corrodens has a propensity toward formation of an abscess in any location, whether alone or in concert with other organisms. Such formation is a hallmark of central nervous system infection.[3] Of intraabdominal infections reported by Danziger and associates, 15 of 19 patients had abscesses.[9] In two cases of orbital cellulitis reported by Hemady and coworkers, both patients had subperiosteal abscesses.[19] Deep or superficial skin abscesses reported in drug addicts[17] or in clenched-fist injury from fistfighting[16] often recur, even after presumed adequate drainage.[40]

CLINICAL MANIFESTATIONS

Infections with *E. corrodens* are indolent. The time from inoculation to onset of symptoms generally is 1 week or longer.[4] Many cases show initial improvement with treatment but relapse days later, even with appropriate therapy.[18,28,38,42] The head and neck are the most common sites of infection at all ages.[37]

Infection of periodontal sites may be associated with rapid progression and bone resorption thought to be secondary to surface-associated materials of *E. corrodens* and other organisms of periodontitis.[33] Craniofacial and neck infections tend to have prolonged morbidity; many require repeated drainage procedures and long courses of antimicrobial agents.[42] Central nervous system infections often are preceded by sinus infections but also have been seen in children with congenital heart disease.[2,50]

Pleuropulmonary infections are marked by fever, cough, and chest pain. Necrotizing pneumonia with multiple abscesses sometimes is seen. Effusions or empyema are noted in 30%, and cavitation is seen in 8%. Children with a predisposition toward aspiration may be at higher risk.[27] In one case, a bedridden 16-year-old girl developed a bronchopleural-cutaneous fistula complicating necrotizing pneumonia with empyema.[52]

Endocarditis is associated with large, friable vegetations and frequent emboli and often requires valve replacement.[13] Intravenous drug use has been implicated in approximately half of reported cases.

Abdominal *E. corrodens* infections are seen most commonly as complications of ruptured appendicitis but also have been associated with abdominal trauma and surgery. The clinical course is protracted.[9]

Chorioamnionitis leading to premature delivery has been documented.[14,24,26,29,47] In one case, the infection precipitated the birth of twins at 23 weeks' gestation and led to the demise of one twin.[29]

Soft tissue infections tend to be severe. Many require wide debridement and skin grafting. Infection of underlying joints, tendons, or bones is not infrequent and can be necrotizing and even lead to amputation.[40]

DIAGNOSIS

Definitive diagnosis rests on recovery of *E. corrodens* in culture, which can be a difficult task because of the organism's slow growth. *Eikenella* tends to be overgrown by hardier species when it is part of a polymicrobial process and may be missed, especially if the isolate does not pit the agar. All the HACEK organisms can pit agar, although not with the regularity of *E. corrodens.*[5]

Many bacteriology laboratories have difficulty identifying and separating catalase-negative, oxidase-positive, gram-negative rods. Not surprisingly, one report noted that of 100 isolates of *E. corrodens* identified by the National Collection of Type Cultures, only 21 were sent in as probable *E. corrodens.*[5] Organisms that *E. corrodens* may be mistaken for include the other HACEK organisms, *Aggregatibacter* (formerly *Haemophilus*) *paraphrophilus, Moraxella atlantae,* and *Actinobacillus ureae.* Novel identification techniques such as matrix-assisted desorption ionization-time of flight mass spectrometry (MALDI-TOF)[8] and 16S sequencing have significantly improved the ability of the clinical lab to identify these organisms.[11]

TREATMENT

E. corrodens has a very unusual antimicrobial susceptibility pattern: although most isolates are sensitive to penicillin and ampicillin, they are resistant to semisynthetic penicillins, such as methicillin and nafcillin.[46] Additionally these organisms uniformly are resistant to clindamycin and metronidazole, drugs commonly used to treat anaerobic infections.[22] They also variably are resistant to aminoglycosides.

Most isolates are susceptible to piperacillin, second- and third-generation cephalosporins, carbapenems, second- and third-generation fluoroquinolones, and tetracycline. In one report, all of 31 *Eikenella* isolates derived from normal oral flora were susceptible to azithromycin in vitro, though resistant to other macrolides.[34] Although penicillin often is cited as the drug of choice, some strains produce β-lactamases. One report associated the β-lactamase with a transposon[31] and another with a plasmid[44]; one report found a chromosomal enzyme that was not inducible.[30] In addition, there are reports of intermediate resistance to penicillin, even in isolates that do not produce a β-lactamase.[15]

Incision and drainage of abscesses and debridement of necrotic tissue are essential to recovery from these infections. Therapy should be prolonged after patients apparently have recovered because early cessation of antibiotic therapy tends to be associated with relapse. If patients continue to have fever or other signs of infection days after appropriate therapy has been started, obtaining more images of the infected area may be prudent to detect early reaccumulation of purulence.

Acknowledgments

We thank Dr. William Gruber and Dr. Thomas Boyce for their invaluable assistance with earlier versions of this chapter.

NEW REFERENCES SINCE THE SEVENTH EDITION

8. Couturier MR, Mehinovic E, Croft AC, et al. Identification of HACEK clinical isolates by matrix-assisted laser desorption ionization-time of flight mass spectrometry. *J Clin Microbiol.* 2011;49(3):1104-1106.
11. de Melo Oliveira MG, Abels S, Zbinden R, et al. Accurate identification of fastidious gram-negative rods: integration of both conventional phenotypic methods and 16S rRNA gene analysis. *BMC Microbiol.* 2013;13:162.

The full reference list for this chapter is available at ExpertConsult.com.

124 *Elizabethkingia* and *Chryseobacterium* Species

Jeffrey M. Bender • Randall G. Fisher

Members of the genus *Chryseobacterium* (formerly *Flavobacterium*) seldom are associated with human infection. Most disease occurs after exposure to a contaminated environmental source. In 1944, Shulmann and Johnson reported a case of meningitis caused by a previously unidentified, gram-negative bacillus isolated from a 9-day-old premature infant.[54] The term *Flavobacterium meningosepticum* was proposed for this organism by King in 1959, based on her studies of bacterial isolates associated primarily with neonatal meningitis and septicemia.[30] Although neonatal meningitis is the most common manifestation of human disease caused by this genus, sepsis, endocarditis, pneumonia, septic arthritis with penetrating trauma or prosthesis, and skin infection occur in individuals beyond the newborn period.

BACTERIOLOGY

The taxonomy of these organisms is confusing because of frequent changes. All but one of the clinically relevant species of the original genus *Flavobacterium* were reclassified to the genus *Chryseobacterium* in 1994.[63] Phylogenetic analysis based on 16S rRNA sequencing demonstrated that the organisms formerly classified as *Chryseobacterium meningosepticum* and *Chryseobacterium miricola* represent a separate lineage. Researchers proposed that these two organisms be moved to a new genus, named *Elizabethkingia* after the microbiologist who first described them.[29] The former *Flavobacterium odoratum,* rarely responsible for human disease, has been divided into two species (*odoratus* and *odoratimimus*) reclassified as members of the genus *Myroides.*[62] *Chryseobacterium indologenes* is the species isolated most frequently from human specimens, but it usually is not associated with significant disease.[28] Therefore this chapter focuses mainly on *Elizabethkingia meningosepticum,* which can cause severe infections, especially in newborns. These organisms are long, thin, catalase-positive, gram-negative rods with slightly swollen ends; they are nonmotile, oxidase-positive, weakly fermentative, and proteolytic and grow on solid agar as 1- to 2-mm, convex, glistening colonies of buttery consistency.[30] Yellow pigmentation is seen occasionally. Colonies do not demonstrate hemolysis on blood agar but may produce a lavender-green color in the surrounding media as a result of extensive proteolytic enzyme activity. *Elizabethkingia* is unable to grow on *Salmonella-Shigella* agar or Simmons citrate and lacks motility. These characteristics distinguish *Elizabethkingia* from *Pseudomonas,* with which it often is confused.[14] Similarly, the use of glucose in an open tube of oxidation-fermentation media distinguishes *Elizabethkingia* from *Achromobacter faecalis.*[14] The clinically relevant species *E. meningosepticum* (also referred to interchangeably in the current literature by its old name *Chryseobacterium meningosepticum* and in the older literature as *Flavobacterium meningosepticum*) and *Flavobacterium IIB* (renamed *Flavobacterium balustinum*) are differentiated by the former's consistent liquefaction of gelatin and early use of mannitol and maltose and the latter's lack of these abilities.[30] *Myroides odoratus* and *Myroides odoratimimus (F. odoratum),* which have been identified most commonly as saprophytes in skin wounds, characteristically are nonsaccharolytic and produce a fruity odor when they are grown on standard media.[25]

EPIDEMIOLOGY

Elizabethkingia spp. and Chryseobacterium are distributed widely as saprophytes in fresh and salt water, as well as in the soil. *E. meningosepticum* has been identified as a pathogen in birds.[61] In hospitals, these organisms have been found to be ubiquitous colonizers of the patient's environment and have been isolated from flower vases,[59] ice machines,[57] vials of intravenous drugs,[44] and nebulizers.[15] In addition, tap water,[15] eyewashes,[48] tube feedings,[15] sink traps,[8] and hand cultures of hospital personnel[15] have yielded this organism. In some instances, these reservoirs have been implicated in nosocomial outbreaks of patient colonization and invasive disease.

Neonatal infection caused by *E. meningosepticum* has been reported frequently in the literature, often in association with nursery epidemics.[2,7,50] As with other neonatal pathogens, infants who are premature and small for gestational age seem to be at particular risk for infection. More than 50% of infected infants weigh less than 2500 g. Almost all cases occur within 3 weeks of birth, and more than 50% of these infants manifest illness before they are 7 days old.[14]

Nosocomial epidemics have occurred sporadically since the nursery outbreak reported by Brody and colleagues in 1958.[2,5,7,8] Cabrera and Davis reported such an outbreak in detail in 1960.[8] During a 3-month period, the bacteria were isolated from a total of 44 infants, of whom 14 had overt infection. Most colonized infants had organisms isolated from the nasopharynx. The only reservoir of infectious bacteria discovered was a faulty sink trap, beneath which cleaning materials for the nursery were stored. Repair of the defective trap and thorough cleansing and repainting of the nursery coincided with termination of the epidemic. In one situation, respiratory tract colonization developed in four premature neonates, but none of them developed disease; routine infection control measures ensured that no further infants were colonized.[40]

Nursery outbreaks of *E. meningosepticum* have been traced to saline used to flush infants' eyes after administration of silver nitrate,[48] and organisms have been recovered from washbasins, sinks, disinfectants, and suction devices in other epidemics.[8] Colonization of patients in a surgical intensive care unit was associated with tap water, sinks, ice machines, and washbasins yielding the bacteria.[15] Ribotyping and random amplified polymorphic DNA fingerprinting (RAPD) offer promise for more precise characterization of epidemics.[12,13] Use of these techniques has also demonstrated that, in some cases, isolates in what appears to be an outbreak may be unrelated. In one case, isolates from the surrounding environment were also all unrelated to the types found in the patients.[64]

In 2016, Wisconsin and surrounding states experienced an outbreak of *Elizabethkingia anopheles* infections that affected primarily older adults with underlying medical conditions. Centers for Disease Control–reported cases numbered 65 at time of publication, with 20 deaths. The age range was 19 to 104 years. No children were reported at the time. This species has been associated with significant morbidity and mortality.[31]

PATHOPHYSIOLOGY

Elizabethkingia spp. and *Chryseobacterium* spp. generally are of low virulence. Rabbits administered 1-mL intravenous infections of 24-hour-old broth cultures demonstrated no mortality or morbidity; death rates were less than 30% in mice inoculated intracerebrally with "barely turbid" preparations.[30]

Most cases of invasive human disease are thought to be caused by environmental contamination with high numbers of *E. meningosepticum*, with spread to the compromised newborn or debilitated older patient. Some neonatal infections may be caused by colonization of the infant during passage through the birth canal of a colonized mother.[13] Intrapartum infection is supported by occurrence of symptoms as early as 10 hours after birth.[14] However, only 0.3% of genital swabs submitted from patients with suspected sexually transmitted infection yielded the organism.[44] Continuing reports of *E. meningosepticum* as a cause of neonatal infection in developing countries have been speculated to be related to use of contaminated groundwater for bathing of newborn infants and feminine genital hygiene.[14] The propensity for this organism to produce meningitis in the newborn is not understood, but infection may occur in association with heavy nasopharyngeal colonization, leading to subsequent bacteremia and seeding of the meninges.

Cases in older children have been related to insulin-dependent diabetes mellitus,[9] thalassemia major with splenectomy,[46] and oncologic disease with indwelling catheters.[43] Peritonitis in patients undergoing continuous ambulatory peritoneal dialysis, including a case series of 30 patients, also has been reported.[47]

In older individuals, *E. meningosepticum* and *Chryseobacterium* primarily play the role of opportunists.[39] Heavy nosocomial colonization combined with a blunted immune response probably accounts for the immunocompromised patient's poor capacity to handle this otherwise noninvasive bacterium.

CLINICAL MANIFESTATIONS

Neonatal sepsis and meningitis caused by *E. meningosepticum* share signs and symptoms in common with other forms of neonatal bacterial infection. However, the development of meningitis may be insidious, and several days of illness often pass before its presentation[14,50]; this factor is consistent with the low virulence of *E. meningosepticum* in contrast to other agents of neonatal sepsis. Prognosis is extremely poor, and mortality rates may exceed 60%.[34] Fifty percent of survivors develop significant neurologic complications, often in association with hydrocephalus.[35]

These organisms are uncommon pathogens in adults, and childhood disease occurring beyond the newborn period is extremely rare. Among the 24 initial isolates of *E. meningosepticum* identified by King, organisms were identified in a throat culture from an adult patient and in cerebrospinal fluid (CSF) from an 8-month-old infant.[30] Bacteria formerly classified as *Flavobacterium IIB* (now known as *F. balustinum*) were isolated from the blood and CSF of several adult patients without clinical information.[26] Since their initial identification in 1959, these agents have been implicated as causes of meningitis,[39,50] postoperative bacteremia,[3,45] bacterial endocarditis,[65] pneumonia,[58,59] catheter-associated infection, septic arthritis, and skin infection.[18] *E. meningosepticum* is the clinically relevant species most commonly isolated, but *C. balustinum, M. odoratus,* and *M. odoratimimus (F. odoratum)* and other *Chryseobacterium* spp. have been implicated in human disease. *Elizabethkingia* and *Chryseobacterium* spp. accounted for 0.25% of infections in a large consecutive series of patients with human immunodeficiency virus infection. Risk factors included low CD4 counts and leukopenia.[38]

E. meningosepticum meningitis beyond the neonatal period typically occurs in immunocompromised patients. Adults with preexisting leukemia,[50] glomerulonephritis,[39] and squamous cell carcinoma[21] have been described as having meningitis caused by this organism. In a 56-year-old woman, meningitis with *E. meningosepticum* developed after she underwent transsphenoidal hypophysectomy[10]; in an 8-month-old male child with preceding severe neurologic damage, meningitis developed with bacteria designated by the Centers for Disease Control and Prevention as *Flavobacterium*-like organisms. In a 6-week-old infant, *E. meningosepticum* bacteremia and meningitis developed in association with a strangulated hernia.[14]

Elizabethkingia and *Chryseobacterium* spp. were isolated frequently from tracheal aspirates of patients in intensive care during a 70-month observation period; yet during that time, none of more than 2000 critically ill patients developed pneumonia attributable to these microbes.[15] However, true respiratory tract infection was identified in an intubated pediatric patient and in adults receiving aerosolized medications.[6,59]

Sporadic cases of bacteremia have been reported in adult patients.[21,27,33,36] Two reviews of adult bacteremia in Taiwan have been published.[27,36] The largest of these included 118 patients at a single center over a 7-year period. The incidence of *E. meningosepticum* bacteremia increased from 7.5/100,000 admissions in 1999 to 35.6 per 100,000 in 2006. The vast majority of these infections were nosocomial, and 60% were acquired in intensive care units. Approximately a third of the patients had malignancy, and a fourth suffered from diabetes mellitus. The 14-day mortality rate was 23.4%. The main risk factor for mortality was acquisition of infection in an intensive care unit setting (odds ratio, 4.23). Rapid institution of appropriate antibiotic therapy reduced mortality.[27] Infection in immunocompromised patients can occur as a complication of relatively benign invasive procedures or as a localized infection.[33,55] Endocarditis was documented in intravenous drug abusers and patients undergoing dialysis.[17,65] Postoperative bacteremia in eight adult patients was linked to contaminated intravenous medications infused during anesthesia.[44] Contaminated arterial catheters were implicated in an epidemic of *Chryseobacterium* bacteremia.[57] Four patients, including a 7-year-old boy, became bacteremic in an outbreak associated with contamination at the time of intracardiac surgery.[3] This organism also has been associated with bacteremia in pediatric burn patients.[53]

Chryseobacterium spp. also have been isolated from infected skin lesions manifesting as papules, sheetlike lesions, plaques, and deep panniculitis.[18] One fatal case of necrotizing fasciitis in a patient with diabetes mellitus and chronic heart failure was reported.[32] Infection may have been related to wound contamination during repair of an orthopedic injury. A woman with pemphigus vulgaris developed cellulitis and sepsis.[56]

DIAGNOSIS

Rapid identification of infection with these organisms is urgent, not only to ensure providing proper therapy for the patient, but also to hasten initiating appropriate infection control measures to forestall epidemic outbreaks. Identification of *E. meningosepticum* is hindered by characteristically long periods required for oxidation of carbohydrates and weak or delayed indole production. Cultures may be misidentified as species of *Achromobacter* or *Pseudomonas.*[14] Clinical isolation of an unidentified gram-negative rod that is catalase- and oxidase-positive and that shows multiple antibiotic resistance should raise suspicion of *E. meningosepticum* infection. Cultures should be kept for several days for observation for typical carbohydrate reactions, which confirm the diagnosis.[14,49]

Identification of *Elizabethkingia* and *Chryseobacterium* species have improved with novel microbiology laboratory techniques. Matrix-assisted laser desorption ionization-time of flight mass spectrometry (MALDI-TOF) was used to quickly identify *C. meningosepticum* in an immunocompetent adult significantly reducing the time to identification and appropriate therapy.[23] 16S sequencing has become the routine definitive reference method in difficult to identify organisms such as *Elizabethkingia* and *Chryseobacterium* species.[52] Pulse-field gel electrophoresis of DNA was used successfully to identify recurrence of intravenous catheter-associated infection in a 6-year-old boy with non-Hodgkin lymphoma.[51] In 2016, clinical isolates of *E. anopheles* in Wisconsin were initially characterized using MALDI-TOF and subsequently confirmed to be associated with a multistate outbreak through whole-genome sequencing techniques.[42]

TREATMENT

Unfortunately, treatment of *E. meningosepticum* meningitis represents an especially difficult challenge for the physician. The organism is paradoxically likely to be sensitive to drugs commonly employed against gram-positive organisms (i.e., rifampin, vancomycin, clindamycin, and trimethoprim-sulfamethoxazole) and resistant to those used to treat gram-negative infections (i.e., aminoglycosides, cephalosporins, tetracyclines, and carbapenems). Most *Elizabethkingia* and *Chryseobacterium* spp. produce broad-spectrum metallo-β-lactamases. In *E. meningosepticum,* the enzyme is highly efficient at hydrolyzing carbapenems. Inactivation of cephalosporins displays a remarkable variability that is based on the affinity of the enzyme for the different compounds.[63] Delay in establishing a specific identification of the organism has historically led to ineffectual therapy as isolates of *E. meningosepticum* are almost uniformly resistant to common empiric gram-negative meningitis antibiotics such as third-generation cephalosporins or ampicillin and an aminoglycoside. Moreover antimicrobial susceptibilities determined by disk diffusion must be interpreted with caution. Aber and associates found clinical isolates in which specific strains were sensitive to gentamicin and rifampin by disk diffusion but were resistant by agar gel dilution susceptibility testing.[1] Therefore more direct methods of measuring the minimal inhibitory concentration than disk diffusion sensitivity should be used to determine the optimal microbial agents for therapy.

Probably as a consequence of difficulties encountered in providing rapid and effective antibacterial therapy, these organisms frequently persist for prolonged periods in CSF. Average persistence of *E. meningosepticum* in CSF is 19 days,[14] in contrast to the 3.9 days described by McCracken[41] for most cases of gram-negative neonatal bacterial meningitis.

Studies of in vitro susceptibility data forced a reappraisal of the idea that vancomycin is a good first-line choice for the treatment of *Chryseobacterium* infection. In one report, a literature review showed that only 65% of historic isolates were susceptible to vancomycin[4]; in another, a thorough search for a susceptible organism among 58 clinical isolates met with failure.[19] Clinically drugs that have been used alone or in combination with some success have included erythromycin, vancomycin, trimethoprim-sulfamethoxazole, fluoroquinolones (especially levofloxacin), and rifampin.[60] Some of these agents have the potential disadvantage of poor penetration of CSF. Combined use of many of these drugs renders interpreting therapeutic response difficult. The 3 survivors among the 12 patients reported by George and associates all received vancomycin intravenously, intrathecally, or both, as a part of their regimen.[20] Hawley and Gump reported a case of *E. meningosepticum* meningitis in a neonate who responded to systemic vancomycin after unsuccessful treatment with multiple antibiotics, including erythromycin.[22]

Intraventricular erythromycin[16,50] or rifampin[11,34,35,50] has been used in conjunction with systemic administration of these drugs. In particular, Lee and associates reported no deaths in seven infants with *E. meningosepticum* meningitis who were treated with intraventricular rifampin through an Ommaya reservoir at a dosage of 2 to 5 mg every 24 hours combined with 40 mg/kg per day administered intravenously.[35] Intraventricular administration continued until the CSF was sterile. However, colonization of the Ommaya reservoir was a common finding, and formation of a porencephalic cyst occurred in one patient. Chandrika and Adler reported sterilization of ventricles in one afflicted neonate within 48 hours after institution of therapy with intraventricular and intravenous rifampin.[11] Erythromycin has been used intraventricularly with limited success at 5 to 10 mg/day.[16,50] Rios and associates reported the successful addition of intraventricular rifampin to a failing regimen of intravenous and intraventricular erythromycin.[50] Development of resistance during therapy has been demonstrated with erythromycin and rifampin; persistence of organisms in the CSF despite administration of presumably adequate therapy should alert the physician to test for this possibility.[16,50] Addition of trimethoprim-sulfamethoxazole may be of benefit with such an occurrence; this agent effected a bacteriologic cure in eight of nine infants with meningitis.[37] This agent usually is not recommended in the neonatal period because of possible displacement of bilirubin from albumin-binding sites. Bacterial eradication was achieved in 48 hours in two patients with meningitis who were treated with clindamycin, rifampin, and cefotaxime systemically and rifampin intraventricularly.[7]

As with other types of gram-negative meningitis, antimicrobial therapy should be continued for at least 2 weeks after sterilization of ventricular fluid has been achieved. Time to sterilization is frequently prolonged; most patients therefore require 4 to 6 weeks of antimicrobial therapy. Complications of hydrocephalus and the potential use of intraventricular therapy render the neurosurgeon an essential part of the management team. Historically mortality has been in excess of 70%, no doubt in part because of delays in identifying the organism and the limited antibiotic spectrum available for effective therapy. More recent series of patients, although small, suggest some improvement in this statistic, but the rate of hydrocephalus and neurologic deficits remains high.

Recovery has been the rule in immunocompetent older individuals infected with contaminated materials, often despite treatment with antibiotics to which the organism was insensitive, a finding highlighting the very low virulence of these organisms in immunocompetent adults.[39] However, significant mortality and morbidity often occur in immunocompromised individuals with bacteremia or meningitis. Use of chloramphenicol, vancomycin, levofloxacin, erythromycin, or rifampin has achieved some success in these patients, but the choice of antibiotic must be based on a detailed examination of the organism's susceptibility.[24,53]

Acknowledgments

We thank Dr. William Gruber and Dr. Thomas Boyce for their invaluable assistance with earlier versions of this chapter.

NEW REFERENCES SINCE THE SEVENTH EDITION

23. Hayek SS, Abd TT, Cribbs SK, et al. Rare *Elizabethkingia meningosepticum* meningitis case in an immunocompetent adult. *Emerg Microbes Infect.* 2013;2(4):e17.
31. Lau SK, Chow WN, Foo CH, et al. *Elizabethkingia* anophelis bacteremia is associated with clinically significant infections and high mortality. *Sci Rep*. 2016;6: 26045.
42. Nicholson AC, Whitney AM, Emery BD, et al. Complete genome sequences of four strains from the 2015-2016 *Elizabethkingia anophelis* outbreak. *Genome Announcements*. 2016;4(3).
52. Shailaja VV, Reddy AK, Alimelu M, et al. Neonatal meningitis by multidrug resistant *Elizabethkingia meningosepticum* identified by 16S ribosomal RNA gene sequencing. *Intl J Pediatr*. 2014;2014:918907.

The full reference list for this chapter is available at ExpertConsult.com.

Pseudomonas and Related Genera

125

Monica I. Ardura • Amy Leber

The genus *Pseudomonas* is large and complex, containing a significant number of bacterial species, most of which are found in the environment as saprophytes and not associated with human or animal infections. Early attempts at better understanding the taxonomy of this diverse group of organisms led to placement of *Pseudomonas* spp. into five species clusters of genetically related organisms, also known as ribosomal RNA (rRNA) homology groups (designated groups I to V).[158] This genus since has undergone extensive revision using DNA-DNA hybridization, 16S rRNA sequencing, and related techniques, with four of the five homology groups reclassified into different genera (Table 125.1).[219] The taxon *Pseudomonas* was retained for organisms in rRNA homology group I with *P. aeruginosa* as the type species. Although they can cause infections in otherwise healthy individuals, they are more commonly opportunistic human pathogens causing disease in patients with burn wounds, cystic fibrosis (CF), malignancy, or immunodeficiency, as well as in individuals who are malnourished, are receiving immunosuppressive therapy, or have indwelling devices. The most important species by far relating to human disease is *P. aeruginosa*; however, some other related organisms are less commonly associated with specific clinical syndromes in both children and adults. This chapter will focus on *Pseudomonas* spp. (classic rRNA group I organisms) and *Burkholderia, Ralstonia, Cupriavidus*, and *Pandoraea* spp. (classic rRNA group II and related organisms) of primary clinical significance in pediatric patients.

TABLE 125.1 Taxonomic Changes Associated With *Pseudomonas* spp. and Related Organisms Causing Disease in Humans

RNA Homology Group	Previous Species Designation	Current Species Designation
I		*Pseudomonas aeruginosa*
		Pseudomonas fluorescens
		Pseudomonas putida
		Pseudomonas monteilii
		Pseudomonas mosselii
		Pseudomonas veroniii
		Pseudomonas stutzeri
		Pseudomonas mendocina
		Pseudomonas pseudoalcaligenes
		Pseudomonas alcaligenes
	Chryseomonas luteola	*Pseudomonas luteola*
	Flavimonas oryzihabitans	*Pseudomonas oryzihabitans*
II	*Pseudomonas cepacia*	*Burkholderia cepacia*
	Pseudomonas gladioli	*Burkholderia gladioli*
	Pseudomonas mallei	*Burkholderia mallei*
	Pseudomonas pickettii	*Ralstonia pickettii*
	Pseudomonas pseudomallei	*Burkholderia pseudomallei*
III	*Pseudomonas acidovorans*	*Delftia acidovorans*
	Pseudomonas testosteroni	*Comamonas testosteroni*
	Pseudomonas delafieldii	*Acidovorax delafieldii*
	Hydrogenomonas facilis	*Acidovorax facilis*
IV	*Pseudomonas diminuta*	*Brevundimonas diminuta*
	Pseudomonas vesicularis	*Brevundimonas vesicularis*
V	*Xanthomonas maltophilia*	*Stenotrophomonas maltophilia*

Based on Henry DA, Speert DP. Pseudomonas. In: Versalovic J, Carroll KC, G Funke, et al., editors. *Manual of Clinical Microbiology*, 10th ed. Washington, DC: ASM Press; 2011.

ETIOLOGY

Pseudomonas spp. and related genera (pseudomonads) are nonfastidious, nonfermentative, obligate aerobic (i.e., metabolize carbohydrates oxidatively and thus require molecular oxygen as the terminal hydrogen/electron acceptor), catalase positive, generally cytochrome oxidase positive and motile, non–spore-forming, gram-negative bacilli. Some species, including *P. aeruginosa*, may grow anaerobically in the presence of nitrates or other nonorganic compounds as terminal hydrogen/electron acceptors. This has clinical relevance for CF, allowing *P. aeruginosa* to grow in the relatively anaerobic atmosphere within the sputum and mucous of such patients.[1,204,395] Because pseudomonads can metabolize a wide variety of carbon sources, including simple and complex carbohydrates, alcohols, and amino acids, they can survive and multiply in almost any moist environment containing minimal amounts of organic compounds.

Among the *Pseudomonas* species (former rRNA homology group I organisms), a division is made into two groups on the basis of production of fluorescent pigments. The "fluorescent pseudomonads" include six clinically relevant members: *P. aeruginosa, P. putida, P. fluorescens*, and less commonly encountered species, *P. veronii, P. monteilii*, and *P. mosselii*. The nonfluorescent group includes six clinically relevant species: *P. stutzeri* and *P. mendocina* (stutzeri group), *P. alcaligenes* and *P. pseudoalcaligenes* (alcaligenes group), and *P. luteola* and *P. oryzihabitans* (yellow-pigmented group).[165] The fluorescent pseudomonads generally produce the water-soluble yellow-green fluorescent pigment pyoverdin (fluorescein), whereas many clinical isolates of *P. aeruginosa* also produce the water-soluble blue phenazine pigment pyocyanin. These pigments diffuse into and color the medium surrounding the colonies. The pyoverdin and pyocyanin produced by *P. aeruginosa* combine to give the bright-green to blue-green color characteristic of this organism on certain clear laboratory media, particularly Mueller-Hinton agar. Some strains of *P. aeruginosa* may produce other pigments, such as dark red (pyorubin) or brown-black (pyomelanin) pigment.

P. aeruginosa is readily recovered from clinical specimens and usually is recognized easily on laboratory media such as sheep blood agar by its characteristic flat-spreading colonies with a metallic-sheen, an irregular edge, and production of β-hemolysis; however, atypical colony types such as smooth-round, mucoid, or small colony variants may occur, particularly in patients with CF. These atypical colony types are likely due to the impact of previous antibiotic therapy on synthetic biochemical pathways. It is common to recover a mixture of colony types in such patients. On selective and differential MacConkey agar, *P. aeruginosa* produces colorless colonies because lactose is not used as a sole carbohydrate source and there is no change in pH of the medium. When pigment production and typical metallic-sheen colony type are combined with a positive cytochrome oxidase test, *P. aeruginosa* can be identified with high certainty without further testing.[72] Many laboratories rely on commercial biochemical identification systems for identifying gram-negative rods suspected of being *P. aeruginosa*, particularly those with atypical colony morphology. Most such systems are highly accurate (>90%) for identification of *P. aeruginosa*, but less accurate for identification of other *Pseudomonas* spp. Such systems for identification of *P. aeruginosa* isolates from patients with CF are less accurate, particularly for slow-growing or variant colony types. Some systems may have difficulty separating the three closely related fluorescent pseudomonads, and thus definitive identification may require additional testing. Although growth is optimal at 35° to 37°C (95°F–98.6°F), *P. aeruginosa* grows at 42°C (107.6°F) and *P. fluorescens* and *P. putida* do not. In addition, most isolates of *P. aeruginosa* reduce nitrogen to gas, whereas the other two fluorescent *Pseudomonas* spp. do not. Additional biochemical characteristics of *P. aeruginosa* include a reaction of alkaline over no change in triple sugar iron agar; production of acid oxidatively from glucose and xylose but not lactose, sucrose, or maltose; and a positive reaction for arginine dihydrolase. In practice, these latter tests are generally not used because they do not clearly differentiate among the fluorescent pseudomonads. Most strains are motile by one or more polar flagella and also display surface pili. Most isolates also carry the genes required to synthesize the extracellular mucopolysaccharide alginate, whose overproduction results in the mucoid colony type; however, such colony types are almost exclusively isolated from the respiratory tract of patients with CF.[240]

Among the nonfluorescent group *Pseudomonas* spp., *P. luteola* and *P. oryzihabitans* are somewhat unique because they are cytochrome oxidase negative and produce an intracellular yellow, nondiffusible pigment. Most isolates of *P. stutzeri* produce a distinctive dry, wrinkled colony on agar media, and the colonies can adhere tenaciously to the agar. In contrast, *P. mendocina* produces smooth colonies with a brown-yellow pigment. Isolates of *P. alcaligenes* and *P. pseudoalcaligenes* do not produce distinctive colony types and are rarely encountered in clinical specimens. As a group, these organisms are identified with variable accuracy by commercial biochemical identification systems. Depending on the clinical situation, an identification of *Pseudomonas*-like gram-negative rod or *Pseudomonas* spp., not *aeruginosa,* with a request to contact the laboratory for further identification and antimicrobial susceptibility testing may be sufficient. When definitive identification is required, nucleic acid–based methods for identification of culture isolates of *Pseudomonas* spp. have proved useful. These methods include sequencing of the genes coding for 16S rRNA or the use of specific nucleic acid probes or polymerase chain reaction (PCR) assays, such as assays targeting the exotoxin A or other *P. aeruginosa*–specific gene sequences. Peptide nucleic acid fluorescence in situ hybridization has also been shown to be sensitive and specific for identification of *P. aeruginosa,* including identification in positive blood culture bottles. As will be mentioned later, newer techniques such as matrix-assisted laser desorption ionization–time of flight mass (MALDI-TOF) spectrometry have been shown to be reliable and accurate in providing identifications of these organisms.

The former rRNA homology group 2 and related organisms currently comprise a diverse group of bacteria in the genera *Burkholderia, Ralstonia, Cupriavidus,* and *Pandoraea.* Like the *Pseudomonas* spp., they are found in a wide variety of environmental habitats as saprophytes, plant pathogens, and opportunistic animal and human pathogens and are nutritionally versatile. The more well-studied organisms in the group belong to the genus *Burkholderia,* which now contains more than 60 species. Members of this genus can be divided into two major groups: the *B. cepacia* complex and non–*B. cepacia* complex organisms. There are currently 18 named *B. cepacia* complex organisms with all but one having been recovered from human specimens.[220] The most important species in the complex are *B. multivorans* and *B. cenocepacia* because of their role as colonizers and opportunistic pathogens in patients with CF; they compromise approximately 80% of *B. cepacia* complex infections in the United States.[220] Of the non–*B. cepacia* complex *Burkholderia* spp., those of human clinical significance include *B. gladioli* and *B. pseudomallei. B. gladioli* is an important agent of respiratory tract colonization and infection in patients with CF and chronic granulomatous disease.[329] *B. pseudomallei* causes melioidosis and has also been recovered from the respiratory tract of patients with CF. *Burkholderia mallei* is an important animal pathogen causing glanders in horses.

The genera *Ralstonia, Cupriavidus,* and *Pandoraea* all contain species of clinical significance, but they are recovered in culture at lower rates than *Burkholderia* spp. The genus *Ralstonia* includes at least five species, with the following species known to cause human infections: *R. pickettii, R. insidiosa,* and *R. mannitolitytica.*[75,77] *R. mannitolilytica* has been reported as causing meningitis and nosocomial outbreaks.[93,176] The genus *Cupriavidus* contains at least 11 species, including *C. gilardii, C. respiraculi, C. taiwanensis,* and *C. pauculus,* the latter of which have been recovered from patients with CF.[372] The genus *Pandoraea* contains at least five named species (i.e., *P. apista, P. pulmonicola, P. pnomenusa, P. sputorum,* and *P. norimbergensis*) and several unnamed species.[76] *P. apista, P. pnomenusa,* and *P. sputorum* have been recovered from patients with CF.[122] As a group, these organisms are of low virulence and infection in healthy individuals is uncommon. They have been associated with catheter-related bloodstream infections and other health care–associated infections in immunocompromised patients and with colonization and infection in those with CF.

As a group, these organisms grow well but slowly on most standard laboratory media such as sheep blood, chocolate, and MacConkey agars and appear as small, smooth, raised colonies. They may appear as colorless colonies or, with prolonged incubation, pink to dark-red colonies because of the slow usage of lactose, as is usually the case with *B. cepacia* complex organisms. They are all cytochrome oxidase weak or strong positive, gram-negative, motile rods, except for *B. gladioli* and *Pandoraea* spp., which are oxidase variable. A majority of *B. cepacia* complex isolates are lysine decarboxylase positive, a helpful feature in identification of this group. Isolation of *B. cepacia* complex organisms from clinical specimens with mixed bacterial flora, particularly the respiratory tract of patients with CF, is enhanced by using selective and differential media with the ability to inhibit the growth of *P. aeruginosa* and other gram-negative rods. In addition, recovery may be improved if culture plates are incubated at least 3 days at 35°C to 37°C (95°F–98.6°F). Several selective agar media are commercially available, including oxidative-fermentative base–polymyxin B–bacitracin–lactose (OFPBL),[386] "*P.*" *cepacia* (PC), and *B. cepacia*–selective (BCSA) agars.[159,397] These media take advantage of the fact that *Burkholderia* spp. and some related organisms are generally resistant in vitro to the polymyxin antibiotics, whereas *P. aeruginosa* and most commonly isolated enteric bacteria are susceptible (*Serratia* spp. are a notable exception) and therefore inhibited on such media. Several studies have shown differences in the ability of these media to recover *B. cepacia* complex organisms or to inhibit the growth of other bacterial flora, with BCSA being equivalent or superior to the other media for this purpose.[159,397] Some of these media are also useful for the recovery of *B. gladioli* from patients with CF.

B. pseudomallei grows on agar media commonly used for isolation of gram-negative bacteria. The colonies develop slowly (over a week) and have a characteristic "daisy-head" appearance. α-Hemolysis is noted on sheep blood agar. Ashdown selective medium, which contains crystal violet and gentamicin, can increase the recovery rate of *B. pseudomallei* from clinical specimens containing mixed bacterial flora, including throat, rectal, and sputum specimens.[14] *B. pseudomallei* produces a dry, wrinkled, violet-purple colony with a pungent, earthy odor on Ashdown medium.[220] Other selective media, including a recently described *B. pseudomallei*–selective agar (BPSA) and selective media for *B. cepacia* (BCSA, PC, and OFPBL), have been evaluated against Ashdown medium for the recovery of *B. pseudomallei.*[144,278] Ashdown medium remains the recommended medium for recovery of *B. pseudomallei* in endemic areas, but commercially available selective agars for *B. cepacia,* particularly PC agar, are acceptable media in nonendemic areas. Selective enrichment broths also have been developed for the recovery of *B. pseudomallei* from superficial sites. Such broths have been shown to improve the recovery of the organism when used in addition to direct plating onto Ashdown medium. Because of the potential of *B. pseudomallei* as an agent of bioterrorism via inhalation, isolation of the organism from patients with no travel history to endemic sites should immediately be reported to public health.

Accurate identification of the rRNA group II and related organisms may be difficult using either traditional biochemical or commercially available biochemical test systems.[137,198,297,299] Few of these species are found in the databases of such systems, and none of these systems is able to clearly differentiate among the various species in the *B. cepacia* complex. As with *P. aeruginosa,* molecular methods including amplification of the 16S rRNA gene followed by sequencing have been most widely used for this purpose; however, such methods may not always discriminate among closely related pseudomonads. Special emphasis should be given to accurate identification of such organisms when recovered from patients with CF because of the clinical significance and patient management implication of a *B. cepacia* complex or related organisms in such patients. An initial, probably biochemical, identification of *B. cepacia* complex for a patient with CF should be confirmed with a molecular method capable of determining the exact species identification. To this end, the Cystic Fibrosis Foundation established a *B. cepacia* reference laboratory at the University of Michigan for phenotypic characterization and genotypic species identification for suspected *B. cepacia* complex and related organisms.

MALDI-TOF spectrometry is quickly supplanting phenotypic methods and is becoming the standard bacterial identification method for many laboratories. It is capable of identifying a wide variety of bacteria, including the difficult to identify organisms recovered from the respiratory tract of patients with CF.[5,98,118,231] MALDI-TOF allows for the analysis of biomolecules such as nucleic acids, proteins, and sugars, as well as other large organic molecules that may be fragile and fragment when ionized by more conventional ionization methods. It has been shown to provide accuracy to the genus and, in most cases, species or subspecies level, which is very useful for organisms in the rRNA groups II through V.

EPIDEMIOLOGY

P. aeruginosa is a ubiquitous environmental organism found in soil, water, and on vegetation, including the surface of many raw fruits and vegetables. Its minimal nutritional requirements and ability to grow in a wide variety of physical environments enhance the organism's ability to survive in numerous ecologic niches. *P. aeruginosa* may be found as colonizing flora in a small percentage of healthy humans.[154] Sites of colonization include moist body sites and mucosal surfaces such as throat, nasal mucosa, axillae, and perineum. Carriage rates in the gastrointestinal tract have been reported as high as 24% based on selective culture of stool. The gastrointestinal tract may be the site of transient colonization after ingestion of food or liquids containing *P. aeruginosa*. Despite the ability to colonize skin and mucosal surfaces, it rarely results in persistent colonization. The respiratory tract is a common site of colonization of patients who have been hospitalized for extended periods, have foreign bodies in place (i.e., endotracheal tubes or tracheostomies), have poor mucociliary clearance, or have received broad-spectrum antibiotics or chemotherapy.

P. aeruginosa is best classified as an opportunistic pathogen whose pathogenic potential is manifest in situations in which the host's immune defenses are diminished or lacking. Such situations include children with poor mucociliary clearance (CF), neutropenia (secondary to cancer chemotherapy), or damaged skin barrier (burn wound).The organism generally does not invade intact skin or mucous membranes.

P. aeruginosa frequently enters the hospital environment on the clothes and shoes of patients, visitors, or hospital personnel and also from the same individuals with skin, gastrointestinal tract, or respiratory tract colonization. It may also enter the hospital on plants or flowers. As a result, the organism may be found growing in any moist hospital environment, including hospital kitchens and laundries, mops, shower heads, whirlpools, antiseptic solutions, eye drops, distilled water sources, irrigation fluid, dialysis fluid, and equipment used for dialysis and respiratory care or inhalation therapy. It tolerates elevated temperatures and can grow in distilled water sources containing only inorganic compounds. *P. aeruginosa* commonly is found on the surface of many types of plants and flowers, raw fruits, and vegetables. Consumption of these foods by profoundly immunosuppressed children can result in colonization of the gastrointestinal tract and potentially can lead to invasive disease. In hospitalized patients, the likelihood of colonization increases with duration of hospitalization. Transmission of *P. aeruginosa* from patient to patient or from hospital personnel to patient often is assumed but rarely documented.[11,12,103,388] Although clear evidence exists of patient-to-patient transmission of "epidemic strains" of *P. aeruginosa* among the CF population, the relative importance of this mode of acquisition as opposed to acquisition from environmental sources is unclear.[4,147,218] Environmental sources of *P. aeruginosa* outside the hospital that may result in colonization with subsequent infection include swimming pools, water slides, hot tubs, contact lens solutions, cosmetics, illicit injectable drugs, and the inner soles of sneakers.

Various typing systems have been used to characterize strains of *P. aeruginosa* for epidemiologic purposes; these can be classified as either phenotypic or genotypic typing methods. Historically the phenotypic method of serologic typing based on the O-polysaccharide component of lipopolysaccharide was used most often, but some strains of *P. aeruginosa* lack the O-polysaccharide. Other phenotypic typing methods include phage and pyocin typing. These methods have limited ability to differentiate strains, particularly from chronic infections, because of the variability of gene expression in this organism. Phenotypic methods have been replaced by genotypic methods, including restriction fragment length polymorphism (RFLP) analysis, pulsed-field gel electrophoresis (PFGE), random amplified polymorphic DNA (RAPD) analysis, multilocus sequence typing (MLST), and others.[81,345] Each of these methods has certain advantages and disadvantages in terms of cost, complexity, and discriminatory power. They have proved helpful in demonstrating, for example, that patients with CF were usually infected with unique strains of *P. aeruginosa* that they harbored for extended periods rather than being replaced by other strains.

The environmental distribution of the other *Pseudomonas* spp. is similar to that of *P. aeruginosa*, and hospitalized as well as nonhospitalized individuals can become transiently colonized. Infection may infrequently occur, particularly in individuals who are immunocompromised. *P. fluorescens* can be isolated from the skin.[327] *P. fluorescens* has been responsible for bloodstream infections, with most cases being iatrogenic, attributable to transfusion with contaminated blood products or infusion equipment.[322,327] In addition, contamination of blood with *P. fluorescens* during the blood culture collection process has been responsible for outbreaks of pseudobacteremia.[193,336] *Pseudomonas pseudoalcaligenes* has one of the more unusual environmental habitats—industrial metalworking fluid consisting of a mixture of water and petroleum products. Although metalworkers with long-term exposure to aerosols containing high concentrations (>10^5 organisms/mL) of *P. pseudoalcaligenes* develop high antibody titers to the organism, they do not have clinical evidence of acute or chronic respiratory or systemic disease.[233] Limited data exist on typing systems for *Pseudomonas* spp. other than *P. aeruginosa*.

B. cepacia complex and related organisms are ubiquitous in nature and can be found in water, soil, decaying organic matter, and as plant pathogens.[171,211,373] Unlike *P. aeruginosa, B. cepacia* complex organisms are infrequently encountered in the hospital environment or nonhospital sites such as swimming pools, sinks, and showers. As a group, these organisms are intrinsically resistant to disinfectants and a wide range of antimicrobial agents, including the aminoglycosides and carboxypenicillins (e.g., ticarcillin and carbenicillin). Moreover resistance can be acquired to quinolones, extended-spectrum penicillin/β-lactamase inhibitor compounds, third- and fourth-generation cephalosporins, and carbapenem antibiotics. *B. cepacia* can survive for extended periods in moist environments, even in the presence of disinfectants, including povidone-iodine.[9] These organisms have been identified as agents of sporadic nosocomial outbreaks of infection in medical intensive care units. When such outbreaks occur, they have been traced to contaminated instruments and solutions, such as in automated peritoneal dialysis machines, blood gas analyzers, mouthwashes, ultrasound gels, medications, and skin antiseptics, including povidone-iodine and chlorhexidine.[29,30,157,341] In patients with CF, colonization of the respiratory tract, sometimes associated with lower respiratory tract and disseminated infection, is of major clinical significance because of the association of this organism group with increased morbidity and mortality.[147,172,220] Although acquisition of *B. cepacia* complex organisms from the environment is the more common mode of transmission, as evidenced by the fact that the majority of infected patients harbor genetically distinct strains, epidemiologic investigations have clearly demonstrated "epidemic strains" and interpatient transmission in the CF population.[20,34] Most data suggest that, once colonized with a specific strain, replacement of that strain with another strain occurs infrequently.[31] *B. cepacia* complex organisms also have become more important as a cause of infection and complications in patients with chronic granulomatous disease[346] and sickle-cell hemoglobinopathies.[32]

B. gladioli, like *B. cepacia* complex organisms, is a plant pathogen found in water and soil. It is associated with infections in immunocompromised patients, including patients with chronic granulomatous disease and in patients with CF. In fact, it is recovered more frequently from patients with CF than most *B. cepacia* complex species other than *B. cenocepacia* and *B. multivorans*. *B. pseudomallei,* the causative agent of melioidosis, and the closely related species *B. thailandensis,* are found in soil and surface water in the tropical and subtropical areas of Southeast Asia and northern Australia, including rice paddy surface waters in rice-growing areas of Thailand, Cambodia, Vietnam, and Laos.[63,87,342] *Ralstonia, Cupriavidus,* and *Pandoraea* spp. are also found in soil and water sources, but their epidemiology has not been well studied. Unlike some *B. cepacia* complex species, person-to-person transmission of other *Burkholderia* spp. or *Ralstonia, Cupriavidus,* and *Pandoraea* spp. has been rarely reported. The first documented spread of *P. pulmonicola* was reported in a CF center in France; the index patient was chronically colonized, and the infection spread to five other individuals.[95]

Genotypic typing systems have been applied to epidemiologic investigations of *B. cepacia* complex organisms, other *Burkholderia* spp., and species of other genera in this group.[220]

PATHOGENESIS

Among the *Pseudomonas* spp., the pathogenesis of infections with *P. aeruginosa* has been well studied. Pathogenesis is multifactorial,[26,224] and the outcome of *P. aeruginosa*–host encounters depends on a variety of organism-specific and host factors. To establish lung infection, for example, *P. aeruginosa* must contend with the mucociliary clearance mechanism and innate immunity, including antibacterial peptides such as lactoferrin, and the action of phagocytic cells.[309] The large genome of the organism provides it with the metabolic flexibility to adapt to various host environments. A large number of varied and redundant virulence factors include cell-associated (bound to the bacterial cell surface) and extracellular proteins and other macromolecules, which are either injected directly into the host cell cytoplasm or secreted into the general extracellular environment.[374] These factors, along with intrinsic and acquired resistance to antimicrobial agents, allow the organism to colonize, resist host defense mechanisms, produce local tissue damage, and, in some situations, invade and result in disseminated infection despite the host immune response.[374,390]

Expression of virulence factors is under tight regulatory control and depends on the body site and type of infection. Different factors may be expressed in acute versus chronic infections. Two major types of regulatory systems promote organism survival and proliferation. The first system type involves one- or two-component transcriptional regulatory secretion of exoproteins. One-step systems promote direct delivery of preformed exoproteins, whereas two-step systems synthesize exoproteins as precursor molecules requiring cleavage before exporting outside the cell.[146] In either case, exoproteins are delivered across the inner and outer cell membranes and peptidoglycan cell wall layer to the periplasmic space. The second regulatory system type involves quorum-sensing regulatory systems that help coordinate gene expression throughout the bacterial population to aid the organism in adapting to environmental conditions. Quorum-sensing systems involve cell-to-cell signaling by production of small diffusible molecules known as autoinducers. Quorum sensing plays an important role in promoting the formation of biofilms on mucosal surfaces and internalized medical devices. Such biofilms are important for survival of the organism and contribute to persistent and chronic infections. Interestingly, macrolide antibiotics, which do not inhibit growth of *P. aeruginosa* in vitro, may inhibit quorum sensing and biofilm formation.[363,374]

P. aeruginosa displays virtually all known classes of microbial virulence factors. Cell-associated virulence factors include flagella, pili, and endotoxin (lipopolysaccharide). Flagella and pili play an important role in establishment of initial infection because of their functions of providing motility and binding to specific epithelial cell surface receptors. *P. aeruginosa* has one or more polar flagella that allow for motility and appear to be important in initial stages of lung colonization. The flagella themselves do not appear to enhance binding to epithelial cells, but they do bind to respiratory mucin produced in response to infection and may contribute to other cell-binding mechanisms. Decreased clearance of mucin in the lung of some individuals may contribute to establishment of infection. Flagellar proteins contribute to excess activation of proinflammatory cytokines. Once infection is established in the lung, flagella are generally no longer produced, and they are usually not found in organisms associated with biofilms. Strains of *P. aeruginosa* that lack flagella are less capable of dissemination from wounds and less likely to cause bacteremia and pneumonia in animal models.[13,106,120] Pili, like flagella, are also found at the poles of the *P. aeruginosa* rod. They promote adherence to mucosal epithelial cells by binding to specific cell-surface glycolipids.[378] They also mediate twitching motility, which appears to be important in biofilm formation, as demonstrated by in vitro models.

Other cell surface adhesions likely exist, including outer membrane proteins and oligosaccharides that work in complement with flagella and pili to promote initial colonization of cell surfaces by *P. aeruginosa*. The CF transmembrane conductance regulator (CFTR) protein also may play an important role as an epithelial cell receptor for *P. aeruginosa*. The CFTR protein appears to be involved with bacterial internalization and clearance from the lung.[326] Diminished internalization of bacteria in murine and primate models of CF might provide some basis for hypersusceptibility of CF patients to infections with *P. aeruginosa*.[326]

P. aeruginosa endotoxin is not as potent as are the endotoxins produced by other gram-negative organisms, including *Escherichia coli* (2 to 3 mg is needed to kill a 20-g mouse). The oligosaccharide side chain of *P. aeruginosa* endotoxin prevents lysis by complement and the lipid moiety triggers cytokine pathways that lead to the sepsis syndrome and shock. The virulence of *P. aeruginosa* in a mouse burn model was found to be related directly to lipopolysaccharide integrity.[83] Deficiency of the O side chain of lipopolysaccharide reduced virulence markedly.[285]

Extracellular virulence factors of *P. aeruginosa* include numerous exotoxins with proteolytic or lipolytic activity. These include the elastolytic proteases LasA protease and elastase (LasB), collagenase, gelatinase, caseinase, alkaline protease, fibrinolysin, phospholipase C (a thermolabile hemolysin), lecithinase, exotoxin A, and a group of exoenzymes including ExoS, ExoT, ExoU, and ExoY. The proteolytic enzymes may be responsible for localized necrosis of the skin or lung tissue and for corneal ulceration. The various proteases also can degrade plasma proteins, including complement and coagulation factors.[396] Solubilization and destruction of lecithin (surfactant) may play a role in the atelectasis seen in pulmonary infections caused by *P. aeruginosa*. Fibronectin protects epithelial cells from bacterial attachment, but its ability to do so is reduced in patients with CF because of the high level of proteases in respiratory secretions and also after cellular injury from trauma, intubation, or postviral infection.

Exotoxin A is an adenosine-5′-diphosphate ribosyltransferase enzyme that inhibits eukaryotic cell protein synthesis by a mechanism similar to the action of diphtheria toxin. Specific exotoxin A–deficient mutants of *P. aeruginosa* have reduced virulence in mouse and rat models of corneal and lung infection.[263,394] Exotoxin A also diminishes the activity of host phagocytes. Passive or active immunization against exotoxin A significantly protects against experimental infection with exotoxin A–producing strains of *P. aeruginosa*. Phospholipase C degrades phospholipids, which are plentiful in eukaryotic but not prokaryotic cell membranes. The hemolysis produced by *P. aeruginosa* may be caused by heat-labile phospholipase C and by a heat-stable moiety.

The exoenzymes S, T, U, and Y have multiple enzymatic and chemical functions. Their secretion is regulated by a type III secretion system commonly found in other bacterial pathogens. This system is associated with acute infections, requires pilin-mediated contact with target epithelial cells, and allows the organism to directly inject these products into the host cell cytoplasm rather than simply into the general environment. ExoS and ExoT are bifunctional proteins that display GTPase activation and ADP-ribosyltransferase activity. They confer antiphagocytic activity by depolarizing actin filaments and thus disrupting normal cytoskeletal organization. ExoS also inhibits interleukin production by alveolar macrophages and induces tumor necrosis factor-α production. Production of ExoS is associated with invasive disease in burn patients. *P. aeruginosa* growing on the burn wound but not on intact skin produces ExoS,[258] and ExoS can be found in the blood of patients who develop *P. aeruginosa* sepsis before the bacteria can be detected. *P. aeruginosa* strains that do not produce ExoS are less able to cause invasive disease.[319] ExoU is a potent cytotoxin possessing phospholipase A2 activity and causing rapid damage to cell membranes and cell death. ExoY has adenylate cyclase activity, but its specific role in virulence is unclear.

The importance of type III secretion proteins in the pathogenicity of *P. aeruginosa* has been demonstrated in animal model systems. Neutralization of these proteins has been shown to prevent septic shock and improve survival in a mouse model system. Similarly antibodies against PcrV, a protein involved in translocation of the exoenzymes, resulted in complete survival of the animals. Rabbit model studies of *P. aeruginosa*–induced septic shock after lung injury also showed the protective effect of antibodies to PcrV.

Among the vast array of proteases produced by *P. aeruginosa,* the elastolytic enzymes LasA and LasB cause direct damage to lung tissue (elastin accounts for 30% of the protein of lung tissue) and can also interfere with immune clearance of *P. aeruginosa* from the lungs. Berger and associates[27] noted that elastase treatment of isolated polymorphonuclear leukocytes severely impaired their ability to kill opsonized *P. aeruginosa.* They demonstrated proteolytic degradation of C3b receptors and suggested that it may contribute to the inability of patients with CF to eradicate *P. aeruginosa* from their lungs. Because several cell types, including macrophages, monocytes, B lymphocytes, and some T lymphocytes, carry the same C3b receptor, the proteolytic activity may cleave this molecule from all these cells, thereby decreasing the phagocytic activity of monocytes and macrophages in these patients. Berger and colleagues[27] also demonstrated that optimal interaction between the complement-derived opsonic ligands C3b and iC3b and their respective receptors does not occur in the milieu of the lungs of patients with CF who are infected with *P. aeruginosa.* They suggested that both *P. aeruginosa* and host proteases may contribute to the initiation of a cycle of events in which neutrophils entering the infected lung actually impair phagocytosis rather than eradicate the source of infection. Breakdown of elastin in the walls of blood vessels might be responsible for the intrapulmonary hemorrhage noted in individuals with CF.

P. aeruginosa also produces siderophores, including pyoverdin and pyochelin; these are iron-scavenging compounds that allow the organism to replicate in an iron-deficient environment. Iron in host tissue is tightly bound to transferrin or lactoferrin in the lungs. Siderophores bind iron efficiently and then are taken up by the bacterium through cell-specific receptors. Siderophores also play a role in control of expression of other virulence factors.

Mucociliary clearance is impeded in patients with CF, and, as a consequence, they fail to cleanse the bronchopulmonary epithelium of inhaled particles, including bacteria.[201,250] *P. aeruginosa* adherence to the airways of children with CF may be enhanced by the acidic environment that results from the hyperacidification of the trans-Golgi network from the dysfunctional CFTR protein in lung epithelial cells.[289] The specific colonizing strain or strains of *P. aeruginosa* may reflect exposure to other colonized individuals in health care facilities, CF camps, or at home, as well as by selective pressure by the use of mist tents, inhalation therapy, and continuous broad-spectrum antibiotic therapy.[200,413]

The evolution of colonization from the nonmucoid to the mucoid phenotype of *P. aeruginosa* can be correlated with the patient's age, clinical score, extent of pulmonary function abnormalities, severity of changes on chest radiographs, and serum immunoglobulin levels.[68,71] The specific lung environment of a patient with CF is believed to trigger a switch to a cluster of genes that code for abundant production of alginate, thereby giving rise to the mucoid phenotype.[68,348] Strains of *P. aeruginosa* expressing the mucoid phenotype are rarely recovered from patients without CF (0.5%–1.7%). Chronic infection of the lungs in patients with CF selects for additional genetic adaptations by *P. aeruginosa,* including the loss of genes coding for virulence factors (primarily proteins) required for initiation of acute infections.[337] The loss of such virulence factors may contribute to a decrease in the immunogenicity of the organism, a diminished effective immune response, and the inability of the host to eradicate *P. aeruginosa* from the airways.

Persistence of *P. aeruginosa* within the respiratory tract is aided by growth of the organism in microcolonies embedded in a biofilm of alginate.[164,167,279] This biofilm allows nutrients to pass while protecting the organism from host defense mechanisms, antibodies, and antibiotics.[203] In addition, investigators have noted that rabbit alveolar macrophages fail to phagocytize and kill the organism in the presence of serum from patients with CF. This phenomenon suggests that these patients have a specific, local defect in pulmonary resistance to *P. aeruginosa.*

The mucoid strains of *P. aeruginosa* isolated from the respiratory secretions of patients with CF produce large quantities of the mucopolysaccharide alginate, which is composed of acetylated D-mannuronic acid and L-glucuronic acid.[68,347] This polysaccharide polymer not only gives *P. aeruginosa* a mucoid appearance on agar medium but also has antiphagocytic activity. Alginate elicits a significant inflammatory immune response in the lungs of patients with CF and may contribute to the lung damage that occurs in chronic *P. aeruginosa* lung infection.[235] Because of its viscous nature, alginate contributes to the thick bronchial secretions in the lungs of children with CF; these secretions obstruct small airways and impair mucociliary clearance and movement of phagocytic cells. Production of alginate by *P. aeruginosa* is regulated and inducible. Mucoid isolates of *P. aeruginosa* lose the mucoid trait when serially cultured on laboratory media. Nonmucoid isolates convert to the mucoid phenotype when inoculated into the lung in a rat model.[319] Alginate also inhibits the action of antibiotics.[163]

The predilection for *P. aeruginosa* to colonize and infect the respiratory tract of patients with CF may partially be the result of decreased oxygen tension within the hyperviscous mucous layer.[395] Epithelial cells in individuals with CF have increased oxygen usage, which is responsible for the decreased oxygen tension.[395] This local hypoxia results in a change in the phenotype of *P. aeruginosa* resulting in alginate production, decreased motility (loss of flagella), and biofilm production.[395] Once these phenotypic changes occur, eradication of *P. aeruginosa* from the lungs of individuals with CF is nearly impossible.

The pathogenicity of *P. aeruginosa* also depends on its ability to resist or overwhelm host cell defense mechanisms. Fick and Reynolds[123,124] noted that in patients with CF, the opsonic function of IgG was reduced as a result of a molecular change in the Fc portion of the immunoglobulin (Ig)G molecule. This deficit was magnified in the lungs of patients with CF infected with *P. aeruginosa* because bacterial proteases can fragment IgG and further impair its opsonic activity. The persistence of *P. aeruginosa* in the lungs of patients with CF also may be related to the presence of one or more factors in their respiratory secretions that interfere with the bactericidal activity of fresh normal human serum against *P. aeruginosa.* These "blocking factors" have been shown to be IgG antibody that inhibit the normal bactericidal activity of human sera IgM antibody.[282,325]

Concentrations of IgG subclass immunoglobulins have been studied in patients with CF and compared with values obtained in age-matched healthy children and adults. Pressler and associates[290] noted that, in 52% of patients with CF, at least one of the four IgG subclasses had an elevated serum concentration in contrast to controls. A significant correlation of elevated serum concentrations of IgG2 (and to a lesser extent IgG3) with decreased forced expiratory volume at 1 second was noted. Moss[251] found that patients with CF who are infected with *P. aeruginosa* have markedly elevated serum concentrations of IgG antibodies to the opsonic immunodeterminant, type-specific lipopolysaccharide. This elevation was distributed among all four IgG subclasses with a significant shift toward IgG3. Sera from patients with CF who were colonized with *P. aeruginosa* had diminished opsonic capacity, but complement-dependent human neutrophil phagocytosis was not impaired. Serum concentrations of IgG4 but not IgG1, IgG2, or IgG3 are correlated inversely with opsonic capacity. On the basis of these data, Moss[251] suggested that high levels of IgG4 antibody to opsonic immunodeterminants may inhibit normal pulmonary clearance of *P. aeruginosa* by pulmonary macrophages in vivo. In addition to alterations in humoral immune responses to *P. aeruginosa,* it appears that dysfunctional CFTR also alters the bacterial activity of macrophages against *P. aeruginosa.*[96]

Infection of the lower respiratory tract in patients with CF results in massive infiltration of lung tissue with neutrophils.[78,105] The neutrophils release elastolytic enzymes that overwhelm the ability of protease-inhibiting compounds of the lung to protect against tissue damage. This results in destruction of lung tissue and accumulation of large amounts of extracellular nucleic acid and cell cytosol matrix, which contributes to airway viscosity.

Virulence factors of other *Pseudomonas* spp., *B. cepacia* complex, and related organisms have been less well studied but include their ability to adhere to indwelling devices and elaboration of exoenzymes such as elastase and gelatinase.[253] *B. cepacia* complex has numerous important virulence factors, some of which play a specific role in the clinical syndromes seen in patients with CF. *P. aeruginosa* enhances subsequent adhesion to epithelial surfaces by *B. cepacia*,[313] suggesting a synergistic relationship between the two bacterial pathogens, particularly in patients with CF.[344] Additionally, *B. cepacia* complex strains from CF patients with the most severe progression bind most avidly to mucin.[316] *B. cepacia* also resists nonoxidative neutrophil killing.[346] These organisms are intrinsically resistant to many antimicrobial agents. The following host-specific factors increase the risk for colonization with these organisms, as well as progression from colonization to infection: (1) prolonged hospitalization, especially in intensive care settings; (2) administration of broad-spectrum antibiotics[348]; (3) malignancy, particularly if associated with immunosuppressive therapy and neutropenia[195,348]; and (4) breaks in mucocutaneous defense barriers, chiefly by instrumentation or the use of invasive devices.[195]

As with most pathogens, the pathogenicity of *B. pseudomallei* is related to both virulence factors of the organism and the host's immune response to infection and in many ways resembles the types of infections and clinical outcomes associated with *P. aeruginosa* and to some extent *B. cepacia* complex organisms. As a saprophyte associated with soil and surface waters, the organism can survive harsh environmental conditions, including extremes of temperature, pH, and levels of moisture.[63] Moreover the organism also resists the action of many antiseptics, disinfectants, and antibiotics. Altered phenotypes of the organism may be found in culture of clinical material, including small-colony variants with increased antibiotic resistance, as are seen in chronic infection with *P. aeruginosa*.

B. pseudomallei produces a variety of exoenzymes secreted into the environment, including proteases, lipases, lecithinase, phospholipase C, and hemolysins.[63] The organism also has type III secretion systems, as are found in many pathogens, including *P. aeruginosa*. These systems allow for delivery of effector molecules directly into host cells and may allow the organism to survive in phagosomes and promote tissue invasion. Interestingly the closely related *B. thailandensis* does not have type III secretion systems and is significantly less virulent. Cell-associated virulence factors include extracellular polysaccharide capsule, lipopolysaccharide, and outer membrane proteins and proteins associated with flagella and pili. As a group, these factors contribute to attachment to epithelial cells and protection against host immune responses, and they may contribute to biofilm formation. Notwithstanding a wide array of virulence factors, *B. pseudomallei* generally has a low potential for causing disease in humans, as evidenced by the high rates of seropositivity in asymptomatic individuals in endemic areas and the increased likelihood of causing disease in individuals with predisposing factors.[63]

CLINICAL MANIFESTATIONS

Previously Healthy Children

P. aeruginosa can produce disease in previously healthy, immunocompetent children.[119,232,264,302,376,392,399] When such infections occur, the source of the organism is water, soil, or vegetative or related contaminated material, and the organism has gained entry through the skin or mucous membrane by a minor or penetrating wound. After entry, the organism may produce a localized infection with cellulitis that may progress to abscess formation and may be associated with a green or blue-green exudate. The skin lesions, whether caused by direct inoculation or secondary to septicemia, begin as pink macules that progress to small cutaneous hemorrhagic nodules and eventually to areas of necrosis, with eschar formation surrounded by an intense red areola (ecthyma gangrenosum, Fig. 125.1).[252,414] In addition to skin infections, previously healthy children may experience localized and systemic infections, including corneal infection, dacryocystitis, otitis externa, mastoiditis, mastitis, urinary tract infection (UTI), septicemia, endocarditis, bone and joint infections, peritonitis, meningitis, pneumonia, and necrotizing fasciitis.

Outbreaks of dermatitis (folliculitis; "hot tub syndrome"), plantar nodules ("hot foot syndrome"), otitis externa, mastitis, and UTIs caused by *P. aeruginosa* have been reported in normal, healthy children after the use of community swimming pools, water slides, recreational whirlpools, or family-owned hot tubs.[117,127,149,317,381] Several outbreaks have been described among children using wading pools.[127,398] Pruritic or painful skin lesions (5 to 30 mm) develop several hours to 5 days or longer (mean, 48 hours) after contact with these water sources. Subcutaneous involvement, including mastitis, has been reported.[138] Skin lesions may be erythematous, macular, or pustular. In some cases, very tender nodules have been observed. Illness may vary from a few scattered lesions in some patients to extensive truncal involvement in others. The rash is most severe in areas occluded by snug-fitting bathing suits. In some children, malaise, fever, otitis externa, vomiting, sore throat, conjunctivitis, rhinitis, pyuria, abdominal cramps, and swollen breasts may be associated with the dermal lesions. Rarely this recreational

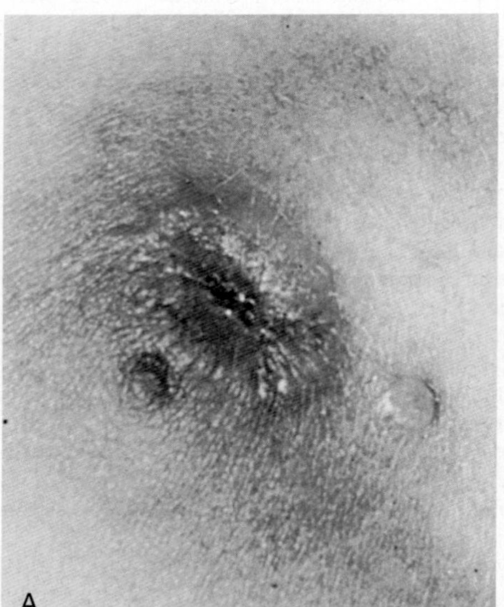

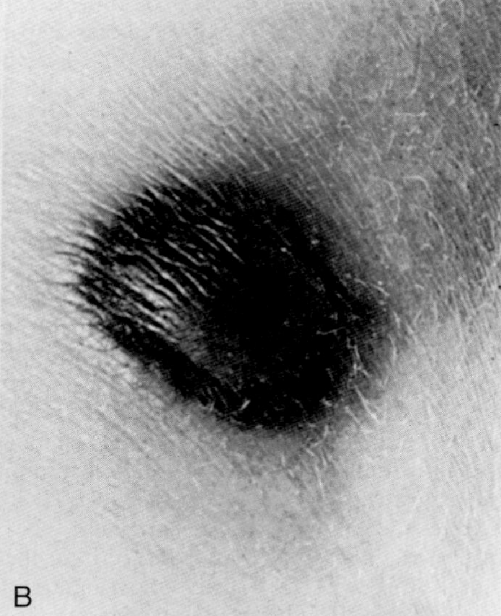

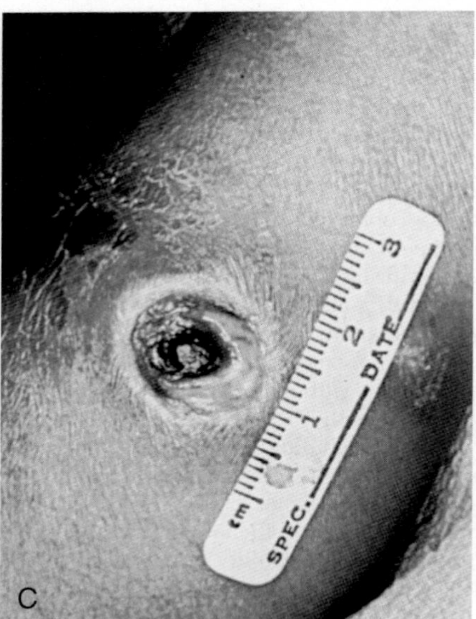

FIG. 125.1 Skin lesion caused by septicemic *Pseudomonas aeruginosa* infection. (A) A large macule has begun to undergo central necrosis and is surrounded by two smaller macules. (B) Small cutaneous nodule representing the skin lesion of septicemic *P. aeruginosa*. (C) Final stage of ecthyma gangrenosum in which a cutaneous hemorrhagic nodule has undergone central necrosis and eschar formation.

water–associated *P. aeruginosa* infection can present with an acute onset of exquisitely painful plantar nodules.[127,407] Skin biopsy of the tender nodules reveals perivascular and perieccrine neutrophilic infiltrate and microabscesses. Laboratory evaluations reveal leukocytosis with increased proportions of neutrophils and elevations of the sedimentation rate and C-reactive protein.

Multiple serotypes of *P. aeruginosa* have been associated with these outbreaks. The use of whirlpool baths usually involves soaking in water for variable periods. Superhydration of skin and exposure to *P. aeruginosa* result in primary cutaneous infection. Whirlpool water is heated to temperatures above 37.8°C (100°F) and frequently is not filtered, thereby allowing for the persistence of desquamated skin. Both of these factors are conducive to growth of *P. aeruginosa*.

Otitis externa caused by *P. aeruginosa* has been reported in healthy competitive swimmers who swim repetitively in a pool contaminated with *P. aeruginosa*.[296] The organism also has been associated with a more malignant form of otitis externa manifested as high fever, necrosis of portions of the external ear, facial nerve paralysis, mastoiditis, and osteomyelitis of the temporal bone and basilar skull.[169,254] Rarely *P. aeruginosa* meningitis results from progression of this infection.[293] Malignant otitis externa usually is associated with predisposing factors such as malnutrition, leukopenia (a disorder of leukocyte function), malignancy, or diabetes mellitus. Successful management of malignant otitis externa requires surgical debridement in addition to appropriate systemic antibiotic therapy.

P. aeruginosa is a common agent of chronic suppurative otitis media (with or without cholesteatoma) and acute and chronic mastoiditis.[245] Chronic suppurative otitis media is a complication of inadequately treated acute otitis media and is manifested as a perforated tympanic membrane with persistent otorrhea. Chronic suppurative otitis media also occurs in children with surgically induced perforations of the tympanic membrane by tympanostomy tubes and incompletely or inadequately treated otitis media. The microbial agents of acute otitis media in children with tympanostomy tubes differ from those in children with intact tympanic membranes. *P. aeruginosa* has been recovered from 12% of children with acute otitis media and tympanostomy tubes.[301] When tympanostomy tubes become colonized with *P. aeruginosa*, eradication may be complicated by the production of a biofilm.[42] The presence of a biofilm will reduce effectiveness of conventional systemic and topical antimicrobial therapy. Outpatient therapy with oral antibiotics frequently is unsuccessful because of a lack of oral antimicrobial agents with antipseudomonal activity. Topical ciprofloxacin with or without dexamethasone has been shown to be effective and superior to oral amoxicillin-clavulanic acid in the treatment of acute otitis media in children with otorrhea through tympanostomy tubes.[101] Intravenous antibiotics targeting the bacterial agents isolated from middle ear aspirates may be needed to cure chronic suppurative otitis media. This therapy may preclude the necessity of performing tympanomastoid surgery, which becomes essential in those with extensive granulation tissue and osteitis in the mastoid.[51]

P. aeruginosa wound infections of the ear have occurred after commercial ear piercing, resulting in perichondritis. Upper ear cartilage is more commonly involved than lobe piercing. In one report reuse of a "single-use" disinfectant bottle contaminated at a sink harboring *P. aeruginosa* was implicated.[190]

P. aeruginosa infections of the eye usually occur after minor trauma or surgery, with deposition of a large inoculum topically, or by hematogenous spread. The use of contaminated contact lens solution or the use of tap water during contact lens care, as well as endotracheal suctioning without covering the eyes of sedated or comatose patients have been implicated in dacryocystitis, keratitis, and blepharoconjunctivitis.[47,160] Use of topical steroids, exposure to contaminated ocular medications, and prior ocular irradiation can predispose to keratitis. Infection of the cornea can result in ulceration, which may progress to more invasive disease, including endophthalmitis.[173] Most cases of endophthalmitis in children result from penetrating ocular injuries or as a postoperative complication of surgery. Loss of vision may result, even if appropriate antimicrobial therapy is administered promptly.

UTI caused by *P. aeruginosa* occurs rarely in healthy children. More typically, pseudomonal UTI occurs in children who are catheterized, have had instrumentation or surgery on their urinary tract, who are receiving prophylactic antibiotics, or who were immunocompromised.[145,230] UTI resulting from *P. aeruginosa* primarily occurs as a result of ascending infection; however, the urinary tract may become infected secondary to bacteremia. The symptoms of pseudomonal UTI are not usually different from those of UTI caused by other bacteria. Because of differing antibiotic susceptibilities of *P. aeruginosa* and the underlying medical condition of the child with a pseudomonal UTI, antimicrobial therapy and clinical response to therapy may differ.

P. aeruginosa is the most common cause of osteomyelitis/osteochondritis after puncture wounds of the foot and is responsible for more than 90% of cases.[45,113,243] The calcaneus or metatarsal bones commonly are affected. Symptoms may be present for 2 to 40 days (mean, 9 days) before diagnosis is made and hospitalization is needed. Pain and swelling are the most common symptoms; fever and wound drainage rarely are noted. Leukocytosis (white blood cell count >10,000/mm^3) and an elevated erythrocyte sedimentation rate are present in most patients.[82] Radiographs of the affected foot usually show evidence of osteomyelitis at some time during the period of evaluation and treatment. Bone scan results almost universally are abnormal and frequently yield evidence of osteomyelitis before positive findings on radiographs. The inner pad of sneakers has been implicated as a possible source of *P. aeruginosa* in these patients; however, *P. aeruginosa* osteomyelitis of the foot bones has developed when the puncture occurred through other types of footwear or while the child was barefoot.[128]

Other *P. aeruginosa* infections of bones and joints are uncommon findings in children. When they do occur, they are the result of hematogenous spread of *P. aeruginosa* in patients who are intravenous drug abusers, have urinary tract or pelvic infections, or are immunocompromised. Although any bone or joint may be associated with an episode of bacteremia, *P. aeruginosa* has proclivity for the vertebrae, sternoarticular joints, pelvis, and symphysis pubis. The clinical course of *P. aeruginosa* osteomyelitis or septic arthritis is more indolent than that occurring after infection with *Staphylococcus aureus*. Contiguous spread can occur after penetrating trauma, surgery, or overlying soft tissue infections, especially decubitus ulcers.

P. aeruginosa may produce serious infections in healthy neonates. Septicemia may be noted in the earliest hours of life and is associated with high morbidity and mortality. In utero acquisition of the organism resulting in intraamniotic infection (amnionitis), neonatal sepsis, and death has been described.[260,306,368] The clinical course is similar to that of any other form of gram-negative septicemia, with hypotension, respiratory distress, and skin lesions being the predominant manifestations and high mortality. Late-onset neonatal *P. aeruginosa* infection is more frequent and usually occurs as a nosocomial infection (i.e., bacteremia, UTI, and pneumonia) associated with a foreign body (e.g., indwelling urinary or vascular catheter or endotracheal tube) in hospitalized infants. Outbreaks of *P. aeruginosa* infections in neonatal intensive care units have been associated with infections in health care workers and contaminated milk.[320,409] Maternal colonization after the use of a hot tub for relaxation during labor was responsible for *P. aeruginosa* meningitis and bacteremia in an 11-day-old infant.[380]

Other pseudomonads (except *B. pseudomallei*) rarely cause disease in healthy persons. Reports in normal, healthy children, particularly when the children have been hospitalized in an intensive care unit, include pneumonia, keratitis, and abscesses caused by *B. cepacia* complex organisms; abscesses caused by *P. fluorescens;* and otitis media, pneumonia, and osteomyelitis caused by *P. stutzeri*.[54,142] A penetrating lawn dart injury resulted in a mixed-flora brain abscess with *Sphingomonas paucimobilis*.[365] Peritonitis and septicemia caused by *B. cepacia* complex organisms have been associated with contamination of equipment used for peritoneal dialysis.[30]

Melioidosis is a disease endemic to a large part of South and East Asia and northern Australia.[389] Sporadic cases have been described outside of endemic regions, including Africa, Central and South America, and the Caribbean. The causative agent is *B. pseudomallei*, an environmental saprophyte of soil and water in the tropics, particularly in rice paddies. Patients with poorly controlled diabetes, renal disease, or immunocompromised conditions caused by collagen vascular disease, hematologic malignancies, or immunosuppressive therapy appear to have an increased risk for development of disease after infection with *B. pseudomallei*.[216]

The predominant mode of transmission is via percutaneous inoculation after contact of abrasions or wounds with contaminated soil or water. Infection may also occur after inhalation of contaminated dust or ingestion of contaminated water. An increase in melioidosis cases presenting as pneumonias has been noted after natural disasters associated with heavy rain and winds and during the rainy season.[67] In the United States, the majority of melioidosis cases have been reported among persons traveling to endemic areas or after occupational exposure, though an autochthonous case has been described in Arizona.[25,352] Transmission from animals to humans is rare; possible zoonotic cases have been described in endemic areas.[69] *B. pseudomallei* has also been isolated from abscesses of pet iguanas.[410] An outbreak of melioidosis in Australia was traced to a potable water source from a water treatment plant that had irregularities in purification.[171]

Most infections with *B. pseudomallei* remain subclinical.[216] Melioidosis can have a broad spectrum of clinical signs, and symptoms may be latent for months or years before the disease becomes clinically apparent. Classic manifestations of melioidosis include pneumonia and localized skin infections. The initial clinical finding may be a single primary skin lesion (i.e., vesicle, pustule, bulla, or urticaria) in a patient with no underlying disease. Hematogenous spread may follow local infection and multiple abscesses may be noted in every organ of the body. The acute septicemic illness is indistinguishable from other types of septicemia caused by gram-negative organisms. Overall mortality approaches 40%.[389] Meningitis; encephalitis; arthritis; nodular pulmonary densities; abscesses of liver, lung, spleen, kidney, and bones; and endophthalmitis have been observed in both normal and compromised hosts after or concomitant with an episode of septicemia.

B. pseudomallei can cause myocarditis, pericarditis, endocarditis, intestinal abscess, cholecystitis, acute gastroenteritis, UTI, septic arthritis, paraspinal abscess, osteomyelitis, hilar lymphadenopathy, and cervical lymphadenopathy. Parotitis was documented in 38% of 126 children with melioidosis in Thailand, none of whom had any apparent predisposition to infection.[88]

Subacute melioidosis generally is characterized by an illness lasting weeks to months. Pulmonary infection in this form of disease is a common occurrence and may mimic tuberculosis. The disease can vary from mild bronchitis to severe, fulminant pneumonitis, and lung consolidation and cavitations occur frequently.[238]

Although sepsis and community-acquired pneumonia are common clinical manifestations in adults, children most frequently present with primary cutaneous melioidosis.[236] Cases of neonatal melioidosis have been reported presenting with bacteremia, meningitis, or both caused by *B. pseudomallei*.[364] The mode of transmission to these newborn infants is not always clear. Vertical transmission of *B. pseudomallei* has been reported in a woman receiving prednisone for exacerbation of underlying ulcerative colitis during a vacation in Thailand who 6 weeks later gave birth to an infant with sepsis and lung abscess. The infant's blood and endotracheal aspirate cultures yielded *B. pseudomalleii*.[3] Review of placental histology revealed microabscesses, and postpartum cultures of the mother's cervix grew *B. pseudomallei*. Pulsed-field gel electrophoresis confirmed isolates in the mother and neonate to be a single strain. Cases of mother-to-infant transmission during breastfeeding have also been described in lactating mothers with mastitis.[292]

Chronic melioidosis is defined by symptoms persisting beyond 2 months, most commonly from recent acquisition but can also occur from reactivation.[85] Chronic melioidosis may involve every organ in the body, including the brain.[206] Melioidosis may become dormant, with exacerbations occurring years after primary infection when host defenses are impaired as a result of steroid use, burns, diabetes mellitus, or other processes. The longest latent period (24 years) was reported by Kingston.[197]

Melioidosis should be considered in any person who has been to Southeast Asia or northern Australia at any time and has fever of unknown origin, overwhelming sepsis, single or multiple abscesses, pneumonia not responding to antibiotic therapy, or any tuberculosis-like illness. The diagnosis is established by culture of blood, skin lesions, or purulent material from an abscess cavity or from other sites of infection.[162]

Burn Wounds

The surface of burn wounds and skin grafts are frequently colonized by pseudomonads and other gram-negative organisms.[119] Colonization does not always progress to infection, but it is a necessary prerequisite to development of invasive disease. Gram-negative bacteria predominate after the fifth day, with *P. aeruginosa* isolated most frequently.[18,70] Septicemia with *P. aeruginosa* is a major problem in burn patients, with the mortality rates of burn wound sepsis approaching 78%.[237] Systemic involvement may be related to multiplication of organisms in devitalized surface areas with subsequent invasion of healthy tissue and dissemination, or it can be associated with prolonged use of intravenous or urinary catheterization required for the care of these patients. In addition, the hydrotherapy that is provided to burn patients promotes colonization of the burned area and other body sites.[366]

In burn patients, abnormalities in neutrophil function that precede the onset of septicemia have been described, and killing of *P. aeruginosa* by neutrophils is impaired.[189] Burn injury is also associated with abnormal responses to microbial antigens, delayed rejection of homografts, abnormal vascular responses, impaired delayed hypersensitivity responses, diminished uptake of foreign substances particles by the reticuloendothelial system, and altered antimicrobial pharmacokinetics. Contamination of wounds with high concentrations of bacteria in excess of 10^5 colony-forming units per gram of tissue impedes contraction and healing of the wound.[276] In addition, *P. aeruginosa* produces numerous substances that can further inhibit the natural healing process of burns and wounds. Exogenous plasminogen activators and proteases break down proteins such as fibrin and halt the contraction process.[283] *P. aeruginosa* ExoA, a protein synthesis inhibitor, also contributes to retardation of wound healing.[155] Secondary bacterial infection results in nearly 25% of skin graft loss after full- or split-thickness skin grafts.[369] *P. aeruginosa* was responsible for nearly 60% of the infections that resulted in skin graft loss. Skin graft loss was more common when the skin grafts were performed on the lower extremities and when grafts were applied at multiple sites. Furthermore infections of skin grafts with *P. aeruginosa* were more severe and resulted in a fourfold increase in reoperation rates.

Cystic Fibrosis

CF is the most common life-shortening inherited disease among Caucasian children and is caused by mutations in the CFTR gene.[79] The course and prognosis of disease are determined largely by chronic infection and inflammation of the airways with opportunistic bacteria and death usually resulting from destructive pneumonitis and chronic obstructive pulmonary disease. *P. aeruginosa*, along with *S. aureus*, is one of most prevalent respiratory bacterial pathogens recovered from patients with CF.[318] A U.S. surveillance study of patients included in the Cystic Fibrosis Foundation reported that 52.5% of patients had *P. aeruginosa* recovered from sputum cultures.[218] The prevalence varied by age, ranging from 25% for children younger than 5 years to 80% for adults in the 25- to 34-year-old group. Contemporary analysis of the microbiology of sputum in patients with CF also describes an increasing prevalence of aminoglycoside resistance among *P. aeruginosa* isolates.[111] Initial recovery of *P. aeruginosa* from the respiratory tract of a child with CF may represent colonization and not infection. Colonization is followed by infection, which is intermittent and usually associated with multiple strains of *P. aeruginosa*. At some point, colonization and subsequent infections by a single strain that expresses the mucoid phenotype is the norm, and eradication of the organism with antimicrobial therapy is impossible.[125,143]

Infection in patients with CF is limited almost entirely to the respiratory tract, and pulmonary exacerbations with endobronchial disease are a common finding.[90,166] Infection of the pulmonary parenchyma rarely occurs. Rather the epithelium of the airways and the submucosa are edematous and contain infiltrates of chronic inflammatory cells. Documentation of a pulmonary exacerbation in CF relies heavily on clinical impression (e.g., increase in the frequency of productive cough; increase in volume or a change in characteristics of the sputum; increase in the respiratory rate or dyspnea; and decrease in appetite, activity, or exercise tolerance). Fever and leukocytosis are present in a minority of patients and are associated with poorer pulmonary function test results and a worse prognostic score.[339] However, pulmonary function abnormalities may be present even in the absence of symptoms. Concentrations of *P. aeruginosa,* host cell DNA (derived from polymorphonuclear leukocytes and to a lesser extent from respiratory epithelial cells), and total protein in sputum are increased during pulmonary exacerbations and decrease significantly after antimicrobial therapy.[339] Bronchitis, bronchiolitis, and bronchiectasis can occur. Eventually local necrotizing pneumonitis may be noted, in contrast to the overwhelming generalized necrotizing pneumonitis seen in immunosuppressed patients. Septicemia is a rare occurrence, but *P. aeruginosa* bacteremia may develop in patients with indwelling venous catheters. Colonization of lungs with *P. aeruginosa* after lung transplantation in patients with CF is common and occurs in the early posttransplantation period.[205]

B. cepacia complex organisms have emerged as agents of asymptomatic colonization, pneumonia, and septicemia in patients with CF. *B. cenocepacia* and *B. multivorans* are the species most frequently isolated from patients with CF in the United States, with *B. multivorans* accounting for the majority of cases. Some members of the complex are more commonly associated with acute clinical deterioration (cepacia syndrome), in particular *B. cenocepacia*[179,229]; however, other species, such as *B. multivorans,* have also been associated with the cepacia syndrome,[37] and *B. dolosa,* an uncommonly encountered species, is associated with a rapid deterioration in lung function and decreased survival.[53,183]

The prevalence of infection with *B. cepacia* complex organisms in the United States generally ranges from 3% to 4%, with rates as high as 8% having been reported.[218] Overall the prevalence rates of infection from *B. cepacia* complex in patients with CF have been decreasing.[218,318] The higher frequency of colonization of the respiratory tract with *B. cepacia* complex in patients with CF has been associated with increased morbidity and mortality rates in some CF centers since the 1980s. The risk for colonization with *B. cepacia* complex increases with the severity of underlying disease and increasing age.[359] The source or mode of transmission of the organism has not been defined adequately,[222,223,360] but person-to-person transmission has been documented.[148,221] Nosocomial transmission (i.e., patient-to-patient and contaminated inhalation therapy equipment–to-patient) within CF centers and social contact, particularly at summer camps, is one mode of acquisition of new infection. Nonetheless the majority of new infections with *B. cepacia* complex organisms are likely to be the result of acquisition of unrelated strains from the natural environment.

Once colonization with *B. cepacia* complex has been identified in patients with CF, three distinct clinical patterns have been noted: (1) chronic asymptomatic carriage, usually in association with *P. aeruginosa;* (2) progressive deterioration over many months with recurrent acute pulmonary exacerbations accompanied by fever, progressive weight loss, leukocytosis, and an elevated erythrocyte sedimentation rate; and (3) rapid, usually fatal deterioration in pulmonary function associated with necrotizing pneumonia and sometimes bacteremia ("cepacia syndrome").[172,179,229,253,344] The last complication can occur even in patients whose respiratory status was affected only mildly before acquiring *B. cepacia* complex infection.

Malignancy, Immunosuppression, and Other Predisposing Conditions

Immunosuppressive agents may be used in the management of malignancies, transplantation, or collagen vascular disease. The location of the infectious process and the type of causative organisms depend somewhat on the underlying disease. Infection by *P. aeruginosa,* particularly pneumonia and septicemia, occurs more commonly in children receiving immunosuppressive therapy than in the normal, healthy population.

Children with leukemia, particularly those receiving chemotherapy and those who have neutropenia, are susceptible to septicemia caused by *P. aeruginosa* and other pseudomonads.[119] Some pseudomonads, including *P. putida,* have been reported as causes of septicemia in children with malignancy.[8] Infection generally results from invasion of the bloodstream by a colonizing *Pseudomonas* spp. (e.g., from the gastrointestinal tract). Anorexia, malaise, nausea, vomiting, diarrhea, and fever may be noted. Generalized vasculitis develops, and hemorrhagic necrotic lesions can be found in all organs, including the skin, where they appear as purple nodules or ecchymotic areas that become gangrenous.[295] Other invasive *P. aeruginosa* infections noted in children receiving immunosuppressive chemotherapy include hemorrhagic gangrenous perirectal cellulitis or abscess, typhlitis, preseptal cellulitis, and necrotizing fasciitis.[241,377] Contemporary mortality rates of 30% have been reported (range, 10–60%).[281]

Children undergoing treatment for malignancies are particularly vulnerable to bacterial infection. The depth of the absolute neutrophil count nadir and duration of severe neutropenia are directly related to the risk of invasive bacterial infection and infection-related mortality in this population. Chemotherapy and radiation therapy also predispose to infections by disrupting protective mucocutaneous barriers and facilitating translocation of pathogens. Fergie and associates[415] described 98 children and adolescents with cancer in whom *P. aeruginosa* bacteremia developed; the rate of bacteremia was highest in patients with leukemia. Most cases occurred when patients had absolute neutrophil counts of less than 100/mm^3. Mortality associated with *P. aeruginosa* bacteremia was higher in patients with solid tumors, an absolute neutrophil count of less than 100/mm^3, perineal skin lesions, and bacteremia during remission or induction therapy rather than during a relapse.

P. aeruginosa is a major cause of health care–associated infections leading to central line–associated bloodstream infections, catheter-associated UTIs, ventilator associated pneumonias, and surgical site infections.[335] In children, infections are associated with the use of implantable medical devices. Infections of intrathecal baclofen pumps used to manage spasticity have been associated with wound infections and meningitis.[400] Delayed infections in cochlear implant recipients with *P. aeruginosa* have been reported.[140] *P. aeruginosa* has also been described as a prevalent pathogen causing invasive infections in children with extracorporeal ventricular assist devices.[52,133] In many cases of device-associated infection, removal of the device is important for successful management of the infection.

P. aeruginosa is a leading cause of nosocomial respiratory tract infection in children receiving inhalation therapy or undergoing mechanical ventilation.[161,203] Asymptomatic colonization of the upper and lower airways occurs commonly and should be distinguished from respiratory tract disease, tracheitis, and pneumonia. In patients receiving mechanical ventilation, with new or progressive infiltrates on serial chest imaging, respiratory specimens obtained from the endotracheal tube demonstrating a predominance of gram-negative bacilli with an abundance of polymorphonuclear leukocytes on Gram stain in conjunction with a positive culture for *P. aeruginosa,* support the role of *P. aeruginosa* as the causative agent for the lower respiratory tract infection. Absence of *P. aeruginosa* from lower respiratory tract secretions markedly reduces the likelihood that *P. aeruginosa* is in the lower respiratory tract.

Health care–associated *P. aeruginosa* septicemia occurs with increased frequency in children with indwelling vascular or urinary catheters.[335,355] *Pseudomonas* bloodstream infections associated with the use of contaminated heparin/saline solutions used to flush central venous catheters have also been described in children with underlying malignancies.[56] *P. aeruginosa* was the second most common pathogen implicated in catheter-associated UTIs, accounting for 11.33% of all cases in the US National Healthcare Safety Network (NHSN) surveillance study from 2009 to 2010.[335] These *P. aeruginosa* strains causing health care–associated UTIs had high antimicrobial resistance rates. An international surveillance study of *P. aeruginosa* clinical isolates from intensive care unit patients from countries in Africa, Asia, Latin America, and Europe reported even higher resistance rates, including 37% resistance to carbapenems.[303] UTIs also have been associated with cystoscopic examination. In addition, septicemia may occur in children with congenital or acquired neutropenia or in persons with a functional deficit in polymorphonuclear leukocyte function. *P. aeruginosa* is a cause of abscesses and meningitis in children with dermoid sinus tracts or dermoids extending down to or communicating with the meninges or neural tissue and in children with myelomeningocele.

Endocarditis caused by *P. aeruginosa* must be considered in children and adolescents with prosthetic valves or other intracardiac synthetic material. The organism also may produce acute or subacute endocarditis in children with congenital cardiac lesions before or after cardiac surgery and on both native and prosthetic heart valves. Tricuspid valve involvement occurs most commonly, but involvement of multiple valves is possible with *P. aeruginosa;* the manifestations are typical of subacute endocarditis. If the left side of the heart is involved (i.e., aortic or mitral valves), the patient has acute and more fulminant disease. Fever and heart murmur are almost universal findings. Overall infective endocarditis due to *P. aeruginosa* is rare in children. Although traditionally associated with the use of intravenous drugs, hospital-associated *P. aeruginosa* endocarditis is not uncommon.[21,217,249] Other *Pseudomonas* spp. have been rarely associated with post–cardiac surgery infections.[129]

P. aeruginosa needs to be considered in children and adolescents at risk for acquiring human immunodeficiency virus (HIV) infection, primarily after severe immunodeficiency has occurred.[130,267,300,343] Risks for acquiring *P. aeruginosa* infection in HIV-infected individuals include hospital exposure, declining $CD4^+$ cell count, and the use of dapsone or trimethoprim-sulfamethoxazole (TMP-SMX); azithromycin use was protective.[343] Bacteremia may occur with or without the presence of an indwelling vascular catheter. Fever, hypotension, skin lesions (i.e., papules or ecthyma gangrenosum), and pneumonia are common manifestations.[130] Children with other severe immune defects are also at risk, and infection may be the initial manifestation of a primary immunodeficiency.[22] *P. aeruginosa* supraglottitis has been reported in a 6-month-old child with severe combined immunodeficiency syndrome.[209] Mortality rates can be high, particularly when empiric antimicrobial therapy is inadequate for the treatment of severe, invasive *P. aeruginosa* infection.

B. cepacia complex organisms can cause opportunistic infections in patients other than those with CF, primarily in hospitalized or immunocompromised patients. These include nosocomial pneumonia in patients on ventilation, bacteremia, wound infections, UTIs, meningitis, endocarditis, and skin lesions. *B. cepacia* complex organisms are also an important cause of infections in patients with chronic granulomatous disease (CGD) because of the organism's ability to resist killing by defective neutrophils using nonoxidative pathways.[304] An 11-year-old Puerto Rican boy with X-linked CGD had documented *B. pseudomallei* lymphadenitis and mediastinitis.[104] Bacteria that cause most infections in CGD are catalase-positive organisms. The CGD-affected neutrophil can kill numerous microorganisms despite its defects because most microorganisms endogenously produce hydrogen peroxide, which the CGD-affected neutrophil can modify and use against the organism in the phagosome. Whereas both *P. aeruginosa* and *B. cepacia* are catalase-positive organisms, the former is a rare pathogen in CGD because CGD neutrophils can kill *P. aeruginosa* organisms by means of nonoxidative mechanisms. Fortunately all of these infections are uncommon findings in children.

P. putida has been primarily associated with health care–associated infection, particularly in the neonatal intensive care unit. Most cases present as bacteremia or as cutaneous infections.[43,97,210,284,403,405] Cutaneous manifestations reported in neonates with *P. putida* may have an appearance similar to that of staphylococcal scalded skin syndrome.[210] Mortality rates after infection with *P. putida* are high because of vulnerability of the patients and inappropriate empirical antibiotic therapy. *P. putida* is typically susceptible to antipseudomonal β-lactam antibiotics and carbapenems but not reliably susceptible to aminoglycosides.

P. fluorescens causes disease primarily in immunocompromised patients who have been inadvertently exposed to contaminated infusion fluids, disinfectants, and drinking water.[110,141,168,194,391] Most infections result in fever; systemic reactions of sepsis and mortality have been reported but are not typical. *P. fluorescens* is usually susceptible to carbapenems, aminoglycosides, and tetracycline; however, *P. fluorescens* is less likely to be susceptible to third-generation cephalosporins and trimethoprim.[168] Mupirocin, a topical antibiotic, is produced through fermentation of *P. fluorescens.*

P. stutzeri has been responsible for a diverse group of clinical conditions, with wound infections being the most common presentation.[257] Bacteremia is the second most common presentation and usually results from exposure to contaminated fluids. *P. stutzeri* causing suppurative arthritis and nosocomially acquired brain abscess have been reported in children.[244,404] Pneumonia, UTI, and skin and eye infections have also been reported. Most patients with presumed *P. stutzeri* infections are hospitalized and have predisposing conditions that make them vulnerable to opportunistic organism.[257] *P. stutzeri* are typically susceptible to antipseudomonal penicillins and cephalosporins, aminoglycosides, and TMP-SMX.

P. mendocina is a recently described opportunistic pathogen.[259] Bacteremia, osteomyelitis, subphrenic abscess, meningitis, and wound infections have been reported.[66,177,259] *P. mendocina* is typically susceptible to carbapenems, third-generation cephalosporins, aminoglycosides, and ciprofloxacin; however, resistance to some or all of these antibiotics has been reported.

P. fulva has been isolated from raw foods and natural environments including rice and petroleum fields but has also recently described as a human pathogen leading to bloodstream and central nervous system (CNS) infections.[112,331] A *P. fulva* VIM-2 carbapenemase-producing strain causing meningitis was described in a 2-year-old after placement of a drainage system for a neuroectodermal tumor.[7] Integration of the VIM-2 genes on mobile gene cassettes in this isolate raises concern for possible transmission of resistance cassettes across different *Pseudomonas* species.

Ralstonia spp., especially *R. pickettii,* have caused infections in immunocompromised patients and in those with CF.* *Ralstonia* spp. infections such as catheter-associated bloodstream infections or health care–associated pneumonia have been reported in association with contamination of infusion fluids or respiratory equipment.[55,57,176,192,208,280] *Ralstonia* spp. have been reported to be susceptible to antipseudomonal β-lactams, ciprofloxacin, and TMP-SMX, and some isolates susceptible to aminoglycosides.[92,411] However, some strains may be resistant to antibiotics typically considered active. Susceptibility testing on clinical organisms is important to guide appropriate therapy. Catheter-associated bloodstream infections may require catheter removal to affect a cure.[199]

Most infections with *Cupriavidus* and *Pandoraea* have occurred in immunocompromised individuals or in those with CF. *Cupriavidus* spp. has resulted in bacteremia, skin and wound infections, and respiratory tract colonization or infection.[17,184,187,212,353,370] *Pandoraea* spp. have been associated with severe lung disease and systemic infection in persons with CF.[178,180,356] Transmission among patients with CF has been documented.

DIAGNOSIS AND DIFFERENTIAL DIAGNOSIS

The diagnosis of *P. aeruginosa* and other pseudomonad infections depends on recovery of the organism from a normally sterile body site such as blood, cerebrospinal fluid (CSF), joint fluid, peritoneal or peritoneal dialysis fluid, or deep tissue obtained in a manner that avoids contamination by cutaneous flora (see previous discussion on etiology). Diagnosis of UTI often requires suprapubic aspiration or urethral catheterization for young children. Purulent material associated with subcutaneous abscesses or areas of cellulitis should be obtained by needle aspiration. A diagnosis of *P. aeruginosa* pneumonia can be made by invasive procedures (i.e., needle aspiration of the lung) and, less convincingly, by recovery of the organism from sputum in a child with CF. Recovery of the organism from the surface of the skin or the throat, a tracheal aspirate, or bronchial secretions may reflect colonization and is not necessarily diagnostic of infection. The validity of a positive culture is enhanced when it is associated with a typical clinical syndrome (e.g., *P. aeruginosa* recovered from a skin lesion typical of "whirlpool" folliculitis). Isolation of *P. aeruginosa* from the respiratory tract, particularly when obtained from an endotracheal tube in an intubated patient, is not an unusual occurrence. Differentiating colonization from infection is clinically important. Gram stain of respiratory secretions obtained by endotracheal suction typically reveals abundant gram-negative rods and polymorphonuclear leukocytes in the setting of a true lower respiratory tract infection caused by *P. aeruginosa* (tracheitis or pneumonitis). An absence of gram-negative rods or the presence of squamous epithelial cells rather than polymorphonuclear leukocytes indicates that either the patient does not have a lower respiratory tract

*References 40, 55, 57, 92, 176, 192, 196, 199, 208, 280, 311, 351, 379, 384, 393.

infection or, if an infection is present, the etiologic agent is not likely to be *P. aeruginosa*.

The presence of bluish, nodular skin lesions and the ulcers with ecchymotic and gangrenous centers and bright areolae (ecthyma gangrenosum) have been considered virtually pathognomonic of *P. aeruginosa* infection. However, ecthyma gangrenosum may be a cutaneous manifestation of other nonpseudomonal bacterial or fungal invasive infections.[371,385] For example, skin lesions that are clinically indistinguishable from those caused by *P. aeruginosa* have been described after septicemia secondary to *E. coli* and *Aeromonas hydrophila*.[269,332] Cutaneous or disseminated mold infections, most frequently with *Aspergillus* and *Fusarium* spp. in immunocompromised patients, also can cause the necrotic skin lesions of ecthyma gangrenosum.

Isolation of *Pseudomonas, Burkholderia,* and other related species other than *P. aeruginosa* from clinical specimens occurs far less frequently. Recovery of these organisms from sites that normally are sterile, such as blood or blood product containers, always should be considered clinically significant unless proved otherwise.

Serologic testing is not clinically useful for the diagnosis of acute *P. aeruginosa* infection. In contrast, serologic tests may be a useful diagnostic adjunct in melioidosis, particularly in latent or asymptomatic forms of this disease.[6,256] Hemagglutination, indirect hemagglutination, complement fixation, enzyme linked immunosorbent assay (ELISA), and immunoblot assays have been used.[15,64,151,152,215] Diagnostic sensitivity of these serologic tests is highly variable. False-negative serology may occur in the setting of acute sepsis. High rates of seropositivity in populations in endemic areas also limit specificity.[15,64,65,401] Hemagglutination A antibodies generally are present within 7 to 14 days after onset of the illness, whereas the complement fixation test yields positive results in 4 to 6 weeks. Maximal titers for both tests are reached in 4 to 6 months, and detectable antibodies may persist for months to years after initial infection. The indirect hemagglutination test, although not currently available commercially, is a validated and widely accepted assay, used by the Centers for Disease Control and Prevention (CDC) for the diagnosis of melioidosis.[62] The test uses sheep red blood cells sensitized with *B. pseudomallei* antigens in a microwell format.

The interpretation of all serologic tests for melioidosis is complicated by the fact that there are no generally accepted cutoff values defining acute infection or exposure. Serologic tests are of limited value in patients living in endemic areas because of the rate of seropositivity of such individuals. In fact, the diagnostic performance characteristics of the indirect hemagglutination test has been defined by studies utilizing different cutoffs to take account of the variable rates of background positivity.[277] Serology may be valuable in individuals who do not reside in but have recently traveled to endemic areas. Paired sera should be tested whenever possible, but a single high-titer serum sample collected from a patient with a relevant travel history and a clinically consistent clinical presentation may be helpful. Because some individuals with culture-proved melioidosis do not have detectable antibodies, a negative serologic test does not rule out infection.[153]

Several direct antigen detection assays have been developed for the rapid detection of *B. pseudomallei* in clinical specimens. These include latex agglutination, ELISA, or direct fluorescent antibody detection on purulent discharges, blood, or body fluid specimens.[10,340,402] As with many other antigen detection assays, the sensitivity of these assays precludes their use as stand-alone tests. Reagents for antigen detection tests for *B. pseudomallei* are not available commercially. Gram stain and immunofluorescent stains are simpler and cheaper than antigen detection assays.

PCR and other molecular methods have been used to detect *P. aeruginosa* directly in clinical specimens, particularly in respiratory specimens from patients with CF.[99,227] Some studies suggest that PCR may be useful in detecting *P. aeruginosa* in sputa of CF patients several months before culture diagnosis and at a time before establishment of chronic infection. This would allow for earlier aggressive antibiotic therapy to eradicate the organisms at a time when eradication may be possible. More recently the application of a quantitative PCR-based protocol directly to samples has been explored. This theoretically will allow sensitive detection along with quantitation of the organism.[35,214] Other studies have suggested that PCR performed directly on clinical specimens does not significantly increase detection of *P. aeruginosa* in contrast to culture. In addition, it is difficult to interpret the clinical significance of a positive PCR and a negative culture on the same sample; a false-positive PCR result cannot easily be ruled out. Subsequent culture-confirmed colonization occurring weeks to months later may or may not be due to colonization by the same strain initially "detected" by PCR.

PCR-based and other molecular assays also have been applied to direct detection of pseudomonads other than *P. aeruginosa,* including *B. cepacia* complex organisms and *B. pseudomallei.* The same difficulty in interpreting PCR results for *P. aeruginosa* in patients with CF applies to *B. cepacia* complex organisms. There have been more studies on the diagnostic accuracy of nucleic acid amplification methods for direct detection of *B. pseudomallei* in clinical specimens.[59,135,182,358] Sensitivity of PCR is highest when performed on specimen types such as body fluids and purulent discharges than on blood, reflective of the bacterial load in the specimen. PCR, when available, may be used as an adjunct to but not a replacement for culture. In addition, molecular detection of resistant genes in *P. aeruginosa* isolates, for example those that produce carbapenemase, is an attractive option for more timely and targeted antimicrobials; however, additional performance and utility data are required.[126] At this point, molecular assays for the pseudomonads are considered investigational.

TREATMENT

Selection of Antimicrobial Therapy

Suspected or proved systemic infections with *P. aeruginosa* should be treated promptly with empirical antimicrobial therapy. It remains unclear, however, whether monotherapy or combination therapy given as either empiric or definitive treatment is associated with improved clinical outcomes. Although in vitro synergy tests and animal studies have shown potential benefits of combination therapy, much of the clinical data demonstrating that combination therapy is superior to monotherapy are retrospective and have varied design, heterogeneous populations, or methodology flaws including lack of statistical power, or importantly, used suboptimal aminoglycoside therapy in the monotherapy study arm. Contemporary meta-analyses do not find a clinical advantage to combination therapy for pseudomonal infections.[38,44,270–275] One meta-analysis did not find a mortality benefit to combination therapy, but, when a subanalysis was restricted to *P. aeruginosa* bacteremia in five studies, there was a trend toward reduced mortality with combination therapy; of note, the majority of studies included utilized aminoglycosides in the monotherapy arm.[310] This effect was not found in other meta-analyses of randomized trials involving 7462 patients, including those with underlying malignancy, fever, and neutropenia; in fact, monotherapy with a broad spectrum β-lactam provided similar survival with less adverse events.[273]

The optimal choice of monotherapy versus combination antibiotics remains controversial and the lack of high quality data hampers informed management decisions. In general, however, empiric combination therapy directed at *P. aeruginosa* is a prudent approach for high-risk patients (e.g., patients with neutropenia or burns) who are critically ill or with severe disease (e.g., bacteremia) until the culture and in vitro susceptibility results are known. Mortality rates among patients with infections caused by multidrug-resistant *P. aeruginosa* strains are two- to threefold higher when compared with non–multidrug-resistant strains.[361] Additionally delayed initiation of appropriate empiric antimicrobial therapy for *P. aeruginosa* bacteremia beyond 2 days directly increased 30-day mortality rates.[247] As such, combination therapy is warranted if the individual patient has a history of previous infection or colonization with a multidrug-resistant *P. aeruginosa* strain or if local institutional rates of antimicrobial resistance are high. Two agents with different mechanisms of action, a β-lactam antibiotic and either an aminoglycoside or a fluoroquinolone, are generally chosen for combination therapy. Combination therapy with two β-lactam antibiotics is inappropriate for serious *Pseudomonas* infections because the induction of β-lactamase by one of the agents may result in resistance to both antibiotics. Once antimicrobial susceptibility profiles are available, monotherapy with a β-lactam agent such as cefepime, piperacillin-tazobactam, or a carbapenem should be considered in the setting of simple *P. aeruginosa* bacteremia, even in patients with malignancies and neutropenia.[134] Definitive combination therapy may be warranted for certain infections, such as endocarditis.[21]

Community-acquired *P. aeruginosa* infections are typically susceptible to antipseudomonal penicillins, including penicillin and β-lactamase inhibitor combinations; ceftazidime; cefepime; carbapenem antibiotics, including meropenem, imipenem, and doripenem, but not ertapenem; aminoglycosides; and quinolone antibiotics, including ciprofloxacin and levofloxacin.[191] Susceptibility is less predictable for aztreonam, a monobactam. Strains of *P. aeruginosa* causing health care–associated infections are more likely to be antibiotic-resistant than strains causing community-acquired infections.

Prior use of a specific antibiotic for treatment of infections caused by *P. aeruginosa* may be associated with emergence of resistance.[109,268] Specifically monotherapy with antipseudomonal β-lactam antibiotics (i.e., antipseudomonal penicillins, cephalosporins, and carbapenems), as well as with the fluoroquinolones, has resulted in selection of resistant mutants during therapy, including selection of multidrug-resistant mutants.[24,94,268,328]

Table 125.2 provides some of the more commonly prescribed antipseudomonal antibiotics. The dosages of some of these antibiotics may vary with different clinical situations and patient populations. Once-daily administration of an aminoglycoside may decrease nephrotoxicity and improve clinical efficacy. Aminoglycoside doses must be decreased, preferably by increasing the dosing interval, in patients with diminished creatinine clearance (e.g., renal impairment, neonates). Significantly higher doses (e.g., gentamicin or tobramycin 7 to 12 mg/kg per day) may be required for patients with increased total plasma clearance, such as those with CF and burns. Therefore aminoglycoside therapy must be individualized and doses guided by pharmacokinetic information.

Extended-infusion of β-lactam antibiotics (e.g., piperacillin-tazobactam, cefepime) has been used to extend the time the free drug concentration remains above the minimum inhibitory concentration (MIC) of *P. aeruginosa*, thereby theoretically enhancing bacterial killing.[188] In one series of critically ill patients with *P. aeruginosa* infections, in whom 102 patients received extended infusion dosing of piperacillin/tazobactam versus standard intermittent dosing in 92 patients, the 14-day mortality rate was significantly lower in the extended infusion group compared with the standard intermittent dosing (12% vs. 21%, respectively; $P = .04$).[225] Noncontrolled data suggest a clinical benefit to this approach but require further prospective study.[23,115,156,225]

TABLE 125.2 Antimicrobial Agents Active Against *Pseudomonas aeruginosa*

Penicillin plus β-lactam inhibitor	Ticarcillin-clavulanate Piperacillin-tazobactam
Third-generation cephalosporin	Ceftazidime
Fourth-generation cephalosporin	Cefepime
Monobactam	Aztreonam
Fluoroquinolones	Ciprofloxacin
Carbapenems	Meropenem Doripenem Imipenem[a]
Aminoglycosides	Gentamicin Tobramycin Amikacin
Other	Colistin Polymyxin b Fosfomycin[b]
Newer agents	Ceftolozane/tazobactam Ceftazidime/avibactam Ceftobiprole

[a]Highest propensity to develop resistance during treatment.
[b]Uncomplicated lower urinary tract infections only.

Endocarditis caused by *P. aeruginosa* requires aggressive medical and surgical therapy. Despite combination therapy with maximal β-lactam and aminoglycoside antibiotics, valve replacement (i.e., native and prosthetic) frequently is required for cure. Quinolones should be reserved for patients who are intolerant of aminoglycosides or whose bacteria are resistant to aminoglycosides and has been used in adults for long-term suppression of *P. aeruginosa* prosthetic valve endocarditis.

Meningitis or brain abscess resulting from *P. aeruginosa* may be treated with ceftazidime or cefepime and should be guided by in vitro susceptibility results. The initial empirical addition of the aminoglycoside or fluoroquinolone should be guided by local susceptibility patterns. Meropenem has good penetration into CSF and can be used as an alternative agent when the *P. aeruginosa* is resistant to cephalosporins. Meropenem is the preferred carbapenem because the high doses of imipenem required to treat CNS infections may be associated with CNS toxicity. Fluoroquinolones such as parenteral ciprofloxacin or the monobactam aztreonam are possible alternative therapies for *P. aeruginosa* CNS meningitis, but experience with these agents for CNS infections in children is limited.[258,357,367]

Ocular infection with *P. aeruginosa* can be serious and sight-threatening. *P. aeruginosa* corneal ulcerations or keratitis may be seen in contact lens wearers or in intubated, sedated patients in intensive care units. Topical therapy with ticarcillin, piperacillin, tobramycin, gentamicin, amikacin, ciprofloxacin, or ofloxacin may be used and is effective. Clinical efficacy is improved by frequently clearing inflammatory debris and topical application of antibiotics. Initially antibiotic solutions should be administered every 15 to 30 minutes. The frequency can be decreased gradually to four to six times per day when clinical improvement is apparent.

P. aeruginosa endophthalmitis frequently occurs after invasive eye surgery or penetrating ocular injuries. Systemic, topical, and intraocular (i.e., anterior chamber and vitreous cavity) routes may all be required.[349] Acute endophthalmitis is a medical emergency, and, even with aggressive medical intervention, return of retinal function is not a common occurrence. The prognosis is worse when initiation of therapy is delayed. Cultures of the vitreous should be obtained as soon as endophthalmitis is suspected. Initial intravitreal therapy for *P. aeruginosa* endophthalmitis should include combination therapy pending culture results. Ceftazidime, imipenem, and ciprofloxacin have greater intraocular penetration than do the aminoglycosides.[108,167] Adjunctive systemic antibiotics may be required for severe cases.

Chronic suppurative otitis media may be due to a variety of organisms, including *P. aeruginosa*. Obtaining cultures from the middle ear is extremely valuable in determining optimal antimicrobial therapy. In most cases, therapy with a fluoroquinolone available as a topical otic compound (i.e., ciprofloxacin, ofloxacin, or besifloxacin) with or without steroids is effective.[375] Because middle ear drainage typically represents perforation of the tympanic membrane, aminoglycoside including neomycin-containing topical therapy should not be used because of potential aminoglycoside ototoxicity. Malignant otitis externa and chronic mastoiditis caused by *P. aeruginosa* require systemic antipseudomonal antibiotic therapy. Surgical debridement also may be required for effective management.

P. aeruginosa folliculitis and plantar nodules generally are self-limited after removal of the exposure and do not usually require specific antimicrobial therapy.[127] Skin abscesses or abscesses in other locations caused by *P. aeruginosa* should be incised and drained.[295] Failure to do so may result in a poor response despite prolonged systemic antibiotic treatment. *P. aeruginosa* may be part of multiorganism infections causing necrotizing fasciitis. Empirical therapy for necrotizing fasciitis should include antibiotics with activity against *P. aeruginosa*. Skin lesions consistent with ecthyma gangrenosum always require empiric antipseudomonal antibiotics.

Osteomyelitis of foot bones from *P. aeruginosa* (e.g., osteochondritis after a puncture wound) requires surgical debridement. Appropriate antipseudomonal antibiotics with a β-lactam or fluoroquinolone for 7 to 14 days after surgery appear to be adequate if infected tissue has been completely removed.[174] Oral ciprofloxacin is an appropriate alternative antibiotic to complete antimicrobial therapy after surgery and evidence of *P. aeruginosa* as a causative agent. The adequacy of surgical debridement of the foot bones and clinical improvement can be monitored by serial sedimentation rates.[82] *P. aeruginosa* infection of foreign bodies (e.g., vascular, peritoneal, and CNS catheters) may require removal of the foreign material to cure the infection, particularly if a tunnel or exit-site infection exists.

Management of UTIs caused by *P. aeruginosa* will depend on the clinical situation of the infected child, that is, presence or absence of septicemia, instrumentation, and the anatomic location of the infection. In patients with chronic indwelling bladder catheters, isolation of *P. aeruginosa* in a urine specimen may be indicative of bacteriuria alone. In these patients, the bladder catheter should be removed. Whether antibiotics are warranted will depend on results of the new culture and evaluation for consistent symptoms. Symptomatic pseudomonal UTIs should be treated. In patients who are clinically stable and not immunocompromised, a single antibiotic is usually adequate. Antibiotic choices should be guided by antimicrobial susceptibilities. Extended-spectrum cephalosporins, aminoglycosides, carbapenems, aztreonam, and fluoroquinolones are reasonable antibiotic options. In children, more experience exists with extended-spectrum cephalosporins and aminoglycosides. Oral fluoroquinolones may be considered in situations with no systemic infection and an interest in providing nonparenteral therapy. Duration of appropriate antibiotic therapy will vary depending on whether the treatment is for cystitis (5 days) or bacteremia and pyelonephritis (10 to 14 days). Longer duration of therapy may be needed in the presence of systemic infection, complicated pyelonephritis, presence of renal abscesses, or in patients with anatomic or functional abnormalities.

P. aeruginosa may be responsible for lower respiratory tract infections in neonates, infants, children, and adolescents in a variety of settings. The most common manifestations are involvement of the airways in patients with CF and health care–associated tracheitis or pneumonitis in intubated patients. In children without CF with *P. aeruginosa* ventilator-associated tracheitis or pneumonia, shorter courses of antimicrobial therapy, 7 and 8 days, respectively, have proven to be effective.[61,362] Antimicrobial therapy in CF is aimed at either early eradication of *P. aeruginosa*, treatment of acute pulmonary exacerbations, or maintenance therapy for chronic infections.[287] In patients with CF experiencing an exacerbation of pulmonary disease and in critically ill intubated patients in whom *P. aeruginosa* infection is suspected, combination therapy with a β-lactam antibiotic and an aminoglycoside is recommended as empirical treatment. In these patients with a pulmonary exacerbation, combination therapy of a β-lactam plus an aminoglycoside compared with β-lactam therapy alone resulted in longer clinical remission and prolonged time to hospital readmission with a new pulmonary exacerbation.[338] Of note, emergence of tobramycin resistance occurred in both groups, but was more frequent in the combination therapy arm.

The choice of which β-lactam antibiotic and which aminoglycoside to use should be based on the patient's previous antibiotic experience and knowledge of the usual antibiotic susceptibility pattern in the patient's clinical environment. Once susceptibility testing results are known, at least two effective antibiotics should be included in the patient's regimen. The dose and pharmacotherapeutics of the chosen antibiotics should be optimized. If the patient fails to respond to appropriate antibiotic therapy, as evidenced by clinical deterioration, acquisition of antibiotic resistance should be anticipated and additional bacterial cultures should be obtained; one or more of the newer antibiotics should be substituted pending additional susceptibility test results.

After years of antibiotic exposure, patients with CF commonly are infected with strains of *P. aeruginosa* resistant in vitro to achievable blood concentrations of many if not all of the common classes of antimicrobial agents. Moreover penetration of aminoglycosides from blood into respiratory secretions is poor.[28] The administration of antibiotics by aerosolization, particularly the aminoglycosides, provides much higher concentrations in respiratory secretions. Inhaled antibiotics have been found to be safe and effective for chronic *P. aeruginosa* lung infections in patients with CF.[228] Administration of aerosolized aminoglycosides to patients with CF resulted in improvement in pulmonary function tests, decreased concentrations of *P. aeruginosa* in sputum, and no significant apparent toxicity. This aerosol treatment did not increase the isolation of *B. cepacia* complex, *Stenotrophomonas maltophilia*, or *Alcaligenes xylosoxidans;* however, isolation of *Candida albicans* and *Aspergillus* spp. increased.[49]

Aerosolized tobramycin may be used to yield concentrations in respiratory secretions in the range of 100 to 200 μg/mL. Some strains of *P. aeruginosa* resistant to blood concentrations of tobramycin may be susceptible to achievable concentrations in respiratory secretions. In vitro susceptibility testing of these organisms may be performed to determine the exact MIC.[143,248] Limited data exist on the correlation of such in vitro test results and clinical outcome; therefore, in practice, such testing is not commonly performed. In addition to management of resistant *P. aeruginosa*, aerosolized tobramycin given over a prolonged period (>1 year) may have the potential to eradicate *P. aeruginosa* temporarily from CF patients who have newly acquired this organism.[294] In patients with CF 6 years of age and older with *P. aeruginosa* persistently present in respiratory airway cultures, the Cystic Fibrosis Foundation recommends the chronic use of inhaled tobramycin in an effort to improve lung function and reduce pulmonary exacerbations.[131] For similar reasons, chronic azithromycin is recommended in children 6 years of age and older.[131] Although the precise mechanism of action of macrolides used for chronic suppressive therapy is unclear, azithromycin seems to have more antiinflammatory properties, including reducing the production of virulence factors, decreasing biofilm production, and having bactericidal effects on *P. aeruginosa* when it is in its stationary (biofilm) phase.[202] A randomized, double-blind, controlled trial assessing thrice weekly azithromycin versus placebo demonstrated that children with *P. aeruginosa* who received azithromycin had improvement in their pulmonary FEV_1, less pulmonary exacerbations, and gained more weight than patients who received placebo.[314] These results did not hold true for children with CF who received azithromycin but were not infected with *P. aeruginosa*.[312]

Although aztreonam is not approved for use in pediatric patients, inhaled aztreonam has been shown to provide benefit to patients with CF who are colonized with *P. aeruginosa* by improving lung function (improvements in FEV_1), health-related quality of life, and weight.[234,262,382] Reductions also occurred in bacterial density in sputum. Inhalation of aztreonam had minimal effect on the susceptibility of the patient's *P. aeruginosa* isolates to aztreonam after a course of treatment; however, increases in susceptibility to tobramycin were observed.[261] Inhaled administration of aztreonam can provide local concentrations of aztreonam in pulmonary mucus that is more than 100 times the MIC_{50} of the patient's *P. aeruginosa* isolates.[16]

Increasing rates of respiratory and invasive infections with multidrug-resistant *P. aeruginosa* in patients with CF and immunodeficient patients, particularly those with malignancies, have resulted in the need to expand antimicrobial options, including reconsideration of older antibiotics. Although the use of polymyxin B and colistin (polymyxin E) has been superseded largely by less toxic agents, they may be useful in selected patients who are infected with strains resistant to the other agents. *P. aeruginosa* is almost always susceptible to these agents (*B. cepacia* complex organisms are resistant). Colistin is available as colistin sulfate, a topical agent or oral preparation (poorly absorbed from the gastrointestinal tract), and colistimethate sodium for parenteral administration. Colistin has retained antimicrobial activity against some multidrug-resistant gram-negative bacteria, including *P. aeruginosa*. During early use of colistin, high rates of nephrotoxicity dampened interest in the drug; however, more recent studies have documented lower rates of nephrotoxicity.[114,286] Studies in adults have shown safety and efficacy in selected populations against *P. aeruginosa* and other multidrug-resistant gram-negative bacteria.[33,41,136,150,185,266,307]

In the United States, fluoroquinolones are approved for use in patients younger than 18 years of age to treat complicated UTIs, pyelonephritis, and postexposure treatment for inhalation anthrax. Among the quinolones, ciprofloxacin and levofloxacin are considered antipseudomonal and have been evaluated most often for the treatment of acute and chronic *P. aeruginosa* infection in adolescents and adults with CF.[305,350] Ciprofloxacin, which may be given orally or intravenously, proved to be effective, as judged by clinical scores and results of pulmonary function tests. Ciprofloxacin may be considered in selected children including the treatment of multiresistant strains of *P. aeruginosa* and the substitution of an oral quinolone to avoid long-term intravenous therapy requiring an indwelling catheter.

Determining the optimal antibiotic therapy for patients with CF may be problematic. Respiratory cultures often yield different colony morphotypes of *P. aeruginosa*. The various morphotypes may have significantly different antibiotic susceptibility patterns. It is common practice for laboratories supporting the management of patients with CF to individually test multiple morphotypes to include both mucoid and nonmucoid strains.

Antibiotic therapy for *B. cepacia* complex infection is challenging and should be guided by results of in vitro susceptibility testing. Unfortunately, *B. cepacia* is frequently resistant to many commonly used antipseudomonal antibiotic agents, particularly the aminoglycosides. Antibiotics that may have activity against *B. cepacia* include TMP-SMX, minocycline, ceftazidime, antipseudomonal penicillins, antipseudomonal quinolones, and carbapenems; meropenem has greater in vitro activity against *B. cepacia* than imipenem. Typically *B. cepacia* isolates from patients with CF are more antibiotic-resistant than isolates from other patient populations. Combination therapy with two or three antibiotics may be required to achieve a clinical response. Combinations of β-lactam agents with aminoglycosides might provide synergy clinically, even when the *B. cepacia* strain isolated is aminoglycoside-resistant. *B. cepacia* may be susceptible to minocycline.[207] Minocycline may be considered to have an adjunctive role in the management of *B. cepacia* infection in patients with CF.

The most active antibiotics against *B. pseudomallei* are imipenem, piperacillin-tazobactam, piperacillin, ceftazidime, ticarcillin-clavulanate, ampicillin-sulbactam, tetracycline, and chloramphenicol.[342] Piperacillin, ceftazidime, and imipenem are not bactericidal in vitro. Ciprofloxacin seems to be of limited value because of a high rate of resistance. For acute systemic melioidosis, ceftazidime or meropenem is preferred.[387] When third-generation cephalosporins have been used, cefoperazone and ceftazidime have shown greater activity against *B. pseudomallei* than have other third-generation cephalosporin agents. Ceftazidime was compared with chloramphenicol, doxycycline, and TMP-SMX for the treatment of severe melioidosis and was associated with a 50% lower overall mortality rate in contrast to that of other forms of therapy.[387] Although the optimal duration of intensive therapy is unknown, generally treatment for a minimum of 14 days is recommended. Intensive therapy lasting 4 to 8 weeks should be provided to patients who are critically ill, with complicated pulmonary disease, with visceral abscesses, and in those with osteoarticular or CNS involvement.

Intensive treatment is followed by eradication therapy with TMP-SMX for at least 12 to 20 weeks to prevent early recrudescence or later relapses of melioidosis.[86] Some eradication regimens might use amoxicillin-clavulanate, oral fluoroquinolones, or doxycycline, but these portend higher rates of relapse than TMP-SMX-based eradication therapy. Recurrent melioidosis may occur as result of a true relapse or from reinfection and required reinitiation of intensive intravenous therapy, followed by eradication therapy.[60] Chronic melioidosis can be treated with chloramphenicol, tetracycline, or doxycycline over a period of many months. TMP-SMX was recommended previously, but many strains are resistant.

Mechanisms of Antibiotic Resistance and In Vitro Susceptibility Testing

Antibiotic resistance is an important factor in management of patients with serious pseudomonal infections that do not respond to antibiotic therapy. *P. aeruginosa* shows intrinsic resistance to some antibiotics generally effective against enteric gram-negative rods. This is partly due to the relative impermeability of the outer membrane of *P. aeruginosa*. This membrane is a selective barrier to the uptake of antibiotics. The major porin channel of *P. aeruginosa*, OprF, has a limited number of large channels and other porins, including OprB and OPrD, and this limits the rate of passage of molecules the size of antibiotics.[268] Aside from the importance of porin channels in resistance or reduced susceptibility to antibiotics, *P. aeruginosa* may show intrinsic resistance to a wide variety of antibiotic classes by the presence of multiple efflux pumps, particularly the resistance modulation systems MexAB-OprM and MexXY-OprM. Multidrug efflux systems exist in *P. aeruginosa* that can result in expulsion of β-lactams, chloramphenicol, fluoroquinolones, macrolides, novobiocin, sulfonamides, tetracycline, trimethoprim and aminoglycoisdes.[121] Finally upregulation and overexpression of the intrinsic, inducible chromosomal AmpC β-lactamase renders the organism resistant to ampicillin, amoxicillin, amoxicillin-clavulanate, and first- and second-generation cephalosporins, as well as cefotaxime and ceftriaxone.[165] Thus the high level of intrinsic resistance to antimicrobial agents in *P. aeruginosa* is a combination of several mechanisms acting concurrently.[46,374]

Aside from intrinsic resistance, *P. aeruginosa* may acquire resistance genes by horizontal transfer from other bacteria by conjugation, transformation, or transduction, as well as by mutational events in the bacterial genome.[80] For example, *P. aeruginosa* may acquire resistance via acquisition of plasmid-mediated β-lactamases, including extended-spectrum β-lactamases such as the TEM, SHV, VEB, GES, and PER types of enzymes, and metallo-β-lactamases (carbapenemases) such as the IMP and VIM types of enzymes or aminoglycoside-inactivating enzymes (AAC [6′]-I and APH [3′]-II). Similarly, mutational events in the genome of *P. aeruginosa* may lead to clinical resistance. Hyperproduction of AmpC β-lactamase (encoded by the *ampC* gene) may result from a mutation in the *ampD* gene, whose protein product controls the activity of the AmpR regulator protein. Mutations in genes coding for antibiotic target enzymes such as DNA gyrase/topoisomerase II (*gryA* and *gyrB*) and topoisomerase IV (*parC* and *parE*) may yield enzymes with reduced fluoroquinolone-binding activity and clinical resistance. Furthermore overexpression of the MexAB-OprM efflux pump as a result of a mutation in the *mexZ* gene may lead to clinical resistance to aminoglycoside, fluoroquinolone, and select antipseudomonal β-lactam antibiotics.[288,408]

The most clinically relevant β-lactamases produced by *P. aeruginosa* are chromosomally encoded Ambler class C cephalosporinases,[298] whose synthesis may be increased on exposure to a number of β-lactam antibiotics (derepression of the *ampC* gene).[321] The propensity to induce *ampC* β-lactamase varies among the β-lactam antibiotics, with both cefoxitin and imipenem being strong inducers.[19,84,107] All antipseudomonal penicillins, cephalosporins (including cephamycins such as cefoxitin), and aztreonam are inactivated to varying degrees by the AmpC β-lactamase produced by *P. aeruginosa,* but cefepime and, to a greater extent, the carbapenems are relatively stable to inactivation.[255] *P. aeruginosa* strains harboring the *ampC* gene may produce only low levels of β-lactamase in vitro on initial isolation, and such strains may appear susceptible to β-lactam antibiotics on initial in vitro testing. Once patients colonized or infected with these strains are exposed to β-lactam antibiotics during therapy, induction of β-lactamase production may lead to emergence of resistance. For this reason, repeat in vitro susceptibility testing of additional clinical isolates of *P. aeruginosa* obtained after 48 to 72 hours of appropriate therapy is warranted.

Clavulanate and tazobactam are β-lactamase inhibitors effective against plasmid-encoded Ambler class A β-lactamases, including extended-spectrum β-lactamases found in *P. aeruginosa* and other gram-negative bacteria. However, these β-lactamase inhibitors are not only ineffective against the common AmpC β-lactamase of *P. aeruginosa,* but also are potent β-lactamase inducers. Use of these β-lactamase inhibitors will not enhance the activity of ticarcillin-clavulanate or piperacillin-tazobactam against *P. aeruginosa* and might actually increase the likelihood of emergence of resistant strains.

Whereas imipenem, meropenem, and doripenem resist the β-lactamases commonly produced by *P. aeruginosa,* resistance to carbapenems can result through the loss of an outer-membrane porin that allows carbapenems to enter *Pseudomonas*.[50] The permeability of other β-lactam antibiotics also may be reduced when this outer-membrane porin is lost. Although chemically distinct from imipenem or meropenem, fluoroquinolones such as ciprofloxacin may induce decreased permeability to both antibiotics.[291] Plasmid-mediated metallo-β-lactamases that confer resistance to imipenem have been described.[242,330,383] Fortunately these metallo-β-lactamases are identified only rarely in *P. aeruginosa*.

Ciprofloxacin and levofloxacin are the most effective of the quinolones against *P. aeruginosa*. Alteration of the binding site of DNA gyrase (plasmid-borne quinolone resistance determinant, gnr) and decreased penetration of ciprofloxacin through the *Pseudomonas* cell membrane can result in resistant strains.[107,213,354]

Tobramycin is the most active aminoglycoside against *P. aeruginosa*, and amikacin induces the lowest frequency of resistant strains. Resistance to aminoglycosides usually results from enzyme-mediated antibiotic modification.[100] The various aminoglycoside-modifying enzymes have different substrate affinities. Therefore resistance to one aminoglycoside through aminoglycoside-modifying enzymes does not predict resistance to others necessarily. Resistance is less common to amikacin than to other aminoglycosides.[139,406] Aminoglycoside-modifying enzymes usually are coded by plasmid-mediated genes, but they occasionally can be coded by genes on the bacterial chromosome.[100] Plasmid-encoded resistance supports rapid transference among strains within an institution. *P. aeruginosa* also can become resistant to aminoglycosides by decreasing the intracellular uptake of aminoglycosides or by modification of intracellular ribosomal attachment.[91,107] These mechanisms of resistance generally cause cross-resistance for all aminoglycosides.

In addition to antibiotic resistance, other clinical factors can adversely affect aminoglycoside activity against *Pseudomonas*. The acidic environment in tissue infected with *P. aeruginosa* can inactivate aminoglycosides.[39] Aminoglycosides may fail to reach therapeutic tissue levels because of poor penetration into bronchial secretions and lung tissue.[28] For patients with tracheitis (e.g., intubated patients) or endobronchial disease (e.g., CF), aminoglycosides and, less frequently, colistin have been administered by aerosol.[323] This route of delivery allows for greater availability of the antibiotic at the site of the infection, with enhanced safety because of negligible absorption into the systemic circulation. Resistance may emerge after prolonged courses.

Some studies have reported on the accuracy of automated or semiautomated antimicrobial susceptibility test systems and their potential for reporting errors for susceptibility of *P. aeruginosa* to various antibiotics, particularly β-lactam agents.[81,181,308] The problem appears to be more pronounced with rapid systems that generate a susceptibility result in less than the 18- to 24-hour incubation period used in conventional testing. Such systems have difficulty in detecting resistance against β-lactam agents that may require a minimum time for expression of resistance to a level detectable by phenotypic methods relying on detection of growth. In general, more traditional antimicrobial susceptibility test systems, which include incubation for at least 18 to 24 hours, such as disk diffusion, broth or agar dilution, or epsilometer test (E-test), produce more reliable results. In one large multicenter study, the agar diffusion methods of disk diffusion and E-test performed acceptably in contrast to a reference broth microdilution method for both mucoid and nonmucoid isolates of *P. aeruginosa* from patients with CF.[48] In the same study, mucoid isolates were generally found to be more susceptible than nonmucoid isolates. This finding agreed with several other, but not all, studies. The clinical significance of these in vitro findings is difficult to interpret given that the mucoid phenotype is thought to be primarily associated with biofilms where antibiotic penetration is compromised. In fact, the role of routine in vitro antibiotic susceptibility testing in children with CF as it relates to clinical response and short-term outcomes has been questioned.[170] Not surprisingly, the role of in vitro antibiotic synergy testing for multidrug-resistant *P. aeruginosa* has also been questioned because of the lack of standardized testing methods and good outcome data.[2,132]

The current disk diffusion and MIC interpretative standards (MIC breakpoints) from Clinical Laboratory Standards Institute (CLSI) for susceptibility to *P. aeruginosa*, reflect changes in the breakpoints for piperacillin, ticarcillin, piperacillin-tazobactam, and ticarcillin-clavulanate and breakpoints for the antipseudomonal carbapenem antibiotics (imipenem, meropenem, and doripenem).[74] The MIC breakpoints for the antipseudomonal penicillin (piperacillin) and penicillin and inhibitor combination antibiotics (piperacillin-tazobactam, ticarcillin-clavulanate) have been changed from the previous breakpoints of 64 μg/mL or less = susceptible (S) and 128 μg/mL or more = resistant (R) to 16 μg/mL or less = S, 32 to 64 μg/mL = intermediate (I), and 128 μg/mL or greater = R. This change was prompted by studies indicating that the likelihood of achieving blood levels of these drugs above 32 or 64 μg/mL for 50% of the time between doses was zero.[225] Indeed some studies suggest that monotherapy for serious *P. aeruginosa* infection is often ineffective with organisms with such elevated MICs.[58] Of note, the drug ticarcillin-clavulanate is no longer manufactured in the United States, and, as of the date of writing, there are no new sources of the drug. A newer combination drug, ceftolozane-tazobactam, is available with CLSI breakpoints of 4 μg/mL or less = S, 8 μg/mL = I, and 16 μg/mL or more = R.[74,116] Similarly the MIC breakpoints against *P. aeruginosa* for doripenem, imipenem and meropenem have been changed from the previous breakpoints of 4 μg/mL or less = S, 8 μg/mL = I, and 16 μg/mL μg/mL or more = R to 2 μg/mL or less = S, 4 μg/mL = I, and 8 μg/mL or more = R. The revised and more conservative carbapenem breakpoints reportedly allow for better detection of "nonsusceptibility" among isolates of *P. aeruginosa*.

It is important to note that CLSI has published separate MIC breakpoints for other *Pseudomonas* spp. and nonfastidious, glucose-nonfermenting, gram-negative rods, as well as specific MIC breakpoints for *B. cepacia, B. pseudomallei,* and selected other related organisms.[73] In most cases, breakpoints are available only for a limited number of antibiotics and may not include disk diffusion breakpoints. In general, MIC methods are preferred for such organisms.

PREVENTION

Prevention of infection with pseudomonads depends in part on a continuous surveillance program of the hospital environment that is designed to identify and subsequently eradicate sources of pseudomonads as quickly as possible. Recent updated guidelines provide recommendations for preventing transmission of infectious agents in health care settings and in special populations, such as patients with CF.[315,334] Transmission of health care–associated *P. aeruginosa* can frequently be traced back to colonization of the health care institution's water distribution system. Biofilm colonization of faucets can be particularly problematic. Pseudomonads can grow to a concentration of 10^6 organisms per milliliter in distilled water that appears to be perfectly clear. Growth of pseudomonads in distilled water, disinfectants, and medications is the factor most commonly incriminated in single-source outbreaks of *Pseudomonas* infection in hospitals. Management of *P. aeruginosa* and other multidrug-resistant organisms in health care settings remains challenging. Recent data from US hospitals report the incidence of *P. aeruginosa* multidrug resistance (MDR) to be 22% among pneumonia isolates and 15% among bloodstream isolates, with MDR isolates being more prevalent than carbapenemase resistant isolates.[412] Thus it is imperative to follow strict infection prevention measures, including good hand hygiene, use of personal protective equipment, and appropriate disinfection and cleaning of equipment and supplies.

Outbreaks of *Pseudomonas* infection in newborn nurseries have been reported.[175] Generally infection has been transmitted by the hands of personnel from washbasin surfaces and suction catheter rinse solution to the newborn infants. Strict attention to hand washing, particularly with a liquid iodophor hand washing agent before and between contact with newborn infants, may prevent or interdict epidemic disease. Daily replacement of all apparatus used for intravenous administration greatly reduces the hazard of extrinsic contamination by *Pseudomonas* and other gram-negative organisms. In addition, meticulous care is required in the preparation of solutions for total parenteral alimentation and in the insertion and care of catheters.

The risk for developing *Pseudomonas* infection in a burn patient also can be minimized by careful protective isolation and by the topical application of silver nitrate (0.5%) solution or 10% mafenide acetate cream. Debridement for removal of devitalized tissue is also imperative. *Pseudomonas* infection of dermal abnormalities that communicate with the cerebrospinal axis can be prevented by careful evaluation and early surgical repair. Providing antibiotic prophylaxis of *Pseudomonas* UTI is difficult without a suitable oral antipseudomonal antibiotic for children. Identification and surgical correction of obstructive lesions of the urinary tract minimize or prevent the development of *Pseudomonas* infection of the urinary tract.

In patients with CF and certain immunocompromised patients, high rates of *P. aeruginosa* colonization and infection and ever-increasing antibiotic resistance render active or passive immunization (or both) against *P. aeruginosa* desirable. In the past 2 decades, an understanding of the human immune response to *P. aeruginosa* and the immune responses that may provide protection against infection or disease has increased considerably. Naturally occurring immunity generally is ineffective. Certain naturally generated antibodies may even be detrimental.[348] These antibodies may form antigen-antibody complexes that increase pulmonary inflammation and direct lung damage. Even if neutralizing antibodies could be administered passively or developed after vaccine administration, the large quantities of mucoid exopolysaccharide produced by *P. aeruginosa* may mask many of the antigens targeted for antibody neutralization or opsonization.

A vaccine against *P. aeruginosa* is a potential preventative strategy for young children with CF but one that, despite years of study, remains a challenge.[102,333] The significant genotypic and phenotypic variability among *P. aeruginosa* isolates has required testing of multiple antigens. Purified bacterial proteins, including flagellar antigen, outer-membrane proteins, lipopolysaccharide-O, several inactivated bacterial toxins, high-molecular-weight polysaccharide antigen and glycoconjugate, and killed whole-cell vaccine preparations, have been tested. Children with CF infected with *P. aeruginosa* have high levels of IgA, IgG, and IgM antibodies in bronchoalveolar fluid and serum against a variety of potential vaccine antigens compared to uninfected children with CF and healthy control subjects.[246] Paradoxically this may interfere with vaccine response. The presence of antibody alone may not be protective enough to prevent infection. The potential impact of a *P. aeruginosa* vaccine also has been suggested as a possible method for preventing or delaying pseudomonal disease in patients with acute leukemia or CF. However, to date, evidence of protective efficacy in humans has not been definitively established for candidate vaccines.

PROGNOSIS

The prognosis of *P. aeruginosa* infection depends on factors related to the host, clinical site of infection, and nature of the underlying disease process. Overall mortality for patients with *P. aeruginosa* bacteremia is approximately 30%, but ranges from 10% to 60%.[186,265] Risk factors associated with increased risk of mortality from *Pseudomonas* bloodstream infection include: (1) the development of septic shock, (2) inappropriate antibiotic therapy, (3) neutropenia (absolute neutrophil count <500/mm^3), and (4) the development of septic metastases.[36,226,239,324] Some studies have also implicated the presence of multidrug-resistant *P. aeruginosa* strains to negatively impact patient outcomes, although this may also be a surrogate for inappropriate antibiotic therapy.[89,247,361] Despite an expanded antibiotic armamentarium and improvement in supportive care strategies, *P. aeruginosa* bacteremia continues to be associated with high mortality rates.

NEW REFERENCES SINCE THE SEVENTH EDITION

1. Aanaes K, Rickelt LF, Johansen HK, et al. Decreased mucosal oxygen tension in the maxillary sinuses in patients with cystic fibrosis. *J Cystic Fibrosis*. 2011;10(2): 114-120.
5. Alby K, Gilligan PH, Miller MB. Comparison of matrix-assisted laser desorption ionization-time of flight (MALDI-TOF) mass spectrometry platforms for the identification of gram-negative rods from patients with cystic fibrosis. *J Clin Microbiol*. 2013;51(11):3852-3854.
7. Almuzara MN, Vazquez M, Tanaka N, et al. First case of human infection due to *Pseudomonas fulva*, an environmental bacterium isolated from cerebrospinal fluid. *J Clin Microbiol*. 2010;48(2):660-664.
17. Aydin B, Dilli D, Zenciroglu A, et al. A case of newborn with community acquired pneumonia caused by *Cupriavidus pauculus*. *Tuberk Toraks*. 2012;60(2): 160-162.
18. Azzopardi EA, Azzopardi SM, Boyce DE, et al. Emerging gram-negative infections in burn wounds. *J Burn Care Res*. 2011;32(5):570-576.
21. Baltimore RS, Gewitz M, Baddour LM, et al. Infective endocarditis in childhood: 2015 update: a scientific statement from the American Heart Association. *Circulation*. 2015;132(15):1487-1515.
23. Bauer KA, West JE, O'Brien JM, et al. Extended-infusion cefepime reduces mortality in patients with *Pseudomonas aeruginosa* infections. *Antimicrob Agents Chemother*. 2013;57(7):2907-2912.
25. Benoit TJ, Blaney DD, Gee JE, et al. Melioidosis cases and selected reports of occupational exposures to *Burkholderia pseudomallei*: United States, 2008–2013. *MMWR Surveill Summ*. 2015;64(5):1-9.
35. Billard-Pomares T, Herwegh S, Wizla-Derambure N, et al. Application of quantitative PCR to the diagnosis and monitoring of *Pseudomonas aeruginosa* colonization in 5–18-year-old cystic fibrosis patients. *J Med Microbiol*. 2011;60(Pt 2):157-161.
38. Bliziotis IA, Petrosillo N, Michalopoulos A, et al. Impact of definitive therapy with beta-lactam monotherapy or combination with an aminoglycoside or a quinolone for *Pseudomonas aeruginosa* bacteremia. *PLoS ONE*. 2011;6(10):e26470.
44. Bowers DR, Liew YX, Lye DC, et al. Outcomes of appropriate empiric combination versus monotherapy for *Pseudomonas aeruginosa* bacteremia. *Antimicrob Agents Chemother*. 2013;57(3):1270-1274.
52. Cabrera AG, Khan MS, Morales DL, et al. Infectious complications and outcomes in children supported with left ventricular assist devices. *J Heart Lung Transplant*. 2013;32(5):518-524.
61. Chastre J, Wolff M, Fagon JY, et al. Comparison of 8 vs 15 days of antibiotic therapy for ventilator-associated pneumonia in adults: a randomized trial. *JAMA*. 2003;290(19):2588-2598.
62. Cheng AC. Melioidosis: advances in diagnosis and treatment. *Curr Opin Infect Dis*. 2010;23(6):554-559.
67. Chierakul W, Winothai W, Wattanawaitunechai C, et al. Melioidosis in 6 tsunami survivors in southern Thailand. *Clin Infect Dis*. 2005;41(7):982-990.
69. Choy JL, Mayo M, Janmaat A, et al. Animal melioidosis in Australia. *Acta Trop*. 2000;74(2-3):153-158.
70. Church D, Elsayed S, Reid O, et al. Burn wound infections. *Clin Microbiol Rev*. 2006;19(2):403-434.
72. Clinical Laboratory Standards Institute (CLSI). *Abbreviated identification of bacteria and yeast: approved guidelines*. CLSA documetn M35-A2. Wayne, PA: CLSI; 2008.
74. Clinical Laboratory Standards Institute (CLSI). *Performance standards for antimicrobial susceptibility testing: 26th informational supplement M100-S26*. Wayne, PA: CLSI; 2016.
86. Currie BJ, Fisher DA, Howard DM, et al. Endemic melioidosis in tropical northern Australia: a 10-year prospective study and review of the literature. *Clin Infect Dis*. 2000;31(4):981-986.
89. Dantas RC, Ferreira ML, Gontijo-Filho PP, et al. *Pseudomonas aeruginosa* bacteraemia: independent risk factors for mortality and impact of resistance on outcome. *J Med Microbiol*. 2014;63(Pt 12):1679-1687.
93. De Baere T, Steyaert S, Wauters G, et al. Classification of *Ralstonia pickettii* biovar 3/'*thomasii*' strains (Pickett 1994) and of new isolates related to nosocomial recurrent meningitis as *Ralstonia mannitolytica* sp. nov. *Intl J Syst Evolution Microbiol*. 2001;51(Pt 2):547-558.
95. Degand N, Lotte R, Deconde Le Butor C, et al. Epidemic spread of *Pandoraea pulmonicola* in a cystic fibrosis center. *BMC Infect Dis*. 2015;15(1):583.
98. Desai AP, Stanley T, Atuan M, et al. Use of matrix assisted laser desorption ionisation-time of flight mass spectrometry in a paediatric clinical laboratory for identification of bacteria commonly isolated from cystic fibrosis patients. *J Clin Pathol*. 2012;65(9):835-838.
102. Doring G. Vaccine development for patients with cystic fibrosis. *Exp Rev Vaccine*. 2012;11(3):259-261.
104. Dorman SE, Gill VJ, Gallin JI, et al. *Burkholderia pseudomallei* infection in a Puerto Rican patient with chronic granulomatous disease: case report and review of occurrences in the Americas. *Clin Infect Dis*. 1998;26(4):889-894.
112. Estepa V, Rojo-Bezares B, Torres C, et al. Genetic lineages and antimicrobial resistance in *Pseudomonas* spp. isolates recovered from food samples. *Foodborne Pathog Dis*. 2015;12(6):486-491.
114. Falagas ME, Kasiakou SK. Toxicity of polymyxins: a systematic review of the evidence from old and recent studies. *Crit Care*. 2006;10(1):R27.
116. Farrell DJ, Flamm RK, Sader HS, et al. Antimicrobial activity of ceftolozane-tazobactam tested against Enterobacteriaceae and *Pseudomonas aeruginosa* with various resistance patterns isolated in U.S. Hospitals (2011–2012). *Antimicrob Agents Chemother*. 2013;57(12):6305-6310.
118. Fehlberg LC, Andrade LH, Assis DM, et al. Performance of MALDI-ToF MS for species identification of Burkholderia cepacia complex clinical isolates. *Diagn Microbiol Infect Dis*. 2013;77(2):126-128.
121. Fernandez L, Hancock RE. Adaptive and mutational resistance: role of porins and efflux pumps in drug resistance. *Clin Microbiol Rev*. 2012;25(4): 661-681.
126. Findlay J, Hopkins KL, Meunier D, et al. Evaluation of three commercial assays for rapid detection of genes encoding clinically relevant carbapenemases in cultured bacteria. *J Antimicrob Chemother*. 2015;70(5):1338-1342.
131. Flume PA, O'Sullivan BP, Robinson KA, et al. Cystic fibrosis pulmonary guidelines: chronic medications for maintenance of lung health. *Am J Resp Crit Care Med*. 2007;176(10):957-969.
133. Fragasso T, Ricci Z, Grutter G, et al. Incidence of healthcare-associated infections in a pediatric population with an extracorporeal ventricular assist device. *Artificial Org*. 2011;35(11):1110-1114.

134. Freifeld AG, Bow EJ, Sepkowitz KA, et al. Clinical practice guideline for the use of antimicrobial agents in neutropenic patients with cancer: 2010 update by the infectious diseases society of america. *Clin Infect Dis*. 2011;52(4):e56-e93.
142. Ghazal SS, Al-Mudaimeegh K, Al Fakihi EM, et al. Outbreak of *Burkholderia cepacia* bacteremia in immunocompetent children caused by contaminated nebulized sulbutamol in Saudi Arabia. *Am J Infect Control*. 2006;34(6):394-398.
145. Goldman M, Rosenfeld-Yehoshua N, Lerner-Geva L, et al. Clinical features of community-acquired *Pseudomonas aeruginosa* urinary tract infections in children. *Pediatr Nephrol*. 2008;23(5):765-768.
151. Hara Y, Chin CY, Mohamed R, et al. Multiple-antigen ELISA for melioidosis: a novel approach to the improved serodiagnosis of melioidosis. *BMC Infect Dis*. 2013;13:165.
156. Heil EL, Lowery AV, Thom KA, et al. Treatment of multidrug-resistant *Pseudomonas aeruginosa* using extended-infusion antimicrobial regimens. *Pharmacotherapy*. 2015;35(1):54-58.
161. Hocevar SN, Edwards JR, Horan TC, et al. Device-associated infections among neonatal intensive care unit patients: incidence and associated pathogens reported to the National Healthcare Safety Network, 2006–2008. *Infect Control Hosp Epidemiol*. 2012;33(12):1200-1206.
162. Hoffmaster AR, AuCoin D, Baccam P, et al. Melioidosis diagnostic workshop, 2013. *Emerg Infect Dis*. 2015;21(2).
165. Hoiby N, Ciofu O, Bjarnsholt T. *Pseudomonas*. In: Jorgensen JH, Pfaller MA, Carrroll KC, et al, eds. *Manual of Clinical Microbiology*. 11 ed. Washington, DC: ASM Press; 2015.
175. Jefferies JM, Cooper T, Yam T, et al. Pseudomonas aeruginosa outbreaks in the neonatal intensive care unit: a systematic review of risk factors and environmental sources. *J Med Microbiol*. 2012;61(Pt 8):1052-1061.
176. Jhung MA, Sunenshine RH, Noble-Wang J, et al. A national outbreak of *Ralstonia mannitolilytica* associated with use of a contaminated oxygen-delivery device among pediatric patients. *Pediatrics*. 2007;119(6):1061-1068.
186. Kang CI, Kim SH, Kim HB, et al. *Pseudomonas aeruginosa* bacteremia: risk factors for mortality and influence of delayed receipt of effective antimicrobial therapy on clinical outcome. *Clin Infect Dis*. 2003;37(6):745-751.
188. Kaufman SE, Donnell RW, Hickey WS. Rationale and evidence for extended infusion of piperacillin-tazobactam. *Am J Health Syst Pharm*. 2011;68(16):1521-1526.
189. Kawasaki T, Nakamura K, Jeschke MG, et al. Impaired ability of burn patient neutrophils to stimulate beta-defensin production by keratinocytes. *Immunol Cell Biol*. 2012;90(8):796-801.
202. Kohler T, Dumas JL, Van Delden C. Ribosome protection prevents azithromycin-mediated quorum-sensing modulation and stationary-phase killing of *Pseudomonas aeruginosa*. *Antimicrob Agents Chemother*. 2007;51(12):4243-4248.
204. Kolpen M, Hansen CR, Bjarnsholt T, et al. Polymorphonuclear leucocytes consume oxygen in sputum from chronic *Pseudomonas aeruginosa* pneumonia in cystic fibrosis. *Thorax*. 2010;65(1):57-62.
214. Le Gall F, Le Berre R, Rosec S, et al. Proposal of a quantitative PCR-based protocol for an optimal *Pseudomonas aeruginosa* detection in patients with cystic fibrosis. *BMC Microbiol*. 2013;13:143.
215. Limmathurotsakul D, Chantratita N, Teerawattanasook N, et al. Enzyme-linked immunosorbent assay for the diagnosis of melioidosis: better than we thought. *Clin Infect Dis*. 2011;52(8):1024-1028.
216. Limmathurotsakul D, Peacock SJ. Melioidosis: a clinical overview. *Br Med Bull*. 2011;99:125-139.
217. Lin TI, Huang YF, Liu PY, et al. *Pseudomonas aeruginosa* infective endocarditis in patients who do not use intravenous drugs: analysis of risk factors and treatment outcomes. *J Microbiol Immunol Infect.[Wei mian yu gan ran za zhi]*. 2014.
220. LiPuma JJ, Currie B, et al. *Burkholderia, Stenotrophomonas, Ralstonia, Cupriavidas, Pandoraea, Brevundimonas, Comamonas, Delfia*, and *Acidovoax*. In: Jorgensen JH, Pfaller MA, Carrol KC, et al, eds. *Manual of Clinical Microbiology*. 11 ed. Washington, DC: ASM Press; 2015.
226. Lodise TP Jr, Patel N, Kwa A, et al. Predictors of 30-day mortality among patients with Pseudomonas aeruginosa bloodstream infections: impact of delayed appropriate antibiotic selection. *Antimicrob Agents Chemother*. 2007;51(10): 3510-3515.
228. Maiz L, Giron RM, Olveira C, et al. Inhaled antibiotics for the treatment of chronic bronchopulmonary *Pseudomonas aeruginosa* infection in cystic fibrosis: systematic review of randomised controlled trials. *Expert Opin Pharmacother*. 2013;14(9):1135-1149.
230. Marcus N, Ashkenazi S, Samra Z, et al. Community-acquired *Pseudomonas aeruginosa* urinary tract infections in children hospitalized in a tertiary center: relative frequency, risk factors, antimicrobial resistance and treatment. *Infection*. 2008;36(5):421-426.
236. McLeod C, Morris PS, Bauert PA, et al. Clinical presentation and medical management of melioidosis in children: a 24-year prospective study in the Northern Territory of Australia and review of the literature. *Clin Infect Dis*. 2015;60(1):21-26.
239. Micek ST, Lloyd AE, Ritchie DJ, et al. *Pseudomonas aeruginosa* bloodstream infection: importance of appropriate initial antimicrobial treatment. *Antimicrob Agents Chemother*. 2005;49(4):1306-1311.
244. Miron D, Keness Y, Bor N, et al. *Pseudomonas stutzeri* knee arthritis in a child: case report and review. *J Pediatr Orthoped*. 2007;16(6 Pt B):419-421.
245. Mittal R, Lisi CV, Gerring R, et al. Current concepts in the pathogenesis and treatment of chronic suppurative otitis media. *J Med Microbiol*. 2015;64(10):1103-1116.
246. Moore R, Kyd JM, Carzino R, et al. Mucosal and systemic antibody responses to potential *Pseudomonas aeruginosa* vaccine protein antigens in young children with cystic fibrosis following colonization and infection. *Hum Vaccine Immunotherapeut*. 2013;9(3):506-514.
247. Morata L, Cobos-Trigueros N, Martinez JA, et al. Influence of multidrug resistance and appropriate empirical therapy on the 30-day mortality rate of *Pseudomonas aeruginosa* bacteremia. *Antimicrob Agents Chemother*. 2012;56(9):4833-4837.
249. Morpeth S, Murdoch D, Cabell CH, et al. Non-HACEK gram-negative bacillus endocarditis. *Ann Intern Med*. 2007;147(12):829-835.
265. Osmon S, Ward S, Fraser VJ, et al. Hospital mortality for patients with bacteremia due to *Staphylococcus aureus* or *Pseudomonas aeruginosa*. *Chest*. 2004;125(2):607-616.
267. Parkins MD, Gregson DB, Pitout JD, et al. Population-based study of the epidemiology and the risk factors for *Pseudomonas aeruginosa* bloodstream infection. *Infection*. 2010;38(1):25-32.
269. Pathak A, Singh P, Yadav Y, et al. Ecthyma gangrenosum in a neonate: not always pseudomonas. *BMJ Case Rep*. 2013;2013.
270. Paul M, Benuri-Silbiger I, Soares-Weiser K, et al. Beta lactam monotherapy versus beta lactam-aminoglycoside combination therapy for sepsis in immunocompetent patients: systematic review and meta-analysis of randomised trials. *BMJ*. 2004;328(7441):668.
271. Paul M, Leibovici L. Combination antibiotic therapy for *Pseudomonas aeruginosa* bacteraemia. *Lancet Infect Dis*. 2005;5(4):192-193, discussion 193–4.
272. Paul M, Leibovici L. Combination antimicrobial treatment versus monotherapy: the contribution of meta-analyses. *Infect Dis Clin N Am*. 2009;23(2):277-293.
274. Paul M, Soares-Weiser K, Grozinsky S, et al. Beta-lactam versus beta-lactam-aminoglycoside combination therapy in cancer patients with neutropaenia. *Cochrane Database Syst Rev*. 2003;(3):CD003038.
277. Peacock SJ, Cheng AC, Currie BJ, et al. The use of positive serological tests as evidence of exposure to *Burkholderia pseudomallei*. *Am J Trop Med Hyg*. 2011;84(6):1021-1022, author reply 1023.
281. Pena C, Suarez C, Ocampo-Sosa A, et al. Effect of adequate single-drug vs combination antimicrobial therapy on mortality in *Pseudomonas aeruginosa* bloodstream infections: a post hoc analysis of a prospective cohort. *Clin Infect Dis*. 2013;57(2):208-216.
287. Pittman JE, Ferkol TW. The evolution of cystic fibrosis care. *Chest*. 2015; 148(2):533-542.
293. Ramphal GPaR. *Pseudomonas aeruginosa*. In: Mandell GL, Dolin JBR, eds. *Principles and Practice of Infectious Diseases. Vol. 2*. 7th ed. Philadelphia: Churchill Linvingstone; 2010:2835-2860.
303. Rosenthal VD, Bijie H, Maki DG, et al. International Nosocomial Infection Control Consortium (INICC) report, data summary of 36 countries, for 2004–2009. *Am J Infect Control*. 2012;40(5):396-407.
304. Ross JP, Holland SM, Gill VJ, et al. Severe *Burkholderia (Pseudomonas) gladioli* infection in chronic granulomatous disease: report of two successfully treated cases. *Clin Infect Dis*. 1995;21(5):1291-1293.
310. Safdar N, Handelsman J, Maki DG. Does combination antimicrobial therapy reduce mortality in gram-negative bacteraemia? A meta-analysis. *Lancet Infect Dis*. 2004;4(8):519-527.
312. Saiman L, Anstead M, Mayer-Hamblett N, et al. Effect of azithromycin on pulmonary function in patients with cystic fibrosis uninfected with *Pseudomonas aeruginosa*: a randomized controlled trial. *JAMA*. 2010;303(17):1707-1715.
314. Saiman L, Marshall BC, Mayer-Hamblett N, et al. Azithromycin in patients with cystic fibrosis chronically infected with *Pseudomonas aeruginosa*: a randomized controlled trial. *JAMA*. 2003;290(13):1749-1756.
315. Saiman L, Siegel JD, LiPuma JJ, et al. Infection prevention and control guideline for cystic fibrosis: 2013 update. *Infect Control Hosp Epidemiol*. 2014;35(suppl 1):S1-S67.
318. Salsgiver EL, Fink AK, Knapp EA, et al. Changing epidemiology of the respiratory bacteriology of patients with cystic fibrosis. *Chest*. 2016;149(2): 390-400.
320. Sanchez-Carrillo C, Padilla B, Marin M, et al. Contaminated feeding bottles: the source of an outbreak of *Pseudomonas aeruginosa* infections in a neonatal intensive care unit. *Am J Infect Control*. 2009;37(2):150-154.
322. Scales BS, Dickson RP, LiPuma JJ, et al. Microbiology, genomics, and clinical significance of the *Pseudomonas fluorescens* species complex, an unappreciated colonizer of humans. *Clin Microbiol Rev*. 2014;27(4):927-948.
324. Schechner V, Gottesman T, Schwartz O, et al. *Pseudomonas aeruginosa* bacteremia upon hospital admission: risk factors for mortality and influence of inadequate empirical antimicrobial therapy. *Diagn Microbiol Infect Dis*. 2011;71(1):38-45.
331. Seok Y, Shin H, Lee Y, et al. First report of bloodstream infection caused by *Pseudomonas fulva*. *J Clin Microbiol*. 2010;48(7):2656-2657.
333. Sharma A, Krause A, Worgall S. Recent developments for *Pseudomonas* vaccines. *Hum Vaccines*. 2011;7(10):999-1011.

334. Siegel JD, Rhinehart E, Jackson M, et al. 2007 Guideline for isolation precautions: preventing transmission of infectious agents in health care settings. *Am J Infect Control*. 2007;35(10 suppl 2):S65-S164.
335. Sievert DM, Ricks P, Edwards JR, et al. Antimicrobial-resistant pathogens associated with healthcare-associated infections: summary of data reported to the National Healthcare Safety Network at the Centers for Disease Control and Prevention, 2009–2010. *Infect Control Hosp Epidemiol*. 2013;34(1):1-14.
349. Sridhar J, Kuriyan AE, Flynn HW Jr, et al. Endophthalmitis caused by *Pseudomonas aeruginosa:* clinical features, antibiotic susceptibilities, and treatment outcomes. *Retina*. 2015;35(6):1101-1106.
352. Stewart T, Engelthaler DM, Blaney DD, et al. Epidemiology and investigation of melioidosis, Southern Arizona. *Emerg Infect Dis*. 2011;17(7):1286-1288.
354. Strahilevitz J, Jacoby GA, Hooper DC, et al. Plasmid-mediated quinolone resistance: a multifaceted threat. *Clin Microbiol Rev*. 2009;22(4):664-689.
357. Sullins AK, Abdel-Rahman SM. Pharmacokinetics of antibacterial agents in the CSF of children and adolescents. *Paediatr Drugs*. 2013;15(2):93-117.
361. Tam VH, Rogers CA, Chang KT, et al. Impact of multidrug-resistant *Pseudomonas aeruginosa* bacteremia on patient outcomes. *Antimicrob Agents Chemother*. 2010;54(9):3717-3722.
362. Tamma PD, Turnbull AE, Milstone AM, et al. Ventilator-associated tracheitis in children: does antibiotic duration matter? *Clin Infect Dis*. 2011;52(11):1324-1331.
364. Thatrimontrichai A, Maneenil G. Neonatal melioidosis: systematic review of the literature. *Pediatr Infect Dis J*. 2012;31(11):1195-1197.
367. Tunkel AR, Hartman BJ, Kaplan SL, et al. Practice guidelines for the management of bacterial meningitis. *Clin Infect Dis*. 2004;39(9):1267-1284.
370. Uzodi AS, Schears GJ, Neal JR, et al. *Cupriavidus pauculus* bacteremia in a child on extracorporeal membrane oxygenation. *ASAIO J*. 2014;60(6):740-741.
371. Vaiman M, Lazarovitch T, Heller L, et al. Ecthyma gangrenosum and ecthyma-like lesions: review article. *Eur J Clin Microbioll Infect Dis*. 2015;34(4):633-639.
385. Weiel JJZCZ, Smith JA, et al. Clinicopathologic aspects of ecthyma gangrenosum in pediatric patients: a case series and review of the literature. *J Clin Anatom Pathol*. 2013;1(101):1-5.
389. Wiersinga WJ, Currie BJ, Peacock SJ. Melioidosis. *N Engl J Med*. 2012; 367(11):1035-1044.
391. Wong V, Levi K, Baddal B, et al. Spread of *Pseudomonas fluorescens* due to contaminated drinking water in a bone marrow transplant unit. *J Clin Microbiol*. 2011;49(6):2093-2096.
395. Worlitzsch D, Tarran R, Ulrich M, et al. Effects of reduced mucus oxygen concentration in airway *Pseudomonas* infections of cystic fibrosis patients. *J Clin Invest*. 2002;109(3):317-325.
398. Wu DC, Chan WW, Metelitsa AI, et al. *Pseudomonas* skin infection: clinical features, epidemiology, and management. *Am J Clin Dermatol*. 2011;12(3):157-169.
404. Yee-Guardino S, Danziger-Isakov L, Knouse M, et al. Nosocomially acquired *Pseudomonas stutzeri* brain abscess in a child: case report and review. *Infect Control Hosp Epidemiol*. 2006;27(6):630-632.
410. Zehnder AM, Hawkins MG, Koski MA, et al. *Burkholderia pseudomallei* isolates in 2 pet iguanas, California, USA. *Emerg Infect Dis*. 2014;20(2):304-306.
414. Zomorrodi A, Wald ER. Ecthyma gangrenosum: considerations in a previously healthy child. *Pediatr Infect Dis J*. 2002;21(12):1161-1164.

The full reference list for this chapter is available at ExpertConsult.com.

126 *Stenotrophomonas (Xanthomonas) maltophilia*

Katherine Y. King

Stenotrophomonas maltophilia is an opportunistic pathogen that rarely causes infection in immunocompetent children but causes significant morbidity and mortality among immunocompromised, medically fragile, and interventionalized patients. This organism is notable for its intrinsic resistance to many antimicrobial agents.

BACTERIOLOGY AND PATHOGENESIS

A gram-negative bacillus, *S. maltophilia* was previously classified in the *Pseudomonas* and subsequently the *Xanthomonas* genus. It was reassigned as *Stenotrophomonas* in 1993.[100] *S. maltophilia* is an aerobic, nonfermentative, gram-negative bacillus that is lysine decarboxylase–positive. It is generally thought to be oxidase negative; however, up to 20% of isolates were described recently to be oxidase positive.[17] Other key features that allow identification of *S. maltophilia* include oxidation of glucose and maltose, and a positive DNase reaction.[52] Optimal growth occurs at 35°C (95°F); on sheep blood agar, colonies appear rough and lavender green and have a distinct ammonia-like odor. Morphologically the organism is a straight bacillus, 0.7 to 1.8/μm long, that is motile by means of multiple polar flagella. It grows well on standard culture media, including blood and chocolate agar, and in standard broth blood culture systems. Because of the hardy nature of this organism, standard collection, transport, and storage procedures are sufficient. Isolation from polymicrobial specimens can be achieved by growth on selective media such as MacConkey agar and by the addition of antibiotics such as imipenem, vancomycin, and amphotericin B to the media.[73]

New molecular techniques for the identification of *S. maltophilia* include use of 16S rDNA sequencing and matrix-assisted laser desorption ionization–time of flight (MALDI-TOF) rapid diagnosis. Early studies suggest that 16S rDNA sequencing provides improved specificity over standard biochemical identification.[63,84,87,95] In patients with cystic fibrosis (CF), *S. maltophilia* is occasionally misidentified as *Bordetella cepacia* due to their similar biochemical profiles.[14] Because of the serious clinical implications of misidentification in this group of patients, molecular analysis of the isolates should be considered if biochemical results remain uncertain even after repetition.[132]

EPIDEMIOLOGY

S. maltophilia is a free-living, ubiquitous organism that naturally lives in water, soil, and plants. Its hearty nature allows it to persist in the hospital environment; it has been cultured from contaminated dialysis fluids,[12] intraocular rinsing solution,[65] ventilators and other respiratory equipment,[32,74,109] and preoperative surgical brushes.[99] Several reports have linked nosocomial outbreaks of *S. maltophilia* to contamination of hospital water sources such as faucet aerators,[130] taps,[110] and sinks,[74] as well as disinfectant solutions.[133] Cases of pseudoinfection caused by contamination of blood collection tubes have been described.[112] Person-to-person transmission can occur; cases of nosocomial cross-infection occurring in neonatal and pediatric intensive care units have been described.[48,57,79] Intestinal colonization with *S. maltophilia* in hospitalized oncology patients with diarrhea could represent a potential source of nosocomial infection.[6] Because nosocomial outbreaks have been reported, infection control offices should be notified if *S. maltophilia* is isolated.

Predisposing factors associated with colonization and infection by *S. maltophilia* include the presence of a severe, debilitating underlying illness, particularly malignancy; immune suppression (including human immunodeficiency virus infection); hematopoietic stem cell transplantation; exposure to broad-spectrum antibiotics (particularly to carbapenems, quinolones, or broad-spectrum cephalosporins); prolonged exposure to antibiotics; the presence of a central venous catheter (CVC); neutropenia; severe mucositis; prolonged hospital stay; stay in an intensive care unit; tracheostomy; mechanical ventilation; chronic obstructive pulmonary disease; or a combination of these factors.*

Among children, predisposing factors are similar to those found in adults.[111] Infection with *S. maltophilia* generally is hospital acquired or health care–associated and is found at higher prevalence in patients with CF.[49,70,111] *S. maltophilia* is being isolated from clinical samples with increasing frequency.* This increase may be related to the increased number and survival of patients with chronic or complex illness and the increased use of broad-spectrum antibiotics.[5]

PATHOGENESIS

Like many pseudomonads, *S. maltophilia* is an organism with low virulence and limited invasiveness. An intact host immune system is an important deterrent to acquisition of a severe and even life-threatening infection; septicemia and death occur in patients with underlying debilitating illnesses. *S. maltophilia* elaborates a range of extracellular enzymes, including DNase, RNase, fibrinolysin, lipase, hyaluronidase, protease, and elastase, which may play a role in the pathogenesis of disease processes associated with *S. maltophilia.*[31] The pathogenesis of *S. maltophilia* infection also may be related to the development of cytotoxic activity.[44] A few specific virulence factors have been studied including YajQ, a cyclic di-GMP binding protein that affects adherence and virulence in a murine infection model.[4] In addition, *S. maltophilia* has been found to adhere to plastic materials, including intravenous catheters, and to produce biofilm that limits access to both phagocytes and antibiotics, properties that may account for the relatively high incidence of catheter-related bloodstream infections caused by this organism.[35,31,40] Differences in the rpf gene cluster that encodes for the organism's quorum sensing system may account for strain differences in virulence.[45,66] The *S. maltophilia* genome was published in 2008 and may facilitate future pathogenesis research.[26]

Colonization with *S. maltophilia,* especially in the respiratory tract, is not an uncommon finding. In debilitated patients, exposure to broad-spectrum antimicrobials, many of which are ineffective against this bacterium, may allow overgrowth of colonizing organisms that subsequently gain access to sterile body sites and cause infection. Portals of infection include indwelling devices such as CVCs, peritoneal dialysis or urinary tract catheters, the respiratory tract, and the gastrointestinal tract. Pathogenesis may also be attributable to the effects of *S. maltophilia* on other bacteria, for example by altering biofilm formation and toxin production by *Pseudomonas aeruginosa.*[106]

DIAGNOSIS AND CLINICAL SYNDROMES

The diagnosis of infection is established by isolating the organism from normally sterile sites in the presence of a compatible clinical picture. Importantly, because this organism can survive in the environment and even in hospital equipment such as blood collection tubes and antiseptic solutions, it is important to consider whether growth of *S. maltophilia* in culture represents contamination, colonization, or true infection.

Pneumonia is the most common clinical manifestation of *S. maltophilia* infection. While most pulmonary isolates of *S. maltophilia* represent colonization rather than infection, *S. maltophilia* pneumonia can occur even in the presence of mixed cultures, and it can cause ventilator-associated pneumonia.[1,46,51,85] Pneumonia can be complicated by septic shock, multiorgan dysfunction, and high mortality, especially if it is accompanied by bacteremia, where attributable mortality has been reported to be 30% to 40%.[24,38,76,113,114]

S. maltophilia bloodstream infections are usually catheter associated.[13,74,77,93,125] In a series of 32 episodes of bacteremia in children, 22 were catheter associated.[111] Primary catheter-associated bacteremia has a good response rate to CVC removal and antibiotic therapy; but secondary bacteremia, which generally occurs in patients who are neutropenic, have concurrent pneumonia, or are critically ill, is associated with a significantly worse outcome.[13] Bacteremia with this organism has also been reported in patients following hematopoietic stem cell transplant[127] and as a complication in burn patients.[81,119]

Bloodstream infections caused by *S. maltophilia* can be severe. In a pediatric series, 31% of the patients presented in septic shock, and the attributable mortality rate was 6.3%.[111] In another pediatric series of 32 episodes of bacteremia occurring in 31 children, the crude mortality rate was 40.6%.[134] In children, the severity of illness appears to be similar regardless of whether *S. maltophilia* is isolated in a monomicrobial or mixed blood culture.[111] However, the death rate associated with *S. maltophilia* bloodstream infection is, in general, higher in adults.[74,75,90,93]

Skin and soft tissue infections caused by *S. maltophilia* have occurred in patients who have had work-related injuries and wounds contaminated with soil and plant material, such as lawnmower injuries.[27,37,54] In the hospital setting, *S. maltophilia* frequently is cultured from wounds and surgical sites, but the clinical significance of this organism in children, particularly when it is isolated in mixed culture, can be difficult to determine.[111] Tender, erythematous nodular skin lesions have been described in neutropenic cancer patients in association with *S. maltophilia* bacteremia and probably represent metastatic infectious foci.[117,124,134] *S. maltophilia* has been implicated in the development of ocular infections, including conjunctivitis and keratitis in the setting of ocular surface compromise resulting from trauma, the use of soft contact lenses, or previous infection with human herpes simplex virus.[104] Endophthalmitis and scleritis occurring after ophthalmologic surgical interventions and trauma also have been described.[21,22,64,71,107]

Other clinical syndromes that have been reported to occur rarely include liver abscesses, cellulitis, meningitis, endocarditis, endophthalmitis, sinusitis, necrotizing ulcerative gingivitis, mastoiditis, chronic diarrhea, peritonitis in patients undergoing peritoneal dialysis, cholangitis, osteochondritis, bursitis, osteomyelitis, and urinary tract infection.* Meningitis is an extremely rare occurrence and may be associated with infection of intraventricular devices,[96,103] but spontaneous meningitis has been described in a preterm infant.[82]

S. maltophilia is the fourth most common organism isolated from the bronchial secretions of patients with CF, after *Pseudomonas aeruginosa, Staphylococcus aureus,* and *Haemophilus influenzae.*[120] The incidence and prevalence of *S. maltophilia* isolated from the respiratory secretions of patients with CF are increasing.[36,72,108,116] *S. maltophilia* is recovered from the sputum of an estimated 12% of patients with CF in the United States and from as many as 25% of CF patients in Europe.[108,128] The origin of the bacterium is uncertain; evidence suggests that it may be acquired both in the hospital and in the community.[29] Colonization may be transient or persistent, with chronic colonization occurring more frequently in older patients.[120] Case-control studies identified greater exposure to antipseudomonal antibiotics, oral ciprofloxacin, inhaled aminoglycosides, and oral corticosteroids, as well as more hospitalization days and isolation of *Aspergillus fumigatus* from the sputum as risk factors for colonization with *S. maltophilia.*[34,86,116] Unlike with *Burkholderia cepacia* infection, no evidence of patient-to-patient transmission of *S. maltophilia* has been found, nor does the organism appear to be associated with rapid deterioration of pulmonary function in patients with CF.[33,55] Indeed S. maltophilia colonization has not been shown to affect 3-year survival in CF patients.[56]

However, *S. maltophilia* colonization has been associated with pulmonary exacerbations in CF patients; patients with chronic *S. maltophilia* infection had a significantly increased risk of pulmonary exacerbation requiring hospitalization and antibiotics compared with patients with no history of *S. maltophilia* (relative risk, 1.63; $P = .0002$).[129] Thus the clinical significance of isolation of *S. maltophilia* from the sputum of patients with CF and its role in the deterioration in lung function are unclear. Its presence may represent more of a marker of severe, advanced disease rather than a causative agent of respiratory deterioration.[30,56]

PREVENTION

The rate of person-to-person transmission is low; most transmission occurs to due to environmental spread. Therefore environmental

*References 7, 8, 15, 16, 31, 38, 39, 47, 75, 88, 89, 92, 97, 98, 108, 111, 121, 126, 135.

*References 9, 10, 28, 59–62, 78, 91, 94, 101–103, 105, 115, 123, 136.

TABLE 126.1 Clinical and Laboratory Standards Institute 2016 Minimum Inhibitory Concentration (MIC) Interpretive Criteria

Agent	Susceptible	Intermediate	Resistant
Trimethoprim-sulfamethoxazole[a]	≤2/38 μg/mL		≥4/76 μg/mL
Ceftazidime	≤8 μg/mL	16 μg/mL	≥32 μg/mL
Chloramphenicol	≤8 μg/mL	16 μg/mL	≥32 μg/mL
Levofloxacin	≤2 μg/mL	4 μg/mL	≥8 μg/mL
Minocycline	≤4 μg/mL	8 μg/mL	≥16 μg/mL
Ticarcillin-clavulanate[a]	≤16/2 μg/mL	32/2 to 64/2 μg/mL	≥128/2 μg/mL

[a]Susceptibility for each drug in the combination is noted in the dosage.

decontamination and hospital practices are key in prevention of hospital-associated infections.

TREATMENT

S. maltophilia is inherently resistant to several classes of antibiotics, particularly β-lactams and aminoglycosides.[24] Resistance to β-lactams and cephalosporins is mediated by inducible expression of two β-lactamases: L1, a class 3a metallo-β-lactamase, and L2, a serine active-site broad-spectrum cephalosporinase. L1 hydrolyzes a broad range of β-lactam antibiotics, including carbapenems such as imipenem and meropenem.[31] Other mechanisms of resistance include reduced antibiotic uptake, the main mechanism of aminoglycoside resistance, and an antibiotic efflux system that confers multidrug resistance.[3,138] The activity of early fluoroquinolones such as ciprofloxacin and ofloxacin varies widely, and emergence of resistance during treatment has been reported.[23] Newer quinolones, including levofloxacin and gatifloxacin, appear to have better activity in vitro against *S. maltophilia*,[11,43,69,80,131]

Trimethoprim-sulfamethoxazole (TMP-SMX) has been the treatment of choice for *S. maltophilia*[3,19]; however, it is bacteriostatic and may not be sufficient for some infections or some hosts. Furthermore, due to acquisition of *sul1* and *sul2* genes contained on mobile genetic elements, TMP-SMX resistance has also emerged globally with a recent incidence reported at 17%.[2,24,42,118] The agents with the best in vitro activity against TMP-SMX–resistant strains are minocycline, tigecycline, and colistin.[24] In vitro studies have also suggested that combination therapy using tigecycline and colistin can be synergistic; however, clinical studies have not been done, clinical experience in children is limited, and the proportion of susceptible isolates varies across studies.[41,42,53,67,68] In vitro antibiotic susceptibility testing is plagued by numerous methodologic problems. Several factors, including the time of incubation and the composition of the medium, affect the interpretation of test results. Furthermore poor reproducibility among different testing methods has been described.[18,58] Despite these limitations, in cases of serious infection such as bacteremia or severe pneumonia, combination antibiotic therapy should be considered when in vitro and in vivo evidence suggests that rapid emergence of resistance may occur during treatment.[50,93,122,137]

In cases of catheter-related bloodstream infection, removal of the catheter has been associated with improved outcome, in some circumstances irrespective of the appropriateness of antibiotic therapy, and should be considered for severely ill patients.[20,38,111,135] Nonetheless successful treatment without removal of the catheter[93] has been described.

The Clinical and Laboratory Standards Institute (CLSI) has established standards for antibiotic susceptibility testing, including testing by both disk diffusion and broth or agar dilution (minimum inhibitory concentration [MIC] evaluation).[25] For the disk diffusion method, CLSI recommends testing only TMP-SMX, levofloxacin, and minocycline. In the case of broth or agar dilution, 2016 CLSI MIC interpretive criteria are listed in Table 126.1.

Regardless, no controlled clinical studies have determined the most effective antibiotic regimen or duration of treatment, although one study simply concludes that it requires longer treatment than PA or methicillin-resistant *Staphylococcus aureus* (MRSA).[83]

NEW REFERENCES SINCE THE SEVENTH EDITION

4. An SQ, Caly DL, McCarthy Y, et al. Novel cyclic di-GMP effectors of the YajQ protein family control bacterial virulence. *PLoS Pathog.* 2014;10(10):e1004429.
5. Ansari SR, Hanna H, Hachem R, et al. Risk factors for infections with multidrug-resistant *Stenotrophomonas maltophilia* in patients with cancer. *Cancer.* 2007;109(12):2615-2622.
19. Chang YT, Lin CY, Chen YH, et al. Update on infections caused by *Stenotrophomonas maltophilia* with particular attention to resistance mechanisms and therapeutic options. *Front Microbiol.* 2015;6:893.
24. Church D, Lloyd T, Peirano G, et al. Antimicrobial susceptibility and combination testing of invasive *Stenotrophomonas maltophilia* isolates. *Scand J Infect Dis.* 2013;45(4):265-270.
45. Fouhy Y, Scanlon K, Schouest K, et al. Diffusible signal factor-dependent cell-cell signaling and virulence in the nosocomial pathogen *Stenotrophomonas maltophilia. J Bacteriol.* 2007;189(13):4964-4968.
62. Hellmig S, Ott S, Musfeldt M, et al. Life-threatening chronic enteritis due to colonization of the small bowel with *Stenotrophomonas maltophilia. Gastroenterology.* 2005;129(2):706-712.
63. Homem de Mello de Souza HA, Dalla-Costa LM, Vicenzi FJ, et al. MALDI-TOF: a useful tool for laboratory identification of uncommon glucose non-fermenting gram-negative bacteria associated with cystic fibrosis. *J Med Microbiol.* 2014;63(Pt 9):1148-1153.
66. Huedo P, Yero D, Martinez-Servat S, et al. Two different rpf clusters distributed among a population of *Stenotrophomonas maltophilia* clinical strains display differential diffusible signal factor production and virulence regulation. *J Bacteriol.* 2014;196(13):2431-2442.
76. Lai CH, Chi CY, Chen HP, et al. Clinical characteristics and prognostic factors of patients with *Stenotrophomonas maltophilia* bacteremia. *J Microbiol Immunol Infect.* 2004;37(6):350-358.
83. Magnotti LJ, Croce MA, Zarzaur BL, et al. Causative pathogen dictates optimal duration of antimicrobial therapy for ventilator-associated pneumonia in trauma patients. *J Am Coll Surg.* 2014;212(4):476-484.
84. Mahboubi MA, Carmody LA, Foster BK, et al. Culture-based and culture-independent bacteriologic analysis of cystic fibrosis respiratory specimens. *J Clin Microbiol.* 2015;54(3):613-619.
106. Pompilio A, Crocetta V, De Nicola S, et al. Cooperative pathogenicity in cystic fibrosis: Stenotrophomonas maltophilia modulates Pseudomonas aeruginosa virulence in mixed biofilm. *Front Microbiol.* 2015;6:951.
113. Senol E, DesJardin J, Stark PC, et al. Attributable mortality of *Stenotrophomonas maltophilia* bacteremia. *Clin Infect Dis.* 2002;34(12):1653-1656.
114. Sumida K, Chong Y, Miyake N, et al. Risk factors associated with *Stenotrophomonas maltophilia* bacteremia: a matched case-control study. *PLoS ONE.* 2015;10(7):e0133731.
127. Wang L, Wang Y, Fan X, et al. Prevalence of resistant gram-negative bacilli in bloodstream infection in febrile neutropenia patients undergoing hematopoietic stem cell transplantation: a single center retrospective cohort study. *Medicine (Baltimore).* 2015;94(45):e1931.

The full reference list for this chapter is available at ExpertConsult.com.

Aggregatibacter Species

127

Suzanne Whitworth • Morgan A. Pence • Richard F. Jacobs

The relatively new genus of *Aggregatibacter* consists of some former members of the *Haemophilus* and *Actinobacillus* species, including *Aggregatibacter actinomycetemcomitans*, *Aggregatibacter aphrophilus*, and *Aggregatibacter segnis*. *Haemophilus aphrophilus* and *Haemophilus paraphrophilus* were combined into a single species, *Aggregatibacter aphrophilus*, because they were shown to differ only in their requirement for nicotinamide adenine dinucleotide (NAD), also known as V factor. Because the two species were combined into a single species, some *A. aphrophilus* isolates (i.e., formerly *H. paraphrophilus*) are V factor dependent, and others (i.e., formerly *H. aphrophilus*) are not.[11]

Species of the genus *Aggregatibacter* are nonhemolytic and capnophilic; however, isolates of *A. actinomycetemcomitans* with overexpression of leukotoxin may exhibit a zone of hemolysis. These organisms are involved in a variety of infections, including endocarditis and central nervous system infections. *A. actinomycetemcomitans* is a copathogen in many cases of actinomycosis. It is also strongly implicated as a pathogen in periodontal disease.

These organisms are members of the HACEK group of organisms that have a propensity for infecting heart valves.[20] The HACEK group includes *Haemophilus* spp. (except *Haemophilus influenzae*), *Aggregatibacter* spp., *Cardiobacterium* spp., *Eikenella corrodens*, and *Kingella* spp. Endocarditis caused by these organisms usually is insidious, with fever occurring in fewer than 50% of cases.[9] *A. aphrophilus* is also an important cause of brain abscesses.[11] These topics are covered in detail in Chapters 26 and 134 on HACEK endocarditis and *Aggregatibacter aphrophilus*.

AGGREGATIBACTER ACTINOMYCETEMCOMITANS

A. actinomycetemcomitans (formerly *Actinobacillus actinomycetemcomitans)* is a fastidious, non–spore-forming, nonmotile, facultatively anaerobic gram-negative coccobacillus that frequently complicates actinomycosis caused by *Actinomyces israelii*. It is a copathogen in at least 30% of these infections.[9] Failure to recognize this organism and treat it adequately has resulted in clinical relapse and deterioration of patients infected with actinomycosis.[10,18]

In addition to being associated with actinomycosis, *A. actinomycetemcomitans* has been implicated as a pathogen in periodontal disease and is part of the oral flora. Periodontitis constitutes a group of oral diseases affecting the supporting soft tissues of the teeth and alveolar bone. Aggressive periodontitis is a group of less frequently occurring but more rapidly progressive forms of periodontitis. These entities are characterized by early age at onset during childhood or adolescence, and there is a propensity for familial involvement. Molar and incisor teeth are affected first in localized aggressive periodontitis that is associated with *A. actinomycetemcomitans*.[15] This is particularly problematic in regions of the world with poor general health.

This organism makes a cytolethal distending toxin, which is an exotoxin that affects mammalian cells by inhibiting cell division and causing apoptosis.[5] It also makes a leukotoxin that activates and lyses human leukocytes and induces release of interleukin-1β from macrophages.[6] One highly virulent clone is the JP2 genotype, which has highly leukotoxic activity and is strongly associated with aggressive periodontitis.[3] *A. actinomycetemcomitans* is also an important pathogen in Papillon-Lefèvre syndrome, an autosomal recessive disorder characterized by prepubertal periodontitis and palmar-plantar hyperkeratosis.[14]

A. actinomycetemcomitans can cause pericarditis, meningitis, brain abscess, parotitis, synovitis, osteomyelitis, urinary tract infection, pneumonia, and empyema.[9] Cases of endophthalmitis,[1,16] facial cellulitis, and cavernous sinus infection also have been reported.[7,17] There is increasing evidence of an association between periodontal and cardiovascular diseases. Periodontitis may be an independent risk factor for cardiovascular disease. One study revealed the presence of *A. actinomycetemcomitans* by polymerase chain reaction (PCR) in atheromatous plaques obtained from carotid endarterectomies.[4] *A. aphrophilus* is also an important cause of brain abscesses.[12]

Most *Aggregatibacter* spp. can be cultured on blood and chocolate agar, but the organisms grow poorly or not at all on MacConkey agar. Some *Aggregatibacter* isolates are cultivatable only on chocolate agar. Cultures require incubation in an enhanced carbon dioxide atmosphere. Since the evolution of continuously monitored blood culture systems with enriched media, extended incubation of blood cultures in cases of HACEK endocarditis is no longer necessary.[13] The standard 5-day incubation for blood culture bottles is sufficient to detect *Aggregatibacter* spp. and other HACEK organisms. On Gram stain, the organism appears coccoid to coccobacillary.

Aggregatibacter spp. are identified in the laboratory using automated systems, miniaturized biochemical methods (e.g., Remel RapID NH System) or matrix-assisted laser desorption ionization time of flight (MALDI-TOF) mass spectrometry. 16S rDNA sequencing of heart valve tissue in cases of culture-negative endocarditis has also been used.[19] Because of the frequency of coinfection with this organism in cases of actinomycosis, attempts always should be made to isolate the organism in these patients.

A. actinomycetemcomitans is typically susceptible to the cephalosporins, rifampin, trimethoprim-sulfamethoxazole, aminoglycosides, quinolones, tetracycline, azithromycin, and chloramphenicol. There has been one case report of a brain abscess successfully treated with prolonged meropenem.[8] *A. actinomycetemcomitans* is also susceptible to penicillin and ampicillin in vitro, but test results do not necessarily correlate with clinical outcomes. Vancomycin, erythromycin, and clindamycin have no activity against this organism. Treatment of aggressive periodontal disease consists of local debridement and antibiotic therapy. Metronidazole and amoxicillin appear to be effective in suppressing *A. actinomycetemcomitans* to below the level of detection.[2]

NEW REFERENCES SINCE THE SEVENTH EDITION

3. Ennibi OK, Benrachadi L, Bouziane A, et al. The highly leukotoxic JP2 clone of *Aggregatibacter actinomycetemcomitans* in localized and generalized forms of aggressive periodontitis. *Acta Odontol Scand*. 2012;70:318-322.
5. Höglund ÅC, Antonoglou G, Haubek D, et al. Cytolethal distending toxin in isolates of *Aggregatibacter actinomycetemcomitans* from Ghanaian adolescents and association with serotype and disease progression. *PLoS ONE*. 2013;8: e65781.
6. Höglund ÅC, Haubek D, Kwamin F, et al. Leukotoxic activity of *Aggregatibacter actinomycetemcomitans* and periodontal attachment loss. *PLoS ONE*. 2014;9: e104095.
8. Maraki S, Papadakis I, Chronakis E, et al. *Aggregatibacter aphrophilus* brain abscess secondary to primary tooth extraction: case report and literature review. *J Microbiol Immunol Infect*. 2016;49:119-122.
11. Nørskov-Lauritsen N. Classification, identification, and clinical significance of *Haemophilus* and *Aggregatibacter* species with host specificity for humans. *Clin Microbiol Rev*. 2014;27:214-240.

12. Rahamat-Langendoen J, van Vonderen M, Engstrom L, et al. Brain abscess associated with *Aggregatibacter actinomycetemcomitans*: case report and review of literature. *J Clin Periodontol.* 2011;38:702-708.
13. Revest M, Egmann G, Cattoir V, et al. HACEK endocarditis: state-of-the-art. *Expert Rev Anti Infect Ther.* 2016;14:523-530.
15. Shaddox L, Huang H, Lin T, et al. Microbiological characterization in children with aggressive periodontitis. *J Dent Res.* 2012;91:927-933.
19. Westling K, Vondracek M. *Actinobacillus (Aggregatibacter) actinomycetemcomitans* (HACEK) identified by PCR/16S rRNA sequence analysis from the heart valve in a patient with blood culture negative endocarditis. *Scand J Infect Dis.* 2008;40:981-983.
20. Yew HT, Chambers ST, Roberts SA, et al. Association between HACEK bacteraemia and endocarditis. *J Med Microbiol.* 2014;63:892-895.

The full reference list for this chapter is available at ExpertConsult.com.

128 Brucellosis

Edward J. Young

Brucellosis is a disease of animals that is transmittable to humans (zoonosis).[98] Humans are accidental hosts, and human-to-human transmission is rare.[113] Brucellosis is distributed worldwide, and it is estimated that 500,000 human cases occur annually.[39,101] Programs to eradicate the disease in animals have reduced the incidence of human infection in many countries; however, brucellosis remains enzootic in large parts of the world.[39,152] Although human brucellosis was once considered rare in childhood, it is now recognized that persons of all ages are susceptible, especially in areas where *Brucella melitensis* is endemic.[133]

HISTORY

Brucellosis was one of many indistinguishable fevers until 1859, when J.A. Marston, a Royal Army Medical Corps (RAMC) physician, provided the first accurate description of the disease among troops stationed on Malta during the Crimean War. He also observed, "When this form of fever attacks children (which it frequently does), it is apt to leave behind it an enlarged condition of the spleen, difficult to remove."[81]

During the 19th century, brucellosis was known by various names, including Mediterranean fever, Malta fever, and undulant fever.[93] Although the disease caused considerable morbidity and mortality among British military personnel stationed throughout the Mediterranean, the cause was not immediately apparent. In 1886, David Bruce, another RAMC surgeon, isolated a microorganism from spleen tissue of victims of Malta fever.[22] Called *Micrococcus melitensis* (later renamed *B. melitensis*), the organism could be found in the blood, urine, and feces of patients with Malta fever. Between 1904 and 1907, Bruce headed the Mediterranean Fever Commission, which studied aspects of the disease in Malta. Themistocles Zammit, a Maltese physician working with the Commission, first identified native goats as the reservoir of brucellosis and their unpasteurized milk as the vehicle of transmission to humans.[143] When fresh goat's milk was replaced with tinned condensed milk in the military mess, the incidence of brucellosis among military personnel declined precipitously.[128] In 1897, Almroth Wright applied the newly devised agglutination assay to the serologic diagnosis of Malta fever.[147]

Unlike *B. melitensis*, which was initially isolated from human tissue, other *Brucella* species were recognized because of the diseases they cause in animals. In 1897, Bernhard Bang, a Danish veterinarian, isolated the "abortion bacillus" (later called *Brucella abortus*) from placental tissue of cattle with contagious abortions. *Brucella suis* was isolated from swine in about 1914 by Jacob Traum at the Bureau of Animal Industry.[63] In 1918, the bacteriologist Alice Evans recognized the relatedness of these disparate bacteria.[49] After Evan's work was confirmed, K.F. Meyer and E.B. Shaw proposed the name *Brucella* for the genus to honor Bruce.[59]

Additional species were isolated from sheep *(Brucella ovis)*, from desert wood rats *(Brucella neotomae)*, and from voles (*Brucella microti*), but none of them have been linked to disease in humans. In 1966, Carmichael and Brunner[26] identified *Brucella canis* as a cause of abortions in kennel-bred dogs; however, it appears to be a rare cause of infection in humans.[144] In the 21st century, previously unrecognized *Brucella* species have been recovered from marine mammals.[21,57,65] Tentatively named *Brucella cetaceae* (dolphin and porpoise isolates) and *Brucella pinnipediae* (seal isolates), their roles as human pathogens remain to be clarified.[32,82,123] Another novel strain of *Brucella (B. inopinata)* was isolated from a woman with an infected breast implant.[41,145] With the availability of molecular genetic techniques, it is likely that additional *Brucella* species will be discovered, and the taxonomy of the genus will need continued revision.[18,51]

ETIOLOGY

The brucellae are small, fastidious, nonmotile, non–spore-forming, gram-negative coccobacilli that lack native plasmids. The outer cell membrane resembles that of other gram-negative bacilli with a dominant lipopolysaccharide (LPS) component. Their metabolism is oxidative, and all strains are aerobic. Some strains require carbon dioxide for growth, especially for primary isolation. Brucellae are always catalase positive, but oxidase activity varies among biovars. Most strains reduce nitrate to nitrite, but some do not. Production of hydrogen sulfide also varies, as does urease activity. A variety of media support the growth of brucellae, including chocolate, trypticase soy, and serum dextrose agars. Growth in vitro is characteristically slow; when brucellosis is suspected, the cultures should not be discarded before 28 days.

Brucellae belong to the α_2-subdivision of the Proteobacteria; they are phylogenetically related to plant pathogens and symbionts such as *Agrobacterium* and *Rhizobium* and to intracellular animal parasites such as *Bartonella* and *Rickettsia*.[33] On the basis of DNA-DNA hybridization and genome sequencing, the genus *Brucella* comprises a single species.[42,60,102] Despite genetic homology greater than 90%, the *Brucella* nomen species show a remarkable preference for certain natural hosts. Consequently, the traditional nomen species classification is retained for epidemiologic purposes (Table 28.1).

EPIDEMIOLOGY

Historically in the United States, brucellosis was linked to the livestock industry, and *B. abortus* was the predominant species causing human illness. Farmers, ranchers, abattoir workers, and veterinarians were at highest risk for infection, usually through direct contact with infected animals. With the virtual elimination of bovine brucellosis by way of test-and-slaughter methods and immunization of susceptible cattle, the epidemiology of brucellosis changed, especially in states that border Mexico. *B. melitensis* replaced *B. abortus* as the major cause of human disease, and foodborne transmission replaced direct contact with animals as the primary mode of infection.[29,138] On the Mexican border, human brucellosis occurs at a rate eight times greater than the national average, and unpasteurized goat's milk cheese is a common

TABLE 28.1 Nomenspecies Classification of *Brucella* spp.

Species	Biovars	Natural Hosts	Pathogenicity for Humans
B. abortus	1-6, 9	Cattle, other Bovidae	Yes
B. melitensis	1-3	Goats, sheep	Yes
B. suis	1-3	Swine	Yes
	4	Reindeer, caribou	Yes
	5	Rodents	Yes
B. canis		Dogs, other canines	Yes
B. neotomae		Desert wood rats	No
B. ovis		Sheep	No
B. pinnipediae		Pinnipeds	Unresolved
B. cetaceae		Cetaceans	Unresolved
B. inopinata		Unresolved	Unresolved (single isolate)
B. microti		Voles, foxes	No

vehicle of transmission.[47,152,158] Human infection caused by *B. suis* has traditionally been an abattoir-associated infection, but in recent years, hunting of feral swine has become a risk when hunters are contaminated with the blood of infected animals.[28,131] Personnel working in clinical or research laboratories are also at risk, and brucellosis continues to be the most commonly reported laboratory-associated bacterial infection.[109,148]

Brucellosis once was thought to be uncommon or mild in children, but susceptibility now is recognized in persons of all ages.[120] Conditions for the transmission of brucellosis from animals to humans vary among countries and cultures. Where farm animals traditionally are raised in the home, contact with children occurs frequently. Foodborne infection is not limited to any age or sex and can occur without direct contact with animals. Childhood brucellosis occurs more commonly in locations where *B. melitensis* is enzootic, and multiple cases often occur within families.[11,79,155]

The clinical manifestations of brucellosis in children are not different from those in adults, although unfamiliarity with the disease can delay the diagnosis.[7,30,121,133] Human-to-human transmission of brucellosis is rare, but venereal transfer has been documented.[113,130] Rare cases associated with blood or bone marrow transplantation have also been reported.[2,5,10] Few cases of brucellosis have been reported in patients infected with the human immunodeficiency virus.[90]

Spontaneous abortion is a common manifestation of brucellosis in animals when brucellae localize within the reproductive organs of both sexes. Brucellosis in pregnant women can lead to abortion if unrecognized and untreated.[111] In a retrospective study from Saudi Arabia, intrauterine death and spontaneous abortion occurred in 46% of 92 women with brucellosis.[70] This rate was significantly higher than the rate of spontaneous abortion in women without brucellosis. When diagnosed early, pregnant women can be treated successfully without compromising their ability to carry to term or to conceive again.[73] On rare occasions, transplacental transmission can lead to neonatal brucellosis.[24,86,91]

PATHOGENESIS

The incubation period for brucellosis varies, but symptoms typically appear within 2 to 3 weeks after infection. Disease caused by *B. melitensis* or *B. suis* tends to be more severe than that caused by *B. abortus* or *B. canis*.[138] Morbidity can be considerable, but death occurs in only about 1% of cases, usually from complications such as neurobrucellosis or endocarditis.[27,152] Although no racial or genetic differences in susceptibility are known in humans, innate immunity has been demonstrated in various animals.[46]

The brucellae lack the usual virulence factors of other bacteria. LPS, the immune-dominant antigen of the cell wall, appears to be the principal mediator of pathogenesis of brucellosis.[25] Although 10 to 100 times less toxic than conventional enterobacterial endotoxins such as *Escherichia coli* toxin brucella LPS functions through the same toll-like receptor 4 (TLR4) pathway and contributes to the organism's ability to survive and replicate within naive mononuclear phagocytes.[76] The distinctive characteristics of *Brucella* LPS containing long-chain fatty acids have been shown to confer stealth pathogenesis by minimizing the host TLR4-mediated innate immune response.[25,76,140]

Although humoral antibodies play some role in resistance to infection, the principal mechanism of recovery involves cellular immunity.[122] Intracellular killing of brucellae occurs when macrophages become activated by specifically committed $CD4^+$ and $CD8^+$ T lymphocytes. This helper T-cell type 1 (Th1) response involves cytokines, including interferon-γ, interleukin-2, and tumor necrosis factor.[149]

CLINICAL MANIFESTATIONS

The spectrum of human brucellosis ranges from subclinical (diagnosed by serology) to chronic (characterized by recurrent symptoms over many years).[156] The disease is characterized by a plethora of nonspecific somatic complaints, such as fatigue, anorexia, nausea, weight loss, sweats, and depression. In contrast, there is a paucity of physical findings, which include fever and occasionally hepatosplenomegaly. The infection can involve any organ or organ system of the body. Sometimes, symptoms related to a single organ predominate, in which case the disease is called *localized*.[36] Localization often involves organs rich in elements of the reticuloendothelial system.

Osteoarticular complications are the most frequent localized manifestations of brucellosis, and in children, symptoms of monoarticular arthritis involving the hips, knees, ankles, and sacroiliac joint predominate.[19,135,137,161] Spondylitis, osteomyelitis, and inflammatory arthropathy have also been described but occur less often in children than adults.[37,125] Despite advances in imaging techniques, serology and culture remain important for diagnosis.[66]

Neurobrucellosis comprises a variety of nervous system complications, including meningitis or encephalitis, myelitis, radiculitis, peripheral and cranial neuropathies, and demyelinating syndromes.[53,58,83,116,141] Vasculitis is common,[156] and rare cases of brain abscess and intracerebral granuloma can mimic a neoplasm of the central nervous system.[48,117] Although most patients complain of headache and weakness, direct invasion of the central nervous system occurs in fewer than 5% of cases.[20,92] Analysis of cerebrospinal fluid (CSF) in cases of *Brucella* meningitis reveals a lymphocytic pleocytosis, elevated protein levels, and normal or low glucose levels. Organisms are rarely seen on Gram stain or cultured from CSF; however, antibodies to *Brucella* are present, and their finding in CSF is diagnostic.[12] Where available, polymerase chain reaction (PCR) assay of CSF can also confirm the diagnosis.[35]

Gastrointestinal complaints are common in uncomplicated brucellosis and include anorexia, nausea, vomiting, abdominal discomfort, and weight loss.[89,119] Rare cases of ileitis,[104] colitis,[67,132] and peritonitis[3] have been reported. As the largest organ of the reticuloendothelial system, the liver is likely always involved in brucellosis even though transaminase levels are only mildly elevated and can be normal.[36,77] Rarely, acute hepatitis occurs with hepatic enzyme levels resembling viral hepatitis.[4] Liver histology in patients infected with *B. abortus* is characterized by epithelioid granulomas indistinguishable from sarcoidosis.[129] In contrast, infection with *B. melitensis* can result in a spectrum of lesions ranging from diffuse hepatitis to granulomas.[150,153,157] Infection with *B. suis* and *B. melitensis* can also result in a suppurative abscess that may become chronic.[17,38,142]

Genitourinary tract involvement usually manifests as orchitis or epididymo-orchitis and can be mistaken for testicular cancer.[61,95] Rare cases of interstitial nephritis, membranous nephropathy, and glomerulonephritis also have been reported.[160]

Respiratory tract localization of brucellosis is reported in about 7% of cases.[97,100,136] Lung lesions attributed to *Brucella* include hilar adenopathy, lobar pneumonia, lung nodules, pleural effusion, and thoracic empyema.[78] Pleural fluid adenosine deaminase levels may be elevated but are difficult to distinguish from those of tuberculosis.[44]

Cardiovascular lesions of brucellosis include endocarditis, myocarditis, pericarditis, and aneurysms of the aorta and cerebral blood vessels.[107] Native and prosthetic valve forms of endocarditis have been described, with the aortic valve involved most often.[43,64] Delays in making a diagnosis can result in life-threatening complications, such as valve rupture, myocardial abscess, and sinus of Valsalva fistulas. Treatment of *Brucella* endocarditis usually requires antibiotics plus valve replacement surgery.[69,118]

Ocular lesions, most notably uveitis, have been described in patients with brucellosis. Other eye lesions that have been reported include endophthalmitis, optic neuritis, episcleritis, nummular keratitis, and chorioretinitis. The pathogenesis of some lesions is a matter of conjecture because brucellae are rarely isolated from the eye.[68,110,134]

Cutaneous lesions attributed to brucellosis include contact dermatitis, rashes, abscess, and vasculitis.[87,88] Occasionally, brucellae have been cultured from subcutaneous papules[79] and from abscesses.[108] Rarely, brucellosis can result in myositis.[71,72] Mastitis caused by *Brucella* is not unusual in animals, and it has recently been recognized in humans.[41,96]

Hematologic abnormalities such as anemia, leukopenia, and thrombocytopenia are common in the course of brucellosis.[31,40] These changes typically are mild and resolve promptly with antimicrobial therapy. Occasionally, thrombocytopenia can be severe, resulting in hemorrhage into the skin and from mucosal sites.[159] The cause of this complication is likely multifactorial, including hypersplenism, disseminated intravascular coagulation, bone marrow suppression and hemophagocytosis, and immune mechanisms.

DIAGNOSIS

Because the symptoms of brucellosis are nonspecific, the importance of obtaining a detailed history, including occupation, avocations, travel, animal exposure, and food habits, cannot be overemphasized. Routine laboratory tests usually are not helpful, but in the right setting, characteristic hematologic findings (i.e., normal or low white blood cell count) can suggest the possibility of brucellosis.[8]

A definitive diagnosis of brucellosis is made by isolating a specific species of *Brucella* from blood, bone marrow, or other tissue. The rate of positive blood cultures varies from 15% to 70%, depending on the methods used and the period of in vitro incubation.[56,115] Bone marrow culture is reported to be more sensitive than blood cultures before the introduction of newer isolation techniques.[45,85] Nucleic acid amplification tests using a variety of gene sequences are being applied with some success to the rapid diagnosis of brucellosis.[6,55,94,106,146]

In the absence of bacteriologic confirmation, a presumptive diagnosis can be made by measuring the titer of specific antibodies in serum.[151] Human brucellosis is characterized by an initial production of immunoglobulin M (IgM) antibodies followed by a switch to IgG synthesis within the second week of infection. Treatment results in a gradual decline in both antibody isotypes; however, the persistence of IgG antibodies is associated with relapse or chronic infection.[103] The pattern of immunoglobulin isotypes is important for differentiating active from treated disease.[52,151] This is accomplished by performing the serum agglutination test (SAT) in tandem with 2-mercaptoethanol or dithiothreitol; the latter are disulfide-reducing agents used to block agglutinability by IgM while preserving agglutination by IgG.[23,151] Alternatively, a more direct way to measure IgM and IgG antibodies is the indirect enzyme-linked immunosorbent assay (ELISA) employing anti-IgM and anti-IgG conjugates.[80,84] Because of problems with commercial IgM enzyme assays, the Centers for Disease Control and Prevention recommends that positive ELISA results be confirmed by agglutination.[28]

Most serologic tests for brucellosis employ smooth lipopolysaccharide (S-LPS) that can detect antibodies to all smooth species (e.g., *B. abortus, B. melitensis, B. suis*). Because *B. canis* is naturally rough (i.e., lacks S-LPS), antibodies to this organism require a test using antigen prepared from a rough species (*B. canis* or *B. ovis*).[105] A variety of other cell wall or cytoplasmic proteins have been studied as potential serodiagnostic antigens,[54] but none has proved superior to LPS-based assays. A latex agglutination assay using S-LPS has been shown to be simple to run, to be rapid, and to have good sensitivity and specificity.[1]

TREATMENT

Antimicrobial therapy lessens morbidity, shortens the course of illness, and reduces the incidence of complications of brucellosis.[154] Many drugs are active against *Brucella* spp., but the results of in vitro sensitivity tests do not always correlate with clinical effectiveness. Because the rate of relapse with single-drug therapy is high, successful treatment requires combination therapy for a prolonged time.[126,154] The tetracyclines remain the most effective antibiotics against brucellae with minimal inhibitory concentrations less than 1 μg/mL. In vitro killing of brucellae by numerous antibiotics can be enhanced by the addition of an aminoglycoside (i.e., streptomycin or gentamicin).[114] Traditionally, the combination of tetracycline administered for 6 weeks plus streptomycin given for 2 to 3 weeks provided the highest cure rates in patients with brucellosis.[13] Currently, the preferred regimen is doxycycline (200 mg/day given orally for 45 days) plus gentamicin (5 mg/kg per day) as a single daily intramuscular dose for the first 7 to 10 days.[14,112,124]

Rifampin also shows good in vitro activity against *Brucella* spp., and in 1986, the World Health Organization (WHO) recommended the combination of doxycycline (200 mg/day) plus rifampin (600–900 mg/day) orally for 45 days as the treatment of choice. Although successful for uncomplicated brucellosis, subsequent studies have shown the superiority of the combination of doxycycline plus an aminoglycoside, especially for osteoarticular complications.[16,127]

Children older than 8 years can be treated similar to adults; however, because tetracycline is contraindicated for children younger than 8 years and for pregnant women, alternative treatments have been sought.[139] Trimethoprim-sulfamethoxazole (TMP-SMX) in a fixed combination of 80 mg of TMP and 400 mg of SMX (i.e., cotrimoxazole) given twice daily for 45 days plus gentamicin (5 mg/kg/day) as a single daily dose for 7 days has yielded satisfactory results.[120] Alternatively, the combination of TMP-SMX plus rifampin (15 mg/kg) once daily administered for 6 or 8 weeks gave comparable results.[112] Similarly, pregnant women can be treated successfully with TMP-SMX plus rifampin without adverse drug effects on the newborn.[70]

The quinolones are active against *Brucella* spp. in vitro, but the minimal inhibitory concentration values vary for each compound and, to some extent, for *Brucella* isolates.[50] In clinical practice, however, the results have been disappointing.[74,75,154] Consequently, quinolones are not recommended as monotherapy for treating brucellosis, and their role in combination therapy awaits well-designed clinical trials.

The optimal treatment of complications of brucellosis such as meningitis and endocarditis has not been defined with certainty.[99] Doxycycline crosses the blood-brain barrier more effectively than generic tetracycline, and it has been used in combination with other drugs (e.g., rifampin, TMP-SMX) for neurobrucellosis.[83,92] Third-generation cephalosporins achieve high concentrations in CSF, but the sensitivity of brucellae varies and, in general, β-lactam drugs are not effective when used alone.[74] Some patients with *Brucella* endocarditis have been treated successfully with the usual antibiotic combination; however, most cases have required additional valve replacement surgery.[9] For both complications, prolonged therapy is advised.

RELAPSE AND CHRONIC BRUCELLOSIS

Most patients with brucellosis recover completely within a few weeks to months after receiving adequate therapy. Despite appropriate treatment, some patients suffer a relapse characterized by recurrence of symptoms and repeat isolation of brucellae from their blood.[15] Relapse is more common if the full course of treatment is not completed, and taking oral antibiotics for 6 weeks can tax a patient's compliance. With few exceptions, relapse is *not* caused by antibiotic-resistant strains of *Brucella*.[13,62]

Even with appropriate treatment, some patients experience a delayed recovery and continue to have nonspecific complaints, notably fatigue. These patients have no objective evidence of infection (e.g., fever), and their antibody titers decline as expected. Whether this represents a variant of the chronic fatigue syndrome is not clear, but additional antibiotic therapy does not improve recovery.[34] Rarely, chronic brucellosis results from a persistent focus of infection such as osteomyelitis or a deep tissue abscess. These patients have fever or other objective signs of infection, and levels of IgG antibodies in the serum remain elevated. Scanning techniques (e.g., scintigraphy with technetium-99m or gallium-67, computed tomography, magnetic resonance imaging) can be useful in localizing an occult focus of infection.

NEW REFERENCES SINCE THE SEVENTH EDITION

18. Banai M, Corbel M. Taxonomy of *Brucella*. *Open Vet Sci J*. 2010;4:85-101.
19. Bosilkovski M, Urosevic VK, Cekovska Z, et al. Osteoarticular involvement in childhood brucellosis: experience with 133 cases in an endemic region. *Pediatr Infect Dis J*. 2013;32:815-819.
28. Centers for Disease Control and Prevention (CDC). Public health consequences of a false-positive laboratory test result for *Brucella*—Florida, Georgia, and Michigan, 2005. *MMWR Morb Mortal Wkly Rep*. 2008;57:603-605.
51. Ficht T. *Brucella* taxonomy and evolution. *Future Microbiol*. 2010;5:859-866.
62. Hasanjani Roushan MR, Moulana Z, Mohseni Afshar Z, et al. Risk factors for relapse of human brucellosis. *Global J Health Sci*. 2015;8:77-82.
71. Kraniotis P, Marangos M, Lekkou A, et al. Brucellosis presenting as piriformis myositis: a case report. *J Med Case Rep*. 2011;5:125-129.
72. Kojan S, Alothman A, Althani Z, et al. Granulomatous myositis associated with brucellosis: a case report and literature review. *Muscle Nerve*. 2012;45:290-293.
86. Mesner O, Eiesenberg K, Bilar N, et al. The many faces of human-to-human transmission of brucellosis: congenital infection and outbreak of nosocomial disease related to an unrecognized clinical case. *Clin Infect Dis*. 2007;45:e135-e140.
96. Nemenqani D, Yaqoob N, Khoja H. Breast brucellosis in Taif, Saudi Arabia: cluster of six cases with emphasis on FNA evaluation. *J Infect Dev Ctries*. 2009;3:255-259.
140. Tsolis RM, Young GM, Solnic JV, et al. From bench to bedside: stealth of enteroinvasive pathogens. *Nat Rev Microbiol*. 2008;6:883-892.
157. Young EJ, Hasanjani Roushan MR, Shafae S, et al. Liver histology of acute brucellosis caused by *Brucella melitensis*. *Human Pathol*. 2014;45:2023-2028.

The full reference list for this chapter is available at ExpertConsult.com.

Pertussis and Other *Bordetella* Infections 129

James D. Cherry • Ulrich Heininger

Pertussis (i.e., whooping cough) is an acute infectious illness of the respiratory tract caused by *Bordetella pertussis* and, less frequently, by *Bordetella parapertussis* and *Bordetella holmesii*.[89,95,113,123,256,367,399,428,452,617] The illness occurs worldwide and affects all age groups, but it is recognized most often in children, and it is most serious in young, unprotected infants.[89,106,113,142,251,367,414,426,427,602]

Pertussis due to *B. pertussis* infection is a truly unique contagious respiratory disease.[109,105,121,269,355,367] The illness (unless complicated by a concomitant or secondary infection) is noninflammatory in nature, and it occurs without significant fever. The paroxysmal cough is different from the cough in all other infectious diseases; it is nonproductive (except for posttussive phlegm), and it is followed by periods of total respiratory normalcy.

HISTORY

Unlike other severe epidemic infectious diseases of children (e.g., smallpox, poliomyelitis, measles), pertussis lacks an ancient history.[269] The first observation of pertussis occurred in France in 1414, and the first epidemic was reported in Paris in 1578.[113,131,319] This epidemic and the clinical characteristics of the cases were described in 1640 by Guillaume de Baillou.

Pertussis was described as the *kink* (a Scottish term synonymous with "fit" or "paroxysm") and *kindhoest* (a Teutonic word meaning "child's cough") in the Middle Ages.[98,269] In 1669, Sydenham named the illness *pertussis* (meaning "violent cough").[319] Isolation of *B. pertussis,* the main causative agent of pertussis, was reported by Bordet and Gengou in 1906.[49,50]

Vaccines consisting of killed, whole *B. pertussis* organisms were developed soon after the bacterium was isolated, and the first results of protection were reported by Madsen in 1925.[352] The mouse protection test, developed and reported by Kendrick and collaborators[298] in 1947, allowed vaccine production to be standardized. Comprehensive studies conducted by the British Medical Research Council[376] in the 1940s and 1950s demonstrated a correlation between the potency of pertussis vaccines as determined by the mouse protection test and their clinical efficacy in children. As a consequence, immunization against pertussis, most commonly in combination with diphtheria and tetanus toxoids (i.e., DTP vaccine), became part of routine vaccination programs in many countries throughout the world.

Concern about a relationship between pertussis vaccination and temporally associated serious adverse events (i.e., sudden infant death syndrome [SIDS] and a variety of neurologic illnesses) led to a sharp decline in vaccination rates in Japan and several European countries during the 1970s.[89,95,109,113,303] Along with well-documented high rates of unpleasant local effects (e.g., swelling, induration) and systemic reactions (mainly fever), concerns about adverse events led to the development of acellular vaccines.

During the 20th century, *B. pertussis* was extensively studied in animal model systems, and many toxins and protective antigens were described.[109,367,379] A leader in *B. pertussis* research was Margaret Pittman, who was at the National Institutes of Health (NIH) and Food and Drug Administration (FDA) from 1936 to 1990. She published two papers about pertussis toxin (PT) and the concept that pertussis was a toxin-mediated disease.[453,455] Pittman's views led to the idea that less reactogenic acellular vaccines could be produced. Sato, who trained at NIH and FDA and was influenced by Pittman, returned to Japan and with colleagues developed the first acellular vaccines (i.e., DTaP vaccines).[109,494] His goal was to produce a PT toxoid vaccine, but the initial vaccines developed in Japan contained (in addition to toxoided PT) filamentous hemagglutinin (FHA), pertactin (PRN), and fimbria 2 (FIM 2). Although evidence exists that pertussis is not a PT-only illness, the idea persists.[473,474,552] The most compelling evidence that pertussis from *B. pertussis* infection is not a PT disease is that an identical illness results from infection with *B. parapertussis*, which does not express PT.[92,256]

In the 1980s, several DTaP vaccines were developed, and phase 2 studies were carried out. In the early 1990s, eight efficacy trials were carried out in Europe and Senegal. The trial vaccines contained different concentrations of one to five antigens. However, all of them were virtually free of lipopolysaccharide (LPS) (i.e., endotoxin), and they were less reactogenic than the whole-cell DTP vaccines. Acellular vaccines (i.e., DTaP vaccines) have been used in Japan since 1981 and in many developed countries since the mid-1990s.[70,168,244,303,583]

B. bronchiseptica, which causes illness with a cough in several animals and in humans, was first isolated in about 1910 by Ferry[181], McGowan,[372] and perhaps others who were studying dogs with distemper.[367] *B. parapertussis* was isolated first from children with pertussis in the 1930s, and *Bordetella holmesii* was found in nasopharyngeal specimens from patients with pertussis-like illnesses in Massachusetts from 1995 through 1998.[52,171,170,368,617]

MICROBIOLOGY

The genus *Bordetella* contains 10 species: *B. pertussis, B. parapertussis*$_{hu}$ (adapted to humans), *B. parapertussis*$_{ov}$ (ovine-adapted), *B. bronchiseptica, Bordetella avium, Bordetella hinzii, B. holmesii, Bordetella trematum, B. ansorpii,* and *Bordetella petrii.*[137,217,256,299,309,367] *B. pertussis* infects exclusively humans. *B. parapertussis* is a human pathogen, but it has also been

TABLE 129.1 Selected Differential Characteristics of *Bordetella* Species That Cause Respiratory Illnesses in Humans

	CHARACTERISTIC				
Organism	**Catalase**	**Oxidase**	**Nitrate Reduction**	**Urease Production**	**Motility**
B. pertussis	+	+	−	−	−
B. parapertussis	+	−	−	+	−
B. bronchiseptica	+	+	+	+	+
B. holmesii	+[a]	−	−	−	−

+, Activity; −, not present.
[a]Results for 10% to 89% of strains are positive.
From Wirsing von Konig CH, Riffelmann M, Coenye T. *Bordetella* and related genera. In: Versalovic J, ed. *Manual of Clinical Microbiology, vol 1.* Washington, DC: ASM Press; 1970:739–50.

recovered from sheep (i.e., ovine strains).[456] Both *B. pertussis* and *B. parapertussis* are respiratory pathogens. *B. bronchiseptica* is primarily an animal pathogen that causes atrophic rhinitis and pneumonia in pigs, kennel cough in dogs, pneumonia in cats, and respiratory illnesses in other animals.[137,206,536] This organism also is the occasional cause of respiratory illness in humans.[51,126,149,219,424,519,536,537,612] *B. avium* is an important cause of respiratory illness in turkeys and other birds.[300]

In addition to *B. pertussis*, *B. parapertussis*, and *B. bronchiseptica*, five other species have been recognized to infect or colonize humans.* *B. holmesii* and *B. hinzii* have been isolated from blood cultures, primarily in patients with underlying chronic illness. *B. holmesii* also has been isolated from the human respiratory tract, as has *B. hinzii* and *B. petrii* in patients with cystic fibrosis, and *B. trematum* has been found in wounds and ear infections. *B. ansorpii* has been isolated from a cyst in an immunocompromised 19-year-old girl.[309] *B. petrii* has been isolated from the environment and is capable of anaerobic growth.[573]

The genus *Bordetella* consists of gram-negative, pleomorphic, aerobic bacilli that are grouped together on the basis of genotypic characteristics; species are differentiated by phenotypic characteristics. Selected differential characteristics of the four *Bordetella* spp. that cause respiratory illnesses in humans are given in Table 129.1. All species have relatively simple requirements, but *B. pertussis* is quite fastidious and is inhibited by constituents in common laboratory media such as fatty acids, metal ions, sulfides, and peroxides.[563,605] For laboratory growth, *B. pertussis* requires the addition of protective substances such as charcoal, blood, or starch. Other species are less fastidious and may grow in blood or MacConkey agars.

More than a decade ago, the genomes of representative strains of *B. pertussis, B. parapertussis,* and *B. bronchiseptica* were sequenced.[68,446,460] The genome sizes are as follows: *B. pertussis* has 4,086,186 base pairs (bp); *B. parapertussis* has 4,773,551 bp; and *B. bronchiseptica* has 5,338,400 bp. *B. pertussis* has 3816 predicted genes, whereas *B. parapertussis* and *B. bronchiseptica* have 4404 and 5007 predicted genes, respectively. Pseudogenes occur most commonly in *B. pertussis* (358) and *B. parapertussis* (220) and are uncommon in *B. bronchiseptica* (18). *B. pertussis* has three insertion sequence (IS) elements: IS 481 (238 copies), IS 1002 (6 copies), and IS 1663 (17 copies). *B. parapertussis* has IS 1001 (22 copies) and IS 1002 (90 copies). The sequenced *B. bronchiseptica* RB50 strain contained no IS elements, but studies of other *B. bronchiseptica* strains found strains with IS 481, IS 1001, and IS 1663.[157,192,344,468,546] Recently, the genomes of other *B. pertussis* strains and strains of *B. holmesii, B. avium,* and *B. hinzii* have been sequenced.[240,403,445,467]

ETIOLOGY OF PERTUSSIS (WHOOPING COUGH)

B. pertussis and *B. parapertussis* are the usual etiologic agents of pertussis, but 86% to 95% of illnesses are caused by *B. pertussis.*[123,208,256,459] In rare instances, *B. bronchiseptica,* which normally is enzootic in pigs, dogs, cats, rodents, and other animals, has been isolated from humans with pertussis-like illnesses.[51,126,149,219,424,519,536,537,612] From 1995 to 1998, *B. holmesii* was isolated from the nasopharynx of 33 individuals in Massachusetts with suspected pertussis; most of them were adolescents or young adults.[368] Since then, *B. holmesii* has been identified by polymerase chain reaction (PCR) from the nasopharynx of coughing patients in an increasing number of countries.[451,452] Unlike all other *Bordetella* spp., this organism is susceptible to cephalexin, an antibiotic that frequently is added to *Bordetella* culture media.[431] This addition may explain why the organism was not previously identified in patients with pertussis in culture-based laboratory studies.

Adenoviruses have been isolated from children with pertussis, and some researchers have suggested that several adenoviral types may on occasion cause a pertussis-like illness.[26,130,132,420] However, the data of Nelson and associates[420] and Baraff and coworkers,[26] as well as our own observations, lead us to suggest that mixed infections are occurring and that the classic symptoms are caused by *B. pertussis* and not by infection with an adenovirus. Similarly, coinfection with respiratory syncytial virus (RSV) may occur, but the classic symptoms are caused by *B. pertussis.*[245] Wirsing von König and associates[606] observed pertussis-like illnesses caused by viral or *Mycoplasma pneumoniae* infections in 83 patients for whom pertussis laboratory studies were negative. The authors serologically identified 33 adenoviral illnesses, 18 illnesses caused by parainfluenza viruses, 15 illnesses caused by *M. pneumoniae,* and 14 caused by RSV. Wang and colleagues[577] retrospectively studied prolonged illness with cough in 179 children and found that 37% had evidence of *B. pertussis* infection and 13% had *M. pneumoniae* infections. The cough duration in those with *M. pneumoniae* was significantly shorter (median, 39 days) than in children with *B. pertussis* infections (median, 118 days). In young infants, coinfection with an adenovirus and perhaps RSV may lead to more severe disease.[36,328] Zouari and associates[624] identified *B. pertussis* and *M. pneumoniae* coinfections in three fatal cases in young infants.

Infection with human bocavirus also may cause an illness with a paroxysmal cough.[19] Of 54 children with laboratory-confirmed bocavirus infections, 85% had cough and 19% had paroxysmal coughing episodes.

Physicians often suggest that *Chlamydia trachomatis* can cause a pertussis-like illness. However, the repetitive cough of *C. trachomatis* is distinctly different from the paroxysmal cough of *B. pertussis* infection, and illnesses caused by the two agents usually should not be confused clinically. Infections with *Chlamydia pneumoniae* and *M. pneumoniae* also cause long-lasting illness with cough.[145,228,571,606] Although infection with these agents in older children and adults can be confused with *B. pertussis* infection, true paroxysms typical of pertussis rarely occur.

ANTIGENIC AND BIOLOGICALLY ACTIVE COMPONENTS OF *BORDETELLA PERTUSSIS*

B. pertussis contains a variety of components that are thought to be antigenic or biologically active.* All known virulence factors produced

*References 20, 135, 146, 161, 193, 194, 239, 279, 292, 294, 296, 322, 337, 341, 368, 398, 399, 418, 420, 444, 516, 518, 541, 561, 594, 617.

*References 1, 13, 14, 17, 29, 62, 105, 92, 113, 121, 137, 139, 179, 204, 237, 241, 244, 258, 260, 264–266, 284, 299, 342, 343, 349, 354, 359, 360, 365, 367, 387, 400, 421, 438, 495, 506, 555, 558, 569, 575, 589, 597, 621.

TABLE 129.2 Biologically Active and Antigenic Components of *Bordetella pertussis* That Have a Role in Human Infections or Illness

Component	Characteristic
Pertussis toxin (PT) (i.e., lymphocytosis-promoting factor)	A classic bacterial toxin with an enzymatically active A subunit and a B oligomer-binding protein; effects in an animal model system include histamine sensitization, promotion of lymphocytosis, stimulation of insulin secretion, and adjuvant and mitogenic activity; the envelope protein is also an important adhesin; it adversely affects host immune cell function
Adenylate cyclase toxin (ACT)	Calmodulin-activated RTX[a] family toxin with dual adenylate cyclase and hemolysin activity; acts as an antiphagocytic factor during infection
Fimbriae (FIMs)	Serologic types 2 and 3; antibody to specific types causes agglutination of the organism; organisms may contain FIM 2, FIM 3, FIMs 2 and 3, or neither form
Filamentous hemagglutinin (FHA)	220-kd surface-associated and secreted protein; highly immunogenic
Lipopolysaccharide (LPS) (i.e., endotoxin)	An enveloped toxin with activities similar to endotoxins of other gram-negative bacteria; a significant cause of reactions to whole-cell pertussis vaccines; antibody to LPS causes agglutination of the organism
Autotransporters	
Pertactin (PRN)	69-kd outer-membrane protein that allows the organism to resist neutrophil-mediated clearance; antibody to pertactin causes agglutination of the organism
Vag8	95-kd outer-membrane protein
BrkA	73-kd surface-associated N-terminal passenger domain with 30-kd outer-membrane C-terminal protein; confers serum resistance and protection against antimicrobial peptides in *B. pertussis*
SphB1	Subtilisin-like Ser protease or lipoprotein required for FHA maturation
Tracheal colonization factor (i.e., *tcfA* gene product)	60-kd secreted protein

[a]The RTX toxin superfamily is a group of cytolysins and cytotoxins produced by bacteria. The name RTX (i.e., repeats in toxin) refers to the glycine- and aspartate-rich repeats at the C-terminus that facilitate toxin export.

by *B. pertussis* are regulated by the single genetic locus *bvgAS*.[137] Under certain conditions, such as an environmental temperature of 37°C, *bvgAS* is active, toxins and biologically active surface proteins are produced, and the organism is virulent in a mouse model (i.e., bvg^+ phase). In the bvg^- phase, a different set of genes (i.e., *vrg* and *vir* repressed genes) are expressed, and *B. pertussis* is avirulent in mice in this phase.[588] The switch from bvg^+ to bvg^- is a phenomenon common to all *Bordetella* spp. and is associated with a change in phenotype. An intermediate phase with reduced virulence and expression of specific proteins also has been characterized. It has been speculated that the intermediate phase may have some function in transmission of the organism.[137,525] Since its original isolation in 1906, *B. pertussis* has been extensively studied by microbiologists, molecular microbiologists, epidemiologists, and clinicians.[49,106,109,121,367,379,444] Vast numbers of studies were carried out in mice. Of most importance were the studies of what now is called PT during the past 65 years. During the past 45 years, additional biologically active proteins, which were thought to be virulence factors, were discovered. The various alleged toxins and virulence factors have been described on numerous occasions, including the previous edition of this textbook. However, we have come to realize that many of the biologically active proteins or toxins that were studied in mice do not have a clear role in human infection or illness.

Antigenic factors or toxins that are thought to have no significant roles in human infections or illnesses are filamentous hemagglutinin (FHA), the type III secretion system, dermonecrotic toxin (DNT), and tracheal cytotoxin (TCT). Significant biologically active proteins of *B. pertussis* are listed in Table 129.2.

Pertussis Toxin

PT is an adenosine diphosphate–ribosylating toxin that is synthesized and secreted exclusively by *B. pertussis.* It is an A-B toxin with an enzymatically active A subunit (S_1) and a B oligomer ($S_{2\text{-}5}$) binding portion.* PT inactivates G proteins, a process that disrupts signaling pathways and leads to histamine sensitization, enhancement of insulin secretion in response to regulatory signals, and suppressive and stimulatory immunologic effects in animal model systems.[367]

The various effects of PT in animal model systems and in humans have been reviewed in depth by Cherry.[113,367] In contrast to animal studies, histamine sensitization does not appear to occur in children, but PT does cause an increase in plasma insulin levels.[113,367] PT also is responsible for leukocytosis with lymphocytosis in *B. pertussis* infections. PT is a strong adjuvant in several immunologic systems in animals, but in DTP-vaccinated persons (who have received small amounts of active toxin in the vaccine), only the enhancement of serum antibody responses to antigens of other vaccines has been demonstrated. In mouse and rat models, PT inhibits chemotaxis and migration of neutrophils, monocytes or macrophages, and lymphocytes to infection sites, and PT functions as an adhesin in the adherence of *B. pertussis* to human macrophages and ciliated respiratory epithelial cells.

PT contributes to morbidity in *B. pertussis* infections, as indicated by the severity of illness, which tends to be greater than that caused by *B. parapertussis* infection. The frequent finding of extreme leukocytosis caused by PT in neonates and young infants with fatal pertussis is noteworthy.[122,367,414,426,427,443,602]

Adenylate Cyclase Toxin

Adenylate cyclase toxin (ACT) is an extracytoplasmic enzyme that impairs host immune cell function.[62,113,137,266,302,367,569,590] ACT enters phagocytic cells (particularly polymorphonuclear neutrophils), where it is activated by calmodulin and catalyzes the production of supraphysiologic amounts of cyclic adenosine monophosphate from adenosine triphosphate, which intoxicates these cells.[367]

Fimbriae

Fimbriae (FIM) are protein projections on the surface of *B. pertussis.*[367,394,401,459,477,478] They are highly immunogenic, and antibody to them and to other antigens causes agglutination of the organism. Two fimbrial antigens (i.e., FIM 2 and 3) are the main agglutinogens; LPS and PRN also are agglutinogens.[92,477]

In the past, typing of *B. pertussis* strains was based on the agglutination patterns observed with specific antisera.[92,169,459,477] Six specific agglutinogens were recognized, and typing was based on the presence or absence

*References 13, 14, 17, 18, 63, 113, 137, 196, 285, 325, 343, 367, 454, 453, 557.

of agglutination with each specific antiserum. Researchers later recognized that two of the agglutinogens (i.e., agglutinogens 2 and 3) are fimbrial in location (i.e., FIM 2 and FIM 3) and that agglutinogens 4, 5, and 6 are minor antigens.[459,477] All *B. pertussis* strains contain agglutinogen 1; the nature of this agglutinogen is unknown.[477] It could be LPS or PRN, but because the original serotyping scheme was based on heat-labile antigens, it probably was not LPS.[53,329,543]

The fimbriae function as adhesins, but some studies suggest that they are not the primary adhesins in infection but serve to sustain the attachment established by other attachment factors.[113,478,555,589] An in vitro study by Rodriguez and associates[479] suggested that the effect of antibody to fimbriae on attachment was the result of bacterial agglutination. In the mouse model system, immunization with purified fimbriae resulted in protection against infection when challenged with *B. pertussis*.[293] Data from two trials in which serologic correlates of immunity were studied indicated that antibody to fimbriae is important in protection.[114,529]

Filamentous Hemagglutinin

FHA is a component of the cell wall of all *Bordetella* species.[1,43,113,137,260,304,354,367,555,569] It is highly immunogenic and is the dominant attachment factor for *Bordetella* in animal model systems.[367,495,505] However, because FHA is released in large amounts from the cell surface, its role as an adhesin must be questioned. Adhesins typically remain associated with the bacterial surface to promote maximum attachment. FHA is a component of most acellular component vaccines (i.e., DTaP and Tdap).[167] However, the importance of antibody to FHA and protection from disease is not clear. Some data indicated that the efficacy of vaccines containing both PT and FHA was greater than that of a vaccine containing only toxoided PT.[527] However, the PT/FHA-containing vaccines also likely contained some PRN and FIM 2. In two studies in which serologic correlates of immunity were evaluated, FHA made no contribution to protection.[114,529] One whole-cell component DTP vaccine in which vaccinees did not mount an antibody response to FHA was nonetheless highly efficacious.[249,520]

Autotransporters

Pertactin

PRN is a 69-kd outer-membrane protein that plays an important role in *B. pertussis* pathogenesis by allowing the organism to resist neutrophil-mediated clearance.[43,284,325,431,432] Antibody to PRN has a strong protective effect in aerosol-challenge studies in mice.[87,506] In the two vaccine efficacy trials in which serologic correlates of immunity were evaluated, researchers found that antibody to PRN was most important in protection.[114,529] In the vaccine efficacy trials conducted in the 1990s, in which mild disease and typical disease were evaluated, DTaP vaccines that contained PRN in addition to PT and FHA were significantly more effective.[96,120,222,367] Another study revealed that anti-PRN antibodies were required for efficient phagocytosis of *B. pertussis* by host immune cells.[259] A recent disturbing finding is the circulation of PRN-deficient mutants in the United States.[361,447]

Other Autotransporters

In addition to PRN, 16 other autotransporters are encoded in the genome of *B. pertussis*.[446] Four that have been studied in animal models are described in Table 129.2.[1] All likely play an important active role in *B. pertussis* infection by interfering with the innate immune response.

Lipopolysaccharide (Endotoxin)

The LPS of *B. pertussis* is somewhat similar to the endotoxins of other gram-negative bacteria.[85,113,137] Its function in disease is unknown, but it may act as an adhesin.[149] LPS is a major cause of reactions to whole-cell pertussis vaccines.[23] LPS is a significant agglutinogen. Antibody to LPS reduces colonization of *B. pertussis* in the lungs and trachea of mice after aerosol challenge.[409]

Polysaccharide Capsule

A *B. pertussis* capsule was identified in the prevaccine era but confirmed only recently.[423] Conover and associates[133] and Ganguly and associates[199] studied the capsule and found it functions in adhesion and protects against complement-mediated killing.

EPIDEMIOLOGY

Pertussis is an extremely infectious disease with an estimated R_0 of 12 to 17. R_0 is the expected number of secondary cases produced by a typical primary case in an entirely susceptible population.[11,116,182]

Considerable misinformation has been circulating with regard to the epidemiology of pertussis.[55,56,106,109,105,324,480,481,586] The main reason for misinformation is failure to recognize the significant differences in the dynamics of reported pertussis compared with *B. pertussis* infections.[101,99] Reported clinical pertussis and *B. pertussis* infection have different epidemiologies.

Reported Pertussis Cases

Rates of reported pertussis depend on surveillance programs in the reporting countries, states, or counties.[539] For example, in Switzerland and three bordering countries (i.e., Germany, Italy, and Austria), the rates of reported pertussis for 1998 to 2002 varied by as much as 70-fold.[65] Because of the proximity of the four countries and the fact that their immunization practices were somewhat similar, the rate differences are explained by the rigorousness of the respective surveillance programs and not by any unique epidemiology by country.

Incidence

The incidence of reported pertussis and its mortality rate are affected markedly by the use of pertussis vaccine. In the prevaccine era in the United States, the average attack rate of reported pertussis was 157 cases per 100,000 people.[89]

After the introduction and widespread use of pertussis vaccines, the attack rate of reported pertussis in the United States fell approximately 150-fold between 1943 and 1976. For the 7-year period from 1976 to 1982, the attack rate in the United States remained between 0.5 and 1.0 case per 100,000 people. From 1982 to 2015, the attack rate curve shifted modestly upward and reached a rate of 15.2 cases per 100,000 in 2012 (Fig. 129.1). In 2012, there were 48,277 cases of reported pertussis; this was the largest number of reported cases in the United States since 1955. Possible reasons for the resurgence of reported pertussis cases are (1) increased vaccine failures resulting from genetic changes in *B. pertussis,* (2) increased vaccine failures related to vaccines of lessened potency, (3) waning immunity, (4) greater awareness of pertussis, and (5) the availability of better laboratory tests.[101,99,120,123,128,212,222] Among these possibilities, we think that greater awareness is the most important.

In the early 1980s, much attention was given to real and perceived reactions to DTP vaccines; later in the decade, there were many reports about the development of DTaP vaccines.* In the 1990s, the efficacy trials with DTaP vaccines were carried out and resulted in numerous publications and general overall pertussis awareness.†

In the current decade, there has been much attention to the general inferiority of DTaP vaccines compared with DTP vaccines.‡

Use of PCR is also important for diagnosis.[122] PCR is considerably more sensitive than culture and is less likely to be adversely affected by delay in getting specimens to the laboratory. Single-serum serologic testing for pertussis is the preferred method for confirming pertussis in adults. The number of cases and the attack rate among adolescents and adults will increase when single-serum serologic diagnosis becomes routine.[124] Data indicate that waning immunity is a major factor.§

Fig. 129.1 shows two periods. During the first period, the increase in cases correlates mainly with increased awareness. In addition to increased awareness, the sharp peaks in 2004 to 2005 and in 2010, 2012, and 2014 are most likely due to DTaP vaccine failure, waning immunity, and the use of PCR and single-serum serology for diagnosis.

There has been considerable debate regarding the role of genetic change as a cause of vaccine failure.[124,153,401,433,500] Over time, genetic changes in PT, PRN, and fimbriae have occurred. In 1965, Preston[458]

*References 4, 6, 22, 23, 25, 37, 109, 90, 91, 92, 113, 129, 303, 350, 351, 384, 388, 389, 385, 429, 439, 494, 508.
†References 3, 93, 120, 148, 168, 212, 222, 223, 248, 249, 332, 358, 520, 553.
‡References 2, 35, 105, 108, 109, 305, 306, 397, 544, 600, 601, 607, 608.
§References 2, 35, 305, 306, 371, 397, 544, 600, 601, 607, 608.

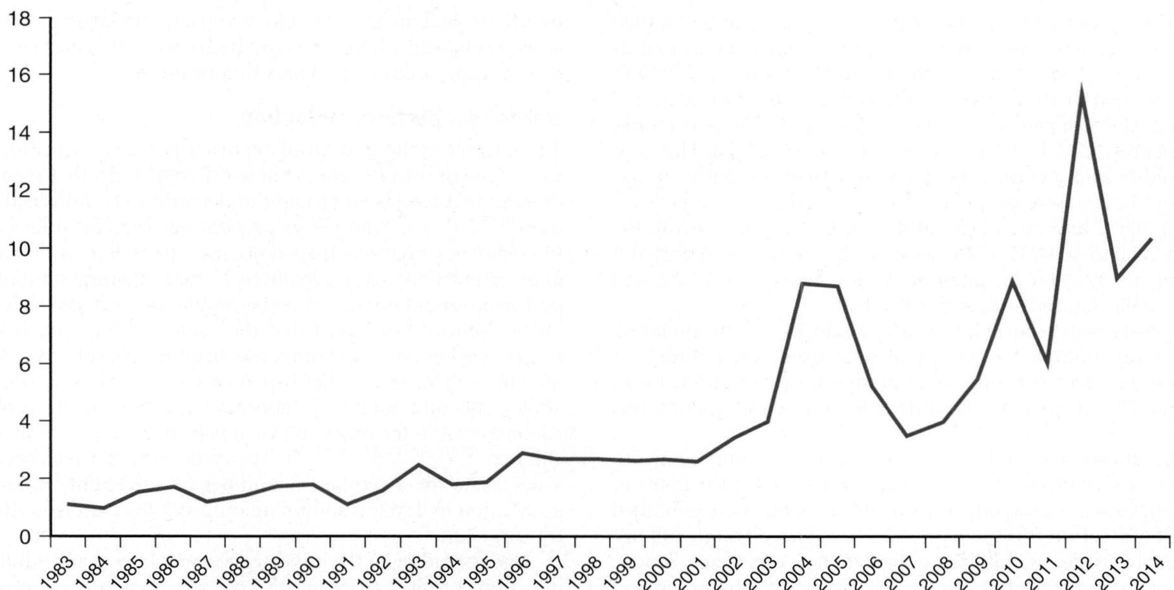

FIG. 129.1 Annual pertussis incidence per 100,000 people in the United States, 1983–2014. (Data from Centers for Disease Control and Prevention. National Center for Health Statistics, Pertussis Cases by Year (1922-2014), and Summary of notifiable diseases: United States, 2014. Available at http://www.cdc.gov/pertussis/surv-reporting/cases-by-year.html.)

observed that the British vaccines at the time contained only agglutinogen 2 (i.e., FIM 2) and that circulating *B. pertussis* strains contained agglutinogen 3 (FIM 3). However, this vaccine-driven genetic change had no demonstrated adverse effect on vaccine efficacy at that time. Currently, genetic changes in *B. pertussis* include *ptx* P1 allele to *ptx* P3 allele, an increase in *fim* 3B strains in the United States, and the circulation of PRN-deficient mutants. Because whole-cell DTP vaccines contain multiple antigens, genetic changes are unlikely to lead to vaccine failure in DTP-vaccinated children. However, DTaP vaccines contain a maximum of five proteins, and genetic change would likely contribute to vaccine failure.

Studies in the Netherlands suggested that the change from *ptx* P1 to *ptx* P3 resulted in an increase in pertussis and an increase in the severity of illness.[401] However, this does not appear to be accurate. In Denmark, physicians have been exclusively using a PT toxoid vaccine since 1997, and there is no evidence of an increase in pertussis incidence or severity.[282,547]

The increase in *fim* 3B strains in the United States has occurred gradually over many years, and because FIM 2 is the dominant FIM antigen, this is unlikely to contribute to vaccine failure to any great degree. In contrast, the circulation of PRN-deficient mutants is a significant problem.[361,447] It would be a greater problem in recipients three-component vaccinees (i.e., PT, FHA, and PRN) compared with five-vaccines (i.e., PT, FHA, PRN, and FIM 2/3). However, any difference in the effectiveness of the two vaccines types has not become apparent, probably because antibody to the B subunit of PT provides considerable efficacy against typical pertussis. To show a difference in effectiveness, a study involving mild illness and typical pertussis in DTaP vaccine failures would need to be carried out. Vaccine failure is discussed later in this chapter.

Pertussis epidemics in the prevaccine era occurred at 2- to 5-year intervals (average, 3.2 years in the United States), and these cycles have continued in the vaccine era. As reported by Fine and Clarkson,[184,185] this continuity indicates that although immunization has controlled disease, it has not reduced transmission of the organism in the population.[89,94,97]

In the prevaccine era, the following percentages of cases by age were reported in Massachusetts: younger than 1 year, 7.5%; 1 to 4 years, 41.1%; 5 to 9 years, 46.0%; 10 to 14 years, 4.1%; and 15 years and older, 0.9%.[49] Associated with the marked reduction in reported cases of pertussis in the United States resulting from widespread pediatric immunization, a major shift occurred in the percentages by age category in the United States.[49] During the period from 1978 to 1981, the age distribution was as follows: younger than 1 year, 53.5%; 1 to 4 years, 26.5%; 5 to 9 years, 8.2%; 10 to 14 years, 5.4%; and 15 years or older, 6.5%. In contrast, U.S. data for 2010 revealed the following pattern: younger than 1 year, 15%; 1 to 6 years, 22%; 7 to 10 years, 18%; 10 to 19 years, 20%; and 20 years or older, 25%. Today, pertussis among adolescents and adults is an important source of *B. pertussis* infection for unimmunized or partially immunized children.* The disease in adolescents and adults usually is not recognized as pertussis, although the cough frequently is paroxysmal and illness may persist for weeks.[97,155,358,457,503]

In a study of university students, members of our group found that about 13% of students with an illness involving cough for 6 or more days had *B. pertussis* infections, none of which had been diagnosed correctly clinically.[393] The study findings led to the suggestion that *B. pertussis* infections are endemic among adults and are responsible for cyclic outbreaks among susceptible children. Other studies in the United States, Germany, and elsewhere support this hypothesis.[45,97,99,101,150,156,401,503,604,616]

Morbidity and Mortality

During the first 30 years of the 20th century, pertussis was an important cause of death in the United States.[319] The number of deaths from pertussis between 1926 and 1930 was 36,013,[208] mostly children younger than 1 year of age. The pertussis death rate curve in the United States declined throughout the 20th century. Among infants, the mortality rate decreased approximately fivefold between 1900 and 1944. During the next 35 years, it declined more than 85-fold.[406,407] Today, most of the deaths caused by pertussis affect unimmunized infants younger than 4 months of age.[221,225,367,414,572,615,622] Currently in the United States, 10 to 20 deaths are reported each year.[74,79,76,221,572,615]

Deaths caused by pertussis frequently are misdiagnosed as deaths from other respiratory tract infectious illnesses.[89,253,425] For example, in England and Wales during the epidemic from 1977 to 1979 and at the beginning of the epidemic in 1982, 32 deaths were reported to be caused by pertussis.[89] However, when the excess deaths from other respiratory tract infectious illnesses were examined, approximately 362 additional deaths appeared to be caused by pertussis. Additional pertussis deaths were reported as SIDS.[425]

*References 46, 82, 97, 101, 99, 111, 317, 339, 340, 405, 419, 560, 592.

The morbidity caused by pertussis in recent years can be gleaned from numerous reports. The numbers of pertussis-related hospitalizations, complications, and deaths in the United States during 1990 to 1996 were reviewed in 1999 by Güris and colleagues.[221] Of the 31,837 cases analyzed, 31.7% of patients were hospitalized, 9.5% had pneumonia, 1.4% had seizures, 0.2% had encephalopathy, and 0.2% died. The most severe morbidity rate was for infants younger than 6 months of age. Of this group, 72.2% were hospitalized, 17.3% had pneumonia, 2.1% had seizures, 0.5% had encephalopathy, and 0.5% died. During the period from 2000 to 2004, 12,174 cases among infants were reported.[82] Of this group, 62.8% were hospitalized, 55.8% had apnea, 12.7% had pneumonia, 1.5% had seizures, and 0.8% died.

In adolescents with reported pertussis, 0% to 2% are hospitalized, and 2% have pneumonia.[81] A review of data from seven studies of adult pertussis reported the following findings: hospitalization, 3% to 12%; seizures, 0% to 0.6%; rib fracture, 0% to 4%; and pneumonia, 0.6% to 8%.[82]

A pertussis surveillance system was introduced in conjunction with a large pertussis vaccine efficacy trial in several regions of Germany in 1990. The initial results of this ongoing surveillance study were published in 1993.[247] Of 601 culture-proven cases, 12.3% occurred among infants, and 86.2% occurred among children younger than 6 years of age. Serious complications were reported in 22 of 275 patients with follow-up and included pneumonia in 5.5%, apnea in 2.2%, and cardiorespiratory failure in 0.4%.

In a follow-up report of the same study, 1 of 185 culture-confirmed cases among infants was fatal.[251] In another German study from 1993 to 1996, Herzig and associates[262] reported 116 hospitalized pertussis patients with the following complications: pneumonia in 81%, apnea requiring assisted ventilation in 15%, seizures in 14%, encephalopathy in 5%, and death of 2%. In Canada from 1991 to 1997, Halperin and colleagues[235] analyzed the complications of pertussis in 1082 hospitalized children younger than 2 years of age and found that 9.4% had pneumonia, 3% had atelectasis, 2.3% had seizures, 0.59% had encephalopathy, 0.8% had inguinal or umbilical hernias, 1.3% had more than a 5% weight loss, and 0.9% died.

Since 2010, several studies in California have examined risk factors for death in young infants.[413,426,602] These studies are discussed in later sections.

Season, Geography, Race, Ethnicity, and Sex

Pertussis occurs throughout the world, but data from large parts of Asia and Africa are less detailed than data from the United States, Canada, Australia, and Europe.[106,109,113,538] Historically, epidemic pertussis had no seasonal pattern.[89] However, in the current vaccine era in North America, pertussis usually occurs in the summer and fall.[123,177,207,221,367,419] The incidence of pertussis is usually greater among female than male patients.[89,177,207,221,584] In 2004, 25,827 cases were reported in the United States; 11,199 (45%) of these patients were male, and 13,879 (55%) were female; sex was not identified in 749 cases.[78] In 2010, 55% of the reported cases occurred in females. In a large study in Germany, 1263 (50.7%) of the 2493 patients were female.[251]

Reported pertussis rates were higher among American Indians and Alaska Natives and whites than among Asians and Pacific Islanders and blacks in 2010.[74] Attack rates for infants are higher among Hispanics than non-Hispanics.

Transmission

Transmission is thought to occur by droplets from a coughing or sneezing patient that reach the upper respiratory tract of a susceptible person. Indirect spread also may occur. A symptomatic patient could contaminate the environment with respiratory secretions; the hands of another person could make contact with the secretions and then inoculate the respiratory tract.[113] Attack rates among susceptible household contacts range from 70% to 100%.[89,113] Antibody studies indicate that asymptomatic infections also occur among contacts.[150,346,347] These asymptomatic infections are likely to be short lived and probably are not important with regard to contagion.

Transmissibility is greatest early in the illness, occurring during the catarrhal and early paroxysmal phases. Young children with primary infections shed more bacteria for a longer period than do older children, adolescents, and adults who have had a pervious infection (recognized or not recognized) or previous immunization.

Bordetella pertussis Infection

The current cyclic pattern of reported pertussis is similar to what it was in the prevaccine era[367] but is different from that seen with other diseases that have been brought under control by universal immunization.[97,101,99,393] For example, as measles was brought under control, the interepidemic cycle lengthened because circulation of the measles virus in the population had been reduced. In contrast, immunization controlled pertussis but did not decrease the circulation of *B. pertussis*.[185,186] In the 1970s, Nelson[419] observed that the source of *B. pertussis* infection in hospitalized infants most often was an adult. This observation led many investigators to suspect that *B. pertussis* infections were endemic among adolescents and adults.[97,393] Sporadic infection in the adolescent and adult reservoir is the major source of *B. pertussis* infections in nonimmune children.[109,511,46,141,142,314,367,566,592] The cyclic pattern occurs because it takes a few years for a significant number of susceptible members of the population to develop and for an outbreak to result from the sustained transmission.

Understanding of the importance of adolescent and adult *B. pertussis* infections resulted from the ability to diagnose infection serologically by measuring immunoglobulin (Ig) G and IgA antibodies to PT by enzyme-linked immunosorbent assay (ELISA).[99,101,124,367,393,462] During the past 30 years, numerous studies of adolescent and adult populations have contributed to the understanding of *B. pertussis* epidemiology.

Studies of prolonged illnesses with cough in adolescents and adults suggest that about 13% of the illnesses are caused by *B. pertussis* infection.* Many studies have looked at overall infection rates by determining significant IgG or IgA titer rises in response to PT in persons who have two or more serum samples collected over extended periods.[99,101,140,156,267,367,483,579] These studies suggest that between 1.0% and 6.6% of adolescents and adults have a *B. pertussis* infection each year. A large study in the Netherlands that used a combination of serologic surveys estimated an incidence of infection of 6.6% per year for persons between the ages of 3 and 79 years.[154] The incidence among children 3 to 4 years of age was 3.3%. It then increased gradually to a peak of 10.8% among those 20 to 24 years of age. Other age-specific incidences were 6.5% for persons 25 to 55 years old and 4.0% for those older than 55 years of age.

The rates of illnesses with cough caused by *B. pertussis* were determined in two prospective, specific population-based studies.[532,578] In the first study, the rate was 500 cases per 100,000 people (0.5%), and in the second, it was 370 cases per 100,000 people (0.37%). These figures underestimated the rates because of observer bias.[118] In both studies, the study physicians or nurses were supposed to document all patients with cough illnesses of 7 days or longer who were not improving. If the physicians or nurses did not follow the protocol but made decisions based on their opinions, many mild cases would be missed, and there is evidence of this error in both studies. The retrospective serologic analysis of a respiratory disease study of adults older than 65 years of age suggested a rate as high as 1.5%.[267] This high value assumes that all respiratory illnesses with cough during the 4-month periods of seroconversion were the result of *B. pertussis* infection.

With increased clinical surveillance and more complete use of the laboratory (i.e., PCR and serologic study), and with the diagnosis of mild cases in children, adolescents, and adults of all ages, the current cyclic pattern of reported pertussis for the most part will disappear. The pattern of reported pertussis has already lost some of its predictable regularity in some European countries with rigorous surveillance systems in place.

PATHOLOGY

Data on the pathology of *B. pertussis* infections have been determined mainly by postmortem study of fatal cases.[89,113,121,126,319,338,355,443,512] However,

*References 45, 99, 101, 201, 291, 367, 393, 422, 485, 503, 532, 571, 604, 616.

some information about uncomplicated pertussis can be gleaned from experiments done more than 80 years ago using rhesus and ringtail monkeys.[319,496] Pure cultures of *B. pertussis* were obtained from between the cilia of the smaller bronchi and bronchioli. Endobronchitis and peribronchitis were identified, and the bronchi contained leukocytes, mucus, and debris.

In a study of autopsy material from 15 infants (≤4 months of age), the consistent histopathologic features were necrotizing bronchiolitis and pneumonia, intraalveolar hemorrhage and fibrinous edema, and abundant intraalveolar macrophages.[443] Angiolymphatic aggregates of mixed leukocytes in the intralobular septa and pleurae were seen in 86% of the specimens. Intact *Bordetella* organisms were found in cilia of the trachea, bronchi, and bronchioles and within airways and alveoli. They also were seen intracellularly in alveolar macrophages and respiratory epithelium. Despite the fact that all patients had severe pneumonia, the ciliated respiratory epithelial cells appeared relatively normal. More than 100 years ago, Mallory and Horner[355] also found that the ciliated epithelial cells in the trachea, bronchi, and bronchioles were relatively normal. Six of the 15 deaths studied had evidence of coinfections with one or more other agents (i.e., cytomegalovirus, 1 child; RSV, 2 children; *Streptococcus pneumoniae,* 2 children; *Streptococcus pyogenes,* 2 patients; *Moraxella catarrhalis,* 1 child; and viridans streptococci, 1 child). It is likely that many of the pathologic findings described earlier resulted from concomitant and secondary viral or bacterial infections and not from the *B. pertussis* infection.[121]

Pathologic changes in the brain and liver have been described. Microscopic or gross cerebral hemorrhage may be seen, and cortical atrophy has been observed. These changes most likely are the result of anoxic brain damage. In some studies of pertussis encephalopathy, findings suggested meningoencephalitis, with perivascular cuffs of lymphocytes in cerebral gray matter and pleocytosis.[611] However, the studies in which inflammation was demonstrated were performed before modern virologic techniques became available. The neurologic findings in these instances probably were caused by interactions with neurotropic viruses or other infectious agents and were not the result of *B. pertussis* infection.[113] Fatty infiltration of the liver has been recognized in patients with pertussis encephalopathy.

PATHOGENESIS AND IMMUNITY

After a patient is exposed to an infectious agent, the pathogenesis of infection usually depends on four important steps: attachment, evasion of host defenses, local damage, and systemic disease.[113,137,204,264,367,409,411,416,459,589] However, illness due to *B. pertussis* infection is unique because there is no systemic disease and, except in young infants, there is no local damage.[109,105,121] The biologically active antigenic components of *B. pertussis* listed in Table 129.2 have various roles in pathogenesis. During the past 2 decades, hundreds of research publications have explored the effects of various *B. pertussis* proteins in animal model systems. These studies have revealed a large amount of information, but what is missing for the most part is the degree of correlation with pathogenesis in human infections.*

Infection is initiated in the respiratory tract by the attachment of *B. pertussis* organisms to the cilia of ciliated epithelial cells.[589] Adhesins (e.g., PT, FIM, LPS) facilitate attachment.[411] Because of the redundancy of protein adhesins, determining the importance of the individual proteins and ascertaining a primary adhesin or adhesins have been difficult.[367] For the attachment proteins, data about human infection are available only for FIMs. In the two trials that looked at serologic correlates of immunity, researchers found that antibody to fimbriae was important.[111,529] Antibodies to fimbriae provided protection against colonization with *B. pertussis* in the murine respiratory tract.[596]

In many publications, PRN and other autotransporters are described as adhesins, which is mostly incorrect. Although antibody to PRN is associated with lack of attachment, PRN and other autotransporters have other specific biologic activities in infection.[29,259,359,360,430,438,597] The two household contact studies of serologic correlates of protection found that antibody to PRN was most important in preventing pertussis.[114,529] PRN and all of the other autotransporters that have been studied adversely affect the innate immune response.

ACT and PT adversely affect immune cell function and therefore allow infection to continue after initiation.[13,14,62,113,266,411,569] PT prevents migration of lymphocytes and macrophages to areas of infection and adversely affects phagocytosis and intracellular killing. ACT enters phagocytic cells and catalyzes excessive production of cyclic adenosine monophosphate, which intoxicates neutrophils and decreases phagocytosis.

TCT and DNT have been suggested to be contributors to local tissue damage in the respiratory tract.[113,204,416] However, there are no data indicating tissue damage in human infections due to these two proteins.

Pertussis is a unique illness in that fever does not occur, and it has only one manifestation of systemic disease in uncomplicated infection: leukocytosis with lymphocytosis caused by PT.[113,256,281] T and B lymphocytes increase to a similar extent in the circulation.[41] Unlike the situation in *B. pertussis* infection, leukocytosis with lymphocytosis is not a characteristic of *B. parapertussis* infection because the organism does not liberate PT. Clinical experience and recent studies indicate that PT is the major causative factor in deaths in young infants.[414,443,602,622] PT inhibits G proteins, causing leukocytosis with lymphocytosis. It has been suggested that the extreme leukocytosis results in obstruction in small pulmonary vessels, which leads to severe pulmonary hypertension.[443] However, it is possible that the inhibition of G proteins in other cells in the lung or heart is the cause of death.[414,622] An important systemic complication of pertussis is encephalopathy, for which the mechanism is unknown. The most likely explanation is anoxia associated with coughing paroxysms.

It has been suggested that pertussis is a toxin-mediated disease caused by PT.[454,453] Although some researchers continue to entertain this idea,[473,474] little evidence supports it. PT is a fascinating protein with activities in experimental animals such as histamine sensitization, promotion of lymphocytosis, effects on glucose metabolism, and induction of adjuvant and mitogenic activity.[79,145,284,326] However, in human infections, the main effects that appear to be caused by PT are leukocytosis with lymphocytosis and mild, compensated hyperinsulinemia. PT has been suggested as the cause of the prolonged cough in pertussis, but this hypothesis should be refuted because persistent cough is a major manifestation of *B. bronchiseptica* infection in dogs and of *B. parapertussis* and *B. holmesii* infection in humans and because none of these organisms liberates PT.[256,367,432]

The hallmark of *B. pertussis* illness is paroxysmal cough, and the cause (i.e., cough toxin) is unknown.[105,109,121] The paroxysmal cough is unique because of its long duration. Because there is memory of the cough, it may return when people have subsequent respiratory tract viral infections. Hewitt and Canning[263] suggested that bradykinin plays a role in the initiation of the cough. During *B. pertussis* infection, bradykinin production is increased and has a prolonged half-life in the airways, and responsiveness to bradykinin reception activation is increased. Bradykinin activates sensory nerves implicated in cough. What is not known is the *Bordetella* antigen (i.e., cough toxin) that stimulates the unique coughing process.

Cell-mediated immune responses (i.e., T-cell response) in *B. pertussis* infection and after immunization were observed more than 2 decades ago and in one of the vaccine efficacy trails of the 1990s.* In a marine model, Mills and colleagues found that infection or DTP immunization resulted in a helper T-cell type 1 (Th1) response, whereas vaccination with a DTaP vaccine resulted in a Th1/Th2 response. Because the antibody responses with the DTaP vaccines were good, the T-cell response findings were ignored by most people involved with pertussis vaccine studies in the 1990s.

However, recent findings of a diminished duration of efficacy in DTaP vaccine recipients compared with DTP vaccine recipients have led to renewed interest in cellular immunity after infection and vaccination. Studies using the baboon pertussis model have confirmed and expanded the findings of Mills and associates.[390,391,490] Warfel and Merkel[580]

*References 1, 13, 14, 29, 62, 63, 133, 137, 151, 180, 187, 197, 259, 260, 299, 359, 360, 367, 379, 411, 430, 438, 459, 479, 555, 569, 589, 597, 618.

*References 21, 353, 390, 391, 392, 397, 486, 489, 490, 620, 551, 595.

and Warfel and colleagues[581] found that infection and DTP vaccination induced a Th17 and Th1 immune memory response, whereas the response to DTaP was a Th1/Th2 response. The Th17 and Th1 response prevents infection and disease, and it gives longer protection than a Th1/Th2 response.

Various antibodies develop after exposure of the human host to infection with *B. pertussis.* The development of agglutinins, hemagglutination-inhibiting antibodies, and bactericidal antibodies has been described.[89] ELISA techniques have demonstrated class-specific antibodies (i.e., IgA, IgE, IgG, and IgM) to many of the specific proteins of *B. pertussis.*[243,356,441] The antibodies develop after infection and, with the exception of IgA antibodies, after immunization. Neutralizing antibody to PT develops after infection and immunization.[231,441] Specific IgA antibodies to PT and FHA also can be demonstrated in nasopharyngeal secretions and saliva.[210,619]

B. pertussis infection and immunization with whole-cell or acellular pertussis vaccines elicit protection to various degrees and durations against pertussis. The prevailing opinion in the past century was that immunity acquired from having *B. pertussis* infection was lifelong, whereas vaccine-induced immunity was relatively short. Although the latter is true,[185] studies performed by members of our research group suggest that the former opinion regarding infection-induced immunity is wrong.[95,98,112,367,503,568] Proceeding from the knowledge that IgA antibodies to pertussis antigens (i.e., PT, FHA, and PRN) result from infection and not from primary vaccination, our group studied the prevalence of these antibodies in the sera of young German and American men of similar ages.[112] In Germany, routine childhood immunization was not carried out during the 1970s and 1980s, and pertussis was epidemic. To our surprise, the rate and mean values of IgA antibodies in the two populations were similar, suggesting that adult infection rates were similar. However, levels of IgG antibody to PT, FHA, PRN, and FIM 2 were significantly higher in young American men than in German men of similar ages. In another study in Germany, we found that *Bordetella* infections were common occurrences in adults, often in persons with a known history of childhood pertussis.[503]

In our studies of cases of pertussis in adults in the United States and Germany, we observed that the Germans (primed by past infection) tended to have more typical pertussis than the Americans (primed by DTP vaccination). The nature of immunity in pertussis is unknown. The consensus is that serum antibodies greater than some unknown concentration to one or more of the pertussis antigens are responsible for protection.[150] Antibodies to PT, FHA, and PRN are protective in animal model systems,[43,139,325,495,506] but no serologic correlates of immunity were established until the 1990s, although several large vaccine trials were carried out in the late 1980s and early 1990s.[3,212,222,332,509,520,553]

In a nested household contact study, our group was able to evaluate the roles of IgG antibodies to PT, FHA, PRN, and FIM 2 by determining preexposure imputed values in children at the time of household exposure to *B. pertussis* infection by using a classification tree and logistic regression methods.[114] The imputed geometric mean antibody values to PT, PRN, and FIM 2 were higher for noncases than for cases. In the classification tree analysis, however, only antibodies against PRN contributed significantly to protection. Subjects with an imputed PRN value of less than 7 ELISA units (EU) per milliliter had a 67% likelihood of infection. Logistic regression analysis found that PRN values of 8 EU/mL or more were associated with protection from illness after household exposure. In accordance with our findings, data from a Swedish study, which had greater power, indicated that antibody values of 5 EU/mL or more to PRN and FIM 2/3 correlated with protection.[529] The data from these two studies suggest that antibody to PRN and FIM are most important in protection. However, what is difficult to understand is why some children get pertussis despite large amounts of antibody to PRN or FIM or both.[117,552] Data from a study by Weiss and associates[591] suggested that high antibody values to PT might block the protective effect of antibody to the more important antigens.

Immunity developed after *B. pertussis* infection or vaccination with a whole-cell pertussis vaccine does not protect against illness caused by *B. parapertussis,* and infection with *B. parapertussis* does not induce protection against disease caused by *B. pertussis.*[320,542] However, the results of our vaccine efficacy trial in Germany provided evidence that the acellular, multicomponent pertussis vaccine, which contained a large amount of FHA, offered some protection against *B. parapertussis* infections, whereas the whole-cell vaccine, which contained minimal amounts of FHA, did not.[254] Although *B. pertussis* infection is a localized infection involving ciliated cells of the respiratory tract, bacteremia has occurred in immunocompromised adults.[77,290,554]

CLINICAL MANIFESTATIONS

The clinical manifestations of *B. pertussis* infection have considerable variation that depends on age, previous immunization or infection, the presence of passively acquired antibody, and other factors such as the degree of exposure, host genetic and acquired factors, and the genotype of the organism. The incubation period for pertussis is 6 to 20 days; in most cases, onset occurs 7 to 10 days after exposure. However, after household exposure, 22% of secondary cases had an onset of more than 4 weeks after the onset of illness in the primary case.[249]

Classic Illness

Classic illness occurs as a primary infection in unimmunized children between the ages of 1 and 10 years.[98,113,124,208,439] The illness usually lasts 6 to 12 weeks and has three stages: catarrhal, paroxysmal, and convalescent. The initial illness is characterized by rhinorrhea, lacrimation, and mild cough suggesting a common cold. Body temperature usually is normal. The severity of the cough gradually increases over 1 to 2 weeks, but pertussis usually is not suspected until the cough becomes paroxysmal.

After the catarrhal period, the coughing increases in severity and number of attacks. Repetitive series of 5 to 10 or more forceful coughs can occur during a single expiration. The paroxysms are followed by a sudden, massive inspiratory effort, and a characteristic whoop may occur as air is forcefully inhaled through a narrowed glottis. Cyanosis, bulging eyes, protrusion of the tongue, salivation, lacrimation, and distention of neck veins occur during paroxysms. Several paroxysmal coughing episodes with their associated massive inspiratory effort may occur sequentially. Purulent sputum is not produced. Posttussive vomiting is a common occurrence. Paroxysms may strike several times per hour, and they occur during both day and night.

The paroxysmal episodes are exhausting, and patients frequently appear dazed and apathetic. Weight loss may occur as a result of vomiting, and eating and drinking may be resisted because they trigger attacks. Attacks also may be triggered by yawning, sneezing, or physical exertion. Between attacks, the patient may appear normal and usually is in no distress.

Common and important complications of classic pertussis include pneumonia, otitis media, seizures, and encephalopathy. Pneumonia in all but young infants is caused by secondary bacterial or viral invaders. Atelectasis may develop as a result of the mucus plugs. The forcefulness of the paroxysms can rupture alveoli and produce interstitial or subcutaneous emphysema.

Otitis media is a common occurrence and frequently is caused by *S. pneumoniae.* Pertussis also has been associated with activation of latent tuberculosis. Convulsions and coma may be observed. Findings may reflect cerebral hypoxia related to asphyxia. Rarely, subarachnoid and intraventricular hemorrhage may occur. Tetanic seizures may be associated with the severe alkalosis that results from the loss of gastric contents caused by persistent vomiting.

Other complications include ulcer of the frenulum of the tongue, epistaxis, melena, subconjunctival hemorrhage, subdural hematoma, spinal epidural hematoma, rupture of the diaphragm, umbilical hernia, inguinal hernia, rectal prolapse, dehydration, meningoencephalitis, the syndrome of inappropriate secretion of antidiuretic hormone, apnea, rib fracture, and nutritional disturbances.[66,98,287,366,457,514,585]

The convalescent stage, which usually lasts 1 to 2 weeks, is characterized by a decreasing frequency and severity of coughing episodes, whooping, and vomiting. However, some patients continue to have pertussis-like coughing spells for several months. Most patients with classic pertussis caused by primary infection have leukocytosis associated with lymphocytosis. Fever, pharyngitis, and wheezing are not usual manifestations in pertussis, and a search for a secondary cause should be undertaken when these findings occur. Except for the observation of typical paroxysmal cough and detection of the complications previously described, physical examination of patients with pertussis usually is unrewarding. Diffuse rhonchi may be elicited on auscultation.

Infection with *B. parapertussis* causes an illness that is similar to that caused by *B. pertussis*. However, it is usually less severe and has a shortened duration.[255,333,364]

Mild Illness and Asymptomatic Infection

Mild, nonclassic illness is common in *B. pertussis* infection.[150,247,251,498] It occurs in previously vaccinated individuals and as a primary infection in unvaccinated children. In a study in which physicians were encouraged to send nasopharyngeal specimens from ill children with cough, regardless of whether the illness was typical of pertussis, to our laboratory, 247 culture-positive cases were identified. Of these patients, 47% had a total duration of cough of 28 days or less. For 26%, the duration of cough was less than 3 weeks. Most of these patients were unvaccinated children. In a similar 6-year study involving 2592 culture-positive, previously unvaccinated children, 38% had a duration of cough of 28 days or less, and for 17%, it was 21 days or less.[251] In a study in which both culture and PCR were used for establishing the diagnosis of *B. pertussis* infection, many mild cases were found to be PCR positive and culture negative.[498] Of these, only 68% had a cough lasting 4 weeks or longer, and only 57% and 32% had paroxysmal cough and whoop, respectively.

In studies of household contacts, asymptomatic infections in family members are common occurrences.[150,346,347] Deen and associates[150] found that 52 (46%) of 114 household contacts who remained well had laboratory evidence of *B. pertussis* infection. In another study, 21 of 399 healthy infants who were control subjects had PCR-positive nasopharyngeal samples.[250]

Infants

Pertussis in infancy is a unique experience.[367,414,602] Its spectrum of clinical manifestations varies by age, immunization, and the magnitude of transplacentally acquired antibody.* Most deaths resulting from *B. pertussis* infection affect neonates and or occur during early infancy, and morbidity is most severe in infants.† From 1997 through 2000, 8276 cases of pertussis were reported for infants in the United States.[76] Of this group, 59% of the infants were hospitalized, 11% had pneumonia, 1% had seizures, 0.2% had encephalopathy, and 0.7% died. Eighty-seven percent of these patients were children younger than 6 months of age.

B. pertussis infection in neonates is particularly severe, with a death rate of 1% to 3%.[36,127,221,253,255,274,336,373] Clinical characteristics of pertussis in early infancy are presented in Box 129.1. A common initial finding is apnea with or without typical coughing. Seizures associated with apnea caused by hypoxia occur frequently. Severe pulmonary hypertension is a relatively common problem in pertussis in the first 4 months of life.[147,160,209,218,227,443,449,517,598] The severity of disease and the risk for death correlate directly with high white blood cell (WBC) counts, particularly the number of lymphocytes.[36,127,147,218,253,373,383,443,449] WBC counts in the range of 30,000 to more than 100,000 cells/mm^3 are common findings.

Two California Department of Public Health studies have provided useful information about risk factors for pulmonary hypertension and death.[414,602,622] The first study involved 31 infants 90 days of age or younger with pertussis who were admitted to a pediatric intensive care unit in Southern California. Infants with pulmonary hypertension or who died had higher WBC counts, had more rapid pulse and respiratory rates, and were more likely to have early onset pneumonia than those who did not have pulmonary hypertension or who died.

In a second Californian study in which 53 fatal pertussis cases from 1998 to 2010 were matched with 183 nonfatal pertussis cases of hospitalized patients older than 120 days of age, the findings in the previous California study were confirmed.[413,602] Additional risk factors for death

*References 36, 89, 113, 127, 173, 177, 253, 314, 373, 419, 425.

†References 30, 36, 64, 127, 141, 142, 147, 182, 200, 209, 218, 221, 225–227, 250, 253, 255, 274, 328, 367, 370, 373, 383, 414, 417, 419, 425, 426, 443, 449, 455, 482, 488, 497, 510, 512, 513, 517, 540, 572, 598, 602, 622.

BOX 129.1 Clinical Features of Pertussis in Young Infants

- Infant looks deceptively well initially; coryza, sneezing, clearing throat, no fever, mild cough
- Paroxysmal stage: gagging, gasping, eye bulging, bradycardia (tachycardia in severe illness), cyanosis, vomiting
- Leukocytosis with lymphocytosis
- Apneic episodes
- Seizures
- Respiratory distress
- Pneumonia and pulmonary hypertension
- Shock or hypotension with renal failure and/or other organ failure
- Death associated with pulmonary hypertension and pneumonia
- Adenovirus or respiratory syncytial virus coinfection confuses picture

were lower birth weight, lower gestational age, and onset of symptoms at an earlier age. Factors associated with survival were paroxysmal cough and the receipt of DTaP vaccine. Treatment characteristics associated with death included the recipient of steroids or nitric oxide and the use of intubation, exchange blood transfusion, and extracorporeal membrane oxygenation (ECMO). The use of macrolide antibiotics correlated with survival.

In a stepwise logistic regression model, indicators of death were low birth weight, extremely high WBC count, and pulmonary hypertension. When treatment characteristics were analyzed in the multivariate, stepwise logistic regression model, only intubation and nitric oxide use were related to death. The association of death with exchange blood transfusion is misleading. All of the patients who died were in cardiovascular shock, and many also had organ failure before the procedure. In another California study, of 10 infants who received exchange blood transfusion, five died and five survived.[426] All five infants who died were in shock, and four of five had organ failure before the procedure was attempted. In the five survivors, the procedure was done before shock or organ failure occurred.

Coinfection with respiratory viruses (e.g., RSV, adenovirus, influenza viruses) and respiratory bacterial pathogens (e.g., *S. pneumoniae*, *Haemophilus influenzae*) is relatively frequent.[16,36,136,142,144,245,313,328,396,443,512]

B. pertussis infection has been associated with SIDS, but a cause-and-effect relationship is unlikely.[250,255,336,425] In a study in England, Nichol and Gardner[425] found that many deaths attributed to SIDS were instead related to *B. pertussis* infection. Using PCR, we found *B. pertussis* DNA in nasopharyngeal specimens from 9 (18%) of 51 infants who had sudden, unexpected deaths.[255] In a subsequent study, we collected specimens for PCR from 254 infants who had sudden, unexplained deaths and from 441 healthy matched controls.[250] The rate of PCR-positive results for the sudden death cases was 5.1%; it was 5.3% for the controls. In a careful follow-up histopathologic study with unique immunohistochemical staining of specimens from a subset of these fatal cases, we found no evidence of specific *B. pertussis* pulmonary infection or pathologic features.[122]

The source of infection in infants usually is a family member.[30,46,142,150,173,314,591] In a study of 616 infant cases, the source was identified for 43%.[46] A family member was the source for 75% of cases, and the mother was the most common source (32%). Of the sources, 56% were adults, and 20% were 10 to 19 years of age. In contrast to previous studies, a Centers for Disease Control and Prevention (CDC) study found that siblings were the most common source of transmission to infants.[511]

Adults

There has been increased awareness of adult pertussis since the 1970s.* Unrecognized adult pertussis cases often are the source from which

*References 45, 46, 78, 79, 81, 82, 97, 101, 99, 106, 109, 103, 116, 124, 150, 154–156, 177, 201, 221, 267, 289, 291, 317, 367, 395, 393, 419, 422, 457, 476, 485, 503, 532, 548, 579, 604, 616.

infants and children become infected.[36,46,97,127,253,373,419,531,592] All adults were previously exposed to *B. pertussis* antigens by immunization or infection, or both,[112,150,156,367] and exposure tends to modify their illness. In a US study, several cough characteristics were observed in 31 university students with laboratory evidence of *Bordetella* infection. The median duration was 21 days before initial evaluation, 94% had one or more coughing episodes per hour, and 90% of the coughs had a staccato or paroxysmal quality.[393] Despite these findings, pertussis was not suspected in any of the students. Clinical diagnoses by the primary care providers included upper respiratory tract infection (39%), bronchitis (48%), and other diagnoses (16%). Although specific records were not available, most of the students probably were vaccinated as children and almost certainly had previous, unrecognized infections.[112,150]

In contrast to the US findings, German adults were found to be more likely to have typical pertussis, even though the epidemiologic data suggested that all had a previous infection and 26% of 64 patients with laboratory evidence of infection recalled having had pertussis during childhood.[112,503] Rates of clinical manifestations in the 64 laboratory-confirmed cases were paroxysms (70%), whoop (38%), posttussive phlegm (66%), and posttussive vomiting (17%). The clinical diagnosis for 39% was definite or probable pertussis; only 14% were thought not to have pertussis. The clinical diagnosis was not made by primary care physicians but by a small team of specially trained central investigators who were alert to the possibility of pertussis.

Similar findings were reported in a German household contact study: 80% of 79 adults with laboratory-confirmed *B. pertussis* infection coughed for 3 or more weeks, and 63% had spasmodic cough for 3 or more weeks.[457] In 53% of patients, coughing was followed by choking or vomiting. However, only 8% of the adults in this study had whoops. Complications included pneumonia, rib fracture, inguinal hernia, and severe weight loss. Unique sweating episodes are reported in approximately 5% of adults, and fainting can be associated with coughing.[103,165,480]

DIFFERENTIAL DIAGNOSIS

In typical pertussis, the clinical diagnosis should be apparent based on the paroxysmal cough with posttussive vomiting and whooping and a lack of significant fever. However, the cause of the illness can be *B. pertussis, B. parapertussis, B. holmesii,* and perhaps *B. bronchiseptica.* A history of contact with a known case helps to establish the diagnosis for a patient with mild or atypical illness. Leukocytosis with lymphocytosis in a child with a cough or apnea in an infant is a strong indication that the illness is caused by *B. pertussis* rather than another *Bordetella* spp. In a matched-control comparison, none of 11 children with culture-proven *B. parapertussis* infection versus 7 (32%) of 22 with *B. pertussis* infection had lymphocytosis of 10,000 cells/mm^3 or more.[256] Lymphocytosis of 10,000 cells/mm^3 or more is observed in few other illnesses that manifest with a cough.

Many other infectious agents cause illnesses with prolonged and repetitive cough that can be confused with *B. pertussis* infections.[367] In particular, *M. pneumoniae, C. pneumoniae,* adenoviruses, bocavirus, and other respiratory viruses can cause a prolonged cough.[19,26,89,113,130,132,145,228,420,606] Coughing episodes also may be seen in children with asthma, bronchiolitis, bacterial pneumonia, cystic fibrosis, *Coccidioides immitis* infection, and other fungal pulmonary infections and tuberculosis. Another problem is the cough associated with sinusitis, which can be confused with *B. pertussis* infection. The cough associated with gastroesophageal reflux also can be confused with pertussis, as can cough associated with a foreign body in the airway.

DIAGNOSIS

The diagnosis of pertussis relies on the combination of clinical and laboratory findings. A laboratory diagnosis of pertussis caused by *B. pertussis* or other *Bordetella* spp. can be made by culturing the organisms on appropriate media, by PCR, and by demonstrating a specific antibody titer rise or a high single-serum antibody titer. *Bordetella* spp. can be recovered from nasopharyngeal specimens, with the highest rate of isolation occurring within the first 3 weeks of cough.[247,531] Specimens for culture can be collected by swabbing the nasopharynx, by nasopharyngeal washing, or by nasopharyngeal aspiration.[113,229] Nasopharyngeal aspiration typically gives the highest yield of positive cultures, and nasopharyngeal wash is the least sensitive.

B. pertussis and *B. parapertussis* are recovered most easily by direct plating of the specimen from the patient onto selective media.[113,115,271,345] Specific swabs (i.e., calcium alginate or Dacron) and media (i.e., Regan-Lowe or Bordet-Gengou agar and modified Stainer-Scholte broth) are required, and laboratory personnel should be experienced in isolating the organisms. If cultures cannot be inoculated directly, the use of Regan-Lowe transport medium is recommended. In classic disease, the culture is positive in approximately 80% of cases if the specimen is obtained within 2 weeks of the onset of cough and antibiotics have not been administered previously[248,441]

Direct fluorescent antibody testing has been used for the diagnosis of pertussis caused by *B. pertussis* or *B. parapertussis* during the past 50 years.[367,410,521] It is rapid and inexpensive, but it lacks sensitivity and specificity; it does not employ amplification for sensitivity, and it lacks specificity because of cross-reactions with other organisms of the nasopharyngeal flora.[175] Because of the lack of sensitivity and specificity, its use is no longer recommended for diagnosis.[124,552,605]

Since the late 1980s, numerous PCR assays with primers derived from many different chromosomal regions of the organism have been developed for the diagnosis of *B. pertussis, B. parapertussis, B. holmesii,* and *B. bronchiseptica* infections, and they have been evaluated in multiple studies by comparison with culture and clinically typical pertussis.*

PCR has the advantage of having much higher sensitivity than that of conventional culture. In a prospective study in which swabs for PCR and culture were obtained simultaneously from 555 ill patients with cough, the use of PCR increased the identification of *B. pertussis* infection almost fourfold, from 28 to 111.[498] Only a few studies have been reported in which the sensitivity and the specificity of PCR for the diagnosis of *B. pertussis* infection were determined by comparison with serologically identified cases.[252,331,335,469,565] In one study,, we compared PCR results with serologic diagnosis and found that PCR had a sensitivity of 61% and a specificity of 88%.[185] Similar findings have been reported from other studies.[331,335,470,565]

The most commonly used primers for the diagnosis of pertussis include IS 481 and IS 1001.[123,344,367,546] IS 481 occurs in the genomes of *B. pertussis* (>50 copies) and *B. holmesii* (8–10 copies) but not in *B. parapertussis.* IS 1001 occurs in the genomes of *B. parapertussis* and *B. holmesii* (about 20 copies) but not in *B. pertussis.* The genome of *B. bronchiseptica* usually contains neither IS 481 nor IS 1001. However, in later studies, *B. bronchiseptica* strains were found to contain IS 1001 in their genomes (in the form of an IS 1001–like element called hIS 1001).[15,192,468,546]

False-positive results are a potential problem with the use of PCR for establishing the diagnosis of pertussis and other respiratory illnesses.[5,374,410] False-positive results can occur if specimens are opened in the pertussis laboratory before transport to the PCR laboratory.[367] False-positive results also can result from contamination of the air in a room in which the previous patient had pertussis and in a room where pertussis vaccine was administered.[357,545] Moreover, *B. bronchiseptica* can be mistaken for *B. parapertussis* when the IS 1001 primer is used.[192,468] Rigorous internal and external laboratory controls are necessary, and because insertion sequence elements are somewhat promiscuous, nucleic acid amplification tests should be accompanied with conventional culture.

Obtaining a routine laboratory diagnosis of *B. pertussis* infection for adults or in other atypical cases is hampered by the problem that medical care usually is not sought until the third or fourth week of the illness and antibiotics frequently have been administered before the possibility of pertussis was considered.[124,393,503] During the past 30 years, the most significant advance in the diagnosis of pertussis has been the development of ELISA.[367]

Natural infection with *B. pertussis* is followed by a rise in serum concentrations of IgA, IgG, and IgM antibodies to specific

*References 12, 123, 124, 162, 174, 178, 203, 215, 224, 242, 252, 278, 307, 330, 331, 335, 344, 357, 363, 374, 435, 468–470, 484, 498, 499, 545, 546, 552, 565, 564, 567, 605.

antigens of the organism and to preparations of the whole organism.[134,191,233,356,382,393,441,520,570] In contrast to natural infection, primary immunization of children induces mainly IgM and IgG antibodies and not IgA antibodies.

Serologic testing for *B. pertussis* infection in the clinical setting is not well standardized but is widely available in Europe and North America.[124] In the research setting, the use of ELISA contributed significantly to establishing the diagnosis of *B. pertussis* infection in many patients with negative cultures.[156,230,346,347,395,393,503,616] Most useful was the determination of IgG and IgA antibodies to PT and FHA. The most reliable proof of acute infection is the demonstration of a significant increase in antibody values between acute phase and convalescent phase serum specimens. Frequently, because collection of acute phase specimens is delayed and the acute phase values already are elevated, significant increases between first and second serum specimens cannot be demonstrated. However, a diagnosis can usually be established on the basis of a high value or values on a single serum specimen.[150,393,503,603,616] Because *B. parapertussis* infection induces cross-reacting antibodies to *B. pertussis* FHA, the use of this antigen alone cannot differentiate *B. pertussis* from *B. parapertussis* infection.[211,520]

Measurement of agglutinating antibodies also is useful for establishing the diagnosis of *B. pertussis* infection, and because the test is simple, inexpensive, and accurate, it can be used in the clinical setting.[150,257,393,441,503] Unfortunately, its sensitivity is low.

In clinical practice, the laboratory diagnosis of pertussis should be approached as follows. In all cases in which the cough is of less than 2 weeks' duration in adolescents and adults or 3 weeks' duration in children, a nasopharyngeal specimen should be obtained for culture or PCR. For adults who have had cough for more than 2 weeks' duration, single-serum ELISA is the preferred method provided they have not been immunized against pertussis in the previous 12 months.[124] This method also can be used for children if they have not been immunized within a year.

Many commercial laboratories offer single-serum diagnostic tests for *B. pertussis,* and almost all of the offered tests lack specificity. Any test that employs the whole organism is fraught with false-positive results. Tests that report specific IgM antibodies also are unreliable. The greatest sensitivity and specificity for the serologic diagnosis of *B. pertussis* infection are achieved by ELISA or an ELISA-like test with the measurement of IgG and IgA antibodies to PT. Single high values of IgG or IgA antibodies to PT indicate infection.[367] A sensitive and specific test in North America is available from Focus Diagnostics (Cypress, CA).[461] The performances of several European commercial serum ELISA kits for the diagnosis of *B. pertussis* illness have been evaluated by Riffelmann and associates.[472] They found that three kits that used PT as the antigen had specificities and sensitivities from 80% to 90%.

Not all infected persons develop antibody responses to PT. Approximately 25% of children lack an adequate response, as do approximately 10% of adolescents and adults (J. Cherry, unpublished observation).[520]

An ELISA has been developed for the detection of IgA antibody to *B. pertussis* in nasopharyngeal secretions as an indicator of recent infection.[205,210,619] *B. pertussis* IgA appears in nasopharyngeal secretions during the second or third week of illness and persists for at least 3 months.[205] However, the appearance of secretory IgA may be delayed in children younger than 1 year of age.[415] This antibody is not induced by primary parenteral *B. pertussis* vaccination. Detection with the use of ELISA of *B. pertussis* IgA in secretions may be a diagnostic aid for culture-negative patients whose symptoms have persisted for longer than 3 weeks. To our knowledge, this test is not clinically available.

TREATMENT

Several antibiotics have in vitro efficacy against *B. pertussis.*[26,33,32,34,40,80,272,275-277] The first choice for treatment since the 1970s has been oral erythromycin. It ameliorates the symptoms if it is given early during the course of the illness and eliminates viable organisms from the nasopharynx within a few days, thereby shortening the period of contagiousness. Unlike culture, PCR may remain positive for prolonged periods, especially in infants.[40,44,158,526] The dose for children is 40 to 50 mg/kg per day given every 6 hours for 14 days; the dose for adults is 2 g/day given every 6 hours for 14 days. A 7-day course of erythromycin estolate was shown in a large Canadian study to be as efficacious as 14 days of treatment.[232]

The newer macrolides also can be expected to be effective.[9,80] Azithromycin is given as 10 mg/kg on day 1 and 5 mg/kg on days 2 to 5 as a single dose for 5 days for children and 500 mg on day 1 and 250 mg on days 2 to 5 for adults. Clarithromycin is given as 15 to 20 mg/kg per day in two divided doses for 7 days for children and 1 g/day in two doses for 7 days for adults.

Although rare, the use of erythromycin in young infants is associated with hypertrophic pyloric stenosis, and parents need to be educated about the symptoms of this potential risk.[75,270] Because of the risk, the CDC recommends treating neonates with azithromycin rather than erythromycin.[80]

The CDC's recommended azithromycin dose is 10 mg/kg for 5 days. However, we are not aware of data that support this recommendation rather than what is also suggested for children beyond the neonatal period (10 mg/kg on day 1, followed by 5 mg/kg on days 2 to 5). Pyloric stenosis has been reported in 2 neonates who had received azithromycin (10 mg/kg for 5 days) and we think the reduced dose should be used in neonates on days 2 through 5 of treatment. In a study using the military health system database, erythromycin and azithromycin use within the first 42 days of life had the risk of inducing pyloric stenosis.[164] The erythromycin risk was about 1.5-fold greater than that of azithromycin. Trimethoprim-sulfamethoxazole can be used as an alternative agent in those who cannot tolerate erythromycin or azithromycin.[276]

The first erythromycin-resistant strain of *B. pertussis* was isolated from a 2-month-old male infant in Yuma County, Arizona, in June 1994.[328] The isolate was highly resistant, with a minimal inhibitory concentration (MIC) greater than 64 μg/mL (the usual MIC of erythromycin is 0.02 to 0.1 μg/mL). Four more resistant *B. pertussis* strains were recovered from cases in California, Utah, and Minnesota.[220,312,323] In France, macrolide resistance developed during illness in a neonate. In Japan, six *B. pertussis* strains were found to have high-level resistance to nalidixic acid and decreased susceptibilities to fluoroquinolones.[434] No evidence of a pattern of emerging macrolide resistance has been seen, but because PCR rather than culture has become the diagnostic method of choice in most laboratories, the chance of missing resistant strains is possible.

Patients infected with *B. parapertussis* and *B. holmesii* should be treated with macrolides, but *B. bronchiseptica* usually is resistant to macrolides, and alternative therapy is necessary.[367] *B. bronchiseptica* strains usually are sensitive to aminoglycosides; extended-spectrum, third-generation penicillins; tetracyclines; quinolones; and trimethoprim-sulfamethoxazole.

Historically, no infectious disease has a greater list of remedies lauded as beneficial but without objective evidence of effectiveness than pertussis.[42,102] Supportive care includes avoidance of factors that provoke attacks of coughing and maintenance of hydration and nutrition. In the hospital, gentle suction to remove secretions and well-humidified oxygen may be required, particularly in infants with pneumonia and significant respiratory distress. For severe infections in neonates and young infants, assisted ventilation is often necessary. However, infants who develop pulmonary hypertension with respiratory and cardiovascular failure respond poorly to aggressive therapy (i.e., pulmonary artery vasodilators and ECMO) and have high mortality rates. Because data suggest that the refractory pulmonary hypertension results from the extreme leukocytosis with lymphocytosis, which is always present in fatal cases, we think that leukocyte-reducing measures such as exchange transfusion should be implemented.[121,159,218,449,482] Exchange transfusion may be better than leukofiltration because it removes PT and reduces the WBC count.

The use of corticosteroids has received attention in the treatment of pertussis.[42,625] Cortisone treatment in the murine model of pertussis increased the mortality rate.[283] In a study by Roberts and associates,[475] dexamethasone treatment did not shorten the course of hospitalization compared with untreated controls.

The use of salbutamol was suggested as having some value, but no benefit was found in three studies reviewed by Bettiol and coworkers.[42,54] Pillay and Swingler[450] reviewed the symptomatic treatment of pertussis and found no statistically significant benefit for the use of diphenhydramine, dexamethasone, or salbutamol.

PROGNOSIS

The prognosis for pertussis is related to the patient's age. For older children and adults, the prognosis is good, but infants have a significant risk of death and development of encephalopathy.* Long-term follow-up suggests that apnea or seizures at the time of disease in children may be associated with subsequent intellectual impairment.[535] A Danish study found that the risk of epilepsy was increased among children with hospital-diagnosed pertussis infection compared with the general population.[440] The current availability of pediatric intensive care units and assisted ventilation has reduced the rate of mortality among infants who receive medical care.[253] Unfortunately, many deaths occur outside the hospital. No evidence has shown that pertussis impairs ventilatory function later in life.[253]

PREVENTION

Vaccine Efficacy

Whole-Cell Vaccines

The first pertussis vaccines were developed in the 1920s, and effective vaccines have enjoyed worldwide use since the 1940s.[89,88,113,367] After World War II, extensive vaccine trials were organized by the British Medical Research Council.[375–377] Based on these studies and smaller studies in England, the United States, and other countries, DTP vaccine use became routine in many countries.[186] The pertussis attack rate was relatively constant in the United States in the prevaccine era between 1922 and 1942. From 1943 to 1976, a 150-fold reduction in the attack rate was associated with widespread childhood pertussis immunization.

The relationship between vaccine use and disease control also was supported by data from England and Wales. The pertussis attack rate declined between 1958 and 1973 and increased dramatically between 1977 and 1983 after a marked decrease occurred in the number of vaccinations administered beginning in 1974.[89] The attack rate decreased with the widespread use of vaccine and increased when vaccine use decreased. Moreover, the attack rate after the decrease in vaccine use was increased most markedly in the newly susceptible cohort of children younger than 4 years of age.

In the 1980s, numerous household contact studies were performed.[67–69,150,442] In a study from 1982 to 1983 involving 440 household contacts between the ages of 6 months and 9 years, the secondary attack rate among unvaccinated contacts was compared with the rate for children who had received three or more DTP doses. Vaccine efficacy was 91.4%. A similar study conducted during the period of 1979 to 1981 revealed an efficacy of 82.4%.

In another study, Onorato and associates[442] found that the calculated efficacy varied markedly according to the clinical case definition. Efficacy against any cough was 63%, whereas it was 83% if a cough duration of 21 or more days was required.

In the 1990s, the most definitive studies of vaccine efficacy of DTP and DTaP were performed in four countries.[212,222,249,335,502,509,520] In these trials, the efficacy of the candidate DTaP vaccines was compared with the efficacy of DTP vaccines; the controls were subjects who received DT. With the exception of one lot of one DTP vaccine (Connaught, USA) that had poor immunogenicity, the DTP vaccines were more efficacious than the DTaP vaccines. The poor efficacy of the Connaught DTP vaccine probably was the result of an unusual low-potency lot of this vaccine rather than a generic problem with the vaccine.[367] In a case-control study in the United States, the efficacy of the Connaught vaccine was similar to that of the Wyeth-Lederle DTP vaccine, which in the controlled trial in Germany had a high level of efficacy.[47] In a large comparative trial, the DTP vaccine from England (Evans vaccine) had long-term efficacy greater than those of the three DTaP vaccines with which it was compared.[437]

Acellular Vaccines

Research in the 1970s showed that three *B. pertussis* antigens (i.e., PT, FHA, and LPS) were liberated into the medium during culture and that the antigens could be concentrated and separated by density-gradient centrifugation.[113,264] This finding enabled development and production of vaccines by six manufacturers in Japan.[119,303,429,494] All six vaccines had minimal or no endotoxin but different amounts of PT and FHA. Some of the vaccines were found to contain FIM 2 and PRN.

Despite limited proof of efficacy, the six vaccines were put into routine use in Japan in 1981, and they have controlled to some degree reported epidemic pertussis during the ensuing decades. However, because adequate data were not available on any single vaccine or on vaccine use in young infants, many extensive trials were performed subsequently in Europe, Africa, and Japan.[3,212,222,249,332,408,509,520]

After extensive analysis of the data from the original efficacy trial in Sweden in the mid-1980s, it was found that calculated efficacy varied significantly, depending on the clinical case definition and the laboratory methods.[3,48,230,527,528,530] Researchers decided that a universal primary case definition should be developed for use in all subsequent efficacy trials so that different vaccines in different trials could be compared.

A World Health Organization (WHO) committee met in Geneva in January 1991, and a primary case definition was developed.[613] This definition and minor variations of it were used in the efficacy trials in the 1990s. The WHO case definition was as follows:

1. An illness with 21 days or more of spasmodic cough and either culture-confirmed infection with *B. pertussis* or serologic evidence of infection with *B. pertussis* as indicated by a significant rise in IgA or IgG antibody by ELISA against PT or FHA in paired sera *or*
2. Contact with a case of culture-confirmed pertussis in the household with onset within 28 days before or after the onset of cough in the study vaccinee.

Not all members of the WHO committee, including Cherry, agreed with this primary case definition because its use results in the elimination of many laboratory-confirmed cases from efficacy calculations.[96,247,251,527,528,530] With this definition, vaccines that lessen the severity of disease but are poor at preventing mild disease were overrated.

In 1994 and 1995, seven efficacy trials with candidate DTaP vaccines in four countries were completed,[212,222,332,502,509,520,553] and an additional trial in Sweden was completed in 1997.[437] As shown in Table 129.3, the nine vaccines are different in the number of antigens that they contain and in the concentrations of the specific antigens. In all efficacy studies, confounding factors may affect the results. Double-blind studies with placebo and whole-cell vaccine controls are ideal. However, placebo control was not ethical in countries in which DTP vaccine was recommended. Studies in Germany and Senegal therefore used various methods to obtain efficacy data despite the lack of a blinded diphtheria-tetanus (DT) toxoid group. Observer bias can affect the results of all studies, including those with a double-blind control. For example, a less efficacious vaccine that prevents typical disease but not mild disease can be determined to be more efficacious than it actually is if the study observers believe they "know pertussis" and dismiss atypical cases as being other respiratory tract illnesses and do not obtain cultures or conduct proper follow-up.[118]

Household contact studies, unless they are nested analyses in prospective cohort studies, also are subject to observer bias, and case-control studies result in significantly inflated efficacy percentages.[96,118,120,183,186,408] In cohort studies, observer bias by parents can be reduced by frequent prospective telephone contact with study families. A serologic diagnosis and a diagnosis by culture increased the identification of mild cases, which are more likely to occur in vaccinees than in control subjects.

A summary of the efficacy data for 10 acellular pertussis vaccines evaluated in the eight trials performed in the 1990s and the earlier 1980s' Swedish trial is presented in Table 129.4. The data in this table indicate that three- and four-component vaccines (i.e., vaccines containing PRN. FIM, PT, and FHA) have greater efficacy against *B. pertussis* illness (i.e., mild and typical) than do the PT or PT/FHA vaccines. The apparent high efficacy of the two-component vaccine (Tripedia) in the Munich study[332] can be explained by the type of study (i.e., case-control study), significant observer bias, the vaccine contents (i.e., PRN, FIM, PT, and FHA), and the lack of serologic diagnosis.

The study done in Stockholm was a comparative study without a DT control group.[436] In this trial, in which vaccines were administered to children at 3, 5, and 12 months of age, the efficacy of CCL DTaP5

*References 30, 36, 127, 141, 142, 176, 177, 200, 218, 221, 274, 370, 373, 383, 414, 417, 426, 455, 482, 488, 497, 510, 512, 540, 572, 602, 622.

TABLE 129.3 Pertussis Antigens in Nine Diphtheria–Tetanus–Acellular Pertussis Vaccines Evaluated in Eight Efficacy Trials (1990–97)

Vaccine Product	Pertussis Toxin (μg/Dose)	Filamentous Hemagglutinin (μg/Dose)	Pertactin (μg/Dose)	Fimbriae (μg/Dose)
Certiva[a]	40			
Tripedia[a,b]	23.4	23.4		
Triavax	25	25		
SKB-2[c]	25	25		
Acelluvax	5	2.5	2.5	
Infanrix[a]	25	25	8	
Acel-Immune[a]	3.5	35	2	0.8[d]
Daptacel[a]	10	5	3	5[e]
CCL DTaP5[f]	20	20	3	5[e]

[a]Licensed in the United States.
[b]This vaccine was subsequently found to contain pertactin and fimbriae.
[c]No product name.
[d]Fimbriae 2.
[e]Fimbriae 2 and 3.
[f]No product name; however, this vaccine is available in Canada with inactivated polio vaccine (IPV) as Quadracel and in Canada and the United States with IPV and *Haemophilus influenzae* type b (Hib) vaccine as Pentacel.

TABLE 129.4 Vaccine Efficacy Data for 10 Acellular Pertussis Vaccines Evaluated in Eight Trials Performed in the 1990s and Earlier 1980s Swedish Trials

				EFFICACY	
Study Location	**Study Design**	**Vaccine**	**Schedule**	**Typical Pertussis (%)**	**Mild and Typical Pertussis (%)**
Stockholm, Sweden[1,34,407]	Double-blind, prospective cohort	JNIH-6 JNIH-7	2 doses (2–3 mo apart starting at 5–11 mo of age)	84[a] 90	42 −7
Göteborg, Sweden[428,b]	Double-blind, prospective cohort	Certiva	3 doses (3, 5, 12 mo)	71	54
Stockholm, Sweden[168]	Double-blind, prospective cohort	SKB-2 Daptacel	3 doses (2, 4, 6 mo)	59 85	42 78
Rome, Italy[160]	Double-blind, prospective cohort	Acelluvax Infanrix	3 doses (2, 4, 6 mo)	84 84	71 71
Erlangen, Germany[401]	Prospective cohort	Acel-Immune	4 doses (3, 4.5, 6, 15–18 mo)	83	72
Mainz, Germany[387]	Household contact	Infanrix	3 doses (3, 4, 5 mo)	89	81
Munich, Germany[256,c]	Case-control	Tripedia	4 doses (2, 4, 6, 15–25 mo)	80, 93	—
Senegal[394,d]	Household contact	Triavax	3 doses	31, 74	—

[a]Efficacy against typical pertussis based on positive culture without serologic analysis.
[b]Significant observer bias occurred in this trial.[56]
[c]Laboratory diagnosis based on culture only; 80% efficacy was against illness with cough of 21 or more days, and 93% efficacy was against the World Health Organization (WHO) case definition.
[d]Thirty-one percent efficacy based on 21 days or more of illness with cough; 74% efficacy was against the WHO case definition.

(i.e., five-component vaccine) was significantly better than that of Acelluvax (i.e., three-component vaccine) and was not significantly different from that of the comparative DTP vaccine (i.e., Evans vaccine) for the initial 3 years of follow-up. Acelluvax had greater efficacy than did the two-component vaccine SKB-2.

Follow-up studies of the various efficacy trials have been done in Sweden, Italy, and Germany, and all suggest sustained protection.[223,348,436,492,493] In a study by Gustafsson and associates,[222] members of a large cohort vaccinated at 3, 5, and 12 months in the 1993 to 1996 trial were observed from October 1997 to September 2004. Overall, good protection lasted for approximately 5 years. The tabular data in this report suggest that Acelluvax had efficacy similar to that of CCL DTaP5. However, when all the data from the original trial and the follow-up data were combined, the overall attack rate for children who had received CCL DTaP5 was lower (47.5 cases/100,000 people) than that for children who had received Acelluvax (59.7 cases/100,000 people). This difference was not significantly different, however. The Evans DTP vaccine had greater sustained efficacy than Acelluvax or CCL DTaP5. It appeared that DTaP vaccines that contained PRN had relatively good efficacy for approximately 5 years but that (with the exception of one lot of one DTP vaccine) DTP vaccines usually were more efficacious.[212,222,332,437,492,502,509,520]

In 2005, two acellular pertussis component, diphtheria, and tetanus toxoid vaccines (i.e., Tdap vaccines) became available for use in adolescents and adults.[81,82,100,189,190,246] The components of the Adacel and Boostrix vaccines are given in Table 129.5. After a single dose, both vaccines elicit vigorous antibody responses to the antigens that they contain. These responses are significantly greater than those observed in infants at 7 months of age after they have received three doses of the DTaP vaccines (i.e., Daptacel and Infanrix) of the two manufacturers.

In a double-blind efficacy trial enrolling adolescents and adults, an acellular pertussis vaccine (without diphtheria and tetanus toxoids) with the same concentrations of PT, FHA, and PRN as Boostrix had an efficacy of 92%.[578] However, the data safety monitoring board allowed the removal of one case that occurred in a vaccinee. If this case is included, the efficacy is approximately 78%. No similar efficacy trial

TABLE 129.5 Antigenic Composition of Adacel and Boostrix per 0.5 mL of Vaccine

Antigen	Adacel	Boostrix
Diphtheria toxoid	2 Lf	2.5 Lf
Tetanus toxoid	5 Lf	5 Lf
Pertussis toxin toxoid	2.5 μg	8 μg
Filamentous hemagglutinin	5 μg	8 μg
Pertactin	3 μg	2.5 μg
Fimbriae 2, 3	5 μg	—

Lf, Flocculation unit.

BOX 129.2 Factors That Lessen Efficacy of DTaP Vaccines Compared With DTP Vaccines

- A Th1/Th2 response in DTaP vaccinees versus a Th17/Th1 response in DTP vaccinees
- Incomplete antigen package
- Incorrect balance of antigens in the vaccine
- Linked-epitope suppression
- Genetic changes in *B. pertussis*

Th1, Helper T cell type 1; *Th2*, helper T cell type 2; *Th17*, helper T cell type 17.

was done with Adacel or its acellular pertussis components. However, extensive epidemiologic data from Canada, where Adacel has been used since 2003, show a marked reduction of pertussis among adolescents.[295]

The 2010 epidemic of pertussis in California and more recent outbreaks in other states and Australia led to several studies of DTaP and Tdap vaccine failure and vaccine effectiveness.[73,464,587,608] In a study by Wei and associates, Tdap vaccine effectiveness in school children 11 years of age and older was 66%.[587] However, because the sample in this study was small, the result was not statistically significant. In a study of adolescents, Tdap effectiveness was found to be 78%.[465]

Reported cases of pertussis started to increase around 1982 to 1984. This was about 14 years before the universal use of DTaP vaccines. However in the DTaP and Tdap vaccine era, there have been marked peaks in reported pertussis incidence in 2005, 2010, 2012, and 2014. Numerous publications indicated that DTaP vaccines were inferior to DTP vaccines in regard to sustained efficacy.[105,109,305,306,334,397,544,600,601,607] Although a major part of the increase in reported pertussis resulted from greater awareness and the use of PCR and single-serum serologic diagnoses, there are several deficiencies in DTaP vaccines compared with DTP vaccines. Tdap vaccines have efficacy that wanes rapidly during a 3-year period.[35,311]

Box 129.2 shows five factors that contribute to the diminished efficacy of DTaP vaccines compared with DTP vaccines. The first is the type of T-cell response. The difference in T-cell response after infection, DTaP vaccination, and DTP vaccination was described more than 25 years ago by Kingston Mills and associates[486,490] in studies using a mouse model. These findings were largely ignored, but later studies using baboons confirmed and expanded what was previous demonstrated.[580–582] Previously infected baboons and DTP-vaccinated baboons possess strong *B. pertussis*–specific helper T-cell type 17 (Th17) memory and Th1 memory (i.e., Th17/Th1 response), whereas DTaP vaccinees had a Th1/Th2 response. The Th17/Th1 response prevents infection and disease, whereas the Th1/Th2 response prevents only disease. The Th17/Th1 response also gives longer protection than a Th1/Th2 response.

The next factor is an incomplete antigen package. From the vaccine efficacy trials in the 1980s and 1990s, it was clear that increasing the number of proteins in a DTaP vaccine increased its initial efficacy.[96] The two DTaP vaccines currently used in most of the world contain three and five proteins. In contrast, DTP vaccines contain more than 3000 proteins, and it is likely that antibodies to many of them contribute to protection.

Another important factor is the incorrect balance of antigens in the vaccines. Of the eight vaccine efficacy trials of the 1990s, only two were done in such a way that serologic correlates of immunity could be determined.[96,529] The two studies were done independently, but they yielded similar findings. Both found that antibody to PRN and FIM induced protection in about 70% of vaccinees. Both also found that antibody to FHA did not contribute to protection. Both studies confirmed that high levels of antibody to PT blocked the effectiveness of antibody to FIM. This blocking effect was also observed for PT and PRN in the Swedish study (J. Cherry, unpublished data, 2005). Studies by Weiss and colleagues[591] using serum from the adult aP vaccine trial supported the idea that antibody to PT had a blocking effect on antibody to PRN. We suspect the same blocking effect relates to PT and FIM. Two highly effective DTP vaccines produce only low levels of antibody to PT and FHA, whereas the currently used DTaP vaccines produce high levels of antibody to PT and FHA, which may suppress efficacy.

The fourth factor reducing vaccine efficacy is linked-epitope suppression. In conjunction with colleagues in Sweden, we described this in 2010.[117,125] We found that people who received a PT toxoid vaccine but were vaccine failures developed antibody to PT but not to FHA, a nonvaccine antigen. Similarly, when people received a PT/FHA-containing vaccine and were vaccine failures, they developed antibody to PT and FHA but not to PRN and FIM 2/3.

With linked-epitope suppression, memory B cells outcompete naive B cells for access to the *Bordetella* epitopes because they are more numerous and their receptors exhibit a higher antigen affinity. Linked-epitope suppression applies as the immune response to novel epitopes is suppressed by the strong response to initial components if they are introduced together.

Findings by Sheridan and associates[507] in Australia support the linked-epitope suppression hypothesis. They found over a 12-year period that the pertussis attack rate among DTP-primed children was significantly less than it was among DTaP-primed children.

The fifth factor is genetic changes in *B. pertussis* proteins. In the whole-cell vaccine era, this was never a problem because immunizations resulted in an antibody response to multiple antigens. However, it is a potential problem for DTaP vaccines. Three genetic changes have occurred in the era of acellular vaccines: shift in the *ptx* P1 allele to the *ptx* P3 allele, increase in *fim* 3B strains in the United States, and the occurrence of PRN-deficient mutants. Of these, only the circulation of PRN-deficient mutants is important. In the United Sates, almost all circulating strains are PRN deficient. Because the main protective antigen in three-component vaccines is PRN, more vaccine failure with three-component vaccines might be expected, but that has not been demonstrated because antibody to the B subunit of PT provides considerable efficacy against typical pertussis.

A Wisconsin study showed that efficacy of Tdap vaccines waned over a 3-year period.[311] This was a surprise to many people because in the adolescent and adult efficacy trial (APERT), antibody to PRN persisted for about 9 years. This led to the suggestion that administering Tdap about every 10 years would decrease circulation of *B. pertussis*.[321,578] This prediction was wrong. The antibody to PRN determined by ELISA is probably cross-reacting antibody to *Bordetella* sp. and other organisms, and the cross-reacting antibody that was measured did not protect against *B. pertussis* infection.

Adverse Events

Whole-Cell Vaccines

Local reactions and relatively mild systemic complaints are frequent occurrences after pertussis immunization. Less commonly, severe neurologic illness and death have been temporally associated with DTP immunization.

The largest study in the United States, which was designed to assess the risk for relatively common and uncommon reactions to pertussis vaccine, was performed by Baraff and associates.[22–25,129] It was conducted between January 1978 and December 1979. Reactions in children who received DTP or DT immunization were compared. A total of 15,752 DTP immunizations and 784 DT immunizations were given to children 2 months to 6 years of age. They were evaluated for reactions that occurred within 48 hours of vaccine administration. All common local and systemic reactions occurred more frequently in the DTP recipients than in the DT group. Differences between the common reactions in the two groups were all highly significant ($P < .005$).

Redness at the injection site occurred in 37.4% of DTP recipients and in 7.6% of DT vaccinees. Fever (≥38°C [100.4°F]) occurred in 46.5% of DTP recipients. A temperature of 39°C (102.2°F) or higher occurred in 6.1% of DTP recipients but in only 0.7% of DT recipients. Drowsiness, fretfulness, vomiting, anorexia, and persistent crying were other reactions recorded for 3.1% (i.e., persistent crying) to 53.4% (i.e., fretfulness) of DTP recipients versus 0.7% (i.e., persistent crying) to 22.6% (i.e., fretfulness) of DT vaccinees. Rates of local reactions, but not those of systemic reactions (except fever), increased from dose to dose in an immunization series.

Another 0.1% of DTP recipients in this study were reported by the parents to have a high-pitched, unusual cry; 0.06% had convulsions, and 0.06% had hypotonic-hyporesponsive episodes (e.g., shock, collapse). No children in the control group (i.e., DT recipients) had similar reactions; however, the control group was of modest size (784 DT recipients), and statistical significance could not be assigned to any of these relatively uncommon events.

Because convulsions in young children are the result of many different etiologic factors, the cause-and-effect relationship with pertussis vaccine is less clear. However, inasmuch as fever develops in almost one half of all DTP vaccinees and febrile convulsions are not uncommon events, a reasonable assumption is that many convulsions that are temporally associated with DTP vaccination are induced by the immunization. Three studies found a significant association between pertussis immunization and febrile convulsions.[27,508,574] Approximately 1 of 1000 vaccinees older than 6 months of age has a first febrile seizure after receiving pertussis immunization. The concomitant use of acetaminophen (15 mg/kg per dose at the time of immunization and every 4 hours for 24 hours) with DTP vaccination has been suggested as a means of reducing the incidence of febrile convulsions in vaccinees.[327]

Neurologic disease and death temporally associated with pertussis immunization have been major concerns throughout the vaccine era. During last 60 years of the 20th century, several case series and individual cases of neurologic illness occurring after receipt of pertussis immunization were reported, and by 1979, more than 1000 cases of alleged neurologic damage induced by pertussis vaccine were reported.[39,60,86,89,315,362,599] Few of these reports had evidence of an adequate search for other possible causes of the neurologic disease, and in none were data available for rate calculations.

From 1967 to 1980, several attempts were made to determine the frequency of neurologic disease after receipt of pertussis immunization.[4,89,165,166,188,238,524,533] However, because controls were not included in any of the population evaluations, all rate estimates included children with temporally related events that had other causes.

A carefully designed, prospective, case-control study (i.e., National Childhood Encephalopathy Study [NCES]) of all hospital admissions of children 2 to 35 months of age with acute, serious neurologic disorders in England, Wales, and Scotland was undertaken between 1976 and 1979.[6,37,351,384,385,388,389] The results of this study for the first time revealed an apparent statistical association between pertussis immunization and neurologic illness. Researchers found that a child who had received DTP vaccine within the previous 3 to 7 days was two to five times more likely to have neurologic disease than was a child who was not immunized during the same interval. However, the causal relationship between DTP immunization and neurologic illness found in this study must be questioned because cases and controls had an equal frequency of immunization during the month preceding the index date. A more appropriate interpretation of the results is that they do not indicate cause and effect; rather, the DTP immunization highlights something that will occur anyway but moves it forward in time (i.e., trigger effect).[90,91]

Cases of infantile spasms, an identifiable seizure disorder of infancy, usually occur in the 6-month period from 2 to 7 months of age; it is therefore not surprising that some cases occur after DTP immunization. Simple calculations indicate that approximately 12% of all patients destined to have infantile spasms between 2 and 7 months of age will have an onset of illness within 7 days after receiving DTP immunization. The temporal association between DTP immunization and infantile spasms has led many people to assume a cause-and-effect relationship. However, controlled data from the NCES in Great Britain provide strong evidence against a causative role for pertussis vaccine in infantile spasms.[37] In a Danish study, Melchior[378] found that the time of onset of infantile spasms was not altered when the time of pertussis immunization was changed from 5, 6, 7, and 15 months of age to 5 weeks, 9 weeks, and 10 months of age. In both periods, 42% of patients had the onset during the first 4 months of life.

Data from the NCES were reanalyzed with the exclusion of cases of infantile spasm.[385,389] From these analyses, the risk of permanent brain damage occurring from pertussis immunization was suggested to be 1 case per 330,000 vaccine doses, and the risk of encephalopathy has been estimated to be 1 case per 140,000 vaccinations. However, a review of the NCES data by other investigators indicates that both rate estimates are incorrect. Stephenson[523] showed that the 1 case per 140,000 vaccine doses rate for all encephalopathy is an artifact resulting from the inclusion of nine children with febrile convulsions. Similarly, MacRae[350] found that the increased relative risk that was observed within 7 days of receiving immunization (which was used to calculate the risk for brain damage of 1 case per 330,000 immunizations) was offset by a decreased relative risk over the subsequent 3-week period. This finding, similar to the original study data and the infantile spasm data, indicates a redistribution of events over time rather than a cause-and-effect relationship.

In the United States, the major neurologic illness that was temporally associated with DTP immunization was the first seizure of what turned out to be severe epilepsy. By chance, this association may occur 400 times per year in the United States. Four carefully performed studies that included approximately 330,000 children and 1 million immunizations have examined the possibility that pertussis immunization is a causative factor in epilepsy; no evidence of a causative role has been found.[91,198,214,508,574] Two large studies in the United States and Canada found no evidence of a causal association with DTP immunization and encephalopathy.[402,466]

Similar to infantile spasms, SIDS occurs in early life, and cases that occur after administration of DTP immunization are not surprising. Hoffman and associates[268] performed an extensive, prospective, case-control study of risk factors in SIDS from October 1978 through December 1979. In this study of 800 cases, investigators found that DTP immunization was not a risk factor for development of the syndrome. Other good, controlled studies have yielded similar results.[113,213] No evidence has demonstrated that DTP vaccinees have an increased risk of developing asthma later in life.[261]

Acellular Vaccines

An extensive amount of reactogenicity information was generated in phase II and phase III studies with all licensed DTaP vaccines.[148,212,222,332,471,501,556] Because endotoxin has been removed from all DTaP vaccines, it is not surprising that all are less reactogenic than DTP vaccines. In a double-blind study, the reactogenicity of 13 DTaP vaccines was compared with the reactogenicity of a DTP vaccine.[148] This study involved 2200 infants; 113 to 217 received an acellular product, and 370 received the whole-cell vaccine. Study participants received three doses of vaccine at 2, 4, and 6 months of age. Overall, all monitored reactions except vomiting occurred less frequently and were less severe in DTaP recipients than in DTP recipients. Results from this study are presented in Table 129.6. Local redness and swelling and fever increased in frequency from the first to the third dose, whereas the complaint of drowsiness decreased.

In our efficacy trial in Germany with Acel-Immune, we monitored reactions in more than 8000 children after receipt of four doses of vaccine at 3, 4.5, 6, and 15 to 18 months.[504,556] For the first three vaccine doses, the findings were similar to those shown in Table 129.6. After the fourth dose, the frequency of occurrence of local erythema and induration and fever increased considerably compared with their frequencies after the third dose. Ten percent of DTaP recipients had local erythema of 2.4 cm or greater, and 28% had temperatures of 38°C or higher. Other investigators also found an increased frequency and severity of local reactions occurring after administration of the fourth and fifth doses of DTaP vaccines.[248,288,448,471,501] Of particular concern is the observation of extensive swelling of the thigh with booster doses of

TABLE 129.6 Reactogenicity Data From the Nationwide Multicenter Acellular Pertussis Trial

	DTAP VACCINE			DTP VACCINE		
Event	**1st Dose (%)**	**2nd Dose (%)**	**3rd Dose (%)**	**1st Dose (%)**	**2nd Dose (%)**	**3rd Dose (%)**
Local						
Redness	13.5	17.1	21.5	49.4	47.7	47.6
Swelling	8.7	12.1	13.3	39.7	34.1	35.7
Pain	3.8	2.0	2.1	27.3	18.7	15.8
Systemic						
Fever (≥38.6°C [100.1°F])	4.2	11.3	15.8	27.3	34.1	37.7
Fussiness	6.6	7.7	6.7	20.1	23.5	17.3
Drowsiness	29.9	17.6	12.9	43.5	31.0	24.6
Anorexia	9.3	8.9	8.9	19.5	16.5	14.3
Vomiting	6.3	4.5	4.2	7.0	4.5	5.3
Use of antipyretic	39.3	36.7	36.3	60.5	59.8	61.4

DTaP, Diphtheria–tetanus–acellular pertussis; *DTP*, diphtheria-tetanus-pertussis.
Data from Decker MD, Edwards KM, Steinhoff MC, et al. Comparison of 13 acellular pertussis vaccines: adverse reactions. *Pediatrics.* 1995;96:557–66.

TABLE 129.7 Severe Events After Diphtheria–Tetanus–Acellular Pertussis Vaccines in the 1990s Efficacy Trials

Vaccine	**Persistent Crying (≥3 h) (Rate per 1000 Doses)**	**Hypotonic- Hyporesponsive Episodes (Rate per 1000 Doses)**	**Seizures (Rate per 1000 Doses)**
Certiva	0	0	0.4
Tripedia	0.1	0.05	0.02
SKB-2	0.8	0	0.3
Acelluvax	1.9	0.07	0
Infanrix	1.3	0	0.07
Acel-Immune	2.0	0	0.1
Daptacel	1.5	0.1	0

Data from references 160, 168, 256, 428, 431.

some DTaP vaccines.[471,501] Rennels and associates[471] found that swelling occurred more commonly after immunization with DTaP vaccines containing high amounts of diphtheria toxoid. With Acel-Immune, a vaccine with a low diphtheria toxoid content, 15.4% of subjects had induration of more than 5 cm but less than 10 cm after receiving a fifth dose; swelling of the entire limb did not occur.[248]

In five of the efficacy trials in the 1990s, the occurrence of less common, more severe events (i.e., persistent crying, seizures, and hypotonic-hyporesponsive episodes) was monitored. These data are summarized in Table 129.7. Temporally related persistent crying, hypotonic-hyporesponsive episodes, and seizures were rare events after receipt of immunization with DTaP vaccines. In a large active surveillance program (IMPACT), researchers found that risks of having febrile seizures and hypotonic-hyporesponsive episodes after receiving pertussis-containing vaccines decreased significantly after the introduction of DTaP vaccines in Canada.[326] In a Vaccine Safety Datalink study, Huang and coworkers[280] did not observe an increased risk of seizures in children 6 weeks to 23 months of age after DTaP vaccination.

Schedules and Contraindications

Immunizing schedules for whole-cell and acellular pertussis vaccines vary throughout the world.[386] Before the acellular vaccine era, schedules related to DTP vaccines were determined to some measure by concern relating to true and perceived reactions[94,127,180,386] An immunization schedule involving only three doses given to infants at 2, 3, and 4 months of age was quite effective in controlling pertussis-related morbidity and mortality in the United Kingdom.[61,562] However, the five-dose schedule used in the United States resulted in lower attack rates in preschool- and school-aged children.[89,113]

A World Health Organization position paper[614] suggests that countries that have been using DTP vaccines continue to do so. They recommend a three-dose primary series with the first dose administered as early as 6 weeks of age. Subsequent doses are recommended to be given 4 to 8 weeks apart at age 10 to 14 weeks and 14 to 18 weeks.

The recommendation for the DTaP vaccine in the United States is that it be given in the same five-dose schedule as previously recommended for DTP vaccines.[9,70] However, follow-up data from the 1990s efficacy trials and reactogenicity data suggested that this approach could be modified.[212,222,436,492,493,501,543,553] Our findings for Acel-Immune suggested that the current five-dose schedule was appropriate.[348,520] Conversely, data from other trials suggested that administration of the fourth dose of some vaccines could be postponed until the child was 4 to 6 years of age or that the third dose could be moved back to the child's second year of life.[223,436,437,492,493,543,553] These changes would not be expected to decrease efficacy but would decrease troubling local reactions with booster doses. However, the follow-up data for the previously described studies employed passive surveillance techniques, and pertussis attack rates in DTaP recipients were likely underestimated. Data from the 2010 California epidemic show a yearly increase in vaccine failures after the fifth dose of DTaP.[104,601] A DTaP vaccination schedule used in several countries is to administer the vaccine at 3, 5, and 12 months of age.

Acellular pertussis-component quadrivalent (DTaP, IPV), pentavalent (DTaP, IPV, HBV; DTaP, IPV, Hib), and hexavalent (DTaP, IPV, HBV, Hib) vaccines are available in many countries.[168] In the United States, the following multicomponent vaccines are used: DTaP/IPV/HBV (Pediarix) and DTaP/IPV/Hib (Pentacel). Multicomponent vaccine use should be encouraged to reduce the number of injections that a child receives.[9]

In addition to providing childhood immunization, the availability of adolescent and adult Tdap vaccines allows the vaccination of adolescents and adults to be conducted.* The schedule for the use of Tdap vaccines varies in different countries.[189,190,246] The most common recommendation is for universal immunization of preadolescents and adolescents and the selective immunization of adults. We previously thought that a universal program involving all preadolescents or adolescents and adults every 10 years would be necessary to prevent the transmission of *B. pertussis* effectively to unimmunized infants and to prevent the continued circulation of *B. pertussis* in a population. However, the recent findings that Tdap vaccine effectiveness lasted only 3 years indicates our previous opinion was wrong. No country has an effective program for universal immunization of adults, and no country is likely to achieve a universal Tdap booster program with even modest compliance. Because adults are the main source of pertussis for young infants, various cocooning programs have been suggeseted.[9,72,216,559] They include postpartum immunization of the mother and, if possible, the father; attempts to vaccinate grandparents; and immunization of mothers-to-be during the second or third trimesters of pregnancy. Also considered is lowering the age of infant immunization, including a dose shortly after birth.[24,31,38,58,59,236,308,609,610] All of these cocooning programs have numerous logistical difficulties.[463,559]

We think the most promising approach is immunization of the mother during the second and third trimesters of pregnancy. In 2011, the Advisory Committee on Immunization Practices (ACIP) updated its Tdap recommendations to include pregnant women. They suggested giving the vaccine during the third trimester or late second trimester.[72] In 2013, the ACIP made an additional recommendation: Providers of prenatal care should implement a Tdap immunization program for all pregnant women. Tdap should be administered during each pregnancy. Vaccine should be administered between 27 and 36 weeks' gestation.[71] Two studies in England found that Tdap in pregnancy had an effectiveness of more than 90% in preventing pertussis in infants during the first 2 months of life.[10,143]

Tdap immunization in all pregnancies can be expected to prevent virtually all pertussis deaths of infants during the first 2 months of life. Unfortunately, the use of Tdap vaccines in pregnant women in the United States is far from optimal.[110]

Tdap immunization of pregnant women is safe and elicits excellent antibody response to PT and other vaccine antigens.[301,412,534] Tdap immunization during pregnancy blunts the infant's response to DTaP antigens and some conjugate vaccines.[318] However, if booster doses are given early in the second year of the life, this is not a problem.[24,58,107]

Over the years, pertussis vaccine recommendations have undergone many changes. Contraindications to pertussis immunization continue to evolve, but few scientific data support any of the current contraindications. The primary goal of national immunization program in the United States is to vaccinate all infants, children, adolescents, and pregnant women and selected adults. If excessive contraindications and their overinterpretation lead to a large number of unimmunized persons, the programs will fail, and the children in greatest need of protection will contract pertussis. In the United States, the most recent recommendations of the Committee on Infectious Diseases of the American Academy of Pediatrics should be followed.

There is considerable pessimism about DTaP vaccines because of their deficiencies. However, this should be put into perspective. There are about 20-fold fewer cases of pertussis today than in the prevaccine era, and illness in cases of DTaP vaccine failure is less severe than illness in unvaccinated children.[28,105,381,549] We should continue to use DTaP and Tdap vaccines as currently recommended. The DTaP schedule in the United States is 2, 4, 6, and 15 months and at 4 to 6 years of age. However, the first dose can be given at 6 weeks of age, and vaccinating at 6 weeks of age rather than 2 months of age can decrease death, hospitalization, and severe illness. We therefore suggest using this acceleration of the schedule.

Preventing deaths and severe disease in infants too young to be vaccinated is our highest priority. In the past, protecting young infants by maternal postpartum Tdap immunization and immunizing persons who had contact with young infants (i.e., cocooning) was pushed. However, immunizing pregnant women with Tdap between 27 and 36 weeks' gestation at each pregnancy, if universally applied, would prevent virtually all young infant pertussis deaths.

We also recommend giving Tdap every 10 years rather than using Td. It also seems reasonable to immunize some adults with Tdap every 3 years. They include health care workers and others who have contact with young infants.

*References 81, 82, 93, 94, 97, 99, 100, 101, 189, 190, 234, 246, 297, 367, 487.

Isolation and Prophylactic Measures

Erythromycin, azithromycin, or clarithromycin treatment in the index case shortens the duration of communicability of the organisms and limits spread of the disease. During the first few days of treatment, contact with susceptible persons should be avoided. Close contacts (e.g., household members, those in childcare centers, playmates) of the index case should be protected from infection. Protection can be implemented by the prophylactic use of erythromycin for 14 days, azithromycin for 5 days, or clarithromycin for 7 days.[9,80,367,522] Active immunization of all exposed persons (i.e., children, adolescents, and adults) who are not adequately vaccinated should be conducted.

The use of prophylactic antibiotics in adolescents and adults in exposure situations such as classrooms and hospital settings frequently is recommended. This approach often involves many people and considerable expense.

Because of the side effects of erythromycin and other macrolides, adult compliance is poor. These antibiotics should not be used prophylactically in large group settings but should be used for treatment only at the first sign of respiratory illness in those exposed.

OTHER *BORDETELLA* INFECTIONS

Bordetella parapertussis Infection

B. parapertussis infection in children can cause unrecognized infection, mild pertussis, or typical pertussis.[367] We studied 38 children with *B. parapertussis* illnesses and compared their illnesses with those occurring in 76 children with *B. pertussis* illnesses.[256] The results *(B. pertussis/B. parapertussis)* were as follows: cough for longer than 4 weeks, 57%/37% (P = .06); whooping, 80%/59% (P = .07); whooping for longer than 2 weeks, 26%/18% (P = .05); paroxysms, 90%/83%; and posttussive vomiting, 47%/42%. Mean leukocyte and lymphocyte counts were 12,500/mm^3 and 7600/mm^3 and 7800/mm^3 and 3500/mm^3 ($P < .0001$), respectively.

In an Italian study, children with *B. parapertussis* infection had the following findings: cough (100%), paroxysms (76%), whooping (33%), posttussive vomiting (42%), apnea (29%), and cyanosis (12%).[364] All of these rates except cough and paroxysms were lower in children with *B. parapertussis* infections than in children with *B. pertussis* infections. Concomitant infections with *B. pertussis* and *B. parapertussis* can occur.[273,286,380,623]

Before and during the early pertussis vaccine era, pertussis caused by *B. parapertussis* was considerably less common than that caused by *B. pertussis.*[367] For example, during a 16-year period in the Grand Rapids area of Michigan, 4483 cases of pertussis were caused by *B. pertussis,* and 106 cases were caused by *B. parapertussis.*[172] During the DTaP vaccine efficacy trials in Europe, the comparative rates of illness caused by *B. pertussis* or *B. parapertussis* were examined. In a German trial, the rate of pertussis caused by *B. parapertussis* infection in control children was 0.9 cases per 100 person-years.[520] Of 130 culture-confirmed cases, 21% were caused by *B. parapertussis.* The percentage of cases caused by *B. parapertussis* in five other trials varied from 2.1% to 20%.[364]

Until recently, reported pertussis caused by *B. parapertussis* has been an uncommon finding in the United States. During the period of 2008 to 2010, clinical specimens from nine states were tested by PCR for *B. pertussis* and *B. parapertussis* in a commercial laboratory.[123] Of the positive samples, 13.9% were identified as *B. parapertussis.* The *B. parapertussis*–positive samples had no seasonal periodicity, whereas the *B. pertussis*–positive samples occurred between weeks 22 and 38 each year. In this study, the ages of the *B. parapertussis* patients were younger than 5 years (66%), 5 to 10 years (28.7%), 11 to 20 years (3.8%), and 21 years or older (0.4%). In contrast, the *B. pertussis* positivity rates by age were younger than 5 years (38.5%), 5 to 10 years (28.3%), 11 to 20 years (22.%), and 21 years or older (10.9%). In contrast to the lack of the demonstration of cyclic peaks in this United States study, Kurova and associates[316] identified *B. parapertussis* cyclic peaks in 1995, 2000, 2003, and 2007 in Saint Petersburg, Russia.

In Wisconsin from 2011 through 2012, 443 *B. parapertussis* infections were reported.[310] For the 218 patients investigated, it was found that macrolide antibiotic treatment within 0 to 6 days after cough onset significantly shortened the duration of illness. The median duration of the illness in these patients was 10 days, whereas the median duration was 19 days in untreated patients.

In a study in central Ohio carried out in 2010 and 2011, it was found that the *B. parapertussis* cases were significantly younger (mean, 3.5 years of age) than the *B. pertussis* cases (mean, 7 years of age).[515] In a 2009 through 2011 study in Poland, the highest rate of *B. parapertussis* infection was in children 3 to 5 years of age.[550]

B. parapertussis bacteremia has been reported in two 6-year-old boys.[576] One patient had rhinovirus coinfection and had been receiving steroids for asthma, and the other patient had acute lymphoblastic leukemia.

Bordetella bronchiseptica Infection

B. bronchiseptica causes respiratory tract infections in at least 18 mammalian species.[137] Most notable are atrophic rhinitis in pigs, kennel cough (i.e., rhinotracheitis) in dogs, and bronchopneumonia in rabbits and other laboratory animals.

In 1911, McGowan[372] observed that laboratory workers exposed to various animals with *B. bronchiseptica* infections occasionally had respiratory tract illness. In 1926, a 5-year-old girl with a pertussis-like illness was found to be infected with *B. bronchiseptica*.[57] Her illness began 10 to 12 days after she had been given a rabbit with mild "snuffles." Otherwise healthy children who became infected with *B. bronchiseptica* after being exposed to farm animals or pets usually have pertussis-like illnesses.[367]

In 2008, Rath and coworkers[465] described an infant who had recurrent episodes of pertussis-like illness due to *B. bronchiseptica* that cleared after imipenem therapy. In a separate study, another immunocompetent infant with recurrent pertussis-like illness was described.[152]

Occasional infections with *B. bronchiseptica* in humans have been reported during the past 40 years, with most occurring in immunocompromised adults, including patients with acquired immunodeficiency syndrome.[8,163,593,612] Respiratory tract infections have ranged from mild upper respiratory tract illnesses to pneumonia. In patients with acquired immunodeficiency syndrome, the pneumonia frequently is cavitary. Sinusitis and bronchitis also occur. An 11-year-old girl with cystic fibrosis had a *B. bronchiseptica* infection that might have been transmitted from a household cat.[466] An adult patient who had received a kidney-pancreas transplant had pneumonia due to *B. bronchiseptica*.[202] The source of this infection might have been from recently vaccinated dogs. The patient's dogs had received a live attenuated *B. bronchiseptica* intranasal vaccination.

Bordetella hinzii Infection

B. hinzii has occasionally been recovered from sputum cultures from patients with cystic fibrosis.[195,516] The role of these isolates in pulmonary disease in cystic fibrosis is unknown. Some isolates likely represent transient colonization,[516] but one adult patient had the organism recovered during pulmonary exacerbations throughout a 3-year period.[195] *B. hinzii* can cause septicemia and cholangitis in adult patients with immunodeficiencies.[20,135,193,279,296]

Bordetella holmesii Infection

In 1999, Yih and associates[617] reported the isolation of *B. holmesii* from the nasopharyngeal specimens of 33 patients suspected of having pertussis. Twenty-three of the cases were investigated further, and 19 (82%) of the patients were adolescents, 2 (9%) were adults, and 2 (9%) were children. All had cough: 61% had paroxysms, 26% had posttussive vomiting, and 9% had whoop. *B. holmesii* has been isolated from nasopharyngeal specimens from patients with pertussis-like illnesses in France, Canada, and the Netherlands.[399,428]

The incidence of pertussis-like illness due to *B. holmesii* is unknown. *B. holmesii* contains IS 481 and IS 1001. The two insertion sequence elements are routinely used to diagnose *B. pertussis* and *B. parapertussis*, respectively.[15,123,343,428,546] If samples are positive for both IS 481 and IS1001, the illness is caused by *B. holmesii*. However, because infection with both *B. pertussis* and *B. parapertussis* can occur, dual positives can be *B. holmesii* or mixed infections with *B. pertussis* and *B. parapertussis*.[123] Use of *B. holmesii* specific primers has been advocated to avoid false interpretations.[15]

In Canada, Guthrie and associates[224] developed a novel duplex real-time PCR assay for the detection of *B. holmesii*. The target in the PCR assay is a 50-bp segment of the *rec* A gene. They found that the prevalence of *B. holmesii* in Ontario was relatively low; of all swabs from patients with pertussis like illness, less than 1% were positive for *B. holmesii*.

B. holmesii has caused meningitis in a 12-year-old anorectic girl, bacteremia in four asplenic children, pneumonia in a 15-year-old child with relapsing nephrotic syndrome, and septic arthritis in a 15-year-old boy with chronic hemolytic anemia.[161,398,444,561] This agent has also caused bacteremia in children with sickle cell disease.[369]

B. holmesii has been isolated from a 10-month-old boy with bacteremia and from patients with septicemia, endocarditis, and respiratory failure.[138,404,541] In adults, *B. holmesii* has caused prosthetic valve endocarditis, pericarditis in a patient with lymphoma, and meningitis in an asplenic patient with systemic lupus erythematosus.[292,341,418]

Bordetella trematum Infection

B. trematum has been isolated from chronic wounds, ear infections, and blood.[7,146,531] All infections have been in adults with chronic vascular problems, impaired nasal function, and diabetes mellitus.

A 7- month-old infant with *B. trematum* bacteremia was described.[491] This child was developmentally delayed, malnourished, and anemic.

Bordetella ansorpii Infection

B. ansorpii was isolated from an infected epidermal cyst in a 19-year-old girl receiving anticancer chemotherapy.[309]

Bordetella petrii Infection

In adults, *Bordetella petrii* has been associated with suppurative mastoiditis, bronchiectasis, septic arthritis, and osteomyelitis and mandibular osteomyelitis.[194,322,429,518] Long-lasting infection in an adult with bronchiectasis has been described.[322] *B. petrii* has been recovered from respiratory specimens of patients with cystic fibrosis.[516]

Bordetella avium Infection

Bordetella avium is an avian pathogen, but it has been recovered from an adult with pneumonia. A *B. avium*–like strain was recovered from an adult with a 4-month history of productive cough.[239]

NEW REFERENCES SINCE THE SEVENTH EDITION

2. Acosta AM, DeBolt C, Tasslimi A, et al. Tdap vaccine effectiveness in adolescents during the 2012 Washington State pertussis epidemic. *Pediatrics*. 2015;135:981-989.
10. Amirthalingam G, Andrews N, Campbell H, et al. Effectiveness of maternal pertussis vaccination in England: an observational study. *Lancet*. 2014;384:1521-1528.
15. Antila M, He Q, de Jong C, et al. *Bordetella holmesii* DNA is not detected in nasopharyngeal swabs from Finnish and Dutch patients with suspected pertussis. *J Med Microbiol*. 2006;55:1043-1051.
28. Barlow RS, Reynolds LE, Cieslak PR, et al. Vaccinated children and adolescents with pertussis infections experience reduced illness severity and duration, Oregon, 2010–2012. *Clin Infect Dis*. 2014;58:1523-1529.
35. Baxter R, Bartlett J, Rowhani-Rahbar A, et al. Effectiveness of pertussis vaccines for adolescents and adults: case-control study. *BMJ*. 2013;347:f4249.
44. Bidet P, Liguori S, De Lauzanne A, et al. Real-time PCR measurement of persistence of *Bordetella pertussis* DNA in nasopharyngeal secretions during antibiotic treatment of young children with pertussis. *J Clin Microbiol*. 2008;46:3636-3638.
61. Campbell H, Amirthalingam G, Andrews N, et al. Accelerating control of pertussis in England and Wales. *Emerg Infect Dis*. 2012;18:38-47.
73. Centers for Disease Control and Prevention. Invasive cancer incidence—United States, 2009. *MMWR Morb Mortal Wkly Rep*. 2009;62:517-526.

105. Cherry JD. Pertussis: challenges today and for the future. *PLoS Pathog.* 2013;9:e1003418.
106. Cherry JD. Adult pertussis in the pre- and post-vaccine eras: lifelong vaccine-induced immunity? *Expert Rev Vaccines.* 2014;13:1073-1080.
108. Cherry JD. Epidemic pertussis and acellular pertussis vaccine failure in the 21st century. *Pediatrics.* 2015;135:1130-1132.
109. Cherry JD. The history of pertussis (whooping cough); 1906–2015: facts, myths, and misconceptions. *Curr Epidemiol Rep.* 2015;2:120-130.
110. Cherry JD. Tetanus-diphtheria-pertussis immunization in pregnant women and the prevention of pertussis in young infants. *Clin Infect Dis.* 2015;60:338-340.
121. Cherry JD, Paddock CD. Pathogenesis and histopathology of pertussis: implications for immunization. *Expert Rev Vaccines.* 2014;13:1115-1123.
125. Cherry JD, Xing DX, Newland P, et al. Determination of serum antibody to *Bordetella pertussis* adenylate cyclase toxin in vaccinated and unvaccinated children and in children and adults with pertussis. *Clin Infect Dis.* 2004;38:502-507.
133. Conover MS, Redfern CJ, Ganguly T, et al. BpsR modulates *Bordetella* biofilm formation by negatively regulating the expression of the Bps polysaccharide. *J Bacteriol.* 2012;194:233-242.
138. Couturier AP, Dahl K. *Bordetella holmesii* endocarditis: case report and review of literature. *Pediatr Infect Dis J.* 2014;33:661-664.
143. Dabrera G, Amirthalingam G, Andrews N, et al. A case-control study to estimate the effectiveness of maternal pertussis vaccination in protecting newborn infants in England and Wales, 2012-2013. *Clin Infect Dis.* 2015;60:333-337.
158. Dierig A, Beckmann C, Heininger U. Antibiotic treatment of pertussis: are 7 days really sufficient? *Pediatr Infect Dis J.* 2015;34:444-445.
164. Eberly MD, Eide MB, Thompson JL, et al. Azithromycin in early infancy and pyloric stenosis. *Pediatrics.* 2015;135:483-488.
240. Harvill ET, Goodfield LL, Ivanov Y, et al. Genome sequences of nine *Bordetella holmesii* strains isolated in the United States. *Genome Announc.* 2014;2:e00438-14.
245. Heininger U, Burckhardt MA. *Bordetella pertussis* and concomitant viral respiratory tract infections are rare in children with cough illness. *Pediatr Infect Dis J.* 2011;30:640-644.
282. Hviid A, Stellfeld M, Andersen PH, et al. Impact of routine vaccination with a pertussis toxoid vaccine in Denmark. *Vaccine.* 2004;22:3530-3534.
301. Kharbanda EO, Vazquez-Benitez G, Lipkind HS, et al. Evaluation of the association of maternal pertussis vaccination with obstetric events and birth outcomes. *JAMA.* 2014;312:1897-1904.
305. Klein NP, Bartlett J, Fireman B, et al. Comparative effectiveness of acellular versus whole-cell pertussis vaccines in teenagers. *Pediatrics.* 2013;131:e1716-e1722.
306. Klein NP, Bartlett J, Rowhani-Rahbar A, et al. Waning protection after fifth dose of acellular pertussis vaccine in children. *N Engl J Med.* 2012;367:1012-1019.
309. Ko KS, Peck KR, Oh WS, et al. New species of *Bordetella, Bordetella ansorpii* sp. nov., isolated from the purulent exudate of an epidermal cyst. *J Clin Microbiol.* 2005;43:2516-2519.
310. Koepke R, Bartholomew ML, Eickhoff JC, et al. Widespread *Bordetella parapertussis* infections—Wisconsin, 2011-2012: clinical and epidemiologic features and antibiotic use for treatment and prevention. *Clin Infect Dis.* 2015;61:1421-1431.
311. Koepke R, Eickhoff JC, Ayele RA, et al. Estimating the effectiveness of tetanus-diphtheria-acellular pertussis vaccine (Tdap) for preventing pertussis: evidence of rapidly waning immunity and difference in effectiveness by Tdap brand. *J Infect Dis.* 2014;210:942-953.
318. Ladhani SN, Andrews NJ, Southern J, et al. Antibody responses after primary immunization in infants born to women receiving a pertussis-containing vaccine during pregnancy: single arm observational study with a historical comparator. *Clin Infect Dis.* 2015;61:1637-1644.
321. Le T, Cherry JD, Chang SJ, et al. Immune responses and antibody decay after immunization of adolescents and adults with an acellular pertussis vaccine: the APERT study. *J Infect Dis.* 2004;190:535-544.
322. Le Coustumier A, Njamkepo E, Cattoir V, et al. *Bordetella petrii* infection with long-lasting persistence in human. *Emerg Infect Dis.* 2011;17:612-618.
334. Liko J, Robison SG, Cieslak PR. Pertussis vaccine performance in an epidemic year-Oregon, 2012. *Clin Infect Dis.* 2014;59:261-263.
355. Mallory FB, Hornor AA. Pertussis: the histological lesion in the respiratory tract. *J Med Res.* 1912;27:115-124.
361. Martin SW, Pawloski L, Williams M, et al. Pertactin-negative *Bordetella pertussis* strains: evidence for a possible selective advantage. *Clin Infect Dis.* 2015;60:223-227.
371. McGirr A, Fisman DN. Duration of pertussis immunity after DTaP immunization: a meta-analysis. *Pediatrics.* 2015;135:331-343.
379. Melvin JA, Scheller EV, Miller JF, et al. *Bordetella pertussis* pathogenesis: current and future challenges. *Nat Rev Microbiol.* 2014;12:274-288.
381. Mertsola J. Editorial commentary: pertussis is less severe in vaccinated than in unvaccinated patients. *Clin Infect Dis.* 2014;58:1530-1532.
397. Misegades LK, Winter K, Harriman K, et al. Association of childhood pertussis with receipt of 5 doses of pertussis vaccine by time since last vaccine dose, California, 2010. *JAMA.* 2012;308:2126-2132.
403. Moreno LZ, Knobl T, Grespan AA, et al. Draft genome sequence of *Bordetella avium* Nh1210, an outbreak strain of lockjaw syndrome. *Genome Announc.* 2015;3:e00120-15.
412. Munoz FM, Piedra PA, Glezen WP. Safety and immunogenicity of respiratory syncytial virus purified fusion protein-2 vaccine in pregnant women. *Vaccine.* 2003;21:3465-3467.
413. Murray EL, Nieves D, Bradley JS, et al. Characteristics of severe *Bordetella* pertussis infection among infants ≤90 days of age admitted to pediatric intensive care units—Southern California, September 2009-June 2011. *J Pediatric Infect Dis Soc.* 2013;2:1-6.
426. Nieves D, Bradley JS, Gargas J, et al. Exchange blood transfusion in the management of severe pertussis in young infants. *Pediatr Infect Dis J.* 2013;32:698-699.
427. Nieves D, Heininger U, Cherry JD. *Bordetella pertussis* and other *Bordetella* spp. infections. In: Wilson CB, Nieves D, Maldonado Y, et al, eds. *Remington and Klein's Infectious Diseases of the Fetus and Newborn Infant.* 8th ed. Philadelphia: Elsevier; 2016.
440. Olsen M, Thygesen SK, Ostergaard JR, et al. Hospital-diagnosed pertussis infection in children and long-term risk of epilepsy. *JAMA.* 2015;314:1844-1849.
445. Park J, Zhang Y, Buboltz AM, et al. Comparative genomics of the classical *Bordetella* subspecies: the evolution and exchange of virulence-associated diversity amongst closely related pathogens. *BMC Genomics.* 2012;13:545.
446. Parkhill J, Sebaihia M, Preston A, et al. Comparative analysis of the genome sequences of *Bordetella* pertussis, *Bordetella parapertussis* and *Bordetella bronchiseptica. Nat Genet.* 2003;35:32-40.
447. Pawloski LC, Queenan AM, Cassiday PK, et al. Prevalence and molecular characterization of pertactin-deficient *Bordetella pertussis* in the United States. *Clin Vaccine Immunol.* 2014;21:119-125.
451. Pittet LF, Emonet S, Schrenzel J, et al. *Bordetella holmesii*: an under-recognised *Bordetella* species. *Lancet Infect Dis.* 2014;14:510-519.
452. Pittet LF, Posfay-Barbe KM. *Bordetella holmesii* infection: current knowledge and a vision for future research. *Expert Rev Anti Infect Ther.* 2015;13:965-971.
463. Quinn HE, Snelling TL, Habig A, et al. Parental Tdap boosters and infant pertussis: a case-control study. *Pediatrics.* 2014;134:713-720.
467. Register KB, Ivanov YV, Harvill ET, et al. Draft genome sequences of six *Bordetella hinzii* isolates acquired from avian and mammalian hosts. *Genome Announc.* 2015;3:e00152-15.
483. Ronn PF, Dalby T, Simonsen J, et al. Seroepidemiology of pertussis in a cross-sectional study of an adult general population in Denmark. *Epidemiol Infect.* 2014;142:729-737.
486. Ross PJ, Sutton CE, Higgins S, et al. Relative contribution of Th1 and Th17 cells in adaptive immunity to *Bordetella pertussis*: towards the rational design of an improved acellular pertussis vaccine. *PLoS Pathog.* 2013;9:e1003264.
490. Ryan M, Murphy G, Ryan E, et al. Distinct T-cell subtypes induced with whole cell and acellular pertussis vaccines in children. *Immunology.* 1998;93:1-10.
507. Sheridan SL, Ware RS, Grimwood K, et al. Number and order of whole cell pertussis vaccines in infancy and disease protection. *JAMA.* 2012;308:454-456.
511. Skoff TH, Kenyon C, Cocoros N, et al. Sources of infant pertussis infection in the United States. *Pediatrics.* 2015;136:635-641.
515. Spicer KB, Salamon D, Cummins C, et al. Occurrence of 3 *Bordetella* species during an outbreak of cough illness in Ohio: epidemiology, clinical features, laboratory findings and antimicrobial susceptibility. *Pediatr Infect Dis J.* 2014;33:e162-e167.
534. Sukumaran L, McCarthy NL, Kharbanda EO, et al. Association of Tdap vaccination with acute events and adverse birth outcomes among pregnant women with prior tetanus-containing immunizations. *JAMA.* 2015;314:1581-1587.
538. Tan T, Dalby T, Forsyth K, et al. Pertussis across the globe: recent epidemiologic trends from 2000 to 2013. *Pediatr Infect Dis J.* 2015;34:e222-e232.
544. Tartof SY, Lewis M, Kenyon C, et al. Waning immunity to pertussis following 5 doses of DTaP. *Pediatrics.* 2013;131:e1047-e1052.
547. Thierry-Carstensen B, Dalby T, Stevner MA, et al. Experience with monocomponent acellular pertussis combination vaccines for infants, children, adolescents and adults—a review of safety, immunogenicity, efficacy and effectiveness studies and 15 years of field experience. *Vaccine.* 2013;31:5178-5191.
549. Tiwari TS, Baughman AL, Clark TA. First pertussis vaccine dose and prevention of infant mortality. *Pediatrics.* 2015;135:990-999.
550. Tomialoic R, Stefanoff P, Paradowska-Stankiewicz I, et al. Incidence and factors predicting whooping cough due to parapertussis diagnosis among patients referred to general practitioners, Poland, 2009-2011. *Eur J Clin Microbiol Infect Dis.* 2015;34:101-107.
559. Urwyler P, Heininger U. Protecting newborns from pertussis—the challenge of complete cocooning. *BMC Infect Dis.* 2014;14:397.
576. Wallihan R, Selvarangan R, Marcon M, et al. *Bordetella parapertussis* bacteremia: two case reports. *Pediatr Infect Dis J.* 2013;32:796-798.
580. Warfel JM, Merkel TJ. *Bordetella pertussis* infection induces a mucosal IL-17 response and long-lived Th17 and Th1 immune memory cells in nonhuman primates. *Mucosal Immunol.* 2013;6:787-796.
581. Warfel JM, Papin JF, Wolf RF, et al. Maternal and neonatal vaccination protects newborn baboons from pertussis infection. *J Infect Dis.* 2014;210:604-610.
582. Warfel JM, Zimmerman LI, Merkel TJ. Acellular pertussis vaccines protect against disease but fail to prevent infection and transmission in a nonhuman primate model. *Proc Natl Acad Sci USA.* 2014;111:787-792.

591. Weiss AA, Patton AK, Millen SH, et al. Acellular pertussis vaccines and complement killing of *Bordetella pertussis*. *Infect Immun*. 2004;72:7346-7351.
600. Winter K, Glaser C, Watt J, et al. Pertussis epidemic—California, 2014. *MMWR Morb Mortal Wkly Rep*. 2014;63:1129-1132.
601. Winter K, Harriman K, Zipprich J, et al. California pertussis epidemic, 2010. *J Pediatr*. 2012;161:1091-1096.
602. Winter K, Zipprich J, Harriman K, et al. Risk factors associated with infant deaths from pertussis: a case-control study. *Clin Infect Dis*. 2015;61:1099-1106.
607. Witt MA, Arias L, Katz PH, et al. Reduced risk of pertussis among persons ever vaccinated with whole cell pertussis vaccine compared to recipients of acellular pertussis vaccines in a large US cohort. *Clin Infect Dis*. 2013;56:1248-1254.
608. Witt MA, Katz PH, Witt DJ. Unexpectedly limited durability of immunity following acellular pertussis vaccination in preadolescents in a North American outbreak. *Clin Infect Dis*. 2012;54:1730-1735.
609. Wood N, McIntyre P, Marshall H, et al. Acellular pertussis vaccine at birth and one month induces antibody responses by two months of age. *Pediatr Infect Dis J*. 2010;29:209-215.
614. World Health Organization (WHO). Pertussis vaccines: WHO position paper, August 2015—recommendations. *Vaccine*. 2016;34:1423-1425.
623. Zouari A, Smaoui H, Brun D, et al. Prevalence of *Bordetella pertussis* and *Bordetella parapertussis* infections in Tunisian hospitalized infants: results of a 4-year prospective study. *Diagn Microbiol Infect Dis*. 2012;72:303-317.

The full reference list for this chapter is available at ExpertConsult.com.

130 *Klebsiella granulomatis*

Mariam R. Chacko

Klebsiella granulomatis (formerly *Calymmatobacterium granulomatis*) is the causative organism for a chronic genital ulcer disease called granuloma inguinale or donovanosis, and it was first isolated in 1905 by Donovan in India.[35,53] The organism is an encapsulated gram-negative rod measuring 1.5 × 0.7 μm, and for many decades, it was considered a unique species belonging to the subclass Proteobacteria.[24,35,36] However, using DNA hybridization techniques and 16S rDNA sequencing, the organism was reclassified under the genus *Klebsiella*.[35]

Transmission electron microscopy shows the organism has a complex cell envelope with an outer membrane, middle electron-opaque layer, and an inner plasma membrane. In addition to its regular bacterial structure (i.e., mesosome, ribosomes, and nuclear material), the cytoplasm contains electron-dense granules. The organisms are enclosed mainly in large histiocytic cells and occasionally in polymorphonuclear cells and plasma cells. They multiply intracellularly to approximately 30 organisms, eventually causing cell rupture.[9,35]

EPIDEMIOLOGY

Granuloma inguinale occurs predominantly in young and older adults (20 to 40 years of age) and is a cause of endemic genital ulcerative disease in tropical and subtropical regions of the world today, including Papua New Guinea, South Africa, India, Brazil, and Australia.[5,10,37,42,51] As with all genital ulcerative diseases, granuloma inguinale has been given greater attention as a risk factor for development of human immunodeficiency virus (HIV) infection. A rapid test for donovanosis was introduced in Durban, South Africa, in the early 1990s, which facilitated increased diagnosis of this disease in HIV and other sexually transmitted infections (STIs) initiatives in South Africa and Australia.[5,16,33] In developed countries, case reports of granuloma inguinale emerged in the 1990s among immigrants living in metropolitan areas such as Toronto, Rome, and London.[21,32,47] The most recent case report from Milan, Italy, was in 2012 of an 18-year-old, pregnant girl from Bolivia.[27]

In the United States during the preantibiotic era, the estimated population prevalence of granuloma inguinale in the United States was 5000 to 10,000 cases,[35] with more than 1000 cases reported per year to the Centers for Disease Control and Prevention (CDC). Since the introduction of antibiotics, the prevalence of this disease has declined rapidly, with 75 cases reported in 1977 and 17 cases reported in 1982. No cases have been reported through standard surveillance reports by the CDC in recent years. However, case reports have been published: one case in 1985 in California[19] and one case in 1991 in Texas.[31] Cases from Chicago in 2006[45] and Charlottesville, Virginia, in 2009 and in 2012 have been reported.[2] Although the prevalence of the disease is low, this disease needs to be suspected in North America and Europe because of international travel and immigration.

Granuloma inguinale is a rare occurrence in children. In the early 1950s, 4% of 1- to 4-year-old children in a Papua New Guinea population had granuloma inguinale. Although the mode of transmission in adolescents and adults is considered to be sexual, the mode of disease transmission in these children was thought to be by skin-to-skin contact from sitting on the laps of infected adults.[35] Cases published since 1997 report otitis media, ear polyps, mastoiditis, neck mass, cervical lymphadenopathy, and meningitis as the initial manifestations of donovanosis in infants and children.[1,4,17,18,43] The modes of transmission in these cases were thought to be perinatal and by skin-to-skin contact.[1,4,17,18,43]

The risk factors and mode of transmission of granuloma inguinale are not clear. It is considered a sexually transmitted disease. Coexistence of granuloma inguinale with other STIs occurs commonly. Syphilis has been described in as many as 23% of patients with granuloma inguinale. In one report, HIV-1 antibodies were found in as many as 8% of male patients with granuloma inguinale.[31,42] O'Farrell and associates[41] found that Zulu men and women with granuloma inguinale and secondary syphilis were more likely to have had sexual intercourse compared with those with other genital ulcer diseases. It is usually more common in males than in females, but among adolescents in Durban, South Africa, the disease occurred more commonly in girls than in boys, probably indicating sexual activity between adolescent girls and adult men.[34] Anal intercourse also has been associated with rectal and penile lesions of granuloma inguinale.[28] The disease has been diagnosed in 12% to 50% of marital or steady sexual partners.[35,40] Studies from India and South Africa have reported a preponderance of granuloma inguinale cases among uncircumcised male patients with poor genital hygiene.[34,35]

PATHOGENESIS AND PATHOLOGY

K. granulomatis organisms invade mononuclear endothelial cells. Extensive acanthosis and dense dermal infiltrates of mainly plasma cells and histiocytes have been observed in the indurated nodules, the initial clinical presentation of the disease. Polymorphonuclear cell infiltration also occurs, but lymphocytes are rare findings when secondary infection develops. The pathognomonic feature of granuloma inguinale is a large, infected mononuclear cell that is 25 to 90 μm in diameter and contains many intracytoplasmic cysts filled with deep-staining Donovan bodies. Metastatic spread to the bones, joints, liver, and lymphatics occasionally occurs.[35]

A possible link between human leukocyte antigen B57 (HLA-B57) and granuloma inguinale infection may exist. Class I, class II, and DQ antigens have been detected in the genital ulcers of individuals with granuloma inguinale.[38] Circulating lymphocytes and tissue-level lymphocyte subpopulations in granuloma inguinale have been studied.[49,50] T-lymphocyte and B-lymphocyte infiltration in tissues is almost identical, without any significant difference in ulcerogranulomatous and hypertrophic variants of granuloma inguinale. Total leukocyte, absolute lymphocyte, and total T lymphocytes counts; CD4, CD8, and CD22 levels; and the CD4/CD8 ratio are all increased significantly in the ulcerogranulomatous variant of granuloma inguinale. In contrast, the hypertrophic variant causes a significant elevation only in the CD4/CD8 ratio. This finding suggests a greater cell-mediated immune response in the ulcerogranulomatous variant of granuloma inguinale and is consistent with the paucity of Donovan bodies in smears obtained from patients with this variant.[50,49]

CLINICAL MANIFESTATIONS

The incubation period of granuloma inguinale usually is less than 2 weeks, but it can be as long as 3 months. The disease begins as one or more subcutaneous nodules that erode through the skin to produce clean, large, beefy-red, granulomatous ulcers that bleed easily. The lesions are sharply defined and painless, and the ulcers feel hard when palpated. The disease usually is limited to local tissue, and constitutional symptoms are therefore unlikely. Autoinoculation is a common manifestation that produces kissing lesions. The genitalia are involved in 90% of cases, the inguinal region in 10%, the anal region in 5% to 10%, and extragenital sites (usually involving the head and neck), in 1% to 5%. Regional (inguinal) lymphadenopathy is not associated with granuloma inguinale.

The morphology of the cutaneous lesions of granuloma inguinale can vary, depending on the stage of the disease. The exuberant or hypertrophic stage appears before secondary infection develops. It consists of large, vegetating masses with overgrowth of granulation tissue, usually in the perianal region. The ulcerative stage is accompanied by secondary infection. In this stage, large, spreading, shallow necrotic ulcers with a foul odor may be observed. The cicatricial stage results after prolonged healing and is characterized by fibrosis, scarring, depigmentation, keloid formation, elephantiasis, and stenosis of the vagina, urethra, and anus. Although lymphadenopathy is an unusual occurrence in granuloma inguinale, pseudobuboes and pseudoelephantiasis of the genitals (i.e., massive edema) may be seen. Pseudobuboes are the result of deep, inguinal granulomas; pseudoelephantiasis is caused by cutaneous extension of lesions and inflammation.[13,31,35]

In male patients, lesions usually occur on the prepuce, coronal sulcus, and frenulum of the penis.[10,35,36] Multiple sites of genital ulceration (i.e., vulva, vagina, and cervix) have been observed only in nonpregnant women (Fig. 130.1).[2,13,34,36] The most common clinical manifestation in women is vulvar ulcerations in pregnant and nonpregnant women, followed by genital tract bleeding reported for nonpregnant women (20%).[3] Extragenital sites may be involved in up to 6% of cases through hematogenous spread, and lesions are reported in the mouth, chin, axillae, abdomen, pelvic cavity, and foot.[12,14,20,26,29,35,44,48,52] These distant sites usually are associated with a primary lesion in the genital area.[35] Lesions in the oral cavity have been described after apparently successful treatment of genital lesions.[12] Donovanosis ulcers may take longer to heal in HIV-positive individuals, and greater destruction of tissue may occur.[20,35,36]

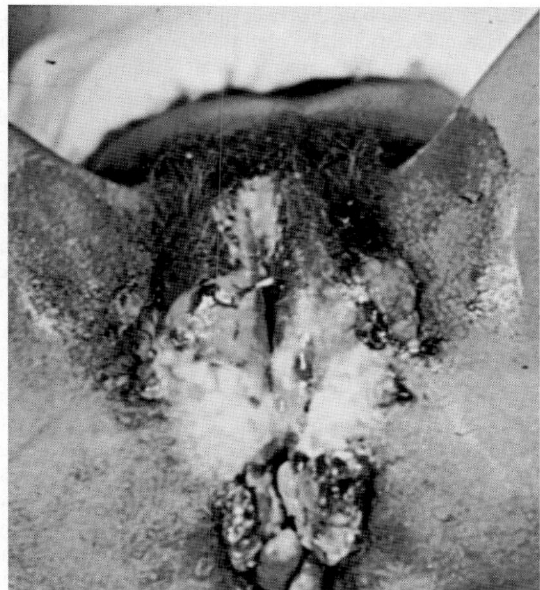

FIG. 130.1 Granuloma inguinale.

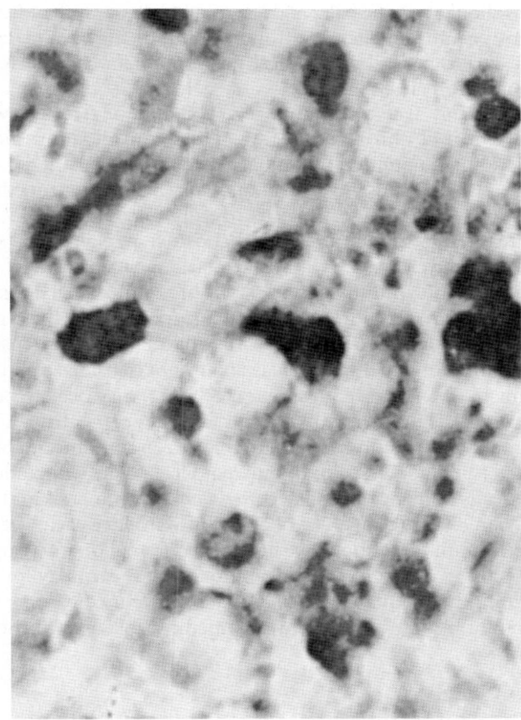

FIG. 130.2 Donovan bodies.

DIAGNOSIS

Granuloma inguinale usually is diagnosed clinically. In contrast to other genital ulcers, the ulcers are larger in granuloma inguinale, are painless, bleed easily in response to touch, and usually are not associated with inguinal lymphadenopathy.[46] The CDC STI surveillance case definition for granuloma inguinale of a confirmed case is a clinically compatible case that is laboratory confirmed.[8]

If donovanosis is suspected, a swab for this condition should be taken before swabs for other organisms to allow an adequate amount of cellular material to be obtained. Examination of appropriately stained specimens from active lesions remains the most reliable diagnostic test using Wright-Giemsa or Warthin-Starry blue-black stain. A modified Giemsa stain (i.e., Rapi-Diff) can also yield rapid results in a busy clinic.[35] Dark-staining Donovan bodies in large, histiocytic cells on a stained crush specimen from the lesion are identified (Fig. 130.2). A biopsy specimen, preferably stained with Giemsa or silver, is recommended for very early, very sclerotic, or heavily superinfected specimens.[23,39,35] Donovan bodies have been identified on Papanicolaou smears from the cervix.[11]

Although *K. granulomatis* has been successfully isolated by culture in South Africa and Australia, this method is not used due to difficulties in isolating the organism.[6,53] Polymerase chain reaction (PCR) techniques for *K. granulomatis* have been developed, and a genital ulcer disease multiplex PCR test has been developed in Australia.[35] No molecular tests for detection of *K. granulomatis* DNA have been cleared by the US Food and Drug Administration, but such an assay can be useful when undertaken by a laboratory that has conducted a Clinical Laboratories Improvement Amendments (CLIA) verification study.[53] A serologic test for granuloma inguinale using the indirect immunofluorescence was developed in the 1990s in South Africa and found to be highly sensitive but not specific.[15]

TREATMENT

Antibiotics with strong activity against *K. granulomatis* are those effective in the treatment of gram-negative bacilli or those whose lipid solubility ensures good intracellular penetration. The CDC recommends treatment of adolescents with 1 g of azithromycin taken orally weekly or 500 mg taken daily for at least 3 weeks until all lesions have completely healed.[53] Alternative regimens include 100 mg of doxycycline taken orally twice each day for at least 3 weeks, or 750 mg of ciprofloxacin taken orally twice each day for at least 3 weeks, or 500 mg of erythromycin base taken orally four times each day for at least 3 weeks, or one double-strength tablet (i.e., 160 mg/800 mg) of trimethoprim-sulfamethoxazole taken orally twice per day for at least 3 weeks. All of these regimens should be prescribed until all lesions have completely healed. [53] A clinical response to antibiotics should be noticed within a week of treatment; the lesions should become paler and less friable. After a week of treatment, the lesions become smaller, and total healing of the area takes 3 to 5 weeks.[35] Ceftriaxone is a possible treatment option for chronic, recurrent granuloma inguinale.[30]

Pregnant and lactating adolescents should be treated with an azithromycin or erythromycin regimen, and consideration should be given to adding a parenteral aminoglycoside such as 1 mg/kg of gentamicin given intravenously every 8 hours. Doxycycline and trimethoprim-sulfamethoxazole are contraindicated during pregnancy.[53]

The treatment regimen for an HIV-positive person is the same as for an HIV-negative person. Treatment can fail in patients with coexisting HIV infection and immunosuppression; in contrast to HIV-negative patients, the mean duration to complete ulcer healing in these patients is significantly longer (25.7 days vs. 16.8 days).[22] More intensive and prolonged antibiotic therapy such as an aminoglycoside (e.g., 1 mg/kg of gentamicin given intravenously every 8 hours) may need to be added if improvement is not evident within a few days of treatment.

Treatment information for children with granuloma inguinale is limited and is not addressed in the current CDC treatment guidelines.[53] The American Academy of Pediatrics *Red Book* recommends for children younger than 8 years of age, 1 g of azithromycin once each week for at least 3 weeks until the lesions have healed, and for children 8 years of age or older, 100 mg of doxycycline taken orally twice each day for at least 3 weeks until the lesions have healed. Alternative medications include suspension forms of trimethoprim-sulfamethoxazole or erythromycin.[25]

PROGNOSIS

Healing is complete in patients who seek treatment early in the course of the disease and who comply with their medication and follow-up regimens.[30,34] Relapse occurs in approximately 10% of cases, especially if use of the antibiotic is discontinued before the primary lesion has healed completely. Donovan bodies may reappear within 7 to 10 days.[35] Up to one third of patients are reported to recover completely without a recurrence after receiving daily doses of ceftriaxone for 7 to 10 days.[30,34]

Complications of granuloma inguinale include pseudoelephantiasis, urethral stricture, and pelvic abscess, which may require surgery. Vulvectomy is reserved for infections that have not responded to antibiotic treatment or for patients with severe vulvar elephantiasis.[13,35]

The severe, mutilating complications of granuloma inguinale are primarily a result of delayed treatment or poor compliance with medication. In Durban, South Africa, almost one half of the male patients had ulcerations for 1 to 6 months before they sought medical care, and 16% had ulcerations for 1 to 3 weeks. In contrast, approximately 25% of female patients had ulcerations for 1 to 6 months, and 50% had ulcerations for 1 to 3 weeks.[30] Delayed medical attention may be related to limited education, ignorance of STIs, absence of suitable medical facilities, or embarrassment in seeking treatment because of extensive genital lesions. Another complication is the acquisition of HIV infection, especially when patients with ulcerations that are left untreated for a prolonged period have sexual contact with an HIV-positive partner.[30,35]

PREVENTION

Sexual partners of persons with the disease who have had sexual contact within 60 days before onset of symptoms should be traced, examined, and treated. However, the value of treating an asymptomatic partner has not been established.[53] Treatment of granuloma inguinale when the nodule first appears is associated with a benign course. Community-based eradication that targets men with granuloma inguinale in endemic areas should be implemented. Neonates whose mothers have granuloma inguinale should have their ears, umbilicus, and genitalia carefully cleansed and should be given a course of prophylactic antibiotics.[46]

Programs should be aimed at early suspicion and identification of lesions, access to care, provision of early treatment, and prevention of severe complications. Teaching the importance of personal genital hygiene, such as instruction on simple retraction of the foreskin in men and cleansing the penis with soap and water, also is effective.[34,35] The CDC and the US Public Health Service provide technical instructions on required examinations and standard treatment regimens to panels of physicians and consular officers evaluating the health of aliens applying for entry into the United States.[7]

NEW REFERENCES SINCE THE SEVENTH EDITION

1. Ahmed N, Pillay A, Lawler M, et al. Donovanosis causing lymphadenitis, mastoiditis, and meningitis in a child. *Lancet.* 2015;385:2644.
25. Kimberlin DW, Brady M, Jackson MA, Long SS. American Academy of Pediatrics Red Book Online 2015: report of the Committee on Infectious Diseases. http://www.redbook.solutions.aap.org.
27. Liverani CA, Lattuada D, Mangano S, et al. Hypertrophic donovanosis in a young pregnant woman. *J Pediatr Adolesc Gynecol.* 2012;25:e81-e83.
43. Ramdial PK, Sing Y, Ramburan *A, et al. Infantile donovanosis presenting as external auditory canal polyps: a diagnostic trap. *Am J Dermatopathol.* 2012;34:818-821.
53. Workowski KA, Bolan GA, Centers for Disease Control and Prevention. Sexually transmitted diseases treatment guidelines, 2015. *MMWR Recomm Rep.* 2015;64(RR-03):1-137.

The full reference list for this chapter is available at ExpertConsult.com.

Campylobacter jejuni

131

Ramia Zakhour • Gloria P. Heresi • James R. Murphy

Campylobacter jejuni is a frequent cause of enteritis and less often of extraintestinal infection in humans. Since it first was recognized as a common human pathogen in the 1970s, appreciation of this agent's importance as a cause of disease has increased steadily. *C. jejuni* is one of the most frequent bacterial causes of human enteritis in the United States, and it is a leading cause of bacterial foodborne diarrheal disease throughout the world.[6,43] Immunoreactive complications may develop after infection.[252,270]

Although they are not isolated as frequently as *C. jejuni* and *Campylobacter coli,* other *Campylobacter* spp. are gaining recognition as human pathogens. At least 25 species of *Campylobacter* have been identified.[201] *Campylobacter fetus,* a classic cause of perinatal infection, also is an infrequent cause of bacteremia in immunocompromised hosts. *Campylobacter upsaliensis, Campylobacter lari, Campylobacter hyointestinalis,* and *Campylobacter concisus* are associated primarily with diarrheal disease. Normal and immunosuppressed hosts are affected by these species. Other less common *Campylobacter* spp. have been isolated from blood or stool or involved in periodontal disease. The clinical spectrum of these organisms is expanding as the testing for them becomes more widely available.

HISTORY

The pathologic consequences of infection with *Campylobacter* were recognized first in 1909 from studies of abortions in sheep,[206] although it might have been identified in 1886, when Theodore Escherich described nonculturable, spiral-shaped bacteria.[298] A few years later, Smith[306] reported their association with bovine abortion and gave them the name *Vibrio fetus.* Although never confirmed microbiologically, these organisms are thought to have been *C. fetus* according to current nomenclature.[169] In 1947, the sheep abortion–associated organism *V. fetus* was isolated from a blood culture from a pregnant woman who had an influenza-like illness and delivered a stillborn infant with a necrotic, infarcted placenta.

In 1957, King hypothesized that *V. fetus*–related organisms might be associated with human enteric disease.[37,173] In addition to pregnancy, gastrectomy, tooth extraction, heart disease, diabetes, and cirrhosis were predisposing conditions in King's 1957 review of 15 patients with *V. fetus* bacteremia.[173] Butzler and colleagues[37] showed that bacteria similar to *V. fetus* were present in the stools of children with diarrhea. This observation was confirmed rapidly and repeatedly.[24,39,107,304,324]

Major differences in biochemical activities, growth characteristics, and DNA base nucleotide content between true *Vibrio* and *V. fetus* led to the establishment of the new genus *Campylobacter* by Sebald and Vernon in 1967.[347] The genome of a representative *C. jejuni* was published in 2000.[248] Information gleaned from this and comparative analyses of additional isolates have markedly advanced knowledge of these agents.[101,136]

Many reports describing new *Campylobacter* spp. were published in the 1980s and early 1990s. *C. upsaliensis* was reported to be a pathogen in dogs and humans in 1983 and 1985, respectively.[248,283] *C. lari,* a common isolate from healthy seagulls, was found to be a cause of gastrointestinal and extraintestinal disease in humans.[19,323] Originally identified in the intestines of swine with proliferative ileitis, *C. hyointestinalis* was reported first as a human pathogen in a homosexual man with proctitis.[79] The hydrogen-requiring *C. concisu,*[341] *C. rectus,*[268] and *Campylobacter curvus; Campylobacter showae;* and *Campylobacter gracilis* have been associated with periodontal disease. *Campylobacter sputorum* has been identified in abscesses, in bacteremia,[56,139] and gastroenteritis,[201] and *Campylobacter mucosalis* was reported in two children with diarrhea.[84] *Campylobacter ureolyticus,* initially known as *Bacteroides ureolyticus,* was first described associated with genital tract infections and later found to be isolated from stools.[34,89]

Once called *Campylobacter*-like organisms 1 and 2, *Helicobacter cinaedi* and *Helicobacter fennelliae* are now classified in the *Helicobacter* genus.[237] These pathogens cause enteritis and proctocolitis in homosexual men and occasionally cause bacteremia.[247,337] *Campylobacter*-like organism 3, which also was described as causing enterocolitis, was recently identified for the first time as a cause of bacteremia.[227] Two former *Campylobacter* spp., *Arcobacter butzleri* and *Arcobacter cryaerophilus,* are associated with abortion and enteritis in cattle and pigs, in addition to bacteremia and diarrhea in humans.[172]

ORGANISM

The *Campylobacter* genus belongs to the family Campylobacteraceae, the order Campylobacterales, the class Epsilonproteobacteria, and the phylum Proteobacteria. The genus *Campylobacter* consists of 34 species and 14 subspecies (http://www.bacterio.cict.fr/c/campylobacter.html); about one half of them cause disease in humans. *Campylobacter* is a Greek word meaning "curved rod."

Members of this genus are fastidious, non–spore forming gram-negative rods that are curved, S-shaped, or spiral (Fig. 131.1). They may vary in width from 0.2 to 0.9 μm and in length from 0.5 to 5.0 μm. Although most grow at 37°C (98.6°F), *C. jejuni* grows best in cultures maintained at 42°C (107.6°F). The thermophilic cluster of the genus *Campylobacter* includes *C. jejuni, C. coli, Campylobacter upsaliensis, Campylobacter insulaenigrae,* and C. *lari.* Most *Campylobacter* spp. require microaerophilic growth conditions (i.e., 5%–10% oxygen). *Campylobacter* spp. usually are motile, with a single polar flagellum or two flagella, one at each end of the rod. Exceptions include *C. gracilis,* which is nonmotile, and *C. showae,* which has multiple flagella. Campylobacters are oxidase positive and reduce nitrates but do not ferment or oxidize carbohydrates.[250]

Some species, including *C. sputorum, C. concisus, C. mucosalis, C. curvus, C. rectus,* and *C. hyointestinalis,* may require hydrogen for primary isolation and growth. Many media selective for isolation of *Campylobacter* spp. have been developed, but because of species differences in antibiotic resistance patterns, no single formulation allows isolation of all species

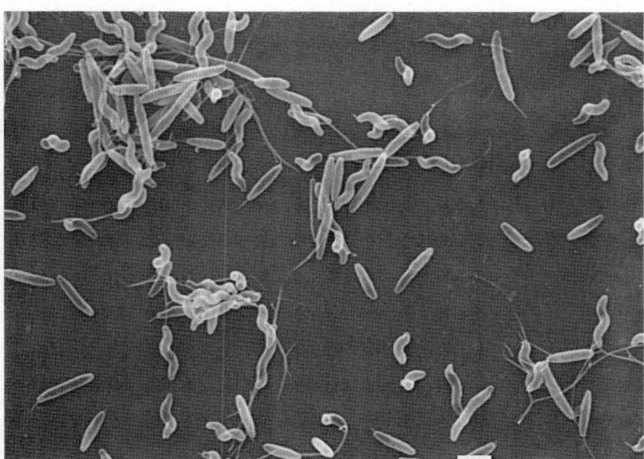

FIG. 131.1 Scanning electron microscopy of *Campylobacter jejuni* strain 20-01. (From Baqar S, Rice B. *Campylobacter jejuni* enteritis. *Clin Infect Dis.* 2001;33:901–5.)

TABLE 131.1 **Growth and Biochemical Characteristics of Species of the Genus *Campylobacter***

	GROWTH							
***Campylobacter* Species**	**25°C**	**37°C**	**42°C**	**Anaerobic Conditions**	**In CO_2 Inhibitor**	**Glycine 1%**	**Bile 1%**	**Charcoal Casein Deoxycholate**
C. lari	–	+	+	+	+	+	+	+
C. upsaliensis	–	+	+	+	+	–	+	+
C. fetus	+	+	(–)	–	+	+	–	–
C. hyointestinalis	(+)	+[a]	+	+	+	+	NA	NA
C. concisus	–	+	+	+	+	+	NA	NA
C. mucosalis	+	+	+	+	+	+	NA	NA
C. sputorum[b]	–	+	+	+	+	+	+	+

[a]Best at 35°C (95°F).
[b]*C. sputorum* has three biovars with different biochemical characteristics.
+, Positive; –, negative; (+), most strains positive; (–), most strains negative; *H_2S*, hydrogen sulfide gas; *NA*, data not available or found; *R*, resistant; *S*, susceptible; *TSI*, triple sugar iron agar.

of clinical importance.[113] For example, *C. jejuni* and *C. coli* are resistant to cephalothin, whereas *C. fetus* is susceptible. A filtration method with nonselective media may be used to complement direct culture on selective media for the detection of antibiotic-susceptible *Campylobacter* spp. Because of their small size and motility, campylobacters may pass through filters with pores of 0.45 to 0.65 μm, whereas other enteric organisms are retained.[39]

Although colonies may appear on plates within 24 to 48 hours, growth of campylobacters from stool may take as long as 72 to 96 hours. Primary isolation from blood may require 2 weeks.[7] Gram stains of young cultures reveal vibrioid forms, and longer incubation may yield spherical or coccoid bodies. Colonies are not pigmented. *Campylobacter* spp. usually can be distinguished from one another on the basis of biochemical tests and growth characteristics (Table 131.1). Although the significant pathogens *C. jejuni, C. coli,* and *C. lari* cannot be discriminated reliably by the use of 16S rDNA data, these sequences provide a substantially improved basis for the identification and differentiation of *Campylobacter* spp.[110] Many investigators have applied molecular techniques to identify enteric campylobacters directly from stool.

C. jejuni belongs to rRNA superfamily VI, a specialized subgroup of gram-negative bacteria that also includes *Arcobacter* and *Helicobacter*. The species *C. jejuni* has two subspecies, *C. jejuni jejuni* and *C. jejuni doylei*. *C. jejuni doylei* can be differentiated from *C. jejuni jejuni* by the failure of *C. jejuni doylei* to grow at 42°C (107.6°F), lack of nitrate reduction, and sensitivity to cephalothin. For brevity, we refer to *C. jejuni jejuni* as *C. jejuni*.

C. jejuni has a circular chromosome of 1.64 million base pairs (i.e., 30.6% guanosine and cytosine).[246] Marked differences in pathogenic surrogates (i.e., motility, colonization of chicks, invasion, and translocation of cultured cells) are associated with variable chromosomal sequences in different passage sequences for a single isolate, and unique chromosomal sequences are associated with known pathogenic isolates of *C. jejuni*. Genomic analyses demonstrate that substantial differences exist among organisms classified by conventional means and that some of these differences are associated with the capacity to cause disease in humans.[101,136,245] Genomic sequence analyses have yielded a catalog of phase-variable surface structures (including lipooligosaccharide and capsule) that appear to relate to pathogenesis and immunity,[90,246] a lack of classical operon structure, repetitive DNA, and an unexpected capacity to produce polysaccharide.[246] Populations of *C. jejuni* are nonclonal, and interstrain exchange of genetic material occurs.[56]

EPIDEMIOLOGY

Human infection with *C. jejuni* occurs worldwide.[23] *C. jejuni* persists in zoonotic niches (Table 131.2), and most human infections are thought to arise from these reservoirs. Chickens and contaminated water are the main sources of campylobacteriosis in developed countries. The organism is a common commensal of the gastrointestinal tract of cattle, pigs, dogs, cats, and most birds used as human food,[25,265] and transmission from these sources occurs. A meta-analysis showed a prevalence of *Campylobacter* among petting zoo animals of 6.5% and a prevalence of 24.7% among household pets.[257] Raw milk and unpasteurized milk products have also been incriminated in outbreaks of *Campylobacter* infections.

Freshwater bathing sites may yield *Campylobacter* organisms that are epidemiologically linked to human infections.[235,292,293] Drinking water directly from a river, stream, or lake also increases the risk of *Campylobacter* infections[199] and waterborne outbreaks have been reported.[167]

In the United States, *C. jejuni* infection peaks in late summer and early fall (Fig. 131.2). In a study from Philadelphia, June and July were shown to be the 2 months with the highest incidence of disease. A study from Switzerland reported peak incidence of *Campylobacter* cases during July and August over several years, with a shorter peak noted in December and January.[289] Reports from Australia and Sweden also suggest increased number of campylobacteriosis cases in summer months.[88,128] Dairy cows in the United Kingdom have higher concentrations of *Campylobacter* organisms in spring and autumn, but the concentration of *Campylobacter* organisms in beef cattle at slaughter does not change with season; as many as 90% of beef cattle may have stools positive for *Campylobacter*.[313] In subtropical areas, the peak incidence of isolation of *C. jejuni* often is associated with the rainy season. In most tropical climates, rates of isolation are similar throughout the year. Overall increases in temperature and humidity are associated with a higher risk of disease. Cooler river water was associated with a higher risk of disease. Lower water temperature has been associated with longer environmental persistence of *Campylobacter*.[354]

Studies of volunteers show an incubation period of 2 to 4 days after challenges ranging from 800 to 2×10^9 colony-forming units.[22] Fecal shedding of *C. jejuni* by humans may last a median of 2 to 3 weeks, with a range of 3 days to several months.[39,169,240]

The distribution of *C. jejuni* infections within populations is linked to the level of industrialization. In industrialized countries, *C. jejuni* infection is often found in children and adults with enteritis and seldom in healthy individuals.[321] In less industrialized areas, *C. jejuni* is isolated frequently from children, even in the absence of enteritis (Tables 131.3 and 131.4). In industrialized countries, *C. jejuni* has been isolated from 1% to 13% of children with diarrhea, and the prevalence of infection among healthy individuals has been 0% to 1.5%.[24,37,272,304]

A 5-year, laboratory-based national surveillance of *Campylobacter* spp. showed an isolation rate of 5.5 cases per 100,000 person-years (with *C. jejuni* accounting for 99% of the *Campylobacter* isolates) (Fig. 131.3).[326] Population-based isolation rates of *Campylobacter* in the United States range from 28 to 1560 per 100,000 annually. In 2014, FoodNet identified 6486 cases of *Campylobacter* infection in 10 sites from the United States from a total of 19542 cases of foodborne infections, with an incidence of 13.45 cases per 100,000 people, which was higher than the rate reported for 2006 to 2008. The number of hospitalizations attributed to *Campylobacter* infection during that year was 1080 (17% of cases), and 11 deaths were reported (case-fatality rate of 0.2%).[53] The estimated rate of death attributable to *Campylobacter* in the United States is between 100 and 124 per year. The case-mortality rate is between 0.10% and 0.23%.[131]

						SUSCEPTIBILITY	
Oxidase	**Catalase**	**Urease**	**Hippurate**	**Nitrate**	**H_2S (TSI)**	**Nalidixic Acid**	**Cephalothin**
+	+	−	−	+	−	R	R
+	(−)	−	−	+	−	S	S
+	+	−	−	+	−	R	S
+	+	−	−	+	+	R	S
+	−	−	−	+	+	R	R
+	−	−	−	+	+	R	S
+	−	−	−	+	+	R	S

TABLE 131.2 Isolation of *Campylobacter jejuni* From Animal Sources

Animal	Sample	Location and Reference	Sample Size	Positive[a]
Chicken	Processing plants, shops	Japan[333]	156	67.9
	Flocks on farms	England[145]	49	76.0
	Flocks on farms	Russia[314]	370	31.5
	Giblets	Egypt[171]	50	23.5
	Eggs from 23 farms	United States[14]	276	0.0
	Live birds	United States[14]	10	90.0
	Processing plants, carcasses	United States[308]	325	78.5
	Backyard chicken farms	Finland,[260]	457	60
Duck	Giblets	Egypt	50	19.0
	At reservoir	United States[239]	113	73.0
Goose	At reservoir	United States[239]	94	5.0
Turkey	Giblets	Egypt[171]	50	14.5
	Feces	United Kingdom[294]	5000	100.0
Squab	Giblets	Egypt[171]	50	4.0
Crane	At reservoir	United States[239]	91	81.0
Pig	Pork at processing plants, shops	Japan[333]	94	2.1
Cow	Beef at processing plants, shops	Japan[333]	52	0.0
	Rectal swabs	United Kingdom[144]	668	72.0
	Farms	Canada[350]	78	13.0
	Milk cows	United States[64]	78	68.0
	Milk, bulk tanks	United States[64]	108	0.9
	Milk, bulk tanks	Netherlands	19	84.0
	Housed indoors, feces	Switzerland[35]	395	38.5
	Outdoors, feces	Switzerland[35]	395	13.3
Goat	Rectal swabs	Ghana[2]	72	33.3
Sheep	Rectal swabs	Ghana	13	23.0
Sheep	Liver	New Zealand[51,105]	272	66.2
Cat	Domestic, rectal swabs	United States[105]	430	1.0
	Zoo, rectal swab (species positive)	United States[105]	15	6.7
	Feces	United States[134]	206	1.0
Monkey	Stool	United States[220]	50	77.0
	Stool	Indonesia[220]	50	36.0
Dog	Rectal swabs of puppies	Denmark[121]	72	22.2
	Fecal culture of puppies	United States[356]	100	4.0
	Fecal swabs	Sweden [138]	180	67
Birds	Feces of migrating passerines	Sweden[242]	101	3.0
	Gulls	Scotland	990	4.8
	Wild birds feces from children's playgrounds	New Zealand	192	12.5
	Crane feces and contaminated peas	Alaska[99]	16	44.4
Pigeons, feral	Rectal swabs, feces	Norway[196]	200	3.0
Penguin	Feces	South Georgia Island[31]	100	3.0
Llama	Not available	Not available[257]	1	1.0
Horses	Not available	Not available[257]	613	4.0
Zoo animals	Tamarins, tapirs, maned wolf, red panda, red kangaroo feces	United Kingdom[315]	44	25.0

[a]Percent positive. In instances in which studies reported ranges of percent positive, the highest rate is recorded.

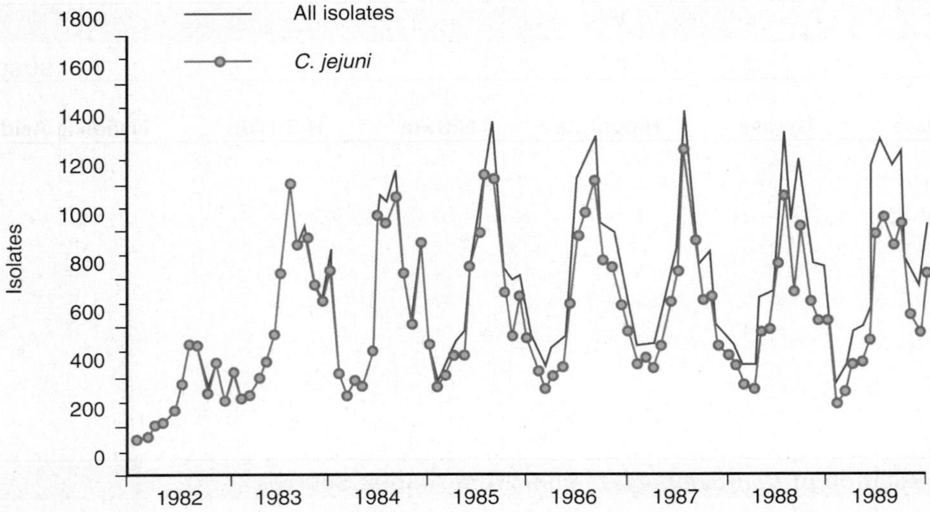

FIG. 131.2 Reported human *Campylobacter* isolates by month in the United States, 1982–89. (From Tauxe RV. Epidemiology of *Campylobacter jejuni* infections in the United States and other industrialized countries. In: Nachamkin I, Blaser MJ, Tompkins LS, eds. *Campylobacter jejuni: Current Strategy and Future Trends*. Washington, DC: American Society for Microbiology; 1992:9–19.)

TABLE 131.3 Longitudinal Studies of the Frequency of *Campylobacter jejuni* Infection in Children

		ISOLATION OF *C. JEJUNI* FROM CHILDREN[a]	
Location and Reference	**No. of Children**	**With Diarrhea (%)**	**Without Diarrhea (%)**
Guatemala[267]	321	12.1	8.1
Czechoslovakia[137]	5831	10.1	NR
Mexico[39]	179	0.4	1.7
Thailand[328]	411	0.4	1.1
Peru[192]	442	8.3	4.9
Bangladesh [320]	147	11.3	NR

[a]Results are reported as percent of stools that were positive for *C. jejuni*.
NR, Not reported.

The World Health Organization (WHO) reported 92 million cases of *Campylobacter* infections globally in 2010 of 550 million cases of diarrheal illness. *Campylobacter* was only second in frequency to norovirus in causing foodborne diarrheal illness. *Campylobacter* resulted in 21,374 (95% confidence interval [CI], 14,604–32,584) deaths annually.[129] Almost 50% of cases of campylobacteriosis globally occurred in children younger than 5 years of age. Guillain-Barré syndrome (GBS) occurred in 31,700 (95% CI, 25,400–40,200) of campylobacteriosis cases.[174] A registry-based study demonstrated fivefold and twofold increases in mortality rates for the first 30 days or first year, respectively, after developing *Campylobacter* infection.[131]

A study from Botswana revealed isolation of *Campylobacter* from stools of children admitted to the hospital with diarrhea to be associated with longer hospital stay and higher mortality rates.[254] A Canadian report showed a 5.1% hospitalization rate for *Campylobacter* infections between 2001 and 2004, with highest rates at extremes of age (<1 year and >59 years). A UK population-based study conducted in 2008 through 2009 showed that *Campylobacter* resulted in 0.5 million cases of intestinal infections yearly and was the most common bacterial pathogen to cause such an infection. The median estimated costs to patients and the health service for *Campylobacter* was £50 million (95% CI, £33m–£75m), the cost per case of *Campylobacter* infection was estimated to be £85, and

TABLE 131.4 Cross-Sectional Studies of *Campylobacter jejuni* Infection in Children

	FREQUENCY OF ISOLATION OF *C. JEJUNI* FROM STOOLS OF CHILDREN	
Location and Reference	**Children With Diarrhea % (No.)**	**Children Without Diarrhea % (No.)**
South Africa[28]	35.0 (78)	16.0 (63)
Zaire[58]	14.4 (416)	3.0 (200)
Rwanda[58]	9.3 (150)	0.0 (58)
Zaire[37]	8.6 (70)	0.0 (30)
Cameroon[180]	7.7 (272)	3.2 (157)
Bangladesh[125]	25.5 (102)	8.6 (93)
China[362]	18.7 (48)	8.6 (104)
China[62]	11.9 (303)	4.6 (953)
China[366]	13.9 (461)	13.9 (461)
Kuwait[367]	7.0 (621)	0.0 (152)
India[229]	4.0 (607)	0.9 (529)
Saudi Arabia[49]	1.0 (7369)	0.1 (1130)
Belgium[108]	5.1 (800)	1.3 (1000)
Canada[240]	4.3 (1004)	0.0 (176)
Chile[83]	10.0 (299)	6.0 (304)
Pakistan[309]	7.0 (8032)	NA
Canada[368]	32.8 (5068)	NA
Uganda[223]	9.3 (226)	NA
Bulgaria[154]	3.6 (51,607)	NA
Korea[47]	0.1 (84,406)	3 (58)
Canada[152]	29 (442)	NA
Taiwan[361]	6.8 (894)	1.6 (256)
South Africa[282]	12.8 (39)	NA
Guatemala[159]	30.8 (289)	NA
Palestine[3]	5 (150)	NA
Sudan[369]	2 (437)	NA
Egypt[71]	3.7 (13)	3.1 (11)
Botswana[254]	14 (95)	NA
Thailand[370]	8.6 (13)	NA

NA, Not available.

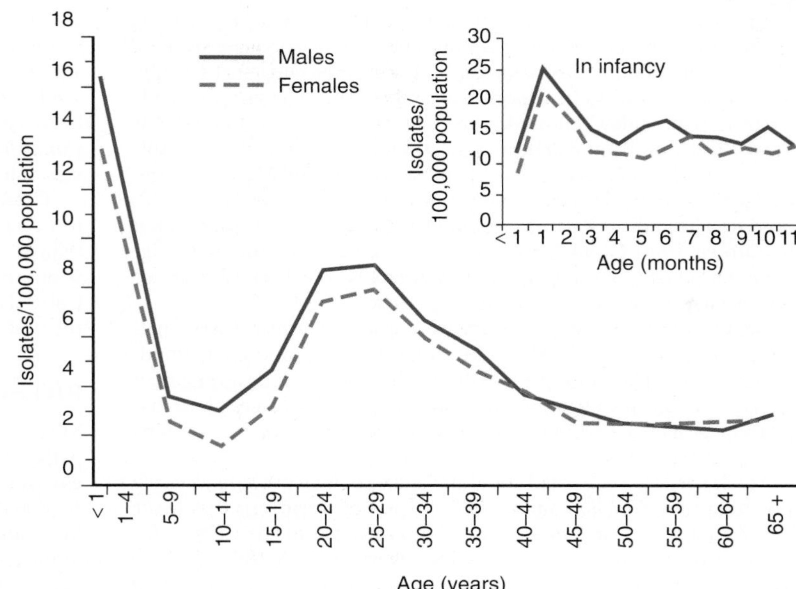

FIG. 131.3 Annual isolation rates of *Campylobacter* by age and sex in the United States, 1982–86. (From Tauxe RV, Hargrett-Bean N, Patton CM, et al. *Campylobacter* isolates in the United States, 1982-1986. *MMWR CDC Surveill Summ.* 1988;37:1–13.)

the cost of a GBS hospitalization related to *Campylobacter* was £1.26 million.[319]

Population-based studies in England, the United States, and Sweden showed a bimodal age distribution, with a peak of illness occurring in children younger than 5 years and a second peak at 15 to 29 years of age.[278,324] The highest isolation rate occurs in the first year of life (see Fig. 131.3). Reports from the United Kingdom suggest a decrease in incidence of campylobacteriosis in the younger age groups in more recent years compared with an increase in the population older than 60 years of age.[106] Similarly, most recent reports from Switzerland show an increase in overall cases of campylobacteriosis (about 150 cases per 100,000 people in 2012) with a decrease, however, in cases for those younger than 5 years of age.[289] An increase in the number of campylobacteriosis has been seen in Norway.[51] A report from Sydney, Australia showed that *Campylobacter* accounted for 22% of diarrheal episodes and was the most common cause of diarrhea in all age groups except in children younger than 5 years of age, for whom viruses were the leading cause of diarrhea.[88] A report on foodborne illnesses in Japan revealed an incidence rate of *Campylobacter* infection of 92.5 (95% CI, 55.2–154.5) per 100,000 people.[181] Doubling of the quantity of chicken meat produced since 2000 may account for increasing numbers of reported campylobacteriosis in the industrialized world in recent years.[303]

A male predominance of campylobacteriosis is seen, which has been reproducible in an animal model, suggesting physiologic differences in response to infection between the genders.[317] In young adults (20–24 years old), however, it has been suggested that there is a female predominance in disease, which may result from higher contact and exposure of females in that age group to children.[289]

In industrialized regions, most sporadic cases occur because of handling, preparing, and consuming contaminated raw or undercooked poultry or beef.[24,38,57,98,296,307,324] Raw milk and contaminated water are less common sources.[141,148,210,327,352] Poor kitchen hygiene plays a role in transmission[59,98]; the risk for acquiring infection is inversely related to the frequency of using soap to clean cutting boards.[324] Barbecues represent a special hazard because they permit easy transfer of bacteria from raw meat to hands and other food and from there to the mouth.[39,199] Other identified risk factors are eating at restaurants and takeaways.[54,59,98] Increased number of chicken meals has been identified as a risk factor for sporadic infection with *Campylobacter* spp. in children.[17] Eating fruits and vegetables has been found to be protective against the acquisition of campylobacteriosis.[17,199]

Cases of *Campylobacter* infections in children have also been associated with contact with pets from the household or petting zoos.[257] Contact with dogs and living on farms with livestock is a risk factor for sporadic cases.[199] An estimated 17% of enteric illnesses due to *Campylobacter* in the United States result from contact with animals and their environment.[122] Eating cantaloupe and queso fresco and Hispanic ethnicity have been identified as risk factors for sporadic *Campylobacter* infection in a study from Arizona.[259] Current or recent use of proton pump inhibitors is associated with higher rates of campylobacteriosis in adults.[359]

Sporadic cases of *C. jejuni* infection occur much more frequently than outbreaks. Hospital outbreaks associated with food provided from the hospital kitchen have been reported.[158] A rural setting and higher income have been associated with higher numbers of infections.[21,85]

Campylobacter has been reported as an important agent in bacterial travelers' diarrhea, mainly travelers returning from Asia.[133,187,279] In a report from the FoodNet, 42% of enteric diseases related to travel were caused by *Campylobacter*; high numbers of cases were reported from Asia, South America, Central America, Europe, and Africa.[170] Outbreaks of *C. jejuni* infections in men having sex with men have been identified.[100] An outbreak due to inadequate milk pasteurization was reported in 2015.[81]

In less industrialized regions, *Campylobacter* is associated with childhood diarrhea in 8% to 45% of cases, but it is isolated at similar rates from healthy children.[39,52,102] The highest rates of *Campylobacter* isolation are for children younger than 5 years of age.[39] As many as 75% of *Campylobacter* infections occurring during the first year of life are asymptomatic.[52] The Global Enteric Multicenter Study (GEMS) looked at children 0 to 59 months old with diarrhea from centers in Africa and Asia and found that *Campylobacter* infections from the Asian centers only caused 6.6% to 16.1% of cases of diarrhea, depending on the center and age group.[179] In the Malnutrition and Enteric Disease (MAL-ED) study, which recruited 2145 children from eight sites in Africa, Asia, and South America, *Campylobacter* was the leading cause of diarrhea in the first and second years of life and was isolated from 30% to 40% of diarrheal stools and at a lower frequency from nondiarrheal stools.[258]

Usually, a contaminated food or a water vehicle transmits *Campylobacter*. However, direct transmission of the agent may occur, usually to individuals with direct exposure to reservoir animals or to those who process contaminated animal products.[34] Person-to-person spread may occur in areas of high contamination, such as where diapered children are present.[249] In one study, increased number of children in the household and diaper use were associated with higher odds of occurrence of campylobacteriosis in children.[17] Intrapartum transmission also has been documented.[36,348] Asymptomatic mothers may transmit the infection to their newborns.[36]

In developing countries, transmission is multifactorial. Free-roaming poultry, toddlers, unsafe water supply, and lack of adequate disposal of excreta are documented sources.[111] However, proving that *Campylobacter* causes disease in regions where the agent is environmentally pervasive is difficult. Confounders include statistically indistinguishable rates of isolation from diarrhea cases and matched controls (see Table 131.3), and direct evidence that the presence in a household of *Campylobacter* shared between humans and chickens is associated with protection from diarrhea. Improved knowledge of the immune responses that protect from *Campylobacter* infection and disease and knowledge of the components of *Campylobacter* required to cause disease are needed to understand the agent's epidemiology better.

Because of the biochemical inactivity of campylobacters, discriminating species and subspecies by conventional chemotaxonomic methods is problematic. The consequences of this difficulty include ambiguities in epidemiologic investigations and low resolution in studies of mechanisms of virulence and immunity. Effort is being invested in devising genotyping schemes.[63,353]

Much needs to be learned about the epidemiology of *Campylobacter* spp. other than *C. jejuni* and *C. coli,* a group of organisms that made up only about 1% of *Campylobacter* spp. reported to the Centers for Disease Control and Prevention (CDC) from 1982 to 1986.[324] These organisms are gaining ground as etiologic agents of undiagnosed gastroenteritis. Non-*jejuni,* non-*coli Campylobacter* spp. also have been associated with extraintestinal disease, especially bacteremia in patients with comorbidities affecting the immune system.

Age-specific isolation rates of *C. fetus* parallel those of *C. jejuni* and *C. coli;* rates peak in infancy and increase in young adulthood, and *C. fetus* increases substantially in elderly persons. Seasonal distribution patterns of *C. jejuni, C. coli,* and *C. fetus* are similar, with peaks occurring in warm months. In a surveillance study, *C. jejuni* and *C. coli* isolates were predominantly from stool, whereas 54% of *C. fetus* isolates with a known source were from blood.[324] The epidemiology and antimicrobial susceptibilities of 111 *C. fetus* strains isolated from 103 patients from 1983 to 2000 in Quebec, Canada, were determined.[339] The isolation site was blood in 69% of the patients, stool in 20%, and other body fluids, including fluid surrounding the aorta, bile, synovial fluid, cerebrospinal fluid, tubo-ovarian abscess, ascites, and pleural fluid, in 11% of these patients.[339]

C. fetus, an important cause of sporadic abortion in cattle and sheep, may be isolated from the intestines and genital tracts of these animals.[250] Contaminated food and water are the suspected sources of infection for sheep, cattle, and other animals, including goats, pigs, cats, dogs, hamsters, guinea pigs, antelopes, chickens, and turkeys.[92]

C. fetus bacteremia usually occurs in immunosuppressed hosts (especially elderly men), pregnant women, and neonates[272,335]; however, cases in immunocompetent hosts have been reported.[212,226] Predisposing conditions include alcoholism or cirrhosis, diabetes mellitus, heart disease, malignancy, splenectomy, and corticosteroid or other immunosuppressive therapy.[65,150,277] *C. fetus* is not considered a major cause of gastroenteritis, perhaps because of the failure of this organism to grow in stool specimens evaluated by routine laboratory methods for *C. jejuni* and *C. coli.*[250,324] In addition to raw milk,[355] raw beef liver[310] and nutritional therapy (i.e., raw fruit, vegetable juice, calves' liver, coffee enemas) are associated with *C. fetus* infection.[42]

First associated with human disease in a homosexual man with proctitis, *C. hyointestinalis* (from *hyos* meaning "hog" and *intestinalis* meaning "pertaining to the intestines") originally was isolated from the intestines of swine with proliferative ileitis.[79,250] *C. hyointestinalis* also has been isolated from the stool of persons with nonbloody, watery diarrhea.[70]

C. lari is frequently isolated from apparently healthy seagulls, although seagulls do not play a direct role in its epidemiology.[325] Epidemiologically and microbiologically similar to *C. jejuni, C. lari* has been reported to cause enteritis in patients with and without a history of animal exposure and bacteremia in two elderly patients with multiple myeloma and permanent pacemakers.[1,218,225,301,325] A waterborne outbreak of *C. lari*–associated gastroenteritis also has been reported.[30]

The *C. upsaliensis* group is associated with gastroenteritis, breast abscess, spontaneous abortion, and bacteremia in normal hosts and with opportunistic infections in immunocompromised persons.[119,123,248] Conditions predisposing to *C. upsaliensis* bacteremia include gallbladder surgery, ectopic pregnancy, kwashiorkor, and acquired immunodeficiency syndrome (AIDS).[248] Young puppies and kittens are potential transmitters of *C. upsaliensis.*[121] In one study *C. upsaliensis* accounted for 77% of *Campylobacter* species isolated from fecal swabs of dogs. An outbreak in a childcare center suggested direct transmission between humans.[108,161]

C. concisus has been implicated in gastrointestinal disease. In contrast to *C. jejuni,* disease distribution occurred throughout the year rather than at certain seasons. Patients most commonly affected were children younger than 1 year of age and elderly people. *C. concisus* has been isolated from oral flora of 3-year-old children and found to be part of the oral microbiota protective against caries.[195]

PATHOLOGY

Most *C. jejuni* infections are not associated with illness or notable pathologic features. When illness does occur, watery diarrhea, invasive enteritis, or systemic infection may result. The spectrum of pathology reflects this range of manifestations. Acute watery diarrhea may occur in the absence of grossly visible pathologic features. Acute inflammation of the colon and rectum is the hallmark of *C. jejuni* invasive enteritis,[200] although hemorrhagic jejunitis and ileitis may also occur.[68,74,169]

In patients who have undergone proctoscopy, normal mucosa is found in approximately 50%; in the remainder, mucosal edema, congestion, friability, and granularity are seen. The spectrum of histologic changes ranges includes minimal edema with acute and chronic inflammatory cells and no vascular congestion, moderate inflammation and cryptitis, and crypt abscess formation. Acute appendicitis, mesenteric lymphadenitis, and ileocolitis have been reported in patients who have undergone appendectomies while they were infected with *C. jejuni.*[22]

At low concentrations of *C. jejuni* organisms, infection is a precursor to immunoreactive complications in which disease results from immunologic effectors generated in response to infection that damages neurons. After adjustments for comorbidities, the demonstration that *Campylobacter* infection is associated with increased mortality rates over the course of a 1-year period after infection suggests that unidentified severe late disease occurs.[131]

C. jejuni is one of a few microbes that have been hypothesized to trigger a common mechanism leading to lymphomas.[116] *C. jejuni* has also been associated with cases of immunoproliferative small intestinal disease, alone or in conjunction with other microbial overgrowth.[76,211]

PATHOGENESIS

The mechanisms by which *C. jejuni* causes diarrhea, dysentery, and less frequently, systemic disease are not well understood. Campylobacters invade different cell lines. Motility, adherence, and invasion of cells and ability to produce toxins have been associated with the capacity to cause disease,[12,13,94,96,132,166,201,217] but the pattern of their expression in disease-associated isolates is not uniform. Dogs,[264] rhesus macaque (*Macaca mulatta*),[86] rabbits,[312] mice,[86] and hamsters[147] have been evaluated as models of *Campylobacter* enteritis, but none faithfully reproduces the disease seen in humans. A mouse intranasal challenge model[16] has been developed for use in studies of *C. jejuni* invasiveness, and a ferret model[18] has been developed for studies of *C. jejuni*–induced diarrhea. Studies in mice mainly have served as disease models associated with *Campylobacter* spp.[201] As few as 500 to 800 colony-forming units have the potential to cause disease.[157]

Capsular polysaccharides produced by *C. jejuni* increase adherence to human intestinal epithelia (i.e., jejunum, ileum, and colon) and provide resistance against some epithelial antimicrobial peptides, including β-defensin and lysozyme. The structural diversity of outer membrane lipooligosaccharides is an important virulence factor of *C. jejuni.* Sialylated lipooligosaccharides have been associated with more severe gastroenteritis and development of GBS.[143] Flagella help overcome peristalsis and allow entry into the mucous layer. Secreted flagellar and nonflagellar proteins are required for adhesion and invasion. Absence of flagellin A (flaA) has been associated with decreased motility and virulence.

Cytolethal distending toxin (CDT) is the best-characterized toxin associated with *Campylobacter*. CDT has three subunits: CdtA and CdtC play a role in binding to host cells and allowing delivery of CdtB, which has a DNAse I–like activity and plays a role in host cell cycle arrest and apoptosis leading to disruption of the mucosal barrier. Type IV and VI secretion systems are associated with various *Campylobacter* species. *C. fetus* and *C. rectus* have a surface layer that makes them more resistant to lysis and phagocytosis than other *Campylobacter* spp. In addition to *cdt*, other genes that confer virulence to *Campylobacter* include those that encode the *Campylobacter* invasion protein *(ciaB)*, *Campylobacter* adhesin to fibronectin F *(cadF)*, and heat survival and stress response proteins (*htrB* and *clpP*).[103]

Survival of *Campylobacter* spp. is facilitated by the ability to form biofilms.[151] Formation of mixed bacteria biofilms may be one strategy for *Campylobacter* to escape host immunity or cause asymptomatic intestinal colonization.[151] *Campylobacter* also relies on other bacteria for iron uptake because its growth depends on iron uptake, but it is not able to produce its own siderophores.[151] In vitro studies demonstrate a capacity to disrupt tight junctions of intestinal epithelial cell monolayers and preferentially induce proinflammatory cytokine responses through activation of nuclear factor-κB (NF-κB) and production of interleukin-18 (IL-18). These capacities and the demonstrated microtubule-dependent eukaryotic cell evasion mechanism[177] may contribute to establishment and maintenance of *C. jejuni* in the gut.[46]

Campylobacter induces an inflammatory cascade and results in activation of innate immunity and recruitment of T and B lymphocytes and neutrophils. Matrix metalloproteinase-2 (MMP-2) plays a role in mediating the immunopathogenesis of *C. jejuni* in mice.[9] Another murine model showed that *Campylobacter* induced phosphatidylinositol 3-kinase to play an important role in neutrophil recruitment and intestinal inflammation. *C. jejuni* GD1a-like sialylated glycan interacts with macrophage sialoadhesins and promotes a proinflammatory and type I interferon (IFN) response. Sialylated lipooligosaccharides also stimulate type I IFN production by dendritic cells and promote B-cell responses through CD14-dependent production of IFN-β and tumor necrosis factor-α (TNF-α).[143] *Campylobacter* also induces production of IL-1β through activation of the NLRP3 inflammasome without a cytotoxic effect.[29]

Susceptibility of different *Campylobacter* strains to the bactericidal effects of normal human sera may dictate which strains are more likely to manifest with bacteremia. For example, *C. concisus* is very sensitive to such effects, whereas *C. fetus* is resistant.[174]

IMMUNITY

The preponderance of evidence of protective acquired immune responses to *C. jejuni* comes from studies of children in developing countries. These children have more frequent symptomatic infections at younger ages; with increasing age, the rate of symptomatic infection decreases. The number of *C. jejuni* organisms excreted per gram of stool of infected individuals also declines with increasing age,[328] as does the duration of excretion of the organism.[326]

These phenomena parallel increasing titers of *Campylobacter*-specific antibodies.[25,26,163,203,318,328,332] Serum *Campylobacter* immunoglobulin A (IgA) and IgM increase within a week of the infection and disappear within 2 to 3 months, whereas IgG levels increase several weeks after infection and last significantly longer.[130] Specific IgA can be isolated from the stools of infected subjects. Additional evidence for the effect of antibodies is provided by breast-feeding, which is associated with a reduced frequency of *C. jejuni* diarrhea.[281,336] Adult volunteers who became ill after a first challenge were protected from illness after a repeat challenge with a homologous strain,[22] and resistance was related to the presence of anti-*Campylobacter* antibodies.

A study challenging adult volunteers with *C. jejuni* CG8421 reported lack of immunity after the first challenge and development of symptomatic infection with a second challenge, suggesting that immunity to *Campylobacter* depends on the strain and repeated exposure.[175] A Canadian study showed recurrence rate of *C. jejuni* infection within 5 years after an initial infection to be 1.2%, suggesting that immunity against *C. jejuni*, at least in developed countries where the environmental load of *Campylobacter* may not be very high, is not persistent or sufficient to protect from subsequent infections.[11]

Prolonged, severe, and sometimes recurrent infections occur in immunodeficient patients.[204,207] Hypogammaglobulinemic patients have difficulty clearing *Campylobacter* organisms. Patients with late-stage AIDS are at increased risk for severe relapsing *Campylobacter* infection; patients with early stages of human immunodeficiency virus (HIV) infection and high CD4 counts are not at risk.

Immunity to disease may not protect against asymptomatic colonization. The bacterial components against which the protective immune responses are directed are unknown, although several potential immunogenic antigens and virulence factors have been investigated.[232] The sum of this evidence forms the basis for attempts to develop *C. jejuni* vaccines.

Very little information is available on cellular immune responses to *C. jejuni*. Cellular responses may play an important role in facilitating the formation of antibody and in clearing intracellular *C. jejuni* from eukaryotic cells.[157]

An in vitro organ culture model system using human gut showed that microcolonies of *C. jejuni* adhere more frequently to small intestine tissue than to colon tissue, despite similar cytokine responses in the tissues. Significant increase in production of interferon -γ (IFN-γ) and IL-22 was noticed in the presence of *C. jejuni* along with IL-23 and to a lesser extent IL-17 production, inferring the presence of an innate and adaptive helper T lymphocyte type 1 and 17 (Th1/Th17) immune response to *C. jejuni*. Findings from the use of mice models suggested that innate immunity and nitric oxide production play important roles in response to *C. jejuni* infection.[321]

Despite the mass of evidence indicating protective roles for immune responses, the *Campylobacter* components against which protective immune responses are targeted are unknown. Similarly, attempts to relate classic serotyping schemes, flagellar types, or presence or absence of virulence factors with disease-causing capacity have yielded associations of poor strength. The completion of the genome sequence of *C. jejuni* (NCTC 11168) in 2000[246] enabled studies to be pursued that are beginning to explain the relationships between bacterial components and immune responses. The *Campylobacter* glycome is remarkably plastic,[168] and *Campylobacter* spp. produce a surprising variety of carbohydrates (i.e., about 8% of the genome is dedicated to the biosynthesis of surface carbohydrates). Multiple mechanisms exist for sequence variation for genes encoding the glycome. In a clinical trial, researchers demonstrated that passage of *C. jejuni* in volunteers could be associated with phase variation in lipooligosaccharides.[263]

CLINICAL MANIFESTATIONS

C. jejuni produces a spectrum of manifestations, the most common of which is enteritis. Bacteremia, other systemic manifestations, and perinatal infections occur infrequently.

Enteritis

Children with *Campylobacter* enteritis may have unformed stools, watery diarrhea, inflammatory diarrhea, or a combination of these manifestations.[7,24,39,169,240,304] Inflammatory diarrhea can be so severe that it is misdiagnosed as inflammatory bowel disease.[304] Inflammatory diarrhea is a more common occurrence in industrialized countries, and secretory watery diarrhea more typically occurs in developing areas. Patients developing diarrhea abroad tend to keep the presentation that is common in their country of origin.[365] Patients with ciprofloxacin-resistant strains have a longer duration of diarrhea than patients infected with sensitive strains,[231] although a study from Finland shows opposite results.[80]

Most cases of enteric illness subside within 7 days, but 20% to 30% last for 2 weeks, and 5% to 10% may persist longer, with a relapsing course lasting for weeks.[169,240] In one third to one half of patients, the initial symptoms are periumbilical cramping, intense abdominal pain, malaise, myalgia, and headache. An acute abdomen or appendicitis may be suspected at first[45] because acute abdominal pain occasionally may be the only initial symptom; pseudoappendicitis or mesenteric adenitis and terminal ileitis can be found.[253] The pain may be mild and intermittent for several weeks, and vomiting is a common occurrence.

Secretory diarrhea with 10 or more profuse, watery stools per day may occur. Because this course commonly occurs in younger children, dehydration frequently (10%) is an outcome. Relapse of symptoms may occur.

The symptoms of inflammatory diarrhea are similar to those caused by *Shigella*, invasive *Escherichia coli*, and *Salmonella* and consist of generalized malaise, fever, abdominal cramps, tenesmus, bloody stools, and fecal leukocytes seen on light microscopy.[200] Fever without other symptoms may develop and can be associated with febrile seizures.[358] Toxic megacolon with massive bleeding may occur.[114,164,290] In neonates, blood-streaked formed stools or hematochezia may be associated with the isolation of *C. jejuni*.[114,164] The abdomen is tender, especially in the right lower quadrant. Splenomegaly occurs rarely.

C. upsaliensis and *C. concisus* are the two most common emerging campylobacters to cause gastroenteritis, although reported cases of gastroenteritis associated with *C. fetus, C. hyointestinalis, C. insulaenigrae, C. lari, C. mucosalis, C. sputorum,* and *C. ureolyticus* exist.[201] These emerging *Campylobacter* spp. may have an important role in gastroenteritis without an identifiable cause. In a study from Ireland, *C. fetus* accounted for 2.4% of cases of intestinal campylobacteriosis.

C. upsaliensis was the only organism isolated from 83 patients in a large stool culture survey using a filtration system for *Campylobacter* in Belgium.[108] Ninety-two percent of patients had acute-onset diarrhea. Vomiting (14%) and fever (7%) were uncommon and symptoms usually abated in less than a week. Gross or occult blood was identified in 25% of cases, and neutrophils were seen on fecal smear in approximately 20%. Erythromycin (11 patients) or amoxicillin (2 patients) eradicated the organism, with resolution of symptoms in all 13 patients treated with antibiotics.[108] An Australian study identified *C. upsaliensis* in 19 (0.1%) of 18,516 stool specimens from August 1992 to March 1999 at the Royal Children's Hospital in Melbourne.[161] Infection with *C. upsaliensis* was associated with milder disease than infection with *C. jejuni*; patients with *C. upsaliensis* infection had significantly less fever, diarrhea, and rectal bleeding.

C. concisus has been associated with gastroenteritis in children. In an older study, *C. concisus* was isolated from 13.2% of stools of 174 children with diarrhea compared with 9% of 958 children without gastrointestinal manifestations.[201] A later study from Denmark showed *C. concisus* to be the second most common bacterial isolate from stools of 8302 patients studied, and the annual incidence was reported to be 35 cases per 100,000 inhabitants. In this study, healthy controls did not have *C. concisus* in their stools, which contradicts previous studies that questioned the true pathologic role of *C. concisus*, especially in children. Four genomospecies of *C. concisus* exist that may have different virulence and clinical manifestations.[189,233]

Six clinical *C. lari* isolates were referred to the national *Campylobacter* reference laboratory at the CDC in 1982 and 1983.[325] Clinical illness associated with these isolates included enteritis in four patients, severe crampy abdominal pain in a 7-year-old girl, and terminal bacteremia in a 71-year-old man with multiple myeloma and chronic renal failure. The ages of the four patients with enteritis were 8 months, 3 years, 22 years, and 39 years. Diarrhea was watery or mucoid, and fever was an unusual occurrence. Potential exposure included consuming chicken, having contact with house pets, drinking untreated surface water, and eating raw oysters. *C. lari* colitis also developed in an HIV-infected woman.[75]

C. hyointestinalis has been isolated from the stool specimens of adult and pediatric patients experiencing nonbloody, watery diarrhea[70] and a rectal culture from a homosexual man with proctitis.[79] Over a 4-year period, 20 strains of *C. curvus* were isolated from two separate and distinct clinical settings, a hospital survey of infectious causes of bloody diarrhea, and an outbreak of Brainerd (chronic) diarrhea in northern California.[1]

A study from Ireland was the first to report isolation of *C. ureolyticus* from diarrheal stools; the organism accounted for 23.8% of 349 stool samples that were positive for *Campylobacter*. Of eight patients who were followed clinically, only two were children (1 and 6 years of age). All eight patients presented with abdominal cramping and had symptoms of more than 5 days' duration. Three of the patients were immunosuppressed; two were diabetic, and one had HIV-associated lymphoma.[34]

Extraintestinal Infections

Bacteremia with *C. jejuni* occurs much less commonly than enteritis. Bacteremia was recognized first in malnourished children, patients with chronic illness or immunodeficiency, and patients at the extremes of age.[4,115,207,269] Cirrhosis, cancer, immunosuppressive therapy, and HIV infection commonly are underlying conditions in patients with bacteremia.[256] These findings led to the view that *C. jejuni* bacteremia was a disease of relatively immunocompromised patients. However, most *C. jejuni* blood isolates are from healthy individuals who often have histories of recent gastrointestinal disease.[305]

The average incidence of *Campylobacter* bacteremia in England and Wales is 1.5 cases per 1000 intestinal *Campylobacter* infections. The CDC reports that only 0.4% of *C. jejuni* isolates in the United States are obtained from blood cultures.[324]

Most *C. jejuni* strains are susceptible to killing by serum, a finding that perhaps explains the transient nature of the bacteremia and its tendency to resolve without specific therapy. In HIV-infected patients, *Campylobacter* bacteremia occurs more frequently and with increased morbidity and higher mortality rates,[202,256,329] although these numbers have improved with combined antiretroviral therapy. Fatal cases have been reported in the absence of enteric disease.[202]

In a Danish study reporting 46 cases of *Campylobacter* bacteremia over a 10-year period, the incidence of bacteremia was estimated at 2.9 cases per 1 million person-years. Only one case was reported for a child. Patients with bacteremia tended to be older than patients with isolated enteritis, and enteritis was detected in 59% of patients with bacteremia. *C. jejuni* accounted for 37 cases; *C. coli, C. fetus,* and *C. lari* were responsible for the rest. The mortality rate associated with bacteremia was 4%. Patients who survived had no recurrence within a 365-day follow-up period.

A study from Spain reported an incidence of 4.7 cases per 1 million person-years over a 23-year period (i.e., 71 episodes of bacteremia). Of these events, 31% originated extraintestinally, and 26% were primary infections. Isolates included *C. jejuni* (66%), *C. coli* (19%), and *C. lari* (12%). The mortality rate was 16.4%. The recurrence rate was 5%. In the Danish and Spanish studies, patients had comorbidities, including major gastrointestinal surgeries, alcoholism, HIV, immunodeficiency, and malignancy.[82]

In the largest published series on *Campylobacter* bacteremia, 183 episodes were reported from France from 178 patients in a 5-year period. Only seven patients were younger than 15 years of age. Fever was the only presenting symptom in 42% of cases. *C. fetus* accounted for 57% of cases. Other isolated *Campylobacter* spp. included *C. jejuni, C. coli,* and *C. lari*.[238] *C. fetus* is the most common *Campylobacter* leading to bacteremia.[349] Bacteremia is one of the most common manifestations of uncommon *Campylobacter* species (Table 131.5).

Increased recognition of extraintestinal *Campylobacter* infections has resulted from the growing application of appropriate microbiologic culture methods. The incidence of *C. jejuni* bacteremia probably remains underestimated. Typically, blood cultures are not performed for individuals with a primary complaint of diarrhea. Rarely, cholecystitis,[118,262] urinary tract infection,[55] pancreatitis,[97] hepatitis,[178] splenic abscess,[295] osteomyelitis, myocarditis,[224,243] myositis,[95] and meningitis[65,332] can result from *Campylobacter* infection. A case report of *C. jejuni* prosthetic joint infection in an older man was reported.[345]

C. fetus is the non-*jejuni*, non-*coli* *Campylobacter* species that most commonly causes disease in humans. It causes perinatal disease but is otherwise rare in healthy children. More commonly, it can cause bacteremia in adults with other comorbidities, especially immune suppression. Typically, illness begins with fever, malaise, and headache. Chills and night sweats are prominent, as is weight loss in prolonged illness. Diarrhea, nausea, vomiting, and abdominal pain occur in as many as 38% of cases, and hepatosplenomegaly or jaundice develops in two thirds.[115,360] Pulmonary involvement is a rare finding.[27,115] *C. fetus* also has a tropism for the vessels.

Three patterns of invasive *C. fetus* disease have been described.[277] Clinical manifestations of the first localized infection accompanied by septicemia include meningitis,[32,193,344] endocarditis,[78,271] pericarditis,[219] thrombophlebitis,[40] mycotic aneurysm,[77,277] cellulitis,[40,91] gluteal abscess,[61]

TABLE 131.5 Clinical Features Associated With Extraintestinal Infection by Atypical *Campylobacter* Species

Campylobacter Species	Extraintestinal Clinical Features
C. fetus	Bacteremia, sepsis, meningitis, vascular infections, septic abortion, spondylitis
C. upsaliensis	Bacteremia, abscesses, abortion, hemolytic uremic syndrome
C. lari	Bacteremia
C. hyointestinalis	Bacteremia
C. sputorum	Pulmonary, perianal, groin, knee, and axillary abscesses, bacteremia
C. concisus	Periodontitis, brain abscess, bacteremia
C. curvus	Liver abscess, bronchial abscess, bacteremia
C. gracilis	Periodontitis, brain abscess, head and neck infection, fatal bacteremia
C. rectus	Periodontitis, necrotizing soft tissue infections, empyema thoracis, vertebral abscess
C. showae	Intraorbital abscess, bacteremia, cholangitis
C. ureolyticus	Oral and perianal abscesses, soft tissue and bone infections
C. insulaenigrae	Bacteremia
C. hominis	Bacteremia
C. rectus	Bacteremia, skin infections, vertebral, septic cavernous sinus thrombosis
C. volucris	Bacteremia

septic arthritis,[185] salpingitis,[32] spondylitis [44,48] and peritonitis.[120,322] The second form is transient, asymptomatic bacteremia, which may be self-limited.[115,272,276] Prolonged and recurrent bacteremia, with waxing and waning symptoms as spontaneous relapses and remissions occur, is the third pattern of invasive *C. fetus* infection.[27,50,155,360]

C. curvus has been associated with polymicrobial liver and lung abscesses in two patients with cancer. *C. rectus* was reported in a polymicrobial breast abscess in a patient with lymphoma.[1] *C. concisus, C. curvus, C. gracilis, C. lari, C. mucosalis, C. rectus, C. showae, C. sputorum,* and *C. ureolyticus* can be isolated from the oral cavity. *C. rectus* and *C. gracilis* are thought to be associated with periodontitis.[201] Fatal cases of bacteremia with *C. upsaliensis* and *C. gracilis* have been reported.[228,297] *Campylobacter volucris* bacteremia was reported for the first time in an immunocompromised patient.[186] The extraintestinal clinical features of uncommon *Campylobacter* spp. are presented in Table 131.5.

Perinatal Infections

Occasionally, abortion or stillbirth, premature labor, neonatal sepsis, and meningitis caused by *C. jejuni* have been described, although these manifestations have been more commonly associated with *C. fetus*.[251] *Campylobacter*-associated second-trimester abortion usually is preceded by mild gastroenteritis.[221,300] The placenta may have areas of necrosis, infarction, microabscesses, and inflammation. The most likely route of placental or fetal infection is through the bloodstream, although a case with possible ascending spread has been reported.[60] Maternal blood, placenta, cervix, vaginal, and stool cultures have yielded *C. fetus* in reported perinatal cases.[193,300,357]

Infected infants often are premature. Illness in neonates typically is mild or asymptomatic, but symptomatic gastroenteritis and asymptomatic bloody diarrhea caused by *C. jejuni* have been reported in newborn infants.[33,240] Bacteremia and meningitis also may occur.[109,332,340] Hemorrhagic infarction, necrosis, and cystic degeneration of the cerebral cortex are the cerebral lesions most commonly reported in *Campylobacter* meningitis.[357] A case of second-trimester intrauterine growth restriction associated with *C. coli* has been described,[182] and *C. curvus* has been incriminated in a premature birth.[208] The source of the organism usually is the mother, who may be symptomatic or asymptomatic at the time of delivery.[33,299]

Immunoreactive and Other Complications

An episode of *C. jejuni* infection may be followed by immunoreactive complications such as GBS,[126,127,214,273] Reiter syndrome,[162,261] reactive arthritis,[69,262,286] and erythema nodosum.[10,93,311,312] A preceding *C. jejuni* infection was documented by serologic methods or stool culture in 12% to 60% of patients with GBS.[6,126,127,142,214] *C. jejuni* infection is the most commonly identified causal factor for GBS.[270] However, the risk for development of this syndrome after having a *C. jejuni* infection is less than 1%.[6] *Campylobacter*-associated GBS is associated with axonal degeneration and poorer outcome than in GBS associated with other causes.[270]

During the 2 months after a symptomatic episode of *C. jejuni* infection, the likelihood of GBS is approximately 100 times (30.4 cases/100,000 people) higher than the risk in the general population (0.3 cases/100,000 people).[205] In a nested case-control study conducted from 1991 to 2001 using data from the United Kingdom General Practice Research Database, 20% of GBS cases were associated with *Campylobacter*.[319] A case-control study from India found that 27.7% of patients with GBS had evidence of a recent *Campylobacter* infection.[165] A study from Bangladesh showed higher rates of *Campylobacter* infection preceding GBS with positive serology in 57% of cases. Patients with *Campylobacter* infection were more likely to have an axonal variant, greater disability, and higher mortality rates; they also had higher titers of antibodies to gangliosides GM_1 and CD1a.[153]

GBS appears to be an age-related risk. One study found no cases among patients younger than 20 years of age, 14 cases per 100,000 patients 20 to 59 years of age, and 248 cases per 100,000 infections in those older than 60 years of age.[205] Certain serotypes of *C. jejuni* (e.g., O:19) are associated more frequently with the subsequent development of GBS.[8,183] A study from Pakistan identified the *wlaN* gene in *C. jejuni* that encodes β-1,3-galactosyl transferase, which converts the GM_2-like lipooligosaccharide structure to a GM_1-like structure that is associated with development of GBS.[234]

The molecular mimicry between GM_1 ganglioside and *C. jejuni* lipooligosaccharide is one of the triggers of GBS.[363] A positive correlation of serologic evidence of *C. jejuni* and antibody to GM_1 has been described.[112,156] Lipopolysaccharide extracted from *C. jejuni* had a core oligosaccharide resembling the human ganglioside GM_1. Pure motor neuropathy with a tendency for more distal weakness and sparing of the cranial nerves have been associated with *C. jejuni* infection in patients with anti-GM_1 antibody.[5]

Campylobacter carrying the *cst-II* sialy transferase gene is associated with the development of GBS and Fisher syndrome, and gene polymorphisms may determine which syndrome develops after having *C. jejuni* enteritis.[363] Cases of Miller-Fisher syndrome, a polyneuritis variant characterized by ophthalmoplegia, areflexia, and cerebellar ataxia, and Bickerstaff brainstem encephalitis, a Miller-Fisher variant with impaired consciousness, also have been associated with *C. jejuni* infection.[117,149] These patients often have antibodies to ganglioside Q_{1b} (GQ_{1b}), which may be helpful in confirming the diagnosis.[117] Chaperone molecules (i.e., human peripheral nerve heat shock proteins [HSPs]) have high sequence homology with components of *Campylobacter*, suggesting their potential involvement in the development of autoimmunity in the setting of GBS.[197]

Reactive arthritis may be associated with *Campylobacter* enteritis, especially in adults with human leukocyte antigen-B27 (HLA-B27).[69,286] *Campylobacter*-reactive arthritis can occur in 1% to 5% of patients infected.[262] The arthritis starts a few days to several weeks after an episode of diarrhea. Involvement of joints can be monarticular or multiple and migratory, and the large and small joints can be affected. Synovial fluid is sterile, and fever and leukocytosis are absent. The duration ranges from 1 week to several months, the course is self-limited, and the prognosis is good.[124] A study from Oregon that included 6379 culture-confirmed *Campylobacter, Salmonella, Yersinia, Shigella,* and *E. coli* O157 infections showed an incidence of 2.1 cases of reactive arthritis per 100,000 patients after *Campylobacter* infection. Women, adults, and patients with more severe illness were at higher risk for this complication. No association with HLA-B27 was found.[338]

C. jejuni and other campylobacters may be associated with the development of inflammatory bowel disease (IBD) in children, although Jess and colleagues[160] attribute increased rates of *Campylobacter* infections around the first episode of IBD to a possible detection bias. In one study, *C. concisus* was isolated from 65% (35 of 54) of stools from children with Crohn disease, and 12 other samples were positive for other non-*jejuni Campylobacter* (i.e., *C. rectus, C. gracilis, and C. showae*).[201] A study looking at bacterial DNA in the mucosa and lymph nodes of patients with Crohn disease found *Campylobacter* to be uncommon in that patient population, whereas *E. coli* was more commonly detected. However. a metaanalysis looking at the role of *Helicobacter* and *Campylobacter* species in IBD found *Campylobacter* species (specifically *C. concisus* and *C. showae*) to be associated with an increased risk of IBD.[41]

It has been postulated that *Campylobacter* enteritis can cause functional gastrointestinal disorders in children, including irritable bowel syndrome and dyspepsia.[284] Moreover, *Campylobacter* has been associated with the development of Barrett esophagus. A study investigating 1753 cases of gastroenteritis, including 738 cases of *Campylobacter,* found that infection with *Campylobacter* increased the risk of celiac disease.[275]

Severe, persistent, and relapsing *C. jejuni* infections have been reported in patients with immune deficiencies, including congenital and acquired hypogammaglobulinemia and malnutrition.[4,140,207] Patients with AIDS have increased frequency and severity of *C. jejuni* infections; the severity correlates inversely with the CD4 count.[194]

A report from Peru showed that symptomatic and asymptomatic campylobacteriosis was associated with decreased weight gain by children (0–6 years of age) over the 3 months after infection. Severe episodes of symptomatic infection were associated with a significant decrease in linear growth over the 9 months after infection.[192]

DIAGNOSIS

The initial characteristics of *C. jejuni* enteritis are not sufficiently distinctive to permit the diagnosis to be established on clinical grounds. The differential diagnosis includes *Shigella, Salmonella,* invasive *E. coli, E. coli* O157:H7, *Yersinia enterocolitica, Aeromonas, Vibrio parahaemolyticus,* amebiasis, and pseudomembranous colitis caused by *Clostridium difficile.* Fecal leukocytes are found in as many as 75% of cases of *Campylobacter* enteritis; gross or occult fecal blood is identified in 50%.[22,24,200] White blood cell counts usually are normal, although a shift to the left in the differential count can indicate a high number of immature white blood cells. Mild elevations in alanine aminotransferase and alkaline phosphatase levels and the sedimentation rate are observed in as many as 25% of patients. *C. jejuni* intestinal infection has been suggested as a cause of thrombocytopenia, leukopenia, or pancytopenia.[1,266,287]

Methods for demonstrating *C. jejuni* include direct microscopy,[241,244] bacteriologic culture, antigen detection by electroimmunoassay (EIA) or enzyme-linked immunosorbent assay (ELISA),[135,288,334] DNA probes,[330] polymerase chain reaction (PCR),[156,190,343] and serology. A rapid immunochromatographic assay received US Food and Drug Administration (FDA) approval in 2009. ELISA using recombinant P18 and P39 as antigens has demonstrated 91.9% sensitivity and 99% specificity.[288] However, those results have not been consistent across studies.

The CDC 2015 definition of a confirmed case of campylobacteriosis relies on a positive culture, whereas culture-independent detection tests (CIDTs) support only the diagnosis of a probable case. Culture on selective media and incubation at 42°C under microaerobic conditions for 72 hours is the traditional gold standard for the diagnosis of *Campylobacter* infection. PCR enables some culture-negative *Campylobacter* infections to be diagnosed.[190,191] In a prospective, multicenter study comparing four *Campylobacter* culture–selective media, four commercially available antigen detection CIDTs, and PCR, the sensitivity, specificity, and positive predictive value of antigen CIDTs were 79.6% to 87.6%, 95% to 99.5%, and 41.3% to 84.3%, respectively. Of 209 samples that tested positive by at least one CIDT, only one was positive by all antigen CIDTs.[87] In the same study, a combination of two culture media for *Campylobacter*—cefoperazone, vancomycin, and amphotericin B (CVA) agar and modified charcoal, cefoperazone, and deoxycholate (CCD) agar—resulted in a higher yield of culture results. Serologic tests appear useful for epidemiologic investigations but are not recommended for routine diagnosis.

C. jejuni can be detected by darkfield and phase-contrast examination of fresh suspensions of stool. The distinguishing characteristic of *Campylobacter* is darting motility. Gram stain of stool showing *Vibrio* forms is useful for making a presumptive diagnosis.[285] Using the direct carbol-fuchsin Gram stain method, Wang and Murdoch[351] reported 89% sensitivity and 99.7% specificity when examining stool samples of *Campylobacter*-infected patients. The indirect fluorescent antibody test can be used for identification of *Campylobacter* on smears, but standardized reagents for this procedure are not available from commercial sources.

Establishing a definitive diagnosis of *Campylobacter* infection requires demonstration of the organism in stool or in a tissue sample. Unfortunately, not all laboratories culture for *Campylobacter,* despite its frequency, and not all laboratories use the same culture technique.[213] Culture of *Campylobacter* from stool requires special methods and media. It can be accomplished with media that contain antibiotics[72] to which *Campylobacter* organisms are resistant. If culturing is done on a medium free of antibiotics, diluted stool samples should be passed through a cellulose acetate membrane filter with a pore size of 0.65 μm to reduce the number of other enteric microorganisms.[72] Inoculated plates should be incubated in 5% oxygen and 10% carbon dioxide at 37°C to 42°C (98.6°F–107.6°F). Colony formation may not be grossly visible until 72 hours after plating. Identification of colonies as *C. jejuni or coli* is based on a Gram stain showing characteristic morphology and positive catalase and oxidase reactions. Hydrolysis of hippurate establishes an isolate that meets the conventional inclusion criteria for *C. jejuni.*

Routine media usually are adequate for isolation of *Campylobacter* from normally sterile body fluids and tissues. There are no specific media for culture from blood samples, and not many studies have investigated isolation of *Campylobacter* species from blood using automated blood culture systems. However, *C. jejuni* may take more than the standard 5-day period to grow from a routine blood culture.[198]

PCR analysis performed on fixed, routinely processed colon biopsies is an excellent diagnostic method for detecting *Campylobacter* from focal active colitis cases. An advantage of the PCR on tissue samples is that it can be done retrospectively from the paraffin block.[291] Multiplex PCR assays for detection of multiple diarrheogenic agents, including *Campylobacter,* have been studied and show promising results. In one study, positive agreement between the assay and culture or EIA for *Campylobacter* was 97%.[176] Another study suggested the benefit of such assays in detecting *Campylobacter* 5 days or more after onset of symptoms, when cultures may be negative.[255]

TREATMENT

Azithromycin is considered the drug of choice in adults and children.[67,184] Most patients with *C. jejuni* enteritis have mild symptoms and do not require antibiotic therapy. For these patients, oral rehydration and replacement of electrolytes are sufficient. Patients who may benefit from antibiotic therapy have extraintestinal infections, fever, bloody stools, and symptoms lasting longer than a week.[7] Patients with HIV infection or other immunodeficiency syndromes should be treated.

Most *C. jejuni* organisms are susceptible to macrolides, aminoglycosides, fluoroquinolones, chloramphenicol, imipenem, and clindamycin and are resistant to cephalosporins, tetracyclines, rifampin, penicillins, trimethoprim, and vancomycin.[302,342] However, resistance to macrolides is starting to emerge, and cases have been reported worldwide.[104] Patterns of antibiotic resistance by *C. jejuni* show regional differences. In the past, quinolones were used as empiric therapy for adult traveler's diarrhea because of their good microbiologic activity against *Campylobacter, Shigella,* and *Salmonella* strains.[6,66] However, since the late 1980s, *Campylobacter* strains have become increasingly resistant to

TABLE 131.6 Antibiotic Resistance Pattern of *Campylobacter jejuni* Isolates

Location and Reference	Study Years	No. Tested	PERCENTAGE OF ISOLATES RESISTANT TO THE DRUG			
			Erythromycin	Fluoroquinolones	Tetracycline	Gentamicin
Netherlands[288]	1994–97	1315	2	11–29	7–15	ND
Minnesota[278]	1994–98	4953	ND	1.3–10.2	ND	ND
Barcelona, Spain[371]	1995–98	909	5	81	72	1
Canada[73]	1995–97	158	0	12.7	56	ND
Spain[372]	1997–98	537	3.2	75	ND	0.4
Taiwan[361]	1994–96	93	10	52	95	1
Thailand[184]	1995	57	ND	84	ND	ND
South Africa[282]	2003–05	98	95	11	35	21
Taiwan[361]	2003–05	61	3.3	90.2	93.4	ND
Cambodia[209]	2004–06	87	2	31	25	ND
Portugal[372]	2003–07	123	ND	80.5	ND	ND
Chile[373]	2002–07	73	0	32.4	ND	ND
Poland[280]	2000–07	251	0.4	49.5	17.5	ND
Thailand[374]	2012	9	12.5	66.7	ND	ND
Japan[374]	2012	20	0	90	ND	ND
UK[316]	1994–2014	5953	2.2	29	ND	ND
Qatar[103]	2005–13	174	8.6	63.2	ND	0

ND, No data.

fluoroquinolones worldwide, except in Australia (Table 131.6). A UK study looking at samples collected between 1994 and 2014 showed an increase in fluoroquinolones resistance from 12.8% to 49.9% of isolates, whereas macrolide resistance was steadily low.[316]

The emergence of fluoroquinolone resistance has been associated with the use of quinolones such as sarafloxacin, difloxacin, and enrofloxacin in veterinary medicine in Europe and the United States.[73,146] The association of human infection with fluoroquinolone-resistant *Campylobacter* spp. and consumption of poultry prompted the FDA to withdraw enrofloxacin for use in poultry, effective September 2005.[230] Despite this measure, it will take time for fluoroquinolone-sensitive *Campylobacter* spp. to be reestablished in the environment. A study comparing infection with erythromycin-resistant and erythromycin-susceptible isolates in children did not show any clinical difference in the course of disease or clinical presentation.

Although fluoroquinolone-resistant *Campylobacter* is thought to cause more severe disease, recent studies show opposite results. A study from Chile showed *C. jejuni* strains from animal and human samples to be more susceptible to antimicrobials than *C. coli* strains, but they exhibited a higher number of virulence genes.[188] Other positive and negative interactions between virulence genes and resistance to ciprofloxacin and erythromycin have been described.[103]

Fluoroquinolone resistance in *C. jejuni* infections appears to be related to mutations in the genes encoding subunits of DNA gyrase, especially *gyrA*.[139] Resistance to tetracycline is mediated through the *tetO* gene. The frequency of erythromycin-resistant *Campylobacter* isolates is low (see Table 131.6). Macrolide resistance is induced by mutations in 23S rRNA genes. *Campylobacter* possess three copies of those genes; mutation of two copies results in macrolide resistance.[236]

A study from Iran looked at 30 food samples and 15 clinical samples of *Campylobacter.* The results showed high resistance to imipenem (86.49% of isolates).[15]

Whole-genome sequencing of two multidrug-resistant *C. coli* strains isolated from poultry in Colombia showed genes that encode proteins conferring antimicrobial resistance to aminoglycosides (Aph3′-III), lincosamides (InuC), fluoroquinolones (GyrA and GyrB), and tetracyclines (EF-G and TetO); genes that encode efflux pump components (CmeA, CmeB, TolC, MATE, MFS, MacA, MacB, RND, AcrB, and OM); and genes affecting CmeA-BCR operon regulation, which is associated with increased multidrug resistance.[20] A U.S. study looking at gentamicin-resistant isolates from humans and chicken meat described nine variants of gentamicin resistance genes. Human isolates were more genetically diverse and displayed more resistance: 98.7% were resistant to tetracycline, 58.2% were resistant to quinolones, and 45.6% were resistant to macrolides.[364]

Data on antibiotic treatment are controversial. A meta-analysis of the effects of antibiotic treatment on duration of symptoms caused by *Campylobacter* spp. looked at 11 randomized, controlled trials. It concluded that antibiotic therapy (with erythromycin, ciprofloxacin, or norfloxacin) shortened the duration of intestinal symptoms by less than 2 days, especially if the drugs were given early in the course of disease.[331] Antibiotic therapy shortened the excretion of *Campylobacter* spp. from feces.[331] There are concerns about antimicrobial resistance and alteration of the intestinal microbiome that may predispose to chronic intestinal inflammation, especially with self-medication by travelers. However, antimicrobial therapy may be more important than previously thought for children because *Campylobacter* infection may stunt weight gain and linear growth in the months after infection. All immunocompromised and bacteremic patients with *C. jejuni* infections should be treated with an appropriate antibiotic such as gentamicin, imipenem, or both drugs.

Synergistic combination therapy is indicated for patients with meningitis and endocarditis, for which bactericidal activity is critical.[216] Patients with *Campylobacter* in their stool who are being treated for an extraintestinal *Campylobacter* infection with gentamicin should be prescribed supplemental oral therapy because gentamicin is ineffective against *Campylobacter* in the gut.[7] Carbapenems are essential for treatment of meningitis, and prolonged courses of treatment up to 6 weeks have been suggested for these infections.[344]

Prolonged antimicrobial therapy and follow-up blood cultures are warranted for patients with *C. fetus* bacteremia because of the relapsing nature of the illness.[219] Chloramphenicol should be used with caution in treating *C. fetus* meningitis because clinical outcomes and in vitro susceptibility results for this drug have been disappointing.[193,216]

PREVENTION

Tactics for prevention of campylobacteriosis include breast-feeding and avoidance of raw food and food that has been cooked under conditions that permit the survival of bacteria or that has been handled in such a way that bacterial contamination can occur. Risks for foodborne illnesses, including campylobacteriosis transmitted by restaurant-prepared meals, may be reduced by mandating that food-service employees obtain training in food safety, such as handwashing with soap and water after handling raw poultry or meat, cooking poultry to 82°C (180°F) or until meat is no longer pink and juices run clear, and separating raw poultry from other foods during preparation.

A 24-month (2002–04), population-based, surveillance case-control study by FoodNet in the United States evaluated infants with laboratory-confirmed *Campylobacter* infection and identified risk factors associated with their infection. Identified risk factors include drinking well water, eating fruits and vegetables prepared at home, having a pet with diarrhea in the home, visiting or living on a farm, riding in a shopping cart next to meat or poultry, and traveling outside the United States.[96] Prevention measures should then be targeted at the potential source. Selected microorganisms may displace *Campylobacter* from its ecologic niches. This finding may prove useful in reducing *Campylobacter* contamination of food animals.[215,222]

Attempts to develop vaccines against campylobacteriosis continue. A recombinant protein vaccine and a killed whole-cell and flagellin subunit recombinant vaccine have failed phase II trials. A capsule-conjugate vaccine that demonstrated efficacy against diarrheal disease in nonhuman primates is in phase I human trials, and a DNA vaccine is in the preclinical stage of development.[274] The next step is to develop combination vaccines targeting different diarrheal agents.[346]

NEW REFERENCES SINCE THE SEVENTH EDITION

9. Alutis ME, Grundmann U, Hagen U, et al. Matrix metalloproteinase-2 mediates intestinal immunopathogenesis in *Campylobacter jejuni*-infected infant mice. *Eur J Microbiol Immunol (Bp)*. 2015;5:188-198.
17. Bassal R, Ovadia A, Bromberg M, et al. Risk factors for sporadic infection with *Campylobacter* spp. among children in Israel: a case-control study. *Pediatr Infect Dis J*. 2016;35:249-252.
20. Bernal JF, Donado-Godoy P, Valencia MF, et al. Whole-genome sequences of two *Campylobacter coli* isolates from the antimicrobial resistance monitoring program in Colombia. *Genome Announc*. 2016;4:e00131-16.
29. Bouwman LI, de Zoete MR, Bleumink-Pluym NM, et al. Inflammasome activation by *Campylobacter jejuni*. *J Immunol*. 2014;193:4548-4557.
48. Choi HS, Shin SU, Bae EH, et al. Infectious spondylitis in a patient with chronic kidney disease: identification of *Campylobacter fetus* subsp. *testudinum* with 16S ribosomal RNA sequencing. *Jpn J Infect Dis*. 2016;69:517-519.
53. Crim SM, Griffin PM, Tauxe R, et al. Preliminary incidence and trends of infection with pathogens transmitted commonly through food—Foodborne Diseases Active Surveillance Network, 10 U.S. sites, 2006-2014. *MMWR Morb Mortal Wkly Rep*. 2015;64:495-499.
71. El-Shabrawi M, Salem M, Abou-Zekri M, et al. The burden of different pathogens in acute diarrhoeal episodes among a cohort of Egyptian children less than five years old. *Prz Gastroenterol*. 2015;10:173-180.
76. Ewers EC, Sheffler RL, Wang J, et al. Immunoproliferative small intestinal disease associated with overwhelming polymicrobial gastrointestinal infection with transformation to diffuse large B-cell lymphoma. *Am J Trop Med Hyg*. 2016;94:1177-1181.
77. Fagan P, Morgan M. Re: mycotic abdominal aortic aneurysm caused by *Campylobacter fetus*: a case report and literature review. *Ann Vasc Surg*. 2015;29:1332.
81. Fernandes AM, Balasegaram S, Willis C, et al. Partial failure of milk pasteurization as a risk for the transmission of *Campylobacter* from cattle to humans. *Clin Infect Dis*. 2015;61:903-909.
87. Fitzgerald C, Patrick M, Gonzalez A, et al. Multicenter evaluation of clinical diagnostic methods for detection and isolation of *Campylobacter* spp. from stool. *J Clin Microbiol*. 2016;54:1209-1215.
88. Fletcher S, Sibbritt D, Stark D, et al. Descriptive epidemiology of infectious gastrointestinal illnesses in Sydney, Australia, 2007-2010. *Western Pac Surveill Response J*. 2015;6:7-16.
95. Fujiki Y, Kotani T, Takeuchi T, et al. Systemic myositis due to *Campylobacter* infection. *Scand J Rheumatol*. 2014;43:78-80.
100. Gaudreau C, Rodrigues-Coutlee S, Pilon PA, et al. Long-lasting outbreak of erythromycin- and ciprofloxacin-resistant *Campylobacter jejuni* subspecies *jejuni* from 2003 to 2013 in men who have sex with men, Quebec, Canada. *Clin Infect Dis*. 2015;61:1549-1552.
103. Ghunaim H, Behnke JM, Aigha I, et al. Analysis of resistance to antimicrobials and presence of virulence/stress response genes in *Campylobacter* isolates from patients with severe diarrhoea. *PLoS ONE*. 2015;10:e0119268.
117. Guisset F, Ferreiro C, Voets S, et al. Anti-GQ1b antibody syndrome presenting as acute isolated bilateral ophthalmoplegia: report on two patients and review of the literature. *Eur J Paediatr Neurol*. 2016;20:439-443.
118. Gupta A, Tse L. Successful conservative management of campylobacter cholecystitis occurring post chemotherapy and rituximab: a rare disease entity. *N Z Med J*. 2015;128:110-112.
128. Harvala H, Ydring E, Brytting M, et al. Increased number of *Campylobacter* bacteraemia cases in Sweden, 2014. *Clin Microbiol Infect*. 2016;22:391-393.
133. Herbinger KH, Alberer M, Berens-Riha N, et al. Spectrum of imported infectious diseases: a comparative prevalence study of 16,817 German travelers and 977 immigrants from the tropics and subtropics. *Am J Trop Med Hyg*. 2016;94:757-766.
138. Holmberg M, Rosendal T, Engvall EO, et al. Prevalence of thermophilic *Campylobacter* species in Swedish dogs and characterization of *C. jejuni* isolates. *Acta Vet Scand*. 2015;57:19.
143. Huizinga R, van Rijs W, Bajramovic JJ, et al. Sialylation of *Campylobacter jejuni* endotoxin promotes dendritic cell-mediated B cell responses through CD14-dependent production of IFN-beta and TNF-alpha. *J Immunol*. 2013;191:5636-5645.
151. Indikova I, Humphrey TJ, Hilbert F. Survival with a helping hand: *Campylobacter* and microbiota. *Front Microbiol*. 2015;6:1266.
174. Kirk KF, Nielsen HL, Nielsen H. The susceptibility of *Campylobacter concisus* to the bactericidal effects of normal human serum. *APMIS*. 2015;123:269-274.
175. Kirkpatrick BD, Lyon CE, Porter CK, et al. Lack of homologous protection against *Campylobacter jejuni* CG8421 in a human challenge model. *Clin Infect Dis*. 2013;57:1106-1113.
176. Knabl L, Grutsch I, Orth-Holler D. Comparison of the BD MAX® Enteric Bacterial Panel assay with conventional diagnostic procedures in diarrheal stool samples. *Eur J Clin Microbiol Infect Dis*. 2016;35:131-136.
179. Kotloff KL, Nataro JP, Blackwelder WC, et al. Burden and aetiology of diarrhoeal disease in infants and young children in developing countries (the Global Enteric Multicenter Study, GEMS): a prospective, case-control study. *Lancet*. 2013;382:209-222.
181. Kumagai Y, Gilmour S, Ota E, et al. Estimating the burden of foodborne diseases in Japan. *Bull World Health Organ*. 2015;93:540C-9C.
182. Kuperman-Shani A, Vaknin Z, Mendlovic S, et al. *Campylobacter coli* infection causing second trimester intrauterine growth restriction (IUGR): a case report and review of the literature. *Prenat Diagn*. 2015;35:1258-1261.
186. Kweon OJ, Lim YK, Yoo B, et al. First case report of *Campylobacter volucris* bacteremia in an immunocompromised patient. *J Clin Microbiol*. 2015;53:1976-1978.
187. Laaveri T, Antikainen J, Pakkanen SH, et al. Prospective study of pathogens in asymptomatic travellers and those with diarrhoea: aetiological agents revisited. *Clin Microbiol Infect*. 2016;22:535-541.
188. Lapierre L, Gatica ML, Riquelme V, et al. Characterization of antimicrobial susceptibility and its association with virulence genes related to adherence, invasion, and cytotoxicity in *Campylobacter jejuni* and *Campylobacter coli* isolates from animals, meat, and humans. *Microbial Drug Resist*. 2016;22:432-444.
192. Lee G, Pan W, Penataro Yori P, et al. Symptomatic and asymptomatic *Campylobacter* infections associated with reduced growth in Peruvian children. *PLoS Negl Trop Dis*. 2013;7:e2036.
195. Lif Holgerson P, Ohman C, Ronnlund A, et al. Maturation of oral microbiota in children with or without dental caries. *PLoS ONE*. 2015;10:e0128534.
197. Loshaj-Shala A, Regazzoni L, Daci A, et al. Guillain Barré syndrome (GBS): new insights in the molecular mimicry between *C. jejuni* and human peripheral nerve (HPN) proteins. *J Neuroimmunol*. 2015;289:168-176.
198. Louwen R, van Baarlen P, van Vliet AH, et al. Campylobacter bacteremia: a rare and under-reported event? *Eur J Microbiol Immunol (Bp)*. 2012;2:76-87.
199. MacDonald E, White R, Mexia R, et al. Risk factors for sporadic domestically acquired *Campylobacter* infections in Norway 2010-2011: a national prospective case-control study. *PLoS ONE*. 2015;10:e0139636.
208. Mendz GL, Petersen R, Quinlivan JA, et al. Potential involvement of *Campylobacter curvus* and *Haemophilus parainfluenzae* in preterm birth. *BMJ Case Rep*. 2014;2014:pii: bcr2014205282.
211. Mesnard B, De Vroey B, Maunoury V, et al. Immunoproliferative small intestinal disease associated with *Campylobacter jejuni*. *Dig Liver Dis*. 2012;44:799-800.
212. Mikals K, Masel J, Gleeson T. *Campylobacter fetus* bacteremia in an immunocompetent traveler. *Am J Trop Med Hyg*. 2014;91:766.
213. M'Ikanatha NM, Dettinger LA, Perry A, et al. Culturing stool specimens for *Campylobacter* spp., Pennsylvania, USA. *Emerg Infect Dis*. 2012;18:484-487.
226. Nagy MT, Hla SM. *Campylobacter fetus* sepsis in an immunocompetent patient with haematological complication. *BMJ Case Rep*. 2013;2013:pii: bcr2013008610.
227. Nakamura I, Ohkusu K, Nakagami Y, et al. First case report of bacteremia due to '*Campylobacter*-like organism 3'. *Int J Infect Dis*. 2016;42:51-53.
228. Nakamura I, Omori N, Umeda A, et al. First case report of fatal sepsis due to *Campylobacter upsaliensis*. *J Clin Microbiol*. 2015;53:713-715.
232. Nielsen LN, Luijkx TA, Vegge CS, et al. Identification of immunogenic and virulence-associated *Campylobacter* jejuni proteins. *Clin Vaccine Immunol*. 2012;19:113-119.
233. Nielsen H, Steffensen R, Ejlertsen T. Risk and prognosis of campylobacteriosis in relation to polymorphisms of host inflammatory cytokine genes. *Scand J Immunol*. 2012;75:449-454.
234. Noreen Z, Abrar M, Siddiqui F, et al. Antibiotic susceptibility and molecular characterization of *Campylobacter jejuni* strain isolated from a Guillain-Barré syndrome child. *Indian J Pediatr*. 2016;83:728.

243. Panikkath R, Costilla V, Hoang P, et al. Chest pain and diarrhea: a case of *Campylobacter jejuni*-associated myocarditis. *J Emerg Med.* 2014;46:180-183.
254. Pernica JM, Steenhoff AP, Welch H, et al. Correlation of clinical outcomes with multiplex molecular testing of stool from children admitted to hospital with gastroenteritis in Botswana. *J Pediatr Infect Dis Soc.* 2016;5:312-318.
255. Petterson J, York V, Ward P, et al. The value of a multiplexed gastrointestinal pathogen panel in 2 distinct patient populations. *Diagn Microbiol Infect Dis.* 2016;85:105-108.
257. Pintar KD, Christidis T, Thomas MK, et al. A systematic review and meta-analysis of the *Campylobacter* spp. prevalence and concentration in household pets and petting zoo animals for use in exposure assessments. *PLoS ONE.* 2015;10:e0144976.
258. Platts-Mills JA, Babji S, Bodhidatta L, et al. Pathogen-specific burdens of community diarrhoea in developing countries: a multisite birth cohort study (MAL-ED). *Lancet Glob Health.* 2015;3:e564-e575.
259. Pogreba-Brown K, Baker A, Ernst K, et al. Assessing risk factors of sporadic *Campylobacter* infection: a case-control study in Arizona. *Epidemiol Infect.* 2016;144:829-839.
260. Pohjola L, Rossow L, Huovilainen A, et al. Questionnaire study and postmortem findings in backyard chicken flocks in Finland. *Acta Vet Scand.* 2015;57:3.
266. Rai B, Ray R. *Campylobacter jejuni* gastroenteritis complicated by pancytopenia. *Indian Pediatr.* 2014;51:505.
271. Reid MJ, Shannon EM, Baxi SM, et al. Steak tartare endocarditis. *BMJ Case Rep.* 2016;2016:pii: bcr2015212928.
274. Riddle MS, Guerry P. Status of vaccine research and development for *Campylobacter* jejuni. *Vaccine.* 2016;34:2903-2906.
275. Riddle MS, Murray JA, Cash BD, et al. Pathogen-specific risk of celiac disease following bacterial causes of foodborne illness: a retrospective cohort study. *Dig Dis Sci.* 2013;58:3242-3245.
279. Ross AG, Olds GR, Cripps AW, et al. Enteropathogens and chronic illness in returning travelers. *N Engl J Med.* 2013;368:1817-1825.
289. Schmutz C, Mausezahl D, Jost M, et al. Inverse trends of *Campylobacter* and *Salmonella* in Swiss surveillance data, 1988-2013. *Euro Surveill.* 2016;21. http://www.eurosurveillance.org/ViewArticle.aspx?ArticleId=21375.
295. Seng P, Quenard F, Menard A, et al. *Campylobacter jejuni*, an uncommon cause of splenic abscess diagnosed by 16S rRNA gene sequencing. *Int J Infect Dis.* 2014;29:238-240.
303. Skarp CP, Akinrinade O, Nilsson AJ, et al. Comparative genomics and genome biology of invasive *Campylobacter jejuni. Sci Rep.* 2015;5:17300.
316. Stockdale AJ, Beeching NJ, Anson J, et al. Emergence of extensive fluoroquinolone resistance in *Campylobacter* gastroenteritis in Liverpool, UK. *J Infect.* 2016;72:398-400.
319. Tam CC, O'Brien SJ. Economic Cost of *Campylobacter*, norovirus and rotavirus disease in the United Kingdom. *PLoS ONE.* 2016;11:e0138526.
320. Taniuchi M, Sobuz SU, Begum S, et al. Etiology of diarrhea in Bangladeshi infants in the first year of life analyzed using molecular methods. *J Infect Dis.* 2013;208:1794-1802.
340. Tsoni K, Papadopoulou E, Michailidou E, et al. *Campylobacter jejuni* meningitis in a neonate: a rare case report. *J Neonatal Perinatal Med.* 2013;6:183-185.
344. van Samkar A, Brouwer MC, van der Ende A, et al. *Campylobacter fetus* meningitis in adults: report of 2 cases and review of the literature. *Medicine (Baltimore).* 2016;95:e2858.
345. Vasoo S, Schwab JJ, Cunningham SA, et al. *Campylobacter* prosthetic joint infection. *J Clin Microbiol.* 2014;52:1771-1774.
346. Venkatesan MM. A novel protein-based subunit *Shigella* vaccine candidate. *Immunol Cell Biol.* 2015;93:603-604.
364. Zhao S, Mukherjee S, Chen Y, et al. Novel gentamicin resistance genes in *Campylobacter* isolated from humans and retail meats in the USA. *J Antimicrob Chemother.* 2015;70:1314-1321.

The full reference list for this chapter is available at ExpertConsult.com.

Tularemia 132

Gordon E. Schutze

Tularemia is an acute febrile illness caused by *Francisella tularensis.* Although it is primarily a disease of animals, humans also are highly susceptible hosts.

HISTORY

McCoy[101] published the first documented evidence of tularemia in 1911, when he described a plague-like disease in ground squirrels *(Citellus beecheyi)* that occurred in Tulare County, California. Within 2 years, McCoy and Chapin[102] isolated and characterized the organism *Bacterium tularense* from naturally infected ground squirrels. They detailed the pathologic process produced in ground squirrels, defined the susceptibility of other animal species to *B. tularense,* and identified fleas as vectors for the plague-like disease in 1912.

The first description of tularemia in humans was provided by Homma Soken, a court physician in eastern Japan. In 1837, he described an illness as "hare meat poisoning." Almost a century later, Vail[144] and Wherry and Lamb[152] independently reported the first etiologically proved case of tularemia in humans in 1914. Thereafter, knowledge of the organism, susceptible hosts, modes of transmission, and clinical manifestations of disease was acquired rapidly, and retrospective information was assessed in light of this new information.

Much of the current understanding of the disease in humans originated from the work of Edward Francis,[52,53] a US Public Health Service surgeon. Intrigued by the new diseases, which were called "deer fly fever" by Pearse[109] in 1911 and "plague-like disease" by McCoy,[101] Francis relocated to Utah in 1919 and established his laboratory in an unused coal shed.[52,53,54,55,56] He soon recognized the singular cause of these two diseases and renamed them *tularemia* because of isolation of *B. tularense* from blood. He isolated the organism from humans and jackrabbits[52] and demonstrated transmission of the organism by the deer fly.[54]

A more complete historical review was provided in the classic paper by Edward Francis,[53] "A Summary of the Present Knowledge of Tularemia." Almost 9 decades later, this article remains accurate and contains most of the knowledge essential for understanding tularemia.

ETIOLOGY

The causative agent of tularemia is *F. tularensis,* named in honor of Edward Francis. *F. tularensis* is a small (0.2 to 1.0 × 1 to 3 μm), nonmotile, non–spore-forming, pleomorphic, gram-negative coccobacillus. It is a strict anaerobe that infects as a facultative intracellular bacterium.

Electron microscopic studies confirmed the presence of a delicate, almost transparent cell wall and the presence of pili on the surface of the organism. Wild strains of *F. tularensis* have a lipid-rich capsule with neither toxic nor immunogenic properties, although capsule loss has been associated with decreased virulence.

The outstanding growth characteristic of these fastidious organisms is their requirement for cysteine or sulfhydryl compounds in amounts exceeding those usually present in nutrient media. Although *F. tularensis* grows best on cysteine-glucose-blood agar and on coagulated egg yolk medium and less well in thioglycolate broth, it can be isolated in routine cultures and on enriched chocolate agar.[89] Hornick[68] suggested that the addition of cycloheximide and penicillin facilitates isolation of the organism from the respiratory tract or skin ulcers. In a study by Johansson and colleagues,[75] an Amies agar medium with charcoal and a Thayer-Martin medium with antibiotics were equal in preserving bacterial viability for 1 week, in contrast to saline or Stuart medium.

F. tularensis is killed readily by heat. Exposure to a temperature of 56°C (132.8°F) for 10 minutes is sufficient for killing. The organisms are not destroyed by freezing and may remain viable in frozen animal carcasses for as long as 3 years. However, adequate cooking renders the meat of game birds and animals harmless. Treatment with tricresol solution (1%) for 2 minutes also kills organisms in tissue; organisms from cultures are killed in 24 hours by 0.1% formalin.

Despite serologic homogeneity, four distinct subspecies of tularemia have been identified. *F. tularensis* subsp. *tularensis* (type A) accounts for approximately 90% of organisms isolated in North America and has been seen in Europe, whereas the less virulent subsp. *holarctica* (type B) is found primarily in Europe and Asia.[18,83] These two strains can coexist in the same ecosystem.[99] *F. tularensis* subsp. *mediasiatica* has been isolated primarily in central Asian republics of the former Soviet Union.[108] *Francisella novicida,* which is isolated rarely and can be found worldwide, is the fourth subspecies. but this designation is not accepted by all.[77]

Through the use of molecular typing techniques, type A isolates can be divided into two distinct clades, A1 and A2.[130] These clades have been further subdivided (i.e., A1a, A1b, A2a, and A2b) based on data from pulsed-field gel electrophoresis and global single-nucleotide polymorphism analysis.[83,87,108] No differences have been found between infections caused by A2a and A2b; therefore, only three type A genotypes (i.e., A1a, A1b, and A2) appear to be clinically important. A1 isolates are mainly found in the eastern United States, and A2 strains occur in the western United States. Infections with A1b have significantly higher mortality rates than do infections from A1a, A2, or B.[87]

F. tularensis can survive and replicate within antigen-presenting cells such as macrophages or dendritic cells, correlating with the organism's high level of virulence. The organism also can invade human erythrocytes, which may shield the pathogen from antimicrobials.[69] *F. tularensis* does not produce any exotoxin, but pharmacologic tests indicate that the organism contains a lipopolysaccharide (LPS) similar to that of gram-negative bacilli. Unlike LPS of other gram-negative enteric organisms, the LPS of *F. tularensis* is 1000-fold less potent and does not activate macrophages or endothelial cells to release proinflammatory cytokines through toll-like receptors.[3,119,137,148] The O antigens of the major subspecies *F. tularensis* that are pathogenic to humans are identical in their carbohydrate content and structure, a finding implying that the differences in virulence among subspecies probably is not the result of the O antigen.[116,141,147,149]

An electron-dense surface material resembling a capsule has been demonstrated with electron microscopy. This capsule-like complex is not always visible, suggesting it may be upregulated under specific conditions.[7]

EPIDEMIOLOGY

Tularemia has been reported throughout the United States, in East Asia, and in Europe.[18,83,97,140,153] *F. tularensis* has been found in Canada and Mexico but has not been reported in South America or Africa. In the United States, the disease most commonly occurs in the south central region. From 2001 to 2010, three states (Arkansas, Missouri, and Oklahoma) accounted for approximately 40% of all reported cases (Fig. 132.1).[21]

In the United States, the incidence of tularemia has been recorded since 1927. Data from a highly endemic region found an average annual incidence of 0.4 cases per 100,000 people.[20] The number of human cases declined steadily from 1939 (2291 cases) until 1975 (129 cases). Since then, the number of reported cases of tularemia has remained consistent, with a range between 90 and 310 cases annually.[22] This range probably is a gross underestimate of the actual incidence. In 1968, in a serologic survey of 1936 subjects in California, approximately 1% of this population had antibody against *F. tularensis.*[44] Using skin test antigens, Casper and Phillip[19] showed that 6.6% of 365 people in eastern Montana had evidence of previous infection with *F. tularensis.* Of those for whom skin test results were positive, 80% had no previous history of the disease, a finding indicating a high number of subclinical or self-limited infections. The number of deaths of humans infected with tularemia ranges from 0 to 4 per year.[22]

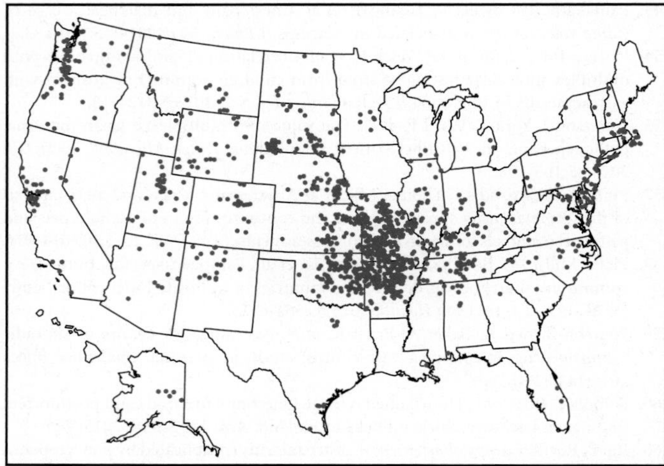

FIG. 132.1 Reported cases of tularemia in the United States, 2001–10. One dot is placed randomly within the county of residence for each reported case. Cases were reported from 47 states. Six states accounted for 59% of reported cases: Missouri (19%), Arkansas (13%), Oklahoma (9%), Massachusetts (7%), South Dakota (5%), and Kansas (5%). (From Centers for Disease Control and Prevention [CDC]. *MMWR Morb Mortal Wkly Rep.* 2013;62:963–6.)

Persons especially at risk are hunters, trappers, meat processors, muskrat farmers,[155] cooks, lawn mowers and brush cutters,[48] sheep herders and shearers,[74] and laboratory workers.[125,145] The incidence of tularemia among American Indians and Native Alaskans (0.3 deaths per 100,000) is significantly higher than that among whites (0.04) and African Americans (<0.01), and in all age groups, boys and men have a higher incidence of tularemia than girls and women.[21]

From 2001 to 2010, the average annual incidence of tularemia ranged from approximately 0.05 to 0.07 cases per 100,000 boys (0.01 to 0.06 cases per 100,000 girls) 0 to 14 years of age, with the highest incidence occurring among boys 5 to 9 years of age. Adults older than 75 years of age have an incidence of tularemia higher than that of children.[21] Children acquire tularemia by the same routes as adults: vector bites, animal bites, and ingestion of infected, inadequately cooked meat.

Tularemia occurs throughout the year, but peaks occur in the summer and winter months, depending on the region. May through August accounted for 77% of all cases of tularemia onset from 2001 to 2010.[21] Tularemia occurs more commonly in the central and southern states during the summer months, when ticks are more prevalent. The incidence in the northern and eastern states peaks in the winter months during the hunting season.

The most common sources of human infection are contact with infected animals or their carcasses and bites by ticks or tabanid flies (i.e., deer flies). Less commonly, people acquire the disease from the bite of a diseased animal or one in which the mouth has been contaminated by the ingestion of a diseased animal. Numerous outbreaks of human tularemia have occurred by water transmission in water contaminated by voles, beavers, lemmings, and muskrats.[10,23,73,80,90] Infection also may occur by aerosolization of the organisms, especially in laboratory workers,[81,145] lawn mowers and brush cutters,[48] farm workers (i.e., inhalation of dust and threshing material contaminated by voles and other rodents),[36,67] and those cleaning infected animals.[64] Person-to-person transmission has not been documented.

Hopla,[67] in describing the ecology of tularemia, states that "rarely does one encounter a zoonotic disease of such complexity." To understand the development of epizootics and transmission to humans, the role of numerous vertebrates (i.e., humans and wild and domestic animals) and many invertebrates must be considered.

Approximately 100 species of wild mammals, nine species of domestic animals, 25 species of birds, and several species of fish and amphibians can be infected naturally,[107] but probably fewer than a dozen species of mammals are important in the transmission of *F. tularensis.*[67] Lagomorphs (i.e., rabbits and hares) and some rodents (i.e., muskrats and voles) are highly susceptible to *F. tularensis.* Sheep and domestic rabbits are also susceptible but have low sensitivity to the organism, particularly in areas where *F. tularensis* is endemic.[88] Domestic dogs and cats can also transmit disease to humans after contact with an infected animal or tick bite.[93,118,156]

Vertebrate animals are called *reservoirs,* but they rarely are true reservoirs because most of them become sick and die or recover, with elimination of the organism. The varying hare (i.e., snowshoe rabbit) is less susceptible to *F. tularensis* and may serve as a reservoir because of its high natural resistance and carrier state.[51] Protozoa, which serve as reservoirs for many other intracellular pathogens, may do the same for *F. tularensis.*[1]

Many invertebrates can be infected experimentally by *F. tularensis,* but relatively few are infected naturally. In 1924, ticks were first described as vectors for *F. tularensis* infection in guinea pigs. However, the role of ticks in the spread of the human disease was not recognized until 1949, when Washburn and Tuohy[150] reported that 56% (391 of 704) of tularemia cases in Arkansas were associated with exposure to ticks. Ticks remain the most common vectors for *F. tularensis* in the United States.

At least 13 species of ticks are infected naturally by *F. tularensis.*[67,153] The main species involved in transmission to humans are *Dermacentor andersoni* (wood tick), *Dermacentor variabilis* (dog tick), and *Amblyomma americanum* (Lone Star tick). A fourth tick, *Haemaphysalis leporispalustris* (rabbit tick) does not transmit tularemia directly to humans, but it perpetuates the cycle of infection by acting as the sylvatic vector between rabbits.

When the tick feeds on an infected animal, the organisms penetrate the gut into the hemolymph and are disseminated throughout the body, including the salivary glands. The tick then transmits the organisms by injecting them with saliva when it feeds on another animal. Transmission by tick fecal contamination also is likely. Ticks, biting flies (i.e., deer flies), and fleas probably are responsible for the continuing endemic disease in susceptible animals and for epizootic disease.[16] Infrequently, mosquitoes and mites may transport *F. tularensis* mechanically from animal to animal or from animal to human.[67,153] Humans act as terminal hosts of *F. tularensis* because they do not transmit it to other humans or to other mammals.

A few cases of tularemia acquired by cat bite have been reported.[5,17,88,93,150,156] Because cats rarely are infected by *F. tularensis,* transmission may be the result of mechanical transmission from the contaminated teeth or claws of a cat that has come into contact with or has fed on an infected animal. Cat bites may be an important source of disease in children.

Ecogenetic analysis of *F. tularensis* in North America shows that the subspecies have specific geographic distributions across the continent.[47,130] *F. tularensis* subsp. *holarctica* was found along the northwestern coast and along the tributaries of the Mississippi River. In contrast, the subspecies *tularensis* spanned the region from the east coast to Arkansas, Oklahoma, Texas, and Louisiana in the south; South Dakota in the north; and the Sierra Nevada in the west. Genetic analysis of the subspecies *tularensis* in this vast region revealed that type A1 is found primarily in the eastern United States, whereas most type A2 clusters to the West.[83,87,130] This spatial separation of subspecies *tularensis* clades A1 and A2 coincides with the distribution of vectors *A. americanum* and *D. variabilis* in the East and *D. andersoni* and *Chrysops discalis* (deer fly) in the West. The spatial clustering of A1 and A2 also coincides with the distribution of an important host, cottontail rabbits, *Sylvilagus floridanus* and *Sylvilagus nuttallii,* respectively.[47]

Whole-genome sequencing of A1 isolates has revealed three major subgroups whose names are consistent with phylogenetic nomenclature within *F. tularensis.* All strains of A1a belong to the AI.12 subgroup, with A1b distributed among AI.3, AI.8, and AI.12. Using this method, it appears that the geographic origin of the A1 group as a whole may be the central United States.[11]

PATHOGENESIS

Bacterial and Host Interactions

Much of the knowledge regarding interactions between *F. tularensis* and the host was derived from experimental studies using live attenuated strains. During World War II, live attenuated strains of *F. tularensis* were developed in the Soviet Union in an effort to produce a vaccine.[114,142] In 1956, a mixture of attenuated strains of *F. tularensis* subsp. *holarctica* was transferred from the Soviet Union to the United States. From this mixture, a strain of suitable virulence was selected, tested for safety and efficacy, and designated *F. tularensis* live vaccine strain (LVS).[38,40,72] This strain has been used extensively in experimental studies on the development of immunity in humans.

Capsulated *F. tularensis* organisms are thought to be opsonized by human macrophages and dendritic cells through the activation of complement, especially C3, and binding to the complement receptor 3 (CD11b/CD18).[9] The interaction of complement-coated *Francisella* with the macrophage membrane initiates an actin-dependent process that engulfs the bacterium in an asymmetric, spacious pseudopod loop that forms the phagosome.[25,27] The organism is able to survive and replicate within macrophages (i.e., *looping phagocytosis*).[25] The phagosomes are surrounded by a dense, fibrillar coating that begins to disintegrate approximately 3 to 4 hours after infection, a process that allows bacteria free access to the cytoplasm.[26] Approximately 24 hours after infection, replication of cytosolic *Francisella* induces apoptosis that leads to cell death and release of bacteria.

Tularemia is followed by effective immunospecific protection of the host; reinfection has been documented.[15] Studies in which the infecting bacteria were suppressed by the use of a bacteriostatic agent such as tetracycline showed that protective immunity seems to be activated approximately 2 weeks after onset of the disease. When tetracycline treatment was initiated on the day of onset of tularemia and was given for 10 days, early relapses were common occurrences. When tetracycline treatment was administered for 14 days, relapses occurred less frequently, indicating that protective immunity had begun to arise.[121]

Innate immunity involving interferon-γ (IFN-γ), tumor necrosis factor-α (TNF-α), and interleukin-12 (IL-12) and the cells that produce these cytokines (i.e., natural killer cells, neutrophils, and macrophages) are thought to help control the initial phase of primary infection by curtailing the replication of *F. tularensis.*[28] Approximately 2 to 3 weeks after infection, *F. tularensis* elicits humoral and cell-mediated immune responses. Both responses reach maximal levels during the second week after infection.[24]

Because *F. tularensis* is described as a facultative intracellular parasite, the general consensus is that long-term control and clearance ultimately depend on cell-mediated immunity, as they do in infections with *Listeria monocytogenes* and *Mycobacterium tuberculosis.*[85,133,157] This finding was confirmed by several trials showing that vaccination with killed tularemia preparations, despite inducing agglutinating serum antibodies, provided poor protection.[15,72,120] Numerous studies showed that passive transfer of mononuclear leukocytes from infected animals to noninfected animals conferred resistance when the nonimmunized animals were challenged with a virulent strain.[126] Ultimately, tularemia-specific $CD4^+$ and $CD8^+$ T lymphocytes are responsible for clearance of the bacteria.[31,33,42,154]

Infection with LVS disrupts the production of proinflammatory cytokines from human macrophages and endothelial cells.[50,138] This event is consistent with the lack of increase in proinflammatory cytokines, with the exception of a slight increase in IFN-γ during the early phase of the infection, in humans with ulceroglandular disease.

The importance of the humoral immune response in tularemia has recently been recognized.[85] Although the presence of immunoglobulin A (IgA) antibodies in nasal secretions correlates with resistance to infection by aerosolized organisms, earlier work by Bellanti and associates[8] showed that humoral immunity plays a an important role, especially in pulmonary tularemia. Specific antibodies probably are involved initially in delaying the infection, allowing time for the induction of cytokine production and specific T-cell–mediated immunity. This is consistent with the observation that although neutrophils have only a minor role in resistance to infection, mice depleted of $CD4^+$ T cells or $CD8^+$ T cells, or both, remained capable of controlling and partly resolving a primary sublethal *F. tularensis* infection.[31] Antibodies may function as opsonins for macrophages and neutrophils, but the level of anti-tularemia antibody does not correlate with protection.[136] Elkins and associates[41] showed that mice deficient in B cells do not succumb to sublethal doses of tularemia during a primary infection. However, in secondary infection, the cytokines from B cells modulate the response of neutrophils against tularemia-infected hepatocytes and prevent the uncontrolled degranulation of neutrophils that may lead to severe tissue damage and poor clinical outcome.[14,30,35]

The role of neutrophils in the control of *Francisella* infection is thought to be minor but necessary. McCaffrey and Allen[100] showed that neutrophils, like macrophages and dendritic cells, rapidly opsonize *Francisella* but are prevented from mounting the respiratory burst to kill the organism. The organisms then escape to the cytosol of the neutrophils and replicate. However, studies in which neutrophils were depleted from mice showed that mice given a sublethal dose of the LVS or mice chronically infected with LVS became susceptible to infection and died.[125] Although the mechanism of action of neutrophils in these cases is unclear, it may involve direct lysis of LVS-infected hepatocytes.[30]

Persistence of immunity to *F. tularensis* depends on the T-cell response to a variety of antigens; the response may not be seen for as long as 2 weeks after exposure. Poquet and associates[115] showed that virulent strains of *F. tularensis* produce high levels of phosphoantigens that cause a proliferation in γ/δ T cells to a greater extent than does exposure to the LVS. The reduced number of this T-cell subtype in vaccinated individuals could explain the lack of complete protection seen in vaccinated laboratory workers. As with membrane proteins stimulating an α/β T-cell response, heat shock protein chaperones such as DnaK and Cpn60 also create a nonimmunodominant proliferation of T cells in immunized individuals.[45] Denaturation of the protein or carbohydrate of a macromolecular antigen of *F. tularensis* showed that T-cell reactivity was associated with only protein determinants, whereas human immune serum reacts mostly with carbohydrate determinants of the organism.[2,39]

Invasion and Disease Production

A single *F. tularensis* organism of a virulent strain can produce fatal infection in susceptible animals such as mice, guinea pigs, and hamsters.[158] As few as 10 organisms of a virulent strain injected intradermally or 25 organisms given by aerosol can produce systemic disease in human volunteers.[72] The organism gains access to the human body through the skin, conjunctiva, oropharynx, respiratory tract, or gastrointestinal tract. It spreads by the lymphatics or hematogenously, and bacteremia usually develops during the first week of infection (3 to 12 days).[81] Infection commonly involves the skin, regional lymph nodes, liver, spleen, and lungs. Rarely, the gastrointestinal tract and the central nervous system also are involved.

Histopathologic examination of mammals experimentally infected with *F. tularensis* indicates that the organism disseminates and causes cellular changes in a manner typical of intracellular parasites. After the organism is introduced into a susceptible host, multiplication occurs locally, with early spread to regional lymph nodes occurring within 48 to 96 hours.[40,49] The developing cutaneous ulcer or soft tissue focus goes through a series of changes in which polymorphonuclear leukocytes are replaced by macrophages. In time, necrosis, epithelioid cell infiltrates, giant-cell formation, and true granulomas may develop.[62,103,123] Organisms are difficult to demonstrate in tissue but occasionally are found at the periphery of lesions. In addition to the development of classic necrotic and granulomatous lesions, degeneration of the parenchyma in the liver and spleen may occur, as may marked hyperplasia of the reticuloendothelial system. Granulomas can organize to form microabscesses and abscesses.

The pace of the illness depends on the virulence of the strain, inoculum size, portal of entry, and immune status of the host.[66] When organisms enter the blood circulation, typical endotoxemia may ensue, sometimes in association with acute rhabdomyolysis.[79]

Autopsies of fatal cases of tularemia in humans have confirmed the findings in experimental animals.[60,94,111] Lymph nodes from patients with nonfatal disease have shown follicular hyperplasia with conglomerates of macrophages and caseating granulomas.[85,94,96,130] These findings are similar to those seen in miliary tuberculosis. Tularemia and tuberculosis may be histopathologically distinguishable only because of the difference in timing of the development of tissue changes,[86] a difference related to the rapid replication of *F. tularensis*.

CLINICAL MANIFESTATIONS

Regardless of the portal of entry, the mode of onset of tularemia and the general features of the disease are the same. The usual incubation period of tularemia is 3 to 4 days, with a range of 1 to 21 days. The onset of symptoms is abrupt. Symptoms include fever, with a temperature usually higher than 39.4°C (103°F), chills, headache, myalgia, anorexia, vomiting, and occasionally photophobia. Fever may be continuous or biphasic, with an intermittent period of defervescence. In untreated patients, fever may persist for longer than 3 weeks. Physical findings usually include lymphadenopathy, hepatosplenomegaly, pharyngitis, and skin lesions. Temperature-pulse dissociation has been described in as many as 42% of cases.[46,57] A variety of skin rashes (e.g., maculopapular, vesicular, and pustular rashes; erythema nodosum,[112] erythema multiforme[124]) may appear during the second week of illness and can last for a few days to several weeks.[6,81,134]

Laboratory studies, including a complete blood cell count, erythrocyte sedimentation rate, and urinalysis, usually are not helpful in diagnosing tularemia. Sterile pyuria has been reported in 22% to 32% of patients with tularemia.[46,110] Sterile pyuria combined with a history of fever, dysuria, or low back pain led to an erroneous diagnosis of urinary tract infection in 11% of the patients reported by Evans and associates.[46] Increased liver function test values with jaundice and atypical lymphocytosis also have been described.[58,61] The six clinical syndromes of tularemia can be classified by the portal of entry: ulceroglandular, glandular, oculoglandular, typhoidal, oropharyngeal, and pneumonic.

Ulceroglandular and Glandular Tularemia

Ulceroglandular and glandular tularemia are the most common forms of the disease in children and adults.[21,20,71,97,153] In ulceroglandular disease, the organism gains access through the skin, and approximately 2 days after the onset of general symptoms, the patient reports tender, swollen lymph nodes, most commonly in the axillary or inguinal areas.

Within 24 hours, the portal of entry may become evident when a painful, swollen papule develops distal to the regional node. This papule ruptures and leaves a punched-out ulcer with raised edges. The ulcer is indolent and, in untreated cases, may persist for longer than a month. The skin over the involved nodes may be inflamed. In untreated cases, approximately 50% of the lymph nodes suppurate and drain. In other cases, the nodes remain firm, enlarged, and tender for several months. Mild, generalized lymphadenopathy and enlargement of the liver and spleen may occur.

Glandular tularemia is almost identical to the ulceroglandular form, except that the portal of entry cannot be identified. The consensus is that the portal is an insignificant break in the skin. Isolated cases of cervical lymphadenopathy have been related causally to *F. tularensis* infection.

Oropharyngeal Tularemia

The infection is introduced into the oropharyngeal mucosa through infected, inadequately cooked meat or contaminated water.[82,90,140] The organisms may enter the body through abrasions or aerosolization during chewing or swallowing. Local involvement consists of acute tonsillitis with cervical adenitis.[13,82] The tonsils may be covered by an exudate or membrane that extends in all directions and may resemble a diphtheritic membrane. Complaints of sore throat usually are out of proportion to the visible pathologic features, but ulcers sometimes form.

The cervical lymph nodes may suppurate. Infrequently, *F. tularensis* invades the lower portions of the gastrointestinal tract, in which case vomiting, diarrhea, and abdominal pain are prominent symptoms. Awareness of the ability of *F. tularensis* to cause oropharyngeal involvement is important for physicians caring for children.[70,82,92,140]

Oculoglandular Tularemia

In oculoglandular tularemia, which accounts for approximately 1% of all cases, the portal of entry is the conjunctival sac, which may become inoculated by rubbing with contaminated fingers, having contact with infected water, splashing of infected liquids, or inhaling infected aerosols. The eyelids may become edematous, and the conjunctivae may be inflamed and painful. Numerous, small, sharply defined, yellowish nodules and ulcers may develop on the palpebral conjunctivae.[129] In some cases, corneal ulceration occurs.

As seen in cat-scratch disease, the Parinaud complex of unilateral preauricular lymph node involvement and conjunctivitis can result.[129,131] The regional lymph nodes, the preauricular nodes, and the submaxillary and cervical nodes are swollen, tender, and painful.[112] In severe cases, the axillary nodes may be involved.[53]

Typhoidal Tularemia

Typhoidal tularemia may manifest as a fever of unknown origin. The symptoms are those of acute septicemia, with no localized skin lesions and often without lymphadenopathy. Patients are seriously ill, and shock may develop. The symptoms and signs of typhoidal tularemia are toxemia, continuous fever, myalgia, and severe headache. Patients may be delirious and may exhibit meningismus. Patients often complain of having severe pharyngeal pain, but pharyngeal lesions may not be evident. Diarrhea occurs in this form of tularemia in adults and children. Patients sometimes have a dry cough and retrosternal pain. Pleuropulmonary involvement is a common finding in adults with typhoidal tularemia.[37]

In children, typhoidal tularemia can be the result of ingestion of the causative agent, and necrotic lesions may occur throughout the bowel.[37] Inhalation of aerosolized organisms is a more common mode of acquisition in adults (e.g., laboratory workers, farmers).

Pneumonic Tularemia

The pneumonic form of the disease occurs most commonly in laboratory workers and is the most severe form of the tularemia. Pneumonic tularemia may be acquired by the aerogenic route,[36,48,139] or it may be associated with other forms of tularemia, particularly the typhoidal type. Dienst[37] and Miller and Bates[105] published outstanding descriptions of pleuropulmonary tularemia. Miller and Bates stressed that the symptoms and signs of pleuropulmonary tularemia are nonspecific and vary with the location and degree of pulmonary involvement.

The various radiographic features may be confused with those of tuberculosis, mycotic infection, common bacterial pneumonia, lymphoma, or carcinoma of the lung. In the series of 29 patients by Miller and Bates,[105] pleural effusion developed in 6 patients. Pleural effusions can contain more than 3 g of protein/100 mL and more than 1000 white blood cells/mm^3 with a lymphocytic predominance.[59] Because of the necrotizing nature of the pathologic process, the lung may heal with residual fibrosis or calcification. In other instances, the disease is so fulminant that death occurs before the pathologic features can progress fully.

Additional Clinical Manifestations

Subcutaneous nodules resembling those seen in sporotrichosis can be found on physical examination. The nodules usually are distributed on the anterior or posterior surface of the arm and may extend from the primary lesion to the regional lymph nodes. Initially, these nodules are firm and movable, but they later become fixed to the skin and may suppurate. They vary in size from less than a centimeter to more than several centimeters if they become confluent. Other unusual manifestations of tularemia include pericarditis, appendicitis, peritonitis, liver abscess, cerebellitis with ataxia, meningitis, encephalitis, osteomyelitis, rhabdomyolysis, and venous thrombosis.[32,65,117]

The incidence of these forms among children is somewhat different from that for adults. Although the pneumonic form previously was thought to be rare in children,[92] it has been shown that the occurrence of pneumonic tularemia is not uncommon. In a 1985 study by Jacobs and associates,[71] 14% of pediatric tularemia cases were the pneumonic form. This percentage contrasts with the absence of pulmonary involvement in a series of 48 children with tularemia reported by Levy and associates[92] in 1950.

The distribution of these forms of tularemia also varies with the geographic location. In a report of 67 children with tularemia in Finland, 79% of cases were of the ulceroglandular form and 8% were glandular.[143] This distribution is significantly different from that in the United States. In the study by Jacobs and associates,[71] who reported 28 cases of tularemia among children, 45% were ulceroglandular, and 25% were glandular. Later from the same region, of the 30 cases described, 57% were ulceroglandular disease.[128] The authors of the Finnish study attributed the higher proportion of the ulceroglandular form in their study to heightened awareness of the disease and early diagnosis. The differences also could be explained by the different strains of *F. tularensis* and different vectors in the two regions.

F. tularensis also can occur in the setting of an immunocompromised host. The pneumonic form of tularemia was reported in a patient with chronic granulomatous disease requiring lobectomy.[98] Pneumonic tularemia also was seen in a patient who previously had undergone peripheral blood stem cell transplantation for acute myelogenous leukemia (it resulted in a solitary pulmonary nodule), in a patient infected with human immunodeficiency virus (HIV),[61,106] in a kidney transplant recipient,[84] and in a patient with graft-versus-host disease.[151] Pneumonic tularemia was identified in a patient with a ventriculoperitoneal shunt.[113] Impairment of normal immunity can prevent adequate protection from *F. tularensis* and necessitate more prolonged therapy.

DIAGNOSIS

The diagnosis of tularemia is established by a thorough history of possible exposure, clinical manifestations, and serial serologic tests. Obtaining a careful family history often is rewarding because several family members commonly are infected simultaneously. In some instances, however, a positive history never is elicited.

Tularemia has no absolute pathognomonic features. In diagnosing tularemia, the physician must account for the endemic rate of the disease in the area, season of the year, clinical manifestations of the disease, precise epidemiologic setting,[132] and unresponsiveness of the disease to antibiotics that are not effective against tularemia.

The diagnosis is confirmed by the standard agglutination test, which is available commercially and is reliable. Unfortunately, it may not provide an early diagnosis because agglutinating antibodies may not be detectable until the second week of illness. Occasionally, seroconversion is not confirmed until the patient has experienced 4 to 6 weeks of illness. In rare cases, agglutinating antibody may never be detected.

A fourfold increase in convalescent titer confirms the diagnosis (with an initial minimum titer of 1 : 160), but a presumptive diagnosis should be considered in patients with acute titers of 1 : 160 or greater. This titer may indicate current or past infection, but in a clinically suspicious case, it should be considered an indication for presumptive therapy. Titers of 1 : 1280 or greater often develop in patients with active disease as the initial manifestation of seroconversion. The agglutination test is specific, but cross-reaction with *Brucella* spp., *Legionella* spp., or other gram-negative bacteria can occur. Antibiotic therapy does not prevent the development of agglutinating antibodies. A single titer of 1 : 128 or greater determined by microagglutination or with a fourfold increase with convalescent testing is also considered positive. Commercially developed enzyme-linked immunosorbent assay (ELISAs) have also been found to be a useful tool.[23]

Polymerase chain reaction (PCR)–based assays are used for early detection of *F. tularensis* infection.[12,78,95] The PCR test is effective in establishing the diagnosis of tularemia even when samples of a tularemic ulcer are obtained 1 to 14 days after infection.[127] When PCR and culture of the wound and blood were compared with agglutination tests, the sensitivity of PCR was 75%, and the sensitivity of culture was 62%.[75] In addition to increasing the safety for laboratory personnel, the PCR method was more sensitive and detected infection at earlier stages. In contrast to conventional PCR-based assays, real-time PCR (rt-PCR) is more specific and 10 times more sensitive.[146] These assays are not widely commercially available.

In a Norwegian field study, a rapid immunochromatography assay proved inexpensive, time efficient, and portable in contrast to PCR and ELISA, but this method was less sensitive than PCR.[10] This assay could accelerate identification and treatment decisions in clinical practice.

Gram-stained smears of patient specimens such as exudate and sputum usually do not reveal the organism. However, collecting the specimens poses no danger, and examination of direct smears helps rule out other causative agents. Specimens should not be cultured for *F. tularensis* in the usual hospital or diagnostic laboratory because isolation of the organisms in facilities other than a level P3 laboratory is hazardous to laboratory personnel. If confirmation by culture is indicated, physicians should notify the laboratory of the potential for the specimen to contain *F. tularensis,* so that appropriate laboratory precautions can be taken.

The differential diagnosis of tularemia depends on the clinical form of the disease. Ulceroglandular and glandular tularemia must be differentiated from disease caused by ordinary bacterial pathogens such as *Streptococcus* and *Staphylococcus,* from disease caused by *M. tuberculosis* and atypical mycobacteria such as *Mycobacterium marinum*, and from anthrax, HIV infection, and cat-scratch disease. In older patients with inguinal lymphadenopathy, lymphogranuloma venereum, granuloma inguinale, and other sexually transmitted infections should be considered. Occasionally, sporotrichosis and infectious mononucleosis are diagnosed in these patients.

Oculoglandular fever is somewhat more distinctive, but the possibility of disease caused by common bacterial pathogens such as *L. monocytogenes* infection, herpes zoster, inclusion conjunctivitis, and keratoconjunctivitis must not be ruled out. Oropharyngeal tularemia must be differentiated from streptococcal tonsillopharyngitis and corynebacterial disease. Typhoidal tularemia can be confused with ordinary bacteremia and must be differentiated from the more common bacterial and enteric disease and from malaria, miliary tuberculosis, brucellosis, and typhoid fever. Tularemic pneumonia must be differentiated from other bacterial and nonbacterial pneumonia, including tuberculosis, *Mycoplasma* infection, legionnaires' disease, psittacosis, viral pneumonia, Q fever, fungal infection, and chemical pneumonitis.

TREATMENT

Gentamicin is recommended for the treatment of tularemia.[153] The dosage for children is 5 mg/kg daily in two divided doses administered intravenously or intramuscularly. The duration of therapy is usually 7 to 10 days, with more severe disease requiring a longer duration of treatment. In mild to moderate cases in which patients become afebrile within 48 hours of starting antimicrobial therapy, a 5- to 7-day course can be used. Defervescence and alleviation of other signs and symptoms usually occur within several days. Response may be delayed if the lymph nodes have progressed to suppuration requiring drainage.

If available, streptomycin given intramuscularly can be used. The recommended dose of streptomycin is 30 to 40 mg/kg per day administered intramuscularly in two divided doses for 7 days. If a patient has mild symptoms initially or responds dramatically to therapy, an alternative streptomycin regimen of 30 to 40 mg/kg per day for 3 days followed by 15 to 20 mg/kg per day for 4 days may be given intramuscularly. In severe cases or if a child does not become afebrile and asymptomatic within a few days of starting therapy, extension of treatment beyond 7 days is indicated. Streptomycin-resistant strains of tularemia are reported, but they are rare. Other aminoglycosides (e.g., tobramycin) are ineffective in treating tularemia and should not be used.

Bacteriostatic agents such as tetracycline (or doxycycline) and chloramphenicol have been used to treat tularemia, with cure rates of 88% and 77%, respectively. However, these agents are considered suboptimal for the treatment of tularemia because of a high incidence of relapse after therapy is stopped.[43]

Although in vitro susceptibility testing indicates that the third-generation cephalosporins may be effective against *F. tularensis,* one report showed treatment failure in eight children given ceftriaxone.[34] Treatment with other antibiotics has been reported sporadically in the literature.[63,91] Fluoroquinolones have been used with success when treating infections caused by the subspecies *holartica*.[4,104,106,122,135] An efficacy trial in Sweden of ciprofloxacin demonstrated successful outpatient management of *F. tularensis* in 10 of 12 patients 1 to 10 years of age.[76] The dosage used was 15 to 20 mg/kg per day given in two divided doses for a 10- to 14-day course of therapy. Defervescence occurred on the fourth day of treatment. The lack of successful treatment data for the subspecies *tularensis* and the issues related to the use of fluoroquinolones in children younger than 18 years of age limit the use of these medications in North American children.[153]

Hearing screening should be considered before initiation of streptomycin or gentamicin therapy. If the child has preexisting hearing loss, the alternative streptomycin regimen or gentamicin therapy can be considered, with close monitoring of serum levels in severe cases. In these cases, audiologic evaluation is indicated after therapy is initiated.

Bed rest and supportive therapy are indicated. In a severely ill patient who shows signs of endotoxic shock, appropriate monitoring and admission to an intensive care unit are indicated, and corticosteroid therapy should be considered. Suppurative lymph nodes may require surgical drainage even after an appropriate course of therapy. In most cases, this does not represent a treatment failure and does not require additional antimicrobial therapy. Complicated cases (e.g., meningitis) may require treatment with more than one antimicrobial agent.

Before the advent of effective antimicrobial therapy, tularemia often was a protracted illness that lasted weeks or months. Subsequently, a long period of convalescence was necessitated by debility. Antibiotics have interrupted the natural history of the disease. When the disease is diagnosed promptly, the course usually is less than a month. As a result of administering appropriate antibiotic therapy, the mortality rate has declined from 5% to 30% to less than 1%, except in cases of fulminant pneumonic and typhoidal disease.

PREVENTION

Prevention of human tularemia depends on prevention of exposure to the vectors or contaminated animal tissue. Children living in areas of tick endemicity should have their skin and hair checked frequently for ticks. Ticks should be removed carefully with tweezers (not with fingernails) by pulling perpendicular to the skin where the ticks have attached. Care should be taken not to squeeze the ticks between the fingers. Persons living in tick-infested areas should wear clothing with tightly fitting cuffs at the wrists and ankles when staying outdoors. Tick repellents should be used with caution on children. Prophylaxis with antimicrobial agents has not proved effective in preventing disease in children with tick bites.

Children should be warned against handling sick or dead rodents or rabbits. Incineration or burial should be used to dispose of rabbits caught by household pets. Rubber gloves should be worn for preparing game animals, and the meat should be cooked thoroughly before eating. Hunters, especially rabbit hunters, should take precautions against contracting tularemia.

A wide range of approaches to vaccine development is being evaluated, but no vaccine against tularemia has been licensed.[29]

NEW REFERENCES SINCE THE SEVENTH EDITION

11. Birdsell DN, Johansson A, Öhrman C, et al. *Francisella tularensis* subsp. *tularensis* group A.1, United States. *Emerg Infect Dis.* 2014;20:861-865.
12. Birdsell DN, Vogler AJ, Buchhagen J, et al. TaqMan real-time PCR assays for single-nucleotide polymorphisms which identify *Francisella tularensis* and its subspecies and subpopulations. *PLoS ONE.* 2014;9:e107964.
18. Carvalho CL, Lopes de Carvalho I, Zé-Zé L, et al. Tularemia: a challenging zoonosis. *Comp Immunol Microbiol Infect Dis.* 2014;37:85-96.
21. Centers for Disease Control and Prevention. Tularemia: United States, 2001-2010. *MMWR Morb Mortal Wkly Rep.* 2013;963-966.
88. Larson MA, Fey PD, Hinrichs SH, et al. *Francisella tularensis* bacteria associated with feline tularemia in the United States. *Emerg Infect Dis.* 2014;20:2068-2071.
90. Larssen KW, Bergh K, Heier BT, et al. All-time high tularemia incidence in Norway in 2011: report from the national surveillance. *Eur J Clin Microbiol Infect Dis.* 2014;33:1919-1926.
97. Mailles A, Vaillant V. 10 years of surveillance of human tularemia in France. *Euro Surveill.* 2014;19:20956.
118. Salit IE, Liles WC, Smith C. Tularemia endocarditis from domestic cat exposure. *Am J Med.* 2013;126:e1.
124. Şenel E, Satilimiş Ö, Acar B. Dermatologic manifestations of tularemia: a study of 151 cases in the mid-Anatolian region of Turkey. *Int J Dermatol.* 2015;54:e33-e37.
140. Tezer H, Ozkaya-Parlakay A, Aykan H, et al. Tularemia in children, Turkey, September 2009–November 2012. *Emerg Infect Dis.* 2015;21:1-7.
151. Weile J, Seibold E, Knabbe C, et al. Treatment of tularemia in patient with chronic graft-versus-host disease. *Emerg Infect Dis.* 2013;19:771-773.
153. World Health Organization. WHO guidelines on tularemia. http://apps.who.int/iris/handle/10665/43793.

The full reference list for this chapter is available at ExpertConsult.com.

Haemophilus influenzae

133

Stephen J. Barenkamp

Relatively few species of the genus *Haemophilus* are pathogenic to humans, and most that cause human disease are encapsulated or unencapsulated strains of *Haemophilus influenzae.* The latter bacteria are small, gram-negative pleomorphic coccobacilli that are considered to be normal constituents of the microbial flora of the upper respiratory tract of humans.[237,268] Strains without polysaccharide capsules often cause infections of mucosal surfaces, such as otitis media, bronchitis, conjunctivitis, sinusitis, and types of pneumonia.[289,295] Encapsulated strains, especially *H. influenzae* type b (Hib), cause invasive diseases such as septicemia, meningitis, septic arthritis, cellulitis, epiglottitis, pneumonia, and empyema. Before Hib vaccines became widely available, *H. influenzae* was the leading cause of bacterial meningitis in the United States and most other countries, and it was an important cause of other bacteremic illnesses, primarily in young children.[50,258,473]

The organism now known as *Haemophilus influenzae* first was described in 1892 by Robert Pfeiffer, who isolated it from the lungs and sputum of patients during the 1889 to 1892 pandemic of influenza. He proposed that the organism was the cause of influenza, and it initially was known as the Pfeiffer influenza bacillus.[333]

The bacteria were difficult to culture on routine media until investigators appreciated that supplementation with X (i.e., hemin) and V (i.e., nicotinamide adenine dinucleotide [NAD]) factors was required for its growth. By the turn of the century, the organism had been recovered from the blood and cerebrospinal fluid (CSF) of young children with meningitis. Although doubts remained about the etiologic role of the Pfeiffer bacillus as the cause of influenza, not until the influenza pandemic of 1918 was its etiologic role questioned seriously.

In 1920, the organism was renamed *Haemophilus influenzae* to acknowledge its inappropriate historic association with influenza and to emphasize its requirement of blood factors for growth (from the Greek *haemophilus*, or "blood loving").[475] In 1933, the viral cause of influenza was discovered, which refuted any remaining confusion about the erroneous association between *H. influenzae* and influenza virus.

Key concepts relevant to the development of treatment and prevention modalities were derived from the pioneering work of Margaret Pittman in the early 1930s.[339,338] Paralleling earlier research on the pneumococcus, she defined two major categories of *H. influenzae*: encapsulated and unencapsulated strains. Among the encapsulated strains, she characterized six distinct serotypes (i.e., designated a through f), which now are known to differ biochemically in the composition of their polysaccharide capsules (Table 133.1). She observed that *Haemophilus influenzae* type b (Hib) strains were recovered primarily from the blood and CSF of young patients with meningitis and that unencapsulated strains and other *H. influenzae* serotypes were recovered primarily from respiratory tract secretions.

TABLE 133.1 Structures of *Haemophilus influenzae* Capsular Polysaccharides

Type	Structure
a	4)-β-D-Glc-(1→4)-D-ribitol-5-(PO_4→
b	3)-β-D-Rib-(1→1)-D-ribitol-5-(PO_4→
c	4)-β-D-GlcNAc-(1→3)-α-D-Gal-1-(PO_4→ 3 ↑ R = OAc | H R
d	4)-β-D-GlcNAc-(1→3)-β-D-ManANAc-(1→ 6 ↑ | R = L-serine | L-threonine R L-alanine
e	3)-β-D-GlcNAc-(1→4)-β-D-ManANAc-(1→
e′	3)-β-D-GlcNAc-(1→4)-β-D-ManANAc-(1→ 3 ↑ 2 β-D-fructose
f	3)-β-D-GalNAc-(1→4)-α-D-GalNAc-1-(PO_4→ 3 ↑ Oac

Pittman demonstrated that antibody to Hib capsule conferred type-specific protection against lethal infection in rabbits. This observation led to the use of antiserum prepared by immunization with formalin-killed Hib, initially in horses and later in rabbits, as the first treatment of disease. Before this development, Hib meningitis and other forms of invasive Hib disease were almost always fatal.[431] However, not until the late 1930s did treatment of children with meningitis with Hib antiserum and sulfonamides substantially reduce the case-fatality rate.[6,7]

In 1933, Fothergill and Wright[130] described the age-related risk of acquiring *H. influenzae* meningitis, which affected mostly children younger than 5 years of age. They noticed the correlation between the age-related risk of disease and the absence of bactericidal antibodies. Later researchers identified antibody to Hib capsule as the major antibody contributing to the protective activity of bactericidal serum.[202,380] These observations suggested that naturally acquired type b anticapsular antibody is protective and that early stimulation of protective immunity with vaccines might be possible.

Unfortunately, the advent of effective antimicrobial agents focused attention away from the need for primary prevention. Even with effective antimicrobial therapies and excellent hospital care, significant mortality (approximately 5%) and neurologic morbidity (approximately 20%) remained.[98,99] Ultimately, appreciation that the morbidity and mortality of the disease could never be eliminated completely by treatment gave impetus to the development of vaccines for prevention.

In the early 1970s, investigators purified and characterized the type b capsular polysaccharide (i.e., polyribosylribitol phosphate [PRP]) and proposed it as a vaccine candidate. Subsequently, the protective efficacy of a PRP vaccine against invasive Hib disease was demonstrated in older children in a 1974 field trial conducted in Finland.[326] This and other studies culminated in the licensure of PRP vaccine in the United States in 1985, rendering it the first vaccine available for the prevention of Hib disease.[62] Unfortunately, this vaccine induced variable immune responses and incomplete protection in older children and provided no protection for young infants, those who had the greatest risk of acquiring Hib disease.[461] Improved vaccines used polysaccharide-protein conjugate techniques, and four such vaccines were licensed for use in children. Three of these vaccines were shown to protect young infants against Hib disease,[37,370,444] and with the universal immunization of young infants, invasive Hib disease has been almost eliminated in many populations.[80,143,193] Unfortunately, Hib disease continues to be a significant cause of morbidity and mortality among children in resource-poor countries around the world where access to Hib vaccines is still limited.[282,464,484]

MICROBIOLOGY

Morphologic and Cultural Characteristics

H. influenzae is a small, gram-negative coccobacillus that in clinical specimens can appear filamentous or pleomorphic, especially when obtained from patients who previously have received antibiotics. The nonmotile, non–spore forming, and facultatively anaerobic organism requires two supplemental factors for in vitro growth.[237] The X factor (i.e., hemin) is a heat-stable, iron-containing protoporphyrin essential for activity of the electron transport chain, which is important for aerobic growth. The heat-labile V factor is the coenzyme NAD. Both factors occur in erythrocytes and are released by appropriate heating or enzyme lysis of the red blood cells, which permits growth on chocolate agar. The requirement for these factors for growth remains the primary basis for the laboratory differentiation of *H. influenzae* from other *Haemophilus* species[20,237]

The growth of *H. influenzae* is fastidious, and clinical specimens need to be inoculated promptly onto appropriate media, such as chocolate agar.[237] The organism can be grown in most enriched liquid or solid media supplemented with X and V factors. Although not mandatory for growth, 5% to 10% carbon dioxide makes some strains grow better. In blood or liquid media, *H. influenzae* may not grow to sufficient quantity to result in visual turbidity, and to detect positive cultures, blood and CSF cultures should be assayed for release of carbon dioxide or routinely subcultured at 24 to 48 hours.

After overnight incubation on solid media, colonies appear that are 0.5 to 1.5 mm in diameter and usually rough or granular in appearance. Encapsulated strains typically produce slightly larger colonies that are mucoid or glistening. Fermentation reactions and other metabolic activities vary and therefore are not particularly useful for identification. However, a biotyping scheme based on the metabolism of indole, urea, and ornithine decarboxylase activity has been used to subtype strains.[237]

Capsular Polysaccharides

Several surface structures of *H. influenzae* contribute to the organism's pathogenicity, but one of the most important is the capsular polysaccharide. Strains can express one of six unique polysaccharide capsules (i.e., a, b, c, d, e, or f) (see Table 133.1) or lack capsule expression completely (i.e., nontypeable strains). The Hib capsule is of particular clinical, pathogenic, and immunologic importance because Hib accounts for 95% of all strains that cause invasive disease in nonimmunized populations.[50,258,265] The Hib polysaccharide consists of a repeating polymer of ribosyl and ribitol phosphate (PRP) that has a 1-1 linkage.[102]

The genes involved in production of the Hib capsule have been cloned and consist of two repeating 17-kb DNA fragments separated by a 1-kb bridge region (i.e., *bex A*)[188,222]; 98% of Hib organisms tested contain this duplication.[222] Encapsulation often is unstable, with loss of capsule production associated with loss of one 17-kb repeat.[221] These strains produce the type b capsule, but in barely detectable amounts. Release of the Hib capsular antigen in the body fluids of infected individuals can be detected by specific immunologic techniques (i.e., latex agglutination) that are useful for rapid diagnosis.[207,463] The other capsular serotypes are composed of hexose rather than pentose sugars,[102,103,435,436] and these strains occasionally result in invasive disease.[53,95,228,439]

Noncapsular Cell Wall Antigens: Proteins

The cell envelope of *H. influenzae* is typical of other gram-negative bacteria, consisting of a cytoplasmic membrane, a peptidoglycan layer, and an outer membrane that represents the outermost layer of the envelope. The outer membrane contains an array of proteins, lipopolysaccharides (LPSs), and phospholipids, many of which serve important functional roles for the organisms. Over the past 2 decades, significant advances have been made in our understanding of these many outer membrane components and their contributions to the pathogenesis of disease.[289,295]

Early laboratory investigations of *H. influenzae* identified and characterized a number of major and minor outer membrane proteins of the organism.[32,287,288,294,310,396] However, an understanding of the functional roles of most of these proteins was lacking. Subsequent studies have helped to clarify the roles in disease pathogenesis of an increasing number of these proteins. Several proteins are important for attachment of *H. influenzae* to host respiratory mucosal tissues.[55,59,84,195,285,429] Other surface proteins play a central role in bacterial acquisition of iron, a phenotypic trait critical for survival of the organism in the human host.[5,199,215,267,283,480] Studies have identified bacterial surface proteins important in resistance of *H. influenzae* to components of the host innate immune system, the first line of defense in the nonimmune host.[96,174,175,177,266,415] The availability of the completed genomes of several representative *H. influenzae* strains has also helped to increase the rate of discovery of other proteins important in disease pathogenesis.[91,110,152,304,447]

Noncapsular Cell Wall Antigens: Lipooligosaccharide

Early studies of *H. influenzae* lipooligosaccharide (LOS) demonstrated that although it differed chemically and structurally from the LPS of *Enterobacteriaceae*, it shared several biologic properties with the latter molecule. LOS purified from Hib produced a dermal Schwartzman reaction, was lethal to mice, caused a febrile response in rabbits, evoked polyclonal B-cell activation, and had limulus lysate activity.[128] Human leukocytes incubated with *H. influenzae* LOS generated potent procoagulant activity,[280] a property that may be relevant to understanding the mechanisms responsible for intravascular coagulation in severe infection.

Over the past 20 years, knowledge concerning the genetics, structure, biosynthesis, and role in pathogenesis of the *H. influenzae* LOS has increased greatly. The structure of *H. influenzae* LOS consists of a conserved triheptose inner core linked by a single 2-keto-3-deoxyoctulosonic acid molecule to lipid A, from which there are oligosaccharide extensions (i.e., outer core), mainly hexose sugars that vary from one strain to another.[172,262,263,420] *H. influenzae* LOS lacks the repetitive side chains typical of gram-negative enteric bacteria but displays great complexity in its outer core sugars and other substituents such as phosphorylcholine[465,466] and sialic acid.[9,46] Several of these sugars and nonsugar substituents of *H. influenzae* LOS are phase variable.[170,171,466] Phase variation is mediated by translational switching of genes that contain tetranucleotide repeats within the 5′ ends of the respective reading frames.[172,194,466] Phase-variable expression of several LPS components contributes to the pathogenesis of disease (discussed later).

IgA Proteases

IgA proteases are bacterial enzymes whose only known substrate is human IgA1. These secreted enzymes cleave the IgA heavy chain at specific sites.[218] IgA proteases are regarded as potentially important virulence factors because mucosal defense is in part IgA mediated. *H. influenzae* produces at least two distinct types of IgA protease that cleave different peptide bonds within the IgA1 hinge region.[286,340] *H. influenzae* isolated from patients with disease express higher levels of IgA protease than strains isolated from asymptomatic carriers,[449] suggesting that IgA protease is an important virulence factor for *H. influenzae*. Investigators have identified and characterized another IgA protease gene that occurs in about 40% of *H. influenzae* strains.[120,296] This gene, designated *igaB*, is distinct from the previously characterized IgA protease gene, and it is associated with higher levels of IgA protease expression and with a greater likelihood of causing disease,[120] particularly in patients with chronic obstructive pulmonary disease.[297] Products of both genes appear to be expressed simultaneously in the course of human infection caused by *H. influenzae*.[296]

Population Structure

Powerful typing techniques have been developed for identifying individual *H. influenzae* strains and defining the relationships between strains.[276,306,332] These techniques have provided valuable information for a variety of epidemiologic studies and have defined the population structure for *H. influenzae* organisms as a whole.[210,382]

Encapsulated *H. influenzae* can be grouped into two distinct primary phylogenetic divisions.[306] The population structure of encapsulated *H. influenzae* is clonal. Most the invasive disease worldwide is caused by serotype b strains from a limited number of clones.[222] Strains producing serotype c, e, and f capsules belong to single divisions and have no close genetic relationships to strains of other serotypes.[306]

Serotype a and b strains occur in both primary phylogenetic divisions, probably as a result of transfer and recombination of serotype-specific sequences of the cap region between clonal lineages.[223,306] In contrast to the encapsulated strains, the unencapsulated or nontypeable *H. influenzae* strains demonstrate substantial genetic diversity.[91,107,210,305,332,382] Contributing to the genetic diversity of the nontypeable *H. influenzae* are apparently high rates of recombination between individual bacterial strains.[77,82,142,276,421]

Antibiotic Resistance

Another important feature of *H. influenzae* is development of antibiotic resistance. Resistance to a wide variety of antibiotics (e.g., sulfonamides, trimethoprim-sulfamethoxazole, erythromycin, tetracycline, penicillin) has been described, but these antibiotics are not essential for therapy. Of greater importance is resistance to ampicillin, which was first identified in the mid-1970s,[265] because it was the primary antibiotic used for the treatment of disease. Since then, ampicillin resistance has become widespread, and between 5% and 40% of all isolates in various parts of the world are now resistant.[29,86,185,398]

The mechanism of resistance usually involves the production of plasmid-mediated β-lactamase enzyme, and resistant strains often are characterized by their plasmid or β-lactamase enzyme content.[204] Non–β-lactamase–mediated ampicillin and ampicillin-clavulanic acid resistance have been reported among an increasing percentage of isolates from around the world, particularly for nontypeable *H. influenzae*.[23,86,150,205,322] The resistance in these stains appears to be mediated primarily by alterations in specific penicillin-binding proteins.[29] Resistance to chloramphenicol usually is mediated by the enzyme chloramphenicol acetyltransferase.[360,453] Although chloramphenicol-resistant strains are rare in the United States, they are more prevalent in some areas of the world, and strains resistant to both ampicillin and chloramphenicol have been reported.[61,320,438]

Third-generation cephalosporins currently are the mainstays of therapy for invasive disease. Concern about the potential for increasing resistance to these highly effective agents further emphasizes the need for means to prevent disease.[434]

PATHOGENESIS

Acquisition and Carriage of Organisms

Illness caused by *H. influenzae* infection results from a series of pathogenic events beginning with exposure to the organism and followed by colonization of respiratory mucosal membranes.[131] Under natural conditions, *H. influenzae* is exclusively a pathogen of humans, and it usually is transmitted asymptomatically from person to person by transfer of respiratory secretions.[185,318,324] The incubation period is unknown because many transmission cycles may occur before a susceptible person becomes ill. In some individuals, the organism can be carried in the upper respiratory tract for many months before it causes disease.[87,350,401]

Typeable and nontypeable organisms may be part of the normal flora of the upper respiratory tract.[198] As many as 80% of individuals are colonized at some point with nontypeable strains.[185,324,337,347] In the prevaccine era, Hib carriage rates were lowest among adults and young infants and highest among preschool-age children.[437] In a prevaccine era study conducted at a childcare center in Dallas where no invasive infections occurred, the average rate of colonization with Hib was 10%.[298] During the 18 months of the study, 71% of the children 18 to 35 months of age and 48% of the children 36 to 71 months of age were colonized at some time. Carriage rates were substantially higher in households or childcare centers in which a case occurred. For example, colonization prevalence rates among children in childcare centers where a case of invasive disease had occurred were as high as 58% to 91%.[161,460] Within families in which a case of invasive disease occurred, rates of colonization of 60% to 70% among siblings and 20% among parents were observed.[56,460] Whether the high carriage rates in these exposed semiclosed populations were the cause or the result of disease was not clear.[268,279] Close contact among exposed susceptible individuals, as occurs within families and childcare centers, facilitated the risk of transmission and acquisition of disease.

Despite a low point prevalence of Hib pharyngeal carriage (1–5%) in the prevaccine era, most young children became colonized with Hib during the first 2 to 5 years of life,[268,437] and specific Hib immunity developed in these colonized children.[168,380] Hib strains were demonstrated to persist in the nasopharynx for months[279,298] and often were not eliminated by treatment with antimicrobial agents that did not penetrate into respiratory secretions.[390,391]

The relationship between carriage of Hib and the subsequent development of disease and immunity is not well understood. Factors that influence the efficiency of transmission and the ability of the organism to establish colonization also are poorly understood. Two factors that probably potentiate the risk for acquiring infection and invasive disease are the size of the bacterial inoculum[411] and the presence of a concomitant viral infection.[220]

Data derived from animal models of infection may elucidate the dynamic nature of the colonization process. Inoculation of Hib organisms into the nose of infant animals results in local infection.[284,363] In this model system, rhinorrhea was not observed, but nasopharyngeal washings revealed numerous polymorphonuclear leukocytes and organisms that reached maximal density in approximately 24 hours. Shortly thereafter, bacteremia could be detected in the animals.

With colonization of humans, Hib is found on the surface of the respiratory mucosa. Rarely, an organism can be observed by electron microscopy penetrating through a nasal mucosal epithelial cell.[411] An acute inflammatory response to the submucosal bacteria occurs, but it is not marked. The exact mode of entrance of the organisms into the vascular compartment is unknown, but it is assumed that they enter through the lymphatics, probably carried by phagocytic cells, which are found in the submucosa. In support of this hypothesis, Rubin and Moxon[363] detected early transient bacteremia in rats after nasal inoculation.

Pathogenesis of Mucosal Infections

Mucosal colonization and mucosal infections occur much more frequently than do invasive bacteremic infections, particularly in populations in which Hib vaccine is in widespread use. Mucosal infections, most of which are caused by nontypeable *H. influenzae*, still cause considerable morbidity and are associated with substantial health care costs.[371,413,424]

Mucosal infections usually involve direct movement of organisms through the nasal ostia to the sinuses and up the eustachian tubes, where they cause otitis media, and down the bronchi, where they cause bronchitis and pneumonia. Bacteremia rarely is involved, and the infections typically are not life-threatening. These infections appear to be enhanced by antecedent viral infection,[68,323] Eustachian tube malfunction,[418] foreign bodies, or mucosal damage from smoking or other irritants.[367]

Much research has focused on better understanding the molecular pathogenesis of mucosal surface infections caused by nontypeable *H. influenzae*. The same principles apply to the early steps in mucosal colonization by encapsulated *H. influenzae*. A model has been proposed to explain early events in the process.[183] After transmission from an *H. influenzae* carrier to a new host,[87] bacteria come in contact with the upper respiratory tract, where they must overcome the nonspecific mucociliary defenses if colonization is to persist.[386] *H. influenzae* major outer membrane proteins P2 and P5 and probably other factors promote bacterial binding to mucus and help establish an early foothold for the bacteria in the upper respiratory tract.[351,411] Local elaboration of LPS and other bacterial products then causes damage to ciliated cells and further impairs mucociliary function.[456] Adhesins, including HMW1, HMW2, Hia, Hap, pili, protein E, and others, help mediate direct adherence to nonciliated epithelial cells.[25,33,124,146,147,399,412]

Cleavage of IgA,[120,296,297] invasion into cells and the subepithelial space,[129,411,419] and phase and antigenic variation of surface antigens facilitate evasion of local immune mechanisms.[21,22,70,90] Binding and uptake of iron and heme allow organisms to persist on the respiratory mucosa despite the relative scarcity of these nutrients.[267,385,471] In the setting of a viral infection, allergic disease, or exposure to cigarette smoke, bacteria spread from the nasopharynx to other sites within the respiratory tract and produce symptomatic disease.[68,323,418]

Pathogenesis of Invasive Disease

After mucosal colonization with *H. influenzae* type b and other potentially invasive strains has been established, dissemination may occur from the upper respiratory tract mucosa to the bloodstream and then elsewhere in the body.[363] The incidence of invasive disease is a small fraction of the carrier rate for *H. influenzae* type b.[298] When dissemination does occur, the organism appears to invade the mucosa by separating the apical tight junctions of the columnar epithelium and moving intercellularly.[411] The resulting bacteremia initially is low in concentration but steadily increases over the course of hours.[319] The dynamics between bacterial proliferation and clearance is influenced by antibody, complement, and phagocytes, all of which have an effect on the magnitude of the bacteremia.[468] The polysaccharide capsule of Hib is antiphagocytic and a major virulence factor. In the absence of anticapsular antibody, bacteremia increases steadily over a period of hours.[169] When the bacterial concentration exceeds 10^4 organisms per milliliter, metastatic seeding occurs, especially to the meninges through the choroid plexus. Although meningitis is the most frequently recognized manifestation of invasive Hib disease, other potential metastatic sites include the lungs, joint synovium, pleura, peritoneum, and pericardium.[50,431]

The pathogenic events that lead to pneumonia, cellulitis, and epiglottitis are less well understood, even though these invasive infections are associated with bacteremia. Presumably, pneumonia occurs after the aspiration of a critical number of virulent organisms, epiglottitis involves focal infection of the epiglottis, and cellulitis occurs by secondary seeding of deep subcutaneous tissues through the bloodstream.[148] With all forms of invasive Hib disease, invasion of the bloodstream occurs as a primary or secondary event.

Viral interactions enhance the pathogenesis of Hib.[309,423] Influenza virus infection reduces neutrophil chemotaxis, bacterial killing, systemic macrophage function, the number of circulating T cells, T-cell blastogenesis, and expression of delayed cutaneous hypersensitivity.[1,2,78] Reduced bacterial killing may result from a defect in phagosome-lysosome fusion, a defect that is maximal 5 to 7 days after viral infection and inoculation of Hib.

Meningitis

Bacteremia precedes the development of meningitis, except for rare situations in which direct extension of infection from adjacent sinuses or an ear infection occurs. Data from experimental studies of infant rats and infant monkeys support this hypothesis.[284] The magnitude and duration of bacteremia are probably the primary determinants of invasion of the central nervous system (CNS). After a critical bacterial concentration is exceeded in blood, Hib appears to enter the CNS through the choroid plexus.[404]

This theory of CNS invasion is supported by several facts: The earliest histopathologic lesion seen in the CNS is choroid plexitis, the choroid plexus is one of the foci seeded from the bloodstream, and bacterial density early in infection is greater in the lateral cerebral ventricles than in other CSF compartments.[404] Pulse-chase experiments using tracer strains show that organisms enter the CSF through the choroid plexus and that inflammation of the choroid plexus is a uniform feature of meningitis. Subsequently, organisms infect the CSF and the arachnoid villi of the leptomeninges and cause blockage of CSF return, thereby increasing bacterial density and CSF pressure.[404] The magnitude of CSF bacterial density correlates with the severity of clinical illness.[117,375] Egress of CSF from the subarachnoid space is by flow through the subarachnoid villi, and bacterial density in CSF can be increased or decreased by manipulating CSF egress, which occurs in meningitis by inflammatory responses. The inflammatory response of the choroid plexus is followed by pachymeningitis, which also inhibits CSF reabsorption and increases pressure. Phlebitis of the cerebral blood vessels and thrombosis can occur. All these events contribute to decreased blood flow to the cortex. The resulting increased bacterial density, inflammation, edema, cranial nerve damage, and overall increased CSF pressure are responsible for the morbidity and mortality associated with meningitis.[99,116,404] Parenchymal invasion of the brain rarely occurs.

IMMUNOLOGY

Resistance to *H. influenzae* infection depends on successful integration of a wide variety of host defenses, including mucosal factors that prevent the organism from attaching and penetrating the respiratory epithelium[238,405,409]; activation of the alternative and classic complement pathways, which leads to killing of the organism and initiation of other inflammatory responses[410,474]; induction of antibody formation[159,163]; phagocytosis and killing by macrophages and polymorphonuclear cells in tissues, the circulation, and the reticuloendothelial system[35,303,478]; and cell-mediated immunity.[100] Assessing the role of each of these immunologic mechanisms independently or determining which mechanisms are most important in host defense is difficult.

Although antibodies are not the sole defense against bacteremia, it has been the research emphasis of vaccine development.[159] The goal has been to induce antibodies that are bactericidal, opsonophagocytic, and ultimately protective. Usually only antibody is measured in these studies, but other immune factors are induced and probably play important roles in protection.

Anticapsular Antibody

Initially, antibody activity was assessed by measuring agglutinin and bactericidal titers of serum. In 1933, Fothergill and Wright[130] suggested that bactericidal activity was responsible for immunity to Hib meningitis and that acquisition of this immunity correlated with the age of the individual. Although antibodies to several surface antigens of *H. influenzae* play roles in conferring immunity to Hib,[392] antibody to Hib capsular polysaccharide appears to be of primary importance.[359] Newborns and young infants are at low risk for infection, presumably because they have maternally acquired antibody. Young children at highest risk of acquiring disease have low or undetectable levels of antibody, whereas older children at lower risk have higher antibody levels. By 5 years of age, most children have naturally acquired anticapsular antibody that appears to provide protection,[168,380] although natural exposure also induces antibodies to outer membrane proteins (OMPs), LPS, and other surface antigens of the bacteria that contribute to natural immunity. The evidence that anticapsular antibodies protect humans from the acquisition of invasive Hib disease is considerable. They activate complement,[410,474] are opsonophagocytic[312] and bactericidal,[130,312] and protect animals from lethal Hib challenge.[414] Passive prophylaxis with serum preparations containing anticapsular antibody protects agammaglobulinemic patients[359] and high-risk children from the acquisition of invasive Hib disease.[369] In the pre-antibiotic era, immune serum was an effective therapy for Hib disease.[6,339] However, the most compelling evidence for the protective efficacy of PRP antibody is the clinical protection achieved in older children vaccinated with purified PRP vaccine[326] and younger infants immunized with Hib conjugate vaccines.[258,327] Induction of antibody to Hib polysaccharide is the immunologic basis of all Hib vaccines.

A precise minimal level of anti-PRP antibody that is protective has not been established.[159] Data from passive protection of agammaglobulinemic children, challenge experiments in infant rats, and studies of naturally acquired antibody levels in healthy individuals of various ages suggest that the minimal serum concentration of anti-PRP antibody that provides protection ranges from 0.05 μg/mL in animals[381] to 0.15 to 1.00 μg/mL in humans.[213,326] These estimates are crude and do not take into account the different functional properties of different immunoglobulins.[163,253] or the contribution of antibodies to other Hib antigens.

Antibody levels decline over time, and a given peak level may not reflect levels at the time of exposure, which would predict long-term protection better.[14,326] In a Finnish PRP vaccine trial, an antibody level greater than 1.0 μg/mL 1 month after immunization correlated with clinical protection for a minimum of 1 year.[326] However, this antibody level may not be extrapolated readily to the immunogenicity data evaluated in different studies or with different Hib conjugate vaccines.

Class- and Subclass-Specific Antibody

Several studies have shown variable immunoglobulin class, isotype, idiotype, and immunoglobulin G (IgG) subclass responses to PRP polysaccharide after natural Hib exposure, disease, and immunization.[214,381] Most individuals respond with IgG antibodies after receiving PRP immunization, although some children have predominantly IgA or IgM responses.[214]

Schreiber and associates[381] showed that IgG antibody is bactericidal, opsonic for polymorphonuclear leukocytes in the presence of complement, and protective for animals. IgM antibody is equally protective and more bactericidal than IgG in the presence of complement, but it opsonizes poorly. IgA antibody is not bactericidal, opsonic, or protective for animals. Some researchers have hypothesized that IgA-specific antibody blocks the activity of other more functional antibodies and thereby may depress immunity.[301]

Data from experiments in mice and humans suggest that polysaccharide antigens induce restricted IgG subclass responses.[357] The findings of increased susceptibility to Hib disease in IgG subclass–deficient patients (predominantly IgG2 and IgG4 deficiencies)[321,383] and the low levels of IgG2 in children younger than 2 years of age[389] suggest that differences exist in the role of subclass-specific anticapsular antibodies. In adults, natural exposure or immunization with PRP vaccine results in a predominantly IgG2 subclass response.[348] In children, IgG1 and IgG2 antibodies develop after PRP immunization, but IgG1 antibodies predominate after immunization with Hib conjugate vaccines.[11,189,211]

Human anti-PRP antibodies express predominantly κ light chains[426] and may be grouped as a few restricted clonotypes. These clonotypes and antibody specificities have been characterized by idiotype analysis[251,254,397] and amino acid sequencing of the immunoglobulin light chain.[426] Individuals of different ages produce different proportions or repertoires of antibody.[252] Some differences in binding specificity and affinity have been described for the different anti-PRP antibodies,[253,254,377] but whether the antibodies have different degrees of protective potency or are substantially different in proportion in individuals given different vaccines is not clear.

The role of mucosal immunity in killing Hib or inhibiting adherence or penetration of the mucosa is understood poorly, although studies of secretory IgA antibody to the Hib capsule have been conducted.[335,336] Moreover, Hib strains produce IgA proteases that can inactivate mucosal antibody.[120,286,296] The observation of reduced carriage of Hib in children given Hib conjugate vaccines suggests that mucosal immunity may be important in reducing transmission of the disease.[121,181,198,300,316]

Genetic Factors

Compared with protein vaccines, the immune responses to most polysaccharide antigens vary and can be influenced by genetic factors. Several studies have shown associations between the immune responses to PRP vaccine and genetically determined factors such as red cell antigens, human leukocyte antigen, and immunoglobulin allotypes.[10,165,388,470] However, because many factors influence immunogenicity, whether these associations have relevance is not known, and establishing controls for them is difficult. The antibody differences may or may not be clinically important. No single genetic relationship regulating susceptibility or the immune responses to polysaccharide antigens has been demonstrated convincingly.

Complement

The importance of complement components in host defense against Hib is substantiated by elimination of the bactericidal activity of serum by heat, the susceptibility of complement-depleted animals to Hib disease, and the increased susceptibility of patients with specific congenital complement deficiencies.[85,410,474] Hib can activate both the classic and alternative complement pathways,[85,410] thereby initiating opsonophagocytosis and cell killing and eliciting other inflammatory responses. Whereas the alternative pathway probably is most important early in the course of infection in a nonimmune host, the antibody-dependent classic complement pathway is more likely to predominate as a defense mechanism at a later stage of infection.[474]

Encapsulated and unencapsulated organisms activate complement, underscoring the importance of noncapsular antigens in host defense.[302,303,478] Although the Hib capsule is a poor activator of the alternative complement pathway, antibody to the capsule activates the classic and alternative pathways.[410] Other cell wall antigens activate the alternative pathway, and antibody to these antigens activates the classic pathway.[85,410,474] In this way, antibodies to capsular and noncapsular antigens activate the complement system, primarily through the classic pathway. Activation of the terminal complement components mediates the bactericidal activity of serum.

Careful studies have explored the contribution of LPS structure to the susceptibility of *H. influenzae* to complement-dependent serum bactericidal activity.[122,172,256,465] Phase-variable structural modifications to the core LPS structure, including additions of phosphorylcholine,[72,466] sialic acid,[387] and other carbohydrate moieties,[105,235,481] influence the susceptibility of these organisms to complement-mediated killing. Related studies in animal models of infection have demonstrated the importance of these phase-variable LPS modifications to disease pathogenesis in vivo.[46,122,200,234,432]

Work by Hallstrom and Riesbeck focused on the ability of *H. influenzae*, particularly nontypeable strains, to modulate activation of the complement cascade by interacting with human complement regulatory proteins.[177] In the presence of human serum, nontypeable *Haemophilus influenzae* are able to bind the C4B binding protein,[175] the human complement inhibitor factor H,[179,233] and vitronectin.[178,400,415,416] The presence of these proteins on the bacterial surface protects the organisms against complement-mediated attack and contributes to the survival of *Haemophilus influenzae* in the presence of human serum and serum components.[176]

Phagocytosis

Opsonization leading to phagocytosis and killing of *H. influenzae* is an important determinant of host defense.[302,303,414,477,478] Impairment of phagocytic function or a reduction in the number of phagocytes results in increased susceptibility to disease, as does loss of the spleen or impairment of its function (e.g., hemoglobinopathies).[66,342] The opsonic activity of serum is influenced greatly by the roles of complement and antibody. Opsonization and phagocytosis of Hib appear to depend on IgG binding, antibody activation of the classic complement pathway with deposition of C3b on the bacterial surface, and direct bacterial activation of the alternative complement pathway.[314] Relatively little is known about direct cell-mediated killing of *H. influenzae*.[100]

EPIDEMIOLOGY

Haemophilus influenzae Type b

Humans are the only natural host for *H. influenzae*, and asymptomatic nasopharyngeal carriage, usually by unencapsulated strains, is a common finding.[113,151,268,347] In the era before widespread use of Hib conjugate vaccines, nasopharyngeal acquisition of Hib strains was common, increased after infancy, and persisted for weeks to months. Most children were colonized at some time during the first 5 years of life.[268] Colonization rates greater than 70% occurred after recent exposure in closed populations, such as among family members or childcare center contacts of a patient with disease.[298] Person-to-person transmission occurred through respiratory droplets, and fomites also played a role. As Hib conjugate vaccine administration has become part of the routine infant immunization schedule in many countries, there has been an associated and pronounced drop in the rate of nasopharyngeal carriage of Hib strains.[181,198,250,299,316,422]

Before the development of immunization, invasive Hib disease was a leading infectious disease problem worldwide that affected primarily the young[454,469,473] (Table 133.2). Hib strains were responsible for more than 95% of invasive *H. influenzae* infections in children. According to population-based studies, an estimated 20,000 to 25,000 people acquired invasive Hib disease annually in the United States, 85% of which occurred in children younger than 5 years of age.[50] The incidence of Hib meningitis and all invasive Hib disease was 40 to 69 cases and 67 to 130 cases per 100,000 children younger than 5 years, respectively. Invasive Hib disease developed in an estimated 1 per 200 children in the United States during

TABLE 133.2 Worldwide Incidence of Invasive *Haemophilus influenzae* Type b (Hib) Disease Before the Use of Hib Vaccines in Children Younger Than 5 Years

Region	Years	Hib Meningitis[a]	All Hib Disease[a]
Australia and New Zealand	1985–87	25–53	39–92
United States and Canada	1959–91	40–69	67–130
Europe	1985–90	15–26	33–60
Israel	1985–90	18	34
Africa	1980s	36–60	NA
South America	1989–90	15–25	21–43
Asia	1990s	1.3–1.9	1.9–2.7

[a]Annual incidence per 100,000 children younger than 5 years.
NA, not available.
Modified from Vadheim CM, Ward JI. Epidemiology in developed countries. In: Ellis RW, Granoff DM, eds. *Development and Clinical Uses of Haemophilus b Conjugate Vaccines.* New York: Marcel Dekker; 1994:231–45; Bijlmer HA. Epidemiology of *Haemophilus influenzae* invasive disease in developing countries and intervention strategies. In: Ellis RW, Granoff DM, eds. *Development and Clinical Uses of Haemophilus b Conjugate Vaccines.* New York, Marcel Dekker; 1994:247–64.

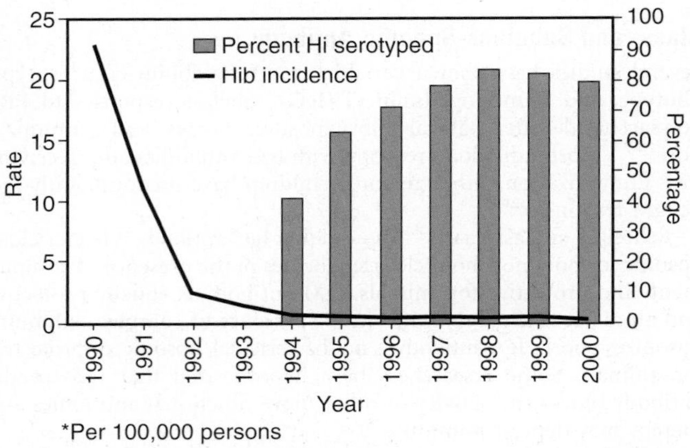

FIG. 133.1 Incidence of *Haemophilus influenzae* type b (Hib) invasive disease per 100,000 people and the percentage of *H. influenzae* (Hi) isolates serotyped for children younger than 5 years in the United States between 1990 and 2000. (From Centers for Disease Control and Prevention. Progress towards elimination of *Haemophilus influenzae* type b invasive disease among infants and children—United States, 1998-2000. *MMWR Morb Mortal Wkly Rep* 2002;51:234–37.)

the first 5 years of life.[75] Hib pneumonia was estimated to cause as many as 15% of cases of ambulatory pneumonia in children younger than 6 years old, but the true incidence was unknown because microbiologic diagnosis is difficult.

Overall, the incidence of Hib disease in the prevaccine era was similar to that of paralytic poliomyelitis during its peak epidemic years before immunization. A bimodal seasonal pattern had been observed in several studies, with one peak occurring between September and December and a second peak between March and May.[352,469] The attack rate of Hib was slightly higher among boys.[260]

The widespread use of Hib conjugate vaccines altered the epidemiology of invasive Hib disease dramatically (Fig. 133.1).[258] The first Hib conjugate vaccine was licensed in the United States in 1987 for use in children 18 months or older.[48] Subsequently, decreases in the incidence of Hib disease were seen among older children and unexpectedly among unimmunized infants and children. This finding was attributed to a direct effect of vaccination on nasopharyngeal carriage, which decreased the environmental burden of Hib infection and ultimately decreased transmission of disease. In late 1990, Hib conjugate vaccines were approved for use in infants beginning at 2 months of age, which heralded a dramatic decline in the incidence of invasive Hib disease in all children.[48] In populations in which immunization rates are high, the development of invasive Hib disease has been eliminated almost completely.[229,258]

Some population-based studies of the incidence of *H. influenzae* disease have been conducted outside the United States, primarily in Western Europe, and they showed an incidence approximately one third to two thirds that in the United States.[328,368,407] The incidence of Hib disease is especially high among certain ethnic groups, including Aboriginal children in central Australia,[182,198] Navajo Native Americans, Native Alaskans, and Apache, Yakima, Athabascan, and Canadian Native Americans.[249,258,462,483] *H. influenzae* appeared to rank as a leading cause of bacterial meningitis in several developing countries.[8,406,457,482] As seen in the United States, a substantial reduction in Hib disease has occurred with the implementation of widespread vaccination programs.[193,395]

Children between the ages of 6 and 18 months are at highest risk for invasive Hib disease[260]; however, the age distribution of specific clinical syndromes of the disease varies. The peak incidence of Hib meningitis occurs in children 6 to 9 months of age and declines markedly after 2 years of age.[134,425] Hib cellulitis tended to occur during the first year of life, whereas epiglottitis occurred in unimmunized children older than 2 years of age. Invasive *H. influenzae* disease was much less common in adults because of the development of protective antibodies over time, but it occurred more frequently in immunocompromised patients. Nonetheless, Hib caused pneumonia and meningitis in adults,[114,330] and disease caused by other serotypes and nontypeable strains, especially pneumonia, otitis media, bronchitis, and sinusitis, are common findings in all age groups.[79,80,258,346] Most adults in whom invasive *H. influenzae* disease develops were not immunized as children and have an underlying condition such as chronic obstructive pulmonary disease, human immunodeficiency virus (HIV) infection, alcoholism, pregnancy, or malignancy.[114,346,448]

The development of invasive Hib disease in a given individual is the consequence of a complex interaction of a variety of factors, including the risk of exposure, the characteristics of the organism, and the host.[132] In populations with a high incidence of disease, such as Native Americans, the age-specific incidence peaked in a younger age group (<6 months), presumably because of early or intense exposure to Hib at home or in the community.[255] Several factors that may reflect environmental exposure to the organism, such as household size,[160] crowding,[441] childcare attendance,[76,196] low family income,[28,133,134] and low parental education level,[133,134] are risk factors for the acquisition of disease, whereas breastfeeding appears to be protective.[331] Several underlying medical conditions are associated with an increased risk for the acquisition of Hib disease, including HIV infection,[60,376] sickle cell anemia,[342] asplenia or splenectomy,[66] antibody[115] and complement deficiency syndromes,[123] and malignancy.[467]

Although the direct contagiousness of invasive Hib disease is limited, small outbreaks and direct secondary transmission of disease can occur.[56,459,460] Numerous studies have estimated the risk of developing secondary disease in household contacts in the 30 days after the onset of disease in an index case. Overall, the attack rate for contacts of all ages in the prevaccine era was 0.3%, which represents a risk approximately 600-fold higher than the age-adjusted risk for the general population.[56,459] However, attack rates varied inversely with age, with children younger than 4 years being at greatest risk. Among household contacts, almost two thirds of secondary cases occurred within the first week after the onset of disease in the index patient.[425] Controversy exists about the degree of risk for the development of secondary Hib disease in childcare center contacts exposed to a child with invasive Hib disease. The risk for unimmunized children younger than 2 years of age ranged from 0% to 3.2%,[28,318] whereas for those older than 2 years, it was less than 1%.

A concerning trend several years ago was the reappearance or persistence of Hib disease in highly immunized populations.[24,198,227,258,402] The factors contributing to these problems are still the subject of debate, but with the reemergence of Hib disease in the United Kingdom in the late 1990s, attention focused on the lack of a booster dosing of infants as part of the regular immunization series and the decreased immunogenicity of combination vaccines in which the Hib conjugate vaccine was combined with acellular pertussis vaccine components.[227,274] The Alaskan experience raised different concerns,[402] but unique characteristics of Hib nasopharyngeal carriage in the rural population and variability in the antibody response of young infants to different Hib vaccines appeared to explain persistent Hib disease in the native Alaskans population.[258,401,402]

Non–type b Encapsulated *Haemophilus influenzae*

Haemophilus influenzae expressing one of the five non–type b capsular types are also carried in the nasopharynx of a small percentage of the population.[87,268] With the success of the Hib conjugate vaccine in preventing invasive disease caused by type b organisms, there was initial concern that disease caused by other encapsulated strains might become more prevalent.[48] Several clusters of invasive disease caused by *Haemophilus influenzae* type a have been reported over the past decade,[4,52,53,208,355] along with occasional cases of disease caused by other serotypes.[206,229,317,366] However, surveillance studies for the most part have failed to document a sustained increase in the incidence of disease caused by non–type b serotypes after introduction of the Hib conjugate vaccines.[206,229,258,271] These data suggest that the concern about serotype replacement may be more theoretical than real.

Nontypeable *Haemophilus influenzae*

Asymptomatic colonization of the mucous membranes of the upper respiratory tract by nontypeable *H. influenzae* strains occurs in 60% to 90% of young children.[224] Infants often become colonized with nontypeable *H. influenzae* early during the first year of life.[111] Nasopharyngeal colonization is a dynamic process characterized by relatively rapid turnover of individual strains and often by simultaneous carriage of several distinct clones.[30,87,113,226,382] With increasing age, nasopharyngeal carriage of nontypeable *H. influenzae* becomes less common, but it still occurs in a significant percentage of the population.[224,382] Nontypeable *H. influenzae* are sometimes associated with invasive disease,[79,81,106,393,448] but they are a much more common cause of mucosal surface infections such as otitis media, sinusitis, bronchitis, and occasionally pneumonia.[240,289,295,334]

CLINICAL MANIFESTATIONS

Bacteremia

Occult bacteremia (i.e., not associated with a primary focus of infection) is not a common occurrence with Hib, but bacteremia does precede essentially all invasive Hib infections. In the prevaccine era, Hib was the second leading cause, after *Streptococcus pneumoniae*, of occult bacteremia primarily affecting children 6 to 36 months of age.[15] Most children initially have fever and peripheral leukocytosis. Unlike some cases of *S. pneumoniae* bacteremia, the condition is not benign. In approximately 30% to 50% of children with occult Hib bacteremia, a focal infection such as meningitis, pneumonia, or cellulitis develops.[83,219]

Meningitis

Meningitis is the most serious manifestation of invasive Hib disease, but no clinical feature differentiates Hib meningitis from other causes of bacterial meningitis in children.[116] The onset of disease can be fulminant,[197] but more commonly the signs and symptoms are nonspecific (particularly in young infants) and may include irritability, fever, lethargy, poor feeding, and vomiting. Children younger than 18 months often do not have nuchal rigidity. Older children are more likely to have findings of headache, photophobia, and meningismus. With fulminant Hib meningitis, very rapid neurologic deterioration may occur with increased intracranial pressure, seizures, coma, and respiratory arrest.[116] Between 10% and 20% of children with meningitis have other foci of infection, such as cellulitis, arthritis, or pneumonia,[7,125] and essentially all have concomitant bacteremia.

CSF examination typically reveals a pleocytosis (mean, 4000–5000 white blood cells/μL) with a predominance of polymorphonuclear leukocytes.[99] Approximately 75% of patients have hypoglycorrhachia, and about 90% have an elevated CSF protein concentration. Eighty percent of meningitis cases caused by Hib will have a positive CSF Gram stain. As with other types of bacterial meningitis, previous antimicrobial therapy significantly decreases the concentration of Hib organisms in the CSF and diminishes the sensitivity of Gram staining.[38] Previous treatment does not affect the total blood cell count and differential, glucose concentration, or protein level substantially, permitting a diagnosis of meningitis. In more than 90% of cases, capsular antigen can be detected in CSF or serum.[463] Anemia, leukocytosis, thrombocytosis, and thrombocytopenia also are observed frequently.[116]

Complications of Hib meningitis include seizures, cerebral edema, subdural effusions or empyema, inappropriate secretion of antidiuretic hormone, cortical infarction (often manifested by focal neurologic abnormalities), cerebritis, intracerebral abscess, hydrocephalus, and rarely, cerebral herniation.[43,99,116,341] Computed tomography and magnetic resonance imaging of the head should not be performed routinely for Hib meningitis, but these studies may be helpful to explore focal neurologic findings or if the clinical course becomes complicated. Small subdural effusions are common findings but are not usually of clinical significance.[116]

Even with prompt intensive care, the mortality rate for Hib meningitis is approximately 5%, and significant long-term morbidity, including sensorineural hearing loss, delay in language acquisition, developmental delay, gross motor abnormalities, vision impairment, and behavior abnormalities, may occur in 15% to 30% of survivors.[98,99,116,341,428] A substantial proportion of such abnormalities may resolve over time, emphasizing the need for long-term monitoring of these patients.[116]

Pneumonia

Hib pneumonia is clinically indistinguishable from other bacterial pneumonias.[149,452] Most patients have a preceding upper respiratory tract infection, fever, and cough accompanied by peripheral leukocytosis with a predominance of polymorphonuclear leukocytes. Radiologically, Hib pneumonia may be segmental, lobar, interstitial, or diffuse, and many cases have evidence of pleural or pericardial involvement on radiographic examination. Cavitation and pneumatoceles are rare occurrences but have been reported.[13,67] Computed tomography or magnetic resonance imaging can be useful adjuncts to the evaluation of complicated disease caused by Hib.[74]

Blood, pleural fluid, tracheal aspirate, and lung aspirate cultures are positive in 75% to 90% of cases. Detection of capsular polysaccharide in pleural fluid, serum, or urine can establish the diagnosis, particularly if antimicrobial therapy had been instituted previously. Although fever may persist for several days while the patient is receiving adequate therapy, uncomplicated Hib pneumonia rarely is associated with long-term pulmonary dysfunction. In the developing world, in addition to disease caused by Hib, pneumonia caused by nontypeable *H. influenzae* is a continuing problem that is associated with significant morbidity and mortality.[140,192,239]

Epiglottitis

Acute upper airway obstruction caused by Hib infection of the epiglottis and supraglottic tissues occurred in the prevaccine era primarily in children 2 to 7 years of age.[34,275] Its onset usually is abrupt, with high fever, sore throat, dysphagia, and sepsis. Antecedent upper respiratory tract infection with cough occurs in approximately 50% of patients.[49,248] The child may drool because of an inability to swallow oropharyngeal secretions, and progressive respiratory distress with tachypnea, stridor, cyanosis, and retractions may develop over a period of hours. The child usually is agitated and may sit forward with the chin extended to maintain an open airway. In children younger than 2 years, Hib epiglottitis may manifest in an atypical fashion, with low-grade fever and a cough suggesting croup.[248]

The most important aspect of the management of a child with epiglottitis is maintenance of a patent airway. Nasotracheal intubation is preferable to tracheostomy because it is equally effective, is not permanent or disfiguring, and has fewer inherent risks.[34] Between 70% and 90% of patients with epiglottitis have positive blood cultures; tissue for culture of the inflamed epiglottis should be obtained only after the airway has been secured. A lateral neck radiograph revealing dilation of the hypopharynx and the thumbprint sign (i.e., swollen epiglottis)[45] can be helpful if the clinical findings are subtle, but in most cases, diagnostic studies should not delay intubation and direct inspection of the epiglottis in controlled surroundings. The mortality rate is 5% to 10% and is almost always related to abrupt airway obstruction.

Joint Infection

Before the routine use of Hib conjugate vaccines, Hib was the leading cause of septic arthritis in children younger than 2 years of age.[125] It affects a single large joint at the knee, ankle, elbow, or hip in more than 90% of cases. Contiguous osteomyelitis occurs in 10% to 20%.[125,236]

No feature clearly distinguishes septic arthritis caused by Hib from that of other bacterial causes. Patients initially are febrile, and more than two thirds have decreased range of motion, local warmth, and swelling.[88,125,236] Usually, pain, swelling, and erythema of the involved joint are preceded by a nonspecific upper respiratory illness. The clinical features may be subtle, with only decreased range of motion of the joint or abnormal gait as the initial finding. Hib capsular antigen concentrations are very high in the infected joint fluid of children with septic arthritis, and rapid detection of antigen is useful diagnostically.

Septic arthritis of the hip requires surgical drainage. Resolution usually is rapid, but long-term cartilage damage may result from Hib arthritis despite adequate therapy.[428]

Cellulitis

Cellulitis is a relatively uncommon form of Hib disease and was seen in the prevaccine era almost exclusively in children younger than 2 years of age. Most cellulitis (74%) is located in the cheek (i.e., buccal cellulitis), periorbital region, and neck[88] and rarely on the extremities. Facial cellulitis occurs most commonly in infants and manifests as acute fever and a unilateral, raised, warm, tender, and indurated area that may progress to a violaceous hue, although this finding is not unique to Hib disease.[430]

Aspirate cultures of the point of maximal swelling usually yield the organism, and bacteremia is a typical finding.[126,191] A secondary focus (including meningitis) may occur in 10% to 15% of patients.[27] Orbital cellulitis usually is a complication of ethmoid sinusitis and consequently can be caused by non-Hib strains. An etiologic diagnosis can be established by blood culture or aspiration of subcutaneous tissues.

Antibiotics always are indicated. The need for surgical drainage depends on the degree of involvement of the tissues within the orbit.

Pericarditis

Hib pericarditis usually is a complication of adjacent pneumonia and is characterized by fever, an ill appearance, respiratory distress, and tachycardia.[65,101,356] The radiographic or clinical diagnosis can be confirmed by two-dimensional echocardiography[479] and may be suggested by finding capsular polysaccharide in serum or pericardial fluid or in Gram-stained pericardial fluid. Cultures of pericardial fluid are positive in more than 70% of cases.[88]

Early drainage is an important part of the management of this illness. Early pericardectomy or pericardiostomy is preferred over repeated pericardiocentesis.[281,356]

Neonatal Disease

H. influenzae causes 2% to 8% of neonatal early-onset sepsis.[57,79,187] Most of these cases are caused by nontypeable strains, most of which are concordant with those isolated from the maternal genital tract.[455] The precise pathogenesis is unknown, but neonatal disease often is associated with prematurity, low birth weight, premature rupture of membranes, and maternal chorioamnionitis; several cases have occurred after cesarean delivery, suggesting in utero transmission.[364] Clinical manifestations include pneumonia, bacteremia, and conjunctivitis. More than two thirds of neonatal *H. influenzae* disease occurs on the first day of life, with an overall mortality rate of 55%.[137]

Other Invasive Infections

Other invasive Hib infections include endophthalmitis,[427] CSF shunt infections,[242,353] necrotizing fasciitis, pyomyositis,[308] peritonitis,[71,136] scrotal abscess,[247] brain abscess,[119] polyserositis,[277] tenosynovitis,[307] epididymitis,[167] lung abscess,[246] periappendiceal abscess,[270] and bacterial tracheitis.[58] Invasive disease also may be characterized by fever alone, fever with petechiae, or fever of unknown origin.[51,446]

Diseases Caused by Non–Type b *H. influenzae*

Respiratory tract infections associated with nontypeable *H. influenzae* are a major cause of morbidity and mortality in developed and nonindustrialized nations.[81,239,454] Previously, invasive disease caused by nontypeable *H. influenzae* was rare and typically associated with underlying medical conditions such as prematurity, malignancy, cystic fibrosis, asthma, CSF leakage, CNS shunts, congenital heart disease, lymphoproliferative disorders, and immunoglobulin deficiency.[112,144,313] With a decline in the rate of infections caused by Hib, other *H. influenzae* serotypes such as types a, e, and f and nontypeable strains have become relatively more common causes of mucosal surface infection and invasive disease,[53,81,206,229,232,439] although it is unclear whether the absolute incidence of disease has increased.[258]

There have been several reports of invasive disease clusters caused by *H. influenzae* type a.[4,52,53,180,439] One suggested that an IS1016-bexA deletion in the chromosome of the recovered type a strains, a deletion similar to that in many Hib strains,[222] might be a marker for more virulent type a clones.[4]

Other serotypes have also been reported as causing cases of non–type b invasive disease.[206,229,258,317] Urwin and associates[440] identified 91 cases of invasive *H. influenzae* type f disease in a multistate area over the course of a 6-year period. The incidence of invasive type f disease was 0.5 cases per 1 million people in 1989 and 1.9 cases per 1 million people in 1994. Among children, pneumonia and meningitis each accounted for 40% of the total cases. The overall mortality rate for type f *H. influenzae* disease was 21% for children. Serotype f also has been reported as a cause of endocarditis[135] and septic arthritis[153] in healthy, normal children.

Invasive disease in children caused by nontypeable *H. influenzae* has been reported by several groups.[81,106,232,448] Heath and associates[186] conducted an active prospective surveillance study of *H. influenzae* infections in the United Kingdom and Republic of Ireland. During the study period (October 1992–December 1998), 102 cases of invasive disease caused by nontypeable *H. influenzae* were reported. Children with nontypeable *H. influenzae* infection were compared with those who had Hib disease. The former were more likely to be younger (16 vs. 22 months) and more likely to have pneumonia and bacteremia ($P < .001$) than were those with Hib disease. In 1998, the incidence of non–type b *H. influenzae* disease among all children younger than 5 years of age in the United Kingdom was 1.3 cases per 100,000, compared with 0.6 per 100,000 children for Hib disease. Most non–type b strains isolated were nontypeable.

Mucosal Infections

Unencapsulated or non-Hib strains cause a variety of mucosal infections, including otitis media, sinusitis, conjunctivitis, and bronchitis.[217,240,295] Nontypeable *H. influenzae* otitis media has clinical features similar to otitis media caused by other common middle ear pathogens, including fever, symptoms referable to the upper respiratory tract, and nonspecific symptoms such as irritability, vomiting, and diarrhea.[241] Data suggest that nontypeable *H. influenzae* is the most common cause of acute otitis media and persistent or recurrent otitis media in children who have received the pneumococcal conjugate vaccine.[39,203,334,472]

Sinusitis caused by nontypeable *H. influenzae* may manifest as common cold symptoms that are persistent or more severe than usual.[450,451] Older children and adults are more likely to complain of headache and paranasal, dental, or facial pain. Other common symptoms are a daytime cough that may worsen at night or reactive airway disease unresponsive to therapy. Rarely, chronic otitis or sinusitis may result in the development of mastoiditis or a parameningeal abscess.[209] Conjunctivitis usually is bilateral and purulent and may occur in outbreaks.[40–42] Although common, these mucosal infections rarely are life-threatening and are not associated with bacteremia in most cases.

DIAGNOSIS

A high index of suspicion for the possibility of Hib disease must be maintained when evaluating children with appropriate clinical manifestations and findings. The primary criterion for the diagnosis of *H.*

influenzae infection is Gram stain or isolation of the organism from an infected focus (e.g., CSF, pleural fluid, sputum, blood).

Because most invasive Hib disease is associated with bacteremia, blood cultures should be performed for any febrile child with potential Hib disease.[219] The specimens need to be processed immediately because the organism is fastidious. Although most commercial blood culture media support the growth of *H. influenzae*, the inoculum should be applied, when possible, directly to chocolate agar or a semisynthetic medium containing heme and NAD.[139,237,329] In liquid medium, growth may not be sufficient to result in turbidity; therefore, for blood cultures, advanced detection systems or subcultures should be performed.[237] Selective media that suppress the growth of gram-positive organisms may increase the recovery of *H. influenzae* from upper respiratory tract specimens.[64] Identification of an isolate as *H. influenzae* relies on its dependence on heme and NAD.[237]

Determination of the capsular type expressed by *H. influenzae* is important for clinical and epidemiologic purposes. Traditionally, this has been performed by slide agglutination with capsular type-specific antisera and suspensions of bacterial organisms.[237] Polymerase chain reaction (PCR) techniques that target the capsular gene locus have been developed that accurately identify strains expressing the six recognized capsular types.[257,311]

Other techniques that may assist in microbiologic diagnosis include rapid antigen detection, staining techniques, and immunofluorescence.[207,264,463] These techniques are useful in the context of a patient whose cultures are sterile because of previous antibiotic therapy, or they can confirm the clinical diagnosis before bacterial growth occurs. The three techniques most commonly used in the past for antigen detection were latex particle agglutination (LPA), countercurrent immunoelectrophoresis (CIE), and coagglutination (CoA). False-positive results on CSF were rare for all three tests but did occur when testing serum and urine. LPA appeared to be the most sensitive of the three tests and is the only one that remains in common use today. False-positive results can occur in the urine of children with nasopharyngeal carriage of the organism or, more commonly, for several days after immunization with Hib conjugate vaccine.[408]

Acridine orange is a fluorescent stain that binds to cellular nucleic acids and may be useful for smaller bacterial concentrations.[216] Immunofluorescent staining of purulent specimens from patients with partially treated disease also has been useful.[73]

TREATMENT

Invasive Disease

Bacteremia plays a central role in the pathogenesis of invasive Hib disease, and occult invasion of the CNS always must be considered in the context of any manifestation of Hib infection.[148,219] Severe Hib disease often is fatal if not treated adequately. Elimination of Hib bacteremia and its complications requires antimicrobial therapy that can penetrate the blood-brain barrier to achieve bactericidal concentrations and is of adequate duration to sterilize the primary and potential secondary foci.

The choice of specific antibiotic therapy must take into account the local antibiotic susceptibility patterns of invasive isolates (Table 133.3). *H. influenzae* resistance to several antimicrobials, including ampicillin, chloramphenicol, trimethoprim-sulfamethoxazole, rifampin, and certain second-generation cephalosporins, has been increasing in several areas of the world.[95,184,354,434]

For proven or suspected Hib meningitis, cefotaxime or ceftriaxone is recommended until the antibiotic susceptibility of the organism is known or an alternative diagnosis is established.[12,116] Both antibiotics have bactericidal activity against Hib strains, including those that produce β-lactamase, and they penetrate well into infected CSF and are well tolerated. Cefuroxime should not be used for the treatment of *H. influenzae* meningitis because delayed sterilization of CSF may be at least twofold more common than with ampicillin plus chloramphenicol or with the third-generation cephalosporins.[18,403] Ampicillin, formerly a mainstay of therapy for this infection, should not be used empirically to treat infections caused by Hib because as many as 50% of Hib isolates in the United States are resistant, usually through plasmid-mediated β-lactamase production.[204,237]

TABLE 133.3 Selected Antimicrobial Agents for Treatment of *Haemophilus influenzae* Infections

Antimicrobial Agent	Total Daily Dose (mg/kg)	Dose Frequency
Parenteral Antibiotics[a]		
Ampicillin[b]	200–400	q4–6h
Cefuroxime[c]	100–200	q8h
Cefotaxime	200–225	q4–8h
Ceftriaxone	50–100	q12–24h
Oral Antibiotics		
Amoxicillin[d]	40–90	tid/bid
Amoxicillin-clavulanate	40–90	tid/bid
Trimethoprim-sulfamethoxazole[d]	8 (trimethoprim)	bid
Clarithromycin[d]	15	bid
Azithromycin[d]	10	qd
Cefuroxime axetil	30	bid
Cefprozil	30	bid
Cefpodoxime	10	bid
Cefixime	8	qd
Cefdinir	14	qd

[a]Other parenteral agents may be used in special circumstances, but they should not be considered first-line drugs. They include ureidopenicillins, carbapenems, and fluoroquinolones.
[b]Not to be used presumptively because of the prevalence of resistant strains.
[c]Not to be used for suspected meningitis.
[d]Do not use these oral agents if resistance is suspected or prevalent in your area.

Chloramphenicol, another medication that frequently was used in the past to treat Hib disease,[278,365] is rarely used now because safer antibiotics with greater activity are available. Although adequate bactericidal blood and CNS levels of chloramphenicol can be achieved, even with oral administration,[118,372] its use requires monitoring of drug levels. Dose-dependent, reversible bone marrow toxicity may occur, particularly in neonates, in patients with liver disease, or in those who require prolonged treatment.[278] Idiosyncratic aplastic anemia, a dose-independent complication of chloramphenicol use, is extremely rare.

Cefuroxime has good activity against *H. influenzae* and is useful for empiric treatment of nonmeningitic infections such as pneumonia, periorbital cellulitis, and septic arthritis.[445] Other parenteral agents that have activity against *H. influenzae* include meropenem, ampicillin-sulbactam, aztreonam, and other third-generation cephalosporins such as ceftazidime.[237,269] The spectrum of activity of the latter agents is too broad for routine use for pediatric infections in which Hib is an important pathogen.

Children with occult Hib bacteremia need to be reevaluated carefully because focal disease may develop in 30% to 50% of patients who are clinically well.[83,219] The duration of therapy is determined by the site of infection and the clinical response. Children with uncomplicated Hib meningitis can be treated for 10 days.[12,116] Children with Hib cellulitis can be switched to oral therapy after several days of parenteral therapy, provided that they have had a satisfactory clinical response and do not have meningitis. Patients with septic arthritis should receive at least 10 to 14 days of therapy,[125] whereas children with pericarditis, empyema, or osteomyelitis may require longer courses of antibiotic treatment (i.e., 3 to 6 weeks).[65,125] These patients often can be switched to oral antibiotics after documenting susceptibility, observing a good therapeutic response, and ensuring compliance.

Equally important in the overall management of a child with invasive Hib disease is supportive care. For Hib meningitis, several studies have shown that adjunctive therapy with dexamethasone moderates the inflammatory cascade and may decrease the likelihood of hearing loss.[315] The recommended dose is 0.6 mg/kg per day given every 6 hours for 4 days, with the first dose administered just before or concurrently with the first antibiotic dose.[12,315,343] Management of a child with meningitis requires continuing careful evaluation for complications such as the development of shock, inappropriate secretion of antidiuretic hormone, seizures, subdural empyema, and secondary foci of infection.[98,99,341] Prolonged fever is a common occurrence, with approximately 10% of children remaining febrile for at least 10 days.[116] Repeat lumbar puncture to document sterility of the CSF is not necessary in uncomplicated cases.

In children with epiglottitis, protection of the airway is the most important component of therapy and should be initiated even before the administration of antimicrobials.[45] Endotracheal intubation or tracheostomy is performed optimally in the operating room by personnel experienced with these procedures in children. Before establishing the airway, care should be taken not to precipitate laryngospasm by attempting to examine the epiglottis or by performing procedures such as venipuncture.[34,45] Blood should be obtained for culture and intravenous antibiotics initiated as soon as possible after the airway has been secured.

Patients with subdural empyema, pericarditis, or pleural empyema usually require percutaneous or surgical drainage.[65,99] Infected joint fluid should be aspirated from children with septic arthritis to confirm the diagnosis and reduce pressure.[125] Repeated aspirations or placement of a surgical drain also may be needed. Infection of the hip requires surgical incision and drainage to decompress the joint; failure to do so may result in avascular necrosis of the femoral head.[125]

Noninvasive Disease

Noninvasive *H. influenzae* infections, usually caused by nontypeable strains, include otitis media, sinusitis, conjunctivitis, bronchitis, and pneumonia. Numerous orally administered antimicrobials are available to treat these infections (see Table 133.3). Despite the increasing prevalence of β-lactamase–producing organisms, amoxicillin remains the drug of choice for empiric treatment of otitis media in most areas because of its low cost and proven safety.[12,245] Several other antimicrobials with activity against *H. influenzae* are available and include amoxicillin-clavulanate, trimethoprim-sulfamethoxazole,; a macrolide such as azithromycin, and second- and third-generation cephalosporins such as cefuroxime, cefpodoxime, and cefdinir.[237] The quinolone antibiotics, such as ciprofloxacin, also are active but are not administered in children routinely for upper respiratory infections. In the context of poor clinical response or isolation of β-lactamase–producing organisms, amoxicillin-clavulanate (Augmentin), cefpodoxime, and cefdinir appear to be the most useful.[12,245]

Most mucosal infections are treated presumptively without obtaining definitive cultures, and consequently, the duration of therapy and the need for alternative antibiotics are based on assessment of the clinical response. Otitis media usually is treated for 7 to 10 days, and sinusitis should be treated for at least 1 week beyond the resolution of symptoms.[12,245,450] If resistance is suspected and leads to failure of treatment, an empiric change in antibiotics is indicated.[24]

PREVENTION

The near elimination of invasive Hib disease in the United States and other countries is a direct result of the routine use of Hib conjugate vaccines and represents a remarkable success story.[258] Prevention with hyperimmunoglobulin also is effective in high-risk populations, but it is costly, has short-lived benefit, and is not licensed for general use.[369] Antimicrobial prophylaxis is effective for the prevention of secondary Hib disease, but it represents only a minor proportion of the overall disease burden.[12,28]

Active Immunization

The first Hib vaccine was the PRP polysaccharide vaccine, which is composed of purified Hib capsular polysaccharide PRP.[19,361] In 1985, it became the first vaccine to be licensed for the prevention of Hib disease in children older than 18 months of age. Children younger than 18 months of age had inadequate immune responses with PRP vaccination.[16,212] PRP vaccine has immunologic properties similar to those of some other polysaccharide vaccines, which are considered to be T-cell–independent immunogens.[3] The antibody responses are limited and of short duration, particularly in young children, and no booster response occurs with repeated administration of the vaccine. The induced antibody may have reduced functional qualities (i.e., primarily IgM and low avidity).[358,389]

Licensure of PRP vaccine was based on the findings of a large, randomized clinical trial conducted in Finland in 1974[325,326] that suggested a protective efficacy of 90% for children who were immunized between 18 and 71 months of age. After licensure of this vaccine in the United States, it became apparent that routine use of the vaccine resulted in efficacy less than that determined in the Finnish vaccine trial (0–88%).[461] This vaccine is mainly of historic significance because its role has been supplanted by development and licensure of the PRP-protein conjugate vaccines.

Hib conjugate vaccines were developed in an effort to enhance immune responses to the PRP antigen. Basic to all conjugate vaccines is the use of a covalently linked (conjugated) immunogenic protein carrier that confers on the PRP polysaccharide hapten recognition by T cells and macrophages and stimulation of T-cell–dependent immunity.[231,461] Four Hib conjugate vaccines have been developed and evaluated in infants, and all use PRP polysaccharide or oligosaccharides derived from it as the primary immunogen (Table 133.4): PRP-D (i.e., diphtheria toxoid), HbOC (i.e., mutant diphtheria toxin), PRP-OMP (i.e., major OMP of *Neisseria meningitidis* serogroup B), and PRP-T (i.e., tetanus toxoid).

The immune response after administration of Hib conjugate vaccination has several characteristics. It is quantitatively enhanced, particularly in younger infants; repeat administration of vaccine elicits booster responses; and maturation of class-specific immunity with a predominance of IgG antibody and probably enhanced functional properties occurs.

The first Hib conjugate vaccine licensed was PRP-D, but it was less immunogenic than the conjugate vaccines developed subsequently, and it is not currently used in the United States. In children 15 months of age or older who received PRP-D, high antibody concentrations were achieved with a single dose.[36,189] However, antibody levels greater than 1 μg/mL developed in less than one half of infants, even after receiving three doses.[92,211] Numerous case-control studies demonstrated that a single dose of vaccine was at least 80% efficacious in preventing disease in children 18 months or older. In infants who received vaccine at 3, 4, 6, and 14 to 18 months of age, the protective efficacy after three doses was 94% in Finland.[108] In contrast, a trial conducted with Native Alaskan infants found no evidence of protection for that high-risk population.[458]

TABLE 133.4 Characteristics of *Haemophilus influenzae* Type b Conjugate Vaccines

Vaccine	Polysaccharide Size	Protein Carrier	Linkage	Trade Name[a]
PRP-D	Medium	Diphtheria toxoid	Protein with 6-carbon spacer	ProHIBiT
HbOC	Small	CRM_{197} (mutant diphtheria toxin)	PS without a spacer	HibTITER
PRP-OMP	Medium	*Neisseria meningitidis* outer-membrane protein complex	Protein and PS with bigeneric spacer	PedvaxHIB
PRP-T	Large	Tetanus toxoid	PS with 6-carbon spacer	ActHIB, Hiberix

[a]PRP-OMP is also available in combination with hepatitis B vaccine (Comvax), and PRP-T is available in combination with diphtheria-tetanus–acellular pertussis (Pentacel) and MenCY (MenHibRix). The PRP-D and HbOC vaccines are no longer commercially available.

HbOC, Mutant diphtheria toxin; *PS*, polysaccharide;.*PRP-D*, diphtheria toxoid; *PRP-OMP*, major outer-membrane protein of *N. meningitidis* serogroup B; *PRP-T*, tetanus toxoid.

A single dose of HbOC was highly immunogenic in children older than 18 months of age,[189,259] and after the administration of three doses in infancy, high antibody levels were achieved.[92,361] Two prospective clinical studies demonstrated that two or three doses of HbOC administered in the first 6 months of life provided a high degree of protective efficacy. In the Kaiser Permanente northern California region population, HbOC was 100% efficacious after two doses administered in infancy.[37] The vaccine also was evaluated in Finland in infants who received vaccine at 4, 6, and 14 to 18 months of age, and efficacy was 95% after two doses.[109] Data from a third postlicensure study in infants in Los Angeles County suggested a protective efficacy of 89% after two doses and 94% after three doses.[443] Although used for a number of years in the United States, the HbOC vaccine is no longer available for use in children in this country.

PRP-OMP induces an immune response that is less age dependent than the response to the other Hib conjugate vaccines. Adults and children respond to a single vaccine dose with high antibody levels.[362] In infants as young as 6 to 8 weeks, a single dose of PRP-OMP induces a good antibody response.[54] The antibody levels achieved after two doses are higher than those after two doses of any of the other conjugate vaccines,[54,92] and a third dose does not enhance the response. PRP-OMP was evaluated in a randomized, double-blind, placebo-controlled trial involving high-risk Navajo Native American infants[370] who received vaccine at 2 and 4 months of age; an overall efficacy of 95% was reported. Additional data from a population-based, case-control study in Los Angeles County suggested a level of effectiveness similar to that seen for HbOC.[442]

PRP-T is highly immunogenic in adults and older children,[69,379] and high concentrations of antibody are achieved in infants with a three-dose immunization series at 2, 4, and 6 months of age.[92] The protective efficacy of PRP-T was evaluated in two large, prospective, randomized trials that were terminated prematurely because of the licensure of other Hib conjugate vaccines for infants. More than 12,000 infants were enrolled in studies in southern California and North Carolina, and no cases of invasive Hib disease occurred in the vaccinated children compared with five cases in the control groups.[138,444] Efficacy subsequently was shown in a study in England; after three doses in infancy, the efficacy of PRP-T was estimated to be 100%.[44] In Finland, during the first 2 years of its general use, more than 100,000 infants were immunized, and only two cases of invasive Hib disease occurred in vaccinees, both after a single dose.

Direct comparisons of Hib conjugate vaccines must be considered in the context of the various study designs, differences in vaccine lots, and different laboratory and statistical methodologies that were used in the clinical trials. Despite these uncertainties, certain principles are evident. First, all Hib conjugate vaccines are safe in infants. Second, PRP-D is the least immunogenic conjugate vaccine. Third, only PRP-OMP induces a good immune response after one dose in young infants, but antibody levels are lower than those induced by multiple doses of HbOC and PRP-T vaccine. Fourth, PRP-OMP, HbOC, and PRP-T appear to be efficacious, but no direct comparison of the protective efficacy of these vaccines has been completed. Mixed administration sequences of Hib vaccines (e.g., PRP-OMP followed by HbOC or PRP-T) may enhance the antibody response,[157,166] and simultaneous or prior receipt of other non-Hib vaccines may affect the antibody response,[162,164,244] presumably due to effects of the carrier proteins. Better understanding of the biologic basis for these observations awaits future studies.

Investigation of the feasibility of administering Hib vaccines in combination with other vaccines has been the focus of much research effort over the past 15 years. Early studies by Schmitt and associates[378] assessed the impact and effectiveness of DTaP (IPV)-Hib combination vaccines in Germany. Although combination DTaP-Hib vaccines elicited lower anti-Hib titers than separate vaccines, the investigators were able to show that combination vaccines were effective in reducing the incidence of Hib disease.[378] Subsequent data from Canada also suggested that a multicomponent Hib-containing combination vaccine was safe and effective in preventing invasive type b *Haemophilus* disease in young children.[373,374] These studies and others led to the subsequent licensing of a five-component combination vaccine (DTaP-IPV-Hib) that has been approved for use in the primary Hib vaccination series for US children since 2008.[63,156]

The phenomenal success of the Hib vaccination strategy has been related to the effectiveness of Hib conjugate vaccines in preventing colonization. Fernandez and associates[121] reported that the anti-Hib capsular polysaccharide antibody concentration required to prevent colonization was greater than that needed for protection against invasive disease. Whether concentrations in the range that Fernandez and associates suggested was important (>5 μg/mL) can be achieved and sustained by using conjugate vaccines in all population groups remains a subject of investigation. Studies of some high-risk population groups (e.g., Alaskan natives) have documented that invasive disease is prevented best by the use of PRP-OMP Hib vaccine,[401,402] at least for the first dose of vaccine, and that even the use of PRP-OMP Hib vaccine in these individuals may not eliminate carriage of the organism in the population.[94,141] Use of combination vaccines in this population is unlikely to be as effective as use of PRP-OMP Hib conjugate vaccine.[48,402]

Currently used *H. influenzae* vaccines are based on immunity to the Hib capsule. Antibodies to other components of the bacterium also have been shown to be bactericidal, opsonophagocytic, and protective in animal studies.[26,31,93,104,173,225,288,292,293,476] Vaccines containing other bacterial antigens could in theory provide supplemental protection against Hib, although this protection does not appear to be necessary in most individuals based on the efficacy of the available Hib conjugate vaccines. Even so, alternative vaccines could provide immunity to non-Hib strains, which are ubiquitous colonizers of the upper respiratory tract of humans.[113,224]

A problem that must be overcome in the development of these vaccines is the known diversity of many of the candidate vaccine antigens.[31,145] Because of the known strain-to-strain variation in a number of these antigens,[97] finding an antigen relevant to all or most strains has been a challenge.[31,290] Human trials have reported limited success in preventing cases of *H. influenzae* otitis media with a pneumococcal polysaccharide–*H. influenzae* protein D conjugate vaccine,[344,345,433] and several other candidate vaccine antigens remain the subject of active preclinical research.[291]

Passive Immunization

Although active immunization is preferred for the control of Hib disease, passive immunization has potential utility in some settings: selected high-risk groups with a risk of acquiring disease soon after birth and too young to respond to vaccination (i.e., Eskimos or Native Americans), functionally asplenic patients, immunocompromised patients, and for prevention of secondary disease in households, childcare centers, or institutions.

A human hyperimmunoglobulin from adult Hib-immunized donors called bacterial polysaccharide immunoglobulin has been prepared,[394] but it is not commercially available. Pharmacologic studies show that high levels of antibody can be achieved after intramuscular injection, and significant protective efficacy against invasive Hib disease has been demonstrated in Apache children given three doses during the first year of life.[369] The use of concurrent active immunization with bacterial polysaccharide immunoglobulin also may be an effective strategy.[243] Another possible approach is maternal Hib immunization[154] to induce transplacental antibody, but questions remain regarding the safety and acceptability of vaccinating pregnant women and the inability to immunize women who do not receive prenatal care.

Impact of *H. influenzae* Type b Vaccination

The impact of widespread vaccination with Hib conjugate vaccine in the United States has been dramatic[48,258] and has been reproduced in many other countries throughout the world.[47,127,384,395,417] The decrease in the incidence of disease has exceeded expectations given the estimated proportion of the population completely immunized. In essentially all of these populations, a significant decrease in the incidence of disease was observed among infants before the licensure and recommended use of vaccines in that age group. These findings probably are explained by a reduction in Hib carriage as a result of vaccination[300,422] and decreased transmission from immunized children to unimmunized young children and infants.

Immunization schedules vary in different countries to parallel immunization practices for other vaccine-preventable diseases. The age-specific incidence of disease also varies in different countries. Initially in the United Kingdom, the occurrence of disease was such that physicians felt justified to use only a three-dose schedule at 2, 3, and 4 months of age and not to provide a booster dose in the second year of life. This schedule, introduced in the United Kingdom in 1993, appeared to coincide with the reappearance of type b disease in older children observed in the late 1990s.[17,201,230,227,273,349] The experience emphasizes the importance of giving a fourth dose when children are between 12 and 18 months of age if circumstances permit.

Chemoprophylaxis

Secondary disease accounts for less than 2% of all cases of invasive Hib disease. Chemoprophylaxis can protect susceptible people from acquiring Hib by eliminating Hib colonization in close contacts. Children younger than 4 years have a 600-fold increased risk of acquiring Hib disease after household contact with a case.[459] Risk also appears to be increased in childcare center settings, but this risk is less well defined.[158,318] Adults and older children who are colonized can transmit Hib to susceptible children even though they have little risk of acquiring invasive disease themselves.

Antimicrobial agents effective for chemoprophylaxis must achieve bactericidal levels intracellularly and in mucosal secretions. Rifampin, which achieves high concentrations in respiratory secretions,[272] is the most effective antimicrobial agent for eradicating Hib from the nasopharynx. Rifampin in a dosage of 20 mg/kg once daily (maximal daily dose, 600 mg) for 4 days eradicates Hib carriage in 95% or more of household[28,155] or childcare center[161] contacts of a case. Cohort studies have shown the effectiveness of rifampin prophylaxis in preventing secondary Hib disease in household contacts and childcare center attendees.[155,161,261] Antimicrobials effective in the treatment of Hib disease, such as ampicillin, trimethoprim-sulfamethoxazole, erythromycin-sulfisoxazole, and cefaclor, have been ineffective for antimicrobial prophylaxis.[190] They eliminated Hib carriage in less than 70% of culture-positive contacts and are not recommended for chemoprophylaxis.

The US Public Health Service Advisory Committee on Immunization Practices[48] and the American Academy of Pediatrics Committee on Infectious Diseases[12] recommend rifampin prophylaxis for all household contacts, including adults, and for the index patient (i.e., therapeutic antibiotics do not eradicate Hib from the nasopharynx consistently) if the household has a contact younger than 4 years who is not fully immunized. Prophylaxis should be instituted as soon as possible because the risk of acquiring secondary disease is greatest during the few days after the onset of disease in the index patient and within 2 weeks of the onset of disease. No consensus exists concerning the need for chemoprophylaxis in the childcare setting because of uncertainty about the magnitude of the risk of acquiring secondary Hib disease in this setting. Some investigators recommend chemoprophylaxis if classroom contacts include children younger than 2 years of age, whereas others think that recommendations should be individualized.[89,318] Virtually all experts recommend prophylaxis if two or more cases of Hib disease have occurred among attendees within 60 days.[12,48]

In all situations in which the potential for secondary disease exists, this risk should be explained to families, with an emphasis on the importance of seeking prompt medical attention for febrile illnesses. Clinicians should not obtain pharyngeal cultures to determine whether prophylaxis should be administered because doing so only delays the prompt administration of chemoprophylaxis.

CONCLUSIONS

The perspective on *Haemophilus* disease has changed dramatically in recent years. Before the availability of Hib conjugate vaccines, invasive Hib was one of the most important bacterial pathogens of children. It was the leading cause of bacterial meningitis and an important cause of other bacteremic illnesses. The spectrum of illness is broad, morbidity and mortality are significant, and subtleties in making an early diagnosis and instituting appropriate management exist. Because most antibiotic use worldwide is for upper respiratory tract infections, including otitis media and *H. influenzae* causes a significant proportion of these illnesses, it still must be considered a very important pediatric pathogen.

The most important aspect of work on *H. influenzae* has been disease prevention by routine immunization of infants with polysaccharide-protein conjugate vaccines. This achievement is the culmination of more than 100 years of research. Although historically there were many technologic problems and misunderstandings about the organism and its pathogenesis, much has been accomplished. The impact of routine infant immunizations with Hib conjugate vaccines has been dramatic. The public health benefits parallel the eradication of polio and the control of other vaccine-preventable childhood diseases. Widespread Hib immunization virtually has eliminated Hib disease in the United States and in many developed countries where it is used routinely. The degree of disease control exceeded all expectations and is in excess of what the known levels of immunization would have predicted.

Some progress has been made at the preclinical level in the development of vaccines against other *H. influenzae* serotypes and nontypeable strains.[291] Control of infection caused by these organisms will have an important public health impact, and use of these vaccines may have a role in the health of adolescents and adults. The technologies that led to the development of Hib conjugate vaccines served as a prototype for vaccines to prevent disease caused by other encapsulated bacteria, including the pneumococcus, meningococcus, and group B *Streptococcus*. The lessons learned in the quest to eliminate Hib disease have had important implications in the control of many other bacterial diseases.

Acknowledgements

This chapter was adapted and updated from earlier versions authored by Joel M. Ward, MD.

NEW REFERENCES SINCE THE SEVENTH EDITION

12. American Academy of Pediatrics. *Haemophilus influenzae* infections. In: Kimberlin DW, Brady MT, Jackson MA, Long SS, eds. *Red Book: 2015 Report of the Committee on Infectious Diseases*. 30th ed. Elk Grove Village, IL: American Academy of Pediatrics; 2015:368-376.
21. Atack JM, Srikhanta YN, Fox KL, et al. A biphasic epigenetic switch controls immunoevasion, virulence and niche adaptation in non-typeable *Haemophilus influenzae*. *Nat Commun*. 2015;6:7828.
22. Atack JM, Winter LE, Jurcisek JA, et al. Selection and counterselection of Hia expression reveals a key role for phase-variable expression of Hia in infection caused by nontypeable *Haemophilus influenzae*. *J Infect Dis*. 2015;212:645-653.
23. Bae SM, Lee JH, Lee SK, et al. High prevalence of nasal carriage of beta-lactamase-negative ampicillin-resistant *Haemophilus influenzae* in healthy children in Korea. *Epidemiol Infect*. 2013;141:481-489.
48. Briere EC, Rubin L, Moro PL, et al. Prevention and control of *Haemophilus influenzae* type b disease: recommendations of the advisory committee on immunization practices (ACIP). *MMWR Recomm Rep*. 2014;63(RR-01):1-14.
53. Bruce MG, Zulz T, DeByle C, et al. *Haemophilus influenzae* serotype a invasive disease, Alaska, USA, 1983-2011. *Emerg Infect Dis*. 2013;19:932-937.
70. Clark SE, Eichelberger KR, Weiser JN. Evasion of killing by human antibody and complement through multiple variations in the surface oligosaccharide of *Haemophilus influenzae*. *Mol Microbiol*. 2013;88:603-618.
79. Collins S, Litt DJ, Flynn S, et al. Neonatal invasive *Haemophilus influenzae* disease in England and Wales: epidemiology, clinical characteristics, and outcome. *Clin Infect Dis*. 2015;60:1786-1792.
80. Collins S, Ramsay M, Campbell H, et al. Invasive *Haemophilus influenzae* type b disease in England and Wales: who is at risk after 2 decades of routine childhood vaccination? *Clin Infect Dis*. 2013;57:1715-1721.
81. Collins S, Vickers A, Ladhani SN, et al. Clinical and molecular epidemiology of childhood invasive nontypeable *Haemophilus influenzae* disease in England and Wales. *Pediatr Infect Dis J*. 2016;35:e76-e84.
82. Connor TR, Corander J, Hanage WP. Population subdivision and the detection of recombination in non-typable *Haemophilus influenzae*. *Microbiology*. 2012;158:2958-2964.
90. Davis GS, Marino S, Marrs CF, et al. Phase variation and host immunity against high molecular weight (HMW) adhesins shape population dynamics of nontypeable *Haemophilus influenzae* within human hosts. *J Theor Biol*. 2014;355:208-218.
91. De Chiara M, Hood D, Muzzi A, et al. Genome sequencing of disease and carriage isolates of nontypeable *Haemophilus influenzae* identifies discrete population structure. *Proc Natl Acad Sci USA*. 2014;111:5439-5444.
95. Desai S, Jamieson FB, Patel SN, et al. The epidemiology of invasive *Haemophilus influenzae* non-serotype b disease in Ontario, Canada from 2004 to 2013. *PLoS ONE*. 2015;10:e0142179.
110. Eutsey RA, Hiller NL, Earl JP, et al. Design and validation of a supragenome array for determination of the genomic content of *Haemophilus influenzae* isolates. *BMC Genomics*. 2013;14:484.

143. Georges S, Lepoutre A, Dabernat H, et al. Impact of *Haemophilus influenzae* type b vaccination on the incidence of invasive *Haemophilus influenzae* disease in France, 15 years after its introduction. *Epidemiol Infect*. 2013;141:1787-1796.
151. Giufre M, Daprai L, Cardines R, et al. Carriage of *Haemophilus influenzae* in the oropharynx of young children and molecular epidemiology of the isolates after fifteen years of *H. influenzae* type b vaccination in Italy. *Vaccine*. 2015;33:6227-6234.
152. Giufre M, De Chiara M, Censini S, et al. Whole-genome sequences of nonencapsulated *Haemophilus influenzae* strains isolated in Italy. *Genome Announc*. 2015;3:e110-e115.
181. Hammitt LL, Crane RJ, Karani A, et al. Effect of *Haemophilus influenzae* type b vaccination without a booster dose on invasive *H influenzae* type b disease, nasopharyngeal carriage, and population immunity in Kilifi, Kenya: a 15-year regional surveillance study. *Lancet Glob Health*. 2016;4:e185-e194.
192. Howie SRC, Morris GAJ, Tokarz R, et al. Etiology of severe childhood pneumonia in The Gambia, West Africa, determined by conventional and molecular microbiological analyses of lung and pleural aspirate samples. *Clin Infect Dis*. 2014;59:682-685.
193. Howie SR, Oluwalana C, Secka O, et al. The effectiveness of conjugate *Haemophilus influenzae* type b vaccine in The Gambia 14 years after introduction. *Clin Infect Dis*. 2013;57:1527-1534.
195. Ikeda M, Enomoto N, Hashimoto D, et al. Nontypeable *Haemophilus influenzae* exploits the interaction between protein-E and vitronectin for the adherence and invasion to bronchial epithelial cells. *BMC Microbiol*. 2015;15:263.
205. Kakuta R, Yano H, Hidaka H, et al. Molecular epidemiology of ampicillin-resistant *Haemophilus influenzae* causing acute otitis media in Japanese infants and young children. *Pediatr Infect Dis J*. 2016;35:501-506.
232. Langereis JD, de Jonge MI. Invasive disease caused by nontypeable *Haemophilus influenzae*. *Emerg Infect Dis*. 2015;21:1711-1718.
233. Langereis JD, de Jonge MI, Weiser JN. Binding of human factor H to outer membrane protein P5 of non-typeable *Haemophilus influenzae* contributes to complement resistance. *Mol Microbiol*. 2014;94:89-106.
234. Langereis JD, Stol K, Schweda EK, et al. Modified lipooligosaccharide structure protects nontypeable *Haemophilus influenzae* from IgM-mediated complement killing in experimental otitis media. *MBio*. 2012;3:e79-e12.
235. Langereis JD, Weiser JN. Shielding of a lipooligosaccharide IgM epitope allows evasion of neutrophil-mediated killing of an invasive strain of nontypeable *Haemophilus influenzae*. *MBio*. 2014;5:e01478-14.
291. Murphy TF. Vaccines for nontypeable *Haemophilus influenzae*: the future is now. *Clini Vaccine Immunol*. 2015;22:459-466.
296. Murphy TF, Kirkham C, Jones MM, et al. Expression of IgA proteases by *Haemophilus influenzae* in the respiratory tract of adults with chronic obstructive pulmonary disease. *J Infect Dis*. 2015;212:1798-1805.
304. Mussa HJ, VanWagoner TM, Morton DJ, et al. Draft genome sequences of eight nontypeable *Haemophilus influenzae* strains previously characterized using an electrophoretic typing scheme. *Genome Announc*. 2015;3:e01374-15.
322. Park C, Kim KH, Shin NY, et al. Genetic diversity of the *ftsI* gene in beta-lactamase-nonproducing ampicillin-resistant and beta-lactamase-producing amoxicillin-/clavulanic acid-resistant nasopharyngeal *Haemophilus influenzae* strains isolated from children in South Korea. *Microb Drug Resist*. 2013;19:224-230.
337. Pickering J, Smith-Vaughan H, Beissbarth J, et al. Diversity of nontypeable *Haemophilus influenzae* strains colonizing Australian Aboriginal and non-Aboriginal children. *J Clin Microbiol*. 2014;52:1352-1357.
346. Puig C, Grau I, Marti S, et al. Clinical and molecular epidemiology of *Haemophilus influenzae* causing invasive disease in adult patients. *PLoS ONE*. 2014;9:e112711.
347. Puig C, Marti S, Fleites A, et al. Oropharyngeal colonization by nontypeable *Haemophilus influenzae* among healthy children attending day care centers. *Microb Drug Resist*. 2014;20:450-455.
384. Scott S, Altanseseg D, Sodbayer D, et al. Impact of *Haemophilus influenzae* type b conjugate vaccine in Mongolia: prospective population-based surveillance, 2002-2010. *J Pediatr*. 2013;163(suppl):S8-S11.
395. Sigauque B, Vubil D, Sozinho A, et al. *Haemophilus influenzae* type b disease among children in rural Mozambique: impact of vaccine introduction. *J Pediatr*. 2013;163(suppl):S19-S24.
415. Su YC, Jalalvand F, Morgelin M, et al. *Haemophilus influenzae* acquires vitronectin via the ubiquitous protein F to subvert host innate immunity. *Mol Microbiol*. 2013;87:1245-1266.
416. Su YC, Mukherjee O, Singh B, et al. *Haemophilus influenzae* P4 interacts with extracellular matrix proteins promoting adhesion and serum resistance. *J Infect Dis*. 2016;213:314-323.
417. Sultana NK, Saha SK, Al-Emran HM, et al. Impact of introduction of the *Haemophilus influenzae* type b conjugate vaccine into childhood immunization on meningitis in Bangladeshi infants. *J Pediatr*. 2013;163(suppl):S73-S78.
429. Tchoupa AK, Lichtenegger S, Reidl J, et al. Outer membrane protein P1 is the CEACAM-binding adhesin of *Haemophilus influenzae*. *Mol Microbiol*. 2015;98:440-455.
433. Tregnaghi MW, Saez-Llorens X, Lopez P, et al. Efficacy of pneumococcal nontypable *Haemophilus influenzae* protein D conjugate vaccine (PHiD-CV) in young Latin American children: a double-blind randomized controlled trial. *PLoS Med*. 2014;11:e1001657.
439. Ulanova M, Tsang RS. *Haemophilus influenzae* serotype a as a cause of serious invasive infections. *Lancet Infect Dis*. 2014;14:70-82.
447. VanWagoner TM, Morton DJ, Seale TW, et al. Draft genome sequences of six nontypeable *Haemophilus influenzae* strains that establish bacteremia in the infant rat model of invasive disease. *Genome Announc*. 2015;3:e01374-15.
471. Whitby PW, VanWagoner TM, Seale TW, et al. Comparison of transcription of the *Haemophilus influenzae* iron/heme modulon genes in vitro and in vivo in the chinchilla middle ear. *BMC Genomics*. 2013;14:925.
478. Winter LE, Barenkamp SJ. Naturally acquired HMW1- and HMW2-specific serum antibodies in adults and children mediate opsonophagocytic killing of nontypeable *Haemophilus influenzae*. *Clin Vaccine Immunol*. 2016;23:37-46.

The full reference list for this chapter is available at ExpertConsult.com.

134 Other *Haemophilus* Species (*Ducreyi, Haemolyticus, Influenzae* Biogroup *Aegyptius, Parahaemolyticus,* and *Parainfluenzae*) and *Aggregatibacter (Haemophilus) aphrophilus*

Stephen J. Barenkamp

Most serious pediatric infections caused by organisms of the *Haemophilus* genus are caused by *H. influenzae*. However, other *Haemophilus* species can cause disease occasionally. Among the other species that have been reported to cause disease in pediatric and adolescent patients are *H. aegyptius*, *H. ducreyi*, and *H. parainfluenzae*. *Aggregatibacter aphrophilus*, until recently known as *Haemophilus aphrophilus*, is also an occasional cause of infections in pediatric patients. *H. aegyptius* is currently classified as a member of the species *H. influenzae* (*H. influenzae* biogroup *aegyptius*), but given the unique characteristics of this organism and the distinctive illness with which it is associated, it is discussed in this chapter. Other *Haemophilus* species such as *H. haemolyticus* and *H. parahaemolyticus*, rarely cause illness in the pediatric population,[12,153] so they are not discussed in detail here. However, *H. haemolyticus* has been the subject of a several reports in the literature because nonhemolytic strains of *H. haemolyticus* are sometimes misidentified as *H. influenzae* unless careful and thorough microbiologic testing is performed.[142,155,170,215]

Members of the *Haemophilus* genus are gram-negative coccobacillary bacteria that are facultatively anaerobic. They demonstrate optimal growth when they are incubated in a humid atmosphere containing

TABLE 134.1 Differential Characteristics of *Haemophilus* Species

Species	Factor Requirement		Hemolysis of Horse Blood	FERMENTATION OF				Presence of Catalase	CO_2 Enhancement of Growth
	X[a]	V		Glucose	Sucrose	Lactose	Mannose		
Haemophilus influenzae[b]	+	+	−	+	−	−	−	+	+
Haemophilus haemolyticus	+	+	+	+	−	−	−	+	−
Haemophilus ducreyi	+	−	−	−	−	−	−	−	−
Haemophilus parainfluenzae	−	+	−	+	+	−	+	D	D
Haemophilus parahaemolyticus	−	+	+	+	+	−	−	+	−
Aggregatibacter aphrophilus	−	−	−	+	+	+	+	−	+

[a]As determined by the porphyrin test.
[b]Includes biogroup *aegyptius*.
CO_2, Carbon dioxide; *D*, differences encountered.

5% to 10% carbon dioxide.[112,122,154] Most species have fastidious nutritional requirements and require special media, supplements, or both for optimal growth.[112,122] X factor (hemin), V factor (nicotinamide adenine dinucleotide), or both are required for in vitro growth.[165] Organisms with the "para-" prefix require V factor only. The specific nutritional requirements of *Haemophilus* isolates are among the characteristics used to subclassify these organisms into the different species (Table 134.1).

AGGREGATIBACTER (HAEMOPHILUS) APHROPHILUS

Bacteriology

H. aphrophilus was described first by Khairat[111] in 1940 in association with a fatal case of endocarditis. He suggested the species name *aphrophilus* because the organism required relatively high concentrations of carbon dioxide for isolation on the usual media. In earlier times, a well-known manifestation of carbon dioxide was the formation of bubbles of gas in fermenting wine (i.e., froth, or *aphros*).[26,111] Although the organism originally was classified as a *Haemophilus* species because of the growth requirement for X factor, more recent studies suggested that it can grow independent of this factor.[112,160,213] Given this latter characteristic and based on other more recent analyses,[52] the organism has now been placed in the genus *Aggregatibacter* and is known as *Aggregatibacter aphrophilus.*[158,243]

Epidemiology and Pathogenesis

A. aphrophilus is a component of the normal oral flora. Using a selective medium, Kraut and coworkers[115] isolated the organism from gingival scrapings and interdental material of one-third of the healthy adults they examined. With respect to disease pathogenesis, it has been suggested that dental disease or manipulation predisposes to transient bacteremia, which results in seeding of distant tissue sites where localized infection subsequently develops.[26,82,157,160,187] In addition, several case reports of patients with *A. aphrophilus* disease reported an association between human infection and contact with or bites from dogs and cats.[67,99,157,160,226] However, a causal relationship has been difficult to confirm, and the human mouth and respiratory tract probably are the portals of entry for most infections.

Clinical Manifestations

A. aphrophilus is a relatively rare cause of infection and disease in pediatric patients, with fewer than 50 cases reported in the literature.* Brain abscesses and endocarditis are the pediatric infections reported most commonly.* Other reported sites of infection in children include the oropharynx,[26] the abdominal cavity,[26,108] and various superficial soft tissue sites.[160,233,234] Infections with *A. aphrophilus* do not appear to be associated with any distinctive clinical features compared with infection caused by other organisms at the same sites. However, *A. aphrophilus* infections frequently are associated with underlying conditions predisposing the host to infection, such as congenital heart disease, trauma, and immunosuppression.[26,63,67,95,149,160,169,233]

Treatment

Antimicrobial susceptibility testing has not been well standardized for this organism, and disk-diffusion testing, in particular, has been found to be unreliable.[26,94,160,213] Tube or agar dilution testing generally is considered to be the preferred testing method. Older reports found that *A. aphrophilus* was uniformly susceptible to several antibiotics, including chloramphenicol and the aminoglycosides.[26,160,213] Susceptibility to penicillins has been variable. Even so, penicillin has been used successfully for treatment of susceptible organisms,[26,82,160,226] at times in combination with aminoglycosides and other antimicrobials. Some reports document the usefulness of ampicillin or ceftriaxone for treatment of infection.[22,146,157,181] Several different antibiotics probably can be used to treat *H. aphrophilus* infections successfully. The choice for treatment should be guided by appropriate in vitro susceptibility testing.

HAEMOPHILUS DUCREYI

Bacteriology

In 1889, Ducrey first identified *H. ducreyi* in purulent material recovered from genital ulcers of patients with soft chancre or chancroid.[54] Although unable to culture the organism in vitro, Ducrey was able to establish the specificity of the infectious agent by serial cutaneous inoculations.[54,151] *H. ducreyi* originally was assigned to the *Haemophilus* genus because of its requirement for hemin (X-factor) and a guanosine plus cytosine content within the expected range for *Haemophilus* species.[4,221] However, more recent studies, including genetic transformation and DNA hybridization analyses, suggest that *H. ducreyi* is not related to the true haemophili, such as *H. influenzae,* and possibly should be placed in a separate genus.[4,221]

Since the 1990s, significant advances have been made in the understanding of bacterial components that contribute to disease pathogenesis. Two cytotoxins, a hemolysin, a diffusible cytolethal distending toxin,

*References 14, 22, 26, 61, 67, 98, 99, 108, 149, 167, 233, 234.

*References 22, 26, 32, 61, 67, 93, 99, 138, 149, 160, 167.

and two classes of serum resistance proteins have been identified; their respective genes have been cloned, and their potential contributions to disease pathogenesis have been investigated.* The lipooligosaccharide of *H. ducreyi* has been characterized in much greater detail, and relevant biosynthetic genes have been cloned and studied.[3,18,65,145,212,222,240,130,172,204] Genes encoding the major outer membrane proteins of the organism have been cloned and the corresponding proteins characterized,[113] and a novel class of pili expressed by *H. ducreyi* has been identified.[37] *H. ducreyi* requires heme for growth, and several of the critical molecules required for heme acquisition and use have been identified.[57,58,123,209,216] The knowledge gained from molecular characterization of these important bacterial components should enhance efforts to understand the pathogenesis of disease more clearly.

Epidemiology

Chancroid is a genital ulcerative disease that is found throughout the world. It is seen frequently in Africa, Asia, and Latin America, where it may be a more common cause of genital ulcer disease than syphilis.[4,23–25,151,218,221] Although generally considered a relatively uncommon cause of illness in the United States, chancroid continues to be diagnosed, particularly among patients, including adolescents, who present with genital ulcer disease in large urban areas.[28,87,92,147,148,195] Furthermore, data suggest that chancroid may be more common in the United States than suspected because it can be difficult to diagnose correctly using traditional clinical and laboratory means.[53,152,221] Symptomatic disease among patients in the United States has been reported most commonly among nonwhite heterosexual male patients.[28,68,87,151] However, symptomatic disease is not restricted to men, and female prostitutes have been implicated as important sources of infection in several of the outbreaks reported in the United States.[28,87,151]

H. ducreyi has been the subject of renewed medical and scientific interest since the early 1980s. This interest followed from epidemiologic studies, primarily from Africa, demonstrating that the presence of genital ulcer disease (much of which was chancroid) was strongly associated with an increased risk of heterosexual transmission of human immunodeficiency virus (HIV) infection.[2,9,104,116,117,152,171,229] Mechanisms proposed to explain this enhanced transmission included an increased shedding of HIV through the ulcers,[116,221] an increased number of HIV-susceptible cells (e.g., CD4 T lymphocytes) in genital ulcers of a person being exposed to HIV,[205,221] or an increased viral load in the blood and semen of persons coinfected with HIV and *H. ducrei.*[56]

Pathogenesis

As noted earlier, significant progress has been since the 1990s in better understanding the pathogenesis of *H. ducreyi* infection.[8,102,201,221] Several useful in vivo models of *H. ducreyi* infection have been developed. These include a temperature-dependent rabbit model of dermal infection,[173] a primate model of genital chancroid infection in adult pigtailed macaques,[219] a swine model of dermal infection,[96] and an experimental model of human infection.[10,11,17,19,103,163,201,206] Several putative virulence factors have been identified, and their contributions to the pathogenesis of disease are being investigated using several in vitro and in vivo model systems. Some of the molecules and characteristics studied include bacterial lipooligosaccharide,[20,39,130,204,242] pili,[3,8,21,66,80,193,202,211,222] the cytolethal distending toxin,[†] an hemolysin,[6,55,162,164,220,236,241] serum resistance proteins,[1,44,75,125,126] lectin binding proteins[1,101,225,228] and the ability to adhere specifically to epithelial cells of genital origin.[5,121] The contribution of these proposed virulence factors to the pathogenesis of natural infection in humans is still being defined.[102] However, it is known that strains deficient in expression of several of these factors are attenuated in their ability to cause disease in the experimental model of human infection.[9,33,70,73,101–103,182,203] Ongoing investigations of *H. ducreyi* undoubtedly will define the virulence mechanisms of the organism more clearly and should enhance efforts to develop protective vaccines.[2,10,45,50,74,88,124]

*References 1, 6, 44, 46, 75, 100, 125, 126, 161, 164, 225.
†References 48, 47, 72, 77, 83, 120, 131, 133, 174, 175, 208, 239.

Clinical Manifestations

The incubation period of chancroid usually is between 4 and 7 days. It rarely is less than 3 days or more than 10 days.[7,151,185,186] Typically the first lesion noted is a small inflammatory papule surrounded by a zone of erythema. Within 2 or 3 days, a pustule forms that soon ruptures, leaving a sharply circumscribed ulcer with ragged undermined edges *without* induration.[128,151,185] The base of the ulcer usually has a granular appearance and always is painful. In male patients, the most common sites of appearance of the ulcers are on the distal prepuce, on the mucosal surface of the prepuce on the frenulum, and in the coronal sulcus. In female patients, most lesions are at the entrance to the vagina.[128,151,185] Painful, tender, inguinal adenopathy is present in up to 50% of patients and usually is unilateral. The involved lymph nodes rapidly may become fluctuant and rupture, with the formation of inguinal ulcers.[151,185]

The combination of a painful ulcer and tender inguinal adenopathy is suggestive of chancroid and, when accompanied by suppurative inguinal adenopathy, is almost pathognomonic.[237] However, a significant percentage of patients with *H. ducreyi* infection may have ulcers that can be confused with other genital ulcer diseases, such as herpes or syphilis.[76,128,151,185] Furthermore, as many as 10% of patients with chancroid may be coinfected with *Treponema pallidum* or herpes simplex virus.[237] Thus it becomes mandatory to establish a definitive diagnosis by laboratory means if one is to be confident about the diagnosis.

Chancroid has also been described as a cause of chronic lower extremity skin ulcers in children in the South Pacific area[139,150,224] and, more recently, in central Africa.[79] These are areas of the world in which yaws, caused by the spirochete *T. pallidum* subsp. *pertenue,* is endemic and where this organism was previously thought to be the primary cause of such ulcers. However, in a more recent study of children with chronic skin ulcers in one endemic region, the incidence of infection caused by *H. ducreyi* exceeded that of infection caused by *T. pallidum* subsp. *pertenue.* Furthermore, a small percentage of children actually had infection with both organisms simultaneously.[150,184,200]

Diagnosis

As noted earlier, diagnosing chancroid on clinical grounds alone is difficult because the clinical presentation often is not classic, and many clinicians do not have much experience with the disease.[221,237] Definitive diagnosis of chancroid requires isolation of the organism from a genital ulcer or from involved lymph nodes. However, the organism is fastidious and is difficult to isolate, even under the best of circumstances.[151] To obtain specimens for culture, a swab should be used to obtain material from the purulent base of an ulcer, or a fluctuant inguinal lymph node should be aspirated directly. Gram stain of purulent material may reveal gram-negative rods in the characteristic "school-of-fish" pattern, but this appearance probably is more characteristic of in vitro propagated organisms.[151] However, even with use of the selective media now recommended for isolation of *H. ducreyi*, it has been estimated that the sensitivity of culture is no higher than 80%.[128,237]

Given the low sensitivity of culture, alternative non–culture-based diagnostic tests have been evaluated. Early studies examined the utility of diagnosing chancroid serologically with an enzyme-linked immunosorbent assay using either an outer membrane protein preparation or a lipooligosaccharide preparation of *H. ducreyi.*[7] More recent studies have used slightly altered antigen preparations and serum preparation techniques meant to improve the sensitivity and specificity of the assay.[42] Although these modifications did lead to improvement in the performance characteristics of the assay, the ability of the modified assay to aid in the diagnosis of acute infection remains limited because many patients do not develop a serum antibody response until several weeks after onset of infection.[42,218] More recent work has focused on the use of recombinant proteins as test antigens for a serologic test.[59] This latter assay does appear to show promise for seroprevalence studies, but its utility in the diagnosis of acute infection has yet to be demonstrated. Another more recently described diagnostic test relies on detection of *H. ducreyi* with monoclonal antibodies directed against the hemoglobin receptor, but it has yet to undergo extensive field testing.[166]

Nucleotide-based diagnostic methods also have been described.[105,188,221] Perhaps most promising are the polymerase chain reaction–based techniques. These assays demonstrate high sensitivity and appear to identify some patients with chancroid, from whom bacterial cultures for *H. ducreyi* are negative.[218,221,150] Multiplex polymerase chain reaction assays that can amplify and subsequently detect DNA from *H. ducreyi*, *T. pallidum*, and herpes simplex virus from genital ulcer specimens simultaneously are undergoing field trials and have shown early promise.[136,159,221]

Even if chancroid is diagnosed definitively, it is recommended that patients also be tested for HIV at the time of diagnosis. In addition, up to 10% of patients with chancroid may be coinfected with *T. pallidum* or herpes simplex virus.[237] Appropriate testing for these other pathogens should be strongly considered when a patient presents with any form of genital ulcer disease.

Treatment and Prevention

Successful antimicrobial treatment of genital ulcers caused by *H. ducreyi* cures the infection, resolves clinical symptoms, and prevents transmission to others. However, in cases of extensive ulcerative disease, scarring may result, despite successful antimicrobial therapy.[237] The Centers for Disease Control and Prevention currently recommend one of four antibiotic regimens for treatment of chancroid in adolescents and adults.[128,194,237] These regimens are: (1) azithromycin, 1 g orally in a single dose, (2) ceftriaxone, 250 mg intramuscularly in a single dose, (3) ciprofloxacin, 500 mg orally twice a day for 3 days, or (4) erythromycin base, 500 mg orally three times a day for 7 days.[194,237] All four regimens are generally effective for treatment of chancroid among patients without HIV infection.[194] A successful response to therapy usually is apparent within 48 to 72 hours, as shown by decreased ulcer tenderness and pain.[185,194,237] Complete healing of ulcers may take up to 28 days but often is achieved in 7 to 14 days.[185] Healing of fluctuant adenopathy is slower than that of the ulcers and may require needle aspiration through adjacent intact skin or incision and drainage to achieve a successful response to therapy.[62,194]

Patients with HIV infection must be monitored closely because they may require longer courses of antimicrobial agents than the standard regimens just outlined.[194,237] Treatment failures have been noted with several of these regimens,[31,194,223] and there is some suggestion that persons who are most immunosuppressed are at the greatest risk for failure of standard regimens.[223] Some experts recommend using the erythromycin 7-day regimen for treating all HIV-infected patients because of good experience with this regimen in the HIV-infected population and limited successful experience with the alternative regimens.[194]

Identifying all sexual contacts of infected persons is critical to prevent further spread of *H. ducreyi* disease. The Centers for Disease Control and Prevention recommend that all persons who have had sexual contact with a patient with proven *H. ducreyi* infection within the 10 days before onset of the patient's symptoms be examined and treated.[237] Contacts should be examined and treated even in the absence of symptoms.

In the longer term, alternative strategies for control of chancroid should be examined. If feasible, vaccination for prevention of *H. ducreyi* infection would be a worthy goal. Data generated in animal models of infection are somewhat encouraging.[2,50,88,191] Protective immunity to both homologous and heterologous challenge has been reported after immunization of rabbits with cell-surface extracts of *H. ducreyi*.[88] In other work, a purified pilus preparation also was reported to induce immunity in that same model.[50] More recently, immunization with the hemoglobin receptor protein was reported to protect against infection in the swine model of chancroid.[2,74,124] These data suggest that prevention of chancroid by vaccination may be an achievable goal. However, data from the experimental human model of infection suggest that development of a protective vaccine for human use may not be a straightforward process.[10,103]

HAEMOPHILUS INFLUENZAE BIOGROUP AEGYPTIUS (HAEMOPHILUS AEGYPTIUS)

Bacteriology

H. influenzae biogroup *aegyptius* (*H. aegyptius*) was described originally by Koch[114] in 1883 in Egyptian patients with conjunctivitis. A more detailed description of the organism and the clinical characteristics of disease followed 3 years later in the work of Weeks.[231] The Koch-Weeks bacillus has continued to be an important cause of conjunctivitis since these initial reports. Because of several reportedly unique characteristics,[141] the Koch-Weeks bacillus originally was designated as a unique species of the *Haemophilus* genus (*H. aegyptius*) distinct from *H. influenzae*. However, more recent phenotypic and phylogenetic studies, including DNA relatedness analyses, have raised questions about the validity of this separation.[36,214] The organism is known currently as *H. influenzae* biogroup *aegyptius*, although debate continues in the literature about the appropriateness of this designation.[132]

This organism became the subject of intense scientific study in the 1980s as a result of its association with a newly described fulminant and often fatal disease called Brazilian purpuric fever.[34,35] *H. influenzae* biogroup *aegyptius* was isolated from 9 blood cultures and 1 hemorrhagic cerebrospinal fluid culture collected from 10 clinically ill children in Serrana, São Paulo State, Brazil.[35] The *H. influenzae* biogroup *aegyptius* strains causing Brazilian purpuric fever were initially believed to be members of a single virulent clone.[36,214] This clone was characterized by the presence of several unique features, including a 24-MDa plasmid with a characteristic restriction endonuclease pattern,[36] a unique multilocus electrophoretic enzyme typing pattern,[156] one of two rRNA gene restriction fragment length polymorphisms,[36,51] a single sodium dodecyl sulfate–polyacrylamide gel electrophoresis profile for whole-cell lysates,[36] specific reactivity with monoclonal antibodies recognizing epitopes unique to Brazilian purpuric fever strains,[127,214] agglutination with antisera specific for the Brazilian purpuric fever clone,[36] and conservation of certain major outer membrane proteins.[179] Although most Brazilian purpuric fever–associated strains of *H. influenzae* biogroup *aegyptius* appeared to be members of a unique clone, a few Brazilian purpuric fever–associated strains were identified that lacked some of the defining characteristics.[214,217] Furthermore, two cases of Brazilian purpuric fever reported from Australia were associated with strains clearly distinct from the Brazilian purpuric fever clone.[132,214] An excellent review of the epidemiologic, clinical, and laboratory aspects of the disease and its investigation has been published, and the reader is referred to that work for additional information.[91]

Epidemiology

In the United States, *H. influenzae* biogroup *aegyptius* has remained an important cause of conjunctivitis, with disease most commonly reported from the southern states.[90] The United States experienced only one reported case of possible Brazilian purpuric fever.[227] In Brazil, the epidemiology of Brazilian purpuric fever became more clearly defined with time.[90,91] The median age of patients with Brazilian purpuric fever was 2 to 3 years, with an overall age range of 3 months to 10 years.[34,35] Brazilian purpuric fever appeared to occur with the onset of warmer temperatures and was less likely during the Brazilian winter.[90] Furthermore, it appeared to be more common in small agricultural towns than in larger cities.[34,35,90] Case-control studies attempting to identify risk factors for development of disease identified a history of preceding conjunctivitis as being associated strongly with the development of Brazilian purpuric fever.[34,35,90] (although many of the control subjects also gave a history of conjunctivitis) and suggested that day care center attendance was an additional risk factor.[35] There have been no additional reported cases of Brazilian purpuric fever since the early 1990s. The reasons for the apparent disappearance of the disease remain unclear.[91]

Pathogenesis

Efforts to identify unique virulence factors of *H. influenzae* biogroup *aegyptius* responsible for the fulminant nature of Brazilian purpuric fever have been ongoing since the initial descriptions of the illness. Progress to date has been limited,[40,91] but several more recent genome-based studies demonstrated clear differences between *H. influenzae* biogroup *aegyptius* prototype strains and other *H. influenza* strains.[129,144,199] Brazilian purpuric fever clone strains express certain novel or unique surface molecules or secreted proteins that theoretically could result in enhanced virulence.[36,40,127,132,190,235] Distinctive lipooligosaccharide phenotypes,[40,190] immunoglobulin A proteases,[40,132,143] pili,[18,177,178,235] secreted proteins,[235] and adhesins[196,210] have been reported for Brazilian purpuric fever strains. However, none has been shown to have a specific dominant role in bacterial virulence. One study suggested that the risk of developing Brazilian purpuric fever correlated with the lack of serum bactericidal activity against the Brazilian purpuric fever clone, but this observation needs further confirmation.[189] In more recent work using a comparative genomic approach, investigators identified differences in known autotransporter adhesins as well as adhesins unique to the Brazilian purpuric fever clone that may play a role in pathogenesis.[210]

Both in vitro and in vivo models were developed for further investigating the pathogenesis of Brazilian purpuric fever.[176,190,232] In these model systems, Brazilian purpuric fever–associated strains demonstrated increased virulence compared with control strains not associated with Brazilian purpuric fever, but again, the specific molecular correlates of this increased pathogenicity have yet to be identified clearly.[176,190]

Clinical Manifestations

The clinical presentation of Brazilian purpuric fever is distinctive and dramatic.[34,35,90,91] The syndrome initially manifests as purulent conjunctivitis without distinguishing characteristics. Symptoms of Brazilian purpuric fever typically appear 3 to 15 days later, after the conjunctivitis has resolved. Affected children experience the acute onset of fever, which may be associated with vomiting and abdominal pain. Death frequently ensues within 48 hours after the development of disseminated purpura, vascular collapse, and hypotensive shock. The precise pathophysiologic mechanisms responsible for progression from conjunctivitis caused by the Brazilian purpuric fever clone to full-blown Brazilian purpuric fever are unknown. The overall case-fatality rate since Brazilian purpuric fever first was recognized is estimated to be 70%.[90] Children may develop conjunctivitis with the Brazilian purpuric fever clone and, after recovery from the conjunctivitis, have no further problems.[90] The risk factors that predispose only some children to develop Brazilian purpuric fever are not well understood.

Treatment

Data from the limited number of Brazilian purpuric fever cases studied suggest that early antimicrobial therapy may improve survival.[35] One suggested regimen is high-dose ampicillin and chloramphenicol. The small number of patients treated to date does not permit a comparison of the efficacy of different antibiotic regimens.[35] Most of the patients who developed Brazilian purpuric fever in the Brazilian studies were treated with topical antimicrobials for conjunctivitis, yet they still developed systemic disease.[35] This finding suggests that local topical therapy is ineffective in eradicating the organism from the host. One study examined the relative efficacy of oral rifampin and topical chloramphenicol in eradicating conjunctival carriage of the Brazilian purpuric fever clone.[168] Although the number of patients who actually carried the Brazilian purpuric fever clone was small, rifampin was shown to be significantly better in eradicating carriage of the Brazilian purpuric fever clone than was topical chloramphenicol.

HAEMOPHILUS PARAINFLUENZAE

Bacteriology

H. parainfluenzae was identified first as a species distinct from *H. influenzae* by Rivers in 1922.[183] Both organisms are fastidious, gram-negative coccobacilli, but with in vitro culture, *H. parainfluenzae* can be propagated on nutrient agar plates with supplemental factor V alone (hence the "para" designation), rather than with both factor X and factor V, which are required by *H. influenzae* isolates (see Table 134.1). Testing for hemolysis on blood-containing media differentiates *H. parainfluenzae* from hemolysis-producing species, such as *H. haemolyticus* and *H. parahaemolyticus.*[112,122] Recovery of *H. parainfluenzae* organisms from blood cultures is enhanced by routine subculturing of all specimens. The organisms tend to grow as small colonies along the side walls of the blood bottles or in the red blood cell mass, thus leaving the broth clear. Routine subculturing to supplemented chocolate agar and incubation with supplemental carbon dioxide should allow recovery of any *H. parainfluenzae* organisms that are present.[43,86]

Epidemiology and Pathogenesis

H. parainfluenzae is found commonly in the oropharyngeal flora of normal children.[85,119,135] The organism can be recovered from oropharyngeal cultures of one-fourth or more of healthy children. Of children who develop serious invasive disease caused by *H. parainfluenzae*, more than one-half give histories of identifiable preceding illnesses, such as upper respiratory tract infection, otitis media, and dental infections,[15,27,85,97] a finding suggesting that local inflammation in the upper respiratory tract may predispose to transient bacteremia with this organism, which allows for seeding of other sites, such as the meninges and the heart valves. No specific virulence factors of the organism have been identified to date.

Clinical Manifestations

H. parainfluenzae remains an uncommon cause of infection in pediatric patients, but an increasing number of cases have been reported since the 1970s.[27] The most commonly reported infection is meningitis.* The clinical courses of the patients described with *H. parainfluenzae* meningitis are not remarkably different from those typical of acute bacterial meningitis caused by other organisms. However, the average age of affected children is 2.2 years,[27] an age significantly greater than that of the typical pediatric patient with bacterial meningitis.

The next most commonly reported infection is endocarditis.[27,29,30,38,60,64,78,134,135,197] *H. parainfluenzae* endocarditis has several unique features. The reported cases of pediatric endocarditis usually occur in adolescents and involve girls more commonly than boys.[27] The clinical presentation often is subacute and frequently is not associated with localizing signs on physical examination (i.e., pathologic murmurs), at least initially.[43,134,135] Another unique feature of *H. parainfluenzae* endocarditis is the high incidence of major arterial occlusion secondary to release of large emboli from the heart.[27,43,78,134,207] This high incidence of embolization is thought to reflect the particularly friable nature of the vegetations.[27,78] Another characteristic feature noted by several investigators is the relatively slow and variable response to antimicrobial therapy of endocarditis caused by this organism.[27,43,134,135]

Other *H. parainfluenzae* infections reported in pediatric patients include brain abscesses,[85,137] septic arthritis,[27] urinary tract infection,[13,27,89] peritonitis,[140] and sepsis in neonates.[41,81,110,180]

Treatment

H. parainfluenzae usually is susceptible in vitro to multiple antibiotics, including chloramphenicol, aminoglycosides, trimethoprim-sulfamethoxazole, and third-generation cephalosporins.[27,43,106,135] Although most isolates in the past were susceptible to penicillins, more recent studies have documented an increasing incidence of β-lactamase–producing strains resistant to penicillin and ampicillin.[27,192] For β-lactamase–negative penicillin-susceptible organisms, administration of ampicillin with an aminoglycoside has been recommended for serious *H. parainfluenzae* infections.[43,154] Individual case reports document successful treatment with a variety of other antimicrobials, including ampicillin alone, cephalosporins, chloramphenicol, and trimethoprim-sulfamethoxazole.[38,43,107,135] At present, pending results of susceptibility testing, it would be reasonable to initiate therapy for serious *H. parainfluenzae* infections with a third-generation cephalosporin, perhaps in combination with an aminoglycoside.

NEW REFERENCES SINCE THE SEVENTH EDITION

12. Anderson R, Wang X, Briere EC, et al. *Haemophilus haemolyticus* isolates causing clinical disease. *J Clin Microbiol.* 2012;50:2462-2465.
13. Ariza Jimenez AB, Moreno-Perez D, Nunez Cuadros E, et al. Invasive disease caused by *Haemophilus parainfluenzae* III in a child with uropathy. *J Med Microbiol.* 2013;62:792-793.
32. Bogdan M, Zujic Atalic V, Hecimovic I, et al. Brain abscess due to *Aggregatibacter aphrophilus* and *Bacteroides uniformis. Acta Med Acad.* 2015;44(2):181-185.
75. Fusco WG, Elkins C, Leduc I. Trimeric autotransporter DsrA is a major mediator of fibrinogen binding in *Haemophilus ducreyi. Infect Immun.* 2013;81(12):4443-4452.

*References 15, 16, 49, 69, 71, 84, 85, 97, 109, 118, 137, 198, 230, 238.

79. Ghinai R, El-Duah P, Chi KH, et al. A cross-sectional study of "yaws" in districts of Ghana which have previously undertaken azithromycin mass drug administration for trachoma control. *PLoS Negl Trop Dis.* 2015;9:e0003496.
81. Govind B, Veeraraghavan B, Anandan S, et al. *Haemophilus parainfluenzae*: report of an unusual cause of neonatal sepsis and a literature review. *J Infect Dev Ctries.* 2012;6(10):748-750.
93. Hidalgo-Garcia L, Hurtado-Mingo A, Olbrich P, et al. Recurrent infective endocarditis due to *Aggregatibacter aphrophilus* and *Staphylococcus lugdunensis*. *Klin Padiatr.* 2015;227(2):89-92.
110. Kaushik M, Bober B, Eisenfeld L, et al. Case report of *Haemophilus parainfluenzae* sepsis in a newborn infant following water birth and a review of literature. *AJP Rep.* 2015;5(2):e188-e192.
138. Maraki S, Papadakis IS, Chronakis E, et al. *Aggregatibacter aphrophilus* brain abscess secondary to primary tooth extraction: case report and literature review. *J Microbiol Immunol Infect.* 2016;49(1):119-122.
139. Marks M, Chi KH, Vahi V, et al. *Haemophilus ducreyi* associated with skin ulcers among children, Solomon Islands. *Emerg Infect Dis.* 2014;20(10):1705-1707.
150. Mitja O, Lukehart SA, Pokowas G, et al. *Haemophilus ducreyi* as a cause of skin ulcers in children from a yaws-endemic area of Papua New Guinea: a prospective cohort study. *Lancet Glob Health.* 2014;2(4):e235-e241.
153. Morton DJ, Hempel RJ, Whitby PW, et al. An invasive *Haemophilus haemolyticus* isolate. *J Clin Microbiol.* 2012;50(4):1502-1503.
154. Murphy TF. *Haemophilus* species, including *H. influenzae* and H. ducreyi (chancroid). In: Mandell GL, Bennett JE, Dolin R, eds. *Mandell, Douglas, and Bennett's Principles and Practice of Infectious Diseases.* 8th ed. Philadelphia: Churchill Livingstone; 2015:2575-2583.
170. Pickering J, Richmond PC, Kirkham LA. Molecular tools for differentiation of non-typeable *Haemophilus influenzae* from *Haemophilus haemolyticus*. *Front Microbiol.* 2014;5:664.
181. Revest M, Egmann G, Cattoir V, et al. HACEK endocarditis: state-of-the-art. *Expert Rev Anti Infect Ther.* 2016;14:523-530.
182. Rinker SD, Gu X, Fortney KR, et al. Permeases of the sap transporter are required for cathelicidin resistance and virulence of *Haemophilus ducreyi* in humans. *J Infect Dis.* 2012;206(9):1407-1414.
184. Roberts SA, Taylor SL. *Haemophilus ducreyi*: a newly recognised cause of chronic skin ulceration. *Lancet Glob Health.* 2014;2(4):e187-e188.
191. Samo M, Choudhary NR, Riebe KJ, et al. Immunization with the *Haemophilus ducreyi* trimeric autotransporter adhesin DsrA with alum, CpG or imiquimod generates a persistent humoral immune response that recognizes the bacterial surface. *Vaccine.* 2016;34(9):1193-1200.
200. Spinola SM. *Haemophilus ducreyi* as a cause of skin ulcers. *Lancet Glob Health.* 2014;2(7):e387.
237. Workowski KA, Bolan GA. Sexually transmitted diseases treatment guidelines, 2015. *MMWR Recomm Rep.* 2015;64(RR-03):1-137.

The full reference list for this chapter is available at ExpertConsult.com.

135 Helicobacter pylori

Aldo Maspons • Mark A. Gilger

The discovery of *Helicobacter pylori* in 1983 as the bacterial cause of peptic ulcer disease revolutionized the understanding, diagnosis, and treatment of acid peptic disease.[115] *H. pylori* appears to infect approximately 50% of the world's population, thus rendering it one of the most common bacterial infections in humans.[15,83] An understanding of *H. pylori* is important to pediatricians because this infection usually is acquired in childhood.[61] This chapter details current consensus and understanding of this important pathogen.

BACKGROUND

The presence of bacteria in the gastric mucosa has been known for more than 100 years. In 1874, Böttcher[1] observed bacteria in the human stomach. Bizzozero[47] described spirochetes in the stomach of dogs in 1893. In 1938, Doenges[68] explored the issue of gastric spirochetes and their clinical relevance. He reported a 43% prevalence of spiral organisms in the human stomach in an autopsy review of 242 patients without known gastrointestinal disease. Specimen autolysis, however, rendered interpretation of the pathologic significance of the gastric spirochetes impossible. Freedberg and Barron[46] verified the findings of Doenges in 1940, when they identified spirochetes in the stomachs of 37% of patients who had undergone partial gastric resection for carcinoma or ulcer disease. Work on the clinical significance of gastric spiral bacteria continued until a report by Palmer[107] was published in 1954. In an attempt to confirm the findings of spirochetes in the gastric mucosa, Palmer performed an exhaustive review of gastric fundus biopsies from 1000 adult patients, 80% of whom were being evaluated for upper gastrointestinal complaints and 20% of whom were healthy control volunteers. Palmer noted, "None of the 1180 specimens was found to contain spirochetes or any structure which could reasonably be considered to be of spirochetal nature."[107] He concluded that spirochetes are not part of the human gastric mucosa in health or illness. Palmer, a prominent researcher in gastritis, inadvertently may have curtailed further research into the role of gastric spiral bacteria.

In 1975, Steer,[126] using electron microscopy, noted curved bacteria in stomach biopsy specimens from patients with gastric ulcers. A few years later, Warren, an Australian pathologist, noted the appearance of spiral bacteria overlying inflamed gastric mucosa. He and Marshall began a series of culture experiments using *Campylobacter*-specific methods because the organism looked like a *Campylobacter*. In an attempt to fulfill the remainder of Koch's postulates, Marshall and associates[93] and Morris and Nicholson[93] independently ingested pure cultures of *H. pylori,* and symptomatic acute gastritis developed in both groups. The organism subsequently was recovered from the gastric mucosa by endoscopy and successfully cultured, thus completing Koch's postulates.

MICROBIOLOGY AND PATHOPHYSIOLOGY

H. pylori initially was named *Campylobacter pyloridis* because of its resemblance to *Campylobacter* spp.,[73] and the name was later changed to *Campylobacter pylori.* However, it became clear that the bacterium did not belong to any known genus. An entirely new genus, *Helicobacter,* was created, with *helico* describing the spiral shape and *pylori* denoting its typical location. *H. pylori* is a spiral-shaped, gram-negative bacterium with four to seven unipolar sheathed flagella (Fig. 135.1).[11,105] It is 0.5 μm wide and 3 to 5 μm long and has a smooth surface.[3,88] It generally is S-shaped in vivo but can take on many forms, from U-shaped to cocci to rodlike.[95]

H. pylori inhabits a unique ecologic niche—the submucosa of gastric epithelium. Several attributes, including adherence, shape, microaerophilism, urease production, and motility, allow adaptation to the acidic gastric environment. *H. pylori* overlies the intercellular tight junctions of epithelial cells, beneath the mucous layer. Specific adhesion molecules appear to be tropic to gastric mucus-producing cells.[95] This adherence allows the organism to maintain colonization despite the rapid gastric cell turnover.[78] The spiral shape may allow the organism to corkscrew through the gastric mucus (see Fig. 135.1). This spiral movement has been demonstrated in vitro with methylcellulose solutions.[78] *H. pylori* is microaerophilic and grows slowly in culture media (Table 135.1).[12,106] Translucent colonies of 1 mm grow after 5 to 7 days on blood-supplemented or serum-supplemented media with a low concentration of oxygen and carbon dioxide at a temperature of 37°C (98.6°F), which promotes optimal growth. This microaerophilism is well suited to the low oxygen levels of the gastric submucosa.[77] *H. pylori* is the most potent urease producer of any known microbe; researchers have estimated that as much as 10% of its total protein production is urease, and the organism appears to surround itself in a cloud of ammonia.[9] The urea is converted to ammonium and bicarbonate.[11,53] Little evidence supports the notion that the ammonium produced is cytotoxic to gastric epithelium.[62] The bicarbonate creates an alkaline environment in the gastric submucosa. *H. pylori* produces several other enzymes, including mucinase,[124] lipase,[69] catalase,[84] hemolysin, and cytopathic toxin.[82] The multiple, unipolar flagella (see Fig. 135.1) provide motility that may enable the organism to escape the acid lumen of the stomach and evade host immune responses.[77,78]

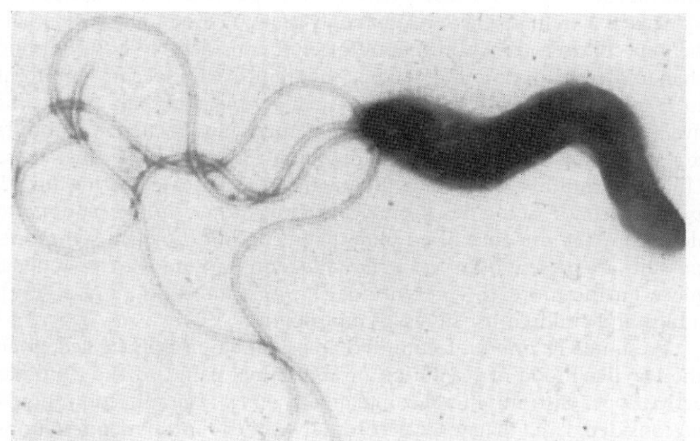

FIG. 135.1 Electron microscopy of *Helicobacter pylori* demonstrating the multipolar flagella and the typical spiral shape.

TABLE 135.1 Examples of Gastric Biopsy Cultures

Culture Media	Incubation Period (Days)	Conditions
Brucella chocolate agar with 7% sheep blood[85]	7	Microaerobic
Preserved in brain-heart infusion broth with 5% glycerin inoculated onto Columbia agar plates with 5% fresh defibrinated sheep blood[128]	3	Microaerophilic
Columbia III agar with 5% sheep blood[23]	10–14	Microaerophilic

H. pylori may be more akin to normal gastrointestinal flora because the bacterium and the host can coexist for decades without apparent problems.[54] *H. pylori* infection produces inflammation, although in most cases the host is asymptomatic.[14] The inflammatory response is characterized by infiltration of polymorphonuclear leukocytes, monocytes, lymphocytes, and plasma cells into the lamina propria (Fig. 135.2).[84] A significant immune response, including the production of antibodies, is generated by the host, but it does not clear the organism in most cases.[82] *H. pylori* produces a chronic infection that persists for decades, possibly for life.[84] This lifelong colonization is accomplished by the same features that allow survival in the gastric mucosa, namely, high urease production, flagellar motility, spiral shape, microaerophilism, and adherence.[84]

Numerous potential virulence factors, such as urease, catalase, cytotoxin, and lipopolysaccharide, have been identified, although whether any of these substances actually contribute to symptomatic disease is unknown. The urease of *H. pylori* is a potent antigen that induces elevations in antiurease immunoglobulin (Ig) G and IgA.[84] Interestingly, the ammonia produced by the urease does not appear to have a significant role in pathogenesis.[56] Catalase, another *H. pylori* enzyme, prevents the formation of oxygen metabolites from hydrogen peroxide in neutrophils,[33] a feature that may provide an ability to evade host destruction. A vacuolating cytotoxin has been identified in many *H. pylori* strains,[33] although whether it is more common in patients with symptomatic disease is unclear. *H. pylori* has a peculiar lipopolysaccharide outer membrane. Unlike most gram-negative bacteria, its lipopolysaccharide coat is a significantly less potent inducer of the host complement cascade, some 1000-fold less potent than that of the Enterobacteriaceae.[84] This low biologic activity of the outer membrane of *H. pylori* may be another adaptive mechanism allowing gastric colonization.[13]

The most pathogenic strain of *H. pylori* contains a cytotoxin-associated gene pathogenicity island (Cag PAI).[118,119] The Cag PAI encodes a type IV secretion system with a pilus that directly injects Cag A into the host's cytoplasm. Cag A affects gastric epithelial functions that include cell proliferation and suppression of apoptosis, as well as affecting intercellular junctions.[7] Cag A–positive strains are considered more virulent because of Cag A involvement in the intestinal cell transdifferentiation of gastric epithelial cells, a precursor to carcinogenesis.[101,102]

EPIDEMIOLOGY

H. pylori infection is one of the most common bacterial infections in humans, with an estimated 1 billion people in the world infected.[15,73] It is estimated that in developing countries more than 80% of the population is infected with *H. pylori*, whereas in industrialized countries

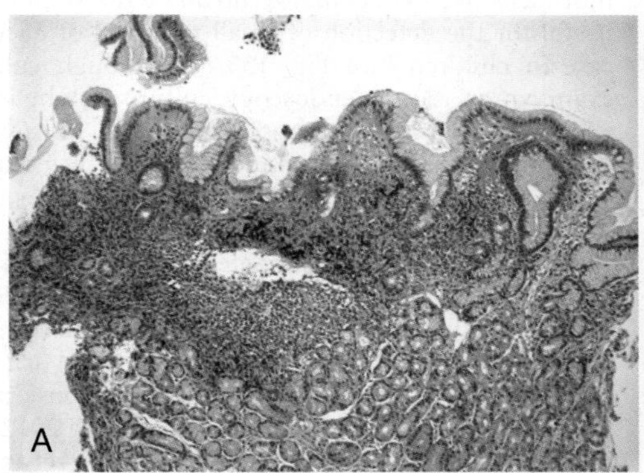

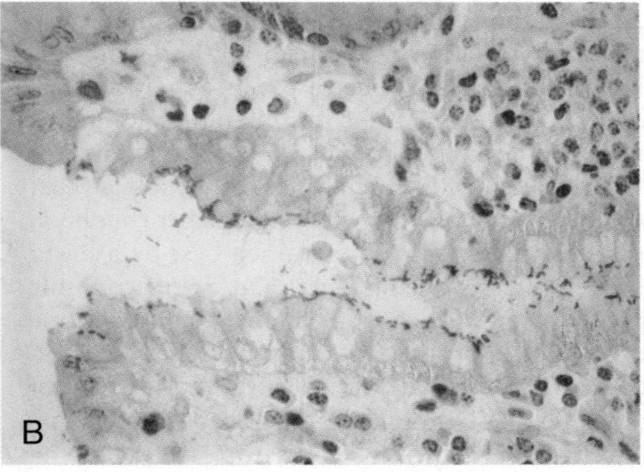

FIG. 135.2 (A) Chronic active gastritis. Corpus mucosa displays a large lymphoid infiltrate (magnification ×100; hematoxylin and eosin stain). (B) *Helicobacter pylori* are abundant at the surface and line the mucous glands of the gastric pit (magnification ×640; silver stain). (Courtesy Dr. Milton J. Finegold, Baylor College of Medicine, Texas Children's Hospital, Houston, TX.)

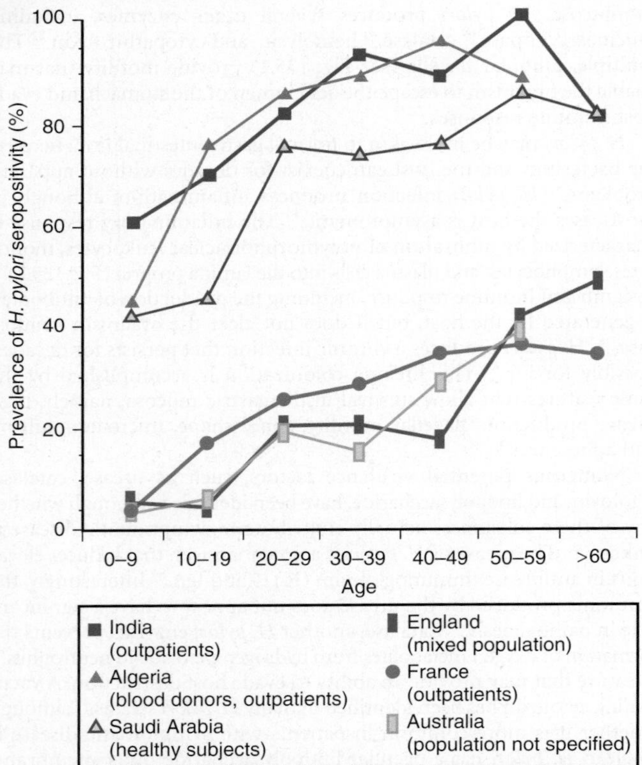

FIG. 135.3 Seroepidemiology of *Helicobacter pylori* infection demonstrating the difference in disease prevalence between developing and developed countries. (Data from Graham DY, Adam E, Reddy GT, et al. Seroepidemiology of *Helicobacter pylori* infection in India: comparison of developing and developed countries. *Dig Dis Sci.* 1991;36:1084–1088.)

the infection rate remains lower than 40% (Fig. 135.3).[109] Transmission appears to be from person to person.[79,130] Transmission through the fecal-oral route is the primary mode of infection. The presence of pets may be a risk factor for *H. pylori* infection, given that the bacterium has been isolated from domestic animals.[16,28] Interestingly, breastfeeding appears to increase the risk for acquiring *H. pylori* infection, possibly secondary to close contact with infected mothers, and breast milk does not protect against infection.[116,138] *H. pylori* usually is acquired in childhood,[24] and humans appear to be natural reservoirs for infection.[55] Environmental sources of *H. pylori* infection, such as municipal water sources, have been confirmed in Peru and Mexico.[87,96]

Children are important factors in the transmission of *H. pylori* infection, which clusters within families with children.[31,91,103] Family clustering emphasizes the role of crowding and personal hygiene in the person-to-person spread of infection. The prevalence of infection increases with age. In the United States, for example, only approximately 20% of persons younger than 30 years of age are infected, in contrast to 50% of those older than 60 years.[94] Infection in young children is rare in the United States and developed nations. The phenomenon of increasing prevalence with age most likely reflects a cohort effect; that is, the high prevalence in older persons simply reflects a higher childhood infection rate.[84] This cohort effect may be explained best by a lower standard of living of older persons during childhood. Socioeconomic status varies inversely with the prevalence of infection, with low-income persons having the highest rates of infection.[41] Conversely, Ozen and associates[106] found that low household population and a history of antibiotic use during the previous 6 months served as protective factors against infection. A higher prevalence of infection exists in developing countries than in developed countries (see Fig. 135.3),[95] and the prevalence of infection varies greatly around the world. In Nigeria, for example, 58% of children younger than 1 year of age and 91% of children older than 10 years of age were infected.[64] Such differences have been attributed to socioeconomic factors, hygiene, and the number of household occupants.[123] *H. pylori* is more prevalent in blacks and Hispanics than in whites in the United States.[125]

The rate of *H. pylori* reinfection in the pediatric population ranges from 2.4% to approximately 20% per year.[70,116] Magista and colleagues[90] demonstrated that the difference in reinfection rate depends primarily on the socioeconomic status of the family and the local prevalence of *H. pylori*. These investigators and others[39,40] also noted that living in an area with a high prevalence of *H. pylori* resulted in a fourfold higher risk of reinfection.

CLINICAL MANIFESTATIONS

Gastritis develops in most *H. pylori*–infected patients, but complications associated with infection develop in only a few.[15] This finding is especially true in children, in whom peptic ulcer is considerably less common than in adults. To confound matters, children have no specific symptoms of *H. pylori* infection.[115] Symptoms such as epigastric pain, nighttime awakening with abdominal pain, hematemesis, and recurrent vomiting are suggestive but in no way predictive of infection.[72] Because these clinical symptoms are typical of peptic ulcer disease, testing for *H. pylori* infection alone has no relevance but rather should be done to determine the presence of an underlying condition.[75] Such symptoms possibly are present only if *H. pylori* infection is found with a duodenal ulcer. Furthermore, the presence of *H. pylori* infection alone in both adults and children usually is asymptomatic.[27,59]

Presumed H. *pylori* infection should not be empirically treated, given the low likelihood of resolution of abdominal pain.[76] If the child has active upper gastrointestinal complaints, then *H. pylori* infection should be considered and diagnosed accordingly. Other clinical manifestations of *H. pylori* include protein-losing enteropathy and iron deficiency anemia.[20,22] Indeed, successful treatment of *H. pylori* infection improves iron stores.[18] Eradication of the bacteria should always be the goal, given that the infection is the most consistent risk factor for gastric cancer.[92]

DIAGNOSIS

The gold standard for diagnosis of *H. pylori* infection is culture of the organism from gastric biopsy samples or histologic review. Upper gastrointestinal endoscopy and other invasive means are necessary to obtain such biopsy specimens. In children, upper endoscopy can be quite helpful in that it often reveals a distinct nodularity at the antrum (Fig. 135.4), but findings also may appear normal. This nodularity is found in two-thirds of infected children but only rarely in adults.[17] Histologically, prominent lymphoid follicles are seen. Routine staining with hematoxylin and eosin may be adequate but must be performed properly to see the bacteria clearly. Alternative staining techniques, such as acridine orange, silver stains, and the "triple" stain, improve visualization.[49,89] The triple, or Genta, stain (Steiner, hematoxylin and eosin, Alcian blue) may offer some distinct advantages because it is significantly more sensitive than hematoxylin and eosin staining and is particularly useful for the detection of small numbers of bacteria, as often is the case in children (see Fig. 135.2). Although culture and histologic examination require endoscopy, culture may be important, especially when considering the increase in antibiotic resistance worldwide.[6,26] In cases of recurrent *H. pylori* infection in which antibiotic resistance is suspected, culture allows in vitro antibiotic susceptibilities to be determined.

Noninvasive methods for detection of *H. pylori* infection are detailed in Table 135.2 and include serology, varying methods for detection of urease production, detection of salivary antibody, stool culture, stool antigen, polymerase chain reaction (PCR), and urine ammonia production. The carbon-13 (^{13}C)–urea breath test is considered the best available noninvasive diagnostic test in children.[15,36] In 2012, it was approved by the US Food and Drug Administration to detect and monitor *H. pylori* infection in pediatric patients 3 to 17 years of age. Serology, conversely, is not useful. Measurement of *H. pylori* stool antigen can be performed by either a polyclonal or monoclonal antibody technique.[35,71] This test detects the presence of antigen, thus providing evidence of active infection for both primary diagnosis or proof of cure. It appears to be as accurate as the urea breath test.

H. pylori infection induces a vigorous neutrophilic and lymphocytic (T-cell and B-cell) response that fails to clear the infection. The humoral immune response produces antibodies that can be detected in gastric secretions, as well as systemically. Some *H. pylori* antigens have been determined with the use of bacterial cell wall sonicates, urease, or membrane extracts as the capture antigen. Some commercial assays have been found to have inappropriate positive and negative cutoff values for use in children.[25] Care must be taken to ensure that the serologic tests performed have been verified for use in children. Although detection of IgA, polymeric IgA, and IgM antibodies against haptoglobin can be performed, such detection is not reproducible and thus has no clinical value. Serologic diagnosis, although simple and widely available, does not indicate symptomatic disease.

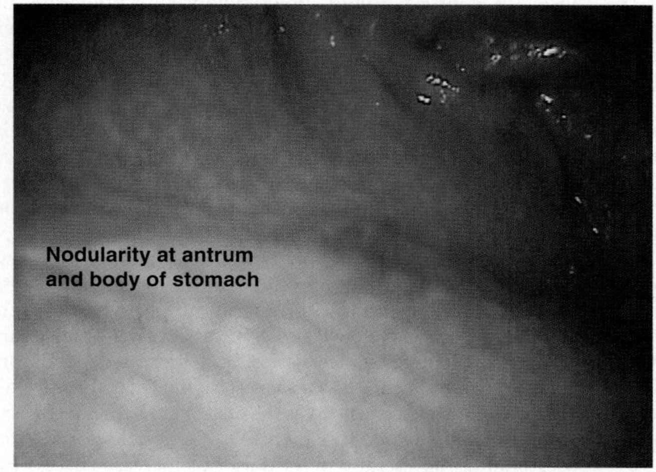

FIG. 135.4 Endoscopic view of the gastric antrum and body demonstrating marked nodularity of the gastric surface.

H. pylori is a vigorous producer of urease. This characteristic has been used to create a variety of tests to detect the presence of urease. The urea breath test uses a labeled carbon of urea, either radioactive ^{14}C[10] or a nonradioactive, stable isotope ^{13}C.[57] Patients fast for 4 to 8 hours and then drink the labeled carbon accompanied by a meal to delay gastric emptying; then the amount of labeled carbon dioxide in the breath is measured. Only patients with gastric *H. pylori* present (and thus gastric urease activity to degrade the labeled urea) are identified. Urea breath testing is useful for both initial diagnosis and determination of successful treatment because the results rapidly return to normal after eradication of the bacterium. The radioactive ^{14}C method does not deserve consideration for use in children. The stable isotope ^{13}C method currently is the simplest and most accurate noninvasive test available for detection of *H. pylori* infection. Its usefulness remains limited, however, because of the need for specialized equipment for analysis.

The urease production of *H. pylori* can be measured directly in gastric biopsy specimens with a variety of commercial assays.[3] A portion of the gastric biopsy specimen is placed into a urea medium, and hydrolysis of urea leads to a color change in the medium from tan to pink. False-negative results have been noted in children because of the low numbers of organisms.[32] Such testing is useful for establishing a

TABLE 135.2 **Summary of Methods for Detecting *Helicobacter Pylori***

Method	Sensitivity (%)	Specificity (%)	Advantages	Disadvantages
Invasive				
Histology	93–99	95–99	Widely available; detection best with special stains; can evaluate underlying mucosal damage; gold standard	Expensive; at least two biopsies required; observer error; recent antibiotics or proton pump inhibitor use can lead to false-negative results
Culture of biopsy specimens	77–92	100	In vitro antibiotic susceptibility can be determined	Expensive; organism requires special transfer and culture technique; requires up to 1 week for results; recent antibiotics or proton pump inhibitor use can lead to false-negative results
Rapid urease test (CLO test, hpFast, PyloriTek)	89–98	93–98	Rapid results; easy to perform; less expensive than other invasive techniques	Formalin, simethicone, local anesthetic spray, recent antibiotics, bismuth, or proton pump inhibitor use can lead to false-negative results; poor technique or handling affects results
Noninvasive				
Urea breath test (^{13}C, ^{14}C)	90–100	89–100	Inexpensive; represents entire mucosa (not subject to biopsy sampling bias)	Antibiotics or proton pump inhibitor use can lead to false-negative results; presence of ulcer disease not determined; can be difficult to collect in children <2 y old
Serology (ELISA; HM-CAP, Pylori.STAT)	44–99	89–95	Widely available; inexpensive	Not useful after treatment
Rapid serology (FlexSure, QuickVue)	92–93%	75–88%	In office diagnostic kit, widely available	Not useful after treatment
Stool antigen testing	85–94	97.7	Inexpensive; more accurate than serology; may become the test of choice in children	Stool must be collected
Saliva	71–93	82–92	Easy to collect; inexpensive;	Low sensitivity, especially in children <2 y old
Urine (anti-*H. pylori* IgG antibodies in urine)	90	100	rapid results; easy to perform; does not require large bacterial load	Length of time needed to prove eradication not known

CLO, Campylobacter-like organism; *ELISA*, enzyme-linked immunosorbent assay; *HM-CAP*, high-molecular-weight, cell-associated protein; *IgG*, immunoglobulin G.
Data from references 51, 104, and 117.

rapid diagnosis during endoscopy but requires gastric biopsy. Urease activity also can be detected by measurement of another nonradioactive, stable isotope, ammonium, in the urine after oral ingestion.[140] This noninvasive test has not proved to be accurate. *H. pylori* has been identified in saliva and dental plaque by culture[74] and PCR.[21] Other investigators have identified salivary antibody to *H. pylori* with an indirect immunofluorescence assay.[65] The saliva test is not accurate in young children and cannot be recommended.[51] Viable *H. pylori* organisms have been cultured from feces in Gambian children.

Proton pump inhibitors (PPIs) should be stopped, ideally, at least 2 weeks before testing because PPI use can lead to a decrease in the bacterial load and raise the possibility of a false-negative result. Histamine H_2 blockers can do the same, but to a lesser extent. After 2 weeks, the bacterial load begins to increase.

TREATMENT

The first-line therapy for *H. pylori* infection in children has long been a twice-daily, three-drug regimen that includes amoxicillin, clarithromycin, and a PPI given for 14 days.[50] Table 135.3 presents a variety of suggested regimens for the treatment of *H. pylori* infection in children.

Confirmation of successful treatment has been defined as the absence of detectable organisms by tissue biopsy, urea breath test, or stool antigen testing at least 1 month after completion of treatment.[50] Because tissue biopsy is invasive, urea breath testing or stool antigen detection is helpful for determination of successful treatment. Serologic tests are not useful for detection of cure because of the prolonged elevation of titers, which remain elevated for 6 months to 1 year or longer after treatment. Moreover, not all serologic tests are equivalent.

A growing body of evidence indicates that acquisition of *H. pylori* infection in childhood is a significant risk factor for the development of gastric cancer such as adenocarcinoma (Fig. 135.5).[66,133] An estimated two- to sixfold increased risk for the development of gastric cancer exists among *H. pylori*–infected patients.[30,132] Patients in whom gastric cancer develops appear already to have atrophic gastritis or metaplasia at baseline.[43,139] This finding argues for treatment of *H. pylori* infection in childhood, before the onset of atrophic gastritis. The location of the infection within the stomach may influence the outcome. For example, antral-predominant infection more commonly leads to increased acid secretion, which results in duodenal peptic ulcers and a low risk for gastric cancer. In contrast, fundus-predominant infection leads to decreased acid secretion, which results in atrophic gastritis and a higher risk for gastric cancer.[81] Treatment of gastric lymphoma with antibiotics directed at *H. pylori* results in regression of the tumor.[5]

Some researchers argue that the risk for developing either lymphoma or adenocarcinoma provides cause for the treatment of all children infected with *H. pylori*. Because the risk for development of cancer cannot be predicted accurately and because most children with *H. pylori* infection have no clinical symptoms, no current rationale exists for treating all children infected with *H. pylori*.

In children, the most common anti-*Helicobacter* therapy is legacy triple therapy, which includes amoxicillin, clarithromycin, and a PPI (see Table 135.3). Resistance to clarithromycin, however, has led to a decline in efficacy from 34% to 66% and eradication rates of less than 80%.[42,134] Clarithromycin resistance varies, and success depends on resistance rates. When resistance is less than 10%, then clarithromycin-containing regimens are recommended as the first-line treatment; efficacy of the regimen can be increased by 8% to 12% if a double-dose PPI is given, and extending the therapy to 14 days can increase success by 5%.[92] Eradication rates greater than 90% were demonstrated when *H. pylori* susceptibility testing was performed in children.[4,127] Antimicrobial evasion to clarithromycin, for example, has been attributed to three

TABLE 135.3 Suggested Treatment Regimens for *Helicobacter Pylori* Infection in Children

Medications	Dosage	Duration (Days)
Triple Therapy		
Amoxicillin[a]	50 mg/kg/day twice daily (max, 1 g twice daily)	7–14
Clarithromycin	15 mg/kg/day twice daily (max, 50 mg)	7–14
Proton pump inhibitor[b] (i.e., omeprazole)	1 mg/kg/day twice daily	7–14
Amoxicillin[a]	50 mg/kg/day twice daily (max, 1 g twice daily)	7–14
Metronidazole	20 mg/kg/day twice daily (max, 500 mg twice daily)	7–14
Proton pump inhibitor[b] (i.e., omeprazole)	1 mg/kg/day	7–14
Quadruple Therapy		
Bismuth subsalicylate[c]	15 mL (17.5 mg/mL) four times daily	10–14
Metronidazole	20 mg/kg/day twice daily (max, 500 mg twice daily)	10–14
Tetracycline[d]	50 mg/kg/day twice daily (max, 1 g twice daily)	10–14
Proton pump inhibitor[b] (i.e., omeprazole)	1 mg/kg/day (max, 20 mg twice daily)	10–14
Amoxicillin[a]	50 mg/kg/day twice daily (max, 1 g twice daily)	10–14s
Clarithromycin	15 mg/kg/day twice daily (max, 500 mg twice daily)	10–14
Metronidazole	20 mg/kg/day twice daily (max, 500 mg twice daily)	10–14
Proton pump inhibitor (i.e., omeprazole)	1 mg/kg/day	10–14
Sequential Therapy		
First 5 Days		
Amoxicillin[a]	50 mg/kg/day twice daily (max, 1 g twice daily)	
Proton pump inhibitor (i.e., omeprazole)	1 mg/kg/day	
Second 5 Days		
Clarithromycin	15 mg/kg/day twice daily (max, 500 mg twice daily)	
Tinidazole	20 mg/kg/day bid (max, 500 mg bid)	
Proton pump inhibitor (i.e., omeprazole)	1 mg/kg/day	

[a]In patients allergic to penicillin, amoxicillin may be replaced with metronidazole.
[b]Comparable proton pump inhibitors such as lansoprazole and rabeprazole can be substituted at appropriate doses.
[c]Bismuth produces black stools and has the potential complication of salicylate toxicity. Salicylates also pose the risk for Reye syndrome.
[d]Tetracycline is not recommended for children younger than 8 years.
Modified from Gilger MA. Treatment of *Helicobacter pylori* infection in children. *Curr Pharm Des.* 2000;6:370–84; additional data from Gatta L, Vakil N, Leandro G, et al. Sequential therapy or triple therapy for *Helicobacter pylori* infection: systematic review and meta-analysis of randomized controlled trials in adults and children. *Am J Gastroenterol.* 2009;104:3069–79.

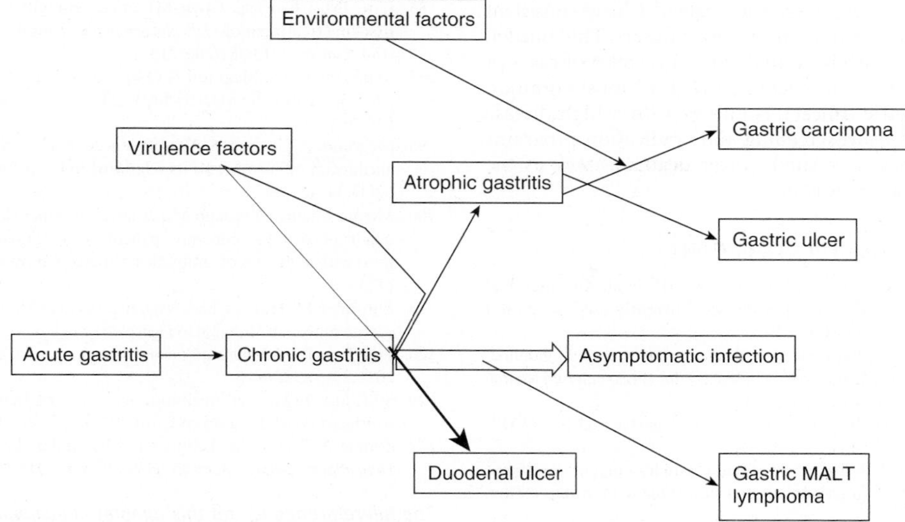

FIG. 135.5 Timeline of possible outcomes of *Helicobacter pylori* infection starting from the acute acquisition of infection and possible sequelae. *MALT,* Mucosa-associated lymphoid tissue. (Courtesy Dr. D. Graham, personal data.)

point mutations: A2143G, A2142G, and A2142C in domain V of 23S ribosomal RNA.[45,134] Clarithromycin-containing therapy should be used if the area resistance rate is low (<10%).[73] Clarithromycin resistance rates of 15% to 20% should dissuade clinicians from using this drug. Increasing resistance has prompted newer treatment regimens, such as sequential therapy, which was shown to be superior to legacy triple therapy in treatment-naïve cases, as well as in clarithromycin-resistant and metronidazole-resistant cases.[45,48,52,67,142] Sequential therapy consists of 5 days of a PPI and one antibiotic, usually amoxicillin, followed by 5 days of a PPI and two other antibiotics, such as clarithromycin and tinidazole (see Table 135.2). The general consensus is that if there is low clarithromycin resistance, clarithromycin-containing regimens and bismuth-containing regimens should be considered the first line of treatment.

Persistence and Resistance

Compliance and resistance are proven factors in the success or failure of a treatment regimen. Knowing the local susceptibilities and prevalence of antibiotic resistance allows for an increased rate of eradication and thus should be the guiding principle when choosing a treatment regimen.[58] Some developing countries, for example, have metronidazole resistance rates as high as 80%,[60] and pockets of Europe have clarithromycin resistance rates of 26%.[99] Therefore, treatment regimens should be regional specific. A clarithromycin resistance rate of 15% to 20% has been used to separate regions of high and low resistance.[92]

The prevalence of clarithromycin resistance is on the rise and varies among countries and regions; in some instances, it is more common in children. Resistance has been associated with the endoscopic finding of an ulcer.[97]

Methods of Testing Resistance

Gastric biopsy culture. Table 135.1 provides examples of gastric biopsy cultures.

Molecular methods. PCR is being used as an alternative to culture. PCR on gastric biopsies can detect mutations responsible for resistance to antibiotics such as clarithromycin and fluoroquinolone.[80,98] Stool-based PCR testing has been shown to be as effective as and in some instances more effective than culture of gastric biopsies.[131,135] Stool-based PCR sensitivities varies from 63% to 97% and specificity of 100% for *H. pylori* detection. Detection of clarithromycin resistance had a sensitivity of 83% and specificity of 100%.[122] Oral-based PCR detection methods are also being studied.

Metronidazole, to which the *H. pylori* organism has been highly susceptible, has a high rate of resistance because of its overuse for other infections.[113] In cases of antimicrobial resistance, rifabutin, furazolidone,[34,38,61,110,111,141] and fluoroquinolones, such as ciprofloxacin, along with rifampin and streptomycin, have been reported as options in treating resistant *H. pylori* infection.[37,44,121] These second-line regimens have no particular advantage over the first-line antibiotics and should be considered only when drug resistance is suspected. No single antibiotic agent given alone provides effective therapy against *H. pylori.*[114,120]

When cure of infection has been obtained, the long-term rates of reinfection are as low as 1% per year in developed countries but much higher in developing nations.[108] However, reinfection may be more likely to occur in families, especially when small children are the first infected.[8] Hence, in recurrence, all family members should be tested. No conclusive evidence currently exists, however, to recommend routine treatment of the entire family.[103]

Vaccination against *H. pylori* infection appears possible and also cost effective.[19,29] Vaccination has cleared *H. pylori* infection in animal models.[136] Human models, however, have proved more difficult. The inactivated whole-cell *H. pylori* vaccine failed to eradicate preexisting infection.[86] Although the live-vector, urease-based vaccines did not completely clear all of the preexisting infections, they showed promise and demonstrated a T-cell–mediated response to infection.[2,136] Success in human subjects was demonstrated with an antibody response to signaling, which is believed to regulate immune and inflammatory responses and has been shown to be important to the vaccine response.[136,137] Despite this progress, the cellular response to bacterial colonization is not completely understood.[129] Prophylactic and therapeutic vaccination is needed because current antibiotic therapy does not eradicate *H. pylori* infection in approximately 20% of affected patients. Despite vaccination successes in treatment and prevention, the failure to achieve sterilization immunity in animal models has led to continued disease secondary to *H. pylori*. A truly effective vaccine has thus far remained elusive.[100]

FUTURE DIRECTIONS

H. pylori is a major cause of peptic ulcer disease in children and adults, and this knowledge has caused a dramatic reappraisal of many previous notions about ulcer disease. Although the dictum "No acid, no ulcer" still holds, many other previous considerations, such as genetic predisposition, must be reexamined. Fig. 135.5 demonstrates a proposed *H. pylori* timeline. It emphasizes the acquisition of an acute infection in childhood, persistent chronic gastritis, and the possible progression to ulcer, atrophic gastritis, and, potentially, gastric carcinoma and lymphoma.

Treatment regimens that use local resistance data to achieve consistent eradication rates of 90% can eliminate disease burden. This burden includes gastric cancer; *H. pylori* is estimated to cause 89% of cases of noncardia gastric carcinoma.[112] To decrease the third most common cause of cancer death (gastric cancer), countries with a high disease burden could consider *H. pylori* screening and eradication programs to assess the overall impact on related cancer deaths as well as the economic burden of such an endeavor.[63]

NEW REFERENCES SINCE THE SEVENTH EDITION

23. Cuadrado-Lavin A, Salcines-Caviedes JR, Carrascosa MF, et al. Antimicrobial susceptibility of *Helicobacter pylori* to six antibiotics currently used in Spain. *J Antimicrob Chemother*. 2012;67(1):170-173.
58. Graham DY, Lee YC, Wu MS. Rational *Helicobacter pylori* therapy: evidence-based medicine rather than medicine-based evidence. *Clin Gastroenterol Hepatol*. 2014;12(2):177-186.e173, discussion e112-173.
63. Herrero R, Parsonnet J, Greenberg ER. Prevention of gastric cancer. *JAMA*. 2014;312(12):1197-1198.
76. Lacy BE, Talley NJ, Locke GR 3rd, et al. Review article: current treatment options and management of functional dyspepsia. *Aliment Pharmacol Ther*. 2012;36(1):3-15.
85. Liou JM, Chen CC, Chen MJ, et al. Sequential versus triple therapy for the first-line treatment of *Helicobacter pylori:* a multicentre, open-label, randomised trial. *Lancet*. 2013;381:205-213.
92. Malfertheiner P, Megraud F, O'Morain CA, et al. Management of *Helicobacter pylori* infection: the Maastricht IV/ Florence Consensus Report. *Gut*. 2012;61(5): 646-664.
98. Megraud F, Coenen S, Versporten A, et al. *Helicobacter pylori* resistance to antibiotics in Europe and its relationship to antibiotic consumption. *Gut*. 2013; 62(1):34-42.
100. Molina-Infante J, Romano M, Fernandez-Bermejo M, et al. Optimized nonbismuth quadruple therapies cure most patients with *Helicobacter pylori* infection in populations with high rates of antibiotic resistance. *Gastroenterology*. 2013;145(1):121-128. e121.
113. Plummer M, Franceschi S, Vignat J, Forman D, de Martel C. Global burden of gastric cancer attributable to *Helicobacter pylori*. *Int J Cancer*. 2015;136(2):487-490.
120. Ruggiero P. *Helicobacter pylori* infection: what's new. *Curr Opin Infect Dis*. 2012;25(3):337-344.
129. Su P, Li Y, Li H, et al. Antibiotic resistance of *Helicobacter pylori* isolated in the southeast coastal region of China. *Helicobacter*. 2013;18(4):274-279.
132. Tonkic A, Tonkic M, Lehours P, Megraud F. Epidemiology and diagnosis of *Helicobacter pylori* infection. *Helicobacter*. 2012;17(suppl 1):1-8.

The full reference list for this chapter is available at ExpertConsult.com.

136 *Kingella kingae*

Eric A. Porsch • Joseph W. St. Geme III

Kingella kingae is being recognized increasingly as an important cause of invasive disease in young children, thus reflecting improved cultivation methods and new molecular diagnostics for this fastidious organism. Other members of the *Kingella* genus include *K. denitrificans, K. oralis,* and *K. potus. K. denitrificans* and *K. oralis* are commensals in the human oral cavity and are uncommon pathogens. *K. potus* is a commensal in the oral cavity of arboreal mammals and has been isolated from a human wound caused by an animal bite.[67]

HISTORY

K. kingae was first isolated in 1960 from blood, joint fluid, bone exudates, and throat swabs by Elizabeth O. King, a bacteriologist at the Centers for Disease Control and Prevention. King's initial studies suggested that this organism was a novel *Moraxella* spp., thereby prompting shipment of samples to Henriksen and Bovre at the University of Oslo, Norway, for their opinion.[51] Work by these investigators confirmed King's initial impressions and led to a publication describing the new species, which they named *Moraxella kingii* in honor of King.[51] Additional studies in the late 1960s and 1970s established significant differences between *M. kingii* and other members of the *Moraxella* genus and resulted in reclassification as a novel genus and renaming of the organism as *Kingella kingae* in 1976.[22,52]

Until the 1990s, *K. kingae* was largely ignored as a human pathogen because of its infrequent recovery in association with disease, generally in young patients with septic arthritis, osteomyelitis, or endocarditis.[37,39,63,66,75,80,86,91,96] As novel culture-based isolation techniques were developed in the early 1990s,[108] the frequency of reported infections caused by *K. kingae* increased. Numerous studies using polymerase chain reaction (PCR)-based diagnostic techniques have shown that *K. kingae* is present in a significant percentage of culture-negative joint fluid and bone samples from patients with suspected osteoarticular infection.[26,27,34,36,54,73,89,93,97] More recent evidence indicates that *K. kingae* is the leading cause of septic arthritis in children 6 to 36 months of age, more common even than *Staphylococcus aureus*.[36]

MICROBIOLOGY

K. kingae is a gram-negative bacterium that belongs to the Neisseriaceae family and is only distantly related to other members of this family. It is a facultative anaerobic, β-hemolytic, small bacillus (0.6 to 1 μm × 1 to 3 μm) that appears as pairs or short chains with tapered ends (Fig. 136.1) and often resists decolorization, thus sometimes resulting in misidentification as a gram-positive organism.[51,98] *K. kingae* produces acid from glucose and maltose but not from other sugars and is oxidase positive and catalase, urease, and indole negative. Growth is supported on blood and chocolate agar but not on Krigler or MacConkey agar. Optimal growth occurs at 37°C (98.6°F) in a 5% to 10% carbon dioxide–enhanced atmosphere, but few strains are truly capnophilic.[98] Colonies from growth on solid agar appear as three distinct types: spreading/corroding, nonspreading/noncorroding, and domed.[59,62,102] The spreading/corroding colony type produces marked indentations on the agar surface, develops a peripheral fringe around the small central raised colony, and is associated with high-density piliation. The nonspreading/noncorroding colony has a smaller fringe with a large, flat, central colony and is associated with low-density piliation. The domed colony produces no fringe and is nonpiliated.[62] *K. kingae* is most easily differentiated from *K. denitrificans, K. oralis, K. potus,* and *Neisseria* spp. by a distinct narrow zone of β-hemolysis surrounding colonies on blood agar plates.

The partial or complete genome sequences of multiple *K. kingae* isolates are now publicly available. The genome size ranges from approximately 1.95 to approximately 2.15 megabases (Mb), has 46.6% to 46.8% GC content, and encodes approximately 1820 to approximately 2170 polypeptides (the range likely reflects the fact that some genomes are only partially sequenced). Genomic comparisons have revealed remarkably conserved synteny across *K. kingae* strains and an overall lack of synteny with other Neisseriaceae family members, a finding that highlights the classification of *K. kingae* as a unique taxonomic unit.[47,58] With regard to extrachromosomal DNA, Banerjee and colleagues[6] identified an approximately 15-kb R-plasmid and a 50-kb or greater

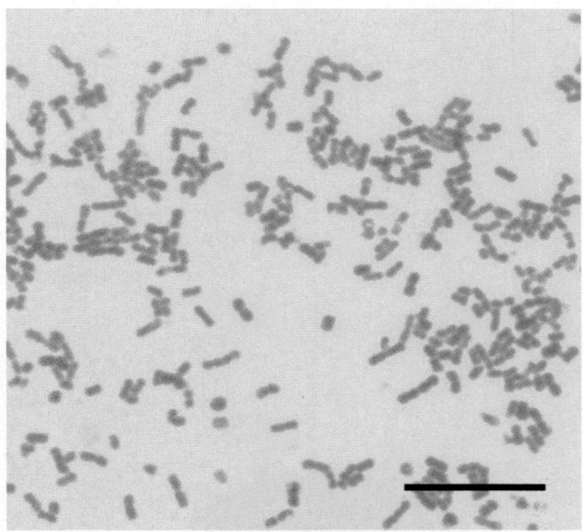

FIG. 136.1 Gram stain of *Kingella kingae* strain 269-492, a septic arthritis isolate. Scale bar = 10 μm.

plasmid harboring a TEM-1 β-lactamase in 12 *K. kingae* strains. In addition, Rouli and colleagues[83] identified an approximately 15.5-kb plasmid encoding a TEM-1 β-lactamase and a streptomycin kinase in *K. kingae* strain KK247. Various studies have demonstrated that the *K. kingae* population structure is clonal.

To date, *K. kingae* has never been isolated from a nonhuman source, a finding suggesting that the organism is human specific.

EPIDEMIOLOGY

Carriage and Transmission

K. kingae is a human commensal that colonizes the posterior pharynx asymptomatically in a subset of the population and occasionally invades the bloodstream to produce invasive disease. Using a novel vancomycin-containing medium developed in the early 1990s for isolation of *K. kingae* from the pharynx[108] or PCR assays, several studies have examined carriage rates in the healthy population.[29,98,105,109,114] Based on studies conducted primarily in Israel and Europe, colonization with *K. kingae* begins at approximately 6 months of age and increases to a rate of 9% to 12% in children 12 to 24 months of age.[3,29,45,105,109] The carriage rate gradually decreases in older persons, a finding suggesting that immune system development in healthy hosts may be responsible for upper respiratory tract clearance.[105,109]

To achieve a better understanding of the transmission of *K. kingae* strains circulating in the community, multiple genotyping techniques have been developed, including pulsed field gel electrophoresis (PFGE),[109] random amplification of polymorphic DNA (RAPD),[110] multilocus sequence typing (MLST),[4,10,16] *por* gene sequencing,[6] *rtxA* gene sequencing,[4,16] and DNA uptake sequence typing (DUST).[10] In a study that compared upper respiratory tract isolates from a cohort of healthy persons and a set of invasive isolates over a 15-year period,[109] genotypically indistinguishable strains were clustered in geographic regions and households, thereby suggesting person-to-person transmission among family members and close contacts. In agreement with this hypothesis, a study of intrafamilial oropharyngeal transmission revealed that 55% of patients with *K. kingae* osteoarticular infection and 40% of asymptomatic carriers had siblings who were colonized with *K. kingae*.[56] High rates of person-to-person transmission have also been documented in day care facilities.[88] In addition, many strains circulating among healthy persons matched historical strains recovered from sites of invasive disease, thus indicating that certain strains may persist in the population.[109]

Yagupsky and colleagues[110] examined paired isolates from the pharynx and bloodstream in three children with *K. kingae* bacteremia and found that the pharyngeal and blood isolates were genotypically identical in each case based on PFGE typing and RAPD; this finding provided evidence that colonization of the posterior pharynx is a precursor to invasive disease. Similarly, Basmaci and associates[13] reported isolation of *K. kingae* from the pharynx in children with confirmed *K. kingae* septic arthritis.

Ceroni and colleagues[31] examined *K. kingae* oropharyngeal colonization density in healthy carriers and in children with invasive *K. kingae* disease by using real-time PCR and observed no differences. This finding suggested that colonization density does not directly influence the development of invasive *K. kingae* disease.

Invasive Disease

The most comprehensive study to date on the epidemiology of invasive disease was a multicenter study in Israel that examined a total of 321 cases of *K. kingae* disease.[40] In this report, 296 of the 321 pediatric cases involved children younger than 4 years of age, thus representing an annual incidence of 9.4 of 100,000 children from birth to 4 years of age. Only four cases involved children younger than 6 months of age.[40] Children younger than 4 years of age who were diagnosed with *K. kingae* disease were generally otherwise healthy,[40] whereas older children and adults who developed *K. kingae* disease usually had underlying predisposing conditions, including malignant disease, immunosuppression, or cardiac valve pathologic processes. The 321 total cases included 140 cases of septic arthritis, 19 cases of osteomyelitis, 7 cases of osteomyelitis with septic arthritis of the adjacent joint, and 3 cases of tenosynovitis, for a total 169 skeletal infections (53% of 321). The remaining cases included 140 cases of bacteremia without a focus (44% of 321), 4 cases of bacteremia and lower respiratory tract infection, and 8 cases of endocarditis.[40] Other reports have described *K. kingae* as a rare cause of pericarditis,[71] meningitis,[92] peritonitis,[21] urinary tract infection,[79] and ocular infection.[23,74]

Studies in France and Switzerland that used sensitive molecular approaches have added to our understanding of the epidemiology of *K. kingae* osteoarticular infection. In France, a 2-year prospective study of osteoarticular infections in children 15 years of age or younger found that *K. kingae* was present in the blood, bone, or joint samples in 52% of patients.[45] In Switzerland, a 3-year study of *K. kingae* carriage and invasive disease found the highest incidence of *K. kingae* disease in children 7 to 12 and 13 to 24 months of age and a progressively lower incidence in children between 24 and 48 months of age.[5]

In Israel, invasive *K. kingae* disease occurs throughout the year and is most common during November and December and least common between February and April.[40,41] In contrast, the occurrence of carriage is more uniform throughout the year, a finding suggesting that the seasonal distribution of invasive *K. kingae* disease cannot be readily explained by the epidemiology of pharyngeal carriage. In Switzerland, invasive disease is most common in autumn, whereas carriage is roughly uniform throughout the year.[5]

The presence of two distinct pediatric populations serviced by the same medical system in southern Israel enabled Amit and colleagues[1] to study the epidemiology of *K. kingae* disease in this setting. Interestingly, the incidence of invasive disease in Westernized Jews (12.21 of 100,000) was significantly higher than the incidence of invasive disease in the Bedouin population (5.83 of 100,000). These findings differ from observations with other respiratory pathogens, such as *Streptococcus pneumoniae*, which have been shown to produce more morbidity in the Bedouin population.[1]

In a study presenting findings in patients with *K. kingae* disease, Yagupsky and colleagues[109] found that approximately 50% of children display symptoms of upper respiratory tract infection, 15% to 20% have stomatitis, and 15% to 20% have diarrhea, thereby raising the possibility that concomitant viral infection contributes to development of invasive disease. In agreement with these findings, a study in France observed that 19 of 21 patients with proven *K. kingae* osteoarticular infection and only 3 of 8 patients with non–*K. kingae* osteoarticular infection had at least one respiratory virus present in throat swabs that were collected at the time of admission.[12] Using a PCR array to detect 18 different respiratory viruses, human rhinovirus (12 of 21), coronavirus OC43 (four of 21), parainfluenza virus 1, 2, 3, or 4 (three of 21), enterovirus (two of 21), and adenovirus (two of 21) were identified in the upper respiratory tract of patients with concurrent *K. kingae* osteoarticular infection.[12]

El Houmami and associates[44] described a series of nine *K. kingae* osteoarticular infections (five epidemic and four sporadic) in a French hospital occurring between April and October 2013. Of the seven patients younger than 24 months of age, five had antecedent hand, food, and mouth disease, and two had antecedent stomatitis. Both patients older than 24 months of age did not have evidence of oral manifestations. Retrospective analysis of an 11-month-old child who presented with arthritis with antecedent hand, food, and mouth disease revealed the presence of *K. kingae* DNA in stored joint fluid and coxsackievirus-A6 in a stored stool specimen.[44] These studies strongly support the hypothesis that upper respiratory tract viral infection contributes to the development of *K. kingae* invasive disease and suggest a possible link between the emerging European coxsackievirus-A6 epidemic and *K. kingae* disease.

Day Care Facility Attendance

A longitudinal study in Israel in the mid-1990s aimed to evaluate the transmission of *K. kingae* strains among day care facility attendees.[88] Fifty isolates were collected over an 11-month period by sampling two cohorts of day care facility attendees every 2 weeks. These isolates were compared with a collection of 60 epidemiologically diverse respiratory tract and invasive isolates. Based on a variety of typing techniques, children were found routinely to carry the same strain continuously or intermittently for weeks or months. Different strains were periodically able to replace the originally detected strain. Interestingly, a single strain represented 28% of the isolates and was most prevalent over the first 6 months of the study, and a different strain represented 46% of the isolates over the remaining 5 months.[88] Epidemiologically unrelated strains showed much greater variability in relatedness than isolates from the day care facility cohorts. A study examining the prevalence of *K. kingae* colonization in young children in Israel found that day care facility attendance is a risk factor for colonization.[2]

To date, 10 reports of day care facility outbreaks of invasive *K. kingae* disease have been described: two in the United States, two in France, and six in Israel.[20,42,43,64,85,101,100,103,106] The first reported *K. kingae* outbreak occurred in Minnesota in 2003 and involved three cases of osteomyelitis or septic arthritis in children from the same classroom of 16- to 24-month-old children.[64] Carriage analysis of other attendees of the same facility revealed an overall colonization rate of 13% (15 of 122) and a peak colonization rate of 45% (nine of 20) in the classroom of 16- to 24-month-old children. All three children with invasive disease had concurrent or antecedent upper respiratory tract illness. In North Carolina in 2007, a case of confirmed *K. kingae* endocarditis and potential meningitis and a case of suspected intervertebral diskitis and osteomyelitis were identified in a 2-week period in children who attended the same day care facility.[85] A 2011 outbreak in France had an overall attack rate of 20.4% (5 of 24) and a carriage rate of 85% (11 of 13) among classmates available for sampling,[20] and a subsequent outbreak in 2013 had an attack rate of 23.8% (5 of 21) and a classmate carriage rate of 93.3% (14 of 15).[42]

In Israel in 2005, one confirmed and two suspected cases of *K. kingae* skeletal infections were diagnosed in children from the same day care facility, and four of 11 classmates were colonized.[106] PFGE demonstrated that the pharyngeal and invasive isolates from the source day care facility were genotypically identical and that pharyngeal isolates from a control facility were genotypically distinct.[106] In 2012, one confirmed case of bacteremia and 1 presumed case of septic arthritis were identified in the same day care facility, with an overall classroom attack rate of 5.6% (two of 36) and a classmate carriage rate of 11.8% (four of 34).[101]

Another two cases of confirmed septic arthritis were identified in a classroom in a 2013 outbreak with an attack rate of 15.4% (two of 13) and a carriage rate among classmates of 45.4% (five of 11).[101] In 2014, three additional outbreaks in Israel were identified.[43,103] Each of these outbreaks had a classroom attack rate of 14.3% to 16.7% and a carriage rate among classmates of 33.3% to 58.3%.[43,103] The 2005 and the three 2014 outbreaks in Israel occurred in so-called closed communities, with three outbreaks occurring on military bases and one occurring in a "kibbutz" commune, findings suggesting that the social communalities represented in these environments facilitate circulation of *K. kingae* among children in the susceptible age range.[103]

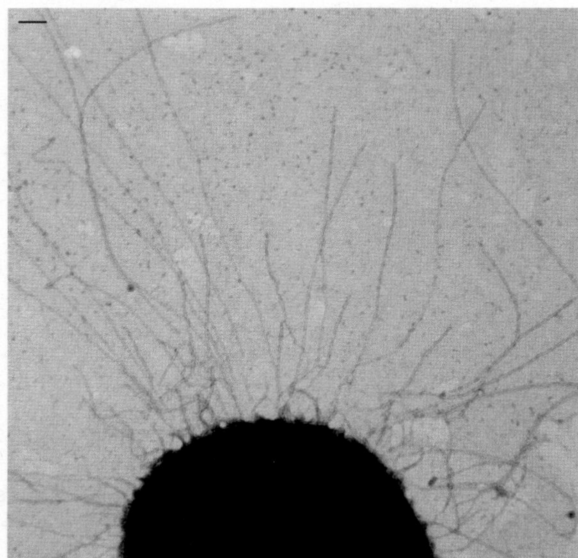

FIG. 136.2 Transmission electron micrograph of type IV pili emanating from the surface of *Kingella kingae* strain 269-492. The sample was negatively stained with uranyl acetate. Scale bar = 100 nm.

PATHOGENESIS AND IMMUNITY

The pathogenesis of disease caused by *K. kingae* is believed to begin with colonization of the posterior pharynx.[98,111] The process of colonization likely involves adherence to respiratory epithelial cells, which is mediated in vitro in part by polymeric surface pili (Fig. 136.2).[59-61] *K. kingae* pili are classified as type IV pili and are composed primarily of a major pilin subunit, PilA1.[60] In addition, *K. kingae* pili contain two pilus-associated proteins, called PilC1 and PilC2, that appear to play complementary roles in promoting pilus assembly and in mediating adherence to respiratory epithelial cells.[60] PilC1 and PilC2 differentially modulate type IV pili–mediated twitching motility because PilC1 mediates robust motility through a calcium ion binding–dependent mechanism, and PilC2 mediates modest twitching motility through a calcium ion binding–independent mechanism.[77] Consistent with the conclusion that pili promote *K. kingae* colonization, examination of a collection of pharyngeal isolates of *K. kingae* demonstrated that most are piliated and express abundant pili.[61]

K. kingae also produces a nonpilus adhesive protein called Knh, which is essential for full-level adherence to cultured respiratory epithelial cells.[78] Knh shares homology with the *Neisseria meningitidis* NhhA adhesin and belongs to the trimeric autotransporter family of proteins. Like other trimeric autotransporters, Knh has an N-terminal signal sequence, a characteristic C terminus, and a modular internal passenger domain that is ultimately surface localized. The passenger domain contains a series of 19 YadA-like head domains with similarity to the β-roll that has been implicated in the adhesive activity of the *Yersinia* YadA trimeric autotransporter and a stalk that contains seven Trp ring domains, three neck domains, three KG domains, and an iSneck2 domain. Disruption of the gene encoding Knh results in an approximately 50% decrease in adherence in in vitro assays.[78] A study by Rempe and colleagues[81] demonstrated that Knh is modified with hexose residues by an unconventional N-linking glycosyltransferase and that glycosylation is essential for the adhesive properties of the protein.

After colonization of the posterior pharynx, *K. kingae* must translocate across the pharyngeal epithelium to enter the bloodstream. Given that patients with invasive *K. kingae* disease frequently have manifestations of viral respiratory tract infection, evidence of herpetic gingivostomatitis, or signs of aphthous stomatitis, it is possible that virus-induced damage to the respiratory mucosa facilitates *K. kingae* invasion of the bloodstream.[42,44,98,111] Beyond the role of viral coinfection, *K. kingae* produces a potent extracellular toxin that belongs to the RTX (repeat in toxin) family of toxins and is capable of lysing epithelial, synovial, and macrophage cells.[62] In vitro studies have shown that the RTX toxin is able to form 1.9-nm pores in artificial membranes and can be delivered to host cells by outer membrane vesicle secretion.[7,70] By using an infant rat infection model, an isogenic RTX-deficient mutant was shown to be attenuated in virulence compared with the parental strain, a finding suggesting that the toxin may play a role in the pathogenesis of *K. kingae* invasive disease.[33] This toxin may facilitate disruption of the respiratory epithelium, perhaps with an increased effect in the setting of viral coinfection. The *K. kingae RTX* locus resembles the *RTX* locus in *Moraxella bovis* and *N. meningitidis* and was likely acquired through horizontal transfer.[62]

Once in the bloodstream, *K. kingae* must be able to evade a variety of host defense mechanisms. Similar to other bacterial pathogens that produce bacteremic disease in children, *K. kingae* produces an extracellular polysaccharide capsule (Fig. 136.3).[17,78,90] By analogy to other encapsulated bacteria, encapsulation of *K. kingae* may facilitate resistance to serum killing activity and opsonophagocytosis and thereby promote intravascular survival and dissemination to distant sites.[111] Analysis of a large collection of invasive and carrier isolates revealed a total of four different capsule types: type a (polymer of GalNAc-Kdo), type b (polymer of GlcNAc-Kdo), type c (polymer of ribose-Kdo), and type d (polymer of GlcNAc-galactose). Interestingly, strains expressing the type c or type d capsule are almost exclusively carrier isolates, and strains expressing the type a and type b capsules account for approximately 96% of invasive disease isolates; this finding suggests that the latter two capsule types may play a role in the development of *K. kingae* invasive disease.[116,117] In addition to the capsular polysaccharide, *K. kingae* has been shown to secrete a linear galactofuranose exopolysaccharide with antibiofilm activity.[17,90]

In patients in whom *K. kingae* is able to persist in the bloodstream, the organism may produce uncomplicated bacteremia or may instead disseminate to joints, bones, or the endocardium.[98,111] Analysis of a large collection of *K. kingae* systemic isolates demonstrated that strains recovered from the blood of patients with uncomplicated bacteremia were generally piliated but typically expressed relatively few pili.[61] In contrast, strains recovered from joint fluid, bone aspirates, or the blood of patients with endocarditis were generally nonpiliated.[61] It is possible that low-density piliation facilitates a tropism for joints, bones, and the endocardium and potentiates an inflammatory response, which then selects against piliated organisms. Consistent with this possibility, pili promote efficient adherence to cultured synovial cells. Similar to type IV pili expressed by other pathogens, *K. kingae* pili are regulated by a

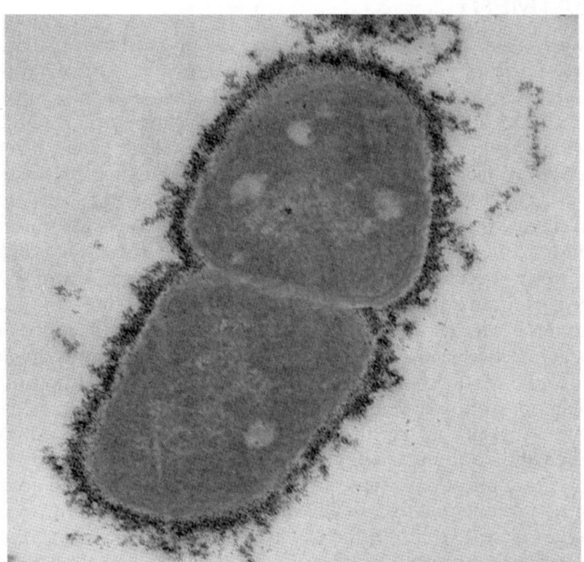

FIG. 136.3 Transmission electron micrograph of thin-sectioned, cationic ferritin-stained *Kingella kingae* strain 269-492. The dark layer of electron density on the surface of the bacteria is caused by cationic ferritin interacting with the polysaccharide capsule. Scale bar = 500 nm.

transcription factor called σ54 and by a two-component sensor/regulator system termed PilS/PilR.[60] Mutations in the PilS sensor result in a reduced density of pili, similar to the relative decrease in density of pili in isolates recovered from the bloodstream in contrast to the posterior pharynx. Conversely, mutations in the PilR response regulator result in elimination of piliation, similar to the absence of pili in isolates from joints and bones.[60] It is unclear which environmental factors influence σ54, PilS, and PilR activity and control the density of *K. kingae* piliation. The three different colony morphologies that are detectable on agar plates and correlate with the level of piliation may reflect mutations in PilS and PilR.[61]

To investigate the role of the host immune system in development of *K. kingae* disease in healthy persons, Slonim and colleagues[87] examined serum immunoglobulin (Ig) A and IgG levels against outer membrane proteins in 19 children with invasive disease. As expected, children convalescing from invasive disease had significant increases in IgA and IgG levels. Further analysis has demonstrated that the age incidence of disease is inversely correlated with serum IgA and IgG levels in healthy persons. Infants younger than 6 months of age have undetectable serum IgA but high serum IgG levels, a finding suggesting that protection from invasive disease in this age group results from maternally derived IgG.[87] Children between 6 and 18 months of age have the highest age incidence of disease and the lowest serum IgG levels.[40] Children 24 months of age and older have a progressively decreasing incidence of disease and progressively increasing IgG and IgA levels, thus suggesting that carriage or exposure to *K. kingae* during the first 2 years of life may be an immunizing event. However, *K. kingae* outer membrane protein epitopes are polymorphic from strain to strain; this property raises the possibility that the immune response is strain specific and may not prevent recolonization by an antigenically distinct strain.[112]

CLINICAL MANIFESTATIONS

Osteoarticular Infections

Septic arthritis caused by *K. kingae* is monoarticular and most often involves the knee, hip, or ankle.[98] Other joints that may be affected include the wrist, shoulder, elbow, sternoclavicular, metacarpophalangeal, and tarsal joints. Fever is present in approximately 85% of patients with *K. kingae* arthritis. Arthrocentesis reveals purulent synovial fluid with a mean white blood cell count of approximately 130,000/mm^3 (range ~5000–300,000/mm^3) and a differential that contains more than 90% neutrophils.[41] Other laboratory measurements include a mean peripheral white blood cell count of 14,800/mm^3 (range, 6000–28,450/mm^3), a mean C-reactive protein of 3.7 mg/dL (range, 0.2–17.0 mg/dL), and a mean erythrocyte sedimentation rate of 44.1 mm/h (range, 5–140 mm/h).[39]

Osteomyelitis resulting from *K. kingae* usually involves long bones such as the femur and tibia.[98] However, *K. kingae* also has an unusual predilection to produce disease in small bones, including the calcaneus and talus.[40,98] Children with *K. kingae* osteomyelitis often present with a limp and have a significantly more prolonged course of symptoms before presentation in contrast to patients with septic arthritis (9.2 ± 9.4 vs. 3.2 ± 3.0 days). Laboratory measurements include a mean peripheral white blood cell count of 13,888/mm^3 (range, 5860–2,000/mm^3), a mean C-reactive protein of 1.8 mg/dL (range, 0.2–4.3 mg/dL), and a mean erythrocyte sedimentation rate of 40.0 mm/h (range, 12–85 mm/h).[40]

Among patients younger than 4 years of age with spondylodiskitis, at least one-fourth have *K. kingae* infection.[28,32,48] In order of frequency, infection involves the lumbar, thoracolumbar, cervical, thoracic, and lumbosacral intervertebral spaces. Patients with *K. kingae* spondylodiskitis can have a limp, back pain, refusal to sit or walk, or neurologic symptoms, but the symptoms are often mild. Fever is present in two-thirds of patients but rarely exceeds 39°C (102.2°F). Other skeletal infections caused by *K. kingae* include dactylitis[35] and tenosynovitis.[42,44,98]

K. kingae bacteremia without evidence of endocarditis or other localizing signs is being increasingly recognized in young children. The duration of symptoms before diagnosis ranges from 1 to 7 days, and the mean maximal fever is 39°C (102.2°F).[41,98] Occasional patients have a maculopapular rash resembling the rash in early meningococcal or gonococcal infection.[49,91] Laboratory evaluation often reveals an elevated peripheral white blood cell count (mean, 12,700/mm^3; range, 7120–47,040/mm^3), modest elevation of C-reactive protein (mean, 2.2 mg/dL, range 0.6–13.4 mg/dL), and significant elevation of erythrocyte sedimentation rate (mean 50 mm/h; range, 14–115 mm/h).[40]

K. kingae is included in the HACEK (*Haemophilus, Actinobacillus, Cardiobacterium, Eikenella,* and *Kingella* spp.) group of bacteria accountable for 3% to 5% of cases of bacterial endocarditis. In contrast to other *K. kingae* infections, *K. kingae* endocarditis is most common in older children and adults.[98] In approximately 50% of cases, infection involves a native valve, often related to a predisposing cardiac malformation or rheumatic heart disease.[18,76,82,95,98,115] Disease usually involves the left side of the heart, most often the mitral valve.[98,111] Patients with *K. kingae* endocarditis typically have fever and elevated C-reactive protein and erythrocyte sedimentation rate.[40] Complications can be severe and include congestive heart failure, septic shock, mycotic aneurysm, pulmonary infarction, meningitis, and stroke, and the overall mortality rate is approximately 16%.[18,46,53,68,82,85,95,115]

DIAGNOSIS

The recovery of *K. kingae* from purulent specimens seeded onto solid culture media is poor, often resulting in a lack of growth. The yield of cultures is improved significantly by inoculating specimens into Isolator 1.5 microbial tubes or aerobic blood culture vials from a variety of automated blood culture systems such as BacTec, BacT/Alert, and Hemoline DUO.[98] When positive blood culture vials are subcultured onto routine solid media, *K. kingae* grows readily, a finding suggesting that exudates may inhibit growth and that dilution of purulent material in a large volume of broth may decrease the concentration of inhibitory factors, thereby improving the recovery of this fastidious organism.[98] In studies in which blood culture vials were routinely used for culturing synovial fluid aspirates from young children with suspected joint infections, *K. kingae* was isolated in almost one-half of the patients who ultimately had culture-proved bacterial disease.[73,102] Matrix-assisted laser desorption ionization–time of flight mass spectrometry has been shown to be effective for the identification of *K. kingae*.[38]

Studies published since the 1990s have demonstrated that PCR dramatically enhances detection of *K. kingae* in bone and joint fluid samples in contrast to routine cultures and blood culture vials. Some studies have used universal 16S rRNA primers,[24,72,89] and others have used specific primers that amplify either the *K. kingae cpn60* gene[36] or the *K. kingae rtxA* gene.[24,27,34,54,69,72] As an example, Chometon and coworkers[36] sequentially analyzed bone and joint samples by using blood culture vials, conventional PCR with universal primers, and real-time PCR with primers derived from the *K. kingae cpn60* gene and achieved a *K. kingae* detection rate that increased from 29% of all microbiologically proved cases with blood culture, to 41% with conventional PCR with universal primers, to 45% with *K. Kingae*–specific PCR, thus accounting for approximately 80% of microbiologically proved cases in children younger than 3 years of age.[36] *K. kingae*–specific PCR approaches are typically more sensitive than PCR assays using broad-range16S rRNA primers.

Given the fastidious nature of *K. kingae* and the difficulty in isolation of the organism from the blood and sites of infection, the clinical value of oropharyngeal PCR detection of *K. kingae* in pediatric patients with suspected osteoarticular infection has been investigated.[25,30] During a 3-year prospective study in a Swiss hospital, a total of 10 patients 6 to 48 months of age had magnetic resonance imaging evidence consistent with spondylodiskitis. Each patient presented with mild to moderate clinical symptoms and inflammatory responses, and all blood culture results were negative. PCR detection of *K. kingae* in peripheral blood was positive in 20% (two of 10) of the patients, but PCR analysis of oropharyngeal swabs was 100% (10 of 10) positive; these results provided reasonable suspicion that *K. kingae* was responsible for the spondylodiskitis.[25]

In a separate study, 123 6- to 48-month-old patients with osteoarticular complaints were screened for oropharyngeal *K. kingae*.[30] Forty patients met the case definition of osteoarticular infection: 30 had *K. kingae* osteoarticular infection, one had another organism, and nine had no microbial diagnosis. All 30 patients with *K. kingae* osteoarticular infection, and eight of the 84 patients without osteoarticular infection or with osteoarticular infection caused by another organism tested positive for oropharyngeal *K. kingae*, thus resulting in a sensitivity of 100% and a specificity of 90.5%.[30] All nine patients with osteoarticular infection with no microbial diagnosis tested positive for oropharyngeal *K. kingae*, were treated for *K. kingae* osteoarticular infection, and demonstrated clinical improvement after treatment.[30]

Plain radiographs often complement culture and PCR-based diagnostic methods; they demonstrate soft tissue swelling and joint effusions in approximately 50% of patients with septic arthritis and show lytic lesions or disk space narrowing in 95% of cases of osteomyelitis or spondylodiskitis.[98] Technetium-99m bone scans may be helpful in diagnosing *K. kingae* osteomyelitis during the early course of disease, before abnormalities are present on plain radiographs.[48,49] Echocardiography is helpful in diagnosing *K. kingae* endocarditis and often reveals large vegetations, especially in patients who have had symptoms for a prolonged period or have clinical evidence of embolization.

Given that gram-positive cocci such as *S. aureus* and *Streptococcus pyogenes* are the other main pathogens responsible for osteoarticular infections in the pediatric population, several studies have investigated various approaches to distinguish infection with these organisms from infection with *K. kingae*. Because of the typically mild to moderate clinical and biologic features of *K. kingae* osteoarticular infection compared with osteoarticular infection caused by gram-positive cocci, Ceroni and colleagues[26] proposed a predictive score system using four variables: body temperature lower than 38°C, serum C-reactive protein lower than 5.5 mg/L, white blood cell count lower than 14,000/mm^3, and band forms lower than 150/mm^3. In their study population, a total of 96.7% of patients with *K. kingae* osteoarticular infection met at least three criteria, whereas only 10% of patients with other pathogens met at least three criteria. However, Basmaci and colleagues[14,15] found that this scoring system was not able to distinguish between *K. kingae* and *S. aureus* osteoarticular infection effectively in a different study population, and the only significant differentiating factor was younger age for the patients with *K. kingae* osteoarticular infection. Simultaneous targeted *K. kingae* and *S. aureus* real-time PCR on synovial fluid samples was shown to be effective in detecting *K. kingae* but was less sensitive than culture in detecting *S. aureus*.[50] A study comparing the early magnetic resonance imaging characteristics of osteoarticular infection caused by *K. kingae* versus gram-positive cocci found that bone reaction was less frequent and soft tissue reaction was less severe in infection with *K. kingae*.[57] In addition, epiphysis cartilage abscesses were present only in *K. kingae* osteoarticular infection.[57]

TREATMENT

K. kingae is almost always susceptible to second- and third-generation cephalosporins, aminoglycosides, macrolides, trimethoprim-sulfamethoxazole, tetracyclines, fluoroquinolones, and chloramphenicol.[55,65,98,107] Most *K. kingae* isolates are susceptible to penicillins, although in vitro susceptibility to oxacillin is relatively reduced. There are increasing reports of β-lactamase production with varying degrees of activity.[11,55,65,99,105,113] Two studies described a series of *K. kingae* isolates with relatively low-level β-lactam resistance; one study reported minimum inhibitory concentrations of 0.094 to 2 μg/mL for penicillin,[113] and the other study reported minimum inhibitory concentrations of 0.25 to 8 μg/mL for amoxicillin.[11] Studies have revealed that the TEM-1 β-lactamase can also be chromosomally or plasmid encoded in *K. kingae*.[8,9,19] Between 40% and 100% of isolates are resistant to clindamycin,[99,107] and virtually all isolates are resistant to trimethoprim and glycopeptide antibiotics, including vancomycin.[41,107]

Given the lack of controlled studies, no detailed guidelines for preferred antibiotic and length of treatment course have been developed for *K. kingae* infections. Typically, treatment varies based on accepted measures for other pathogens. Given the reduced susceptibility of many *K. kingae* isolates to oxacillin and clindamycin and the increasing recognition of β-lactam resistance, administration of a β-lactamase–resistant penicillin or a second-generation or third-generation cephalosporin is appropriate for suspected skeletal infections while laboratory results are pending.[94,99,98] In areas where methicillin-resistant *S. aureus* is common, addition of vancomycin is recommended.[84] Once *K. kingae* is identified and β-lactam resistance is excluded, antibiotic therapy is commonly changed to amoxicillin or cefuroxime. The switch from intravenous to oral antibiotic therapy should be evaluated based on clinical response and assessment of acute-phase reactants such as C-reactive protein.

The length of antibiotic treatment for *K. kingae* disease has varied based on specific type of infection. Treatment has generally varied from 2 to 3 weeks for *K. kingae* arthritis, from 3 to 6 weeks for *K. kingae* osteomyelitis, and from 3 to 12 weeks for *K. kingae* spondylodiskitis.[98] Patients with septic arthritis usually respond well to antibiotic therapy and do not require repeated joint aspirations or invasive surgical procedures.[98]

Patients with *K. kingae* bacteremia typically have a relatively benign course and are usually treated initially with an intravenous β-lactam antibiotic and are then switched to oral therapy once the clinical condition has improved. Antibiotic therapy is generally continued for a total of 1 to 2 weeks.[104]

Children with *K. kingae* native valve endocarditis are usually treated intravenously with a β-lactam agent alone or in combination with an aminoglycoside.[98] Typically, the length of treatment is 4 to 7 weeks.[98] Because of the potential risk for life-threatening valve damage resulting from endocarditis, patients who do not respond to antibiotic therapy may require early surgical intervention.[82,95,115]

PREVENTION

In the reported cases of day care outbreaks, oral antibiotics were administered to contacts of the infected children to prevent further spread. The antibiotic courses varied and included either rifampin, 2 mg/kg up to 600 mg per dose twice daily for 2 days; rifampin, 10 mg/kg twice daily for 2 days[20]; a combination of rifampin, 10 mg/kg and amoxicillin, 40 mg/kg twice daily for 2 days[85]; or a combination of rifampin, 20 mg/kg twice daily for 2 days and amoxicillin, 80 mg/kg twice daily for 4 days.[106] A wide range of antibiotic prophylaxis efficacy has been reported. For example, a combination of rifampin, 20 mg/kg twice daily for 2 days, and amoxicillin, 80 mg/kg per day for 2 days, was prescribed to classroom contacts in three Israeli day care facility outbreaks for which postprophylactic treatment carriage rates were reported. In two of these outbreaks, complete eradication of carriage in contacts (4 of 11 to 0 of 11[106] and 5 of 11 to 0 of 11[101]) was reported, and in the other outbreak the carriage rate was reduced from 11.8% (4 of 34) to 5.6% (2 of 36).[101] Treatment with only rifampin, 10 mg/kg up to 600 mg per dose twice daily for 2 days, appears less efficacious, with one study showing a 0% reduction of colonized contacts after prophylaxis[20] and another study showing only a 14.2% reduction in colonized contacts after prophylaxis.[42]

Currently no measures are available to prevent *K. kingae* infection in the general population. Given that *K. kingae* expresses a capsular polysaccharide,[17,78] it is possible that a polysaccharide-conjugate vaccine would be a viable approach to prevention of disease, similar to the situation with *Haemophilus influenzae* type b, *S. pneumoniae,* and *N. meningitidis*. The observation that two capsule types account for more than 95% of invasive disease isolates suggests that the development of a polysaccharide-conjugate vaccine may be a feasible strategy to prevent *K. kingae* disease.

NEW REFERENCES SINCE THE SEVENTH EDITION

1. Amit U, Dagan R, Porat N, et al. Epidemiology of invasive *Kingella kingae* infections in 2 distinct pediatric populations cohabiting in one geographic area. *Pediatr Infect Dis J*. 2012;31(4):415-417.
2. Amit U, Dagan R, Yagupsky P. Prevalence of pharyngeal carriage of *Kingella kingae* in young children and risk factors for colonization. *Pediatr Infect Dis J*. 2013;32(2):191-193.
3. Amit U, Flaishmakher S, Dagan R, et al. Age-dependent carriage of *Kingella kingae* in young children and turnover of colonizing strains. *J Pediatric Infect Dis Soc*. 2014;3(2):160-162.
4. Amit U, Porat N, Basmaci R, et al. Genotyping of invasive *Kingella kingae* isolates reveals predominant clones and association with specific clinical syndromes. *Clin Infect Dis*. 2012;55(8):1074-1079.
5. Anderson de la Llana R, Dubois-Ferriere V, Maggio A, et al. Oropharyngeal *Kingella kingae* carriage in children: characteristics and correlation with osteoarticular infections. *Pediatr Res*. 2015;78(5):574-579.
6. Banerjee A, Kaplan JB, Soherwardy A, et al. Characterization of TEM-1 β-lactamase producing *Kingella kingae* clinical isolates. *Antimicrob Agents Chemother*. 2013; 57:4300-4306.
7. Barcena-Uribarri I, Benz R, Winterhalter M, et al. Pore forming activity of the potent RTX-toxin produced by pediatric pathogen *Kingella kingae*: Characterization and comparison to other RTX-family members. *Biochim Biophys Acta*. 2015;1848(7):1536-1544.
8. Basmaci R, Bidet P, Bercot B, et al. First identification of a chromosomally located penicillinase gene in *Kingella kingae* species isolated in continental Europe. *Antimicrob Agents Chemother*. 2014;58(10):6258-6259.
9. Basmaci R, Bidet P, Jost C, et al. Penicillinase-encoding gene blaTEM-1 may be plasmid borne or chromosomally located in *Kingella kingae* species. *Antimicrob Agents Chemother*. 2015;59(2):1377-1378.
10. Basmaci R, Bidet P, Yagupsky P, et al. Major intercontinentally distributed sequence types of *Kingella kingae* and development of a rapid molecular typing tool. *J Clin Microbiol*. 2014;52(11):3890-3897.
11. Basmaci R, Bonacorsi S, Bidet P, et al. Genotyping, local prevalence and international dissemination of beta-lactamase-producing *Kingella kingae* strains. *Clin Microbiol Infect*. 2014;20(11):O811-O817.
12. Basmaci R, Bonacorsi S, Ilharreborde B, et al. High respiratory virus oropharyngeal carriage rate during *Kingella kingae* osteoarticular infections in children. *Future Microbiol*. 2015;10(1):9-14.
14. Basmaci R, Ilharreborde B, Lorrot M, et al. Predictive score to discriminate *Kingella kingae* from *Staphylococcus aureus* arthritis in France. *Pediatr Infect Dis J*. 2011;30(12):1120-1122.
15. Basmaci R, Lorrot M, Bidet P, et al. Comparison of clinical and biologic features of *Kingella kingae* and *Staphylococcus aureus* arthritis at initial evaluation. *Pediatr Infect Dis J*. 2011;30(10):902-904.
16. Basmaci R, Yagupsky P, Ilharreborde B, et al. Multilocus sequence typing and *rtxA* toxin gene sequencing analysis of *Kingella kingae* isolates demonstrates genetic diversity and international clones. *PLoS ONE*. 2012;7(5):e38078.
19. Bidet P, Basmaci R, Guglielmini J, et al. Genome analysis of *Kingella kingae* strain KWG1 reveals how a beta-lactamase gene inserted in the chromosome of this species. *Antimicrob Agents Chemother*. 2015;60(1):703-708.
20. Bidet P, Collin E, Basmaci R, et al. Investigation of an outbreak of osteoarticular infections caused by *Kingella kingae* in a childcare center using molecular techniques. *Pediatr Infect Dis J*. 2013;32(5):558-560.
24. Carter K, Doern C, Jo CH, et al. The clinical usefulness of polymerase chain reaction as a supplemental diagnostic tool in the evaluation and the treatment of children with septic arthritis. *J Pediatr Orthop*. 2016;36:167-172.
25. Ceroni D, Belaieff W, Kanavaki A, et al. Possible association of *Kingella kingae* with infantile spondylodiscitis. *Pediatr Infect Dis J*. 2013;32(11):1296-1298.
30. Ceroni D, Dubois-Ferriere V, Cherkaoui A, et al. Detection of *Kingella kingae* osteoarticular infections in children by oropharyngeal swab PCR. *Pediatrics*. 2013;131(1):e230-e235.
31. Ceroni D, Llana RA, Kherad O, et al. Comparing the oropharyngeal colonization density of *Kingella kingae* between asymptomatic carriers and children with invasive osteoarticular infections. *Pediatr Infect Dis J*. 2013;32(4):412-414.
33. Chang DW, Nudell YA, Lau J, et al. RTX toxin plays a key role in *Kingella kingae* virulence in an infant rat model. *Infect Immun*. 2014;82(6):2318-2328.
38. Couturier MR, Mehinovic E, Croft AC, et al. Identification of HACEK clinical isolates by matrix-assisted laser desorption ionization-time of flight mass spectrometry. *J Clin Microbiol*. 2011;49(3):1104-1106.
42. El Houmami N, Minodier P, Dubourg G, et al. An outbreak of *Kingella kingae* infections associated with hand, foot and mouth disease/herpangina virus outbreak in Marseille, France, 2013. *Pediatr Infect Dis J*. 2015;34(3):246-250.
43. El Houmami N, Minodier P, Dubourg G, et al. Patterns of *Kingella kingae* disease outbreaks. *Pediatr Infect Dis J*. 2016;35:340-346.
44. El Houmami N, Mirand A, Dubourg G, et al. Hand, foot and mouth disease and *Kingella kingae* infections. *Pediatr Infect Dis J*. 2015;34(5):547-548.
45. Ferroni A, Al Khoury H, Dana C, et al. Prospective survey of acute osteoarticular infections in a French paediatric orthopedic surgery unit. *Clin Microbiol Infect*. 2013;19:822-828.
46. Foster MA, Walls T. High rates of complications following *Kingella kingae* infective endocarditis in children: a case series and review of the literature. *Pediatr Infect Dis J*. 2014;33(7):785-786.
47. Fournier PE, Rouli L, El Karkouri K, et al. Genomic comparison of *Kingella kingae* strains. *J Bacteriol*. 2012;194(21):5972.
50. Haldar M, Butler M, Quinn CD, et al. Evaluation of a real-time PCR assay for simultaneous detection of *Kingella kingae* and *Staphylococcus aureus* from synovial fluid in suspected septic arthritis. *Ann Lab Med*. 2014;34(4):313-316.
53. Holmes AA, Hung T, Human DG, et al. *Kingella kingae* endocarditis: a rare case of mitral valve perforation. *Ann Pediatr Cardiol*. 2011;4(2):210-212.
56. Kampouroglou G, Dubois-Ferriere V, De La Llana RA, et al. A prospective study of intrafamilial oropharyngeal transmission of *Kingella kingae*. *Pediatr Infect Dis J*. 2014;33(4):410-411.
57. Kanavaki A, Ceroni D, Tchernin D, et al. Can early MRI distinguish between *Kingella kingae* and gram-positive cocci in osteoarticular infections in young children? *Pediatr Radiol*. 2012;42(1):57-62.
58. Kaplan JB, Lo C, Xie G, et al. Genome sequence of *Kingella kingae* septic arthritis isolate PYKK081. *J Bacteriol*. 2012;194(11):3017.

68. Le Bourgeois F, Germanaud D, Bendavid M, et al. *Kingella kingae* sequence type 25 causing endocarditis with multiple and severe cerebral complications. *J Pediatr*. 2016;169:326-326.e1.
70. Maldonado R, Wei R, Kachlany SC, et al. Cytotoxic effects of *Kingella kingae* outer membrane vesicles on human cells. *Microb Pathog*. 2011;51(1-2):22-30.
72. Morel AS, Dubourg G, Prudent E, et al. Complementarity between targeted real-time specific PCR and conventional broad-range 16S rDNA PCR in the syndrome-driven diagnosis of infectious diseases. *Eur J Clin Microbiol Infect Dis*. 2015;34(3):561-570.
74. Munoz-Egea MC, Garcia-Pedrazuela M, Gonzalez-Pallares I, et al. *Kingella kingae* keratitis. *J Clin Microbiol*. 2013;51(5):1627-1628.
77. Porsch EA, Johnson MD, Broadnax AD, et al. Calcium binding properties of the *Kingella kingae* PilC1 and PilC2 proteins have differential effects on type IV pilus-mediated adherence and twitching motility. *J Bacteriol*. 2013;195(4):886-895.
81. Rempe KA, Spruce LA, Porsch EA, et al. Unconventional N-linked glycosylation promotes trimeric autotransporter function in *Kingella kingae* and *Aggregatibacter aphrophilus*. *MBio*. 2015;6:e1206-e1215.
83. Rouli L, Robert C, Raoult D, et al. *Kingella kingae* KK247, an atypical pulsed-field gel electrophoresis clone A strain. *Genome Announc*. 2014;2:e01228-14.
90. Starr KF, Porsch EA, Heiss C, et al. Characterization of the *Kingella kingae* polysaccharide capsule and exopolysaccharide. *PLoS ONE*. 2013;8(9):e75409.
94. Weiss-Salz I, Yagupsky P. *Kingella kingae* infections in children: an update. *Adv Exp Med Biol*. 2011;719:67-80.
99. Yagupsky P. Antibiotic susceptibility of *Kingella kingae* isolates from children with skeletal system infections. *Pediatr Infect Dis J*. 2012;31(2):212.
101. Yagupsky P. Outbreaks of *Kingella kingae* infections in daycare facilities. *Emerg Infect Dis*. 2014;20(5):746-753.
100. Yagupsky P. Risk for invasive *Kingella kingae* infections and day-care facility attendance. *Pediatr Infect Dis J*. 2012;31(10):1101.
103. Yagupsky P, Ben-Ami Y, Trefler R, et al. Outbreaks of invasive *Kingella kingae* infections in closed communities. *J Pediatr*. 2016;169:135-139 e131.
113. Yagupsky P, Slonim A, Amit U, et al. Beta-lactamase production by *Kingella kingae* in Israel is clonal and common in carriage organisms but rare among invasive strains. *Eur J Clin Microbiol Infect Dis*. 2013;32(8):1049-1053.

The full reference list for this chapter is available at ExpertConsult.com.

137 Legionnaires' Disease, Pontiac Fever, and Related Illnesses

Paul H. Edelstein

Legionnaires' disease (LD) is an acute pneumonic illness caused by gram-negative bacilli of the genus *Legionella*. Pontiac fever is a febrile, nonpneumonic, systemic illness closely associated with, if not caused by, *Legionella* spp. infection.

HISTORY

LD first was recognized as a distinct clinical entity when it caused an epidemic of pneumonia at an American Legion convention in Philadelphia in 1976 where 221 people were affected and 34 died.[83] Investigators were unable to determine the exact cause of the outbreak immediately, and this mystery provoked considerable fear and widespread speculation about the cause. Approximately 6 months later, two investigators at the Centers for Disease Control and Prevention (CDC), Joseph McDade and Charles Shepard, announced that they had discovered the etiologic agent, a fastidious gram-negative bacillus.[141] Researchers determined subsequently that both the organism and the disease had been studied previously as long ago as the 1940s, but had been forgotten.[47,65,191] Because of the historical association with the American Legion convention, this disease now is called LD, and the etiologic agents belong to the family Legionellaceae.

ETIOLOGIC AGENT

Legionella is the only genus in the family Legionellaceae. Sixty different species of *Legionella* are now recognized (Table 137.1). The closest pathogenic relative of the Legionellaceae is *Coxiella burnetii*, the agent of Q fever. *Legionella pneumophila* was responsible for the 1976 Philadelphia epidemic and causes most cases of LD.[47,52,65,122,130,191] *L. pneumophila* serogroup 1 is estimated to cause 70% to 90% of all cases of LD in previously healthy people.[54,137] *Legionella* spp. other than *L. pneumophila*, and serogroups other than *L. pneumophila* serogroup 1, cause 25% to 40% of nosocomial outbreaks of LD; of these, *L. pneumophila* serogroups 4 and 6, *Legionella micdadei*, and *Legionella dumoffii* are the most common.[104,211] *L. pneumophila* and *Legionella longbeachae* are the only two *Legionella* spp. that normally infect nonimmunocompromised patients.

The Legionellaceae are obligately aerobic, mesophilic, motile, L-cysteine auxotrophic gram-negative bacilli with variable oxidase and catalase reactions.[64] Genomes of multiple *Legionella* spp. strains have been sequenced, revealing that these bacteria harbor certain eukaryotic-like genes, several secretion systems, remarkable plasticity, and the presence of mobile elements.[27,91,132] Approximately 10% of the approximately 3.5-Mb genome is devoted to strain-specific genes.[25,38,41]

Antigenic relationships among different *Legionella* spp. and among serotypes of the same species are complex.[191] The serologic typing scheme is based on surface antigens (O antigens), which primarily are lipopolysaccharides. These surface antigens are shared by different species and, in rare cases, by other gram-negative bacilli, such as *Pseudomonas* spp. Identifying an unknown strain by use of serologic methods alone may lead to incorrect identification. Cross-reactions also may be observed in testing for human antibodies to *Legionella* spp. Patients with infections caused by some *Pseudomonas* spp. strains, *Campylobacter jejuni*, and other gram-negative bacilli may develop antibodies to *Legionella* spp.[61]

Identification of *Legionella* spp. other than *L. pneumophila* often requires the capabilities of a research, or national reference, laboratory that performs molecular-based identification. However, isolation and presumptive identification of *L. pneumophila* should be within the capabilities of most clinical laboratories.[64]

Legionella bacteria are ubiquitous in the aqueous environment and can be found, often in high concentrations, in lake water, ponds, bathing water, hot water tanks, hot water plumbing, and air conditioning cooling towers.[191] Optimal growth temperature ranges from 28° to 40°C (82°–104°F). The natural hosts and reservoirs of environmental *Legionella* bacteria are freshwater amebae, such as *Acanthamoeba* and *Hartmannella*.[78] Factors that promote the environmental growth of *Legionella* include the presence of other microorganisms, the use of plumbing materials that promote bacterial growth, stagnation, and warm temperatures.[191] In the home, older municipal water distribution systems, the use of electric rather than gas water heaters, and the use of well water all appear to promote the presence of *Legionella* in water.[78,185] In the particular case of *L. longbeachae*, amebae-laden potting soil exposed to warm temperatures allows multiplication of the bacterium to high concentrations.[206] Most newly discovered *Legionella* spp. have been environmental isolates not associated with clinical illness.[78]

Many bacterial virulence factors have been described, the most important of which is the Dot/Icm complex. This complex comprises 26 genes that form a type IV secretion system that is required for *L.*

TABLE 137.1 *Legionella* Species and Serogroups

Species	No. of Serogroups	Implicated in Human Disease
adelaidensis	1	No
anisa	1	Yes
beliardensis	1	No
birminghamensis	1	Yes
bozemane	2	Yes
brunensis	1	No
busanensis	unknown	No
cardiaca	unknown	Yes
cherrii	1	No
cincinnatiensis	1	Yes
drancourtii	unknown	No
dresdenensis	1	No
drozanskii	unknown	No
dumoffii	1	Yes
erythra	2	No
fairfieldensis	1	No
fallonii	unknown	No
feeleii	2	Yes
geestiana	1	No
gormanii	1	Yes
gratiana	1	No
gresilensis	1	No
hackeliae	2	Yes
impletisoli	unknown	No
israelensis	1	No
jamestowniensis	1	No
jordanis	1	Yes
lansingensis	1	Yes
londiniensis	1	No
longbeachae	2	Yes
lytica	unknown	Yes
maceachernii	1	Yes
massiliensis	unknown	No
micdadei	1	Yes
moravica	1	No
nagasakiensis	1	Yes
nautarum	1	No
norrlandica	unknown	No
oakridgensis	1	No
parisiensis	1	Yes
pneumophila	16	Yes
quateirensis	1	No
quinlivanii	2	No
rowbothamii	unknown	No
rubrilucens	1	No
sainthelensi	2	Yes
santicrucis	1	No
saoudiensis	unknown	No
shakespearei	1	No
spiritensis	2	No
steelei	unknown	No*
steigerwaltii	1	No
taurinensis	1	No
thermalis	unknown	No
tucsonensis	1	Yes
tunisiensis	unknown	No
wadsworthii	1	Yes
waltersii	1	No
worsleiensis	1	No
yabuuchiae	unknown	No

*Isolated from humans but unlikely to have caused disease.

pneumophila growth within macrophages. *L. pneumophila* is not killed actively by macrophages. The Dot/Icm complex allows the bacterium to evade normal phagolysosomal trafficking and bacterial destruction by injecting effectors into the host macrophage within minutes of the time of initial bacterial-macrophage contact. More than 300 injected effectors of *L. pneumophila* have been described, but only a few have been fully characterized functionally.[81,109,156] Other *Legionella* spp. have different predicted effectors, with at least 5800 different predicted effectors, and only seven predicted effectors shared among 38 different species.[27] The end result is that the normal host processes are hijacked into providing an intracellular compartment for the bacterium that associates with endoplasmic reticulum.[43,150,175] Other bacterial virulence factors include a variety of enzymes, iron binding proteins, miscellaneous proteins enhancing intracellular growth, and survival or invasion.[43] An important virulence factor for *L. pneumophila* serogroup 1 is a lipopolysaccharide 8-O-acetylase of unknown pathogenic mechanism of action; bacterial strains with this acetylase constitute the majority of *L. pneumophila* clinical isolates yet are uncommon in the environment.[37]

Availability of intracellular iron appears to play a key role in the growth of intracellular *L. pneumophila*. Interferon-γ, the production of which is increased during *L. pneumophila* infection of macrophages, downregulates the number of iron-binding receptors on macrophages, which has the effect of decreasing the availability of intracellular iron and hence limiting intracellular growth of the bacterium.[29]

L. pneumophila is serum resistant.[191] High-titer antibody promotes phagocytosis but may not enhance killing. Macrophage activation factors possibly are more important than is antibody in promoting phagocytosis and bacterial killing.[107]

EPIDEMIOLOGY

Incidence and Frequency

National passive LD surveillance has been initiated through the CDC by using serologic, culture, and mainly urine antigen testing. Cases reported to the CDC from 2000 through 2009 included a total of 22,418 cases, of which there were 204 (1%) pediatric cases, with 39% of those in children less than age 10 years.[39] In an earlier CDC report spanning 1990 to 2005, 375 pediatric cases were reported, comprising 1.7% of the total number of reported cases. The most pediatric cases, 44.3%, were in the 15- to 19-year age group, followed by those younger than 1 year of age, at 18.1%.[155] In 2015, the CDC reported 5315 cases of LD, a number reflecting an approximate doubling of reported cases from the prior decade.

Pediatric LD rarely appears to be the cause of pneumonia in otherwise healthy children.* Fewer than 20 well-documented cases of LD have been reported in otherwise normally healthy children older than a month, and fewer than 100 culture-confirmed cases have been reported in immunosuppressed children.†

A CDC study on the epidemiology of LD in children from 1984 through 2004 found that 66 of 6575 cases (1%) of LD reported during the period occurred in children younger than 19 years of age. The median age was 11 years; 72% reported a health care exposure, 30% had at least one risk factor for the infection, 26% of cases were associated with an outbreak, and 22% died.[3] The very low frequency of LD in US children has also been observed in children with pneumonia in China, Kenya, Gabon, and Germany.[23,40,124,205]

A retrospective serosurvey of 500 patients with pneumonia, 83% of whom did not need hospitalization, found that only five of the 132 patients younger than 15 years of age had significant antibody titers against *L. pneumophila*, and none developed seroconversion.[82] The estimated incidence of LD in the overall population was approximately 12 per 100,000 per year. Several prospective serologic studies of children with pneumonia found that LD constitutes approximately 1% of the diagnosed causes of pneumonia.[45,159,173] This rate is approximately the same as the 0.5% to 4% frequency found in the adult population.[47,137,191] LD is not a major cause of pneumonia in either children or adults.

*References 6, 13, 21, 33, 34, 45, 51, 85, 105, 108, 126, 144, 165, 181, 190.
†References 1, 9, 21, 22, 32–34, 45, 48, 69, 76, 93, 94, 112, 119, 121, 123, 128, 129, 154, 163, 169, 182, 194, 198, 207.

The frequency of LD in immunosuppressed children is unknown, although it is clear that immunosuppressed children can be at high risk for this disease. LD has been reported in children with acute leukemia or chronic granulomatous disease, after bone marrow or solid organ transplantation, or after treatment with corticosteroids for other reasons.[‡] Nosocomial or community-acquired LD has been reported in several "immunologically normal" infants, who may have had some degree of immunocompromise that predisposed them to this disease.[46,77,85,105,106,115,126,154,169] Neonates appear to be at increased risk for acquiring nosocomial, water birthing–related, and community-acquired LD.[84,94,129,146,167,179,189,196,204,209] *Legionella*-contaminated nursery and home humidifiers have been implicated as environmental sources in both nosocomial and sporadic LD cases in neonates and infants.[21,209] Neonatal LD acquired from formula made with tap water has also been reported.[204] As much as possible, neonates should be protected from environmental sources of *Legionella* that can be inhaled or aspirated.

More than 100 cases of Pontiac fever in children have been reported in outbreaks of this disease.[26,90,110,113,133] The risk for acquiring Pontiac fever was found to be greater for younger people in one outbreak,[110] which was just the opposite finding of another outbreak investigation.[113] The true frequency of Pontiac fever in children is difficult to know because the diagnosis is impossible to make with certainty in the sporadic form. One hotel hot tub–related outbreak of both LD and Pontiac fever in families and attendees of a youth athletic event found that the median ages of patients with LD and Pontiac fever were 6.5 and 15 years, respectively.[26]

Several serosurveys found asymptomatic elevations of *L. pneumophila* antibody in widely varying frequency. In one study, about one-half of 52 children studied developed an increase in antibody titer unrelated to acute illness over a period of several years.[6] Another study found that 15% of 126 children sampled had antibody titers to *L. pneumophila* of 256 or higher, a finding that was not significantly different from titers seen in an adult control population.[149] The striking finding was that the antibody titers rose with age, doubling each year until age 3 years, when the values plateaued; this finding held even when patients with pneumonia were excluded. The significance of these elevated antibody titers in children without documented pneumonia is unclear, and it can be interpreted as cross-reactions to other colonizing or infecting bacteria, asymptomatic infection, or atypical disease.

Several investigators have examined the question whether atypical disease caused by *Legionella* occurs in children using poorly specific serologic tests. Italian physicians found that two children with acute, reversible cerebellar ataxia developed significant antibody titer changes to *L. pneumophila*.[158] Another Italian study found two children with pericarditis who had significant antibody changes.[183] None of 140 British infants with sudden death had measurable antibodies to *L. pneumophila*, despite suggestions that they could be linked.[202] Three studies have shown that children with cystic fibrosis have higher antibody levels to *Legionella* than do normal children, although these data are suspect because of known cross-reactions between *Legionella* and *Pseudomonas aeruginosa*.[44,67,116] Thus despite several epidemiologic surveys, the prevalence of atypical *Legionella* infections in children is unclear.

In adults LD incidence figures vary widely, most likely related to the insensitivity of passive reporting systems and the vigor of diagnostic testing. The highest reported incidence rates, between 187 and 375 LD cases per million population per year, were reported from a 2008 prospective study of community-acquired pneumonia in Germany, where special efforts were made to capture all cases and to use sensitive diagnostic tests.[199] A significantly lower incidence has been reported in France (20 cases/million per year), where surveillance is passive but disease reporting is mandatory.[31] The reported rate in the United States, 17 cases per million per year, is lower, most likely because of a reliance on passive surveillance and limited diagnostic testing for the disease.[39] Estimates based on serologic surveys range from 20 to 200 cases per million population per year.[47,171,191] A prospective study in Ohio found that the incidence of LD requiring hospitalization was approximately 60 per million per year, in what is thought to be a geographic region with an above-average frequency of the disease.[138] Estimates of the proportion of adult pneumonias caused by LD range from 1% to 25%, with a reasonable mean of 3%.[137] Mild or atypical *Legionella* infection certainly occurs in adults, although the exact incidence is unknown. On the basis of serosurveys, asymptomatic infection may occur in adults. Neither oropharyngeal colonization nor a carrier state has been documented.[24]

Although LD is often thought of as an epidemic disease, it is actually more common as a sporadic disease. One European study showed that sporadic cases represented approximately 92% of all 5960 reported LD cases from 2007 through 2008, similar to the findings in the United States.[39,114]

Risk factors for acquisition of LD can be divided into two main categories: those that increase exposure to contaminated water and those that suppress pulmonary defense mechanisms.[47,191] Included in the former category are occupational or residential exposure to warm or stagnant water, traveling and residence in hotels, and stays in hospitals with contaminated water distribution systems; a risk factor for residential acquisition of disease is the use of well water.[185] Weather may be a risk factor in some regions, with increased humidity or rain implicated in a few studies.[80] Included in risk factors that suppress pulmonary defense mechanisms are surgical procedures requiring general anesthesia, administration of glucocorticosteroids, cigarette smoking, chronic lung disease, and diseases or therapies that compromise the innate or cellular immune systems. Use of biologic response modifiers, especially tumor necrosis factor antagonists, is a significant risk factor for LD.[135,195] Alemtuzumab treatment is also a likely significant risk factor for LD. Male patients are more than twice as likely as female patients to develop the disease, perhaps as a result of the greater male prevalence of cigarette smoking and chronic lung disease. Middle-aged and older people also are at significantly higher risk than are younger people, as exemplified by data from the United States for 2000 to 2009; the incidence rates (per million/year) were 0.2, 0.3, 1.3, 3.6, 8.1, 14.4, and 26.6 for people younger than 9, 10 to 19, 20 to 29, 30 to 39, 40 to 49, 50 to 59, and older than 80 years of age, respectively.[39] Other than exposure to aerosols of contaminated water, no particular predisposing factors for the development of Pontiac fever have been identified. LD is not contagious, and transmission from patients to staff or other patients has never been documented.

Disease Outbreaks

Multiple epidemics of LD and Pontiac fever have been recognized.[22,47,90,191] In the case of LD, most outbreaks have occurred in residents, employees, or visitors to large buildings; or in urban settings with exposure to aerosolized water from fountains and cooling towers. Hotels, hospitals, museums, factories, retail stores, office buildings, and housing complexes have all been implicated in LD epidemics. Nosocomial LD has been reported in hospitals throughout the world. Disease reservoirs and disseminators have been potable water distribution systems, air conditioning cooling towers, hot tub spas, decorative fountains, industrial water systems, and others.[47,191] Outbreaks have been ended by disinfection of water and cooling tower systems through hyperchlorination or pasteurization.[47,191] In some of these outbreaks, disease occurred for many years until effective disinfection procedures were used. Attack rates in LD epidemics consistently have been less than 5% overall. Incubation periods ranging from 2 to 19 days have been observed, with median incubation periods of 4 to 6 days and average ranges from 2 to 10 days.

Pontiac fever outbreaks generally have been associated with exposure to an aerosol of warm water contaminated with *Legionella*.[89,118,191] Examples include whirlpool baths, an engine assembly plant using contaminated water to cool machine lathes, and a health department building in which condensate in the air conditioning system was contaminated. The attack rates in Pontiac fever outbreaks have been high, in the range of 95% to 100%. The incubation period is short, from 12 to 36 hours.[89]

PATHOLOGY, PATHOGENESIS, AND IMMUNITY

Very good, but indirect, epidemiologic and pathologic evidence suggests that LD infection results from inhalation of an aerosol.[47,191] The bacterial form that causes infection is unknown, with possibilities including a

‡References 48, 69, 99, 112, 119, 121, 127, 163, 164, 176, 178, 186, 192.

sporelike form, intra-amebal bacteria, bacteria enmeshed in biofilm, and bacteria released from biofilm.[78,87,125] Some patients have acquired LD after aspiration of *Legionella*-contaminated tap water, rather than by aerosol inhalation.[19,111,136,197]

In guinea pigs infected by the aerosol route, multiplication of *L. pneumophila* begins within 16 hours.[49] Bacterial multiplication occurs within the alveolar macrophage, although growth in respiratory epithelial cells may also occur. Cell culture studies show that multiplication occurs only in cells and not in the extracellular tissue culture medium.[107] This intracellular location of bacteria protects them from serum factors such as antibody and complement, as well as from the effects of those antimicrobial agents that are not concentrated in cells. Killing of *L. pneumophila* within macrophages in cell culture is limited by failure of phagolysosomal acidification and fusion.[107]

L. pneumophila avoids macrophage killing by injecting phagosomal maturation-altering compounds into its host cell within minutes of initial contact by using the Dot/Icm type IV secretion system.[109] An additional mechanism involves shedding of bacterial flagellin into the host cytosol, which acts through the innate immune system to alter macrophage killing of the bacteria.[172] In the late phases of bacterial multiplication in macrophages, the bacteria change phenotype to enable infection of the next susceptible macrophage, thereby becoming highly motile, quite small, and more resistant to antimicrobial agents.[10,145] The *L. pneumophila*–containing vacuole becomes huge, occupying almost the entire volume of the macrophage, over a period of a few days. The bacteria escape from the presumably nutrient-depleted macrophage by inducing cellular apoptosis and can then infect available uninfected macrophages.[2] Innate macrophage resistance to bacterial infection may be mediated by Toll-like receptors, in particular TLR-2 and TLR-5, and perhaps TLR-4.[100–102] Acquired macrophage resistance to infection derives from activation by interferon-γ and the resultant downregulation of available iron stores.[28] Tumor necrosis factor-α plays a very important role in host defense to infection.[142]

Polymorphonuclear leukocytes neither ingest nor kill the organism effectively in vitro, although animal studies suggest that they may form the bulwark of initial host defenses.[49] Clinical evidence suggests that leukopenic hosts without concomitant macrophage dysfunction are not high-risk candidates for LD, although they may be at higher risk than is the normal population.[35,65]

Lung histopathologic findings in LD show intense intra-alveolar inflammation.[191] Airways larger than the terminal bronchioles are not affected. The interstitial spaces generally are uninvolved, although necrosis of alveoli may bridge the interstitial spaces. The alveoli contain a variable mixture of polymorphonuclear leukocytes, alveolar macrophages, and necrotic debris. Hemorrhage is observed, as are microabscesses. Later, fibrin formation and a histiocytic predominance occur.

Gross lung changes evolve in the classic pattern of lobar pneumonia, with first red and then gray hepatization.[191] Lymph nodes are involved occasionally. The lung segments involved may be subpleural, a finding that sometimes suggests septic or bland infarction to the clinician. The pleural space is involved variably and seemingly is more prone to infection in immunosuppressed patients. One of the most striking pulmonary findings is the usual absence of significant intrabronchial exudate. This absence of intrabronchial exudate and the lack of bronchial inflammation may mislead clinicians to exclude bacterial pneumonia.

Despite frequent signs and symptoms of extrapulmonary disease in patients with LD, no specific extrapulmonary pathologic findings have been identified.[191] In fatal cases, organisms often can be recovered or detected in the liver or spleen. Occasionally, patients have nonbacterial endocardial vegetations. Some patients have hilar and paratracheal adenitis. Patients may have metastatic foci with abscesses in almost any location, including the myocardium, pericardium, peritoneum, brain, kidney, bowel wall, perirectal region, prosthetic and native heart valves, muscle and skin, and hemodialysis shunts (Box 137.1).[65,161,191] Bacteremia is rarely detected, although molecular studies and clinical findings suggest that it is common.[65,151,191] Elaboration of toxins by *Legionella* has been postulated to account for some aspects of the systemic disease, but supporting evidence is not convincing.[191]

Host cytokine production in response to *L. pneumophila* infection likely causes most of the acute toxicity of the disease. Cell culture and animal experiments show that tumor necrosis factor, interferon-γ, and other cytokines are produced during *L. pneumophila* infection.[14,208] Humans infected with *L. pneumophila* have been shown to produce several cytokines during infection, as well as inflammatory markers such as procalcitonin, neopterin, and C-reactive protein.[50,75,188]

BOX 137.1 Diseases Caused by *Legionella*

Pneumonia (Legionnaires' Disease)

Associated With Pneumonia

Bacteremia
Bowel wall abscess
Brain abscess
Colitis
Endocarditis
Hemodialysis shunt infection
Myopericarditis
Myositis, cellulitis
Peritonitis
Perirectal abscess
Pleural empyema
Renal abscess

Not Associated With Pneumonia

Colitis
Lymphadenitis
Peritoneal dialysis–related peritonitis
Pleural empyema
Endocarditis
Sepsis syndrome
Sinusitis
Soft tissue infections
Wound infection
Pontiac Fever (toxin mediated?)

Episodes of recurrent or relapsing LD in patients with elevated antibody titers support experimental evidence suggesting that the humoral immune system plays a minor role in this disease.[65] Also supporting this evidence is the rarity of LD case reports in patients with hypogammaglobulinemia or other diseases in which the humoral immune system primarily is deficient. The rise of specific antibody levels does not seem to have any clinical correlates, nor does the absolute antibody level.[65] Patients may recover from LD without any significant increase in antibody levels, again providing indirect evidence of the limited role of the humoral immune system.

Several studies showed that passive or active immunization is protective against intraperitoneal and subcutaneous chamber infection in rats, mice, and guinea pigs.[7,68,103,174] Preopsonization of *L. pneumophila* before intratracheal inoculation of hamsters was found to be partially protective, but several investigators showed that active immunization fails to protect against pneumonia after intratracheal, aerosol, or intranasal inoculation of large numbers of *L. pneumophila* bacteria.[11,55,68] Protective immunity to pulmonary challenge in the guinea pig can be achieved after sublethal infection or infection with an avirulent mutant strain and by vaccination with an *L. pneumophila*–derived metalloprotease or outer membrane protein.[15,16,18,203]

Evidence for the importance of the cellular immune system in preventing infection largely is indirect and is based on the greater prevalence of LD in immunosuppressed patients with cellular immunodeficiencies.[65,191] Curiously, LD in patients with acquired immunodeficiency syndrome (AIDS) has been reported infrequently, although one epidemiologic survey showed that patients with AIDS had a disease attack rate approximately 40 times greater than that in the normal population.[17,18,137,203]

The pathogenesis of Pontiac fever is not understood. No differences have been detected between an *L. pneumophila* strain isolated from an outbreak of Pontiac fever and strains isolated from outbreaks of LD; these studies have included examination of virulence in an animal model, toxin production, and biochemical characteristics.[191] The lack of detailed clinical studies of patients with Pontiac fever makes it difficult to produce an experimental model of this disease. Because Pontiac fever has a short incubation time, which can be as brief as 12 hours, this disease likely does not represent widespread bacterial multiplication within the body and more likely it is a toxin-induced or allergic disease. In fact, the link between *Legionella* and Pontiac fever is circumstantial; entirely possible is that other microbes, or their toxins, coexisting with *Legionella* may cause the disease.[89,118] The clinical syndromes most like Pontiac fever are bath-water fever, humidifier fever, and extrinsic allergic alveolitis; these syndromes are thought to be caused either by the direct toxic activity of inhaled endotoxin or by an allergic reaction to microorganisms, most particularly amebae such as *Naegleria* spp.[66,148,177] *L. pneumophila* makes a poorly active endotoxin, a finding suggesting that if inhaled endotoxin is the cause of Pontiac fever, then the endotoxin comes from non-*Legionella* bacteria. Support for inhaled endotoxin as the cause of Pontiac fever is found in two studies of endotoxin present at outbreaks of the disease.[36,79] Both Pontiac fever and LD have been reported from the same disease outbreaks, thus raising the questions whether Pontiac fever is a very mild form of LD, whether it is caused by non-*Legionella* toxins or bacteria present in the same aerosols, and why some people develop LD and others Pontiac fever.[4,70,157]

CLINICAL MANIFESTATIONS OF LEGIONNAIRES' DISEASE

Signs and Symptoms

LD usually manifests as pneumonia.[65] The pneumonia is atypical in that usual pathogenic bacteria generally are not isolated from respiratory tract secretions or blood, and patients do not respond, except fortuitously, to antimicrobial agents commonly used to treat pneumonia in adults (e.g., penicillins, cephalosporins, and aminoglycosides). Beyond this, considerable speculation and controversy continue over whether a distinct clinical syndrome exists. Several prospective studies of both community-acquired and nosocomial LD failed to demonstrate any clinical, radiographic, or nonspecific laboratory features that distinguish LD from other common causes of pneumonia.[57,74,96] The classic clinical findings are reviewed because many physicians consider that they are distinctive for *Legionella* pneumonias. Whether LD in children mimics the clinical findings in adults is unknown because of the rare instances of well-documented pediatric cases and the possibility of spectrum bias.

The onset of pneumonia may be either insidious or abrupt. Recurrent chills, abdominal pains, myalgia, headache, malaise, anorexia, and severe fatigue are common findings. Diarrhea, consisting of loose, nonbloody stools several times a day, occurs in 30% to 40% of patients. Fever may be low grade or absent initially. Over the course of a day to several days, these nonspecific symptoms gradually worsen, often resulting in severe debilitation. These symptoms gradually increase in severity, as measured by the median time of 4 to 5 days to present for hospital care, at which time the patient can be quite ill. Noteworthy is the frequent absence of symptoms referable to the respiratory system. Rash, splenomegaly, adenopathy, and rhinorrhea are exceptionally uncommon findings. Physical examination early in the illness generally is remarkable for a paucity of localizing findings and the frequent impression that the patient has an influenzal or typhoidal illness.

Within a day to several days after onset, the patient usually, but not always, develops a high fever. Respiratory complaints, especially dyspnea and pleuritic chest pains, may become prominent. Cough usually is not a major complaint, although it is common. The sputum is hardly ever frankly purulent; blood-streaked sputum or frank hemoptysis is observed in 20% to 30% of patients. Many patients experience confusion, cerebellar ataxia, lethargy, agitation, or some other neurologic disorder. Severe abdominal or back pain may occur, sometimes with localization. Physical examination at this time reveals a "toxic" febrile patient with apparent multisystem disease. Chest examination usually discloses findings of consolidating pneumonia. Depending on the location and stage of consolidation, rales may or may not be heard. Pleural friction rubs or signs of pleural effusion can be observed. Despite frequent symptoms of abdominal pain, signs of peritoneal irritation, such as decreased bowel sounds or rebound tenderness, seldom are detected. Signs of meningeal irritation occur rarely.

Most previously healthy patients recover without specific therapy, usually by day 7 to 10 of illness. Patients with mild disease not requiring hospital admission appear to do quite well without antibiotic therapy.[199] Patients who do not recover usually die of progressive respiratory failure, along with failure of other organ systems. Empyema, pulmonary cavitation, renal failure, memory loss, fatigue, and neurologic disorders all are potential complications and may persist for weeks to months after onset of the disease. Various extrapulmonary diseases may very rarely occur as the result of LD; the most common of these disorders are pancreatitis,[143] hepatitis, and myopericarditis.[8,139] Myositis, as measured by elevated serum creatine kinase levels, occurs commonly, with severe muscle disease such as rhabdomyolysis a rare complication.[117,201] Most of these extrapulmonary diseases improve rapidly with resolution of the pneumonia.

Focal infection without pneumonia is a very rare manifestation of *Legionella* spp. infections, with only a handful of cases reported (Box 137.1). Direct inoculation of bacteria into surgical or traumatic wounds is the usual mode of pathogenesis, although bacteremia and bacteremic metastatic infection have been reported.[140,168] *Legionella* spp. were implicated by polymerase chain reaction (PCR) testing as a cause of persistent cervical lymphadenitis in children, often after hot tub exposure. Because the involved lymph nodes were stain and culture negative for *Legionella*, and because the patients failed to improve with macrolide therapy, the study needs verification.[42]

Radiographic Findings

The radiographic hallmark of LD is an acinar filling pattern with consolidation.[47,65,191] There is no distinctive predilection for any lung region; pleural-based consolidation and bilateral infiltrates may occur. Nodular infiltrates may be seen, as may cavitation in the areas of original consolidation. Purely interstitial infiltrates are distinctly uncommon findings in established disease, but they rarely occur very early in the disease process; these interstitial infiltrates rapidly progress to consolidating infiltrates within a day or so. High-resolution computed tomography of lungs of patients with LD often reveals a mixture of ground-glass opacities and consolidation, and in the convalescent phase an organizing pneumonia pattern may be seen.[98,210] Pleural effusion, with or without parenchymal infiltrates, is a common finding in chest computed tomography scans and is less commonly visualized in plain films. Pleural effusion has been documented as the only chest finding in patients treated early with specific antibiotic therapy.

Laboratory Findings

Nonspecific abnormal laboratory results are common in patients with LD.[47,65] Hematologic abnormalities may include leukocytosis or leukopenia, usually with a left shift; lymphopenia; thrombocytosis; and disseminated intravascular coagulation. Proteinuria and pyuria are common findings; myoglobinuria also may be present. Hyponatremia and hypophosphatemia commonly occur, as do elevations of aminotransferase enzymes, bilirubin, alkaline phosphatase, lactate dehydrogenase, and creatine kinase. Elevated ferritin is also seen. Severe azotemia occurs, although rarely. Elevation of cold agglutinin titers, cold agglutinin–induced hemolytic anemia, and elevation of complement fixation titers to *Mycoplasma pneumoniae* may also occur. Arterial oxygenation usually is depressed in relation to the extent of pneumonia.

Laboratory diagnosis of LD is best accomplished by urine antigen testing, but results of this test can be falsely negative. Recovery of *Legionella* from sputum or other lower respiratory tract secretions or tissues requires specialized laboratory testing and is insensitive.[64] Other specific diagnostic methods are detection of *L. pneumophila* antigen by immunofluorescent microscopy and detection of *Legionella* DNA in respiratory tract specimens by using PCR. Serologic diagnosis is of uncertain value in children, but it is useful in adults.

Sputum is plated on buffered charcoal yeast extract medium supplemented with α-ketoglutaric acid (buffered charcoal yeast extract [BCYE-α]) and on BCYE-α supplemented with antibiotics.[64] *Legionella* organisms grow on these media 3 to 7 days after inoculation and incubation at 35°C in air. Culture diagnosis has a higher yield than does immunofluorescent microscopy or serology and yields no false-positive results. Sputum culture yield depends on the severity of illness; it is close to 100% for LD affecting immunocompromised patients and patients with ventilator dependent pneumonia, but can be as low as 10% to 25% in mild LD. Blood and pleural fluid cultures have very low yield, less than 5% to 10%, with blood culture positive only in severely ill, usually immunocompromised, patients.

Immunofluorescent microscopy for *L. pneumophila* is a rapid and highly specific (99.9%), but insensitive (50–70% sensitivity), technique for diagnosis.[62] It can be performed on sputum or lung tissue in 1 to 2 hours after receipt of the specimen. The test is technically demanding, requiring extensive expertise and training; use of the test by inexperienced technologists yields more false-positive than true-positive findings. Because of these difficulties, few laboratories perform this testing.

Serologic testing is of most value in epidemiologic studies and of least value in the short-term diagnosis of sporadic cases.[61] As many as 25% of patients with culture-documented disease fail to undergo seroconversion against the homologous serotype; this failure is not related solely to early treatment or immunosuppression, although these factors may cause failure of antibody formation. As long as 3 months may be required for antibody levels to increase after onset of illness; the median time is approximately 2 weeks. Moreover, as with any other means of immunologic diagnosis of this disease, the multiplicity of antigenic types renders serologic testing extremely cumbersome. Because between 5% and more than 25% of the normal population have antibody titers as high as 1:512 to *Legionella*, only a fourfold rise in titer is considered significant. The specificity is highest for *L. pneumophila* serogroup 1 and much lower for other species. Commercial testing kits can yield false-positive results, and they may also be insensitive in comparison with reference laboratory tests. Only paired samples, drawn 3 to 6 weeks apart and tested in parallel, should be tested. Specimens taken up to 9 to 12 weeks after onset of the disease should be tested if earlier samples reveal no changes. A negative serologic test result does not exclude disease.

The specificity of seroconversion to *L. pneumophila* serogroup 1 ranges from 95% to 99%.[61] Cross-reactive antibodies may be found in the serum of patients with leptospirosis, melioidosis, *Bacteroides fragilis* infections, *P. aeruginosa* infections, *C. jejuni* enteritis, and possibly *Haemophilus influenzae* or enteric bacterial infections. However, even 99% specificity is not sufficient for certainty of diagnosis of a sporadic case. If the estimated 1% prevalence of LD in children is correct, fewer than 50% of all seroconversions yield truly positive results (positive predictive accuracy of 45%). This observation, combined with the studies cited previously showing age-related elevations of anti-*Legionella* antibody in young asymptomatic children, renders serologic diagnosis of pediatric LD highly suspect.

Detection of soluble bacterial antigen in urine can be used to diagnose *L. pneumophila* serogroup 1 infections successfully, and it is the most sensitive and fastest test for community-acquired LD.[62,60] The major drawback of this test is that it preferentially detects only *L. pneumophila* serogroup 1 infections. Otherwise, it has an excellent sensitivity (90–99% versus culture and 60–70% in patients with community-acquired LD) and extraordinary specificity (at least 99.9%). The antigen test may be positive when the result of sputum culture for *L. pneumophila* serogroup 1 is negative, especially in previously treated patients and in epidemics of LD. In nosocomial LD and in LD of immunocompromised patients, the antigen test is less sensitive because other serogroups and other *Legionella* spp. become likely in these groups. Although the antigen test detects 60% to 70% of patients with community-acquired LD, fewer than 40% of patients with nosocomial disease test positive. A negative urine antigen test result should not be used as the sole reason to stop therapy for LD.[56]

The PCR test has been used to detect *L. pneumophila* in sputum, serum, and urine. Whereas both sensitive and specific PCR tests are available, none are commercially available in the United States. Several US reference laboratories perform home brew PCR assays. PCR testing appears to add approximately 11% additional yield to that obtained by urine antigen testing.[53] In regions where LD caused by *L. longbeachae* is common, such as Australia and New Zealand, PCR testing can be significantly more sensitive than urine antigen testing.[152] The same can be said of diagnosis of LD in immunosuppressed patients and in patients with nosocomial disease, especially when there is not local expertise with respiratory tract culture for *Legionella* spp.

With the exception of the urine antigen and the PCR test, none of the nonculture tests is as sensitive as is culture diagnosis. Culture should be performed in every case; if desired, the other tests can be used to provide same-day answers. Because none of the *Legionella*-specific tests is 100% sensitive, the clinician sometimes must treat for LD in the absence of confirmatory laboratory tests. One or 2 days of therapy with erythromycin apparently does not affect the sensitivity of the diagnostic tests, although therapy with azithromycin or levofloxacin can affect culture yield. Therapy should not be withheld pending results of laboratory tests.

TREATMENT

No adequately sized prospective clinical studies of antimicrobial therapy for LD have been performed. All recommendations regarding therapy are based on retrospective and small prospective clinical studies in adults, as well as laboratory studies.

Because of the superiority of newer fluoroquinolone agents and azithromycin in experimental nonhuman studies, and in large retrospective studies of these agents in adults with LD, the current recommendation is that adults with severe LD and immunocompromised patients with the disease be given either azithromycin or fluoroquinolone therapy, rather than erythromycin or clarithromycin therapy. In one prospective observational study in adults that compared levofloxacin-treated patients with patients who received the less effective macrolides, erythromycin and clarithromycin, patients who received levofloxacin had a significantly shorter time to defervescence and a shorter length of hospital stay than did patients treated with erythromycin or clarithromycin.[153] However, other studies have shown no significant differences in outcome for patients treated with clarithromycin or levofloxacin.[72,95] A retrospective cohort analysis of clinical outcomes in 3152 patients hospitalized for LD showed no significant differences in outcomes between patients treated with either quinolones or azithromycin, including patients with severe disease.[88] The results of this study were confirmed in another retrospective propensity-adjusted, single-hospital study that also showed that clarithromycin therapy was associated with a longer length of stay.[212] A recent retrospective study of critically ill French patients showed that fluoroquinolone therapy, as opposed to therapy with a macrolide other than azithromycin, was associated with a lower mortality rate. In addition, this study showed that combination antiinfective therapy was not superior to fluoroquinolone monotherapy.[213] Taken together, these three studies provide reasonably strong evidence that either levofloxacin, or another highly active fluoroquinolone, or azithromycin should be used for hospitalized patients, that clarithromycin or erythromycin administration should be avoided in such patients, and that combining a macrolide with a fluoroquinolone for severe disease provides no substantial benefit. Nonhospitalized patients with mild LD can be treated equally well with any of the specific therapies, including doxycycline, newer fluoroquinolones, azithromycin, clarithromycin, or erythromycin.[58,59,134] No inherent reason, other than age-specific drug toxicity, precludes these guidelines for children.

Fluoroquinolone antimicrobial agents generally are contraindicated in children, although the evidence suggests that the risk for toxicity from short courses of therapy is low. On the basis of minimal, if any, significant differences in outcomes in adults treated with either azithromycin or fluoroquinolones, fluoroquinolone therapy should be reserved for special cases such as drug allergy, potential for cardiac toxicity, availability, and drug interactions.

Clarithromycin (7.5 mg/kg every 12 hours) may be used in place of erythromycin, although good laboratory and reasonable clinical data show that this drug is no more effective for LD than is erythromycin.[20,162] Clarithromycin is not approved by the US Food and Drug Administration (FDA) for the treatment of LD. Azithromycin has largely replaced erythromycin as the drug of choice for the treatment of LD in children primarily because of the adverse effects associated with erythromycin, especially gastrointestinal effects and severe phlebitis when the drug is given intravenously.

Azithromycin, which is approved for use in children in the United States, is as active against *Legionella* bacteria as are the newer fluoroquinolone agents, thus making it a candidate for the drug of choice for severe pediatric LD or for LD in immunocompromised children. The drug dose for children for this type of pneumonia has not been studied, but on the basis of extrapolation from adults, a dose of 10 mg/kg (maximum, 500 mg) given once daily for 3 to 5 days should be sufficient in most cases, with extended duration of therapy (7–10 days) for severely immunocompromised patients. Azithromycin is available in both intravenous and oral forms and is approved by the FDA for use in adults with LD. All macrolide/azalide antimicrobial agents, including azithromycin, have the potential for causing QT prolongation. Two studies of deaths resulting from cardiovascular causes in adults who were administered azithromycin gave diametrically opposed results. One study showed that azithromycin was associated with a higher death rate than in patients given amoxicillin, but not levofloxacin, particularly when the patients had significant risk factors for cardiovascular disease.[170] The other study showed that patients without a high risk of cardiovascular disease had no increased death risk with azithromycin when compared with the risk of penicillin administration, a finding suggesting that infection by itself increases the risk of death from cardiovascular causes.[187] A study of pneumonia mortality rates in 74,000 adults showed that those patients receiving azithromycin had lower mortality rates than did patients receiving other antimicrobial agents, although a slight increase in myocardial infarctions was reported in azithromycin-treated patients.[147] Patients with risk factors for cardiac arrhythmias are probably at somewhat increased risk for heart block when they are given macrolides/azalides, as well as fluoroquinolone antimicrobial agents, but the risk is relatively low.[131]

Newer fluoroquinolone agents, along with azithromycin, are considered to be the drugs of choice for the treatment of severe LD in adults. Levofloxacin is used commonly in the United States to treat this disease, in a dosage of 500 to 750 mg daily for 10 to 14 days. No dosage guidelines exist for the treatment of pediatric LD because of the potential for drug toxicity in this population. Levofloxacin is the only available quinolone agent approved by the FDA for the treatment of LD in adults; neither ciprofloxacin nor moxifloxacin is approved for this indication. Ciprofloxacin appears to be effective for this indication on the basis of case reports, and moxifloxacin may be effective on the basis of limited laboratory studies and case reports.[86] Combining a macrolide with a fluoroquinolone has been reported to be no more effective than a fluoroquinolone alone.[213]

Alternative drugs to macrolides or quinolones include doxycycline and possibly cotrimoxazole. Neither of these agents has been approved for this use by the FDA, although limited clinical and experimental data support their effectiveness, more for doxycycline than for cotrimoxazole. Cotrimoxazole should be used only if there is no possibility of using a macrolide, tetracycline, or fluoroquinolone drug because of the lack of clinical reports of its successful use for the treatment of LD. Doxycycline, because of its high lipid solubility, may be more effective than is tetracycline, although whether this is true remains conjecture. The dosage of doxycycline used in children is 2 to 4 mg/kg per day, given in one or two doses. The use of tetracyclines is associated with the risk for dental staining in children younger than 8 years of age. The daily cotrimoxazole dosage is 15 to 20 mg/kg of the trimethoprim component and 75 to 100 mg/kg of the sulfamethoxazole component in three divided doses; cotrimoxazole use in newborns may cause kernicterus. The duration of therapy for these drugs is the same as that for erythromycin.

Rifampin therapy for LD is not recommended, whether the drug is given by itself or in combination with another agent. The use of this drug for treatment of LD is not approved by the FDA. A small, nonrandomized study showed that adult patients treated with combination rifampin and clarithromycin had significantly longer hospital lengths of stay than did patients treated with clarithromycin alone, with a trend to worse outcome in other outcome measures in those patients given combined therapy.[92] Rifampin therapy induces the metabolism of macrolides for many weeks, so that when rifampin therapy is stopped, macrolide serum and lung levels will be quite low.[166,200] No good clinical or laboratory evidence indicates that combining rifampin with either azithromycin or a fluoroquinolone is beneficial.

Treatment of extrapulmonary foci of infection does not appear to differ from treatment of LD without extrapulmonary disease. The duration of therapy and indications for surgical drainage need to be assessed individually in these cases.

Response to Treatment

Most patients improve dramatically within a few days after initiation of specific therapy.[47,57,65,191] Response may be as rapid as 6 hours after administration of the first dose of therapy. Patients regain their appetite, lose symptoms of myalgia and fatigue, and feel better overall within a few days. Up to a week may be required for a patient to become completely afebrile, with longer periods sometimes required for severely immunosuppressed patients. The chest radiograph changes slowly and even may appear to worsen despite overall clinical improvement; progressive consolidation after 3 to 4 days of antimicrobial therapy is unusual. Because very severe immunocompromise can impair the ability of the cellular immune system to clear infection completely, some of these patients are prone to relapses of disease once antimicrobial therapy has been stopped, even after a long course of therapy.[97,180] The relapses can be insidious and manifest only with renewed immunosuppression. Profoundly immunosuppressed patients with LD who do not have recovery of immune function may benefit from prolonged suppressive antimicrobial therapy until they recover sufficient cellular immune function.

Failure to respond to appropriate therapy can result from severe underlying disease, advanced pneumonia at presentation, coinfection with another microorganism, mistaken diagnosis, and complications of pneumonia. These complications can include pulmonary embolism, empyema, pancreatitis, myopericarditis, hepatitis, and soft tissue infections.

The mortality rate in otherwise healthy adults who are treated promptly is approximately 5%, whereas in treated immunosuppressed patients it is approximately 20%. Untreated fatality rates range from 15% to 20% in normally healthy patients and upward of 80% in immunosuppressed patients. However, very mild community-acquired LD in healthy adults who do not require hospitalization appears to have a negligible mortality risk, and patients may not require specific antibiotic therapy, although such a course may not be advisable.[199] Even in previously healthy patients, delayed therapy and development of respiratory failure are exceptionally poor prognostic factors.[71,160,193]

DIFFERENTIAL DIAGNOSIS

Other causes of atypical, or culture-negative, pneumonia may closely resemble LD. Mycoplasma pneumonia usually is a milder illness not requiring hospitalization. Cough is a prominent symptom in mycoplasma pneumonia, whereas it is not in LD. Neither rash nor otitis is found in LD, nor is postpneumonia reactive airways disease. Laboratory abnormalities also are found more commonly in LD. Serologic testing may provide positive results for both diseases, a confusing finding that can be clarified by performing specific laboratory testing. Fortunately the treatment is the same for both diseases.

Psittacosis and Q fever may closely resemble LD. A history of bird or cattle exposure may be helpful, but the absence of such exposure does not exclude either of these zoonoses. An interstitial rather than an acinar-filling infiltrate on chest radiograph would be a point against LD. Pathogen-specific laboratory tests help in this differential diagnosis. A tetracycline can be used successfully for all three of these diseases.

Early in their evolution, some diseases may resemble LD. They include typhoid fever, acute coccidioidomycosis, influenza, the typhus or spotted fevers, and leptospirosis. Distinguishing these diseases on the basis of their clinical evolution, the laboratory results, and the exposure or travel history generally is easy.

Tularemia may pose a problem in the differential diagnosis because immunologic test results for LD can be falsely positive in tularemia and because some of the growth characteristics of *Francisella tularensis* closely resemble those of *Legionella*. In regions endemic for tularemia, clinicians must work closely with the laboratory to facilitate this differential diagnosis. One case record of tularemia misdiagnosed as LD reported that the patient responded to erythromycin therapy.

Dual infection sometimes occurs in LD. Coexistence of LD with pneumonia caused by *Mycobacterium tuberculosis*, pneumococcus, *H. influenzae*, *Neisseria meningitidis*, *Pneumocystis jiroveci*, *Moraxella catarrhalis*, and various viral agents has been reported. Thus dual infection should be suspected in patients not responding to therapy for LD. Pathogen-specific laboratory tests often are useful in these cases.

CLINICAL SYNDROMES CAUSED BY OTHER *LEGIONELLA* SPECIES

Relatively few cases have been reported of disease caused by the non–*L. pneumophila Legionella* spp., with the major exception of *L. longbeachae*.[5,73,206] These reported cases have few differences in clinical findings, diagnostic methods, or treatment. Almost all cases of LD caused by to *Legionella* spp. other than *L. pneumophila* or *L. longbeachae* have been reported to occur in immunocompromised patients, and because of these patients' underlying diseases and immunocompromise, the pneumonia severity and rapidity of response to therapy may be compromised. Disease caused by *L. longbeachae* appears to very similar to that caused by *L. pneumophila* in terms of clinical findings and response to therapy.[214] The lower frequency of these infections in normal hosts most likely reflects the decreased virulence of the bacteria. *L. longbeachae* has a different mechanism of transmission than does *L. pneumophila* because *L. longbeachae* infections do not appear to be transmitted from water sources, but rather from nonsterile potting soil.[30,120,184] Exposure to potting soil that has been exposed to high ambient temperatures, not washing hands after using the soil, and cigarette smoking are the major risk factors for this disease. The mode of spread and nosocomial reservoirs of the *Legionella* spp. other than *L. pneumophila* and *L. longbeachae* are not well defined. These infections are unlikely to be diagnosed by immunologic means, except for *L. longbeachae* infection in endemic regions (Australia and New Zealand) because few laboratories routinely test for all possible species. Laboratory testing by culture is the preferred test for all these non–*L. pneumophila* species, although genus- and species-specific PCR testing may also have good yield.[12,152] As with *L. pneumophila*, and even more so for the non–*L. pneumophila Legionella* spp., treatment sometimes must be based solely on clinical suspicion without the benefit of confirmatory laboratory tests.

PONTIAC FEVER

Clinical Manifestations

Fever, myalgia, malaise, chills, and headache are the most common symptoms of Pontiac fever.[89] The symptoms may begin suddenly or may have a more gradual onset for several hours. Many symptoms are respiratory, such as dry and nonproductive cough, chest pain, and pharyngitis. Nausea is a common manifestation, but diarrhea and vomiting are less frequent. Neurologic symptoms including dizziness, confusion, and poor coordination also have been reported. Pontiac fever symptoms usually are at their worst within a day after the onset of illness and gradually resolve over a 2- to 7-day period. Physical examination shows only tachycardia and fever. Leukocytosis has been the only laboratory abnormality reported. Chest radiographs show no abnormalities. Pulmonary function testing has not been performed in patients with Pontiac fever. Rechallenge by return to the contaminated building in the original Pontiac outbreak produced only a mild illness compared with first exposure; the length of time between first and second exposures was not stated clearly.

Diagnosis

The diagnosis of Pontiac fever primarily is one of exclusion.[47,191] Significant rises in anti-*Legionella* antibody level, combined with characteristic symptoms and isolation of *Legionella* from an aerosol source, are the diagnostic criteria. Rarely, *L. pneumophila* urinary antigen may be detected.[63] Detailed epidemiologic and environmental studies must be performed to diagnose Pontiac fever specifically because of the nonspecificity of the symptoms and the ubiquitous presence of environmental *Legionella*. Definitive diagnosis of sporadic cases is difficult.

Treatment

Antimicrobial therapy is not effective for the treatment of Pontiac fever. Removal of the patient from the area of the contaminated water source and symptomatic therapy as needed are the best means of management.

Acknowledgment

William Mason provided excellent suggestions for improvements in the manuscript.

NEW REFERENCES SINCE THE SEVENTH EDITION

4. Ambrose J, Hampton LM, Fleming-Dutra KE, et al. Large outbreak of Legionnaires' disease and Pontiac fever at a military base. *Epidemiol Infect*. 2014;142(11):2336-2346.
12. Benitez AJ, Winchell JM. Clinical application of a multiplex real-time PCR assay for simultaneous detection of *Legionella* species, *Legionella pneumophila*, and *Legionella pneumophila* serogroup 1. *J Clin Microbiol*. 2013;51(1):348-351.
21. Bonilla Escobar BA, Montero Rubio JC, Martinez JG. Neumonía por *Legionella pneumophila* asociada al uso de un humidificador doméstico en una niña inmunocompetente. *Med Clin (Barc)*. 2014;142(2):70-72.
33. Canpolat M, Kumandas S, Yikilmaz A, et al. Transverse myelitis and acute motor sensory axonal neuropathy due to *Legionella pneumophila*: a case report. *Pediatr Int*. 2013;55(6):778-782.
62. Edelstein PH. Legionella. In: Murray PR, Baron EJ, Jorgensen JH, Landry ML, Pfaller MA, eds. *Manual of Clinical Microbiology*. Vol. 9. Washington, DC: ASM Press; 2006:835-849.
70. Euser SM, Pelgrim M, den Boer JW. Legionnaires' disease and Pontiac fever after using a private outdoor whirlpool spa. *Scand J Infect Dis*. 2010;42(11-12):910-916.
84. Fritschel E, Sanyal K, Threadgill H, et al. Fatal legionellosis after water birth, Texas, USA, 2014. *Emerg Infect Dis*. 2015;21(1):130-132.
86. Garau J, Fritsch A, Arvis P, et al. Clinical efficacy of moxifloxacin versus comparator therapies for community-acquired pneumonia caused by *Legionella* spp. *J Chemother*. 2010;22(4):264-266.
131. Lu ZK, Yuan J, Li M, et al. Cardiac risks associated with antibiotics: azithromycin and levofloxacin. *Expert Opin Drug Saf*. 2015;14(2):295-303.
146. Moran-Gilad J, Lazarovitch T, Mentasti M, et al. Humidifier-associated paediatric Legionnaires' disease, Israel, February 2012. *Euro Surveill*. 2012;17(41):20293.
147. Mortensen EM, Halm EA, Pugh MJ, et al. Association of azithromycin with mortality and cardiovascular events among older patients hospitalized with pneumonia. *JAMA*. 2014;311(21):2199-2208.
157. Nicolay N, Boland M, Ward M, et al. Investigation of Pontiac-like illness in office workers during an outbreak of Legionnaires' disease, 2008. *Epidemiol Infect*. 2010;138(11):1667-1673.
166. Peters J, Eggers K, Oswald S, et al. Clarithromycin is absorbed by an intestinal uptake mechanism that is sensitive to major inhibition by rifampicin: results of a short-term drug interaction study in foals. *Drug Metab Dispos*. 2012;40(3):522-528.
167. Phin N, Cresswell T, Parry-Ford F, et al. Case of Legionnaires disease in a neonate following a home birth in a heated birthing pool, England, June 2014. *Euro Surveill*. 2014;19(29):2014.
187. Svanstrom H, Pasternak B, Hviid A. Use of azithromycin and death from cardiovascular causes. *N Engl J Med*. 2013;368(18):1704-1712.
189. Teare L, Millership S. *Legionella pneumophila* serogroup 1 in a birthing pool. *J Hosp Infect*. 2012;82(1):58-60.
200. Wallace RJ Jr, Brown BA, Griffith DE, et al. Reduced serum levels of clarithromycin in patients treated with multidrug regimens including rifampin or rifabutin for *Mycobacterium avium-M. intracellulare* infection. *J Infect Dis*. 1995;171(3):747-750.
204. Wei SH, Chou P, Tseng LR, et al. Nosocomial neonatal legionellosis associated with water in infant formula, Taiwan. *Emerg Infect Dis*. 2014;20(11):1921-1924.
209. Yiallouros PK, Papadouri T, Karaoli C, et al. First outbreak of nosocomial *Legionella* infection in term neonates caused by a cold mist ultrasonic humidifier. *Clin Infect Dis*. 2013;57(1):48-56.
212. Garcia-Vidal C, Sanchez-Rodriguez I, Simonetti AF, et al. Levofloxacin versus azithromycin for treating *Legionella* pneumonia: a propensity score analysis. *Clin Microbiol Infect*. 2017. Epub ahead of print.
213. Cecchini J, Tuffet S, Sonneville R, et al. Antimicrobial strategy for severe community-acquired legionnaires' disease: a multicentre retrospective observational study. *J Antimicrob Chemother*. 2017;72(5):1502-1509.
214. Isenman HL, Chambers ST, Pithie AD, et al. Legionnaires' disease caused by *Legionella longbeachae*: clinical features and outcomes of 107 cases from an endemic area. *Respirology*. 2016;21(7):1292-1299.

The full reference list for this chapter is available at ExpertConsult.com.

138 *Streptobacillus moniliformis* (Rat-Bite Fever)

Kara A. DuBray • Carol A. Glaser

Rat-bite fever is an acute febrile illness usually acquired by humans from the bite of a rat. The disease may be caused by two different bacteria both known to colonize rats. Although both *Streptobacillus moniliformis* and *Spirillum minus* are causative agents of rat-bite fever, these organisms have different epidemiology, incubation periods, and clinical presentation. *S. moniliformis* accounts for most cases of rat-bite fever reported in published reports and is the focus of this chapter. *S minus*, reportedly more common is Asia, is discussed in Chapter 143.

Rat-bite fever caused by *Streptobacillus* is typically characterized by fever, rash, and arthritis. Although it is frequently attributed to the bite of a rat, other animals may be infected, and modes of transmission other than a bite have been documented. Haverhill fever, for example, is acquired after ingestion of contaminated food or water. *S. moniliformis* is a zoonosis with worldwide distribution,[50,141] and it is the leading cause of rat-bite fever in the United States.

HISTORY

The first description of rat-bite fever is found in the 2500-year-old Indian *Compendium of Medicine,* the *Susruta Samhita.*[26] In this text, a description of the illness is given that remains valid today: "The blood of any part of the human body coming in contact with the semen of rats or scratched with their nails or teeth is vitiated and gives rise to the appearance of nodes, swellings, eruptions of circular erythematous patches on skin, pustules, violent and acute erysipelas, breaking pain in the joints, extreme pain in the body, fever, anemia, aversion to food, shivering, and horripilation." The disease also was known in ancient Japan, where treatment consisted of the local application of herbs and dynamite to cause an "explosion in the wound."[26]

The first modern accounts of the disease are found in a lecture by Professor Eli Ives at Yale University in 1831.[47] In 1900, Miyake[83] gave a detailed description of the disease, which he named *sodoku,* from the Japanese *so* ("rat") and *doku* ("poison"). The first case report was published in 1839.[138] Schottmüller,[117] Blake,[13] and Levaditi and colleagues[68] were the first to isolate and describe the causative agent of streptobacillary rat-bite fever in 1914, 1916, and 1925, respectively. The organism has been known as *Streptothrix muris ratti* and *Streptobacillus muris minus* but currently is referred to as *S. moniliformis.*[59]

EPIDEMIOLOGY

Rats are estimated to compose one-third of the mammalian population of the world, with numbers of approximately 10 billion.[50] More than 2 million animal bites are reported annually in the United States, and rat bites account for a small number (<1%), although the incidence is probably underreported.[38,50,53] A review of animal bites in Maryland during a 3-year period found that approximately 4.7% were caused by rats or lagomorphs.[32] According to another report, 40,000 rat bites are reported annually.[27] Among bitten patients, the risk for rat-bite fever developing is significant, with reported rates between 4% and 11%.[102,137]

Between 10% and 100% of laboratory rats and between 50% and 100% of wild rats carry *S. moniliformis* as normal nasopharyngeal flora and excrete it in their urine.[5,50,126] The disease also has been transmitted to humans from mice,[100] squirrels,[81] weasels,[34] gerbils,[139] and rat-eating carnivores such as cats,[52,82] dogs,[90,103] and pigs.[136] In addition, *S. moniliformis* can cause disease in turkeys,[84] guinea pigs,[65] koalas,[111] spinifex hopping mice,[61] and nonhuman primates (rhesus monkey).[130] In one study looking at colonization in dogs with confirmed rat contact, 3 of 10 animals had evidence of *S. moniliformis* by polymerase chain reaction (PCR) using mouth swabs.[140] Because many of these animals prey on rodents, they could pose a potential source of infection for humans.

Children living in crowded urban centers or rural impoverished areas have traditionally thought to be at the highest risk.[32,60,99,133] However, given the changing perception of rats as family pets, rat-bite fever in the United States is shifting from a disease of poverty to a disease of pet owners, particularly children.[33,87] Children are generally reported to account for at least 50% of rat-bite fever cases, and indeed, one-half of all *S. moniliformis* isolates identified at the California state Microbial Diseases Laboratory between 1970 and 1998 involved children younger than 9 years of age.[56] A 2014 *Morbidity and Mortality Weekly Report* review of 17 cases showed a median age of 10 years.[1]

In addition, over the last few years in the United States, most cases are now reported among pet owners. To demonstrate the changing epidemiology, a 2007 review of 65 cases going back as far as 1938 showed 26 patients (40%) with wild rat exposure, eight (12%) with laboratory rat exposure, and three (5%) with pet shop rat exposure. Twenty-two (34%) of the patients described an exposure not relating to a bite or a rat.[40] However, among 11 US cases published since 2012, 10 were associated with pet rats.[1,11,16,19,43,66,69,71,134,142] Moreover, a review of 17 cases in San Diego from 2010 to 2012 demonstrated that 94% of cases were associated with pets. Although 44% of the patients in this cases series reported having handled a rat, only 38% reported being bitten.[1] An estimated 0.1% of US households owned one or more pet rats during 2011.[1] Some authors have related this figure to the increasing popularity of rats as pets driven by popular culture.[134,142]

Pet owners include those who keep rats, as pets as well as those who keep rats to feed other pets, such as snakes and large reptiles.[5,8,30,43,66,69,70,131] Some cases of rat- bite fever have involved laboratory personnel who handle rats.[1,7] Although rat-bite fever is often reported after the bite of a rat, it also may be transmitted by rat scratches, contact with a break in the skin, mucosal contact (kissing a rat), or simply handling an animal.[21,30,45,58,96,112]

Rat-bite fever has been reported worldwide; however, it is not a reportable disease. The actual incidence is unknown, although it is widely believed to be underreported. A report from the California state Microbial Disease Laboratory from 2001 reported an incidence of approximately 1.5 cases per year from 1970 to 1998, with more than one-half of the reported cases occurring after 1990. The report cited a possible increase in incidence after 1990; however, this is largely speculative because the numbers represent only confirmed cases.[56] Difficulty in isolating the organism, improved detection techniques, and an increase in physicians' awareness of the disease all may influence the reported rates. The mortality rate of rat-bite fever has been reported to be 7% to 13% if the disease is left untreated[33,40,50]; however, the number of patients with mild or subclinical disease is not known.

BACTERIOLOGY

S. moniliformis is a pleomorphic, microaerophilic, nonmotile, nonencapsulated, non–acid-fast, gram-negative bacillus. It measures 1 to 5 μm in length.[59] The organism is oxidase and catalase negative and ferments glucose, maltose, fructose, galactose, and salicin.[59] *S. moniliformis* is facultatively anerobic,[44,50] and it is the only species in its genus.

The organism is fastidious and requires special handling for isolation. Optimal growth is achieved in trypticase soy agar or broth supplemented with 20% horse or rabbit serum.[89] Alternatively, brain-heart infusion broth supplemented with "Panmede" (a papain digest of ox liver) also has been shown to support the growth of *S. moniliformis.*[121] Sodium polyanethol sulfonate, which is added to most aerobic blood culture bottles at a concentration of 0.05%, inhibits the growth of *S. moniliformis* at concentrations as low as 0.0125%.[121] Blood culture bottles without sodium polyanethol sulfonate added should be used for primary isolation of *S. moniliformis* when rat-bite fever is suspected. Another option is to inoculate twice the amount of blood than recommended by the manufacturer into the blood culture bottle.[51] Anaerobic cultures may be more likely to yield the organism.[29] Material from lymph nodes, abscesses, and synovial fluid also may be useful material for isolation of the organism.[51] One other alternative is to inoculate citrated blood directly into broth. Cultures should be incubated at 35° to 37°C (95°F–98.6°F) in a humid environment with a partial pressure of carbon dioxide between 8% and 10%.

The morphologic characteristics of the bacterium depend on the environment.[87] In favorable media, the typical appearance is that of short rods that may grow in chains. In other conditions, the organism tends to grow in long, interwoven filaments that commonly contain beaded and fusiform swellings throughout their length. The Latin term *moniliformis* translates to "in the form of a necklace." In broth culture, colonies usually appear in 2 to 10 days.[59] The colonies are white, soft "puffballs" measuring 1 to 2 mm in diameter.[5] On blood agar plates, the colonies are round, gray, and glistening and measure 1 to 2 mm in diameter after 2 to 3 days of incubation.[59]

Stable L forms of the organism develop spontaneously in vivo or in vitro. These cell wall–deficient forms have a "fried egg" appearance with dark centers and lacy edges when they are grown on solid media.[59,92] The L form is considered nonpathogenic, even though spontaneous conversion between the two forms has been reported in vitro and may be responsible for relapses and resistance to therapy, although this is not certain.[40,49,119] L forms are resistant to penicillin and other antibiotics active against the bacterial cell wall. These variants may be deposited in tissues and prolong the symptoms of illness.[36]

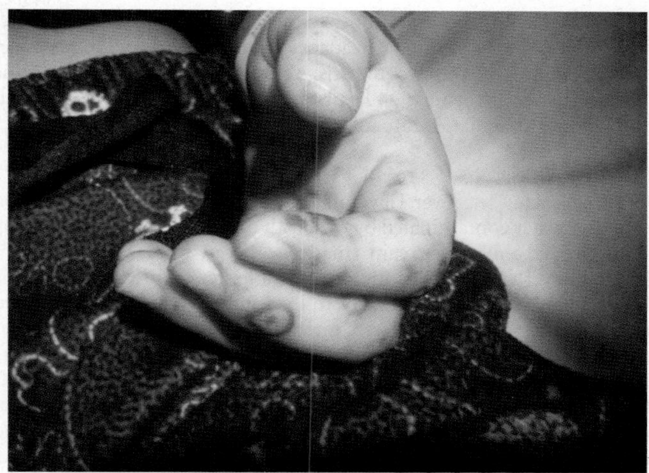

FIG. 138.1 An 8-year-old child with fever, rash, and arthritis with confirmed rat-bite fever from contact with a pet rat. (Courtesy S. Islam, A. Petru, and A. LaBeaud, Children's Hospital and Research Center, Oakland, CA.)

CLINICAL MANIFESTATIONS

Streptobacillary rat-bite fever often has an incubation period of less than a week, usually ranging from 3 to 10 days, although an incubation period of up to 3 weeks has been documented.[4] Young children may have shorter incubation times. Typically the bite or scratch site, if known, is well healed (as opposed to spirillary rat-bite fever) and often is not evident on examination. Most patients have evidence of contact with a rat, often as a pet, although not necessarily a bite history. Up to 30% or more of patients are reported to have no history of a bite or scratch.[22]

A review of 65 patients showed an age range of 2 months to 87 years. Symptoms described included fever (92%), polyarthralgias (66%), rash (61%), nausea and vomiting (40%), headache (34%), myalgias (29%), and sore throat (17%). White blood cell counts were often normal, with polymorphonuclear cell and band form predominance. Only 5 patients (8%) demonstrated white blood cell counts higher than 15,000/mm.[4,40] Hypertension is also reported.[19,70]

Rash develops usually within a few days of fever onset (range, 1–8 days) in approximately 75% of patients. The rash may be generalized, but more often it is prominent on the extremities and frequently involves the palms and soles (Fig. 138.1).[2,30,77,92] The characteristics of the rash are variable, and the rash has been described as maculopapular, petechial, purpuric, pustular, hemorrhagic, vesicular, and bullous.[4,11,31,40,50,62,66] Desquamation is reported in approximately 20% of patients, and the rash may take several weeks to resolve.[50]

Arthralgia or arthritis with or without joint effusion also develops in more than 50% of patients, classically within the first week of illness. Arthritis usually involves large joints but also may affect small joints, and it tends to be migratory, nonsymmetric, and extremely painful.[7,45,60,118] Arthritis may be monarthric or polyarticular and acute or subacute. Although multiple joints are usually affected, at least two cases of monarthric involvement in children have been described involving the hip joint.[37,57] With untreated infection, persistent or recurrent episodes of fever and arthritis may be experienced.[46,128]

The arthritis from rat-bite fever is often nonsuppurative with sterile joint fluid cultures. Investigators have hypothesized that *Streptobacillus* may cause both direct infective arthritis and an immune-mediated phenomenon, although this is not well understood.[33] At least two reviews of septic arthritis caused by *S. moniliformis* (defined by isolation from joint or synovial fluid) with at least 17 individual cases have been reported.[33,135] Rash was present in a minority of patients only. Arthritis may manifest as a septic hip in children and may mimic rheumatoid arthritis in older patients with peripheral joints affected.[67,86] Patients with underlying osteoarthritis may be predisposed to this complication. *Streptobacillus* has also been reported as a cause of culture-negative arthritis in patients with human immunodeficiency virus infection.[24] The prognosis is quite favorable overall, with all patients in these series recovering with treatment.[33,135]

Complications of *S. moniliformis* infection include anemia,[106] cutaneous or subcutaneous abscess formation,[20,57,92,132] interstitial pneumonia,[79,119] mastoiditis,[93] meningitis,[8,119] pericardial effusion,[18] pancreatitis, prostatitis,[141] septic arthritis,[33,58,73,109,113,135] and overwhelming sepsis.[1,22,88,119] Children presenting with sepsis may not have rash or typical findings.[1,22,119] Abscess formation in several different organs, including the brain,[35] the female genital tract,[92] and the spleen,[25] has been reported. Unusual and potentially devastating complications include chorioamnionitis,[41] periarteritis nodosa,[98] and endocarditis. Rapid acute kidney injury has also been described[19] as well as osteomyelitis (first reported in a toddler in 2013).[43] Vertebral osteomyelitis[114] and vertebral spondylodiskitis[86] have also been reported in adults.

The most frequent serious complication is bacterial endocarditis, with a nearly 50% mortality rate.[9,23,77,101,104,110,124] At least 25 cases of endocarditis have been reported in publications, with more than one-half of the cases reported before 1968.[23,40,42,72,74,110,123] Many patients reported had underlying valvular disease.[40] In a review of 17 cases, the majority of patients (12) had systemic symptoms, including fever, rash, and arthritis.[110] Of 14 cases in which patients' clinical symptoms were reported, murmur was noted in 100%, petechiae in 13%, Osler's nodes in 13%, hepatosplenomegaly in 33%, anemia in 33%, and cardiac dysrhythmia in 13%.[110] At least six cases have involved children younger than 18 years of age, with the youngest just 2 months of age.[79,97,107,110,119,124,127] Of the six children, five died during the acute illness. The three most recent reported cases of endocarditis were reported from Spain in 2010, India in 2013, and the United Kingdom in 2014, all involving adults with native mitral valve endocarditis.[42,72,74]

At least eight fatal pediatric cases have been reported, the majority with endocarditis. Most deaths were described in the 1930s and 1940s among older children with endocarditis. In the 1980s, two separate cases of infant deaths related to rat-bite fever were described. One case involved a 3-month-old infant with endocarditis, and the other was a 2-month-old infant with disseminated disease. In 2011, another fatal case in a 14-month-old infant with disseminated disease was described, with autopsy findings similar to those of the 2-month-old infant, including interstitial pneumonitis, meningitis (with isolation of the organism from cerebrospinal fluid [CSF]), and hepatomegaly.[10,59,87,106] In 2013, a 10-year-old previously healthy child with pet rats died after a 2-day history of fever and nonspecific symptoms. He initially experienced rigors, fevers, vomiting, headaches, and leg pains, and the disorder was misdiagnosed as gastroenteritis. The child collapsed and became unresponsive over the next 24 hours; he had evidence of disseminated intravascular coagulation on autopsy.[1]

Haverhill Fever

Unlike typical rat-bite fever, Haverhill fever is transmitted by the ingestion of food or water contaminated by rats, with previous outbreaks involving unpasteurized milk, ice cream (made from raw milk), and water.[78,94] Haverhill fever was reported first in 1926 after an outbreak of epidemic illness in Haverhill, Massachusetts. In that outbreak, 86 cases developed and were traced to contaminated, unpasteurized milk.[94] The illness was referred to as *erythema arthriticum epidemicum*. Although this was the first published outbreak, in 1925 approximately 400 cases of a similar illness were reported in Chester, Pennsylvania.[40] The causative organism was isolated, described in detail by Parker and Hudson[89] in 1926, and given the name *Haverhillia multiformis*. It was later shown to be identical to *S. moniliformis*. The first outbreak in Britain was described in 1983 at a boarding school in Essex and affected more than 200 students; it was also believed to be related to contaminated raw milk.[91,122] Haverhill fever is similar to streptobacillary rat-bite fever, with an abrupt onset of fever and chills (100%), rash (95%), and arthritis (97%).[3,78] Generally, the incubation period is 1 to 3 days. Upper respiratory and gastrointestinal problems are common. Multiple recurrences of fever are found rarely, and the rash tends to be small and uniform in size.[79]

PATHOPHYSIOLOGY AND PATHOLOGY

Factors influencing the virulence of *S. moniliformis* are not well described. The organism has an affinity for synovial tissue in both animals and humans, but the mechanisms by which *S. moniliformis* produces arthritis are unknown.[54,55,60,63,73,115,129] Studies performed in mice indicate that *S. moniliformis* is only slightly immunogenic and produces mild leukocytosis and minimal homologous antibody production.[115,116] In addition, the organism is resistant to phagocytic destruction.[115] These factors may allow chronic infection to develop. Because the organism may spontaneously convert to the cell wall–deficient form (or L form), this has been speculated to be responsible for relapsing disease.

The pathologic features of streptobacillary rat-bite fever have been described in a limited number of autopsy reports. Common features include ulcerative endocarditis with secondary septic embolization in the liver and spleen, septic arthritis, and interstitial pneumonia.[13,119] Mononuclear meningitis and erythrophagocytosis also have been reported.[119] In a pediatric autopsy report, in which *Streptobacillus* grew from the cerebrospinal fluid, mild flattening of the cerebral gyri with mild collapse of the ventricular system was seen, but no major histopathologic changes were noted in the brain. The kidneys had findings consistent with disseminated intravascular coagulopathy. The small and large intestine, liver, thymus, thyroid gland, larynx, and heart showed mild to moderate autolysis, but no other major histopathologic changes.[10] In most reports, the site of the bite reveals little histologic evidence of inflammation.[79]

DIAGNOSIS

Three fatal cases reported in the Centers for Disease Control and Prevention (CDC) *Morbidity and Mortality Weekly Report* highlight the importance of considering rat-bite fever in the differential diagnosis.[1,22] The diagnosis of rat-bite fever requires a high index of suspicion on the part of the physician. The diagnosis is suggested in a febrile patient with a history of exposure to rats, but in most clinical settings, the exposure history is not elucidated until after the diagnosis is made. This diagnosis should be considered in patients who present with fever, rash, and arthritis.[125]

Nonspecific laboratory findings may include the following: elevation in the white blood cell count,[13] usually in the range of 10,000 to 30,000 cells/mm^3 with a left shift; mild anemia; and a false-positive serologic test result for syphilis, which may occur in 25% of patients.[106] Direct visualization of the organism on Giemsa stain of blood or joint fluid may suggest the diagnosis. Serologic assays are not currently available for humans. An enzyme-linked immunosorbent assay has been developed to monitor infection in rodent colonies.[14]

Molecular techniques may be an effective means for detection of *S. moniliformis* from humans and animals and may offer an alternative to traditional culture methods.[6,12,15,47] Broad-range PCR amplification of a part of the 16S rRNA gene followed by sequencing allowed the detection and identification of *S. moniliformis* in blister fluid of a patient reported in 1991.[12] A PCR assay specific for *S. moniliformis* was described by Boot and colleagues[15] by using primers designed on the basis of 16S rRNA gene base sequence data of human and rodent strains of *S. moniliformis*, and similar assays have been used subsequently.[85,140] PCR testing is becoming more refined; a 2008 publication described new primers to amplify the 16S rRNA gene of *Streptobacillus* spp. more specifically than prior tests.[64] Since 2008 multiple reports have noted detection of *S. moniliformis* by PCR from blood, bite wounds, and synovial fluid.[17,19,24,31,43,71,85] Although PCR testing using 16s rRNA is becoming more readily available through tertiary care centers and reference laboratories, it is still not widely used in the community hospital setting.[19]

S. moniliformis has been cultured from blood, joint fluid, abscesses, pericardial fluid, meninges, and tissues obtained at autopsy.[10,21] The organism has strict growth requirements, and the choice of culture media and technique is of critical importance for optimal growth of the bacterium (see the earlier discussion of bacteriology). Whenever this agent is suspected, it is helpful to alert the laboratory that will be performing isolation. In general, routine aerobic blood cultures are not satisfactory for isolation. If the organism is isolated, it may be identified rapidly by gas-liquid chromatography. *S. moniliformis* has a characteristic fatty acid profile, with major peaks of palmitic, linoleic, oleic, and stearic acid.[92,108] Electrophoretic protein patterns also have been described that can distinguish Haverhill fever strains from rat-bite fever strains.[28]

The differential diagnosis for streptobacillary rat-bite fever includes illness caused by *S. minus* (see Chapter 142). It also includes all relapsing fevers, such as *Borrelia recurrentis* infection, malaria, and typhoid. Rocky Mountain spotted fever must be considered[76] as well as other infectious entities, including leptospirosis, Lyme disease, disseminated gonococcal infection, meningococcemia, brucellosis, and syphilis. Viral infections also may be mistaken for rat-bite fever. Acute rheumatic fever should be considered as well. The frequent symmetric involvement of small joints of the hands can be particularly suggestive of rheumatoid arthritis.[60] Other noninfectious entities include drug reactions, collagen vascular disease, and other rheumatologic conditions. With the emergence of outbreaks of Coxsackievirus A6 in the United States as recently as 2011, clinicians must also be wary of misdiagnosing rat-bite fever as atypical hand, foot, mouth disease.[43,75]

TREATMENT AND PREVENTION

Although fatal in some cases, streptobacillary rat-bite fever is a very treatable disease that is usually responsive to a variety of antibiotics. The treatment of choice for *S. moniliformis* is penicillin G. Either procaine penicillin intramuscularly or aqueous penicillin intravenously is acceptable.[4,98] Tests of *S. moniliformis* antibiotic susceptibility usually demonstrate sensitivity to penicillins, cephalosporins, carbapenems, aztreonam, clindamycin, tetracyclines, and vancomycin; intermediate susceptibility to aminoglycosides, fluoroquinolones, amikacin, and chloramphenicol; and resistance to trimethoprim-sulfamethoxazole.[39,141] Only one penicillin-resistant *S. moniliformis* strain has been demonstrated, and that was more than 50 years ago.[40] A 1965 study noted the rapid response to penicillin was in stark contrast to other regimens.[98] Penicillin is also the drug of choice for Haverhill fever; however, Haverhill fever has also been successfully treated with tetracycline.[121]

Traditionally in adults, the dosage of penicillin has been recommended at no less than 400,000 to 600,000 IU/day of intravenous aqueous penicillin G continued for at least 7 days and up to 10 to 14 days.[40,48,62,87,104] Treatment with penicillin for up to 28 days or more has been reported in cases of presumed septic arthritis and osteomyelitis.[43,135] If no response is seen within 2 days, the dosage should be increased to 1.2 million IU/day.[98] Children have been treated successfully with 20,000 to 50,000 IU/

kg/day of intravenous penicillin, up to a maximum of 1.2 million IU/day.[120] In children, some investigators suggest that after 5 to 7 days of intravenous therapy with goal response, treatment may be completed by oral penicillin.[22,40,62]

No controlled studies have been conducted on the duration of intravenous versus oral therapy, and increasingly more patients are being treated with shorter durations of intravenous therapy. Case reports have shown success with as little as 48 to 72 hours or less of intravenous therapy in patients without severe disease.[80,105,134] Both adults and children have also been treated successfully as outpatients with regimens including oral penicillin, amoxicillin, cephalexin, clarithromycin, and doxycycline (in the case of penicillin-allergic patients).[21,31,69,70,131,142] Oral penicillin VK, 1 to 2 g/day in divided doses, may be given.[48,120] Other successful regimens have included aminoglycosides, cephalosporins, chloramphenicol, and gentamicin.[19,21,30,58,95,104,110,118] The suggested dose is oral tetracycline, 500 mg four times per day, or intramuscular streptomycin, 7.5 mg/kg twice daily.[94] Treatment failure with oral erythromycin has been reported.[57]

Optimal therapy for *S. moniliformis* endocarditis is based on case reports, given the rarity of disease. High-dose aqueous intravenous penicillin G or procaine penicillin intramuscularly is the treatment of choice. Some experts suggest using penicillin in combination with streptomycin or gentamicin for up to 2 weeks, although data are limited.[40,72] For adults, daily administration of intramuscular procaine penicillin G at 4.8 million IU has been recommended if the isolate is susceptible (0.1 μg/mL).[40,110] If the isolate is more resistant, intravenous penicillin G at 20 million IU/day should be used.[110] In children, the dosage is intravenous aqueous penicillin, 160,000 to 240,000 IU/kg/day (96–144 mg/kg per day), up to the adult maximum of 20 million IU/day.[40,110,120] Treatment should be continued for at least 4 weeks up to 6 weeks on the basis of treatment of other types of bacterial endocarditis.[40] Successful treatment of endocarditis with ceftriaxone in combination with gentamicin has been reported.[104] In a review of 16 patients with endocarditis, four patients who did not receive specific antimicrobial therapy died, as did three patients who received less than 1 million IU/days of penicillin; only two patients who received more than 1 million IU/day of penicillin died, and oneof those patients died suddenly 4 months after valve replacement.[110] Although endocarditis is more common in patients with artificial valves, the three most recently reported published cases since 2010 all had native valve endocarditis.[42,72,74]

PREVENTION

Rat-bite fever can be prevented by controlling rodents in urban areas, properly handling rodents including pets, and avoiding unpasteurized milk products. Persons who own rats and those who work with rodents should receive anticipatory guidance regarding the handling of these animals and the signs and symptoms of rat-bite fever. If a rat bites a person, prophylactic antibiotics, such as amoxicillin or amoxicillin-clavulanic acid, may prevent rat-bite fever, but current data do not support the routine use of antibiotics after all rat bites. Some researchers suggest that because of the serious nature of rat-bite fever in young infants, infants younger than 3 months of age who are bitten by a rat should receive antibiotic prophylaxis.[76]

Acknowledgment

We thank Carrie L. Byington, MD, for her work on this chapter in the previous edition of the text.

NEW REFERENCES SINCE THE SEVENTH EDITION

1. Adam JK, Varan AK, Pong AL, McDonald EC, Centers for Disease Control and Prevention (CDC). Notes from the field: fatal rat-bite fever in a child—San Diego County, California, 2013. *MMWR Morb Mortal Wkly Rep*. 2014;63(50):1210-1211.
11. Barsky M, Higgins HW, Lee KC, Robinson-Bostom L, Muglia JJ. Acrally distributed purpuric and necrotic lesions with pustular features. *Arch Dermatol*. 2012;148(12):1411-1416.
16. Brown CM, Tsai G, Sanchez-Flores X. Oh rats! Fever, rash and arthritis in a young woman. *BMJ Case Rep*. 2015;2015:2015212240.
17. Budair B, Goswami K, Dhukaram V. Septic arthritis secondary to rat bite fever: a challenging diagnostic course. *BMJ Case Rep*. 2014;2014:2014204086.
19. Carr JP, McCloskey KM, Campbell J, Efron D. Fever, rash and acute kidney injury in a 10-year-old girl. *Pediatr Infect Dis J*. 2014;33(2):227-231.
24. Chean R, Stefanski DA, Woolley IJ, Francis MJ, Korman TM. Rat bite fever as a presenting illness in a patient with AIDS. *Infection*. 2012;40(3):319-321.
29. Crews JD, Palazzi DL, Starke JR. A teenager with fever, rash, and arthralgia: *Streptobacillus moniliformis* infection. *JAMA Pediatr*. 2014;168(12):1165-1166.
31. Danion F, Bui E, Riegel P, Goichot B. *Streptobacillosis* characterised by palmoplantar pustulosis. *Lancet Infect Dis*. 2013;13(1):96.
42. Fenn DW, Ramoutar A, Jacob G, Bin Xiao H. An unusual tale of rat-bite fever endocarditis. *BMJ Case Rep*. 2014;2014:2014204989.
43. Flannery DD, Akinboyo I, Ty JM, Averill LW, Freedman A. Septic arthritis and concern for osteomyelitis in a child with rat bite fever. *J Clin Microbiol*. 2013;51(6):1987-1989.
66. Kwon CW, Somers K, Scott G, Mercurio MG. Rat bite fever presenting as palpable purpura. *JAMA Dermatol*. 2016;152:723-724.
69. Lewis BK, Vanderhooft S. Rat bite fever: fever, arthritis, and rash in a 4-year-old boy. *Pediatr Dermatol*. 2012;29(6):767-768.
70. Lu H, van Beers EJ, van den Berk GE. Pythons and a palmar rash. *Neth J Med*. 2012;70(5):230-233.
71. Mackey JR, Melendez EL, Farrell JJ, et al. Direct detection of indirect transmission of *Streptobacillus moniliformis* rat bite fever infection. *J Clin Microbiol*. 2014;52(6):2259-2261.
72. Madhubashini M, George S, Chandrasekaran S. *Streptobacillus moniliformis* endocarditis: case report and review of literature. *Indian Heart J*. 2013;65(4):442-446.
74. Maroto F, Gallego S, Pérez C, Colon C. [Infectious endocarditis in rat bite disease]. *Med Intensiva*. 2011;35(5):317-318.
75. Mathes EF, et al. "Eczema coxsackium" and unusual cutaneous findings in an enterovirus outbreak. *Pediatrics*. 2013;132(1):e149-e157.
80. McKee G, Pewarchuk J. Rat-bite fever. *CMAJ*. 2013;185(15):1346.
86. Nei T, Sato A, Sonobe K, et al. *Streptobacillus moniliformis* bacteremia in a rheumatoid arthritis patient without a rat bite: a case report. *BMC Res Notes*. 2015;8:694.
88. Okamori S, Nakano M, Nakamura M, et al. A Japanese patient with a rare case of *Streptobacillus moniliformis* bacteremia. *J Infect Chemother*. 2015;21(12):877-878.
105. Rosser A, Wiselka M, Pareek M. Rat bite fever: an unusual cause of a maculopapular rash. *Postgrad Med J*. 2014;90(1062):236-237.
114. Sato R, Kuriyama A, Nasu M. Rat-bite fever complicated by vertebral osteomyelitis: a case report. *J Infect Chemother*. 2016;22:574-576.
134. Vetter NM, Feder HM Jr, Ratzan RM. Rat bite fever caused by a kiss. *Am J Emerg Med*. 2016;34:1190.e3-1190.e4.
142. Zerbib LD, Steele RW. A Harry Potter fan. *Clin Pediatr (Phila)*. 2013;52(1):96-98.

The full reference list for this chapter is available at ExpertConsult.com.

139 *Bartonella* Infections

Leigh M. Howard • Kathryn M. Edwards

DEFINITION

Bartonella species cause infection in both zoonotic and human hosts and give rise to a wide spectrum of acute or chronic disease symptoms. The development of different manifestations of *Bartonella* disease depends on the immune status of the host. Until 1993, only three human diseases were known to be caused by *Bartonella* species.[2] However, advances in molecular techniques have led to the reclassification of several pathogens within the family Bartonellaceae, genus *Bartonella,* expanding to include more than 30 validated species.[11] Several of these species have been associated with human disease (Table 139.1). The current *Bartonella* genus was created by merging with the genus *Rochalimaea* on the basis of both DNA-DNA hybridization data and comparison of 16s rRNA gene sequences.[12] Of the members of the genus *Rochalimaea* that have been reclassified as *Bartonella* spp., *Bartonella henselae,* the cause of cat-scratch disease (CSD), is the most common *Bartonella*-associated infection in children. *Bartonella* infections other than CSD seldom occur in children and are discussed briefly later in the chapter.

MICROBIOLOGY

Comparisons of the 16s rRNA-encoding genes have shown that the *Bartonella* genus is most closely related to *Brucella* and *Agrobacterium. Bartonella* are small, gram-negative, fastidious coccobacilli or slightly curved rods that grow best on enriched blood–containing media in 5% carbon dioxide. Colony morphology varies from small, dry, gray-white colonies to smooth, creamy yellow colonies. Although the optimal growth temperature for *B. bacilliformis* is 28°C, optimal temperatures for other *Bartonella* species range from 35° to 37°C. Even with optimal conditions, these organisms require 1 to 6 weeks to grow in culture.[13] Increasingly, the presence of *Bartonella* organisms is detected by molecular methods. Organisms of the *Bartonella* genus may colonize human endothelial cells or may persist as intraerythrocytic parasites in the host.[24]

CAT-SCRATCH DISEASE

CSD, caused by *Bartonella henselae,* is an acute, self-limited infection that begins as a papule or nodule at the site of a scratch or bite by a cat, followed by regional lymphadenopathy. In a small number of patients, more serious systemic complications result, including involvement of the central nervous system, liver, spleen, bone, heart, eyes, or skin. Although CSD was recognized as a clinical entity in the 1930s, the first written report, by Debré from France, was not published until 1950.

Etiology

For more than 40 years, numerous unsuccessful attempts were made to isolate an organism from nodes of patients with CSD. The first clue emerged in 1983, when Wear and colleagues,[83] using Warthin-Starry silver stain, demonstrated small, pleomorphic, gram-negative bacilli in lymph nodes and skin papules from patients with CSD. Then, in 1988, an organism was isolated by English and associates[25] from the lymph nodes of patients with CSD and was subsequently termed *Afipia felis.* However, the discovery of bacillary angiomatosis and its association with *B.* (formerly *Rochalimaea*) *henselae* suggested that it could be the agent responsible for CSD.[67] In 1992, Regnery and coworkers,[66] using indirect fluorescent antibody (IFA) assays, demonstrated elevated antibodies to *B. henselae* in serum samples from patients with suspected CSD. We and others,[2,3] using enzyme-linked immunosorbent assays demonstrated that patients with CSD had significant serologic responses to *B. henselae* and *Bartonella quintana* but not to *A. felis.*[58,79] These data further supported that the causative agent of CSD was related antigenically to the *Bartonella* genus and not to *Afipia.*[79] In a physician survey to identify cases of CSD occurring during a 13-month period in cat owners in Connecticut, Zangwill and colleagues[85] demonstrated that of 45 patients with clinical CSD, 38 had antibody titers of 1:64 or higher to *B. henselae* as compared with only 4 of 112 samples from controls ($P < .001$). Finally, the use of polymerase chain reaction (PCR)

TABLE 139.1 ***Bartonella* Species Causing Human Disease**

Bartonella Species	Country of First Cultivation	Year of Description	Reservoir Host/Vector	Human Disease
B. alsatica	France	1999	Rabbit	Endocarditis, lymphadenopathy
B. bacilliformis	—	1909	Human/sand fly	Carrión disease, Oroya fever, verruga peruana
B. clarridgeiae	—	1996	Cat/cat flea	Cat-scratch disease
B. elizabethae	United States	1993	Rat	Endocarditis, neuroretinitis
B. grahamii	United Kingdom	1995	Rat, insectivore	Neuroretinitis
B. henselae		1990	Cat/cat flea	Cat-scratch disease, endocarditis, bacillary angiomatosis, bacillary peliosis hepatis, Parinaud oculoglandular syndrome, neuroretinitis, osteomyelitis, arthropathy, bacteremia with fever
B. koehlerae	United States	1999	Cat	Endocarditis
B. mayotimonensis	United States	2009	Unknown	Endocarditis
B. melophagi	United States	2006	Unknown	Bacteremia
B. quintana		1920	Human/body louse	Trench fever, endocarditis, bacillary angiomatosis
B. rochalimae	United States	2007		Bacteremia, fever, splenomegaly
B. tamiae	Thailand	2008		Febrile illness
B. vinsonii subsp. arupensis	United States	1999	Dog, rodent/ticks	Bacteremia with fever, endocarditis
B. vinsonii subsp. berkhoffii	United States	1999	Dog	Endocarditis
B. washoensis	—	2000	Ground squirrel	Myocarditis

Modified from Rolain JM, Rauoult D. *Bartonella* infections. In: Goldman L, Schafer AI, et al, eds. *Cecil Medicine.* 24th ed. Philadelphia: Elsevier; 2012:1907.

confirmed the causative agent of CSD as *B. henselae*.[3] Eventually, PCR amplification was used to detect *B. henselae* not only in purulent material aspirated from involved nodes but also in CSD skin test material.[1,35,74] Subsequently, *B. henselae* has been cultured from lymph nodes obtained from patients with CSD.[32]

Transmission

Domesticated house cats are healthy carriers of *B. henselae,* and cat fleas *(Ctenocephalides felis)* play a major role in cat-to-cat transmission. Approximately 90% of patients with CSD have a history of exposure to cats, particularly a scratch or bite from a kitten with fleas. Although cats remain asymptomatic, they serve as a persistent reservoir for *B. henselae.* Reported *B. henselae* seroprevalence rates in cats vary. The southeastern United States, Hawaii, and coastal California have the highest seroprevalence in cats (40–54.7%), whereas rates are much lower (3.7–6.7%) in the Rocky Mountain and Midwestern regions.[43] In another study, blood was collected from a convenience sample of 271 pet cats 3 months to 2 years of age in four areas of the United States (southern California, Florida, metropolitan Chicago, and metropolitan Washington, DC). Overall, 65 (24%) cats had *B. henselae* bacteremia, and 138 (51%) cats were seropositive for *B. henselae.* Regional prevalences for bacteremia and seropositivity were highest in Florida (33% and 67%, respectively) and California (28% and 62%, respectively) and lowest in the Washington, DC (12% and 28%, respectively) and Chicago (6% and 12%, respectively) areas.[37] In another report, blood samples obtained from domestic and impounded cats in the San Francisco Bay region grew *B. henselae* 27% of the time; kittens were 4.7 times more likely to have a very high bacterial load than were young adult cats.[27] Investigators reported that *Bartonella* spp. were isolated from the blood of 4 of 14 (29%) mountain lions and from 7 of 19 (37%) bobcats living in the wild.[20] *B. henselae* also was detected in fleas from infected cats by both direct culture and PCR, although no data support flea-to-human transmission.

Interestingly, Chang and colleagues[18] found that *Ixodes pacificus* and *Dermacentor* ticks from five of six California counties were also PCR positive for *B. henselae.* Coinfections with *B. henselae* and *Borrelia burgdorferi* were described in three patients in New Jersey.[26] *Ixodes* ticks obtained from two of the three households of patients with CSD were PCR positive for *B. henselae.* More recently, potentially zoonotic strains from six *Bartonella* species were detected in samples from patients who had chronic, subjective symptoms and who reported tick bites. Three strains were *B. henselae,* and three were from other animal-associated *Bartonella* spp. (*B. doshiae, B. schoenbuchensis,* and *B. tribocorum*). This investigation identified three novel *Bartonella* spp. strains with human pathogenic potential and showed that *Bartonella* spp. may be the cause of undifferentiated chronic illness in humans who have been bitten by ticks.[81] Thus clinicians should consider *Bartonella* infection in humans after tick bites, although the frequency of transmission is unknown.

Epidemiology

CSD most commonly affects children and young adults worldwide, with regional variations. The Centers for Disease Control and Prevention estimate that, overall, more than 22,000 cases of CSD occur each year in the United States. Using a national inpatient database, Reynolds and coworkers[70] estimated that 437 pediatric hospitalizations for CSD (0.60 per 100,000 population) occurred in 2000, with 60% between July and October. Rates were higher in children younger than 5 years of age and higher in the southern states, findings underscoring the regional differences. Zangwill and colleagues[85] suggested that the seasonality of CSD could be explained by the breeding patterns of cats and fleas. Cats often become pregnant in late spring or early fall, and after a 9-week gestation period, kittens are born in early fall or midwinter. Flea breeding peaks during the late summer months.

Pathobiology

Histopathologic examination of the primary inoculation lesion demonstrates dermal necrosis, with variable numbers of histiocytes and occasional multinucleated giant cells accompanied by scattered microabscesses with neutrophils, eosinophils, lymphocytes, and plasma cells. The epidermal changes are nonspecific and consist of parakeratosis, hyperkeratosis, edema, and exocytosis of inflammatory cells. Characteristic findings in the lymph nodes, similar to the primary lesion, include follicular hyperplasia, focal cortical necrosis, and necrotizing granulomas with central microabscesses and palisading histiocytes. A perivascular neutrophilic infiltrate may also be present. Subsequently, the lesions progress to "stellate microabscesses" within small cortical granulomas. Warthin-Starry or Steiner silver impregnation stains may reveal pleomorphic bacilli in clusters or short chains within the areas of central necrosis or around small vessels, particularly in early lesions. Granulomas with microabscess formation also can be found in the liver, spleen, and bone. Because other organisms such as the cause of tularemia, fungi, and mycobacteria may have similar histopathologic characteristics, the histopathologic findings must be correlated with the clinical findings and other laboratory studies, including serology, culture, or PCR.

In vitro studies have identified several additional properties of *B. henselae.* When *B. henselae* infects endothelial cells, it induces activation of nuclear factor-κB and expression of adhesion molecules, an important step in the pathogenesis of CSD and bacillary angiomatosis.[18,33] Animal studies have shown that interferon-γ–mediated activation of macrophages is involved in clearing *B. henselae* infection and that microbicidal activity is mediated to a large extent by nitric oxide.[56] A role for cell-mediated immunity in CSD is suggested by the positive skin test reaction to injected material aspirated from cat-scratch nodes and the granulomatous lesions noted in biopsy specimens.

Clinical Manifestations and Course

The most common clinical manifestation, often referred to as *typical CSD,* is a gradually enlarging regional lymph node occurring 1 to 3 weeks after a scratch or bite from a cat. An inoculation site, which often appears as a red papule 3 to 5 mm in diameter, can be detected in two-thirds of patients. Constitutional symptoms of malaise, fatigue, anorexia, emesis, and headache are common but usually are mild. Fever occurs in less than one-half of the patients with typical CSD, thus rendering the common name "cat-scratch fever" inexact. Physical examination generally reveals a skin papule at the inoculation site and regional lymphadenopathy (Fig. 139.1). In approximately 50% of cases, lymphadenopathy is the only manifestation of the disease and occurs most commonly in the upper extremity (axillary or epitrochlear lymph nodes, 46.1%), the head and neck area (cervical or submandibular, 26.1%), and the lower extremities (femoral or inguinal, 17.5%).[15] Supraclavicular lymphadenopathy, which often raises concern for malignant neoplasm, occurs rarely (2% of typical CSD cases). Suppuration of the involved lymph nodes occurs in approximately 10% of patients (Fig. 139.2). More unusual manifestations of CSD include neuroretinitis, subacute iritis, optic neuritis, focal chorioretinitis, and the oculoglandular syndrome of Parinaud (Fig. 139.3). Patients with this syndrome have painful conjunctivitis without eye drainage and

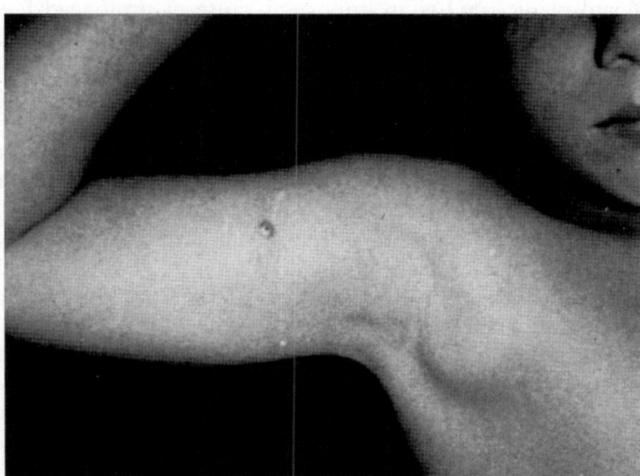

FIG. 139.1 Cat-scratch disease involving an axillary lymph node with a primary granuloma of the upper part of the arm. Note that the primary lesion is within the line of a healed scratch. (Courtesy Hugh A. Carithers, MD.)

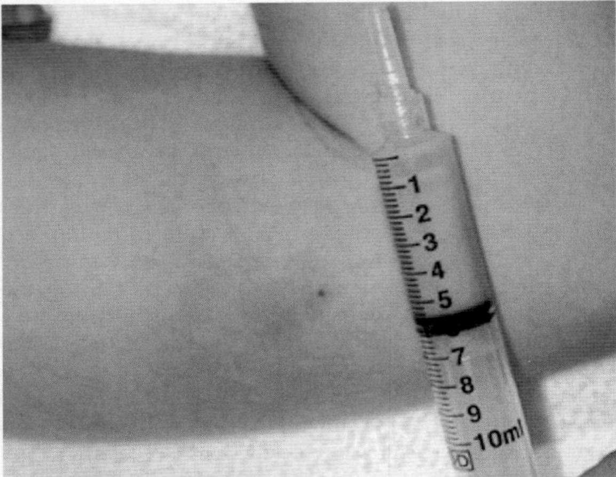

FIG. 139.2 Purulent material aspirated from an epitrochlear lymph node of a child with cat-scratch disease. The primary lesion was on the index finger.

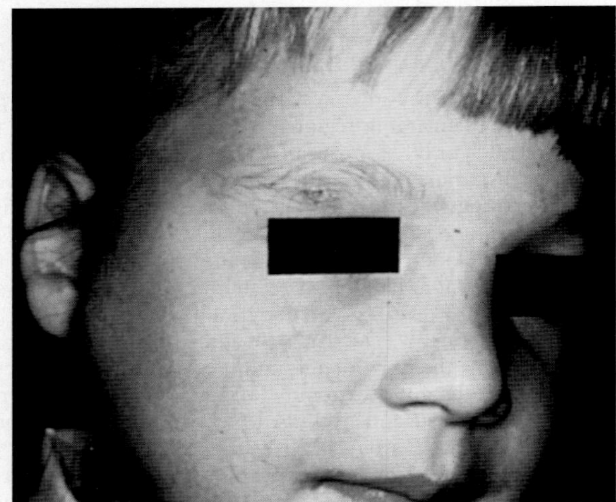

FIG. 139.3 Child with the oculoglandular syndrome of Parinaud as a manifestation of cat-scratch disease. Note the parotid swelling and the primary site in the right eyebrow. (Courtesy James D. Cherry, MD.)

preauricular adenopathy. Recovery is spontaneous without sequelae within 2 to 4 months after onset.

Hepatosplenic CSD is an important cause of prolonged fever in children and should be included in the differential diagnosis of fever of unknown origin. Often these children have fever for several weeks (mean, 3 weeks), abdominal pain (occurring in about two-thirds of patients),[5,23] joint pain, headache, weight loss, and chills. Significant lymphadenopathy is lacking in more than 50% of cases, thus rendering the diagnosis problematic. Hepatic or splenic enlargement (or both) is found in one-half of these children, but hepatic transaminase levels usually are normal. Erythrocyte sedimentation rates invariably are elevated and frequently are greater than 100 mm/h. Abdominal imaging usually demonstrates typical granulomatous lesions in the liver or spleen that often are diagnostic of this entity (Fig. 139.4). Although both ultrasonography and computed tomography (CT) demonstrate these lesions, some reports suggest that ultrasound evaluation is more sensitive than CT.[48,51] As is the case with other infections causing hepatosplenic granulomas, late calcification has been described.

Neurologic complications have been reported in approximately 2% of CSD cases, with an estimated 51 pediatric hospitalizations in 2000.[70] Encephalopathy, the most common manifestation, typically occurs 1 to 6 weeks after the onset of lymphadenopathy. Fever and seizures

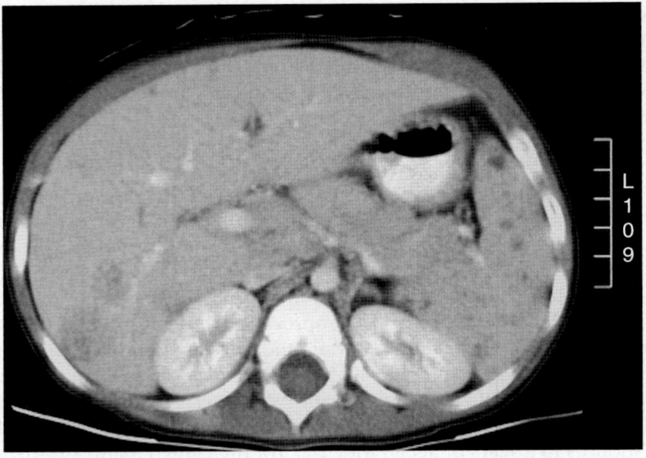

FIG. 139.4 Multiple hypodense lesions in the liver and spleen seen on computed tomography in a child with prolonged fever, abdominal pain, and positive *Bartonella henselae* serologic findings.

develop abruptly, followed by confusion, disorientation, and, occasionally, combativeness. Status epilepticus is well described. Results of cerebrospinal fluid examination frequently are normal, but occasional mild pleocytosis or an elevated protein level is seen. Electroencephalographic findings frequently are abnormal, with diffuse slowing or focal abnormalities. CT findings of the head generally are normal. Resolution of seizures and normalization of mental status often occur as suddenly as does the onset. Neurologic recovery commonly occurs within weeks and almost always is complete within a year. Persistent deficit or a need for prolonged anticonvulsant therapy has been reported in only a few cases.[38,68] Two immunocompetent children were reported to have central nervous system infection associated with *B. quintana* with a similar symptom constellation.[59]

Osteomyelitis caused by *B. henselae* is well described in publications, with one report documenting its occurrence in 2 of 1200 cases. With improved imaging, serologic methods, and PCR for diagnosis, it is now clear that *B. henselae* osteomyelitis can occur as part of a disseminated infection, in the setting of otherwise typical CSD, or as a seemingly isolated manifestation.[41,82] The pathogenesis is not clear, but it probably represents hematogenous spread, although local spread from a lymph node or abscess has been reported. Although the presentation of osteomyelitis may be acute, many patients have weeks to months of pain and intermittent fever before the diagnosis is made. A high proportion of reported cases involves the axial skeleton, most commonly the vertebral column. In a review of 47 cases by Hajjaji and colleagues,[39] lesions in the vertebrae or pelvic girdle were present in more than 50% of cases. Involvement of the long bones of the limbs, the sternum, and the skull has also been described. Although single-site involvement is typical, multifocal involvement was present in 28% of the cases in the review by Hajjaji and colleagues.[39] Most commonly, the bony lesions identified by plain film, CT, or magnetic resonance imaging are osteolytic. Magnetic resonance imaging also may show periosteal reactions, marginal sclerosis, and bone marrow lesions without cortical destruction, which are seen as hyperintense foci on T2-weighted images.

Patients with CSD also may have skin lesions other than at the inoculation site, including maculopapular rash, erythema nodosum, and petechiae secondary to thrombocytopenia. Molecular techniques have also documented hepatitis, hemolytic anemia, atypical pneumonia, pulmonary nodules, an infectious mononucleosis–like syndrome, and disseminated bartonellosis. Bacillary angiomatosis (mixed neovascular and inflammatory lesions in the skin or viscera), bacillary peliosis (dilated capillaries or multiple blood-filled cavernous spaces in the liver, spleen, or lymph nodes), and relapsing fever with bacteremia caused by *B. henselae* also can develop in immunocompromised subjects.[53]

Hemophagocytic lymphohistiocytosis, an uncommon multisystem disorder that may be triggered by infection, was also reported following

B. henselae infection, in an 11-year-old immunocompromised renal transplant recipient. Early recognition of hemophagocytic lymphohistiocytosis allowed for more directed therapy with eventual resolution.[62] CSD has also been reported in patients undergoing immunomodulatory therapy for rheumatologic diseases.[75,88]

ENDOCARDITIS

Epidemiology

Bartonella spp. have been reported as the cause of endocarditis in more than 100 cases,[64] with most cases in adults and several in adolescents. Often the culture results are negative.[7,61,63,77] In a series from a large referral laboratory in France, *Bartonella* species accounted for 28% of cases of culture-negative endocarditis, whereas in another report *Bartonella* accounted for only 3% of culture-negative cases. *B. quintana* predominates and accounts for roughly 75% of cases of endocarditis. *B. henselae* causes most of the remaining cases, and other species (*Bartonella elizabethae* and *Bartonella vinsonii*) have been reported in isolated cases. The epidemiologic characteristics of the patients differ considerably between the main two causative species. *B. quintana* endocarditis is highly associated with homelessness, chronic alcoholism, and body lice and is less likely to occur in the setting of cat exposure and underlying valvular heart disease. Endocarditis cases resulting from *B. quintana* infection also have been described in persons immunocompromised by infection with human immunodeficiency virus (HIV).[63,76] In contrast, *B. henselae* endocarditis occurs most often in patients with underlying valvulopathy (90%) and clearly is linked to exposure to cats or fleas.[30]

Clinical Manifestations

Bartonella endocarditis has a subacute presentation with fever, heart murmur, and often evidence of heart failure. Prolonged fever, night sweats, and profound weight loss also may occur. The aortic valve usually is affected; right ventricular or prosthetic valve involvement is an unusual finding. Valvular surgical intervention is needed in many cases, often because of a delay in diagnosis.

BARTONELLOSIS (CARRIÓN DISEASE)

Bartonellosis is a term that has been used to describe a distinct disease seen in Peru, Ecuador, and Colombia and that is caused by *Bartonella bacilliformis. B. bacilliformis* causes two distinct illnesses: Oroya fever, a severe type of febrile hemolytic anemia; and verruga peruana, an eruption of hemangioma-like lesions.

The first written account of bartonellosis is attributed to Gago de Vadillo, who published a treatise on the subject in 1630. Then, in 1764, Cosme Bueno first described the vector of this disease and of cutaneous leishmaniasis as the uta or sand fly.[40] In the mid-1800s an epidemic occurred that took the lives of hundreds.[73]

In 1885, a Peruvian medical student (Carrión) was collecting data on the geographic distribution and clinical features of verruga peruana. To study disease symptoms in the pre-eruption period of verruga, he inoculated himself with material taken from a patient with verruga. Within 21 days after inoculation he became symptomatic, developed classic Oroya fever, and died. In 1905, Alberto Barton, a Peruvian physician, described the etiologic agent *(Bartonella bacilliformis)*, but several years passed before this organism was accepted as the cause of Oroya fever and named in his honor.

Epidemiology

Historically, the distribution of bartonellosis has been restricted to the mountain valleys of the Andes Mountains in Peru, Ecuador, and Colombia between the altitudes of 500 and 3200 m above sea level and primarily in valleys that are at right angles to the prevailing wind. The distribution of disease reflects the presence of the sand fly vector *Lutzomyia verrucarum,* which is seen only at these altitudes. The disease is usually acquired at twilight or soon thereafter because of the feeding habits of the insects. Within the region, the disease is endemic, but with sporadic epidemic outbreaks.[36,46]

Pathobiology

After inoculation by the sand fly, *Bartonella* organisms enter the endothelial cells of the blood vessels, where they proliferate. Microscopically, masses of organisms are noted within the cytoplasm of the cells lining the blood vessels and lymph channels, thus causing the lumen of the vessel to bulge. The organisms may also be found in reticuloendothelial cells in the lymph nodes, liver, and spleen, as well as within the bone marrow, kidneys, adrenals, pancreas, and rarely, the skin, heart, and lungs of infected patients.[9] They also parasitize erythrocytes and cause indentations and deformation of the erythrocyte membrane, membrane fusion, and entrance of the organisms into intracellular vacuoles, where they replicate.[10] Severe anemia results from destruction of the parasitized cells, with as many as 90% of the erythrocytes involved. However, all parasitized cells are not destroyed, and no hemolysins or agglutinins have been recovered.[69] Cuadra and Takano[22] showed that the parasites are located predominantly within cells, rather than on the surface. In the recovery phase, the rod-shaped organisms change to a more coccoid form and rapidly disappear from the blood.

A patient who survives the acute phase of Oroya fever may or may not experience cutaneous manifestations of the disease, which appear as nodular, hemangiomatous lesions ranging from a few millimeters to several centimeters. Light microscopy reveals angioblastic and histiocytic hyperplasia of the dermis. Numerous newly formed small vessels with endothelial cell proliferation are found. Mast cells, lymphocytes, and macrophages are present.[4] Electron microscopy demonstrates that the bacterial organisms are located within the verruga, extracellular in the fine fibrous interstitium.[65] In vitro studies have shown that *B. bacilliformis* stimulates endothelial cells, and in vivo studies have shown angiogenic activity. This finding may explain the similar pathologic findings of verruca and bacillary angiomatosis produced by other *Bartonella* spp.[4] One article summarized the current state of knowledge on *B. bacilliformis* and reviewed its host-cell parasitism, molecular pathogenesis, phylogeny, sand fly vectors, diagnostics, and prospects for control.[55]

Clinical Manifestations

The incubation period of bartonellosis varies from 2 to 14 weeks, with a mean of 3 weeks. Some patients are totally asymptomatic, and disease is detected only by blood culture or on serologic survey. In a population-based cohort study, 0.5% of participants had asymptomatic bacteremia.[17] Other patients develop only headache, malaise, and occasional fever, with *B. bacilliformis* recovered from blood cultures. Still others have severe anemia (Oroya fever), are febrile, and are deeply apathetic, with a peculiar discoloration of their skin and sclerae.[71] Tachycardia and soft murmurs are noted; occasionally, peripheral vascular collapse occurs. Clouding of the sensorium and delirium are common findings; these effects usually are mild but may progress to overt psychosis. The body temperature usually fluctuates between 37.5°C and 38.5°C (99.5°F and 101.3°F). Physical examination discloses generalized lymphadenopathy and nonpainful hepatomegaly.[50]

Laboratory studies reveal anemia that is macrocytic and hypochromic, with anisocytosis and poikilocytosis. The erythrocyte count may drop to as low as 500,000/mm^3 in the first 2 to 4 weeks of illness, with reticulocytes increasing to 50%. The pathognomonic sign of the disease is the presence of *B. bacilliformis* within Giemsa-stained erythrocytes as red-violet rods. The leukocyte count may be normal, low, or elevated.

The "critical stage" of the anemia is the period of transition when the organism suddenly disappears from the erythrocytes. In as many as 40% of patients, the illness becomes more severe, with the development of an intercurrent infection, particularly with *Salmonella.*[21] In the preeruptive stage, patients may complain of pain in their joints, bones, and muscles, as well as cramps and paresthesias, but the anemia and lymphadenopathy of the invasive stage disappear.

The appearance of red cutaneous nodules, or verruga, is pathognomonic of the disease in the eruptive stage. Usually, these nodules are present in the skin, but they may also be found in mesenchymatous tissue. They vary greatly in number and size, from small, asymptomatic nodules to disfiguring zonular (hemangioma-like) lesions. This stage may last from several months to a year and may be the sole manifestation of the disease, particularly in school-aged children in endemic areas.

TRENCH FEVER

Epidemiology

Trench fever (from *B. quintana*) was first described in Russia during World War I, when more than 1 million troops were infected.[9] The human body louse, *Pediculus humanus* var. *corporis*, is the vector, with humans the only known reservoir.

Clinical Manifestations

After an incubation period that is extremely variable (from 4 to 35 days, with an average of 22 days), one of four major fever patterns results: (1) a single febrile episode; (2) a single febrile period lasting 4 to 5 days; (3) three to eight recurrent febrile episodes, each lasting 4 to 5 days (sometimes for a year or more); or (4) persistent fever lasting 2 to 6 weeks.[29,78] Associated signs and symptoms include conjunctival injection, retroorbital pain, myalgias, arthralgias, headache, bone pain (especially in the shins), and splenomegaly. Chronic bacteremia following clinical improvement is common.[29]

BACILLARY ANGIOMATOSIS AND BACILLARY PELIOSIS HEPATIS

Etiology

Both *B. henselae* and *B. quintana* can cause vasculoproliferative disorders, which typically occur in immunocompromised persons, primarily adults with acquired immunodeficiency syndrome (AIDS) and with very low $CD4^+$ counts, and, to a lesser extent, in adults with cancer or recipients of organ transplants. Although these infections are exceptionally rare in children, reports have described bacillary angiomatosis in a child infected with HIV,[19] a child undergoing chemotherapy,[57] and, more rarely still, children who are thought to be immunocompetent.[86] Vasculoproliferation can also manifest as cutaneous or subcutaneous lesions (bacillary angiomatosis, caused by *B. henselae* or *B. quintana*) and pathologically can resemble the verruga of *B. bacilliformis* infection or solid organ lesions (bacillary peliosis hepatis, caused only by *B. henselae*).

Clinical Manifestations

Characteristically, the vasoproliferative lesions of bacillary angiomatosis are red with a collarette of scale, but the clinical findings can be diverse. Deep soft tissue masses may develop, and trauma may result in ulceration or bleeding. Osseous lesions occur in the long bones and can be very painful. The central nervous system, bone marrow, and mucosal surfaces of the gastrointestinal and respiratory tracts may also be involved.

Bacillary peliosis hepatis is seen primarily in HIV-infected adults who have fever and abdominal pain. In these patients, vascular proliferative lesions develop, primarily in the liver and spleen, although the abdominal lymph nodes and bone marrow may also be involved. This disease has not been reported in children.

DIAGNOSIS

Cat-Scratch Disease

Until recently, the clinical diagnosis of CSD required the presence of at least three of the following: a history of contact with a cat and the presence of a scratch or a primary lesion; a positive skin test result using material obtained from a purulent node from a patient with CSD; regional lymphadenopathy with negative studies for other potential causes of lymphadenopathy; and characteristic histopathologic findings on a biopsy specimen. The difficulty in isolating organisms from routine cultures of lymph nodes or other tissue specimens from patients with suspected CSD required the use of this strict clinical definition. In addition, an intradermal skin test composed of heated purulent lymph node material from patients with CSD was used for many years as a skin test reagent. Although the skin test was 90% to 98% sensitive and specific for the diagnosis of CSD, the material was not readily available, was not standardized, and was not licensed for routine use. In addition, the potential for transmission of other infectious agents with this test currently prohibits its use.

Specific diagnostic tests to assess serum antibodies against *B. henselae* such as IFA, enzyme-linked immunosorbent assay, and PCR amplification to identify *B. henselae* DNA sequences in tissues have reduced the need for the skin test and for invasive diagnostic procedures. Giladi and colleagues[34] developed a new enzyme immunoassay (EIA) for immunoglobulin (Ig) M and IgG that uses *N*-lauroylsarcosine–insoluble outer membrane antigens from agar-grown *B. henselae* and demonstrated increased sensitivity. This study determined the EIA sensitivity to be 75% for anti–*B. henselae* IgG alone, 48% for IgM alone, and 85% overall when positive IgG, IgM, or both were accepted as diagnostic. Another study[54] evaluated the kinetics of anti–*B. henselae* IgM and IgG antibodies by using EIA. Forty-eight (92%) of the 52 IgM-positive patients became IgM negative within 3 months after the onset of disease;208 (93%) of 223 serum samples tested positive for anti–*B. henselae* IgG. Beyond 6, 12, and 24 months, 35%, 25%, and 25% of serum samples (and patients), respectively, remained IgG positive. Some investigators have suggested that a single IgG titer greater than 1:256 is reliably diagnostic of acute infection. For any manifestation of CSD, detection of a significant rise in titer between acute and convalescent sera is confirmatory. However, cross-reactions between antibodies directed toward *B. henselae, B. quintana,* and *Chlamydia* spp. can render interpretation problematic. Cross-adsorption and Western immunoblotting can overcome this problem.[42]

Histopathologic examination of cat-scratch tissue includes granuloma formation with microabscesses and follicular hyperplasia. A Warthin-Starry stain and culture (ideally plated on both chocolate and rabbit blood agar and co-cultivated with eukaryotic cells) may be performed, although neither has high sensitivity. Very strain-specific assays involving PCR amplification of the 16S rRNA gene, the citrase synthase gene *(gltA)*, or the *htrA* gene of *B. henselae* offer improved sensitivity over culture and can be useful in establishing a diagnosis when purulent lymph node aspirates or other infected tissues are obtained.[28]

One report described a new detection method that combines enrichment culture and molecular amplification, which increases the testing sensitivity. This method detected DNA from at least 1 *Bartonella* species in 32 (28%) of the 114 veterinary subjects.[47] After DNA sequencing, the *Bartonella* species were determined for 27 of the 32 infected subjects, including *B. henselae* in 15 (56%), *B. vinsonii* subsp. *berkhoffii* in 7 (26%), *B. koehlerae* in 6 (22%), and a *B. volans*-like sequence in 1 (4%). This study suggests that cryptic *Bartonella* bloodstream infection may be more frequent in humans than previously recognized.

The differential diagnosis of CSD includes other forms of bacterial adenitis, typical or atypical mycobacterial infections, lymphogranuloma venereum, infectious mononucleosis, tularemia, plague, sporotrichosis, blastomycosis, histoplasmosis, syphilis, HIV infection, neoplasm, and sarcoidosis.

Endocarditis

The diagnosis of endocarditis is generally made with the use of serologic or PCR techniques; however, among patients with culture-negative endocarditis, a single IgG titer of 1:800 or higher has a 95.5% positive predictive value for *Bartonella* as the cause.[31] Because results of PCR of blood rarely are positive, PCR of valvular tissue is the most sensitive method to diagnose endocarditis. Special culturing techniques, including the use of Isolator tubes, and prolonged incubation may be helpful, in addition to serologic tests, histopathologic examination of valvular tissue, and PCR.[87]

Bartonellosis

The diagnosis of bartonellosis is made on the basis of clinical manifestations, Giemsa-stained blood smears showing typical organisms, or positive blood culture results. The presence of typical verruga in patients from an endemic area is pathognomonic of the disease. IgM antibody may be present in both stages of the disease, as well as in some asymptomatic persons.[36,44] Persons with typical Oroya fever who are treated with antibiotics may not have an antibody response.[36,44] An IFA assay has shown promise for evaluating patients in both the acute and convalescent phases of the disease.[16] The differential diagnosis in the initial phase includes typhoid fever, malaria, tuberculosis, leptospirosis, brucellosis, and meningitis, as well as hematologic malignant disease and aplastic or hemolytic anemia. The eruptive phase may resemble hemangiomas, bacillary angiomatosis, Kaposi sarcoma, and other nodular diseases.

Trench Fever

In a nonepidemic situation, establishing the diagnosis of trench fever is very difficult because the manifestations are not distinctive. The relapsing form can mimic malaria or *Borrelia recurrentis* relapsing fever. A history of body louse infestation or association with an epidemic should heighten suspicion. *B. quintana* can be cultured from blood by using a modification that includes culturing on epithelial cells. Serologic testing is available; however, cross-reactions with *B. henselae* occur.

Bacillary Angiomatosis and Bacillary Peliosis Hepatis

Given the difficulty with culture and the poor reliability of serologic studies, the diagnosis of these diseases relies on direct visualization of the organisms in tissue samples on electron microscopy or with Warthin-Starry stain or, increasingly, on detection of the organism in the affected tissue by PCR. The differential diagnosis of bacillary angiomatosis includes Kaposi sarcoma, pyogenic granuloma, verruga peruana, and multiple other opportunistic infections. The differential diagnosis of bacillary peliosis hepatis includes hepatic Kaposi sarcoma, lymphoma, extrapulmonary pneumocystosis, and infection with *Mycobacterium avium-intracellulare.*

TREATMENT

Cat-Scratch Disease

In an immunocompetent host, typical CSD is self-limited and resolves spontaneously in 1 to 2 months without the use of antibiotics. Application of moist soaks and local heat, use of analgesics, limitation of activity of the affected limb, and aspiration of fluctuant material in the nodes (in some instances, done serially) may relieve the pain and resolve the inflammation. Excisional biopsy of chronically involved lymph nodes also can be performed occasionally to rule out other treatable causes. However, conflicting data exist in publications regarding whether antibiotic therapy is ever helpful in normal hosts. Macrolides, fluoroquinolones, trimethoprim-sulfamethoxazole (TMP-SMX), doxycycline, and β-lactam agents all have in vitro activity against the organism, but gentamicin and rifampin appear to be the only bactericidal agents. Because in vitro susceptibility testing is technically challenging, lacks standards for interpretation of results, and produces minimum inhibitory concentrations that have correlated poorly with clinical efficacy, it often is not useful.[72] In Margileth's[52] retrospective review of 202 patients treated with antibiotics for CSD, rifampin was more effective than ciprofloxacin, gentamicin, or TMP-SMX. Another prospective, randomized, double-blind, placebo-controlled study using oral azithromycin for 5 days was effective in reducing lymph node volume measured by three-dimensional ultrasonography.[8] Adults and children weighing more than 100 lb were given an initial single dose of 500 mg azithromycin on day 1 of treatment and 250 mg on days 2 to 5 as single daily doses. Patients weighing less received the liquid preparation of 10 mg/kg on day 1 and 5 mg/kg on days 2 to 5.

No randomized, prospective, controlled studies have evaluated therapy for the systemic manifestations of CSD. In one retrospective review, children with hepatosplenic CSD who were given rifampin, 20 mg/kg per day in two doses for 14 days, either alone or in combination with another agent, experienced a decreased duration of fever.[5] In the same retrospective review, gentamicin or TMP-SMX also led to defervescence within 5 days, but penicillins, cephalosporins, tetracycline, and erythromycin had minimal or no clinical efficacy. In 2004, evidence-based treatment recommendations for *Bartonella* infections were published, and no recommendations for typical CSD, hepatosplenic CSD, or osteomyelitis were presented.[72] Outcomes of hepatosplenic disease and osteomyelitis caused by *B. henselae* generally have been excellent with or without antibiotic therapy or surgical intervention. Suggested therapy for central nervous system disease includes doxycycline and rifampin; however, no data suggest that antibiotic treatment of CSD encephalopathy is beneficial. Reports of the duration of antibiotic therapy have varied from 5 days in immunocompetent patients to 6 weeks in patients with atypical CSD or in immunocompromised patients.

Corticosteroid therapy has been reported in a small number of cases, including patients with typical CSD, retinal involvement, hepatosplenic disease, or encephalopathy, as well as in a single immunocompromised patient with fever and diffuse lymphadenopathy.[14,15,49,84] Because the pathogenesis of CSD with prolonged symptoms may include a postinfectious, inflammatory process,[14,72] corticosteroids appear to have some theoretical role. Despite the reported anecdotal successes, however, corticosteroids are not recommended for routine treatment of any manifestation of CSD.

Endocarditis

Initial empiric treatment of culture-negative endocarditis with ceftriaxone and gentamicin is effective for *Bartonella* organisms. A retrospective analysis of 101 adult patients with endocarditis showed a benefit with the use of an aminoglycoside as part of a treatment regimen for a minimum of 14 days. If a *Bartonella* infection is proven, doxycycline in combination with gentamicin is recommended. The recommended duration of ceftriaxone or doxycycline therapy is 6 weeks, with gentamicin combination therapy for the first 14 days.[6]

Bartonellosis

B. bacilliformis is sensitive to many antibiotics, including penicillin, tetracycline, streptomycin, and chloramphenicol. With treatment, the fever usually abates by 24 hours; the rod-shaped organisms change to more coccoid forms and soon disappear from the blood. The choice of antibiotic may be guided by considerations other than simple eradication of *B. bacilliformis*, including the risk for developing intercurrent infection. Chloramphenicol is considered to be the drug of choice because it also is useful in the treatment of salmonellosis.[80] Occasionally patients need the addition of another antibiotic, usually a β-lactam agent.[72] Blood transfusions may be helpful during the period of severe anemia, especially if blood is obtained from patients who have recently recovered from the disease.[69]

Treatment of verruga peruana usually is not necessary unless particularly large zonular lesions interfere with function; in these persons, surgical treatment may be necessary. Treatment is considered when there are more than 10 cutaneous lesions, when lesions are particularly erythematous or violaceous, or when the onset of lesions was more than 1 month before presentation. Oral rifampin, ciprofloxacin, or tetracycline with or without gentamicin may be used to aid in healing of the cutaneous lesions.[11,51,72]

Trench Fever

No controlled trials of treatment of trench fever have been performed, but dramatic defervescence has been noted with the use of tetracycline and chloramphenicol.[45,78] Recommended therapy for *B. quintana* bacteremia is doxycycline in combination with gentamicin.[11]

Bacillary Angiomatosis and Bacillary Peliosis Hepatis

Both bacillary angiomatosis and bacillary peliosis hepatis have been treated successfully with antimicrobial therapy, including erythromycin, azithromycin, or clarithromycin for 3 months for bacillary angiomatosis or for 4 months for bacillary peliosis hepatis.[45,60,78] The duration of therapy is critical to prevent relapses. Doxycycline may be used as an alternative regimen.

PROGNOSIS AND PREVENTION

Arthropod control should be recommended for prevention of transmission of *Bartonella* species to humans, particularly with regard to pet ownership for immunocompromised patients. Routine veterinary visits and control of flea and tick infestations in young kittens are the current practical preventive measures for CSD. Currently, no vaccine is available to prevent *Bartonella* infections in animals or humans.

Typically, the prognosis of CSD is excellent without any sequelae. Although patients with atypical findings and involvement of other organs may have a prolonged course and antibiotics may be used, the prognosis is good. Reinfection occurs only rarely. Although the mortality rate in patients with *Bartonella* endocarditis has been reported to be as high as 30%, more recent series have shown lower rates (7%). The mortality rate in untreated bartonellosis in the past was estimated at approximately 40%. However, the fatality rate was reported as approximately 9% in hospitalized patients and 0.7% in a population-based study.[44,46] Intercurrent *Salmonella* infection increases the mortality rate. Treatment with chloramphenicol improves prognosis, and permanent immunity develops in most patients. Treatment of trench fever with antimicrobial therapy improves outcomes and prevents progression to more severe disease, such as endocarditis. Antibiotics are usually effective for bacillary angiomatosis and bacillary peliosis hepatis, although prolonged courses are needed.

NEW REFERENCES SINCE THE SEVENTH EDITION

20. Chomel BB, Molia S, Kasten RW, et al. Isolation of *Bartonella henselae* and two new *Bartonella* subspecies, *Bartonella koehlerae* subspecies *boulouisii* subsp. nov. and *Bartonella koehlerae* subspecies *bothieri* subsp. nov. from free-ranging Californian mountain lions and bobcats. *PLoS ONE*. 2016;11(3):e0148299.
24. Eicher SC, Dehio C. *Bartonella* entry mechanisms into mammalian host cells. *Cell Microbiol*. 2012;14(8):1166-1173.
27. Fleischman DA, Chomel BB, Kasten RW, et al. *Bartonella* infection among cats adopted from a San Francisco shelter, revisited. *Appl Environ Microbiol*. 2015;81(18):6446-6450.
37. Guptill L, Wu CC, HogenEsch H, et al. Prevalence, risk factors, and genetic diversity of *Bartonella henselae* infections in pet cats in four regions of the United States. *J Clin Microbiol*. 2004;42(2):652-659.
47. Lantos PM, Maggi RG, Ferguson B, et al. Detection of *Bartonella* species in the blood of veterinarians and veterinary technicians: a newly recognized occupational hazard? *Vector Borne Zoonotic Dis*. 2014;14(8):563-570.
55. Minnick MF, Anderson BE, Lima A, et al. Oroya fever and verruga peruana: bartonelloses unique to South America. *PLoS Negl Trop Dis*. 2014;8(7):e2919.
58. Not T, Canciani M, Buratti E, et al. Serologic response to *Bartonella henselae* in patients with cat scratch disease and in sick and healthy children. *Acta Paediatr*. 1999;88(3):284-289.
62. Poudel A, Lew J, Slayton W, Dharnidharka VR. *Bartonella henselae* infection inducing hemophagocytic lymphohistiocytosis in a kidney transplant recipient. *Pediatr Transplant*. 2014;18(3):E83-E87.
75. Singh N, Sinclair LL, IJdo J. Cat-scratch fever and lymphadenopathy in a rheumatoid arthritis patient on tocilizumab. *J Clin Rheumatol*. 2015;21(1):40.
81. Vayssier-Taussat M, Moutailler S, Féménia F, et al. Identification of novel zoonotic activity of *Bartonella* spp., France. *Emerg Infect Dis*. 2016;22(3):457-462.
88. Zhou Y, Yin G, Tan C, Liu Y. Cat scratch disease during infliximab therapy: a case report and literature review. *Rheumatol Int*. 2015;35(5):911-913.

The full reference list for this chapter is available at ExpertConsult.com.

SUBSECTION VI Treponemataceae

140 Lyme Disease

Sunil K. Sood • Peter J. Krause

Lyme borreliosis or Lyme disease is caused by a group of spirochetal bacteria (genus *Borrelia*) that are transmitted by several hard-bodied ticks of the genus *Ixodes*. It is found in the temperate zones of North America and Eurasia and is the most common tick-borne disease in these regions. The name Lyme disease dates from the late 1970s, but the first description of the disease was published in 1883, when a German physician described the chronic skin manifestation later named acrodermatitis chronica atrophicans (ACA).[14,92] The hallmark expanding erythema chronicum migrans (ECM) rash of acute Lyme disease was first reported by a Swedish physician in 1909.[2] About half a century later, a Wisconsin physician provided the first description of the disease in the New World and reported successful treatment with penicillin.[78] A small cluster of cases of ECM observed in 1975 in Connecticut and Massachusetts occurred in the same year the Connecticut Health Department and Yale University rheumatologists responded to reports from the public of several children with arthritis in and around the towns of Lyme, Old Lyme, and East Haddam in southeastern Connecticut.[39,56] Ultimately 51 cases of arthritis (39 children and 12 adults) associated with ECM rash were documented and given the name *Lyme arthritis*.[98] Lyme arthritis was subsequently recognized to be part of a multisystem disease that was named *Lyme disease*.

ORGANISMS

The microbial etiology of Lyme disease was established in 1983 when Willy Burgdorfer discovered spirochetes in *Ixodes* ticks from Shelter Island, New York[15] and when the same organism was isolated from cultures of blood, skin lesions, and cerebrospinal fluid (CSF) of patients from Connecticut and Long Island, New York.[11,97] The pathogen was named *Borrelia burgdorferi* and was soon linked to the ECM rash in European patients, which is now called *erythema migrans*.[44] The name *Borrelia burgdorferi* sensu lato ("sensu lato" meaning "in a broad sense") indicates that other genospecies are included under this group name (Table 140.1). At least three other genospecies (*B. afzelii*, *B. garinii*, and *B. bavariensis*) are established causes of Lyme disease in Eurasia and account for variation in the clinical presentation on that continent. *B. afzelii* is strongly associated with ACA and is a common cause of erythema migrans; *B. garinii* is associated with neurologic infection. In addition, there are a few reports of *B. bissettii*, *B. lusitaniae*, *B. spielmanii*, and *B. valaisiana* isolates from Lyme disease patients.[77] In North America, Lyme disease is caused by the genospecies *B. burgdorferi* sensu stricto ("meaning in a narrow sense"). *B. burgdorferi* is a slow-growing bacterium with a cell membrane that is covered by a loosely associated outer membrane and by flagella that account for the coiled shape of the microorganism and provide motility. In 2016, a new genospecies of *Borrelia* was found to cause Lyme disease in the United States and was named *B. mayonii* after the site of its discovery at the Mayo Clinic. The likely vector is *Ixodes scapularis,* the same as for *B. burgdorferi*.[68]

EPIDEMIOLOGY

Lyme disease is the most commonly reported vector borne illness in the United States and was the sixth most common Nationally Notifiable Disease in 2015. In that year, 28,453 confirmed and 9616 probable cases were reported to the Centers for Disease Control and Prevention (CDC; incidence 8.9 cases per 100,000 population), but the actual number of infections is estimated at 10- to 12-fold higher.[18,47,57,58,95] Lyme disease–endemic areas in the United States are primarily located in the Northeast and northern Midwest. (Fig. 140.1). Almost all (95%) of the confirmed cases in 2015 were reported from 14 states in these regions

TABLE 140.1 Principal Vector Tricks and Spirochetes Associated With Lyme Borreliosis

Tick Species	Distribution	Genotype of *Borrelia burgdorferi*
Ixodes scapularis	Eastern North America	*B. burgdorferi* sensu stricto
Ixodes pacificus	Western North America	*B. burgdorferi* sensu stricto
Ixodes ricinus	Western and central Europe[a]	*B. garinii, B. afzelii, B. burgdorferi* sensu stricto
Ixodes persulcatus	Central Europe and Asia	*B. garinii, B. afzelii*

[a]*B. spielmanii, B. lusitaniae,* and *B. valaisiana* occasionally isolated from humans; *B. garinii* serotype 4 also known as *B. bavariensis.*

From Piesman J, Humair P-F. The spirochetes and vector ticks of Lyme borreliosis in nature. In: Sood SK, editor. *Lyme Borreliosis in Europe and North America.* Hoboken, NJ: John Wiley & Sons; 2011.

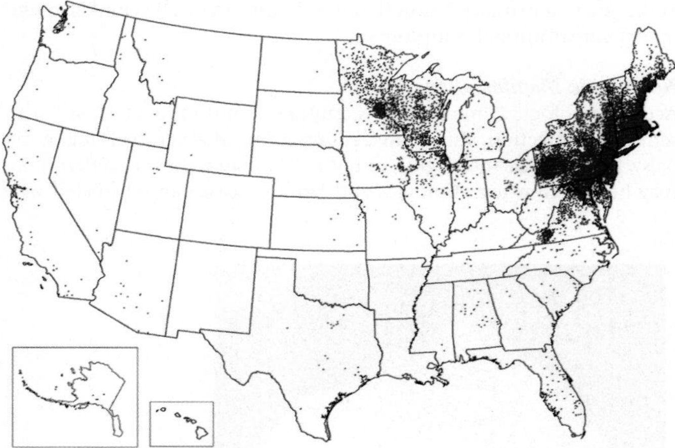

FIG. 140.1 Reported cases of Lyme disease–United States, 2015. One dot represents one case of Lyme disease and is placed randomly in the patient's county of residence. The presence of a dot in a state does not necessarily mean that Lyme disease was acquired in that state. The place of residence is sometimes different from the location where the patience became infected. (From Centers for Disease Control and Prevention. National Center for Emerging and Zoonotic Infectious Diseases, Division of Vector-Borne Diseases.)

(Connecticut, Delaware, Maine, Maryland, Massachusetts, Minnesota, New Hampshire, New Jersey, New York, Pennsylvania, Rhode Island, Vermont, Virginia, and Wisconsin).[18] Far fewer cases are reported from the northern Pacific Coast region.[31]

In Europe the incidence varies among countries, in part because of different reporting methods and because of travel. The highest incidence is generally in the temperate zone between latitudes 42 and 62 degrees North.[92] Lyme disease is more common among children than adults, presumably because of their increased exposure to *Ixodes* ticks, with about one-fourth of all reported cases occurring in children younger than 14 years.[9,90]

Lyme disease is a zoonotic infection that involves multiple hosts and reservoirs.[54] *Ixodes* ticks take a blood meal from a vertebrate host in each of the three active stages during their 2-year life cycle (larva, nymph, and adult). Spirochetes are ingested during a blood meal from an asymptomatic infected reservoir host and transmitted to other reservoir hosts or to humans by the nymphal or adult stages during a subsequent blood meal. The primary reservoir hosts are the white-footed mouse (*Peromyscus leucopus*) in the Northeast and Midwest and the western gray squirrel and western fence lizard in the Pacific Coast region. Other small mammals such as chipmunks and some species of birds may also serve as reservoir hosts.[66] White-tailed deer (*Odocoileus virginianus*) provide an important habitat for adult ticks during the winter season. They do not become infected with *B. burgdorferi* but amplify the tick population by providing an area for procreation and a blood meal for adult ticks. An increase in the deer population over the past few decades is an important factor in the increase in the *I. scapularis* population and in the number of Lyme disease cases in the United States.[70] Domestic animals such as the dog may carry adult *Ixodes* ticks but do not appear to be important reservoir hosts for the tick, even though dogs can be infected with *B. burgdorferi.* The tick vectors in Europe have a greater variety of reservoir hosts, including ground-feeding birds such as blackbirds, small mammals such as *Apodemus* mice, and medium-sized mammals such as hedgehogs.[92]

PATHOGENESIS

Borrelia spirochetes are deposited in the skin during tick feeding. The organism does not produce toxins, so disease is primarily a result of the immunologic host response. Major antigens of the bacteria include the outer-surface lipoproteins (Osp) A, B and C, as well as the flagellar protein. Outer surface proteins are important for survival both in the tick and in mammalian hosts.[69,103] Innate immune activation begins with spirochete binding to pattern recognition receptors such as toll-like receptors on dendritic cells and macrophages in the dermis.[13,40,53,74] This initiates signal transduction pathways that result in production of chemokines and cytokines by macrophages and dendritic cells.[53,75] Spirochetes are ingested by macrophages and neutrophils and degraded within phagocytic vacuoles.[75] Degradation products bind to intercellular pattern recognition receptors that further amplify the inflammatory response.[75] Adaptive immune responses also help to clear spirochetes. *Borrelia*-specific T cells are activated. These aid in macrophage killing and help B cells differentiate into antibody-producing plasma cells.[69] Patients with Lyme arthritis typically have higher *Borrelia*-specific antibody titers than do patients with other manifestations of Lyme disease.[24] Despite a vigorous immune response, the spirochetes are not immediately killed, partly owing to immune evasion strategies, such as downregulation of expression of outer surface proteins and antigenic variation from the variable major protein-like sequence expression locus (VlsE).[26,69] *B. burgdorferi* produces specific proteins that inhibit complement activity.[51]

Surviving *Borrelia* can disseminate from the skin to other tissues through blood and possibly also through tissue planes. During dissemination within humans, *B. burgdorferi* attach to certain host integrins. This elicits a proinflammatory response that includes production of both matrix glycosaminoglycans and extracellular matrix proteins, which may explain the organism's tropism for particular tissues (e.g., collagen fibrils in the extracellular matrix of the heart, nervous system, and joints).[69] Dissemination appears to be genotype or strain dependent, with some strains more likely to disseminate than others.[107,108] Furthermore, infection with specific *B. burgdorferi* genotypes may result in unique clinical manifestations of disease. For example, only the European species *B. afzelii* causes chronic skin lesions of ACA. Long-term immunity is incomplete because episodes of Lyme disease may reoccur in some people. Reinfection has been found in about 3% of children and 10% of adults.[33,58,111,112]

Several lines of evidence suggest that persistent symptoms do not result from active infection. Synovial tissue from patients with Lyme arthritis typically shows hypertrophy, vascular proliferation, and a marked mononuclear cell infiltrate, but joint cultures in patients with recurrent arthritis are negative.[13,96] Some adult patients with Lyme arthritis, particularly those with HLA-DRB1 alleles, will develop a chronic, antibiotic refractory, autoimmune arthritis.[96] Antibiotic refractory Lyme arthritis may be due to *B. burgdorferi* breakdown components that can persist near cartilaginous tissue and induce an inflammatory response after treatment is completed.[13] Meningitis results from direct invasion of the subarachnoid space by *B. burgdorferi,* as shown by the presence of spirochetes in cultures of CSF. *B. burgdorferi* infiltrates the connective tissue sheath surrounding each bundle of peripheral nerve fibers in the peripheral nervous system in a monkey model.[73] There is no evidence to suggest that long-term neurologic symptoms are due to persistent *Borrelia* infection, however.

CLINICAL MANIFESTATIONS

The clinical presentation of Lyme disease in children includes a few well-characterized manifestations that are classified as early or late. Early manifestations are defined as those that begin within 8 weeks after the tick bite and are further characterized as early localized or early disseminated disease.[81,105] In North America, about 90% of children have erythema migrans, either as a single lesion or as multiple erythema migrans. The remainder present with arthritis, facial palsy, aseptic meningitis, or carditis.[33] Some children with early Lyme disease present with more than one manifestation. In Europe, neurologic manifestations are significantly more common in children (17–38% of cases) than in adults, and Bannwarth polyradiculoneuritis is more common.[19,90] Borrelial lymphocytoma only occurs in Europe and is common in children.[59,67]

Early Localized Disease

Erythema Migrans

The initial disease manifestation of Lyme disease is a single erythema migrans lesion that begins at the site of the tick bite and appears after an incubation of about 1 to 31 days (mean of 10 days) (Fig. 140.2A–C). This generally consists of a flat red rash that expands over days. The bull's-eye shape with central clearing is firmly entrenched in both the lay and medical literature but occurs in only two-thirds of skin biopsy or culture-proven erythema migrans.[61] Although the lesion is usually painless, there may be mild stinging, warmth, pruritus, hyperesthesia, or dysesthesia. Vesicular, urticarial, scaling, purpuric, and noncircular variants are well documented.[61,86] There can be alternating rings of lighter and darker erythema or triangular lesions in areas like the inguinal region. Patients with erythema migrans often have mild constitutional symptoms including low-grade fever. Because small ring-shaped lesions from insect bites are common in children, practitioners should not rush to diagnose erythema migrans in a child with a focal rash of that type. Close follow-up will establish the diagnosis if the lesion attains a diameter of at least 5 cm, the minimum diameter required to meet the CDC 2017 surveillance case definition of erythema migrans. Rashes that suggest erythema migrans have been observed in nonendemic southern states and recently in a child on Long Island, New York, following bites of Lone Star ticks.[16,29] This entity has been given the name *southern tick-associated rash illness* (STARI), and although not due to *B. burgdorferi* infection, the causative organism is unknown.

Early Disseminated Disease

Spirochetemia can occur shortly after the tick bite, leading to disseminated skin, neurologic, cardiac, and musculoskeletal manifestations.

Multiple Erythema Migrans

Multiple erythema migrans are the most common form of early disseminated Lyme disease (Fig. 140.2D).[6,87] Lesions can be distinguished from erythema multiforme by the fact that all are morphologically similar, although they vary in size. A single secondary lesion may occur at the site of a primary lesion that has disappeared. The child also may report constitutional symptoms.

Neurologic Manifestations

Acute neurologic Lyme disease is another common form of early disseminated infection, almost always presenting as seventh cranial nerve palsy, lymphocytic meningitis, or both.[10,88] Because these manifestations may be due to other etiologies and Lyme disease can be treated with

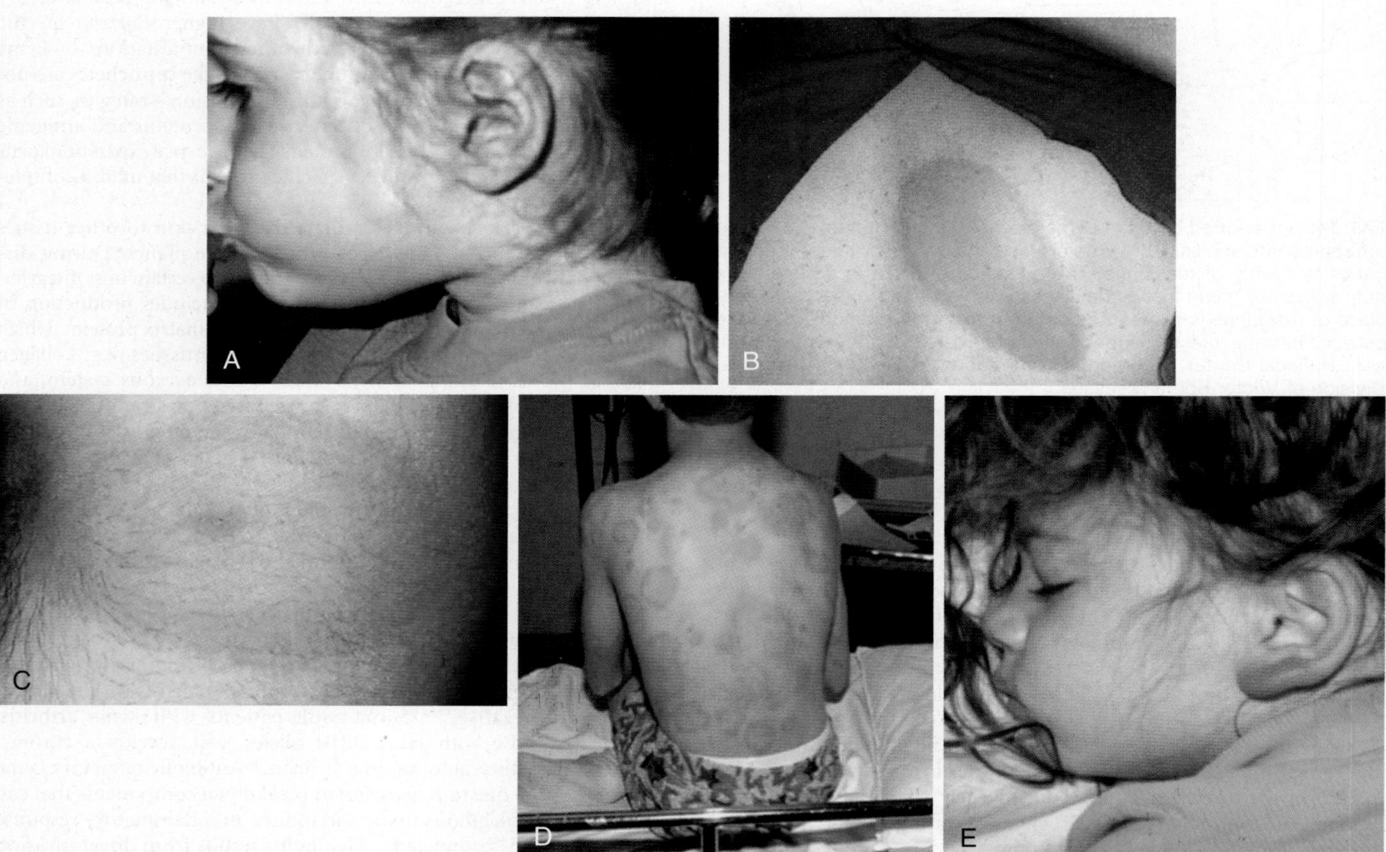

FIG. 140.2 (A) Erythema migrans scalp lesion only partially visible on the face. (B) Erythema migrans oval lesion. (C) Erythema migrans dark annular lesion. (D) Multiple erythema migrans. (E) Borrelial lymphocytoma. Five-year-old girl from southern California who, while visiting Norway in August 2006, had a tick removed from her left ear lobe. (From Sood SK, editor. *Lyme Borreliosis in Europe and North America*. Hoboken, NJ: John Wiley & Sons; 2011. A–C, Courtesy Vijay Sikand, MD; D, courtesy Lorry Rubin, MD; E, courtesy Mark Salzman, MD.)

antibiotics, a specific etiology of Lyme disease should be sought in children who present with these symptoms in endemic areas. Facial palsy should always raise the diagnostic possibility of Lyme disease. Children with facial palsy should be assessed for meningitis and the need for lumbar puncture, especially when there is neck stiffness or severe headache.[82] If a lumbar puncture is performed and shows CSF pleocytosis consistent with meningitis, treatment should consist of an antibiotic administered intravenously rather than orally.

Because Lyme meningitis and enteroviral meningitis are common in Lyme disease–endemic areas, it is important to appreciate characteristic clinical and laboratory features of each, in the absence of an erythema migrans rash. The presentation of Lyme meningitis is more indolent.[27,80] Children with Lyme meningitis often experience several days of headache, lethargy, and neck pain symptoms before seeing a physician. Evidence of meningismus, such as Kernig and Brudzinski signs, is less pronounced. The CSF pleocytosis consists predominantly of mononuclear cells (mostly lymphocytes), compared with the relative prominence of neutrophils early in the course of viral meningitis. In one study, the negative predictive value for Lyme meningitis was 99% when neutrophils composed more than 10% of the cells in the CSF.[80] Clinical prediction algorithms based on these features have been developed to help in the diagnosis of Lyme meningitis.[8,20] One of these was termed the "rule of 7s."[20] Children with meningitis in whom all three of the following were present: 7 or more days of headache, 70% or more mononuclear cells, and presence of seventh (or other) cranial nerve palsy, had a 77% likelihood of Lyme meningitis, while absence of all of these predictors was highly sensitive (96%) for identifying a low risk for Lyme meningitis. Another important difference between Lyme meningitis and viral meningitis is the more frequent complication of increased intracranial pressure that is associated with Lyme meningitis. This is important because such elevated intracranial pressure is sometimes associated with transient or permanent loss of vision.[63,72] Almost all published reports of raised intracranial pressure in Lyme disease have been in children, and the complication has been observed in the absence of meningitis.[45,90] Headache is prominent in these children. It is important to examine the optic discs of every child with acute disseminated Lyme disease for papilledema even though this is a rare complication. Opening CSF pressure should be measured as part of the lumbar puncture, and if elevated, treatment to lower intracranial pressure should be initiated immediately.

Other neurologic signs or symptoms are very uncommon in children. Bannwarth syndrome, a neurologic manifestation of Lyme disease in Europe, consists of inflammation of peripheral nerves.[65] It should be considered in children who have recently traveled to Europe or Asia and present with neuralgia, paresthesia, and motor or sensory impairment, mostly affecting cervical and thoracic dermatomes. A true association of Lyme disease with optic neuritis, Guillain-Barré–like syndrome, or acute meningoencephalitis in published reports is very uncertain.

Carditis

Lyme carditis is a rare early dissemination manifestation of Lyme disease. It usually occurs in association with involvement of the skin and nervous system but may be the sole manifestation, presenting with syncope and malaise. Abnormalities include first-, second-, or third-degree atrioventricular conduction block or bundle branch block.[32,36] An electrocardiogram should be considered in a child with acute disseminated Lyme disease because cardiac conduction abnormalities are often asymptomatic. Rare presentations of Lyme carditis are myocarditis, myopericarditis, left ventricular dysfunction, or cardiomegaly. Patients with Lyme carditis almost invariably have positive *B. burgdorferi* serology acutely or at follow-up.[5] The outcome in children who receive appropriate antibiotic therapy for Lyme carditis is excellent.

Acute Generalized Illness

Investigators in Connecticut tested the hypothesis that early Lyme disease can present with a nonspecific illness without focal manifestations. Five of 24 untreated children who presented to their primary care physicians with "flu-like illness" of less than 3 weeks' duration without identifiable cause were found to have serologic evidence of acute *B. burgdorferi* infection.[28] Less than 10% of children with *B. burgdorferi* infection are estimated to present in this way. Antibiotic treatment should not be prescribed for children with nonspecific illness without *B. burgdorferi*–specific laboratory confirmation of Lyme disease. Because babesiosis, human granulocytic anaplasmosis, ehrlichiosis , and *Borrelia miyamotoi* infection can have a similar generalized clinical presentation, these infections also should be considered in evaluating any child thought to have tick-borne illness who presents with nonspecific findings.[48]

Borrelia mayonii *Infection*

Six patients (three children and three adults) were described in the initial report of *Borrelia mayonii* infection. All resided in Minnesota, North Dakota, or Wisconsin. Disease manifestations differed from those of *B. burgdorferi* sensu lato because all presented with prominent constitutional symptoms, and some patients had diffuse macular rash or lymphopenia, thrombocytopenia, or elevated hepatic transaminases. All patients had a high level of spirochetemia. Five were treated with doxycycline and one with ceftriaxone. Infection resolved in all the patients without complications.[68]

Late Disseminated Disease

Arthritis

Arthritis develops as the first symptom of Lyme disease weeks to months after the tick bite. The mean incubation period is about 4 months.[102] Arthritis usually presents in children who do not receive appropriate antibiotics for acute Lyme disease because the tick bite or rash goes unnoticed. Many children report intermittent and migratory arthralgias or mild periarticular inflammation in the weeks leading up to development of frank arthritis. Lyme arthritis presents as a monoarthritis in two-thirds of cases and as an oligoarthritis (fewer than four joints) in the remainder.[35] The knee is the most common presenting joint and is involved in 90% of the cases. There usually is obvious joint swelling and effusion with greater stiffness than expected, given mild to moderate associated pain. Children most often continue to walk and are not immediately taken for emergency care. It is not unusual for the swelling to be attributed to an acute traumatic event and for a child to be initially evaluated by an orthopedic surgeon. These clinical features distinguish Lyme arthritis from septic arthritis (which usually presents in a more fulminant manner), despite similar laboratory findings of neutrophil-predominant exudate in synovial fluid and elevated acute phase reactants. An effusion typically reaccumulates if arthrocentesis is performed, consistent with the pathogenesis of a reactive arthritis. Active inflammation persists for several weeks even after appropriate treatment. Both the severity and duration of arthritis are increased in adolescents.[41] Recurrent episodes can involve the same joint or a different joint, another pattern that is consistent with reactive arthritis.

Late Neurologic Disease

Follow-up studies of children who previously had Lyme disease have demonstrated an excellent neuropsychological outcome.[1] Low-grade encephalopathy and sensorineural peripheral neuropathy have been described infrequently as late sequelae of Lyme disease in adults. In contrast, late neurologic disease is rarely, if ever, encountered in children. Occasionally, cognitive disorders, processing deficits on neuropsychological tests, or persistent fatigue in children are erroneously attributed to Lyme disease. Even if *B. burgdorferi* antibodies are detected in a child with these symptoms, this is almost always evidence of previously resolved infection that is unrelated to neurologic symptoms. There is very little evidence that incidentally detected nonspecific white matter changes on magnetic resonance imaging of the brain are due to Lyme disease. Assays of CSF for culture, *B. burgdorferi* DNA, antibody, or antigen detection are not useful in children with suspected *B. burgdorferi*–induced neurologic disease because they have very poor specificity and sensitivity.[37]

Other Manifestations

Asymptomatic Seroconversion

Asymptomatic seroconversion refers to the development of antibodies to *B. burgdorferi* infection in the absence of a recognized illness. This is well documented and common in endemic areas.[47] The ratio of symptomatic infection to asymptomatic Lyme disease was about 9:1 in a prospective study in an endemic area.[99] Children remain well, indicating successful clearance of the spirochete rather than latent infection. There is no evidence that children with asymptomatic seroconversion should be treated with antibiotics if they have continued to be well at the time of this diagnosis.

Acrodermatitis Chronica Atrophicans

ACA is a late chronic skin manifestation of Lyme borreliosis that occurs in Europe.[59] The lesions are painful, blue-red discolored areas of swelling on the extremities, usually accompanied by a sensory peripheral neuropathy. Although rarely encountered in children, it is important to include ACA in the differential diagnosis of discolored skin lesions so that atrophic and neural sequelae can be minimized by early treatment.[110]

Borrelial Lymphocytoma

Borrelial lymphocytoma is a localized manifestation of disseminated Lyme disease that is seen in Europe. It mimics a benign tumor of the skin, usually on the earlobes or breast areolae.[21] The lesion is a painless solitary blue-red plaque or nodule 1 to 5 cm in diameter, which develops 1 to 6 months after the tick bite (Fig. 140.2E).

Coinfection With Other Ixodes Tick-Borne Pathogens

Human babesiosis and human granulocytic anaplasmosis (HGA) are tick-borne diseases that may be cotransmitted with *B. burgdorferi* in areas where these infections are endemic. Between 3% and 13% of Lyme disease patients may experience babesiosis or HGA coinfection, or both, in areas where these infections are endemic.[23,48,50,76] Coinfection with babesiosis or HGA is associated with an increase in acute symptoms compared with Lyme disease alone and may result in a more extended period of illness. Physicians caring for patients with moderate to severe Lyme disease should consider obtaining diagnostic tests for babesiosis and anaplasmosis in regions where these diseases are zoonotic. This is especially important when the response to antibiotic treatment is inadequate. There are no data indicating that Lyme disease complications are increased as a result of coinfection.

Lyme Disease in Pregnancy

There has been concern that untreated Lyme disease during pregnancy could result in fetal or neonatal disease, even though maternal-to-fetal transmission appears to be very rare, if it occurs at all. Large epidemiologic investigations have failed to show an association between mothers' exposure during pregnancy and fetal death, prematurity, or congenital malformations.[34,100,101] To date, there have been no proven cases of *B. burgdorferi* causing fetal wastage, fetal malformations, or persistent neonatal infection.[25,55]

DIAGNOSIS

Most persons who acquire Lyme disease do not recall a tick bite because the tick is small, the bite is painless, and the tick falls off after feeding. Lyme disease is primarily diagnosed by clinical manifestations, most commonly an erythema migrans rash, with supportive epidemiologic evidence, and laboratory confirmation for manifestations other than erythema migrans. The CDC developed a clinical case definition for Lyme disease that was initially intended for epidemiologic surveillance purposes. When used in conjunction with the US Food and Drug Administration (FDA) guidelines for diagnostic tests, this case definition has been widely accepted as a way to standardize the clinical diagnosis of Lyme disease. A patient is considered to have Lyme disease by the CDC case definition if they have an erythema migrans rash, or at least one objective sign of early disseminated or late disease (musculoskeletal, nervous, or cardiovascular signs), in addition to a positive laboratory test result that confirms infection with *B. burgdorferi*. Laboratory testing is not required or recommended for a patient who has erythema migrans.

Erythema migrans is defined as a skin lesion that begins as a red macule or papule and expands over a period of days to weeks to form a large round lesion, often with partial central clearing. For CDC surveillance purposes a single primary lesion must reach at least 5 cm in size. Epidemiologic evidence includes visiting a wooded, brushy, or grassy area where Lyme disease is endemic, 1 to 32 days before onset of the rash. A deer tick bite at the site of the rash may or may not have been identified. Positive *B. burgdorferi* serology is not necessary for the diagnosis of erythema migrans. Early disseminated neurologic manifestations include cranial neuritis (particularly facial palsy) or lymphocytic meningitis, alone or in combination. Encephalomyelitis must be confirmed by demonstration of antibody production against *B. burgdorferi* in the CSF with a higher titer of antibody in the CSF than in the serum. Early disseminated cardiovascular system manifestations include acute onset of a high-grade second- or third-degree atrioventricular conduction defect that resolves in days to weeks and is sometimes associated with myocarditis. Late musculoskeletal manifestations consist of objective joint swelling in one or a few joints.

Serology is the primary laboratory test used to confirm the diagnosis of Lyme disease because unlike most other bacterial illnesses, Lyme disease is very seldom diagnosed by culture, polymerase chain reaction (PCR), or microscopic visualization of the organism.[52,109] Antibodies to *B. burgdorferi* begin to develop during early localized infection. The immune response intensifies in patients with early disseminated or late disease.[5] A patient with erythema migrans may become *B. burgdorferi* antibody positive during therapy. This does not constitute treatment failure because approximately one-fourth of patients with erythema migrans are antibody positive when diagnosed and an additional one-half become positive during therapy. In contrast to syphilis where a falling VDRL titer indicates successful therapy, *B. burgdorferi* antibodies may remain elevated for years in a successfully treated patient. Serial *B. burgdorferi* serology should not be used to monitor effectiveness of treatment of Lyme disease.

A two-tier approach is recommended for the detection of antibodies to *B. burgdorferi*.[5,17] The first test consists of one of several FDA-approved enzyme-linked immunosorbent assay (ELISA) tests for total immunoglobulin M (IgM) and IgG antibodies to the antigens of *B. burgdorferi* spirochete. The ELISA is a very sensitive assay, and false-positive results are common, primarily from cross-reacting antibodies against microorganisms that share antigenically similar proteins with *B. burgdorferi*. Therefore sera that are positive or equivocal by ELISA are then tested using separate IgM and IgG Western immunoblot assays to confirm the ELISA results. The Western immunoblot is more specific than the ELISA because it identifies antibodies in the patient's serum to individual polypeptides of *B. burgdorferi*. They are visualized and reported as "bands" according to their molecular weight expressed in kilodaltons (kD). Based on extensive laboratory testing, the CDC has defined a positive *B. burgdorferi* IgM immunoblot result as the presence of at least two of three following bands: 23, 39, and 41 kD. A blot for IgG is considered positive if at least five of the following 10 bands are present: 18, 23, 28, 30, 39, 41, 45, 58, 66, and 93 kD.[17] Only the IgG response should be used to support the diagnosis after the first month of infection. After that time, an IgM response alone is very likely to represent a false-positive result.[79] Immunoblot interpretation should only be performed in qualified laboratories that follow CDC-recommended evidence-based guidelines on immunoblot interpretation. The use of immunoblot alone for diagnosis of Lyme disease is not recommended.

As with any diagnostic test, the predictive value of serologic tests for Lyme disease depends on the probability that the patient has Lyme disease, based on epidemiologic and clinical history and the physical examination (the "pretest probability" of Lyme disease). Use of serologic tests to "rule out" Lyme disease in patients with a low probability of the illness will result in a very high proportion of test results that are falsely positive.[43] Therefore antibody tests for Lyme disease should not be used as screening tests, as has become common practice in children with nonspecific fevers, arthralgias, headaches, or fatigue. Even in areas with a high prevalence of Lyme disease, patients with only nonspecific signs and symptoms are not likely to have Lyme disease.[30,83] Physicians should avoid requesting *B. burgdorferi* serology on such patients because they have a very low pretest probability of disease and false-positive results cause patient anxiety, unnecessary antibiotic treatment, and the possibility of missing another diagnosis.[30]

Patients with erythema migrans should not have serologic testing because they frequently are seronegative at this early stage of the infection, and a typical erythema migrans rash is pathognomonic for Lyme disease. If the rash is atypical, the patient is not treated, and serology is negative or equivocal, a second specimen should be obtained within 2 to 4 weeks. Patients with early neurologic manifestations of Lyme disease have demonstrable serum antibodies to *B. burgdorferi*, but the response may be limited to IgM antibodies.[20,42] Patients with Lyme carditis almost always have positive *B. burgdorferi* serology acutely or at follow-up.[4,5] Patients with Lyme arthritis invariably have positive *B. burgdorferi* serology for IgG antibodies.[5] The presence of a positive serologic result does not guarantee that a medical condition is due to *B. burgdorferi* infection, however, because the positive serology may be due to previous infection or to a false-positive test result. The background *B. burgdorferi* seropositivity in areas that are highly endemic for Lyme disease may exceed 4%.[49]

Additional tests to confirm *B. burgdorferi* infection in clinical specimens have been used primarily in research settings. For CSF, these include measurement of CSF-to-serum antibody ratios to document specific intrathecal antibody production, *B. burgdorferi* DNA detection by PCR testing, and *B. burgdorferi* culture of CSF, skin biopsies, and joint fluid.[109] Because of limited availability, expense, poor sensitivity, and insufficient evidence of value in the management of most patients, these tests should be reserved for special situations in which the pretest probability of Lyme disease is high but manifestations are atypical. Tests to detect antigens of *B. burgdorferi* in urine are not FDA approved, and they have no current role in the diagnosis or management of Lyme disease.

TREATMENT AND PROGNOSIS

The current standard for treatment of Lyme disease in children is the evidence-based Infectious Diseases Society of America Practice Guideline.[106] Treatment recommendations are listed in Table 140.2, and selected treatment principles are discussed here. *Borrelia burgdorferi* is highly susceptible to β-lactam antibiotics and tetracyclines. Consequently, treatment of Lyme disease is effective at all stages of the infection, and treatment failures are very uncommon. First-line antibiotics are β-lactams or doxycycline, the latter drug being effective for treatment of HGA (although not for babesiosis) that may simultaneously occur with Lyme disease.

Doxycycline and amoxicillin are equivalent choices for treatment of early Lyme disease. Doxycycline usually is prescribed for children 8 years or older and amoxicillin for children younger than 8 years. Ceftriaxone is the treatment of choice for early disseminated Lyme disease presenting as meningitis or advanced atrioventricular heart block. If a child presenting with Lyme facial palsy is assessed for concomitant meningitis, presence of CSF pleocytosis would suggest the use of parenteral ceftriaxone rather than an oral antibiotic. Children experiencing carditis who have second- or third-degree atrioventricular block and those with first-degree heart block when the PR interval is prolonged to 30 milliseconds or longer should be hospitalized and continuously monitored. This is because the degree of block may fluctuate and worsen very rapidly. Patients experiencing advanced heart block should have a consultation with a cardiologist. A temporary pacemaker may be required. Fortunately, cardiac arrhythmias and heart block due to Lyme disease usually resolve within a few days.

Children with Lyme arthritis are treated with doxycycline or amoxicillin. For those who have persistent or recurrent joint swelling after antibiotic therapy, retreatment with a 4-week course of oral antibiotics or with a 2- to 4-week course of ceftriaxone should be considered. If persistent synovitis is associated with significant pain or limitation of function, nonsteroidal antiinflammatory agents, intraarticular corticosteroids, disease-modifying antirheumatic drugs such as hydroxychloroquine, or arthroscopic synovectomy provides symptomatic relief.[104] Ongoing knee pain is often due to patellofemoral joint disease rather than arthritis.

The prognosis for children given appropriate antibiotic therapy for Lyme disease is excellent. This includes children with arthritis, even though recurrent episodes of arthritis can occur.[104] In one study, parents were telephoned 2 to 12 years after their child had experienced Lyme disease. Four of 90 children had ongoing musculoskeletal complaints, but none had evidence of arthritis.[35] The incidence of chronic arthritis was higher in children in Germany, where about half of 55 children treated for a previous diagnosis of Lyme arthritis had chronic arthritis either at onset or during their follow-up.[91] A poorer outcome was associated with older age and female gender.

Despite resolution of the objective manifestations of Lyme disease, children on rare occasions may continue to experience fatigue, musculoskeletal pain, or difficulties with concentration or short-term memory. There is no evidence that these are attributable to persistent *B. burgdorferi* infection.[85] The pathogenesis of these symptoms is not well defined but is probably similar to other postinfectious conditions in which persistent immune-mediated inflammation occurs in the absence of active infection. There is no evidence that prolonged courses of antibiotic treatment that exceed 1 month are effective for adults with

TABLE 140.2 Treatment of Lyme Borreliosis

Manifestation	First-Line Drugs	Alternate Drugs	Second-Line Drugs
Early localized erythema migrans	Amoxicillin PO 14 days or doxycycline PO 10 days	Cefuroxime axetil PO[a] 14 days	Azithromycin PO 7–10 days
Multiple erythema migrans	Amoxicillin PO 14 days or doxycycline PO 10 days	Cefuroxime axetil PO[a] 14 days	Azithromycin PO 7–10 days
Facial palsy or spinal radiculopathy	Amoxicillin PO 14 days or doxycycline PO 14 days		Azithromycin PO 7–10 days
Meningitis	Ceftriaxone IV 14 days or cefotaxime IV 14 days	None, although trials in Europe demonstrated efficacy of doxycycline PO	
Cardiac[b]	Amoxicillin PO 14–21 days or doxycycline PO 14–21 days *or* ceftriaxone IV 14–21 days or cefotaxime IV 14–21 days		
Arthritis	Amoxicillin PO 28 days or doxycycline PO 28 days		
Persistent arthritis after course of oral therapy	Retreat with one of above oral regimens	Ceftriaxone[c] IV 14–28 days or cefotaxime[c] IV 14–28 days	
Asymptomatic seroconversion or acute constitutional illness	Amoxicillin PO 14 days or doxycycline PO 14 days		Azithromycin PO 7–10 days

[a]Cefuroxime axetil was tested in children age ≥12 years.
[b]First-degree block with PR interval <0.3 s, PO therapy; PR >0.3 s or higher grade, IV initially then PO if there is a rapid response.
[c]For oral therapy failures only.
IV, Intravenously; *PO*, orally.
Doses:

- Doxycycline PO 2–4 mg/kg/day divided into 2 doses, up to adult dose of 100 mg twice a day.
- Amoxicillin PO 50 mg/kg/day divided into 3 doses, up to adult dose of 2 g/day.
- Cefuroxime axetil PO 30 mg/kg/day divided into 2 doses, up to adult dose of 500 mg twice a day.
- Azithromycin 10 mg/kg once daily, up to 500 mg/day.
- Ceftriaxone IV 100 mg/kg/day once daily, up to adult dose of 2 g/day.
- Cefotaxime IV 180 mg/kg/day, up to adult dose of 2 g q8h.

ongoing symptoms after Lyme disease, based on at least four prospective controlled antibiotic trials.[12,30] There also are no data to suggest that children differ from adults in this regard. As with adults, it is not appropriate to prescribe an antibiotic for a child who has positive serology in the absence of accompanying or recent specific clinical manifestations. The term *chronic Lyme disease* has been used by a small number of practitioners to describe patients whom they believe have persistent *B. burgdorferi* infection, a condition they suggest requires long-term antibiotic treatment and may even be incurable.[30] The assumption that chronic, subjective symptoms are caused by persistent infection with *B. burgdorferi* is not supported by carefully conducted laboratory studies or by controlled treatment trials.[7]

PREVENTION AND MANAGEMENT OF *IXODES* TICK BITES

Prevention of Tick Bites

It is obviously best to keep free of tick-infested vegetation such as brush and wooded areas, but recreational, occupational, and residential habits make it difficult to avoid tick exposure for most people living in endemic areas.[38] Ticks are often present in grassy areas and in leaf litter on personal property and can attach during even brief exposure. Use of repellents is very helpful in preventing tick bites. Light-colored clothes (to make crawling ticks more visible), long-sleeved clothing, and socks tucked or taped into pants are somewhat effective, and more so if used in conjunction with repellents. The repellent DEET (N,N-diethyl-m-toluamide, or N,N-diethyl-3-methylbenzamide) is the most effective but is underutilized because of exaggerated concerns about potential toxicity. Very little DEET is absorbed after topical application, and it is rapidly metabolized and eliminated. In very young children care should be taken to avoid application near mucosal surfaces. Certain DEET-sunscreen combinations and topical retinoids can enhance the absorption of DEET, however, and the use of combination DEET-sunscreen preparations is not recommended.[46,71] A 30% formulation provides about 6 hours of protection. The use of higher concentrations has been discontinued in Canada. Permethrin is a highly effective acaricide and repellent that can be applied to or impregnated in clothing, shoes, and fomites and affords additional protection.[46]

Tick checks under bright lighting should be performed at the end of each day of exposure. Use of a washcloth or tweezers with special attention to armpit, groin, back, and scalp areas may dislodge unattached ticks. Studies have demonstrated that early removal of an *Ixodes* tick minimized the risk for acquiring *B. burgdorferi* infection.[60,93]

The geographic range of *Ixodes* tick species is expanding beyond previously endemic regions, and practitioners should be knowledgeable about the incidence of Lyme disease where they practice. Most Lyme disease occurs in the peridomestic environment. Landscape-management measures, such as keeping grass mowed, removing leaf litter, using plantings that do not attract deer, deer fences, spraying areas of high tick density with acaricidal formulations, and using dry pebble or wood chip borders between lawns and surrounding vegetation may help reduce the risk for tick-borne infections.[38] The elimination of deer populations sharply reduces the risk for infection but is difficult to implement. Public education about the risks and characteristic symptoms of tick-borne diseases is an important component of prevention.

Preventing Infection After an *Ixodes* Tick Bite

The risk for acquiring *B. burgdorferi* infection following an *Ixodes* tick bite is low, even in endemic areas. The incidence was 1.2% to 4.4% in US studies.[3,22,84] Nevertheless, considerable apprehension accompanies tick bites, and practitioners tend to overprescribe antibiotic prophylaxis.[64]

The use of an evidence-based approach will serve to allay anxiety, decrease indiscriminate use of antibiotics, and prevent some cases of *B. burgdorferi* infection. A tick should be removed with an ordinary pair of thin-tipped tweezers or forceps. The tick should be grasped by the mouth end and gently pulled straight upward. There is no evidence that residual embedded mouth parts or crushing the tick increase risk for transmission. Other removal techniques are ineffective and can be dangerous.[62] Most important, the patient should save the tick in any dry vessel for identification because almost one-third of suspected deer ticks are a different species or not ticks at all.[93] By referring to images on the Internet, a practitioner should be able to distinguish a six-legged insect from an eight-legged tick, differentiate a dog tick or a Lone Star tick from a deer tick, and differentiate a nymphal from an adult female deer tick.[89] Most commercial laboratories and health departments in endemic areas perform tick identification. Patient requests to have a tick analyzed for *B. burgdorferi* DNA should be discouraged because this testing may be unreliable and does not correlate with transmission risk. More important are the developmental stage of the tick and the duration of attachment. Most cases of Lyme disease are transmitted by nymphal deer ticks.[60] Duration of attachment is critical because there is a 36- to 72-hour delay between the onset of feeding and the migration of spirochetes from the tick midgut to saliva and transmission to the host. The incidence of infection increases 20-fold for ticks attached for 72 hours or longer compared with those attached for less than 72 hours.[93] Tick identification and assessment of engorgement can be used to help define a small, high-risk subset of people who should benefit from antibiotic prophylaxis.

A single dose of doxycycline was shown to be 87% effective in prevention of Lyme borreliosis in a study in a Lyme disease hyperendemic area of the United States, where an *I. scapularis* tick was analyzed within 72 hours of the bite and duration of attachment of 72 hours was documented by an entomologist.[60] Adverse effects occurred in 30% of doxycycline recipients, however. If the tick species, stage, and duration of attachment cannot be determined, a "wait and watch" approach is appropriate, given the overall low risk for Lyme borreliosis. This is the standard approach in Europe.[94] Serologic testing does not benefit management decisions after a tick bite and is not recommended. In sum, routine use of antibiotics to prevent Lyme disease in persons who are bitten by a deer tick is not recommended, even in highly endemic areas. Persons who have removed attached ticks from themselves can submit the tick for identification and should be monitored closely for signs and symptoms of Lyme disease (and other tick-borne diseases) for up to 1 month. Those who develop a rash at the site of the tick bite or multiple skin lesions elsewhere, or a generalized nonspecific illness, should promptly seek medical attention.

NEW REFERENCES SINCE THE SEVENTH EDITION

23. Diuk-Wasser MA, Vannier E, Krause PJ. Coinfection by Ixodes tick-borne pathogens: ecological, epidemiological, and clinical consequences. *Trends Parasitol.* 2016;32(1):30-42.
31. Forrester JD, Brett M, Matthias J, et al. Epidemiology of Lyme disease in low-incidence states. *Ticks Tick Borne Dis.* 2015;6(6):721-723.
32. Forrester JD, Mead P. Third-degree heart block associated with Lyme carditis: review of published cases. *Clin Infect Dis.* 2014;59(7):996-1000.
49. Krause PJ, Narasimhan S, Wormser GP, et al. *Borrelia miyamotoi* sensu lato seroreactivity and seroprevalence in the northeastern United States. *Emerg Infect Dis.* 2014;20(7):1183-1190.
52. Lantos PM, Auwaerter PG, Nelson CA. Lyme disease serology. *JAMA.* 2016;315(16):1780-1781.
57. Mead PS. Epidemiology of Lyme disease. *Infect Dis Clin North Am.* 2015;29(2):187-210.
63. Patterson-Fortin J, Kohli A, Suarez MJ, et al. Ocular Lyme borreliosis as a rare presentation of unilateral vision loss. *BMJ Case Rep.* 2016;2016.
64. Perea AE, Hinckley AF, Mead PS. Tick bite prophylaxis: results from a 2012 survey of healthcare providers. *Zoonoses Public Health.* 2015;62(5):388-392.
68. Pritt BS, Mead PS, Johnson DK, et al. Identification of a novel pathogenic *Borrelia* species causing Lyme borreliosis with unusually high spirochaetaemia: a descriptive study. *Lancet Infect Dis.* 2016;16(5):556-564.
76. Sanchez E, Vannier E, Wormser GP, et al. Diagnosis, treatment, and prevention of lyme disease, human granulocytic anaplasmosis, and babesiosis: a review. *JAMA.* 2016;315(16):1767-1777.
77. Schutzer SE, Fraser-Liggett CM, Qiu WG, et al. Whole-genome sequences of *Borrelia bissettii, Borrelia valaisiana,* and *Borrelia spielmanii. J Bacteriol.* 2012;194(2):545-546.
81. Shapiro ED. Clinical practice. Lyme disease. *N Engl J Med.* 2014;370(18):1724-1731.
111. Krause PJ, Foley DT, Burke GS, et al. Reinfection and relapse in early Lyme disease. *Am J Trop Med Hyg.* 2006;75(6):1090-1094.
112. Nadelman RB, Hanincová K, Mukherjee P, et al. Differentiation of reinfection from relapse in recurrent Lyme disease. *N Engl J Med.* 2012;367(20):1883-1890.

The full reference list for this chapter is available at ExpertConsult.com.

Relapsing Fever

141

Peter J. Krause • Kenneth M. Boyer

Relapsing fever is an arthropod-borne infection caused by several species of spirochetes in the genus *Borrelia*.* Two major types of relapsing fever are classified according to their arthropod vector, tick-borne (TBRF) relapsing fever and louse-borne (LBRF) relapsing fever. TBRF may further be classified into soft tick-borne relapsing fever (STBRF) and hard tick-borne relapsing fever (HTBRF). Each category of arthropod vector transmits a different *Borrelia* species or group of species, but all cause relapsing fever (Fig. 141.1). Illness is characterized by recurring episodes of fever and nonspecific symptoms that include headache, shaking chills, myalgia, arthralgia, and abdominal distress, separated by periods of well-being or minor symptoms.[22,24,53] The characteristic relapse of symptoms is caused by recurrent spirochetemia and the associated immune responses. After a *Borrelia* relapsing fever strain infects a person, its proliferation in blood is curtailed by antibody and other immune factors. The *Borrelia* subsequently change surface antigens so that a new variant (serotype) emerges and the cycle is repeated.[2,4,5,46,56,65] A single organism can produce as many as 40 antigenic variant membrane proteins, and six or more relapses may occur over several months.[22] The clinical presentation is highly variable, with some patients experiencing a viral-like illness, some gastrointestinal symptoms, and others meningitis or meningoencephalitis.[16] Although the disease may be severe, the fatality rate in treated STBRF patients is less than 5%.[23] The fatality rate for treated LBRF patients is about 5%; however, it may exceed 40% in large LBRF epidemics among nutritionally and immunosuppressed populations caught up in war or famine.[11,23,63] During the last great LBRF epidemic in North Africa and Europe during WWII, an estimated 50,000 patients died of the illness.[11,23,27] Both HTBRF and LBRF occur worldwide, but only LBRF is currently confined to northern Africa and Europe (through refugees).

ORGANISM

Borrelia are spirochetal bacteria whose spiral shape enhances their motility and whose loose coiling helps distinguish them from other spirochetes such as *Leptospira* and *Treponema* (Fig. 141.2).[6,26,34,72] They have inner and outer membranes and several internal flagella that are not surface exposed. The flagella are responsible for shape and motility. *Borrelia* spp. are divided into two major groups: the Lyme borreliosis group that are transmitted exclusively by hard-bodied ticks, and the relapsing fever group that are primarily transmitted by soft-bodied ticks but also by hard-bodied ticks and lice.[6,26,72]

The genome of the STBRF spirochete relapsing fever *Borrelia hermsii* contains a linear chromosome of about 1 million base pairs and one copy each of several types of linear and circular plasmids. There are 5 to 10 identical genomes in each organism.[5,6] Numerous surface lipoproteins of the outer membrane called *variable major proteins* (Vmps) determine variant or serotype identity.[2] A change in the expression of Vmps allows the relapsing fever *Borrelia* to survive in the highly diverse environments of mammal and tick and allows the organism to escape immune attack within mammalian hosts.[2,3,4,5,46,50,56,65] The HTBRF *Borrelia* (*Borrelia miyamotoi*) genome consists of a linear chromosome of about 1 million base pairs and eight complete linear plasmids. It also contains incomplete plasmids, including up to five putative incomplete circular plasmid and one linear plasmid.[74]

Relapsing fever *Borrelia* are microaerophilic and can be cultivated in cell-free media but have complex nutritional requirements for growth.[6,72] They may no longer be able to infect laboratory animals after several passages in vitro and may lose their ability to infect ticks after prolonged passage in laboratory animals.

*References 6, 11, 22–24, 26, 27, 32, 34, 36, 41, 54, 72.

TRANSMISSION

Relapsing fever is transmitted in almost all cases by an infected tick or louse (see Fig. 141.1). Rare causes of transmission include blood transfusion, intravenous drug use, laboratory worker accidents, and transplacental transmission from mother to fetus.[6,28,64,72]

Currently, most reported cases of relapsing fever are transmitted by soft-bodied (*Ornithodoros*) ticks. Transmission begins within minutes of the start of a blood meal that takes from 15 to 90 minutes.[6,23] The ticks usually feed at night, and most relapsing fever patients are unaware of being bitten. The *Borrelia* and the ticks are maintained in a tick-mammalian host life cycle in which rodents and other small mammals become asymptomatically infected and provide a blood meal for the ticks.[22,23,26] Nymphal and adult ticks are the most common source of transmission, but in some tick species larvae may be infected through transovarial transmission whereby an adult female transmits infection to her eggs.[23] Humans are a dead-end host for TBRF and do not contribute to the transmission cycle. The recently discovered HTBRF *Borrelia* (*Borrelia miyamotoi*) has been found in hard-bodied (ixodid) ticks in North America and Eurasia.[29,51,62] About 15% of the spirochetes found in *Ixodes scapularis* (the tick vector for Lyme disease, babesiosis, and anaplasmosis) are *B. miyamotoi*.[62]

LBRF occurs when an infected louse feeds on a human, the sole known host.[36] In contrast to TBRF, humans are the reservoir host for LBRF and are responsible for perpetuating the infection cycle. Transmission occurs when the louse is wounded or crushed by scratching and infected hemolymph or feces contaminate the bite site. LBRF is most common when large numbers of people gather in one area and hygiene is compromised.

EPIDEMIOLOGY

Twelve different species of *Borrelia* have been shown to cause TBRF (Table 141.1).[6] In the United States, the most common species is *Borrelia hermsii* followed by *Borrelia turicatae* and *Borrelia parkeri*.[6,23] Cases are reported most frequently from California, Washington, and Colorado.[75] Cases most commonly occur in the summertime among people who have slept in rustic cabins or caves in forested areas.[1,8,17,18,19,67,68] TBRF is very widespread outside the United States, and cases have been described in Canada, Mexico, Central and South America, Africa, Asia, and Europe.[1,23] Human cases of *B. miyamotoi* relapsing fever have been described in the United States, Europe, and Asia. The discovery of this spirochete in a variety of ixodid ticks greatly expands the potential geographic distribution of relapsing fever, and it is likely that *B. miyamotoi* will be found wherever Lyme disease is endemic.[30,39,33,21,40,58,35,43,51,62] In contrast, LBRF is caused by a single species of *Borrelia*, *Borrelia recurrentis*. It has been found worldwide but is currently only significantly endemic in Ethiopia and Sudan.[53,54] Cases have been reported from European countries in recent years among refugees from North Africa.[76,77]

PATHOGENESIS AND PATHOLOGY

Relapsing fever *Borrelia* enter the bloodstream after tick transmission and rapidly multiply. Based on animal experiments and human studies with LBRF and STBRF, it is estimated that bacterial concentrations reach 100,000 to 1 million spirochetes per milliliter of blood during symptomatic disease.[11,23,65] This accounts for their characteristics visualization on Wright-stained peripheral blood smears (Fig. 141.2).[8,76] *Borrelia* are initially phagocytized in the bloodstream by neutrophils, macrophages, and dendritic cells that cause the release of cytokines and other immune

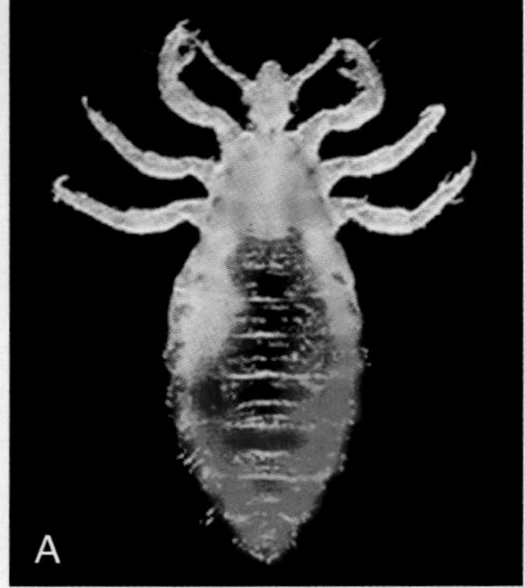

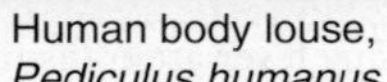

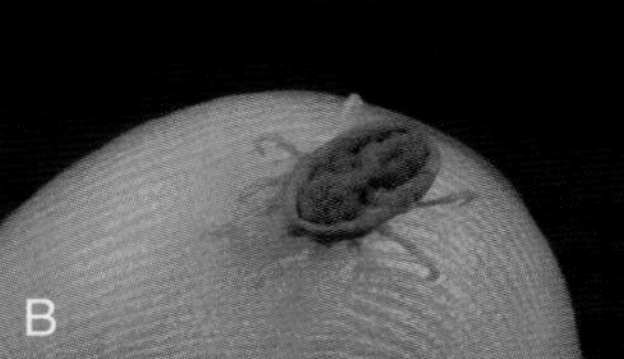

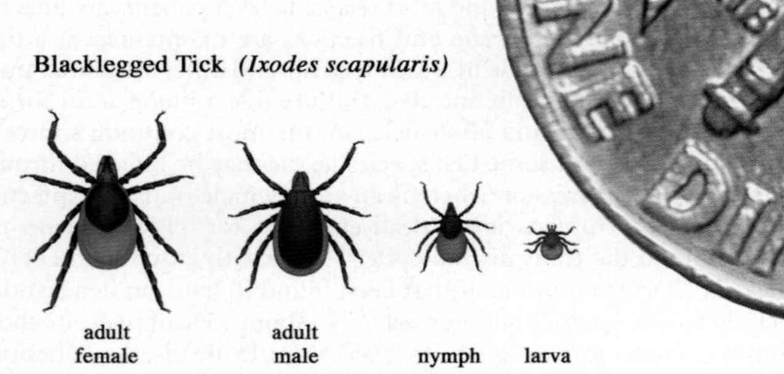

FIG. 141.1 Examples of vectors of relapsing fever. (A) Louse-borne relapsing fever (human body louse *Pediculus humanus*). (B) Soft tick-borne relapsing fever (*Ornithodoros hermsii*). (C) Hard tick-borne relapsing fever (*Ixodes scapularis*). (From Centers for Disease Control and Prevention. https://www.cdc.gov/relapsing_fever/symptoms/index.html.)

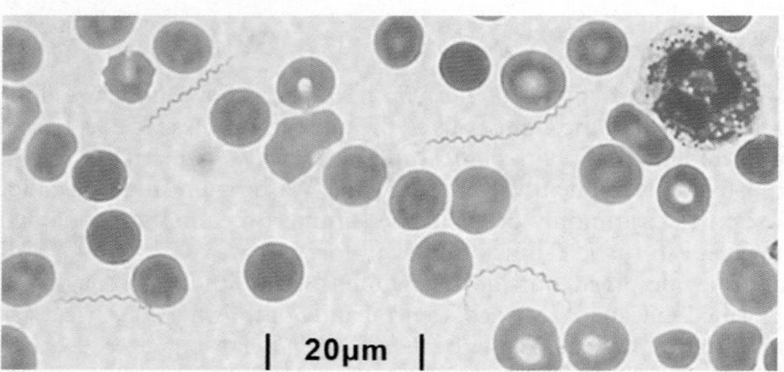

FIG. 141.2 *Borrelia hermsii* spirochetes in the peripheral blood smear of a patient with tick-borne relapsing fever (Wright stain, ×1000). (From Centers for Disease Control and Prevention. https://www.cdc.gov/relapsing fever/symptoms/index.html.)

TABLE 141.1 Important *Borrelia* Causing Relapsing Fever, Their Vectors, and Their Current Geographic Distribution

Borrelia Species	Vector	Geographic Distribution
Louse-Borne Relapsing Fever		
B. recurrentis	*Pediculus humanus humanus*	Ethiopia, Sudan
Soft Tick-Borne Relapsing Fever		
B. caucasica	*Ornithodoros verrucosus*	Iraq, central Russia
B. crocidurae	*Ornithodoros erraticus* (small variant)	North Africa, Middle East
B. duttonii	*Ornithodoros moubata*	Eastern and Central Africa
B. hermsii	*Ornithodoros hermsi*	Western United States and Canada
B. hispanica	*Ornithodoros erraticus* (large variant)	Spain, western North Africa
B. latyschewii	*Ornithodoros tartakowskyi*	Iran, central Asia
B. mazzottii	*Ornithodoros talaje*	Mexico, Central America
B. parkeri	*Ornithodoros parkeri*	Western United States
B. persica	*Ornithodoros tholozani*	Middle East, western Asia
B. turicatae	*Ornithodoros turicata*	Southwestern United States, Mexico
B. venezuelensis	*Ornithodoros rudis*	Northern South America
Hard Tick-Borne Relapsing Fever		
B. miyamotoi	*Ixodes scapularis, Ixodes pacificus, Ixodes ricinus, Ixodes persulcatus,*	Northeastern, northern Midwestern, and Pacific Coast United States; central Russia, Europe, Japan

factors, resulting in symptoms.[13,15,52,70,73] Antibody (especially immunoglobulin M [IgM]) plays a central role in bacterial eradication, and most *Borrelia* are cleared from the bloodstream after 2 to 3 days.[23,65] Surviving *Borrelia* are able to change outer membrane proteins so that the original IgM antibodies are no longer effective. A new antigenic variant emerges and causes recurrence of fever and other symptoms.[2-5,38,46,56,59,65] The same process repeats itself for several cycles in untreated patients. Because there is some antibody cross-reactivity, subsequent spirochetemia and clinical manifestations usually are milder.[9] *Borrelia* antigenic variation is a result of new outer surface Vmps that are encoded by alternative *vmp* genes found on linear plasmids.[2-5,59] There is a copy of silent and expressed genes on the same or different plasmids within each borrelial microorganism. Antigenic switching occurs when a silent *vmp* gene begins to encode for protein while the existing *vmp* gene is shut down. The stimulus for antigenic switching is unknown. Recent data suggest that the antigenic switching that occurs when relapsing *Borrelia* move from mouse to tick is induced by the temperature change from the warm-blooded host to the cooler tick vector.[59]

Relapsing fever *Borrelia* are not confined to the bloodstream but also infect the nervous system, eyes, lung, liver, kidney, heart, and spleen.[20,23,24,27,36] They may persist in these tissues.[6] There is evidence in animal models that the same serotype antigenic variation that is seen in the blood also occurs in brain tissue, where *Borrelia* have been shown to persist for up to 3 years.[6] Tissue damage in fatal human cases has been noted in the central nervous system (meningitis, degenerative lesions, hemorrhage, and perivascular infiltrates), heart (myocarditis), lung (pneumonia), gastrointestinal tract (hemorrhage), liver (enlargement, hepatic necrosis), and spleen (splenic abscess).[27,36] Relapsing fever *Borrelia* can cross the placenta or be transmitted during birth, causing abortion, premature birth, or severe perinatal infection.[28,64]

CLINICAL MANIFESTATIONS

Initial clinical manifestations may consist of the characteristic recurring fever and accompanying symptoms of headache, chills, and fatigue or may reflect rapid dissemination to the central nervous system, gastrointestinal tract, or lungs.* Symptom type and severity depend on the species and strain of infecting *Borrelia* and the age and immune status of the host. Although TBRF and LBRF have similar clinical manifestations, tick-borne illness generally is less severe (Table 141.2). *B. recurrentis* (LBRF) and *Borrelia duttonii* (STBRF) are associated with severe disease. Pregnant women often experience severe disease.[22,28,64]

*References 8, 11, 16, 20, 22–24, 32, 38, 41, 53, 67, 68, 72.

TABLE 141.2 Characteristics of Tick-Borne Relapsing Fever and Lyme Disease

	FREQUENCY	
Characteristic[a]	**Tick-Borne Relapsing Fever**	**Lyme Disease**
Fever relapses	Common	Rare/none
Fever ≥39°C	Common	Rare
Focal skin rash	Rare/none	Common
Arthritis	Rare/none	Common
Neurologic involvement	Occasional	Occasional
Spirochetes on blood smear	Common	Rare/none
Jarisch-Herxheimer reaction	Common	Occasional

[a]Clinical characteristics of untreated patients in the United States.

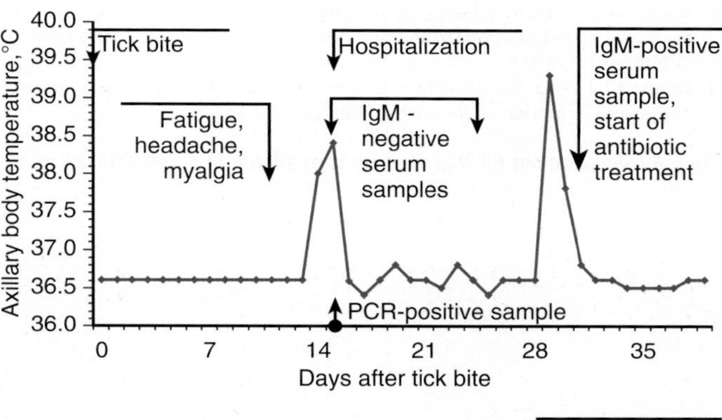

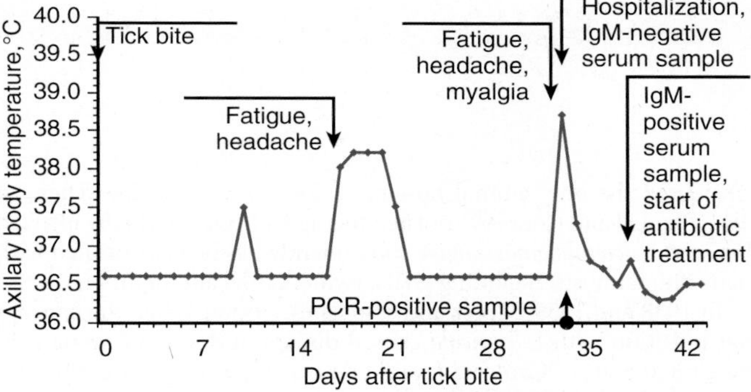

FIG. 141.3 Examples of relapsing fever episodes in two patients with *Borrelia miyamotoi* infection. *Arrows* indicate the timing of tick bite, hospital admission, polymerase chain reaction (PCR) testing, anti-*Borrelia* immunoglobulin M (IgM) testing, and initiation of antimicrobial drug therapy. (From Platonov AE, Karan LS, Kolyasnikova NM, et al. Humans infected with the relapsing fever spirochete *Borrelia miyamotoi*, Russia. *Emerg Infect Dis.* 2011;17:1816-1823.)

For STBRF, the mean incubation period is 7 days, with a range of 4 to 18 days. Symptoms generally last 3 to 6 days (range, 12 hours to 17 days) for the first episode in untreated patients. This is followed by a week (range, 3 to 36 days) of well-being or mild nonspecific symptoms before the next febrile episode (Fig. 141.3).[23] The duration of symptoms and asymptomatic intervals are several days longer for LBRF. As many as six relapses have been noted in TBRF patients, but the average number is three to five in untreated patients.[8,22,23,51] The duration of symptoms decreases and the time between relapses increases with each episode, although this is not always the case.[67]

STBRF may be associated with fatal hypotension and shock, usually at the end of the first episode of fever. Gastrointestinal manifestations such as nausea, vomiting, diarrhea, hepatomegaly, or splenomegaly occur in more than one-half the cases; dry cough in about one-fourth of cases; a macular, papular, or petechial rash in about one-fifth of cases; and meningitis in about 3% of cases.[22,23] Ocular manifestations are seen in less than 10% of STBRF, patients and include eye pain, photophobia, and conjunctival injection. Pregnant women are subject to more severe disease with high fever and associated miscarriage and congenital infection.

The clinical presentation of HTBRF is similar to that of STBRF. The typical presentation consists of fever that may exceed 140°C, fatigue, headach, myalgia, arthralgia, and chills. Relapses were reported in 11% of the first cases from Russia reported by Platonov et al. (Fig. 141.3).[51] Other symptoms included nausea, vomiting, and neck stiffness.[43,51] Meningoencephalitis has been reported in immunocompromised people.[30,33,78]

DIAGNOSIS AND DIFFERENTIAL DIAGNOSIS

A history of travel to wooded areas, especially rustic cabins or caves with exposure to small rodents and ticks, is helpful in making the diagnosis of STBRF, whereas residence in or travel to a Lyme disease–endemic area is required for diagnosis of hard HTBRF. A definitive diagnosis of STBRF or LBRF generally is made by examination of a Wright-stained thick or thin blood smear (see Fig. 141.2). Use of a buffy coat smear using Giemsa stain, acridine orange stain, or darkfield examination increases diagnostic sensitivity.[61] *Borrelia* are rarely found during afebrile periods.

An initial enzyme-linked immunosorbent assay (ELISA) or immunofluorescent antibody (IFA) assay followed by an immunoblot test is often used to test for antibody in acute and convalescent sera.[40,55,60,] Serology testing is compromised by alternating outer surface protein (antigenic switching) and by cross-reactivity of relapsing fever *Borrelia* antibody against other spirochetes, such as the causative agents of Lyme disease and syphilis. Glycophosphoryl diester phosphodiesterase (GlpQ) protein (produced with recombinant DNA technology) has been identified in relapsing fever spirochetes but not in the Lyme disease or syphilis spirochetes.[60] GlpQ protein–based ELISA assays are superior to those that use whole-cell preparations of cultured bacteria such as *B. hermsii*.[60] Other tests that have been developed to diagnose TBRF include *B. hermsii* and *B. miyamotoi* polymerase chain reaction, in vitro cultivation, or amplification of organisms by mouse inoculation followed by microscopic visualization.[37,51,69]

TBRL and LBRF are frequently misdiagnosed. The differential diagnosis is broad and includes enterovirus infection, dengue, hepatitis, influenza, leptospirosis, malaria, and typhoid fever. Other tick-borne illnesses need to be considered, including anaplasmosis, babesiosis, Colorado tick fever, ehrlichiosis, Lyme disease, and Rocky Mountain spotted fever. Periodic fever syndromes such as PFAPA (periodic fever, aphthous ulcers, pharyngitis, and adenitis), hyper IgD syndrome, and familial Mediterranean fever have longer intervals between febrile episodes.[23,42,47]

TREATMENT

Several antibiotics have been shown to be effective in treatment of relapsing fever, including doxycycline, tetracycline, erythromycin, penicillin, and chloramphenicol.[7,44,48,49,57] For older children, doxycycline or tetracycline are the antimicrobial therapies of choice. Erythromycin is the drug of choice for children younger than 8 years because penicillin is probably less effective, doxycycline and tetracycline are associated with teeth staining, and chloramphenicol may suppress the bone marrow. For older children, doxycycline or tetracycline are the antimicrobial therapies of choice. A proposed management approach for febrile children is to substitute oral phenoxymethyl penicillin (a single low dose of 7.5 mg/kg) or intravenous penicillin G (10,000 U/kg infused over a period of 30 minutes) as initial treatment on the first day in order to minimize the potential problem of the Jarisch-Herxheimer reaction.[12,56,70] Patients with this reaction experience an acute exacerbation of symptoms following the first dose of antibiotic.[10,12,14,25,45,66,71] Data suggest that large numbers of bacteria are abruptly fragmented and killed with antibiotic therapy, exposing antigen that elicits an intense cytokine response. Penicillin may result in less rapid destruction of spirochetes than tetracycline or doxycycline. In one large study, 54% of patients treated for

STBRF experienced the Jarisch-Herxheimer reaction, with more than one-half experiencing high fever (≥40°C), chills, rigors, diaphoresis, and hypotension.[23] Associated symptoms are even worse with LBRF. Fortunately, children generally experience milder reactions than adults. Regardless, they still should be monitored closely for the first 12 hours after the initial dose of antibiotic in the emergency department or hospital with intravenous access in place. Therapy consists of supportive measures, such as volume expansion and antipyretics. A 10-day course of oral erythromycin (40 mg/kg per day divided every 6 hours, maximum 500 mg/dose) or doxycycline (4 mg/kg per day divided every 12 hours, maximum 100 mg/dose) should then be given to eradicate tissue spirochetes and prevent relapse. Preventive measures for STBRF include the use of doxycycline tick bite prophylaxis and acaricidal spraying of tick-infested bedding and sleeping areas.[8,31]

Therapy for HTBRF is the same as for Lyme disease, specifically doxycycline, amoxicillin, and ceftriaxone (for meningoencephalitis).[30,33,43,51,79] HTBRF can be prevented by avoiding areas where ticks, deer, and mice are known to thrive, using protective clothing, applying diethyltoluamide, checking for and removing ticks, managing landscape (keeping grass mowed, clearing leaf litter, spraying property with acaricides), and reducing the number of deer.[79]

NEW REFERENCES SINCE THE SEVENTH EDITION

21. Chowdri HR, Gugliotta JL, Berardi VP, et al. *Borrelia miyamotoi* infection presenting as human granulocytic anaplasmosis: a case report. *Ann Intern Med*. 2013;159:21-27.
30. Gugliotta JL, Goethert HK, Berardi VP, et al. Meningoencephalitis from *Borrelia miyamotoi* in an immunocompromised patient. *N Engl J Med*. 2013;368:240-245.
33. Hovius JW, de Wever B, Sohne M, et al. A case of meningoencephalitis by the relapsing fever spirochaete *Borrelia miyamotoi* in Europe. *Lancet*. 2013; 382:658.
35. Jahfari S, Herremans T, Platonov AE, et al. High seroprevalence of *Borrelia miyamotoi* antibodies in forestry workers and individuals suspected of human granulocytic anaplasmosis in the Netherlands. *New Microbes New Infect*. 2014;2:144-149.
39. Krause PJ, Narasimhan S, Wormser G, et al. Human *Borrelia miyamotoi* infection in the United States. *N Engl J Med*. 2013;368:291-293.
40. Krause PJ, Narasimmhan S, Wormser GP, et al. *Borrelia miyamotoi* sensu lato seroreactivity and seroprevalence in the Northeastern United States. *Emerg Infect Dis*. 2014;20:1183-1190.
43. Molloy PJ, Telford SR 3rd, Chowdri HR, et al. *Borrelia miyamotoi* disease in the United States: a case series. *Ann Intern Med*. 2015;163:91-98.
58. Sato K, Takano A, Konnai S, et al. Human infections with *Borrelia miyamotoi*, Japan Emerg. *Infect Dis*. 2014;20:1391-1393.
74. Kingry LC, Replogle A, Batra D, et al. Toward a complete North American *Borrelia miyamotoi* genome. *Genome Announc*. 2017;5:e01557-16.
75. Centers for Disease Control and Prevention. Tickborne relapsing fever–United States, 1990-2011. *MMWR Morb Mortal Wkly Rep*. 2015;64:58-60.
76. von Both U, Alberer M. *Borrelia recurrentis* infection. *N Engl J Med*. 2016;375:e5.
77. Cutler SJ. Refugee crisis and re-emergence of forgotten infections in Europe. *Clin Micrbiol Infect*. 2016;22:8-9.
78. Boden K, Lobenstein S, Hermann B, Margos G, Fingerle V. *Borrelia miyamotoi*-associated neuroborreliosis in an immunocompromised person. *Emerg Infect Dis*. 2016;22:1617-1620.
79. Krause PJ, Fish D, Narasimhan S, Barbour AG. *Borrelia miyamotoi* infection in nature and in humans. *Clin Microbiol Infect*. 2015;21:631-639.

The full reference list for this chapter is available at ExpertConsult.com.

142 Leptospirosis

Delma J. Nieves

Leptospirosis is considered an emerging zoonosis due to increased contact between animals and humans and the resulting human encroachment into wildlife habitat. Climate changes of global warming and environmental shifts can affect the degree of transmission. Early detection is important to prevent morbidity and mortality most effectively. In June 2012, leptospirosis was reinstated as a Nationally Notifiable Condition in the United States. This has aided in further investigation of incidence, distribution, and risk factors associated with human cases.[112] Worldwide research efforts continue to dedicate additional resources and improve understanding of this fascinating organism, which continues to contribute to human morbidity and mortality. Thus far, leptospirosis is far from controlled.

HISTORY

Weil[286] is credited with providing the first description of leptospirosis in 1886, although it had likely been previously described under various names.[244] Not until 1915, however, was the causal agent, originally known as *Spirochaeta icterohaemorrhagiae*, identified by Inada and associates.[126] Eight years earlier, Stimson[242] unknowingly had identified the same organism within sections of kidney obtained from a patient in whom yellow fever had been diagnosed incorrectly.

Inada and associates demonstrated the role of the rat as a carrier in 1916.[126] Noguchi[182] first recovered this organism from a Norway rat in 1917. Although the etiology of Weil syndrome in British Army troops in Flanders was found to be spirochetes and a possible connection with rats was suspected, the route of acquiring infection was not understood. In 1922, *Leptospira icterohaemorrhagiae* was isolated from the blood of a laboratory worker who developed jaundice after an accidental needlestick containing the serum of an infected rat.[281] For many years the rat was considered the only animal host of *L. icterohaemorrhagiae.* Then, in 1944, Randall and Cooper[197] isolated this agent from a naturally infected dog, and *L. icterohaemorrhagiae* subsequently has been associated with many animal hosts, including goats, swine, cattle, and hamsters.

In 1938 and 1939, Meyer and associates[163] popularized the concept that infection with *L. canicola* caused disease in dogs and humans in the United States. "Canicola fever" first was reported in Great Britain in 1946[20]; in 1951, 40% of the dogs in Great Britain were noted to be seropositive.[45] Surveys have confirmed the presence of *L. canicola* infection in species other than dogs.[220,271]

In 1950, Gochenour and colleagues[103] identified *L. pomona* as the agent responsible for leptospirosis in cows. Widespread *L. pomona* infection among cattle in the United States was recognized quickly, and in time this finding stimulated extensive epidemiologic investigations in livestock. Infections of cattle with *L. hebdomidis* and *L. grippotyphosa* were identified, and, concomitantly, infections of swine and horses with *L. pomona* were documented.[121] In Europe, *L. pomona* was identified as the agent responsible for "swineherd disease," and it was recovered from other domestic animals as well. In 1951, the first human cases of *L. pomona* infection were identified.

Many new serotypes of leptospires were recognized in the early 1950s after the establishment of serologic diagnostic services for leptospires by the Centers for Disease Control and Prevention (CDC) and the Walter Reed Army Institute of Research. Along with the identification of additional leptospiral serotypes, the spectrum of clinical disease associated with infection by leptospires was elucidated. Patients with autumnal fever (a disease in Japanese peasants and potters) and Fort Bragg fever (a febrile illness associated with pretibial eruptions described in army recruits) were shown to suffer from leptospirosis caused by *L. autumnalis.*[102,212] "Mud fever," "pea-pickers disease," and "European swamp fever," names that were used to describe a disease of undetermined etiology in eastern Germany, the Far East, and western Poland, respectively, were shown to be examples of leptospirosis caused by *L. grippotyphosa.*[51] Seven-day fever in Japan, Wycon fever and Bushy Creek fever in the United States, cane field fever in Australia, and swineherd disease in Europe were identified as examples of infection caused by *L. hebdomidis, L. canicola, L. pomona, L. australis,* and *L. pomona,* respectively.[26,32,39,63,121]

Leptospirosis is a disease now thought to be caused by a single family of organisms that has multiple serogroups and serotypes[4] and is characterized by a broad spectrum of clinical findings.[190] More than 300 strains, called serovars (serotypes), which are divided into serogroups on the basis of common antigens, have been identified. These are divided into two species: *L. interrogans* sensu lato, which contains the pathogenic strains; and *L. biflexa* sensu lato, which contains the saprophytic strains.[118] Using a newer classification based on DNA relatedness, the genus *Leptospira* can be classified into 22 species. Identified thus far are 10 species of pathogenic *Leptospira,* five intermediate species that may cause mild clinical manifestations, and seven saprophytic species that are environmental but do not cause disease in humans or animals.[38] Serovars of the same group may be distributed between different species.[54] Leptospirosis is now often described as the most widespread and prevalent zoonotic disease worldwide. The organism's ability to survive outside the host as well as establish a chronic carrier state in rodents promotes its survival and promulgation. Global warming and increased rainfall are predictors of increased incidence. In 2003, the World Health Organization (WHO) reported a worldwide incidence of 0.1 to 1 case per 100,000 population per year in temperate climates, more than 10 cases per 100,000 population in humid subtropical region, and more than 100 cases per 100,000 population during outbreaks.[118] However, the difficulty in diagnosing and identifying chronic infection leads to underestimation.[3] Traxler and colleagues analyzed US hospital discharge records for 1998–2009 and estimated an annual rate of leptospirosis-associated hospitalizations of 0.6 per 1 million population. But this is just the peak of the iceberg in terms of describing the true incidence of leptospirosis in the United States, where national surveillance ceased from 1994 to 2013.[259] Outbreaks in poor urban slums with rat infestations have contributed to its title as a neglected infection of poverty in the United States.[122] It is also considered an infection of adventure seekers with outdoor recreational exposure and international travel.[145,185,215] WHO established the Leptospirosis Burden Epidemiology Reference Group (LERG), which is focused on better estimating the global burden of disease.[291] In September 2015, LERG published findings from a systematic literature review of the data on leptospirosis morbidity and mortality, estimating annually 1.03 million cases and 58,900 deaths due to leptospirosis worldwide.[67]

EPIDEMIOLOGY

Animal Reservoirs

Among mammals, rodents are the most important reservoir of leptospires, but nearly all mammals may be infected and can transmit the disease.[257] Leptospires also have been isolated in reptiles and birds, but the epidemiologic significance of these animals in terms of maintenance of the organism in nature or transmission of disease to humans is not clear. For many species, infectivity rates of 10% to 50% have been reported frequently.[121,200] During epizootics, the circulation of leptospires among many species of animals (including rats, cows, dogs, swine, mongoose) living within a given biocenosis has been well recognized.[19,71,130,166,210,217]

The failure of leptospires to elicit a significant systemic antibody response in certain animal species may be due to the development of local immunity within their kidney tubules.[21,250] Some animals fail to develop homologous antibody titers but harbor leptospires in their kidneys for extended periods.[250] Thus lack of a positive titer to leptospires, as determined during the course of serologic surveys of animal populations, does not indicate absence of infection, leaving the true incidence of infection unknown.

A particular host species may serve as a reservoir for one or more serotypes of leptospires, and a particular serotype may be hosted by many different animal species. Turner[264,267] stressed that a particular animal species commonly serves as a reservoir for selected serotypes but temporarily may be infected and serve as an incidental host for other serotypes with which it usually is not infected.

Transmission of Leptospires to Humans

Leptospires are transmitted to humans either by contact with blood, urine, tissues, or organs of infected animals or by exposure to an environment that has been contaminated by leptospires. Humans usually represent a dead end in the chain of infection because although person-to-person transmission is possible theoretically, it is rare. After direct exposure of humans to infected animals, leptospires may enter breaks in the skin or may penetrate the mucous membranes, including the conjunctiva, nasopharynx, and vagina.[26,74,211,267] Human-to-human transmission via human milk has been reported in a breast-fed infant from a lactating mother who was infected with *L. interrogans.*[36]

Indirect transmission of leptospires to humans (from soil or water) depends on the presence of an environment that favors the survival of leptospires outside the animal host. A warm climate (25°C [77°F]), the presence of moisture, and pH values of soil or surface water between 6.2 and 8.0 are optimal conditions for survival of leptospires. These conditions prevail in many tropical regions throughout the year and in temperate climates during the late spring, summer, and autumn. Smith and Self[231] demonstrated survival of leptospires in cultures of infected soil for 43 days. In a survey of leptospirosis in Hawaii from 1999 to 2008, among 177 cases where exposure was determined, 45% were from recreational exposure (freshwater swimming, hiking, camping), 44% were occupational (taro farming), and 11% were from exposure around the home (gardening).[138] A study of human leptospirosis in the Caribbean from 1997 to 2005 found that in cases of suspected leptospirosis the highest seropositivity was found among 1- to 20-year-old and 31- to 40-year-old males, and its occurrence was higher during the wet season.[5] Ingestion or exposure from contaminated water sources, such as through infected rat or cattle urine, is a well-described source of leptospirosis in humans.[47,101,267] The importance of occupation as related to the risk for leptospirosis was emphasized in 1965.[121] Disease appeared to occur most frequently in people with occupations that required exposure to cattle or swine or to water contaminated by rat urine. The urine of infected cows may contain as many as 100 million leptospires per milliliter. If conditions are favorable, surface water contaminated by the urine of infected cattle may remain infectious for several weeks.[48] The largest reported outbreak of leptospirosis in the United States occurred in 1998 in Springfield, Illinois, after a triathlon that was preceded by heavy rains. There were 66 laboratory-confirmed cases of leptospirosis after the event, which included a swimming portion in a lake that received runoff from nearby livestock farms. Fifty-two of these cases occurred in triathlon participants, and 11 cases involved nonparticipants who came in contact with lake water near the event.[170] In a study performed in Detroit, 90% of rats carried *L. icterohemorrhagiae.*[77] Strain-specific tests comparing antibody titers in the sera of inner-city and suburban children were performed. Thirty-one percent of inner-city children had antibodies against *L. icterohaemorrhagiae;* 10% of suburban children also had antibodies to this organism. Lau and colleagues have studied the patterns of global climate change, flooding, and urbanization to predict that an increase in leptospirosis can be expected.[144]

Venereal transmission of leptospirosis is important in rodents and can occur in livestock. Leptospires have been recovered from the semen of bulls and have been transmitted by artificial insemination and by coitus. The possibility of seminal transmission in humans remains speculative. Transplacental infection of the fetus in utero is well documented in livestock and other animals and may occur in humans.[50,59,60,64,74,265,267]

During the past several decades, the number of cases acquired during outdoor recreation has increased. In developed countries, an increasing percentage of cases of leptospirosis are from travelers returning from areas of high endemicity and are often related to water activities.[145] In California, from 1982 to 2001, 59% of reported cases of leptospirosis were due to recreational exposure (often to contaminated freshwater), increasing to 85% in the 1997 to 2001 period.[161]

The dog, including the immunized pet dog, has been incriminated as an important vector and as a reservoir of leptospirosis.[106,249] Although immunization of dogs against leptospirosis is possible, it is important to remember that (1) immunization may not prevent the dog from having renal carriage and excreting the organism, (2) canine immunity after immunization may wane after just 1 year, and (3) immunity, when established, is effective only for serotypes present in the canine vaccine.[21]

In one survey of suburban and urban areas, however, between 15% and 40% of dogs were found to be infected.[31] Harkin and coworkers found that irrespective of health status, 8.2% of dogs were shedding pathogenic leptospires.[117] Rojas and colleagues found that 7.05% of dogs had urinary shedding.[204] Dogs were implicated in 58% of the 820 known cases of leptospirosis reported between 1962 and 1971.[53]

Asymptomatic renal colonization in humans has been shown. Using a 16S rDNA hybridization assay technique to identify *Leptospira* DNA in urine, Ganoza and associates identified a long-term renal shedder group (interestingly all women) among persons asymptomatically infected with pathogenic and intermediately pathogenic *Leptospira*. Almost 5% of healthy people living in a rural Amazonian community were urinary shedders of *Leptospira* but did not have serologic or clinical evidence of recent infection.[99] It is not understood if this could play a role in human-to-human transmission or some subtle degree of kidney disease.

A recent review of the literature found that a large proportion of cases (48%) and deaths (42%) were estimated to occur in adult males 20 to 49 years of age, and the highest estimates of disease morbidity and mortality were observed in the Global Burden of Disease regions of South and Southeast Asia; Oceania; Caribbean, Andean, central, and tropical Latin America; and east sub-Saharan Africa.[67] Another study estimated that globally approximately 2.90 million disability-adjusted life years are lost per annum from the approximately annual 1.03 million cases.[256] A study reviewing the literature and focusing specifically on African countries reported that acute human leptospirosis ranged from 2.3% to 19.8% in hospital patients with febrile illness.[10]

PATHOPHYSIOLOGY

After almost 100 years since the discovery of the causative organism of leptospirosis, the understanding of mechanisms of pathogenesis has come a long way. Leptospires are thin and highly motile spirochetes with two periplasmic flagella responsible for their movement.[88] They have a double-membrane structure, making it unique and similar to both gram-positive and gram-negative bacteria. Describing the membrane from inside out, leptospires have an inner cytoplasmic membrane, a peptidoglycan cell well, periplasm, outer membrane with outer-membrane proteins (OMPs), phospholipids, and lipopolysaccharide (LPS).[69,70]

The era of genomics with the data generated by the *Leptospira* Genome Project has provided new insights into potential virulence factors as well as host response to disease.[148,155,176] Valuable information has been obtained by the use of animal models of acute and chronic disease, by observing the interactions of leptospires with various cell lines, and by employing molecular genetic tools. Because of their inherent ability to revolve rapidly in a corkscrew fashion, it had been suggested in early studies that the organism bores through connective tissue.[238] Since then, the specific factors responsible for invasiveness of leptospires have been extensively studied and are better understood.[85,95,240] In vitro studies have shown that leptospires bind to a wide range of extracellular matrix components. They have been shown to bind to several different cells, including endothelial cells, monocytes, macrophages, kidney epithelial cells, and fibroblasts.[43] They can translocate through polarized MDCK cells, suggesting a possible intracellular component to its life cycle.[27] Goeijenbier and colleagues found that plasma level of soluble E (sE)-selectin and von Willebrand factor (VWF) was strongly increased in patients with severe leptospirosis, sE-selectin was significantly elevated in survivors, endothelial cells exposed to virulent *Leptospira* showed increased VWF expression, and soluble Fas-ligand and soluble interleukin-2 (IL-2) receptor were strongly associated with mortality.[105] These findings show that endothelial cell activation and immune activation were associated with disease severity in leptospirosis patients. Pathogenic *Leptospira* may inhibit the activation of the complement system through the secretion of proteases that cleave and inactivate key complement proteins.[96] The ability of spirochetes to interact with the host fibrinolytic system may contribute to the degradation of the extracellular matrix components, immune evasion, and tissue penetrations and invasion.[275]

Leptospiral immunoglobulin-like proteins (Lig), surface proteins found in pathogenic leptospires, are believed to be involved in cell adhesion[92] and are among those that have been studied as potential vaccine candidates.[169] Lig-bound plasmin was shown to cleave fibrinogen and the complement proteins C3b and C5, which may allow for invasion and complement immune system evasion by *Leptosira.*[52]

Specific factors responsible for the virulence of leptospires, although better understood, still remain unclear. Some of these virulence factors that continue to be a subject of investigation include LPS, hemolysins, OMPs, surface proteins, and adhesion molecules.[85] An animal model of disease showed caspase-3 reactive renal epithelial cells, alveolar cells, and liver cells, suggesting that *L. interrogans* induce activation of apoptosis in later phases of the infection process.[153] The completion of the *Leptospira* genome sequence has revealed several proteins suspected to play a role in pathogenesis.[7,61,198] Comparative analysis of *Leptospira* proteomes looking at different serovars of pathogenic organisms, nonpathogenic organisms, clinical isolates, and acute lethal infection versus chronic carrier infection has elucidated potential virulence factors and vaccine candidates.[61,69,180,181,254] Hemolysin-like proteins have been identified, including sphingomyelinases that are present in pathogenic but not saprophytic leptospires. Surface-exposed proteins that might have potential roles in adhesion and pathogenesis include OmpL36, OmpL37, OmpL47, and OmpL54.[191] OmpL1 displayed significant adhesin activity binding to glycosaminoglycans and monolayers of human cells in vitro and may be a promising component for a subunit vaccine.[203] The outer surface proteins LigA, LigB, and LigC contain immunoglobulin-like domains[156] found in virulence factors such as intimin and invasin. Leptospiral endostatin-like proteins (Len) have been identified that have been shown to be involved in the organism's ability to evade the complement system.[240]

LipL32 is the major OMP of *Leptospira* shown to bind collagens, laminin, and fibronectin and is highly conserved in pathogenic species.[114,120,263] It is the most abundant protein in the cell and is highly immunogenic.[280] LipL32 stimulates a strong antibody response during natural infection, yet vaccination studies using LipL32 have yielded mixed results.[175] A study of *Leptospira* from urine of infected rats showed acetylation or trimethylation of the highly abundant LipL32 in comparison with culture-grown *Leptospira,* which did not result in a lysine modification, suggesting that LipL32 modifications may alter protein recognition by the immune response, perhaps contributing to bacterial persistence during infection.[290]

Loa22 is a lipoprotein that is upregulated during acute infection and appears to be necessary for virulence in animal models of disease.[181,202] However, the specific roles and functions in pathogenesis for many of these molecules are not entirely understood. A significant amount of redundancy in functional virulence proteins is suspected.

The possible role played by animal hosts in determining the virulence of leptospires for humans remains speculative. Faine[86] compared the fate of virulent and nonvirulent strains of *L. icterohaemorrhagiae* in guinea pigs. Both strains behaved similarly after intraperitoneal infection, but virulent organisms survived and multiplied, whereas avirulent strains did not. Both virulent and avirulent strains were taken up by fixed phagocytes in reticuloendothelial tissues in vivo. Faine[87] also showed that the severity of lesions correlated positively with the number of organisms present and that a discrete number of organisms were required to cause death. He hypothesized that virulence results from the selective multiplication of virulent leptospires in vivo. This hypothesis was supported by the fact that maximum virulence can be regained after a single animal passage that follows isolation in culture. Virulence may be lost in culture by mutation to nonvirulent forms.

The humoral response is the main mechanism of resistance against leptospirosis. Immunoglobulin G (IgG) and IgM antibodies are detected in patients who have recovered from infection. Antibodies are produced against leptospiral LPS. LPS vaccines are effective, but immunity is limited to homologous serovars.[85] Wang and associates[283] demonstrated that polymorphonuclear leukocytes are not an efficient defense factor for pathogenic leptospires in nonimmune hosts. The virulence of leptospires appears to be related to their ability to resist killing both by serum and by neutrophils.

A toxic and pathogenic potential in vivo for lipid products of leptospiral metabolism has been suggested.[2] The cell wall of the leptospire is high in lipid content; component fatty acids vary among leptospiral strains. Lipids are used as a source of energy by leptospires.[2] Saprophytic leptospires invariably possess lipase activity, whereas pathogenic leptospires may be lipase positive or lipase negative.[2] Kasarov and Addamiano[137] investigated the lipolytic activity of leptospires on serum lipoproteins. On the basis of their ability to attack these lipoproteins, leptospires can be divided into three groups: (1) strains that degrade lecithin and sphingomyelin, (2) strains that degrade neither lecithin nor sphingomyelin, and (3) strains that degrade lecithin but not sphingomyelin. Virulent leptospires behaved as group 1 and 2 strains, whereas saprophytic leptospires behaved as a group 3 strain.

Pathophysiology as seen and understood of the clinical disease processes seen in leptospirosis is outlined in Box 142.1. Hemolytic anemia, jaundice, hepatic and renal injury, pulmonary injury, and cardiovascular, nervous system, ocular, and musculoskeletal findings have been extensively studied and described.

CLINICAL MANIFESTATIONS

Leptospirosis is an acute systemic infection characterized by extensive vasculitis. Serologic surveys in human populations indicate that a large number of subclinical infections also occur. Surveys of veterinarians and packinghouse and abattoir workers reveal positive leptospiral titers in 5% to 16% of people tested.[131,165,171,255] A low index of suspicion for this disorder by physicians, coupled with the diversity and nonspecificity of its manifestations, accounts for the significant number of cases that go unrecognized. In one series of 483 proven cases, only 17% were diagnosed initially as leptospirosis.[32]

The incubation period generally is 7 to 12 days, but a range of 2 to 20 days has been noted.[216,238,266] The incubation period does not vary significantly among serotypes and is not of prognostic significance. Variability in incubation period may be attributed to the dose of virulent organisms to which the host is exposed and to the portal of entry of the organism.[216,238,266]

The clinical course of leptospirosis varies, but generally it is predictable: both anicteric leptospirosis and icteric leptospirosis follow a biphasic course (Fig. 142.1).

The first stage (septicemic phase) is characterized by acute systemic infection. The onset of symptoms is abrupt. This phase terminates after 4 to 7 days; symptomatic improvement and defervescence coincide with disappearance of leptospires from the blood, CSF, and all other tissues, with the exception of the aqueous humor and renal parenchyma. Antibody titers to leptospires develop rapidly; this immune response

BOX 142.1 Pathophysiology of Specific Clinical Findings in Leptospirosis

Hemolytic Anemia, Jaundice, and Hepatic Injury

- Presence of a hemolysin in the supernate of leptospiral cultures[9,30,123,172,206]
- Cloned hemolysin of *L. interrogans* serovar Lai demonstrated cell membrane pore-forming activity in vitro[147]
- Thrombocytopenia, depletion of serum prothrombin, depletion of host vitamin K[51,62,81,110,196,201,283]
- Capillary injury perhaps by toxin[15]
- Hemorrhage of skin or mucosal surfaces and rarely gastrointestinal or into a vital organ[110]
- Hepatic manifestations, including jaundice, most likely are the result of hepatocellular injury[14,15,34,81,196,281]
- Hemolysis possibly contributing to jaundice[81,253]
- One or more toxins by leptospires or release of various products after lysis possibly injuring hepatocytes[16,109,198]

Renal Injury

- Tubular epithelial cell necrosis, acute vasculitis, segmental thickening of basement membrane, and interstitial edema
- Infiltrates of lymphocytes, monocytes, plasma cells, and neutrophils
- Cells lining the lumen of the renal tubules distended, disorganized, and contain hyaline, granular, epithelial, and bile casts
- Glomeruli showing mesangial hyperplasia, focal fusion of foot processes, swelling of the epithelium in Bowman capsule, and thickening of the basement membrane[14,16,59,66,76,125,142,229,292]
- Renal potassium wasting by increased secretion of aldosterone and cortisol[1]
- Tubulointerstitial nephritis the most common lesion associated with chronic infection[14,125]
- Leptospires demonstrated in the liver, renal tubules, and the interstices of the renal cortex[14,81,142]
- Leptospires evading the renal immune system, including absence of complement, downregulation of antigens, delayed lymphocyte infiltration, and delayed colonization of renal tubules[167,168]
- Impaired renal blood flow leading to nephropathy[15,16,34,66,81,84,146]
- Host response to infection possibly inducing damage as B cells and T cells induce inflammation in the liver and kidneys via a TLR-independent pathway[108,194,287,288]

Pulmonary Involvement

- Pulmonary lesions generally the result of hemorrhage rather than acute inflammation[17,189,226,293]
- Leptospires visualized directly in lung parenchyma[226]
- Alveolar septal deposition of immunoglobulin and complement[76,179,218,293]

Cardiovascular Findings

- Hypovolemia or hypotension from dehydration, bleeding, or third spacing[18,81,93,189,293]
- Vascular collapse seen with adrenal insufficiency secondary to hemorrhage[147]
- Hypoperfusion, focal hemorrhagic myocarditis, acute coronary arteritis, pericarditis, aortitis, cardiac arrhythmias, congestive heart failure, hypertension, hypovolemia, electrolyte imbalance, or uremia[14,75,223,234,248]
- Epicardium, endocardium, and myocardium all possibly involved[14,15,81,109,253]

Nervous System Findings

- Meningeal reaction occurs only after the development of antibody, leptospiral meningitis suggested to be a reflection of an antigen-antibody reaction[14,17,21,62,110]
- Uncommon features of leptospirosis include encephalitis, myelitis, radiculitis, and peripheral neuritis[14,81,100,104,142,164]
- Neurologic manifestations attributed to subarachnoid, peripapillary, and subdural hemorrhages[46,48]

Ocular Involvement

- Possibly direct *Leptospira*-mediated injury to eye structures, but suggestion that cross-reacting antibodies play a role in *Leptospira*-associated recurrent uveitis[143,274]

Musculoskeletal Findings

- Myalgia an early clinical feature concurrent with leptospirosis septicemic stage, correlating with the timing of the histologic changes in muscle that often quickly resolves
- Muscle pain that subsides after leptospiral agglutinin titers develop[35,81,129,146,224,235,253]
- Bone involvement in leptospirosis not a significant feature[127]

Other

- No characteristic lesions noted in the adrenal glands, lymph nodes, spleen, gastrointestinal tract, pancreas, ureter, or bladder
- Interstitial edema with monocytic and lymphocytic infiltrates found in testicular tissue associated with impaired spermatogenesis[104]

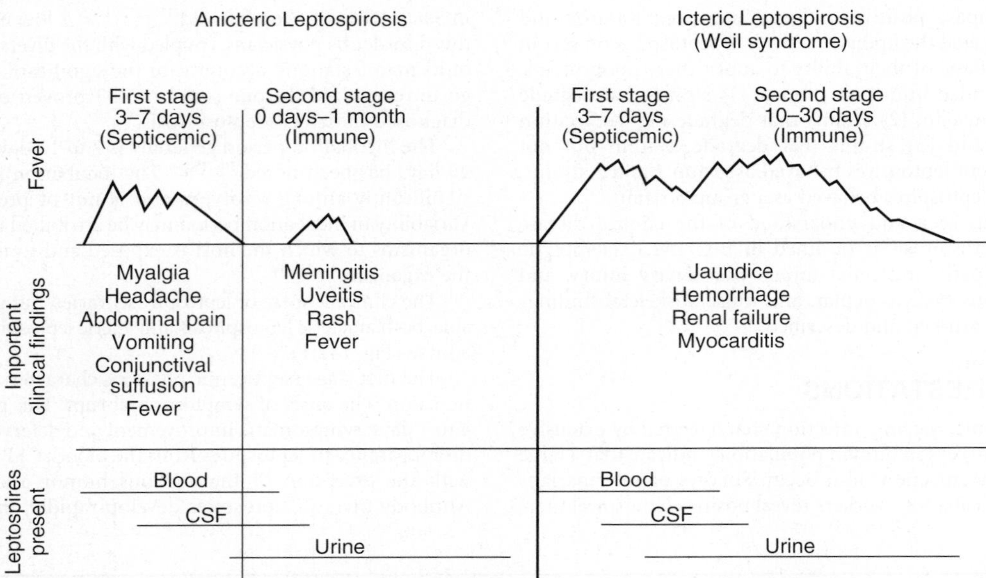

FIG. 142.1 Clinical course of leptospirosis: anicteric and icteric disease. *CSF,* Cerebrospinal fluid.

heralds the second, or "immune," stage of the illness, which lasts 4 to 30 days. Leptospiruria is prevalent and continues for 1 week to 1 month; generally, it is unaffected by antibiotic therapy. Meningitis or hepatic or renal manifestations, when present, reach their peak intensity during this stage of the disease.

There is also a more recently described severe pulmonary form of leptospirosis that may occur in the absence of jaundice or as an elevated Weil syndrome and carries a high mortality (see later).[152]

Leptospirosis manifestations in children are similar and can be very severe as well.[58,134,135,262,273,274,276] During the 2001 outbreak of leptospirosis in Mumbai, India, 32% of children admitted in a 2-month period had leptospirosis.[135] A year earlier in the same city, following floods, leptospirosis was found in 34% of children screened who had abrupt onset of fever, contact with flood water, conjunctival suffusion, abdominal pain, or rash.[134]

Anicteric Leptospirosis

Ninety percent or more of all patients with leptospirosis are anicteric. They frequently escape definitive diagnosis because jaundice and azotemia are absent. The onset of the septicemic phase of anicteric leptospirosis is abrupt[82] and heralded by fever, malaise, headache, myalgia, and occasionally prostration and circulatory collapse.[158] Chills, remittent fever, headaches, severe myalgia, and abdominal pain are prominent for 4 to 7 days. Fever defervesces by lysis, and other symptoms resolve. Death is an extraordinarily rare occurrence in the first stage of anicteric illness. Some patients with anicteric leptospirosis do not experience a biphasic illness and remain asymptomatic after the first week.[82]

The second phase of anicteric disease may be characterized by fever, uveitis, rash, headache, and meningitis. If present, fever usually is of brief duration and has a lower peak than that of the septicemic phase.[81,82,121] Maximum temperatures range from 38.2°C to 40.6°C (100.8°F–105°F), with one or more daily peaks. Recurrence of fever 2 or 3 weeks after leptospirosis resolves is not unusual, but no reports of the isolation of leptospires from blood document relapse on these occasions. Relapse generally occurs when the immune response of the host is peaking and at a time of maximal leptospiruria, which suggests an allergic or immune basis for the febrile episodes.[34] Headache may be intense and usually is not controlled well by analgesics. Typically, it is frontal in distribution and characterized as bitemporal or occipital. It may be associated with retrobulbar pain.[65,81,82] Persistence or recurrence of headache after termination of the septicemic phase of disease generally indicates the onset of meningitis. The factors responsible for headache in the septicemic phase of leptospirosis are unknown.

Restlessness, nocturnal confusion, mood disturbances, and mild alterations in consciousness usually occur briefly and commonly in both stages of leptospirosis.[81,121] Delirium, hallucinations, psychotic behavior, and suicidal tendencies have been reported.[81,121,222]

Anorexia, nausea, vomiting, and abdominal pain may be reported in both stages of anicteric disease. Constipation, diarrhea, and gastrointestinal hemorrhage also have been documented.[81,158,182] Generally, hemorrhagic complications are associated exclusively with icteric disease.

Physical examination during the septicemic stage may reveal dehydration, muscle tenderness, conjunctival suffusion, generalized lymphadenopathy, hepatosplenomegaly, and rashes that may be macular, maculopapular, erythematous, urticarial, petechial, purpuric, hemorrhagic, or desquamating. Skin lesions are most prominent over the trunk, but any area of the body may be affected. Pretibial eruptions have been noted in patients with infection caused by *L. autumnalis,* but other serotypes also may cause disease with pretibial eruptions. Recurrent, transient urticarial eruptions have appeared for many days after resolution of the other manifestations of leptospirosis. Pharyngitis, rales, arthritis, and nonpitting edema occur less commonly.* Tachycardia is a common occurrence, and cardiac arrhythmias are noted occasionally.[188,234] Hypotension rarely occurs in anicteric leptospirosis.[82]

Muscle pain and tenderness may be generalized, but the muscles of the calf, lumbosacral spine, and abdomen are affected most frequently. Tenderness and rigidity of the abdominal wall may suggest the possibility of an acute surgical abdomen. Tenderness of the muscles adjacent to the cervical spine often causes nuchal rigidity in patients without meningeal involvement. The muscle tenderness usually subsides with termination of the septicemic stage of the disease.

Conjunctival suffusion, photophobia, ocular pain, and conjunctival hemorrhage are more specifically helpful diagnostic signs. Chemosis and inflammatory exudates generally are absent despite marked conjunctival infection. In anicteric disease, conjunctival infection involves primarily the bulbar conjunctiva only. It appears by the third day of illness and disappears 3 days to 3 weeks later.

Abdominal pain and tenderness, when associated with vomiting and hypoactive bowel sounds, clearly suggest the possibility of a surgical abdomen and present a challenging diagnostic problem because acute intraabdominal catastrophes may complicate the natural history of this disease. Nonobstructive toxic dilation of the gallbladder requiring cholecystotomy has been noted repeatedly in children with leptospirosis

*References 11, 14, 33, 65, 82, 121, 129, 158, 207, 260, 266,

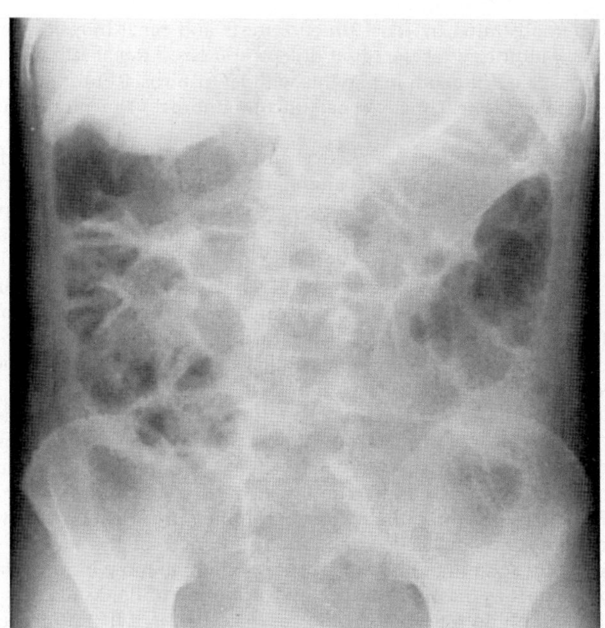

FIG. 142.2 Nonobstructed toxic dilation of the gallbladder in a child with leptospirosis. Radiograph demonstrates a dilated, opaque gallbladder protruding from the inferior margin of the liver.

(Fig. 142.2). Pain of this type must be differentiated from myositis, subperitoneal or subserosal hemorrhage, abdominal wall causalgia, or pancreatitis, all of which may occur in some children with anicteric or icteric disease.

Pulmonary involvement may be observed in anicteric patients, generally during the septicemic phase, and usually is manifested as a dry, hacking cough, occasionally productive of blood-stained sputum, or by the finding of infiltrates on a chest radiograph.[33,193,226] Hemoptysis, chest pain, respiratory distress, and cyanosis appear rarely during anicteric disease.[193] Hemoptysis, when present, clears in 3 to 5 days. Physical examination of the chest may reveal rales, evidence of consolidation, or a pleural or pericardial friction rub.

Chest radiographs may show (1) confluent infiltrates or massive consolidation representing larger areas of pulmonary hemorrhage; (2) small, patchy, snowflake-like lesions in the periphery of the lung fields that are restricted to a few intercostal spaces or disseminated widely; and (3) solitary, patchy lesions with ill-defined margins.[193,282] Of these radiographic appearances, the second is most common. Small pleural effusions are rare occurrences in anicteric disease,[282] and hilar adenopathy has not been described. Although the chest radiograph may help delineate the extent of pulmonary disease, it does not provide information that could be considered pathognomonic of leptospirosis.

Other signs and symptoms of the septicemic phase of anicteric leptospirosis that have been reported include parotitis,[29] orchitis,[243] epididymitis,[121] prostatitis,[121] otitis media,[33] arthralgia,[33,81,121] and monoarticular or polyarticular arthritis.[76]

The hallmark of the immune phase of anicteric leptospirosis is meningitis, and it is reflected by CSF pleocytosis with or without meningeal symptoms or signs. During the leptospiremic phase, leptospires may be found in the subarachnoid space unassociated with the presence of inflammatory cells. As an antibody titer develops, leptospires are cleared rapidly from CSF, and an inflammatory response develops.[81] If CSF is examined during the second week of illness in all patients with anicteric leptospirosis, a meningeal reaction can be demonstrated in more than 80%, but only 50% of these patients have clinical signs and symptoms of meningitis.[49,81] The severity of meningitis varies and does not correlate with the severity of other clinical manifestations of leptospirosis. Symptoms referable to the nervous system usually subside within 1 or 2 days but rarely persist for 2 or 3 weeks. The CSF pleocytosis may persist for 2 to 3 months but generally disappears within 7 to 21 days.[81] In some cases, patients do not have symptoms during the septicemic phase of leptospirosis but seek medical attention during the immune phase because of headache, vomiting, and nuchal rigidity. Papilledema rarely has been observed in patients with leptospirosis.[46]

Lumbar puncture may reveal CSF pressures varying from normal to 350 mm H_2O. Mean values generally are less than 200 mm H_2O.[124] Cell counts within CSF vary from normal to more than 500 cells/mm^3; generally, fewer than 500 cells have been reported.[81,121] Polymorphonuclear leukocytes predominate early in the immune phase, but mononuclear cells subsequently predominate. Protein concentrations within CSF range from normal to 300 mg/dL. In some cases, protein values have been elevated in the absence of pleocytosis. Abnormal values may persist for several weeks after the clinical symptoms resolve.[33,49,121,159,160] Glucose concentrations within CSF generally are normal.[49,82,159]

Encephalitis, focal weakness, spasticity, paralysis, nystagmus, peripheral neuritis, cranial nerve paralysis, seizures, radiculitis, visual disturbances, myelitis, Guillain-Barré syndrome, or acute disseminated encephalomyelitis may appear with or subsequent to the immune stage of anicteric disease.[12,25,55,81,84,121,159,164,272] Generally, these symptoms resolve, but complete resolution may require several weeks to months. Neurologic sequelae secondary to central nervous system hemolysis may occur.[46,48]

The anterior uveal tract may be affected as early as the third week of illness, but symptoms may be found up to 1 year after the onset of leptospirosis. Conjunctival suffusion (characteristic during the septicemic phase) is not found in the immune stage of the disease. Rather, iritis, iridocyclitis, and, occasionally, chorioretinitis are noted.[32,81,82,121] Uveal involvement may be unilateral or bilateral and may occur as a single, self-limited episode, as recurrent episodes, or as a chronic unrelenting process.[41,81] The severity of the uveitis does not correlate with the severity of other clinical manifestations. When uveitis is transient or self-limited, complete healing is the rule; however, in some cases, blindness and cataract formation are noted.

The precise incidence of involvement of the uveal tract is unclear because symptoms may be minimal or may not appear until after other clinical manifestations have resolved completely. The generally benign course of uveitis may be attributable to the capacity of leptospires to survive in the aqueous humor without eliciting an intense inflammatory response.[82] Despite the presence of high titers of specific antibodies to leptospires in serum, antibodies to leptospires are absent or found in low titer in the aqueous humor.

Leptospiruria is the rule during the immune stage of anicteric leptospirosis, and it is not associated with impaired renal function. In contrast to many animal species, humans do not serve as a reservoir for leptospires; leptospiruria is transient. In anicteric patients, proteinuria, pyuria, microscopic hematuria, and mild to moderate azotemia may be observed.[33]

The white blood cell count may be low, normal, or elevated. Neutrophilia is the rule, regardless of the total white blood cell count. Leukocytosis generally is associated with hepatic involvement. Anemia is an inconsistent finding; when present, it may be attributable to blood loss, vascular damage, or hemolysis. In the absence of blood loss, significant anemia is not a manifestation of anicteric cases. The erythrocyte sedimentation rate is elevated consistently.

Icteric Leptospirosis (Weil Syndrome)

The term *Weil syndrome* should be applied to define a form of leptospirosis that is distinctive in clinical expression but nonspecific with respect to serotypic etiologic agents. In addition to having the symptoms and signs of anicteric leptospirosis, Weil syndrome is set apart by the presence of impaired hepatic and renal function, vascular collapse, hemorrhage, severe alterations in consciousness, and a high mortality rate.

Weil syndrome may be heterogeneous in its manifestations, and the course may be dominated by symptoms of renal, hepatic, or vascular dysfunction. Jaundice and azotemia may be so severe that the biphasic course of illness is not observed. Fever may persist without defervescence between the septicemic and immune stages and is more prominent and of longer duration during the immune stage than in anicteric cases. The mortality rate, despite adequate supportive care, is between 5% and 10%.

Jaundice remains the hallmark of Weil syndrome. The intensity of jaundice varies; a maximum total serum bilirubin concentration in the range of 60 to 80 mg/dL has been reported.[159] Usually, the bilirubin concentration is less than 20 mg/dL. Both direct- and indirect-reacting bilirubin levels increase, but an increase in the direct fraction usually accounts for most of the elevation in bilirubin.[239] Jaundice may occur as early as the third day of illness or may not appear until the second week.[17,82] The serum bilirubin concentration peaks within the first 7 days after the onset of jaundice in 85% of cases.[196]

Modest elevations in serum alkaline phosphatase level and depressed activity of plasma prothrombin are noted occasionally.[196] Hypoprothrombinemia responds uniformly to parenteral administration of vitamin K. The serum albumin level may be depressed; concentrations of 2.0 to 2.5 g are not uncommon.[239] Aspartate aminotransferase and alanine aminotransferase values are elevated minimally, rarely exceeding 100 and 200 units, respectively. The urine may contain bilirubin and urobilinogen.

Hepatomegaly is found in approximately 24% of patients, a frequency that is no greater than that in anicteric cases.[81] Transient biliary obstruction, probably intrahepatic, may occur, but no evidence that obstructive phenomena are the primary mechanism of impaired hepatic function exists. Even in severely icteric cases, acholic stools generally are not observed.[81,121] Pruritus has been reported rarely in patients with leptospirosis.[81] The presence of abnormal urinary urobilinogen values in the absence of acholic stools suggests patency of the biliary tract in most cases.[196]

In some reports of children with leptospirosis, acalculous cholecystitis has been seen in 55% of cases.[241] In these patients, right upper quadrant pain, tenderness, and a palpable mass were present. Abdominal radiographs confirmed the presence of a mass in the region of the gallbladder. When cholecystotomy was performed, a massively distended gallbladder containing colorless bile was noted. Routine aerobic and anaerobic cultures of bile were negative, but cultures for leptospires were positive.

Hepatic dysfunction is not an important cause of death in patients with leptospirosis. It is present, however, in most patients who die of this disease;, conversely, a fatal outcome is extremely rare in the absence of hepatic dysfunction.[33] Renal dysfunction, cardiovascular collapse, and hemorrhagic complications occur most often in patients whose icterus is most prominent.

Renal dysfunction may be observed in all forms of leptospirosis, regardless of the severity of disease or the serotype causing infection.[33,81,121] Symptoms attributable to functional renal impairment generally are observed only during icteric leptospirosis.[17,33,81,82,266] In the leptospiremic phase, abnormal urinalysis results are noted in as many as 80% of cases.[33,81,241] Proteinuria is the most frequent abnormality and generally is mild. Hyaline or granular casts and cellular elements (red and white blood cells) may be found in the urinary sediment. Microscopic or gross hematuria is seen in many patients and most likely reflects the presence of a hemorrhagic diathesis rather than glomerular injury.[272]

Fatal cases of icteric leptospirosis in which urinalysis results were normal have been reported.[17] The abnormalities in urinary sediment and proteinuria may persist for weeks in patients without significant azotemia.[28]

Oliguria or anuria may be noted as early as the third day of illness but occurs more commonly after the first week. Generally, blood urea nitrogen values remain below 100 mg/dL, but values may exceed 300 mg/dL in some cases.[121,183] The height of the blood urea nitrogen value is not of prognostic value in individual cases, although in groups of patients it correlates well with outcome.[253]

Azotemic patients with leptospirosis can be divided into two groups: (1) those with decreased renal perfusion (ratio of urine osmolality [U_{Osm}] to plasma osmolality [P_{Osm}] of about 2:1) and a good response to fluid administration; and (2) those with a U_{Osm}/P_{Osm} ratio close to 1:1, with impaired resorption of sodium and water from the renal tubules and no response to administration of fluids. The manifestations of the second group of patients are those of acute tubular necrosis. The factors responsible for oliguria in the first group of patients (those with prerenal azotemia), including hypotension, shock, and volume depletion, if uncorrected, ultimately may progress to acute tubular necrosis as well.

Anuria is an ominous sign, whereas diuresis is a good prognostic omen.[17] The impairment in renal function may persist, and fatalities have been recorded after the onset of diuresis.[183] Hyposthenuria can persist for months in some cases.[81] Some evidence of renal disease has been demonstrated by renal function tests and renal biopsies for as long as 6 months after the onset of leptospirosis.[23] Renal failure is the principal cause of death in patients with leptospirosis, but it generally is reversible in time. Usually, renal function improves by 6 months after acute infection.[72]

Cardiac involvement is a relatively infrequent occurrence, but when it is present, congestive heart failure and cardiovascular collapse may occur.[82,129] Electrocardiographic changes are seen in all forms of leptospirosis.[188] In one series of patients, electrocardiograms obtained during the first week of illness were abnormal in 90% of patients at a time when none had signs or symptoms of congestive failure, pericarditis, or hypotension.[188] The electrocardiographic abnormalities disappeared by 10 days in most cases. The electrocardiographic changes that have been described often are nonspecific findings common to many infectious diseases or attributable to fever alone.[188,208]

Cerebrovascular accidents may occur in patients with leptospirosis.[149] In a study of 21 cases in which postmortem examination was performed, subarachnoid hemorrhage was described in 1 case, cerebral hemorrhage in 2, and recent cerebral infarction in 1.

Hyponatremia is a rather consistent finding in patients with severe icteric leptospirosis. The hyponatremia appears to be the result of (1) failure of the sodium pump, which causes sodium to move intracellularly in exchange for potassium; and (2) redistribution of fluid such that the extracellular fluid space is expanded at the expense of the intracellular space. Hyponatremia in these patients may be unresponsive to either sodium replacement or fluid restriction. It is treated best by fluid restriction, which can be continued unless systemic blood pressure falls. Clinical improvement in the patient generally follows a spontaneous increase in serum sodium level, which may occur before any other evidence of clinical improvement is noted.

Most patients with leptospirosis recover without long-term sequelae.[214] However, given the evidence of prolonged urinary shedding, it has been speculated that there may be a chronic form of leptospirosis.[122] A prospective study in São Paulo, Brazil, followed patients who had been hospitalized with leptospirosis[236]: two of 47 patients reported continuing symptoms, one with profound malaise without a defined reason and one with new diagnosis of panic disorder. A study[294] in a *Leptospira*-endemic town reported that subjects with a microscopic agglutination test (MAT) titer of 400 or greater showed a decreased renal function compared to those with lower titers. And, two subjects with persistently high MAT titers and positive urine *Leptospira* DNA had worsening renal function during the study period of 2 years.

Severe Pulmonary Form of Leptospirosis

A recently described severe pulmonary form of leptospirosis may occur in the absence of jaundice or as an elevated Weil syndrome. It carries a mortality rate of greater than 50%[152] and manifests as dyspnea, chest pain, and cough with hemoptysis.

The chest radiograph shows small nodular opacities that may progress into larger coalescent areas of consolidation.[78] High-resolution computed tomography shows bilateral ground-glass opacities, areas of consolidation, airspace nodules, and small pleural effusions. On gross pathology, extensive pulmonary hemorrhage with numerous bleeding foci of different sizes can be seen. Histologic sections usually demonstrate pulmonary congestion, pulmonary edema, and several foci of interstitial and intraalveolar bleeding, with varying degrees of severity.[152] Treatment involves maintaining hemodynamic stability and respiratory support. Corticosteroids and platelet transfusions have been used.[225] Because the pathogenesis of the severe pulmonary form of leptospirosis is thought to likely be immune mediated, immunosuppression has been used in its treatment, including plasma exchange, cyclophosphamide, desmopressin, dexamethasone, and recombinant factor.[152]

INDICATORS OF PROGNOSIS

Attempts have been made to identify prognostic factors associated with leptospirosis. Such studies, which aimed to evaluate the prognostic significance of certain clinical and laboratory variables at different stages of disease, have produced variable results. Hypotension, oliguria, hyperkalemia, the development of pulmonary rales or rhonchi, and electrocardiographic repolarization abnormalities each have been associated with a poor prognosis,[73,79,80,151,186,252] although conflicting data exist about the implications of hypotension.[80] In a small series of 12 patients, Truccolo and colleagues[261] reported death of all patients with a leptospiral load greater than 10^4 organisms/mL as determined by quantitative polymerase chain reaction (PCR). Chang and colleagues,[57] in a series of 11 patients with late leptospirosis, reported mortality in all patients with hepatitis and a disproportionate aspartate aminotransferase level, as defined by a ratio of peak aspartate aminotransferase to peak alanine aminotransferase greater than 3. Respiratory failure, hemoptysis, metabolic acidosis, and thrombocytopenia also have been associated with increased mortality rates.[252] In Marotto and coworkers' prediction model, serum potassium, serum creatinine, respiratory rate, presenting shock, and Glasgow Coma Scale score less than 15 were independently associated with development of leptospirosis-associated pulmonary hemorrhage syndrome.[154] Advancing age, renal involvement, pulmonary involvement, and multiple organ dysfunction have been repeatedly found to be associated with increased mortality.[195] A case of severe leptospirosis complicated by Epstein-Barr virus reactivation has been described.[136] A case has also been described of an HIV-infected man on antiretroviral therapy and with a history of hepatitis C who developed fever and hepatitis and was found to have leptospirosis and acute or recurrence of occult hepatitis C.[90] These cases point to the need to consider concomitant infections in severe cases of leptospirosis.

LABORATORY DIAGNOSIS

Whenever possible, the physician should use laboratory facilities in which culture and serologic tests for leptospirosis are performed routinely. It is recommended that specimens be sent to the standard reference laboratory, the National Leptospirosis Laboratory at the CDC in Atlanta. Despite proper collection and handling of specimens, obtaining laboratory confirmation of cases of leptospirosis may be difficult, even for facilities with skill in this area.

A confirmed case of leptospirosis, as defined by the US Department of Health and Human Services, fulfills one of the following criteria: (1) clinical specimens that are culture positive for leptospires or (2) clinical symptoms compatible with leptospirosis and either seroconversion or a fourfold or greater rise in the MAT titer between acute and convalescent serum specimens obtained 2 or more weeks apart and studied at the same laboratory. PCR has been shown to be effective for detecting pathogenic *Leptospira* but may not be commercially available.

Presumptive leptospirosis is defined as the presence of clinical symptoms that are compatible with leptospirosis and an MAT titer of 1:100 or greater, a positive slide MAT reaction on a single serum specimen obtained after the onset of symptoms, or a stable MAT titer of 1:100 or greater in two or more serum specimens obtained after the onset of symptoms.

Identification by Culture

Leptospires can be recovered from blood or CSF obtained from patients during the septicemic stage of illness or from urine during the immune stage. Other than these body fluids, only tissue sections obtained by biopsy or at necropsy are sources from which organisms can be recovered. Rarely, organisms are isolated from intraocular fluid obtained during convalescence.[8]

Media for the cultivation of leptospires generally contain a buffered solution, with or without peptone and with or without 0.1% to 0.2% agar to which rabbit serum has been added to provide a final concentration in the medium of 5% to 10%. In addition, a pH between 7.2 and 7.8 appears to be essential. Clinical material obtained for culture frequently is contaminated; antimicrobial agents, including neomycin, vancomycin, or bacitracin, added to leptospiral media in low concentration have been found to be effective in reducing contamination and exert little if any effect on leptospires.

For routine use, Fletcher semisolid medium[94] or EMJH semisolid medium[132,238] is recommended. Stuart medium[245] has been used to prepare and maintain antigens for serologic tests. Tween 80–albumin medium (OAC) was developed not long ago and is available commercially. This medium seems to be superior for primary isolation of leptospires.

Several solid media are available but appear to be most useful for isolation and purification of leptospires from contaminated natural material such as water.[246,265] Preparation, use, and maintenance of these solid media and other media are described in other works.[162,246,265]

Multiple cultures should be obtained from patients with leptospirosis because the concentration of organisms in blood at any point in time is low.[132] Freshly drawn blood is most desirable, but leptospires may remain viable in anticoagulated blood for as long as 11 days.[245] Blood should be inoculated into several tubes of semisolid media. The number of drops of blood placed into each tube should be varied (one to four drops). Excessive amounts of blood inhibit the growth of leptospires; hence a small inoculum yields the best results.[94] Cultures are incubated at 28°C to 30°C in the dark for 6 weeks or longer.

In semisolid media, leptospires grow in a concentrated ring about 0.5 to 1 cm below the surface. Growth may not be detected in Fletcher semisolid medium for several weeks but may occur earlier in polysorbate medium.

Contaminated specimens or suspensions of primary cultures in which contamination is suspected may be inoculated into hamsters. When an animal dies, phlebotomy or necropsy is performed, and sections of liver, kidney, and brain then are recultured in appropriate semisolid media.

If collected during the septicemic phase, CSF may be cultured in the same manner as blood.

Urine serves as the main source from which leptospires can be isolated during the immune and convalescent phases of leptospirosis. Prolonged urinary shedding after infection is possible in humans. Chow and coworkers reported a 10-year-old girl who shed leptospires in urine for 6 weeks after exposure.[58] Clean-voided urine may be inoculated directly into an appropriate semisolid medium. Urine specimens must be diluted with sterile, buffered saline solution to ensure growth.[253] Best results are obtained by adding 0.1 mL of urine to 0.9 mL of buffered saline before inoculation into 5 mL of semisolid medium. This procedure can be continued with four additional dilutions. Other bacterial contaminants that may be present in undiluted urine cultures generally do not survive in these cultures after dilution.[246]

Identification by Means Other Than Culture

The morphologic appearance of all members of the genus *Leptospira* is similar. They are slender, threadlike organisms about 0.1 µm in diameter and 6 to 12 µm in length, tightly coiled on their long axis. Like other spirochetes, they cannot be seen in wet preparations by lightfield microscopy, but on darkfield examination they may be observed readily. For the detection of one leptospire per high-power field by darkfield examination, a concentration of 10,000 to 20,000 leptospires per milliliter of fluid is needed.[265] At best, darkfield examination should be considered an aid that may suggest but not establish a diagnosis of leptospirosis.

Leptospires can be stained by several silver impregnation techniques.[44,140,162,246,265] The modified method of Van Orden has been used at the CDC for demonstrating organisms in sections of liver, kidney, or other tissues. Infecting serotypes cannot be differentiated by silver impregnation techniques. Leptospiral antigen also has been detected with the use of an immunoperoxidase staining procedure.[91]

Fluorescent antibody techniques may be applied successfully to the detection of leptospires in urine or tissue.[173,174,246,265] This test is based on specific antigen-antibody reactions using fluorescence-tagged antisera. In theory, the fluorescent antibody reaction should demonstrate distorted and fragmented, as well as whole, organisms, but caution is required. Control specimens that have been treated with unlabeled antiserum before the addition of fluorescein-labeled antiserum should be used.[162] The control specimen should not fluoresce. The fluorescent antibody technique may provide the physician with useful information in the course of the disease in some patients. Positive results, however, are considered only presumptive evidence of infection.

In addition to this technique, DNA hybridization techniques or nucleic acid amplification procedures, including PCR protocols using *Leptospira*-specific cDNA probes or oligonucleotide primers, can be used to detect the presence of leptospires in body fluids or culture supernatants.[37] These techniques are being developed in the laboratories of the Leptospirosis Branch at the CDC, but proof of their superiority in terms of sensitivity or specificity in detecting leptospiral organisms in body fluids or other clinical samples has not been established.

The reference method for serovar identification is considered to be the cross-agglutinin absorption test (CAAT) but requires maintenance of large panels of reference antisera and live antigens. Multilocus sequence typing has been applied to provide strain information but is limited to a few species.[178] Pulse-field gel electrophoresis can be used to identify *Leptospira* to the serovar level, is applicable to all pathogenic species, and can rapidly identify new serovars.[97]

Serologic Tests

Evaluation of serologic findings to supplement clinical and epidemiologic information generally is recommended as a first step in establishing a diagnosis of leptospirosis. One of the most widely used specific serologic tests for leptospirosis has been the MAT, in which live antigen is used. This test is time-consuming and potentially hazardous to the technician but is considered the reference test against which all other tests are evaluated. Formalinized antigens can be used for the MAT, and they are preferred in some laboratories, but the titers obtained are lower than those obtained with live antigen, and more cross-reactions with heterologous serotypes occur. Generally, serum is used for the MAT or other agglutination tests, but CSF, urine, bile, or aqueous humor may be used as well.[162]

The CDC uses a standard panel of commonly occurring serovars for routine performance of the MAT. However, because of geographic differences in serovar distribution, serovars are added or changed depending on the region where exposure occurred and the location from which specimens were obtained. Killed antigens remain stable for at least 12 months and are available commercially either individually or in pools. Sulzer and associates[246] have provided detailed descriptions of methods for performance of the MAT. Modifications of the MAT have been developed and include the semi-micromethod and microtiter techniques.[98]

A newer serologic test involving diffusion in gel, the enzyme-linked immunosorbent assay (ELISA), has been compared with the MAT for the serologic diagnosis of leptospirosis.[71,279] The results suggest that this test is a viable alternative to the MAT because of its sensitivity, potential for standardization, and simplicity. Variations of this test have been developed; rapid serodiagnosis of leptospirosis with the use of an IgM-specific dot ELISA has proved to be as sensitive and specific as MAT.[277,284] The dot ELISA is inexpensive, simple to perform, and uses minute volumes of leptospiral antigens.

The IgM-PK ELISA, an assay for IgM using a proteinase K–treated antigen, was compared with the Leptoteste-S macroagglutination test and with the MAT for the diagnosis of leptospirosis. All three tests were comparable in their ability to detect the presence of leptospirosis. Both the IgM-PK ELISA and the Leptoteste-S differed statistically from the MAT in terms of the positivity of acute phase sera. Thirty-eight percent of patients with leptospirosis were identified earlier with either test than when the MAT was used. The IgM-PK ELISA, which had a sensitivity of 89.9% and a specificity of 97.4%, has been suggested as the test of choice for laboratories that are equipped to perform ELISA.[199]

A slide agglutination test available commercially has been compared with the ELISA IgM and has yielded equivalent results for the diagnosis of leptospirosis. The slide agglutination test is inexpensive and can be performed more quickly and more easily than ELISA, thus rendering it a useful test for laboratories that are less well equipped than those in which IgM ELISA currently is performed.[42]

The Lepto Dipstick, a dipstick assay for detection of *Leptospira*-specific IgM antibodies in serum, has been studied as a method for the diagnosis of leptospirosis in situations in which laboratory facilities may not be available.[232] This test's results correlated well (80–96.7% observed agreement; κ value, 0.62–0.92) with results obtained by the IgM ELISA leptospiral antigen detection method.[24,113] A 93.2% agreement (κ value, 0.66) was reported between the Lepto Dipstick and MAT, along with a high number of false-positive results as well.[24] The dipstick test is a valuable and useful tool for rapid screening for leptospirosis and may be useful in the field for detecting and monitoring outbreaks of leptospirosis. Leptocheck, a simple and rapid commercially available immunochromatographic test (which can be used on serum or urine) has also been proved helpful in early diagnosis of leptospirosis cases, which should then be confirmed with other serologic methods later.[192]

Other tests that may be used for the serologic diagnosis of leptospirosis include a complement fixation assay, a hemolytic test, an indirect immunofluorescent test, an erythrocyte-sensitizing substance test, countercurrent immunoelectrophoresis, and flow cytometry light scatter analysis.[56,177,258,295] These tests are genus specific and may yield positive results earlier in the course of leptospirosis than the agglutination tests do. Their results also revert to negative earlier; therefore these tests are of little value for serologic surveys. They may be of value in distinguishing current from past infections when agglutination test results are equivocal.[245,246]

An indirect hemagglutination test offers the advantage of detecting antibodies as early as the fourth day after the onset of illness. It is genus specific, is less time-consuming, and requires just one antigen in the test system. It has excellent sensitivity and specificity, and some investigators have suggested that it may replace the MAT as the screening test of choice.[246] Effler and colleagues,[83] however, reported discouraging results when this test was used for the diagnosis of leptospirosis in Hawaii.

Agglutination tests have been considered to be serotype specific. Because of the antigenic complexity of leptospires, however, cross-agglutination reactions occur; serotypes that belong to the same serogroup cross-react at high titers. Early in the course of leptospirosis, heterologous reactions may be stronger than homologous reactions. Because of these paradoxical cross-reactions, one should not depend on serologic determination alone to define the infecting serotype. When agglutination tests are performed on serial specimens over the course of time, the homologous reaction becomes the dominant one in most cases. Performance of agglutination absorption studies may be necessary to define the infecting serotype in some cases. The antigen (serotype) that absorbs out agglutinin to all the serotypes in a serogroup most likely is the infecting serotype.[162,239,268]

A passive microcapsule agglutination test that uses chemically stable microcapsules instead of sheep erythrocytes has been developed.[17] When compared with the MAT, the passive microcapsule agglutination test showed a relatively greater degree of genus specificity and 4- to 32-fold higher titers. The sensitized microcapsules were stable for at least 1 year. This test is simple to perform and reproducible and can be used readily in the routine laboratory. Moreover, the test appears to be more sensitive than is the MAT in the early stages of leptospirosis.[221]

A positive leptospiral agglutination reaction generally is not found until the 6th to 12th day of illness, and maximal levels are reached between 21 and 28 days. After recovery, low titers may persist for many years. One blood sample should be obtained early in the course of illness, and a second one should be obtained at the end of 1 month. Negative reactions in serial samples do not exclude the possibility of leptospirosis because patients may be infected with a serotype not included in the battery of test antigens or with a previously unrecognized serotype. Moreover, the titer may have peaked before the acute-phase specimen was collected. Antibiotic therapy also may suppress the development of positive titers or delay their appearance.[111,162] Peak MAT titers of 1 : 3000 to 1 : 100,000 usually are reached during the third week of illness.[81,268] An unchanging titer of 1 : 100 on two successive serum specimens has been defined as sufficient for making a presumptive diagnosis of leptospirosis. A fourfold increase in titer between acute and convalescent sera is indisputable evidence of active leptospirosis. The global criterion for laboratory confirmation of a current *Leptospira* infection is usually defined as seroconversion or a fourfold rise in titer in paired serum samples or set at a single MAT titer greater than 1 : 400 in the presence of clinical signs and appropriate history of animal contact.[88] Goris and colleagues have recently evaluated the performance of MAT and ELISA in a population in the Netherlands, where positive culture was used as a reference. They also concluded that the sensitivities of MAT and IgM ELISA are low at the acute stage of illness and require a follow-up sample for confirming seroconversion or a significant titer rise, but rather than waiting 2 to 4 weeks for convalescent titers, these could be done much sooner in urgent cases because significant antibody rise was seen in some cases as early as 2 days later, allowing for earlier diagnosis and proper treatment.[107]

Leptospira DNA may be detected by PCR at a minimum detection limit of two to three cells per sample.[150,233] Nonradioactive, arbitrarily primed PCR assays can be used to discriminate species of *Leptospira.* Romero and colleagues reported that PCR was more likely to facilitate the early diagnosis of leptospiral aseptic meningitis than was either the IgM ELISA or the MAT test.[205] Another recent study exploring the use of 16S ribosomal RNA for development of PCR-based diagnostics for human leptospirosis found promising results, perhaps superior to traditional DNA-based PCR.[22]

PCR, IgM ELISA, latex agglutination, the Lepto Dipstick assay, and an antibody-based urine antigen assay each may be more sensitive than the MAT early in the course of disease.[139,184,209]

Unbiased next-generation sequencing aided in diagnosing a case of neuroleptospirosis in a 14-year-old boy with severe combined immunodeficiency who had gone undiagnosed for a period of 4 months with fever and headache worsening to hydrocephalus and seizures. PCR and serologic testing at the CDC subsequently confirmed *L. santarosai* infection, which he had likely contracted on a trip to Puerto Rico.[289]

TREATMENT

To be of maximum therapeutic benefit, an antimicrobial agent would have to be administered before invading organisms damage the endothelium of blood vessels and various organs or tissues. One of the problems in evaluating the efficacy of treatment is the fact that, generally, leptospirosis is a self-limited disease with a favorable prognosis. Even patients with severe icteric leptospirosis may recover without specific treatment.

Most claims of the beneficial value of antimicrobial agents in human leptospirosis are based on the response of individual patients rather than on controlled studies. Hall and associates[116] compared the effects of penicillin, chloramphenicol, chlortetracycline, and oxytetracycline with placebo in 67 confirmed cases of leptospirosis. No appreciable effect of antibiotics could be demonstrated on the duration or severity of illness or on the prevention or amelioration of central nervous system, hepatic, renal, or hemorrhagic complications of this disease. Moreover, the duration of leptospiremia and the persistence of organisms in CSF were not altered by treatment. Kocen[141] compared the effects of penicillin administered on the fourth day of illness to 28 patients with a control group of 33 who were given only supportive care and reported that the duration of fever was shorter and the incidence of jaundice, meningismus, renal involvement, and hemorrhagic manifestations was diminished in the treated group.[141] None of these controlled studies was entirely satisfactory with respect to randomization of patients.

McClain and associates[157] studied the therapeutic efficacy of doxycycline in military recruits who contracted leptospirosis while training at the Jungle Operations Training Center in Panama. Twenty-nine patients with anicteric disease were treated in a randomized, double-blinded fashion with doxycycline 100 mg orally twice a day or with placebo. Therapy was administered for 7 days in the hospital, after which patients were monitored for 3 weeks. The duration of illness before therapy and the severity of illness were similar in both study groups. Doxycycline shortened the duration of illness by 2 days and favorably influenced fever, malaise, headache, and myalgia. Treatment also prevented leptospiruria, and no significant adverse effects of doxycycline administration were observed.

In another randomized, double-blinded, placebo-controlled field trial at the same military training site, Takafuji and associates[251] demonstrated that doxycycline in a 200-mg oral dose given weekly or at the completion of jungle training was highly effective in preventing the onset of clinical leptospirosis. Twenty cases of disease were documented in the placebo group (attack rate, 4.2%) as opposed to only one case in the treatment group (attack rate, 0.2%), findings supporting the prophylactic utility of doxycycline in this setting.

Watt and associates[285] reported the results of a trial in which a 7-day course of intravenous penicillin with 6 million units per day was compared with placebo in a randomized, double-blinded trial involving 42 patients. All the patients had severe, advanced disease. Every measurable aspect of the disease was affected favorably by penicillin. The duration of fever was shortened significantly ($P < .005$) in the group receiving penicillin. Penicillin therapy decreased the number of days of hospitalization and prevented the development of leptospiruria. These investigators concluded that intravenous penicillin should be given to patients with severe leptospirosis, even if therapy can be initiated only late in the course of their disease. Subsequently, Costa and associates[68] reported the contrary. Two hundred fifty-three patients with leptospirosis and longer than 4 days of symptoms were randomized to receive 6 million units of penicillin for 7 days or placebo (mean pretreatment duration of symptoms of 6.6 days and 6.5 days, respectively). Neither the number of days of hospitalization nor the in-hospital case-fatality rate differed significantly between the two groups.

Limited data exist comparing the use of alternative antimicrobial agents with penicillin. Panaphut and colleagues[187] reported no difference in time to resolution of fever, mortality, or duration of organ dysfunction between patients randomized to receive a 7-day course of penicillin or intravenous ceftriaxone. A subsequent study[247] comparing penicillin, doxycycline, and cefotaxime reported no significant differences among the three groups with regard to mortality, time to defervescence, or time to resolution of abnormal laboratory test results.

Empiric treatment with penicillin or a tetracycline (to be avoided in children younger than 9 years) *early* in the course of disease can be used if a diagnosis of leptospirosis is suspected. Parenteral aqueous penicillin G 6 to 8 million units/m^2 per day in six divided doses should provide optimal blood and tissue concentrations of penicillin. For patients sensitive to penicillin, tetracycline 25 to 50 mg/kg per day orally in four divided doses (up to 3 g/day) or doxycycline 5 mg/kg per day orally in two divided doses (up to 200 mg/day) for 1 week, should be provided.

Management of leptospirosis requires careful attention to supportive care. Fluid and electrolyte balance requires meticulous attention. Dehydration, cardiovascular collapse, and acute renal failure may necessitate prompt and specific treatment. In some cases, acute renal failure may be prevented by ensuring adequate renal perfusion and appropriate fluid administration early in the course of disease, when prerenal azotemia and shock may be seen.[28,227] If prerenal azotemia is suspected, diuresis should be attempted promptly with administration of a fluid or colloid load designed to expand extracellular volume and replace extracellular fluid deficits.[28] In patients who do not respond to such therapy, acute tubular necrosis may be suspected, and appropriate fluid restriction should be initiated. If azotemia is severe or prolonged, peritoneal dialysis or hemodialysis should be instituted.[13,89,270] The use of exchange transfusion has been suggested in patients with marked hyperbilirubinemia and acute renal failure and may be associated with lower mortality.[174,183,195,228]

The use of corticosteroids in the treatment of severe cases has not been evaluated critically, but their use in patients with impending hepatic coma has been suggested.[82] Anecdotal reports also suggest that corticosteroids may be of value in patients with profound hypotension or shock.

PREVENTION

Prevention of leptospirosis, as with many other infections, invokes hygienic practices, immunizations, and prophylaxis after potential exposures. Benches in rat-infested, fish-gutting sheds and sewers may be decontaminated. Hygienic conditions should be encouraged in slaughterhouses, farmyard buildings, and bathing pools. Public health prevention campaigns in Australia emphasize the "cover-wash-clean up" strategy for reducing the incidence of leptospirosis. "Cover" exposed skin and mucous membranes that might come in contact with animals or animal secretions, "wash" hands or shower after a potential contamination, and "clean up" areas that might be contaminated or might attract rodents.[230] Given the rise of leptospirosis acquired during recreation or international travel, travelers should be advised about preventive measures such as avoiding flood waters, wearing protective clothing and boots, and covering up cuts and abrasions on their skin when engaging in outdoor activities.[145] Monitoring water for infection, whether for consumption or recreation, could help prevent exposure. Zhou and colleagues describe a PCR-based DNA microarray system for waterborne pathogen detection in water samples, including *L. interrogans.*[296] Identifying contaminated water sources can aid in the prevention of further spread.

In addition to hygiene, prevention of leptospirosis primarily depends on immunization of animals. Human immunization has generally been restricted to individuals with high-risk occupations and in response to epidemics or following natural disasters. Immunization of workers at high risk for acquiring leptospirosis has been used successfully in those working in mines in Japan and Poland, in rice fields in Italy and Spain, and in sewers in Paris.[115,267] Leptospire bacterins are available commercially and have been evaluated for safety and efficacy in laboratory animals and domestic livestock.[40,133,213,237] The degree of protection attained depends largely on the antigenic potential of the immunizing agent. Requirements for the *L. pomona* vaccine used in cattle are such that not more than $\frac{1}{800}$ of the dose recommended for cattle must protect 80% of hamsters challenged intraperitoneally 14 to 18 days after vaccination with a dose of 100 hamster LD_{50}. In contrast, most dogs are immunized with a vaccine that is but $\frac{1}{10}$ of the potency of that used for cattle. Most dogs thus immunized have been protected against disease but not necessarily from carrying and excreting leptospires in their urine. Trends documenting that many cases of leptospirosis in children have been associated with contact with dogs suggest that more stringent requirements for the immunization of pet dogs are needed. The challenge in vaccine efforts has been production of a safe and efficacious vaccine that promotes cross-protection against various pathogenic serovars that will eliminate infection and prevent chronic renal carriage.[297] Much of leptospirosis research efforts continue to focus on identification of potential vaccine candidates.[6] The availability of the genome sequence of *Leptospira* has facilitated this search and provided grounds for continued attempts at finding the ideal vaccine.[119,169] A detailed review of the literature on vaccines against leptospirosis was recently published. Adler[6] concludes that despite extensive research and increased knowledge of leptospirosis, the only vaccine licensed for use in animals and humans are inactivated bacterins not very different from those first used 90 years ago. There have been and continue to be active attempts at identifying leptospiral proteins that are able to elicit cross-protective immunity, but true success has yet to be reached. Promising candidates under judicious study include LipL32 and LigA.[6] The search for the perfect vaccine continues.[128,269,278]

A randomized trial of doxycycline versus placebo was undertaken to assess the efficacy of doxycycline prophylaxis in the prevention of infection and disease caused by leptospires during outbreaks in North Andaman.[219] Leptospiral infection was not prevented, but the patients who received doxycycline and in whom disease subsequently developed had lower morbidity and mortality rates.

NEW REFERENCES SINCE THE SEVENTH EDITION

6. Adler B. Vaccines against leptospirosis. *Curr Top Microbiol Immunol.* 2015;387:251-272.
10. Allan KJ, Biggs HM, Halliday JE, et al. Epidemiology of leptospirosis in Africa: a systematic review of a neglected zoonosis and a paradigm for "One Health" in Africa. *PLoS Negl Trop Dis.* 2015;9(9):e0003899.
19. Ayral F, Zilber AL, Bicout DJ, et al. Distribution of *Leptospira interrogans* by multispacer sequence typing in urban Norway rats *(Rattus norvegicus):* a survey in France in 2011–2013. *PLoS ONE.* 2015;10(10):e0139604.
22. Backstedt BT, Buyuktanir O, Lindow J, et al. Efficient detection of pathogenic leptospires using 16S ribosomal RNA. *PLoS ONE.* 2015;10(6):e0128913.
38. Bourhy P, Collet L, Brisse S, et al. *Leptospira mayottensis* sp. nov., a pathogenic species of the genus *Leptospira* isolated from humans. *Int J Syst Evol Microbiol.* 2014;64(Pt 12):4061-4067.
52. Castiblanco-Valencia MM, Fraga TR, Pagotto AH, et al. Plasmin cleaves fibrinogen and the human complement proteins C3b and C5 in the presence of *Leptospira interrogans* proteins: a new role of LigA and LigB in invasion and complement immune evasion. *Immunobiology.* 2016.
67. Costa F, Hagan JE, Calcagno J, et al. Global morbidity and mortality of leptospirosis: a systematic review. *PLoS Negl Trop Dis.* 2015;9(9):e0003898.
90. Ferraz RV, Pereira NR, Carvalho C, et al. Hepatitis C and leptospirosis: simultaneous acute infections or recurrence of occult hepatitis C. *BMJ Case Rep.* 2015;2015.
96. Fraga TR, Courrol Ddos S, Castiblanco-Valencia MM, et al. Immune evasion by pathogenic Leptospira strains: the secretion of proteases that directly cleave complement proteins. *J Infect Dis.* 2014;209(6):876-886.
105. Goeijenbier M, Gasem MH, Meijers JC, et al. Markers of endothelial cell activation and immune activation are increased in patients with severe leptospirosis and associated with disease severity. *J Infect.* 2015;71(4):437-446.
107. Goris MG, Leeflang MM, Boer KR, et al. Establishment of valid laboratory case definition for human leptospirosis. *J Bacteriol Parasitol.* 2012;3(2):8.
112. Guerra MA. Leptospirosis: public health perspectives. *Biologicals.* 2013;41(5):295-297.
115. Haake DA, Levett PN. Leptospirosis in humans. *Curr Top Microbiol Immunol.* 2015;387:65-97.
128. Jacobs AA, Harks F, Hoeijmakers M, et al. Safety and efficacy of a new octavalent combined *Erysipelas, Parvo* and *Leptospira* vaccine in gilts against *Leptospira interrogans* serovar Pomona associated disease and foetal death. *Vaccine.* 2015;33(32):3963-3969.
130. Jobbins SE, Sanderson CE, Alexander KA. *Leptospira interrogans* at the human-wildlife interface in northern Botswana: a newly identified public health threat. *Zoonoses Public Health.* 2014;61(2):113-123.
136. Karrasch M, Herfurth K, Klaver M, et al. Severe leptospirosis complicated by Epstein-Barr virus reactivation. *Infection.* 2015;43(6):763-769.
143. Koshy JM, Koshy J, John M, et al. Leptospiral uveitis. *J Assoc Physicians India.* 2014;62(11):65-67.
148. Lehmann JS, Matthias MA, Vinetz JM, et al. Leptospiral pathogenomics. *Pathogens.* 2014;3(2):280-308.
153. Marinho M, Taparo CV, Oliveira-Junior IS, et al. Tissue apoptosis in mice infected with *Leptospira interrogans* serovar Icterohaemorrhagiae. *J Venom Anim Toxins Incl Trop Dis.* 2015;21:22.
155. Martins-Pinheiro M, Schons-Fonseca L, da Silva JB, et al. Genomic survey and expression analysis of DNA repair genes in the genus *Leptospira. Mol Genet Genomics.* 2016;291(2):703-722.
166. Miraglia F, Moreno LZ, Morais ZM, et al. Characterization of *Leptospira interrogans* serovar Pomona isolated from swine in Brazil. *J Infect Dev Ctries.* 2015;9(10):1054-1061.
175. Murray GL. The lipoprotein LipL32, an enigma of leptospiral biology. *Vet Microbiol.* 2013;162(2-4):305-314.
176. Murray GL. The molecular basis of leptospiral pathogenesis. *Curr Top Microbiol Immunol.* 2015;387:139-185.
185. Pages F, Larrieu S, Simoes J, et al. Investigation of a leptospirosis outbreak in triathlon participants, Reunion Island, 2013. *Epidemiol Infect.* 2016;144(3):661-669.
192. Podgorsek D, Cerar T, Logar M, et al. Evaluation of the immunochromatographic (Leptocheck) test for detection of specific antibodies against leptospires. *Wien Klin Wochenschr.* 2015;127(23-24):948-953.
203. Robbins GT, Hahn BL, Evangelista KV, et al. Evaluation of cell binding activities of *Leptospira* ECM adhesins. *PLoS Negl Trop Dis.* 2015;9(4):e0003712.
210. Samir A, Soliman R, El-Hariri M, et al. Leptospirosis in animals and human contacts in Egypt: broad range surveillance. *Rev Soc Bras Med Trop.* 2015;48(3):272-277.
215. Schreiber PW, Aceto L, Korach R, et al. Cluster of leptospirosis acquired through river surfing in Switzerland. *Open Forum Infect Dis.* 2015;2(3):ofv102.
217. Schuller S, Arent ZJ, Gilmore C, et al. Prevalence of antileptospiral serum antibodies in dogs in Ireland. *Vet Rec.* 2015;177(5):126.
218. Schuller S, Callanan JJ, Worrall S, et al. Immunohistochemical detection of IgM and IgG in lung tissue of dogs with leptospiral pulmonary haemorrhage syndrome (LPHS). *Comp Immunol Microbiol Infect Dis.* 2015;40:47-53.
244. Stokes A, Ryle JA. A note on Weil's disease (spirochaetosis ictero-haemorrhagica) as it has occurred in the army in Flanders. *Br Med J.* 1916;2(2908):413-417.
256. Torgerson PR, Hagan JE, Costa F, et al. Global burden of leptospirosis: estimated in terms of disability adjusted life years. *PLoS Negl Trop Dis.* 2015;9(10):e0004122.
259. Traxler RM, Callinan LS, Holman RC, et al. Leptospirosis-associated hospitalizations, United States, 1998-2009. *Emerg Infect Dis.* 2014;20(8):1273-1279.
269. Umthong S, Buaklin A, Jacquet A, et al. Immunogenicity of a DNA and recombinant protein vaccine combining LipL32 and Loa22 for leptospirosis using chitosan as a delivery system. *J Microbiol Biotechnol.* 2015;25(4):526-536.
275. Vieira ML, Nascimento AL. Interaction of spirochetes with the host fibrinolytic system and potential roles in pathogenesis. *Crit Rev Microbiol.* 2015;1-15.
278. Vijayachari P, Vedhagiri K, Mallilankaraman K, et al. Immunogenicity of a novel enhanced consensus DNA vaccine encoding the leptospiral protein LipL45. *Hum Vaccin Immunother.* 2015;11(8):1945-1953.
280. Vivian JP, Beddoe T, McAlister AD, et al. Crystal structure of LipL32, the most abundant surface protein of pathogenic Leptospira spp. *J Mol Biol.* 2009;387(5):1229-1238.
289. Wilson MR, Naccache SN, Samayoa E, et al. Actionable diagnosis of neuroleptospirosis by next-generation sequencing. *N Engl J Med.* 2014;370(25):2408-2417.
290. Witchell TD, Eshghi A, Nally JE, et al. Post-translational modification of LipL32 during *Leptospira interrogans* infection. *PLoS Negl Trop Dis.* 2014;8(10):e3280.
294. Yang HY, Hung CC, Liu SH, et al. Overlooked risk for chronic kidney disease after leptospiral infection: a population-based survey and epidemiological cohort evidence. *PLoS Negl Trop Dis.* 2015;9(10):e0004105.

The full reference list for this chapter is available at ExpertConsult.com.

Spirillum minus (Rat-Bite Fever)

143

Kara A. DuBray

Spirillum minus is one of the two known causative agents of rat-bite fever. Rat-bite fever also may be caused by *Streptobacillus moniliformis* (see Chapter 138). *S. minus* is a spirochete that was first isolated in 1917 and was reported to be a common cause of rat-bite fever in Asia, although few reports exist in the English literature to confirm its prevalence.[5,9] Few cases of spirillary rat-bite fever have been reported in the American literature in the past 4 decades, with most cases reported in the early 1900s.[3,5,13] No confirmed cases have been reported in the last 25 years. Many reports discuss both etiologies simultaneously, although the two types of rat-bite fever are distinct with different epidemiology and clinical presentations.

BACTERIOLOGY

S. minus is a short, rigid, aerobic, gram-negative, flagellated spirochete measuring 2 to 5 μm in length. The organism is thicker and more rigid than *Treponema pallidum* and usually contains two to three regular sharp turns along its length. On darkfield microscopy, the organism moves quickly with the use of a terminal flagellum.[5] *S. minus,* like other spirochetes, does not grow on artificial media and requires animal inoculation for successful isolation.[15] However, two reports in the literature describe the isolation of *S. minus* in broth,[8,14] but these cases may have represented other infectious illnesses.

EPIDEMIOLOGY AND PATHOLOGY

Like streptobacillary infection, disease appears to be transmitted primarily through rat bites. In 1928 approximately 25% of rats were carriers of *S. minus* in the nasopharynx, and rats with conjunctivitis were shown to have *S. minus* in the eye discharge that drained into their mouths.[11] Disease has not been reported after oral ingestion of the organism. Human-to-human transmission has not been reported but conceivably could occur during blood transfusions.

Gunning[6] gave an excellent description of the pathologic changes associated with *S. minus* infection. The infection provokes edema, mononuclear leukocyte infiltration, and necrosis at the site of inoculation. Regional lymph nodes are hyperplastic. The relapsing symptoms are associated with invasion of the blood by spirilla. Toxic, hemorrhagic, or necrotic changes may occur in the liver and kidney.

CLINICAL MANIFESTATIONS

The original description by Futaki and colleagues[5] described "the clinical symptoms of rat-bite fever are inflammation of the bitten parts, paroxysms of fever of the relapsing type, swelling of the lymph glands, and eruption of the skin, all occurring after an incubation period usually from 10 to 22 days, or longer." The incubation period of spirillary rat-bite fever typically is longer than that of the streptobacillary form, with an average of 14 to 18 days and a range of 1 to 36 days.[2] The disease is heralded by the appearance of an indurated lesion at the site of the initially healed bite, which coincides with the onset of fever and chills. Chancre formation or ulceration may occur at the site, and regional lymphadenopathy is a common finding. The temperature may reach 41°C (105.8°F) in a stepwise fashion over the course of 2 to 4 days and then fall abruptly.[6]

Six to eight regularly occurring relapses of fever may occur, separated by afebrile periods lasting 3 to 7 days. During febrile periods, the patient also may experience myalgia, headache, and vomiting. In approximately 50% of patients, a purple to red-brown rash develops and consists of large macules with occasional indurated erythematous plaques or urticarial lesions.[15] In contrast to streptobacillary rat-bite fever, joint manifestations are rare occurrences. In untreated cases, the illness may persist for 3 to 8 weeks, but relapses have occurred after months or years.[13]

Spontaneous cure is the general rule, but several untreated cases persisted for more than 1 year.[15] The untreated mortality rate was reported to be 6.5% in 1942.[2] In protracted, untreated cases, severe complications included endocarditis,[8] meningitis,[10] myocarditis, hepatitis, and nephritis.[4] Anemia, weight loss, and severe diarrhea were common complications in infants and children. Epididymitis, nuchal rigidity, headache, pleurisy, pleural effusion, and splenomegaly also were reported.[12] Mortality was noted to be significantly lower than in streptobacillary rat-bite fever.[13] Herxheimer reactions were reported in patients treated with arsenic-based therapies used before penicillin.[13]

The differential diagnosis includes streptobacillary rat-bite fever as well as many other infectious and noninfectious diseases (see Chapter 138).

DIAGNOSIS

Definitive diagnosis requires isolation and identification of the spirochete. The organism rarely may be seen on a peripheral blood smear with Giemsa or Wright stain[1,3] or darkfield examination of ulcer exudate.[7] Animal inoculation usually is required for isolation. Blood or wound aspirates are injected intraperitoneally into guinea pigs or mice. The spirochetes then may be recovered in 5 to 15 days from the animals' blood, which is examined under darkfield microscopy. This process is time consuming and may not be available in most centers. In addition, the inoculated animals must be screened carefully for previous *Spirillum* carriage.

Nonspecific diagnostic criteria include a false-positive test for syphilis in 50% of patients, white blood cell count between 10,000 and 20,000 cells/mm,[3] and moderate anemia.[2,15] No specific serologic tests are available for *S. minus*. Molecular methods, such as polymerase chain reaction, may offer hope in the future for detection of *S. minus*.[4]

TREATMENT

Before penicillin, *S. minus* was treated successfully with arsenic therapy; however, response was slower, with reported relapses and even death.[13] In general, *S. minus* is considered more sensitive to penicillin than *S. moniliformis,* and penicillin is the drug of choice for both forms of the disease. Doses as low as 24,000 U/day for 5 days were shown to be effective.[13] However, because distinguishing spirillary disease from streptobacillary disease may be difficult, it is important to treat initially with higher dosages effective against *S. moniliformis* (see Chapter 138).

The full reference list for this chapter is available at ExpertConsult.com.

144 Syphilis

Simon R. Dobson and Pablo J. Sánchez

Syphilis was recognized first at the end of the 15th century in Europe, where it appeared seemingly as an emerging infectious disease. It rapidly spread to reach epidemic proportions. Its European origins are a mystery that will not be solved easily, with theories ranging from its being a disease introduced from the New World by the returning crew of Columbus to its being a virulent form of the endemic yaws and bejel of African peoples that appeared later as virulent syphilis in a susceptible European population.

Syphilis initially was called the *Italian disease,* the *French disease,* and the *great pox* (as distinguished from smallpox). Its venereal transmission was not recognized until the 18th century. Delineation of characteristics of syphilis was hindered by the confusion of its symptoms with those of gonorrhea. In 1767, Hunter, a great English experimental biologist and physician, inoculated himself with urethral exudate from a patient with gonorrhea. The patient also had syphilis, and the subsequent symptoms experienced by Hunter convinced two generations of physicians of the unity of gonorrhea and syphilis. The separate natures of gonorrhea and syphilis were shown in 1838 by Ricord, who reported his observations on more than 2500 human inoculations. Recognition of the stages of syphilis followed; in 1905, Schaudinn and Hoffman discovered the causative agent. The following year, Wassermann introduced the diagnostic blood test that bears his name.

ORGANISM

Morphologic characteristics are the primary features by which members of the family Spirochaetaceae are placed into a single taxon. Spirochetes are helix-shaped, heterotrophic bacteria. These organisms are slender, coiled, and flexible, with one or more complete turns in the helix. Spirochetes are motile, their corkscrew motility resulting from the action of axial fibrils known as *endoflagella.* The family Spirochaetaceae has five genera, of which only *Treponema, Borrelia,* and *Leptospira* spp. cause major human illnesses. Differentiation among genera of the family Spirochaetaceae is based primarily on the morphology of the organism.

The name *Treponema* is derived from the Greek words meaning "turning thread." Individual organisms are 5 to 15 μm in length and 0.092 to 0.5 μm in diameter and have finely tapered ends. Whole cells appear to have a flat wave with one or more planes per cell, giving the appearance of a helical coil. Each cell has 8 to 14 evenly distributed waves. They exhibit a sluggish mobility, with drifting motion and graceful flexuous movements.[73] The internal structure of *Treponema pallidum* subsp. *pallidum* generally is similar to that of other spirochetes. An outermost thin three-layered membrane surrounds the protoplasmic cylinder of the cell. Intracytoplasmic microtubules have been described, and such structures may be specific for *Treponema* spp.

The six axial fibrils or endoflagella are long, flagella-like, intracellular organelles that originate at either end of the cell from knoblike structures and extend toward the other end. Axial fibrils vary in length but overlap one another near the middle of the cell. These fibrils are thought to determine the spiral shape of the cells and are responsible for the characteristic motility along the longitudinal axis exhibited by members of Spirochaetaceae.

The complete genome of *T. pallidum* subsp. *pallidum* (Nichols strain) was sequenced by the whole-genome rapid sequencing method.[47] The *T. pallidum* genome is a circular chromosome and is small compared with most bacteria at 1.14 Mb that encode 1041 predicted proteins. By polyacrylamide gel electrophoresis technique, the major constituent proteins of *T. pallidum* have been characterized and include integral membrane proteins with apparent molecular masses of 47, 34, 17, and 15 kDa.[102] These lipoprotein antigens are highly immunogenic in laboratory animals and humans.[7,65]

Virulent strains of *T. pallidum* are propagated by intratesticular inoculation of rabbits, and the inability to propagate the organisms in vitro has hampered study of these microorganisms. The time required for division of the organism to occur in rabbits is slow, at approximately 30 hours. Velocity sedimentation employing discontinuous gradients of radiocontrast medium (Hypaque) successfully has purified and concentrated treponemes extracted from infected rabbit testes. These organisms retain the antigens for the fluorescence test, although motility is lost.

Limited cultivation of *T. pallidum* on monolayers of baby hamster kidney cells in 7% carbon dioxide has been reported. Research with in vitro characteristics of these organisms also has resulted in the description of adherence of virulent *T. pallidum* to primary cell cultures of rabbit testicular cells and to an established continuous line of human epithelial cells (HEp-2). To date, however, direct in vitro culture for establishing the diagnosis of *T. pallidum* disease has not been possible. In vitro growth is hindered by the reliance of *T. pallidum* on glycolysis alone for adenosine triphosphate synthesis, its sensitivity to oxygen, and its sensitivity to growth temperature.[73]

Other pathogenic *Treponema* organisms cause characteristic clinical diseases and now are known to be genetically different from *T. pallidum* subsp. *pallidum.* These are *T. pallidum* subsp. *carateum* (pinta), *T. pallidum* subsp. *endemicum* (bejel or endemic syphilis), and *T. pallidum* subsp. *pertenue* (yaws). Several nonpathogenic treponemes also inhabit the oral cavity and intestinal tract.[19]

TRANSMISSION

Acquired Syphilis

Syphilis is not a highly contagious disease. An individual who has had sexual contact with an infected partner has approximately a 30% chance of acquiring disease. The median infective dose to humans experimentally has been estimated to be 57 organisms. *T. pallidum* has the capability to invade the intact mucous membrane or microabrasions of the skin. Direct inoculation from contact with an infected individual is necessary for infection to occur because survival of the organism outside the host is very limited. The organism is killed easily by heat, drying, soap, and water. Sexual contact is the common method of transmission of acquired disease, and the site of inoculation usually is on the genital organs—the vagina or cervix in females and the penis in males. Other sites include lips, breast, tongue, and abraded areas of the skin. Examining physicians and pathologists may be infected by contact if appropriate barrier protection is not used.

Congenital Syphilis

Congenital syphilis usually results from transplacental infection of the developing fetus from spirochetes in the maternal bloodstream. *T. pallidum* becomes widely disseminated to many tissues in an adult soon after initial infection occurs even if clinical manifestations are delayed by months. Maternal spirochetemia and placental infection are not surprising findings.[9] A neonate occasionally may be infected at delivery by contact with an infectious lesion present in the birth canal or perineum. Intrauterine transmission is supported by isolation of the organism from umbilical cord blood and amniotic fluid,[52,99,127,149] detection of spirochetes in the placenta and umbilical cord in association with typical histopathologic changes,[41,46,112] and detection of specific immunoglobulin M (IgM) antibody to *T. pallidum* in neonatal serum obtained at birth.[82,91,124,127] The isolation of *T. pallidum* from 74% of amniotic fluid specimens obtained from women with early syphilis also suggests that the organism is capable of traversing the fetal membranes, gaining access to the amniotic fluid and resulting in fetal infection.[83] Breastfeeding is not associated with transmission of syphilis, unless the mother has a chancre on her breast.

Transmission of syphilis to the fetus can occur throughout pregnancy. Occasional reports in the literature describing treponemes in fetal tissue or placentas before the fifth month of gestation were disputed for decades.[40] The thought was that the Langhans cell layer of the cytotrophoblast formed a placental barrier against treponemal invasion of the fetus. Researchers subsequently showed, however, that the layer of Langhans cells in the placenta persisted throughout pregnancy.

In 1976, Harter and Benirschke[57] visualized spirochetes by Warthin-Starry silver stain and immunofluorescence in tissue from two aborted fetuses at gestational ages of 9 and 10 weeks. The expected inflammatory response was not observed in these two fetuses, but such changes have been found in infected fetuses after the 15th week of pregnancy. These investigators noted that researchers describing syphilitic fetuses or placentas in the older literature worked with the products of spontaneous abortions. Such fetal loss caused by syphilis occurred only after 18 weeks of gestation, implying that the fetal loss was a reflection of damage incurred as a result of the host response to the organism. The observation of sequential acquisition by the fetus of the ability to respond to a variety of antigens suggests that inflammation can be present only after the fetus acquires the immunologic ability to recognize the treponeme.[136] The detection of spirochetes in amniotic fluid obtained by amniocentesis from a woman with early syphilis at 14 weeks of pregnancy has shown that the fetus can be infected with *T. pallidum* in early pregnancy.[98] The rate of vertical transmission does increase with advancing gestation, however.

Vertical transmission is related directly to the maternal stage of syphilis, with early syphilis resulting in significantly higher transmission rates than late latent infection. Generally, the greater the time that has elapsed since the woman's primary or secondary infection, the less likely she is to transmit disease to the fetus. Ingraham[62] reported in 1950 that among 251 women with syphilis having a duration of 4 years or less, 41% of their infants were born alive and had congenital syphilis; 25% were stillborn; 14% died in the neonatal period; 21% had low birth weight, but no evidence of syphilis; and 18% were normal full-term infants. In contrast, only 2% of infants born to mothers with late disease had congenital syphilis. In 1952, Fiumara and colleagues[44] reported that untreated primary or secondary syphilis resulted in 50% of infants having congenital syphilis, whereas the other half were stillborn or premature or died in the neonatal period. With early latent infection, 40% of the infants had congenital syphilis, whereas only 10% with late latent disease developed syphilis. These data are supported by a more recent study of Sheffield and colleagues,[132] in which mothers with primary, secondary, early latent, and late latent infection had transmission rates of 29%, 59%, 50%, and 13%, respectively.

Syphilis is an ulcer-causing disease that is associated with increased sexual transmission of human immunodeficiency virus (HIV). In this regard, increasing numbers of neonates who are infected with congenital syphilis also are born to mothers with HIV, and vice versa. The contribution of maternal coinfection with *T. pallidum* and HIV to vertical transmission of either syphilis or HIV has not been elucidated fully. Virulent *T. pallidum* can promote the induction of HIV gene expression in macrophages, possibly resulting in increased systemic HIV levels and more rapid progression of the HIV infection.[144] A more recent study noted higher rates of congenital syphilis in infants born to coinfected mothers, but the diagnosis of congenital syphilis was based on a surveillance definition used by the Centers for Disease Control and Prevention (CDC) and not on strict diagnostic criteria.[129]

EPIDEMIOLOGY

The introduction of penicillin in 1942, and its subsequent widespread use in the 1950s, resulted in a marked decline in the occurrence of syphilis in the United States. After an increase in the number of cases occurred in the early 1960s, the rates again declined in the 1970s, only to have a dramatic resurgence from 1986 to 1991.[21,30,117] The rapid increase during these years in the rate and numbers of cases of primary and secondary syphilis in adults, specifically among women of childbearing age, resulted in a significant increase in rates of congenital syphilis. Rates of syphilis were greatest among blacks and Hispanics residing in large urban centers. The disease was centered in populations in which substance abuse, particularly crack cocaine, was common and where there was involvement with the sex trade industry often in exchange for drugs.[21]

Other factors that may have contributed to the increased rates of syphilis included underfunded and overwhelmed public health resources; use of spectinomycin for treatment of penicillinase-producing *Neisseria gonorrhoeae* because spectinomycin is ineffective against incubating syphilis; and failure to implement safer sexual practices, especially among adolescents and young adults. Generally, individuals who acquire syphilis characteristically are young and often have had contact with an average of five individuals during the incubation period. Because of the high rate of dual infection (8%) with *N. gonorrhoeae,* some individuals identified and treated for gonorrhea with ceftriaxone also are treated for syphilis while in the preprimary stage of disease.

Strenuous attempts were made to control syphilis, and the lowest rate ever reported in the United States was reached in 2000, with the rate of primary and secondary syphilis declining by 90% between 1990 and 2000 to 2.1 per 100,000 population.[23] The reasons for this decline included (1) wider screening practices secondary to medical and public awareness of the syphilis epidemic of the late 1980s that led to identification and treatment of infected individuals; (2) increased state and local funding for syphilis control programs such as partner notification, community-based screening and presumptive treatment strategies, and risk-reduction counseling; (3) introduction of HIV prevention programs that target prevention of other sexually transmitted infections (STIs); (4) decrease in crack cocaine use and trading sex for drugs behaviors; and possibly (5) development of acquired immunity to syphilis among high-risk populations that resulted in less reacquisition of infectious syphilis.

The concentration of cases in the United States to a few geographic areas, especially in the southeastern United States, led to an optimistic "National Plan to Eliminate Syphilis" announced by the CDC in 1999.[140] The plan had to be restated in 2006 in the presence of resurgent rates.[23] A gender gap has been noted, with rates of primary and secondary syphilis in men increasing from 3 per 100,000 in 2001 to 5.7 per 100,000 in 2006. The increase in male rates has been explained partly by cases in men who have sex with men and attributed to high-risk sexual behaviors and coinfection with HIV. In 2006, there also was an increase in rates in women from 0.8 per 100,000 in 2004 to 1 per 100,000. With the rates increasing in heterosexuals, the rates of congenital syphilis also have rebounded.

In 1987, the reported rate of congenital syphilis was 10.5 cases per 100,000 live births. By 1991, there were 4398 cases of congenital syphilis (107 per 100,000 live births). These rates reflect a reporting surveillance case definition that was changed in 1988[21,156] and resulted in an almost fourfold increase in the number of cases reported to the CDC.[30] There also was a genuine increase, however, in the number of actual cases and case rates secondary to the increase in early syphilis among women.[70] Canadian rates had followed a similar trend where it was notable that delayed access to antenatal care was a key factor, in that all women who were delivered of infants with congenital syphilis had histories of substance abuse and street involvement.[137]

In 1988, investigators recognized that prior definitions of congenital syphilis that had been used for surveillance and for treatment decisions had been difficult to apply to the clinical setting because they required a diagnosis that often could be established only over weeks or months. During that period, many children were lost to follow-up and were neither treated nor reported.[30] Because of the high incidence of congenital disease in infants born to inadequately treated mothers, current definitions of congenital syphilis for a presumptive case (which should be reported and treated) require only (1) that the infant be born to a mother with untreated or inadequately treated syphilis or (2) that the child have physical or laboratory signs of congenital syphilis. A summary of the surveillance case definition used since 1988 is provided in Box 144.1.

Minor differences exist among case definitions of congenital syphilis as formulated by several agencies and experts.[122] Some experts would consider as a presumptive case a neonate who is well clinically but was born to a mother who had contact within 90 days before delivery with an individual with primary or secondary syphilis and who had not been treated or had been treated inadequately, even if the mother has nonreactive serology. Although recommendations for therapy commonly have assumed that adequate therapy given to a mother with primary or secondary syphilis during pregnancy would prevent congenital syphilis with a high degree of reliability, reasons to doubt this premise have emerged.[3,88,155] In particular, treatment failures in which the infant

BOX 144.1 Surveillance Case Definition for Congenital Syphilis

A *confirmed case* of congenital syphilis is when *Treponema pallidum* is identified by darkfield microscopy, fluorescent antibody, or other specific stains in specimens from lesions, placenta, umbilical cord, amniotic fluid, or autopsy material.

A *presumptive case* of congenital syphilis can occur in either of the following:

A. Any infant whose mother had untreated or inadequately treated[a] syphilis at delivery, regardless of findings in the infant, *or*
B. Any infant or child who has a reactive treponemal test for syphilis and any one of the following:
   1. Any evidence of congenital syphilis on physical examination, *or*
   2. Any evidence of congenital syphilis on long bone radiograph, *or*
   3. Reactive cerebrospinal fluid VDRL, *or*
   4. Elevated cerebrospinal fluid cell count or protein (without other cause), *or*
   5. Quantitative nontreponemal serologic titers that are fourfold higher than the mother's (both drawn at birth), *or*
   6. Reactive test for FTA-ABS-19S-IgM antibody

A *syphilitic stillbirth* is defined as a death of a fetus weighing >500 g or having a gestational age >20 weeks in which the mother had untreated or inadequately treated syphilis at delivery.

[a]Inadequate treatment consists of any nonpenicillin therapy or penicillin given <30 days before delivery.

FTA-ABS, Fluorescent treponemal antibody absorption; *IgM,* immunoglobulin M; *VDRL,* Venereal Disease Research Laboratory.

Modified from Centers for Disease Control. Congenital syphilis, New York City, 1986–1988. *MMWR Morb Mortal Wkly Rep.* 1989;38:828.

BOX 144.2 Circumstances in Which Maternal Therapy for Syphilis May Be Subtherapeutic or Inadequate

Treatment with a nonpenicillin regimen (including macrolide antibiotics)
History of maternal treatment was not documented fully or verifiable
Treatment during the month before delivery
Treatment in HIV-infected women
Serial posttherapy assays of maternal nontreponemal antibody titers were not performed
Serial posttherapy assays of maternal nontreponemal antibody titers did not show a fourfold decline in titers after treatment of early syphilis, not permitting assessment of adequacy of therapy, and suggesting possibility of failure to eradicate infection
Serial posttherapy assays of maternal nontreponemal antibody titers show a fourfold increase in titers, suggesting reinfection or relapse

developed syphilis despite maternal therapy have been reported when the mother was treated first within 30 days of delivery.[10,14,87,101,121]

An infant born to a mother who was treated within 30 days of delivery is considered to have been treated inadequately, and the infant should receive appropriate therapy. Box 144.2 lists the various circumstances in which maternal therapy may be presumed to be subtherapeutic. The consequences of inadequate therapy for the mother are shown in data in Table 144.1. In that experience, 13% of children born to inadequately treated mothers had congenital syphilis, all of which was neurosyphilis.[120]

Substantial underreporting of infected infants did occur previously,[37] but the revised surveillance definition does not represent diagnostic criteria. Rather, it reflects the public health burden of the disease because these infants require medical and public health interventions. Notwithstanding this change in reporting guidelines, the number of cases of congenital syphilis had continued to decline from a peak of 107 per 100,000 live births in 1991. In the United States, the rate of congenital syphilis decreased during 1991–2005 but increased slightly during

TABLE 144.1 Clinical Findings of 148 Infants Whose Mothers Had Syphilis

	MATERNAL TREATMENT		
Infant Findings	***None (n = 72)***	***Inadequate (n = 31)***	***Adequate (n = 45)***
Clinical disease	3	0	0
Positive CSF-VDRL test	7	4	0
Abnormal bone radiograph	6	0	0
Stillbirth	6	0	0
Total (any abnormality)	22 (31%)	4 (13%)	0

CSF, Cerebrospinal fluid; *VDRL,* Venereal Disease Research Laboratory.

From Reyes MP, Hunt N, Ostrea EM, et al. Maternal/congenital syphilis in a large tertiary care urban hospital. *Clin Infect Dis.* 1993;17:1041-1046.

2005–08. The overall rate of reported congenital syphilis decreased from 10.5 to 8.4 cases per 100,000 live births during 2008–12, and then increased to 11.6 cases per 100,000 live births in 2014, the highest congenital syphilis rate reported since 2001. From 2012–14, reported cases and rates of congenital syphilis increased across all regions of the United States, reflecting a parallel 22% national increase in the rate of primary and secondary syphilis among women during the same period. Lack of prenatal care remained the most important factor.[12]

Worldwide, syphilis remains a considerable public health problem. Mother-to-child transmission cannot be easily measured globally because definitive diagnosis is difficult. Estimating the burden of disease must rely on modeled data. In 2007 the World Health Organization (WHO) reported global estimates for congenital syphilis burden based on a review of published data from 1997 through 2003. They estimated that annually there were 2,036,753 syphilis infections among pregnant women, of which 65% (1,323,889; range, 728,547–1,527,565) resulted in adverse pregnancy outcomes, including early fetal loss, stillbirths, and neonatal deaths.[128] In 2007, WHO launched an initiative to eliminate congenital syphilis that set targets of at least 90% of pregnant women being tested for syphilis and at least 90% of seropositive pregnant women receiving adequate treatment by 2015.[152] To facilitate assessment of the initiative's progress, a more up-to-date model was developed using global and regional health services delivery data to estimate the burden of syphilis in pregnancy in 2008. An active syphilis infection occurred in 1.4 million pregnant women, 80% of whom had attended antenatal care services. Infection caused 520,000 adverse outcomes in 2008, including 215,000 stillbirths or fetal deaths, 90,000 neonatal deaths, 65,000 preterm or low-birth-weight infants, and 150,000 infants with congenital disease. Almost two-thirds of the adverse effects occurred in women who had attended antenatal care but were either not tested or not treated for syphilis. For those tested at antenatal clinics, regional seropositivity rates among antenatal care attendees were Africa 2.13%, Asia 0.62%, Europe 0.16%, and the Americas 0.84% (Fig. 144.1).[100]

Congenital syphilis is a disease that should be amenable almost fully to eradication if currently available prenatal health measures were implemented completely. Table 144.2 presents two studies in the United States of prenatal care of women who were delivered of infants with congenital syphilis and indicates the hurdles that control of the disease will have to overcome.[31,88] Lack of optimal prenatal care is the most important one.[35,90,147] National surveillance data analyzed by the CDC in 2002 highlight the fact that cases of congenital syphilis still occur even when prenatal care is implemented if the mother's response to treatment is inadequate or if the infant's evaluation is not thorough (Fig. 144.2).[22]

Globally, the WHO initiative has been acted on with emphasis on (1) ensuring advocacy and sustained political commitment, (2) increasing access to maternal and newborn services, (3) screening and treating pregnant women and their partners, and (4) establishing surveillance, monitoring, and evaluation systems. The last is especially important in terms of allowing for a process to validate countries as being free of mother-to-child transmission of syphilis.[66,153] Several countries have now achieved this status, including Cuba (2015) and Thailand, Moldova, Armenia, and Belarus (2016).

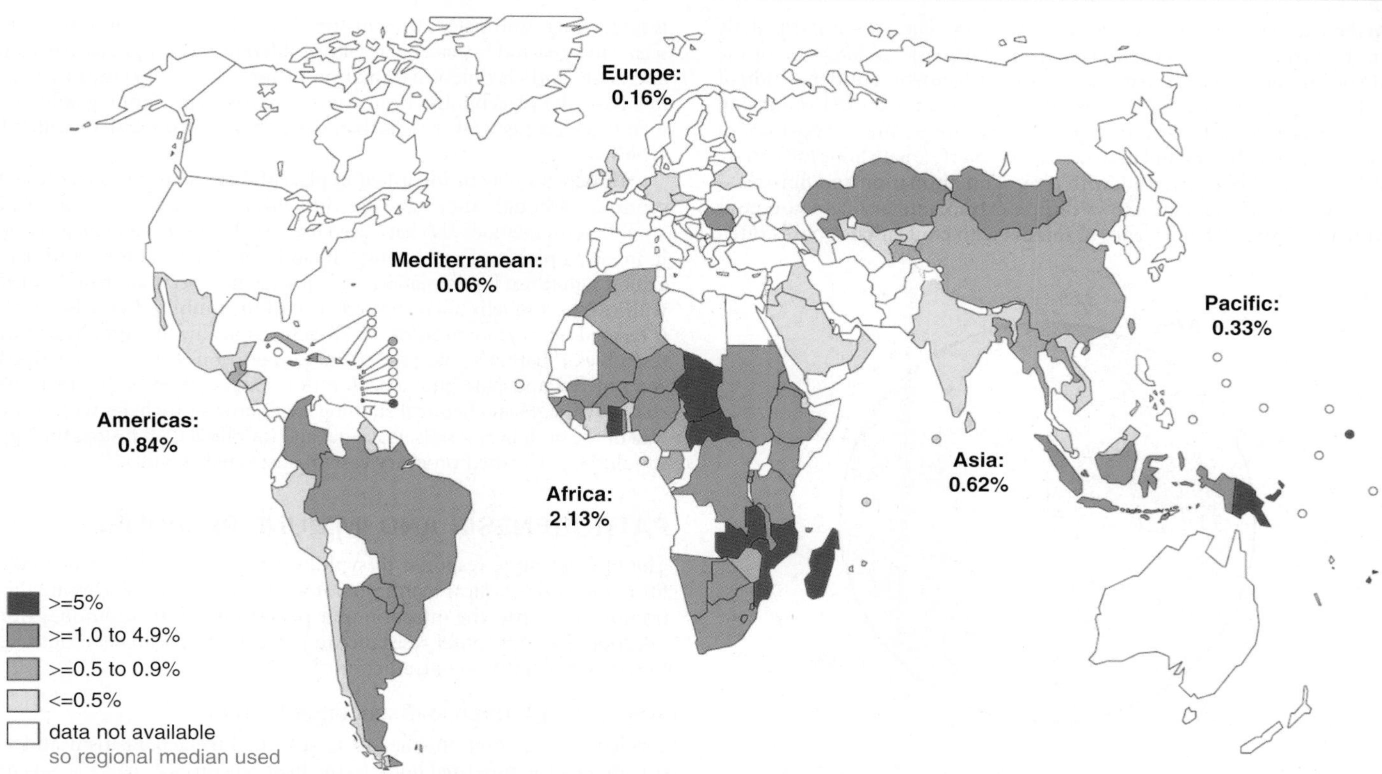

FIG. 144.1 Syphilis seropositivity among antenatal care attendees reported by countries through the World Health Organization HIV Universal Access reporting system in 2008 or 2009, and regional median for nonreporting countries. (From Newman L, Kamb M, Hawkes S, et al. Global estimates of syphilis in pregnancy and associated adverse outcomes: analysis of multinational antenatal surveillance data. *PLoS Med.* 2013;10[2]:e1001396.)

TABLE 144.2 Prenatal Care and the Occurrence[a] of Congenital Syphilis in Infants

Prenatal Care	Mascola et al., 1984[87] (*n* = 50)	Coles et al., 1995[31] (*n* = 318)
No prenatal care	56	46
First prenatal test negative; testing not repeated in late pregnancy	6	14
Medical mismanagement	6	10
Failure of conventional prenatal syphilis treatment of mother	8	5
Negative maternal syphilis test at delivery	14	—
Infection late in pregnancy or no prenatal care until late in pregnancy	—	20
Mother not tested	8	3
Laboratory error	2	—

[a]Numbers represent percentage of total cases in study.

Modified from Gutman LT. Congenital syphilis. In: Mandell GL, ed. *Atlas of infectious disease. Vol. 5. Sexually transmitted diseases.* Philadelphia: Current Medicine; 1996.

PATHOLOGY

Syphilis often is a lifelong infection that progresses in three clear characteristic stages (Fig. 144.3). After initial invasion occurs through mucous membranes or skin, the organism undergoes rapid multiplication and is disseminated widely. Spread through the perivascular lymphatics and then through the systemic circulation probably occurs even before the clinical development of the primary lesion. Ten to 90 days later, usually within 3 to 4 weeks, the patient manifests an inflammatory response to the infection at the site of the inoculation. The resulting lesion, the chancre, is characterized by the profuse discharge of spirochetes; accumulation of mononuclear leukocytes, lymphocytes, and plasma cells; and swelling of capillary endothelia. The regional lymph nodes are enlarged, and the cellular infiltrate resembles that of the primary lesions. Resolution of the primary lesion occurs by fibrosis.

Secondary lesions develop when tissues of ectodermal origin, such as skin, mucous membranes, and central nervous system (CNS), participate in an inflammatory response. Mucous patches in the mouth are caused by local vasculitis. The cellular infiltrate resembles that of the primary lesion, with the predominance of plasma cells. Little or no necrosis is present, and healing is without scarring but may include pigmentary changes.

Tertiary syphilis may involve any organ system and often is asymmetric. Gummas are lesions typified by extensive necrosis, a few giant cells, and a paucity of organisms. They commonly occur in internal organs, bone, and skin. The other major form of tertiary lesion is a diffuse chronic inflammation, with plasma cells and lymphocytes but without caseation, which may result in an aneurysm of the aorta, paralytic dementia, or tabes dorsalis. Chronic swelling of the capillary endothelium and fibrosis result in the characteristic tissue changes.

Congenital syphilis is a result of hematogenous infection and the disseminated involvement of almost all viscera. The intense inflammatory response occurs in the perivascular framework and interstitial stroma, rather than in the parenchyma.[97] Bone, liver, pancreas, intestine, kidney, and spleen are involved most reproducibly and severely. Other tissues, such as the brain, pituitary gland,[14] lymph nodes, and lungs, also may be infected. The gastrointestinal tract shows a pattern of mononuclear cell infiltration in the mucosa and submucosa, with subsequent widening of the submucosa by the ensuing fibrosis. This event is most prominent in the small bowel. In the kidney, a perivascular inflammation, particularly in the juxtamedullary region, is evident. The basic architecture of the tissue influences the ultimate pattern of involvement. The deposition of collagen around arteries of the spleen produces a typical onionskin appearance. Periosteum and epiphyses are the most affected portions of bone, and syphilitic granulation tissue may interfere with bone formation. Pancreatitis also is observed, with typical inflammation and fibrosis.

The fetus or neonate shows diffuse extramedullary hematopoiesis in many tissues. The placenta of infants with congenital syphilis often is large, thick, and pale. Three histopathologic features commonly are seen: enlarged and hypercellular villi, proliferative fetal vascular changes, and acute and chronic inflammation of the villi.[50,132] Erythroblastosis involving the placenta has been seen more frequently among stillborn infants with congenital syphilis than in live-born infants with or without syphilis.[132]

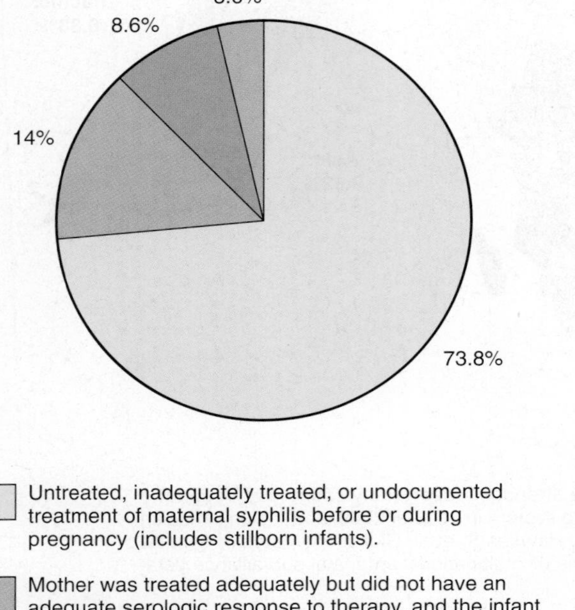

Untreated, inadequately treated, or undocumented treatment of maternal syphilis before or during pregnancy (includes stillborn infants).

Mother was treated adequately but did not have an adequate serologic response to therapy, and the infant was evaluated inadequately for CS.

Mother was treated adequately but did not have an adequate serologic response to therapy, and infant's evaluation revealed signs of CS.

Other

FIG. 144.2 Maternal treatment history of 451 cases of congenital syphilis *(CS)* reported in 2002. (From Centers for Disease Control and Prevention. Congenital syphilis—United States, 2002. *MMWR Morb Mortal Wkly Rep.* 2004;53:716-719.)

Spirochetes may be identified in placental tissue using conventional staining, although they may be difficult to visualize. Nucleic acid amplification methods also have been used to identify *T. pallidum* genome in involved placental specimens.[50] In addition, the umbilical cord may exhibit significant inflammation, with abscess-like foci of necrosis located within Wharton jelly and centered around the umbilical vessels, which is termed *necrotizing funisitis.*[46,133] Macroscopically, the umbilical cord resembles a "barber's pole"; the edematous portions have a spiral striped zone of red and pale blue discoloration, interspersed with streaks of chalky white. Histochemical staining may show spirochetes within the wall of the umbilical vessels. Placental and umbilical cord histopathology should be performed on every case of suspected syphilis.[133]

PATHOGENESIS AND IMMUNE RESPONSE

The host immune response to syphilis is vigorous and is responsible for many of the clinical manifestations seen in the disease. Despite this immune response, the infection may persist for life. In addition, prior infection does not confer resistance to reinfection. Researchers continue to try to explain this contradiction.[107]

Treponemal Virulence–Associated Factors

Virulent *T. pallidum* attaches to host cells during parasitism and is oriented by the proximal hook to the host cell surface. There seems to be a ligand-receptor adherence mechanism involving the treponemal outer membrane proteins. Virulent strains attach to metabolically active mammalian cells, and treponemes are capable of multiplication only during attachment. Fetal and infant cells seem to support treponemal growth maximally, and capillary cells are the prime target of parasitism. Virulent treponemal strains produce hyaluronidase, which may facilitate the perivascular infiltration that is apparent by histopathologic study. These strains also may invade the ground substance that joins capillary endothelial cells.

Virulent *T. pallidum* is coated with fibronectin of host origin. This coating seems to protect the organism from antibody-mediated phagocytosis; allows the organism to adhere to the surface of host phagocytes with only limited ingestion of the organisms; may block complement-mediated lysis of the coated treponemes; and, finally, may allow the treponemes additionally to acquire physiologically active host proteins, such as ceruloplasmin and transferrin, on which they are dependent.[108]

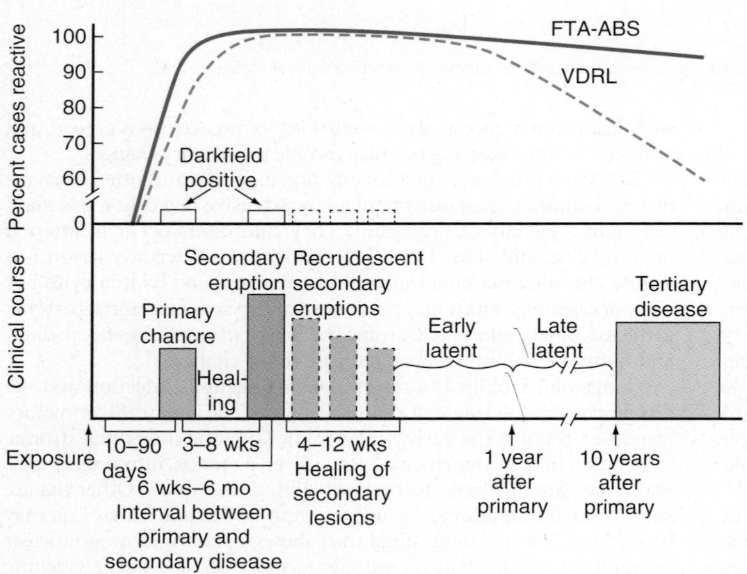

FIG. 144.3 The course of untreated syphilis. *FTA-ABS,* Fluorescent treponemal antibody absorption; *VDRL,* Venereal Disease Research Laboratory.

Host Response

Treponemes seem to persist in extracellular loci with little or no inflammatory response elicited. Polymorphonuclear leukocytes ingest virulent treponemes, incorporate them into phagocytic vacuoles, degranulate, and digest *T. pallidum*. In addition, phagocytosis occurs slowly and is facilitated by the presence of immune serum.[4] Large numbers of treponemes are needed to elicit this response, however, and small numbers may escape recognition.[94] Although there are few surface-exposed transmembrane proteins, one more recently described, Tpr K, seems to act as a porin.[26] It has been shown to elicit an opsonic antibody response in the rabbit model. Variable regions of the protein are explained by diversity in the encoding genes. This antigenic variation could explain the success of the treponeme in evading the host response.[25,78,92] Innate immunity through toll-like receptor 4 is activated by lipoproteins under the outer membrane and may be important in orchestrating the overall immune response to *T. pallidum*.[17,114,123]

Alterations in host cell-mediated immunity occur during primary and secondary stages of syphilis. During early stages of disease, all aspects of cell-mediated immunity, including responses to nonspecific T-cell mitogens, are suppressed. Blastogenesis to treponemal antigens is not demonstrable until late in the course of secondary disease. Natural killer cell activity is increased during early primary syphilis and depressed in secondary and latent syphilis.[64] Some evidence supports the idea that lymphocytes from previously infected animals confer moderate protection to nonimmune animals. In human disease, $CD4^+$ T cells and macrophages predominate in primary chancres, whereas $CD8^+$ cells predominate in secondary syphilis lesions. In primary and secondary syphilis lesions, helper T cell type 1 (Th1) cytokines are present.[110,123,145] Some investigators have suggested that increased apoptosis of peripheral blood lymphocytes and $CD4^+$ cells by a Fas-mediated pathway that occurs during the secondary stage of infection may explain the failure to clear the organism and set up a chronic infection.[39] Alterations in the immune environment of the mother during pregnancy may alter the balance of containment of the organism, allowing transplacental passage to the fetus.[154]

During the initial infection with *T. pallidum,* humoral IgG and IgM antibodies are detectable by the time the chancre appears. In primary syphilis, the main IgG subclass is IgG1, whereas IgG1 and IgG3 predominate in secondary syphilis.[8] If the patient is treated adequately, IgM antibody declines during the next 1 to 2 years, but IgG antibody usually persists through the lifetime of the patient. The stages of syphilis evolve, despite humoral antibody response.

Individuals with untreated syphilis have only a relative resistance to reinfection, so the development of a chancre with reinfection is unusual and probably depends on the challenge inoculum. After reexposure, untreated individuals may develop an increased humoral antibody level.

In individuals who have been treated for syphilis, especially if treatment was provided during the secondary or earlier stages, the protective effect of prior disease is minor, and active disease frequently occurs after reinfection, regardless of whether the patient maintains a reactive nontreponemal antibody test (serofast) or is sero-nonreactive. Patients who have been treated for congenital syphilis also may acquire symptomatic disease.[43,106] Although active or prior syphilis modifies the response of a patient to subsequent reinfection, protection is only relative and is unreliable.

Secondary syphilis and congenital infection may be accompanied by the nephrotic syndrome. The nephrosis characteristically responds rapidly to penicillin, and light microscopy reveals membranous glomerulonephritis with glomerular mesangial cell proliferation. The subendothelial basement membrane deposits contain IgG and C3 or only globulin. Acute syphilitic glomerulonephritis seems to be an immune complex disease.[16,49,67] In infants with congenital syphilis, analysis of circulating immune complexes using immunoblotting methods showed the presence of an 83-kDa *T. pallidum* antigen.[36] Findings have been similar with secondary syphilis.

CLINICAL MANIFESTATIONS

The course of untreated syphilis characteristically progresses through three or four stages over many years. Information on the natural history of untreated syphilis comes primarily from follow-up studies of almost 2000 untreated syphilitic patients who were seen initially between 1891 and 1910 in the clinic of Boeck. The subsequent studies of these patients by Bruusgaard and by other epidemiologists later provided the basis for most of our concepts of the consequences of syphilis. Clark and Danbolt[29] published a summary of some of these studies. Fig. 143.3 depicts some of the characteristics of an untreated course of disease.

Acquired Syphilis

Most recognized syphilitic disease in children is congenital. Acquired syphilis in prepubertal children seldom is reported and is assumed to resemble the clinical course of acquired syphilis in adulthood. Children with acquired syphilis should be assumed to have been infected through contact during child sexual abuse, unless another method of transmission is identified. All patients with syphilis should be tested for HIV infection.[24]

The decision to screen for syphilis during the medical evaluation of a child who is suspected of having been sexually abused should be made on an individual basis. Situations in which screening is recommended include the following: the perpetrator has an STI or is at high risk for having one, such as residing in a community or being of a social setting in which the prevalence of STIs is high; multiple perpetrators are involved; the child is infected with another STI, such as HIV infection, or has physical signs of sexual abuse; STIs have been diagnosed in siblings, other children, or adults in the household; the patient is postpubertal; or screening is a matter of patient or family preference.[11,75,134,135] Darkfield examination of chancre fluid, if present, should be performed, as well as serologic tests at the time of abuse and 6, 12, and 24 weeks later because the initial test may not detect incubating syphilis.

Primary Disease

The chancre of primary syphilis typically is a single reddish lesion, nontender and firm, with a clean surface and raised border. It may be overlooked by women because it frequently is situated on the cervix or vaginal wall. Systemic signs or symptoms are absent, but adjacent lymph nodes frequently are enlarged and nontender. Gutman[54] provides depictions of children with acquired primary syphilis.

Secondary Disease

The patient may experience secondary disease 2 to 10 weeks after the primary lesions manifest. Prominent findings include fever, sore throat, muscle aches, generalized lymphadenopathy, headache, and rash. The palms and soles frequently are involved, in contrast to many other dermatologic conditions. On mucous membranes, the lesions may appear as white mucous patches. Condylomata lata occur around moist areas, such as the anus and vagina. All secondary lesions of the skin and mucous membranes are highly infectious. In their review, Baughn and Musher[9] give a full description of the manifestations of secondary syphilis. Acquired syphilis in early childhood may reveal minimal dermal findings.[1]

Latent Disease

After the clinical signs of secondary disease resolve, the patient enters the stage of latent disease. *Latent syphilis* refers to infection in individuals who have reactive serologic tests for syphilis but no clinical manifestations. The first year after infection is considered *early latent infection,* and the subsequent period is considered *late latent syphilis.* Early latent syphilis originally was classified as syphilis occurring within 4 years of the acquisition of infection, based on the time when mucocutaneous lesions may recur. More recent classification of early latent syphilis is based on the time period of highest communicability, which is in the first year after infection is acquired. Treponemes still can be present in the blood intermittently, however, and pass across the placenta to the fetus during latent syphilis in a pregnant woman.

If the duration of infection with syphilis cannot be determined, the disease is classified as syphilis of unknown duration; clinical management and treatment should be the same as that for late latent infection. If therapy for syphilis is given first during the latent stage, the patient is unlikely to show regression of nontreponemal antibody determinations. Approximately 60% of untreated patients in the late latent stage continue to have an asymptomatic course, whereas 30% to 40% develop symptoms of late or tertiary disease. Progression of disease from late latent to late symptomatic syphilis usually is prevented if appropriate antimicrobial therapy is given at this stage. The reader is referred to the article by Gutman[54] for depictions of children with acquired secondary syphilis.

Tertiary Disease

Three to 10 years after the last evidence of secondary disease has occurred, the patient may develop nonprogressive, localized nodules of the dermal elements or supporting structures of the body, called *gummas*. These nodules are granulomatous and can have central necrosis. Because these lesions are relatively quiescent, the term *benign tertiary syphilis* often is used. Spirochetes are extremely sparse or absent. The gummatous reaction is primarily a pronounced immunologic reaction of the host.

Neurosyphilis

During the early stage of syphilis, approximately one-third of all patients have involvement of the CNS. If untreated, only half of these patients develop late neurosyphilis. The interval between primary disease and late neurosyphilis usually is more than 5 years. Of the few children recognized to have acquired (vs. congenital) late neurosyphilis, several have developed symptomatic disease at a very early age. It is possible that the disease progresses more rapidly in children than in adults.

Late neurosyphilis may be asymptomatic or, if symptomatic, may occur in a variety of ways. Classic presentations include paralytic dementia, tabes dorsalis, amyotrophic lateral sclerosis, meningovascular syphilis, seizures, optic atrophy, and gummatous changes of the cord. Neurosyphilis may resemble virtually any other neurologic disease.

Cardiovascular Syphilis

Ten to 40 years after having primary syphilis, an untreated patient may develop signs of cardiovascular involvement. Most frequently involved are the great vessels of the heart, where syphilitic aortic and pulmonary arteritis develop. One complication of this development is aortic regurgitation. The inflammatory reaction also may cause stenosis of the coronary ostia, with resulting angina, myocardial insufficiency, and death.

Syphilis in Pregnancy

Pregnancy has no known effect on the clinical course of syphilis. Untreated syphilis can affect profoundly the outcome of the pregnancy, however, resulting in spontaneous abortion, stillbirth, nonimmune hydrops fetalis,[6,18] premature delivery, perinatal death, or two characteristic syndromes of congenital disease, early and late congenital syphilis (see later discussion).[53,125] The outcome of untreated fetal infection varies. Intrauterine death occurs in an estimated 25% of infections, with abortion usually occurring after the first trimester. Perinatal death may occur in another 25% to 30% of untreated infected infants.[97] In a study of the perinatal outcome of congenital syphilis, the fatality rate was 464 per 1000 infected births. Of the fatalities, 27% were neonatal deaths and 73% were stillbirths.[121] Currently, most infected infants, if not hydropic at birth, survive the neonatal period, most likely because of early identification and treatment of infected infants and improved neonatal care.

The investigations of Taber and Huber[143] illustrate the importance in pregnant women of recognition of the disease and administration of appropriate therapy. In this study, 22 women with syphilis were undiagnosed during pregnancy and did not receive prenatal therapy. Eleven infants were followed without initial therapy. At delivery, all were asymptomatic clinically, four had a reactive Venereal Disease Research Laboratory (VDRL) test, five had a nonreactive VDRL test, and two were not tested. All these infants were readmitted with obvious disease involving multisystem infection, three with proven spirochetal hepatitis, two with nephrotic syndrome, and three with CNS involvement. This experience emphasizes the importance of recognition of transmission of infection late in gestation, leading to delivery of infants who are well clinically but whose disease emerges in the weeks after delivery if untreated.[38]

Congenital Syphilis

At the onset of congenital syphilis, *T. pallidum* is liberated directly into the circulation of the fetus, resulting in spirochetemia with widespread dissemination. The clinical, laboratory, and radiographic abnormalities of congenital syphilis are a consequence of active infection with *T. pallidum* and the resultant inflammatory response induced in various body organs and tissues. The severity of these manifestations varies and can range from overwhelming involvement of multiple organs and body systems, as is seen in fetal hydrops, to only laboratory or radiographic abnormalities. Most of the infants born to mothers with untreated syphilis seem completely normal at birth and have no clinical or laboratory evidence of infection at birth. These infants may develop manifestations of disease several months to years later if left untreated.[28] The signs and symptoms of congenital syphilis are divided arbitrarily into early manifestations, which appear in the first 2 years of life, and late manifestations, which emerge at any time thereafter, usually near puberty.

Early Congenital Syphilis

The abnormal physical and laboratory findings in early congenital syphilis are varied and unpredictable.[115] Table 144.3 lists the major physical and laboratory findings from 310 reported cases of early congenital syphilis.[33,67,77,103,121,143] These results undoubtedly are minimal rates for each finding. The onset occurs between birth and approximately 3 months of age, with most cases occurring within the first 5 weeks of life.

Skeletal system. Bone involvement is the most common manifestation of congenital syphilis, occurring in 60% to 80% of infants with clinical signs of syphilis. In addition, it may be the only abnormality seen in infants born to mothers with untreated syphilis. Because of their frequency and early appearance, the radiographic changes in the bones, termed *osteochondritis* and *periostitis,* are of diagnostic value.[33] The femur and humerus are involved most often. Radiographically, accumulating calcified matrix is seen at the epiphyseal margin, which may be smooth or serrated. The serrated appearance is known as *Wegner sign* and represents points of calcified cartilage along the nutrient cartilage canal.

A zone of rarefaction at the metaphysis that represents syphilitic granulation tissue containing a few scattered calcified remnants and a mass of connective tissue containing areas of perivascular infiltration of small round cells may be seen. Irregular areas of increased density and rarefaction produce the moth-eaten appearance of the radiograph. The demineralization and osseous destruction of the upper medial tibial metaphysis are called *Wimberger sign.* Previously thought to be specific for syphilis, Wimberger sign also may occur in osteomyelitis and hyperparathyroidism. Epiphyseal separation may occur as a result of a fracture of the brittle layer of calcified cartilage. Irregular periosteal thickening also is a common finding. The changes usually are present at birth but may appear in the first few weeks of life. The bony changes are self-limited and usually are healed in the first 6 months, even in the absence of specific therapy. They may be painful lesions, and pain on motion often leads an affected infant to appear to have a limb paralysis, termed *pseudoparalysis of Parrot.*

TABLE 144.3 Findings in 310 Cases of Early Congenital Syphilis

Findings	No. Patients
Hepatomegaly	100
Skeletal abnormalities	91
Birth weight <2500 g	51
Skin lesions	45
Hyperbilirubinemia	40
Pneumonia	51
Splenomegaly	56
Severe anemia, hydrops, edema	50
Snuffles, nasal discharge	27
Painful limbs	22
Pancreatitis	14
Cerebrospinal fluid abnormalities	21
Nephritis	11
Failure to thrive	10
Testicular mass	1
Chorioretinitis	1
Hypoglobulinemia	1

Data from references 41, 76, 89, 91, 95–98.

Rhinitis. Rhinitis, coryza, or snuffles are likely to mark the onset of congenital syphilis. Usually, it appears in the first week of life and seldom later than the third month. The snuffles are more severe and persist longer than the common cold. The nasal discharge is white and often bloody, and the snuffles frequently are associated with laryngitis. Secondary bacterial superinfection may result in a purulent appearance. The nasal discharge is teeming with spirochetes and should be examined by darkfield microscopy to confirm its diagnosis.

Rash. The syphilitic rash usually appears 1 to 2 weeks after rhinitis manifests. The typical eruption is maculopapular and consists of small spots that are dark red-copper. If the rash is present at birth, it often is widely disseminated and bullous and is called *pemphigus syphiliticus.* It is most severe on the hands and feet. The bullous fluid contains many spirochetes. The rash erupts slowly, taking 1 to 3 weeks, and is followed by desquamation and crusting. As the rash fades, the lesions become coppery or dusky red, and pigmentation may persist. The reader is referred to the article by Gutman[54] for depictions of a variety of cutaneous manifestations of early congenital syphilis.

Fissures and mucous patches. Fissures and mucous patches are not seen often but are highly characteristic features of congenital syphilis. The fissures develop around the lips, nares, and anus. They bleed readily and heal with scarring. A cluster of scars radiating around the mouth is called *rhagades* and is a characteristic of late congenital syphilis. Mucous patches may be found on any of the mucous membranes, especially in the mouth and genitalia. Condylomata lata are raised, moist lesions appearing on areas of the skin where there is moisture or friction. They are highly infectious because they contain many spirochetes.

Hematologic findings. Congenital syphilis is characterized by anemia, thrombocytopenia, hemolytic processes, and leukopenia and leukocytosis.[77] The hemolytic process is Coombs test negative and often accompanied by cryoglobulinemia, immune complex formation, and macroglobulinemia. The hemolysis, similar to the liver disease, is refractory to therapy and may persist for weeks. Paroxysmal nocturnal hemoglobinuria is a late manifestation of congenital syphilis.

Central nervous system involvement. In the era before the introduction of penicillin therapy, approximately 15% of infants with congenital syphilis developed manifestations of meningovascular disease. These findings included meningitis, meningeal irritation, bulging fontanelle, cranial nerve palsies, seizures, and hydrocephalus.[61] In addition, involvement of the pituitary gland in congenital syphilis is a common manifestation, occurring in approximately 40% of autopsy cases,[103] and consists of interstitial inflammation and fibrosis with formation of gumma in the anterior lobe. Clinical disease in affected infants is manifested by persistent hypoglycemia and diabetes insipidus.[34,101]

Most infants infected with *T. pallidum* are completely symptom free, and involvement of the CNS is inferred from abnormalities of the cerebrospinal fluid (CSF), such as reactivity on a VDRL test, pleocytosis, and elevated protein content. Because of the wide range of normal values for CSF protein, red blood cells, and white blood cells in the neonatal period, defining the proportion of infants with congenital syphilis who have abnormalities of these laboratory values has been difficult. Current consensus identifies an abnormal CSF white blood cell count in infants being evaluated for possible congenital syphilis as greater than 25 cells/mm^3 and protein as greater than 150 mg/dL (>170 mg/dL if infant is premature). A reactive CSF VDRL test is considered to be specific for neurosyphilis in older children and adults. In neonates, the significance of a reactive CSF VDRL test is suspect, however, because maternal nontreponemal IgG antibodies can pass from maternal serum to fetal and neonatal serum and then diffuse into the CSF. Children may fail to have a reactive VDRL test on initial examination and still develop later signs of neurosyphilis.

Using rabbit infectivity testing, which involves the inoculation of CSF into rabbits to determine the presence of the spirochete in the CSF specimen, Michelow and coworkers[91] found that invasion of the CNS with *T. pallidum* occurs in 41% of infants who have clinical, laboratory, or radiographic abnormalities of congenital syphilis. None of these infants had clinical signs of neurologic disease. Compared with isolation of spirochetes in CSF by rabbit inoculation, the sensitivity and specificity in CSF of a reactive VDRL test, elevated white blood cell count, and elevated protein were 54% and 90%, 38% and 88%, and 56% and 78%, respectively. These investigators also documented CNS infection in three infants who had normal CSF studies. Using current methods, the best indicator of CNS infection in neonates is an abnormal evaluation consisting of abnormal findings on physical examination, anemia, thrombocytopenia, CSF abnormalities, and abnormal bone radiographs. A normal evaluation renders CNS infection rare.

Pneumonia. Syphilitic pneumonia is a common occurrence in congenital syphilis, particularly in developing countries. The classic radiographic appearance is one of complete opacification of both lung fields and is termed *pneumonia alba.* More commonly today, a fluffy, diffuse infiltrate involving all lung areas is seen on the chest radiograph. At autopsy, pneumonia alba consists of a focal obliterative fibrosis with scarring and thickening of alveolar walls and loss of alveolar spaces. Follow-up evaluation of children who have recovered from congenital syphilis has shown that at least 10% may have chronic pulmonary disease, particularly if they were premature and required mechanical ventilation.

Hepatosplenomegaly. Hepatomegaly is the most common clinical sign in congenital syphilis. Its occurrence in the fetus has been documented by ultrasonography, and it may be a marker of inadequate treatment of the fetal infection despite maternal treatment during pregnancy.[58] Hepatosplenomegaly often is caused by extramedullary hematopoiesis. Hepatomegaly may occur in the absence of splenomegaly; but in contrast to congenital cytomegalovirus, the reverse does not. Neonatal syphilitic hepatitis is associated with visible spirochetes on biopsy specimens of liver tissue, jaundice, and cholestasis. Aspartate aminotransferase, alkaline phosphatase, and alanine aminotransferase determinations often are elevated, and direct hyperbilirubinemia is a common finding. The prothrombin time may be delayed. The liver disease often resolves slowly, even after administration of apparently adequate therapy, and may be exacerbated by penicillin therapy before improving.[131]

Ectodermal changes. Ectodermal changes in syphilitic infants include suppuration and exfoliation of the nails, loss of hair and eyebrows, choroiditis, and iritis.

Other findings. Other clinical manifestations of congenital syphilis include nonimmune fetal hydrops, possibly intrauterine growth restriction, generalized lymphadenopathy, fever, failure to thrive, nephrotic syndrome, and myocarditis. Involvement of the eyes has been manifested by chorioretinitis, cataract, glaucoma, and chancre of the eyelid. Gastrointestinal presentations include rectal bleeding caused by syphilitic ileitis, necrotizing enterocolitis, malabsorption secondary to fibrosis of the gastrointestinal tract, and fetal bowel dilation seen on antenatal ultrasonography.[116,121] Some children with symptomatic congenital syphilis also may have sepsis caused by other bacteria, including *Escherichia coli,* group B streptococci, and *Yersinia* spp. Neonates and infants with congenital syphilis may resemble infants with other illnesses peculiar to neonates, including toxoplasmosis, rubella, cytomegalovirus infection, herpes simplex virus infection, "sepsis" of the newborn, blood group incompatibilities, battered child syndrome, "periostitis" of prematurity, neonatal hepatitis, and osteomyelitis.

Late Congenital Syphilis

Late manifestations or stigmata of congenital syphilis are the result of scarring from the early systemic disease or reactions to persistent inflammation and include involvement of the teeth, bones, eyes, and eighth cranial nerve; gummas in the viscera, skin, or mucous membranes; and neurosyphilis (Table 144.4).[45] Approximately 40% of surviving and untreated infected infants, as reported in the early literature, develop late manifestations of infection. Some of these changes can be prevented by treating the mother during pregnancy or the infant before the child reaches 3 months of age. In contrast, treatment of 15 children at 4 months of age or later showed seven with dental changes.[111] Other stigmata (e.g., keratitis, saber shins) may occur or progress, despite the infants being administered appropriate therapy. Nonspecific sequelae of congenital syphilis have not been described well because follow-up studies of children with congenital syphilis are minimal. It has been the experience of one of the authors (P.J.S.), however, that infants who are diagnosed with congenital syphilis and treated appropriately in the neonatal period generally do well at least through early childhood. There is every reason to be hopeful and optimistic with the families of these children, even if they are symptomatic and have CNS involvement at the time of diagnosis.

TABLE 144.4 Stigmata of Late Congenital Syphilis[a]

Stigmata	Percentage of Total Patients
Frontal boss of Parrott	87
Short maxilla	84
High palatal arch	76
Hutchinson triad	75
Higouménakis sign	73
Relative protuberance of mandible	65
Saddle nose	63
Interstitial keratitis	39
Rhagades	26
Mulberry molars	9
Saber shin	7
Eighth nerve deafness	4
Hutchinson teeth	3
Scaphoid scapulae	0.7
Clutton joint	0.3

[a]Analysis of 271 patients.
Modified from Fiumara NJ, Lessell S. Manifestations of late congenital syphilis. *Arch Dermatol.* 1970;102:78-83.

Dentition. Characteristic changes are found in the permanent upper central incisors, which have a notched appearance of the biting edges; radiographic study leads to diagnosis, even while deciduous teeth are in place. These are Hutchinson teeth, which also are small and hypoplastic and widely spaced with abnormal enamelization. If first molars show maldevelopment of the cusps, the finding is called *mulberry* or *moon molars.*

Interstitial keratitis. Interstitial keratitis is the most common late lesion. It may appear at any age between 4 and 30 years or later but characteristically appears when the patient is close to puberty. A ground-glass appearance may develop in the cornea, accompanied by vascularization of the adjacent sclera. These changes become bilateral and usually lead to blindness. It has been seen in adolescent patients despite their having received previous and appropriate penicillin therapy during infancy. At the time of its occurrence, keratitis is not affected by penicillin therapy, but it may respond transiently to corticosteroid treatment.

Central nervous system. The same manifestations of neurosyphilis seen in acquired syphilis may occur in congenital syphilis. Paresis is seen more frequently and tabes dorsalis less frequently in the congenital form than in the acquired form of the disease. Cranial nerve palsies and optic atrophy are prominent.

Eighth cranial nerve deafness. Hearing loss usually is sudden and occurs when the child reaches 8 to 10 years of age. It often accompanies interstitial keratitis. The constellation of eighth cranial nerve deafness, interstitial keratitis, and Hutchinson teeth is called the *Hutchinson triad.* The hearing loss usually involves the higher frequencies, and normal conversational tones become affected later. This hearing loss may respond to long-term corticosteroid treatment.

Bone and joint changes. Bone changes include the sclerosing lesions, saber shin, and frontal bossing, which are sequelae of periostitis that involved the frontal bone and tibia. Periosteal reaction of the sternoclavicular portion of the clavicle may lead to swelling, known as the Higouménakis sign. The gummatous or destructive lesions include saddle-nose deformity, which occurs as a sequela of rhinitis. Perforation of the hard palate is almost pathognomonic of congenital syphilis. Clutton joints are uncommon findings and represent painless arthritis of the knees and, rarely, other joints.

Cutaneous lesions. Rhagades represent scars resulting from persistent rhinitis during infancy and rarely are seen today.

DIAGNOSIS

The vagaries of the maternal history and signs or lack of signs in the infant at birth (i.e., timing of the mother's initial syphilis infection before or during pregnancy, adequacy and documentation of her treatment, an infant who is infected and symptomatic at birth, an infant who is asymptomatic at birth but may not remain so because infection has occurred, and an infant who is asymptomatic and not infected) demand a "safety first" approach to diagnosis and treatment. Efforts to diagnose infectious syphilis suffer from the lack of a method to culture the organisms on laboratory media. Methods that are used in establishing the diagnosis of syphilis include (1) direct visualization of the organism by darkfield microscopy or fluorescent antibody technique of infected fluids or lesions, (2) demonstration of the organism by special stains on histopathologic examination of tissue,[56,119] (3) animal inoculation (rabbit infectivity test), (4) demonstration of serologic reactions typical of syphilis, and (5) detection of *T. pallidum* DNA in a clinical specimen.[20]

The rabbit infectivity test is still the gold standard for the identification of viable *T. pallidum* in clinical specimens, having a sensitivity of less than 10 organisms.[84,85] It involves intratesticular inoculation of the specimen into a rabbit and awaiting serologic seroconversion and orchitis with subsequent visualization of motile spirochetes by darkfield microscopy in testicular tissue. The rabbit infectivity test is performed only in research laboratories and may take several months for identification of the organism. *T. pallidum* DNA has been detected by polymerase chain reaction (PCR) in body fluids such as amniotic fluid and infant blood, CSF, and endotracheal aspirate.[52,91] The new genetic information about *T. pallidum* may lead to development of novel diagnostic tools.

In the clinical setting, the diagnosis of syphilis is established by visualization of the spirochete by darkfield microscopy or special staining and serology. Patients with a primary syphilis lesion (chancre) and with active secondary lesions may be diagnosed by darkfield microscopy. Because this diagnosis depends on direct visualization of motile spirochetes, the organisms must be active and viable. Prior use of many antibiotics rapidly destroys the motility of the organisms, as do many topical disinfectants. Serous fluid from the base of the lesion should be collected for darkfield examination. Syphilitic lesions of the mouth may harbor indigenous treponemes, of which the morphologic similarity to pathogenic species can confuse the interpretation of findings.

Direct darkfield examination is particularly helpful in establishing a diagnosis early in the course of the disease, before the development of seroreactivity. If a darkfield microscope is unavailable, a direct fluorescent antibody stain for *T. pallidum* may be made.[18] Exudate is collected in capillary tubes or slides and stained with specific antibody. Amniotic fluid may be examined for the presence of spirochetes using darkfield microscopy or fluorescent antitreponemal staining; the finding of spirochetes may be a marker for more severe fetal disease.[51,148] On a practical basis, however, the diagnosis is established by serologic methods.[81,150]

Serologic Tests

The two types of serologic tests for syphilis are the nontreponemal antibody tests and the treponemal antibody tests (Table 144.5). Although the latter tests indicate experience with a treponemal infection in the past, they cross-react with the antigens of other treponemal diseases, such as the antigens causing yaws and pinta. No test is specific for syphilis, and no test is completely sensitive. Efforts to produce a more sensitive and more specific test are continuous. A promising approach is the use of recombinant clones expressing immunogenic proteins of *T. pallidum* to investigate pathogen-specific antigens.[63] Some of these products are being investigated for use as diagnostic material.[127]

Point of care testing is becoming a feasible reality for low resource settings, usually linked to HIV testing using immunochromatographic strips. These tests can be done during antenatal visits, do not require the laboratory infrastructure necessary for conventional tests, and can be performed on fingerstick blood samples. They are easy to perform, results are easily interpreted, and there is a quick turnaround time of 20 minutes or so. They have good sensitivity and specificity, comparable to those of conventional treponemal and nontreponemal tests.[15,74]

Nontreponemal Tests

The original test for syphilis, as described by Wassermann, used syphilitic tissue as complement-fixing antigen to detect the presence of antibody

TABLE 144.5 **Standard Serologic Tests for Syphilis**

		SENSITIVITY BY STAGE OF INFECTION (%)				
Type	**Test**	***Primary***	***Secondary***	***Latent***	***Late/Tertiary***	**Specificity (%)**
Nontreponemal						
Extracts of tissue (cardiolipin-lecithin-cholesterol)	VDRL	78	100	96	71	98
	RPR	86	100	98	73	98
Treponemal						
Treponema pallidum	MHA-TP[a]	76	100	97	94	99
	FTA-ABS	84	100	100	96	97
	EIA	100	100	100	-	99
	CIA	98	100	100	100	99

[a]MHA-TP has been replaced with *Treponema pallidum* particle agglutination (TP-PA) test.
CIA, Chemiluminescence immunoassay; *EIA,* enzyme immunoassay; *FTA-ABS,* fluorescent treponemal antibody absorption; *MHA-TP,* microhemagglutination assay–*Treponema pallidum; RPR,* rapid plasma reagin; *VDRL,* Venereal Disease Research Laboratory.
Modified from Seña AC, White BL, Sparling PF. Novel *Treponema pallidum* serologic tests: a paradigm shift in syphilis screening for the 21st century. *Clin Infect Dis.* 2010;51(6):700-708.

(reagin) that is induced by *T. pallidum.* Extracts of other normal tissue, such as beef heart, had similar properties, and purification and standardization of these materials led to the use as antigen of a preparation containing cardiolipin and lecithin in cholesterol.

Two tests currently using cardiolipin, lecithin, and cholesterol are the VDRL and rapid plasma reagin (RPR) tests. These tests measure mostly IgG, but also IgM antibodies nondiscriminatively. The tests provide similar clinical information and have similar advantages. The RPR titer often is one to two dilutions higher than the titer obtained using the VDRL test, so caution must be exercised when making clinical decisions on the basis of results obtained from these two tests performed on the same patient. Both are inexpensive to perform and show increasing and decreasing antibody titers that often correlate with adequacy of therapy and the clinical status of a patient. A fourfold increase in RPR or VDRL titers indicates active disease, whereas a fourfold decrease suggests adequate therapy. Disadvantages include a high proportion of biologic acute and chronic false-positive reactors and an increasing proportion of false-negative reactions in the later stages of untreated syphilis. The main technical difficulty is a negative reaction owing to the prozone phenomenon, which occurs in 1% to 2% of individuals, usually patients with secondary syphilis, and is due to an excess amount of reagin antibody present in the patient's undiluted serum that prevents flocculation. Diluting the serum sample before testing overcomes the inhibition and results in the positive reaction. Because the RPR test generally is more sensitive than is the VDRL test, it is preferred for screening pregnant women. The VDRL test is recommended for use on CSF, however.

The RPR test is used frequently to screen pregnant women for possible infection with *T. pallidum.* Transplacental passage of IgG antibodies to the infant means that mothers with reactive RPR tests usually transmit these antibodies to their infants. Taber and Huber[90] reviewed the relationship of maternal to newborn VDRL tests in their study of mothers who were undiagnosed and untreated. Although 12 of 22 mothers had VDRL test results two to four times that of their infants, 6 of these women and their infants had nonreactive serology at the time of delivery. These and other data showed that it was unusual for an infant to have a VDRL test of greater titer than the mother's, even if the infant was incubating congenital syphilis.[139] Nonetheless, the finding of a titer in the infant serum fourfold higher than that seen in the maternal serum when both are obtained at the same time is indicative of active infection in the infant. Even if the infant is asymptomatic, a 10-day course of penicillin therapy should be administered.

Treponemal Tests

The most significant development of the past 4 decades in the serologic study of syphilis was the detection of treponemal antibody by fluorescein-labeled antihuman antibody and indirect agglutination. These tests are used to confirm the validity of a positive nontreponemal test and to diagnose late stages of syphilis. The tests are sensitive and reliable. More recently, newer versions of these tests, such as the *T. pallidum* enzyme immunoassay (TP-EIA) and chemiluminescence immunoassay (CIA), have been automated, enhancing simplicity and ease of use. As a result, the TP-EIA and CIA tests are increasingly used to screen for syphilis rather than as confirmatory tests with a reversal in the order of testing so that a positive treponemal immunoassay test requires confirmation using the nontreponemal tests (reverse sequence screening).[130]

The advantages and disadvantages of this reversal of the usual testing algorithm and how it is being used in the WHO elimination of mother to child transmission of syphilis is well summarized in a recent review.[74]

Fluorescent treponemal antibody absorption (FTA-ABS) tests use lyophilized Nichols strain organisms as antigen and measure IgG and IgM antibodies. Antigen is fixed to a slide, and the test serum is applied, allowing reaction of antitreponemal antibody with antigen to occur. The slide is layered with fluorescein isothiocyanate–labeled antihuman gamma globulin, and the presence or absence of antibody is determined by fluorescent microscopy.

Test sera are preabsorbed with sorbent to eliminate group-reactive antibody. The test is rendered specific for disease with virulent treponemal species, usually *T. pallidum.* The FTA-ABS test is expensive and time-consuming, however. It is recommended not for general screening but for confirmation of positive nontreponemal tests and for establishing the diagnosis of later stages of syphilis in which the results of nontreponemal tests may be negative.

Microhemagglutination tests, and specifically the *T. pallidum* particle agglutination (TP-PA) test, depend on the passive hemagglutination of erythrocytes or latex particles that have been sensitized with Nichols strain *T. pallidum.* The test has been automated and is easy to perform technically and inexpensively. The TP-PA test has largely replaced the FTA-ABS test as the most efficient specific test for antibody to *T. pallidum.* The TP-PA test is as sensitive as is the FTA-ABS test, except in primary syphilis. The test is positive in 75% to 85% of patients with primary syphilis and in 100% of patients with secondary syphilis. Similar to the FTA-ABS test, the TP-PA test is unlikely to revert to a nonreactive state after treatment of the patient, unless treatment is given very early.

IgM Tests

In the diagnosis of congenital syphilis, having a means to differentiate between passive transplacental transfer of maternal antibody to the fetus and production by the fetus of endogenous antitreponemal antibody would be most helpful. Because antibodies of the IgM class do not cross the placenta, detection of IgM antibody in the fetal or neonatal serum would indicate antibody production by the fetus because of active fetal infection. No IgM assay currently is commercially available that is sufficiently sensitive and specific to recommend for routine use in the evaluation of infants born to mothers with syphilis. The fluorescent treponemal antibody that measures IgM antitreponemal antibodies, the IgM-FTA-ABS test, has been associated with false-positive and false-negative results. When the test was refined further by use of the IgM fraction of neonatal serum only, it had a sensitivity of 73%.[141] The test also is insensitive when the onset of disease is delayed. Occasional false-positive IgM-FTA-ABS tests occur because of the presence of an IgM anti-IgG antibody or rheumatoid factor. For these reasons, the CDC has recommended that the IgM-FTA-ABS test be suspended for diagnostic testing of neonates, and the test is available only as a provisional test.

Efforts to develop a sensitive and specific serologic test for congenital syphilis have led to the identification of antigenic components of *T. pallidum* that are epitopes for the immune response. A 34-kDa membrane protein is a dipoprotein[142] and the target of IgM antibody formation in the sera of some congenitally infected infants.[37] The Captia Syphilis-M test is an enzyme-linked immunosorbent assay that uses this treponemal protein; it is commercially available but showed a sensitivity of only 88% among infants with clinical and laboratory findings of congenital syphilis.[79,141]

Immunoblotting has been used to characterize the specific neonatal IgM antibody responses to *T. pallidum*. Specific IgM antibodies directed against *T. pallidum* antigens with apparent molecular masses of 72, 47, 45, 42, 37, 17, and 15 kDa have been detected in sera of fetuses[60] and infants with clinical findings of congenital syphilis and in 20% to 40% of asymptomatic infants born to mothers with untreated syphilis.[37,82,90,124,126,127] IgM reactivity against the 47-kDa antigen, a membrane lipoprotein of the organism, has been the most consistent finding. Similar reactivities also have been seen in CSF of infants with congenital syphilis.[82,126] One study showed that a reactive serum IgM immunoblot identified all 17 infants in whom spirochetes were detected in their CSF by rabbit infectivity testing.[90] Efforts to develop rapid diagnostic tests have been based on these findings.[75] In addition, immunoblotting has been used to detect similar IgA reactivities among infants with congenital syphilis.[126]

Polymerase Chain Reaction Assay

The PCR assay has been used on neonatal blood and CSF for establishing the diagnosis of congenital syphilis.[52,91,127] Compared with isolation of the organism by rabbit infectivity testing, the sensitivity and specificity of PCR on CSF was 65% to 71% and 97% to 100%, respectively.[91,124] Among 17 infants who had spirochetes detected in their CSF by rabbit inoculation, blood PCR test was the best predictor of CNS infection with *T. pallidum*.[91] This finding supports further the concept that spirochetes gain access to the CNS by a hematogenous route. Further research is needed on PCR assays that will reliably detect *T. pallidum* DNA in neonatal clinical specimens.

False-Positive Reactions

All of the available serologic tests for syphilis produce occasional reactive results in patients who have no other evidence of syphilitic infection. These reactions usually are called *biologic false-positive* (BFP) reactions and are distinct from positive reactions owing to technical errors. Most BFP reactions occur with nontreponemal tests; approximately 1% of normal adults have a BFP reaction by nontreponemal antigen tests. These reactions probably are more common in pregnant women than in the general population. Reaginic antibody is reactive with at least 200 antigens other than those of *T. pallidum*, and although the specific stimulus for this antibody in syphilis and other diseases is unknown, it may represent antibody to cellular lipoidal antigens of the host that are liberated during various diseases. For clinical purposes, BFP reactions may be classified as acute, in which the reactivity resolves within 6 months, or chronic, in which reactivity is persistent.

Acute biologic false-positive reactions. Most BFP reactions are detected by nontreponemal tests and occur in patients with other acute illnesses, especially pneumonia, hepatitis, and viral exanthematous disease, or after receiving vaccinations. The prognosis for the patient's health is not affected by the finding. The titer of antibody usually is low (<1:8), and in most instances the FTA-ABS or TP-PA test is nonreactive. Approximately two-thirds of patients with BFP reactions have acute reactions, and reactivity subsides within 6 months.

Chronic biologic false-positive reactions. Many patients with chronic BFP reactions have or develop systemic disease. Drug addiction, chronic hepatitis, old age, leprosy, and collagen vascular disease, especially systemic lupus erythematosus, are associated highly with chronic BFP reactions. A familial predisposition to this finding may exist. The antibody detected by the VDRL test in chronic BFP reactions predominantly is IgM, whereas it mainly is IgG in syphilis. Patients with chronic BFP reactions and systemic lupus erythematosus commonly also have a reactive FTA-ABS test.[80] The triosephosphate isomerase test may be helpful in the differential diagnosis in these instances. A finding of particular concern is that there seems to be a relative increase in acute and chronic BFP reactions in women who are infected with HIV.

Screening with EIA/CIA treponemal tests has resulted in some individuals having a reactive EIA/CIA test but a nonreactive nontreponemal test. If the individual does not have a history of adequately treated syphilis, a second treponemal test (TP-PA preferred) should be performed, and if it is negative, the positive EIA/CIA is more likely to represent a false-positive test.

Evaluation and Diagnosis of Early Congenital Syphilis

The diagnosis of congenital syphilis is suggested by results of serologic tests, physical examination, laboratory tests including CSF examination, and radiographs of long bones and is established by the observation of spirochetes in body fluids or tissue. Examination of the placenta or umbilical cord using specific fluorescent antitreponemal antibody staining is recommended.[50,112] The decision to evaluate and ultimately to treat an infant for congenital syphilis is based on clinical, serologic, and epidemiologic considerations. The evaluation includes an assessment of the mother for general risk factors for increased rates of syphilis (Box 144.3), followed by an evaluation of the mother's current known serologic status (Box 144.4). If the mother has been treated, the clinician must assess the adequacy of the therapy.

BOX 144.3 General Maternal Risk Factors Associated With Increased Rates of Early Syphilis in Pregnancy

- Infection with HIV
- Adolescent or unmarried status
- History of sexually transmitted disease
- Substance abuse, especially cocaine
- Inadequate or absent prenatal care
- Prostitution or promiscuity
- Localized populations or geographic areas
- Treatment of gonorrhea with ciprofloxacin or spectinomycin
- Poor communication among medical personnel regarding maternal/infant status

Data from references 42, 46, 48, and 49.

BOX 144.4 Components of Epidemiologic Evaluation of a Mother for Possible Syphilis That Aid in Evaluation and Treatment of Her Infant

- Evaluate mother for prior history of syphilis or major risk factors for syphilis (see Box 144.3).
- If mother received treatment for syphilis, evaluate course of therapy for adequacy in the treatment of congenital syphilis (see Box 144.2).
- Evaluate current maternal status with a nontreponemal test (e.g., Venereal Disease Research Laboratory, rapid plasma reagin) and, if reactive, a treponemal test (e.g., fluorescent treponemal antibody absorption, *Treponema pallidum* particle agglutination test).
- If mother is identified clinically or through contact tracing as having early syphilis during the 3 months after delivery, reevaluate the infant and consider therapy at that time.
- Higher maternal titers to nontreponemal tests are associated with failure of maternal therapy to prevent congenital disease.[89]
- Unknown duration of maternal syphilis is associated with failure of maternal therapy to prevent congenital disease.[89]

If the mother's serologic assays have been positive, the infant must be assessed for clinically apparent disease. The nontreponemal (RPR) and treponemal (TP-PA; EIA) tests measure IgG antibody and do not distinguish disease of the infant from maternally derived antibody. Many infants are born to women who have had syphilis in the past, received therapy, and remained seroreactive. Their infants also are seroreactive. Ensuring that the infant does not have congenital disease in the immediate neonatal period may be impossible.

Fig. 144.3 and Table 144.6 present an approach to the evaluation of infants born to mothers with reactive serologic tests for syphilis. Testing of all pregnant women with syphilis for coinfection with HIV is recommended strongly, even though infants born to coinfected mothers do not require any different evaluation for syphilis.[79] All infants born to mothers with reactive serologic tests for syphilis should have a serum quantitative nontreponemal test performed and a thorough physical examination that focuses on finding evidence of congenital syphilis. The nontreponemal test that is performed on the infant should be the same as the test done on the mother to be able to compare serologic titers. Although it is an uncommon finding, a serum quantitative nontreponemal titer that is fourfold or greater than the corresponding maternal titer is diagnostic of congenital syphilis; when it has occurred, one of the authors (P.J.S.) has isolated spirochetes from blood or CSF in all infants.

The CDC recommends that the infant's serologic test be performed on serum and not umbilical cord blood because false-positive test results have been reported with the use of umbilical cord blood secondary to contamination of the specimen with maternal blood and Wharton jelly. Some clinicians continue to use umbilical cord blood, however, because it is readily available and easily collected; appropriate care should be taken during collection to minimize contamination with maternal blood. In addition, false-negative test results may occur when the maternal titer is low dilution, which argues for maternal screening rather than screening of infant serum.

Infants who have (1) an abnormal physical examination that is consistent with congenital syphilis, (2) a serum quantitative nontreponemal serologic titer that is fourfold or greater than the mother's, or (3) a positive darkfield or fluorescent antibody test of body fluid should have a complete blood cell count and platelet count performed and

TABLE 144.6 Treatment Guidelines for Congenital Syphilis

Scenario	Maternal Stage/Treatment	Evaluation	Antimicrobial Regimen
Infant age ≤28 d with proven or highly probable disease: (a) Abnormal physical examination (b) Abnormal evaluation[a] (c) Serum nontreponemal titer ≥4 times maternal titer (d) Visualization of spirochetes in clinical specimen	Any or none	CSF analysis: VDRL, cell count, and protein; CBC and platelet count; other tests as clinically indicated (e.g., long bone radiographs, liver function tests, ophthalmologic examination, hearing evaluation, neuroimaging)	Aqueous penicillin G 50,000 U/kg IV q12h (≤1 wk old), q8h (>1 wk old, ≤4 wk old), q6h (>4 wk old) × 10 d, *or* Procaine penicillin G 50,000 U/kg IM × 10 d (≤4 wk old)
Infant age ≤28 d with possible congenital syphilis: normal physical examination and serum quantitative nontreponemal titer the same or less than fourfold the maternal titer[b]	Any stage of infection and: mother (a) was not treated, inadequately treated, or has no documented treatment; (b) was treated with erythromycin or other nonpenicillin regimen; or (c) received appropriate treatment but ≤4 wk before delivery	CSF analysis for VDRL, cell count, and protein; CBC and platelet count; long bone radiographs[b]	If complete evaluation normal: (a) benzathine penicillin G 50,000 U/kg IM × 1[c] *or* (b) aqueous penicillin G 50,000 U/kg IV q12h (≤1 wk old), q8h (>1 wk old, ≤4 wk old), q6h (>4 wk old) × 10 days, *or* (c) procaine penicillin G 50,000 U/kg IM × 10 d (≤4 wk old)
Infant age ≤28 d with congenital syphilis less likely: normal physical examination and serum quantitative nontreponemal titer the same or less than fourfold the maternal titer	Mother with: (a) adequate therapy >4 wk before delivery, and appropriate for stage of infection; *or* (b) nontreponemal titers remained stable and low for late syphilis and no evidence of reinfection or relapse	No evaluation	Benzathine penicillin G 50,000 U/kg IM × 1 (preferred), *or* Clinical, serologic follow-up
Infant age ≤28 d old with congenital syphilis unlikely: normal physical examination and serum quantitative nontreponemal titer the same or less than fourfold the maternal titer	Mother with adequate therapy before pregnancy and nontreponemal serologic titer remained low and stable during pregnancy and at delivery	None	None
Congenital syphilis in infant age >28 d	Any or none	CSF analysis: VDRL, cell count, protein; CBC and differential; platelet count. As clinically indicated: radiographs of long bones, liver function tests, neuroimaging (cranial ultrasonography), eye examination, hearing evaluation	Aqueous penicillin G, 50,000 units/kg q4–6h × 10 d[d]

[a]CSF examination (VDRL test, cell count, protein), bone radiographs, CBC, platelets.
[b]If the infant's nontreponemal test is nonreactive, no evaluation is required, but the infant should receive a single IM dose of benzathine penicillin G 50,000 U/kg.
[c]Clinical and serologic follow-up must be certain.
[d]Some experts prefer prolonged therapy by administration of a single dose of benzathine penicillin G after the 10-day course of IV aqueous penicillin G.
From American Academy of Pediatrics. Syphilis. In: Kimberlin DW, ed. *Red Book: 2015 Report of the Committee on Infectious Diseases.* 30th ed. American Academy of Pediatrics, Elk Grove Village, IL: American Academy of Pediatrics; 2015:755; and Workowski KA, Bolan GA, CDC. Sexually transmitted diseases treatment guidelines, 2015. *MMWR Recomm Rep.* 2015;64(RR-3):1-138.

examination of the CSF for cell count, protein content, and VDRL test. Other tests, such as bone and chest radiographs, liver function tests, cranial ultrasonography, ophthalmologic examination, and auditory brainstem response, should be performed as clinically indicated. These infants are considered to have proven or highly probable disease; spirochetemia with invasion of the CNS occurs in 40% to 50% of these infants.[16] Although these infants must receive a full course of penicillin therapy, which treats possible neurosyphilis, it is beneficial for follow-up purposes to establish CNS abnormalities at presentation. Nonetheless, the diagnosis of congenital neurosyphilis is difficult to establish (see Clinical Manifestations). The presence of red blood cells in the CSF as a result of a traumatic lumbar puncture can produce a false-positive serologic reaction. Examination of the CSF for *T. pallidum* DNA by PCR may prove more useful for diagnosing congenital neurosyphilis.[52,91,127]

For infants who have a normal physical examination and a reactive serum quantitative nontreponemal test that is less than fourfold the maternal titer (possible congenital syphilis), further evaluation and treatment depend on the maternal treatment history and stage of infection (see Fig. 144.3 and Table 144.6). Whether to perform a complete evaluation (lumbar puncture, radiographs of the long bones, and complete blood cell and platelet counts) on the infant depends on the maternal treatment history and planned treatment of the infant (see Treatment). If the mother did not receive any prior treatment for syphilis, or the treatment was inadequate, a complete evaluation must be performed and be normal if a single intramuscular dose of benzathine penicillin G therapy is administered. Although it is preferred to help establish a diagnosis of congenital syphilis, a complete evaluation is unnecessary if a full 10-day course of parenteral penicillin is provided because such therapy would treat for the possibility of congenital infection.[13,93]

A full evaluation also is not needed if the infant's nontreponemal test is nonreactive and the physical examination is normal because it is unlikely to reveal any abnormalities that would require prolonged penicillin therapy.

The need to perform a lumbar puncture has been questioned because the yield of abnormal findings from examination of the CSF has been very low in some experiences and appreciable in others.[10,42,120] A primary benefit of obtaining CSF studies from infants who are receiving a 10-day parenteral course of aqueous or procaine penicillin therapy is identification of infants for whom follow-up of abnormal CSF results should be done. Likewise, radiographs of long bones are abnormal in approximately 65% of infants with clinical findings of syphilis but only in a few asymptomatic infants. The finding of osteochondritis or periostitis in an infant born to a mother with reactive serologic tests for syphilis indicates congenital syphilis, and the infant requires a full course of penicillin therapy for highly probable disease. Such an infant is likely to have CNS infection, however, even in the absence of clinical signs of neurosyphilis, and close clinical and serologic follow-up would be indicated.[91]

After the neonatal period, children with syphilis should have a lumbar puncture performed for evaluation of the CSF to detect asymptomatic neurosyphilis. In addition, birth and maternal records should be reviewed to assess whether such children have acquired or congenital syphilis.[28] Children with acquired syphilis should be evaluated for the possibility of sexual abuse.[72]

TREATMENT

T. pallidum is extremely sensitive to penicillin, as defined by experimental animal work. The minimal inhibitory concentration of penicillin is approximately 0.004 units/mL (or 0.0025 μg/mL). There is no evidence of increasing resistance to penicillin by the spirochetes, but such evidence would come only from the recognition of therapeutic failures. Effective treatment of syphilis must maintain a minimal inhibitory concentration of 0.03 units/mL of penicillin in serum (or CSF) for 7 to 10 days. Therapy is designed to achieve and maintain several times the necessary inhibiting levels and to avoid penicillin-free intervals during therapy. Penicillin remains the drug of first choice because of its established efficacy and minimal toxicity.[22]

Acquired Syphilis

Early syphilis (i.e., primary, secondary, and early latent infection) is treated with benzathine penicillin G, 50,000 units/kg up to the adult dose of 2.4 million units IM in a single dose. Late latent syphilis requires benzathine penicillin G, 150,000 units/kg up to the adult dose of 7.2 million units, administered as 50,000 units/kg up to the adult dose of 2.4 million units at 1-week intervals for 3 weeks. When the duration of infection is unknown, the patient should be treated as for late latent disease.

All patients with syphilis should be tested for HIV infection at diagnosis, although HIV-infected individuals are managed in the same manner as HIV-negative patients. Quantitative nontreponemal serologic tests should be repeated at 6, 12, and 24 months. A CSF examination should be performed if (1) neurologic or ophthalmic signs or symptoms are present or develop, (2) the patient has tertiary syphilis, (3) a sustained (>2 weeks) fourfold increase or greater in titer is observed and reinfection unlikely, (4) an initially high titer (≥1:32) fails to decline at least fourfold within 12 to 24 months of therapy, or (5) signs or symptoms attributable to syphilis persist, recur, or develop following therapy. In such circumstances, patients with CSF abnormalities should be treated for neurosyphilis.[24] Benzathine penicillin does not produce inhibitory CSF levels of penicillin reliably.[139] Shorter acting penicillins must be employed for neurosyphilis. In evaluating a patient for neurosyphilis, a CSF specimen without contamination by peripheral blood is needed.[66]

The recommended therapy for neurosyphilis is aqueous crystalline penicillin G, 18 to 24 million units/day, administered as 3 to 4 million units intravenously every 4 hours or continuous infusion for 10 to 14 days. An alternative regimen consists of procaine penicillin, 2.4 million units IM once daily, plus probenecid, 500 mg orally four times per day, for 10 to 14 days. Because these regimens are of shorter duration than is the regimen used for late latent syphilis, some experts recommend the additional administration of benzathine penicillin G, 2.4 million units IM once per week for up to 3 weeks after completion of the 10- to 14-day course. Older children with definite acquired syphilis and a normal neurologic and CSF examination may be treated with benzathine penicillin G, 50,000 units/kg IM to a maximal dose of 2.4 million units. Children with neurosyphilis should receive aqueous penicillin G, 200,000 to 300,000 units/kg per day intravenously administered as 50,000 units/kg every 4 to 6 hours for 10 days. Similar to the procedure with adults, an additional dose of benzathine penicillin G, 50,000 units/kg IM, may be given following the 10-day intravenous penicillin treatment.

The evaluation and treatment of early syphilis in HIV-infected individuals are the same as for individuals not infected with HIV except that they may be at increased risk for developing neurologic complications and have a higher risk for experiencing treatment failure. Close serologic follow-up of HIV-infected individuals is mandatory to detect treatment failure and the need for examination of CSF and retreatment.

Data to support the use of alternatives to penicillin in the treatment of syphilis are limited. Any history of penicillin allergy should be documented clearly, and, whenever possible, patients should receive skin testing, desensitization, and therapy with penicillin.[24] Doxycycline 100 mg orally twice daily and tetracycline 500 mg four times daily have been used for 14 days for treatment of early syphilis and 28 days for late latent infection and syphilis of unknown duration. Close serologic follow-up is mandatory. Neither of these therapies is recommended for children younger than 8 years. Ceftriaxone 100 mg/kg per day (maximum of 1 g daily) given either intravenously or IM for 10 to 14 days may be effective for treating early syphilis, but neither the optimal dose nor the duration of treatment has been defined.[59] Preliminary data also suggest that azithromycin as a single dose of 2 g may be effective in adults, but treatment failures have been described, as has emergence of resistance.[24] Because experience with these alternative antibiotics in HIV-infected individuals is limited, they should be used with caution.

Two to 12 hours after receiving treatment for syphilis, a variable proportion of patients develop an acute systemic (Jarisch-Herxheimer) reaction usually consisting of headache, malaise, fever (≥38°C [100.4°F]), and resolution within 1 day. The reaction is observed most frequently in the early stages of syphilis, probably represents a reaction to liberated endotoxin,[48] and does not affect the course of recovery. In the later stages of syphilis, fewer than one in four patients develop the reaction. Most reactions in late syphilis clinically are insignificant, but an occasional reaction may produce damage to the CNS or cardiovascular system.

Syphilis in Pregnancy

Pregnant women with reactive serologic tests for syphilis should be considered infected unless an adequate treatment history is documented and sequential nontreponemal antibody titers have declined. They should receive the penicillin regimen appropriate for the stage of syphilis.[24,150] For early syphilis, some experts recommend that an additional dose of benzathine penicillin G be provided 1 week after the initial dose. Management and treatment decisions may be guided further by the use of fetal ultrasonography. Evidence of fetal infection may require additional doses of benzathine penicillin G until resolution of fetal abnormalities has been achieved. The Jarisch-Herxheimer reaction may complicate treatment and result in preterm labor and fetal decelerations, although concern for its occurrence should not delay initiation of treatment.[71,96] No alternative to penicillin is available; pregnant women who have a history of penicillin allergy should undergo skin testing, desensitization, and treatment with penicillin.[151] Neither erythromycin nor azithromycin is recommended; infants have been born with congenital syphilis after maternal treatment with both agents. Any therapy other than penicillin is considered to be inadequate fetal therapy.[41,109]

Women who are coinfected with syphilis and HIV should receive treatment regimens corresponding to their stage of syphilis. The follow-up on treated HIV-infected women must be thorough and frequent.[55,95]

Patients who received therapy for gonorrhea with ceftriaxone have a high rate of cure of preprimary syphilis, but failures have occurred, and efficacy in pregnancy is not well studied.[59] This regimen cannot be assumed to have provided adequate therapy for syphilis in pregnancy.

Congenital Syphilis

Infants With Proven or Highly Probable Disease

Infants who have findings on physical examination that are consistent with congenital syphilis, such as a serum quantitative nontreponemal serologic titer that is at least fourfold greater than the mother's titer or spirochetes visualized or detected by PCR in body fluids or lesions, should be treated with aqueous crystalline penicillin G, 50,000 units/kg/dose intravenously every 12 hours during the first 7 days of age and every 8 hours thereafter for 10 days, or with procaine penicillin G, 50,000 units/kg/dose administered IM in a single daily dose for 10 days (see Table 144.6).[24] Although the concentration of penicillin that is achieved in the CSF during procaine therapy is lower than the levels seen with intravenous penicillin treatment, the clinical significance is unclear.[5] No treatment failures have been reported after procaine penicillin therapy. If more than 1 day of penicillin therapy is missed, the entire course should be restarted.

During a penicillin shortage in the United States, ceftriaxone was recommended as an alternative agent, although data are insufficient for its routine administration (see http://www.cdc.gov/std/treatment/drugnotices/penicilling.htm). When possible, a full 10-day course of penicillin is preferred even if ampicillin or another agent was provided initially for possible sepsis. Infants born to mothers coinfected with syphilis and HIV do not require more intense or prolonged treatment for syphilis than is recommended for all infants.

Infants With a Normal Physical Examination and a Serum Quantitative Nontreponemal Serologic Titer the Same or Less Than Fourfold the Maternal Titer

Treatment decisions for "asymptomatic" infants are based on the maternal history of syphilis and past treatment. The following situations are associated with a high likelihood that the infant may be infected with *T. pallidum* and should receive treatment: (1) mother was not treated, was inadequately treated, or has no documentation of having received treatment[113]; (2) mother was treated with erythromycin or other nonpenicillin G regimen; or (3) mother received recommended treatment *less than* 4 weeks before delivery.[14] If the infant's nontreponemal test is reactive, the infant should be evaluated with a complete blood cell count and differential; platelet count; radiographs of long bones; and CSF analysis for VDRL test, cell count, and protein content (Fig. 144.4 and Table 144.6).[24] If the entire evaluation is normal and follow-up is certain, the infant may receive benzathine penicillin G, 50,000 units/kg as a single IM dose.

If any part of the evaluation is abnormal or not done, or follow-up is uncertain, treatment should consist of aqueous penicillin G or procaine penicillin G (see earlier discussion) for 10 days. If the infant's nontreponemal serum test is nonreactive, the evaluation may be omitted, but the infant should be treated with a single intramuscular dose of benzathine penicillin for the possibility of incubating syphilis. Some experts prefer that all infants born to mothers with untreated syphilis receive parenteral penicillin therapy for 10 days because even if the evaluation is normal, these infants are at increased risk for being infected with *T. pallidum*, especially if the mother has secondary syphilis at delivery.[24]

Some studies have reevaluated the efficacy of treatment regimens for asymptomatic infants who are born to mothers in whom the treatment for possible syphilis was suboptimal.[105,110] Paryani and colleagues[105] randomly assigned 152 infants to receive either one injection of benzathine penicillin or a 10-day course of parenteral procaine penicillin. All study infants were asymptomatic on physical examination and had normal CSF evaluation, normal radiographic studies of long bones, and no visceral abnormalities. The results of both forms of therapy were excellent, with no treatment failures. This study indicates that single-dose therapy may have a high rate of success when an infant has negative studies and no symptoms.

Failure of a single administration of intramuscular benzathine penicillin G in three infants has been reported; however, the frequency seems to be low.[10,155] None of the three infants who developed clinical signs of congenital syphilis several weeks after having received a single intramuscular dose of benzathine penicillin was fully evaluated for congenital syphilis at birth. The concern has been that infected but symptom-free infants may have CNS infection and fail therapy with benzathine penicillin because benzathine penicillin does not achieve treponemicidal concentrations in CSF.[139] Using rabbit inoculation, Michelow and colleagues[91] showed that invasion of the CNS is an infrequent occurrence among these infants who have normal results on clinical, laboratory, and radiographic evaluations.

An infant does not require any evaluation in the following situations: (1) the mother was treated during the pregnancy, treatment was appropriate for the stage of infection, and treatment was administered more than 4 weeks before delivery; and (2) the mother has no evidence of reinfection or relapse. The CDC recommends, however, that these infants receive a single dose of benzathine penicillin G, 50,000 units/kg IM.[69,24] Infection of the fetus may occur despite administration of appropriate maternal therapy during pregnancy; failure rates of maternal treatment for prevention of fetal infection have been reported to be 2% to 14% and are more common with maternal secondary syphilis.[2,32,98,132] Treating the infant at birth may prevent the development of clinical disease if these infants were infected in utero. Some specialists would not treat the infant, however, but would provide close serologic follow-up only.

If the mother's treatment was adequate before pregnancy, and the mother's nontreponemal serologic titer remained low and stable during pregnancy and at delivery, no evaluation or treatment is recommended by the CDC. Some specialists would provide a single intramuscular dose of benzathine penicillin, however, if follow-up were uncertain for the remote possibility that the mother was reinfected. These infants are at very low risk for having congenital syphilis; for the most part, these mothers are serofast.

After the neonatal period, all children who are diagnosed with congenital syphilis should be evaluated with a complete blood cell count and differential, platelet count, and examination of the CSF for VDRL, cell count, and protein. Other tests, such as auditory brainstem responses, long bone radiographs, and neuroimaging, should be performed as clinically indicated. These children and children with late congenital syphilis should be treated with 200,000 to 300,000 units/kg per day of aqueous crystalline penicillin G, given as 50,000 units/kg every 4 to 6 hours for a minimum of 10 to 14 days. However, if the infant or child

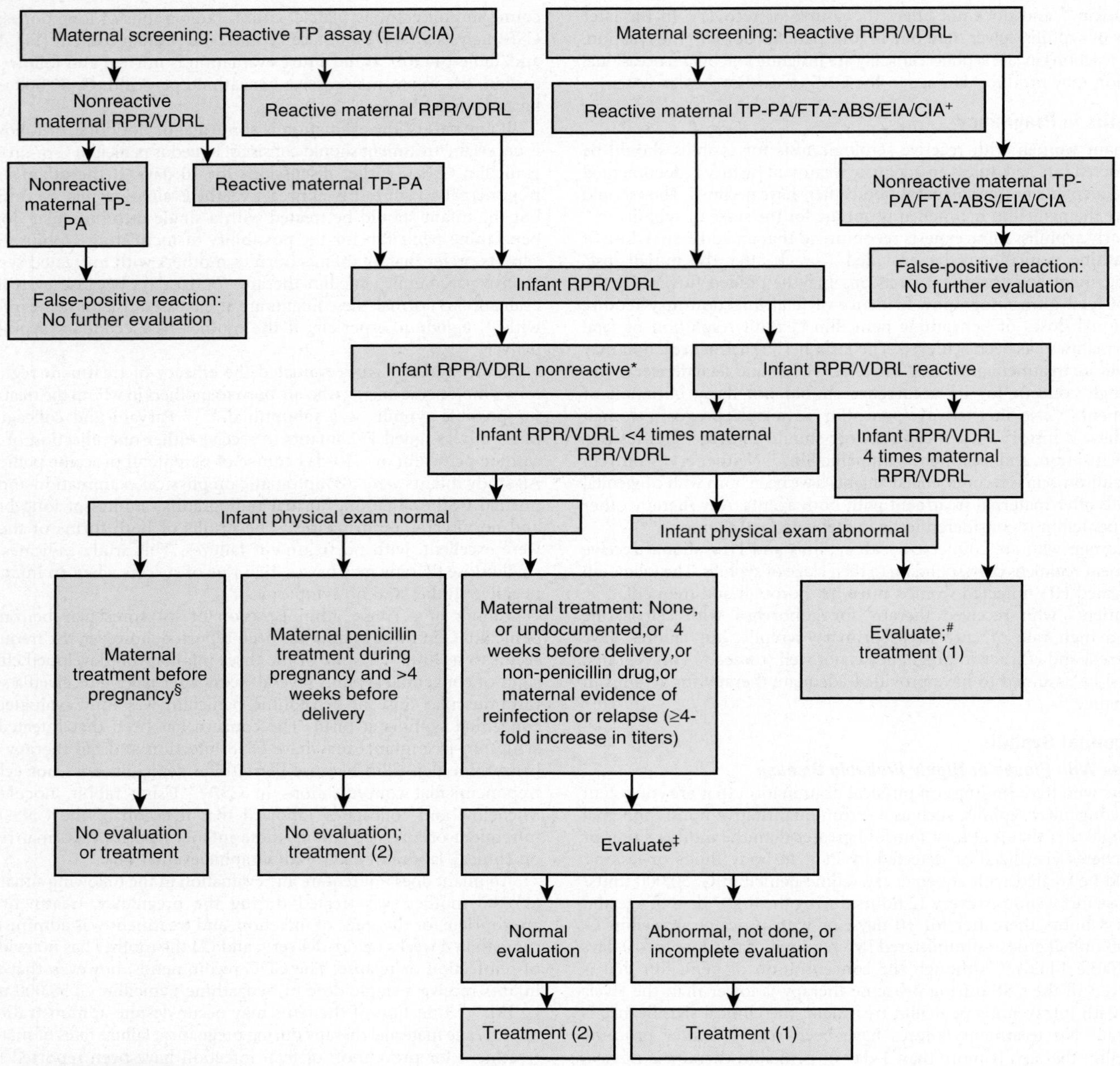

TREATMENT:

(1) Aqueous penicillin G 50,000 U/kg IV q 12 hr (1 wk of age), q 8 hr (>1 wk), or procaine penicillin G 50,000 U/kg IM single daily dose, x 10 days

(2) Benzathine penicillin G 50,000 U/kg IM x 1 dose

FIG. 144.4 Algorithm for evaluation and treatment of infants born to mothers with reactive serologic tests for syphilis. +, Test for HIV antibody. Infants of HIV-infected mothers do not require different evaluation or treatment. *If the mother has had no treatment, undocumented treatment, treatment ≤4 weeks before delivery, or evidence of reinfection or relapse (fourfold or higher increase in titers) *and* the infant's physical examination is normal, *then* treat infant with a single intramuscular injection of benzathine penicillin (50,000 U/kg). No additional evaluation is needed. §Women who maintain a VDRL titer ≤1:2 (RPR ≤1:4) beyond 1 year after successful treatment are considered serofast. #Evaluation consists of CBC, platelet count; CSF examination for cell count, protein, and quantitative VDRL. Other tests as clinically indicated: long-bone x-rays, neuroimaging, auditory brainstem response, eye examination, chest radiograph, liver function tests. ‡CBC, platelet count; CSF examination for cell count, protein, and quantitative VDRL; long-bone radiographs. Treatment regimens are as follows: (1) aqueous penicillin G 50,000 units/kg IV every 12 hours (≤1 week old) or every 8 hours (>1 week old) or procaine penicillin G 50,000 units/kg IM single daily dose × 10 days; (2) benzathine penicillin G 50,000 units/kg IM × 1 dose. *CBC,* Complete blood count; *CIA,* chemiluminescence; *CSF,* cerebrospinal fluid; *EIA,* enzyme immunoassay; *RPR,* rapid plasma reagin; *TP, Treponema pallidum; TP-PA, Treponema pallidum* particle agglutination; *VDRL,* Venereal Disease Research Laboratory.

has no clinical manifestations of congenital syphilis and the evaluation (including the CSF examination) is normal, treatment with up to 3 weekly doses of benzathine penicillin G, 50,000 U/kg IM can be considered. In addition, a single dose of benzathine penicillin G 50,000 units/kg IM up to the adult dose of 2.4 million units in a single dose can be considered after the 10-day course of IV aqueous penicillin to provide more comparable duration of treatment in those who have no clinical manifestations and normal CSF.

The Jarisch-Herxheimer reaction may complicate the treatment of congenital syphilis. It rarely is seen in newborns, although it occurs more commonly when syphilis is treated later in infancy. It is manifested usually by fever, but cardiovascular collapse and seizures also have been reported.

FOLLOW-UP EVALUATION

Box 144.5 summarizes recommendations concerning follow-up of infants after they have been treated for congenital syphilis and of seroreactive infants who were not treated because of the presumed adequacy of the management of the mother's serologic status.[60,61,113] Infants born to mothers with syphilis should have serial quantitative nontreponemal tests performed until the test results show nonreactivity.[56,118] Similarly, infants who are seronegative but whose mothers acquired syphilis late in gestation should be followed with serial testing after penicillin therapy is instituted.

Follow-up for infants who received appropriate penicillin therapy for possible syphilis can be incorporated into routine pediatric care at 2, 4, 6, 12, 15, and 24 months. These infants should show a fourfold decrease in nontreponemal serologic titers. In infants with congenital syphilis, nontreponemal serologic tests become nonreactive within 6 to 12 months after they have received appropriate treatment. Uninfected infants usually become seronegative by the time they reach 6 months of age.[27] Infants with persistently low, stable titers of nontreponemal tests beyond 1 year of age may require retreatment.

BOX 144.5 Recommended Follow-up of Infants Born to Mothers With Syphilis

1. Nontreponemal test (e.g., RPR):
   a. *Treated infant:* Perform at 2, 4, 6, 12, 15, and 24 months old (or after therapy) until nonreactive. Nontreponemal test titer should decrease fourfold within 6 months after treatment and be nonreactive by 6 to 12 months. If test remains reactive ≥12 months after treatment, consider reevaluation and retreatment. If nontreponemal test titer increases fourfold, full reevaluation and retreatment for proven disease is required.
   b. *Untreated infant:* Perform at 1, 2, 4, 6, 12, 15, and 24 months old (or after therapy) until nonreactive. Nontreponemal test titer should decrease fourfold within 6 months after treatment and be nonreactive by 6 months. If nontreponemal assay is reactive at 6 months, reevaluate child (including CSF examination) and treat. If nontreponemal test titer increases fourfold, full evaluation and treatment for proven disease are required.
2. Treponemal test (e.g., TP-PA): Perform at 12 months. If reactive, repeat at ages 18 and 24 months.[a]
3. Abnormal CSF examination at diagnosis: Repeat CSF examination (VDRL, cell count, protein content) at age 6 months (or after therapy). If abnormal and no other explanation found, retreat infant.
4. Monitor yearly for neurologic, hearing, and ophthalmic disorders.
5. Monitor developmental status and assess school function.

[a]Approximately 30% of infected children maintain a reactive treponemal test beyond age 18 months. This finding confirms the diagnosis of congenital syphilis. If child was not previously treated, treatment for proven congenital syphilis is mandatory.

CSF, Cerebrospinal fluid; *RPR,* rapid plasma reagin; *TP-PA, Treponema pallidum* particle agglutination; *VDRL,* Venereal Disease Research Laboratory.

Modified from Ikeda MK, Jenson HB. Evaluation and treatment of congenital syphilis. *J Pediatr.* 1990;117:843–852; and Rathbun KC. Congenital syphilis: a proposal for improved surveillance, diagnosis and treatment. *Sex Transm Dis.* 1983;10:102-107.

Untreated infants may benefit from having a nontreponemal test performed at 1 month of age. Untreated infants whose nontreponemal test remains reactive by the time they are 6 months old may need to be reevaluated clinically and treated. If the nontreponemal titer increases fourfold in any infant during follow-up, full evaluation and treatment are indicated. All infants and children should be evaluated thoroughly for the extent of disease if there is serologic evidence of failure of treatment or of recurrent disease. At a minimum, such evaluation should consist of CSF examination and complete blood cell count and platelet count. Other tests, such as long bone radiographs, liver function tests, hearing evaluation, and ophthalmologic evaluation, can be performed as clinically indicated.

A reactive treponemal test in infants who are 18 months or older when they have lost all maternal antibody confirms the diagnosis of congenital syphilis. A nonreactive treponemal test at that time indicates the lack of active and ongoing infection, but it does not exclude a previously infected child who was treated adequately in the neonatal period. Seroreversion of the treponemal test has been seen in some infants with treated congenital syphilis as documented by the detection of spirochetes in blood or CSF. However, if the child did not receive treatment previously and the treponemal test remains reactive at 18 months or older, a full evaluation and treatment are indicated.

Infants with abnormal CSF findings should have a repeat lumbar puncture performed 6 months after therapy. A reactive CSF VDRL test result or an abnormal protein content or cell count at that time is an indication for retreatment.

Adults and older children with primary or secondary syphilis should be examined clinically and serologically at least at 6 and 12 months after treatment. Failure of nontreponemal titers to decrease fourfold within 6 to 12 months of treatment indicates possible treatment failure. These individuals should be reevaluated for HIV infection, and consideration should be given to performance of a lumbar puncture for detection of unrecognized neurosyphilis and retreatment. For latent syphilis, subsequent follow-up with quantitative serology at 6, 12, and 24 months is recommended. Failure of a fourfold decrease in initially elevated nontreponemal serologic titers (1:32) within 12 to 24 months of therapy is an indication for examination of CSF and retreatment. Retreatment for syphilis also is recommended when clinical signs or symptoms persist or recur, or if there is a sustained fourfold increase in titer of a nontreponemal serologic test. Patients with neurosyphilis require examinations and repeat CSF examinations every 6 months until the CSF results are normal. After 2 years of follow-up, a reactive CSF VDRL test or abnormal CSF index that persists and cannot be attributed to other ongoing illness requires retreatment for possible neurosyphilis.

In most patients receiving appropriate therapy during the primary or secondary stages, active disease is arrested totally and permanently. Persistent seroreactivity as measured by a treponemal test may be avoided if treatment is given during the preprimary stage, but seldom thereafter. Nonetheless, progression to tertiary disease seldom, if ever, occurs. Similarly, therapy administered during early or late latent syphilis averts the development of symptomatic tertiary disease. Antimicrobial therapy for symptomatic neurosyphilis, optic neuritis, and cardiovascular syphilis may not be followed by significant clinical improvement, and established damage to vital organs may fail to resolve.

PREVENTION

Methods to control the spread of syphilis have relied extensively on treatment of case contacts. Individuals with active syphilis are interviewed to identify all sexual contacts that may have occurred at (1) 3 months plus duration of symptoms for primary syphilis, (2) 6 months plus duration of symptoms for secondary syphilis, and (3) 1 year for early latent syphilis. The contacts are examined, tested serologically, and treated appropriately even if they are seronegative. Advantage is taken of the long incubation period of syphilis by preventing disease in contacts before they can transmit infection.

Adverse outcomes of pregnancy and congenital infection can be prevented effectively by performing routine prenatal serologic screening and providing penicillin treatment to infected women and their sexual partners.[138,146] All pregnant women should have a serologic test for syphilis at the first prenatal visit. For communities and populations in which the prevalence of syphilis is high or for patients at increased risk for contracting disease, serologic testing should be performed at 28 to 32 weeks' gestation and at delivery because some women may acquire syphilis during pregnancy.[4] When epidemiologic, clinical, or serologic evidence of infection is present, or the diagnosis of active infection cannot be excluded, treatment should be instituted.

For years, nontreponemal antibody testing has been recommended for antepartum syphilis screening. Recently, treponemal antibody testing is being used increasingly by many laboratories as a cost-cutting measure for screening pregnant women (reverse sequence screening). If a treponemal EIA or CIA test is used for antepartum syphilis screening and is positive, a quantitative nontreponemal test (RPR or VDRL) should then be performed. If the nontreponemal test is reactive, then a diagnosis of past or present syphilis is made and the management of the mother and infant should be as discussed previously. However, if the nontreponemal test is negative, then the results are considered discrepant and a second treponemal test (TP-PA preferred) should be performed, preferably on the same specimen. If the second treponemal test is positive, current or past syphilis infection is confirmed. For women with a history of adequately treated syphilis, no further treatment is necessary. Women without a history of treatment should be staged and treated accordingly with a recommended penicillin regimen. If the second treponemal test is negative, the positive EIA/CIA is more likely to represent a false-positive test result in low-risk women with no history of treated syphilis.[104]

Serologic screening tests should be performed on maternal serum and not on the infant's serum or umbilical cord blood.[116] An infant's nontreponemal serologic titer usually is one to two dilutions less than that of the mother's titer; an infant may have a nonreactive serologic test for syphilis when the maternal titer is of low dilution. Some of these infants, especially infants born to mothers with no prior treatment for syphilis, require treatment for prevention of late-onset disease. They would be missed if only infant screening were performed.

Limitations of current screening practices also exist. A false-negative nontreponemal test can occur from a prozone phenomenon. Also, a negative maternal nontreponemal test at delivery does not exclude incubating syphilis or even primary syphilis if nontreponemal and treponemal antibodies have not yet reached detectable concentrations.[38,125] Infants born to such mothers may be infected and develop clinical disease in the ensuing 3 to 14 weeks. Repeat screening of mothers who reside in areas with a high prevalence of syphilis or engage in high-risk behaviors may be advisable at the first postpartum visit.

It is a policy statement of the CDC that no infant should leave the hospital without the serologic status of the infant's mother having been documented at least once during pregnancy and preferably again at delivery.[24,86] In this era of early and very early discharge from the hospital after deliveries, fulfilling the policy goal may require careful planning and advocacy by the clinician.

All syphilis cases must be reported to the local public health department. This practice allows for contact investigation, appropriate follow-up, and identification of core environments and populations in which the greatest transmission of syphilis is occurring in a particular community. Despite great progress in recent years, the prevention, control, and even elimination of endemic syphilis in the United States remain an elusive goal in public health policy and on a global scale in countries where resources may be limited and the practicalities of serologic screening and treatment in prenatal care settings are challenging. However, as discussed in the Epidemiology section, the WHO initiative to achieve global elimination of congenital syphilis is making progress. Linking to a dual integrated strategy of eliminating mother-to-child HIV transmission affords the opportunity of synergistic benefits. The median proportion of pregnant women receiving at least one antenatal care visit is now 90% in 58 reporting countries, and there have been notable successes in declaring some countries free of mother-to-child transmission of syphilis.[68]

NEW REFERENCES SINCE THE SEVENTH EDITION

15. Bonawitz RE, Duncan J, et al. Assessment of the impact of rapid syphilis tests on syphilis screening and treatment of pregnant women in Zambia. *Int J Gynaecol Obstet.* 2015;130(suppl 1):S58-S62.
24. CDC, Workowski KA, et al. Sexually transmitted diseases treatment guidelines, 2015. *MMWR. Recommendations and reports.* 2015;64(RR-03):1-137.
66. Kamb ML, Newman LM, et al. A road map for the global elimination of congenital syphilis. *Obstet Gynecol Int.* 2010;312798.
68. Kiarie J, Mishra CK, et al. Accelerating the dual elimination of mother-to-child transmission of syphilis and HIV: Why now? *Int J Gynaecol Obstet.* 2015;130(suppl 1):S1-S3.
69. Kimberlin DW. Syphilis. In: Kimberlin DW, ed. *The Red Book: 2015 Report of the Committee on Infectious Diseases.* Elk Grove Village, II, The American Academy of Pediatrics; 2015:755.
74. Lago EG. Current perspectives on prevention of mother-to-child transmission of syphilis. *Cureus.* 2016;8(3):e525.
100. Newman L, Kamb M, et al. Global estimates of syphilis in pregnancy and associated adverse outcomes: analysis of multinational antenatal surveillance data. *PLoS Med.* 2013;10(2):e1001396.
104. Park IU, Chow JM, et al. Screening for syphilis with the treponemal immunoassay: analysis of discordant serology results and implications for clinical management. *J Infect Dis.* 2011;204(9):1297-1304.
128. Schmid GP, Stoner BP, et al. The need and plan for global elimination of congenital syphilis. *Sex Transm Dis.* 2007;34(7 suppl):S5-S10.
130. Sena AC, White BL, et al. Novel *Treponema pallidum* serologic tests: a paradigm shift in syphilis screening for the 21st century. *Clin Infect Dis.* 2010;51(6):700-708.
152. WHO. *The global elimination of congenital syphilis: rationale and strategy for action.* Geneva, Switzerland.: WHO, Department of Reproductive Health and Research; 2007.
153. WHO (2014). Elimination of mother-to-child transmission (EMTCT) of HIV and syphilis. Global guidance on criteria and processes for validation. Available at http://www.who.int/reproductivehealth/publications/rtis/9789241505888/en/.

The full reference list for this chapter is available at ExpertConsult.com.

145 Nonvenereal Treponematoses

David C. Hilmers

Pinta, yaws, and endemic syphilis (bejel) are the three chronic granulomatous diseases that constitute the pathogenic nonvenereal treponematoses of humans. These diseases are caused by morphologically indistinguishable treponemes found almost exclusively in underdeveloped areas of the tropics and bordering arid regions. The pathogenic treponemes have been given subspecies designations as follows: syphilis, *Treponema pallidum* subsp. *pallidum (T. pallidum);* yaws, *T. pallidum* subsp. *pertenue (T. pertenue);* and endemic syphilis, *T. pallidum* subsp. *endemicum (T. pallidum).* The designation for the causative agent of pinta remains *Treponema carateum* (Table 145.1).[40]

Although neither sexually nor congenitally acquired, agents responsible for the nonvenereal treponematoses are transmitted person to person by means of skin or mucous membrane contact. Close contact with children or young adults, traumatized areas of skin, lack of clothing, and poor personal hygiene are important factors in the transmission of these diseases. All three nonvenereal treponematoses are potentially

TABLE 145.1 **Comparison of the Treponematoses**

	Syphilis	Yaws	Endemic Syphilis	Pinta
Organism	*T. pallidum* subsp. *pallidum*	*T. pallidum* subsp. *pertenue*	*T. pallidum* subsp. *endemicum*	*T. carateum*
Distribution	Worldwide	Tropics, Africa, Asia, Pacific	Arid areas of Africa, Arabia	Tropical Central, South America
Peak ages affected	All ages	1–12 y	<15 y	15–20 y
Route of entry	Mucous membranes	Skin	Oral mucosa, fomites	Skin
Incubation period	2–10 wk	3–9 wk	3 wk	2–3 wk
Experimental hosts	Rabbit, primate, guinea pig, hamster	Rabbit, hamster	Rabbit, hamster	Primate only
Sexual transmission	Yes	No	No	No
Congenital transmission	Yes	No	No	No
Skin infection	Yes	Yes	Yes	Yes
Bone involvement	5–10%	20–40%	20–40%	0
Neurologic involvement	Yes	No	Rare	No
Cardiologic involvement	Yes	No	Rare	No

debilitating diseases that have enormous social and economic implications within endemic areas.[25] The worldwide prevalence was reduced considerably by means of seroepidemiologic and mass treatment campaigns sponsored by the World Health Organization (WHO) and the United Nations International Children's Emergency Fund (UNICEF) in the 1950s and 1960s. A new campaign for eradication of yaws has recently been formulated by the WHO (the Morges strategy) in which single-dose azithromycin to treat entire communities is used.[5] This strategy also includes follow-up assessment of efficacy using serologic surveys at 6-month intervals. The goal is to eradicate at least one of these diseases, yaws, by the year 2020. There are no specific plans for eradication of endemic syphilis and pinta because more epidemiologic and molecular data are required before an eradication strategy can be promulgated for these less well-characterized diseases. As for now, all three remain public health problems in areas of the world where sporadic outbreaks continue to occur.[40]

Since the termination of the mass treatment campaigns in the 1960s, lack of attention to these diseases and diversion of resources to other public health problems, such as human immunodeficiency virus, malaria, and tuberculosis, led to a resurgence in the nonvenereal treponematoses in some parts of the world. Because of a lack of vigilance and awareness of these diseases, they probably are underreported. Data reported by WHO in 1997 estimated that there were more than 2.5 million cases worldwide.[18] The potential effectiveness of a determined treatment and surveillance program was demonstrated in a region of northern Ecuador where no new cases of yaws were reported from 1993 to 1998.[2] Before the inception of this program there was a prevalence of clinical cases of 16.5% in the area's population. A focused effort in India has also been successful, and no new cases have been reported since 2004.[4] There is great hope that a determined and organized campaign using a single dose of azithromycin can successfully eliminate these diseases.[46]

The history, development, and global spread of treponemal diseases have been the subject of widespread debate.[56] Because the primary reservoirs for these organisms are humans, their history is intertwined within the economic, cultural, and social framework of humanity. One theory postulates that all treponemal diseases originated from pinta or yaws, first found in Central Africa. This view states that treponemes spread widely from there, and the various disease processes that we know today are a result of mutations caused by the adaptation of the organisms to environmental and development changes in their hosts. Supporters of the pre-Columbian existence of syphilis in Europe point to radiocarbon dating of skeletons in 14th-century England that appear to bear the stigmata of syphilis. Critics of this evidence point to possible inaccuracies in methods and lack of peer review.[3,66] The Columbian theory suggests that treponemes began as nonvenereal pathogens in Africa that spread to the Americas via Asia thousands of years ago while mutating into endemic syphilis as they crossed Africa and Asia. In North America, they developed into the venereally transmitted form of disease caused by *T. pallidum* that we know today as syphilis. Syphilis was carried to Europe by Columbus and his men on his return voyage from the Americas. Supporters of this theory point to skeletal evidence of syphilis found in the Dominican Republic before the arrival of Columbus on the island and to evidence of nonvenereal treponemal infections, but not syphilis, in England during the same period.[73] More recent investigations in Guyana found an isolated tribe with treponemal infections that had characteristics of both yaws and syphilis. Phylogenetic analysis of this strain lends support to the Columbian theory of the origin of syphilis and the Old World roots of the nonvenereal species.[30,74,75]

On morphologic examination, the treponemes are thin, tightly coiled organisms that do not stain or stain poorly with the usual aniline dyes. They contain 4 to 14 spirals and are actively motile by virtue of periplasmic flagella. The organisms are quite fragile and sensitive to drying, atmospheric oxygen, and temperatures greater than 35°C. The organisms can be stored in either 15% glycerol at −70°C or liquid nitrogen and still retain their virulence for long periods. Although limited multiplication of *T. pallidum* subsp. *pallidum* has been achieved in a tissue-culture system,[19] it has not been accomplished as yet with the nonvenereal pathogenic treponemes. No human pathogenic treponemes have been cultured in or on artificial media. Because they measure 10 to 13 μm in length but only 0.15 μm in width, they are below the resolution of light microscopy and must be identified by darkfield microscopy in infected skin or mucous membrane lesions.

Sequencing of the yaws and endemic syphilis genomes has identified targets for molecular diagnostics that can differentiate venereal syphilis from yaws and bejel.[11,64] For example, yaws and syphilis treponemes have been shown to differ by less than 0.2% of the genome sequence.[10] It has also been shown that there is heterogenecity within strains at certain gene sites. [9] Clinical and epidemiologic features of each disease state from which the treponeme is recovered constitute the primary method of differentiation. Although not practical, further differentiation is based on the response of animal models to experimental infection.[29,33,54,60,61] Each of the pathogenic treponemes stimulates cross-reactive antibodies assayed in the serologic diagnosis of the human diseases by nontreponemal and treponemal tests. Various degrees of homologous resistance and cross-immunity exist after infection occurs with any of these spirochetes.[29,31,37,41,42,60,68] Rabbit models have shown complete immunity against reinfection with homologous pathogens but only incomplete or nonexistent protection against other subspecies.[67] No specific antigenic differentiation has been found among species to explain these findings. Despite differences in methods of transmission, clinical disease, geographic distribution, and rare reports of resistant cases, all human treponemes remain sensitive to penicillin.[7,18]

PINTA

Pinta (mal del pinto, carate, enfermedad azul) is a chronic, contagious, nonvenereally transmitted treponemal disease that normally is the mildest of these disorders. Although it affects primarily patients in the first 2 decades of life, it can affect children and adults of all age groups, producing dyschromic skin lesions without pathogenic involvement of deeper organ structures. Pinta is not a fatal disease, but a disfiguring one, which results in social ostracism and an inability to adjust to an urban society.

Biology and Immunology

Pinta is caused by *T. carateum.* The organism is characterized primarily by its isolation from patients with clinically apparent pinta and by its lack of pathogenicity in small laboratory animals. Only chimpanzees have been shown to be susceptible to experimental infection.[34,35] Human studies by Medina[42] suggest that *T. carateum* induces significant protection against homologous reinfection and cross-immunity against the treponemes of yaws and syphilis; however, these two subspecies of *T. pallidum* fail to confer cross-protection against *T. carateum.*[42]

Epidemiology

Pinta is found primarily in tropical Central and South America among underprivileged Indians and in the Caribbean. It occurs in major river basins of Mexico, Venezuela, Colombia, Brazil, Peru, and Ecuador. Cases also have been reported in Argentina, Chile, Haiti, Guatemala, Dominican Republic, Honduras, Nicaragua, and Bolivia. Pinta rarely occurs at higher elevations in the mountain regions of these countries. In the early 1920s, approximately 500,000 cases occurred throughout Latin America; however, as a result of seroepidemiologic and mass treatment campaigns, few cases, if any, are being reported today. The possibility of underreporting exists because a 20% clinical prevalence was reported in 1982 in a village in Panama.[52] A case of pinta in Austria in a visitor from Cuba was reported in 1999.[73]

The disease is found where poor hygienic and crowded conditions exist. Although endemic areas basically are rural, tribal tradition allows very close contact among its members to occur. These tropical societies, with their absence of shoes and clothes, continually subject exposed skin to trauma and to contact with infectious lesions. Transmission of *T. carateum* occurs primarily by intimate skin-to-skin contact; a break in the skin is required for invasion of the treponeme. Pinta is not acquired congenitally or by blood transfusion. Transmission of the disease by insect vectors has been proposed but not proved[42]; insects probably initiate disease by producing the necessary breaks in the skin.[16] Pinta is distributed equally between males and females and among all races in endemic areas. It is acquired primarily by individuals aged 15 to 20 years,[53] frequently spreading to family members because of crowded living conditions.

Pathogenesis and Pathology

T. carateum penetrates skin through breaks in the epidermis, with resultant damage restricted to the dermal and epidermal tissues. The organisms multiply in these layers, eliciting cellular proliferation and plasma cell, lymphocyte, and Langerhans cell infiltration. The resulting primary lesions (one to three) may appear on any area of exposed skin but usually occur on the legs, the dorsum of the feet, the forearms, or the back of the hands.[53] A lesion enlarges as a result of continual progression and direct extension or by coalescence with adjacent primary lesions; occasionally, regional lymphadenopathy develops. Secondary lesions, known as *pintids,* may arise years later from treponemal dissemination and exhibit a cellular proliferation and infiltration similar to that of the primary lesion. In contrast to venereal syphilis, blood vessels remain intact and do not show proliferation. The dyschromic or multicolored nature (brown, slate blue, black, or gray) of the primary and secondary lesions is more characteristic of older than of younger lesions, in which pigmentary changes usually are minimal. The variously pigmented older lesions may show hyperkeratosis or parakeratosis. Large numbers of treponemes can be found throughout the dermis and epidermis in the highly contagious primary and secondary lesions.

Late pinta is characterized by pigmentary changes, from dyschromic treponeme-containing lesions to achromic treponeme-free lesions. This depigmentation process occurs at different rates even within the same lesion, which gives rise to different degrees of hypochromia and atrophy around dyschromic and achromic lesions.[53] A concomitant paucity of hair follicles and sebaceous glands may occur.[15]

Clinical Manifestations

Pinta is characterized by a continuing production of early infectious lesions from either direct extension or dissemination and by the concomitant presence of lesions in various stages of dyschromia and achromia. The lesions are not well delineated, often merge, and may be accompanied by regional lymphadenopathy. Primary, secondary, and tertiary stages may or may not occur simultaneously.

The early stage of pinta includes the initial lesions, occasional regional lymphadenopathy, and secondary lesions resulting from dissemination of treponemes. A primary lesion (not always evident) develops after an incubation period of 3 days to 2 months, usually 2 to 3 weeks. The primary lesion begins as one or more small erythematous papules that may appear scaly and indurated. The papules progressively enlarge over 1 to 3 months, often coalescing, becoming pigmented, more erythematous, and scaly while developing heaped-up margins. Occasionally, an accompanying regional lymphadenopathy is present. The lesion may disappear in several months or may continue to enlarge for several years, forming larger psoriasiform plaques that coalesce further.

The primary lesions of pinta generally overlap development of the secondary lesions or pintids, which appear months to years after infection occurs. During this stage, dissemination ensues and almost any area of the skin can be involved. The lesions occur typically on exposed areas of skin and are variously pigmented. The degree of pigmentation is related to the state of development of the lesion, the age of the lesion, the degree of exposure to sun, and the host's natural pigmentation. Pintids begin as small, scaly papules that gradually enlarge and coalesce. Several colors may exist within the same lesion. Initially, pintids usually are red to violaceous; later, they become slate blue, gray, or black as a result of photosensitization. Lesions on the legs typically are yellowish brown or dark brown.

The late stage of pinta is characterized by the development of depigmented lesions. Achromia usually begins several years after the onset of the disease but may appear 3 months after onset. Areas of depigmentation spread slowly, leaving large achromic lesions, reminiscent of vitiligo, as the end result. Early achromia tends to be asymmetric, whereas later depigmented lesions are symmetric. Characteristic of the Cuban form of pinta is the development of hyperkeratosis of the palms and soles. Many chronic dermatologic entities characterized by scaly, psoriasiform lesions or by dyschromia or depigmentation can be confused with pinta in endemic areas. Maculopapulosquamous diseases, including psoriasis, parapsoriasis, and lichen planus, and dyschromic dermatologic diseases such as vitiligo, ochronosis, and argyria must be taken into consideration.[17,62]

Prognosis

Pinta is not a fatal disease; it produces changes related only to the skin. There is no involvement of the central nervous system, the cardiovascular system, or other internal organs. If the disease is not treated, the patient frequently develops large achromic cutaneous blemishes. The major resulting problem is one of social ostracism from the community. Infected individuals are removed from the urban society and find refuge in the rural areas. This isolation separates the patient farther from the principal sources of medical therapy.[16]

YAWS

Yaws (frambesia, pian, buba, bouba) is a communicable, nonvenereally transmitted treponematosis of the tropical zones. The disease is characterized by its early acquisition (usually before puberty) and its chronic, relapsing pattern of early benign lesions separated by periods of latency that terminate with late destructive lesions of skin, bones, and cartilaginous tissues. A very prevalent disease in the early part of the 20th century, yaws was estimated to have affected more than 50 million people. Although seroepidemiologic and mass treatment campaigns sponsored by WHO and UNICEF have reduced its overall prevalence dramatically, endemic areas of concern continue to exist.[4,23,47,61,68] Data showing the efficacy of single-dose azithromycin at 30 mg/kg gives hope of eradicating the disease with a goal of the year 2020.[46]

Biology and Immunology

T. pallidum subsp. *pertenue*, the etiologic agent of yaws, is morphologically identical to other pathogenic treponemes. The presence of infection with either yaws or syphilis strains was previously distinguishable only by epidemiologic and clinical means but now is possible by molecular probes.[11] The genomes of three strains of *T. pallidum* subsp. *pertenue* were completely sequenced and compared with four strains of *T. pallidum* in an attempt to find differences between the genomic structures of syphilis and yaws. The two genomes were found to have a 99.8% concordance. This is important in differentiating between childhood congenital syphilis and yaws, a distinction that can be clinically problematic.[9,10]

Although not clinically useful, animal models can be used to distinguish between syphilis and yaws. Rabbits and hamsters have been infected experimentally by both diseases, with resultant lymphadenopathy and visible lesions. Characteristic differences in the distribution, form, and number of lesions can be used to distinguish the identity of the infectious agent. On the basis of human and experimental studies, the organism stimulates a significant degree of homologous resistance to reinfection and superinfection and cross-immunity to *T. pallidum* subsp. *pallidum* and *endemicum*.[29,33,60,67]

Epidemiology

Yaws is a disease of tropical countries found primarily among rural populations. It exists in the warm, moist, endemic areas of rural Africa, Southeast Asia, the Caribbean, South America, the Pacific, and central and southern Africa. As indicated, seroepidemiologic and mass treatment campaigns have resulted in a significant reduction in prevalence of the disease in most of these areas. The failure of many countries to integrate active control measures into the functions of local health services has led, however, to a gradual buildup and extension of reservoirs of yaws, with the emergence of significant numbers of new, active cases since 1974 in Ghana, Togo, Benin, Indonesia, Papua New Guinea, and the Ivory Coast.[4] In a WHO survey in the Central African Republic, Congo, and Gabon, clinical yaws was detected in more than 20% of the Pygmy population and reactive serologic tests were obtained in 80%. Health care workers in the periurban settlements of Port Moresby, Papua New Guinea identified 494 cases between April 2000 and September 2001. A 2001 survey in the Solomon Islands showed that yaws was the sixth leading cause of morbidity and that the prevalence was 4106 cases per 100,000 population.[65] In Lihir Island in Papua New Guinea, the prevalence of active yaws was found to be 2.4% and that of latent yaws in children was 18.3% before treatment.[46] In Latin America, cases still occur in Brazil, Colombia, Haiti, Venezuela, and Suriname.[17,43] Intense surveillance and eradication efforts in India, however, appear to have been successful, with no new cases reported since 2004.[4]

Poor hygiene, close crowding among children (especially in sleeping areas), and lack of protective clothing facilitate transmission of the disease by direct skin-to-skin contact, whereby *T. pallidum* subsp. *pertenue* enters traumatized exposed areas from an infected lesion. The usual portals of entry are the lower extremities, head, face, and mouth. The presence of treponemal antibodies and the isolation of treponemes (most probably *T. pallidum* subsp. *pertenue* from West African monkeys)[8,20] suggest that primates in this area may act as a reservoir for spread of the disease.

Yaws usually is acquired before puberty and is most prevalent among children. Because such a large percentage of the population contracts the disease in infancy, young children represent the primary reservoir. Older children and adults generally are not infectious; therefore, congenital and sexual transmission does not occur. Boys and girls are affected equally.

Pathogenesis and Pathology

T. pallidum subsp. *pertenue* enters the host through abraded skin, most frequently below the knees. The organisms multiply locally and in the regional lymph nodes. Epithelial hyperplasia and plasma cell, lymphocytic, and macrophage infiltration are elicited. The end result is the formation of a primary lesion and lymphadenopathy containing numerous treponemes. Shortly after their introduction into the host, organisms are carried to skin, bone, and cartilage through the circulation. Disseminated treponemes in these tissues multiply, eliciting a chronic inflammatory response similar to that seen in the primary lesion. They produce distant papillomas, lymphadenopathy, hyperkeratosis, and bone involvement that develop without interruption until they are reversed by either immune mechanisms or treatment. In contrast to those associated with venereal syphilis, vascular changes are discrete or do not occur in cutaneous yaws.[71]

Untreated primary and secondary cutaneous lesions generally heal with only minimal scarring, unless they are complicated by secondary bacterial infection. The healing process and maintenance of latency seem to involve humoral and cellular mechanisms of immunity.[59] Relapses may occur during latency and, together with late disease, may be caused by a breakdown in the immune state, the development of antigenic variation by the treponeme, or both.

The late gummatous lesions presumably are caused by a hypersensitivity-induced mechanism similar to that postulated for the syphilitic gumma. Bone changes in late stages of yaws most often involve the long bones and manifest as hypertrophic periostitis, gummatous periostitis, osteitis, and nodular or generalized osteomyelitis.[26] Juxtaarticular nodules occur near major joints and are characterized as nonspecific granulomas.[14]

Clinical Manifestations

Yaws is a chronic, debilitating disease characterized by early infectious lesions; periods of latency and relapse; and late destructive lesions of cutaneous, subcutaneous, cartilaginous, and bony tissue. After an incubation period of 9 to 90 days (usually about 3 weeks), the primary lesion forms at the site of inoculation and is accompanied by regional lymphadenopathy. The lesion typically appears as a raised papule on the lower extremity that enlarges to become a hyperkeratotic papilloma measuring 2 to 5 cm in diameter, referred to as a *mother yaw.* It undergoes shallow ulceration and persists a few months to 3 years, at which time healing occurs with a resultant hypopigmented scar and surrounding dark margins.[14]

Before healing of the mother yaw or weeks to months thereafter, crops of secondary, generalized, nondestructive papular lesions appear together with lymphadenopathy and malaise. These lesions tend to form near areas with mucous membranes, such as the nose and mouth, and may resemble condylomata lata. Some papules fade, whereas others enlarge to become papillomatous lesions referred to as *satellite secondaries* or *daughter yaws.* The multiple papillomas are circular, raised, red-yellow lesions with a granular, lobulated, and verrucous surface. They contain numerous treponemes, usually measure 1 to 3 cm in diameter, and produce a yellow discharge that dries to form a black scab. Hyperkeratotic involvement of the palms and soles occurs commonly. Painful fissuring of the soles may cause the patient to walk on the sides of the feet, producing the characteristic gait of "crab" yaws. Bone pain may be severe, and nondestructive long bone lesions, including periostitis, osteitis, and osteomyelitis, may occur.[14,26]

Untreated secondary lesions may persist for longer than 6 months, at which time, owing to the development of host immune mechanisms, they usually heal without scars or residual defects, unless ulceration caused by secondary bacterial infection occurs. During the dry season, early yaws lesions often are atypical, tending to be macular and fewer in number; papillomas, which are small, scanty, dry, flat, and grayish in appearance and of short duration (about 1 month), are confined mainly to the hidden, protected, moist skinfolds.[49,53,69]

Despite healing, some treponemes evade the immune process and persist in the affected tissues (latency). Latency frequently is interrupted by relapses, which tend to occur several times over a 3- to 5-year period. Fewer lesions are produced with each relapse, and they tend to be localized to the periaxillary, perianal, or circumoral area. On cessation of the relapses and usually after a latent period of 3 to 10 years, tertiary lesions occur in 10% of patients; the latent state persists in the remaining patients for their lifetime.[53]

The tertiary lesions characteristically are solitary and destructive; they involve skin, subcutaneous tissue, bone, or cartilage and most commonly occur after the onset of puberty. Painful hyperkeratosis of the palms and soles similar to that seen in early yaws frequently occurs. Other lesions develop as ulcerating, subcutaneous nodules and may heal spontaneously to form scars or extend widely from their margins. The scarring results in depigmentation and sometimes contractions. Bone deformities of late-stage yaws include chronic hypertrophic periostitis, osteitis, gummatous periostitis, and osteomyelitis, each of which may ulcerate through the skin. Gangosa, or rhinopharyngitis mutilans, the destructive gummatous ulceration of the skin and bones of the central face, and juxtaarticular nodules, ganglions of tendon sheaths, and saber tibiae also may occur as manifestations of the late stages of the disease.[27] Gondou, a disfiguring hypertrophic osteitis of the frontal processes of the maxillae, previously reported among western Africans with yaws, seems to have disappeared.[38] Other diseases that must be differentiated from the skin lesions of yaws include vitamin deficiencies, early stages of leprosy, venereal syphilis, tinea versicolor, molluscum contagiosum, scabies, lichen planus, plantar warts, tungiasis, psoriasis, and cutaneous leishmaniasis. Sickle cell disease, tuberculosis, and bacterial osteomyelitis may produce clinical manifestations that mimic the osseous lesions of yaws.[28]

Prognosis

Yaws is not a benign disease. If left untreated, it can produce destructive, disfiguring lesions of the face, feet, and hands and painful and disabling lesions of the fingers and long bones. Ulcers near joints may result in crippling contractures. Secondary bacterial infection of ulcers and of protruding bone lesions can result in further permanent damage to skin and bone tissues. Pathologic fractures generally do not occur.

ENDEMIC SYPHILIS

Endemic syphilis (bejel, njovera, siti, dichuchwa) is a chronic, nonvenereally transmitted disease of prepubescent children. It occurs in the warm, dry, arid regions of the world[53]; lesions are confined to the skin, bone, and cartilage.[53] The disease, known to exist for centuries in Africa, has been recorded in epidemic proportions in areas where conditions among children allow transmission. As with yaws, although seroepidemiologic and mass treatment campaigns have reduced its overall prevalence drastically,[70] endemic areas of concern continue to exist and include the region bordering the southern Sahara Desert, Botswana, and the Arabian Peninsula.[50,53,72]

Biology and Immunology

T. pallidum subsp. *endemicum,* the etiologic agent of endemic syphilis, morphologically is identical to the other pathogenic treponemes. *T. pallidum* subsp. *endemicum* exhibits similarity to syphilis and yaws by producing visible lesions and generalized lymphadenopathy in rabbits and hamsters experimentally infected by the intratesticular and intradermal routes.[29,61] The degree of induration of lesions, distribution and number of lesions, and characteristic lymphadenopathy can be used to differentiate among the species. On the basis of experimental studies in inbred hamsters, *T. pallidum* subsp. *endemicum* stimulates a high degree of homologous resistance to reinfection and cross-immunity to *T. pallidum* subsp. *pallidum* and *T. pallidum* subsp. *pertenue.*[61,67] The genome of the treponeme has been sequenced and was found to be very similar to yaws. However, it was also found to have some loci previously only seen in venereal syphilis.[64]

Epidemiology

Endemic syphilis continues to persist in the warm, drier desert areas bordering the tropical belt. It is prevalent primarily among the seminomadic rural populations in the Arabian peninsula and along the southern border of the Sahara Desert in Africa known as the Sahel region[50,53]; a significant resurgence occurred in Mali, Mauritania, Niger, and the upper Volta during the 1970s.[47] More than 1000 cases were reported in Senegal in 1980.[43] Although scattered endemic foci did exist in central Asia, Australia, Bosnia, and India, they have been virtually eliminated from these areas by mass treatment campaigns.[50,53]

As with pinta and yaws, endemic syphilis propagates under conditions of poor hygiene, crowding, and wearing of little or no clothing. Transmission by oral mucous membranes is favored through contaminated objects, such as drinking vessels and kitchen utensils, and through contact with saliva-contaminated fingers and mouth-to-mouth contact.[13,18,32] Fomites are thought to play a role. Transmission may occur through direct contact of the oral lesion to skin.[53] Occasionally, a previously uninfected nursing mother develops a primary lesion on or near the nipple after the transfer of treponemes from her infected infant.[23,72] Congenital transmission does not seem to occur. Recent analysis of pre-Columbian European skeletons found no endemic syphilis despite significant contact with cases during combat in the Crusades. The conclusions drawn from this analysis are that adults are not susceptible to transmission from other adults and furthermore that adults cannot transmit endemic syphilis.[57] The role of insect vectors, such as flies, has been suggested, but it may be caused by creating a portal of entry by breaks in the skin after itching. Endemic syphilis occurs predominantly among children, with onset usually occurring in children younger than 15 years and with equal sex distribution. Spread occurs most commonly within the family, and active disease can be manifest in more than one family member at any given time.

Pathogenesis and Pathology

T. pallidum subsp. *endemicum* usually enters the host through the oral mucosa. The small number of treponemes introduced into a susceptible host normally precludes the local multiplication and host inflammatory response required to produce a visible primary buccal lesion.[23] When a primary lesion does occur, it appears as a papule or ulcer resulting from a chronic inflammatory response to the proliferating organisms consisting of plasma cell, lymphocytic, and macrophage infiltration. Endothelial cell swelling of small blood vessels also is evident.

The organisms are carried to the regional lymph nodes within a few hours of entry, commonly through the oral mucosa portal. They multiply and elicit epithelial hyperplasia and plasma cell, lymphocytic, and macrophage infiltration, with resultant lymphadenopathy. Dissemination occurs through the circulation, and the organisms are carried to the skin, bone, oral mucosa, axillae, and anogenital regions, where they multiply and elicit a chronic inflammatory response characterized by a cellular infiltration, as seen in the lymph nodes. Vascular changes and perivascular cuffing are prominent.

The untreated early lesions heal as a result of mechanisms thought to involve humoral and cellular immune responses by the host,[58] and the disease enters into a state of latency. Maintenance of latency is thought to involve similar mechanisms. The occurrence of infectious relapses during the latent period still is uncertain.

The late lesions of endemic syphilis are strikingly similar to those of late-stage yaws. Late-stage disease and relapses (if they occur) may be caused by a hypersensitivity-induced mechanism similar to that postulated for the syphilitic gumma.[21,23] Juxtaarticular nodules may occur and represent a nonspecific granulomatous response occurring near major joints.[14] The rarity of cardiovascular and neurologic manifestations may be due to the slow acquisition of small numbers of organisms over a long time, which results in the immunologic protection of the heart and nervous system.[23,36]

Clinical Manifestations

Endemic syphilis is a chronic, often debilitating disease characterized by early infectious secondary lesions; variable periods of latency; and late destructive lesions of cutaneous, subcutaneous, and bone tissues. As mentioned, primary lesions are rare. They appear usually on the breast or nipple as a papule or shallow ulcer similar to that seen in primary venereal syphilis after an approximate 3-week incubation period[1]; they may persist for years before healing.[32]

Even without the appearance of a primary lesion, generalized infection occurs as a result of early dissemination. The onset begins after an incubation period of 3 to 6 months and is characterized by the presence of highly infectious, relatively painless, ulcerative patches on the oropharyngeal mucosa, including the tongue, lips, palate, tonsils, and larynx, with accompanying regional lymphadenopathy. Involvement of the larynx usually results in hoarseness.[14] Split papules or angular stomatitis occurs at the angles of the mouth. Osteoperiostitis of the long bones of the lower extremities, similar to that seen in yaws, is a common early manifestation causing nocturnal leg pains.[14] Occasionally, axillary and anogenital secondary-type lesions result and consist of condylomata similar to those of yaws or dry papillomatous annular patches, with accompanying axillary and inguinal lymphadenopathy. Disseminated papules that are indistinguishable from the papules seen in secondary venereal syphilis may occur. Other forms of cutaneous lesions can occur but are rare.

Untreated secondary lesions may persist for 6 to 9 months, at which time healing occurs because of the development of host immunity. This period of latency varies and, similar to yaws, may last for several years.

Most patients develop tertiary manifestations. Late lesions generally occur during adolescence or adult life and may resemble lesions seen in either late yaws or late-stage venereal syphilis. Gummas may affect any part of the body but commonly occur in the nasopharynx, skin, and bone, resulting in destructive, disfiguring, chronic ulcerations characteristic of gangosa or gangosa-like lesions. Late gummatous lesions can occur during childhood, possibly as a result of superinfection in an already infected host.[24] Bone involvement also is a common finding and results in painful lesions. This condition involves osteitis with gumma formation and, similar to yaws, periostitis affecting most frequently the long bones of the lower extremities. Bilateral synovitis, especially of the knees, occasionally may occur with concomitant juxtaarticular nodules.[24] The cardiovascular and neurologic findings common to venereal syphilis rarely occur in endemic syphilis; when clinical manifestations do occur, they usually are atypical and very mild.[12,50]

Endemic syphilis reportedly has become "clinically attenuated" in Saudi Arabia. Previously florid, the classic disease seems to have been replaced by a milder form in which the number, severity, and duration of early and late lesions are reduced and seroreactive latent infection is increased.[50] The most common late manifestation observed in one study was painful osteoperiostitis of the legs affecting mainly the tibia and fibula. Researchers have postulated that attenuation is a result of improvement in hygienic conditions, better nutrition, and medical care.[50] This indicates the importance of attention to public health measures and the use of antibiotics in the eradication of the disease.

Prognosis

The main complication of endemic syphilis is the destructive gummatous lesions of the face and bones. Severely disfiguring and disabling, these lesions prevent the patient from working effectively in the community. Many of the bone lesions are extremely painful and incapacitating.

DIAGNOSIS

The development of point-of-care treponemal and nontreponemal antibody tests (described later) is an important advance in the clinical diagnosis of nonvenereal treponematoses in the field.[6] However, differentiating the treponematoses from one another solely on the basis of serologic testing is currently untenable because of shared antigens.[48] Although tests based on molecular probes have been developed, these are still mostly research tools. A presumptive diagnosis is based largely on clinical presentation of the disease in an endemic area. Although darkfield examination of early lesions and lymph nodes permits visualization of treponemes, late lesions usually contain few, if any, organisms. The diagnosis of yaws in nonendemic areas or during periods of latency is difficult to make. The coexistence of yaws and endemic syphilis in certain geographic locations, together with their often identical clinical manifestations, renders darkfield and serologic assays useless for differentiating these diseases in such areas.[53] Similar limitations are applicable in differentiating venereal syphilis from yaws or endemic syphilis in nonendemic areas. Under these circumstances, the diagnosis can be based only on a careful history and epidemiologic data.[53]

In tropical areas, numerous other diseases may be confused with yaws.[28,53] Impetigo and chronic tropical ulcers are found frequently and may respond to penicillin or macrolide therapy. Ecthyma may produce ulcers that occasionally are similar to the ulcerative papillomas of yaws. The bacteria *Haemophilus ducreyi* has also been shown to produce lesions indistinguishable on examination to yaws.[39]

Serologic testing is used in the diagnosis of both venereal and nonvenereal treponematoses. The rapid plasma reagin and Venereal Disease Research Laboratory tests are useful but may be nonreactive in early lesions. They are nonspecific nontreponemal studies using cardiolipin antigens that produce similar results in the presence of each disease and cannot be used to differentiate between them. Care must be taken in the interpretation of nontreponemal tests in establishing the diagnosis because of the possibility of obtaining false-positive reactions among patients with nontreponemal diseases or conditions.[45] These tests are quantitative, however, and false-positive results usually have a titer of less than 1:4. After treatment has been given, a twofold or greater drop in titers usually signifies a successful outcome.

The treponemal tests, such as the fluorescent treponemal antibody absorption test, the *T. pallidum* immobilization test, and the *T. pallidum* hemagglutination assay, are specific but normally remain positive for life, and used alone they may not be helpful in diagnosing active cases. Combining nontreponemal and treponemal tests is helpful in establishing the diagnosis when there is a high pretest suspicion, when a false-positive nontreponemal test is likely, when a treponemal test is negative, or when there is a low pretest probability. In pinta, both types of tests may not become reactive until 4 months after the development of the initial lesion, whereas in yaws and endemic syphilis, both tests become reactive within the first few weeks of illness.

Although it may be less practical than serologic testing in remote and resource-poor areas, darkfield examination of fluid obtained from the initial serous exudates from cutaneous or mucous membrane lesions generally reveals the presence of treponemes. As the lesions become more chronic, treponemes become difficult to find. Silver impregnation of biopsy material from skin lesions or lymph nodes may reveal the organisms, but care must be taken in differentiating treponemes from tissue artifact.

The sequencing of the genomes of *T. pallidum pertenue* and *T. pallidum endemicum* has led to the development of polymerase chain reaction (PCR)-based molecular probes for the diagnosis of yaws and endemic syphilis. Another PCR assay has been developed to screen for point mutations in the 23S ribosomal RNA genes that are associated with macrolide resistance in strains of venereal syphilis. As yet, the genome for pinta has not been sequenced.[11,64] Although PCR is highly sensitive and specific, it is not readily available to clinicians in remote areas. Newer treponemal tests using enzyme-linked immunosorbent assays (ELISA), chemiluminescence immunoassay (CIA), and enzyme immunoassay (EIA) have also been developed.[48] Point-of-care tests using fingerstick blood have been developed that employ the CIA technique. These have been shown to be accurate in the identification of antibodies to both treponemal and nontreponemal antigens. Point-of-care tests such as this will be an integral part of the WHO strategy to eradicate yaws because they eliminate the need for sophisticated laboratory equipment and transport of blood specimens, will aid in rapid diagnosis and differentiate between conditions causing similar symptoms, and can demonstrate response to treatment.[6]

TREATMENT AND PREVENTION

For decades, the treatment of choice for all treponemal infections was intramuscular benzathine penicillin G. Although effective, challenges in its use included the need for refrigeration and for intramuscular injection. A noninferiority trial of a single dose of 30 mg/kg of azithromycin versus benzathine penicillin in Papua New Guinea in children aged 6 months to 15 years with confirmed diagnoses of yaws showed that yaws can be cured in its early stages and can prevent transmission with both drugs.[47] Renewal of flagging efforts toward eradication with a single dose of an oral medication overcomes some of the disadvantages of the standard treatment with benzathine penicillin. Sterile protocols for intramuscular injections are not always easy to follow in remote areas, trained medical personnel are needed to administer the injections, penicillin allergy is often encountered, and penicillin requires refrigeration. Oral penicillin also is effective but requires 10 days of treatment, which makes compliance problematic. As a result, azithromycin at 30 mg/kg (up to 2 g maximum) is now the treatment of choice for yaws. Although not yet demonstrated in clinical trials, it is likely that endemic syphilis and pinta are similarly susceptible.

The efficacy and ease of administration of azithromycin led the WHO to adopt the Morges strategy in 2012 to eradicate yaws.[5] There are two parts to this plan. First, mass treatment of all members of at-risk communities with azithromycin is performed. This has the advantage of treating both active and latent cases of yaws, the latter of which can be difficult to detect. Second, surveys are to be conducted every 6 months after mass treatment in order to verify efficacy and to identify and treat persons with active yaws and their contacts.[63] The efficacy of this strategy in a geographically defined area was tested in a large clinical trial on an island of Papua New Guinea between 2013 and 2014. Within a population of 16,092, 82% of the population received a single dose of azithromycin. The prevalence of active yaws decreased from 2.4% to 0.3% one year after treatment, and the prevalence of latent yaws with high titer antibody positivity went from 18.3% to 6.5%. The treatment was generally well tolerated, and there was no evidence of resistance against azithromycin.[46] This study provided evidence that the Morges strategy is effective and can be used in future programs to eradicate yaws. Although no resistance to macrolides was noted, this still remains a concern. Another study looked at the prevalence of yaws in districts of Ghana where population treatment programs with azithromycin had previously been performed for trachoma. In patients examined, there was no evidence of yaws, indicating that the treatment programs may have interrupted the spread of yaws in these previously endemic areas. It was also encouraging that there was no evidence of the development of drug resistance to azithromycin.[22]

For those with macrolide allergies or inability to tolerate these medications, intramuscular benzathine penicillin remains an effective treatment. Patients older than 10 years with clinical disease, those in a period of latency or in the incubatory stages, and contacts of cases should receive 1.2 million units of benzathine penicillin G intramuscularly in a single dose; children younger than 10 years of age should receive 600,000 units in a single dose by the same route.[40] Tetracycline is another alternative treatment for penicillin-allergic patients older than 8 years and not pregnant. The recommended dosage is 500 mg by mouth 4 times daily for 15 days (total dose of 30 g); children aged 8 to 15 years old may be given half the dose.[53] Although the newer tetracyclines have been used and are assumed to be equally effective, no information is available about clinical outcomes.

Therapy for yaws renders early lesions noninfectious in a few days, with complete healing achieved in 7 to 10 days. Recurrences after treatment may occur as a result of reinfection.[28] Late lesions heal more slowly after therapy and may require surgery. In endemic syphilis, infectious lesions disappear rapidly and relapses usually are prevented after therapy. The clinical response to therapy is remarkably slow in pinta. Primary and early secondary lesions take 4 to 6 months to disappear, whereas late secondary lesions require 6 to 12 months for complete healing to occur.[55] Hyperchromic lesions heal without residua, and hypochromic lesions often result in depigmented areas. Old achromic lesions usually remain intact without repigmentation.

In yaws and endemic syphilis, nontreponemal serologic titers may revert to nonreactive if the patient is treated early in the course of the disease. The longer the patient remains untreated, however, the more slowly conversion to seronegativity occurs, and treatment during the later stages may result in the persistence of high titers.[51] Generally, the serologic response to therapy is absent or slow in pinta; nontreponemal tests may take years to decline after adequate therapy has been given.[44] In each of these diseases, treponemal tests remain reactive for life after the patient has received adequate therapy.

Improvement of living conditions and the general hygiene of the community, mass treatment of patients and contacts, and seroepidemiologic campaigns contribute significantly to the prevention of yaws. The Morges strategy formulated by the WHO recommends treatment of an entire endemic community for yaws irrespective of the number of clinical cases and treatment of all active clinical cases and their contacts discovered on resurvey. When implemented, community-wide strategies have been remarkably effective, such as seen in an eradication program in Ecuador and the successful program in India. This underscores the need for accurate epidemiologic data throughout the world to properly identify and treat affected populations.[62,63]

FUTURE CONSIDERATIONS

It is a tragedy that such easily curable diseases have yet to be eradicated. There remains a dearth of epidemiologic data because many governments have stopped collecting prevalence data since the presence of these diseases implies poor health conditions. The immigration of large numbers of people from endemic areas to developed countries means that clinicians everywhere must have an awareness of these diseases and keep them in their differential diagnosis of skin lesions. Important advances have been made strategically with the adoption of the Morges protocol by the WHO, diagnostically with the development of molecular probes and point-of-care dual antibody testing, and clinically with the confirmation that mass treatment with single dose azithromycin is both efficacious and practical. For eradication programs to succeed, prevalence data must be compiled, public health resources in affected countries need to be marshaled, and funding must be obtained. Simple measures, such as improved hygiene, education, and better access to health care in concert with other economic and public health programs, can greatly ameliorate the prevalence and severity of disease. The effective eradication campaigns of the 1950s and 1960s show that such programs can ultimately succeed given adequate resources and international cooperation.

NEW REFERENCES SINCE THE SEVENTH EDITION

5. Asiedu K, Fitzpatrick C, Jannin J. Eradication of yaws: historical efforts and achieving WHO's 2020 target. *PLoS Negl Trop Dis*. 2014;8(9):e3016.
9. Cejkova D, Strouhal M, Norris SJ, Weinstock GM, Smajs D. A Retrospective study on genetic heterogeneity within Treponema strains: subpopulations are genetically distinct in a limited number of positions. *PLoS Negl Trop Dis*. 2015;9(10):e0004110.
11. Chi KH, Danavall D, Taleo F, et al. Molecular differentiation of *Treponema pallidum* subspecies in skin ulceration clinically suspected as yaws in Vanuatu using real-time multiplex PCR and serological methods. *Am J Trop Med Hyg*. 2015;92(1):134-138.
22. Ghinai R, El-Duah P, Chi KH, et al. A cross-sectional study of "yaws" in districts of Ghana which have previously undertaken azithromycin mass drug administration for trachoma control. *PLoS Negl Trop Dis*. 2015;9(1):e0003496.
39. Marks M, Mitja O, Solomon AW, Asiedu KB, Mabey DC. Yaws. *Br Med Bull*. 2015;113(1):91-100.
40. Marks M, Solomon AW, Mabey DC. Endemic treponemal diseases. *Trans R Soc Trop Med Hyg*. 2014;108(10):601-607.
46. Mitja O, Houinei W, Moses P, et al. Mass treatment with single-dose azithromycin for yaws. *N Engl J Med*. 2015;372(8):703-710.
48. Morshed MG, Singh AE. Recent trends in the serologic diagnosis of syphilis. *Clin Vaccine Immunol*. 2015;22(2):137-147.
62. Stamm LV. Pinta: Latin America's Forgotten Disease? *Am J Trop Med Hyg*. 2015;93(5):901-903.
63. Stamm LV. Yaws: 110 Years after Castellani's discovery of *Treponema pallidum* subspecies pertenue. *Am J Trop Med Hyg*. 2015;93(1):4-6.
64. Staudova B, Strouhal M, Zobanikova M, et al. Whole genome sequence of the *Treponema pallidum* subsp. *endemicum* strain Bosnia A: the genome is related to yaws treponemes but contains few loci similar to syphilis treponemes. *PLoS Negl Trop Dis*. 2014;8(11):e3261.
66. Tampa M, Sarbu I, Matei C, Benea V, Georgescu SR. Brief history of syphilis. *J Med Life*. 2014;7(1):4-10.

The full reference list for this chapter is available at ExpertConsult.com.

Clostridial Intoxication and Infection

146

Martha Muller • Gary D. Overturf

Clostridia are obligate anaerobic, endospore-forming bacilli that usually are positive on Gram stain. Of the more than 200 species of *Clostridium*, at least 30 are potential pathogens in humans, mostly by virtue of their biologically active proteins (toxins). More than 25 lethal toxins produced by species of *Clostridium* have been defined in humans, including neurotoxins, enterotoxins, cytotoxins, necrotizing toxins, and enzymatic toxins.[13,89] These ubiquitous organisms frequently are found in soil, sewage, decaying tissue, and the intestinal tract of humans and other animals.[19] Clostridial species flourish in tissue with impaired vascularity and decreased oxygen tension.[53] The genus *Clostridium* has undergone significant revisions in taxonomy since 1994, which has resulted in a proposal for definitions of several clusters based on 16S rRNA gene sequences.[5] Human disease caused by *Clostridium tetani* is discussed in Chapter 148.

BOTULISM

Botulism is an acute descending flaccid paralysis that results from the neurotoxin of *Clostridium botulinum*, which blocks neuromuscular transmission. Four naturally occurring clinical forms of botulism occur: (1) classic foodborne botulism, an intoxication caused by the ingestion of preformed botulinal toxin (BoNT) in contaminated food; (2) wound botulism, which results from elaboration of botulinal toxin in vivo after growth of *C. botulinum* in an infected wound; (3) infant botulism, in which botulinal toxin is produced in vivo in the gastrointestinal tract; and (4) botulism resulting from intestinal colonization in children and adults.[5,25,50] Inhalational and iatrogenic forms of botulism have also been reported.[62] Recently, the potential use of botulinum toxin as a bioterrorist agent has become an important concern. The Centers for Disease Control and Prevention (CDC) characterizes the toxin as a Category A biothreat item.[57] Infant botulism is discussed in Chapter 147.

Epidemiology and Etiology

Antigenically distinct types of botulinum toxins are designated by the letters A through H.[36] More than 40 years after the last toxin characterization, type H toxin was described in 2013 after its recovery from a patient with infant botulism.[9,33] Disease in humans is caused by toxin types A, B, E, F (rarely), and possibly G.[2,22,28,36,41,49,58,60] Types C and D cause botulism in animals.[40,90] From 1973 to 1996, a median of 24 cases of foodborne botulism, three cases of wound botulism, and 71 cases of infant botulism were reported annually to the CDC.[87] This trend has continued recently; in 2009, the Centers for Disease Control and Prevention reported 10 cases of foodborne, 83 infant, and 25 wound or other source botulism cases.[24] In the United States, approximately 50% of foodborne cases are caused by toxin A and 25% each by toxins E and B. Type A occurs primarily in western states, and type B is seen more commonly in eastern states. Type E outbreaks occur more frequently in Alaska and the Great Lakes region. In addition, unique strains of clostridial organisms, other than *C. botulinum*, can produce botulinal neurotoxins and include *C. butyricum*, *C. barati*, and *C. argentinense*.[92]

BoNT is considered the most potent and lethal of all naturally occurring compounds; the intravenous lethal dose for BoNT has been estimated to be 0.1 to 0.5 ng per kilogram of body weight, or an oral dose of 0.2 to 1 μg/kg. BoNT consists of a simple dichain composed of a heavy 100-kDa chain joined by a disulfide bond to a 50-kDa light chain. The toxin's light chain is a Zn^{2+}-containing endopeptidase that blocks acetylcholine-containing vesicles from fusing with the terminal membrane of the motor neuron, thereby resulting in flaccid paralysis.[54] It is heat-labile; 5 minutes of boiling destroys the toxin, and little remains after 30 minutes of exposure at 80°C (176°F). Neurotoxins are produced by *C. botulinum* at all temperatures at which growth occurs (3í to 48° C [37.4° F]). BoNT also is formed at all pH values at which growth occurs (pH 4.8 to 8.5), but it is unstable at pH values higher than 7.0. Toxin thus is produced only during active growth and released during lysis of bacterial cells. The presence of organisms in improperly processed acidic food, however, can allow toxin production to occur.[41,90] Type E BoNT may be produced quickly in small fragments of fish exposed to air and at lower pH values and cooler temperatures than noted with other BoNT types.[40]

Most outbreaks of botulism in the United States are traceable to home-processed foods; however, in recent years the proportion of cases that result from restaurant-associated outbreaks has increased significantly.[87] The most important food vehicles are vegetables, fish, fruits, and condiments. Type E botulism almost always is traceable to fish and fish products, but types A and B also may be involved in outbreaks related to this type of food. Recent outbreaks have been traced to unusual foods, such as potato salad and sautéed onions served by restaurants and commercial frozen pot pies mishandled at home.

Wound botulism results from infection of traumatized tissue by *C. botulinum* type A or B and subsequent production of toxin.[69] In the United States, approximately 80% of cases are caused by toxin A and 20% by toxin B.[87] Although infrequently reported, wound infection is a disease of pediatric concern; approximately half of the cases in the United States that occurred before 1991 involved children and teenagers, most of whom were boys with compound extremity fractures. In recent years, however, most new cases have occurred in users of contaminated injectable black tar heroin.[5,28,87]

Pathophysiology

Botulinum toxin is absorbed from the proximal part of the intestine or an infected wound and is distributed hematogenously to the neuromuscular junction of motor neurons. The toxin irreversibly binds to presynaptic membranes, where it penetrates the plasma membrane by receptor-mediated endocytosis and the light chain of toxin (50 kDa) is internalized into the nerve cell through a protein channel. BoNT specifically cleaves proteins involved in vesicle trafficking of neurotransmitters, and exocytosis of acetylcholine is prevented. The prevention of neurotransmission results in clinically flaccid paralysis.[40,41,90] The cranial nerves are affected earliest and often most severely. Death occurs mainly from respiratory muscle paralysis (asphyxia) or its complications, such as cardiac arrhythmia, aspiration, and pneumonia.[29] The clinical hallmark of botulism is an acute flaccid paralysis that begins with bilateral cranial nerve impairment of the muscles of the eye, face, head, and pharynx, descending symmetrically to involve muscles of the thorax and extremities.[95] BoNT, unlike tetanus toxin, does not enter the central nervous system (CNS). Recovery occurs by regeneration of terminal motor function and the formation of new motor end-plates. The lethal dose of botulinum toxin for humans is not known but can be estimated from primate studies; the dose of crystalline toxin lethal to a 70-kg human would be approximately 0.09 to 0.15 μg intravenously (or intramuscularly), 0.70 to 0.90 μg by inhalation, and 70 μg orally.[86]

Clinical Manifestations

Because the pathogenesis of botulism involves the systemic absorption of BoNT and hematogenous dissemination with subsequent involvement of cholinergic synapses, virtually all forms of botulism have identical neurologic signs. The signs and symptoms of botulism are summarized in Table 146.1.[8] The onset of illness varies from 12 to 72 hours after the implicated food is ingested, but it has been documented to occur as late as 108 hours after ingestion in some epidemics.[8]

Foodborne illness, or classic botulism, may be preceded by abdominal cramps, nausea, vomiting, or diarrhea. The neurologic illness begins as mentioned previously, as a descending symmetric motor paralysis first affecting muscles supplied by the cranial nerves.[8,38] No sensory disturbance occurs, although vision may be impaired and hearing distorted because of cranial nerve involvement. Mental processes remain clear, but anxiety and agitation may be present. Fever is absent unless a secondary bacterial infection occurs. The triad of bulbar palsies (including a sluggish or absent pupillary response to light), lucid sensorium, and absent fever always should bring botulism to mind. Common symptoms include blurred vision, diplopia, dysarthria, and dysphagia. The degree of ocular involvement is quite variable; in severe cases, the pupils may become fixed and dilated. The mucous membranes of the mouth, tongue, and pharynx may be so dry that pain results, which may lead to the mistaken diagnosis of pharyngitis. Dizziness or vertigo may occur. Urinary retention may be seen, occasionally with stress incontinence.

Two thirds of patients have no gastrointestinal symptoms. In those who do, with type A or type B botulism the gastrointestinal manifestations are primarily abdominal pain, cramps, fullness, and diarrhea. However, after an initial period of diarrhea, constipation or obstipation may be noted and, indeed, is more typical of the disease. In contrast to those with the other types, most patients with type E botulism first have gastrointestinal symptoms, including nausea, vomiting, substernal burning or pain, abdominal distention, and decreased bowel sounds. The most common signs encountered in botulism are respiratory impairment; specific muscle weakness or paralysis; eye muscle involvement, including ptosis; dry throat, mouth, or tongue; dilated, fixed pupils; and ataxia. Respiratory involvement, even aside from aspiration pneumonia, is a fairly common occurrence. Vital capacity is a more sensitive indicator of respiratory compromise than is measurement of blood gas. Postural hypotension, nystagmus, and somnolence may be noted.

TABLE 146.1 Symptoms and Signs of Foodborne Botulism Types A and B

	% of Cases
Symptoms	
Dysphagia	96
Dry mouth	93
Double vision	91
Dysarthria	84
Fatigue	77
Arm weakness	73
Constipation	73
Leg weakness	69
Blurred vision	65
Nausea	64
Dyspnea	60
Vomiting	59
Dizziness	51
Sore throat	54
Abdominal cramps	42
Diarrhea	19
Paresthesia	14
Signs	
Alert mental status	90
Arm weakness	75
Ptosis	73
Leg weakness	69
Gaze paralysis	65
Facial palsy	63
Diminished gag reflex	58
Tongue weakness	58
Pupils dilated or fixed	44
Hyporeflexia or areflexia	40
Nystagmus	22
Ataxia	17

The usual interval (incubation period) between the ingestion of food and the onset of symptoms is 18 to 36 hours, but it may be as short as 2 hours or as long as 8 days. In general, patients with shorter incubation periods are affected more severely and have a poorer prognosis. The shortness of the incubation period and the severity of illness correlate with the amount of BoNT ingested. Although the syndrome is similar for each toxin type, type A toxin has been associated with more severe disease and a higher mortality rate than has either type B or type E toxin.[104]

The symptoms of wound botulism are similar to those of food botulism, but some important differences may occur.[69] Fever may or may not be present. Constipation occurs, but nausea and vomiting do not. Unilateral sensory changes in association with the trauma or infection may be noted. The wound itself may have grossly purulent drainage, but sometimes the wound shows no evidence of infection. The incubation period of wound botulism usually is 4 to 14 days.

In the event of intentional foodborne poisoning with BoNT, the signs and symptoms probably would resemble those of naturally occurring foodborne botulism.[8,87] If the aerosolized BoNT from a bioterrorist attack were to be inhaled, the incubation period might be slightly longer, and gastrointestinal symptoms might not occur.[8,87]

Differential Diagnosis

The differential diagnosis of botulism includes myasthenia gravis, cerebrovascular accidents, Guillain-Barré syndrome (particularly the Miller-Fisher variant), tick paralysis, paralytic shellfish poisoning, chemical intoxication, diphtheritic polyneuritis, psychiatric disease, and the Eaton-Lambert syndrome.[40,90]

Ordinary bacterial food poisoning generally is not a problem in the differential diagnosis because of the absence of cranial nerve involvement. Chemical food poisoning may cause neurologic manifestations, but the signs almost always appear within minutes or at most hours after consumption of contaminated food. Atropine poisoning has a very rapid onset and is distinctive because of facial flushing and hallucinations. Shellfish and fish poisonings have a rapid onset and often cause characteristic paresthesias, tremors, and other signs. Mushroom poisoning results in severe abdominal pain, violent vomiting, diarrhea, and coma.

Myasthenia gravis usually spares pupillary oculomotor function. An edrophonium (Tensilon) test should be performed. Guillain-Barré syndrome can mimic botulism but usually shows ascending peripheral paralysis and, later, cranial nerve involvement. Muscle cramps, paresthesias, and an elevated protein content in cerebrospinal fluid (CSF) in the absence of cells help distinguish this disease. Electromyography may be extremely useful in differentiating botulism from atypical cases of Guillain-Barré syndrome. Because BoNT does not enter the CNS, abnormalities of the CSF are virtually never present.

The problem of identifying a case is complicated by reports of patients with features not characteristic of either botulism or the action of botulinum toxin, such as paresthesias, asymmetric weakness of the extremities, asymmetric ptosis, slightly elevated CSF protein, and a positive response to edrophonium. Some of these symptoms may be a consequence of the high anxiety that prevails in persons who know that they have eaten a food containing BoNT.

Specific Diagnosis

Confirmation of the diagnosis of botulism depends primarily on detection of botulinum toxin or the organism in the patient or in the implicated food or wound.[40,90] Specimens to be examined for botulinum toxin include serum, gastric contents or vomitus, feces (at least 20 to 50 g when possible), and exudates from wounds and tissues. These specimens, particularly blood specimens, should be obtained as soon as possible and before antitoxin is given. When feasible, at least 15 to 20 mL of blood should be drawn into a large vacuum tube and sent without separation of the serum to the nearest laboratory capable of performing the mouse neutralization test and other tests for toxin. On suspicion of clinical botulism, state health departments and the CDC should be consulted immediately regarding appropriate specimen collection and transport and the appropriate laboratories to which samples can be sent. The CDC can be contacted for general information at 800-232-4636, available Monday through Friday, 8 AM to 8 PM Eastern time, and the CDC Emergency Operations Center is also available for consultation and provision of therapeutic materials at 770-488-7100 (current information available at http://www.cdc.gov).

Specimens should be refrigerated (4°C [39.2°F]) and be examined as quickly as possible after collection. Whenever feasible, suspect food should be kept sealed in the original container. Sterile unbreakable containers should be used for other food samples. Specimens to be shipped to laboratories must be placed in leak-proof containers; packed with dry ice in a second leak-proof, insulated container; and marked "Danger, hazardous material." Extreme caution should be used in handling material that may contain botulinum toxin because even minute quantities of toxin acquired by ingestion, inhalation, or absorption through the eye or a break in the skin may cause profound intoxication and death.

Laboratory confirmation of suspected botulism should be attempted, even late in the clinical course. Detection of the organism itself may be achieved by culture or a variety of molecular methodologies. However, the most reliable assay for BoNT remains the mouse bioassay with type-specific neutralization of toxin with specific antitoxins.[29]

Botulinum neurotoxin is detected in serum or stool specimens in approximately 46% of clinically diagnosed cases. When stool specimens also are cultured for *C. botulinum*, confirmatory evidence is obtained in approximately 70% of botulism cases.[87,104] Thus, detection of C. botulinum toxin or organisms in the stool of a symptomatic person should be considered diagnostic.

Treatment

The mainstay of therapy for all forms of botulism is meticulous supportive care, with particular attention paid to the respiratory and nutritional needs of the patient and to anticipation of potential complications.[40,41] Symptomatic persons known to have ingested toxin-containing food should be hospitalized, with careful monitoring of respiratory and cardiac function.

In cases of foodborne botulism, if the patient is seen early, protected induced emesis and gastric lavage may be considered to reduce the amount of unabsorbed toxin; in the absence of ileus, cathartic agents may be helpful. Magnesium-containing cathartic agents should be avoided because they may enhance the action of botulinum toxin.

Heptavalent antitoxin (types A to G; i.e., H-BAT) of equine origin frequently is considered in the management of foodborne botulism in adults, although conclusive evidence of its efficacy is lacking.[40,95] In the past, trivalent (A, B, and C) and bivalent (A and B) were available, but since 2010 only the hepatavalent material is provided by the CDC. Antitoxin is provided to neutralize circulating botulinum toxin molecules that are not yet bound to nerve endings. This material has been "despeciated" by the removal of the Fc fragment of the immunoglobulins, resulting in a material which is more than 90% Fab and F (ab) immunoglobulin fragments. Although antitoxin is recommended for treatment, the paralysis caused by irreversible binding of the neurotoxin cannot be reversed by administered antitoxins. The dose currently recommended in adults is one vial per patient as a single dose.[87] Recommendations for children will accompany the full instructions included from public health and CDC authorities. Hypersensitivity reactions have been reported in approximately 9% of persons treated with equine sera, so skin testing should be performed before administration of the antitoxin (recommendations for testing are provided by the CDC). Treatment of a single patient with suspected or proved foodborne botulism requires immediate notification of state and federal (CDC) health officials, who also are the antitoxin source, and the food responsible for the index patient's illness still may be available to other persons. The appropriate initial contact is via the state health department. If this agency cannot be reached, the CDC should be contacted immediately (see the CDC telephone numbers in the earlier discussion of diagnosis). Presently, a human-derived botulinum antitoxin is available in the United States exclusively for the treatment of infantile botulism and is discussed in Chapter 147.

In the event of a potential exposure to a suspected contaminated food, the following procedures should be implemented. Locate all persons who ate the suspect food and determine whether anyone has signs or symptoms of botulism.[40] If patients are seen soon after the suspect meal, the use of gastric lavage, emetics, and cathartics deserves consideration. Antitoxin should be made available. Any samples of the suspect food that may remain should be collected and refrigerated. The health authorities should assist the clinician with these tasks. The fecal and serum specimens needed to establish the diagnosis should be obtained. If neurologic signs are present, one should try to identify defective neuromuscular transmission by electromyelography. If neurologic signs are absent, the patient and family should be informed of the early signs of botulinum intoxication and be instructed to return at the first manifestation of ptosis, diplopia, blurred vision, dysphonia, dysarthria, or dysphagia. Because of the serious side effects of equine botulinum antitoxin, prophylactic administration of it to asymptomatic persons who have ingested food known to contain botulinum toxin generally is not recommended.[5]

When wound botulism is suspected, exploration and débridement of the site must be undertaken, ideally after the administration of antitoxin has begun. Arrangements should be made to obtain material for anaerobic culture in the operating room and antibiotic therapy begun there. High-dose penicillin 250,000 to 400,000 U/kg per day for 10 to 14 days is the drug of choice. Guanidine, aminopyridine, steroids, and intravenous immunoglobulin have been used to treat a small number of cases of foodborne and wound botulism, but convincing evidence of their efficacy is lacking. Metronidazole has been suggested as an alternative for penicillin, based on studies suggesting its enhanced efficacy in tetanus, but evidence for its effectiveness in botulism is not available.

Prognosis

With an emphasis on mechanical ventilation and intensive supportive care, the mortality rate from botulism has decreased steadily from 60% in the 1950s to 3% to 5%, and a mortality of less than 1% among hospitalized patients. It is lower with type B and type C disease than with type A19 and lower with any type in individuals younger than 20 years. An important factor is the dose of toxin ingested as reflected by the length of the incubation period. The longer the incubation period, the better the prognosis, whereas shorter incubation periods are associated with ingestion of larger doses and higher rates of morbidity and mortality. Thus, if the index case in an outbreak can be detected early, other patients exposed to the same food will have a much better prognosis. Recovery may be prolonged, and some symptoms (e.g., fatigability) may persist for as long as 1 year. Most patients recover entirely.

Prevention

Local and state health authorities and the CDC should be notified immediately of all suspected cases of botulism so that timely investigations can be undertaken. Although commercial products still are responsible for botulism occasionally, control measures taken by industry have done a great deal to prevent botulism from this source. Home canners still must be instructed regarding appropriate means for sterilizing containers and food preservation and for adequate cooking of food before serving.[40,90] In canning, a pressure cooker must be used to obtain temperatures well above boiling to destroy spores of *C. botulinum* types A and B. For certain foods, a temperature of 116°C (240.8°F) is recommended. Spores of *C. botulinum* are destroyed at 120°C (248°F) after 30 minutes. Pressure cookers set at 15 lb will achieve this temperature, but correction for higher altitudes must be made. Home-canned foods should be boiled for 10 minutes before serving. Food containers that appear to bulge may contain gas produced by *C. botulinum* and should not be opened. The pentavalent botulinum toxoid vaccine has been used in military personnel to protect them from biologic warfare assault; given in three subcutaneous doses, it leads to detectable antibodies in 83% of subjects.[28]

CLOSTRIDIAL INFECTIONS

Clostridia are encountered less commonly in infections than are non–spore-forming anaerobic bacteria, but these spore formers rarely may produce devastating disease. Overall, clostridia are present in 5% to 10% of anaerobic or mixed (aerobic and anaerobic) infections.[17,34,40,97] Table 146.2 depicts the relative frequency of clostridial species from clinically significant infections at a single academic hospital.[5] Surgical or traumatic events are reported to precede 90% of cases of clostridial infections.[84]

Clostridium perfringens is the species encountered most commonly. It may be isolated in pure culture but more commonly is part of a mixed flora involving other anaerobes and nonanaerobes. Other species important clinically or encountered commonly (or both) include *C. novyi*, *C. septicum*, *C. bifermentans*, *C. histolyticum*, and *C. sordellii* (together with *C. perfringens*, these species commonly are referred to as the "gas gangrene group"); *C. tetani* (see Chapter 147); *C. difficile*, a major pathogen in pseudomembranous colitis; and a group of clostridia important in infections other than gas gangrene or myonecrosis (wound infection, abscesses, bacteremia, etc.)—*C. perfringens*, *C. ramosum*, *C. bifermentans*, *C. sphenoides*, *C. sporogenes*, and others.

Clostridia may be involved in a wide variety of infections throughout the body. Certain of these infections have a distinctive clinical picture and are discussed in this chapter. Many other infections, including peritonitis, intraabdominal infection, wound infection, soft tissue infection, and, occasionally, pleuropulmonary infection, CNS infection, and urinary tract infection, are not distinctive and will not be discussed specifically here. Emphysematous cholecystitis involving *C. perfringens* has distinctive features, but it is not encountered in the pediatric age group and thus is not discussed. Bacteremia involving *C. perfringens* may or may not have characteristic features. The distinctive intravascular hemolysis that may occur with *C. perfringens* bacteremia is discussed in connection with female genital tract infections caused by this organism.

Clostridial infections in children have revealed diverse species among 113 isolates in 107 specimens, including (in order of frequency) unidentified *Clostridium* spp. (33%), *C. perfringens* (12%), *C. inoculum* (5%), *C. ramosum* (4%), *C. botulinum* (3%), *C. difficile* (2%), and *C. butyricum* (2%), as well as single isolates of *C. bifermentans*, *C. clostridioforme*, *C. limosum*, and *C. parputrifucum*.[18] Most were from abscesses, peritonitis, bacteremia, and chronic otitis media, and many children had underlying conditions such as immunodeficiency, malignancy, diabetes, trauma, presence of foreign bodies, and prior surgery. Clostridia were isolated from 7% of all specimens processed for anaerobic bacteria, with frequent coisolation of *Bacteroides* spp., *Escherichia coli*, *Prevotella* spp., *Porphyromonas* spp., and *Fusobacterium* spp.

TABLE 146.2 *Clostridium* Species Most Frequently Encountered in Clinical Specimens at Indiana University Hospital Anaerobe Laboratory (1989–2001)[a]

	ISOLATES	
Species[b]	**No.**	**% of Total**
C. perfringens	515	20
C. clostridioforme	421	16
C. inoculum	380	15
C. ramosum	357	14
C. difficile	287	11
C. butyricum	113	4
C. cadaveris	99	4
C. bifermentans	53	2
C. sporogenes	49	2
C. glycolicum	44	2
C. septicum	42	2
C. tertium	39	2
C. sordellii, *C. subterminale*, *C. paraputrificum*, *C. symbiosum*, and *C. baratii*	15-30	1

[a]The 2555 isolates do not include 270 isolates that did not belong to a recognized species (total of 2825 isolates), nor do they include *C. difficile* from fecal specimens.
[b]Six or fewer isolates each of *C. beijerinckii*, *C. botulinum*, *C. carnis*, *C. celatum*, *C. coccoides*, *C. cochlearium*, *C. ghoni*, *C. hastiforme*, *C. histolyticum*, *C. indolis*, *C. limosum*, *C. malenominatum*, *C. novyi*, *C. putrefaciens*, *C. putrificum*, and *C. sphenoides*.

Epidemiology

The vast majority of clostridial infections are of endogenous origin. Even those secondary to trauma and contamination of a wound with foreign bodies usually involve *C. perfringens* or other clostridia from the host's flora, chiefly the intestinal tract. *Clostridium* spp. are ubiquitous in nature, with habitats in soil and the intestinal tracts of many animals, including humans and most other mammals. Clostridia even may be isolated from infant intestine as early as the first week of life, and by 6 to 20 months of age, the feces of infants contain approximately the same number of *C. perfringens* organisms as that of adults.[5]

Pathophysiology

The principal sites of normal carriage of *C. perfringens* and many other clostridial species in humans are the colon and vagina.[5,40,41] These organisms may gain access to tissues through wounds, by perforation of abdominal viscera, or because of local disease such as tumor. The organism then may grow in tissues if the oxidation-reduction potential is low, host defense mechanisms are impaired, or both. Factors favoring anaerobic growth include the presence of abundant necrotic tissue, a poor blood supply, presence of foreign bodies, or previous multiplication of other bacteria in the wound leading to a lowered oxidation-reduction potential.

As noted, *Clostridium* spp. produced a wide range of toxins.[51,92] *C. perfringens* produces at least a dozen different extracellular toxins or other factors that account for its pathogenicity.[40] The most important of the five major lethal toxins is α-toxin, a lecithinase and the main toxin responsible for destruction of tissue, hemolysis, and death. Other important factors include collagenase, hyaluronidase, leukocidin, deoxyribonuclease, and fibrinolysin. The enterotoxins produced by some strains of *C. perfringens* and *C. difficile* are important in the pathogenesis of certain gastrointestinal diseases.[63,67] Gas gangrene, or clostridial myonecrosis, is characterized by profound toxicity, necrosis of muscle, edema, thrombosis of small vessels, gas bubbles in tissues, and minimal infiltration of leukocytes (probably caused by destruction of leukocytes at the site).

Clinical Manifestations

Gas Gangrene or Myonecrosis

Although other clostridia also are involved in gas gangrene, *C. perfringens* is the single causative species in approximately 90% to 95% of cases associated with trauma. Gas gangrene usually results from contamination of open wounds with contiguous injured muscle. Tissue destruction in gas gangrene is related to profound attenuation in blood flow as a result of activation of platelet responses by the α-toxin of *C. perfringens*.[20] Clostridial myonecrosis may occur in the absence of a traumatic wound, so-called spontaneous myonecrosis, and is caused by bacteremic seeding of muscle with either *C. perfringens*, *C. tertium*, or *C. septicum*.[100,103] The last species is almost entirely associated with the spontaneous form of gas gangrene.[61] In spontaneous myonecrosis, the source of the organism typically is the bowel, and the usual predisposing factors are mucosal tumors of the bowel or ulcerations produced by cytotoxic chemotherapy.[40] Additional reported risk factors for the development of spontaneous myonecrosis are intramuscular or subcutaneous inoculations, malignancies, immunocompromising conditions, and leukopenia.[70] Only a handful of cases of spontaneous myonecrosis in children have been described.[70]

The typical case of clostridial myonecrosis is manifested by sudden appearance of pain in the region of a wound.[40] The pain increases in severity but remains localized to the infected area. Subsequently, local swelling and edema occur, and a thin hemorrhagic exudate appears. The pulse is very rapid, out of proportion to the mild elevation in temperature. Initially, the skin is tense, white, somewhat colder than normal, and very tender. Bronze discoloration appears and increases with time. The process extends and becomes more severe, and the patient becomes toxemic. The skin becomes dusky or bronzed, and bullae filled with dark-red or purple fluid appear. Crepitus caused by gas may be noted, but the amount of gas produced generally is small. A peculiar sweet smell may be noted in some cases. Occasionally, a fetid odor that probably reflects the presence of a *Clostridium* organism other than *C. perfringens* may be present.[40] Toxic delirium and, later, overwhelming prostration and toxemia may develop. Some patients are alert and apprehensive, whereas others are apathetic. Later in the course of the disease, shock supervenes. At surgery, early changes in muscle consist primarily of edema and pallor, but increased reddening with mottled purple is present. The consistency of the muscle may be pasty or mucoid, and contractility disappears. Eventually, the muscle becomes diffusely gangrenous, dark greenish-purple or black, friable, and even liquefied. When bacteremia supervenes, mortality rates often exceed 50%.

Gram stain of the drainage or fluids or tissue obtained by biopsy is usually definitive, revealing gram-positive rods and a lack of inflammatory cells. Indeed, a paucity of inflammatory cells in tissue stains is highly indicative of infection with *Clostridium*.[1] However, recent studies indicate that the marked tissue destruction and absence of neutrophils with *C. perfringens* gas gangrene are caused by α-toxin-induced occlusion of blood vessels by platelets and neutrophils.[19] The margin between healthy and necrotic tissue often advances several inches per hour despite appropriate antibiotic therapy, and radical amputation or debridement of necrotic infected tissue remains the best life-saving treatment. Hyperbaric oxygen has also been used as additional therapy,[39] but its efficacy is controversial, and its use often makes other supportive treatment difficult.

Soft Tissue Infection

C. perfringens and other clostridia also may be involved in less dramatic and less serious infections ranging from minor superficial infections to anaerobic cellulitis and necrotizing fasciitis.[40] Clostridial organisms in these infections may occur as single isolates, as part of a mixed flora consisting solely of anaerobic bacteria, or as part of a mixed anaerobic-aerobic bacterial flora. The clinical picture in these various infections is no different from that noted with other types of organisms and thus is not discussed further here.

Bacteremia and Sepsis

Clostridium spp. are important causes of sepsis, although infrequent in children. *C. septicum* is isolated only rarely from feces of healthy individuals but may be found in the appendixes of normal individuals, and more than 50% of persons whose blood is positive for this organism have some gastrointestinal anomaly such as colonic diverticulae or Meckel diverticulum. Additionally, malignancy has been reported in 50% to 90% of cases of *C. septicum* sepsis.[79] Many of the conditions most frequently predisposing to clostridial sepsis, such as gastrointestinal malignancy, vascular insufficiency or atherosclerosis, cirrhosis, neutropenia and pancreatitis, or uncontrolled diabetes, are rare in children and therefore, clostridial sepsis is rare in children.

Septic Abortion and Puerperal Sepsis

C. perfringens infections of the uterus usually occur after incomplete or traumatic abortions and are induced under nonsterile conditions.[40] More recently, *C. sordellii* has been more frequently associated with these infections. Occasionally, this type of infection will develop after spontaneous abortion, prolonged labor, ruptured membranes, or operative interference with pregnancy. Early symptoms include uterine bleeding, suprapubic and back pain, and chills, but often with little or no fever.[40,41] The incubation period after the precipitating event usually is several days, but it may be less than 24 hours. In addition to vaginal bleeding, a foul-smelling, brown vaginal discharge containing necrotic tissue often is present. The uterus is tender, and the lower abdominal wall may be tense. Nausea, vomiting, and diarrhea may occur. Generalized peritonitis may complicate the picture. The most striking systemic manifestation of the disease, however, is massive intravascular hemolysis with hemoglobinemia, hemoglobinuria, and jaundice. Shock and acute renal failure may complicate the picture. Intrauterine gas formation may be detected. Postnatal uterine infections resulting in gas gangrene of uterus are often rapidly fatal.

Neonatal Sepsis and Meningitis

A small number of cases of sepsis or meningitis (or both) caused by *Clostridium* spp. have been reported in newborns.[42,44,71,72,93] Although some of these neonatal cases have been associated with invasive procedures or devitalized tissue, others have not had an obvious source.[44,52,71] In several of these cases, the systemic infection involved both the mother and infant. The typical clinical picture in neonatal infections is one of fulminant septic shock, intravascular hemolysis, respiratory distress, and rapid death. Pneumocephalus may occur in the presence of meningitis.

Pseudomembranous Colitis (C. difficile)

Clostridium difficile is increasing as a pathogen in children despite high carriage rates in asymptomatic newborns and infants younger than 2 years. In addition, the epidemiology of *C. difficile* in children has been increasingly defined in recent years.[7,15,58] The organism is the major cause of antibiotic associated diarrhea and pseudomembranous colitis.[45] Pathogenesis of this colitis is the production of two toxins, toxin A and B.[35,37,98] Treatment and management of infections in children has been adapted from adult standards.[105] See Chapter 45 for a detailed description of the organism, current epidemiology in children, pathogenesis, and treatment of disease in children.

Food Poisoning and Other Enteric Infections

A usually mild, self-limited, and very common form of food poisoning may be caused by *C. perfringens*. Meat and meat products are the most common vehicles for such outbreaks.[40,41,77] Food poisoning is caused by a heat-labile enterotoxin produced by *C. perfringens* type A. Disease is the result of ingestion of 10^8 or more vegetative cells that sporulate in the alkaline environment of the small intestine, producing the enterotoxin. The incubation period after ingestion of contaminated food varies from 6 to 30 hours but usually is 8 to 12 hours. The major symptoms are crampy abdominal pain and diarrhea. Stools are liquid but do not contain blood or mucus. Nausea may be noted on occasion, but vomiting and fever seldom are present. The illness typically lasts less than 24 hours but may be more severe in the very young or elderly.[16]

Rarely, *C. perfringens* also may produce a very severe type of enteritis known as enteritis necroticans. Although food poisoning is produced by *C. perfringens* type A, necrotizing enteritis involves the β-toxin of *C. perfringens* type C.[60] Consumption of excessive amounts of rich food by people normally on a low-protein diet who have decreased levels of digestive proteases seems to be an important background factor. Additionally, proteases may be blocked by ingestion of trypsin inhibitors found in sweet potatoes. In some cases, consumption of contaminated canned meat is involved. In Papua New Guinea, where this condition is known as "pigbel," enteritis necroticans in children is associated with traditional pig-feasting activities in which large quantities of pork are consumed. The disease is characterized by abdominal cramps, vomiting, shock, diarrhea (sometimes bloody), and acute inflammation of the small intestine with areas of necrosis and gangrene, particularly in the jejunum.[81] A 12-year-old diabetic boy in whom enteritis necroticans developed after the ingestion of pig intestines (chitterlings) has been reported.[80]

Miscellaneous Infections Caused by Clostridia

Fewer than 40 cases of septic arthritis attributable to *Clostridium* spp., including several pediatric patients, have been reported.[48] Anaerobic osteomyelitis caused by *Clostridium* also is a rare finding.[43] Aggressive surgical debridement and prolonged antibiotic therapy are warranted in the treatment of anaerobic musculoskeletal infections.[88]

The clinical spectrum of clostridial bacteremia ranges from an asymptomatic patient with an incidental positive blood culture to fulminant sepsis syndrome.[23] Bacteremia with *C. septicum* is considered a unique syndrome associated with malignancies, particularly leukemia and colon cancer, and it has a devastating clinical course.[47,64] Infections with this organism also have been linked to children with cyclic neutropenia.[5,10,11,75] In a recent review of 28 pediatric patients with *C. septicum* bacteremia, Caya[25] noted that all of them had underlying cancer or gastrointestinal disease. The overall mortality rate was 72%. Several cases of *C. septicum* infection occurring after *E. coli* O157–induced hemolytic-uremic syndrome have been described.[6,12,55,66,82,83,102]

Clostridium sordellii infections have been associated with high fatality rates and most often have occurred after trauma, childbirth, and routine gynecologic procedures. They have been reported after medically induced abortions and intravenous drug injections. In one review of 45 cases, eight (18%) occurred after normal childbirth and five occurred (11%) after medically induced abortions, with a 100% case-fatality rate in this group.[4] A few cases have occurred in children, including a 4-year-old child with arm trauma, a 17-year-old adolescent with omphalitis, a 12-year-old child with ear infection, an 18-year-old adolescent with a medically induced abortion, an 8-month-old with a pericarditis and associated pyopericardium with tamponade, and a 12-year-old boy with tuberous sclerosis.[3,27]

Panophthalmitis involving *C. perfringens* or, occasionally, other clostridia is secondary to penetrating injury, usually with retention of a foreign body, but can also be seen without foreign bodies.[40,101] Pain and loss of vision occur within 12 hours after the injury. By 18 hours, evidence of fulminating panophthalmitis is present and consists of chemosis and brawny swelling of the lids, proptosis, hypopyon, increased intraocular tension, gas bubbles in the anterior chamber, and necrosis of the wound margins. Intracranial infections involving *Clostridium*, usually as a result of penetrating trauma with items such as a lawn dart or an arrow, have been described.

Pneumatosis cystoides intestinalis can be produced in animals by *C. perfringens*, and this organism has been recovered from this process in humans.[40,41] Pneumatosis cystoides intestinalis may be found in conjunction with toxic megacolon and neonatal necrotizing enterocolitis and as a complication of ileal bypass for obesity. Evaluation regarding the associating between *Clostridium* species and necrotizing enterocolitis and ultimate outcomes is ongoing.[31,32] *Clostridium septicum* has been reported as causative of enterocolitis.[26]

Clostridial species have also been implicated in infections after musculoskeletal allograft placement.[57]

Clostridium has also been described as the causative agent of pyogenic liver abscess, especially sustained after blunt abdominal trauma. *Clostridium novyi*, *Clostridium clostridioforme*, *Clostridium bifermentans* and *Clostridium perfringens* have all been reported from pediatric patients with liver abscesses.[2,68,73,76]

Specific Diagnosis

The diagnosis of gas gangrene must be made on clinical grounds. The presence of a gas-forming infection and recovery of *C. perfringens* from the wound do not establish the diagnosis of gas gangrene. The key to this diagnosis is demonstration of myonecrosis. Clostridial myonecrosis must be differentiated from other gas-forming soft tissue infections, which may or may not involve *C. perfringens*, and from other causes of myonecrosis. The sudden onset, extreme toxemia, and severe pain that are noted in clostridial myonecrosis represent important differential features. Entities such as anaerobic cellulitis and streptococcal myonecrosis have a gradual onset, slight toxemia, and less pain than seen with clostridial myonecrosis. Synergistic nonclostridial aerobic-anaerobic myonecrosis is a severe infection characterized by discrete areas of blue-gray necrosis of skin, along with extensive involvement of the underlying soft tissue and muscle and foul "dishwater" pus. Anaerobic cellulitis typically has much more gas and does not involve muscle.

In streptococcal myonecrosis, edema of the muscle is present initially, followed later by a hemorrhagic appearance.[40] Specimens for Gram staining and culture should be obtained from involved muscle rather than from the surface of the wound. Large gram-positive rods will be demonstrated on Gram stain in clostridial myonecrosis; no white blood cells may be demonstrable, or the white blood cells present may be distorted significantly as a result of the toxin of *C. perfringens* acting on them. Anaerobic-aerobic mixed cellulitis typically shows a mixture of organisms, which may include *C. perfringens*. Streptococcal myonecrosis reveals anaerobic streptococci, sometimes along with group A streptococci, *Staphylococcus aureus*, and other organisms.[30] In synergistic nonclostridial anaerobic-aerobic myonecrosis, *Bacteroides* organisms seem to be key pathogens, together with anaerobic cocci and aerobic gram-negative bacilli.[40] Of importance when obtaining material for culture is to place it under anaerobic conditions or designated anaerobic transport media or devices for transport to the laboratory. Anaerobic blood cultures also should be performed.

Uterine infection by *C. perfringens* varies in severity from secondary invasion of necrotic material into the uterus or a dead fetus to invasion of intact uterine muscle producing myonecrosis and physometra.[40] Although bacteremia is a relatively uncommon finding in gas gangrene, uterine infection with *C. perfringens* frequently is accompanied by sepsis, which leads to the dramatic picture of intravascular hemolysis described earlier. Demonstration of severe hemolytic anemia in association with uterine infection essentially is diagnostic. Anaerobic blood cultures should be performed.

Clostridia, particularly *C. perfringens*, occasionally are isolated from the blood of a patient with a clinically benign course. The usual scenario is that a hospitalized patient has a single fever spike of unclear etiology and blood cultures are performed as part of the evaluation; by the time the culture becomes positive, no evidence of an infectious process is present. This transient and benign bacteremia probably originates from the colonic flora.[15,21]

C. perfringens food poisoning usually is seen in the setting of a sizable outbreak.[40] The organism grows to high counts in the responsible food and then sets up an infection in the host, with production of enterotoxin in the colon of patients. Demonstration of large numbers ($>10^5$/g) of *C. perfringens* in the implicated food and demonstration of the same serotype of *C. perfringens* in the stool of affected individuals and in the food are important in documenting the nature of the food poisoning. Enterotoxin also may be found in the stool of affected individuals, and the *C. perfringens* recovered from stool or food can be demonstrated to produce enterotoxin in vitro. Necrotizing enteritis caused by *C. perfringens* may be suspected by virtue of the dramatic clinical picture and confirmed by demonstration of *C. perfringens* type C in the stool or suspect food or demonstration of serum antibody to the β-toxin of the organism.

C. difficile–associated diarrhea should be suspected in children with diarrhea who have received antibiotics within the previous 2 months or whose diarrhea begins 72 hours after hospitalization.[7,15,38,45,47,58,59,74] Typically, toxin testing of a single stool specimen will establish the diagnosis, but, occasionally, repeat testing or endoscopy may need to be performed. The finding of exudative plaques (pseudomembranes) and a hyperemic, friable mucosa by direct endoscopic visualization suggests the diagnosis of pseudomembranous colitis. Although *C. difficile* is isolated conveniently with use of a selective medium, distinction between toxigenic and nonpathogenic strains cannot be made. Its toxin B (cytotoxin) is identified most easily by tissue culture assay, which remains the gold standard for diagnosis of antibiotic-associated diarrhea.[40] A simple latex particle agglutination test for detection of *C. difficile* is available, although it is considered relatively insensitive and nonspecific and, for that reason, no longer is recommended.[67,94,96]

In recent years, commercially available enzyme immunoassay (EIA) kits that detect toxin B or both toxin A and B have become the preferred method of diagnosis.[14,96] The EIAs in general are easy to perform, relatively inexpensive, and specific. Polymerase chain reaction amplification tests for toxins A and B have been designed but are not available commercially.[37,85,98]

Interpreting the significance of finding *C. difficile* or its toxins in very young patients with diarrhea is difficult because infants and toddlers have a high rate of asymptomatic carriage.[35,56,99] Quantitation of toxin or organisms has not correlated with the presence or absence of symptoms. Consequently, once the possible presence of other diarrhea-producing pathogens (e.g., rotavirus, *Salmonella*) has been excluded, effort should be made to stop the presumptive precipitating antibacterial agent. If diarrhea with mucus or blood persists, endoscopy should be considered and specific therapy begun.

Treatment

The most important aspect of treating clostridial myonecrosis is immediate surgical intervention consisting of radical debridement and drainage and decompression of the fascial compartments.[40,41] The wound should not be closed after surgery. Of crucial importance is that all bits of necrotic muscle and other tissue be removed. Polyvalent gas gangrene antitoxin was never established firmly as being beneficial in the context of modern therapy, and this product no longer is available in the United States. Hyperbaric oxygen is recommended enthusiastically by some physicians, but no definitive evidence that its use reduces mortality rates has been shown. It does facilitate demarcation of a limb with impaired vascular supply, and it appears to slow or arrest local spread of the gangrenous infection. Clearly, however, hyperbaric oxygen must not be used as a substitute for any of the important principles of surgical management. Antimicrobial therapy also is important as an adjunct, with high-dose penicillin G (250,000 to 400,000 U/kg per day) being the drug of choice.[40,41] In individuals allergic to penicillin G, clindamycin or metronidazole may be used. In addition, chloramphenicol is routinely active against all clostridia. The combination of penicillin and clindamycin has been used widely on the basis of experimental animal models that have shown enhanced efficacy with such a combination.[91]

Clostridial cellulitis is treated by incision plus drainage and antimicrobial therapy. Radical débridement is not necessary, but it is important to lay the tissues open to effect proper drainage and permit removal of all necrotic tissue.[40,41]

Uterine curettage should be performed for diagnosis and treatment of postabortal or puerperal clostridial infections.[41] Hysterectomy may be required if the myometrium is involved and if the patient's condition is deteriorating. At times, perforation of the uterus may be present without the typical clinical findings. Exchange transfusion has been recommended for sepsis caused by *C. perfringens* when significant intravascular hemolysis is present.

Food poisoning caused by *C. perfringens* is self-limited and requires no therapy. Antitoxin to the β-toxin produced by *C. perfringens* type C has been of considerable benefit in the treatment of necrotizing enteritis caused by this organism.

In any serious infection caused by *C. perfringens* or other clostridia, the usual supportive measures for shock, dehydration, anemia, and renal insufficiency are implemented as indicated.

Treatment of *C. difficile*–associated disease involves discontinuation of the offending antibiotic regimen when feasible. Isolates of *C. difficile* are susceptible to metronidazole and vancomycin. Oral or intravenous metronidazole 30 mg/kg per day in four divided doses is considered the drug of choice. With the recent and rapid increase in the recovery of vancomycin-resistant enterococci, many experts and the CDC suggest that oral vancomycin 40 mg/kg per day in four divided doses be used to treat *C. difficile*–induced diarrhea only in patients who are critically ill or those who do not respond to metronidazole.[38,78,105] Intravenous vancomycin has not been shown to consistently effective. Orally administered bacitracin also may be useful, although some experts suggest that it may be less effective than metronidazole or vancomycin. Antimicrobial agents typically are administered for 10 days, but as many as 20% of patients may experience a relapse requiring a second course of treatment.[65] The use of cholestyramine or probiotics, such as *Saccharomyces* or *Lactobacillus*, in adult patients with multiple relapses has been advocated by some physicians, but such treatment has not been evaluated in children with disease caused by *C. difficile*.

Prognosis

The mortality rate in patients with gas gangrene varies between 15% and 35% and is worse when large muscle groups, such as those of the buttock, thigh, leg, and shoulder, are involved or when areas that are difficult to débride, such as the viscera and pelvis, are involved with disease. Clostridial cellulitis has a much better prognosis, but aggressive therapy still is important to minimize mortality rates. The mortality rate in postabortal clostridial sepsis remains 50% to 85%. *C. perfringens* food poisoning has an excellent prognosis, but mortality rates are significant with necrotizing enteritis caused by *C. perfringens* type C.

Prevention

Wounds involving areas with large muscle masses are particularly prone to gas gangrene, as are compound fractures, severe crush injuries, and injuries secondary to high-velocity missiles. Extensive laceration or devitalization of muscle tissue, impairment of the main blood supply to a limb or large muscle group, and contamination by dirt or bowel contents all predispose to the development of clostridial myonecrosis. The most important aspect of prophylaxis by far is early and adequate surgical management.[40,41] All devitalized tissue must be débrided; meticulous hemostasis is very important. Primary closure and tight packing of the wound should be avoided. All aspects of the wound must be drained adequately. If a cast must be applied, it should be bivalved from the outset. Hyperbaric oxygen is not indicated prophylactically. Antimicrobial prophylaxis, however, definitely is indicated. Penicillin is the drug of choice and should be given as early as possible after the injury occurs. Of emphasis is that antimicrobial prophylaxis is strictly adjunctive and far from adequate by itself. Bathing, particularly showering, and application of a compress wet with an iodophor for 15 minutes have been shown to reduce the skin count of *C. perfringens* significantly and minimize the likelihood of postoperative gas gangrene developing. This type of decontamination, of course, also may be useful in the management of traumatic wounds.

Prevention of clostridial uterine infection involves ensuring that all products of conception are removed during abortion and that retained portions of placenta are removed immediately after the third stage of labor. Prolonged labor should be anticipated when possible and analgesics administered judiciously. During labor, particularly with ruptured membranes, pelvic and rectal examinations should be kept to a minimum. During delivery, trauma should be minimized and lacerations repaired according to accepted surgical principles.

Proper sanitation in food-preparing facilities and adequate refrigeration are important safeguards against acquisition of *C. perfringens* food poisoning. In areas where necrotizing enteritis caused by *C. perfringens* type C is found with some frequency (such as in Papua New Guinea), a *C. perfringens* type C toxoid has been given with encouraging results.

Contact isolation for the duration of the illness is recommended for hospitalized children with *C. difficile*–associated diarrhea. Meticulous hand washing, the use of gloves for handling contaminated objects and fomites, environmental cleaning and disinfection, and limiting the use of antimicrobial agents have been advocated widely to control the transmission of *C. difficile* in health care facilities.[46]

NEW REFERENCES SINCE THE SEVENTH EDITION

1. Abd Rashid AH, Ramli R, Ibrahim S. *Clostridium perfringens* surgical site infection after osteotomy for knee deformity correction in a non-immunocompromised child. *Surg Infect (Larchmt)*. 2014;15:656-658.
2. Abdel-Haq NM, Chearskul P, Salimnia H, et al. Clostridial liver abscess following blunt abdominal trauma: case report and review of the literature. *Scand J Infect Dis*. 2007;39:734-737.
3. Abdulla A, Yee L. The clinical spectrum of *Clostridium sordellii* bacteraemia: two case reports and a review of the literature. *J Clin Pathol*. 2000;53:709-712.
9. Barash JR, Arnon SS. A novel strain of *Clostridium botulinum* that produces type B and type H botulinum toxins. *J Infect Dis*. 2014;209:183-191.
11. Barnes C, Gerstle JT, Freedman MH, et al. *Clostridium septicum* myonecrosis in congenital neutropenia. *Pediatrics*. 2004;114:e757-e760.
26. Chang YJ, Wu CT, Chiu CH, et al. Fulminant *Clostridium septicum* infection mimicking appendicitis in a healthy child. *Trop Paediatr*. 2007;27:91-94.
27. Chaudhry R, Verma N, Bahadur T, et al. *Clostridium sordellii* as a cause of constrictive pericarditis with pyopericardium and tamponade. *J Clin Microbiol*. 2011;49:3700-370230.
31. de la Cochetiere MF, Piloquet H, des Robert C, et al. Early intestinal bacterial colonization and necrotizing enterocolitis in premature infants: the putative role of *Clostridium*. *Pediatr Res*. 2004;56:366-370.
32. Dittmar E, Beyer P, Fischer D, et al. Necrotizing enterocolitis of the neonate with *Clostridium perfringens*: diagnosis, clinical course, and role of alpha toxin. *Eur J Pediatr*. 2008;167:891-895.
33. Dover N, Barash JR, Hill KK, et al. Molecular characterization of a novel botulinum neurotoxin type H gene. *J Infect Dis*. 2014;209:192-202.
36. Fan Y, Barash JR, Lou J, et al. Immunological characterization and neutralizing ability of monoclonal antibodies directed against botulinum neurotoxin type H. *J Infect Dis*. 2016;213:1606-1614.
39. Fielden MP, Martinovic E, Ells AL. Hyperbaric oxygen therapy in the treatment of orbital gas gangrene. *J AAPOS*. 2002;6:252-254.
49. Hart GB, Lamb RC, Strauss MB. Gas gangrene. *J Trauma*. 1983;23:991-1000.
53. Hill BJ, Skerry JC, Smith TJ, et al. Universal and specific quantitative detection of *botulinum* neurotoxin genes. *BMC Microbiol*. 2010;10:267.
55. Hunley TE, Spring MD, Peters TR, et al. *Clostridium septicum* myonecrosis complicating diarrhea-associated hemolytic uremic syndrome. *Pediatr Nephrol*. 2008;23:1171-1175.

57. Kainer MA, Linden JV, Whaley DN, et al. *Clostridium* infections associated with musculoskeletal-tissue allografts. *N Engl J Med.* 2004;350:2564-2571.
62. Lindstrom M, Korkeala H. Laboratory diagnostics of botulism. *Clin Microbiol Rev.* 2006;19:298-314.
66. Martin SE, Allen SD, Faught P, et al. A 2-year-old boy with hemolytic uremic syndrome and pneumocephalus. *Brain Pathol.* 2012;22:121-124.
68. Mera CL, Freedman MH. *Clostridium* liver abscess and massive hemolysis. Unique demise in Fanconi's aplastic anemia. *Clin Pediatr (Phila).* 1984;23:126-127.
73. Nachman S, Kaul A, Li KL, et al. Liver abscess caused by *Clostridium bifermentans* following blunt abdominal trauma. *J Clin Microbiol.* 1989;27:1137-1138.
75. Ogah K, Sethi K, Karthik V. *Clostridium clostridioforme* liver abscess complicated by portal vein thrombosis in childhood. *J Med Microbiol.* 2012;61:297-299.
76. O'Hanrahan T, Dark P, Irving MH. Cyclic neutropenia-unusual cause of acute abdomen. Report of a case. *Dis Colon Rectum.* 1991;34:1125-1127.
77. Pelletier JP, Plumbley JA, Rouse EA, et al. The role of *Clostridium septicum* in paraneoplastic sepsis. *Arch Pathol Lab Med.* 2000;124:353-356.
81. Poka H, Duke T. In search of pigbel: gone or just forgotten in the highlands of Papua New Guinea. *P N G Med J.* 2003;46:135-142.
82. Randall JM, Hall K, Coulthard MG. Diffuse pneumocephalus due to *Clostridium septicum* cerebritis in haemolytic uraemic syndrome: CT demonstration. *Neuroradiology.* 1993;35:218-220.
83. Sadarangani SP, Batdorf R, Buchhalter LC, et al. *Clostridium septicum* brain abscesses in a premature neonate. *Pediatr Infect Dis J.* 2014;33:538-540.
84. Salvador C, Kropshofer G, Niederwanger C, et al. Fulminant *Clostridium perfringens* sepsis during induction chemotherapy in childhood leukemia. *Pediatr Int.* 2012;54:424-425.
100. Wiersema BM, Scheid DK, Psaradellis T. A rare trifocal presentation of *Clostridium septicum* myonecrosis. *Orthopedics.* 2008;31:2746.
101. Wiles SB, Ide CH. *Clostridium perfringens* endophthalmitis. *Am J Ophthalmol.* 1991;111:654-656, 7.
102. Williams EJ, Mitchell P, Mitra D, et al. A microbiological hazard of rural living: *Clostridium septicum* brain abscess in a child with *E coli* 0157 associated haemolyic uraemic syndrome. *BMJ Case Rep.* 2012.
103. Wong SN, Lau YL, Lo RN, et al. *Clostridium clostridiforme* infection in a postoperative cardiac patient. *Pediatr Infect Dis J.* 1992;11:52-54, 9.

The full reference list for this chapter is available at ExpertConsult.com.

147 Infant Botulism

Jessica M. Khouri • Stephen S. Arnon

Of the three main forms of human botulism (foodborne, wound, and infant), infant botulism is the most recently recognized (1976) and since 1980 the most common form in the United States. Now recognized globally,[76] infant botulism results from a unique pathogenesis. Ingested spores of *Clostridium botulinum* germinate, colonize the infant's colon, and produce botulinum neurotoxin within it. The toxin is then absorbed, binds to peripheral cholinergic synapses, and causes flaccid paralysis. Knowledge of this intestinal pathogenesis resulted in discovery of novel pathogenic strains of *Clostridium baratii* and *Clostridium butyricum,* each of which produces a botulinum neurotoxin and causes infant botulism. Discovery of these strains enlarged the number of organisms known to cause the "intestinal toxemias of infancy," of which infant botulism is the prototype. Parenthetically, adults and older children rarely may become susceptible to infant-type (i.e., intestinal toxemia) botulism after broad-spectrum antibiotic treatment, intestinal surgery, or inflammatory bowel disease,[9,35,45,52,60,136] or in association with a Meckel diverticulum[49,118] or bone marrow transplantation.[126]

HISTORY

Infant botulism is not a new disease but instead is a relatively recently recognized "emerging" infectious disease. The first laboratory-proven case of human infant botulism occurred in California in 1931, although it was misdiagnosed at the time.[18] Decades later and well before the etiology of the disease was apparent, the characteristic clinical features of infant botulism had become evident to discerning observers. In 1974, Grover and associates[58] described nine patients from Pennsylvania with a neurologic syndrome of undetermined cause that from today's perspective almost certainly was infant botulism. The same idiopathic syndrome was recognized in southern California and was reported by Ramseyer and colleagues in 1976 to have a characteristic electromyographic pattern.[114] A year later, Clay and associates linked their eight southern California patients to infant botulism.[36]

The first report of botulism in infancy was provided by Pickett and colleagues in 1976.[112] Although the source of botulinum neurotoxin for their two patients was undetermined, the possibility of its in vivo production was suggested.[92,112] The diagnosis of botulism in these and other California patients was established by identification of *C. botulinum* toxin and organisms in the infants' feces.[92] Evidence also was obtained that ingested spores of *C. botulinum* had produced the toxin in the infants' intestinal tract.[13,92,152]

In subsequent years the clinical spectrum of infant botulism was found to include mild outpatient cases and, in some but not all[30] locations, sudden unexpected death indistinguishable from typical sudden infant death syndrome.[14,100,105,111] In 1985, a *C. baratii* strain that produced a type F botulinum neurotoxin was recognized belatedly as the true cause of a case of infant botulism that occurred in New Mexico in 1979,[59,65] and in 1986, a *C. butyricum* strain that produced a type E botulinum neurotoxin was recognized as the cause of two cases of infant botulism in Rome, Italy.[19] In 2014, a *C. botulinum* strain that produced both type B and a novel type H botulinum toxin was reported.[22,41,46] These latter three novel clostridia were discovered only because they caused human infant botulism (rather than foodborne or wound botulism); their existence suggests that others like them await discovery.

ETIOLOGIC AGENT

Clostridium botulinum is a gram-positive, spore-forming, obligate anaerobe whose natural habitat worldwide is the soil. Consequently, *C. botulinum* is as ubiquitous as the dust on which it may travel; hence, its spores commonly are present on fresh fruits, vegetables, and other agricultural products such as honey. Members of the *C. botulinum* species are so diverse in their biochemical capabilities and nucleic acid profiles that they would not be grouped as a single species except for the similar neurotoxin molecule that each strain produces.[63,135] The species *C. botulinum* is subdivided into four groups (I to IV) based on metabolic characteristics.[63,135] Almost all cases of infant botulism in the United States have been caused by group I proteolytic type A or type B strains. However, unusual strains of *C. baratii* and *C. butyricum* that make botulinum toxins E and F also cause infant botulism.[19,24,43,47,59,108,140,149] The entire 3.9-megabase (Mb) chromosome and a 16.3-kilobase (kb) plasmid within a *C. botulinum* type A strain were sequenced and found to contain 3650 and 19 predicted genes, respectively,[124] thereby launching the era of comparative genomic studies of this special bacterium.[74,89,132,153] Whole genome sequencing has enabled comparison of *C. botulinum* strains at the nucleotide level.[63,74,89,153]

In general, each vegetative cell of *C. botulinum* produces just one of eight distinguishable toxins, which have been arbitrarily assigned the letters A to H.[22,41,46,87,110,135] A ninth toxin type of uncertain in vivo pathogenicity identified by genome database review and designated "serotype X" was recently reported.[154–156] The eight toxin types are operationally distinguished by polyclonal monovalent antitoxins raised against each of the toxin types; each monovalent antitoxin does not protect against any of the other seven toxin types. Hence, effective treatment of botulism occurs only when the antitoxin type (A-H) matches the toxin type (A-H) that matches the patient's illness. The different toxin types serve as convenient epidemiologic and clinical markers. Strains that produce two toxins have been isolated from patients (e.g., Ab, Af, Ba Bf, Bh); the capital letter indicates the toxin produced in greater amount.[22,38,39,132] Subtypes of several toxin types have been identified by immunologic methods,[71,72,77,144] by neutralization studies using monoclonal antibodies,[6,134] and by toxin gene nucleic acid investigations.[63,64,134] Each toxin molecule is a simple protein consisting of two polypeptide chains of approximately 100,000 (heavy chain) and 50,000 (light chain) daltons joined by a disulfide bond. The gene for botulinum toxin, *bont*, is part of an operon termed the "toxin gene cluster," which is a mobile genetic element that may be located in the chromosome, a plasmid, or a bacteriophage.[63,131,132]

Botulinum toxin is the most poisonous substance known.[53] For this reason and because of the ease with which it may be produced, transported, and disseminated, the Centers for Disease Control and Prevention (CDC) has listed botulinum toxin as a Tier 1 ("mass casualty capable") potential bioweapon agent.[1,16] By extrapolation from studies involving adult primates, the lethal dose in the bloodstream of humans is approximately 1 ng/kg body weight.[16,53] The potency of the toxin for infants may be even higher because of the narrowness of their pharyngeal airway.[147]

The basis of the phenomenal potency of the botulinum (and tetanus) toxins is enzymatic. The light chain of each neurotoxin is a zinc-containing protease that hydrolyzes one or more of three intracellular proteins needed for vesicle fusion and release of acetylcholine into the synaptic cleft.[120] The specificity of the toxins for peripheral cholinergic neurons results from their expression of a low-affinity ganglioside cell surface receptor to which the toxin attaches first that is then followed by its attachment to a second, high-affinity protein receptor that uniquely appears from the interior of the synaptic vesicle when it fuses with the terminal membrane to release acetylcholine.[34,68,106,116]

PATHOGENESIS

Infant botulism is not the diminutive form of foodborne botulism, and, hence, the disease is not "infantile botulism." Rather, infant botulism results from a unique infectious disease pathway and was so named to emphasize that fact.[13,92,152] Ingested spores of *C. botulinum* germinate, colonize the infant's colon, and produce botulinum neurotoxin in it.[13,61,94,96,152] The toxin subsequently is absorbed and carried by the bloodstream to peripheral cholinergic synapses, where it binds and is endocytosed. The light chain then passes into the cytosol of the neuron, where it blocks the release of acetylcholine by enzymatic cleavage of "fusion complex" proteins.[120] Clinically, the most important peripheral cholinergic synapse is the neuromuscular junction; the toxin's action here results in flaccid paralysis and hypotonia. Preganglionic cholinergic synapses in the autonomic nervous system may also be affected.[83,120]

By use of a mouse model system of intestinal colonization (in which the animals paradoxically remained free of symptoms), Sugiyama and colleagues[29,96,141,142] demonstrated that the intestinal microbiome of adult animals ordinarily prevents colonization of the gut by *C. botulinum*. Administration of 10^6 type A spores failed to colonize the intestine of normal adult mice, whereas after treatment for 2.5 days with a combination of oral erythromycin and kanamycin, half the mice could be colonized by just 2×10^4 spores. When the antibiotic-treated mice were placed in cages with normal mice, they lost their susceptibility to intestinal colonization after 3 days.[29] (Mice normally exhibit coprophagia.) In addition, adult germ-free mice could be colonized intestinally by just 10 *C. botulinum* type A spores. When the germ-free adult animals were placed in a room with conventional mice (but not in the same cages), in 3 days the formerly germ-free animals became resistant to colonization by 10^5 spores.[96]

In contrast to the experimental work with adult mice, normal infant mice were susceptible to intestinal colonization by *C. botulinum* spores.[141] Like human infants, the normal infant mice were subject to colonization for only a limited period (7 to 13 days of age).[11,141] Susceptibility of the infant mice peaked between days 8 and 11 in a pattern reminiscent of the peaking of susceptibility seen between 2 and 4 months of age in human infant botulism (e-Fig. 147.1). The infective dose of spores for infant mice was much smaller than that of their antibiotic-treated adult counterparts; the 50% infective dose for normal infants was only 700 spores. In one experiment, just 10 spores were needed to colonize an infant mouse.[141] The minimum infective dose of *C. botulinum* spores for human infants is not known, but from exposure to spore-containing honey, it has been estimated to be as low as 10 to 100.[15]

Recognition of the central role of the host's intestinal microbiome in determining susceptibility or resistance to colonization by *C. botulinum* has directed attention to its composition and to factors that may influence it.[128] Diet may be the most important of these factors. When compared to adult-type intestinal flora, the infant flora is simpler, with fewer genera and species.[78,81,138,139] The dominant members vary, depending in part on whether the infant is fed only breast milk, only formula milk, or a mixture of the two.[138,139] In addition, the composition of the intestinal microbiome is changed if solid foods, such as cereals, become part of the infant's diet. The normal human infant microbiome contains several bacterial species, mainly *Bifidobacterium* and *Bacteroides,* that in vitro can inhibit the multiplication of *C. botulinum*.[143]

The onset of infant botulism occurs at a significantly younger age in formula-fed infants (7.6 weeks) than in breast-fed infants (13.7 weeks),[12] perhaps reflecting the earlier availability in formula-fed infants of suitable ecologic niches[12,84,138,139] and the formula-fed infants' lack of the immune factors (e.g., secretory IgA, lactoferrin, leukocytes) contained in human milk.[7,8,50,55] Moreover, introduction of solid foods may "perturb" the intestinal microbiome[139] and thereby assist in colonization with *C. botulinum*.[8,11,84,139]

An additional physiologic risk factor for infant botulism is slower gut motility, as measured by the frequency of defecation before the onset of illness.[123,137] Less than one bowel movement per day is a risk factor for both breast-fed and formula-fed infants, but this factor occurred in just 50% of cases.[123] Whether a Meckel diverticulum may predispose to the development of infant botulism caused by *C. botulinum,* as it appears to do for infant botulism caused by *C. butyricum,* is not known.[47,49,118]

EPIDEMIOLOGY

Any discussion of the epidemiology of infant botulism should be prefaced by the caveat that almost all presently available information is derived from study of only part of the clinical spectrum, namely, hospitalized patients. Accordingly, current perspectives may need to be modified as the outpatient and sudden death parts of the clinical spectrum become more completely characterized. In addition, the perceived incidence remains more a reflection of physician awareness and access to diagnostic testing than the actual occurrence of disease. Somewhat more than one third (37.8%) of US cases have been reported from California, which has the largest number of births of any state. However, California does not have the highest incidence of infant botulism once adjustment is made for differences in annual births (Table 147.1). Notably, eight of the 12 states with the highest incidence are located west of the Rocky Mountains, and six of the eight are contiguous. The four eastern states with the highest incidence also are contiguous.

A unique epidemiologic feature of infant botulism is its age distribution, which, perhaps coincidentally, is virtually identical to the age distribution of sudden infant death syndrome (see e-Fig. 147.1).[11,14,31,137] Almost all US cases (99.7%) of infant botulism reported to date have occurred in children younger than 1 year old. Some 88.7% of cases have occurred in the patients' first 6 months of life, 11.0% were distributed over the subsequent 6 months, and just 0.3% have occurred between 53 and 72 weeks of age. The youngest known patient was only 38 hours old at onset (and had illness caused by *C. baratii* type F toxin),[24] whereas the oldest was 72 weeks old at onset. The illness has occurred in all major racial and ethnic groups and in approximately equal proportions in males and females. A national seasonality is not evident. In California more cases have occur in the six warmer, drier months (May to October, 58%) than in the six cooler, wetter months (November to April, 42%).

Infant botulism has been reported from all inhabited continents except Africa. In the United States, with 53 exceptions (1.5% of cases), all hospitalized cases known as of December 2015 were caused by either type A or type B botulinum toxin. All 50 states have reported infant

TABLE 147.1 Cases and Incidence of Infant Botulism: Top 12 States in Incidence, United States (1977–2014)

State	Cases (*N*) 1977–2014	Incidence[a] 1977–2014
Delaware	58	14.2
Utah	127	7.5
Hawaii	52	7.4
Pennsylvania	413	7.1
California	1247	6.4
New Jersey	174	4.2
Washington	105	3.6
New Mexico	36	3.5
Oregon	57	3.4
Montana	15	3.3
Idaho	24	3.2
Maryland	82	3.2

[a]Per 100,000 live births per year.

botulism; California (1976) was the first and Rhode Island (2008) was the last. In general, the distribution of cases by toxin type has paralleled the distribution of toxin types in US soil,[90,129] with type B cases predominating from the Great Plains eastward and type A cases from the Rocky Mountains westward.

The 53 exceptional cases resulted from a variety of toxin types. Three cases in California and in Iowa, two in Colorado and Ohio, and one each in Idaho, Massachusetts, New Mexico, Texas, Virginia, Washington, and Wisconsin resulted from type F toxin produced by neurotoxigenic *C. baratii* strains.[24,59,65,97,108] Twenty-three cases were caused by *C. botulinum* that produced mostly type B and some type A toxin (designated type Ba), and 11 cases resulted from Bf strains. One case caused by both *C. botulinum* type A and type B from today's perspective probably resulted from either a Ba or Ab strain.[132] Five patients with Bf illness lived in California,[21] one lived in New Mexico, and four lived in Texas, whereas the 11th patient had traveled from California through New Mexico to Texas immediately before onset of the illness. Two type Bf cases occurred in the United Kingdom.[133] The only *C. baratii* type F cases reported outside the United States occurred in Canada and Hungary.[149] In Illinois in 2008, a type E case caused by *C. botulinum* occurred,[86] and in Arizona in 2006 a type E case caused by *C. butyricum* was recognized.[43] Five *C. butyricum* type E infant botulism cases were reported from Italy, two from Ireland, and one each from the United Kingdom and Japan.[3,19,47-49,125]

Potential environmental sources of *C. botulinum* spores have been identified in many locales. The soil in Pennsylvania,[84] soil and cistern water in Australia,[99] untreated well water in Japan,[75] vacuum cleaner dust in Finland,[105] and soil and vacuum cleaner dust in California[11] obtained from case homes were found to contain *C. botulinum*, with the toxin type (A or B) in each instance matching the toxin type of the infant's illness. In addition, *C. butyricum* type E isolated from pet terrapin samples and their commercial food was associated with two cases in Ireland.[125] However, despite the foregoing, it deserves emphasis that for most cases of infant botulism, no source of *C. botulinum* spores is ever identified, even circumstantially. In these cases illness probably was acquired by swallowing spores adherent to airborne microscopic (invisible) dust.

Approximately one fifth (876 of 4302; 20.4%) of all known global infant botulism cases between 1976 and 2015 have been recognized from 34 countries other than the United States.[76] Of these cases, Argentina has reported the largest number (610),[85] followed by Australia (42), Canada (41), Italy (32), Japan (31), Spain (22), United Kingdom (16), Germany (14), France (8), Denmark (7), and Israel (5). The remaining countries have reported five or fewer cases each.[76] The non-US cases occurred in Europe (18 countries), Asia (3), the Middle East (5), North America (2), South America (3), and Australia.[88] The small number of reported cases from most non-US countries most likely reflects limited physician awareness of the disease and limited access to specialized diagnostic testing laboratories, as well as actual variation in disease incidence.[76]

Geographic clustering has been noted.[38,89] In Pennsylvania, 43 of 53 cases in the period 1977 to 1983 occurred in four suburban counties that form an arc bordering the city of Philadelphia.[82,84] In Colorado, three type A cases occurred in three separate families in a small town with approximately 30 annual births over a 3-year period. Two of the infants had used the same crib sequentially; environmental samples, including the crib, soil, and household dust, yielded *C. botulinum* type A.[67]

In a 35-year surveillance period in California both geographic (2 type A, 3 type B) and geographic-temporal (2 type A, 3 type B, 1 type A(B)) clustering was recognized (e-Figs. 147.2, 147.3, and 147.4).[38] In addition, two type A cases occurred 5 years apart in the children of two California families who lived one house apart. In another California family two successive infants each acquired type A infant botulism, but the third child born in sequence did not. Soil and dust specimens from the house where all three infants lived contained *C. botulinum* type A.

The role of breast-feeding and formula-feeding as factors possibly predisposing to illness remains unsettled. All studies to date have identified an association between being breast-fed and being hospitalized for infant botulism.[7,12,82-84,98,137,146] This finding has resulted in one perspective that holds that breast-feeding predisposes to the development of illness,[82-84,137] whereas the other perspective holds that breast-feeding slows its onset sufficiently to permit hospitalization to occur.[7,8,11,12] Among hospitalized patients in California, the mean age at onset of botulism in formula-fed infants (7.6 weeks) was significantly younger and about half that of breast-fed infants (13.7 weeks).[12] In addition, all California patients with fulminant-onset infant botulism who stopped breathing and died at home were formula fed.[12] The relative susceptibilities of formula-fed and breast-fed infants to infant botulism and the resultant severity of their disease may reflect differences in availability ecologic niches for *C. botulinum* in the intestinal microbiome, differences in immune factors (e.g., lactoferrin and secretory IgA) contained in human milk but not in formula milk,[55] or other differences not identified yet.

Probably few, if any, patients with infant botulism acquire *C. botulinum* spores from infant formula, despite isolation in the United Kingdom of *C. botulinum* type B from powdered infant formula consumed by a patient with type B infant botulism.[28,70] However, the capacity of powdered infant formula (a nonsterile product) to serve as a vehicle of clostridial spores was identified in a study of US commercial powdered infant formulas that found a dozen different clostridial species in them, including *Clostridium sporogenes* (the functional equivalent of atoxigenic proteolytic *C. botulinum*).[23] In addition, the possibility that an infant patient may have foodborne botulism needs to be kept in mind because foodborne botulism caused by home-prepared baby food has occurred.[5,25]

Honey is the one dietary reservoir of *C. botulinum* spores thus far definitively linked to infant botulism by both laboratory and epidemiologic evidence.[11,15,20,62,66,73,93,104,117,142] More than 35 instances worldwide are known in which *C. botulinum* spores have been found in the actual honey fed to the affected infant before the onset of illness. In each instance, the toxin type (A or B) of the spores in the honey matched the toxin type of the *C. botulinum* that caused the infant's illness; the probability that such perfect concordance occurred by chance is less than 1 in 10 billion. Occasionally, *C. botulinum* has been isolated from honey in which the spore toxin type in the honey did not match the toxin type of the infant's illness[20,47]; in such instances, the conclusion is that the honey was not the source of the infective spores.

C. botulinum spores have been found in honey from the United States, Argentina, Australia, Brazil, Canada, China (Taiwan also), Denmark, Finland, Hungary, Italy, Mexico, Norway, Spain, Japan, and Central America,[15,20,62,66,73,93,101-104,121,142] and recently, in the United Kingdom in honeys fed to two patients with infant botulism.[2,57,130]

In general, only low concentrations of *C. botulinum* spores have been found in honey (≤1 spore/g),[93,102] with the occasional higher concentrations (e.g., 36–60 spores/g) thought to result from multiplication of *C. botulinum* in dead bees and bee pupae.[101] Toxin type A, B, C, and F spores all have been found in honey, with some of these toxin types linked to the geographic origin of the honey.[102] For these reasons and because honey is not nutritionally essential, all major pediatric, public health, and honey industry agencies in the United States have joined in the recommendation that honey not be fed to infants. In 2000, several brands of honey sold in the United States began to carry a warning not to feed honey to infants; an equivalent label first appeared on British honey in 1996.

In addition to honey, hundreds of traditional and nontraditional infant food items, including formula milk, have been examined and found not to contain *C. botulinum.*[91] However, in instances not associated with illness, *C. botulinum* spores have been found in raw sugar and molasses but not in refined sugar[103] and in herbal (chamomile) tea[26] and other herbal preparations.[27,76]

Discussion of the possible role of corn syrup in infant botulism is necessitated by two reports. In 1982, the US Food and Drug Administration (FDA) found *C. botulinum* type B spores in approximately 0.5% (5 of 961) of previously unopened retail samples of light and dark corn syrup[76]; the manufacturer then made changes in the production process. In 1989, the federal CDC reported the results of a 2-year epidemiologic study of US cases from all states except California.[137] By subgrouping patients by age and using logistic regression modeling techniques, a statistical association was obtained among the triad of exposure to corn syrup, breast-feeding, and age at onset of 2 months or older.[107,137]

In contrast to these reports, a 1988 Canadian survey found no *C. botulinum* spores in 43 samples of corn syrup.[62] A 1991 FDA market survey of 783 syrups (354 of which were light corn syrup and 271 were dark corn syrup) concluded that none contained *C. botulinum* spores.[79] A California study (unpublished) of 103 corn syrups, 72 of which had been fed to infants who subsequently became ill with infant botulism, did not find *C. botulinum* in any sample. Moreover, a 1979 epidemiologic study that simply compared rates of exposure to corn syrup in 41 cases and 107 control infants identified feeding of corn syrup as a significant protective factor against type A infant botulism.[15] The explanation offered for the latter observation was that if a parent chose corn syrup as a sweetener for the infant, the child was unlikely to have been fed honey as a second sweetener. Thus, on the basis of the available evidence, corn syrup appears not to constitute a source of *C. botulinum* spores or a risk factor for the development of infant botulism.

CLINICAL MANIFESTATIONS

Like other infectious diseases, infant botulism displays a spectrum of clinical severity.[8,11,14,83,84,94,111,122,146] To date, almost all patients with recognized disease have been sufficiently hypotonic and weak to require hospitalization. Consequently, the present picture of infant botulism is derived from hospitalized patients. However, outpatients who displayed only a few days of lethargy, poor feeding, and some decrease in frequency of bowel movement have been detected by alert physicians familiar with the more "classic" illness. At the opposite end of the clinical spectrum are patients whose "catastrophic presentations" obscured and delayed establishment of the correct diagnosis[95,105] and those few cases for which the history and clinical findings were indistinguishable from typical cases of sudden infant death syndrome (SIDS, crib death),[14,105,111] approximately one in 20 of which (in California) appears to result from fulminant infant botulism.[11,14]

The onset of infant botulism ranges from the insidious to the abrupt. At one extreme are patients who were nursing normally 6 hours before becoming so floppy that acute meningitis was the diagnosis at initial evaluation, and at the other extreme are patients who returned to their physicians four times in a week as the signs of illness gradually became apparent. Although rare, illness caused by *C. baratii* type F appears to be generally characterized by the triad of very young age at onset, rapid onset, and profound paralysis.[24,97,108] Equally rare, illness caused by *C. butyricum* type E may be manifested as a paradoxically rigid abdomen and associated bowel colonization with *Clostridium difficile.*[47,48]

In the "classic" case of infant botulism, the first sign of illness almost always is constipation (defined as 3 or more days without defecation in a previously regular infant), yet the constipation often is overlooked. A few patients (<5%) will not have a history of constipation. Usually, a mother first notices listlessness, lethargy, and poor feeding, together with breast engorgement if the infant had been nursing. The increasing weakness over the ensuing 1 to 4 days typically brings the infant to medical attention.

Botulism is manifested clinically as a symmetric, descending paralysis. Early in the course, weakness and hypotonia characterize the illness, and the remainder of the physical examination not involving the neuromuscular system is normal. The first signs of illness are found in the cranial nerves; a patient cannot have infant botulism without having bulbar palsies. The typical patient has an expressionless face, a feeble cry, ptosis (evident when the eyelids must work against gravity), poor head control, and generalized weakness and hypotonia (Fig. 147.1). Eye muscle paralysis varies, with the pupils often at mid position and initially briskly reactive. However, fatigability of the pupillary light reflex and extraocular motility is also often present; these are pathognomonic signs and should be sought at presentation (Box 147.1).[8] The gag, suck, and swallow reflexes are impaired, as is the corneal reflex if tested repetitively. Deep tendon reflexes frequently are normal at initial evaluation and diminish subsequently as the paralysis extends and increases. The "frog's legs" sign is often observed. Patients are afebrile unless a secondary infection (e.g., aspiration pneumonia) is present.

Most laboratory and clinical studies are normal. At admission, the child may have evidence of mild dehydration and fat mobilization because of diminished oral intake. Occasionally at admission, the cerebrospinal fluid (CSF) protein concentration becomes elevated because of the mild dehydration. If infant botulism is suspected soon after admission, electroencephalography, computed tomography, and magnetic resonance imaging are seldom required. However, if performed, these examinations yield nonspecific or normal results. Electromyography may offer rapid bedside confirmation of the clinical diagnosis.[40,44]

The definitive diagnostic laboratory study is examination of feces for the presence of *C. botulinum* organisms and toxin, which is the only certain way to identify the toxin type (A, B, or other) responsible for the illness. Small amounts (<5 mouse LD_{50}/mL) of botulinum toxin can sometimes be identified in serum specimens if collected early in the course of illness.[19,47,61,85,109,145,148] In one US report almost one patient in eight had toxin demonstrable in serum.[61] Clinically suspected cases that lack an identified toxin type are not included in official tallies of infant botulism.[33,32,76]

The usual hospital course of *untreated* infant botulism has certain general features.[8,69,84,122] After the increasing weakness has necessitated admission, the weakness and hypotonia continue to progress and usually become generalized. The deep tendon reflexes, which may be normal at admission, may diminish or disappear temporarily. The nadir of paresis and paralysis in untreated patients usually occurs within 1 to 2

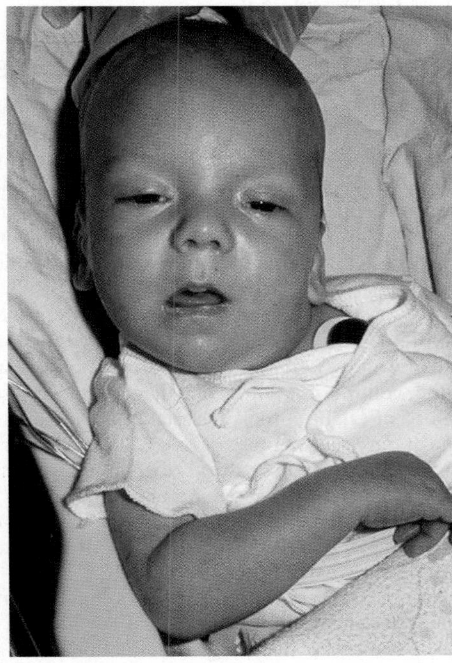

FIG. 147.1 Mildly affected 7-week-old infant with botulism. Note the minimal signs, including ptosis, mildly disconjugate gaze, expressionless face, slack jaw, and neck and arm hypotonia.

BOX 147.1 Neurologic Signs Helpful in the Diagnosis of Infant Botulism

1. Take the patient to a dark room. Shine a bright light into the eye; note the quickness of pupillary constriction. Remove the light when the constriction is maximal; let the pupil dilate. Then immediately repeat with the light, continuing thus for 1 to 3 minutes. The initially brisk pupillary response may become sluggish and the pupil unable to constrict maximally. *Fatigability with repetitive muscle contraction is the clinical hallmark of botulism.*
2. Shine a bright light onto the fovea and keep it there for 1 to 3 minutes, even if the infant tries to deviate the eyes. Latent ophthalmoplegia may be elicited, purposeful efforts to avoid the light may diminish, or both may occur.
3. Place a clean fifth finger in the infant's mouth while taking care to not obstruct the airway. Note the strength and duration of the reflex sucking. The suck is weak and poorly sustained. The gag reflex strength also may be quickly checked (if the infant has not been fed recently).

Modified from Arnon SS. Infant botulism. *Annu Rev Med.* 1980;31:541–560.

BOX 147.2 Complications of Infant Botulism

Adult respiratory distress syndrome
Anemia
Aspiration
Blood pressure instability
Clostridium difficile colitis
Fracture of the femur and humerus
Inappropriate secretion of antidiuretic hormone
Misplaced or plugged endotracheal tube
Necrotizing enterocolitis
Otitis media
Pneumonia
Recurrent atelectasis
Respiratory arrest
Seizures secondary to hyponatremia
Sepsis
Subglottic stenosis
Tension pneumothorax
Tracheal granuloma
Tracheal stenosis
Tracheitis
Tracheomalacia
Transfusion reaction
Urinary tract infection

weeks after admission; such patients often remain at their nadir for as long as 1 to 3 weeks before showing signs of improvement. However, once strength and tone begin to return, the improvement continues steadily and gradually over the ensuing weeks in the absence of complications (Box 147.2). In contrast, patients treated with human botulism immune globulin (BIG-IV) have a mean hospital stay of approximately 2 weeks (see Treatment).[17]

In the California experience, infant botulism does not have a relapsing or biphasic course and perceived "relapses" have been found, in retrospect, to be an indication of premature discontinuation of gavage feeding or respiratory support, of the onset of a complication (see Box 147.2), or of premature discharge. However, the clinical experience elsewhere with regard to relapses has been different.[47,54,115,122] The patient is ready for discharge when gag, suck, and swallow are sufficiently strong both to protect the airway against accidental aspiration and to ensure adequacy of oral intake. Parents also may be taught to feed by gavage at home. In either situation, discharge may occur safely while head lag and constipation are still present.

DIFFERENTIAL DIAGNOSIS AND DIAGNOSIS

When initially brought to medical attention, patients with infant botulism are often so mildly weak and hypotonic that the illness is not considered. Even today, more than 40 years after the disease first was recognized, suspected sepsis remains the most common admission diagnosis. A careful history (constipation is commonly overlooked) and physical examination (especially evaluation of cranial nerve function) usually can identify patients with infant botulism correctly and render unnecessary most additional testing for other entities typically suspected (Table 147.2). A review of entities that so closely mimicked infant botulism that BIG-IV was administered soon after admission identified spinal muscular atrophy type I, mitochondrial disorders, and a small number of other conditions as the actual diagnoses (see Table 147.2).[51]

The diagnosis of infant botulism is established by identification of *C. botulinum* (or, rarely, of neurotoxigenic *C. butyricum* or *C. baratii*) organisms in the feces or enema effluent of an infant with clinical signs consistent with the paralyzing action of botulinum toxin.[69,92,113] Extensive studies have demonstrated that *C. botulinum* is not part of the normal resident microbiome of infants or adults.[11,61,138,139] If the fecal specimen is obtained sufficiently early in the course of the illness, it also will contain botulinum toxin. Because of the patient's constipation, an enema with sterile, nonbacteriostatic water (not saline) is often needed to obtain a fecal specimen for diagnostic examination. The mouse neutralization test remains the "gold standard" assay for detection of botulinum toxin and diagnosis of infant botulism.[32,80] However, mass spectrometry for detection of botulinum toxins[71,72,151] and nucleic acid-based methodologies for detection of botulinum toxin genes[74,89,105,132] are being increasingly applied. Laboratory diagnosis that identifies the type of toxin responsible for the illness is essential for the case to be registered as infant botulism[76] and is important for prognosis; mean hospital stay is significantly longer in untreated type A cases than in untreated type B cases (see Treatment).[8,17] Physicians are reminded that in all states, botulism or suspected botulism (all types) is an immediately reportable illness.

Bedside electromyography sometimes can be helpful in ambiguous situations, in that when a clinically weak muscle is tested, electromyography often discloses a pattern known by its acronym BSAP (*b*rief, *s*mall, *a*bundant motor unit action *p*otentials).[13,37,44,56,114,122,127] The edrophonium (Tensilon) test is unnecessary because congenital myasthenia gravis can be excluded by the history and because the immaturity of the infant's immune system precludes the occurrence of de novo myasthenia at this age. Likewise, Guillain-Barré syndrome that is well documented by consistently elevated CSF protein concentration is of negligible occurrence in infancy. In infant botulism the CSF protein concentration is normal unless the patient is mildly dehydrated.

TREATMENT

BIG-IV is approved in the United States as the specific therapy for infant botulism, and its use to treat patients hospitalized with suspected infant botulism constitutes current standard of care. BIG-IV was licensed following a 5-year, randomized, double-blind, placebo-controlled treatment trial in California that demonstrated its safety and efficacy.[10,17] Use of BIG-IV reduced mean hospital stay per case from 5.7 weeks to 2.6 weeks ($P < .001$) and reduced mean hospitalization cost per case by more than $99,000 (2015 dollars; $P < .001$).[17] In a 6-year, follow-on open-label study, treatment with BIG-IV within 7 days of hospital admission reduced mean hospital stay to 2.2 weeks.[17] Since licensure of BIG-IV in October 2003, its use in more than 1400 US infant botulism patients has resulted in more than 85 years of avoided hospital stay and more than $125 million of avoided hospital costs. Treatment with BIG-IV should be started as early in the illness as possible to maximally neutralize the toxemia and should not be delayed for laboratory confirmation of the clinical diagnosis. BIG-IV may be obtained from the California Department of Public Health

TABLE 147.2 Working Differential Diagnosis of Infant Botulism

Most Common Admission Diagnoses	Inpatient Working Diagnoses	Clinical Mimics[a]	
Rule-out sepsis	Amino acid metabolic disorder	Acute disseminated encephalomyelitis	Likely resolved sepsis
Dehydration	Brain stem encephalitis	Acute transverse myelitis	Long-chain 3-hydroxyacyl-CoA dehydrogenase deficiency
Viral syndrome	Guillain-Barré syndrome	Carnitine deficiency	Miller-Fisher variant of Guillain-Barré syndrome
Pneumonia	Heavy metal poisoning (Pb, Mg, As)	Chiari malformation	Mitochondrial disorders
Idiopathic hypotonia	Hirschsprung disease	Congenital disorder of glycosylation	Nemaline rod myopathy
Failure to thrive	Hypothyroidism	Cystic fibrosis and hypovitaminosis A	Parainfluenza and macrocephaly
	Medium-chain acyl-CoA dehydrogenase deficiency	Dystonia	Parechovirus encephalitis
	Metabolic encephalopathy	Global developmental delay	Polio-like enterovirus
	Myasthenia gravis	Hemophilia A, cervical epidural hemorrhage	Polyradiculopathy
	Poliomyelitis	Human metapneumovirus pneumonia/bronchiolitis	Roseola
	Spinal muscular atrophy	Hypothyroidism	Spinal muscular atrophy
	Viral polyneuritis	Leukodystrophy	Urea cycle defect

[a]Patients with conditions so indistinguishable from infant botulism at admission that they were treated with human botulism immune globulin (BIG-IV). Modified from Khouri JM, Payne JR, Arnon SS. More Clinical Mimics of Infant Botulism. *J. Pediatr.* 2017 (in press).

as a public service (i.e., not-for-profit) orphan drug (24-hour telephone: 510-231-7600; www.infantbotulism.org).

Successful management of infant botulism also depends on meticulous supportive care and the anticipation and avoidance of potentially fatal complications (see Box 147.2). Feeding and breathing generally require the most attention. At admission, patients should receive cardiac, respiratory, and transcutaneous blood gas monitoring (especially carbon dioxide pressure) until it becomes clear that paralysis is no longer progressing. An endotracheal tube is often necessary to maintain and protect the airway even if mechanical ventilation is not needed. Avoidance of nosocomially acquired *C. difficile* colitis is particularly important.[48,119]

A third cornerstone of management is forbearance. Antibiotics should be reserved to treat secondary infections (principally pneumonia, urinary tract infection, and otitis media). Otherwise, their use may result in lysis of intraluminal *C. botulinum* with liberation of neurotoxin into the gut with subsequent absorption. This potential problem may be avoided by prompt treatment with BIG-IV because its substantial antitoxin content and long (28-day) half-life enable it to neutralize all circulating and newly absorbed toxin.

Tracheostomy is not necessary.[4] Improved management of the airway can be accomplished by two simple positioning measures. First, to expand the thoracic cage and assist diaphragmatic function, patients should be placed in a crib with a rigid bottom mattress that can tilt the entire body to a 30-degree angle. Second, to tip the head back, and to maintain normal curvature of neck and airway, a soft cloth should be rolled to the thickness of about three fingers and placed under just the child's neck. This maneuver allows oral secretions to drain away from the trachea and into the posterior pharynx where they are most easily swallowed.

Intravenous feeding (hyperalimentation) is discouraged because of potential secondary infections and because it is unnecessary. Nasogastric or post-pyloric tube feeding works well. Mother's milk is the nutritional fluid of choice. Isolation measures or "enteric precautions" are not required, but meticulous hand washing and standard precautions are. Soiled diapers should be autoclaved because some of them will contain botulinum neurotoxin, as well as viable spores and vegetative cells of *C. botulinum*. For this reason staff with open lesions on their hands should not handle the diapers.

OUTCOME AND PROGNOSIS

Recovery from infant botulism occurs through regeneration of the toxin-poisoned terminal unmyelinated nerve endings. The newly synthesized nerve twigs then induce the formation of new motor endplates that are indistinguishable functionally and morphologically from the original ones.[40,42] In experimental animals and in human infants, completion of this process takes several weeks.[42] Consequently, in the absence of hypoxic cerebral complications, full and complete recovery of strength and tone is the expected outcome. In addition, because botulinum toxin does not cross the blood-brain barrier to any functional degree, the child's intelligence and personality remain intact. Parents often need reassurance on this latter point. Reinfection with the same or a different toxin type of *C. botulinum* has not occurred. In the United States, the case-fatality ratio of hospitalized patients is less than 1%, a reflection of, and tribute to, the high quality of intensive care given to these critically ill infants.[150] In other countries the experience has not been as fortunate.[76]

PREVENTION

At present the most important way to prevent infant botulism is not to feed honey to infants, and all major pediatric and public health agencies have endorsed this recommendation. Avoidance of untreated well water[75] and of pet terrapins and their commercial food[125] may also prevent some cases. In addition, breast-feeding may help moderate the rapidity of onset and the severity of illness.[12] Persuasive evidence that links infant botulism to the ingestion of corn or other syrups is lacking. In the pre–BIG-IV era, the patient with the most protracted illness was hospitalized in 1988 for 10 months at a cost of more than $1.8 million (2015 dollars). Mean hospital costs for the placebo-treated patients in the 1992 to 1997 randomized clinical trial of BIG-IV were $207,500, which were reduced in the BIG-IV group to $108,000, a net cost savings of $99,500 (2015 dollars).[17] These economic facts combine with humanitarian considerations to make a compelling case for the prevention and effective treatment of infant botulism.

SUGGESTED READING

Rummel A, Binz T. eds. *Botulinum neurotoxins. Curr Top Microbiol Immunol.* 2013;364:1-321.

Smith LD, Sugiyama H. *Botulism: The Organism, Its Toxins, the Disease.* 2nd ed. Springfield, Ill: Charles C Thomas; 1988.

NEW REFERENCES SINCE THE SEVENTH EDITION

1. 42 Code of Federal Regulations Part 73; 2012.
2. Abdulla CO, Ayubi A, Zulfiquer F, et al. Infant botulism following honey ingestion. *BMJ Case Rep.* 2012;2012.
3. Abe Y, Negasawa T, Monma C, et al. Infantile botulism caused by *Clostridium butyricum* type E toxin. *Pediatr Neurol.* 2008;38(1):55-57.
22. Barash JR, Arnon SS. A novel strain of *Clostridium botulinum* that produces type B and type H botulinum toxins. *J Infect Dis.* 2014;209(2):183-191.

27. Bianco MI, Lúquez C, De Jong LI, et al. Linden flower (*Tilia* spp.) as potential vehicle of *Clostridium botulinum* spores in the transmission of infant botulism. *Rev Argent Microbiol*. 2009;41(4):232-236.
33. Centers for Disease Control and Prevention. Botulism (*Clostridium botulinum*): 2011 Case Definition. Available at: https://wwwn.cdc.gov/nndss/conditions/botulism/case-definition/2011/.
38. Dabritz HA, Hill KK, Barash JR, et al. Molecular epidemiology of infant botulism in California and elsewhere, 1976-2010. *J Infect Dis*. 2014;210(11):1711-1722.
39. de Jong L, Fernández RA, Pareja V, et al. First report of an infant botulism case due to *Clostridium botulinum* type Af. *J Clin Microbiol*. 2015;53(2):740-742.
41. Dover N, Barash JR, Hill KK, et al. Molecular characterization of a novel botulinum neurotoxin type H gene. *J Infect Dis*. 2014;209(2):192-202.
43. Dykes JK, Lúquez C, Raphael BH, et al. Laboratory investigation of the first case of botulism caused by *Clostridium butyricum* type E toxin in the United States. *J Clin Microbiol*. 2015;53(10):3363-3365.
45. Fagan RP, Neil KP, Sasich R, et al. Initial recovery and rebound of type F intestinal colonization botulism after administration of investigational heptavalent botulinum antitoxin. *Clin Infect Dis*. 2011;53(9):e125-e128.
46. Fan Y, Barash JR, Lou J, et al. Immunological characterization and neutralizing ability of monoclonal antibodies directed against botulinum neurotoxin type H. *J Infect Dis*. 2016;213(10):1606-1614.
50. Field CJ. The immunological components of human milk and their effect on immune development in infants. *J Nutr*. 2005;135(1):1-4.
55. Goldman AS. The immune system in human milk and the developing infant. *Breastfeed Med*. 2007;2(4):195-204.
57. Grant KA, McLauchlin J, Amar C. Infant botulism: advice on avoiding feeding honey to babies and other possible risk factors. *Community Pract*. 2013;86(7):44-46.
60. Hannett GE, Schaffzin JK, Davis SW, et al. Two cases of adult botulism caused by botulinum neurotoxin producing *Clostridium baratii*. *Anaerobe*. 2014;30c:178-180.
71. Kalb SR, Lou J, Garcia-Rodriguez C, et al. Extraction and inhibition of enzymatic activity of botulinum neurotoxins/A1, /A2, and /A3 by a panel of monoclonal anti-BoNT/A antibodies. *PLoS ONE*. 2009;4(4):e5355.
72. Kalb SR, Santana WI, Geren IN, et al. Extraction and inhibition of enzymatic activity of botulinum neurotoxins/B1, /B2, /B3, /B4, and /B5 by a panel of monoclonal anti-BoNT/B antibodies. *BMC Biochem*. 2011;12(1):58.
74. Kenri T, Sekizuka T, Yamamoto A, et al. Genetic characterization and comparison of *Clostridium botulinum* strains isolated from botulism cases in Japan between 2006 and 2011. *Appl Environ Microbiol*. 2014;80(22):6954-6964.
75. Kobayashi T, Haginoya K, Morimoto T, et al. A case of infant botulism infection due to consumption of untreated well-water. *J Pediatr*. 2014;164(4):931-933.
78. Lee SA, Lim JY, Kim BS, et al. Comparison of the gut microbiota profile in breast-fed and formula-fed Korean infants using pyrosequencing. *Nutr Res Pract*. 2015;9(3):242-248.
81. Liu Z, Roy NC, Guo Y, et al. Human breast milk and infant formulas differentially modify the intestinal microbiota in human infants and host physiology in rats. *J Nutr*. 2016;146(2):191-199.
87. Maslanka SE, Lúquez C, Dykes JK, et al. A novel botulinum neurotoxin, previously reported as serotype H, has a hybrid-like structure with regions of similarity to the structures of serotypes A and F and is neutralized with serotype A antitoxin. *J Infect Dis*. 2015;213:6.
89. McCallum N, Gray TJ, Wang Q, et al. Genomic epidemiology of *Clostridium botulinum* isolates from temporally related cases of infant botulism in New South Wales, Australia. *J Clin Microbiol*. 2015;53(9):2846-2853.
90. Meyer KF, Dubovsky BJ. The distribution of the spores of *B. botulinus* in the United States. *J Infect Dis*. 1922;31(6):559-594.
97. Moodley A, Quinlisk P, Garvey A, et al. Notes from the field: infant botulism caused by *Clostridium baratii* type F—Iowa, 2013. *MMWR Morb Mortal Wkly Rep*. 2015;64(14):400.
110. Pellett S, Tepp WH, Bradshaw M, et al. Purification and characterization of botulinum neurotoxin FA from a genetically modified *Clostridium botulinum* strain. *mSphere*. 2016;1(1):e100-e115.
116. Rummel A. Double receptor anchorage of botulinum neurotoxins accounts for their exquisite neurospecificity. *Curr Top Microbiol Immunol*. 2013;364:61-90.
121. Schocken-Iturrino R, Carneiro M, Kato E, et al. Study of the presence of the spores of *Clostridium botulinum* in honey in Brazil. *FEMS Immunol Med Microbiol*. 1999;24(3):379-382.
125. Shelley EB, O'Rourke D, Grant K, et al. Infant botulism due to *C. butyricum* type E toxin: a novel environmental association with pet terrapins. *Epidemiol Infect*. 2015;143(3):461-469.
128. Shirey TB, Dykes JK, Lúquez C, et al. Characterizing the fecal microbiota of infants with botulism. *Microbiome*. 2015;3(54).
130. Smith JK, Burns S, Cunningham S, et al. The hazards of honey: infantile botulism. *BMJ Case Rep*. 2010;2010.
132. Smith TJ, Hill KK, Xie G, et al. Genomic sequences of six botulinum neurotoxin-producing strains representing three clostridial species illustrate the mobility and diversity of botulinum neurotoxin genes. *Infect Genet Evol*. 2014;30:102-113.
136. Spiegelman J, Cescon DW, Friedman Y, et al. Bowel loops and eyelid droops. *Can Med Assoc J*. 2008;179(9):927-929.
151. Wang D, Baudys J, Krilich J, et al. A two-stage multiplex method for quantitative analysis of botulinum neurotoxins type A, B, E, and F by MALDI-TOF mass spectrometry. *Anal Chem*. 2014;86(21):10847-10854.
153. Williamson CH, Sahl JW, Smith TJ, et al. Comparative genomic analyses reveal broad diversity in botulinum-toxin-producing *Clostridia*. *BMC Genomics*. 2016;17(1):180.
154. Kakinuma H, Maruyama H, Takahashi H, Yamakawa K, Nakamura S. The first case of type B infant botulism in Japan. *Acta Paediatr Jpn*. 1996;38(5):541-543.
155. Yamakawa K, Karasawa T, Kakinuma H, et al. Emergence of *Clostridium botulinum* type B-like nontoxigenic organisms in a patient with type B infant botulism. *J Clin Microbiol*. 1997;35(8):2163-2164.
156. Zhang S, Masuyer G, Zhang J, et al. Identification and characterization of a novel botulinum neurotoxin. *Nat Commun*. 2017;8:14130.

The full reference list for this chapter is available at ExpertConsult.com.

148 Tetanus

James D. Cherry • Myke Federman

Tetanus is caused by the anaerobic, spore-forming bacillus *Clostridium tetani*, an organism present in soil and in human and animal feces. The clinical symptoms are not caused by infection but result from a specific toxin, tetanospasmin, that is produced at the site of injury and acts primarily on the spinal cord but also on the brain, motor end plates, and autonomic nerves. The disease may appear as a local form or as a more generalized syndrome. It is characterized by tonic spasms of skeletal muscles, little or no fever, and occasional spasms of the glottis and larynx. Bilateral trismus is the most common sign. Active immunization is highly protective. Although tetanus is controlled well today in developed countries throughout the world, it remains a major cause of death in developing countries.[6,32,30,87,92,97,132,141]

In the present era, there has been an increase in unvaccinated children due to personal belief exemptions. In 2012, two cases of tetanus in home-schooled children were noted.[66] One of those children was in the intensive care unit for 18 days and was hospitalized for approximately 2 months.

HISTORY

The first description of tetanus in recorded medical history probably was written by Hippocrates.[62] A vivid picture of the clinical course of the disease was recorded by Aretaeus the Cappadocian in the second century,[8] but very little of importance was added to this knowledge during the next 18 centuries. Transmissibility of tetanus was demonstrated by Carle and Rattone[26] in 1884. They reported that when the sciatic nerves of rabbits were injected with the contents of a human "pustule," the characteristic disease developed in the animals in 2 to 3 days; inoculation of tissue obtained from their nervous systems into healthy rabbits produced a similar syndrome. The role of soil in the pathogenesis of tetanus was demonstrated by Nicolaier[94] in 1884; although he saw the organism, he was unable to recover it.

The bacterium responsible for the disease was identified first by Rosenbach,[113] who described a bacillus containing a round terminal spore in pus obtained from a human case; tetanus developed when the purulent exudate was injected into animals. *C. tetani* was isolated by Kitasato,[70] who fulfilled Koch's postulates with it in 1889. One year later, von Behring and Kitasato[135] reported the appearance of specific antitoxin in the serum of animals given injections of the tetanus toxin produced by the organism. This finding was followed, in 1926, by the development of toxoid, injections of which produced immunity.

MICROBIOLOGY

The vegetative form of *C. tetani* is a gram-positive, spore-forming, motile, anaerobic bacillus that measures 0.3 to 0.5 µm in width and 2.0 to 2.5 µm in length; in culture, long filament-like cells develop.[15,25,112,125,139] *C. tetani* is a strict anaerobe that grows best at 33°C to 37°C (91.4°F to 98.6°F); it can be cultured in many different routine media used for anaerobic organisms, such as thioglycolate, casein hydrolysate, and cooked meat. Enhanced growth occurs in medium supplemented with reducing substances and maintained at neutral or alkaline pH. With growth, gas with a fetid odor usually is produced.

The first step in the process of spore formation is the development of a bulge at one end of the organism; this bulge contains the spore and is responsible for the characteristic drumstick or tennis racquet appearance. As sporulation progresses, the organism decreases in length and the spores are extruded. They stain poorly by the Gram method. Sporulation occurs in tissues as well as in vitro and is dependent on the composition of the medium and the temperature of the culture. Enhanced sporulation occurs in the presence of oleic acid, phosphates, 1% to 2% sodium chloride, and manganese salts.[15,25,112] In vivo, sporulation is enhanced by lactic acid and other substances toxic to cells. Sporulation is inhibited by high and low temperatures (>41°C and <25°C [>105.8°F and <77°F]), glucose, fatty acids, and potassium salts. The metabolic activity of *C. tetani* is limited; carbohydrates and proteins are digested poorly, and the vegetative, nonsporulated forms are killed easily by heat and numerous disinfecting agents. In contrast, the spores are resistant to boiling and phenol, cresol, 1 : 1000 bichloride of mercury, and other disinfectants; however, they are destroyed by heating at 120°C (248°F) for 15 to 20 minutes. If not exposed to sunlight, the spores may survive in soil for months to years. They also may constitute part of the normal intestinal microflora of some horses, cows, guinea pigs, sheep, dogs, cats, rats, chickens, and humans.

Three nonpathogenic clostridia are present in soil and in human and animal feces: *Clostridium tetanomorphum, Clostridium tertium,* and *Clostridium tetanoides*. Diagnostic confusion may occur because they are morphologically similar to the organism responsible for tetanus. *C. tetani* is recovered much more commonly from cultivated than from virgin or uncultivated soil. Rural dwellers and people engaged in agricultural occupations have a higher rate of intestinal, skin, and oral carriage of the organism than do city dwellers. Dust and dirt from houses, streets, and operating rooms, as well as solutions of heroin used by injection drug users, have been found to be contaminated with the organism.

EPIDEMIOLOGY

Source of Exposure

The predominant reservoir of *C. tetani* is the soil; it is also part of the normal flora of the intestinal tract of animals, both herbivores and omnivores.[112] Intestinal spores and bacilli are shed in the feces of animals and contribute to the soil reservoir.

The worldwide morbidity and mortality attributable to tetanus is related inversely to adequate immunization with tetanus toxoid and directly to suboptimal hygiene, childbirth practices, and wound care.[6,112] Throughout the world, tetanus has a seasonal trend; more cases occur in the summer or in "wet" seasons. Rates of illness are highest in countries that are located near the equator and have fertile soil.

Acute wounds, including relatively minor ones, are the site of most *C. tetani* infections leading to tetanus. In addition, infection may occur after parenteral drug use and surgical procedures. In many cases the source of exposure is unknown. The source of infection in neonatal tetanus is the umbilical cord or stump as a result of unsterile delivery conditions and unhygienic cultural rituals involving the umbilical stump.[63,64,106]

Incidence

The incidence of tetanus in the vaccine era is related inversely to the degree to which effective immunization programs have been implemented in a population.[112] In the early 1980s an estimated 2 million cases of tetanus occurred throughout the world, with 1 million fatal neonatal cases and 122,000 to 300,000 nonneonatal fatal cases.[53,54]

Although neonatal tetanus is of very minor importance in developed areas of the world, it has been and still is a major cause of death in infants in developing countries.[31,30,73,74,82,124,132,141] In 1993, an estimated 515,000 deaths worldwide were caused by neonatal tetanus.[30] These deaths occurred predominantly in Southeast Asia (34.2%); Africa (28.2%); the western Pacific, including China (21.4%); and the eastern Mediterranean region (15.7%). The global mortality rate in 1993 was estimated to be 4.1 per 1000 live births. The very high frequency of neonatal tetanus in these areas was related to conditions surrounding the birth of infants.[52] Most babies were born in very unhygienic environments; delivery rarely took place in an adequate hospital. In addition, unclean instruments were used to sever the umbilical cord, rags—often contaminated with soil or feces—were used as dressings, and mud and manure were applied directly to the umbilical stump. In a study in Senegal that examined risk factors for the development of neonatal tetanus, the major source of *C. tetani* was found to be the hands of the birth attendant, and the mode of contamination of the infant was related to the method that the birth attendant and the mother used to dress the umbilical cord stump.[74] In rural Pakistan, the ritual of bundling (wrapping the baby for prolonged periods in a sheepskin cover after the application of cow dung) was a significant risk factor for the acquisition of neonatal tetanus.[13] In a case-control study of risk factors for neonatal tetanus in Karachi, Pakistan, the following risks were identified: application of substances (e.g., mustard oil, ghee, or surma) to the umbilical cord, home delivery, and illiterate mothers.[106]

In 2002, deaths worldwide caused by tetanus were estimated at 213,000, with approximately 180,000 occurring in neonates, and there were 15,000 to 30,000 maternal cases.[141] Most maternal cases are the result of unclean delivery or abortion practices. In 2008, 59,000 neonatal deaths occurred as a result of tetanus.[73] In 2013, the World Health Organization (WHO) established that 49,000 newborns died from neonatal tetanus.[142]

The reported incidence of tetanus and tetanus-related deaths in the United States from 1947 to 2008 is presented in Fig. 148.1, and the reported cases and fatal cases and their incidence are presented by age group for 1998 to 2000 in Fig. 148.2.[34,99] From 1947 through 1976, the incidence of tetanus fell tenfold; since 1976, the continued decrease in incidence has been less than twofold. During the same period, mortality rates fell from 91% in 1947 to 44% in 1976 to 18% in 1998 to 2000.

In the period 1998 to 2000, 36% of the cases occurred in patients 60 years or older, 55% in patients aged 20 to 59 years, and only 9% in those younger than 20 years. During this period, the vaccination status was known in only 50 of the patients (38%). Of this group, eight (16%) had received three or more doses of tetanus toxoid, with the last dose being received less than 10 years before the onset of tetanus. None of these eight patients sought medical care for the injury before the onset of tetanus, and three were younger than 20 years. The outcome of the illness was available for only 18 of the 50 patients with a known immunization history, and one death occurred—in an injection drug user whose last dose of tetanus toxoid was 11 years before the onset of tetanus.

During the period 1998 to 2000, 60% of the cases occurred in males.

PATHOGENESIS

Tetanus is, by strictest definition, not a true infection. Spores introduced at a site of injury remain harmless until they are converted, after being stimulated by a variety of factors, to vegetative forms that multiply but do not produce injury to tissue or provoke an inflammatory response. The clinical syndrome is caused entirely by toxin elaborated in the area where the vegetative cells are growing. *C. tetani* produces two exotoxins:

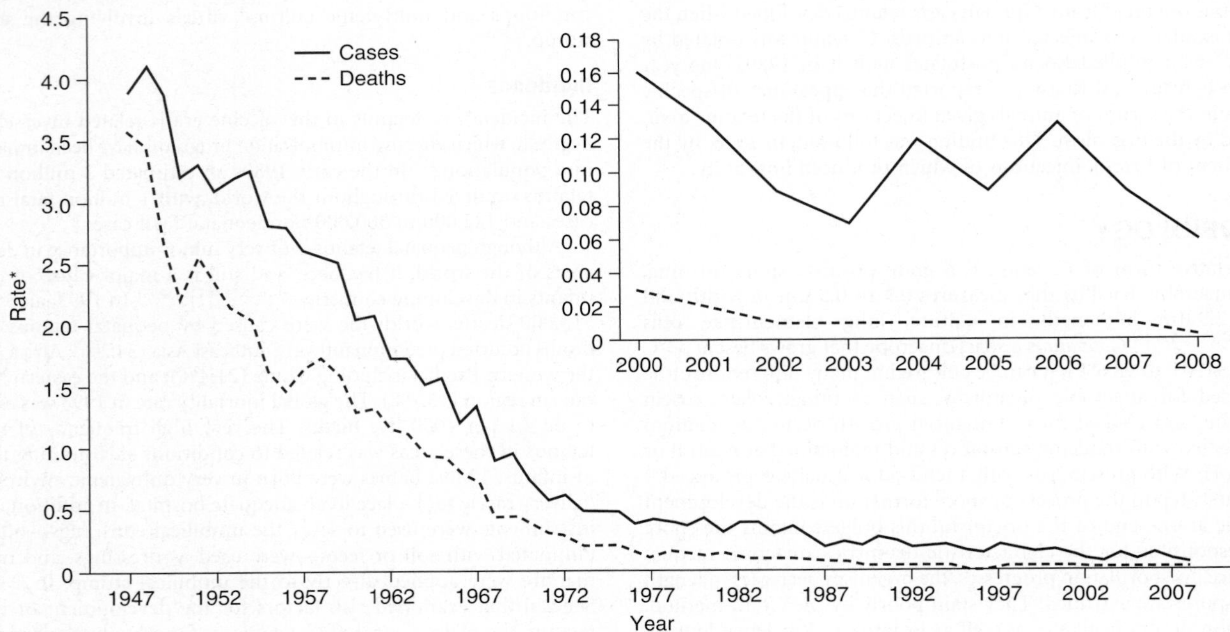

FIG. 148.1 Reported incidence of tetanus and tetanus-related deaths in the United States, 1947–2000. (From Centers for Disease Control and Prevention. Tetanus surveillance: United States, 2001-2008. *MMWR Morb Mortal Wkly Rep.* 2011;60:365–369.)

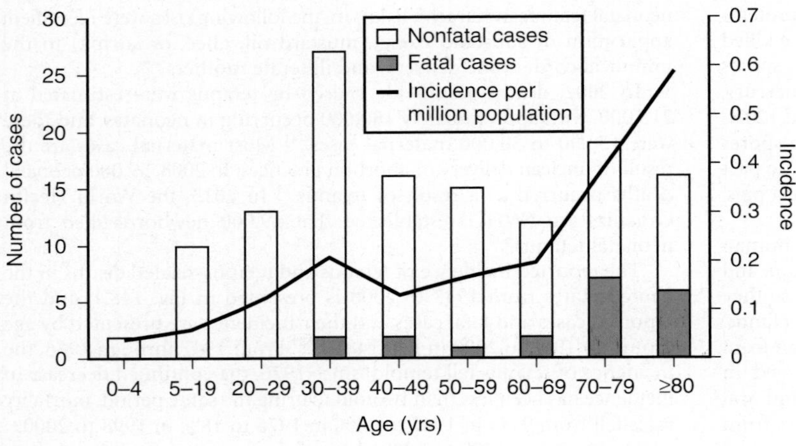

FIG. 148.2 Reported tetanus cases and incidence rates by age group in the United States, 1998–2000. (From Pascual FB, McGinley EL, Zanardi LR, et al. Tetanus surveillance: United States, 1998-2000. *MMWR Surveill Summ.* 2003; 52:1–8.)

tetanolysin and tetanospasmin.[102] Tetanolysin induces hemolysis but plays no role in the disease. The activity of tetanospasmin is responsible for the clinical features of the disease. This toxin has a molecular weight of 150 kDa and is activated by proteolytic cleavage into two polypeptides, a heavy (100 kDa) and a light (50 kDa) chain that are linked by a disulfide bond.[24] One milligram contains 6,400,000 lethal doses for mice; 0.00001 mg may kill a 20-g mouse in 2 hours. With the exception of the toxin produced by *Clostridium botulinum,* tetanospasmin currently is the most potent known poison. Humans are most susceptible to this agent and require only $\frac{1}{2500}$ and $\frac{1}{350,000}$ of the dose that is fatal for cats and chickens, respectively.

C. tetani is introduced into an area of injury as the spore, the form usually present in soil and intestinal contents. Disease does not develop until the spores are converted to the toxin-elaborating bacillus, which does not follow the simple inoculation of spores. When these spores are injected with very sharp needles into animals so that tissue is not injured but merely separated, tetanus does not develop. However, the addition of a small quantity of calcium chloride to a suspension of spores before injection leads to development of the typical disease. Such development is not caused by a specific effect of the cation on conversion of the spore to the vegetative form of the organism but is related to the necrosis of tissue produced by it, which leads to a reduction in oxidation-reduction potential and oxygen tension, factors involved in vegetation of the spore; the same effects are produced by the presence of a foreign body, trauma, or a localized suppurative process.

The pathway by which toxin elaborated at the site at which *C. tetani* is multiplying reaches the central nervous system (CNS) has been a matter of controversy. Researchers first thought that tetanospasmin was absorbed chiefly by motor nerve endings and then traveled along axis cylinders to the anterior horn cells.[103] Symptoms of the disease were thought to appear only after the toxin had reached the nervous system, with the initial tetanic contractions occurring first in the injured extremity, then in the opposite limb, and finally, as the toxin diffused through the spinal cord, in all the muscles. A small amount of toxin was suggested to be absorbed into the lymph and carried to the bloodstream, from which it was taken up by motor nerve endings in various parts of the body.[84]

Abel and associates[1] postulated that toxin reached the nervous system via the arterial circulation and suggested the following series of events. Some of the toxin diffuses from the local site of injury into adjacent skeletal muscle and acts on neuromuscular organs to produce a state of maintained contraction—local tetanus. Some toxin also enters the lymphatics and bloodstream, from which it is taken up by specifically reactive cells in the spinal cord, medulla, and the motor end-organs of muscle.

Friedlander[52] noted that tetanus toxin did not penetrate the blood-brain barrier and therefore questioned hematogenous transmission. This finding led researchers to focus attention on transport of tetanospasmin in nerves. Wright and coworkers[143] observed that direct injection of toxin into the vagal, facial, or hypoglossal nerves of rabbits led, within 24 hours, to the development of a syndrome characteristic of involvement of the brain stem, as indicated by the appearance of strabismus, immobility of hairs in the nasal cavity, salivation, bradycardia, and torticollis. Inoculation of the vagus nerve resulted in the successive development of these manifestations; those dependent on innervation from motor nuclei in close proximity to the nerve tended to appear early. This hypothesis is supported by observations indicating that a variety of substances, including India ink and radioactive compounds, migrate along peripheral nerves to the CNS after intraneural injection.[49] This observation, together with the demonstration by numerous investigators that toxin is present in the peripheral nerves closest to the site of inoculation, supports the concept of transport of tetanospasmin in the tissues of the nervous system.

Knowledge of the specific mechanisms involved in the absorption of tetanus toxin and its mechanisms of action on body cells is incomplete. Most of the evidence presently available indicates that some element of the peripheral nerve is involved. Whether transport occurs in the axis cylinder, the perineural space, or the lymphatics remains unsettled. Tetanus toxin is carried to the neurons of the sciatic nerve via the neurofibrillae in axis cylinders at a rate of approximately 3.35 mm/h.[111]

PATHOPHYSIOLOGY

Tetanospasmin exerts its effects in four areas of the nervous system: (1) the motor end plates in skeletal muscle, (2) the spinal cord, (3) the brain, and (4) the sympathetic nervous system (in some cases).[21-23,27,40,65,68,83,120,133,145]

Motor End Plates in Skeletal Muscle

Tetanus toxin has been noted to interfere with neuromuscular transmission. Release of acetylcholine from the nerve terminals in muscle is inhibited. The presence of tetanospasmin in the transverse and terminal sacs of the longitudinal elements of the sarcotubular system of skeletal muscles suggests that it acts by interfering with contraction coupling or with the mechanisms involved in contraction and relaxation. These phenomena probably are involved in the pathogenesis of local tetanus.

Spinal Cord

The effects of the toxin on the spinal cord are practically identical to those produced by strychnine. It does not act on reflex arcs that include only sensory and motor neurons (two-neuron or monosynaptic reflexes). However, the toxin profoundly alters the activity of the more complex polysynaptic reflexes involving interneurons, thereby leading to the inhibition of antagonists. Hyperpolarization of the membranes of neurons, a mechanism normally operating when direct inhibitory pathways are stimulated, is suppressed. The depolarization associated with excitation is not affected. Whether tetanospasmin blocks inhibitory synapses by preventing release of the inhibitory transmitter substance or by suppressing the action of this substance on the membrane of motor neurons is unknown. Selective blocking of inhibitory synapses in the CNS appears adequate to account for the primary phenomena of tetanus. Unchecked and uncoordinated excitatory impulses multiply and traverse reflex pathways to produce the characteristic tetanic spasms of muscles.

Brain

Some investigators have suggested that the action of tetanospasmin on the brain may be responsible for the typical seizures of tetanus.[21] This hypothesis is supported, in part, by the observation that cerebral gangliosides fix the toxin. The antidromic inhibition of evoked cortical activity is decreased. The effects of tetanospasmin on the brain are the same as those on the spinal cord, as well as those that occur after exposure to strychnine.

Sympathetic Nervous System

Manifestations indicating dysfunction of the sympathetic nervous system have been observed in some patients with tetanus. Signs and symptoms include profuse sweating, peripheral vasoconstriction, labile hypertension, cardiac arrhythmias, tachycardia, increased output of carbon dioxide, elevated urinary concentration of catecholamines, and hypotension late in the course of the disease.

CLINICAL MANIFESTATIONS

Although it may be as short as 1 day or as long as several months, the incubation period of tetanus usually is 3 to 21 days. A direct relationship may exist between the distance of the site of invasion by *C. tetani* from the CNS and the length of the interval between injury and the onset of disease; the greater the distance between the local area and the CNS, the longer, in general, the incubation period. Sustained or separate, repeated tonic spasms of isolated or multiple muscles are the characteristic clinical feature of the disease. Tetanus may appear in two forms: local and generalized.

Local Tetanus

The occurrence of local tetanus most likely is more common than recognized. Although local tetanus is thought to occur infrequently, it probably is so because it may be uncommon as an isolated syndrome or because by the time that diffuse involvement has occurred, the spasms in the muscles in the area of the site of entry of the organism cannot be separated from the generalized spasms. Local manifestations frequently precede development of the generalized disorder. The characteristic abnormality in local tetanus is unyielding, persistent, painful rigidity of the group of muscles that lie in close proximity to the site at which *C. tetani* was introduced. Local tetanus often is present when a dose of antitoxin has been given that is adequate to inactivate circulating toxin but insufficient to neutralize what has accumulated at the site of injury. Symptoms may persist for several weeks or months and finally disappear without leaving any residua.[85,107] Local tetanus may be the only manifestation, usually is mild, and has a fatality rate of approximately 1%.

Cephalic tetanus is a variant of local tetanus. It generally occurs after the introduction of *C. tetani* in the course of injuries to the scalp, eye, face, ear, or neck; in conjunction with chronic otitis media; and rarely, after tonsillectomy.[5,10] Insect bites on the face or head, especially if secondarily infected by pyogenic organisms, also may serve as portals of entry for the organism. The incubation period of this syndrome is short, frequently no more than 1 to 2 days. The principal distinctive clinical features are palsies of cranial nerves III, IV, VII, IX, X, and XII; they may be involved singly or in any combination. Dysfunction may persist for days or many months. In general, the prognosis for survival is poor. However, if death does not intervene, complete recovery without residual neurologic dysfunction is the rule. In some, but not all, instances, generalized tetanus may develop during the course of the cephalic form of the disease.

Generalized Tetanus

Generalized tetanus is the most common manifestation of the disease.[109,137] Despite the general impression that inoculation of the organism is associated most frequently with deep penetrating injury, the portal of entry in approximately 80% of cases is an insignificant wound.[103] Burns, injuries induced by blank cartridges, deep punctures, furunculosis, dental extraction, embedded splinters, decubitus ulcers, hypodermic injections, and compound fractures complicated by chronic active osteomyelitis are typical situations in which tetanus may develop because the environment in the tissues is optimal (decrease in oxidation-reduction potential and tension of oxygen) for conversion of spores to the toxin-producing vegetative organisms. Iatrogenic disease has occurred after the use of smallpox vaccine and surgical sutures contaminated with the spores of *C. tetani*. It also has occurred as a postoperative complication in patients exposed to the organisms present in the dust in operating rooms.[105,108,119]

Very minor injuries, such as penetration by "clean" sewing needles and bites by chiggers, bees, and scorpions, have been recorded as portals of entry. Tetanus also has occurred after induced abortion, usually one performed under poor asepsis.

The initial manifestation in more than 50% of cases of generalized tetanus is trismus; it may be unilateral early in the disease but becomes bilateral within a short time. In some cases, it may be absent during the entire course of the illness or appear only after other abnormalities have become evident. In some instances, the only symptoms and signs may be irritability, restlessness, stiffness of the neck, difficulty swallowing, and rigidity of the abdominal or thoracic muscles; these symptoms may be present singly or in various combinations. The diagnostic importance of trismus cannot be overemphasized, despite the fact that it may be associated with numerous disorders unrelated to tetanus. Among these disorders are postmeasles encephalitis, trichinosis, suppurative and other types of parotitis, tender cervical lymphadenopathy, infected impacted upper molar teeth, and exposure to phenothiazine drugs.

As the activity of tetanospasmin persists, groups of muscles other than the masseters may become involved, including tonic spasms of the jaw, neck, back, and abdomen. Unrelenting trismus leads to the development of a characteristic facial expression, the sardonic smile (risus sardonicus). The abdominal and spinal muscles may become rigid. Intense and sustained contraction of the muscles of the chest and back results in persistent opisthotonos; in young children, this condition may be so severe that the youngster lies on one side with the soles of the feet resting on top of the head.

Generalized seizures, or tetanospasms, are unique in their appearance and peculiar to this disease. Characteristically, a sudden burst of tonic contractions of all groups of muscles occurs and leads to the development of opisthotonos, flexion and abduction of the arms, clenching of the fists on the chest, and extension of the legs. Pain in the spastic muscles usually is severe. Glottal and laryngeal spasm with the chest in the position of full inspiration may develop in some patients. During such an episode, the face becomes florid, the neck veins are distended markedly, and cyanosis develops. The features of this syndrome are consistent with an intense and sustained Valsalva maneuver; unless the tonic contraction of the glottis and larynx subsides or a tracheostomy is performed, death results. Dysphagia and hydrophobia may develop as isolated phenomena in the absence of a generalized tetanospasm. Dysuria or urinary retention also may occur.

Autonomic nervous system dysfunction commonly occurs in tetanus.[76,127,136] Manifestations include labile or persistent hypertension or hypotension, persistent sinus tachycardia, tachyarrhythmia or bradycardia alternating with tachycardia, and profuse sweating.

Electroencephalographic studies of patients have indicated involvement of the brain. Of 106 patients studied by Luisto,[78] 76% were found to have abnormal electroencephalograms. When patients of the same age and sex who had not had tetanus were compared with 40 individuals who had contracted the disease 7 years earlier, the latter were found to have more muscle fatigue and cramps; difficulty in speech, balance, and memory; and more peripheral paresis, muscular atrophy, decreased or absent tendon reflexes, and impaired mental capacity.[69]

The generalized seizures of tetanus often are triggered by very slight external stimuli, such as a light breeze, talking, a bump on the bed, or slight touching of the patient. The intense work generated by sustained or frequently repeated tetanospasms often leads to increases in body temperature of 1°C to 3°C (33.8°F to 37.4°F) or more.

The intense suffering of patients with the generalized tonic seizures of tetanus and the total frustration of the physician, who in ancient times had to stand by helplessly, unable to alter the course of the disease, were described best by Aretaeus[8] in the second century BCE; no better description has ever appeared:

> An inhuman calamity! An unseemly sight! A spectacle painful even to the beholder, an incurable malady! Owing to the distortion, not to be recognized by the dearest friends; and hence the prayers of the spectators, which formerly would have been reckoned not pious, now becomes good, that the patient may depart from life, or being a deliverance from the pains and unseemly evils attendant on it. But neither can the physician, though present and looking on, furnish any assistance, as regards life, relief from pain or from deformity. For if he should wish to straighten the limbs, he can do so only by cutting and breaking those of a living man. With them, then, who are overpowered by this disease, he can merely sympathize. This is the great misfortune of the physician.

Injection Drug Users

When generalized tetanus develops in injection drug users, many of the clinical features differ from those present in people who do not use drugs.[75] Among such features are much higher levels of fever; absence of trismus at onset and throughout the course of the disease or its appearance at some time after other manifestations have been present; marked stiffness of the neck and back, which in the absence of trismus may be confused with meningitis (the normal cerebrospinal fluid in patients with tetanus excludes this possibility); and early onset of coma. Prophylaxis is less effective in injection drug users than in non–injection drug users. The fatality rate approaches 100%.

Neonatal Tetanus

Neonatal tetanus usually begins 3 to 14 days after birth and is characterized by poor sucking and excessive crying.[52,137] Manifestations include trismus, difficulty swallowing, other tetanic spasms, and, frequently, marked opisthotonos.

A study by Salimpour[115] of the causes of death in patients with neonatal tetanus indicated pulmonary disease to be most common. Bronchopneumonia or hemorrhage in the lungs (or both) was the most frequent finding at autopsy. Among the nonpulmonary disorders responsible for a fatal outcome were hepatitis, omphalitis, cerebral hemorrhage, thrombosis, and rupture of the renal vein. As has been noted not only in infants but also in older children and adults with tetanus, any gross or histologic abnormalities are very uncommon findings. The complications described by Salimpour,[115] especially those involving the lungs, probably are related to aspiration associated with the laryngoglottal spasm characteristic of the disease. Newborns who survived tetanus in rural Kenya often had evidence of brain damage.[11] Indicators of a poor prognosis for neonates include age younger than 10 days when admitted to the hospital, symptoms of less than 5 days' duration, and the presence of risus sardonicus and fever.[80]

DIAGNOSIS

Differential Diagnosis

The differential diagnosis depends on the major clinical manifestations of the illness.[112] Cephalic tetanus may be confused with Bell palsy, trigeminal neuritis, and encephalitis, whereas generalized tetanus can be confused with rabies, strychnine poisoning, and phenothiazine reactions. An 11-year-old boy with neuromyotonia (Isaac syndrome) was diagnosed as having tetanus.[98] Trismus can result from dental problems, tonsillitis, peritonsillar abscess, temporomandibular joint dysfunction, and parotitis. Tetany caused by hypocalcemia or hyperventilation should be considered as well.

Specific Diagnosis

The diagnosis of tetanus is established on the basis of the history of an injury, particularly one in which either soil or fecal material has been introduced. In a small number of cases, especially those in which a relatively long incubation period has occurred, the site of entry of the organism may be healed and undetectable. In a review of 130 cases that occurred in the United States between 1998 and 2000, 94 (72%) were related to an acute injury[99]—47 puncture wounds, 31 lacerations, and eight abrasions. In 34 cases not involving an acute injury, the following associations were noted: abscess, seven cases; ulcer, seven cases; gangrene, two cases; cellulitis, one case; gingivitis, three cases; and other infections, two cases. In 12 cases, no injury or other source location was identified. One of the 130 patients was a neonate, and 18 of the nonacute injury cases occurred in patients with a history of injection drug use. Laboratory studies are of little help. Peripheral leukocytosis may or may not be present. The characteristic gram-positive rods, some of which may contain subterminal spores, may be seen occasionally in stained material obtained from the wound that has served as the portal of entry. Anaerobic cultures of exudate or necrotic tissue may grow typical sporulated rods and vegetative forms, but the yield of positive findings tends to be low.[38]

Low or undetectable levels of serum antitoxin at the time of onset of the illness are supportive of the diagnosis, but, occasionally, serum antitoxin is present.[112] Rises in antitoxin titer occur uncommonly after infection, so the use of paired sera for retrospective diagnosis generally is not helpful; in addition, this form of serologic diagnosis is not possible when therapy included active immunization. In selected cases, electrophysiologic studies of the masseter muscle may be helpful.[12] A characteristic absence or shortening of the silent period occurs as a result of failure of Renshaw cell inhibition; exaggerated F responses indicating hyperexcitability also may be noted.

TREATMENT

Management of generalized tetanus is directed at the following goals:

1. Neutralization of toxin still present in the blood before it comes in contact with the nervous system. Neutralization is accomplished by the administration of antitoxin as soon as the possibility of the disease is suspected or confirmed.[7,15] However, no acceptable evidence has shown that toxin can be inactivated by antitoxin once the toxin is fixed to tissues. In fact, the effectiveness of even large doses of antitoxin in reducing the fatality rate has been questioned.
2. Surgical removal of the site of entry of the organism, when possible, to eliminate the "factory" in which tetanospasmin is being produced. Omphalectomy has been performed with good results in children with neonatal tetanus.[41] Hysterectomy has been recommended when the disease has complicated induced and often septic abortions; however, patients in whom the infected uterus is not removed occasionally may survive. When the surgical procedure may be mutilating, as is the case with lesions on the face, it should not be performed.
3. Constant and meticulous intensive care unit monitoring and nursing care, with particular attention to fluid, electrolyte, and caloric balance because these frequently are abnormal, especially in patients with high temperature and repeated seizures, as well as in those unable to take food or liquids because of severe trismus, dysphagia, or hydrophobia.
4. Management of muscle spasm and autonomic instability.

The slightest external stimulus may precipitate potentially lethal seizures in persons with diffuse disease. For this reason, all therapeutic and other manipulations should be coordinated and carefully scheduled so that the risk for producing a tetanospasm is reduced to a minimum. All maneuvers are performed best after patients have received optimal sedation and relaxation. A quiet, darkened room in which the light is subdued and the doors padded, removed as far as possible from the mainstream of hospital traffic, is ideal, but at the same time the patient requires constant monitoring and observation in an intensive care environment.

The antitoxin of choice for the treatment of tetanus is human tetanus immune globulin (TIG) at a dose of 3000 to 6000 U intramuscularly; a second dose does not appear to be necessary. When TIG is not available, equine antitoxin (EA) may be used, but it should be avoided if at all possible. The dose of EA is 100,000 U; half is injected intramuscularly after appropriate tests to rule out sensitivity to horse serum have been performed. If EA is well tolerated, the remainder is given slowly intravenously. Patients sensitized to horse serum must be desensitized. An intramuscular injection of 80,000 units of EA produces maximal concentrations of antibody in the blood in 48 to 72 hours; very good levels may be maintained for 7 days.[57,130,131] Intravenous administration of the same dose yields concentrations of 40 U or more of antitoxin per milliliter of serum after 6 hours; it may persist for approximately 48 hours. Essentially no difference in circulating quantities of antitoxin exists 7 days after it is given by either route. Local instillation of antitoxin around the known or suspected wound may be of value if excision cannot be performed; it also has been recommended before surgical removal of the injured area.

Intravenous immune globulin (IVIG) contains antibodies to tetanus toxin.[7] The Committee of Infectious Diseases of the American Academy of Pediatrics suggests using IVIG in a dose of 200 to 400 mg/kg if TIG is not available.

Although reports[93,94] have documented that intrathecal administration of antitetanus serum did not improve the rate of survival in neonatal tetanus, the results of a study by Mongi and colleagues[90] led them to recommend this form of therapy. They found that intrathecal serotherapy may be of great value in the management of tetanus. Their experience indicated that the death rate from this disease in patients given intrathecal therapy was 45%; in those who did not receive this agent, it was 82%.[2] In a controlled trial in Brazil involving 120 adolescents and adults, 58 patients received TIG intrathecally and intramuscularly and 62 received TIG only by the intramuscular route.[86] The patients who received intrathecal and intramuscular treatment had better clinical progression than did those who were treated by only the intramuscular route. Two smaller pediatric-specific reports also suggest a morbidity and mortality benefit from intrathecal versus intramuscular administration of TIG or antitoxin. Ahmad and colleagues demonstrated a reduction in mortality and hospital stay in 35 neonates treated with intrathecal TIG compared to 35 neonates who received antitetanus serum via the intramuscular route.[3] A retrospective analysis by Geeta and colleagues of 66 children who received intrathecal TIG also suggested a morbidity and mortality reduction compared to intramuscular treatment alone.[55]

Two meta-analyses have been performed in an effort to establish the true benefit of intrathecal therapy, but unfortunately, they found conflicting results. The results of one meta-analysis led Abrutyn and Berlin[2] to conclude that intrathecal therapy with either EA or TIG is not of proved benefit and, therefore, should be given only during well-designed, controlled therapeutic trials.

A meta-analysis that involved 942 patients in 12 trials was reported.[67] In this analysis, the overall relative risk for mortality with intrathecal (antitetanus serum or TIG) versus intramuscular therapy was 0.71 (95% confidence interval, 0.62–0.81). Subcategory analyses for both adults and neonates and for high- and low-dose intrathecal therapy also indicated the beneficial effect of intrathecal therapy.

Penicillin kills the vegetative forms of *C. tetani*. Parenteral administration of penicillin G, 100,000 U/kg/day intravenously every 6 hours for 10 days, has been recommended in the past in all cases of tetanus. Observations have suggested that penicillin may act as an agonist to tetanospasmin by inhibiting the release of γ-aminobutyric acid (GABA).[112] Because of this possibility and the results of a controlled study in Indonesia, metronidazole has become the antimicrobial treatment of choice.[4,7] The metronidazole dosage is 30 mg/kg/day intravenously every 6 hours after an initial dose of 15 mg/kg. The usual duration of therapy is 10 to 14 days.

The spasticity and seizures of tetanus are caused by exaggerated reflex responses to afferent stimuli as a result of suppression of balancing central inhibition. Several classes of drugs that act at different sites along the reflex pathway are useful for control of these manifestations. Among them are hypnotics and sedatives, which reduce sensory input and generalized excitability; general anesthetics, which produce broad depression of the CNS; centrally acting muscle relaxants or spinal depressants, which lower reflex activity and decrease motor output from the spinal cord; and neuromuscular blocking agents, which inhibit the transmission of excess motor nerve activity to effector muscles.

Historically many different drugs have been used for the patient with tetanus. The use of diazepam was first reported in *The Lancet* in 1965, shortly after the drug was introduced clinically.[61] Since then the benzodiazepines have become the preferred drugs for the spasms and rigidity associated with tetanus.[39,96,126,134] They also have the advantage of being potent anticonvulsants and sedative hypnotic agents. Additionally, they are GABA agonists, perhaps partially overcoming the effect of tetanospasmin interfering with the normally inhibitory effect of GABA.[133] Diazepam (Valium) and lorazepam (Ativan) have been the most frequently used benzodiazepines for tetanus. Lorazepam has a somewhat longer half-life and may be preferred for this reason. Very large total daily doses (500 mg) of diazepam or lorazepam (200 mg) may be required. [120] Both drugs are formulated in propylene glycol solution for intravenous dosage, and the large doses required may result in significant propylene glycol toxicity, including a metabolic acidosis. For this reason, an enteral preparation that is free of propylene glycol should be given enterally if at all possible.[17]

Midazolam (Versed) is a short-acting benzodiazepine that is soluble in water and thus does not include propylene glycol in its parenteral formulation. Because of its short half-life, it should be administered as a continuous infusion and an initial infusion dose of 0.1 to 0.3 mg/kg per hour may be required. The benzodiazepines all induce tachyphylaxis and will require escalation of the dosage with time. The dosage should be titrated to prevent tetanic spasms and provide adequate sedation instead of being a specified dose. To avoid withdrawal symptoms after long-term use, the benzodiazepines should be tapered over the course of several weeks.

Magnesium sulfate has been advocated by some authors as first-line therapy for tetanus.[9,104,129] Magnesium was first reported as a therapy for tetanus, given intrathecally, more than 100 years ago.[16] Magnesium is a muscle relaxant and has been well tolerated at high doses in the obstetric population. In addition, magnesium reduces catecholamine release and lowers heart rate and vascular tone, stabilizing some of the effects of autonomic instability seen in tetanus. The largest trial of magnesium therapy for severe tetanus was reported in *The Lancet.*[129] This was a randomized, double-blind, placebo-controlled trial of 256 Vietnamese patients over the age of 15 years. Magnesium was given as a loading dose of 40 mg/kg followed by an intravenous infusion titrated to maintain serum levels of 2 to 4 mmol/L. There was no difference in the requirement for mechanical ventilation, although the patients receiving magnesium required less benzodiazepine and neuromuscular blockade and also were less likely to require treatment for cardiovascular instability. A smaller, less well-controlled clinical trial of magnesium has reported a decreased incidence of the need for mechanical ventilation.[121] Case reports in the pediatric population are somewhat limited,[28,104] although both reports advocate the use of magnesium as part of the therapeutic regimen for tetanus.

If benzodiazepines and magnesium are unable to control the spasms and rigidity associated with tetanus, intrathecal baclofen should be considered. Baclofen is a GABA receptor agonist that directly stimulates the postsynaptic GABA β receptors on synapses blocked by tetanus toxin, thereby restoring physiologic inhibition of the α motor neuron. Numerous centers have described the efficacy of intrathecal baclofen for treating tetanus, although its safety and efficacy have not been established in children younger than 4 years.[18,44,45,117] When magnesium, benzodiazepines and intrathecal baclofen are unable to control the spasms and rigidity associated with tetanus, neuromuscular blockade is indicated. Although succinylcholine has been used in the past,[51] newer agents have supplanted it. Additionally, theoretical reasons provide the basis to avoid the use of succinylcholine. With functional denervation of the motor end plate in neuromuscular junctions directly affected by tetanospasmin, succinylcholine may result in exaggerated release of potassium and hyperkalemia. This condition has been associated with cardiac arrhythmias and death in other denervating conditions. For this reason, nondepolarizing agents should be used. Potential agents include pancuronium, vecuronium, atracurium, cisatracurium, rocuronium, and pipecuronium—the agent of choice in a large tetanus treatment center in Vietnam.[129]

Neuromuscular blocking drugs should be used only by physicians experienced in their use in a critical care environment, typically anesthesiologists or intensivists.[72] Although neuromuscular blockers formerly were used at low doses to preserve diaphragmatic function and spontaneous respiration, current thought is that they should be administered in conjunction with tracheostomy or endotracheal intubation and ventilatory support. Remembering that neuromuscular blocking drugs have no effect on cortical function and have no sedative effect is critical. The benzodiazepines are good sedatives and have a significant amnestic effect. They are not, however, analgesics, and if pain is present (such as from previous muscle spasms), morphine sulfate is an effective analgesic. It also may be helpful in treating sympathetic hyperactivity. If sympathetic overactivity remains problematic, a combined α- and β-receptor blocker such as labetalol should be used. The use of a β-blocker such as propranolol alone should be avoided because the unopposed α-mediated vasoconstriction could lead to significant hypertension. Several alternative therapies have been suggested, but their use is not widespread, so it is difficult to draw conclusions regarding their efficacy. Clonidine and dexmedetomidine, both α_2-adrenoreceptor agonists, have shown potential benefit in controlling both muscle spasm and hemodynamic instability.[56,58,88] A combination of epidural bupivacaine and sufentanil has been used by some physicians to treat the sympathetic overactivity.[11] Finally, isolated case reports have shown success with dantrolene, ketamine, and propofol in combination with the agents described earlier.[14,19,36,88,95]

The management approach to a patient with tetanus spasms or rigidity should be one of escalation of therapy based on need. Benzodiazepines should be administered initially, with high doses often being required. If the benzodiazepines are not effective, infusion of magnesium to decrease muscle spasms and cardiovascular instability should be considered.[129] If control of the spasms or rigidity is still not achieved, intrathecal baclofen may be used.[44,45] If these therapies are inadequate or result in airway compromise or inadequate ventilation, endotracheal intubation should be performed with a nondepolarizing neuromuscular blocking agent.

Sixty-six percent of 103 children aged 1 to 12 years with severe tetanus studied by Wesley and Pather[138] required management with total muscle paralysis and intermittent positive-pressure ventilation. The death rate in this group was 14.5%.

PROGNOSIS

The average fatality rate associated with tetanus ranges from 25% to 70%, but mortality rates can be reduced to 10% to 30% with modern intensive care.[110,112] The risk for death occurring in patients with tetanus neonatorum is particularly high; it was reported to be 99.5% in a group of 5794 infants in 1930.[62] With modern treatment and high-intensity supportive care, the mortality rate associated with neonatal tetanus can be reduced to approximately 25%.[112] Injection drug users are highly susceptible to the development of very severe disease and are likely to die.[69,75]

A variety of other factors play an important role in determining the outcome of tetanus.[60,128] Patients in the second and third decades of life have a higher rate of recovery than the elderly. An inverse relationship exists between the length of the incubation period and risk, as first pointed out by Hippocrates. The risk for death is approximately 58% when the interval between injury and the onset of tetanus is 2 to 10 days. When the interval is 11 to 22 days or longer, fatality rates have been 35% to 17%, respectively. A relationship also appears to exist between the period elapsing from the time of appearance of the first signs of tetanus and development of the first seizure or maximal intensity of the disease; the shorter this interval, the poorer the prognosis.[38]

The clinical form of tetanus also influences the outcome.[77] Cephalic tetanus and tetanus neonatorum are associated with the highest incidence of death. In contrast, local tetanus, unless complicated by development of the generalized syndrome, has an excellent prognosis. Early administration of prophylactic antitoxin markedly increases the frequency of survival.

Cause of Death

Because the clinical course of tetanus may be prolonged and the therapy used is complex and potentially dangerous, the cause of death often is not clear. Animals may die after the injection of toxin without any recognizable signs of the disease appearing.[50] Studies in parabiotic rats suggest that tetanospasmin exerts a lethal effect on the respiratory center.[118] Involvement of the medulla has been observed in experimental animals and humans, in whom episodes of respiratory failure, often in the absence of seizures, have been described.[72,143] The action of the toxin on brain tissue has been postulated to be the cause of hyperpyrexia, tachycardia, hypotension, bulbar palsy, and cardiac arrest.[91] Myocardial damage also may occur, and both histologic and electrocardiographic abnormalities have been described.[101]

Death may occur during a seizure, but the specific mechanisms involved are not clear in all cases. Laryngospasm and disturbances in electrolyte balance may play important roles. Pneumonia complicating aspiration, induced by an inability to swallow and oversedation, occurs commonly. It may be directly responsible for death or may contribute to a fatal outcome by increasing the degree of anoxia of the respiratory center.

PREVENTION

As noted in Fig. 148.1, tetanus in the United States has decreased dramatically, and this decline can be attributed to routine universal use of tetanus toxoid and improved wound management, including the use of tetanus prophylaxis in emergency departments.

Active Immunization

For complete information regarding tetanus immunization, the reader is referred to the most recent recommendations of the Advisory Committee on Immunization Practices of the US Public Health Service,[29,30,33] the recommendations of the Committee on Infectious Diseases of the American Academy of Pediatrics,[7] and product information from vaccine manufacturers.

In the United States, primary immunization against tetanus is performed in conjunction with immunization against diphtheria and pertussis in the form of diphtheria and tetanus toxoids and acellular pertussis vaccine adsorbed (DTaP). The schedule involves an initial series of three doses of vaccine at 2, 4, and 6 months of age; a reinforcing dose at 12 to 18 months of age; and a booster dose at 4 to 6 years of age. After the initial series, additional booster doses of adult-type diphtheria and tetanus toxoids adsorbed (Td) are recommended at 10-year intervals.[41,43] In 2005, two adult-type diphtheria and tetanus toxoids and acellular pertussis vaccine adsorbed (Tdap) were approved for use in the United States.[32,33] In adolescents and adults, Tdap should be the routine vaccine. At present, Tdap vaccines are FDA approved for only one dose, but our opinion is that an every-10-year boosting schedule with Tdap rather than Td will maintain protective antitoxin levels and be less confusing for the physician. It is anticipated that a boosting schedule of Tdap will be similar to that recommended for Td (every 10 years). The minimal serum level of antitoxin needed for protection is 0.01 IU/mL.[42,79,80,122] After the initial three-dose series, the reinforcing dose, and the booster dose, levels of antitoxin 100- to 1000-fold higher than 0.01 IU/mL are attained, and levels higher than 0.01 IU/mL persist in nearly all vaccinees until the scheduled subsequent dose.

Although protection against tetanus by immunization is long-lasting in most children and adults, some immunocompromised children and adults may need more frequent booster doses.[37,71,87,89]

Tetanus Prophylaxis in Wound Management

Antimicrobial prophylaxis against tetanus is neither practical nor useful in managing wounds.[20,144] Cleaning of the wound, debridement when indicated, and proper immunization are important factors. The need for tetanus toxoid (active immunization), with or without TIG (passive immunization), depends on both the condition of the wound and the patient's vaccination history (Table 148.1).[7,29,35] Rarely has tetanus occurred in persons with documentation of having received a primary series of toxoid injections.

A thorough attempt must be made to determine whether a patient has completed primary vaccination. Patients with unknown or uncertain previous vaccination histories should be considered to have had no previous tetanus toxoid doses. Patients who have not completed a primary series may require tetanus toxoid and passive immunization at the time of wound cleaning and debridement (see Table 148.1).

The evidence available indicates that complete primary vaccination with tetanus toxoid provides long-lasting protection for 10 or more years in most recipients. Consequently, after complete primary tetanus vaccination, boosters—even for wound management—need to be given only every 10 years when wounds are minor and uncontaminated. For other wounds, a booster is appropriate if the patient has not received tetanus toxoid within the preceding 5 years.[100] Antitoxin antibodies develop rapidly in persons who have received at least two doses of tetanus toxoid.

Tdap is the preferred preparation for active tetanus immunization in the wound management of patients aged 7 years or older. Because a large proportion of adults are susceptible, this plan enhances diphtheria protection. Thus, by taking advantage of acute health care visits, such as for wound management, some patients can be protected who otherwise would remain susceptible. For routine wound management in children younger than 7 years of age who are not vaccinated adequately, DTaP should be used instead of Td. Td may be used if there is a valid contradiction to pertussis vaccine. For patients of all ages who are inadequately vaccinated, completion of primary vaccination at the time of discharge or at follow-up visits should be ensured. Presently, Tdap rather than Td is recommended for wound management in adolescents and adults.[32,33]

If passive immunization is needed, human TIG is the product of choice. It provides protection longer than that of antitoxin of animal origin and causes fewer adverse reactions.[81,114,123] The TIG prophylactic dose currently recommended for wounds of average severity is 250 U intramuscularly. When tetanus toxoid and TIG are given concurrently, separate syringes and separate sites should be used. If TIG is not available, intravenous immune globulin should be used.

Neonatal Tetanus

Several approaches have been taken to reduce the incidence and fatality rate of neonatal tetanus in developing areas of the world. Among these approaches are (1) educating pregnant women concerning the danger of using contaminated materials for cutting the umbilical cord and covering the stump, (2) training midwives in the application of modern techniques of obstetric asepsis, (3) developing hospitals in which babies are born under strict asepsis, and (4) immunizing all women of child-bearing age or, if such immunization is not possible, all who are pregnant. Studies performed by the WHO have demonstrated

TABLE 148.1 Summary Guide to Tetanus Prophylaxis in Routine Wound Management

	CLEAN, MINOR WOUNDS		ALL OTHER WOUNDS[a]	
History of Adsorbed Tetanus Toxoid (Doses)	**DTaP, Tdap, or Td[b]**	**TIG[c]**	**DTaP, Tdap, or Td[b]**	**TIG[c]**
Unknown or <3	Yes	No	Yes	Yes
≥3[d]	No if <10 y since last tetanus-containing vaccine dose Yes if ≥10 y since last tetanus containing vaccine dose	No	No[e] if <5 y since last tetanus-containing vaccine dose Yes if ≥5 y since last tetanus-containing vaccine dose	No

DTaP, Diphtheria and tetanus toxoids and acellular pertussis vaccine; *Td,* adult-type diphtheria and tetanus toxoids vaccine; *TdaP,* tetanus toxoid, reduced diphtheria toxoid, and acellular pertussis vaccine; *TIG,* tetanus immune globulin (human).

[a]Such as, but not limited to, wounds contaminated with dirt, feces, soil, and saliva; puncture wounds; avulsions; and wounds resulting from missiles, crushing, burns, or frostbite.

[b]For children <7 years, DTaP (unless there is a pertussis contraindication vaccine) is preferred to tetanus toxoid alone. For persons ≥7 years, Tdap is preferred to Td alone.

[c]Intravenous immune globulin should be used when TIG is not available.

[d]If only three doses of fluid toxoid have been received, a fourth dose of toxoid, preferably an adsorbed toxoid, should be given.

[e]More frequent boosters are not needed and can accentuate adverse effects.

Data from Centers for Disease Control and Prevention (CDC). Diphtheria, tetanus and pertussis: recommendations for vaccine use and other preventive measures; recommendations of the Immunization Practices Advisory Committee (ACIP). *MMWR Recomm Rep.* 1991;40(RR-10):2-28; CDC. *Tetanus in Epidemiology and Prevention of Vaccine-Preventable Diseases: The Pink Book—Course Textbook.* 13th ed. Atlanta, 2015, CDC. Available at http://www.cdc.gov/vaccines/pubs/pinkbook/tetanus.html; and American Academy of Pediatrics. Tetanus. In Kimberlin DW, Brady MT, Jackson MA, Long SS, eds. *Red Book: 2015 Report of the Committee on Infectious Diseases.* 30th ed. Elk Grove Village, IL: American Academy of Pediatrics; 2015:775.

that such immunization is practical and leads to an appreciable reduction in the incidence of neonatal tetanus.[48,47,46,124,132,141] Babies born to mothers who have been immunized during pregnancy have adequate levels of circulating antibody and are protected against acquiring the disease. The level of protective antibody in newborns and the magnitude of the transfer rate of passive immunity to tetanus depend directly on the level of tetanus antitoxin in maternal serum. Mothers who had tetanus antitoxin levels of 1.28 IU/mL or greater could transfer protection to almost all the newborns (97–100%), irrespective of the doses of tetanus toxoid administered. Mothers who had received two doses of tetanus toxoid during pregnancy not only conferred good protection but also transferred high antitoxin levels to their newborns.[116]

In 1989, the WHO adopted a resolution to eliminate neonatal tetanus worldwide,[120,121] and in 1990, the World Summit for Children issued a declaration for global elimination of neonatal tetanus by the end of 1995.[30,140] In 1993, the WHO's goal was defined as elimination of neonatal tetanus as a public health problem by reducing its case incidence to less than one per 1000 live births for all health districts.[59]

From 1989 to 1993, the rate of vaccination coverage with two or more doses of tetanus toxoid administered to pregnant women in areas at risk increased from 27% to 45%. To achieve and maintain elimination of neonatal tetanus, 80% or more of infants need to be protected at birth through vaccination of their mothers with at least two doses of tetanus toxoid or through clean delivery and cord-care practices.[59] Considerable progress has been made in the reduction of maternal and neonatal tetanus, but the goal to reduce the rate of neonatal tetanus cases to less than one per 1000 live births in all geographic areas has not been achieved.[132] In 2003, 57 countries still remained in which neonatal tetanus had not been eliminated in all districts.

NEW REFERENCES SINCE THE SEVENTH EDITION

3. Ahmad A, Qaisar I, Naeem M, et al. Intrathecal anti-tetanus human immunoglobulin in the treatment of neonatal tetanus. *J Coll Physicians Surg Pak.* 2011;21(9):539-541.
5. Alhaji MA, Abdulhafiz U, Atuanya CI, et al. Cephalic tetanus: a case report. *Case Rep Infect Dis.* 2011;2011:780209.
6. Alhaji MA, Bello MA, Elechi HA, et al. A review of neonatal tetanus in University of Maiduguri Teaching Hospital, North-eastern Nigeria. *Niger Med J.* 2013;54(6):398-401.
19. Borgeat A, Popovic V, Schwander D. Efficiency of a continuous infusion of propofol in a patient with tetanus. *Crit Care Med.* 1991;19(2):295-297.
35. Centers for Disease Control and Prevention. Tetanus. In: Atkinson W, Hamborsky J, Wolfe S, eds. *Epidemiology and Prevention of Vaccine-Preventable Diseases.* 12th ed. Washington, DC: Public Health Foundation; 2012:291-300.
36. Checketts MR, White RJ. Avoidance of intermittent positive pressure ventilation in tetanus with dantrolene therapy. *Anaesthesia.* 1993;48(11):969-971.
37. Choudhury SA, Matin F. Subnormal and waning immunity to tetanus toxoid in previously vaccinated HIV-infected children and response to booster doses of the vaccine. *Int J Infect Dis.* 2013;17(12):e1249-e1251.
55. Geeta MG, Krishnakumar P, Mathews L. Intrathecal tetanus immunoglobulins in the management of tetanus. *Indian J Pediatr.* 2007;74(1):43-45.
56. Girgin NK, Iscimen R, Gurbet A, et al. Dexmedetomidine sedation for the treatment of tetanus in the intensive care unit. *Br J Anaesth.* 2007;99(4):599-600.
58. Gregorakos L, Kerezoudi E, Dimopoulos G, et al. Management of blood pressure instability in severe tetanus: the use of clonidine. *Intensive Care Med.* 1997;23(8):893-895.
66. Johnson MG, Bradley KK, Mendus S, et al. Vaccine-preventable disease among homeschooled children: two cases of tetanus in Oklahoma. *Pediatrics.* 2013;132(6):e1686-e1689.
71. Kwon HJ, Lee JW, Chung NG, et al. Assessment of serologic immunity to diphtheria-tetanus-pertussis after treatment of Korean pediatric hematology and oncology patients. *J Korean Med Sci.* 2012;27(1):78-83.
87. Mishra K, Basu S, Kumar D, et al. Tetanus—still a scourge in the 21st century: a paediatric hospital-based study in India. *Trop Doct.* 2012;42(3):157-159.
88. Miya K, Shimojo N, Koyama Y, et al. Efficacy of concomitant use of dexmedetomidine and propofol in tetanus: report of a case. *Am J Emerg Med.* 2015;33(12):1848.e3-e4.
89. Modarresi M, Gheissari A, Sattari M. Protective status of end-stage renal disease children against tetanus and diphtheria vaccination. *Int J Prev Med.* 2013;4(4):420-424.
92. Narang M, Khurana A, Gomber S, et al. Epidemiological trends of tetanus from East Delhi, India: a hospital-based study. *J Infect Public Health.* 2014;7(2):121-124.
93. Neequaye J, Nkrumah FK. Failure of intrathecal antitetanus serum to improve survival in neonatal tetanus. *Arch Dis Child.* 1983;58(4):276-278.
95. Obanor O, Osazuwa HO, Amadasun JE. Ketamine in the management of generalised cephalic tetanus. *J Laryngol Otol.* 2008;122(12):1389-1391.
97. Oyedeji OA, Fadero F, Joel-Medewase V, et al. Trends in neonatal and post-neonatal tetanus admissions at a Nigerian teaching hospital. *J Infect Dev Ctries.* 2012;6(12):847-853.
125. Stevens DL. *Manual of Clinical Microbiology.* vol. 1. 11th ed. Washington, DC: ASM Press; 2015.
142. World Health Organization. Maternal and Neonatal Tetanus (MNT). www.who.int/immunization/disease/MNTE_initiative/en/.

The full reference list for this chapter is available at ExpertConsult.com.

149 Actinomycosis

Suzanne Whitworth • Morgan A. Pence • Richard F. Jacobs

Human actinomycosis is a clinical illness with typical histologic findings that is caused by a variety of pathogens. Actinomycetes are a group of aerobic and anaerobic bacteria in the order Actinomycetales. The name *actinomycosis* means "ray fungus," and the organisms may resemble fungi because of their filamentous appearance.[66] Actinomycosis is often polymicrobial, and *Aggregatibacter* (formerly *Actinobacillus*) *actinomycetemcomitans* is frequently a co-pathogen. It is endogenous worldwide, with sporadic cases reported annually. Occurrence of the disease is unrelated to age, sex, season, or occupation, although it is an uncommon event in the pediatric population. These organisms have the ability to spread locally without regard to fascial planes or other anatomic barriers. Actinomycosis is characterized by localized swelling with suppuration, abscess formation, and draining sinuses. The abscesses have fibrous walls and are filled with pus and characteristic sulfur granules. The three most common types of actinomycosis are oral/cervicofacial, abdominal/pelvic, and pulmonary. However, involvement of the liver, female reproductive tract, and brain has been described. Definitive diagnosis of the infection rests on isolation of the organism from pus or identification of sulfur granules on histopathologic sections of biopsy material. Adequate treatment generally consists of surgical removal of the lesion, prolonged antibiotic therapy, or a combination of both.

MICROBIOLOGY

The clinical entity of actinomycosis has historically been attributed to species of the genera *Actinomyces* and *Propionibacteriu.* Over time and with improved methods of detection this definition has broadened to include other genera, including *Actinobaculum, Cellulomonas,* and *Trueparella,* Other actinomycosis-related genera include *Actinotignum* and *Varibaculum.*[26] Human actinomycosis most often is caused by *Actinomyces israelii,* although over 20 species of *Actinomyces* are reported to cause human disease, including more commonly, *Actinomyces gerencseriae*, *Actinomyces naeslundii*, *Actinomyces viscosus*, *Actinomyces odontolyticus*, *Actinomyces meyeri*, *Actinomyces radicidentis*, *Actinomyces neuii*, *Actinomyces radingae*, *Actinomyces turicensis*, and *Actinomyces graevenitzii*.[22,54] *Propionibacterium propionicum* is the only species in the *Propionibacterium* genus that is a cause of human actinomycosis.

These bacteria are irregular, non–spore-forming, non–acid-fast, non–motile, gram-positive rods. They grow in most rich culture media and have various oxygen requirements. For example, *A. israelii* requires anaerobic conditions for growth. *A. viscosus*, however, grows in an aerobic environment with carbon dioxide. These species ferment carbohydrates as their source of energy for growth.[18] These organisms are now firmly classified as prokaryotic bacteria, although they originally were thought to be fungi because of the mycelial appearance of the organisms in sulfur granules and their branching morphology. They are also members of the endogenous flora of mucous membranes. *A. israelii* is always found in the oral cavity when the appropriate anaerobic culture technique is used. It also has been found in the gastrointestinal tract, bronchi, and female genital tract.[53]

A. actinomycetemcomitans is a fastidious, non–spore-forming, nonmotile, facultatively anaerobic gram-negative coccobacillus that frequently complicates actinomycosis caused by *A. israelii*.[20,21,37,44,56,59] Further information about this organism is detailed in Chapter 127.

PATHOGENESIS

The organisms that cause actinomycosis normally are found in the oral flora from infancy to adulthood. Actinomycetes are primary colonizers that can initiate the formation of plaque and set the stage for the development of infectious disease, as well as predispose to the formation of caries.[4,9,12] These bacteria adhere tenaciously to both the hard and soft tissue surfaces of the oral cavity.[69] Disruption of this mucous membrane probably is the initiating event for oral and cervicofacial disease.[1] The organisms then invade locally and spread without regard to fascial planes. The exact mechanism of this spread is unknown but may be related to the ability of these organisms to suppress part of the host immune system. Organisms of the *Actinomyces* genus have been shown to be chemotactic, to activate lymphocyte blastogenesis, and to stimulate the release of lysosomal enzymes from polymorphonuclear leukocytes and macrophages.[18,45] In addition, the co-pathogens involved in this infection may reduce local oxygen tension. Dental extractions are associated with mucosal breaks and tissue necrosis and may predispose to oral or cervicofacial actinomycosis.[47] Hematogenous dissemination can occur eventually but is an uncommon development. Gastrointestinal disease is likely associated with disruption of the mucosal barrier, similar to oral and cervicofacial disease.[53] Organisms causing pulmonary actinomycosis most likely reach the lungs through aspiration. Thoracic actinomycosis usually is a complication of localized pulmonary parenchymal infection. Actinomycetes produce enzymes and thus are able to spread by extension into the lungs, pleura, and chest wall without regard to tissue planes.[61] Numerous reports in the literature associate actinomycosis with intrauterine devices (IUDs), and some question exists regarding the association of foreign bodies with actinomycosis.[5,14]

PATHOLOGY

Actinomycosis is most commonly manifested as a chronic infection with single or multiple indurated swellings. These lesions eventually soften, become fluctuant, and suppurate. The walls are fibrous and firm and often described as wooden, which frequently results in their confusion with neoplasms. Over the course of time, sinus tracts form and extend through the overlying skin or to adjacent bones or tissues. The overlying skin may have a bluish hue.[53]

Histologically, a typical lesion has a central purulent area containing neutrophils and sulfur granules, surrounded by an outer zone of granulation with collagen fibers and fibroblasts. The sulfur granules are firm, yellowish granules containing the organisms and are virtually diagnostic of actinomycosis, although they can be seen in nocardiosis and botryomycosis. In addition to neutrophils, lymphocytes and plasma cells frequently are seen in the lesions; eosinophils and multinucleated giant cells occasionally are seen.[53]

CLINICAL MANIFESTATIONS

Actinomycotic infection occurs in three important sites. The order of frequency of occurrence is oral/cervicofacial, abdominal/pelvic, and pulmonary. Actinomycosis resembles several other chronic inflammatory diseases and must be differentiated from mycotic infections, tuberculosis, appendicitis, *Yersinia enterocolitica* pseudoappendicitis, osteomyelitis, amebiasis, hepatic abscess, and other chronic bacterial infections, including nocardiosis.

Because oral and cervicofacial actinomycosis occurs after disruption of the mucous membranes in the mouth or oropharynx, patients who have this type of actinomycosis may have a history of oral surgery, dental procedures, or trauma to the mouth. Clinical findings may include pain, trismus, firm swelling, and fistulae with drainage that contains the characteristic sulfur granules (Figs. 149.1 and 149.2). Patients most commonly have a chronic disease course but may be seen acutely with cellulitis. Infection may spread through the sinus tracts to the cranial bones, which gives rise to meningitis. Bone is not involved early in the disease, but periostitis may develop later. The marked ability of the organisms in this disease to burrow through tissue planes and even bone differentiates actinomycosis from nocardiosis and is an important characteristic of this infection. The cervicofacial type of actinomycosis, or "lumpy jaw," has the best prognosis. With surgical debridement and excision as an adjunct to proper antibiotic therapy, the disease usually is cured. At least two cases of thyroiditis secondary to actinomycosis have been reported in pediatric patients.[24,68]

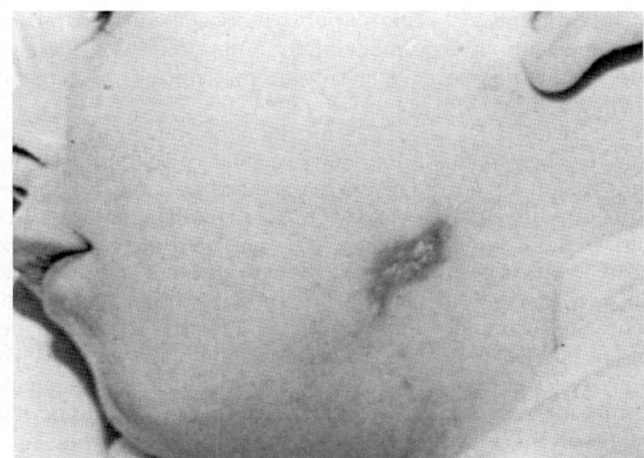

FIG. 149.1 Cervicofacial disease with draining sinus tracts caused by *Actinomyces israelii.*

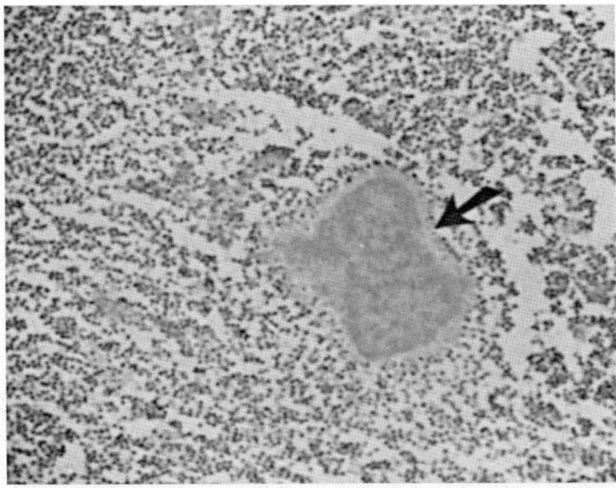

FIG. 149.2 Abscess containing an actinomycotic granule surrounded by purulent exudate. The peripheral clubbing *(arrow)* is stained by eosin (hematoxylin and eosin, ×52).

Abdominal actinomycosis is the result of disruption of the mucosa of the gastrointestinal tract, and thus, patients may have a history of gastrointestinal surgery, diverticulitis, or appendicitis. The patient also may have a history of trauma to the abdomen. Patients may have chills, fever, night sweats, and weight loss. The course is indolent and similar to that of tuberculous peritonitis. Because appendicitis is the most common predisposing event, on physical examination patients may have a hard, irregular mass in the ileocecal area that softens and then drains to the outside. Extension from such foci usually is by direct continuity (or, rarely, hematogenously) and involves any tissue or organ, including muscle, liver, spleen, kidney, fallopian tubes, ovaries, uterus, testes, bladder, esophagus, or rectum.[2,3,10,28,33,50] A delayed diagnosis of actinomycosis involving the abdomen or pelvis is typical and is frequently confused with malignancy.[29]

Hepatic involvement occurs in approximately 15% of cases of abdominal actinomycosis. Involvement of the liver can occur through direct extension from a subdiaphragmatic or subhepatic abscess. It also is a common finding in disseminated actinomycosis.[53] Occult disruption of the gastrointestinal mucosa with spread of organisms through the portal vein may provide a portal of entry for the organisms in cases of primary or isolated hepatic disease. Initial symptoms may include fever, abdominal pain, anorexia, weight loss, nausea, vomiting, shoulder pain, back pain, or diarrhea. The course is usually indolent, with 1 to 6 months of symptoms. On physical examination, the patient commonly has fever, abdominal tenderness, and hepatomegaly. A palpable abdominal mass, jaundice, or draining sinuses may be present. Disseminated intravascular coagulation has been reported.[65] Hepatic actinomycosis has been found in children who have undergone appendectomies.[38] Thrombotic thrombocytopenic purpura has been described in association with hepatic actinomycosis in an adult.[50] Other causes of liver masses included in the differential diagnosis are pyogenic abscess, amebiasis, and malignancy.

Women with IUDs are at risk for the development of pelvic actinomycosis. These patients may have vaginal discharge, pelvic pain, abdominal pain, menorrhagia, fever, a pelvic mass, a history of pelvic inflammatory disease, or a history of prolonged IUD use (Fig. 149.3). The risk is more significant if the IUD has been in place for longer than 2 to 3 years. These devices are thought to cause an inflammatory response in the endometrium with focal necrosis. This anaerobic environment encourages the growth of *A. israelii*. In such patients, removal of the IUD plus treatment with antibiotics is necessary.[14] Pelvic actinomycosis can develop in both men and women; it can appear as a tumorlike mass and be confused with malignancy. A urachus or urachal remnant is also a risk factor.[36]

Establishing the diagnosis of pulmonary actinomycosis depends on having a high index of suspicion because neither the clinical nor the radiographic findings are specific. Patients may have a history of or risk factors for aspiration. Adults with thoracic actinomycosis usually have abnormal local defenses, such as chronic bronchitis, bronchiectasis, or emphysema; however, pediatric patients have been shown to have predisposing factors less often.[30,61] This type of actinomycosis also occurs after the introduction of a colonized foreign body. Patients with oral, cervicofacial, or abdominal actinomycotic infections are at risk for the development of pulmonary infection from direct or hematogenous spread. A history of these preexisting infections should heighten the index of suspicion. Pulmonary actinomycosis may be manifested as an endobronchial infection, a tumorlike lesion, diffuse pneumonia, or a pleural effusion.[8,11,46] The presence of chronic pleural effusion, underlying lung changes, and periosteal rib involvement is indicative of actinomycosis but seldom is reported.[67] The principal symptoms include chest pain, fever, productive cough, and weight loss. Hemoptysis has been reported.[48] The infection frequently dissects along tissue planes and may extend through the chest wall or diaphragm and produce multiple sinuses (Figs. 149.4 and 149.5). These characteristic sinus tracts contain small abscesses and purulent drainage. Empyema necessitans has been reported in one child.[62] The differential diagnosis of pulmonary actinomycosis includes tuberculosis, lung abscess, nocardiosis, fungal infection, and botryomycosis.

Laryngeal actinomycosis rarely has been reported in older teenagers.[41] Colonization of the oropharynx with these organisms may be involved in the development of obstructive tonsillar hypertrophy.[47] Several adult cases of pericardial actinomycosis are reported in the literature.[15] Bacteremia is reported in all age groups, including neonates.[7,15,25,34] Septic arthritis has been reported.[31] Brain abscess has occurred in a child with complex congenital heart disease (Fig. 149.6).[42] A case has been reported of purulent meningitis caused by *Actinomyces* species.[23] Actinomycetes

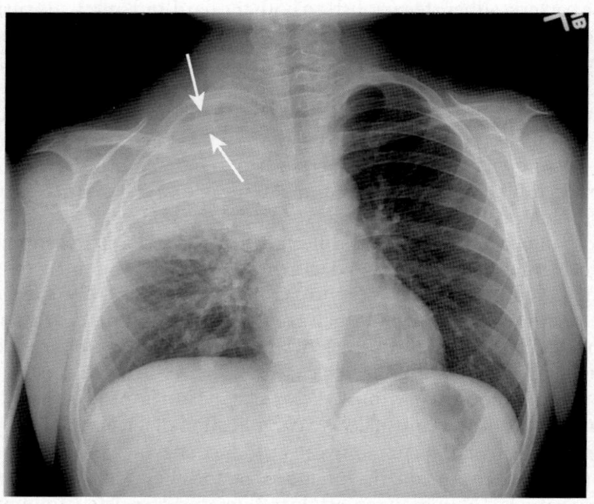

FIG. 149.4 Chest radiograph of a 10-year-old child with chronic pneumonia whose lung biopsy revealed sulfur granules and bacteria in the actinomycoses species.

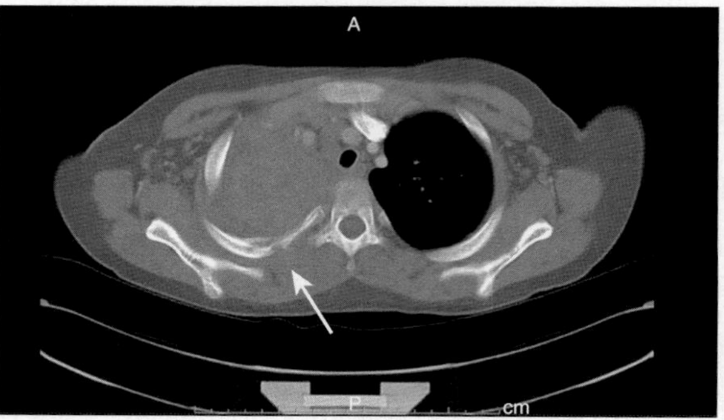

FIG. 149.5 Computed tomographic image of the same child in Fig. 149.4 revealing bony erosion *(arrow)* of the ribs next to the infiltrate.

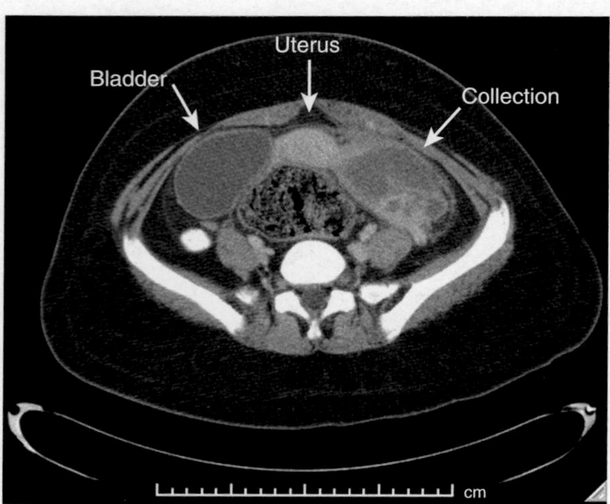

FIG. 149.3 Pelvic abscess that grew *Actinomyces turicensis*.

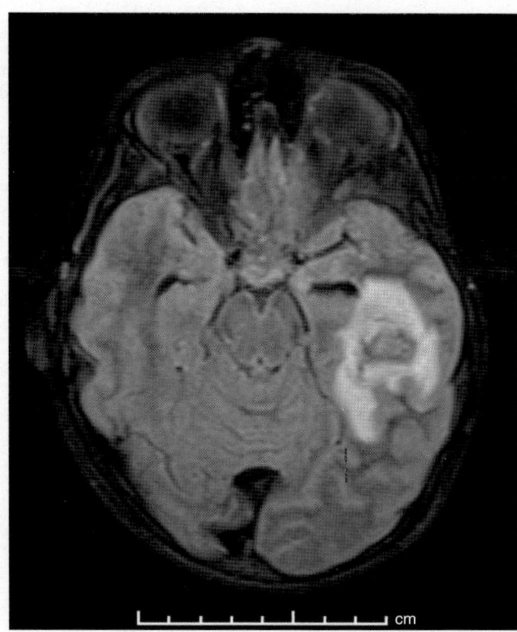

FIG. 149.6 Brain abscess that grew *Actinomyces turicensis.*

have been isolated from nearly every organ in the body, including the kidneys, brain, heart, breasts, mastoids, male genitourinary tract, and eyes.[12] Osteomyelitis is reported in children, often involving the mandible, but other bones have been infected as well.[51] It has been associated with brain abscesses in patients with hereditary hemorrhagic telangiectasia.[27] Ocular canaliculitis in pediatric patients has been recently reported.[70] *Trueparella pyogenes* has been implicated only rarely as a cause of human infection, but cases of septicemia, endocarditis, meningitis, arthritis, empyema, pneumonia, otitis media, cystitis, mastoiditis, appendicitis, and cutaneous infection have been reported.[13,17]

Actinomycosis does not seem to be associated commonly with human immunodeficiency virus infection. Thoracic, esophageal, oral, and anal cases have been reported, however, and all immunocompromised hosts should be monitored closely for this potential group of pathogens.[2,3,43,64] Actinomycosis has been reported in patients with chronic granulomatous disease, including cervicofacial, pulmonary, and hepatic infection.[49] Primary cutaneous actinomycosis caused by *Actinomyces bovis* has been reported in a patient with common variable immunodeficiency.[35]

A. actinomycetemcomitans is a pathogen in at least 30% of actinomycotic infections[37] (see Chapter 127). Failure to recognize this organism and treat it adequately has resulted in clinical relapse and deterioration in patients infected with actinomycosis.[40,69]

DIAGNOSIS

To establish a definitive diagnosis of actinomycosis, the clinician must isolate the causative organism from tissue or pus from a normally sterile body site, such as the lungs. Isolation of the organism from the oral cavity or the female genital tract without clinical evidence of disease, therefore, is not diagnostic. Because the organisms that cause actinomycosis are exquisitely sensitive to antibiotics, clinical specimens must be obtained before initiating their use. The specimens should be processed carefully to maintain anaerobic conditions. They should undergo routine Gram stain, which will reveal pleomorphic gram-positive rods with or without branching.[18] Gram stain is more sensitive than culture, particularly if the patient has been given antibiotics. Immunofluorescence is available for confirmation of organisms in biopsy specimens with suggestive Gram stains. Growth on media usually appears within 5 to 7 days but may take 2 to 4 weeks.[53] Identification methods include RapID ANA II kits (Remel), matrix-associated laser desorption ionization time-of-flight (MALDI-TOF) mass spectrometry, and 16S rDNA sequencing.[16,32,57]

True microbiologic identification of these organisms occurs uncommonly, and the diagnosis most often rests on the clinical picture, along with identification of the characteristic sulfur granules. The sulfur granules may be found by drawing pus from a lesion, on the bandage covering the lesion, or in surgical specimens (see Fig. 149.2). Pus that is poured down the side of a glass will leave sulfur granules adhering to the sides so that the granules can be identified more easily. On hematoxylin and eosin stain, the granules are eosinophilic or variably surrounded by a radiating fringe of eosinophilic clubs. The formation of granules is a hallmark of actinomycosis and is related to a bacterial secretion that cements elements of *Actinomyces* spp. together. However, the formation of granules related to various nonfilamentous bacteria such as *Staphylococcus aureus* or *Pseudomonas* spp. is termed botryomycosis or bacterial pseudomycosis, and they can look grossly similar to the typical sulfur granules of actinomycosis.[11] Washed, crushed actinomycotic granules or well-mixed pus in the absence of granules is cultured on a rich medium, such as brain-heart infusion blood agar, blood or chocolate agar if aerotolerant, or anaerobic blood agar if anaerobic. The plates are then incubated anaerobically and aerobically with added carbon dioxide. Plates can be examined after 24 hours and should be held 5 to 7 days for recovery of *Actinomyces* spp.[18]

Various imaging modalities have been useful in diagnosing and characterizing actinomycosis. Computed tomography has been shown to help differentiate between inflammatory masses and tumors. In addition, the location, extension, and relationship between the mass and surrounding structures can be defined better. Ultrasonography has been shown in one report to reveal a mass with an ill-defined margin that was hypoechoic with intrinsic hyperechoic spots.[55] Magnetic resonance imaging has been used for diagnosing actinomycotic brain abscess, as well as actinomycosis of the chest, spine, soft tissues, and mandible.[30,42,51]

Because of the frequency of coinfection with this organism in cases of actinomycosis, attempts always should be made to isolate *A. actinomycetemcomitans* in these patients. Further details are found in Chapter 127.

TREATMENT

The mainstays of therapy for actinomycosis remain surgical debridement or removal of the lesion and prolonged antimicrobial therapy. Most experts still recommend drainage of abscesses, fistulotomy, sinus tract excision, and debulking of large masses, although numerous successful outcomes with antimicrobial therapy alone are reported in the literature.[38,52,53] The option to treat medically and observe for clinical response seems reasonable in a stable, noncritical patient.

The traditionally recommended total duration of therapy ranges from 6 to 12 months. There are, however, numerous reports in the literature of successful treatment with various combinations of intravenous followed by oral therapy for much shorter periods of time. Thoracic actinomycosis has been treated successfully with a total duration of therapy of only 4 months.[58] Two studies in adults with thoracic actinomycosis revealed good success rates with less than 14 days of intravenous therapy followed by prolonged oral treatments. Some of those patients required surgery.[6,63] Another study in adults with cervicofacial disease reported good success rates with surgical debridement and intravenous penicillin and metronidazole followed by oral therapy for a total duration of 2 to 4 weeks.[39] Because the disease is an uncommon occurrence in children and no significant randomized prospective treatment trials have been performed, most authors still recommend a few weeks of intravenous therapy followed by prolonged oral therapy. The total duration of therapy is based on clinical and radiographic follow-up. Certainly in cases for which surgical debridement or incision and drainage have been performed, a shorter duration of therapy would be reasonable provided that close clinical follow-up can be ensured. Osteomyelitis may require longer therapy.[51] Failure to respond to adequate treatment has been noted in patients with underlying malignancy.

The antibiotic of choice for treatment of actinomycosis is penicillin. For patients who are allergic to penicillin, tetracycline or erythromycin is acceptable. Other alternatives are clindamycin and the third-generation cephalosporins.[58] Susceptibility breakpoints have been established for linezolid and meropenem for aerotolerant *Actinomyces*. Most isolates are clearly resistant to ciprofloxacin and metronidazole.[19,60] Administration of daily ceftriaxone for 3 weeks followed by prolonged administration of ampicillin was effective treatment in one case.[61]

A. actinomycetemcomitans is susceptible to the third-generation cephalosporins, rifampin, trimethoprim-sulfamethoxazole, aminoglycosides, quinolones, tetracycline, azithromycin, and chloramphenicol. It also is susceptible to penicillin and ampicillin in vitro, but test results do not necessarily correlate with clinical outcome. Vancomycin, erythromycin, and clindamycin have no significant activity against this organism.

NEW REFERENCES SINCE THE SEVENTH EDITION

1. Alani A, Seymour R. Aggressive periodontitis: how does an understanding of the pathogenesis affect treatment? *Dent Update*. 2011;38:511-521.
6. Choi J, Koh WJ, Kim TS, et al. Optimal duration of IV and oral antibiotics in the treatment of thoracic actinomycosis. *Chest*. 2005;128:2211-2217.
16. Figuero E, Sanchez-Beltran M, Cuesta-Frechoso S, et al. Detection of periodontal bacteria in atheromatous plaque by nested polymerase chain reaction. *J Periodontol*. 2011;82:1469-1477.
21. Hsieh CJ, Hwang KP, Kuo KC, Hsueh PR. Facial cellulitis because of *Aggregatibacter (Actinobacillus) actinomycetemcomitans* and *Capnocytophaga* species in an immunocompetent patient. *J Microbiol Immunol Infect*. 2011;44:149-151.
22. Hwang SS, Park SD, Jang IH, et al. *Actinomyces graevenitzii* bacteremia in a patient with alcoholic liver cirrhosis. *Anaerobe*. 2011;17:87-89.
23. Imamura K, Kamitani H, Nakayasu H, Asai Y, Nakashima K. Purulent meningitis caused by *Actinomyces* successfully treated with rifampicin: a case report. *Intern Med*. 2011;50:1121-1125.
26. Könönen E, Wade WG. Actinomyces and related organisms in human infections. *Clin Microbiol Rev*. 2015;28:419-442.
27. Koubaa M, Lahiani D, Mâaloul I, et al. Actinomycotic brain abscess as the first clinical manifestation of hereditary hemorrhagic telangiectasia—case report and review of the literature. *Ann Hematol*. 2013;92:1141-1143.
33. Lin CH, Chen AC, Lin HC, et al. Abdominal actinomycosis complicated with hydronephrosis. *J Formos Med Assoc*. 2005;104:666-669.
39. Moghimi M, Salentijn E, Debets-Ossenkop Y, Karagozoglu KH, Forouzanfar T. Treatment of cervicofacial actinomycosis: a report of 19 cases and review of the literature. *Med Oral Patol Oral Cir Bucal*. 2013;18:e627-e632.
61. Snape PS. Thoracic actinomycosis: an unusual childhood infection. *South Med J*. 1993;86:222-224.
64. Spadari F, Tartaglia GM, Spadari E, Fazio N. Oral actinomycosis in acquired immunodeficiency syndrome. *Int J STD AIDS*. 1998;9:424-426.
70. Yuksel D, Hazirolan D, Sungur G, Duman S. *Actinomyces canaliculitis* and its surgical treatment. *Int Ophthalmol*. 2012;32:183-186.

The full reference list for this chapter is available at expertconsult.com.

150 *Bacteroides, Fusobacterium, Prevotella,* and *Porphyromonas*

Catherine Foster • Lucila Marquez • Steven C. Buckingham

The most clinically important anaerobic gram-negative bacilli include *Bacteroides, Fusobacterium,* and *Prevotella,* along with *Porphyromonas*. These bacteria, like other anaerobes, normally colonize the skin and mucosal surfaces of humans. Anaerobic gram-negative rods can cause infections of various body sites in children, although their importance as pediatric pathogens has historically been underappreciated. Many infections with these and other anaerobic pathogens are never diagnosed as such because clinicians fail to use appropriate methods for collection or transportation of specimens or because laboratories fail to use appropriate methods for the isolation and identification of anaerobic bacteria.

BACTERIOLOGY AND TAXONOMY

Bacteria belonging to the genera *Bacteroides, Fusobacterium, Prevotella,* and *Porphyromonas* are obligately anaerobic gram-negative bacilli. The taxonomic classification of these and other anaerobic bacteria has undergone considerable revision in recent decades, based largely on the characterization of the bacteria with the use of nucleic acid analyses.

Bacteroides Species

Bacteroides spp. are strictly anaerobic, nonmotile gram-negative rods, about 0.5 to 2.0 × 1.6 to 12 μm, with rounded ends. In general, these bacteria are nonpigmented, saccharolytic, and bile resistant, and on blood agar they form smooth, white to gray colonies that are 1 to 3 mm in diameter. In the 1980s, the genus *Bacteroides* comprised a large and heterogeneous group of anaerobic gram-negative bacilli, but over the past 3 decades, many species formerly assigned to this genus have been reassigned to other genera.[119] The most notable taxonomic shift occurred between 1988 and 1990, when numerous *Bacteroides* spp. were reclassified into the newly created genera *Prevotella* and *Porphyromonas*.[116,117,118] Historically, the *Bacteroides* spp. most frequently recovered in clinical specimens have been collectively classified as the so-called *Bacteroides fragilis* group, consisting of *Bacteroides fragilis, Bacteroides distasonis, Bacteroides ovatus, Bacteroides thetaiotaomicron, Bacteroides vulgatus,* and others. Taxonomic revisions based on nucleic acid analyses have disrupted even this close-knit group, because *B. distasonis, B. goldsteinii,* and *B. merdae* have been reclassified under the genus *Parabacteroides* and *Bacteroides forsythus* has been renamed *Tannerella forsythensis*.[112,113] Today, most previously recognized *Bacteroides* spp. that were not members of the *B. fragilis* group have been moved to other genera. In 2010, *Bacteroides ureolyticus* was reclassified as *Campylobacter ureolyticus*.[134]

Resistance to multiple classes of antibiotics is a hallmark of *Bacteroides* spp., and resistance even to drugs traditionally considered to have broad activity against anaerobes has increased substantially over the past 2 decades. Most *Bacteroides* spp., and virtually all members of the *B. fragilis* group, produce a class 2e cephalosporinase, encoded by the *cepA* gene, which confers broad resistance to penicillins and first- and third-generation cephalosporins. This β-lactamase, however, is uniformly neutralized by the β-lactamase inhibitors clavulanate, sulbactam, and tazobactam. Another, less frequently encountered β-lactamase, encoded by *cfxA*, confers resistance to cefoxitin. Resistance to β-lactams also can result, less commonly, from alterations in the penicillin-binding proteins, PB1 and PB2, or from porin mutations, which alter the permeability of the bacterial outer membrane to β-lactams.[62,74,95,119]

Resistance to carbapenems remains rare among *Bacteroides* spp., although recent reports from Turkey and Taiwan reported resistance rates of 6% to imipenem and 8% to meropenem among *B. fragilis* group isolates.[91,95,132] Carbapenem resistance results from production of a class B metallo-β-lactamase encoded by either *cfiA* or *ccrA*. Expression of these genes requires the presence of special insertion sequences upstream of the gene, which act as promoters. The resulting β-lactamase renders the organism resistant not only to carbapenems but also to all β-lactams, including the penicillin/β-lactamase inhibitor combinations (i.e., amoxicillin-clavulanate, ampicillin-sulbactam, and piperacillin-tazobactam).[74,95,133]

Resistance to clindamycin, which has been increasingly documented among *Bacteroides* isolates in recent decades, usually results from MLS-type ribosomal alterations coded by various *erm* genes, although other mechanisms apparently account for resistance in some isolates.[74,95] Metronidazole resistance, which remains rare, results from the production of nitroimidazole reductases encoded by any of seven known *nim* genes. Expression of these genes requires the presence of upstream insertion sequences, which act as promoters. In some cases, metronidazole resistance has been documented in *Bacteroides* isolates lacking *nim* genes, following prolonged exposure to the drug.[62,74,95] Resistance to moxifloxacin, which has increased rapidly since the late 1990s, results either from alterations in the DNA gyrase genes *gyrA* and *gyrB* or from increased production of efflux pumps.[74,95] Most *B. fragilis* group isolates are resistant to tetracycline, owing to ribosomal alterations encoded by *tetQ, tetM,* or *tet36* genes. Tigecycline has much better activity against *Bacteroides* spp., although some isolates are resistant by virtue of their production of a tetracycline-degrading mono-oxygenase encoded by *tetX*.[95]

Prevotella Species and *Porphyromonas* Species

The genus *Prevotella* includes more than 40 recognized species, all of which are moderately saccharolytic, bile-sensitive gram-negative bacilli that were formerly classified under the genus *Bacteroides.* Some species are pigmented (e.g., *Prevotella corporis, Prevotella denticola, Prevotella intermedia, Prevotella loescheii, Prevotella melaninogenica,* and *Prevotella nigrescens*), whereas others are nonpigmented (e.g., *Prevotella bivia, Prevotella disiens, Prevotella oris, Prevotella buccae,* and *Prevotella heparinolytica*).[80,119]

Compared with the *B. fragilis* group, *Prevotella* spp. are generally more susceptible to antibiotics. Resistance to penicillin is frequently observed, owing to the production of β-lactamases coded by *cfxA* or other genes, although most isolates remain susceptible to third-generation cephalosporins, cefoxitin, carbapenems, and penicillin/β-lactamase inhibitor combinations.[74,95] Resistance to metronidazole, which is mediated by *nim*-encoded production of nitroimidazole reductases, occurs infrequently. Clindamycin resistance, which has increased in prevalence in recent years, is associated with *ermF*- or *ermG*-mediated ribosomal modification.[95] Data on moxifloxacin's activity against *Prevotella* spp. are sparse, but available studies indicate that most isolates are susceptible.[68,72,89,91,141] *Prevotella* spp. are frequently resistant to tetracycline, owing to ribosomal alterations encoded by the *tetQ, tetM,* or *tetW* genes. Available data suggest that tigecycline, however, is highly active against *Prevotella* strains.[95]

The genus *Porphyromonas* consists of pigmented or nonpigmented gram-negative bacilli that, like *Prevotella* spp., were formerly classified under the genus *Bacteroides.* Unlike *Prevotella* spp., *Porphyromonas* spp. are asaccharolytic or only weakly saccharolytic.[80,119] In contrast to *Bacteroides* and *Prevotella* spp., antibiotic resistance is unusual among *Porphyromonas* spp. Penicillin resistance, mediated by *cfxA*-encoded β-lactamase production, occurs in a minority of clinical specimens but is somewhat more frequent in animal-derived specimens.[74,95,119] Carbapenems and penicillin/β-lactamase inhibitor combinations are uniformly active against *Porphyromonas* spp. Resistance to clindamycin, associated with *ermF* and *ermG* genes, occurs in fewer than 10% of strains. Resistance to metronidazole and tetracycline, although described, is only rarely observed.[95]

Fusobacterium Species

Fusobacterium spp. are nonmotile, thin, long, filamentous anaerobic gram-negative rods that metabolize peptones or carbohydrates to produce butyric acid. Since the early 1980s, several new *Fusobacterium* spp. have been described (*Fusobacterium periodonticum, Fusobacterium simiae, Fusobacterium ulcerans, Fusobacterium equinum,* and *Fusobacterium canifelinum*), whereas two long-standing members of the genus have been reclassified to other genera (*Fusobacterium plautii* and *Fusobacterium prausnitzii*). Moreover, three newly described species were subsequently reclassified to other genera (*Fusobacterium alocis, Fusobacterium sulci,* and *Fusobacterium polysaccharolyticum*), and another (*Fusobacterium pseudonecrophorum*) was described but found to be identical to *Fusobacterium varium.*[119] The type species, *Fusobacterium nucleatum,* is the one most frequently recovered from clinical specimens.[12]

Fusobacterium spp. are usually susceptible to penicillin, third-generation cephalosporins, clindamycin, and moxifloxacin, and more than 90% of strains are susceptible to cefoxitin, penicillin/β-lactamase inhibitor combinations, carbapenems, and metronidazole. In one study, all isolates of *F. nucleatum* and *Fusobacterium necrophorum* were susceptible to imipenem, amoxicillin-clavulanate, cefoxitin, and clindamycin. Isolates of the *Fusobacterium mortiferum/varium* group, however, demonstrated reduced susceptibility rates to imipenem (85%), amoxicillin-clavulanate (90%), and clindamycin (55%).[138] Tetracycline resistance, associated with *tetW* and *tetM* genes, is unusual among *Fusobacterium* spp. but has been described.[74,95] Erythromycin has unreliable activity against *Fusobacterium* spp., but limited data suggest that azithromycin is active against more than 90% of isolates in vitro.[67,71,80,88,136]

EPIDEMIOLOGY

A variety of aerobic and anaerobic bacteria normally colonize the skin and mucosal surfaces of healthy human hosts and are collectively referred to as the human microbiome. The human microbiome is an area of active scientific investigation. Through the use of advanced bacterial sequencing technologies, significant progress has been made in identifying the numerous microorganisms that comprise the microbiome, although a full understanding of the factors that influence colonization and the complex interactions between microbiota and hosts regarding health and disease has not been reached. In the oral cavity, gastrointestinal tract, and female genital tract, anaerobes vastly outnumber aerobes; in the colon, where hundreds of different anaerobic species are found, anaerobes account for more than 99.9% of all bacteria present.[42,95]

The predominance of anaerobes among the normal microbial flora stands in stark contrast to the infrequency with which these organisms are identified in clinical specimens. Nonetheless, several types of infections routinely involve anaerobic bacteria, such as sinogenic infections, odontogenic infections, human and animal bite-associated infections, aspiration pneumonia, peritonitis in the presence of a ruptured viscus, amnionitis, endometritis, necrotizing infections of soft tissues, and abscesses of the brain, lung, tubo-ovarian tract, and perirectal area. Underlying conditions that predispose patients to anaerobic infections include trauma, foreign bodies, malignancy, recent surgery, shock, colitis, vascular disease, and current or recent infection with aerobic or facultative organisms.[50] In general, anaerobic infections occur less frequently in children than in adults, probably because children are less likely than are adults to have these types of predisposing conditions.

Taxonomic revisions aside, organisms traditionally classified as belonging to the *B. fragilis* group comprise much of the normal human colonic flora and also form part of the normal flora of the female genital tract. *Bacteroides* spp., which are the most frequently recovered anaerobic bacteria from clinical specimens, are frequently found in intraabdominal infections, especially abscesses, and occasionally in extraabdominal infections, such as aspiration pneumonia, chronic otitis media, and brain abscesses.[67,80]

Prevotella spp. and *Porphyromonas* spp. are normal inhabitants of the oral cavity, gastrointestinal tract, and female urogenital tract of humans. These organisms are associated with infections in a diverse range of body sites, most commonly including abscesses of the head and neck region, chronic otitis media, sinusitis, aspiration pneumonia, and intraabdominal infections. In a series of 504 pediatric clinical isolates of *Prevotella* and *Porphyromonas* spp., the most frequently recovered organisms were *Prevotella melaninogenica* (32%), *Prevotella intermedia* (21%), *Porphyromonas asaccharolytica* (17%), *Prevotella oris-buccae* (11%), and *Prevotella oralis* (11%).[33] *Prevotella bivia* and *Prevotella disiens* have been associated with genital tract infections in female adults, although they may also be recovered from oral infections. *Prevotella intermedia, Porphyromonas gingivalis,* and *Porphyromonas endodontalis* are particularly involved in adult periodontal disease and various dental infections.[67,80]

Fusobacterium spp. also constitute part of the normal flora of the human oral cavity and gastrointestinal tract, and they are associated with a range of pediatric infections similar to those involving *Prevotella* spp. and *Porphyromonas* spp. The *Fusobacterium* spp. most commonly isolated from clinical specimens is *F. nucleatum,* followed by *F. necrophorum;* organisms of the *F. varium-mortiferum* group are rarely recovered from clinical specimens. The virulent pathogen *F. necrophorum* is occasionally isolated from peritonsillar abscesses and is the principal cause of Lemierre disease (see later discussion).[28,67,80,95,44]

PATHOGENESIS

For the most part, anaerobic bacteria and humans enjoy a mutually beneficial relationship. The colon, for example, provides a home for the billions of anaerobic bacteria that make up the normal intestinal flora of humans. In turn, the presence of *Bacteroides* spp. and other colonizing anaerobic flora serve beneficial functions for humans, through such mechanisms as occupying an ecologic niche that might otherwise be invaded by enteric pathogens (a process known as colonization resistance); inducing tolerance to microbial epitopes, thereby serving to regulate the immune system; and breaking down otherwise indigestible plant polysaccharides while also producing vitamin K. Infections with anaerobic bacteria usually arise either because mucosal surfaces become disrupted, allowing these opportunistic pathogens access to normally sterile tissues, or because anaerobes are directly inoculated into such tissues, as occurs with traumatic or bite wounds.[95,142] Pathologic characteristics of anaerobic infections include suppuration, abscess formation, tissue destruction, foul odor, and, occasionally, formation of gas.

The pathogenesis of anaerobic infections reflects a complex interaction among bacterial virulence factors, host defense mechanisms, and synergy with other organisms. The elucidation of the complete genome sequence of *B. fragilis, B. thetaiotaomicron, F. nucleatum,* and *Porphyromonas gingivalis* has facilitated the identification of a host of genes encoding putative virulence determinants. These include gene sequences encoding fimbriae, hemagglutinins, proteinases (e.g., immunoglobulin proteases and collagenases), and hemolysins, which collectively serve to enhance pathogenicity by facilitating adherence to other bacteria and to host cells, thus disrupting the integrity of host tissues and interfering with host immune responses.[56,75,81,87,98,101,142]

Another key virulence factor for these bacteria is their possession of a capsule, which allows the organisms to evade phagocytosis and which is important to abscess formation.[24,33,98,101] The genomes of *B. fragilis* and *Porphyromonas gingivalis* also include aerotolerance operons, which encode proteins that allow the organisms to survive despite exposure to limited quantities of oxygen.[98,129] Moreover, enterotoxin-producing *B. fragilis* isolates have been identified in livestock and humans, and the presence of these bacteria has been associated with cases of diarrhea in children and adults.[75,95,139]

Anaerobic infections are typically polymicrobial and often involve multiple species of both aerobic and anaerobic flora. Experiments in mice, which evaluated mixed aerobic-anaerobic infections involving *Bacteroides* spp., *Prevotella* spp., and *Porphyromonas* spp., demonstrated that while the growth of both aerobes and anaerobes is enhanced in such infections, the enhancement of the aerobes' growth is by far more pronounced. The factors responsible for aerobic-anaerobic synergism are not fully understood. Some have postulated that the bacterial species involved assist one another by providing essential growth factors, interfering with phagocytic uptake and killing, secreting β-lactamase into the extracellular milieu, or altering the oxidation-reduction potential of infected tissue.[22,33]

CLINICAL MANIFESTATIONS

Serious anaerobic infections are seen more frequently in compromised hosts or in neonates than in otherwise healthy children. Outcomes of severe anaerobic infections are tied to patients' underlying disease states and to the promptness with which appropriate antimicrobial therapy is started.

Bacteremia and Endocarditis

Anaerobic bacteremia is unusual in children; when it does occur, it usually arises from a primary focal anaerobic or mixed aerobic-anaerobic infection. The risk for anaerobic bacteremia is elevated in patients compromised by a variety of conditions, including recent gastrointestinal or gynecologic surgery, dental manipulation, malignancy, immunosuppression, neonatal status, diabetes mellitus, and asplenia.[18,36,42,95] Among neonates, risk factors for anaerobic bacteremia include premature birth, maternal perinatal complications (e.g., premature rupture of membranes), and necrotizing enterocolitis.[27]

Overall, *B. fragilis* is the most frequently identified anaerobic bloodstream isolate. The specific anaerobes recovered from blood cultures vary depending on the entry portal: when the primary focus is in the gastrointestinal tract, *Bacteroides* spp. and *Clostridium* spp. predominate; in cases associated with oropharyngeal or pulmonary foci, pigmented *Prevotella* and *Porphyromonas* spp., *Fusobacterium* spp., and anaerobic gram-positive cocci are more likely. The presenting features of anaerobic bacteremia in children are similar to those associated with bacteremia caused by aerobic organisms. Fever, chills, and leukocytosis are frequently encountered, whereas hypotension, shock, and disseminated intravascular coagulation are less common findings. Mortality rates of 5% to 10% have been reported among children with anaerobic bacteremia.[18,36,42,95] Among neonates, reported mortality is higher among those with bacteremia caused by *Bacteroides* spp. (34%) than with other anaerobic species (17%).[27]

Although exceedingly uncommon among the pediatric population, there are case reports of anaerobic endocarditis. The most common source for *B. fragilis* group endocarditis is the gastrointestinal system, whereas the head and neck are the most common origin for *Fusobacterium* and *Bacteroides* species endocarditis. Anaerobic endocarditis due to *F. necrophorum* has been observed as a rare complication of Lemierre syndrome and has a strong association with thromboembolic events. The mortality rate for patients with anaerobic infective endocarditis is high and ranges from 21% to 43%.[41,110,115]

Head and Neck Infections

Odontogenic Infections

Anaerobes are usually involved in infections of dental origin, such as gingivitis, periodontitis, and periapical and dental abscesses. The most commonly implicated anaerobes in such infections are *Prevotella* spp. (particularly *P. melaninogenica*) and *Porphyromonas* spp. (particularly *P. gingivalis*).[42,95] Often these are found in mixed infections along with oral aerobic flora, including *Streptococcus salivarius* and microaerophilic streptococci. *Fusobacterium* spp. can also be recovered in odontogenic infections and are particularly associated with the ulcerative form of gingivitis known as Vincent angina (trench mouth).[42]

Perioral Infections

Prevotella and *Porphyromonas* spp. are also frequently recovered from various suppurative perioral infections, such as retropharyngeal and peritonsillar abscesses, cervical lymphadenitis, deep neck abscesses, thyroiditis, parotitis, infected cysts, and postsurgical wound infections involving the oral cavity. Occasionally, these infections also involve *Fusobacterium* spp., *Bacteroides* spp., and/or anaerobic gram-positive cocci, along with oral and nasopharyngeal aerobic flora.

Tonsillitis

Anaerobes likely play a role in the pathogenesis of acute tonsillitis.[45] A prospective study compared bacterial culture results from patients with peritonsillar abscesses undergoing acute tonsillectomy to patients undergoing elective tonsillectomy and found that *Fusobacterium necrophorum* and *Streptococcus* group A (GAS) were isolated significantly more frequently from the tonsillar cores of patients with peritonsillar abscesses than from the tonsillar cores of patients who underwent elective tonsillectomy. Additionally, the peritonsillar abscess patients had the same incidence of *F. necrophorum* from the abscessed tonsil as from the contralateral, nonabscessed tonsil, suggesting that the growth of *F. necrophorum* is not a result of an overgrowth phenomenon once the abscess is formed, but that *F. necrophorum* is a pathogen in both peritonsillar abscesses and acute tonsillitis.[83] Anaerobes, including *Prevotella, Porphyromonas,* and *Fusobacterium* spp., are also thought to be involved in the pathogenesis of recurrent or chronic tonsillitis, and production of β-lactamase by these organisms has been postulated to explain the failure of penicillin to eradicate pharyngeal carriage of *Streptococcus pyogenes* in some children.[42]

Lemierre Disease

Rarely, pharyngotonsillitis and tonsillar abscesses can be complicated by Lemierre disease (also known as postanginal sepsis or human necrobacillosis), a syndrome characterized by bacteremia, septic thrombophlebitis of the internal jugular and facial veins, and metastatic emboli to the lung and other distant organs. *F. necrophorum* is responsible for more than 80% of all cases. Occasionally, *F. nucleatum* or other *Fusobacterium* spp. are involved, often in combination with other anaerobic or aerobic flora. Lemierre disease is most common among adolescents and young adults but can occur in patients of any age. In the preantibiotic era, most patients with this syndrome died of overwhelming sepsis; more recently, mortality rates of 4% to 22% have been reported.[95,108,140]

Deep Neck Infections

Deep neck infections are usually polymicrobial and tend to follow oral, dental, and pharyngeal infections. The predominant organisms are *S. aureus*, group A β-hemolytic streptococci, and anaerobic bacteria of oral origin, including *Prevotella, Porphyromonas,* and *Fusobacterium* spp.[43] In an analysis of 634 patients with deep neck infections, 32% had both aerobic and anaerobic bacteria isolated. The most common aerobic bacteria were *Streptococcus pyogenes* and *Staphylococcus aureus,* and the most common anaerobic bacteria were *Peptostreptococcus* followed by *Prevotella*.[53]

Otitis Media and Mastoiditis

Although anaerobic gram-negative bacilli have not been implicated in the pathogenesis of acute otitis media, these organisms are present in up to 50% of middle ear fluid cultures from patients with chronic suppurative otitis media or infected cholesteatomas and in nearly all patients with chronic mastoiditis. The microbial pathogens recovered from such patients include *Prevotella, Porphyromonas, Bacteroides,* and *Fusobacterium* spp., along with anaerobic gram-positive cocci and various aerobes, most notably *Staphylococcus aureus* and *Pseudomonas aeruginosa*.[42,47] Fusobacterium spp. have been isolated from children with acute mastoiditis. In an Israeli study, seven children were diagnosed with complicated mastoiditis with abscess formation caused by *F. necrophorum*. Four patients were found to have epidural abscess, three patients had evidence of osteomyelitis beyond the mastoid bone, and four children had imaging evidence of sinus vein thrombosis. All seven children underwent cortical mastoidectomy with tympanostomy tube insertion, and two required multiple surgical interventions.[145]

Rhinosinusitis

Anaerobes are not usually associated with acute bacterial rhinosinusitis, but they are frequently implicated as pathogens in children with chronic sinusitis (symptoms for >30 days). In one study, sinus aspirate cultures from 37 children with chronic sinusitis yielded an average of 2.7 anaerobes and 0.6 aerobes per patient. Anaerobic pathogens associated with chronic sinusitis include *Prevotella, Porphyromonas,* and *Fusobacterium* spp., along with members of the *B. fragilis* group.[20,28,42] Additionally, anaerobes are well-recognized pathogens in the setting of complications of sinusitis, including orbital abscesses and intracranial extension.

Central Nervous System

Anaerobes can be isolated from the majority of intracranial abscesses that arise in association with sinusitis, otitis media, or dental infection. In one study, cultures of brain abscess specimens from 23 children yielded 11 aerobic and 44 anaerobic isolates, and cultures of subdural empyema fluid from 16 children yielded six aerobic and 35 anaerobic isolates. Anaerobic gram-positive cocci were the anaerobes most frequently recovered from these patients, followed by *Fusobacterium* spp. (especially *F. nucleatum*), *Bacteroides* spp. (including *B. fragilis* group members), *Prevotella* spp., and *Actinomyces* spp.[26] A similar range of anaerobes have been isolated, alone or along with aerobes, from epidural abscesses found in patients (primarily boys aged 10 to 14 years) with frontal sinusitis complicated by a Pott puffy tumor.[4,5,65] *B. fragilis* group members have been particularly associated with temporal lobe abscesses arising from chronic otitis media.[2]

Fusobacterial central nervous system infection in children can occur in relation to chronic sinusitis or Lemierre disease. In a pediatric study performed in Israel, 27 children with fusobacterial infections were found to have a high frequency of neurologic manifestations at presentation, including most commonly seizures (30%). Frequent thrombotic complications were also observed. Fifteen children (56%) underwent brain imaging, and in seven of these children, a thrombus was identified either in a sinus vein or in an internal jugular vein.[94]

Anaerobic meningitis occurs rarely in children. The symptoms, signs, and laboratory characteristics of children with anaerobic meningitis are similar to those of children with meningitis caused by more common bacterial pathogens. Unlike most anaerobic infections, meningitis is often monomicrobial, and mixed infections involving aerobes and anaerobes are unusual. The anaerobes most frequently recovered from cerebrospinal fluid cultures are *B. fragilis,* other *Bacteroides* spp., *F. necrophorum,* other *Fusobacterium* spp., and *Clostridium* spp. Meningitis caused by *Bacteroides* spp. generally occurs as a complication of a preceding anaerobic infection of the oropharynx or lower respiratory tract or of an underlying gastrointestinal insult (e.g., recent surgery or necrotizing enterocolitis). Meningitis caused by *F. necrophorum* in children is frequently associated with an otogenic focus.[38]

Intraabdominal Infections

Secondary peritonitis occurs when the intestinal wall is disrupted (e.g., by perforation of an inflamed appendix or surgical misadventure) and enteric bacteria consequently gain access to the peritoneal cavity. Over time the peritoneal infection may evolve, resulting in the formation of one or more intraabdominal abscesses.[42,95] Secondary peritonitis and intraabdominal abscesses are almost always polymicrobial processes involving a mixed flora of anaerobes and anaerobes. *B. fragilis* and other members of the *B. fragilis* group are recovered in most cultures of peritoneal or abscess fluid from patients with such infections; *Prevotella* and *Fusobacterium* spp. are also frequently implicated. Other anaerobic bacteria, including *Clostridium* spp., *Lactobacillus* spp., and anaerobic gram-positive cocci, are also commonly involved. The aerobic flora most frequently recovered in these infections include *Escherichia coli,* viridans streptococci, *Klebsiella* spp., *P. aeruginosa,* and *Enterococcus* species.[9,19,90,96,123]

Anaerobic gram-negative bacilli are also frequently present, as part of a mixed aerobic-anaerobic flora, in abscesses of the liver, spleen, and retroperitoneal space. The anaerobic bacteria most frequently recovered from liver abscesses are anaerobic gram-positive cocci, followed by *Bacteroides* spp., *Fusobacterium* spp., and *Prevotella* spp.[33,49,106] Splenic abscesses are associated with a similar range of anaerobic flora.[33] In a study of retroperitoneal abscess cultures in children, the most frequently isolated anaerobes were *Bacteroides* spp., followed by gram-positive cocci and *Prevotella* spp.[35]

Sexually active adolescent females are at risk for pelvic inflammatory disease and its complications (e.g., tubo-ovarian abscess). In addition to aerobic sexually transmitted organisms (e.g., *Chlamydia trachomatis* and *Neisseria gonorrhoeae*), these infections frequently involve anaerobic gram-negative bacilli, which originate from the normal vaginal flora and include *Prevotella* species (especially *P. bivia, P. disiens,* and *P. melaninogenica*), *Porphyromonas* spp., and *B. fragilis* group organisms. Anaerobic gram-positive cocci and *Clostridium* spp. may also be involved.[42,95]

Skin and Soft Tissue Infections

Cutaneous abscesses in children can be polymicrobial, involving both aerobic and anaerobic bacteria. Aerobes (particularly *S. aureus*) predominate in infections of the hand, neck, leg, and trunk regions, whereas anaerobes are more frequently recovered in infections of the vulvovaginal, buttocks, perirectal, finger, nail bed, and head regions.[48] A similar regional distribution of aerobes and anaerobes also occurs in cases of cellulitis.[30] The anaerobes most likely to be recovered from infections near the perirectal area include, not surprisingly, *B. fragilis* group and *Clostridium* spp.; infections closer to the oropharynx usually involve oral flora, such as *Prevotella* spp., *Porphyromonas* spp., *Fusobacterium* spp., and anaerobic gram-positive cocci. A wide variety of aerobic and anaerobic flora, including anaerobic gram-negative bacilli, can be isolated from sundry skin infections such as paronychia, infected burn wounds, pilonidal cysts, gastrostomy or tracheostomy site infections, and secondary infections of scabies lesions.[21,29,31,42,46,50] Anaerobes are also a part of the normal soil flora, and thus can be isolated from wounds complicated by heavy dirt or soil contamination. In the pediatric population, such wounds can include traumatic lawn-mower injuries.[40,52] Bacteria of the normal oral flora of humans and animals figure prominently in infected bite wounds. Such infections are frequently polymicrobial and usually involve a mix of aerobic and anaerobic bacteria. In infected human bite wounds, the most commonly involved anaerobes are *Fusobacterium* spp. (especially *F. nucleatum*) and *Prevotella* spp. (especially *P. melaninogenica, P. buccae,* and *P. intermedia*), whereas the predominant aerobic pathogens are *Streptococcus anginosus, Staphylococcus aureus,* and *Eikenella corrodens.*[127] In infections arising from dog and cat bite wounds, the most frequently isolated anaerobes are *Fusobacterium* spp. (especially *F. nucleatum*), *Bacteroides* spp. (especially *B. pyogenes,* previously designated *B. tectum*), *Porphyromonas* spp., and *Prevotella* spp. (especially *P. heparinolytica*), whereas the most frequently isolated aerobes are *Pasteurella* spp., *Staphylococcus* spp., and *Streptococcus* spp.[128] Anaerobic gram-negative bacilli are occasionally involved in complicated skin and soft tissue infections. Crepitant cellulitis is a superficial infection that is associated with less systemic toxicity but more noticeable crepitus than clostridial myonecrosis. The usual causative pathogen is *Clostridium perfringens,* but crepitant cellulitis can also result from infection with combinations of aerobic bacteria with *B. fragilis* and/or other anaerobic pathogens. Necrotizing fasciitis is a dreaded soft tissue infection that can be rapidly progressive. In one type of necrotizing fasciitis, anaerobes such as *Bacteroides* spp. and anaerobic gram-positive cocci are frequently recovered, usually in association with various aerobic enteric flora. This type should be distinguished from necrotizing fasciitis caused by *S. pyogenes* (or, less frequently, by groups B, C or G streptococci), in which anaerobes are generally not involved.[60,95]

Bone and Joint Infections

Septic arthritis caused by anaerobic bacteria is rare in both children and adults and, unlike most anaerobic infections, is usually not polymicrobial. Most cases result from anaerobic bacteremia with gram-negative rods (especially *Fusobacterium* spp. or the *B. fragilis* group) or anaerobic gram-positive cocci. In some cases, the presence of anaerobes is suggested by foul-smelling synovial fluid, gas under pressure within the joint, negative synovial fluid cultures in the clinical picture of septic arthritis, or an anaerobic infection elsewhere in the patient.[37,95]

Anaerobic osteomyelitis is also quite uncommon in children. When it does occur, it generally results from direct extension from a contiguous focus, rather than via hematogenous seeding. In a series of 26 children with culture-proven anaerobic osteomyelitis, all had preexisting anaerobic infections at adjacent sites or other predisposing conditions for anaerobic infection. Culture results reflected those of the underlying anaerobic infection or of the normal flora of the nearest mucous membrane surface. Anaerobic gram-positive cocci were isolated most frequently, followed by pigmented *Prevotella* and *Porphyromonas* spp., *Fusobacterium* spp., *Clostridium* spp., *Prevotella oralis,* and *Bacteroides* spp. All but two patients had polymicrobial infections; in 10 patients, aerobic flora were also recovered. In contrast to acute hematogenous osteomyelitis, these cases presented insidiously; the mean duration of symptoms before presentation was 21 days.[23,37]

Pleuropulmonary Infections

Anaerobic infections of the lower respiratory tract are rare in healthy children. They are, however, relatively common in children with tracheoesophageal malformations or central nervous system abnormalities that impair cough reflexes. Such children are predisposed toward aspirating not only food, milk, and vomitus but also their oropharyngeal secretions. Thus, aspiration pneumonia is usually a polymicrobial process involving both aerobic and anaerobic flora of the oral cavity. The risk for pneumonia is further elevated in children with poor oral hygiene, gingivitis, or periodontitis. If untreated, aspiration pneumonia can follow a progressive course with the development of single or multiple lung abscess and/or pleural empyema. The predominant anaerobes recovered from children with aspiration pneumonia (including those with and without associated lung abscesses) are anaerobic gram-positive cocci, followed by *Prevotella* and *Porphyromonas* spp., *F. nucleatum, B. fragilis* group members, and other *Bacteroides* spp. The major aerobic copathogens implicated in these infections include *P. aeruginosa, Streptococcus pneumoniae, E. coli, Klebsiella pneumoniae,* and *S. aureus.*[39,95]

Anaerobes are occasionally isolated from pleural fluid cultures of patients with pleural empyema, and it is possible that they account for at least some cases of empyema in which routine bacterial cultures are negative. In a study of 104 children with pleural empyema, anaerobes were isolated from five adolescents, in all cases along with other aerobic or anaerobic oral flora. Predisposing conditions in these patients were pneumonia in four and alcohol intoxication in one.[64] In another study of 72 neurologically impaired children with empyema, anaerobic bacteria were recovered in 24% of patients. Anaerobic pleural empyema was associated with the presence of other anaerobic infections in or near the respiratory tract, including aspiration pneumonia, lung abscess, subdiaphragmatic abscess, and dental or oropharyngeal abscess. Anaerobes isolated from these patients included *B. fragilis* group members, pigmented *Prevotella* and *Porphyromonas* spp., *Fusobacterium* spp., and anaerobic gram-positive cocci.[25,39]

Anaerobes are occasionally isolated from lower respiratory tract specimens of children with ventilator-associated pneumonia.[32,34] In one study, anaerobes were recovered from nine of 10 sputum culture specimens obtained using protective brush catheters, either alone (three children) or as part of a mixed infection with aerobic bacteria (six children). The anaerobic flora recovered in these children included pigmented *Prevotella* and *Porphyromonas* spp. (five children), anaerobic gram-positive cocci (four children), *Fusobacterium* spp., and members of the *B. fragilis* group (two children).[32]

DIAGNOSIS

As with other anaerobic infections, the diagnosis of infections caused by anaerobic gram-negative bacilli requires a high index of suspicion. For the most part, these infections must be suspected based on the clinical presentation and then diagnosed using microbiologic methods. When anaerobic infections are suspected, specimens for culture should be collected without contamination from the endogenous flora of adjacent mucous membranes. In general, acceptable specimens for anaerobic culture include blood; aspirates of normally sterile body fluids, abscesses, or deep wounds; and surgically obtained specimens. Optimum specimens include aspirates and tissue, not swabs. In the setting of pneumonia, specimens should be obtained via a protected brush or catheter.[7] Gram-stained smears of aspirated material should be examined and interpreted in the context of culture results.

Specimens submitted for anaerobic culture should be rapidly transported to the laboratory in anaerobic transport devices and promptly inoculated into appropriate media in an oxygen-free environment (e.g., anaerobic jar or glove box). Media that support cultivation of anaerobes are supplemented with reducing substances (e.g., thioglycolate, dithiothreitol, cysteine, iron shavings, or chopped meat) and antibiotics to suppress the growth of facultative bacteria. Even before inoculation, such media must be prepared and stored under anaerobic conditions to prevent generation of superoxide or hydrogen peroxide.[42,102,130] In one hospital, improvements in techniques for recovery of anaerobes (i.e., media and transport conditions) and education of clinicians and microbiologists were associated with dramatic reductions in health care costs and mortality among patients with anaerobic infections.[6]

Bacterial isolates that grow anaerobically should be tested for aerotolerance to confirm whether they are obligate or facultative anaerobes. This process necessarily lengthens the time to reporting of culture reports to the clinician; however, the morphologic characteristics of certain anaerobes (e.g., *B. fragilis* group, pigmented *Prevotella* and *Porphyromonas* spp.) are sufficiently distinctive to allow preliminary reporting of presumptive results before aerotolerance testing, at least in experienced laboratories. Definitive identification of anaerobic isolates is performed using biochemical tests, gas-liquid chromatography of fermentation reaction products, direct immunofluorescence, molecular genetic methods, or a combination of these.[42,130] At a minimum, anaerobic bacteria should be tested for the production of β-lactamase. Detailed antimicrobial susceptibility testing of anaerobes is possible using broth dilution, agar dilution, or E-test methods, but these procedures are not routinely performed in most hospital laboratories today.[42,70,95,51] Recently, advances in molecular detection methods, especially polymerase chain reaction (PCR) technologies and 16S RNA gene sequencing, have improved detection, identification, and quantitation of anaerobes. Sequence-based identification offers several advantages over culture-based methods, including improved accuracy over phenotypic identification and more rapid recognition of species.[124] Additionally, novel next-generation DNA sequencing technology is beginning to be available for clinical laboratories.[114]

TREATMENT

Appropriate therapy for anaerobic infections is both surgical and medical. In general, abscesses should be drained (and their contents sent for routine and anaerobic cultures). Debridement of necrotic tissue is critical to survival in severe infections such as necrotizing fasciitis.[42,95] Hyperbaric oxygen has been used, in addition to debridement and antibiotics, in some children with clostridial myonecrosis or necrotizing fasciitis, but definitive recommendations as to its use cannot be made based on this limited experience.[42]

Patients with anaerobic infections should promptly receive appropriate antibiotic therapy (Table 150.1). Delays in the initiation of antianaerobic therapy have been associated with increased morbidity, mortality, and duration of hospitalization in patients with severe infections involving anaerobes.[62] In certain situations (e.g., peritonitis with a perforated viscus, brain abscess related to chronic mastoiditis), the clinician should assume that anaerobes are present and include agents active against these organisms in the initial antimicrobial regimen. For many anaerobic bacteria, there is no particular drug of choice, because many different antibiotics (alone or in combination) might be reasonable for a given patient. Because anaerobic infections often involve a mixed flora of aerobic and anaerobic bacteria, the selection of antimicrobial therapy must also take into account the likely aerobic bacteria involved in a given infection. Often it is this consideration that drives the selection of one antianaerobic drug over another, as in the choice of meropenem or piperacillin-tazobactam (active against most aerobic Enterobacteriaceae as well as *B. fragilis* group organisms and other anaerobes) over metronidazole (active against most anaerobes but inactive against aerobes) for treatment of a complicated intraabdominal infection. Other factors to consider include the toxicity, tolerability, tissue penetration, and cost of various available antibiotics.[42,95]

Complicating matters, many anaerobic gram-negative bacilli have demonstrated increasing rates of resistance to penicillin, clindamycin, and other drugs in recent decades. Not surprisingly, resistance among anaerobic bacteria has been identified as a risk factor for clinical failure in the treatment of these infections.[62,95] Because most hospital laboratories do not routinely perform antimicrobial susceptibility testing for anaerobes, and because geographically relevant surveillance data on anaerobic susceptibility patterns are usually not available, clinicians often lack guidance (beyond that available in review articles and textbook chapters) as to the optimal selection of antibiotics for anaerobic infections in their patients.[93] Nonetheless, some general principles still apply. For example, aminoglycosides, monobactams (e.g., aztreonam), and older fluoroquinolones all have uniformly poor activity against anaerobes, whereas macrolides and older tetracyclines are only modestly more reliable. Several classes of antibiotics (see later discussion), traditionally considered as antianaerobic drugs, vary in their activity against different anaerobes, including *Bacteroides, Prevotella, Porphyromonas,* and *Fusobacterium* spp. (see Table 150.1). Serious anaerobic infections should be treated with intravenous antimicrobial agents at maximum dosages to optimize their penetration into devitalized tissue and abscesses.[42,57,71]

Penicillins and Penicillin/β-Lactamase Inhibitor Combinations

Penicillin G, ampicillin, and amoxicillin are active against most anaerobes that do not produce β-lactamase, including most isolates of *F. nucleatum, F. necrophorum,* and *Porphyromonas* spp. These drugs are less reliable against *Prevotella* spp. and virtually devoid of activity against *Bacteroides* spp. and thus should no longer be considered first-line agents for initial treatment of anaerobic infections in any body site. Their use should be limited to selected infections where source control has been achieved and involvement of β-lactamase–producing organisms (especially *B. fragilis* group members) has been excluded or where clinical suspicion of such organisms is low.

Combinations of penicillins with β-lactamase inhibitors, on the other hand, achieve broad-spectrum activity against anaerobic and aerobic bacteria, including anaerobic gram-negative bacilli. These agents are particularly well suited for treatment of intraabdominal infections, in which β-lactamase–producing gram-negative bacilli are uniformly present. A clinical practice guideline, published in 2010, endorses (among other options) the use of piperacillin-tazobactam for antimicrobial treatment of complicated intraabdominal infections in children.[123] Ampicillin-sulbactam and amoxicillin-clavulanate are active against most anaerobic and aerobic oropharyngeal flora and thus are suitable parenteral and oral antibiotics, respectively, for treatment of most anaerobic infections arising in the head, neck, and chest (although their use as single agents may be limited by their lack of activity against methicillin-resistant *S. aureus*). In recent years, increasing resistance to amoxicillin-clavulanate and piperacillin-tazobactam among *B. fragilis* group isolates has been noted in Europe, indicating that continued vigilance for emerging resistance to this class of antibiotics will be required.[95]

TABLE 150.1 Percentages of Anaerobic Gram-Negative Bacilli Susceptible to Selected Antimicrobial Agents in Recent Reports

	Bacteroides fragilis group[a]	*Prevotella* spp.[b]	*Fusobacterium* spp.[c]	*Porphyromonas* spp.[d]
Penicillin G	0–13	16–69	85–100	74–100
Amoxicillin	0–21	55–88	80–100	88–100
Amoxicillin-clavulanate	82–90	93–100	89–100	100
Cefoxitin	60–90	93–100	91–100	95–100
Ceftriaxone	15–32	71–97	80–100	95–100
Chloramphenicol	97–100	100	96–100	
Clindamycin	48–80	62–97	85–100	90–100
Imipenem	94–100	94–100	92–100	100
Meropenem	92–100	99–100	92–100	100
Metronidazole	93–100	94–100	93–100	94–100
Moxifloxacin	52–89	71–88	80–88	96
Piperacillin-tazobactam	92–100	98–100	100	100
Tigecycline	73–100	100	100	

[a]References 1, 11, 66, 68, 72, 77, 82, 84, 85, 89, 91, 93, 96, 97, 99, 100, 109, 111, 121, 122, 126, 132, 133, 135, 138, 141.
[b]References 1, 3, 13, 14, 68, 72, 77, 79, 84, 85, 86, 88, 89, 91, 93, 99, 100, 107, 109, 131, 135, 136, 138, 141.
[c]References 1, 13, 59, 68, 72, 76, 77, 84, 85, 86, 88, 91, 93, 99, 109, 131, 135, 136, 138, 141.
[d]References 1, 3, 72, 76, 77, 78, 79, 84, 86, 88, 99, 100, 136, 138.

Cephalosporins

First-generation cephalosporins have antianaerobic activity similar to that of penicillin G, and third-generation cephalosporins are only moderately more active. Ceftriaxone is active against most isolates of *Prevotella, Porphyromonas,* and *Fusobacterium* spp., but most *B. fragilis* group isolates are resistant. The most active cephalosporins against anaerobes are the second-generation agents cefoxitin, cefotetan, and cefmetazole; of these, cefoxitin has the best activity against *B. fragilis* group members.[42] Cefoxitin is recommended, among other options, as surgical prophylaxis for abdominal procedures involving entry into a hollow viscus and single-agent therapy for adults with community-acquired complicated intraabdominal infections of mild to moderate severity (but not for adults with severe disease or high-risk conditions).[15,123] Increasing resistance to cefoxitin has been documented in recent years, however, suggesting that its use as monotherapy for intraabdominal infections should be approached with caution.[95] Cefoxitin remains useful for perioperative antimicrobial prophylaxis in surgical procedures involving the abdomen.[16] Moreover, it is recommended as a first-line agent, in combination with doxycycline, for parenteral therapy for pelvic inflammatory disease.[55]

Carbapenems

The carbapenems are parenterally administered β-lactams with broad coverage against both aerobes and anaerobes, including many cephalosporin-resistant gram-negative enteric pathogens. Because of this broad-spectrum activity, carbapenems are well suited for single-agent therapy for a variety of infections involving anaerobes, including complicated intraabdominal infections.[123] Resistance to carbapenems has been documented among *B. fragilis* group organisms but remains rare, affecting less than 2% of isolates in most surveys. Resistance is exceptionally rare among isolates of *Prevotella* and *Fusobacterium* spp., and such resistant isolates have not been observed in the United States. Of the available carbapenems, meropenem is the preferred agent for use in children, because it is less likely to induce seizures than imipenem-cilastatin.[92,103]

Metronidazole

Metronidazole has excellent activity against anaerobic gram-negative bacilli, including *B. fragilis* group members that are frequently resistant to other classes of antibiotics. Resistance to this agent has begun to emerge among *B. fragilis* group strains and *Prevotella* spp. in the developing world and in Europe, but such isolates remain exceptionally rare in the United States.[1,72,91,95,100,121] Of note, metronidazole is less reliable in its activity against many gram-positive anaerobes, and virtually all aerobic bacteria are inherently resistant to it. Because most anaerobic infections are polymicrobial, metronidazole is generally not used alone but in combination with other antibiotics active against aerobic bacteria. For example, a recent practice guideline lists combination therapy with metronidazole plus either cefepime, a third-generation cephalosporin, or an aminoglycoside (with or without ampicillin) as an appropriate antimicrobial strategy for therapy of complicated intraabdominal infections in children.[123] Among the many advantages of metronidazole are that it is generally well tolerated; penetrates well into many tissues, including those of the central nervous system; and can be administered orally.

Clindamycin

Over the past 2 decades, resistance to clindamycin has increased substantially among members of the *B. fragilis* group, with resistance rates exceeding 50% in some series.[68,77,89,95] Because clindamycin is now less reliable than carbapenems, penicillin/β-lactamase inhibitor combinations, or metronidazole against these organisms, it should no longer be considered a first-line agent for treatment of complicated intraabdominal infections. However, clindamycin continues to have good activity against most other anaerobic bacteria, including most strains of *Prevotella, Porphyromonas,* and *Fusobacterium* spp. and gram-positive anaerobes. Thus, today clindamycin is better suited for treatment of infections involving oropharyngeal anaerobes than for those involving intestinal flora.

Clindamycin achieves comparable serum levels whether administered orally or intravenously and penetrates well into most tissues and fluids, including bones, joints, and abscesses. Clindamycin does not penetrate well into cerebrospinal fluid and thus should not be used for treatment of central nervous system infections.[57] For treatment of polymicrobial infections, clindamycin should be combined with a β-lactam or other antibiotic active against aerobic gram-negative bacilli (e.g., *Pasteurella multocida* in animal bite wounds or *Eikenella corrodens* in human bite wounds). Although clindamycin has traditionally been particularly associated with *Clostridium difficile*–induced pseudomembranous colitis, many other antibiotics can also induce this complication.[42]

Quinolones

In contrast to earlier generations of fluoroquinolones, newer agents such as moxifloxacin possess significant in vitro activity against many anaerobic bacteria.[63,72] Unfortunately, resistance to moxifloxacin among *B. fragilis* group organisms rapidly emerged in the late 1990s, and has continued to increase globally, thereby limiting the usefulness of newer quinolones for treatment of complicated intraabdominal and other anaerobic infections.[10,69,95] However, a recent pooled analysis with four well controlled clinical trials published in 2013 evaluated the use of moxifloxacin for the treatment of adults with complicated intraabdominal infections. Of the pretherapy anaerobes from the moxifloxacin-treated group, 561 (87.4%) were susceptible at 2 mg/L or less, 34 (5.3%) were intermediate at 4 mg/L, and 47 (7.3%) were resistant at 8 mg/L or more. Moxifloxacin achieved similar clinical success rates against all anaerobes, including those isolated from patients infected with *Bacteroides fragilis, Bacteroides thetaiotaomicron,* and *Clostridium* species. For all anaerobes combined, the clinical success rate was 83.1% (466 of 561 patients) for a minimum inhibitory concentration (MIC) of 2 mg/L or less, 91.2% (31 of 34 patients) for an MIC of 4 mg/L, 82.4% (14 of 17 patients) for an MIC of 8 mg/L, 83.3% (5 of 6 patients) for an MIC of 16 mg/L, and 66.7% (16 of 24 patients) for an MIC of 32 mg/L or greater.[73] These results suggest that moxifloxacin can be considered for the treatment of mild to moderate intraabdominal infections.[51] Moxifloxacin's activity against other anaerobic gram-negative bacilli has not been as well studied, but available data suggest that resistance occurs among a substantial minority of *Prevotella* and *Fusobacterium* spp. isolates.

Therapeutic advantages of the quinolones include their wide distribution in tissues and fluids and their good absorption after oral administration.[104] Newer quinolones may provide options for treating anaerobic infections in selected children, such as older adolescents. Nonetheless, the quinolones' role in pediatrics remains limited because concern lingers over their potential toxicity, because other agents with established safety profiles have equal or better activity against anaerobes, and because bacterial resistance to quinolones will likely continue to rise, owing to their continued widespread use in adults.

Tetracyclines

Most *B. fragilis* group organisms are resistant to tetracycline, as are a substantial proportion of *Prevotella* and *Fusobacterium* spp. isolates. Tigecycline is a newer antibiotic, belonging to the glycylcycline class, which has vastly improved activity against anaerobic gram-negative bacilli. Tigecycline is listed, among other options, as an appropriate single-agent therapy for adults with community-acquired complicated intraabdominal infections of mild to moderate severity (but not for adults with severe disease or high-risk conditions).[123] However, a recent meta-analysis of randomized controlled trials revealed that tigecycline is associated with increased mortality compared to other antimicrobial regimens.[144] Tigecycline's safety and efficacy in children have not been established. Additionally, *Pseudomonas aeruginosa* has been identified in up to 35% of children with intraabdominal infections, and more than 90% of *Pseudomonas* strains are resistant to tigecycline.[123,125] In addition, the high rates of gastrointestinal side effects (e.g., pancreatitis) associated with this drug will likely limit its use in pediatric patients.[61]

Oxazolidinones

Linezolid possesses surprisingly good in vitro activity against anaerobic gram-negative bacilli. In a study of isolates in Belgium from 2003 through 2005, susceptibility rates to linezolid were 99% among *B. fragilis* group members, 98% among *Prevotella* spp., and 100% for *Fusobacterium* spp.[141] In another study from Germany, 100% of 80 *Fusobacterium* isolates were susceptible to linezolid.[59] Moreover, earlier studies also found overall excellent activity of oxazolidinones against many types of anaerobic bacteria, including *B. fragilis* group members.[8,58,105,143] Although experience with the clinical use of this agent for anaerobic infections is limited, a case report described microbiologic cure and clinical improvement with linezolid therapy in a patient with sepsis caused by a *B. fragilis* strain resistant to metronidazole, penicillin/β-lactamase inhibitors, carbapenems, and tetracyclines.[137] In another patient, an extensive soft tissue infection of the leg with *B. fragilis* resistant to clindamycin, metronidazole, cefoxitin, carbapenems, piperacillin-tazobactam, and tigecycline was successfully cured after combination therapy with linezolid and moxifloxacin.[120] The role of linezolid in therapy for complicated anaerobic infections merits further investigation.

PREVENTION

The prevention of infections caused by *Bacteroides, Prevotella, Porphyromonas,* and *Fusobacterium* spp. hinges on measures that serve to limit the introduction of these bacteria into healthy tissues. Such methods include, but are not limited to, cleaning and debriding wounds properly, removing foreign bodies promptly, maintaining good dental and oral hygiene, avoiding disruption of the intestinal wall during surgery, appropriately prescribing perioperative antibiotic prophylaxis, and following recommendations for prevention of nosocomial pneumonia.[16,17,42,54]

Acknowledgment

We thank Dr. Steven C. Buckingham for his extensive contributions to this chapter in previous editions of this text.

NEW REFERENCES SINCE THE SEVENTH EDITION

7. Baron EJ, Miller JM, Weinstein MP, et al. A guide to utilization of the microbiology laboratory for diagnosis of infectious diseases: 2013 recommendations by the Infectious Diseases Society of America (IDSA) and the American Society for *Microbiology* (ASM)(a). *Clin Infect Dis.* 2013;57(4):e22-e121.
15. Bratzler DW, Dellinger EP, Olsen KM, et al. Clinical practice guidelines for antimicrobial prophylaxis in surgery. *Surg Infect (Larchmt).* 2013;14(1):73-156.
19. Brook I. Bacterial studies of peritoneal cavity and postoperative surgical wound drainage following perforated appendix in children. *Ann Surg.* 1980;192:208-212.
40. Brook I. Recovery of anaerobic bacteria from wounds after lawn-mower injuries. *Pediatr Emerg Care.* 2005;21(2):109-110.
41. Brook I. Infective endocarditis caused by anaerobic bacteria. *Arch Cardiovasc Dis.* 2008;101(10):665-676.
43. Brook I. Anaerobic bacteria in upper respiratory tract and head and neck infections: microbiology and treatment. *Anaerobe.* 2012;18(2):214-220.
44. Brook I. Fusobacterial infections in children. *Curr Infect Dis Rep.* 2013;15(3):288-294.
45. Brook I. Spectrum and treatment of anaerobic infections. *J Infect Chemother.* 2016;22:1-13.
51. Brook I, Wexler HM, Goldstein EJ. Antianaerobic antimicrobials: spectrum and susceptibility testing. *Clin Microbiol Rev.* 2013;26(3):526-546.
52. Campbell JR. Infectious complications of lawn mower injuries. *Pediatr Infect Dis J.* 2001;20(1):60-62.
53. Celakovsky P, Kalfert D, Smatanova K, et al. Bacteriology of deep neck infections: analysis of 634 patients. *Aust Dent J.* 2015;60(2):212-215.
73. Goldstein EJ, Solomkin JS, Citron DM, et al. Clinical efficacy and correlation of clinical outcomes with in vitro susceptibility for anaerobic bacteria in patients with complicated intra-abdominal infections treated with moxifloxacin. *Clin Infect Dis.* 2011;53(11):1074-1080.
82. Karlowsky JA, Walkty AJ, Adam HJ, et al. Prevalence of antimicrobial resistance among clinical isolates of *Bacteroides fragilis* group in Canada in 2010-2011: CANWARD surveillance study. *Antimicrob Agents Chemother.* 2012;56(3):1247-1252.
83. Klug TE, Henriksen JJ, Fuursted K, et al. Significant pathogens in peritonsillar abscesses. *Eur J Clin Microbiol Infect Dis.* 2011;30(5):619-627.
93. Marchand-Austin A, Rawte P, Toye B, et al. Antimicrobial susceptibility of clinical isolates of anaerobic bacteria in Ontario, 2010-2011. *Anaerobe.* 2014;28:120-125.
94. Megged O, Assous MV, Miskin H, et al. Neurologic manifestations of *Fusobacterium* infections in children. *Eur J Pediatr.* 2013;172(1):77-83.
110. Rodrigues C, Siciliano RF, Zeigler R, et al. *Bacteroides fragilis* endocarditis: a case report and review of literature. *Braz J Infect Dis.* 2012;16(1):100-104.
114. Salipante SJ, Hoogestraat DR, Abbott AN, et al. Coinfection of *Fusobacterium nucleatum* and *Actinomyces israelii* in mastoiditis diagnosed by next-generation DNA sequencing. *J Clin Microbiol.* 2014;52(5):1789-1792.
115. Samant JS, Peacock JE Jr. *Fusobacterium necrophorum* endocarditis case report and review of the literature. *Diagn Microbiol Infect Dis.* 2011;69(2):192-195.
124. Song Y. PCR-based diagnostics for anaerobic infections. *Anaerobe.* 2005;11(1-2):79-91.
125. Stein GE, Craig WA. Tigecycline: a critical analysis. *Clin Infect Dis.* 2006;43(4):518-524.
126. Székely E, Eitel Z, Molnár S, et al. Analysis of Romanian *Bacteroides* isolates for antibiotic resistance levels and the corresponding antibiotic resistance genes. *Anaerobe.* 2015;31:11-14.
135. Veloo AC, van Winkelhoff AJ. Antibiotic susceptibility profiles of anaerobic pathogens in The Netherlands. *Anaerobe.* 2015;31:19-24.
144. Yahav D, Lador A, Paul M, et al. Efficacy and safety of tigecycline: a systematic review and meta-analysis. *J Antimicrob Chemother.* 2011;66(9):1963-1971.
145. Yarden-Bilavsky H, Raveh E, Livni G, et al. *Fusobacterium necrophorum* mastoiditis in children—emerging pathogen in an old disease. *Int J Pediatr Otorhinolaryngol.* 2013;77(1):92-96.

The full reference list for this chapter is available at ExpertConsult.com.

Index

Page numbers followed by "*f*" indicate figures, "*t*" indicate tables, "*b*" indicate boxes, and "*e*" indicate online content.

A

B

F

G

H

J

K

L

N

P

Q

R

S

V

W

Feigin and Cherry's *Textbook of* Pediatric Infectious Diseases

Feigin and Cherry's

Textbook of Pediatric Infectious Diseases

EIGHTH EDITION

JAMES D. CHERRY, MD, MSc
Distinguished Research Professor of Pediatrics
David Geffen School of Medicine at UCLA;
Attending Physician
Pediatric Infectious Diseases
Mattel Children's Hospital UCLA
Los Angeles, California

GAIL J. HARRISON, MD
Professor
Department of Pediatrics
Section of Infectious Diseases
Baylor College of Medicine;
Attending Physician
Infectious Diseases Service
Texas Children's Hospital
Houston, Texas

SHELDON L. KAPLAN, MD
Professor and Executive Vice-Chair
Head, Section of Infectious Diseases
Department of Pediatrics
Baylor College of Medicine;
Chief, Infectious Disease Service
Head, Department of Pediatric Medicine
Texas Children's Hospital
Houston, Texas

WILLIAM J. STEINBACH, MD
Professor of Pediatrics
Professor in Molecular Genetics and Microbiology
Chief, Pediatric Infectious Diseases
Director, Duke Pediatric Immunocompromised Host Program
Director, International Pediatric Fungal Network
Duke University School of Medicine
Durham, North Carolina

PETER J. HOTEZ, MD, PhD
Dean, National School of Tropical Medicine
Professor, Pediatrics and Molecular & Virology and Microbiology
Head, Section of Pediatric Tropical Medicine
Baylor College of Medicine;
Endowed Chair of Tropical Pediatrics
Center for Vaccine Development
Texas Children's Hospital;
Professor, Department of Biology
Baylor University
Waco, Texas;
Baker Institute Fellow in Disease and Poverty
Rice University
Houston, Texas;
Co-Editor-in-Chief, *PLoS Neglected Tropical Diseases*

ELSEVIER

ELSEVIER

1600 John F. Kennedy Blvd.
Ste 1800
Philadelphia, PA 19103-2899

FEIGIN AND CHERRY'S TEXTBOOK OF PEDIATRIC INFECTIOUS DISEASES, EIGHTH EDITION ISBN: 978-0-323-37692-1

Hookworm and tick images courtesy of Anna Grove Photography. Staphylococcus aureus image from CDC Public Health Image Library (provided by Frank DeLeo, National Institute of Allergy and Infectious Diseases). Mosquito scanning electron micrograph from DCD Public Health Imaging Library (provided by Dr. Paul Howell, CDC).

ISBN: 978-0-323-37692-1

Senior Acquisitions Editor: Kate Dimock
Senior Content Development Specialist: Jennifer Shreiner
Publishing Services Manager: Patricia Tannian
Senior Project Manager: Carrie Stetz
Design Direction: Maggie Reid

Printed in China

Last digit is the print number: 9 8 7 6 5 4 3 2 1

To my wife, Jeanne M. Cherry, who passed away on June 2, 2017
To my children, James Cherry, Jeffrey Cherry and Kass Hogan,
Susan Cherry, and Kenneth and Jennifer Cherry
To my grandchildren, Ferguson, Dennis, and Siena Rose Cherry
James Cherry

To my husband, Neil Harrison
To my children and sons-in-law, Emily Wolfe and Josh Wolfe,
Kelly Green and Daniel Green, Matthew Demmler, Amy Demmler,
Anna Rose Demmler, and Haley Harrison
To my grandchildren, Jensen Wolfe and William Green
To my brother, Loddie Naymola
Gail Harrison

To my wife, Marsha Kaplan
To my children, Lauren Kaplan, Mindy Kaplan Langland,
and son-in-law Lance Langland
To my grandchildren, Reece and Macy Langland
Sheldon Kaplan

To my wife, Sandy Steinbach
To my children, Amelia Steinbach, Aidan Steinbach, and Conner Franzen
To my parents, Charles and Kathy Steinbach
William Steinbach

To my wife, Ann Hotez
To my children, Matthew, Emily, Rachel, and Daniel Hotez
To my mother, Jean Hotez, and mother-in-law, Marcia Frifield
To the memories of my father, Ed Hotez, and father-in-law, Don Frifield
Peter Hotez

Ralph D. Feigin, MD

April 3, 1938–August 14, 2008

This eighth edition of the *Textbook of Pediatric Infectious Diseases* is dedicated to Ralph D. Feigin. As everyone in pediatrics and, in particular, pediatric infectious diseases, knows, Ralph was an extraordinary individual, and his untimely death in 2008 leaves a void that will never be filled.

Ralph Feigin was born in New York City on April 3, 1938. He graduated from Columbia College in New York City in 1958 and received his M.D. from Boston University School of Medicine in 1962. He married Judith S. Zobel, a childhood friend, in 1960 while in medical school. Ralph completed his first two years of pediatric residency at Boston City Hospital and his third year at the Massachusetts General Hospital. He then fulfilled his military service requirement at the United States Army Research Institute of Infectious Diseases, Ft. Detrick, Frederick, Maryland. While at the United States Army Research Institute, he participated in significant studies relating to circadian periodicity and susceptibility to infections, as well as other studies that resulted in eight publications for which he was the first author. After completing his service commitment, he was Chief Resident at Massachusetts General Hospital during the 1967-68 academic year.

Ralph was recruited to Washington University in St. Louis by Phil Dodge in 1968, and soon thereafter he and one of us (JDC), who was then at St. Louis University, got together and forged an academic and personal friendship that continued until the time of his death. Over 40 years ago, Ralph and Jim recognized the need for a comprehensive book on pediatric infectious diseases, but because of their busy schedules the plan was put on hold, and in 1973 Jim moved to California. In 1976, the pediatric research meetings were held in St. Louis, and at this time Jim and Ralph met with W. B. Saunders representatives, and the book was conceived. The first edition of the textbook was published 5 years later in the fall of 1981. In comparison with this 8th edition, it was a modest effort, with 44 chapters and 124 contributors.

At Washington University and St. Louis Children's Hospital, Ralph developed one of the finest infectious diseases divisions in the country. His "Feigin Rounds" were an unparalleled learning experience and were legendary among medical students and residents. In 1977, Ralph moved to Houston, Texas, to accept the challenge of being the Chair of Pediatrics for Baylor College of Medicine and the Physician-in-Chief at Texas Children's Hospital. During the ensuing 30 years, the Department grew from 43 faculty members to almost 500. One of us (SLK) came under Ralph's spell in St. Louis and moved to Houston with him. Another one of us (GJH), an intern in Houston in 1977, was waiting for Dr. Feigin when he arrived.

In Houston, Ralph served as the Chair of Pediatrics for Baylor College of Medicine and the Physician-in-Chief at Texas Children's Hospital for 31 years. For 7 years of his tenure, he also served as President and CEO of Baylor College of Medicine. In addition to his commitments in Houston, Ralph served in leadership roles on more than 100 local, regional, and national committees and professional societies. His efforts in persuading government officials of all ranks helped children in Texas, the United States, and in all parts of the world. Many consider him to have been the foremost pediatrician in the world.

Not only was Dr. Feigin a powerhouse of energy, speed, and unsurpassed accomplishments, but he also was a gentleman, full of compassion, warmth, and kindness, and a man who kept people and patients first in his heart and mind. He was a loving husband to his wife, Judy, and a proud father to his three children, Susan, Debra, and Michael; doting grandfather to his six grandchildren, Rebecca, Matthew, Sarah, Rachel, Jacob, and Eli; and a mentor to so many in the field of pediatrics and pediatric infectious diseases. Ralph Feigin is missed by everyone who knew him, particularly by Judy Feigin and the family as well as by the present editors of this eighth edition of Feigin and Cherry.

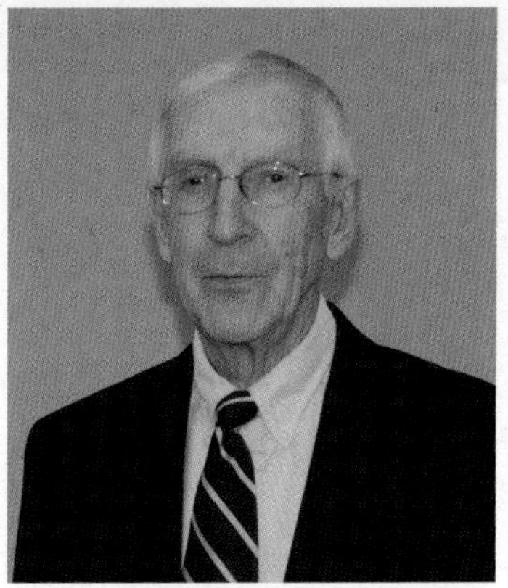

James D. Cherry, MD, MSc
Distinguished Research Professor of Pediatrics
David Geffen School of Medicine at UCLA;
Attending Physician
Pediatric Infectious Diseases
Mattel Children's Hospital UCLA
Los Angeles, California

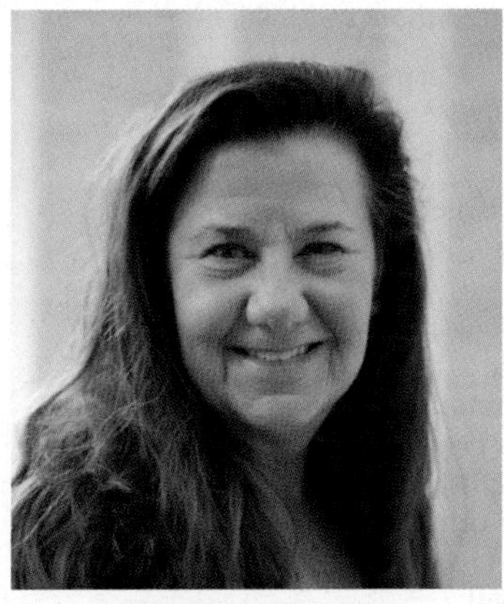

Gail J. Harrison, MD
Professor
Department of Pediatrics
Section of Infectious Diseases
Baylor College of Medicine;
Attending Physician
Infectious Diseases Service
Texas Children's Hospital
Houston, Texas

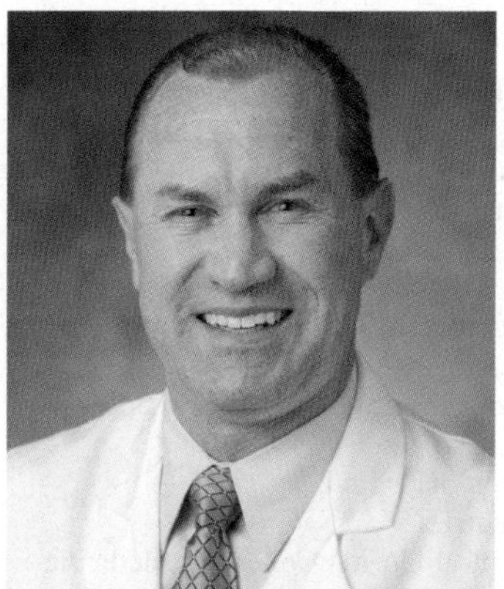

William J. Steinbach, MD
Professor of Pediatrics
Professor in Molecular Genetics and Microbiology
Chief, Pediatric Infectious Diseases
Director, Duke Pediatric Immunocompromised Host Program
Director, International Pediatric Fungal Network
Duke University School of Medicine
Durham, North Carolina

Sheldon L. Kaplan, MD
Professor and Executive Vice-Chair
Head, Section of Infectious Diseases
Department of Pediatrics
Baylor College of Medicine;
Chief, Infectious Disease Service
Head, Department of Pediatric Medicine
Texas Children's Hospital
Houston, Texas

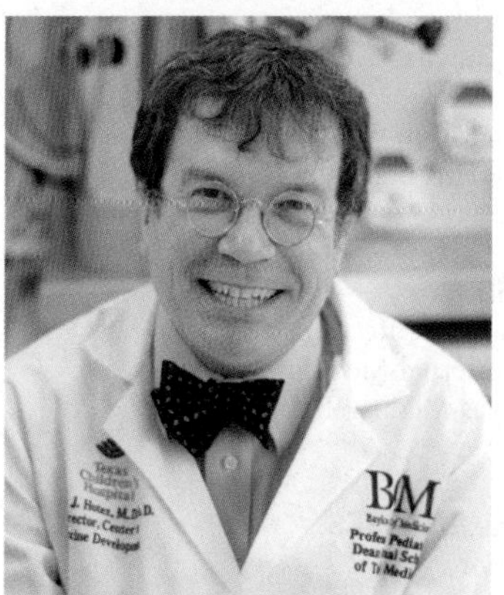

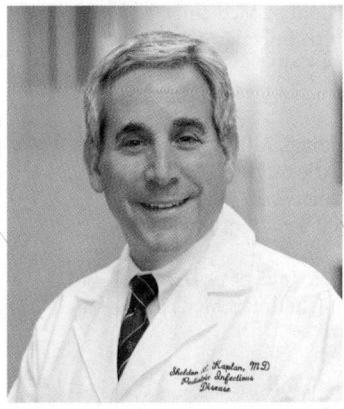

Peter J. Hotez, MD, PhD
Dean, National School of Tropical Medicine
Professor, Pediatrics and Molecular & Virology and Microbiology
Head, Section of Pediatric Tropical Medicine
Baylor College of Medicine;
Endowed Chair of Tropical Pediatrics
Center for Vaccine Development
Texas Children's Hospital;
Professor, Department of Biology
Baylor University
Waco, Texas;
Baker Institute Fellow in Disease and Poverty
Rice University
Houston, Texas;
Co-Editor-in-Chief, *PLoS Neglected Tropical Diseases*

Contributors

John Aaskov, BSc, PhD, FRCPath
World Health Organization Collaborating Centre for Arbovirus Reference and Research
Institute of Health and Biomedical Innovation
Queensland University of Technology
Brisbane, QLD, Australia

Kristina Adachi, MD, MA
Clinical Instructor
Department of Pediatrics
Division of Infectious Diseases
David Geffen School of Medicine at UCLA
Los Angeles, California

Christoph Aebi, MD
Professor of Pediatrics and Infectious Diseases
Chairman, Department of Pediatrics
University of Bern
Bern, Switzerland

Kenneth A. Alexander, MD, PhD
Chief
Division of Allergy, Immunology, Rheumatology, and Infectious Diseases
Nemours Children's Hospital;
Professor of Pediatrics
University of Central Florida College of Medicine
Orlando, Florida

Ghada N. Al-Rawahi, MD, DTM&H (London), D(ABMM), FRCPC
Medical Microbiologist
Children's and Women's Health Centre of British Columbia;
Medical Lead, Infection Prevention & Control
BC Cancer Agency;
Clinical Associate Professor
University of British Columbia
Vancouver, BC, Canada

Duha Al-Zubeidi, MD
Children's Mercy Hospital
Kansas City, Missouri

Seher Anjum, MD
Professor, Division of Infectious Disease
Department of Internal Medicine
University of Texas Medical Branch
Galveston, Texas

Monica I. Ardura, DO, MSCS
Associate Professor
Department of Pediatrics
Ohio State University;
Medical Director, Host Defense Program
Department of Pediatrics, Infectious Diseases, and Immunology
Nationwide Children's Hospital
Columbus, Ohio

Stephen S. Arnon, MD, MPH
Founder and Chief
Infant Botulism Treatment and Prevention Program
California Department of Public Health
Richmond, California

Amy Arrington, MD, PhD
Section Chief, Global Biologic Preparedness
Department of Pediatrics
Baylor College of Medicine and Texas Children's Hospital;
Assistant Professor
Department of Pediatric Critical Care Medicine
Baylor College of Medicine
Houston, Texas

Ann M. Arvin, MD
Lucile Salter Packard Professor of Pediatrics
Professor of Microbiology and Immunology
Stanford University School of Medicine
Stanford, California

Robert L. Atmar, MD
Professor
Department of Medicine
Baylor College of Medicine
Houston, Texas

Amira Baker, MD
Fellow, Pediatric Infectious Diseases
Mattel Children's Hospital
University of California–Los Angeles
Los Angeles, California

Carol J. Baker, MD
Professor
Departments of Pediatrics and Molecular Virology & Microbiology
Baylor College of Medicine
Houston, Texas

Robert S. Baltimore, MD
Professor
Departments of Pediatrics and Epidemiology
Yale University School of Medicine;
Associate Director of Infection Control
Yale-New Haven Hospital
New Haven, Connecticut

Stephen J. Barenkamp, MD
Professor of Pediatrics and Molecular Microbiology
Department of Pediatrics
St. Louis University School of Medicine;
Director
Division of Pediatric Infectious Diseases
Cardinal Glennon Children's Medical Center
St. Louis, Missouri

Elizabeth D. Barnett, MD
Attending Physician
Boston Medical Center
Boston, Massachusetts

Theresa Barton, MD
Associate Professor
Department of Pediatrics
Baylor College of Medicine
Houston, Texas

Gil Benard, MD, PhD
Medical Researcher
Departamento Dermatologia
Faculdade de Medicina;
Laboratorio de Micologia Medica
Instituto de Medicina Tropical
Universidade de São Paulo
São Paolo, Brazil

Jeffrey M. Bender, MD
Assistant Professor
Department of Pediatrics
Division of Pediatric Infectious Diseases
Children's Hospital Los Angeles;
Assistant Professor of Pediatrics and Pediatric Infectious Diseases
University of Southern California
Los Angeles, California

Gregory J. Berry, PhD, D(ABMM)
Assistant Medical Director
Division of Infectious Disease Diagnostics
Northwell Health Laboratories;
Assistant Professor of Pathology and Laboratory Medicine
Hofstra Northwell School of Medicine
Lake Success, New York

Amit Bhatt, MD
Assistant Professor
Department of Ophthalmology
Baylor College of Medicine;
Pediatric Ophthalmology Subsection
Texas Children's Hospital
Houston, Texas

Charles D. Bluestone, MD
Distinguished Professor Emeritus of Otolaryngology
University of Pittsburgh School of Medicine
Pittsburgh, Pennsylvania

Jeffrey L. Blumer, PhD, MD
Professor and Chairman
Department of Pediatrics
The University of Toledo
Toledo, Ohio

Claire Bocchini, MD, MS
Texas Children's Hospital
Houston, Texas

Kenneth M. Boyer, MD
Professor and Woman's Board Chair
Department of Pediatrics
Rush Medical College of Rush University;
Clinical Associate
Department of Pediatrics
University of Chicago
Chicago, Illinois

John S. Bradley, MD
Professor and Chief
Division of Infectious Diseases
Department of Pediatrics
University of California–San Diego School of Medicine
San Diego, California

Patricia Brasil, MD, PhD
Clinical Researcher
Instituto Nacional de Infectologia
Fundação Oswaldo Cruz
Rio de Janeiro, Brazil

William J. Britt, MD
Charles A. Alford Professor of Pediatric Infectious Diseases
Department of Pediatrics
University of Alabama
Birmingham, Alabama

David E. Bronstein, MD, MS
Department of Pediatrics
Southern California Permanente Medical Group
Palmdale, California

David A. Bruckner, ScD
Professor Emeritus
Department of Pathology & Laboratory Medicine
David Geffen School of Medicine at UCLA
Los Angeles, California

Kristina A. Bryant, MD
Professor of Pediatric Diseases
Department of Pediatrics
University of Louisville
Louisville, Kentucky

Steven C. Buckingham, MD, MA[†]
Associate Professor
Department of Pediatrics
University of Tennessee Health Science Center
Memphis, Tennessee

Carrie L. Byington, MD
Vice Chancellor, Health Services
Senior Vice President, Health Sciences Center
Jean and Thomas McMullin Professor and Dean
College of Medicine
Texas A&M University and System
Bryan, Texas

Miguel M. Cabada, MD, MSc
Assistant Professor
Department of Internal Medicine
Division of Infectious Diseases
University of Texas Medical Branch
Galveston, Texas

Adriana Cadilla, MD
Physician
Department of Pediatric Infectious Disease
Nemours Children's Hospital
Orlando, Florida

Judith R. Campbell, MD
Professor
Department of Pediatrics
Section of Infectious Diseases
Baylor College of Medicine;
Attending Physician
Infectious Disease Service
Texas Children's Hospital
Houston, Texas

Justin E. Caron, MD
Pathology Resident
Department of Pathology
University of Utah School of Medicine
Salt Lake City, Utah

[†]Deceased.

Maria Carrillo-Marquez, MD
Assistant Professor
Department of Pediatrics
University of Tennessee Health Science Center
Memphis, Tennessee

Janet R. Casey, MD
Director of Research
Legacy Pediatrics;
Clinical Associate Professor of Pediatrics
Department of Pediatrics
University of Rochester
Rochester, New York

Luis A. Castagnini, MD, MPH
Assistant Professor
Department of Pediatrics
Baylor College of Medicine/Children's Hospital of San Antonio
San Antonio, Texas

Mariam R. Chacko, MBBS
Professor
Department of Pediatrics
Section of Adolescent Medicine and Sports Medicine
Baylor College of Medicine and Texas Children's Hospital;
Medical Director, Adolescent Medicine
Baylor Teen Health Clinics
Houston, Texas

Lakshmi Chandramohan, PhD, D(ABMM)
Senior Scientist
Biopharma Division
NeoGenomics Laboratories
Houston, Texas

Louisa E. Chapman, MD, MSPH†
Medical Epidemiologist
Centers for Disease Control and Prevention
Atlanta, Georgia

Remi N. Charrel, MD, PhD
UMR "Emergence des Pathologies Virales"
Aix Marseille Université;
Fondation IHU Mediterranée Infection
APHM Public Hospitals of Marseille
Marseille, France

Elsa Chea-Woo, MD
Professor
Department of Pediatrics
Universidad Peruana Cayetano Heredia
Lima, Peru

Ira M. Cheifetz, MD, FCCM, FAARC
Chief Medical Officer
Children's Services
Duke Children's Hospital;
Associate Chief Medical Officer
Duke University Hospital;
Division Chief, Pediatric Critical Care Medicine
Professor, Departments of Pediatrics and Anesthesiology
Duke University Medical Center
Durham, North Carolina

†Deceased.

Tempe K. Chen, MD
Assistant Clinical Professor
Department of Pediatrics
University of California Irvine School of Medicine
Irvine, California

James D. Cherry, MD, MSc
Distinguished Research Professor of Pediatrics
David Geffen School of Medicine at UCLA;
Attending Physician
Pediatric Infectious Diseases
Mattel Children's Hospital UCLA
Los Angeles, California

Javier Chinen, MD, PhD
Associate Professor
Pediatrics, Allergy, and Immunology
Baylor College of Medicine and Texas Children's Hospital
Houston, Texas

Natascha Ching, MD
Assistant Clinical Professor
Department of Pediatrics
John A. Burns School of Medicine at the University of Hawaii;
Physician
Department of Pediatric Infectious Diseases
Kapiolani Medical Center for Women and Children
Kapiolani Medical Specialists
Honolulu, Hawaii

Ivan K. Chinn, MD
Assistant Professor
Department of Pediatrics
Baylor College of Medicine and Texas Children's Hospital
Houston, Texas

John C. Christenson, MD
Professor of Clinical Pediatrics
Ryan White Center for Pediatric Infectious Disease and Global Health
Indiana University School of Medicine
Indianapolis, Indiana

Susan E. Coffin, MD, MPH
Professor of Pediatrics
Associate Chief
Division of Infectious Diseases
UPENN School of Medicine;
Associate Hospital Epidemiologist
Children's Hospital of Philadelphia
Philadelphia, Pennsylvania

Armando G. Correa, MD
Assistant Professor
Department of Pediatrics
Baylor College of Medicine;
Attending Physician
Texas Children's Hospital
Houston, Texas

Elaine G. Cox, MD
Professor of Clinical Pediatrics
Ryan White Center for Pediatric Infectious Disease and Global Health
Indiana University School of Medicine
Indianapolis, Indiana

Jonathan D. Crews, MD, MS
Assistant Professor
Department of Pediatrics
Baylor College of Medicine;
Attending Physician
Pediatric Infectious Diseases
Children's Hospital of San Antonio
San Antonio, Texas

Andrea T. Cruz, MD, MPH
Assistant Professor
Department of Pediatrics
Baylor College of Medicine
Houston, Texas

Zev Davidovics, MD
Department of Pediatric Gastroenterology, Digestive Diseases, Hepatology, and Nutrition
Connecticut Children's Medical Center
Hartford, Connecticut;
Assistant Professor of Pediatrics
University of Connecticut School of Medicine
Farmington, Connecticut

Walter N. Dehority, MD, MSc
Associate Professor
Department of Pediatrics
University of New Mexico Health Sciences Center
Albuquerque, New Mexico

Xavier de Lamballerie, MD
Professor
Emergence des Pathologies Virales
Aix-Marseille Université;
IRD French Institute of Research for Development
EHESP French School of Public Health
Laboratory of Virology
IHU Mediterranée Infection
APHM Public Hospitals of Marseille
Marseille, France

Penelope H. Dennehy, MD
Director
Division of Pediatric Infectious Diseases
Hasbro Children's Hospital;
Professor and Vice Chair for Academic Affairs
Department of Pediatrics
Alpert Medical School of Brown University
Providence, Rhode Island

Minh L. Doan, MD, COL, MC, USA
Chief, Division of Pediatric Pulmonology
Brooke Army Medical Center
San Antonio, Texas

Simon R. Dobson, MD, FRCPC
Medical Director, Infection Prevention and Control
Antimicrobial Stewardship Consultant
Sidra Medical and Research Center
Qatar Foundation
Doha, Qatar

Jan E. Drutz, MD
Professor
Department of Pediatrics
Baylor College of Medicine and Texas Children's Hospital
Houston, Texas

Kara A. Dubray, MD
Clinical Instructor
Pediatric Infectious Disease
Lucile Packard Children's Hospital
Palo Alto, California

Andrea Duppenthaler, MD
Pediatric Infectious Diseases
Children's University Hospital
Bern, Switzerland

Christopher C. Dvorak, MD
Professor & Chief
Department of Pediatric Allergy, Immunology, & Bone Marrow Transplant
University of California–San Francisco Benioff Children's Hospital
San Francisco, California

Paul H. Edelstein, MD
Professor Emeritus of Pathology and Laboratory Medicine
University of Pennsylvania Perelman School of Medicine
Philadelphia, Pennsylvania

Kathryn M. Edwards, MD
Sarah H. Sell and Cornelius Vanderbilt Chair in Pediatrics
Department of Pediatrics
Vanderbilt University School of Medicine
Nashville, Tennessee

Morven S. Edwards, MD
Professor of Pediatrics
Baylor College of Medicine;
Attending Physician
Pediatric Infectious Diseases Section
Texas Children's Hospital
Houston, Texas

Samer S. El-Kamary, MBChB, MS, MPH
Associate Professor
Department of Epidemiology and Public Health
University of Maryland School of Medicine;
Associate Professor
Department of Pediatrics
University of Maryland School of Medicine
Baltimore, Maryland

Janet A. Englund, MD
Professor
Department of Pediatrics
University of Washington/Seattle Children's Hospital
Seattle, Washington

Jessica Ericson, MD, MPH
Assistant Professor
Department of Pediatrics
Division of Pediatric Infectious Diseases
Pennsylvania State University College of Medicine
Hershey, Pennsylvania

Leland L. Fan, MD
Professor Emeritus
Department of Pediatrics
University of Colorado School of Medicine
Aurora, Colorado

Myke Federman, MD
Associate Professor of Pediatrics
Division of Pediatric Critical Care
University of California–Los Angeles
Los Angeles, California

Pedro Fernando da C. Vasconcelos, MD, PhD
Chief, Department of Arbovirology and Hemorrhagic Fevers
Coordinator, National Reference Laboratory of Arboviruses
Director, National Institute of Science and Technology for Viral Hemorrhagic Fevers
Director, PAHO-WHO CC for Research and Diagnostic Reference on Arbovirus
Instituto Evandro Chagas
SVS/Ministry of Health
Ananindeua, Brazil

Philip R. Fischer, MD
Professor of Pediatrics
Mayo Clinic
Rochester, Minnesota

Brian T. Fisher, DO, MPH, MSCE
Assistant Professor of Pediatrics and Epidemiology
Perelman School of Medicine at the University of Pennsylvania;
Division of Infectious Diseases
Children's Hospital of Philadelphia
Philadelphia, Pennsylvania

Randall G. Fisher, MD
Professor
Department of Pediatrics
Eastern Virginia Medical School;
Medical Director
Division of Pediatric Infectious Diseases
Children's Hospital of The King's Daughters
Norfolk, Virginia

Douglas S. Fishman, MD
Director of Gastrointestinal Endoscopy and Pancreaticobiliary Program
Texas Children's Hospital;
Associate Professor of Pediatrics
Baylor College of Medicine
Houston, Texas

Anthony R. Flores, MD, MPH, PhD
Assistant Professor
Department of Pediatrics
Section of Infectious Diseases
Texas Children's Hospital
Baylor College of Medicine
Houston, Texas

Catherine Foster, MD
Clinical Postdoctoral Fellow
Pediatrics, Section of Infectious Diseases
Baylor College of Medicine
Houston, Texas

Ellen M. Friedman, MD
Professor
Department of Otolaryngology
Texas Children's Hospital;
Director
Center for Professionalism in Medicine
Baylor College of Medicine
Houston, Texas

Claudia Raja Gabaglia, MD, PhD
Assistant Professor
Biomedical Research Institute of Southern California
Oceanside, California

Lynne S. Garcia, MS, CLS, BLM, FAAM
Director
LSG & Associates
Santa Monica, California

Gregory M. Gauthier, MD, MS
Associate Professor
Department of Medicine
University of Wisconsin
Madison, Wisconsin

Anne A. Gershon, MD
Professor
Department of Pediatrics
Columbia University College of Physicians and Surgeons
New York, New York

Francis Gigliotti, MD
Professor and Chief of Infectious Diseases
Department of Pediatrics
Associate Chair for Academic Affairs
University of Rochester School of Medicine and Dentistry
Rochester, New York

Mark A. Gilger, MD
Pediatrician-in-Chief
Children's Hospital of San Antonio;
Professor and Vice Chair
Department of Pediatrics
Baylor College of Medicine
Houston, Texas

Susan L. Gillespie, MD, PhD
Associate Professor
Department of Pediatrics
Baylor College of Medicine
Houston, Texas

Carol A. Glaser, DVM, MPVM, MD
Pediatric Infectious Diseases
Permanente Medical Group
Oakland Medical Center
Oakland, California

David L. Goldman, MD
Associate Professor
Department of Pediatrics
Children's Hospital at Montefiore/Albert Einstein College of Medicine
New York, New York

Jennifer L. Goldman, MD
Department of Pediatrics
Children's Mercy Hospitals and Clinics
Kansas City, Missouri

Nira A. Goldstein, MD, MPH
Professor and Attending Physician
Department of Otolaryngology
State University of New York Downstate Medical Center
New York, New York

Blanca E. Gonzalez, MD
Assistant Professor of Pediatrics
Cleveland Clinic Lerner College of Medicine of Case Western Reserve University
Center for Pediatric Infectious Diseases
Cleveland Clinic Children's
Cleveland, Ohio

Michael D. Green, MD, MPH
Professor
Department of Pediatrics, Surgery, & Clinical and Translational Research
University of Pittsburgh School of Medicine
Division of Pediatric Infectious Diseases
Children's Hospital of Pittsburgh of UPMC
Pittsburgh, Pennsylvania

Andreas Groll, MD
Professor
Department of Pediatric Hematology/Oncology
University Children's Hospital
Muenster, Germany

Charles Grose, MD
Professor
Department of Pediatrics
Director of Infectious Diseases
Children's Hospital
University of Iowa
Iowa City, Iowa

Duane J. Gubler, ScD, FAAAS, FIDSA, FASTMH
Emeritus Professor
Programme in Emerging Infectious Diseases
Duke-NUS Medical School
Singapore;
Chair, Global Dengue and Aedes Transmitted Diseases Consortium
International Vaccine Institute
Seoul, Korea

Javier Nieto Guevara, MD, MPH
Infectious Diseases Specialist
Panama City, Panama

Caroline B. Hall, MD[†]
Formerly Professor
Department of Pediatrics and Medicine
University of Rochester School of Medicine and Dentistry
Rochester, New York

Roy A. Hall, BSc(Hons), PhD
Professor
School of Chemistry and Molecular Biosciences
University of Queensland
St Lucia, QLD, Australia

Scott B. Halstead, MD
Adjunct Professor
Preventive Medicine and Biostatistics
Uniformed Services University of the Health Sciences
Bethesda, Maryland

Shinjiro Hamano, MD, PhD
Professor
Department of Parasitology
Institute of Tropical Medicine
Nagasaki University
Nagasaki, Japan

Margaret R. Hammerschlag, MD
Professor of Pediatrics and Medicine
SUNY Downstate Medical Center
New York, New York

Nicole L. Hannemann, MD
Chief Resident and Clinical Instructor
Department of Pediatrics
Baylor College of Medicine and Texas Children's Hospital
Houston, Texas

I. Celine Hanson, MD
Professor
Department of Pediatrics
Baylor College of Medicine
Houston, Texas

Nada Harik, MD
Associate Professor
Department of Pediatrics
Division of Pediatric Infectious Diseases
George Washington University School of Medicine and Health Sciences
Children's National Medical Center
Washington, DC

Kathleen H. Harriman, PhD, MPH, RN
Chief
Vaccine Preventable Diseases Epidemiology Section
Immunization Branch
California Department of Public Health
Richmond, California

Gail J. Harrison, MD
Professor
Department of Pediatrics
Section of Infectious Diseases
Baylor College of Medicine;
Attending Physician
Infectious Diseases Service
Texas Children's Hospital
Houston, Texas

C. Mary Healy, MB BCh, BAO, MD
Associate Professor
Department of Pediatrics
Division of Infectious Diseases
Baylor College of Medicine and Texas Children's Hospital
Houston, Texas

Ulrich Heininger, MD
Chair, Pediatric Infectious Diseases
University of Basel Children's Hospital;
Member, Medical Faculty
University of Basel
Basel, Switzerland

Maria Hemming-Harlo, MD, PhD
Medical Researcher
Vaccine Research Center
University of Tampere
Tampere, Finland

Sheryl L. Henderson, MD, PhD
Assistant Professor
Department of Pediatrics
University of Wisconsin School of Medicine and Public Health
American Family Children's Hospital
Madison, Wisconsin

[†]Deceased.

Gloria P. Heresi, MD
Professor
Department of Pediatrics
University of Texas Medical School at Houston
Houston, Texas

Peter W. Hiatt, MD
Associate Professor of Pediatrics
Section Head, Pediatric Pulmonology
Baylor College of Medicine;
Chief, Pulmonary Medicine
Texas Children's Hospital
Houston, Texas

Harry R. Hill, MD
Professor
Departments of Pediatrics, Pathology, and Internal Medicine
University of Utah
Salt Lake City, Utah

David C. Hilmers, MD, EE, MPH
Professor
Departments of Internal Medicine and Pediatrics
Baylor Global Initiatives
Baylor Center for Space Medicine
Baylor College of Medicine
Houston, Texas

Jill A. Hoffman, MD
Associate Professor
Department of Pediatrics
Keck School of Medicine
University of Southern California;
Attending Physician
Division of Infectious Diseases
Children's Hospital Los Angeles
Los Angeles, California

Peter J. Hotez, MD, PhD
Dean, National School of Tropical Medicine
Professor, Pediatrics and Molecular & Virology and Microbiology
Head, Section of Pediatric Tropical Medicine
Baylor College of Medicine;
Endowed Chair of Tropical Pediatrics
Center for Vaccine Development
Texas Children's Hospital;
Professor, Department of Biology
Baylor University
Waco, Texas;
Baker Institute Fellow in Disease and Poverty
Rice University
Houston, Texas;
Co-Editor-in-Chief, *PLoS Neglected Tropical Diseases*

Leigh M. Howard, MD, MPH
Assistant Professor
Department of Pediatric Infectious Diseases
Vanderbilt University Medical Center
Nashville, Tennessee

Kristina G. Hulten, PhD
Assistant Professor
Department of Pediatrics
Baylor College of Medicine
Houston, Texas

Romney M. Humphries, PhD
Chief Scientific Officer
Accelerate Diagnostics
Tucson, Arizona

David A. Hunstad, MD
Associate Professor
Departments of Pediatrics and Molecular Microbiology
Washington University School of Medicine
St. Louis, Missouri

W. Garrett Hunt, MD, MPH, DTM&H, FAAP
Associate Professor
Department of Pediatrics
Section of Infectious Diseases
Nationwide Children's Hospital/Ohio State University
Columbus, Ohio

W. Charles Huskins, MD, MSc
Professor of Pediatrics
Mayo Clinic School of Medicine;
Chair, Division of Pediatric Infectious Diseases
Mayo Clinic;
Vice Chair of Quality and Health Care Epidemiologist
Mayo Clinic Children's Center
Rochester, Minnesota

David Y. Hyun, MD
Senior Officer
Antibiotic Resistance Project
Pew Charitable Trusts
Philadelphia, Pennsylvania

Mary Anne Jackson, MD
Director, Infectious Diseases
Children's Mercy Kansas City
Professor of Pediatrics
UMKC School of Medicine
Kansas City, Missouri

Michael R. Jacobs, MB BCh, PhD
Professor of Pathology and Medicine
Department of Pathology
Case Western Reserve University;
Director of Clinical Microbiology
Department of Pathology
University Hospitals Cleveland Medical Center
Cleveland, Ohio

Richard F. Jacobs, MD, FAAP
Robert H. Fiser Jr, MD, Endowed Chair in Pediatrics
Pediatrician-in-Chief
Department of Pediatrics
Arkansas Children's Hospital;
Chairman and Professor
Department of Pediatrics
University of Arkansas for Medical Sciences
Little Rock, Arkansas

Ravi Jhaveri, MD
Associate Professor
Department of Pediatrics
University of North Carolina at Chapel Hill School of Medicine
Chapel Hill, North Carolina

Audrey R. Odom John, MD, PhD
Associate Professor
Departments of Pediatrics and Molecular Microbiology
Washington University School of Medicine
Saint Louis, Missouri

Samantha H. Johnston, MD, MPH
Associate Physician
Pediatric Infectious Diseases
UCSF Benioff Children's Hospital Oakland
Oakland, California

Meena R. Julapalli, MD
Assistant Professor
Department of Dermatology
University of Colorado
Denver, Colorado

Sheldon L. Kaplan, MD
Professor and Executive Vice-Chair
Head, Section of Infectious Diseases
Department of Pediatrics
Baylor College of Medicine;
Chief, Infectious Disease Service
Head, Department of Pediatric Medicine
Texas Children's Hospital
Houston, Texas

Gregory L. Kearns, PharmD, PhD
President
Arkansas Children's Research Institute
Senior Vice President and Chief Research Officer
Arkansas Children's;
Ross and Mary Whipple Family Distinguished Research Scientist
Professor of Pediatrics
University of Arkansas for Medical Sciences
Little Rock, Arkansas

Jessica M. Khouri, MD
Senior Medical Officer
Infant Botulism Treatment and Prevention Program
California Department of Public Health
Richmond, California

Kwang Sik Kim, MD
Professor and Director
Department of Pediatric Infectious Diseases
Johns Hopkins University School of Medicine;
Professor
Department of Molecular Microbiology and Immunology
Johns Hopkins University Bloomberg School of Public Health
Baltimore, Maryland

Yae-Jean Kim, MD, PhD
Associate Professor
Department of Pediatrics
Samsung Medical Center
Sungkyungkwan University School of Medicine
Seoul, Korea

Katherine Y. King, MD, PhD
Assistant Professor
Department of Pediatric Infectious Diseases
Baylor College of Medicine
Houston, Texas

Louis V. Kirchhoff, MD, MPH
Professor
Department of Internal Medicine (Infectious Diseases), Psychiatry, and Epidemiology
Carver College of Medicine and College of Public Health
University of Iowa
Iowa City, Iowa

Martin B. Kleiman, MD
Ryan White Professor Emeritus of Pediatrics
Ryan White Center for Pediatric Infectious Disease and Global Health
Indiana University School of Medicine
Indianapolis, Indiana

Bruce S. Klein, MD
Gerard B. Odell and Shirley S. Matchette Professor of Pediatrics
Professor of Internal Medicine and Medical Microbiology and Immunology
University of Wisconsin–Madison
Madison, Wisconsin

Stephan A. Kohlhoff, MD
Associate Professor
Departments of Pediatrics and Medicine
State University of New York Downstate Medical Center
New York, New York

Tobias R. Kollmann, MD, PhD
Professor of Pediatrics
Interim Head, Division of Infectious Diseases
University of British Columbia
Vancouver, BC, Canada

Poonum S. Korpe, MD
Assistant Scientist
Department of Epidemiology
Johns Hopkins Bloomberg School of Public Health
Baltimore, Maryland

Margaret Kosek, MD
Assistant Professor
Department of International Health
Johns Hopkins University Bloomberg School of Public Health
Baltimore, Maryland

Michael P. Koster, MD
Division of Pediatric Hospital Medicine
Hasbro Children's Hospital;
Associate Professor, Clinical Educator
Department of Pediatrics
Alpert Medical School of Brown University
Providence, Rhode Island

Peter J. Krause, MD
Senior Research Scientist
Yale School of Public Health
Yale School of Medicine
New Haven, Connecticut

Leonard R. Krilov, MD
Chairman, Department of Pediatrics
Chief, Pediatric Infectious Disease
Children's Medical Center
NYU Winthrop Hospital
Mineola, New York;
Professor of Pediatrics
State University of New York Stony Brook School of Medicine
Stony Brook, New York

Paul Krogstad, MD
Professor
Departments of Pediatrics and Molecular and Medical Pharmacology
David Geffen School of Medicine at UCLA
Los Angeles, California

Damian J. Krysan, MD, PHD
Associate Professor
Departments of Pediatrics and Microbiology/Immunology
University of Rochester School of Medicine and Dentistry
Rochester, New York

Edward Kuan, MD, MBA
Resident Physician
Department of Head and Neck Surgery
David Geffen School of Medicine at UCLA
Los Angeles, California

Thomas Kuhls, MD
Department of Pediatrics
Norman Pediatric Associates
Norman, Oklahoma

Sarah M. Labuda, MD, MPH
Pediatric Infectious Diseases Fellow
Tulane School of Medicine
New Orleans, Louisiana

Paul M. Lantos, MD
Assistant Professor
Division of Pediatric Infectious Diseases
Division of General Internal Medicine
Duke University School of Medicine
Duke Global Health Institute
Durham, North Carolina

Timothy R. La Pine, MD
Professor
Department of Pediatrics and Pathology
University of Utah;
Director of Neonatology
St. Mark's Hospital
Salt Lake City, Utah

Suvi Heinimäki, PhD
Project Researcher
Vaccine Research Center
University of Tampere
Tampere, Finland

Jerome M. Larkin, MD
Division of Infectious Diseases
Rhode Island Hospital
Associate Professor, Clinical Educator
Department of Medicine
Alpert Medical School of Brown University
Providence, Rhode Island

Matthew B. Laurens, MD, MPH
Associate Professor
Institute for Global Health
University of Maryland School of Medicine
Baltimore, Maryland

Charles T. Leach, MD
Professor and Chief of Infectious Diseases
Department of Pediatrics
Baylor College of Medicine/Children's Hospital of San Antonio
San Antonio, Texas

Amy Leber, PhD
Director, Clinical Microbiology and Immunoserology
Department of Pathology and Laboratory Medicine
Nationwide Children's Hospital
Columbus, Ohio

Robert J. Leggiadro, MD
Adjunct Professor
Departments of Biology and Geography and the Environment
Villanova University
Villanova, Pennsylvania;
Adjunct Clinical Professor
Department of Pediatrics
Donald and Barbara Zucker School of Medicine at Hofstra/Northwell
Hempstead, New York;
Adjunct Attending Physician
General Pediatrics
Cohen Children's Medical Center
New Hyde Park, New York

Deborah Lehman, MD
Professor
Department of Pediatrics
David Geffen School of Medicine at UCLA
Los Angeles, California

Diana R. Lennon, MB CHB, FRACP
Professor of Population Health, Child, and Youth
Department of Pediatrics
University of Auckland;
Pediatrician in Infectious Diseases
Department of Pediatrics
Starship and KidzFirst Children's Hospital
Auckland, New Zealand

Daniel H. Leung, MD
Associate Professor of Pediatrics
Division of Gastroenterology, Hepatology, and Nutrition
Baylor College of Medicine;
Director of Clinical Research
Medical Director, Viral Hepatitis Program
Texas Children's Hospital
Houston, Texas

Moise L. Levy, MD
Chief, Pediatric/Adolescent Dermatology
Dell Children's Medical Center;
Professor of Pediatrics and Medicine (Dermatology)
Dell Medical School
University of Texas
Austin, Texas;
Clinical Professor of Dermatology and Pediatrics
Baylor College of Medicine
Houston, Texas

W. Matthew Linam, MD, MS
Medical Director of Infection Prevention and Hospital Epidemiology
Associate Professor, Department of Pediatrics
Division of Pediatric Infectious Diseases
Arkansas Children's Hospital
University of Arkansas for Medical Sciences
Little Rock, Arkansas

Latania K. Logan, MD
Chief, Pediatric Infectious Diseases
Department of Pediatrics
Rush University Medical Center
Associate Professor
Rush Medical College
Chicago, Illinois

Timothy E. Lotze, MD
Associate Professor of Pediatrics and Neurology
Division of Child Neurology
Baylor College of Medicine and Texas Children's Hospital
Houston, Texas

Yalda C. Lucero, MD, PhD
Pediatric Gastroenterologist
Assistant Professor
Microbiology and Mycology Program
Institute of Biomedical Sciences
Faculty of Medicine
University of Chile and Northern Campus Department of Pediatrics
Santiago, Chile

Debra J. Lugo, MD
Fellow, Pediatric Infectious Diseases
Mattel Children's Hospital
University of California–Los Angeles
Los Angeles, California

Berkley Luk, BSc
PhD Candidate
Program in Integrative Molecular and Biomedical Sciences
Baylor College of Medicine;
Department of Pathology
Texas Children's Hospital
Houston, Texas

Susan A. Maloney, MD, MHSc
Global Tuberculosis Coordinator
Division of Global Migration and Quarantine
National Center for Infectious Diseases
Centers for Disease Control and Prevention
Atlanta, Georgia

Michelle C. Mann, MD
Assistant Professor
Department of Pediatrics
Baylor College of Medicine
Houston, Texas

Lucila Marquez, MD, MPH
Assistant Professor of Pediatrics, Section of Infectious Diseases
Associate Medical Director, Infection Control and Prevention
Baylor College of Medicine and Texas Children's Hospital
Houston, Texas

Kimberly C. Martin, DO, MPH
Assistant Professor of Pediatrics
Division of Pediatric Infectious Diseases
University of Oklahoma School of Community Medicine
Tulsa, Oklahoma

Laurene Mascola, MD, MPH, FAAP
Epidemiology Consultant
Acute Communicable Disease Program
Los Angeles County Department of Public Health
Los Angeles, California

Edward O. Mason Jr, PhD
Professor
Department of Pediatrics
Baylor College of Medicine
Houston, Texas

Aldo Maspons, MD
CEO/Cofounder
VeMiDoc, LLC;
Maspons Pediatric Gastro
Pediatric Gastroenterology
El Paso, Texas

Marc A. Mazade, MD
Consultant
Pediatric Infectious Disease
Cook Children's Medical Center
Fort Worth, Texas

Holly E. McBride, MPH, MHS, PA-C
Physician Assistant
Internal Medicine
University of Colorado Health
Loveland, Colorado

Jonathan A. McCullers, MD
Chair
Department of Pediatrics
University of Tennessee Health Science Center
Memphis, Tennessee

Kenneth McIntosh, MD
Professor
Department of Pediatrics
Harvard Medical School;
Senior Physician
Department of Medicine
Children's Hospital
Boston, Massachusetts

James E. McJunkin, MD
Professor of Pediatrics
Department of Pediatrics
West Virginia University Health Sciences Center
Charleston, West Virginia

Kelly T. McKee Jr, MD, MPH
Vice President
Department of Public Health and Government Services
QuintilesIMS
Durham, North Carolina

Ross McKinney Jr, MD
Professor Emeritus
Department of Pediatrics
Duke University School of Medicine
Durham, North Carolina;
Chief Scientific Officer
Association of American Medical Colleges
Washington, DC

J. Chase McNeil, MD
Assistant Professor
Department of Pediatrics
Section of Infectious Diseases
Baylor College of Medicine
Houston, Texas

Rojelio Mejia, MD
Assistant Professor of Infectious Diseases and Pediatrics
National School of Tropical Medicine
Baylor College of Medicine
Houston, Texas

Asuncion Mejias, MD, PhD
Associate Professor of Pediatrics
Ohio State University College of Medicine
Department of Pediatrics
Division of Infectious Diseases
Nationwide Children's Hospital
Columbus, Ohio

Maria José Soares Mendes Giannini, PhD
Full Professor
Department of Clinical Analysis
Laboratory of Clinical Mycology
São Paulo State University-UNESP
Araraquara, São Paulo, Brazil

Marian G. Michaels, MD, MPH
Professor
Department of Pediatrics and Surgery
University of Pittsburgh School of Medicine
Division of Pediatric Infectious Diseases
Children's Hospital of Pittsburgh of UPMC
Pittsburgh, Pennsylvania

Ian C. Michelow, MD, DTM&H
Division of Pediatric Infectious Diseases
Hasbro Children's Hospital
Associate Professor
Department of Pediatrics
Alpert Medical School of Brown University
Providence, Rhode Island

Marjorie J. Miller, DrPH
Senior Specialist, Virology
Department of Pathology and Laboratory Medicine
UCLA Medical Center
Los Angeles, California

James N. Mills, PhD
Adjunct Faculty
Population Biology, Ecology, and Evolution Group
Emory University
Atlanta, Georgia

Leena B. Mithal, MD, MSCI
Attending Physician
Department of Pediatric Infectious Diseases
Ann & Robert H. Lurie Children's Hospital of Chicago;
Instructor, Department of Pediatrics
Northwestern University Feinberg School of Medicine
Chicago, Illinois

Kathryn S. Moffett, MD
Professor of Pediatrics
Section Chief, Infectious Diseases
Department of Pediatrics
West Virginia University
Morgantown, West Virginia

Martin Montes, MD
Assistant Professor
Instituto de Medicina Tropica "Alexander von Humboldt"
Universidad Peruana Cayetano Heridia
Lima, Peru;
Assistant Professor
Department of Medicine
Division of Infectious Diseases
University of Texas Medical Branch
Galveston, Texas

Martha Muller, MD
Associate Professor
Department of Pediatrics
University of New Mexico
Albuquerque, New Mexico

Randy George Mungwira, MBBS, MPH
Blantyre Malaria Project
Blantyre, Malawi

James R. Murphy, PhD
Professor
Department of Pediatrics
University of Texas
Houston, Texas

Santhosh M. Nadipuram, MD
Postdoctoral Fellow
Department of Microbiology, Immunology, & Molecular Genetics
University of California–Los Angeles
Los Angeles, California

James P. Nataro, MD, PhD, MBA
Benjamin Armistead Shepherd Professor and Chair
Department of Pediatrics
University of Virginia School of Medicine;
Physician-in-Chief
University of Virginia Children's Hospital
Charlottesville, Virginia

Heather Needham, MD, MPH
Assistant Professor of Pediatrics
Section of Adolescent Medicine & Sports Medicine
Baylor College of Medicine and Texas Children's Hospital
Houston, Texas

Karin Nielsen-Saines, MD, MPH
Professor of Clinical Pediatrics
Division of Pediatric Infectious Diseases
David Geffen School of Medicine at UCLA;
Director, Center for Brazilian Studies
Los Angeles, California

Delma J. Nieves, MD
Assistant Clinical Professor
Department of Pediatric Infectious Diseases
University of California–Irvine School of Medicine
Children's Hospital of Orange County
Orange, California

Richard Oberhelman, MD
Professor and Chair
Global Community Health & Behavioral Sciences
Tulane School of Public Health and Tropical Medicine;
Professor of Pediatrics
Tulane School of Medicine
New Orleans, Louisiana

Theresa J. Ochoa, MD
Associate Professor
Department of Pediatrics
Instituto de Medicina Tropical "Alexander von Humboldt"
Universidad Peruana Cayetano Heredia
Lima, Peru;
Associate Professor
Division of Epidemiology, Human Genetics, and Environmental Sciences
Center for Infectious Diseases
School of Public Health
University of Texas Health Science Center at Houston
Houston, Texas

Rosemary M. Olivero, MD
Clinical Associate Professor of Pediatrics and Human Development
Michigan State College of Human Medicine;
Attending Physician
Section of Pediatric Infectious Diseases
Helen DeVos Children's Hospital
Grand Rapids, Michigan

Miguel O'Ryan, MD
Professor, Pediatric Infectious Disease
Millennium Institute of Immunology and Immunotherapy
Faculty of Medicine
Microbiology and Mycology Program
Institute of Biomedical Sciences
University of Chile
Santiago, Chile

Gary D. Overturf, MD
Professor Emeritus
Departments of Pediatrics and Pathology
University of New Mexico School of Medicine;
Medical Director, Infectious Diseases
TriCore Reference Laboratories
Albuquerque, New Mexico

Debra L. Palazzi, MD, MEd
Associate Professor of Pediatrics
Section of Infectious Diseases
Baylor College of Medicine;
Chief, Infectious Diseases Clinic
Texas Children's Hospital
Houston, Texas

Pia S. Pannaraj, MD, MPH
Associate Professor
Pediatrics and Molecular Microbiology and Immunology
University of Southern California/Children's Hospital Los Angeles
Los Angeles, California

Janak A. Patel, MD
Professor and Division Director
Department of Pediatrics
Division of Pediatric Infectious Disease and Immunology
University of Texas Medical Branch
Galveston, Texas

Mary E. Paul, MD
Associate Professor
Department of Pediatrics
Baylor College of Medicine
Chief, Retrovirology and Global Health
Texas Children's Hospital
Houston, Texas

Stephen I. Pelton, MD
Professor of Pediatrics and Epidemiology
Department of Pediatrics
Boston University Schools of Medicine and Public Health;
Chief, Section of Pediatric Infectious Diseases
Department of Pediatrics
Boston Medical Center
Boston, Massachusetts

Morgan A. Pence, PhD, D(ABMM)
Clinical Microbiologist
Department of Laboratory and Pathology
Cook Children's Medical Center
Fort Worth, Texas

John R. Perfect, MD
James B. Duke Professor of Medicine
Duke University Medical Center
Durham, North Carolina

C.J. Peters, MD
Department of Microbiology and Immunology
University of Texas Medical Branch
Galveston, Texas

William A. Petri Jr, MD, PhD
Chief
Division of Infectious Disease and International Health
University of Virginia Health System;
Wade Hampton Frost Professor of Epidemiology
University of Virginia
Charlottesville, Virginia

Yen H. Pham, MD
Assistant Professor
Department of Pediatric Gastroenterology, Hepatology, and Nutrition
Baylor College of Medicine and Texas Children's Hospital
Houston, Texas

Francisco P. Pinheiro, MD
Department of Arbovirus
Instituto Evandro Chagas
FNS
Ministry of Health
Belem, Brazil

Benjamin A. Pinsky, MD, PhD
Associate Professor
Departments of Pathology and Medicine (Infectious Diseases)
Stanford University School of Medicine;
Medical Director
Clinical Virology Laboratory
Stanford Health Care and Stanford Children's Health
Stanford, California

Alice Pong, MD
Department of Pediatric Infectious Diseases
University of California–San Diego;
Department of Pediatric Infectious Diseases
Rady Children's Hospital San Diego
San Diego, California

Eric A. Porsch, PhD
Department of Pediatrics
Children's Hospital of Philadelphia
Philadelphia, Pennsylvania

Joan S. Purcell, MD
Adolescent Medicine and Pediatrics
STEP Pediatrics
Woodlands, Texas

Natalie M. Quanquin, MD, PhD
Research Fellow
Department of Microbiology, Immunology, and Molecular Genetics
University of California–Los Angeles
Los Angeles, California

Kevin K. Quinn, MD
Physician
Department of Pediatric Infectious Diseases
Southern California Permanente Medical Group
Fontana, California

Susan M. Abdel-Rahman, PharmD
Chief, Section of Therapeutic Innovation
Clinical Pharmacology, Medical Toxicology & Therapeutic Innovation
Children's Mercy–Kansas City;
Professor of Pediatrics
University of Missouri–Kansas City School of Medicine
Kansas City, Missouri

Octavio Ramilo, MD
Henry G. Cramblett Chair in Medicine
Professor of Pediatrics
Ohio State University College of Medicine
Department of Pediatrics
Chief, Division of Infectious Diseases
Nationwide Children's Hospital
Columbus, Ohio

Ramya Ramraj, MD, MBBS
Affiliate Assistant Professor
Oregon Health and Sciences University;
Attending Pediatrician and Pediatric Gastroenterologist
Doernbecher Children's Hospital and Kaiser NW Permanente
Portland, Oregon

Paula A. Revell, PhD
Assistant Professor
Departments of Pathology and Immunology and Pediatrics
Baylor College of Medicine;
Director of Microbiology and Virology
Texas Children's Hospital
Houston, Texas

Anne W. Rimoin, PhD, MPH
Associate Professor
Department of Epidemiology
UCLA Fielding School of Public Health
Los Angeles, California

José R. Romero, MD
Horace C. Cabe Professor of Infectious Diseases
Department of Pediatrics
University of Arkansas for Medical Sciences;
Director, Pediatric Infectious Diseases Section
Department of Pediatrics
Arkansas Children's Hospital;
Director, Clinical Trials Research
Arkansas Children's Hospital Research Institute
Little Rock, Arkansas

Lawrence Ross, MD, DTM&H
Professor Emeritus
Division of Pediatric Infectious Diseases
Children's Hospital of Los Angeles
Keck School of Medicine at the University of Southern California
Los Angeles, California

Anne H. Rowley, MD
Professor
Department of Pediatrics and Microbiology/Immunology
Northwestern University Feinberg School of Medicine
Attending Physician, Division of Infectious Diseases
Department of Pediatrics
Ann & Robert H. Lurie Children's Hospital of Chicago
Chicago, Illinois

Charles E. Rupprecht, VMD, MS, PhD
Chief Executive Officer
LYSSA, LLC
Atlanta, Georgia

Xavier Saez-Llorens, MD
Professor of Pediatrics
Head of Infectious Diseases
Hospital del Niño "Dr. José Renán Esquivel"
Distinguished Investigator, SNI, Senacyt
Panama City, Panama

Julia Shaklee Sammons, MD, MSCE
Assistant Professor of Clinical Pediatrics
Division of Infectious Diseases
Perelman School of Medicine at the University of Pennsylvania;
Medical Director and Hospital Epidemiologist
Infection Prevention and Control
Children's Hospital of Philadelphia
Philadelphia, Pennsylvania

Pablo Sánchez, MD
Prinicipal Investigator
Center for Perinatal Research
Fellow, Infectious Diseases
Fellow, Neonatology
Nationwide Children's Hospital
Columbus, Ohio

Linette Sande, MD
Assistant Professor of Pediatrics
Department of Pediatric Infectious Diseases
Loma Linda University;
Attending Physician
Department of Pediatric Infectious Diseases
Loma Linda University Children's Hospital
Loma Linda, California

Javier Santisteban-Ponce, MD
Attending Physician
Pediatric Infectious Disease Unit
Department of Pediatrics
Hospital Nacional Edgardo Rebagliati Martins-EsSalud;
Lima, Peru

Laura A. Sass, MD
Assistant Professor
Department of Pediatrics
Eastern Virginia Medical School;
Attending Physician
Department of Pediatric Infectious Diseases
Medical Director, Infection Prevention and Control, Antiobiotic Stewardship
Children's Hospital of The King's Daughters
Norfolk, Virginia

Stephen J. Scholand, MD
Associate Professor
Department of Medicine
Frank Netter School of Medicine
Quinnipiac University
North Haven, Connecticut

Danica J. Schulte, MD
Assistant Professor in Residence
Department of Pediatrics
University of California–Los Angeles;
Assistant Professor
Departments of Pediatrics, Pediatric Infectious Diseases, Immunology and Allergy
Cedars-Sinai Medical Center
Los Angeles, California

Jennifer E. Schuster, MD, MSCI
Assistant Professor
Department of Pediatrics
Children's Mercy Kansas City
Kansas City, Missouri

Gordon E. Schutze, MD, FAAP
Professor of Pediatrics
Executive Vice Chairman
Martin I. Lorin, MD, Endowed Chair in Medical Education
Department of Pediatrics
Baylor College of Medicine;
Vice President, International Programs
Baylor International Pediatric AIDS Initiative at Texas Children's Hospital
Houston, Texas

Patrick C. Seed, MD, PhD
Assistant Professor
Department of Pediatrics/Pediatric Infectious Diseases
Duke University School of Medicine;
Assistant Professor
Department of Molecular Genetics and Microbiology
Duke University School of Medicine
Durham, North Carolina

Jose A. Serpa, MD, MS
Associate Professor
Department of Medicine
Baylor College of Medicine
Houston, Texas

Samir S. Shah, MD, MSCE
Professor
Department of Pediatrics
University of Cincinnati College of Medicine;
Director, Division of Hospital Medicine
Attending Physician
Divisions of Infectious Diseases and Hospital Medicine
James M. Ewell Endowed Chair
Cincinnati Children's Hospital Medical Center
Cincinnati, Ohio

Eugene D. Shapiro, MD
Professor
Departments of Pediatrics, Epidemiology of Microbial Diseases, and Investigative Medicine
Yale University
New Haven, Connecticut

Nina L. Shapiro, MD
Professor, Department of Head and Neck Surgery
Director, Division of Pediatric Otolaryngology
David Geffen School of Medicine at UCLA
Los Angeles, California

William T. Shearer, MD, PhD
Professor of Pediatrics and Pathology and Immunology
Distinguished Service Professor
Baylor College of Medicine;
Allergy and Immunology Service
Texas Children's Hospital
Houston, Texas

Robyn Shimizu-Cohen, CLS(ASCP)
Specialist
Department of Pathology and Laboratory Medicine
University of California–Los Angeles
Los Angeles, California

Stanford T. Shulman, MD
Chief Emeritus, Division of Infectious Diseases
Ann & Robert H. Lurie Children's Hospital of Chicago
Virginia H. Rogers Professor of Pediatric Infectious Diseases
Northwestern University Feinberg School of Medicine
Chicago, Illinois

Kareem W. Shehab, MD
Assistant Professor
Department of Pediatrics
Section of Infectious Disease
University of Arizona
Tucson, Arizona

Ziad M. Shehab, MD
Professor of Pediatrics and Pathology
University of Arizona
Tucson, Arizona

Constantine Simos, DMD
Attending Surgeon
Oral and Maxillofacial Surgery
Robert Wood Johnson University Hospital
Saint Peter's University Hospital
New Brunswick, New Jersey;
Assistant Clinical Professor
Oral and Maxillofacial Surgery
Columbia University College of Dental Medicine
New York, New York

Michael A. Smit, MD, MSPH
Division of Pediatric Infectious Diseases
Hasbro Children's Hospital
Assistant Professor
Department of Pediatrics
Alpert Medical School of Brown University
Providence, Rhode Island

P. Brian Smith, MD, MPH, MHS
Professor of Pediatrics
Duke University Medical Center
Duke Clinical Research Institute
Durham, North Carolina

Priya R. Soni, MD
Fellow, Pediatric Infectious Disease
Mattel Children's Hospital
University of California–Los Angeles
Los Angeles, California

Sunil K. Sood, MBBS, DCH, MD
Professor
Departments of Pediatrics and Family Medicine
Hofstra Northwell School of Medicine
Hempstead, New York;
Chair of Pediatrics
Southside Hospital, Northwell Health
Bay Shore, New York;
Attending Physician
Pediatric Infectious Diseases
Cohen Children's Medical Center
New Hyde Park, New York

Mary Allen Staat, MD, MPH
Professor
Department of Pediatrics
University of Cincinnati College of Medicine;
Director
International Adoption Center
Cincinnati Children's Hospital Medical Center
Cincinnati, Ohio

Damien Stark, MSc, PhD, FASM, FACTM
Associate, Department of Medical and Molecular Biosciences
University of Technology Sydney
Broadway, NSW, Australia;
Senior Hospital Scientist
Department of Microbiology
St. Vincent's Hospital
Darlinghurst, NSW, Australia

Jeffrey R. Starke, MD
Professor
Department of Pediatrics
Baylor College of Medicine
Houston, Texas

Victoria A. Statler, MD, MSc
Assistant Professor
Department of Pediatric Infectious Diseases
University of Louisville
Louisville, Kentucky

Barbara W. Stechenberg, MD
Pediatric Infectious Diseases Specialist
Department of Pediatrics
Baystate Children's Hospital
Springfield, Massachusetts;
Professor Emerita of Pediatrics
Department of Pediatrics
Tufts University School of Medicine
Boston, Massachusetts

William J. Steinbach, MD
Professor of Pediatrics
Professor in Molecular Genetics and Microbiology
Chief, Pediatric Infectious Diseases
Director, Duke Pediatric Immunocompromised Host Program
Director, International Pediatric Fungal Network
Duke University School of Medicine
Durham, North Carolina

Joseph W. St. Geme III, MD
Professor of Pediatrics and Microbiology
Chair, Department of Pediatrics
Perelman School of Medicine at the University of Pennsylvania;
Chair, Department of Pediatrics
Physician-in-Chief
Children's Hospital of Philadelphia
Philadelphia, Pennsylvania

Jeffrey Suen, MD
Private Practice
Bakersfield, California

Lillian Sung, MD, PhD
Professor
Division of Haematology/Oncology
Hospital for Sick Children
Toronto, ON, Canada

Douglas S. Swanson, MD
Associate Professor of Pediatrics
Department of Pediatric Infectious Diseases
Children's Mercy Kansas City;
Associate Professor of Pediatrics
University of Missouri–Kansas City
Kansas City, Missouri

Tina Q. Tan, MD
Professor
Department of Pediatrics
Feinberg School of Medicine
Northwestern University;
Infectious Diseases Attending Physician
Department of Pediatrics
Ann & Robert H. Lurie Children's Hospital
Chicago, Illinois

Ruston S. Taylor, PharmD
Department of Pharmacy
Legacy Community Health
Houston, Texas

Michael A. Tolle, MD, MPH
Assistant Professor
Department of Pediatrics
Retrovirology and Global Health Section
International Pediatrics AIDS Initiative (BIPAI)
Baylor College of Medicine Children's Foundation
Texas Children's Hospital
Houston, Texas;
Tanzania Buganda Medical Centre
Mwanza, Tanzania

Philip Toltzis, MD
Professor
Department of Pediatrics
Rainbow Babies and Children's Hospital
Cleveland, Ohio

Stuart R. Tomko, MD
Division of Child Neurology
Texas Children's Hospital
Houston, Texas

Michael F. Tosi, MD
Professor of Pediatrics
Division of Pediatric Infectious Diseases
Mount Sinai School of Medicine
New York, New York

Leidy J. Tovar Padua, MD
Fellow
Division of Pediatric Infectious Diseases
Mattel Children's Hospital of UCLA
Los Angeles, California

Amelia P.A. Travassos da Rosa, BSc
Research Associate
Center for Tropical Diseases
Department of Pathology
University of Texas Medical Branch
Galveston, Texas

Theodore F. Tsai, MD, MPH
Senior Vice President, Scientific Affairs
Novartis Vaccines
Cambridge, Massachusetts

Andrew M. Vahabzadeh-Hagh, MD
Resident
Department of Head and Neck Surgery
David Geffen School of Medicine at UCLA
Los Angeles, California

Jorge J. Velarde, MD, PhD
Instructor
Division of Infectious Diseases
Boston Children's Hospital
Boston, Massachusetts

Jesus G. Vallejo, MD
Associate Professor
Department of Pediatric Infectious Diseases
Baylor College of Medicine
Houston, Texas

John A. Vanchiere, MD, PhD
Professor and Chief
Section of Pediatric Infectious Diseases
Louisiana State University Health Sciences Center
Shreveport, Louisiana

Robert S. Venick, MD
Associate Professor
Departments of Pediatrics and Surgery
David Geffin School of Medicine at UCLA
Los Angeles, California

Sanjay Verma, MBBS, MD
Additional Professor of Pediatrics
Advanced Pediatrics Centre
Postgraduate Institute of Medical Education and Research
Chandigarh, India

James Versalovic, MD, PhD
Pathologist-in-Chief
Department of Pathology
Texas Children's Hospital;
Milton J. Finegold Professor
Department of Pathology and Immunology
Baylor College of Medicine
Houston, Texas

Timo Vesikari, MD, PhD
Director
Vaccine Research Center
University of Tampere
Tampere, Finland

Ellen R. Wald, MD
Chair, Department of Pediatrics
University of Wisconsin School of Medicine & Public Health;
Pediatrician-in-Chief
American Family Children's Hospital
Madison, Wisconsin

Thomas J. Walsh, MD
Director, Transplantation-Oncology Infectious Diseases Program
Weill Cornell Medical Center of Cornell University
New York, New York

Mark A. Ward, MD
Associate Professor
Department of Pediatrics
Baylor College of Medicine
Houston, Texas

Rachel L. Wattier, MD, MHS
Assistant Clinical Professor
Department of Pediatrics
University of California–San Francisco
San Francisco, California

Sing Sing Way, MD, PhD
Professor of Pediatrics
Pauline and Lawson Reed Chair
Division of Infectious Diseases
Cincinnati Children's Hospital
University of Cincinnati College of Medicine
Cincinnati, Ohio

Jill Weatherhead, MD
Assistant Professor of Infectious Diseases and Pediatrics
National School of Tropical Medicine
Baylor College of Medicine
Houston, Texas

Michelle Weinberg, MD, MPH
Medical Epidemiologist
Immigrant, Refugee, and Migrant Health Branch
Division of Global Migration and Quarantine
Centers for Disease Control and Prevention
Atlanta, Georgia

Nicholas Weinberg, MD
Assistant Professor
Department of Emergency Medicine
Geisel School of Medicine
Dartmouth-Hitchcock Medical Center
Hanover, New Hampshire

Melanie Wellington, MD, PhD
Associate Professor
Department of Pediatrics
University of Rochester Medical Center
Rochester, New York

Robert C. Welliver Sr, MD
Professor of Pediatrics
Division of Pediatric Infectious Diseases
University of Oklahoma Health Sciences Center
Oklahoma City, Oklahoma;
Emeritus Professor of Pediatrics
Division of Pediatric Infectious Diseases
SUNY at Buffalo and Children's Hospital
Buffalo, New York

J. Gary Wheeler, MD, MPS
Professor of Pediatrics
Division of Infectious Diseases
University of Arkansas for Medical Sciences
Little Rock, Arkansas

A. Clinton White Jr, MD
Professor, Division of Infectious Disease
Department of Internal Medicine
University of Texas Medical Branch
Galveston, Texas

Suzanne Whitworth, MD
Medical Director
Department of Pediatric Infectious Diseases
Cook Children's Healthcare System
Fort Worth, Texas

Bernhard L. Wiedermann, MD, MA
Professor
Department of Pediatrics
George Washington University School of Medicine and Health Sciences;
Attending Physician
Division of Infectious Diseases
Children's National Health System
Washington, DC

John V. Williams, MD
Professor and Chief
Pediatric Infectious Diseases
Henry L. Hillman Chair in Pediatric Immunology
Children's Hospital of Pittsburgh of UPMC
Pittsburgh, Pennsylvania

Natalie M. Williams-Bouyer, PhD, D(ABMM)
Associate Professor, Department of Pathology
Associate Director, Division of Clinical Microbiology
University of Texas Medical Branch;
Clinical Consultant, Clinical Laboratory Services
Shriners Hospitals for Children
Galveston, Texas

Charles R. Woods Jr, MD, MS
Professor and Vice Chair for Faculty Development
Department of Pediatrics
University of Louisville School of Medicine
Louisville, Kentucky

Terry W. Wright, PhD
Associate Professor
Department of Pediatrics
University of Rochester Medical Center
Rochester, New York

Nave Yeganeh, MD, MPH
Assistant Professor
Department of Pediatrics
Division of Pediatric Infectious Diseases
David Geffen School of Medicine at UCLA
Los Angeles, California

Edward J. Young, MD
Professor of Medicine
Baylor College of Medicine
Houston, Texas

Ramia Zakhour, MD
Clinical Instructor
Department of Pediatrics and Adolescent Medicine
Division of Pediatric Infectious Diseases
American University of Beirut
Beirut, Lebanon

Theoklis Zaoutis, MD, MSCE
Professor of Pediatrics and Epidemiology
Perelman School of Medicine at the University of Pennsylvania;
Associate Chief
Division of Infectious Diseases
Children's Hospital of Philadelphia
Philadelphia, Pennsylvania

Preface

Morbidity and mortality rates related to infectious diseases decreased dramatically during the first half of the 20th century in the developed world because of major improvements in public health (e.g., clean water, adequate sanitation, and vector control) and personal health. Further major reductions occurred in the second half of that century following the introduction of antimicrobial therapy, as well as active and passive immunization efforts. Despite these advances, infectious diseases in the developed world remain the leading cause of morbidity in infants and children in the 21st century. Children in the United States continue to experience three to nine respiratory infections and one to three gastrointestinal illnesses annually, requiring visits to physicians that outnumber the visits made for the purpose of well-child care. Infectious diseases are also the most common cause of school absenteeism.

Children in low and middle income countries also experience high rates of respiratory and gastrointestinal infections, which are often more severe and more frequent than those in children in the developed world. In addition, in the developing world there are great morbidity and mortality due to parasitic and vector-borne diseases. Also of importance are "spillover" infectious diseases such as Ebola, which because of increased urbanization resulted in an extensive epidemic in three African countries in 2014–15. In addition, mosquito-borne diseases such as Zika and Chikungunya have increased in prevalence in the Americas.

In more recent years, the emergence of resistance to multiple antibiotics by a large number of bacterial microorganisms (e.g., community-associated methicillin-resistant *Staphylococcus aureus*) has contributed to this infection-related morbidity and mortality, as have new infectious agents (e.g., SARS and MERS coronaviruses) and changes in the clinical manifestations and severity of established infectious agents (e.g., enterovirus 71, swine influenza).

The first edition of *Textbook of Pediatric Infectious Diseases* was written because Drs. Feigin and Cherry and many of their colleagues were concerned that no single reference text existed that comprehensively covered infectious diseases in children and adolescents. With each subsequent edition, including this one, the goal has been to provide comprehensive coverage of all subjects pertinent to the study of infectious diseases in children. Any attempt to summarize our present understanding of infectious diseases for serious students of the subject is a formidable task. In many areas, new information continues to accrue so rapidly that material becomes dated before it can appear in a text of this magnitude. Nevertheless, in this edition the editors and their author colleagues have endeavored to provide the most comprehensive and up-to-date discussion of pediatric infectious diseases ever compiled. This new edition is available online as well as in print. Purchasers can access the online version by registering their personal identification number (PIN) (found on the inside front cover of the book) at expertconsult.inkling.com. Online access includes not only fully searchable text, photos, illustrations, and tables, but also references linked to PubMed.

To provide a text as comprehensive and authoritative as possible, we, the editors, have enlisted contributions from a large number of individuals whose collective expertise is responsible for whatever success we may have had in meeting our objective. We offer our most profound appreciation to the 307 fellow contributors from nearly 100 universities or institutions in 18 countries for their professional expertise and devoted scholarship. Their cooperation and willingness to work with us leave us deeply in their debt. Of note is the fact that 10 authors (Carol Baker, Ken Boyer, Jim Cherry, Morven Edwards, Chuck Grose, Scott Halstead, Maggie Hammerschlag, Shelly Kaplan, Ed Mason, and Barbara Stechenberg) have contributed to all eight editions of *Textbook of Pediatric Infectious Diseases.*

Once again, infectious diseases are discussed according to organ systems that may be affected, as well as individually by microorganisms. In all sections in which diseases related to specific agents are discussed, emphasis has been placed, to the greatest extent possible, on the specificity of clinical manifestations that may be related to the organism causing the disease. Detailed information regarding the best means to establish a diagnosis and explicit recommendations for therapy are provided. In the present era of instant information, we have noted that historical perspectives relating to disease categories, as well as specific agents, are ignored. Because history is an important teacher, we have retained relevant historical details in this eighth edition.

Throughout the 37 years and eight-edition history of the *Textbook of Pediatric Infectious Diseases,* a number of classic chapters exist (e.g., measles, rubella, enteroviruses, and mycoplasma infections). The data in these chapters are unavailable in any other single-source publication.

The entire text of this eighth edition has been revised extensively. The seventh edition contained almost 4000 pages even though we included only new references in the print edition, which is close to the maximum that can be included in a two-volume book. Therefore, with this eighth edition, we were faced with a major dilemma: specifically, how to include new important material that had become available since the seventh edition but not to substantially increase the size of the book. We approached this dilemma in two ways. One problem in previous editions was redundancy, which we have addressed by combining information in some previous separate chapters into more concise single presentations and by shortening some chapters. The second way, which we introduced in the last edition, is to print only new references. The electronic version of the text contains all references.

This edition continues the format that was initiated in the fourth edition, in that infections with specific microorganisms have been organized to provide appropriate emphasis on the common features that may relate specific microorganisms to one another. Thus, all gram-positive coccal organisms are presented sequentially and are followed by gram-negative cocci, gram-positive bacilli, enterobacteria, gram-negative coccobacilli, Treponemataceae, anaerobic bacteria, and so forth. In addition, special sections of the text have been devoted to discussions of each of the following: molecular determinants of microbial pathogenesis; immunologic and phagocytic responses to infection; metabolic response of the host to infections; interaction of infection and nutrition; pathogenesis and treatment of fever; the human microbiome; epidemiology and biostatistics of infectious diseases; infections of the compromised host; Kawasaki disease; chronic fatigue syndrome; international travel issues for children; infectious disease problems of international adoptees and refugees; nosocomial infections; prevention and control of infections in hospitalized children; pharmacology and pharmacokinetics of antibacterial, antiviral, antifungal, and antiparasitic agents; immunomodulating agents; active and passive immunizing agents; public health considerations; infections in day care environments; and use of the bacteriology, mycology, parasitology, virology, and serology laboratories. The section on infections in the compromised host has again been expanded. This expansion has been necessitated by the large number of children, particularly transplant recipients, who have many infectious disease problems and constitute a large part of the consulting practice of many pediatric infectious disease physicians.

With some sadness, we have retained a section on bioterrorism, which is necessitated by the current state of world affairs. The section on immunomodulating agents and their potential use in the treatment of infectious diseases has been expanded because information on this subject has become more extensive since the publication of the last edition. We have also expanded the section on Ebola virus and included a new chapter on Zika virus.

This project could not have been brought to fruition without the help and assistance of many people whose names do not appear in the text. No words are sufficient to adequately convey our gratitude appropriately; we hope that they know they have our heartfelt thanks.

We would like to single out certain individuals for specific mention. First and foremost, we convey our appreciation to Laura Wennstrom Sheehan for the many hours she devoted to this edition. In her spare time between her position as Manager of Research Administration for the UCLA Department of Family Medicine and raising her young daughter, she coordinated the overall process of moving the book forward. She tended to numerous details relating to copyediting, transcribing, references, timing, and communication between the editors and Elsevier. Her expertise in EndNote was invaluable to the authors, editors, and publishing team for the organization of countless references throughout this edition. We are extremely grateful to have her as a part of our team. We would also like to acknowledge the hard work of Jordan Mann who assisted Laura throughout this process.

The following students at UCLA played a key role in processing chapters and in particular helping with references: Lauren M. Nguyen, David Dang, and Jewel Powe. We would also like to thank Nathaniel Wilder Wolf at Baylor who coordinated all the parasite chapters.

Of course this eighth edition of *Textbook of Pediatric Infectious Diseases* would not have been possible without Elsevier. We have been particularly fortunate to have been able to work with Kate Dimock, Executive Content Strategist, Clinical Solutions at Elsevier throughout the whole process relating to this eighth edition. In addition, the initial planning contribution by Lauren Elise Boyle, Content Development Specialist, was invaluable. This was followed-up by the day-to-day contributions of Margaret Nelson, also a Content Development Specialist at Elsevier. Margaret kept everyone on track in meeting deadlines.

Finally, we thank the Baylor College of Medicine and Texas Children's Hospital in Houston, Texas, the David Geffen School of Medicine at UCLA and the Mattel Children's Hospital UCLA in Los Angeles, California, and Duke University School of Medicine in Durham, North Carolina for providing an environment that is supportive of intellectual pursuits.

James D. Cherry, MD
Gail J. Harrison, MD
Sheldon L. Kaplan, MD
William J. Steinbach, MD
Peter J. Hotez, MD

Contents

VOLUME ONE

PART I Host-Parasite Relationships and the Pathogenesis of Infectious Diseases

PART II Infection of Specific Organ Systems

SECTION 1 Upper Respiratory Tract Infections

SECTION 2 Lower Respiratory Tract Infections

SECTION 3 Infections of the Heart

SECTION 4 Central Nervous System Infections

SECTION 5 Genitourinary Tract Infections

Classification and Nomenclature of Viruses

151

Marjorie J. Miller

Viruses originally were differentiated from other microorganisms by their small size and their filterability. Initial efforts to classify viruses were based on disease, pathogenesis, organ tropisms, and epidemiologic characteristics rather than on physicochemical properties of the virus particle. During the 1950s and 1960s, many new viruses were being discovered while evidence of virus structure and composition also was emerging, thereby prompting proposals that viruses be grouped on the basis of shared virion properties. The herpesvirus,[1] myxovirus,[2] and poxvirus[6] groups were among the first taxonomic groups delineated. As more information concerning the physicochemical characteristics of viruses accumulated, the need for a universal system of classification and nomenclature became apparent.

The International Committee on Nomenclature of Viruses was established in 1966 at the International Congress of Microbiology in Moscow, some 20 years after a bacterial taxonomy first was published and 75 years after the discovery of viruses. In 1973, the International Committee on Nomenclature of Viruses became the International Committee on Taxonomy of Viruses (ICTV), which operates under the auspices of the Virology Division of the International Union of Microbiological Societies. The ICTV classifies viruses isolated from vertebrates, invertebrates, plants, fungi, protozoa, bacteria, and mycoplasmas and publishes periodic reports summarizing the most recent developments in viral taxonomy.[5,7,8,10,11,13,17–19] Interim updates were published in *Intervirology* and more recently in *Archives of Virology.* The most updated information on virus taxonomy can be accessed through the Internet (http://www.ICTVonline.org and http://www.ncbi.nlm.nih.gov).

The hierarchical levels of virus taxonomy consist of order, family, subfamily, genus, and species and are based on the structural, physicochemical, biologic, and replicative properties of viruses.[13] Structural characteristics include size, shape, presence or absence of an envelope, and capsid symmetry. Physicochemical characterization is based on type, strandedness, and the number of segments of nucleic acid, as well as the number and size of proteins and their functional activities. Biologic properties include host range, serologic relationships, pathogenicity, and transmission; replicative properties include nucleic acid replication, transcription, and translation.

Virus orders comprise groups of families that share common characteristics (e.g., biochemical composition, viral replication strategy, particle structure, and general genomic organization) distinguishable from those of other orders and families. Virus orders are designated with the suffix *-virales.* Currently, the ICTV has approved six orders, four comprising viruses affecting humans: *Herpesvirales*, family *Herpesviridae*; *Mononegavirales*, which includes the families *Paramyxoviridae*, *Rhabdoviridae*, and *Filoviridae*; *Nidovirales*, which comprises the families *Coronaviridae* and *Arteriviridae*; and *Picornavirales*, family *Picornaviridae.*

Virus families represent groups of genera that share common characteristics distinct from those of other families. Virus families are designated with the suffix *-viridae.* Most families have unique virion morphology, genome structure, or strategies of replication (Fig. 151.1). Virus subfamilies are designated with the suffix *-virinae* and have been introduced in seven families: *Coronaviridae* (*Coronovirinae*, *Torovirinae*), *Herpesviridae* (*Alphaherpesvirinae*, *Betaherpesvirinae*, *Gammaherpesvirinae*), *Paramyxoviridae* (*Paramyxovirinae*, *Pneumovirinae*), *Parvoviridae* (*Parvovirinae*), *Poxviridae* (*Chorodopoxvirinae*), *Reoviridae* (*Sedoreovirinae*, *Spinareovirinae*), and *Retroviridae* (*Orthoretrovirinae*, *Spumaretrovirinae*) (Table 151.1).

Virus genera consist of groups of species that share common characteristics different from those of members of other genera. Common properties within a genus include viral replication strategy, genome size, organization, numbers of segments, sequence homologies, and vector transmission. Virus genera are designated with the suffix *-virus.*

The species taxon is the most fundamental unit in biologic classification, but the viruses have proved to be the most difficult to classify, and years elapsed before a definition of virus species was accepted internationally. In 1991, the ICTV accepted the definition of a virus species proposed by van Regenmortel[14]: "A virus species is defined as a polythetic class of viruses that constitutes a replicating lineage and occupies a particular ecological niche." Members of a polythetic class have several properties in common, although no single common attribute is present in all members, thereby accommodating the inherent variability of viruses. Common species properties include genome rearrangement, sequence homologies, serologic relationships, vector transmission, host range, pathogenicity, tissue tropism, and geographic distribution.[8,17] Some properties of viruses used in taxonomy are listed in Box 151.1.[13]

The ICTV also has established criteria for formal virus nomenclature[8,9,17] and recommended abbreviations for virus names.[4,8,9,17] In formal taxonomic usage, the names of orders, families, subfamilies, genera, and species are printed in italics, and the first letter of the name is capitalized. This form applies when using a species name to refer to a taxonomic category (e.g., in the Materials and Methods section of a paper when describing the particular virus used in the study). Some examples of formal taxonomic terminology are *Poliovirus*, genus *Enterovirus*, family *Picornaviridae* or *Human herpesvirus 1* (herpes simplex virus type 1) and genus *Simplexvirus*, subfamily *Alphaherpesvirinae*, family *Herpesviridae.* Thereafter, vernacular names can be used throughout the publication. In informal vernacular usage when referring to virions or virus particles or if used as an adjective, italics and capital initial letters are not required and the names are written in lowercase Roman script (e.g., "poliovirus cytopathic effect" or "picornaviruses/polioviruses were inoculated into cell culture").[8,9,15,16] Viruses with uncertain taxonomic status are considered "tentative" species, and names are not italicized, although the initial letter is capitalized. Although not part of the formal international code, abbreviations also have been recommended by the ICTV for every virus name to reduce the possibility of duplication when new abbreviations are proposed[4,8,17] (see Table 151.1).

Fig. 151.2 is a schematic diagram showing the basic forms and composition of viruses.[3] The type of nucleic acid, capsid symmetry, presence or absence of an envelope, and peplomers (spikes) all are characteristics used in classification. Fig. 151.1 is a more detailed diagram not only illustrating the relative shapes and sizes of families and genera of vertebrate viruses but also indicating the type and nature (single-stranded [ss], double-stranded [ds], sense [+/–]) of the nucleic acid, presence of reverse transcriptase (RT), and presence or absence of an envelope.

Fig. 151.3 and Fig. 151.4 show classification of DNA and RNA virus families,[12] respectively, by some of the taxonomic characteristics listed in Box 151.1. Representative DNA and RNA viruses affecting humans are listed in Table 151.1, which uses the most recent nomenclature reported by the ICTV (for a complete listing, see King and colleagues[8]).

The full reference list for this chapter is available at expertconsult.com.

Families and Genera of Viruses Infecting Vertebrates

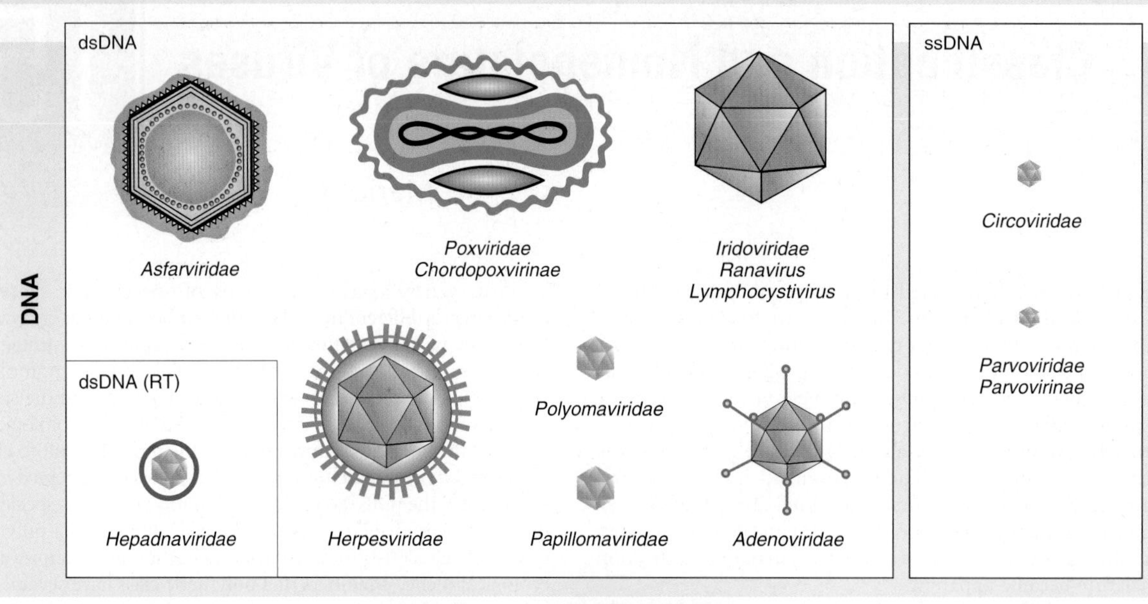

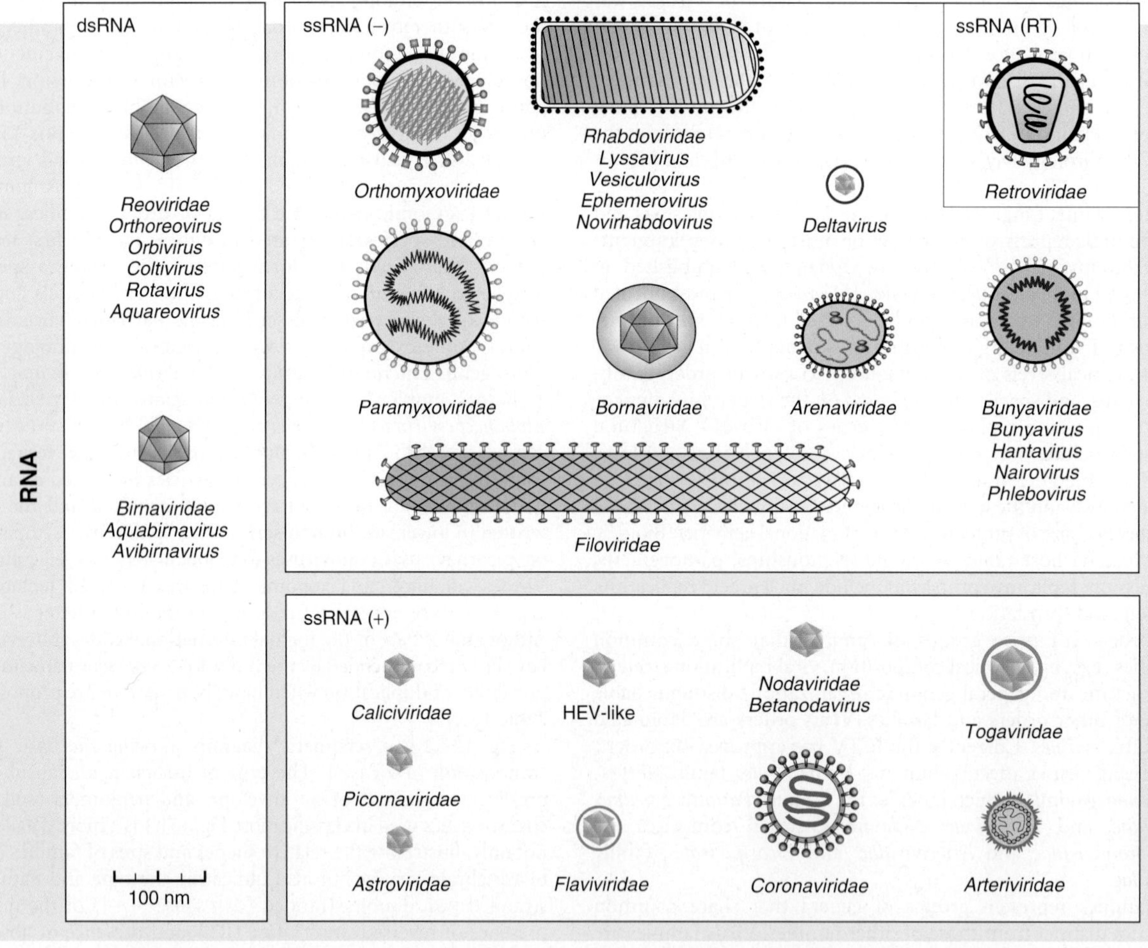

FIG. 151.1 Shapes and relative sizes of animal viruses of the major families. (From Van Regenmortel MHV, Fauquet CM, Bishop DHL, et al, editors. *Virus taxonomy: classification and nomenclature of viruses. Seventh report of the International Committee on Taxonomy of Viruses.* San Diego, CA: Academic Press; 2000:30.)

TABLE 151.1 **Classification and Nomenclature of Representative Viruses Affecting Humans**

Family	Subfamily	Genus	Representative Species Pathogenic for Humans (Abbreviation, Common Examples, Disease, Synonym, or No. of Members)
DNA Viruses			
Poxviridae	*Chordopoxvirinae*	*Orthopoxvirus*	Vaccinia virus (VACV)
			Variola virus (VARV)
		Parapoxvirus	Orf virus (ORFH, contagious pustular dermatitis)
			Pseudocowpox virus (PCPV, milker's nodule)
		Molluscipoxvirus	*Molluscum contagiosum* virus (MOCV)
		Yatapoxvirus	Yaba monkey tumor virus, tanapox virus (YMTV, TANV)
Herpesviridae	*Alphaherpesvirinae*	*Simplexvirus*	Human herpesvirus 1 (HHV-1, herpes simplex virus type 1)
			Human herpesvirus 2 (HHV-2, herpes simplex virus type 2)
			Macacine herpesvirus 1 (McHV-1, monkey B virus)
		Varicellovirus	Human herpesvirus 3 (HHV-3, varicella-zoster virus)
	Betaherpesvirinae	*Cytomegalovirus*	Human herpesvirus 5 (HHV-5, cytomegalovirus)
		Roseolovirus	Human herpesvirus 6A and 6B (HHV-6, human B lymphotropic virus)
			Human herpesvirus 7 (HHV-7)
	Gammaherpesvirinae	*Lymphocryptovirus*	Human herpesvirus 4 (HHV-4, Epstein-Barr virus)
		Rhadinovirus	Human herpesvirus 8 (HHV-8, Kaposi sarcoma–associated herpesvirus)
Adenoviridae		*Mastadenovirus*	Human mastadenovirus A (HAdV-A; 12, 18, 31)
			Human mastadenovirus B (HAdV-B; 3, 7, 11, 14, 16, 21, 34, 35, 50, 55)
			Human mastadenovirus C (HAdV-C; 1, 2, 5, 6, 57)
			Human mastadenovirus D (HAdV-D; 8–10, 13, 15, 17, 19, 20, 22–30, 32, 33, 36–39, 42–49, 51, 53, 54, 56)
			Human mastadenovirus E (HAdV-E; 4)
			Human mastadenovirus F (HAdV-F; 40, 41)
			Human mastadenovirus G (HAdV-G; 52)
Papillomaviridae		*Alphapapillomavirus*	Alphapapillomavirus 7 (HPV 18, 39, 45, 59, 68, 70, 85, 97)
			Alphapapillomavirus 9 (HPV 16, 31, 33, 35, 52, 58, 67)
		Betapapillomavirus	Betapapillomavirus 1 (HPV 5, 8, 12, 14, 19–21, 25, 36, 47, 93)
		Gammapapillomavirus	Gammapapillomavirus 1 (HPV 4, 65, 95)
Polyomaviridae		*Polyomavirus*	BK polyomavirus (BKPyV, polyomavirus hominis 1)
			JC polyomavirus (JCPyV, polyomavirus hominis 2)
Parvoviridae	*Parvovirinae*	*Bocaparvovirus*	Human bocavirus (HBoV)
		Erythroparvovirus	Human parvovirus B19 (B19V, erythema infectiosum or fifth disease)
Hepadnaviridae		*Orthohepadnavirus*	Hepatitis B virus (HBV)
Hepeviridae		*Hepevirus*	Hepatitis E virus (HEV, enterically transmitted non-A, non-B)
RNA Viruses			
Reoviridae	*Sedoreovirinae*	*Orbivirus*	Changuinola virus (CGLV); Great Island virus (GIV)
		Rotavirus	Rotavirus A–H (RV)
	Spinarevirinae	*Coltivirus*	Colorado tick fever virus (CTFV)
Bornaviridae		*Bornavirus*	Borna disease virus (BDV)
Paramyxoviridae	*Paramyxovirinae*	*Henipavirus*	Hendravirus, Nipahvirus
		Morbillivirus	Measles virus (MeV)
		Respirovirus	Human parainfluenza virus 1 and 3 (HPIV-1, HPIV-3)
		Rubulavirus	Mumps virus (MUV), human parainfluenza virus 2 (HPIV-2) and 4 (HPIV-4a and b)
	Pneumovirinae	*Pneumovirus*	Human respiratory syncytial virus (HRSV)
		Metapneumovirus	Human metapneumovirus (HMPV)
Rhabdoviridae		*Vesiculovirus*	Vesicular stomatitis Indiana virus (VSIV)
		Lyssavirus	Rabies virus (RABV)
Filoviridae		*Marburgvirus*	Marburg marburgvirus (LVMARV, Lake Victoria)
		Ebolavirus	Zaire ebolavirus (ZEBOV), Reston ebolavirus (REBOV)
Orthomyxoviridae		*Influenzavirus A*	Influenza A virus (FLUAV)
		Influenzavirus B	Influenza B virus (FLUBV)
		Influenzavirus C	Influenza C virus (FLUCV)
Bunyaviridae		*Orthobunyavirus*	Bunyamwera virus (BUNV, Bunyamwera serogroup), California encephalitis virus (CEV, California serogroup) (mosquito and culicid fly transmitted)
		Hantavirus	Hantaan virus (HTNV, Korean hemorrhagic fever or hemorrhagic fever with renal syndrome), Sin Nombre virus (SNV, Four Corners hantavirus, hantavirus pulmonary syndrome), and others (rodent associated)
		Nairovirus	Crimean-Congo hemorrhagic fever virus (CCHFV; tick transmitted)
		Phlebovirus	Sandfly fever Naples virus (SFNV), Rift Valley fever virus (RVFV) (sandfly-borne primarily); Uukuniemi virus (UUKV) (phlebotomine, tick, and mosquito transmitted)
Arenaviridae		*Mammarenavirus*	Lymphocytic choriomeningitis mammarenavirus (LCMV)
			Lassa mammarenavirus (LASV)
			Junin mammarenavirus (JUNV, Argentine hemorrhagic fever virus)
			Machupo mammarenavirus (MAVC, Bolivian hemorrhagic fever virus)

Continued

TABLE 151.1 Classification and Nomenclature of Representative Viruses Affecting Humans—cont'd

Family	Subfamily	Genus	Representative Species Pathogenic for Humans (Abbreviation, Common Examples, Disease, Synonym, or No. of Members)
Picornaviridae		*Aphthovirus*	Foot-and-mouth disease virus
		Enterovirus	Enterovirus A (EV-A, 25 serotypes; coxsackieviruses A2, 8, 10, 12, 14, 16; enterovirus A 71, 76, 89–92, 114, 119–121)
			Enterovirus B (EV-B, 63 serotypes; coxsackieviruses B1–B6; coxsackievirus A9, 23; echovirus 1–21, 24–27, 29–33; enterovirus B, 28 serotypes)
			Enterovirus C (EV-C, 23 serotypes; coxsackieviruses A1, 11, 13, 17, 19–22, 24; PV, polioviruses 1–3; human enterovirus C, 11 serotypes)
			Enterovirus D (EV-D, 5 serotypes; enterovirus D68, 70, 94, 111, 120)
			Rhinoviruses A , B, and C (RV-A, B, C; 167 serotypes)
		Parechovirus	Parechovirus A (HPeV, 1–16; human parechovirus 1, formerly echovirus 22; human parechovirus 5, formerly echovirus 23)
		Hepatovirus	Hepatovirus A (HAV, enterovirus 72)
Caliciviridae		*Norovirus*	Norwalk virus (NoV, genogroups I, II, IV; >25 genotypes)
		Sapovirus	Sapporo virus (SaV, genogroups I, II, IV, V)
Astroviridae		*Mamastrovirus*	Mamastrovirus 1, 6, 8, 9 (MAstV)
Coronaviridae	*Coronavirinae*	*Alphacoronavirus*	Human coronavirus 229E (HCoV-229E); human coronavirus NL63 (HCoV-NL63)
		Betacoronavirus	Human coronavirus HKU1 (HCoV-HKU1); human coronavirus OC43 (HCoV-OC43); severe acute respiratory syndrome–related virus (SARS-CoV); Middle East respiratory syndrome (MERS-CoV)
Flaviviridae		*Flavivirus*	St. Louis encephalitis virus (SLEV), yellow fever virus (YFV), dengue virus (DENV), and West Nile virus (WNV), Zika virus (ZIKV) group B arboviruses (mosquito-borne)
			Kyasanur Forest disease virus (KFDV), tick-borne encephalitis virus (TBEV) (tick-borne)
			Vector-unassociated viruses
		Hepacivirus	Hepatitis C virus (HCV, parenterally transmitted non-A, non-B hepatitis)
Togaviridae		*Alphavirus*	Western, Eastern, and Venezuelan equine encephalitis viruses (WEEV, EEEV, VEEV); Ross River and Sindbis viruses (RRV, SINV; group A arboviruses, mosquito-borne)
		Rubivirus	Rubella virus (RUBV)
Retroviridae	*Orthoretrovirinae*	*Deltaretrovirus*	Primate T-cell lymphotropic viruses 1–3 (simian T-lymphotropic viruses, STLV 1–3; human T-lymphotropic viruses, HTLV 1–3)
		Lentivirus	Human immunodeficiency viruses 1 and 2
Subviral Agents (Satellites, Viroids, and Agents of Spongiform Encephalopathies)			
Prions			Kuru, Creutzfeldt-Jakob disease (CJD), Gerstmann-Sträussler-Scheinker syndrome (GSS), fatal familial insomnia (FFI)
Unclassified Viruses			
		Deltavirus	Hepatitis delta virus (HDV)

BOX 151.1 Representative Properties Used in Virus Taxonomy

Virion Properties
Size
Shape
Presence, absence of envelope and peplomers
Capsid structure, symmetry

Physical Properties
Molecular mass
Buoyant density
Sedimentation coefficient
pH stability
Thermal stability
Solvent, detergent stability
Cation (Mg^{2+}, Mn^{2+}) stability
Radiation stability

Genome
Type of nucleic acid, DNA or RNA
Strandedness, single- or double-stranded
Linear or circular
Sense: positive, negative, or ambisense
Number of segments
Size
Presence or absence and type of 5′ terminal cap
Nucleotide sequence comparisons

Protein Properties
Number
Size
Functional activities
Amino acid sequence comparisons

Lipids
Presence or absence
Nature

Carbohydrates
Presence or absence
Nature

Genome Organization and Replication
Organization
Strategy of replication
Characteristics of transcription
Characteristics of translation and posttranslational processing
Site of accumulation of assembly, maturation, and release

Antigenic Properties
Serologic relationships
Mapping epitopes

Biologic Properties
Host range
Pathogenesis
Tissue tropisms, pathology
Mode of transmission
Vector relationships
Geographic distribution

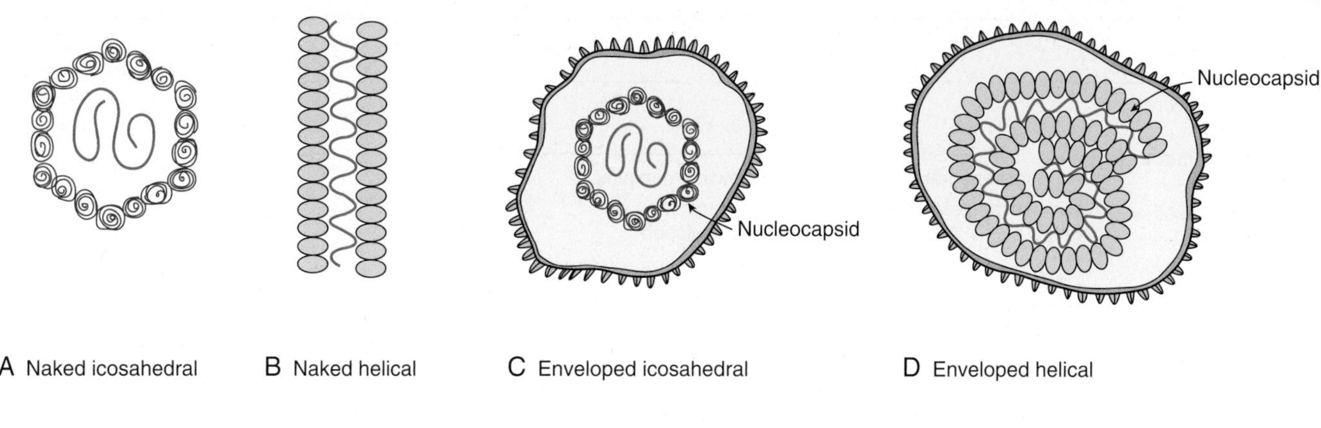

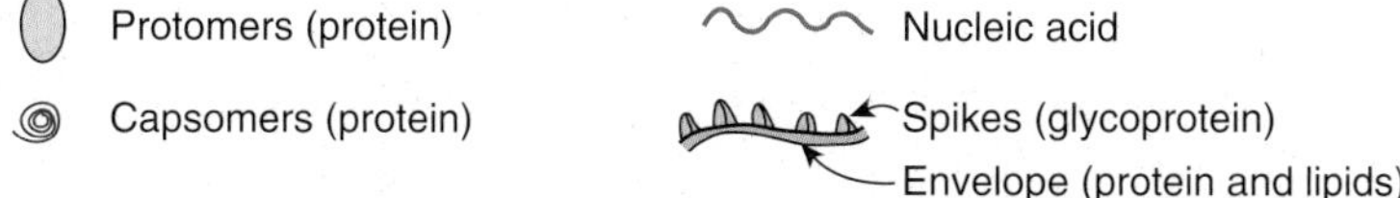

FIG. 151.2 Simple forms of virions and their components. The naked icosahedral virions resemble small crystals; the naked helical virions resemble rods with a fine regular helical pattern in their surface. The enveloped icosahedral virions are composed of icosahedral nucleocapsids surrounded by the envelope; the enveloped helical virions are helical nucleocapsids bent to form a coarse, often irregular, coil within the envelope. (From Davis BD, Dulbecco R, Eisen HN, et al. *Microbiology.* 4th ed. Philadelphia: JB Lippincott; 1990:772.)

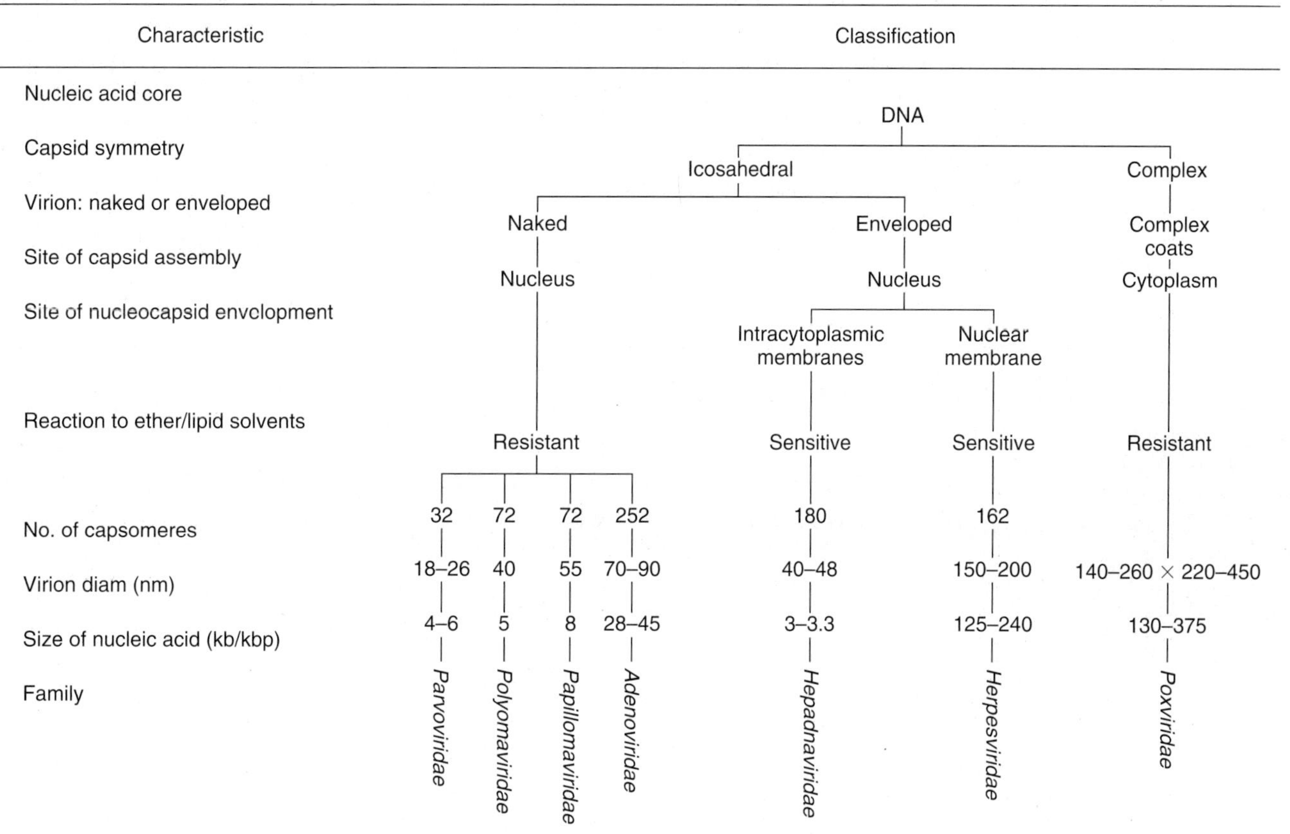

FIG. 151.3 Classification of major DNA-containing viruses affecting humans.

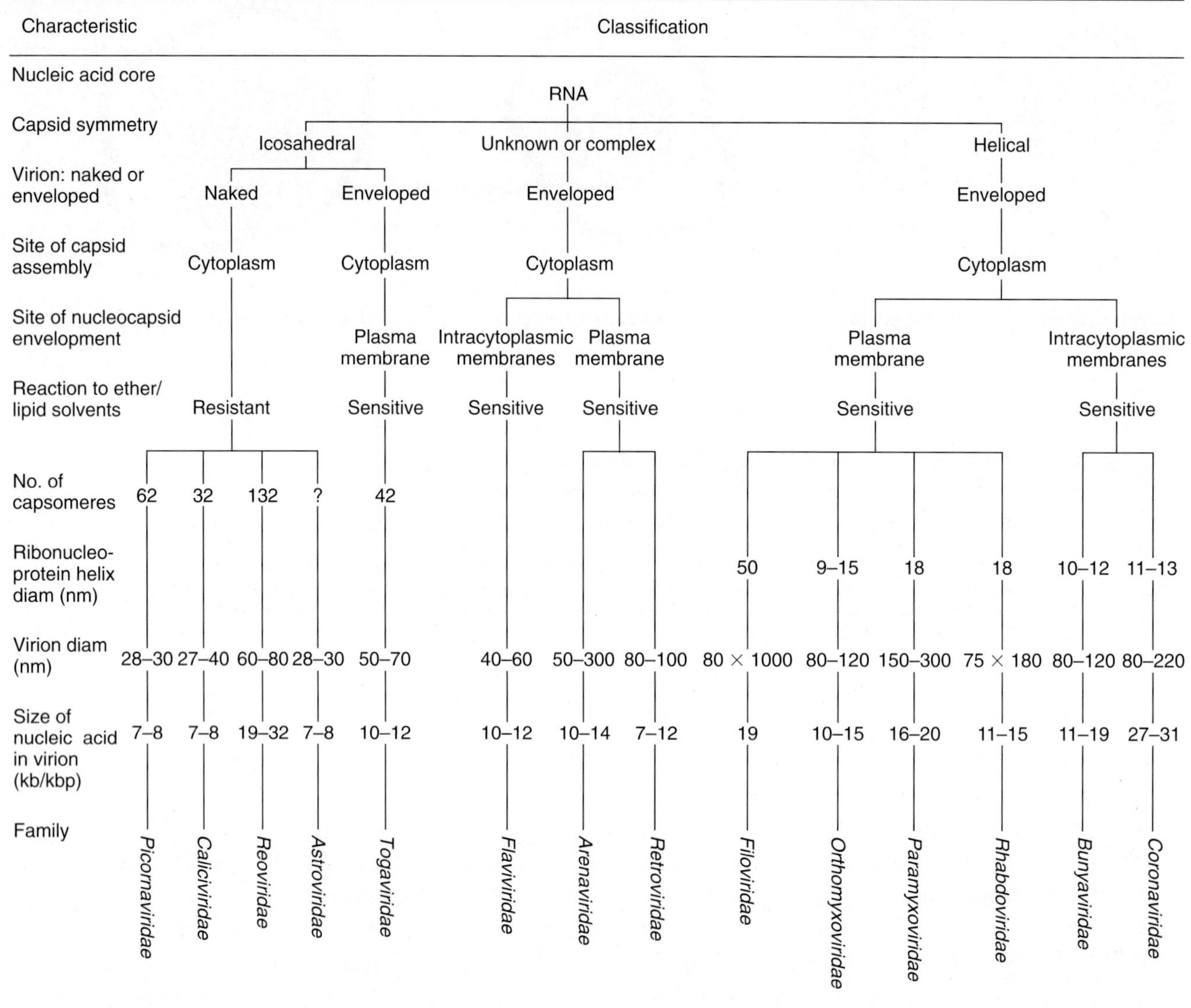

FIG. 151.4 Classification of major RNA-containing viruses affecting humans.

SUBSECTION I DNA—*Parvoviridae*

152 Human Parvovirus B19

Danica J. Schulte

The family *Parvoviridae* includes two subfamilies: *Parvovirinae* and *Densovirinae*.[353,482] The subfamily *Parvovirinae* has six genera: Erythrovirus, Parvovirus, Dependovirus, Bocavirus, Amdovirus, and Parv4; the subfamily *Densovirinae* has five genera: Brevidensovirus, Pefudensovirus, Densovirus, Iteravirus, and Centravirus. Densonucleosis viruses (*Densovirus* spp.) infect insect hosts and have not been found in humans or mammals,[37,391] whereas the *Parvovirinae* are viruses of vertebrates.[54]

Currently, human parvovirus B19 is the only member of the genus *Erythrovirus* that infects humans; however, two other genera of the subfamily *Parvovirinae* (Parv4 and Bocavirus) also cause human infection.[444] Originally, B19 virus was classified in the genus *Parvovirus*. Despite the reclassification, the contemporary literature still refers to this Erythrovirus as parvovirus B19. This virus is autonomous and does not require the presence of a helper virus.

Three human parvovirus B19 genotypes have been defined based on isolates with greater than 10% divergence in overall DNA sequence, all causing human disease.[54,416] In 1999, Erythrovirus V9, a member of genotype 3, was found to be clinically significant.[194,198,200,382,443] V9 virus was found in the serum and bone marrow of a 6-year-old boy with transient aplastic anemia[360]; however, routine testing for B19 virus failed to identify the V9 virus[194] because it has more than 11% % variation from the published B19 genome, with nucleotide discrepancies encompassing the entire genome.[198,200,444]

B19 typically is well conserved, with less than 2% sequence variability among isolates.[198,200,360,484] The prevalence of each genotype varies with geographic origin, population, and sample type. Genotype 1 is present worldwide, whereas genotype 3 is prevalent in Africa, and genotype 2[139,444,546] primarily circulates in Europe and North America and is very limited.[170,444]

More recently, two additional members of the *Parvovirinae* subfamily have been discovered. One of these, human bocavirus, is discussed in Chapter 153. The other virus, Parv4, was found in plasma samples from pooled plasma collections,[159,300,473] placentally,[80] and in persons screened for acute human immunodeficiency virus (HIV) infection.[231,312]

Erythema infectiosum is the most common clinical manifestation of infection with parvovirus B19. Other clinical findings include arthralgia and arthritis, aplastic crisis in patients with red blood cell defects, chronic anemia in immunocompromised patients, fetal hydrops, cardiac disease, neurologic disease, and a variety of other significant illnesses.

HISTORY

The first parvoviruses to be discovered infecting humans were found in stool specimens by electron microscopy.[392] These fecal parvoviruses have been linked with gastrointestinal symptoms, often in outbreaks associated with the consumption of shellfish.[123,491] Their precise pathogenic role remains unclear because these viruses also may be found in the feces of asymptomatic individuals.[392]

In 1974, a second type of parvovirus, human parvovirus B19, was found in the serum of asymptomatic blood donors.[54,104,194] Discovered by chance as an agent responsible for false-positive results in the counterimmunoelectrophoresis tests then in use for detection of hepatitis B surface antigen, it was revealed by electron microscopy to be uniform icosahedral particles with a mean diameter of 23 nm.

Preliminary studies of the physiochemical nature of this agent suggested its probable identity as a member of the family *Parvoviridae*.[104] In the following years, reports concerning this virus named it variously as human parvovirus–like agent, serum parvovirus–like virus,[96] and B19[450] after one of the original isolates. After its chemical properties were elucidated in 1983,[91,469] the virus was referred to as human parvovirus—or human serum parvovirus—to denote that it is distinct from the fecal viral particles. Today, the virus most commonly is called human parvovirus B19 or simply B19 virus.[9,97,247]

For many years after its discovery, infection with B19 virus appeared to be either asymptomatic or associated with a nonspecific febrile illness.[450] However, in the early 1980s, the central role of B19 virus in the etiology of aplastic crisis in patients with chronic hemolytic anemia was identified.[87,122,236,412,442] Soon thereafter came the appreciation that erythema infectiosum (fifth disease) is the common manifestation of infection with B19 virus.[16] Over 20 years ago, the association between B19 virus infection in pregnancy and fetal death was observed; during the past few decades, the clinical spectrum of B19 virus infection has broadened considerably.*

Although human parvovirus B19 was not discovered until 1974, its most common clinical disease (erythema infectiosum) was described more than 200 years ago.[48] Tschamer's report in 1889 was considered by most reviewers to be the first description of erythema infectiosum.[487] However, Boysen[48] noted that the English dermatologist Robert Willan had reported the illness first in 1799 and then more completely in 1840.

*References 8, 42, 83, 194, 197, 210, 238, 239, 352, 397, 434, 439, 528, 546.

After Tschamer's report came a succession of Austrian and German reports of the illness.[48] Tschamer thought that erythema infectiosum was a manifestation of rubella, but a few years later Escherich[141] suggested that it was a specific disease. Stricker,[467] in 1899, gave the name erythema infectiosum to the clinical entity.

In 1905, Shaw,[449] after having observed cases of erythema infectiosum in Austria, published the first account in the American literature. Herrick[206] was the first to document in detail an outbreak in the United States; however, cases of erythema infectiosum had been observed previously in St. Louis[551] and in Hamburg, New York.[206] Over the past century, numerous outbreaks and epidemics have been described in North America.* Erythema infectiosum frequently is referred to as fifth disease; in the past, it also was called ring rubella, large-spotted disease, and epidemic megaloerythema.

PROPERTIES OF THE VIRUS

Human parvovirus B19 is a naked icosahedral virus with a mean diameter of 23 nm and a mean buoyant density in cesium chloride of 1.43 g/dL.[104] The capsid is formed from two major structural proteins (VP1 and VP2) discernible by sodium dodecyl sulfate–polyacrylamide gel electrophoresis.[91] VP2 is the major structural protein, with a molecular weight of 58 kDa; VP1 has a molecular weight of 84 kDa. A total of 96% of the capsid is VP2, and 4% is VP1. The structure of VP2 has been determined by x-ray crystallography.[194,234] The major nonstructural protein (NS1) has a molecular weight of 77 kDa and acts as a strong transcription activator by recruiting cellular transcription factors and participating in viral replication.[444]

The genome consists of a single molecule of single-stranded DNA approximately 5.6 kb in length.[112] The DNA in B19 virus occurs as both plus and minus strands in approximately equal numbers.[238] When virions are disrupted with protease, the two complementary strands anneal to form a stable duplex.[469] At each end of the molecule are palindromic sequences forming hairpin loops. The hairpin at the 3′ end of the genome serves as a primer for DNA polymerases. The hairpin duplex at the 5′ end of the molecule consists of sequences that are neither complementary to those at the 3′ end, as is found in dependoviruses, nor as highly complementary within this 5′ end as are those at the 3′ end.[72] Folding of the VP1 and VP2 proteins creates α-helical loops that appear on the surface of the capsid and are available to the host immune system. The unique region of VP1 is external to the capsid; it contains linear epitopes recognized by neutralizing antibodies and elicits a more efficient immune response than the VP2 region,[546] but antibodies against the VP2 capsid protein are maintained.[98] NS1 can activate tumor necrosis factor-α, interleukin-6, nuclear factor κB, and TP53 and influences signaling pathways involved in the antiviral response.[98] Moreover, B19 DNA can activate Toll-like receptor 9 into erythroid cells, leading to inhibition of cell growth.[444]

Parvovirus infectivity is relatively heat stable, tolerant of a wide range of pH, and resistant to ether.[19] Successful replication of parvoviruses can be accomplished only in a dividing cell because of the absolute requirement for the host-cell function or functions found in late S phase.[190] Human parvovirus B19 can be propagated only in human erythropoietic cells from bone marrow, erythroid cells from a patient with erythroleukemia, human umbilical cord, and peripheral blood and in primary fetal liver culture.[58,194,238,386,391,462,463,476] It grows only in dividing cells; therefore, all the aforementioned tissue culture systems require the addition of erythropoietin and are regulated by STAT5A and MEK signaling.[79]

The cellular receptor for B19 virus infection is the blood group P antigen, which is a globoside and a neutral glycolipid.[55] The P antigen also requires a cellular coreceptor, $\alpha_5\beta_1$ integrin, for sufficient entry of parvovirus B19 into human cells.[517] In cooperation with P antigen, B19 virus can also bind to Ku80 autoantigen, expressed on B and T lymphocytes, to mediate efficient cell entry.[98] P antigen is found on erythroblasts, megakaryoblasts, endothelial cells, and fetal myocytes.[55] People who lack P antigen are resistant to infection with B19 virus, and

*References 3, 20, 24, 25, 30, 50, 70, 78, 89, 93, 99, 125, 153, 158, 166, 173, 194, 249, 283, 284, 296, 333, 354, 398, 399, 413, 453, 506, 507, 522, 525, 546, 547.

in vitro studies demonstrate that the erythroid precursors from people lacking P antigen cannot be infected, even in the presence of high concentrations of virus.[57,194,294]

Antigenically, this human erythrovirus is distinct from the parvovirus-like particles found in feces[393] and from the human dependoviruses and autonomous animal parvoviruses.[104] However, the nucleotide sequence and hybridization results reported by Turton and associates[491] suggest that the viruses from gastroenteritis cases in 1977 and 1986 are similar to B19 virus. In contrast to animal parvoviruses, no hemagglutinin has been demonstrated.

The degree to which B19 virus is related to other mammalian parvovirus types has been investigated by DNA-DNA hybridization. Although no relationship is discernible with the human dependoviruses, a distant evolutionary relationship to the genomes of the autonomous parvoviruses of rodents is apparent. Interestingly, this relationship is closer than that between B19 virus and the parvoviruses infecting domestic animals (bovine, feline, and canine parvoviruses).[105] Shackelton and Holmes[447] studied the evolutionary dynamics and phylogenetic history of the *Parvoviridae* and observed a high rate of evolutionary change, with 10^{-4} nucleotide substitutions per site per year.

Many recent studies have examined genetic variability in parvovirus B19 isolates.[42,138,160,204,229,247] Hemauer and associates[204] suggested that greater genome variability occurs in isolates from patients with persistent infection than in isolates from patients with acute infection. Erdman and colleagues[138] noted that geographically defined genetic lineages of parvovirus B19 existed but that no particular genotype was associated with a specific clinical manifestation.

EPIDEMIOLOGY

Outbreaks of erythema infectiosum have been observed throughout the world, but most reports have come from nontropical regions. The epidemic pattern of erythema infectiosum is surprisingly similar to that of rubella. Community epidemics are most prevalent in the winter and spring, and they usually last for 3 to 6 months. In a review of 30 well-described epidemics,* 26 had their onset in the period from December through May and 23 of the 30 peaked in March, April, or May. When the North American literature for a 50-year period is examined, a cyclic pattern is evident, with peaks in disease activity occurring approximately every 6 years. The peak periods last for an average of 3 years. A longitudinal study of aplastic crisis in persons with sickle-cell anemia in Jamaica suggested that peaks in incidence occur every 2 to 3 years in that island population.[442]

The case-to-case interval of erythema infectiosum is reported to be between 4 and 14 days[3,16,125,173,404,506,525] In an epidemic in an elementary school, Greenwald and Bashe[173] noted that the mean case-to-case interval was 8.7 days. Ager and associates[3] in their studies noted clustering of intervals between cases of 7 to 11 days. The data of Wilcox and Evans[525] on multiple cases in households suggest that the case-to-case interval usually is closer to 12 to 14 days. In a volunteer study in which adults were inoculated intranasally, the incubation time until onset of the rash was 17 to 18 days.[13] From this study, the case-to-case interval in the community would be expected to be between 6 and 12 days because shedding of virus occurs between days 5 and 12 of infection. This prediction accords well with intervals in the studies noted earlier, as well as intervals observed in patients with hematologic diseases and aplastic crisis.[340]

In epidemics, the attack rate is high. Lauer and colleagues[283] noted an overall attack rate of 24.3% in schoolchildren in kindergarten through the eighth grade. Similar attack rates were noted in three other school-related outbreaks.[125,168,173] In the community as a whole, the attack rate is highest in children 5 to 14 years of age,[2,3] but secondary cases occur in preschool children, teachers, and parents. In the home, secondary cases are reported more commonly in mothers than in fathers.[3] In school epidemics, the attack rate is considerably higher in girls than in boys.[125,283] Prevalence studies of serum IgG antibody to B19 virus have noted that 40% to 60% of adults older than the age of 20 years, up to 85% of the elderly, and only 2% to 21% of children younger than age 11 years are seropositive.[9,17,15,444] The rate of transmission among household contacts is nearly 50%.[496]

*References 3, 10, 20, 25, 48, 50, 78, 89, 93, 99, 125, 153, 161, 206, 249, 283, 284, 296, 354, 399, 413, 453, 474, 506, 521, 525, 556.

Nosocomial infections do occur; most often, the index case is an unrecognized, chronically infected patient.[2,269,401] During community outbreaks, the risk for acquisition by hospital workers is no greater than that in other community residents.

Although erythema infectiosum long had been postulated to be transmitted by droplet via the respiratory tract,[3] proof of this route was not obtained until a group of volunteers were infected successfully with B19 virus after intranasal inoculation. One week after inoculation, virus was excreted from the respiratory tract for 6 days.[13]

The role of human leukocyte antigen (HLA) class I and II alleles was investigated by Kerr and associates[242] in northwestern England. Thirty-six patients with symptomatic B19 infection and 900 controls were studied. The frequency of HLA alleles DRB1*01, DRB1*04, and DRB1*07 was significantly higher in patients with B19 infection than in control subjects.

In a cohort study of 169 children with severe anemia in Papua New Guinea, a strong association between severe anemia and B19 infection was observed; however, the authors were unable to show a combined deleterious effect of malaria and B19 infection.[522] They and others demonstrated that 60% of the children were infected with B19 before reaching 2 years of age and that more than 90% were infected by 6 years of age.[179,390,430,526]

Parvovirus B19 infection also can be transmitted by blood transfusion and clotting factor concentrates.* One case of transmission of B19 DNA via peripheral blood progenitor cell transplantation that resolved after treatment with intravenous immune globulin (IVIG) has been reported.[18] Hayakawa and colleagues[191] reported a case of parvovirus B19 infection that they thought was transmitted by IVIG. Researchers have described donor-transmitted parvovirus infection in transplant patients.[535]

PATHOGENESIS AND PATHOLOGY

The pathogenesis of erythroviral disease involves two quite separate components. The first is caused by the lytic infection of susceptible dividing cells and the second by interaction with products of the immune response.

As stated earlier, parvoviruses replicate only in dividing cells. Thus, infection of an organ or tissue in which a significant proportion of the cells are dividing may give rise to organ-specific disease. This condition is seen clearly in canine and feline parvovirus infections, in which replication of virus in the crypt cells of the intestine gives rise to a severe and often fatal enteritis.[184,306]

Parvovirus B19 is thought not to infect cells of the gastrointestinal tract; virus could not be detected in the feces of volunteers,[13] nor have viruses of this type been found in stool specimens.

After gaining entry via the respiratory tract, the virus sets up a systemic infection with copious viremia (Fig. 152.1) in which 10^{10} or 10^{11} virus particles per milliliter of blood is not an uncommon finding.[13,406]

Parvovirus infection results in profound reticulocytopenia for some 7 to 10 days, commencing during viremia.[13,546] In vitro studies on cultured bone marrow and peripheral blood have shown that B19 virus inhibits the formation of blast-forming erythroid colonies, thus suggesting that an early erythrocyte precursor cell is susceptible to infection with the virus. B19-associated damage to cells of the erythroid lineage is due to the cytotoxicity mediated by viral proteins, whereas the apoptotic features mediated by caspase 3 are induced by NS1.[81,86] Overexpression of NS1 has been found to trigger signaling cascades that help promote pro-apoptotic and apoptotic processes, resulting in anemia, acute fulminant liver failure, placental insufficiency, and myocarditis.[532] In addition to profound erythroid hypoplasia, giant pronormoblasts typically are seen in the bone marrow at the height of transient aplastic crises and normoblasts have characteristic intranuclear eosinophilic inclusion bodies, termed *Lampion* or *lantern cells*.[63]

*References 18, 120, 194, 322, 342, 403, 429, 461, 531, 537, 549.

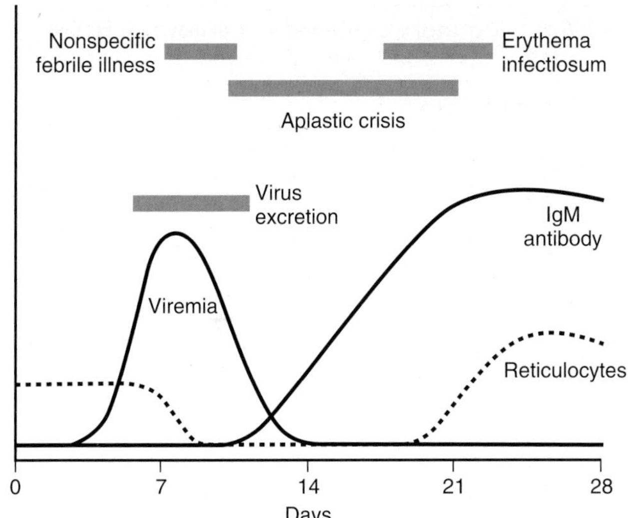

FIG. 152.1 Selected virologic, immunologic, hematologic, and clinical events in parvovirus B19 virus infection.

Granulocytes and megakaryocytes are unaffected by virus in these in vitro systems. However, during B19 virus infection in a normal host, clinically insignificant lymphopenia and neutropenia occur, as does a drop in platelet number.[13,404] The mechanisms of loss of these cells from peripheral blood remain to be determined. Srivastava and associates[462] noted that B19 virus infection of bone marrow cells in culture results in suppression of megakaryocyte colony formation. In this study, tropism of B19 virus for cells other than erythroid progenitor cells appeared to take place, although viral DNA replication did not occur in the megakaryocyte-enriched fractions. They suggested that the virus might be toxic to cell populations that are nonpermissive of viral DNA replication.

As noted in Fig. 152.1, viremia ends at the time of appearance of specific immunoglobulin M (IgM) antibody. In addition, researchers have found that the appearance of antibody neutralizes the inhibitory effect of B19 virus on formation of erythrocyte colonies in vitro.[547] The early IgM response is almost entirely VP2 specific. IgG antibody first appears approximately 2 weeks after exposure and later becomes the major antibody subclass; in contrast to the initial IgM response, the IgG response is directed at VP1 rather than VP2. The role of cellular immunity in recovery from infection is unclear. Most patients with persistent infection have T-cell as well as other immune defects, thus suggesting a cellular component in the host response.[42] Von Poblotzki and associates[504] showed that the T cells of persons with parvovirus B19 antibody had HLA class II–restricted responses against B19 structural proteins. Franssila and colleagues[156] demonstrated virus-specific helper T-cell proliferation in recently and remotely infected patients. Their data suggested that B cells that recognize the viral capsid (VP1 and VP2) receive class II–restricted help from $CD4^+$ T lymphocytes. While investigating a parvovirus B19 vaccine, this same group demonstrated that VP1 contains important B-cell epitopes required for protective B-cell immunity; they concluded that VP2, the major structural protein of B19 virus, appears to provide the major target for B19-specific helper T cells years or decades after initial infection occurs.[154,155] A persistent, activated B19-specific $CD8^+$ T-cell repertoire with maintained effector function occurs in healthy patients who successfully clear the B19 virus. Researchers have hypothesized that these activated $CD8^+$ T cells may play a prominent role in controlling acute B19 infection.[222,233,297,370] Additionally, Kerr and colleagues[240,245] reported that circulating cytokine and chemokine levels in acute B19 disease may correlate with clinical disease.

The most common result of infection with B19 virus is erythema infectiosum. Fig. 152.1 shows that the symptoms of this disease begin 17 or 18 days after inoculation and that approximately 1 week after inoculation virus can be detected in either throat swabs or blood. Skin biopsy results have been reported in three studies.[30,174,212] In three skin biopsy specimens from regions of reticulated eruption, Bard and Perry[30] noted either normal skin or very mild inflammatory changes. Hoffman[212] described edema in the epidermis and perivascular infiltration with mononuclear cells; he also noted swelling of the endothelium of superficial vessels and the presence of cleavage spaces between the epidermis and dermis. The histopathology in 10 cases was investigated by Grimmer and Joseph.[174] They reported dilation of blood vessels with lymphocytic and occasional plasma cell perivascular infiltration. However, the clinical manifestations of many of the cases in the epidemic that Grimmer and Joseph[174] studied were quite atypical.

Virus-specific IgM is present at the time of onset of the rash in erythema infectiosum; thus, although the mechanisms of production of the rash (and arthralgia) of erythema infectiosum remain to be elucidated, postulating an immune-mediated pathogenesis is not unreasonable.[546] The perivascular infiltrations noted by Hoffman[212] would support this suggestion. However, Schwarz and colleagues[438] have found both viral capsid proteins and viral DNA in a skin biopsy specimen of the rash from a patient with erythema infectiosum. They suggest that the rash may be a direct effect of the virus rather than being immune complex mediated.

Intrauterine infection results in infection of the fetus and, frequently, abortion.* The main finding in infected fetuses is hydrops fetalis, which results from the anemia caused by infection of the erythrocyte precursor cells. Intranuclear inclusions are seen in nucleated red blood cells; viral particles are identified in the same cells by electron microscopy.[75] The mechanism responsible for hydrops fetalis stems from severe anemia, and cardiogenic failure results in generalized ascites, edema, pericardial and pleural effusions, and a thick hydropic placenta.[157] Concomitant myocarditis also occurs, which complicates the clinical picture because the blood group P antigen is expressed on fetal cardiac myocytes.[55,86] The shorter half-life of fetal erythrocytes also exacerbates the disease.[86]

In immunocompromised patients, persistent infection with B19 virus often occurs[274] as a result of failure to produce effective neutralizing antibodies.[86,444] Patients taking immunosuppressive calcineurin inhibitors may be unable to clear B19 virus because these medications inhibit interleukin-2 production and the patients are unable to mount an effective T-helper cell type 1 response.[86,335]

CLINICAL MANIFESTATIONS

Infection with human parvovirus B19 results in a spectrum of clinical manifestations; classic cases of erythema infectiosum occupy a central position in this spectrum. Other major manifestations include arthritis and arthralgia, intrauterine infection and hydrops fetalis, transient aplastic crisis in patients with a variety of underlying hemolytic illnesses, and persistent infection with chronic anemia in patients with immunodeficiencies. In addition, subclinical, nonexanthematous infection occurs, especially in children.[13,404]

Other less common illnesses include myocarditis, vasculitis, glomerulonephritis, hepatitis, and neurologic disease. In addition to the established parvovirus B19 disease associations is an ever-expanding list of categories of illness in which evidence of parvovirus B19 infection has been found (Box 152.1).

Erythema Infectiosum

Although a search of the literature related to outbreaks of erythema infectiosum reveals a conspicuous absence of prodromal symptoms in patients, infected volunteers have had febrile episodes with nonspecific symptoms of headache, chills, myalgia, and malaise accompanying the viremic phase of infection with B19 virus (see Fig. 152.1).[13] These symptoms last for 2 to 3 days and coincide with excretion of virus from the pharynx. This phase is followed by a period of 7 days, during which individuals are free of symptoms before onset of the second, or exanthematous, phase of illness. Most likely, the relatively long period between symptoms in this biphasic illness prevented recognition of the link between these nonspecific prodromal symptoms and erythema infectiosum.

*References 8, 9, 70, 75, 110, 166, 194, 252, 409, 418, 436, 528, 545, 546.

BOX 152.1 Reported Unusual Clinical Findings in Patients With Laboratory Evidence of Parvovirus B19 Virus Infection

Persistent Arthritis

Juvenile rheumatoid arthritis[84,254,377]
Rheumatoid arthritis[98,364,464,477]
Adult Still disease[298,407]

Neurologic Disease

Encephalitis[26,119,149,199,242,465]
Meningitis[72,267,383,471,474]
Stroke[175,311]
Postinfectious neuralgic amyotrophy[28,394]
Guillain-Barré syndrome[28,329]
Transverse myelitis[28]
Facial palsy[313]
Carpal tunnel syndrome[28,426]
Numbness and tingling of fingers[4,28,143]
Myofasciitis[217]

Myocarditis[a]

Cutaneous Manifestations

Papular-purpuric gloves-and-socks syndrome[b]
Vesiculopustular exanthema[357]
Erythema multiforme[164]
Henoch-Schönlein syndrome[88,501]
Petechial and purpuric rashes[1,100,121,216,287,321]
Pruritus without rash[305]

Hematologic Manifestations

Thrombocytopenic purpura[5,40,150,221,289,543]
Pancytopenia[185,268,346]
Hemophagocytic syndrome[47,346,460,490,495,515,548]
Neutropenia[318,440]
Diamond-Blackfan syndrome[318,480]
Splenic sequestration[309]

Other Manifestations

Sepsis[23]
Glomerulonephritis[219,225,267,337,523]
Nephrotic syndrome[379]
Kawasaki disease[213,363]
Behçet disease[253]
Polyarteritis nodosa[502]
Wegener granulomatosis[365]
Leukocytoclastic vasculitis[101]
Giant-cell arteritis[161]
Systemic sclerosis[146,147,382]
Systemic vasculitis[109]
Systemic lupus erythematosus[114,207,218,362]
Hepatitis[121,124,189,281,367,459,542]
Raynaud phenomenon[186]
Pseudoappendicitis or mesenteric lymphadenitis[338]
Necrotizing lymphadenitis[230]
Cervical lymphadenopathy[255,489]
Parotitis[313]
Pneumonia[339,465,512]
Pulmonary emboli[19]
Acute respiratory distress syndrome[145]
Mixed cryoglobulinemia[85]
Chronic infection without immunosuppression but with chronic hemolytic anemia[246]
Persistent arthralgia[247]
Chronic fatigue syndrome[226,243,244,247,255,315,319]
Recurrent paresthesias[142]
Fibromyalgia[36]

[a]References 6, 33, 43, 44, 62, 113, 116, 134, 232, 270, 271, 280, 349, 361, 389, 423, 550.
[b]References 7, 12, 22, 39, 131, 183, 214, 325, 384, 454, 485, 497.

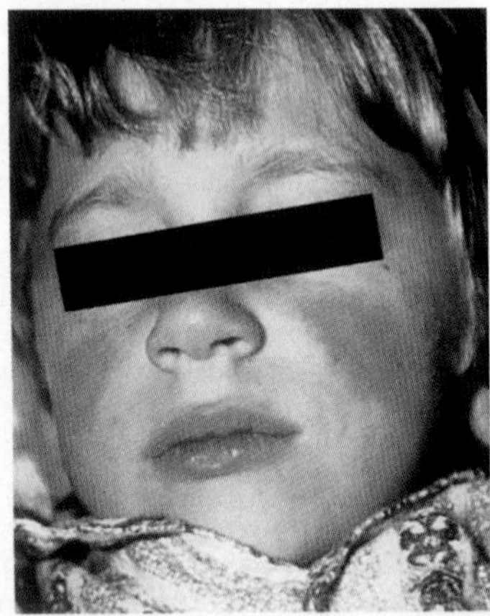

FIG. 152.2 Slapped-cheek appearance with a relative circumoral maculopapular rash in erythema infectiosum.

The exanthem in classic cases of erythema infectiosum occurs in three stages.* The first stage begins 18 days after the acquisition of infection and is characterized by a fiery red rash on the cheeks (Fig. 152.2; "slapped-cheek" appearance). The edges of the involved areas may be raised slightly, and a relatively circumoral pallor is present. At this stage, the appearance may be suggestive of scarlet fever, drug sensitivity or other allergic reactions, or collagen vascular disease. The facial exanthem is aggravated by the transition from outdoors to a warm room.

The second stage of the exanthem occurs 1 to 4 days after the onset of facial involvement and consists of the appearance of an erythematous, maculopapular rash on the trunk and limbs. This rash is discrete initially but spreads to involve large areas. Toward the end of this stage, central clearing of the rash from these areas gives the characteristic lacy or reticular pattern (Fig. 152.3).

The third stage of the exanthem is highly variable in duration (i.e., lasting from 1 to 3 or more weeks) and is characterized by marked changes in the intensity of the rash, with periodic complete evanescence and recrudescence. These fluctuations are related to environmental factors, such as exposure to sunlight and temperature (a hot bath may result in recrudescence in an apparently recovered child).

The rash often is pruritic, especially in adults, and it generally is more prominent on the extensor surfaces; the palms and soles rarely are affected. Slight desquamation has been noted in a small number of patients in most reviews.

Although classic cases of erythema infectiosum are easy to recognize clinically, especially during outbreaks, wide variation in the form of the exanthem can be noted—from a very faint, fleeting rash to a florid exanthem that is confluent over large areas (Fig. 152.4). In many cases, the illness may be indistinguishable from rubella. Yermalovich and colleagues published the experience in Belarus following the institution of a national screening program in 2005 for B19 virus in patients with

*References 3, 24, 50, 78, 84, 89, 173, 449, 496, 507, 508, 506.

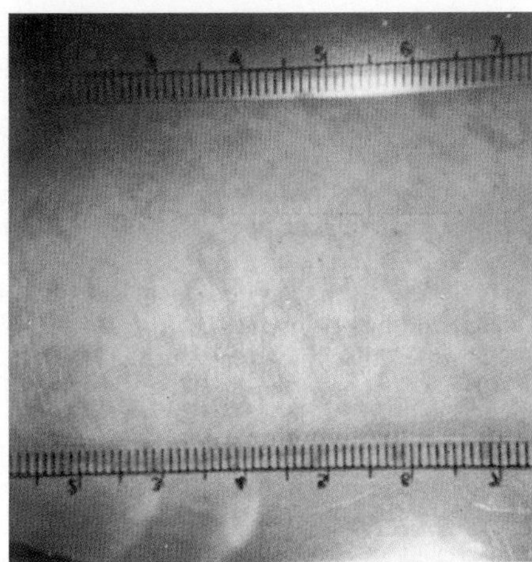

FIG. 152.3 Rash with a lacelike, or reticular, pattern in erythema infectiosum.

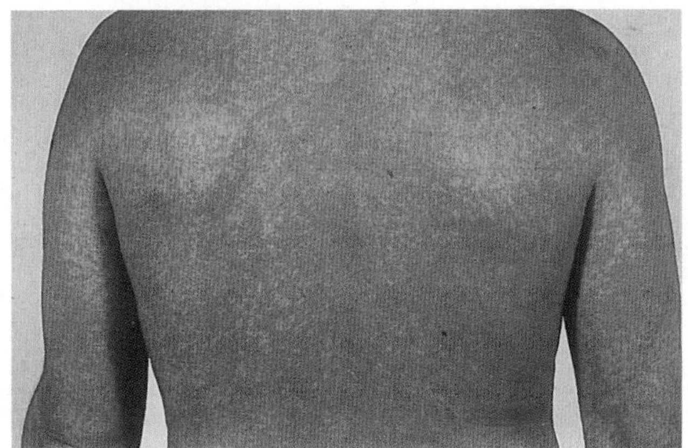

FIG. 152.4 Confluent exanthem in a patient with human parvovirus infection.

fever and rash who were measles and rubella negative and reported that more than 35% of patients were B19 positive.[539]

The overwhelming majority of cases of erythema infectiosum have no exanthem. Kerr and Marsh[249] and Condon[99] noted a few children with pharyngitis.

Other symptoms and signs occur uncommonly in erythema infectiosum (Table 152.1). In general, complaints are expressed more frequently by adults than by children. Headache is reported in approximately a fifth of childhood cases and about half of afflicted adults. Joint pain and swelling and myalgia are particularly troublesome in adults.

Routine laboratory studies are of little use in erythema infectiosum. The leukocyte count usually is normal, although mild eosinophilia is noted occasionally.[24,48,507,508]

The most common complication of erythema infectiosum is joint involvement; it is relatively rare in children (<10% of cases) but is the norm in adults and occurs in 80% or more of cases.* A range of severity from mild arthralgia to frank arthritis is observed. The joints most commonly involved are the knees, ankles, and proximal interphalangeal joints; symptoms generally are bilateral. The joint involvement usually is transient and lasts only a few days. In some individuals, symptoms may persist for some weeks or, rarely, months. When joint involvement occurs after an exanthem, the diagnosis may be inferred, but such is not invariably the case. As with rubella, the frequency of arthralgia and arthritis is higher in women than in men.[98]

Other Exanthems

Grimmer and Joseph[174] described cases in which the rashes were morbilliform, hemorrhagic, urticarial, vesicular, and resembled erythema multiforme. Their studies were conducted during an epidemic of

*References 9, 15, 16, 24, 192, 197, 355, 414, 417, 509, 522.

TABLE 152.1 Frequency of Symptoms and Signs in Erythema Infectiosum

	% OCCURRENCE	
Sign or Symptom	***Children***	***Adults***
Rash	100	100
Pruritus	15	50
Headache	20	50
Fever	15	25
Sore throat	15	15
Coryza	10	15
Cough	8	8
Sore eyes	10	10
Anorexia	15	22
Nausea	7	26
Vomiting	4	7
Diarrhea	4	12
Abdominal pain	10	15
Joint pain	10	70
Joint swelling	5	60
Myalgia	4	50

Data from references 3, 125, 173, 507.

erythema infectiosum in Berlin, Germany, in which an estimated 50,000 persons were affected. The cases with markedly unusual manifestations quite possibly were not of the same etiology as the typical cases. Other authors also have noted papular, purpuric, petechial, vesicular, urticarial, and morbilliform eruptions.*

García-Tapia and associates[164] described a 5-year-old girl with erythema multiforme bullosum but without other systemic manifestations. Her serum had B19 virus–specific IgM antibody. Additionally, a papular-purpuric or petechial "glove-and-sock" syndrome has been reported with acute B19 infection.† It is more commonly seen in adults but has been noted in children. B19 virus has been identified in the endothelium of cutaneous biopsy specimens from these patients.[127,427] This unique rash is characterized by petechiae and purpura, with painful or pruritic edema of the hands and feet extending proximally with less severity, and it is self-limited.[7,188,214,220,325] Henoch-Schönlein syndrome and other vasculitic rashes also have been reported.[1,88,101,121,202,382,393,434,501]

Grimmer and Joseph[174] stated that most of their patients in the Berlin epidemic had dark red spots on the pharynx, gums, soft palate, and uvula. These cases, again, must be regarded with some suspicion because the investigators also noted genital lesions and conjunctivitis in a few patients.

Aplastic Crisis

In individuals with chronic hemolytic anemia, the profound reticulocytopenia of human parvovirus B19 infection results in depression of hemoglobin concentrations to critical levels.‡ With resolution of the infection, reticulocytes reappear in the peripheral blood, and hemoglobin concentrations return to the normal steady-state values for these patients. This transient arrest in production of erythrocytes is termed *aplastic crisis* and may occur in any individual whose erythrocytes have a short life span. Examples of such conditions include sickle-cell anemia,[169,307,442,455,555] hereditary spherocytosis,[77,140,185,236,373,378,519] thalassemia,[287,288,412] glucose-6-phosphate dehydrogenase deficiency,[167] and pyruvate kinase deficiency.[122] However, there are case reports of aplastic anemia secondary to B19 virus developing in immunocompetent patients without underlying diseases.[178,235,303,330,410,520]

Serjeant and coworkers[441] studied the epidemiology of B19 virus infection over time in 308 children with homozygous sickle-cell disease and in 239 controls with normal hemoglobin. B19 virus infection

*References 78, 99, 100, 151, 216, 287, 309, 321, 357, 399, 534.
†References 4, 7, 9, 22, 39, 131, 183, 214, 216, 452, 454, 485, 496, 497.
‡References 9, 11, 70, 122, 167, 169, 185, 236, 237, 287, 340, 373, 378, 412, 421, 442, 455, 469, 519, 545, 547, 555.

accounted for all 91 episodes of aplastic crisis that occurred. Twenty-three additional patients with sickle-cell disease had B19 virus infections; of these, 10 had mild hematologic changes and 13 had no changes. By 15 years of age, approximately 40% of the sickle-cell group and the control group had IgG antibody to B19 virus, thus indicating equal infection rates in the two groups. No patient or control subject had two infections caused by B19 virus.

Smith-Whitley and associates[455] studied a cohort of 633 patients with sickle-cell disease (including patients with various sickle-cell disease genotypes—SS-, SC-, and Sβ-thalassemia—as well as those receiving chronic transfusions and hydroxyurea) for complications attributable to acute B19 infection. At study entry, 29.8% of the cohort had IgG antibody to B19 virus. The secondary attack rate in the group of children who had siblings with sickle-cell disease was 56%. Thirty-five percent of the total patient population with B19 infection did not have worsening anemia; however, transient red cell aplasia developed in 50% of the children, with those with SC- or Sβ-thalassemia genotypes characterized by less severe disease. Neutropenia developed in 18% of patients and thrombocytopenia in 27%. In only one of seven patients receiving chronic transfusions did transient red cell aplasia develop, potentially because of the lower red cell turnover in these patients.

Rao and colleagues[411] found that 70% of patients with transient aplastic crisis admitted to their hospitals during a 7-year period had B19 viral infections. No patients had chronic or recurrent infections. In a study of 48 patients with aplastic crises, Mallouh and Qudah[310] found 91% to be infected with B19 virus. In addition to the anemia, 21% of the patients had leukopenia, 27% had neutropenia, and 42% had thrombocytopenia. The same investigators noted acute splenic sequestration together with aplastic crisis in three patients with sickle-cell disease and B19 virus infection.[309] Lowenthal and associates[301] noted three young adults with sickle-cell acute chest syndrome associated with B19 virus infection. Yetgin and colleagues[541] reported a case of a 10-year-old child with severe, refractory aplastic anemia ultimately requiring bone marrow transplantation, which resolved the symptoms. Seo and colleagues reported 13 patients, over a 5-year period, with pure red cell aplasia with associated neutropenia diagnosed with B19 virus on bone marrow biopsy.[440]

Interestingly, reports of exanthematous illness occurring after aplastic crisis are rare.[237,519] However, patients with aplastic crisis require transfusion with packed cells; rashes occurring after such treatment possibly would be regarded as transfusion reactions. Joint symptoms occur fairly frequently in patients with conditions such as sickle-cell anemia; thus, although the symptoms may occur as a result of B19 infection, they may be diagnosed as "painful crises."

As noted earlier, human parvovirus B19 infection does not result in aplastic crisis invariably in a chronic hemolytic anemic patient. Some individuals escape this complication if they have undergone transfusion recently,[11] possibly because of a protective effect of transfused antibody (>60% of donors are immune), the substitution of longer-lived, donated erythrocytes for the patients' own fragile ones, or a combination of these two mechanisms.

In populations in which aplastic crisis does occur, the severity of the episode varies among individuals, perhaps reflecting the variation in erythrocyte life span among these patients.[11] In 2013, Gupta and colleagues studied the prevalence of B19 infection in previously healthy, immunocompetent pediatric patients with acquired aplastic anemia.[178]

Other Hematologic Manifestations

In addition to pure red blood cell aplasia, numerous other hematologic manifestations, including thrombocytopenic purpura, pancytopenia, hemophagocytic syndrome, neutropenia, and Diamond-Blackfan syndrome, have been observed in association with B19 virus infection.* Thrombocytopenia has been noted as an isolated event; however, idiopathic thrombocytopenic purpura may be associated with aplastic crisis.[5,150,221,289,352,543] Thrombocytopenia is most commonly related to a decrease in megakaryocytes in bone marrow as a result of the inhibitory effect of the virus on granulocyte-megakaryocyte colony-forming-units,[5,405,519] although acquired pure amegakaryocytic thrombocytopenic purpura with resultant absence of bone marrow megakaryocytes secondary to B19 virus also has been described.[40]

Pancytopenia has been observed in association with aplastic crisis, and hemophagocytosis often is demonstrated.* Yufu and coauthors[548] described a 15-year-old girl with hemophagocytic syndrome and lymphadenopathy resembling histiocytic necrotizing lymphadenitis (Kikuchi disease).

McClain and colleagues[318] studied 19 children with immune-mediated neutropenia and found by polymerase chain reaction (PCR) assay of bone marrow specimens that 15 had evidence of B19 virus infection.

*References 5, 47, 143, 150, 185, 194, 195, 197, 221, 239, 268, 286, 289, 292, 318, 346, 352, 408, 480, 490, 495, 515, 543.

Arthritis and Arthralgia

As noted earlier, acute arthritis and arthralgia occur commonly in patients with erythema infectiosum. In most instances, the joint symptoms subside within a few weeks, but the arthralgia and arthritis persist occasionally. Researchers also have observed that the joint manifestations caused by B19 virus infection can occur without any exanthem or with an exanthem not typical of erythema infectiosum, and autoantibodies may be produced.[464,477,500] These findings have led to investigations related to the role of B19 virus in rheumatoid arthritis (RA).†

Nocton and associates[368] described the clinical characteristics of 22 children seen in their rheumatology clinic with joint complaints and evidence of recent B19 virus infection. Of this group, 16 were girls and 6 were boys. The youngest patient was 2 years old, and the oldest was 19 years old. Seven of the patients had associated rashes, but none had typical erythema infectiosum. One of these children had a petechial rash on the lower extremities, and another child had a past history of urticaria. Fever, anorexia, malaise, or fatigue occurred in 11 of the patients.

Of the 22 patients, 20 had arthritis and 2 had only arthralgia. The knee joints were most commonly involved. The following frequency of specific joint involvement was reported: knees, 82%; ankles and wrist, 41%; elbows, 32%; neck, small joints of the hands and feet, and hips, 27%; shoulders, 23%; and sternoclavicular joints, 9%. Ten of the patients had involvement of five or more joints, and in 12 patients the pattern was pauciarticular, with four or fewer joints involved. Two patients had only a single joint involved, and two patients had migratory illness.

The duration of the arthritis or arthralgia was less than 6 weeks in 50% of the children and less than 4 months in 64%. Of the 11 children with illness lasting longer than 2 months, 6 had manifestations that fulfilled the criteria for the diagnosis of juvenile rheumatoid arthritis (JRA). Selected laboratory results were as follows: the erythrocyte sedimentation rate was greater than 25 mm/h in 32% of the children, antinuclear antibody titers were greater than 1:40 in 7 of 21 of the patients, and 3 of 6 children had a low total hemolytic complement (CH_{50}) value.

The relationship between B19 virus infection and JRA, RA, and adult Still disease has been studied extensively during the past 15 years, but the findings are difficult to interpret.‡ Clearly, B19 virus can cause illnesses that fulfill the criteria for a diagnosis of JRA[60,368,377,522] and adult Still disease.[239,298] However, three possible scenarios need to be considered: (1) B19 virus causes a similar illness, (2) B19 virus infection triggers the onset of an illness caused by another condition, and (3) B19 virus directly causes JRA, adult Still disease, and RA.

In one study involving patients with refractory RA and refractory polyarticular JRA, researchers found that both groups had a significantly higher frequency of IgG B19 virus antibody as determined by enzyme-linked immunosorbent assay (ELISA) than did aged-matched controls.[328] However, when the data in this study were examined, the prevalence of antibody in the control population clearly was less than expected. In another study, Kishore and colleagues[254] studied IgM antibody to B19 virus by ELISA and found that 28% of patients with JRA, 8% of controls, and none of the patients with RA had positive values. They

*References 47, 185, 197, 239, 268, 282, 346, 352, 487, 495, 515, 548.

†References 73, 98, 152, 182, 197, 210, 238, 239, 254, 328, 334, 364, 368, 407, 458, 464, 477.

‡References 42, 60, 64, 109, 197, 238, 290, 291, 298, 304, 326, 328, 347, 348, 355, 368, 377, 396, 407, 458, 477, 494, 522.

interpreted their JRA findings to be either triggering B19 virus infections or perhaps concurrent infections in patients with established JRA. In a provocative study, Takahashi and coworkers[477] found B19 virus DNA in the synovial tissue of 30 of 39 patients with RA. The data suggested that the virus identified in synovial tissue was active and led to their conclusion that B19 virus is involved in the initiation and perpetuation of RA synovitis. In contrast, Nikkari and associates[364,366] in Finland performed extensive studies and noted that chronic rheumatoid-like arthropathies triggered by B19 virus occasionally occur. However, their data do not support a general role for B19 virus in the etiology or pathogenesis of RA. Varache and colleagues investigated the utility of routine viral screening in patients with early RA and determined that the seroprevalence of B19 was not increased compared with the general population.[500] B19 infection can lead to increased circulation of immune complexes, endothelial injury, inflammation, and exacerbation of underlying vasculitic disease.[63]

Tyndall and colleagues[492] described an adult woman with erosive polyarthritis associated with B19 virus infection, and Samii and coworkers[426] reported two adults with bilateral carpal tunnel syndrome associated with B19 virus infection. Berg and colleagues[36] could find no association with either IgG or IgM antibody to B19 virus and fibromyalgia in a study of 26 adult women and matched controls. Guillaume and colleagues[176] reported a case of chronic arthropathy in the lumbar facet joints after B19 infection.

Other rheumatic and vasculitic syndromes have been noted in association with parvovirus B19 infection; however, the strength of these associations is unclear. These associated syndromes include fibromyalgia,[358] systemic lupus erythematosus,[102,114,207,218,445] Kawasaki disease, leukocytoclastic vasculitis, polyarteritis nodosa, Wegener granulomatosis,[126] chronic fatigue syndrome,[243,244,319] systemic sclerosis,[146,381,380] giant-cell arteritis, transient anticardiolipin syndrome and transient antiphospholipid syndrome,[19] hemophagocytic syndrome,[47,460] mixed cryoglobulinemia,[85] Henoch-Schönlein purpura,[88,202,382] uveitis with and without associated systemic disease,[203] myofasciitis,[217] and Raynaud phenomenon.*

Infection in Immunocompromised Patients

Immunocompromised patients may suffer chronic B19 virus infections.† These patients have persistent anemia caused by continuous lysis of red cell precursors. Lackner and colleagues reviewed 1059 consecutive patients with various hematologic and oncologic diseases and characterized 35 patients diagnosed with B19 infection.[278] B19 infection has been commonly seen in children with acute lymphocytic leukemia.‡

Other immune deficiency states in which chronic B19 virus was documented include Nezelof syndrome, acute myeloid leukemia, chronic myeloid leukemia, Burkitt lymphoma, lymphoblastic lymphoma, myelodysplastic syndrome, astrocytoma, Wilms tumor, HIV infection,[90,356] severe combined immunodeficiency, bone marrow transplantation,[193,250,402,468] other organ transplants,[34,76,128,272,335,385] systemic lupus erythematosus,[470] and patients receiving chemotherapy.[126,144,201,273] The immune deficiency in the aforementioned conditions can be a primary event or a secondary event related to treatment.

Eid and colleagues[129] reviewed 98 transplant recipients in whom acute parvovirus B19 infection developed after transplantation. The median time to B19 disease was 7 weeks after transplantation. Anemia developed in 99%, leukopenia in 38%, thrombocytopenia in 21%, and allograft loss or dysfunction in 10%. Three patients died of myocarditis and cardiogenic shock as a result of B19 infection. B19 virus was associated with chronic renal allograft injury.[32]

Patients with chronic anemia have high persistent concentrations of B19 virus in their serum, although the values (10^8 particles/mL) are less than those seen in primary infections (10^{10}–10^{11} particles/mL) in healthy individuals and in patients with hemoglobinopathies.

Viremia and anemia may, if untreated, persist for years. Fatigue and pallor are the most common clinical symptoms; other findings of B19 virus infection, such as exanthem and arthralgia, occur rarely. Because of immunodeficiency, IgM antibody studies generally are not useful in making the diagnosis. Therefore, the diagnosis of persistent B19 virus infection depends on demonstration of specific B19 antigen or DNA in blood.[63]

In immunocompromised patients, persistent infection with B19 virus often occurs as a result of failure to produce effective neutralizing antibodies.[63,86,268] Intravenous immunoglobulin (IVIG) preparations have been used successfully for the treatment of B19 virus in immunocompromised patients.* Patients taking immunosuppressive agents, especially calcineurin inhibitors, may be unable to clear B19 virus because these medications inhibit interleukin-2 production, and the patients are unable to mount an effective T-helper cell type 1 response.[86,335] It may be necessary to reduce the dose of immunosuppressive agents in addition to IVIG treatment to successfully eradicate B19 virus.[31,130,295] LaMonte and associates[279] reported five children (three HIV-infected children and two otherwise normal children) with chronic infections without B19-associated anemia.

Intrauterine Infection

Although a large epidemiologic study of an outbreak of erythema infectiosum over 40 years ago failed to reveal evidence of teratogenicity, virologic and serologic studies conducted during the past 25 years indicate that B19 virus crosses the placenta and causes infection in the fetus.† Infection in pregnancy results in fetal hydrops because of severe anemia and leads to cardiac failure, fetal death, and miscarriage.[86,115,314,375]

Bonvicini and colleagues followed 72 pregnancies complicated by B19 infection. Vertical transmission was documented in 39% of the pregnancies, B19 fetal hydrops in 11.9%, and overall fetal demise in 10.2%, with the highest rate of congenital infection and fatal outcome with maternal infection prior to 20 weeks of gestation.[45]

To determine the rate and outcome of fetal involvement after infection in pregnant women, two prospective studies were performed in England during a 3.5-year period from January 1985 to June 1988[409] and from 1992 to 1995.[327] These two studies included 427 pregnant women infected with B19 virus; 367 infants survived, and 129 of them had follow-up examinations at 7 to 10 years of age.[327] The excess rate of fetal loss was 9%; such loss occurred only during the first 20 weeks of gestation. Seven cases of fetal hydrops occurred. Three of these fetuses survived; two of the three received intrauterine transfusions. None of the surviving infants in the two studies had abnormalities attributable to B19 virus infection, and no later effects were found at 7 to 10 years of age. Of the infants exposed in utero after 20 weeks of gestation, more than half were infected, but no clinical effects were identified. In a study by Nyman and colleagues,[376] the frequency of first-trimester fetal loss associated with B19 virus was 3%, with 12% occurring in the second trimester. Maternal B19 seroconversion during pregnancy was not associated with lower birth weight or reduced length of gestation in live-born children in a study of 35,940 pregnant women in Norway.[428]

In a study in Connecticut related to a large outbreak of erythema infectiosum in which 39 infected pregnant women were monitored, two miscarriages occurred.[419] The frequency of fetal loss caused by B19 virus infection was estimated to be 5%. In another study in Spain, fetal loss occurred in only 1 of 60 women infected with B19 virus during pregnancy.[172] Enders and colleagues[136] studied 1018 pregnant women with acute parvovirus infection. The overall rate of fetal loss was 6.3%, with a rate of 11% if the B19 infection occurred in the first 20 weeks of gestation. The overall rate of hydrops fetalis was 3.9%; the peak incidence occurred between 17 and 24 weeks of gestation.

De Jong and colleagues[111] investigated the neurodevelopmental impairment in children treated with intrauterine transfusion for fetal anemia due to B19 infection. Twenty-eight children were evaluated at a median age of 5 years, and the study showed increased impairment when compared with the general population.

*References 91, 147, 161, 186, 213, 226, 239, 362, 363, 415, 548.
†References 9, 38, 46, 52, 82, 106, 181, 197, 209, 238, 261, 263, 275, 308, 344, 351, 365, 372, 400, 433, 446, 448, 544–546.
‡References 69, 106, 133, 144, 162, 180, 201, 241, 261, 275, 540.

*References 31, 42, 60, 117, 197, 205, 223, 238, 261, 446.
†References 3, 8, 9, 49, 52, 56, 70, 110, 115, 118, 132, 165, 166, 172, 196, 197, 228, 238, 252, 256, 257, 259, 260, 277, 314, 317, 320, 327, 331, 371, 374, 383, 397, 409, 418–420, 425, 456, 483, 498, 499, 516, 527–531, 533, 545, 554.

Koch and colleagues[259] performed follow-up examinations on 19 infants born to mothers who had serologically confirmed B19 virus infection between the 4th and 38th weeks of gestation. In none of these infants did hydrops develop during pregnancy, and all were normal after birth. One child whose mother had erythema infectiosum at approximately the 20th week of gestation had a persistent asymptomatic infection for at least the first 7 months of life. Donders and coworkers[118] noted a child in whom a sonogram demonstrated fetal hydrops at 30 weeks of gestation. Cordocentesis revealed a hemoglobin concentration of 2.4 g/dL. One week later, a hydropic 1550-g infant was delivered by cesarean section. The neonate's bone marrow showed an arrest in erythropoiesis with giant pronormoblasts. The infant received multiple transfusions for the first 4 months of life, and B19 viral DNA was identified in the infant's blood at 19 weeks of age. At 2 years of age, this child was found to be clinically, hematologically, and immunologically normal. In contrast to the case just noted, Brown and associates[56] reported an infant with a similar exposure and delivery history who had persistent anemia and, despite therapy, was dependent on transfusions at 4 years of age. In addition, Brown and associates[56] reported two other infants who had received intrauterine transfusions for fetal hydrops and had persistent anemia after birth.

Candotti and colleagues[65] studied plasma samples from 885 pregnant women from Ghana and found that, contrary to the high rate of B19 transmission during primary viremia in pregnancy, pregnant women with B19-specific IgG and low levels of B19 DNA by PCR did not transmit virus to the fetus. Weiffenbach and colleagues[516] determined B19 viral DNA and anti-B19 viral antibody titers in maternal and fetal blood samples obtained from 41 pregnancies complicated by prenatal B19 viral infection and determined that anemia or hydrops due to B19 virus is most likely due to a limited maternofetal transfer of IgG and a poor fetal antibody response.

At the present time, a large number of infants who were exposed to the B19 virus in utero have been studied, with no convincing evidence of specific congenital malformations.[252,341,409,418,419,528] However, van Elsacker-Niele and associates[499] noted B19 virus infection in cells other than those of the erythroid series in two aborted fetuses. Ocular malformation was found in one, and evidence of extensive inflammatory reactions in all fetal and placental tissues was noted in both. Fishman and associates report a case of fetal cardiomyopathy with atrioventricular nodal disease.[148] Carlsen and colleagues suggest a higher mortality rate in B19-infected fetuses with fetal trisomy.[66]

Tiessen and colleagues[483] reported an aborted fetus with a bilateral cleft lip, alveolus, and palate; micrognathia; and webbed joints. In another aborted fetus, ocular abnormalities similar to those seen in congenital rubella were observed.[518] In a neonate with anemia, blueberry muffin rash, and hepatomegaly, parvovirus B19 viral gene sequences were found in the liver and placenta.[451] Gulen and associates[177] described a premature infant born at 29 weeks of gestation with leukoerythroblastosis associated with B19-specific IgM and IgG antibody in both the mother and infant.

Yeh and colleagues[538] described severe, transient dyserythropoietic anemia in a puerperal woman with preeclampsia and eclampsia with concomitant B19 infection.

Neurologic Illness

Parvovirus B19 has been linked with various clinical syndromes, including neurologic manifestations.[29] Douvoyiannis and colleagues[119] reviewed the literature of 81 cases of neurologic disease associated with B19 virus from 1966 to 2008. The median patient age was 9 years, the majority were immunocompetent patients, and there were no differences in the prevalence of sequelae noted between immunocompetent patients and patients with altered immunity. There were also no differences in sequelae between patients with central nervous system manifestations who received intravenous immunoglobulin with or without corticosteroids and those patients with central nervous system manifestations who did not.

Two children with encephalitis in association with erythema infectiosum were noted in the era before discovery of the causative role of B19 virus in erythema infectiosum.[26,51] In the present era, a number of cases of aseptic meningitis and encephalitis have been reported in association with B19 virus infection in both children and adults.* These cases have been documented by the demonstration of specific B19 virus IgM antibody or the presence of B19 viral DNA in cerebrospinal fluid. Bilge and colleagues[41] reported a 12-year-old boy with a history of renal transplantation who had recurrent episodes of encephalopathy and focal neurologic defects associated with B19 DNA in blood and bone marrow and on skin biopsy specimens. He was treated successfully with IVIG. Nolan and colleagues[369] reported an HIV-positive patient in whom parvovirus B19 encephalitis developed during immune reconstitution while receiving highly active antiretroviral therapy. Chorea-encephalopathy, with parvovirus B19 DNA in both serum and cerebrospinal fluid, developed in a previously healthy 8-year-old girl.[149]

Other neurologic illnesses associated with B19 virus infection[28] include postinfectious neuralgic amyotrophy,[394] Guillain-Barré syndrome,[329,481] parainfectious myelitis,[431] acute bilateral carpal tunnel syndrome,[302,426] mononeuritis multiplex,[4,293] stroke,[175,311] transverse myelitis,[472] cerebellitis,[493] and numbness and tingling of the fingers.[143]

Myocarditis

Myocarditis in association with parvovirus B19 infection has been observed in immunocompetent children and adults.* B19-associated myocarditis can progress to chronic dilated cardiomyopathy.[227,270,271,280,299,387,388,552] In a study of 3345 patients who underwent cardiac biopsy for suspected myocarditis or dilated cardiomyopathy, Pankuweit and colleagues[388] found B19 DNA by PCR in 17.6% of patients with dilated cardiomyopathy without significant inflammation, and inflammatory heart disease, ventricular dilation, and reduced ejection fraction were noted in 33.3% of patients. In 2012, Molina and colleagues[332] published a retrospective study characterizing the outcomes of 19 children with B19 myocarditis. They noted a varied presentation from subclinical illness, subacute congestive heart failure to fulminant myocardial involvement. Kühl and associates[271] showed that viral persistence in the setting of myocarditis or dilated cardiomyopathy was associated with progressive deterioration of the left ventricular ejection fraction whereas elimination of virus resulted in significant improvement in left ventricular function.

In a study by Wang and colleagues,[511] B19 virus was detected by nested PCR in cardiac tissues in 7 of 42 patients with congenital heart disease and in none of the 38 controls, thus suggesting a correlation between B19 virus and congenital heart disease.

Enders and associates[134] described two children with life-threatening myocarditis. One of these children died, and the second received a cardiac transplant. The illnesses in both these children occurred in the spring; one had joint pain and urticarial lesions on the flexor surfaces of both arms, erythematous macules on the abdomen and upper part of the chest, and purpuric lesions on the back. Both children had B19 viral DNA identified in the heart and B19-specific IgM antibody.

Nigro and colleagues[361] noted three young children—aged 7, 12, and 18 months—with acute lymphocytic myocarditis and parvovirus B19 infection. Two of these children exhibited full cardiac recovery, but chronic persistent myocarditis developed in the other child. Papadogiannakis and coworkers[389] reported a healthy 11-month-old child who had severe respiratory distress and died of sudden cardiac arrest within 3 hours of admission because of parvovirus-associated lymphocytic myocarditis. Zack and associates[550] reported a 5-year-old girl who suddenly collapsed and died of acute myocarditis secondary to parvovirus B19 infection. Significant lymphocytic infiltration of the sinoatrial node and perivascular infiltration around the atrioventricular node probably resulted in conduction disturbances and death. Jonetzko and colleagues[232] reported a case of fatal parvovirus B19–associated myocarditis in a liver transplant recipient. Parvovirus B19 infection also can mimic acute myocardial infarction[62,270] and isolated diastolic dysfunction in adults.[488]

It is hypothesized that the blood group P antigen on the endothelial cells of coronary vessels is a portal for infection and that such infection results in endothelial dysfunction, impairment of the coronary microcirculation, and inflammation of the myocardium.[28,270,280,532] The blood

*References 28, 41, 72, 149, 187, 197, 199, 238, 248, 264, 369, 383, 465, 471, 474, 514, 536.

*References 33, 44, 62, 113, 116, 134, 265, 270, 280, 299, 332, 349, 361, 387–389, 395, 423.

group P antigen is not present on the myocytes of children and adults; however, it is present on fetal myocytes.[55,268,270,280]

Acute Hepatitis

Acute hepatitis has been noted as a manifestation of B19 virus infection.[189,266,459,542] Yoto and coworkers[542] described seven children with acute hepatitis in association with B19 virus infection. They carefully studied and ruled out other common causes of acute hepatitis. Sokal and associates[459] reported fulminant hepatitis in four children younger than 5 years of age in association with parvovirus B19 infection. Their patients had a distinct clinical pattern consisting of low serum bilirubin concentrations and rapid recovery of liver function without transplantation. Nobili and colleagues[367] reported a case of autoimmune hepatitis followed by severe autoimmune hemolytic anemia in a 1-month-old boy with parvovirus B19 infection. Treatment with cyclosporine and prednisone resulted in resolution of his symptoms.

Hsu and associates[215] studied 54 patients with B19 virus infection in addition to hepatitis B virus (HBV) infection and 51 patients with hepatitis C virus (HCV) infection who were not taking immunosuppressive drugs. The study found that the prevalence of parvovirus B19 DNA was high in patients with HBV (85.2%) or HCV (70.6%). Coinfection with B19 and HBV or HCV did not increase the frequency of liver dysfunction in these patients with chronic hepatitis.[215,285] Additionally, in a study by Wong and associates,[530] there was no significant difference in the prevalence of parvovirus B19 DNA in liver biopsy specimens from patients with fulminant hepatitis or hepatitis-associated aplastic anemia and those with HBV or HCV infection. However, Dwivedi and colleagues showed that pediatric patients with fulminant hepatic failure who had high prevalence of B19 associated with coinfection of other hepatitis viruses had relatively severe disease and poor outcome.[124]

Other Illnesses

One adult patient had chronic red cell aplasia for a 10-year period that was treated with regular blood transfusions.[276] After a diagnosis of persistent B19 virus infection, the patient was treated with IVIG, which resulted in an apparent cure. A presumably immunologically normal woman had recurrent episodes of paresthesia over the course of a 4-year period in conjunction with persistent B19 viral DNA in her blood.[142] Evidence of persistent infection in immunologically normal patients has been noted in other studies.[246,350]

Kerr and associates[247] studied 53 patients who had contracted acute B19 virus illnesses. Seven of those studied had B19 viral DNA demonstrated in serum specimens 26 to 65 months after their acute illnesses. All seven were women, and four were asymptomatic. Of the other three, one had chronic hemolytic anemia, one had persistent arthralgia of the knees, and the last had arthralgia and chronic fatigue syndrome.

Multiple case reports have described patients with chronic fatigue syndrome and persistent parvovirus B19 DNA in their serum.[226,243,244,315,319] In 2002, Kerr and colleagues[243] described three patients with chronic fatigue syndrome and chronic B19 virus infection treated with IVIG. Such treatment resulted in the clearance of B19 viremia, improvement of symptoms, and resolution of cytokine dysregulation.

Faden and associates[142] described a nurse with recurrent episodes of paresthesia who had B19 viral DNA demonstrated in her serum for almost a 4-year period. This woman also had persistent serum IgM antibody to B19 virus.

Lymphadenitis associated with parvovirus B19 infection has been described by many authors. Tsuda and coworkers[489] reported five young adults with cervical lymphadenopathy associated with B19 virus infection. All had fever, one had arthralgia, and all had leukopenia. Morinet and colleagues[338] described a 27-year-old man with pseudoappendicitis or acute mesenteric lymphadenitis and serologic evidence of B19 virus infection. A 16-month-old boy had peripheral facial palsy, parotitis, and intraparotid lymphadenitis with evidence of parvovirus B19 IgM antibody and IgG antibody seroconversion.[313] Johnson and associates[230] described an 18-year-old woman with parvovirus B19 resulting in necrotizing lymphadenitis, and Knösel and colleagues[255] reported unilateral cervical lymphadenopathy in a 16-year-old girl. In both cases, parvovirus B19 DNA was detected by PCR on lymph node biopsy specimens.

Parvovirus B19 infection also has been shown to induce proliferative glomerulonephritis, usually endocapillary or mesangioproliferative (or both), with hypocomplementemia and spontaneous recovery.[219,225,337,379,478,479,513] Ieiri and colleagues[219] studied 10 patients with acute glomerulonephritis associated with human parvovirus B19 infection. These authors found that this specific renal disease characterized by endocapillary hypercellularity was associated with hypocomplementemia, leukopenia, positive antinuclear antibody, and a female preponderance (9 of 10 patients). Ohtomo and associates[379] reported a healthy 8-year-old boy with erythema infectiosum and glomerulonephritis with immune complex deposits associated with B19 virus diagnosed by both monoclonal antibody against human parvovirus B19 antigen and nested PCR on renal biopsy. The association between parvovirus B19 and sepsis also has been reported by multiple authors. These patients exhibited shock, severe respiratory distress, and parvovirus B19 infection.[23,145,339,389,512] Parvovirus B19 infection has also been linked to generalized edema in 2 previously healthy women.[503,524]

DIFFERENTIAL DIAGNOSIS

Because the exanthem of erythema infectiosum is unique, its diagnosis should be easy. During epidemics, no difficulties should arise, but sporadic cases can be a problem. In the differential diagnosis, rubella and scarlet fever are of most concern. Because rubella virus has been recovered from some patients with illness thought to be erythema infectiosum[26] and because an erythema infectiosum–like illness was observed in volunteers who underwent intranasal administration of a rubella virus strain recovered from a patient with erythema infectiosum–like illness,[432] this diagnostic possibility always should be considered. When the risk for development of congenital rubella is a possibility, rubella-specific diagnostic tests should be performed (see Chapter 174).

Erythema infectiosum can be differentiated from scarlet fever by the usual lack of pharyngitis in the former and a positive culture for *Streptococcus pyogenes* in the latter. Other differential diagnostic considerations are other infectious exanthems (see Chapter 58), collagen vascular diseases, drug reactions, and allergic responses to environmental substances.

Although a presumptive diagnosis of B19 virus infection may be made by exclusion of other etiologic possibilities, a definitive diagnosis can be made only by specific serologic tests or identification of B19 antigens or DNA in blood or tissue specimens.

Aplastic crisis in a patient with chronic hemolytic anemia can be diagnosed by finding a hemoglobin concentration that is 2 g/dL or more below the steady-state value for that patient, together with a reticulocyte count either less than 0.2% of the steady-state value or elevated above the steady-state value (indicative of hyperplasia of erythrocyte precursors in the recovery phase). Although B19 virus infection is the most common cause of aplastic crisis, moderate to severe degrees of hypoplasia may be associated with systemic bacterial infections (e.g., *Salmonella, Streptococcus pneumoniae*) or marrow-suppressive drugs.[323,442]

DIAGNOSIS

Several tests have been developed and refined that allow a reliable serologic diagnosis of acute and past B19 virus infection to be established and B19 virus in blood and tissues to be demonstrated.* IgM and IgG antibody can be detected by enzyme immunoassay, hemadherence, radioimmunoassay, or immunofluorescence; antigen can be detected by DNA hybridization, PCR, or electron microscopy.

In a normal host, acute or recent infection is determined best by demonstration of specific IgM antibody. In immunocompromised patients with suspected acute or chronic infection, the diagnosis is made by detection of antigen in blood. Similarly, detection of antigen also can be performed early in aplastic crisis and to study aborted fetal tissues. Gallinella and colleagues[163] recommend both specific IgM and B19 DNA PCR to establish a diagnosis of B19 infection. Past infection

*References 9, 14, 21, 35, 59, 61, 67, 71, 74, 92, 94, 95, 107, 108, 137, 157, 163, 208, 211, 251, 258, 262, 324, 336, 359, 424, 435, 437, 475, 510, 529, 553.

and immunity to B19 virus are determined by demonstration of specific serum IgG antibody.

Some caution should be observed in accepting the results of IgM serology and antigen detection in unusual clinical circumstances.[53] The sensitivity and specificity of the various serologic tests vary, and additional false-positive and false-negative results can be expected, depending on the skill of workers in individual laboratories.[61,94,486,496] Antigen-detection systems can be contaminated, and such contamination may not be discernible by conventional controls. When the results of tests on specimens from patients with unusual illnesses are positive, repeating the tests in a different laboratory is worthwhile.

Söderlund and associates[457] reported an IgG avidity assay that is highly sensitive and specific for the identification of recent primary infection with parvovirus B19. Enders and coworkers[135] also recommended VP1 IgG avidity or VP2 epitope–type specificity assays in the presence of low-level IgM or B19 DNA to confirm or refute the diagnosis of B19 infection during pregnancy. Because there is a window of 7 days after initial infection occurs until the development of IgM-specific B19 antibody and because IgM can be negative or low in the presence of overt hydrops fetalis, both serology and B19 DNA PCR are recommended on both maternal and fetal sera (or cord blood).[128]

Beersma and colleagues[35] demonstrated the superiority of B19 VP2 IgM ELISA by showing high correlation with elevated levels of B19 DNA in sera. Persistent infection may be determined by the presence of IgG antibody to NS1.[505]

If parvovirus B19 infection is suspected in pregnancy, ultrasound should be performed to assess for fetal anemia and hydrops (excess of fluid in at least two body compartments of the fetus).[128] The use of middle cerebral artery peak systolic velocity for the detection of fetal anemia may be a useful adjunct to ultrasound scanning.[103,343]

TREATMENT AND PROGNOSIS

No specific treatment of B19 virus infection exists. Symptomatic therapy for erythema infectiosum rarely is necessary, especially in children. Starch baths may be helpful in reducing pruritus. Arthralgia or arthritis may be troublesome and may be treated with analgesics.

The outlook in virtually all cases of erythema infectiosum is excellent. If patients with aplastic crisis receive transfusions with packed erythrocytes when necessary, the prognosis for these patients also is excellent. If B19 virus infection occurs during pregnancy, the pregnancy should be monitored carefully. At delivery, examination of cord blood or blood from the neonate for detection of virus and IgM antibody will reveal whether the virus has crossed the placenta and infected the neonate. When infection has occurred, the child should be examined carefully for any defect and monitored for some years to exclude the possibility of delayed sequelae.

Some researchers have suggested that pregnant women with symptomatic B19 virus infection be observed for fetal aplastic crisis by monitoring maternal serum for elevated levels of α-fetoprotein.[68] If levels are found to be elevated, serial ultrasonography can be performed to detect hydrops fetalis. Fetal hydrops can be treated by in utero transfusions[139,171,422]; however, there is a risk for infection and the potential for congenital malformations with cordocentesis and fetal transfusion. Enders and colleagues[136] reported that 84.6% of those with severe hydrops fetalis survived to delivery. In 2005, Matsuda and colleagues[316] successfully treated a B19-infected fetus with hydrops at 21 weeks of gestation with two injections of B19 IgG-rich immunoglobulin injected into the fetal peritoneal cavity. The fetal ascites and pericardial effusion resolved completely 8 days after the initial injection, and a healthy infant was born at 38 weeks of gestation without evidence of cardiac dysfunction or B19 DNA detected in serum. Therapeutic abortion is not indicated for pregnant women with documented B19 virus infection.

Patients with chronic myocarditis caused by B19 virus and acute heart failure caused by B19 have been treated successfully with IVIG.[6,466] Chronic myocarditis secondary to B19 also has been treated with immunosuppressive agents, including corticosteroids and cyclosporine.[280,349,423] Ito and associates[224] described a patient with baseline refractory autoimmune hemolytic anemia who was taking immunosuppressive medications while infected with B19 virus. The patient had a complicated course of illness; persistent pure red cell aplasia subsequently developed but resolved after treatment with cyclosporine and IVIG.

Immunocompromised patients with chronic B19 virus infection can be treated successfully with IVIG preparations,[42,60,117,197,203,223,238,261,446] as can other patients without demonstrated immune deficiencies who have chronic infections.[142,224,226,345,466] Although the amount of specific B19 virus antibody varies among different IVIG products, all contain significant concentrations.[117] No formal treatment studies have been performed, and several different treatment programs have been used. Even though some cures have been achieved with single-dose IVIG therapy, we favor an initial 4-day course with 500 mg/kg per day. After the patient has received treatment, the viremia should cease and clinical improvement should occur. Some immunocompromised patients have required repeated treatment courses.

PREVENTION

B19 virus is spread by the oral and respiratory routes, and virus shedding during routine infection occurs when patients are not aware of their illness. Because B19 virus infections occur in outbreaks, the virus can be widespread in a community, with many infections going unrecognized.

Patients with erythema infectiosum do not need to be isolated because they have passed their period of infectivity. Although patients with aplastic crisis also usually are past the period of virus shedding, they should be isolated because some will be shedding virus at the time of initial evaluation. All patients with chronic infection should be considered contagious until treated with IVIG and demonstrated to be nonviremic.

Pregnant women are of particular concern during an outbreak.[70,166] The rate of parvovirus seropositivity is approximately 50% in women of childbearing age; thus, no risk exists in approximately half of those who might become exposed. Determining an IgG antibody titer can allay the fear in those who are antibody positive. Cartter and associates[70] examined occupational risk factors for B19 virus infection in pregnant women. They found the following rates of infection: school teachers, 16%; daycare workers, 9%; homemakers, 9%; and women working outside the home, 4%. In another study, Gillespie and colleagues[166] found that the greatest risk for infection occurred in school and daycare personnel. These results suggest that in certain circumstances (in older women and those with past fertility problems), having women in high-risk occupations avoid the workplace during the outbreak period might be reasonable.

Technological advances have led to the development of experimental recombinant vaccines that show considerable promise for effective prevention.[27,97,139,155,194,546] These vaccines could be useful in selected populations, such as patients with hemoglobinopathies and seronegative women of childbearing age.

NEW REFERENCES SINCE SEVENTH EDITION

6. Alberti L, Loffi M, Fragasso G, et al. Acute heart failure caused by parvovirus B-19 myocarditis treated with human immunoglobulin. *Case Rep Cardiol.* 2012;2012:180871.
29. Barah F, Whiteside S, Batista S, et al. Neurological aspects of human parvovirus B19 infection: a systematic review. *Rev Med Virol.* 2014;24(3):154-168.
77. Cefalo MG, Arlotta A, Maurizi P, et al. Human parvovirus B 19 and Epstein-Barr virus co-infection in a child with hereditary spherocytosis. *Eur Rev Med Pharmacol Sci.* 2012;16(2):265-269.
102. Cooray M, Manolakos JJ, Wright DS, et al. Parvovirus infection mimicking systemic lupus erythematosus. *CMAJ.* 2013;185(15):1342-1344.
179. Gupta V, Saini I, Nath G. Prevalence of parvovirus B 19 infection in children with aplastic anemia. *Indian Pediatr.* 2013;50(5):489-491.
227. Jain P, Jain A, Khan DN, et al. Human parvovirus B19 associated dilated cardiomyopathy. *BMJ Case Rep.* 2013;2013.
235. Kawakami C, Kono Y, Inoue A, et al. Severe bone marrow failure associated with human parvovirus B19 infection in a case with no underlying disorder. *Int J Hematol.* 2012;96(6):820-821.
265. Koehl B, Oualha M, Lesage F, et al. Fatal parvovirus B19 myocarditis in children and possible dysimmune mechanism. *Pediatr Infect Dis J.* 2012;31(4):418-421.
266. Koliou M, Karaoli E, Soteriades ES, et al. Acute hepatitis and myositis associated with erythema infectiosum by parvovirus B19 in an adolescent. *BMC Pediatr.* 2014;14:6.

277. Kyeong KS, Won HS, Lee MY, et al. Clinical features of 10 fetuses with prenatally diagnosed parvovirus b19 infection and fetal hydrops. *Fetal Pediatr Pathol.* 2015;34(1):49-56.
307. Makhlouf MM, Elwakil SG, Ibrahim NS. Molecular and serological assessment of parvovirus B-19 infection in Egyptian children with sickle cell disease. *J Microbiol Immunol Infect.* 2015;S1684–1182(15):914-917.
332. Molina KM, Garcia X, Denfield SW, et al. Parvovirus B19 myocarditis causes significant morbidity and mortality in children. *Pediatr Cardiol.* 2013;34(2):390-397.
470. Suzuki M, Yoto Y, Ishikawa A, et al. Acute transverse myelitis associated with human parvovirus B19 infection. *J Child Neurol.* 2014;29(2):280-282.
481. Terhes G, Jenei M, Bereg E, et al. Neurologic consequence of a parvovirus B19 infection. *J Clin Virol.* 2013;56(2):156-158.
493. Uchida Y, Matsubara K, Morio T, et al. Acute cerebellitis and concurrent encephalitis associated with parvovirus B19 infection. *Pediatr Infect Dis J.* 2012;31(4):427.
503. Vlaar PJ, Mithoe G, Janssen WM. Generalized edema associated with parvovirus B19 infection. *Int J Infect Dis.* 2014;29:40-41.
520. Wen JQ, Zhou N, Li D, et al. Study on clinical characteristics and follow-up visit of acquired aplastic anemia associated with parvovirus B19 infection. *Indian J Pediatr.* 2012;79(6):741-746.
524. Wiggli B, Imhof E, Meier CA, et al. Water, water, everywhere. Acute parvovirus B19 infection. *Lancet.* 2013;381(9868):776.
552. Zedtwitz-Liebenstein K, Robak O, Burgmann H, et al. Retrospective evaluation of antibody index of human parvovirus B19 as a prognostic factor in patients with dilated and ischemic cardiomyopathy. *J Med Virol.* 2013;85(6):1111-1114.

The full reference list for this chapter is available at ExpertConsult.com.

Human Bocaviruses 153

Jennifer E. Schuster • John V. Williams

Human bocavirus (HBoV) was discovered in 2005 by Allander and colleagues.[3] Studies have shown that HBoV infection is ubiquitous worldwide and that nearly all adults are seropositive. HBoV has been detected in respiratory specimens from persons with acute respiratory illness and in stool specimens from patients with gastroenteritis. However, controlled studies do not always show a consistent association between HBoV and acute respiratory disease, and prolonged shedding of HBoV further clouds the issue of causality. Much remains to be elucidated about the biology and epidemiology of this virus.

HISTORY

Allander and colleagues discovered HBoV using a novel molecular virus discovery approach on nasopharyngeal aspirates collected from patients with acute respiratory illness.[3] The method consisted of pooling clinical specimens, concentrating virus particles by ultracentrifugation, depleting human DNA, amplifying viral DNA by random polymerase chain reaction (PCR), sequencing the PCR products, and aligning the sequences to published databases. The group tested nasopharyngeal aspirates collected from patients with acute respiratory illness. Novel parvovirus-like sequences were identified that most closely aligned with *bo*vine parvovirus (BPV)[26] and minute virus of *ca*nines (MVC)[11]; thus, the new virus was designated HBoV. Related bocaviruses have been discovered in pigs,[13] gorillas,[79] and sea lions.[97]

PROPERTIES

HBoV is a member of the *Parvoviridae* family, subfamily *Parvovirinae*, genus *Bocaparvovirus*. Like other parvoviruses, HBoV is a small, nonenveloped virus with a single-stranded, linear DNA genome of ~5 kb. The capsid size is ~22 to 28 nm.[61] The genomic organization of HBoV closely resembles that of the other known bocaviruses BPV and MVC. Like all members of the *Parvovirinae* subfamily, there are two major open reading frames (ORFs) encoding a nonstructural protein (NS1) and two capsid proteins (VP1 and VP2), respectively. However, like BPV and MVC, HBoV also has a third ORF. In BPV and MVC, this ORF encodes a nonstructural protein with unknown function, NP1.[26,139] HBoV has ~42% amino acid identity of both major ORFs to BPV and MVC and thus represents a distinct virus. Other HBoV genotypes have been identified and tentatively designated species HBoV2, HBoV3, and HBoV4.[8,80,81] Some of these may have arisen from recombination events among different HBoV species.[53,80,84] Nucleotide identity among these different HBoVs ranges from 73% to 88%.[29,80] There is evidence of some antigenic cross-reactivity among these viruses,[76] and the biological significance of the different types is not clear.

HBoV has been cultivated in well-differentiated primary airway epithelial cell cultures.[41–43] No cytopathic effects were observed, but increasing amounts of HBoV DNA and RNA in cell cultures suggested active viral replication. In one study, HBoV-infected cells exhibited loss of cilia, disruption of tight junctions, and loss of transepithelial resistance.[42] Moreover, supernatant from infected cells could successfully pass infection to a new cell monolayer, confirming production of infectious viral particles.

HBoV exhibits a complex transcriptional strategy, with multiple monocistronic, polycistronic, and variably spliced mRNAs.[25,43] The overall transcription profile of HBoV is similar to that of BPV and MVC.[128,145] The cellular site of HBoV replication is not known, though viral proteins NS1 and NP1 localize to the nucleus.[25,98] NP1 interferes with innate immune responses by blocking interferon beta production via interferon regulatory factor 3 signaling, is required for mRNA splicing and expression of viral capsid proteins, and induces apoptosis in host cells.[144,155,158] VP2 modulates interferon beta signaling.[105] No animal model of infection has been identified. However, a reverse genetics system has been established for HBoV, which will enhance study of the biology and pathogenesis of this virus.[66]

EPIDEMIOLOGY

HBoV infections have been identified in humans worldwide. Following the discovery of the virus in pooled respiratory specimens, a number of groups tested convenience sample sets collected from patients with acute respiratory illness. HBoV was detected by PCR in these specimens at rates between 5% and 20%.[5,9,51,52,83,92,106–108,142] The virus is detected most frequently in children less than 2 years old. Australian investigators detected HBoV in 18 (6%) of 324 specimens collected during autumn and winter in a single season from children with acute respiratory illness.[141] HBoV was present in 18/318 (6%) Japanese children with lower respiratory infection.[106] Investigators in Connecticut tested 425 hospital laboratory specimens collected from children younger than 2 years and detected HBoV in 22 (5%), all between October and April.[83] HBoV was detected in hospitalized children with acute respiratory illness in Vietnam (78/1082 [7%]),[147] Thailand (39/304 [13%]),[64] and China (386/3022 [13%]).[104] A South African study found HBoV in 49 of 517 (10%) HIV-infected and 125 of 943 (13%) HIV-uninfected children hospitalized with lower respiratory illness.[120]

A recent study tested monthly saliva specimens collected from 87 children followed from birth to 18 months of age.[112] Almost all children had HBoV detected at least once, and 66 (76%) had a primary detection event. Primary detection was statistically associated with the presence of new cough symptoms within 14 days, though this included the 7 days prior to HBoV detection. This association was stronger when restricted to those with a high viral load, supporting some studies that link viral load with clinical disease (discussed later).

Most published studies include only patients with symptomatic respiratory illness, while those including asymptomatic controls offer conflicting findings. Several studies reported lower rates of HBoV detection in controls compared to cases with respiratory illness.[2,55,83,107] However, most of the controls were not well age matched or season matched, or they comprised different types of respiratory specimens collected from cases and controls. Large prospective studies in Canada, Denmark, and The Netherlands with age-matched and season-matched controls have found similar rates of HBoV in asymptomatic subjects and children with ARI.[102,148,151] A prospective study in Thailand reported four-fold higher HBoV detection in all respiratory illness cases compared to controls. However, HBoV was not detected significantly more often in either hospitalized pneumonia cases or outpatients with influenza-like illness than in controls when considering only HBoV-positive patients without co-detection of other viruses and controlling for age and month.[52] In a prospective 1-year cohort study of 119 daycare attendees, HBoV was detected in 20 (44%) of 45 asymptomatic subjects at enrollment.[110] In a prospective pneumococcal vaccine trial cohort of 221 children in Papua New Guinea, HBoV was detected in 53 of 273 (19%) asymptomatic children and in 18 of 80 (22%) children with acute respiratory illness.[28] A prospective Swedish study of children hospitalized for community-acquired pneumonia found HBoV in 14 of 121 (15%) cases and 50 of 240 (21%) age-, gender-, and season-matched asymptomatic controls.[131]

HBoV is detected year round, though detection is more common during the winter months.[2,6,9,30,52,54,55,83] It should be noted that this period is when most respiratory specimens are collected due to the seasonality of other acute respiratory viruses. HBoV infections are reported in immunocompromised hosts.[21,39,74,91,136,137] HBoV was uncommon in adults with chronic obstructive pulmonary disease exacerbations.[133]

Seroprevalence studies using diverse methods have reported seroprevalence of 74% to 99% among adults.[47,58,63,68,71,75,76,96,99] A prospective serosurvey of 109 Finnish children found that all seroconverted by age 6 years.[113] One factor that complicates the interpretation of prior seroepidemiology is the recent discovery of serologic cross-reactivity between HBoV1, HBoV2, HBoV3, and HBoV4.[76] This study used HBoV viruslike particles to deplete cross-reactive antibodies, and the investigators found that the seroprevalence of HBoV2, HBoV3, and HBoV4 in adults was 34%, 15%, and 2% and in children aged 1 to 2 years 25%, 10%, and 5%, respectively. The HBoV1 seroprevalence among adults decreased from 96% to 59% after depletion of HBoV2, HBoV3, and HBoV4-reactive antibodies. A similar Chinese study reported that the seroprevalence of HBoV1, HBoV2, HBoV3, and HBoV4 in adults was 67%, 49%, 39%, and 1%, respectively; in children, the seroprevalence was 50%, 37%, 29%, and 1%, respectively.[60] Thus, serologic data suggest that HBoV1 is the most frequent bocavirus type infecting humans.

PATHOGENESIS

The method of transmission of HBoV is not known. However, because the virus is present in the nasopharynx in high concentrations, a reasonable conclusion is that its spread is similar to that of other respiratory viruses.[70] This spread could involve contact transmission with droplet nuclei or by fomites. Parvovirus B19 can be transmitted via respiratory secretions.[4,37,57] A few nosocomial infections have been reported.[18,31,45,83] Parvoviruses are resistant to disinfectants, which could contribute to environmental persistence.[49]

A unique feature of HBoV respiratory infections is the high frequency of mixed infections with other established pathogenic respiratory viruses. Several potential reasons for the high rates of co-detection have been postulated: bocavirus may be an asymptomatic passenger agent, function as a helper virus during respiratory viral co-infection, or be activated by inflammation induced by other viruses.[138] Studies have identified high rates of 20% to 90% co-infection with HBoV and other viruses, including influenza, human metapneumovirus (MPV), parainfluenza viruses (PIV), and respiratory syncytial virus (RSV).* Manning and colleagues[108] detected HBoV in 47 (8.2%) of 574 specimens from subjects with acute respiratory illness, 43% of which were co-infected with another virus. Co-infection with another virus—including influenza, PIV, or RSV—was detected in 90% of outpatients with influenza-like illness in Thailand.[52] A prospective study of daycare attendees found another established respiratory virus in 72% of HBoV-positive acute respiratory infection episodes during the study.[110] This high rate of co-detection of other viruses with HBoV is similar to other reports of 60% to 90% co-detection.[2,15,19,35,52,69,102,122,148] The presence of established respiratory pathogens makes it difficult to assign a causal role to HBoV in these reports.

Several studies have shown an association between HBoV single infection and respiratory symptoms, and several suggest that a higher HBoV viral load in the nasopharynx correlates with symptomatic disease.[17,33,56,72,83,95,124,156,157] Kantola and associates demonstrated the occurrence of IgM antibody responses and titer increases of IgG antibody in children with respiratory illnesses.[75] Concurrent detection of HBoV in nasopharyngeal samples and blood has also been suggested to correlate with acute respiratory illness.[33,143] However, HBoV has also been detected in the serum of healthy blood donors.[14,96]

Another unusual feature of HBoV is prolonged shedding and intermittent detection of HBoV over weeks to months.[12,17,95,151] Martin and colleagues[110] documented prolonged shedding (up to 75 days) in 20 subjects, with intermittent detection several months apart in 18 other children. However, prolonged shedding was not detected during single HBoV infections but only during co-infections with other viruses, suggesting that HBoV may cause either acute short-term infection or a more indolent long-shedding infection.[111] The aforementioned longitudinal saliva specimen study from the same group reported a median duration of HBoV shedding of 50 days, with a maximum of 402 days.[112] Several groups detected HBoV in tonsil and adenoid tissues from surgical specimens, suggesting long-term persistence.[32,36,59,103,123,126,127] Interestingly, the rates of detection were higher in adenoids (24–56%) than tonsils (5–16%). Moreover, HBoV mRNA was detected, indicating active viral replication, and viral mRNA correlated with the detection of HBoV DNA in blood.[126] One study detected HBoV in 18 of 102 (18%) sinus mucosal biopsy specimens from patients with histories of chronic sinusitis but without acute illnesses; 17 of these had HBoV-negative nasopharyngeal swabs and blood.[50] Prolonged detection of HBoV in stool has been reported,[82,136] and HBoV can persist as episomal DNA within gastrointestinal tissue.[78] Thus, prolonged detection of HBoV in humans appears to reflect the viral capacity to establish persistent infection, though the compartment, mechanisms, and nature of this infection are not clear.

HBoV is rarely detected in other tissues. HBoV DNA has been detected in heart tissue from patients undergoing cardiac surgery without evidence of virus-associated cardiomyopathy.[90] HBoV has not been associated with any systemic illness or anemia. HBoV has not been detected in amniotic fluid or fetal tissues,[46,132] in contrast to BPV, MVC, and B19, which can cause intrauterine infections in animals or humans.[65,109] HBoV was not detected in skin or synovial tissues.[119]

CLINICAL MANIFESTATIONS

Respiratory Illness

HBoV has been detected in nasopharyngeal specimens from children with both upper and lower respiratory tract illnesses. Most studies focus on hospitalized cohorts with predominantly lower tract disease. Many investigations have compared the signs and symptoms associated with HBoV infection with those caused by other respiratory viruses.† These comparative studies show that the clinical findings associated with HBoV infections are similar to those of viral infections caused by RSV, MPV, adenoviruses, influenza viruses, PIV, and rhinoviruses. Laboratory findings associated with HBoV infection are non-specific. White blood cell counts ranged from 3000 to 31,000 cells/mm^3 in several studies, with means of 11 to 14,000, while C-reactive protein levels ranged from 0.2 to 11.4 mg/dL with median values of 0.4 to 1.2 mg/dL.[6,106,150]

*References 2, 20, 52, 64, 87, 104, 107, 108, 111, 112, 130, 147.

†References 2, 5, 6, 9, 30, 51, 52, 55, 83, 106–108, 142, 151.

Upper Respiratory Tract Infections

In one study, 86% of 49 HBoV infections without co-infection with other agents were classified as upper respiratory illnesses.[48] In contrast, only 42% of 50 children in this study who had HBoV and a co-infecting virus were diagnosed with an upper respiratory illness. Pharyngitis was observed in 55% of the cases in which HBoV was the single agent identified. Of the children with HBoV infections without co-infections, 18% had acute otitis media and 12% had sinusitis. In another study, otitis media was reported in 61% of all HBoV infections.[102]

In a large study, Arnold and associates[6] noted the following findings at the time of presentation: fever, 68%; rhinorrhea, 67%; cough, 85%; conjunctivitis, 7%; vomiting, 30%; diarrhea, 21%; and rash, 7%. Of interest was that the cough was paroxysmal in 19% of the HBoV-infected children, whereas paroxysmal cough was much less common in adenovirus infections (7%) and MPV infections (5%).

In one Korean study, three of 36 (8.3%) children infected with HBoV had croup.[30] In a study in Canada, two of 58 (3%) HBoV-infected children had croup,[10] and in a study in Japan, one of 18 (6%) had laryngotracheitis.[106]

Lower Respiratory Tract Infections

Longtin and colleagues[102] noted that 42% of children with HBoV infections had pneumonia and that 42% had bronchiolitis. In a large study in San Diego, California, involving 82 children with HBoV infections, 76 children with adenoviral infections, and 87 children with MPV infections, the investigators were able to compare the rates of various clinical findings.[7] In this study, the following rates of events were noted in HBoV-infected children: hospitalization, 69%; need for oxygen administration, 44%; admission to intensive care unit, 11%; intubation, 4%; clinical lower respiratory tract disease, 61%; hypoxia, 41%; increased work of breathing, 59%; abnormal lung findings, 51%; "atelectasis versus infiltrate," 11%; "infiltrate" or "pneumonia," 9%; and bronchiolitis, 46%. Comparatively, adenovirus-infected children had less lower respiratory tract disease, less hypoxia, less increased work of breathing, and they were more likely to have normal chest radiographic findings than were children with HBoV and MPV infections.

In a study in Korea, 53% of HBoV-infected children had rales noted on chest auscultation and 42% had wheezing.[30] The clinical diagnoses in this study were bronchiolitis (25%), pneumonia (56%), exacerbation of asthma (11%), and croup (8%). In a study in Germany, 32 children with lower respiratory tract disease were studied.[152] The diagnoses were bronchitis (16%), wheezing bronchitis (14%), bronchiolitis (3%), and pneumonia (18%). Ten of the 11 patients in this study with pneumonia had co-infections with other respiratory viruses. In a study in Canada involving 58 bocavirus infections, 40% had bronchiolitis and 22% had pneumonia.[10] In a study of 18 children in Japan, the lower respiratory tract diagnoses were wheezy bronchitis (33%), pneumonia (33%), bronchiolitis (11%), bronchitis (11%), and asthmatic attack (6%).[106]

Gastrointestinal Illness

Gastroenteritis has been associated with HBoV infections, and HBoV has been detected in stool[92,93,149,154] by PCR, but the biological significance of this is not clear. Similar to the acute respiratory infection data, established gastrointestinal pathogens are co-detected frequently with HBoV, and HBoV is detected in stool specimens from asymptomatic subjects.[8,81,118,134] In one study in Hong Kong, diarrhea was noted in 11% of 79 patients with respiratory symptoms.[92] In the same study, HBoV was identified in fecal samples of 25 children with gastroenteritis. Of these children, 16% had blood in the stool, 8% had mucus in the stool, 32% had vomiting, and 68% had fever. The following respiratory findings were noted in these children with gastroenteritis: coryza (56%), acute bronchitis (16%), and pneumonia (12%). Co-pathogens were identified in 56% of the children: rotavirus (36%), *Salmonella* spp. (8%), *Campylobacter* spp. (4%), *Staphylococcus aureus* (4%), and *Clostridium difficile* (4%).

In a study of 962 stool samples from children with acute gastroenteritis in Seoul, Korea, a viral agent was found in 44.4% of the specimens, including rotavirus (25.7%), norovirus (13.7%), adenovirus (3.0%), astrovirus (1.1%), and HBoV (0.8%).[93] In Brazilian children with gastroenteritis, HBoV1 was detected in 2% to 10% of stool samples, often with other viruses, and viral load did not correlate with disease.[1,125] One study detected HBoV1 in 12% in asymptomatic South Korean subjects.[86]

Several studies suggest that the newer bocaviruses HBoV2, HBoV3, and HBoV4, which were discovered in stool specimens, may be more likely to be associated with diarrhea than HBoV1.[8,22,62,67,81,85,118,134,146] HBoV2 is the most frequent type detected in stool from gastroenteritis at 3% to 5%, but in several studies, it is detected at similar rates in asymptomatic controls.[27,81,118,134,154] A study of Finnish subjects with acute respiratory illness with or without gastroenteritis symptoms found that HBoV1 to HBoV3 were not associated with gastrointestinal illness.[121]

Infections in Immunocompromised Patients

Koskenvuo and associates[89] described three children with acute lymphoblastic leukemia with detection of HBoV in respiratory specimens collected during acute febrile illness. In addition to fever, one of these children had cough, rhinitis, and otitis media, and another child had vomiting and diarrhea. The third child had five consecutive febrile episodes during the course of a 6-month period; with each of these episodes, HBoV was found in nasal swab samples. Another report described prolonged detection of HBoV for up to 3 months in children with various immunodeficiencies.[136] Other cases of HBoV infection in immunosuppressed children and adults have been reported, none fatal.[6,21,39,74,91,107,108,137,142] A series of 53 pediatric stem cell transplant recipients testing only serum specimens found no episodes of HBoV viremia.[129]

Other Clinical Findings

In addition to respiratory and gastrointestinal signs and symptoms, numerous other clinical findings and diagnoses have been observed in children with HBoV infections. Arnold and colleagues[6] noted four children with maculopapular erythematous rashes, and exanthems have been noted in other studies.[34,92,116] In three studies, the rate of exanthema varied between 5% and 9% in the children studied.

Three studies detected HBoV in respiratory or fecal samples from children clinically thought to have Kawasaki disease (KD).[7,24,92] However, a case-control study of 12 children with KD and 33 age- and gender-matched controls found equal serum levels of HBoV-specific IgA and IgG in both groups, while none in either group was HBoV IgM-positive.[94] None of the KD cases and only one control had HBoV DNA in the serum. Another study performed HBoV PCR on endothelial cells from 22 cases of KD, including 18 with coronary artery lesions; none was positive for HBoV.[16]

Other events noted in temporal association with HBoV infection include intussusception,[23,92] aseptic meningitis,[92] and nephritic syndrome.[92] There are isolated reports of HBoV DNA detection in the cerebrospinal fluid of patients with encephalitis, but the biologic and clinical implications of this finding are not clear.[114,115,153]

DIAGNOSIS

Differential Diagnosis

The clinical features of HBoV respiratory infections are similar to those of other common respiratory viruses, including adenovirus, influenza virus, MPV, PIV, rhinovirus, and RSV. Similarly, gastroenteritis associated with HBoV infection cannot be differentiated from rotavirus infections and illness associated with other viral and bacterial agents.

Specific Diagnosis

Presently, the only diagnostic method for the demonstration of HBoV infection is PCR. Specimens for PCR may be obtained from respiratory secretions, stool, and blood. Primer sets used target the NP1 region 4 and the NS1 region of the genome.[3,141] A real-time PCR assay targeting the NS1 gene is capable of detecting all four known HBoV types.[77] Some commercially available multiplex molecular assays include HBoV.[38,135]

Some authors argue that serodiagnosis, the measurement of HBoV viral load, or a combination of serologic testing and blood PCR provides a more accurate diagnosis of acute infection versus asymptomatic shedding.[33,75,88,113,140,143] Some studies report confirmation of primary HBoV infection using paired acute and convalescent sera, which would not be useful during an acute illness.[44,75,113,117,143] There are no commercial reagents for serodiagnosis of HBoV at present.

TREATMENT

No specific antiviral treatment for HBoV infections is known. General care should be similar to that employed for other respiratory or gastrointestinal viral infections. Humans develop $CD4^+$ T-cell and antibody responses against HBoV.[100,101,143] Moreover, antigenic epitopes on the HBoV capsid have been identified using monoclonal antibodies, and recombinant virus-like particles were immunogenic in mice.[40,73] Thus, the potential for vaccine development exists if warranted.

PROGNOSIS

Although the full spectrum of HBoV infections and possible sequelae are not known presently, nearly all HBoV infections appear to be self-limited. There are rare reports of severe disease or fatalities in persons with chronic underlying conditions.

NEW REFERENCES SINCE THE SEVENTH EDITION

11. Binn LN, Lazar EC, Eddy GA, et al. Recovery and characterization of a minute virus of canines. *Infect Immun.* 1970;1(5):503-508.
13. Blomstrom AL, Belak S, Fossum C, et al. Detection of a novel porcine boca-like virus in the background of porcine circovirus type 2 induced postweaning multisystemic wasting syndrome. *Virus Res.* 2009;146(1-2):125-129.
20. Calvo C, Garcia-Garcia ML, Pozo F, et al. Respiratory syncytial virus coinfections with rhinovirus and human bocavirus in hospitalized children. *Medicine (Baltimore).* 2015;94(42):e1788.
21. Campbell AP, Guthrie KA, Englund JA, et al. Clinical outcomes associated with respiratory virus detection before allogeneic hematopoietic stem cell transplant. *Clin Infect Dis.* 2015;61(2):192-202.
38. Costa E, Rodriguez-Dominguez M, Clari MA, et al. Comparison of the performance of 2 commercial multiplex PCR platforms for detection of respiratory viruses in upper and lower tract respiratory specimens. *Diagn Microbiol Infect Dis.* 2015;82(1):40-43.
41. Deng X, Li Y, Qiu J. Human bocavirus 1 infects commercially available primary human airway epithelium cultures productively. *J Virol Methods.* 2014;195:112-119.
42. Deng X, Yan Z, Luo Y, et al. In vitro modeling of human bocavirus 1 infection of polarized primary human airway epithelia. *J Virol.* 2013;87(7):4097-4102.
40. Deng ZH, Hao YX, Yao LH, et al. Immunogenicity of recombinant human bocavirus-1,2 VP2 gene virus-like particles in mice. *Immunology.* 2014;142(1): 58-66.
44. Don M, Soderlund-Venermo M, Valent F, et al. Serologically verified human bocavirus pneumonia in children. *Pediatr Pulmonol.* 2010;45(2):120-126.
45. Durigon GS, Oliveira DB, Vollet SB, et al. Hospital-acquired human bocavirus in infants. *J Hosp Infect.* 2010;76(2):171-173.
53. Fu X, Wang X, Ni B, et al. Recombination analysis based on the complete genome of bocavirus. *Virol J.* 2011;8:182.
56. Ghietto LM, Majul D, Ferreyra Soaje P, et al. Comorbidity and high viral load linked to clinical presentation of respiratory human bocavirus infection. *Arch Virol.* 2015;160(1):117-127.
58. Guido M, Zizza A, Bredl S, et al. Seroepidemiology of human bocavirus in Apulia, Italy. *Clin Microbiol Infect.* 2012;18(4):E74-E76.
59. Gunel C, Kirdar S, Omurlu IK, et al. Detection of the Epstein-Barr virus, human Bocavirus and novel KI and KU polyomaviruses in adenotonsillar tissues. *Int J Pediatr Otorhinolaryngol.* 2015;79(3):423-427.
63. Hao Y, Gao J, Zhang X, et al. Seroepidemiology of human bocaviruses 1 and 2 in China. *PLoS ONE.* 2015;10(4):e0122751.
64. Hasan R, Rhodes J, Thamthitiwat S, et al. Incidence and etiology of acute lower respiratory tract infections in hospitalized children younger than 5 years in rural Thailand. *Pediatr Infect Dis J.* 2014;33(2):e45-e52.
66. Huang Q, Deng X, Yan Z, et al. Establishment of a reverse genetics system for studying human bocavirus in human airway epithelia. *PLoS Pathog.* 2012;8(8):e1002899.
68. Hustedt JW, Christie C, Hustedt MM, et al. Seroepidemiology of human bocavirus infection in Jamaica. *PLoS ONE.* 2012;7(5):e38206.
73. Kailasan S, Garrison J, Ilyas M, et al. Mapping antigenic epitopes on the human bocavirus capsid. *J Virol.* 2016;90(9):4670-4680.
79. Kapoor A, Mehta N, Esper F, et al. Identification and characterization of a new bocavirus species in gorillas. *PLoS ONE.* 2010;5(7):e11948.
84. Khamrin P, Okitsu S, Ushijima H, et al. Complete genome sequence analysis of novel human bocavirus reveals genetic recombination between human bocavirus 2 and human bocavirus 4. *Infect Genet Evol.* 2013;17:132-136.
86. Kim S. Prevalence of human bocavirus 1 among people without gastroenteritis symptoms in South Korea between 2008 and 2010. *Arch Virol.* 2014;159(10):2741-2744.
88. Korppi M. Polymerase chain reaction in respiratory samples alone is not a reliable marker of bocavirus infection. *Pediatr Pulmonol.* 2014;49(5):515-516.
96. Li H, He M, Zeng P, et al. The genomic and seroprevalence of human bocavirus in healthy Chinese plasma donors and plasma derivatives. *Transfusion.* 2015;55(1):154-163.
97. Li L, Shan T, Wang C, et al. The fecal viral flora of California sea lions. *J Virol.* 2011;85(19):9909-9917.
98. Li Q, Zhang Z, Zheng Z, et al. Identification and characterization of complex dual nuclear localization signals in human bocavirus NP1: identification and characterization of complex dual nuclear localization signals in human bocavirus NP1. *J Gen Virol.* 2013;94(Pt 6):1335-1342.
100. Lindner J, Karalar L, Zehentmeier S, et al. Humoral immune response against human bocavirus VP2 virus-like particles. *Viral Immunol.* 2008;21(4):443-449.
101. Lindner J, Zehentmeier S, Franssila R, et al. CD4+ T helper cell responses against human bocavirus viral protein 2 viruslike particles in healthy adults. *J Infect Dis.* 2008;198(11):1677-1684.
104. Lu QB, Wo Y, Wang HY, et al. Epidemic and molecular evolution of human bocavirus in hospitalized children with acute respiratory tract infection. *Eur J Clin Microbiol Infect Dis.* 2015;34(1):75-81.
105. Luo H, Zhang Z, Zheng Z, et al. Human bocavirus VP2 upregulates IFN-beta pathway by inhibiting ring finger protein 125-mediated ubiquitination of retinoic acid-inducible gene-I. *J Immunol.* 2013;191(2):660-669.
111. Martin ET, Fairchok MP, Stednick ZJ, et al. Epidemiology of multiple respiratory viruses in childcare attendees. *J Infect Dis.* 2013;207(6):982-989.
112. Martin ET, Kuypers J, McRoberts JP, et al. Human bocavirus 1 primary infection and shedding in infants. *J Infect Dis.* 2015;212(4):516-524.
115. Mori D, Ranawaka U, Yamada K, et al. Human bocavirus in patients with encephalitis, Sri Lanka, 2009-2010. *Emerg Infect Dis.* 2013;19(11):1859-1862.
117. Nascimento-Carvalho CM, Cardoso MR, Meriluoto M, et al. Human bocavirus infection diagnosed serologically among children admitted to hospital with community-acquired pneumonia in a tropical region. *J Med Virol.* 2012;84(2):253-258.
119. Norja P, Hedman L, Kantola K, et al. Occurrence of human bocaviruses and parvovirus 4 in solid tissues. *J Med Virol.* 2012;84(8):1267-1273.
120. Nunes MC, Kuschner Z, Rabede Z, et al. Clinical epidemiology of bocavirus, rhinovirus, two polyomaviruses and four coronaviruses in HIV-infected and HIV-uninfected South African children. *PLoS ONE.* 2014;9(2):e86448.
121. Paloniemi M, Lappalainen S, Salminen M, et al. Human bocaviruses are commonly found in stools of hospitalized children without causal association to acute gastroenteritis. *Eur J Pediatr.* 2014;173(8):1051-1057.
125. Proenca-Modena JL, Martinez M, Amarilla AA, et al. Viral load of human bocavirus-1 in stools from children with viral diarrhoea in Paraguay. *Epidemiol Infect.* 2013;141(12):2576-2580.
126. Proenca-Modena JL, Paula FE, Buzatto GP, et al. Hypertrophic adenoid is a major infection site of human bocavirus 1. *J Clin Microbiol.* 2014;52(8):3030-3037.
129. Rahiala J, Koskenvuo M, Norja P, et al. Human parvoviruses B19, PARV4 and bocavirus in pediatric patients with allogeneic hematopoietic SCT. *Bone Marrow Transplant.* 2013;48(10):1308-1312.
131. Rhedin S, Lindstrand A, Hjelmgren A, et al. Respiratory viruses associated with community-acquired pneumonia in children: matched case-control study. *Thorax.* 2015;70(9):847-853.
135. Salez N, Vabret A, Leruez-Ville M, et al. Evaluation of four commercial multiplex molecular tests for the diagnosis of acute respiratory infections. *PLoS ONE.* 2015;10(6):e0130378.
144. Sun B, Cai Y, Li Y, et al. The nonstructural protein NP1 of human bocavirus 1 induces cell cycle arrest and apoptosis in Hela cells. *Virology.* 2013;440(1):75-83.
147. Tran DN, Nguyen TQ, Nguyen TA, et al. Human bocavirus in children with acute respiratory infections in Vietnam. *J Med Virol.* 2014;86(6):988-994.
148. van de Pol AC, Wolfs TF, Jansen NJ, et al. Human bocavirus and KI/WU polyomaviruses in pediatric intensive care patients. *Emerg Infect Dis.* 2009;15(3):454-457.
153. Yu JM, Chen QQ, Hao YX, et al. Identification of human bocaviruses in the cerebrospinal fluid of children hospitalized with encephalitis in China. *J Clin Virol.* 2013;57(4):374-377.
156. Zhao B, Yu X, Wang C, et al. High human bocavirus viral load is associated with disease severity in children under five years of age. *PLoS ONE.* 2013;8(4):e62318.
157. Zhou L, Zheng S, Xiao Q, et al. Single detection of human bocavirus 1 with a high viral load in severe respiratory tract infections in previously healthy children. *BMC Infect Dis.* 2014;14:424.
158. Zou W, Cheng F, Shen W, et al. Nonstructural protein NP1 of human bocavirus 1 plays a critical role in the expression of viral capsid proteins. *J Virol.* 2016;90(9):4658-4669.

The full reference list for this chapter is available at ExpertConsult.com.

Human Polyomaviruses 154

John A. Vanchiere

The human polyomaviruses are a diverse group of viruses that are believed to have existed in the human population for thousands of years, but their ability to cause disease in modern humans is largely limited to opportunistic diseases in severely immunocompromised patients. The acquired immunodeficiency syndrome (AIDS) epidemic and increasing use of immunosuppressive therapies for the treatment of oncologic, neurologic, autoimmune, and rheumatologic disorders brought the family of *Polyomaviridae* to the foreground of biomedical science since the 1980s. With the increasing use of deep-sequencing methods, numerous human polyomaviruses with unique tissue tropisms have been detected since 2000, highlighting the need to understand the natural history and disease potential of these diverse agents. While the polyomaviruses derive their name from "poly," meaning many, and "oma," which refers to their ability to induce tumors in laboratory animals, the story of their emergence as opportunistic causes of both malignant and nonmalignant diseases is continuing to unfold. Their colorful history and critical role in the elucidation of fundamental cellular and molecular pathways has immortalized them as research tools.

HISTORY

The recognition of progressive multifocal leukoencephalopathy (PML) as a clinical entity in 1958 marks the beginning of our knowledge of the human polyomaviruses.[16] Richardson and colleagues described three cases of progressive neurologic disease in patients receiving chemotherapy for leukemia. At autopsy, they found many foci of demyelination, including oligodendrocytes with intranuclear inclusions and astrocytes that were enlarged with bizarre nuclear changes, defining the classic histopathologic features of PML.[16] Richardson subsequently reported a larger series of PML cases and proposed a viral etiology associated with immunosuppression.[176] In 1965, papovavirus-like particles were observed by electron microscopy of brain tissue from patients with PML and, in 1971, JC virus (JCV) was isolated from primary human fetal glial cell cultures that had been inoculated with a brain extract from a patient with PML.[158,239] In the same year, another human polyomavirus, BK virus (BKV), was cultivated from the urine of a renal transplant patient.[73] Each virus was named with the initials of the patient from whom it was isolated.

Between 2000 and 2015, 11 additional human polyomaviruses were discovered, each with unique features that have challenged our understanding of polyomavirus biology. The respiratory polyomaviruses, KI polyomavirus (KIPyV) and WU polyomavirus (WUPyV), were discovered in 2007 by interrogation of respiratory secretions using deep-sequencing methods.[4,74,91,155] The St. Louis and Malawi polyomaviruses were discovered in fecal specimens and have also been detected in tonsil tissue, but no clinical disease has been associated with these unique viruses.[134,154,165] The visualization of the trichodysplasia spinulosa polyomavirus (TSPyV) by electron microscopy marked the beginning of the characterization of cutaneous polyomaviruses in the human population, an area of intense study due to the more recent discovery of the Merkel cell polyomavirus (MCPyV) and several additional cutaneous polyomaviruses in the human population.[65,183,197,220,221]

Simian virus 40 (SV40), the prototype polyomavirus, was isolated in 1960 by Sweet and Hilleman as a contaminant of secondary rhesus monkey kidney cell cultures that were used to produce early polio vaccines.[209] Additionally, several early adenovirus vaccines and a respiratory syncytial virus vaccine were contaminated with SV40.[131,148] Although rhesus monkey kidney cells showed no cytopathic effect, when supernatants from vaccine cultures were used to inoculate green monkey kidney cells, a pronounced cytopathic effect was observed, thus giving rise to the original name of SV40, vacuolating virus. By that time, millions of doses of both live and killed preparations of polio vaccine containing SV40 had been given to humans in the United States and Europe. Soon after its identification, the demonstration that SV40 induced tumors in neonatal rodents prompted great concern about its potential effects in humans.[83] Serologic studies showed that the formaldehyde-inactivated Salk poliovirus vaccine, but not the live-attenuated Sabin poliovirus vaccine, induced high-titer, SV40-specific antibody responses.[76] Although the live-attenuated poliovirus vaccine preparations contained higher titers of infectious SV40 virus, they failed to induce virus-specific antibodies in vaccinees despite prolonged shedding in stool.[144] A 30-year follow-up of infants possibly exposed to SV40 between 1955 and 1962 via inactivated poliovirus vaccine preparations showed no excess risk of cancer, but such epidemiologic studies have significant limitations.[64,203,205] Despite numerous reports of the detection of SV40 in human tumors, tissues, and excretions, whether SV40 is the cause of human diseases—including malignancies—remains controversial.[33] Since the 1960s, the mechanism of SV40-induced tumorigenesis has been intensely studied and, as a result of SV40-related research, many facets of cell and molecular biology have been elucidated, including transcriptional regulation, alternative splicing, eukaryotic DNA replication, tumor suppressor proteins, nuclear localization signals, and viral effects on cell cycle control.[45]

VIROLOGY

Polyomaviruses are classified in the family *Polyomaviridae*, which has been separated into four genera: *Alphapolyomaviruses*, *Betapolyomaviruses*, *Gammapolyomaviruses*, and *Deltapolyomaviruses*. More than 100 polyomaviruses are now known, each with a limited host range in which one or several closely related species can be infected.[204,223] Primate, rodent, and avian polyomaviruses are the most studied members of the family *Polyomaviridae*, but the rapid detection of unique polyomaviruses in other species may offer unique insights into viral evolution and virus-host coevolution that could challenge long-held concepts. Based on their similar genomic structure and replication strategies, it is likely that the polyomaviruses and papillomaviruses evolved from a common progenitor virus. Human polyomaviruses are 45 nm in diameter with a genome approximately 5200 base pairs in length; papillomaviruses are somewhat larger, 55 nm in diameter with a genome approximately 8000 base pairs in length. The genomic organization of the polyomaviruses and papillomaviruses differs in that polyomaviruses use both DNA strands to encode proteins, whereas papillomaviruses use just one DNA strand. Viruses in both families cause infection in immunocompetent and immunodeficient hosts and also have been associated with malignancies.

Based on their tissues' tropisms, the human polyomaviruses can be divided into three groups: a nephrotropic group, including JCV and BKV; a respiratory group, including WUPyV and KIPyV; and a cutaneous group, including TdSPyV, MCPyV, and other cutaneous PyVs (Table 154.1). Among the nephrotropic human polyomaviruses, the nucleotide sequence of JCV has approximately 75% overall homology with BKV and 69% homology with SV40.[45] WU and KI are distant outliers among

TABLE 154.1 Human Polyomviruses

ICTV Name[37]	Alternate Name	Genus	Tissue Tropism
HPyV1	BK virus	Beta-PyV	Kidney, GI
HPyV2	JC virus	Beta-PyV	Kidney, GI, brain
HPyV3	KI polyomavirus	Beta-PyV	Lungs
HPyV4	WU polyomavirus	Beta-PyV	Lungs
HPyV5	Merkel cell polyomavirus	Alpha-PyV	Skin
HPyV6	—	Delta-PyV	Skin
HPyV7	—	Delta-PyV	Skin
HPyV8	Trichodysplasia spinulosa polyomavirus	Alpha-PyV	Skin
HPyV9	Human polyomavirus 9	Alpha-PyV	Skin
HPyV10	MW polyomavirus	Delta-PyV	GI
HPyV11	STL polyomavirus	Delta-PyV	GI
HPyV12	—	Alpha-PyV	Skin
HPyV13	New Jersey polyomavirus	Alpha-PyV	Vascular endothelium, skin

GI, Gastrointestinal; ICTV, International Committee on the Taxonomy of Viruses.

the primate polyomaviruses, sharing only 30% to 40% nucleotide identity with BKV and JCV in the late region. Despite the high degree of divergence of the respiratory polyomaviruses from the nephrotropic polyomaviruses, both of these subgroups are members of the genus *Betapolyomavirus*.[37] In contrast, the MCPyV and several other cutaneous polyomaviruses (HPyV-8, -9, -12, and -13) are more closely related to nonhuman primate and rodent polyomaviruses, whereas the STL and MW polyomaviruses cluster among *Deltapolyomavirus* with bovine polyomaviruses.[37,65,223]

Several decades of studies of the biology of BKV, JCV, and SV40 have contributed to the current understanding of the biology of human polyomaviruses, principles of which may be challenged by ongoing studies of the more recently identified respiratory and cutaneous polyomaviruses that apparently lack a regulatory agnoprotein gene.[80,223] All polyomaviruses share a characteristic circular genome that can be divided into structural, nonstructural, and regulatory regions. The structural (late) region of the viral genome encodes VP1, VP2, and VP3, the capsid proteins that envelop the viral genome. VP1 is the major capsid protein, accounting for more than 70% of the virion mass; it participates in host-cell recognition and stimulation of the host immune response. VP2 and VP3 are smaller, less abundant capsid proteins. The nonstructural (early) region of the polyomavirus genome encodes the large T antigen, the best studied of the polyomavirus proteins; this protein initiates viral DNA replication, stimulates cellular entry into S phase, and influences cellular and viral transcription. The small t antigen is produced by alternative splicing of the early viral mRNA and promotes G_1 cell cycle progression; it is not required for viral growth in cultured cells. The large T antigen of SV40 is responsible for the transformation of cells in vivo and in vitro, but the T antigens of other primate polyomaviruses are generally less adept at eliciting transformation. The large T antigen is a multifunctional protein that contains binding sites for the cellular pRb and p53 proteins. By binding to pRb, the large T antigen allows E2F-mediated progression of the cell cycle, thus providing the right environment for replication of viral DNA. Through its association with p53, a cellular tumor suppressor protein, the large T antigen blocks p53-induced cellular gene expression, thereby leading to genomic instability.[32] In addition to its interaction with host proteins, the large T antigen has enzymatic activities that may be useful sites for targeting antiviral compounds.[188] Similarly, the large T antigens of JCV and BKV can interact with a variety of cellular proteins, including the p53 and pRb family proteins.[103] The large T antigen of MCPyV has been shown to interact with pRB but not p107 or p130 proteins, and the genome of MCPyV is frequently found integrated into the genome of Merkel cell carcinomas.[65,95] The regulatory region of the polyomavirus genome contains both the origin of replication and the viral promoter. The origin is recognized by the large T antigen, in concert with host-cell factors, including cellular DNA polymerase, and viral DNA replication is initiated. Both early and late viral transcription is mediated by cellular RNA polymerase. T antigen binding to viral DNA autoregulates the production of early mRNA and, by interaction with cellular factors, stimulates late transcription. Polyomaviruses have either an archetypal (single-enhancer) or rearranged (complex) regulatory region that can alter the efficiency of virus replication in vitro.[30,32,85,103]

Variants of BKV and JCV with complex regulatory regions are common in immunocompromised patients and, at least for JCV in PML, these variants are considered the pathogenic virus.[66] While regulatory region variants of BKV may impact viral replication in vitro, there is no clear evidence that such changes are necessary or sufficient for the pathogenesis of BK virus–associated nephropathy (BKVAN) in at-risk patients.[30] Recent data on the virology of PML-associated strains of JCV suggests that mutations in the viral coat proteins may alter the tissue tropism of JCV and facilitate its dissemination into the central nervous system.[84] Another important advance in the current understanding of polyomavirus replication has been the discovery of virus-produced micro-RNAs that regulate gene expression and may play a role in the immunologic control of polyomavirus persistence.[206] The clinical importance of this novel regulatory mechanism in the pathogenesis of polyomavirus-associated diseases is an area of intense investigation that may soon provide new targets for therapeutic intervention.[41,42]

EPIDEMIOLOGY

Polyomaviruses are ubiquitous in the human population, and the prevalence of virus-specific antibodies increases with age, beginning in early childhood. BKV seroconversion occurs in 50% of children by the time they reach the age of 3 to 4 years.[157,191] Population-based seroprevalence data suggest that more than 80% of adults have been infected with BKV.[111,232] In contrast to earlier data, recent studies suggest that only about 50% to 70% of the adult population has been infected with JCV.[5,27,68,111,116,157,166,191,217,232] BKV seroconversion has been associated with mild upper respiratory tract illnesses in a small number of children, and BKV viruria has been reported in a child with acute tonsillitis.[87,207] To date, no distinct clinical syndrome has been associated with BKV infection of healthy children. The prevalence of antibodies in humans directed against SV40 has not been well established, primarily due to the variability in methods used by different research laboratories. Several studies have reported seroprevalences of 2% to 11% for SV40 using a plaque neutralization assay.[34,36,179] However, other studies have suggested that much SV40 reactivity may be due to cross-reactivity with BKV.[39,116,171,233] Whether BKV-reactive antibodies provide significant cross-protection against SV40 infection (or vice versa) has not been determined. As with the nephrotropic human polyomaviruses, the seroprevalence data for the respiratory and cutaneous polyomaviruses suggests that these viruses are ubiquitous in the human population, with infections occurring throughout life and more than 70% of humans having detectable specific antibodies to MCPyV, WUPyV, KIPyV, STL-PyV and MW-PyV.[24,43,111,133,222,232]

Humans are the only known reservoir for JCV and BKV, which persist in the kidney, uroepithelium, and gastrointestinal tract.[12,15,54,139,175,218,224–226] Their persistence in other organ systems is less certain but may include B lymphocytes and oligodendrocytes.[20,55,59,123] The exact mechanism of transmission of JCV and BKV is not known, but several studies have shown that fecal excretion of BKV may be common in infancy and adulthood, suggesting that fecal-oral transmission could explain the ubiquity of early childhood infection.[225–227] As described earlier, SV40 was introduced inadvertently into humans as a contaminant of early polio vaccines; however, such direct exposure cannot account for the SV40 seropositivity in children born more recently than 1962, suggesting continued human-to-human spread of the virus, albeit at low levels. In the pediatric population, one SV40 seroprevalence survey found nearly 6% of hospitalized children with antibodies to SV40.[35] Among kidney transplant patients in the cohort, 40% had evidence of SV40 infection, but whether such infection was related to immunosuppressive medications or the underlying kidney disease was not clear.[35] SV40 DNA sequences have been detected in kidney tissue from several pediatric renal transplant recipients and in tonsil tissue from immunocompetent children.[35,164]

In immunocompetent individuals, persistence of JCV and BKV in the kidney and uroepithelium is asymptomatic, and point prevalence studies suggest that intermittent shedding of JCV in urine is more common than shedding of BKV.[2,192] Viral DNA (JCV or BKV) can be found in 30% to 50% of kidney samples from immunocompetent adults taken at surgery or autopsy.[44,93,216] The frequency of JCV excretion in urine increases with age, while the prevalence of BKV excretion is approximately 2% to 5% in healthy adults.[54,60,115] Recent data from a longitudinal study suggest that BKV excretion may be more common than previously thought, having been detected in over 19% of specimens collected daily from 7 of 20 women over a 2-month period.[113]

JCV is lymphotropic, and the finding of JCV in plasma and peripheral blood mononuclear cells generally correlates with immune status in that it is noted less frequently in immunocompetent patients and increases in frequency in HIV-infected patients with lower CD4 counts.[52,72,117] Several conditions, including pregnancy and autoimmune disorders, are associated with excretion of BKV or JCV in urine.[137,143,208,210,211] The immunologic and virologic factors regulating initiation and maintenance of persistence remain largely unknown.

CLINICAL MANIFESTATIONS

Central Nervous System Manifestations

PML is a clinical syndrome characterized by progressive neurologic impairment in severely immunocompromised patients. In PML, the host immune system fails to maintain viral latency, and acquired mutations in the VP1 and regulatory region of JCV facilitate neurotropism that leads to central nervous system invasion.[66,84] JCV replicates in and lyses oligodendroglia and causes destruction of cerebral white matter in a multifocal or patchy distribution (Fig. 154.1). PML most commonly occurs in adult patients with AIDS, in whom approximately 5% will develop PML in the absence of antiretroviral therapy.[19–21,89] Other immunosuppressed individuals who are at high risk for PML include patients receiving chemotherapy, solid organ or hematopoietic stem cell transplant (HSCT) recipients, and those with primary T-cell defects. Numerous immunosuppressive agents used in the treatment of malignancies, autoimmune disease, and inflammatory disorders have been associated with an increased risk of PML, including rituximab, natalizumab, efalizumab, and others.[18,25,38,119,160] For JCV-seropositive patients receiving natalizumab, the risk of PML is approximately 1% after 24 to 59 months of natalizumab treatment.[25] PML is rare in HIV-infected children compared to adults and has not been reported in association with monoclonal antibody therapies that predispose to PML in adults.[23,202] At present, serologic testing for JCV-specific IgG antibodies is the only clinical test that may be useful for risk stratification of patients receiving prolonged immunosuppression. In addition to JCV seropositivity, both the duration of natalizumab therapy and a history of prior immunosuppressant therapy were associated with increased risk of PML among multiple sclerosis patients.[25] PML has also been reported in patients with relatively mild immunosuppression and without any known immunocompromise, although such cases are rare.[81]

Clinical manifestations of PML can include behavior changes; blindness, deafness, and other cranial nerve dysfunctions; motor and cognitive deficits; and incoordination as a result of cerebellar involvement.[22] The onset of symptoms usually is insidious, and associated systemic signs such as fever and headache are uncommon. Progression of symptoms occurs over a period of several weeks to months, and the condition is inevitably fatal. The diagnosis of PML is largely clinical and based on the history, physical examination, and characteristic findings on neuroimaging studies. Computed tomography and magnetic resonance imaging of the brain show focal demyelination and white matter edema with relative sparing of the gray matter. The magnetic resonance image of a child with AIDS and PML is shown in Fig. 154.1.[149] Cerebrospinal fluid (CSF) analysis is often normal in patients with PML, likely a result of impairment or depletion (or both) of T lymphocytes.[22] BKV-associated neurologic disease has been reported in several AIDS patients, and BKV encephalitis has been reported in a patient without known immunodeficiency in association with polyomavirus seroconversion.[28,219,234]

Urinary Tract Manifestations

Asymptomatic polyomaviruria is a common occurrence in immunocompetent adults and children.[40,60,106,115,181,227] Hemorrhagic cystitis temporally associated with BKV viruria has been reported rarely in immunocompetent children, but no other nonmalignant diseases have

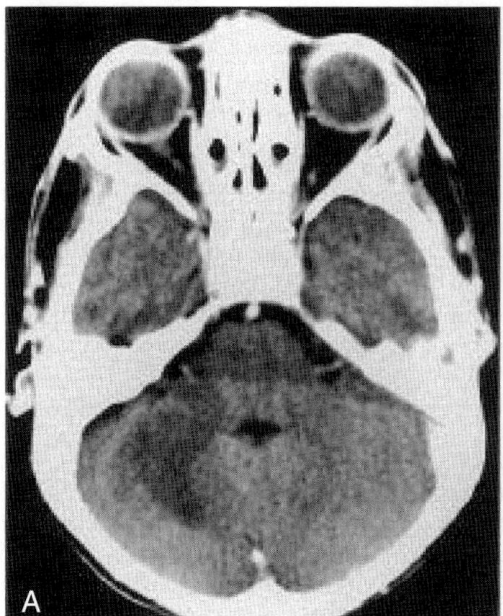

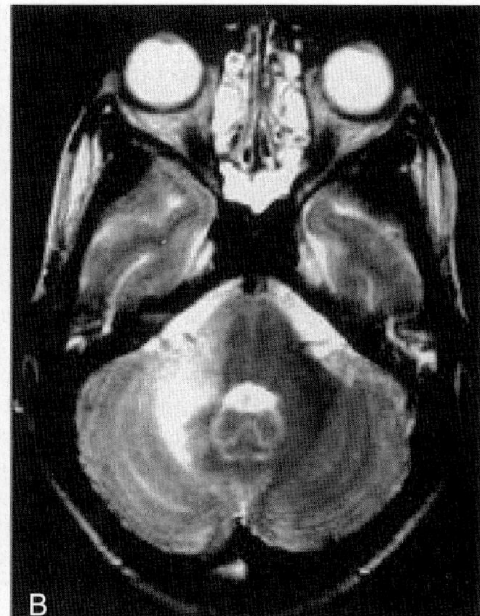

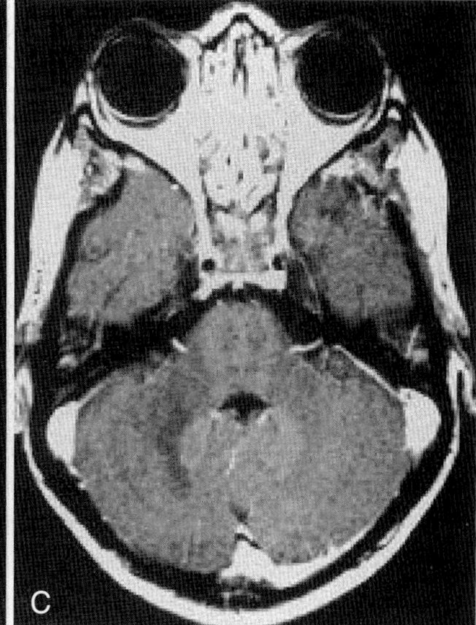

FIG. 154.1 (A) Contrast-enhanced computed tomography of a brain of a child with progressive multifocal leukoencephalopathy showing low-density, nonenhancing, right-sided cerebellar white matter lesion without a mass effect. (B) On T2-weighted magnetic resonance imaging (MRI), the lesion produces a high signal without a mass effect or edema. (C) The lesion gives a low signal on T1-weighted MRI and fails to enhance with intravenous contrast. (From Morriss MC, Rutstein RM, Rudy B, et al. Progressive multifocal leukoencephalopathy in an HIV-infected child. *Neuroradiology*. 1997;39:142–144.)

been linked to polyomavirus infection in immunocompetent children.[184] Urinary excretion of BKV occurs in about 20% to 40% of adult and pediatric renal transplant recipients, approximately one-third to one-half of whom may also have BK viremia.[94,97,98,100,102] Posttransplant polyomaviruria is due predominantly to reactivation of latent infection, and limited data suggest that the reactivated virus is often donor derived, at least for kidney transplant recipients.[230] Excretion of BKV usually begins in the first 2 to 3 months after transplantation. In renal transplant recipients, BKV viruria may be associated with ureteral ulceration and stenosis, sometimes requiring surgical intervention to prevent or relieve obstructive nephropathy. The prognostic significance of polyomavirus reactivation in renal transplant patients has become a topic of great interest, especially as managing immunosuppression has become more sophisticated.

BKV has emerged as the most common infectious cause of renal allograft failure and is increasingly identified as a cause of native-kidney dysfunction in nonrenal transplant recipients (Fig. 154.2).[17] BKVAN affects 1% to 10% of renal transplant recipients, resulting in allograft loss for approximately 60% to 75% of those affected.[194] Initially, case reports linking polyomavirus infection and allograft failure identified BKV as a possible pathogen.[152,163,170] Larger studies have since revealed the pathogenesis of BKVAN as well as the appropriate diagnostic and therapeutic strategies. Retrospective analyses have found that BKVAN may be more commonly associated with the use of tacrolimus and mycophenolate, but BKVAN has been reported in patients receiving other immunosuppressive agents and in nonkidney solid-organ transplant recipients.[1,29] Molecular characterization of BKV isolates from patients with BKVAN has not identified particular strains of BKV that are more likely to cause BKVAN, but some data suggest that the donor is the source of BKV in many BKVAN cases.[187,195] The role of host factors in the pathogenesis of BKVAN remains an area of intense investigation. Importantly, repeat renal transplantation after allograft loss due to BKVAN has been successful without increased risk of BKVAN in the second allograft.[75]

Polyomaviruria, especially that involving BKV, is a common finding after HSCT, occurring in 50% to 80% of patients within 2 to 8 weeks after transplantation.[7,14,190] BKV viruria is associated with hemorrhagic cystitis (BKV-HC) in 15% to 25% of adult and pediatric HSCT recipients.[13,67,82,127–130] BKV-HC is both painful and distressing for HSCT patients, occasionally necessitating erythrocyte transfusions and, rarely, surgical intervention.[82,118] For the majority of patients with BKV-HC, supportive care, including intravenous hydration and erythrocyte transfusions, is adequate management, as T-cell engraftment eventually controls BKV replication and leads to resolution of symptoms. Adenovirus is an important, but less common, cause of hemorrhagic cystitis after HSCT.[3,67,130]

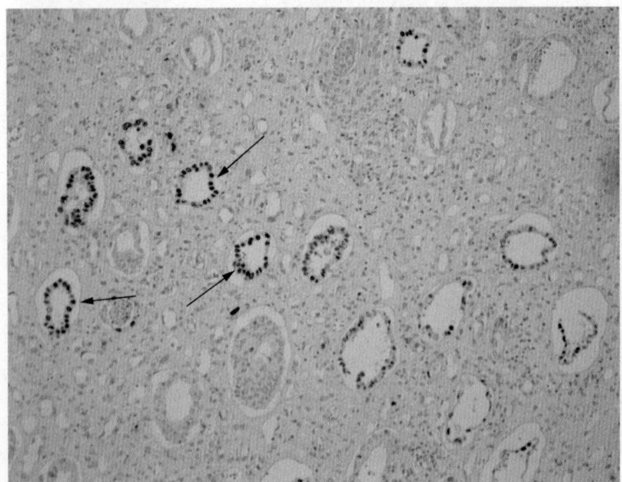

FIG. 154.2 Immunohistochemical detection of the BK virus T antigen in kidney tissue obtained at autopsy from a pediatric patient with disseminated BK virus infection after hematopoietic stem cell transplantation (magnification ×40). *Arrows* indicate positively stained renal tubular epithelial cells. (Courtesy J.A. Vanchiere, MD, PhD.)

Interstitial nephritis caused by BKV has been described in children with various immunodeficiencies, including hyperimmunoglobulin M immunodeficiency and AIDS.[48,180] Renal dysfunction is a common finding in AIDS patients, but its etiology has only rarely been linked to polyomaviruses; one study found SV40 in kidney tissue from several AIDS patients with a collapsing variant of focal segmental glomerulosclerosis, but the pathogenesis of this disease remains uncertain.[132] Several studies of Balkan endemic nephropathy have associated this enigmatic disease in Eastern Europe with polyomaviruses, but further study is needed to establish a causal link.[151,201] One pediatric study observed an association between SV40 seropositivity and renal transplantation and detected SV40 sequences in renal biopsy specimens, suggesting a possible role for SV40 in pediatric renal disease.[34,35]

Cutaneous Manifestations

The clinical manifestations of cutaneous polyomaviruses are evident almost exclusively in immunocompromised patients, especially among those with marked T-lymphocyte suppression. The association of Merkel cell carcinoma and HIV infection was first described in 2002, but it was not until deep-sequencing approaches were used that the causative agent, MCPyV, was discovered.[65] Numerous case series have now established that the MCPyV can be detected in more than 75% (range: 43%–100%) of Merkel cell carcinomas, including tumors in immunocompromised and immunocompetent patients.[10] Mutations in the helicase domain of the large T-antigen are commonly found in MCPyV strains from Merkel cell carcinomas and are believed to be necessary for the oncogenesis of MCPyV.[197] The role of individual immunoresponses to MC-PyV in the pathogenesis of Merkel cell carcinoma is an area of growing interest.[215] Trichodysplasia spinulosa due to TSPyV is predominantly a disease of severely immunocompromised patients, especially solid-organ transplant recipients and patients with hematologic malignancies.[141] This striking disease is characterized by the eruption of erythematous papules with 1-mm to 3-mm keratotic spicules on the nose and chin, with occasional lesions on the trunk and back. In addition, patients often have eyelash and eyebrow loss.[212] To date, approximately 20 cases of virus-associated trichodysplasia spinulosa have been reported in the medical literature.[141] Other cutaneous polyomaviruses remain enigmatic. While they appear to be very common in the human population, they have not yet been associated with malignancy, and only the New Jersey polyomavirus has been associated with acute clinical disease. This unique alphapolyomavirus was the cause of vasculitis in an adult pancreas transplant recipient with neurologic symptoms and necrotic skin lesions.[147]

Pulmonary Manifestations

While some contend that the nephrotropic polyomaviruses can be transmitted in respiratory secretions, there is little evidence to indicate that such transmission, if it does occur, is accompanied by clinical disease of the respiratory tract. Several case reports of BKV-associated pulmonary disease have been published, uniformly in the setting of severe immunosuppression and with poor outcomes.[48,185,219,237] While interstitial pneumonitis in a patient with severe immunocompromise might raise the suspicion of polyomavirus-associated disease, other viral pathogens, such as cytomegalovirus (CMV) and adenovirus, should be considered more likely.

WUPyV and KIPyV can be found in upper and lower respiratory tract secretions from immunocompetent and immunocompromised patients, most often in association with other common respiratory tract pathogens.[4,74,122] Numerous studies have documented that the clinical consequences of WUPyV and KIPyV are minimal, even in the most severely compromised patients.[101,122]

Other Manifestations

BKV-associated retinal necrosis in an AIDS-infected patient has been described, as have elevated hepatic transaminase levels in association with BKV viruria and detection of BKV in normal liver specimens.[28,92,114,156] The clinical significance of these manifestations is unknown.

Malignancies

The polyomaviruses are named for their ability to induce tumors in laboratory animals. Their association with human tumors was noted first in 1974 when Soriano and colleagues isolated SV40 from a metastatic malignant melanoma in a patient with SV40 neutralizing antibodies.[199] SV40 T antigen and capsid antigen were detected in lung, liver, and muscle metastases of the patient but not in normal tissue.[199] Since that time, polyomaviruses have been linked to a variety of neoplasms in humans, frequently analogous to the tumor types produced by SV40 in rodents. SV40 has been detected in association with human cancers much more frequently than have JCV and BKV. SV40 T antigen or DNA has been detected in a significant number of meningiomas, ependymomas, choroid plexus tumors, astrocytomas, pleural mesotheliomas, and osteosarcomas.[11,104] Several studies reported the presence of SV40 in non-Hodgkin lymphomas.[140,178,231] In the case of pleural mesotheliomas, which also have been associated with asbestos exposure, the presence of SV40 may be a negative prognostic indicator.[168] A possible synergistic effect of SV40 and asbestos has been observed in vitro and in case-control studies of human mesothelioma patients, suggesting that the two agents may work in concert as cocarcinogens.[26,47,120] In one study of pediatric patients, JCV DNA was detected in 11 of 23 medulloblastomas, and JCV T-antigen expression was detected by immunohistochemistry in four of 16 samples tested.[121] Other investigators have not detected polyomavirus DNA or protein expression in medulloblastoma tissue.[112,150,236]

JCV has also been detected in colorectal and gastric cancers and in normal tissue samples from the human gastrointestinal tract.[124,174,175] BKV has been detected in both normal and neoplastic prostate tissue, suggesting a potential role for BKV in the pathogenesis of this common cancer of adulthood.[49,50] While Merkel cell carcinoma may be more common among immunocompromised patients, this neuroendocrine tumor occurs in immunocompetent patients as well, though very rarely in children.[46] Not surprisingly, immunocompromised patients tend to have poorer outcomes than immunocompetent patients. As such, the study of cutaneous diseases in immunocompromised patients is a growing area of research.[136,147] Further studies, including evaluation of host immunogenetic factors, will be required to establish whether other polyomaviruses are commonly oncogenic in humans.

LABORATORY DIAGNOSIS

While the suspicion of polyomavirus disease is primarily a clinical one, laboratory techniques are important for making the diagnosis in the proper clinical circumstances. Serologic tests and viral culture are of little use clinically because these tests are laborious and rarely available. Furthermore, serologic data should be interpreted with caution in immunocompromised patients. Polyomaviruses in urine could be considered normal flora among immunocompetent patients, much like CMV detected in urine after infancy. Histologic study of urinary sediment can reveal "decoy cells," which are uroepithelial cells with characteristic polyomavirus inclusions. The presence of decoy cells is a specific and moderately sensitive marker of polyomavirus-associated nephritis in renal transplant patients.[56,58] Detection of specific polyomavirus DNA from urine samples is of little known significance, whereas polymerase chain reaction (PCR) detection from blood samples, especially viremia of greater than 10,000 genomes per milliliter, may correlate with the risk of BKVAN after solid-organ transplantation.[126,153,169] Consensus guidelines suggest routine monitoring of kidney transplant recipients for BKV replication every 1 to 3 months for 1 to 2 years after transplantation, using either urine or plasma (preferred) quantitative PCR.[99,110] Immunohistochemical detection of BKV T antigen in renal biopsy material is the gold standard for diagnosis of BKVAN, although electron microscopic identification of polyomavirus-like particles in renal biopsy material may also be diagnostic.[98,135] The diagnosis of BKV-HC is based on clinical symptoms and the detection of BKV in urine, usually by PCR. Urinary viral loads in patients with BKV-HC and BKVAN can be extremely high, even 10^{12} or 10^{13} genome copies per milliliter.

Detection of JCV DNA in CSF by PCR is the diagnostic test of choice for suspected PML, although CSF PCR may be negative in some patients with PML.[90,117,138,186] In adult patients with AIDS and neurologic symptoms, PCR amplification of JCV DNA from CSF is 99% predictive of PML, whereas brain biopsy has a slightly lower sensitivity.[51] Rare cases of PML with negative JCV PCR of the CSF have been reported.[142] On gross examination, tissue typical of PML has been described as "worm eaten," and microscopic examination reveals multiple foci of demyelination with enlarged oligodendroglia, giant astrocytes, and an intense phagocytic infiltration.[229] Immunohistochemical techniques and other nucleic acid detection methods also can be used to confirm the diagnosis of PML.[107] JC viremia is a general indicator of immunosuppression and is a common finding in HIV-infected patients without PML; thus, its utility in the diagnosis of suspected PML is questionable.[117]

Detection of the cutaneous and respiratory polyomaviruses relies on PCR testing that is performed in research laboratories. With the exception of MCPyV and TdSPyV in immunocompromised patients, there are no clear clinical indications for pursuit of these viruses.[122]

TREATMENT AND PREVENTION

No specific antiviral agents have been studied in randomized trials for the treatment of polyomavirus disease or polyomavirus-associated tumors. Studies in both adult and pediatric patients have demonstrated that routine monitoring of plasma BKV viral loads and preemptive reduction of immunosuppression are useful for the prevention of BKVAN without significant risk of allograft rejection, and routine screening for BKV has been recommended by international panels.[99,110] Several studies have demonstrated the utility of frequent surveillance for reduction of the incidence of BKVAN.[53,61] However, BKV reactivation may persist and lead to chronic renal dysfunction in some patients.[228] BKVAN should be suspected in any renal transplant patient with otherwise unexplained allograft dysfunction. For renal transplant recipients with biopsy-proven BKVAN, reduction of immunosuppression may be helpful for preservation of allograft function, especially among patients with low-grade disease.[57,71] The additional benefit of antiviral agents beyond that of reducing immunosuppression has not been established. Case series have reported variable results with the use of cidofovir and leflunomide in patients with BKVAN.[8,9,63,108,109] Despite its potential nephrotoxicity, low-dose cidofovir has been suggested by an international consensus group as a potential investigational agent for treatment of BKVAN and is probably the most widely used antiviral for treatment of polyomavirus diseases.[98] Intravenous immunoglobulin has been used to treat several patients with BKVAN, with some authors reporting success and some not.[6,189,196,235] A more recent report suggests that intravenous immunoglobulin is safe and effective for treatment of BKVAN in patients with inadequate response to leflunomide.[193] Both leflunomide and cidofovir have been used to treat HSCT recipients with particularly severe hemorrhagic cystitis and/or disseminated disease due to BKV, but immune restoration by T-cell engraftment is likely the most important factor in resolution of BKV-related cystitis. Despite numerous studies attesting to the ability of fluoroquinolone antibiotics to inhibit BKV in vitro and case series suggesting a potential clinical benefit, a well-designed clinical trial of levofloxacin for treatment of BKV viremia in adult kidney transplant recipients failed to demonstrate a benefit of levofloxacin compared to placebo.[125] However, an open-label study of ciprofloxacin and leflunomide in pediatric kidney transplant recipients suggests that this regimen may be advantageous.[238] The prophylactic utility of ciprofloxacin for the prevention of BKV-HC after HSCT is suggested by an open-label study in adult HSCT recipients, but a controlled clinical trial for this indication has not been performed.[70,146] Brincidofovir (formerly CMX001) is a lipid derivative of cidofovir that has in vitro activity against both BKV and JCV.[86,177] Furthermore, this orally bioavailable agent is approximately 100 times more potent than cidofovir and has an improved safety profile in vivo.[69,159] The use of brincidofovir has been reported in several pediatric and adult patients, and controlled clinical trials of its efficacy for the prevention of CMV disease after HSCT are ongoing.[162,173]

Initiation of highly active antiretroviral therapy (HAART) can restore immune function and alleviate the symptoms of PML for AIDS patients.[62,167,214] Despite administration of HAART, PML may develop in some HIV-infected patients due to incomplete immune reconstitution or immune reconstitution inflammatory syndrome.[198,213] Cidofovir has been used successfully in conjunction with HAART in patients with AIDS and PML, but its benefit above that of HAART and in non-AIDS patients with PML has not been determined.[145,182] Though not reported in children, treatment of PML associated with immunomodulatory monoclonal antibody therapies should include consideration of plasmapheresis and/or the use of leukocyte colony-stimulating factors in order to promote restoration of immune function as quickly as possible. Consultation with research centers that study the pathogenesis and treatment of PML is advised, as the modalities being used vary greatly and may change frequently.[105,200] Adoptive transfer of in vitro–stimulated, virus-specific, allogeneic cytotoxic T lymphocytes is a potentially promising prophylaxis and treatment option for patients after HSCT. This novel approach has been used successfully to prevent and treat Epstein-Barr virus–related disease after HSCT and may be useful for other viruses as well.[77–79,96,161] Several potential immune-boosting vaccines for secondary prophylaxis against polyomavirus disease are in development.[31,172] Given the ubiquity and generally benign nature of polyomavirus infections, as well as the paucity of information about the nature of their transmission and clinical significance in immunocompetent patients, specific efforts to prevent polyomavirus transmission are not indicated at this time. Universal precautions are appropriate for care of patients with polyomavirus disease.

NEW REFERENCES SINCE THE SEVENTH EDITION

5. Antonsson A, Green AC, Mallitt KA, et al. Prevalence and stability of antibodies to the BK and JC polyomaviruses: a long-term longitudinal study of Australians. *J Gen Virol*. 2010;91(Pt 7):1849-1853.
8. Araya CE, Garin EH, Neiberger RE, et al. Leflunomide therapy for BK virus allograft nephropathy in pediatric and young adult kidney transplant recipients. *Pediatr Transplant*. 2010;14(1):145-150.
15. Arthur RR, Shah KV, Yolken RH, et al. Detection of human papovaviruses BKV and JCV in urines by ELISA. *Prog Clin Biol Res*. 1983;105:169-176.
19. Berger JR, Houff S. Progressive multifocal leukoencephalopathy: lessons from AIDS and natalizumab. *Neurol Res*. 2006;28(3):299-305.
21. Berger JR, Major EO. Progressive multifocal leukoencephalopathy. *Semin Neurol*. 1999;19(2):193-200.
23. Berger JR, Scott G, Albrecht J, et al. Progressive multifocal leukoencephalopathy in HIV-1-infected children. *AIDS*. 1992;6(8):837-841.
24. Berrios C, Jung J, Primi B, et al. Malawi polyomavirus is a prevalent human virus that interacts with known tumor suppressors. *J Virol*. 2015;89(1):857-862.
31. Buck CB. Exposing the molecular machinery of BK polyomavirus. *Structure*. 2016;24(4):495.
33. Butel J. Patterns of polyomavirus SV40 infections and associated cancers in humans: a model. *Curr Opin Virol*. 2012;2(4):508-514.
37. Calvignac-Spencer S, Feltkamp MC, Daugherty MD, et al. A taxonomy update for the family Polyomaviridae. *Arch Virol*. 2016;161(6):1739-1750.
38. Carson KR, Newsome SD, Kim EJ, et al. Progressive multifocal leukoencephalopathy associated with brentuximab vedotin therapy: a report of 5 cases from the Southern Network on Adverse Reactions (SONAR) project. *Cancer*. 2014;120(16):2464-2471.
41. Chen CJ, Cox JE, Azarm KD, et al. Identification of a polyomavirus microRNA highly expressed in tumors. *Virology*. 2015;476:43-53.
42. Chen CJ, Kincaid RP, Seo GJ, et al. Insights into Polyomaviridae microRNA function derived from study of the bandicoot papillomatosis carcinomatosis viruses. *J Virol*. 2011;85(9):4487-4500.
46. Coursaget P, Samimi M, Nicol JT, et al. Human Merkel cell polyomavirus: virological background and clinical implications. *APMIS*. 2013;121(8):755-769.
56. Drachenberg C, Hirsch HH, Papadimitriou JC, et al. Cost efficiency in the prospective diagnosis and follow-up of polyomavirus allograft nephropathy. *Transplant Proc*. 2004;36(10):3028-3031.
60. Egli A, Infanti L, Dumoulin A, et al. Prevalence of polyomavirus BK and JC infection and replication in 400 healthy blood donors. *J Infect Dis*. 2009;199(6):837-846.
61. Elfadawy N, Flechner SM, Liu X, et al. The impact of surveillance and rapid reduction in immunosuppression to control BK virus-related graft injury in kidney transplantation. *Transpl Int*. 2013;26(8):822-832.
64. Farwell JR, Dohrmann GJ, Marrett LD, et al. Effect of SV40 virus-contaminated polio vaccine on the incidence and type of CNS neoplasms in children: a population-based study. *Trans Am Neurol Assoc*. 1979;104:261-264.
78. Gerdemann U, Katari UL, Papadopoulou A, et al. Safety and clinical efficacy of rapidly-generated trivirus-directed T cells as treatment for adenovirus, EBV, and CMV infections after allogeneic hematopoietic stem cell transplant. *Mol Ther*. 2013;21(11):2113-2121.
80. Gerits N, Moens U. Agnoprotein of mammalian polyomaviruses. *Virology*. 2012;432(2):316-326.
82. Gilis L, Morisset S, Billaud G, et al. High burden of BK virus-associated hemorrhagic cystitis in patients undergoing allogeneic hematopoietic stem cell transplantation. *Bone Marrow Transplant*. 2014;49(5):664-670.
85. Gosert R, Rinaldo CH, Funk GA, et al. Polyomavirus BK with rearranged noncoding control region emerge in vivo in renal transplant patients and increase viral replication and cytopathology. *J Exp Med*. 2008;205(4):841-852.
95. Hesbacher S, Pfitzer L, Wiedorfer K, et al. RB1 is the crucial target of the Merkel cell polyomavirus large T antigen in Merkel cell carcinoma cells. *Oncotarget*. 2016;7(22):32956-32968.
105. Jelcic I, Combaluzier B, Jelcic I, et al. Broadly neutralizing human monoclonal JC polyomavirus VP1-specific antibodies as candidate therapeutics for progressive multifocal leukoencephalopathy. *Sci Transl Med*. 2015;7(306):306ra150.
110. Kasiske BL, Zeier MG, Chapman JR, et al. KDIGO clinical practice guideline for the care of kidney transplant recipients: a summary. *Kidney Int*. 2010;77(4):299-311.
118. Koskenvuo M, Dumoulin A, Lautenschlager I, et al. BK polyomavirus-associated hemorrhagic cystitis among pediatric allogeneic bone marrow transplant recipients: treatment response and evidence for nosocomial transmission. *J Clin Virol*. 2013;56(1):77-81.
119. Kothary N, Diak IL, Brinker A, et al. Progressive multifocal leukoencephalopathy associated with efalizumab use in psoriasis patients. *J Am Acad Dermatol*. 2011;65(3):546-551.
125. Lee BT, Gabardi S, Grafals M, et al. Efficacy of levofloxacin in the treatment of BK viremia: a multicenter, double-blinded, randomized, placebo-controlled trial. *Clin J Am Soc Nephrol*. 2014;9(3):583-589.
133. Lim ES, Meinerz NM, Primi B, et al. Common exposure to STL polyomavirus during childhood. *Emerg Infect Dis*. 2014;20(9):1559-1561.
134. Lim ES, Reyes A, Antonio M, et al. Discovery of STL polyomavirus, a polyomavirus of ancestral recombinant origin that encodes a unique T antigen by alternative splicing. *Virology*. 2013;436(2):295-303.
136. Ma JE, Brewer JD. Merkel cell carcinoma in immunosuppressed patients. *Cancers (Basel)*. 2014;6(3):1328-1350.
138. Marshall WF, Telenti A, Proper J, et al. Rapid detection of polyomavirus BK by a shell vial cell culture assay. *J Clin Microbiol*. 1990;28(7):1613-1615.
139. Marshall WF, Telenti A, Proper J, et al. Survey of urine from transplant recipients for polyomaviruses JC and BK using the polymerase chain reaction. *Mol Cell Probes*. 1991;5(2):125-128.
142. Mazda ME, Brosch JR, Wiens AL, et al. A case of natalizumab-associated progressive multifocal leukoencephalopathy with repeated negative CSF JCV testing. *Int J Neurosci*. 2013;123(5):353-357.
147. Mishra N, Pereira M, Rhodes RH, et al. Identification of a novel polyomavirus in a pancreatic transplant recipient with retinal blindness and vasculitic myopathy. *J Infect Dis*. 2014;210(10):1595-1599.
150. Munoz-Marmol AM, Mola G, Ruiz-Larroya T, et al. Rarity of JC virus DNA sequences and early proteins in human gliomas and medulloblastomas: the controversial role of JC virus in human neurooncogenesis. *Neuropathol Appl Neurobiol*. 2006;32(2):131-140.
154. Nicol JT, Leblond V, Arnold F, et al. Seroprevalence of human Malawi polyomavirus. *J Clin Microbiol*. 2014;52(1):321-323.
161. Papadopoulou A, Gerdemann U, Katari UL, et al. Activity of broad-spectrum T cells as treatment for AdV, EBV, CMV, BKV, and HHV6 infections after HSCT. *Sci Transl Med*. 2014;6(242):242ra283.
162. Papanicolaou GA, Lee YJ, Young JW, et al. Brincidofovir for polyomavirus-associated nephropathy after allogeneic hematopoietic stem cell transplantation. *Am J Kidney Dis*. 2015;65(5):780-784.
165. Peng J, Li K, Zhang C, et al. MW polyomavirus and STL polyomavirus present in tonsillar tissues from children with chronic tonsillar disease. *Clin Microbiol Infect*. 2016;22(1):97.e91-97.e93.
172. Ray U, Cinque P, Gerevini S, et al. JC polyomavirus mutants escape antibody-mediated neutralization. *Sci Transl Med*. 2015;7(306):306ra151.
173. Reisman L, Habib S, McClure GB, et al. Treatment of BK virus-associated nephropathy with CMX001 after kidney transplantation in a young child. *Pediatr Transplant*. 2014;18(7):E227-E231.
187. Schmitt C, Raggub L, Linnenweber-Held S, et al. Donor origin of BKV replication after kidney transplantation. *J Clin Virol*. 2014;59(2):120-125.
193. Shah T, Vu D, Naraghi R, et al. Efficacy of intravenous immunoglobulin in the treatment of persistent BK viremia and BK virus nephropathy in renal transplant recipients. *Clin Transpl*. 2014;109-116.
194. Sharif A, Alachkar N, Bagnasco S, et al. Incidence and outcomes of BK virus allograft nephropathy among ABO- and HLA-incompatible kidney transplant recipients. *Clin J Am Soc Nephrol*. 2012;7(8):1320-1327.
195. Sharma AP, Moussa M, Casier S, et al. Intravenous immunoglobulin as rescue therapy for BK virus nephropathy. *Pediatr Transplant*. 2009;13(1):123-129.
198. Sidhu N, McCutchan JA. Unmasking of PML by HAART: unusual clinical features and the role of IRIS. *J Neuroimmunol*. 2010;219(1-2):100-104.
200. Sospedra M, Schippling S, Yousef S, et al. Treating progressive multifocal leukoencephalopathy with interleukin 7 and vaccination with JC virus capsid protein VP1. *Clin Infect Dis*. 2014;59(11):1588-1592.

202. Stoner GL, Walker DL, Webster HD. Age distribution of progressive multifocal leukoencephalopathy. *Acta Neurol Scand*. 1988;78(4):307-312.
215. Thakuria M, LeBoeuf NR, Rabinowits G. Update on the biology and clinical management of Merkel cell carcinoma. *Am Soc Clin Oncol Educ Book*. 2014;e405-e410.
218. Tsai RT, Wang M, Ou WC, et al. Incidence of JC viruria is higher than that of BK viruria in Taiwan. *J Med Virol*. 1997;52(3):253-257.
220. van der Meijden E, Bialasiewicz S, Rockett RJ, et al. Different serologic behavior of MCPyV, TSPyV, HPyV6, HPyV7 and HPyV9 polyomaviruses found on the skin. *PLoS ONE*. 2013;8(11):e81078.
225. Vanchiere JA, Carillo B, Morrow AL, et al. Fecal polyomavirus excretion in infancy. *J Pediatric Infect Dis Soc*. 2016;5(2):210-213.
238. Zaman RA, Ettenger RB, Cheam H, et al. A novel treatment regimen for BK viremia. *Transplantation*. 2014;97(11):1166-1171.

The full reference list for this chapter is available at ExpertConsult.com.

155 Human Papillomaviruses

Adriana Cadilla • Kenneth A. Alexander

The human papillomaviruses (HPVs) are members of the virus family *Papillomaviridae*. More than 200 HPV genotypes have been identified. The double-stranded DNA genome of the HPV genome is approximately 8000 base pairs; intact virions are approximately 55 nm in diameter. Although most HPV infections are benign, HPVs can cause malignant transformation of squamous epithelia in both immunocompetent and immunodeficient hosts. HPVs also can cause a variety of benign cutaneous proliferations, including common skin warts. HPVs also have been associated with respiratory papillomatosis, which is a histologically benign but potentially life-threatening process. Our understanding of the complex role that HPVs play in these diverse clinical conditions remains incomplete, and management of these diseases remains an ongoing challenge. The licensure of two prophylactic vaccines against HPVs provides hope that the public health impact of these viruses will decrease.

HISTORY

Warts, or papillomas, have been recognized for centuries to occur at a variety of different body sites, in particular, the skin, genital tract, oral cavity, conjunctiva, and respiratory tract. The viral etiology of warts was demonstrated in 1907, when human volunteers were inoculated experimentally with a cell-free extract prepared from wart tissue.[71] These early experiments also suggested that warts were transmissible from person to person. When electron microscopy became available in the 1940s, virus particles were visualized, initially in skin warts and subsequently in genital warts, thereby confirming the viral etiology of these lesions. However, despite the abundance of virus particles seen in some lesions, virologic investigation of HPV-associated disease processes was hampered by the inability to propagate papillomaviruses in either cell culture or laboratory animals. The limited amount of information available from the study of virus particles obtained directly from wart tissue led in the 1960s to speculation that HPVs were composed of a single virus type. Scientists further theorized that the specific body site and epithelium involved, rather than the virus type, were responsible for the characteristic morphology and disease process.[299] With the advent of molecular biologic techniques in the 1970s, however, more than 70 different types of HPVs were described, and researchers quickly recognized that specific clinical diseases were associated with infection with specific HPV types. Most recently, HPV infection of the genital tract has been recognized as the most prevalent sexually transmitted infection, and a causal link between HPV infection and squamous carcinomas of the cervix is now well accepted. Challenges for the future revolve around developing effective treatment strategies because current measures are palliative at best and most lesions recur. New antiviral chemotherapeutic agents are being developed, and immunomodulators such as interferon provide promise for the treatment of serious disease caused by HPVs.

VIROLOGY

The family *Papillomaviridae* consists of small, nonenveloped viruses with a diameter of about 55 nm and includes the HPVs. *Papillomaviridae* viruses have a capsid composed of 72 capsomeres arranged in icosahedral symmetry. The papillomavirus genome is composed of double-stranded circular DNA that is approximately 8 kb in length. The complete nucleotide sequence is available for all clinically relevant HPVs, and partial sequence information is available for more than 120 HPV types.[91] Sequence conservation between the many HPV types is substantial. The papillomavirus genome is divided into three regions: an early region that encodes the proteins required for viral replication (E1, E4), transcription control (E2), and cell transformation (E5, E6, E7; Table 155.1); a late region that encodes the viral major and minor capsid proteins (L1 and L2); and the viral long control region, which contains the origin of replication and many control elements for viral transcription and replication.[111,135,193,269,270,271] The virus appears to replicate solely in the nucleus of the cell in association with low-molecular-weight histones.[197,388]

Papillomaviruses display a high degree of species, tissue, and cellular specificity. HPVs appear to infect only humans; most animal papillomaviruses do not infect other species as well. Although all HPVs infect epithelial surfaces, each HPV type has a tropism for specific epithelia.[124,352,380,381] The more than 200 HPV types that have been recognized may be classified according to the type of epithelia they infect (cutaneous or mucosal).[273] The mucosal HPV types are further subclassified according to the oncogenic potential of each virus (Table 155.2). The common cutaneous HPV types are found in a variety of skin warts (e.g., palmar warts, plantar warts, flat warts) and are uniformly benign.[35,36,279,350,372] The mucosal HPVs occur mainly in the anogenital tract but also infect and produce disease at mucosal sites in the respiratory tract, the oropharyngeal cavity, and the conjunctiva. The mucosal HPVs also are subgrouped into low-, high-, and intermediate- or moderate-risk types, depending on the frequency with which they are found in invasive cancers.[30,202,304,340,367] A third group of HPVs cause cutaneous diseases in a small group of patients with epidermodysplasia verruciformis (EV, also known as Lewandowsky-Lutz dysplasia or Lutz-Lewandowsky epidermodysplasia verruciformis), an extremely rare autosomal recessive disorder marked by extreme warty growths, particularly on the skin of the extremities.[282] These EV-associated viruses (most commonly HPV types 5 and 8, but there are others) have variable oncogenic activity and can underlie the development of squamous tumors in sun-exposed areas.[41,211,255,336,388]

The life cycle of HPVs is intimately entwined with the cell cycle and differentiation of epithelial cells.[105] HPV infection occurs after damage to the mucosa, allowing introduction of the virus into basal keratinocytes. Early infection is marked by E2 protein–regulated transcription of the viral early proteins. HPV infections are maintained in basal keratinocytes.

TABLE 155.1 **Major Human Papillomavirus Genes**

Gene	Protein Products and Function
Early (E) Region	
E1	Viral regulatory protein that initiates viral DNA replication
E2	Viral regulatory protein that controls replication and inhibits or activates early transcription of the viral genome
E3	Unknown
E4	A late viral protein that controls viral maturation; expressed in terminally differentiated keratinocytes
E5	Major transforming protein; causes cellular proliferation
E6	Major transforming oncoprotein; associates with the cellular target, TP53, a tumor suppressor protein, and promotes its proteolytic degradation; causes cellular proliferation and perturbation of keratinocyte differentiation
E7	Major transforming protein; associates with the cellular target pRB and inactivates its cell cycle restriction function; causes cellular proliferation and perturbation of keratinocyte differentiation
E8	Unknown; perhaps regulates viral DNA replication
Late (L) Region	
L1	Major structural viral capsid protein
L2	Minor structural viral capsid protein

Within basal keratinocytes, two forms of HPV DNA replication occur: maintenance replication and vegetative replication. Maintenance replication occurs in nondifferentiating basal keratinocytes at low levels sufficient only to ensure that HPV DNA is propagated to daughter keratinocytes; viral protein expression is minimal and limited to the viral early proteins. Vegetative replication occurs in differentiating keratinocytes as they enter the stratum spinosum. In the stratum spinosum, high-level viral replication occurs, with expression of the late proteins and production of complete virions. Progeny viruses are not released until fully differentiated keratinocytes are sloughed from the epithelial surface.[239,377]

Interestingly, the HPV genome does not encode any viral DNA or RNA polymerase, rendering the virus wholly dependent on host enzymes for replication. In view of this absolute dependence on host cell DNA and RNA polymerases, replication of papillomaviruses must occur at a time in the host cell cycle during which cellular polymerases, replication factors, and nucleoside triphosphates are in abundance (i.e., S phase). To drive host cells from G0 into S phase, HPVs express the E6 and E7 oncoproteins. Although the E6 and E7 oncoproteins have many identified biochemical activities,[305,358,379] the dominant activities of E6 and E7 are as follows. The E7 oncoprotein activates the cell cycle by displacing the E2F regulatory factor from the retinoblastoma tumor suppressor (pRB). This displacement of E2F from pRB allows E2F entry into the nucleus, where E2F activates genes that trigger cell cycle progression from G0 into S phase, with consequent activation of cellular (and viral) DNA replication. To attenuate the normal cellular protective response to unscheduled DNA replication (p53-induced cellular apoptosis), papillomaviruses express the E6 oncoprotein. The E6 oncoprotein forms a stable complex with the p53 tumor suppressor. This E6:p53 complex is then bound by the E6-associated protein (E6-AP), a ubiquitin ligase that, by ubiquitinating p53, earmarks p53 for destruction on the proteasome. By displacing E2F from pRB and by then degrading p53, papillomaviruses, in effect, "activate the engine" of cell proliferation and then "take away the brakes." The oncogenic activity of HPVs lies largely with the E6 and E7 oncoproteins. Although E6 and E7 expression appear to be tightly regulated in HPV infection, HPVs can integrate, apparently at random, into the host cell genome, leading to unregulated E6 and E7 expression. Most, but not all, HPV-induced malignancies contain chromosomally integrated copies of the HPV genome.[32,238,377]

Because full epithelial cell differentiation and keratinization of squamous epithelial cells are required for the HPVs to replicate completely, and because such differentiation is not achieved in conventional cell culture, HPVs cannot be propagated using standard tissue culture methods. Limited propagation of HPVs in keratinocyte raft cultures that recapitulate the structure of a differentiating epithelium is now performed routinely in research laboratories but has no clinical application. Research laboratories have also propagated papillomaviruses successfully by inoculating virion extracts into susceptible tissue (typically human foreskins) and transplanting this tissue into athymic nude mice.[167,184] Nonetheless, the laboratory and clinical study of HPVs and HPV-associated diseases has been and remains heavily dependent on the use of molecular biology techniques—in particular, polymerase chain reaction (PCR) assay.

EPIDEMIOLOGY

Among humans, HPVs are ubiquitous and, as a group, are the cause of the most common sexually transmitted infection. Although HPVs infect nearly all individuals of both sexes at some point in their lives, most infections are asymptomatic; only a minority of HPV infections come to medical attention. Even though a large proportion of HPV infection is subclinical and does not cause significant disease, the importance of HPV infection lies in the ability of HPVs to cause malignant transformation of squamous epithelial mucosal surfaces, potentially leading to significant cancer morbidity and mortality. Recently developed HPV vaccines have made important strides toward preventing HPV-associated neoplasias and malignancies.[104,136]

HPVs are transmitted by direct skin-to-skin contact, with most sexually transmitted infection resulting from penetrative vaginal and/or anal intercourse. Other types of sexual contacts, such as oral sex, and even indirect genital contact, can also transmit the virus.[136,387] Common body warts are transmitted by direct contact, often after minor skin trauma.[200] There is also evidence of latent epithelial disease activation in immunocompromised individuals, including solid-organ transplant recipients and individuals with human immunodeficiency virus (HIV) infection.[201,302,303] After vaginal births, HPV DNA can be detected in the mouths of up to 30% of neonates.[55,292,351] Associations between the types of HPV DNA found in maternal and paternal oral and genital mucosa and that in infant's oral mucosa have been made, although there is a high rate of HPV genotype discordance.[69,176,240,258] Perinatal infection after vertical transmission during childbirth is implicated in recurrent respiratory papillomatosis (RRP) as well as hepatitis in some cases.[98,264,317,392] There have been strong associations found between RRP in children and genital warts present in the mother at the time of delivery.[2,55,349]

The incubation period for HPV infection varies greatly but is approximately 3 months.[203] Nonetheless, disease can appear weeks to years after exposure, with invasive cancers typically developing after a decade or more.

It is estimated that, at any given time, nearly 20 million Americans are infected with HPV, with approximately 6 million new cases occurring each year, and about the same number of individuals clearing their infection each year. Most individuals with HPV infection do not show any signs or symptoms of infection; most infections are transient and cleared uneventfully, with median time to clearance of 8 months.[159] Seventy percent of infections are cleared by 12 months; more than 80% of genital HPV infections clear spontaneously by 24 months. HPV-16 is associated with increased persistence but still with a high rate (70%) of clearance within 24 months.[18,68,159,177,234,294] For men and women, the lifetime risk for developing a genital HPV infection exceeds 50%; estimates are that 80% of individuals will have had a genital HPV infection by age 50 years. The highest rates of HPV infection are seen in females younger than 25 years old.[51,166] Higher prevalence of HPV 6 and 11 is found in girls and young women 14 to 19 years old, whereas a higher prevalence of HPV 16 and 18 is found in those 20 to 24 years old.[23,24,26,100,225,231,232,291] Most HPV infections are acquired within the first few years after sexual debut. Not surprisingly, the risk for HPV infection is proportional to the number of sexual contacts. Recently, however, data are emerging that indicate that normal adolescents who have never been sexually active can be infected with mucosal HPV types.[94,162,326]

Other important risk factors for HPV infection include age older than 30 years, parity, smoking status, use of oral contraceptives, single marital status, and immunosuppression.[56,161,298,300]

TABLE 155.2 **Human Papillomavirus (HPV) Types and Associated Clinical Conditions**

Condition	Usual Location	Morphology	HPV Type
Cutaneous (Skin) Warts			
Common (verruca vulgaris)	Hands, lips, extremities	Multiple, dome shaped	2, 4
Plantar (verruca plantaris)	Bottom of feet	Single, painful	1
Flat (verruca plana)	Arms, face, knees	Multiple	3, 10, 28, 41
Filiform	Face, neck	Multiple, threadlike	2, 4
Mosaic	Feet, hands	Multiple, superficial	7
Butcher's	Hands	Multiple, dome shaped	7
Epidermodysplasia verruciformis	Face, trunk, extremities	Multiple flat warts or reddish-brown plaques	5, 8, 9, 12, 14, 15, 17, 19–25, 36–38, 47, 49
Immunosuppressed patients	Face, trunk, extremities	Dome-shaped or epidermodysplasia verruciformis–like plaques; may be persistent or progressive	1–5, 8, 10, 20, 23, 28, 49
Mucosal (Anogenital) Warts			
Subclinical	Cervix	Asymptomatic	6, 11, 13, 16, 18, 30–35, 39, 40, 42–45, 51–59
Condylomata acuminata	Cervix, vulva, urethra, anus, penis, scrotum	Multiple exophytic, pink, gray	6, 11, 16
Flat condylomata	Cervix	Asymptomatic, flat plaques	6, 11, 16, 18, 31
Giant condylomata acuminata (Buschke-Löwenstein tumors)	Perirectal area	Large, tumorlike	6, 11
Bowenoid papulosis	Penis, vulva, perirectal area	Multiple, large	16
Cervical cancer	Cervix	Asymptomatic; pigmented papillomas; erythematous or white plaques; ulcerations; mass lesion	Strong association: 16, 18, 31, 45 Moderate association: 30, 33, 35, 39, 51, 52, 56, 58, 59, 68 Weak association: 6, 11, 26, 34, 40, 43, 44, 53–55, 57, 62, 66, 74
Vaginal cancer	Vagina	Asymptomatic; ulcerative mass lesions; vascular pattern with punctation and mosaicism	16
Vulvar cancer	Vulva	Asymptomatic; pigmented papillomas; erythematous or white plaques; ulcerations; mass lesion	16
Penile cancer	Penis	Painless, ulcerative mass lesion	16
Anal cancer	Perianal area, anal canal	Asymptomatic; pigmented papillomas; erythematous or white plaques; ulcerations; mass lesion	16, 18, 31
Ovarian cancer	Ovaries	Unknown	6?, 16?, 18?
Mucosal (Other) Warts			
Respiratory papillomatosis	Larynx, trachea, bronchi, lungs	Multiple papillomas	6, 11
Nasal and paranasal papillomas	Nose, paranasal sinuses	Single or multiple papillomas	6, 11, 57, 57b
Focal epithelial hyperplasia (Heck disease)	Oral cavity	Discrete, multiple nodules	13, 32
Oral cavity papillomas	Gums, buccal mucosa, soft palate, tonsils	Single or multiple papillomas	6, 11, 16
Conjunctival papillomas	Conjunctivae	Single or multiple papillomas	6, 11, 16
Giant cell hepatitis	Liver	Unknown	6?

The clinical presentation of HPV infection depends on the anatomic location and the type of HPV with which an individual is infected. Males and females infected with HPV experience similar clinical disease processes with related cutaneous warts while experiencing differing manifestations of anogenital condyloma and cancers based on anatomy. In both genders, rates of HPV-associated oropharyngeal and anogenital cancers are increasing.[45]

The Centers for Disease Control and Prevention (CDC) estimates that, in the United States, nearly 30,000 cases of HPV-associated cancers occur annually, with two-thirds of those cases affecting females. Cervical cancer is the most common HPV-associated cancer overall; the second most common group of HPV-associated cancers comprises those of the oral cavity and the oropharynx. HPV-associated cancer rates vary greatly by state in both males and females, with higher rates (11 to 16/100,000) seen in southern, southeastern, and mideastern seaboard cities and states (e.g., Louisiana, Kentucky, Tennessee, and the District of Columbia). Rates of HPV-associated cancers in other parts of the country (e.g., Colorado, Utah, and Maryland) are lower (4 to 8/100,000).[59]

Female-Specific HPV-Associated Malignancies

In females, HPV infections can progress to vulvar, vaginal, and cervical cancers. Persistent HPV infection is associated with increased risk for progressive epithelial pathologic process and cancer.

Although the incidence of cervical cancer has declined significantly in the United States in the past 50 years (largely through the development of universal cervical cytology screening programs), cervical cancer remains the second leading cause of cancer death in women worldwide, with more than 80% of cases occurring in the developing world.[40] Most cervical cancers are diagnosed in females older than 30 years. In contrast to vulvar and vaginal cancer, essentially all cervical cancer is HPV associated.[59,359] In the United States, Hispanic (12/100,000) and black (10/100,000) females have higher rates of cervical cancer than females of all other races (7/100,000). Approximately 4000 females die annually of cervical cancer.[19,59,359] Worldwide, the mortality to incidence ratio of cervical cancer is 52%. Globally, nearly 300,000 women die of cervical cancer each year, the majority of whom are in developing countries.[260,325,378]

The most studied relationship between HPV and cancer risk is cervical cancer and its preceding grades of dysplasia.[239,241,245,309,357] It is estimated that approximately 10% of all women in the world have a cervical HPV infection at any given time, with prevalence of infection being higher in the developing world. Some of the highest rates of infection are seen in Eastern Africa, whereas some of the lowest rates are seen in Southeast Asia. In all developed and developing countries, the prevalence of HPV infection is highest among young women; infection rates decline in younger middle-aged women, with a second resurgence of HPV infection in the perimenopausal age range. The cause for this perimenopausal resurgence of HPV infection phenomenon is not known but may be due to changes in sexual behaviors and acquisition of new HPV infection in middle age, reactivation of latent infection, or a high-exposure population promoting a cohort effect.[157,180,188,245,283,284,344,345,347]

HPV-16 is the most common HPV type in cervical dysplasias and malignancies. HPV-18 is the second most prevalent, with some intercontinental variation seen between Europe, Asia, and the Americas.[90,144,172] HPV-16 is the most oncogenic, responsible for nearly half of all cervical cancer. In women with invasive cervical cancer, HPV-16 and HPV-18 together contribute to approximately 70% of all cases.[74]

Since 1986, in the United States, the rate of vulvar cancers has increased. In the United States, the overall incidence rate of vulvar cancers is 2.3 per 100,000 females. Each year, there are approximately 3000 new cases of vulvar cancer. Half of these cases are HPV associated.[89,136,163] Worldwide, vulvar cancer contributes to approximately 4% of all gynecologic cancers.[12,41]

Vaginal cancer is much rarer than vulvar cancer and occurs most often in females older than 80 years. In the United States, HPV-associated vaginal cancer cases account for over 700 (65%) new cases annually.[7] Vaginal cancers affect black females (0.7/100,000) disproportionately more than females of all other races (~0.4/100,000).[59,136]

Male-Specific HPV-Associated Malignancies

There are nearly 1700 new cases (and 250 deaths) of HPV-associated anal cancers diagnosed in males annually. Black males (1.6/100,000) are disproportionately more affected than males of all other races (0.2 to 1.0/100,000).[59,136] Men who have sex with men are a unique population at high risk for persistent low- and high-grade anal lesions that can progress to invasive cancer.[142,371]

Penile cancer is very rare and occurs most commonly in males older than 60 years of age. Approximately 1000 cases of penile cancer occur in the United States each year, of which 35% are believed to be HPV associated. Penile cancers affect Hispanic males (1.3/100,000) disproportionately more than males of all other ethnicities (0.7/100,000).[59,136] The incidence of penile cancer is much lower than that of cervical cancer. Penile circumcision affords some degree of protection against penile cancers.

In addition to gender-specific HPV-associated invasive disease, other common HPV-associated disease processes, including cutaneous warts, anogenital warts, and oropharyngeal cancers, affect both sexes similarly.

A progressively higher prevalence of mucosal disease occurs in adolescence and young adulthood. In both males and females, anogenital warts (condylomata acuminata) occur in and around the genitalia and anus.[146] All anogenital warts are caused by HPV, with more than 90% caused by HPV types 6 and 11.[142] Every year in the United States, there are approximately 1 million new cases of anogenital condylomata diagnosed, often first noticed within weeks or months of exposure. The majority of infections last longer than 4 months.[189] Individuals will have varying clinical courses, some with very few lesions lasting only a few months and some with progressive lesions increasing in size and number and causing significant morbidity.[40,131,248]

HPV-Associated Malignancies in Males and Females

Similar to cervical cancer, nearly all new cases (90%) of anal cancer are HPV associated.[6] In US women, there are 3000 new cases (and 500 deaths) of HPV-associated anal cancers annually. HPV-associated anal cancers affect white females (2/100,000) disproportionately more than females of all other races (0.4 to 1.4/100,000). The incidence of anal cancers in females in the general population is increasing at a rate of nearly 2% per year.[59,136] Among HPV-positive females, the prevalence of HPV-related anal cancers is even higher than that for cervical cancer.[260,262]

HPV-Associated Oral and Oropharyngeal Cancers

Cancer of the oral and oropharyngeal cavities has gained increasing attention because its relationship to HPV infection has more recently been elucidated. HPV-16 DNA has been detected in up to 82% of head and neck cancers.[244] Historically, oropharyngeal cancer risk has been associated with advanced age and with alcohol and tobacco use (alcohol- and tobacco-associated oropharyngeal cancers are often HPV negative). In contrast, HPV-associated oropharyngeal cancers occur in younger adults without strong histories of alcohol or tobacco use.

Although the incidence of non–HPV-associated oral and oropharyngeal cancers is declining, the incidence of HPV-associated cancers is increasing at a rate of approximately 5% per year.[61,171] Among all oropharyngeal cancers, the prevalence rates of HPV-associated oropharyngeal cancers have risen from 33% of new cases in the 1980s to 70% in the 1990s and over 80% in the 2000s, particularly among white males.[46] In the United States, there are nearly 12,000 (60%) new HPV-associated oropharyngeal cancer cases annually. HPV-associated oral cancers affect males (9300 cases) more than females (2300 cases), with much lower rates found in Asian/Pacific Islander males (3/100,000) and females (0.5/100,000) compared with males and females of all other races (6/100,000 and 0.5/100,000, respectively).[359] In the 1980s, HPV was associated with approximately 16.3% of oropharyngeal squamous cell carcinomas; in the 2000s, this number rose to 72.7%.[63] In the United States in 1999, the incidence of cancer in the oral cavity or pharynx was 6.4 per 100,000 for females and 16.3 per 100,000 for males; in 2013, the incidence in females was 6.3 per 100,000, and in males it was 17.4 per 100,000.[361]

In both males and females, the incidence of HPV-associated oral and oropharyngeal cancers increases dramatically after 50 years of age.[47,136,209] Those at increased risk for developing HPV-associated head and neck cancer compared with those with HPV-negative disease are generally white, younger, and of a higher socioeconomic status and have a higher education and more lifetime oral sex partners.[21,137]

HPV-associated malignancies likely arise as an unusual consequence of oral HPV infection. The prevalence of oral HPV infection is estimated to be between 2% and 3% of young adults (18–30 years old).[275] Those with concurrent HIV infection and those who are smokers have a higher prevalence of oral HPV.[61,62,72,73] Even though white males experience the majority of HPV-associated oropharyngeal disease burden, they also show improved survival over females.[254] Rates of HPV-associated oropharyngeal disease have increased so markedly within the past 20 years in the United States that by 2020 it is anticipated that the number of HPV-associated oropharyngeal cancers will exceed the number of incident cervical cancers.[62,229]

HPV-associated head and neck cancers occur in younger persons (<60 years of age), with a preponderance of cases diagnosed in white males. In contrast, tobacco- and alcohol-related HPV-negative head and neck malignancies occur most frequently in older African American men.[63]

A recent study determined that presence of HPV-16 in the oral cavity preceded incidence of oropharyngeal cancer.[4] It remains unclear what effect HPV vaccine will have in head and neck cancer incidence, as it will take years for currently vaccinated children to reach the age at which head and neck cancer presents itself. However, it is speculated that the vaccine will afford protection, and a decline in head and neck cancer should occur.

HPV-Associated Malignancies in Persons With HIV

In 1993, the CDC added cervical cancer as an AIDS-defining malignancy. Since then, our understanding of the association between HPV malignancy and HIV has continued to grow. In the United States, the incidence of cervical cancer is two- to 22-fold greater among HIV-positive females than in HIV-negative females. Similarly, vulvar intraepithelial neoplasia has been reported to occur 29 times more frequently in HIV-positive women when compared with HIV-negative women.[290] Most striking is the increasing incidence of anal cancer. The incidence of anal cancers has been on the rise, with a yearly estimated increase of 1.7% among men. However, among HIV-positive men, the rise is greater, at 3.4% per year.[44]

Penile cancer also seems to affect HIV-positive men more frequently than it does HIV-negative men, as HIV-positive men have a two- to threefold increased risk.[290] Curiously, and in contrast with other AIDS-defining malignancies, there have not been decreases in the rates of HPV-associated malignancies in HIV-infected people despite the institution of highly active antiretroviral therapy (HAART). For example, pre-HAART (1992–95), the incidence of anal cancer among HIV-positive males and females was 19 per 100,000 person-years. This increased to 48 per 100,000 person-years post HAART (1996–99) and increased further to 78 per 100,000 person-years from 2000 to 2003.[259] Ongoing studies are needed to better understand the association between HIV infection and HPV-associated malignancies. Current studies show conflicting results and no clear correlation between CD4 counts and the risk of HPV-associated malignancies. Improved universal screening guidelines are needed.

HPV and Sexual Abuse

The detection of mucosal (i.e., genital) HPV types in children may raise the suspicion of sexual abuse. Both vertical and horizontal transmission have been described (including perinatal transmission, heteroinoculation (e.g., during diaper changes and autoinoculation).[296] Contributing to the uncertainty of timing of infection is the delay in presentation of clinical disease. The occurrence of anogenital disease resulting from perinatal infection may be delayed up to 24 months; the development of symptomatic laryngeal papillomatosis (which also arises from perinatal infection) may be delayed up to 5 years.[327] To date, few studies have addressed HPV in sexual abuse. One report attributed sexual abuse as the source of genital warts in 31% to 58% of children 14 years of age and younger.[296] Unger et al. found a high prevalence of genital HPV in children with evidence of possible, probable, or definite sexual abuse. However, these authors also found genital HPV in children without evidence of sexual abuse.[363] Further, universal use of HPV vaccine may continue to alter the presence of clinical/microbiologic disease. Nonetheless, with an estimated 702,000 children in the United States suffering from abuse and neglect in 2014, of whom 8.3% were sexually abused,[360] the discovery of a mucosal HPV type in a child older than 2 years should prompt investigation into the possibility of child maltreatment.[147,179]

CLINICAL MANIFESTATIONS

Cutaneous Warts

Common cutaneous skin warts, or verrucae, have variable morphology and may appear at any location on the skin.[64,320] Common skin warts, or verrucae vulgaris, present as well-demarcated, dome shaped papules with multiple conical projections (papillomatosis) that give the surface of the wart a rough appearance and texture. Flat warts, or verrucae planae, in contrast, do not have papillomatosis or hyperkeratosis and often occur in clusters. Warts occasionally have a mosaic appearance; such warts occur most commonly on the plantar surface of the feet and spread superficially over the skin. Warts may also be filiform and appear as threadlike warts on the face and neck.[53]

Common warts generally occur on the hands, especially the dorsum of the fingers, but they also are seen frequently between the fingers. Warts on the hands and feet may occur periungually and on the palms.[169,301] Plantar warts, also called verrucae plantares, occur most commonly in adolescents and young adults.[84,168] Plantar warts generally are single lesions and have a highly thickened corneal layer, or hyperkeratosis, with areas of punctate bleeding. Plantar warts may be painful because they typically are found on pressure-bearing points on the plantar surface of the foot. Flat warts are more common findings in young children and occur most frequently on the arms, face, and knees.[84] Butcher's warts are a form of cutaneous wart seen in meat and poultry handlers who suffer repeated minor trauma to the hands.[87] Although the clinical appearance of cutaneous warts almost always is diagnostic, the differential diagnosis of warty lesions includes other skin disorders, such as molluscum contagiosum, actinomycosis, blastomycosis, sporotrichosis, leishmaniasis, chronic vegetating pyoderma, atypical mycobacterial infection (e.g., swimming pool granuloma), and tuberculosis verrucosa cutis (warty tuberculosis). Giant verrucae or warts also must be differentiated from squamous cell carcinoma.[252]

Epidermodysplasia Verruciformis

Epidermodysplasia verruciformis (EV) is a very rare skin disorder initially manifested in infancy or early childhood. It is characterized by the inability to resolve HPV-induced, cutaneous wart-like lesions.[210] Patients with EV have both nonspecific and HPV-specific defects in cell-mediated immunity, especially T-cell defects; and some patients will have developmental disabilities.[49,79,139,165,211–213,330,353,368] Although the lesions seen with EV are polymorphic, two clinical types of warts are seen primarily in these patients: flat warts and red or reddish-brown macular plaques. Both the flat warts and plaques appear first on the face, trunk, and extremities. They slowly become confluent and then appear to disseminate. Occasionally, the plaques may be achromatic with pigmented borders and resemble pityriasis versicolor. Histopathologically, EV lesions may appear as an in situ or invasive carcinoma.[165] These EV-related carcinomas generally do not metastasize unless exposed to co-carcinogens, such as radiation.[257]

Patients with EV may be infected with multiple types of HPVs, including HPV-3 and HPV-10, HPV types associated with flat warts in healthy individuals.[8,210,250,320] The HPV types most commonly associated with lesions in patients with EV (HPV types 5, 8, 17, and 20) do not usually cause lesions in immunocompetent individuals; however, HPV-8 antibodies have been found in healthy individuals, and HPV-5 DNA and HPV-8 DNA have been detected in refractory warts and skin carcinomas in immunocompromised patients, such as renal allograft recipients.[85,143,204,272,338] EV-like skin lesions also may be seen in individuals who are immunocompromised as a result of HIV infection, as well as in transplant recipients, those receiving cancer chemotherapy, and other immunosuppressed patients.[29,31,72]

Infections of Male and Female Genital Tracts

Genital tract HPV is the most common clinical manifestation of mucosal HPV disease and is, in both sexes, the most common viral sexually transmitted infection. Genital tract HPV infection carries high rates of morbidity and mortality to both males and females by its oncogenic potential. However, condylomata acuminata, or genital warts, are the most common genital tract clinical manifestation and rarely develop into dysplastic lesions or invasive carcinoma.[285,375] Persistent HPV infection is required for the development of neoplasia. Oncogenic HPV types establish persistent infection and express the E7 oncogenes that drive the epithelial cell from G0 into S phase while simultaneously disrupting the apoptotic machinery of epithelial cells. This driving infected cells into S phase and the inhibition of the normal apoptotic response to unscheduled cell division lead to disorganized and uninhibited cell proliferation and disruption of the normal keratinocyte maturation process. HPV persistence is seen before the appearance and even after the regression of cytologic pathology.[57,310] Early HPV infection manifests as mucosal dysplasia. Grading systems for intraepithelial neoplasias (INs) are similar for the different anatomic areas, increasing in severity going from grade 1 through grade 3, with carcinoma in situ being the most severe. Dysplasia can be further classified into mild (one-third thickness), moderate (two-thirds thickness), or severe (full thickness) based on the extent to which the cervical epithelium is involved with abnormal cells. The majority of mild dysplastic lesions will regress. Moderate and severe dysplasias are considered premalignant lesions. Invasive carcinomas are preceded by a precursor lesion, a carcinoma in situ that morphologically resembles the adjacent invasive squamous carcinoma.[243,312]

More common than dysplasia and invasive disease in both males and females are condylomata acuminata, or genital warts. Ninety percent of genital warts are caused by HPV types 6 and 11; a small proportion are caused by HPV-16.[112,190]

Generally, genital warts occur in multiples as flesh-colored, pink, and/or purple-gray papules. Warts, which can also be pedunculated, are covered by an acanthotic squamous epithelium. Giant condylomata acuminata (also known as Buschke-Lowenstein tumors) occur in similar areas as other condylomata but are large, tumor-like lesions that may cause, albeit rarely, inguinal lymphadenopathy, fistulous tracts, inflammation, hemorrhage, and fibrosis of the surrounding tissue. Buschke-Lowenstein tumors can progress to squamous carcinoma.[278]

In females, genital warts are found on the vulva and in and around the vagina, the perineum, inner thighs, and anus. Although physically visible and palpable, most lesions are asymptomatic. However, genital warts can cause burning, itching, and pain. Intravaginal and cervicovaginal condylomata, usually in the form of less easily visualized flat warts, are also found and have a higher rate of progression to low- or high-grade dysplastic intraepithelial lesions than external lesions.[113] Anogenital flat warts are most frequently caused by HPV types 6, 11, 16, 18, and 31.[16] During pregnancy, genital warts can increase in size and quantity but often regress after delivery. In males, genital warts can be found on the penis, scrotum, groin and upper thighs, perineum, and anus. Similar to in females, lesions are often asymptomatic but can cause burning, itching, and dyspareunia. Bowenoid papulosis, another clinical manifestation of HPV infection of both the male and female genital tracts—characterized by multiple, large erythematous, maculopapular lesions that can take on a red, purple, or brown color with a smooth, velvety surface—occurs typically in individuals younger than 40 years old. Bowenoid papules may regress spontaneously or may persist as high-grade intraepithelial lesions and are most commonly associated with HPV-16.[39]

Adolescents can develop genital warts within 1 to 2 months of sexual exposure. Children can have genital and anal warts as a consequence of sexual abuse or from perinatal transmission.[146,148]

The differential diagnoses of anogenital warts include condylomata lata associated with secondary syphilis, molluscum contagiosum, epithelial papillae, enlarged sebaceous cysts, seborrheic keratosis, lentigo, pigmented nevi, skin tags, hemorrhoids, Crohn disease, and carcinoma.

Female-Specific Disease

Beyond condylomata acuminata, female-specific genital tract disease involves the cervix, vulva, and vagina. Early infection manifests as dysplasia of varying degrees that most often regresses spontaneously but can progress to invasive cancer. The site at which the majority of cervical neoplasias develop (90%) is the squamocolumnar junction. The squamocolumnar junction, located on the face of the cervix in adolescents and later receding into the cervical os in adult women, is the transition zone between the squamous epithelium of the cervix and the columnar epithelium that lines the uterus.[39]

Cervical epithelial lesions identified by Papanicolaou screening are described using the Bethesda system, which classifies precursor lesions into low-grade squamous intraepithelial lesion (often correlating with the presence of cervical intraepithelial neoplasia [CIN] grade 1 lesions) or moderate/high-grade squamous intraepithelial lesion (HSIL, which often correlates with the presence of CIN grade 2 or 3 lesions).[243] The majority (approximately 60%) of CIN grade 1 lesions regress spontaneously; only 10% progress to CIN grade 3, and only about 1% progress to cervical cancer. In contrast, higher grade lesions have a higher rate of cancer progression. Only one-third of CIN grade 3 lesions are likely to regress, and up to 10% to 12% of untreated cases progress to cervical cancer.[256] The risk for progression of CIN grade 3 lesions to cervical cancer increases with age, with 0.5% per year of CIN grade 3 lesions in young women 20 to 24 years old progressing to cervical cancer; this rate of progression increases to up to 10% per year in women 80 years old.[230,235] HPV types 16, 18, 31, and 45 are the types most strongly associated with cervical cancer. Cervical cancer occurs occasionally due to HPV types 33, 35, 39, 51, 52, 56, 58, 59, and 68 and only rarely due to HPV types 6 and 11.

Using a colposcope, cervical dysplasias and carcinomas appear as pigmented papular or plaque-like lesions and as leukoplakic or, if advanced, larger and/or ulcerated lesions. Cervical dysplasia may or may not be visible to the naked eye. Common clinical characteristics of cervical carcinoma include atypical nonbranching vessels (e.g., corkscrew, comma shape), ulcerations, raised irregular surface, yellow hue to epithelium, and firmness to palpation.

Vulvar intraepithelial neoplasias (VINs) are named to distinguish lesion morphologies. VIN lesions include VIN, usual type; VIN, warty type; VIN, basaloid type; VIN, mixed (warty/basaloid) type; and VIN, differentiated type. VIN is often asymptomatic and is discovered at the time of gynecologic examination and/or during evaluation for other lesions, such as anogenital warts or cervical dysplasias. VIN lesions are flat or rough elevated papules, are often multicentric, and can occur anywhere on the vulva, including the periurethral and perianal areas. VIN, warty type, is most associated with high-risk HPV, most often HPV type 16. Regression of VIN is common; progression to malignancy most often occurs with the basaloid type. Because of the high frequency of multicentric vulvar disease, patients with suspected VIN should receive a full examination looking for disease of the cervix and vagina. Up to 50% of women with VIN will have an antecedent or concomitant lower genital tract dysplasia, including cervical or vaginal intraepithelial neoplasia.[366] As VIN progresses, a more distinct vulvar tumor evolves. The most common characteristics of vulvar carcinoma include red, pink, or white bumps, often with rough or eroded surfaces; persistent, nonhealing ulcer with bleeding; intense vulvar pruritus; burning; and dysuria.[41,318]

For vaginal disease, the IN classification is employed, using the term *vaginal intraepithelial neoplasia* (VaIN). VaIN is divided into grades 1, 2, and 3 to describe the severity of a lesion. As with cervical and vulvar dysplasia, VaIN is usually asymptomatic, but it can present as abnormal vaginal discharge and/or with spontaneous or postcoital bleeding. VaIN usually affects the posterior upper third of the vagina and presents as single or multicentric lesions[38] and cannot be seen without use of a colposcope. VaIN lesions typically have a vascular pattern with punctation and mosaicism. The vascular pattern can become more unusual as lesions become more invasive. Progression of VaIN to vaginal cancer is more unpredictable than other female genital intraepithelial lesions. Fortunately, less than 10% of VaIN lesions progress to invasive cancer.[268] Vaginal cancer is rare. In contrast, VaIN is a disease of younger women and is associated with HPV infection. HPV-negative vaginal cancers occur most often in elderly women.

Male-Specific Disease

Male-specific genital tract dysplasia and invasive cancer affect the penis. As in all other genital tract dysplasias, the IN system is used to describe the histologic stage of each lesion (penile intraepithelial lesion [PIN] grades 1, 2, and 3 and penile carcinoma in situ). Penile dysplasia and invasive disease present most often as a lump or nodule and sometimes as an ulcerative or erythematous lesion. Penile dysplasia can also present as phimosis, penile pain, and bleeding along with a foul-smelling discharge. Because of social stigma and psychological stress surrounding penile pathology, clinical presentation is often late.[50,86] Squamous cell carcinoma is the most common type of neoplasia of the penis, with several different types described: classic, basaloid, verrucous, sarcomatoid, and adenosquamous.[332] About half of penile carcinomas are HPV associated, most often the warty-basaloid type. HPV-16 and less so HPV-18 are most commonly associated with HPV-associated PIN and invasive penile cancer. Invasive cancer is localized to the glans most commonly, then the prepuce, with the least amount of disease seen on the coronal sulcus and shaft. If penile carcinoma in situ involves the glans, it is also known as erythroplasia of Queyrat; if disease involves the shaft, it is also known as Bowen disease. In Bowen disease, inguinal lymph node involvement is common.

Recurrent Respiratory Papillomatosis

RRP is a rare, potentially life-threatening condition caused by HPV types 6 and 11.[91,119,155,183,370] Worldwide, RRP probably is the most common tumor of the larynx in children, with an incidence of 0.1 to 2.8 per 100,000 observed.[342,364] In the United States, the estimated incidence of RRP in children is 0.6 to 4.3 per 100,000 and up to 1.8 per 100,000 in adults.[88] RRP is newly diagnosed in an estimated 1500 patients each year.[88,236,364] The disease may be seen in both children and adults. Approximately two-thirds of cases of RRP are seen in children; the disease is then referred to as juvenile-onset recurrent respiratory papillomatosis (JORRP).[76] In children, approximately a fourth of the cases will be present before age 1 year; half are present by age 5 years, and the other half by age 11 years. Adult-onset RRP is most often first seen in patients between 20 and 40 years of age, but occasionally RRP may be seen in adolescents.[119,237,320]

Infants and children with JORRP most likely acquire HPV infection perinatally during passage through an HPV-infected birth canal. Thirty percent to 60% of mothers of children with JORRP have a history of genital warts, compared with less than 5% of mothers of children who do not have JORRP; children with JORRP rarely are born by cesarean section.[28,265,280,321] Risk factors for JORRP include vaginal delivery, being firstborn, and maternal age younger than 20 years.[322] HPV types 6 and 11, the HPV types most commonly associated with genital warts seen in women, also underlie most cases of JORRP.[37,107,320] Although HPV DNA has been detected in the oropharynx of infants born to mothers with genital HPV infection,[320] RRP develops in only a small proportion of infants born to mothers with genital warts or subclinical HPV infection.[293] The presence of HPV DNA in human breast milk renders this mode of transmission also a possibility for some infants.[306] The mode of transmission of HPV types 6 and 11 in adult-onset RRP is unknown.

The most common initial symptom of RRP and JORRP is hoarseness or a change in voice. Infants and toddlers may have a hoarse cry, stridor, airway obstruction, respiratory distress, or difficulty in phonation. They also may have a crouplike illness. The most common site for RRP and JORRP is the true vocal cord of the larynx. Supraglottic and subglottic extension of the lesions also may occur. In addition, the disease may involve the trachea, bronchi, palate, nasopharynx, paranasal sinuses, and lungs. When the lungs are involved, pulmonary nodules, atelectasis, and secondary bacterial pneumonia may occur (Fig. 155.1). The disease also may produce permanent lung damage with bronchiectasis and cavitations (Fig. 155.2). In 2% to 3% of patients, progression to invasive squamous papillomatosis and even malignant transformation to squamous cell carcinoma will occur, with invasion of the soft tissues of the neck, esophagus, and lung parenchyma; such an exceptionally aggressive disease course may occur in association with infection by HPV type 16 (Fig. 155.3).[331,383] The incidence of progression to squamous carcinoma increases to 14% in patients who received the radiation therapy that was commonly used previously to treat RRP.[78,133,214,313] Smoking and severe recurrent disease are also risk factors for development of malignant transformation in adolescents and adults. Clinical courses of RRP and JORRP are highly variable and characterized by common and unpredictable remissions and exacerbations, even despite apparently successful removal of the lesions. Longitudinal studies of JORRP show that infection with HPV type 11 and age younger than 3 years at initial diagnosis are associated with more aggressive tracheal disease requiring frequent surgical debulking.[78,281,383] Sudden and unexpected death may also occur from airway obstruction if the lesions obstruct the laryngeal lumen.[333]

The mainstay treatment of RRP is surgical debulking, with the goal of reducing tumor burden, decreasing spread of disease, maintaining airway patency, and prolonging time between surgical procedures. Because of the recurrent nature of disease, adjuvant pharmacotherapy is used in some cases. Use of interferon alpha has shown mixed results, with remission demonstrated in some patients and no benefit to others.[370] Interferon alpha binds cell receptors and produces antiviral, antiproliferative, and immunomodulatory effects. Cidofovir has been used, mostly intralesionally, with a few additional reports of inhaled delivery.[370] Studies with intralesion administration have reported complete resolution in up to 57% of patients and partial resolution in 35%.[123] Both interferon alpha and cidofovir have significant toxicities that need to be taken into account when considering their use. Other pharmacotherapies are being investigated, including indole 3 carbinol, a substance from cruciferous vegetables that has been found to decrease papilloma growth through alterations of estrogen metabolism. Also being investigated is a therapeutic vaccine, HSPE7 (a recombinant protein combining heat shock protein 65 of *Mycobacterium bovis* with E7 protein of HPV-16), which, when administered subcutaneously as an adjuvant to surgery, has shown a decrease in the number and frequency of papilloma debulking surgeries required.[370] Intralesional mumps vaccine has shown prolonged remission in children[370] and continues to be studied. COX-2 inhibitors are being tested.[385] Bevacizumab (a vascular endothelial growth factor inhibitor) is also being investigated as adjunctive therapy.[385] Last, initial studies have shown an added benefit to antireflux therapy.[370]

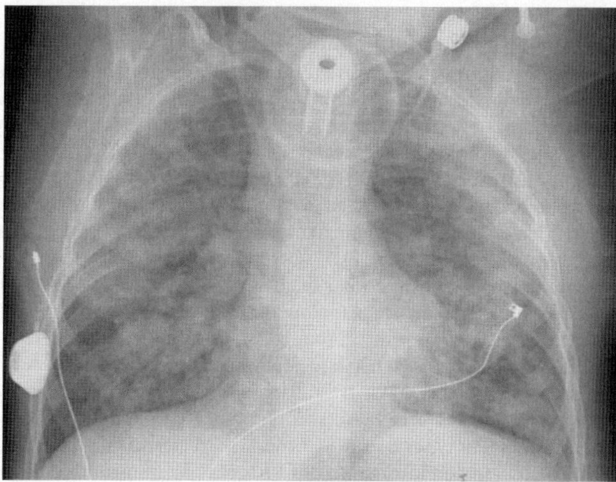

FIG. 155.1 Chest radiograph of a 6-year-old girl with severe, recurrent, and progressive respiratory papillomatosis since 1 year of age.

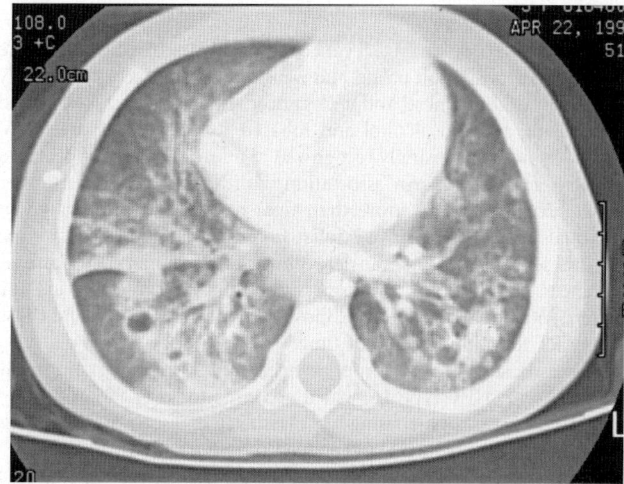

FIG. 155.2 Computed tomographic chest scan of a 6-year-old girl with severe, recurrent, and progressive respiratory papillomatosis shows pulmonary nodules, bronchiectasis, and cavitations.

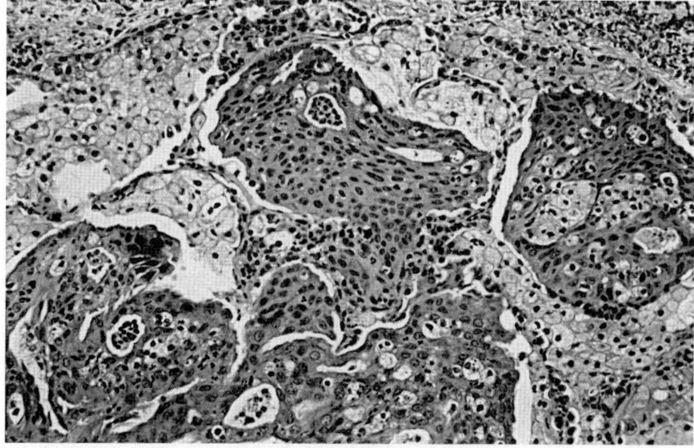

FIG. 155.3 Lung biopsy tissue from a 6-year-old girl with severe, progressive, recurrent respiratory papillomatosis. This specimen demonstrates invasive squamous papillomatosis. The squamous cells are growing along preformed pulmonary structures, but no evidence of malignancy is apparent at this time because of the absence of invasion of lung tissue (hematoxylin and eosin stain, ×50 original magnification, light microscopy). (Courtesy Dr. Claire Langston, Department of Pathology, Baylor College of Medicine and Texas Children's Hospital, Houston, TX.)

Upper Respiratory Tract Papillomas

Nasal papillomas or warts are rare tumors that may develop at any age, including childhood, and may occur as solitary lesions or in combination with papillomas elsewhere in the respiratory tract.[41,289] Histologically, they usually resemble the laryngeal papillomas seen in RRP. They most commonly are caused by HPV types 6 and 11, although HPV types 16, 57, and 57b also have been detected in nasal papillomas. Cocaine snorting is one risk factor for the development of nasal papillomas.[316,339] Papillomas also may involve the paranasal sinuses.[42,289]

Conjunctival papillomas occur in all age groups but are exceedingly rare (Fig. 155.4). Conjunctival papillomas may be asymptomatic initially but with increasing size can cause a constant foreign body sensation or chronic conjunctivitis. When large, they appear as pink mulberry- or cauliflower-like growths that may cause pain or interfere with lid closure. In most children and some adults, conjunctival papillomas appear to be caused by HPV types 6 and 11, which characteristically infect the genital tract and, therefore, similar to RRP, may be transmitted during birth.[191,223] HPV type 16, another HPV that commonly infects the genital tract, also has been associated with conjunctival and lacrimal sac carcinoma in adults.[207,222]

Gastrointestinal Disease

Oropharyngeal Cancer

HPV-associated oropharyngeal cancers typically occur within the base of the tongue, tonsils, soft palate, and walls of the pharynx. As previously mentioned, although head and neck cancer risk has been closely linked to increasing age and alcohol and tobacco use, persistent oral HPV infection is now increasingly recognized as a leading cause of oral and oropharyngeal cancers. An association with having a higher number of oral sexual partners (more than five) has been demonstrated in individuals with HPV-positive exfoliative cells within their oropharynx; thus, oral sexual behaviors translate into risk for oropharyngeal disease and cancer. Individuals at risk for persistent oral HPV infection include smokers, individuals of older age, those with low CD4 count, and those on HAART for a long period of time.[47,75]

HPV-associated oral and oropharyngeal cancers are most commonly associated with HPV type 16, which accounts for over 90% of HPV-associated disease.[43] This rising HPV-associated disease prevalence is most striking in the United States and less so in Europe and other areas.[64] Not only have HPV-associated oropharyngeal cancers been increasing in incidence overall, but, anatomically, this increase is seen particularly within the palatine and lingual tonsils.[80,153] HPV targets the specialized reticulated epithelium lining the tonsillar crypts.[221] HPV-associated cancer most commonly occurs next within the soft palate and Waldeyer's ring (the uninterrupted ring of lymphoid tissue including the tubal, pharyngeal, palatine, and lingual tonsil). HPV-associated malignancy can also occur in other head and neck regions.[185,246,346,355,369]

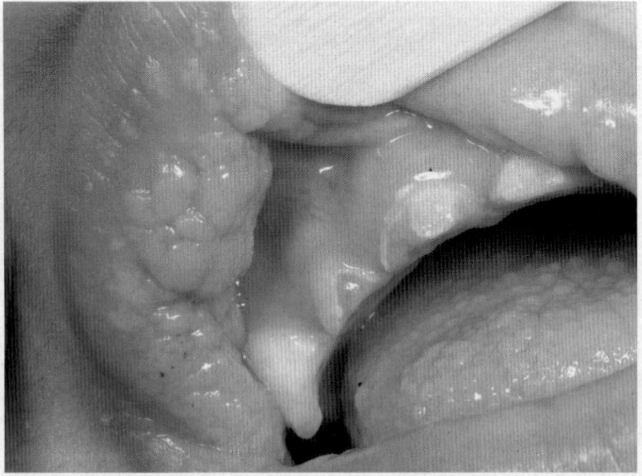

FIG. 155.4 Focal epithelial hyperplasia of the oral gingiva and mucosa (Heck disease). Patient was a 3-year-old Hispanic boy with a history of orthotopic liver transplantation and mild acute organ rejection who had an extensive eruption of painless, rounded, soft nodules present on the tongue, buccal mucosa, and gingivae. (Courtesy Dr. Federico Laham, Department of Pediatrics, Baylor College of Medicine and Texas Children's Hospital, Houston, TX.)

Cancer of the oral cavity and oropharynx often presents with delayed clinical signs. Clinical signs and symptoms can include persistent odynophagia, dysphagia, palpable or visible lump in throat or mouth, changes in voice, increased cough, and otalgia.[92] Most often, individuals have a nonhealing ulcer or sore.[15,295,356] Given the increasing prevalence of HPV-associated head and neck cancers, an adult with a later neck mass must be assumed to have an HPV-associated malignancy until proven otherwise.[128]

Interestingly, individuals with HPV-associated head and neck cancer have better clinical outcomes after therapy compared with those with HPV-negative head and neck cancers. This is likely due to a host of factors, including greater local-regional control of HPV-positive lesions and a higher intrinsic sensitivity of HPV-positive lesions to radiation and cisplatin therapies.[10] HPV-associated cancers are also found to have less cancer recurrence.[254] It is possible that identification of HPV in the oral cavity could serve as a biomarker for monitoring of early disease, disease progression and regression, tumor staging, and continued post-therapeutic surveillance.[221]

Anal Cancer

While anal cancers remain uncommon, the incidence of anal cancers is increasing at approximately 2% per year.[319] Importantly, there are groups with increased incidence of anal disease and cancer, particularly women with HPV-associated cervical disease, men who have sex with men, solid-organ transplant recipients, and individuals with concurrent HIV infection.[73,114,263]

Like the cervix, the anus has a squamocolumnar junction, and, like the cervix, it is this squamocolumnar junction that is most susceptible to HPV infection and is most prone to the development of dysplasia. HPV types 16 and 18 (and 31 less so) are most commonly associated with anal cancer. Even though anal warts are largely associated with HPV types 6 and 11, anal warts are still associated with invasive anal disease, perhaps because of their association with other sexual risk behaviors and predisposition to other, more oncogenic HPV types.[116,142,187,247,260]

Similar to all other intraepithelial lesions and cancers, the IN grading system is used, applying the term *anal intraepithelial lesion* (AIN) and a number (i.e., AIN 1 to 3) for classifying the severity of anal disease. Similar to other grade 1 lesions at other sites, AIN 1 is not considered a precancerous lesion. Higher grade lesions (AIN 2 or 3) can progress to invasive cancer.[66] AIN lesions are often warty and white but can be gray and/or pigmented. At the anal verge, lesions are often associated with epithelial stalks, each containing a single-looped capillary. Anal tags can have AIN and are often mistaken as hemorrhoids.

The age of anal cancer diagnosis in females is most often in the mid to late 60s. Women with related anogenital disease and intraepithelial neoplasia have a higher risk for developing anal cancer. Approximately 30% of women with VIN have involvement of the anal canal with AIN.[260] The average age at anal cancer diagnosis in males is the mid to late 50s.[260] In men who have sex with men, in particular, there is a high incidence and prevalence of anal disease and cancer found in both HIV-positive and HIV-negative individuals, with age-related prevalence approximately 60% across all age groups.[142] HIV-positive men who have sex with men are at highest risk for HPV infection and its sequelae.[150,362] Interestingly, despite the introduction of HAART, the incidence of HPV-associated anal disease and cancer in the HIV-positive men who have sex with men has continued to increase. It is postulated that because individuals are living longer on HAART, there is more time for slowly progressing AIN to develop into invasive disease, all the while with unchanged levels of surveillance for anal disease in this surviving population.[99,266,276]

LABORATORY DIAGNOSIS

Although most HPV infections are asymptomatic, the typical appearance of verrucae vulgaris on the skin and condylomata acuminata in the anogenital area in otherwise healthy individuals usually is sufficient to establish the clinical diagnosis of HPV infection. Laboratory confirmation of HPV-associated lesions may be necessary for unusual manifestations in healthy individuals, for immunocompromised patients, and for patients with suspected malignant lesions. Because HPVs cannot be grown in cell culture monolayers, a variety of molecular methods, used alone or in combination, are used in research and clinical settings.[392] Cytologic and histologic approaches also are helpful in diagnosing HPV-associated cancers.

Electron Microscopy

Although not used clinically, electron microscopy can be used to detect virions with typical papillomavirus morphology in cutaneous warts. Such virions are difficult to detect in tissue from patients with RRP, JORRP, genital warts, or in histologically diagnosed cancers.

Cell Culture

HPVs have not been propagated in cell culture monolayer. Therefore, the routine viral cultures available in most diagnostic virology laboratories will not detect the presence of HPVs.

Serology

HPV serologies are not used clinically and are not available in most diagnostic laboratories. Serologic methods have been used extensively in recent clinical trials of HPV vaccines; however, in natural infection, only 60% of women with proven genital HPV infections mount a detectable type-specific IgG response.*

Cytology

Since the 1960s, the Papanicolaou technique for obtaining and staining exfoliated cervical cells (i.e., the Pap smear) has been a procedure used widely as a screening method for detection of dysplastic and malignant cervical epithelial cells. Despite its relative insensitivity, the widespread and consistent use of the Pap smear has reduced dramatically the incidence of invasive squamous cell carcinoma of the cervix in nations with robust screening programs. Although screening guidelines vary by country and evolve constantly, cervical cytology screening is generally recommended at 1- to 3-year intervals for sexually active women. Current cervical cytology screening recommendations from the American College of Obstetrics and Gynecology are as follows:

- Screening should occur every 3 years between ages 21 and 29 years. HPV testing is not recommended.
- Women aged 30 to 65 years should have a Pap test and an HPV test (co-testing) every 5 years (preferred). It also is acceptable to have a Pap test alone every 3 years.
- Women who have a history of cervical cancer, are infected with HIV, have a weakened immune system, or who were exposed to diethylstilbestrol before birth may require more frequent screening and should not follow these routine guidelines.
- Having an HPV vaccination does not change screening recommendations. Women who have been vaccinated against HPV still need to follow the screening recommendations for their age group.
- Sexually active adolescents should be counseled and tested for sexually transmitted infections and counseled about safe sexual practices and about contraception.[164]

The operator characteristics of cervical Pap smear screening are dependent on the expertise of the physician who obtains the specimen and of the cytologist who performs the cytologic analysis.[233] Because most cervical neoplasias arise at the junction of the squamous and columnar epithelium of the cervix (transformation zone), care must be taken to obtain cells from this region. Substantial interobserver variability also occurs among cytologists who read Pap smears.[25]

The cytologic abnormalities identified on Pap smears reflect the cytopathic effects of HPV infection in cervical epithelial cells. The cytologic abnormality characteristic of HPV infection is koilocytosis (derived from the Greek word *koilos,* which means "hollow" or "cavity"). Koilocytotic cells display fat, swollen, wrinkled, or raisin-like nuclei surrounded by a halo, giving infected cells an owl's eye–like appearance. Other cytologic abnormalities—including dyskeratosis, parakeratosis, and hyperkeratosis—may occur but are considered secondary or nonspecific. In women screened by Pap smears consistently, the prevalence of cytologic abnormalities has been estimated at 2% to 3%.[158,314] Reflecting the spontaneous resolution rate of HPV infections, most cytologic abnormalities detected on Pap smears resolve spontaneously in 3 to 6 months. Nonetheless, cytologic abnormalities evolve in some patients, reflecting progression from infection through dysplasia to cervical squamous cell carcinoma. As HPV infection progresses to disease, the koilocytosis typically diminishes and the cervical epithelial cells begin to display dysplastic changes and nuclear abnormalities. While several Pap smear grading systems have been developed, the Bethesda system is used in the United States.[1] In the Bethesda system, the cytologic abnormalities seen on Pap smears are graded into four categories: (1) atypical squamous cells (this category is subdivided into atypical squamous cells of uncertain significance, ASC-US, and atypical squamous cells–cannot exclude high-grade squamous intraepithelial lesion, ASC-H); (2) low-grade squamous intraepithelial lesion; (3) HSIL; and (4) squamous cell carcinoma.[243,312]

Colposcopy

Evaluation by cervical colposcopy typically follows for women with abnormal Pap smears or external anogenital warts. Gynecologists, urologists, and family practitioners, as well as pediatricians who are specialists in adolescent medicine, usually perform the procedure. Briefly, the cervix, vulva, and anus in females or the urethral meatus, penis, scrotum, and anus in males are visualized under magnification with a colposcope to identify lesions, with special attention paid to their topography, the presence of abnormal whitening, and their vascular architecture. The area then is soaked in acetowhite (3–5% acetic acid) and reexamined for the presence of previously undetected lesions that appear as whitened plaques. Although whitening with acetowhite treatment is useful for detection of lesions, whitening after application of acetic acid is not specific for HPV infection or disease. Therefore, biopsy is required for definitive diagnosis. Tissue biopsy specimens are sent for histologic examination and for detection of HPV DNA by molecular techniques. Anal colposcopy, referred to as anoscopy, is similar to cervical colposcopy and is used to screen men and women at high risk for anal HPV infection.

Histology

HPV infection most often occurs in histologically normal tissue and is detectable only by molecular methods that detect viral DNA. Benign and asymptomatic HPV infection also may cause koilocytosis. Condylomata acuminata lesions display koilocytosis and other histopathologic characteristics of active HPV infection, such as hyperkeratosis, parakeratosis, acanthosis, and lengthening of the rete pegs. Atypical features, including mitotic figures above the basal layer, dysplastic cells, and single-cell keratinization, indicate higher grades of dysplasia. Precancerous and cancerous lesions of the cervix, vulva, vagina, penis, and anus also may be graded as low-grade or high-grade squamous intraepithelial lesions and invasive squamous cell carcinoma. In like manner, HPV-associated oral and oropharyngeal lesions are graded according to cellular atypia and invasion.

Molecular Methods That Detect Human Papillomavirus DNA

A nonradioactive, chemiluminescent liquid hybridization assay (hybrid capture assay) is commercially available and detects as many as 14 HPV types divided into high-risk (types 16, 18, 31, 33, 35, 45, 51, 52, 56) and low-risk (types 6, 11, 42, 43, 44) groups on the basis of association with cervical cancer.[209,211,311] This DNA hybrid capture assay is relatively rapid and simple to perform and is used typically as a reflex test to detect and classify (high-risk or low-risk) HPV DNA in abnormal cervical cytology specimens. Although this DNA hybridization/amplification method is in widespread clinical use, the laboratory and clinical use of other HPV DNA detection methods—including dot-blot, slot-blot, Southern blot, and in situ hybridization—have largely been supplanted by PCR.* Commercially available PCR-based assays capable of identifying

*References 14, 35, 54, 117, 118, 143, 156, 160, 194, 213, 297, 337, 389.

*References 58, 145, 152, 216, 249, 251, 267, 348, 374, 376, 390, 391.

and distinguishing 37 high- and low-risk mucosal HPV types are used in clinical trials but are not yet approved for diagnostic use in the United States.

More recently, a variety of PCR-based HPV detection methods have become available commercially (e.g., see http://www.mayomedicallaboratories.com/test-catalog/Clinical+and+Interpretive/62599). These tests are designed to detect broad arrays of oncogenic HPV types, and provide genotype identification. This is a rapidly evolving area of molecular diagnostics. While these methods are valuable for epidemiologic studies of HPV, and have proven very useful in vaccine clinical trials, how type-specific identification of HPVs assists in clinical management remains controversial.

In Situ Hybridization

In situ tissue DNA hybridization assays are performed directly on fresh or fixed tissue sections or on cytologic specimens. In situ assays offer the unique advantage of allowing the examiner to correlate histopathologic abnormalities with the location of HPV DNA. In situ assays may be performed with radioactive or enzyme-labeled probes. Commercial reagents and kits are available. Given the greater sensitivity and ease of detection, immunohistochemical detection of p16 antigen appears to be a sensitive and specific surrogate for tumor HPV positivity.[35,82,328]

TREATMENT

In healthy individuals, most HPV-associated lesions will regress spontaneously in 1 to 2 years. Treatment may be desirable if the lesions are large, multiple, or recurrent; if they cause pain or discomfort; or if they are undesirable cosmetically. Treatment is required if the lesions are life threatening, such as laryngeal papillomas that obstruct the airway, or lead to cervical cancer. A variety of treatment strategies are available, but none produces a universally effective or permanent cure. Rather, currently available approaches seek reduction of the clinically apparent lesion, and most require repetitive application. Clinically significant HPV-associated lesions also usually require care by a specialist. For example, a dermatologist should be consulted to assist in the management of a patient with severe recalcitrant cutaneous warts, a gynecologist for patients with cervical dysplasia, an oncologist for patients with cervical cancer, a colorectal surgeon for patients with anal dysplasia or carcinoma, an ophthalmologist for patients with conjunctival papillomas, and an otolaryngologist and pulmonologist for children and adults with severe RRP. The role of the infectious disease specialist in the management of HPV-associated disease is evolving and is principally to ensure that high-risk patients under their care (i.e., patients who are immunocompromised, posttransplant, HIV infected, or have had multiple sexually transmitted infections) are referred regularly for screening and treatment. Infectious disease physicians will become more directly involved in the care of HPV-associated diseases when HPV-specific antiviral chemotherapy becomes available for clinical trial and eventually for routine clinical use in patients.

Surgical techniques used to treat papillomas include traditional local excision, cryotherapy with liquid nitrogen or dry ice, electrocautery and curettage, and ultrasonication.[17,33,34,109,170,219,329] Newer ablative surgical techniques that use carbon dioxide laser vaporization and flash-lamp pulsed-dye laser therapy allow more precise and complete removal of visible papillomas and are becoming widely used to treat genital and laryngeal papillomas.[108,287,343] Surgical excision by knife remains the mainstay of HPV treatment, however, because excision provides tissue for a histopathologic diagnosis, as well as removal or debulking of large lesions. Ablation by cryotherapy with liquid nitrogen, electrocautery, or laser vaporization may be used to remove small, single, or multiple lesions or may be performed in combination with surgery for large or difficult lesions.[226,308,309] These surgical therapies also may release viral antigens, evoking a local and systemic immunologic response that may assist in eradicating the lesions. Disadvantages of these physical methods of wart and papilloma removal include pain, scarring, and disfigurement. These methods also are relatively invasive and impractical for patients with disseminated disease. Furthermore, recurrent treatments usually are necessary. In addition, laser vapors contain HPV DNA and may be a vehicle for spreading the infection in the patient or to the treating physician or surgeon; thus, the vapors or smoke plume should be contained.[129,307] Recurrence of lesions after treatment occurs commonly and most likely is due to the presence of HPV DNA sequences in clinically and histologically normal epithelium adjacent to and beyond the treatment area.[110] The mainstay of treatment for RRP and JORRP is repeated surgical debulking of obstructing papillomas augmented by immunomodulators and antiviral therapies.[141,155] Surgical rates tend to decrease over time in many patients; however, those patients infected with HPV type 11 may eventually require more frequent, more extensive, and more prolonged surgical procedures.[281,384]

Warts and papillomas also may be disrupted physically and removed by using chemical ablatives applied topically to the lesion. Simple organic acids such as bichloracetic acid, trichloracetic acid, or salicylic acid applied twice daily for several days have shown some success in the localized treatment of skin and genital warts.[120] They are caustic substances that produce a white slough that peels off, and they can be applied weekly until the lesion is destroyed.[120] Antimitotic agents such as podophyllin or the newer preparation podophyllotoxin can be applied twice daily for several weeks. Antimetabolites such as bleomycin, cantharidin, and 5-fluorouracil also have shown efficacy when administered locally once or twice a week because they inhibit the cellular proliferation induced by HPV infection.[182,274] These topical chemicals are easily applied to skin and genital warts but may cause local pain, redness, swelling, irritation, blisters, and scarring.[182] Moreover, antimetabolites are not virus specific, and recurrences are common. Antimetabolites are impractical for extensive lesions and may be toxic if used in certain circumstances. For example, they may damage the cornea if used to treat conjunctival papillomas. Antimetabolites should not be used on pregnant women.[226] The systemically administered antitumor agent methotrexate also has been administered to individual patients with disseminated HPV disease, with variable success.

Immunomodulation is another treatment strategy for HPV-associated disease. A systemic immunologic response probably is responsible for the spontaneous regression frequently observed in cutaneous and mucosal warts. Therefore, stimulation of the immune system with immunomodulators also may produce remission in patients with HPV-associated disease. Interferons have antiviral, antiproliferative, and immunomodulating properties. Decades of clinical experience have accrued in treating HPV-associated disease with interferon administered topically, intralesionally, or systemically by subcutaneous injection. Both lymphoblastoid and fibroblast interferon have been used with some success to treat patients with genital warts and respiratory papillomatosis topically, locally, and systemically.[103,115,122,155,286,315,320] However, interferon-γ has not been shown to be beneficial. Both recombinant and natural-source interferon-α preparations have been demonstrated in placebo-controlled trials to be effective and are approved by the US Food and Drug Administration (FDA) for the intralesional treatment of genital warts.[103,104] A 25- to 30-gauge needle is used to inject approximately 0.1 mL (1×10^6 units) at the base of up to five warts at a time for a total dose of 5×10^6 units at each visit. This dose is repeated two to three times weekly for 3 weeks. Maximal effect usually is seen within 4 to 8 weeks. Repeat injections may be given if the warts are persistent or recurrent. Interferon therapy also may be effective if used alone or in combination with laser surgery to treat patients with RRP.[152,156,195,205] Fever, headache, chills, and myalgia frequently occur with local and systemic interferon treatment. Severe and persistent fatigue, nausea, and leukopenia are other fairly common adverse reactions, especially with systemically administered interferon. Systemic natural leukocyte interferon also causes regression of warts and reduction of the virus load in tissues in patients with EV.[9] Cimetidine, an immunomodulator that alters lymphocyte function, has been used in an attempt to treat children with recalcitrant cutaneous warts.[253]

Topical immunotherapeutic agents provide alternative treatment options for HPV-associated disease in some patients.[130,132,178,227,320] Imiquimod, also known as imidazoquinoline, is a first-generation member of a class of immune response modifiers approved for topical treatment of genital and perianal warts.[130,132,178,227] Imiquimod is a synthetic compound that is a topically active Toll-like receptor–7 agonist. It activates innate immune cells to produce interferon-α and other cytokines to enhance antigen presentation and promote antigen-specific T-helper type 1 cell-mediated immune responses. Imiquimod is marketed as a 5% cream that is applied to lesions and appears to be effective in some patients. Resiquimod and other related second-generation imidazoquinoline analogs also are in clinical development.

Retinoids and retinoic acid, which are analogs of vitamin A, can regulate the growth and differentiation of malignant, premalignant, and even normal cells.[5,288] Clinically, retinoids have a documented effect against squamous cell carcinoma.[198,199] For these reasons, anecdotal reports and small series of patients have emerged in which retinoic acid was used to treat HPV-associated disease, especially RRP. In these reports, retinoids were used with varying success, primarily as adjuvant agents with surgical therapy, to treat adult patients with severe refractory RRP.[20,101] The combination of interferon and retinoic acid has been shown to be synergistic against breast cancer cells in vitro and potentially may be useful in refractory cases of RRP.[220]

Unique aspects of HPV infection and disease render designing specific antiviral therapies a challenge. For example, HPV disease usually is focal, viral replication is tied intricately to the host cell's life cycle, and HPV has great diversity with more than 70 genotypes. The inability to grow HPVs readily in cell culture also hampers our ability to study the antiviral properties and cellular toxicities of candidate compounds. Molecular assays that isolate individual viral functions, therefore, have been used to evaluate the ability of antiviral compounds to inhibit each individual step in the virus life cycle. Furthermore, animal models for HPV-associated disease are lacking. Despite these challenges, the in vitro antiviral activity and clinical efficacy of a variety of compounds have been studied. Ribavirin, a purine nucleoside analog with a broad antiviral spectrum, has been used in clinical trials for the treatment of laryngeal papillomatosis.[224] As noted before, cidofovir, an antiviral compound effective against serious disease caused by cytomegalovirus, also appears to have activity against HPVs, and possible clinical benefit for certain HPV-associated disease has been shown. For example, repeated intralesional administration of cidofovir directly into the site of papillomas and also submucosally at the sites of resected papillomas is associated with partial or complete regression of lesions, improvement of voice quality and airway status, and decreased need for repeat surgery. Published studies report a wide variety of intralesional doses (2–57 mg of a 5 mg/mL cidofovir concentration solution), frequency of injections (every 2–8 weeks), and duration of treatment (4 months to 4 years). Rarely, cidofovir has been administered intravenously in patients with refractory, disseminated papillomatosis.[155] The greatest benefits have most often been documented after the fourth series of injections, and benefit appears to plateau after the eighth series of injections in most patients.[67,70,96,125,151,215,323,324] However, because most published reports are single-center, uncontrolled case series with relatively small numbers of patients, controlled, multicenter trials with larger numbers of patients are necessary to accurately determine the benefits of cidofovir therapy and the optimal dose, frequency, and duration of therapy for RRP and JORRP.[354]

PREVENTION

Secondary prevention by cytologic screening remains an essential component of cancer prevention programs. Historically, screening practices for HPV-associated diseases have focused on cervical cytology. Today, most cases of invasive cervical cancer are preventable with regular screening for precancerous lesions (e.g., by Pap smear) and close follow-up of abnormal results. As mentioned earlier, cervical cytology screening is a continuously evolving process, with the largest changes to the most recent recommendations advocating for screening starting at age 21 years.[3,13,164]

Data analyses from the National Health Interview Survey find overall cervical cancer screening rates of just over 80%, with lower rates among Asian, American Indian/Alaska Native, Hispanic, and foreign-born women. Higher rates of cervical cancer seen among black and Hispanic women are likely multifactorial but are, in large part, related to reduced access to screening and/or follow-up care. In these same disproportionately affected ethnic groups, the disparity of HPV and cancer rates will likely continue to grow if these groups are undervaccinated.[99,266]

Anal cancer shares many similarities with cervical cancer. As such, more aggressive screening (similar to cervical cancer screening) is needed to decrease its incidence.[261] Anal cytology serves as the primary screen and is described according to the Bethesda system for cervical cytology (normal, atypical squamous cells of undetermined significance, low-grade squamous intraepithelial lesion, HSIL, and atypical squamous cells, cannot rule out HSIL).[121] Individuals with anal cytologic abnormalities should be referred for high-resolution anoscopy (HRA) with biopsy. HRA is similar to cervical colposcopy and can be done in the ambulatory setting. The utility of HRA is highly dependent on the expertise and proficiency of the operator. An anoscope is inserted and a colposcope is used for visualization of the squamocolumnar junction, the distal anal canal, and the anal margin. Acetic acid and Lugol's iodine are applied to the mucosa and biopsies are obtained from abnormal sites.[121,261] HRA, similarly to colposcopy, can be used in conjunction with ablative therapies for treatment of HPV-associated anal dysplasias. Anal histology is graded based on mucosal dysplasia: mild dysplasia is graded as anal intraepithelial neoplasia I (AIN I; low-grade dysplasia) and moderate dysplasia is graded as anal intraepithelial neoplasia II or III (AIN II or III; high-grade dysplasia).[121]

Quadrivalent HPV Vaccine

In June 2006, the FDA approved the first vaccine to prevent HPV-associated dysplasias and malignancies. This quadrivalent recombinant vaccine against serotypes 6, 11, 16, and 18, given as a series of three 0.5-mL intramuscular injections at 0, 2, and 6 months, is now approved for females and males ages 9 through 26 years old. The vaccine, prepared using purified viruslike particles (VLPs) of the capsid (L1) protein of HPV types 6, 11, 16, and 18, stimulates humoral and cellular immune responses to HPV L1 capsid proteins.

The quadrivalent HPV vaccine is indicated for prevention of the following HPV-associated diseases *due to vaccine types* in females:

- Cervical, vulvar, vaginal, and anal cancer
- Genital warts
- CIN grades 1/2/3 and cervical adenocarcinoma in situ (AIS)
- VIN grades 2/3
- VaIN grades 2/3
- AIN grades 1/2/3

The quadrivalent HPV vaccine is indicated for the prevention of the following HPV-associated diseases *due to vaccine types* in males:

- Anal cancer
- Genital warts
- AIN grades 1/2/3

Quadrivalent HPV Vaccine Efficacy

Quadrivalent HPV vaccine efficacy has been assessed in six double-blinded, randomized controlled trials, together evaluating over 28,000 males and females ages 16 through 26 years. Among these trials, the FUTURE I/II trials of vaccine efficacy and safety provided most of the efficacy and safety data submitted to support vaccine licensure.[14,117,118,174,217]

Females. Primary analysis of efficacy regarding HPV types 6, 11, 16, and 18 were conducted in the per protocol efficacy (PPE) population, which consisted of women ages 16 through 26 years, who were HPV naïve to the relevant strains 1 month before the first dose, remained negative until 1 month after the third dose, received all three doses within 1 year, and had no protocol violations. Detection of CIN grades 2/3, AIS, VIN grades 2/3, and VaIN grades 2/3 were the efficacy endpoints to assess prevention of cervical, vulvar, and vaginal cancer. Presence of external genital lesions was the efficacy endpoint to assess prevention of genital warts. Anal disease and anal cancer were not endpoints in the female studies.

In combined analysis from all clinical trials, efficacy was 98%, 100%, and 100% against HPV type 16 or type 18–related CIN grades 2/3 + AIS, VIN grades 2/3, and VaIN grades 2/3, respectively. By HPV type, vaccine prevented 98% of HPV type 16–related lesions and 100% of HPV type 18–related lesions. The vaccine prevented 99% of anogenital condyloma infections related to HPV types 6, 11, 16, and 18.[46,48]

Secondary analysis approximated the impact on the general population of young American females. This intention-to-treat analysis looked at vaccine efficacy in those receiving at least one dose of the vaccine in both HPV-naïve females and females regardless of HPV status. Females who were HPV naïve at day 1 were found to have reduction of genital warts, CIN grades 2/3 + AIS, and VIN + VaIN grades 2/3 by 83%, 43%, and 77%, respectively. Females regardless of HPV status were found to have reduction of genital warts, CIN grades 2/3 + AIS, and VIN + VaIN grades 2/3 by 63%, 18%, and 51%, respectively.[14,22,117,118,126,362]

Males. To assess the efficacy of the quadrivalent vaccine for the prevention of genital warts in males, primary analysis of efficacy against disease due to HPV types 6, 11, 16, and 18 was conducted in the per protocol efficacy population, which consisted of males ages 16 through 26 years who were HPV naïve to the relevant strains 1 month before the first dose, remained negative until 1 month after the third dose, received all three doses within 1 year, and had no protocol violations. Presence of external genital warts and penile/perineal/perianal intraepithelial neoplasia (PIN) grades 1/2/3 were the efficacy endpoints to assess prevention of penile/perineal/perianal cancers. Vaccine efficacy for prevention of anal disease was assessed in a substudy population of men who have sex with men derived from the larger per protocol efficacy male population.

In combined analyses from all clinical trials, quadrivalent vaccine efficacy was 100% and 78% for prevention of HPV types 6, 11, 16, and 18-related PIN grades 1/2/3 and AIN grades 1/2/3, respectively. The quadrivalent vaccine prevented 90% of anogenital condylomas related to HPV types 6, 11, 16, and 18.[138]

Secondary analysis approximated the impact on the general population of young American males. This intention-to-treat analysis assessed vaccine efficacy in men receiving at least one dose of the vaccine in both HPV-naïve males and males regardless of HPV status. Males who were HPV naïve at day 1 were found to have reduction of external genital lesions, genital warts, PIN grades 1/2/3, and AIN grades by 76%, 80%, 21%, and 77%, respectively. Males, regardless of HPV status, were found to have reduction of external genital lesions, genital warts, PIN grades 1/2/3, and AIN grades 1/2/3 by 67%, 68%, 0.3%, and 50%, respectively.

Bivalent HPV Vaccine

In 2009, 3 years after FDA approval of the quadrivalent HPV vaccine, the FDA licensed a second vaccine to prevent HPV-associated diseases due to HPV types 16 and 18. The bivalent vaccine is an HPV-16/18 VLP-based, AS04-adjuvanted vaccine given as a series of three 0.5-mL intramuscular injections given at 0, 1, and 6 months. The bivalent vaccine is FDA approved for use in girls and young women aged 9 through 25 years. The vaccine is prepared by combining adsorbed VLPs (L1 proteins) of HPV types 16 and 18 together with a novel AS04 adjuvant system (3-*O*-decasyl-4′-monophosphoryl lipid A [MPL] adsorbed onto aluminum) in sodium chloride, sodium dihydrogen phosphate dihydrate, and water to stimulate a humoral immune response (IgGs against HPV-L1 capsid proteins).[60]

The vaccine is used for prevention of the following HPV-associated diseases *due to vaccine type* HPVs in females:

- Cervical cancer
- CIN grades 1/2/3 and AIS

Bivalent Vaccine Efficacy

The efficacy of the bivalent vaccine was assessed in two double-blinded, randomized controlled trials, together evaluating over 19,000 young women aged 15 to 25 years, most notably the PATRICIA (PApilloma TRIal against Cancer In young Adults) trial of vaccine efficacy for both according to protocol (ATP) and total vaccinated cohort (TVC) populations.[154,194] Presence of CIN grades 1/2/3 or AIS served as efficacy endpoints to assess prevention of cervical cancer. Persistence of infection past 12 months served as the virologic endpoint.

Primary analysis included an ATP population, or HPV-naïve population, consisting of women ages 15 through 25 years who received all three vaccine doses, who were HPV naïve to HPV-16 and HPV-18 at baseline and at 6 months, and for whom all efficacy measures were available. Vaccine efficacy for the prevention of HPV type 16– or 18–related CIN grades 2/3 or AIS and CIN grades 1/2/3 or AIS was 93% and 92%, respectively. Also within the ATP cohort, the vaccine reduced persistence of infection at 12 months by 91%.[154,194]

Further analysis included HPV-naïve and nonnaïve females (those with current infection and/or previous exposure) and the TVC, including females who received at least one vaccine dose, for whom all efficacy measures were available, regardless of HPV status. Females who were HPV naïve (negative for 14 oncogenic HPV types 6, 18, 31, 33, 35, 39, 45, 51, 52, 56, 58, 59, 66, and 68) at day 1 were found to have vaccine efficacy for CIN grades 1/2/3 or AIS, CIN grades 2/3 or AIS, and CIN grade 3 or AIS of 97%, 98%, 100%, respectively. Females regardless of vaccine-type HPV status were found to have vaccine efficacy for CIN grades 1/2/3 or AIS, CIN grades 2/3 or AIS, and CIN grade 3 or AIS of 56%, 53% and 34%, respectively. Females regardless of all-type (vaccine + nonvaccine) HPV status were found to have vaccine efficacy for CIN grades 1/2/3 or AIS, CIN grades 2/3 or AIS, and CIN grade 3 or AIS of 22%, 30%, and 33%, respectively.[154,194]

9-Valent Vaccine

To increase the scope of protection against the range of oncogenic mucosal HPV types, a 9-valent L1 vaccine has been produced by the manufacturer of the quadrivalent vaccine.[242,277]

The 9-valent HPV vaccine contains the same L1 virus-like particles as the quadrivalent vaccine (based on HPV types 6, 11, 16, and 18) plus L1 virus-like particles based on HPVs types 31, 33, 45, 52, and 58. In clinical trials, the efficacy of the 9-valent HPV vaccine for prevention of the combined endpoint of HPV 31-, 33-, 45-, 52-, and 58-related CIN2/3, AIS, cervical cancer, VIN2/3, VaIN2/3, vulvar cancer and vaginal cancer was 96.7%.[127] In many regions, including North America and Europe, use of the 9-valent vaccine is now supplanting use of the bivalent and quadrivalent vaccines.

Two-Dose HPV Vaccination Regimens

While the initial licensure trials of the bivalent, quadrivalent, and 9-valent HPV vaccines all used 3-dose immunization regimens, immunogenicity studies of all 3 vaccines suggest that a 2-dose regimen, with the first and second dose administered 6 months apart, induces a noninferior antibody response to all vaccine antigens.[93,192,335]

The possibility of an effective 2-dose HPV vaccination regimen improves the prospects for widespread HPV vaccine use in the low- and middle-income countries. It should be noted, however, that licensure of HPV vaccines has been based on proven efficacy for prevention of HPV-associated diseases. To date, the rationale for 2-dose vaccine regimens is based solely on immunogenicity noninferiority; vaccine efficacy data are not yet available. As such, widespread implementation of two-dose vaccine regimes warrants some degree of caution.[95]

Population Effectiveness of HPV Vaccines

Data from several national vaccination programs suggest that widespread HPV immunization leads to substantial reductions in the prevalence of genital warts and in the prevalence of HPV infection. For examples, see Canvin et al.[52] and Markowitz et al.[218]

HPV vaccines also appear to induce substantial herd immunity, conferring protection to nonimmunized population members.[97]

HPV Vaccine Safety

From the perspective of vaccine safety, HPV vaccines stand as some of the most widely studied vaccines in history. While there have been substantial concerns about HPV vaccine safety expressed on the Internet and in the lay press, large, well-designed postmarketing vaccine safety surveillance studies of HPV vaccine safety have confirmed findings of the vaccine licensure trials; most HPV vaccine-associated adverse events are at the immunization site and are predominantly pain, swelling, and erythema.[127,60] Postlicensure studies have shown that syncope and possibly skin infections are associated with HPV vaccination. Surveillance for serious adverse events—such as adverse pregnancy outcomes, autoimmune diseases (including Guillain-Barré syndrome and multiple sclerosis), anaphylaxis, venous thromboembolism, and stroke—were extensively studied and have shown no increase in the incidence of these events compared with background rates.[11,134,206,208,341,373]

HPV Vaccine Immunogenicity in Immunocompromised Patients

Studies of HPV vaccine immunogenicity in immunocompromised hosts have demonstrated a very slightly lower rate of seroconversion in comparison to immunocompetent patients. However, antibody response in immunocompromised patients is still robust. A number of studies have been published in the HIV-positive population. In children 7 to 12 years of age, 97% to 100% seroconversion was observed in children vaccinated with the quadrivalent vaccine.[196] However, a decrease in titers 72 weeks following administration of the last vaccine (>76% antibody seropositivity persisted) was noted in another study, raising the question that perhaps booster doses may be beneficial in this population.[382] In HIV-positive men, greater than 95% seroconversion of all 4 vaccine types occurred with administration of the quadrivalent vaccine (this study population had a median CD4 count of 517; 97% had a viral load less than 10,000 copies per mL).[386] Recently, Faust[106] demonstrated a 100% seroconversion in HIV-positive subjects following administration of a bivalent HPV vaccine. In comparison, vaccination with a quadrivalent vaccine led to 95% to 100% seroconversion of types 6, 11, and 16 and 73% seroconversion of type 18.[106] Studies in other immunocompromised populations are scant. Results show a lesser response to vaccine; nonetheless, seroconversion was demonstrated. In patients with systemic lupus erythematosus, vaccination with quadrivalent HPV vaccine showed a 76% seroconversion rate.[228] In adult solid-organ transplant patients, 52.6% to 68.4% seroconversion was noted depending on HPV type (only 47% had evidence of seroconversion to all 4 types).[186] Most studies noted lower antibody titers in immunocompromised subjects than in immunocompetent hosts, though it remains unclear if antibody concentration is clinically significant. More studies of HPV vaccine immunogenicity and effectiveness in immunocompromised patients are needed.

Vaccine Limitations

With widespread use, HPV vaccines offer the exciting prospects of substantial reductions in HPV-associated morbidity and mortality. However, as with other vaccines, quadrivalent and bivalent HPV vaccines have specific limitations. It is important to consider the following limitations when giving these vaccines:

- HPV pseudovirion-based vaccines do not eliminate the need for continued routine cervical and anal cancer screening.
- HPV vaccines do not provide protection against or change the natural history of established infections due to vaccine and nonvaccine HPV types. Although, interestingly, while virus-like, particle-based HPV vaccines are considered preventive (as opposed to therapeutic), previous quadrivalent HPV vaccination of women who had surgical treatment for HPV-related disease significantly reduced the incidence of subsequent HPV-related disease, including high-grade disease.[173]
- The vaccines are not intended to treat active external genital lesions; any intraepithelial lesion type; or cervical, vulvar, vaginal, and anal cancers.

Although most HPV-associated head and neck malignancies are attributable to HPV type 16 and 18 infections, there are currently no data demonstrating that HPV immunization impacts the incidence or course of HPV-associated head and neck malignancies. Similarly, although it is anticipated that HPV immunization with the quadrivalent vaccine will reduce the incidence of HPV type 6– and HPV type 11–associated laryngeal papillomatosis, there are no data indicating that the quadrivalent vaccine will prevent or alter the clinical course of laryngeal papillomatosis at this time.

The overall personal and public health and economic benefits of vaccination have been well demonstrated in both males and females.[65,102,181] The importance of both male and female prevention efforts resides in the fact that not only is there disease burden in women and men alone but there is also significant opportunity for transmission and infection of the other, potentially leading to significant morbidity and mortality (e.g., as evidenced by the increased frequency of CIN in females with partners with penile lesions).[77,140,149,163,175,334,365]

Vaccine benefits vary according to the population immunized. In populations that are provided regular cervical cytology screening, HPV immunization serves largely to prevent high-grade dysplasia and to reduce the economic and emotional costs associated with treatment of premalignant disease. In resource-poor populations that are unscreened, HPV vaccines benefit by preventing cervical cancer and its associated economic and emotional expenses.[77,83]

Based on trends in sexual behaviors, age of sexual debut, knowledge that acquisition of HPV infection occurs within first few years of sexual debut, and the fact that vaccination is most efficacious in HPV-naïve individuals, initiating vaccination prior to any sexual contact (vaginal, anal, oral, digital) will prevent the most infections and their sequelae.[27] It becomes the responsibility of any primary care provider of children, adolescents, and young adults to discuss HPV infection with both patients and their caregivers and to offer vaccination to patients as early as possible to prevent as much disease as possible.[81]

NEW REFERENCES SINCE THE SEVENTH EDITION

4. Agalliu I, Gapstur S, Chen Z, et al. Associations of oral α-, β-, and γ-human papillomavirus types with risk of incident head and neck cancer. *JAMA Oncol.* 2016 Jan 21. [Epub ahead of print].
6. Alemany L, Saunier M, Alvarado-Cabrero I, et al.; HPV VVAP Study Group. Human papillomavirus DNA prevalence and type distribution in anal carcinomas worldwide. *Int J Cancer.* 2015;136(1):98-107.
7. Alemany L, Saunier M, Tinoco L, et al.; HPV VVAP study group. Large contribution of human papillomavirus in vaginal neoplastic lesions: a worldwide study in 597 samples. *Eur J Cancer.* 2014;50(16):2846-2854.
11. Angelo MG, Zima J, Tavares Da Silva F, et al. Post-licensure safety surveillance for human papillomavirus-16/18-AS04-adjuvanted vaccine: more than 4 years of experience. *Pharmacoepidemiol Drug Saf.* 2014;23(5):456-465.
44. Brickman C, Palefsky JM. Human papillomavirus in the HIV-infected host: epidemiology and pathogenesis in the antiretroviral era. *Curr HIV/AIDS Rep.* 2015;12:6-15.
52. Canvin M, Sinka K, Hughes G, et al. Decline in genital warts diagnoses among young women and young men since the introduction of the bivalent HPV (16/18) vaccination programme in England: an ecological analysis. *Sex Transm Infect.* 2016 Jun 30. [Epub ahead of print].
60. Cervarix [package insert]. Rixensart, Belgium: GlaxoSmithKline Biologicals; 2016.
63. Chaturvedi AK, Engels EA, Pfeiffer RM, et al. Human papillomavirus and rising oropharyngeal cancer incidence in the United States. *J Clin Oncol.* 2011;29(32):4294-4301.
89. de Sanjosé S, Alemany L, Ordi J, et al.; HPV VVAP study group. Worldwide human papillomavirus genotype attribution in over 2000 cases of intraepithelial and invasive lesions of the vulva. *Eur J Cancer.* 2013;49(16):3450-3461.
90. de Sanjose S, Quint WG, Alemany L, et al.; Retrospective International Survey and HPV Time Trends Study Group. Human papillomavirus genotype attribution in invasive cervical cancer: a retrospective cross-sectional worldwide study. *Lancet Oncol.* 2010;11(11):1048-1056.
93. Dobson SR, McNeil S, Dionne M, et al. Immunogenicity of 2 doses of HPV vaccine in younger adolescents vs 3 doses in young women: a randomized clinical trial. *JAMA.* 2013;309(17):1793-1802.
94. Doerfler D, Bernhaus A, Kottmel A, et al. Human papilloma virus infection prior to coitarche. *Am J Obstet Gynecol.* 2009;200(5):487.e1-487.e5.
95. Donken R, Knol MJ, Bogaards JA, et al. Inconclusive evidence for non-inferior immunogenicity of two- compared with three-dose HPV immunization schedules in preadolescent girls: a systematic review and meta-analysis. *J Infect.* 2015;71(1):61-73.
97. Drolet M, Bénard É, Boily MC, et al. Population-level impact and herd effects following human papillomavirus vaccination programmes: a systematic review and meta-analysis. *Lancet Infect Dis.* 2015;15(5):565-580.
106. Faust H, Toft L, Sehr P, et al. Human papillomavirus neutralizing and cross-reactive antibodies induced in HIV-positive subjects after vaccination with quadrivalent and bivalent HPV vaccines. *Vaccine.* 2016;34:1559-1565.
112. Forman D, de Martel C, Lacey CJ, et al. Global burden of human papillomavirus and related diseases. *Vaccine.* 2012;30(suppl 5):F12-F23.
121. Gaisa MM, Goldstone SE. Diagnosis and treatment of anal intraepithelial neoplasia and condylomata. *Semin Colon Rectal Surg.* 2011;22(1):21-29.
123. Gallagher TQ, Derkay CS. Recurrent respiratory papillomatosis: update 2008. *Curr Opin Otolaryngol Head Neck Surg.* 2008;16:536-542.
127. Gardasil 9 [package insert]. Whitehouse Station, NJ: Merck & Co., Inc.; 2014.
128. Garden AS, Gunn GB, Hessel A, et al. Management of the lymph node-positive neck in the patient with human papillomavirus-associated oropharyngeal cancer. *Cancer.* 2014;120(19):3082-3088.
131. Garland SM, Steben M, Sings HL, et al. Natural history of genital warts: analysis of the placebo arm of 2 randomized phase III trials of a quadrivalent human papillomavirus (types 6, 11, 16, and 18) vaccine. *J Infect Dis.* 2009;199(6):805-814.

134. Gee J, Weinbaum C, Sukumaran L, Markowitz LE. Quadrivalent HPV vaccine safety review and safety monitoring plans for nine-valent HPV vaccine in the United States. *Hum Vaccin Immunother*. 2016;12(6):1406-1417.
144. Guan P, Howell-Jones R, Li N, et al. Human papillomavirus types in 115,789 HPV-positive women: a meta-analysis from cervical infection to cancer. *Int J Cancer*. 2012;131(10):2349-2359.
162. Houlihan CF, de Sanjosé S, Baisley K, et al. Prevalence of human papillomavirus in adolescent girls before reported sexual debut. *J Infect Dis*. 2014;210(6):837-845.
172. Joura EA, Ault KA, Bosch FX, et al. Attribution of 12 high-risk human papillomavirus genotypes to infection and cervical disease. *Cancer Epidemiol Biomarkers Prev*. 2014;23(10):1997-2008.
173. Joura EA, Garland SM, Paavonen J, et al.; FUTURE I and II Study Group. Effect of the human papillomavirus (HPV) quadrivalent vaccine in a subgroup of women with cervical and vulvar disease: retrospective pooled analysis of trial data. *BMJ*. 2012;344:e1401.
186. Kumar D, Unger E, Panicker G, et al. Immunogenicity of quadrivalent human papillomavirus vaccine in organ transplant recipients. *Am J Transplant*. 2013;13(9):2411-2417.
189. Lacey CJ, Lowndes CM, Shah KV. Chapter 4: Burden and management of non-cancerous HPV-related conditions: HPV-6/11 disease. *Vaccine*. 2006;24(suppl 3):S3/35-S3/41.
192. Lazcano-Ponce E, Stanley M, Muñoz N, et al. Overcoming barriers to HPV vaccination: non-inferiority of antibody response to human papillomavirus 16/18 vaccine in adolescents vaccinated with a two-dose vs. a three-dose schedule at 21 months. *Vaccine*. 2014;32(6):725-732.
196. Levin MJ, Moscicki AB, Song LY, et al.; IMPAACT P1047 Protocol Team. Safety and immunogenicity of a quadrivalent human papillomavirus (types 6, 11, 16, and 18) vaccine in HIV-infected children 7 to 12 years old. *J Acquir Immune Defic Syndr*. 2010;55(2):197-204.
206. Macartney KK, Chiu C, Georgousakis M, et al. Safety of human papillomavirus vaccines: a review. *Drug Saf*. 2013;36(6):393-412.
208. Mahajan D, Dey A, Cook J, et al. Surveillance of adverse events following immunisation in Australia annual report, 2013. *Commun Dis Intell Q Rep*. 2015;39(3):E369-E386.
218. Markowitz LE, Liu G, Hariri S, et al. Prevalence of HPV after introduction of the vaccination program in the United States. *Pediatrics*. 2016;137(3):e20151968.
228. Mok CC, Ho LY, Fong LS. Immunogenicity and safety of quadrivalent human papillomavirus vaccine in patients with systemic lupus erythematosus: a case-control study. *Ann Rheum Dis*. 2013;72(5):659-664.
244. Ndiaye C, Mena M, Alemany L, et al. HPV DNA, E6/E7 mRNA, and p16INK4a detection in head and neck cancers: a systematic review and meta-analysis. *Lancet Oncol*. 2014;15(12):1319-1331.
259. Palefsky J. Human papillomavirus-related disease in people with HIV. *Curr Opin HIV AIDS*. 2009;4(1):52-56.
261. Palefsky JM. Practising high-resolution anoscopy. *Sex Health*. 2012;9:580-586.
277. Pils S, Joura EA. From the monovalent to the nine-valent HPV vaccine. *Clin Microbiol Infect*. 2015;21(9):827-833.
290. Reusser NM, Downing C, Guidry J, et al. HPV carcinomas in immunocompromised patients. *J Clin Med*. 2015;4(2):260-281.
296. Rogstad KE, Wilkinson D, Robinson A. Sexually transmitted infections in children as a marker of child sexual abuse and direction of future research. *Curr Opin Infect Dis*. 2016;29:41-44.
305. Sano D, Oridate N. The molecular mechanism of human papillomavirus-induced carcinogenesis in head and neck squamous cell carcinoma. *Int J Clin Oncol*. 2016. [Epub ahead of print].
319. SEER Stat Fact Sheets: Anal Cancer. http://seer.cancer.gov/statfacts/html/anus.html. Accessed 29 April 2017.
326. Shew ML, Weaver B, Tu W, et al. High frequency of human papillomavirus detection in the vagina before first vaginal intercourse among females enrolled in a longitudinal study cohort. *J Infect Dis*. 2013;207(6):1012-1015.
327. Sinclair KA, Woods CR, et al. Anogenital and respiratory tract human papillomavirus infections among children: age, gender, and potential transmission through sexual abuse. *Pediatrics*. 2005;116(4):815-825.
335. Stanley MA, Sudenga SL, Giuliano AR. Alternative dosage schedules with HPV virus-like particle vaccines. *Expert Rev Vaccines*. 2014;13(8):1027-1038.
341. Stillo M, Carrillo Santisteve P, Lopalco PL. Safety of human papillomavirus vaccines: a review. *Expert Opin Drug Saf*. 2015;14(5):697-712.
358. Tulay P, Serakinci N. The route to HPV-associated neoplastic transformation: a review of the literature. *Crit Rev Eukaryot Gene Expr*. 2016;26(1):27-39.
360. U.S. Department of Health & Human Services, Administration for Children and Families, Administration on Children, Youth and Families, Children's Bureau; 2014. http://www.acf.hhs.gov/programs/cb/research-data-technology/statistics-research/child-maltreatment. Accessed 29 April 2017.
361. U.S. Department of Health and Human Services, C. f.; 2015. United States Cancer Statistics: 1999–2013 Incidence and Mortality Web-based Report. www.cdc.gov/uscs. Accessed 6 July 2016.
363. Unger ER, Fajman NN, Maloney EM, et al. Anogenital human papillomavirus in sexually abused and nonabused children: a multicenter study. *Pediatrics*. 2011;128(3):e658-e665.
373. Vichnin M, Bonanni P, Klein NP, et al. An overview of quadrivalent human papillomavirus vaccine safety: 2006 to 2015. *Pediatr Infect Dis J*. 2015;34(9):983-991.
379. Wallace NA, Galloway DA. Novel functions of the human papillomavirus E6 oncoproteins. *Annu Rev Virol*. 2015;2(1):403-423.
382. Weinberg A, Song LY, Saah A, et al.; IMPAACT/PACTG P1047 Team. Humoral, mucosal, and cell-mediated immunity against vaccine and nonvaccine genotypes after administration of quadrivalent human papillomavirus vaccine to HIV-infected children. *J Infect Dis*. 2015;206:1309-1318.
385. Wilcox LJ, Hull BP, Baldassari CM, et al. Diagnosis and management of recurrent respiratory papillomatosis. *Pediatr Infect Dis J*. 2014;33(12):1283-1284.
386. Wilkin T, Lee JY, Lensing SY, et al. Safety and immunogenicity of the quadrivalent human papillomavirus vaccine in HIV-1 infected men. *J Infect Dis*. 2010;202(8):1246-1253.

The full reference list for this chapter is available at ExpertConsult.com.

SUBSECTION III DNA—*Adenoviridae*

156 Adenoviruses

Tempe K. Chen • James D. Cherry

Adenoviruses, which are responsible for a varied array of illnesses in children,* are associated most commonly with respiratory illness and gastroenteritis, but cardiac, neurologic, cutaneous, urinary, and lymphatic manifestations also occur frequently. Although many of the clinical manifestations of adenoviral infections are distinctive, the specific viral etiologic agent rarely is recognized by physicians.

Adenoviruses were noted first in explant cultures of human adenoid tissue; this finding, plus the observation of their apparent general affinity for lymphatic tissue, led to the designation of their name.[178,186,214,585]

*References 2, 3, 70, 72, 107, 176, 214, 308, 315, 392, 574, 589, 621, 673.

HISTORY

The first adenoviral strains were not isolated until 1953, when tissue culture techniques became available, although epidemic disease caused by adenoviruses had been observed throughout the first half of the 20th century. Epidemic keratoconjunctivitis first was noted and reported in Austria by several physicians in 1889.[4,220,563,599,632] Major outbreaks of epidemic keratoconjunctivitis were reported in Bombay in 1901, in Madras in 1920 and 1928, in Hawaii in 1941, and on the West Coast of the United States in 1942.[290,311,312,378,727]

Epidemics of illness such as pharyngoconjunctival fever were observed throughout the 20th century. Béal[37] in 1907 was the first to report the syndrome; in the 1920s, epidemics associated with swimming in public pools and in lakes were noted in Germany and the United States.[30,523] Initial studies by Rowe and colleagues[585] revealed cytopathic changes in explant tissue cultures of human adenoids that had been removed surgically. Fluid from these cultures caused distinctive cytopathologic changes in other tissue cultures, and antiserum prepared in hyperimmunized rabbits neutralized the effect. In 1954, Hilleman and Werner[305] isolated similar cytopathic agents from the throat washings of military recruits with febrile acute respiratory disease. Shortly thereafter, epidemic keratoconjunctivitis and pharyngocon junctival fever were seen to be illnesses of adenoviral etiology.[139,142–144,335]

Initially, adenoviruses were known by the following names: adenoid degeneration (AD) agent because of its recovery in human adenoid tissue explants[585]; respiratory illness patient number 67 (RI-67) agent, which was recovered from a military recruit with primary atypical pneumonia during an epidemic of acute respiratory disease[304,305]; adenoidal-pharyngeal-conjunctival (APC) agent[321]; and acute respiratory disease (ARD) agent.[122] In 1956, investigators in the field selected the term *adenovirus* for the new group of viruses. The name suggested the characteristic involvement of lymphadenoid tissue, as well as the tissue from which the organism was first isolated.[178]

Because of considerable morbidity and major economic considerations related to adenoviral epidemic respiratory disease in military recruits, the development of vaccines received early attention. Initially, inactivated vaccines were produced, and they achieved some degree of success.[266,303,406] Later, live viral preparations grown in diploid human fibroblast tissue culture became available and proved quite successful in controlling specific adenoviral infections in the military services.*

In 1975, enteric adenoviruses (adenovirus types 40 and 41) first were reported.[182,601,713] They were demonstrated by electron microscopy and subsequently were shown to be a significant cause of diarrhea in children.[70,116,391,472,524,655,669,673] Particularly important today are adenoviral infections in immunocompromised hosts, particularly transplant recipients.[383]

PROPERTIES OF THE VIRUS

Classification

Adenoviruses that infect humans are placed in the family *Adenoviridae* and the genus *Mastadenovirus*.[197,313,463,604] At present, more than 70[271,421,435] immunologically distinct adenoviral types have been recovered from humans.† Additional adenoviral types have been isolated from monkeys, cattle, dogs, mice, and chickens.[293,295–297] Mammalian adenoviruses have a common generic antigen that can be identified by complement fixation and enzyme linked immunosorbent assay (ELISA).[342,539,576,715] Individual serotypes are identified by neutralization.[274,279,375] Adenovirus type 52, the first human adenovirus identified based on genetic analysis, was also classified as a novel species human adenovirus G. Subsequent types have been identified by bioinformatic analysis of genomic sequences.[421]

Adenoviruses originally were subclassified on the basis of four hemagglutination patterns with rat and rhesus monkey red blood cells.[581] This subclassification is updated in Table 156.1. In 1962, researchers found that adenovirus type 12 could cause tumors in hamsters, and soon thereafter, investigators realized that adenoviruses also could be classified by their oncogenic potential in rodents.[319,662] Grouping by oncogenic potential was similar, with few exceptions, to grouping by hemagglutination properties: organisms in hemagglutination group I had moderate oncogenic potential, group II and group III organisms had low or no potential, and group IV organisms had high oncogenic potential.[245,314,327]

Adenoviruses also have been subclassified (A to G) on the basis of the percentage of guanine plus cytosine in their DNA and other biochemical and biophysical criteria[299,373,546,600,696–698] (Table 156.2). In general, subgroup A organisms are the same as hemagglutination group IV; subgroup B, the same as hemagglutination group I; subgroups C, E, and F, the same as hemagglutination group III; and subgroup D, the same as hemagglutination group II. Restriction enzyme analysis has resulted in genomic typing of specific adenoviral serologic types.[416] In particular, numerous genotypes of adenovirus type 7 have been identified, and the severity of disease may relate to the genotype.

*References 166, 168, 255, 271, 351, 407, 421, 434, 451, 572, 573, 580, 620, 656, 659.

†References 107, 130, 141, 168, 207, 208, 210, 212, 213, 228, 263, 425, 494, 495, 506.

TABLE 156.1 Separation of Human Adenoviruses Into Subgroups by Ability to Agglutinate Rhesus Monkey and Rat Erythrocytes

Subgroup	Characteristic	Type
I	Complete agglutination of monkey erythrocytes	3, 7, 11, 14, 16, 21, 34, 35, 50
II	Complete agglutination of rat erythrocytes	8–10, 13, 15, 17, 19, 20, 22–30, 32, 33, 36–39, 42–49, 51
III	Partial agglutination of rat erythrocytes	1, 2, 4–6, 40, 41
IV	No or little agglutination of monkey or rat erythrocytes	12, 18, 31

Data from references 147, 293, 299, 307, 310, 358, 373, 406, 508, 509, 600, 716.

TABLE 156.2 Human Adenoviral Serotypes Based on Biochemical and Biophysical Criteria

Subgroup	Adenovirus Type(s)	Location and Manifestations of Infection
A	12, 18, 31, 61	Gastrointestinal; may cause disease in children
B:1	3, 7, 16, 21, 50, 55, 66	Respiratory, eye, and gastrointestinal symptomatic infections
B:2	11, 14, 34, 35	Urinary and respiratory; symptomatic urinary tract infections (particularly in immunosuppressed patients) and symptomatic respiratory infections
C	1, 2, 5, 6, 57	Respiratory and gastrointestinal; symptomatic respiratory infections and hepatitis in immunosuppressed patients
D	8–10, 13, 15, 17, 19, 20, 22–30, 32, 33, 36–39, 42–49, 51, 53, 54, 56, 58–60, 63–67	Eye and gastrointestinal; symptomatic eye infections, gastrointestinal infections in HIV-infected patients
E	4	Symptomatic eye and respiratory infections
F	40, 41	Symptomatic gastrointestinal infections
G	52	Symptomatic gastrointestinal infections

Data from references 147, 299, 314, 373, 406, 421, 425, 546, 571, 573, 600, 697, 704.

Physical Properties

Adenoviruses are nonenveloped DNA viruses 65 to 80 nm in diameter.[197,245,313,314,327,382,463] The virion consists of a protein capsid composed of 252 capsomeres and a nucleoprotein core that contains the DNA viral genome and two to four internal proteins.[554] The virion is roughly spherical in the form of an icosahedron; each of the 20 sides is an equilateral triangle, with the vertices of each converging in groups of five and resulting in 12 pentagonal vertices.[70,214,313] Each vertex capsomere contacts five other capsomeres and is designated a penton. Each penton contains a base plate and a rodlike projection, the fiber. The virion has 240 nonvertex capsomeres that occur in groups of six and are known as hexons.[382,509,672] Hexons contain the generic complement-fixing antigen.[214] Each capsomere has a diameter of 8 nm and a central hole that is 2 to 3 nm in diameter.[721] The capsomeres constitute 87% of the dry weight of the virion.

The central core of the virion, which accounts for 12% to 14% of its dry weight, is composed of linear double-stranded DNA (molecular mass, 23.85 × 10^6 Da for adenovirus type 2) and two to four basic proteins.[222,314,721]

Adenoviruses are highly stable in general.[151,214,243,327,409] They are resistant to lipid solvents and retain activity at pH values ranging from 2 to 10. They can be inactivated upon exposure to sodium hypochlorite for 10 minutes or to 85% ethanol for at least 2 minutes.[452]

At 24°C, maximal infectivity is maintained between pH 6 and 9.5. Adenoviruses are stable at room temperature for 2 weeks, at 36°C for 7 days, and at 4°C for at least 70 days. Infectivity is destroyed by heating to 56°C for 30 minutes. Sodium dodecyl sulfate (0.25%) inactivates virus by disruption of the capsid.[382] Hydrogen peroxide vapor has been shown to inactivate adenoviruses[51] and free chlorine is effective in controlling adenoviruses in drinking water.[525] Adenovirus serotypes 2, 10, 40, and 41 are highly resistant to ultraviolet radiation, and, therefore, they can be used as markers of the quality of water treatment practices.[302]

Antigenic Composition

The antigenic determinants of adenoviruses are contained on the protein structural subunits (hexons, pentons, and fibers).[672] The hexon antigen (alpha component) carries the generic antigenic component that is common to all mammalian adenoviruses and is measured by complement fixation or ELISA. Another hexon antigen (epsilon component) reacts with neutralizing antibodies lacking hemagglutination-inhibiting activity. The antigen related to viral fiber also induces the production of type-specific neutralizing antibody for some adenoviral types. Minor antigens are related to the pentons. One of them (the cell-detaching factor) causes rounding and clumping of tissue culture cells.

Gerna and associates,[241] using the immunoperoxidase antibody technique, found that the early antigens of all serotypes belonging to one group (see Table 156.1) react strongly with all type-specific immune sera of the same group.

Tissue Culture Growth

Although adenoviruses can be grown in a wide variety of cells of human epithelial origin, primary or diploid cultures of human embryonic kidney are preferable for recovery of agents from clinical specimens.[409] Continuous cell lines such as HeLa and HEp-2 also are quite sensitive.[288,327,570,586] Adenoviruses will grow in monkey kidney tissue culture, but evolution of the cytopathic effect is considerably slower than that occurring in cells of human origin. In addition, the cytopathic effect is more variable in monkey kidney tissue culture, and many isolates will be missed.

Enteric adenoviruses have been detected in human feces by electron microscopy.* These enteric adenoviruses, identified as types 40 and 41, usually do not grow in standard tissue culture systems. Both viral types will grow in Graham 293 cells (a human embryonic kidney cell line transformed by adenovirus type 5); type 40 also will grow in tertiary monkey kidney cells, and some strains of type 41 will grow in HEp-2, Chang conjunctiva cells, and tertiary cynomolgus cells.[646,699] Grabow and associates[258] noted that the PLC/PRG/5 cell line was 100 times more sensitive to a laboratory strain of adenovirus type 41 and 10 times more sensitive to a laboratory strain of adenovirus type 40 than were Graham 293 cells.

Specimens for viral culture may be obtained from the eye, pharynx, blood, lungs, pleural and pericardial fluid, liver, stool, intestinal epithelium, lymph nodes, cerebrospinal fluid (CSF), brain, urine, and renal tissue. For best isolation rates, clinical specimens should be inoculated in cell culture within 6 hours of being collected. Tissue culture tubes are incubated best at 37°C, and rolling offers no advantage over stationary incubation.[409] Although the cytopathic effect has considerable variability, the most consistent finding is marked rounding and clumping of cells, often in grapelike clusters.[554,558] A cytopathic effect may be noted as early as 1 to 2 days after inoculation, but it may be delayed as long as 4 weeks. Use of the shell viral technique, in which infected cells in a specimen are centrifuged onto HEp-2 tissue culture cells, yields positive cultures in 1 to 2 days.[183] The cytopathic effect characteristically is followed by detachment of the entire cell sheet from the glass of the tissue culture tube within 2 to 4 days.[263,290,540,583,586]

Virus Multiplication

Initial attachment of adenoviruses to cells is relatively slow, with up to 6 hours being required.[140,244,327] The fiber protein of the virus mediates attachment to the cellular receptor.[606] An important adenovirus receptor is the coxsackievirus and adenovirus receptor (CAR) protein. It is a high-affinity receptor for all adenoviral subgroups except subgroup B. Penetration into the host cell occurs rapidly, either by phagocytosis or by direct entry through the plasma membrane.[327,430] The eclipse period with adenoviruses varies from 11 to 21 hours, depending on the serotype.[244,327] During eclipse, viral DNA uncoating requires approximately 2 hours when determined biochemically.[327] After uncoating, the viral DNA rapidly enters the nucleus of the cell and disassociates from its internal protein.[140,245,430] After the eclipse period, viral DNA accumulates, often doubling the content of the infected cell and becoming part of the typical inclusion bodies of the infected cells.[245]

Characteristic cytopathic changes in tissue culture, as demonstrated by light microscopy of hematoxylin and eosin–stained material or by electron microscopy, appear as early as 8 to 24 hours after infection occurs.[66,68,274] Two types of intranuclear alterations may be seen. In the first type, early, small, discrete eosinophilic inclusions are observed. They gradually enlarge, become more prominent, and then form a large crystalline central mass surrounded by a clear zone or halo.[66,252] This type of early cytopathic effect appears to take place in cells that contain only small amounts of infectious virus.[67] The second type of intranuclear alteration, which generally occurs later, consists of large basophilic intranuclear inclusions.[66] Occasionally, giant forms measuring greater than 14 mm across are noted.[66] These mature inclusions may expand the nucleus of the cell so greatly that the cell's DNA content is 10 times larger than that of an uninfected cell. They contain a large amount of viral antigen and infective virus. Cytopathic changes vary considerably with the different adenoviral serotypes.[68,382]

In general, virus remains within the nucleus of intact, infected cells, with less than 1% of the total viral content of a culture being free within the extracellular fluid at any one time.[382]

Animal Susceptibility

Human adenoviruses usually do not produce clinical illness in laboratory animals, although infections with several different serotypes have occurred in selected animals.[327] When adenoviral strains were administered intranasally to young, "pathogen-free," colostrum-deprived pigs or 1-month-old cotton rats, pneumonia developed in the animals, and intranuclear inclusions were observed microscopically in their lungs.[327,522] An adenovirus type 5 strain was injected intravenously into a rabbit, and the virus was recovered from the animal's spleen when removed 2 months later. Many adenoviral strains will propagate in a variety of different animal tissue cultures. In addition, in some cultures, marked cytopathic effects are observed, but little infectious virus is produced.

Adeno-Associated Viruses

Adeno-associated viruses are a group of small, replication-defective, single-stranded, nonenveloped DNA-containing, nonpathogenic virus-like particles of the *Parvoviridae* family that replicate in tissue culture only in the presence of adenoviruses.[60,105,140,214,327,368,596,621] Twelve natural serologic types have been identified; however, only types 2, 3, 5, 6, and 9 have been recovered from humans.[214,382,596] These agents have been isolated from throat and anal swab specimens of children from whom adenoviral strains also were isolated.[60] Approximately 30% of children have complement-fixing antibody to adeno-associated virus types 2 and 3; most of these children have had evidence of adenoviral infection as well.[61] Neutralizing antibody to adeno-associated virus types 2 and 3 is noted in the sera of 60% to 80% of children 8 to 14 years of age.[532] The specific relevance of adeno-associated viruses is unknown. Adeno-associated viruses reliably insert genetic material at a specific site on chromosome 19. Research on their potential as viral vectors in recombinant gene therapy for disorders such as lysosomal storage diseases, spinal muscular atrophy, glycogen storage diseases, leukodystrophies, Parkinson disease, Alzheimer disease, and age-related macular

*References 70, 132, 148, 342, 373, 562, 575, 669, 697, 715.

degeneration is ongoing.[596,617] To date, adeno-associated viral vectors have been successfully used as gene therapy in the treatment of hemophilia B, inherited night blindness, and lipoprotein lipase deficiency.[357] A replication-competent, genetically engineered oncoloytic adenovirus VCN-01 has demonstrated a potent antisarcoma effect with possible therapeutic application in combination with chemotherapy for treatment of osteosarcoma.[446]

EPIDEMIOLOGY

General Prevalence

Adenoviral infections account for 2% to 10% of all respiratory illnesses.* In children, adenoviruses are estimated to be responsible for 2% to 35% of respiratory viral illnesses,† and they are implicated in 5% to 17% of upper respiratory tract infections, 4% to 10% of cases of pharyngitis, 3% to 9% of cases of croup, 5% to 11% of cases of bronchitis, 2% to 16% of cases of bronchiolitis, and 4% to 11% of cases of pneumonia.[69,87,98–100,216,233,330,486,534] Enteric adenoviral infections are the cause of 2% to 15% of acute diarrheal illnesses in children.‡ Specific categories of illness caused by adenoviruses vary with respect to viral serotype, patient age, socioeconomic status, and environmental conditions.[95,126,270,289,343,741] Adenoviruses have a predilection for infants and children younger than 5 years who spend portions of their days in closed environments, such as daycare centers, orphanages, and other institutions.[44,47,95,280,429,694] Epidemics of disease caused by adenoviral infection have been associated with swimming pools, daycare centers, resident schools, certain industries, hospitals, physicians' offices, and early basic military training centers in young recruits.§ Adenoviruses are recovered commonly from children in tropical countries and in situations characterized by crowding, such as lower socioeconomic settings.[95,100,119,343,741]

Age, Incidence, and Prevalence

Although adenoviral infections occur in all age groups, the incidence of infection generally is related inversely to age.[126,382] More than 90% of newborn infants have transplacentally acquired complement-fixing adenoviral serum antibody.[499,633] Most infants have neutralizing antibody to one or more of the common adenoviral types, which appears to be protective during the first 6 months of life. When adenoviral infection does occur in a neonate, it often is severe and occasionally fatal.[18,190,749] By the sixth month of life, only 14% of infants have demonstrable adenoviral complement-fixing antibody. By the time children reach 1 year of age, complement-fixing adenoviral antibody is observed in 44% to 50% of sera tested.[321,504]

The incidence of adenoviral infection peaks in infants and children between 6 months and 5 years of age.[114,470,541] By the time that they are 5 years of age, 70% to 80% of children have neutralizing antibody to adenovirus types 1 and 2, and 50% have antibody to adenovirus type 5.[150,212,321,332,533,541,676]

Adenoviral infections also occur commonly in grade school– and junior high school–aged children, but the incidence diminishes in high school–aged adolescents. Adenoviral infections occur in only 1% to 2% of college students, and they are noted infrequently in civilian adults.[184,185,187,262,636] Approximately 1% of adults with a respiratory infectious illness will have adenoviral infection; in hospitalized adults, the incidence is approximately 4%.[262] The most common adenoviral respiratory infections in children are caused by types 1, 2, 3, and 5.[1,13,44,405,676,688,694] Types 6 and 7 are the next most frequent isolates associated with childhood respiratory infection. Adenovirus types 40 and 41 are the most common causes of diarrhea.[116,389,413]

Military Recruits

Epidemic adenoviral disease occurs commonly in military recruits, with virtually all illness developing during the first 8 weeks of basic training.[211,384,439,461,588,590,678,679] The attack rate has varied between 40% and 90%.[211,263,439,677] Adenoviruses account for 30% to 70% of acute respiratory disease, 67% of common cold-like illnesses, 62% to 77% of cases of acute febrile pharyngitis and tonsillitis, 67% of cases of bronchitis, and 24% of cases of pneumonia.[50,210] Some adenoviral infections are associated with minimal or no symptoms.[210,263]

A vaccine against adenovirus serotypes 4 and 7 was developed for use in military basic training centers and effectively prevented outbreaks of adenovirus. Routine vaccination began in 1971, but the sole manufacturer of the vaccine ceased its production in 1995. The first large post–vaccine era outbreak of adenovirus serotypes 3 and 7 occurred in naval recruits in Great Lakes, Illinois, in 1997.[590] Subsequent adenoviral epidemics occurred in military recruits in Fort Jackson, South Carolina, in 1998 with type 4, and in Lackland Air Force Base in San Antonio Texas, in 2007 with serotype 14.[75,650,693]

The last remaining stocks of vaccine were depleted or expired by 1999. Because of continued outbreaks, vaccine development was reinitiated, leading to the development of a live oral vaccine against adenovirus 4 and 7. The vaccine was licensed for military personnel ages 17 to 50 years in March 2011. It is currently manufactured by Barr Labs and distributed via Teva Pharmaceuticals.[667] A full review of eight deaths caused by adenovirus infection in military recruits from 1999 to 2010 was published by Potter and colleagues. All eight deaths occurred after the cessation of the immunization program in 1999. In contrast, there were no deaths due to adenovirus in US military members from 1975 to 1998 while this program was in place.[553] Koren and colleagues[387] conducted an observational, longitudinal study of 1536 children and adults under 65 years of age at five US-based military medical centers from September 2009 through May 2014. They found that adenovirus accounted for 2.8% of cases of influenza-like illness that was described as relatively mild (e.g., no hospitalizations or deaths reported). Coinfection was identified in 51.1% of cases, with 27.3% of coinfections identified in adults. Kajon and coworkers[350] sought to describe the molecular epidemiology of adenovirus type 21 causing febrile respiratory illness among US military recruits from 1997 to 2011. Adenovirus type 21 is the predominant source of adenoviral illness when circulation of adenovirus types 4 and 7 is well controlled by vaccination. As such, it is possible that it may become an active pathogen again following reintroduction of the vaccine.

Geographic Distribution

Adenoviral infections have been noted throughout the world.* Epidemic, endemic, and sporadic infections all occur.

Seasonal Patterns

Sporadic infections with adenoviruses occur throughout the year.[212,217,251,307,320,428,440,476,486] Epidemic adenoviral respiratory disease usually occurs in the winter, spring, and early summer.† Seasonal patterns depend on serotypes, population groups, and exposure. Epidemics of disease in military recruits commonly associated with adenovirus types 4 and 7 occur most frequently in the winter and spring.[62,211,210,303] Epidemics of pharyngoconjunctival fever have been noted most commonly in the summer months in school-aged children in association with summer camps or swimming pools.[447,680,721] No seasonal pattern has been identified for adenoviral gastroenteritis.[132,372,575,669]

Host and Social Factors

The overall incidence of adenoviral illnesses is higher in males.[126,290] In a study involving 3313 adenovirus isolates, the male-to-female ratio was 1.3 : 1.[126]

Susceptibility to adenoviral infection apparently does not vary by race. More severe disease has been noted in infants of native and Indian populations in New Zealand and Canada.[9,40,253] However, the relationship of these findings to socioeconomic conditions was not identified initially.

*References 90, 117, 118, 125, 188, 212, 213, 371, 435, 541.

†References 69, 90, 98, 100, 313, 428, 440, 498, 557, 561, 603, 692.

‡References 116, 132, 322, 341, 413, 472, 524, 562, 568, 669, 673, 719.

§References 31, 110, 135, 190, 260, 335, 337, 381, 384, 411, 447, 521, 535, 548, 567, 588, 590, 618, 731, 744.

*References 31, 98, 102, 134, 193, 208, 214, 219, 222, 253, 289, 298, 307, 325, 332, 334, 343, 360, 368, 371, 379, 381, 382, 393, 397, 476, 477, 531, 607, 613, 628, 633, 632, 640, 647, 675–678, 680, 721, 731, 738, 741.

†References 13, 62, 69, 214, 280, 312, 332, 393, 531, 552, 557, 676, 679.

The incidence of adenoviral infection is greatest in lower socioeconomic population groups.[343] Spread of infection has been observed in daycare centers, schools, children's homes, hospitals, clinics, physicians' offices, and certain industrial settings.* Acute overwhelming illness, including bronchiolitis and pneumonia with severe pulmonary residua, has been reported in neonates, small infants, and occasionally, adults.[18,289,412] Adenoviral infections are a significant problem in immunocompromised hosts; when they occur, they frequently are severe and occasionally are fatal.†

Spread of Infection

Adenoviruses frequently are isolated from the conjunctiva, throat, and stool. Despite the ease of isolating the virus, the effectiveness of spread of infection in the general population varies considerably.[100] Adenovirus types 1, 2, 3, 5, and 7 are effective spreaders; however, they are not as highly contagious as varicella, measles, and influenza viruses.[99,100] Close contact appears to be necessary for infection to spread from one person to another.[633] Illness does not spread rapidly in the usual school setting but does spread dramatically in closed environments.[47,99,280,320] Although adenovirus type 4 spreads less effectively in the general population, spread is rapid in nonimmune military recruits who live in close contact with each other.[112] In an outbreak of adenovirus type 7 in a children's home, 84% of the residents were shown to be infected.

Transmission of virus occurs by droplets reaching the conjunctiva, nose, or throat or, alternatively, by the fecal-oral route. In volunteer studies, adenoviruses have been shown to spread by small-droplet aerosols and, to a lesser degree, by large droplets.[21,127,128] Adenovirus type 4 has been recovered from room air and cough samples of patients with the virus in their throats.[22] A study by Russell and colleagues[587] of 341 military recruits and support personnel at the Marine Corps training center in San Diego, California, demonstrated that more than 79% of incoming recruits were susceptible to adenoviral infection in the postvaccine era. They identified incoming recruits with prolonged asymptomatic shedding of adenovirus and the presence of adenoviruses on multiple living quarter surfaces as potential sources of transmission. They also found evidence of extended pharyngeal shedding of adenovirus over the course of several days among recruits who had febrile respiratory illnesses.

In epidemics of pharyngoconjunctival fever, the virus appears to spread from contaminated swimming pool water to the eyes of recipients. In non–swimming-associated outbreaks of adenoviral respiratory illness with appropriate serotypes, conjunctivitis occurs only rarely.[31,47,208,280,345,379] This fact, in conjunction with the finding that pharyngoconjunctival fever occurred after conjunctival administration of virus, but not after nasopharyngeal application in volunteers,[43,621,708] suggests that the conjunctiva must be inoculated directly for the syndrome to occur. Epidemics of keratoconjunctivitis have occurred as a result of contact with contaminated ophthalmic instruments and fingers.[33,142,304,335,337,360,381,476,626] In daycare centers, orphanages, and the military, transmission probably occurs most commonly through small-droplet aerosols in crowded quarters.[548] An alternative in children is the fecal-oral route. Enteric adenoviruses have been identified in fecal specimens for approximately 8 days after the onset of gastroenteritis.[372]

Family members may excrete adenoviruses in their feces intermittently for prolonged periods after initial infection.[72,212] In one study, 20% of persons excreted adenoviruses in stool for longer than 3 months. Intrahousehold spread appears to continue as long as susceptible family members are present.[212] Infants born into households in which members are adenoviral fecal excreters often become infected, presumably through the fecal-oral route. In general, 50% of susceptible household members will experience infection, although the rate varies inversely with age and also depends on the serotype of adenovirus. Reinfection with specific adenoviral serotypes occurs, but most are asymptomatic or associated with only minimal illness.

Nosocomial spread of both respiratory and enteric adenoviruses is a common occurrence and has been the cause of fatal illnesses in infants and immunocompromised patients.[5,153,203,386,618,749] DNA viruses are known to be more stable than RNA viruses and have been considered a good indicator of viral contamination when assessing the quality of cleaning of environmental surfaces in the hospital environment, even in a nonoutbreak setting.[526] Ganime and colleagues[230,231] analyzed 480 fomite samples collected over a 1-year period from the neonatal intensive care unit and general pediatric ward for both adenoviruses and rotavirus species A. They found that adenovirus was detected more frequently in the pediatric ward (38% in pediatric ward vs. 3.2% in neonatal intensive care unit). They attributed this difference to the fact that adenoviruses are more stable in the environment and can remain viable for 7 to 90 days, thereby highlighting a possible role for fomite transmission in the healthcare setting. They emphasized the importance of assessment of hand hygiene adherence, as well as regular assessment of the efficacy of disinfectant solutions and cleaning practices in the healthcare setting.

*References 44, 47, 50, 97, 110, 190, 270, 274, 337, 521, 524, 535, 618, 673, 744.
†References 88, 91, 136, 141, 204, 264, 383, 431, 468, 513, 625, 749.

PATHOGENESIS AND PATHOLOGY

Adenoviral infections usually are acute and self-limited, and, therefore, opportunities to study the pathogenesis and pathologic process have been infrequent. Study of the pathologic mechanisms has been performed in human volunteers, tissue and organ culture systems, and recent murine model systems and by examination of specimens from persons dying of adenoviral disease.

Viral Infection

In general, the characteristics of adenoviral infection depend on the host and the serotype of the agent.* The route of infection with adenoviruses that are capable of causing pharyngoconjunctival fever determines the pathologic manifestations. In most respiratory illnesses, initial viral infection occurs in the respiratory tract and involves the mucous membranes of the nose, oropharynx, and conjunctiva. Adenoviral agents have been isolated from sputum and oral secretions from 2 days before the onset of clinical illness to up to 8 days after the onset of symptoms. Deeper respiratory involvement of the trachea, pleurae, and lungs may result from initial small-particle aerosol, from progression of local infection, or perhaps as a result of viremia. Gastrointestinal infection in conjunction with respiratory infection also occurs early and probably is the result of swallowed virus. Stool isolates of respiratory viral types frequently are noted concomitantly with respiratory tract infection. However, in contrast to the upper respiratory infection, the virus may persist for a long time in the lower gastrointestinal tract. Infection with enteric adenoviral types is presumed to involve intestinal epithelial cells. In one fatal infection, adenoviral antigen was demonstrated in jejunal cells.[562,714]

In experimental studies with aerosolized adenovirus type 4, recovery of virus from throat specimens occurred on day 5 or 6, progressed to a maximum concentration on day 11 or 12, and was seen uncommonly after day 20. Maximal recovery of adenovirus type 4 from anal specimens occurred on day 13, and shedding continued for longer than 3 weeks. Adenovirus types 26 and 27 inoculated into the conjunctiva resulted in short-term isolation of virus from the eyes on days 3 to 7 and, less frequently, from the throat on day 4.[359] Isolation of virus from the rectum was common beginning at the end of the first week. Maximal fecal shedding occurred during the second and third weeks.

Like other DNA viruses, adenoviruses can establish latent infection in lymphoid tissues, particularly in T lymphocytes.[236] Garnett and colleagues[237] studied adenoidal and tonsillar tissue from children 1 to 19 years of age undergoing elective tonsillectomies for tonsillar hypertrophy, recurrent bacterial infections, or recurrent otitis media. Among 243 samples from 203 patients, they detected species C adenovirus DNA in 78% of samples, with peak detection at age 4 years, followed by decreasing frequency with increasing donor age. Interestingly, although adenoviral DNA was detected, infectious virus was isolated from culture in only 12.2% of samples. Not surprisingly, adenoviruses were more commonly found in adenoidal tissue when compared to tonsillar tissue. Faden and colleagues[189] subsequently conducted a prospective study of 59 children undergoing elective tonsillectomy and adenoidectomy. They also noted

*References 49, 72, 77, 121, 247–249, 499, 549, 629, 713, 726.

a very high rate of asymptomatic infection in the adenoids and tonsils of such children. Viruses were detected in 70.9% of tonsils and 94.7% of adenoids, with adenovirus being the most common virus detected overall and the most commonly detected virus in adenoids (71.4%). The authors theorized that chronic stimulation of both tonsillar and adenoidal tissue is associated with obstructive airway disease. Alkhalaf and colleagues[14] conducted a similar study and proposed that DNA methylation of adenoviral DNA might contribute to establishment of latency, which ultimately was not confirmed. Yeshuroon-Koffler and coworkers[737] compared adenotonsillar tissue of 56 patients who underwent tonsillectomy and adenoidectomy for obstructive sleep apnea or recurrent throat infections. Viral DNA was detected in 50% of samples removed from patients with obstructive sleep apnea, but none in the recurrent infection group, thereby highlighting a possible role for adenoviral infection in the pathogenesis of obstructive sleep apnea.

Viremia is a common finding in uncomplicated adenoviral respiratory infections in children. In a study involving 68 children, adenoviral DNA was noted in acute-phase serum samples from 28 (41%) of these children.[2] In the children with primary infection, 72% (21 of 29) had adenoviral DNA in their acute-phase serum samples. Other evidence of the presence of adenoviruses in the bloodstream early in disease is the occurrence of maculopapular, morbilliform, or petechial exanthems (or any combination of such rashes), as well as recovery of virus from multiple organs such as the brain, kidney, urinary bladder, lymphoid tissue, and liver and at postmortem examination.* The virus has been cultured from the mononuclear cells of heparinized blood.[17]

Coinfections

With the expanded use of direct fluorescent assays and PCR, investigators are discovering a common prevalence of coinfections of adenoviruses with multiple serotypes,[36] with other viruses,[152,160,301,402,705] and with bacteria.[57] As technology is improving and made more available, the epidemiology of coinfection, as well as its impact on disease, is becoming clearer. Calvo and colleagues[87] conducted a prospective study of children admitted to the hospital with acute respiratory infections. Adenovirus was detected in 403 out of 2371 confirmed viral infections with a 62% rate of coinfection. Approximately 49% experienced coinfection with RSV and 24% experienced coinfection with enterovirus and rhinovirus. A large international cohort study of 3717 influenza-like illness episodes in 2421 pediatric patients ages 6 months to 10 years in 17 sites in eight countries found adenovirus coinfection with bocavirus to be most frequent.[652] Studies by Song and colleagues have demonstrated that 55% to 63% of pediatric patients have respiratory adenovirus coinfection.[623,624]

Pathology

Early pathologic changes are observed in the epithelium of the respiratory tract. The severity of adenoviral involvement varies with the different serotypes. In tracheal organ cultures, growth of adenovirus type 7 was characterized by an initial focal cytopathologic effect at 100 hours that quickly progressed to involve the whole epithelium.[130] Frequently, the cilia of inclusion-bearing cells were noted to be intact. In contrast to the findings with adenovirus type 7, a type 12 strain resulted in only a mild cytopathologic effect on the organ culture system.[130]

Microscopic examination of autopsy material from patients dying of adenoviral pneumonia revealed a loss of cilia in the tracheal epithelium, proliferation of other respiratory epithelial cells, and the presence of intranuclear inclusions.[39,49,77,101,219,717,722,725,752] In severe pneumonia, total destruction along with necrotizing bronchitis, bronchiolitis, and pneumonia is observed (Fig. 156.1). Mononuclear cellular infiltration is seen, and hyaline membranes and necrosis are present. Cilia and goblet cells are absent, and muscle fiber bundles and elastic fibers are dispersed. Frequently, epithelial cells have a characteristic appearance with adenoviral infection. These infected cells are enlarged grossly and lose their nuclear membranes; the nuclear material has migrated into the cytoplasm.[549] Blood vessels show edema, separation of filaments in their walls, and occasionally thrombosis.[752]

*References 17, 18, 49, 63, 77, 101, 253, 265, 269, 432, 450, 608.

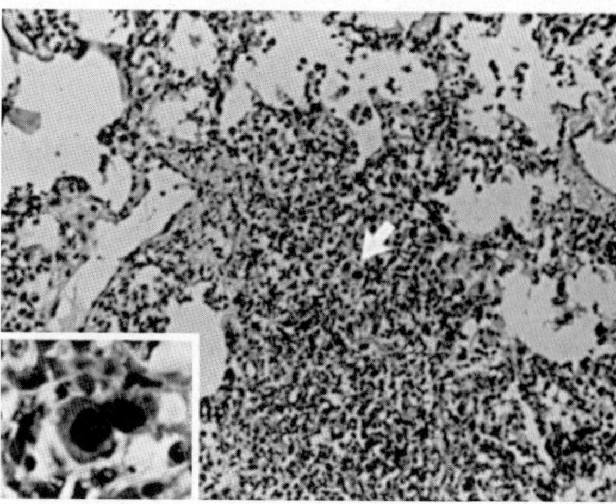

FIG. 156.1 The lung of a 17-month-old infant with adenoviral pneumonia. The infant died 10 days after the onset of illness, with no other contributing disease. The adenovirus isolated was not typed. A patchy pneumonia is present, and the *arrow* indicates two cells with nuclear inclusions. *Inset,* Two similar cells with typical adenoviral nuclear inclusions at higher magnification (hematoxylin and eosin staining, ×190; inset, ×770). (Courtesy Dr. David D. Porter, Department of Pathology, David Geffen School of Medicine at UCLA.)

In cases of pharyngoconjunctival fever, conjunctival biopsy specimens in volunteer studies revealed an inflammatory response with lymphocytic infiltration of the submucosal layer.[42,43] Biopsy material from palatine tonsils of infected volunteers revealed hypertrophy and hyperplasia of the lymphoid tissue, with congestion and edema of the surrounding connective tissue.

On histologic examination, adenoviral inclusions are characterized by small eosinophilic and larger basophilic intranuclear bodies.[39,219,499,629]

Hepatic involvement in adenoviral infection has been reported frequently.[4,22,49,91,219,549,625] In addition to isolation of virus from the liver, focal areas of liver necrosis accompanied by characteristic hepatic intranuclear inclusions have been demonstrated.[4,91,749] Electron microscopic examination has revealed adenoviral particles within the intranuclear inclusions.[4,49,549,717,749] Hematogenous spread to the central nervous system (CNS) has been observed.[613] Most patients with adenoviral CNS infection have had an associated pneumonia.[131,612] In CNS disease, the brain is edematous and congested. On microscopic examination, a perivascular accumulation of lymphocytes is noted, along with gigantic nuclear inclusions in the cortical neurons. Viral particles have been observed within these nuclear inclusions by electron microscopy.[115]

In epidemic keratoconjunctivitis caused by adenovirus type 8, the walls of the conjunctival vessels are damaged, and aneurysms are present. The surrounding conjunctival connective tissue is edematous. The virus has been suggested to penetrate the cornea along nerves deep into the epithelial layers in a manner similar to that occurring in herpes simplex virus (HSV) infection.[690]

Adenoviral strains have been isolated from and intranuclear inclusions have been demonstrated in renal tubular epithelium, lymph nodes, muscle, and gastrointestinal epithelium.[46,91,714,746,747,749]

Immunologic Events

The local response in adenoviral infection depends on the site of viral inoculation, the method of transmission, the viral serotype, the concentration of inoculum, and the antibody status of the host. Three days after infection develops, when virus can be recovered from the nasopharynx, marked transudation of proteins from serum into the respiratory tract occurs, along with the production of secretory IgA antibody.[457] Approximately 7 days after the onset of illness, serum-neutralizing, hemagglutination-inhibiting, and complement-fixing antibodies appear.[140,408,551] At the same time, the nasal secretions contain specific IgA and IgG antibodies.[48] In general, neutralizing antibody is the most sensitive indicator of adenoviral infection, hemagglutination-inhibiting antibody is less sensitive, and complement-fixing antibody is the least sensitive.[381,524] Antibody titers peak in 2 to 3 weeks; complement-fixing antibody declines in 2 to 3 months but may persist for up to a year.[140,551] Neutralizing antibody persists for a longer period and is measurable in many instances for periods as long as 10 years. Reinfection with the same adenoviral serotype is rare because of type-specific immunity.[43,584]

Although alterations in leukocytes are not common findings, a decrease in the number of lymphocytes has been observed before or at the onset of clinical illness and an increase in neutrophils early in the disease, followed by a decrease later. Neutropenia may develop in severe disseminated illness and is attributed to a direct toxic effect of virus on leukocytes, marrow reserves, or both.[163] The erythrocyte sedimentation rate (ESR) of children has been normal or elevated to 55 mm/h.[633,632]

Studies by Ginsberg and associates[247–249] in murine adenoviral pneumonia model systems noted that tumor necrosis factor-α, interleukin-1, and interleukin-6 were elaborated during the first 2 to 3 days of infection. However, only tumor necrosis factor-α played an early role in the initial phase of pathogenesis. The second phase of the inflammatory response is caused by the infiltration of cytotoxic T cells. In an extensive study, Kawasaki and colleagues[362] compared numerous clinical and laboratory test results in children with adenoviral infections with those in children with influenza and respiratory syncytial virus (RSV) infections. They found that the children with adenoviral infections had higher white blood cell (WBC) counts with a greater number of neutrophils than did children with influenza or RSV infections (12,322, 7638, and 8460 WBCs/mm,[3] respectively). The children with adenoviral infections also had more atypical lymphocytes and higher C-reactive protein (CRP) and ESR values. The mean serum interleukin-6 concentration was significantly higher in the children with adenoviral infections than it was in those with influenza and RSV infections (131.0, 26.7, and 15.0 pg/mL, respectively).

Mistchenko and coworkers[471] studied cytokines and adenovirus-specific circulating immune complexes in 38 children with adenoviral infections. They placed the patients into three groups based on the severity of their respiratory illnesses: moderate illness, severe illness, and fatal illness. Serum interleukin-1 was not detected in children with moderate illness but was found in 7 of 12 with severe illness and in 13 of the 16 children who died. Tumor necrosis factor-α frequently was present in the sera of fatal cases, it was not present in the sera of moderately ill children, and it was detected in the sera of only 2 of 12 patients with severe but nonfatal illness. Interleukin-8 was noted in all sera, but values were highest in children with fatal illness. Serum immune complexes (containing IgG) were found in 7 of the 16 children who died. Finally, patients with increased concentrations of interleukin-6, interleukin-8, and tumor necrosis factor-α were those with hypoperfusion, febrile peaks, seizures, and a manifestation of septic shock. Five of 10 children with severe or fatal illness had serum autoantibodies specific for smooth muscle.

Matsubara and associates[449] noted the participation of peripheral blood $CD8^+$ T cells and $HLA\text{-}DR^+$, $CD8^+$ T cells in children with adenoviral infection. One child with severe adenoviral type 7 pneumonia had a marked increase in $HLA\text{-}DR^+$ $CD8^+$ T cells, serum levels of interferon-γ, and peripheral blood interferon-γ–producing T cells.

CLINICAL MANIFESTATIONS

Adenoviral infections are exceedingly common events, and the spectrum of disease is quite broad (Table 156.3). As noted in Table 156.3, some specific adenoviral diseases exist; however, the overall majority of infections involve a variety of anatomically associated illnesses. In many instances, similar illnesses are caused by other respiratory viruses, and the clinical spectra of the various adenoviral serotypes frequently overlap. Certain specific adenoviral types do have clinical characteristics that facilitate etiologic diagnosis, however.

Respiratory Tract

Common Cold

Although adenoviruses frequently receive etiologic consideration in colds, they are, in fact, associated only rarely with this illness.[345] In one report, 3% of common colds in children were attributed to adenovirus,[541] and in another study, 6.4% of children with coryza had adenoviral isolates.[176] Respiratory tract infections with adenoviruses usually are associated with fever and, frequently, with some degree of pharyngitis; therefore, when strict clinical criteria are applied, they do not qualify as colds.[320,636] Occasionally, adenoviruses, particularly types 1, 2, 3, 5, and 7, have been recovered from patients with typical colds.

Nasopharyngitis, Pharyngitis, and Tonsillitis

Adenoviral pharyngitis is an acute illness characterized by fever, sore throat, extensive exudative tonsillitis, and frequently, cervical adenopathy.[162,176,345,477,621] In two studies involving 74 children with adenoviral pharyngitis, Ruuskanen and associates[589] described the pharyngeal findings. Most commonly, only mild inflammation and redness were observed. When exudates were present, they found them to be thick and membranous, thin and follicular, or thin and spotty; most typical were follicular and spotty exudates. Associated symptoms include malaise, headache, myalgia, chills, and cough. In infants and preschool children, nasal congestion and discharge are noticeable, and abdominal pain is a common complaint.[676] Children with adenoviral acute febrile pharyngitis also frequently have laryngotracheitis, bronchitis, or pneumonia.[738] The usual duration of illness varies from 5 to 7 days, although occasionally, symptoms persist well into the second week.[589]

Acute febrile pharyngitis is the most common adenoviral illness in children and is particularly important as an epidemic illness in closed environments.[47,621,633,738] For example, in an epidemic in a children's home, 63% of the residents were infected with adenovirus type 7a.[280] Moffet and colleagues[477] noted that adenoviruses were the etiologic agents recovered most commonly from hospitalized preschool children with febrile exudative pharyngitis; 23% of the children studied had adenoviral infections. In a university student health service study, 2.4% of illnesses with acute febrile pharyngitis were caused by adenoviruses.[491] Adenoviruses account for 37% to 75% of cases of nonstreptococcal pharyngitis in military recruits.

In children, 86% of cases of febrile pharyngitis are associated with adenovirus types 1, 2, 3, 5, and 7.[280,320,477]

On occasion, adenovirus types 7a, 9, 14, 15, and the intermediate strain 21/H21+35[300,621,633] also have been noted in association with pharyngitis. In military recruits, adenovirus types 4 and 7 are the main etiologic agents.

Acute Respiratory Disease

ARD is an epidemic disease that occurs predominantly in military recruit populations. This illness was studied extensively during World War II by the Commission on Acute Respiratory Diseases, and although individual cases were quite undifferentiated, the epidemiologic aspects of the outbreaks clearly indicated a specific etiologic agent.[31,122,246,621,639,675] The disease is an acute, febrile respiratory illness of short duration with constitutional and localized respiratory symptoms.[193] After an incubation period of 5 to 7 days, fever (mean temperature of 39.5°C), pharyngitis, laryngitis, tracheitis, and a nonproductive cough develop.[59,138,246,533] The initial dry, hacking cough may progress to paroxysms. Malaise, myalgia, chills, headache, dizziness, rhinitis, conjunctivitis, abdominal pain, and local cervical lymphadenopathy are common complaints.[138] The inflammatory process may spread to the bronchi, the bronchioles, and the parenchyma of the lungs. In epidemics, as many as 67% of those affected wheeze and have other evidence of small airway obstruction; pneumonia occurs in 10% to 20%.[303,412,483] The illness gradually resolves over the course of an 8- to 36-day period.[217] Early in the illness, the total WBC count may be slightly elevated, with a small increase in the percentage of polymorphonuclear leukocytes.

In experimental aerosol-induced ARD, the incubation period ranged between 6 and 13 days.[128] Typical illness included fever to 39°C, rhinitis, prostration, malaise, myalgia, and headache. Pneumonia occurred occasionally. The virus was recovered from throat culture specimens 5 days after inoculation, from the nose at 6 days, and after 9 days in fecal specimens. Serum-neutralizing antibody responses occurred between the third and fourth weeks. All ill volunteers had leukopenia and an elevated ESR during the illness.

TABLE 156.3 Clinical Spectrum of Adenoviral Infections

System/Organ	Illness Category	Epidemic Occurrence	Frequency	Adenoviral Type(s)
Respiratory	Common cold	No	Rare	1, 2, 3, 5, 7
	Nasopharyngitis, pharyngitis, and tonsillitis	Yes	Common	1,[a] 2,[a] 3,[a] 4, 5,[a] 7,[a] 7a, 14, 15, (21/H21+35)[b]
	Acute respiratory disease	Yes (in military recruits)	Very common	2, 3, 4,[a] 5, 7,[a] 8, 11, 14, 21
	Acute laryngotracheitis	No	Occasional	1, 2, 3, 5, 6, 7
	Acute bronchiolitis	No	Occasional	3, 7, 21, 60
	Pneumonia (civilian population)	Yes	Common	1, 2, 3,[a] 4, 5, 7,[a] 7a,[a] 8, 11, 14, 14p1, 21,[a] (21/H21+35),[b] 35, 55, 56
	Atypical pneumonia in military recruits	Yes	Common	4,[a] 7,[a] 14, 21
	Pertussis-like syndrome	No	Rare	1, 2, 3, 5, 12, 19
	Bronchiolitis obliterans	No	Rare	2, 3, 7, 21
	Unilateral hyperlucent lung	No	Rare	7, 21
Eye	Acute follicular conjunctivitis	Yes	Common	1, 2, 3, 4, 6, 7, 8, 9, 10, 11, 15, 16, 17, 19, 20, 22, 31, 34, 37
	Pharyngoconjunctival fever	Yes	Common	1, 2,[a] 3,[a] 4,[a] 5, 6, 7,[a] 7a,[a] 8, 14,[a] 37
	Epidemic keratoconjunctivitis	Yes	Occasional	2, 3, 4, 5, 7, 8,[a] 10, 11, 13, 14, 15, 16, 17, 19, 23, 29, 37, 54, 56
Skin	Morbilliform and rubelliform exanthem	Rare	Occasional	3, 4, 7, 7a
	Roseola-like	No	Occasional	1, 2
	Stevens-Johnson syndrome	No	Rare	7
	Petechial exanthem	No	Rare	7
Genitourinary	Acute hemorrhagic cystitis	No	Rare	7, 11, 21
	Nephritis	No	Rare	3, 4, 7a
	Orchitis	No	Rare	Unknown
	Oculogenital syndrome	Yes	Rare	19, 37
Gastrointestinal	Gastroenteritis	Yes	Common	1, 2, 3,[a] 5, 7,[a] 11, 12, 15, 17, 31,[a] 32, 33, 40,[a] 41[a]
	Mesenteric lymphadenitis	No	Rare	1, 2, 3, 5, 7
	Intussusception	No	Rare	1, 2, 3, 5, 6, 7
	Appendicitis	No	Rare	1, 2, 7
	Hepatitis	No	Rare	1, 2, 3, 5,[a] 7, (11+35/H11+35)[b]
Heart	Myocarditis	No	Rare	3, 7, 7a, 21
	Pericarditis	No	Rare	7
Neurologic	Encephalitis and meningitis	No	Rare	1, 2, 3, 4, 5, 6, 7, 11, 12, 26, 32, 41
	Transient encephalopathy	No	Rare	3
	Acute flaccid paralysis	Yes	Rare	21
Joint	Arthritis	No	Rare	7
Auditory	Deafness	No	Rare	3
Endocrine	Thyroiditis	No	Rare	Unknown

[a]Most common.
[b]Intermediate strain.

The syndrome occurs most commonly in military recruits early in basic training; illness has been documented in as many as 90% of new trainees within the first 8 weeks of arrival at a training site.[303] The usual etiologic agents are adenovirus types 4 and 7. Occasionally, epidemics have been associated with adenovirus types 3, 11, 14, and 21,[75,214,650,693] and sporadic cases have been noted in connection with adenovirus types 2, 5, and 8.[303,533] The peak seasons of illness are winter and spring.[303]

Because of the magnitude of the problem of ARD in military recruits, live attenuated adenoviral vaccines against types 4 and 7 were developed and used in all branches of the U.S. military beginning in the early 1970s.[35,261] These vaccines were used successfully until the early 1990s, when production delays occurred; subsequently, in 1995, the vaccine manufacturer stopped production. From 1999 to 2011, no vaccine was available, and epidemic disease returned to military training bases.[75,384,587,590,650,693] Although illness may occur in civilian adults, it is an uncommon event and not epidemic. In volunteer studies, subjects with serum antibody to a particular adenoviral type are protected against disease with that type of adenovirus induced by intranasal inoculation.[43,128]

Epidemic ARD has not been described in children. However, a sporadic comparative illness, usually clinically identified as acute bronchitis, is commonly the result of adenoviral infection.[741] Adenovirus type 7 is the etiologic agent most frequently found in these cases.

Acute Laryngotracheitis

On occasion, adenoviruses have been implicated as a cause of acute laryngotracheitis. In general, the croup caused by adenoviruses is not severe and often is manifested only as a barking, brassy cough. Laryngotracheitis frequently is seen in association with febrile pharyngitis, bronchiolitis, and pneumonia.[669] Epidemics have not been observed. Adenovirus types 1, 2, 3, 5, 6, and 7 have been implicated as etiologic agents.

Acute Bronchiolitis

Adenoviruses account for approximately 5% to 18% of cases of bronchiolitis in infants.[233,722] In a recent study of 143 children with adenoviral infections, the admitting diagnosis was bronchiolitis in 24%.[574] The bronchiolitis caused by adenoviral infection is sporadic and usually similar to illness associated with other viral agents. Occasionally, adenoviral bronchiolitis occurring early in infancy has been fatal or has resulted in serious residual lung damage and chronic disease.[711] This severe illness has been associated with serotypes 3, 7, and 21.

Pneumonia

Young children. Adenoviruses are common isolates in children with pneumonia. The overall frequency of adenoviruses as a cause of nonbacterial pneumonia in children is less than that of RSV and parainfluenza virus type 3, but an alarming number of fatal illnesses have been noted. Severe and fatal illnesses in infants and young children have occurred in association with adenovirus types 1, 2, 3, 4, 5, 7, 7a, 7h, 7i, 8, 19, 21, 35, and the intermediate strain 21/H21+35.* The more severe cases of pneumonia have been linked to types 3, 7, 14, 21, and 55.[86,242,250,435,614,649,725] Adenoviral pneumonia has been epidemic and sporadic.[94,101,112,182,415]

Severe pneumonia occurs most commonly in neonates and young children aged 3 to 18 months.† The onset of illness is acute, with persistent cough and fever (>39°C). On physical examination, moderate to severe dyspnea is apparent, as is the associated tachypnea. Inspiratory and expiratory wheezes and rales are heard on auscultation. Other signs and symptoms include lethargy, diarrhea and vomiting, pharyngitis, and occasionally, conjunctivitis. Extrapulmonary complications that occur commonly are meningitis, encephalitis, seizures, splenomegaly, hepatomegaly and hepatitis, myocarditis, nephritis, bleeding tendency, and exanthems.[49,77,101,124,397,612,614,629,632] Chest radiographs reveal diffuse infiltrates, which usually are bilateral and may be bronchial, peribronchial, or interstitial.[39,397,574,718] Hyperinflation and lobar collapse occur frequently.[253] Rarely, pleural effusions or mediastinal lymphadenopathy has been described.[397] In surviving infants, symptoms persist for 2 to 4 weeks, and radiographic changes resolve slowly, frequently being present at the 3-week follow-up examination.[101,112,614] Recovery often is gradual, and exacerbations occur commonly.[331,531]

Serious sequelae often result from adenoviral lower respiratory disease, particularly in association with adenovirus types 3, 7, 7a, 21, and 21a.[28,40,93,190,253,271,331,397,614] Such sequelae include bronchiectasis, bronchiolitis obliterans, and unilateral hyperlucent lung.‡ An estimated 14% to 60% of children with documented adenoviral lower respiratory tract disease have some degree of permanent pulmonary sequelae.[253,397,613,614] In a study of 27 children conducted 10 years after they had documented adenoviral type 7 pneumonia, 12 had radiographic evidence of bronchiectasis or residual pulmonary changes; 16 children had abnormal results on pulmonary function studies.[613]

Hakansson and coworkers[272] previously demonstrated increased binding of adherent *Streptococcus pneumoniae* to cultured human respiratory tract epithelial A549 cells in the presence of infection with adenovirus types 1, 2, 3, and 5, thereby postulating that adenovirus infection upregulated receptors for *Streptococcus pneumoniae*. Lebel and colleagues[404] subsequently reported 7 cases of adenoviral infection with secondary bacteremia in hospitalized children over an 8-year period, the majority (6 of 7) being immunocompetent and previously healthy. They highlighted the importance of considering secondary bacteremia as a possible complication of adenoviral infection in immunocompetent children.

Macek and associates[436] have suggested that persistent adenoviral infection may be the cause of chronic obstructive airway disease in children. They noted adenoviral antigen in bronchoalveolar lavage specimens from 31 of 34 patients with chronic disease but in no bronchoalveolar specimens from a control group. Wurzel and colleagues[730] performed adenovirus genotyping on bronchoalveolar lavage fluid samples of 245 children found to have protracted bacterial bronchitis and mild bronchiectasis (evidence of chronic endobronchial suppuration). Species C adenoviruses were the most common viruses detected comprising 23 of 24 adenovirus-positive lavage specimens.

On occasion, severe and fatal adenoviral pneumonia has been related to malnutrition, environmental crowding, or a preceding severe viral disease such as measles.[28,40,39,253,393,499,614]

Severe adenoviral pneumonia associated with adenovirus types 3 and 7 also has been reported occasionally in previously healthy adults.[537,548,619] One adult had severe pneumonia caused by adenovirus type 21 that was associated with myalgia, rhabdomyolysis, and myoglobinuria.[726] Hage and colleagues[271] reported on six cases of severe pneumonia between 2005 and 2013 in Germany due to human adenovirus type 21a, the difference from adenovirus type 21 being a unique 15–amino acid sequence deletion and a 2–amino acid sequence in the RGD loop resembling the RGD loop of adenovirus types 3 and 7.

Atypical pneumonia in military recruits. Approximately 7% to 20% of cases of pneumonia in military recruits are associated with adenoviral infection.[80,210,239] Primary atypical adenoviral pneumonia commonly occurs in the winter months and generally is caused by adenovirus types 4, 7, and 21.[210] The illness is associated with fever, cough, sore throat, rhinorrhea, and chest pain. Other common symptoms include nausea, vomiting, myalgia, headache, and diarrhea. On physical examination, rales and pharyngitis are present in almost all cases. Rhinitis and generalized lymphadenopathy are observed in approximately half of those afflicted, and occasionally conjunctivitis is noted. Chest radiographs reveal a bilaterally mottled appearance, most prominent in the lower lobes; they remain abnormal for 4 to 36 days.[80] Although serum cold agglutinins are observed, titers of 1:32 or higher are detected in only 18% of patients.[80,239]

Fatal pneumonia, absolute leukopenia, and disseminated disease have been reported in four previously healthy military trainees. Adenovirus type 7 was the etiologic agent in three of these cases, and the fourth illness was caused by adenovirus type 4.[169,412]

Pertussis-like syndrome. A pertussis-like illness has been noted in association with several adenoviruses, including types 1, 2, 3, 5, 12, and 19.[121,123,280,503,516] The illness occurs commonly in children younger than 36 months. The onset of illness is insidious and initially suggestive of a cold. The cough becomes progressively worse and, by 1 to 2 weeks, is paroxysmal. Severe recurrent episodes of paroxysms result in the production of mucus, posttussive fatigue, and vomiting.[123] Approximately 50% of children have a typical whoop, and cyanosis occurs with the paroxysms. Peripheral leukocytosis with WBC counts ranging from 25,000 to 125,000 cells/mm^3, along with lymphocytosis and thrombocytosis, is the usual finding.[121,516] The recovery time ranges from 4 to 10 weeks from the onset of illness.[123] Radiologic evidence of bronchiolitis is present in most children; interstitial pneumonia occurs occasionally. In our opinion most, and probably all, of these pertussis-like illnesses are indeed *Bordetella pertussis* infections in which adenovirus is a coinfecting agent (see Chapter 129). In young infants, coinfection (adenovirus plus *B. pertussis*) may lead to more severe disease.[41,414,453]

Bronchiolitis obliterans. Bronchiolitis obliterans is a chronic bronchiolitis that initially was described in 1901 by Lange.[398] It has been noted to occur after measles, influenza, and pertussis, as well as after the inhalation of toxic substances.[28,40,722] Adenovirus types 2, 3, 7, and 21 have resulted in a bronchiolitis obliterans–type chronic illness.[6,28,40,93,474,544,711,722] These adenoviruses cause a severe necrotizing bronchiolitis that heals with fibrosis and predominantly obliterates the small airways.[35] The onset of disease is characterized by an acute febrile illness, cough, and respiratory distress. Disease may wax and wane for several weeks or months and is associated with recurrent episodes of atelectasis, pneumonia, and wheezing. Although some children recover from these episodes, the remainder have chronic pulmonary disease, including irreversible atelectasis, bronchiectasis, or hyperlucent lung syndrome.[40,711,722]

Castro-Rodriguez and colleagues[93] conducted a 5-year follow-up study of 38 children hospitalized with adenoviral pneumonia during an outbreak in Santiago, Chile, in 1998. Bronchiolitis obliterans developed in almost 50% of these children. Nosocomial acquisition of adenoviral infection was found to be associated more significantly with the development of bronchiolitis obliterans than community-acquired infection was. Murtagh and colleagues conducted a retrospective review of 415 children with lower respiratory infection caused by adenoviruses. They found that risk factors for the development of bronchiolitis obliterans included prolonged hospitalization (>30 days), multifocal pneumonia, and hypercapnia.[490] Wu and colleagues[728] identified hypoxemia as an independent predictor of bronchiolitis obliterans in a retrospective study of 544 hospitalized children with acute respiratory infection due to adenovirus in China.

Unilateral hyperlucent lung. Unilateral hyperlucent lung is a well-defined syndrome characterized by increased translucency of all or part of one

*References 17, 39, 40, 49, 77, 78, 101, 112, 146, 153, 232, 253, 305, 331, 352, 353, 374, 375, 377, 393, 401, 432, 450, 474, 475, 488, 512, 531, 544, 545, 565, 612, 614, 629, 632, 725.

†References 39, 40, 77, 78, 93, 124, 153, 190, 253, 352, 377, 397, 450, 545, 565.

‡References 28, 40, 93, 190, 397, 437, 474, 544, 614, 722.

lung, along with a reduction in lung size.[133,437] The unilateral hyperlucency is associated with a decrease in the size and number of pulmonary vessels, as observed on pulmonary angiograms, and an absence of peripheral filling at bronchography.[437] Although the disease may have a number of causes, including pneumonia secondary to other viruses, it has been noted to occur after severe necrotizing bronchiolitis and pneumonia caused by adenovirus types 7 and 21.[437,722]

Eye

Acute Follicular Conjunctivitis

Acute follicular conjunctivitis is the most common and benign of the adenoviral infections of the eye. The infection in this disease is confined to the eye, generally is unilateral, and is manifested by follicular lesions on the palpebral conjunctival surface. Symptoms occur after an incubation period of 5 to 7 days and include lacrimation, itching, burning, a foreign body sensation, and conjunctival erythema.[150] It should be noted that, although the preceding symptoms increase the likelihood of viral infection, rather than bacteria, the diagnosis by clinical symptoms alone can be difficult to make. Examination shows erythema and lymphoid follicular hyperplasia in the conjunctiva in association with serous drainage and increased lacrimation. Occasionally, adenopathy of the preauricular lymph nodes is seen. Symptoms resolve in 10 days to 3 weeks, with recovery usually complete.[127,150] Adenovirus types 1, 2, 3, 4, 6, 7, 8, 9, 10, 11, 15, 16, 17, 19, 20, 22, 30, 31, 34, and 37 have been isolated from the eyes of afflicted patients.[64,124,150,190,443,597,604,668]

Pharyngoconjunctival Fever

By definition, pharyngoconjunctival fever is a syndrome characterized by fever, pharyngitis, and conjunctivitis. During epidemics, not all patients have the complete syndrome triad. For purposes of this discussion, all descriptions of frequency of signs and symptoms are calculated from the starting point of 100% fever, pharyngitis, and conjunctivitis.

Tables 156.4 and 156.5 summarize the frequencies of specific symptoms and signs.* The usual onset of illness is abrupt, with sore throat, generalized aches and pains, eye irritation or pain, and fever. Throat complaints vary from mild to severe. On examination, the tonsils and pharyngeal lymphoid tissue are hypertrophied with pharyngeal redness varying considerably from patient to patient. Approximately one-third of affected patients have follicular exudative lesions that cannot be differentiated from streptococcal disease on clinical grounds. Hypertrophy of the adenoids occurs, which may result in nasal blockage. Coryza and posterior nasal discharge are common, leading to cough in many instances.

With respect to conjunctivitis, most patients note some aching or soreness; photophobia and lacrimation are unusual. The appearance of the palpebral conjunctiva usually is granular. The lesions may be almost microscopic or 2 to 3 mm in diameter. Hemorrhages occasionally are noted on the bulbar surface. Frequently, involvement starts in one eye and does not involve the other eye until 2 or 3 days later. Occasionally, the involvement is restricted to one eye.

Compared with other respiratory viral infections, the duration of illness with pharyngoconjunctival fever is long. In most patients, the fever is sustained or remittent for 3 to 4 days. However, approximately 10% of patients have fever that lasts longer than 7 days. Throat and eye findings usually are improved considerably by the seventh day of illness, but these findings and nasal complaints, fatigue, and headache may persist for 14 days.

In epidemic pharyngoconjunctival fever, the most likely etiologic agent is adenovirus type 3.† The next most prevalent adenovirus associated with epidemic disease is type 7.[85,172,209,735] One or more epidemics also have been noted with adenoviruses 2, 4, 7a, 11, and 14.[11,16,43,135,177,180,500,680,741] Sporadic occurrences of pharyngoconjunctival

*References 11, 16, 20, 31, 34, 42, 43, 47, 120, 172, 180, 208, 209, 222–225, 320, 334, 344, 345–348, 369, 379, 380, 464, 500, 515, 518, 633, 632, 634, 676, 680, 700, 708.

†References 34, 43, 45, 47, 120, 215, 223, 225, 334, 347, 348, 361, 380, 447, 460, 515, 535, 632, 680, 734, 741.

TABLE 156.4 Frequency of Symptoms in Epidemic Pharyngoconjunctival Fever

Symptoms	Frequency
Throat Complaints	++++
Soreness	++++
Cough	++
Foreign body sensation	++
Dry feeling	+
Eye Complaints	+++
Aching or soreness	+++
Burning sensation	++
Lacrimation	+
Photophobia	+
Nasal Complaints	+++
Coryza	++
Stuffiness or blockage or both	++
Sneezing	+
Epistaxis	+
Other Complaints	++++
Headache	++++
Anorexia	+++
Malaise	++
Generalized aches and pains	++
Nausea	++
Vomiting	+
Diarrhea	+
Abdominal pain	+

++++, 76–100%; +++, 51–75%; ++, 26–50%; +, 1–2%.
Data from References 20, 42, 85, 209, 223, 347, 369, 376, 447, 535, 621, 680.

TABLE 156.5 Frequency of Signs in Epidemic Pharyngoconjunctival Fever

Signs	Frequency
Throat Findings	++++
Erythema and infection	++++
Hypertrophied lymphatic tissue	++++
Particulate exudate	++
Eye Findings	++++
Erythema and infection of palpebral and bulbar conjunctiva	++++
Edema	+++
Granular and follicular involvement	++
Eyes unequally affected	++
Superficial punctate keratitis	+
Lymph Node Enlargement	++++
Cervical	++++
Preauricular	+
Generalized	+
Fever	++++
≥39°C (≥102.2°F)	+++
Other	
Flushed face	+++
Enlarged liver or spleen or both	+

++++, 76–100%; +++, 51–75%; ++, 26–50%; +, 1–25%.
Data from References 20, 42, 85, 209, 223, 278, 376, 535, 621, 680.

fever have been observed in association with infections with adenoviruses 1, 2, 3, 4, 5, 6, 7, 7a, 8, 14, 19, and 13/30 (an intermediate type).*

Epidemic Keratoconjunctivitis

Epidemic keratoconjunctivitis is caused most commonly by adenovirus type 8, but it also has resulted from infection with adenovirus types 2, 3, 4, 5, 7, 10, 11, 13, 14, 15, 16, 17, 19, 22, 23, 29, 37, 53, 54, and 56.† Currently, adenovirus type 37 is the virus most commonly recovered from patients with epidemic keratoconjunctivitis in the United States and Europe. The most severe disease is associated with adenovirus types 5, 8, and 19.[137] More recently in Japan, adenovirus 54 and 56 have been recovered from patients with epidemic keratoconjunctivitis.[10,326]

The illness occurs most commonly in adults, but a few cases have been reported in children.[281,476,647] It has no seasonal pattern. Although transmission of the viral agent from the respiratory tract to the eye occurs in sporadic cases, the usual method of viral spread is by contaminated ophthalmic instruments and eye solutions, hand-to-eye contact by medical personnel and others, swimming pools, or hands or fomites in close-contact situations, such as in families and in industry.‡ The incubation period typically is 5 to 10 days but ranges from as short a period as 2 days to as long as 2 weeks.[139,381] The initial symptom generally is unilateral, acute, follicular conjunctivitis that suggests the presence of a foreign body. Photophobia, lacrimation, discharge, hyperemia, and edema of the conjunctiva are notable. Preauricular adenopathy occurs in as many as 90% of patients, and 50% of those afflicted have pharyngitis and rhinitis. Spread to the other eye may occur in 2 to 7 days. Seven to 10 days after onset of the disease, the conjunctivitis resolves, and painful, superficial, punctate epithelial opacities appear in the center of the cornea. These lesions frequently extend subepithelially and then heal, with subepithelial infiltrates left behind that may persist for months. In severe cases, hazy vision may continue for several years.[33]

An infantile form of epidemic keratoconjunctivitis has been described that usually affects children younger than 2 years old.[181] This pseudomembranous or membranous conjunctivitis generally is accompanied by high fever, pharyngitis, otitis media, diarrhea, and vomiting. Preauricular lymphadenopathy typically is absent.[647]

Virus can be recovered from the eye for a usual period of approximately 2 weeks but has been detected for 2 to 3 years in patients with chronic papillary conjunctivitis.[137,543] In acute illness, conjunctival scrapings obtained during the first 10 days of infection reveal characteristic inclusion bodies when stained with Giemsa.[291] Virus-specific fluorescent antibody staining is diagnostic in epidemic keratoconjunctivitis.[602] Preparations of corneal and conjunctival epithelia reveal adenoviral particles when examined with the electron microscope.[144]

Skin

Adenovirus types 1, 2, 3, 4, 7, and 7a, plus several unknown types, have been noted in connection with exanthematous disease.[106] The cutaneous manifestation most commonly associated with adenoviral infection is an erythematous maculopapular rash that appears while the child is febrile. In many instances, children with this illness have been thought to have either measles or rubella.[393] In most adenoviral infections with exanthems, other clinical findings more characteristic of adenoviruses, such as conjunctivitis, rhinitis, pharyngitis, and lymphadenopathy, also are present. In some instances, the exanthem truly is morbilliform with a characteristic confluence, but Koplik spots do not occur.

A widespread erythematous rash often is present early in the course of severe pneumonia in infants.[253] Chany and colleagues[101] noted a measles-like rash in five patients who died of adenovirus type 7a pneumonia. One report describes a child with an adenovirus type 7 infection and illness suggestive of meningococcemia.[592] This patient had fever, vomiting, diarrhea, and a petechial exanthem. Rocholl and associates[574] noted that rash occurred in 10 percent of 143 adenoviral illnesses in children.

*References 31, 42, 43, 104, 214, 225, 280, 290, 320, 345, 369, 379, 464, 597, 602, 633, 634, 640, 674, 676, 691, 707.

†References 33, 64, 83, 97,128, 137, 139, 142, 144, 145, 181, 193, 270, 276, 281, 335, 337, 360, 364, 367, 435, 462, 476, 479, 505, 507, 597, 626, 631, 648, 738.

‡References 33, 83, 97, 137, 139, 142, 207, 335, 381, 447, 476, 479, 647, 709.

On several occasions, illness characterized by fever and defervescence and then the appearance of a maculopapular rash suggesting the diagnosis of roseola infantum has been observed.[208,222,333,334,504] Adenoviral infections also are confused with rubella. However, the respiratory symptoms and the degree of fever associated with adenoviral infection should clarify the diagnosis. With rubella, respiratory complaints and fever are minimal. On occasion, severe disease with Stevens-Johnson syndrome has been noted. Such patients frequently have pneumonia, and the illness is quite similar to that caused by *Mycoplasma pneumoniae*.

Lähdeaho and associates[396] have noted that serum antibodies to the E1b protein–derived peptides of the enteric adenovirus type 40 are associated with dermatitis herpetiformis. Keyes and coworkers[370] reported a case of a woman who underwent T-cell–depleted peripheral blood hematopoietic stem cell transplant that was complicated by EBV-associated posttransplant lymphoproliferative disorder and disseminated adenovirus infection. She underwent skin punch biopsy for a pruritic, burning rash described as 2- to 3-mm erythematous papules on the palms, some having a vesicle-like appearance, which, on closer inspection, revealed a firm keratotic plug. Biopsy demonstrated epidermal hyperplasia with a column of parakeratosis. Underlying and adjacent keratinocytes had focal acantholytic dyskeratosis with several keratinocytes having hyperchromatic nuclei. Mild interface dermatitis was also present. Immunohistochemical staining of the hyperchromatic nuclei was positive for adenovirus.

Genitourinary Tract

Acute Hemorrhagic Cystitis

Acute hemorrhagic cystitis is an uncommon manifestation of adenoviral infection in immunocompetent children and is characterized by a sudden onset of dysuria and frequency, with hematuria developing 12 to 24 hours later.[403,407,441,484,485,510] Occasionally, fever, suprapubic pain, and enuresis occur. Antecedent upper respiratory tract infection is noted in some children. Symptoms persist for a few days to 2 weeks, with the usual duration being approximately 5 days. Acute hemorrhagic cystitis has been reported in both the United States and Japan. It occurs primarily in children, most often boys, and usually is associated with adenovirus type 11. Occasionally, adenovirus types 7 and 21 have been implicated. Adenoviral antigen has been identified by immunofluorescence in exfoliated bladder cells. Although no sequelae have been reported, the long-term prognosis is unknown.[484] Montaruli and colleagues[478] reported the case of a 14-year-old boy who underwent allogeneic bone marrow transplantation for refractory acute lymphoblastic leukemia. He developed acute hemorrhagic cystitis 4 weeks after transplant, complicated by adenovirus-induced obstructive uropathy and acute renal failure. The child eventually recovered but required temporary placement of a double J stent in order to relieve the obstruction.

Nephritis

Hematuria occasionally has been reported in infants with severe pneumonia and disseminated adenoviral infection. Red blood cells and, at times, red blood cell casts also have been noted in the urine of some children with upper respiratory illnesses caused by adenoviruses and specifically in patients with pharyngoconjunctival fever associated with adenovirus types 3, 4, and 7a.[621,630,676,680] In one instance, a young boy had a maculopapular and petechial exanthem and thrombocytopenia associated with adenovirus type 7 infection. Hematuria also was present.

Orchitis

Orchitis developed in one child who had a 5-day history of pain and fever, erythema, and swelling of the right testicle.[502] The testicular involvement resolved in several days, and the illness was associated with a 16-fold rise in adenoviral complement-fixation antibody titer.

Oculogenital Syndrome

In 1977, Laverty and associates[403] reported a woman who, in addition to pharyngoconjunctival fever, had cervicitis and paresthesia of the legs; a type 19 adenovirus was recovered from this woman's cervix. In Perth, Australia, adenovirus type 19 was recovered from the genital tracts of 59 men and women being examined for genital HSV infection in a clinic for sexually transmitted diseases.[325] Several of the patients also had conjunctivitis, and in two, adenovirus type 19 was isolated from conjunctival specimens. Similar oculogenital illnesses have been noted in association with adenoviral types 2, 8, and 37.[96,597,642]

Hemolytic-Uremic Syndrome

Two 2-year-old children with hemolytic-uremic syndrome in association with adenoviral infections have been described.[58]

Hemorrhagic Fever With Renal Syndrome

A 22-year-old woman with an adenovirus type 11 infection and hemorrhagic fever with renal syndrome has been reported.[671]

Gastrointestinal Tract

Gastroenteritis

Infantile diarrhea has been associated with epidemic and sporadic adenoviral diseases such as acute upper respiratory tract infection, severe pneumonia, and pharyngoconjunctival fever.[208,397,621,634,714] Outbreaks of diarrhea characterized by acute abdominal pain followed by diarrhea, nausea and vomiting, fever, headache, and pharyngitis have been associated with adenovirus type 3 and 7 infections.[235,633] Other symptoms occurring in patients with diarrhea include conjunctivitis, rhinitis, pharyngotonsillitis, hepatomegaly, and cervical adenitis.[634] In two patients who had diarrhea and upper respiratory illness in association with adenovirus type 15 infection, viral particles were visualized within the nuclei of mucosal cells at autopsy by electron microscopy.[170]

The widespread use of electron microscopy for the study of rotaviral diarrhea led to the finding of previously unrecognized adenoviruses that were fastidious and could not be grown in routine cell cultures.[182,601] These adenoviruses, now identified as types 40 and 41, subsequently were shown to be important causes of gastroenteritis in children.* In enteric adenoviral infection, diarrhea is the most prominent symptom.[668] In children with adenovirus type 40 infection, Uhnoo and colleagues[669] found that the mean duration was 8.6 days, as opposed to 12.2 days in those infected with adenovirus type 41. Most illnesses occur in children younger than 3 years old: the mean age for adenovirus type 40 diarrhea was 15.2 months, whereas it was 28.3 months in type 41 illnesses. Most patients had mild vomiting that lasted approximately 2 days. When compared with illnesses caused by established respiratory adenoviruses, fever occurred less commonly, was less severe, and had a shorter duration in enteric adenoviral infections. Upper respiratory symptoms and signs, such as pharyngitis, coryza, cough, and otitis media, were observed in 21% of children with enteric adenoviral infection. Brandt and colleagues[71] noted that dual infections with respiratory viruses (such as RSV and enteric adenoviruses) are common occurrences, so caution should be observed in attributing respiratory symptoms to enteric adenoviruses. Chhabra and colleagues[109] conducted active population-based surveillance of 782 children under 5 years of age presenting with acute gastroenteritis to hospitals, emergency departments, and primary care clinics as compared to 499 healthy controls in Ohio, New York, and Tennessee. Adenovirus was detected in 11.8% of children with gastroenteritis versus 1.8% of healthy controls. Coinfection was seen in 13.1% of specimens, with *Norovirus* being the most frequently associated virus.

Yolken and Franklin[743] found that enteric adenoviruses were an important cause of nosocomial diarrhea in infants who had previously undergone gastrointestinal surgery for necrotizing enterocolitis. Stockmann and colleagues[635] evaluated stool pathogens via multiplex PCR assay among 779 children with 1089 diarrheal episodes. Adenovirus types 40 and 41 were the second most commonly detected virus, with 6% detected in hospitalized patients, 5% detected in the outpatient setting, and 10% detected in the emergency department. Liu and coworkers[424] reanalyzed data from the Global Enteric Multicenter Study of moderate to severe diarrhea in children younger than 5 years in Africa and Asia. Not surprisingly, they found a greater pathogen incidence using molecular techniques for diagnosis (5 times the originally reported incidence). The attributable incidence of adenovirus 40/41 infection in infants was 3.9 epsiodes per 100 child-years and 1.8 episodes per 100 child-years in toddlers. Mhaissen and colleagues[467] conducted a study of 114 episodes of diarrheal illness in 93 pediatric oncology patients. Ninety-five percent of patients had one or more enteropathogens with adenovirus identified among 15% of patients. They found that patients with more than one pathogen had a longer duration of illness and greater likelihood of dehydration.

*References 72, 76, 116, 154, 155, 254, 389, 391, 472, 514, 524, 575, 655, 669, 673.

Mesenteric Lymphadenitis

Adenoviral serotypes 1, 2, 3, 5, and 7 have been recovered from lymph nodes and the appendix in cases of mesenteric lymphadenitis.[46,63,379] Patients with mesenteric lymphadenitis often have abdominal pain and other symptoms similar to those of acute appendicitis. Pharyngitis is a frequently related finding. Mesenteric adenitis often is associated with concurrent or recent adenoviral illness.[124,555] Frequently, the peak incidence of mesenteric lymphadenitis occurs when adenoviral illness is common in the community.

Intussusception

The suggestion that adenoviruses could be an etiologic factor in intussusception arose because these agents frequently can be recovered from throat, stool, and mesenteric lymph node specimens obtained from children who undergo surgery for intussusception.* Most children with intussusception were younger than 2 years old; some had preceding respiratory symptoms.[582,746] Adenovirus serotypes 1, 2, 3, 5, 6, and 7 have been implicated. Typical adenoviral intranuclear inclusions have been demonstrated in cells in stool, intestinal epithelia (ileum), and the appendix by electron microscopy.[511,746,747] Mesenteric lymph nodes often are enlarged at surgery.[523] Increases in antibody titer to adenoviruses have been observed in children after the development of intussusception. Ukarapol and coworkers[670] conducted a prospective cohort study of patients with intussusception using patients with acute gastroenteritis as controls. Viral infection was identified in 16 of 40 cases of intussusception seen over a 2-year period. Of the 16 cases where viral infection was implicated, adenovirus subtype C infection was identified in 12 cases (30%). They found that adenovirus infection was higher in the intussusception group as compared to the acute gastroenteritis group, which was statistically significant. Investigators have suggested that bowel wall hypermotility caused by direct viral involvement or by hypertrophy of lymphatic tissue is the lead point for the intussusception.[46,119,234,511,552,582,746,747]

Appendicitis

Adenoviruses have been associated with both acute and chronic appendicitis.[63] Right iliac fossa abdominal pain in conjunction with sore throat is a common finding. The virus has been isolated from the appendix and mesenteric lymph nodes at surgery. During acute infection, lymphoid follicles of the ileum, appendix, and mesenteric lymph nodes are infected with virus. In chronic infection, adenovirus remains in cells; on microscopic examination, slight inflammation is seen in the appendix.

Hepatitis

Hepatitis in association with adenoviral infection has been reported many times in small infants, in children with overwhelming disseminated disease, and in immunocompromised patients.[4,22,49,77,91,375,749] In one study, 27 of 30 persons thought to have sporadic infectious hepatitis were found to be infected with adenovirus type 5.[282] Adenovirus types 1, 2, and 3 were isolated from the stool specimens of 12 children younger than 3 years old in an outbreak of infectious hepatitis on a Native American reservation in Arizona.[284]

In one report, three children with severe, fatal adenovirus type 7 pneumonia had associated findings that simulated Reye syndrome: lethargy, diarrhea, seizures, elevated CSF pressure, myocarditis, hepatitis, and disseminated intravascular coagulation.[395] Edwards and colleagues[175] reported three children with Reye syndrome and adenoviral infection. They suggested that adenoviruses might be an important agent in initiating the syndrome. Few cases of adenovirus hepatitis in immunocompetent pediatric patients have been reported, with two reports of death due to fulminant hepatic failure, one with associated encephalopathy.[488,538,574]

*References 46, 52, 119, 234, 317, 511, 548, 582, 746, 747.

Matoq and Salahuddin[448] reported the case of a previously healthy immunocompetent 23-month-old who developed acute noncholestatic hepatitis, hypoalbuminemia, anasarca, and pancytopenia associated with adenovirus infection and who eventually improved with supportive care. Ronan and colleagues[578] conducted a review of 89 cases of adenovirus hepatitis among transplant recipients reported in the English literature from 1960 to 2012. They noted that 90% of infections occurred within 6 months after transplant, with 47% of infections occurring within the first month after transplant. Biopsy-confirmed histologic findings included hepatic necrosis (94%), intranuclear inclusions (72%), and smudge cells (21%). They highlighted the potential for the development of fatal fulminant hepatic failure due to adenovirus in solid organ transplant recipients that mimics that of fulminant hepatic disease due to herpes simplex virus infection. Kawashima and colleagues[363] noted that elevation of γ-glutamyltransferase (GGT) without any specified causes preceded adenoviral hepatitis by 2 weeks in their case review, concluding that GGT may be a useful sentinel marker for adenoviral hepatitis. Van Montfrans and coworkers[683] postulated that intestinal viral infection prior to transplant was a predictor for the development of acute intestinal graft-versus-host disease in 48 patients undergoing allogeneic hematopoietic stem cell transplantation. Among 15 of 48 patients with viruses detected in stool by PCR, 60% of cases had adenovirus infections.

Heart

Myocarditis

In children, myocarditis has been noted in association with severe pneumonia and disseminated disease caused by adenovirus types 7, 7a, and 21.[287,292] Similar cardiac involvement has been seen in military recruits with severe ARD.[101,112,287,621] One case of sudden death in an 11-year-old boy due to myocarditis with adenovirus type 3 has been documented.[661]

The use of polymerase chain reaction (PCR) assays has led to recognition of adenovirus as the cause of many cases of acute myocarditis.[65,73,267,433,445] In an extensive study of myocarditis and dilated cardiomyopathy, Bowles and coworkers[65] analyzed 773 endomyocardial biopsy samples obtained from patients of all ages. In this large group, 624 patients had myocarditis, and adenoviral DNA was identified by PCR in 142 (23%) of the endomyocardial biopsy samples. There were 26 neonates, 37 infants, 20 toddlers, 25 older children, 11 adolescents, and 23 adults. The results of this study suggest that adenoviruses are the leading viral cause of myocarditis, with enteroviruses being the second most common association (14%). On histopathologic examination, only 57 (40%) of the enterovirus-positive samples were found to be acute myocarditis. Simpson and colleagues[615] conducted a multicenter study of 21 pediatric patients with clinical myocarditis looking for detectable blood viral PCR within 6 weeks of symptom onset. They noted that 89% of positive blood viral PCRs were found in infants 12 months and younger with clinical myocarditis versus 3.5% of control patients. Nine patients had detectable viral PCR with one due to adenovirus (~11%).

Dilated Cardiomyopathy

In the study by Bowles and associates,[65] specimens from 149 patients exhibited dilated cardiomyopathy. Of this subgroup, 18 (12%) had adenoviral DNA demonstrated by PCR in the endomyocardial biopsy specimen. Of these 18 samples, 2 were from neonates, 2 from infants, 2 from toddlers, 4 from older children, 2 from adolescents, and 6 from adults. In a study in adults, 28 explanted hearts from patient undergoing transplant for dilated cardiomyopathy yielded adenovirus type 3 in 25% of cases by nested PCR.[651]

Pericarditis

Pericarditis has been associated with severe adenoviral pneumonia. In a patient with adenovirus type 7 pneumonia, electrocardiographic changes consistent with pericarditis were demonstrated, and the virus was isolated in high titer from pericardial fluid at postmortem examination.[499] In 1995, Mistchenko and coworkers[473] reported a 10-month-old boy with fatal pericarditis caused by adenovirus type 7. In serum and pericardial fluid from this child, interleukin-6, tumor necrosis factor-α, and adenovirus-specific immune complexes were identified.

Nervous System

Although CNS disease in adenoviral infection is an uncommon finding, a variety of clinical manifestations have been observed. Both meningitis and encephalitis have been noted as the major manifestations of adenoviral infection or in association with severe disease at other body sites.[508,512] Huang and coworkers[318] found that 3.3% of 3298 children less than 18 years of age with positive throat cultures for adenovirus between 2000 to 2008 had symptoms of CNS infection with seizure, altered level of consciousness, headache, and visual hallucinations. Adenovirus types 1, 2, 3, 5, 6, 7, 12, 26, and 32, in isolated instances, have been recovered from both brain and CSF.*

Reyes-Andrade and colleagues[564] reported a case of adenovirus meningoencephalitis in a previously healthy 15-month-old girl whose presentation mimicked that of bacterial sepsis with petechial rash. They reviewed 18 publications on presumed CNS disease due to adenovirus over the past 4 decades. Among the 92 children involved, there were 57 cases of encephalitis, 12 cases of encephalopathy, 13 cases of meningitis, 9 cases of meningoencephalitis, and 1 case of cerebellitis. Meningoencephalitis often occurs as part of disseminated adenoviral disease in immunocompromised patients, with the most commonly associated serotypes being 2, 3, 5, and 7. Adenovirus serotype 26 DNA was identified in peripheral blood, CSF, urine, and postmortem brain tissue of a 28-year-old woman undergoing radiation therapy for medulloblastoma; progressive neurologic deterioration developed, followed by her eventual death as a result of disseminated adenoviral infection.[165] In two children with respiratory and CNS symptoms, adenoviruses were recovered from spinal fluid.[194] One child was convalescing from herpes zoster and the other from varicella. Adenovirus type 7 was recovered from brain tissue cultures from an elderly patient with chronic schizophrenia.[432] In another instance, adenovirus type 32 was recovered from the brain of a man with lymphosarcoma and subacute encephalitis.[115,579] In an epidemic of adenoviral infection caused by type 7, 25% of the hospitalized patients had symptoms referable to the CNS.[612,614] Many of the patients died; those who survived had little residual effect.

Too few cases are reported in the literature to predict the prognosis of CNS disease in children accurately. Adenovirus type 2 was isolated from a muscle biopsy specimen from a patient with inclusion body myositis.[469] Ooi and colleagues[517] reported eight children with adenovirus serotype 21–associated acute flaccid paralysis in the setting of an enterovirus 71–mediated hand, foot, and mouth disease outbreak in Sarawak, Malaysia, in 1997. Of these eight children, four had upper limb monoparesis, two had lower limb monoparesis, and two had paraparesis. Four of the children experienced complete recovery, one was improving at hospital discharge, and three had residual flaccid weakness and wasting. Seven children with initially appearing typical adenoviral infections had transient encephalopathy.[637] All these children were infected with adenovirus type 3. On initial evaluation, five had pneumonia, one had follicular tonsillitis, and one suffered from diarrhea. Three of the children were lethargic, two were stuporous, and two were obtunded. All had elevated serum aspartate aminotransferase values (range, 39 to 401 U/L), and CSF evaluations were within normal limits. The neurologic findings resolved in all patients in about 1 week.

Syrbe and colleagues reported a case of adenovirus-associated opsoclonus-myoclonus syndrome due to adenovirus type 3.[643] Awosika and colleagues[27] reported a fatal case of adenovirus meningoencephalitis that rapidly progressed to myeloradiculitis in an adult patient 6 months after umbilical cord stem cell transplantation for T-cell polymorphic leukemia. Naselli and coworkers[501] reported a case of acute postinfectious cerebella ataxia mimicking myositis due to human herpesvirus-6 and adenovirus in a previously healthy 4-year-old boy who presented with acute onset of lower extremity pain and refusal to walk.

Infection in Immunocompromised Hosts

Adenovirus types 1, 2, 3, 4, 5, 6, 7, 7a, 11, 29, 31, 32, 34, and 35 have been recovered from children and adults who were immunocompromised by

*References 103, 124, 131, 165, 194, 228, 366, 529, 542, 579, 632, 640, 679.

immunodeficiency diseases, malignancies, steroid therapy, immunosuppressive therapy, radiation therapy, and transplantation procedures.* Adenoviral infections occur more frequently in pediatric than in adult hematopoietic stem cell and solid organ transplant recipients.[32,308,316] Infection is thought to occur as a result of transmission from the donor, reactivation of latent infection, or newly acquired infection.[392] McLaughlin and colleagues[459] examined the incidence of adenovirus infection in 146 children who underwent liver and intestinal transplants. They found that adenoviral infection occurred in 4.1% of liver transplant recipients and 20.8% of intestinal transplant recipients.

In a study of eight children with liver and small bowel transplants and six with just small bowel transplants, Pinchoff and coworkers[547] noted that all had evidence of adenoviral infection of the graft. In eight of the children, histologic evidence of infection (adenoviral intranuclear inclusions) developed, and these eight had received intensive corticosteroid therapy, had virus isolated from multiple sites, and had persistent positive viral cultures. In a retrospective review of 110 small bowel and liver (combined) transplants in 98 children by Florescu and colleagues, adenovirus infection was found in 38 transplants. Twenty-three of these developed invasive disease, and over 80% occurred within the first year of transplant. In this series, the presence of adenovirus did not have an effect on all-cause mortality.[205] For most solid organ transplants, the source of invasive adenoviral disease often is thought to be the transplanted organ.

Kampmann and colleagues[355] conducted a prospective study on 155 pediatric stem cell transplant recipients and identified 17% with adenoviremia (26/155). Their study showed that early detection of adenoviremia, withdrawal of immunosuppression, and early antiviral therapy led to resolution of adenoviremia in 81% of the patients. de Mezerville and collaborators[149] retrospectively identified 28 solid organ transplant recipients and 27 hematopoietic stem cell transplant recipients with adenovirus infection at the Hospital for Sick Children in Toronto, Canada. Their study found a similar rate of posttransplant adenoviral infection in solid organ transplant recipients (50.9%) and hematopoietic stem cell transplant recipients (49.1%). de Mezerville's group found a much higher mortality rate in the group of hematopoietic stem cell transplant recipients (30% mortality rate vs. 0% in the solid organ transplant group). Using PCR, Bil-Lula and colleagues reviewed adenovirus infection in 116 patients (98 children, 18 adults) who underwent stem cell transplant. Infection was found in 52 patients (44.8%). Although overall mortality in infected patients was 19%, this did not differ significantly from uninfected patients.[56,179]

Control of adenovirus infection is thought to be T-cell mediated, and patients receiving T-cell–suppressive regimens are thought to be at greater risk for adenovirus disease.[710] Myers and colleagues[492] demonstrated an increased risk for the development of adenoviral infection in bone marrow transplant recipients receiving alemtuzumab (Campath 1H), a monoclonal antibody used for T-cell depletion, in comparison to patients receiving antithymocyte globulin (ATG), which was composed of polyclonal antibodies directed toward T cells. Avivi and colleagues[26] demonstrated that the most important risk factors for progression of adenovirus disease included severe lymphocytopenia (absolute lymphocyte count of less than 200/mm^3) and continued immunosuppression. They also found a correlation between lack of cytomegalovirus (CMV) prophylaxis with ganciclovir and risk of progression of adenovirus disease.

Ahmad and coworkers[8] reported a case of severe adenovirus pneumonia developing after infused infliximab (Remicade) was used to treat a 35-year-old man with Crohn's disease. Infliximab is a monoclonal antibody directed against tumor necrosis factor-α that is used frequently in the treatment of autoimmune and rheumatologic diseases. Ahmad's group emphasized the fact that tumor necrosis factor-α antagonists can impair cell-mediated immunity, an essential component of recovery from adenoviral infection in immunocompromised hosts and therefore can predispose patients to the development of viral pneumonia.

*References 4, 32, 38, 88, 91, 115, 136, 141, 192, 198, 204, 238, 264, 273, 285, 294, 349, 365, 420, 431, 491, 506, 513, 530, 547, 579, 607–610, 616, 625, 663, 689, 717, 742, 749.

Other groups have demonstrated that having low lymphocyte counts at the time of development of adenovirus infection was predictive of adenovirus viremia and that clearance of infection and host survival were dependent on recovery of adenovirus-specific CD4$^+$ T-cell responses.[285,685,710] Lankester and colleagues[400] showed that isolation of adenovirus from multiple sites was associated with the development of adenovirus disease. Lins' group[419] demonstrated an association between isolation of adenovirus in peripheral blood and progression or dissemination (or both) of adenovirus disease. High levels of adenovirus viremia (i.e., detection of PCR product at 100-fold or greater dilution of template DNA) have been correlated with fatal outcomes in children receiving allogeneic stem cell transplants.[598,684]

Baldwin and colleagues[32] studied the outcome and clinical course of 105 adenoviral infections in 100 patients after they received bone marrow transplants. The incidence was higher in unrelated donor transplants than in matched sibling donor transplants. Diarrhea and fever were the most common initial findings. Six deaths were attributed to the adenoviral infections; five of the six patients had pneumonia, and four had associated graft-versus-host disease. Three additional patients had severe disease.

In a study involving 532 recipients of hematopoietic stem cell transplants, a 12% incidence of adenoviral infection was noted.[316] Forty-one patients had infections classified as "invasive," and mortality was 76% in this group. Recipients of allogeneic transplants were more likely to have adenoviral infections than autologous stem cell recipients were.

The most common manifestation of adenoviral infection in pediatric patients with bone marrow transplants at St. Jude Children's Research Hospital was hemorrhagic cystitis, followed by gastroenteritis, pneumonitis, and liver failure.[190] Adenovirus-induced acute hemorrhagic cystitis is a complication encountered after hematopoietic stem cell transplantation and, more rarely, after renal transplantation.[199,309] Gorczynska and colleagues[257] examined the incidence of virus-induced hemorrhagic cystitis in 102 children and adolescents who underwent allogeneic stem cell transplantation. Hemorrhagic cystitis occurred in 25.5% of these children, with 3.9% of the cases attributed to adenoviruses. Another retrospective review of 266 adults undergoing stem cell transplant showed the incidence of adenoviral hemorrhagic cystitis to be 9.8%. Increased risk of cystitis was linked with underlying disease (cancer other than acute leukemia), and T-cell purging with antithymocyte globulin or alemtuzumab. Patients with acute graft-versus-host disease had a decreased incidence of hemorrhagic cystitis.[480]

Shirali and coworkers[609] noted that demonstration of the adenoviral genome in endomyocardial biopsy specimens from heart transplant recipients was a predictor of graft loss in children. Graft loss with concomitant adenovirus infection has been described in renal transplant patients.[385,390] Scattered reports have found an association between adenoviral infection and viruria and hemorrhagic cystitis in patients with renal transplants.[202,398] Fatal and severe cases of subacute meningoencephalitis caused by an adenovirus have been described in bone marrow transplant recipients.[141,218] Severe necrotizing pneumonia with pulmonary hemorrhage due to adenovirus in a lung transplant patient has been described.[454]

Lion and coworkers[423] conducted prospective quantitative adenovirus PCR screening in weekly stool and peripheral blood samples of 153 allogeneic stem cell transplants in pediatric patients from 1999 to 2005. They found that increased stool adenovirus copy number (greater than 10^6 copies per gram of stool) preceded detectable viremia in the peripheral blood by almost a week. This permitted early diagnosis of impending invasive infection with a sensitivity of 100% and specificity of 83%. Srinivasan and colleagues[627] also looked at the ability of stool adenovirus load to predict adenoviremia in 117 patients undergoing hematopoietic stem cell transplantation. Their data supported the conclusions of Lion et al., but they found stool adenovirus load of greater than 10^6 copies per gram of stool demonstrated a sensitivity and specificity of 82%. By using a cut-off of greater than 10^7 copies per gram of stool, sensitivity decreased to 73% while specificity increased to 86%. Kosulin and colleagues[388] sought to evaluate persistence and reactivation of adenoviruses in the gastrointestinal tract. They evaluated biopsies from 143 nontransplant pediatric patients undergoing endoscopy and found persistence of adenovirus in the GI tract in 31% of children (11% of biopsies), with the highest prevalence in the lymphoid cells from the lamina propria of the terminal ileum (61%). Viral proliferation, in contrast, was found to occur in epithelial cells in patients after hematopoietic stem cell transplant. Feghoul and colleagues[196] found that umbilical cord blood transplantation, in vitro T-cell depletion, and graft-versus-host disease grade III and IV were significant risk factors for systemic adenoviral infection. They supported prospective monitoring of adenoviral stool viral load to identify candidates for preemptive treatment to control adenoviral replication and prevent systemic spread of infection. Additional reported risk factors have included grafts from unrelated donors or umbilical cord blood, as well as absence of adenovirus-specific T cells.[421]

In many instances, a fulminant, bacterial, sepsis-like picture with high fever, cough, and lethargy is associated with adenoviral infection in compromised patients.[749] Severe pneumonia often is demonstrated, both clinically and radiologically, and hepatic involvement with disseminated intravascular coagulation also is a frequent occurrence. Fatalities are reported, and recovery often is slow.

Other Manifestations

Arthritis

Arthritis has been noted in association with adenovirus type 7 infection.[527] The illness was characterized by fever, acute respiratory symptoms, erythematous macular rash, aseptic meningitis, and inflammatory arthritis of both knees.

Thyroiditis

In 1964, Swann[641] reported five patients with acute thyroiditis and thyroid enlargement in whom serologic study revealed greater than fourfold rises in titer of adenoviral complement-fixing antibody.

Adrenal Insufficiency

Rai and colleagues[559] reported a case of transient adrenal insufficiency associated with adenovirus type 40 infection in a previously healthy 6-year-old boy who required mineralocorticoid and glucocorticoid supplementation for 8 weeks, confirming known adrenotropic potential of adenoviruses. Adenoviruses have been demonstrated to induce inflammatory cytokines, enhance adrenal hormone production, and impair adrenal gland steroidogenesis.

Deafness

Deafness of sudden onset was reported in an adult with a 2-day history of sore throat, low-grade fever, rhinorrhea, and cough. Adenovirus type 3 was isolated from the patient's throat, and a greater than fourfold rise in neutralizing antibody titer to this virus was observed.[328]

Obesity

Studies have shown that exposure to human adenovirus serotype 36 is associated with increased adiposity in chickens, mice, and nonhuman primates.[156–158] Continuing work in mouse models shows that adenovirus 36 infection increased macrophage infiltration into adipocytes[497] and impairs insulin signaling, thus altering glucose metabolism.[340] Paradoxically, reduced serum cholesterol and serum triglycerides are seen in the same animal models. Atkinson and colleagues[24,686] proposed that adenovirus serotype 36 directly affects adipocytes by increasing the number and size of preadipocytes. Vangipuram and associates[687] explored the possible mechanisms by which adenovirus types 36 and 37 increase adiposity in animal models. They performed ex vivo experiments in human adipocytes and a murine preadipocyte cell line (3T3-L1) and in vivo experiments in the rat model, which demonstrated suppression of leptin mRNA expression, decreased leptin secretion, and increased glucose uptake. In vitro studies show that adenovirus 36 infection causes upregulation of adipogenesis-related genes, along with inflammation that leads to lipid accumulation in cells.[496] Fatty acid oxidation was also shown to be impaired in in vitro models.[706] Additional studies have noted possible associations between in vitro infection with adenovirus types 5, 9, and 31 and obesity.[53–55,695]

Based on studies that adenoviruses increase adiposity in animal models, Atkinson and coworkers[24] screened 502 subjects for neutralizing antibodies to adenovirus 36. They detected antibodies to adenovirus 36 in as many as 30% of obese study subjects as opposed to 11% of nonobese subjects. Similarly, they found paradoxically decreased serum cholesterol and triglycerides in patients with antibodies to adenovirus 36. Subsequent studies have shown mixed results. Several studies have shown a correlation between seropositivity to adenovirus 36 and obesity,[12,23,25,227,664,732] but a longitudinal study from childhood to adulthood among a Finnish cohort failed to demonstrate a causal relationship.[591] In a study of adults, Na et al.[495] showed that while seropositivity to adenovirus 36 did correlate with overweight body mass index (BMI) (23–25), this relationship did not hold when examining obese individuals (BMI >25). A study completed in Holland and Belgium by Goossens and colleagues[256] in active-duty US military personnel[74] failed to show correlations between adenovirus 36 seropositivity and BMI. Interestingly, Trovato and colleagues showed that adenovirus 36 seropositivity was correlated with greater decrease in BMI and reduction of insulin resistance when subjects were placed on diet and exercise programs.[665] One study has shown increased serum cholesterol and triglycerides in children with antibodies against adenovirus 36.[494] Ponterio and colleagues demonstrated the presence of adenovirus type 36 DNA in adipose tissue biopsies of 4 out of 21 overweight and obese adults.[550] Shang and colleagues[605] conducted a meta-analysis of 11 case-control studies (2508 cases, 3005 controls) looking at adenovirus 36 infection and obesity. They identified a strong association with adenovirus 36 infection and significantly increased risk of development of obesity, especially in children and those with a BMI of 30 or greater, when compared to nonobese controls. Xu and coworkers[732] showed that adenovirus 36 infection was associated with the status of obesity but did not find an association with weight gain through analysis of BMI or BMI z-scores. Additional studies by Whigham and colleagues[712] demonstrated that human adenovirus serotype 37 also is associated with an increase in adipocyte differentiation and reduced serum triglycerides but increased serum cholesterol.

Congenital and Neonatal Infections

Neonatal and congenital adenoviral infections reflect disseminated infection with the involvement of multiple organs.[3,77,113,190,377,519,632] Major manifestations include hepatosplenomegaly, progressive pneumonia, hepatitis, and thrombocytopenia. Towbin and colleagues[660] reported intrauterine adenoviral myocarditis manifested as nonimmune hydrops fetalis. Illnesses frequently appear initially as an early-onset sepsis syndrome. An infant was reported with a congenital pleural effusion from which type 3 adenovirus was recovered.[466]

A recent study by Couroucli and associates[129] has noted an association between adenoviral infection and bronchopulmonary dysplasia (BPD). They found a significant increase in the frequency of adenovirus genome in tracheal aspirates from patients with BPD versus controls.

DIAGNOSIS

Differential Diagnosis

The differential diagnosis of adenoviral infection must be subcategorized on the basis of the major clinical manifestations. In many instances, specific clinical symptoms such as pharyngoconjunctival fever or epidemic keratoconjunctivitis can lead to strong suspicion of the adenoviral etiology. With other, more general respiratory diseases such as pharyngitis, bronchitis, croup, bronchiolitis, and pneumonia, the adenoviral etiology cannot be established on clinical grounds. Fever in adenoviral respiratory infections tends to be higher than that occurring in parainfluenza and RSV infections but similar to that in influenza A and B viral infections.[556] High and prolonged fever occurs as commonly in adenoviral infections as it does in bacterial respiratory infections. Because the symptom triad of fever, pharyngitis, and conjunctivitis is virtually unique to pharyngoconjunctival fever, establishing the diagnosis of this disease should be easy. Generalized diseases that occasionally might be confused with pharyngoconjunctival fever include leptospirosis, psittacosis, *Mycoplasma pneumoniae* infection, Q fever, Newcastle disease virus infection, and prodromal measles.

In pharyngitis, adenoviral infection must be differentiated both from other viral diseases, such as those caused by Epstein-Barr virus, parainfluenza and influenza viruses, and enteroviruses, and from streptococcal disease. In a young child, follicular pharyngitis is more likely to be caused by adenoviral than by streptococcal infection.

Adenoviral pneumonia in young children frequently is not distinguishable on clinical grounds from that caused by bacteria. In older children and adolescents, in particular, adenoviral pneumonia often can be differentiated from bacterial disease by its bilateral nature. Differentiating adenoviral illness from disease caused by *M. pneumoniae* is more difficult; however, cold agglutinin titers generally are higher and more persistently positive in mycoplasmal disease.

Adenoviral eye disease must be differentiated from that caused by viruses of the herpes group, enteroviral epidemic conjunctivitis (acute hemorrhagic conjunctivitis),[418,739,740] and *Chlamydia* spp. and bacteria, including *Neisseria gonorrhoeae*.

Diarrhea caused by enteric adenoviruses can be differentiated from other viral diarrheas by electron microscopy, by identification with ELISA, and by specific culture of the enteric agents in Graham 293 cell culture. Enteric bacterial and parasitic agents also must be considered in the differential diagnosis.

The high, relatively prolonged fever occurring in association with lymphadenopathy, exanthem, and enanthem noted with adenoviral infection often causes confusion with Kawasaki disease.[574] Because Kawasaki disease must be treated early with intravenous immunoglobulin, adenoviral infections should be considered early and appropriate studies performed. Jordan-Villegas and colleagues[346] conducted a study of almost 400 children diagnosed with Kawsaki disease in a 10-year period. They found that patients with concomitant respiratory viral infections diagnosed by DFA and/or viral culture had a higher frequency of coronary artery aneurysms. Jaggi and colleagues[329] highlighted challenges in interpreting detection of adenovirus by respiratory viral PCR among patients meeting criteria for complete or incomplete Kawasaki disease. They cautioned that detection may represent viral shedding and persistence, however, noting that adenovirus was detected in 8.8% to 25% of patients meeting criteria for complete and incomplete Kawasaki disease, respectively. Song and collaborators[622] noted that the most common clinical feature between adenovirus and Kawasaki disease was conjunctivitis. They found that features most consistent with conjunctivitis due to adenovirus included unilateral onset, prominent tearing (as compared to purulence), and follicular hyperplasia; CRP was consistently higher among their subjects with Kawasaki disease; and lower viral burden was more likely to be associated with complete Kawasaki disease.

Specific Diagnosis

Adenoviral infection can be diagnosed specifically by isolation of virus in an appropriate tissue culture system, direct antigen detection assay, or by DNA PCR. Most adenoviral types can be recovered from clinical specimens in primary or diploid cultures of human embryonic kidney.[409] The enteric viral types 40 and 41 can be grown in Graham 293 cells.[646,699] The rapidity of detection of adenoviruses by culture is enhanced by centrifugation of specimens in shell vials or plastic-welled plates.[171,183,438]

Direct identification of adenoviruses in respiratory secretions by radioimmunoassay, immunofluorescence techniques, and ELISA now is performed widely.[79,438,465,560,574,589,593,654] However, in general, the sensitivity, when compared with that of virus isolation, is relatively low; on the other hand, the specificity is high (>95%). Rocholl and colleagues[574] demonstrated the impact of rapid diagnosis of adenoviral respiratory disease with an adenoviral direct fluorescent antibody technique by noting discontinuation of empiric antibiotic use in a retrospective analysis of hospitalized patients with respiratory cultures positive for adenovirus. Rapid techniques for the identification of enteric adenoviruses in general have been sensitive and specific.[7,259,277,291,594,671,724] However, in newborns, false-positive results with a latex agglutination test have been reported.[324] Several techniques using DNA probes have been studied for the rapid identification of both respiratory and enteric adenoviral infection.[82,323,645] PCR assay also is useful for the rapid detection of adenoviral infection and is rapidly becoming the gold standard of diagnosis alongside tissue culture isolation.* PCR assay is particularly useful for identifying adenoviral DNA in formalin-fixed, paraffin-embedded tissues and other biopsy and postmortem specimens.[65,267,433,445,609,666]

Several groups have demonstrated the utility of PCR detection of adenoviral DNA in acute respiratory infections in immunocompetent patients.[2,191,574,608,733] The first multiple PCR assay for detection of respiratory viruses (Luminex xTAG Respiratory Viral Panel) was approved in January 2008, and more than nine commercially available assays have been approved since then.[751] Kuypers and colleagues[394] demonstrated significantly increased sensitivity of quantitative real-time PCR assay over fluorescent antibody detection of adenoviruses. They showed that 77.7% of respiratory specimens that were negative for adenovirus by fluorescent antibody detection were positive by PCR detection of adenovirus DNA. This increased sensitivity was replicated by Stroparo and colleagues.[638] Multiple PCR assays have been developed to detect multiple serotypes of adenovirus.[419,733] Buckwalter and colleagues developed real-time PCR for qualitative detection of 57 serotypes of adenovirus with high sensitivity and specificity in a variety of clinical samples.[81] Others have demonstrated similar multiplex assays for adenovirus although narrower in scope.[520] Aberle and colleagues[2] were able to detect adenoviral DNA with a nested PCR assay in acute-phase sera collected within the first week after the onset of symptoms in 72% of immunocompetent children experiencing their first adenoviral infection and in 25% of those experiencing recurrent infection.

It is important to note that the commercially available multiplex PCR assays to detect respiratory viral pathogens, particularly the BioFire Film Array Respiratory Panel (BioFire Diagnostics; Salt Lake City, Utah), had lower sensitivity for adenovirus group C, serotypes 2 and 6.[29] The package insert recommended testing of negative specimens using alternate methods to detect adenovirus when infection is clinically suspected. In April 2013, version 1.7 was released. Doern and colleagues[161] specifically looked at the Film Array assay's ability to detect adenoviruses. They found that version 1.7, which includes a second adenovirus assay, demonstrated improved sensitivity in both retrospective and prospective studies with improvements in sensitivity from 66.6% to 90.5% and from 42.7% to 83.3%, respectively. However, Song and colleagues[624] analyzed 4750 nasopharyngeal specimens for respiratory viruses in a large pediatric cohort and found that 146 (3.1%) of specimens were positive for adenovirus using version 1.7. They noted an additional 220 specimens that were negative by version 1.7 to be positive for adenovirus by a laboratory-developed adenovirus-specific PCR, representating a 4.6% increase in adenovirus detection. They found that the adenovirus-specific PCR had lower limits of detection, had difficulty with detection of nonrespiratory species, and confirmed the manufacturer's data that species A and F (serotypes 18, 31, 40, and 41) were detected with very low sensitivity. The group cautions use of this assay when evaluating immunocompromised patients for adenoviral infection for diagnostic, therapeutic, and epidemiologic concerns.

Interpretation of a positive result from nasopharyngeal specimens is challenging, however, as prior studies have shown that adenovirus can be detected in up to 11% of healthy, asymptomatic children by PCR versus 0.6% by culture. Additionally, interpretation of the clinical significance of a positive PCR specimen for species F adenoviruses (subtypes 40 and 41) from a respiratory specimen remains unclear. Song and collaborators[623] suggest the use of both viral load quantitation as well as species/serotype identification when using PCR-based testing to aid in assessment of the clinical significance of a positive PCR result. Other groups have demonstrated the utility of using serum PCR assays to diagnose and monitor adenoviral infection and disease in immunocompromised hosts.[400,598] Lion's group[422] developed a species-specific real-time quantitative PCR assay that allows detection and quantification of 51 human adenovirus subtypes. They showed that detection of adenovirus DNA in the peripheral blood of allogeneic bone marrow transplant recipients preceded the onset of clinical symptoms of disseminated adenoviral disease by a median of 3 weeks. Two other groups[410,702] have used real-time quantitative PCR assays to detect adenoviral DNA load to aid in both the diagnosis and management of disseminated adenoviral infections in immunocompromised patients. Ebner and colleagues[173] presented a two-stage PCR algorithm for diagnosis in immunosuppressed patients. Although algorithms for detection and

---

*References 2, 15, 65, 173, 174, 191, 198, 286, 338, 339, 394, 400, 410, 422, 459, 481, 482, 530, 574, 598, 608, 702, 733.

typing of adenoviruses have been used in the past,[173,456] the use of type-specific PCR and other techniques such as reverse-line-blot has made serotyping more efficient.[81,89]

Multiplex PCR to detect multiple different viruses in a clinical sample (respiratory secretions, stool, blood, etc.) are now becoming widely available. Commercial as well as "home-made" assays can now test for up to 13 different viruses with fast turnaround (1–4 hours) and excellent sensitivity and specificity.[195,226,268,275,301,405,444,682] The availability of cheap, reliable, and fast PCR kits has raised the question of whether the detection of viral genetic material can be attributed to true infection or shedding of dead virus from a past event. Kalu and colleagues[354] showed in a cohort of 76 children with 581 episodes of upper respiratory infection that adenoviruses of the same type and strain would persistently be detected by PCR in nasopharyngeal washes of the same host for over 200 days. The authors caution that clinical interpretation of PCR test results is necessary, as most practitioners do not have access to phylogenetic analysis. Respiratory viral coinfection has also made interpretation of positive results challenging, with studies showing 55% to 63% of patients having adenovirus coinfection.[623,624] Manji and colleagues[442] conducted a prospective multicenter study of the Adenovirus R-gene assay (Argene/bioMérieux; Verniolle, France) at three major US medical centers from September 2010 through November 2011. They tested 395 nasopharyngeal aspirates and 1186 nasopharyngeal swabs obtained from patients who had symptoms of a respiratory illness. This real-time PCR assay detects but does not different among adenovirus serotypes. They found overall sensitivity for nasopharyngeal aspirates and nasopharyngeal swabs to be 100% and 98.9%, specificity 100% and 98.9%, positive predictive value 97.6% and 100%, and negative predictive value 100% and 99.9%, respectively.

Many hospitals relied on fluorescent antibody staining, shell vial culture, and viral culture to identify adenovirus infection. Multiplex PCR, especially for the diagnosis of respiratory viral illness, as well as single-plex adenovirus PCR is quickly taking the place of these methods.

Acute infection also can be diagnosed serologically by the expression of specific serum IgM antibody.[465] Infection can be confirmed serologically by the demonstration of a rise in antibody titer in two sequential serum samples. Antibody response to the adenovirus group antigen can be detected by complement fixation or ELISA. Type-specific antibodies can be determined by neutralization, ELISA, or hemagglutination inhibition.

Currently, there are 13 available commercial GI multiplex PCR assays, but only two are FDA-approved syndromic multiplex assays for detection of bacterial, viral, and parasitic pathogens causing gastroenteritis (Luminex xTAG GPP, BioFire Film Array GI Panel).[751] Ye and coworkers[736] conducted a prospective pilot study of five healthy asymptomatic infants in whom weekly stool samples were collected over the first 2 years of life. Stool samples were tested for six enteric viruses including adenovirus. Approximately 40% of samples were positive for virus detection by PCR with adenovirus detected most frequently in 25.6% of samples. They noted frequent asymptomatic shedding of adenoviruses as detected by PCR for up to 3 months in infants without gastrointestinal symptoms. Buss and coworkers[84] showed a sensitivity of greater than or equal to 94.5% and specificity greater than or equal to 97.1% for all 22 panel targets.

TREATMENT

During the febrile period of illness, adequate hydration should be maintained and excessive activity discouraged. The fever may be controlled with acetaminophen. In children with eye involvement, careful attention should be paid to the possibility of secondary bacterial infection. If local purulence develops, specimens should be procured for culture and topical antimicrobial therapy started. The use of steroid-containing ophthalmic ointments should be avoided.

A consistent, safe, and effective therapy to treat adenovirus infection has yet to be established. Whereas vidarabine, ribavirin, and cidofovir demonstrate good activity against adenoviruses in vitro, several studies have shown only limited success with the use of vidarabine, ribavirin, ganciclovir, and cidofovir in treating adenovirus disease in humans.[426,487] The potential beneficial effects must be weighed carefully against the adverse side effects of these antiviral agents, including myelosuppression, pancytopenia, and nephrotoxicity. Walls and coworkers[703] conducted a retrospective study of 26 patients undergoing hematopoietic stem cell transplantation. They were unable to demonstrate a direct correlation among adenoviral DNA load, clinical features, and severity of disease. They also identified two children who experienced low-level adenoviral viremia after undergoing hematopoietic stem cell transplantation; the children cleared the virus without treatment. Williams and colleagues[720] created an algorithm to risk-stratify pediatric oncology and stem-cell transplant patients with adenovirus infection to determine who would benefit from cidofovir therapy without unnecessary risk of nephrotoxicity. They determined high-risk patients to be those with recent transplant (<60 days allogeneic or <180 days autologous), those with graft-versus-host disease, and those on immunosuppressive therapy. These patients would benefit from cidofovir, while those without these risk factors would do well without treatment. Their algorithm was validated in a small prospective cohort of 11 patients.[720] Matthes-Martin and colleagues developed an algorithm for preemptive antiviral therapy for adenovirus infection based on weekly monitoring of adenovirus viral load in blood and stool. Based on their review of existing literature, they suggest treatment when greater than or equal to 10^2 copies/mL adenovirus is detected in peripheral blood or greater than or equal to 10^6 copies/g feces are detected. They also advised reduction in immune suppression if possible until the serum adenoviral load is less than 10^2 copies/mL.[452]

Ribavirin is a guanosine nucleoside analogue used for the treatment of severe RSV infection in its inhaled form and for the treatment of chronic hepatitis C infection. In a number of instances, immunocompromised patients with disseminated adenoviral infection have been treated with ribavirin administered intravenously, and successful outcomes have been reported.[19,356,417,455,489,569,729] In one instance, a loading dose of 30 mg/kg per day divided into three doses was followed by maintenance therapy with 15 mg/kg per day.[455] Gavin and Katz[238] reported complete clinical recovery in two of five patients with severe adenovirus disease. A later study by Lankester and associates[399] demonstrated no effect on plasma adenoviral DNA load despite initiation of treatment with ribavirin at the first onset of clinical symptoms in four pediatric patients receiving allogeneic stem cell transplants. Intravenous ribavirin is available in the United States only as an emergency investigational drug as it is not approved by the FDA. Data on its use, efficacy, and safety are still very limited.[569]

The antiviral agent with the most promise to date has been cidofovir (Vistide), a cytosine nucleoside analogue with efficacy against several DNA viruses, including CMV, HSV, polyomaviruses, and adenoviruses. Cidofovir was used successfully in treating a 17-year-old boy who had received a stem cell transplant and had severe adenoviral gastroenteritis.[566] Ljungman and colleagues[427] conducted a study of cidofovir for the Infectious Diseases Working Party for Blood and Marrow Transplantation (EMBT). They demonstrated successful treatment of adenovirus infections in 69% of allogeneic hematopoietic stem cell transplant recipients, primarily with a 5-mg/kg dose of cidofovir given intravenously one time per week for the first 3 weeks and every other week after that, along with concomitant use of probenecid and intravenous fluid hydration. Other studies have shown a similar effect with reduced dosing of cidofovir at 1 mg/kg per dose given three times a week.[283,426,487] A case report by Fanourgiakis and colleagues[192] demonstrated successful treatment of severe (grade IV) hemorrhagic cystitis in a 34-year-old man by intravesical instillation of 5 mg/kg of cidofovir in 100 mL saline twice daily. This method avoided the known nephrotoxicity associated with cidofovir. Saquib and colleagues reported on two adult renal transplant patients with adenovirus viremia successfully treated with cidofovir along with intravenous immune globulin and concurrent reduction in immune suppressive therapy.[595] Yusuf and coworkers[748] reported complete resolution of clinical symptoms in 57 of 58 pediatric hematopoietic stem cell transplant recipients treated with cidofovir. Wallot and colleagues[701] had some success using reduced-dose cidofovir, inhaled nitric oxide, and decreased immunosuppression to treat two liver transplant recipients with disseminated adenoviral disease and acute respiratory distress syndrome. Lugthart and coworkers[434] evaluated cidofovir efficacy in 36 pediatric allogeneic hematopoietic stem cell transplant recipients who developed adenoviremia. While they noted rapid decline in adenoviral load and clearance from peripheral blood with cidofovir treatment, they noted that this coincided with T-cell and natural killer–cell reconstitution. They cautioned that cidofovir efficacy may be overestimated if the contribution of T cells, and possibly natural killer cells, reconstitution is not considered as well. Hydration and coadministration of probenecid may help minimize cidofovir-induced nephrotoxicity.

Caruso Brown and coworkers[92] reported the safety of a single dose of cidofovir in an open-label, nonrandomized pilot study of 12 pediatric hematopoietic stem cell transplant recipients with symptomatic adenovirus infection, nucleoside-resistant CMV or HSV, and/or human papovavirus infections. Four of seven patients with adenovirus infection were successfully treated and eventually cleared their infections. Two patients in their cohort developed evidence of acute kidney injury after a single dose of cidofovir (one recovered, one progressed to chronic kidney disease), and two patients developed late nephrotoxicity. Ganapathi and colleagues[229] conducted a retrospective chart review of 16 patients who received 19 courses of cidofovir for asymptomatic viremia as well as probable and definite adenovirus disease in hematopoietic stem cell transplant recipients and multiple solid organ transplant recipients (including lung, heart, combined kidney and liver, and multiple visceral transplants). Patients experienced an average 50% increase in creatinine from baseline. However, this was found to be a transient effect as creatinine normalized upon discontinuation of cidofovir.

Mynarek and colleagues[493] reported data prospective monitoring of serum adenovirus PCR in 238 consecutive pediatric allogeneic hematopoietic stem cell transplant recipients over a 9-year period. They found that peak blood adenovirus levels greater than 10^4 copies/mL was an independent risk factor for poor survival. Additionally, peak serum adenovirus levels greater than or equal to 10^4 copies/mL was associated with peak stool viral loads greater than 10^6 copies/mL. Using univariate and multivariate logistic regression analysis, they found that detection of adenovirus in peripheral blood before day +50 and age less than 6 years at transplant was associated with adenoviremia greater than 10^4 copies/mL. They recommend preemptive antiviral therapy in patients with serum adenovirus PCR greater than 10^4 copies/mL, those with at least two samples greater than 10^3 copies/mL, and those with increasing viral loads. They also recommended treating end-organ infection as early as possible irrespective of blood viral load.

Brincidofovir (3-hexadecyloxy-1-propyl-cidofovir) is a new oral antiviral drug made by Chimerex and is a lipid conjugate of cidofovir. The lipid moiety allows entry into the cell, and intracellular phospholipase cleavage prevents easy exit from the cell. Brincidofovir is less nephrotoxic than cidofovir as it does not accumulate in renal tubules due to the fact that it is not a substrate for renal organic anion transporter 1. It has broad activity against five double-stranded DNA viruses in vitro including BK polyomavirus, vaccinia, and molluscum contagiosum.[111] Brincidofovir is currently undergoing phase III clinical trials to treat adenovirus infections in allogeneic hematopoietic stem cell transplant recipients (Phase III, Open-labeled, Multicenter Study of Safety and Efficacy of Brinciofovir [CMX001] in the Treatment of Early Versus Late Adenovirus Infection [the AdVise Study]). Subjects receive 100 mg BCV biweekly (or 2 mg/kg biweekly for subjects under 50 kg) for 12 weeks and are assessed for adenovirus clearance from blood, respiratory secretions, urine, and stool.[723] Evaluation of treatment of poxviruses in mouse models is also ongoing.[164]

Paolino and colleagues were the first to report successful recovery from disseminated adenovirus infection in a pediatric stem cell transplant patient using brincidofovir after treatment failure with cidofovir.[528] McKillop and coworkers[458] reported successful treatment of disseminated adenovirus disease complicated by progressive necrotizing hepatitis with one dose of cidofovir and an 8-month course of brincidofovir 4 mg/kg per dose two times a week.

Florescu and colleagues retrospectively reviewed salvage treatment of adenovirus infection with brincidofovir (after failure with cidofovir) in 13 solid organ and stem cell transplant patients; 9 patients had a significant lowering of viral load, whereas 4 patients did not. The former group did have a statistically longer survival time, and no patients were discontinued due to drug side effects.[206]

Further studies into possible immunotherapies for the treatment of adenovirus infections also have been investigated. Feuchtinger and associates[201] were able to perform successful and safe adoptive transfer of adenovirus-specific, T-cell immunity in five of six patients with documented adenovirus infection after allogeneic hematopoietic stem cell transplantation. This effect was found to be independent of the T-cell dose. Furthermore, the adenovirus-specific T-cell expansion was sustainable, and proliferation of the adenovirus-specific T cells was unimpaired by adenovirus viremia, in contrast to the myelosuppressive effects seen with CMV viremia. Currently, emphasis of study is on the efficient and effective in vitro manufacturing of cytotoxic T-lymphocytes for use in immunocompromised individuals.[9,221,240,611,750] Di Nardo and coworkers[159] reported successful treatment of a 10-year-old boy with congenital amegakaryocytic thrombocytopenia who underwent T-cell–depleted haploidentical hematopoietic stem cell transplantation. He developed severe adenovirus respiratory disease requiring extracorporeal membrane oxygenation. Despite treatment with cidofovir, he developed hemorrhagic cystitis. Adoptive T-cell transfer of adenovirus-specific T cells was performed, allowing the patient to come off extracorporeal membrane oxygenation in 7 days and off the mechanical ventilator in 10 days. They noted that absolute lymphocyte count increased following infusion and C-reactive protein declined, while central memory and effector memory $CD4^+$ T cells increased and NK cells decreased. Feucht and colleagues[200] conducted a clinical trial of donor-derived adoptive T-cell transfer in 30 hematopoietic stem cell transplant patients with adenovirus viremia or disease refractory to antiviral therapy after 2 weeks. They utilized hexon-specific T cells, primarily of the T-helper (Th1) phenotype and late effector T-cell stage, isolated via the interferon gamma (IFN-γ) capture technique. Infusions were well tolerated with no significant side effects or development of or worsening of alloreactivity (e.g., graft-versus-host disease). Sustained and protective T-cell responses were detected up to 6 months after adoptive T-cell transfer. Patel and colleagues[536] reported the case of a 26-month-old male recipient of a liver transplant for hepatoblastoma who developed adenoviremia as well as adenovirus-associated gastroenteritis and hepatitis. The child was able to recover with reduced immune suppression alone without antiviral therapy, thereby highlighting the importance of reduced immunosuppression.

Teuchner and colleagues[653] studied *N*-chlorotaurine (NCT), a compound produced by monocytes and granulocytes during the oxidative burst, in a double-blind investigation of adult patients with epidemic keratoconjunctivitis. Among the group of 60 patients, 33 were treated with a 1% aqueous solution of NCT, and 27 were treated with gentamicin. They analyzed both subjective and objective scores. In the total study group, the NCT-treated subjects were subjectively better than the gentamicin-treated patients at day 8, but there were no objective differences. However, in severe infections, both the subjective and objective scores were better on days 4 and 8 in the NCT-treated patients. They concluded that NCT treatment was well tolerated and that it shortened the duration of illness. A study of the use of 1% cidofovir eye drops with and without 1% cyclosporine eye drops to treat adenovirus-associated keratoconjunctivitis was conducted by Hillenkamp and colleagues.[306] This study demonstrated significant local toxicity in the skin of the eyelids and conjunctiva but a decreased frequency of severe corneal opacities associated with the use of cidofovir. A novel drug, NVC-422, has shown good in vitro activity against adenovirus types 5, 8, 19, and 37.[336] This compound is an analogue of NCT that has been modified to gain better stability in solid-state solution. A phase II clinical trial for adenoviral conjunctivitis is ongoing.[745]

Human fibroblast–derived interferon, applied topically, was used to treat epidemic adenoviral keratoconjunctivitis in a comparative trial.[577] The duration of illness was reduced in the patients treated with interferon, but many of the control patients received dexamethasone. A child with combined immunodeficiency and severe, diffuse adenovirus type 7a pneumonia improved dramatically after receiving a large dose of high-titer adenovirus type 7a immune serum globulin.[136]

PREVENTION

Serious incapacitating epidemics caused by adenoviruses in military recruits in basic training led to the development of adenoviral vaccines.[18,406] The initial vaccines were formalin-inactivated preparations of monkey kidney tissue culture-grown virus and were administered parenterally.[17,266,303] These vaccines achieved only limited success because of variable degrees of potency in different vaccine lots.[40] An inactivated adenoviral vaccine that contained types 3, 4, and 7 was prepared in monkey tissue culture for trial in children.[681] Three doses of this vaccine resulted in high levels of neutralizing antibody to the three viral types, and this antibody persisted in most infants for at least 1 year. Many of the initial lots of inactivated adenoviral vaccine were found to contain live simian adenoviruses that were capable of producing neoplasms in suckling hamsters. Because of this finding, inactivated vaccine trials were discontinued. Next, a live, attenuated adenovirus type 4 vaccine that was cultivated in human diploid tissue culture was developed and administered orally by enteric-coated capsule to volunteers. Asymptomatic gastrointestinal infection occurred, and a good serum-neutralizing antibody response was elicited.[266,620,628] Most recipients of live oral vaccine excrete virus in stool for several days to a month after being vaccinated. With military use of the vaccine, shedding in stool was not associated with transmission of the virus to nonimmune contacts.[483] In other studies of married couples and families with children, virus was transmitted to nonimmune contacts.[483,629] Transmission usually occurred without illness.[483]

The administration of live, enteric-coated, type 4 and 7 adenovirus vaccine resulted in a significant decrease in the incidence of ARD in military recruits.[168,255,644] Unfortunately, adenoviral vaccines no longer are available, and the incidence of ARD in military recruits again is a significant problem.[33,261,384,590] This vaccination program was terminated in 1999. However, after a subsequent rise in the incidence of acute respiratory disease and deaths in military servicemen,[553] vaccination was resumed. A new live oral vaccine for type 4 and 7 human adenoviruses is now licensed and in use since 2011.[667] Few attempts have been made to protect children with live adenoviral vaccines. In one study, live enteric-coated adenovirus type 4 vaccine was given to children aged 5 to 11 years. Asymptomatic gastrointestinal infection resulted from administration of the vaccine. Because the major cause of pharyngoconjunctival fever caused by adenoviruses is swimming in contaminated water, discretion in bathing locations is advised. Swimming pool water should be chlorinated adequately, and pool filtration systems should be inspected daily. Ill individuals should be excluded from swimming pools during their illness and for at least 2 weeks after recovery.

PROGNOSIS

The overall prognosis of adenoviral infection generally is excellent. Secondary bacterial complications, if untreated, can result in prolongation of illness and permanent sequelae in some instances. The prognosis of adenoviral infection in the very young and in immunocompromised patients must be guarded.

NEW REFERENCES SINCE THE SEVENTH EDITION

12. Aldoon-Hainerova I, et al. Clinical and laboratory characteristics of 1179 Czech adolescents evaluated for antibodies to human adenovirus 36. *Int J Obes.* 2014;38:285-291.
14. Alkhalaf MA, et al. Prevalence and quantitation of adenovirus DNA from human tonsil and adenoid tissues. *J Med Virol.* 2013;85:1947-1954.
27. Awosika OO, et al. Fatal adenovirus encephalomyeloradiculitis in an umbilical cord stem cell transplant recipient. *Neurology.* 2013;80:1715-1717.
29. Babady NE. The FilmArray respiratory panel: an automated, broadly multiplexed molecular test for the rapid and accurate detection of respiratory pathogens. *Expert Rev Mol Diagn.* 2013;13:779-788.
55. Bil-Lula I, et al. Infectobesity in the Polish population—evaluation of an association between adenovirus type 5, 31, 36, and human obesity. *Int J Virol Mol Biol.* 2014;3:1-8.
54. Bil-Lula I, et al. Adenovirus type 9 enhances differentiation and decreases cytokine relase from preadipocytes. *J Med Virol.* 2015;87:230-239.
53. Bil-Lula I, et al. An infection of human adenovirus 31 affects the differentiation of preadipocytes info fat cells, its metabolic profile, and fat accumulation. *J Med Virol.* 2016;88:400-407.
84. Buss SN, et al. Multicenter evaluation of the BioFire FilmArray gastrointestinal panel for etiologic diagnosis of infectious gastroenteritis. *J Clin Microbiol.* 2015;53:915-925.
87. Calvo C, et al. Eight year prospective study of adenovirus infections in hospitalized children, comparison with other respiratory viruses. *PLoS ONE.* 2015;10(7):1-10.
92. Caruso Brown AE, et al. Pharmacokinetics and safety of intravenous cidofovir for life-threatening viral infections in pediatric hematopoietic stem cell transplant recipients. *Antimicrob Agents Chemother.* 2015;59:3718-3725.
93. Chen R, Lee C. Adenoviruses types, cell receptors, and local innate cytokines in adenovirus infection. *Int Rev Immunol.* 2014;33:45-53.
109. Chhabra P, et al. Etiology of viral gastroenteritis in children <5 years of age in the United States, 2008-2009. *J Infect Dis.* 2013;208:790-800.
159. Di Nardo M, et al. Adoptive immunotherapy with antigen-specific T cells during extracorporeal membrane oxygenation (ECMO) for adenovirus-related respiratory failure in a child given haploidentical stem cell transplantation. *Pediatr Blood Cancer.* 2014;376-379.
161. Doern CD, et al. Evaluation and implementation of FilmArray version 1.7 for improved detection of adenovirus respiratory tract infection. *J Clin Microbiol.* 2013;51:4036-4039.
189. Faden H, et al. The ubiquity of asymptomatic respiratory viral infections in the tonsils and adenoids of children and their impact on airway obstruction. *Int J Pediatr Otorhinolaryngol.* 2016;90:128-132.
196. Feghoul L, et al. Adenovirus infection and disease in paediatric haematopoietic stem cell transplant patients: clues for antiviral pre-emptive treatment. *Clin Microbiol Infect.* 2015;21:701-709.
200. Feucht J, et al. Adoptive T-cell therapy with hexon-specific Th1 cells as a treatment of refractory adenovirus infection after HSCT. *Blood.* 2015;125:1986-1994.
229. Ganapathi L, et al. Use of cidofovir in pediatrics patients with adenovirus infection. *F1000Res.* 2016;5:758.
230. Ganime AC, et al. Viability of human adenovirus from hospital fomites. *J Med Virol.* 2014;86:2065-2069.
231. Ganime AC, et al. Dissemination of human adenoviruses and rotavirus species A on fomites of hospital pediatric units. *Am J Infect Control.* 2016;44:1411-1413.
236. Garnett CT, et al. Prevalence and quantitiation of species C adenovirus DNA in human mucosal lymphocytes. *J Virol.* 2002;76:10608-10616.
237. Garnett CT, et al. Latent species C adenoviruses in human tonsil tissues. *J Virol.* 2009;83:2417-2428.
250. Girouard G, et al. Adenovirus serotype 14 infections, New Brunswick, Canada, 2011. *Emerg Infect Dis.* 2013;19(1):119-122.
271. Hage E, et al. A human adenovirus species B subtype 21a associated with severe pneumonia. *J Infect.* 2014;69:490-499.
272. Hakansson A, et al. Adenovirus infection enhances in vitro adherence of *Streptococcus pneumoniae*. *Infect Immun.* 1994;62:2707-2714.
318. Huang YC, et al. Adenovirus infection associated with central nervous system dysfunction in children. *J Clin Virol.* 2013;57:300-304.
329. Jaggi P, et al. Human adenovirus infection in Kawasaki disease: a confounding bystander. *Clin Infect Dis.* 2013;56:58-64.
330. Jain S, et al. Community-acquired pneumonia requiring hospitalization among U.S. children. *N Engl J Med.* 2015;372:835-845.
336. Jekle A, et al. Broad-spectrum virucidal activity of (NVC-22) N,N-dichloro-2,2-dimethyltaurine against viral ocular pathogens in vitro. *Invest Ophthalmol Vis Sci.* 2013;54:1244-1251.
346. Jordan-Villegas A, et al. Concomitant respiratory viral infections in children with Kawasaki disease. *Pediatr Infect Dis J.* 2010;29:770-772.
350. Kajon AE, et al. Molecular epidemiology of adenovirus type 21 respiratory strains isolates from US military trainees (1996-2014). *J Infect Dis.* 2015;212:871-880.
351. Kajon AE. Identification of a novel intertypic recombinant species D human adenovirus in a pediatric stem cell transplant receipient. *J Clin Virol.* 2014;61:496-502.
357. Karda R, et al. Gene therapy with adeno-associated virus for cystic fibrosis. *Am J Respir Crit Care Med.* 2016;193:234-236.
363. Kawashima N, et al. Fulminant adenovirus hepatitis after hematopoietic stem cell transplantation: retrospective real-time PCR analysis for adenovirus DNA in two cases. *J Infect Chemother.* 2015;21:857-863.
370. Keyes A, et al. Cutaneous involvement of disseminated adenovirus infection in an allogeneic stem cell transplant recipient. *Br J Dermatol.* 2016;174:885-888.
387. Koren MA, et al. Type-specific clinical characteristics of adenovirus-associated influenza-like illness at five US military medical centers, 2009-2014. *Influenza Other Respir Viruses.* 2016;10:414-420.
388. Kosulin K, et al. Persistence and reactivation of human adenoviruses in the gastrointestinal tract. *Clin Microbiol Infect.* 2015;22:381.e1-381.e8.
404. Lebel A, et al. Secondary bacteremia following adenovirus infection. *Infect Dis.* 2016;48:403-405.
423. Lion T, et al. Monitoring of adenovirus load in stool by real-time PCR permits early detection of impending invasive infection in patients after allogeneic stem cell transplantation. *Leukemia.* 2010;24:706-714.
421. Lion T. Adenovirus infections in immunocompetent and immunocompromised patients. *Clin Microbiol Rev.* 2014;27:441-462.
424. Liu J, et al. Use of quantitative molecular diagnostic methods to identify causes of diarrhea in children: a reanalysis of the GEMS case-control study. *Lancet.* 2016;388:1291-1301.
434. Lugthart G, et al. The effect of cidofovir on adenovirus plasma DNA levels in stem cell transplantation recipients without T cell reconstitution. *Biol Blood Marrow Transplant.* 2015;21:293-299.

435. Lynch JP, Kajon AE. Adenovirus: epidemiology, global spread of novel serotypes, and advances in treatment and prevention. *Semin Respir Crit Care Med*. 2016;37:586-602.
442. Manji R, et al. Multi-center evaluation of the adenovirus R-gene US assay for the detection of adenovirus in respiratory samples. *J Clin Virol*. 2014;60:90-95.
446. Martinez-Velez N, et al. The oncolytic adenovirus VCN-01 as therapeutic approach against pediatric osteosarcoma. *Clin Cancer Res*. 2015;2217-2225.
448. Matoq A, Salahuddin A. Acute hepatitis and pancytopenia in healthy infant with adenovirus. *Case Rep Pediatr*. 2016;2016:8648190.
451. Matsushima Y, et al. Genome sequence of a novel virus of the species human adenovirus d associated with acute gastroenteritis. *Genome Announc*. 2013;1(1):e00068-12. doi:10.1128/genomeA.00068-12.
452. Matthes-Martin S, et al. Diagnosis and treatment of adenovirus infection in immunocompromised patients. *Expert Rev Anti Infect Ther*. 2013;11:1017-1028.
458. McKillop SJ, et al. Adenovirus necrotizing hepatitis complicating atypical teratoid rhabdoid tumor. *Pediatr Int*. 2015;57:974-977.
467. Mhaissen MN, et al. Epidemiology of diarrheal illness in pediatric oncology patients. *J Pediatric Infect Dis Soc*. 2016;[epub ahead of print].
478. Montaruli E, et al. Adenovirus-induced obstructive uropathy with acute renal failure in an immunodeficient child. *Urology*. 2014;83:217-219.
493. Mynarek M, et al. Patient, virus, and treatment-related risk factors in pediatric adenovirus infection after stem cell transplantation; results of a routine monitoring program. *Biol Blood Marrow Transplant*. 2014;20:250-256.
501. Naselli A, et al. Acute post-infectious cerebellar ataxia due to co-infection of human herpesvirus-6 and adenovirus mimicking myositis. *Ital J Pediatr*. 2014;50:98.
526. Pankhurst L, et al. Routine monitoring of adenovirus and norovirus within the health care environment. *Am J Infect Control*. 2014;42:1229-1232.
536. Patel RR, et al. A case of adenovirus viremia in a pediatric liver transplant recipient with neutropenia and lymphopenia: who and when should we treat? *J Pediatric Infect Dis Soc*. 2015;4:e1-e5.
538. Peled N, et al. Adenovirus infection in hospitalized immunocompetent children. *Clin Pediatr (Phila)*. 2004;43:223-229.
550. Ponterio E, et al. Adenovirus 36 DNA in human adipose tissue. *Int J Obes*. 2015;39:1761-1764.
559. Rai B, et al. Transient acute adrenal insufficiency associated with adenovirus serotype 40 infection. *BMJ Case Rep*. 2014.
564. Reyes-Andrade J, et al. Meningoencephalitis due to adenovirus in a healthy infant mimicking severe bacterial sepsis. *Pediatr Infect Dis J*. 2014;33:416-419.
572. Robinson CM, et al. Molecular evolution of human adenoviruses. *Sci Rep*. 2013;3:1812.
573. Robinson CM, et al. Predicting the next eye pathogen: a novel adenovirus. *MBio*. 2013;4(2):e00595-12.
578. Ronan BA. Fulminant hepatitis due to human adenovirus. *Infection*. 2014;42:105-111.
591. Sabin MA, et al. Longitudinal investigation of adenovirus 36 seropositivity and human obesity: the Cardiovascular Risk in Young Finns Study. *Int J Obes (Lond)*. 2015;39:1644-1650.
596. Saraiva J, et al. Gene therapy for the CNS using AAVs: the impact of systemic delivery by AAV9. *J Control Release*. 2016;241:94-109.
605. Shang Q, et al. Serological data analyses show that adenovirus 36 infection is associated with obesity: a meta-analysis involving 5739 subjects. *Obesity (Silver Spring)*. 2014;22:895-900.
615. Simpson KE. High Frequency of detection by PCR of viral nucleic acid in the blood of infants presenting with clinical myocarditis. *Pediatr Cardiol*. 2016;37:399-404.
617. Singh A, Dwaipayan S. Therapeutic value of adeno associated virus as a gene therapy vector for Parkinson's disease—a focused review. *Curr Gene Ther*. 2016.
622. Song E, et al. Clinical and virologic characteristics may aid distinction of acute adenovirus disease from kawasaki disease with incidental adenovirus detection. *J Pediatr*. 2016;170:325-330.
623. Song E, et al. Diagnosis of pediatric acute adenovirus infections: is a positive PCR sufficient? *Pediatr Infect Dis J*. 2016;35:827-834.
624. Song E, et al. Performance characteristics of FilmArray Respiratory Panel v1.7 for detection of adenovirus in a large cohort of pediatric nasopharyngeal samples: one test may not fit all. *J Clin Microbiol*. 2016;54:1479-1486.
627. Srinivasan A, et al. Impact of adenoviral stool load on adenoviremia in pediatric hematopoietic stem cell transplant recipients. *Pediatr Infect Dis J*. 2015;34:562-564.
635. Stockman C, et al. Detection of 23 gastrointestinal pathogens among children who present with diarrhea. *J Pediatric Infect Dis Soc*. May 2016;[epub ahead of print].
643. Syrbe S, et al. Opsoclonus-myoclonus syndrome after adenovirus infection. *Springerplus*. 2015;4:636.
652. Taylor S, et al. Respiratory viruses and influenza-like illness: epidemiology and outcomes in children aged 6 months to 10 years in a multi-country population sample. *J Infect Dis*. Sep 2016;[epub ahead of print].
670. Ukarapol N, et al. Adenovirus infection: a potential risk for developing intussuception in pediatric patients. *J Med Virol*. 2016;88:1930-1935.
683. van Montfrans J, et al. Viral PCR positivity in stool before allogeneic hematopoietic cell transplantation is strongly associated with acute intestinal graft-versus-host disease. *Biol Blood Marrow Transplant*. 2015;21:768-774.
695. Voss JD, et al. Role of adenoviruses in obesity. *Rev Med Virol*. 2015;25:379-387.
723. Wold W, Toth K. New drug on the horizon for treating adenovirus. *Expert Opin Pharmacother*. 2015;16(14):2095-2099.
728. Wu P, et al. Hypoxemia is an independent predictor of bronchiolitis obliterans following respiratory viral infection in children. *Springerplus*. 2016;5:1622.
730. Wurzel DF, et al. Adenovirus species C is associated with chronic suppurative lung diseases in children. *Clin Infect Dis*. 2014;59(1):34-40.
732. Xu M, et al. Human adenovirus 36 infection increased the risk of obesity: a meta-analysis update. *Medicine (Baltimore)*. 2015;94:e2357.
736. Ye S, et al. Detection of viruses in weekly stool specimens collected during the first 2-years of life: a pilot study of five healthy Australian infants in the rotavirus vaccine era. *J Med Virol*. 2016;[Epub ahead of print].
737. Yeshuroon-Koffler K, et al. Detection of common respiratory viruses in tonsillar tissue of children with obstructive sleep apnea. *Pediatr Pulmonol*. 2015;50:187-195.
751. Zhang H, Morrison S, Tang YW, Multiplex PCR. Tests for detection of pathogens associated with gastroenteritis. *Clin Lab Med*. 2015;35:461-486.

The full reference list for this chapter is available at ExpertConsult.com.

SUBSECTION **IV** DNA—*Hepatoviridae*

Hepatitis B and D Viruses 157

Yen H. Pham • Daniel H. Leung

HEPATITIS B VIRUS

Hepatitis B virus (HBV) infection remains a significant health problem worldwide. Review of worldwide seroprevalence data shows a decrease in prevalence of chronic HBV infection, from 4.2% to 3.7%, but an increase in absolute numbers of persons chronically infected, from 223 million to 240 million between 1990 and 2005 despite the availability of the HBV vaccination. In the United States, the total number of persons with chronic hepatitis B is estimated at 2 million, although acute cases have dropped to only 0.9 cases per 100,000 persons in 2014.[158,222,307] Individuals chronically infected with HBV are at risk for developing cirrhosis and hepatocellular carcinoma (HCC). Worldwide mortality is still estimated at 0.5 to 1.2 million deaths per year.[170] Most individuals with chronic HBV infection acquired the virus through vertical transmission, which can now be prevented in the majority of cases by active and passive immunization.

Biology

HBV is the prototype of a family of deoxyribonucleic acid (DNA) viruses called *hepadnaviruses* (hepatotropic DNA viruses). This group consists of enveloped, coated, double-stranded DNA viruses with similar structure and genome organization. All primarily infect the livers of their respective hosts and can cause acute and chronic infections.

The three types of particles found in the sera of HBV-infected people—the Dane particle and two subviral particles, one spherical and the other filament shaped—have influenced how we serologically monitor for HBV. All three types share a common surface antigen, hepatitis B surface antigen (HBsAg), but only one, the Dane particle, contains viral DNA and is capable of replication. The Dane particle, or whole virion, is 42 nm in diameter and contains a core, or nucleocapsid, enclosing the DNA. The outer shell is composed of large amounts of hepatitis B surface proteins in a lipoprotein envelope, which is derived from host cells. Inside this shell is the nucleocapsid, an icosahedral structure composed of 240 core protein subunits with regular penetrating channels. These nucleocapsid proteins are detected serologically as hepatitis B core antigen (HBcAg). Within this nucleocapsid are also contained the viral genome and polymerase. Hepatitis B envelope antigen (HBeAg), a marker of viral replication, is a soluble antigen produced from the same open reading frame as is HBcAg. However, unlike core antigen, e antigen is secreted into serum, where it is thought to have a role in induction of tolerance to HBV. The viral genome is composed of double-stranded circular DNA that can be relaxed or closed depending on the stage in the reproduction cycle.

The subviral particles (spheres and filaments) are composed of envelope proteins and host-derived lipid components.[254] Neither the filament nor the sphere contains nucleic acid. These particles are abundant in the serum of infected individuals (10^6–10^{14} particles/mL), and they are highly immunogenic, stimulating the production of neutralizing antibodies. One hypothesis is that they absorb neutralizing antibodies, thus shielding the intact virion from the host immune response. Subviral particles were used to produce the first effective HBV vaccine.[280]

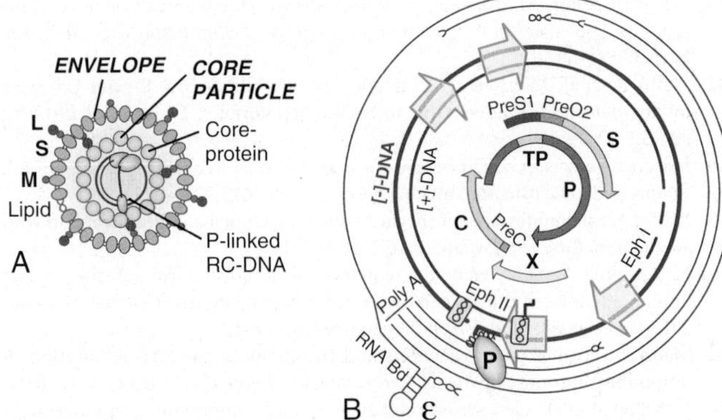

FIG. 157.1 Molecular features of hepatitis B virus. (A) Virion structure. Infectious virions consist of an outer envelope with the lipid-embedded surface proteins small (S), medium (M), and large (L), and an icosahedral inner nucleocapsid harboring the viral genome as a relaxed circular (RC)-DNA. (B) Genome organization. *Outer lines* denote viral transcripts, *arrowheads* denote transcription starts, and ε symbolizes the RNA encapsidation signal on pregenomic (pg)RNA. The two DNA strands are shown as present in RC-DNA to highlight the relative positions of RC-DNA–typical features; however, the viral RNAs encoding the open reading frames (ORFs) depicted in the center are transcribed from covalently closed circular DNA. (From Nassal M. HBV cccDNA: viral persistence reservoir and key obstacle for a cure of chronic hepatitis B. *Gut.* 2015;64[12]:1972–1984.)

Molecular Virology

The compact partially double-stranded viral genome contains four open reading frames (ORFs): (1) precore/core (preC/C), which encodes the e antigen (HBeAg) and core protein (HBcAg); (2) P for polymerase (reverse transcriptase); (3) PreS1/PreS2/S for surface proteins (three forms of HBsAg, small [S], middle [M], and large [L]); and X for a transcriptional transactivator protein (Fig. 157.1).

Nine HBV genotypes and multiple subgenotypes have been identified by use of polymerase chain reaction (PCR)-restriction fragment length polymorphism analysis of the complete viral genome.[140,180] They have been designated A through I and differ in genome length, the size of ORFs and proteins translated, and the development of various mutations.[160] Genotype and subgenotype predominance varies by geographic location. Genotype A is found in northwestern Europe, North America, and Africa. Genotypes B and C are characteristic of southeast Asia. Genotype D has a worldwide distribution but predominates in the Mediterranean area. Genotype E is found in Africa, and genotypes F and H are found in South and Central America.[180,278,309] In a US study, a strong statistical association has been found between genotype and ethnicity and genotype and place of birth: genotypes A and D were detected more often in whites, whereas Asian carriers were infected with genotypes B and C; 77% of carriers born in the United States were infected with genotype A, but the genotype of carriers born outside the United States reflected their place of origin.[279,309]

The clinical differences among HBV genotypes are being elucidated. Infection with genotype C was found in Taiwanese adults to be associated with more severe liver disease and HCC in those older than 50 years of age, whereas genotype B is associated with HCC in younger persons.[139] In a study of 487 Chinese HBV-infected children, genotype C was more common (76.4%) than genotype B (22.3%) or genotype D (1.3%). Children with chronic HBV B2 had less severe inflammation and fibrosis than those with HBV C2.[329] An association of genotype with response to interferon-α (IFN-α) treatment also has been demonstrated. A study from Taiwan analyzed the responses of 58 patients with chronic HBV infection genotypes B and C to treatment with IFN-α. The patients with genotype C had higher aminotransferase levels at baseline. After 48 weeks of follow-up, only 15% of those with genotype C were HBeAg negative and HBV DNA negative as compared with 42% of those with genotype B.[142] The genotype of HBV can influence the outcome of HBV infection in children because it can affect the frequency of HBeAg positivity, the age at which HBeAg loss occurs, and the mode of transmission.[141,161,201]

Mutations affecting all ORFs of the HBV genome have been described. Most viral genomes carry more than one mutation, and most individuals are infected with more than one variant. Some of the mutations are thought to contribute to viral latency, level of infection, severity of liver disease, and vaccine escape. Mutations in the core gene, the precore region, and the promoter for *C* have become clinically important. The group best studied is the precore mutants, which result in lack of HBeAg production, even in the presence of active viral replication, the so-called HBe antigen–negative infection. In contrast to the situation in persons with wild-type virus, in whom absence of HBeAg usually signifies absent HBV replication and mild liver disease (see later discussion), in HBeAg-negative hepatitis, HBV DNA levels are high, antibody to hepatitis B e antigen (anti-HBe) is detected, and liver disease may be severe. Sporadic cases and outbreaks of fulminant HBV infection have been attributed to precore mutants. Mutations in the *S* or *pre-S* gene, which encode envelope protein, have been reported in patients infected after vaccination and in individuals who received monoclonal antibody to HBV after liver transplantation. This variant contains a missense mutation in the surface antigen. Subsequently, these mutants were demonstrated in chronic HBV carriers even without these immune pressures. This mutation causes an infection in which HBsAg is undetectable but in which HBeAg and HBV-DNA are found, in contrast to the typical serologic pattern (see later discussion).

The role of X protein is not fully understood, but it is required for establishment of infection in vivo although not for transfection of cells in vitro.[23,55] X protein is a regulatory protein involved in transcriptional activation during viral replication[172]; it has also has been shown to transactivate the promoters of other viruses, such as human immunodeficiency virus (HIV) and human T-lymphotropic virus type 1.[247] In addition, the X protein appears to be involved in the development of HCC.[19]

Viral Life Cycle Overview

Viral binding and cell entry. Infection of the target cells begins at the plasma membrane of hepatocytes, where viral envelope proteins interact with specific cellular receptors (Fig. 157.2). While the identity of the receptors is unknown, the N-terminal region of the large envelope protein (pre-S1) appears to be essential and to mediate cell fusion interactions. Monoclonal antibodies to these proteins prevent infection and are a possible therapeutic strategy.[149] This process is thought to be triggered by low pH and/or proteolytic cleavage of envelope protein.[190]

After uncoating/release into the cytoplasm and transport of the nucleocapsid to the nucleus, the partially double-stranded viral relaxed circular DNA (rcDNA) is repaired by both viral and cellular enzymes. Specifically, the incomplete plus-strand of the rcDNA is completed by the viral polymerase; in another step, the viral polymerase and ribonucleic acid (RNA)-primers used for DNA plus-strand synthesis are removed by cellular enzyme. In the nucleus, the genomic DNA is converted to a covalently closed circular DNA (cccDNA) form that serves as a template for reverse transcription.[152] cccDNA's fundamental role is to act as a template for all viral RNAs and, consequently, progeny virion. This stable episomal plasmid-like molecule is the virologic key to the persistent reservoir of HBV that contributes to the difficulty in clearing HBsAg with currently available treatment even after prolonged treatment and the frequent rebound of viral replication upon withdrawal of DNA therapy or immunosuppression. A few copies of cccDNA per liver can (re)initiate full-blown infection and persist for the lifespan of the hepatocyte. A cure for chronic HBV requires elimination of cccDNA.[210]

Genomic Replication

The first step in HBV genomic replication is the encapsidation of the genomic RNA template.[277] Pregenomic RNA (pgRNA) is encapsidated together with the P protein.[86] Inside the nucleocapsid, pgRNA is reverse transcribed into negative-strand DNA. rcDNA is generated by plus-strand synthesis from negative-strand DNA. The nucleocapsids are either reimported to the nucleus for cccDNA amplification or enveloped and released via the endoplasmic reticulum (ER).

Viral Assembly and Release

The 20-nm subviral particles are assembled between the ER and Golgi apparatus.[125] These 20-nm particles contain predominantly S HBsAg proteins, which are synthesized in the ER.[109] In addition, these particles may contain M subunits but generally do not have L HBsAg proteins.[116] The assembly process is encoded totally in the S domain.[169] Assembled particles are transported through the secretory pathway and traverse the Golgi complex.[144,275] The S protein carries out the entire assembly process without the involvement of other viral proteins.[4] Therefore, subviral particles containing only envelope proteins are released. In vitro studies have shown that overexpression of L proteins gives rise to filamentous viral particles in the ER.[60] The overabundance of L, M, and S aggregates apparently is cytopathic to hepatocytes in vitro. Similar cytopathic features have been seen in human infections with HBV, yet the role of envelope protein expression in hepatocyte injury remains to be determined.[4]

The assembly of the Dane particle differs from the assembly of the 20-nm particles in that all three proteins—L, M, and S—are present.[116] Studies of HepG2 cell lines transfected with HBV mutants have shown that no virus budding occurs if the envelope proteins are not present (mutations in S) and that for virion formation and release, both L and S proteins are needed.[36] M proteins apparently are not necessary for viral assembly.

Immunopathogenesis

HBV is not directly cytopathic, and the variability in liver damage is due to host immune responses. Although HBV preferentially infects hepatocytes and replicates therein, it can infect other liver cells, such as cholangiocytes, as well as cells in extrahepatic tissue, such as peripheral blood lymphocytes, pancreatic acinar cells, cornea, spleen, thyroid gland, kidney, adrenal gland, and smooth muscle.[13,331]

Responses to HBV infection and the likelihood of developing chronic infection are dependent on both age at the time of acquisition and immune competence. Of infants born to mothers who are HBeAg positive, 90% become chronically infected with HBV compared with only 5% of those infected as adults. The production of antibodies to pre-S and S antigens by B cells, as well as cytotoxic T-lymphocyte (CTL) responses, mediates recovery from acute HBV infection. Individuals who clear HBV have a strong polyclonal human leukocyte antigen class I–restricted CTL response to multiple epitopes in the HBV envelope, nucleocapsid, and polymerase regions. This CTL response can be reactivated many years after clearance of all detectable evidence of HBV infection.[184]

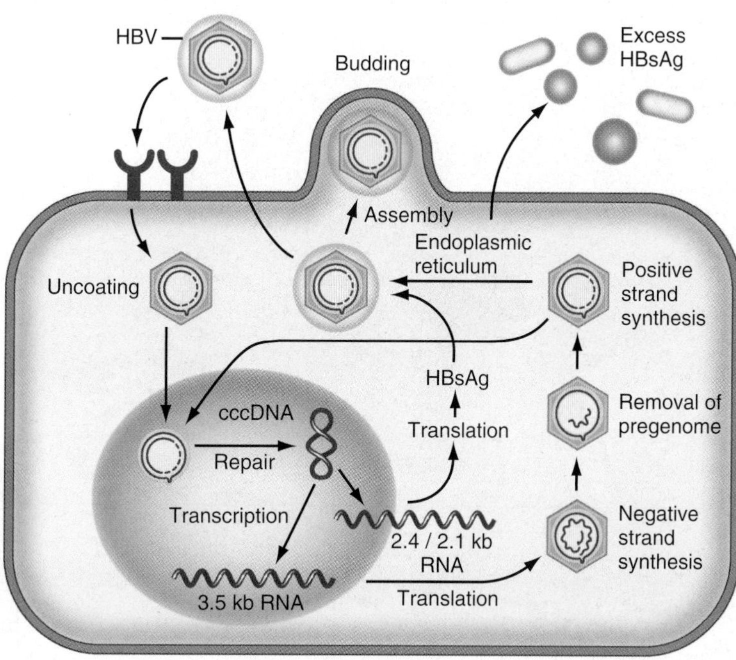

FIG. 157.2 Hepatitis B (HBV) virus infectious cycle. *HBsAg,* Hepatitis B surface antigen. (From Wells JT, Perillo R. Hepatitis B. In: Feldman M, Friedman LS, Brandt LJ, eds. *Sleisenger and Fordtran's Gastrointestinal and Liver Disease.* 10th ed. Philadelphia: Elsevier; 2016.)

Infants infected perinatally are at the highest risk for development of chronic HBV infection. During childhood, those infected as neonates characteristically have high circulating levels of HBV DNA but low disease activity, with very low rates of HBeAg seroconversion, either spontaneously or after treatment with IFN.[184] Researchers have offered numerous hypotheses as to why immune tolerance develops in neonates. One theory proposes that transplacental passage of HBeAg induces $CD4^+$ anergy and, therefore, no CTL responses to HBeAg develop. However, HBeAg-specific T-cell proliferation eventually is detected in those who subsequently seroconvert, rendering clonal deletion an unlikely mechanism.[184]

The development of chronic infection is either a failure of host immune responses or a testament to the ability of HBV to evade that response. As the virus replicates within hepatocytes, viral antigens appear on the cell surface. Subsequently, CTLs directed against HBcAg infiltrate the liver and cause hepatocyte necrosis.[75] In addition, HBV interferes with the production of cytokines of the Th1 response, especially IFNs that would otherwise elicit class II major histocompatibility complex antigen expression and enhance viral clearance. For reasons not fully understood, both the HBV-specific CTL response and the $CD4^+$ helper T-cell response are weak in chronic HBV infection. The high HBV viral load may lead to depletion of peripheral T-cell responses.[94] However, HBeAg—produced in large amounts in chronic HBV infection—and HBsAg share T-cell epitopes. HBeAg may enter the thymus and induce immune tolerance to both HBsAg and HBeAg by decreasing the production of HBV-specific cytotoxic T lymphocytes. However, these cells can be reactivated in patients who undergo a spontaneous or IFN-induced HBeAg seroconversion.[241] Soluble HBeAg may itself contribute to persistence of HBV; there is some evidence that HBeAg favors production of T-helper–cell type 2 cytokines rather than T-helper–cell type 1 cytokines, which have a greater role in noncytolytic control of HBV.[94]

Fulminant hepatitis is seen in less than 1% of infected individuals and has a high mortality rate. It is characterized by a brisk immune response and viral clearance. Those who survive will clear HBV and do not develop chronic HBV infection. A higher incidence of fulminant hepatitis occurs in those patients infected with HBV mutants that do not produce the HBeAg, suggesting either an increased rate of replication or lack of immune detection of the mutant HBV.[156]

Epidemiology and Transmission

Although HBV occurs throughout the world, marked geographic differences exist, with highest endemicity levels in sub-Saharan Africa and prevalence below 2% in regions such as tropical and Central Latin America, North America, and Western Europe (Fig. 157.3).[222]

Areas of high, intermediate, and low endemicity, as reflected by carrier status, have been identified. Highly endemic areas are those where more than 8% of the population is infected. Examples include Southeast Asia, Africa, Commonwealth of Independent States, and China. More than 70% of the world's population lives in these high-endemicity areas. The Middle East, Central and South America, and parts of Eastern Europe are examples of intermediate-endemicity regions, where infection is found in 2% to 7% of the population. The United States, Australia, and Western Europe are areas of low endemicity, with chronic infection rates of less than 2% of the total population.[299] In countries where HBV infection is highly endemic, perinatal or vertical transmission is very common. In areas of low endemicity, acute infections occur more commonly in adults, which, although causing significant morbidity, are less likely to result in chronic carriage than are asymptomatic infections in children.

In the United States, the prevalence of chronic HBV infection (HBsAg positive) among the general population was 0.27% from 1999 to 2006. During this time, 4.7% of the US population had evidence of either past or chronic infection with HBV.[307] The most recent National Health and Nutrition Examination Survey (NHANES) covering 2007 to 2012 reports a stable overall prevalence of 0.3% in the United States. Since 1999, an estimated 10.8 million people have been infected with HBV.[245]

The rates among ethnic groups vary, with non-Hispanic blacks having the highest rates (12.2%) compared with non-Hispanic whites (2.8%) and Mexican Americans (2.9%). The prevalence rate of chronic HBV infection was higher among foreign-born children (0.89%) than US-born children (0.16%).[307]

HBV may be transmitted vertically, horizontally, parenterally, or sexually. Vertical transmission of HBV occurs in the perinatal setting when an infected mother transmits the infection to her child. If a mother is seropositive for both HBeAg and HBsAg, the risk for transmission of HBV to her child is 85% to 90% without immunoprophylaxis.[14]

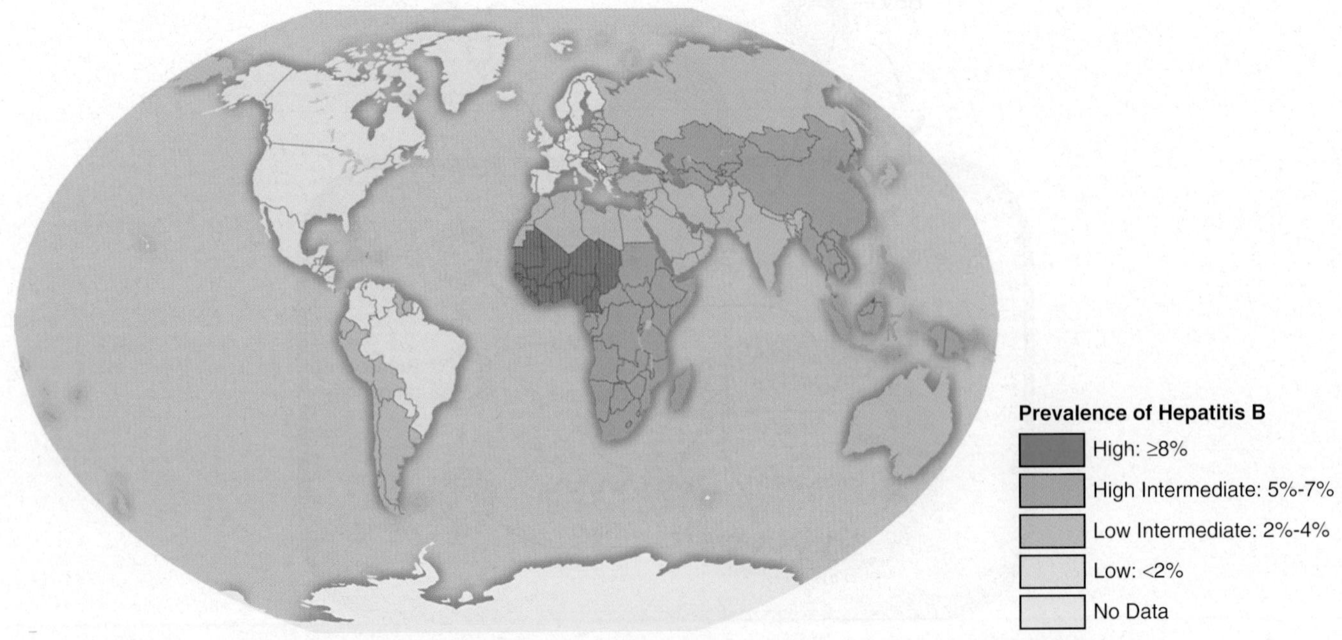

FIG. 157.3 Global prevalence of hepatitis B virus infection among adults. (From Centers for Disease Control and Prevention. Infectious diseases related to travel. Available at: http://wwwnc.cdc.gov/travel/yellowbook/2016/infectious-diseases-related-to-travel/hepatitis-b.)

Horizontal transmission occurs among children in groups with moderate to high endemicity[83] who were not infected at birth.

The most common risk factors for acquisition of acute HBV in adults in the United States were heterosexual exposure or having multiple sexual partners (27%), intravenous drug use (18%), men who have sex with men (13%), household contact (3.6%), and occupational exposure (16%).[106] Approximately one-third of people reported no risk factors during the study period.[106]

Within the United States, the number of reported cases of acute hepatitis B decreased 81% between 1990 and 2006 to the lowest rate ever recorded (0.9 per 100,000 population).[306] Hepatitis B elimination strategies—such as screening of pregnant women, universal immunization of infants, and catch-up immunization of older children—are credited with the reduced incidence in children.

The experience from Taiwan, the first country to implement mass vaccination against HBV, is encouraging. Since 1986, all neonates have been vaccinated against HBV. Seroprevalence of HBsAg declined from 9.8% before this strategy to 0.6% 20 years later.[211] There was a significant decrease in the incidence of HCC, from 0.54 to 0.20 per 100,000 children, between 1986 and 2000, and the proportion of infants and children with hepatitis B as a cause of fulminant hepatic failure in Taiwan decreased from 82% before mass vaccination to 57%.[53]

Researchers have estimated that only 45% of the expected 20,000 HBsAg-positive women giving birth in the United States between 1993 and 1996 were identified.[265] This low figure may be due to numerous factors; women likely to be infected often do not receive prenatal care[263] or women may be tested but the information not conveyed to the place of birth or to the pediatrician caring for the child.[14] Attention to this aspect of care is extremely important because the reduction in rate of transmission from mother to child with use of hepatitis B immunoglobulin (HBIG) and hepatitis B vaccine is as high as 90%.[274] HBsAg can be found in the breast milk of HBV-infected mothers. However, in studies performed in Taiwan and England, breastfeeding by HBsAg-seropositive mothers did not significantly increase the risk for neonatal acquisition of HBV infection.[230] A study of 230 infants in China demonstrated that breastfed infants had similar response rates to HBV vaccination and failure rates to HBV immunoprophylaxis as bottle-fed infants.[305] Effective immunoprophylaxis should allow for safe breastfeeding.

Natural History

Individuals infected with HBV can develop acute or chronic infection. Acute HBV infection is most common in young men older than 19 years and women older than 40 years,[78,106] but most do not develop chronic disease. Children infected perinatally rarely develop acute hepatitis, but fulminant hepatic failure has been reported, particularly in infants born to HBeAg-negative mothers.[53] The clinical and serologic findings of chronic hepatitis B are shown in Fig. 157.4.

After infection with HBV, most patients either develop immunity and clear the infection or become chronic carriers. A lower percentage will develop liver disease or chronic active hepatitis with an increased risk of developing cirrhosis, liver cancer, or both. Chronic HBV infection progresses nonlinearly through four phases (Fig. 157.5): immune-tolerant phase (high viral load, normal alanine transaminase [ALT]), immuno-clearance phase (elevated viral load and ALT), inactive chronic carrier phase (low viral load, normal ALT), and reactivation of viral replication, which is observed only rarely. However, interplay among stages differs among patient groups.

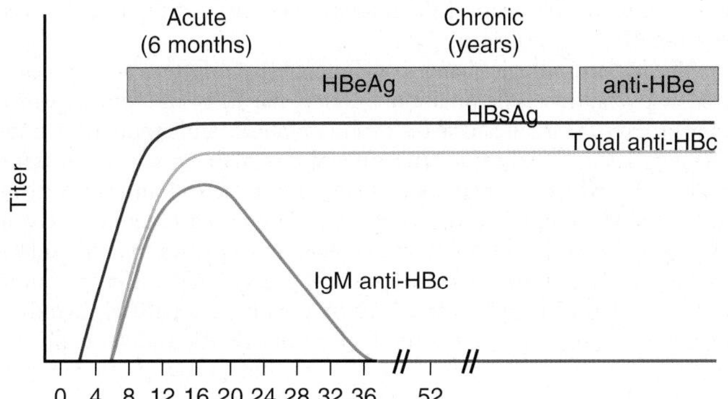

FIG. 157.4 Progression to chronic hepatitis B virus infection. *HBc*, Hepatitis B core antigen; *HBeAg*, hepatitis B envelope antigen; *HBsAg*, hepatitis B surface antigen; *IgM*, immunoglobulin M.

The risk for acquiring chronic hepatitis B is related to a number of factors, such as very young age, other medical conditions, and other infections. The likelihood of progression to chronic infection is inversely related to age at the time of infection (Fig. 157.6). Approximately 90% of infants infected perinatally become chronic carriers unless vaccinated at birth. The risk for chronic HBV infection decreases to 30% of children infected between ages 1 and 4 years and to less than 5% of persons infected as adults. If an infected person has other medical problems, such as end-stage renal disease requiring hemodialysis, or is coinfected with HIV, the risk for development of chronic HBV infection increases. The risk for development of HCC is increased in all HBV chronic carriers but especially those with active viral replication.[17] Four of 99 children in an Italian study had HBeAg-positive cirrhosis; after 14.5 ± 6.1 years of follow-up, two developed HCC and two had lost histopathologic features of cirrhosis.[31,33]

Most Chinese children, in whom chronic HBV usually is perinatally acquired, remain HBeAg positive, with very high levels of viral replication yet only minimal clinical liver disease.[182,183] In contrast, children in the West with chronic HBV infection frequently clear HBeAg and HBV DNA from serum during the first 2 decades.[32] In extended follow-up of the Italian study above, of 89 children who cleared HBeAg, four experienced reactivation, three of whom had HBeAg-negative hepatitis.[33] Those who lost HBeAg tend to have higher ALT levels early in life, indicating more active liver disease. Some of the children (15.4%) became seronegative for HBsAg as well.[33]

Children born to Asian and Afro-Caribbean mothers in the United Kingdom who acquired HBV infection perinatally had a much lower (29%) rate of HBeAg seroconversion than white children in the U.K. study (80%)[34] or Italy (98%).[33] These differences are ascribed to the older age at acquisition of HBV in Western children which is associated with a more efficient immune response. These observations influence the management and counseling of children with chronic HBV infection as well as the design and interpretation of therapeutic trials.

Extrahepatic manifestations of both acute and chronic HBV infection occur more commonly in adults. Up to 25% of adults with acute HBV infection have extrahepatic manifestations, such as arthralgia and even serum-like sickness. Vasculitides can develop in both acute and chronic HBV infections; examples include polyarteritis nodosa, renal disease, and mononeuritis.[202] Membranoproliferative glomerulonephritis is an extrahepatic manifestation of chronic HBV infection in some children.[148,272] There is a case report of epididymitis related to acute hepatitis B in a 12-year-old boy.[284]

Carcinogenesis

HCC is a recognized sequela of chronic infection with HBV; worldwide, most cases of HCC are linked to HBV infection. In Taiwan, the incidence of HCC in chronically infected individuals was 200 to 812 cases per 100,000 person-years compared with 10 to 30 cases per 100,000 person-years in the general population. In those with liver cirrhosis secondary to chronic HBV infection, the incidence increased to 1000 to 5000 cases per 100,000 person-years (1–5% per year).[54] Prior to effective therapies, the lifetime risk for development of HCC in a chronically infected person was estimated at 40% to 50%.[17] The incidence of HCC is associated with serum HBV DNA levels in a dose-response relationship.[59] The risk for HCC after treatment is not clear; most treated individuals remain HBsAg positive and remain at some risk.

The detection of integrated HBV sequences in both human HCC and animal models has led to numerous theories regarding the mechanisms leading to HCC. Current hypotheses center on the integration of viral DNA into host genome, which may be associated with activation of oncogenes, deactivation of tumor suppressor genes, or other genetic instability. The finding that HCC cells in an infected individual contain

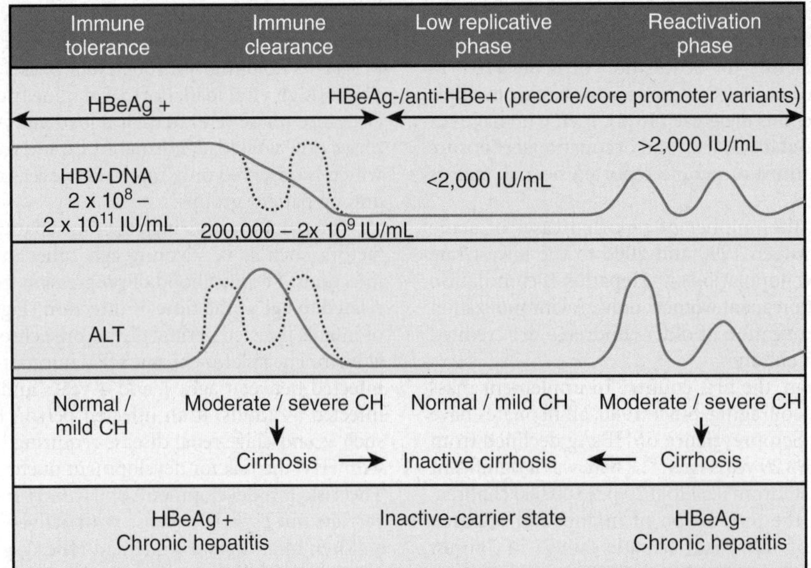

FIG. 157.5 Phases of chronic hepatitis B virus (HBV) infection: immune tolerant phase (high viral load, normal alanine aminotransferase [ALT]), immunoclearance phase (elevated viral load and ALT), inactive chronic carrier phase (low viral load, normal ALT), and reactivation of viral replication. *CH,* Chronic hepatitis; *HBeAg,* hepatitis B envelope antigen. (From Gish RG. Diagnosis of chronic hepatitis B and the implications of viral variants and mutations. *Am J Med.* 2008;121[12 Suppl]:S12–S21.)

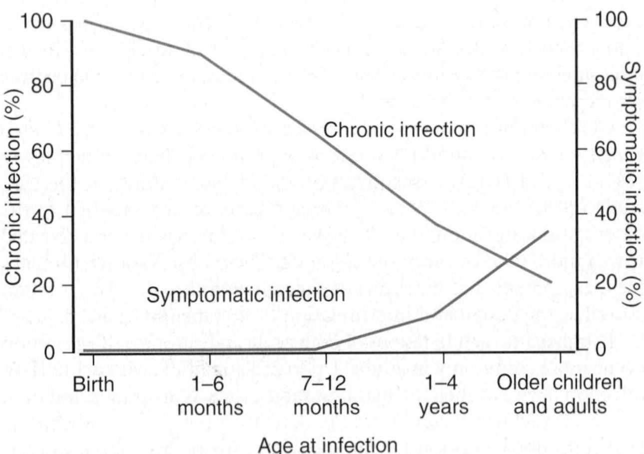

FIG. 157.6 Outcome of hepatitis B virus infection by age at infection.

HBV DNA in discrete rather than random sites, indicating clonal expansion of tumor cells, supports this theory.[236] The frequency and significance of integration of viral DNA into the host genome are unresolved issues in childhood HBV infection; some studies have shown early integration, whereas others describe it as a rare event.[15,49,107,257,310] HBsAg loss has been associated with decreased risk of HCC, particularly if it occurs before the development of cirrhosis. Recent studies showed that high levels of HBV viremia are associated with an increased risk of cirrhosis, HCC, and liver-related mortality. Genotype of HBV may be an indirect marker of HCC risk. Genotype C with TCC at codon 15 of the precore region is associated with an increased risk for HCC in a Hong Kong population with cirrhosis.[43]

Prevention of HBV infection and eradication of existing infection remain the most effective measures to prevent HCC. After a nationwide hepatitis B vaccination program implemented in Taiwan in 1984, there was a significant decrease in the incidence of HCC, from 0.54 to 0.23 per 100,000 children between 1986 and 2000.[47,211] A recent review of 1509 patients age 6 to 26 years from two Taiwan HCC registries diagnosed with HCC from 1983 to 2011 demonstrated a significant difference in incidence of HCC among vaccinated and unvaccinated cohorts: 0.23 and 0.92 per 100,000 people, respectively.[51] Incomplete immunization was the most important risk predictor of HCC among vaccinated infants.[48,53] The 5-year survival rate in children with HCC is less than 30% despite treatment.[321]

The age at which surveillance for HCC should commence and the optimal frequency have not been determined.[186] Although HCC is detected most often after at least 20 years of chronic HBV infection, cases in children as young as 8 months old have been reported.[103,283,314] Childhood HCC associated with HBV infection has been described in both Asian[52,283] and Western[103,232] populations. Because most cases are reported retrospectively, data regarding incidence are not available. No guidelines have been developed for prospective monitoring of children with chronic HBV infection for development of HCC, although periodic measurement of serum α-fetoprotein levels combined with hepatic ultrasound evaluations are recommended in adults.

Histopathologic Features

The purposes of obtaining a liver biopsy in chronic HBV infection are to quantify the severity of fibrosis, to rule out other causes of liver disease, and to monitor disease severity after treatment. In typical acute viral hepatitis, a liver biopsy usually is not required or indicated. If performed, the findings are liver cell degeneration and necrosis, with lobular disarray. The acute injury to hepatocytes is manifested as both ballooning and acidophilic degeneration, either of which can resolve or progress to cell death. Inflammatory cell infiltration and liver cell regeneration are also seen.[121]

The histopathologic changes of chronic HBV infection are characterized by portal tract inflammation, interface hepatitis, and fibrosis, which may progress to architectural distortion of lobules and eventual cirrhosis (see Fig. 157.7).[121] Chronic HBV infection is characterized by "ground glass" cells, which are hepatocytes containing HBsAg and most easily identified by staining with orcein, Victoria blue, or aldehyde fuchsin. However, these cells also are found in other liver diseases, and the pattern of staining is important. In hepatitis B, ground glass cells are found either singly or in clusters arranged in a haphazard pattern. "Sanded" liver nuclei are caused by accumulation of HBcAg and generally are identified by electron microscopy[127] or immunoperoxidase techniques (see Fig. 157.7).

Histopathologic staging and grading systems are used to allow standardization and meaningful comparisons in chronic hepatitis. One such system is the Knodell-Ishak score, which evaluates four

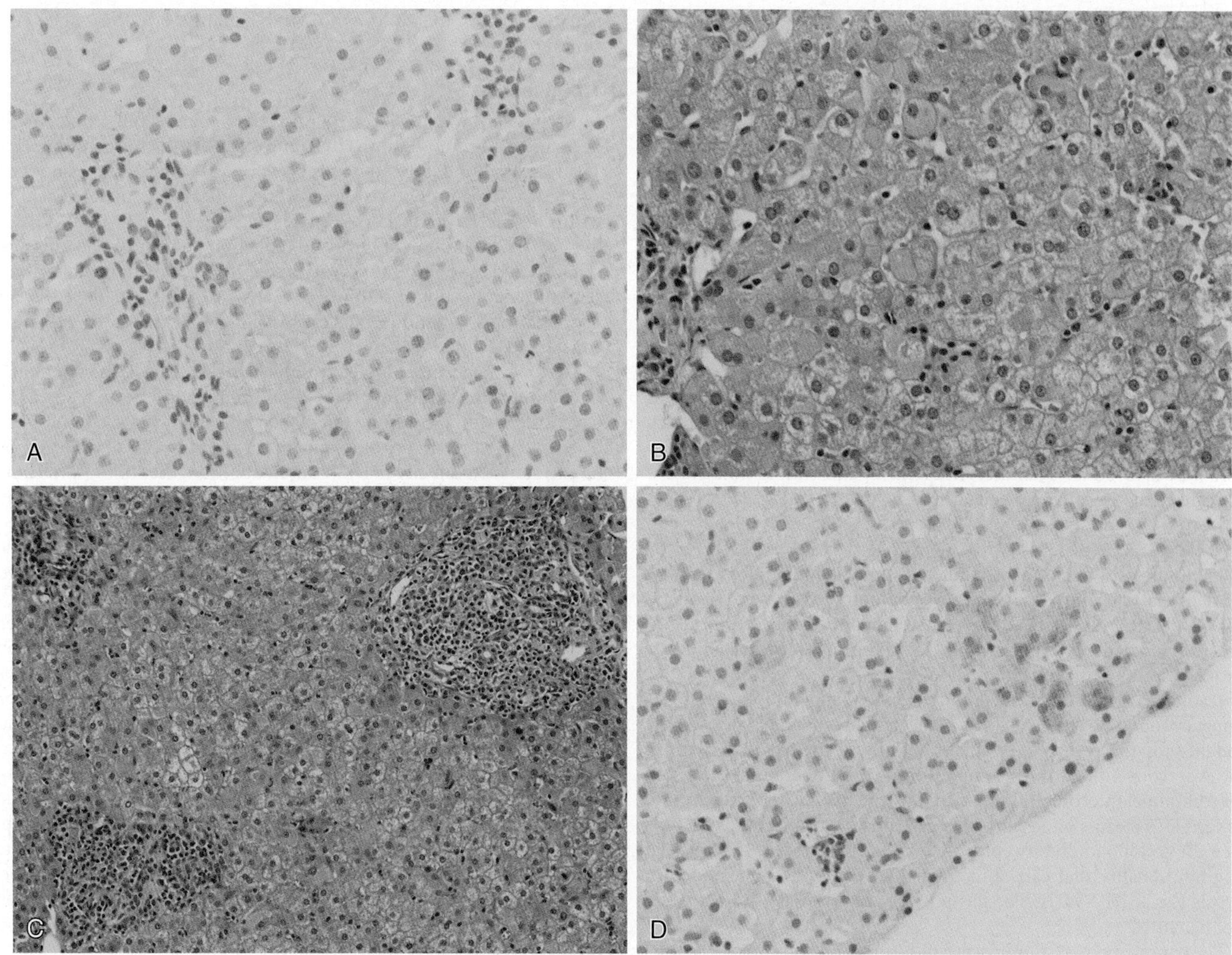

FIG. 157.7 Liver histology in hepatitis B infection. (A) Core antigen (HBcAg) immunohistochemical stain demonstrating nuclear staining of scattered hepatocytes at ×40. (B) Scattered hepatocytes with ground glass, finely granular cytoplasmic inclusions with focal displacement of the nucleus to the periphery at ×40. (C) Portal tracts with moderate lymphoplasmacytic inflammation and minimal interface activity at ×20. Occasional hepatocytes show ground glass, finely granular cytoplasmic inclusions. (D) Hepatitis B surface antigen (HBsAg) immunohistochemical stain shows occasional hepatocytes with cytoplasmic staining at ×40.

histopathologic features, each scored using specific criteria.[150] This system has proved reproducible, is now in common use, and is also known as the modified histologic activity. Other systems are the Batts-Ludwig[16] system and the METAVIR system, which categorizes liver fibrosis into 4 stages (F0, no fibrosis; F1, portal fibrosis without septa [mild]; F2, portal fibrosis with few septa [moderate]; F3, numerous septa without cirrhosis [severe]; and F4, cirrhosis).[250] The systematic classifications are useful in estimating progression of disease and response to therapy and for comparing outcomes in therapeutic trials. More recent studies of patients with chronic HBV showed improvement and even reversal of hepatic fibrosis[157] and histologic activity index after treatment with antivirals.

Biomarkers

The rapid onset of liver disease in some children (i.e., HBV, genotype C) indicates a need to identify early markers of liver fibrosis to help facilitate early intervention. Serum chemistries used to assess hepatic inflammation and injury are not reliable. Empirically identified markers identified by genomic, proteomic, and metabolomic technologies, as well as targeted serum marker analysis, offer new strategies with which to diagnose and predict outcomes in pediatric liver diseases.[92,218,225,270] Preliminary studies in children with fibrotic liver diseases have identified specific markers reflecting matrix remodeling, hepatic stellate cell activation, and chemoattractant expression in this age group.[218–220,270] Collagen markers and micro-RNA are also among the biomarkers of fibrosis being investigated for viral hepatitis.

No single marker has yet proven useful in children with chronic HBV infection, but serum noninvasive models using a combination of serum markers and enzyme immunoassays to predict hepatic fibrosis have been studied in adults and children with viral hepatitis with promising results.[171,238] Fibrotest (Biopredictive), which includes alpha2-microglobulin, haptoglobin, gamma-glutamyl peptidase, total bilirubin, ALT, and apolipoprotein A1 to provide a score of 0 to 1, with a conversion to the stages of fibrosis has been widely studied and proven to be a good biomarker for fibrosis[74,233] in viral hepatitis. The Enhanced Liver Fibrosis (ELF) test (Siemens Healthcare Diagnostics Inc.) is another panel of biomarkers comprised of hyaluronic acid, tissue inhibitor of matrix metalloproteinase-1, and aminoterminal propeptide of procollagen type III, derived from studies in patients with a range of chronic liver diseases including chronic hepatitis B.[246] A study looking at ELF in a cohort of 182 patients with chronic hepatitis B who underwent liver biopsies showed areas under the receiver operating characteristic curve (AUROC) of 0.77, 0.82, 0.80, and 0.83 for detecting METAVIR fibrosis stages $F \geq 1$, $F \geq 2$, $F \geq 3$, and F4, respectively, suggesting that ELF has good performance in detection of liver fibrosis in patients with chronic hepatitis B.[291]

Aspartate aminotransferase (AST)-platelet ratio index (APRI) and fibrosis index based on the four-factor (platelets, ALT, AST, and age) fibrosis-4 (FIB-4) calculation are the most useful serum biomarkers in identifying advanced or severe liver fibrosis in patients with chronic hepatitis C.[110,259,297] However, their clinical utilities in patients with chronic hepatitis B have been controversial.[40,258,286,292,304,320] Recent studies have shown APRI and FIB-4 to be useful for the diagnosis of fibrosis, with similar accuracy in predicting significant and severe fibrosis.

For prediction of significant fibrosis, severe fibrosis, and cirrhosis, the AUROCs of FIB-4 were 0.646, 0.670, and 0.715, respectively, and 0.656, 0.653, and 0.639, respectively, for APRI in a 2016 study looking at 1543 consecutive chronic hepatitis B patients who underwent liver biopsies from 2006 to 2010. Further subgroup analysis demonstrated that the diagnostic accuracy of FIB-4 and APRI in patients with normal ALT was higher than that in patients with elevated ALT.[328] A systematic review and meta-analysis in 2015 showed that APRI and FIB-4 can identify hepatitis B–related fibrosis with moderate sensitivity and accuracy in adult patients.[315] In children with chronic hepatitis B, APRI has also been shown to be an accurate, inexpensive, and simple noninvasive index in predicting advanced liver fibrosis.[71,200]

Imaging

Other noninvasive techniques studied in adults and children include transient elastography, shear wave elastography (SWE), and acoustic radiation force impulse (ARFI).[18] These modalities appear promising in identifying patients with normal or near-normal ALT but significant fibrosis who might benefit from therapy.[146]

Traditional gray-scale ultrasound imaging (sonography) uses high-frequency sound waves to view soft tissues and organs and is an excellent modality for the pediatric population, limiting the use of radiation. However, conventional ultrasound is limited by operator experience and technique, interpretation bias, and by the inability to differentiate between liver steatosis and fibrosis, a particularly important distinction given the childhood obesity epidemic.[57,104] Furthermore, a noninvasive imaging modality that can differentiate between mild and moderate fibrosis (i.e., F1/F2 vs. F2/F3) has not yet been validated in pediatric viral hepatitis.

The complementary noninvasive ultrasound advancement, elastography, measures the inherent elasticity of the liver, which may be altered by pathologic processes such as inflammation, tumor, and, importantly, fibrosis.[38,217,319] Elastography has the ability to assess small changes in pliability of liver tissue across the entire liver. Elasticity of tissue in the context of elastography is the ratio of tension (stress) needed to produce a relative change in length (strain) and quantifies how much pressure must be placed on tissue in order to cause elastic deformation.[45,282] Two types of elastography are widely used in imaging, transient elastography (TE) and SWE. TE—that is, FibroScan (EchoSens)—requires mild compression with the ultrasound transducer with some limitations gaining access to the liver due to overlying ribs. SWE is a reproducible technology that assesses tissue stiffness by measuring the speed of a shear wave through tissue, measured in units of speed in the United States and pressure (kilopascals) in Europe, neutralizing operator variability. Recent publications have reported that SWE is more accurate than TE in the detection of significant liver fibrosis (greater than F2). Similarly, ARFI imaging allows for the assessment of tissue stiffness by evaluating the wave propagation speed[204] using a conventional probe without the need for external compression, which reduces operator dependency. The generated wave scan provides qualitative (imaging by Virtual Touch Tissue Imaging; Siemens) or quantitative (wave velocity values, measured in m/s using Virtual Touch Tissue Quantification; Siemens) responses. Studies comparing TE and ARFI demonstrate that both methods yield reliable assessment of liver fibrosis. ARFI is being used with promising results in studies to evaluate liver fibrosis in children with diffuse liver diseases and biliary atresia before and after transplantation.[114,115]

Normal values of SWE and ARFI have been established for the liver and other organs in the body, showing much promise as a tool to distinguish normal from abnormal tissue in adults and children.[10,97,113]

Elastography and ARFI allow for a more global assessment of liver fibrosis than a single core of liver tissue and are being used to detect hepatic fibrosis in adults with viral hepatitis[5,93,108] but not yet in children.

Treatment

Most patients with acute HBV infection recover fully and develop permanent immunity (anti-HBs), and treatment is purely supportive. The role of antiviral therapy in fulminant HBV infection has not been studied systematically. Treatment, when indicated, is directed at those with chronic HBV infection. In this setting, the long-term goals of therapy are eradication of HBV and reduction of cirrhosis, development of HCC, and mortality. Intermediate goals for treatment include HBeAg seroconversion, suppression of HBV DNA to undetectable levels, and normalization of aminotransferase values. Clearance of HBsAg is considered a functional cure.

To date, no agents completely fulfill all of these goals in either adults or children, but significant progress has been made. Children and adults have differences in immune tolerance and rate of progression of liver disease. Therefore, studies of treatments of chronic HBV in adults cannot be extrapolated directly to children. In addition, the timing and choice of therapeutic agent are crucial because of differences in age, maturity, stage in natural history, and comorbidities.

A child being considered for treatment should have serologic evidence of chronic HBV infection, such as HBsAg for at least 6 months, as well as evidence of active HBV replication, HBeAg, or HBV DNA (in the case of eAg-negative HBV infection). In addition, children with consistent ALT elevation of at least twice the upper limit of normal or active disease on liver biopsy are more likely to benefit from treatment. Because therapy may be indefinite, a liver biopsy should be considered before the start of therapy to provide evidence of chronic hepatitis, to stage the disease, and to rule out other processes.

In most studies performed before the high prevalence of HBeAg-negative infections, seroconversion from HBeAg to anti-HBe in serum was used as the primary outcome variable for response to therapy. Therapeutic trial results must be compared with the "background rate" of spontaneous conversion from HBeAg positive to anti-HBe, which in children younger than 3 years is very low (<2% per year) but increase with age so that in children older than 6 years, the yearly clearance rates vary from 14.3% to 35.3%.[46]

Quantitative HBsAg and quantitative HBeAg are being investigated as predictors for treatment responses. Varying levels of quantitative HBsAg have been documented over the natural course of HBV infection and among different genotypes.[129] Levels of HBsAg decrease with increasing age and progression of disease with increased fibrosis.[128] These values may be helpful in determining treatment strategies and algorithms for stopping therapy.[44,173]

First-line antiviral treatment options for HBV-infected children include IFN-α and the nucleos(t)ide analogs entecavir and tenofovir. In the United States, interferon (IFN-α) is approved for children after the age of 1 year and lamivudine and entecavir after 2 years. Adefovir and tenofovir have been approved for use in children 12 years and older. IFN, lamivudine, and adefovir are no longer recommended first-line treatments for adults with HBV due to availability of other agents with better side effect profile and resistance rate. Clinical trials using pegylated IFN-α2a and tenofovir in children with chronic HBV are under way.

Interferon

IFNs are a family of cytokines with immunomodulatory, antiproliferative, and direct antiviral actions. IFN induces the display of human leukocyte antigen class I molecules on hepatocyte membranes, which, in turn, promotes lysis by $CD8^+$ cytotoxic lymphocytes. At the same time, it directly inhibits viral protein synthesis.[172] IFN-α has been the primary form used in the treatment of chronic HBV infection; IFN-α2a and IFN-α2b have been licensed in the United States for use in children. Peginterferon-α, in which the IFN molecule is attached to polyethylene glycol to allow for once weekly versus three times weekly injections, is the preferred form in adults but has not yet been approved in the United States for children with chronic HBV. Clinical trials of a combination of pegylated IFN plus entecavir in children with immune-tolerant chronic HBV are under way.

Loss of HBV DNA or development of HBeAg seroconversion was achieved with IFN-α treatment in 20% to 58% (compared to 8–17% in the control group) of European and 3% to 17% of Asian children in early studies.[164,296] The difference may be due to higher rates of perinatally acquired infections in the Asian countries studied. A large multinational, randomized control led trial of IFN-α2b later showed similar loss of HBsAg between children born in Asian countries (22%) and those from Europe and North America (26%) if aminotransferase values were elevated.[267] Ten percent of treated adults and children lose HBsAg, compared with 1% of untreated patients.[155,267] Long-term (1.1–11.5 years) follow-up of adult responders to IFN-α showed a significantly reduced incidence of HCC compared with either treated nonresponders or untreated control patients.[179] The long-term outlook for treated children is not yet clear. In a Turkish study, none of the 23 treatment nonresponders developed cirrhosis or HCC at a mean follow-up of 4.5 years.[151] A second study compared long-term (5.6 ± 3.1 years) outcome in two groups of 37 children: one group was treated with IFN-α2β and the second control group of children age matched for age, sex, and baseline ALT level received no treatment. At time of follow-up, the rates of HBeAg and HBsAg loss were 54.1% (20/37) and 8.1% (3/37) in treated children compared with 35.1% (13/37) and 2.7% (1/37), respectively, in untreated children (not significant). Histologic outcomes in children with chronic HBV treated with IFN-α for 20 weeks have been reported in 93 children, average age 7.1 years, in Poland. Liver biopsy samples were obtained before treatment and 12 months after the end of the treatment and graded for fibrosis and inflammation using three different scoring systems. Over a third of children underwent HBeAg/anti-HBe seroconversion. Liver fibrosis did not improve regardless of responder status, but inflammatory activity was decreased after treatment in both responders and nonresponders.[312] Two meta-analyses of treatment of chronic HBV in children with IFN-α have been conducted. Each concludes that treatment leads to a higher rate of HBeAg seroconversion than would occur spontaneously.[290,295] Unfortunately, two-thirds of children treated with IFN-α show no sustained response to therapy.

Children with evidence of active immunologic responses to HBV (i.e., low/high alternation levels of viral replication [HBV DNA]) and high ALT values (greater than twice normal) are more likely to have a response to therapy with IFN-α.[290] A study from Sweden demonstrated that pretreatment HBV DNA levels were associated with sustained virologic response.[266] Children who acquired disease by vertical transmission are more likely to have established immune tolerance and may be less likely to respond to treatment. Children with very low HBV DNA levels may be in the process of spontaneous seroconversion; therefore, an expectant policy may be prudent.

Side effects of IFN-α include a transient influenza-like syndrome (fever, myalgia, headache, arthralgia, and anorexia) that occurs in virtually all patients at the start of therapy. Bone marrow suppression, especially neutropenia, is a common side effect, seen in 39% of children in one series.[126] Changes in personality, irritability, and temper tantrums are reported more frequently in children than in adults and may interfere with compliance.[126,267] These problems resolve once treatment is withdrawn. Febrile seizures and marked elevation of aminotransferase levels have also been reported. Quality of life is impaired in children during IFN therapy compared with their pretreatment levels because of medication side effects and fear of injections. However, within 3 months of cessation of treatment, these effects are reversed.[126]

HBV Polymerase Inhibitors

This class of agents includes the nucleoside and nucleotide analogs that inhibit HBV polymerase by incorporation into viral DNA, leading to termination. They are administered orally and generally well tolerated[189] and presented in the order they were approved by the US Food and Drug Administration.

Lamivudine

Lamivudine (2′,3′-dideoxycytosine), also known as 3TC, is an oral nucleoside analog. It is triphosphorylated intracellularly to an active intermediate that is incorporated into the growing DNA chain, thereby terminating the chain and inhibiting viral replication.

There are a number of large randomized studies demonstrating benefit of lamivudine in children and adults.[79,163] Treatment with lamivudine achieved clearance of HBV DNA and HBeAg in 23% compared with 13% in the placebo group ($P < .05$). However, 19% of the treatment group developed the primary mutation associated with lamivudine resistance (i.e., tyrosine-methionine-aspartate-aspartate) in the first 48 weeks of therapy. Higher response rates were observed in those with positive HBeAg and higher ALT levels, as had been noted with IFN.[212] Longer duration of treatment (3 years) improved response rate but also showed increased development of resistant mutants (up to 58%). Mutations induced by lamivudine often confer resistance to the newer antiviral agents. The virologic response to those with the tyrosine-methionine-aspartate-aspartate variant was only 5% (5/100) compared with 49% (34/70) in those with wild-type HBV.[269] The use of lamivudine has largely been replaced in adult HBV treatment by newer agents with more favorable resistance profiles. The same has been true within pediatrics. While no longer considered a first-line treatment option, lamivudine has utility in the prevention of vertical transmission of HBV in developing countries and may be considered in restricted circumstances.

No serious side effects of lamivudine were reported. However, lamivudine is excreted by the kidneys, and use in patients with renal failure requires dose reduction. On cessation of therapy, patients need to be monitored for the occurrence of "lamivudine withdrawal flare" presenting with elevation of serum ALT of up to three times baseline (as compared with 8% of placebo-treated patients) possibly progressing to jaundice and incipient liver failure.[119]

Studies of combination therapy with IFN-α and lamivudine have been performed in both children and adults. In adults with HBeAg-positive chronic HBV, peginterferon-α2a either alone or in combination with lamivudine for 48 weeks was superior to lamivudine alone, achieving HBeAg seroconversion, normalization of ALT, and HBV DNA suppression in 21% compared with 23% of those who received peginterferon plus placebo and 10% who received lamivudine alone.[168] A complete response rate of 34% has been reported in children on combination therapy.[7,162]

Adefovir Dipivoxil

Adefovir dipivoxil (ADV) is a synthetic nucleotide analog of adenosine monophosphate[326] that was first approved in 2002 but is no longer considered first-line therapy for HBV infection. Previous studies have demonstrated efficacy in patients with HBeAg-positive and HBcAg-negative chronic HBV infection, showing significant virologic, biochemical, and histologic improvement after 48 weeks of treatment in adults and children.[112,134] A study of ADV in 173 children with HBeAg-positive chronic hepatitis B showed that 23% of children aged 12 to 18 years were able to achieve a normal ALT and HBV DNA less than 1000 copies/mL compared with no subjects treated with placebo.[134] However, approximately 30% of patients display primary nonresponse to ADV, defined as a less than $2\log_{10}$ drop in serum HBV DNA after 6 months of treatment.

Various mutations (including N236T and A181V) have already been described to confer resistance to ADV, with resistance rates up to 29% after 5 years of treatment. Also of concern is that HBV isolates with N236T and A181V mutations in in vitro studies have decreased susceptibility to the newer agent tenofovir by 4-fold and 3.2-fold, respectively,[181,298,302,332] making adefovir a less desirable treatment for HBV.

Tenofovir

While tenofovir disoproxil fumarate (TDF), a nucleotide analog reverse-transcriptase inhibitor, was approved for children more than 2 years when used as a component of antiretroviral therapy in 2001, it had only recently been approved in September 2012 for monotherapy of chronic HBV in children over 12 years of age in the United States. A randomized, placebo-controlled trial using tenofovir in adolescents demonstrated potent antiviral effects with acceptable safety. A total of 106 patients were enrolled to take either tenofovir 300 mg or placebo once daily for 72 weeks. Normalization of the ALT value occurred in 74% of patients taking tenofovir and 31% (relative risk [RR], 2; 95% CI, 1.4–2.9) of patients taking placebo with significantly higher HBV DNA suppression (RR, 92.4; 95% CI, 5.8–146.7).[209] The study did not show any evidence of TDF resistance at the end of 72 weeks, a significant advantage of TDF.[209] This finding was also confirmed in adult open-label phase III studies in which 238 HBeAg-positive patients receiving TDF monotherapy were able to maintain effective suppression of HBV DNA through 288 weeks of treatment with no evidence of TDF resistance.[147] Furthermore, tenofovir appears to be an effective rescue therapy in chronic HBV patients who failed previous nucleoside analog treatments.[159] Baseline HBV DNA may be a significant predictive factor for a virologic response to TDF mono-rescue therapy for multidrug-resistant chronic HBV.[174]

Adverse events were not common in either group, but TDF was associated with a small risk in decreased bone mineral density compared to placebo, especially in patients with HIV who are at risk for osteoporosis.[207,209] Clinical trials to examine the safety and efficacy of TDF in children age 2 to less than 12 years as well as tenofovir alafenamide are currently under way (ClinicalTrials.gov NCT01651403).

Entecavir

Entecavir (ETV) is a cyclopentyl guanosine analog that inhibits HBV polymerase that was approved by the Food and Drug Administration for use in March 2014 to treat children age 2 years and older with chronic HBV. ETV for 48 weeks suppresses HBV DNA levels in both HBeAg-positive and HBeAg-negative adults at higher rates compared with lamivudine.[120,133,136,185,187,311]

In one cohort study of 1980 adult patients with chronic HBV and cirrhosis followed for a mean of 52 months, ETV versus control reduced the risk of HCC (RR, 0.3; 95% CI, 0.1–0.5) and death (RR, 0.6; 95% CI, 0.3–0.98). A randomized control led trial comparing ETV versus placebo in 228 children with chronic HBV from North America, South America, Europe, and Asia demonstrated higher ALT normalization (RR, 2.9; 95% CI, 1.8–4.7), HBV DNA suppression (RR, 14.8; 95% CI, 3.7–58.3), and HBeAg seroconversion (RR, 2.4; 95% CI, 1.1–5.5) at 48 weeks. Longer duration of treatment (96 weeks) resulted in persistently statistically significant HBeAg seroconversion (RR, 1.8; 95% CI, 1.0–3.4). More recent studies of patients with chronic HBV treated with ETV showed improvement and even reversal of hepatic fibrosis.[157,303] Long-term follow-up studies of ETV in children are forthcoming.

In children with baseline HBV DNA less than 8 log_{10} IU/mL, the virologic response rates were similar between children (83%) and adults (79%). The virologic response was lower (28%) at 48 weeks when HBV DNA was greater than or equal to 8 log_{10} IU/mL) but increased to 64% with 96 weeks of ETV therapy. A 2016 report by Chang et al.[50] described nine children with chronic HBV treated with ETV at 0.015 mg/kg/day (maximum dose, 0.5 mg daily) for at least 52 weeks, five of whom (55.6%) demonstrated a complete viral response. These children had undetectable HBV DNA levels at 1 year after study entry, which was significantly higher than the control group (11.1%).

Furthermore, ETV has been shown to have low resistance rates in adults and children and is able to suppress both lamivudine-resistant and adefovir-resistant viruses, although a higher dose of the medication is indicated in the lamivudine experienced. In a randomized control led trial in children, ETV was well tolerated with no observed differences in adverse events or changes in growth compared with placebo.[132] A clinical trial using combination pegylated IFN and ETV in children with chronic HBV is under way (ClinicalTrials.gov NCT01368497, Phase III).

Hepatitis B in Special Populations

Hepatitis B and Human Immunodeficiency Virus Coinfection

Although the prevalence varies from region to region, approximately 5% to 10% of HIV-infected adults worldwide also have chronic HBV infection. HIV/HBV coinfection in some sub-Saharan African populations is believed to be significantly higher.[37,197,287] The prevalence of HBV infection among HIV-positive individuals is significantly higher than in HIV-negative individuals, an expected finding due to the common transmission routes (perinatal, horizontal, parenteral, sexual).[6,195] The prevalence of HBV/HIV-coinfected pregnant women in Africa ranges from 0.4% to 7.1%. It is estimated that three million people from sub-Saharan Africa are coinfected with HIV and HBV, many of whom may be immunotolerant children.[234,248]

The prevalence and course of HBV infection in adults who are coinfected with HIV have been examined in numerous studies. Of 181 HIV-infected adults in Greece, 71.8% of men who have sex with men and 91.7% of intravenous drug users had evidence of HBV infection.[81] In a study from Australia conducted between 1985 and 1989, men with HIV infection were more likely to have chronic HBV infection than were HIV-negative men.[24] In Western Europe and the United States, among HIV-infected persons, 6% to 14% have chronic hepatitis B, including 4% to 6% of heterosexuals, 9% to 17% of men who have sex with men, and 7% to 10% of injection drug users.[8] A recent study in Thailand found the prevalence of HBV coinfection in perinatally HIV-infected adolescents to be 3.3%.[12]

In HIV-positive patients—even those on combination antiretroviral therapy (cART), including lamivudine—low CD4 counts are associated with a higher rate of detectable HBV viremia.[271] Conversely, chronic HBV does not seem to alter the progression of HIV infection and does not influence HIV suppression or CD4 cell responses following cART. No evidence has been found for direct interaction between HBV and HIV. HIV/HBV-coinfected individuals have higher circulating levels of HBV DNA but not worse hepatic necroinflammation.[66] In patients with HBV and HIV coinfection, there are higher rates of HBV persistence, HBV relapse (reemergence of HBsAg), and more severe and rapid progression of liver disease. Spontaneous HBeAg seroconversion rarely occurs in this group.

In adults with coinfection, the progress and complications from HBV hepatitis occur at an increased rate. Patients with HIV, especially those with a lower number of CD4 cells, are up to six times more likely to develop chronic hepatitis B after acquiring infection than those without HIV. Furthermore, coinfected adults have more severe liver fibrosis with an increased risk of development of cirrhosis and end-stage liver disease in spite of evidence of less hepatic necroinflammatory pathology and lower ALTs.[67,100,111,235,288,289] Follow-up of over 5000 adult men in the Multicenter AIDS Cohort Study for a mean of 10.5 years found that those coinfected with HIV/HBV had an eightfold greater risk of mortality due to liver disease compared with those with HIV infection only and a 19-fold greater increase compared with those with HBV infection only. Immune reconstitution hepatitis can occur after initiation of cART, which may lead to anti-HBeAg seroconversion and loss of HBsAg or severe hepatic decompensation and death.[85,199] Furthermore, patients with coinfection are at risk for HBV reactivation following withdrawal of cART, which includes HBV-active agents.[84]

Limited longitudinal studies of HBV/HIV coinfection in children show that the mean HIV-1 RNA level was higher and the CD4 percentage was lower in children who had detectable HBV DNA levels, suggesting that children with more active HIV disease have less immune control of HBV. Adolescents with more severe immune suppression had higher levels of HBV DNA and were more likely to be HBsAg positive and have a significantly lower clearance rate.[249,251] Extrapolating from adult data, there is concern that HBV/HIV-coinfected children may have more active liver disease and progress more quickly to hepatic fibrosis and cirrhosis than monoinfected children.

HIV-infected children may be unprotected from HBV even after receiving the full three-dose immunization series, due to a less robust initial immunologic response and waning of anti-HBs antibody tiers.[3,231,264] In a study conducted by the International Maternal Pediatric Adolescent AIDS Clinical Trials group, only 24% of 204 HIV-infected cART-treated children (median age, 9 years) with a history of previous immunization with three doses of HBV vaccine had protective anti-HBsAg antibody levels prior to receiving a booster vaccine. Forty-five percent of the children became seropositive 8 weeks after a booster vaccine. Vaccine response was greatest in those children with higher CD4 counts and undetectable viral loads. Lao-Araya et al. [165,166] reported on 64 HIV-infected children (median age, 10 years) on cART for a median of 31 months with a previous history of routine infant HBV immunization. Eighty-seven percent had no measurable anti-HBsAg antibody prior to revaccination. The response rate to a repeat HBV immunization series was 17% after the first vaccine, 82.5% after the second, and 92% after the third. After 3 years, 71% of these children maintained protective anti-HBsAg antibody levels, suggesting that

HIV-infected children will benefit from a repeat HBV vaccine series after initiation of cART.

Extrapolating from data in adults, IFN-α may be less effective in coinfected children, particularly in those with significant HIV-associated immune suppression. Nevertheless, IFN-α is the preferred treatment, particularly in younger children and in those who meet indications for HBV but not HIV treatment.[80,143]

Lamivudine has an excellent safety profile for extended use in HIV- and HBV-infected children and is recommended as a part of a combination antiretroviral regimen for coinfected children who require both HIV and HBV treatment. However, therapy with lamivudine as the only anti-HBV agent is problematic due to the high risk of development of HBV resistance mutations after prolonged therapy in monoinfected adults and children and in coinfected adults with uncontrolled HBV viremia. Thus, lamivudine should not be used for treatment of HBV in coinfected individuals in the absence of additional antiretroviral agents. Options for treating HIV/HBV-coinfected children would be to initiate LMV-sparing cART in those who would not otherwise require HBV treatment or to include additional anti-HBV medications in the cART regimen.[206]

Adefovir has minimal anti-HIV activity. Therefore, it could be used in older coinfected children who require HBV but not HIV treatment.[135] Several small studies in HIV/HBV-coinfected adults failing previous anti-HBV treatment have similarly shown significant decreases in HBV DNA after the addition of ETV.[226,239] While insufficiently potent to be considered an HIV therapy, entecavir has activity against HIV such that monotherapy ETV results in the development of the M184V mutation and should not be used as monotherapy in HIV-coinfected individuals in the absence of additional antiretroviral agents.[199] Adult treatment guidelines recommend inclusion of tenofovir plus lamivudine in the antiretroviral therapy regimen for coinfected adults who require treatment for HIV.[35,143] Tenofovir has recently been labeled for treatment of HIV-infected children down to 2 years of age. As with lamivudine, tenofovir also has significant HIV activity and should not be used as a single agent in coinfected individuals without additional antiretroviral agents.

Due to concerns of hepatic flares after initiating cART in coinfected individuals, adult guidelines recommend that HBV-active agents be included in any cART regimen for coinfected adults regardless of stage of HBV disease.[143] Specifically, tenofovir plus lamivudine or emtricitabine (another nucleos(t)ide analog not labeled for treatment of HBV) are recommended to decrease the risk of HBV mutations. However, up to 25% of HBV/HIV-coinfected adults experience hepatic flares after starting cART.[85,199]

Hepatitis B in Solid-Organ Transplant Recipients

Chronic HBV infection became a relative contraindication to liver transplantation after initial poor results. In the 1970s and 1980s, more than 80% of patients became reinfected quickly, and 55% died within 60 days of surgery. Patients who had recurrence of HBV infection after liver transplantation (LT) developed a characteristic histologic lesion, termed *fibrosing cholestatic hepatitis,* which eventually led to loss of the allograft.[20] The term *de novo HBV infection* is defined as HBV infection occurring in HBsAg-negative liver recipients who become HBsAg positive after transplant. In a retrospective study of 71 HBsAg-negative Taiwanese children who received orthotopic LT, 15.3% of patients developed de novo HBV infection. In this study, higher HBsAb titers (>200 mIU/mL) were thought to be sufficient to possibly prevent de novo HBV infection in LT patients.[276] The demonstration in the 1990s that HBIG is efficacious in decreasing infection of the allograft has allowed successful transplantation. The use of long-term HBIG decreases the risk for recurrence to 30% at 12 months and increases patient survival to greater than 90% at 12 months after transplantation.[253] The allograft reinfection rate is even lower if the patient does not have active HBV replication at the time of transplantation. The cost of HBIG is a major factor, and duration of therapy appears to be lifelong to maintain protective HBs titer.

HBV infection is the fourth most common cause of acute liver failure in adults in the United States.[221] Rarely, however, does a child in the United States with HBV need a liver transplant for either acute or chronic liver failure.[273] Of 215 children who underwent transplantation between 1986 and 1992 at a major French center, only 4 had HBV-associated disease.[194]

All patients with HBV-decompensated cirrhosis should be commenced on nucleos(t)ide analogs (NAs), regardless of viral load and ALT activity. Such patients should be selected for LT if they present hepatic dysfunction.[61,208] The application of NAs prompted a new era for LT of HBV-decompensated cirrhotic patients, because they reduced the rates of recurrence remarkably and improved their prognosis dramatically (survival rates up to 90% over 5 years after LT).[73] All data suggest that an effective pretransplant anti-HBV therapy prevents posttransplant HBV recurrence.[223] ETV administration in HBV-decompensated cirrhotic patients improved mortality. Those treated with ETV for 24 weeks had greater reduction in ALT levels and Model for End-Stage Liver Disease score compared to those on lamivudine.[56] In adults, ETV and tenofovir are the recommended first-line NAs in patients with HBV-decompensated cirrhosis.

After LT, HBV DNA of 20,000 IU/mL or greater and HBeAg positivity at the time of LT are associated with high risk of HBV recurrence, while HBV DNA clearance and fulminant HBV and hepatitis D virus coinfection pose less risk of HBV recurrence.[167] To date, the combination of an NA with a low dose of HBIG is the preferred therapeutic regimen.[62]

Patients treated with HBIG and lamivudine had more frequent recurrence than those who received HBIG and adefovir. The combination of HBIG and ETV or TDF is the best prophylaxis, almost eliminating posttransplant HBV recurrence (<2%).[63]

The course of HBV infection in heart transplant recipients was examined in a French study in which 69 of 874 heart transplant patients were infected with HBV, most through nosocomial infection during endomyocardial biopsies. HBV infection had little impact on 5-year survival.[192] In a group of 120 lung transplant recipients in Israel, 11 patients with either chronic hepatitis B or receipt of an organ from an HBcAb-positive donor were given lamivudine prophylaxis. Only one patient developed resistance, which responded to treatment with adefovir. Two patients had reactivation of HBV infection with high aminotransferase levels and high HBV DNA levels.[261]

In a study from Taiwan, overall patient and allograft survival after kidney transplantation were not affected by HBV infection despite increased hepatic morbidity.[124] Of the 113 patients who received kidney transplants between 1986 and 1998, 20 patients were HBsAg positive and nine were positive for both HBsAg and HCV antibody. Of the 20 who were infected with HBV alone, four developed fulminant hepatic failure and died within 2 years of renal transplantation (RT), two developed cirrhosis, and two others developed HCC.[124] Overall, however, the 5-year survival was not dissimilar in those infected with HBV and those not infected.

Patients with HBV-compensated cirrhosis are at risk for hepatic decompensation after RT. Patients with HBV-decompensated cirrhosis require combined liver and kidney transplantation.[64] Antiviral treatment has significantly improved graft survival and mortality.[69,318] Patients with HBsAg positivity should be started on NAs prior to RT, regardless of the baseline liver histology and serum HBV DNA level.[145] NAs should be continued after RT to retain viral load clearance and prevent liver decompensation and fibrosis.[88]

Immunosuppressive therapy after RT predisposes HBV-infected patients to rapidly progressive fibrosis cholestatic hepatitis, even if the underlying liver disease was mild before RT.[229] Antiviral prophylaxis is recommended for HBV-infected patients who undergo RT.

The child most likely to be treated successfully with today's agents is one who acquired HBV beyond infancy, has evidence of immune responsiveness to HBV, and has mild to moderate inflammatory changes on liver biopsy. The child ideally has no other medical problems, and child and family can comply with the regimen and monitoring. A perinatally infected infant may still respond to therapy as long as there is evidence of immune activation, indicated primarily by ALT values consistently at least 1.5 times the upper limit of normal.[131]

Even if the child has some success with treatment but remains HBsAg positive, the child is still at risk for HCC or reactivation to HBeAg and HBV. Yearly follow-up of virologic status, determination of α-fetoprotein level, and ultrasonography are recommended by most experts even though clear evidence to support this practice is lacking.

Immunoprophylaxis

A comprehensive strategy to prevent HBV infection, both acute hepatitis B and the sequelae of chronic HBV infection, can eliminate transmission that occurs during infancy, childhood, and adulthood. It has been clearly demonstrated that HBV transmission cannot be prevented through vaccination strategies targeting only the groups considered at highest risk for developing infection. A comprehensive immunization strategy is currently recommended by the Centers for Disease Control and Prevention (CDC).

Two types of products are available for prophylaxis against HBV infection. HBIG provides antibody to HBsAg, which gives temporary (3–6 months) protection by means of passive immunity; it is indicated only in certain postexposure settings. Hepatitis B vaccine evokes active immunity and is recommended for both preexposure and postexposure prophylaxis.

Hepatitis B Immunoglobulin

HBIG is prepared from plasma known to contain a high titer of anti-HBs. The human plasma from which HBIG is prepared is screened for antibodies to HIV and HCV; the process used to prepare HBIG inactivates and eliminates live viruses from the final product. HBIG is used in the postexposure prophylaxis of neonates of HBV-infected women and for susceptible individuals with sexual, needle-stick, or mucosal exposures. It is administered intramuscularly. The dose for infants with perinatal HBV exposure is 0.5 mL/kg. The dose for adults is 0.06 mL/kg. Efficacy ranges from 70% to 95%.[14] HBIG in large doses is used after LT in HBV-infected patients to prevent infection of the allograft. HBIG is typically administered together with the HBV vaccine; however, nucleos(t)ide therapy is the mainstay of treatment even after LT.

Hepatitis B Vaccine

Hepatitis B vaccines are available as single-antigen formulations or are combined with other vaccines. The two licensed single recombinant vaccines are produced by using *Saccharomyces cerevisiae* (common baker's yeast), into which a plasmid containing the gene for HBsAg has been inserted. Purified HBsAg is obtained by lysis of the yeast cells and separation of HBsAg by biochemical and biophysical techniques. Hepatitis B vaccines are packaged to contain 10 to 40 μg of HBsAg protein/mL after adsorption to aluminum hydroxide (0.5 mg/mL). See Table 157.1 for recommended dosages. Vaccines available in the United States are Recombivax HB and Engerix-B. Recombinant HBsAg is also used in the three combination vaccines available in the United States: Comvax, Pediarix, and Twinrix. The immunogenicity is similar for all preparations. Oral route of vaccination administration is being studied in mice models by a group of researchers in India using hepatitis B surface antigen (HBsAg)-entrapped polycaprolactone nanoparticles in 60- to 90-nm size range coated with Pluronics F127, showing superior antibody response with a higher titer of anti-HBsAg antibody at 2 months following single oral administration compared to other routes of immunization and conventional alum-based HBsAg vaccine.[82] A recent multicenter, double-blind, comparator-controlled, phase III study (NCT01480258) conducted in Sweden, Italy, and Finland has demonstrated safety and immunogenicity of a hexavalent DTaP5-HB-IPV-Hib vaccine (Infanrix hexa) to be given at 2, 4, and 11 to 12 months of age to be comparable with the analogous component vaccines,[196,262] which may improve hepatitis B vaccination coverage rates.

The recommended series of three intramuscular doses of hepatitis B vaccine induces a protective antibody response (anti-HBs) in more than 90% of healthy adults and in more than 95% of infants, children, and adolescents. Hepatitis B vaccine should be administered into the deltoid muscles of adults and children or the anterolateral thigh muscles of neonates and infants; the immunogenicity is substantially lower when injections are administered into the buttocks. When hepatitis B vaccine is administered to infants at the same time as other vaccines, separate sites in the anterolateral thigh may be used for the multiple injections.

The vaccination schedule used most often for adults and children has been three intramuscular injections, the second and third administered 1 and 6 months after the first. Each of the two available vaccines has been evaluated to determine the age-specific dose at which an optimal antibody response is achieved.

Perinatal transmission of HBV can be prevented effectively if the HBsAg-positive mother is identified and if her infant receives appropriate immunoprophylaxis. Administration of HBIG and the first dose of hepatitis B vaccine within 12 hours of birth prevents 90% of perinatal infections.[137] Serologic testing of infants who receive immunoprophylaxis to prevent perinatal infection should be performed to identify the 5%

TABLE 157.1 Recommended Dosages for Hepatitis B Vaccines

	SINGLE-ANTIGEN VACCINE				COMBINATION VACCINE					
	Recombivax HB		**Engerix-B**		**Comvax**[a]		**Pediarix**[b]		**Twinrix**[c]	
Age Group	***Dose (μg)***[d]	***Volume (mL)***	***Dose (μg)***[d]	***Volume (mL)***	***Dose (μg)***[d]	***Volume (mL)***	***Dose (μg)***[d]	***Volume (mL)***	***Dose (μg)***[d]	***Volume (mL)***
Infants (<1 y)	5	0.5	10	0.5	5	0.5	10	0.5	NA[e]	NA
Children (1–10 y)	5	0.5	10	0.5	5[a]	0.5	10[b]	0.5	NA	NA
Adolescents										
11–15 y	10[f]	1.0	NA	NA	NA	NA	NA	NA	NA	NA
11–19 y	5	0.5	10	0.5	NA	NA	NA	NA	NA	NA
Adults (≥20 y)	10	1.0	20	1.0	NA	NA	NA	NA	20[c]	1.0
Hemodialysis Patients and Other Immunocompromised Persons										
<20 y[g]	5	0.5	10	0.5	NA	NA	NA	NA	NA	NA
≥20 y	40[h]	1.0	40[i]	2.0	NA	NA	NA	NA	NA	NA

[a]Combined hepatitis B-*Haemophilus influenzae* type b conjugate vaccine. This vaccine cannot be administered at birth, before age 6 weeks, or after age 71 months.
[b]Combined hepatitis B-diphtheria, tetanus, and acellular pertussis-inactivated poliovirus vaccine. This vaccine cannot be administered at birth, before age 6 weeks, or at age ≥7 years.
[c]Combined hepatitis A and hepatitis B vaccine. This vaccine is recommended for persons aged ≥18 years who are at increased risk for both hepatitis B virus and hepatitis A virus infections.
[d]Recombinant hepatitis B surface antigen protein dose.
[e]Not applicable.
[f]Adult formulation administered on a 2-dose schedule.
[g]Higher doses might be more immunogenic, but no specific recommendations have been made.
[h]Dialysis formulation administered on a 3-dose schedule at ages 0, 1, and 6 months.
[i]Two 1.0-mL doses administered at one site, on a 4-dose schedule at ages 0, 1, 2, and 6 months.
From Mast EE, Margolis HS, Fiore AE, et al. A comprehensive immunization strategy to eliminate transmission of hepatitis B virus infection in the United States: recommendations of the Advisory Committee on Immunization Practices (ACIP) part 1: immunization of infants, children, and adolescents. *MMWR Recomm Rep.* 2005;54(RR-16):1–31.

of infants who become HBV carriers despite these measures. Testing for anti-HBs and HBsAg in children 12 to 15 months of age determines the success of vaccination and, in the case of failure, identifies HBV-infected infants or those who may require treatment or revaccination. The following are the current recommendations as to timing of immunizations for infants in the United States.[198]

- *Infants born to HBsAg-negative mothers* should receive the first single-antigen vaccine dose at birth or before hospital discharge. The plan thereafter depends on whether a single antigen or combination vaccine is used. For single-antigen vaccine, the second dose should be administered at age 1 to 2 months and the third at age 6 to 18 months. If combination vaccines are used, the first dose should be of a single-antigen vaccine at birth or before hospital discharge. The second dose should be at 2 months, the third at 4 months, and a fourth dose at either 6 months or 12 to 15 months, depending on the combination of vaccines used. Testing for serologic response is not necessary and is not recommended.
- *Infants born to HBsAg-positive mothers* should receive 0.5 mL of HBIG and the first dose of single-antigen hepatitis B vaccine within 12 hours of birth, administered intramuscularly at separate sites. The infant can then complete the immunization series with either single-antigen or combination vaccine. Premature infants of HBV-infected women should receive the vaccine on the same schedule, but those weighing less than 2000 g at birth have a decreased response to hepatitis B vaccination younger than 1 month old. For such infants, the dose given at birth should not be counted as the start of the vaccine series, and three additional doses of vaccine (for a total of four doses) should be administered beginning when the infant reaches 1 month of age.[198]
- *Infants born to mothers whose HBsAg status is unknown* should receive the first dose of vaccine within 12 hours of birth. Meanwhile, a maternal blood sample should be sent for HBsAg testing. If positive, HBIG should be given as soon as possible (no later than 1 week of age). The infant then should complete the routine vaccination schedule. If the infant is preterm and weighs less than 2000 g and the mother's HBsAg is not established within 12 hours of birth, the infant should receive HBIG and single-antigen hepatitis B vaccine and then complete four doses of hepatitis B vaccinations.

Despite the use of hepatitis B vaccine and HBIG in infants born to HBsAg-positive mothers, a portion of infants are still non- or low responders or have immunoprophylaxis failure. A large multicenter study in China demonstrated an immunoprophylaxis failure rate of 3.4% (39/1150). HBeAg-positivity and high viral load (HBV DNA ≥6 $\log_{10}$ copies/mL) were associated with the greatest transmission and highest immunoprophylaxis rate. Antepartum HBIG had no significant effects on HBV mother-to-infant transmission[327] and is currently not recommended for the mother to prevent vertical transmission of HBV. Meta-analysis of 7561 Chinese participants showed estimated rates of immunoprophylaxis failure of infants with HBsAg-positive and HBeAg-positive mothers to be 4.87% and 9.66%, respectively.[178] Zou et al. retrospectively examined 621 infants of HBsAg-positive mothers in Beijing who received three doses of 10 μg HB vaccine (at 0, 1, and 6 months of age) and two doses of 200 IU HBIG (at birth and 2 weeks of age) and found a comparable immunoprophylaxis failure rate of 2.9% (0% and 5.2% for infants of HBeAg-negative and HBeAg-positive mothers, respectively).[330]

Testing for serologic response (HBsAg and anti-HBs) should be done in infants born to HBsAg-positive mothers when the child is 12 to 15 months of age. If anti-HBs response is inadequate (<10 mEq/L) and the child is HBsAg negative, the child should be revaccinated. If the child's anti-HBs titers are greater than 10 mU/L and the child is HBsAg negative, that child is immune and not infected. If the child is HBsAg positive at age 12 to 18 months, the child should be considered as potentially chronically infected and followed appropriately (Box 157.1).

Others who should receive hepatitis B vaccine. All nonimmunized children and young adults younger than 19 years of age should begin HBV vaccination at any health care provider visit. For older children and adolescents aged 11 to 15 years, the routine three-dose schedule may be used, but a two-dose schedule of vaccination also has been approved, using the Recombivax HB vaccine. The adult dose (1.0 mL/10 μg) is administered to the adolescent, and the second dose is given 4 to 6 months later. Short-term (2-year) follow-up in groups immunized by either schedule showed similar rates of anti-HBs decline. Of importance is that a lower dose of vaccine is used in the three-dose schedule; if the original dose is not known, the full three-dose schedule should be used.[42] Immunization also should be offered to high-risk groups, although universal childhood immunization has created an immune adult population for the most part, except immigrants, who comprise the largest reservoir of adult HBV infection in the United States.

In a three-dose schedule, increasing the interval between administrations of the first and second doses of hepatitis B vaccine has little effect on immunogenicity or final antibody titer. The third dose confers optimal protection, acting as a booster dose. Longer intervals between the last two doses (4–12 months) result in higher final titers of anti-HBs antibodies. Larger vaccine doses (40 μg) or an increased number of doses is required to induce protective antibody in many hemodialysis patients and other immunocompromised persons (e.g., those who take immunosuppressive drugs or who are infected with HIV). Children with end-stage renal disease respond better than do adults to HBV immunization. Ninety percent of pediatric chronic dialysis patients and 100% of children vaccinated before beginning hemodialysis became anti-HBs positive in one study.[96] An immunocompromised person who has previously shown an adequate anti-HBs antibody titer that then falls to less than 10 mIU/mL should receive a booster dose.

Testing for immunity (anti-HBs titer) is advised only for patients whose subsequent clinical management depends on knowledge of their immune status (e.g., infants born to HBsAg-positive mothers, hemodialysis patients and staff, patients with HIV infection, LT recipients). Patients who are immunocompromised or on immunosuppressants have been shown to have reduced durable protection from hepatitis B virus vaccine. A cross-sectional study looking at 160 pediatric LT recipients found that the majority (67%) were nonimmune at mean time of 5.6 years from liver transplant despite having received the full HBV vaccination series prior to transplant.[177]

Postvaccination testing also should be considered for those at occupational risk who may have exposures from injuries with sharp instruments because knowledge of their antibody response helps determine appropriate postexposure prophylaxis.[99]

When revaccinated, 15% to 25% of people who do not respond to the primary vaccine series produce an adequate antibody response after one additional dose, and 30% to 50% do so after three additional doses.[130] Therefore, revaccination should be considered for people who do not respond to the initial series.

The duration of vaccine-induced immunity has been evaluated in long-term follow-up studies of both adults and children. The duration of response from neonatal or later immunization is still not clear, but studies in both Asian and European children vaccinated in infancy

BOX 157.1 Recommended Physician Visits for Children With Chronic Hepatitis B Virus Infections

Every 6 Months

Blood work: AST/ALT, CBC, HBsAg, anti-HBs, HBeAg, anti-HBe, HBV DNA

Annual

History taking
Physical examination (including growth parameters)
Review of risk factors for transmission
Liver ultrasound evaluation (in patients with genotype C or with family history of HCC, may consider repeating every 6 months)
α-Fetoprotein level (optimum frequency not yet clear)

ALT, Alanine aminotransferase; *AST,* aspartate aminotransferase; *CBC,* complete blood cell count; *HBeAg,* hepatitis B e antigen; *HBsAg,* hepatitis B surface antigen; *HCC,* hepatocellular carcinoma.

demonstrate that immune memory persisted at least 10 years in Italy,[325] was 12 years in Hong Kong,[322] but started to wane by 15 years postimmunization in Taiwanese children.[191] Booster doses were administered to the children in the latter study with anti-HBs titers less than 100 mIU/mL, and 4 of 128 demonstrated no response.[191] A previous study from the same group demonstrated excellent response in all subjects to a booster dose at age 10 years in those who were anti-HBs seronegative despite neonatal vaccination after being born to HBsAg- and HBeAg-positive mothers.[122] The timing and necessity of a booster dose are still unclear and not recommended on a population basis.[138]

Therapeutic vaccination—that is, immunization of those already infected in an effort to boost their HBV-specific T-cell responses—has shown limited clinical success in adults. However, a trial of combination immunization (pre-S2/S vaccine) with IFN-α2b compared with IFN-α2b alone in children with chronic HBV infection did not show any benefit compared with IFN-α2b alone.[117]

Vaccine side effects and adverse reactions. Hepatitis B vaccines are safe for both adults and children. Anaphylaxis is the only serious adverse event in children and adolescents, with a reported observed risk in 2003 of 1.1 per million vaccine doses administered.[26] Pain at the injection site (3–29%) and a temperature greater than 37.7°C (99.9°F; 1–6%) have been the side effects most frequently reported, but they were reported no more frequently among vaccinees than among subjects receiving a placebo.[41,280] In the United States, surveillance from the CDC of adverse reactions has shown a possible association between Guillain-Barré syndrome and receipt of the first dose of plasma-derived hepatitis B vaccine in adults; plasma-derived HBV vaccine is no longer in use.[41] Reports of multiple sclerosis developing after vaccination for HBV led to concern that the vaccine might cause multiple sclerosis in previously healthy subjects, a theory later refuted in a study of large cohorts, as no association was found.[11,68]

Until 1999, hepatitis B vaccines were prepared with thimerosal (sodium ethylmercuric thiosalicylate) to prevent bacterial and fungal contamination, which aroused public concern regarding mercury toxicity. No adverse outcomes were associated clearly with thimerosal use, but HBV vaccination of neonates was temporarily suspended in 1999 until thimerosal-free vaccines became available. Two thimerosal-free hepatitis B vaccines are now available in the United States for use in infants. Thus, parents can be reassured about the lack of exposure to mercury in hepatitis B vaccines.

Contraindications. There are only a few clinical situations in which hepatitis B vaccine is not recommended: those with a history of anaphylaxis to the vaccine and those with history of acute hypersensitivity to yeast. Vaccination should be deferred in those with an intercurrent moderate to severe illness. Pregnancy is not a contraindication to immunization.[198]

Recommendations to Prevent Household Transmission

When a person is found to have acute or chronic infection with HBV, immunization of household contacts is recommended. Guidance on universal precautions should be provided. Parents of infected children and siblings should learn to treat bodily fluids, especially blood, as potentially infectious. All bloody emissions and blood-soiled items should be handled with gloves, and any blood-stained items should be either cleaned with bleach or disposed of carefully. Both the infected person and others in the house should cover skin abrasions with waterproof bandages. Razors and toothbrushes never should be shared. If needle sharps are in use, they should be secured and disposed of according to local guidelines. Schools, workplaces, and health care providers should practice universal precautions for all individuals regardless of whether HBV status is known.

Future Strategies/Targets for Treatment

As new technologies and better understanding of the HBV lifecycle are developed, potential treatments for HBV infection continue to emerge. Several new agents that focus on viral and host targets are under development to cure HBV, including new polymerase inhibitors. Agents targeting cccDNA, such as engineered site-specific nucleases and RNA interference therapeutics, could eliminate cccDNA or silence cccDNA transcription. Inhibitors of HBV nucleocapsid assembly suppress capsid formation and prevent synthesis of HBV DNA. The HBV entry inhibitor, Myrcludex-B, has been shown to effectively inhibit amplification of cccDNA and the spread of intrahepatic infection. Agents targeting host factors that enhance innate and adaptive immune responses, including the lymphotoxin-β receptor agonist, toll-like receptor agonist, immune checkpoint inhibitors, and adenovirus-based therapeutic vaccine, could play a critical role in the elimination of HBV-infected cells.

Despite advances in treatment, prevention of new infections must remain at the forefront of all therapeutic endeavors. Vertical transmission of HBV to children can be prevented by proper antenatal testing, careful follow-up of results, and availability of immunization programs to infants.

HEPATITIS D

Hepatitis D virus (HDV) is a subviral particle that requires a helper virus, HBV, to establish infection. As a subviral particle, HDV, which also is known as the delta agent or virus, does not encode its own envelope protein and requires HBV envelope production to become an infectious virion. HDV first was described in 1977 when a new antigen was described in the hepatocytes of patients infected with HBV. Transmission experiments demonstrated that the antigen was indeed a new virus.[242] Infection with HDV and HBV can be contracted at the same time (coinfection), or HDV can be contracted as a new infection in a person previously infected with HBV (superinfection). There are currently eight major genotypes (clades) of HDV.[237,244] There is geographic variation in both incidence and genotype distribution.[260] HDV genotype 1 is the most frequent genotype found worldwide, but HDV genotypes 2 and 4 are found in the Far East and are associated with milder disease.[175] HDV genotype 1 infection appears to be associated with a more fulminant hepatitis in acute infection and increased rates of cirrhosis and HCC compared with genotype 2.[313]

Virology

HDV is a spherical particle with a diameter of 36 nm.[205] When the envelope is degraded, a nucleocapsid containing hepatitis D antigen (HDAg) and the HDV RNA genome is released. The two forms of HDAg are the small s-HDAg, which is 195 amino acids in length and is required for replication, and the larger l-HDAg, which is 214 amino acids long, is required for virion assembly, and inhibits HDV replication.[205] s-HDAg is a nuclear protein that undergoes phosphorylation by protein kinase C, and inhibitors of protein kinase C inhibit HDV replication in cell culture systems.[58] The ratio of the two forms of HDAg found in patients may vary.

The HDV RNA genome is single stranded and circular, with a length of 1679 nucleotides. During viral replication, the genomic RNA serves as a template for complementary RNA, which, in turn, is a template for more genomic RNA. A host-derived RNA polymerase is required.[285] Each copy of the genome and antigenome contains ribozyme activity that cleaves RNA and is required for HDV replication.[205] Posttranscriptional modification of the RNA leads to the production of the l-HDAg in addition to the s-HDAg already transcribed.[58,285]

To leave the host cell, HDV RNA and HDAg must be packaged into virions. The l-HDAg undergoes isoprenylation of a cysteine residue near its C terminus to allow virion assembly. Inhibition of this isoprenylation interferes with viral production by preventing interaction with HBsAg.[58] Once this interaction occurs, HBsAg and host cell membrane lipids enclose HDV RNA, l-HDAg, and s-HDAg to form virions. Noninfectious HDV particles, which contain only l-HDAg and HBsAg, can be found in serum.[205]

Epidemiology

The epidemiology of HDV infection parallels that of HBV infection, for obvious reasons. Modes of transmission of HDV also are similar to those for HBV and include direct or indirect parenteral exposure to blood or body fluids and sexual and perinatal transmission. Sexual transmission is less efficient than that of HBV, as evidenced by the relatively low frequency of HDV infection in men who have sex with men.[255] Perinatal transmission can occur but is rare because HBV carrier mothers also infected with HDV usually are anti-HBe positive and thus less infectious. Intrafamilial transmission of HDV has been demonstrated in endemic areas, such as southern Italy, by means of a combined epidemiologic and molecular study, which demonstrated that within family units, the HDV strains were nearly identical.[213] Transmission of HDV infection has also been documented among residents of institutions for the developmentally disabled.

The geographic differences in HDV endemicity in the world are great, and four levels have been characterized. High endemicity (i.e., HDV is found in more than 20% of asymptomatic HBV carriers and more than 60% of HBV carriers with chronic liver disease) is seen in northern South America and Africa as well as in Romania.[47] In these populations, HDV superinfection of HBV carriers is a significant cause of chronic liver disease and causes outbreaks of fulminant hepatitis. In these areas, HDV infection is seen commonly in both children and adults, and household transmission has been implicated. Parts of the Middle East, Africa, some Pacific Islands, and parts of Asia report intermediate HDV endemicity (in 10–20% of asymptomatic HBV carriers and 30–60% of HBV carriers with chronic liver disease). Infection in these regions occurs predominantly in adults, and outbreaks are uncommon, but HDV is an important cause of chronic liver disease. Low endemicity (in 3–9% of asymptomatic HBV carriers and 10–25% of HBV carriers with chronic liver disease) is observed in most developed countries, including the United States, but subpopulations in these countries, such as parenteral drug abusers and prostitutes, have a high infection rate. In areas of low HBV endemicity, transmission of HDV appears to be mainly by the percutaneous route, with higher rates of HDV infection found in intravenous drug users and hemophiliacs than in other HBV high-risk groups. HDV is considered only a moderately important cause of chronic liver disease in developed countries.[310] Finally, for as yet unexplained reasons, certain subpopulations have a high carriage rate of HBV but virtually no HDV infection; they include American Indians, Alaska Natives, and residents of some Asian countries.

Within the U.S. blood donor population, the prevalence of HDV infection is low; only 1.4% to 8% of donors are infected or have evidence of prior infection.[9] Estimates from the CDC for 1990 indicate that among the approximately 250,000 cases of acute HBV infection each year, 7500 simultaneously acquire HDV infection. There are about 70,000 carriers of HDV in the United States, where about 1000 deaths per year are caused by chronic HDV and 35 by fulminant HDV. In certain regions, the prevalence of HDV infection appears to be decreasing. In Italy, the prevalence of HDV infection in HBsAg carriers decreased from 23% in 1987 to 14% in 1992 and 8.3% in 1997.[98,252] Corresponding data for the United States are not available.

Immunopathogenesis

Unlike HBV, HDAg is found only in the liver or serum.[101] The mechanism by which HDV infection leads to hepatic injury has not been elucidated. Despite some evidence that HDV can be directly cytopathic, cytopathic viruses seldom result in chronic infections. In addition, some HDV carriers have no evidence of hepatic cell damage. Both cellular and humoral components of the host immune system are involved in the response to HDV, although the relative contribution of each is controversial. Investigations into the humoral response to HDV demonstrated that HDAg contains epitopes or immunogenic domains to which sera from acutely infected humans and woodchucks react. The predominantly recognized epitopes are not exposed on the virion surface; thus, antibodies that recognize these epitopes cannot neutralize virus particles, which may explain why no association exists between the humoral response and clinical outcome.[205] Autoantibodies, especially liver-kidney microsomal type 3 antibodies and anti–basal cell layer antibody, are found occasionally in people with HDV infection. The significance of these antibodies is unclear, but they may play a role in the immunopathogenesis of HDV.

Cellular immune responses to HDV also have been demonstrated. Both $CD4^+$ and $CD8^+$ lymphocytes have been found in the liver of patients infected with HDV; it is not clear whether these cells contribute to hepatitis or aid in control of HDV infection.[205] Patients with HDV superinfection of chronic HBV who had peripheral $CD4^+$ cells that reacted to four epitopes on HDAg were seronegative for HDV IgM, implying inactive disease.[213] Such $CD4^+$ T-cell clones produce IFN-γ and may be directly cytopathic. Individuals without these specific $CD4^+$ cells had active HDV disease.[216] These epitopes are in highly conserved regions of HDV, which is encouraging for the prospect of vaccine development.

An unusual mechanism of HDAg presentation by hepatocytes has been reported. The processing of HDAg peptide appears to occur outside the cell, where the peptide is cleaved into smaller fragments that bind to class II major histocompatibility complex molecules of all three human leukocyte antigen types found on hepatocytes and mononuclear cells. This form of antigen presentation could have many possible effects on T-cell responses: amplification of T-cell response to HDAg, stimulation of cytotoxic T cells to kill uninfected hepatocytes, or exhaustion of T-cell responses to HDAg, allowing infected cells to escape detection.[205]

The relationship of HBV infection status to pathogenesis of HDV is also unclear. Patients with active HBV replication (i.e., HBV DNA and HBeAg seropositive) have high levels of HDV viremia.[242,243] Conversely, in HBV and HDV carriers without liver disease or with minimal inflammatory hepatic lesions, markers of HBV replication are absent and HDV viremia is low.[27,243] In coinfected LT recipients, HDV reinfection can occur without evidence of active HBV replication, but necroinflammatory activity does not develop until HBV infection is reactivated.[72]

Diagnosis

Establishing the diagnosis of either acute or chronic HBV infection is a prerequisite for the diagnosis of HDV infection, which is made by detection of antibody to HDV (anti-HDV). HDV antigen can be measured in serum, but it is usually present only transiently during acute infection and in immunosuppressed individuals.[175] Radioimmunoassay or enzyme immunoassay kits for the detection of both IgM and IgG anti-HDV are available.

HDV infection may occur at the same time as HBV infection, a pattern that is termed *coinfection*. If an individual has acute, resolving hepatitis B, the HDV infection also will resolve.[76] In this instance, anti-HDV is found in the IgM form during the acute illness and persists for 2 to 6 weeks. Subsequently, IgG anti-HDV is found in serum, but it also diminishes to undetectable levels when the HBV infection resolves (Fig. 157.8). In HDV superinfection, both IgM and IgG anti-HDV are detected. Most often, superinfection with HDV leads to chronic HDV infection, diagnosed by persistence of both IgM and IgG anti-HDV. Anti-HDV becomes predominantly IgG after about 6 weeks and persists if infection does not resolve; titers correlate well with ongoing viral replication.

Real-time PCR assay quantification of HDV RNA is also now commercially available that can detect all eight genotypes.[153] Owing to the variability of the HDV genome sequence, HDV RNA assays may yield false-negative results if inadequate primers are used. Therefore, HDV IgM should be tested in patients with negative HDV RNA levels if there is a clinical suspicion for HDV infection or high-risk exposures. Furthermore, quantitative assays of HDV in serum do not correlate with disease activity, although serial measurement of HDV may be useful in monitoring response in treatment.[324]

Histopathologic features of HDV infection are very similar to those of isolated HBV infection (see earlier discussion). HDAg can be identified in nuclei and, to a lesser extent, in the cytoplasm of infected hepatocytes. Liver biopsies are recommended in adult patients with HDV to grade inflammation and stage liver fibrosis due to the rapid progression to more severe liver disease.[224] There is a lack of substantial pediatric series to make definitive recommendations in children with HDV. In a child with HBV/HDV coinfection with persistently elevated ALT or clinical deterioration out of proportion to known disease, a liver biopsy may guide clinical decision making (more aggressive HBV therapy, primary HDV treatment, or LT consideration).[317]

Clinical Manifestations

In general, coinfection with HDV infection does not have clinical features that distinguish it from HBV infection alone. Symptoms develop 2 months after exposure, are similar to those of acute HBV infection, and usually resolve by 4 months after exposure. However, two peaks in

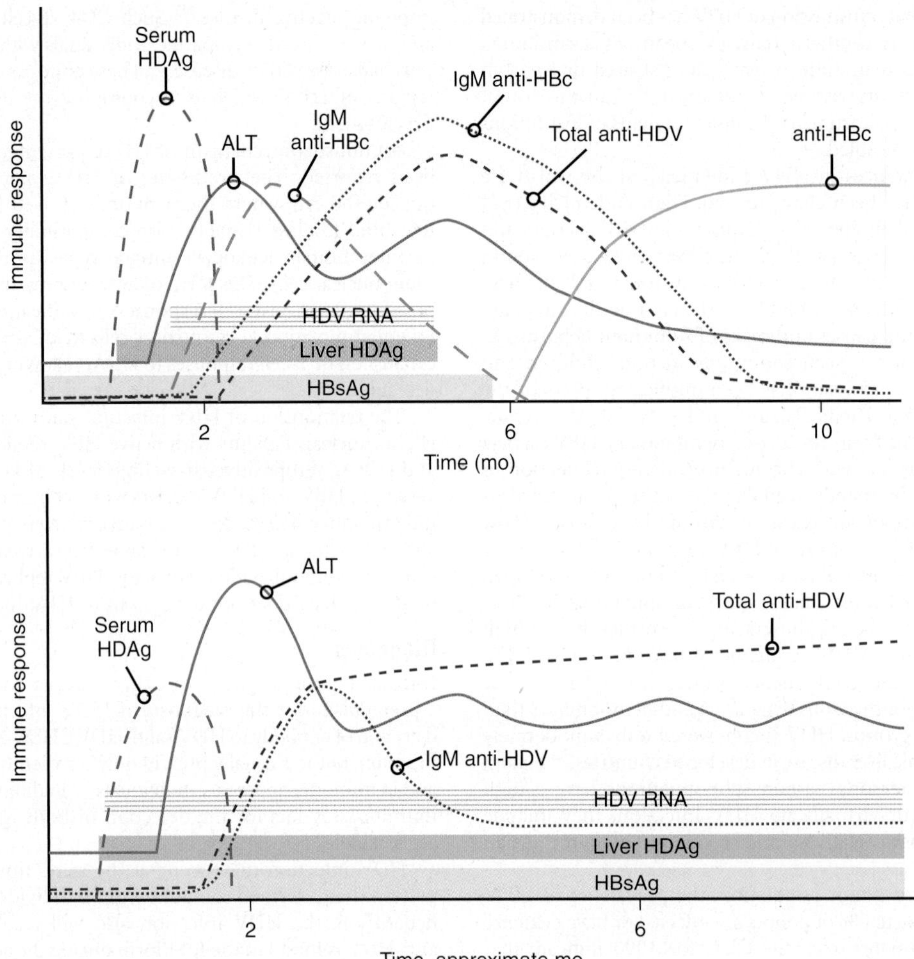

FIG. 157.8 Hepatitis D virus (HDV) serology. Typical serologic course of hepatitis B virus (HBV)-HDV coinfection *(top)* and HBV-HDV superinfection *(bottom)*. *ALT,* Alanine transaminase; *anti-HDV,* HDV antibody; *HBc,* hepatitis B core antibody; *HBsAg,* hepatitis B virus surface antigen; *HBV,* hepatitis B virus; *HDAg,* hepatitis delta antigen; *HDV,* hepatitis D virus; *IgM,* immunoglobulin M. (From Xue MM, Glenn JS, Leung DH. Hepatitis D in children. *JPGN* 2015;61:271–281.)

aminotransferase levels often are noted, a pattern that is unusual in HBV infection alone. The infections resolve together.[77] Coinfection with both viruses does not increase the risk for development of chronic HBV infection.[188]

HDV superinfection in individuals with chronic HBV infection has different manifestations. HDV infection becomes persistent in most individuals, and the predominant clinical pattern of chronic HDV infection varies by geographic location. In the United States and Europe, HDV superinfection leads to chronic liver disease in more than 90% of cases, whereas in some Pacific Island and African populations, most individuals with chronic HDV are asymptomatic.[243] When chronic liver disease does occur, the progression to cirrhosis is rapid; in studies in both adults and children, cirrhosis has been noted to occur in as few as 2 to 10 years. The cirrhosis associated with HDV infection has two patterns: in a minority of patients, especially the high-risk drug users, it progresses rapidly to hepatic failure and portal hypertension. In others, more stable cirrhosis occurs, with little inflammatory component, compatible with prolonged survival.[32] In a small minority of those who are superinfected, a self-limited hepatitis develops, and subsequently both HBV and HDV infections are cleared. HDV infection has been demonstrated to lead to HCC at a younger age and a higher rate than does HBV infection alone.[243] In a study of 166 patients with HBV and HDV from Romania, the median survival after the diagnosis of HDV-compensated cirrhosis was 58.3 months.[102] A multicenter European study of 200 HBsAg-positive patients with compensated cirrhosis found that 39 (20%) were anti-HDV positive. Those with HDV, HBV, and cirrhosis were younger than those with only HBV and cirrhosis; indeed, HDV infection may lead to the development of cirrhosis 15 years earlier.[91] In this study, HDV infection increased the risk for HCC three times and risk for mortality twofold compared with those with HBV and cirrhosis.[91] The natural history in those without cirrhosis is difficult to establish. In a study of 13 institutions for those with development disabilities in Illinois, 67 of 238 (28%) of HBsAg carriers also had anti-HDV antibodies.[118] Long-term (20 years) follow-up information was available on 65 of 66 anti-HDV– and HBsAg–positive individuals and 166 persons who were HBsAg positive. Liver-related deaths occurred in 7 of 65 (11%) anti-HDV–positive persons but only 1 in 166 anti-HDV–negative persons.[2] Hepatitis D was associated with both a higher rate of chronic liver disease and a higher liver-related mortality rate.[2]

A retrospective study of 188 chronically HDV-infected individuals in Italy was performed over an 8-year period. At presentation, 44% of patients had chronic hepatitis, and 56% had cirrhosis. A fourth of the patients with chronic hepatitis progressed to cirrhosis during the study period. In 40 patients, the viremia resolved either while on therapy or spontaneously. Nine percent of patients were diagnosed with HCC during the 8-year follow-up period.[215]

Children with HDV infection follow a course similar to that of adults. In one European series, the subset of children chronically infected with HBV who also were infected with HDV had more advanced liver disease, and the prevalence of HDV infection increased in parallel with the activity of hepatitis. During the study period, disease progressed more rapidly in children infected with both viruses.[90] Testing for HDV infection is recommended in any child with chronic hepatitis B and unusually severe liver disease or an acute exacerbation of stable liver disease.

HDV infection after LT can appear without apparent HBV reinfection of either the graft or serum. However, use of PCR assay has demonstrated that low levels of HBV infection do, in fact, occur in patients with recurrent HDV infection, and this replication of HBV is sufficient to permit replication of HDV. The HDV virion found in such infections shares the characteristics of typical HDV infection.[30]

Treatment

The goal of treating HDV infection is a sustained HDV virologic response as defined by undetectable HDV RNA 6 months after the end of treatment. This may be achieved via the eradication of HBV infection and clearance of HBsAg.[317] Currently approved regimens include nucleos(t)ide analogs (NAs) and IFN-α, usually in its pegylated form (PEG-IFN). For hepatitis D, PEG-IFN represents the only available treatment option with limited success.

Trials in adults in both Europe and the United States have shown that treatment with either 9 million units three times weekly or 5 million units daily of IFN-α results in normalization of serum aminotransferase levels, decrease or disappearance of HDV RNA from serum, and improvement in hepatic inflammation in about 50% of cases.[90] However, most patients experienced a relapse shortly after treatment was discontinued. Response maintained after treatment was noted primarily in individuals who became HBsAg negative.

PEG-IFN has been increasingly favored due to its longer half-life, allowing for once weekly dosing. PEG-IFN-α2b has shown promise as a treatment for chronic HDV in small trials. Fourteen patients were treated with PEG-IFN-α2b 1.5 μg/kg weekly for 12 months, and 6 (43%) had a sustained virologic response.[39] A recent randomized trial compared a 48-week treatment regimen of PEG-IFN-α2a plus adefovir, PEG-IFN-α2a alone, and adefovir alone in 31 patients with HDV. Twenty-three percent of patients treated with combination therapy and 24% of those treated with PEG-IFN-α2a monotherapy cleared HDV RNA. No patients treated with adefovir alone cleared HDV RNA at 48 weeks.[308] Treatment with NAs—including famciclovir, ribavirin, tenofovir, and entecavir alone or in combination with PEG-IFN—has not been proven to be more effective than PEG-IFN alone due to their inability to efficiently eradicate HBsAg, which is necessary and sufficient for enabling the continuous spread of HDV infection.[1,214,240]

No factors predictive of response have been identified. Prognosis in nonresponders to IFN-α and in those who relapse has been poor. The author of an editorial in *Hepatology* recommended continuation of IFN-α or pegylated IFN-α2b in patients with a decline in HDV RNA as long as possible, until HDV RNA and HBsAg disappear.[89]

Currently, no recommendations have been established regarding the use of IFN-α or PEG-IFN-α2b for the treatment of chronic HDV infection in children. A trial in seven children in Greece treated with IFN-α in a dosage of 3 million units/m^2 of body surface area three times a week for 1 year yielded disappointing results. All remained anti-HDV IgM positive, and four of the seven had persistent HDV RNA in serum. A significant reduction in serum aminotransferase values was noted after 1 year of treatment, but there was no significant improvement in liver histology.[70] A study of eight children from Germany also found no effect of IFN-α on replication of HDV. However, serum aminotransferase values improved, and children underwent earlier anti-HBe seroconversion compared with historical controls.[256]

Some children and adults require LT for management of end-stage HDV-associated liver disease. Patients coinfected with HDV and HBV have lower rates of HBV infection of the allograft than do those in patients with isolated HBV infection. These data were reported in a series of 58 patients with HBV infection, 25 of whom also had HDV infection and underwent LT between 1984 and 1996 in Belgium. Fifty-two patients survived longer than 3 months, and median follow-up was 74 months. HDV infection improved survival at 5 years: 96% ± 4% compared with 63% ± 10% for those infected with HBV alone.[176] As yet, no explanation has been given for the better outcome of transplantation in individuals who have both HBV and HDV infections. Administration of HBIG is required before and after transplantation, as in those patients with HBV infection alone.

Future Therapies

Alternative antiviral agents are being studied for the treatment of HDV infection.[294] Farnesylation inhibitors, which inhibit protein farnesyltransferase, are presently being developed to inhibit viral assembly and secretion.[28,29,65,105,228] In a phase IIa double-blinded, randomized, placebo-controlled study (ClinicalTrials.gov, NCT01495585), the oral farnesyltransferase inhibitor lonafarnib, given as 200 mg or 400 mg daily in two doses for 28 days, showed a dose-dependent anti-HDV activity with a 0.74 log (200 mg arm) to 1.54 log (400 mg arm) decrease in HDV RNA.[154] However, although serum HBsAg levels did not change, HDV RNA returned to baseline in all patients after discontinuing therapy, and the more effective 400-mg bid dose was accompanied by substantial gastrointestinal side effects. Longer treatments with lower doses (200–300 mg twice daily for 12 weeks) and ritonavir boosted regimens (100 mg twice daily + ritonavir for 8 weeks) are currently being investigated.[323]

The discovery of the sodium taurocholate cotransporting polypeptides (NTCPs) as the main receptor for HBV and HDV entry has also opened doors for the development of new drugs and strategies to inhibit viral entry and propagation. High-dose conjugated bile salts inhibit NTCP-mediated HDV entry into hepatocytes in vitro but have no impact on serum HDV RNA in chronically HDV-infected individuals.[300] Cyclosporine A, which irreversibly binds NTCP, and the cholesterol absorption inhibitor ezetimibe, which acts as a transport substrate for NTCP, both inhibit HBV/HDV entry in cell culture models.[294] Myrcludex B, a myristylated PreS1 peptide that competes with HBV/HDV for binding to NTCP, has been shown to prevent HBV/HDV entry and to impair viral dissemination in mice.[193,227] A phase IIa trial conducted in 40 HBeAg-negative noncirrhotic CHB patients showed a dose-dependent effect on HBV DNA, with greater than 1 $\log_{10}$ HBV DNA decline in 6 of 8 (75%) patients receiving 10 mg subcutaneously (SC) per day of Myrcludex B for 24 weeks but no change in serum HBsAg levels. Treatment was generally well tolerated.[294] In a subsequent phase IIa substudy in HBV/HDV-coinfected patients, Myrcludex B at 2 mg SC daily for 24 weeks was associated with anti-HDV activity (6/7 patients >1 $\log_{10}$ HDV RNA decline, 2 patients HDV RNA negative, 2 patients below the limit of quantification, and 4 patients ALT normalization at week 24).[25] Oral administration of a liposomal formulation of Myrcludex B has been recently reported.[293] The future role for Myrcludex B remains unclear due to the limited efficacy as monotherapy for HBV. The impact on bile acid metabolism may limit the long-term treatment with Myrcludex B.[21,22,316] NTCP co-receptors have been identified, including heparan sulfate proteoglycans and, more recently, Glypican 5,[301] but their potential value as new targets for HBV entry inhibition strategies remains to be established. Other strategies aim to target HBV cccDNA production and processing; viral replication and viral protein expression are being explored. Pediatric trials studying novel HDV therapies are being considered.

Immunoprophylaxis

Passive or active immunization specifically against HDV infection is not available. HDAg itself is highly immunogenic, but antibodies are not neutralizing. Description of a T-cell response to several HDV epitopes in individuals with less severe disease activity has stimulated speculation about possible vaccine development, but studies are preliminary. A DNA-based HDV vaccine successfully induced cellular responses in an animal model and also was successful when used with an HBV vaccine.[123] A trial of vaccine derived from B-cell epitopes of HDAg and HDAg p24 expressed in *Escherichia coli*, yeast, or baculovirus in woodchucks provoked a specific antibody response but did not protect against HDV superinfection.[95]

At the present time, individuals with chronic HBV infection who are at risk for acquiring HDV cannot be protected from HDV infection except by avoidance of high-risk behaviors and exposures. However, prevention of HBV infection in susceptible individuals will prevent HDV coinfection and will be the most important mechanism for decreasing the prevalence of HDV infection in a population. The current strategy aimed at decreasing susceptibility to HBV infection by universal immunization of neonates and catch-up immunization of older children and adolescents should reduce substantially the risk for subsequent development of HDV infection during young adulthood. In Italy, the decrease in HDV prevalence in those with chronic HBV infection from 23% in 1987 to 8.3% in 1997 has led to speculation that chronic hepatitis D may be a "vanishing disease."[98]

Acknowledgment

We thank Dr. Deborah Schady, Assistant Professor of Pathology and Immunology at Texas Children's Hospital and Baylor College of Medicine, for providing histologic images and comments that greatly improved the manuscript.

NEW REFERENCES SINCE THE SEVENTH EDITION

1. Abbas Z, Memon MS, Umer MA, Abbas M, Shazi L. Co-treatment with pegylated interferon alfa-2a and entecavir for hepatitis D: A randomized trial. *World J Hepatol.* 2016;8(14):625-63129.
3. Abzug MJ, Warshaw M, Rosenblatt HM, et al. International Maternal Pediatric Adolescent AIDS Clinical Trials Group P1024 and P1061s Protocol Teams. Immunogenicity and immunologic memory after hepatitis B virus booster vaccination in HIV-infected children receiving highly active antiretroviral therapy. *J Infect Dis.* 2009;200(6):935-946.
5. Adebajo CO, Talwalkar JA, Poterucha JJ, et al. Ultrasound-based transient elastography for the detection of hepatic fibrosis in patients with recurrent hepatitis C virus after liver transplantation: a systematic review and meta-analysis. *Liver Transpl.* 2012;18:323-331.
6. Adesina O, Oladokun A, Akinyemi O, et al. Human immuno-deficiency virus and hepatitis B virus coinfection in pregnancy at the University College Hospital, Ibadan. *Afr J Med Med Sci.* 2010;39(4):305-310.
7. Al-Mahtab M, Rahman S, Akbar SM. Combination therapy of lamivudine and interferon-alpha in pediatric patients with chronic hepatitis B in Bangladesh: a safe and effective therapeutic approach for pediatric CHB patients in developing countries. *Int J Immunopathol Pharmacol.* 2010;23(2):659-664.
10. Arda K, Ciledag N, Aktas E, et al. Quantitative assessment of normal soft-tissue elasticity using shear-wave ultrasound elastography. *AJR Am J Roentgenol.* 2011;197:532-536.
13. Balmasova IP, Yushchuk ND, Mynbaev OA. Immunopathogenesis of chronic hepatitis B. *World J Gastroenterol.* 2014;20(39):14156-14171.
18. Belei O, Sporea I, Gradinaru-Tascau O, et al. Comparison of three ultrasound based elastographic techniques in children and adolescents with chronic diffuse liver diseases. *Med Ultrason.* 2016;18(2):145-150.
20. Blank A, Eidam A, Haag M, et al. Combination of the hepatitis B/D entry inhibitor Myrcludex B and tenofovir: assessment of the effect on plasma bile acid profiles and tenofovir pharmacokinetics. *J Hepatol.* 2016;64:S164.
21. Blank A, Markert C, Hohmann N, et al. First-in-human application of the first-in-class hepatitis B and hepatitis D virus entry inhibitor Myrcludex B. *J Hepatol.* 2016;65(3):483-489.
24. Bogomolov P, Alexandrov A, Voronkova N, et al. Treatment of chronic hepatitis D with the entry inhibitor Myrcludex B – first results of a phase Ib/IIa study. *J Hepatol.* 2016;65(3):490-498.
27. Bordier BB, Marion PL, Ohashi K, et al. A prenylation inhibitor prevents production of infectious hepatitis delta virus particles. *J Virol.* 2002;76:10465-10472.
28. Bordier BB, Ohkanda J, Liu P, et al. In vivo antiviral efficacy of prenylation inhibitors against hepatitis delta virus. *J Clin Invest.* 2003;112:407-414.
34. Brook G, Main J, Nelson M, et al; BHIVA Viral Hepatitis Working Group. British HIV Association guidelines for the management of coinfection with HIV-1 and hepatitis B or C virus 2010. *HIV Med.* 2010;11(1):1-30.
37. Burnett RJ, François G, Kew MC, et al. Hepatitis B virus and human immunodeficiency virus co-infection in sub-Saharan Africa: a call for further investigation. *Liver Int.* 2005;25(2):201-213.
38. Castera L, Bernard PH, Le Bail B, et al. Transient elastography and biomarkers for liver fibrosis assessment and follow-up of inactive hepatitis B carriers. *Aliment Pharmacol Ther.* 2011;33:455-465.
39. Celikbilek M, Dogan S, Gursoy S, et al. Noninvasive assessment of liver damage in chronic hepatitis B. *World J Hepatol.* 2013;5(8):439-445.
43. Chan HL, Wong GL, Wong VW. A review of the natural history of chronic hepatitis B in the era of transient elastography. *Antivir Ther.* 2009;14:489-499.
50. Chang KC, Wu JF, Hsu HY, et al. Entecavir treatment in children and adolescents with chronic hepatitis B virus infection. *Pediatr Neonatol.* 2016;57(5):390-395.
51. Chang MH, You SL, Chen CJ. Long-term effects of hepatitis B immunization of infants in preventing liver cancer. *Gastroenterology.* 2016;151(3):472-480.
52. Chen CH, Lin CL, Hu TH, et al. Entecavir vs. lamivudine in chronic hepatitis B patients with severe acute exacerbation and hepatic decompensation. *J Hepatol.* 2014;60:1127-1134.
56. Chen CH, Lin ST, Yang CC, et al. The accuracy of sonography in predicting steatosis and fibrosis in chronic hepatitis C. *Dig Dis Sci.* 2008;53:1699-1706.
60. Cholongitas E, Germani G, Burroughs AK. Prioritization for liver transplantation. *Nat Rev Gastroenterol Hepatol.* 2010;7:659-668.
61. Cholongitas E, Goulis J, Akriviadis E, Papatheodoridis GV. Hepatitis B immunoglobulin and/or nucleos(t)ide analogues for prophylaxis against hepatitis B virus recurrence after liver transplantation: a systematic review. *Liver Transpl.* 2011;17:1176-1190.
62. Cholongitas E, Papatheodoridis GV. High genetic barrier nucleos(t)ide analogue(s) for prophylaxis from hepatitis B virus recurrence after liver transplantation: a systematic review. *Am J Transplant.* 2013;13:353-362.
63. Chopra A, Cantarovich M, Bain VG. Simultaneous liver and kidney transplants: optimizing use of this double resource. *Transplantation.* 2011;91:1305-1309.
64. Ciancio A, Rizzetto M, Lin S, et al. Chronic hepatitis D at a standstill: where do we go from here? *Nat Rev Gastroenterol Hepatol.* 2014;11:68-71.
66. Colin JF, Cazals-Hatem D, Loriot MA, et al. Influence of human immunodeficiency virus infection on chronic hepatitis B in homosexual men. *Hepatology.* 1999;29(4):1306-1310.
68. Cosconea S, Fontaine H, Méritet JF, et al. Benefits associated with antiviral treatment in kidney allograft recipients with chronic hepatitis B virus infection. *J Hepatol.* 2012;57:55-60.
70. Lebensztejn DM, Skiba E, Sobaniec-Lotowska M. A simple noninvasive index (APRI) predicts advanced liver fibrosis in children with chronic hepatitis B. *Hepatology.* 2005;41(6):1434-1435.
72. Degertekin B, Han SH, Keeffe EB, et al. Impact of virologic breakthrough and HBIG regimen on hepatitis B recurrence after liver transplantation. *Am J Transplant.* 2010;10:1823-1833.
73. Degos F, Perez P, Roche B, et al. Diagnostic accuracy of FibroScan and comparison to liver fibrosis biomarkers in chronic viral hepatitis: a multicenter prospective study (the FIBROSTIC study). *J Hepatol.* 2010;53:1013-1021.
77. Di Martino V, Thevenot T, Colin JF, et al. Influence of HIV infection on the response to interferon therapy and the long-term outcome of chronic hepatitis B. *Gastroenterology.* 2002;123(6):1812-1822.
82. Dinda AK, Ghat M, Srivastava S, et al. Novel nanocarrier for oral hepatitis B vaccine. *Vaccine.* 2016;34(27):3076-3081.
83. Dore GJ, Soriano V, Rockstroh J, et al; SMART INSIGHT study group. Frequent hepatitis B virus rebound among HIV-hepatitis B virus-coinfected patients following antiretroviral therapy interruption. *AIDS.* 2010;24(6):857-865.
84. Drake A, Mijch A, Sasadeusz J. Immune reconstitution hepatitis in HIV and hepatitis B coinfection, despite lamivudine therapy as part of HAART. *Clin Infect Dis.* 2004;39(1):129-132.
87. Mast EE, Margolis HS, Fiore AE. A comprehensive immunization strategy to eliminate transmission of hepatitis B virus infection in the United States: recommendations of the Advisory Committee on Immunization Practices (ACIP) part 1: immunization of infants, children, and adolescents. *MMWR.* 2005;54(RR16):1-23.
88. European Association for the Study of the Liver. EASL clinical practice guidelines: Management of chronic hepatitis B virus infection. *J Hepatol.* 2012;57:167-185.
92. Feldstein AE, Nobili V. Biomarkers in nonalcoholic fatty liver disease: a new era in diagnosis and staging of disease in children. *J Pediatr Gastroenterol Nutr.* 2010;51:378-379.
93. Ferraioli G, Tinelli C, Dal Bello B, et al. Accuracy of real-time shear wave elastography for assessing liver fibrosis in chronic hepatitis C: a pilot study. *Hepatology.* 2012;56:2125-2133.
96. Fontanilla T, Cañas T, Macia A, et al. Normal values of liver shear wave velocity in healthy children assessed by acoustic radiation force impulse imaging using a convex probe and a linear probe. *Ultrasound Med Biol.* 2014;40:470-477.
98. Gara N, Abdalla A, Rivera E, et al. Durability of antibody response against hepatitis B virus in healthcare workers vaccinated as adults. *Clin Infect Dis.* 2015;60(4):505-513.
99. Gatanaga H, Yasuoka A, Kikuchi Y, et al. Influence of prior HIV-1 infection on the development of chronic hepatitis B infection. *Eur J Clin Microbiol Infect Dis.* 2000;19(3):237-239.
103. Giorgio A. Ultrasound in the diagnosis of steatosis and fibrosis of chronic liver diseases. *Dig Liver Dis.* 2007;39:391-392.
104. Glenn JS, Watson JA, Havel CM, et al. Identification of a prenylation site in delta virus large antigen. *Science.* 1992;256:1331-1333.
108. Gou YZ, Liu B, Jiang W, et al. The diagnostic value of ultrasound elastography in patients with hepatitis B virus infection: a prospective study. *J Int Med Res.* 2010;38:2117-2125, 73.
109. Güzelbulut F, Çetınkaya ZA, Sezıklı M, et al. AST-platelet ratio index, Forns index and FIB-4 in the prediction of significant fibrosis and cirrhosis in patients with chronic hepatitis C. *Turk J Gastroenterol.* 2011;22(3):279-285.
110. Hadler SC, Judson FN, O'Malley PM, et al. Outcome of hepatitis B virus infection in homosexual men and its relation to prior human immunodeficiency virus infection. *J Infect Dis.* 1991;163(3):454-459.
112. Hanquinet S, Courvoisier D, Kanavaki AM. Acoustic radiation force impulse imaging normal values of liver stiffness in healthy children. *Pediatr Radiol.* 2013;43:539-544.

113. Hanquinet S, Rougemont AL, Courvoisier D. Acoustic radiation force impulse (ARFI) elastography for the noninvasive diagnosis of liver fibrosis in children. *Pediatr Radiol.* 2013;43(5):545-551.
115. Hanquinet S, Courvoisier DS, Rougemont AL. Contribution of acoustic radiation force impulse (ARFI) elastography to the ultrasound diagnosis of biliary atresia. *Pediatr Radiol.* 2015;45(10):1489-1495.
119. Hosaka T, Suzuki F, Kobayashi M, et al. Long-term entecavir treatment reduces hepatocellular carcinoma incidence in patients with hepatitis B virus infection. *Hepatology.* 2013;58:98-107.
132. Jonas MM, Chang MH, Sokal E. Randomized, controlled trial of entecavir versus placebo in children with hepatitis B envelope antigen-positive chronic hepatitis B. *Hepatology.* 2016;63(2):377-387.
133. Jonas MM, Chang M-H, Sokal E, et al. Randomized controlled trial of entecavir versus placebo in children with HBeAg-positive chronic hepatitis B. *Hepatology.* 2015;81.
135. Jonas MM, Kelly D, Pollack H, et al. Safety, efficacy, and pharmacokinetics of adefovir dipivoxil in children and adolescents (age 2 to <18 years) with chronic hepatitis B. *Hepatology.* 2008;47(6):1863-1871.
136. Jonas MM, Lok AS, Mohammed K, et al. Antiviral therapy for chronic hepatitis B viral infection in children: a systematic review and meta-analysis. *Hepatology.* 2016;63:307-318.
141. Kao JH. Hepatitis B viral genotypes: clinical relevance and molecular characteristics. *J Gastroenterol Hepatol.* 2002;17:643-650.
143. Kaplan JE, Benson C, Holmes KH, et al. Guidelines for prevention and treatment of opportunistic infections in HIV-infected adults and adolescents: recommendations from CDC, the National Institutes of Health, and the HIV Medicine Association of the Infectious Diseases Society of America. *MMWR Recomm Rep.* 2009;58(RR-4):1-207.
145. Kidney Disease: Improving Global Outcomes (KDIGO) Transplant Work Group. KDIGO clinical practice guideline for the care of kidney transplant recipients. *Am J Transplant.* 2009;9(suppl 3):S1-S155.
147. Kitrinos KM, Corsa A, Liu Y, et al. No detectable resistance to tenofovir disoproxil fumarate after 6 years of therapy in patients with chronic hepatitis B. *Hepatology.* 2014;59(2):434-442.
153. Kodani M, Martin A, Mixson-Hayden T, et al. One-step real-time PCR assay for detection and quantitation of hepatitis D virus RNA. *J Virol Methods.* 2013;193:531-535.
154. Koh C, Canini L, Dahari H, et al. Oral prenylation inhibition with lonafarnib in chronic hepatitis D infection: a proof-of-concept randomised, double-blind, placebo-controlled phase 2A trial. *Lancet Infect Dis.* 2015;15:1167-1174.
157. Kose S, Tatar B, Gül S. The effect of long-term entecavir therapy on liver histopathology in patients with chronic viral hepatitis B. *Acta Clin Belg.* 2016;71(4):244-249.
158. Kowdley KV, Wang CC, Welch S, et al. Prevalence of chronic hepatitis B among foreign-born persons living in the United States by country of origin. *Hepatology.* 2012;56:422-433.
159. Kozielewicz D, Halota W, Wietlicka-Piszcz M, et al. Tenofovir rescue therapy in chronic hepatitis B patients who failed previous nucleoside analogue treatment. *Hepatol Int.* 2016;10(2):302-309.
161. Kramvis A, Kew MC. Relationship of genotypes of hepatitis B virus to mutations, disease progression and response to antiviral therapy. *J Viral Hepat.* 2005;12:456-464.
160. Kramvis A. Genotypes and genetic variability of hepatitis B virus. *Intervirology.* 2014;57:141-150.
162. Kuloğlu Z, Kansu A, Erden E. Efficacy of combined interferon alpha and long-term lamivudine therapy in children with chronic hepatitis B. *Turk J Pediatr.* 2010;52(5):457-463.
165. Lao-Araya M, Puthanakit T, Aurpibul L, et al. Antibody response to hepatitis B re-vaccination in HIV-infected children with immune recovery on highly active antiretroviral therapy. *Vaccine.* 2007;25(29):5324-5329.
166. Lao-Araya M, Puthanakit T, Aurpibul L, et al. Prevalence of protective level of hepatitis B antibody 3 years after revaccination in HIV-infected children on antiretroviral therapy. *Vaccine.* 2011;29(23):3977-3981.
167. Laryea MA, Watt KD. Immunoprophylaxis against and prevention of recurrent viral hepatitis after liver transplantation. *Liver Transpl.* 2012;18:514-523.
174. Lee S, Park JY, Kim do Y, et al. Prediction of virologic response to tenofovir mono-rescue therapy for multidrug resistant chronic hepatitis B. *J Med Virol.* 2016;88(6):1027-1034.
177. Leung DH, Ton-That M, Economides JM, et al. High prevalence of hepatitis B nonimmunity in vaccinated pediatric liver transplant recipients. *Am J Transplant.* 2015;15(2):535-540.
178. Lin X, Guo Y, Zhou A. Immunoprophylaxis failure against vertical transmission of hepatitis B virus in the Chinese population: a hospital-based study and a meta-analysis. *Pediatr Infect Dis J.* 2014;33(9):897-903.
181. Locarnini S, Qi X, Arterburn S, et al. Incidence and predictors of emergence of adefovir resistant HBV during four years of adefovir dipivoxil (ADV) therapy for patients with chronic hepatitis B (CHB). *J Hepatol.* 2005;42(suppl 2):17.
187. Lok AS, McMahon BJ, Mohammed K, et al. Antiviral therapy for chronic hepatitis B viral infection in adults: a systematic review and meta-analysis. *Hepatology.* 2016;63:284-306.
190. Lu X, Block TM, Gerlich WH. Protease-induced infectivity of hepatitis B virus for a human hepatoblastoma cell line. *J Virol.* 1996;70:2277-2285.
193. Lutgehetmann M, Mancke LV, Volz T, et al. Humanized chimeric uPA mouse model for the study of hepatitis B and D virus interactions and preclinical drug evaluation. *Hepatology.* 2012;55:685-694.
195. Mamadou S, Ide M, Maazou AR, et al. HIV infection and hepatitis B seroprevalence among antenatal clinic attendees in Niger, West Africa. *HIV AIDS (Auckl).* 2012;4:1-4.
196. Marshall GS, Adams GL, Leonardi ML, et al. Immunogenicity, safety, and tolerability of a hexavalent vaccine in infants. *Pediatrics.* 2015;136(2):e323-e332.
197. Martín-Carbonero L, Poveda E. Hepatitis B virus and HIV infection. *Semin Liver Dis.* 2012;32(2):114-119.
199. Matthews GV, Avihingsanon A, Lewin SR, et al. A randomized trial of combination hepatitis B therapy in HIV/HBV coinfected antiretroviral naive individuals in Thailand. *Hepatology.* 2008;48(4):1062-1069.
200. McGoogan KE, Smith PB, Choi SS, et al. Performance of the AST-to-platelet ratio index as a noninvasive marker of fibrosis in pediatric patients with chronic viral hepatitis. *J Pediatr Gastroenterol Nutr.* 2010;50(3):344-346.
201. McMahon BJ. The influence of hepatitis B virus genotype and subgenotype on the natural history of chronic hepatitis B. *Hepatol Int.* 2009;3:334-342.
204. D'Onofrio M, Crosara S, De Robertis R. Acoustic radiation force impulse of the liver. *World J Gastroenterol.* 2013;19(30):4841-4849.
206. Mofenson LM, Brady MT, Danner SP, et al; Centers for Disease Control and Prevention; National Institutes of Health; HIV Medicine Association of the Infectious Diseases Society of America; Pediatric Infectious Diseases Society; American Academy of Pediatrics. Guidelines for the Prevention and Treatment of Opportunistic Infections among HIV-exposed and HIV-infected children: Recommendations from CDC, the National Institutes of Health, the HIV Medicine Association of the Infectious Diseases Society of America, the Pediatric Infectious Diseases Society, and the American Academy of Pediatrics. *MMWR Recomm Rep.* 2009;58(RR-11):1-166.
207. Mugwanya KK, Baeten JM. Safety of oral tenofovir disoproxil fumarate-based pre-exposure prophylaxis for HIV prevention. *Expert Opin Drug Saf.* 2016;15(2):265-273.
209. Murray KF, Carithers RL. AASLD practice guidelines: Evaluation of the patient for liver transplantation. *Hepatology.* 2005;41:1407-1432.
210. Nassal M. HBV cccDNA: viral persistence reservoir and key obstacle for a cure of chronic hepatitis B. *Gut.* 2015;64:1972-1984.
216. Nitta Y, Kawabe N, Hashimoto S, et al. Liver stiffness measured by transient elastography correlates with fibrosis area in liver biopsy in patients with chronic hepatitis C. *Hepatol Res.* 2009;39:675-684.
218. Nobili V, Alisi A, Torre G, et al. Hyaluronic acid predicts hepatic fibrosis in children with nonalcoholic fatty liver disease. *Transl Res.* 2010;156:229-234.
220. Nobili V, Marcellini M, Giovannelli L, et al. Association of serum interleukin-8 levels with the degree of fibrosis in infants with chronic liver disease. *J Pediatr Gastroenterol Nutr.* 2004;39:540-544.
222. Ott JJ, Stevens GA, Groeger J, Wiersma ST. Global epidemiology of hepatitis B virus infection: new estimates of age-specific HBsAg seroprevalence and endemicity. *Vaccine.* 2012;30:2212-2219.
223. Papatheodoridis GV, Cholongitas E, Archimandritis AJ, et al. Current management of hepatitis B virus infection before and after liver transplantation. *Liver Int.* 2009;29:1294-1305.
224. Pascarella S, Negro F. Hepatitis D virus: an update. *Liver Int.* 2011;31:7-21.
225. Pereira TN, Lewindon PJ, Smith JL, et al. Serum markers of hepatic fibrogenesis in cystic fibrosis liver disease. *J Hepatol.* 2004;41:576-583.
226. Pessôa MG, Gazzard B, Huang AK, et al. Efficacy and safety of entecavir for chronic HBV in HIV/HBV coinfected patients receiving lamivudine as part of antiretroviral therapy. *AIDS.* 2008;22(14):1779-1787.
227. Petersen J, Dandri M, Mier W, et al. Prevention of hepatitis B virus infection in vivo by entry inhibitors derived from the large envelope protein. *Nat Biotechnol.* 2008;26:335-341.
228. Petersen J, Thompson AJ, Levrero M. Aiming for cure in HBV and HDV infection. *J Hepatol.* 2016;65(4):835-848.
229. Pham PT, Pham PA, Pham PC, et al. Evaluation of adult kidney transplant candidates. *Semin Dial.* 2010;23:595-605.
231. Pippi F, Bracciale L, Stolzuoli L, et al. Serological response to hepatitis B virus vaccine in HIV-infected children in Tanzania. *HIV Med.* 2008;9(7):519-525.
233. Poynard T, Morra R, Halfon P, et al. Meta-analyses of Fibrotest diagnostic value in chronic liver disease. *BMC Gastroenterol.* 2007;7:40.
234. Puoti M, Manno D, Nasta P, et al. Hepatitis B virus and HIV coinfection in low-income countries: unmet needs. *Clin Infect Dis.* 2008;46(3):367-369.
235. Puoti M, Torti C, Bruno R, et al. Natural history of chronic hepatitis B in co-infected patients. *J Hepatol.* 2006;44(suppl 1):S65-S70.

239. Ratcliffe L, Beadsworth MB, Pennell A, et al. Managing hepatitis B/HIV co-infected: adding entecavir to truvada (tenofovir disoproxil/emtricitabine) experienced patients. *AIDS*. 2011;25(8):1051-1056.
245. Roberts H, Kruszon-Moran D, Ly KN, et al. Prevalence of chronic hepatitis B virus (HBV) infection in U.S. households: National Health and Nutrition Examination Survey (NHANES), 1988-2012. *Hepatology*. 2016;63:388-397.
246. Rosenberg WMC, Voelker M, Thiel R, et al. Serum markers detect the presence of liver fibrosis: a cohort study. *Gastroenterology*. 2004;127:1704-1713.
248. Rouet F, Chaix ML, Inwoley A, et al. Programme Enfant Yopougon (Agence Nationale de Recherches sur le SIDA et les Hépatites Virales B et C 1244/1278). Frequent occurrence of chronic hepatitis B virus infection among West African HIV type-1-infected children. *Clin Infect Dis*. 2008;46(3):361-366.
249. Rouet F, Chaix ML, Kpozehouen A, et al. Relationship of CD4+ T-cell counts and plasma HIV-1 RNA levels with serological HBeAg/anti-HBe patterns obtained in West-African HBV–HIV-1-co-infected children. *J Trop Pediatr*. 2009;55(6):409-412.
251. Ruta SM, Matusa RF, Sultana C, et al. High prevalence of hepatitis B virus markers in Romanian adolescents with human immunodeficiency virus infection. *Med Gen Med*. 2005;7(1):68.
258. Selinger CP, Leong RW. Noninvasive liver fibrosis assessment: why does the APRI not work for hepatitis B? *Hepat Mon*. 2011;11(7):556-557.
259. Shaheen AA, Myers RP. Diagnostic accuracy of the aspartate aminotransferase-to-platelet ratio index for the prediction of hepatitis C-related fibrosis: a systematic review. *Hepatology*. 2007;46(3):912-921.
262. Silfverdal SA, Icardi G, Vesikari T, et al. A Phase III randomized, double-blind, clinical trial of an investigational hexavalent vaccine given at 2, 4, and 11-12 months. *Vaccine*. 2016;34(33):3810-3816.
264. Simani OE, Leroux-Roels G, François G, et al. Reduced detection and levels of protective antibodies to hepatitis B vaccine in under 2-year-old HIV positive South African children at a paediatric outpatient clinic. *Vaccine*. 2009;27(1):146-151.
270. Song Z, Dong R, Fan Y, Zheng S. Identification of serum protein biomarkers in biliary atresia by mass spectrometry and ELISA. *J Pediatr Gastroenterol Nutr*. 2012;55(4):370-375.
271. Soriano V, Mocroft A, Peters L, et al. EuroSIDA. Predictors of hepatitis B virus genotype and viraemia in HIV-infected patients with chronic hepatitis B in Europe. *J Antimicrob Chemother*. 2010;65(3):548-555.
278. Sunbul M. Hepatitis B virus genotypes: global distribution and clinical importance. *World J Gastroenterol*. 2014;20(18):5427-5434.
279. Swenson PD, Van Geyt C, Alexander ER, et al. Hepatitis B virus genotypes and HBsAg subtypes in refugees and injection drug users in the United States determined by LiPA and monoclonal EIA. *J Med Virol*. 2001;64:305-311.
282. Talwalkar JA, Kurtz DM, Schoenleber SJ, et al. Ultrasound-based transient elastography for the detection of hepatic fibrosis: systematic review and meta-analysis. *Clin Gastroenterol Hepatol*. 2007;5:1214-1220.
286. Teshale E, Lu M, Rupp LB, et al. APRI and FIB-4 are good predictors of the stage of liver fibrosis in chronic hepatitis B: the Chronic Hepatitis Cohort Study (CHeCS). *J Viral Hepat*. 2014;21(12):917-920.
287. Thio CL, Seaberg EC, Skolasky R Jr, et al. Multicenter AIDS Cohort Study. HIV-1, hepatitis B virus, and risk of liver-related mortality in the Multicenter Cohort Study (MACS). *Lancet*. 2002;360(9349):1921-1926.
288. Thio CL. Hepatitis B and human immunodeficiency virus coinfection. *Hepatology*. 2009;49(suppl 5):S138-S145.
287. Thio CL. Hepatitis B in the human immunodeficiency virus-infected patient: epidemiology, natural history, and treatment. *Semin Liver Dis*. 2003;23(2):125-136.
291. Trembling PM, Lampertico P, Parkes J, et al. Performance of Enhanced Liver Fibrosis test and comparison with transient elastography in the identification of liver fibrosis in patients with chronic hepatitis B infection. *J Viral Hepat*. 2014;21:430-438.
292. Ucar F, Sezer S, Ginis Z, et al. APRI, the FIB-4 score, and Forn's index have noninvasive diagnostic value for liver fibrosis in patients with chronic hepatitis B. *Eur J Gastroenterol Hepatol*. 2013;25(9):1076-1081.
293. Uhl P, Helm F, Hofhaus G, et al. A liposomal formulation for the oral application of the investigational hepatitis B drug Myrcludex B. *Eur J Pharm Biopharm*. 2016;103:159-166.
294. Urban S, Bartenschlager R, Kubitz R, et al. Strategies to inhibit entry of HBV and HDV into hepatocytes. *Gastroenterology*. 2014;147:48-64.
297. Vallet-Pichard A, Mallet V, Nalpas B, et al. FIB-4: an inexpensive and accurate marker of fibrosis in HCV infection. Comparison with liver biopsy and fibrotest. *Hepatology*. 2007;46(1):32-36.
298. Van Bommel F, de Man R, Stein K, et al. A multicenter analysis of antiviral response after one year of tenofovir mono-therapy in HBV-monoinfected patients with prior nucleos(t)ide analog experience. *J Hepatol*. 2008;48(suppl 2):S32.
300. Veloso Alves Pereira I, Buchmann B, Sandmann L, et al. Primary biliary acids inhibit hepatitis D virus (HDV) entry into human hepatoma cells expressing the sodium-taurocholate cotransporting polypeptide (NTCP). *PLoS ONE*. 2015;10(2):e0117152.
301. Verrier ER, Colpitts CC, Bach C, et al. A targeted functional RNA interference screen uncovers glypican 5 as an entry factor for hepatitis B and D viruses. *Hepatology*. 2016;63:35-48.
302. Villet S, Pichoud C, Billioud G, et al. Impact of hepatitis B virus rtA181V/T mutants on hepatitis B treatment failure. *J Hepatol*. 2008;48:747-755.
304. Wang H, Xue L, Yan R, et al. Comparison of FIB-4 and APRI in Chinese HBV-infected patients with persistently normal ALT and mildly elevated ALT. *J Viral Hepat*. 2013;20(4):e3-e10.
303. Wang JL, Du XF, Chen SL. Histological outcome for chronic hepatitis B patients treated with entecavir vs lamivudine-based therapy. *World J Gastroenterol*. 2015;21(32):9598-9606.
309. Westland C, Delaney W, Yang H, et al. Hepatitis B virus genotypes and virologic response in 694 patients in phase III studies of adefovir dipivoxil1. *Gastroenterology*. 2003;125:107-1664.
311. Wong GL-H, Chan HL-Y, Mak CW-H, et al. Entecavir treatment reduces hepatic events and deaths in chronic hepatitis B patients with liver cirrhosis. *Hepatology*. 2013;58:1537-1547.
315. Xiao G, Yang J, Yan L. Comparison of diagnostic accuracy of aspartate aminotransferase to platelet ratio index and fibrosis-4 index for detecting liver fibrosis in adult patients with chronic hepatitis B virus infection: a systematic review and meta-analysis. *Hepatology*. 2015;61(1):292-302.
316. Xinfeng H, Fengfeng M, Zhiyi J, et al. Inactivation of NTCP causes gallbladder disease in mice; October 4-8, 2015. 2015 International Meeting on Molecular Biology of Hepatitis B Viruses, Bad Nauheim, Germany, Abstract O-177 (personal communication).
317. Xue MM, Glenn JS, Leung DH. Hepatitis D in children. *JPGN*. 2015;61:271-281.
318. Yap DY, Tang CS, Yung S, et al. Long-term outcome of renal transplant recipients with chronic hepatitis B infection-impact of antiviral treatments. *Transplantation*. 2010;90:325-330.
319. Ye XP, Ran HT, Cheng J, et al. Liver and spleen stiffness measured by acoustic radiation force impulse elastography for noninvasive assessment of liver fibrosis and esophageal varices in patients with chronic hepatitis B. *J Ultrasound Med*. 2012;31:1245-1253.
320. Yilmaz Y, Yonal O, Kurt R, et al. Noninvasive assessment of liver fibrosis with the aspartate transaminase to platelet ratio index (APRI): usefulness in patients with chronic liver disease—APRI in chronic liver disease. *Hepat Mon*. 2011;11(2):103-106.
323. Yurdaydin C, Borochov N, Kalkan C, et al. Hepatitis delta virus kinetics under the prenylation inhibitor lonafarnib suggest HDV-mediated suppression of HBV replication. *J Hepatol*. 2016;64:S587.
324. Zachou K, Yurdaydin C, Drebber U, et al; for the HIDT-1 Study Group. Quantitative HBsAg and HDV-RNA levels in chronic delta hepatitis. *Liver Int*. 2010;30:430-437.
327. Zhang L, Gui XE, Teter C. Effects of hepatitis B immunization on prevention of mother-to-infant transmission of hepatitis B virus and on the immune response of infants towards hepatitis B vaccine. *Vaccine*. 2014;32(46):6091-6097.
328. Zhang Z, Wang G, Kang K. The diagnostic accuracy and clinical utility of three noninvasive models for predicting liver fibrosis in patients with HBV infection. *PLoS ONE*. 2016;11(4):e0152757.
330. Zou H, Chen Y, Duan Z, Zhang H. Protective effect of hepatitis B vaccine combined with two-dose hepatitis B immunoglobulin on infants born to HBsAg-positive mothers. *PLoS ONE*. 2011;6(10):e26748.
331. Zou ZQ, Wang L, Wang K. Innate immune targets of hepatitis B virus infection. *World J Hepatol*. 2016;8(17):716-725.
332. Zoulim F, Buti M, Lok AS. Antiviral-resistant hepatitis B virus: can we prevent this monster from growing? *J Viral Hepat*. 2007;14(suppl 1):29-36.

The full reference list for this chapter is available at ExpertConsult.com.

Herpes Simplex Viruses 1 and 2

158

Gail J. Harrison • Benjamin A. Pinsky • Ann M. Arvin

Herpes simplex virus (HSV) types 1 and 2 are in the family of nine human herpesviruses, which also includes cytomegalovirus (CMV), Epstein-Barr virus (EBV), varicella-zoster virus (VZV), and human herpesviruses (HHV) types 6A, 6B, 7, and 8.

HSV-1 is the prototype of the α-herpesvirus subfamily, which includes HSV-2 and VZV.[334] These viruses are ubiquitous and neurotropic and establish latency in sensory ganglia; persistence is associated with periodic reactivation and reappearance of infectious virus at mucocutaneous sites. Most individuals infected with HSV-1 and HSV-2 do not have clinical manifestations, either at the time of initial acquisition or during episodes of reactivation. When HSV-1 or HSV-2 causes disease, the illness may range from minor, such as "fever blisters," to life threatening, as exemplified by HSV encephalitis or neonatal disease. Proper management of HSV-1 and HSV-2 infection depends on clinical recognition of the common and atypical syndromes caused by these viruses, knowledge of laboratory methods that are useful for proving the diagnosis, and early and appropriate antiviral therapy.

THE VIRUSES

HSV-1 and HSV-2 virions consist of an icosahedral protein capsid enclosing a core of double-stranded DNA, surrounded by a protein tegument, and enclosed in a lipid-containing envelope.[334] The genomic DNA of HSV-1 and HSV-2 has substantial sequence homology (approximately 50%), but the viruses also have unique sequences that encode variant proteins, and they differ biologically in their patterns of replication in vitro and in vivo. Tegument proteins are located between the capsid and the viral envelope. The envelope has glycoproteins that are important targets of the humoral and cellular immune responses (gB, gC, gD, and gG). The glycoproteins gE and gI function as immunoglobulin (Ig) Fc receptors. Other glycoproteins include gH and gL, which form a complex with gB that plays a role in cell entry and spread; gK, which is required for viral exocytosis; and gM, which has a role in capsid envelopment and exocytosis. These glycoproteins are found in both HSV-1 and HSV-2 and exhibit a high degree of amino acid similarity. The gG of HSV-2 is larger than its HSV-1 homologue and has unique sites that are recognized by virus-specific host responses. Both forms of HSV can infect either oral or genital sites; however, HSV-1 usually causes infections of oral mucocutaneous sites, and most genital mucocutaneous infections are caused by HSV-2.[123,334] HSV-1 is more likely to recur at oral sites, and HSV-2 reactivates more frequently in the genital area, even in persons who were infected initially at both oral and genital sites with HSV-1 or HSV-2.[234]

HSV attaches to and penetrates cells via gB and gD through specific cell surface herpes family receptors. This process also involves gH and gL. The herpes family coreceptors belong to the tumor necrosis factor family (Hve-A), the immunoglobulin superfamily of receptors (nectins), and the 3-*O*-sulfated heparin sulfates.[334] After the virion enters the cell, an orderly expression of immediate early, or α, genes occurs that triggers viral gene transcription and inhibits host cell function; early, or β, viral genes that encode regulatory proteins and DNA replication enzymes, including thymidine kinase and viral DNA polymerase; and finally, late, or γ, genes that encode structural proteins. Replication of viral DNA and accumulation of structural proteins allow assembly of the virion capsid in the cell nucleus and envelopment by modified cellular membranes that are incorporated into the virion envelope during virion egress. Infectious virions are released from the infected cell or can spread to adjacent cells via membrane fusion.

Human HSV replicates in tissue culture cells derived from many mammalian species and various laboratory animals, including rodents, rabbits, and primates. Lack of restriction of the host range distinguishes HSV-1 and HSV-2 from the other human herpesviruses. HSV-1 and HSV-2 replication progresses rapidly in cell culture and causes characteristic focal cytopathologic effects. Confirmation that these effects are caused by HSV can be accomplished by staining the infected cells with specific antisera or monoclonal antibodies that differentiate HSV-1 from HSV-2 and from other viral pathogens.

Like other herpesviruses, HSV-1 and HSV-2 have gene products that inhibit intrinsic cellular responses that interfere with replication and facilitate the avoidance of immune surveillance during primary infection, latency, and reactivation.[53] Among others, these mechanisms include elaboration of virally encoded IgG Fc receptors formed by gE/gI and complement receptors that bind host immune components; downregulation of major histocompatibility complex (MHC) class I antigen, which prevents recognition of infected cells by $CD8^+$ T cells; interference with upregulation of MHC class II molecules by interferon-γ, which inhibits $CD4^+$ T-cell–mediated adaptive immune responses; and inhibition of the lytic activity of natural killer cells.[334]

TRANSMISSION

Infectious HSV-1 and HSV-2 virions are released into the oral or genital secretions of infected but asymptomatic persons who are experiencing primary or recurrent infection. This phenomenon is referred to as viral excretion or *viral shedding* and results in periodic opportunities for the virus to be transferred to susceptible contacts. Most HSV-1 and HSV-2 transmission is caused by silent infections, and transmission occurs with equivalent frequency regardless of whether the individual who is shedding the virus has ever had symptoms of oral or genital herpes.

Although HSV-1 and HSV-2 are highly infectious after inoculation of mucocutaneous sites, they are not transmitted casually from person to person. The enveloped virions are unstable outside mammalian cells, and close interpersonal contact is required for transfer of infectious virus particles. In most circumstances, transmission requires direct apposition of infected with uninfected mucous membranes or skin during intimate contact such as kissing or sexual contact. Outbreaks associated with gingivostomatitis have occurred at daycare centers.[365] If uninfected exposed skin or mucous membranes are damaged, the risk for transmission appears to be enhanced. Although skin is less susceptible to direct inoculation than the mucous membranes are, transmission via inoculation of skin may be increased by local trauma. For example, affected areas are more susceptible in burned patients[140] and infants with diaper rash. Children with eczema are at risk for contracting serious disseminated HSV infections (Kaposi varicelliform eruption).[14,450] Transfer of HSV-1 between wrestlers (herpes gladiatorum)[370] and between rugby players (herpes rugbeiorum or "scrumpox")[372] probably takes place after the abrasion of saliva-contaminated skin. One outbreak at a wrestling camp involved 60 of 175 participants.[38,79] Health care workers may acquire HSV infections of the paronychial region (herpetic whitlow), presumably from direct contact of ungloved hands with oropharyngeal secretions.[148,337] Medical personnel can transfer HSV to their patients. Children acquire HSV whitlow in the course of primary HSV-1 gingivostomatitis through nail biting or thumb sucking. When herpetic whitlow develops in persons who are not health care workers, HSV-2 is a common cause and often is associated with primary genital HSV infection.[150] The usual route of transmission to neonates is by exposure during passage through an HSV-infected birth canal. Genital and anal HSV infections are transmitted through direct contact with infected genitalia or from orogenital or oroanal contact.

Newly acquired HSV-1 and HSV-2 infections are associated with shedding of high titers of infectious virus, regardless of whether the individual is symptomatic. In addition, active recurrent HSV-1 or HSV-2 lesions contain substantial titers of virus, which may increase the likelihood of transmission occurring during close contact with a susceptible individual.

The incidence of acquisition of HSV-2 is 5% to 15% per year in individuals who are HSV-1 and HSV-2 seronegative or HSV-1 seropositive but HSV-2 seronegative and whose sexual partners have recurrent genital herpes.[272,273] In studies of discordant couples, transmission occurred in 10% of partners, with higher transmission from men (17%) than from women (4%). In women lacking antibodies to HSV-1 and HSV-2, the rate of transmission was 32%; if they had antibodies to type 1, the rate was 9%.[272] Studies of patients by HSV-2-specific serology show that many individuals remain uninfected despite having long-term contact with a person who is infected with HSV-2.[229] The extent to which HSV-1 immunity protects against HSV-2 infection is not clear, but the evidence is that symptoms of new HSV-2 infection may be prevented if the exposed individual has HSV-1 immunity, whereas subclinical infection frequently is not blocked.[48,62] Information about whether HSV-1 or HSV-2 acquired earlier interferes with the acquisition of infection by unrelated HSV-1 or HSV-2 strains is limited, but a few individuals with multiple sexual partners have been found to shed HSV-2 viruses that are genetically distinct.

HSV has been isolated from the hands of patients with oral lesions and has been shown to persist for several hours on inanimate objects or in distilled water. Nonetheless, inanimate sources have not been implicated as important reservoirs of HSV persistence and spread.[291,421] HSV transmission from transplanted organs[124] and inseminated donor sperm has been reported.[277]

When HSV-1 and HSV-2 shedding has been evaluated prospectively in seropositive individuals with or without a history of symptoms, the usual frequency of detection of virus in oral or genital secretions is 1% to 2%.[16,334] In patients with known genital herpes, silent excretion has been documented as often as 10% of the time when they appear to be lesion free. Twelve percent of women with primary HSV-1 genital infection and 18% with primary genital HSV-2 infection subsequently shed virus asymptomatically, especially in the first 3 months after resolution of the primary infection.[218] Two percent of women attending a sexually transmitted disease clinic shed HSV-2 asymptomatically.[227] In partner studies, 70% of HSV-2 transmissions were associated with sexual contact during periods of asymptomatic viral shedding.[273]

Polymerase chain reaction (PCR) is considerably more sensitive than is culture for detection of HSV on mucosal surfaces, and the use of this technology has improved understanding of the extent of HSV viral shedding. However, it is important to recognize that the detection of segments of the viral genome by PCR does not necessarily mean that infectious virus is present. PCR detects subclinical shedding of HSV-2 on 20% to 25% of days. Factors that influence the magnitude and frequency of shedding include the site of infection, immune status of the patient, and time of acquisition of the virus.[342] Previous studies using viral cultures rarely reported isolation of HSV-2 from the mouth, but recent quantitative PCR studies detected asymptomatic oral HSV-2 reactivation from 40% of men with HSV-2 genital herpes. Oral HSV-2 shedding frequently is concurrent with genital HSV-2 shedding.[210]

Investigation of HSV-1 transmission is less extensive, but the high prevalence of asymptomatic HSV-1 infection in the population and its acquisition in early childhood suggest a similar pattern of spread by exposure to virus present in oral secretions from asymptomatic individuals.

Both HSV-1 and HSV-2 can be transmitted to a neonate. Approximately 4% of neonatal herpes cases are acquired in utero, 86% around the time of birth, and 10% postnatally. Three fourths of natal/postnatal cases of neonatal herpes infection are caused by HSV-2, and the remainder are caused by HSV-1 strains.[299] Virtually all neonatal HSV-2 infections probably are acquired from mothers having an active genital herpes infection by contact with infected genital secretions at or during delivery from an asymptomatic mother who acquired her first episode of genital herpes infection in the third trimester or near the time of delivery.[299,403,462,472] The majority of neonates with HSV appear to acquire the infection by contact with infected genital secretions at or during delivery from an asymptomatic mother who acquired her first episode of genital herpes infection in the third trimester or near the time of delivery.[54,56,58-60] Because 60% to 80% of mothers who have newborns with HSV have no signs or symptoms of genital herpes at the time of labor and delivery and have a negative past history of genital herpes or contact with a partner who had a genital vesicular rash, some experts recommend routine serologic screening of pregnant women and their partners to identify potential at-risk mothers.[54,56,264,454,458,459] However, based on the low accuracy of currently available serologic tests for HSV-2, and the potential harm of false-positive HSV-2 serologic tests, as well as the lack of randomized clinical trials to show that antiviral medication reduces transmission risk in asymptomatic seropositive individuals, the 2016 US Preventive Services Task Force Recommendation Statement from 2016 recommended against serologic screening for genital HSV-2 infection in asymptomatic adolescents and young adults, including those who are pregnant.[135,424]

Neonates with HSV-1 infection can acquire the virus from several sources: maternal genital tract, oral contact with mother, breast lesions,[54,56,59,126,254,402,474,473] oral herpes in the father or other family members,[122,403,473,474] or health care–associated transmission from other infected infants or health care workers.[167,255] Although HSV-1 cold sores and asymptomatic oral shedding may be common findings in nursery personnel,[176,177] transmission to a neonate from this source appears to be rare.[333,425] Male neonates may also contract HSV infection after out-of-hospital ritual circumcision.[83] In a recent report, 11 neonates were reported infected with HSV after orthodox Jewish ritual circumcision that included metzitzah b'peh, a practice in which the circumciser uses his mouth to apply direct orogenital suction to the newly circumcised penis to clean the blood away from the wound.[83]

EPIDEMIOLOGY

Understanding HSV epidemiology requires distinguishing between the prevalence of infection, which is high, and the frequency of HSV-related disease, which is low. These viruses maintain their persistence in the human population through their capacity to persist and reactivate in the individual host. The prevalence of HSV-1 and HSV-2 is a consequence of efficient transmission to susceptible close contacts and the continuous presence of a large pool of infected persons in the population. Because HSV-1 and HSV-2 are not cleared after primary infection but instead establish latency and reactivate frequently in an infected host, opportunities for viral spread to new susceptible persons are common. Seroepidemiologic studies have shown that HSV infections are found in all human populations, even in the most remote and isolated communities. HSV-1 and HSV-2 have no seasonal pattern because the mechanism of transmission is by intimate contact, which occurs year round. Individuals who have been infected with HSV-1 or HSV-2 remain a reservoir for infectious virus throughout their lifetimes and, as intermittent shedders, are sources of virus that spreads to susceptible contacts. Most transmission is from asymptomatic infection, and most acquisition is asymptomatic. For example, the rate of subclinical shedding of HSV-2 in individuals with no reported history of genital herpes was similar to that in subjects with such a history (3.0% vs. 2.7%).[440] Shedding of HSV-1 in oral secretions is equally prevalent.

When symptoms of a new HSV-1 infection do occur, the source of the infection rarely is identified because the susceptible individual usually has many infected contacts. The first symptomatic episodes of HSV-1 or HSV-2 often represent reactivations of earlier infections.

The average age at acquisition and the prevalence of HSV-1 and HSV-2 infection are influenced by the virus type. Although neonatal HSV infections are usually acquired from maternal genital infection and usually are caused by HSV-2, HSV-1 acquisition predominates in childhood. Depending on social and economic factors, 20% to 40% of young children are seropositive by the time they reach 5 years of age, with higher rates of acquisition in lower socioeconomic groups, non-Hispanic blacks, and children born outside the United States.[471] Earlier acquisition of HSV-1 may be influenced by whether the mother, or other major caregivers, has HSV-1 infection. Attendance at child care centers, which brings children together in close contact, may increase the likelihood of acquiring HSV-1 at an earlier age.[232,365] Acquisition of HSV-1 continues with age at an average rate of 1% to 2% per year throughout the childhood and adult years; by later ages, 70% to 90% of individuals have been infected by HSV-1.[379] Seroepidemiologic studies of higher socioeconomic groups have reported HSV-1 infection in 30% to 46% of university students.[147]

The prevalence of HSV-2 is highly variable and depends on the country, region, sex, age, population subgroup, and whether a population is "high risk."[376] Because transmission of HSV-2 is associated with sexual activity, the prevalence of HSV-2 begins to increase with adolescence. It is estimated that one in six individuals between ages 14 and 49 years will transmit genital HSV.[424] Now that serologic methods can be used to differentiate HSV-1 and HSV-2 infection, the seroprevalence of HSV-2 in adults has been shown to range from 20% to 60%. Continuing comprehensive investigation of HSV-2 epidemiology in the United States by the National Health and Nutrition Examination Survey (NHANES) documented a 30% increase in prevalence from the 1970s to the 1990s, which resulted in HSV-2 infection in approximately 20% of adults in the period between 1988 and 1994.[78,139,199] Since that time, HSV-2 seroprevalence has decreased to approximately 16% in individuals 14 to 49 years of age.[81] High HSV-2 infection rates are documented in higher as well as lower socioeconomic groups, with estimated transmission occurring in one of every six individuals.[48,227,229,401,477] Rates are *consistently* higher in women, non-Hispanic blacks, and individuals with multiple sexual partners. However, despite the high prevalence of seropositivity and transmission rates, serologic screening is not recommended based on the US Preventive Services Task Force Recommendation Statement because there is a high false-positive rate for HSV serologic test results, which have resulted in psychosocial harm and distress related to false-positive results. Furthermore randomized clinical trial data to support preventive antiviral treatment for seropositive individual are lacking.[135]

Changes in the epidemiology of symptomatic HSV-2 infection have been suggested by rising numbers of medical visits for genital herpes. The extent to which the increase in symptomatic cases of HSV-2 infection reflects a true increase in the prevalence of HSV-2 or a higher likelihood that HSV-2 infection will result in symptoms is not certain. The decrease in the number of young adults with HSV-1 infection acquired in childhood could be associated with loss of cross-reactive HSV immunity and an increased risk for the development of symptomatic genital herpes. A higher risk for contracting genital HSV-2 infection is associated with lower socioeconomic status, early age at first intercourse, increased numbers of sexual partners, female gender, previous marriage, urban living, black race, and incidents of trichomoniasis, bacterial vaginosis, and other sexually transmitted diseases.[139,155,198]

A retrospective analysis of genital HSV cultures obtained from a group of college students over the course of a 9-year period showed that HSV-1 is an increasingly common cause of genital herpes in some populations in the United States. In this particular population, HSV-1 accounted for more than 70% of positive genital cultures by the end of the study period, as compared with approximately 30% at the beginning.[331]

Symptomatic disease occurs after newly acquired HSV infection at an estimated incidence of 10 to 20% or less. However, silent infections can give rise to symptoms that appear months or years later as a result of viral reactivation. The epidemiology of HSV-1 or HSV-2 reactivation as a cause of symptomatic illness depends on the prevalence of these infections in the population as a whole, but it also is influenced by host factors that perturb the balance between the virus and the infected individual. For example, HSV-related symptoms may be triggered by exposure to sunlight (ultraviolet), febrile illnesses, immunosuppression from illness or necessary therapies, and other variables. These variables are cofactors that affect the frequency of HSV-related disease within the infected cohort but not the epidemiologic pattern of infection.

HSV infections may be transmitted from the mother to her fetus and neonate. Fulminant or disseminated primary HSV disease may occur in pregnancy, but whether it develops more often than in nonpregnant women is not clear.[235] A review[308] of seven such cases revealed (1) infection during the third trimester in all; (2) four beginning as a genital HSV infection and three as oral disease; (3) hepatitis in six, encephalitis in two, and pancreatitis in two; (4) maternal death in three (43%)—two from hepatitis and one from encephalitis; and (5) three instances of fetal death—each secondary to severe maternal systemic illness rather than direct infection with HSV. Postpartum HSV endometritis may also occur and result in disseminated infection in both mother and neonate.[142,268]

An increased rate of spontaneous abortion occurs in women with primary genital herpes during early pregnancy, regardless of socioeconomic status.[58,170,171,284] Premature delivery does not occur more commonly in prospectively monitored women with recurrent genital herpes,[170,299,429,468] but most reports of neonatal herpes cases find a greater preponderance of premature infants than in the general population.[299,462,473] This finding, however, may reflect a higher susceptibility of premature infants to HSV infection secondary to a lack of transplacentally acquired IgG neutralizing antibodies rather than being a cause of the prematurity. Recurrent genital herpes in middle-class pregnant women is no more severe or frequent than in nonpregnant ones,[170,429,468] but older studies demonstrated more frequent and longer episodes in women of lower socioeconomic groups.[284,292] Between 74% and 88% of middle-class pregnant women with a history of genital herpes had at least one clinical recurrence during an observed pregnancy.[170,429,468] A mean of 2.7 to 3.0 episodes occurred during gestation, and HSV was isolated from lesions in 56% to 75% of the recurrences and in 0.6% to 12% of concomitant cervical cultures obtained during the recurrence. Asymptomatic shedding of HSV from the cervix, either between clinical recurrences or in a history-positive woman with no episodes during the observed pregnancy, was detected in 0.5% to 2.3% of the cultures obtained. Importantly, the presence of HSV shedding during the latter weeks of pregnancy was not predictive of shedding at the time of delivery.[16,468]

The number of cases of neonatal herpes occurring in the United States each year is far less than one would expect from the probable number of pregnancies complicated by genital herpes. Of the 3.5 to 4 million annual pregnancies, 7000 to 200,000 of these women have genital herpes at some time during the pregnancy and 3500 to 14,000 have positive HSV cultures at the time of delivery.[46,157,171,409,429,458,468] The actual number of cases of neonatal herpes per year in Seattle and Atlanta (0.1 and 0.3 per 1000 live births, respectively) would project to a national estimate of 350 to 1,050 per year in the United States.[403] An estimate of the incidence of neonatal HSV is between 1 in 3,000 and 1 in 20,000 and may vary with the demographics and geographic location of the population. Because asymptomatic HSV infection of the neonate rarely, if ever, occurs, subclinical cases or missed diagnoses probably do not account for the differences between the estimated number of maternal and neonatal infections. More likely, neonatal infection rates in the neonates of mothers with genital herpes are far lower than currently assumed, possibly because of the preventive measures used. The estimated infection rates quoted most often currently are (1) a 33% to 50% rate for infants vaginally delivered by mothers with primary genital herpes, (2) a 3% to 5% rate for infants vaginally delivered by mothers with recurrent lesions, and (3) less than 3% for those delivered by mothers with recurrent asymptomatic shedding at the time of delivery.[46,54,97,299,468] In the early 1970s,[284] the following neonatal infection rates in neonates born to mothers with genital herpes during pregnancy were reported: (1) 33% in mothers with primary disease after the 32nd week of gestation, (2) 3% in mothers with recurrent episodes after 32 weeks, and (3) 42% in mothers with virus-positive lesions at the time of delivery (primary vs. recurrent episodes not specified). More recent studies have determined a significant risk for neonatal herpes occurring in neonates born to mothers with asymptomatic shedding at the time of vaginal delivery: 33% with subclinical first episodes and 0 to 3% with recurrent shedding.[54,72-74,300,318] Accurate knowledge of the actual neonatal infection risk is important for making decisions about management (e.g., cesarean section, prophylactic antiviral therapy). Researchers and experts have estimated that as many as 75% of neonates with HSV disease are born to mothers with no history or clinical findings suggestive of active HSV infection during pregnancy, labor, or delivery.[5,54,72-74]

Several factors influence the risk for acquiring neonatal herpes and the severity of neonatal disease once the infection develops. The greater risk for transmitting neonatal infection by mothers with primary, as opposed to recurrent, vesicular or ulcerative lesions at the time of delivery is well established. Also, a woman with virus-positive recurrent lesions at the time of delivery is likely to be at greater risk than is a woman who is asymptomatic and shedding virus identified by HSV surveillance cultures. Other aspects of the anatomic site and the severity of maternal genital herpes also may be associated with a greater risk for development of neonatal disease: (1) maternal cervical as opposed to vulvar or buttock skin involvement—resulting in more virus being shed into vaginal secretions; (2) multiple as opposed to single vesicles or ulcers—again, more virus from multiple lesions; (3) higher titer of virus in vaginal secretions—cultures positive sooner or more intensely positive in the diagnostic virology laboratory; and (4) longer duration of fetal exposure to infected vaginal secretions because of prolonged rupture of membranes or of fetal scalp monitors.[97,297-299]

Investigations by Yeager and associates[473,474,] indicate that no anti-HSV antibody or a low titer of such antibody in maternal and neonatal serum is associated with a greater risk for acquisition of neonatal infection and more serious disease and that high-titer antibody is associated with a lower risk. Studies of HSV antibody titers in neonates do not show an association between antibody titer and outcome of disease. More investigations are required, therefore, to determine the potential protective role of maternal transplacental anti-HSV antibody.

Premature infants have accounted for 40% to 50% of cases of neonatal herpes,[413,454,465] in contrast to the usual prematurity rates of 6% to 18% reported in the general maternal population. Whether the increased frequency of prematurity among neonates with herpes indicates a greater propensity of mothers with genital herpes to deliver prematurely or a greater susceptibility of premature infants to HSV infection is not known. Premature infants appear more likely to have a fatal outcome.[74,454,455]

Instrumentation of the neonate, particularly scalp electrodes for fetal monitoring, is known to increase the risk for acquiring neonatal HSV infection.[127,207,303] Mortality rates appear to be higher in neonates with HSV-2 than in those with HSV-1 infection, probably because of the greater proportion of HSV-2–infected infants with dissemination.[455] In neonatal herpes survivors, neurologic damage occurs much more frequently in infants with HSV-2 infection than in those with HSV-1 infection.[101,455] Infants with disseminated infection (liver, lungs, adrenals), with or without central nervous system (CNS) involvement, have the highest mortality rates (70–80%); those with encephalitis have only intermediate rates (30–40%); and those with infection limited to the skin, eye, or mouth have the lowest rates (0%).[465] Rarely, neonatal HSV has been implicated as a cause of sudden unexpected death in infancy.[446]

The prevalence of HSV infection in febrile neonates presenting to an acute pediatric emergency treatment center appears similar to that of bacterial meningitis, suggesting that HSV infection should be in the differential of neonatal fever and evaluated accordingly.[72-74] Factors associated with neonatal HSV infection in febrile or hypothermic neonates presenting to acute care centers include history of peripartum maternal fever, history of maternal primary HSV infection, prematurity, vaginal delivery, neonatal seizures, vesicular rash, respiratory distress, thrombocytopenia, elevated hepatic enzymes, and cerebrospinal fluid (CSF) pleocytosis.[72-74] Because the presentation of neonatal HSV is nonspecific, and delay in diagnosis and treatment is associated with significant morbidity and mortality, some experts recommend all neonates younger than 21 days of age receive evaluation for HSV infection and early empirical treatment with acyclovir.[72-74,260]

PATHOGENESIS AND PATHOLOGY

HSV-1 and HSV-2 exhibit particular tropism for cells of ectodermal origin, including skin and neuronal cells. Initial viral replication is thought to occur at the portal of entry, usually in mucous membranes or skin. In symptomatic cases, the incubation period for primary infection appears to vary from 2 to 20 days. In contrast to varicella, HSV viremia is difficult to detect by culture in a normal host, although it may be found in some immunocompromised patients.[164,390] HSV DNA in plasma and peripheral blood mononuclear cells in HSV-infected neonates has been detected with PCR techniques.[116] HSV DNA has also been detected in approximately 25% of patients with confirmed primary genital HSV infection. Women are more likely to be viremic than men, and viremia is detected more frequently early after infection.[200]

If mucocutaneous lesions are induced during primary or recurrent infection, the pathologic cell changes caused by HSV-1 or HSV-2 replication include cytoplasmic enlargement and nuclear alterations. Cell fusion may lead to the formation of multinucleated giant cells. The nuclei of infected cells often have eosinophilic intranuclear inclusions and marginated nuclear chromatin. As the cells manifest injury, a local inflammatory response ensues, intercellular edema develops, and vesicles form. The vesicles become visible as they enlarge and usually are surrounded by an erythematous margin. At later stages, the vesicles become pustular and then dry and crust. HSV lesions typically are superficial and do not scar. Vesicles that form on mucous membranes are transient, with rapid sloughing of the superficial layer, and are seen first as shallow ulcers.

HSV-1 and HSV-2 establish latency in neurons of the sensory ganglia by mechanisms that are as yet unidentified. The viruses persist in this latent state for various intervals, although frequent asymptomatic reactivation is common; reactivation induces viral replication with the production of infectious virus at mucosal or other sites. Persons who have recurrent HSV infections frequently describe tingling sensations, itching, and burning at the site of recurrence beginning several hours before the appearance of clusters of vesicles. Persons who have recurrent genital herpes may experience severe shooting pain in their legs and even urinary retention in connection with recurrence. Occasionally, recurrent HSV skin eruptions may occur in a zosteriform pattern in a distribution reflecting the sensory innervation of a particular dermatome.

Replication at the portal of entry appears to result in infection of sensory nerve endings, followed by transport of the virus to the cranial and dorsal root ganglia along neuronal axons. Latency is established regardless of whether the primary infection is symptomatic, and it appears to be an invariable consequence of HSV infection with either virus type.[29,332,334] HSV-1 and HSV-2 persist in neuronal cells of the sensory ganglia, with substantial numbers of these cells harboring latent virus, as demonstrated by the detection of latency-associated transcripts. The latency-associated transcripts overlap the viral genes *ICPO* and *ICP34.5* in an antisense direction.[102,334,392] The role of these transcripts in the establishment or maintenance of latency remains to be clarified.[53] The presence of latency-associated transcripts appears to be necessary for establishment of latency and efficient reactivation of viral production in some animal models in vivo.[310] Viral particles are not produced in latently infected cells. HSV-1 persists most predominantly in the cranial nerve ganglia, whereas HSV-2 latency occurs in the lumbosacral ganglia. Cocultivation techniques have been used to recover HSV from the dorsal root ganglia innervating the areas of skin in which persons have experienced recurrent herpes lesions. HSV-1 has been found in trigeminal ganglia, and HSV-2 has been recovered from sacral ganglia.[32] Once latency is established in the sensory ganglia, antiviral drugs cannot eradicate the latent virus from infected neurons. Because the latent virus does not multiply, it is not susceptible to drugs that affect viral DNA synthesis, such as acyclovir. When reactivation is triggered, HSV-1 or HSV-2 is transported back down axons to mucocutaneous sites, where it replicates and releases infectious virus into secretions.[29,104,332,334] Individuals with symptomatic recurrent HSV infections almost always have HSV lesions in the identical or a directly adjacent site. Reactivation is not prevented by adaptive immunity, although whether symptoms occur and whether the virus disseminates may be influenced by the host response.

The stimulus for reactivation of latent virus may be provided by iatrogenic or naturally occurring episodes of immunosuppression and by endocrine (e.g., menstruation) or exogenous (e.g., trauma, sun, acupuncture, emotional stress) factors. Ultraviolet irradiation of the usual site of recurrence of persons who have a history of recurrent oral herpes reliably induces recurrence either quickly (within 48 hours) or 2 to 7 days later.[380] Skin subject to recurrent HSV infection has been transplanted elsewhere on the body and exchanged with skin taken from the site of graft placement and previously not involved in HSV infections. Subsequent recurrence of HSV infection was found to be localized to the original site, not to the original skin. These studies and others strongly suggest that latent virus does not reside in skin cells.

Primary HSV infection elicits humoral and cellular immunity, which can be detected shortly after the appearance of lesions in individuals in whom symptoms develop. Based on animal models and some human studies, the initial host response is mediated by innate, nonspecific mechanisms, followed by the acquisition of virus-specific adaptive immunity.[219] The nonspecific response consists of mobilization of polymorphonuclear leukocytes and monocytes to the site of infection, release of interferon-γ and other cytokines, and activation of macrophages and natural killer cells. The innate response is followed by the production of antiviral antibodies that can be detected 2 to 12 weeks after infection occurs. HSV-specific antibodies mediate neutralization of virus, complement fixation, and cellular or complement cytotoxicity. Induction of specific cellular immunity is detected by measuring T-cell recognition of HSV proteins in proliferation and cytotoxicity assays and production of interleukin-2 and interferon-γ. Failure of virus-specific, cell-mediated immunity to develop, as may occur in neonates and children with genetic immunodeficiencies, immunocompromised children, and other high-risk populations, can be associated with life-threatening dissemination of HSV-1 or HSV-2. Disseminated HSV can infect and destroy cells in many organs (e.g., the lungs, liver, adrenals, and brain), with multiple-organ hyperinflammation leading to massive apoptosis, with catastrophic effects. It is likely that disseminated HSV in the neonate and in the older child and adult causes a systemic inflammatory response syndrome that often leads to a fatal outcome. One case report reported the sequential changes of hyperinflammation in a neonate with disseminated HSV disease. As the HSV DNA copies rose in the patient's serum, an increase in the biomarker concentrations of first high-mobility group box 1 and then cytochrome c was observed. Antiinflammatory interventions with prednisolone, high-dose immunoglobulin, blood exchange, and high-dose acyclovir were used for treatment, and the patient survived.[282] A small group of immune-seronegative individuals with HSV-specific T-cell responses has been described. None of these individuals had clinical symptoms of oral or genital HSV. All had exposure to HSV-2-positive sexual partners, but HSV was never isolated by culture or PCR assay from these exposed individuals, even after extensive sampling over a prolonged period.[316] Studies are in progress to determine whether genetic immunologic determinants of disease or mutations in HSV entry receptors alter susceptibility to HSV infection.[398]

Symptomatic HSV-1 and HSV-2 recurrences are less severe than are primary lesions in immunologically intact persons. In persons previously infected with one type of virus (e.g., HSV-1), new infections with the second type (e.g., HSV-2) more often are silent, or the symptoms are less severe than in a host who has never been infected with either virus. When reinfection with unrelated strains has been identified, symptoms also have been mild and, without molecular analysis of viral DNA, would be attributed to reactivation of endogenous virus.[65] The immune response to symptomatic reactivation is not associated with a significant increase in the production of antibody, although fourfold rises and reemergence of IgA and IgM antiviral antibody may occur. Natural killer cell activity and cytokine production increase. Relative defects in these and HSV-specific T-cell responses may predispose the individual to frequent or severe symptomatic recurrences. A cohort of patients with severe eczema, sinopulmonary infections, elevated serum IgE levels, eosinophilia, and cutaneous viral infection (including severe HSV) caused by DOCK8 deficiency has been described.[476] Patients who have diseases or are being treated with agents that reduce cell-mediated immunity, such as those undergoing antitumor chemotherapy or individuals with acquired immunodeficiency syndrome (AIDS), often have frequent HSV recurrences that are longer in duration and more severe, but dissemination rarely occurs.

Viral encephalitis is the most severe consequence of HSV infection in an otherwise healthy host. HSV-1 is the pathogen in almost all these cases, and the pathologic mechanism is thought to be ascending infection along neuronal pathways from the cranial nerve ganglia to the brain.[109] Encephalitis may accompany or develop after primary HSV infection, but it also occurs as a consequence of reactivation of latent virus. When the virus reaches brain parenchymal cells, it replicates efficiently and induces widespread hemorrhagic necrosis and vascular compromise. The neuroimmune response to infection contributes to brain inflammation and subsequent sequelae. Activated glial cells (astrocytes and microglia) respond to HSV infection with the production of cytokines and chemokines.[259] HSV encephalitis has been associated with an acute-phase elevation in β_2-microglobulin, neopterin, interleukin-6, and interferon-γ in CSF.[22,23] During convalescence, increased levels of soluble CD8, β-microglobulin, neopterin, and specific anti-HSV IgG have been detected. How these markers relate to the pathogenesis of disease has not been established.

Genetic heterogeneity involving a collection of inborn errors of immunity to HSV may predispose to herpes encephalitis. To date, signal transducer and activator of transcription-1 (STAT1), UNC93B, Toll-like receptor-3 (TLR3), and TNF receptor-associated factor-3 (TRAF3) deficiencies and nuclear factor-κB (NF-κB) essential modulator mutations have been found in a few children with herpes encephalitis.[21,70,477] Most recently, TIR-domain-containing adapter-inducing interferon-β (TRIF) deficiency has been reported in children with herpes encephalitis, demonstrating the importance of TRIF for the TLR3-dependent production of antiviral interferons in the CNS during primary infection with HSV-1 in childhood.[352] A recent genetic epidemiology survey suggests that childhood HSV encephalitis, although sporadic, may result from mendelian predisposition (from autosomal recessive susceptibility in particular), at least in some children.[1]

HSV may be transmitted to the neonate in utero either by a transplacental (congenital infection) or ascending route, at the time of birth (natal infection), or after birth (postnatal infection).[413] Congenital infection probably results from transplacental transmission of virus secondary to leukocyte-associated viremia in a mother with genital herpes, but no direct evidence supports this hypothesis. HSV-2 viremia has been documented in two women with primary genital herpes.[201] A report of 13 neonates with intrauterine HSV infection indicated that primary genital herpes was present during pregnancy in four mothers, recurrent disease was present in one, and no history of genital herpes was elicited in the remaining eight.[375] In the fetus, HSV appears to be transmitted directly from the placenta through the bloodstream to target organs. Because of the known tropism of HSV for the CNS, one is not surprised that most infants with congenital infection have evidence of brain involvement at birth.[375] Intrauterine infection also may occur by an ascending route from an infected maternal genital tract, and such transmission is supported by the development of clinical signs of HSV infection in the first 5 days of life.

The natal infection presumably is acquired secondary to aspiration of infected vaginal secretions into the nares, oropharyngeal cavity, conjunctivae, and upper respiratory tract of the infant. Other portals of entry for natal infection include the scalp, skin, and umbilical cord. In postnatal HSV infection, no evidence supports the genital tract as a source of virus. Most postnatally acquired infections appear to result from contact with saliva from persons with oral herpes or with virus carried on the hands of personnel. After natal or postnatal acquisition of HSV occurs, initial replication of the virus occurs at the portal of entry, which most often may be the conjunctivae or oral mucosa, with subsequent viremic dissemination to viscera. Involvement of the CNS occurs either from hematogenous spread to the brain in infants with disseminated disease, which results in meningoencephalitis and multiple areas of cortical hemorrhagic necrosis, or from retrograde axonal transport of the virus to the CNS from localized, superficial replication in the skin, eye, or mouth.

CLINICAL MANIFESTATIONS

Most HSV-1 and HSV-2 infections do not cause symptoms, but when infection is symptomatic the clinical manifestations usually are self-limited and not severe. If symptoms occur, the disease associated with primary infection tends to be much more extensive than are the minor, localized lesions at mucocutaneous junctions caused by viral reactivation.

Nonetheless, prospective studies document that new HSV infections can be as mild as symptomatic recurrences, and, as a result, definitive differentiation of primary from recurrent infection is not possible with clinical criteria.

Gingivostomatitis

Gingivostomatitis is the most common form of HSV-induced primary illness in children. A history of such symptoms has been reported in as few as 1% to as many as 31% of seropositive children, the higher percentage being from a study involving the Navajo Indians. It usually is seen in young children between 10 months and 3 years of age. In those younger than 10 months old, residual maternal antibody probably modifies or prevents the appearance of recognizable symptoms in association with primary HSV-1 infection. Although acute gingivostomatitis caused by HSV is a relatively infrequent occurrence, it is sufficiently common that most pediatricians are familiar with the condition and learn to distinguish this infection from herpangina.[302,334]

The illness begins with irritability and fever. Despite these systemic symptoms, HSV is not cultured from blood during this period[164]; however, investigators have detected HSV-1 DNA by PCR assay in whole blood or plasma early in the course of illness in approximately a third of young children with primary HSV-1 gingivostomatitis.[169] The infant usually refuses to eat and may refuse fluids. Thereafter, vesicular lesions appear around and on the lips, along the gingiva, on the anterior tongue, and on the anterior (hard) portion of the palate (Figs. 158.1 and 158.2).

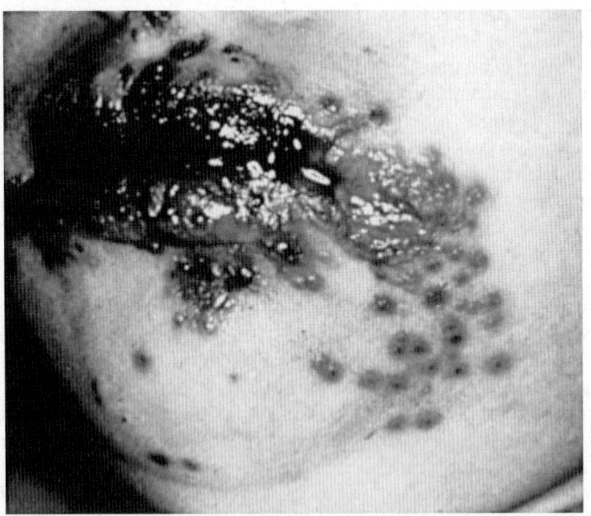

FIG. 158.1 Primary herpes simplex virus gingivostomatitis in a normal toddler: ulcerative-vesicular stage. (Courtesy Dr. Theodore Rosen, Department of Dermatology, Baylor College of Medicine, Houston.)

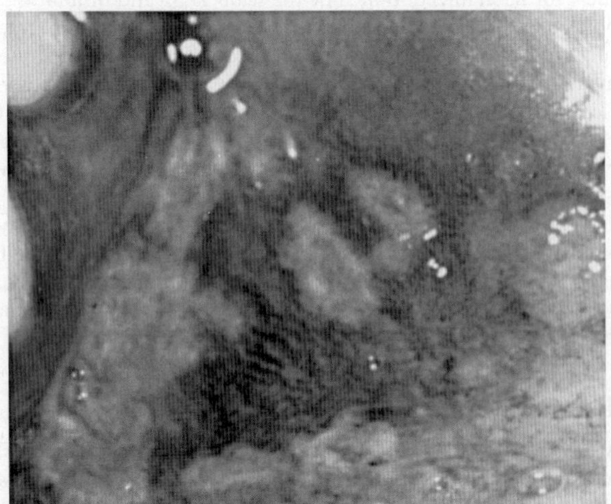

FIG. 158.2 Primary herpes simplex virus gingivostomatitis with ulcers of the oral mucosa in a 6-year-old child.

The vesicles break down rapidly, and, when seen, lesions usually appear as 1- to 3-mm shallow gray ulcers on an erythematous base. The gums are erythematous, mildly swollen, and ulcerated. They may appear friable and bleed on contact. The child experiences extreme discomfort, will not eat, and, if fluids are refused as well, may require hospitalization to ensure that adequate hydration is maintained. The risk for dehydration is compounded by the fever that generally accompanies this syndrome. Vesicles often extend around the lips and chin or down the neck in an immunologically intact child. The child frequently has foul-smelling breath (fetor oris). The lesions bleed easily and may become covered with a black crust. The cervical and submental nodes usually are swollen and tender. The clinical signs continue to evolve for 4 to 5 days, and the process of resolution requires at least an additional week. In an analysis of the natural history of HSV gingivostomatitis in 36 children, oral lesions persisted for an average of 12 days, most children had extraoral lesions, fever lasted for 2 to 6 days, and difficulty taking liquids was noted for 4 to 10 days. The duration of viral shedding was 7 days (range, 2 to 12 days).[7] Herpetic epiglottitis[47] and acute otitis media[89] and severe hepatitis[88] are unusual complications. In addition, transverse myelitis and severe acute disseminated encephalomyelitis have occurred after herpetic gingivostomatitis.[355]

HSV gingivostomatitis is differentiated from herpangina, a manifestation of enteroviral infection, by the location of ulcers in the anterior portion of the oropharynx. Herpangina generally causes posterior pharyngeal ulcers. In addition, unlike HSV infection, herpangina often has a more acute onset, a shorter duration, and seasonal occurrence.[302] Whereas enterovirus-associated hand, foot, and mouth disease can manifest as oral ulcers and a vesicular eruption on the distal portions of extremities, its bilateral distribution should differentiate it from HSV gingivostomatitis and concurrent HSV autoinoculation of a digit. Severe Stevens-Johnson syndrome (erythema multiforme) may mimic HSV infection, but the generalized macular rash accompanied by bull's-eye lesions is characteristic of erythema multiforme. Rarely, recurrent HSV infection can be associated with erythema multiforme (see later discussion). Impetigo may be confused with the lesions of HSV infection, and misdiagnosis is reinforced because colonization of skin by *Staphylococcus aureus* may be identified in bacterial cultures and be considered causative.

Parents and caregivers are familiar with "cold sores" or "fever blisters" but may not know that these lesions are caused by HSV. Because HSV infection may be thought of as a sexually transmitted disease, the physician is advised to anticipate confusion and anxiety when making the diagnosis of HSV oral infection and to address these concerns by explaining the normal mode of acquisition of oral HSV infection by young children.

Pharyngitis, Tonsillitis, Epiglottitis, Supraglottitis, Laryngotracheitis

In adolescents, primary HSV-1 infection can be seen initially as ulcerative, exudative tonsillopharyngitis.[270] Characteristic findings are shallow tonsillar ulcers with a gray exudate. HSV infection of the tonsils may be HSV type 1 or 2 and must be differentiated from streptococcal and Epstein-Barr virus infection and rarely from diphtheria, acute human immunodeficiency virus (HIV) infection, and tularemia-induced pharyngitis. In one study of college students of a higher socioeconomic level, HSV was the most common etiologic agent of acute pharyngitis (24%).[149] Another study of 613 college students with upper respiratory tract complaints documented an incidence of 5.7% with positive HSV cultures. Twelve of the 35 students with positive cultures had vesicular lesions on their lips, throat, or gums, and 29 of the 35 had a primary diagnosis of pharyngitis that was indistinguishable from other causes of pharyngitis.[270] In some cases, acute pharyngitis is caused by HSV-2; the symptoms and clinical course appear to be similar to HSV-1, but also may be severe, and viral cultures or PCR tests are required to identify the type of infecting virus.[336]

Acute, prolonged, atypical laryngotracheitis or herpetic croup, often nonresponsive to steroids, also may be caused by HSV types 1 or 2, in both normal and immunocompromised patients of all ages.[86] The diagnosis can be made by laryngoscopy with appropriate viral HSV culture and PCR studies and tissue immunohistochemistry for HSV antigens.

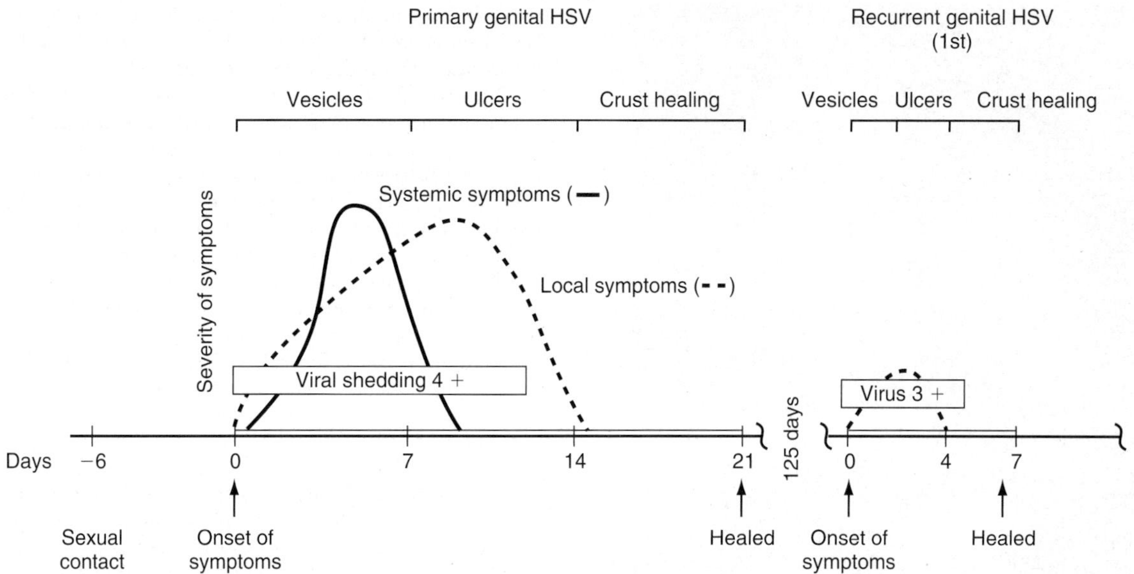

FIG. 158.3 Course of primary and recurrent herpes simplex virus *(HSV)* genital infection. The days illustrated are for average cases.

Epiglottitis, now a relatively rare disease in children, may rarely be caused by HSV in neonates, as well as older children, and should be included in the differential diagnosis of causes of epiglottitis, in addition to the usual *Haemophilus influenzae* and *Staphylococcus aureus* bacterial causes.[263]

Vulvovaginitis, Genital Herpes Infections

Primary herpetic vulvovaginitis occurs rarely in infants and children. HSV-1 may cause this clinical syndrome, perhaps if inadvertently introduced when the genital area is touched by a caregiver with HSV on the hands. Progression of the infection may be limited to a few lesions, or it may resemble symptomatic primary genital herpes caused by HSV-2. Obtaining material for culture to identify the type of infecting virus is important because HSV-1 infection is less likely to recur and HSV-2 infection may reflect sexual abuse of the child. Genital HSV infection in young children warrants a careful and sensitive appraisal of the circumstances that possibly led to the infection. Children infected with HSV-2 in the neonatal period have had genital lesions later in childhood.

Pediatricians are likely to encounter genital herpes in their adolescent patients.[190] Reports on the incidence of genital herpes in which data are provided for subgroups of children and adolescents are limited, but a rate of three per 100,000 in the 10- to 14-year-old age group and 76 per 100,000 in the 15- to 19-year-old age group was reported in a Minnesota study of a predominantly white, middle-class population of northern European ethnicity.[90] Older NHANES studies reported the prevalence in 12- to 19-year-old subjects to be 5.6%.[139] Recent NHANES data (2005 to 2008) show a decrease in HSV-2 seroprevalence in this age group, most recently to 1.4% in 14- to 19-year olds.[472] In one report of 379 adolescents aged 14 to 19 years who were treated at a sexually transmitted disease or urban community clinic, 12% had HSV-2 antibodies and only 22% of these patients had a history of genital herpes. HSV-2 seropositivity correlated with black race or female gender but not with condom use, the number of sexual partners in the previous 2 months, or a previous history of a sexually transmitted disease, thus indicating that prevalence was related to demographic rather than behavioral variables.[399]

Prospective studies have documented that many infections are subclinical and that new genital HSV-2 infections have a wide range of manifestations.[242,273] Variation is common with respect to the extent and severity of lesions; whether the lesions are bilateral or localized; the presence or absence of systemic symptoms such as malaise, myalgia, headache, and fever; dysuria; and regional lymphadenopathy. Symptoms can be mild enough to suggest recurrent infection or may be those of severe, "classic" primary genital herpes. In such cases in adults, local genital symptoms include severe pain (in 95% of men and 99% of women), itching, dysuria (44% of men and 83% of women), vaginal or urethral discharge, and tender inguinal adenopathy (80%). The lesions begin as vesicles or pustules and progress to wet ulcers and then to healing ulcers with or without crusts (Figs. 158.3 to 158.5). Crusting usually occurs only on squamous epithelium. Lesions tend to last for 2 to 3 weeks (mean, 19 days) before complete healing occurs. They may spread in a wavelike fashion from the initial site to the thighs, buttocks,

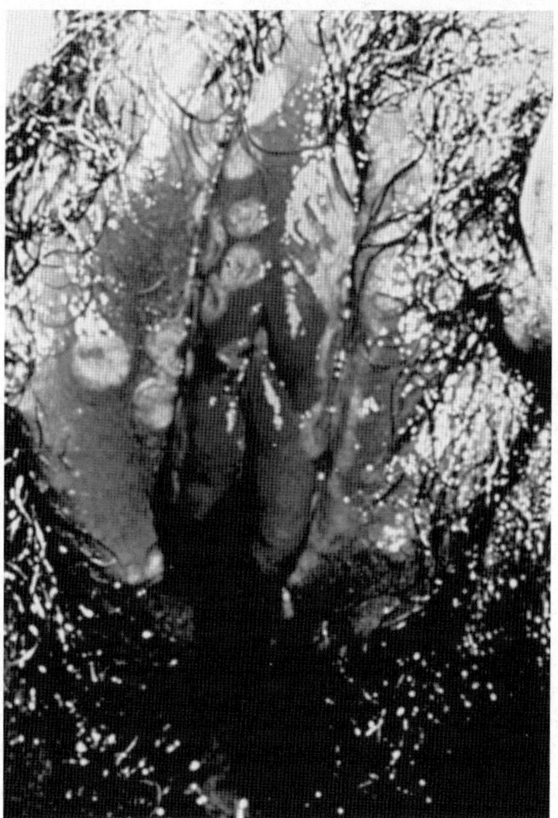

FIG. 158.4 Primary genital herpes in a female. (Courtesy Dr. Theodore Rosen, Department of Dermatology, Baylor College of Medicine, Houston.)

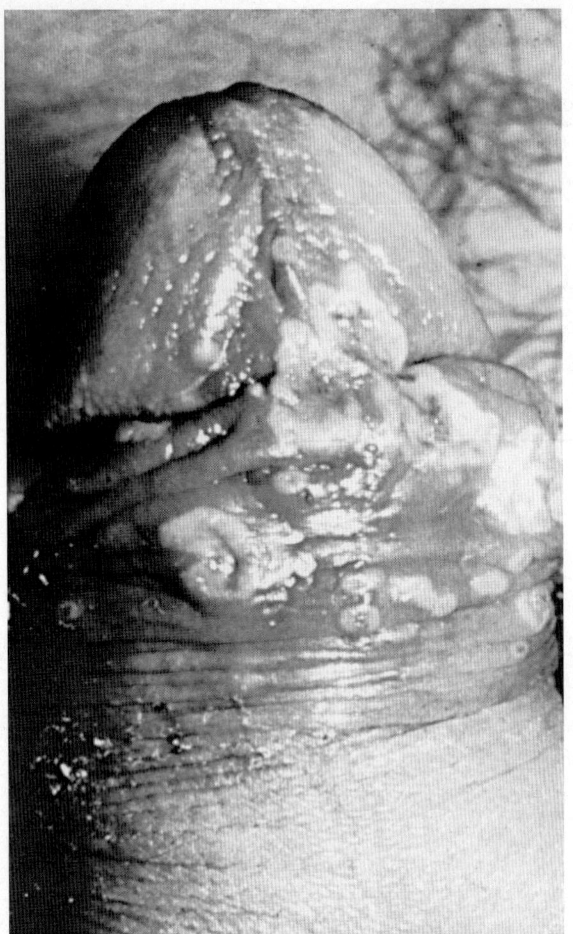

FIG. 158.5 Primary genital HSV infection in a male. (Courtesy Dr. Theodore Rosen, Department of Dermatology, Baylor College of Medicine, Houston.)

and urethra. Virus shedding generally persists for 1 to 2 weeks or longer. Some primary infections are associated with atypical lesions (e.g., fissures, furuncles, excoriations), and extragenital lesions, typically on the buttocks, may be observed.[40,227]

When evaluating potential primary genital herpes in a sexually active adolescent, the history may reveal recent contact with a partner who is known to have recurrent genital herpes. When exposure can be documented, the incubation period is estimated to be 2 to 14 days. However, most episodes will not be associated with a known exposure. It is important to recognize that as many as two thirds of first-reported episodes of symptomatic genital herpes actually are caused by reactivation. The exposure may have occurred months or years before the signs of HSV-2 infection appear. In some adult series, 50% to 60% of persons without a history of HSV infection can identify symptoms consistent with previous infection after receiving education about the typical signs, but many have not had any previous episodes.[240] HSV-1 accounts for 5% to 25% of primary genital HSV infections in the United States. Up to 50% of cases diagnosed in other geographic areas, such as England and Japan, are caused by HSV-1. Indications are that HSV-1 is becoming a more common primary genital isolate in the United States. In recent years, HSV-1 has been isolated from genital cultures more often than HSV-2 has in some populations.[331] Patients with primary HSV-1 genital infection occasionally exhibit lesions elsewhere (25%), typically on the hands and face.[40]

Primary genital HSV-2 infections may be associated with viral meningitis. It also may be associated with recurrent aseptic lymphocytic meningitis, or Mollaret meningitis.[286,317] This complication is manifested as fever, stiff neck, headache, and photophobia with a CSF lymphocytic cellular response and usually a normal glucose level.[180,411] HSV-2 can be isolated in cell culture or detected by PCR from CSF obtained in the early phase of the illness. HSV-2-associated meningitis differs from HSV-1 encephalitis in that it is almost always mild, self-limited, and not associated with neurologic sequelae.

Other complications of primary HSV genital infection include sacral autonomic nervous dysfunction, which is manifested as poor rectal sphincter tone, constipation, sacral anesthesia, urinary retention, or impotence. Extragenital lesions may be present. These are more frequent in women and occur on the buttocks, groin, thighs, or, less commonly, the fingers or conjunctiva, generally in the second week of disease. In addition, secondary yeast infections in women, and pharyngitis, which usually is associated with fever, malaise, myalgia, headache, tender anterior cervical adenopathy, and a mildly erythematous to diffusely ulcerative or exudative posterior pharyngitis may be seen. Most patients have throat cultures positive for HSV. HSV has been associated uncommonly with acute salpingitis[249] and inguinal lymphadenitis.[407] Transmission to the fetus or neonate is an important and very serious complication of primary or recurrent genital herpes in women of child-bearing age.

Of critical importance is the association of previous HSV infection with an increased incidence of HIV infection.[388] Investigators have considered the possibility that the risk for infection with HIV is enhanced by mucosal ulcers or that the increase in local CD4$^+$ lymphocytes resulting from HSV infection offers a greater number of target cells for HIV attachment and entry. Conversely, individuals with HIV infection reactivate HSV frequently and also have HIV present in mucosal ulcers.[437] A study from Kenya showed that HSV shedding was associated with significantly higher vaginal and cervical HIV shedding, even after controlling for plasma HIV load and CD4$^+$ count.[28] Although all patients with HSV-2 genital infection appear to be at higher risk for acquiring HIV infection, those with recent HSV-2 seroconversion appear to be more susceptible.[329,415] This finding has been confirmed in other populations.[206]

Genital herpes creates significant psychological difficulties for many patients. Whereas many people cope well with the illness and the likelihood of recurrent disease, a syndrome of profound depression, poor self-esteem, complete abstention from sexual activities, and general withdrawal develops in some. This reaction, or "leper syndrome," must be anticipated and discussed in a sensitive and caring manner. Information about the high prevalence of these infections in the population may be helpful, with emphasis placed on the fact that most infected people do not realize that they are infected and shed the virus intermittently, just like those who have had symptoms, as well as effective treatment options.

Primary Herpetic Skin Infections

Mucocutaneous junction areas are common sites of HSV infection, and damaged skin often provides a portal of entry for HSV. Vesicular lesions spread throughout the affected skin and usually crust and resolve in approximately 1 week. The illness accompanying eczema herpeticum can be severe (Fig. 158.6) and even fatal, and this condition is often referred to as Kaposi varicelliform eruption. Predisposing skin conditions such as epidermolysis bullosa also may predispose infants and children to severe skin super infections with HSV and Kaposi varicelliform eruption.[186] However, most cases of uncomplicated eczema herpeticum in otherwise healthy children resolve and leave no sequelae. Increased use of topical calcineurin inhibitors has raised concern regarding possible immune suppression and an increase in cases of eczema herpeticum. One study showed the incidence density of herpesvirus skin infections to be similar in infants who received 1% pimecrolimus cream and those who received the vehicle without active drug.[304] However, of those children characterized as having eczema herpeticum (more extensive skin involvement), all infants were in the group receiving 1% pimecrolimus cream. Further studies are needed to determine the magnitude of risk, if any, of the use of topical calcineurin inhibitors in the development of eczema herpeticum. Current recommendations include discontinuing topical calcineurin inhibitor therapy and beginning appropriate antiviral therapy expeditiously if eczema herpeticum develops.[304] Topical steroids may also predispose to eczema herpeticum.

Widespread herpetic lesions may occur in skin altered by thermal or chemical burns. In this situation, a secondary fever may occur, usually 1 week to several weeks after the initial insult. Careful inspection of

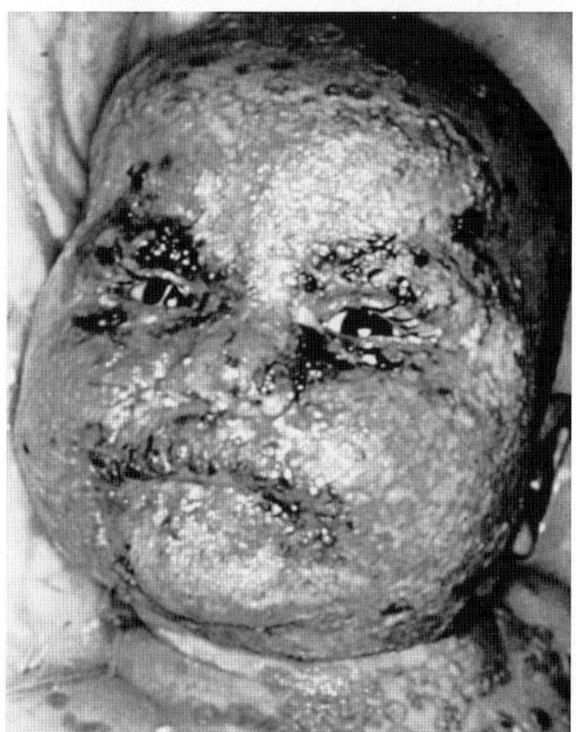

FIG. 158.6 Extensive herpes simplex virus infection in an infant with atopic eczema (Kaposi varicelliform eruption). (Courtesy Dr. Theodore Rosen, Department of Dermatology, Baylor College of Medicine, Houston.)

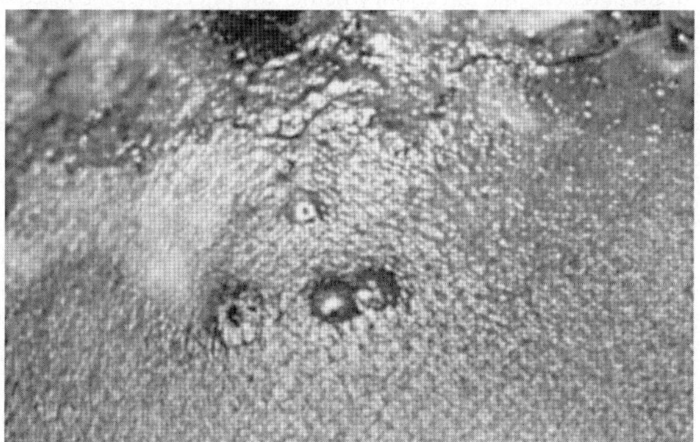

FIG. 158.7 Secondary herpes simplex virus infection at a burn site in a 2-year-old child. Note the vesicles at the border of the burn.

the burn site or adjacent normal tissue may reveal vesicles (Fig. 158.7) or nonspecific ulcerative lesions. Without therapy, these patients may die of disseminated HSV infection.[140] A similar syndrome occurs rarely in children after they have incurred simple skin abrasions (Fig. 158.8). Herpetic recurrences may follow in these cases, but recurrences are localized to the area of skin that was affected initially. HSV can even cause minor or severe infection at the site of common diaper rash.[195]

Herpetic whitlow is a painful, erythematous, swollen lesion that occurs on the terminal phalanx, sometimes associated with a damaged cuticle.[36,134,148,337] The fingers (69%) and thumb (21%) are involved most frequently.[148] Less commonly, the palm may be the site of inoculation and major involvement.[359] The digit is swollen, and the painful white swelling appears to be filled with pus but, when opened for drainage, is found to contain little fluid and no purulent material. The white appearance is caused by the presence of necrotic epithelial cells. Occasionally, the whitlow, which may persist for 7 to 10 days, is accompanied initially by a few vesicles that may give a clue to the etiologic agent of the primary infection. Less commonly, the whitlow is associated with fever, lymphadenopathy, and lymphangitis.[353]

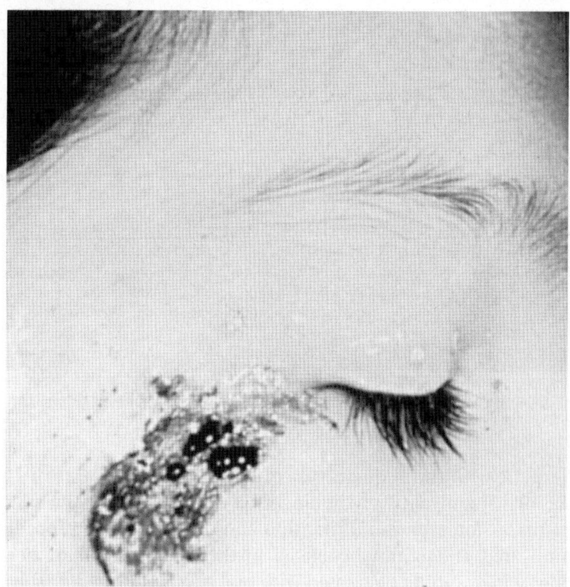

FIG. 158.8 Facial herpes simplex virus infection in a young girl after a mild abrasion. (Courtesy Dr. Johnie Frazier, Department of Pediatrics, University of Texas Medical School, Houston.)

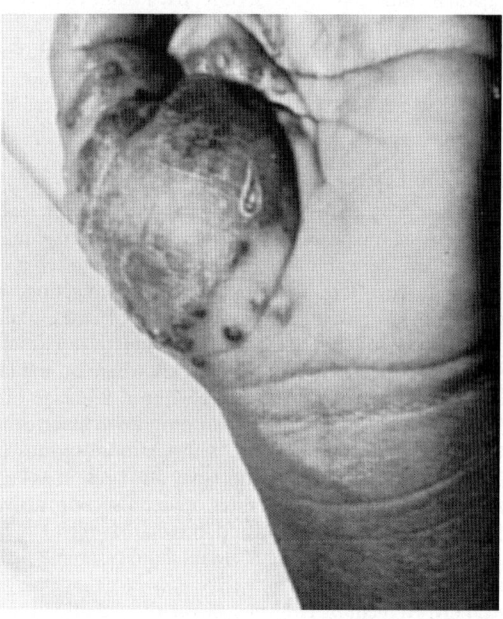

FIG. 158.9 Extensive herpetic whitlow in a toddler with oral herpes simplex virus infection.

Whitlow is seen in four typical situations.[134] Most commonly, infants with primary herpetic gingivostomatitis autoinoculate their fingers (Fig. 158.9). At times, whitlow is encountered in infants without obvious oral disease, and sometimes it may be caused by adults kissing their children's fingers. In these settings, the viral isolate almost always is HSV-1.[36,148] In sexually active patients, the whitlow more commonly is a manifestation of concurrent genital disease, which should be sought by appropriate history and physical examination.[150] These infections are caused most frequently by HSV-2. In the fourth setting, persons such as dentists, respiratory therapists, nurses, and pediatricians who examine oral cavities or handle secretion-contaminated material without wearing gloves are at risk for acquiring herpetic whitlow (Fig. 158.10).[134] In addition, health care–associated transmission of HSV to other patients, especially in intensive care settings, may occur if careful attention to use of gloves and other personal protective equipment is not practiced.[3]

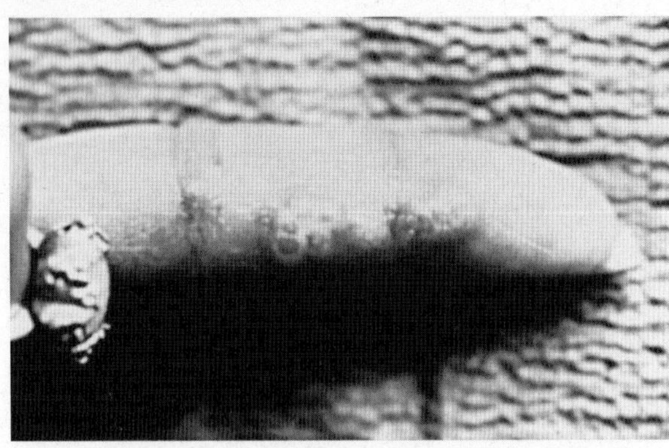

FIG. 158.10 Recurrent herpetic whitlow in a pediatrician.

Herpetic whitlow frequently is confused with bacterial felon, paronychia, or osteomyelitis of the fingertip. Such confusion may lead to the incorrect intervention of incision and drainage. This procedure is not indicated and is not beneficial in the management of herpetic whitlow, which should be treated with oral acyclovir. Needle aspiration and bacterial and viral cultures provide the diagnosis of whitlow, and initiation of antiviral therapy can be based on clinical signs.

In several sports, cutaneous (especially facial) HSV infection is a hazard, particularly in sports with close physical contact such as wrestling (herpes gladiatorum) and rugby (scrum pox, a name derived from the lineup of rugby players, the "scrum" or "scrummage").[38,79,370,372,451] Frequently, the initial lesions are misdiagnosed as impetigo. HSV infection develops in approximately 3% of wrestlers in high school, typically on the head and neck but also on the extremities and trunk and in the eyes.[79]

Infection of the Eye

Ocular herpes occurs as a result of primary infection or reactivation of virus in the trigeminal ganglion. Primary infection may manifest as blepharitis or follicular conjunctivitis. The symptoms often are accompanied by preauricular lymphadenopathy, corneal injection, watering, discharge, itching, lid swelling, and, in a third of cases, malaise and fever. If the infection is restricted to the conjunctivae (which can be accompanied by vesicular herpetic lesions elsewhere on the face or in the nose or mouth), it usually resolves without sequelae or specific features. Herpetic infection of the eye may progress to involve the cornea and progress to keratoconjunctivitis, with far more serious potential consequences. Neonatal HSV infection may also present as keratoconjunctivitis and has been reported after cesarean section delivery over intact chorioamniotic membranes and in twin deliveries.[145,442] For this reason, an ophthalmologic consultant always should examine and evaluate these cases.

Corneal involvement by HSV may be manifested initially as minute vesicles at the corneal margin. Progression of the corneal infection (best seen with the use of topical fluorescein dye) is marked by the appearance of branching lesions (a dendritic pattern) or the less diagnostic irregular (ameboid or geographic) ulcer.[37,106] The child complains of severe photophobia often accompanied by blurred vision, chemosis, and lacrimation. Primary eye infection may include stromal involvement, uveitis, and, rarely, retinitis.[305] Retinitis is manifested as multiple whitish yellow, punctate retinal lesions. Spontaneous healing, which generally requires 2 to 3 weeks, can be speeded by the application of topical antiviral therapy. Corticosteroids are contraindicated. The risk for visual impairment caused by direct viral damage, immunopathologic reactions, or both is enhanced greatly with recurrences. With each bout of infection, the corneal ulcers become more extensive and can result in scarring and impairment of sight. Herpetic infection of the eye recurs in approximately 32% of patients who have primary symptomatic infection and occurs more commonly in younger patients.[467] Recurrences may be manifested as blepharitis, follicular conjunctivitis with or without lid lesions, or ulcers and keratitis, which more often are accompanied by ulcerations deeper into the corneal stroma (diskiform or necrotizing keratitis) with resultant extensive scarring, irregular astigmatism, and even corneal perforation.[467] Children with dendritic ulcers have a better prognosis for good vision than do those with geographic or diskiform keratitis.[37]

Rarely, HSV eye infection results in acute retinal necrosis. HSV-2 is the most common cause of acute retinal necrosis identified in childhood. Most affected children have a history of congenital or perinatal herpes infection.[239] Acute retinal necrosis may also be a late sequela of HSV-1 encephalitis.[105] Many patients have preexisting chorioretinal scars. Reactivation is triggered by periocular trauma or occurs with immunosuppression, such as during treatment with systemic corticosteroids.[417] Symptoms include eye irritation and photophobia.

Very infrequently, an oculoglandular syndrome of conjunctivitis and preauricular adenopathy may be caused by HSV infection.[69]

Infections of the Central Nervous System

HSV is the most common identifiable cause of serious or life-threatening sporadic, endemic encephalitis.[252] It accounts for 2% to 5% of all cases of encephalitis in the United States and for as many as 20% of all cases with an etiologic diagnosis (60–70% of cases of encephalitis have no established cause).[325] With the advent of immunization for measles, mumps, rubella, and varicella, the relative incidence of HSV in cases of encephalitis has increased, although absolute numbers remain stable in children.[224,252,325] The case-fatality rate associated with untreated HSV encephalitis is approximately 70%,[464] and survivors generally have severe and permanent neurologic disability. Both HSV-1 and HSV-2 have been implicated in the etiology of CNS infection by HSV, but typical HSV encephalitis in patients outside the neonatal age range is caused by HSV-1.[1,102,334,358] Spread of HSV-1 to the CNS seems to proceed either via neurogenic pathways or by hematogenous dissemination, or perhaps through the cribriform plate from infected nasopharyngeal mucosa during primary infection. Recurrent infection probably results from spread via sensory neurons. HSV-2 meningitis is not associated with brain parenchymal infection; whether the infection is a consequence of hematogenous delivery or spread along neuronal pathways is not known.

Although HSV encephalitis may involve virtually any area of the brain, or even the entire brain and spinal cord, this infection has a striking tendency to involve the orbital region of the frontal lobes and, with particular frequency, portions of the temporal lobes. The predilection of HSV to involve regions of the brain governing olfaction suggests that a pathogenetic pathway proceeds from the nasal-respiratory mucosa via the olfactory bulbs and along the subsequent tracts into the brain.[198] Other researchers have suggested that reactivated virus travels from the trigeminal ganglia via fifth nerve fibers to the meninges of the anterior and middle fossae.[109,110] HSV brain stem encephalitis also occurs and may be associated with neuroophthalmologic findings and cranial nerve deficits.[309] Studies in children involving diagnosis by PCR assay and magnetic resonance imaging (MRI) have defined cases with more diffuse cerebral involvement.[334,360,430]

HSV encephalitis must be differentiated from primary or recurrent HSV meningitis (Mollaret meningitis), which usually is caused by HSV-2 and is a complication of primary genital or oropharyngeal infection. In HSV meningitis, symptoms and signs of meningitis, including headache, photophobia, and stiff neck, appear before or shortly after genital or oropharyngeal lesions are noted. The signs are similar to those of other acute viral meningitides such as enteroviral meningitis. This syndrome may occur in children and adolescents as well as in adults.[119] HSV-2 meningitis is reported in the absence of lesions[362] and rarely in neonates.[361] Seizures and focal CNS findings generally are absent. Examination of CSF reveals lymphocytosis (with 300 to 2600 white blood cells) and may demonstrate low glucose levels. In cases of HSV meningitis, in contrast to HSV encephalitis, virus is often cultured from CSF,[16,18,102,180] and HSV PCR assay also is diagnostic.[362] Recovery usually is complete without specific therapy, but with the availability of effective antiviral agents, HSV meningitis should be treated with acyclovir. HSV meningitis may reappear with or without obvious genital recurrences. Studies using PCR DNA detection analysis have shown that HSV is the major agent responsible for benign recurrent lymphocytic meningitis.[408] These adult patients had three to nine attacks of recurrent lymphocytic meningitis, with 48 to 1600 cells/L, normal glucose, and

TABLE 158.1 **Historical and Clinical Findings in Herpes Simplex Virus Encephalitis**

Historical Finding	Initial Clinical Finding (%)
Alteration of consciousness	97
Memory loss	92
Personality changes	85
Fever	81
Dysphasia	76
Persistent seizures	71
Headache	67
Autonomic dysfunction	60
Personality change	46
Ataxia	40
Seizures	38
Focal	28
Generalized	10
Vomiting	33
Cranial nerve defects	32
Hemiparesis	24
Visual field loss	14
Papilledema	14

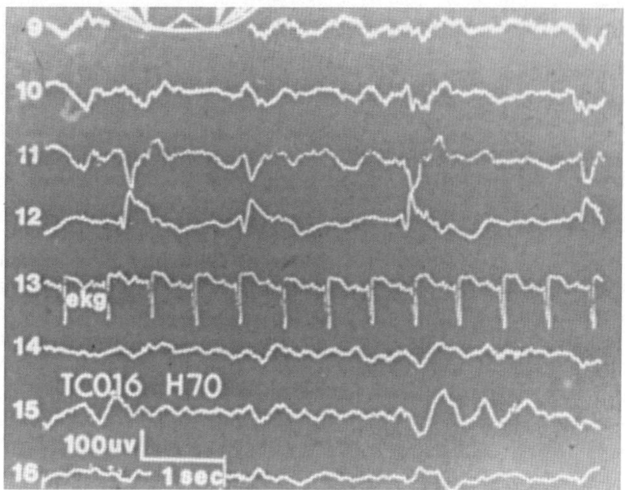

FIG. 158.11 Electroencephalogram in a 9-month-old infant with herpes simplex virus encephalitis. Note the paroxysmal discharges, especially in lead 12.

protein concentrations of 41 to 240 mg/dL in CSF. PCR analysis detected HSV-2 and, less commonly, HSV-1. Acute viral meningitis caused by reactivation of HSV-1 also has been described in a preadolescent child.[96]

HSV encephalitis is a highly lethal disease caused by HSV-1 in 93% to 96% of cases.[25,285,334,452,456] It may be a result of primary (30%) or recurrent (70%) infection.[285,334] Although no specific data exist, researchers have suggested that HSV encephalitis is more likely to be associated with primary infection in younger persons because new infections occur more commonly in this age group. One report suggests that primary infection is more likely to be associated with fatal encephalitis. Of 113 cases of biopsy-documented HSV encephalitis, 31% occurred in patients younger than 20 years, and 6% to 10% of patients were between 6 months and 10 years of age.[374,375] Unlike most other common forms of viral meningoencephalitis such as enterovirus or arbovirus infection, HSV encephalitis is not seasonal. It is an acute illness characterized by fever, headache, malaise, irritability, and nonspecific symptoms lasting 1 to 7 days, with progression to the signs and symptoms of CNS involvement in 3 to 7 days and, finally, to coma and death (Table 158.1). A biphasic illness consisting of initial improvement followed by worsening may occur. The signs of HSV encephalitis resemble those of other viral encephalitides, with initial fever and altered behavior.[172] Meningeal signs are uncommon findings. No correlation exists between isolation of HSV from sites extrinsic to the CNS (e.g., the oropharynx or genital tract) and the diagnosis of HSV encephalitis.[285,453] Thus, the presence of oral or genital lesions is of no help in establishing or excluding the diagnosis of HSV encephalitis. Nonetheless, if a patient has HSV encephalitis, identical viruses have been isolated from the brain and oral secretions.[460] Herpes simplex encephalitis has also been reported as a rare complication of neurosurgical procedures, craniotomy, and stereotactic radiotherapy.[193]

The CSF in herpes encephalitis generally reveals pleocytosis, usually (80% of the time) more than 50 white blood cells/mm^3, with as many as 2000 white blood cells/mm^3 in some cases. In 90% of cases, more than 60% of the cells are lymphocytes. Early in the course of infection, neutrophils may predominate and there will be few or no red cells. In advanced cases, red blood cells, reflecting the hemorrhagic necrosis, may be seen in the CSF. Between 5% and 25% of patients have hypoglycorrhachia, and 80% to 88% have elevated protein levels in CSF (median, 80 mg/dL), which rise to striking levels as the disease progresses if untreated. Two to 3% of patients with early HSV encephalitis have normal CSF.[225,285] Repeat analysis of CSF usually reveals abnormalities consistent with encephalitis. HSV is rarely cultured in cell culture from lumbar CSF in patients outside the neonatal age range and rarely has been grown from ventricular fluid.[141] Thus, whereas CSF examination is helpful, it is not at all diagnostic of HSV encephalitis. When the CSF of patients with HSV encephalitis is compared with that of patients undergoing biopsy for suspected HSV but with another resultant diagnosis, no differentiating characteristics of CSF are found that could allow one to predict HSV infection accurately. HSV DNA can be detected by the use of PCR assay of the CSF of patients who have HSV encephalitis and is currently the diagnostic test of choice.[9,24,115,120,236,339,418]

Neurodiagnostic tests may support the diagnosis of herpes encephalitis. One useful test for early changes associated with herpes encephalitis is the electroencephalogram (EEG) (Fig. 158.11).[52] A "typical" pattern of unilateral or bilateral (poor prognosis) periodic focal spikes against a background of slow (flattened) activity (paroxysmal lateral epileptiform discharges [PLEDs]) has been associated with HSV encephalitis.[209] These findings are suggestive but not pathognomonic. Other findings include large-amplitude, irregular slow activity, sharp waves, and variable spikes. In 80% to 90% of patients, the EEG is not only abnormal but also localizing. In many cases in the pediatric and adult age groups, the EEG may be one of the earliest localizing laboratory tests.[117,156,223] Less commonly, the results of a radionuclide or computed tomographic (CT) scan are abnormal and localizing (50–60% of cases).[205,250]

CT results may be characteristic late in the illness and consist of low-density, contrast-enhanced lesions in the temporal area, mass effect, edema, and hemorrhage (Fig. 158.12); early in the illness, when establishing the diagnosis is critical, CT results more often are unremarkable.[156,223,279] Abnormal CT results are a poor prognostic factor.[279]

MRI findings are more likely to be abnormal at initial evaluation for HSV encephalitis because of its high sensitivity to changes in brain water content[367] (Fig. 158.13), and MRI is more sensitive than is CT for detection of HSV encephalitis.[114,319] Findings include hyperintensity of the temporal and brain stem areas on T2-weighted MR images, and imaging results may be normal if performed in the early stages of the disease.[4,209]

Focal abnormalities in HSV encephalitis are significantly more likely to be observed on EEG, CT, or MRI than in other illnesses confused with it. All these findings are biased by the current concept of HSV encephalitis as a focal encephalitis, with very few biopsy data available on the etiology of nonfocal encephalitis. Studies using EEG, MRI, and PCR technology have identified cases with multifocal brain involvement.[469,250,360]

Clinical and laboratory evaluations of patients with suspected HSV encephalitis are valuable only for increasing the index of suspicion, not for confirming the diagnosis. In one series of 24 children with HSV encephalitis diagnosed by PCR assay and compared with 38 children in whom HSV encephalitis was excluded by PCR, no significant differences were found in clinical manifestations at onset or in CSF cell counts, protein, or glucose.[189] However, more children with HSV encephalitis had localizing findings detected by CT (75% vs. 31%), whereas 36% of those without HSV encephalitis had EEG abnormalities as opposed to no EEG abnormalities detected in those with HSV encephalitis.

The differential diagnosis of HSV encephalitis is large (Box 158.1). Especially in the pediatric age range, the ability to discriminate HSV encephalitis from other etiologic agents mimicking it is poor (50% in the national collaborative series in 71 patients <20 years and 42% in a smaller series of 12 patients <12 years).[223] Confirmation of the specific diagnosis of HSV encephalitis remains essential, both to provide optimal aggressive therapy for that condition and, of equal importance, to achieve a diagnosis for the 50% to 60% of patients without HSV infection, roughly 16% of whom would benefit from other specific therapies.[117,223,279,453] In most cases, the diagnosis can be established by PCR analysis of CSF.[9,24,159,236,339,360,362,423] Large studies show PCR analysis to be 98% sensitive and 94% specific when compared with brain biopsy.[159,236]

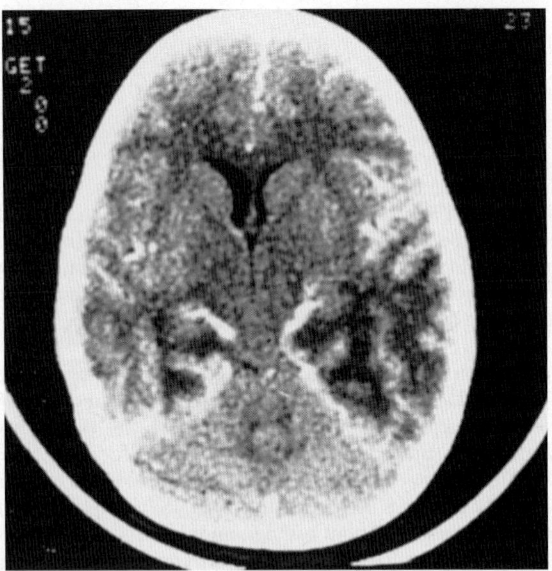

FIG. 158.12 Computed tomographic scan 1 week after the onset of herpes simplex virus encephalitis in a 6-year-old child. Note the bilateral temporal low-density areas with dye enhancement and the greater mass effect on the patient's left side compared with the right side.

PCR analysis may yield positive results by 1 day after the onset of symptoms.[159] However, a negative PCR result obtained soon after the onset of symptoms does not exclude the diagnosis of HSV encephalitis. In two small series of patients, repeat testing of CSF 4 to 7 days after an initial negative HSV PCR assay showed positive PCR results.[447] HSV DNA persists in most specimens for a week or more, even after antiviral therapy.[418,452] PCR primers must be chosen to detect HSV-2, as well as HSV-1, because 4% to 6% of HSV encephalitis cases may be caused by HSV-2.[25]

If PCR results are negative in a patient who has symptoms and signs of HSV encephalitis, repeat CSF HSV PCR analysis should be performed. If this is still negative, and the patient's condition is progressively worsening, brain biopsy may be contemplated, in addition to other diagnostic tests on CSF. A negative HSV PCR on the CSF does not exclude the diagnosis of HSV encephalitis. In the national collaborative study of 432 biopsies, six complications occurred after brain biopsy (hemorrhage in three patients and poorly controlled brain edema in three, for a 1.4% complication rate).[456] Roughly 2% to 3% of brain biopsies yielded false-negative results, usually because of biopsy of the wrong site.[456] Decision analysis suggests that performing a biopsy is especially critical in a patient with low CSF glucose levels.[356]

Quantitative PCR analysis may have value as a prognostic tool and as a method of assessing the response to antiviral therapy in patients with HSV encephalitis.[15,452] In 16 patients, those with high copy numbers of HSV DNA in CSF tended to have abnormal CT scans, be older, and exhibit more severe sequelae. HSV DNA levels were found to decrease during acyclovir therapy in seven patients; the exception was a patient whose copy numbers increased and who subsequently had a fatal infection.

A less acute form of HSV encephalitis, with indolent presentation, in immunocompromised patients has been reported. Also less commonly, HSV has been implicated in brain stem encephalitis.[129]

Relapse occurs in approximately 5% of treated patients.[223] Choreoathetosis may be an initial sign of relapse.[230,441] Reports of a postherpetic encephalomyelitis caused by a probable autoimmune or demyelinating etiologic factor have appeared[2,13,220]; moreover, virus-positive recurrence of HSV encephalitis has been described months after patients have undergone apparently successful therapy.[118] HSV encephalitis may recur, after successful treatment and suppression, in neonates, as well as in children and adolescents.[178]

Infection of the Gastrointestinal Tract in Normal Hosts

Whereas infection of visceral organs is well recognized in immunocompromised hosts, case reports of such infection in apparently healthy

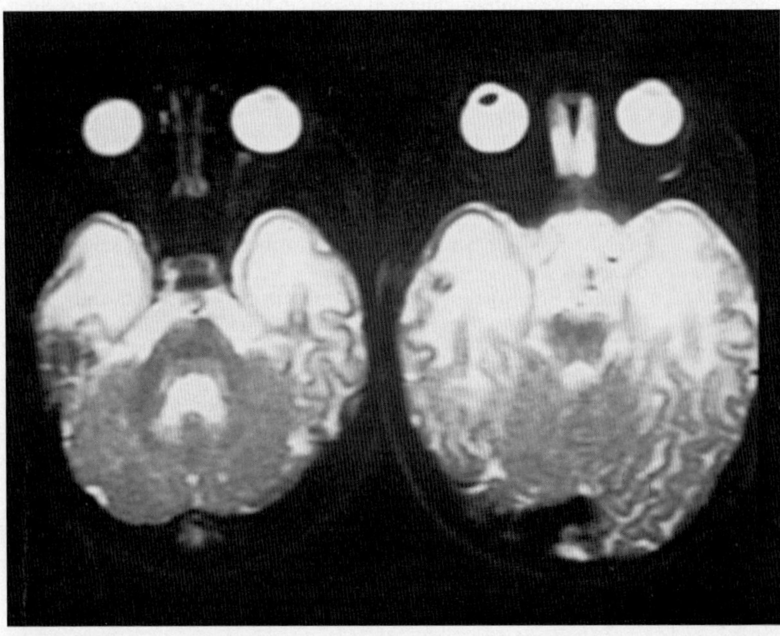

FIG. 158.13 Magnetic resonance image in a patient with herpes simplex virus encephalitis. Note the increased signal intensity bilaterally in the temporal lobes. (From Kohl S. Herpes simplex virus encephalitis in children. *Pediatr Clin North Am.* 1988;35:465–483.)

BOX 158.1 Differential Diagnosis of Herpes Simplex Virus Encephalitis

Infections

Fungal

Cryptococcus spp.
Coccidioides immitis
Histoplasma spp

Bacterial

Abscess, cerebritis
Listeria monocytogenes meningitis
Borrelia burgdorferi meningitis
Subdural, epidural empyema
Mycobacterium tuberculosis meningitis
Bacterial endocarditis
Bacterial meningitis (e.g., *Neisseria meningitidis, Haemophilus influenzae, Streptococcus pneumoniae*)
Mycoplasma pneumoniae encephalitis

Protozoal

Toxoplasmosis
Amebic meningoencephalitis
Rickettsial

Viral

Mumps virus
Coxsackievirus, echovirus
Arbovirus (St. Louis, California, eastern and western equine encephalitis, West Nile virus)
Influenza
Reye syndrome
Lymphocytic choriomeningitis virus
Rabies virus
Epstein-Barr virus
Human herpesvirus–6
Rubella virus
Cytomegalovirus
Adenovirus
Tick-borne encephalitis virus
Powassan virus
Subacute sclerosing encephalitis (measles virus)
Progressive multifocal leukoencephalopathy
Acute disseminated encephalomyelitis

Noninfectious Disorders

Tumor
Vascular disease
Arteriovenous malformations
Toxins
Alcoholic encephalopathy
Leukemia
Cerebral infarction
Subdural or epidural hematoma
Adrenal leukodystrophy

persons are less common. Nonetheless, HSV esophagitis has been described in patients, including several children who were 11 months to 17 years of age.[19,31,67,144,278,301] Esophagitis has recently been reported as complication of wrestling.[208] HSV-1 is the usual pathogen, and the syndrome is associated with primary infection.[122] Initial symptoms include fever, severe odynophagia, retrosternal and subxiphoid pain, and an inability to eat. Oral lesions may be present, but skin lesions generally are absent. Esophagoscopy reveals ulcerations and fibrinous and, at times, hemorrhagic exudate. Distal involvement may be more extensive than the proximal esophageal findings suggest. Double-contrast esophagography may be diagnostic, although endoscopy and biopsy usually are necessary for establishing a definitive diagnosis. Symptoms generally remit in 5 to 7 days after the administration of acyclovir and nonspecific therapy such as antacids, histamine-2 blockers, and hydration.[19,67,278] Perforation of the esophagus is a rare complication.

HSV infection can manifest as an anorectal infection in males who have sex with males.[153,321] In most series of HSV proctitis, cases are in younger adolescent males involved in passive anal intercourse. This syndrome occasionally affects women practicing passive anal intercourse. Initial symptoms include severe anorectal pain, discharge, tenesmus, hematochezia, and, in particular, fever, difficulty urinating, sacral paresthesias, constipation, and (in 50–70% of patients) ulcers or vesicles in the perianal or distal rectal area.[153] The duration of symptoms is 2 to 3 weeks. Primary HSV infection accounts for proctitis in this group in 25% to 30% of cases. Syphilis and infection with *Giardia lamblia, Entamoeba histolytica, Campylobacter fetus, Shigella* spp., other enteric bacteria, and *Neisseria gonorrhoeae* also must be considered in the differential diagnosis of this entity. Appropriate cultures and histologic analysis are crucial for establishing a specific diagnosis.

HSV is a rare cause of hepatitis and represents a broad spectrum of disease from mild elevation of aminotransferases to fulminant liver failure and death. HSV-1 and HSV-2 should always be considered in the differential diagnosis of acute liver failure.[427] HSV hepatitis occurs in all ages from neonate to adult, in pregnancy, and in both immunocompetent and special hosts.[30,269,275] In one review of the literature describing 35 patients who had HSV-associated hepatitis, 14% had no underlying condition. The remainder had various immunocompromising conditions such as transplantation, corticosteroid administration, pregnancy, burns, primary immunodeficiency, or cancer. These patients tended to have fulminant hepatic necrosis, extremely elevated serum aminotransferase levels, disseminated intravascular coagulation, and a mortality rate of 86%.[85] In a prospective study of healthy young adults with genital herpes (primary or recurrent), 14% had mild elevations in liver enzyme tests.

Recurrent Infections

HSV-1 and HSV-2 have the characteristic capacity of herpesviruses to establish latency and undergo episodes of reactivation despite the presence of an apparently adequate immune response. Persistence is facilitated because latent infection of neurons occurs in an immunologically "privileged" site. Reactivation of HSV infection with viral shedding generally causes no lesions. HSV can be recovered from the pharynx and genital sites of asymptomatic persons. It has been found in the tears of persons with a history of recurrent ophthalmic disease, even in the absence of eye lesions or symptoms. All HSV-2–seropositive women from whom samples of vaginal secretions were obtained for more than 100 days had documented asymptomatic viral shedding, and shedding occurred on 1% of the days on which cultures were performed.[440]

Patterns of HSV reactivation include asymptomatic reactivation after silent primary infection, asymptomatic reactivation after symptomatic primary infection, and symptomatic recurrence after either silent or symptomatic primary infection. The risk for having symptomatic recurrences may be higher in individuals who have symptomatic primary infections. When reactivation causes disease, the clinical manifestations of recurrent HSV infection depend on the area involved. Most HSV recurrences are milder than the primary illness, although patients may have symptomatic recurrences without having had clinically apparent primary disease. Recurrent infection in a normal host also may be more severe than is the primary infection. This pattern is particularly evident in HSV infection of the eye, in which recurrent illness is associated with deep stromal damage and scarring.[315,475] This enhanced severity may be related to a greater extent to a more exuberant immune response than to viral damage. HSV encephalitis, which may be a manifestation of viral reactivation, is devastating.[285,334]

The most common manifestation of recurrent HSV infection is herpes labialis ("cold sores," "fever blisters"). Recurrences are observed in 25% to 50% of persons who have had symptomatic primary HSV-1 oral infection but in only 24% of those who had primary HSV-2 oral

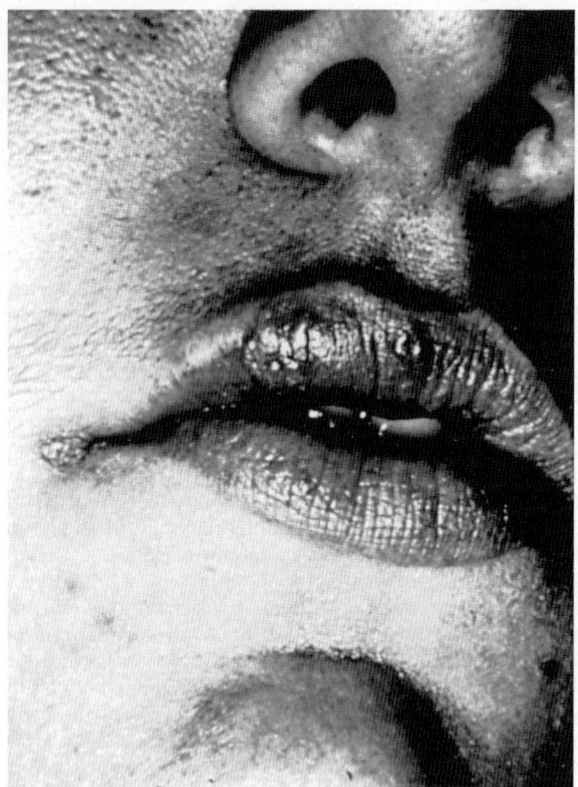

FIG. 158.14 Recurrent herpes labialis (cold sore) in an adolescent.

infection. The mean rate of recurrence after symptomatic primary HSV-1 infection in adults is approximately 0.1 per month. These recurrences often are associated with a variety of febrile illnesses, local trauma, sun exposure, or menstruation.[27,382,385] Whether acquisition of HSV-1 in childhood is less likely to be associated with recurrent herpes labialis is not known.

Most persons with herpes labialis experience a prodrome (pain, burning, tingling, or itching) at the site that lasts a few hours to several days. Subsequently, an orderly progression ensues from papules (lasting 12 to 36 hours) to vesicles (usually gone by 48 hours) and finally to ulcers and crusting (lasting 2 to 4 days) (Fig. 158.14). The typical lesion measures 35 to 80 mm. The majority of outbreaks are healed by 5 to 10 days (mean, 200 hours). Most pain occurs during the vesicular stage. Virus is isolated readily from vesicles (80–90% of the time) and less commonly from ulcers and crusts (34% of the time). Maximal virus titers (10^7 to 10^8) in lesions are detected in the first 1 or 2 days, and virus generally is not isolated after 120 hours.[27,385] Virus is detected in the saliva and on the hands of persons with herpes labialis.

Recurrences tend to affect the same location or closely related areas. In general, they occur on the lips, mucocutaneous junction, or other parts of the face. Recurrent lesions found inside the mouths of normal hosts rarely are caused by HSV and more likely are aphthous lesions. When HSV recurrences are within the mouth, they tend to be on tissue adjacent to bone, such as the gums or palate, and not on the lips or buccal mucosa.[380] A differential diagnosis of the condition also includes pemphigus, lichen planus, ulcers caused by cyclic neutropenia, and ulcers associated with celiac disease, ulcerative colitis, Crohn disease, pernicious anemia, and Behçet syndrome.

Recurrent genital herpes is the second most common manifestation of HSV. Studies have elucidated several factors that increase the risk for recurrent genital disease after symptomatic primary genital infection. Recurrence rates are much higher after primary HSV-2 (90%) than after primary HSV-1 (25–55%) infection.[234,326] The mean rate of recurrence is 0.02 to 0.1 per month after primary genital HSV-1 infection and 0.3 per month after primary HSV-2 genital infection.[234,326] Recurrences are seen more commonly in men than in women and more commonly after a recurrent lesion than after a first attack.[326]

Only 5% to 12% of persons with recurrent genital herpes have constitutional symptoms. Local symptoms include pain (average, 4–6 days), itching, dysuria (10–30%), adenopathy (20–30%), and lesions (average, 50–60 mm) lasting 4 to 5 days until crusting, with healing taking place by 9 to 11 days (range, 4–29 days) (see Fig. 158.3). Symptoms in females tend to be more severe than those in males. Virus is shed for an average of 3 to 4 days (but in some cases as long as 20 days). Virus generally is shed with titers of 10^2 to 10^4 per lesion. Vesicles are seen in dry areas, but in wet areas the vesicles rapidly break down into ulcers. Symptoms generally are milder and of shorter duration than those in primary genital disease.[55] New crops of lesions commonly occur during the course of recurrence. The severity of recurrence is quite variable; in some cases, several discrete recurrences blend into a single, prolonged recurrence, and in rare cases, patients have almost continuous recurrences.[160] In one study of patients who were HSV-2 seropositive with no history of genital herpes, 62% had recognized herpetic lesions at later evaluation.[440] Recurrences in the previously asymptomatic group were shorter (3 vs. 5 days) and less frequent (3.0 vs. 8.2 per year) when the pattern of recurrence in this cohort was compared with that of subjects with a known history of genital herpes.

With endonuclease restriction analysis, researchers have clear evidence that, whereas most recurrences represent endogenous reactivation of the same latent virus, reinfection with a new homologous virus (i.e., HSV-2 and new HSV-2), as well as heterologous virus (i.e., HSV-2 and then HSV-1 or vice versa), is possible.[65] How common this occurrence is remains to be ascertained and must depend to some degree on the sexual activity and number of partners of the persons studied.[364]

Other cutaneous recurrences may develop at each anatomic site of primary infection. HSV infection may recur on the face or trunk in a typical dermatome distribution, such as that associated with VZV. Indeed, frequent repeated attacks of zosteriform lesions on any part of the body in a normal host suggest HSV and not VZV infection.

Erythema Multiforme

Erythema multiforme is thought to be an immune-mediated, "allergic" response to recurrent HSV infection.[138,185,276,296,449] It has been associated with the presence of human leukocyte DQw3 antigen.[204] In several series, approximately 15 to nearly 100% of patients who have erythema multiforme, especially those with recurrent erythema multiforme, gave a history of recurrent HSV infection before the skin eruption, which may be macular or urticarial.[185] In one series, five of 80 patients who had recurrent oral HSV infection experienced a rash (presumably erythema multiforme) that manifested 8 to 14 days after the onset of a cold sore.[385] Studies in adults and children have documented HSV antigen-antibody immune complexes and HSV DNA (detected by PCR analysis and in situ hybridization) in the skin of patients who had erythema multiforme after having HSV infection.[49,50,296] In a series of 20 children with erythema multiforme (10 who had antecedent herpes), 16 were documented to have HSV DNA at the site of the rash.[449] The mechanism of transport of viral DNA fragments is not clearly understood. Recent studies suggest that $CD34^+$ cells play a role in transport of HSV DNA fragments to lesional skin.[295]

The skin manifestations may last 14 to 21 days, and therapy generally is directed toward the allergic and not the viral component of the illness. Suppression of HSV recurrences prevents the associated episodes of erythema multiforme. Indeed, suppressive treatment of erythema multiforme with acyclovir, even in the absence of recurrent HSV infection, completely suppresses clinical manifestations.[366,406] In one series, the syndrome developed in 12 children at a mean age of 8 years within 4 days after the appearance of herpes labialis lesions and symptoms lasted for an average of 10 days; nine children had recurrent erythema multiforme, with an average of 2.6 episodes per year.[449] Detection of HSV by PCR assay of skin biopsy tissue was described in all cases. None of three children given acyclovir suppressive therapy had recurrences during treatment for at least 6 months, but erythema multiforme with recurrent HSV developed in one child when use of the drug was discontinued, thus supporting a causative role of HSV in the syndrome.

HSV Infection in Immunocompromised Hosts

As the practice of pediatrics continues to include more patients with severe acquired immunodeficiency states brought about by expanding

BOX 158.2 Conditions Contributing to Unusually Severe Herpes Simplex Virus Infections

Neonatal period
Malnutrition
Malignancy
Immunosuppressive therapy:
- Antineoplastic
- Transplantation
- Corticosteroids or adrenocorticotropic hormone

Primary immunodeficiency:
- Agammaglobulinemia
- Wiskott-Aldrich syndrome
- Ataxia-telangiectasia
- Severe combined immunodeficiency syndrome
- Nucleoside phosphorylase deficiency
- Thymoma and hypogammaglobulinemia
- Common variable agammaglobulinemia
- Chronic mucocutaneous candidiasis
- Natural killer cell defect
- Acquired immunodeficiency syndrome
- DOCK8 deficiency

Pregnancy
Burns
Trauma
Skin abnormalities:
- Atopic eczema
- Bullous impetigo
- Burns
- Darier disease
- Ichthyosiform erythroderma
- Pemphigus

Viral infection:
- Measles

Bordetella pertussis
Tuberculosis
Severe bacterial infection
Haemophilus influenzae meningitis
Sarcoidosis

application of bone marrow and organ transplantation, HIV infection, and increasingly intensive therapy for malignancies, tumors, and primary immune deficiency disorders, the prevalence of severe HSV infection in immunocompromised hosts is increasing.[271] Box 158.2 lists conditions associated with unusually severe HSV infections. Aside from several cases of HSV encephalitis in patients with agammaglobulinemia (who also had concomitant infections with enterovirus),[256] common links in these varied groups are either skin abnormalities (eczema, burns) or immunologic defects, primarily in the cell-mediated components of the immune system.[43,140,179,312,387,410] The critical defects have not been defined and may involve one or a combination of inadequate functions (e.g., of $CD4^+$ T cells, $CD8^+$ T cells, natural killer cells, macrophage antigen processing, or other factors).

The incidence of severe HSV infection in children with diseases that predispose them to these complications (see Box 158.2) is defined poorly but, in limited series, was similar to that seen in adults.[143,151,323,334] Most infections are caused by reactivation, as would be expected given the relative frequency of primary and recurrent infections.

In series of pediatric or adult patients who have received renal, bone marrow, or cardiac transplants, 70% to 90% of seropositive persons excreted HSV, usually from the oropharynx and generally at the time of peak immunosuppression (in the first month after transplantation).[287] HSV disease usually occurs within 2 to 3 weeks of solid organ or hematopoietic transplantation in patients who do not receive antiviral prophylaxis.[151] Of 68 children who underwent renal transplantation, a herpesvirus was isolated in 43%, with 28% of the isolates being HSV.[416] HSV in cardiac transplant cases causes symptomatic illness in 45% to 85% of seropositive patients, depending on the intensity of immunosuppression. HSV was the virus most commonly isolated in children who underwent bone marrow transplantation (23%).[444] HSV has been suggested to be one of the etiologic agents of the interstitial pneumonitis that can develop after bone marrow transplantation.[290,324] In children with leukemia, HSV infection occurs more commonly in those with myelocytic leukemia than in those with lymphocytic leukemia, and the risk for the development of infection increases with neutropenia and chemotherapy. HSV infection was the most common serious viral infection in children with leukemia. Whereas most infections occurred during periods of remission, on a per-day basis, the risk for development of infection was seven times higher during induction.[469]

In Africa, patients suffering from underlying malnutrition and concomitant measles infection may contract fatal disseminated HSV infection; such events rarely occur in industrialized nations.[34,215,410]

In children with HIV infection, HSV causing chronic mucocutaneous ulcers (persisting for more than 1 month), bronchitis, pneumonitis, and esophagitis is an AIDS-defining condition.[80] Chronic ulcerative HSV lesions often develop in children with HIV infection.[351] Chronic HSV mucocutaneous disease or widespread organ involvement was reported as the AIDS-defining condition in seven of 789 (0.9%) HIV-infected children in one analysis.[420] In another series of children with AIDS, five to 29% contracted HSV opportunistic infection.[143] Many of these children have perianal ulcers from which HSV-1 is isolated. In HIV-infected patients, dissemination is a rare occurrence.[20] Multiple recurrences of infection are common as the immunodeficiency worsens. In patients with AIDS, HSV can cause a typical[165,428] or more indolent encephalitis. HSV usually does not result in mortality in HIV-infected patients, but it causes significant morbidity.[217] HSV genital ulcer disease increases the risk for acquisition of HIV.[182] Studies show that suppression of clinical and subclinical reactivation of HSV is associated with a decrease in HIV viral load.[357] In one recent study, daily acyclovir therapy did not reduce the risk for transmission of HIV-1, despite a reduction in plasma HIV-1 RNA and a 73% reduction in the occurrence of genital ulcers due to HSV-2, suggesting that a more substantial reduction in plasma HIV-1 RNA is necessary to reduce transmission.[77]

Several major syndromes are attributable to HSV in immunocompromised patients, with some overlap and occasionally progression from one to another. The first and most common manifestation is a local, chronic, often extensive cutaneous or mucocutaneous infection. The second form is infection involving a single organ (e.g., esophagitis or pneumonitis). The most serious illness is characterized by more widespread dissemination involving distant areas of the skin or visceral organs (e.g., the lungs, liver, adrenal glands) and the CNS. Although data are limited, disseminated disease probably most often represents primary infection except in the most severely immunocompromised patients. More localized syndromes may be a manifestation of either primary infection or recurrent illness.[271]

The typical localized HSV infection begins in the mouth or about the lips, often appearing innocuously as recurrence of ordinary herpes labialis. Over the course of several days, the papules and vesicles progress to bullae, frequently with hemorrhagic fluid. The bullae or vesicles evolve into huge, chronic, bloody, coalescing, ulcerated, oozing lesions eroding into subcutaneous tissue and occasionally destroying underlying structures. The tissue is malodorous, and the lesions are painful (Fig. 158.15). The lip and palate are the sites most commonly affected. Oral lesions account for approximately 60% of HSV infections in children undergoing transplantation.[416] A similar syndrome, usually caused by HSV-2 infection, may be seen in the perianal or vaginal area and is one of the characteristic syndromes that occur in males who have sex with HIV-infected males (Fig. 158.16). If untreated, the lesions may lead to death because of local destruction and hemorrhage, or they may regress as the immune status of the host improves or as antiviral chemotherapy is administered. A syndrome of herpetic geometric glossitis has been reported in HIV-infected patients.[158] Affected patients have a tender tongue accompanied by dorsal longitudinal crossed and branching fissures.

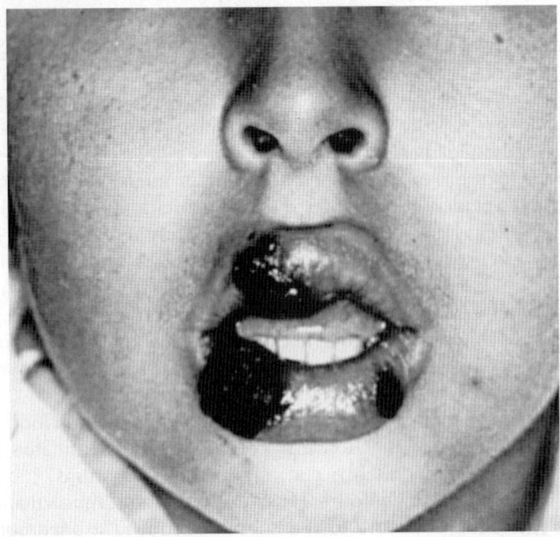

FIG. 158.15 Chronic hemorrhagic herpes simplex virus infection in a girl with leukemia who had received a bone marrow transplant.

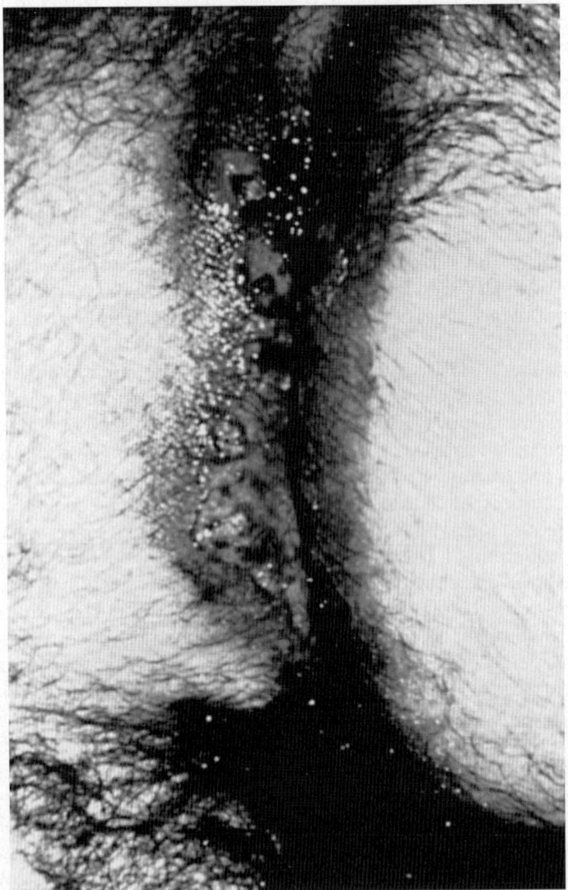

FIG. 158.16 Herpes simplex virus proctitis and rectal infection in a homosexual male with AIDS. (Courtesy Dr. Victor Fainstein, Department of Internal Medicine, MD Anderson Cancer Center, Houston.)

Extensive HSV skin infections may occur in patients with burns, eczema, pemphigus, or abrasions, often with conversion of second-degree tissue damage to third-degree damage (see Figs. 158.6 and 158.7). Of 179 children with eczema, herpes skin infections developed in 10, seven of whom required hospitalization.[108] Although rare, local infection may progress to dissemination in some cases, possibly as a result of the more severe immunodeficiency occurring with several of these conditions. The widespread necrotizing lesions are known commonly as *Kaposi varicelliform eruption* or *eczema herpeticum* (see Fig. 158.6). The predisposition to severe HSV-1 infection in children with atopic eczema appears to be due to the cutaneous abnormalities because these children have T-cell responses to HSV, as well as high HSV IgG antibody titers.[154] Studies have looked at the role of the cathelicidin family of antimicrobial peptides in protecting children with atopic dermatitis against disseminated skin infection with HSV. Variable skin expression of cathelicidin peptide LL-37 may explain why eczema herpeticum develops in some children with atopic dermatitis and others appear to be at lower risk.[154,183] One study evaluating phenotypic risks for eczema herpeticum demonstrated that children with severe atopy and greater T-helper type 2 (Th2) polarity (as demonstrated by an increase in Th2 chemokines) were at increased risk for HSV and *Staphylococcus aureus* skin infections.[33]

Herpes skin lesions must be differentiated from bacterial infections caused by gram-positive or gram-negative organisms, chronic fungal infections (as seen with *Mucor* or *Blastomyces*), other viral infections (vaccinia, varicella), mycobacterial infection, and various noninfectious lesions such as pyoderma gangrenosum, chemotherapy-induced ulcers, or Sweet syndrome.

HSV esophagitis rarely has been reported in normal children,[31,67,208] but it is a relatively common finding in immunocompromised patients. Pathologic studies have suggested that approximately 25% of cases of autopsy-proven esophagitis (1–6% of all autopsies) are secondary to HSV infection (14 of 55 cases).[289] Underlying conditions included burns, aplastic anemia, malignancies, transplantation, a variety of other serious medical problems, and postoperative trauma induced by nasogastric tubes.[67,262,289] Twenty to 50% of these patients have HSV involvement elsewhere (the lungs, trachea, and, less commonly, the skin). The esophagitis may be asymptomatic or associated with dysphagia, odynophagia, epigastric discomfort, and retrosternal pain. Characteristic findings in the esophagus are ulcers with raised granular margins. The ulcers often are covered with fibrinous exudate and, in advanced cases, are confluent, with progression to complete mucosal loss in large segments of the esophagus. Typically, visceral herpes infection is not suspected before the patient's death, but, uncommonly, involvement of adjacent gastric tissue can be documented. Diagnostic evaluation should include a barium swallow, which may demonstrate edema, nodules, and ulceration of the esophagus; however, barium studies cannot differentiate HSV from other etiologic agents of esophagitis. Esophagoscopy accompanied by biopsy and viral culture is diagnostic and helps exclude other common causes of this syndrome, including *Candida*, CMV, and possibly other fungi and bacteria or chemotherapy-induced changes.[66,67,289] Although the oral cavity, esophagus, and rectum are the usual sites of HSV infection in the gastrointestinal tract of immunocompromised patients, HSV-2 colitis has been reported in a young child after combined liver and small bowel transplantation.[113]

HSV pneumonia is an unusual condition, but lung involvement has been described in neonates[41] and immunocompromised hosts. This diagnosis frequently is made post mortem almost exclusively in immunocompromised patients. In one series of 1000 consecutive autopsies,[288] HSV pneumonia was identified in 10 cases. HSV pulmonary infection occurred in 3% of children who had undergone renal transplantation.[416] In most adult cases, the process is a result of endogenous viral mucocutaneous reactivation and involvement of lung tissue by contiguous spread, which causes focal pneumonia (60% of the time), or involvement by hematogenous spread from an oral or genital site, which results in diffuse pneumonitis.[324] Although the largest series consisted primarily of adult patients, three of the patients were aged 7 years or younger (with Down syndrome and congestive heart failure, rhabdomyosarcoma, and pneumococcal pneumonia and a seizure disorder).[187] Patients had cough, dyspnea, fever, and hypoxia; and 50% had rales. Most had other concomitant pulmonary infections with bacteria, *Candida, Aspergillus,* and CMV. HSV pneumonia cannot be diagnosed by the association of upper airway cultures and radiographic abnormalities. It must rest on an aggressive approach involving culture and histopathologic examination of involved lung tissue obtained by either biopsy or bronchoscopy.

HSV meningoencephalitis is not a common occurrence in immunocompromised patients. It may occur as a component of widely disseminated disease, or it may be a localized condition. Several cases have been reported in patients who had agammaglobulinemia in association with concomitant enteroviral infection of the brain.[256] The meningoencephalitis may be fulminant, such as occurs in a normal host. An interesting case that followed an atypical subacute course accompanied by bilateral brain involvement has been reported in an anergic patient who had Hodgkin disease. HSV encephalitis may also involve the brain stem.[257] Although HSV does not appear to have a predilection for CNS infection in immunocompromised hosts, patients with AIDS are an exception and may have ascending myelitis, acute transverse myelitis, and encephalitis.[143,146,165,428]

Hepatitis caused by HSV has been reported most commonly after solid organ or bone marrow transplantation[85,197,231] and during pregnancy.[216] Signs include fever, abdominal pain, and elevated liver enzyme levels. Hepatitis usually occurs during the first 3 weeks after transplantation, unless prophylactic acyclovir is given. The mortality rate is very high (67–100%). In at least one case, orthotopic liver transplantation resulted in survival.[371] HSV is reported as the most frequently identified viral etiology of hepatitis on one series of patients with systemic lupus erythematosus.[323]

The most severe form of HSV in an immunocompromised host is widely disseminated disease that can involve the liver, adrenals, lungs, spleen, kidney, and often the brain. In studies from South Africa and Kenya,[34,215,410] measles and severe malnutrition were frequent cofactors in children who had widely disseminated HSV infection. These illnesses represented fatal primary infections. Similar syndromes have been described; they and other underlying conditions are listed in Box 158.2. Dissemination has been reported coincident with *Bordetella pertussis, Haemophilus influenzae* meningitis,[194] and other bacterial infections.[34] Disseminated HSV infection occurred in 10% and 25% of children who had HSV infection and underwent bone marrow and renal transplantation, respectively.[287,444]

Disseminated HSV infection initially usually manifests as initial fever and skin or mucocutaneous involvement in 80% of cases, but instead of healing as expected, the infection disseminates. The cutaneous dissemination may involve a widespread vesicular eruption that looks much like varicella, or it may involve more local, large hemorrhagic vesicles and bullae. Involvement of the major target organs, as noted previously, gives rise to syndromes of hepatitis, pneumonia, shock, bleeding, disseminated intravascular coagulopathy, seizures, coma, renal failure, hypothermia, and death in days to weeks. Laboratory examination may reveal leukopenia, thrombocytopenia, elevated liver function test values, hyponatremia, azotemia, pneumonitis, hypoglycemia, CSF pleocytosis, abnormal EEG results, and electrocardiographic abnormalities. Death occurs commonly in this syndrome (90%), even after the institution of antiviral chemotherapy. Because the liver frequently is involved and biopsy may be precluded by the tenuous condition of the patient, HSV infection should be considered in all high-risk groups (see Box 158.2) with fulminant hepatitis.

Fetus and Newborn

HSV may infect the fetus before delivery (congenital or in utero infection), infect the newborn during delivery (perinatal or natal infection), or infect the infant after birth (postnatal infection).

The clinical spectrum in infants with in utero acquired, congenital HSV infection is different from that observed in infants with natal or postnatal disease. The classic triad of cutaneous findings, CNS disease, and ophthalmologic disease is seen in approximately one third of neonates with congenital HSV.[265] The most prominent and most common features of congenital infection are vesicular rash, bullae, or cutaneous scars present at birth or within a few days of birth. In some cases, the extent and severity of these lesions may result in an initial diagnosis of epidermolysis bullosa. At least one case report of limb hypoplasia, similar to congenital varicella syndrome, has been shown to be caused by HSV-2.[196] Two thirds of infants demonstrate extensive involvement of the CNS at birth, either clinically or from autopsy findings: diffuse brain damage, microcephaly, or intracranial calcifications. In some infants, eye findings have been noted, including chorioretinitis, microphthalmos, retinal scars and retinal dysplasia, and cataracts.

The three general patterns of natal or postnatal neonatal HSV infection are categorized by the extent of disease: (1) disseminated infection with or without CNS involvement, present in 25% of cases; (2) infection localized to the CNS, in 30% of cases; and (3) infection localized to the skin, eye, or mouth, in 45% of cases.

Infants with natal or postnatal HSV infection commonly have a clinical picture resembling that of bacterial sepsis: alterations in temperature, lethargy, respiratory distress, anorexia or vomiting, and cyanosis. In febrile neonates presenting to an acute care treatment center, HSV infection should be considered in the differential diagnosis of neonatal fever, especially in the presence of mononuclear CSF pleocytosis, hypothermia, or sepsis-like syndrome.[72-74] If skin involvement is present, then skin vesicles or mucous membrane ulcers may be apparent. If the conjunctivae or cornea is involved, then nonexudative conjunctivitis, tearing, and pain will be present. If the CNS is involved, then seizures may occur.[442] The frequency of disseminated disease has decreased after a high of 51% reported in the years 1973 to 1981; this decrease probably represents earlier diagnosis and treatment of localized infection before dissemination occurs.[457] The disseminated form of infection in the earlier years of recognition presented in infants between 9 and 11 days of age and usually involved the liver, where it caused fulminant hepatitis with disseminated intravascular coagulation, and the adrenal glands, and it most closely resembled the picture of bacterial sepsis.[427] Current reports show disseminated neonatal HSV may present as early as the first week of life, without cutaneous or localizing signs, similar to bacterial sepsis, and confirm that HSV remains an important cause of neonatal morbidity and mortality. A disseminated infection can affect multiple organs, including the brain, larynx, trachea, lungs, esophagus, stomach, lower gastrointestinal tract, spleen, kidneys, pancreas, and heart. Pneumonia occurs in 37% of infants. Markedly elevated aminotransferase levels, direct hyperbilirubinemia, coagulopathy, and thrombocytopenia are common findings late in the disease process. From 60% to 75% of infants with disseminated disease have hematogenously acquired CNS involvement and meningoencephalitis, as manifested by irritability, a bulging fontanelle, localized or generalized seizures, flaccid or spastic paralysis, opisthotonos, decerebrate rigidity, or coma. Importantly, 39% of infants with disseminated disease do not have skin vesicles or eye lesions at initial evaluation, and vesicles do not develop during the acute HSV disease; only 56% initially have fever, and many are hypothermic on presentation.

CNS disease from retrograde axonal transmission of virus presents later than does disseminated disease, usually when the infant is 11 to 17 days old but occasionally when the infant is as old as 4 to 6 weeks of age. Typically, these infants have focal seizures that subsequently generalize. Examination of CSF demonstrates mononuclear pleocytosis with a predominance of lymphocytes, a moderately low glucose concentration, and elevated protein levels. A normal cell count, glucose, and protein concentration, however, may be found on the initial lumbar puncture, if performed early in the disease process. An elevated red blood cell count secondary to hemorrhagic brain involvement may be present but by itself is an unreliable sign. Fever is present at initial evaluation in only 44% of infants with HSV encephalitis, and 32% of infants do not have skin vesicles either initially or during the course of their illness. Neonatal HSV encephalitis can be disseminated to all parts of the brain, multifocal in many parts of the brain, or limited to only the temporal lobes, brain stem, or cerebellum; and watershed distribution ischemia may be seen in some cases.[309,430] Delayed recurrence of HSV infection of the central nervous system may occur once the newborn recovers and has completed 6 months of antiviral suppressive therapy.[178] Recurrence in the CNS has been reported to occur as long as 7 years after neonatal herpes simplex virus CNS disease.[26,178]

Localized skin, eye, or mouth disease usually presents within the infant's first 7 to 10 days of life. Approximately 83% of these neonates have skin lesions: usually single vesicles, occasionally vesicle clusters, and rarely a zoster-like rash. As many as 46% to 80% of neonates with skin lesions have one to 12 recurrences during the first 6 to 12 months of life. Thirteen to 25% of infants have eye involvement; disease is limited to only the eye in one third of these cases, but the risk for disseminated disease is significant.[442] Common manifestations include eye pain and eyelid swelling, fussiness, tearing, nonexudative conjunctivitis, keratitis, and chorioretinitis. As many as 83% of infants are afebrile initially. One third of all infants have evidence of herpetic mouth lesions.

Unusual manifestations of HSV infection in the neonate, from perinatal or postnatal sources, also include conjunctivitis with keratitis, laryngotracheobronchitis, pneumonitis, and epiglottitis.[263]

DIAGNOSIS

Clinical findings may suggest a probable diagnosis of HSV infection, but obtaining a definitive laboratory diagnosis is necessary or useful in many circumstances and should always be sought in neonates and patients with severe disease.[17,75] Accurate laboratory diagnosis requires giving attention to obtaining the correct specimens necessary for identifying the etiology of the clinical syndrome. Appropriate interpretation of the laboratory results is the second critical factor. Evaluation of mucocutaneous lesions in high-risk patients guides the use of antiviral therapy if the lesion is herpetic. However, because HSV often is shed in immunosuppressed and otherwise healthy individuals, finding HSV in oropharyngeal secretions does not mean that the clinical condition is caused by HSV. In general, the virus must be isolated from the relevant tissue or involved end organ for confirmation of the diagnosis. The test selected also is important (e.g., HSV is rarely found in CSF cultures of patients outside the neonatal age group with HSV encephalitis but often is present in aseptic lymphocytic meningitis caused by HSV). Detection of HSV DNA in CSF by PCR assay or by brain biopsy is indicated to prove the diagnosis and exclude other treatable causes of encephalitis. Laboratory diagnosis also is valuable when HSV infections are not life threatening.[75] For example, establishing that a genital lesion is caused by HSV-1 or HSV-2 facilitates decisions about antiviral therapy and allows initiation of appropriate counseling regarding the risk for recurrences and measures that may reduce transmission of HSV to contacts and during pregnancy to the neonate.

Viral Culture

The original gold standard for HSV diagnosis was recovery of infectious virus in cell culture. HSV replicates rapidly in cell culture, typically in 1 to 2 days, and produces a characteristic cytopathic effect (CPE) (Fig. 158.17).[75,238,350] A variety of cell lines (human fibroblasts, A549, and many others) support HSV replication and are used by diagnostic laboratories to isolate HSV. Although the presence of HSV is suggested by the cell types infected as well as the character and timing of the CPE, definitive identification of the infecting virus is accomplished via microscopy of fixed cells with immunofluorescence assay with HSV-1– and HSV-2–specific antibodies.

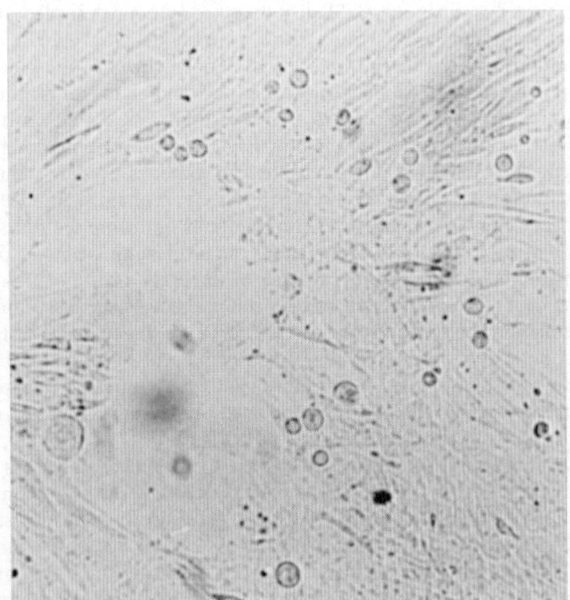

FIG. 158.17 Culture of herpes simplex virus on human fibroblasts demonstrating disruption of the cell monolayer and rounding and enlargement of cells to show the cytopathic effect.

Several culture methods that do not rely on the evaluation of CPE have been devised that provide more rapid diagnosis of HSV than traditional culture. One approach is the use of a genetically modified baby hamster kidney cell line containing a reporter gene encoding β-galactosidase under control of an HSV-specific promoter (enzyme-linked viral inducible system [ELVIS]).[103,245] Addition of a colorimetric reporter substrate after centrifugation-enhanced infection and overnight incubation allows identification of cells infected with HSV. Similarly, the shell vial method uses centrifugation-enhanced infection of cell monolayers and overnight incubation, followed by immunofluorescence assay staining with HSV-specific antibodies.[133,188,311,419] Although these methods may reduce the time to result, they are typically less sensitive than traditional cell culture.[84,201]

HSV culture methods, both traditional and rapid, are being phased out by many diagnostic laboratories and replaced by type-specific nucleic acid amplification tests for HSV-1 and HSV-2 DNA. These tests do not show definitively that infectious virus is present in the specimen but suggest that it is or may have been shortly before the specimen was obtained.

Direct Detection of HSV-Infected Cells

Direct detection methods allow a diagnosis of HSV infection to be established more rapidly than any available HSV culture method.[17,107,245,363] Direct immunofluorescent assay of cells taken from mucocutaneous lesions is the procedure most commonly used.[280] Specimens are obtained by unroofing the lesion, swabbing the exposed base to remove infected cells, and transferring the swab to viral transport media. The collected cells are centrifuged and washed, applied to a glass slide, then fixed and stained with fluorescently labeled, HSV-specific antibodies. This method, the direct viral examination or direct fluorescent antibody (DFA) testing, yields sensitivities, when compared with traditional viral culture, in the range of 61% to 80% with few false-positive reactions.[75,84] To optimize DFA performance, diagnostic laboratories set criteria for specimen adequacy (e.g., requiring a certain number of basal, parabasal, and intermediate cells from lesion sites), thereby emphasizing the importance of proper specimen collection. Despite these precautions, direct detection of HSV by immunofluorescence remains less sensitive than by culture. Because of this, it is recommended that DFA-negative lesional samples be tested by a more sensitive method to rule out false-negative results.[75]

HSV antigens can be detected directly in clinical specimens by a variety of additional methods including enzyme-linked immunosorbent assays (ELISAs) and immunoperoxidase assays.[8,51,95,245,280,294,363,426] However, these assays have been replaced in the diagnostic laboratory by nucleic acid amplification tests.

Nonspecific methods such as Papanicolaou (Pap) staining or the Tzanck test have been used in the past to suggest possible HSV infection. Even though these methods may show cytologic changes in specimens obtained from suspected HSV lesions, the diagnosis of HSV should not rely on these methods in current practice because rapid, specific methods are available. Although cytologic examination of HSV lesions reveals typical giant cells and, less commonly, Cowdry type A intranuclear inclusions, these changes also are seen with CMV and VZV. Cytologic changes are identified in approximately 70% of culture-positive specimens, but sensitivity is dependent on the experience of the examiner and may be low.[283,378] Electron microscopy of vesicular fluid or tissue preparations may reveal the characteristic virus of the herpes family (Fig. 158.18). However, the microscopist cannot differentiate HSV from other herpesviruses, and this diagnostic approach rarely is available as a rapid method. Because selection of antiviral therapy for herpesviruses requires specific identification of the infecting virus, nonspecific methods have limited clinical value in the current era of specific antiviral therapy.

Polymerase Chain Reaction Assays

Type-specific HSV nucleic acid amplification assays, particularly PCR assay, have become the gold standard for HSV diagnosis and have replaced virus culture and direct examination in many diagnostic laboratories. The detection of HSV DNA by PCR is more sensitive than the isolation

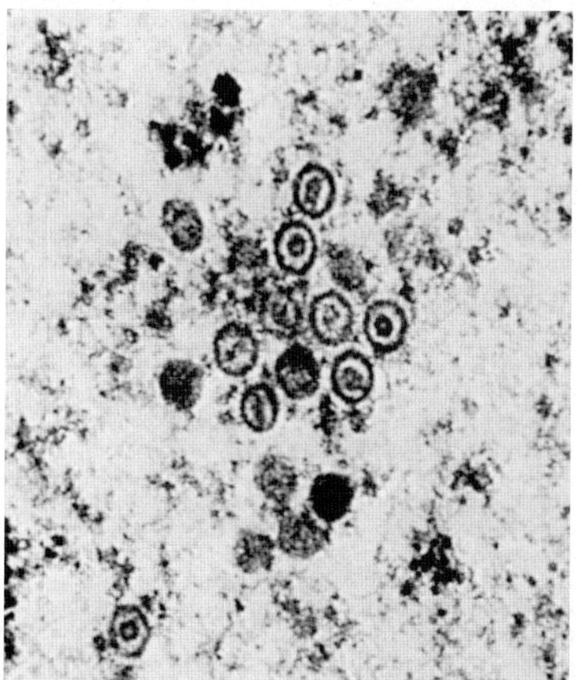

FIG. 158.18 Electron microscopic demonstration of herpes simplex virus (HSV) particles in a brain biopsy specimen from a 9-month-old infant with HSV encephalitis.

of virus by culture.[9,25,181,339,347] In one study of mucosal specimens, the ratio of PCR positivity to virus culture ranged from 3.8 : 1 in the winter to 8.8 : 1 in the summer. PCR does not require the presence of infectious virus for detection, and this is one of the great advantages and disadvantages of HSV DNA testing. Given the high sensitivity of HSV PCR, false-positive results may occur, particularly if original specimen contamination occurs at time of collection or if cross-contamination between specimens occurs during performance of PCR assay. However, the implementation of careful molecular diagnostic workflows and the development of the real-time PCR methodology have considerably reduced the risk for false-positive reactions.

The clinical utility of HSV PCR was first demonstrated for the diagnosis of HSV encephalitis.[25,71,159,213,320,328,339,374,418] Given its high negative predictive value, HSV PCR testing of CSF is often used to rule out HSV infection in patients with suspected herpes encephalitis. However, it is important to recognize that HSV DNA may not be detectable in CSF early in the course of disease.[447] A single negative test should not exclude the diagnosis of HSV when there is high clinical suspicion, and sequential testing of CSF by PCR has rendered the use of brain biopsy unnecessary in most situations. In one study, HSV DNA was detected by PCR in the CSF of 53 (98%) of 54 patients with biopsy-proven herpes simplex encephalitis and was detected in all 18 CSF specimens obtained before brain biopsy was performed on patients with proven herpes encephalitis.[236] Testing febrile neonates with CSF pleocytosis using CSF HSV PCR assay and empirically treating with acyclovir until PCR test results are known has also been shown to save lives and be cost effective.[74]

PCR assay also has demonstrated the presence of HSV DNA in plasma or whole blood and has been used to diagnose HSV viremia in neonates and in immunocompetent patients with eczema herpeticum and primary herpetic gingivostomatitis, as well as in immunocompromised patients with disseminated disease. PCR analysis also may demonstrate prolonged presence of HSV DNA in genital lesions.[94] The sensitivity of the PCR method is adequate for detecting asymptomatic shedding of HSV.[68,93,168] HSV PCR also has utility when the clinical diagnosis is difficult to make, as illustrated by detection of HSV in vitreous fluid[173] and in unusual mucocutaneous lesions in patients with AIDS.[244] HSV DNA may also be quantitated in clinical specimens using PCR-based methods and used to predict severity of disease, especially in hepatitis and encephalitis, and to follow virologic response in these patients.[35,68]

Serologic Diagnosis

Serologic methods are used to assess HSV immune status and document whether an individual has been infected with HSV. Because these viruses cause persistent infections, the presence of HSV IgG antibodies may only signify that the individual has latent HSV-1 or HSV-2 (or both) in sensory ganglia and that the virus can be expected to reactivate and intermittently shed. Clinical laboratories use ELISA or immunoblot methods to detect HSV-1 and HSV-2 type-specific IgG antibodies in patient sera. These assays use specific HSV gG antigens and can be used to show whether an individual is infected with HSV-1, HSV-2, or both, but not when the infection was acquired.[128,175,246,379,401,434] If paired sera are available, these assays are capable of demonstrating type-specific seroconversion, even if a patient is already exposed to a single type. The sensitivities of commercial gG type-specific HSV serology tests range from 90% to 98%, with specificities greater than 94% when compared with Western blot analysis.[434] As with any serologic test, false-negative results are more likely early in the course of infection, and false-positive results may occur in patients with a low pretest probability of exposure.

If a patient is seronegative at the onset of symptoms or at initial evaluation, primary HSV infection can be documented by demonstrating seroconversion with paired sera.[203,222] However, serologic tests are not useful for evaluating HSV recurrence, because IgG antibody titers often do not rise during viral reactivation. On the other hand, increases in IgG antibody titer may occur in the absence of recurrent disease. In addition, testing for IgM antibodies does not improve the serologic diagnosis. HSV IgM assays cannot be used to distinguish primary from recurrent infection because reactivation can also induce the production of IgM antibody.[174]

Local production of HSV IgG in CSF samples can be used to document HSV encephalitis in some patients, but a 2- to 4-week interval is required to demonstrate this change, and it cannot be used to guide antiviral therapy.[285,418,423] Testing CSF for HSV IgM antibodies has no demonstrated diagnostic value.

Genetic Analysis for Molecular Epidemiology

HSV DNA from epidemiologically unrelated isolates has a specific cleavage pattern when digested by endonuclease restriction enzymes and subjected to gel electrophoresis (Fig. 158.19).[64] This restriction fragment length polymorphism (RFLP) method is primarily used for epidemiologic purposes to demonstrate relatedness among isolates during the evaluation of apparent outbreaks or nosocomial transmission events.[64,65,166,255,460] In addition, RFLP analysis has contributed to our understanding of exogenous reinfection versus recurrence and the possibility that individuals may harbor more than one latent virus strain. This method is laborious and not typically performed in diagnostic laboratories. Precise differentiation of HSV strains requires genomic sequencing, which is performed on a research basis.

Antiviral Drug Susceptibility Testing

The persistence of lesions, emergence of new lesions, or increasing plasma viral load despite appropriate antiviral therapy is suggestive of treatment failure and should prompt laboratory evaluation of antiviral resistance. This testing may be useful to guide selection of an alternative therapy, but, unfortunately, testing is not readily available in clinical practice or even in large reference laboratories. Although resistance is uncommon in immunocompetent patients (prevalence 0.1–0.7%), immunocompromised patients, many of whom receive long-term HSV prophylaxis or treatment, are at relatively high risk for the development of resistance (prevalence 2.5–11%).[314] The gold standard method for HSV antiviral susceptibility testing is the plaque reduction assay. This phenotypic assay uses Vero cells (African green monkey kidney cells) inoculated with a standardized viral inoculum and incubated for 48 to 72 hours in the presence of serial drug concentrations and no drug controls.[322,404,448] After incubation, the cells are fixed and stained, the number of plaques or focal areas of cytopathic effect is counted, and the concentration of drug that reduces the plaque number by 50%

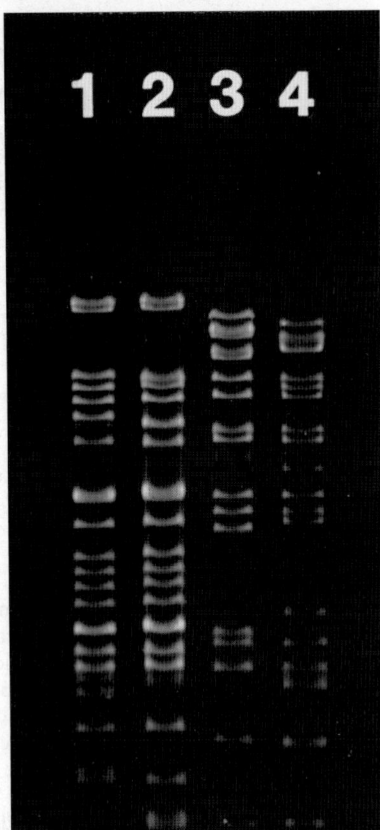

FIG. 158.19 Electrophoretic separation of the DNA fragments of four herpes simplex virus (HSV) isolates by size, produced by restriction endonuclease enzyme digestion using the BamHI enzyme. Lanes 1 and 2 are two different HSV-2 clinical isolates, whereas lanes 3 and 4 are two different HSV-1 clinical isolates. The origin of the gel is at the top. (Courtesy Dr. Saul Kit, Division of Biochemical Virology, Baylor College of Medicine, Houston.)

(IC_{50}) is calculated. The plaque reduction assay has well-described breakpoint values of 2 µg/mL or greater for acyclovir and 100 µg/mL or greater for foscarnet. Other phenotypic susceptibility methods utilize a variety of techniques to measure HSV replication in culture, including dye uptake, ELISA, DNA hybridization, and PCR assay.[243,314,412,448] Specific breakpoint values will vary based on the assay. Although laborious, phenotypic evaluation remains the primary approach to HSV susceptibility testing in clinical laboratories. Sequence analysis of the genes encoding thymidine kinase *(UL23)* and DNA polymerase *(UL30)*, the targets of HSV antiviral agents acyclovir and foscarnet, have revealed a large number of resistance mutations as well as polymorphisms that do not contribute to the resistance phenotype.[251,314,349] Genotypic susceptibility testing is primarily utilized as a research tool to understand the mechanism of antiviral resistance and is not generally performed for clinical purposes.

PROGNOSIS, COMPLICATIONS, AND SEQUELAE

Most HSV infections occurring beyond the fetal and neonatal periods cause minor morbidity but may be life threatening if brain or other internal organs are involved. The introduction of antiviral drugs that inhibit HSV replication has changed the management and outcome of these infections. Even before these drugs were available, eczema herpeticum resolved without sequelae in most cases. Despite administration of antiviral therapy, HSV encephalitis can be fatal or be associated with serious consequences ranging from moderate to extensive and permanent neurologic disability.[443] The case-fatality rate for untreated encephalitis may be as high as 75%,[464] and progressive neurologic damage may occur.[118,163,221] In a series of PCR-diagnosed cases, a Glasgow Coma Scale score lower than 11 was associated with a poor outcome, and the youngest cohort, those younger than 3 years, had higher morbidity and mortality rates.[189] Genital herpes causes significant physical and psychological morbidity. In immunocompromised patients, disseminated HSV infection can result in fatal or serious illness. HSV is one of the most common infectious causes of blindness in developed countries.

TREATMENT

HSV-1 and HSV-2 infections are treated with acyclovir or related drugs. Acyclovir is a nucleoside analog that is a competitive inhibitor of HSV DNA polymerase, and it terminates DNA chain elongation. Acyclovir is an inactive agent. Inhibition of viral DNA synthesis by blocking viral DNA polymerase and DNA chain elongation requires phosphorylation of acyclovir. HSV-1 and HSV-2 viral thymidine kinases are much more active than are mammalian cell kinases, and acyclovir becomes a specific antiviral agent in the presence of viral thymidine kinase.

Because the oral bioavailability of acyclovir is only approximately 20%, efficacy with oral administration requires high and frequent dosing. Concentrations of acyclovir achieved in CSF are approximately 50% of plasma levels. Acyclovir is excreted by glomerular filtration, so doses must be reduced in patients with impaired renal function. Acyclovir has been an exceptionally safe drug in clinical practice, but adverse reactions, including rash, nausea, vomiting, diarrhea, abdominal pain, headache, and neutropenia, can occur. Neurotoxicity may occur with an overdose, usually when the dose is not adjusted for poor renal clearance. Acyclovir also can cause acute renal insufficiency by precipitation in the renal tubules in dehydrated patients with high plasma concentrations or by rapid infusion of the drug. Valacyclovir, the L-valine ester of acyclovir, is converted to acyclovir[422] and has much higher bioavailability after oral administration, with plasma concentrations similar to those obtained after intravenous administration of acyclovir. Famciclovir is an oral prodrug of penciclovir[112]; it also is well absorbed orally and is metabolized to the active form on absorption. The major advantage of these agents is that less frequent dosing is required than with acyclovir. HSV-1 and HSV-2 seldom are resistant to acyclovir or related drugs in the immunocompetent host (<1%). Resistance can occur in up to 10% of isolates from immunocompromised patients who receive prolonged antiviral therapy. HSV isolates resistant to acyclovir usually have mutations in the gene encoding viral thymidine kinase *(UL23)* and less often to *UL30*, which encodes for the viral target DNA polymerase enzyme. Foscarnet or, in some cases, cidofovir is an alternative for the treatment of acyclovir-resistant HSV.[44] Resistance to foscarnet and cidofovir has been reported.[314,470]

Oral HSV Infection

Although published experience is limited, administration of oral acyclovir to children with gingivostomatitis is appropriate and can be expected to modify the duration of symptoms if it is initiated early in the clinical course.[184] Several small placebo-controlled trials of primary herpes gingivostomatitis in young children have been reported.[6,11] In one study, the pain and hypersalivation resolved more quickly in acyclovir-treated patients.[125] In a larger study, symptoms resolved more rapidly with a 10-day course of oral acyclovir 600 mg/m^2 four times a day; differences were observed in drooling (4 vs. 8 days with placebo), gum swelling (5 vs. 7 days), speed of healing of intraoral lesions (6 vs. 8 days), appearance of new lesions (57% vs. 94%), and viral shedding in saliva (4 vs. 10 days). Therapy had no effect on the subsequent development of cold sores.[11] A comparison of oral acyclovir suspension, 15 mg/kg five times a day for 7 days, and placebo started within 72 hours documented that drug recipients had a shorter duration of oral lesions (median of 4 vs. 10 days [difference, 6 days; 95% confidence interval (CI), 4.0–8.0]) and earlier resolution of other symptoms, including fever (1 vs. 3 days [difference, 2 days; CI, 0.8–3.2]), extraoral lesions (0 vs. 5.5 days [difference, 5.5 days; CI, 1.3–4.7]), difficulty eating (4 vs. 7 days [difference, 3 days; CI, 1.31–4.69]), and difficulty drinking (3 vs. 6 days [difference, 3 days; CI, 1.1–4.9]).[6] Treatment also decreased the period of viral shedding (1 vs. 5 days [difference, 4 days; CI, 2.9–5.1]). Symptomatic therapy includes antipyretics and oral hydration. The use of oral anesthetics is not recommended and has resulted in self-injury as a result of children chewing on anesthetized oral mucosa or lips.

Although the duration of symptoms is shorter with recurrences, children with frequent or severe recurrences may benefit from treatment with oral acyclovir as soon as new lesions appear. Topical acyclovir has been licensed for the treatment of recurrent oral herpes labialis based on experience in adults. However, its benefits on clinical symptoms are minimal. If treatment in children is indicated, oral acyclovir is the best option. Studies in adult patients with herpes labialis show that patient-initiated, high-dose, short-duration treatment with valacyclovir or famciclovir initiated at the onset of symptoms significantly reduces the time to healing and hastens resolution of pain and tenderness when compared with placebo.[381,384]

Several studies have produced conflicting results regarding the use of topical acyclovir for the treatment of oral herpes recurrences. Topical acyclovir can decrease the duration of HSV shedding from 2 to 3 days with placebo treatment to 1 to 2 days,[386] and the effect on symptoms is either none or subtle (1 less day with vesicles and a 2- to 3-day acceleration of healing). Although no controlled studies have been conducted, acyclovir therapy should be used for the treatment of rare cases of HSV esophagitis in normal hosts.[144]

HSV Keratitis

Children with HSV keratitis should be referred for immediate evaluation by an ophthalmologist who is familiar with this illness and its progressive, sight-threatening forms and with optimal antiviral therapy.[442] The use of cycloplegic and antiinflammatory agents, which may be necessary, requires specialized experience. Topical preparations have been shown to have a beneficial effect on HSV keratitis and probably other superficial ocular HSV infections such as conjunctivitis and blepharitis.[253] These preparations include idoxuridine (Stoxil), vidarabine (Vira-A), trifluridine (Viroptic), and acyclovir. Neonates with ocular involvement with HSV should also receive both a topical ophthalmic drug and parenteral acyclovir or other antiviral treatment. Orally administered acyclovir also has been used to treat dendritic keratitis, with effects that were similar to those achieved with topical acyclovir in the treatment of dendritic corneal ulceration. Several series suggest that oral acyclovir is therapeutic in patients who have stromal keratitis or keratouveitis.[247,368] When given in conjunction with topical antiviral therapy, the response to oral acyclovir is good, even in those who had failed topical therapy.[369] Oral therapy also is useful for prophylaxis against viral reactivation in those with stromal keratitis,[466] and prophylaxis is associated with decreased recurrence of corneal disease.[475]

HSV Encephalitis

Intravenous acyclovir is the drug of choice for HSV encephalitis.[452] For children 3 months to 12 years of age, 10 to 15 mg/kg per dose every 8 hours is recommended. For children older than 12 years of age and for adults, 10 mg/kg per dose every 8 hours is recommended.[192] Renal function and hydration status should both be monitored closely while the patient is receiving intravenous acyclovir. The recommended duration of therapy ranges from 14 to 21 days or longer and should be determined by clinical response and HSV DNA PCR levels in CSF. Neonates with any form of HSV infection, including encephalitis, should receive parenteral acyclovir until HSV DNA PCR assay of the CSF is negative. Thereafter, oral acyclovir suppressive therapy should be administered at a dose of 300 mg/m^2 per dose every 8 hours for 6 months, to improve neurodevelopmental outcomes and prevent skin recurrences.[214]

Two well-controlled clinical studies in Sweden and the United States that compared vidarabine with acyclovir 30 mg/kg per day in three divided doses for 10 to 12 days provided evidence that acyclovir is significantly more effective than vidarabine in treating HSV encephalitis.[375,453] In the Swedish study, the early mortality rate was 19% in the acyclovir-treated group and 50% in the vidarabine-treated group.[375] The National Institutes of Health collaborative study[453] generated similar data. As was observed in the earlier vidarabine studies,[464] younger age and less severe neurologic signs at initiation of therapy markedly influence the outcome of HSV encephalitis treated with acyclovir. Lethargic patients have a 15% mortality rate, whereas comatose patients have a 40% mortality rate.

In addition to antiviral therapy, intensive care is required for optimizing the outcome of these patients. Fluid management for the prevention of overhydration or underhydration is critical. Frequently, direct measurement of intracranial pressure is necessary for effective monitoring of increased pressure and treatment with diuretic agents. Anticonvulsant therapy for management of the often severe and prolonged seizures, as well as ventilatory support, usually is necessary at some time during the illness.

Genital HSV Infection

Recommended antiviral therapies for genital herpes simplex infection include acyclovir, famciclovir, and valacyclovir (Box 158.3), but acyclovir remains the best studied drug in children.[82,112] Although topical acyclovir was the first antiviral therapy used to treat genital herpes, it has been replaced by the oral agent. Some benefit was observed with the topical drug, but it is difficult to use, and its effectiveness is limited when compared with oral acyclovir; treatment decreased the mean duration of viral shedding (4.1 vs. 7.0 days with placebo) and time to crusting of lesions (7.1 vs. 10.5 days).[99] In the treatment of recurrent genital disease, topical acyclovir generally tended to have a minor effect on the duration of viral shedding (from 1–2 days in treated patients vs. 2–3 days in placebo recipients), with little or no effect on symptoms.[261,327] These results were not improved markedly with the immediate use of topical ointment. Early studies in which intravenous acyclovir was given to patients with primary genital HSV infection also were performed.[98,274] When used in a placebo-controlled, double-blind study at a dose of 5 mg/kg every 8 hours for 5 days, acyclovir decreased the duration of viral shedding (2 vs. 8 to 13 days in placebo-treated patients), shortened the duration of local and systemic symptoms by 2 to 5 days, and decreased the time to healing by 7 to 12 days. Complications such as extragenital lesions or urinary retention were reduced significantly.[307]

Oral acyclovir has therapeutic effects on both primary and recurrent HSV infection in adults and should be given to adolescents with these infections. The major effect of intravenous acyclovir therapy on the first episode of genital HSV infection is seen in those who have true

BOX 158.3 Recommended Treatment Regimens for Adults and Adolescents With Genital Herpes Simplex Virus Infection

First Clinical Episode

Acyclovir 400 mg orally 3 times a day for 7–10 days
or
Acyclovir 200 mg orally 5 times a day for 7–10 days
or
Famciclovir 250 mg orally 3 times a day for 7–10 days
or
Valacyclovir 1 g orally twice a day for 7–10 days

Suppressive Therapy

Acyclovir 400 mg orally twice a day
or
Famciclovir 250 mg orally twice a day
or
Valacyclovir 500 mg orally once a day
or
Valacyclovir 1 g orally once a day

Episodic Therapy[a]

Acyclovir 400 mg orally 3 times a day for 5 days
or
Famciclovir 125 mg orally twice a day for 5 days
or
Valacyclovir 500 mg orally twice a day for 3 days

[a]Additional dosing recommendations can be found in the guidelines referenced.

From Centers for Disease Control and Prevention: Sexually transmitted disease treatment guidelines 2010. *MMWR Recomm Rep.* 2010;59(RR-12);1–109.

primary disease, as opposed to those who have HSV-1 immunity and are experiencing new HSV-2 infection.[307] The intravenous route of administration has been replaced by oral therapy with acyclovir and related agents. In either case, optimal benefit requires early intervention. In a double-blind, placebo-controlled study of patients with primary genital infection, acyclovir at a dose of 200 mg five times per day for 5 to 10 days significantly reduced viral shedding (1–6 days vs. 13–15 days with placebo), lesion formation after 48 hours (0–4% vs. 43–44%), the duration of lesions (10–12 vs. 16–21 days), and the duration and severity of symptoms.[63] In similar studies of adult patients with recurrent genital HSV infection, acyclovir 200 mg five times per day for 5 days decreased the duration of virus shedding (1–2 vs. 2–4 days), time to healing (5–6 vs. 6–7 days), and development of new lesions (2–10% vs. 19–25%), especially when administered early in the recurrence.[293]

In these short-term studies in which patients were cautioned regarding hydration, no significant side effects were observed. Furthermore, no cytogenetic effects were noted.[91] Studies of virus from either placebo or acyclovir recipients showed that 4% to 15% of viruses isolated after therapy were more resistant to acyclovir, regardless of therapy.[92] Neither oral nor intravenous acyclovir reduces the rate of recurrence when used to treat either primary or recurrent genital infection. Oral antiviral agents are appropriate for patients who have primary genital HSV infection, HSV proctitis,[82,335] and frequent recurrent disease. Intravenous acyclovir should be reserved for patients who have severe local or disseminated disease with pneumonitis, hepatitis, or meningoencephalitis or complications such as urinary retention or aseptic meningitis syndrome.[82,307]

In adults, valacyclovir administered two times a day was as effective as acyclovir administered five times a day in the treatment of first-episode genital herpes.[136] When compared with placebo, valacyclovir is as effective as acyclovir in suppressing HSV viral replication as measured by culture and HSV PCR assay.[162] Similarly, famciclovir is efficacious in the treatment of first-episode and recurrent genital HSV infection.[12,341]

Symptomatic therapy for HSV lesions should be directed toward reduction of local discomfort, promotion of healing, and prevention of autoinoculation and superinfection. Nonspecific creams and ointments probably delay healing and increase risk for the development of maceration and infection. Keeping lesions clean and dry probably is the most important local measure. Urinating sometimes is painful and can be made less so if done in a bathtub or sitz bath. Some experts advise Burow solution sitz baths or short compress treatments. Prolonged soaking delays healing.

Mucocutaneous HSV Infection in Immunocompromised Hosts

Acyclovir and related drugs given orally or intravenously are the agents of choice for serious mucocutaneous HSV-1 or HSV-2 infection in high-risk hosts. Early initiation of treatment provides the best outcome. Given the limited oral bioavailability of acyclovir, higher plasma concentrations can be achieved with valacyclovir or famciclovir, but clinical experience with these drugs remains limited in children. If the infection is considered potentially life threatening, intravenous acyclovir is the treatment of choice. Therapeutic responses to HSV infection in immunocompromised hosts have been difficult to study because of the variable nature of the disease. The historical experience with vidarabine demonstrated the benefits of antiviral therapy initially. In a randomized, controlled, crossover study of mucocutaneous HSV infection, vidarabine 10 mg/kg per day intravenously in a 12-hour infusion was shown to decrease pain and induce defervescence in patients older than 40 years. In none of the 85 patients in this study did visceral dissemination of HSV develop. However, these observations are of historical interest now because the drug is not available and has been replaced by acyclovir. Acyclovir ointment appears to have some minor effects on pain, viral shedding, and time to complete healing of lesions in immunocompromised persons with mild, non-life-threatening mucocutaneous HSV infection,[461] but oral acyclovir is more effective for mild illness.

Patients with more severe illness should receive care in a hospital setting with the intravenous preparation. Intravenous acyclovir has been analyzed extensively in immunocompromised patients with mucocutaneous HSV infection.[143,334] When used early, acyclovir arrests the progression of infection. In several double-blind, placebo-controlled studies, acyclovir has been shown to be highly effective. It decreased the time to cessation

TABLE 158.2 Guidelines for Dosing Intervals of Acyclovir in Patients With Renal Impairment[a]

Creatinine Clearance (mL/min/1.7 M²)	Dose	Dosing Interval (H)
≥50	Normal	8
25–50	Normal	12
10–25	Normal	24
0–10	50% of normal	24

[a]A dose should be administered after each dialysis session in patients undergoing hemodialysis.

of new lesions (1 vs. 3 days with placebo), time to lesion crusting (3–7 vs. 9–14 days), time to lesion healing (12–14 vs. 18–28 days), cessation of pain (4–10 vs. 7–16 days), and termination of viral shedding (3 vs. 14–17 days).[433] Acyclovir administered intravenously is the most effective agent and the drug of choice for treating HSV in an immunocompromised host. The dosage is 250 mg/m^2 or 5 to 10 mg/kg per dose every 8 hours infused over a 1-hour period. In patients with severe disease, the dose may be doubled. The major toxic effect has been renal, with reversible obstructive nephropathy and transient rises in serum creatinine levels (5–10% of patients). Adequate hydration, keeping urine specific gravity measurements less than 1.010, usually prevents this problem. Dosage guidelines have been established in patients who have impaired renal function (Table 158.2). From 1% to 5% of patients may experience nausea and vomiting. Less commonly (1%), reversible neurologic symptoms (lethargy, agitation, tremor, disorientation, coma, transient hemiparesthesia) and laboratory abnormalities (abnormal EEG, increased CSF myelin basic protein) have developed in bone marrow transplant recipients. These patients usually had received interferon and CNS chemoprophylaxis for leukemia.[432] Other less serious problems include phlebitis (14%) and hives (5%).

Several studies have focused on the use of oral acyclovir in this patient population.[396] The IC_{50} of acyclovir generally is 0.1 to 0.5 μg/mL for HSV-1 and 0.5 to 2 μg/mL for HSV-2. Many studies use molar concentrations; in the case of acyclovir, the dose in micromoles divided by 4 equals the dose in micrograms per milliliter. Whereas peak serum levels with intravenous acyclovir vary from 8 to 15 μg/mL, the levels achieved with oral therapy are considerably lower (1 to 2 μg/mL). In preliminary studies of relatively small populations of immunocompromised adults, oral acyclovir at doses of 200 mg five times per day effectively promoted the healing of lesions and inhibited viral shedding.[396] Pediatric studies have used oral doses of 600 mg/m^2 given four times per day.[400] The relative efficacies of oral and intravenous acyclovir have not been compared in this setting. The choice of route of administration requires clinical judgment about the degree of immunosuppression, assessment for evidence of dissemination, and frequent reevaluation if oral drug is given.

Preliminary pharmacokinetic information regarding valacyclovir in immunocompromised children is available.[281] Valacyclovir was administered to 28 immunocompromised children aged 5 to 12 years in an open-label, randomized, dose-ranging study. Doses of valacyclovir administered were 250 or 500 mg twice a day or 500 mg three times a day. Pharmacokinetic evaluation has estimated that the bioavailability of oral valacyclovir is twofold to fourfold greater than that of oral acyclovir. The information provided in this study provides preliminary guidance for dosing of oral valacyclovir in children; however, more studies are needed to determine efficacy and safety in children. Recently published data regarding the pharmacokinetics of valacyclovir suspension in children suggest that valacyclovir oral suspension at doses of 10 and 20 mg/kg administered two to three times daily in children 3 months to 12 years of age produces drug levels similar to doses of 500 mg and 1000 mg caplets, respectively in adults.[212] Pharmacokinetics of famciclovir in children are also being evaluated with a recently proposed dosing scheme that awaits formal clinical evaluation.[45]

All studies of acyclovir in immunosuppressed patients have documented the propensity of recurrent lesions to reappear when therapy is withdrawn. Whether acyclovir reduces the humoral and cellular immune responses to HSV is not certain.[431]

Neonatal Herpes Simplex Virus Infection

Antiviral therapy for neonatal HSV disease significantly improves mortality rates and long-term outcomes of infected neonates. Historically, vidarabine was the first commercially available drug for the treatment of neonatal HSV disease. Placebo-controlled trials demonstrated that vidarabine at doses of 15 or 30 mg/kg per day given as a 12-hour infusion significantly reduced the mortality rate from 62% in historic cases and placebo controls to 35% in treated cases and increased the percentage of normal survivors from 19% to 43%. Results were best in infants with disseminated infection and disease localized to the CNS, with the mortality rate being reduced from 70% to 40% and the percentage of normal survivors increased from 10% to 30%. No difference was found between the 15 mg and the 30 mg dose in side effects, but the higher dose appeared to inhibit more effectively the progression of disease from skin-eye-mouth involvement to disseminated or CNS disease. None of the 49 treated patients had significant adverse clinical reactions or laboratory abnormalities attributable to the drug. On the negative side, 21% of infants progressed to more serious disease while receiving therapy and serious neurologic sequelae developed in 27% of the total. Fifteen percent of infants with disseminated or CNS disease continued to excrete HSV in the throat after 10 days of therapy.

The results of a vidarabine-acyclovir comparison trial in the treatment of neonatal herpes did not show any difference in efficacy and safety between the two drugs.[454] When the results with vidarabine and vidarabine-acyclovir were combined, the mortality rate was reduced from 49% in untreated historical controls to 17% in treated patients. Normal survivors increased from 26% to 67%. Although the results in the total group of patients were encouraging, the outcome in the group of patients with disseminated disease was not: a mortality rate of 54% in treated patients versus 76% in untreated historical controls and normal development in 59% of treated survivors versus 54% of controls. Factors that predicted mortality and their relative risk were as follows: disseminated disease, 33; CNS disease, 5.8; semicoma or coma, 5.2; disseminated intravascular coagulation, 3.8; prematurity, 3.7; and pneumonitis, 3.6.[455] Factors significantly associated with neurologic sequelae in survivors and their relative risk in these studies were as follows: skin-eye-mouth disease with three or more recurrent skin lesions after completion of acute therapy, 21; skin-eye-mouth disease caused by HSV-2, 14; HSV-2 infection, regardless of disease category, 4.9; CNS disease, 4.4; and seizures, 3.0. In infants with HSV disease limited to the skin, eye, or mouth, neonates with HSV-1 infection were all normal developmentally at 1 year of age as compared with 86% of those with HSV-2 infection. Among the latter infants, those with impaired neurologic outcome were significantly more likely to have had three or more skin recurrences in the first 6 months of life.

Because of greater ease of administration, intravenous acyclovir has supplanted vidarabine as the drug of choice for the treatment of neonatal HSV infection. Vidarabine no longer is available commercially. Because mortality and morbidity in neonates with HSV infection remained high using standard (30 mg/kg per day) dosing of acyclovir for 10 days, intermediate-dose (45 mg/kg per day) and high-dose (60 mg/kg per day) intravenous acyclovir for 21 days in 79 neonates was evaluated to treat neonatal HSV infection. Data were compared with those of a previous study in which all infants received standard doses of acyclovir (30 mg/kg per day) for 10 days. Overall, after stratification for disease category, the survival rate for patients treated with high-dose acyclovir was significantly higher than that for patients treated with the standard dose. Specifically, in neonates who received high-dose acyclovir, those with disseminated disease but not encephalitis had a significantly higher survival rate. The mortality rate at 24 months for patients with disseminated disease who received 21 days of high-dose acyclovir was 31%, compared with 57% for patients who received an intermediate dose for 21 days and 61% for those who received the standard dose for 10 days in the earlier study. For encephalitis, the mortality rate of infants at 24 months was 6% with high-dose acyclovir, 20% with the intermediate dose, and 19% with the standard dose. In addition, recipients of high-dose acyclovir had less morbidity than did historical control infants who received the standard dose of acyclovir. Patients treated with high-dose acyclovir were 6.6 times as likely to have normal development at 12 months of age. Among infants with encephalitis, however, 31% of high-dose acyclovir recipients were developing normally at 12 months compared with 29% of patients treated with the standard dose. With respect to toxicity in the high-dose acyclovir recipients, 21% had a transient neutropenia that resolved either during continuation of high-dose acyclovir or after its cessation. Nephrotoxicity occurred in four (6%) infants who had disseminated disease. Because acyclovir is eliminated by the kidneys, the dose should be adjusted for renal disease. High-dose acyclovir did not impede the development of an adequate antibody response to HSV in infected infants.

These studies have led to the current recommendation for the use of intravenous acyclovir at a dose of 60 mg/kg per day for a minimum of 21 days to treat neonatal CNS and disseminated HSV disease and a minimum for 14 days for skin-eye-mouth disease.[5] In addition, infants with ocular involvement should receive a topical ophthalmic drug (1–2% trifluridine, 1% idoxuridine, or 3% vidarabine), in addition to systemic acyclovir. Consultation with an ophthalmologist is also recommended to assist in the management of ocular HSV in the neonate, because corticosteroids and other medications may be indicated in some patients to preserve vision. All patients with HSV CNS infection should have a repeat lumbar puncture performed at the completion of acyclovir therapy to determine resolution of abnormal CSF parameters and to document whether the CSF specimen is HSV culture and/or HSV DNA PCR negative. A positive result from a CSF HSV PCR assay at the end of 21 days is an indication for continuing intravenous acyclovir therapy and, if clinically indicated, for performing repeat neuroimaging studies to evaluate the extent of CNS damage. Repeat samples of blood and CSF should be obtained weekly until HSV studies are negative.[191]

Concern has been raised that some infants may have progressive neurologic injury after acquiring neonatal herpes encephalitis. In addition, infants who have three or more skin recurrences with HSV-2 in the first 6 months of life have been shown to be at increased risk for having neurodevelopmental abnormalities at follow-up, whether as a consequence of previously undetected CNS infection or because of CNS dissemination during skin reactivation. Suppression of HSV skin reactivation by the administration of acyclovir (300 mg/m^2 per dose given orally three times daily) for 6 months is recommended.[5] Oral suppression for 6 months also improves neurodevelopmental outcome in neonates with all forms of HSV infection. The infant's blood cell counts should be monitored while receiving long-term oral acyclovir therapy because documented suppressive therapy resulted in neutropenia in 50% of treated infants. In addition, emergence of acyclovir-resistant HSV isolates has been documented. Acyclovir suppression also has been used after development of HSV eye infection in which reactivation might imperil vision.

General supportive measures, such as maintenance of fluid and electrolyte balance, correction of hypoglycemia, management of disseminated intravascular coagulation and shock, control of seizures with anticonvulsants, mechanical support of the respiratory system, nutritional support, and antimicrobial therapy for complicating bacterial infections, also are critical in improving the outcome for neonates with HSV infection. Because neonates with a disseminated form of HSV with hepatitis and hepatic necrosis may have secondary peritonitis and gram-negative bacteremia or sepsis, administration of antibiotics is also recommended. In severe cases of hepatic failure associated with neonatal disseminated HSV infection, liver transplantation has been effective treatment for some infants.[275,330]

Acyclovir-Resistant HSV Infection

Despite its widespread use, acyclovir remains an effective antiviral compound. In immunocompetent hosts, acyclovir resistance has been an unusual problem, even with prolonged courses of suppressive therapy. Mutant, thymidine kinase-negative virus strains have been recovered in 3% to 10% of patients treated with acyclovir, but acyclovir-resistant virus also can be recovered in placebo-treated patients, thus indicating that subpopulations of HSV are present in the lesions.[92] Thymidine kinase-negative HSV recurrences in immunocompromised patients have been documented well, with demonstration of the ability of these viruses to establish latency and recur. These viral mutants are less virulent in animal models. Patients who were culture positive for such mutants often have thymidine kinase-positive HSV isolates recovered from lesions during their next recurrence.[373]

Acyclovir-resistant virus occasionally has been shed by immunocompetent patients before, during, or after receiving therapy, yet it usually has not been associated with treatment failure.[161,226,248,397] In pretreatment patients, 3.6% of isolates (31 of 870) were resistant to acyclovir (not inhibited by 3 µg/mL). A similar percentage (3.1%) of resistant isolates was recovered from 663 immunocompetent patients after administration of acyclovir therapy.[92] An immunocompetent patient was reported who had an acyclovir-resistant virus containing an altered thymidine kinase that caused multiple recurrences of genital herpes unresponsive to acyclovir therapy.[226] In another immunocompetent patient receiving prophylactic acyclovir for recurrent genital herpes and long-term prednisone therapy for chronic urticaria, recurrent genital lesions with acyclovir- and penciclovir-resistant HSV-2 developed.[228] To date, these occurrences remain rare findings in the immunocompetent patient population. Acyclovir-resistant HSV has also been documented in neonates treated for HSV infection.[252]

Drug resistance occasionally is a problem in the acyclovir-treated immunocompromised population. Cases of acyclovir-resistant virus causing local invasive disease and, less commonly, dissemination and acyclovir-unresponsive meningoencephalitis have been reported.[143,146,258,344] Recurrences with acyclovir-resistant HSV-1 may be encountered, as described in a child with Wiskott-Aldrich syndrome.[348,349] Of the three mechanisms of altered sensitivity of HSV to acyclovir (absent thymidine kinase [TK$^?$], altered thymidine kinase [TK^A], and altered viral DNA polymerase), the TK$^?$ type is encountered in the vast majority of cases.[92,143,146] These viruses cannot phosphorylate acyclovir and convert it to the active triphosphate. Among bone marrow transplant recipients receiving multiple courses of acyclovir, acyclovir-resistant virus was recovered from 2% of patients during initial therapy and from 9% after treatment of a second recurrence. In a tertiary care center, acyclovir-resistant, clinically significant virus was recovered from 5% of immunocompromised patients (usually after receiving acyclovir) but not from any immunocompetent hosts.[130] Illness caused by acyclovir-resistant viruses was more severe in pediatric patients and occurred more commonly in very immunocompromised patients, such as those with AIDS or those who had undergone bone marrow transplantation.[131] Among bone marrow transplant recipients and patients with AIDS who were tested after receiving acyclovir therapy, 18% (105 of 582) had isolates that were acyclovir resistant.[92] In vitro viral susceptibility of HSV has been highly associated with clinical response to acyclovir in HIV-infected patients.[345] Acyclovir-resistant isolates are resistant to penciclovir and ganciclovir, which also require phosphorylation. Foscarnet has been used and is associated with successful clinical response and cessation of viral shedding. The most common side effects of foscarnet are nephrotoxicity (azotemia), alterations in serum calcium and phosphorus, and neutropenia, which has been observed in 10 to 25% of patients.[202,344] Foscarnet therapy is indicated for an immunocompromised patient who has HSV infection unresponsive to acyclovir. Viral susceptibility testing may aid in clinical management.[314,346]

In patients receiving chronic or multiple courses of foscarnet, foscarnet-resistant HSV isolates (IC_{50} >100 µg/mL) have been recovered from lesions failing to respond to foscarnet.[345,346] Of note, these lesions often responded to acyclovir, alone or in combination with foscarnet.[346] Perhaps the mutation in DNA polymerase responsible for foscarnet resistance was in an area not related to acyclovir activity. Other experimental strategies used to treat acyclovir-resistant viruses have included high-dose, continuous-infusion acyclovir (1.5 to 2.0 mg/kg per hour) or intravenous cidofovir,[61,130,237,377] although recent cases of cidofovir-resistant isolates have been reported.[470] In the case of acyclovir- and foscarnet-resistant viruses, topical 3-hydroxy-2-phosphonomethoxypropyl cytosine (HPMPC or cidofovir) or a combination of topical trifluorothymidine and interferon-α[42,343,348] has been used successfully in patients with chronic mucocutaneous lesions.

Prevention and Infection Control

Because HSV infection is ubiquitous in the human population and intermittent asymptomatic shedding is extremely common, preventing transmission of HSV is difficult. By diminishing the passage of infectious HSV-2, condoms offer moderate protection and should be recommended routinely.[266,436] Circumcised males are also less likely to acquire HSV-2 infection compared with uncircumcised controls.[414]

HSV is sensitive to heat and lipid solvents, so the use of antiseptics, soap and hot water, or chlorine decreases the risk for transfer of virus in settings such as the home, spas, pools, wrestling meets, and hospitals. In addition, appropriate use of gloves and other personal protective wear, by all health care personnel who come in contact with potentially infected body secretions or rashes should decrease the acquisition and health care–associated transmission of HSV. Health care workers with an active herpetic whitlow should wear gloves and not have direct patient care responsibilities for neonates and immunocompromised patients.[5] Health care workers with active oral herpes lesions should practice good hygiene and precautions, and reassignment to non–patient care areas should be made on an individual basis. Health care providers should wear gloves and wash carefully before and after contact with respiratory or genital tract secretions. Parents and caretakers of infants with eczema or severe diaper rash should be especially careful to avoid making direct or indirect contact of this altered skin with an active HSV lesion. Burn patients should be protected against exposure to or direct contact with personnel or visitors who have active HSV lesions. Immunosuppressed patients with evidence of HSV infection usually are experiencing reactivation of latent virus. Primary HSV infections in immunosuppressed persons, as in neonates, may be especially severe, and protecting these susceptible patients against exposure to HSV lesions is important. Wrestlers and rugby players who have exposed skin lesions caused by HSV should be excluded from competition.

The major approaches to the prevention of neonatal herpes involve interruption of transmission from sites of HSV infection and disease at the time of delivery and postnatally from a variety of potential sources. Because in utero transplacental congenital infection occurs so infrequently and predicting the occurrence of congenital infection during pregnancy is not possible, no standard recommendations for prophylaxis are available.

Cesarean delivery within 4 hours of rupture of fetal membranes in a mother with active genital herpes at the time of delivery is recommended to reduce the risk for natal infection. Because serial vaginal cultures taken during the latter stages of pregnancy have failed to predict shedding at the time of delivery, such monitoring is not recommended. Cesarean delivery is recommended only for women with active vesicular or ulcerative lesions at the time of delivery.[5] Cesarean delivery is not always 100% protective, even if the membranes are intact. Between 1.2% and 3% and, in one study, up to 33% of neonates with HSV infection are delivered by cesarean delivery. The cost-effectiveness of performing a cesarean delivery in women with recurrent lesions at delivery has been questioned by some experts, but it remains the current recommendation in the United States. Multiple clinical trials have shown that administration of prophylactic acyclovir and valacyclovir beginning at 36 weeks' gestation reduces the risk for clinically apparent HSV genital vesicles and ulcers at delivery, reduces the risk for HSV viral shedding at delivery, and also reduces the incidence of cesarean delivery. However, although the hope is that the risk for HSV disease in the neonate also would be reduced, in none of these studies was sufficient power or evidence available to determine the effect of peripartum prophylaxis on the incidence of neonatal HSV. No adverse effects have been seen in infants exposed to maternal acyclovir during pregnancy. Because fetal scalp electrode monitor, forceps, and maneuvers that might cause a break in the infant's skin during delivery appear to increase the risk for acquisition of neonatal HSV, they should be used only with clear indication and a careful assessment of the risk-to-benefit ratio.

The results of antenatal genital HSV cultures from pregnant women with a history of genital herpes do not predict the infant's risk for exposure to HSV at delivery. Because 60% to 80% of mothers of infants with neonatal herpes are asymptomatic or have unrecognized infection, the optimal approach may be to perform a screening test to identify women shedding or likely to shed HSV at the time of delivery. Although HSV rapid antigen-detection tests continue to be developed commercially, their sensitivity in *asymptomatic* women still is only 60% to 75%. Screening of pregnant women for non–type-specific HSV antibody would be confounded by the presence of HSV-1 antibody, which is present in 60% to 80% of the population. The presence of HSV-1 antibody probably represents oral herpes, which poses little risk to the neonate. Although type-specific antibody assays are available to identify pregnant women infected with HSV-2, such an approach would miss women with genital HSV-1 infection or those with asymptomatic primary HSV-2 infection near the time of delivery before antibody is detectable. Its use has been recommended in identifying discordant couples, that is, women with no history of having genital HSV infection but whose sexual partner has had previous infection, so barrier precautions may be used before delivery to decrease the chance of development of a maternal primary infection that poses a greater risk to her infant. Culturing the genital tract of women at the time of vaginal delivery would identify infants exposed to HSV and allow anticipatory management. However, because genital HSV infection rates are only 0.1% to 0.4%, this approach likely would not be practical or cost effective for *all* women. Culturing of *selected* women at delivery could focus on (1) positive or partner-discordant HSV-2 serologic tests, (2) those women with a history of genital herpes in themselves or their sexual partners, (3) those women with a history of another sexually transmitted disease or multiple sexual partners, and (4) mothers with a history of maternal fever in labor. However, routine or selective serologic screening, although recommended by some experts, is not currently a standard recommendation, and further investigation is required to determine whether screening of pregnant women to prevent neonatal herpes is beneficial, practical, and cost effective.

No studies have been conducted on the optimal management of asymptomatic infants exposed to maternal HSV infection at delivery, although guidelines on maternal and neonatal evaluation and prophylactic or anticipatory antiviral therapy are available.[211] A recently published algorithm for the evaluation of asymptomatic neonates following vaginal or cesarean delivery to women with active genital herpes lesions recommends the following approach:

1. Obstetricians who note a visible lesion should obtain a swab for HSV culture and HSV PCR and determine maternal history of genital HSV preceding pregnancy.
2. If there is a positive maternal history of prior genital HSV, HSV surface cultures and PCR, and blood PCR should be obtained from the asymptomatic infant at 24 hours of age. If the mother has recurrent infection, the risk of neonatal disease is probably less than 3% to 5%. Acyclovir does not need to be initiated if the infant remains asymptomatic. If the laboratory studies from the infant are negative, then the family is educated regarding signs and symptoms of neonatal HSV disease and the infant is followed closely. If any of the infant testing is positive, then further evaluation is performed and intravenous acyclovir is initiated.
3. If there is no maternal history of prior genital HSV, then it is recommended that type-specific serology for HSV-1 and HSV-2 antibodies be sent from the mother. At 24 hours of age, HSV surface cultures and HSV PCR, HSV blood PCR, CSF studies, and serum ALT should be obtained from the infant. Intravenous acyclovir at 60 mg/kg per dose in three divided doses is then initiated pending results of maternal serology. The duration of treatment is dependent on whether maternal lesion culture and PCR are positive and whether maternal serology reflects first episode primary, first episode nonprimary, or recurrent infection. If maternal serology is consistent with primary or first episode nonprimary infection at delivery, the neonatal infection rate may be as high as 30% to 50%.

It is recommended that this management algorithm be used only in facilities where access to PCR and type-specific serologic testing is readily available and turnaround time for test results is reasonably short. In addition, evaluation and treatment is indicated in any infant before 24 hours of age if signs and symptoms of HSV disease are present. Immediate evaluation and treatment may be considered if infant is preterm (≤37 weeks' gestation) or there was prolonged rupture of membranes (>4–6 hours). Situations that increase the risk for neonatal transmission despite maternal recurrent disease include prematurity, the use of a scalp electrode monitor, or skin lacerations. All infants should be monitored closely for any clinical evidence of HSV infection. Any positive culture or the occurrence of signs or symptoms suggesting HSV infection in the neonate suggests that a full virologic evaluation, including blood and CSF analysis for HSV by PCR, should be performed and antiviral therapy initiated. Antiviral therapy also should be administered to neonates with positive HSV cultures of mucosal sites, and these neonates should not be assessed as being merely colonized, because all require intravenous acyclovir therapy.[5] Breast-feeding is contraindicated only if the mother has a vesicular lesion on her breast. Physicians also have recommended that circumcision be delayed for 1 month in infants at highest risk for transmission.

Prevention of postnatally acquired neonatal infection needs to take into account the potential sources of HSV: (1) maternal oral herpes or breast lesions; (2) household member, such as father or sibling, or other close contact, such as grandparent or caretaker, with oral herpes or herpetic gingivostomatitis; and (3) health care–associated transmission from other infected infants or health care workers. Transmission to the neonate from family members with oral herpes lesions can be interrupted by education, avoidance of kissing and nuzzling of the neonate if they have oral herpes ulcers or history of "cold sores," and avoidance of touching the neonate if they have a herpetic skin lesion or whitlow, as well as common-sense personal hygiene, including hand washing. Health care–associated transmission can be reduced by contact isolation and hospital infection control measures, as well as universal precautions and good hand washing techniques. Personnel with herpetic whitlow should not have direct patient care responsibilities until the lesion has healed. Infants with HSV infection should be placed in contact isolation for the duration of the illness.[5] The median duration of viral shedding from skin vesicles and mucosal sites in infants receiving acyclovir is 5 to 8 days. Asymptomatic but high-risk infants born to mothers with herpes at delivery also should be in contact isolation; alternatively, they may room in with the mother in a private room.

Immunoprophylaxis and Chemoprophylaxis

The development of vaccines is a long-term objective that has significant potential to ameliorate the disease burden associated with HSV-1 and HSV-2.[15] However, to date, attempts to create effective HSV vaccines have met with limited success.[39,272,338,389] In one early report, a vaccine containing the recombinant glycoprotein D of HSV-2 (gD_2) was used in patients who had established recurrent genital herpes infections, and vaccine recipients had a third fewer genital herpes recurrences than those experienced by placebo recipients during the study year.[393] However, experience with the use of recombinant vaccines to prevent primary HSV infections has yielded mixed results. Recombinant HSV-2 gD_2 and gB_2 have been demonstrated to induce high humoral and cell-mediated immune responses in seronegative and seropositive recipients.[241] Some vaccines may protect women who have no HSV immunity at baseline.[389] In a study of discordant couples, an HSV-2 gD_2 subunit vaccine with alum and monophosphoryl lipid adjuvant was approximately 73% effective in preventing symptomatic genital HSV-2 disease in women who were seronegative for both HSV-1 and HSV-2.[391] However, when the same vaccine was given to 8323 women who were negative for antibodies to HSV-1 and HSV-2 in a randomized double-blind efficacy field trial, the vaccine was not efficacious, presumably owing to differences in the populations studied.[39] These studies illustrate that high levels of neutralizing antibody do not guarantee protection against infection. Other vaccine types in early stages of development include disabled infectious single-cycle virus vaccines, live genetically attenuated vaccines, and naked DNA.[389,463] No adequate controlled trials of high-dose intravenous immune globulin as an intervention to suppress frequently recurring genital herpes have been reported, and this method is not likely to be effective because infected patients have high titers of HSV-specific antibodies.[267]

Intramuscular human interferon-α administered before and after surgery on the trigeminal nerve root significantly decreased the incidence of HSV shedding and clinical reactivation.[306] In similar studies, interferon had no significant effect on HSV shedding or reactivation in renal transplant patients.[87]

Intravenous acyclovir has been shown to prevent reactivation of HSV almost completely in immunosuppressed patients receiving a bone marrow transplant or antileukemic chemotherapy.[354] In patients with bone marrow transplants, intravenous therapy is begun at the onset of immunosuppression and continued through the immediate transplant period, and then therapy is switched to oral acyclovir for several months.[151] Oral acyclovir administered chronically markedly suppressed recurrence in immunodeficient patients.[405] The use of prophylactic acyclovir is indicated in HSV-seropositive, immunosuppressed pediatric patients. Long-term use of suppressive prophylactic acyclovir appears to prevent the emergence of drug-resistant HSV disease in hematopoietic stem cell transplant recipients.[112,132]

Oral acyclovir 200 mg two to five times per day administered chronically can prevent reactivation of genital HSV nearly completely in patients with frequent recurrences. Recurrences decreased by 50% to 70%, and the time to recurrence changed from 14 to 25 days in patients receiving placebo to 100 to 125 days in those receiving acyclovir.[121,397] Breakthrough recurrences tended to be mild and to have less viral shedding and rarely were caused by acyclovir-resistant virus. When acyclovir was discontinued (after 12 to 15 weeks of administration), HSV recurrences reverted to the pretreatment frequency. Higher doses of acyclovir suppressed recurrences in patients experiencing a "breakthrough" with more conventional doses. In patients receiving therapy for 5 years, the number of recurrences declined from the first year (1.7) to the fifth year (0.8). From 20% to 25% of patients are recurrence free for 4 to 5 years.[152] After prophylactic therapy ended, suppressive therapy no longer was warranted in some patients because of longer periods between recurrences.[137,394] Patients who had resistant virus exhibited re-isolation of acyclovir-sensitive virus. Thus, acyclovir suppressed recurrences without eliminating latent virus. One study has reported that acyclovir does not seem to change the rate of asymptomatic viral shedding.[395] A subsequent study demonstrated that acyclovir 400 mg twice a day resulted in a 95% reduction in subclinical viral shedding when compared with placebo in women with genital herpes.[439] Side effects of chronic acyclovir therapy include an increase in mean corpuscular volume and hemoglobin concentration without anemia or megaloblastic changes, neutropenia and asthenia, and mild gastrointestinal upset.[397] Valacyclovir and famciclovir also can be used to suppress frequently recurring genital herpes effectively, and they suppress both symptomatic and asymptomatic HSV shedding.[111,162,340,438] Both drugs are more expensive than is acyclovir. The decision of whether to use episodic or suppressive therapy for individuals with recurrent genital HSV infection depends on the frequency of recurrences. Those with a recent primary infection and frequent recurrences may prefer long-term suppressive therapy. If episodic therapy is used, it should be initiated as soon as symptoms begin. Oral herpetic recurrences were prevented in skiers given a brief course of acyclovir during their ski trip.[383]

Chronic antiviral suppressive therapy with valacyclovir reduced genital HSV transmission in heterosexual HSV-2-discordant couples in one study.[100] Once-daily suppressive therapy with valacyclovir or placebo was given to the HSV-2-seropositive partner. Acquisition of HSV-2 occurred in four of 743 susceptible partners given valacyclovir and 16 of 741 susceptible partners given placebo (hazard ratio, 0.52). HSV was identified in genital secretions 2.9% of days in source partners receiving valacyclovir and 10.8% of days in placebo recipients. Use of condoms and abstinence during symptomatic outbreaks still are recommended. Use of HSV type-specific serologic testing to identify HSV-seropositive individuals and disclosure of HSV status, in combination with condom use, risk reduction counseling, and long-term suppressive antiviral therapy have the potential to control the spread of HSV-2 infection.[155,435] The US Preventive Services Task Force Recommendation Statement from 2016 however recommended against routine serologic screening for genital HSV-2 infection in asymptomatic adolescents and young adults because serologic screening results in many false positive results which may cause psychosocial harm and distress, and antiviral prophylaxis has not been shown in randomized clinical trials to prevent transmission of HSV-2.[135,424] The potential utility of antiviral therapy against herpes simplex however is being evaluated as a strategy for prevention of HIV infection.[76,77]

The role of antiviral therapy during pregnancy to prevent neonatal HSV infection is undergoing evaluation for safety and efficacy. In one randomized, blinded trial, women with recurrent genital HSV received either acyclovir, 400 mg three times a day, or placebo from 36 weeks' gestation until delivery. Genital lesions were present at delivery in 14% of women receiving placebo and 5% of women taking acyclovir (P = .08). A significant decrease in HSV culture and PCR positivity was noted in the acyclovir group near the time of delivery. No significant difference in delivery by cesarean section was found between the groups. Suppressive acyclovir treatment decreased but did not eliminate genital lesions or HSV viral detection at delivery.[445] Another randomized, placebo-controlled study evaluated the effect of daily valacyclovir suppression initiated at 36 weeks' gestation. Women receiving valacyclovir had fewer recurrences of genital HSV; however, valacyclovir suppression did not decrease the number of women who had viral shedding or lesions near delivery. A limited sample size may have contributed to failure to observe a significant difference in groups treated with drug versus placebo.[10] Neonatal HSV infection may still occur after maternal acyclovir suppression, as illustrated by a recently published case series.[313]

Experience with acyclovir prophylaxis for reactivation of HSV in children is limited. Prophylactic oral acyclovir 30 to 60 mg/kg per day in three to five doses for 1 week has been shown to decrease seroconversion effectively and to eradicate symptomatic cases of HSV gingivostomatitis in a nursery setting in which outbreaks of primary HSV infection were occurring.[233] Suppression, at doses of 300 mg/m^2 three times daily, has been effective in infants with frequent recurrences of HSV after neonatal HSV infection and has been safe, although prolonged use has been associated with reversible neutropenia. To date, prolonged suppressive therapy in adults has not resulted in serious side effects[137,152,394] or an increase in the problem of drug-resistant HSV in a healthy host.

NEW REFERENCES SINCE THE SEVENTH EDITION

13. Armangue T, Moris G, Cantarin-Extemera V, et al. Autoimmune post-herpes simplex encephalitis of adults and teenagers. *Neurology*. 2015;85(20):1736-1743.
26. Bache M, Andrei G, Bindl L, et al. Antiviral drug-resistance typing reveals compartmentalization and dynamics of acyclovir-resistant herpes simplex virus type-2 (HSV-2) in a case of neonatal herpes. *J Pediatric Infect Dis Soc*. 2014;3(2):e24-e27.
53. Brown JC. Herpes simplex virus latency: the DNA repair-centered pathway. *Adv Virol*. 2017;2017:7028194.
86. Chauhan N, Robinson J, Guillemaud J, El-Hakim H. Acute herpes simplex laryngotracheitis: report of two pediatric cases and review of the literature. *Int J Pediatr Otorhinolaryngol*. 2007;71(2):341-345.
88. Chen C, Su S, Huang Y. Herpetic gingivostomatitis with severe hepatitis in a previously healthy child. *J Microbiol Immunol Infect*. 2012;45:324-325.
135. Feltner C, Grodensky C, Ebel C, et al. Serologic screening for genital herpes: an updated evidence report and systematic review for the US preventive services task force. *JAMA*. 2016;316(23):2531-2543.
178. Henderson B, Kimberlin D, Fije S. Delayed recurrence of herpes simplex infection in the central nervous system after neonatal infection and completion of six months of suppressive therapy. *J Pediatric Infect Dis Soc*. 2017; [Epub ahead of print].
186. Huguen J, Fraitag S, Misery L, et al. Kaposi varicelliform eruption in a patient with epidermolysis bullosa simplex generalized severe. *JAAD Case Rep*. 2016;2(3):209-211.
190. Jaichnankar D, Shukla D. Genital herpes: insights into sexually transmitted infectious diseases. *Microb Cell*. 2016;3(9):438-450.
191. James SH, Kimberlin DW. Neonatal herpes simplex virus infection: epidemiology and treatment. *Clin Perinatol*. 2015;42(1):47-59.
193. Jaques D, Bagetakou S, L'Hullier A, et al. Herpes simplex encephalitis as a complication of neurosurgical procedures: report of 3 cases and review of the literature. *Virol J*. 2016;18:83.
196. Johansson AB, Rassart A, Blum D, et al. Lower-limb hypoplasia due to intra-uterine infection with herpes simplex virus type 2: possible confusion with intrauterine varicella-zoster syndrome. *Clin Infect Dis*. 2004;38:e57-e62.
209. Kim Y-S, Hyng K-H, Lee S-T, et al. Prognostic value of initial standard EEG and MRI in patients with herpes simplex encephalitis. *J Clin Neurol*. 2016;12(2):224-229.
211. Kimberlin DW, Baley J. Committee on Infectious Diseases, and Committee on Fetus and Newborn: Guidance on management of asymptomatic neonates born to women with active genital herpes lesions. *Pediatrics*. 2013;131:383-386.
263. Machin N, Morgan D, Turner A, et al. Neonatal herpes simplex 2 infection presenting with supraglottitis. *Arch Dis Child*. 2013;98(8):611-612.
271. Mean M, Schaller M, Asner S, et al. Thymoma, immunodeficiency, and herpes simplex virus infections. *Med Mal Infect*. 2009;39(5):344-347.
286. Nakamura Y, Nakajima H, Kano Y, et al. Herpes simplex virus type 2-associated recurrent aseptic meningitis (Mollaret's meningitis) with a recurrence after 11 year interval: a case report. *Rinsho Shinkeigaku*. 2016;56(11):785-787.

317. Poulikakos P, Sergi E, Margaritis A, et al. A case of recurrent benign lymphocytic (Mollaret's) meningitis and review of the literature. *J Infect Public Health.* 2010;3(4):192-195.
336. Rosain J, Froissart A, Estrangin E, et al. Severe acute pharyngotonsillitis due to herpes simplex virus type2 in a young woman. *J Clin Virol.* 2015;63:63-65.
355. Sarioglu B, Kose S, Saritas S, et al. Severe acute disseminated encephalomyelitis with clinical findings of transverse myelitis after herpes simplex virus infection. *J Child Neurol.* 2014;29(11):1519-1523.
424. US Preventive Services Task Force, Bibbins-Domingo K, Grossman DC, et al. Serologic screening for genital herpes infection: US Preventive Services Task force Recommendation statement. *JAMA.* 2016;316(23):2525-2530.
457. Whitley RJ, Corey L, Arvin A, et al. Changing presentation of herpes simplex infection in neonates. *J Infect Dis.* 1988;158:109.

The full reference list for this chapter is available at ExpertConsult.com.

159 Cytomegalovirus

Gail J. Harrison

Cytomegalovirus (CMV) is a ubiquitous agent that commonly infects persons of all ages from all parts of the world and from all socioeconomic and cultural backgrounds. Although most CMV infections are asymptomatic, certain patient groups are at risk for acquiring serious, even life-threatening illness. Discerning which role CMV is playing in a particular patient requires a thorough understanding of the epidemiology, virology, and pathophysiology of the virus and can be difficult, even for the most experienced clinicians.

HISTORY

The recorded history of CMV probably began when Ribbert[421] described in 1881 and then reported in 1904 "protozoan-like cells" in the organs of an infant who died of presumed congenital syphilis. In 1921, Goodpasture and Talbot[202] hypothesized that these swollen cells, or "cytomegalia," were host cells that had been injured by a virus. During the first half of the 20th century, CMV was recognizable only by the pathologic changes that it produced in infected cells; because these cells frequently were seen in the salivary glands of animals and humans, CMV originally was called the "salivary gland virus."

In 1956, human CMV was isolated in tissue culture by independent investigators Rowe and colleagues,[435] Smith,[461] and Weller and associates.[530] Because several human and animal viruses subsequently were found to replicate in salivary glands, the descriptive name *cytomegalovirus* was proposed by Weller in 1960. The ability to cultivate CMV in tissue culture led to the development of serologic techniques, which in the 1960s and 1970s resulted in many important clinical and epidemiologic observations. For example, CMV was found to infect people of all ages throughout the world. By 1962, CMV was established as a significant pathogen of the fetus and neonate that was capable of producing a spectrum of clinical manifestations and neurologic sequelae.[529] In 1966, Kaariainen and colleagues[259] presented evidence supporting CMV as a cause of posttransfusion mononucleosis syndrome.

The molecular biology of the virus was explored during the 1970s and 1980s and continues to be studied by many investigators. In addition, during the 1970s and 1980s, CMV emerged as a major cause of morbidity and mortality in immunosuppressed patients, especially those who underwent organ or marrow transplantation or who had acquired immunodeficiency syndrome (AIDS) or a congenital primary combined immune deficiency syndrome.

In 1976, the first clinical trial of the live, attenuated CMV vaccine Towne 125 was reported; since then, more than 500 renal allograft recipients, as well as healthy young men and women, have received the vaccine under investigational protocols.[177,388] In addition, research on a glycoprotein B subunit vaccine based on one of the glycoproteins of the virus began in the 1980s; and in the 1990s and the early part of the 21st century, other recombinant vaccines were developed and tested in human volunteers. Beginning in 2000, clinical trials with other vaccines, such as DNA vaccines, alphavirus replicon particles, and live, attenuated viral vaccines using chimeric viruses constructed from Towne strain and Toledo strain of CMV, were conducted.[13,490]

However, after decades of research, a successful CMV vaccine remains elusive. In 1999, the Institute of Medicine of the National Academy of Sciences assigned a high priority for a vaccine to prevent CMV infection, an action that was quickly endorsed in 2000 by the National Vaccine Advisory Committee, based on the lifetime costs to society and the human suffering associated with CMV disease in neonates and immunocompromised individuals.[29,267]

Attempts by clinicians to treat CMV disease began in the late 1960s and early 1970s,[167] and now CMV infection is a treatable disease; several specific and effective antiviral agents, including ganciclovir (licensed in 1989), foscarnet (licensed in 1991), and cidofovir (licensed in 1996), are available to clinicians to treat seriously ill patients.[83] In addition, valganciclovir, an oral form of ganciclovir available in tablets and solution, has facilitated long-term, outpatient treatment for CMV disease and CMV prophylaxis in immunocompromised pediatric patients and infants with congenital CMV infection.[273,380,510]

In 2000 to 2017, immunomodulating agents, such as CMV hyperimmune globulin and adoptive immunotherapies using CMV-specific cytotoxic T lymphocytes, have been evaluated in clinical trials as adjuncts to available antiviral therapies to prevent or treat CMV infection and disease in immunocompromised transplant recipients and in pregnant women to reduce risk for CMV transmission to the fetus.[193,257,408,419]

A resurgence of awareness of CMV from public health officials and the lay community began in 2004, providing hope that prevention and treatment of CMV disease may become a priority for research, education, and public health policy.[88] In 2013, the first groundbreaking CMV public health legislation was passed in Utah. This law, "Rule R398-4. Cytomegalovirus Public Education and Testing" [H.B. 81 (2013 General Session) UCA 26-10-10] directed the Utah Department of Health to create a public education program to inform pregnant women and women who may become pregnant about the occurrence of CMV, the transmission of CMV, the birth defects that are caused by CMV, methods of CMV diagnosis, and available preventative measures. This law also directs medical practitioners to test infants who fail newborn screening for congenital CMV and inform the parents about the possible birth defects caused by CMV.[142,549]

Since the Utah law passed, at least 6 states have enacted CMV laws that create public education programs for pregnant women or women who may become pregnant, or create targeted newborn testing programs for congenital CMV for newborns who fail their newborn hearing screens; 6 additional states have CMV legislation proposed, and an additional 12 states have CMV legislation in discussion.[549] In addition, evidence shows that universal newborn screening for congenital CMV may be cost effective, and the debate continues as more research unfolds about adding congenital CMV to the recommended uniform screening panel for newborn screening.[192]

VIROLOGY

CMV is a member of the Herpesviridae family of DNA viruses. This family contains many important human pathogens and is subdivided into three subfamilies: (1) Alphaherpesvirinae, fast-growing, cytolytic viruses that are latent in neurons and include herpes simplex virus (HSV) types 1 and 2 and varicella-zoster virus (VZV); (2) Betaherpesvirinae, slow-growing, cytomegalic viruses that contain the CMVs; and (3) Gammaherpesvirinae, herpesviruses that preferentially grow in lymphocytes and sometimes transform them into malignant states; this subfamily includes Epstein-Barr virus and human herpesviruses 6, 7, and 8.

CMV is the largest member of Herpesviridae. The genome is double-stranded DNA 240 kb in size (150 × 106 daltons; guanine + cytosine [G + C] content, 58%), and it has a unique long sequence and a unique short sequence, both of which are bounded by repetitive sequences that are inverted relative to each other. The genome, therefore, can assume four isomeric forms. The viral particle has a 110-nm icosahedral capsid composed of 162 capsomeres. The entire virion is enclosed by a lipid envelope, which yields a final diameter of approximately 200 nm.[484]

Replication of CMV is slow compared with that of HSV. Whereas it takes herpes simplex only 4 to 8 hours to produce infectious progeny virus, CMV requires at least 24 hours. The CMV genome is transcribed slowly in a regulated sequence; on the basis of the appearance of different classes of CMV-specific proteins, the replicative cycle can be divided into three periods: immediate-early, early, and late. The immediate-early period is defined as the first 4 hours after infection occurs. During this period, specific segments of the DNA genome undergo restricted transcription and certain regulatory proteins are produced that allow the virus to take control of host-cell macromolecular synthesis. The early period of replication begins after the immediate-early phase and persists for almost 20 hours. This period is characterized by replication of viral DNA, synthesis of infected cell proteins, and production of progeny virus. The late period usually is considered to occur 24 hours after infection develops. During this period, the structural components of the virus are produced, and infectious virus is released from the cell. Monoclonal antibodies against the various immediate-early, early, and late proteins produced by CMV have been used as rapid viral diagnostic tools. Cytomegalovirus entry into fibroblasts differs from entry into epithelial cells. CMV also spreads cell to cell and can induce syncytia. This cell-to-cell spread of CMV is sensitive to antibody inhibition in epithelial cells but not fibroblasts.[125]

CMV has no distinct serotypes. However, strain relatedness or differences can be determined by molecular analysis of viral DNA. Restriction enzyme analysis of DNA extracted from CMV isolates that are linked epidemiologically (e.g., serial isolates from the same person, mother-infant pairs, or family members experiencing temporally related CMV infections) shows identical or similar DNA fragment mapping patterns. This technique or modifications of this technique have been applied to the epidemiology of CMV in a variety of patients, such as transplant recipients, congenitally infected infants, and patients whose CMV was transmitted from person to person in hospitals, child care centers, and residences. Polymerase chain reaction (PCR) methodology has determined CMV genotypes exist, by showing differences in the a sequence, major immediate-early, glycoprotein B (gB or UL55), H (gH or UL75), N (gN or UL73), and UL144 regions of the viral genome.* The four gB genotypes (gB1, gB2, gB3, gB4) have been characterized, and although all genotypes cause congenital and acquired infections, studies suggest that adverse outcomes after CMV infection may be linked to infection with a specific gB genotype, but none has been conclusive. Infection with the CMV gB3 genotype appears to be associated more commonly with fatal infections in bone marrow transplant recipients and hearing loss in congenitally infected neonates, and CMV gB2 and gB4 genotypes appear to be more often fatal in patients with AIDS, in some studies.[42,190,404,548,555] Some studies have suggested neonates with gN-4 genotype may have higher risk for sequelae, whereas others have not confirmed this association.[239,383,384] Mixed gB genotype infections in transplant recipients may be associated with higher viral loads and delayed viral clearance.[314]

*References 42, 138, 213, 239, 241, 350, 383, 384.

Pregnant women, neonates with congenital CMV infection, healthy toddlers, and immunocompromised patients may also harbor more than one CMV genotype (gB, gH, or gN) and may have different genotypes in different compartments of the body.[141,213,335,350,434]

EPIDEMIOLOGY

Seroepidemiologic studies have shown that infection with CMV occurs commonly in all parts of the world and usually is inapparent.[26,54,278,513,519,565,525] However, the burden of CMV infection and severe disease may be increasing in certain high-risk groups, such as neonates and premature infants and older children and adults with immune deficiencies as well as transplant recipients.[386,452,492] The incidence of CMV infection does not appear to be seasonal. However, the prevalence of CMV immunoglobulin G (IgG) antibody is influenced by many factors, including the age, geographic location, cultural and socioeconomic status, race or ethnicity, and child-rearing practices of the group. For example, in developed countries such as the United Kingdom and the United States, the prevalence of CMV antibody is 40% to 60% in adult populations of middle to upper socioeconomic status and more than 80% in lower socioeconomic status groups.[210,478,564] CMV seroprevalence in the United States also may differ by race and ethnicity, with reports of 51% of non-Hispanic white individuals being CMV seropositive compared with 76% of non-Hispanic black individuals and 82% of Hispanic or Mexican Americans.[117,148,481] In contrast, in developing countries, 80% of children acquire CMV by the time they reach 3 years of age, and almost all persons have been infected by adulthood.[19,30,523] In countries with high HIV prevalence, CMV remains a common cofactor and an important pathogen in disease.[54] Studies on the age-related prevalence of infection with CMV in the United States suggest three periods of increased incidence of acquisition: early childhood, adolescence, and the childbearing years.[19,532,563]

Pregnancy

Between 45% and 100% of women of childbearing age will be CMV seropositive, depending on age, race, ethnicity, and geographic location.[92,295,405,406,525] Seroprevalence of CMV in women of childbearing age is higher usually in developing countries than in Europe or North America. In one study of US women of childbearing age, a higher CMV seroprevalence was associated with higher parity, with higher number of live births, younger age at first sexual intercourse, higher number of lifetime sexual partners, race/ethnicity of Hispanic origin, poverty index, and lower level of education.[295] Annual seroconversion rates among CMV-seronegative pregnant women vary between 1% and 7%, with an average of 2.3%.[241,254] Certain groups of women may be at higher risk for primary CMV infections. For example, women who work in child care centers have higher annualized seroconversion rates of 8% to 20%.[5] Women who have a toddler who attends child care and is actively excreting CMV at the time have been observed to have a 45% annualized seroconversion rate.[374] Although most CMV infections in pregnancy are asymptomatic, up to 50% of maternal CMV infections may have nonspecific clinical symptoms and only will be detected with specific serologic testing.[341] The risk for intrauterine transmission of CMV infection from mother to fetus during pregnancy appears to vary with type of maternal infection.[304,313] Maternal CMV infection that is either primary or recurrent during pregnancy can result in an infant who is infected congenitally with CMV. However, the rate of intrauterine infection with recurrent infection in the mother is less than 1%, whereas transmission to the fetus occurs in 32% to 50% of mothers who are infected primarily with CMV during pregnancy.[266,478] Naturally occurring immunity to CMV infection reduces the risk for congenital CMV infection in future pregnancies by at least 69%.[185] Symptoms and sequelae are also much more likely to occur in infants congenitally infected as a result of the mother's primary infection during pregnancy than in infants congenitally infected from a recurrent maternal infection.[221] However, even though symptoms are more likely in neonates congenitally infected as a result of a maternal primary infection, congenitally infected neonates from maternal recurrent CMV infections, resulting from reactivation of endogenous strain or reinfection with a new strain, may also experience long-term sequelae, including hearing loss and neurologic

BOX 159.1 Sources of Cytomegalovirus Infection

Congenital (acquired before birth from maternal source)
Perinatal (acquired at or around time of birth from maternal sources)
- Breast milk
- Cervicovaginal secretions

Postnatal (acquired after birth from nonmaternal sources)
- Blood product transfusions
- Organ transplantation
- Stem cell transplantation
- Person-to-person transmission (close contact such as sharing food or drink, kissing, sexual contact)

disease.[105] In one study from Finland, symptomatic congenital CMV infections were more commonly due to maternal nonprimary infection than proven maternal primary infections with CMV, and resulted in significant morbidity to the newborn.[398]

Congenital Infection

Approximately 1% of all neonates are born congenitally infected with CMV; ranges of 0.18% to 6.1% have been reported, varying between countries and the social demographics of the population.[266,313,560] Congenital infections arise from maternal source through vertical transmission (Box 159.1). Birth prevalence of congenital CMV infection is higher in developing countries than in Europe and North America in most studies because of the higher maternal CMV serologic seroprevalence ranging from 84% to 100% in developing countries.[293,525] An estimated 30,000 to 40,000 neonates with congenital CMV infection are born annually in the United States.[47,99,437] Less than 20% (estimated 5–15% in most studies) of children with congenital CMV infection show obvious clinical signs at birth, resulting in an estimated 8000 to 10,000 children annually in the United States who have long-term neurologic and sensory sequelae of hearing and vision disorders from congenital CMV disease.[516,296] Although most neonates congenitally infected with CMV do not have symptoms, up to 20% of apparently symptom-free neonates with congenital CMV have hearing loss by 18 years of age—either congenital hearing loss or later onset, progressive sensorineural hearing loss.[292]

Perinatal Infection

CMV can be transmitted perinatally from a mother to her infant[386] (see Box 159.1). The virus can be shed in the CMV-seropositive mother's cervicovaginal secretions, urine, saliva, and breast milk. The most common and most efficient routes of perinatal transmission are ingestion or aspiration of cervicovaginal secretions at the time of delivery or ingestion of fresh breast milk after delivery. CMV-seropositive mothers, especially mothers with high levels of CMV IgG antibody, frequently shed CMV in their breast milk; and as many as 53% of children who are breast-fed with milk that contains infectious virus or CMV DNA can become infected with CMV.[158,252,360,520] These infections usually are benign in full-term infants but may be extremely serious in preterm, very-low-birth-weight neonates, associated with prolonged hospitalization, bronchopulmonary dysplasia, and mortality rates of 9%.[265,291,318,518] In addition, as many as 57% of neonates whose mothers shed CMV at or around the time of delivery become infected with CMV.[420]

Postnatal Infection in Childhood

Children not congenitally or perinatally infected with CMV may be infected during the toddler or preschool years through person-to-person transmission[386] (see Box 159.1). The acquisition of CMV by children between 1 and 3 years of age is influenced by home exposure to the virus, by the socioeconomic status or country of origin of the family, and by group child care exposure.[91] Weller and Hanshaw[529] suggested that the child-rearing practices in Sweden, where group child care was common practice, accounted for the relatively high prevalence of CMV infection in Swedish children compared with children in the United States and Great Britain, where child care centers were not common at that time.

Pass and colleagues[370] first reported the prevalence of CMV in child care centers in the United States in 1982. They found that 51% of children who attended a child care center in Alabama excreted CMV in their saliva or urine. In this study, the prevalence of CMV excretion varied with age; 83% of children aged 13 to 24 months shed virus, as opposed to only 9% of children younger than 1 year old. Pass and colleagues concluded that the high prevalence of CMV infection probably was due to horizontal spread between the children in child care. Subsequent studies have confirmed a high prevalence of CMV excretion in children in child care centers across the United States. Overall prevalence rates of 11% to 57% have been observed in many other studies in the United States and other countries, with the highest prevalence of active CMV infection (29–78%) found in children 1 to 3 years of age.[4,255,340,354,355] Child care homes may have lower prevalence of CMV excretion in children (8–15%); however, CMV seroconversion in home child care providers appears similar to that of child care providers in larger centers.[43,370,373,372] Children who attend child care centers also shed high titers of virus (up to 10^5 median tissue culture infective dose per milliliter), with a mean duration of viral shedding of 13 months in urine and 7 months in saliva.[339] This prolonged, generally asymptomatic shedding of large quantities of virus, coupled with mobility and the less than hygienic daily habits notorious in toddlers, no doubt facilitates the transmission of CMV in child care centers.

Several studies support the idea that the high prevalence of CMV infection in young children who attend child care centers is due to horizontal transmission; these studies used molecular fingerprinting techniques to show that infected children in contact with each other shed strains of CMV with similar or identical restriction enzyme banding patterns and that predominant strains of CMV appeared to circulate during a given period in a given child care center.[5,4,238] Reinfection with a genetically different strain of CMV also has been observed and may be important in child-to-child transmission of CMV in the child care center environment.[9] The importance of horizontal spread of CMV has been shown in special care centers for mentally retarded children as well.[455] CMV also has been isolated from plastic toys and from the hands of child care center workers.[165,238,370]

CMV-infected children may transmit the virus to the child care center workers.[5,7] In addition, children who attend child care centers may transmit CMV to their CMV-seronegative parents. In one study of parents of children who attended one of three child care centers in Alabama, 14 of 67 parents (21%) whose children attended group child care seroconverted, compared with none of 31 parents whose children were cared for at home.[374] Excretion of CMV by the child clearly was a key risk factor for parental seroconversion because none of the seroconversions occurred in parents whose children attended the child care center but did not shed CMV. Moreover, this study revealed a strong trend toward a greater risk for acquiring CMV infection (seroconversion rate, 45%) in the parents of children 18 months or younger. Additional evidence implicating young children who attend child care centers as a source of CMV infection for their parents was provided by a study in Virginia child care centers, in which the parents of children in child care shed CMV strains identical to the strains shed by their children.[6] Furthermore, CMV strains from child care settings, when transmitted from toddlers to their pregnant mothers, may be the source of congenital infection.[340]

Whereas infancy, toddlerhood, and early childhood probably are the most rapid periods of acquisition of CMV, seroprevalence of CMV IgG antibody between 1 and 5 years of age has been estimated at 20% (range, 14–28%).[294] Annual seroconversion rates of 3% to 6.2% have been observed in older children aged 3 to 10 years in the United States and other countries, thus reflecting an age-related plateau in the acquisition of CMV. One identified risk factor for the acquisition of CMV infection in a school-aged child has been recent or active CMV infection in a family member.[117,140,148,481,482,563]

Infection in Adolescents

In support of these early findings, a seroepidemiologic study of CMV infection in sexually active adolescent girls found a strong association between indicators of sexual activity and serologic evidence of CMV infection and concluded that sexual activity is an important risk factor for the acquisition of CMV infection in adolescent girls.[103,468] Early cross-sectional epidemiologic studies of CMV implied that a gradual increase in CMV antibody prevalence occurs during the teenage years, and this period of rapid acquisition was attributed to the intimate physical contact that commonly occurs during the teenage years.[19,428] However, these studies were conducted primarily in lower socioeconomic groups. In a seroepidemiologic study of several groups in Houston, Texas, on the acquisition of CMV infection in late childhood and adolescence, the prevalence of antibody increased with age in subjects of nonwhite races, as it did according to previous studies, but the prevalence of antibody in white subjects did not increase with age.[532]

In one recent study, however, of sexually active African American adolescents, CMV infection as measured by CMV IgG seroprevalence was not associated with sexual activity (34% in sexually active adolescents compared with 21% in sexually inactive adolescents).[187]

Vertical transmission of CMV acquired during the teenage years may result in congenital infection with CMV in infants born to teenage mothers. In 1984, Kumar and colleagues[280] studied primary CMV infection in more than 3000 pregnant adolescents in Ohio. They found that 57% were CMV seropositive, that 1% of susceptible pregnant adolescents acquired CMV, and that the risk for intrauterine transmission was 50% if primary CMV infection occurred during pregnancy. Information provided by the National Congenital Cytomegalovirus Disease Registry and the National Center for Health Statistics suggests that adolescents who are pregnant actually may be at higher risk than are older mothers for giving birth to an infant with congenital CMV disease because 34% of mothers who give birth to an infant with congenital CMV disease are younger than 20 years old; however, this age group represents only 16% of the mothers giving birth in the United States.[132,243]

Intrafamilial Transmission

CMV also can be transmitted within the family setting. Evidence for intrafamilial transmission of CMV has been provided in the form of case reports, seroepidemiologic studies, and accounts in which molecular analysis of CMV strains was used to trace the transmission of CMV in family members or extended family members with temporally related CMV infections. In most studies, the index case was a child; when a CMV-infected child entered a household, attack rates were 47% to 53%.[494,502,556]

Three patterns of intrafamilial transmission have been observed: transmission between siblings, transmission between parents, and transmission between children and parents. Additional support for the intrafamilial transmission of CMV has been provided by published studies in which molecular analysis was performed on CMV isolates from family members or extended family members who experienced temporally related CMV infections. In each of these studies, restriction enzyme analysis of viral DNA from CMV isolates in family members showed that the strain of CMV was the same within each family.[156,375,476,556] New molecular techniques based on PCR amplification of a hypervariable region of the CMV genome also have corroborated the observation that genetically similar strains of CMV can be transmitted between family members over the course of time.[469]

Sexual Transmission

CMV also appears to be transmitted by heterosexual and homosexual contact. The evidence to support sexual transmission is anecdotal, virologic, serologic, and molecular and, taken together, suggests that sexual transmission of CMV is important in certain groups. However, because the virus is shed in saliva, cervicovaginal secretions, and semen, which form of intimate contact results in transmission between sex partners is unclear.[135,290,420]

Several observations support the idea that CMV can be transmitted sexually. For example, CMV antibody prevalence increases with age; CMV antibody is more prevalent in sexually active women than in celibate women; CMV antibody is associated with indices of sexual activity, such as recent infection with *Chlamydia trachomatis* or *Neisseria gonorrhoeae;* and a strikingly high annual incidence (37%) of primary CMV infection has been observed in young women with a recent first sexual experience.[104,116,130,184,256,468,482,539] In addition, in a longitudinal study of the site-specific shedding of CMV in human immunodeficiency virus (HIV)–seropositive homosexual and bisexual men, CMV was cultured from semen more frequently than from other body sites or fluids.[423] Moreover, molecular analysis of viral DNA has shown strains of CMV isolated from sex partners to be identical in most cases analyzed.[135,223]

Infection of the genital tract can recur by reactivation of an endogenous strain or by reinfection with an exogenous or different strain of CMV.[468] The consequences of such reinfections are unknown but may have important implications for transmission, especially if a CMV vaccine is used to control congenital CMV disease in the future. Sexual debut and recent sexual activity significantly influence CMV seroprevalence among women of childbearing age. In addition, engaging in sexual activity within 2 years of delivery of an infant adds increased risk for delivering a congenitally infected infant. Because sexual activity appears to influence CMV seroprevalence and congenital CMV infection rates in some groups, strategies to reduce sexual transmission of CMV may be important.[184,482]

Nosocomial Health Care–Related Transmission

CMV can be transmitted in the hospital setting by transfusion of blood products, by bone marrow and organ transplantation, and, rarely, by person-to-person transmission (see Box 159.1). Despite numerous studies that have used serologic, virologic, and molecular epidemiologic techniques, transmission of CMV from a CMV-infected patient to a health care worker has not been documented.[10,38,44,75,137,157,236] Therefore, even though health care workers are exposed to CMV-infected patients, their risk for acquiring CMV appears to be no greater than that of the general population. In addition, unlike homes and child care centers, hospitals routinely perform rigorous infection-control procedures, including universal precautions, which probably accounts for the relatively low risk for acquiring CMV as well as other infections in the hospital setting. However, infant-to-infant transmission has been shown to occur, albeit infrequently, in crowded hospital units with a high prevalence of CMV excretion in patients.[137,472] CMV also can survive on plastic surfaces and has been cultured from inanimate objects in contact with CMV-infected patients in the hospital setting.[137,472]

Blood products are a well-established source of CMV infection, and donor-to-recipient transmission of CMV has been documented by restriction enzyme analysis of viral DNA.[501] Posttransfusion CMV mononucleosis can be seen in adults who receive large volumes of fresh whole blood.[259] In addition, 15% to 17% of CMV-seronegative neonates who receive blood products from CMV-seropositive donors acquire CMV.[556,557] Posttransfusion CMV infection in neonates, especially premature infants, can cause a syndrome of shock, lymphocytosis, and pneumonitis; CMV infection also appears to hasten the progression to bronchopulmonary dysplasia in these patients.[442,557]

CMV apparently is transmitted in the residual leukocytes found in whole blood, packed red blood cells, and platelet fractions as well as by pure leukocyte transfusions. The risk for development of posttransfusion CMV infection is approximately 3% per unit transfused, and the risk for symptomatic infection is much higher in CMV-seronegative recipients than in CMV-seropositive recipients.

Extremely low-birth-weight infants in the neonatal intensive care unit have a risk for acquiring CMV infection when fed fresh or refrigerated breast milk from CMV-seropositive donors, and they may develop serious illness associated with the infection. CMV infection through breast milk may be reduced, but not eliminated, in these vulnerable neonates by feeding freeze-thawed breast milk, and likely can be prevented through pasteurization of breast milk.[561]

Immunosuppressed Patients

Primary and reactivation infections, as well as reinfection with CMV, occur commonly in children receiving anticancer chemotherapy,[222] in children who are solid organ and marrow transplant recipients, and in infants with primary immune deficiency syndromes that involve T-cell or natural killer (NK)-cell dysfunction, severe combined immunodeficiency (SCID), or acquired immune deficiency from HIV infection or AIDS.[222,521] The health care burden of severe CMV disease appears to be increasing in these special pediatric patient groups.[452] Active infection with CMV occurs in almost all organ and marrow transplant recipients and usually is manifested clinically and virologically 30 to 90 days after transplantation. Rarely, CMV retinitis can occur years after a patient has undergone transplantation and generally is associated with chronic CMV viremia.[173] CMV can be transmitted to the recipient by the transplanted organ, by transfused blood products, and, theoretically, also by intimate contact with persons actively infected with CMV.

Infections with CMV are primary when they occur in CMV-seronegative recipients who receive transplants or blood products from CMV-seropositive donors. Recipients who are CMV seropositive before undergoing transplantation can experience reactivation of their own endogenous strain of CMV. In addition, CMV-seropositive transplant recipients may be superinfected by strains of CMV present in the donor organ.[109] In fact, in one study of renal transplant recipients in the United Kingdom, proven superinfection with the donor's strain of CMV occurred more frequently than did proven reactivation of the recipient's strain of virus.[215] Although reactivation, reinfection, and primary CMV infection all can produce symptoms in immunosuppressed transplant recipients, primary CMV infections are much more likely to be severe and even fatal.[394]

The type of transplant also appears to influence the type of CMV disease expressed. For example, the most severe and lethal form of CMV interstitial pneumonitis is seen in bone marrow transplant recipients, especially those experiencing a graft-versus-host reaction. CMV pneumonia also is a common occurrence after heart, lung, or renal transplantation, and severe CMV hepatitis is a special problem after liver transplantation.[18]

The iatrogenic immunosuppression essential for graft maintenance probably is responsible for the common occurrence of reactivation infection after transplantation, as well as the increased incidence of severe and symptomatic infection seen after primary CMV infection in transplant recipients. Cytotoxic drugs such as cyclophosphamide and azathioprine, in addition to corticosteroids, have been associated with reactivation of latent CMV infection, and the addition of antilymphocyte globulin to an immunosuppressive regimen can increase the morbidity of CMV infections.[376] The use of cyclosporine as the primary immunosuppressive agent, even in conjunction with corticosteroids, does not appear to reduce the risk for acquiring CMV infection compared with a regimen of azathioprine and corticosteroids; however, it may decrease the incidence of severe, symptomatic CMV disease in some transplant recipients.[154] The use of OKT3 to treat rejection in certain transplant patients increases the risk for dissemination in those with primary CMV infection.[458]

The frequency and morbidity of CMV infection in patients with malignant neoplasms are not as high as in patients who have undergone marrow and organ transplantation; however, the use of chemotherapy, especially for leukemia, is associated with significant CMV disease, particularly pneumonitis and persistent fever with viral dissemination. CMV-seropositive patients receiving immunosuppressive therapy for connective tissue disease also can have significant reactivation infection with CMV.[149]

The progressive and profound immunosuppression in adults and children with AIDS also is associated with CMV infection and disease. Although the source of CMV infection in adults with AIDS most likely is heterosexual or homosexual contact, sources of CMV infection in young children with AIDS have not been determined. It is likely, however, that many of these infections are acquired from the mother, either congenitally or perinatally. Infants infected perinatally with HIV who also acquire CMV congenitally appear to be at significant risk for experiencing rapid progression of disease in the first 18 months of life, as well as debilitating neurologic disease.[150,279,451] Patients with AIDS also may be infected with multiple strains of CMV.[153,473]

Infants with primary immune deficiency syndromes involving T-cell or NK-cell function may have persistent CMV infection and progressive, life-threatening CMV disease. They often will have very high levels of CMV DNA levels by quantitative PCR in their blood or plasma, and present with hepatosplenomegaly, pneumonitis, colitis, retinitis, meningitis, thrombocytopenia, or elevated aminotransferase levels.[493] Because prompt diagnosis and management of possible underlying immune disorder and specific antiviral therapy against CMV are important in these patients, most centers will screen newborns with SCID for evidence of active CMV infection.[330]

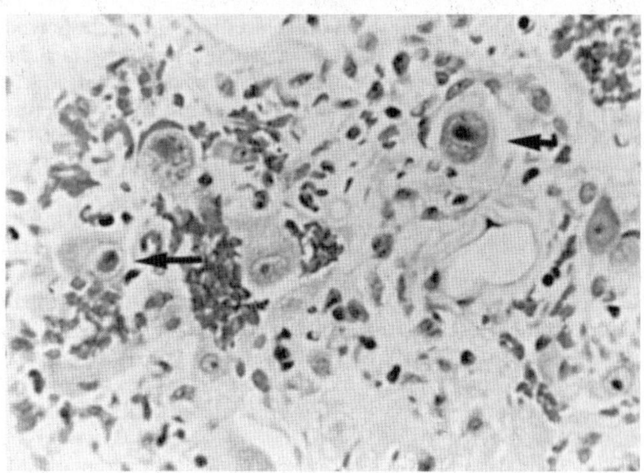

FIG. 159.1 Typical cytomegalic inclusion cells seen in lung tissue obtained by open-lung biopsy from a bone marrow transplant recipient with fatal cytomegalovirus pneumonitis (×640). (Courtesy Dr. Milton J. Finegold, Department of Pathology, Texas Children's Hospital, Houston.)

PATHOLOGY, PATHOGENESIS, AND IMMUNITY

CMV infection causes characteristic type A Cowdry intranuclear inclusions and massive enlargement of the affected cells (Fig. 159.1). It is this property of "cytomegaly" from which CMV acquired its name. The cytomegalic cells (25–40 µm in diameter) are two to four times larger than normal cells, and the nucleus usually is more than 10 µm in diameter. The intranuclear inclusion also is large (up to 10 µm in diameter) and is surrounded by an intranuclear halo and then the nuclear membrane, which gives a characteristic "owl's eye" appearance. Basophilic, granular, intracytoplasmic inclusions (2–4 µm in diameter) also may be present in cells that have intranuclear inclusions. These large cells represent productive virus infection, and both the nuclear and cytoplasmic inclusions contain viral nucleocapsids and express virus-specific antigens.[230] These cytomegalic cells frequently are associated with epithelial cells, and their presence generally indicates a productive and symptomatic infection with CMV. Cells also may be infected latently with CMV. These cells may express virus-specific antigen and contain viral nucleic acid without producing typical cytomegaly or a cytopathic effect. The significance of these cells must be considered carefully within the clinical context of the patient.

With severe, disseminated CMV disease, involvement can be seen in virtually all organ systems. The salivary glands frequently are infected in both symptomatic and asymptomatic infections, and the ductal epithelium usually is the site of pathologic involvement. The kidneys also are infected frequently in both symptomatic and asymptomatic CMV infection. In the kidneys, cytomegalic cells are most pronounced in the proximal tubules and interstitial cellular infiltrates, and even immune complex deposits can be seen in the glomeruli.

CMV infection often causes prolonged viruria, but it rarely results in significant renal dysfunction. Virions of CMV shed in urine have a reversible block to epithelial cell entry and may be highly resistant to antibody neutralization.[124] In the lungs, cytomegalic cells are seen in alveolar and bronchial epithelium and are associated with mononuclear cell inflammation. Pulmonary alveolar macrophages also may express viral antigen and contain CMV DNA. The brain parenchyma can be involved, and a variety of pathologic processes can be observed and include sensorineural hearing loss. Other organs that can be infected or diseased with CMV include the liver, pancreas, adrenals, eyes, lymph nodes, heart, skin, bone, male and female genital tracts, esophagus, stomach, intestine, and placenta.

Infections with CMV can be latent and nonproductive, productive yet asymptomatic, or productive and symptomatic. Therefore determination of whether a patient is "sick with CMV" or "sick from CMV" sometimes is difficult. Viral strain differences have not been shown to date to influence pathogenicity. However, immune responses, including maturity of the immune response, appear to be a major factor in virulence of the infection because CMV disease occurs more frequently in fetuses, premature neonates, transplant recipients, and patients with AIDS than in older healthy infants, children, and adults with acquired CMV infection.

The cell-mediated immune response, both specific and nonspecific, is thought to be important in host defense against CMV. The nonspecific immune mechanisms of NK cells and interferon production occur soon after the development of CMV infection, when early antigens are being produced and before infectious virus is released from the cell. The generation of cytotoxic T cells against CMV early antigens probably is the most important specific host immune response to CMV, and patients who are defective in this T-cell response are at high risk for acquiring serious CMV disease.[211]

Clinical and laboratory evidence also supports the concept of CMV as an immunosuppressive agent. The proliferative response of T cells to stimulation with mitogens and CMV antigen is suppressed in patients with CMV mononucleosis, and immunosuppressed patients with active CMV disease frequently have other opportunistic infections.[422] In addition, CMV pneumonitis in bone marrow transplant recipients has been hypothesized to result from host cell–mediated events produced in response to chronic viral replication.[566] Homology between certain CMV proteins and class I and class II major histocompatibility complex products has been observed. This "molecular mimicry" implies that the severe tissue destruction seen in CMV pneumonitis may be partly an autoimmune phenomenon in these patients.

Humoral immunity, on the other hand, although contributory, does not appear to be the key factor in the host's defense against CMV infection. For example, the fetus can be infected by intrauterine transmission as a result of reactivation of CMV infection in a woman who is CMV seropositive before pregnancy, and infants frequently are infected perinatally from infected cervicovaginal secretions or breast milk in the presence of passive maternal antibody.[478] In addition, CMV-seropositive transplant recipients can be reinfected with a new strain of CMV from the donor organ, and viruria and viremia occur in transplant recipients despite high titers of neutralizing antibody against the specific strain of CMV.[109,110] The presence of CMV antibody, therefore, should be considered a marker of previous or current infection with the virus rather than a measure of immunity per se.

Although humoral immunity does not appear to prevent infection with CMV, it does appear to lessen the severity of associated symptoms. Infants congenitally infected with CMV as a result of reactivation of infection in their mother almost always are asymptomatic, whereas perinatally infected infants rarely have significant symptoms. Primary infections in transplant recipients are more likely to be symptomatic than is reinfection or reactivation. One hypothesis regarding how CMV eludes host humoral defenses is that the virus binds to the host protein β_2-microglobulin and masks the antigenic determinants that are important for neutralization by antibody.[321]

CLINICAL MANIFESTATIONS

Fetal and Congenital Infections

The fetus with in utero CMV infection may show ultrasonographic abnormalities, including signs of abnormal somatic or head growth, enlarged liver or spleen, echogenic bowel patterns, and hepatic calcifications, as well as biologic findings such as fetal thrombocytopenia and lymphopenia and elevated liver enzymes and elevated CMV-specific IgM antibody levels. In addition, cerebral fetal ultrasonography may show enlarged ventricles in the fetal brain, intracranial calcifications, or microcephaly or mimic a Dandy-Walker malformation in severe cases.[35,217,307]

Annually, 30,000 to 40,000 infants are born with congenital CMV infection, and they may be symptomatic or asymptomatic at birth (Box 159.2). Of these infants, as many as 10% have severe, classical "cytomegalic inclusion disease," characterized by intrauterine growth retardation, jaundice, hepatosplenomegaly, thrombocytopenia with petechiae and purpura, pneumonia, and severe central nervous system (CNS) damage with microcephaly, intracerebral calcifications, chorioretinitis, and sensorineural hearing loss[296] (Box 159.3). Another 5% have atypical involvement, such as ventriculomegaly, periventricular leukomalacia, periventricular cystic malformations with or without calcifications, polymicrogyria, neuronal migration abnormalities, cerebral thrombosis, strabismus, optic atrophy, long bone osteitis characterized by fine vertical metaphyseal striations, isolated and transient thrombocytopenia and petechiae, cutaneous vasculitis, hemolytic anemia, ascites, chronic hepatitis, and intrahepatic cholestatic disease.[20,32,114,176,250,354] Newborns with congenital CMV infection may also exhibit a primary neurophenotype, presenting with microcephaly, neonatal seizures, and abnormal brain imaging, without the somatic manifestations of classic congenital CMV disease in other organs. Fetal brain disruption sequence (FBDS), also associated with congenital Zika virus syndrome and genetic disorders, can be seen in rare cases associated with congenital CMV disease of the CNS (Fig. 159.2). Brain involvement in these other asymptomatic infants includes polymicrogyria and other cortical maldevelopment syndromes and migration disorders of the developing brain, and neurologic sequelae are common (Fig. 159.3). As many as

BOX 159.2 Categories of Congenital Cytomegalovirus (CMV) Infection

Asymptomatic at Birth

Asymptomatic with normal hearing at birth
Asymptomatic with congenital sensorineural hearing loss (unilateral or bilateral) at birth
Asymptomatic with normal hearing at birth, with later-onset sensorineural hearing loss

Symptomatic at Birth

Classic "cytomegalic inclusion disease"
Symptomatic congenital CMV infection
Primary neurophenotype congenital CMV infection

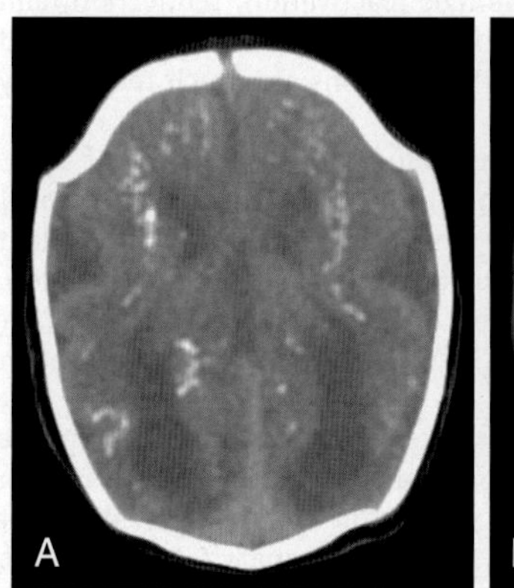

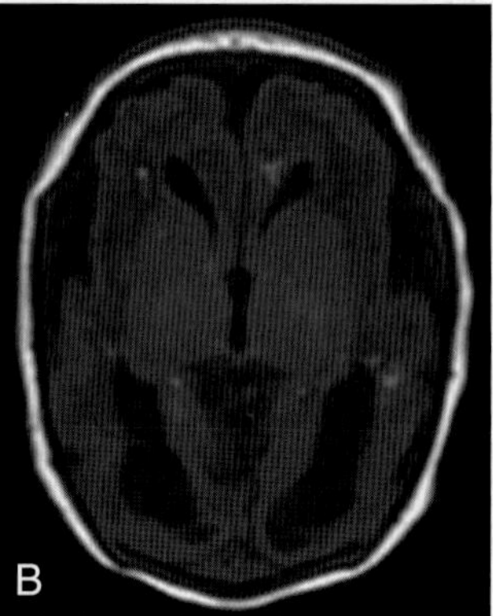

FIG. 159.2 Congenital CMV, virologically confirmed on day 1 of life, with primary neurophenotype presentation including developmental brain malformation compatible with fetal brain disruption or fetal brain arrest syndrome. (A) Computed tomography scan with unenhanced noncontrast and (B) magnetic resonance image of brain of newborn showing severe simplification of the supratentorial gyral pattern with diffiuse polymicrogyria, multiple punctate areas of periventricular calcifications, prominence of the ventricles, and cerebral volume loss. Also present on imaging was mild atrophy of the brainstem and left cerebellar hemisphere, and an abnormal corpus callosum, with a decreased craniofacial ratio compatible with the clinical finding of microcephaly. Diagnosis was suspected prenatally, when routine anatomy scan at 20 weeks' gestation showed abnormalities in the fetus and maternal serologies showed evidence of a primary cytomegalovirus infection. The baby was born at term, 38 weeks' gestation, and had profound microcephaly (head circumference, 29.5 cm), overlapping sutures, and scalp rugae. As an infant, the patient later exhibited seizures, strabismus, sensorineural hearing loss, cortical vision impairment, cerebral palsy, and severe global developmental delay.

BOX 159.3 Clinical, Laboratory, and Brain Imaging Findings Associated With Symptomatic Congenital Cytomegalovirus (CMV) Infection

Clinical Findings

Small for gestational age
Jaundice at birth
Petechiae or purpura
Hepatosplenomegaly
Ascites
Mycarditis
Enterocolitis
Lethargy and poor sucking ability
Hypotonia
Viral sepsis syndrome
Hemophagocytic lymphohistiocytosis syndrome
Pneumonitis
Chorioretinitis, optic atrophy, cortical vision impairments, delayed vision maturation
Seizures
Hemolytic anemia
Microcephaly
Fetal brain sequence disruption or arrest syndrome (extreme microcephaly, overriding sutures, flattened cranium, and scalp rugae)
Sensorineural hearing loss (unilateral or bilateral)

Laboratory Findings

Thrombocytopenia
Elevated liver transaminases
Elevated direct and indirect serum bilirubin
Hemolytic anemia
Neutropenia
Lymphopenia
Lymphocytosis
Leukemoid reaction
Elevated CSF protein levels
CMV detected by polymerase chain reaction or culture in saliva, urine, blood, or CSF
CMV immunoglobulin M antibody elevation

Brain Imaging Findings

Microcephaly
Intracranial calcifications (periventricular most common location)
Ventriculomegaly
Ventricular septations or adhesions
Periventricular leukomalacia
Periventricular cystic abnormalities/malformations
Lenticulostriate vasculopathy
Migration abnormalities (unilateral or bilateral polymicrogyria, pachygyria, lissencephaly)
Vasculitis or stroke
Cerebral atrophy
Dysgenesis of corpus callosum
Cerebellar hypoplasia
Fetal brain sequence disruption or arrest syndrome

CSF, Cerebrospinal fluid.

90% of these infants who are symptomatic at birth with classic somatic manifestations also later may have neurologic sequelae, vision loss, or progressive deafness. However, the range of severity of these sequelae appears to be broad, and severity may be predicted by head circumference, prenatal fetal and postnatal neonatal head ultrasound, and computed tomography (CT) and magnetic resonance imaging (MRI) findings in

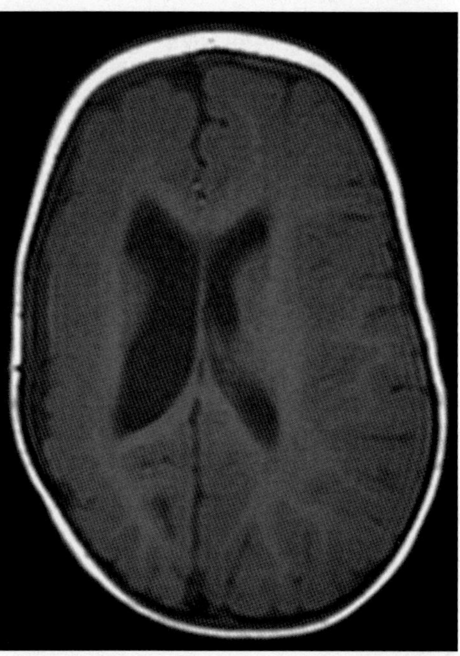

FIG. 159.3 Congenital cytomegalovirus (CMV) with primary neurophenotype presenting with microcephaly, left hemiparesis, left sensorineural hearing loss, and seizures. Magnetic resonance imaging of brain shows abnormal right cerebral hemisphere, smaller than the left, with cortical polymicrogria of the right frontal, temporal, and parietal lobes; volume loss of cerebral white matter; enlargement of the right lateral ventricle; and small right brainstem. The cerebellum and corpus callosum appeared normal. Newborn was born premature at 36 weeks' gestation, with mild microcephaly. Diagnosis of congenital CMV was not suspected until later in infancy, when microcephaly was apparent, and was confirmed retrospectively by detection of CMV DNA by polymerase chain reaction on newborn screening dried blood spots, retrieved with parental permission from the state newborn screening laboratory.

the fetus prenatally and in the newborn at birth.[33,70,89,352,362] In addition, CMV viremia and high levels of CMV DNA by PCR analysis in the blood or plasma in congenitally infected neonates is associated with symptomatic disease and hearing loss at birth. Development of hearing loss in newborns with asymptomatic congenital CMV infection has been associated with CMV DNAemia levels higher than 17,000 copies/mL.[179] These studies suggest that the level of virus contributes to disease severity in some newborns with congenital CMV.[69,74]

The differential diagnosis of symptomatic congenital CMV disease includes congenital Zika virus syndrome, congenital toxoplasmosis, congenital HSV infection, congenital syphilis, congenital rubella syndrome, congenital infection with lymphocytic choriomeningitis virus, and congenital HIV infection (Box 159.4). In addition, noninfectious causes, such as genetic disorders, metabolic disease, and maternal exposure to drugs and toxins, should be considered.

Most infants who are infected congenitally with CMV are asymptomatic at birth (see Box 159.2). However, 10% to 17% of these infants later may have unilateral or bilateral deafness at birth or develop later differences in higher-level auditory function.[118,478,538] Progressive or late-onset hearing loss also may occur in these infants, with up to 20% of children born with asymptomatic congenital CMV infection by 18 years of age having hearing loss, and with 2% of them with severe hearing loss requiring cochlear implant devices.[292] It is therefore likely that universal neonatal hearing screening programs, even if paired with targeted testing for congenital CMV infection, will miss rather than detect many of these children.[181,292,353] Small retinal lesions may occur as well in children born with asymptomatic congenital CMV infection, but they are rarely sight threatening.[114,253] Earlier studies suggested that developmental problems may occur in asymptomatically infected children, but more recent studies suggest that cognitive outcome, at least as measured by intelligence quotients and achievement testing, appears to be normal compared with uninfected children.[263]

BOX 159.4 Differential Diagnosis of Symptomatic Congenital Cytomegalovirus Infection, Including Isolated Neurophenotype

Other Congenital and Neonatal Viral Infections

- Zika virus
- Herpes simplex virus
- Rubella virus
- HIV
- Lymphocytic choriomeningitis virus
- Hepatitis A, B, or C
- Epstein-Barr virus (rare)
- Enterovirus
- Adenovirus
- Congenital toxoplasmosis
- Neonatal bacterial sepsis

Genetic and Metabolic Disorders

- Tuberous sclerosis
- Sturge-Weber syndrome
- Galactosemia
- Urea cycle deficiencies
- Organic acidemias
- Lysosomal storage disorders
- Peroxisomal disorders

In Utero Toxin or Drug Exposure

- Fetal alcohol syndrome
- Cocaine and other substance abuse
- Isotretinoin (oral)

Other Conditions

- Biliary atresia
- α^1-Antitrypsin deficiency
- Ischemia
- Venous thrombosis
- Hemophagocytic lymphohistiocytosis syndrome

Very-low-birth-weight infants who are infected congenitally with CMV may experience pulmonary and systemic deterioration temporally associated with corticosteroid therapy.[506]

Neonates and infants younger than 6 months with persistently high levels of CMV viremia or high levels of CMV DNA by PCR analysis in the blood or plasma, or infants who have significant rebound of their CMV DNA levels after antiviral treatment, may have a primary immune disorder of T-cell function, such as SCID, or a disorder of NK-cell function. Prompt diagnosis and management of the underlying immune disorder, as well as specific antiviral therapy against CMV, are important in these patients.

Perinatal Infections

Perinatally acquired infections in healthy infants usually manifest when the child is between 4 and 16 weeks of age, but most such infections are asymptomatic. However, as many as one third of infants exposed to CMV perinatally may have signs and symptoms of disease associated with CMV infection, most often self-limited lymphadenopathy, hepatosplenomegaly, hepatitis, or pneumonitis.[282] Perinatally acquired infection with CMV also can cause a viral, sepsis-like syndrome or severe, protracted pneumonitis that has been associated with the development of bronchopulmonary dysplasia in premature infants.[318,442] A limited number of studies suggest that these infections, however, do not appear to cause neurodevelopmental sequelae or deafness.[283] Infants with primary immune deficiency of T-cell or NK-cell function, or AIDS from perinatally acquired HIV infection, who acquire CMV perinatally may have CMV viremia, high levels of CMV DNA by PCR analysis in blood or plasma, and associated hepatosplenomegaly, thrombocytopenia, viral sepsis, pneumonia, retinitis, meningitis, or colitis. Prompt diagnosis of an underlying primary immune disorder, as well as antiviral therapy, is life-saving management in these patients. The differential diagnosis includes other perinatally acquired infections, such as *Chlamydia* pneumonitis, hepatitis B virus infection, and infection with HIV, as well as postnatally acquired infections with enteroviruses, adenovirus, and a variety of bacterial pathogens.

Mononucleosis Syndrome

CMV-induced mononucleosis occurs as a primary infection in both immunocompetent and immunosuppressed persons, in pregnant women, and, occasionally, as a reactivation infection in immunosuppressed patients.[304] It can result from person-to-person transmission of the virus as well as from transmission by blood products or by organ or marrow transplantation. Although originally described in adults and most often occurring in patients between 20 and 40 years of age, it also can be seen in adolescents, children, and even infants.[312,368] Typical CMV-induced mononucleosis is characterized by fever and strikingly severe malaise of 1 to 4 weeks' duration, peripheral lymphocytosis with atypical lymphocytes, and mildly elevated liver enzymes. In some patients, headache, myalgia, and abdominal pain with diarrhea are prominent symptoms. In premature infants with transfusion-acquired CMV mononucleosis, prominent manifestations include shock, hepatosplenomegaly, pneumonitis, thrombocytopenia, and renal failure.[472] In contrast to Epstein-Barr virus–induced mononucleosis, CMV-induced mononucleosis rarely causes pharyngitis, tonsillitis, or significant splenomegaly, and it does not result in production of heterophil antibodies.[115,237] However, like Epstein-Barr virus–induced mononucleosis, it can be associated with morbilliform rash after administration of ampicillin, elevated erythrocyte sedimentation rate, polyclonal hypergammaglobulinemia, and production of other antibodies such as rheumatoid factor, cold agglutinins, and antinuclear antibodies. Complications rarely occur but include interstitial pneumonitis, myocarditis, pericarditis, hemolytic anemia, thrombocytopenia with or without petechiae or purpura, hemophagocytic syndrome, arthralgias and arthritis, maculopapular rashes, adrenal insufficiency, splenic infarction, ulcerative colitis and proctitis, Guillain-Barré syndrome, and meningoencephalitis.[102,115,127,172,237,276,277,303] Severe, icteric hepatitis and granulomatous hepatitis also can occur, but hepatic necrosis and liver failure caused by CMV have not been documented convincingly in normal hosts.[67,115,237,277,415]

The differential diagnosis of CMV-induced mononucleosis includes mononucleosis induced by other viruses such as Epstein-Barr virus, hepatitis A or B virus, and HIV. In addition, acquired toxoplasmosis can produce a mononucleosis syndrome in healthy persons.

Interstitial Pneumonitis

CMV is a major cause of interstitial pneumonia in both adults and children who are immunosuppressed because of congenital primary immunodeficiency of T-cell or NK-cell function, AIDS, organ or marrow transplantation, or malignant disease. In recipients of bone marrow transplants, CMV accounts for 17% to 70% of cases of interstitial pneumonitis in adult patients but only 10% of cases in patients younger than 21 years.[528,529] Pneumonia also can occur in apparently immunocompetent young infants with perinatally acquired CMV infection and in healthy children, adolescents, and adults with CMV-induced mononucleosis.[269,282,477,534] Whereas the pneumonia in immunocompetent hosts almost always is benign and self-limited, CMV pneumonia in immunosuppressed patients is a serious, often fatal illness, especially in bone marrow transplant recipients, who have a mortality rate of up to 90%. It also can be particularly troublesome after pediatric heart and lung transplantation.[351] CMV pneumonitis usually occurs 1 to 3 months after the patient has undergone transplantation and begins with symptoms of fever and a dry, nonproductive cough. It then can progress during the course of 1 to 2 weeks to dyspnea, retractions, wheezing, and hypoxia, which require ventilatory support. It may occur as the only disease manifestation or be part of a disseminated CMV infection. The radiographic appearance of CMV pneumonia usually is diffuse, interstitial infiltrates, but peribronchial infiltrates with hyperinflation and nodular pulmonary infiltrates also have been described

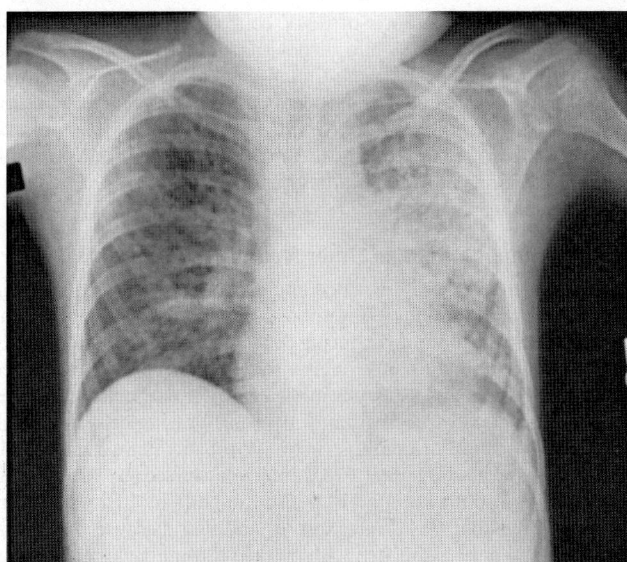

FIG. 159.4 Chest radiograph of a bone marrow transplant recipient with rapidly fatal cytomegalovirus pneumonitis. An open-lung biopsy specimen showed numerous cytomegalic inclusion cells, exhibited cytomegalovirus early antigens by immunoperoxidase staining, and grew cytomegalovirus after inoculation into tissue culture.

(Fig. 159.4).[269,496] Unusual central peribronchial patterns with organizing pneumonia that results in bronchiectasis and chronic lung damage have also been reported with CMV pneumonia in patients who received T-cell–depleted allogeneic stem cell transplantation.[123] Coinfection with other pathogens, especially gram-negative enteric bacteria and fungal pathogens in transplant recipients and in patients with *Pneumocystis jiroveci* infection and AIDS, can occur.[524] A quantitative assessment of CMV DNA viral load in bronchoalveolar lavage (BAL) specimens may be helpful in providing circumstantial evidence that CMV pneumonitis is present.[240]

Congenitally infected infants also may be born with CMV pneumonitis, which often is sufficiently severe to require ventilatory support and usually is part of a multisystemic CMV disease process. Very low-birth-weight infants who are infected congenitally with CMV may experience CMV pneumonitis in temporal association with corticosteroid therapy.[506]

The differential diagnosis of CMV pneumonitis in immunocompromised patients, including neonates, is extensive. It includes infection with other viruses, such as HSV, VZV, measles virus, respiratory syncytial virus, influenza A and B viruses, parainfluenza viruses, and adenoviruses; bacterial pneumonia caused by a variety of gram-positive and gram-negative organisms; infection with protozoa, such as *P. jiroveci* and *Toxoplasma gondii;* infection with *Chlamydia* and *Mycoplasma;* and fungal pneumonia, caused especially by *Candida* and *Aspergillus.* Noninfectious causes of pneumonitis, such as pulmonary hemorrhage, aspiration pneumonia, rejection, and pulmonary damage from chemotherapeutic agents, also should be considered.

Retinitis and Other Eye Abnormalities

Chorioretinitis as well as optic atrophy, cortical visual impairment (also called cortical blindness), and strabismus occur in 17% to 41% of neonates with symptomatic congenital CMV infection and rarely in children born with asymptomatic congenital CMV infection.[68,114,253,296,437] Although most retinal lesions in congenitally infected infants appear to be inactive at birth, some observations suggest that progression of preexisting lesions and late-onset new lesions resulting in vision loss may occur rarely in both symptomatic and asymptomatic congenitally infected infants.[68,119] Retinitis does not seem to be a prominent part of perinatally or early postnatally acquired infection in immunologically normal infants but has been rarely reported to occur.[283,382] Infants with primary immune disorders involving T-cell or NK-cell dysfunction, on the other hand, often have CMV viremia, usually at persistently high titers, and CMV retinitis, which may be severe and necrotizing.[363] CMV retinitis historically was a rare manifestation of CMV disease in solid-organ transplant recipients undergoing chronic immunosuppression for more than a year and in patients receiving chemotherapy for malignant disease.[173] In the 1980s, CMV retinitis emerged as a frequent manifestation of CMV disease in patients with severe immunosuppression, especially bone marrow transplant recipients and patients with AIDS. It probably is a result of hematogenous spread of the virus to the retina, with continued local viral replication. Despite the common occurrence of CMV retinitis in adults with AIDS, however, it is not often reported in children with AIDS.[306]

CMV produces characteristic white, perivascular infiltrates and hemorrhage, with a necrotic, rapidly progressive retinitis. It descriptively has been called "cottage cheese" retinitis and "ketchup" or "brushfire" retinitis.[64] Early, peripheral retinitis can be asymptomatic, or the complaints may be minimal and nonspecific; it is especially difficult to ascertain in infants and young children. It does not cause eye pain, photophobia, or conjunctivitis. When the retinitis has progressed, it can cause blurred vision, decreased visual acuity, visual field defects, and blindness. Young children and infants who have suffered visual loss as a result of CMV retinitis may exhibit strabismus or failure to fix and follow objects within their visual field. CMV retinitis also can progress rapidly to total blindness if the macula is involved. Immunosuppressed children from any cause who have CMV disease or persistently high levels of CMV DNA in their blood or plasma should receive regular expert ophthalmologic examinations to monitor for the development of sight-threatening retinitis. Establishing the diagnosis early may allow prompt institution of antiviral therapy, which may be sight saving.[306]

The ophthalmoscopic appearance of CMV retinitis usually is characteristic. However, in patients in whom the appearance of the retina is not typical or in whom the retinitis has progressed despite specific antiviral treatment, other causes of retinal lesions that should be considered include cotton-wool spots associated with hypertension, diabetes, connective tissue disease, anemia and leukemia, ocular toxoplasmosis, and candidal infection of the retina as well as syphilis, HSV infection, lymphocytic choriomeningitis virus infection, and VZV infection. Detection of the virus by culture or its DNA by a PCR-based method in vitreous fluid may help establish the diagnosis in difficult or atypical patients.[169] CMV antibodies also have been detected in the tears of patients with active ocular infections, including retinitis.[436]

CMV also has been associated in some studies with other unusual eye abnormalities. In coincidentally congenitally infected infants, microphthalmos, anophthalmia, optic nerve hypoplasia and coloboma, optic nerve atrophy, Peter anomaly, and irregular retinal pigment have been observed.[189] However, the role that CMV is playing in these anomalies is unclear and unsubstantiated by prospective studies.[114] CMV does not appear to cause congenital cataracts.[457] CMV also has been isolated from tears and has been associated with conjunctivitis in patients with CMV mononucleosis and AIDS as well as with corneal epithelial keratitis and disk neovascularization.[300]

Hepatitis

CMV hepatitis usually is manifested as mild to moderate hepatomegaly and mildly to moderately elevated serum hepatic enzyme levels in neonates with congenital CMV disease; in children who are bone marrow, heart, and lung transplant recipients; in patients with cancer or AIDS; in infants with primary immune deficiency of T-cell or NK-cell function; in patients with autoimmune disorders; and even in healthy infants and children experiencing a primary CMV infection.[498] Infants with primary immune disorders of T-cell and NK-cell function may have progressive hepatomegaly, increasing aminotransferase levels, and the presence of CMV evident on histopathology in the liver. CMV hepatitis commonly occurs in conjunction with fever, thrombocytopenia, and lymphopenia or lymphocytosis. Jaundice and hyperbilirubinemia may occur, severe hepatitis or cirrhosis is exceedingly rare, and hepatic necrosis and liver failure caused by CMV hepatitis have not been documented convincingly in these patients. CMV infection also has been associated with granulomatous hepatitis.[67,415] In addition, CMV hepatitis is a unique and prominent problem in children who have undergone liver transplantation.[77,511] Most CMV hepatitis occurs 1 to 2 months after the patient has undergone transplantation, but it may be noted as early as 2 weeks or as long as 4 months afterward.[79] It is more common and more severe after a primary CMV infection and is associated with liver transplantation from a CMV-seropositive donor and the use of OKT3 antibodies for severe rejection.[459] CMV hepatitis in liver transplant recipients is characterized by prolonged fever, leukopenia, thrombocytopenia, elevated levels of liver enzymes, hyperbilirubinemia, and liver failure. Distinguishing between CMV hepatitis and acute rejection often is difficult, even with a liver biopsy, and the two commonly coexist. CMV infection also has been associated with ascending cholangitis, chronic rejection, and the vanishing bile duct syndrome in liver transplant recipients.[79,357]

Infants with congenital CMV disease also may have hepatitis. The liver usually is smooth and nontender and commonly extends 3 to 5 cm below the right costal margin. Ascites may be present prenatally and may persist postnatally for 1 to 2 weeks. The hepatomegaly usually resolves by the time the infant is 3 months of age, and persistence beyond 1 year is highly unusual. Mild hepatitis generally is present, and aminotransferase levels in neonatal hepatitis caused by CMV rarely exceed 500 IU. Hyperbilirubinemia is present at birth in approximately one-third of neonates with congenital CMV and may be striking, with conjugated (direct) bilirubin levels up to 30 mg/dL.[243] The abnormal results of liver function tests gradually resolve during the course of the first few weeks of life, and chronic hepatitis as a result of congenital infection with CMV is an unusual occurrence. Congenital CMV disease also has been associated with intrahepatic and extrahepatic biliary atresia in some studies, but the direct role of CMV in neonatal cholestatic disease is unclear.[20,176,250] A neonate or infant with congenital CMV disease and recurrent, persistent or progressive hepatomegaly and hepatitis, despite antiviral treatment, may have an underlying primary immune deficiency of NK-cell or T-cell function.

The differential diagnosis of CMV hepatitis includes other causes of viral hepatitis, such as hepatitis A virus, hepatitis B virus, hepatitis C virus, Epstein-Barr virus, HSV, enterovirus, and adenovirus, as well as toxoplasmosis; other infections, such as bacterial ascending cholangitis; and noninfectious causes, such as ischemic injury, vascular thrombosis, hemolysis, rejection, and hepatitis induced by drugs or toxins. In neonates with a significant and persistent direct hyperbilirubinemia, the diagnosis of neonatal giant cell hepatitis or biliary atresia should be considered as well.

Gastrointestinal Disease

Serious gastrointestinal disease causing esophagitis, gastritis, gastric ulcers, gastric outlet obstruction, gastroenteritis, pyloric and small bowel obstruction, duodenitis, colitis, proctitis, pancreatitis, hemorrhage, and acalculous cholecystitis has been associated with CMV infection in immunocompromised persons, especially patients with AIDS or neoplastic disorders, patients with refractory autoimmune disorders receiving steroids and immunomodulators, and those who have undergone bone marrow, kidney, intestinal, or liver transplantation.[145,319,332,361,397,512] Rarely, self-limited CMV gastroenteritis, colitis, and proctitis have been associated with CMV mononucleosis syndrome in apparently normal individuals.[18,115,145,237,332,400,401] CMV enterocolitis has also been reported as a cause of intractable diarrhea, which often is bloody, in infants with congenital and postnatal CMV disease.[144,145,186,242,319,397,399,427] Characteristic signs and symptoms in infants and children include nausea, vomiting, dysphagia, epigastric pain and tenderness, delayed gastric emptying, watery guaiac-positive stools or gastrointestinal hemorrhage, and disaccharide and monosaccharide intolerance.[319,332,512] Severe disease may cause dehydration and failure to thrive. Endoscopy with biopsy is required to establish a definitive diagnosis and usually shows linear, localized, or punctate ulcers. Hemorrhagic lesions or diffuse erosion can occur in severe disease. Characteristic cytomegalic inclusion cells can be seen in the gastrointestinal endothelium, epithelium, and glandular tissue; CMV may be cultured from stool or biopsy specimens; or CMV DNA may be detected by PCR-based methods.[201] In addition, these patients often are viremic with CMV DNA by PCR detectable in their blood or plasma and occasionally have evidence of disseminated CMV infection with involvement of the lungs and retina. Infants with severe end-organ disease caused by CMV should receive an immunologic workup to exclude primary immune deficiency of T-cell or NK-cell function.

The differential diagnosis of CMV colitis includes infection with other viruses, especially HSV and adenovirus, and infection with bacteria, particularly *Salmonella, Shigella, Campylobacter,* and *Yersinia,* as well as *Clostridium difficile* and *Mycobacterium avium-intracellulare.* Parasitic infection with *Cryptosporidium, Giardia,* and amebae also should be excluded. The differential diagnosis of CMV esophagitis and gastritis includes HSV infection, *Candida* esophagitis, reflux esophagitis, and peptic ulcer disease.

Meningoencephalitis and Other Neurologic Disorders

CNS involvement is well described and occurs relatively frequently in infants with symptomatic congenital CMV infection. Although the severity of damage to the CNS during congenital infection varies greatly, postmortem examination of severely affected infants has demonstrated necrotizing encephalitis, especially in the deep periventricular structures, and scattered areas of necrosis and inclusion-bearing cells. Although direct viral infection of neural structures probably plays a major role in CNS disease in congenital CMV infection, infectious ventriculitis and vasculitis also may occur. FBDS also can be associated with severe forms of congenital CMV infection. In addition, because congenital CMV disease can be associated with marked thrombocytopenia, intracranial hemorrhage can contribute to CMV-related CNS injury.[41,86,226,516] Clinical manifestations of this disease process include microcephaly, cerebral palsy, intracerebral calcifications, seizures, hemiparesis, developmental delay, ventriculomegaly, paraventricular cysts, intraventricular strands, periventricular leukomalacia, lissencephaly-pachygyria, porencephaly, schizencephaly, cortical malformations such as polymicrogyria, multifocal deep white-matter lesions and gliosis, atrophy from cerebral volume loss, parenchymal and ependymal cysts, periventricular cysts, cerebellar lesions, meningoencephalitis, and sensorineural deafness (Figs. 159.2, 159.3, and 159.5).[105,285,354,491,508] Remarkably, despite the well-documented neuropathologic process in congenital disease, isolation of CMV from the cerebrospinal fluid (CSF) of a congenitally infected child is an extremely unusual finding.[248] CMV DNA has been detected in the CSF of congenitally infected infants, and its presence at birth appears to identify infants at risk for a poor neurodevelopmental outcome.[31]

The differential diagnosis of symptomatic congenital CMV infection with neurologic disease includes congenital Zika virus syndrome, congenital toxoplasmosis, congenital HSV infection, congenital rubella syndrome, congenital infection with lymphocytic choriomeningitis virus, brain tumors such as craniopharyngioma, and calcified hematoma. In addition, congenital CMV disease involving the CNS also may be mimicked by genetic disorders such as tuberous sclerosis, Sturge-Weber syndrome, and Aicardi syndrome; metabolic conditions such as hyperthyroidism; α_1-antitrypsin deficiency; galactosemia; peroxisome disorders such as Zellweger syndrome, neonatal adrenoleukodystrophy, and infantile Refsum disease; urea cycle deficiencies; organic acidemias; and liposomal storage disorders.[40] Maternal exposure to drugs and toxins, especially isotretinoin, cocaine, and alcohol, also is included in the differential diagnosis. The presence or absence of intracerebral calcification and the pattern of calcifications when they are present may be helpful in distinguishing among these disorders. In addition, the appropriate microbiologic studies, chromosome analysis, metabolic studies, and drug screens should be performed.

In postnatal life, CMV meningoencephalitis appears to be rare yet well documented.[39] It may occur as a complication of CMV mononucleosis, as an isolated manifestation of primary CMV infection in a normal host, or as a primary or recurrent infection in an immunocompromised patient.[401] In infants, it may be the presenting condition of a primary immune deficiency of T-cell or NK-cell function, or SCID. Symptoms include headache, photophobia, nuchal rigidity, memory deficits, and inability to concentrate. CSF findings include mild mononuclear pleocytosis and slightly elevated protein. Although the virus is isolated from the CSF and brain parenchyma exceedingly rarely, neuropathologic findings of intranuclear inclusions and microglial nodules are characteristic.

CMV encephalitis may complicate adult and pediatric immunocompromised transplant recipients and patients with AIDS.[46] As many as 50% of patients with AIDS may have evidence of CMV infection of

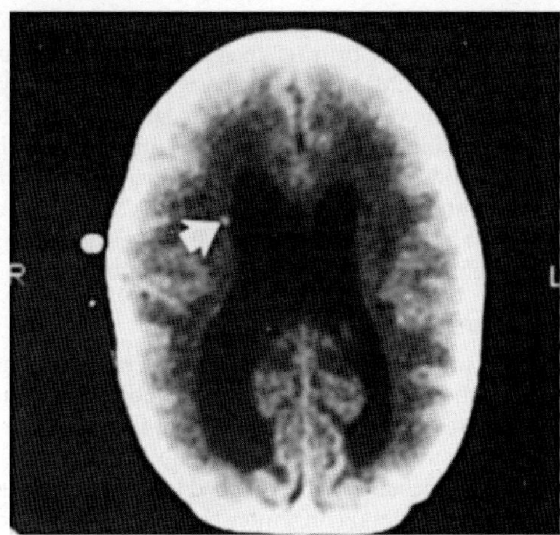

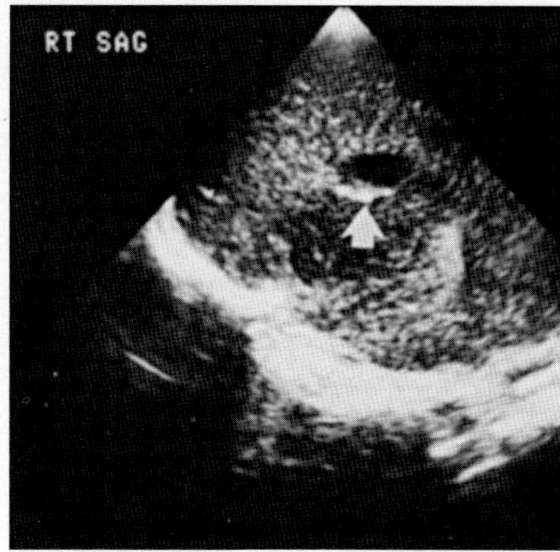

FIG. 159.5 (A) Computed tomography scan and (B) ultrasound examination of the head of an infant with congenital cytomegalovirus disease. Both tests showed moderate asymmetric enlargement of the lateral ventricles with punctate periventricular calcifications.

the CNS at postmortem examination.[344] CMV has been reported to cause a subacute, occasionally progressive encephalitis in patients with AIDS and has been implicated as a cofactor in the pathogenesis of the AIDS dementia complex seen in both adults and children.[126,231,333,462,536] In this disease, CMV may be isolated from CSF, or CMV DNA may be detected in the fluid or brain by PCR-based methods.[204] In children, this syndrome is characterized by weakness, confusion, and loss of developmental milestones.

The differential diagnosis of CMV encephalitis and meningoencephalitis in a normal host includes primarily infection with other neurotropic viruses, such as HSV, Epstein-Barr virus, VZV, enterovirus, and arboviruses. Neurosyphilis and tuberculous meningitis also should be considered. In immunocompromised patients, especially those with AIDS, the following should be added to the differential diagnosis of CNS infection: progressive multifocal leukoencephalopathy caused by papovavirus; HIV encephalitis; fungal CNS infection caused by *Cryptococcus neoformans, Candida* spp., *Aspergillus,* or *Histoplasma;* protozoal infections with *T. gondii* and, rarely, *P. jiroveci* and *Strongyloides stercoralis;* bacterial infections with *M. avium-intracellulare* and *Nocardia asteroides;* noninfectious diseases such as primary cerebral lymphoma and lymphomatoid granulomatosis; and vascular complications such as hemorrhage and infarction.[24] In immunosuppressed patients, more than one of these conditions can coexist in the CNS.

CMV also can invade the peripheral nervous system and cause a painful peripheral neuropathy in patients with AIDS.[191,426,515] Ascending paralysis caused by myelitis, with or without vasculitis or necrosis, also can occur and may appear similar to Guillain-Barré syndrome.[515] In addition, CMV polyradiculopathy has been described in adult patients with AIDS and may occur in older children. This disease usually begins as leg pain and sacral paresthesias and may progress to weakness and flaccid paralysis. The CSF characteristically has a polymorphonuclear pleocytosis and moderately elevated protein level.[270] The association of CMV infection with infantile spasms, Guillain-Barré syndrome, Charcot-Marie-Tooth disease, Huntington disease, Alzheimer disease, myasthenia gravis, and neuropsychiatric diseases (e.g., schizophrenia) has been reported, but a definite causal relationship between CMV and these diseases remains to be proved.[39,275]

Deafness and Other Ear Disorders

Hearing loss is present at birth in 25% to 50% of infants with symptomatic congenital CMV infection and in approximately 10% to 15% of newborn infants with asymptomatic congenital CMV infection.[243] By 18 years of age, up to 20% of children born with asymptomatic congenital CMV infection may develop progressive, sensorineural hearing loss, with 2% of them progressing to bilateral severe hearing loss requiring cochlear implants.[292,296] The sensorineural hearing loss associated with symptomatic congenital CMV disease is often bilateral at birth or during early infancy, whereas hearing loss associated with asymptomatic congenital CMV infection often begins unilaterally but may progress to bilateral hearing loss. In fact, 2% of children born with asymptomatic congenital CMV infection will develop bilateral sensorineural hearing loss by 18 years of age that is severe enough to warrant cochlear implantation.[527] Given that congenital CMV infection affects 30,000 to 40,000 infants annually in the United States, this congenital infection probably is the most common cause of nonhereditary sensorineural deafness. Investigators have estimated that congenital CMV infection may account for as many as 40% of cases of congenital hearing loss.[48,146,214] Progression or fluctuation of the hearing loss occurs in at least two-thirds of these children through the preschool years, and continued progression occurs through the school-aged and adolescent years.[182,538] Although CMV has been detected in the endolabyrinth of infants who died from congenital CMV disease, whether this progressive deafness is caused by continued viral replication in the inner ear, reinfection with a new strain of virus, or a complex cascade of immunopathologic events remains unclear.[129] Mondini dysplasia of the temporal bones has been seen in infants with congenital CMV infection, but the importance of this observation relative to the pathogenesis of the progressive hearing loss commonly seen in congenitally infected infants is unknown at this time.[55] Some studies suggest that higher levels of CMV in urine and blood are present in neonates who develop hearing loss from congenital CMV infection,[27,289,425,522] whereas other studies speculate that genetic mutations or inflammatory genes may play a role in CMV-associated hearing loss.[353,356,433,450]

CMV has been isolated from the middle ear effusions of healthy and immunocompromised children with otitis media.[108,161] In addition, CMV infection, defined serologically, has been associated with sudden-onset deafness, acute labyrinthitis, and Meniere disease.[486,540,541] Older children who were born with asymptomatic congenital CMV infection also may exhibit differences in higher auditory function, even though they do not have sensorineural or conductive hearing loss.[118]

Myocarditis and Other Cardiovascular Disorders

Myocarditis has been described as a rare complication of severe in utero fetal and newborn congenital CMV disease and CMV mononucleosis in presumably otherwise healthy adults and children.[367,500,526,541] CMV myocarditis and myopericarditis, occasionally accompanied by CMV hepatitis, has been reported in immunocompetent patients as well as immunocompromised patients.[170,364] CMV myocarditis also has been seen in renal and heart transplant recipients, usually as part of a disseminated CMV infection and associated with graft rejection treated with high-dose immunosuppressive therapy.[200,395,453] Myocarditis caused by CMV may be present in infants with primary immune deficiency disorders of T-cell and NK-cell function and SCID. Patients can have heart failure, cardiomegaly, electrocardiographic abnormalities, and poor left ventricular function on echocardiography; cytomegalic inclusion cells and the presence of CMV DNA can be documented by myocardial biopsy.

The association of CMV infection with other cardiac disorders such as congenital heart block, structural cardiac anomalies, and pericarditis is anecdotal, and a cause-and-effect relationship is not well documented.[262]

Thrombotic phenomena, often serious and life-threatening, have been associated with primary and active CMV infection in neonates, infants, adolescents, and adults, as well as transplant recipients and patients with HIV/AIDS.[3,131,309] The virus may cause damage to endothelial cells, activate coagulation factors, and induce production of antiphospholipid antibodies.[471]

CMV coronary endotheliitis with superimposed thrombosis and myocardial infarction has been described in adult heart transplant recipients and was reported in an infant who died of disseminated CMV disease with an apical ventricular aneurysm.[331,440] CMV primary or acute infection also has been associated with venous and arterial thrombosis in previously healthy individuals, in patients undergoing solid-organ transplantation (especially renal and heart transplant recipients), and in infants with congenital and early postnatal CMV infection.[2,32,309] Primary CMV infection has been associated with pulmonary embolism and portal vein thrombosis in an adolescent with CMV mononucleosis.[2,3,14,288] CMV infection has been postulated to play a role in the pathogenesis of atherosclerosis and coronary artery disease in animal models, as well as in both normal persons and heart transplant recipients.[206,251,320,324,496] High levels of CMV antibody have also been epidemiologically associated with coronary artery disease in studies in performed in many countries and continents, including India, Finland, the United States, and China.[2,3,14,251,337,338,471]

CMV also has been associated with hypertension in animal (murine) models, but studies definitely linking CMV to hypertension in humans have not been definitive.[107]

Endocrine System

Histopathologic evidence of involvement of the organs of the endocrine system is described well in both congenital and postnatally acquired disseminated CMV infections.[230] Endocrine disorders such as Graves disease and diabetes insipidus have been associated with congenital CMV infection, but these reports may represent coincidental findings.[325,439] Longitudinal studies are required to determine whether the autoimmune endocrinopathies in children with congenital rubella parallel the findings in children with congenital CMV infection. CMV infection also has been associated with autoimmune type 1 diabetes, although a specific cause-and-effect relationship has not been established.[366] In addition, immunosuppressed patients, especially persons with AIDS, may manifest clinical endocrinopathies caused by CMV infection, such as adrenal insufficiency and adrenal necrosis.[207] CMV inclusions also have been found in the pituitary gland of patients with AIDS, all of whom showed evidence of CMV encephalitis or disseminated infection elsewhere in the body.[171] Moreover, involvement of the thyroid and parathyroid glands with CMV has been reported in adults with AIDS.[188]

Genitourinary System

Disease of the male and female genitourinary system as a result of CMV has been reported. Patients with AIDS may have symptomatic epididymitis and cystitis caused by CMV.[57,403,488] Lower urinary tract infections and hemorrhagic cystitis caused by CMV have been diagnosed in patients after they have undergone stem cell and solid-organ transplantation.[365] CMV also commonly yet asymptomatically infects the cervicovaginal secretions and semen of both healthy and immunosuppressed adults.[256,290]

Skin

Cutaneous manifestations of CMV infection are described well and can occur with both congenital and acquired CMV infection.[303] Infants with symptomatic congenital infection may have nonpalpable petechiae, purpura, or bruises, usually as a result of thrombocytopenia. Violaceous or dark magenta infiltrative papules or nodules, called "blueberry muffin" lesions, also may occur, but these lesions are more characteristic of congenital rubella syndrome. The skin lesions associated with acquired CMV infection usually are localized cutaneous ulcers or a widespread, exanthematous, maculopapular eruption, although vesiculobullous lesions also have been described.[378] CMV mononucleosis syndrome in adults and children may be accompanied by a maculopapular, rubelliform rash that may be pruritic. In addition, ampicillin-associated rashes may occur with CMV mononucleosis. CMV also may cause a cutaneous, leukoblastic vasculitis.[441] Well-demarcated, ulcerated lesions that show histopathologic evidence of CMV infection may be seen in immunocompromised patients who have undergone transplantation or in those who suffer from AIDS. Finally, CMV may play a cofactor role with human herpesvirus type 8 in the neoplastic process in Kaposi sarcoma, but definitive proof of a causal relationship remains to be shown.

Unusual Associations

CMV infection, either congenital or acquired, has been detected in association with a wide variety of conditions, including defects in tooth structure and the formation of enamel, arterial or venous thrombosis, atherosclerosis, portal vein thrombosis associated with protein S and protein C deficiency, unexplained fevers in burn patients, bacterial sepsis in burn patients, congenital eventration of the diaphragm, inguinal hernia, and fatal *Staphylococcus epidermidis* infection in very low-birth-weight infants.* CMV infection also may be involved in the genesis and maintenance of immunopathologic phenomena, such as allograft rejection in solid-organ transplant recipients and graft-versus-host disease in bone marrow and stem cell transplant recipients, as well as autoimmune diseases.[284,508] Case reports have linked primary CMV infection with the onset of autoimmune disorders or recurrent CMV infection with worsening of autoimmune disease.[219,381,509] CMV also has been associated with hemophagocytic syndrome in adults and children.[284] However, given the common occurrence of CMV infection, it is difficult to determine whether the relationships are coincidental or comorbid, rather than part of a cause-and-effect relationship.

LABORATORY DIAGNOSIS

Detection of the Infectious Agent

CMV can be isolated in cell culture with fibroblast cell lines such as human foreskin fibroblasts and human embryonic lung fibroblasts.[448] Specimens that contain a high titer of virus, such as those from congenitally infected infants, may show growth in 24 hours. Some specimens, such as those from persons with acquired asymptomatic infection, may require as long as 6 weeks for detectable growth, but most cultures grow in 1 to 2 weeks. CMV has been isolated from a variety of specimens, including urine, saliva, nasopharyngeal and sinus washings, conjunctiva, tears, middle ear fluid, breast milk, semen, cervicovaginal secretions, stool, CSF, peripheral white blood cells and plasma, amniotic fluid, bronchial lavage samples, and biopsy or autopsy specimens. One study also evaluated umbilical cord samples as a method of diagnosis and applied it to newborn screening for congenital CMV.[504] Urine may be collected in a pediatric urine bag or trapped by cotton balls inserted in the diaper.[429] Saliva samples should be collected from the infant's mouth with a swab, allowing the infant to suck on the swab for a short period of time to make sure the swab is saturated with saliva before being placed in viral transport media. Waiting at least 1 hour after breast-feeding is also recommended for saliva swab collection because small amounts of CMV may be present in breast milk and produce a false-positive result in some breast-fed infants.[72] All samples for isolation of viruses (except blood, which should be at room temperature) should be held at 4°C (on wet ice or in a refrigerator) until processed in the virology laboratory. Specimens for isolation of virus should be inoculated within hours of collection for an optimal isolation rate. Although isolation of CMV proves that a productive infection is present, it does not confirm an etiologic relationship with the disease process and requires careful interpretation within the patient's clinical context. The exception is detection of CMV by culture, shell vial assay or CR methods in a sample or urine, saliva, or blood/plasma obtained in the first 21 days of life of a newborn because this will establish that a congenital CMV infection is present. Clinical correlation will then be needed to establish any organ involvement associated with the congenital infection (Box 159.5).

An adaptation of tissue culture is a low-speed centrifugation enhancement, monoclonal antibody culture technique, also called a *shell vial*

*References 2, 14, 28, 32, 56, 218, 260, 281, 288, 308, 311, 479, 496.

BOX 159.5 Virologic Testing to Establish the Diagnosis of Congenital Cytomegalovirus (CMV) Infection

Detection of CMV by culture or polymerase chain reaction in saliva or urine or blood in first 21 days of life
CMV immunoglobulin M antibody (should be confirmed with CMV testing of urine or saliva) at birth
Detection of CMV DNA in newborn screening dried blood spot
Detection of cytomegalic inclusion cells or detection of CMV by immunohistochemical staining in tissue from clinically involved organs from biopsy or autopsy specimens

assay. In this test, inoculated tissue culture cells in small vials are stained with a fluorescein-conjugated monoclonal antibody to either an early or a late CMV antigen (or both). Cells infected with CMV exhibit nuclear and membrane fluorescence 18 to 72 hours after inoculation. This rapid viral diagnostic technique is especially reliable with saliva, urine, and BAL specimens and has been applied with variable results to blood and tissue specimens.[198,385] However, maximal sensitivity and specificity are obtained when shell vials are used as an adjunct to and not in place of routine tissue culture. CMV-infected cells also can be detected by direct immunofluorescence assay on exfoliated cells in BAL specimens or in frozen tissue specimens.[220] These procedures, however, require a laboratory experienced in direct immunofluorescence assay technique.

Real-time PCR-based methods, both quantitative and qualitative, coupled with automated nucleic acid extraction systems, are available in many clinical and reference laboratories for detection and quantitation of CMV DNA in a variety of clinical samples (saliva, urine, blood, amniotic fluid, vitreous samples, and tissue).[62] These very sensitive tests may be used to detect and to quantify CMV DNA in a variety of samples and are useful for diagnosis or prediction of CMV disease, as well as for monitoring response to antiviral treatment.[82,98,128,134,197,462,468,475] Recently, PCR assays for detection of CMV DNA in saliva specimens, urine specimens (liquid urine collected by bags or using cotton balls in diapers), and dried blood spot (DBS) specimens from newborn screening Guthrie cards have been applied as tools to screen newborns for congenital CMV infection[96,432,429,552] (see Box 159.5). Detection of CMV DNA in the CSF of immunocompromised patients with AIDS, of patients with primary immune disorders, and of transplant recipients seems to be a reliable diagnostic method for detection of CMV infection of the CNS, and detection of CMV DNA in the CSF of neonates with congenital CMV disease correlates with poor neurodevelopmental outcome.[31,113,204,546] Similarly, detection of CMV DNA by PCR analysis in vitreous fluid provides persuasive evidence that a patient's retinitis is CMV related.[154] CMV DNA also may be detected in the peripheral white blood cells and plasma of patients with CMV infection, and detection of CMV DNA in the plasma or serum of neonates and immunocompromised patients appears to correlate with severity of disease and viral dissemination.[343,456,474,475] Detection of CMV DNA in amniotic fluid provides prenatal diagnosis of congenital CMV infection and, when correlated with fetal ultrasonography and other clinical evaluations of the fetus, supports the presence of CMV-associated in utero disease.[307] PCR assays also have detected CMV DNA in DBS or Guthrie cards collected, as well as in urine and saliva, as part of neonatal screening programs and used to diagnose congenital CMV infection and disease.[48,51,71,72,522]

Another use for PCR-based diagnosis of CMV infection is the very early diagnosis of CMV infection in high-risk patients, such as transplant recipients, before the development of potentially fatal CMV disease, such as pneumonitis. This approach may allow preemptive antiviral therapy to be initiated when CMV infection appears active but before overt disease is detected.[81,547] CMV quantitative DNA detection by PCR assay is now standard for monitoring a patient's response to antiviral therapy and should be correlated with the resolution of CMV-related clinical symptoms.[150,195]

CMV pp65 antigen also may be detected in the white blood cells of patients with CMV infection and disease, but this CMV antigenemia test is now rarely used by clinical laboratories as a rapid, same-day screen for CMV viremia. Even though it is relatively easy to perform and the degree of antigenemia may be quantitated to monitor response to antiviral therapy, it has been replaced by quantitative PCR assays in most clinical and reference laboratories.[150]

Exfoliated cells in urine or BAL specimens or cells in tissue obtained by biopsy can be examined for histologic evidence of CMV infection. Cells that are infected productively with CMV are enlarged, have type A Cowdry intranuclear inclusions, and occasionally have perinuclear inclusions. The appearance of these cells is characteristic and has been likened to owl's eyes. Immunohistochemical staining with immunoperoxidase can be used to augment the detection of these typical cells. The presence of these cells correlates with the presence of active CMV disease and may be useful clinically. In addition, viral load assessed by quantitative PCR of BAL specimens helps with diagnosis of CMV pneumonitis in immunocompromised patients.[240]

Serology

Standard serologic techniques also can be applied to the diagnosis of CMV infections. CMV IgG antibody can be determined in serum by several different methods, including complement fixation, hemagglutination inhibition, indirect fluorescent antibody assay, anticomplement immunofluorescence assay, enzyme-linked immunosorbent assay (ELISA), and latex agglutination and neutralization tests. ELISA and the indirect fluorescent antibody assay are used most commonly in clinical virology laboratories. The presence of CMV IgG antibody in a single serum specimen implies that the patient at some time has been infected with CMV. On the other hand, a negative IgG antibody determination is good evidence against current or past CMV infection because CMV antibody usually is present at the time of infection and persists for life. Severely immunocompromised patients, especially bone marrow transplant recipients, or infants and children with a primary immune deficiency, however, can lose their ability to make IgG antibody and become CMV seronegative, even though they are infected actively with CMV. This occurrence has a poor prognosis and requires immediate reconstitution with antibody and aggressive antiviral therapy until immune reconstitution is achieved. Primary infection with CMV is documented best by clear seroconversion from negative to positive CMV IgG antibody. A fourfold rise in CMV IgG antibody titer is not diagnostic of a primary infection because reactivation or reinfection also can cause titers to fluctuate. In addition, the height of the titer or ELISA index in a single serum specimen is not diagnostic of a recent infection or indicative of severity of CMV disease.

CMV IgM antibody can be determined in serum by radioimmunoassay, indirect fluorescent antibody assay, or ELISA. Both the indirect fluorescent antibody assay and ELISA are used commonly in clinical laboratories, although some indirect fluorescent antibody assays have a considerable false-positive rate. Accurate interpretation of CMV IgM antibody results requires knowledge of the methods used and careful consideration of the clinical context to exclude diseases that produce cross-reacting antibody or polyclonal responses. Test methods also should remove rheumatoid factor from the test serum, a common cause of false-positive IgM reactions. If the test is performed properly, the presence of CMV IgM antibody implies a current or recent primary CMV infection. In healthy adults, CMV IgM antibody usually persists for 6 weeks and may be present for as long as 3 to 12 months, rarely even longer, after the primary infection.[136] Commercial immunoblot and avidity assays may be used to supplement conventional CMV IgG and IgM serology.[297] The CMV IgG avidity index and IgM immunoblot assay are now available in clinical reference laboratories in many countries and continents, including Europe, Asia, and the United States. This testing may be used to help time a suspected primary infection with CMV (see Box 159.4).[163,298,402,416] A low avidity index (30%) suggests a recent primary infection, usually within 3 months, because low to moderate CMV avidity anti-CMV antibody may persist for 18 to 20 weeks after primary CMV infection.[298] A high avidity index (>60%) suggests a past or recurrent CMV infection.[205] There are several manufacturers of these supplemental CMV assays, and results may vary among manufacturers, so interpretation should be within clinical context and in concert with other CMV testing, if available.[402] In immunocompromised adults experiencing clinically significant reactivation infection with CMV, CMV IgM antibody may be detected for prolonged periods.[345] The sensitivity and specificity of CMV IgM antibody determination in the diagnosis of acquired, primary CMV infection or clinically significant reactivation infection in infants and children have not been studied systematically, although clinicians frequently use this test for this purpose.

Western blot assays using viral structural proteins separated from purified viral particles or from recombinant viral proteins appear to be sensitive and specific for detection of glycoprotein-specific CMV IgG and IgM. Currently, these tests are available only in research or reference laboratories.[299]

Recently, two interferon-γ release assays (IGRAs) that measure cell-mediated immunity against CMV, the cytomegalovirus enzyme-linked immunosorbent spot (ELISOT) and CMV QuantiFERON assays, have been evaluated as potential biomarkers for primary versus nonprimary maternal CMV infections and as predictors of congenital CMV transmission. They also have been used to detect protective, CMV-specific T-cell responses in transplant recipients at risk for CMV infection and CMV disease. These assays are now available in some clinical and reference laboratories, and as more clinical experience evolves on their clinical utility, CMV IGRAs testing may become more common in certain at-risk groups of patients.[1,180,438]

Laboratory Diagnosis of Specific Clinical Syndromes

Pregnancy

Diagnosis of primary maternal CMV infection is best made by de novo seroconversion of virus-specific CMV IgG antibody or by the presence of both CMV IgG antibody and CMV IgM antibody associated with a low IgG avidity index.[559] For timing of the onset of CMV infection (before or in early pregnancy), CMV avidity testing is most helpful if performed during the first or early second trimester.[163] In primary maternal CMV infection, the risk for transmission of CMV to the fetus is approximately 40%, and it is up to 25% overall to the fetus for development of sequelae of some type. A maternal recurrent infection may result from reactivation of the woman's own endogenous strains of CMV or by reinfection with a new strain of CMV. Recurrent CMV infection is difficult to diagnosis prenatally and may be considered if there is a significant rise in CMV IgG antibody, with the presence of IgM and a high avidity IgG index. The diagnosis of recurrent CMV infection in the mother can also be considered if she is CMV IgG antibody positive and CMV IgM antibody negative at the beginning of pregnancy yet gives birth to a congenitally infected but usually symptom-free neonate. Routine serologic screening of pregnant women for CMV infection is controversial; although recommended by some experts, it is not currently performed in the United States or Canada.[304] However, selective serologic screening for diagnosis should be performed for women who request it and for women in high-risk circumstances, including those with clinical evidence of CMV infection, such as mononucleosis during pregnancy or detection of fetal abnormalities on screening ultrasonography suggestive of in utero CMV disease.[147] Serologic screening and counseling may also be considered for child care workers and for women with a young child or toddler in the household. Prenatal diagnosis of in utero CMV infection of the fetus is best accomplished by amniocentesis, which should be done at least 7 weeks after the presumed time of maternal primary CMV infection and after 21 weeks' gestation.[235,430] This interval is important because it may take 5 to 7 weeks (at least 2 weeks) after maternal infection to produce fetal infection and subsequent replication in the kidney for a detectable quantity of CMV to be detected in the amniotic fluid.[235] Amniotic fluid may be sent for CMV culture or detection of CMV DNA by qualitative or quantitative PCR. Quantitative determination of CMV DNA in amniotic fluid that shows very high levels of DNA may predict more serious disease in the fetus and poorer outcome in the neonate. After diagnosis of maternal primary or recurrent CMV infection, monitoring of the fetus by serial ultrasound examinations should be performed every 2 to 4 weeks to detect abnormalities, which may aid in management.

Congenital Infection

Viral culture or CMV culture is the traditional diagnostic test for congenital infection with CMV, but it is being replaced by molecular methods in most clinical laboratories.[132] The diagnosis of congenital CMV infection is established by isolation of the virus or detection by PCR of viral CMV DNA from urine or saliva obtained from the infant during the first 3 weeks of life[429] (see Box 159.5). Cell culture of urine or saliva has been used successfully to screen large numbers of neonates for congenital CMV, as well as diagnose individual patients clinically.[132,138,359,478,564] Urine cultures obtained after 3 weeks of life must be interpreted cautiously because perinatally acquired and transfusion-acquired infections with CMV may be manifested as early as 3 weeks of age.[442] Detection of nuclear inclusion-bearing renal epithelial cells in urinary sediment collected in the first 2 weeks of life also implies the presence of congenital infection. This technique is insensitive, however, compared with cell culture and is important only historically. Detection of CMV DNA in the urine, saliva, blood, or CSF of neonates by DNA PCR amplification techniques correlates with congenital infection and disease, and this method is currently used by most clinicians and laboratories for diagnosis of congenital CMV.[31,80,134,343] Detection of CMV DNA in DBS or Guthrie cards collected for neonatal metabolic screening also has been used for the retrospective and prospective diagnosis of congenital CMV infection and disease.[49,50,52,551] However, this method may not detect all congenitally infected neonates, especially those with silent or asymptomatic infection, because the level of CMV in blood is lower in asymptomatic congenital CMV infection. Studies evaluating real-time PCR assays performed on DNA extracted from DBS samples used to screen neonates for other congenital conditions have mostly shown DBS relatively insensitive for neonatal screening programs when compared with traditional methods but possibly are useful for identification of neonates with symptomatic disease or at high risk for sequelae.[71,302,432,551] Genotyping may be performed by PCR assays on DNA extracted from DBS samples, providing a tool to study the possible association of CMV gB or gH genotype with disease in neonates.[138,141] Real-time PCR assays performed on saliva specimens (both liquid and dried) have shown high sensitivity compared with traditional saliva rapid culture and may be a potential screening tool for diagnosis of congenital CMV in neonates.[49,50,52,72,467,508,553,554] Currently, two approaches to newborn screening for congenital CMV infection have been proposed. One is targeted testing for congenital CMV infection of newborns who fail their newborn hearing screening, by CMV testing of urine or saliva by culture or PCR assays done in the first days of life, because CMV is a cause of congenital hearing loss.[183,225,504] The other approach is universal newborn screening for congenital CMV, testing all newborns for CMV at birth, by detection methods applied to urine, saliva, or DBS from newborn screening Guthrie cards.[225,405] Some birthing centers have adopted targeted newborn testing for congenital CMV, and even two states have laws providing for targeted testing. However, neither approach at this time is adopted by all birthing centers or all states in the United States or all countries in the world, but discussions among CMV experts around the world continues concerning the relative merits of targeted versus universal newborn screening for congenital CMV infection.[405]

Newborns with virologic evidence of congenital CMV infection should receive a thorough clinical, laboratory, and imaging evaluation to determine whether there is end-organ involvement (Box 159.6). Also, neonates with high CMV DNA levels by quantitative PCR methods appear to be at highest risk for severe illness in the neonatal period and for sequelae such as progressive or late-onset hearing loss and therefore are potential candidates for CMV antiviral therapy, especially if ongoing clinical trials show benefit.[289,522]

An in utero CMV infection may be suspected if routine fetal anatomy scans performed at 19 to 20 weeks' gestation show intrauterine growth restriction, microcephaly, echogenic bowel, fetal ascites, hepatosplenomegaly, or malformations of the brain. Fetal condition also can be determined by serial fetal ultrasound examinations or fetal MRI in special circumstances.[113,182,313] Most in utero fetal CMV infections, however, are asymptomatic.[65] The diagnosis of fetal intrauterine CMV disease in single, twin, and multiple births may be established by isolating the virus from amniotic fluid or detecting CMV DNA by

BOX 159.6 Initial Evaluation of Newborn Confirmed to Have Congenital Cytomegalovirus (CMV) Infection (Asymptomatic or Symptomatic at Birth)

Physical, neurologic, and neurodevelopmental examination
Weight, length, and head circumference measurements
Laboratory testing
- CBC, differential platelet count
- Liver function tests (AST, ALT, total and direct bilirubin, GGT)
- Kidney function tests (BUN and creatinine)
- Coagulation studies (select patients)
- Whole blood or plasma for CMV DNA quantitative PCR to establish presence and level of viremia as risk factor for later sequelae
- TRECs newborn screen for severe combined immunodeficiency syndrome (check results if done)

Hearing evaluation by auditory brainstem response
Ophthalmology evaluation
Neuroimaging (one or more of the following, depending on clinical presentation)
- Neonatal head ultrasound
- CT scan, unenhanced
- MRI, unenhanced

ALT, Alanine aminotransferase; *AST,* aspartate aminotransferase; *BUN,* blood urea nitrogen; *CBC,* complete blood count; *CMV,* cytomegalovirus; *CT,* computed tomography; *GGT,* γ-glutamyl transferase; *MRI,* magnetic resonance imaging; *PCR,* polymerase chain reaction; *TRECs,* T-cell receptor rearrangement excision circle.

PCR amplification in amniotic fluid obtained at least 2 weeks after the suspected time of maternal primary infection and after 21 weeks' gestation.[226,430,560] Fetal blood samples that show the presence of CMV DNA by PCR assay, CMV IgM antibody, thrombocytopenia, leukopenia, or elevated liver function test results also provide supportive evidence of CMV-associated fetal disease and may predict severe disease.

Prenatal screening of pregnant women and prenatal diagnosis of congenital CMV infection should be accompanied by consultation with a maternal-fetal medicine specialist as well as a pediatric infectious diseases specialist and a prenatal counselor knowledgeable about all the possible outcomes that can occur and all the options that are available to the parents and physician.[162,346,416]

Standard serologic tests also can be applied to diagnose congenital infection with CMV, but this approach is cumbersome, retrospective, and rarely used clinically. The absence of CMV IgG antibody in cord blood may rule out congenital infection, unless the infant has a primary immune disorder affecting antibody response to CMV, whereas its presence may imply passive transfer from the mother or indicate a congenital infection. Serial serologic specimens also can be obtained when the infant is 1, 3, and 6 months of age. If CMV IgG antibody levels disappear during the infant's first months of life, congenital infection is ruled out. However, if CMV IgG antibody persists, the infant either was infected congenitally or acquired CMV infection perinatally or postnatally. The presence of CMV IgM antibody in cord or infant blood collected in the first 3 weeks of the infant's life suggests the diagnosis of congenital CMV infection.[212,480] However, CMV IgM antibody is insensitive (as low as 22%) compared with urine or saliva CMV culture or CMV DNA detection for the diagnosis of congenital infection.[343] In one study, positive CMV IgM antibody was found in only 49% of newborns with symptomatic congenital CMV infection and 22% of newborns with asymptomatic congenital CMV infection.[60]

Perinatal and Postnatal Infection

The diagnosis of perinatal infection with CMV is difficult to establish but is documented best by a negative CMV viral culture or negative CMV DNA PCR analysis of urine or saliva and negative CMV IgM antibody level at birth or in first 21 days of life, followed by a positive viral culture and positive CMV IgM antibody at 8 to 16 weeks of age and persistence of CMV IgG antibody beyond 4 to 6 months of age. Postnatal primary CMV infection is diagnosed by CMV IgG seroconversion, the presence of CMV IgM antibody, and CMV excretion or "shedding" detected by culture or PCR in saliva, urine, and other body fluids.

Cytomegalovirus Syndromes in Immunocompromised Hosts

In immunocompromised patients, determination of whether serologic or virologic evidence of active CMV infection correlates with disease is difficult because CMV commonly is shed from saliva, urine, and respiratory tract secretions in these patients without clear evidence of a disease process.[222] Therefore detection of a productive virus infection in the organ system suspected to be involved is often necessary to establish the diagnosis of CMV disease in an immunocompromised patient. For example, interstitial pneumonitis caused by CMV is documented best by an open-lung biopsy specimen that shows characteristic CMV histopathologic features and positive viral culture.[122] Detection of CMV in BAL specimens also correlates with lung biopsy results for diagnosis of CMV pneumonitis.[122,197] In addition, CMV viral load in BAL specimens greater than the plasma viral load, associated with signs and symptoms associated with pneumonitis, suggests CMV as the cause of pneumonia in transplant recipients. Similarly, the diagnosis of CMV hepatitis or colitis is documented best by the presence of cytomegalic inclusion cells, isolation of CMV, or detection of CMV by DNA PCR or immunohistochemical stains from biopsy specimens. If biopsy of the suspected organ is not feasible or practical, then detection of CMV viremia or rising titers of CMV DNA by quantitative PCR can support the diagnosis because it often precedes or accompanies serious disease, such as CMV pneumonitis in bone marrow or solid-organ transplant recipients, CMV retinitis or colitis in patients with AIDS, or disseminated disease in infants with primary immune deficiency syndromes.[195,475,514]

Prospective monitoring of high-risk patients by serial samples of blood or plasma for quantitative CMV DNA PCR analysis or, alternatively, by CMV cultures of urine or blood or bronchial lavage samples and collection of serum to detect seroconversion by serologic testing is indicated and often performed because positive tests indicate the need for preemptive therapy with a CMV-specific antiviral agent, such as ganciclovir or valganciclovir, when CMV infection is active but before overt disease develops.[195,407,449,497]

TREATMENT

Antiviral agents with activity against CMV include derivatives of acyclovir, such as ganciclovir and valganciclovir, as well as foscarnet and cidofovir (Fig. 159.6).* Investigational agents, such as maribavir, are in clinical trials to determine safety, antiviral effects, and efficacy for treatment and prevention of CMV infection in transplant recipients and possibly, in the near future, for congenital CMV disease.[34,317,318,542,543] However, the lack of reliable CNS penetration of maribavir may limit its clinical utility in high-risk patients with CMV disease. Acyclovir and valacyclovir also may have limited activity against CMV under certain conditions. In addition, biologic agents such as immune globulin and CMV hyperimmune globulin may benefit selected patients, and novel approaches such as cell-based, cytotoxic T-cell adoptive immunotherapy also are being investigated in clinical trials.[25,63,224,347,393,503] Treatment is beneficial for adult and pediatric immunocompromised hosts as well as for neonates with congenital CMV disease.† Normal hosts with severe CMV disease also may benefit from antiviral therapy.[401]

Treatment of CMV-associated disease, such as retinitis, pneumonitis, hepatitis, colitis, esophagitis, or encephalitis, in immunocompromised hosts, such as those patients with primary immune deficiency disorders, AIDS, or transplant recipients, usually involves a 2- to 3-week period of induction therapy with an intravenous antiviral medication, usually ganciclovir, as first-line treatment.[83,122,143,178,216,245,264,527] In special circumstances, such as suspected drug resistance or marrow suppression, foscarnet or cidofovir may be indicated.[164,489] The administration of ganciclovir plus foscarnet or cidofovir is advocated by some experts

*References 17, 85, 88, 261, 301, 424, 470, 487, 527.
†References 83, 122, 143, 168, 178, 216, 228, 233, 264, 271, 272, 274–276, 305, 349, 410, 413.

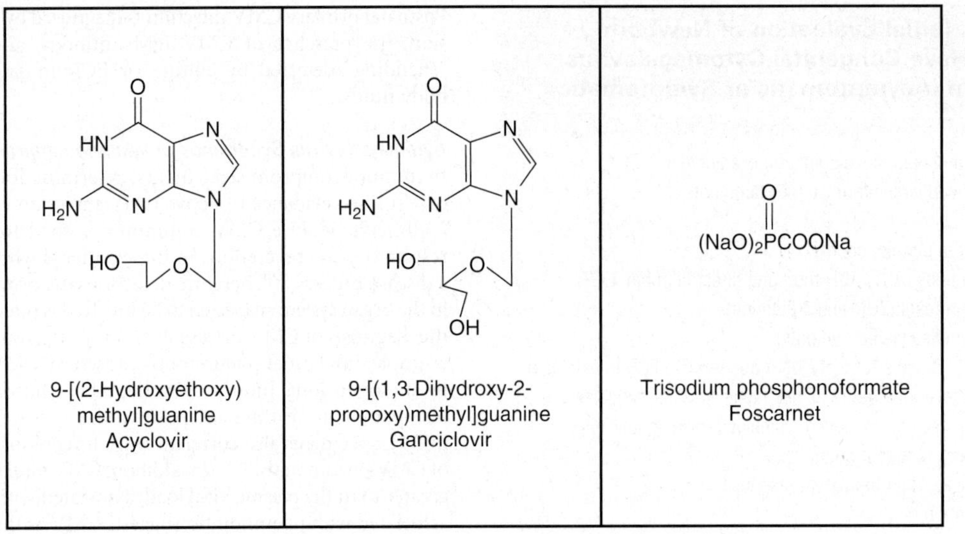

9-[(2-Hydroxyethoxy) methyl]guanine Acyclovir	9-[(1,3-Dihydroxy-2-propoxy)methyl]guanine Ganciclovir	$(NaO)_2PCOONa$ Trisodium phosphonoformate Foscarnet

FIG. 159.6 Structures of acyclovir, ganciclovir, and foscarnet.

for treatment of CMV disease in infants with primary immune deficiency of T-cell or NK-cell function, to avoid emergence of resistant strains, until immune reconstitution is achieved. The induction period should be accompanied by clinical improvement and a virologic response, with reduction in the blood quantitative CMV DNA PCR titers. If the host is expected to remain severely immunocompromised after receiving successful induction therapy, or is awaiting immune reconstitution, maintenance therapy at the same dosage as treatment levels or, alternatively, a reduced dosage schedule, three to five times a week, administered intravenously or orally is indicated through the expected period of immune suppression. In patients with AIDS, primary immune disorders of T-cell or NK-cell function, solid-organ transplant recipients receiving high levels of immunosuppression, and bone marrow/stem cell transplant recipients who have not yet engrafted and shown T-cell function may receive full doses of antiviral medication as maintenance therapy. Such therapy is usually continued indefinitely, or until immune reconstitution or resolution of immune suppression.[151] In patients with AIDS or other immune deficiency conditions who have refractory CMV retinitis, treatment with a ganciclovir implant by an ophthalmologist may augment systemic therapy, but published experience evaluating this approach in infants and children is limited.[94,505] Valganciclovir, an orally bioavailable prodrug of ganciclovir, appears to be as effective as is intravenous ganciclovir for induction therapy for CMV retinitis and for mild to moderate CMV disease in solid-organ transplant recipients.[159,316] Clinical experience has shown valganciclovir is also useful for other CMV-associated illnesses in mild to moderately ill patients. If, despite administration of antiviral therapy, CMV disease persists or progresses or if a virologic response does not occur, drug resistance should be considered. Resistance to ganciclovir has been documented most commonly in patients with AIDS, but it also can occur in patients with primary immune deficiency disorders of T-cell and NK-cell function or malignant neoplasms and in solid-organ and stem cell transplant recipients.[111,244] Most ganciclovir-resistant CMV strains have a mutation in the UL97 phosphotransferase gene, but specific mutations in the UL54 DNA polymerase gene also may occur alone or in combination with UL97 mutations.[100] Most ganciclovir-resistant CMV strains are susceptible to foscarnet but may exhibit cross-resistance to cidofovir, and strains simultaneously resistant to ganciclovir, cidofovir, and foscarnet also rarely may occur.[112,489] Reports of repopulation of previously susceptible wild-type strain of CMV may occur after discontinuation of ganciclovir in patients in whom a ganciclovir strain has emerged.[152] Resistant strains of CMV may compartmentalize in the eye or brain and cause progressive disease, even if plasma and peripheral sites appear to harbor susceptible strains.

The association of CMV immune globulin administration and acute and long-term clinical outcomes in transplantation has not been well defined.[53,160,175] The administration of ganciclovir along with intravenous immune globulin (IVIG) or CMV hyperimmune globulin to bone marrow transplant recipients with CMV pneumonitis has been shown to increase survival over that of historical controls who were treated with a variety of other antiviral regimens, including ganciclovir alone, immune globulin alone, acyclovir, vidarabine, and interferon.[160] However, differences in the method used to diagnose CMV pneumonitis, duration of illness, and treatment regimens between study subjects and historical controls obscure interpretation of these studies.[126,307] Nonetheless, CMV-associated interstitial pneumonitis in bone marrow transplant recipients, and other types of CMV disease in immunocompromised hosts, may be an immunopathologic process, and combination therapy may prevent active virus replication (ganciclovir, foscarnet, cidofovir) while enhancing immune responsiveness of cellular immunity in immune globulin–deficient patients or blunting the immune response to viral antigens already expressed on CMV-infected cells.[246,454] CMV hyperimmune globulin administered to liver transplant recipients has been shown to increase the risk for organ rejection but results in greater long-term graft and patient survival.[175] In pediatric and adult heart transplant recipients, administration of CMV hyperimmune globulin with or without antiviral prophylaxis is also associated with decreased mortality and graft loss.[463,464]

Oral maribavir has been reported in clinical trials to be possibly effective for CMV prophylaxis for prevention of CMV infection in stem cell transplant recipients and treatment of refractory or drug-resistant CMV in transplant recipients.[503,544] Clinical trials for treatment of congenital CMV infection may also be conducted in the future. Standard IVIG or CMV hyperimmune globulin, although possibly beneficial in selected patients when combined with specific antiviral therapy, should not be used alone for the treatment of established CMV infections in immunocompromised patients.[175,323,464] The combination of high-dose corticosteroids with ganciclovir does not appear to improve survival in bone marrow transplant recipients with biopsy-proven CMV pneumonitis.[411] On the other hand, a regimen combining ganciclovir with hematopoietic growth factor may allow ganciclovir to be continued in selected patients with mild marrow toxicity.

CMV hyperimmune globulin or CMV-enriched immune globulin has been shown to be of possible benefit during pregnancy in women experiencing a primary CMV infection, by reducing fetal disease in the CMV-infected fetus and by reducing transmission from mother to fetus.[406] Case series and nonrandomized studies show that CMV hyperimmune globulin appears to reduce the risk for transmission of CMV to the fetus from 40% to 16% when administered during a primary maternal infection during pregnancy, may reverse fetal abnormalities, and may improve outcome in the CMV-infected fetus with in utero disease.[87,286,347,517] One recent randomized clinical trial showed that treatment with hyperimmune globulin reduced the transmission of CMV to the fetus in mothers experiencing a primary CMV infection during pregnancy from 44% to 30%. However, this difference was not statistically significant.[418] Currently, another randomized, double-blind, placebo-controlled clinical trial evaluating CMV hyperimmune globulin for prevention of CMV transmission to the fetus during primary maternal CMV infection is underway in the United States (NCT01376778; www.clinicaltrials.gov).

Treatment of infants with symptomatic congenital CMV infection with the antiviral agent floxuridine was reported first by Feigin and colleagues in 1969 and 1971.[167] More recent reports suggest that antiviral agents, such as ganciclovir and valganciclovir, benefit congenitally infected infants.[84,287,328,329,342,358,359,446,558] Anecdotal reports, case series, and randomized clinical trials have shown clinical and virologic improvement in congenitally infected neonates treated with ganciclovir and valganciclovir.[232,348,359,414,495,506] A multicenter phase I and II study of the pharmacokinetics, antiviral effects, and safety of intravenous ganciclovir was conducted in 47 neonates with symptomatic congenital CMV disease and neurologic involvement.[502,535,567] In this study, a 6-mg/kg dose of ganciclovir administered by a 1-hour infusion every 12 hours for a period of 6 weeks produced a significant reduction in the quantity of urinary virus excretion; however, viral shedding recurred when ganciclovir treatment was discontinued. Neutropenia, thrombocytopenia, and elevated levels of liver enzymes also were observed. Limited clinical follow-up in 30 of the original 47 infants showed that hearing loss improved or stabilized in 16% of the treated infants. Subsequently, a phase III, multicenter, randomized clinical trial enrolled 100 infants and was completed in 1999.[274] In this study, ganciclovir treatment in the neonatal period appeared to have an impact on hearing loss by slightly improving hearing, maintaining normal hearing, or preventing hearing deterioration, as measured when the infants reached 6 and 12 months of age. Because only 44% of the enrolled infants were assessed in follow-up at 1 year of age, a long-term follow-up study of treated infants is needed to determine whether the early beneficial effects last through childhood and adolescence. In addition to an effect on hearing loss, treatment provided more rapid resolution of hepatitis, when present, and improved short-term growth in weight and head circumference and developmental milestones.[358,359] Reversible neutropenia was encountered in 63% of treated infants, and 2% developed reversible and mild drug-associated hepatitis, but otherwise the antiviral treatment was well tolerated.

Valganciclovir treatment for 6 weeks versus 6 months was evaluated in another randomized clinical trial of newborns with symptomatic congenital CMV infection, with and without central nervous system involvement, expanding both the clinical phenotype treated and the duration of antiviral treatment administered to the infants.[273] In this clinical trial, 6 months of oral valganciclovir administered at a dose of 16 mg/kg per dose every 12 hours provided superior benefit over the shorter 6 weeks' duration of treatment, and was more easily administered at home with careful outpatient monitoring. In this trial, hearing outcomes were improved at 1 year of age, and neurodevelopmental scores on the Bayley Scales of Infant and Toddler Development on the language-composite component and the receptive communication scale were superior in the group treated for 6 months compared with the group treated for 6 weeks. Reversible neutropenia occurred during the first 6 weeks in 19% of the infants treated. Therefore monitoring of blood counts should be done regularly in infants treated with valganciclovir.[21,225]

Currently, most experts agree that antiviral treatment is indicated in neonates with moderate to severe congenital CMV disease with or without neurologic involvement or eye disease or sensorineural hearing loss (see Box 159.5). Some experts recommend treatment of all neonates who have symptoms to reduce the risk for late-onset hearing loss and improve neurodevelopmental outcome. For maximum benefit, treatment should begin within the first month of life.[21,225] The decision to administer antiviral therapy to a neonate with congenital CMV disease remains at the discretion of the clinician and should be based on disease severity and risk factors for sequelae.[225,460,487,495,533] Short-term antiviral therapy is likely to benefit infants who have multisystem disease with viremia detected by positive CMV quantitative DNA PCR assay, pneumonia, severe or persistent thrombocytopenia, hepatitis, enterocolitis, or active sight-threatening retinitis.[242] In these clinical circumstances, a reduction in viral load should improve the infant's clinical condition and resolve end-organ disease. However, the sustained effect beyond 1 year of life of short-term treatment on long-term sequelae, such as hearing loss and neurodevelopmental disabilities, is not clear at this time and requires long-term follow-up studies to confirm this benefit.[84] A 6 months' duration or longer of therapy with an oral antiviral agent such as valganciclovir may improve outcomes and reduce the development of long-term sequelae, including hearing loss, in these infants.[23,495,533] Anecdotal reports and phase I pharmacokinetic and pharmacodynamic studies have demonstrated that valganciclovir oral solution provides plasma concentrations and antiviral effects similar to those levels achievable with use of intravenously administered ganciclovir in neonates, and clinical trials have shown that treatment with 6 months of oral valganciclovir provides benefit to some newborns with symptomatic congenital CMV infection.[272,336] Clinical trials evaluating the long-term benefits of prolonged treatment for 1 year or more with oral valganciclovir in congenitally infected infants are needed because the effects of congenital CMV infection, especially on hearing loss, may be lifelong and progressive. Case series of children with asymptomatic congenital CMV infection and hearing loss treated with ganciclovir and valganciclovir have reported improvement in hearing loss with treatment.[228,558] However, routine treatment of newborns with asymptomatic congenital CMV infection with or without congenital hearing loss is not recommended but is considered on an individual basis by some CMV experts.[21,225,405]

In addition to specific antiviral therapy, management of congenitally infected infants includes supportive care, nutritional and feeding support, and control of seizures. If thrombocytopenia is severe and persistent, platelet transfusions and immune globulin also are of benefit. Long-term management includes careful attention to nutrition to ensure adequate growth because many of these infants may have feeding disorders and disorders of growth. In addition, serial hearing tests to detect progressive or late-onset hearing loss should be performed every 3 to 6 months during the first 3 years of life, and then annually thereafter or when clinical changes occur, probably at least through 18 years of age, if not longer.[527] Treatment with hearing aids for sensorineural hearing loss is recommended. Cochlear implants may also benefit children with profound hearing loss caused by CMV. Developmental assessments to evaluate for cognitive and motor disabilities should be done on a regular basis, and physical therapy, occupational therapy, and speech language therapies should be prescribed as needed. Motor and mobility disorders also should be assessed and treated with mobility devices, braces, and if indicated, Botox injections for severe spasticity. Careful orthopedic monitoring for scoliosis and hip displacement is important. Ophthalmologic evaluations to follow up abnormalities present in the neonatal period, such as retinitis, and to monitor for vision-threatening, late-onset sequelae, strabismus, and cortical vision impairment should be performed on a regular basis as well.[253,533,538]

PREVENTION

Prevention of CMV disease is important because it causes significant morbidity and mortality in a variety of patients. In immunocompromised hosts, it also is associated with the development of other complications, such as opportunistic coinfections and graft rejection in transplant recipients, and it increases resource use in transplant programs. In neonates and infants with primary immune deficiency disorders of T-cell and NK-cell function, or SCID, congenital or acquired CMV infection is sight- and life-threatening.[330] In premature neonates, potentially fatal viral sepsis syndromes can occur. Furthermore, congenital infection is a leading cause of deafness, vision loss, and developmental and motor and mobility disabilities in children. Approaches to the prevention of CMV disease include the use of CMV-seronegative blood products, freeze-thawing or pasteurization of maternal breast milk from CMV-seropositive mothers and donors fed to premature newborns, selection of CMV-seronegative donors for transplant recipients, passive immunoprophylaxis with CMV hyperimmune globulin, prophylactic or preemptive use of antiviral agents, active immunization with a CMV vaccine, and behavioral strategies to reduce exposures to CMV-infected secretions.

Blood Product, Human Milk, and Transplant Donor Selection

Transplant recipients who are CMV seronegative and receive solid-organ or bone marrow or stem cell transplants from CMV-seropositive donors are at significant risk for acquiring symptomatic primary CMV infection (see Box 159.6). Therefore, whenever possible, CMV-seronegative recipients should receive transplants from CMV-seronegative donors, and all blood product transfusions should be from CMV-seronegative donors. CMV-seropositive transplant recipients may also experience CMV infection and disease after transplant.

Infection with CMV in seriously ill CMV-seronegative neonates can be prevented by use of blood products from CMV-seronegative donors or by use of frozen deglycerolized red blood cells.[76,557] Saline-washed red blood cells also reduce but do not always prevent the acquisition of CMV infection in neonates, even though as many as 90% of the leukocytes can be removed by this method.[133] An alternative method of preparing leukocyte-depleted blood, filtration through a cotton-wool filter, appears to prevent posttransfusion acquisition of CMV infection in neonates.[196] Many institutions now provide CMV-seronegative or leukocyte-depleted blood products routinely to all neonates or to all low-birth-weight neonates, as well as other immune compromised infants and children, regardless of the CMV serostatus of the mother.

Ingestion of CMV-positive breast milk by premature infants, especially those of less than 28 weeks' gestation, has been associated with illness. Neonatal units may have protocols to test premature neonates with sepsis syndromes with negative bacterial cultures for evidence of CMV infection, to identify them early and institute antiviral treatment if CMV disease is documented and is clinically severe. Donor selection for CMV-seronegative donors or pretreatment through pasteurization or freeze-thaw cycles of human milk administered to extremely premature infants may reduce the risk for acquisition of CMV-associated disease in these infants.[95,252,318,360,518,520] Pasteurization of breast milk is also effective but reduces the immunologic and nutritional benefits of human milk. Healthy term infants may receive fresh breast milk from CMV-seropositive mothers and donors.[379]

Passive Immunoprophylaxis

Although immune globulin, CMV hyperimmune globulin, or CMV-enriched immune globulin should not be used alone for the treatment of established CMV disease in immunocompromised patients, these preparations may be used with antiviral agents to treat CMV disease in selected patients and to prevent the acquisition of serious CMV disease in selected immunocompromised patients. The association of CMV immune globulin administration and acute and long-term clinical outcomes in transplantation has not been well defined, but some studies suggest potential benefit.[53,175]

Passive immunization remains controversial, however, partly because studies or protocols have used different dosages (100–400 mg/kg) administered at varying intervals (1 week before transplantation and every 1 to 3 weeks after transplantation) for varying times (60–120 days). CMV immune globulin has been shown to decrease the incidence of symptomatic CMV disease from 60% to 21% in CMV-seronegative renal transplant recipients who received a kidney from a CMV-seropositive donor.[465] CMV immunoprophylaxis also has decreased the incidence of CMV pneumonitis in CMV-seronegative bone marrow transplant recipients who did not receive granulocyte transfusions.[73,326,409,542] CMV hyperimmune globulin administered to liver transplant recipients has been shown to increase the risk for organ rejection but improves long-term graft and patient survival.[175] In pediatric and adult heart transplant recipients, administration of CMV hyperimmune globulin with or without antiviral prophylaxis is also associated with decreased mortality and graft loss.[463,464] A clinical trial with a CMV-specific monoclonal antibody specific to CMV gH (MSL-109) did not show benefit in a randomized, placebo-controlled, double-blind study in allogeneic stem cell transplant recipients, nor in infants with congenital CMV infection.[65]

The use of immune globulin preparations (CMV hyperimmune globulin, CMV-enriched immune globulin, and standard human IVIG that may contain high titers of CMV IgG) in pregnant women with primary CMV infections to prevent or to ameliorate CMV infection in the fetus has been reported, and results were favorable.[15,16,87,121,346,349,517] CMV immune globulin reduces placental inflammation and thickening, neutralizes virus with high avidity antibodies, and reduces cytokine-mediated cellular immune responses.[10,11,286] In one case-control study, the severity of neurodevelopmental and hearing disabilities in the infants and children of mothers with primary CMV infection who received CMV immune globulin was less compared with those who did not receive CMV immune globulin.[347] However, despite these promising results, definitive recommendations for the routine clinical use of CMV immune globulin immunoprophylaxis in women experiencing primary CMV infection during pregnancy to reduce transmission of CMV to the fetus, or to treat or ameliorate in utero CMV disease in the fetus, await results of randomized clinical trials.[22,334,346,349,393,405]

Prophylaxis and Early Preemptive Therapy With Antiviral Agents

The prophylactic use of antiviral agents in transplant recipients reduces the incidence of serious CMV disease.[159] However, no regimen has been shown to completely prevent the acquisition of CMV infection or disease in recipients of all types of transplants.[379]

Acyclovir is used by some clinicians as prophylaxis for CMV disease in organ transplant recipients, despite evidence that acyclovir is inactive against most strains of CMV and that CMV disease occurs despite such prophylaxis.[459] In one study, intravenous administration of acyclovir 500 mg/m^2 of body surface area per dose every 8 hours for 5 days before and 30 days after transplantation to CMV-seropositive bone marrow transplant recipients appeared to reduce the incidence of CMV disease.[327] High-dose oral acyclovir administered 1 day before and for 12 weeks after transplantation also has been shown to reduce the incidence of CMV disease and infection in renal transplant recipients.[45]

The prophylactic administration of human leukocyte interferon-α has been shown to reduce the incidence of severe CMV disease in renal transplant recipients, but it has no apparent benefit in bone marrow transplant recipients, and it is not used routinely in any patient population.[106,229,234,412]

The prophylactic use of intravenous ganciclovir and oral valganciclovir in solid-organ and bone marrow and stem cell transplant recipients at high risk for acquiring serious CMV disease is now routine and favored over preemptive treatment.[159,268,315] Prophylaxis treatment regimens vary, however, and it is difficult to make recommendations about which regimen is best. Most solid-organ transplant recipients appear to benefit from intravenous ganciclovir 5 to 10 mg/kg per day administered once or twice daily for 2 to 6 weeks after transplantation, usually followed by continuing antiviral prophylaxis with a reduced dose of ganciclovir or with orally administered valganciclovir.[37,507] Administration of a short 2-week course of ganciclovir near the time of transplantation, without continuing antiviral prophylaxis, does not appear to reduce significantly the incidence of CMV disease in most solid-organ transplant recipients studied.[37,507] Antiviral prophylaxis not only reduces the risk for serious CMV disease but also improves solid-organ graft survival and overall patient survival.[159] A duration of prophylaxis with oral valganciclovir extended to 200 days compared with 100 days after transplantation appears to significantly reduce the incidence of CMV disease. However, delayed-onset CMV disease may still occur, and antiviral resistance may emerge in some patients.[268,315]

IVIG or CMV hyperimmune or CMV-enriched immune globulin, when it is given with a prophylactic antiviral agent in solid-organ recipients, improves allograft and patient survival. In bone marrow transplant recipients, the administration of ganciclovir prophylaxis after marrow engraftment reduces CMV disease. In addition, some ganciclovir-treated bone marrow transplant recipients may experience prolonged neutropenia.[203] Even though most transplantation centers have adopted prophylaxis strategies with antiviral agents and CMV hyperimmune globulin to reduce the risk for CMV infection and disease, some experts believe the strategy of preemptive antiviral therapy has certain advantages over strategies that either treat only patients with overt clinical disease or administer prophylactic antiviral agents to many patients at risk, only a few of whom appear to benefit.[194] In addition, preemptive or very early antiviral treatment strategies include viral surveillance of blood, urine, and respiratory samples. Viral surveillance of these samples can be by standard viral culture, viral antigen detection, viral nucleic acid detection by qualitative or quantitative PCR assay, or a combination of these tests. Detection of CMV viremia, or rising quantitative CMV DNA PCR levels, and culture-positive or PCR-positive BAL samples have correlated with the development of serious CMV disease in transplant recipients.[81] In bone marrow, stem cell, and solid-organ transplant recipients, early intervention with intravenous ganciclovir therapy at the time of positive CMV surveillance cultures is beneficial.[203,449,461] Another approach to preemptive therapy that is currently not practiced routinely and that does not entail viral surveillance techniques is to administer an antiviral agent, such as ganciclovir, only during times of rejection, when CMV reactivation is likely to occur. This approach has been modestly successful in high-risk renal transplant recipients.[227] Simultaneous virologic and immunologic follow-up is the best approach for monitoring CMV infection in transplant recipients. Lack of immune reconstitution or presence of graft rejection or graft-versus-host disease usually heralds repeated episodes of recurrent or persistent CMV infection or disease, requiring multiple or prolonged courses of antiviral and immune globulin therapy.[194] Antiviral resistance to single or multiple agents may occur in these high-risk patients and has been increasingly recognized as a significant problem.[100]

In pregnancy, maternal administration of valacyclovir in mothers whose fetus has symptomatic intrauterine CMV infection has been shown to reduce CMV viral load, but not to have direct benefit for the fetus.[247,405,406] It is not routinely recommended but may be evaluated soon in clinical trials.[466]

Active Immunization

Prevention of acquisition of CMV disease through active immunization is a priority for the 21st century.[447,485] Universal vaccination of adolescent females to protect their future children against congenital CMV infection has been determined to be cost effective, if a CMV vaccine with at least 61% efficacy is available.[139] In addition to pregnant women and their fetuses, transplant recipients will benefit greatly if a safe, effective CMV vaccine becomes widely available.[29,258,443,447] The ideal CMV vaccine should be safe, effective, immunogenic, and cost effective. It should prevent the development of primary CMV infection without causing chronic persistent infection. The vaccine also should not be capable of infecting the fetus, and it should not be oncogenic. However, because the optimal composition and strategy for an ideal CMV vaccine that would be licensed for clinical use remains to be discovered, research continues in animal models and human clinical trials.[58,199,209,444,447]

In 1975, Plotkin and associates[390] characterized and reported a candidate CMV vaccine strain, Towne 125, that was isolated originally from the urine of a congenitally infected infant named Towne. Since then, more than 500 subjects, including renal transplant recipients and healthy adult male and female volunteers, received the investigational Towne 125 vaccine.[97,177,258,388-390,392,483] Studies of these subjects showed that Towne 125 is attenuated and relatively safe and that it induces humoral and cellular immunity in both healthy and immunosuppressed subjects.

The Towne 125 vaccine also appeared to be protective in a randomized, placebo-controlled study of 91 immunosuppressed renal transplant recipients.[389] In this study, 30 CMV-seronegative vaccine recipients received a kidney from a CMV-seropositive donor, and the incidence of severe CMV disease was significantly lower in the vaccine group than in the placebo group. However, the CMV infection rate did not differ significantly between the groups, and members of both groups experienced mild to moderate CMV disease. Subsequent studies have confirmed that CMV-seronegative renal transplant recipients who receive a live, attenuated CMV vaccine are more resistant to serious CMV disease.[391] Another vaccine strategy investigated was the development of mutant hybrid strains of CMV that combine the safety of the Towne strain with the more virulent and potentially more immunogenic Toledo strain. Early clinical trials demonstrated enhanced immunogenicity but possibly also enhanced virulence.[12,387,490] Other investigators have evaluated subunit vaccines for CMV that contain purified glycoprotein B (gB) complexed with a powerful adjuvant—alphavirus replicon particle vaccines and live, attenuated CMV vaccines.[78,166,371,490] A CMV gB vaccine with MF59 adjuvant recent showed vaccine efficacy of 50% in adult women and provided proof that vaccination has the potential to decrease maternal and congenital CMV infection.[377,369] However, a similar vaccine, when administered to CMV-seronegative adolescent girls between 12 and 17 years of age, was safe and immunogenic but had an efficacy of only 45%.[59] The cellular immune system has been targeted by "DNA vaccines" that encode gB and appear to induce protective cellular immunity against CMV.[322] Also, the human CMV gH/gL/UL128/UL130/UL131A pentameric complex has been shown to elicit potently neutralizing antibodies and is currently under research and development as a possible vaccine candidate.[531] Finally, adoptive immunotherapy with sensitized T cells has shown promising results for prevention of CMV infection and disease in transplant recipients and is currently being evaluated in clinical trials.[224,445]

Behavioral Strategies to Prevent Primary Cytomegalovirus Infection in Pregnancy

With the current complexities associated with the development of a CMV vaccine and the challenges of administering effective antiviral therapy, an alternative practical option for prevention of CMV infection during pregnancy and other high-risk times of life is education to increase public awareness about CMV and its modes of transmission.[101,132,138,208,249,417,430,562] Surveys have documented that knowledge about CMV around the world is low.[310] Most studies have shown that less than 20% of responders to CMV knowledge surveys have heard of CMV. For example, approximately 7% of men and 13% of women in one study from the 2010 HealthStyles survey had even heard of CMV, even though it is considered a common viral infection.[93,431] Surveys of a variety of groups confirm broad lack of knowledge about CMV in pregnancy and the newborn.[36,61,155,396,499,537,545] Educational materials are available from clinicians, from public health and university websites (e.g., Centers for Disease Control and Prevention: www.cdc.gov/cmv; Baylor College of Medicine: www.bcm.edu/pedi/infect/cmv; and National CMV Foundation www.nationacmv.org), and from nonprofit organizations and social media websites. These sites provide factual information to promote CMV awareness and guidelines for reducing the risk for CMV transmission to pregnant women, women of childbearing age, and other susceptible individuals.[430] Reliable, relatively inexpensive serologic evaluation is available, and some experts recommend that all women contemplating pregnancy should know their CMV serologic status, although it is not routine obstetrical practice to do so.[22,405] In addition, because epidemiologic studies have shown a major source of CMV infection to be close contact with young children, women who are pregnant, especially women who are known to be CMV seronegative, should be aware that a high percentage of young children are infected actively with CMV and that while pregnant they should exercise good hygienic practices when in close contact with young children, especially those who attend child care centers or are known to have an active CMV infection.[90,93,120,372] Studies from the United States and Europe have shown that the incidence of child-to-parent transmission of CMV may be reduced by interventions that identify susceptible pregnant women and educate them about increasing protective behaviors when around young toddles who are likely to be actively shedding CMV in their saliva and urine, such as hand washing after all wet and dirty diaper changes and after wiping tears and nasopharyngeal mucus and decreasing risky behavior for acquiring CMV, such as kissing on or near the mouth and sharing food or sharing eating utensils or cups for drinking.[7,11,120,174] Many experts recommend women of childbearing age should know about CMV and practice recommended hygienic precautions during pregnancy.[90,120,138,208,405,406] Studies have shown that these CMV awareness and prevention precautions, as a "CMV knowledge vaccine," are readily accepted and easily implemented by women in the home.[499] In addition, CMV can be transmitted from husband to wife, and if the spouse or partner experiences a CMV mononucleosis syndrome, a CMV-seronegative woman may wish to consider avoiding pregnancy for an individualized period of time.[135]

Given the proven lack of CMV awareness in women of childbearing age and in the medical community serving women and children, CMV can be considered "the most common virus most people have never

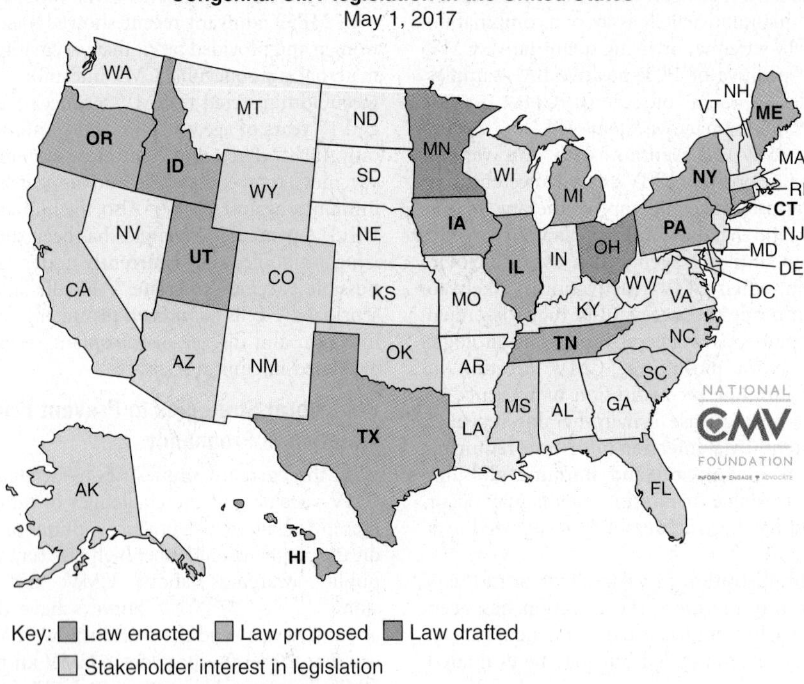

FIG. 159.7 Map of the United States showing states with cytomegalovirus (CMV) legislation enacted, proposed, or in discussion as of May 2017. Addressing CMV awareness and education for pregnant women and health care workers and newborn testing for congenital CMV through public policy can provide greater access to resources to combat the public health problem of congenital CMV. (Courtesy National CMV Foundation; www.nationalcmv.org.)

heard of." Many states in the United States and many countries around the world have now adopted CMV education and CMV testing laws and policies directing their public health departments to provide CMV educational materials to pregnant women and providing for CMV-targeted testing laws for congenital CMV infection for newborns who fail their newborn hearing screens[225,550] (Fig. 159.7).

NEW REFERENCES SINCE THE SEVENTH EDITION

1. Abate D, Saldan A, Mengoli C, et al. Comparison of cytomegalovirus (CMV) enzyme-linked immunosorbent spot and CMV QuantiFERON gamma interferon-releasing assays in assessing risk of CMV infection in kidney transplant recipients. *J Clin Microbiol.* 2013;51(8):2501-2507.
13. Adler S, Manganella A, Lee R, et al. A phase 1 study of 4 live, recombinant human cytomegalovirus Towne/Toledo chimera vaccines in cytomegalovirus-seronegative men. *J Infect Dis.* 2016;214(9):1341-1348.
21. American Academy of Pediatrics. Cytomegalovirus infection. In: Byington C, Maldonaldo Y, eds. *Report of the Committee on Infectious Diseases RedBook.* 30th ed. Elk Grove, IL: American Academy of Pediatrics; 2015:317-322.
22. American College of Obstetrics and Gynecology. Cytomegalovirus, parvovirus B 19, varicella-zoster virus, and toxoplasmosis in pregnancy. Clinical management guidelines for obstetricians and gynecologists. Vol 151, 2015, pp 1-16.
26. Antona D, Lepourtre A, Fonteneau L, et al. Seroprevalence of cytomegalovirus infection in France in 2010. *Epidemiol Infect.* 2017;145(7):1471-1478.
33. Averill L, Kandula V, Akyol Y, Epelman M. Fetal brain magnetic resonance imaging findings in congenital cytomegalovirus infection with post natal imaging correlation. *Semin Ultrasound CT MR.* 2015;36(6):476-486.
36. Baer H, McBride H, Caviness A, Demmler-Harrison G. Survey of congenital cytomegalovirus (cCMV) knowledge among medical students. *J Clin Virol.* 2014;60(3):222-243.
54. Bates M, Brantsaeter A. Human cytomegalovirus (CMV) in Africa: a neglected but important pathogen. *J Virus Erad.* 2016;2(3):136042.
59. Bernstein D, Munoz F, Callahan S, et al. Safety and efficacy of a cytomegalovirus glycoprotein B (gB) vaccine in adolescent girls: a randomized clinical trial. *Vaccine.* 2016;34(3):313-319.
60. Bilavsky E, Watad S, Levy I, et al. Positive IgM in congenital CMV infection. *Clin Pediatr (Phila).* 2017;56(4):371-375.
61. Binda S, Pellegrinelli L, Terraneo M, et al. What people know about congenital CMV: an analysis of a large heterogeneous population through a web-based survey. *BMC Infect Dis.* 2016;16(1):513-517.
62. Binnicker M, Espy M. Comparison of six real-time PCR assays for qualitative detection of cytomegalovirus in clinical specimens. *J Clin Microbiol.* 2013;51(11):3749-3753.
89. Cannie M, Devlieger R, Leyder M, et al. Congenital cytomegalovirus infection: contribution and best timing of prenatal MR imaging. *Eur Radiol.* 2016;26(10):3760-3769.
96. Cardoso E, Jesus B, Gomes L, et al. The use of saliva as a practical and feasible alternative to urine in large-scale screening or congenital cytomegalovirus infection increases inclusion and detection rates. *Rev Soc Bras Med Trop.* 2015;48(2):206-207.
123. Cuardrad M, Ahmed A, Carpenter B, Brown J. Cytomegalovirus pneumonitis complicated by a central peribronchial pattern of organising pneumonia. *Respir Med Case Rep.* 2017;20:184-187.
124. Cui X, Adler S, Schleiss M, et al. Cytomegalovirus virions shed in urine have a reversible block to epithelial cell entry and are highly resistant to antibody neutralization. *Clin Vaccine Immunol.* 2017;24(6):e24-e17.
125. Cui X, Freed D, Wang D, et al. Impact of antibodies and strain polymorphisms on cytomegalovirus entry and spread in fibroblasts and epithelial cells. *J Virol.* 2017;91(13):e01650-16.
142. Diener M, Zick C, McVicar S, et al. Outcomes from a hearing-targeted cytomegalovirus screening program. *Pediatrics.* 2017;139(2):e20160789.
155. Duval M, Park A. Congenital cytomegalovirus: what the otolaryngologist should know. *Curr Opin Otolaryngol Head Neck Surg.* 2014;22(6):495-500.
170. Fernandez-Ruiz M, Munoz-Codoceo C, Lopez-Medrano F, et al. Cytomegalovirus myopericarditis and hepatitis in an immunocompetent adult: successful treatment with oral valganciclovir. *Intern Med.* 2008;47(22):1963-1966.
179. Forner G, Abate D, Mengoli C, et al. High cytomegalovirus (CMV) DNAemia predicts CMV sequelae in asymptomatic congenitally infected newborns born to women with primary infection during pregnancy. *J Infect Dis.* 2015;212(1):67-71.
180. Forner G, Saldan A, Mengoli C, et al. Cytomegalovirus (CMV) enzyme-linked immunosorbent spot assay but not CMV QuantiFERON assay is a novel biomarker to determine risk of congenital CMV infection in pregnant women. *J Clin Microbiol.* 2016;54(8):49-54.
183. Fowler K, McCollister F, Sabo D, et al; for CHIMES Study. A targeted approach for congenital cytomegalovirus screening with newborn hearing screening. *Pediatrics.* 2017;139(2):e20162128.

187. Foxworth M, Wilms I, Brookman R, et al. Prevalence of CMV infection among sexually active adolescents: a matched case-control study. *Adolesc Health Med Ther.* 2014;5:7308.
192. Gantt S, Dionne F, Kozak F, et al. Cost-effectiveness of universal and targeted newborn screening for congenital cytomegalovirus infection. *JAMA Pediatr.* 2016;170(12):1173-1180.
193. Garcia-Gallo L, Fadul G, Laporta R, et al. Cytomegalovirus immunoglobulin for prophylaxis and treatment of cytomegalovirus infection in the (val)ganciclovir era: a single-center experience. *Ann Transplant.* 2015;20:661-666.
221. Hadar E, Dorfman E, Bardin R, et al. Symptomatic congenital cytomegalovirus disease following non-primary maternal infection: a retrospective cohort study. *BMC Infect Dis.* 2017;17(1):31.
222. Han M, Lee HJ, Lee H, et al. Risk factors and clinical features of cytomegalovirus disease in children receiving anticancer chemotherapy. *J Pediatr Hematol Oncol.* 2016;38(3):e113-e119.
225. Harrrison G. Current controversies in diagnosis, management, and prevention of congenital cytomegalovirus: updates for the pediatric practitioner. *Pediatr Ann.* 2015;44(5):e115-e125.
240. Iglesias L, Perera M, Torres-Minana L, Pena-Lopez M. CMV viral load in bronchoalveolar lavage for diagnosis of pneumonia in allogeneic hematopoietic stem cell transplantation. *Bone Marrow Transplant.* 2017;52(6):895-897.
247. Jacquemard F, Yamamoto M, Costa J, et al. Maternal administration of valciclovir in symptomatic intrauterine cytomegalovirus infection. *BJOG.* 2007;114(9):1113-1121.
253. Jin H, Demmler-Harrison G, Coats D, et al. for the Houston Congenital CMV Longitudinal Study Group. Long-term visual and ocular sequelae in patients with congenital cytomegalovirus infection. *Pediatr Infect Dis J.* 2017;[Epub ahead of print].
254. Jin Q, Su J, Wu S. Cytomegalovirus infection among pregnant women in Beijing: seroepidemiological survey and intra uterine transmission. *J Microbiol Biotechnol.* 2017;27(5):1005-1009.
257. Juckstock J, Rothenburger M, Friese K, Traunmuller F. Passive immunization against congenital cytomegalovirus infection: current state of knowledge. *Pharmacology.* 2015;95(5-6):209-217.
265. Kelly M, Benjamin D, Puopolo K, et al. Postnatal cytomegalovirus infection and the risk of bronchopulmonary dysplasia. *JAMA Pediatr.* 2015;169(12):e153785.
273. Kimberlin D, Jester P, Sanchez P, et al; for the National Institute of Allergy and Infectious Diseases Collaborative Antiviral Study Group. Valganciclovir for symptomatic congenital cytomegalovirus disease. *N Engl J Med.* 2015;372(10): 933-943.
278. Korndewal M, Mollema L, Tcherniaeva I, et al. Cytomegalovirus infection in the Netherlands: seroprevalence, risk factors, and implications. *J Clin Virol.* 2015;63:53-58.
293. Lanzieri T, Dollard S, Bialek S, Grosse S. Systematic review of the birth prevalence of congenital cytomegalovirus infection in developing countries. *Int J Infect Dis.* 2014;22:44-48.
291. Lanzieri T, Bialek S, Bennett M, Gould J. Cytomegalovirus infection among infants in California neonatal intensive care units, 2005–2010. *J Perinat Med.* 2014;42(3):393-399.
292. Lanzieri T, Chung W, Flores M, et al. Hearing loss in children with asymptomatic congenital cytomegalovirus infection. *Pediatrics.* 2017;139(3):e20162610.
294. Lanzieri T, Kruszon-Moran D, Amin M, et al. Seroprevalence of cytomegalovirus among children 1 to 5 years of age in the United States from the National Health and Nutrition Examination Survey of 2011 to 2012. *Clin Vaccine Immunol.* 2015;22(2):245-247.
295. Lanzieri T, Kruszon-Moran D, Gambhir M, Bialek S. Influence of parity and sexual history on cytomegalovirus seroprevalence among women aged 20–49 years in the USA. *Int J Gynaecol Obstet.* 2016;135(1):82-85.
296. Lanzieri TM, Leung J, Caviness A, et al. Long-term outcomes of children with symptomatic congenital cytomegalovirus disease. *J Perinatol.* 2017;[Epub ahead of print].
322. McVoy M, Lee R, Saccoccio F, et al. A cytomegalovirus DNA vaccine induces antibodies that block viral entry into fibroblasts and epithelial cells. *Vaccine.* 2015;33(51):7328-7336.
330. Miguel V, Mejias A, Ramillo O, et al. Cytomegalovirus meningitis in an infant with severe combined immunodeficiency. *J Pediatr.* 2016;173:235-237.
335. Mujtaba G, Khurshid A, Sharif S, et al. Distribution of cytomegalovirus genotypes among neonates born to infected mothers in Islamabad, Pakistan. *PLoS ONE.* 2016;11(7):e0156049.
341. Naing Z, Scott G, Shand A, et al. Congenital cytomegalovirus infection in pregnancy: a review of prevalence, clinical features, diagnosis and prevention. *Aust N Z J Obstet Gynaecol.* 2016;56(1):9-18.
362. Oosterom N, Nijman J, Gunkel J, et al. Neuro-imaging findings in infants with congenital cytomegalovirus infection: relation to trimester of infection. *Neonatology.* 2015;107(4):289-296.
363. Ozcan P, Celik H, Sonmez K, Celik M. Necrotizing retinitis secondary to congenital cytomegalovirus infection associated with severe combined immunodeficiency. *Case Rep Ophthalmol Med.* 2016;2016:1495639.
364. Padala SK, Kumar A, Padala S. Fulminant cytomegalovirus myocarditis in an immunocompetent host: resolution with oral valganciclovir. *Tex Heart Inst J.* 2014;41(5):523-529.
367. Palmeira M, Ribeiro U, Lira G, et al. Heart failure due to cytomegalovirus myocarditis in immunocompetent young adults: a case report. *BMC Res Notes.* 2016;9:9-12.
380. Peled O, Berkovitch M, Rom E, et al. Valganciclovir dosing for cytomegalovirus prophylaxis in pediatric solid-organ transplant recipients: a prospective pharmacokinetic study. *Pediatr Infect Dis J.* 2017;36(8):745-750.
385. Pinniinti S, Ross S, Shimamura M, et al; for the CHIMES Study. Comparison of saliva PCR assay versus rapid culture for detection of congenital cytomegalovirus infection. *Pediatr Infect Dis.* 2015;34(5):536-537.
396. Price S, Bonilla E, Zador P, et al. Educating women about congenital cytomegalovirus: assessment of health education materials through a web-based survey. *BMC Womens Health.* 2014;14:144.
398. Puhaka L, Renko M, Helminen M, et al. Primary versus non-primary maternal cytomegalovirus infection as a cause of symptomatic congenital infection–register-based study for Finland. *Infect Dis (Lond).* 2017;49(6):445-453.
405. Rawlinson W, Boppana S, Fowler K, et al. Congenital cytomegalovirus infection in pregnancy and the neonate: consensus recommendations for prevention, diagnosis, and therapy. *Lancet Infect Dis.* 2017;17(6):e177-e188.
406. Rawlinson W, Hamilton S, van Zuylen W. Update on treatment of cytomegalovirus infection in pregnancy and of the newborn with congenital cytomegalovirus. *Curr Opin Infect Dis.* 2016;29(6):615-624.
408. Rea F, Potena L, Yonan N, et al. Cytomegalovirus hyperimmunoglobulin for CMV prophylaxis in thoracic transplantation. *Transplantation.* 2016;100 Suppl 3:S19-S26.
418. Revello M, Lazzarotto T, Guerra B, et al. A randomized trial of hyperimmune globulin to prevent congenital cytomegalovirus. *N Engl J Med.* 2014;370(14):1316-1326.
419. Revello M, Lazzarotto T, Guerra B, et al. for the CHIP Study Group. A randomized trial of hyperimmune globulin to prevent congenital cytomegalovirus. *N Engl J Med.* 2014;370(14):1316-1326.
432. Ross S, Ahmed A, Palmer A, et al. Newborn dried blood spot polymerase chain reaction to identify infants with congenital cytomegalovirus-associated sensorineural hearing loss. *J Pediatr.* 2017;184:57-61.
429. Ross S, Ahmed A, Palmer A, et al. Urine collection method for the diagnosis of congenital cytomegalovirus infection. *Pediatr Infect Dis J.* 2015;34(8): 903-905.
438. Saldan A, Forner G, Mengoli C, et al. Comparison of the cytomegalovirus (CMV) enzyme-linked immunosorbent spot and CMV QuantiFERON cell-mediated assays in CMV-seropositive and -seronegative pregnant and non pregnant women. *J Clin Microbiol.* 2016;54(5):1352-1356.
445. Schleiss M. Cytomegalovirus vaccines under clinical development. *J Virus Erad.* 2016;2(4):198-207.
466. Society for Maternal-Fetal Medicine (SMFM), Hughes B, Gyamfi-Bannerman C. Diagnosis and antenatal management of congenital cytomegalovirus infection. *Am J Obstet Gynecol.* 2016;214(6):B5-B11.
493. Szczawinska-Poplonyk A, Joricyk-Potoczna K, Ossowska L, et al. Cytomegalovirus pneumonia as the first manifestation of severe combined immunodeficiency. *Cent Eur J Immunol.* 2014;39(3):392-395.
498. Tezer H, Yuksek K, Gulhan B, et al. Cytomegalovirus hepatitis in 49 pediatric patients with normal immunity. *Turk J Med Sci.* 2016;46:1629-1633.
499. Thackeray R, Magnusson B. Women's attitudes toward practicing cytomegalovirus prevention behaviors. *Prev Med Rep.* 2016;4:517-524.
504. Uematsu M, Haginoya K, Kikuchi A, et al. Asymptomatic congenital cytomegalovirus infection with neurological sequelae: a retrospective study using umbilical cord. *Brain Dev.* 2016;38(9):819-826.
510. Varela-Fascinetto G, Benchimol C, Reyes-Acevedo R, et al. Tolerability of up to 200 days of prophylaxis with valganciclovir oral solution and/or film-coated tablets in pediatric kidney transplant recipients at risk of cytomegalovirus disease. *Pediatr Transplant.* 2017;21(1).
511. Verma A, Palinswamy K, Cremonini G, et al. Late cytomegalovirus infection in children: high incidence of allograft rejection and hepatitis in donor negative and seropositive liver transplant recipients. *Pediatr Transplant.* 2017;21(3).
513. Vilibic-Cavlek T, Kolaric B, Beader N, et al. Seroepidemiology of cytomegalovirus infections in Croatia. *Wien Klin Wochenschr.* 2017;129(3-4):129-135.
519. Voigt S, Schaffrath R, Mankertz A, et al. Cytomegalovirus seroprevalence among children and adolescents in Germany: data from the German Health interview and examination survey for children and adolescents (KiGGS), 2003–2006. *Open Forum Infect Dis.* 2016;3(1):ofv193.
521. Vora B, Englund J. Cytomegalovirus in immunocompromised children. *Curr Opin Infect Dis.* 2015;28(4):323-329.
525. Wang S, Want T, Zhang W, et al. Cohort study on maternal cytomegalovirus seroprevalence and prevalence and clinical manifestations of congenital infection in China. *Medicine (Baltimore).* 2017;96(5):e6007.
531. Wen Y, Monroe J, Linton C, et al. Human cytomegalovirus gH/gL/UL128/UL130/UL131A complex elicits potently neutralizing antibodies in mice. *Vaccine.* 2014;32(30):3796-3804.

537. Willame A, Blanchard-Rohner G, Combescure C, et al. Awareness of cytomegalovirus infection among pregnant women in Geneva, Switzerland: a cross-sectional study. *Int J Environ Res Public Health*. 2015;12(12):15285-15297.
545. Wizman S, Lamarre V, Coic L, et al. Awareness of cytomegalovirus and risk factors for susceptibility among pregnant women, in Montreal, Canada. *BMC Pregnancy Childbirth*. 2016;16:54.
552. Yamaguchi A, Oh-Ishi T, Arai T, et al. Screening for seemingly healthy newborns with congenital cytomegalovirus infection by quantitative real-time polymerase chain reaction using newborn urine: an observational study. *BMJ Open*. 2017;7(1):e013810.
549. Utah Department of Health. Cytomegalovirus Public Health Initiative. health.utah.gov/cshcn/programs/cmv.html.
550. National CMV Foundation. Only 9% of women know about CMV. http://www.nationalcmv.org.
561. Yoo H, Sung S, Jung Y, et al. Prevention of cytomegalovirus transmission via breast milk in extremely low birth weight infants. *Yonsei Med J*. 2015;56(4):998-1006.

The full reference list for this chapter is available at ExpertConsult.com.

160 Epstein-Barr Virus

Luis A. Castagnini • Charles T. Leach

Epstein-Barr virus (EBV) is an extremely common herpesvirus that is the etiologic agent of classic infectious mononucleosis (IM).[596] Evidence continues to mount that the virus also plays a principal role in the development of certain lymphoproliferative diseases and epithelial malignant neoplasms. Its ability to remain in a dormant (latent) state after infection allows reactivation and recurrence of disease, especially under immunosuppressive conditions. Unfortunately, antiviral agents have little effect on EBV-associated diseases, but progress is being made toward improved treatment of the malignant types. Eventually, vaccination may provide protection for those persons at highest risk for development of severe disease manifestations.

This chapter reviews progress in understanding of the immunobiology of EBV and its disease associations. Enhanced understanding of EBV is leading to newer diagnostic methods and improved management of EBV-associated diseases.

HISTORY

Four distinct periods of history are identified with IM and its etiologic agent, EBV[169,558]: (1) early descriptions of IM, (2) identification of the heterophile antibody test associated with IM, (3) discovery of EBV in Burkitt lymphoma (BL) cells, and (4) association of acute EBV infection with heterophile-positive IM.

Credit for the original description of a disease consistent with what is now called infectious mononucleosis commonly is given to a German physician named Pfeiffer,[499] who in 1889 described relatively mild illness characterized by fever and lymphadenopathy; later, his report was translated into English.[418] The illness came to be known as Drüsenfieber, or glandular fever. Although some cases of glandular fever were typical of what is now recognized as IM, certain characteristics of this illness, including its predominance in children and familial clustering, did not fit. In England, glandular fever and IM have become synonymous, yet many experts consider glandular fever to be a different illness.

In the early 1900s, numerous case descriptions of illnesses epidemiologically and clinically compatible with IM appeared.[77,252,306] However, because the illness now recognized as IM had not yet been described and these illnesses were suggestive of leukemia, most of them were reported erroneously as acute leukemia with spontaneous cure. Although the term *infectious mononucleosis* was used first in one of these case reports,[306] the illness was not distinguished from leukemia until Sprunt and Evans published their landmark paper in 1920.[587] These authors described a series of patients with clinical syndromes consistent with typical IM, including classic hematologic findings. A subsequent report by Downey and McKinlay provided a more detailed description of the hematologic manifestations.[147]

Although most cases of IM could be identified by hematologic and clinical findings, not until a specific serologic test was identified in 1932 could classic IM be better defined. In the course of investigating heterophile antibodies in serum from patients with rheumatic fever and other diseases, Paul and Bunnell[489] noted high titers of heterophile antibodies in serum from a control patient. Further investigation revealed that the control patient was a medical student with IM. Evaluation of sera from three other patients confirmed the presence of high titers of heterophile antibodies during acute IM. Over the next few decades, extensive research continued in a quest to identify the agent responsible for IM. However, no organisms could be cultivated from patients with IM, and attempts at transmitting disease to animals were unsuccessful.

In 1958, Dennis Burkitt, an English surgeon, described 38 cases of "round-cell sarcoma" developing in children and adolescents living in one region of Uganda, Africa.[75] The tumors were later determined to be lymphomas, not sarcomas. After a seminar at Middlesex Hospital, London, wherein Burkitt described his findings regarding the new tumor in Ugandan children, he met a pathologist, M.A. Epstein, and a collaboration was established.[1] Shipments of lymphoma tissues began appearing in Epstein's laboratory, and eventually Epstein and a lab assistant (B. Achong)[161] successfully cultivated and evaluated tumor cells by electron microscopy. Particles were noted with ultrastructural characteristics similar to those of herpes simplex virus (HSV), which had been described a few years earlier. Further work established this virus as the fourth human herpesvirus (after HSV-1, HSV-2, and cytomegalovirus [CMV]).

The association between this new herpesvirus and IM was noted serendipitously in 1968 when an IM-like illness developed in a technician working in the laboratory of Gertrude and Werner Henle at Children's Hospital of Philadelphia.[272] Stored, preillness serum from this technician contained neither heterophil nor EBV antibodies, but both heterophil and EBV antibodies appeared 6 days after the onset of symptoms. In addition, virus was cultivated from the technician's peripheral white blood cells. Subsequent testing of serial specimens from other patients with IM also demonstrated seroconversion to EBV in all cases. This work as well as studies from Yale University,[172,458] among others, firmly established EBV as the cause of IM. Investigators subsequently showed that EBV has the capacity to transform (immortalize) human B lymphocytes in vitro, which allows the derivation of EBV-transformed B-lymphoblastoid cell lines capable of being propagated indefinitely in tissue culture.[267,506]

VIROLOGY

EBV is in the order Herpesvirales, family Herpesviridae, subfamily Gammaherpesvirinae, and genus *Lymphocryptovirus*. Its closest relative, human herpesvirus 8 (also known as Kaposi sarcoma–associated herpesvirus), is also a gammaherpesvirus, in a separate genus. The taxonomic name for EBV was recently changed from human herpesvirus type 4 to human gammaherpesvirus 4.[135]Although the original taxonomic name is used by many bibliographic search services, most scientists and physicians use the historic name.

Structure and Genome[410]

The structure of the EBV is typical for a member of the herpesvirus family; it displays an inner core of DNA surrounded by a nucleocapsid, tegument, and envelope.[162] Within the core, which measures approximately 45 nm, exist approximately 184 kilobase pairs (kbp) of double-stranded DNA coding for nearly 100 proteins. The surrounding nucleocapsid displays icosahedral symmetry (162 capsomeres) and measures approximately 100 nm in diameter. Outside the capsid lies the tegument, which is an amorphous substance consisting of numerous proteins common to all human herpesviruses, several proteins specific to the gammaherpesviruses, as well as cell proteins such as actin and β-tubulin, likely involved with reenvelopment.[324] The tegument in turn is surrounded by the viral envelope containing glycoprotein spikes. The complete virion measures approximately 150 to 220 nm.

The sequence of the entire EBV genome was first published in 1984.[35] Eleven more EBV genomes were reported through 2015, when Palser et al.[481] provided the complete sequences of an additional 71 genomes and analyzed the 83 cumulative genomes. The structure of EBV is characteristic of all the herpesviruses, with short and long sections of "unique" sequences (U_S and U_L, respectively) separated by a major internal repeat region (IR_1) generally consisting of six to 12 direct repeats of a 3-kbp sequence.[138] The virus also has numerous other regions of repeated nucleotide sequences, including direct repeat of a 0.5-kbp sequence at its termini.

Molecular Biology

Much of the early information about the molecular biology of EBV comes from laboratory strains derived from BL tumor cell lines (e.g., HR-1)[280] and marmoset lymphoid cell lines transformed by viral strains infecting human beings (e.g., B95-8). Sequencing information on 83 complete genomes has recently added to the amount of information available for studying the molecular biology of EBV.[481]

Replication

EBV infection of B cells is initiated by attachment of EBV envelope glycoprotein gp350 to a cell surface receptor (CR2, CD21) found primarily on B lymphocytes. It has long been recognized that CD21 is not necessary for B-cell fusion, and recently another B-cell receptor for EBV has been identified: CR1, or CD35.[468] Fusion of the host B cell first requires assembly of the core fusion machinery, common to all herpesviruses: EBV glycoproteins gB and gH, as well as gL (necessary for the unfolding and transport of gH). This complex then requires activation via interactions with human leukocyte antigen (HLA) class II protein, which is mediated by the binding of gp42 to gH/gL, thus forming the complex gp42/gH/gL. Because epithelial cells do not possess CD21 receptor, an alternative mechanism for fusion exists, involving EBV glycoproteins gH/gL binding to integrins αvβ6 and αvβ8.[104]After entering the B lymphocyte, the virus is transported through the cytoplasm and is stripped of its envelope in endocytic vesicles.[456] Subsequently, the viral genome circularizes and is maintained in the cell nucleus as a multicopy plasmid (or episome).[405]

Epithelial cells recently were conjectured as playing a much larger role in oropharyngeal replication and shedding of EBV, based on biologic data and mathematical reasoning.[248] The initial and predominantly replicative (lytic) EBV infection probably occurs in epithelial cells of the oropharynx and adjacent structures,[577,671] with virus then transmitted to circulating B cells passing through these lymphoepithelial tissues. Although lytic genes may be found in EBV-associated tumors (e.g., posttransplant lymphoproliferative disease [PTLD]),[443] the overall proportion of replicating cells is far surpassed by latently infected B cells. In contrast, after infection of epithelial cells occurs, active replication develops and leads to lysis and death of the cell. Alternating replication of viral glycoproteins in B cells and epithelial cells appears to modify the viral tropism, allowing virus from replicating B cells to infect epithelial cells more efficiently, and vice versa.[64] There are also data suggesting that monocytes may play an important role as a reservoir for EBV and could provide an important link for the transfer of virus from B cells to the oral epithelium.[634] Proteins synthesized during viral replication are important for viral gene regulation, replication of the genome, production of mature particles, and modulation of the immune system.

Latency

Latently infected B cells are the primary reservoir of EBV in the body. In a typical healthy EBV-seropositive adult, 1 to 50 per million B cells are infected with EBV, and this condition remains relatively constant for many years.[31] Although more than 80 gene products may be expressed during active viral replication, only a limited number are expressed during viral latency. This is one method by which the virus limits cytotoxic T-cell recognition of EBV-infected cells. The EBV gene products that may be expressed during latency include six nuclear proteins (EBV nuclear antigens [EBNAs] 1, 2, 3A, 3B, and 3C and a leader protein [EBNA-LP]); three membrane proteins (latent membrane proteins [LMPs] 1, 2A, and 2B); two small, nonpolyadenylated (noncoding) RNA molecules (EBV-encoded RNAs [EBERs] 1 and 2); the Bam H1A rightward transcripts (BARTs); and microRNAs (miRNAs).

On the basis of in vitro genetic and somatic cell hybrid experiments, three different patterns of latent gene expression can exist in EBV-infected cells from patients with EBV-associated disease.[138,336,366,410,605,623,680,686] Type I latency, exemplified by cells derived from BL and gastric carcinoma, exhibits a limited repertoire of genes consisting of EBNA-1, EBERs, BARTs, and BART miRNAs. Type II latency typically is observed in cells derived from EBV-positive Hodgkin lymphoma (HL), nasopharyngeal carcinoma (NPC), and T-cell lymphomas. Besides EBNA-1, EBERs, BARTs, and BART miRNAs, these cells also express all three latent membrane proteins (LMP-1, LMP-2A, and LMP-2B). Lymphoblastoid cell lines as well as tissues from patients with IM and PTLD display the broadest pattern of latent gene expression (type III), wherein all genes associated with latency are expressed[366,555,620,685] as well as both BART and BHRF1 miRNAs.[362] Type 0 latency occurs within circulating EBV-infected memory B cells from healthy persons, wherein only EBERs and BARTs are expressed.[410] Although these latency expression pattern categories may be useful for histopathologic characterization, significant heterogeneity among histopathologically similar tumors can occur.

A brief description of latency-associated EBV genes follows.

EBNA

EBNA-1 is required for replication and maintenance of EBV episomal DNA in latently infected cells.[366] It also interacts with various viral promoters in regulating transcription of the EBNAs (including itself) as well as LMP-1. As mentioned previously, amino acid repeat structures in the EBNA-1 protein protect it from proteosomal degradation, thereby stabilizing protein levels and possibly preventing presentation by major histocompatibility complex class I molecules.[395] The protein's contribution to the transformation of B cells was recently reported, and evidence continues to accumulate supporting EBNA-1's role in oncogenesis.[193] EBNA-2 resides in the cellular nucleoplasm, chromatin, and nuclear matrix. It is clearly a viral oncogene that is essential for cellular transformation. The ability of type 1 EBV genotypes (discussed in the section on EBV genome variation) to more efficiently transform B cells is attributable to differences in the EBNA-1 region of the genome. It transcriptionally activates several viral genes (e.g., LMP-1, LMP-2A) and cellular genes (e.g., CD21 and CD23) by its interaction with the DNA-binding protein RBP-Jκ (Jκ recombination-binding protein).[272] All three EBNA-3 proteins (A, B, and C) are transcriptional regulators of key cellular and viral promoters, but only 3A and 3C have proved to be indispensable for in vitro B-cell transformation.[627] The primary regulatory functions of EBNA-3 proteins, like those of EBNA-2, occur through interactions with RBP-Jκ.[534] Moreover, EBNA-3C is able to overcome the arrest of the retinoblastoma (Rb) gene cell cycle and increases expression of LMP-1.[402] The exact mechanistic contribution of EBNA-LP (also called EBNA-5) to B-cell immortalization is not well understood. Although EBNA-LP is not required for transformation of B cells, the absence of EBNA-LP drastically reduces the efficiency of transformation.[422] EBNA-LP possibly contributes to immortalization by enhancing EBNA-2–mediated transcriptional activation of the LMP-1 gene.[493] Also, previous studies have demonstrated that EBNA-LP cooperates with EBNA-2 in driving cells into the G_1 cell cycle phase by binding and inactivating the tumor suppressors Rb and p53.[609]

Latent Membrane Proteins

Like EBNA-2, LMP-1 (a viral oncogene) is essential for EBV transformation of B cells and appears to be the main transforming protein of EBV.[87] LMP-1 displays pleiotropic effects when it is expressed in EBV-infected cells. Most prominently, LMP-1 mimics the CD40 B-cell receptor, which plays a key role in the activation and differentiation of B cells.[353] The protein also induces expression of antiapoptosis genes (e.g., BCL-2 and A20) as well as activation and adhesion of B cells.[558] LMP-2 consists of two transmembrane proteins: LMP-2A contains two intracytoplasmic domains (at the amino and carboxy termini) and 12 integral membrane domains; LMP-2B differs by the lack of the amino-terminal cytoplasmic domain. LMP-2 generally is recognized as a modifier of normal B-cell development, promoting maintenance of viral latency.[686] LMP-2A mimics the B-cell receptor and alters normal B-cell signal transduction by inducing a range of genes involved in cell cycle induction, inhibition of apoptosis, and suppression of cell-mediated immunity. Functions of LMP-2B are less well described, due to lack of any specific antibody reagents. Nevertheless, it appears that its main role is to serve as a negative regulator of LMP-2A.[544]

EBERs

These two small nonpolyadenylated (noncoding) RNAs are the most abundant viral transcripts, consistently found in latently infected EBV cells (approximately 10^7 copies per cell) and, indeed, serve as important diagnostic tools through the use of in situ hybridization (see later section on diagnosis, EBV nucleic acid). Studies indicate that EBERs may play important roles in viral persistence and oncogenesis for some tumors. However, conflicting laboratory results have made it difficult to confirm any specific roles for EBERs, with further careful studies to settle these discrepancies anticipated.[410]

BHRF1 and BALF1

BHRF1 is a virally-coded homologue of bcl-2 (an antiapoptosis protein), and can protect EBV-infected cells from apoptosis. BALF1 also is antiapoptotic, and recent studies indicate that it can enhance tumor formation as well as potentiate metastases.[295]

BARTs

These consist of a family of differentially spliced RNAs, first identified in NPC and later found in other EBV-associated malignant diseases.[580] BART mRNAs are found at low levels in all forms of latent and lytic EBV infections. Four proteins are encoded by BART mRNAs: BARF0, RK- BARF0, A73, and RPMS1. However, none of these proteins have been identified in EBV-infected cells.

MicroRNAs

MicroRNAs (miRNAs) are recently discovered, small (19-24 nucleotides) noncoding RNAs that posttranscriptionally regulate mRNA translation.[369] The EBV genome produces at least 44 mature miRNAs, located in three clusters (one adjacent to the BHRF1 gene, and two within BART transcripts).[362] Research on EBV miRNAs is in its infancy, yet several key targets have been identified. Studies to date indicate that most of EBV's miRNAs are involved in sustaining latent infected cells. Other functions include contributing to the transformation to B lymphocyte latency, regulation of apoptosis, and immune evasion.[180,362]

Transformation

In vitro, resting human B cells infected with EBV develop into lymphoblastoid cell lines. These cells are described as immortalized or transformed because instead of following one of two normal pathways (differentiation or apoptosis [programmed cell death]), they proliferate continuously.[340] Current evidence suggests that EBV proteins coded by six latency-associated genes (described previously) are important for this cell transformation process: EBNA-2 and LMP-1 are absolutely essential; EBNA-1, EBNA-3A, EBNA-3C, and EBNA-LP also play critical roles.[410] The remaining latency-associated viral gene products, although not essential for transformation, are involved in the initiation and maintenance of cell transformation.

EBV generally transforms relatively mature B lymphocytes, secreting a complete immunoglobulin product (heavy chain plus light chain).[70,461] EBV also is capable of infecting and transforming B cells in earlier stages of development (e.g., pre-B cells [producing only μ chains] and lymphoid precursors lacking immunoglobulin gene rearrangement)[198,199,340,350]; mature plasma cells cannot be infected by EBV. Tumor cells and cell lines from BLs are B cells that generally express small amounts of immunoglobulin, which may be detected as surface immunoglobulin molecules, cytoplasmic/secreted molecules, or both. The major heavy-chain isotype expressed by Burkitt tumors appears to be μ chain (IgM), although other isotypes can be observed.[461] Similarly, the EBV-infected cells observed in the blood of persons with mononucleosis and the tumor cells found in immunodeficient hosts with EBV-associated lymphoproliferative diseases and lymphoma are B lymphocytes; these EBV-infected cell populations may include cells producing any of the major classes of human immunoglobulin (IgG, IgA, or IgM).[70,461,535,536] EBV-related malignant lymphoproliferations in immunosuppressed patients may be polyclonal, oligoclonal, or monoclonal; the lymphoproliferations probably are polyclonal at first but eventually progress to monoclonality.[139] BLs, on the other hand, always appear to be monoclonal at initial evaluation.[48,461]

EBV Genome Variation

Two genotypes of EBV (EBV-1 and EBV-2, or type A and type B) were first identified in the 1980s on the basis of marked differences in several genes, including EBNA 2 and EBNA 3A, 3B, and 3C.[545,552] EBV types 1 and 2 have only 70% DNA sequence homology in the EBNA2 gene, whereas EBV isolates with the same genotype share more than 95% of sequences in this region. Subsequent studies identified geographic differences in the prevalence of these genotypes.[98,176,179] Recent analysis of 83 sequenced EBV genomes has indicated that there is diversity throughout the genome, but the highest degree of diversity occurs among the latency genes, particularly EBNA2 and the EBNA3 family,[481] with the type 1 and type 2 classification being the major form of EBV variation.[481]

EBV-1 is the most common genotype worldwide and is the main genotype in regions with predominantly Caucasian or Asian populations. EBV-2 can only be found at rates comparable to EBV-1 in equatorial Africa, Papua New Guinea, and Alaska. Most EBV-infected persons harbor one genotype, but coinfections can occur. There is some evidence that immunocompromised populations are coinfected at higher rates.[122,123,164,480,677]

Besides DNA sequence variability, EBV genotypes also differ in certain in vitro biologic properties. Most notably, type 1 viruses display more efficient transformation of B lymphocytes as well as a faster growth rate.[530] EBV-2, in contrast to EBV-1, can spontaneously enter the lytic cycle when incubated with B lymphocytes.[73]

Early studies suggested that healthy and immune-compromised patients harbored only one or two EBV isolates (or strains). Since then, more powerful methods have made it possible to distinguish EBV isolates with relatively minor differences in DNA sequence. Subsequent studies have revealed that multiple infections can exist in healthy as well as immunosuppressed patients.[105,159,370,589,649] Some studies have demonstrated that multiple strains are typically acquired early in the infection, and that strains generally remain stable over time within each compartment (e.g., mouth, PBMCs, plasma), although there is some degree of movement among compartments.[370,572] It is important to note that there is neither convincing scientific evidence that a specific EBV genotype or strain is responsible for specific lymphoproliferative diseases, nor such evidence that one causes higher proportions of any recognized EBV-related diseases.[98,513]

IMMUNOPATHOGENESIS

Infectious Mononucleosis

EBV elicits a wide range of immunologic responses in humans, partly because of its propensity to infect B lymphocytes. In a normal host, immunologic effects are generally believed to be responsible for EBV-associated disease manifestations. Both cellular and humoral immunity develop in response to EBV infection. Detection of humoral antibodies directed against viral capsid and nuclear proteins is important for establishment of the diagnosis of acute infection. However, the responsibility for effective control of EBV infection lies primarily with the cellular immune system.[226]

As discussed earlier, during the incubation period for IM, EBV can be detected in the mouth as early as 1 week prior to disease. Low-level EBV viremia can begin up to 3 weeks prior to onset of symptoms,[151] although high blood levels do not appear until near the onset of symptoms. In conjunction with the onset of symptoms, a massive expansion of CD8$^+$ T cells ensues. In college students developing primary EBV infection, increased NK cells were observed, in addition to predicted increases in CD8$^+$ T cells and EBV viremia.[38] Moreover, higher CD8$^+$ and NK cell numbers, as well as an increased level of EBV in blood, were all associated with the severity of illness. This challenges the long-held belief that IM symptoms simply resulted from an immunopathologic process primarily involving CD8$^+$ T cells. As symptoms abate, the level of EBV in blood also abates, although low-level viremia can extend past 6 months.[38] In contrast, high concentrations of virus can remain in saliva for many months.[38,173]

In adults the proliferation of CD8$^+$ T cells causes a temporary inversion of the normal CD4$^+$/CD8$^+$ T-cell ratio; however, CD8$^+$ T-lymphocyte expansion is less marked in children.[655] After this T-cell response, the number of EBV-infected B cells falls dramatically during the next 4 to 6 weeks to concentrations of approximately one per 1 million circulating B cells.[537] During convalescence, HLA-restricted cytotoxic T lymphocytes keep EBV in check, primarily by targeting the latently expressed EBNA-3 protein.[612]

During the acute stages of IM, despite a brisk immune system response to EBV, widespread and extensive impairment in general cell-mediated and humoral immunity also exists. For example, low or absent delayed-type hypersensitivity reactions develop in response to tuberculin and other antigens.[249,421] In addition, T cells from patients with IM display unusually weak proliferative responses when they are exposed to recall antigens (e.g., *Candida albicans*, tetanus toxoid).[444,618] Although EBV-specific cytotoxic and suppressor T cells appear during acute infection, the T-cell response is primarily nonspecific and HLA unrestricted.[361,486,524] Furthermore, a polyclonal humoral response occurs during acute infection with EBV.[542] Each B cell committed to one isotype continues to produce that isotype after transformation of EBV, thereby leading to secretion of all classes of immunoglobulins, although primarily IgM.[603,672] In addition, at least 16 EBV proteins and RNAs (e.g., LMP1, LMP2, EBERs) have been identified as suppressing various functions of the immune response.[410]

Once primary infection occurs, EBV, like other herpesviruses, is able to persist in a latent state in a human host throughout that person's lifetime. For EBV, the cellular site for latency is the memory B-cell. The ability to remain undetected for the lifetime of its host indicates that EBV exerts some influence on the immune response to prevent its complete eradication. With its large genome, this process of immune system evasion is carried out primarily through the coding of functional homologues of many cellular factors that are involved in cell cycle regulation, signal transduction, and inhibition of programmed cell death (apoptosis).

Epstein-Barr Virus–Associated Tumors

In normal hosts, cellular immune responses are adequate for control and sequestration of EBV-infected cells. However, cellular immune deficiency may allow uncontrolled proliferation of EBV-infected B cells to occur during primary or reactivated (recrudescent) EBV infection. Such an excessive EBV-associated production of B cells may be histologically pleomorphic (such as B-cell lymphoproliferative diseases) or relatively uniform (monomorphic, such as B-cell lymphomas). In organ transplant recipients, no consistent chromosomal translocations are associated with the lymphomas. Many of these lesions regress once immunosuppressive therapy initiated after transplantation is withdrawn.[685] In rare, severe cases, B cells harboring EBV DNA and expressing EBNA may become disseminated throughout the body as plasmacytoid cells visible on peripheral blood smears and as B-lymphoid cells potentially invading all organs of the body. Life-threatening EBV infections also may be correlated with an overly strong virus-induced T-cell proliferation that might cause autoaggressive activity, producing hypogammaglobulinemia or other major organ dysfunctions.[46]

The pathogenesis of EBV-associated malignant disorders in some settings may be multifactorial and involve a mixture of virologic, genetic, and environmental factors. NPC, which occurs predominantly in a specific geographic locale, has been linked etiologically with EBV.[269,283] The identification of epithelial cells as potential targets for EBV infection, thereby allowing a lytic (productive) infection, has strengthened this relationship.[577] Further studies have revealed that NPC is a monoclonal proliferation that develops subsequent to EBV infection, with EBV gene products required for tumor growth.[487] However, NPC also clearly has a genetic association, inasmuch as strong linkage to a specific HLA type exists.[389] Furthermore, early EBV gene expression can affect profoundly the growth of infected cells, with full malignant potential reached when mutations occur on chromosomes 3 or 9 (presumably affecting tumor suppressor genes).[296,297] These mutations possibly result from adverse environmental conditions (e.g., exposure to chemical carcinogens, such as the volatile nitrosamines and polycyclic hydrocarbons in salted fish).[322] Furthermore, miRNAs also appear to play a key role in the carcinogenetic process.[413]

The EBV genome and expression of EBNA-1 are present in more than 95% of BL cells derived from African patients with BL (endemic BL), with the genome existing as circular episomes. In contrast, only 15% to 30% of cases of nonendemic (or sporadic) BL occurring in Europe and the United States contain EBV DNA.[299,693] In addition, EBV is present in more than 95% of primary lymphomas of the central nervous system (CNS) in patients with acquire immunodeficiency syndrome (AIDS).[415] BL cells, but not the lymphoid cells found in IM, exhibit characteristic chromosomal alterations associated with enhanced malignant potential. Approximately 90% of BL tumors exhibit a reciprocal translocation involving the long arms of chromosomes 8 and 14, t(8;14); most of the remainder have t(8;2) and t(8;22).[360,546] These translocations place the c-*myc* oncogene under the control of an immunoglobulin promoter,[131,617] which results in transcriptional deregulation and overexpression of the c-*myc* oncogene.[126,384] Malaria is well known to cause chronic B-cell stimulation, providing enhanced opportunities for c-*myc* translocations within germinal centers of lymphatic tissue. Healthy children living in areas with holoendemic malaria may have high viral loads of EBV in peripheral blood, with acute malaria further augmenting the viral load.[684] In addition, Piriou et al.[502] demonstrated that infants living in an area of Kenya with year-round malaria exposure acquired EBV at a younger age, compared to controls with less intense malaria exposure (7.28 months vs, 8.39 months, respectively). Furthermore, these infants had higher levels of EBV viremia, indicating poor control of the virus. This further contributes to the hypothesis that early acquisition of EBV is one important step that, when complemented with malaria-induced B-cell proliferation, and c-*myc* gene rearrangement and activation (and possibly other events), eventually leads to endemic BL.[136]

The differential incidence distribution of HL in children throughout the world corresponds with the age at first EBV infection: it increases in adolescence in developed countries and increases in early childhood in developing countries.[245,325] The association of EBV with HL is based primarily on serologic studies[392,450] and identification of EBV DNA in H-RS cells (the malignant cells characteristic of HL).[350,658] Virtually all cases of HL in developing countries are associated with the presence of EBV, whereas the virus is present in 20% to 50% of patients (age <35) with HL in developed countries.[349] However, in developed countries, EBV is strongly associated with HL in children younger than 10 years and in tumors displaying the mixed cellularity variant.[24,296,479] The precise pathogenetic mechanisms for EBV-associated HL are being unraveled, but evidence indicates that HL is primarily a result of chronic inflammation, with EBV (via latency II gene products and RNAs) contributing to the overproduction of various cytokines and chemokines by H-RS cells and the surrounding inflammatory cells.[177]

PTLD may develop in organ and bone marrow transplant recipients during the intense immunosuppression that occurs after placement of the graft. PTLDs span a spectrum of lymphoproliferation from polyclonal disease to monoclonal, monomorphic disease that often is difficult to distinguish from typical malignant lymphomas developing in patients with intact immune systems. No proof exists that an orderly progression leading to malignant lymphoma occurs; however, one model for the pathogenesis of PTLD proposes that defective immune surveillance after transplantation allows polyclonal proliferation of EBV-infected cells displaying a type III latency pattern (similar to that observed in IM).[117] Subsequently, genetic mutations at various loci (e.g., c-*myc*, p53) may allow progression to full malignant lymphoma.[139]

HISTOPATHOLOGY

Infectious Mononucleosis

Because IM typically is benign and the diagnosis is based primarily on clinical and serologic findings, histopathologic examination of tissues seldom is required.[126,128,219,608] However, histopathologic information is available on some tissues (e.g., lymph nodes, tonsils, spleen) from unusual cases and from patients requiring surgery.[626] For patients in whom lymphoproliferative disease and other serious manifestations of EBV infection develop, a larger amount of information is available from a broader range of tissues.[444]

Lymph nodes are enlarged diffusely during acute IM. On histologic examination, active lymphoid follicles are noted, with lymphoid proliferation extending to the sinuses, blood vessels, trabecula, and capsule.[444] The capsule remains intact despite substantial hyperplasia. The lymphoid response consists primarily of T and B immunoblasts, typically with a pleomorphic pattern and frequent mitoses indicative of rapid cell turnover.[626] Other cells identifiable in lymph node tissues include a substantial number of small lymphocytes, large atypical lymphocytes, plasma cells, histiocytes, and eosinophils. Micronecrosis may be present, although it is less extensive than that observed with herpes lymphadenitis. Tonsillar tissue also contains an active lymphoproliferative response but with more prominent follicles and extensive necrosis.

The spleen is enlarged two to three times its normal weight during acute IM, primarily as a result of hyperplasia of the red pulp. As in the lymph nodes, the cellularity is principally from immunoblasts with substantial pleomorphism. Hemorrhage, primarily subcapsular in location, is identified commonly. The liver typically shows minimal disease; infiltration by lymphocytes and monocytes occurs principally in the portal areas, and possibly minor degenerative changes take place in hepatocytes. Bone marrow may appear relatively normal during IM, but some series have reported hypercellularity and small granulomas.[128] From the relatively few cases of CNS disease associated with EBV infection, histopathology reveals lymphocytic infiltration of the meninges.[13] Less common findings include demyelination, degeneration, focal hemorrhage, congestion, and edema.

Epstein-Barr Virus–Associated Malignant Diseases

The most common form of non-Hodgkin lymphoma (NHL) is BL, which consists of sheets of small non-cleaved cells that are histologically uniform. Most arise from a single infected cell (monoclonality). The majority of CNS NHL tumors display large-cell morphology, with virtually all containing monoclonal EBV DNA. In PTLD, a wide range of histologic findings may be noted. At one extreme, one finds benign lymphoid hyperplasia with normal tissue architecture and a pleomorphic response arising from numerous infected cells (polyclonality). At the other end is observed frank malignant lymphoma.[125] The 2016 WHO classification of lymphoid malignancies recognizes six histologic types of PTLD[606]; polymorphic and monomorphic types of PTLD are the most common in children. Most polymorphic PTLD cases occur less than 1 year after transplantation, and virtually all are linked to EBV; monomorphic PTLD, however, typically presents later and is more heterogeneous, with a slightly lower rate of EBV association. T-cell PTLD is quite rare, occurs very late, and usually is not EBV driven.[667]

HL is unique among cancers, as less than 1% of cells within the tumor are actually neoplastic.[343] HL tissues are characterized by the presence of diffuse inflammatory cell infiltrates admixed with a low level of neoplastic cells: classic Reed-Sternberg cells and mononuclear Hodgkin cells (referred to collectively as H-RS cells). Reed-Sternberg cells are large (15–45 μm), multinucleated cells demonstrated to derive from germinal center-derived B cells.[366] These cells exhibit strongly stained nucleoli surrounded by a characteristic clear area resembling a halo. In the 2016 World Health Organization classification system of lymphoid neoplasms,[606] HL consists of two main subgroups: nodular lymphocytic-predominant HL and classic HL. Within classic HL are four distinctive histologic categories based on the predominant cell type and characteristics of the background cellularity: (1) lymphocyte rich, (2) nodular sclerosis, (3) mixed cellularity, and (4) lymphocyte depleted. In Western countries, EBV can be identified in approximately 40% of HL tissue specimens; mixed cellularity and lymphocyte-depleted types are associated most strongly with EBV. Children most commonly develop the nodular sclerosing variety.

Of the three histopathologic categories of epithelial tumors in the nasopharynx, the most common form in children is the undifferentiated variety, which is associated most strongly with EBV.[29] Examination of these tumors reveals undifferentiated squamous cells, with substantial infiltration by lymphocytes. Malignant cells consistently contain multiple copies of monoclonal EBV DNA within episomes, and several EBV proteins are expressed.[110]

Other Epstein-Barr Virus–Associated Diseases

The tissues involved in hemophagocytic lymphohistiocytosis typically include the bone marrow, spleen, liver, and lymph nodes, but the skin or brain may be affected as well.[186] Early in HLH that is secondary to EBV (or other infectious agents), bone marrow is typically normal; later, abnormalities such as hypocellularity or hypercellularity can be noted.[209] Activated macrophages (or histiocytes) appearing "stuffed" are observed engulfing all bone marrow cellular elements or their precursors or fragments, including erythrocytes, leukocytes, and platelets.[186,533,668] Immunostaining for CD163, a receptor whose upregulation can promote hemophagocytosis, may be useful.[209] Tissues affected by oral hairy leukoplakia (predominantly in adult patients with AIDS)[160] reveal keratin or parakeratin projections, mild hyperparakeratosis and acanthosis, ballooning and hyperplasia of the prickle cell layer, and only a sparse inflammatory cell infiltrate in the subepithelial connective tissue.[233] The principal histologic findings in pulmonary tissue from children infected with human immunodeficiency virus (HIV) and having lymphocytic interstitial pneumonitis are lymphoid nodules and diffuse infiltration of the alveolar septa and peribronchiolar regions by lymphocytic cells, including lymphocytes, plasma cells, plasmacytoid lymphocytes, and immunoblasts.[21] Some lymphoid nodules may be observed as well. The infiltrating lymphocytes consist of B cells and T cells.[334] Necrosis is not observed, and blood vessels are not affected.

EPIDEMIOLOGY

Seroprevalence

Epidemiologic studies of EBV were stimulated by development of reagents for detection of specific anti-EBV antibodies in serum in the mid-1960s. Specifically, tests detecting antibodies to VCA (long-lasting, early in infection) and EA (short duration, early in infection) were used. Henle and Henle,[268] using an immunofluorescence method, first noted a high prevalence of EBV VCA antibodies (100%) in patients with BL, but they also discovered a relatively high prevalence (85%) in normal adults. Subsequent studies, published between 1969 and 1975, in American[210,271,508,595,601] and British[495] populations, established that 80% to 95% of adults have serologic evidence of past EBV infection, with most infections occurring during infancy and childhood. More recently, information from antibody testing of a sampling of the US population (the NHANES study—see below) revealed an EBV antibody prevalence of 89% for 18- and 19-year-olds.

The age at initial (primary) infection varies markedly in different cultural and socioeconomic settings, a fact that has great pertinence to manifestations of disease associated with primary infection. Recently, EBV seroepidemiologic data were published on a statistically representative sample of the U.S. population (National Health and Nutrition Examination Survey [NHANES]),[89] in the age range of 6 to 19 years.[40] Sera collected during four 2-year time periods, between 2003 and 2010, were tested for EBV VCA IgG antibodies. EBV antibody prevalence in the most recent population group (2009-10) showed a significant increase with increasing age: 50% (ages 6–8 years), 55% (9–11 years), 59% (12–14 years), 69% (15–17 years), and 89% (18–19 years). Interestingly, over the course of the study, a significant decline in seroprevalence was noted for the combined age groups (i.e., age 6–19 years): 72% (in 2003) and 65% in 2010 ($P = .027$).[40] Non-Hispanic whites had a lower EBV antibody prevalence (64%) compared to Mexican Americans and non-Hispanic blacks (88% each). Finally, a lower EBV antibody prevalence was observed in each race/ethnicity group with respect to health insurance coverage, increased education, and less household crowding.[40]

In developing countries, EBV infection occurs at an earlier age than in developed countries, with recent studies demonstrating EBV infections in more than 50% of 12-month-old infants.[502,579] HIV-infected infants from Africa have even higher rates of EBV infection.[579] As in developed countries, EBV prevalence in developing countries also varies according to race/ethnicity, geography, and specific socioeconomic factors.[316]

In developing countries, most children with primary EBV infection have clinically silent or mild disease.[55,189,575,601] In developed countries such as the United States, primary infection with EBV typically is delayed. For reasons that remain largely unclear, primary infection in older age groups (e.g., ages 10–30 years) in developed countries is more likely to induce clinical symptoms—most often a mononucleosis syndrome.[92] Possible reasons for this occurrence were recently suggested by Balfour et al.,[37] including (1) lack of recognition of IM in preadolescent children; (2) a higher inoculum of virus via "deep kissing" in adolescents/young adults (a known risk factor for IM)[39,284]; and (3) certain NK T cells identified in the blood of children, but not adolescents/adults, which play an important role in controlling early EBV infection.[30] A recent prospective study involving students from one US university demonstrated that 77% of those acquiring primary EBV infection developed classic IM.[39]

Incidence

The incidence of IM from population-based studies ranges between 50 and 100 cases per 100,000 population.[172,265,266] These studies indicate that the highest incidence rates for IM occur in the age group of 15 to 19 years. The incidence of IM on a college campus was 14.4 cases per 100 person-years at risk.[39] Early reports of higher rates of IM in whites versus other racial/ethnic groups[82,265] are most likely explained by the higher prevalence of EBV antibodies in some nonwhite racial/ethnic groups, including non-Hispanic blacks and Mexican Americans.[40] Since IM is a manifestation of primary EBV infection, a larger proportion of nonwhite populations are already EBV positive and therefore unable to develop IM.[39] No consistent data support any seasonality associated with EBV infections. Although the infection has no clear-cut predilection for males or females, one study noted IM developing in males at a slightly higher rate than in females.[266]

Viral Shedding

In 1971, Chang and Golden[95,96] first described a "leukocyte transforming agent" in throat washings from four adults with IM. Although EBV was suspected, specific laboratory tests could not confirm it at that time.[224] Other investigators, using more specific identification methods, soon identified EBV as the leukocyte transforming agent.[211,407,439,459] Subsequent studies, utilizing virologic and DNA methods, suggested that most patients began shedding EBV in saliva during the acute phase of IM, and then shed virus either intermittently or continuously, with up to 20% of subjects shedding EBV at any one period of time. However, recent studies using much more sensitive polymerase chain reaction (PCR) methods have altered our view regarding EBV shedding.[39,151,248,466] It is now clear that EBV can be detected in the mouth well before IM symptoms occur: EBV first appears at very low levels in saliva 4 to 5 weeks prior to symptoms; later, levels increase dramatically, at approximately 1 week before symptoms[151] Following the acute illness, virus continues to be shed from saliva in more than 95% of subjects. Hadinoto et al.[248] have noted little change in concentrations of virus over short periods of time, but over months to years, large changes up to 4 to 5 $\log_{10}$ can occur. This suggests variability in the infectiousness of EBV-positive patients, depending how much virus is being shed at that time.[466]

After IM, EBV DNA may be found in other biologic fluids or body sites, including the uterine cervix,[576,621] the male reproductive tract,[310,621] breast milk,[335] and urine.[376]

TRANSMISSION

Common Modes of Transmission

Reports in the first half of the 20th century, before widespread acceptance and use of the heterophil antibody test, suggested the occurrence of epidemics of IM.[251,462,625] However, researchers generally thought that the criteria used in most of those reports to establish the diagnosis of IM were inadequate to establish that the outbreaks were indeed associated with EBV.[284] Although some success was reported for transmission of human EBV infections to certain primate species,[329] attempts to experimentally infect humans with EBV collected from the oropharyngeal secretions, blood, urine, and feces of patients with IM generally failed.[167,168,460,583] These experiments, conducted before development of specific EBV antibody tests, presumably were unsuccessful because most experimental subjects were immune as a result of having had a previous EBV infection.

Intimate sharing of oral secretions, typically through kissing, is the major source of EBV transmission in healthy populations.[39,171,284] The fact that EBV infection is extremely common worldwide, especially in underdeveloped regions, suggests that the virus is spread relatively efficiently in the general population. Surprisingly, outbreaks of EBV infection are uncommon events. However, transmission of EBV, even among close contacts of a person with acute EBV infection, may occur slowly. Studies of families of index cases of IM have indicated that EBV is not transmitted efficiently,[91,190,266] and one report[91] describes a lack of EBV transmission from a man with IM to his EBV-seronegative wife after 16 months of follow-up. In addition, data from another family study indicated that after the index IM episode, EBV antibodies (seroconversion) developed in only 35% of the nonimmune sibling contacts after an average observation period of 5.6 contact months.[600] Nonetheless, this same study also noted that the eventual seroconversion event in siblings was more likely to be associated with an IM episode than would be expected in the general population.[600] The complexity of EBV transmission and induction of IM is suggested further by the finding of multiple strains and variability of strains in distinct body compartments of individuals with primary EBV infections.[573]

Evidence has shown that EBV replicates in oropharyngeal epithelial cells[577]; subsequent infection of B cells possibly occurs as a result of contact with these epithelial cells.[6] However, it remains unclear which cells (B cells vs. oral epithelial cells) initially become infected following natural exposure to EBV via the oropharynx. Several models have been brought forward, but the answer remains elusive. Perhaps clues can be gleaned from a recent study involving college students incubating IM. Students had mouthwashes collected early in the course, which were negative for EBV DNA, pointing against lytic epithelial cell infection, and supporting possible early B-cell infection.[151] Perhaps this or other similar clinical studies may soon reveal the answer to this mystery.

The incubation period for typical EBV-associated IM (32–49 days) has long been based on the seminal study of IM by Hoagland.[284] In a case report, a teenager kissed his girlfriend just before her diagnosis of IM and began having symptoms 38 days later.[604] Most recently, a modal incubation period of 42 days was calculated among college students followed prospectively who developed IM.[39]

Transmission via Blood Products or Transplanted Organs

Transmission of EBV via blood transfusion has been reported.[212,274,284,615,678] Also, a recent retrospective study suggests that EBV is associated with posttransplant transfusions in stem cell transplants.[632] Transmission of EBV via transfusion occurs much less commonly than with CMV, however. High levels of immunity, transfer of neutralizing antibodies during transfusion, and limited survival of B cells may account for the rarity of this occurrence.[270] Despite WBCs potentially containing very high concentrations of EBV DNA,[646] only one case of EBV infection due to leukocyte transfusion has been reported, in an immunocompromised adult.[214] In transplant recipients, EBV-positive donor organs may transmit EBV to the recipient.[86,96,262]

Intrauterine and Perinatal Transmission

Because most females reaching child-bearing age already have been infected with EBV, primary infections during pregnancy occur infrequently[187,302,381] (see the later discussion of congenital infection).

EBV has been found commonly in breast milk from various populations. Several series report healthy women carrying EBV in breast milk at rates of 33% to 46%[218,335]; HIV-infected mothers from South Africa had similar rates (27%).[643] In another study from Africa, Daud et al.[133] prospectively measured the rate of EBV positivity and EBV concentration in breast milk from 94 mothers every 4 weeks (6, 10, 14, and 18 weeks) after delivery and noted a significant decrease over time.[133] Despite the presence of EBV in breast milk at substantial rates, and its potential transmissibility,[133] there is no evidence that this biologic material plays a major role in transmission of EBV to infants.[368]

Sexual Transmission

Detection of EBV in genital ulcers,[253,510] the uterine cervix,[52,576] and the male reproductive tract[216,621] raises the possibility of venereal transmission. The first seroepidemiologic study examining EBV as a sexually transmitted agent was conducted by Higgins et al.[278] in 2007 among a group of 2000 college students and indicated possible sexual transmission. However, the low concentrations of EBV in male and female reproductive tracts, compared to levels up to 10^6 copies per mL in saliva,[39] support epidemiologic studies demonstrating saliva as the major vehicle for EBV transmission.[39]

NONMALIGNANT CLINICAL SYNDROMES ASSOCIATED WITH EBV INFECTION

Primary EBV infection in children typically is silent but may result in mild clinical symptoms. Nonspecific clinical symptoms may include prolonged low-grade fever with or without lymphadenopathy, cough, rhinorrhea, fatigue and pharyngitis.[628]

Infectious Mononucleosis

EBV is the most frequent etiologic agent of IM. The signs and symptoms of classic IM[39,93,153,158,185,285,596,598] develop in most adolescents and adults, as well as in some young children, when they experience a primary (initial) EBV infection. Factors determining an asymptomatic versus symptomatic response to EBV infection are largely unknown. The degree of viremia appears to be related to disease severity in some studies,[38,39] but not in others.[569]

The incubation period is followed by a short mild prodrome of 3 to 5 days and may consist of malaise, fatigue, mild headache and possibly fever. At this stage, differentiation of IM from other viral infections is difficult.

Acute Phase

The prodrome is followed by the classic clinical features of IM (i.e., fever, sore throat, malaise, and fatigue), and physical examination reveals lymphadenopathy and tonsillopharyngitis (Table 160.1). The temperature ranges from 38°C (100.4°F) to 40.5°C (104.9°F) (usually <39°C [102.2°F]); the fever usually begins abruptly, is more prominent in the afternoon and evening, and persists for 1 to 2 weeks. On occasion, the fever may last 4 to 5 weeks. Lymphadenopathy occurs in more than 90% of children and adults and typically involves the anterior and posterior cervical lymph nodes. Generalized lymphadenopathy can also be seen and involves the supraclavicular, axillary, epitrochlear, and inguinal chains. The presence of occipital, inguinal, or axillary lymphadenopathy has a higher specificity for the diagnosis of IM when compared to anterior cervical lymphadenopathy alone.[158] Affected nodes are slightly tender, nonerythematous, and moderately enlarged in a symmetric manner. Lymphadenopathy is most prominent during weeks 2 to 4 of the illness. The absence of lymphadenopathy reduces the likelihood of IM the most when compared to other findings.[158] Tonsillopharyngitis develops during the first week of illness and usually resolves abruptly the next week. The presence of palatine petechiae in adolescents and adults with sore throat strongly suggests IM.[158]

Exudative pharyngitis, similar to that found with *Streptococcus pyogenes* pharyngitis, occurs in approximately half of patients (Fig. 160.1). *S. pyogenes* is present in the posterior pharyngeal region of 5% of patients with IM and probably represents carriage rather than simultaneous bacterial tonsillopharyngitis. Individuals with EBV infection shed higher numbers of viral particles if they are colonized with *S. pyogenes*.[636]

Splenomegaly occurs in approximately 50% of patients with IM but more frequently in younger children. Usually only the tip of the spleen

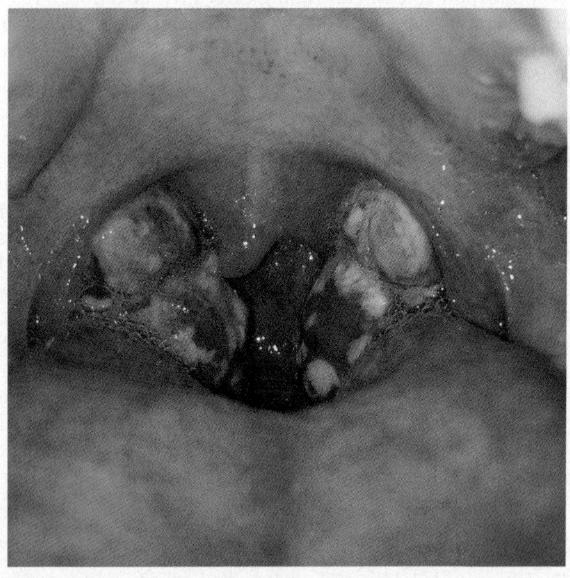

FIG. 160.1 Exudative pharyngitis with palatal petechiae in a young adult patient with infectious mononucleosis. (Courtesy Dr. Lauren Kjolhede, Baylor College of Medicine, Children's Hospital of San Antonio, San Antonio, TX.)

TABLE 160.1 Clinical Manifestations of Infectious Mononucleosis in Children and Adults

	FREQUENCY (%)		
Sign or Symptom	**Age <4 y**	**Age 4–16 y**	**Adults (Range)**
Lymphadenopathy	94	95	93–100
Fever	92	100	63–100
Sore throat or tonsillopharyngitis	67	75	70–91
Exudative tonsillopharyngitis	45	59	40–74
Splenomegaly	82	53	32–51
Hepatomegaly	63	30	6–24
Cough or rhinitis	51	15	5–31
Rash	34	17	0–15
Abdominal pain or discomfort	17	0	2–14
Eyelid edema	14	14	5–34

Data from references 93, 185, 285, 596, 598.

is palpable, with maximal size developing by the end of the second week and typically resolving by the third or fourth week of illness. Massive enlargement of the spleen is very uncommon. Hepatomegaly occurs in approximately 60% of young children with IM and less commonly in older age groups. However, silent inflammation of the liver is a common finding.[291] Cough and rhinitis are noted frequently in children younger than 4 years old with IM, perhaps as a result of other concurrent viral infections. Rash (unassociated with antibiotic administration) develops in less than 15% of adults with IM but occurs more commonly in children and adolescents (18–34%)[598] (Fig. 160.2). The strong correlation in young adults between the administration of ampicillin and the subsequent development of a rash (Fig. 160.3) is not observed in children with IM, possibly overshadowed by the overall increased incidence of cutaneous manifestations in children with IM (see Complications of Infectious Mononucleosis for a detailed discussion of rashes associated with IM). Children are more likely than are adults to have abdominal pain, failure to thrive, otitis media, and recurrent tonsillopharyngitis preceding or following IM.[598] Eyelid edema is described in up to a third of adults but occurs less commonly (15%) in children.[598]

Resolution Phase

The acute phase of IM lasts several days to 3 to 4 weeks, with gradual and uneventful resolution in immunocompetent individuals. On occasion, biphasic illness is observed, with recrudescence of acute symptoms after significant improvement. Organomegaly may persist for 1 to 3 months. The severe fatigue usually resolves within 3 to 4 weeks, but several months may be required for persons with IM to fully resume their pre-illness activity levels.[522] There is evidence, albeit minimal, suggesting that subsequent fatigue-like syndromes in patients with IM may be related to (or predicted by) the presence of preexisting lower physical fitness or prolonged bed rest during convalescence, whereas mood disorders are more related to premorbid psychiatric history.[662]

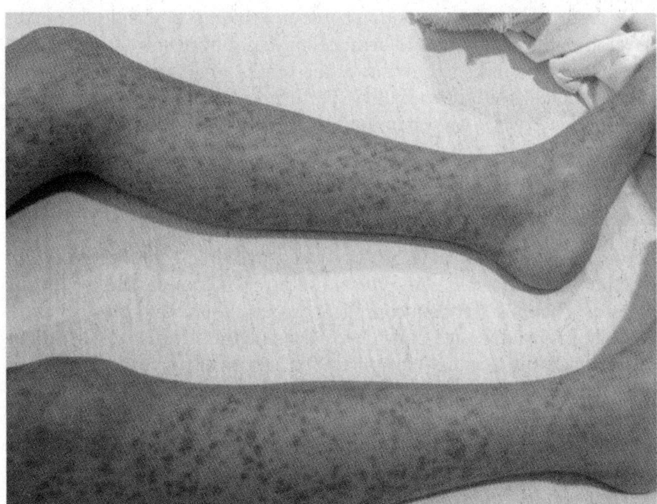

FIG. 160.2 Generalized exanthem on a 10-year-old boy with infectious mononucleosis. (Courtesy Dr. Luis A. Castagnini, Baylor College of Medicine, Children's Hospital of San Antonio, San Antonio, TX.)

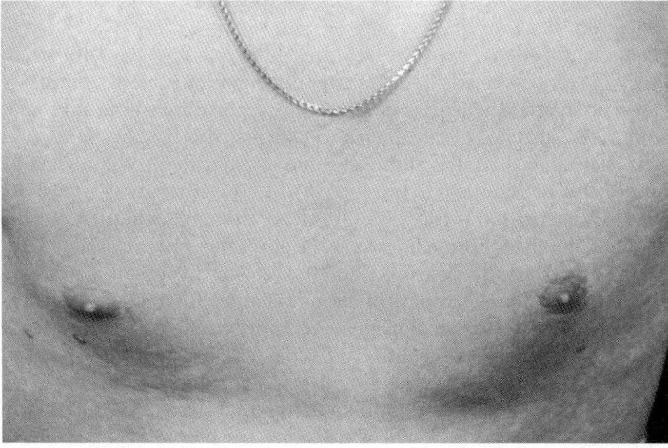

FIG. 160.3 Ampicillin rash occurring in an adolescent with infectious mononucleosis after the administration of amoxicillin. (Courtesy Dr. James Brien, Scott and White Hospital, Temple, TX.)

Infectious Mononucleosis in Young Children

Increasing incidence of EBV-IM or IM-like illness is being reported in very young children, usually accompanied by compatible EBV-specific laboratory testing.[103,146,206,598,599,651] Young children may have less intense EBV-specific serologic responses or not yield these immune responses until later in the disease course. EBV genomic testing by quantitative PCR of peripheral blood mononuclear cells and plasma has been suggested as a laboratory diagnostic aid in some cases.[103]

Disseminated EBV Infection in X-Linked Lymphoproliferative Disease

Overwhelming primary EBV infection, seen rarely in immunocompetent patients, occurs more commonly in children with certain primary immunodeficiency disorders, most notably boys with X-linked lymphoproliferative disease (XLP).[517,594] EBV infection triggers an excessive proliferation of EBV-infected B cells, macrophages, and cytotoxic T cells. Infiltration of tissues by a dysregulated immune system in conjunction with cytokine release causes parenchymal damage of the liver, bone marrow, kidneys, brain, and heart. These patients typically first present with features consistent with IM, including prominent lymphadenopathy and hepatomegaly, but fulminant disease (FIM) leading to death subsequently develops. Thrombocytopenia, anemia, and liver dysfunction are commonly seen early in the course of illness, followed by severe hepatitis, liver necrosis, acute hemorrhage, meningoencephalitis, and liver failure. Mortality rates from FIM exceed 75% in patients with XLP. Survivors usually have hypogammaglobulinemia, aplastic anemia, and B-cell lymphomas later in life.[207,449,624] Widespread, uncontrolled lymphoproliferation and hemophagocytosis are usually found at autopsy. XLP is associated with the deletion or mutation of a specific gene (SLAM-associated protein) located in the chromosomal Xq25 region, which is involved in key cellular signaling pathways for immune responses[116,457,557]; absence of this functional protein permits overwhelming and usually fatal infection from a primary EBV infection.

Hemophagocytic Lymphohistiocytosis

Hemophagocytic syndrome, first described in 1939, is a rare but life-threatening condition characterized by excessive activation of the immune system. Hemophagocytosis (engulfment of erythrocytes, leukocytes, platelets, and their precursors) by activated macrophages is usually seen in bone marrow aspirates as well as in biopsies from liver, lymph nodes, or spleen[543] (Fig. 160.4). Hemophagocytic lymphohistiocytosis (HLH) is characterized primarily by fever, pancytopenia, hepatosplenomegaly, and hemophagocytosis in lymphoreticular tissue. Since the initial description of its association with viral infections in 1979,[533] numerous viral infections, including EBV, have been linked with HLH.[209,477,525] Hereditary (familial) forms of HLH exist, most prominently those occurring in children with XLP (see preceding section).[449] Male patients with EBV-induced HLH should be screened for XLP.[209] A disseminated form of EBV infection with features of HLH may develop in these patients; most other cases are sporadic. In contrast to IM, which involves infection of B cells, primary infection in patients with sporadic HLH results in an EBV-driven T-cell proliferation with proinflammatory cytokines playing a central pathogenetic role.[314] Untreated EBV-associated HLH carries a high mortality rate.

Chronic Active Disease

Horwitz et al. first described patients with persistent or intermittent fever and lymphadenopathy and unusually elevated IgG against viral capsid antigen of EBV in 1975.[292] A similar clinical entity was described

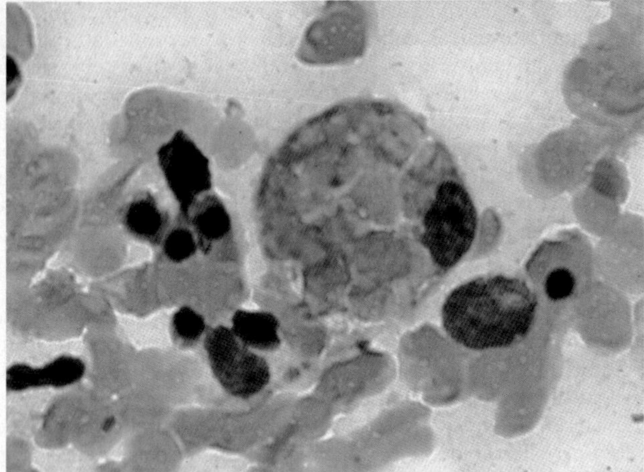

FIG. 160.4 Bone marrow from an 18-year-old woman with Epstein-Barr virus–associated hemophagocytic lymphohistiocytosis revealing a macrophage (center) filled with phagocytosed red blood cells. (From *Blood* 93:1991, 1999. Photo courtesy Dr. Lindsey Baden and Dr. Frank Evangelista, Beth Israel Deaconess Medical Center, Boston. MA.)

by Virelizier et al. in 1978 in a 5-year-old girl with a severe disease characterized by persistent fever, lymph node enlargement, pneumonitis, hepatosplenomegaly, and thrombocytopenia associated with extremely high levels of IgG and IgM against EBV VCA and EA.[644] In 1984, DuBois et al. proposed the term "chronic mononucleosis syndrome" to describe this entity,[149] and later the condition was called chronic, symptomatic EBV infection.[529] Although these reports were published decades ago, chronic active Epstein-Barr virus (CAEBV) infection is not as well characterized as are other EBV-associated diseases.[201] It shares with HLH the central theme of infection and proliferation of non-B cells. CAEBV infection occurs more commonly in Asians,[359] with children affected more frequently than adults. Two forms of the disease have been described, one involving EBV-infected T cells and the other affecting NK cells.[356,357] Patients with the more severe form can be considered to have a chronic version of HLH, with similar symptoms and a uniformly poor prognosis. After having a typical IM-like illness, these patients develop persistent infection of their peripheral T cells ($CD4^+$, $CD8^+$, or both) and do not recover fully. Guidelines for the diagnosis of CAEBV have been proposed[471] and include (1) persistent or recurrent IM-like symptoms, (2) elevated EBV anti-VCA antibodies and anti-EA, and/or detection of increased EBV genomes in affected tissues, including peripheral blood, and (3) chronic illness that cannot be explained by other known disease processes at diagnosis. Patients with suspected CAEBV must fulfill each category. Continuous or intermittent signs and symptoms, persisting for 3 months or longer, typically include fever, hepatosplenomegaly, lymphadenopathy, headache, malaise, and fatigue.[566,664,665] More severe cases display neurologic disease (e.g., encephalitis), malignant disease (e.g., lymphoma or leukemia), hepatic failure, hematologic disease (e.g., hemophagocytosis), cardiovascular disease (e.g., coronary aneurysms, valvular disease, or myocarditis) and disease localized to other organs (e.g., skin eruptions or pneumonitis).[308,359] One distinctive characteristic of these patients is extremely high antibody titers against EBV replicative antigens, including VCA and EA, and low or absent responses to EBNA. Poor prognostic factors include older age and high EBV viral loads.[359] Some cases may be related to mutations in the perforin gene.[330,341] Clonal expansion of EBV-infected T cells probably plays a central role in disease pathogenesis.[359] A second form of the disease, described principally in Japanese patients, is characterized by milder IM symptoms, less extreme EBV serologic abnormalities, granular lymphocytosis, and high IgE levels.[356] Interestingly, these patients also typically develop pronounced skin reactions in response to mosquito bites.[108,309] Large expansions of EBV-infected, CD56-positive NK cells are observed in peripheral blood and in the skin reactions. CAEBV infection should not be confused with chronic fatigue disorder, which has no clear association with EBV.

Congenital Infection

Primary EBV infection during pregnancy is rare, mainly because immunity to EBV exceeds 95% in women of child-bearing age.[381] The role of EBV as a potential cause of fetal infection is uncertain, and evidence of a link between infection and congenital anomalies is lacking. Chang and colleagues[94,97] found only one EBV-infected specimen among 2696 samples of cord blood lymphocytes. However, in a study of more than 700 pregnant women, the persistence of EBV EA was associated with increased risk of adverse pregnancy outcomes, including fetuses with malformations, early fetal death, and prematurity.[302] More recently, investigators have demonstrated rare instances of in utero transmission of EBV confirmed by PCR,[436] but adverse fetal outcomes have not been clearly documented. The strongest evidence of congenital EBV infection comes from case reports of infants with congenital anomalies attributed to EBV infection. Goldberg et al.[223] reported a newborn infant who had bilateral central cataracts, cryptorchidism, hypotonia, and petechial rash. Laboratory evaluation showed thrombocytopenia, and EBNA was detected in the infant's lymphocytes. In 1978 Brown and Stenchever[71] reported an infant born to a mother with confirmed EBV infection; the infant died soon after birth with multiple malformations and a positive antibody titer to EBV on cerebrospinal fluid (CSF). However, confirmation by virologic studies was not possible in either of these cases.

Other Diseases

EBV has been linked with various autoimmune disorders in children and adults, primarily on the basis of seroepidemiologic information. Early reports[78,560] of an association between EBV infection and subsequent development of rheumatoid arthritis have not been substantiated by a recent meta-analysis.[42] On the other hand, large systematic reviews suggest that infection with EBV predisposes to the development of multiple sclerosis[8] and systemic lupus erythematosus.[260]

COMPLICATIONS OF INFECTIOUS MONONUCLEOSIS

Acute EBV infection in a healthy child or adolescent, regardless of whether it is associated with typical IM, rarely is complicated by serious illness.[596] The most frequent complications, exanthems and mild hepatitis, more appropriately are considered part of the normal spectrum of disease.[365] More serious complications involving major organs have been reported regularly since IM first was described as a distinct clinical entity, but they remain rare (for review, see elsewhere[9,317,494,598]). Most complications, including the more severe ones, are transient.

In one prospective study,[598] significant complications involving mainly the pulmonary, neurologic, and hematologic systems were noted in approximately 20% of children with IM. Thrombocytopenia with hemorrhagic manifestations, severe airway obstruction, and neurologic complications developed in children with IM more frequently than in adults; jaundice occurred less frequently.

Exanthems

Ampicillin Rash

Historically, patients with IM were treated frequently with antibiotics, primarily for suspected streptococcal pharyngitis or bacterial lymphadenitis. Soon after the release of ampicillin, reports linked the antibiotic with the occurrence of exanthems in patients with IM. Two large case series have indicated that administration of ampicillin (or amoxicillin) precipitates an exanthem in most (95% to 100%) adolescents and adults with EBV-associated IM,[485,515] but it is less common in children.[598] This phenomenon has become known as the ampicillin rash associated with IM. The rash usually develops 5 to 10 days after treatment is initiated and resolves within a few days of discontinuation. Characteristically, the cutaneous lesions are maculopapular and pruritic and involve the trunk, face, and extremities (see Fig. 160.3).[485] A rash also may develop in patients with IM treated with other antibiotics, including azithromycin[130] and cefprozil,[32] but such rashes do not represent hypersensitivity reactions.

Other Exanthems

An exanthem will develop in approximately 3% to 15% of persons with IM not treated with antibiotics.[34,285,327,425,522,598] These rashes are maculopapular but can be urticarial, scarlatiniform, or erythema multiforme–like (see Fig. 160.2). Rarely, the rash has been described as vesicular or purpuric.[7] Erythema nodosum also has been noted.[61] Although most commonly associated with hepatitis B, some cases of Gianotti-Crosti syndrome (papular acrodermatitis of childhood) also have been related to primary EBV infection.[288]

Cardiac

Mild electrocardiographic abnormalities (mostly nonspecific ST- and T-wave changes) have been observed in 6% to 16% of adults with IM.[153,286] Abnormalities usually are noted during the second or third week of illness and disappear by the fourth week, but they may persist longer. A case of myocarditis heralding typical IM has been noted in a young adult.[648] Mild, asymptomatic and self-limiting pericardial effusion has been reported in children during the acute phase of IM.[482] Serious cardiac complications occur extremely rarely.[197]

Hematologic

Hemolytic Anemia

Hemolytic anemia occurs in 1% to 3% of patients with IM,[152,414,598] and many cases have been reported in children with previously unrecognized hemoglobinopathies. The anemia typically develops during the second or third week of illness and resolves in 1 to 2 weeks. Corticosteroid therapy may hasten resolution.[208]

Aplastic Anemia

This anemia is a rare complication of IM, with only scattered case reports in the literature.[43,380,638,656] Steroids have been beneficial,[236] but bone marrow transplantation has been necessary in some cases.[14,396] Fatalities have been recorded, usually in association with pancytopenia.[3,638]

Thrombocytopenia

Mild thrombocytopenia occurs in 25% to 50% of patients with IM[80,83] and probably is immune mediated, related to the presence of autoantibodies to platelet glycoproteins,[613] although splenic sequestration may contribute. Platelet counts usually return to normal levels 4 to 6 weeks after the onset of illness, only on rare occasions lasting 8 weeks or more.[80] Severe thrombocytopenia (platelet counts $<20 \times 10^3/mm^3$) occurs rarely, with fewer than 40 cases identified in one review.[501] Most cases presented with petechiae, purpura, or bruising, and 30% had epistaxis.[501] The authors noted a complication rate of 27% and a mortality rate of 5% associated with severe thrombocytopenia. Case reports have suggested beneficial effects of corticosteroids[400,611] or intravenous immune globulin[150,613] for severe, life-threatening thrombocytopenia. Platelet transfusions provide only temporary improvement; however, patients who receive transfusions are less likely to develop complications of severe thrombocytopenia.[501]

Neutropenia

Mild to moderate neutropenia occurs frequently during IM.[81,84] Neutrophil counts typically reach their lowest values during the third and fourth weeks of illness but may persist for another month or more. Although severe neutropenia (absolute neutrophil count <200) and agranulocytosis are rare events, with patients recovering uneventfully, death from overwhelming bacterial infection has been reported.[258,455] Antibodies against anti-human neutrophil-specific antigens elicited during EBV-induced polyclonal antibody stimulation probably are the source.[559,683]

Pancytopenia

Pancytopenia has been reported to develop in a small number of children and adults with IM.[371] Fatalities attributable to overwhelming bacterial infection have occurred.[313,638]

Spleen

Detectable splenomegaly develops in up to 50% of patients with IM; one study demonstrated splenic enlargement by ultrasound examination in 100% of patients hospitalized with IM.[145] Patients with a palpable spleen are at risk for having spontaneous rupture. In the United States, splenic rupture occurs in 0.1% to 0.5% of all patients with IM[26,175,419]; male patients are more commonly affected, and about 50% of ruptures occur spontaneously.[419] The rate of splenic rupture in children is unknown but probably is lower. The risk of splenic rupture is not related to the severity of IM.[192] Rupture typically occurs during the first to third week of illness and is heralded by abdominal pain. Signs of hypovolemia occur frequently and include orthostasis, tachycardia, and syncope. Pain in the left shoulder (Kehr sign),[411] caused by diaphragmatic irritation from blood, is observed in approximately 50% of patients with splenic rupture; right shoulder and subscapular pain may develop as well.[554] Splenic infarction following IM occurs rarely, but its presentation mimics splenic rupture and should be considered in patients with left upper quadrant abdominal pain. A recent literature review shows 19 of such cases, 12 of which were in patients 21 years of age or younger.[276] Splenic abscess has been described in a child with IM.[111]

To reduce the risk of splenic rupture, physicians customarily caution patients against engaging in strenuous physical activity and contact sports during recovery from the acute illness and for the period of significant organomegaly.[549,652] Recommendations for reduced activity vary between 3 weeks and 6 months. In one review, the lack of evidence-based information about the timing of return to activity for athletes is acknowledged, and physicians are discouraged from making decisions on the basis of a single parameter.[652] Instead, individualized decisions must be made. In general, if the patient is asymptomatic without a palpable liver or spleen, a gradual return to pre-IM levels of light activity probably is safe. Some authors recommend avoiding contact sports or any strenuous activity associated with increased abdominal pressure (i.e., weight lifting, rowing) for at least 3 weeks after illness onset,[27,419] while others recommend waiting a minimum of 4 weeks before returning to competitive contact sports.[145,196] Some studies have evaluated the role of imaging procedures (e.g., computed tomography or ultrasonography) to assess spleen size and document resolution of splenomegaly, and while some show benefit of serial ultrasonography, [465] imaging is generally not cost effective or accurate in determining the timing for normal activity.[45] Ultrasonography may be considered for asymptomatic athletes desiring to return to play early and for those with ambivalent examination findings.[45,518]

Most cases of splenic rupture require emergency splenectomy.[175] However, in an effort to maintain the patient's hematologic and immunologic competence, practical management of splenic rupture is evolving. At some institutions, selected patients with splenic rupture who meet certain requirements, including hemodynamic stability with low transfusion requirements and a normal level of consciousness, may be managed with medical therapy[26] or endovascular interventional methods[67,241] instead of traditional splenectomy.

Gastrointestinal Tract

Liver

Mild to moderate, subclinical inflammation of the liver occurs in more than 90% of patients with IM.[291] Rarely, more serious cases of hepatic disease, including fulminant hepatic failure in children, have been des cribed.[140,200,264,365,409,416,423] Mellinger and colleagues published a case series of consecutive adults with acute liver failure and found that less than 1% of all cases were related to primary EBV infection; however, the case-fatality rate was high.[434] Rare pediatric cases of EBV-induced acute liver failure treated with liver transplantation have been reported.[182,434] Chronic hepatitis also has been documented.[614]

Other

Other gastrointestinal diseases purportedly associated with IM include pancreatitis, gastritis, typhlitis, proctitis and cholecystitis.[364,365,399,568,688]

Neurologic

Acute neurologic disorders[120,428,570] develop in 1% to 5% of persons with IM.[51,285,428,570] Neurologic complications usually occur at the height of the typical manifestations of IM, but they also may develop during the resolution phase. In addition, some reports document neurologic disease as a heralding event, before the development of typical IM, or even as the sole manifestation of EBV infection, especially in children.[63,141,144,165,448] The most common neurologic complications include those occurring in the CNS, such as aseptic meningitis, meningoencephalitis, and encephalitis; however, other central and peripheral neurologic complications have been described.[428] The pathophysiologic process of CNS manifestations is not well established. Possible mechanisms include direct viral invasion, immunologic mechanisms, and inflammation.[355]

Encephalitis and Aseptic Meningitis

EBV frequently affects the CNS, causing abnormalities in both CSF and electroencephalography, yet most patients exhibit no symptoms.[492] In two large series of patients with encephalitis, EBV was responsible for up to 10% of cases,[143,347] and EBV caused 8% of cases of focal encephalitis.[663] Clinical findings in EBV encephalitis include fever, headache, vomiting, seizures, alteration in mental status, focal deficits (i.e., bilateral leg weakness, leg spasticity, face and arm weakness, asymmetric reflexes) irritability, disorientation, lethargy, and, occasionally, a comatose state.[141,143] Symptoms suggestive of schizophrenia, such as delusions, hallucinations, and extreme agitation, are seen occasionally. Patients with aseptic meningitis typically complain of a stiff neck, headache, fever, and vomiting. Symptoms of IM occur uncommonly in children developing EBV encephalitis. Typical CSF findings in children with EBV encephalitis include mild to moderate pleocytosis (lymphocytic predominance) in 50%, mildly elevated protein levels in half of cases, and normal glucose concentration.[144] EBV antibodies, EBV DNA, and even EBV virions have been identified in the CSF or brain tissue of persons with EBV-associated neurologic complications.[2,143,255,303,328,355,490] Some reports suggest that the immune dysregulation caused by primary EBV infection may act as a triggering mechanism for the development of measles-associated subacute sclerosing panencephalitis.[181,287] Because typical IM symptoms seldom occur in children with EBV encephalitis and clinical findings are not specific, EBV should be considered a possible etiology for any child with acute encephalitis. Fulminant and fatal outcomes have rarely been reported in children with EBV-associated meningoencephalitis.[426,428]

Other CNS Manifestations

EBV-associated cerebellitis is a rare occurrence that develops primarily in children and young adults.[109,114,120,165,220] Full recovery occurs within weeks to months. Cranial nerve palsies, singly or in combination, also occur rarely; the facial nerve is affected most commonly, including bilateral involvement in some cases.[435,619] Other manifestations of cranial nerve involvement include optic neuritis,[143,194] dysarthria from hypoglossal nerve palsy,[687] deafness,[165,666] and ophthalmoplegia.[551] Some cases of brain stem encephalitis,[463,565] radiculomyelitis, and recurrent aseptic (Mollaret) meningitis[227] have been reported.

Non-CNS Neurologic Complications

Guillain-Barré syndrome (ascending polyradiculoneuritis) is the most common neurological complication of EBV infection outside the CNS.[237,238,528] Others include peripheral neuropathy,[155] autonomic dysfunction,[676] hemiplegia,[36] and transverse myelitis.[143,633]

Renal

Silent abnormalities of the urine sediment, including proteinuria and microscopic hematuria, occur commonly in patients with IM.[285,387] However, clinically significant renal disease is an extremely rare event. Tubulointerstitial nephritis, acute tubular necrosis, and nephrotic syndrome have been observed most commonly.[60,438,641] Acute renal failure with and without rhabdomyolysis has been reported.[195,390,464,475,641] Some children and adolescents have developed hemolytic-uremic syndrome related to acute EBV infection.[385,564,571]

Respiratory Tract

Airway Obstruction

Severe airway obstruction is one of the most common indications for hospitalization in children with IM.[317] Alpert and Fleisher[9] observed severe airway obstruction in a fourth of children admitted for complications of IM. Overall, it is estimated that up to 5% of children and adults will develop this complication over the course of their illness.[317] Patients typically have severe tonsillopharyngitis with progressive symptoms of airway obstruction, usually in association with dysphagia and odynophagia. Airway obstruction may occur at any of several levels, including inflammation and hypertrophy in the Waldeyer ring, edema of the epiglottis and pharynx, and development of pseudomembranes in large airways.[219,246] Acute onset of obstructive sleep apnea in children with IM has rarely been reported.[102] Management of airway obstruction has included systemic corticosteroids, tonsillectomy, tracheostomy, and nasopharyngeal airway placement, as well as general supportive measures such as humidification and elevation of the head of the bed.[582,669] Nonsurgical management, including the systemic administration of steroids, usually is beneficial, although tonsillectomy may be necessary in refractory cases.[582,591,669] With the widespread availability of intensive care and mechanical ventilation, mortality from this complication is much lower than previously observed.

Neck Abscesses

Cervical and peritonsillar abscesses have been described in association with IM.[76,259,326,660] This uncommon complication follows severe tonsillopharyngitis in patients with IM and typically is caused by bacteria found in the oral cavity, including alpha-hemolytic streptococci and anaerobes. Appropriate management includes administration of antibiotics and surgical drainage. Some concern exists that corticosteroid therapy of incipient airway obstruction may predispose to the development of an abscess.[76,259] Gold and colleagues reported the case of a 17-year-old girl with IM treated with corticosteroids for the management of airway obstruction who subsequently developed jugular vein suppurative thrombophlebitis (Lemierre syndrome).[221] On the other hand, abscesses may develop in the absence of previous corticosteroid therapy.[205,509]

Pulmonary Disease

Radiographic evidence of pulmonary infiltrates occurs in 0% to 5% of patients with IM,[153,377] yet significant symptoms rarely are present.[153,285,377] Some cases of IM with pulmonary manifestations may represent coinfection with other etiologic agents.[20,184] However, several immunocompetent adults (but few children) with acute EBV infection have been described with pulmonary disease seemingly unrelated to other organisms.[115,254,432,467] Typically, unilateral or bilateral interstitial infiltrates are observed, and pleural effusions may be present.[100,156,363] In some cases, EBV has been detected in lung tissues.[588,639] Recovery is the rule, although mechanical ventilation may be necessary.

Psychiatric

Chronic Fatigue

In the early 1980s, a chronic debilitating disorder, now designated chronic fatigue syndrome or systemic exertion intolerance disease (SEID/CFS),[204] began receiving increased publicity and purportedly was linked etiologically to EBV.[331,593] The syndrome occurs more commonly in middle-aged women and is characterized primarily by at least 6 months of debilitating fatigue leading to a substantial reduction in level of activity. Accompanying symptoms may include low-grade fever, mild lymphadenopathy, pharyngitis, neuropsychological problems, sleep disturbances, headache, and other symptoms.[592] The association with EBV was drawn mainly from epidemiologic features and some abnormal EBV-specific immune responses. Variable general immunologic abnormalities have been described in some cases. However, no consistency exists in these findings, and a plausible pathogenetic association has not been demonstrated. Most experts today do not regard EBV as an etiologic agent in the development of this syndrome, although it may play a contributory role along with other infectious etiologies (e.g., human herpesvirus 6, CMV, Lyme disease, giardiasis).[344] Performing diagnostic tests for infections, including EBV, is not routinely recommended for patients with SEID/CFS. Variably prolonged episodes of fatigue symptoms after IM continue to be reported, particularly among young adult women and those with premorbid mood disorders.[345,496]

"Alice in Wonderland" Syndrome

This unusual syndrome, technically termed metamorphopsia, is a visual illusion manifested as a distortion in size, form, movement, or color, and it is associated most commonly with migraine headaches, epilepsy, and hallucinogenic drugs. Infections have also been associated with the development of this syndrome.[58,453] Copperman[121] first described its association with IM in 1977, and other similar cases also have been described.[112,166,373,374] Onset may occur during or soon after resolution of the clinical IM symptoms, and it may resolve within 4 to 6 weeks. Visual evoked potentials suggest diminished cerebral perfusion in affected patients.[373]

Miscellaneous Complications

Other complications purportedly associated with IM or primary EBV infection include recurrent tonsillitis,[640] sinusitis,[602] periorbital cellulitis,[602] ocular disease,[427] acute dacryocystitis,[215] rhabdomyolysis,[474] genital ulcers,[4,256,510,553] proctitis,[365] and orchitis.[521] EBV has been implicated in the pathogenesis of advanced types of periodontal disease.[578]

MALIGNANT DISEASES ASSOCIATED WITH EPSTEIN-BARR VIRUS

Burkitt Lymphoma

Endemic BL is a rapidly progressive and fatal tumor that predominantly affects young children in central Africa and Papua New Guinea (Fig. 160.5).[75] Approximately 60% of African patients with BL present with jaw masses; abdominal masses are second most common.[689] Jaw involvement occurs more commonly in younger patients (peak incidence at 3–7 years).[441] Less common sites include the CNS and the eye, with bone marrow involvement being rare. In patients with sporadic BL, the abdomen is the most common site involved at presentation (60–80%), with head and neck second most common (e.g., lymph glands, oropharynx and nasopharynx, sinuses).[441] Bone marrow is involved in 20% of patients. In some patients with BL and some with congenital or acquired immunodeficiencies (including AIDS), CNS involvement is present or eventually develops and is characterized by intracranial mass lesions of lymphomatous cells or a CSF pleocytosis consisting of malignant cells, or both.[18,689,691]

Hodgkin Lymphoma[516]

Pediatric HL is divided into two categories: childhood HL (age <14 years), and "AYA" (adolescent/young adult, 14–35 years). HL rarely occurs in children younger than 5 years in Western countries, but it is seen more commonly at younger ages in developing countries. Painless cervical or supraclavicular lymphadenopathy is the most common presentation for both age groups, with obstructive symptoms secondary to mediastinal lymphadenopathy occasionally seen. Constitutional symptoms such as fever, night sweats, and weight loss develop in approximately one fourth of patients with HL, and these symptoms worsen the prognosis. Of the four HL histologic subtypes, AYA patients display one predominant histology—nodular sclerosis (65–80%), whereas 90% of patients with childhood HL have nodular sclerosis or mixed cellularity.

Nasopharyngeal Carcinoma

NPC occurs primarily among adults in east and southeast Asia, accounting for 0.6% of cancers worldwide; the tumor is extremely rare in Western countries.[110] In endemic regions, children younger than 16 years account for only 1% to 2% of all cases of NPC, but this age group accounts for 10% of NPC cases in the United States.[110,305,397] Within the nasopharynx, the fossa of Rosenmüller is typically the tumor's epicenter; from there it invades adjacent organs and anatomic spaces. Symptoms at presentation in children include a painless unilateral neck mass, nasal symptoms (congestion, epistaxis, discharge), auditory symptoms (otalgia, otitis media, hearing loss, tinnitus), headaches, and cranial nerve abnormalities (cranial nerves III, V, VI, and XII most likely).[29,110] Metastasis to cervical lymph nodes occurs in 75% of patients.

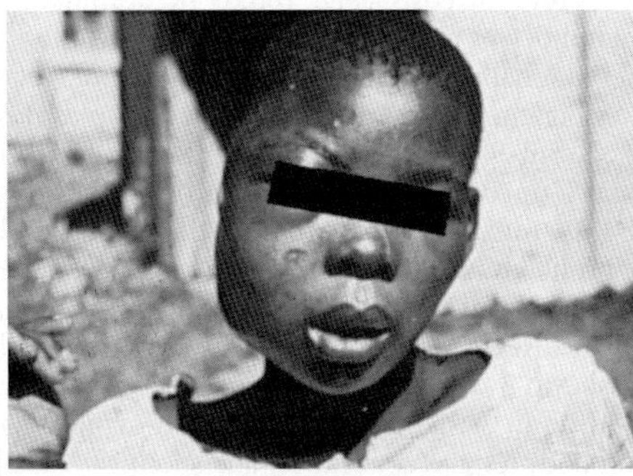

FIG. 160.5 African boy with Burkitt lymphoma involving the jaw. (Courtesy Dr. George Miller, Yale University.)

Posttransplant Lymphoproliferative Disease

Children immunosuppressed for organ transplantation have an increased risk for development of EBV-related lymphoproliferative syndromes and B-cell lymphomas (collectively termed PTLD).[281,367,584] Ho and colleagues[281] reported a greater frequency of lymphoproliferative lesions in pediatric transplant recipients (4%) than in adult transplant recipients (0.8%). Pediatric organ transplant recipients are thought to have an increased risk for development of EBV-related PTLDs because, compared with adult transplant recipients, they are more likely to be seronegative for EBV at transplantation, and primary infection is more likely to progress to PTLD and other severe EBV-associated disorders.[281,282] Recipients acquire EBV via passenger WBCs in the allograft, blood transfusions, or more naturally via exposure to EBV-positive saliva.[231] Some variability exists in the incidence of PTLD according to the specific organ transplanted. The incidence is highest in children receiving intestinal transplants (11%),[228] which is postulated to be attributable to stronger immunosuppressive regimens and greater loads of lymphatic tissue in the grafts. The incidences of PTLD are lower in other pediatric organ transplant populations. One year and 5 years after pediatric solid organ transplantation, the PTLD incidence was 1.3%/2.4% (kidney), 1.6%/5.7% (heart), 2.1%/5.4% (liver), and 4%/16% (heart and heart/lung).[231] After human stem cell transplantation, the 10-year cumulative incidence rate for PTLD is approximately 1% overall.[127]

The clinical history, physical examination findings, and confirmatory virologic laboratory testing are required to establish a diagnosis of PTLD. Symptoms may be nonspecific, especially early in the course, and include fever, malaise, weight loss, abdominal symptoms (bleeding, nausea, vomiting), sore throat, swollen lymph nodes, headache, focal neurologic symptoms, and indications of graft dysfunction.[231] On examination, signs may include lymphadenopathy, large tonsils, hepatosplenomegaly, pallor, subcutaneous nodules, and focal neurologic findings.[231]

Posttransplant EBV-positive smooth muscle tumors (PTSMTs) have been described in children and adults undergoing solid organ transplantation.[332] Interestingly, previous PTLD occurs in approximately 40% of pediatric cases, but in less than 5% of adults.

Lymphoproliferative Disease in Other Immunodeficient Patients

Patients with a wide variety of primary immunodeficiencies (e.g., Wiskott-Aldrich syndrome, ataxia-telangiectasia, Chédiak-Higashi syndrome) as well as iatrogenically immunosuppressed patients (e.g., patients receiving cancer chemotherapy) also are at risk for development of various EBV-associated lymphoproliferative diseases and severe atypical EBV infections.[478] EBV-associated diseases reported in these patients include severe IM, HLH, lymphoproliferative disease, BL, HL, diffuse large B-cell lymphomas (DLCBLs), smooth muscle tumors, and mesenchymal tumors.[478] One should keep in mind, however, that most immunocompromised children with acute EBV infections display minimal symptoms, or have a clinically silent course, similar to immunocompetent persons.[273,281]

Other Malignant Diseases

Gastric carcinomas are more common in Asia, but they are extremely rare in children. EBV is associated with approximately 10% of cases worldwide, but is found in the majority of tissues from patients with gastric tumors displaying an undifferentiated (lymphoepithelioma-like) histopathologic pattern.[352] Aberrant DNA methylation is important in the pathogenesis of EBV-associated cases, with viral proteins and micro RNAs also playing roles.[679]

Other rare lymphoproliferative diseases (B-cell and T-cell) as well as carcinomas have putative associations with EBV. The strengths of these associations is variable. These include pyothorax-associated lymphoma, lymphomatoid granulomatosis, plasmablastic lymphoma, systemic EBV-positive T-cell lymphoma, angioblastic T-cell lymphoma, enteropathy-associated T-cell lymphoma, extranodal T/NK-cell lymphoma (nasal type), and aggressive NK-cell leukemia.[85,148,202,312,657,675]

Epstein-Barr Virus and Human Immunodeficiency Virus

Several studies have indicated that underlying HIV infection is responsible for abnormal responses to EBV infections. These findings probably are attributable to the relative ineffectiveness of T cells from patients with AIDS in controlling EBV-infected lymphocytes.[59] In HIV-infected adults, these unusual reactions include exaggerated antibody responses to certain EBV antigens, including VCA and EA,[520] and enhanced oropharyngeal shedding of EBV.[10,183,320] Oropharyngeal shedding of EBV occurs more commonly in younger HIV-infected children, and children whose HIV disease progressed more rapidly had a substantially higher rate of excretion.[183,320] Infection with EBV develops in HIV-infected children more frequent and at an earlier age and is more likely to involve hepatosplenomegaly and pneumonia compared to HIV-uninfected infants.[491,579] In addition, HIV-infected infants have higher EBV viral loads, are more likely to be coinfected with both EBV genotypes, and are generally poor controllers of EBV viremia.[498,579] Whether EBV contributes directly to the progression of immune deficiency in these patients continues to be a matter of conjecture, although in vitro studies do indicate that some EBV proteins (e.g., LMP, BZLF1) are able to transactivate HIV-1.[257,420]

Certain lymphoproliferative and other diseases develop in HIV-infected patients at rates higher than those in healthy persons.[54,124,472,567] The immune activation triggered by HIV infection is thought to be responsible for B-cell stimulation and EBV-infected cell expansion, which may favor the development of EBV-related lymphoproliferative diseases.[497] In addition, several HIV proteins (e.g. gp120, Tat, and Nef) are able to induce polyclonal B-cell activation.[500] EBV-associated lymphoproliferative diseases include NHL, HL, body cavity lymphoma, smooth muscle tumors, lymphocytic interstitial pneumonitis (LIP), and oral hairy leukoplakia (OHL).

Lymphomas

NHL has remained the most common malignant disease occurring in children with AIDS[54,106] and is an AIDS-defining condition.[88] In the present era of combination antiretroviral therapy (cART), NHL also has surpassed Kaposi sarcoma as the most common malignant disease in adults.[160] In one pediatric study, approximately one third of NHL tumors contained EBV DNA.[431] Primary CNS lymphomas are extremely rare occurrences in healthy children, but they have accounted for 8%[431] to 23%[54] of NHLs in children with AIDS. Primary CNS lymphomas are linked strongly to EBV, with the virus present in virtually every case.[415] Pediatric patients with AIDS and NHL typically have systemic symptoms of fever and weight loss. Signs of extranodal disease include hepatosplenomegaly, abdominal distention, jaundice, bone marrow involvement, and, rarely, CNS symptoms.[430] Although it is not an AIDS-defining condition, HL in adults with HIV infection historically has occurred at rates 5 to 15 times higher than in the general population. HL is an uncommon occurrence in HIV-infected children, but it has been described.[11,431,512] HIV-infected patients, including children,[512] appear more likely than non–HIV-infected patients to present with disseminated disease, sometimes without obvious nodal involvement on physical examination.[505] In patients with HIV infection, including children, the incidence of HL has increased in the cART era.[11,160] Interestingly, HL incidence rates are higher in patients with moderate compared with severe immune suppression, and the increased incidence is postulated possibly to be related to the inability of EBV-infected H-RS cells to recruit sufficient lymphocytes and histiocytes for their survival.[56]

Body cavity lymphoma (or primary effusion lymphoma) is a rare malignant disease that occurs almost exclusively in adult patients with AIDS, but it has been reported in children.[383] Patients typically have immunoblastic lymphomatous effusions without solid tumors in body cavities, such as the peritoneum or pleura.[452] More than 75% of these nonsolid tumors are associated with human herpesvirus 8; however, EBV also is identified frequently in tumor cells. EBV may play a cofactorial role in the pathogenesis of these unusual tumors.[527]

Smooth Muscle Tumor

Leiomyosarcoma is an extremely rare occurrence in healthy patients,[682] but it is the second most common malignant disease in children with AIDS[429,681] and is an AIDS-defining condition (Category B).[88] It also has developed in solid-organ transplant recipients[386] and in patients with other types of immunodeficiency.[437] EBV may be responsible for the unusually high incidence of these smooth muscle tumors found in children with AIDS.[319,431] Leiomyosarcoma tissues from patients with AIDS have high concentrations of EBV (CD21) receptors, contain clonal (or oligoclonal) EBV DNA, and express EBERs and EBNA-1.[319,431] In addition, some tumors demonstrate overexpression of *myc*, a proto-oncogene that leads to cell proliferation.[321] Leiomyosarcoma may develop in any smooth muscle tissue in patients with AIDS, but more typically it is noted first in the gastrointestinal tract and lungs. Tumors can appear simultaneously in multiple locations in the same individual.[137]

Lymphocytic Interstitial Pneumonitis

LIP is a lymphoproliferative disease that occurs primarily in children with AIDS.[19] In the era before cART, the incidence of LIP was 12% to 17% among children[225,561]; in the cART era, this incidence has dropped to less than one case of LIP per 1000 person-years. Previous serologic and virologic evidence pointed to an association with EBV,[19,343,523,547] but the exact role that EBV plays in this lymphoid proliferation is unclear at present. Children with LIP typically present in the second or third year of life.[561] The presence of LIP is generally associated with an improved prognosis for survival.[547] On radiographic examination, diffuse, bilateral reticulonodular and interstitial infiltrates are noted.[503] Many infants are asymptomatic, and whereas some children remain stable for long periods, others may exhibit a slow but relentless progression to chronic lung disease typified by tachypnea, cough, wheezing, and hypoxemia. Generalized lymphadenopathy and chronic parotitis may accompany LIP.[607] Advanced disease is characterized by clubbing, wasting, cor pulmonale, and bronchiectasis.

Oral Hairy Leukoplakia

OHL is a nonmalignant squamous cell proliferation that develops in the oropharynx of HIV-infected patients. Although a common occurrence in adults, it occurs in less than 5% of HIV-infected children.[417] EBV DNA and virus replication can be detected within epithelial cells,[234,581,650] with defective variants possible.[203] OHL lesions are manifested as painless nonremovable gray or white plaques on the lateral surface of the tongue; rarely lesions can develop elsewhere in the mouth. Typical lesions often have vertical corrugations and a shaggy or "hairy" appearance when dry. OHL does not have any malignant potential, and treatment is not routinely necessary.[348,562]

DIAGNOSIS OF INFECTIOUS MONONUCLEOSIS

General Laboratory Findings

Patients with IM typically have an absolute lymphocytosis (defined as absolute count of >4500/μL or >50% lymphocytes), prominent atypical lymphocytes (usually >10% of total leukocytes), and a positive test result for Paul-Bunnell heterophile antibodies (positive differential heterophile).[188] The atypical lymphocytes observed in the blood of patients with mononucleosis (Fig. 160.6) predominantly consist of activated T lymphocytes responding to the B-cell infection.[488] Although often considered a hallmark of IM, atypical lymphocytes also may be observed in association with CMV infection, toxoplasmosis, measles, mumps, roseola, rubella, drug reactions, and other conditions.[107,673]

For a typical uncomplicated case of IM, establishing a specific diagnosis of EBV infection is unnecessary; a complete blood count, differential, and heterophile antibody test are sufficient for diagnostic testing.[57,68,188] The results of these tests are uncommonly normal early in the course of disease, and thus the tests may need to be repeated during the first 2 to 3 weeks before diagnostic results are achieved. In adolescent and adult patients with classic IM symptoms, a positive heterophile antibody test has a sensitivity and specificity of approximately 85% and 100%, respectively.[229] The false-negative rates of the heterophile antibody test can be as high as 25% during the first week of illness, 5%

to 10% in the second week, and 5% in the third week.[157] The specificity of lymphocytosis (>50% of the absolute lymphocyte count) and presence of atypical lymphocytes (>10% of total leukocyte count) is 85% and 92%, respectively.[68,158] The clinician should be aware that very young (<4 years) patients with primary EBV infection frequently have a negative heterophile test result,[599] and only 25% to 50% of children under 12 years of age have a positive test result.[406,414] Some studies suggest that a higher ratio (>0.35) of lymphocytes to white blood cell counts[670] or the detection of lymphatic tissue with fibrinous membranes observed by nasopharyngeal endoscopy[654] may distinguish between IM and acute bacterial tonsillitis.

Heterophile antibodies classically were measured as sheep erythrocyte agglutinins.[489] Beef, ox, and horse red blood cells also are agglutinated by the heterophile antibodies found in the serum of patients with IM, but these heterophile antibodies do not bind to guinea pig kidney antigen extracts. These properties of mononucleosis heterophile antibodies distinguish them from the naturally occurring Forssman heterophile antibodies and from the heterophile antibodies found in serum sickness and other conditions. Thus, traditional tests for Paul-Bunnell heterophile antibodies involve absorption of the test serum with beef or ox red blood cells (which remove Paul-Bunnell heterophile antibodies) and guinea pig extract (which does not remove them). Tests in current use (e.g., mono test, Mono-Diff, Monospot) typically use horse red blood cells, which provide a more sensitive assay than do sheep erythrocytes. However, when horse erythrocyte agglutination tests are performed, the specificity of a positive result always should be confirmed by absorption of the serum with at least guinea pig kidney extract or, preferably, with both guinea pig kidney extract and beef (or ox) red blood cells. Materials for the absorption steps are included in many but not all of the kits available commercially. Another heterophile antibody test, the beef (or ox) erythrocyte hemolysin assay, does not require absorption of the test sera but is somewhat less sensitive than is horse erythrocyte agglutination testing. Other tests[191,250,391,539] using purified forms of heterophile antigen do not seem to offer any significant advantage over the rapid slide test using horse erythrocyte agglutination.

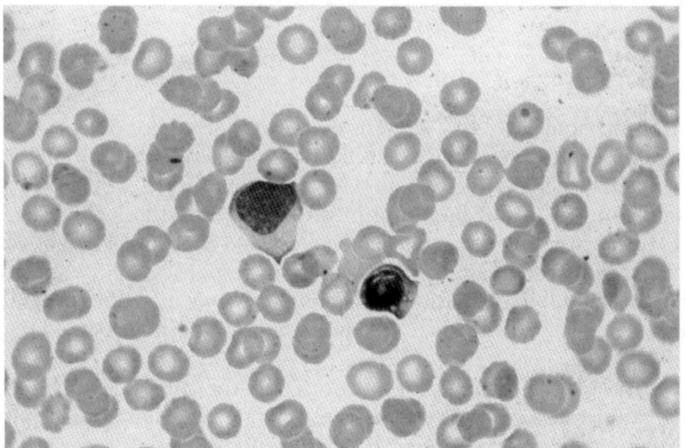

FIG. 160.6 Atypical lymphocytes in the peripheral blood of a patient with infectious mononucleosis. (Courtesy Dr. Margaret Gulley, University of North Carolina, Chapel Hill, NC.)

Other laboratory tests in patients with severe mononucleosis syndromes or in those with atypical clinical manifestations may indicate involvement of major organs, but such involvement rarely is associated with severe complications (see the previous section, Complications of Infectious Mononucleosis). These laboratory abnormalities include elevated transaminase levels, mild hemolytic anemia, and neutropenia.

EBV-specific laboratory testing should be reserved for patients with an EBV-suspected disease (1) lacking a heterophile antibody response, (2) exhibiting atypical, severe manifestations, or (3) associated with significant lymphoproliferative, oncogenic, or chronic findings.[597] In most cases of EBV-associated IM episodes in immunocompetent patients, EBV-specific serology (i.e., antibody determination) is sufficient to affirm the viral-specific diagnosis. Isolation of virus from body secretions, fluids, and tissues (see later section, Virus Isolation) is labor intensive and not widely available. Quantitation or semiquantitation of EBV-specific viral load provides some measure of activity or putative influence of the virus in a variety of EBV-associated diseases. Other laboratory methods demonstrating high concentrations of actively replicating virus or latent antigens (such as immunohistochemical methods for antigen testing or quantitative PCR) may be more useful in associating EBV infection with disease, particularly in immunocompromised patients (Table 160.2).

Epstein-Barr Virus Antibodies

The viral-specific diagnosis of EBV-associated primary infections as IM in immunocompetent individuals (and commonly in immunocompromised patients) usually requires three types of antibody analysis on acute serum: IgG to EB VCA (VCA IgG), IgM to EB VCA (VCA IgM), and IgG to EBNA (EBNA IgG).[597] (The EBNA complex is composed of six nuclear antigens or proteins, principally EBNA-1; the antibody response to the complex will herein be referred to as IgG to EBNA, or EBNA IgG.) The three EBV antibodies can be detected by commercially available immunofluorescent techniques or by various enzyme immunoassays. The need to add the determination of IgG to EB early antigen, a serologic response commonly found early in the primary infection, usually is not necessary for IM-like episodes.

Evolution of the serologic response to EBV antigens after a prototypic EBV-associated IM episode is depicted in Fig. 160.7. By the time clinical evaluation for IM and probably other forms of primary EBV infection is performed, an appreciable antibody response to EBV VCA has developed in most persons.[269,599] In the case of primary infections (e.g., IM), the initial serum sample often contains both IgG and IgM antibodies to VCA. Most children also have (or will develop shortly) antibodies

TABLE 160.2 Summary of Laboratory Tests for Epstein-Barr Virus (EBV)-Associated Diseases

Detection of	Test	Purpose
Antibodies	Heterophile antibody	Detect heterophile antibodies indicating infectious mononucleosis (more reliable in patients >4 y)
	EBV antibodies	Measure antibody response to viral proteins in serum samples; distinguish acute from remote infection
EBV DNA and RNA	Southern blot	Assess clonality of lesions with respect to EBV DNA structure; distinguish latent from replicative infection
	In situ hybridization	
	RNA (EBERs)	Identify EBER transcripts in specific cell types within histologic lesions
	DNA	Identify EBV DNA in specific cell types within histologic lesions
	PCR	Detect and quantitate EBV DNA in blood or CSF to diagnose and monitor disease
EBV proteins	Immunohistochemistry	Identify EBV protein expression in specific cell types within histologic lesions; distinguish latent from replicative infection on the basis of expression profiles
EBV	Virus culture	Detect infectious virions or latently infected B cells; impractical for routine clinical use
	Electron microscopy	Identify whole virions representing replicative infection; impractical for routine clinical use

CSF, Cerebrospinal fluid; *EBER*, EBV-encoded RNA; *PCR*, polymerase chain reaction.
Modified from Gulley ML. Molecular diagnosis of Epstein-Barr virus–related diseases. *J Mol Diagn*. 2001;3:1-10.

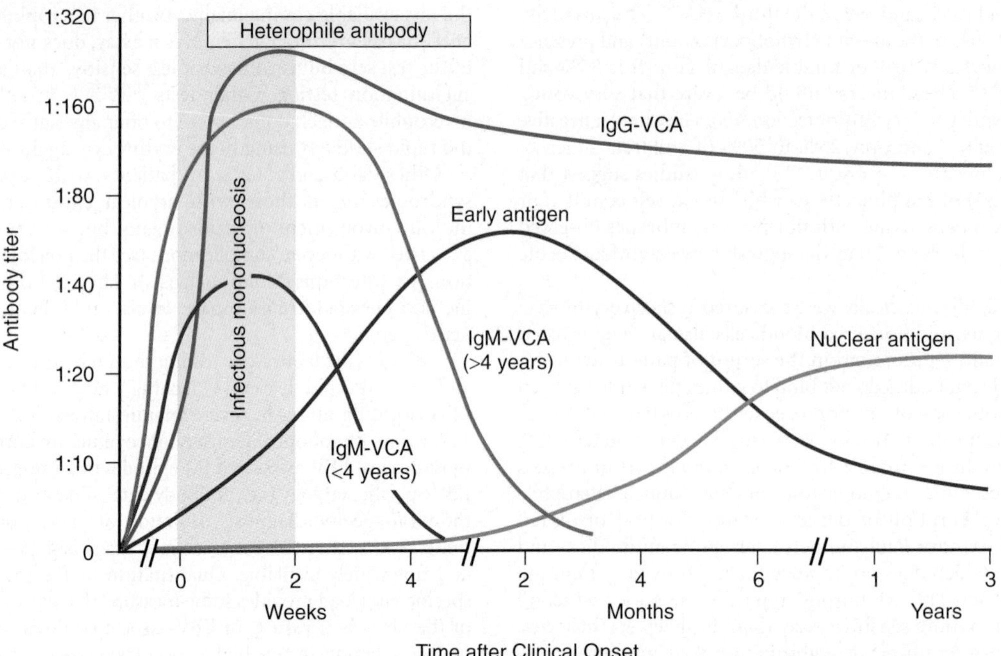

FIG. 160.7 Evolution of antibodies to various Epstein-Barr virus antigens in patients with infectious mononucleosis. The titers are geometric mean values expressed as reciprocals of the serum dilution. The minimal titer tested for viral capsid antigen (VCA) and early antigen (EA) antibodies was 1:10; for Epstein-Barr nuclear antigen (EBNA), it was 1:2.5. The immunoglobulin (Ig) M response to capsid antigen was divided because of the significant differences noted according to age. (From Jenson HB, Ench Y, Sumaya CV. Epstein-Barr virus. In: Rose NR, de Macario EC, Folds JD, et al, editors. *Manual of Clinical Laboratory Immunology*, 5th ed. Washington, DC: American Society for Microbiology; 1997:634-43.)

to the EA complex, which can be measured separately as antibodies to the restricted (R) or diffuse (D) components.[189,599] During the early phase of primary infection, most persons do not have detectable IgG antibodies to EBNA; a few have marginally detectable anti-EBNA titers. Thus, the serologic diagnosis of a recent or current primary EBV infection typically consists of a positive IgG and IgM anti-VCA response and negative anti-EBNA, with positive results in the anti-EA assay, if it is performed.

After the acute primary EBV infection (reflected in IM), IgM antibodies to VCA typically disappear within 2 to 3 months, and IgG antibodies to EA usually disappear within 6 to 12 months after infection (see Fig. 160.7).[597,599] IgG anti-VCA and anti-EBNA antibodies persist for life and are indicative of a typical, chronic virus-carrying state.[599] Some studies also have shown the persistence of anti-EA antibodies for several years after an acute EBV infection and the occasional appearance of anti-EA antibodies in healthy seropositive persons; however, the clinical or virologic importance of this finding is not clear. Heterophile antibodies are detectable during the first or second week of illness and may persist for months and sometimes for a year or more in persons who have recovered from IM; they remain detectable longer (usually more than a year) when the more sensitive horse erythrocyte agglutination and a quantitative method to determine the antibody response are used.

The antibody profile for an acute primary EBV infection, particularly that associated with an IM episode, is relatively clear in comparison with the variability of serologic or antibody profiles found in persons with other EBV-related disorders (Table 160.3). When a disease is not a consequence of primary infection but may be related to persistent or reactivated EBV infection (e.g., BL, NPC, some lymphomas of immunocompromised hosts, some chronic or atypical illnesses), the following serologic profile may be observed: positive IgG anti-VCA, often in high titer; usually negative IgM anti-VCA; often elevated anti-EA titer; and positive anti-EBNA assay (although sometimes at low titer and occasionally undetectable).[259,270,273,318,517,594] Of note is that males with XLP frequently have no or low levels of EBV antibodies in response to EBV infection.[550]

Some studies[424,531,540] suggest that monitoring for decreases in anti-EBNA antibodies or identification of increased immunologic mediators such as interleukin-4 and soluble CD23 and increased circulating EBV may be useful in providing early serologic signs of EBV-associated tumor development in organ and bone marrow transplant recipients. Further, testing for IgA antibody responses to EBV antigens may be helpful in establishing a diagnosis of acute infection in immunocompetent individuals[53] and evaluating the response to therapy for NPC.[337]

Molecular cloning of subregions of the EBV genome into high-expression plasmid vectors can generate large amounts of pure proteins containing EBV-encoded polypeptide sequences for use in immunoblot and enzyme-linked immunosorbent assay (ELISA)-based tests.[74,90,174,279,531,540] These methods have extended the availability and use of EBV laboratory diagnosis and follow-up. There are a growing number of commercially available EBV serologic tests, particularly enzyme immunoassays.[72,277] Yet after several decades of use, immunofluorescent techniques still remain the gold standard in EBV-specific serologic testing because of their overall excellent specificity and sensitivity. However, they require more expensive equipment, time, effort, and experience in interpretation. ELISAs are important alternatives for serologic testing because of their ease of performance and enhanced sensitivity. However, their specificity may be inferior to that of immunofluorescent techniques.[393] It is noteworthy that there is insufficient standardization of antigen preparation, antigen and substrate selection, and cross-comparability of serologic techniques and manufacturers involved with commercially available EBV serologic tests. Therefore, interpretations should be drawn carefully, particularly with serum of young children, an age group that has been less well evaluated.[394]

Improvements in standardization as well as in specificity and sensitivity of commercially available serologic testing would benefit the laboratory diagnosis of primary EBV infections. Current EBV-specific serologic testing for nonprimary infections, particularly in immunocompromised patients, provides more limited diagnostic interpretations. The expanding capacity in the detection and quantitation of EBV viral load in body

TABLE 160.3 Correlation of Clinical Status and Characteristic Serologic Responses to Epstein-Barr Virus (EBV) Infection[a]

Clinical Status	Heterophile Antibodies (Quantitative Test)	RESPONSE TO EBV-SPECIFIC ANTIBODIES				
		IgM-VCA	IgG-VCA	EA-D	EA-R	EBNA
Susceptible	–	–	–	–	–	–
Infectious mononucleosis						
Acute primary infection	++[b]	++/+++	+/+++	+/+++	–[c]	–/+
Recent primary infection	+/–	–/+	++++	+++	–[c]	–
Remote infection	–	–	++	–[d]	–/+	+/++
Reactivation immunosuppressed/immunocompromised	–	–	+++/++++	–[d]	++/+++	–/+++
Burkitt lymphoma	–	–	+++/++++	–[d]	++/+++	+/++
Nasopharyngeal carcinoma	–	–	+++/++++	++/+++	–[e]	++/+++

[a]Antibody response scale is none or negative (–), low (+), average (++), above average (+++), and very high (++++). A scale is used for application to various antibody tests and techniques. This table is modified from numerous studies. Individual responses outside the characteristic range may occur.

[b]Children younger than 4 years may have weak or undetectable heterophil antibody responses as determined by qualitative rapid slide tests.

[c]In some young children and in adults with asymptomatic seroconversion, the anti-EA response may be mainly to the EA-R component.

[d]A minority of individuals will have the anti-EA response mainly to the EA-D component.

[e]A minority of individuals will have the anti-EA response mainly to the EA-R component.

compartments and lesions (see next section) is of growing diagnostic importance in these circumstances.

Epstein-Barr Virus Nucleic Acid (DNA or RNA)

In young patients, EBV serologic testing may reveal false-positive results owing to retained maternal antibodies from the placenta, excessive blood product infusions, or asymptomatic seroconversion. In patients treated with immunosuppressants, a false-negative serologic response to EBV antigens may occur. In such situations, demonstrating EBV nucleic acid in tissue sections or in blood may be necessary for diagnostic purposes.[12] Methods include Southern blotting, in situ hybridization, and detection of EBV DNA by PCR.[69] Besides their utility as diagnostic aids, these tests also are useful for epidemiologic and pathogenetic purposes relevant to EBV infections.

Southern blot hybridization has been useful in demonstrating the association of EBV with disease.[18,69,659] Although it is not as sensitive as PCR, Southern blotting has the advantages of providing additional information about the monoclonality of EBV-associated lesions, detecting lytic EBV processes, and recognizing viral integration into the genome.[233,244,247,519]

Because of their ubiquity in EBV-infected cells (up to 10^7 copies per cell), detection of EBERs in tissues by in situ RNA hybridization has become a standard method for detecting and localizing latent EBV in tissues.[44,243,415] Probes for detection of EBERs (riboprobes) are labeled conveniently by immunoperoxidase methods. Detection of EBV DNA by in situ hybridization also can be performed,[67] although DNA detection is less sensitive because of the lower copy numbers per cell in comparison with EBERs.

Amplification of EBV DNA by PCR has emerged as an important test for establishing the diagnosis and treatment of several EBV-associated diseases. In adult patients with AIDS and primary CNS lymphomas, detection of EBV DNA in CSF has high sensitivity and specificity in most studies.[22,113,415,442] PCR for EBV in CSF, possibly in combination with certain imaging studies,[22,301] may be sufficient to establish the diagnosis of CNS lymphoma and could preclude performance of brain biopsy, which can be associated with complications. On the other hand, lumbar puncture in patients with cerebral lesions also must be considered carefully because of the risk for cerebral herniation.

In stem cell and solid-organ transplant recipients, quantitative PCR for EBV DNA in peripheral blood serves as a useful tool for the diagnosis of PTLD and as a marker during follow-up.[232,388,645,680] Levels of EBV DNA in blood typically are low in healthy control subjects, high in those with PTLD or other EBV-associated diseases, and intermediate in asymptomatic organ transplant patients. A high EBV load in the blood has a clear relationship with development of PTLD,[230] and with successful management, EBV DNA concentrations typically diminish to baseline levels.[230,294,538] Although negative predictive values for these tests are higher than 90%, positive predictive values are substantially lower. Healthy subjects with IM, asymptomatic seroconverters, and transplant recipients with PTLD may have comparably high levels of EBV detected in the blood, thus making it difficult to separate out true PTLD from increases unassociated with PTLD. Detection of EBV within cellular specimens, such as whole blood or peripheral blood mononuclear cells, appears to be more reproducible and accurate than are tests measuring cell-free EBV in plasma or serum. Further studies clearly are necessary to establish quantitative laboratory standards for diagnosis and monitoring of EBV-associated PTLD. Histopathologic evaluation of a suspicious tumor site is much more informative and less controversial regarding diagnostic utility.

Quantitative PCR also may be useful for diagnosis and monitoring of other EBV-associated malignant diseases, including NPC,[382] HL,[389] and NHL.[590] Larger studies are necessary to define better the role of EBV viral load testing in these diseases. PCR testing may also be of assistance in the laboratory testing for EBV-induced disease (as IM) in young children and infants.[103,146] A systematic review on the performance of a quantitative real-time PCR assay for the detection of EBV DNA in immunocompetent children and young adults showed a pooled sensitivity of 77% and a pooled specificity of 98%.[323,504]

Epstein-Barr Virus Proteins

Immunofluorescent techniques may be used to detect the presence of cells carrying EBV proteins in touch imprints of biopsy material or in frozen sections of cryopreserved tissue.[233,415,507,685] Most commonly, tissues are examined for VCA, EBNA-1, and LMP-1 proteins with the use of mouse monoclonal antibodies.

Virus Isolation

EBV from blood or oropharyngeal specimens (rarely, other specimens) can be isolated in tissue culture with a transformation assay.[318] For oropharyngeal specimens, the test requires incubation with fresh cord blood mononuclear cells for as long as 6 weeks. Transforming virus can be identified in peripheral blood by incubating mononuclear cells in the presence of cyclosporine (for inhibition of cytotoxic T cells, which can suppress the growth of EBV-positive B cells). An end-point dilution assay may be used to quantitate the amount of EBV within blood specimens.[537] Virus isolation tests are used primarily for research purposes and are not widely available.

Electron Microscopy

EBV virions also may be detected by electron microscopy, which has been used in patients with oral hairy leukoplakia,[311] NPC,[25] and other EBV-associated lesions. The ultrastructural features of EBV virions, however, are indistinguishable from those of other herpesviruses, and confirmatory tests usually are necessary. Electron microscopy generally is available only at larger research centers and therefore is impractical for routine diagnostic testing.

Imaging Studies

Imaging studies seldom are necessary in typical patients with IM. In one study of patients hospitalized with IM, the most common findings on chest radiography were splenomegaly (47%), hilar adenopathy (13%), and interstitial infiltrates (5%).[377] Imaging studies are used more commonly for evaluation of EBV-associated neurologic disease, especially in immunocompromised patients. Children with EBV-associated encephalitis usually have normal neuroimaging results.[144] However, some patients may display diffuse swelling or patchy low-density lesions by computed tomography, and magnetic resonance imaging (MRI) may reveal increased signal on T2-weighted images as well as atrophy.[144,565] Involvement of one or more anatomic locations of the brain in children with encephalitis may been seen on MRI, including cerebral hemispheres, basal ganglia, cerebellum, brain stem, and thalamus. The most common site of isolated involvement is the cerebellum.[2] Contrast-enhanced computed tomography scans of primary cerebral lymphoma in patients with AIDS typically reveal large (2 to 6 mm) lesions occurring anywhere in the cerebrum with diffuse and homogeneous enhancement[610]; however, some overlap exists with findings observed in other diseases, such as cerebral toxoplasmosis. Thallium-201 single-photon emission computed tomography, in conjunction with magnetic resonance imaging and PCR testing of CSF for EBV DNA, may be useful in distinguishing CNS lymphomas from toxoplasmosis in adult patients with AIDS.[22,301]

Differential Diagnosis

Infectious Mononucleosis

EBV causes an estimated 80% to 95% of IM syndromes.[170,375] Numerous agents have been associated with heterophile-negative IM. CMV is responsible for most cases of heterophile-negative IM with typical clinical and hematologic findings.[293] Certain features of CMV mononucleosis may help distinguish it from EBV (e.g., less common sore throat and lymphadenopathy, less intense atypical lymphocytosis, and prominent splenomegaly), but these characteristics have considerable overlap with EBV-associated IM. Serologic testing consistent with acute CMV infection in the absence of characteristic EBV serologic findings confirms the diagnosis.[375] The remainder of cases may be attributable to infection with *Toxoplasma gondii*, adenoviruses, rubella virus, or hepatitis A virus. Acute HIV syndrome also may mimic IM. However, in children with non-EBV IM, the etiology frequently remains elusive. In heterophile-negative children with mononucleosis and both the clinical and hematologic characteristics of the syndrome, the most likely known agents are EBV and CMV.

Other EBV-Associated Disorders

EBV-associated HLH may be confused with IM, systemic connective tissue disorders, septicemia, and certain hematologic malignant neoplasms.[304] EBV-associated CNS lymphomas in adults with AIDS are difficult to distinguish from cerebral toxoplasmosis on the basis of clinical findings and imaging studies. Historically, a negative *T. gondii* serum antibody test response eliminates toxoplasmosis, whereas a positive test response may necessitate a trial of antitoxoplasmic therapy. Response within a week suggests toxoplasmosis, but a nonresponse indicates the need for stereotactic brain biopsy to establish a diagnosis. Identification of EBV DNA in CSF by PCR may help confirm the diagnosis of lymphoma.[301] Because PTLDs may affect the graft, a high EBV viral load in conjunction with graft abnormalities (e.g., elevated liver enzyme values in a liver transplant recipient) may be confused with graft rejection; histologic evaluation of biopsy tissue from the graft should differentiate PTLD from acute graft rejection.

TREATMENT

Infectious Mononucleosis

Supportive Care

Support, including rest, fluids, and antipyretics, is all that is required for uncomplicated IM. Although clinical trials and case reports dating to the 1950s generally have demonstrated a beneficial effect of short-term use of corticosteroids in patients with severe symptoms (e.g., high fever, severe pharyngitis), [16,49,66] a recent systematic review concluded that there is insufficient evidence of the efficacy of steroids for symptom improvement in patients with IM.[526] Furthermore, some studies have shown adverse effects of such therapy, including respiratory distress, neurologic complications, secondary bacterial infections, and acute-onset diabetes.[221,526,647] Although little controversy exists about the use of corticosteroids for patients with complicated illnesses (e.g., with stridor from massively enlarged tonsils or paratracheal adenopathy, or for those with hematologic or neurologic complications; see Complications of Infectious Mononucleosis earlier), personal experience and clinical judgment largely dictate the use of corticosteroids in practice.[142,622] For example, in a report of patients with IM evaluated as outpatients and inpatients, 45% received systemic corticosteroids, with only a small proportion (<10%) of these patients having airway concerns.[622]

Antiviral Treatment

Numerous antiviral agents inhibit replication of EBV in vitro. Such agents include acyclovir, famciclovir, penciclovir, ganciclovir, and other nucleoside analogues.[33,118,132,222,404,586] None of these agents is capable of eliminating latent EBV present as episomes in infected cells. Five randomized, placebo-controlled trials of acyclovir (with or without corticosteroids) in adolescents and adults with IM demonstrated no beneficial effect in resolving the clinical signs and symptoms associated with illness as well as no reduced rate of complications.[15,17,476,635,637] Moreover, a meta-analysis substantiated these findings.[629] Acyclovir did significantly reduce the rate of EBV shedding in the oropharynx, albeit temporarily.[629] A study reported a decrease in the quantity of EBV DNA in oral washings and blood as well as in illness severity during treatment with valacyclovir.[642]

Epstein-Barr Virus-Associated Malignant Diseases

Providing details about treatment of EBV-associated lymphoproliferative diseases, including lymphomas, is beyond the scope of this chapter. Pediatric oncologists must be involved in the care of children with these malignant diseases. A brief overview of treatment of the principal diseases is provided.

Posttransplant Lymphoproliferative Disease

The most effective therapy for PTLD in transplant recipients is reduction (or complete elimination)[300] of immunosuppression to allow more effective control of rampant EBV infection by the cell-mediated immune system. This measure halts progression of PTLD in approximately two thirds of pediatric solid-organ transplant recipients developing polymorphic PTLD in the first year after undergoing transplantation.[232] Decisions concerning reduction of immunosuppression must be weighed against the risk of graft rejection, and careful follow-up with frequent EBV viral load measurements must be ensured. If no improvement occurs after a trial of reduced immune suppression, other therapeutic modalities must be considered singly or in combination.

Although antiviral agents (acyclovir, ganciclovir, valganciclovir) are used frequently for PTLD, largely on the basis of an anecdotal report published in 1982,[261] no clinical trials have confirmed their efficacy. Because these agents treat lytic EBV infections, yet PTLD primarily involves latent virus, the consensus has been that these agents should have minimal impact on PTLD. However, this view has been challenged by reports in experimental animals suggesting that the small proportion of lytically infected cells within these tumors may contribute to the growth of EBV-associated malignant lesions by enhancing angiogenesis and inducing paracrine B-cell growth factors.[289,290]

There is now considerable experience with the use of rituximab, a chimeric monoclonal antibody directed at CD20, against PTLD.[217,240,630] Although no randomized controlled clinical trials have been conducted to date in children, data from cohort studies, case reports, and a phase II trial indicate that rituximab is safe and effective.[217,240] Most adverse events are mild or moderate and usually are related to the first infusion of the antibody. Despite a profound reduction of circulating B cells in peripheral blood, hypogammaglobulinemia is an uncommon occurrence with rituximab treatment (although more likely in young children), and patients are not at higher risk for development of infectious complications. Most centers now use rituximab as a primary therapeutic agent for PTLD if reduction of immune suppression is unsuccessful.

IFN-α has induced complete remissions in some studies,[134,398] but relapses and graft rejections have occurred. Conventional NHL chemotherapy (CHOP regimen) consisting of cyclophosphamide, daunorubicin, vincristine, and prednisone may have increased toxicity and mortality associated with infection when standard doses are used,[454,586,608] thus leading to investigation of low-dose CHOP regimens consisting of cyclophosphamide and prednisone.[41,239]

Experimental therapy using EBV-specific cytotoxic T lymphocytes has been successful for PTLD in human stem cell transplant recipients,[541] but it is more complicated for solid-organ transplant recipients with PTLD. In contrast to stem cell transplant recipients, whose EBV-associated PTLD tumors are derived from the donor, tumors in solid-organ transplant recipients are invariably derived from the recipient. Therefore, EBV-specific cytotoxic T lymphocytes must be prepared by ex vivo EBV transformation of either the recipient's B cells[62,213,351] or at least partially HLA-matched banked B cells.[263] Surgery and radiation therapy generally are reserved for local complications of tumors, including compression of an airway or gastrointestinal bleeding,[232] but they have been used more widely at some institutions.[119] A multifaceted approach, such as that used by Comoli and colleagues,[119] ultimately may yield the highest response rates against the most aggressive forms of PTLD. Clinical trials of cytotoxic T lymphocytes as prophylaxis and treatment of PTLD continue to show promising results.[62,213]

B-Cell Lymphoma

Endemic (African) BLs, which are highly associated with EBV,[371] are treated primarily with cyclophosphamide-based chemotherapy.[372,690] Favorable responses were observed by Labrecque and coworkers[372] in patients with tumors expressing lytic genes. Treatment of sporadic BL also is based primarily on multiagent chemotherapy that includes cyclophosphamide.[401] Case reports have indicated positive responses to rituximab, and Children's Oncology Group protocols now include rituximab as first-line treatment of BL.[217]

B-cell lymphomas in patients with AIDS are extremely difficult to treat, primarily because of the underlying severe host immune deficiency. Early regimens using standard chemotherapeutic regimens were largely failures, with survival rates lower than those of untreated patients; most patients died of opportunistic infections, drug toxicity, and resistant tumors. Alternative therapeutic strategies have improved outcomes for this malignant disease, yet mortality rates remain substantial.[408] These strategies have included lower doses of standard drugs,[338] hematopoietic growth factors,[379] novel immunotherapies (e.g., interleukin-2),[50] and adoptive immunotherapy,[661] as well as improved management of opportunistic infections and HIV infection. In vitro data indicate the effectiveness of anti-NF-κB treatments, including bortezomib[692] and certain statin drugs,[342] and the hope is that human studies will follow. An exciting emerging area of therapy is termed lytic induction and involves treatment of EBV-positive lymphoma cells with certain agents that induce a transition from latent to lytic infection, thus rendering them susceptible to antiviral therapy (e.g., ganciclovir, zidovudine).[47,129]

AIDS-related primary CNS lymphomas are extremely difficult to treat. Historically, palliative whole-brain radiation therapy in conjunction with corticosteroids was used for treatment, but with disappointing survival rates of only a few months. Combined modality therapy with whole-brain radiation and chemotherapy has been investigated but generally also produces poor outcomes.[339] However, most studies were conducted before wide availability of cART. A minority of healthier patients with AIDS may respond better to combined modality regimens.[339] For patients not already receiving cART, initiation of an appropriate regimen is recommended, because case reports have described improvement. The use of ganciclovir has been shown to decrease EBV DNA load in CSF and improve survival in adult patients with HIV-related primary CNS lymphoma.[65]

Hodgkin Lymphoma

Historically, children with HL were treated with high-dose radiation. However, high rates of skeletal growth inhibition and secondary malignant neoplasms were noted in survivors, so new trials using lower involved-field radiation in conjunction with multiagent chemotherapy were conducted. These trials form the basis for combination treatment regimens used currently in growing children.[298,511] Although the presence of EBV in tumor (more likely in mixed-cellularity types) currently plays no role in pretreatment staging, some studies suggest improved outcomes for patients with EBV-positive tumors.[445,451] However, the presence of pretreatment EBV DNA in peripheral blood has been linked with poor outcomes in patients with HL.[483]

Nasopharyngeal Carcinoma

NPCs are sensitive to radiotherapy as well as to chemotherapy. Surgery usually is not an option because of the location of the primary tumor, although it may be necessary for persistent or recurrent lymph node disease. For early localized disease, radiotherapy generally is indicated, whereas combined modality treatment (radiation and chemotherapy) may be considered for more advanced disease.[5,29] Children whose treatment is failing have a high rate of distant metastases, principally to bone.[28,305]

Nonmalignant Epstein-Barr Virus-Associated Diseases

XLP

In an effort to prevent fulminant IM, intravenous immune globulin is recommended for patients with XLP who display hypogammaglobulinemia, although such therapy is not fully effective.[207] Traditional therapy with antivirals and IFN-α has been disappointing for fulminant IM, but reported success with rituximab (in combination with corticosteroids and other agents) has provided some enthusiasm.[440,452] Males with XLP also can develop lymphomas, which may respond to traditional chemotherapy regimens. Presently, the only definitive cure for XLP is allogeneic hematopoietic stem cell transplantation. Fifteen such transplants were reported between 1986 and 2005, with 10 survivors.[378] Younger age appears to be associated with improved survival in this limited population. Administration of rituximab may be considered a bridge between the diagnosis of XLP and transplantation.[378,563] Now that the gene defect in XLP has been identified, consideration may be given to a gene therapeutic approach.[440]

HLH

Early studies using non–etoposide-containing regimens were largely unsuccessful in significantly reducing the high mortality rate associated with HLH.[23] Chemotherapeutic regimens including etoposide (toxic to macrophages) have reduced the mortality rate significantly. Results of a standardized protocol (HLH-94) developed by the Histiocyte Society have been published.[275,631] Agents in this protocol included etoposide and corticosteroids for initial therapy, followed by etoposide, corticosteroids, and cyclosporine (continuation therapy), leading to *Bone Marrow Transplant.* Patients with CNS involvement, as determined by symptomatology, CSF analysis, or MRI results, also should receive intrathecal chemotherapy with methotrexate and hydrocortisone. A similar standardized protocol (HLH-2004), but including cyclosporine at initiation, currently is being evaluated.[314] Few data are available on salvage therapy for children unresponsive to the HLH-94 protocol, but Janka[314] has summarized anecdotal successes with standard NHL or HL treatment protocols, some monoclonal antibodies (e.g., anti-CD25 and anti-CD52), and treatment with fludarabine (an antiviral agent) of one child who survived until bone marrow transplantation could be performed. For patients with EBV-induced HLH, most experts recommend the use of rituximab 375 mg/m^2 weekly for 1 to 4 weeks.[99,333,440] Chellapandian and colleagues showed improved symptoms, reduced EBV viral loads, and decreased inflammation in patients with EBV-induced HLH when rituximab was added to the standard treatment.[99]

CAEBV Infection

Treatment modalities for CAEBV infection have varied widely, because the rarity of this disease precludes performing proper clinical trials. Resolution of symptoms has been reported in case reports with use of antiviral drugs (e.g., acyclovir, ganciclovir),[307] etoposide,[470] immunomodulatory agents (e.g., corticosteroids, intravenous immune globulin, cytokines),[191,201,346] adoptive transfer of cytotoxic T cells,[556] or combinations thereof. For the most severe forms of disease, stem cell transplantation may be considered.[469]

HIV-Associated Diseases

Oral hairy leukoplakia generally does not require therapy because patients typically are asymptomatic and the lesions have no malignant potential. However, therapy may be required for troubling symptoms or cosmetic or psychological reasons. Small lesions may be treated topically,[446] but large lesions require systemic oral antiherpesvirus agents.[484] Treatment strategies for LIP are not defined well. Supportive care, including supplemental oxygen, may be necessary. Suppression of HIV with effective antiretroviral agents also is logical to improve immune function and to minimize the potential direct effect of HIV infection. Although no controlled studies have documented the value of antiretrovirals, benefit is suggested by the declining prevalence of LIP in children during the cART era.[225] Corticosteroids also may be of benefit.[21,433] Some reports suggest benefit of chloroquine therapy in children with LIP with and without HIV infection.[79,653] No controlled studies have evaluated antiherpesvirus drugs (e.g., acyclovir) for LIP.

PROGNOSIS

The prognosis for healthy persons with IM is extremely good, with mortality considered a rare occurrence. In a series of 30 fatal cases of IM from the 1950s, Lukes and Cox[412] found splenic rupture, Guillain-Barré syndrome, hemorrhage, and secondary infection to be the most common causes of death. In Penman's[494] later study of 20 documented deaths, predominantly of young adults, the causes of death (in decreasing order of frequency) were neurologic complications, splenic rupture, secondary infection, hepatic failure, and myocarditis. EBV-induced aplastic anemia, a rare but dreaded hematologic complication, now is thought to have a better prognosis for eventual recovery if the patient can be supported successfully through the acute stages.[43,380] It has been suggested that older patients are at higher risk for severe EBV-related IM.[616]

The prognosis for patients with EBV-associated lymphoproliferative diseases is variable and depends on the immunologic status of the patient and the type of lymphoproliferation. A registry of 161 males with XLP indicated a mortality rate of 70% by the age of 10 years and 100% by the age of 40 years.[235] HLH has a greater than 90% fatality rate without treatment; most deaths are caused by hemorrhage, overwhelming infection, disseminated intravascular coagulation, or multiorgan failure.[101,315] Etoposide-based treatment has improved outcomes considerably.[314] The median survival rate was 54% at 6 years follow-up in patients treated on the HLH-94 protocol. Patients without neurological involvement and those older than 6 months had higher survival rates (approximately 65%).[275,631] The largest case series of CAEBV infection (from Japan), which included 21 children younger than 18 years, reported a mortality rate of approximately 30% despite various forms of therapy.[358] Historically, PTLD that develops after solid-organ transplantation has carried a relatively high mortality rate (50–80%), with higher mortality rates in bone marrow transplant recipients.[178] Presently, the mortality rate is probably much lower, but more time is necessary to assess the impact of newer therapeutic modalities. The prognosis for healthy children with NHL generally is good, with 5-year relative survival rates of 80%.[532] However, the prognosis for patients with AIDS and NHL is poor. In adults with AIDS, median survival is 2 to 4 months for CNS lymphomas (virtually all of which are EBV associated), with only slightly longer survival noted in patients receiving cART.[339] Childhood HL generally has a very good prognosis, with 5-year survival rates of approximately 95%.[532] With use of combined modality therapy, children with NPC have long-term survival rates in the range of 70% to 90%.[29]

PREVENTION

EBV is shed regularly in saliva, and therefore infection control policies are difficult to develop. In addition, mechanisms for EBV transmission are not well understood, and EBV outbreaks occur rarely if at all. For these reasons, no more than standard infection control precautions are recommended for patients hospitalized with EBV infections, including IM.[354] Although transfusion-associated EBV infection occurs rarely, persons with recent EBV infection of mononucleosis-like illnesses are urged to refrain from donating blood or organs.[354] Because EBV is spread through salivary contact, individuals should avoid sharing food and drinks, especially with someone known to have had a recent EBV infection, if they wish to reduce the risk of acquiring EBV.

Vaccine

Efforts continue in the development of an EBV vaccine. Because of concern about the administration of a vaccine with unknown long-term consequences, including malignant transformation, most efforts have been focused on development of subunit EBV vaccines. A subunit vaccine containing the EBV gp350 protein has proved effective in preventing EBV infection in an experimental animal model.[163,574] A vaccinia virus-based gp350 vaccine has been evaluated in a small number of Chinese patients, eliciting good antibody responses and providing some protection from EBV infection[242]; however, these findings were not corroborated, and this vaccine was not developed further. A recombinant gp350 vaccine with adjuvant has been evaluated in Belgium, with phase I and phase II data published.[447,585] The vaccine was immunogenic, safe, and well tolerated. Although vaccine recipients were not protected from EBV infection, symptoms of IM were reduced compared with controls.[410,585] The EBV vaccine may soon enter phase III trials.[514] An effective vaccine could be considered for persons at high risk for development of EBV-associated lymphoproliferative disease and cancer, such as patients with AIDS, those with XLP, and organ or stem cell transplant recipients. Before such a vaccine is approved, further research must be conducted to address issues such as protection against exogenous superinfection from wild-type EBV strains.[649] Therapeutic vaccines, aimed primarily at latent antigens expressed in EBV-associated malignant diseases such as NPC, also are under investigation.[154,403,573] Virus-like particle-based EBV vaccine candidates are also in preclinical development.[548]

Prevention of Posttransplant Lymphoproliferative Disease

Strategies for prevention of PTLD reflect many of those used for treatment of established PTLD (see earlier section on treatment of PTLD).[440] Children at high risk for development of PTLD (e.g., EBV-seronegative children and infants younger than 12 months) typically are given prophylactic anti-CMV immune globulin and an antiviral after transplantation. A retrospective analysis of a large renal transplant database covering Europe and North America (96% adults) has suggested a beneficial effect of anti-CMV immune globulin (e.g., CytoGam) in the prevention of B-cell lymphomas.[473]

After undergoing transplantation, these children should have frequent EBV viral load testing. If EBV viral loads persist above a significant cutoff value established by the laboratory, preemptive measures should be considered. Although real-time PCR tests are sensitive in predicting development of PTLD, they are not highly specific and lack standardization. Cutoff values for "significant" concentrations of EBV DNA vary from laboratory to laboratory. Once a decision is made that preemptive therapy is warranted, reduction or elimination of immunosuppressive medications should be performed. In addition, rituximab treatment administered preemptively in patients who have significant viremia (>40,000 copies/mL in blood) may respond with resolution of viremia, without development of PTLD.[674]

Adoptive transfer of cytotoxic T lymphocytes specific for EBV, produced from donor peripheral blood mononuclear cells stimulated with EBV target antigens, is also under clinical development as an antiviral prophylactic agent as well as an antiviral treatment agent for EBV-expressing lymphoproliferative diseases in allogeneic hematopoietic stem cell transplant recipients.[62,213]

NEW REFERENCES SINCE THE NEW EDITION

1. Abe H, Kaneda A, Fukayama M. Epstein-Barr virus-associated gastric carcinoma: use of host cell machineries and somatic gene mutations. *Pathobiology*. 2015;82(5):212-223.
2. Abul-Kasim K, Palm L, Maly P, et al. The neuroanatomic localization of Epstein-Barr virus encephalitis may be a predictive factor for its clinical outcome: a case report and review of 100 cases in 28 reports. *J Child Neurol*. 2009;24(6):720-726.
4. Al-Rawahi GN, Dobson SR, Scheifele DW, et al. Severe genital ulceration in an acute Epstein-Barr virus infection. *Pediatr Infect Dis J*. 2011;30(2):176-178.

7. Almagro M, Del Pozo J, Martinez W, et al. Pityriasis lichenoides-like exanthem and primary infection by Epstein-Barr virus. *Int J Dermatol.* 2000;39(2):156-159.
8. Almohmeed YH, Avenell A, Aucott L, et al. Systematic review and meta-analysis of the sero-epidemiological association between Epstein Barr virus and multiple sclerosis. *PLoS ONE.* 2013;8(4):e61110.
11. Alvaro-Meca A, Micheloud D, Jensen J, et al. Epidemiologic trends of cancer diagnoses among HIV-infected children in Spain from 1997 to 2008. *Pediatr Infect Dis J.* 2011;30(9):764-768.
14. Anderlini P, Riggs SA, Korbling M, et al. Syngeneic blood stem cell transplantation for infectious mononucleosis-related aplastic anaemia. *Br J Haematol.* 1999;106(1):159-161.
27. Auwaerter PG. Infectious mononucleosis: return to play. *Clin Sports Med.* 2004;23(3):485-497, xi.
30. Azzi T, Lunemann A, Murer A, et al. Role for early-differentiated natural killer cells in infectious mononucleosis. *Blood.* 2014;124(16):2533-2543.
32. Baciewicz AM, Chandra R. Cefprozil-induced rash in infectious mononucleosis. *Ann Pharmacother.* 2005;39(5):974-975.
37. Balfour HH Jr, Dunmire SK, Hogquist KA. Infectious mononucleosis. *Clin Transl Immunol.* 2015;4(2):e33.
38. Balfour HH Jr, Holman CJ, Hokanson KM, et al. A prospective clinical study of Epstein-Barr virus and host interactions during acute infectious mononucleosis. *J Infect Dis.* 2005;192(9):1505-1512.
39. Balfour HH Jr, Odumade OA, Schmeling DO, et al. Behavioral, virologic, and immunologic factors associated with acquisition and severity of primary Epstein-Barr virus infection in university students. *J Infect Dis.* 2013;207(1):80-88.
40. Balfour HH Jr, Sifakis F, Sliman JA, et al. Age-specific prevalence of Epstein-Barr virus infection among individuals aged 6-19 years in the United States and factors affecting its acquisition. *J Infect Dis.* 2013;208(8):1286-1293.
42. Ball RJ, Avenell A, Aucott L, et al. Systematic review and meta-analysis of the sero-epidemiological association between Epstein-Barr virus and rheumatoid arthritis. *Arthritis Res Ther.* 2015;17:274.
45. Bartlett A, Williams R, Hilton M. Splenic rupture in infectious mononucleosis: a systematic review of published case reports. *Injury.* 2016;47(3):531-538.
47. Bayraktar UD, Diaz LA, Ashlock B, et al. Zidovudine-based lytic-inducing chemotherapy for Epstein-Barr virus-related lymphomas. *Leuk Lymphoma.* 2014;55(4):786-794.
52. Berntsson M, Dubicanac L, Tunback P, et al. Frequent detection of cytomegalovirus and Epstein-Barr virus in cervical secretions from healthy young women. *Acta Obstet Gynecol Scand.* 2013;92(6):706-710.
53. Bhaduri-McIntosh S, Landry ML, Nikiforow S, et al. Serum IgA antibodies to Epstein-Barr virus (EBV) early lytic antigens are present in primary EBV infection. *J Infect Dis.* 2007;195(4):483-492.
57. Biggs TC, Hayes SM, Bird JH, et al. Use of the lymphocyte count as a diagnostic screen in adults with suspected Epstein-Barr virus infectious mononucleosis. *Laryngoscope.* 2013;123(10):2401-2404.
58. Binalsheikh IM, Griesemer D, Wang S, et al. Lyme neuroborreliosis presenting as Alice in Wonderland syndrome. *Pediatr Neurol.* 2012;46(3):185-186.
65. Bossolasco S, Falk KI, Ponzoni M, et al. Ganciclovir is associated with low or undetectable Epstein-Barr virus DNA load in cerebrospinal fluid of patients with HIV-related primary central nervous system lymphoma. *Clin Infect Dis.* 2006;42(4):e21-e25.
68. Brigden ML, Au S, Thompson S, et al. Infectious mononucleosis in an outpatient population: diagnostic utility of 2 automated hematology analyzers and the sensitivity and specificity of Hoagland's criteria in heterophile-positive patients. *Arch Pathol Lab Med.* 1999;123(10):875-881.
73. Buck M, Cross S, Krauer K, et al. A-type and B-type Epstein-Barr virus differ in their ability to spontaneously enter the lytic cycle. *J Gen Virol.* 1999;80(Pt 2):441-445.
79. Campos JM, Simonetti JP. Treatment of lymphoid interstitial pneumonia with chloroquine. *J Pediatr.* 1993;122(3):503.
82. Carson RJ, Reinschmidt JS, Lemon HC. Infectious mononucleosis in American Negroid students. *J Am Coll Health Assoc.* 1967;16(2):174-177.
87. Cen O, Longnecker R. Latent Membrane Protein 2 (LMP2). *Curr Top Microbiol Immunol.* 2015;391:151-180.
88. Centers for Disease Control and Prevention. Revised surveillance case definitions for HIV infection among adults, adolescents, and children aged <18 months and for HIV infection and AIDS among children aged 18 months to <13 years—United States, 2008. *MMWR Recomm Rep.* 2008;572008:1-12.
89. Centers for Disease Control and Prevention (CDC). *NHANES 1999-2000 Public Release File Documentation.* Hyattsville, MD: CDC; 2002.
91. Chang CM, Yu KJ, Mbulaiteye SM, et al. The extent of genetic diversity of Epstein-Barr virus and its geographic and disease patterns: a need for reappraisal. *Virus Res.* 2009;143(2):209-221.
93. Chang RS Infectious mononucleosis. 1980.
95. Chang RS, Blankenship W. Spontaneous in vitro transformation of leukocytes from a neonate. *Proc Soc Exp Biol Med.* 1973;144(1):337-339.
96. Chang RS, Golden HD. Transformation of human leucocytes by throat washing from infectious mononucleosis patients. *Nature.* 1971;234(5328):359-360.
99. Chellapandian D, Das R, Zelley K, et al. Treatment of Epstein Barr virus-induced haemophagocytic lymphohistiocytosis with rituximab-containing chemo-immunotherapeutic regimens. *Br J Haematol.* 2013;162(3):376-382.
100. Chen J, Konstantinopoulos PA, Satyal S, et al. Just another simple case of infectious mononucleosis? *Lancet.* 2003;361(9364):1182.
103. Cheng J. Obstructive sleep apnea (OSA): a complication of acute infectious mononucleosis infection in a child. *Int J Pediatr Otorhinolaryngol.* 2014;78(3): 561-562.
104. Chesnokova LS, Nishimura SL, Hutt-Fletcher LM. Fusion of epithelial cells by Epstein-Barr virus proteins is triggered by binding of viral glycoproteins gHgL to integrins alphavbeta6 or alphavbeta8.[Erratum appears in *Proc Natl Acad Sci U S A.* 2010 Feb 16;107(7):3275]. *Proc Natl Acad Sci USA.* 2009;106(48):20464-20469.
105. Chiang AK, Wong KY, Liang AC, et al. Comparative analysis of Epstein-Barr virus gene polymorphisms in nasal T/NK-cell lymphomas and normal nasal tissues: implications on virus strain selection in malignancy. *Int J Cancer.* 1999;80(3):356-364.
106. Chiappini E, Berti E, Gianesin K, et al. Pediatric human immunodeficiency virus infection and cancer in the highly active antiretroviral treatment (HAART) era. *Cancer Lett.* 2014;347(1):38-45.
108. Chiu TM, Lin YM, Wang SC, et al. Hypersensitivity to mosquito bites as the primary clinical manifestation of an Epstein-Barr virus infection. *J Microbiol Immunol Infect.* 2016;49(4):613-616.
109. Cho TA, Schmahmann JD, Cunnane ME. Case records of the Massachusetts General Hospital. Case 30-2013. A 19-year-old man with otalgia, slurred speech, and ataxia. *N Engl J Med.* 2013;369(13):1253-1261.
110. Chua ML, Wee JT, Hui EP, et al. Nasopharyngeal carcinoma. *Lancet.* 2016;387(10022):1012-1024.
122. Correa RM, Fellner MD, Alonio LV, et al. Epstein-barr virus (EBV) in healthy carriers: Distribution of genotypes and 30 bp deletion in latent membrane protein-1 (LMP-1) oncogene. *J Med Virol.* 2004;73(4):583-588.
123. Correa RM, Fellner MD, Durand K, et al. Epstein Barr virus genotypes and LMP-1 variants in HIV-infected patients. *J Med Virol.* 2007;79(4):401-407.
124. Cote TR, Biggar RJ, Rosenberg PS, et al. Non-Hodgkin's lymphoma among people with AIDS: incidence, presentation and public health burden. AIDS/Cancer Study Group. *Int J Cancer.* 1997;73(5):645-650.
130. Dakdouki GK, Obeid KH, Kanj SS. Azithromycin-induced rash in infectious mononucleosis. *Scand J Infect Dis.* 2002;34(12):939-941.
133. Daud II, Coleman CB, Smith NA, et al. Breast milk as a potential source of Epstein-Barr virus transmission among infants living in a malaria-endemic region of Kenya. *J Infect Dis.* 2015;212(11):1735-1742.
135. Davison A, Pellett P, Stewart J Rename species in the family Herpesviridae to incorporate a subfamily designation. 2016; http://www.ictvonline.org/proposals/2015.010aD.A.v2.Herpesvirales_spren.pdf.
137. Dekate J, Chetty R. Epstein-Barr virus-associated smooth muscle tumor. *Arch Pathol Lab Med.* 2016;140(7):718-722.
143. Doja A, Bitnun A, Jones EL, et al. Pediatric Epstein-Barr virus-associated encephalitis: 10-Year Review. *J Child Neurol.* 2006;21(5):385-391.
149. DuBois RE, Seeley JK, Brus I, et al. Chronic mononucleosis syndrome. *South Med J.* 1984;77(11):1376-1382.
151. Dunmire SK, Grimm JM, Schmeling DO, et al. The incubation period of primary Epstein-Barr virus infection: viral dynamics and immunologic events. *PLoS Pathog.* 2015;11(12):e1005286.
152. Dunmire SK, Hogquist KA, Balfour HH. Infectious mononucleosis. *Curr Top Microbiol Immunol.* 2015;390(Pt 1):211-240.
157. Ebell MH. Epstein-Barr virus infectious mononucleosis. *Am Fam Physician.* 2004;70(7):1279-1287.
158. Ebell MH, Call M, Shinholser J, et al. Does this patient have infectious mononucleosis? The rational clinical examination systematic review. *JAMA.* 2016;315(14):1502-1509.
159. Edwards RH, Sitki-Green D, Moore DT, et al. Potential selection of LMP1 variants in nasopharyngeal carcinoma. *J Virol.* 2004;78(2):868-881.
164. Erickson KD, Berger C, Coffin WF 3rd, et al. Unexpected absence of the Epstein-Barr virus (EBV) lyLMP-1 open reading frame in tumor virus isolates: lack of correlation between Met129 status and EBV strain identity. *J Virol.* 2003;77(7):4415-4422.
168. Evans AS. Infectious mononucleosis and related syndromes. *Am J Med Sci.* 1978;276(3):325-339.
173. Fafi-Kremer S, Morand P, Brion JP, et al. Long-term shedding of infectious Epstein-Barr virus after infectious mononucleosis. *J Infect Dis.* 2005;191(6):985-989.
176. Farrell K, Jarrett RF. The molecular pathogenesis of Hodgkin lymphoma. *Histopathology.* 2011;58(1):15-25.
177. Farrell PJ. Epstein-Barr virus strain variation. *Curr Top Microbiol Immunol.* 2015;390(Pt 1):45-69.
179. Feederle R, Klinke O, Kutikhin A, et al. Epstein-Barr virus: from the detection of sequence polymorphisms to the recognition of viral types. *Curr Top Microbiol Immunol.* 2015;390(Pt 1):119-148.
180. Feldman ER, Tibbetts SA. Emerging roles of herpesvirus microRNAs during in vivo infection and pathogenesis. *Curr Pathobiol Rep.* 2015;3(3):209-217.

182. Feranchak AP, Tyson RW, Narkewicz MR, et al. Fulminant Epstein-Barr viral hepatitis: orthotopic liver transplantation and review of the literature. *Liver Transpl Surg*. 1998;4(6):469-476.
189. Fleisher GR, Collins M, Fager S. Limitations of available tests for diagnosis of infectious mononucleosis. *J Clin Microbiol*. 1983;17(4):619-624.
192. Foreman BH, Mackler L, Malloy ED. Clinical inquiries. Can we prevent splenic rupture for patients with infectious mononucleosis? *J Fam Pract*. 2005;54(6):547-548.
193. Frappier L. EBNA1. *Curr Top Microbiol Immunol*. 2015;391:3-34.
196. Friman G, Wesslen L. Special feature for the Olympics: effects of exercise on the immune system: infections and exercise in high-performance athletes. *Immunol Cell Biol*. 2000;78(5):510-522.
204. Ganiats TG. Redefining the chronic fatigue syndrome. *Ann Intern Med*. 2015;162(9):653-654.
209. George MR. Hemophagocytic lymphohistiocytosis: review of etiologies and management. *J Blood Med*. 2014;5:69-86.
214. Gharpure V, Rubin L, Amlin J, et al. Lymphocytosis of donor origin in cerebrospinal fluid, and marrow aplasia after donor leukocyte infusion for EBV-lymphoproliferative disease. *Bone Marrow Transplant*. 1996;18(1):221-224.
216. Gianella S, Ginocchio CC, Daar ES, et al. Genital Epstein Barr virus is associated with higher prevalence and persistence of anal human papillomavirus in HIV-infected men on antiretroviral therapy. *BMC Infect Dis*. 2015;16:24.
218. Glenn WK, Whitaker NJ, Lawson JS. High risk human papillomavirus and Epstein Barr virus in human breast milk. *BMC Res Notes*. 2012;5:477.
221. Gold WL, Kapral MK, Witmer MR, et al. Postanginal septicemia as a life-threatening complication of infectious mononucleosis. *Clin Infect Dis*. 1995;20(5):1439-1440.
228. Grant D, Abu-Elmagd K, Reyes J, et al. 2003 report of the intestine transplant registry: a new era has dawned. *Ann Surg*. 2005;241(4):607-613.
229. Gray JJ, Caldwell J. Sillis M. The rapid serological diagnosis of infectious mononucleosis. *J Infect*. 1992;25(1):39-46.
231. Green M, Michaels MG. Epstein-Barr virus infection and posttransplant lymphoproliferative disorder. *Am J Transplant*. 2013;13(suppl 3):41-54.
239. Gross JL, Woll NL, Hanson CA, et al. Embolization for pediatric blunt splenic injury is an alternative to splenectomy when observation fails. *J Trauma Acute Care Surg*. 2013;75(3):421-425.
241. Gross TG, Orjuela MA, Perkins SL, et al. Low-dose chemotherapy and rituximab for posttransplant lymphoproliferative disease (PTLD): a Children's Oncology Group Report. *Am J Transplant*. 2012;12(11):3069-3075.
248. Hadinoto V, Shapiro M, Sun CC, et al. The dynamics of EBV shedding implicate a central role for epithelial cells in amplifying viral output. *PLoS Pathog*. 2009;5(7):e1000496.
253. Hall LD, Eminger LA, Hesterman KS, et al. Epstein-Barr virus: dermatologic associations and implications: part I. Mucocutaneous manifestations of Epstein-Barr virus and nonmalignant disorders. *J Am Acad Dermatol*. 2015;72(1):1-19, quiz 19-20.
258. Hammond WP, Harlan JM, Steinberg SE. Severe neutropenia in infectious mononucleosis. *West J Med*. 1979;131(2):92-97.
260. Hanlon P, Avenell A, Aucott L, et al. Systematic review and meta-analysis of the sero-epidemiological association between Epstein-Barr virus and systemic lupus erythematosus. *Arthritis Res Ther*. 2014;16(1):R3.
276. Heo DH, Baek DY, Oh SM, et al. Splenic infarction associated with acute infectious mononucleosis due to Epstein-Barr virus infection. *J Med Virol*. 2016.
278. Higgins CD, Swerdlow AJ, Macsween KF, et al. A study of risk factors for acquisition of Epstein-Barr virus and its subtypes. *J Infect Dis*. 2007;195(4):474-482.
293. Horwitz CA, Henle W, Henle G, et al. Clinical evaluation of patients with infectious mononucleosis and development of antibodies to the R component of the Epstein-Barr virus-induced early antigen complex. *Am J Med*. 1975;58(3): 330-338.
295. Hsu WL, Chung PJ, Tsai MH, et al. A role for Epstein-Barr viral BALF1 in facilitating tumor formation and metastasis potential. *Virus Res*. 2012;163(2):617-627.
301. Hussain FS, Hussain NS. Clinical utility of thallium-201 single photon emission computed tomography and cerebrospinal fluid Epstein-Barr virus detection using polymerase chain reaction in the diagnosis of AIDS-related primary central nervous system lymphoma. *Cureus*. 2016;8(5):e606.
308. Ishihara S, Okada S, Wakiguchi H, et al. Chronic active Epstein-Barr virus infection in children in Japan. *Acta Paediatr*. 1995;84(11):1271-1275.
309. Ishihara S, Yabuta R, Tokura Y, et al. Hypersensitivity to mosquito bites is not an allergic disease, but an Epstein-Barr virus-associated lymphoproliferative disease. *Int J Hematol*. 2000;72(2):223-228.
316. Jansen MA, van den Heuvel D, Bouthoorn SH, et al. Determinants of ethnic differences in cytomegalovirus, Epstein-Barr virus, and herpes simplex virus type 1 seroprevalence in childhood. *J Pediatr*. 2016;170:126-134 e121-126.
321. Jenson HB, Montalvo EA, McClain KL, et al. Characterization of natural Epstein-Barr virus infection and replication in smooth muscle cells from a leiomyosarcoma. *J Med Virol*. 1999;57(1):36-46.
323. Jiang SY, Yang JW, Shao JB, et al. Real-time polymerase chain reaction for diagnosing infectious mononucleosis in pediatric patients: a systematic review and meta-analysis. *J Med Virol*. 2016;88(5):871-876.
324. Johannsen E, Luftig M, Chase MR, et al. Proteins of purified Epstein-Barr virus. *Proc Natl Acad Sci USA*. 2004;101(46):16286-16291.
332. Jonigk D, Laenger F, Maegel L, et al. Molecular and clinicopathological analysis of Epstein-Barr virus-associated posttransplant smooth muscle tumors. *Am J Transplant*. 2012;12(7):1908-1917.
333. Jordan MB, Allen CE, Weitzman S, et al. How I treat hemophagocytic lymphohistiocytosis. *Blood*. 2011;118(15):4041-4052.
336. Kang MS, Kieff E. Epstein-Barr virus latent genes. *Exp Mol Med*. 2015;47:e131.
344. Katz BZ, Jason LA. Chronic fatigue syndrome following infections in adolescents. *Curr Opin Pediatr*. 2013;25(1):95-102.
354. Kimberlin DW, Brady MT, Jackson MA, et al Epstein-Barr virus infections (infectious mononucleosis). *Red Book*, 30th ed.; 2015.
355. Kimiya T, Yagihashi T, Shinjoh M, et al. Presence of Epstein-Barr virus in cerebrospinal fluid from patients with aseptic meningitis appears to be common. *Infection*. 2013;41(5):1045-1046.
357. Kimura H, Hoshino Y, Hara S, et al. Differences between T cell-type and natural killer cell-type chronic active Epstein-Barr virus infection. *J Infect Dis*. 2005;191(4):531-539.
362. Klinke O, Feederle R, Delecluse HJ. Genetics of Epstein-Barr virus microRNAs. *Semin Cancer Biol*. 2014;26:52-59.
364. Kottanattu L, Lava SA, Helbling R, et al. Pancreatitis and cholecystitis in primary acute symptomatic Epstein-Barr virus infection—systematic review of the literature. *J Clin Virol*. 2016;82:51-55.
368. Kusuhara K, Takabayashi A, Ueda K, et al. Breast milk is not a significant source for early Epstein-Barr virus or human herpesvirus 6 infection in infants: a seroepidemiologic study in 2 endemic areas of human T-cell lymphotropic virus type I in Japan. *Microbiol Immunol*. 1997;41(4):309-312.
369. Kuzembayeva M, Hayes M, Sugden B. Multiple functions are mediated by the miRNAs of Epstein-Barr virus. *Curr Opin Virol*. 2014;7:61-65.
370. Kwok H, Chan KW, Chan KH, et al. Distribution, persistence and interchange of Epstein-Barr virus strains among PBMC, plasma and saliva of primary infection subjects. *PLoS ONE*. 2015;10(3):e0120710.
375. Lajo A, Borque C, Del Castillo F, et al. Mononucleosis caused by Epstein-Barr virus and cytomegalovirus in children: a comparative study of 124 cases. *Pediatr Infect Dis J*. 1994;13(1):56-60.
386. Lee MH, Cho KS, Kahng KW, et al. A case of hemolytic uremic syndrome associated with Epstein-Barr virus infection. *Korean J Intern Med*. 1998;13(2):131-135.
402. Lin C-L, Lo W-F, Lee T-H, et al. Immunization with Epstein-Barr Virus (EBV) peptide-pulsed dendritic cells induces functional CD8+ T-cell immunity and may lead to tumor regression in patients with EBV-positive nasopharyngeal carcinoma. *Cancer Res*. 2002;62(23):6952-6958.
406. Linderholm M, Boman J, Juto P, et al. Comparative evaluation of nine kits for rapid diagnosis of infectious mononucleosis and Epstein-Barr virus-specific serology. *J Clin Microbiol*. 1994;32(1):259-261.
410. Longnecker R, Kieff E, Cohen J. Epstein-Barr virus. In: Knipe DM, Howley P, eds. *Fields virology*. 6th ed. Philadelphia: Wolters Kluwer Health/Lippincott Williams & Wilkins; 2013.
413. Lung RW, Tong JH, To KF. Emerging roles of small Epstein-Barr virus derived non-coding RNAs in epithelial malignancy. *Int J Mol Sci*. 2013;14(9):17378-17409.
414. Luzuriaga K, Sullivan JL. Infectious mononucleosis. *N Engl J Med*. 2010;362(21):1993-2000.
426. Mathew AG, Parvez Y. Fulminant Epstein Barr virus encephalitis. *Indian Pediatr*. 2013;50(4):418-419.
428. Mazur-Melewska K, Brenska I, Jonczyk-Potoczna K, et al. Neurologic complications caused by Epstein-Barr virus in pediatric patients. *J Child Neurol*. 2016;31(6):700-708.
432. McManus TE, Coyle PV, Lawson J, et al. Epstein-Barr virus pneumonitis. *Ulster Med J*. 2009;78(2):137-138.
434. Mellinger JL, Rossaro L, Naugler WE, et al. Epstein-Barr virus (EBV) related acute liver failure: a case series from the US Acute Liver Failure Study Group. *Dig Dis Sci*. 2014;59(7):1630-1637.
441. Molyneux EM, Rochford R, Griffin B, et al. Burkitt's lymphoma. *Lancet*. 2012;379(9822):1234-1244.
442. Monforte A, Cinque P, Vago L, et al. A comparison of brain biopsy and CSF-PCR in the diagnosis of CNS lesions in AIDS patients. *J Neurol*. 1997;244:35-39.
453. Nakaya H, Yamamoto T, Takano M, et al. Alice in Wonderland syndrome caused by the 2009 pandemic H1N1 influenza A virus. *Pediatr Infect Dis J*. 2011;30(8):725-726.
464. Norwood VF, Sturgill BC. Unexplained acute renal failure in a toddler: a rare complication of Epstein-Barr virus. *Pediatr Nephrol*. 2002;17(8):628-632.
465. O'Connor TE, Skinner LJ, Kiely P, et al. Return to contact sports following infectious mononucleosis: the role of serial ultrasonography. *Ear Nose Throat J*. 2011;90(8):E21-E24.
466. Odumade OA, Hogquist KA, Balfour HH Jr. Progress and problems in understanding and managing primary Epstein-Barr virus infections. *Clin Microbiol Rev*. 2011;24(1):193-209.
468. Ogembo JG, Kannan L, Ghiran I, et al. Human complement receptor type 1/ CD35 is an Epstein-Barr Virus receptor. *Cell Rep*. 2013;3(2):371-385.

471. Okano M, Kawa K, Kimura H, et al. Proposed guidelines for diagnosing chronic active Epstein-Barr virus infection. *Am J Hematol.* 2005;80(1):64-69.
472. Ometto L, Menin C, Masiero S, et al. Molecular profile of Epstein-Barr virus in human immunodeficiency virus type 1-related lymphadenopathies and lymphomas. *Blood.* 1997;90(1):313-322.
475. Ozgurhan G, Ozcetin M, Vehapoglu A, et al. Acute kidney injury complicated Epstein-Barr virus infection in infancy. *Case Rep Pediatr.* 2015;2015:848959.
478. Palendira U, Rickinson AB. Primary immunodeficiencies and the control of Epstein-Barr virus infection. *Ann N Y Acad Sci.* 2015;1356:22-44.
480. Palma I, Sanchez AE, Jimenez-Hernandez E, et al. Detection of Epstein-Barr virus and genotyping based on EBNA2 protein in Mexican patients with Hodgkin lymphoma: a comparative study in children and adults. *Clin Lymphoma Myeloma Leuk.* 2013;13(3):266-272.
481. Palser AL, Grayson NE, White RE, et al. Genome diversity of Epstein-Barr virus from multiple tumor types and normal infection. *J Virol.* 2015;89(10):5222-5237.
482. Papadopoulou-Legbelou K, Papadopoulou-Alataki E, Fleva A, et al. Cardiac complications and immunophenotypic profile of infectious mononucleosis syndrome in children. *Indian Pediatr.* 2012;49(3):195-198.
483. Park JH, Yoon DH, Kim S, et al. Pretreatment whole blood Epstein-Barr virus-DNA is a significant prognostic marker in patients with Hodgkin lymphoma. *Ann Hematol.* 2016;95(5):801-808.
497. Petrara MR, Cattelan AM, Zanchetta M, et al. Epstein-Barr virus load and immune activation in human immunodeficiency virus type 1-infected patients. *J Clin Virol.* 2012;53(3):195-200.
498. Petrara MR, Penazzato M, Massavon W, et al. Epstein-Barr virus load in children infected with human immunodeficiency virus type 1 in Uganda. *J Infect Dis.* 2014;210(3):392-399.
500. Pinzone MR, Berretta M, Cacopardo B, et al. Epstein-barr virus- and Kaposi sarcoma-associated herpesvirus-related malignancies in the setting of human immunodeficiency virus infection. *Semin Oncol.* 2015;42(2):258-271.
502. Piriou E, Asito AS, Sumba PO, et al. Early age at time of primary Epstein-Barr virus infection results in poorly controlled viral infection in infants from Western Kenya: clues to the etiology of endemic Burkitt lymphoma. *J Infect Dis.* 2012;205(6):906-913.
503. Pitcher RD, Beningfield SJ, Zar HJ. Chest radiographic features of lymphocytic interstitial pneumonitis in HIV-infected children. *Clin Radiol.* 2010;65(2):150-154.
504. Pitetti RD, Laus S, Wadowsky RM. Clinical evaluation of a quantitative real time polymerase chain reaction assay for diagnosis of primary Epstein-Barr virus infection in children. *Pediatr Infect Dis J.* 2003;22(8):736-739.
516. Punnett A, Tsang RW, Hodgson DC. Hodgkin lymphoma across the age spectrum: epidemiology, therapy, and late effects. *Semin Radiat Oncol.* 2010;20(1):30-44.
518. Putukian M, O'Connor FG, Stricker P, et al. Mononucleosis and athletic participation: an evidence-based subject review. *Clin J Sport Med.* 2008;18(4):309-315.
543. Rouphael NG, Talati NJ, Vaughan C, et al. Infections associated with haemophagocytic syndrome. *Lancet Infect Dis.* 2007;7(12):814-822.
553. Sardy M, Wollenberg A, Niedermeier A, et al. Genital ulcers associated with Epstein-Barr virus infection (ulcus vulvae acutum). *Acta Derm Venereol.* 2011;91(1):55-59.
560. Scotet E, David-Ameline J, Peyrat MA, et al. T cell response to Epstein-Barr virus transactivators in chronic rheumatoid arthritis. *J Exp Med.* 1996;184(5):1791-1800.
561. Scott GB, Hutto C, Makuch RW, et al. Survival in children with perinatally acquired human immunodeficiency virus type 1 infection. *N Engl J Med.* 1989;321(26):1791-1796.
563. Shamriz O, Vilk SR, Wolf DG, et al. Hematopoietic stem cell transplantation conditioning with use of rituximab in EBV related lymphoproliferative disorders. *Clin Immunol.* 2014;151(2):79-83.
572. Sitki-Green D, Covington M, Raab-Traub N. Compartmentalization and transmission of multiple epstein-barr virus strains in asymptomatic carriers. *J Virol.* 2003;77(3):1840-1847.
579. Slyker JA, Casper C, Tapia K, et al. Clinical and virologic manifestations of primary Epstein-Barr virus (EBV) infection in Kenyan infants born to HIV-infected women. *J Infect Dis.* 2013;207(12):1798-1806.
589. Srivastava G, Wong KY, Chiang AK, et al. Coinfection of multiple strains of Epstein-Barr virus in immunocompetent normal individuals: reassessment of the viral carrier state. *Blood.* 2000;95(7):2443-2445.
604. Svedmyr E, Ernberg I, Seeley J, et al. Virologic, immunologic, and clinical observations on a patient during the incubation, acute, and convalescent phases of infectious mononucleosis. *Clin Immunol Immunopathol.* 1984;30(3):437-450.
606. Swerdlow SH, Campo E, Pileri SA, et al. The 2016 revision of the World Health Organization classification of lymphoid neoplasms. *Blood.* 2016;127(20):2375-2390.
607. Swigris JJ, Berry GJ, Raffin TA, et al. Lymphoid interstitial pneumonia: a narrative review. *Chest.* 2002;122(6):2150-2164.
614. Tanaka M, Kamijo T, Koike K, et al. Specific autoantibodies to platelet glycoproteins in Epstein-Barr virus-associated immune thrombocytopenia. *Int J Hematol.* 2003;78(2):168-170.
619. Terada K, Niizuma T, Kosaka Y, et al. Bilateral facial nerve palsy associated with Epstein-Barr virus infection with a review of the literature. *Scand J Infect Dis.* 2004;36(1):75-77.
624. Thorley-Lawson DA. Epstein-Barr virus: exploiting the immune system. *Nat Rev Immunol.* 2001;1(1):75-82.
628. Topp SK, Rosenfeldt V, Vestergaard H, et al. Clinical characteristics and laboratory findings in Danish children hospitalized with primary Epstein-Barr virus infection. *Infect Dis (Lond).* 2015;47(12):908-914.
630. Trappe R, Oertel S, Leblond V, et al. Sequential treatment with rituximab followed by CHOP chemotherapy in adult B-cell post-transplant lymphoproliferative disorder (PTLD): the prospective international multicentre phase 2 PTLD-1 trial. *Lancet Oncol.* 2012;13(2):196-206.
631. Trottestam H, Horne A, Arico M, et al. Chemoimmunotherapy for hemophagocytic lymphohistiocytosis: long-term results of the HLH-94 treatment protocol. *Blood.* 2011;118(17):4577-4584.
632. Trottier H, Buteau C, Robitaille N, et al. Transfusion-related Epstein-Barr virus infection among stem cell transplant recipients: a retrospective cohort study in children. *Transfusion.* 2012;52(12):2653-2663.
636. Ueda S, Uchiyama S, Azzi T, et al. Oropharyngeal group A streptococcal colonization disrupts latent Epstein-Barr virus infection. *J Infect Dis.* 2014;209(2):255-264.
643. Viljoen J, Tuaillon E, Nagot N, et al. Cytomegalovirus, and possibly Epstein-Barr virus, shedding in breast milk is associated with HIV-1 transmission by breastfeeding. *AIDS.* 2015;29(2):145-153.
646. Wagner HJ, Kluter H, Kruse A, et al. Determination of the number of Epstein-Barr virus genomes in whole blood and red cell concentrates. *Transfus Med.* 1995;5(4):297-302.
647. Waldo RT. Neurologic complications of infectious mononucleosis after steroid therapy. *South Med J.* 1981;74(9):1159-1160.
650. Walling DM, Etienne W, Ray AJ, et al. Persistence and transition of Epstein-Barr virus genotypes in the pathogenesis of oral hairy leukoplakia. *J Infect Dis.* 2004;190(2):387-395.
653. Waters KA, Bale P, Isaacs D, et al. Successful chloroquine therapy in a child with lymphoid interstitial pneumonitis. *J Pediatr.* 1991;119(6):989-991.
656. Weinblatt ME. Immune thrombocytopenic purpura evolving into aplastic anemia in association with Epstein-Barr virus infection. *Am J Pediatr Hematol Oncol.* 1991;13(4):465-469.
667. Wistinghausen B, Gross TG, Bollard C. Post-transplant lymphoproliferative disease in pediatric solid organ transplant recipients. *Pediatr Hematol Oncol.* 2013;30(6):520-531.
677. Yao QY, Croom-Carter DS, Tierney RJ, et al. Epidemiology of infection with Epstein-Barr virus types 1 and 2: lessons from the study of a T-cell-immunocompromised hemophilic cohort. *J Virol.* 1998;72(5):4352-4363.
679. Yau TO, Tang CM, Yu J. Epigenetic dysregulation in Epstein-Barr virus-associated gastric carcinoma: disease and treatments. *World J Gastroenterol.* 2014;20(21):6448-6456.
681. Yin X, Wu T, Yan Y, et al. Treatment for leiomyosarcoma and leiomyoma in children with HIV infection. *Cochrane Database Syst Rev.* 2010;(5):CD007665.
683. Yokoyama T, Tokuhisa Y, Toga A, et al. Agranulocytosis after infectious mononucleosis. *J Clin Virol.* 2013;56(3):271-273.

The full reference list for this chapter is available at ExpertConsult.com.

161 Human Herpesviruses 6A, 6B, 7, and 8

Charles Grose

Before 1986, five human herpesviruses (HHVs) were known. They were herpes simplex virus (HSV) type 1 (oral) and type 2 (genital), cytomegalovirus (CMV), varicella-zoster virus (VZV), and Epstein-Barr virus (EBV). The herpesviruses are important pathogens causing a variety of childhood diseases that are described in other chapters of this text. An inherent characteristic of herpesviruses is their ability to form a latent infection, in which the viral genome continues to reside within the host. When the virus reactivates, it often causes further symptoms and signs. Thus, herpesviruses cause a spectrum of illnesses during the lifetime of the infected human host.

During the last decades of the 20th century, three novel herpesviruses were discovered. Two of these were originally designated HHV-6 and HHV-7, whereas the newest member of the family has been called either Kaposi sarcoma-associated herpesvirus (KSHV) or HHV-8. In 2012, the decision was made to separate HHV-6 into two distinct species called HHV-6A and HHV-6B. These viruses and the diseases they cause are described in this chapter. A point of particular interest for pediatric infectious disease is the increasingly convincing association of HHV-6B infection with febrile seizures and subsequent epilepsy.

HUMAN HERPESVIRUSES 6A, 6B, AND 7

One unexpected consequence of the epidemic of acquired immunodeficiency syndrome (AIDS) was the discovery of a new human DNA virus. The virus was isolated first from the white blood cells of six patients with lymphoproliferative disorders, two of whom had AIDS.[27] Further electron microscopic characterization of the virus demonstrated properties of a herpesvirus, including (1) an icosahedral capsid composed of 162 capsomers covered by a lipid membrane and (2) an enveloped particle with a diameter of 200 nm (Fig. 161.1). Because the virus was isolated originally from B lymphocytes, the agent was designated human B-lymphotropic virus. However, this apparent tropism for B lymphocytes was not confirmed by other investigators, who found that the virus preferentially infected CD4 T lymphocytes and not B lymphocytes.[20,30] Thus, the initial designation of human B-lymphotropic virus was changed to HHV-6.

The DNA sequence and the deduced amino acid sequence of the HHV-6 genome have been published.[6] Calculation of the percentage of amino acid identity shared by HHV-6 proteins with those in other herpesviruses revealed that HHV-6 proteins most closely resembled those of human CMV. The strains of HHV-6 have been divided into group A and group B. The HHV-6 isolates related to prototype strain U1102 have been called group A, whereas those related to strain Z29 have been designated group B. The genomes of the group A and B viruses exhibit a 90% nucleotide sequence identity. In 1990, while searching for additional strains of HHV-6, Frenkel and coworkers[14] isolated a new T-lymphotropic herpesvirus that was designated HHV-7. HHV-7 is related closely at a genetic level to HHV-6 and to a lesser degree to CMV.[6] In 2012, the International Committee on Taxonomy of Viruses decided to designate HHV-6A and HHV-6B as distinct species.[1] Thus, there are now nine human herpesviruses.

Most people contract their primary HHV-6 infection before reaching the age of 5 years.[3] In the United States, primary HHV-6 infection occurred in 40% of children by the time they reached 12 months of age and in 77% by the age of 24 months.[41] In these young children, HHV-6 strains (now known to be mainly HHV-6B) appear to be a major cause of the disease roseola (exanthem subitum). Roseola is discussed in Chapter 59. Children also may contract a primary HHV-6 infection without manifesting a rash. After acute infection, HHV-6 forms a latent infection, probably in T lymphocytes. In a small number of infants, acute HHV-7 infection appears to cause a roseola illness much like that of acute HHV-6 infection.[17]

Diseases Caused by HHV-6A, HHV-6B, and HHV-7

Studies in Japan first delineated the nature of the illness associated with acute HHV-6 infection in young children.[39] HHV-6 was cultured from the peripheral blood leukocytes of four infants with roseola (exanthem subitum); each subject was 6 months old and had an acute febrile illness followed by a concurrent fall in temperature and the onset of a rash. The blood samples were collected during the febrile stage of the disease. In a subsequent paper by the same group, two infants (6 and 7 months of age) were described who developed HHV-6 infection *without* a rash.[29] Both infants had been seen by physicians because of a 2- to 3-day history of high temperature (38.5–39.5°C). The only abnormal clinical finding was congestion of the throat. In both cases, the temperature rapidly returned to normal around day 3 of illness, but no rash was ever observed. Cultures of peripheral blood cells from both infants were positive for HHV-6.[29] Further seroprevalence studies performed in Japan showed that most Japanese children (86%) contracted HHV-6 infection by the time they were 24 months of age.[40] Thereafter, the increase in seropositivity among the childhood populations was small. These statistics suggest that HHV-6 infection goes unrecognized in most children.

Primary HHV-6 infection has been implicated in a few cases of severe hepatitis. The first case was that of a 21-year-old patient with cystic fibrosis who received a liver transplant.[36] The recipient lacked antibodies to HHV-6, and the organ donor was seropositive. Two weeks after undergoing transplantation, the recipient developed fever and grand mal seizures; her hepatic function deteriorated. HHV-6 was cultured from her peripheral blood cells. The apparent source of infection was the donor liver, from which HHV-6 presumably was reactivated after transplantation. She gradually recovered her hepatic function during the course of several weeks.

A fatal case of fulminant HHV-6 hepatitis has been reported in a 3-month-old boy.[4] The infant was admitted to a hospital because of fever, jaundice, convulsions, and loss of consciousness. His serum bilirubin concentration, liver transaminases, and blood ammonia level were elevated markedly. Within 7 days, he became comatose and died. As part of the diagnostic evaluation, HHV-6 was cultured from his mononuclear cells. Furthermore, HHV-6 DNA was detected in biopsy samples of liver and brain, which were obtained immediately after death.

In a large retrospective review of roseola in association with acute HHV-6 infection, the signs and symptoms were tabulated.[3] The study population included 94 boys and 82 girls, who ranged in age from 3 weeks to 18 months (Table 161.1). As would be predicted, the two most common clinical findings were fever and rash. The temperature often rose to 39°C, and fever persisted for 2 to 4 days. The rash usually appeared when the fever lessened; the rash was papular in 54%, macular in 40%, and maculopapular in the remainder of the children. The exanthem typically persisted for 3 to 4 days and was not followed by desquamation. Diarrhea was a surprisingly frequent occurrence, but it was not severe. An enanthem called *Nagayama spots* in Japan consisted of papules on the mucosa of the soft palate and uvula. Of the total study group, 8% developed febrile seizures. More severe central nervous system (CNS) complications have been documented in children not enrolled in this study. A few children with HHV-6 encephalitis have had abnormal electroencephalographic recordings. Some children with encephalitis have had permanent neurologic sequelae. In the United States in particular, acute HHV-6 infection also appears to be associated with concurrent acute otitis media.[24]

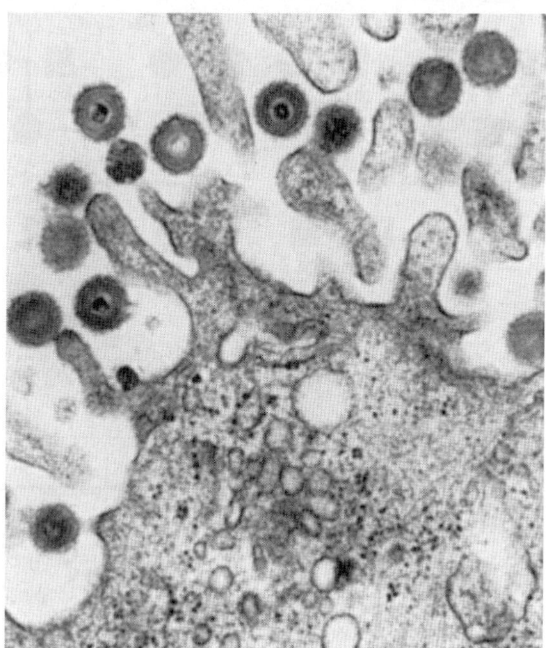

FIG. 161.1 Electron micrograph of cultured mononuclear cells infected with human herpesvirus 6. Several enveloped viral particles are visible in the extracellular area. (Courtesy Dr. Y. Asano.)

TABLE 161.1 **Selected Features in Roseola Associated With Infection in Children**

Clinical Findings	%
Temperature >37.5°C	98
Rash	98
Diarrhea	68
Nagayama spots	65
Cervical adenopathy	31
Edematous eyelids	30
Bulging fontanelle	26
Prodromal symptoms	14
Convulsions	8
Cough	0

Modified from Asano Y, Grose C. Human herpesvirus type 6 infections. In: Glaser R, Jones J, eds. *Herpesvirus Infections*. New York: Marcel Dekker; 1994:227-244.

Reactivation of previous HHV-6 infection has been demonstrated in some healthy children and adults who contracted a second herpes-type infection, such as primary EBV infection (infectious mononucleosis) or primary CMV infection.[3] A similar serologic survey was performed in 10 renal transplant recipients who initially were HHV-6 seropositive.[3] After transplantation, all 10 showed greater than fourfold rises in antibody to HHV-6. Only two of the 10 developed a febrile illness, and both of them also had primary CMV infection.

Among the human herpesviruses, HHV-6 infections are unique in that HHV-6 DNA is integrated into the subtelomeric region of chromosomes in about 1% of the adult population.[1] In a recent survey of 21 cases of integrated HHV-6 infection following transplantation, HHV-6B DNA was found more often among solid organ transplant recipients, whereas integrated HHV-6A was more common among allogeneic hematopoietic stem cell recipients. None of the 21 transplant patients developed clinical symptoms related to the integrated HHV-6 infections.[18] Furthermore, HHV-6 infection is not related causally to Kawasaki disease, nor does HHV-6 infection appear to alter the course of human immunodeficiency virus (HIV) infection.[28]

Whether HHV-7 causes a distinct illness has been the subject of many medical investigations since 1990. In general, HHV-7 antibody is acquired by mid-childhood, but there appears to be no corresponding sentinel illness. However, in two infants with roseola, both isolation of HHV-7 and seroconversion to HHV-7 were documented; in addition, another five children with roseola were found to have undergone seroconversion to HHV-7.[32] HHV-7 also has been isolated from one infant with an acute febrile illness.[25] Therefore, in a small number of young children, acute HHV-7 infection may be associated with fever and sometimes a roseola-like rash.

Finally, congenital infections also can occur in pregnant women already infected with HHV-6. In a survey of 5638 cord blood samples, HHV-6 DNA was detected in 57 samples (1%), but the congenital infections did not cause an identifiable disease in the newborn.[16] Of great interest, congenital HHV-6 infections appear to be caused mainly by chromosomally integrated HHV-6 DNA. Therefore, the HHV-6 genome will be present in all cell types, including tissues in the central nervous system of the newborn. Chromosomal integration during congenital infection appears to occur more commonly with HHV-6A than with HHV-6B strains.

Neurologic Complications

In the preceding paragraphs, CNS symptoms were mentioned briefly. In a large series of clinical studies performed in Japan, seizures were a common feature of acute HHV-6 infection.[3,37] In one series of 105 young children with acute febrile convulsions, 21 had evidence of primary HHV-6 infection, as assayed by either isolation of virus from blood or seroconversion of HHV-6 antibodies. When the age of the patient was assessed, HHV-6 infection was found in 13 of 23 seizure patients younger than 1 year; thus, the seizure group with HHV-6 infection was significantly younger than the seizure group without HHV-6 infection. In addition, the frequency of clustering seizures, long-lasting seizures, partial seizures, and postictal paralysis in children having their first febrile convulsion episode was significantly higher in those with primary HHV-6 infection than in those without HHV-6 infection. One child with fatal acute necrotizing encephalitis and concurrent HHV-6 infection also has been described.[22]

In early studies from Japan, assays for HHV-6 and HHV-7 DNA were performed on cerebrospinal fluid samples from 43 children with CNS symptoms.[38] All children had symptoms compatible with aseptic meningitis. HHV-6 DNA was detected in the peripheral blood cells of 15 and in the cerebrospinal fluid of 7 children; all were HHV-6 variant B. HHV-7 DNA was detected in the peripheral blood cells of 28 and in the cerebrospinal fluid of 6 patients. Thus, the clinical study demonstrated that both HHV-6 and HHV-7 can invade the CNS or, alternatively, frequently reactivate within the CNS during childhood neurologic disease. The results from Japan have been confirmed in a similar large analysis of young children with seizures in Britain and Ireland.[35] Among 156 children hospitalized with febrile seizures, 26 (17%) were associated with acute HHV-6 or HHV-7 infection. The median age for hospitalization in the HHV-6 group was 53 weeks, and the median age for the HHV-7 group was 60 weeks. In turn, the prior results were again confirmed in a prospective study of 199 children between the ages of 1 month and 5 years from the United States, who presented with prolonged febrile seizures. Blood samples were tested for HHV-6A, HHV-6B and HHV-7 DNA and RNA. HHV-6B viremia was detected in 32% and HHV-7 viremia was detected in 7% of the children, whereas no child had HHV-6A viremia.[13]

HHV-6 infection is an important cause of post-transplant acute limbic encephalitis (PALE) after a hematopoietic stem cell transplantation. Among six children who underwent cord blood transplantation for hematological malignancies at one hospital in Australia, all six developed PALE in association with HHV-6 infection.[17] Three patients developed confusion, general impairment of memory, and sporadic seizures. The other three had more severe symptoms, including generalized epilepsy that presented during the third week after the transplant. The diagnosis of HHV-6 infection was made by detection of viral DNA in blood and spinal fluid. The seizures were initially controlled and the HHV-6 infection was treated. However, after another 11 to 18 months, all three patients developed generalized seizures that were much more difficult to control. All three patients experienced a severe regression in their motor and intellectual functioning. HHV-6B infection also may be an important cause of mesial temporal lobe epilepsy.[18] HHV-6B DNA was detected in approximately one fourth of resected brain biopsies from patients with temporal lobe epilepsy. Several of these epilepsy patients had a history of febrile seizures earlier in childhood.

Pathogenesis of HHV-6 and HHV-7 Infection

The pathogenesis of HHV-6 infection certainly includes a viremia while the child is asymptomatic; the total duration of the incubation period is not well defined but may be approximately 10 days. Although these studies were performed before HHV-6A and HHV-6B were distinguished, it is now known that the vast majority of these cases in young children are caused by HHV-6B infection (roseola). The prodrome, which signals the end of the incubation period, includes 2 to 4 days of fever, which precedes the onset of the rash.[3,26] During this period, virtually 100% of peripheral blood cell cultures are positive for HHV-6. By day 3 or 4, when the rash first appears, the viremia is abating. Between 5 and 7 days after the onset of the fever (or 2 to 4 days after appearance of exanthem), viremia persists in less than 20% of the children. Viremia is absent later in convalescence, when the antibody response is detectable. HHV-6 occasionally reactivates from latency throughout the lifetime of an infected human, but usually no apparent illness is present.[7]

The mothers of infants with HHV-6 infection have been studied to determine whether they are the source of the infectious agent.[16] Because most mothers are seropositive, the possibility exists that HHV-6 infection could reactivate in the mother, who would then transmit the infection to her child, possibly through exchange of saliva. Obviously, mothers with an integrated HHV-6 DNA infection can pass the infection to their fetus during gestation.[16] However, for mothers without an integrated infection but with HHV-6 seropositivity, HHV-6 DNA was detected in the vaginal secretions, so perinatal HHV-6 transmission remains a possibility. Older siblings are another possible source of infection within a household.[41]

In contrast with HHV-6, HHV-7 seropositivity occurs in children, but often after the first 2 years of life. HHV-7 transmission has been investigated in large multigenerational Japanese families living in the same household.[31] The results indicated that HHV-7 is transmitted gradually from older generation to younger generation (Fig. 161.2). Transmission often occurs in children before the child enters a traditional primary school at the age of 6 years. Either parent or presumably an older sibling can transmit the virus. A reasonable explanation for this pattern of transmission is repeated exchange of infectious saliva among family members living in the same household during the course of many years.

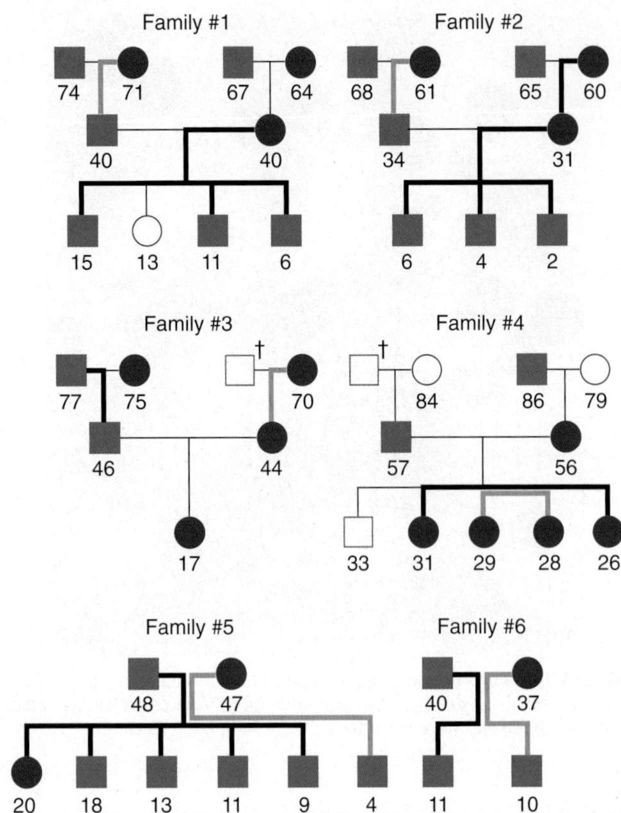

FIG. 161.2 Pedigrees of six families with human herpesvirus (HHV)-7 infection. All families resided in Okayama, Japan. Males and females are indicated as boxes and circles, respectively. Persons from whom HHV-7 was isolated are shaded. A person who was already deceased is marked (†). Members who have similar HHV-7 DNA restriction patterns are connected with bold lines. Numbers under the boxes and circles indicate ages. (From Takahashi Y, Yamada M, Nakamura J, et al. Transmission of human herpesvirus 7 through multigenerational families in the same household. *Pediatr Infect Dis J.* 1997;16:975-978.)

Diagnosis

Infection with HHV-6 can be diagnosed by several means, including (1) measurement of antibody, (2) isolation of virus, (3) detection of viral antigen, and (4) detection of viral DNA. The first method (i.e., the traditional approach for diagnosis of virus infection) usually requires acute and convalescent serum samples for determination of a fourfold or greater rise in titer of virus-specific IgG antibody. The finding of IgM specific for HHV-6 in a single serum sample also would indicate an acute infection in a young child. HHV-6 antibodies usually have been measured by an indirect immunofluorescence method, although neutralization tests also have been performed.[3,4,34]

Isolation of HHV-6 was the original technique for identification of this herpesvirus.[27] The method is more difficult to perform than are those methods commonly used for most herpesviruses (e.g., HSV, CMV, VZV) but is similar to that required for isolation of another herpesvirus, EBV. HHV-6 usually is isolated in a cell substrate consisting of mononuclear cells obtained from cord blood of a newborn infant. The source of virus in the patient also is the peripheral blood mononuclear cell population.[34]

Viral genome can be detected in infected tissues by DNA hybridization techniques.[34] Viral DNA also can be detected in tissue samples by polymerase chain reaction (PCR); for example, in one fatal case of HHV-6 infection,[4] DNA was extracted from postmortem liver and brain samples and amplified by the PCR test. Currently, HHV-6A and HHV-6B infections can be distinguished by PCR amplification technology.[13] Extremely high copy numbers may indicate an integrated HHV-6 infection. Likewise, HHV-7 infection usually is diagnosed by PCR amplification of viral DNA in samples from patients.

Treatment of HHV-6 Infection

In most instances of HHV-6 infection in healthy children, treatment with an antiviral medication is not indicated. Recovery is complete within a few days after onset of the rash, and sequelae rarely occur. However, HHV-6 disease in immunocompromised children may be more persistent or severe (e.g., encephalitis). Several groups have analyzed the in vitro sensitivity of HHV-6 to four antiviral drugs: acyclovir, ganciclovir, phosphonoformic acid, and cidofovir.[1,3] All four compounds have been used in treatment of other herpesvirus infections. Multiplication of HHV-6 in cell culture is inhibited readily by ganciclovir at a concentration of 2 to 10 μg/mL, levels that are easily achievable in humans. Phosphonoformic acid (foscarnet) at a concentration of 6 μg/mL also is effective against HHV-6 infection. On the other hand, HHV-6 is affected by acyclovir only at concentrations of 50 μg/mL, considerably higher levels than those required for treatment of HSV-1, HSV-2, and VZV infections and probably toxic in humans. Likewise, cidofovir has more side effects than ganciclovir and usually would not be recommended for HHV-6 treatment. At present, none of these antiviral drugs has been approved specifically for treatment of HHV-6 infections. One caveat for antiviral therapy for HHV-6 infection is the consideration whether the HHV-6 infection is related to chromosomally integrated HHV-6 DNA; these patients often have high copy numbers of HHV-6

DNA in the blood. Under these circumstances, however, antiviral therapy may exert no demonstrable effect.[18]

KAPOSI SARCOMA HERPESVIRUS (HUMAN HERPESVIRUS 8)

Yet another consequence of the HIV epidemic in the 1980s was the appearance of Kaposi sarcoma in many people with AIDS. The increase in Kaposi sarcoma was especially puzzling because the tumor occurred more frequently in people who acquired HIV by sexual transmission rather than by infusion of infected blood products, such as factor VIII in hemophiliac patients. The question often arose whether a second infectious agent was involved in the etiology of Kaposi sarcoma. The answer to that question was provided by a report published in late 1994. The authors announced the identification of a previously unknown herpesvirus-like DNA sequence collected from patients with AIDS in New York.[9] The viral DNA was called *Kaposi sarcoma-associated herpesvirus* (KSHV). Other virologists prefer that the agent be called *human herpesvirus 8* (HHV-8).

Diseases Caused by Kaposi Sarcoma-Associated Herpesvirus

The authors of the original KSHV report were investigating patients with Kaposi sarcoma. They discovered the herpesvirus-like DNA sequences by using a combination of genetic techniques, including amplification of DNA by PCR and subsequent representational difference analysis.[9] Thereby, they were able to identify and to characterize unique DNA sequences in Kaposi sarcoma that showed close homology to regions of the genome of *Herpesvirus saimiri,* a simian herpesvirus, and to a lesser degree to EBV, the agent that causes infectious mononucleosis. In their study, the authors located one or both of these herpesvirus-like DNA sequences in 20 of 27 different samples of Kaposi sarcoma tissue. The investigators correctly concluded that they had discovered DNA of a previously unknown herpesvirus within Kaposi sarcoma tissues.

Their virology results were confirmed quickly by other groups. In one study from California, investigators detected identical viral sequences in 13 of 13 biopsy specimens of Kaposi sarcoma from patients with AIDS.[2] This study also found the same sequence in the peripheral blood cells collected from 10 of the 13 patients but not in the blood samples of 20 patients with no history of Kaposi sarcoma. A third study from France found the herpesvirus-like DNA in biopsy specimens from five patients with Mediterranean-type Kaposi sarcoma; all five patients were HIV seronegative.[11] In subsequent studies, HHV-8 DNA has been detected in most Kaposi sarcomas (classic) in HIV-seronegative individuals, often men residing in the Mediterranean area.

The authors of the original KSHV report subsequently found the herpesvirus-like DNA sequences in body cavity–based lymphomas from patients with AIDS.[8] HHV-8 DNA also has been found in the B-cell lymphoproliferative disorder known as *multicentric Castleman disease.*[5] Of equal importance, KSHV sequences were not found in several other lymphomas or leukemias (e.g., small-lymphocyte lymphoma, monocytoid B-cell lymphoma, follicular lymphoma, diffuse large-cell lymphoma, Burkitt lymphoma, lymphoblastic lymphoma, anaplastic large-cell lymphoma, multiple myeloma, hairy-cell leukemia, acute lymphoblastic leukemia, or cutaneous T-cell lymphoma). Recently, multicentric Castleman disease has been diagnosed in an HHV-8 infected child, who may have had errors in innate immunity secondary to consanguineous parents.[19]

Transmission of HHV-8 Among Children

One of the most perplexing aspects of HHV-8 epidemiology is the mode of transmission. That the seroprevalence is high among a population of adult men who have sex with men is well known.[23] Yet, the question remains whether larger segments of the population are infected on a worldwide basis and, in particular, whether children are infected. To answer this question, several HHV-8 seroepidemiology studies were surveyed. Two studies provide partial answers to the question of childhood infection.

An early study was performed in a village in French Guiana, South America, among 1337 individuals of African origin.[24] They ranged in age from 2 to 91 years. The serologic data indicated that HHV-8 seropositivity was strongly age dependent. Among 14 children aged 2 to 14 years, 3 of 146 were positive; aged 5 to 9 years, 14 of 278 were positive; aged 10 to 14 years, 31 of 232 were positive; aged 15 to 19 years, 24 of 149 were positive; aged 20 to 29 years, 38 of 236 were positive; aged 30 to 39 years, 16 of 120 were positive; aged 40 to 49 years, 19 of 70 were positive; and older than 50 years, 32 of 106 were positive. These seroprevalence data clearly show a gradual acquisition of infection during early childhood, with a stepwise increment from approximately 5% to 12% at age 10 years.

HIV infection did not play a role in the likelihood of transmission because HIV infection is not a common occurrence in this village. Instead, extensive analyses of intrafamilial relationships demonstrated a highly significant familial correlation in HHV-8 seropositivity between mother and child (especially when children were <10 years) and between siblings. The correlation was highest when the siblings had an age difference of less than 5 years. Of interest, a similarity in transmission appears to exist between HHV-8 and HHV-7, when HHV-7 was studied in multigenerational Japanese households (see Fig. 161.2).

A second large HHV-8 seroepidemiology analysis was performed in Israel.[10] Because the incidence of classic Kaposi sarcoma in Israel is among the highest in the developed world, the investigators undertook a study to ascertain the HHV-8 seroprevalence in Israel and also to investigate HHV-8 intrafamilial transmission. The Israeli data showed that 9% of children aged 2 to 14 years and 9% of adolescents and young adults aged 15 to 24 years were HHV-8 seropositive. Seroprevalence in older adults ranged from 12% to 18%. HHV-8 positivity was more likely to occur in children when at least one of the parents was positive compared with children with neither parent positive. The most important predictor of a child's HHV-8 seropositivity status was maternal seropositivity.

HHV-8 seropositivity rises throughout adolescence and adulthood, regardless of HIV infection status.[33] In a recent review of KSHV infection in endemic countries, the authors reiterated that KSHV infection was spread among children primarily by exchange of saliva.[21] Feeding young children food premasticated by the mother may be a particularly effective means of transmission. In contrast to CMV infection, KSHV infection is not spread via breastfeeding.[21] In nonendemic countries in North America and western Europe, the seropositivity rate among HIV-seronegative adults is considered to be low, approximately 3% to 5%. The reasons for these differences between continents are not completely resolved. Nonetheless, a reasonable hypothesis is a decreased likelihood for transmission within smaller family groups in developed countries.[12] An alternative mode of infection, described next, is transmission by blood transfusion.

Hemophagocytic Lymphohistiocytosis

Hemophagocytic lymphohistiocytosis (HLH) is a rare and sometimes fatal disorder of immune regulation, often associated with mutations in the perforin gene. Even carriers of the mutated gene may require an acute infection to trigger HLH. HHV-8 is one of the triggers. HLH in association with HHV-8 infection has occurred in adults with severe HIV infection or with a recent kidney transplant.[13,19]

HLH has been diagnosed in two identical siblings from Iowa during the first 6 months of life.[15] The siblings were born prematurely and spent several months in intensive care. Both siblings had mutations in the perforin gene. Both siblings had HHV-8 infection. Because the mother of the two was negative for HHV-8 infection, one possible route of transmission was a blood transfusion given while they were in the nursery. In fact, in a large study in East Africa, blood transfusions were shown to transmit HHV-8 infection.[18] Therefore, children who have had multiple blood transfusions may be at risk for acquiring HHV-8 infection.[11]

Diagnosis and Treatment of HHV-8 Infection

Diagnosis of prior HHV-8 infection can be made by serology. More commonly, diagnosis of acute HHV-8 infection can be accomplished by PCR amplification of HHV-8-specific DNA.[9,11,12]

Treatment is not necessary in most healthy hosts because the virus quickly enters latency after the primary infection. No disease has been associated with a latent infection in children, except in those with immunodeficiency. However, acute HHV-8 infection in recent transplant recipients or HIV-seropositive children could be an indication for treatment.[13,19] Some of the same antiviral drugs described for HHV-6 treatment also inhibit HHV-8 replication (e.g., ganciclovir), but currently there are too few clinical data on which to base a standard regimen, so treatment would need to be individualized for each infected patient. Finally, for children coinfected with HIV and KSHV, the use of highly active antiretroviral therapy (HAART) has curtailed HIV infection and thereby caused a sharp decline in the incidence of AIDS-defining syndromes such as Kaposi sarcoma.

NEW REFERENCES SINCE THE SEVENTH EDITION

17. Howell KB, Tiedemann K, Haeusler G, et al. Symptomatic generalized epilepsy after HHV6 post-transplant acute limbic encephalitis in children. *Epilepsia.* 2012;53:122-126.
18. Kawamura Y, Nakayama A, Kato T, et al. Pathogenic role of human herpesvirus 6B infection in mesial temporal lobe epilepsy. *J Infect Dis.* 2015;212:1046-1052.
19. Leroy S, Moshous D, Cassar O, et al. Multicentric Castleman disease in an HHV-8 infected child born to consanguineous parents. *Pediatrics.* 2012;129:199-203.

The full reference list for this chapter is available at ExpertConsult.com.

162 Varicella-Zoster Virus

Anne A. Gershon

Varicella-zoster virus (VZV) causes two diseases: varicella (chickenpox) and zoster (shingles). Varicella, the primary infection, usually occurs in childhood and manifests as a pruritic rash accompanied by fever and other systemic signs and symptoms that usually are mild to moderate. Zoster is primarily a disease of adults, although it can occur in children. It develops when latent VZV, acquired with varicella or at vaccination, reactivates in a setting of low cell-mediated immunity to VZV as a result of disease or the use of various therapies, such as corticosteroids, cancer chemotherapy, organ transplantation, and irradiation. During primary infection, VZV establishes latency in sensory or other ganglia; zoster results when latent VZV reactivates in the neurons of the ganglia. Usually, reactivation results in skin infection and produces a unilateral dermatomal eruption that may be painful or pruritic. On occasion, however, VZV reactivation occurs without producing a rash; symptoms other than rash (such as aseptic meningitis) are the result of reactivation of VZV. Reactivation may also occur in the absence of symptoms.

The origin of the name "chickenpox" is uncertain, but it may have come from the French *pois chiche* (chickpea) or from the domestic fowl (in Old English, *cicen,* and in Middle High German, *kuchen*).[53] *Herpes* is the Greek word meaning "to creep," and *zoster* comes from the Greek and Latin word meaning "girdle" or "belt." Originally VZV was thought to be a poxvirus.

THE ORGANISM

VZV is an alpha herpesvirus. It has a DNA core surrounded by a nucleocapsid composed of 162 hexagonal capsomers that form an icosahedron with a diameter of approximately 100 nm. A tegument surrounds this structure, which in turn is surrounded by a lipid-containing envelope. Enveloped virions have a diameter of approximately 200 nm.[63] The genome of VZV has been sequenced; it contains 71 open-reading frames (ORFs).[65] The linear, double-stranded DNA consists of a long unique segment, U_L, and a short unique sequence, U_S, flanked by internal and terminal repeats.[67,70,228] The genome of the Oka vaccine strain (vOka) also has been sequenced; the molecular basis for attenuation of the strain is still under investigation.[4,107,158,251]

At least six genes of VZV—4, 21, 29, 62, 63, and 66—have been described as being expressed in human ganglia during latent VZV infection. VZV is synthesized by an orderly cascade of gene expression consisting of immediate-early (IE), early (E), and, finally, late (L) lytic genes that encode structural proteins. In *latent* infection there is thought to be a block in the cascade that permits synthesis of only roughly one tenth of the genes that are synthesized in productive or *lytic* infection. The genes expressed during latent infection are IE and E genes; L genes are not expressed. One hypothesis concerning latency is that cellular immunity to VZV normally can control early replication of the virus so that productive or lytic infection does not occur.[49,58-60,120,135-137,165,166]

During productive or lytic infection, VZV synthesizes more than 30 polypeptides; the function of most of these polypeptides remains unknown, but some are structural and others are nonstructural and presumably have regulatory action. VZV synthesizes at least nine glycoproteins (g): gB, gC, gE, gH, gI, gK, gL, gM, and gN.[57,64,111,140] These glycoproteins correspond somewhat to those of herpes simplex virus (HSV), but, unlike HSV, VZV has no equivalent of gD, which is the major glycoprotein of HSV, nor of gG. The major glycoprotein of VZV is gE; it is the most abundant and immunogenic glycoprotein of VZV. The VZV glycoproteins not only provide structures for the virion but also play roles in infectivity, such as mediating adhesion and promoting entry of VZV from an infected cell into another uninfected cell. The glycoproteins also are antigenic, as is the tegument, and immune responses are directed toward these structures.

Just one antigenic type of VZV has been identified. Three major classifications of wild-type (WT) VZV were originally described, referred to as European (E), Japanese (J, for strains homologous to the Oka parental vaccine strain), and Mosaic (M, for strains displaying a combination of European and Japanese genotype-like mutations).[19,163,213,238] Worldwide, six VZV clades have now been described, with three additional putative clades. The clades have differing geographic origins, which have been influenced by worldwide immigration patterns. All six clades have been observed in the United States, although clades 1 and 3 (both E) predominate.[29] vOka is derived from a clade 2 strain, which is mainly found in Asia.

Wild-type VZV DNA can be distinguished from that of vaccine-type (Oka) virus by restriction enzyme analysis of DNA from cultured virus and/or by polymerase chain reaction (PCR) assay and by direct sequencing, particularly of three gene segments at positions 106262, 107252, and 108111 in ORF 62, which contain the major mutations in Oka.[4,107,148,162,171,181,198,210]

VZV replicates in the nuclei of infected cells, where the DNA core and capsid are synthesized. The capsid is enveloped by a complex process in the Golgi apparatus, after which it traverses the cell in cytoplasmic vesicles.[94] In vitro, and in patients with VZV infections, the virus grows rather slowly and is highly cell associated. Its synthetic pathway entraps it in endosomic vesicles, where it is inactivated before it can be released from cells in infectious form. In vivo, however, infectious VZV is released from cells of the superficial epidermis and is highly contagious; this may be the only place in the body where cell free virus is produced. VZV avoids the endosomal route in this particular tissue because of the loss of its receptor (the large calcium-independent mannose-6-phosphate receptor) and thereby it can exit epidermal cells in infectious form by the secretory pathway.[50]

VZV has an extremely limited host range and infects mostly primates. Various strains of guinea pigs, including hairless ones, may be infected with VZV, but either no symptoms are produced or the illness produced is extremely mild, although specific immune responses can be demonstrated.[182] Animal models of latent VZV infection have been described in rodents, including guinea pigs.[48,177,204,250] An in vitro model of latency and reactivation of VZV in intestinal neurons from guinea pigs has recently been developed.[49]

TRANSMISSION

VZV is spread by the airborne route[150] and requires contact with an infected individual for transmission to occur. In varicella, VZV is transmitted mainly from the skin[50,233]; the respiratory tract cannot be excluded but is not likely to be a significant mode of viral spread. VZV is isolated readily from skin lesions, but isolation of the virus from the respiratory tract just before or during rash is extremely rare.[106,187,231] Spread of VZV from varicella patients before the onset of rash in closed communities has been reported, implicating respiratory spread, although early skin lesions could have been overlooked.[31,108] VZV DNA has been detected by PCR assay in the nasopharynx of children during the preeruptive and early stages of varicella.[138,188,208] Investigations of leukemic recipients of live attenuated varicella vaccine have implicated spread of VZV from skin. No transmission to siblings from vaccinees who did not have a rash was found, but a 14% transmission rate occurred when siblings were exposed to a recently immunized child who had a vaccine-associated rash.[233] The chance of transmission occurring was directly proportional to the number of skin lesions present.[233] Observations in children with WT varicella despite their having been immunized indicated that higher transmission rates are associated with greater numbers of skin lesions.[215] Interestingly, an attack rate of more than 20% occurred after medical students were exposed to VZV during the autopsy of a patient with disseminated varicella; clearly, this transmission could not have occurred by the respiratory route.[190] Taken together, these observations suggest that VZV spreads mainly from skin lesions rather than from the respiratory tract. Epidemiologic studies suggest that transmission is most likely to take place in the early stages of varicella.[39,180]

Zoster is not transmissible per se, but the vesicular lesions of zoster contain infectious VZV and can transmit varicella to other individuals who have not yet had primary infection.[32,144] Zoster is perhaps 75% less contagious than is varicella,[201,212] and whether VZV is spread from the respiratory tracts of patients with zoster is unknown. Presumably, however, the major source of contagion, as for varicella, is the skin lesions.[212]

EPIDEMIOLOGY

VZV infections occur worldwide, and both sexes are affected equally. The virus spreads less efficiently in countries with tropical climates than in those with temperate climates,[124] thereby resulting in a high rate of susceptibility in adults reared in tropical countries. In the prevaccine era, approximately 3.8 million cases of chickenpox, an entire birth cohort, occurred annually in the United States. At that time, 8% to 9% of children between the ages of 1 and 9 years contracted the illness annually.[195] These data were collected before many children attended daycare facilities; exposure to VZV in the daycare setting might have led to earlier acquisition of disease. Today there is little varicella disease in the United States owing to widespread routine vaccination. (See the later discussion of the health effects of widespread immunization in the United States.)

The link between varicella and zoster was recognized first about 100 years ago when Bokay[27] appreciated that cases of varicella often occurred after exposure to a patient with zoster. Early in the 20th century, medical investigators inoculated vesicular fluid from zoster patients into varicella-susceptible children, who then contracted chickenpox.[32,144] Weller first successfully isolated VZV in vitro, gave the virus its name, and demonstrated that the viruses isolated from patients with varicella and zoster are identical.[243] Garland proposed that zoster is the result of reactivation of latent VZV.[81] Hope-Simpson presciently recognized the importance of the immune system in preventing reactivation of VZV; he postulated that periodic exposure to varicella (external boosting) and asymptomatic reactivation from latency (internal boosting) stimulate immunity to VZV and that zoster results when despite these boosts, immunity to VZV wanes as the immune system begins to deteriorate during aging.[123] Declining cell-mediated immunity to VZV has been identified as contributing significantly to the development of zoster.[9,21,34,118] With the use of molecular techniques for DNA analysis, researchers have established that the DNA of the viruses causing varicella and zoster is the same, and autopsies and surgical specimens have revealed that latent VZV is detectable in neurons of the sensory ganglia of individuals with a past history of varicella or vaccination.[61,86,136,164,167] Zoster is not acquired by contact with patients who have zoster or chickenpox, but by reactivation of latent VZV.[90] Zoster is said to develop in approximately 30% of the varicella-immune population during their lifetimes, resulting in an annual rate of 1 million cases, but the true incidence of zoster is probably underestimated due to a significant number of cases with very mild, nonexistent, and/or atypical rashes.[186]

Varicella is highly contagious; clinical infection develops in 80% to 90% of susceptible individuals exposed in a household.[202] Secondary varicella cases in a family usually are more severe than primary cases, probably because of intensity of exposure.[194,202] Approximately 75% of American adults with no past history of varicella have detectable antibodies to VZV,[149] thus indicating that subclinical varicella can occur. One epidemiologic study suggests that its incidence is approximately 5%.[202]

Subclinical zoster also may occur, and zoster with dermatomal pain and no rash has been described (zoster sine herpete).[101] Increases in VZV immune responses and episodes of viremia shown by PCR assay in asymptomatic individuals indicate that silent reactivation occurs.[97,112,248] Asymptomatic shedding of infectious VZV is essentially nonexistent.

Second attacks of varicella are uncommon but may happen more frequently in persons who are immunocompromised than in immunologically normal individuals.[98,131] Immunologic boosting to VZV occurs commonly on reexposure to the virus.[8,91,98] Whether exogenous boosting is necessary for long-term maintenance of immunity to VZV is not known for certain. A recent study suggests that exogenous boosting is unlikely to be required, probably because of the phenomenon of internal boosting. The long-term incidence (over a 30-year period) of herpes zoster was found to be similar in isolated communities of people (monks and nuns) compared to individuals living in the general public.[62,78]

Adults and children older than age 2 years with zoster usually have a history of a previous attack of varicella or vaccination.[123,217] Zoster may be due to vaccine type or WT VZV. In vaccinated children with zoster, approximately half of cases are caused by WT VZV.[46,47,79,217,242] Zoster caused by vOka appears to be no less severe than that caused by WT VZV. Zoster is an unusual event in children, but the incidence is increased in young children who had varicella either in utero or before reaching their second birthday.[69] Chickenpox in the first year of life increases the risk for development of childhood zoster by a relative factor between roughly 3 and 21,[113] possibly because of immaturity of the immune response to VZV in young infants. Infants with the congenital varicella syndrome are at greatly increased risk, as high as 18% in the first few years of life, for the development of zoster.[85] In vaccinated children aged 3 to 9 years old, the reported incidence of zoster is 0.39 per 1000 person-years of observation. In children of a similar age with a history of natural varicella the incidence is higher, 1.39 per 1000 person-years. In young vaccinated children the incidence of zoster was reported to be higher than in children of a similar age who were not vaccinated, but this is not a fair comparison because unvaccinated children less than 3 to 4 years old are unlikely to have had varicella and therefore are not at risk to develop zoster. Actually the incidence of zoster is likely to be even lower in vaccinees than after natural infection because of the high incidence of wild-type zoster (50%) in vaccinees who were given only one dose of varicella vaccine. With time, better information on the true incidence of zoster caused by vaccine-type VZV should become available in individuals after the recommended two doses of varicella vaccine.

The incidence of zoster in a population begins to increase sharply at approximately 50 years of age.[123] In healthy young adults the incidence of zoster is roughly two cases per 1000 person-years of observation.

This increases by a factor of 3 to 5 as a population ages. The loss of cell-mediated immunity to VZV that occurs naturally with normal aging contributes to the increased incidence of zoster, as does aging of the population, increases in immunocompromised individuals due to disease and various medications, stress, and other factors.[21,34] A computer modeling study in 2002, of long-term immunity to zoster in young adults in the vaccine era when exposure to wild-type VZV would be decreased, predicted a doubling of the incidence of zoster with significant morbidity.[30] Fortunately evidence collected in the past 13 years has failed to support this hypothesis.[116]

It is now clear that zoster can be prevented by therapeutic immunization of varicella immunes. In a double-blind, placebo-controlled study involving more than 38,000 healthy individuals older than 60 years, immunization with a live attenuated zoster vaccine (Oka strain) reduced the burden of illness of zoster by 61%.[186] Zoster vaccine in the United States contains approximately 20,000 plaque-forming units of VZV, and it is approximately 14 times as potent as monovalent varicella vaccine.[186] Recently, the efficacy and safety of this vaccine in persons between ages 50 and 59 years was demonstrated, although this vaccine is not routinely recommended for healthy persons younger than the age of 60 years.[209] Recent studies of vaccination of healthy older individuals with an adjuvanted (noninfectious) subunit zoster vaccine based on gE of VZV indicated over 90% efficacy of prevention of zoster over a 3-year period.[147] This vaccine has not yet received FDA approval, but when that occurs, it is likely significantly to improve patient care with regard to vaccination against zoster of healthy and immunocompromised individuals.

Zoster also develops with increased frequency in patients with neoplasms and organ transplants[161]; in severely immunocompromised patients with zoster, disseminated infection with viremia also may occur.[74] Spinal trauma, irradiation, diabetes, and corticosteroid therapy may be additional precipitating factors. Children who are infected with human immunodeficiency virus (HIV) and have $CD4^+$ levels less than 15% when varicella develops are at great risk for the development of zoster; in one published series, the incidence of herpes zoster was 70%.[92] HIV-infected children who have received varicella vaccine with relatively normal CD4 cell records, however, rarely experience zoster.[221]

Zoster may develop in healthy children or young adults who are not immunocompromised, presumably the result of a transient fall in cell-mediated immunity to VZV caused by a stimulus such as another viral infection or stress. Zoster does not develop in all immunocompromised persons; the deficiency of cell-mediated immunity to VZV is a necessary but not sufficient requirement for this illness to develop. The distribution of lesions in chickenpox, which primarily involves the trunk and head, is reflected in a proportionately greater representation of these regions in the dermatomal lesions of zoster.[226] Zoster may recur in either the same or a different dermatome; the chance of developing recurrent zoster is similar to the chance of having a first attack for a particular age group and is reported as occurring in 2% to 5% of adults, but this may be an underestimate.[123,199]

Varicella occurs most commonly in the winter and early spring. In contrast, zoster occurs at equal rates during all seasons of the year. VZV may seed ganglia and establish neuronal latency either directly from skin lesions or by viremia.[48]

PATHOGENESIS

The incubation period of varicella ranges from 10 to 23 days (average, 14 days).[108] VZV can be isolated from blood cultures either a few days before the onset of rash or within 1 to 2 days after onset in immunocompetent children.[11] VZV reaches tonsillar keratinocytes soon after infection and infects $CD4^+$ memory T cells that normally circulate through the skin. Overcoming innate immunity in skin accounts for the 2- to 3-week incubation period that follows infection.[142,143]

The skin lesions of VZV infection begin as macules and progress rapidly to papules, vesicles, pustules, and scabs. Histologic changes in the skin lesions are similar for chickenpox and zoster. The hallmarks of each disease are multinucleated giant cells and intranuclear inclusions. In varicella, they are localized primarily in the dermis and epidermis, where ballooning degeneration of cells in the deeper layers is accompanied by intercellular edema. As the edema progresses, the cornified layers and basal layers separate to form a thin-roofed vesicle. An exudate of mononuclear cells is seen in the dermis.[2,243] In zoster, in addition to skin lesions that resemble those of varicella, a mononuclear inflammatory infiltrate is present in the ganglion of the affected dermatome. Hemorrhagic necrosis of ganglion cells and demyelination of the corresponding axon also may be present.[72,121,164]

Both humoral and cell-mediated immune responses to VZV develop within a few days after the onset of varicella. Peak antibody levels are attained 4 to 8 weeks after onset, remain high for approximately 6 months, and then decline. IgG VZV antibody titers are detectable in healthy adults for decades after recovery from varicella.[96,225,247] After active immunization against varicella, antibody titers are lower than after natural infection occurs but persist for as long as 20 years in healthy vaccinees immunized as children.[244] Serum IgG, IgA, and IgM are detectable after both varicella and zoster. Zoster occurs despite high levels of specific antibodies, but significantly higher titers develop during convalescence and are indicative of an anamnestic response to VZV in this secondary infection.[235]

Cell-mediated immune responses (adaptive immunity) are thought to play the major role in host defense against VZV. Cell-mediated immunity to VZV can be demonstrated in vitro by stimulation of lymphocytes with VZV antigens,[118,252] an intradermal skin test,[149] specific lysis of histocompatible target cells by cytotoxic T cells,[6] and an enzyme-linked immunosorbent spot assay.[156] The predominant cell in VZV vesicular lesions is the polymorphonuclear leukocyte. These leukocytes play a role in generating interferon in vesicular lesions, which may be a factor in recovery.[227] Natural killer (NK) cells are also important in host defense (innate immunity) against VZV and other herpesviruses.[126] The importance of NK cells in immune responses to VZV was discovered in children who developed severe wild-type varicella or serious reactions to varicella vaccine who lacked NK cells.[18,24,73,157,185]

Individuals with past varicella may experience boosts in VZV immunity in the absence of symptoms or exposure to the virus, suggesting subclinical reactivation of VZV, which may be important in preserving long-term immunity to the virus.[160,211,248] Cell-mediated immune reactions remain positive for years after varicella, although this response wanes in many individuals older than 50 years.[21,34]

Exactly how immunity to varicella and zoster is mediated is unclear and also complex. Because patients with isolated agammaglobulinemia do not experience either severe or recurrent varicella, researchers long presumed that cell-mediated immunity is more important in host defense than humoral immunity; we now recognize that T-cell cytotoxicity is crucial in recovery from VZV infection and that NK cells also play a part.[7,18,24,73,157,185] The response or responses that prevent clinical illness after reinfection with VZV are presumed to be those of cytotoxic T lymphocytes, but antibodies also may play a role. Elderly individuals with poor cell-mediated immune responses to VZV are not subject to recurrent chickenpox. In addition, specific antibodies must have some importance because passive immunization is used successfully to prevent or to modify varicella in exposed susceptible persons, perhaps by neutralization of cell-free VZV early in the infection. These issues, however, are not straightforward. Varicella may develop in young infants after exposure despite detectable transplacental antibody titers,[14] and modified cases of breakthrough varicella have developed in vaccinated leukemic children despite the presence of humoral or cell-mediated immune responses at exposure to VZV.[95,99] Still, clinical illness is far less likely to develop in individuals with detectable antibody titers or positive cell-mediated immune responses (or both) at exposure to VZV than in those without positive immune responses. Possibly, some forms of cell-mediated immunity and specific antibodies each play roles in host defense against VZV, and there may be some redundancy in the system.

NOSOCOMIAL VARICELLA

Although it is probably less of a problem since licensure of varicella vaccine, nosocomial varicella is a potentially serious and expensive problem in hospitals, where both patients and employees may be susceptible to chickenpox.[110,115,240] Because varicella-susceptible hospital employees may serve as vectors for the spread of VZV to susceptible patients, serologic testing of employees for immunity to chickenpox with no past history of having clinical varicella and offering vaccine to those who are susceptible are standard measures in many hospitals. The results of serologic tests for varicella are often unreliable, however, so another approach is to administer two doses of vaccine at least 1 month apart to health care workers with no history of previous varicella or zoster and not to perform serologic testing. Inadvertent vaccination of immune individuals is not harmful.

The risk for horizontal transmission in maternity wards or the neonatal nursery after hospital exposure to an adult or child is surprisingly low.[85] A few episodes of nursery transmission of varicella have been reported,[77,93,114] but the low incidence of such transmission may be, at least partly, because many infants are in isolettes. Furthermore, most hospital employees and most mothers and their neonates have antibodies to VZV and are at low risk for the development of clinical illness. Even in low-birth-weight infants, antibodies to VZV may be detectable.[176,200]

CLINICAL MANIFESTATIONS

Varicella

Varicella is a highly contagious, usually self-limited systemic infection characterized by fever and a generalized pruritic rash lasting approximately 5 days. A prodromal phase in children is unusual, but malaise and fever for 1 to 2 days before the onset of rash is a common manifestation in adults.[53] The rash is more intense on the trunk and head than on the extremities, and it typically evolves as a series of "crops" during the course of 1 to 3 days in normal hosts. Most children with varicella have 250 to 500 superficial skin lesions, many of which are vesicular (Fig. 162.1).[202] Not uncommonly, a few lesions may develop in the mouth, conjunctiva, or other mucosal sites. Residual scarring is exceptional but can occur, and depigmented areas of skin may develop in dark-skinned patients. A self-limited increase in hepatic transaminase levels without jaundice is not an uncommon occurrence during varicella.[193] Rarely, thrombocytopenia and neutropenia may transiently occur. Severe infections are more likely to develop in adults than in children, presumably because of less robust cell-mediated immune responses to VZV in adults than in children.[82,183] Neonates who acquire varicella from their mothers in the few days before delivery also are at risk for acquisition of severe varicella because of immaturity of the cell-mediated immune response.[85]

Complications of Varicella

The most frequent complications of varicella in normal hosts are bacterial superinfections and central nervous system (CNS) complications. Bacterial superinfection usually involves the skin, lungs, or bones; these are most often caused by *Staphylococcus aureus* or group A β hemolytic streptococci[28,249] CNS complications, which may precede or follow varicella, include transient cerebellar ataxia, severe cerebral encephalitis, aseptic meningitis, and transverse myelitis.[129,130] Recently it was found that the incidence of stroke in children is increased in the months following varicella.[54] An exhaustive study did not find an association of increased stroke incidence in children who were vaccinated against varicella.[66] Encephalopathy as a sequela of Reye syndrome has become a rare complication because aspirin no longer is recommended for children with varicella. Other complications of chickenpox encountered less commonly include arthritis, glomerulonephritis, myocarditis, and purpura fulminans.[243]

Varicella may be severe and even fatal in immunocompromised patients, including those with an underlying malignant neoplasm or congenital or acquired deficits in cell-mediated immunity, such as patients who have undergone organ transplantation or have underlying HIV infection, and in children receiving high doses of corticosteroids for any reason (Fig. 162.2).[76] These patients may be susceptible to progressive varicella, with continuing fever and the development of new vesicular lesions for 2 weeks or longer. Their skin lesions characteristically are large, umbilicated, and hemorrhagic, and primary varicella pneumonia is a frequent complication. Often children with severe varicella will present with severe abdominal pain.[173] This is not surprising because VZV may invade the gastric mucosa.[15] Alternatively, in some immunocompromised patients, an acute form of varicella with disseminated intravascular coagulation develops and is rapidly fatal, at times before antiviral therapy can be instituted. A 30% rate of dissemination with a 7% fatality rate was reported in leukemic children in whom chickenpox developed in the pre-antiviral drug era.[75] Severe varicella has been observed in children with underlying HIV infection, especially those classified as having acquired immunodeficiency syndrome (AIDS).[132] In most HIV-infected children, however, mild to moderate forms of varicella develop, although the illness generally is more severe than that in otherwise healthy children.[92] Varicella does not seem to be a cofactor for clinical progression of HIV infection to AIDS, but in approximately 5% of these children, chronic wartlike hyperkeratotic VZV lesions may develop after varicella, presumably being a chronic form of zoster in which the infection is low grade but persistent.[5]

Primary varicella pneumonia accounts for many of the fatalities ascribed to varicella, particularly in immunocompromised patients and adults.[191] In male military recruits with varicella, radiographic evidence of pneumonia was found in 16%.[241] Symptoms include fever, cough, and dyspnea. Other common symptoms and signs are cyanosis, rales, hemoptysis, and chest pain. The chest radiograph typically reveals a diffuse nodular or miliary pattern that is most pronounced in the perihilar region.[230] Blood gas analyses and pulmonary function tests indicate a diffusion defect that may persist in some cases for months after recovery.[26] The availability of antiviral chemotherapy has greatly improved the outcome of this complication.

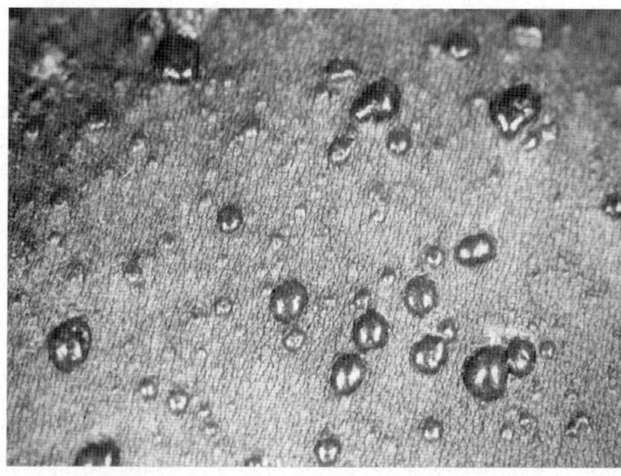

FIG. 162.1 Typical skin lesions of varicella.

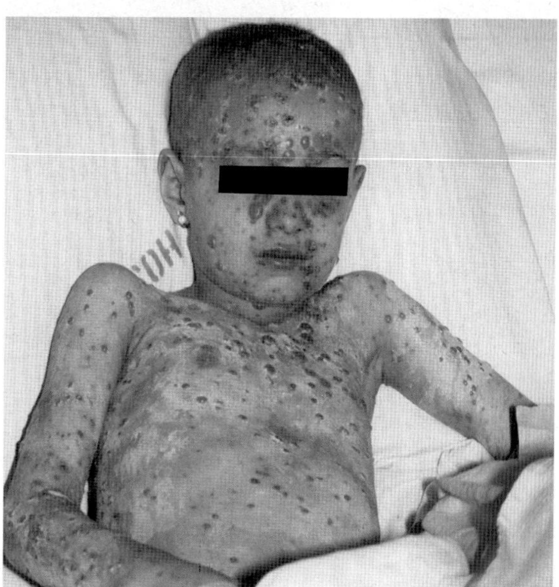

FIG. 162.2 Progressive varicella in a 9-year-old child with underlying leukemia.

Congenital Varicella Syndrome

LaForet and Lynch, who were medical students in 1947, were the first to describe an infant with multiple congenital anomalies after contraction of maternal chickenpox.[146] The infant had hypoplasia of the right lower extremity, clubfoot, and absent right deep tendon reflexes, along with cerebral cortical atrophy, cerebellar aplasia, chorioretinitis, torticollis, insufficiency of the anal and vesical sphincters, and cicatricial cutaneous lesions on the left lower extremity. These manifestations are now recognized to be typical of this syndrome. In 1974, Srabstein and colleagues rediscovered this syndrome, which appeared to have been forgotten.[223] Their report of another case and review of the literature concluded that although the virus could not be isolated from affected infants as with congenital rubella or cytomegalovirus infection, the congenital syndrome consisted of a typical constellation of birth defects as originally described by LaForet and Lynch. This syndrome occurs after maternal VZV infection develops in the first or second trimester of pregnancy; approximately 2% of the offspring of pregnancies complicated by varicella are affected. Approximately 100 affected infants have been described in the literature; 95% occurred after maternal varicella and 5% after maternal zoster. In the pre-vaccine era, approximately 40 affected infants were thought to be born annually in the United States.[85] Today in the vaccine era, this syndrome may once more be forgotten.

Cicatricial scars of the skin, the most prominent stigmata, are reported in more than 60% of cases.[85] Other frequent abnormalities include chorioretinitis, microphthalmos, Horner syndrome, cataract, nystagmus, hypoplastic limbs, cortical atrophy or intellectual disability (or both), and early death. Many of these children develop zoster (in which VZV can be identified) in the early months of life. There is a high correlation between limb abnormalities and a poor outcome in these infants. The Oka strain is not known to cause the congenital syndrome.[85]

Zoster

Zoster usually begins as a localized unilateral vesicular skin eruption involving one to three dermatomal segments (Fig. 162.3). The skin lesions resemble those of varicella but tend more toward confluence and are likely to be painful or pruritic, especially in adults. Zoster generally is a milder disease in children than in adults. Zoster may follow natural varicella or vaccination; however, the incidence of zoster is clearly lower after vaccination than after varicella disease, even in immunocompromised vaccinees.[117,118,232]

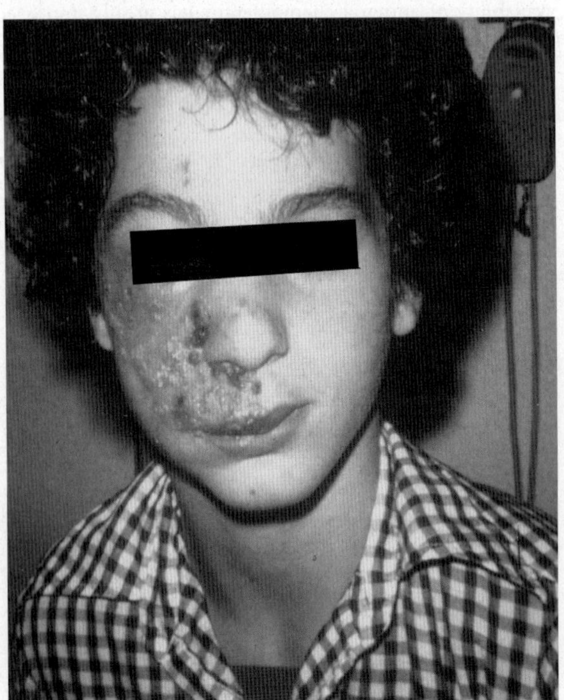

FIG. 162.3 Zoster in an otherwise healthy 10-year-old boy.

Zoster is a considerable cause of morbidity, but death is unusual or rare.[168]

Complications of Zoster

Two kinds of pain are associated with herpes zoster: (1) acute pain that is related to reactivation of VZV in sensory neurons and (2) pain that develops after the acute phase of the illness, often in the area of healed rash. Between 25% and 50% of persons older than 50 years in whom zoster develops may experience late protracted pain, or postherpetic neuralgia, after the rash has healed. Postherpetic neuralgia (PHN) also occurs frequently in immunocompromised patients. Pain may persist for months to years and is described as aching, jabbing, or boring. The cause of PHN is unknown but may be related to healing of injured nerves. Otherwise healthy children rarely experience PHN; both the incidence and duration are related directly to increasing age.[102,103] Zoster may be particularly severe and common after bone marrow transplantation; in the first year after undergoing transplantation, 20% to 70% of recipients develop zoster.[83]

Neurologic complications of zoster in addition to PHN include meningitis, stroke, and various forms of paralysis. Meningitis can present either with or without the presence of a zosteriform rash. It can occur in immunologically normal individuals, in whom the prognosis is good, and in immunocompromised persons, in whom the prognosis can be problematic. The diagnosis is made by demonstration of VZV DNA in cerebrospinal fluid (CSF); it is quite rare to culture VZV from CSF.[128] Stroke is more common after zoster than after varicella. Strokes after zoster are more often seen in adults than children, possibly because zoster is more common in adults than in children, as well as other factors. Strokes that follow zoster are due to vasculopathy and ischemia; VZV particles have been demonstrated in cerebral arteries in strokes associated with zoster, indicating viral replication. Whether treatment with antivirals improves the prognosis of this form of stroke is unknown at present. Other neurologic complications of zoster include various forms of paralysis, retinal necrosis, and giant cell arteritis; in addition to demonstrating VZV DNA in CSF, the diagnosis may be made by the presence of VZV antibodies in CSF.[104,105,172] Immunodeficiency diseases have been unmasked on rare occasions in patients with severe VZV neurologic complications involving vaccine-type VZV following varicella immunization.[203]

Visceral zoster, involving the gastrointestinal tract, may produce severe abdominal symptomatology, at times in the absence of rash; this is ascribed to latent VZV in enteric ganglia with reactivation and local spread of the infection.[48,86,71] If there is no rash, the diagnosis is made much more difficult. Zoster may cause a wide variety of gastrointestinal disorders, including achalasia, gastric and duodenal ulcers, and colonic psuedoobstruction.[71,87,179] At times the diagnosis is made when abdominal pain is the chief complaint and this is accompanied or followed by the typical rash of zoster. At other times the diagnosis is made when gastrointestinal tissue becomes available for study and VZV is demonstrated by molecular studies such as PCR and/or immunofluorescence. Testing saliva for VZV DNA has been used as a screening test for visceral zoster.[87]

DIAGNOSIS

Clinical Diagnosis of Varicella and Zoster

It usually is not difficult to establish a clinical diagnosis of VZV infection because the vesicular rash is so characteristic. In questionable cases of varicella, epidemiologic information, such as a history of recent exposure to varicella or zoster and subsequent transmission of varicella to another person, may be useful. The differential diagnosis of varicella includes generalized HSV infection, enterovirus infections, rickettsialpox, impetigo, allergic reactions (including Stevens-Johnson syndrome and poison ivy), and insect bites.

Zoster rashes are unilateral and often painful or pruritic. There may be some scattered vesicles outside of the dermatome. Rashes of zoster and HSV can resemble each other. In one study of zoster, 13% of clinically diagnosed zoster cases were proven by culture to be caused by HSV infection.[133] The unilateral rash of zoster most frequently appears on the trunk or face. The trigeminal nerve, most commonly the ophthalmic branch, is an especially significant site because the eye may be involved. When skin lesions are absent, diagnosis of zoster has to be made by laboratory testing.

Laboratory Diagnosis

Laboratory diagnosis of VZV infection is facilitated by the presence of VZV in superficial skin lesions, where it is easily accessible for testing. The diagnosis is made best by the demonstration of specific viral antigens or VZV DNA in skin vesicles or scrapings. VZV antigens are demonstrable by immunofluorescence with a commercial monoclonal antibody to VZV that is conjugated to fluorescein.[88] Immunofluorescence testing is highly sensitive and can be completed within approximately an hour. PCR assay is used to demonstrate VZV in skin lesions and also in saliva and CSF when there is CNS involvement with VZV.[87,189] PCR is more sensitive than immunofluorescence and is becoming the preferred method for diagnosis of VZV.[88,236] PCR also may be used to distinguish between vaccine (Oka strain) and wild-type VZV infections.[88,198]

The diagnosis also may be made by isolation of virus from skin lesions very early in the course of illness. Within several days after the onset, vesicular fluid no longer is likely to be infectious, although viable VZV may be present in zoster lesions for a longer period compared to varicella, especially in immunocompromised patients. VZV cannot be isolated from skin lesions that have become pustular or dry. Isolation of VZV is a slow method because at least 48 hours is required before the first signs of a viral cytopathic effect are seen. It is also less sensitive than is immunofluorescence or PCR. VZV rarely is isolated from respiratory secretions or from infected CSF during VZV meningitis.[106] Demonstration of VZV DNA, antigens, or isolation of virus from samples obtained from skin, other sites, or autopsy tissue is diagnostic of a current infection with VZV because, unlike other herpesviruses, no known carrier state or shedding of VZV by asymptomatic individuals exists.[88] VZV infections can also be diagnosed by demonstration of viral DNA in saliva.[87,154,174,175]

Numerous serologic tests, including the fluorescent antibody to membrane antigen (FAMA) method and enzyme-linked immunosorbent assay (ELISA), are useful for measuring antibodies to VZV.[88] Antibody to VZV develops within a few days after the onset of varicella, persists for many years, and is present before the onset of zoster. VZV infections may be documented by a fourfold or greater rise in VZV antibody titer in acute and convalescent serum specimens. Specific IgM in one serum specimen suggests recent VZV infection, either varicella or zoster; false-negative and false-positive reactions, however, are a problem with this assay. Persistence of VZV IgG antibody beyond 8 months of age in an infant is highly suggestive of intrauterine varicella.[93] Immunity to varicella is present if a positive FAMA titer to VZV is demonstrated on a single serum sample after varicella or immunization.[178] Serologic methods, however, particularly commercial ELISAs, may fail to identify individuals who have had natural infection or have been immunized.[88,225] Unfortunately, the FAMA assay is not now readily available.

The value of serologic procedures for the diagnosis of zoster is limited. Heterologous increases in antibody titer against VZV in patients with HSV infection who previously had varicella may occur and have been ascribed to antigens common to the two viruses.[88] Laboratory diagnosis of zoster is best accomplished by PCR assay on skin lesions or in saliva.[87] As has been mentioned, it is possible to differentiate between VOka and WT VZV by molecular methods.

TREATMENT

Traditionally, nonspecific measures, such as frequent bathing to discourage bacterial skin infection, antihistamines given orally, calamine lotion applied locally, oatmeal baths to decrease itching, and cutting fingernails short to discourage scratching, have been used to treat varicella. Fever is controlled best with acetaminophen rather than aspirin, which may predispose to Reye syndrome.[119] The issue of whether treatment with ibuprofen is associated with group A streptococcal superinfection in varicella has not been resolved, and, therefore, avoidance of its use for symptomatic treatment of varicella seems to be the best approach.[35,52,152,254]

Useful specific antiviral therapy for VZV became available in the mid-1980s with the introduction of the nucleoside analogue acyclovir, an inhibitor of DNA polymerase and a DNA chain terminator. The antiviral effect of acyclovir depends on its being phosphorylated in the body by virus-induced thymidine kinases, which accounts for its relative lack of toxicity.[246] Antiviral therapy for varicella and zoster is similar.

Patients with severe or potentially severe VZV infections should be treated with intravenous acyclovir 30 mg/kg per day for adults and adolescents and 1500 mg/m^2 per day for children, both given in three divided doses. Orally administered acyclovir is less reliable for immunocompromised patients because only approximately 20% of this formulation is absorbed from the gastrointestinal tract, and no data on its efficacy in high-risk patients have been published. Because acyclovir is excreted by the kidneys, patients with a creatinine clearance of less than 50 mL/min per 1.73 m^2 should receive one-half to one-third of this dosage. Intravenous acyclovir is infused for at least 1 hour, with maintenance fluids given both before and during the infusion. Providing adequate hydration is important to prevent renal damage from precipitation of the drug in the renal tubules. Other adverse effects of acyclovir include phlebitis, rash, nausea, and neurologic manifestations such as headache and tremor. In general, however, acyclovir is extremely well tolerated.[246]

Early intravenous therapy should be instituted for patients at high risk for development of severe VZV infection, such as leukemic children and those who have undergone organ or bone marrow transplantation, to prevent the dissemination of VZV.[218,245] Not only may this therapy be potentially lifesaving in immunocompromised patients, but it also prevents considerable morbidity from VZV infection. Children thought to be somewhat less immunocompromised, such as those with HIV infection but without AIDS, may be given a treatment trial with oral acyclovir under close medical supervision. In such patients who are not doing well, intravenous therapy should be administered. In zoster patients, the use of intravenous acyclovir is associated with more rapid healing of skin lesions and resolution of acute pain than if no specific treatment is given.[246]

Considerable controversy has ensued about the role of orally administered acyclovir for the treatment of varicella and zoster in otherwise healthy children because most of these infections are self-limited. Customarily, however, adults, who are at greater risk for development of severe infection, are treated. Oral dosages used are 80 mg/kg per day (in four divided doses) for children and 4 g/day (in five divided doses) for adults. Double-blind, placebo-controlled studies in healthy children given oral acyclovir at 80 mg/kg per day for 5 days or placebo beginning within 24 hours of the onset of varicella rash have revealed that the number of chickenpox skin lesions is reduced significantly by acyclovir. A modest benefit was derived from acyclovir; children who received it had fever for approximately 1 day less, but they did not return to school any more rapidly, nor did they have fewer complications of chickenpox.[17,68]

Some evidence indicates that early administration of oral acyclovir may decrease the acute pain associated with zoster.[125] However, the need to administer specific therapy for zoster in otherwise healthy children for whom pain is not a particular problem rarely occurs. Usually however, children with zoster are treated in order to speed recovery.

The newer drug, penciclovir, has an action similar to that of acyclovir.[122] It is administered as famciclovir, a prodrug that when given orally is converted rapidly to penciclovir in the body. A major advantage of famciclovir is that it is administered only three times a day (1500 mg/day for an adult), whereas acyclovir is given four or five times daily. Penciclovir has an antiviral action similar to that of acyclovir. One study suggests that famciclovir given to elderly patients with zoster early in the course of infection decreases the duration of PHN, although not its incidence.[234] No data regarding whether varicella may be treated successfully with famciclovir have been published, nor have any data on the use of famciclovir in immunocompromised patients or in children.

The prodrug of acyclovir, valacyclovir, also is given orally, reaches blood levels that are approximately three to four times higher than those following oral acyclovir and has been shown in one study to be superior to acyclovir for treatment of zoster.[22] Valacyclovir rather than acyclovir may be used in children older than age 2 years with chickenpox.

The dose of valacyclovir is 20 mg/kg per dose orally three times a day for 5 days, not to exceed 1 g per dose 3 times daily.

Of concern about the potential widespread use of acyclovir is that drug resistance may develop. At present, resistance is less a problem with VZV than with HSV, but VZV resistant to acyclovir has been reported in a few patients with underlying AIDS.[127] Two vaccinated children with neuroblastoma who developed zoster caused by the Oka strain that became resistant to acyclovir after prolonged treatment have also been described.[33,155] Foscarnet was licensed by the Food and Drug Administration for the treatment of VZV infections that are resistant to acyclovir and famciclovir. Foscarnet inhibits the synthesis of VZV DNA polymerase.[205,206,220] Intravenous foscarnet is given at a dosage of 180 mg/kg per day in two divided doses, adjusted according to renal function. The main toxicity of foscarnet is renal damage and electrolyte imbalance.[83]

PROGNOSIS

The prognosis of varicella and zoster is excellent in children without underlying health problems. The outlook for immunocompromised patients receiving antiviral chemotherapy also is good, especially if treatment is begun at an early stage of the illness. In general, zoster carries a better prognosis than varicella, possibly because it is a secondary infection. If the disease is diagnosed promptly, complications such as bacterial superinfections usually can be treated successfully with antimicrobial agents. In the pre-vaccine era, despite the availability of antiviral therapy and passive immunization, the Centers for Disease Control and Prevention (CDC) estimated that approximately 100 deaths from varicella occurred annually in the United States, mostly in children with no previous health problems. An epidemiologic study of more than 250,000 health maintenance organization records indicated that the rates of varicella in adolescents and young adults and the complication and hospitalization rates had increased between 1992 and 1995 by a factor of approximately 5.[51]

The widespread use of varicella vaccine in the United States decreased the morbidity and mortality rates from chickenpox substantially. By 2000, in the three sentinel communities in the United States, vaccine coverage among children 19 to 35 months was more than 80%, and reported varicella cases had declined by roughly 70% to 80% compared with the prevaccine era. Hospitalizations for varicella also declined by approximately 80%. The greatest declines occurred in young children.[184] Deaths from varicella have become rare.[170] At present, more than 90% of children in the United States are routinely vaccinated against varicella.[41]

PREVENTION

VZV is such an infectious agent that general measures are not useful for prevention of varicella in susceptible individuals. Some protection, however, can be achieved by isolation of hospitalized patients. Hospitalized patients with active VZV infection should be admitted to a private room, preferably with negative-pressure ventilation, and hospital personnel and visitors should wash their hands before and after entering the room and wear masks, gowns, and gloves while in it. The CDC now recommends postexposure vaccination for healthy varicella-susceptible exposed individuals.[37]

Passive Immunization Against Varicella

Varicella-susceptible children at high risk for development of severe chickenpox should be passively immunized if they are closely exposed to VZV. Passive immunization may be lifesaving; it may modify varicella or prevent it.

Passive immunization is indicated for varicella-susceptible individuals who have been closely exposed to varicella or zoster and are at high risk for development of severe chickenpox. This population includes immunocompromised children and adults, pregnant women, neonates whose mothers have active varicella at the time of delivery, and premature infants of less than 28 weeks' gestation or who weighed less than 1000 g at birth. Children at high risk should be considered to be susceptible to varicella if they have no history of having had chickenpox or vaccination. False-positive antibody test results may occur in immunocompromised individuals, and, therefore, susceptible children may be identified serologically as immune; hence, a history of illness is a preferred indication of these patients' immune status. Passive immunization usually is reserved for VZV-exposed adults only if they have been proved serologically to be susceptible to chickenpox, because most adults with a negative history of varicella raised in the continental United States are immune. Immigrants who came from countries with tropical climates, however, may be presumed to be susceptible without a history of varicella because the disease spreads less readily in tropical countries than in those with temperate climates.

Patients with HIV infection, especially those with AIDS, have some increased risk for development of severe varicella, and their management should be similar to that of immunocompromised children with regard to passive immunization. Even children who are receiving intravenous globulin for treatment of HIV infection should receive passive immunization if they have no past history of varicella and close exposure has occurred.

Infants whose mothers have an onset of chickenpox 5 days or less before delivery or within 48 hours after delivery should be given passive immunization as soon as possible after birth.[85] The transplacental route of infection and the immaturity of the immune system probably account for the severity of varicella in these infants.[85] Attack rates for varicella as high as 50% in infants exposed to mothers who have varicella have been reported, despite their having passive immunization.[85,197] Passively immunized infants should be observed closely, but usually they can be managed as outpatients. Intravenous acyclovir should be reserved for the rare, passively immunized infant with varicella in whom an extensive rash (>200 vesicles) or possible pneumonia develops.[16]

Passive immunization need not be given to full-term infants who are exposed to VZV after they are 48 hours old. Passive immunization is optional for neonates (<1 week old) if their siblings at home have active varicella. Infants exposed to VZV after birth almost always have mild varicella. Although the reported mortality rate from varicella in children younger than 1 year is four times that in older children, both rates are exceedingly low—eight per 100,000 cases and two per 100,000 cases, respectively.[196] The mortality rate for adults and for leukemic children receiving chemotherapy, in contrast, is 20 and 1000 times higher, respectively.[195] Passive immunization is not useful to treat VZV infections or to prevent zoster. Whether it is useful for pregnant varicella-susceptible women who have been exposed to VZV to protect the fetus from developing the congenital varicella syndrome is uncertain but possible.[56]

Historically, varicella-zoster immune globulin (VZIG), was used successfully for passive immunization for many years. Because of limited requests for VZIG since licensure of varicella vaccine, however, VZIG no longer is being produced in the United States. Another product, varicella immune globulin (human), VariZIG, manufactured in Canada, is now used for passive immunization, VariZIG can be obtained from FFF Enterprises (Temecula, CA; 800-843-7477) or ASD Healthcare (Frisco, TX; 800-746-6273). An alternative to VariZIG is intravenous immune globulin 400 mg/kg.

Although passive immunization has been shown to be effective when it is given within 4 days and perhaps as long as 5 days, it should be administered as soon as possible after an exposure to VZV.[3,40] In 2012, the CDC has recommended passive immunization for as long as 10 days after close exposure to VZV (based on limited data) with the possibility that it will have a salutary effect.[43,44] The dose is 1 vial or 125 U for every 10 kg of body weight, with a maximal dosage of 5 vials or 625 U, given intramuscularly. VariZIG should be readministered to high-risk susceptible individuals who are closely reexposed 3 weeks after a first dose.[3]

Active Immunization Against Varicella

A live attenuated varicella vaccine, the Oka strain, was developed in Japan more than 40 years ago.[168] It was licensed in the United States in 1995 for universal immunization of healthy children and adults who are susceptible to varicella[41,36] and has proved to be extremely safe and well tolerated.[25,41,46,79,217] Varicella vaccine is labile. The lyophilized vaccine must be stored frozen at an average temperature of 5°F or colder. The freezer must have its own door; frost-free freezers are acceptable. Prior to use, the vaccine must be diluted with its supplied diluent and administered subcutaneously to the patient within 30 minutes to preserve its potency.[41]

Originally a monovalent formulation of varicella vaccine was licensed in the United States. Currently two licensed varicella vaccine formulations are available in the United States, both produced by Merck. Monovalent varicella vaccine, which contains 1350 plaque-forming units (PFU) at expiry, is recommended for healthy varicella-susceptible persons above the age of 12 months. A combination vaccine, MMRV, which was licensed in 2005, contains a larger amount of VZV than Varivax, approximately 10,000 PFU at expiry. MMRV is recommended for healthy children between 1 and 12 years of age. It should not be given to adults. Varicella vaccines used worldwide are the Oka strain, made and sold by various manufacturers, and appear to be similar to the vaccine used in the United States. The only country in which a different but similar strain of vaccine virus is available is South Korea.[139]

Safety

The most frequent adverse reaction to vaccination is a mild rash that develops several weeks later in approximately 5% of healthy children, particularly after the first dose.[96,100,217,244] These rashes can be serious in immunocompromised children who are vaccinated inadvertently[84,89,217] but usually respond to antiviral therapy. When vaccinees develop rash from the Oka strain, the potential for transmission of the vaccine virus exists, but transmission is extremely rare from healthy individuals, with fewer than 12 reported instances from healthy vaccinated individuals after more than 20 years of routine immunization of more than 80 million American children.[41,79,109,217] In contrast, the rate of transmission of the Oka strain was 14% after household exposure from vaccinees with underlying leukemia who had a rash and exposed their susceptible healthy siblings.[233]

It was observed that the incidence of febrile seizures was double that in children from 1 to 2 years of age in the 5 to 12 days after MMRV compared with monovalent varicella vaccine (one extra febrile seizure for every 2500 vaccinees).[141] After careful consideration the CDC recommended that for the first dose of measles, mumps, rubella, and varicella at age 12 to 47 months, either MMR vaccine and monovalent varicella vaccine or MMRV may be used. Providers are advised to discuss the risks and benefits of each of the two choices with the infant's parent or caregiver, particularly if it is anticipated to give MMRV; the CDC favors giving MMR and varicella vaccines in separate sites. For the second doses, at any age, and if the first dose is given at age 4 years or older, MMRV is preferred.[42]

Few serious neurologic events have been causally demonstrated to be connected to varicella vaccine. There have been nine reports of herpes zoster due to the Oka strain with accompanying meningitis (VZV DNA found in CSF by PCR assay) in a group of healthy and immunocompromised patients, all of whom had a rash and recovered with antiviral therapy.[23] It is well known that meningitis may also accompany herpes zoster caused by wild-type VZV,[45,101,192,222,224] so it is unclear whether these nine patients should be classified as having a vaccine-associated adverse event or not. Because there is no known denominator, the incidence of these complications after vaccination is not known, but it appears to be rare. Transient cerebellar ataxia has been temporally associated with vaccination, but its connection to VZV has not been proven.[79,217]

Effectiveness

Live attenuated varicella vaccine is highly effective in healthy children and adults, but not all vaccinees are completely protected. From 10% to 20% of children given one dose may develop a modified breakthrough illness after intimate exposure to VZV. Varicella vaccine has, however, been 97% effective in preventing severe varicella.[237,236] The vaccine is also highly effective in adults; after two doses, more than 75% are completely protected from varicella after household exposure to the virus.[1,96,207] Severe wild-type varicella in vaccinated adults is very rare.

Originally, it was observed that approximately 85% of healthy children are protected after only one dose of vaccine,[145,237,236,244] and there was little concern about breakthrough varicella because it had been found to be almost always a modified illness. There was no significant waning of immunity in a case-control study with laboratory verification of varicella.[237] Loss of VZV antibodies, moreover, occurs rarely in healthy vaccinated children, some of whom have been monitored for as long as 20 years after immunization.[10,12,55,145,219,239,253]

Beginning in approximately 2000, however, breakthrough varicella became a growing concern in the United States. The incidence of varicella in sentinel geographic areas where active surveillance was being performed revealed that although the incidence of disease fell after 1995, it leveled off at a low rate in about 2000.[214,215] The number of reports of outbreaks of varicella among vaccinated children was, moreover, increasing; some of these studies indicated vaccine effectiveness as low as 44% and 56%, although most showed 80% to 85% effectiveness.[80,151] Also recognized was that children with breakthrough infections could spread wild-type VZV to contacts almost as efficiently as unvaccinated children with varicella.[215] Attempts at outbreak control with second doses of varicella vaccine during outbreaks proved to be expensive and complicated.[169] Finally, one study indicated that the FAMA seroconversion rate after one dose of vaccine could be as low as 76%, indicating an unexpectedly high rate of primary vaccine failure after one dose of vaccine.[178] The fear was that without a second routine dose, a gradual accumulation of susceptible young adults would develop as a result of primary vaccine failure and would be at risk to develop severe chickenpox.

In the light of all these problems, a second dose of varicella vaccine was recommended for all children, not just those older than 12 years, by the CDC in June 2006. Early studies exploring immune responses to two doses had indicated the safety of a second dose and a marked boost in immunity and the seroconversion rate afterward. An interval of 4 to 6 years between the first and second doses was recommended in 2007, but there was flexibility in that the second dose could be administered at any time 1 month after the first dose.[41] Catch-up immunization was also recommended for children who received only one dose of varicella vaccine.[41] With the institution of two routine doses, protection achieved 98% in a case-control study,[216] and the incidence of varicella was reported to have decreased significantly in Connecticut.[134]

Because the risk from wild-type VZV is greater than is the risk from vaccine-type VZV, immunization is recommended for health care workers and persons whose varicella-susceptible family members are immunocompromised or pregnant.[41] Varicella vaccine is recommended only for healthy persons. Vaccinees in whom an extensive VZV rash develops within 2 to 3 weeks after immunization are likely to have wild-type infection.

In such situations, PCR and restriction fragment length polymorphism analysis can be used to differentiate between wild-type and vaccine-type VZV. Passive immunization could be considered for immunocompromised individuals inadvertently exposed to a vaccinee with rash resembling chickenpox that might be caused by wild-type VZV.

Most states now require varicella vaccination for children to attend daycare or school. In geographic areas where vaccine use in children younger than 3 years is 70% or more, the incidence of varicella has decreased sharply, not only in the vaccinated group but also in all age groups, a process indicative of herd immunity.[214,221] As has been mentioned, the incidence of zoster appears to be less of a problem after immunization than after natural infection in vaccinated immunocompromised individuals and in healthy vaccinees.[191,242]

HIV-infected children may be immunized with monovalent varicella vaccine if they are free of symptoms and have 15% or more CD4 T lymphocytes (for children >8 years, a CD4 T lymphocyte level of ≥200 cells/μL is used). For these children, varicella vaccine has been shown to be safe, immunogenic, and effective.[41,221]

Individuals who are immunocompromised should not be given live attenuated varicella vaccine because rare severe and even fatal varicella has been reported in these individuals.[23] It is hoped that immunocompromised persons will be protected by herd immunity. Those who become infected by WT VZV should be promptly treated with intravenous acyclovir. Mortality from VZV has decreased significantly since licensure of the vaccine with little or no evidence of waning immunity.[20,153,170]

Drug Prophylaxis

Prophylaxis of varicella in exposed persons may be achieved by the administration of acyclovir.[13,124,159,229] This approach is not recommended often, however, because the optimal dosage and timing of administration have not been studied in large groups of children, nor is it known whether long-term maintenance of immunity exists in all children. In the United States, prevention of varicella by vaccination is a preferable approach. Long-term acyclovir therapy may be used to prevent the development of zoster in patients who have undergone bone marrow transplantation; however, its value is questionable because zoster commonly develops after administration of acyclovir is stopped.[38]

NEW REFERENCES SINCE THE SEVENTH EDITION

15. Baker CJ, Gilsdorf JR, South MA, et al. Gastritis as a complication of varicella. *South Med J.* 1973;66(5):539-541.
18. Banovic T, Yanilla M, Simmons R, et al. Disseminated varicella infection caused by varicella vaccine strain in a child with low invariant natural killer T cells and diminished CD1d expression. *J Infect Dis.* 2011;204(12):1893-1901.
20. Baxter R, Ray P, Tran TN, et al. Long-term effectiveness of varicella vaccine: a 14-year, prospective cohort study. *Pediatrics.* 2013;131(5):e1389-e1396.
23. Bhalla P, Forrest GN, Gershon M, et al. Disseminated, persistent, and fatal infection due to the vaccine strain of varicella-zoster virus in an adult following stem cell transplantation. *Clin Infect Dis.* 2015;60(7):1068-1074.
24. Biron CA, Byron KS, Sullivan JL. Severe herpesvirus infections in an adolescent without natural killer cells. *N Engl J Med.* 1989;320(26):1731-1735.
30. Brisson M, Gay NJ, Edmunds WJ, et al. Exposure to varicella boosts immunity to herpes-zoster: implications for mass vaccination against chickenpox. *Vaccine.* 2002;20(19-20):2500-2507.
44. Centers for Disease Control and Prevention. Updated recommendations for use of VariZIG-United States, 2013. *MMWR Morb Mortal Wkly Rep.* 2013;62(28): 574-576.
54. Ciccone S, Faggioli R, Calzolari F, et al. Stroke After varicella-zoster infection: report of a case and review of the literature. *Pediatr Infect Dis J.* 2010;29(9):864-867.
66. Donahue JG, Kieke BA, Yih WK, et al. Varicella vaccination and ischemic stroke in children: is there an association? *Pediatrics.* 2009;123(2):e228-e234.
71. Edelman DA, Antaki F, Basson MD, et al. Ogilvie syndrome and herpes zoster: case report and review of the literature. *J Emerg Med.* 2010;39(5):696-700.
73. Etzioni A, Eidenschenk C, Katz R, et al. Fatal varicella associated with selective natural killer cell deficiency. *J Pediatr.* 2005;146(3):423-425.
87. Gershon AA, Chen J, Gershon MD. Use of saliva to identify varicella zoster virus infection of the gut. *Clin Infect Dis.* 2015;61(4):536-544.
104. Gilden D, Nagel M. Varicella zoster virus in temporal arteries of patients with giant cell arteritis. *J Infect Dis.* 2015;212(suppl 1):S37-S39.
105. Gilden D, Nagel MA, Cohrs RJ, et al. The variegate neurological manifestations of varicella zoster virus infection. *Curr Neurol Neurosci Rep.* 2013;13(9):374.
116. Hales CM, Harpaz R, Joesoef MR, et al. Examination of links between herpes zoster incidence and childhood varicella vaccination. *Ann Intern Med.* 2013;159(11):739-745.
128. Jemsek J, Greenberg SB, Taber L, et al. Herpes zoster-associated encephalitis: clinicopathologic report of 12 cases and review of the literature. *Medicine (Baltimore).* 1983;62(2):81-97.
139. Kim JI, Jung GS, Kim YY, et al. Sequencing and characterization of varicella-zoster virus vaccine strain SuduVax. *Virol J.* 2011;8:547.
147. Lal H, Cunningham AL, Godeaux O, et al. Efficacy of an adjuvanted herpes zoster subunit vaccine in older adults. *N Engl J Med.* 2015;372(22):2087-2096.
153. Leung J, Bialek SR, Marin M. Trends in varicella mortality in the United States: data from vital statistics and the national surveillance system. *Hum Vaccin Immunother.* 2015;11(3):662-668.
157. Levy O, Orange JS, Hibberd P, et al. Disseminated varicella infection due to the vaccine strain of varicella-zoster virus, in a patient with a novel deficiency in natural killer T cells. *J Infect Dis.* 2003;188(7):948-953.
160. Ljungman P, Lonnqvist B, Gahrton G, et al. Clinical and subclinical reactivations of varicella-zoster virus in immunocompromised patients. *J Infect Dis.* 1986;153(5):840-847.
170. Marin M, Zhang JX, Seward JF. Near elimination of varicella deaths in the US After implementation of the vaccination program. *Pediatrics.* 2011;128(2): 214-220.
172. Mathias M, Nagel MA, Khmeleva N, et al. VZV multifocal vasculopathy with ischemic optic neuropathy, acute retinal necrosis and temporal artery infection in the absence of zoster rash. *J Neurol Sci.* 2013;325(1-2):180-182.
173. McIlwaine LM, Fitzsimons EJ, Soutar RL. Inappropriate antidiuretic hormone secretion, abdominal pain and disseminated varicella-zoster virus infection: an unusual and fatal triad in a patient 13 months post Rituximab and autologous stem cell transplantation. *Clin Lab Haematol.* 2001;23(4):253-254.
179. Milligan KL, Jain AK, Garrett JS, et al. Gastric ulcers due to varicella-zoster reactivation. *Pediatrics.* 2012;130(5):e1377-e1381.
185. Ornstein BW, Hill EB, Geurs TL, et al. Natural killer cell functional defects in pediatric patients with severe and recurrent herpesvirus infections. *J Infect Dis.* 2013;207(3):458-468.
203. Sabry A, Hauk PJ, Jing H, et al. Vaccine strain varicella-zoster virus-induced central nervous system vasculopathy as the presenting feature of DOCK8 deficiency. *J Allergy Clin Immunol.* 2014;133(4):1225-1227.
211. Schunemann S, Mainka C, Wolff MH. Subclinical reactivation of varicella-zoster virus in immunocompromised and immunocompetent individuals. *Intervirology.* 1998;41(2-3):98-102.
242. Weinmann S, Chun C, Schmid DS, et al. Incidence and clinical characteristics of herpes zoster among children in the varicella vaccine era, 2005-2009. *J Infect Dis.* 2013;208(11):1859-1868.
248. Wilson A, Sharp M, Koropchak CM, et al. Subclinical varicella-zoster virus viremia, herpes zoster, and T lymphocyte immunity to varicella-zoster viral antigens after bone marrow transplantation. *J Infect Dis.* 1992;165(1):119-126.

The full reference list for this chapter is available at ExpertConsult.com.

SUBSECTION VI DNA—Poxviridae

163 Smallpox (Variola Virus)

James D. Cherry

Smallpox is a dreaded febrile exanthematous disease caused by the orthopoxvirus variola virus.[5,6,10,23,26,37] After an extensive decade-long World Health Organization (WHO) program to eradicate smallpox, the world was certified free of smallpox in 1979.[17,95] Increased concern relating to biologic terrorism occurred during the 1990s, and the events of September 11, 2001, and immediately thereafter brought home the potential reality of this threat for the present and future.[3,24,50,49,53,69,72,88,95]

HISTORY*

Evidence suggests that endemic smallpox was occurring before 1500 BCE. Three mummies dating from the 18th to the 20th dynasties in

*References 26, 28, 34, 36, 37, 46, 52, 54, 57, 82, 83, 92.

Egypt had pustular lesions all over their bodies.[36] Reliable written accounts of smallpox first appeared during the 4th century. Smallpox was differentiated from measles in 340 by Ko Hung in China. At that time in China, smallpox was an established endemic disease that had come from the west 300 years earlier. During the period from 340 to 1000, the disease was described in Egypt, India, Korea, Japan, southern Europe, and North Africa. A major contributor to the spread of smallpox was the great Islamic expansion across North Africa and into Spain in the 7th and 8th centuries.

By the year 1000, smallpox probably was endemic in populated areas of Europe, Asia, and the African Mediterranean countries. Smallpox was established further in northern Europe by the population movements related to the Crusades. By the 16th century, smallpox was a serious disease in Europe, as indicated by death statistics in Geneva, London, and Sweden. In London during the 17th century, approximately 10% of yearly deaths were attributed to smallpox.

The disease was introduced into the American colonies in 1507 and into Mexico soon thereafter. Epidemics of smallpox posed serious problems for the colonists as well as for the Native Americans. These epidemics also may have been important in certain stages of the American Revolution.[6,38] Smallpox persisted in the United States and Mexico until the 1940s and 1950s, respectively, despite concerted efforts to eliminate the problem.

Soon after this disease was recognized, the Chinese are reported to have made efforts to prevent it. The technique used presumably was variolation, the intentional intranasal or intracutaneous inoculation of susceptible persons with vesicular fluid or crusts from patients with smallpox. This technique apparently originated in China and subsequently was used in many countries, including the United States. As recently as 1968 and 1969, isolated instances of the use of variolation were noted in remote areas of Africa and Asia.[38,54]

After making his observations in 1796 on the immunity against smallpox that was conferred by inoculation with material obtained from cowpox lesions, Jenner extended his research to include intentional and deliberate exposure of some of those persons immunized with cowpox. This strategy provided convincing evidence of solid protection against smallpox.[60] Encouraged by the results, Jenner predicted in 1801 the ultimate eradication of smallpox, a remarkable prediction indeed.[38,48]

The Intensified Smallpox Eradication Program of the WHO, established in 1967, initiated remarkable progress toward total global eradication of this disease.[52] Several factors responsible for this rapid progress included emphasis on surveillance of disease, with containment rather than routine vaccination; improved vaccines and vaccination technology; and sound administrative and fiscal support.[38,39,51,52,64] Of the more than 30 countries in 1967 in which smallpox was endemic, the disease persisted in only five in 1975 and in two in 1977. The world's last case of endemic smallpox occurred on October 31, 1977, in Merca, Somalia.[31] A year later, in 1978, a photographer working at the University of Birmingham in England was infected with a laboratory strain of smallpox virus and died.[91]

After the worldwide eradication of smallpox was achieved, the World Health Assembly (WHA) in 1980 recommended that all countries cease vaccination.[95] Subsequently, a WHO expert committee recommended that all laboratories throughout the world destroy their stocks of variola virus or transfer them into either of two WHO reference laboratories.[53] The laboratories were the Russian State Research Center on Virology and Biotechnology, Koltsovo, Novosibirsk Region, and the Centers for Disease Control and Prevention (CDC) in Atlanta, Georgia.[9] Reportedly, all countries complied with this recommendation.

The WHO committee at a later date recommended that all variola virus stocks be destroyed by 1999, and the WHA concurred with this recommendation.[11] In 1998, a committee of the Institute of Medicine reviewed the possible importance of retaining variola virus for research purposes.[58] In May 1999, the WHA agreed to postpone the destruction of all variola stocks until 2002.[40] In 2005, the WHA again voted not to destroy smallpox stocks.[85] In May 2011, the WHA agreed to postpone setting a date for destruction of smallpox stocks.[86,94] It was to be considered again at the 67th WHA meeting in 2014. Prior to the WHA meeting a number of significant events and concerns had arisen, and therefore the decision on the fate of the smallpox stocks was again put off until 2016 at the earliest.[70,80] On July 1, 2015, scientists found six vials, labeled "variola" in a storage area in the Food and Drug Administration (FDA). These vials were then shipped to CDC for study. Another WHO concern was whether smallpox virus could be synthesized from scratch by those who might have nefarious intentions. If this were the case, it would be important to preserve the virus stocks so that research could be continued to develop counterviruses against terrorist attacks.[2,29,59]

Also of note was the finding of variola virus DNA in a 300-year-old Siberian mummy.[8,87] In this instance, no intact virus was found; however, finding complete viral genome in other studies of mummies would appear to be a possibility. At the present time, research using the virus is being conducted in the United States and Russia. This research is related to the development of safer vaccines and to antiviral agents.

In the early 1990s, evidence revealed that during the previous 10 years, the Soviet government apparently had developed a successful program to produce variola virus for use as a biologic weapon.[53,84] In the late 1990s, concern increased with regard to bioterrorism and, in particular, with the possibility that Russian expertise and equipment could have fallen into non-Russian hands because financial support for laboratories and workers had declined.

Smallpox was used as a biologic weapon almost 250 years ago.[4,28] In the French and Indian Wars (1754–1767), British forces sent smallpox-contaminated blankets and handkerchiefs to the Native Americans surrounding Fort Pitt in the summer of 1763.

ETIOLOGY

Smallpox is caused by a variola virus, an orthopoxvirus.[37,52,74] The virus particles are brick shaped and measure 250 to 300 × 200 to 250 × 100 nm; the size and shape are similar for all orthopoxviruses. The distinctive appearance is helpful in rapidly identifying members of this virus group by electron microscopy of vesicular fluid or crusts. The virus is stable when dried and may remain viable for long periods in dried crusts and indefinitely under freeze-drying techniques in the laboratory. It is propagated readily on the chorioallantoic membrane of embryonated eggs and in a variety of mammalian cell cultures.

EPIDEMIOLOGY

In infected patients, variola virus was found in respiratory secretions and in vesicular fluid from skin lesions. Transmission usually occurred after close personal contact, but airborne spread also could occur.[7,52,53,91] Patients with smallpox were most infectious from the onset through the first 7 to 10 days of rash.

All persons were susceptible to smallpox unless they previously had been infected with variola virus itself or with cowpox or vaccinia virus. Thus, the occurrence of smallpox depended entirely on the presence of a human source of infection and effective exposure of susceptible persons. The age distribution of cases varied in individual countries, depending largely on vaccination practices. Preschool-aged children often were not vaccinated and thus had the greatest prevalence of disease.

The seasonal influence was substantial and perhaps is shown best by the spread of disease after the winter and spring introduction of smallpox into Europe; spread of infection was more than 30 times as great after the introduction of infection into European nations between December and May, in contrast to substantially less frequent spread after introduction between June and November.[96]

Substantial contrast in case-fatality rates was recognized in different geographic areas; these differences did not seem to depend on the supportive care available and did not appear to be related to ethnic or specific resistance factors. The only logical explanation for these different rates was substantial differences in the virulence of the virus prevalent in the regions. The mildest form of smallpox, described as *variola minor,* or *alastrim,* was prevalent in Brazil, Ethiopia, and adjacent countries. Case-fatality rates of 1% or less were customary, and permanent residual scarring and blindness were most unusual occurrences. In other areas of Africa and Indonesia, the disease appeared to be of intermediate severity, whereas on the Indian subcontinent, case-fatality rates were as high as 30%, with residual permanent scarring, blindness, and other sequelae occurring frequently in those who survived the acute illness.[38]

PATHOLOGY

The characteristic pathologic lesions affected the skin and mucous membranes. They involved the deeper layers of the skin and progressed through macular, papular, vesicular, and pustular stages, with the subsequent formation of crusts. Lesions similar to those on the skin also were found in the lower respiratory and gastrointestinal tracts.

Secondary bacterial infection occurred frequently and often affected the skin and lungs. Hemorrhagic complications (hemorrhagic smallpox) were not uncommon events.

CLINICAL MANIFESTATIONS

After an incubation period of 7 to 17 days, the disease began abruptly with fever (i.e., temperatures between 38.9°C and 40.5°C [102°F and 105°F]), headache, and marked malaise.[11] Backache and muscle pain were prominent symptoms. Nausea, vomiting, and abdominal pain also were present.[34,52,63,73]

After these prodromal signs and symptoms were present for 2 to 4 days, the fever usually decreased, and the characteristic cutaneous eruption appeared. The rash was most extensive on the face and extremities, and the individual lesions passed through the stages of macules and papules; by the third or fourth day, they clearly were vesicular. Lesions in a single area of the body were characteristically at the same stage of development.

By the sixth day, the vesicular fluid usually was cloudy and the individual pustules frequently were umbilicated. Pustules often converged and become confluent. By the tenth day, the individual lesions began to dry and formed characteristic crusts that remained intact for several days before they were shed. The patient's temperature customarily fell during the early appearance of the rash, although the fever usually returned. Significant fever that persisted after the tenth or twelfth day of disease suggested the presence of bacterial superinfection.

Although most cases were similar to this description, which was characteristic of the ordinary type of smallpox, other clinical variations were described. The hemorrhagic type was the most severe form, with a case-fatality rate that approached 100%. In this form, hemorrhagic manifestations appeared during the prodromal stage, with extensive cutaneous extravasation of blood and bleeding from the various body orifices. Death usually occurred within the first week of illness, and, frequently few typical diagnostic lesions appeared on the skin surfaces before death ensued. Fortunately, this form of disease occurred in only 2% or 3% of the total cases of variola major in Asia, and it rarely was seen elsewhere.

A flat variety had been reported in approximately 6% of cases observed in India. In this variety, the cutaneous lesions remained flat and soft to the touch, in contrast to the ordinary variety; these lesions characteristically resolved without pustulation. This form was associated with case-fatality rates of 75% to 96%.[38]

A modified form of disease occurred almost exclusively in previously vaccinated persons. Although the prodromal illness often was severe, skin lesions were few, evolved rapidly, and were more superficial. The prognosis was excellent.

The mildest form of the disease, alastrim, or variola minor, was caused by a specific variola virus having less pathogenicity in humans. Serious forms of the illness, as with variola major, were unusual occurrences. The skin lesions tended to be superficial, and the clinical course resembled that of varicella, with the exception of the distribution of cutaneous lesions. These lesions involved the face and extremities, in contrast to the characteristic central body distribution of varicella. Residual scarring, if it occurred at all, usually reflected secondary bacterial infection of individual lesions.

In recently vaccinated persons, asymptomatic infection with variola virus after exposure had been demonstrated by increases in antibody titer against the virus when acute and convalescent sera were tested. This uncommon event was of neither clinical nor epidemiologic significance.

Complications included hemorrhagic events and various secondary bacterial infections, including impetigo, pneumonia, empyema, and otitis media. Nephritis and arthritis with permanent joint changes were described.

DIFFERENTIAL DIAGNOSIS

The typical course, the characteristic cutaneous lesions, and the presence of other cases after contact 7 to 17 days earlier left little doubt about the etiologic agent. Varicella presented the greatest problem in differential diagnosis, particularly from the variola minor, or alastrim, form of the disease, but the distribution of cutaneous lesions for each condition was characteristic. Generalized vaccinia or eczema vaccinatum was distinguished by a history of exposure to vaccinia virus, previous skin lesions, and the distribution of the rash. Impetigo (especially the bullous variety caused by staphylococcal infection), scabies, secondary syphilis, and yaws were other considerations. Usually, little difficulty was encountered clinically in distinguishing among these infections.

Monkeypox can be clinically similar to smallpox, and, therefore, specific laboratory procedures are required for diagnosis (see Chapter 164). Other conditions included in the differential diagnosis were erythema multiforme, pityriasis rosea, measles, rickettsialpox, disseminated herpes simplex infection, syphilis, enteroviral exanthems, and bacterial, viral, and rickettsial petechial and purpuric rashes.

SPECIFIC DIAGNOSIS

Several laboratory procedures are available to provide specific and accurate diagnosis. Vesicular fluid, crusts, or scrapings from skin lesions reveal the characteristic brick-shaped viral particles of the variola-vaccinia virus group when examined by electron microscopy. These orthopoxviruses differ in appearance from the herpesviruses, which in the past were the agents most frequently confused with smallpox. Electron microscopy is precise and rapid and is preferred when facilities for this examination are available.[27] Smallpox virus DNA also can be identified rapidly by polymerase chain reaction (PCR).[34,35,62,81] PCR has an advantage over electron microscopy in that it can specifically distinguish smallpox virus from the other orthopoxviruses.

Orthopoxviruses may be recovered and propagated on the chorioallantoic membrane of embryonated eggs or in tissue culture.[34] Virus recovery requires more time (3 to 7 days) than the direct antigen-detection tests, but it provides the specific active virus required for differentiation among the various orthopoxvirus types.[75,77] Infection also can be determined serologically by using acute-phase and convalescent-phase sera in enzyme-linked immunosorbent assay (ELISA), Western blotting, or virus neutralization assays.[34]

The specific diagnosis of a disease that does not currently exist anywhere in the world presents unique challenges. Recognizing these challenges, the CDC has a diagnosis and evaluation plan with laboratory testing recommendations (http://emergency.cdc.gov/agent/smallpox/diagnosis).

TREATMENT

Therapy primarily was supportive and symptomatic. The skin was kept clean, the bed linen was changed at regular intervals, and local or systemic therapy was provided for the frequent bacterial complications. Attention given to appropriate fluid and nutritional support was required.

Methisazone, convalescent smallpox serum, and vaccinia immune globulin (VIG) were effective in preventing the disease after exposure, but no evidence showed that these agents altered the course of the disease once symptoms occurred.[61] Idoxuridine was used for corneal lesions.[6]

At the present time the United States has a stockpile of VIG, which is produced by Cangene Corporation in Canada (http://www.cdc.gov/laboratory/drugservice/formulary.html).[93] This product is presently available for the treatment of smallpox vaccination complications (i.e., eczema vaccinatum, vaccinia necrosum, or severe generalized vaccinia). In the event of a biological terrorism smallpox release, it is assumed that VIG would be available for treatment.

Studies with the antivirals cidofovir, ST-246, and CMX001 show broad antiviral activity against orthopoxviruses.[1,24,68,73,78] Through the Project BioShield Act of 2004, 1.7 million doses of ST-246 have been stockpiled.

TABLE 163.1 Rates of Reported Complications Associated With Vaccinia Vaccination (Cases/Million Vaccinations)

Age (y) and Status Total[a]	Inadvertent Inoculation	Generalized Vaccinia	Eczema Vaccinatum	Progressive Vaccinia	Postvaccinial Encephalitis	Total
Primary						
<1	507.0	394.4	14.1	—[b]	42.3	1549.3
1–4	577.3	233.4	44.2	3.2	9.5	1261.8
5–19	371.2	139.7	34.9	—	8.7	855.9
≥20	606.1	212.1	30.3	—	—	1515.2
Overall rates	529.2	241.5	38.5	1.5	12.3	1253.8
Revaccination						
<1	—	—	—	—	—	—
1–4	109.1	—	—	—	—	200.0
5–19	47.7	9.9	2.0	—	—	85.5
≥20	25.0	9.1	4.5	6.8	4.5	113.6
Overall rates	42.1	9.0	3.0	3.0	2.0	108.2

[a]Rates of overall complications by age group include complications not provided in this table, including severe local reactions, bacterial superinfection of the vaccination site, and erythema multiforme.

[b]No instances of this complication were identified during the 1968 10-state survey.

From Lane JM, Ruben FL, Neff JM, et al. Complications of smallpox vaccination, 1968: results of 10 statewide surveys. *J Infect Dis.* 1970;122:303–309.

PREVENTION

Active Immunization

In the 20th century, many strains of vaccinia virus were used in the effective prophylaxis of smallpox, which led to the control and then eradication of smallpox from the world. After smallpox was eliminated from the United States and Western Europe, general concern shifted to morbidity and mortality resulting from smallpox vaccines.[45,66,67] It was realized that the risk for smallpox was remote and that vaccine reactions were significant (Table 163.1). Because of this, routine smallpox vaccination was discontinued in the United States in the 1970s.

In the late 1990s, concerns arose that smallpox could be used as a weapon of bioterrorism. The events of September 11, 2001, and immediately thereafter highlighted the potential reality of this threat.[3,24,50,49,53,72,88] Estimates were that probably less than 20% of the US population had any immunity.[50] These concerns led to recommendations by the Advisory Committee on Immunization Practices (ACIP) for the use of smallpox vaccine to protect persons who may need to work with orthopoxviruses and to prepare for a possible bioterrorism attack.[16] The government took steps to prepare the country in the event of a bioterrorist attack involving smallpox. These measures included building an adequate supply of vaccine, enhancing the laboratory capacity for diagnosis of variola and vaccinia virus infection, and training health care and public health personnel.[44]

Through the *Project BioShield Act,* the United States has an ample supply of smallpox vaccine.[76] This is presently available for immunization of selected people (e.g., first responders and laboratory workers) and would be available if a bioterrorist attack were to occur.[79] This stockpile includes ACAM 2000, which is prepared in cell culture, and a modified vaccinia, Ankara (MVA), a new vaccine. This vaccine is thought to be safer than conventional smallpox vaccines, and it was purchased by the United States to be used in immunocompromised persons if a terrorist smallpox release occurred.[43,49,51,89]

The primary strategy used in the past to control an outbreak of smallpox and to interdict the transmission of virus was known as a *surveillance and containment (ring vaccination)* strategy. This strategy identified infected persons through intensive surveillance and subsequently both isolated the individuals with the disease and vaccinated household and close contacts of the infected patient. Vaccination also was recommended for contacts of the primary contact with the patient (secondary contacts). This strategy was instrumental in the eradication of smallpox as a naturally occurring disease. Depending on the size of any smallpox outbreak and the availability of resources for rapid and thorough contact tracing, ring vaccination was supplemented previously in areas with identified smallpox cases to include voluntary vaccination of all individuals without vaccine contraindications. This strategy was pursued to expand the ring of immune individuals within an outbreak area and to reduce further the chance of any secondary transmission of smallpox to patients before they could be identified and isolated.

The CDC developed protocols to permit rapid, simultaneous delivery of smallpox vaccine to every state in the US territory within 12 to 24 hours. Smallpox response planning at the federal level has been conveyed to state and local health departments to address the rapid distribution of the vaccine if vaccination programs are suggested.

The CDC currently recommends that cases of febrile rash illnesses for which smallpox is considered in the differential diagnosis be reported immediately to local or state health departments or both. After evaluation is performed by local or state health departments, if smallpox laboratory diagnostics are considered necessary, the CDC Rash Illness Evaluation Team should be consulted. At this time, laboratory confirmation for smallpox is available routinely only at the CDC. Both a clinical consultation and a preliminary laboratory diagnosis can be completed within a period of 8 to 24 hours.

In the present bioterrorism era the CDC and the ACIP have devoted considerable effort into the diagnosis of smallpox and have looked at risks and benefits of smallpox immunization programs. To assist public health and other medical personnel in evaluating the possibility of smallpox in patients with febrile rash illnesses, the CDC developed a rash illness assessment algorithm (http://emergency.cdc.gov/agent/smallpox/diagnosis/riskalgorithm/).

Medical evaluation of the risks for acquiring smallpox under current conditions and in the absence of a case of smallpox or a confirmed smallpox bioterrorism threat in contrast to the potential risks for developing vaccine complications was such that the ACIP concluded that vaccination of the general population was not recommended because the potential benefits of vaccination did not outweigh the risks for vaccine complications. In 2001, the ACIP recommended smallpox vaccine for laboratory workers who directly handle (1) cultures or (2) animals contaminated or infected with vaccinia, recombinant vaccinia viruses, or other orthopoxviruses that infect humans (e.g., monkeypox and cowpox).[16] Other health care workers (e.g., physicians and nurses) whose contact with these viruses is limited to contaminated material (e.g., dressings) but who adhere to appropriate infection control measures are at lower risk for inadvertently acquiring infection than are laboratory workers. However, because a theoretical risk for developing infection does exist, vaccination may be considered for this group. Because of the low risk for developing infection, vaccination was not recommended for persons who do not handle virus cultures or materials directly or who do not work with animals contaminated or infected with these viruses. According to available data on the persistence of neutralizing antibody after vaccination, persons working with vaccinia, recombinant vaccinia viruses, or other nonvariola orthopoxviruses should be revaccinated every 10 years.

In 2003, the ACIP and the Healthcare Infection Control Practices Advisory Committee (HICPAC) published supplemental recommendations for using smallpox vaccine in a pre-event vaccination program.[18] A summary of these recommendations is presented here:

To facilitate preparedness and response, smallpox vaccination is recommended for persons designated by public health authorities to conduct investigation and follow-up of initial smallpox cases that could necessitate direct patient contact.[18] The ACIP recommended that each state and territory establish and maintain more than one smallpox response team. The ACIP and the HICPAC recommended that each acute-care hospital identify health care workers who can be vaccinated and trained to provide direct medical care for the first smallpox patients requiring hospital admission and to evaluate and manage patients who are suspected as having smallpox. When feasible, the first-stage vaccination program was to include previously vaccinated health care personnel to decrease the potential for adverse events. Additionally, persons administering smallpox vaccine in this pre-event vaccination program were to be vaccinated.

Side Effects and Adverse Events of Smallpox Vaccines

The risk for adverse events resulting from smallpox vaccine today is presumed potentially to be at least as great, in terms of severity and frequency of events, as during the era when universal vaccinia vaccination was performed.[19,45] One can suspect that the number of adverse reactions may be increased in frequency in the current era in contrast to the 1960s and 1970s because a larger proportion of the population of the United States and the world may have an inherited or acquired a form of immunodeficiency or may be receiving a variety of agents that suppress the immune system. Factors thought to predispose to development of adverse events include pregnancy or breast-feeding, extensive skin eruptions, atopic dermatitis, T-cell immune defect, immunosuppressive therapy, inflammatory or disruptive diseases of the cornea, and age younger than 1 year.[19]

Fever occurs commonly after smallpox vaccination. As many as 70% of children have 1 or more days with a temperature of 37.8°C (100°F) or higher 4 to 14 days after receiving primary vaccination,[22,71] and 15% to 20% have temperatures of 38.9°C (102°F) or higher. After receiving revaccination, 35% of children have temperatures of 37.8°C (100°F) or higher, and 5% have temperatures of 38.9°C (102°F) or higher.[71] Fever after vaccination or revaccination occurs less commonly in adults than in children.

An erythematous or urticarial rash may occur approximately 10 days after receipt of primary vaccination. The vaccinee usually is afebrile, and the rash resolves spontaneously within 2 to 4 days. Rarely, bullous erythema multiforme (Stevens-Johnson syndrome) occurs.[63]

Inadvertent inoculation at other sites, the most frequent complication of vaccinia vaccination, accounts for approximately half of all complications of primary vaccination and revaccination.[17] Inadvertent inoculation usually results from autoinoculation of vaccine virus transferred from the site of vaccination. The most common sites involved are the face, eyelid, nose, mouth, genitalia, and rectum. Most lesions heal without specific therapy, but VIG may be useful for cases of ocular implantation.

Generalized vaccinia in persons who have no underlying illness is characterized by a vesicular rash of varying extent. The rash generally is self-limited and requires little or no therapy, except in patients whose conditions appear to be toxic or in those who have a serious underlying illness.

Other expected systemic symptoms associated with smallpox vaccination include malaise, myalgia, headache, chills, nausea, and fatigue (0.3–37%).[41,42] Soreness at the site of the vaccination is a very common development, as are local lymphadenopathy and erythema surrounding the vaccination site.[44]

Expected local events occurring relatively infrequently require symptomatic treatment. They include satellite lesions within 2.5 cm of the primary lesion, viral lymphangitis, local edema, and intense inflammation surrounding the papule.[41,42,44]

TABLE 163.2 Number of Reported Events Associated With Smallpox Vaccination in the Military: 2002–07

Event Type	Department of Defense Experience[a]	US Military Experience[b]
Inadvertent inoculation	61	Self: 48 Transfer to contact: 21
Generalized vaccinia	43	36
Eczema vaccinatum	1	0
Progressive vaccinia	0	0
Myopericarditis	140	37
Ischemic heart disease	16	NA
Encephalitis	NA	1
Treated with VIG	6	NA
Death[c]	8	0

NA, Not applicable; *VIG*, vaccinia immune globulin.
[a]Department of Defense experience: December 2002 to May 2007, 1.2 million vaccinees.[28]
[b]Experience of US military: December 2002 to May 2003, 450,293 vaccinees.[49]
[c]After review, one death was the result of an acute lupuslike illness that may have been caused by the vaccine, and others were thought to result from other causes.[28]

More severe complications of vaccinia vaccination include eczema vaccinatum, progressive vaccinia, myopericarditis, and postvaccinial encephalitis. These complications, with the exception of myopericarditis, occur at least 10 times more often among primary vaccinees than among revaccinees and more frequently among infants than among older children and adults.[65-67]

The number of adverse events per million doses of primary smallpox vaccination and revaccination is reported in Table 163.1. The rates described are based on surveys of vaccination-associated complications that occurred in the late 1960s in the United States. The high prevalence of immunosuppression in the United States today in contrast to the late 1960s may render the rates of vaccinia necrosum higher than in 1968. The rate of postvaccinial encephalitis in adults was difficult to document in the 1960s because very few adults were primary vaccinees. Studies performed in Europe showed higher rates of postvaccinial encephalitis in adults than in young children. Studies performed since 2002, when efforts were made to vaccinate members of the military and civilians, have shown similar rates of adverse reactions, although cardiac side effects have been more notable (Table 163.2).

Eczema vaccinatum is a localized or systemic dissemination of vaccinia virus in persons who have eczema or a history of eczema and other chronic or exfoliative skin conditions (e.g., atopic dermatitis). The illness often is mild and self-limited but may be severe and occasionally fatal. The most serious cases in vaccine recipients occur in primary vaccinees and appear to be independent of the activity of the underlying eczema.[90] Severe cases also have been observed after contact infection has occurred.

Progressive vaccinia (vaccinia necrosum) is a severe, potentially fatal illness characterized by progressive necrosis in the area of vaccination, often with metastatic lesions. It occurs almost exclusively in persons with cellular immunodeficiency.

In the 1960s, cardiac complications were reported but were not considered significant. Myopericarditis now is thought to be a true adverse event related to smallpox vaccine, although most cases resolve without further complications.[12,32,33,98] Cases of ischemic heart disease occurring after receipt of smallpox vaccination also have been reported. Although this association has not been shown to be causal, the ACIP recommended excluding persons with cardiac disease from participation in current smallpox vaccination programs.[18] The incidence of cardiac events in children is not known because the recent vaccination program has targeted adults.

The most serious complication is postvaccinial encephalitis. Usually, it affected primary vaccinees younger than 1 year. Of affected vaccinees with this complication, 15% to 25% died and 25% had permanent neurologic sequelae.[47,66,67]

Death rarely occurred after receipt of vaccinia vaccination; reports note approximately one to two deaths per million primary vaccinations and 0.1 death per million revaccinations. Death most often was the result of postvaccinial encephalitis or progressive vaccinia.

Vaccinia may be transmitted when a recently vaccinated person has contact with a susceptible person. In the CDC's 10-state survey of complications of smallpox vaccination, the risk for transmission to contacts was 27 infections per million total vaccinations; 44% of these contact cases occurred in children age 5 years or younger.[67] Since 1980, several cases of contact transmission of vaccinia from vaccinated military recruits have been reported and include six cases transmitted by a single vaccine recipient.[15,14,13,97] Nonmilitary secondary and tertiary transmission cases after smallpox vaccination have been noted.[21,55,56]

Since 2001, among 1.2 million vaccinated military personnel, 61 suspected instances of transfer of vaccinia occurred, 36 of which were laboratory confirmed.[30] This number included two cases of tertiary transfer, one from a service member to his wife and then to their breastfeeding baby and another among male sports partners.[20,44] Fetal vaccinia occurs rarely (<40 reported cases), but it is usually fatal.[45]

More than 60% of cases of contact transmission result in uncomplicated inadvertent inoculation. Approximately 30% of these cases result in eczema vaccinatum, which may be fatal.[67] Eczema vaccinatum may be more severe in contacts than in vaccinated persons, possibly because of simultaneous multiple inoculation at several sites.[25,66] Contact transmission rarely results in postvaccinial encephalitis or vaccinia necrosum.

Smallpox Vaccine Availability

The CDC is the only source of smallpox vaccine and VIG for civilians. In the advent of need to carry out smallpox vaccination, procedural information will be available from the CDC.

NEW REFERENCES SINCE THE SEVENTH EDITION

2. Arita I, Francis D. Is it time to destroy the smallpox virus? *Science.* 2014;345(6200):1010.
4. Barras V, Greub G. History of biological warfare and bioterrorism. *Clin Microbiol Infect.* 2014;20(6):497-502.
8. Biagini P, Theves C, Balaresque P, et al. Variola virus in a 300-year-old Siberian mummy. *N Engl J Med.* 2012;367(21):2057-2059.
21. Centers for Disease Control and Prevention. Secondary and tertiary transmission of vaccinia virus after sexual contact with a smallpox vaccinee—San Diego, California, 2012. *MMWR Morb Mortal Wkly Rep.* 2013;62(8):145-147.
29. Damon IK, Damaso CR, McFadden G. Are we there yet? The smallpox research agenda using variola virus. *PLoS Pathog.* 2014;10(5):e1004108.
33. Engler RJ, Nelson MR, Collins LC Jr, et al. A prospective study of the incidence of myocarditis/pericarditis and new onset cardiac symptoms following smallpox and influenza vaccination. *PLoS ONE.* 2015;10(3):e0118283.
43. Frey SE, Winokur PL, Hill H, et al. Phase II randomized, double-blinded comparison of a single high dose (5×10^8 TCID50) of modified vaccinia Ankara compared to a standard dose (1×10^8 TCID50) in healthy vaccinia-naive individuals. *Vaccine.* 2014;32(23):2732-2739.
55. Hsu CH, Farland J, Winters T, et al. Laboratory-acquired vaccinia virus infection in a recently immunized person—Massachusetts, 2013. *MMWR Morb Mortal Wkly Rep.* 2015;64(16):435-438.
56. Hughes CM, Blythe D, Li Y, et al. Vaccinia virus infections in a martial arts gym, Maryland, USA, 2008. *Emerg Infect Dis.* 2011;17(4):730-733.
68. Lederman ER, Davidson W, Groff HL, et al. Progressive vaccinia: case description and laboratory-guided therapy with vaccinia immune globulin, ST-246, and CMX001. *J Infect Dis.* 2012;206(9):1372-1385.
70. McCarthy M. Smallpox samples are found in FDA storage room in Maryland. *BMJ.* 2014;349:g4545.
78. Olson VA, Smith SK, Foster S, et al. In vitro efficacy of brincidofovir against variola virus. *Antimicrob Agents Chemother.* 2014;58(9):5570-5571.
79. Petersen BW, Damon IK, Pertowski CA, et al. Clinical guidance for smallpox vaccine use in a postevent vaccination program. *MMWR Recomm Rep.* 2015;64(RR-02):1-26.
80. Reardon S. "Forgotten" NIH smallpox virus languishes on death row. *Nature.* 2014;514(7524):544.
87. Theves C, Biagini P, Crubezy E. The rediscovery of smallpox. *Clin Microbiol Infect.* 2014;20(3):210-218.
89. von Sonnenburg F, Perona P, Darsow U, et al. Safety and immunogenicity of modified vaccinia Ankara as a smallpox vaccine in people with atopic dermatitis. *Vaccine.* 2014;32(43):5696-5702.
97. Young GE, Hidalgo CM, Sullivan-Frohm A, et al. Secondary and tertiary transmission of vaccinia virus from US military service member. *Emerg Infect Dis.* 2011;17(4):718-721.
98. Zitzmann-Roth EM, von Sonnenburg F, de la Motte S, et al. Cardiac safety of Modified Vaccinia Ankara for vaccination against smallpox in a young, healthy study population. *PLoS ONE.* 2015;10(4):e0122653.

The full reference list for this chapter is available at ExpertConsult.com.

164 Monkeypox and Other Poxviruses

Samantha H. Johnston • Anne W. Rimoin

Smallpox, caused by variola virus (see Chapter 163), at one time was the most important human poxvirus disease, but this disease has been eradicated from the world. Today, only one human poxvirus, molluscum contagiosum virus, causes specific human illness. In addition, at least nine other poxviruses can cause human infections. Eight of these viruses are acquired zoonotically, and the ninth, vaccinia, is acquired by active immunization against smallpox, inadvertently by laboratory accident, or by transfer from a vaccinated person to an unvaccinated person.

PROPERTIES OF THE VIRUSES

Classification

The family *Poxviridae* has two subfamilies: *Chordopoxvirinae* (vertebrate poxviruses) and *Entomopoxvirinae* (insect poxviruses).[55,60,125] Eight genera are included in the *Chordopoxvirinae* subfamily, and four of these genera contain species that infect humans (Table 164.1).

Structure

Poxviruses are the largest animal viruses and are discernible by light microscopy.[15,129] In general, by electron microscopy, orthopoxviruses appear brick shaped, with a length of 350 nm and a width of 270 nm. They contain double-stranded DNA genomes that vary from 130 to 300 kbp, depending on the particular species. A 30-nm lipoprotein bilayer (envelope) surrounds the virus core. The envelope contains seven or more distinct glycoproteins. *Parapoxvirus* organisms have a different structure than do *Orthopoxvirus, Yatapoxvirus,* and *Molluscipoxvirus* organisms. They are ovoid and vary from 260 to 160 nm for orf virus to 300 to 190 nm for pseudocowpox virus.

SPECIFIC VIRUSES AND THEIR ILLNESSES

Monkeypox Virus

Monkeypox is a zoonotic orthopoxvirus that causes a serious smallpox-like illness in humans. Monkeypox virus was first discovered in 1958,

TABLE 164.1 Poxviruses That Can Cause Human Illness

Genus	Species
Orthopoxvirus	Variola virus Monkeypox virus Vaccinia virus Cowpox virus
Parapoxvirus	Orf virus Bovine papular stomatitis virus Pseudocowpox virus Parapox of seals Parapoxvirus of reindeer
Yatapoxvirus	Tanapoxvirus Yabapoxvirus
Molluscipoxvirus	Molluscum contagiosum virus

when it was isolated from the lesions of a generalized smallpox-like vesiculopustular disease among captive monkeys at the State Serum Institute in Copenhagen, Denmark.[181] The disease was not recognized as being distinct from smallpox until 1970, when, after smallpox had been eliminated from many countries, a similar illness continued to circulate in rural regions of the Democratic Republic of Congo (DRC).[46,82,91,129] Between 1970 and 1979, 55 cases of monkeypox were confirmed by the World Health Organization (WHO) in forested areas of Western and Central Africa; 44 of these cases (80%) occurred in the DRC.[14,91,110]

In 1980, smallpox was declared eradicated by the WHO Advisory Committee on Orthopoxvirus Infections. Despite sporadic reports of human monkeypox in Africa, the WHO Advisory Committee also recommended that smallpox vaccination cease globally because of the cost and complexity of sustaining a special vaccination program for what was then a comparatively rare disease.[147] To address the concern that in the absence of smallpox vaccination campaigns monkeypox might have the potential to emerge from central Africa and occupy the niche vacated by smallpox, a WHO-sponsored active surveillance program was carried out in selected districts in the DRC from 1981 to 1986.[153,154] This surveillance program initiated modeling of monkeypox human-to-human transmission patterns. Models predicted that the reproductive number (R_o) was less than 1 and that human-to-human transmission was at low enough levels not to present a significant public health threat. Thus, the WHO recommended against sustained vaccinia vaccination for protection against monkeypox.[77,185]

During this period 338 cases were identified, most cases found in children (mean age, 4.4 years), leading to the hypothesis that smallpox vaccine may confer a degree of immunity in adults.[91,122,129] Since the WHO's initial efforts at monkeypox surveillance began, outbreaks, mostly in the DRC, have been reported in the literature. Monkeypox has since supplanted smallpox as the most important orthopoxvirus affecting humans, and more attention has been directed to understanding the transmission patterns, epidemiology, and control strategies of this illness.

Epidemiology

Epidemiologic studies beginning in 1970 continue to identify outbreaks of human monkeypox, with most cases arising in the DRC. Jezek and associates[95,96] reported disease in 338 patients and found that among patients with primary infection (i.e., cases associated with an animal source), 50% were younger than 4 years and 93% were younger than 14 years. Ninety-six percent of these children were not vaccinated against smallpox.[14] Animal sources were suspected in 245 of the 338 cases, and human-to-human transmission occurred in the remaining 93 cases. Analysis of unvaccinated contacts of the patients showed a secondary attack rate of 9.3%.[14] The longest chain of infection was four generations.[96] Index cases of monkeypox were usually women or children who had frequent contact with animals.[30,41] Since initial pox lesions on the hands or arms indicative of direct inoculation were not described, infection was presumably acquired by inhaling material aerosolized during handling or butchering of an animal. Person-to-person transmission was generally limited to family members and other close contacts, suggesting monkeypox was less transmissible than smallpox, but the small size and low population density of rural villages also may have helped limit the size of outbreaks.[41]

After the end of the active WHO surveillance program in 1986, only 13 cases of human monkeypox were reported until 1995, likely because political instability in the region impeded surveillance activities. In 1996 to 1997, the largest outbreak recorded to date occurred in the Kasai Oriental region of the DRC. During an initial investigation by the WHO and the Centers for Disease Control and Prevention (CDC), 92 cases were identified and a follow-up investigation suggested an additional 419 suspected cases. However, confusion with a concurrent varicella outbreak made precise estimates of the true outbreak size difficult to ascertain.[24,77] Analysis of 320 possible and probable cases showed attack rates of 18% in susceptible individuals, 3% if vaccinated, and 26% if unvaccinated.[77] Eighty-five percent of cases occurred in patients younger than 16 years. The case-fatality rate was 1.5%, lower than the previously reported rate of 10%.[24] The broad case definition used for monkeypox case identification of fever and vesiculopustular rash could have included infections with varicella as well, thus artificially increasing rates of reported secondary transmission as well as artificially decreasing case-fatality rates.[46]

Meyer and colleagues[122] used viral isolation and amplification by polymerase chain reaction (PCR) to detect monkeypox virus after a 2001 outbreak in the DRC. The group found that, as in previous outbreaks, coinfection and cotransmission of varicella could have misrepresented actual cases of monkeypox. Of the seven small outbreaks, two were proved to be the result of monkeypox (16 cases, four deaths); two showed evidence of cocirculating monkeypox and varicella (seven cases, one death); two were the result of varicella-zoster virus (six cases, no deaths); and neither virus was isolated in the final outbreak. Children were the principal victims in all outbreaks.

Rimoin and colleagues[154] conducted active surveillance for human monkeypox in the DRC between 2005 and 2007 to assess the current burden of infection and noted a dramatic increase in monkeypox cases since the 1980s. The most heavily affected health zones showed a 20-fold increase in monkeypox activity in contrast to the 1980s, with an increase in cases from 0.72 to 14.42 per 10,000. Ninety-two percent of cases occurred in those born after smallpox vaccination ended in 1980. The study concluded that risk for monkeypox is "inversely associated with smallpox vaccination."

The burden of monkeypox disease continues to be greatest in the DRC, but outbreaks have also been reported in Sudan (now South Sudan), the Republic of Congo, and the Central African Republic in recent years. Phylogenetic and ecologic analyses indicate that monkeypox infections in South Sudan were more likely due to importation of infected animals or human-to-human transmission, rather than new zoonotic transmission in that area.[10,42,64,111,127]

These surveillance activities have supported the three main factors determining monkeypox burden in enzootic areas: smallpox vaccination, exposure to animal reservoir species, and human-to-human transmission of disease. Smallpox vaccination officially ceased in the DRC in 1982; thus, vaccine-induced herd immunity has waned, partially contributing to increased incidence.[102] Another contribution has been the change in animal contact during this time period. Monkeypox generally occurs in villages in or near tropical rainforest. Clearing of these forests as well as increased reliance on reservoir species for nutrition likely has brought humans into closer contact with reservoir species.[154]

A noted increase in monkeypox incidence in recent years has led to concern that changes in the virus are leading to increased human-to-human transmissibility. Mathematical modeling has demonstrated that changes in viral characteristics and demographics would be required in order for endemic spread of monkeypox to occur in the human population.[11] While analysis of genomic variability among human monkeypox infections in the DRC showed genetic changes that may indicate active evolution toward adaptation and improved transmission between humans, no sustained transmission has yet occurred.[107] In fact, the longest sustained chain of human-to-human transmission has been six events.[111] The effect of increased human-to-human transmission has not been formally investigated, but waning immunity to smallpox is thought to allow more sustained transmission of monkeypox in an increasingly unimmunized population.

Technological advances in diagnosis have made comparison of disease burden over time difficult. Thus ecological niche modeling (ENM) using human case data, satellite imaging, climactic data, and mathematical models has been employed to better define areas of potential disease transmission. ENM has predicted expansion of areas suitable for disease transmission to larger areas of the Congo Basin, which have already been involved in recent outbreaks. These areas are expected to expand in the coming century.[53,128,175]

Two distinct clades of monkeypox virus have been identified, West African (WA) and Congo Basin (CB), with notable differences in transmissibility and clinical features. In animal models, the WA clade demonstrates less transmissibility as compared to the CB clade.[85] In addition, whereas most reports of monkeypox disease are from the DRC, these represent CB virus. There are very few reports of WA clade virus: fewer than 10 between1970 and 2005 from Liberia, Sierra Leone, Côte d'Ivoire, and Nigeria.[149] Several genomic differences have been seen between the WA and CB clades that may account for differences in virulence. These include T-cell suppression and deletion of a complement control protein among WA virus linked to virulence.[2,73,80]

Although monkeypox outbreaks in humans had been reported during the 1970s, few cases have been noted outside of the DRC.[8,149] However, serologic evidence shows that orthopoxvirus, presumably monkeypox, may be circulating in West Africa among multiple species, including humans.[119,150]

Only one known outbreak has occurred outside of Africa. In May of 2003, the CDC reported the first outbreak of monkeypox in humans in the Western Hemisphere among 47 patients with laboratory-confirmed or probable cases.[25,26,27,28,150] No case fatalities and no cases of secondary transmission occurred. Fourteen cases resulted in hospitalization; two of these were severe cases in children. One girl developed encephalitis that resolved over the course of a 14-day hospitalization; a second girl developed diffuse oral and pharyngeal lesions that impaired swallowing, and she also recovered.[26] The outbreak was linked to the distribution of North American prairie dogs as pets that had become ill after being housed with an infected rope squirrel and an infected giant pouched rat shipped from Ghana. Patients were identified in Illinois, Indiana, Kansas, Missouri, Ohio, and Wisconsin.[10,26,27,28,84,148] PCR analysis of tissue obtained from the prairie dogs revealed 100% similarity with the monkeypox virus strain Zaire 96-I-16 that had been isolated previously from the DRC.[103]

The virus is thought to spread to humans by handling of infected animals or by direct contact with an infected animal's body fluids or lesions.[103] While it has been thought that interactions with infected wildlife would be highest risk for infection, one community study pointed to index cases as more likely to be school-aged boys, which may be related to increased susceptibility or activities of boys at this age.[131] Person-to-person spread occurs by large respiratory droplets, although monkeypox transmission is much less efficient than that of smallpox.[30,129,161] A risk factor for secondary transmission is close contact with a primary case, such as sharing food service items and sleeping quarters.[131] Evidence of previous vaccination is thought to be protective, with surveillance programs estimating vaccine efficacy between 80 and 85%.[40,59,154] Mortality rates have varied between 0 and 17% during outbreaks.[3,11,46,62,84,91,94,96,123]

Serologic evidence suggests that many animals, including both arboreal and terrestrial rodents and nonhuman primates, can be infected with monkeypox virus, however, rope squirrels (*Funisciurus anerythrus*) are thought to be the primary host.[46,66,84] Epidemiologic studies from the DRC have implicated squirrels living in agricultural areas as primary candidates to sustain transmission among people in nearby settlements, although no definitive host has been identified. Since 2003, there have been concerns that monkeypox virus could spread through North American rodent populations and serve as a vector for continued zoonotic exposure.[46] However, in the ensuing 14 years, this did not happen.

Clinical Features

The clinical features of human monkeypox virus infection are similar to those of smallpox, but the overall illness tends to be less severe. The characterization of symptoms during outbreaks in Africa has been limited by poor access to medical care, retrospective identification, and civil unrest in areas of outbreaks. The outbreak reported in the Midwestern United States allowed researchers to describe clinical and laboratory parameters of disease.[84]

After a 10- to 14-day period of incubation (range, 1–31 days), a 2-day prodrome of fever, malaise, and lymphadenopathy precedes the manifestation of rash.[14,46,91] Lymphadenopathy occurs in 90% of unvaccinated individuals and is a key feature distinguishing monkeypox from smallpox because lymphadenopathy generally does not occur in smallpox. Affected lymph nodes may be unilateral or bilateral and include submandibular, cervical, postauricular, axillary, inguinal, or any combination of these locations.[12] Other signs and symptoms include chills, sweats, headache, backache, sore throat, cough, and shortness of breath.

The rash usually appears first on the face. As in smallpox, lesions develop and progress together in the same body region through the stages of macules, papules, vesicles, and pustules. Over the course of a 2- to 4-week period, the lesions progress until they finally scab over and desquamate. Most patients have discrete lesions; it is estimated that 23% have semiconfluent lesions and 7% have confluent lesions. Mucous membrane involvement and conjunctivitis are common manifestations.[94,122] Lesions usually are found on the extremities, head, and trunk, as well as on the palms and soles.[82] During the first week of the rash, patients are considered to be infectious.[93] Cases without rash have been described.[83] The presence of rash on the palms and soles and the stages of progression of the rash distinguish this from varicella.

Complications include secondary bacterial infection of the skin; pneumonia; vomiting, diarrhea, and dehydration; keratitis and corneal ulceration; septicemia; and encephalitis. The death rate in nonvaccinated patients was 11% in the study reported by Jezek and associates,[94] and all deaths occurred in children aged 8 years or younger, possibly reflecting protective effect in older individuals who may have received vaccinia immunization.

One case of congenital monkeypox infection has been reported.[90] The child's mother presented with clinical characteristics of monkeypox on August 12, 1983, and the child was born prematurely on September 23, 1983. At birth, the child had generalized skin lesions and died 6 weeks later of malnutrition. No data are available on the clinical course of monkeypox in patients with human immunodeficiency virus and acquired immunodeficiency syndrome (HIV/AIDS) or other immunocompromised states.

Unlike African patients, in whom more severe illness is noted, most of the patients in the United States had what was described as a mild, self-limited febrile rash illness.[28] The majority of patients had localized lesions associated with direct contact with infected animals, and only one patient, a child, had a generalized rash. Nevertheless, the outbreak resulted in 14 hospitalizations among the 47 cases. Differences in the severity of disease may result from differences in virulence among genetically distinct clades of monkeypox viruses: the West African monkeypox virus group and the Congo Basin isolates.[118] Congo Basin isolates have been shown to be more virulent in nonhuman primates and, based on epidemiologic and genetic sequence analyses, are thought to be more virulent in humans as well.[34,55,91,120,160]

Laboratory alterations noted in patients of the Midwestern US outbreak included elevated transaminases in 50% of patients, low blood urea nitrogen (61%), hypoalbuminemia (50%), leukocytosis (45%), and thrombocytopenia (35%).[84]

Diagnosis

All suspect cases should be reported immediately to the local health department. Laboratory confirmation is required for establishing a definitive diagnosis. The CDC case definitions from 2004 can help guide clinicians (Box 164.1).[30] CDC specifies a variety of respiratory, blood, and lesion samples that may be collected from various stages of illness, as well as collection techniques at different disease stages and including respiratory samples (Table 164.2). Samples used for diagnosis include blood and cutaneous tissue from at least two scabs that have been unroofed and collected in a sterile fashion. Once lesions have been unroofed, the base of the vesicle should be swabbed with sterile cotton or polyester swab and the material applied to a clean microscope slide

BOX 164.1 Centers for Disease Control and Prevention Case Definition for Human Cases of Monkeypox (January 2004)

Suspect Case

The patient meets one of the epidemiologic criteria and has fever or unexplained rash and two or more other signs or symptoms with onset of first sign or symptom within 21 days after the last exposure.

Probable Case

The patient meets one of the epidemiologic criteria and has fever and vesicular-pustular rash with onset of the first sign or symptom less than 21 days after the last exposure meeting epidemiologic criteria; or if rash is present but type is not described, the patient demonstrates elevated levels of IgM antibodies reactive with orthopoxvirus between at least 7 and 56 days after the rash onset.

Confirmed Case

The patient meets one of the laboratory criteria.

Clinical Criteria

Rash (macular, papular, vesicular, pustular, generalized or localized, discrete or confluent)

Fever (subjective or measured, ≥37.4°C)

Other signs and symptoms (chills and/or sweats, headache, backache, lymphadenopathy, sore throat, cough, shortness of breath)

Epidemiologic Criteria

Exposure (includes living in a household, petting or handling, or visiting a pet-holding facility such as a pet store or veterinary clinic) to an exotic or wild mammalian pet (including prairie dogs, Gambian giant rats, and rope squirrels, among others to be considered on a case-by-case basis) obtained on or after April 15, 2003, with clinical signs of illness (e.g., conjunctivitis, respiratory symptoms, and/or rash)

Exposure (as described earlier) to an exotic or wild mammalian pet (as described earlier) with or without clinical signs of illness that has been in contact with either a mammalian pet (living in a household or originating from the same pet holding facility as another animal with monkeypox) or a human

Exposure (skin-to-skin or face-to-face contact) to a suspect, probable, or confirmed human case

Laboratory Criteria

Isolation of monkeypox virus in culture

Demonstration of monkeypox virus DNA by PCR testing of a clinical specimen

Demonstration of virus morphologically consistent with an orthopoxvirus by electron microscopy in the absence of exposure to another orthopoxvirus

Demonstration of presence of orthopoxvirus in tissue using immunohistochemical testing methods in the absence of exposure to another orthopoxvirus

Exclusion Criteria

An alternative diagnosis can explain the illness.

or

The case was reported on the basis of primary or secondary exposure to an exotic or wild mammalian pet (as described earlier) or a human subsequently determined not to have monkeypox, provided other possible epidemiologic exposure criteria are not present.

or

A patient without a rash does not develop a rash within 10 days of onset of clinical symptoms consistent with monkeypox.

The case is determined to be negative for nonvariola generic orthopoxvirus by PCR testing of a well-sampled rash lesion by the approved protocol.

The case is determined to have undetectable levels of IgM antibody 7 to 56 days after rash onset.

IgM, Immunoglobulin M; *PCR,* polymerase chain reaction.

Modified from Centers for Disease Control and Prevention: *Updated interim case definition for human monkeypox, Atlanta, 2004, CDC.* Available at http://www.cdc.gov/ncidod/monkeypox/casedefinition.htm; and Centers for Disease Control and Prevention: Update: multistate outbreak of monkeypox—Illinois, Indiana, Kansas, Missouri, Ohio, and Wisconsin, 2003. *MMWR Morb Mortal Wkly Rep.* 2003;52:561-564.

TABLE 164.2 Centers for Disease Control and Prevention Guidance for Preparation and Collection of Specimens

Disease Phase	Specimens to Collect
Prodrome	Tonsillar tissue swab
	Nasopharyngeal swab
	Acute serum and whole blood
Rash[a]	
Macules or papules	Tonsillar tissue swab
	Lesion biopsy
	Acute serum and whole blood
Vesicles or pustules	Lesion fluid, roof, or biopsy
	Electron microscopy grid (if supplies available)
	Acute serum and whole blood
Scabs or crusts	Lesion scab or crust
	Acute serum and whole blood
Post-rash	Convalescent serum

[a]More than one lesion should be sampled, preferably from different locations on the body and/or from different looking lesions.

From http://www.cdc.gov/poxvirus/monkeypox/clinicians/prep-collection-specimens.html#modalIdString_CDCTable_0.

and air dried. The material should be sent to the CDC or a national reference laboratory in the country of origin for diagnostic testing. Other specimens used for analysis include skin biopsy specimens, which may be indistinguishable from those of smallpox lesions, with necrosis of the stratum basale, adjacent dermal papillae, and stratum spinosum. Electron microscopy of the lesions shows abundant large, brick-shaped orthopoxvirus particles in the cytoplasm of infected epidermal cells.[172] Due to limitations in specimen storage and cold chain in affected areas, lesion exudate collected on a swab or crust specimens are likely the most useful specimens.

Blood samples may be analyzed for paired acute-phase and convalescent-phase serum samples; however, serologic testing is limited because of the close antigenic relationship that exists among orthopoxviruses. More specific methods used by the CDC include cell culture or chick chorioallantoic membrane isolation, along with PCR and sequencing to differentiate monkeypox virus from other orthopoxviruses.[41,108,116] PCR also can differentiate between Congo Basin and West African monkeypox strains.[117,159]

Given difficulties of diagnosis in areas most affected by monkeypox, much work has been dedicated to developing rapid, specific, on-site diagnostic techniques. Dumont and colleagues demonstrated on-site deployment of dual PCR testing for monkeypox virus and varicella virus and were able to successfully identify causative viruses in three outbreaks of rashlike illness in the DRC.[49]

Treatment and Prevention

In 1968, investigators reported that monkeys could be immunized against monkeypox virus using smallpox vaccine.[120] In outbreaks in the DRC described by Jezek and colleagues, as well as by more recent surveillance by Rimoin and colleagues,[94,154] prior smallpox inoculation was found to be protective and result in a milder form of disease, often difficult to distinguish from chickenpox. Hammarlund and associates[72] also described protective immunity to monkeypox virus in persons previously vaccinated against smallpox. Vaccine efficacy was estimated to be 85% during surveillance trials in the 1980s and more than 80% for more than 30 years during more recent surveillance.[61,154] However, the smallpox vaccination status did not alter either the severity of illness or hospitalization rates in the Midwestern US outbreak.[82] The CDC recommended vaccination with smallpox vaccine for those without contraindications to vaccination, including health care workers and household contacts of patients with suspected or confirmed monkeypox cases. Preexposure vaccination is preferred, but vaccination can be administered after laboratory confirmation of an infection. Vaccination should be given within 4 days but may be considered protective up to 14 days after exposure.[30] Currently, in the United States, vaccination is recommended for laboratory personnel working with certain orthopoxviruses and for military personnel.[33]

Because of the high frequency of complications associated with administering vaccinia, work has been done to develop safer vaccines (see Chapter 163). Second-generation smallpox vaccines such as ACAM2000 have demonstrated good protection, but also have a high side-effect profile.[74] This vaccine is licensed in the United States and kept in the Strategic National Stockpile. In macaque models, third-generation vaccines using highly attenuated modified vaccinia Ankara (MVA) appear to be very efficacious against both smallpox and monkeypox with lower rates of complications than previous vaccines.[174] This vaccine candidate, IMVAMUNE, was shown to be safe and provide immunity in humans; as of 2010 it had been granted fast track status by the US Food and Drug Administration and is currently stockpiled for use in emergencies.[58] Lc16m8 is an attenuated vaccinia virus vaccine, licensed for use in Japan, which seems to exhibit a more favorable side effect profile than other vaccines and has demonstrated anti-vaccinia, -variola, and -monkeypox neutralizing antibodies.[100,101] A variety of other vaccines intended to elicit more specific antibody responses have been studied in various primate models, and these have also shown promise.[44,52,65,68,76,78] Some groups have also initiated work on recombinant bovine herpesvirus vaccine vectors specifically targeting monkeypox.[65]

Important questions have been raised as to the risks and benefits of testing these vaccines for efficacy and vaccinating humans in monkeypox endemic areas.[152] These concerns may become more relevant global public health issues should monkeypox become established in an animal reservoir outside of Africa or develop more effective human-to-human transmission.

Roess and colleagues[157] evaluated education-based prevention efforts in areas endemic for monkeypox; after a community intervention trial, they found improved disease recognition and transmission and risk-limitation methods in place. Until an effective and inexpensive monkeypox vaccine becomes available, this type of intervention may be the best option to provide some degree of disease prevention.[157]

During the US outbreak, as a potential preventive measure, 28 affected residents (26 adults and two children) received a smallpox vaccine to try to prevent further transmission of monkeypox.[27] No data exist on the effectiveness of vaccinia immunoglobulin; however, it may be considered as a treatment for severe cases of monkeypox infection and as prophylaxis in severely immunocompromised exposed persons.[46]

Of the many compounds that have been investigated as potential treatments of orthopoxvirus infections, three drugs have shown the most promise: cidofovir, brincidofovir (CMX-001), and tecovirimat. Cidofovir and brincidofovir inhibit viral DNA polymerase. Cidofovir has been shown to be active in vitro and in vivo in animal models as a potential treatment,[3,43,144,145] but no reported data on its effectiveness for treating infected humans exists to date. However, the CDC recommends that it be considered as a treatment in severe monkeypox virus infections and in immunocompromised hosts, but should not be used as a prophylaxis because of its significant toxicities.[17] Brincidofovir is a modified form of cidofovir being developed that lacks the nephrotoxicity associated with cidofovir.[63] Tecovirimat (ST-246), a compound with activity against orthopoxviruses by blocking release of intracellular virus from the cell, also has shown promise in treating severe monkeypox virus infection in rodent and nonhuman primate models and may one day be approved for use in humans.[99,162,171] It is maintained in stockpile in the United States and is available under an investigational protocol to treat orthopoxvirus infections. Mitoxantrone, a drug already FDA approved for multiple sclerosis and cancer, recently demonstrated the ability to carry some antiviral effects against monkeypox and cowpox viruses, although less effectively than cidofovir.[1] Other treatments, such as monoclonal antibodies and interferon-beta, are being investigated but remain in the preclinical phases.[37,81,97]

Among hospitalized patients, isolation precautions should be taken because the virus may be transmitted by direct contact or large respiratory droplets that may be airborne.[29,30] Isolation can be discontinued for patients with vesiculopustular rash after all lesions have crusted; however, contact with immunocompromised persons should be limited until all crusts have separated. For patients without rash, isolation should be continued for 7 days after the onset of fever. Asymptomatic contacts should remain under symptom surveillance for 21 days after the last exposure, and temperature should be monitored twice daily. Affected individuals should not donate any body fluids or organs while ill.[30]

Bioterrorism Concerns

Concern over monkeypox virus as an agent of bioterrorism has been raised, but there has been no evidence to suggest that the virus becomes more severe, virulent, or easily transmissible after passages through human hosts.[96] Furthermore, evidence that monkeypox evolved independently from smallpox alleviated some fears that the virus could "evolve back" into smallpox. In addition, low rates of primary infection, limited transmissibility, and low case fatality make monkeypox an unlikely bioterrorist threat.[13] However, some concerns remain about the potential of molecular biologic techniques to manipulate the virus genetically into a more lethal form.[87,163]

Cowpox Virus

Cowpox disease has been recognized for hundreds of years in Europe. The infection causes ulcers on the teats of cows.[55] Those working with infected cows, including milkmaids, often developed similar ulcers on their hands and were known to be immune to smallpox. In May of 1796, this led Edward Jenner to inoculate James Phipps, an 8-year-old boy, with cowpox material obtained from a lesion on a local dairy maid.[8,88,89,90] No infection occurred after exposing him to material from a smallpox lesion.

Cowpox is a rare illness reported throughout western Europe and northern and central Asia with the broadest host range of the poxviruses and, similar to monkeypox, likely to have wild rodents as natural reservoirs.[5,8,15,56,105,138] With broad host and geographic range, groups have investigated varying degrees of virulence among different strains, leading to growing evidence to suggest there are at least several clades of cowpox virus, and even that these should be further divided into separate genera.[39,51]

Baxby[5] reported 12 human patients with illnesses caused by cowpox virus; only five were exposed to infected cows and the other seven reported no direct contact with cows. All patients, however, lived in or had visited rural areas before the onset of illness. Of the 10 patients with lesions, six had lesions on the hand only, three had lesions on the chin or face only, and one patient had lesions on both the face and hand. Most patients had local edema, lymphadenitis, and fever. Initially, lesions were confused with anthrax in two patients. With a growing portion of the population no longer immunized against smallpox, there are increasing numbers of cowpox cases reported in the literature, with a wide variety of suspected animals transmitting to humans.[109] Additional cases of cowpox causing mostly cutaneous infection continue to be reported from various European countries. Most identified cases resolved between 3 weeks and 6 months, but one fatality in an immunocompromised host has been reported.[38] Although cowpox is generally a self-limited infection, immunocompromised hosts and those with atopic skin conditions can develop more severe, even lethal, infections, and a case of lymphadenopathy persisting for 2 years in a child was also reported.[38,133,135] Reports of illness have followed exposure to sick animals, including cats, dogs, wild rats, voles, and other rodents. Complicated ocular infections caused by cowpox have also been reported and associated with orthopoxvirus circulating among rodents in surrounding areas.[6,69,106,164]

As with other poxviruses, PCR has aided in specific diagnosis of the virus. Recent studies have used PCR to detect the etiologic agent of cutaneous findings: Schupp and associates[163] reported a single case of cowpox virus potentially from a cat, causing necrotic ulcers on a 12-year-old boy in Germany. The virus was isolated and detected by PCR.

Similar to monkeypox virus, several compounds have shown antiviral effects for cowpox virus in vitro or in animal models. These include cidofovir, tecovirimat, terameprocol, and mitoxantrone.[4,140,146]

Vaccinia Virus

Vaccinia virus is the live immunizing antigen successfully used in the global program to eradicate smallpox. This orthopoxvirus is different from cowpox virus, the agent that Jenner and others used for vaccination in the early 19th century. Vaccinia virus has been used for vaccination for more than 100 years. Restriction endonuclease studies indicated that various strains of vaccinia virus from different geographic regions are similar to each other but distinctly different from cowpox virus.[55] The origin of vaccinia virus is unknown, but various hypotheses exist regarding its origin,[15] including (1) evolving from variola virus through continual passage in the skin of cows or humans, (2) evolving from cowpox virus through continual passage in the skin of animals, (3) hybridization between cowpox virus and variola virus, and (4) evolving in a an extinct natural animal host.

Vaccinia virus has caused outbreaks in several countries in milk herds; most commonly it has been reported in India and Brazil, with reports published since 1999. An outbreak in India was described in which infected buffaloes were thought to have had contact with vaccinated humans during smallpox eradication programs, rather than the virus being a primary buffalo pathogen.[15,55] In several Brazilian provinces, skin lesions resembling cowpox on dairy cows and their milkers were found to be caused by a variety of vaccinia virus strains belonging to two distinct groups. During the 18th and 19th centuries, cases with vaccinia virus were thought to have evolved from repeated introduction of vaccinia.[177] In addition to cutaneous symptoms, patients reported fever, malaise, myalgia, headache, cough, and adenopathy.[168] Secondary bacterial infection of cutaneous lesions has been reported.

Because of the success of the smallpox eradication program in the United States, routine vaccinia vaccination was discontinued in 1971,[23,158] and by 1976, the recommendation of vaccinating health care workers also was discontinued.[19] However, the Advisory Committee on Immunization Practices (ACIP) continues to recommended vaccinating laboratory workers with ACAM2000 to protect them from possible infection while working with replication-competent vaccinia, recombinant vaccinia, or other orthopoxviruses capable of infecting humans (e.g., cowpox, monkeypox, variola).[62,75,136]

In 1982, the only active licensed producer of vaccinia vaccine in the United States ceased production for general use, and distribution to civilian populations was discontinued in 1983.[22] However, the CDC has continued to provide vaccinia vaccine for laboratory workers.[20,21,124,136] In 1984, the laboratory recommendations were formally included in guidelines for biosafety in microbiologic and biomedical laboratories. This was expanded to include persons working in animal care areas where studies with orthopoxviruses were performed.[165]

Since January 1982, smallpox vaccination has not been required for international travelers, and International Certificates of Vaccination no longer include smallpox vaccination.[186] Military personnel continued to be vaccinated routinely for several years after discontinuation. More recently, only selected groups of military personnel are vaccinated against smallpox; groups include those designated for military action in areas where the threat of biological warfare exists.

Recombinant Vaccinia Virus

Vaccinia virus is the prototype of the genus *Orthopoxvirus*.[55] It is a double-stranded DNA virus that has a broad host range under experimental conditions and is rarely isolated from animals outside the laboratory. Many strains of vaccinia virus exist with various levels of virulence in humans and animals. Some examples include the Temple of Heaven and Copenhagen vaccinia strains, which are highly pathogenic in animals, and the NYCBOH strain, from which the Wyeth vaccine was derived, which has relatively low pathogenicity in animals and humans.[59]

Vaccinia virus can be engineered genetically to contain and express foreign DNA without impairing the ability of the virus to replicate. Such foreign DNA can encode protein antigens that induce protection against one or more infectious agents. These recombinant vaccinia viruses created from several different strains have been engineered to express the immunizing antigens of many viruses, bacteria, parasites, and tumors of veterinary and medical importance.[70,104,169,170,187] In the United States, recombinant viruses have been made from the NYCBOH strain or a mouse neuroadapted derivative, the WR strain. Some recombinant viruses have been made from the Copenhagen and Lister vaccinia strains, which are more pathogenic in animals than the NYCBOH strain. More recently, studies using recombinant vaccinia to vaccinate against prostate cancer, malaria, Middle East Respiratory Syndrome corona virus, tuberculosis, and HIV have used the Ankara strain.[7,71,86,143] Animal studies generally suggest that recombinant viruses may be no more pathogenic than the parent strain of vaccinia virus. However, no consistently reliable laboratory marker or animal test has been able to predict the attenuation of vaccinia virus or a particular recombinant virus for humans.[147] Laboratory-acquired infections with vaccinia or recombinant viruses have been reported[98,139,166]; however, no surveillance system exists to monitor laboratory workers, and thus the risk for acquiring infection in persons who handle virus cultures or contaminated materials is not known.

With the initiation of human and veterinary trials using recombinant vaccines, physicians, nurses, veterinarians, and other personnel may be susceptible to both vaccinia and recombinant agents. This exposure could occur from direct contact with the recombinant virus or contaminated dressings, but the risk for transmission is unknown. To date, no reports of transmission to health care personnel from vaccine recipients have been published. When appropriate infection control precautions are observed, health care workers exposed to smaller volumes and lower titers of virus may be at less risk for acquiring infection in contrast to their laboratory counterparts.[167] However, because the risk for transmission exists in such persons, the ACIP suggests that all those who work or enter laboratories or animal care facilities where vaccinia, monkeypox, or cowpox viruses are being handled demonstrate evidence of vaccination. Vaccination is advised at least every 10 years for those working with vaccinia viruses. Personnel should also observe appropriate biosafety guidelines and infection control procedures.[136,142,158,165,167,183]

Camelpox

Camelpox virus is an orthopoxvirus that is genetically the closest known virus to variola virus (smallpox virus).[50] Its disease is restricted to camels, and it is enzootic in all regions (except Australia) where camel breeding is practiced. The illness in camels is severe, with smallpox-like lesions, and has led to development of vaccines for use in camels.[141] Human cases are occasionally reported in the literature,[9] generally noted in animal handlers in areas where human contact with camels is common. Human illness has been mild and limited to a few cutaneous lesions.

Orf Virus

Orf virus is a member of the genus *Parapoxvirus* (see Table 58.1). Orf disease, also called *ecthyma contagiosum*,[55] is an occupationally acquired disease, with most cases occurring in adults.[67,112] The reservoir hosts of orf virus are sheep and goats, and the virus has worldwide distribution. Human disease is characterized by single or multiple lesions that last approximately 35 to 40 days, progress through six stages, and most often are located on the hands.[67,112] The stages include maculopapular (1–7 days), target (7–14 days), acute (14–21 days), regenerative (21–28 days), papillomatous (28–35 days), and regressive (35 to ≥40 days). Patients may have low-grade fever, but regional lymphadenitis is an uncommon finding. A range of less typical presentations due to orf virus infection has also been reported. Two patients with a widespread papulovesicular eruption, fever, malaise, and lymphadenopathy were described.[184] A giant orf granuloma was described in a 12-year-old boy who lived on a farm.[137] These atypically proliferating giant orf lesions have occurred in both immunosuppressed and immunocompetent individuals. Complications after infection can occur, including erythema multiforme, bullous pemphigoid, swan-neck deformity of a finger, paresthesia, and autoimmune blistering disorders. A burn unit in Turkey reported a nosocomial outbreak involving 13 cases in which orf virus affected damaged and exposed skin.[123] Mortality among flocks of goats and sheep infected with orf virus can be very high, which could be economically damaging.[79]

The CDC reported four unrelated cases of cutaneous, self-resolving orf virus infections in people either exposed to sheep or goats with oral lesions or who had been vaccinated recently with live orf virus vaccine. These cases occurred in New York, Illinois, California, and Tennessee, and patients' ages ranged from 11 to 51 years.[31] Uzel and colleagues[179] reported nine cases of orf virus infection in Turkey related to feasts of sacrifice; adults involved in the preparation of the animals for consumption were found to be at risk. Four additional cases reported in the United States between 2009 and 2011 highlighted the potential for household exposures to the virus, including how food was prepared from infected animals.[32] Orf virus infections generally do not require treatment; however, use of imiquimod in complicated cases in immunocompetent hosts[54] and in immunocompromised patients has been reported.[113]

Until recently, diagnosis of orf virus depended on electron microscopy or serology. In 2001, Torfason and Gunadóttir[176] described a PCR method to detect orf virus that helped make identification of the virus more accessible.[182]

Orf virus has been shown to have immunomodulatory characteristics, antifibrotic as well as antiviral activity against recurrent genital herpes disease in guinea pigs, against hepatitis B and herpes simplex virus 1 in mice, and against hepatitis C in vitro.[134,186] The protection in mice happens by modulating the host innate immune system, inducing phagocytosis, natural killer cell activity, and release of interferon-α, tumor necrosis factor-α, interleukin-2, and granulocyte-macrophage colony-stimulating factor. This finding may have implications for immune therapy for patients with serious infection from these viruses.[182] Furthermore, the low virulence in humans and ability to repeatedly infect has made orf virus a potential backbone for delivery of oncologic treatments.[155]

Other Parapoxviruses

Human infections with pseudocowpox virus and bovine papular stomatitis virus are considered occupational diseases. Pseudocowpox infections occur on the hands of milkers, and infections with bovine papular stomatitis virus have also been reported on the hands of veterinarians and others with close contact with cows.[16,55,121] The initially red lesions of the pseudocowpox nodule are relatively painless, but they may be pruritic and will eventually become purple. They are firm, do not ulcerate, and typically last 4 to 6 weeks. In comparison, the lesions caused by bovine papular stomatitis virus are wartlike and typically last 3 to 4 weeks.

Additionally, reports on humans infected with other parapoxviruses from reindeer and seals are available.[56,57,156] One report noted that in a human infection with sealpox virus, the person had orflike lesions that resolved after biopsy specimens were obtained.[35]

Yatapoxviruses

Tanapox virus, yaba-like disease virus (YLDV), and yaba monkey tumor virus (YMTV) are three viruses found in monkeys that can cause human infection.[41,47,48,55,92] DNA maps of tanapox virus and YLDV are extremely similar, indicating they may be the same. Tanapox in humans first was observed along the Tana River in Kenya in 1957, and outbreaks in Africa, including the DRC, have involved both children and adults.[55,92]

The illness starts with fever, headache, backache, and mild prostration; skin lesions occur 2 to 4 days after onset. Individual lesions start as an itchy path, followed by the development of a pocklike lesion. At 7 days, lesions are approximately 10 mm in diameter with surrounding erythema. Lymphadenitis is both local and regional. The lesions ulcerate during the second week of illness and last approximately 6 weeks. Most patients have a single lesion, but some have 2 to 10 lesions. The prognosis usually is good, although secondary bacterial infection can occur.

Two cases of tanapox were reported in the United States. The first case was a 51-year-old man with papular lesions with general malaise after visiting Tanzania and being exposed to a cat.[173] A second case occurred in a 21-year-old female student from New Hampshire, who developed fever, headaches, malaise, and several papules after being exposed to chimpanzees in the DRC.[36] The symptoms of both patients were diagnosed using PCR techniques and resolved spontaneously. As international travel increases, more case reports of such poxvirus illnesses may surface. PCR techniques to diagnose such infections quickly have been developed,[45,173,188] and these methods will assist in rapid diagnosis of poxvirus illnesses that may be confused with more serious illnesses such as smallpox and monkeypox. Of interest, tanapox virus has been recently been studied in human cancer cell lines in hope of developing an oncolytic viral vaccine to be used therapeutically in a variety of human cancers with minimal side effects.[114]

YMTV was isolated from tumors in monkeys in Nigeria, and animal handlers in primate centers in the United States have become ill as a result of this virus. Human infections have not been identified in the field in Africa. YMTV produces epidermal histiocytomas, tumorlike masses of histiocytic polygonal mononuclear cell infiltrates that may advance to suppurative inflammation.[41]

Molluscum Contagiosum Virus

In contrast to the other zoonotic poxviruses discussed in this chapter, *molluscum contagiosum* virus is a human virus that is a common cause of human skin lesions[55] (see Chapter 60B and Table 58.1). The virus has not been grown in cell culture as yet, but has been extracted from human lesions, and it does not cause infection in experimental animals. Analysis of viral DNA from lesions in geographically different patients indicates existence of two major subtypes and a third, rare subtype. The clinical aspects of molluscum contagiosum virus infection are presented in Chapter 60B.

DIAGNOSIS AND DIFFERENTIAL DIAGNOSIS

Because all but two viruses presented in this chapter are zoonotic agents, careful attention must be given to geographic location and animal exposure. All diseases described here are characterized by local lesions, which easily can be collected for direct identification. All poxviruses can be identified by examination of material from lesions by electron microscopy and by PCR.[130] All viruses except molluscum contagiosum virus grow in one or more tissue culture systems, the chorioallantoic membrane of embryonated eggs, or both. Unusual agents should be referred to specific reference laboratories for species identification.

NEW REFERENCES SINCE THE SEVENTH EDITION

2. Alzhanova D, et al. T cell inactivation by poxviral B22 family proteins increases viral virulence. *PLoS Pathog*. 2014;10(5):e1004123.
6. Becker C, et al. Cowpox virus infection in pet rat owners: not always immediately recognized. *Dtsch Arztebl Int*. 2009;106(19):329-334.
10. Berthet N, et al. Maculopapular lesions in the Central African Republic. *Lancet*. 2011;378(9799):1354.
11. Blumberg S, Lloyd-Smith JO. Inference of R(0) and transmission heterogeneity from the size distribution of stuttering chains. *PLoS Comput Biol*. 2013;9(5):e1002993.
33. Centers for Disease Control and Prevention. Smallpox vaccine guidance. Available at: http://www.cdc.gov/poxvirus/monkeypox/clinicians/smallpox-vaccine.html.
37. Crickard L, et al. Protection of rabbits and immunodeficient mice against lethal poxvirus infections by human monoclonal antibodies. *PLoS ONE*. 2012;7(11):e48706.
38. Czerny CP, et al. Characterization of a cowpox-like orthopox virus which had caused a lethal infection in man. *Arch Virol Suppl*. 1997;13:13-24.
39. Dabrowski PW, et al. Genome-wide comparison of cowpox viruses reveals a new clade related to Variola virus. *PLoS ONE*. 2013;8(12):e79953.
49. Dumont C, et al. Simple technique for in field samples collection in the cases of skin rash illness and subsequent PCR detection of orthopoxviruses and varicella zoster virus. *PLoS ONE*. 2014;9(5):e96930.
51. Duraffour S, et al. Emergence of cowpox: study of the virulence of clinical strains and evaluation of antivirals. *PLoS ONE*. 2013;8(2):e55808.

53. Ellis CK, et al. Ecology and geography of human monkeypox case occurrences across Africa. *J Wildl Dis.* 2012;48(2):335-347.
56. Essbauer S, Pfeffer M, Meyer H. Zoonotic poxviruses. *Vet Microbiol.* 2010;140(3-4):229-236.
63. Florescu DF, Keck MA. Development of CMX001 (brincidofovir) for the treatment of serious diseases or conditions caused by dsDNA viruses. *Expert Rev Anti Infect Ther.* 2014;12(10):1171-1178.
64. Formenty P, et al. Human monkeypox outbreak caused by novel virus belonging to Congo Basin clade, Sudan, 2005. *Emerg Infect Dis.* 2010;16(10):1539-1545.
65. Franceschi V, et al. BoHV-4-based vector single heterologous antigen delivery protects STAT1(−/−) mice from monkeypoxvirus lethal challenge. *PLoS Negl Trop Dis.* 2015;9(6):e0003850.
68. Golden JW, et al. Side-by-side comparison of gene-based smallpox vaccine with MVA in nonhuman primates. *PLoS ONE.* 2012;7(7):e42353.
69. Graef S, et al. Clinicopathological findings in persistent corneal cowpox infection. *JAMA Ophthalmol.* 2013;131(8):1089-1091.
71. Haagmans BL, et al. An orthopoxvirus-based vaccine reduces virus excretion after MERS-CoV infection in dromedary camels. *Science.* 2016;351(6268):77-81.
73. Hammarlund E, et al. Monkeypox virus evades antiviral CD4+ and CD8+ T cell responses by suppressing cognate T cell activation. *Proc Natl Acad Sci USA.* 2008;105(38):14567-14572.
74. Hatch GJ, et al. Assessment of the protective effect of Imvamune and Acam2000 vaccines against aerosolized monkeypox virus in cynomolgus macaques. *J Virol.* 2013;87(14):7805-7815.
80. Hudson PN, et al. Elucidating the role of the complement control protein in monkeypox pathogenicity. *PLoS ONE.* 2012;7(4):e35086.
81. Hughes LJ, et al. A highly specific monoclonal antibody against monkeypox virus detects the heparin binding domain of A27. *Virology.* 2014;464-465:264-273.
85. Hutson CL, et al. Transmissibility of the monkeypox virus clades via respiratory transmission: investigation using the prairie dog-monkeypox virus challenge system. *PLoS ONE.* 2013;8(2):e55488.
97. Johnston SC, et al. In vitro inhibition of monkeypox virus production and spread by Interferon-beta. *Virol J.* 2012;9:5.
101. Kenner J, et al. LC16m8: an attenuated smallpox vaccine. *Vaccine.* 2006;24(47-48):7009-7022.
105. Kinnunen PM, et al. Orthopox virus infections in Eurasian wild rodents. *Vector Borne Zoonotic Dis.* 2011;11(8):1133-1140.
106. Kinnunen PM, et al. Severe ocular cowpox in a human, Finland. *Emerg Infect Dis.* 2015;21(12):2261-2263.
107. Kugelman JR, et al. Genomic variability of monkeypox virus among humans, Democratic Republic of the Congo. *Emerg Infect Dis.* 2014;20(2):232-239.
109. Kurth A, et al. Cowpox virus outbreak in banded mongooses (*Mungos mungo*) and jaguarundis (*Herpailurus yagouaroundi*) with a time-delayed infection to humans. *PLoS ONE.* 2009;4(9):e6883.
111. Learned LA, et al. Extended interhuman transmission of monkeypox in a hospital community in the Republic of the Congo, 2003. *Am J Trop Med Hyg.* 2005;73(2):428-434.
123. Midilli K, et al. Nosocomial outbreak of disseminated orf infection in a burn unit, Gaziantep, Turkey, October to December 2012. *Euro Surveill.* 2013;18(11): 20425.
127. Nakazawa Y, et al. Phylogenetic and ecologic perspectives of a monkeypox outbreak, southern Sudan, 2005. *Emerg Infect Dis.* 2013;19(2):237-245.
128. Nakazawa Y, et al. Mapping monkeypox transmission risk through time and space in the Congo Basin. *PLoS ONE.* 2013;8(9):e74816.
131. Nolen LD, et al. Introduction of monkeypox into a community and household: risk factors and zoonotic reservoirs in the Democratic Republic of the Congo. *Am J Trop Med Hyg.* 2015;93(2):410-415.
133. Pahlitzsch R, Hammarin AL, Widell A. A case of facial cellulitis and necrotizing lymphadenitis due to cowpox virus infection. *Clin Infect Dis.* 2006;43(6):737-742.
134. Paulsen D, et al. Inactivated ORF virus shows antifibrotic activity and inhibits human hepatitis B virus (HBV) and hepatitis C virus (HCV) replication in preclinical models. *PLoS ONE.* 2013;8(9):e74605.
135. Pelkonen PM, et al. Cowpox with severe generalized eruption, Finland. *Emerg Infect Dis.* 2003;9(11):1458-1461.
136. Petersen BW, et al. Use of vaccinia virus smallpox vaccine in laboratory and health care personnel at risk for occupational exposure to orthopoxviruses—recommendations of the Advisory Committee on Immunization Practices (ACIP), 2015. *MMWR Morb Mortal Wkly Rep.* 2016;65(10):257-262.
138. Pfeffer M, et al. Retrospective investigation of feline cowpox in Germany. *Vet Rec.* 2002;150(2):50-51.
141. Prabhu M, et al. Evaluation of stability of live attenuated camelpox vaccine stabilized with different stabilizers and reconstituted with various diluents. *Biologicals.* 2014;42(3):169-175.
142. Supplemental recommendations on adverse events following smallpox vaccine in the pre-event vaccination program: recommendations of the Advisory Committee on Immunization Practices. *MMWR Morb Mortal Wkly Rep.* 2003;52(13):282-284.
149. Reynolds MG, et al. A silent enzootic of an orthopoxvirus in Ghana, West Africa: evidence for multi-species involvement in the absence of widespread human disease. *Am J Trop Med Hyg.* 2010;82(4):746-754.
155. Rintoul JL, et al. ORFV: a novel oncolytic and immune stimulating parapoxvirus therapeutic. *Mol Ther.* 2012;20(6):1148-1157.
158. Rotz LD, et al. Vaccinia (smallpox) vaccine: recommendations of the Advisory Committee on Immunization Practices (ACIP), 2001. *MMWR Recomm Rep.* 2001;50(RR-10):1-25, quiz CE1-7.
164. Schwarzer H, et al. Severe ulcerative keratitis in ocular cowpox infection. *Graefes Arch Clin Exp Ophthalmol.* 2013;251(5):1451-1452.
165. U.S. Department of Health and Human Services. Biosafety in microbiological and biomedical laboratories. HHS Publication No. (NIH) 88-8396. Washington, DC: U.S. Government Printing Office; 1984:78-79.
167. Siegel JD, et al. 2007 guideline for isolation precautions: preventing transmission of infectious agents in health care settings. *Am J Infect Control.* 2007;35(10):S65-S164.
174. Stittelaar KJ, et al. Modified vaccinia virus Ankara protects macaques against respiratory challenge with monkeypox virus. *J Virol.* 2005;79(12):7845-7851.
175. Thomassen HA, et al. Pathogen-host associations and predicted range shifts of human monkeypox in response to climate change in central Africa. *PLoS ONE.* 2013;8(7):e66071.
183. Wharton M, et al. Recommendations for using smallpox vaccine in a pre-event vaccination program. National Emergency Training Center; 2003.

The full reference list for this chapter is available at ExpertConsult.com.

165 Mimiviruses

Ramya Ramraj • Gail D. Harrison

In 1992, while investigating the source of an outbreak of community-acquired pneumonia in a hospital in Bradford, in northern England, investigators discovered a bizarre microorganism.[13,14] The microorganism, resembling a small gram-positive coccus, was found inside a free-living amoeba in a water cooling tower. Researchers initially thought it was a bacterium, but subsequent analysis demonstrated a giant double-stranded DNA virus, and it was reported in 2003 to be a giant virus of amoeba called *Acanthamoeba polyphaga mimivirus* (APMV), more commonly known now as *Mimivirus*. Originally named mimivirus or "mimicking microbe" because it resembled bacteria in Gram-stained smears, it now is designated officially as a quasi-autonomous virus, *Acanthamoeba polyphaga mimivirus.* It is a member of the order Megaviridae, family Mimiviridae (nucleocytoplasmic large DNA viruses), and genus *Mimivirus*, defining a new fourth domain of life containing these nucleocytoplasmic large DNA viruses.[4-6,15] There is now a closely related *Mamavirus* comparable to the complex virus *Mimivirus*, so named because it appears larger than *Mimivirus*, but with similar characteristics.

There are now four new proposed families of giant viruses that have been isolated: Pandoravirus, Pithovirus, Faustovirus, and Mollivirus. The role of these giant viruses in human disease is still unknown. The role of the megavirome in human disease is still emerging.

STRUCTURE AND PROPERTIES

A. polyphaga mimivirus is a giant, double-stranded, icosahedral DNA virus.[34] With a diameter of approximately 650 nm, *Mimivirus* is the fourth largest virus known to date. *Mimivirus* morphologically resembles nucleocytoplasmic large DNA viruses (NCLDVs), such as the iridovirus, asfarvirus, and phycodnavirus.[10,30] However, evolutionary dissimilarities define a new family, the Mimiviridae.[13] *Mimivirus* comprises a central dense core that is surrounded by two lipid membrane layers inside a capsid protein shell covered by fibrils. The 1.2-Mb genome sequence[19,22,25] is complex and possesses genes that are shared by the NCLDV families as well as several that have not been identified previously in viruses. The origins and the various processes[1] involved in shaping gene content of *Mimivirus* are not entirely clear at this time.[13,19] It appears that these giant virus particles contain mRNA and more than 100 proteins; they have gene repertoires that are broad and encode for translation components. The mimiviruses also are infected by virophages, including the satellite virus Sputnik virophage, a 740-Å diameter satellite virus with an icosahedral capsid and a lipid membrane inside a protein shell that infects mamaviruses. Sputnik is thought to have been derived from other viruses, prior to its association with the giant *Mimivirus*.[6,8,28]

The virus can survive on inanimate surfaces for at least 30 days, is resistant to alcohol-based biocidal agents, but is inactivated by free chlorine and glutaraldehyde.[3,10]

VIRAL REPLICATION

In *A. polyphaga*, the replication cycle of *Mimivirus* starts with entry of the virus by phagocytosis, followed by a 4-hour eclipse phase inside the nucleus,[13] and then the formation of the "virus factory" in the cytoplasmic space,[29] ending with cell lysis and virus release 24 hours after infection (Fig. 165.1). The virus factory,[20] where virus replication and assembly occur, is the major site of production of *Mimivirus* DNA and induces profound alteration of the infected cell structure, such as by recruitment of organelles and organization of cellular compartments. Very specific mechanisms and complex interactions between viral and cellular factors that are not entirely clear at this time must be involved to build this remarkably large and efficient virus factory, which can generate this sophisticated microorganism rapidly.[29] The Sputnik virophage infects the giant viruses of the genus *Mimivirus*.[8]

ANIMAL SUSCEPTIBILITY

An experimental model of infection was developed to establish a possible role of *Mimivirus* as a human pathogen. Autopsy specimens of laboratory mice that were inoculated intracardially with infecting units of *Mimivirus* revealed histopathologic evidence of pneumonia, and mimiviruses were reisolated from samples from the lung.[12] Inoculation of human

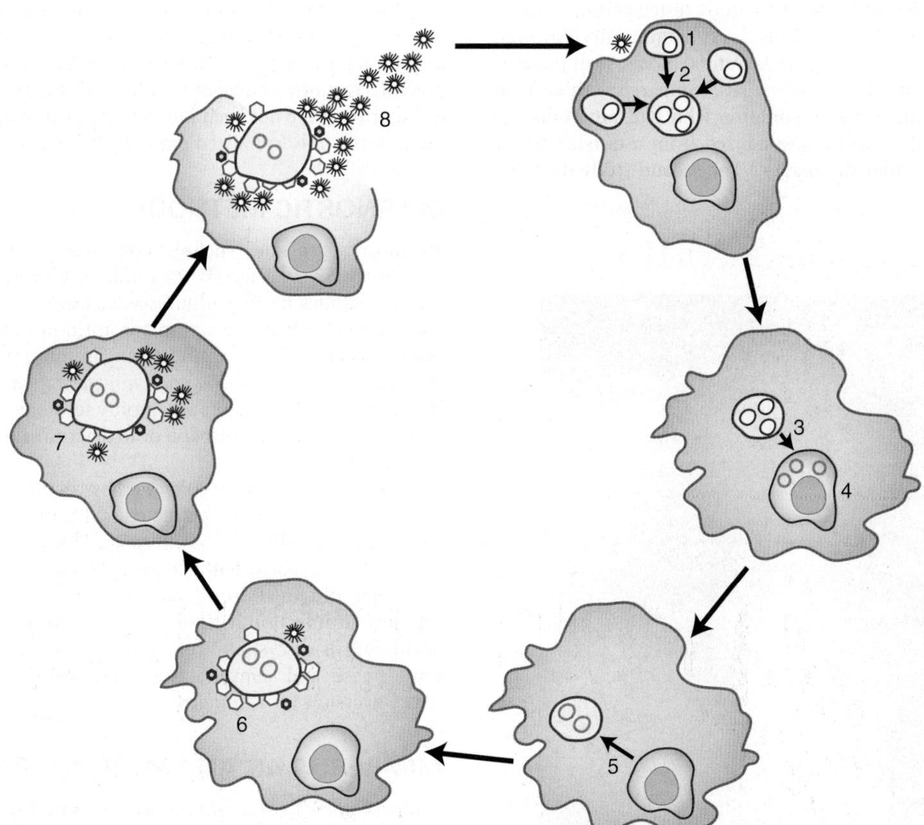

FIG. 165.1 Schematic representation of the *Acanthamoeba polyphaga mimivirus* replication cycle. *1, Mimivirus* entry through a phagocytic vacuole. *2,* Fusion of phagocytic vacuoles and delivery of *Mimivirus* genetic material into the cell cytoplasm *(3)*. *3, Mimivirus* DNA entry into the host nucleus, where the first round of DNA replication could begin *(4)*. *5,* At 3 hours after infection, *Mimivirus* DNA comes from the host nucleus to form the virus factory (VF) replication center. *6,* At 5 hours after infection, the VF size shows a 50% increase, and viral proteins begin to be detected; proviral capsid assembly and viral capsids budding from the VF central core can be observed. *7,* Empty or DNA-filled capsids accumulate near the central core, resulting in a growing VF with viral particles free in the cytoplasm. *8,* Complete viral capsids surrounded by fibrils may be released through cell lysis. (From Suzan-Monti M, La Scola B, Barrassi L, et al. Ultrastructural characterization of the giant volcano-like virus factory of *Acanthamoeba polyphaga mimivirus*. *PLoS One*. 2007;2:e328.)

macrophages with mimiviruses showed evidence of infection, although no evidence of a lytic cycle was observed.[23] Efforts to induce infection in other cell lines were futile, and the target cell in mice remains to be identified.

MIMIVIRUS INFECTION IN HUMANS

In December 2004, a laboratory technician in France developed subacute pneumonia with dry cough, fever, and chest pain.[24] This technician was in charge of performing *Mimivirus* serologic testing and Western blot analysis and thus had handled relatively large amounts of *Mimivirus* antigens. Radiographic examination of his chest revealed bilateral basilar infiltrates (Fig. 165.2). The illness did not respond to amoxicillin-clavulanate treatment prescribed on day 15 after the onset of symptoms, but after an additional 2 weeks, the illness resolved, and the technician made a full recovery. Serum samples screened against pneumonia agents showed seroconversion (<1:50 to 1:3200) only for *Mimivirus,* which was confirmed by testing with two-dimensional Western blotting against 23 identified proteins of *Mimivirus. Mimivirus* has also been isolated from a patient with pneumonia.[26]

Little is known about the host defense relationship of *Mimivirus* with humans. However, studies have shown that it is recognized by the human immune system, and it is able to interfere with the human type 1 interferon system.[27]

Prevalence of Antibodies to *Mimivirus* in Patients With Pneumonia

Three early studies investigated the prevalence of antibodies to *Mimivirus* in specific human populations.[23] The first study tested serum samples obtained from 376 Canadian patients with community-acquired pneumonia and from 511 healthy subjects. A total of 9.66% of patients with pneumonia had antibodies to *Mimivirus,* compared with 2.3% of control subjects.[18] Patients with pneumonia who had antibodies to *Mimivirus* were more likely to be hospitalized from a nursing home and to be rehospitalized after discharge.[16] The second study included 26 patients from Marseille, France, who acquired pneumonia while in an intensive care unit and 50 control serum samples (from blood donors). Antibodies to *Mimivirus* were detected in samples obtained from five patients but in none of the control samples.[16] The third serosurvey involved 157 patients in intensive care units who had pneumonia. Serum specimens obtained from these patients were tested against a panel of antigens from "conventional" pneumonia agents as well as ameba-associated microorganisms, including *Mimivirus.*[2] Evidence of infection with conventional pathogens was found in 28 cases and with ameba-associated pathogens in 18 cases. In the group infected by ameba-associated pathogens, more patients had seroconversion to *Mimivirus* than to any other pathogen (five cases), and seroconversion was more common among patients with ventilator-associated pneumonia than among those with community-acquired pneumonia (31.6% and 10.5% of patients, respectively). Additional serologic studies have shown an association of *Mimivirus* seropositivity and increased duration of mechanical ventilation and prolonged stay in the intensive care unit in adult patients.[32]

However, studies that have used molecular detection techniques of reverse transcription–polymerase chain reaction (RT-PCR) have not detected *Mimivirus* DNA in respiratory secretions of hospitalized adult and pediatric patients with pneumonia.[7,17,32,33] Taken together, these studies reveal a significant rate of seroconversion and seropositivity in hospitalized patients with either community-acquired pneumonia or hospital-acquired pneumonia, but direct detection of the pathogen in clinical respiratory secretions has not been confirmed.[23]

The first isolation of *Mimivirus* from a patient with pneumonia has been reported.[26]

Mimivirus has been detected by molecular and virologic methods to be present on inanimate surfaces in hospital settings, especially in respiratory-isolation units, suggesting that mimiviruses may play a potential role nosocomial or health care–associated infections.[9] However, mimiviruses have not been found to be a cause of ventilatory-associated pneumonia in hospitalized patients in intensive care units.[31]

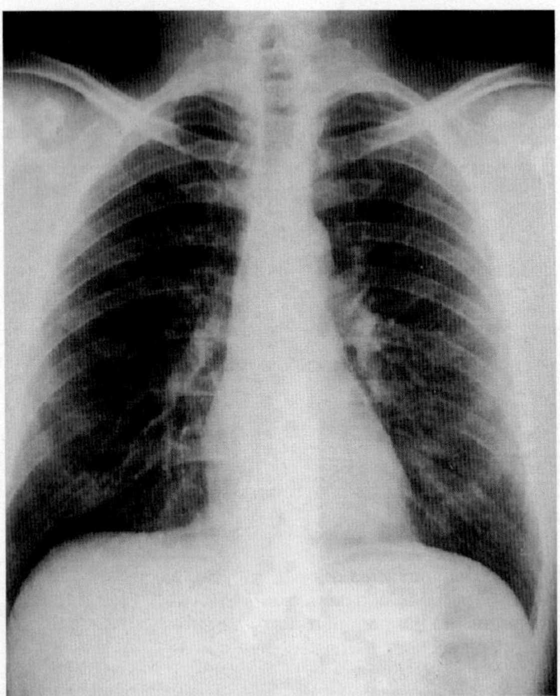

FIG. 165.2 Chest radiograph of a laboratory technician who was infected with *Mimivirus,* with bilateral basilar infiltrates evident. (From Raoult D, La Scola B, Birtles R, et al. The discovery and characterization of *Mimivirus,* the largest known virus and putative pneumonia agent. *Clin Infect Dis.* 2007;45:95–102.)

DIAGNOSTIC METHODS

Diagnostic strategies include collection of nasal wash specimens, bronchoalveolar lavage (BAL) fluid, and serologic samples. Serologic testing includes immunofluorescence assay of samples of acute-phase and convalescent-phase serum for antibodies to proteins specific for *Mimivirus.*[2] However, one study using immunoproteomics showed cross reaction between *Mimivirus* and *Francisella tularensis*, suggesting caution in interpretation of results when only serologic methods are employed to diagnose *Mimivirus* infection or to determine associations of *Mimivirus* and pneumonia.[21]

Mimivirus also can be cultivated by coculture with amoeba.[11] It also can be detected in DNA extracted (QIAamp tissue kit; Qiagen) from BAL samples amplified by a PCR assay.[2] However, real-time PCR methods have failed to consistently detect *Mimivirus* in clinical respiratory secretions obtained from patients with pneumonia. The strongest evidence of infection includes a combination of positive BAL culture, positive PCR assays, and fourfold increase in antibody titer between acute-phase and convalescent-phase serum samples or significant seroconversion for *Mimivirus.*[2]

MIMIVIRUS AS AN EMERGING PATHOGEN

Evidence indicates that *Mimivirus* is a new human pathogen that causes pneumonia.[3] However, *Mimivirus* does not replicate efficiently in coculture with any of the mammalian cells tested to date, and serologic cross reactions among pathogens are observed commonly. Isolation of the virus or DNA detection by RT-PCR from respiratory secretions of patients with pneumonia has not consistently confirmed the presence of the pathogen directly in clinical samples from adults and children.[16,35]

Mimivirus infection in hospitalized children with pneumonia has not been confirmed.[35] However, *Mimivirus* has been isolated from a patient with pneumonia on at least one occasion and has been detected in the blood and lymph node of a child.[26]

NEW REFERENCES SINCE THE SEVENTH EDITION

6. Colson P, LaScola B, Levasseur A, et al. Mimivirus: leading the way in the discovery of giant viruses of amoebae. *Nat Rev Microbiol.* 2017;15(4):243-254.
8. Desnues C, Boyer M, Raoult D. Sputnik, a virophage infection the viral domain of life. *Adv Virus Res.* 2012;82:63-89.
9. Dos Santos Silva L, Arantes T, Andrade K, et al. High positivity of mimivirus in inanimate surfaces of a hospital respiratory-isolation facility, Brazil. *J Clin Virol.* 2015;66:62-65.
11. Khallil J, Andreani J, La Scola B. Updating strategies for isolation and discovering giant viruses. *Curr Opin Microbiol.* 2016;31:80-87.
26. Saadi H, Pagnier I, Colson P, et al. First isolation of mimivirus in a patient with pneumonia. *Clin Infect Dis.* 2013;57(4):e127-e134.
27. Silva L, Almelda G, Oliveira D, et al. A resourceful giant: APMV is able to interfere with the human type 1 interferon system. *Microbes Infect.* 2014;16(3): 187-195.
28. Sun S, La Scola B, Bowman V, et al. Structural studies of the Sputnik virophage. *J Virol.* 2010;84(2):894-897.
31. Vanspauwen M, Schnabel R, Bruggman C, et al. Mimivirus is not a frequent cause of ventilator associated pneumonia in critically ill patients. *J Med Virol.* 2013;85(10):1836-1842.
35. Zhang X-A, Zhu T, Zhang P-H, et al. Lack of mimivirus detection in patients with respiratory disease, China. *Emerg Infect Dis.* 2016;22(11):2011-2012.

The full reference list for this chapter is available at ExpertConsult.com.

SUBSECTION I RNA—Picornaviridae

Enteroviruses, Parechoviruses, and Saffold Viruses 166

James D. Cherry • Paul Krogstad

Enteroviruses (EVs), parechoviruses (PeVs), and Saffold viruses (SAFVs) are members of three distinct genera of the Picornaviridae family of small RNA viruses. Although these viruses have clear differences in their structural features and molecular biology, they have overlapping clinical features and epidemiology and are therefore discussed together in this chapter.

HISTORY

Poliomyelitis, the first enteroviral disease to be recognized and the most important one, has a long history.[894] The earliest record is an Egyptian stele of the 18th dynasty (1403–1365 BCE) that shows a young man with a withered, shortened leg, the characteristic deformity of paralytic poliomyelitis.[503,768] Michael Underwood,[1111] a London pediatrician, published the first medical description in 1789 in *A Treatise on Diseases of Children*. During the 19th century, many reports appeared in Europe and the United States describing small clusters of cases of "infantile paralysis." These investigators were puzzled about the nature of the affliction; not until the 1860s and 1870s was the spinal cord firmly established as the seat of the pathologic process. The contagious nature of poliomyelitis was not appreciated until the late 19th century. Medin, a Swedish pediatrician, was the first to describe the epidemic nature of poliomyelitis (1890), and his pupil Wickman[1163] worked out the basic principles of the epidemiology.

The virus was isolated first in monkeys by Landsteiner and Popper[669] in 1908. The availability of a laboratory animal assay system opened many avenues of research that in the ensuing decades led to the demonstration that an unrecognized intestinal infection was the usual manifestation and the finding that paralytic disease was a relatively uncommon event.

Coxsackieviruses and echoviruses have had a shorter history. Epidemic pleurodynia was described clinically in 1735 by Hannaeus[455] more than 200 years before the coxsackieviral origin of this disease was discovered. In 1948, Dalldorf and Sickles[280] first reported the isolation of a coxsackievirus after inoculation of suckling mice.

In 1949, Enders and associates[333] described the growth of poliovirus 2 in tissue culture, and their techniques paved the way for recovery of a large number of other cytopathic viruses. Most of these "new" viruses failed to produce illness in laboratory animals. Because the relationships of many of these newly recovered agents with human disease were unknown, these agents were called *orphan viruses*.[767] Later, several agents were grouped together and were called *e*nteric *c*ytopathogenic *h*uman *o*rphan viruses, or echoviruses. Two such viruses identified in 1956 by Wigand and Sabin in studies of summer diarrhea were originally classified as echoviruses 22 and 23 but were reclassified into a new genus *(Parechovirus)* in the late 1990s because of features of their structure and replication that distinguish them from EVs.[1045] Similarly, stool cultures of a child evaluated in 1981 for prolonged fever revealed a novel virus that became the first recognized SAFV when molecular methods revealed similarities to known members of the cardiovirus genus of the picornavirus family.[580,1218]

Inactivated and live-attenuated poliovirus vaccines became available in the late 1950s and early 1960s, and the most notable advance since the late 1980s has been a dramatic reduction in worldwide poliomyelitis as a result of the global immunization initiative.[249,527,881,1080] The last case of confirmed paralytic poliomyelitis in the Western Hemisphere caused by a wild-type virus strain occurred in 1991.[953]

Since the 1950s, pandemics of specific nonpolio EV have occurred. These were caused by echovirus 9 in the 1950s, coxsackievirus A16 in the 1960s, and, more recently, EVs 71 and D68. Interestingly, during the period of almost universal use of oral poliovirus vaccines (OPVs) between the 1960s and 2000 there were no nonpolio virus pandemics. In the present era with the switch from OPV to inactivated poliovirus vaccines (IPV) both EV 71 and EV D68 have emerged in much of the developed world.

THE VIRUSES

Classification

EVs, PeVs, and SAFVs are RNA viruses belonging to the family Picornaviridae (*pico*, "small").* These viruses are grouped together because they share certain physical, biochemical, and molecular properties. In electron micrographs, the viruses are seen as 30-nm particles that consist of naked (nonenveloped) protein capsids, constituting approximately 70% to 75% of the mass of particles that contain the genomic RNA.

To bring order to the growing list of poliovirus-like agents, coxsackieviruses, echoviruses, and polioviruses first were categorized together and named in 1957 by a committee sponsored by the National Foundation for Infantile Paralysis.[774] The human alimentary tract was thought to

*References 207, 351, 535, 771, 772, 775, 773, 880, 927, 974, 1044.

TABLE 166.1 **Original Classification of Human Enteroviruses: Animal and Tissue Culture Spectrum**[a]

		CYTOPATHIC EFFECT		ILLNESS AND PATHOLOGY	
Virus	**Antigenic Types**[b]	**Monkey Kidney Tissue Culture**	**Human Tissue Culture**	**Suckling Mouse**	**Monkey**
Polioviruses	1–3	+	+	–	+
Coxsackieviruses A	1–24[c]	–	–	+	–
Coxsackieviruses B	1–6	+	+	+	–
Echoviruses	1–34[d]	+	±	–	–

[a]Many enterovirus strains have been isolated that do not conform to these categories, thus leading to the revised classification scheme shown in Table 166.2.
[b]New types, beginning with type 68, were initially assigned enterovirus type numbers instead of coxsackievirus or echovirus numbers. Types 68 through 71 were identified before the strategy for taxonomy was changed, as described in the text.
[c]Coxsackievirus A23 was found to be the same as echovirus 9.
[d]Echovirus 10 was reclassified as a reovirus; echoviruses 22 and 23 were made the first members of the *Parechovirus* genus within the picornavirus family, and echovirus 28 was reclassified as a rhinovirus.
+, Present; –, absent; ±, variably present.
Modified from Cherry JD. Enteroviruses. In: Remington JS, Klein JO, eds. *Infectious Diseases of the Fetus and Newborn Infant.* 3rd ed. Philadelphia: WB Saunders, 1990:325–66.

be the natural habitat of these agents, and the term *enterovirus* was coined. They were originally distributed into four groups (Table 166.1) on the basis of their different effects in tissue culture and pattern of disease in experimentally infected animals: polioviruses (causal agents of poliomyelitis in humans and nonhuman primates), coxsackieviruses A (associated with herpangina, human central nervous system [CNS] disease, and flaccid paralysis in suckling mice), group B coxsackieviruses (human CNS and cardiac disease, spastic paralysis in mice), and the echoviruses (nonpathogenic in mice and not linked to human disease at first). Although this scheme was useful initially, many strains were isolated subsequently that do not conform to such rigid specificities. For example, several coxsackievirus A strains replicate and have a cytopathic effect in monkey kidney tissue cultures, and some echovirus strains cause paralysis in mice.

For this reason, and to simplify the nomenclature, EVs subsequently were assigned sequential numbers. Following this convention, the prototype EV strains Fermon, Toluca-1, J 670/71, and BrCr (identified between 1959 and 1973) were designated EV 68 through EV 71, respectively. Additional EVs continued to be identified that could not be identified using antisera specific for the classic serotypes. More than 50 distinct additional EVs have been identified by culture and molecular detection methods, although not all have not been linked to human disease.

Since the late 1990s, genetic, biologic, and molecular properties have been used to revise picornavirus taxonomy. Determining the nucleotide sequence encoding the viral VP1 capsid protein plays a major role in this approach and predictably identifies viruses originally classified by serologic means, thus leading to the term *molecular serotyping.*[860,861,915,923] This phylogenetic technique formed the basis for taxonomic reorganization of the EVs known to infect humans into four alphabetically designated species (EV-A, EV-B, EV-C, and EV-D) (Table 166.2). The three polioviruses (PV1–PV3) are members of EV-C, in view of their close molecular relationship with other members of the species.[123]

As noted previously, two of the original echoviruses (echoviruses 22 and 23) were found to have genomic and proteomic differences from the other early "enteroviruses" and were reclassified as first members of the new genus *Parechovirus* as *Human Parechovirus* (HPeV) types 1 and 2.[927,1045,1046] Fourteen additional types of human HPeV have now been identified. Similarly, hepatitis A virus was initially assigned the designation EV 72, but it was reclassified as the prototype of the *Hepatovirus* genus within the picornavirus family because of marked genetic and biologic distinctions from all other picornaviruses.

The *Cardiovirus* genus of the Picornaviridae has been augmented by identification of the SAFVs. Beginning with a strain isolated in 1981 and characterized in 2007, 11 genetically distinct SAFVs have been identified since 2007 and grouped into the Cardiovirus B species.[580]

The application of molecular phylogenetic approaches has also revealed that recombination between circulating picornaviruses is a frequent event and is likely to increase the genetic diversity of EVs,

TABLE 166.2 **Genomic Classification of Enteroviruses**[a]

Species Designation	**Types**
Enterovirus A (EV-A)	Coxsackievirus A2–8, 10, 12, 14, 16
	Enterovirus A71, A76, A89, A90, A91, A114, A119
Enterovirus B (EV-B)	Coxsackievirus A9
	Coxsackievirus B 1–6
	Echovirus 1–9, 11–21, 24–27, 29–33
	Enterovirus B69, B73–75, B77–88, B93, B97, B98, B100, B101, B106, B107
Enterovirus C (EV-C)	Poliovirus 1–3
	Coxsackievirus A 1, 11, 13, 17, 19–22, 24
	Enterovirus C95, C96, C99, C102, C104, C105, C109, C113, C116–C118
Enterovirus D (EV-D)	Enterovirus D68, D70, D94, D111

[a]Coxsackievirus A15 has been reclassified as a strain of coxsackievirus A11, and coxsackievirus A18 has been reclassified as a strain of coxsackievirus A13. Echovirus 34 has been recognized as a variant of coxsackievirus A24.
From King AM, Adams MJ, Carstens EB, et al, eds. Virus Taxonomy: Classification and Nomenclature of Viruses: Ninth Report of the International Committee on Taxonomy of Viruses. San Diego: Elsevier; 2011.

cardioviruses, and PeVs.* This propensity for recombination has played a role in more recent outbreaks of paralytic diseases involving vaccine-derived strains of poliovirus.[615]

Morphology and Replication

EVs, PeVs, and SAFVs have single-stranded, positive-sense RNA genomes that are 7.4 to 8 kb in length.[916] For all three, the genome consists of a 5′ noncoding region followed by a single long open-reading frame, a short 3′ noncoding region, and a poly-A tail. The 5′ noncoding region contains a 450-nucleotide internal ribosome entry site that recruits the translational machinery to an initiation site approximately 740 nucleotides downstream from the 5′ terminus of the viral RNA. The 3′ noncoding region folds into a highly conserved structure that is required for initiation of the synthesis of a minus-sense viral RNA that in turn is the template for the message-sense genomic RNA. This genome is packaged into capsids that exhibit icosahedral symmetry with 20 triangular faces and 12 vertices.

Replication of EVs begins with the adsorption of virions to cell surface receptors; most of those known are integrins or immunoglobulin-like

*References 83, 173, 215, 311, 719–721, 863, 867, 1030, 1062.

TABLE 166.3 Cellular Receptors and Cofactors for Infection of Representative Enteroviruses

Virus	HEV Species	Receptor	Cofactor for Infection[a]
Enterovirus 71	EV-A	PSGL-1, SCARB2	
Coxsackieviruses B1–6	EV-B	CAR	Some group B coxsackieviruses may use CD55 (DAF) or heparan for attachment
Echovirus 9	EV-B	$\alpha_v\beta_3$ integrin (vitronectin receptor)	MAP-70
Echoviruses 1, 8	EV-B	VLA-2 ($\alpha_2\beta_1$ integrin)	Heparan sulfate
Coxsackieviruses A13, 17, 20, 21, 24	EV-C	ICAM-1	
Polioviruses 1–3	EV-C	CD155(PVR)	
Enterovirus 70	EV-D	CD55 (DAF)	

CAR, Coxsackie and adenovirus receptor; *DAF,* decay-accelerating factor; *HEV,* human enterovirus; *ICAM-1,* intercellular adhesion molecule 1; *MAP-70,* microtubule-associated protein 70; *PSGL-1,* P-selectin glycoprotein ligand 1; *Pvr,* poliovirus receptor; *SCARB2,* scavenger receptor class B member 2; *VLA-2,* a human integrin.
[a]The cofactors generally facilitate adhesion to cells, but their sole expression is insufficient to permit infection to occur.

proteins (Table 166.3). The virions penetrate the surface of the cell and undergo conformational changes that release the viral genome, which functions as the messenger RNA that encodes viral polyprotein.[693,1014] This polypeptide contains three domains, P1 to P3, which are cleaved into three or four proteins each. The P1 region is liberated from the polyprotein by the viral 2A protein, a chymotrypsin-like protease. P1 initially is split into three proteins, VP0, VP1, and VP3, by the viral 3C protease. VP0 is subsequently processed during virion maturation into two smaller proteins, VP4 and VP2. Portions of VP1, VP2, and VP3 are exposed at the surface of the virion, whereas VP4 is entirely internal. VP1, VP2, and VP3 have no sequence homology but share the same topology.[927] Specifically, they form an eight-stranded antiparallel β-barrel that is wedge shaped and comprises two antiparallel β-sheets. The amino acid sequences in the loops that connect the β-strands and the N- and C-terminal sequences that extend from the β-barrel domain of VP1, VP2, and VP3 give each EV its distinct antigenicity. The replication of EVs occurs in the cytoplasm in membrane-associated replication complexes and is completed rapidly (5–10 hours). Studies of polioviruses and coxsackieviruses have shown that enteroviral replication is associated with disruption of cellular protein secretion, and host-cell protein synthesis is suppressed because of cleavage of human eukaryotic translation initiation factor 4G (eIF4G) by enteroviral 2A proteases, which abrogates cap-dependent translation. The coxsackievirus 2A protein also cleaves dystrophin, a cytoskeletal protein; this activity has been hypothesized to play a role in damage to the myocardium.[52,301]

The PeVs replicate in a similar fashion.[652] Integrins ($\alpha_v\beta_3$ and perhaps $\alpha_v\beta_1$ and $\alpha_v\beta_6$) are used as receptors, and replication occurs in cytoplasmic structures.[776] However, the P1 portion of the viral polyprotein is processed into only three capsid proteins, and only one protease has been identified in the PeVs. In addition, PeV replication occurs in small, discrete foci in the cytoplasm, rather than in large accumulations of membranous vesicles like the EVs. Moreover, transcription and translation do not appear to be disrupted by the PeVs, thus perhaps explaining their relatively mild and delayed cytopathic effect when they are grown in tissue culture.[1045]

The replication of the Saffold cardioviruses has not been specifically examined, but genetic similarities to Theiler murine encephalomyelitis virus (TMEV) and other murine cardioviruses suggest that they possess a single protease related to the 3C protease of other picornaviruses.[488] The SAFV genome also appears to encode a leader (L) protein at the amino terminus of the viral polyprotein. The L proteins of TMEV and encephalomyocarditis viruses are thought to modulate viral translation, innate immune responses, and cellular apoptosis.[488]

Replication Characteristics and Host Systems

EVs and PeVs are relatively stable viruses in that they retain activity for several days at room temperature and can be stored indefinitely at ordinary freezer temperatures (−20°C [−4°F]). They are inactivated quickly by heat (>56°C [132.8°F]), formaldehyde, chlorination, and ultraviolet light, but they are refractory to ether, ethanol, and isopropanol.[771,775,880,960]

Enteroviral strains grow rapidly when adapted to susceptible host systems and cause cytopathologic features in 2 to 7 days. The typical tissue culture cytopathic effect is shown in Fig. 166.1; characteristic pathologic findings in mice are shown in Figs. 166.2 and 166.3. Final titers of virus recovered in the laboratory vary markedly among different viral strains and the host system used; typically, concentrations of 10^4 to 10^8 infectious units/mL tissue culture fluid or tissue homogenate are obtained. Unadapted viral strains frequently require long periods of incubation. In both tissue culture and suckling mice, evidence of growth usually is visible. Blind passage occasionally is necessary for the cytopathologic features to become apparent.

Although many different primary and secondary tissue culture systems support the growth of various EVs, primary rhesus monkey kidney cultures generally are accepted to have the most inclusive spectrum.[126,1053] Other simian kidney tissue cultures, however, also have the same broad spectrum. Tissue cultures of human origin have a more limited spectrum, but several echovirus types have shown more consistent primary isolation in human than in monkey kidney culture. A satisfactory system for the primary recovery of EVs from clinical specimens would include the following: primary rhesus, cynomolgus, or African green monkey kidney; a diploid, human embryonic lung fibroblast cell strain; rhabdomyosarcoma cell line tissue cultures; and intraperitoneal and intracerebral inoculation of suckling mice younger than 24 hours.[76,464,478,771,775,960,1053]

Antigenic Characteristics

Although some minor cross-reactions exist among several coxsackievirus and echovirus types, common group antigens of diagnostic importance have not been defined well.[770,771,768,775,880] Heat treatment of virions and the use of synthetic peptides have produced antigens with broad enteroviral reactivity.[1082,1083] These antigens have been used in enzyme-linked immunosorbent assay and complement fixation tests to determine immunoglobulin (Ig) G and IgM enteroviral antibodies and for antigen detection. In one study, Terletskaia-Ladwig and colleagues[1082] reported the identification of patients infected with EVs by the use of an IgM enzyme immunoassay. This test used heat-treated coxsackievirus B5 and echovirus 9 as antigens, and it identified patients infected with echoviruses 4, 11, and 30. The sensitivity of the test was 35%. In another study involving heat-treated virus or synthetic peptides, the respective sensitivities were 67% and 62%.[1083] However, both tests lacked specificity. Intratypic strain differences are common findings, and some strains (prime strains) are neutralized poorly by antisera to prototype viruses. In animals, however, these prime strains induce antibodies that neutralize the specific prototype viruses.

The identification of polioviral, coxsackieviral, and echoviral types by neutralization in suckling mice or tissue culture with antiserum pools is relatively well defined. Neutralization is induced by the epitopes on structural proteins VP1, VP2, and VP3; in particular, several epitopes are clustered on VP1. Prime strains do cause diagnostic difficulty because frequently they are not neutralized by the reference antisera, a particular problem with echoviruses 4, 9, and 11 and EV 71. If these types are suspected, in some instances this problem can be overcome by using antisera in less diluted concentrations or antisera prepared against several different strains of problem viruses. Kubo and associates[655] were able to type enteroviral isolates not identified through neutralization by

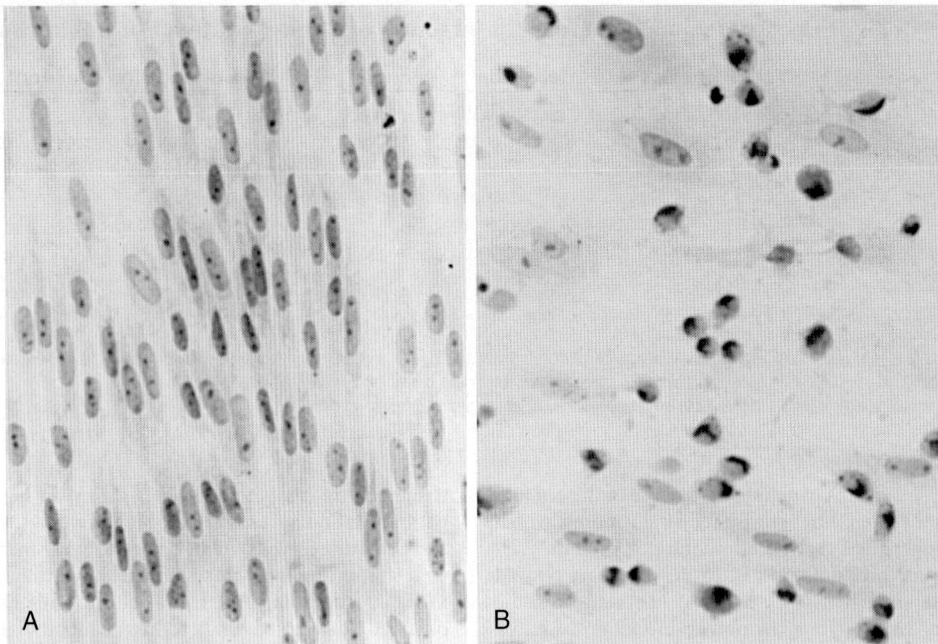

FIG. 166.1 Fetal rhesus monkey kidney tissue culture (HL-8). (A) Uninoculated tissue culture. (B) Echovirus 11 cytopathic effect. (From Cherry JD. Enteroviruses. In: Remington JS, Klein JO, eds. *Infectious Diseases of the Fetus and Newborn Infant.* Philadelphia, PA: WB Saunders; 1976.)

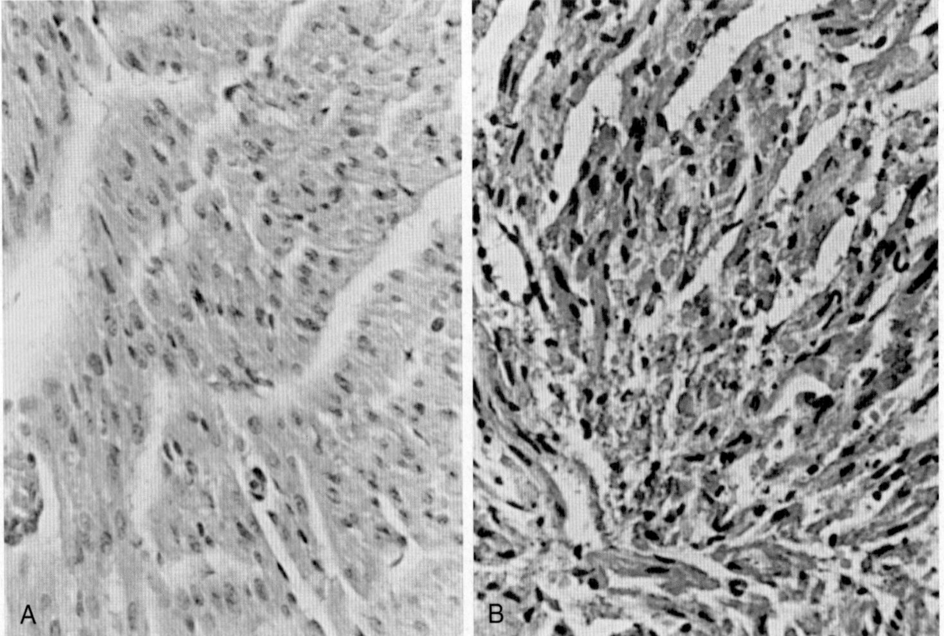

FIG. 166.2 Suckling mouse myocardium. (A) Normal suckling mouse myocardium. (B) Myocardium of a suckling mouse infected with coxsackievirus B1. (From Cherry JD. Enteroviruses. In: Remington JS, Klein JO, eds. *Infectious Diseases of the Fetus and Newborn Infant.* Philadelphia, PA: WB Saunders; 1976.)

nucleotide sequence analysis of the VP4 gene. These investigators specifically identified prime strains of echovirus 18 and EV 71. Sequence analysis of the VP1 gene also is useful for typing enteroviral prime strains not identified by neutralization.[850]

Host Range

Humans are the only natural hosts of polioviruses, coxsackieviruses, and echoviruses.[1,279,399,623,767,1011,1158,1160] However, EVs have been recovered in nature from sewage, flies, swine, dogs, a calf, a budgerigar, a fox, mussels, monkeys, and oysters.[200] In addition, serologic evidence of infection with EVs similar to human strains has been noted in chimpanzees, cattle, rabbits, a fox, a chipmunk, and a marmot.[200] Various EVs that are distinct from the human EVs have been isolated from nonhuman primates.[862] Contamination of shellfish also is interesting because, in addition to a possible role in human infection, shellfish offer a source of enteroviral storage during periods of cold weather.[200] Contaminated food is another possible source of human infection.[200]

EPIDEMIOLOGY

Transmission

The spread of human EVs, PeVs, and also presumably SAVFs, is from person to person by the fecal-oral and possibly the oral-oral (respiratory spread) route. Swimming and wading pools may serve as a means of

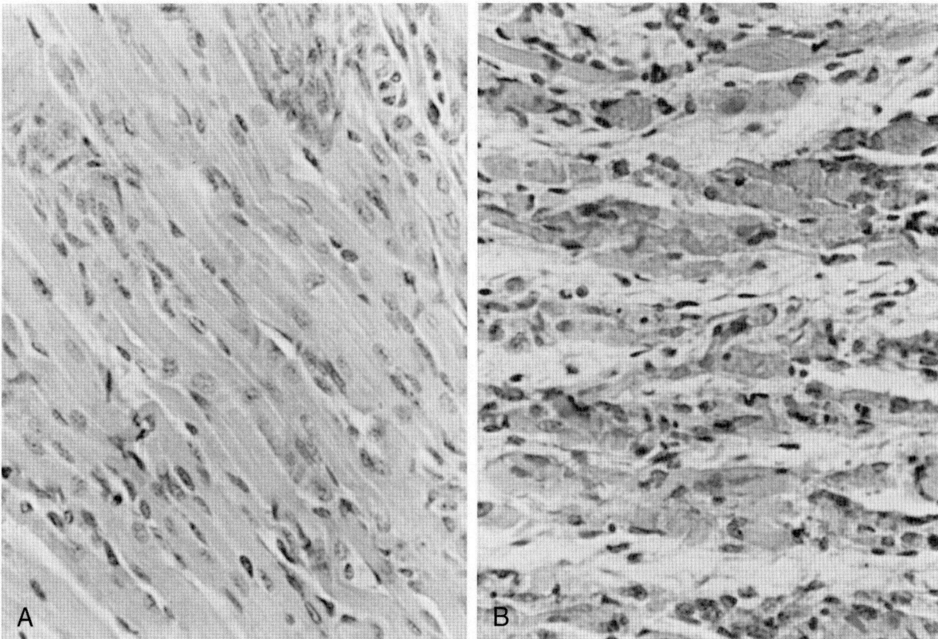

FIG. 166.3 Suckling mouse skeletal muscle. (A) Normal suckling mouse skeletal muscle. (B) Skeletal muscle of a mouse infected with coxsackievirus A16. (From Cherry JD. Enteroviruses. In: Remington JS, Klein JO, eds. *Infectious Diseases of the Fetus and Newborn Infant.* Philadelphia, PA: WB Saunders; 1976.)

spread of EVs during the summer.[611] Oral-oral transmission by way of the contaminated hands of health care personnel and transmission by fomites were documented in a long-term care pediatric ward.[572] EVs have been recovered from trapped flies, and such carriage probably contributes to the spread of human infection, particularly in lower socioeconomic populations with poor sanitation facilities.[200] Between 1972 and 2004, Sinclair and colleagues[1032] noted 13 outbreaks of EV disease related to swimming in lakes, pools, or the ocean. One noteworthy point-source outbreak occurred in a group of travelers to Mexico who swam in contaminated seawater.[71] Of 29 travelers (25 teenagers and four adults) 21 became ill; four had echovirus 30 infection, 11 had coxsackievirus A1 infection, and four had both viruses isolated.

Children comprise the main susceptible cohort; they are immunologically susceptible, and their unhygienic habits facilitate the spread of infection. Spread is from child to child (from feces to skin to mouth) and then within family groups. Recovery of EVs is related inversely to age, but the prevalence of specific antibodies is related directly to age. The incidence of infection and the prevalence of antibodies do not differ between boys and girls.

Geographic Distribution and Season

EVs, PeVs, and SAFVs have worldwide distribution.[200,362,381,399,1218] Neutralizing antibodies for specific viral types have been noted in serologic surveys throughout the world, and most strains have been recovered in global isolation studies. In any given area, frequent fluctuations occur in predominant types. Epidemics probably depend on newly susceptible individuals in the population rather than on reinfection. Epidemics may be localized and sporadic, and they may vary in origin from place to place in the same year. Pandemic waves of infection also occur.

In temperate climates enteroviral infections occur primarily in the summer and fall, but in the tropics they are prevalent all year.[200,399,770] A basic concept in understanding the epidemiology of these illnesses concerns the far greater frequency of unrecognized infection than clinical disease, as illustrated by poliomyelitis, which remained an epidemiologic mystery until researchers appreciated that unrecognized infections were the main source of contagion. Serologic surveys were instrumental in elucidating the problem; in populations living in conditions of poor sanitation and hygiene, epidemics did not occur, but wide dissemination of polioviruses was confirmed by demonstrating the presence of specific antibodies to all three types in almost 100% of children by the time they reached 5 years of age.

Epidemics of poliomyelitis first began to appear in Europe and the United States during the latter part of the 19th century; they continued with increasing frequency in economically advanced countries until the introduction of effective vaccines in the 1950s and 1960s.[104,238,503,894] The evolution from endemic to epidemic follows a characteristic pattern beginning with collections of a few cases, then endemic rates that are higher than usual, followed by severe epidemics with high attack rates. The age group attacked in endemic areas and in early epidemics is the youngest; more than 90% of paralytic cases begin in children younger than 5 years of age. Once this pattern of epidemicity begins, it is irreversible unless preventive vaccination is performed.

As epidemics recur over a period of years, a shift in age incidence occurs whereby relatively fewer cases are seen in the youngest children; the peak often is in the 5- to 14-year-old group, and increasing percentages of cases develop in young adults. These changes are correlated with socioeconomic factors and improved standards of hygiene—when children are protected from immunizing infections in the first few years of life, the pool of susceptible persons builds up, and introduction of a virulent strain often is followed by an epidemic.[503] The extensive use of vaccines since the late 1950s resulted in the elimination of paralytic poliomyelitis from large geographic areas, but the disease remains endemic in various parts of the world. Although seasonal periodicity is distinct in temperate climates, some viral activity does take place during the winter months.[200] Infection and the acquisition of postinfection immunity occur with greater intensity and at earlier ages in crowded, economically deprived populations with less efficient sanitation.

Molecular techniques have allowed researchers to study the genotypes of specific viral types in populations over the course of time.[308,545,706,814] For example, Mulders and colleagues[814] studied the molecular epidemiology of wild poliovirus 1 in Europe, the Middle East, and the Indian subcontinent. These investigators found that four major genotypes were circulating. Two genotypes were found predominantly in Eastern Europe, a third genotype was circulating mainly in Egypt, and the fourth genotype was dispersed widely. All four genotypes were present in Pakistan.

Prevalence of Different Types

The epidemiologic behavior of coxsackieviruses and echoviruses parallels that of polioviruses, in which unrecognized infections far outnumber infections with distinctive symptoms. The agents are disseminated widely throughout the world, and outbreaks caused by one or another type occur regularly. These outbreaks tend to be localized, with different agents prevalent in different years. In the late 1950s, however, echovirus 9 had a far wider circulation; it swept through a large part of the world and infected not only children but also young adults.

Coxsackievirus A16 viral infection with hand-foot-and-mouth disease first was noted in Toronto and New Zealand in 1957.[211] Subsequently, illness caused by this virus was noted throughout the world. Antibody studies and viral isolation studies in 1957 to 1963 in California and Wisconsin indicated that coxsackievirus A16 was a newly circulating virus.[205,211] Since the 1960s, coxsackievirus A16 outbreaks of hand-foot-and-mouth disease continued to occur in the United States. However, since 1968, this virus has not been one of the five most prevalent yearly isolates (Table 166.4).

EV 71 was first isolated in California from patients with aseptic meningitis from 1969 to 1972.[872,1003] Subsequently, this virus has been noted in the United States in association with aseptic meningitis and occasionally with encephalitis. The clinical manifestations of EV 71 changed, and the chronology of this change is presented by Ooi and colleagues.[872] In addition to aseptic meningitis, hand-foot-and-mouth disease and a broad range of encephalitis presentations (e.g., paralytic disease and brainstem encephalitis) occurred. In Japan, in 1973,1977, and 1978, 1031 cases occurred; most patients had hand-foot-and-mouth disease. Since 1997, severe hand-foot-and-mouth disease with paralysis, cardiorespiratory dysfunction, and brainstem encephalitis has had epidemic occurrence in Malaysia, Taiwan, Singapore, Brunei, Japan, China, and other Asian-Pacific countries.[225,226,432,1081]

Although severe EV 71 disease has occurred occasionally in North America and Western Europe, epidemics similar to those occurring in the Asian-Pacific region have not been noted.[53,786,872] The three genotypes of EV 71 are A, B, and C. B and C have subtypes B 1 to 5 and C 1 to 5. However, a clear association does not appear to exist with specific subtypes and the occurrence of more severe disease. Chang and colleagues[179] found that the human leukocyte antigen (HLA)-A33 phenotype was associated with EV 71 infections. This HLA-A33 phenotype is common in Asian populations but is rare in white populations. This finding suggests a possible reason for the difference in epidemic occurrence in the Asian-Pacific region and the United States and Western Europe.

After a long absence, a particular agent may return and circulate among susceptible persons of different ages who have been born since the last epidemic. Other agents remain endemic in a given area and surface as sporadic cases and occasionally in small outbreaks. Multiple types frequently are active at the same time, although one agent commonly is predominant in a given locality.

Listed in Table 166.4 are the five most prevalent nonpolio enteroviral isolations per year in the United States from 1961 through 2013.[3,155,162,164,168,189,190,200,1057]

Most patients from whom viruses were isolated had neurologic illnesses. Other EVs also possibly were prevalent but did not cause clinical disease sufficiently severe enough to induce physicians to submit specimens for study. In addition, probably many coxsackievirus A infections, even in epidemic situations, have gone undiagnosed because inoculation of suckling mice was not performed. Although more than 62 nonpolio EV types and 16 PeV types have been identified, of interest is that in the 53 years covered in Table 166.4, only 26 different virus types are noted. Khetsuriani and associates[166] at the CDC presented an extensive report on enteroviral surveillance in the United States for the period from 1970 to 2005. During this period, the most common enteroviral isolates, in order, were as follows: echoviruses 9, 11, and 30; coxsackievirus B5; and echovirus 6. During the period from 2000 to 2005, the most common isolates, in order, were echoviruses 9, 30, 18, and 13 and coxsackievirus B5. The extensive EV surveillance report (between 1970 and 2005) contained data on both serotype and genomic species designation.[166] Of 49,637 viral isolates, 58 different EV serotypes and 2 PeV serotypes were identified. Of these isolates, 94.6%, 3.1%, 0.3%, and 0.1% were genomic species EV-B, EV-A, EV-C, and EV-D, respectively, and 1.9% were PeVs. Similar serotype and genomic species data are also available for 2006 to 2008.[168] During this period, 15 serotypes were identified, 13 of which were genomic species EV-B.

Similar data for the most common enteroviral isolates in Spain from 1988 to 1997 and in Belgium from 1980 to 1994 are available.[314,1099] The EV isolated most frequently in both countries was echovirus 30. In 1997 and 1998, major epidemic disease caused by EV 71 occurred in Taiwan, Malaysia, Australia, and Japan.[122,176,491,646,759]

Even though the use of live polioviral vaccine has eliminated epidemic poliomyelitis in the United States, determining the effect of polio vaccine viruses on EV ecology has been difficult. In 1970, polioviruses accounted for only 6% of the total number of enteroviral isolations from patients with neurologic illnesses.[200] Although the numbers are not directly comparable, more than one-third of the enteroviral isolations in 1962 from similar patients were polioviruses.[200] However, Horstmann and colleagues[504] studied specimens from sewage and from asymptomatic children during the early vaccine era and noted that the number of yearly polioviral isolations (presumably vaccine strains) was greater than the number of nonpolio EVs. The prevalence of vaccine viruses apparently did not affect the seasonal epidemiology of other EVs.

PATHOGENESIS AND PATHOLOGY

Events During Pathogenesis

Fig. 166.4 diagrams the events in pathogenesis. After initial acquisition of virus by the oral or respiratory route, implantation occurs in the pharynx and the lower alimentary tract.[104,200,200,771,880,979] Within 1 day, the infection extends to the regional lymph nodes. On approximately the third day, minor viremia develops and results in the involvement of many secondary infection sites. In congenital infections, the infection is initiated during the minor viremia phase. Multiplication of virus in secondary infection sites coincides with the onset of clinical symptoms. Illness can vary from minor infection to fatal disease. Major viremia occurs during the period of multiplication of virus in secondary infection sites; this period usually lasts from the third to the seventh day of infection. In many echovirus and coxsackievirus infections, involvement of the CNS apparently occurs at the same time as other secondary organ involvement. Occasionally, the CNS symptoms of enteroviral infections are delayed, thus suggesting that seeding occurred later in association with the major viremic phase.

Cessation of viremia correlates with the appearance of serum antibody. The viral concentration in secondary infection sites begins to diminish on approximately the seventh day. However, infection continues in the lower intestinal tract for prolonged periods.

In Fig. 166.5, clinical and subclinical events in polioviral infections are presented. By 3 to 5 days after exposure, virus can be recovered from blood, the throat, and feces. This finding may be accompanied by symptoms of the "minor illness," or the infection may be unrecognized clinically. The end of the period of viremia coincides with the appearance of antibodies and the onset of clinical signs of CNS involvement. The available evidence favors blood as the main pathway of CNS invasion in natural disease, but experimental infections in monkeys indicated that the virus can travel along the axons of peripheral nerves. Possibly, when tonsillectomy is performed on a child with an inapparent poliovirus infection, the virus enters the nerve fibers exposed during surgery and spreads to the cranial nerve nuclei in the brain, thereby resulting in bulbar paralysis.

Factors That Affect Pathogenesis

The pathogenesis and pathology of EVs, PeVs, and SAFVs infections depend on the virulence, tropism, and inoculum concentration of virus, as well as on many specific host factors. EVs, PeVs, and SAFVs obviously have marked differences in both tropism and virulence. Although some generalizations can be made with regard to tropism, marked differences occur even among strains of specific viral types. Differences in the virulence of specific viral types may be the result of recombination or point mutations.[933,951,992]

Van Eden and associates[1117] studied 17 families during an outbreak of poliomyelitis caused by type 1 virus in the Netherlands. The findings suggested that HLA-related genetic factors were important in the

TABLE 166.4 **Predominant Types of Nonpolio Enteroviral Isolations in the United States, 1961–2013**[a]

	FIVE MOST COMMON VIRAL TYPES PER YEAR				
	First	**Second**	**Third**	**Fourth**	**Fifth**
1961	Coxsackievirus B5	Coxsackievirus B2	Coxsackievirus B4	Echovirus 11	Echovirus 9
1962	Coxsackievirus B3	Echovirus 9	Coxsackievirus B2	Echovirus 4	Coxsackievirus B5
1963	Coxsackievirus B1	Coxsackievirus A9	Echovirus 9	Echovirus 4	Coxsackievirus B4
1964	Coxsackievirus B4	Coxsackievirus B2	Coxsackievirus A9	Echovirus 4	Echovirus 6, coxsackievirus B1
1965	Echovirus 9	Echovirus 6	Coxsackievirus B2	Coxsackievirus B5	Coxsackievirus B4
1966	Echovirus 9	Coxsackievirus B2	Echovirus 6	Coxsackievirus B5	Coxsackievirus A9, A16
1967	Coxsackievirus B5	Echovirus 9	Coxsackievirus A9	Echovirus 6	Coxsackievirus B2
1968	Echovirus 9	Echovirus 30	Coxsackievirus A16	Coxsackievirus B3	Coxsackievirus B4
1969	Echovirus 30	Echovirus 9	Echovirus 18	Echovirus 6	Coxsackievirus B4
1970	Echovirus 3	Echovirus 9	Echovirus 6	Echovirus 4	Coxsackievirus B4
1971	Echovirus 4	Echovirus 9	Echovirus 6	Coxsackievirus B4	Coxsackievirus B2
1972	Coxsackievirus B5	Echovirus 4	Echovirus 6	Echovirus 9	Coxsackievirus B3
1973	Coxsackievirus A9	Echovirus 9	Echovirus 6	Coxsackievirus B2	Coxsackievirus B5, echovirus 5
1974	Echovirus 11	Echovirus 4	Echovirus 6	Echovirus 9	Echovirus 18
1975	Echovirus 9	Echovirus 4	Echovirus 6	Coxsackievirus A9	Coxsackievirus B4
1976	Coxsackievirus B2	Echovirus 4	Coxsackievirus B4	Coxsackievirus A9	Coxsackievirus B3, echovirus 6
1977	Echovirus 6	Coxsackievirus B1	Coxsackievirus B3	Echovirus 9	Coxsackievirus A9
1978	Echovirus 9	Echovirus 4	Coxsackievirus A9	Echovirus 30	Coxsackievirus B4
1979	Echovirus 11	Echovirus 7	Echovirus 30	Coxsackievirus B2	Coxsackievirus B4
1980	Echovirus 11	Coxsackievirus B3	Echovirus 30	Coxsackievirus B2	Coxsackievirus A9
1981	Echovirus 30	Echovirus 9	Echovirus 11	Echovirus 3	Coxsackievirus A9, echovirus 5
1982	Echovirus 11	Echovirus 30	Echovirus 5	Echovirus 9	Coxsackievirus B5
1983	Coxsackievirus B5	Echovirus 30	Echovirus 20	Echovirus 11	Echovirus 24
1984	Echovirus 9	Echovirus 11	Coxsackievirus B5	Echovirus 30	Coxsackievirus B2, A9
1985	Echovirus 11	Echovirus 21	Echovirus 6, 7[b]		Coxsackievirus B2
1986	Echovirus 11	Echovirus 4	Echovirus 7	Echovirus 18	Coxsackievirus B5
1987	Echovirus 6	Echovirus 18	Echovirus 11	Coxsackievirus A9	Coxsackievirus B2
1988	Echovirus 11	Echovirus 9	Coxsackievirus B4	Coxsackievirus B2	Echovirus 6
1989	Coxsackievirus B5	Echovirus 9	Echovirus 11	Coxsackievirus B2	Echovirus 6
1990	Echovirus 30	Echovirus 6	Coxsackievirus B2	Coxsackievirus A9	Echovirus 11
1991	Echovirus 30	Echovirus 11	Coxsackievirus B1	Coxsackievirus B2	Echovirus 7
1992	Echovirus 11	Echovirus 30	Echovirus 9	Coxsackievirus B1	Coxsackievirus A9
1993	Echovirus 30	Coxsackievirus B5	Coxsackievirus A9	Echovirus 7	Coxsackievirus B3
1994	Coxsackievirus B2	Coxsackievirus B3	Echovirus 6	Echovirus 30	Enterovirus 71
1995	Echovirus 9	Echovirus 11	Coxsackievirus A9	Coxsackievirus B2	Echovirus 30, coxsackievirus B5
1996	Coxsackievirus B5	Echovirus 17	Echovirus 6	Coxsackievirus A9	Coxsackievirus B4
1997	Echovirus 30	Echovirus 6	Echovirus 7	Echovirus 11	Echovirus 18
1998	Echovirus 30	Echovirus 9	Echovirus 11	Coxsackievirus B3	Echovirus 6
1999	Echovirus 11	Echovirus 16	Echovirus 9	Echovirus 14	Echovirus 25
2000	Coxsackievirus B5	Echovirus 6	Coxsackievirus A9	Coxsackievirus B4	Echovirus 11
2001	Echovirus 18	Echovirus 13	Coxsackievirus B2	Echovirus 6	Echovirus 4
2002	Echovirus 7	Echovirus 9	Coxsackievirus B1	Echovirus 11	Coxsackievirus B5
2003	Echovirus 9	Echovirus 30	Coxsackievirus B1	Coxsackievirus B4	Coxsackievirus A9
2004	Echovirus 30	Echovirus 9	Coxsackievirus A9	Coxsackievirus B5	Coxsackievirus B4
2005	Coxsackievirus B5	Echovirus 6	Echovirus 30	Echovirus 18	Coxsackievirus B3
2006	Echovirus 6	Echovirus 9	Coxsackievirus A9	Coxsackievirus B5	Coxsackievirus B3
2007	Coxsackievirus B1	Echovirus 18	Echovirus 9	Coxsackievirus B4	Echovirus 11
2008	Coxsackievirus B1	Echovirus 30	Echovirus 6	Echovirus 9	Echovirus 11
2009	Enterovirus D68	Echovirus 30	Coxsackievirus B1, B4	Echovirus 9	Echovirus 18
2010	Parechovirus 3	Echovirus 6	Echovirus 18	Coxsackievirus B5	Echovirus 18
2011	Echovirus 6	Coxsackievirus B3	Echovirus 30	Coxsackievirus B1	Echovirus 18
2012	Coxsackievirus A6	Parechovirus 3	Coxsackievirus A9	Echovirus 11	Coxsackievirus B4
2013	Echovirus 11	Parechovirus 1	Parechovirus 3	Coxsackievirus B4	Echovirus 18

[a]The majority of patients from whom viruses were isolated had neurologic illnesses.
[b]Third and fourth place tie.
Data from references 3, 155, 159, 160, 162, 164, 168, 200, and 1057; J.P. Alexander and L.J. Anderson, LJ, Respiratory and Enterovirus Branch, Centers for Disease Control, personal communication, 1990; H. Gary, Respiratory and Enteric Viruses Branch, CDC, personal communication, 1996; and A. LaMonte-Fowlkes, Epidemiology Branch, Division of Viral Diseases, National Center for Immunization and Respiratory Diseases, Centers for Disease Control and Prevention, personal communication, for the 2005 data.

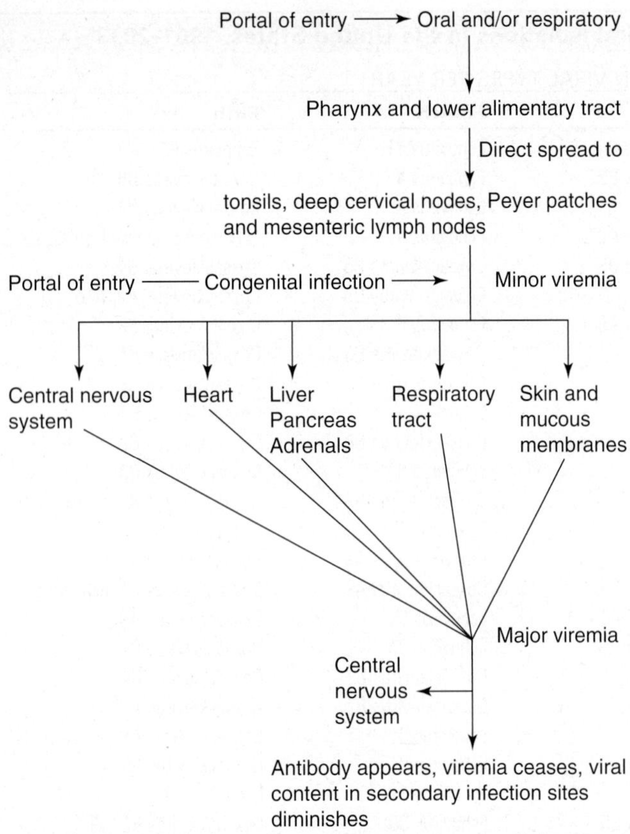

FIG. 166.4 Pathogenesis of enteroviral infections. (From Cherry JD. Enteroviruses. In: Remington JS, Klein JO, eds. *Infectious Diseases of the Fetus and Newborn Infant*. Philadelphia, PA: WB Saunders; 1976.)

occurrence of paralytic disease. In a study of 219 EV 71 cases and 97 control children in Taiwan, Chang and associates[178] found that susceptibility was related to HLA-A33. The phenotypic frequency of HLA-A33 is approximately 17% to 35% in Asian populations, whereas it is only 0% to 1% in white populations. These investigators suggest that this population genetic difference may explain the general lack of severe EV 71 disease (with encephalitis or polio-like syndrome with or without cardiopulmonary failure) in the United States. The greatest risk factor in this study, however, was male sex.

EV and PeV infections in the fetus and neonate generally are thought to be more severe than similar infections in older persons. This situation undoubtedly is the case with coxsackievirus B infection and probably also with coxsackievirus A, echovirus and PeV infections. Although the reasons for this increased severity are unknown, several aspects of neonatal immune mechanisms have been suggested. In addition, the similarity of coxsackievirus B infections in suckling mice to those in human neonates provided a useful animal model system. Heineberg and associates[472] compared coxsackievirus B1 infections in 24-hour-old suckling mice with similar infections in older mice. These investigators noted that adult mice produced interferon in all infected tissues, whereas suckling mice produced only small amounts of interferon in the liver. These researchers thought that the difference in outcome of coxsackievirus B1 infection in suckling and older mice could be explained by the inability of cells of the immature animals to elaborate interferon. Additional studies of abnormalities of innate immunity in neonates may enhance our understanding of the severity of enteroviral infections in newborns.[692]

Other researchers suggested that the increased susceptibility of suckling mice to severe coxsackievirus infections is related to the transplacentally acquired, increased concentrations of adrenocortical hormones.[73,106] Kunin[658] suggested that the difference in age-specific susceptibility could be explained at the cellular level. He showed that various tissues of newborn mice bind coxsackievirus B3, whereas tissues of adult mice are virtually inactive in this regard.[658,657] The

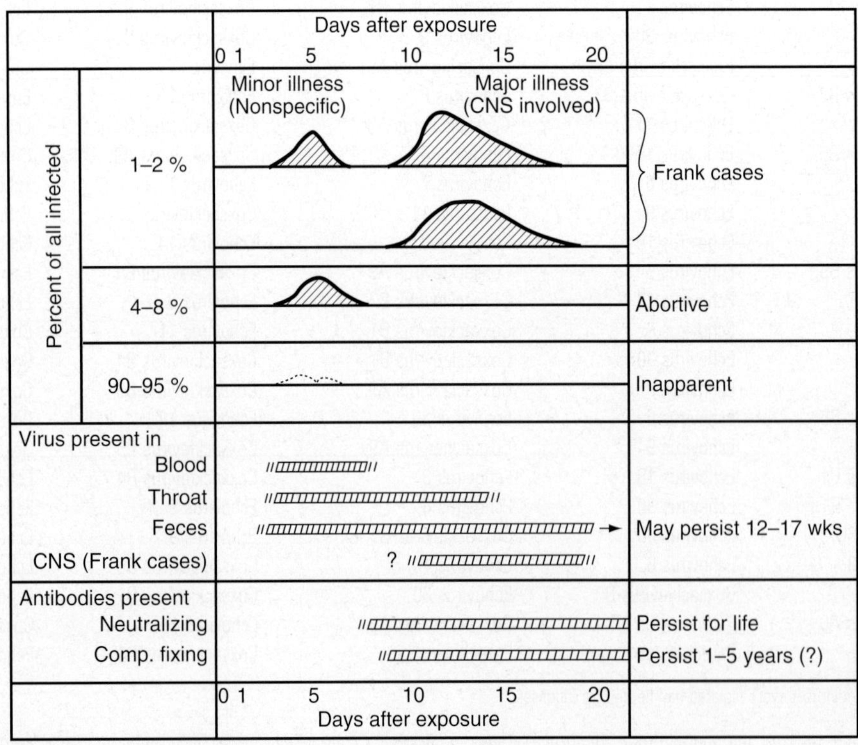

FIG. 166.5 Course of clinical and subclinical forms of poliovirus infection in relation to the presence of virus and the development of antibodies. *CNS*, Central nervous system; *Comp.*, Complement. (From Bodian D, Horstmann DM. Poliomyelitis. In: Horsfall FL, Tamm I, eds. *Viral and Rickettsial Infections of Man*. 4th ed. Philadelphia, PA: Lippincott; 1965:430–473.)

progressive loss of receptor-containing cells with increasing age may be the mechanism that accounts for less severe infections in older animals. Supporting this suggestion, Ito and colleagues[550] showed that expression of coxsackievirus and adenovirus receptor (CAR) decreases with increasing age in rats. In the past, researchers assumed that specific disease in various organs and tissues in enteroviral infections was caused by the direct cytopathic effect and tropism of a particular virus. In more recent years, however, large numbers of studies using murine model systems suggested that host immune responses contribute to the pathologic process.[*] These studies suggested that T-cell–mediated processes and virus-induced autoimmunity cause both acute and chronic tissue damage. In contrast, other studies suggested that the primary viral cytopathic effect is responsible for the tissue damage and that the various T-cell responses are a reaction to the damage and not its cause.[757]

Since the early 1960s, the clinical manifestations caused by several enteroviral serotypes have changed. For example, echovirus 11 infection initially was noted in association with an outbreak of upper respiratory tract infection in a day care center in 1958.[904] Then, in the 1960s, this infection was found to be related to exanthem and aseptic meningitis.[204,210] Following this event and occurring in the 1980s was the association of echovirus 11 infection and severe sepsis-like illness with hepatitis in neonates.[107,200,200,449,579,789,809]

Another example relates to EV 71 infections. Initially, this virus was noted in association with aseptic meningitis, and only a few patients also had exanthem.[609,1003] Since the late 1990s, severe epidemic disease with EV 71 has occurred in Taiwan, Singapore, Australia, Malaysia, and Japan. In these epidemics, hand-foot-and-mouth disease is a major finding, and the neurologic disease is more severe than in the past.[†]

These phenotypic changes could be the result either of point mutations or of recombination among EVs.[173,215,613,719,720,863,992,1030] Chan and AbuBaker[173] presented evidence indicating that a recombination event occurred between EV 71 and coxsackievirus A16.

PATHOLOGY

The clinical signs of enteroviral infection vary widely, so great variations in pathology also exist. Because pathologic material generally is available only from patients with fatal illness, this section discusses only the more severe manifestations. Worth emphasizing, however, is that these fatal infections account for just a small portion of all enteroviral infections. The pathologic findings in children with milder infections, such as nonspecific febrile illness, have not been described.

Coxsackieviruses A

Records of severe illness associated with coxsackieviruses A are rare. Gold and colleagues,[416] in a study of sudden unexpected death in infants, recovered coxsackievirus A4 from the brains of three children. In none of these patients were histologic abnormalities noted in the brain or spinal cord. An adult with a fatal coxsackievirus A7 infection had diffuse pancarditis and organized pneumonitis.[55]

Coxsackieviruses B

Of the nonpolio EVs, group B coxsackieviruses have been associated most frequently with severe and catastrophic disease. The most common findings in these cases have been myocarditis, meningoencephalitis, or both. Involvement of the adrenals, pancreas, liver, and lungs also has been noted.

Heart

Grossly, the heart usually is enlarged, with dilation of the chambers and flabby musculature.[197,346,398,1180] Microscopically, the pericardium frequently contains some inflammatory cells along with thickening and edema, and the endocardium may have focal infiltrations of inflammatory cells. The myocardium (Fig. 166.6) is congested and contains infiltrations of inflammatory cells (i.e., lymphocytes, mononuclear cells, reticulum cells, histiocytes, plasma cells, and polymorphonuclear and eosinophil leukocytes). Involvement of the myocardium often is patchy and focal but occasionally diffuse. The muscle shows loss of striation, as well as edema and eosinophilic degeneration. Muscle necrosis without extensive cellular infiltration is a common finding.

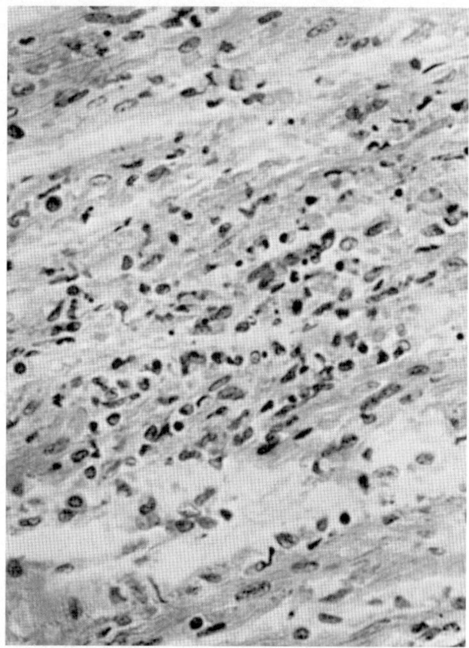

FIG. 166.6 Coxsackievirus B4 myocarditis in a 9-day-old infant. Note the myocardial necrosis and mononuclear cellular infiltration. (From Cherry JD. Enteroviruses. In: Remington JS, Klein JO, eds. *Infectious Diseases of the Fetus and Newborn Infant.* Philadelphia, PA: WB Saunders; 1976.)

Brain and Spinal Cord

The meninges are congested, edematous, and occasionally mildly infiltrated with inflammatory cells.[200,346,798,1180] Lesions in the brain and spinal cord are focal rather than diffuse, but they frequently involve many different areas. The lesions consist of areas of eosinophilic degeneration of cortical cells, clusters of mononuclear and glial cells (Fig. 166.7), and perivascular cuffing. Two children with fatal coxsackieviral B infection (types 2 and 4) had, in addition to typical inflammatory encephalitic lesions, widespread multifocal areas of liquefaction necrosis without inflammation.[337]

Other Organs

The lungs frequently have areas of mild focal pneumonitis with peribronchiolar mononuclear cellular infiltration.[15,123,200,396,798] The liver often is engorged and occasionally contains isolated foci of liver cell necrosis and mononuclear infiltration. In the pancreas, occasional focal degeneration of islet cells occurs. Congestion has been observed in the adrenal glands, along with mild to severe cortical necrosis; inflammatory cells are present.

Echoviruses

Although frequently responsible for illness, echoviruses rarely were associated with fatal infection until relatively recently. In several different reports with eight different echovirus types, hepatic necrosis was a major pathologic finding.[97,200,401,449,789,809,1186] Massive hepatic necrosis has been seen with echoviruses 3, 6, 7, 9, 11, 14, 19, and 21. At autopsy, one infant with echovirus 6 infection had cloudy and thickened leptomeninges, liver necrosis, adrenal and renal hemorrhage, and mild interstitial pneumonitis.[200] One infant with echovirus 9 infection had an enlarged and congested liver with marked central necrosis,[200] and another with

*References 36, 191, 391, 394, 476, 479, 493, 584, 670, 880, 883, 925, 934, 959, 1016, 1177.

†References 142, 174, 176, 180, 181, 183, 184, 193, 225, 226, 229, 375, 432, 491, 508, 513, 516, 517, 546, 591, 646, 697, 701, 704, 703, 705, 716, 743, 758, 848, 871, 917, 1081, 1138, 1139, 1143, 1195.

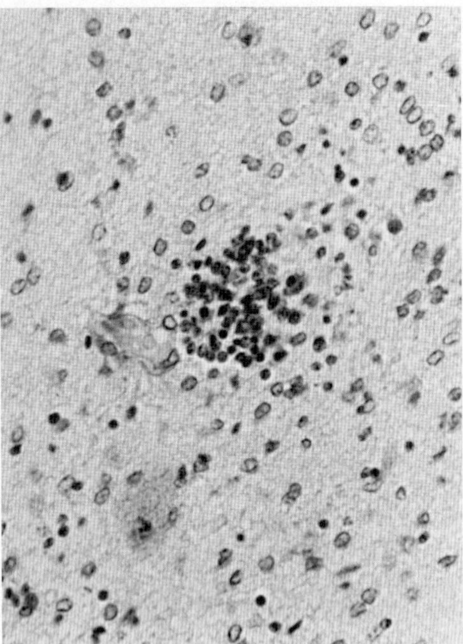

FIG. 166.7 Coxsackievirus B4 encephalitis in a 9-day-old infant with focal infiltration of mononuclear and glial cells. (From Cherry JD. Enteroviruses. In: Remington JS, Klein JO, eds. *Infectious Diseases of the Fetus and Newborn Infant.* Philadelphia, PA: WB Saunders; 1976.)

this virus had interstitial pneumonitis without liver involvement.[200] Three infants with echovirus 11 infection had renal and adrenal hemorrhage and small vessel thrombi in the renal medulla and in both the medulla and inner cortex of the adrenal glands.[818] These patients' livers were normal. Two infants, one with echovirus 6 and the other with echovirus 31 infection, had only extensive pneumonia.[114,200]

Enteroviruses

Enterovirus D68

Kreuter and associates[651] described the pathologic findings in a fatal CNS EV D68 infection in a 5-year-old boy. The lungs were three times the normal weight for age. On microscopic evaluation, mixed pneumonia with hemorrhage was noted. The spleen was twice the normal weight for age; microscopically, follicular hyperplasia was present. The brain had profound edema. On microscopic study, the neurons in the hippocampus were hypereosinophilic with pyknotic nuclei. The meninges, cerebellum, midbrain, pons, medulla, and cervical spinal cord all had lymphocytic meningomyelitis and encephalitis. The motor nuclei demonstrated neurophagia.

Enterovirus 71

Teoh and colleagues[1081] described the clinical characteristics and functional motor outcomes of EV 71 neurologic disease in 61 children. Four precipitous deaths occurred in this group. The pathologic findings of the brain and brainstem in two of the fatal cases were described. Severe inflammation that mainly involved the medulla was noted. Examiners observed numerous perivascular and interstitial activated microglia, macrophages, and lymphocytes. Findings also included scattered microglial nodules and areas of necrosis; rare foci of neuronophagia were seen.

The brain of a child who died of acute encephalitis caused by EV 71 infection was examined.[1193] Grossly, the brain appeared normal, but microscopically, it revealed typical features of acute encephalitis consisting of perivascular cuffing with mixed inflammatory cells, neuronophagia, and inflammatory nodules.

Parechoviruses

Although parechoviral infections have a broad spectrum of clinical manifestations, including encephalitis and sepsis-like neonatal disease, it is surprising that deaths have not been reported, and therefore pathologic data are not available.*

Saffold Virus

SAFV was detected in the myocardium, lung tissue, and blood of a 2-year, 7-month-old previously healthy boy who died unexpectedly after 1 day of low-grade fever.[839] The heart microscopic examination revealed acute lymphocytic myocarditis.

Polioviruses

The neuropathy of poliomyelitis usually is pathognomonic; only certain cells and areas of the neuraxis are susceptible to the virus.[104,238] Neuronal damage is caused directly by virus multiplication, but not all affected neurons are killed. The injury may be reversible, and function may be restored within 3 to 4 weeks after onset. Little histologic evidence of meningeal reaction exists. Perivascular cuffing and some interstitial glial infiltration are present. Histologic sections generally reveal more widespread lesions than would be estimated from the clinical findings. Scattered neurons may undergo considerable destruction without causing clinical disability.

Regions in which neuronal lesions occur are (1) the spinal cord (anterior horn cells chiefly and, to a lesser degree, the intermediate and dorsal horn and dorsal root ganglia), (2) the medulla (vestibular nuclei, cranial nerve nuclei, and the reticular formation that contains the vital centers), (3) the cerebellum (nuclei in the roof and vermis only), (4) the midbrain (chiefly the gray matter but also the substantia nigra and occasionally the red nucleus), (5) the thalamus and hypothalamus, (6) the pallidum, and (7) the cerebral cortex (motor cortex). The viruses spare the following areas: (1) the entire cerebral cortex, except the motor area; (2) the cerebellum, except the vermis and deep midline nuclei; and (3) the white matter of the spinal cord. This distribution of lesions permits the physician to establish a histologic diagnosis of poliomyelitis.

Extraneural disease usually is a secondary phenomenon. Bronchopulmonary changes such as aspiration pneumonia, atelectasis, and purulent bronchitis may be caused by impaired coughing and decreased thoracic movement. Cardiovascular changes may result in hypertension, cardiac failure, and pulmonary edema. Prolonged immobilization leads to negative nitrogen and calcium balance, along with urinary lithiasis, renal failure, hypertension with encephalopathy, and seizures. Treatment itself may cause untoward complications, such as urinary tract infection (after catheterization), decubitus ulcers, and psychotic disturbances. Ulcerations in the alimentary tract may result in serious bleeding and occasional perforation. Respiratory failure culminates in respiratory acidosis and anoxic changes.

CLINICAL MANIFESTATIONS: NONPOLIO ENTEROVIRUSES, PARECHOVIRUSES, AND SAFFOLD VIRUSES

Nonpolio enteroviral, parechoviral, and Saffold viral infections are exceedingly common, and the spectrum of disease is protean. Many of the clinical-virologic associations listed in Tables 166.5 through 166.19 are made on the basis of a limited number of cases. Because EVs, PeVs, and SAFVs frequently are carried asymptomatically in the gastrointestinal tract for relatively long periods, some of the observed illnesses and the viruses concomitantly recovered may not have a cause-and-effect relationship. However, repeated observations since the 1960s have supported many virus-illness associations, even though their occurrence has been sporadic.

Few specific EV, PeV, or SAFV diseases exist, but, rather, various interrelated syndromes and anatomically associated illnesses are reported. Many illnesses and syndromes can be caused by different viral types, and most types are capable of inducing a variety of clinical syndromes. Conversely, certain specific coxsackieviral, echoviral, and enteroviral types have clinical characteristics that facilitate an etiologic diagnosis.

*References 4, 89, 109, 119, 284, 552, 596, 619, 645, 680, 859, 885, 1022, 1038, 1151.

Since the late 1980s, few careful studies (with the exception of clinical experiences with EVs D68 and 71 and PeV 3.) have been conducted in which specific clinical findings were correlated with individual enteroviral types. This paucity of studies was fostered by the expense of serotyping and the lack of using inoculation of suckling mice for isolation of virus. The increased use of polymerase chain reaction (PCR) also has contributed to the lack of identification of manifestations of disease by specific viral type. This situation is unfortunate because the clinical manifestations caused by specific viral types are not constant, and disease severity varies by specific enteroviral type.

Asymptomatic Infection

Because researchers have known that 90% to 95% of poliovirus infections are not recognized clinically, they have assumed that most infections with EVs, PeVs, and SAFVs are asymptomatic. This opinion is strengthened by the finding that these viruses can be recovered frequently from the stools of healthy children. However, relatively few data are available on the rate of asymptomatic infection with nonpolio EVs, PeVs, and SAFVs. All too frequently, isolation of EVs and PeVs from stool is equated with asymptomatic infection. This assumption is an error because illness, if it takes place, occurs shortly after the acquisition of virus and is short-lived; a particular infection may have been associated with a nonspecific illness 2 or 3 months before a stool specimen is obtained in a surveillance program. Unfortunately, in several studies involving controlled population groups in which accurate clinical expression rates could have been determined, clinical observations apparently were of secondary importance to the investigators.[200,399,400,402,644] The data available suggest differences in clinical expression among coxsackieviral and echoviral types.

Table 166.5 lists the approximate frequency of asymptomatic infections with selected coxsackieviruses and echoviruses. As can be seen, the rates vary among the group as a whole and even within specific types. Overall, approximately one-half, and perhaps more, of all nonpolio enteroviral infections appear to be associated with clinical manifestations. In general, the more carefully clinical symptoms are examined, the smaller is the percentage of truly asymptomatic infections. Clinical expression also is related inversely to age. With coxsackievirus A16, asymptomatic infection occurs in only approximately 10% of children younger than 5 years of age, whereas rates are higher in older children and adults.[13,200] Sabin[978] reported no asymptomatic infections in infants with echovirus 18, and Nishmi and Yodfat[845] noted fewer than 20% of infections without illness in children younger than 8 years of age during an echovirus 4 epidemic. At the other extreme, Clemmer and associates[248] reported that 96% of infections with coxsackievirus B3 were asymptomatic. In other studies, the illness rate of coxsackievirus B3 was 60% to 75%. Extensive seroepidemiologic studies by Zoll and colleagues[1218] and Galama and associates[381] of SAFV types 2 and 3 indicate that infection is very common in young children with these viruses. Because other studies have only occasionally noted clinical associations with these viruses, it appears that Saffold viral infections are most often asymptotic.*

Since 2008, EV D68 has caused severe respiratory and neurologic illnesses but the rate of asymptomatic infection with this virus is unknown.†

Similarly, EV 71 has caused hand-foot-and-mouth syndrome and severe neurologic illness, but the rate of asymptomatic infections with this virus also is unknown.‡

Asymptomatic infections in neonates with PeV 1 were noted on three occasions in the late 1960s and 1970.[93,824]

TABLE 166.5 Approximate Frequencies of Asymptomatic Infection With Selected Coxsackieviruses and Echoviruses

Virus	Asymptomatic Infection Frequency (%)
Coxsackieviruses	
A	50
16	50
B	20
B2	11–50
B3	25–96
B4	30–70
B5	5–40
Echoviruses	50
4	Uncommon to 60
6	Rare
9	15–60
18	Rare to 20
20	33
25	30
30	50

Nonspecific Febrile Illness

Nonspecific febrile illness is the most common manifestation of coxsackieviral and echoviral infection (Table 166.6). All viral types cause this clinical finding, but its frequency varies considerably among the individual viruses.

The onset of illness usually is abrupt, without a prodrome. In young children, the initial finding is fever and associated malaise. In older children, headache generally is noted. The temperature ranges between 38.3°C and 40° (101°F and 104°F) and has a mean duration of 3 days. In some instances, the fever is biphasic; it occurs for 1 day, is absent for 2 to 3 days, and then recurs for an additional 2 to 4 days. In many young children, the only manifestation of illness is fever, and its presence is discovered by chance by a parent.

Malaise and anorexia often are related to the degree of temperature elevation, as is headache in older patients. Sore throat is a common complaint, but an inflamed pharynx is not seen on examination. Nausea and vomiting occasionally occur at the onset of illness, as does mild abdominal discomfort. One or two loose stools may be noted. Generalized myalgia also is observed, and children complain of a scratchy feeling in the throat.

Physical examination usually yields benign findings. Minimal conjunctivitis, infection of the pharynx, and cervical lymphadenitis may be present. The duration of illness varies from 24 hours to approximately 6 days, with an average of 3 to 4 days. The white blood cell count (WBC) count is normal. EVs, particularly coxsackieviruses A, are significant causes of febrile seizures in young children.[509] An SAFV was noted in a stool sample from a child with a fever of unknown origin.[580]

Respiratory Manifestations

Common Cold

Although numerous coxsackieviruses and echoviruses have been recovered from children with mild upper respiratory tract infections, only rarely do the illnesses qualify as common colds (see Chapter 7; Table 166.6). (The common cold is an acute illness with nasal stuffiness, rhinitis, no objective evidence of pharyngitis, and no or minimal fever.) In most instances, significant fever (temperature >38.3°C [>101°F]) is associated with enteroviral infections and usually some degree of pharyngitis.

Coxsackievirus A21 is the only EV that clearly qualifies as a common cold virus.[200,569] This agent has produced epidemics of mild respiratory illness in military populations. In adult volunteers, instillation of this virus in the nose has resulted in the common cold syndrome. Epidemic disease has not been observed in children. Other viruses that have been associated with the common cold syndrome include echoviruses 2 and 20 and coxsackieviruses B1 to B6 and A24.[200]

*References 2, 30, 100, 223, 240, 312, 488, 547, 548, 580, 616, 704, 836, 837, 940, 941, 1104, 1105, 1190, 1200.

†References 108, 146, 538, 556, 651, 718, 778, 922, 1007, 1010, 1037.

‡References 53, 142, 174, 176, 180, 184, 193, 225, 226, 229, 375, 403, 432, 491, 508, 513, 518, 519, 546, 591, 646, 697, 701–703, 705, 716, 743, 759, 769, 786, 848, 871–873, 917, 977, 1138, 1139, 1143, 1193, 1195, 1216.

TABLE 166.6 Coxsackieviruses, Echoviruses, Enteroviruses, Parechoviruses, and Saffold Viruses Noted in Association With Nonspecific Febrile Illness and Respiratory Disease

	VIRUS TYPES					
Clinical Categories	**Coxsackieviruses A**	**Coxsackieviruses B**	**Echoviruses**	**Enteroviruses**	**Parechoviruses**	**Saffold Viruses**
Nonspecific febrile illness	All types	All types	All types	All types	All types	All types
Common cold	21, 24	1–6	Mainly 2, 20; rarely other types			
Pharyngitis (pharyngitis, tonsillitis, tonsillopharyngitis, and nasopharyngitis)	Probably all types; mainly 9	Probably all types; mainly 1–5	Probably all types; mainly 2, 4, 6, 9, 11, 16, 19, 25, 30,	71	3, 6	2, 3
Herpangina	1–10, 12, 16, 22	1–5	6, 9, 11, 16, 17, 25	71	1, 6	2, 3, 6
Lymphonodular pharyngitis	10					
Stomatitis and other lesions in the anterior of the mouth	5, 9, 10, 16	2, 5	9, 11, 20	71	1, 6	2, 3, 6
Parotitis	Coxsackievirus A not typed	3, 4		70		
Croup	9	4, 5	4, 11, 21			
Bronchitis		1,4	8, 12-14,	D 68	1	2
Bronchiolitis and infectious asthma	Many types	Many types	Many types	Many types, especially D68	Many types	Unknown
Pneumonia	9, 16	1–6	6, 7, 9, 11, 12, 19, 20, 30	68, 71, 74, 78, especially D68	1	
Pleurodynia	1, 2, 4, 6, 9, 16	1–6	1–3, 6–9, 11, 12, 14, 16–19, 24, 25, 30		2	

Pharyngitis (Pharyngitis, Tonsillitis, Tonsillopharyngitis, and Nasopharyngitis)

Pharyngitis is a common clinical manifestation of coxsackieviral and echoviral infection (see Chapter 9). Probably all EVs on occasion cause mild pharyngitis. The most common coxsackieviruses and echoviruses associated with pharyngitis are as follows: coxsackieviruses A9, B1, B2, B3, B4, and B5; echoviruses 2, 4, 6, 9, 11, 16, 19, 25, and 30; and EV 71.*

Pharyngitis in coxsackievirus and echovirus infections frequently is associated with other clinical findings, such as meningitis, pleurodynia, and exanthem. These other manifestations become more important than pharyngitis in individual cases in the minds of parents as well as clinicians.

Pharyngitis caused by coxsackieviruses and echoviruses usually is abrupt in onset, without a prodrome. Although pharyngeal involvement is present at the onset of disease, the initial complaint usually is fever. The temperature usually ranges between 38.3°C and 40°C (101°F and 104°F), but higher temperatures are not unusual. In general, fever tends to be more pronounced in younger patients. Young children have malaise and anorexia. School-age children complain of headache and myalgia. Sore throat, coryza, and vomiting, diarrhea, or a combination thereof also may be noted.

Examination of the tonsils and pharynx shows varying degrees of erythema. In some cases, only infection is noted, whereas in others, severe pharyngitis with patches of exudate is seen. The usual duration of uncomplicated coxsackieviral or echoviral pharyngitis is 3 to 6 days. Routine laboratory study is of minimal value in enteroviral pharyngitis; the total WBC count may be normal or slightly elevated with a normal differential determination. Throat culture rules out disease caused by group A streptococci.

SAFV 2 was noted in 13 children with pharyngitis and 12 children with tonsillitis in a Japanese study.[547] Also in Japan, two children with SAFV 3 were noted to have tonsillitis.[1105]

*References 200, 208–210, 262, 339, 450, 468, 597, 598, 608, 623, 685–687, 807, 976, 981, 1028.

Other Intraoral Manifestations

Herpangina. The onset of herpangina is typical of most EV infections and is characterized by the sudden awareness of fever.[889,1144,1210,1209] No characteristic prodrome usually exists, but young children may be irritable and occasionally listless and anorexic for a few hours before the febrile state is recognized. The initial temperature can be variable, with a range from normal to 41°C (106°F). In general, the temperature tends to be higher in younger patients. Breese[117] noted that the most common temperature in young children was between 39.5°C and 40°C (103°F and 104°F). Older children frequently complain of headache and backache. Vomiting occurs in approximately 25% of children younger than 5 years of age. In one outbreak of illness caused by coxsackievirus A4,[360] initial symptoms were as follows: anorexia and drooling (100%); sore throat (50%); coryza (45%); headache (18%); and vomiting, diarrhea, or both (36%).

In most instances of herpangina, the oropharyngeal lesions are present on the first examination at the time of fever or shortly after fever is noted. In the coxsackievirus A4 outbreak described by Forman and Cherry,[360] the enanthem was not observed until 24 to 48 hours after the onset of initial nonspecific symptoms. The characteristic lesions in herpangina are small (1–2 mm) vesicles and ulcers. These lesions apparently start as papules, become vesicular, and then ulcerate in a short but variable period. In the experience of one of us (J.D.C.), the lesions most commonly observed are ulcers. Breese[117] noted in some children seen early in the course of the illness that a petechial appearance preceded the appearance of typical vesicular-ulcerative enanthem.

The lesions usually are discrete, with an average of 5 per patient; some patients have only 1 or 2 lesions, whereas others may have 14 or more. When seen early, the vesicular lesions are observed to enlarge from 1 to 2 mm to 3 to 4 mm during a 2- to 3-day period.[889] Each vesicular and ulcerative lesion is surrounded by an erythematous ring that varies in size up to 10 mm in diameter. The most common sites of the lesions are the anterior tonsillar pillars. Lesions also occur on the soft palate, uvula, tonsils, and pharyngeal wall and occasionally on the posterior buccal surfaces. In some cases, additional lesions have been noted on the dorsum or tip of the tongue. However, by definition, cases in which the primary involvement is on the tongue or anterior mouth and in which the lesions are of a general size greater than 5 mm are not considered to be herpangina.

Aside from the specific lesions, the remainder of the throat appears normal, minimally injected, or mildly erythematous. The usual duration of signs and symptoms is 3 to 6 days. Most cases of herpangina are mild and without complications, but aseptic meningitis and other more severe enteroviral manifestations also occur occasionally. Severe neurologic manifestations have been observed in children with herpangina caused by EV 71.[179,182,491,646] During epidemic disease in Taiwan in 1998, children with herpangina and aseptic meningitis, acute flaccid paralysis, and rhombencephalitis were described.[491,518] In one study, a biphasic course was described, with herpangina occurring first and neurologic manifestations 2 to 5 days later.[488]

EVs, PeVs, and SAFVs found in association with sporadic or epidemic herpangina occurrence are presented in Table 166.7.

Acute lymphonodular pharyngitis. In 1962, Steigman and colleagues[1049] reported a unique enanthem associated with coxsackievirus A10 infection. The lesions had the typical distribution of herpangina; they were papular, discrete, 3 mm in diameter, and surrounded by a zone of erythema. The lesions were white to yellow and persisted for 6 to 10 days. This entity has not been reported again, although coxsackievirus A10 has been noted in association with hand-foot-and-mouth disease.[200,1012]

Stomatitis and other lesions in the anterior of the mouth. Historically, the main enteroviral cause of stomatitis and ulcerative lesions in the anterior of the mouth was coxsackievirus A16, and the clinical entity was hand-foot-and-mouth disease. This condition is presented in detail later in this chapter. Worth mentioning here, however, is that occasionally enanthem occurs without the exanthem, and this enanthem also has been associated with other coxsackieviruses (A5, A9, A10, B2, B5), echovirus 33, and in more recent years EV 71.[200,225,226,286,315,356,432,707,1012,1081]

In echovirus 9 infection, Tyrrell and colleagues[1110] reported six children with a unique enanthem: painless whitish dots, ulcers, or vesicles on the buccal surfaces near the Stensen duct. These investigators also noted the occasional occurrence of similar lesions under the tongue.

Deseda-Tous and colleagues[294] reported an adolescent with hemorrhagic vesicular lesions on the pharynx, mucosal surfaces, and tongue in association with an echovirus 11 infection. Clarke and Stott[245] observed reddish macules on the buccal mucosa of a patient with echovirus 20 infection, and Cherry and Jahn[203] noted a child with hand-foot-and-mouth disease in whom the buccal lesions suggested Koplik spots, although the lesions were larger and yellower in this patient.

TABLE 166.7 Etiologic Agents Found in Association With Sporadic or Epidemic Herpangina Occurrence

	OCCURRENCE	
Virus	**Epidemic**	**Sporadic**
Coxsackievirus A		
1	+	
2	+	
3	+	
4	+	
5	+	
6	+	
7		+
8	+	
9		+
10	+	
12		+
16		+
22	+	
Coxsackievirus B		
1	+	+
2		+
3		+
4		+
5		+
Echovirus		
6		+
9		+
11		+
16	+	+
17		+
25	+	
Parechovirus 1 and 6		+
Enterovirus 71	+	
Saffold virus types 2, 3		+

Parotitis

Parotitis in association with herpangina and coxsackievirus A infection was reported in 1957 by Howlett and associates.[512] In 1960, Kraus[650] described two additional cases, and Bertaggia and associates[98] and Winsser and Altieri[1176] noted parotitis in association with coxsackieviruses B3 and B4, respectively. Three patients with acute hemorrhagic conjunctivitis and parotitis caused by EV 70 also have been reported.[997]

Croup

In large studies of respiratory illness in young children, croup is associated sporadically with coxsackieviral and echoviral infection.[187,200,366,407,1161] In general, these illnesses are mild, in contrast to croup caused by parainfluenza and influenza viruses.

An outbreak of croup associated with echovirus 11 in a day care center was reported.[904] In this instance, 17 of 53 ill children were found to be infected with the U strain of echovirus 11. A subsequent study noted the same virus in 4 children with croup.[905] Croup also was reported in outbreaks of coxsackievirus B5 infection.[51,260] Other specific agents associated with croup include coxsackieviruses A9 and B4 and echoviruses 4 and 21.[200]

Bronchitis (Not Including Enterovirus D68)

An acute febrile illness with cough, rhonchi, and referred breath sounds occasionally is a sporadic manifestation of enteroviral infection. A specific association of coxsackieviruses B1 and B4, echoviruses 8, 12, 13, and 14, and PeV 1 has been found.[187,200,260,322,324] SAFV type 2 was noted in one child with bronchitis.[547]

Bronchiolitis and Infectious Asthma (Not Including Enterovirus D68)

Coxsackieviruses and echoviruses have been associated sporadically with bronchiolitis, infectious asthma, and the precipitation of asthmatic attacks in atopic children.[187,200,322,366,407,429,499,1161] Epidemic disease has not been observed, and the illnesses usually have been mild.

Pneumonia (Not Including Enterovirus D68)

In general, studies of respiratory tract infections in children, sporadic coxsackieviruses, and echoviruses have been noted in 1% to 7% of patients with pneumonia and positive viral cultures.[187,200,366,407] Specific virus types include the following: coxsackieviruses A9, A16, B1, B2, B3, B4, B5, and B6; echoviruses 6, 7, 9, 11, 12, 19, 20, and 30; EV 71; and SAFV (type not identified).*

In only three instances can an outbreak of pneumonia caused by specific viruses be suggested to have occurred. During the summer of 1959, Lerner and colleagues[688] noted that 3 of 15 children infected with coxsackievirus A9 had pneumonia. The patients with pneumonia had a vesicular rash, and one of these children died.

Eckert and associates[322] observed six children with coxsackievirus B1 infection and pneumonia during the summer of 1963. These illnesses were not described further, although the mean WBC count in 12 children who had lower respiratory tract infections with group B coxsackieviruses

*References 115, 200, 262, 322, 355, 403, 558, 598, 688, 797, 999, 1028, 1159, 1214.

was reported as 11,383 with a normal differential. All children were hospitalized.

Goldwater[418] reported a coxsackievirus B6 outbreak in south Australia during the summer of 1992 to 1993. Twenty-seven patients had pneumonia associated with high fever and severe cough that lasted several weeks. In addition to the fatal case of coxsackievirus A9 infection described by Lerner and colleagues,[688] deaths have resulted from infection with coxsackieviruses B1, B5, and A16.[355,558,1188]

In the Philippines in 2009, 21 children with EV 68, severe respiratory tract infections, and presumed pneumonia were noted.[537] All children had cough and chest indrawing. Two deaths occurred.

Enterovirus D68 (Bronchitis, Bronchiolitis, and Pneumonia)

In California between October and December 1962, EV D68 was isolated from throat swabs of four children with acute lower respiratory tract illness.[998] All these children had pneumonia and "wheezing characteristic of bronchiolitis." This virus was not noticed in association with respiratory illnesses for about 40 years after 1962.[1007] Between 2005 and 2011, small outbreaks of respiratory disease with EV D68 were observed in Asia, Europe, and the United States.[146,495,537–539,587,717,864,1007] In 2014, EV D68 respiratory illness was widespread throughout the United States and Canada.[266,495,778,781,876,1037] In 2013 and 2014, widespread respiratory illness with EV D68 was noted in Europe and South America.[108,138,1007,1093]

Holm-Hansen[495] reviewed the clinical characteristics of 195 children noted in 19 published papers. She noted the following: cough, 75%; fever, 44%; wheeze, 40%; chest indrawing, 30%; difficulty breathing, 25%; pneumonia, 25%; coryza, 24%; influenza-like illness, 22%; bronchitis, 16%; bronchiolitis, 13%; dyspnea, 12%; respiratory failure, 7%; gastrointestinal symptoms, 15%; and neurologic symptoms, 5%. Midgley and colleagues[780] reviewed 614 US cases in patients admitted to the hospital in 2014 and noted the following: dyspnea, 84%; cough, 81%; wheezing, 70%; and fever, 48%. Fifty-nine percent of these patients were admitted to intensive care units, and 28% received ventilation support. A history of asthma or reactive airway disease was noted in 52%, and these patients were more likely to require care in an intensive care unit. The median age of the patients in this review was 5 years, with an age range from 3 days to 92 years.

Orvedahl and associates[876] reviewed 139 children at St. Louis Children's Hospital in St. Louis, Missouri, and reported the following historical findings: fever, 48%; upper respiratory tract symptoms, 96%; difficulty breathing, 80%; wheezing, 67%; and vomiting, diarrhea, or abdominal pain, or a combination, 37%. Physical examination of these patients elicited these findings: fever (temperature ≥38°C), 9%; rhinorrhea, 24%; rash, 8%; tachypnea, 69%; wheezing, 71%; retractions, flaring, grunting, head bobbing, or abdominal breathing, 65%; tachycardia, 42%; delayed capillary refill, 3%; abnormal abdominal examination, 4%; and abnormal neurologic examination, 3%. Treatment in the St. Louis Children's Hospital patients included the following: oxygen by nasal cannula or face mask, 26%; intravenous fluids, 40%; albuterol, 79%; intravenous or oral antibiotics, 15%; intravenous or oral steroids, 68%; and intravenous magnesium sulfate, 16%.

Neurologic disease has been a significant manifestation of EV D68 infections; this topic is covered later in the neurologic manifestations section of this chapter.*

Pleurodynia (Bornholm Disease)

Epidemic pleurodynia[54,200,279,422,440,623,796,1067,1146] is an illness that was noted first in 1735 by Hannaeus, a Danish physician.[455] Not until the late 19th century, however, did the illness receive further attention in the medical literature. At this time, several epidemics in Scandinavian countries were described.[200,271,354] Although Finsen[354] referred to the disease as *pleurodynia,* other investigators who designated outbreaks used geographic names, such as Skien disease, Bamle disease, Drangedal disease, and Bornholm disease, or descriptive names such as epidemic myalgia, devil's grippe, epidemic diaphragmatic spasm, or epidemic benign pleurisy.[422] In 1933, Sylvest[1067] published the classic monograph on the subject, and from this publication the name Bornholm disease (from Bornholm Island, a Danish island in the Baltic Sea) came to be associated with the illness. The enteroviral origin of epidemic pleurodynia was established in 1949.[270,1155]

Historically, pleurodynia is an epidemic disease, but sporadic cases do occur. A characteristic incubation period of approximately 4 days is followed by the sudden onset of fever and pain. The pain typically is located in the chest or upper part of the abdomen and is muscular in origin and of variable intensity. Occasionally, the pain occurs in other areas of the body. Frequently, the pain is excruciatingly severe and sudden and is associated with profuse sweating, so the patient may appear pale and as though in shock. The pain is spasmodic, with durations varying from a few minutes to several hours. Most commonly, the spasmodic periods last approximately 15 to 30 minutes. During spasms, respirations usually are rapid, shallow, and grunting, suggestive of pneumonia or pleural inflammation. Coughing, sneezing, or deep breathing makes the pain worse. Older children and adults describe the pain as stabbing or knifelike. An older person often fears that a heart attack is occurring.

When pain localizes in the abdomen, it frequently is crampy and suggests colic in a younger child. The child may double over and refuse to walk or move. Occasionally, the abdominal pain in association with a pale, sweaty, shock-like appearance suggests acute intestinal obstruction. Splinting and guarding of the abdomen also lead to consideration of appendicitis and peritonitis.

The fever and pain usually last 1 to 2 days. Frequently, however, the illness is biphasic; after the initial febrile period, the patient is asymptomatic for several days, and then the pain and fever recur. Rarely, patients have several recurrent episodes over the course of several weeks. In these patients, fever is less prominent.

Some degree of tenderness is present in the areas of pain, but frank myositis with muscle swelling is not observed. Pleural friction rubs may be noted on auscultation, and they may appear and disappear with the coming and going of episodes of pain.

In epidemics, both children and adults are afflicted, but most cases occur in persons younger than 30 years of age. Most children have other symptoms of enteroviral infection, such as anorexia, nausea, vomiting, headache, and sore throat. Routine laboratory study is not very helpful. The WBC count varies considerably, but increased percentages of polymorphonuclear neutrophils and band forms are frequent findings. The erythrocyte sedimentation rate also is inconsistent; normal to extremely high values may be observed. The chest radiograph usually is normal.

Complications of pleurodynia seldom develop. Aseptic meningitis has been noted in some patients, and men have experienced orchitis. Cardiac involvement, in the form of myocarditis and pericarditis, also may complicate pleurodynia.

The major etiologic agents in epidemic pleurodynia are coxsackieviruses B3 and B5.[54,200,523,976,1005,1028] Other viruses associated with epidemic disease include coxsackieviruses B1 and B2 and echoviruses 1 and 6.[39,200,317] Agents associated with sporadic occurrences of pleurodynia include the following: coxsackieviruses A1, A2, A4, A6, A9, A16, B1, B2, B3, B4, B5, and B6; echoviruses 1, 2, 3, 6, 7, 8, 9, 11, 12, 14, 16, 17, 18, 19, 24, 25, and 30; and PeV 2.[77,200,260,317,451,590,628,755,796,1065]

Pleurodynia rarely is reported today. Because the EVs that cause pleurodynia still circulate, cases probably are overlooked or misdiagnosed. An outbreak caused by coxsackievirus B1 in football players at a public high school was reported.[536] Unfortunately, no clinical data were presented. In 2005, 28 pediatric patients with pleurodynia were observed in a medical center in Northern Taiwan.[517] This outbreak was caused by coxsackievirus B3.

Gastrointestinal Manifestations

Gastrointestinal manifestations occur commonly in enteroviral and parechoviral infections.* Clinical manifestations in addition to vomiting and diarrhea are varied (Table 166.8).

*References 20, 48, 300, 430, 651, 718, 778, 779, 891, 1109, 1118, 1170.

*References 1, 41, 42, 116, 200, 232, 279, 440, 499, 551, 623, 672, 745, 748, 753, 755, 767, 796, 801, 802, 900–902, 930, 1011, 1042, 1116, 1157, 1158, 1160, 1179.

TABLE 166.8 Coxsackieviruses, Echoviruses, Enteroviruses, Parechoviruses, and Saffold Viruses Noted in Association With Gastrointestinal Complaints

Clinical Categories	VIRUS TYPES: Coxsackieviruses A	Coxsackieviruses B	Echoviruses	Enteroviruses	Parechoviruses	Saffold Viruses
Gastrointestinal, not specified	2, 4, 5, 6, 7, 9, 10, 14, 16	1–5	1–9, 11, 12, 14, 16–21, 24, 25, 30,	D68, 71	1–6, 8, 10, 11	
Nausea and vomiting	9, 16	2–5	2, 4, 6, 9, 11, 16, 18–20, 30		1	
Diarrhea	1, 9, 16	2–5	3, 4, 6, 7, 9, 11–14, 16–21, 25, 30		1	1, 2
Constipation	9	3–5	4, 6, 9, 11			
Abdominal pain	9, 16	2–5	4, 6, 9, 11, 18, 19, 30	D68		
Pseudoappendicitis			1, 8, 14			
Peritonitis		1				
Mesenteric adenitis		5	7, 9, 11			
Appendicitis		2, 5				
Intussusception		3	7, 9			
Hepatitis	4, 9, 10, 20, 24	1–5	1, 3, 4, 6, 7, 9, 11, 14, 20, 21, 30			
Reye syndrome	2	4	14		1	
Pancreatitis	9	3–5				
Diabetes mellitus		1–5				

Early studies paid particular attention to diarrheal disease in children. However, when specific studies of infantile diarrhea were undertaken, the enteroviral association was far from clear.[74,200,421,887,1205] The correlation of infection and disease in these studies was compromised by the problem that the main source of culture in study patients and control subjects was from stool; persistent infection in the bowel rendered separation of control subjects and ill patients impossible.

Infections with all coxsackieviruses and echoviruses frequently have one or more gastrointestinal symptoms as part of the general illness. The intensity and spectrum do vary among the specific agents, however, and also among strains of particular viral types. In a review of World Health Organization (WHO) virus reports covering a 4-year period, Assaad and Cockburn[42] found that the main clinical sign or symptom was gastrointestinal in 12% of coxsackieviral infections and in 6.8% of echoviral infections. In another analysis, Assaad and Borecka[41] noted 16 deaths during the period 1967 to 1975 in patients with coxsackievirus and echovirus infections in whom the principal clinical association was gastrointestinal.

In a 20-year survey in Wisconsin, Nelson and colleagues[828] noted that gastrointestinal symptoms occurred in approximately one-third of all patients from whom these investigators recovered nonpolio EVs. Morens and colleagues[802] reported that in 4% of patients from whom nonpolio EVs were recovered during the 1971 to 1975 period, gastrointestinal disease was the major diagnosis. Horn and coworkers,[499] studying respiratory viral infections, noted that 21.2% of subjects from whom EVs were recovered had gastrointestinal complaints.

Vomiting

Vomiting is a common manifestation of infection with many coxsackieviral and echoviral types, but it rarely is the major complaint of the patient or the parent.* The frequency of vomiting during outbreaks of illness caused by coxsackieviruses and echoviruses depends on the specific types of virus and on the major manifestation during a particular outbreak. Table 166.9 presents the frequency of vomiting by coxsackieviral and echoviral type. In 14 different enteroviral types, vomiting has been noted as a significant aspect of the illness during disease outbreaks. Except for coxsackievirus A16 infections (hand-foot-and-mouth disease), in which it is an uncommon complaint, vomiting occurs in approximately 50% of all patients with epidemic enteroviral disease. Vomiting is noted most commonly in meningitis and least commonly in pleurodynia and uncomplicated exanthematous disease.

*References 13, 40, 200, 208, 209, 222, 262, 263, 292, 349, 350, 422, 444, 450, 451, 457, 593, 597, 598, 608, 626, 636, 685, 735, 737, 845, 910, 914, 937, 954, 973, 978, 981, 991, 1028, 1050, 1092, 1146, 1152, 1162, 1172, 1173.

Diarrhea

Diarrhea occurs commonly in enteroviral, PeV and SAFV infections, but it usually is just one of many manifestations of systemic illness.* Specific studies of diarrheal disease in infants and children have had varied results; some studies indicate an enteroviral origin, whereas others reveal that coxsackieviruses and echoviruses were recovered from well children at the same prevalence.

Ramos-Alvarez and Olarte[931] carried out an extensive study of diarrheal disease in Mexico City and noted that echoviruses were recovered eight times more frequently from children with diarrhea than from control children without diarrhea. These investigators found that echoviruses 6 and 19 predominated, but types 3, 7, 9, 12, 14, 18, and 21 also were recovered. Pelon and colleagues[895] noted an association between coxsackieviruses B4 and B5 and acute diarrhea; these investigators observed a 42% coxsackievirus B isolation rate in children with acute diarrhea and a corresponding rate of only 12% in those without diarrhea. Goodwin and associates[421] noted echoviruses in the stools of children with diarrhea at twice the rate observed in healthy children. In a study by Yow and colleagues,[1205,1206] no association was found between EVs and infantile diarrhea. Echoviruses were recovered twice as frequently from children ill with diarrhea as from children without gastrointestinal illness.[1206] In Canada, McLean and colleagues[753] could find no association between enteroviral infection and gastroenteritis. In a large study of diarrhea in India, coxsackieviruses A9, B3, and B6 and echoviruses 12 and 21 were recovered more commonly from ill patients than from children without diarrhea.[820]

In several studies of specific diarrhea outbreaks, afflicted persons were noted to be actively infected with a particular virus type. Goldwater[417] observed three children younger than 6 months of age who

*References 13, 39, 40, 92, 124, 127, 200, 203, 260–263, 292, 349, 350, 417, 422, 440, 450, 451, 457, 597, 598, 608, 617, 623, 636, 665, 678, 685, 735, 745, 748, 753, 820, 888, 895, 910, 913, 918, 930–932, 954, 976, 978, 1011, 1042, 1043, 1078, 1160, 1173, 1205, 1206, 1214.

TABLE 166.9 Frequency of Vomiting in Outbreaks of Illness Caused by Coxsackieviruses and Echoviruses

Virus Type	Age Group (y)	Vomiting (%)	Main Characteristics of Outbreak	References
Coxsackievirus A9	Mainly children	60–73	Meningitis	200
	Children	14–20	Rash	200, 688
Coxsackievirus A16	Children and adults	3–15	Hand-foot-and-mouth disease	13, 954
Coxsackievirus B2	Mainly children	50	Meningitis	200
	Mainly children	18–66	Febrile illness, respiratory illness	201
Coxsackievirus B3	Adults and children	33	Pleurodynia	200
	Children	9	Febrile illness, respiratory illness	200
	Mainly children	25	Fever, diarrhea	347
Coxsackievirus B4	Mainly children	27	Nonspecific fever	349
Coxsackievirus B5	Adults and children	31–37	Pleurodynia	422, 1028
	Adults and children	50–95	Meningitis	200, 222, 444, 973
	Mainly children	25–33	Nonspecific febrile illness	222, 973, 1173
	Children	45	Febrile illness, respiratory illness	991
	Mainly children	100	Hepatosplenic syndrome	1028
	Children	40	Rash	209
Echovirus 2	Children	12	Respiratory illness, rash	200
Echovirus 4	Mainly children	70–90	Meningitis	597, 937
	Mainly children	9–50	Epidemic disease, including meningitis, minor illness	200, 845
Echovirus 6	Mainly children	55–98	Meningitis	457, 598, 626, 663, 1152
	Mainly children	50–75	Epidemic disease, including meningitis	200, 1173
Echovirus 9	0–4	64–71	Rash, meningitis	200, 981
	5–9	81–83		
	10–19	61–92		
	>20	20–38		
	Mainly children	39–95	Rash, meningitis	200, 914, 1152, 1162
	Mainly children	26	Pharyngitis	200
	Mainly children	71	Epidemic disease, including meningitis	200
Echovirus 11	Not specified	100	Febrile illness, respiratory illness	200
Echovirus 16	Children	30	Rash	450
Echovirus 19	<0.5	25	Meningitis, upper respiratory tract illness, nonspecific febrile illness	200
	0.5–2	31		
	3–5	37		
	6–12	68		
	13–18	61		
	19–25	53		
	26+	43		
Echovirus 20	Children	67	Febrile illness, respiratory illness	262
Echovirus 30	Mainly children	15–91	Meningitis	426, 593, 910, 1092
	<5	50	Febrile illness, respiratory illness	200
	>5	70		

were infected with echovirus 19 and who had gastroenteritis without other signs or symptoms. Klein and colleagues[636] recovered echovirus 11 from the blood of two laboratory workers with acute gastroenteritis. Diarrhea occurred in three of nine volunteers given echovirus 11.[127] Eichenwald and Kotsevalov[326] and Cramblett and colleagues[260] reported epidemic diarrhea caused by echovirus 18 in neonates. An outbreak of diarrhea associated with coxsackievirus A1 was noted in 7 of 14 bone marrow transplant recipients during a 3-week period.[1095]

Table 166.10 presents the frequency of diarrhea in outbreaks of specific coxsackieviral and echoviral illnesses. Diarrhea varied with regard to the viruses represented and in different studies with the same agents. Diarrhea in enteroviral disease rarely is severe. In most instances, loose stools occur for a 2- to 4-day period. The stools rarely are watery, never are bloody, and at most number six to eight per day. In two child care centers, diarrhea associated with a parechoviral infection occurred in 21% of the children during a one-half-year period.[116] The following PeV genotypes have been identified in children with diarrhea: 1, 3, 4, 5, 6, 8, 10, 11.[900–902,1212] SAFVs have been identified in stool samples from children with diarrhea, but a cause-and-effect relationship has not been established.[100,459,616,940,1190]

Constipation

Some degree of constipation is a rather frequent occurrence in many acute infectious illnesses, but evaluation is rendered difficult by the subjective nature of the complaint. In coxsackieviral and echoviral diseases, a short period of constipation may be associated with fever, vomiting, and anorexia early in the course of the illness. This period frequently is followed by mild diarrhea.[127] As noted in Table 166.8, constipation has been reported specifically as a symptom with four coxsackieviral and four echoviral types. Constipation is a particularly common event in children with enteroviral meningitis; it occurs in 10% to 40% of cases.[200,349,350,597,598,662]

Abdominal Pain

Abdominal pain is a common symptom in many coxsackieviral and echoviral infections. Table 166.11 lists the frequency of occurrence of abdominal pain and the main characteristic of the illness by virus type. Approximately 10% of patients with coxsackievirus A16 hand-foot-and-mouth disease report abdominal pain. In approximately one-fourth of patients, many coxsackieviruses and echoviruses associated with meningitis cause abdominal pain.

TABLE 166.10 Frequency of Diarrhea in Outbreaks of Illness Caused by Coxsackieviruses and Echoviruses

Virus Type	Age Group (y)	Diarrhea (%)	Main Characteristics of Outbreak	References
Coxsackievirus A9	Adults and children	7–100	Fever, rash	200, 690
Coxsackievirus A16	Mainly children	4–33	Hand-foot-and-mouth disease	13, 203, 685, 958
Coxsackievirus B2	Mainly children	9–56	Febrile illness, respiratory illness	200
	Mainly children	12	Meningitis	734
Coxsackievirus B3	Mainly children	2–5	Pleurodynia	200
	Children	11	Meningitis	260
	Mainly children	54	Nonspecific febrile illness	347
Coxsackievirus B4	Children	9	Meningitis	261
	Mainly children	8	Febrile illness, respiratory illness	350
Coxsackievirus B5	<1	21	Meningitis and fever, respiratory illness	913
	1–9	15		
	10–29	3		
	Mainly children	5–9	Meningitis	200, 260, 1173
Echovirus 4	Mainly children	5–75	Meningitis	597, 678, 978
	Mainly children	65	Nonspecific febrile illness	678
Echovirus 6	Mainly children	6–12	Meningitis	
Echovirus 9	0–4	14	Meningitis, rash	200, 457, 598, 978
	5–9	10		
	10–19	8		
	<20	0		
	Mainly children	3–40	Meningitis	200, 263, 978
	Children	15	Rash, febrile illness	313
	Mainly children	5–15	Respiratory illness	200
Echovirus 11	Adults	33–100	Gastrointestinal illness	127, 636
	Mainly infants	40	Nonspecific febrile illness	92
Echovirus 13	Children	11	Respiratory illness	200
Echovirus 16	Children	20	Rash	450
Echovirus 17	<1–4	100	Fever, diarrhea	200
Echovirus 18	Infants	100	Diarrhea	325
Echovirus 19	<2	30	Meningitis	200
	2–4	7		
	5–11	7		
	12–17	0		
	>18	9		
	Mainly children	3	Meningitis	417
	Mainly children	10	Respiratory illness	261, 417
	Mainly children	9	Diarrhea	429
Echovirus 20	Children	100	Respiratory, enteric illness	262
Echovirus 30	<5	12	Meningitis	200
	>5	5		
	Adults and children	7–10	Meningitis	451, 910, 1092

The magnitude of abdominal pain as a clinical symptom in coxsackieviral and echoviral infections varies considerably. For example, in aseptic meningitis, headache and other neurologic reports overshadow the abdominal symptoms. In other situations, fever and abdominal pain are diagnostically troublesome because of the possible presence of a surgical abdomen (discussed further in the next paragraph). The pain most frequently is periumbilical; it may be either constant or colicky. The fever is most often higher than 38.3°C (101°F).

Peritonitis, Pseudoperitonitis, Appendicitis, Pseudo-obstruction, Mesenteric Adenitis, and Intussusception

Occasionally, coxsackieviruses and echoviruses are associated with illnesses that suggest severe abdominal involvement. Liebman and St. Geme[698] described two children with abdominal findings suggestive of acute appendicitis (i.e., semirigid, tender abdomen, rebound tenderness, and rectal tenderness) who had associated infections with echoviruses 1 and 14. McLean[752] described a surgical abdomen in one child with coxsackievirus B1 infection. In this case, virus was recovered from the peritoneal exudate; at surgery, this boy was found to have peritonitis, but his appendix was normal. Thomas[1085] reported a 5-year-old boy with coxsackievirus B5 infection who at surgery was found to have excessive clear peritoneal fluid and markedly enlarged mesenteric lymph nodes. A pregnant woman with acute abdominal pain and rebound tenderness associated with echovirus 8 infection was described.[893]

In immunofluorescence studies, Tobe[1090] showed the presence of coxsackievirus B2 and B5 antigens in the mucous membranes and mesenteric lymph nodes of patients with appendicitis more often than in similar studies in control subjects. He suggested that the viral infection acts as a trigger for appendicitis. Bell and Steyn[81] recovered echoviruses 7 and 9 from the mesenteric lymph nodes of children with intussusception.

Hepatitis

Marked liver involvement is not a rare finding in disseminated coxsackieviral and echoviral infections in neonates.*

The association of hepatitis and enteroviral infection in older children is defined less clearly but probably occurs more commonly than generally realized, on the basis of the number of individual cases reported. Caution

*References 14, 171, 186, 279, 507, 623, 672, 677, 737, 801, 802, 807, 858, 999, 1008, 1011, 1028, 1061, 1127, 1142.

TABLE 166.11 Frequency of Abdominal Pain in Outbreaks of Illness Caused by Coxsackieviruses and Echoviruses

Virus Type	Age Group (y)	Abdominal Pain (%)	Main Characteristics of Outbreak	References
Coxsackievirus A9	Mainly children	7	Meningitis	200
	Children	20	Rash	208
Coxsackievirus A16	Mainly children	12	Hand-foot-and-mouth disease	688, 954
Coxsackievirus B2	Mainly children	22	Meningitis	735
Coxsackievirus B3	Children and adults	25–90	Pleurodynia	200
Coxsackievirus B4	Children and adults	10	Meningitis	200
	Mainly children	36	Febrile illness, respiratory illness	350
Coxsackievirus B5	Mainly children	10	Meningitis	200
	Children	13	Febrile illness, respiratory illness	991
	Children and adults	23–67	Pleurodynia	422, 976, 1028
Echovirus 4	Mainly children	28–50	Meningitis	200,597
	Mainly children	13	Febrile illness, respiratory illness	845
Echovirus 6	Mainly children	17–43	Meningitis	200, 457, 598, 626
Echovirus 9	0–4	28	Meningitis, rash	200, 222, 685, 981
	5–9	30		
	10–19	25		
	≥20	0		
Echovirus 11	Adults	38	Gastrointestinal illness	127
Echovirus 16	Children	20	Rash	450
Echovirus 19	<0.5	3	Meningitis	200
	0.5–2	3		
	3–5	27		
	6–12	38		
	13–18	13		
	19–25	9		
	26+	3		
Echovirus 30	Mainly children	17	Meningitis	593, 1092

must be exercised in accepting EVs as the exclusive etiologic agents of hepatitis, however, because hepatitis A virus infection was ruled out in only a few of the available older studies.

Morris and associates[807] described an illness suggestive of a coxsackieviral or echoviral infection in an 18-month-old child who had hyperbilirubinemia and abnormal liver function test results. From this child, coxsackievirus A4 was recovered from blood during the acute illness, and a rise in neutralizing antibody titer to the isolated virus was demonstrated. Chang and Weinstein[186] reported a 3-year-old boy with pharyngitis, urinary abnormalities, and neurologic symptoms who had elevated liver enzyme values (i.e., aspartate transaminase value of 1600 and alanine transaminase value of 1180). Coxsackievirus A9 was recovered from this child's cerebrospinal fluid (CSF), and the child's antibody response to this agent was significant. Coxsackievirus A20 has been associated with clinical hepatitis, and simultaneous infections with coxsackievirus A24 and hepatitis A virus have been demonstrated.[1008]

An adult with a coxsackievirus B1 infection had both myocarditis and liver involvement.[14] A similar illness caused by coxsackievirus B3 in a 19-year-old woman was described.[1061] An 11-month-old boy had a Reye-like syndrome in conjunction with coxsackievirus B2 infection.[602] Reye syndrome has been associated with echovirus 3 infection.[466] Siegel and colleagues[1028] described a hepatosplenic syndrome in which 15 patients had hepatomegaly and coxsackievirus B5 infection. These patients, most of whom were children, had otherwise typical enteroviral illnesses. Liver function studies were performed in only three instances, and the results were normal.

Echoviruses 1, 3, 4, 6, 7, 9, 11, 14, 20, 21, 25, and 30 have been associated with hepatitis.[200,525,623,733,796,999,1178,1199] Hepatomegaly occurs commonly in enteroviral infections.[204,203,347,665,688] During the period from 1971 through 1975, more than 7000 cases of nonpolio enteroviral infection were reported to the Viral Diseases Division at the CDC.[801] In this group were 13 cases of hepatitis and 6 of Reye syndrome; coxsackieviruses A2 and B4 and echoviruses 14 and 22 were associated with Reye syndrome.

Pancreatitis

One of the effects of coxsackievirus B in suckling mice is extensive infection in the pancreas. As with other similarities of infection between suckling mice and human neonates, generalized coxsackievirus B infection in neonates also is accompanied frequently by extensive pancreatic damage. In contrast, pancreatic involvement in older children and adults is not a common occurrence.[141,816,821,1112] Coxsackieviruses B3, B4, B5, and A9 have been noted. Groeneweg and coworkers[441] described a 3-year-old girl with chronic hereditary pancreatitis associated with a serine protease inhibitor Kazal type 1 gene mutation and a high antibody titer to coxsackievirus type 5.

Diabetes Mellitus

A possible relationship between juvenile diabetes mellitus (DM) and the seasonal occurrence of coxsackievirus B4 was suggested in 1969 by Gamble and Taylor.[386] In a second study, Gamble and associates[385] noted that titers of coxsackievirus B4 antibodies in patients with type 1 DM within 3 months of the onset of disease were higher than those in physiologically normal subjects or in patients with chronic diabetes.

Since the 1960s, many studies in animal models and children have looked at the relationship between juvenile-onset, type 1 DM and coxsackieviruses B.* Between 1973 and 1984, 10 case-control studies examined the prevalence of antibody to various group B coxsackieviruses in patients with type 1 DM and control subjects. In eight of these studies, the prevalence was greater in the patients with type 1 DM. In three of these studies, IgM antibody to the group B coxsackieviruses was examined, and the prevalence in each was greater in the patients with type 1 DM than in control subjects. A Finnish study noted that patients with type 1 DM were more likely to have IgA antibodies to coxsackievirus B4 than were control subjects.[532]

*References 28, 43, 57, 58, 172, 246, 268, 299, 371, 372, 427, 461, 473, 482, 487, 489, 505, 585, 589, 631, 712–714, 877, 1002, 1013, 1088, 1114, 1121, 1171.

Helfand and associates[473] performed a well-done case-control study of type 1 DM. These investigators found that new-onset cases of type 1 DM in patients 13 to 18 years of age were more likely than were control subjects to be IgM antibody–positive for 9 of 14 EV serotypes. The serotypes were as follows: coxsackieviruses B2, B3, B4, B5, and B6; coxsackievirus A9; and echoviruses 9, 30, and 34. Green and associates[427] in 2004 performed a systematic review of published case-control studies relating to coxsackievirus B serology and type 1 DM. In 13 studies that looked at antibody to all coxsackievirus B types, seven (54%) had significantly more positive antibody values in the cases than in the control subjects. The findings were less impressive when rates of antibody by specific coxsackievirus B serotypes were compared. However, with coxsackievirus B4, the odds ratio was greater than one in 17 (53%) comparisons, and this finding was significant in six (35%) of the studies.

In an extensive study, Skarsvik and colleagues[1035] noted that children with type 1 DM had an impaired type 1 T-cell response against coxsackievirus B4 in contrast to the response in healthy children. The findings led these investigators to suggest that the defect in T-cell function delayed clearance of coxsackievirus B4 and made damage to β cells more likely. In another study involving adults, Varela-Calvino and coworkers[1121] noted that T-cell proliferative responses against the VP2 protein of coxsackievirus B4 was significantly reduced in patients with type 1 DM, in contrast to the responses in control subjects.

Cudworth and colleagues[268] noted a correlation between HLA-BW15 and coxsackieviruses B1, B2, B3, and B4 antibodies in patients with type 1 DM. In 1979, Yoon and colleagues[1202] reported the recovery of coxsackievirus B4 from the pancreas of a previously healthy 10-year-old boy who died after being in a diabetic coma. Hindersson and coworkers[489] noted the simultaneous onset of type 1 DM in a mother and her 10-year-old son coincident with a coxsackievirus B5 infection.

Clements and coworkers[246] noted that 9 of 14 serum samples from children with new-onset type 1 DM were positive for EV RNA by PCR. In contrast, only 4% of serum samples from control children had evidence of EV RNA. Oikarinen and associates[869] conducted a nested case-control study involving children in Finland who took part in a type 1 DM prediction and prevention study. All case children ($n = 38$) had progressed to clinical type 1 DM. Nondiabetic control children ($n = 140$) were pairwised matched for sex, birth date, hospital district, and HLA-DP-conferred genetic susceptibility. Serum samples (at 3- to 12-month intervals) were examined for EV RNA. EV RNA–positive samples (5.1%) were significantly more frequent among cases than among control subjects (1.9%). In a more recent study involving children in Finland, Sweden, England, France, and Greece it was noted that antibodies against coxsackievirus B1 were more frequent among diabetic children than among control children.[792A] In another study from Finland antibody to coxsackievirus B1 was associated with an increased risk of β-cell autoimmunity.[664] In another Finnish study involving adults, 50% of the patients with type 1 DM had RNA evidence of ongoing enteroviral infection in the gut, whereas none of the control subjects had similar infections.[870]

In a murine model, See and Tilles[1013] found that a diabetogenic strain of coxsackievirus B4 infection resulted in persistent detection of viral RNA in the pancreases of most infected mice. This persistence of antigen was associated with chronic islet cell inflammation and elevated islet cell antibody levels. Stimulated peritoneal macrophages caused lysis of islet cells either directly or by an antibody-dependent mechanism. A study in prediabetic children found that the presence of EV RNA in serum was a risk factor for development of β-cell autoimmunity and type 1 DM.[714] Glutamic acid decarboxylase (GAD_{65}) is one of the major β-cell target antigens in the autoimmune β-cell damaging process that leads to the development of type 1 DM.[712] Antibody and cellular immunity cross-reactivity exists between GAD_{65} and the 2C protein of coxsackievirus B4.[43,712] The results of several studies suggest that enteroviral infections are associated with the development of β-cell autoimmunity and the eventual destruction of islet cells.[135,487,713] Time periods from enteroviral infection to the development of β-cell autoimmunity and the eventual development of type 1 DM from β-cell destruction have a great range that perhaps explains the lack of a more specific seasonally related onset of type 1 DM.

A case of neonatal type 1 DM associated with a maternal echovirus 6 infection has been reported.[877] In Northern Sweden there is a PeV (Ljungan virus) that has been isolated from bank voles.[844] This virus is a separate species in the PeV genus. It was found that captured bank voles developed diabetes, and they had antibodies to Ljungan virus and autoantibodies against glutamic acid decarboxylase 65 (GADA), islet antigen-2 (IA-2), and insulin (IAA). Antibodies to the Ljungan virus were found in the sera in children in Northern Sweden. Children with type 1 DM had higher antibody values to this virus than were found in nondiabetic control children.

Eye Findings

Acute Hemorrhagic Conjunctivitis

Although conjunctivitis has been a frequent finding in nonpolio enteroviral illnesses since the 1950s, its occurrence as a dominant symptom has been observed only since the 1960s.[134,182,404,592]

In June 1969, Chatterjee and associates[188] noted an epidemic of acute hemorrhagic conjunctivitis in Accra, Ghana. This disease was nicknamed Apollo 11 disease because it coincided with the time of the Apollo 11 moon landing. Since 1969, many epidemics of acute hemorrhagic conjunctivitis have been described. In most epidemics, EV 70 has been the etiologic agent, but similar epidemics have been caused by a variant of coxsackievirus A24.[239] More recently, this virus has been the cause of more epidemics than has EV 70.* Most epidemics have occurred in tropical and semitropical countries; however, outbreaks have been observed in Minnesota, as well as in Moscow, London, and other European cities.[661,1198] In the continental United States, epidemic disease has occurred in Florida and North Carolina.[153] During epidemics, all age groups are affected, but the highest attack rate is in school-age children.[1148]

Acute hemorrhagic conjunctivitis has a sudden onset, with severe eye pain and associated photophobia, blurred vision, lacrimation, erythema, and congestion of the eye, as well as edema and chemosis of the lids.[483] Subconjunctival hemorrhages of varying size, frequently transient punctate epithelial keratitis, conjunctival follicles, and preauricular lymphadenopathy are present. The eye discharge initially is serous but becomes mucopurulent with secondary bacterial infection. Systemic symptoms, including fever, are rare manifestations. Within 2 to 3 days after the onset of illness, patients note some improvement, and recovery is usually complete in 7 to 12 days. In a study in American Samoa, researchers found that illness caused by coxsackievirus A24 was somewhat different from that caused by EV 70.[995] In cases caused by coxsackievirus A24, conjunctival hemorrhage was less severe, and upper respiratory and systemic symptoms occurred more frequently. In a study in American Samoa of disease caused by EV 70, researchers found that children 2 to 10 years of age had the highest attack rate, and antibody from previous infection gave only partial protection against symptomatic reinfection.[96]

Occasionally, findings suggestive of pharyngoconjunctival fever have been noted. A few patients have had a poliomyelitis-like illness or polyradiculomyeloneuropathy after EV 70 acute hemorrhagic conjunctivitis.[529,1135] Epidemics are explosive, with spread mainly by the eye-hand-fomite-eye route.

Conjunctivitis Associated With Other Enteroviral Illness

Conjunctivitis is a common minor manifestation of enteroviral illness with several specific agents. Table 166.12 presents the frequency of occurrence of conjunctivitis in selected outbreaks of disease caused by coxsackieviruses and echoviruses. Conjunctivitis was most prevalent in coxsackievirus B3 and B5 and echovirus 9 and 30 infections. In addition to the outbreaks reported in Table 166.12, conjunctivitis has been noted in isolated illnesses associated with echoviruses 1, 6, and 20.[623]

Photophobia

As would be expected, photophobia occurs commonly in aseptic meningitis caused by coxsackieviruses and echoviruses. During epidemic

*References 136, 156, 163, 247, 413, 618, 659, 886, 937, 1079, 1189.

TABLE 166.12 Frequency of Conjunctivitis in Outbreaks of Illness Caused by Coxsackieviruses and Echoviruses

Virus Type	Age Group	Conjunctivitis (%)	Main Characteristics of Illness	References
Coxsackievirus A9	Children	20	Pharyngitis, rash	688
Coxsackievirus A16	Mainly children	0–18	Hand-foot-and-mouth disease	188, 728, 954
Coxsackievirus B2	Mainly children	2	Nonspecific febrile illness, respiratory illness	200
Coxsackievirus B3	Children	2–42	Upper respiratory illness	200
Coxsackievirus B4	Children	25	Upper respiratory illness	200
Coxsackievirus B5	Mainly children	7–50	Rash, meningitis, hepatosplenic illness, respiratory illness, pleurodynia	210, 260, 976, 991
Echovirus 2	Children	25	Rhinorrhea	200
Echovirus 4	Children	Rare	Meningitis	733
Echovirus 9	Mainly children	13–30	Rash, meningitis	154, 200, 981
Echovirus 11	Children	15	Rash	210
Echovirus 16	Children	6–10	Rash	450, 832
Echovirus 30	Mainly children	10–60	Meningitis, nonspecific febrile illness	200, 451, 1092

meningitis, researchers have noted it with the following viruses: coxsackievirus A9 and echoviruses 3, 4, 6, 7, 9, 19, and 30.* It is a most common occurrence with echovirus 9 and 30 infections, but the incidence of this complaint varies greatly in different reports. In one echovirus 30 outbreak, 80% of the patients studied had photophobia.[1092] On average, 20% of patients with meningitis have remarkable photophobia. Photophobia also is associated with pleurodynia caused by coxsackievirus B infections.[976,1146]

Other Eye Findings

Nodular lesions on the palpebral conjunctiva were observed in some patients with coxsackievirus A10 infection and lymphonodular pharyngitis.[1049] A corneal ulcer occurred in one patient with hand-foot-and-mouth disease.[728] Optic neuritis was described in a boy with pleurodynia, although the enteroviral origin of the illness was not confirmed in the laboratory.[1107] Keratoconjunctivitis was noted in two boys with echovirus 13 infections.[630] Periorbital edema was observed in one patient with echovirus 9 meningitis. A woman with panuveitis associated with coxsackievirus B3 infection was described.[361] One report detailed monofocal outer retinitis in a 36-year-old man with hand-foot-and-mouth disease.[445] Five extensive outbreaks of uveitis caused by echoviruses 11 and 19 in hospitalized young children were noted in three Siberian cities.[1122] These cases occurred predominately in infants hospitalized for other illnesses such as bronchitis, pneumonia, gastroenteritis, sepsis, dystrophy, and premature birth. Three normal adult patients with anterior uveitis in whom PeV was identified in ocular fluid have been noted.[287] In the same study an adult positive for human immunodeficiency virus (HIV) had panuveitis. Sore eyes and other unspecified eye complaints also have been noted frequently in patients with coxsackieviral and echoviral infections.[200,343,359,444,678,727,830,993,1000]

Cardiovascular Manifestations

Pericarditis, Myocarditis, and Dilated Cardiomyopathy

Pericarditis or myocarditis or both have been noted in association with 27 different nonpolio EVs. The relative importance of the different serotypes is presented in Table 166.13. The group B coxsackieviruses have been implicated most frequently in heart disease. Coxsackievirus B5 has been the most common causative agent, but types 2, 3, and 4 also have been reported frequently. Of the echoviruses, type 6 has been associated most often with cardiac involvement, but the clinical findings with this agent have been described in only a few cases.

In patients with coxsackievirus B cardiac disease, hepatitis, pneumonia, nephritis, meningitis, and orchitis have been occasional associated findings. In 2007 to 2008, severe neonatal disease (often with myocarditis) associated with coxsackievirus B1 infection was detected.[167,879,1164] These severe cases were caused by a single genetic lineage. Sometimes, arrhythmias are the only clinical manifestations of myocarditis.[206,1106] Constrictive pericarditis occurs occasionally.[746] The mortality rate for acute coxsackieviral and echoviral heart disease is unknown, but it is significant. Unfortunately, proper virologic study rarely is performed in nonfatal disease. In the only published follow-up study, researchers found that patients who survived acute coxsackievirus myocarditis usually recovered completely, without any residual disability.[1059]

The early descriptions of coxsackievirus B infection with myocarditis in the 1950s and early 1960s indicated acute, usually fulminant illnesses in which a coxsackievirus B serotype could be recovered from multiple sites, such as the throat, stool, and CSF, as well as from the heart and other organs at autopsy.[398,438,622,624,1115] Group B coxsackieviruses originally were isolated from suckling mice, and the infection in these mice caused acute, overwhelming fatal infections involving multiple organs, including the heart.[279,576] Coxsackievirus B infections in mice were studied in mouse model systems in the 1950s and 1960s, and researchers found that infections in older mice were affected markedly by the virus strain, mouse genetics, and drugs.[106,511,629] Since the 1970s, studies in mouse model systems have become more sophisticated, but they still depend on specific coxsackievirus B strains and specific mouse strains.*

More recent studies in mouse model systems noted the progression of acute coxsackievirus B infection to chronic infection and cardiomyopathy.[26,492,588,744,925,942] Since the mid-1980s, acute, subacute, and chronic cardiomyopathy has been studied in patients by antigen-detection techniques and newer serologic methods.†

Bowles and colleagues[113] found coxsackievirus B nucleic acid sequences in myocardial biopsy samples from several patients with cardiomyopathy. Muir and colleagues[813] detected EV-specific IgM antibodies in the sera of nine patients with chronic relapsing pericarditis. Fujioka and coworkers[377] reported positive enteroviral PCR results from endomyocardial biopsy specimens in 6 of 31 patients (19%) with dilated cardiomyopathy (DCM). Andréoletti and collaborators[29] noted EV RNA in 18 of 25 samples from the heart tissue of patients with DCM or ischemic cardiomyopathy. However, in two other well-controlled studies, enteroviral RNA could not be identified in endomyocardial biopsy samples or in heart tissue from patients undergoing heart transplantation.[251,699] In 1994, Muir and Archard[810] and Melchers and associates[765] reviewed the evidence for persistent enteroviral infection in chronic medical conditions, including idiopathic DCM. Muir and Archard[810] concluded that persistent enteroviral infection is associated causally with chronic medical

*References 75, 200, 422, 429, 592, 593, 597, 598, 626, 685, 733, 910, 1092.

*References 26, 134, 140, 234, 395, 392, 392, 398, 410, 476, 479, 492, 521, 522, 588, 620, 627, 635, 670, 725, 744, 757, 829, 855, 883, 925, 942, 945, 946, 955, 1015, 1016, 1097, 1100, 1177.

†References 25, 27, 29, 37, 112, 251, 289, 367, 376, 377, 471, 696, 699, 765, 810, 811, 813, 1213.

TABLE 166.13 **Nonpolio Enteroviruses and Parechoviruses Associated With Pericarditis and Myocarditis**

Virus Type		Age Group or Age of Individual Patients	HEART INVOLVEMENT				Other Aspects of Illness	References
			Etiologic Importance	Pericarditis	Myocarditis	Unspecified		
Coxsackievirus	A1	Infants and adults	±	+	+			200, 435
	A2	Adults	±			+		42, 200
	A4	Mainly children	+	+	+		Sudden infant death	42, 416, 436, 1149
	A5	—	±	+				1119
	A7	Adults	±	+	+		Hand-foot-and-mouth disease	55
	A8	—	±			+		435
	A9	Mainly infants	+		+		High fatality rate	436
	A10	—	±			+		42
	A16	Infants and child	±		+		High fatality rate	200, 1142, 1188
Coxsackievirus	B1	Infants, children, and adults	++	+	+		Rare hepatitis	14, 39, 42, 130, 200, 292, 435, 623, 755, 828, 958, 1004, 1158
	B2	Infants, children, and adults	+++	+	+		Occasional pneumonia	39, 42, 129, 130, 200, 292, 352, 440, 507, 623, 647, 755, 828, 958, 1004, 1011, 1149, 1158
	B3	Infants, children, and adults	+++	+	+		Rare hepatitis	42, 49, 79, 129, 130, 200, 292, 440, 508, 623, 647, 694, 828, 958, 1011, 1061, 1144, 1145, 1149, 1158
	B4	Infants, children, and adults	+++	+	+		Occasional pneumonia; myocardial calcifications; rare hepatitis, orchitis, nephritis, hemolytic uremic syndrome	39, 42, 49, 64, 120, 128–130, 200, 292, 352, 440, 508, 623, 647, 828, 938, 958, 1065, 1106, 1110, 1149
	B5	Infants, children, and adults	+++	+	+		Occasional pneumonia, pleurodynia, and meningitis; rare orchitis	39, 41, 54, 109, 130, 200, 404, 422, 470, 475, 647, 711, 755, 805, 828, 854, 909, 913, 920, 1004, 1011, 1149, 1154, 1158, 1173
Echovirus	1	Adolescents	±	+	+			42, 1000, 1158
	4	—	±			+		42, 764
	6	Children and adults	++	+				42, 78, 200, 1158
	7	Children and adults	±			+		42, 200,796
	8	Adolescents	±	+				200, 573, 590
	9	Children and adults	+	+	+			42, 200, 206, 694, 764, 794, 1149
	11	Children and adults	+			+		42, 78, 200, 958
	14	—	±			+		796, 1119
	17	—	±			+		42
	19	Children and adults	±	+	+			78
	25	Children	±		+			77, 78
	30	—	±			+		42, 694
Enterovirus	71			±		+	Encephalitis	491
Parechovirus	1	Children	±		+			734, 975

++++, Most common; ±, rare.

conditions, whereas Melchers and colleagues[765] found no clear evidence for enteroviral persistence and the subsequent development of chronic medical conditions.

Since the mid-1990s, additional studies in humans have been performed, with mixed results with regard to the role of coxsackievirus B in the origin of chronic cardiomyopathy. Bowles and associates[112] studied cardiac samples for PCR analysis from 624 patients of all ages with myocarditis and 149 patients with DCM. Enteroviral genome was found in the cardiac samples of 85 patients with myocarditis and in the samples from 12 patients with DCM. The histopathologic findings in nine of these 12 patients demonstrated borderline or mild findings of inflammatory infiltrates. Another study by investigators in the same group examined 80 explanted hearts from children with end-stage heart disease, and an enteroviral genome was not detected.[367] In another study, Zhang and coworkers[1214] found evidence of enteroviral capsid protein VP1 by immunohistochemical staining in 47 of 89 patients with DCM. In a study performed in Japan, Fujioka and associates[376] detected EV RNA in 7 of 30 American patients (23%) and in 15 of 47 Japanese patients (32%) with DCM. In our opinion, the data in these studies suggest that EVs have a role in some patients with DCM.

The general theme in most contemporary mouse model studies is that damage to the myocardium is not caused by the direct cytopathic effect of the virus, but rather it is caused by the cellular immune response of the host. Unfortunately, the mouse model data and the less than definitive data from human studies have led cardiologists and others to think that the model systems are representative of human disease.[348,710] No adequate follow-up studies of survivors of acute enteroviral myocarditis or pericarditis have been conducted. Levi and colleagues[690] compared follow-up cardiac data on 10 adults who had acute myocarditis associated with coxsackieviral infections 42 to 68 months previously with similar cardiac data from normal age- and sex-matched subjects. No statistically significant differences in the two groups were found in the seven tests evaluated.

Orinius[875] performed cardiac examinations on 53 adults who had coxsackievirus B infections 2 to 11 years previously. The initial diagnoses in these 53 patients were meningitis in 33 cases, encephalitis in three cases, pleurodynia in six cases, pericarditis in two cases, and nonspecific complaints in 9 cases. Of this group, the "possibility of cardiomyopathy was established" in two (4%) cases. Two patients who previously had pericarditis were normal at follow-up.

Sainani and associates[982] performed follow-up studies on 20 adults and two teenagers who had coxsackievirus B myocarditis or pericarditis and found that five (23%) patients had chronic heart failure. Unfortunately, the duration of time since the primary illness of the patients was not reported.

Bergström and colleagues[91] performed follow-up examinations on five patients (two teenagers and three adults) who had had enteroviral myopericarditis and found that none had significant symptoms or physical signs. No follow-up data are available for neonates, infants, and children who have had enteroviral myocarditis.

In 1954, Stürup[1059] reported a follow-up study of patients admitted to the hospital in 1930 to 1932 with pleurodynia. Of nine patients evaluated, including four who had a history of acute pericarditis, none had constructive pericarditis.

Other Cardiac Manifestations

Numerous investigators have studied the possible association of coxsackievirus B infection and myocardial infarction.* In many instances, patients with infarction have been demonstrated to have concomitant coxsackievirus B infection.[328,431,438,674,675,834,843,856,1181,1184] In controlled studies, the results have varied. Nikoskelainen and associates[843] noted that nine of 59 patients with acute myocardial infarction had coxsackievirus B infection, whereas in the control group of 38 patients without infarction, only one patient had evidence of infection. Similarly, Nicholls and Thomas[834] found that 26% of patients had infections, but no infections were found in the control subjects.

In contrast, five other studies failed to show an increased rate of infection in patients with myocardial infarction, in contrast to control subjects.[431,438,856,912,1181] However, two of these studies were performed during a nonenteroviral season,[912,1181] and in a third study, little coxsackievirus B activity occurred in the community during the study period.[431] Analysis of the available studies indicates that coxsackievirus B infection would appear to have a role in myocardial infarction. In one coxsackievirus B5 infection, inferolateral wall myocardial necrosis occurred, but coronary arteriography did not demonstrate obstruction.[293]

Chandy and associates[177] presented data in which antibody to group B coxsackieviruses was related to rheumatic-like valvular heart disease, and Burch and associates[130] demonstrated coxsackievirus B antigens in rheumatic lesions of the heart. Limson and colleagues[700] could find no association between group B coxsackieviruses and rheumatic fever. Soboleva and associates[1039] noted an association between coxsackievirus A13 and rheumatic fever; these investigators reported seven children with concomitant streptococcal and coxsackievirus A13 infection. Children with fulminant EV 71 infection have been noted to have acute left ventricular dysfunction.[176,183,516] A 27-month-old girl who died suddenly was found to have SAFV identified in the CSF, blood, and myocardium.[836]

A 4-month-old boy who had repair of an atrioventricular septal defect was found to have a coxsackievirus B2 endocarditis.[102] This virus was recovered from the excised prosthetic patch.

Genitourinary Manifestations

Orchitis and Epididymitis

Group B coxsackieviruses are second only to mumps as causative agents of orchitis.[39,200,258,369,440,623,802,1011,1065,1158] Coxsackievirus B5 is the virus associated most commonly with this disease, although coxsackieviruses B2 and B4 also have been implicated on many occasions. In almost all instances, orchitis is a secondary event in enteroviral infections. The most common association is with pleurodynia. The illness frequently is biphasic: fever and pleurodynia develop initially, and then apparent recovery is followed by orchitis approximately 2 weeks after onset. Many patients also have epididymitis. In epidemics of disease caused by group B coxsackieviruses, the occurrence of testicular involvement varies considerably. Generally, orchitis occurs infrequently, but in one outbreak of coxsackievirus B2, 17% of postpubertal male patients had orchitis, and 7% also had epididymitis.[200] Orchitis also is associated frequently with pericarditis and myocarditis. In one instance, coxsackievirus B5 was recovered from a testicular biopsy specimen.[258]

In virtually all instances, testicular involvement has occurred in postpubertal patients, mostly in young adults. In addition to coxsackieviruses B2, B4, and B5, other EVs have been implicated: coxsackieviruses B1 and B3[200,623] and echoviruses 6, 9, and 11.[623,1156] Meningitis and exanthem have been associated with orchitis.

Nephritis

Scattered cases of nephritis associated with nonpolio enteroviral infections have been reported. Bayatpour and colleagues[70] noted acute glomerulonephritis in a 9-year-old boy with an extensive coxsackievirus B4 infection. This child had a concomitant rise in antistreptolysin O titer. Yuceoglu and associates[1207] reported twins with echovirus 9 infection and acute glomerulonephritis; Burch and Colcolough[128] observed a patient with progressive fatal pancarditis and nephritis in whom coxsackievirus B4 antigen was found in the kidneys. Mesangiolytic glomerulonephritis associated with an echovirus 6 infection was described in an infant with immune deficiency.[520]

Other Genitourinary Findings

Hemolytic-uremic syndrome has been associated with virologic or serologic evidence of infection with the following: coxsackieviruses A2, A4, A9, A10, A16, A21 and B1 to B6; echoviruses 4, 6, and 7; and PeV 1.[44,290,406,857,938,939] De Petris and colleagues[290] demonstrated titer rises to various EVs in patients with hemolytic-uremic syndrome who tested positive or negative for infections with verocytotoxin-producing *Escherichia coli*. Other abnormal renal or urinary findings in nonpolio enteroviral infections include the following: acute oliguric renal failure

*References 328, 431, 438, 674, 675, 834, 843, 856, 912, 1181, 1184.

with coxsackievirus B5[38]; pyuria, hematuria, or proteinuria with echoviruses 1, 6, and 9 and coxsackievirus B5[200,598,685,981,1000]; and hemorrhagic cystitis.[802] A 7-year-old girl with coxsackievirus A10 infection had vaginal ulcerative lesions,[787] and Wassermann test results have been falsely positive in patients with echovirus 9 and coxsackievirus B5 infections.[924]

Hematologic Findings

In 1968, Horwitz and Moore[506] described an outbreak of infectious lymphocytosis during which 27 mentally handicapped children were studied. The mean WBC count of the study group patients was 57,200; lymphocytes accounted for at least 50% of the total in all cases. Approximately one-half of the patients had low-grade fever, and 15 of 27 had moderate diarrhea. A nontypeable EV suggestive of coxsackievirus group A was recovered from the ill patients, and neutralizing antibody to a strain (EVU-16) of the isolated virus developed in 31% of the patients in whom serologic studies were performed.[442,506]

Letsas and colleagues[689] reported a 17-year-old-boy with fulminant myocarditis and hemophagocytic syndrome. Over the course of a 3-day period, his hematocrit decreased from 40.9% to 31.7%, and his platelet count went from 90,000 to 38,000/mm^3. Examination of the bone marrow revealed many mature histiocytes with active hemophagocytosis. The patient improved dramatically with inotropic and intravenous immunoglobulin (IVIG) treatment. Katsibardi and coworkers[600] reported the occurrence of hemophagocytic syndrome associated with enteroviral infections in three children with malignant diseases; in spite of IVIG and pleconaril treatment, all cases had a fatal outcome.

Muscle and Joint Manifestations

Arthritis

During the period from 1971 to 1975, during which EVs were recovered from 7075 persons in the United States, nine instances of rheumatic disease were reported[802]; although not clearly specified, three patients apparently had arthritis. Blotzer and Myers[101] noted an adult with echovirus 9 infection and the concomitant onset of arthritis that persisted for 3 months. Echovirus 9 was recovered from the synovial fluid of a man with acute monocytic arthritis,[656] and one adult and one adolescent had serologic evidence of coxsackievirus B4 infection in association with the onset of rheumatoid arthritis–like illness.[531]

Myositis

Because group A coxsackieviruses routinely cause myositis in suckling mice, a reasonable approach is to suspect a similar clinical manifestation in people. Myalgia also is a common complaint in illnesses caused by many coxsackieviruses and echoviruses.[39,200,369,451,663,755] However, almost no direct (i.e., demonstration of virus in muscle) or indirect (i.e., elevations in muscle enzymes) evidence of muscle involvement in routine enteroviral illnesses exists. Of the nine patients with rheumatic disease described by Morens and colleagues,[802] six apparently had myositis; in one instance, coxsackievirus A2 was implicated, and in another patient with polymyositis, coxsackievirus A9 was the related agent. Three patients with echovirus 18 infection and polymyositis have been reported.[610] Acute rhabdomyolysis in one adult and myositis, myoglobinemia, and myoglobinuria in another adult have been associated with echovirus 9 infection.[564,582] Christensen and associates[237] noted that children with dermatomyositis were more likely to have serum antibody to one or more group B coxsackieviruses than were control children. Chou and Gutmann[233] noted EV-like particles in the muscles of two patients with fatal dermatomyositis; Tang and colleagues[1076] demonstrated coxsackievirus A9 in the muscles of an 11-year-old girl with chronic myopathy. Using both PCR and dot-blot hybridization assays, Fox and colleagues[364] could not find evidence of persistent enteroviral infection in 32 adults with inflammatory muscle disease (one patient with dermatomyositis and 31 patients with polymyositis).

Yousef and coworkers[1204] reported EV RNA in biopsy specimens from six of 13 patients (46%) with idiopathic polymyositis or dermatomyositis but in no samples from 13 patients with other muscle disorders. Behan and associates[72] looked for picornavirus RNA in biopsy specimens from 41 patients with inflammatory myopathy, but all results were negative.

Dekel and associates[288] reported a 4-year-old girl with localized thigh swelling caused by coxsackievirus A21. On muscle biopsy, perivascular infiltrates were noted, but the muscle fibers were not affected. Widespread edema was found in the muscle.

Skin Manifestations

Nonpolio EVs as a group are a common cause of a variety of skin manifestations.[197,1159,1162] In the summer and fall, these viruses are the leading causes of exanthems. Variation in the clinical expression rate of exanthem and in the age of the host is marked among the various viral types. In general, dermatologic expression is related inversely to the age of the infected patient. The frequency of exanthem and common associated illnesses by viral type are presented in Table 166.14.

Coxsackievirus A2

Rash associated with coxsackievirus A2 has occurred rarely. Febrile illness with exanthem in conjunction with coxsackievirus A2 infection was observed in Cincinnati in 1957; no details of this outbreak were presented.[978] Assaad and Cockburn[42] reviewed approximately 15,000 enteroviral illnesses for the period from 1967 to 1970 that were reported to the WHO and noted that in 45 instances, skin or mucous membrane lesions associated with coxsackievirus A2 infection were the main clinical manifestations.

Coxsackievirus A3

One case was reported, but no details are available.[796]

Coxsackievirus A4

Exanthem has been noted infrequently with coxsackievirus A4 infection.[42,204,360,807,1211] However, many cases may be missed because this virus grows poorly in tissue culture, and suckling mouse inoculation rarely is used in diagnostic laboratories. Six children were observed in one outbreak.[360] All patients initially had herpangina, and then the exanthem appeared concurrently with or after defervescence. It initially was erythematous, maculopapular, and discrete. In some children, the rash resolved within 4 days, but in others it progressed and became vesicular. The vesicular lesions occurred in crops, spread to the extremities, but not the palms and soles, and were yellowish, opaque, and 5 to 10 mm in size. They persisted for 1 to 2 weeks and regressed, with a brownish discoloration. The lesions easily were confused with resolving bug bites. Other manifestations of coxsackievirus A4 infection include an exanthem suggesting combined scarlet fever and rubella,[397] a maculopapular rash that clears with desquamation,[807] and an anaphylactoid, purpura-like rash (Fig. 166.8).[204]

Coxsackievirus A5

During the 4-year period studied by Assaad and Cockburn,[42] coxsackievirus A5 was second only to coxsackievirus A16 in the number of instances for which exanthem or mucous membrane involvement was the main clinical manifestation. Even with this apparent frequency, most instances of exanthem have been sporadic rather than part of an outbreak of exanthematous disease. The most common finding is hand-foot-and-mouth disease, which is not clinically discernible from that caused by coxsackievirus A16.[267,356,360] In one patient, the virus was recovered from vesicular fluid.[356]

Coxsackievirus A6

In the present decade, severe hand-foot-and-mouth disease has been found in coxsackievirus A6 outbreaks in the United States, Taiwan, Finland, Japan, Singapore, New Zealand, China, and the United Kingdom.* Rash and fever were more severe, and hospitalization was more common than that seen in coxsackievirus A16 hand-foot-and-mouth syndrome cases. In the United States, there were 63 cases noted between November 7, 2011 and February 29, 2012.[147] In California, cases continued to occur in the spring and summer of 2012 (C. Glaser, Department of Public Health, California, personal communication, 2013). The rash in coxsackievirus A6 hand-foot-and-mouth disease is

*References 132, 228, 242, 465, 496, 514, 715, 726, 742, 919, 1032.

TABLE 166.14 Frequency of Exanthem in Outbreaks of Illness Caused by Enteroviruses and Parechoviruses

Virus Type		Age Group	Occurrence of Rash	Characteristics of Rash	Associated Manifestations	References
Coxsackievirus	A2	Children	Rare	Maculopapular	Fever	42, 978
	A4	Children	Rare	Maculopapular, vesicular	Fever, herpangina, hepatitis	42, 204, 360, 807, 1211
	A5	Mainly children	Occasional	Hand-foot-and-mouth disease	Fever	42, 267, 356, 360
	A6	Children and adults	Common	Hand-foot-and-mouth disease	Fever	919
	A7	Children and adults	Rare	Morbilliform; hand-foot-and-mouth disease, pancarditis	Meningitis, pneumonia	55, 434
	A9	Mainly children	4%	Maculopapular, vesicular, urticarial, petechial; hand-foot-and-mouth disease	Fever, meningitis, pneumonia	42, 200, 204, 208, 501, 524, 574, 578, 628, 688, 802, 853, 1167
	A10	Mainly children	Occasional	Hand-foot-and-mouth disease	Fever	42, 131, 200, 244, 315, 691
	A16	Children and adults	88%; <5 y 38%; 5–12 y 11%; adults	Hand-foot-and-mouth disease	Fever	13, 21, 33, 39, 42, 124, 200, 203, 204, 340, 360, 373, 397, 415, 414, 484–486, 691, 728, 729, 761, 805, 819, 950, 954, 1089
	B1	Children	Occasional	Maculopapular, vesicular	Fever, meningitis	42, 200, 204, 202, 286, 723
	B2	Children	Rare	Maculopapular, vesicular, petechial	Fever, herpangina, meningitis	39, 42, 360
	B3	Mainly children	Occasional	Maculopapular, vesicular, petechial	Fever, hepatosplenomegaly	39, 42, 139, 200, 256, 347, 458, 523,686
	B4	Mainly children	Occasional	Maculopapular, vesicular, urticarial	Fever, respiratory illness	200, 350, 597, 625
	B5	Mainly children	10%	Maculopapular, petechial, urticarial	Fever, meningitis	42, 109, 200, 209, 256, 292, 444, 469, 828, 847, 909, 913, 991, 1028, 1054, 1058, 1066, 1173, 1191
	B6	Children and adults	20%	Morbilliform	Pneumonia	418
Echovirus	1	Children	Rare	Maculopapular	Conjunctivitis	747
	2	Children	Rare	Macular, maculopapular	Fever, pharyngitis	200, 981, 1047
	3	Children	Rare	Petechial	Fever, meningitis	42, 466, 502
	4	Mainly children	10–20%	Macular, maculopapular, petechial	Fever, meningitis	200, 202, 323, 383, 597, 678, 733, 845, 937, 1043
	5	Infants and adults	Occasional	Macular	Fever	402, 1019
	6	Mainly children	Rare	Maculopapular, macular, papulopustular, vesicular	Fever, meningitis	42, 598, 740, 754, 760, 1128, 1132, 1173
	7	Children	Occasional	Maculopapular	Fever, meningitis	42, 562, 747
	9	Children and adults 41%; 5–9 y 6%; >10 y	57%; <5 y	Maculopapular, petechial, vesicular	Fever, meningitis	42, 89, 200, 243, 254, 263, 283, 343, 357, 384, 387, 467, 501, 560, 574, 586, 623, 625, 638, 662, 682, 727, 756, 802, 828, 841, 914, 921, 935, 972, 981, 1040, 1055, 1071, 1162
	11	Mainly children	Occasional	Maculopapular, vesicular, urticarial	Fever, meningitis	42, 127, 200, 210, 294, 1011
	13	Children	Occasional	Maculopapular		497, 1041
	14	Mainly children	Rare	Maculopapular, scarlatiniform	Fever, meningitis	42, 981
	16	Children	Occasional	Roseola-like	Fever, herpangina	197, 257, 450, 830–833
	17	Children	Occasional	Macular, maculopapular, papulovesicular	Fever, diarrhea, herpangina, meningitis	42, 124, 202, 212
	18	Children and adults	Occasional, epidemic	Rubelliform	Fever, meningitis	610, 763, 802, 828
	19	Children and adults	Occasional	Maculopapular	Fever, meningitis, upper respiratory illness	252, 261, 417
	25	Children	Occasional	Maculopapular, hemangioma-like	Fever, pharyngitis	77, 806, 825
	30	Children and adults	Occasional	Macular, maculopapular	Fever, meningitis	42, 199, 593, 1092, 1192
	32	Children	Rare	Hemangioma-like	Fever	202
	33	—	Rare	—	Meningitis	595, 607
Enterovirus	71	Children	Occasional	Macular, maculopapular, vesicular; hand-foot-and-mouth disease	Fever, meningitis, encephalitis, paralytic disease	18, 53, 403, 546, 609, 769, 786, 788, 872, 977, 1216
Parechovirus	1	Infants	Rare	Morbilliform	Respiratory illness	93
	3	Infants	Rare	—	—	1147
	6	Infants	Rare	—	—	1147

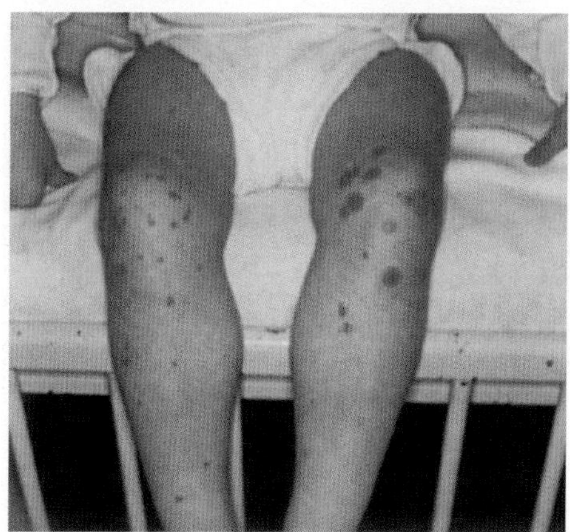

FIG. 166.8 Erythematous, papular, papulovesicular, and petechial lesions suggestive of anaphylactic purpura in a child with coxsackievirus A4 infection.

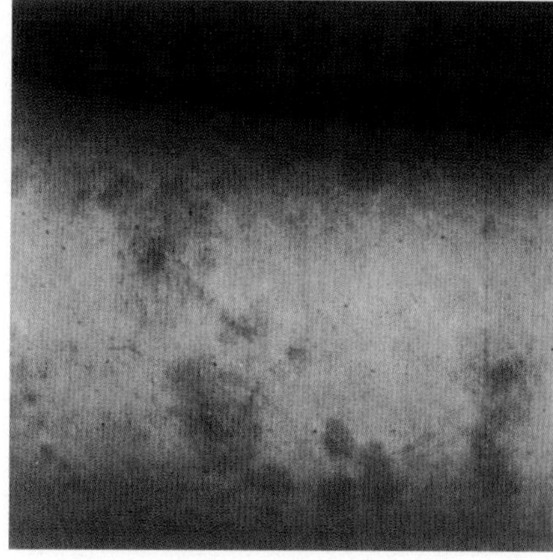

FIG. 166.9 Papular-urticarial lesions in coxsackievirus A9 infection. (From Cherry JD. Newer viral exanthems. *Adv Pediatr.* 1969;16:233–86.)

different ("atypical") from that seen in coxsackievirus A16 and EV 71 infections. In a review of 80 patients it was noted that 99% had a vesiculobullous and erosive eruption.[742] In 55% of the patients, the rash was accentuated in areas of eczematous dermatitis ("eczema coxsackium"). The rash involved more than 10% of the body surface area in 61% of the patients. In 37% of the patients the exanthem was Gianotti-Crosti-like; 17% of the patients had petechial or purpuric lesions. Some of the patients had delayed cutaneous findings including desquamation of the palms and soles and onychomadesis and Beau lines. In the summer of 2015, Banta and colleagues[60] noted an outbreak of coxsackievirus A6 hand-foot-and-mouth disease in 53 military basic trainees at Lockland Air Force Base in Texas. In association with a coxsackievirus A6 outbreak in Marseille, France in 2013 there was an outbreak of osteoarticular infections with *Kingella kingae* in a day care facility involving five toddlers.[329] It was suggested that the enteroviral infections triggered the *K. kingae* outbreak.

Coxsackievirus A7

Coxsackievirus A7 was recovered from one child with a morbilliform rash and aseptic meningitis.[434] An adult with a fatal coxsackievirus 7 infection had pancarditis, pneumonia, and hand-foot-and-mouth disease.[55]

Coxsackievirus A9

Coxsackievirus A9 is a common cause of exanthem (Figs. 166.9 and 166.10).† In contrast to coxsackievirus A16 and echovirus 9, in which rates of clinical exanthem expression are high, the rate of skin manifestations in coxsackievirus A9 infection is low. A review of 259 coxsackievirus A9 infections in 1970 revealed an exanthem rate of 4%.[200] Most cases of coxsackievirus A9 exanthem occur sporadically, although a few outbreaks have been described.[208,686,853]

Skin manifestations in coxsackievirus A9 infection have been interesting and varied. The most common rash illness is characterized by fever and an erythematous, maculopapular rash that starts on the face and neck and spreads to the trunk and extremities. Aseptic meningitis is a common associated finding.

In 1960, Lerner and colleagues[688] reported on 11 children with exanthem associated with coxsackievirus A9 infection. Of the patients, six had vesicular lesions and two patients had associated viral pneumonia. Since 1960, vesicular exanthem has been noted on several occasions.[200,208,524] Most commonly, illnesses have been described as hand-foot-and-mouth disease, but when the reports were analyzed, the rashes were vesicular but not always in a peripheral pattern.

Papular urticaria and large urticarial lesions have been occasional manifestations of coxsackievirus A9 infection (see Fig. 166.9).[204,208] Other manifestations include Stevens-Johnson syndrome and a severe illness simulating meningococcemia (see Fig. 166.10).[204,802]

†References 42, 200, 204, 208, 501, 515, 524, 570, 578, 628, 688, 802, 853, 1169.

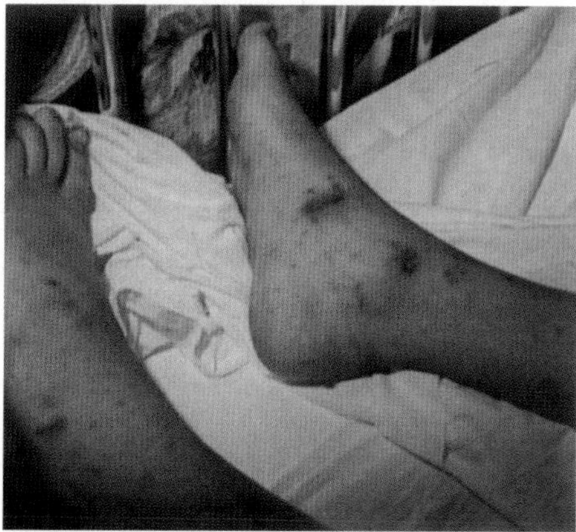

FIG. 166.10 Petechial and purpuric rash in a child with coxsackievirus A9 infection.

Coxsackievirus A10

The most common exanthematous illness associated with coxsackievirus A10 infection is hand-foot-and-mouth disease.[131,200,244,315,549,691] Stevens-Johnson syndrome was associated with coxsackievirus A10 infection in one instance,[200] and a child with ulcerative genital lesions also was reported.[787]

Coxsackievirus A16

In the WHO review of enteroviral infections for the 4-year period from 1967 through 1970, coxsackievirus A16 was associated with almost one-half of all skin or mucous membrane diseases. Coxsackievirus A16 is the major cause of hand-foot-and-mouth disease (Figs. 166.11 through 166.14). Of historical interest is that hand-foot-and-mouth disease apparently was a new clinical entity in 1956.[852] It was noted in sporadic outbreaks until approximately 1963, and since that time it has been a regularly recurring disease throughout the world.* Serologic data suggest that coxsackievirus A16 was not in wide circulation until approximately 1963.[203]

The signs and symptoms of coxsackievirus A16 hand-foot-and-mouth disease are recorded in Table 166.15. All illnesses have a typically enteroviral pattern with a short incubation period (4–6 days) and a summer and fall seasonal pattern. The clinical expression rate of the enanthem-exanthem complex is high—close to 100% in young children, 38% in schoolchildren, and 11% in adults.[803] Exanthem occurs more commonly in children, but in adults, the rash occurs more frequently

*References 13, 21, 33, 39, 124, 200, 203, 236, 340, 360, 373, 397, 412, 414, 415, 484, 485, 691, 728, 729, 761, 803, 826, 950, 954, 1089.

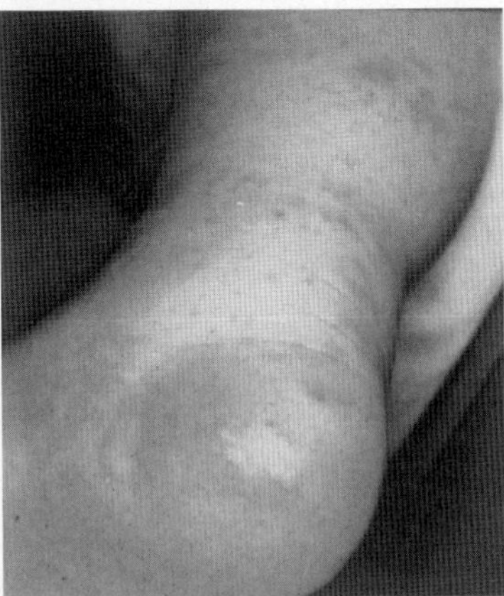

FIG. 166.11 Vesicular and maculopapular lesions on the foot and lower part of the leg as part of hand-foot-and-mouth disease caused by coxsackievirus A16. (From Cherry JD, Jahn CL. Hand-foot-and-mouth syndrome: report of six cases due to coxsackievirus, group A, type 16. *Pediatrics*. 1966;37:637.)

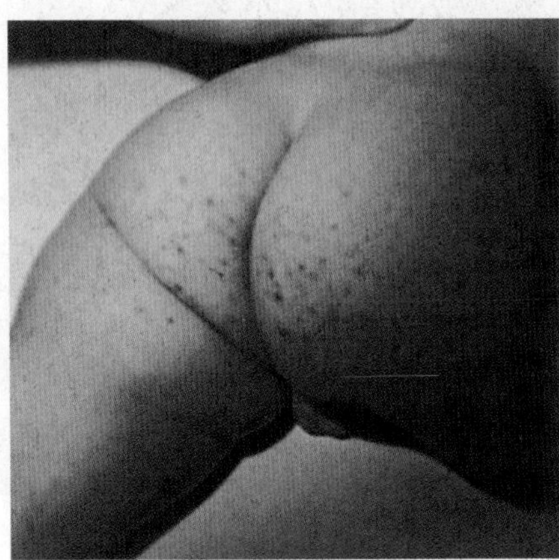

FIG. 166.12 Erythematous maculopapular lesions on the buttocks as part of hand-foot-and-mouth disease caused by coxsackievirus A16. (From Cherry JD, Jahn CL. Hand-foot-and-mouth syndrome: report of six cases due to coxsackievirus, group A, type 16. *Pediatrics*. 1966;37:637.)

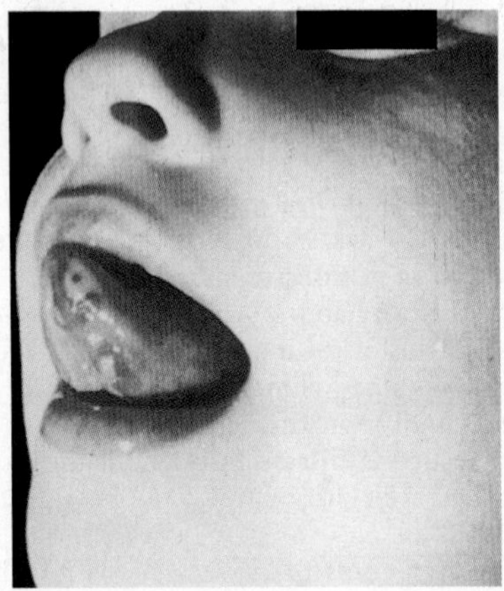

FIG. 166.13 Two large ulcerative lesions on the underside of the tongue in a patient with hand-foot-and-mouth disease caused by coxsackievirus A16.

with coxsackievirus A16 than with any of the other enteroviral agents.

Illness is ushered in with a mild prodromal fever, anorexia, malaise, and frequently a sore mouth. Enanthem occurs 1 to 2 days after the onset of fever, and the exanthem appears shortly thereafter. Of the

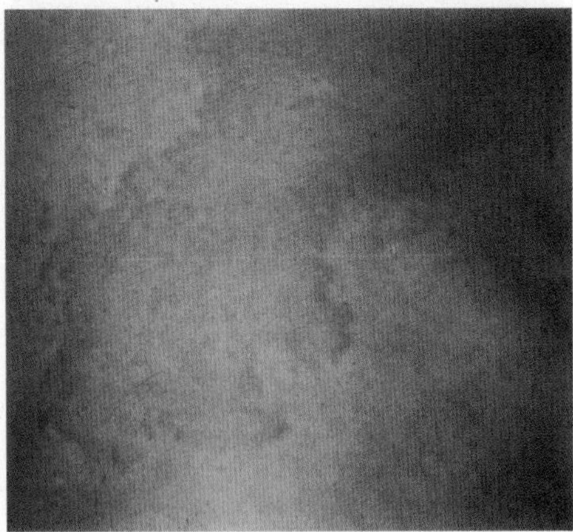

FIG. 166.14 Acute urticaria in a child with hand-foot-and-mouth disease caused by coxsackievirus A16 infection.

TABLE 166.15 Symptoms and Signs of Coxsackievirus A16 Illness (Hand-Foot-and-Mouth Disease)

Symptoms and Signs	Cases (%)
Enanthem	90
Buccal	61
Tongue	44
Palate, uvula, anterior pillars	36
Gums	15
Exanthem	64
Hands	52
Feet	31
Buttocks	31
Legs	13
Arms	10
Face	5
Sore mouth or throat	67
Malaise	61
Anorexia	52
Fever	42
Submandibular and/or cervical adenitis	22
Coryza	11
Cough	11
Diarrhea	10
Nausea and vomiting	3

Data from references 21, 205, 360, 373, 728, 761, 950, 954 and Cherry JD. Newer viral exanthems. *Adv Pediatr*. 1969;16:233–86.

cutaneous lesions, oral lesions are present more consistently than lesions of the skin. Because of this prevalence, illness, particularly in adults, is identified mistakenly as aphthous stomatitis (canker sores) or herpes simplex virus (HSV) infection. The intraoral lesions are ulcerative and average approximately 4 to 8 mm. The tongue and buccal mucosa are involved most frequently.

As noted in Table 166.15, the hands are involved more commonly than the feet. Buttock lesions also occur frequently, but they usually do not progress to vesiculation. The lesions on the hands and feet generally are vesicular and vary in size from 3 to 7 mm; they typically occur more commonly on the dorsal surfaces but frequently on the palms and soles, as well. The vesicles contain virus, but cytologic examination usually does not reveal diagnostic findings. These lesions clear by absorption of the fluid in approximately 1 week.

Of considerable interest is the frequent association of coxsackievirus A16 with subacute, chronic, and recurring skin lesions.[340,826] Evans and

Waddington[340] described an 84-year-old woman with chronic recurring skin lesions of more than 2 years' duration. Nankervis and associates[826] noted both subacute and recurring lesions in children. Higgins and Crow[484] reported a 31-year-old woman with Darier disease who had a Kaposi varicelliform eruption caused by coxsackievirus A16, and a similar illness was noted in a 1-year-old boy with eczema.[819] One child with a Gianotti-Crosti–like eruption (papular acrodermatitis of childhood) associated with coxsackievirus A16 infection was described.[559]

Coxsackievirus B1

Exanthem occasionally occurs in coxsackievirus B1 infections.[42,200,204,202,286,723] The most common cutaneous finding is an erythematous maculopapular eruption that is discrete. Two children with illnesses suggestive of hand-foot-and-mouth disease have been observed.[204]

Coxsackievirus B2

Coxsackievirus B2–associated exanthem is a rare occurrence. Maculopapular, vesicular, and petechial lesions have been noted.[39,42,360]

Coxsackievirus B3

Exanthem occasionally is reported as a sporadic event in coxsackievirus B3 infections, and a small outbreak occurred in one instance.[39,42,139,256,349,458,523,686,1208] Erythematous maculopapular eruptions occur most commonly, but petechial rash illnesses suggestive of meningococcemia also have been observed. Hand-foot-and-mouth disease was reported in one child,[686] and another child had a more generalized vesicular eruption. An adult with recurrent hand-foot-and-mouth disease had a rise in neutralizing antibody titer to coxsackievirus B3.[256]

Coxsackievirus B4

Although cutaneous manifestations with coxsackievirus B4 were noted as frequently as were those associated with coxsackieviruses B1, B2, and B3,[42,200] few clinical descriptions exist.[597,625] Morbilliform, petechial, and urticarial rashes have been described.

Coxsackievirus B5

Of the group B coxsackieviruses, type B5 is noted most frequently to have skin manifestations.* The rash usually is maculopapular; petechial lesions are observed occasionally, and one child with urticaria was reported.[209] Several children studied by Cherry and colleagues[209] had a roseola-like illness pattern. During outbreaks of coxsackievirus B5 illness, approximately 10% of young children have an exanthem. Many patients have concomitant aseptic meningitis. One adult patient with recurrent hand-foot-and-mouth disease had serologic evidence of coxsackievirus B5 infection.

Coxsackievirus B6

Goldwater[418] identified 97 children and adults with coxsackievirus B6 infection. The most prominent finding in these cases was cough and pneumonia. Twenty patients had exanthems; the rash was morbilliform and was associated with high fever and cough.

Echovirus 1

Exanthem and conjunctivitis have been associated with echovirus 1 infection in several children.[747]

Echovirus 2

Exanthem occasionally occurs with echovirus 2 infection.[200,981,1047] The rash has been erythematous macular in some instances but usually is maculopapular and discrete. Most children have had associated fever and pharyngitis.

Echovirus 3

Exanthem was noted in 2 of 29 children with echovirus 3 infection.[466] In both instances, the rashes were petechial; most patients in this outbreak had aseptic meningitis. Details of other echovirus 3 infections and exanthems are lacking.[42,502]

*References 42, 109, 200, 209, 256, 292, 444, 469, 847, 909, 913, 991, 1028, 1054, 1058, 1066, 1173.

TABLE 166.16 Signs and Symptoms in Echovirus 9 Disease

Sign or Symptom	Cases (%)
Fever	92
Headache	85
Nuchal rigidity	83
Nausea and vomiting	71
Pain (neck, back, trunk)	44
Exanthem	35
Nonexudative pharyngitis	28
Cough	24
Sore throat	20
Cervical lymphadenopathy	18
Coryza	18
Abdominal pain	17
Photophobia	16

Data from references 89, 283, 344, 357, 384, 560, 662, 682, 972, 1040, 1162 and Cherry JD. Newer viral exanthems. *Adv Pediatr.* 1969;16:233–86.

Echovirus 4

Echovirus 4 is a common cause of epidemic aseptic meningitis, and exanthem is an associated finding in 10% to 20% of pediatric cases.[204,358,383,597,678,733,845,937,1043] The rash usually is macular or maculopapular, has its onset 1 to 3 days after the initial fever, and lasts 1 to 2 days. A child with a petechial rash was noted.[597]

Echovirus 5

One major outbreak of echovirus 5 infection with exanthem was described.[402] This outbreak, which involved a maternity unit, resulted in a macular rash in 36% of the infants and 14% of the mothers. The rash was most prominent on the limbs and buttocks, appeared 24 to 36 hours after the onset of fever, and lasted 2 days. Selwyn and Howitt[1019] reported a child who had a macular rash with a zoster distribution. A neonate with sepsis-like illness and exanthem was described.[447]

Echovirus 6

Although echovirus 6 has been one of the more prevalent EVs since the late 1970s, it has been associated only sporadically with exanthematous disease. The following manifestations have been observed: morbilliform,[1128] maculopapular,[754,1173] macular,[740] and papulopustular exanthems[598]; Stevens-Johnson syndrome[1132]; and pityriasis rosea in an adult and a child.[598] Meade and Chang[760] reported an interesting zoster-like eruption in a 7-year-old boy in whom echovirus 6 was recovered from several bullae.

Echovirus 7

Echovirus 7 has been associated occasionally with exanthem.[42,272,562,796] In one outbreak of aseptic meningitis, five of 13 patients had erythematous maculopapular rashes that occurred during fever.[562] One child with a discrete maculopapular rash and thrombocytopenia was described.[747] The case of a 37-year-old woman with echovirus 7 infection, leukocytoclastic vasculitis, and palpable purpura was reported.[218]

Echovirus 9

Since the 1960s, echovirus 9 has been the most prevalent nonpolio EV, and exanthem is a common clinical manifestation (Table 166.16, Fig. 166.15).* Nonspecific febrile illness and aseptic meningitis are the usual

*References 42, 89, 200, 243, 254, 263, 283, 343, 357, 374, 384, 387, 419, 467, 501, 560, 570, 586, 623, 625, 638, 662, 682, 727, 756, 802, 841, 914, 921, 935, 972, 981, 1040, 1055, 1071, 1162.

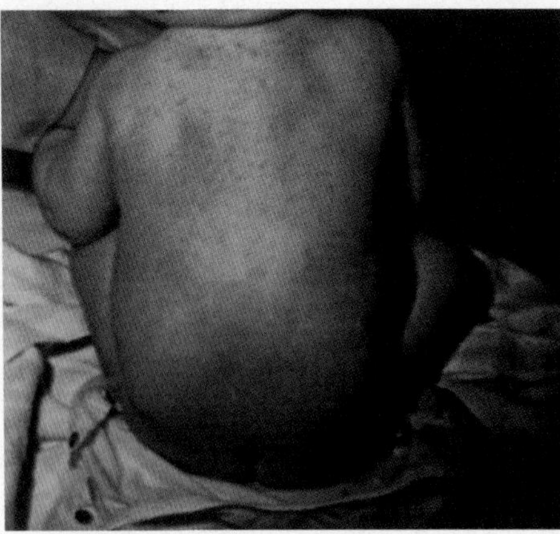

FIG. 166.15 Erythematous, discrete, maculopapular, and petechial rash of echovirus 9 infection. (From Cherry JD. Newer viral exanthems. *Adv Pediatr.* 1969;16:233–86.)

major manifestations of echovirus 9 infection. Exanthem occurs in approximately one-third of cases. The prevalence of exanthem is related inversely to age; 57% of children younger than 5 years of age have a rash, whereas only 6% of those older than 10 years have similar cutaneous findings.[685] The rash usually is rubelliform, but in addition or as the sole manifestation, petechiae are common findings. Rash and fever generally appear at approximately the same time, and frequently the illness closely mimics meningococcemia. The rash usually lasts approximately 3 to 5 days. In one instance, the rash progressed to a vesicular stage.[682] Drago and associates[307] noted a 24-year-old woman with echovirus 9 infection with herpangina and a maculopapular rash with petechiae that was localized to her buttocks.

Echovirus 11

Exanthem occasionally occurs with echovirus 11 infection, and it varies considerably in appearance.[42,127,200,210,294,1011] The most notable lesions have been bug bite–like vesicles and urticaria.[210] A child with subacute recurrent vesicular lesions[210] and a woman with a disseminated vesicular eruption were reported.[294]

Echovirus 13

One child with a maculopapular eruption was described.[497] During an outbreak of echovirus 13 aseptic meningitis in Israel, 15 patients had a concomitant exanthem.[1041]

Echovirus 14

Echovirus 14 is a rare cause of exanthem, and few details are available.[42,981] One child with a scarlatiniform eruption and aseptic meningitis was reported.[981]

Echovirus 16

The first of the enteroviral exanthematous diseases to be described was that caused by echovirus 16. It initially was studied by Neva and Enders[831] and, later, by Neva and colleagues,[832] and the illness was called *Boston exanthem.* Two outbreaks of echovirus 16 infection with exanthem were documented by Neva[830] in 1951 and by Neva and Zuffante[833] in 1954, and another occurred in Paris in 1960.[257] Since then, Boston exanthem has been reported only once. Seven cases were observed in 1974.[450]

The exanthem associated with echovirus 16 infection is erythematous, maculopapular, and discrete and is similar to that of other enteroviral infections. What has been unique with echovirus 16 infection is the relationship of rash with fever. Frequently, the illness resembles roseola in that the rash occurs at the time of or after defervescence.[197,450] Ulcerative lesions on the soft palate and tonsillar pillars (herpangina) sometimes have been observed.

Echovirus 17

Rash is an occasional occurrence in echovirus 17 infection.[42,124,204,212] In one outbreak, transient erythematous rashes were noted.[124] In cases that one of us (J.D.C.) studied, papular, maculopapular, and papulovesicular lesions were noted; two patients had herpangitic enanthems, and one had aseptic meningitis.[204,212]

Echovirus 18

Kennett and associates[610] described an extensive epidemic of echovirus 18 infection in which aseptic meningitis with or without exanthem was the major finding. In 15 patients, exanthem was the chief complaint. The rash was described as rubelliform. Most patients were children, but adults also had exanthem.

Echovirus 19

In one extensive epidemic of echovirus 19 infection, exanthem was a common occurrence.[252] Fifty percent of children younger than 6 months of age had exanthem, and many of these infants presented a picture of septicemia with peripheral circulatory failure. Rash occurred in adults and older children, but the percentage decreased with age. The rash usually was erythematous, maculopapular, and discrete. It started on the face and upper part of the trunk and spread to the extremities. Fever occurred in all cases, and meningitis and signs of upper respiratory tract involvement were noted frequently. In another outbreak of echovirus 19 infection, 33% of those infected had exanthem,[417] whereas in an outbreak studied by Cramblett and colleagues,[261] exanthem was a rare finding.

Echovirus 21

A 19-day-old infant with aseptic meningitis and rash was reported.[231]

Echovirus 24

A 4-month-old infant had rash and aseptic meningitis as a result of echovirus 24 infection.[231]

Echovirus 25

Echovirus 25 has been associated with an array of different skin manifestations.[80,205,443,806,825] In one epidemic of febrile pharyngitis, approximately one third of the patients had exanthem.[806] The rash usually was maculopapular and discrete, but occasionally it displayed a morbilliform confluence. The rash most frequently occurred during the period of defervescence.

Of considerable interest are two children with acute hemangioma-like lesions.[205] The lesions were erythematous and papular and surrounded by a 1- to 4-mm–wide halo of blanched-appearing skin. The center of each lesion had a bright red dot that suggested a dilated capillary or terminal arteriole. The whole lesion blanched with pinpoint pressure applied to its middle.

Echovirus 30

Echovirus 30 is a common cause of epidemic aseptic meningitis, and exanthem occasionally is noted concomitantly. The rash is macular or maculopapular.[42,200,542,593,680,1092,1192]

Echovirus 32

Two children with echovirus 32 infection and hemangioma-like lesions were described by Cherry and colleagues.[202] Some lesions seemed to be composed of many dilated capillaries; they easily blanched with pressure.

Echovirus 33

Four patients with aseptic meningitis and echovirus 33 infection also had exanthem.[595,607] Two adults had vesicular lesions that suggested HSV infection.[286]

Enterovirus 71

Kennett and associates[609] in Australia studied 49 patients with EV 71 infection and noted exanthem in 11. Six patients had aseptic meningitis, and rash was the predominant complaint in 5 patients. The exanthems varied: some were erythematous maculopapular, some vesicular, and some a combination of lesions. Two children had hand-foot-and-mouth disease, and a single child had a florid, diffuse erythematous rash. Since the 1970s, outbreaks and epidemics of hand-foot-and-mouth disease caused by EV 71 have been noted throughout the world.* Most notable have been epidemics in Asian-Pacific countries. In addition to hand-foot-and-mouth disease, these illnesses also have severe encephalitic manifestations.

Parechoviruses

Exanthem has been noted in association with PeV infections on several occasions. In some reports, genotypes have been reported,[93,551,879,1018,1116] whereas in others only PeV is indicated.[59,907,1124,1125,1179] In one study that included 110 PeV infections, 9.1% had unspecified exanthems, and, in addition, 6.4% had hand-foot-and-mouth disease.[551] Genotypes included types 1 and 3. In a study by Selvarangan and associates[1018] of CNS infections with PeV type 3, 60.3% had associated maculopapular exanthems. A morbilliform rash has been described in three infants with genotype 1 infections.[93] Genotypes 1 to 6 have all had infections associated with rash.

Clinical Exanthematous Manifestations and Syndromes

The major clinical exanthematous manifestations and syndromes of coxsackieviruses and echoviruses are presented in Table 166.17. Unusual findings include hemangioma-like lesions with echoviruses 25 and 32, anaphylactoid purpura with coxsackievirus A4 and echoviruses 9 and 18, zoster-like rash with echoviruses 5 and 6, pityriasis-like rash with echovirus 6, and chronic or recurrent rash with coxsackievirus A16 and echovirus 11.

Neurologic Manifestations

Neurologic illness is a frequent manifestation of infection with most EVs and PeV. The most common illness is aseptic meningitis, but encephalitis and other manifestations also occur. Parechoviral neurologic manifestations are particularly common and significant in neonates and during the first 3 months of life (these are discussed in the later section on neonatal infections). The prevalence of nonpolio EVs and PeVs in the various clinical syndromes is presented in Table 166.18.

Aseptic Meningitis

Aseptic meningitis caused by EVs occurs both in epidemics and as isolated cases. The etiologic agents most often associated with epidemic disease are presented in Table 166.19. Epidemic disease has occurred most commonly with coxsackievirus B5, echoviruses 4, 6, 9, 13, and 30 and EV 71. In general, illness occurs more frequently in children, but if a specific outbreak is large, adults also are involved. Virtually all patients have fever and pharyngitis; other respiratory manifestations occur commonly. Rash is a frequent occurrence but varies with the specific viral agents. Between one-third and one-half of all patients with echovirus 9 meningitis have exanthem. Abdominal pain is a common symptom in patients with epidemic enteroviral aseptic meningitis.

Except for rash, herpangina, pleurodynia, or myocarditis, little else occurs clinically to help identify the origin in a sporadic case of aseptic meningitis. Initial symptoms include fever, headache, malaise, nausea, and vomiting. The headache usually is frontal or generalized; adolescents and adults frequently note retrobulbar pain. Pain in the neck, back, and legs occurs commonly. Abdominal pain is noted in approximately one-fifth of patients, but this symptom varies with the specific etiologic viral type. Photophobia is a common occurrence.

Physical examination reveals a temperature in the range of 38° to 40°C (100.4°–104°F). Skin rash occurs often and usually is erythematous, maculopapular, and discrete. Frequently, particularly with echovirus 9 infection, the rash is petechial and suggests meningococcemia. Hand-foot-and-mouth disease is a common event in cases of aseptic meningitis caused by EV 71 infection.[176,183,491,646,759] Pharyngitis occurs frequently. Generalized muscle stiffness or spasm usually is observed, although the degree varies considerably; the Kernig and Brudzinski signs are positive in fewer than half of the cases. Deep tendon reflexes usually are normal. In one study, 9% of children with enteroviral meningitis had the syndrome of inappropriate secretion of antidiuretic hormone.[192] The onset of this syndrome was noted 36 hours after admission to the hospital, and it usually lasted less than 2 days.

Examination of CSF reveals considerable variation among patients and in the same patient on repeated examination. CSF leukocyte counts vary from a few cells to a few thousand per cubic millimeter; the median is in the range of 100 to 500 cells/mm^3. The percentage of neutrophils also varies greatly. Initial examinations frequently reveal a predominance of neutrophils, but rarely more than 90%, as seen in bacterial disease. Usually, a range between 30% and 60% neutrophils is found on initial examination. Repeated examinations of CSF demonstrate an increasing percentage of mononuclear cells. Dagan and colleagues[273] observed that the rate of isolation of virus from the CSF in enteroviral meningitis was directly proportional to the number of leukocytes in the fluid. Dalal and associates[278] found that children with echovirus 4 meningitis had elevated values of interleukin-6 and interferon in the CSF and that the interleukin-6 value correlated with the CSF leukocyte values.

CSF protein levels usually are elevated mildly, and glucose concentrations usually are normal; hypoglycorrhachia rarely occurs.[46,214,327,665,684,736,1020,1029,1033,1060] Occasionally, the CSF findings suggest tuberculosis meningitis with mononuclear pleocytosis, hypoglycorrhachia, and elevated protein levels.[732] A child with coxsackievirus B4 meningitis had eosinophils in the CSF.[213] The results of other routine laboratory studies such as the WBC count occasionally are abnormal but are not helpful diagnostically.

The duration of illness varies significantly. In most patients, the temperature returns to normal within 4 to 6 days, and disability as a result of neurologic involvement lasts 1 to 2 weeks. Occasionally, the pattern of illness is biphasic; an initial period with fever, headache, nausea, vomiting, and muscle aches and pains of a few days' duration is followed by general recovery and then a return to the same symptoms in addition to more pronounced neurologic involvement.

Wilfert and associates[1166] performed a longitudinal assessment of children who had enteroviral meningitis early in life and found that receptive language functioning was significantly worse than that of children in a control group without meningitis. In another study, Sells and colleagues[1017] examined the long-term effects of CNS enteroviral infection in 19 children. Of this group, 11 were free of detectable abnormalities, 5 had possible defects, and 3 had definite neurologic sequelae. In more recent studies, patients who have had meningitis have performed as well as control subjects in follow-up developmental evaluations.[90,961,966]

Encephalitis

In the United States, approximately 2500 cases of encephalitis per year, on average, are reported to the CDC.[154] In this group, only approximately 2% of these patients demonstrate an enteroviral origin of illness. However, the seasonal pattern of disease and the absence of arboviral activity in many geographic locations suggest that 500 to 1000 cases of enteroviral encephalitis actually occur each year in the United States. The prevalence of coxsackieviruses, echoviruses, EVs, PeVs, and SAFVs as etiologic agents in encephalitis is presented in Table 166.18. Echovirus 9 is the most frequent cause of enteroviral encephalitis. Other enteroviral types commonly associated are echoviruses 4, 6, 11, and 30 and coxsackievirus B5. Echoviruses 4, 6, and 11 have been noted most frequently over a long period.

In general, the prognosis in encephalitis caused by enteroviral infection is good, but fatalities do occur. The viral types that have been isolated from the brain or CSF in fatal cases are as follows: coxsackieviruses B3 and B6; echoviruses 2, 9, 17, and 25; and EV 71.[440,623] First noted in Japan in the 1970s were outbreaks of hand-foot-and-mouth disease associated with a diverse array of encephalitic manifestations.[872] Since the mid-1970s, epidemics of hand-foot-and-mouth disease with encephalitis mainly caused by EV 71 have been occurring in Asian-Pacific countries.*

*References 53, 142, 174, 176, 180, 181, 183, 184, 193, 229, 375, 403, 491, 508, 513, 516, 519, 546, 591, 646, 697, 701–703, 705, 716, 743, 759, 769, 786, 848, 858, 871–873, 917, 977, 1143, 1138, 1139, 1193, 1195, 1216.

*References 142, 174,175, 180, 181, 183, 184, 193, 226, 229, 375, 491, 508, 513, 516, 519, 546, 591, 646, 697, 701–703, 705, 716, 743, 758, 759, 848, 871, 873, 917, 1081, 1138, 1139, 1143, 1195.

TABLE 166.17 Clinical Exanthematous Manifestations of Enteroviruses

		ASSOCIATED VIRAL AGENTS AND PREVALENCE OF MANIFESTATIONS		
Clinical Manifestations	**Virus Subgroup**	**Common**	**Occasional**	**Rare**
Macular rash	Coxsackievirus A			
	Coxsackievirus B		1, 2, 5	
	Echovirus and enterovirus		2, 4, 5, 13, 14, 17, 19, 30	18, 71
Maculopapular rash	Coxsackievirus A	9	2, 4, 5, 10, 16	6, 7
	Coxsackievirus B		1–5	
	Echovirus and enterovirus	4, 9	2, 5–7, 11, 16–19, 25, 30, 71	1, 3, 13, 14, 27, 33
Vesicular rash	Coxsackievirus A	5, 6, 16	8–10	4, 7
	Coxsackievirus B			1-3, 5
	Echovirus and enterovirus		11	6, 9, 17, 71
Petechial or purpuric rash	Coxsackievirus A	9	4, 6	
	Coxsackievirus B		2-5	
	Echovirus	9	4, 7	3
Urticarial rash	Coxsackievirus A	9	16	
	Coxsackievirus B		4, 5	
	Echovirus		11	
Erythema multiforme or Stevens-Johnson syndrome	Coxsackievirus A		9	10, 16
	Coxsackievirus B			4, 5
	Echovirus			6, 11
Exanthem and meningitis	Coxsackievirus A		2, 9	7
	Coxsackievirus B		1, 2, 4, 5	
	Echovirus and enterovirus	4, 9	6, 11, 17, 18, 25, 30	3, 14, 33, 71
Exanthem and pneumonia	Coxsackievirus A		9	7
	Coxsackievirus B		6	1
	Echovirus			9, 11
Hand-foot-and-mouth disease	Coxsackievirus A	6, 16	5, 10	7, 9
	Coxsackievirus B			1, 3, 5
	Echovirus and enterovirus	71		
Hemangioma-like lesions	Coxsackievirus A			
	Coxsackievirus B			
	Echovirus			25, 32
Herpangina and exanthem	Coxsackievirus A		4	9
	Coxsackievirus B			2
	Echovirus		16, 17	
Roseola-like illness	Coxsackievirus A			6, 9
	Coxsackievirus B		5	1, 2, 4
	Echovirus		16, 25	9, 11, 27, 30
Anaphylactoid purpura	Coxsackievirus A			4
	Coxsackievirus B			
	Echovirus			9, 18
Zoster-like rash	Coxsackievirus A			
	Coxsackievirus B			
	Echovirus			5, 6
Pityriasis-like rash	Coxsackievirus A			
	Coxsackievirus B			6
	Echovirus			
Chronic or recurrent rash	Coxsackievirus A	16		
	Coxsackievirus B			
	Echovirus			11

In an outbreak in Taiwan in 1998, 30 of 78 (38%) patients with severe illness had encephalitis, and 25 of these patients with encephalitis also had pulmonary edema or hemorrhage, two had myocarditis, and one had acute flaccid paralysis.[491] In another study, 30 of 34 children with CNS involvement had brainstem encephalitis, and 9 of this group (30%) died.[1141] Children who recovered from EV 71 encephalitis associated with cardiopulmonary failure often had neurologic sequelae with delayed neurodevelopment, reduced cognitive function, and attention-deficit/hyperactivity–related problems.[181,389,917,1103]

Paralysis

Paralysis caused by anterior horn cell disease occasionally results from infection with nonpolio EVs. In contrast to the prevalence of poliovirus, which in the prevaccine era resulted in epidemic paralytic disease, paralysis caused by nonpolio EVs usually is a sporadic event. Coxsackievirus A7 has been associated with outbreaks of paralytic disease on three occasions.[437,439,1133] Many cases of illness similar to poliomyelitis have occurred during outbreaks and epidemics of illness caused by EV 71 and by EV D68.* A 6-year-old girl developed acute flaccid paralysis in association with EV C105 infection.[500] Paralytic disease also has been noted during epidemics of acute hemorrhagic conjunctivitis caused by EV 70.[1135,1198]

†References 18, 20, 48, 281, 300, 403, 430, 468, 546, 769, 988, 1081, 1109, 1118.

TABLE 166.18 Neurologic Manifestations of Coxsackieviruses, Echoviruses, Enteroviruses, Parechoviruses, and Saffold Viruses

Clinical Manifestations	ASSOCIATED VIRAL AGENTS AND PREVALENCE OF MANIFESTATIONS				
	Virus Subgroup	Common	Occasional	Rare	References
Aseptic meningitis	Coxsackievirus A	9	7	1–6, 8, 10, 11–14, 16–18, 21, 22, 24	18, 19, 45, 86, 89, 95, 150, 161, 176, 183, 199, 225, 265, 283, 321, 332, 336, 343, 345, 357, 383, 384, 419, 440, 446, 454, 474, 491, 560, 562, 566, 574, 605, 606, 623, 634, 637, 641, 646, 662, 679, 680, 685, 750, 754, 759, 769, 796, 804, 851, 949, 961, 966, 972, 978, 1011, 1020, 1024, 1040, 1041, 1098, 1113, 1131, 1147, 1162, 1167, 1192
	Coxsackievirus B	2, 4, 5	1, 3	6	
	Echovirus	4, 6, 9, 13, 30, 33	3, 11, 12, 14, 16, 18, 19, 25, 31	1, 2, 5, 7, 8, 15, 17, 21, 24, 26, 27, 29, 32	
	Enterovirus	71	75	D68, 77	
	Parechovirus			1, 2, 3	
Encephalitis	Coxsackievirus A		9	2, 4–7, 10, 16	18, 142, 174, 176, 180, 181, 183, 184, 193, 199, 226, 229, 375, 440, 469, 491, 508, 513, 516, 519, 546, 591, 623, 646, 649, 666, 676, 695, 697, 701, 702, 703, 705, 716, 722, 743, 759, 758, 792, 796, 848, 871, 873, 917, 966, 1003, 1081, 1138, 1139, 1139, 1195
	Coxsackievirus B	5	1, 2, 4	3	
	Echovirus	4, 6, 9, 11, 30	3, 25	1, 2, 5, 7, 8, 12, 13, 14, 15, 17–21, 24, 27, 31, 33	
	Enterovirus	71	75		
	Parechovirus			1, 2	
Paralysis (lower motor neuron involvement)	Coxsackievirus A		4, 7, 9	2, 5, 6, 10, 11, 14, 21, 24	5, 7, 10, 15, 18, 20, 21, 27, 42, 48, 176, 183, 189, 199, 232, 266, 281, 300, 318, 353, 358, 403, 411, 430, 433, 437, 439, 440, 468, 491, 500, 546, 623, 646, 648, 728–730, 759, 769, 865, 891, 911, 936, 988, 1011, 1048, 1109, 1118, 1133, 1135, 1198, 1208
	Coxsackievirus B		2, 3	1, 4–6	
	Echovirus		9, 11, 30	1–4, 6–8, 12, 14, 16–19, 25, 27, 31, 33	
	Enterovirus	D68,70, 71		74, 75	
	Parechovirus			1, 6	
Guillain-Barré syndrome and transverse myelitis	Coxsackievirus A		9	2, 4, 5, 6, 19	18, 61, 80, 75, 99, 225, 292, 353, 397, 424, 529, 555, 571, 622, 683, 759, 785, 988, 1069, 1070, 1170
	Coxsackievirus B			1, 4	
	Echovirus		6	5, 7, 19	
	Enterovirus		70		
	Parechovirus			1	
Cerebellar ataxia	Coxsackievirus A		9	4, 7	87, 347, 440, 450, 546, 623, 740, 749, 822, 1211
	Coxsackievirus B			3, 4	
	Echovirus		6, 9	16	
	Enterovirus		71		
Peripheral neuritis	Coxsackievirus A				1011
	Coxsackievirus B				
	Echovirus		9		
Neurologic sequelae and other neurologic illness	Coxsackievirus A		3	9	170, 176, 183, 233, 389, 491, 623, 646, 759, 897, 957, 1011, 1017, 1137, 1140, 1185
	Coxsackievirus B		3	2, 4	
	Echovirus		9	19, 25, 30, 33	
	Enterovirus	71			

Guillain-Barré Syndrome and Transverse Myelitis

As Table 166.18 shows, many coxsackieviruses and echoviruses apparently have been associated with Guillain-Barré syndrome. In general, no specific viral types appear to cause the disease. Rather, the disease occurs sporadically in association with the prevalent enteroviral types. However, in South Wales, United Kingdom, a cluster of atypical Guillain-Barré syndrome cases in adults was temporally associated with EV D68.[1170] Two children also had Guillain-Barré syndrome.

Other Neurologic Illnesses

Cerebellar ataxia has been associated with coxsackieviruses A4, A7, A9, B3, and B4 and echoviruses 6, 9, and 16 (see Table 166.18). A 16-month-old boy with ataxia was found to have SAFV in the CSF and in a fecal sample.[836] Scott[1011] specifically commented on peripheral neuritis with echovirus 9 infection. Coxsackievirus A9 has been associated with focal encephalitis and acute hemiplegia on two occasions,[170,200] and echovirus 25 infection was noted in a 5-year-old boy with focal encephalitis and subacute hemichorea.[897] Coxsackievirus B4 was isolated from the CSF of a 22-year-old woman with intracranial hypertension,[1185] and postencephalitis Parkinson syndrome occurring after an episode of coxsackievirus B2 meningoencephalitis was described.[1137] Coxsackievirus B3 and EV 71 infections have been associated with opsoclonus-myoclonus.[654] The case of a 4-year-old boy with "Alice in Wonderland" syndrome (complex symptoms of perceptual distortion) associated with coxsackievirus B1 infection was described.[1140] A 16 month-old-boy had monosymptomatic ataxia in association with SAFV infection.[836] The virus was recovered from the CSF.

Phillips and colleagues[906] and Barrett and associates[63] noted the simultaneous occurrence of enteroviral and St. Louis encephalitis viral infection in the same community. In six instances, dual infections occurred, and the afflicted children tended to have more serious illnesses. Ribai and colleagues[948] noted an 18-month-old boy with transient cerebral arteriopathy and an enteroviral infection. The child had aphasia, right hemiplegia, and seizures, which occurred intermittently over a 3-day period.

Ergul and associates[334] described a 7-year-old boy with vestibular neuritis from whom enteroviral RNA was found in both the CSF and a nasopharyngeal sample. Multiple attacks of enteroviral aseptic meningitis in the same individuals have been noted occasionally.[639,823]

Woodall and associates[1183] found conserved enteroviral sequences in spinal cords from subjects with sporadic motor neuron disease and from one patient with possible familial motor neuron disease. Berger and associates[88] noted EV RNA sequences in spinal cord specimens from 13 of 17 patients with amyotrophic lateral sclerosis, but Walker and colleagues[1136] could not duplicate these findings in a study of 20 spinal cord specimens from similar patients. Simonsen and coworkers[1031]

TABLE 166.19 **Coxsackieviruses and Echoviruses Associated With Epidemic Aseptic Meningitis**

Virus Type		Age Group	Common Non-neurologic Findings	References
Coxsackievirus	A7	Children and adults	Fever	434
	A9	Mainly children	Fever, rash, pharyngitis	199, 688
	B1	Mainly children	Fever, pharyngitis	199
	B2	Children and adults	Fever, pharyngitis, rhinitis, abdominal pain, diarrhea	199, 735
	B3	Children and adults	Fever, pharyngitis, conjunctivitis	199
	B4	Children and adults	Fever, pharyngitis, rash, conjunctivitis	199, 350
	B5	Mainly children	Fever, pharyngitis, rash, pleurodynia, abdominal pain, diarrhea, rhinitis, myocarditis	54, 199, 209, 222, 444, 752, 913, 973, 1058, 1066, 1068
Echovirus	3	Children	Fever, rash	466
	4	Mainly children	Fever, pharyngitis, abdominal pain, rash, conjunctivitis	199, 359, 383, 592, 597
	6	Children and adults	Fever, pharyngitis, abdominal pain, pleurodynia, cardiac involvement	199, 457, 598, 626, 663
		Children	Fever, rash	562
	9	Mainly children	Fever, rash, abdominal pain, pharyngitis	199, 283, 357, 374, 419, 467, 560, 586, 662, 727, 845, 921, 972, 981, 1040, 1055, 1094, 1152, 1160
	11	Mainly children	Fever, upper respiratory illness, pneumonia	767
	13	Mainly children	Fever	161
	16	Children	Fever, rash	450
	18	Children and adults	Fever, rash	610
	19	Mainly children	Fever, upper respiratory illness, rash	252, 417
	25	Children and adults	Fever, rash	77
	30	Children and adults	Fever, pharyngitis, rhinitis, conjunctivitis, rash, abdominal pain	199, 426, 451, 593, 910, 1192
	31	Children and adults	Fever	679
	33	Children and adults	Fever, rash	595, 607
Enterovirus	71	Mainly children	Fever, rash	176, 183, 491, 609, 646, 759

noted an outbreak of vertigo in Wyoming in August of 1992 in which IgM antibody studies suggested an enteroviral origin.

Chronic Fatigue Syndrome and Fibromyalgia

From molecular techniques and antibody prevalence data, chronic enteroviral infections have been suggested to play a role in the chronic fatigue and postviral fatigue syndromes.[32,137,247,810,1203] However, these findings have not been confirmed by other investigators.[765,782,1064] More recently, Douche-Aourik and associates[304] found enteroviral RNA in muscle biopsies from 4 of 30 (13%) patients with fibromyalgia or chronic fatigue syndrome but in no biopsy samples from 29 healthy subjects. However, in none of the four positive samples could the presence of VP1 enteroviral capsid protein be demonstrated using a specific monoclonal antibody. In another study, Lane and colleagues[671] found enteroviral RNA in muscle biopsy samples of 10 of 48 patients (20.8%) with chronic fatigue syndrome and in no samples from 29 control subjects. These investigators also found that nine of the 10 subjects with positive muscle biopsy results had abnormal lactate responses to exercise in the subanaerobic threshold exercise test. In an editorial relating to these data, Dalakas[275] warned that similar findings in the past were "epiphenomenal" because EVs are ubiquitous in humans, and technical flaws inherently connected to contamination in laboratories working with these viruses are inevitable.

The greatest proponents for a causal role of EV in chronic fatigue syndrome have been Chia and Chia.[217,219] Although these investigators have had extensive experience with chronic fatigue syndrome and have conducted several studies, none of their data had been adequately controlled.[643] They have presented data suggesting that some cases of chronic fatigue syndrome are the result of chronic enteroviral infections of the stomach.[221,220]

Sudden Infant Death

Balduzzi and Greendyke[56] recovered coxsackievirus A5 from the stool of a 1-month-old child who died suddenly. In a similar investigation of sudden infant death, Gold and associates[416] recovered coxsackievirus A4 from the brains of three babies. Coxsackievirus A8 also was recovered from the stool of a child in whom anorexia was noted on the day before death. Coxsackievirus B3 was recovered at the autopsy of an infant who died suddenly on the eighth day of life.[56] In Hong Kong in 2012 two children with sudden deaths and recombinant coxsackievirus A2 viral infections were reported.[1199] Neither child had myocarditis or encephalitis, but one had evidence of viral pneumonia. The viruses were recombinants involving coxsackievirus A2, A4, and EV 71. Morens and colleagues[802] noted sudden infant death eight times in association with enteroviral infection; PeV was found on two occasions. In a subgroup of infants with sudden unexplained death in whom the "clinical, biologic, and histologic" findings suggested viral infection, evidence of enteroviral infection was found more frequently than in infants without findings of viral infection.[425] Specifically, enteroviral RNA was detected in the respiratory tract in 54% of the viral infection group and in none of the group without findings suggestive of viral infection. These results were supported by IgM antibodies to group B coxsackieviruses in 56% of the first group and in none of the second group. Four infants with suspected sudden infant death syndrome were found to have coxsackievirus B3 myocarditis with minimal histopathologic changes.[296] In five instances of crib death in one study, echovirus 11 was isolated from the lungs in two cases, from the myocardium in one case, and from the nose or feces in the other two cases.[97] Drexler and associates[310] noted RNA evidence of genotype 2 SAFV in the CSF of an infant with sudden infant death syndrome.

Chronic Enteroviral Infections in Immunocompromised Patients

Patients with cell-mediated and combined immunodeficiencies are susceptible to chronic and often fatal infections with many viruses.[379] Patients with agammaglobulinemia and normal cell-mediated function generally survive infections with these same viruses. EVs are the exception, however, in that chronic, unusual infections with a variety of EVs have been reported.* The most common illness is meningoencephalitis, but arthritis and polymyositis are other frequent findings. Echovirus 11 has been the most common cause of chronic infection, but the following other EVs also have been causative: echoviruses 2, 3, 5, 6, 7, 9, 13, 14, 15, 17, 18, 19, 21, 24, 25, 26, 29, 30, and 33; coxsackieviruses A11, A15, B1, B2, and B3; and PeV 1.[751] EVs have been recovered from many other body sites, such as the liver, heart, lung, pancreas, lymph nodes, bone marrow, muscle, throat, and stool, in addition to the CSF.

Several patients with X-linked agammaglobulinemia have had polymyositis-like or dermatomyositis-like syndromes caused by echovirus infections; the following echoviruses have been implicated: types 2, 3, 5, 9, 11, 17, 19, 24, 25, 30, and 33.[62,264,762] The case of a 15-year-old boy with X-linked agammaglobulinemia and chronic arthritis caused by echovirus 11 was reported.[12] Three children with X-linked hyper-IgM syndrome and persistent enteroviral meningoencephalitis were described.[269] Persistent enteroviral infections of the CNS were reported in pediatric and adult patients infected with HIV.[320,882] In addition, enteroviral infections caused deaths in bone marrow transplant recipients.[31,380]

Congenital Infections

Abortion

Landsman and associates[668] studied 2631 pregnancies during an epidemic of echovirus 9 and could find no difference in antibody to echovirus 9 in women who aborted and in those who delivered term infants. A similar study in Finland revealed no increase in the abortion rate in women infected in early pregnancy with echovirus 9.[935] Although coxsackieviral infections occur commonly, epidemics with specific viral types involving large populations have not been studied.

Two women with coxsackievirus A16 hand-foot-and-mouth disease had spontaneous abortions.[868] In one instance, coxsackievirus A16 was recovered from the products of conception. Frisk and Diderholm[370] found that 33% of women with abortions had IgM antibody to coxsackieviruses B, whereas only 8% of control subjects had similar antibody. In a second, larger study, the same research group confirmed their original findings.[47]

Ljungan virus (a PeV) is endemic in some rodent populations, and it can cause fetal death in these animals. Krous and Langlois[653] and Samsioe and colleagues[987] suggest that this virus may be the cause of some intrauterine deaths in humans. In one study, both PCR and immunohistochemical staining identified Ljungan virus in specimens from five human intrauterine fetal deaths.[987]

Congenital Malformations

In a large prospective study, Brown and Karunas[121] made a serologic search for selected maternal enteroviral infections in association with congenital malformations. Sera from 630 mothers of infants with anomalies and from 1164 mothers of children without defects were studied carefully. Specifically, serologic evidence of infection with coxsackieviruses B1, B2, B3, B4, B5, and A9 and with echoviruses 6 and 9 was sought during the first trimester and during the last 6 months of pregnancy. In this study, infants were examined for 113 specific abnormalities; these anomalies were grouped into 12 categories for analysis. The investigators demonstrated a positive correlation between maternal infection and infant anomaly with coxsackieviruses B2, B3, B4, and A9. The overall anomaly rate associated with first trimester infection with coxsackievirus B4 was significantly higher than that in control subjects. Maternal coxsackievirus B2 infection throughout pregnancy, coxsackievirus B4 infection during the first trimester of pregnancy, and infection with at least one of the five group B coxsackieviruses during pregnancy were associated with urogenital anomalies in contrast to control subjects. Coxsackievirus A9 infection was associated with digestive anomalies and coxsackieviruses B3 and B4 with cardiovascular defects. When group B coxsackieviruses were analyzed as a group (B1–B5), an overall association with congenital heart disease was found; the likelihood of having cardiovascular anomalies was increased when maternal infection with two or more group B coxsackieviruses occurred.

Gauntt and colleagues[393] found that ventricular fluid from four of 28 babies with severe anatomic defects contained neutralizing antibody to one or more coxsackievirus B types. In one case, specific IgM antibody to coxsackievirus B6 was demonstrated.

In a serologic study in Scotland, Ross and colleagues[962] found no association between maternal coxsackievirus B infection and fetal developmental anomalies. Elizan and associates[330] were unable to find any relationship between maternal infection with group B coxsackieviruses and congenital CNS malformations. In three studies, no association between maternal echovirus 9 infection and congenital malformation was noted.[638,668,935]

Niklasson and associates[842] studied CNS malformations in terminated pregnancies. PeV (Ljungan virus) was diagnosed in nine of 10 cases of hydrocephalus and in five of nine cases of anencephaly, whereas this virus was found in only one of 18 trisomy 21 control subjects.

Prematurity and Stillbirth

Bates[68] reported an 8-month-old stillborn fetus with calcific pancarditis and hydrops fetalis at autopsy. Fluorescent antibody study revealed coxsackievirus B3 antigen in the myocardium. Burch and colleagues[129] reported three stillborn infants who had fluorescent antibody evidence of coxsackievirus B myocarditis, one each with coxsackieviruses B2, B3, and B4. These investigators also described a premature boy who had histologic and immunofluorescent evidence of cardiac infection with coxsackieviruses B2, B3, and B4; he lived only 24 hours.

Freedman[368] reported the occurrence of a full-term stillbirth in a woman infected with echovirus 11. Because the baby had no pathologic or virologic evidence of infection, Freedman attributed the event to a secondary consequence of maternal infection caused by fever and dehydration rather than primary transplacental infection. In another stillbirth in which echovirus 11 was recovered from amniotic fluid, the fetus was found to have evidence of focal encephalitis, massive adrenal hemorrhage, and diffuse subarachnoid hemorrhage.[1036] Echovirus 27 was recovered from amniotic fluid in an intrauterine fetal death at 28 weeks of gestation.[834] A 26-week, 1300-g stillborn fetus with hydrocephalus, fibrotic peritonitis, and hepatosplenomegaly was found by PCR and immunohistochemical study to have an EV 71 infection.[235] A baby of 26 weeks' gestation with nonimmune hydrops fetalis and an intrauterine infection with coxsackievirus B3 was reported by Ouellet and coworkers.[878]

NEONATAL INFECTIONS

Epidemiology and Pathogenesis

Neonatal infection with EVs and PeVs can result from transplacental viral transmission, contact infection during birth, and human-to-human contact after birth. Transplacental passage of coxsackieviruses and echoviruses at term has been noted on many occasions. Benirschke[1220] studied the placentas in three cases of congenital coxsackievirus B disease and could find no histologic evidence of infection. In 1956, Kibrick and Benirschke[1221] reported the first case of intrauterine infection with coxsackievirus B3. In this instance, the infant was delivered by cesarean section and became symptomatic several hours after birth. Brightman and associates[118] recovered coxsackievirus B5 from the placenta and rectum of a premature infant. No histologic abnormalities of the placenta were noted.

Berkovich and Smithwick[94] noted an asymptomatic neonate who had specific IgM PeV 1 antibody in cord blood, thus suggesting intrauterine infection with this virus. Hughes and colleagues[525] reported a newborn infant with echovirus 14 infection who had markedly elevated IgM (190 mg/dL) on the sixth day of life. This child probably also was infected in utero. In addition, echovirus 19 has been noted in a transplacentally acquired infection.[903] Other evidence of intrauterine infection has been presented for coxsackieviruses A4, B1, B2, B3, B4, and B5 and echoviruses 9, 11, and 19.[68,82,107,200,212,338,458,579,594,731,878,903,1084]

Little definitive evidence exists for either ascending infection or contact infection with coxsackieviruses or echoviruses during birth. However, transmission of infection during the birth process seems probable.[196,212,594] The fecal carriage rate of EVs in asymptomatic adult patients varies between 0% and 6% or higher in different population

*References 12, 97, 103, 255, 264, 269, 316, 319, 335, 448, 452, 480, 599, 751, 968, 1120, 1151, 1153, 1165.

groups.[200] Cherry and colleagues[212] reported that in 2 of 55 mothers (4%), EVs were present in feces shortly after delivery.

Coxsackievirus B5 was recovered from the cervices of four women with febrile illnesses during the third trimester of pregnancy.[944] Echovirus 11 was isolated from the cervix of a mother whose baby became ill on the third day of life with fatal echovirus 11 necrotizing hepatitis.[943] Chang and colleagues[185] detected coxsackievirus B3 in breast milk of two symptomatic mothers, and their babies both suffered severe illnesses with hepatic necrosis and meningitis caused by coxsackievirus B3.

Several epidemics with coxsackieviruses and echoviruses in newborn nurseries have been studied.[118,143,777,818] Brightman and associates[118] observed an epidemic of coxsackievirus B5 in a premature nursery. Their data suggested that the virus was introduced into this nursery by an asymptomatic infant who had been infected in utero. Secondary infections occurred in 12 babies and two nurses. The timing of the secondary cases suggested that three generations had occurred and that the nurses had been infected during the second generation. The investigators suggested that the infection had spread from infant to infant and from infant to nurse.

Javett and associates[563] reported an acute epidemic of myocarditis associated with coxsackievirus B3 infection in a Johannesburg, South Africa maternity home. Unfortunately, no epidemiologic investigation or search for asymptomatic infected infants was performed. However, in analyzing the dates of onset of the illnesses, single infections apparently occurred for five generations, and then five children became ill within a 3-day period.

Kipps and colleagues[633] carried out epidemiologic investigations in two coxsackievirus B3 nursery epidemics. In the first epidemic, the initial infection probably was transmitted from a mother to her baby; this baby then was the source of five secondary cases in newborn infants and one illness in a nurse. Four of the five secondary cases were located on one side of the nursery, but only one crib was close to that of the index baby, and this crib did not adjoin the cribs of the three other contact cases. In the second outbreak, a baby who also was infected by his mother probably introduced the virus into the nursery. The three secondary cases were geographically far removed from the primary case.

Cramblett and colleagues[259] reported an outbreak of echovirus 11 disease in four infants in an intensive care nursery. All infants were in enclosed incubators, and three patients became ill within 24 hours; the fourth child became ill 4 days later. Echovirus 11 was recovered from two members of the nursery staff. These data suggest that transmission from personnel to infants occurred because of inadequate washing of hands.

In another outbreak in an intensive care unit, the initial patient was transferred to the nursery because of severe echovirus 11 disease.[818] After transfer, the senior house officer and a psychologist in the unit were infected. The investigators inferred that these infected personnel spread the disease by respiratory droplet to nine other babies. In another nursery outbreak of echovirus 11, Mertens and colleagues[777] found that the infection spread through close contact between infected newborns and the nurses in the unit. Spread of infection was interrupted with the installation of vigorous hygienic and isolation measures. In an outbreak of echovirus 11 in an intermediate care unit, Kinney and colleagues[632] found that gavage feeding, mouth care, and being a twin were risk factors for acquiring illness.

Many other instances of isolated nursery infections and small outbreaks with coxsackieviruses and echoviruses have been reported. The most consistent source of original nursery infection seems to be transmission from a mother to her baby,* but virus can be introduced into the nursery by hospital personnel.[543,673,1066]

In a longitudinal study of neonatal enteroviral infections carried out during the summer and fall of 1981, Jenista andassociates[565] found that the nonpolio enteroviral infection rate was 12.8%. Lower socioeconomic status and lack of breastfeeding were found to be risk factors for acquiring infection. Nonpolio enteroviral infections were determined to be a significant cause for readmission of the cohort neonates to the hospital.

*References 36, 65, 190, 194, 200, 214, 252, 282, 327, 341, 450, 544, 665, 708, 736, 790, 818, 926, 1066, 1075.

During a community outbreak of echovirus 11 disease, Modlin[790] found that passive transplacental passage of antibody to neonates prevented the development of severe disease but not mucosal infection.

Clinical Manifestations

Enteroviral and parechoviral infections in neonates result in a wide variety of clinical manifestations ranging from asymptomatic infection to fatal encephalitis and myocarditis.[200] An overview by illness category and prevalence is presented in Table 166.20.

Inapparent Infection

Although inapparent infection probably occurs occasionally with many different EVs, little documentation of this assumption exists. Cherry and colleagues[212] studied 590 normal neonates during a 6-month period and noted only a single asymptomatic infection. This child was infected in utero or immediately thereafter with coxsackievirus B2. The mother had an upper respiratory tract illness 10 days before delivery.

During a survey of perinatal viral infections, 44 babies were found to be infected with PeV 1 in the study period May to December of 1966 (I. Jack, et al, personal communication, 1967). The prevalence of virus and the incidence of new infections during this period were fairly uniform. No illness was attributed to PeV 1 infection, and the virus disappeared from the nursery in mid-December. Asymptomatic infections with PeV 1 were noted on two other occasions.[93,824] Infections without evidence of illness also have been noted with coxsackieviruses A9, B1, B4, and B5 and echoviruses 3, 5, 9, 11, 13, 14, 20, 30, and 31.[200,325,342,402,543,554,565,673,808,1066]

Mild, Nonspecific Febrile Illness

In a review of 338 enteroviral infections in early infancy, 9% were classified as nonspecific febrile illnesses.[801] Illness may be sporadic or part of an outbreak with a specific viral type. When the illness is part of an outbreak, the clinical manifestations vary, depending on the viral type; some infants have aseptic meningitis and other signs and symptoms, whereas others simply have nonspecific fever. Specific viruses related to nonspecific fever are listed in Table 166.20. Although by definition illness in this category is mild, awareness that viral infection may be extensive is important. When sought, virus may be isolated from the blood, urine, and CSF of infants with mild illnesses.[65,557] In an outbreak of relatively benign illness caused by echovirus 7 in six neonates, all the infants were found to have high C-reactive protein values.[272]

Sepsis-Like Illness

The main diagnostic problem in neonatal enteroviral and parechoviral infections is differentiation of bacterial from viral disease. Even in an infant with mild, nonspecific fever, bacterial disease must be considered strongly. The sepsis-like illness described here always is alarming. Illness is characterized by fever, poor feeding, abdominal distention, irritability, rash, lethargy, and hypotonia.[59,450,463,665,907,1018,1125,1179] Other findings include diarrhea, vomiting, seizures, and apnea. In severe, frequently fatal illnesses, most often caused by echovirus 11 infection, jaundice, hepatitis, disseminated intravascular coagulation (DIC), thrombocytopenia, and hypotension occur.[579,789,809,943]

Sepsis-like illness is a common occurrence. Morens[801] noted its presence in one-fifth of 338 enteroviral infections in infants. In an attempt to differentiate bacterial from viral disease, Lake and associates[665] studied 27 infants with enteroviral infection. WBC counts were not helpful because the total count, the number of neutrophils, and the number of band-form neutrophils were elevated in most cases. Of most importance were historical data. Most mothers had experienced a recent febrile, viral-like illness. In addition, other factors often associated with bacterial sepsis, such as prolonged rupture of membranes, prematurity, and low Apgar scores, were unusual findings in the enteroviral infection group. Bone marrow failure developed in a newborn baby boy with a sepsis-like illness caused by echovirus 11 infection.[1077] The neutropenia resolved spontaneously, and the thrombocytopenia normalized after treatment with IVIG.

Abzug[6] reviewed the prognosis in 16 neonates who had a sepsis-like illness with hepatitis and coagulopathy. The case-fatality rate was 31%. In addition to having hepatitis and coagulopathy, the five patients with fatal cases had myocarditis and three patients had encephalitis. The

TABLE 166.20 Major Manifestations of Neonatal Nonpolio Enteroviral and Parechoviral Infections

Specific Involvement	Common	Rare	References
Inapparent infection		Cox A9, B1, B2, B4, B5	94, 199, 212, 325, 342, 402, 554, 808, 824
	PeV 1	Echo 3, 5, 9, 11, 14, 20, 30, 31	
Mild, nonspecific, febrile illness	Cox B5	Cox B1-B4, A9, A16	33, 65, 85, 92, 110, 199, 212, 282, 327, 402, 462, 557, 595, 708, 795, 818, 1027, 1108
	Echo 5, 11, 33	Echo 4, 7, 9, 17, 30	
		PeV 4	
Sepsis-like illness	Cox B2-B5	Cox B1, A9	9, 35, 86, 97, 105, 107, 195, 199, 200, 224, 252, 259, 282, 3 44, 416, 449, 579, 594, 665, 708, 736, 777, 789, 809, 818, 903, 943, 990, 994, 1051, 1066, 1123, 1188
	Echo 5, 11, 16	Echo 2-4, 6, 9, 14,19, 21	
		PeV 1, 2, 3	
Respiratory illness (general)		Cox B1, B4, B5, A9	212, 477, 525, 554
	Echo 11	Echo 9, 17	
	PeV 1, 3		
Herpangina		Cox A5	190
Coryza		Cox A9	94, 261, 477, 824, 1003
		Echo 11, 17, 19	
		PeV 1	
Pharyngitis		Cox B4	92, 477, 763, 990, 1027
		Echo 11, 17, 18	
Laryngotracheitis or bronchitis		Cox B1, B4	322, 477, 798
		Echo 11	
Pneumonia		Cox B4, A9	94, 199, 224, 282, 344, 477, 554, 783, 1091, 1168, 1176
		Echo 9, 11, 17, 31	
		PeV 1	
Cloud baby		Echo 20	325
Gastrointestinal			
Vomiting or diarrhea		Cox B1, B2, B5	92, 199, 252, 325, 326, 344, 402, 460, 477, 554, 708, 783, 931, 990, 1066
	Echo 5, 17, 18	Echo 4, 6, 8, 9, 11, 16, 19, 21	
		PeV 1	
Hepatitis		Cox A9, B1, B3, B4	185, 199, 200, 508, 579, 623, 789, 809, 1188, 1196
	Echo 11, 19	Echo 6, 9, 14, 21	
Pancreatitis		Cox B3, B4, B5	642, 1176
Necrotizing enterocolitis		Cox B2, B3	665
Cardiovascular			
Myocarditis and pericarditis	Cox B1-B4	Cox B5, A9	64, 129, 199, 325, 343, 397, 449, 507, 530, 544, 554, 563, 594, 622, 624, 625, 633, 795, 798, 1072, 1108, 1188
		Echo 11, 19	
Skin	Cox B5	Cox B1, 3	94, 110, 199, 204, 209, 259, 272, 402, 450, 594, 708, 763, 783, 847, 990, 1084
	Echo 5, 17	Echo 4, 7, 9, 11, 16, 18	
	PeV 1, 3		
Neurologic			
Aseptic meningitis	Cox B2-B5	Cox A9, A14, B1	94, 110, 199, 200, 209, 259, 303, 325, 346, 449, 458, 467, 468, 574, 594, 736, 777, 783, 847, 1001, 1003, 1008, 1051, 1066
	Echo 3, 9, 11, 17	Echo 1, 14, 21, 30	
		EV 71	
Encephalitis	Cox B1-B4	Cox B5	86, 214, 341, 342, 467, 581, 994, 1009, 1188
		Echo 9	
		PeV 2, 3	
Paralysis		Cox B2	574
Sudden infant death		Cox B3, A4, A5, A8	56, 416, 802
		PeV 1	

Cox, Coxsackievirus; *echo*, echovirus; *EV*, enterovirus; *PeV*, parechovirus.

follow-up of six survivors noted normalization of liver function and platelet counts and the absence of subsequent significant medical problems.

Respiratory Illness

Respiratory complaints generally are overshadowed by other manifestations of neonatal enteroviral disease. Only 7% of 338 enteroviral infections in early infancy were classified as respiratory illness in one study.[801] Herpangina has been observed and photographed only once; Chawareewong and associates[190] noted several infants with herpangina and coxsackievirus A5 infection.

Hercík and colleagues[477] reported an epidemic of respiratory illness in 22 neonates associated with echovirus 11 infection. All these infants had rhinitis and pharyngitis, 50% had laryngitis, and 32% had interstitial pneumonitis. Berkovich and Pangan[93] studied respiratory illnesses in premature infants and reported 64 babies with illness, 18 of whom had virologic or serologic evidence of PeV 1 infection. In addition, many had high but constant levels of serum antibody to PeV 1. Some of the infants with high antibody levels probably also were infected with PeV 1. The children with proved PeV 1 infection could not be differentiated clinically from those without evidence of such infection. Ninety percent of the infants had coryza, and 39% had radiographic evidence of pneumonia.

Except for echoviruses 11 and PeV 1, respiratory illness associated with EVs has occurred sporadically. The following other viruses have been noted: coxsackieviruses A5, A9, B1, B4, and B5 and echoviruses

9, 17, 18, 19, 20, 22, and 31. In the review by Morens,[801] only seven of 338 enteroviral infections of infancy were classified as pneumonia. A newborn with an echovirus 11 infection developed meningitis, DIC, and persistent pulmonary hypertension.[1168] Postmortem examination revealed pneumonia, hyaline membranes, pulmonary interstitial emphysema, meningitis, and DIC.

Eichenwald and Kotsevalov[326] recovered echovirus 20 from four full-term infants younger than 8 days of age. Although these infants were asymptomatic, they were found to be colonized extensively with staphylococci, and they disseminated these organisms into the air around them. Because of this ability to disseminate staphylococci, they were called *cloud babies*. The investigators thought these cloud babies contributed to the epidemic spread of staphylococci in the nursery. Because active staphylococcal dissemination occurred only when echovirus 20 could be recovered from the nasopharynx, viral-bacterial synergistic activity was thought to be present.

Gastrointestinal Manifestations

Significant gastrointestinal illness occurs in approximately 7% of enteroviral infections of infancy.[801] Vomiting and diarrhea occur commonly but usually are only part of the overall illness complex and not the major manifestations. In 1958, Eichenwald and associates[325] described epidemic diarrhea associated with echovirus 18 infection. In a nursery unit of premature infants, 12 of 21 babies were mildly ill. Neither temperature elevation nor hypothermia occurred. Six infants were lethargic and listless, and moderate abdominal distention developed in two infants. The diarrhea lasted from 1 to 5 days; these infants had five or six watery, greenish stools per day, occasionally expelled explosively. Two infants had a small amount of blood, but no mucus or pus cells, noted in their stools. Five babies in another nursery also had similar diarrheal illness. Echovirus 18 was recovered from all ill infants.

In 22 infants with epidemic respiratory disease caused by echovirus 11, all had vomiting as a manifestation of the illness.[477] Linnemann and colleagues[708] reported vomiting in 36% and diarrhea in 7% of neonates with echoviral infection. In another study, Lake and associates[665] found diarrhea in 81% and vomiting in 33% of neonates with nonpolio enteroviral infections.

Hepatitis is an important neonatal nonpolio enteroviral illness. Morens[801] reported that 2% of neonates with clinically severe enteroviral disease had hepatitis. Lake and colleagues[665] observed that hepatomegaly was present in 37% of neonates with enteroviral infection, and hepatosplenomegaly was observed by Hercík and associates[477] in 12 of 22 newborns with echovirus 11 respiratory illness.

Severe hepatitis, frequently with hepatic necrosis, has been noted with echoviruses 6, 9, 11, 14, 19, 21, and 30.[92,107,200,449,525,579,789,809,903,908] Echovirus 11 most often has been associated with severe and usually fatal hepatitis; findings include DIC and thrombocytopenia, as well as apnea, lethargy, poor feeding, and jaundice.

Philip and Larson[903] reported three catastrophic neonatal echovirus 19 infections that resulted in hepatic necrosis and massive terminal hemorrhage. One infant, infected in utero, was symptomatic at birth. The Apgar score was 3, and multiple petechiae were observed. Generalized ecchymoses and apneic episodes occurred, and the infant died at 3.5 hours of age. Thrombocytopenia was noted, and echovirus 19 was isolated from the brain, liver, spleen, and lymph nodes. The other two infants who died of echovirus 19 infection were twins. They were normal during the first 3 days of life but then became mildly cyanotic and lethargic. Shortly thereafter, apneic episodes occurred, and jaundice and petechiae developed. Both twins became oliguric, and they died on the eighth and ninth days of life with severe, terminal gastrointestinal bleeding. Both twins were thrombocytopenic, and virus was recovered from systemic sites in both.

Pancreatitis was found in three of four newborns with coxsackievirus B5 meningitis[642] and in a coxsackievirus B4 infection at autopsy.[1176] In other fatal coxsackievirus B infections, pancreatic involvement has been detected, but clinical manifestations rarely have been observed.

Lake and associates[665] reported three infants with necrotizing enterocolitis. Coxsackievirus B3 was recovered from two of these infants, and coxsackievirus B2 was recovered from the third.

TABLE 166.21 Signs and Symptoms of Neonatal Coxsackievirus B Myocarditis

Category	Frequency (%)
Feeding difficulty	84
Listlessness	81
Cardiac signs	81
Respiratory distress	75
Cyanosis	72
Fever	70
Pharyngitis	64
Hepatosplenomegaly	53
Biphasic course	35
Central nervous system signs	27
Hemorrhage	13
Jaundice	13
Diarrhea	8

Modified from Kibrick S. Viral infections of the fetus and newborn. *Perspect Virol.* 1961;2:140–59.

Cardiovascular Manifestations

In contrast to enteroviral cardiac disease in children and adults, in which pericarditis is a common finding, neonatal disease almost always involves the heart muscle. Most cases of neonatal myocarditis are caused by coxsackievirus B infection, and nursery outbreaks have occurred on several occasions. In 1961, Kibrick[622] reviewed the clinical findings in 45 cases of neonatal myocarditis; his findings are summarized in Table 166.21. Of interest is that many of the early experiences, particularly in South Africa, involved catastrophic nursery epidemics. Since the observation in 1972 of five newborns with echovirus 11 infection and myocarditis, no other nursery epidemics have been reported.[309]

The illness caused by group B coxsackieviruses most commonly was abrupt in onset, with symptoms of listlessness, anorexia, and fever. A biphasic pattern was noted in approximately one third of the patients. Progression was rapid, and signs of circulatory failure appeared in a 2-day period. If death did not occur, recovery occasionally was rapid but usually took place gradually over an extended period. Most patients had cardiac findings such as tachycardia, cardiomegaly, electrocardiographic changes, and transitory systolic murmurs. Many patients showed signs of respiratory distress and cyanosis. Approximately one third of the infants had signs suggesting neurologic involvement. Of the 45 cases analyzed by Kibrick,[622] only 12 patients survived.

In an echovirus 11 nursery outbreak reported by Drew,[309] five of 10 babies had tachycardia out of proportion to their fever. Three of these babies had electrocardiograms; supraventricular tachycardia was noted in all, and ST-segment depression was observed in two patients' records. Supraventricular tachycardia also has occurred with coxsackievirus B infection.[554] Echovirus 19 has been associated with myocarditis, and coxsackievirus A9 was noted in a child with pericarditis.[261,1072]

In the 1970s, neonatal myocarditis caused by EVs was seen less commonly than it was in the 1950s and early 1960s. In his review, Morens[801] noted only two instances among 248 severe neonatal enteroviral illnesses. Hoi-shan Chan and Lun[494] reported a neonate with coxsackievirus B4 myocarditis who developed a ventricular aneurysm.

Exanthem

Exanthem as a manifestation of neonatal enteroviral infection has been reported with coxsackieviruses B1, B3, and B5; with echoviruses 4, 5, 7, 9, 11, 16, 17, and 18; and with PeV 1, 3, 4, 5, and 6. In most instances, rash is just a minor manifestation of severe neonatal disease. In 27 infants studied by Lake and colleagues,[665] 41% had exanthem. Cutaneous manifestations generally commence between the third and fifth days of illness. The rash usually is macular or maculopapular. Petechial lesions are noted occasionally. Surprisingly, vesicular lesions have not been described, nor has any rash illness in neonates been associated with coxsackievirus A16. Hall and associates[450] reported two neonates with echovirus 16 infections in which the illnesses resembled roseola. These patients had fever for 2 and 3 days, defervescence, and then the appearance of a maculopapular rash.

A newborn with a vesiculopapular-crusted rash on the face, trunk, and extremities caused by coxsackievirus B3 was reported by Theodoridou and associates.[1084] It was a congenital infection in which new lesions appeared over the course of a 5-day period, and the total duration of the rash was 10 days.

Neurologic Manifestations

As noted in Table 166.20, neurologic illness has been associated with coxsackieviruses B1, B2, B3, B4, and B5, many echoviruses and PeVs. In neonates, differentiating meningitis from meningoencephalitis usually is difficult. Meningoencephalitis occurs commonly in infants with sepsis-like illness, and postmortem studies revealed many infants with disseminated viral disease (heart, liver, adrenal glands) in addition to CNS involvement. In Morens' review,[801] 50% of the patients with enteroviral infection who were analyzed had encephalitis or meningitis.

The initial clinical findings in neonatal meningitis or meningoencephalitis are similar to those in nonspecific febrile illness or sepsis-like illness. Most often, the child is normal and then becomes febrile, anorectic, and lethargic. Jaundice frequently is noted in newborns, and vomiting occurs in neonates of all ages. Less common findings include apnea, tremulousness, and general increased tonicity. Seizures occur occasionally. Extensive white matter injury has been noted in neonatal PeV encephalitis.[1124] This finding can be confused with white matter changes associated with hypoxic-ischemic injuries.

Examination of CSF reveals considerable variation in protein, glucose, and cellular values. In seven newborns with meningitis caused by coxsackievirus B5 studied by Swender and colleagues,[1066] the mean CSF protein value was 244 mg/dL, and the highest value was 480 mg/dL. The mean CSF glucose value was 57 mg/dL, and one of the seven infants had pronounced hypoglycorrhachia (a value of 12 mg/dL). The mean CSF leukocyte count in the seven babies was 1069 cells/mm^3, with 67% polymorphonuclear cells. The highest cell count was 4526 cells/mm^3, with 85% polymorphonuclear cells. In another study involving 28 children younger than 2 months of age in which coxsackievirus B5 was the implicated pathogen, 36% of the infants had CSF leukocyte counts of 500 cells/mm^3 or greater.[736] In this same study, only 13% of the infants had CSF protein values of 120 mg/dL or greater; 12% of the infants had glucose values lower than 40 mg/dL.

In summary, the CSF findings in neonatal nonpolio enteroviral and parechoviral infections frequently are similar to those in bacterial disease. In particular, the most consistent finding in bacterial disease, hypoglycorrhachia, is noted in approximately 10% of newborns with enteroviral meningitis.[214,327,665,736,1066]

Johnson and associates[570] reported a 1-month-old boy with right-sided facial paralysis and loss of abdominal reflexes. The facial paralysis persisted through convalescence; the reflexes returned to normal within 2 weeks. The boy was infected with coxsackievirus B2. Jones and associates[581] noted a neonate with coxsackievirus B1 meningoencephalitis and central diabetes insipidus.

Euscher and associates[338] detected coxsackievirus RNA in placental tissue from six of seven newborn infants with respiratory difficulties and other manifestations at birth. Of these infants, one died shortly after birth, and the other six suffered neurodevelopmental delays.

CLINICAL MANIFESTATIONS: POLIOVIRUS

When a susceptible person has had effective contact with a poliovirus, one of several responses may occur, in the following order of frequency: (1) inapparent infection, (2) minor illness (abortive poliomyelitis), (3) nonparalytic poliomyelitis (aseptic meningitis), and (4) paralytic poliomyelitis.[22,104,198,200,238,510] Paralytic poliomyelitis is the most dramatic expression of the infection and the only one clinically recognizable as caused by a poliovirus; it accounts for not more than 1% to 2% of infections during epidemics and considerably less under endemic conditions (see Fig. 166.5). The aseptic meningitis syndrome is similarly infrequent; nonspecific "minor illness" is estimated to occur in 4% to 8%, and 90% to 95% of those infected have inapparent infections. Factors that determine the type of clinical response are poorly understood, but the degree of virulence of the virus and certain host characteristics are important.

Age has a significant effect on patterns of infection; older patients are more likely to have severe paralytic disease and a higher mortality rate. Pregnancy increases the risk, probably primarily because of hormonal factors but also because pregnant women may be exposed more to young children, who are the main sources of contagion. Tonsillectomy in the presence of inapparent infection can precipitate bulbar poliomyelitis; evidence also suggests that tonsillectomy at any time in the past results in enhanced susceptibility to the bulbar form of the disease. Recent diphtheria-tetanus-pertussis vaccination increases the likelihood of development of paralysis; the site of injection and the site of paralysis appear to be correlated. Physical exertion and trauma around the time of onset also increase the risk for severe paralysis, especially in adults.

Minor Illness (Abortive Poliomyelitis)

The minor illness is mild and nonspecific, with low-grade fever, malaise, anorexia, and sore throat. Physical examination reveals no significant abnormalities, CSF is normal, and recovery occurs within 24 to 72 hours. The illness often is so mild that it goes unrecognized, and patients rarely are seen by a physician.

Nonparalytic Poliomyelitis (Aseptic Meningitis)

The onset of nonparalytic poliomyelitis is associated with vague malaise followed by fever, headache, aching of the muscles, and sometimes hyperesthesia and paresthesia. Anorexia, nausea, vomiting, constipation, or diarrhea also may be present. The temperature rises to 37.8°C to 39.5°C (101°F–103°F); stiffness of the neck, back, and hamstrings soon appears.

Approximately two-thirds of affected children have a short, symptom-free interlude between the first phase (minor illness) and the second phase (CNS or major illness). This two-phase course occurs less commonly in adults, in whom the evolution of symptoms is more insidious. Nuchal and spinal rigidity is necessary for establishing the diagnosis of nonparalytic poliomyelitis during the second phase.

Physical examination reveals nuchal-spinal signs and changes in superficial and deep reflexes. With cooperative patients, the nuchal-spinal signs are sought first by active tests. The child is asked to sit up unassisted. If doing so causes undue effort, if the knees flex upward, and if the patient writhes a bit from side to side while sitting up and uses the hands on the bed for the tripod supporting position, unmistakable spinal rigidity is present. Still sitting, the patient is asked to flex chin to chest and is observed for nuchal rigidity. Alternatively, from the supine position with the knees held down gently, the patient is asked to sit up and kiss the knees. If the knees draw up sharply or if the maneuver cannot be completed adequately, the patient has stiffness of the spine caused by muscle spasm. If the diagnosis still is uncertain, attempts should be made to elicit the Kernig and Brudzinski signs. Gentle forward flexion of the occiput and neck elicits nuchal rigidity, which may precede spinal rigidity. Head drop may be demonstrated by placing the hands under the patient's shoulders and raising the trunk. Normally, the head follows the plane of the trunk, but in poliomyelitis, it often falls backward limply. The frequency of the head-drop sign, even in nonparalytic poliomyelitis, with no subsequent residuals indicates that it is not caused by true paresis of the neck flexors. In struggling infants, distinguishing voluntary resistance from clinically important involuntary nuchal rigidity may be difficult. One may place the infant's shoulders flush with the edge of the table, support the weight of the occiput in the hand, and then flex the head anteriorly. Nuchal rigidity that persists during this maneuver may be interpreted as involuntary. When not closed, the anterior fontanelle also may be tense or bulging.

In the early stages, the reflexes are normally active and remain so unless paralysis supervenes. Changes in reflexes, either increased or depressed, may precede the onset of weakness by 12 to 24 hours; hence detecting such changes is important, especially in nonparalytic patients managed at home. The superficial reflexes (i.e., cremasteric and abdominal and the reflexes of the spinal and gluteal muscles) are usually the first to be diminished. The spinal and gluteal reflexes are elicited by tapping segmentally downward on each side of the spine and buttocks. These reflexes may disappear before the abdominal and cremasteric ones. Changes in the deep tendon reflexes, whether exaggerated or depressed, generally occur 8 to 24 hours after depression of the superficial reflexes and indicate impending paresis of the extremities.

Laboratory findings consist of a normal or slightly elevated WBC count and the characteristic CSF changes of aseptic meningitis—approximately 20 to 300 cells, predominantly lymphocytes, a normal glucose level, and a normal or slightly elevated protein level. If a spinal tap is performed in the first few hours after onset, a predominance of polymorphonuclear leukocytes may be seen, but it shifts in 6 to 12 hours to more than 90% lymphocytes. If no further progression of clinical signs occurs, the disease remains nonparalytic, the temperature falls to normal, and signs of meningeal irritation gradually disappear. Recovery ensues in 3 to 10 days, depending on the severity of the illness.

Paralytic Poliomyelitis

The manifestations of paralytic poliomyelitis are those enumerated earlier for nonparalytic poliomyelitis in addition to weakness in one or more muscle groups, either skeletal or cranial. Patients in whom paralysis is destined to develop often wear an anxious expression; they are extremely alert, restless, and flushed and appear acutely ill. The fever is higher than that in abortive disease, and the patient may have intense muscle pain. Shortly before actual muscle weakness is detected, the superficial and deep reflexes often diminish or disappear on the affected side. Frequently, a symptom-free interlude of several days occurs between the initial illness phase and the recurrence of symptoms that culminate in paralysis.

The onset of paralysis may be extraordinarily sudden and may progress in a few hours to complete loss of motion in one or more extremities. Asymmetric involvement is typical in milder cases. More gradual spread of weakness also occurs and may continue over a period of 3 to 5 days. Bladder paralysis of 1 to 3 days' duration develops in approximately 20% of patients, and bowel atony frequently is noted, occasionally to the point of paralytic ileus. In general, when the fever subsides, no further paralysis is likely to occur. The lower limbs are affected more commonly than are the upper, but in severe cases, quadriplegia and loss of function of the intercostal, abdominal, and trunk muscles with resultant respiratory difficulty may ensue. The superficial and deep reflexes in the affected limbs are lost; twitching of the muscles and diffuse fasciculations may be seen transiently. Sensory abnormalities are rare occurrences.

Flaccid paralysis is the most obvious clinical expression of the neuronal changes. The ensuing muscular atrophy is caused by denervation in addition to the atrophy of disuse. The pain, spasticity, nuchal and spinal rigidity, and hypertonia early in the illness probably are caused by lesions in the brainstem, spinal ganglia, and posterior columns. Respiratory and cardiac arrhythmias, blood pressure and vasomotor changes, and similar manifestations reflect damage to vital centers in the medulla.

On physical examination, the distribution of paralysis characteristically is spotty. To detect mild muscular weakness, one often must apply gentle resistance in opposition to the muscle group being tested. The spinal form has weakness of some of the muscles of the neck, abdomen, trunk, diaphragm, thorax, or extremities. The bulbar form is characterized by weakness in the motor distribution of one or more cranial nerves, with or without dysfunction of the vital centers of respiration and circulation. Patients with bulbar disease often are extremely agitated, even delirious, or they may become stuporous. The tenth cranial nerve nuclei are involved most commonly and result in paralysis of the pharynx, soft palate, and vocal cords. Facial paralysis occurs less commonly; it usually is asymmetric and involves only selected muscle groups. Ocular palsies are unusual findings.

Components of both the bulbar and spinal forms occur together in bulbospinal poliomyelitis. In the encephalitic form of the disease, irritability, disorientation, drowsiness, and coarse tremors not explained by inadequate ventilation are noted. Even during epidemics of poliomyelitis, this form can be recognized only if some peripheral or cranial nerve paralysis coexists or ensues. Hypoxia and hypercapnia caused by inadequate ventilation from respiratory insufficiency may produce disorientation without true encephalitis.

BOX 166.1 Common Sources of Hypoxia and Hypercapnia in Poliomyelitis

1. Cranial nerves IX to XII involved with:
   a. Pharyngeal paralysis and pooling of secretions
   b. Laryngeal involvement, either spasm of laryngeal muscles or paralysis of vocal cords
   c. Lingual paralysis
   d. Tracheal accumulation of secretions from inability to cough
   e. Aspiration of vomitus
2. Vital center involvement with:
   a. Inefficient, irregular respiration
   b. Cardiovascular disturbance
   c. Hyperpyrexia causing increased oxygen consumption
3. Cervical and spinal cord involvement causing paresis of the primary and accessory muscles of respiration
4. Pulmonary complications (e.g., pneumonia, atelectasis, and edema)
5. Contributory factors:
   a. Panic
   b. Gastric dilation
   c. Sedation
   d. Inadequate equipment (e.g., small-bore tracheostomy tubes, unsuitable respirator settings)

From Cherry JD. Enteroviruses. In: Behrman RE, Vaughan VC, eds. *Nelson Textbook of Pediatrics*. 12th ed. Philadelphia: WB Saunders, 1983:791–804.

Numerous components acting together may result in insufficiency in ventilation (Box 166.1). The most serious consequences are hypoxia and hypercapnia, which may produce profound effects on many other systems. Respiratory insufficiency should be detected early to diminish its widespread effects, and because the situation may shift rapidly, continued clinical evaluation is essential. Despite weakness of the respiratory muscles, the patient may respond with so much respiratory effort that normal alveolar ventilation is maintained. In fact, the increased effort (associated with anxiety and fear) actually may produce overventilation at the outset and may result in respiratory alkalosis. Such effort is fatiguing and soon leads to respiratory failure.

For clarity, certain terms characterizing patterns of disease need definition. First, *pure spinal poliomyelitis with respiratory insufficiency* refers to tightness, weakness, or paralysis of the respiratory muscles (chiefly the diaphragm and intercostals) without discernible clinical involvement of the cranial nerves or vital centers. The cervical and thoracic spinal cord segments chiefly are involved. Second, *pure bulbar poliomyelitis* refers to paralysis of the motor cranial nerve nuclei with or without involvement of the vital centers that control respiration, circulation, and body temperature. Involvement of the ninth, tenth, and twelfth cranial nerves is most important because it results in paralysis of the pharynx, tongue, and larynx, with consequent airway obstruction. Third, *bulbospinal poliomyelitis with respiratory insufficiency* refers to involvement of the respiratory muscles with coexisting bulbar paralysis.

The clinical findings resulting from involvement of the respiratory muscles are as follows: (1) an anxious expression; (2) inability to speak without frequent pauses, a situation resulting in short, jerky, "breathless" sentences that can be demonstrated by asking the child to count numbers serially; (3) increased respiratory rate; (4) movement of the alae nasi and the accessory muscles of respiration; (5) inability to cough or sniff with full depth; (6) paradoxical abdominal movements caused by diaphragmatic immobility from spasm or weakness of one or both leaves; and (7) relative immobility of the intercostal spaces, whether segmental, unilateral, or bilateral. When the arms are weak and especially when deltoid paralysis occurs, one should beware of impending respiratory paralysis because the phrenic nerve nuclei are in adjacent areas of the spinal cord. Observing the patient's capacity for thoracic breathing while the abdominal muscles are splinted manually can be performed to assess minor degrees of paresis. Light manual splinting of the thoracic cage helps in evaluating the effectiveness of diaphragmatic movement.

The clinical findings of bulbar poliomyelitis with respiratory difficulty (other than paralysis of the extraocular, facial, and masticatory muscles) include the following:

1. Nasal twang to the voice or cry as a result of palatal and pharyngeal weakness (hard consonant words such as "cookie" or "candy" bring out this condition best).
2. Inability to swallow smoothly that results in an accumulation of saliva in the pharynx and indicates partial immobility (holding the larynx lightly and asking the patient to swallow confirms the immobility).
3. Accumulated pharyngeal secretions, which may cause irregular respiration because each inspiration must be "planned" and cannot be "subconscious" in view of the risk for aspirating; the respirations thus may appear interrupted and abnormal even to the point of falsely simulating intercostal or diaphragmatic weakness.
4. The impossibility of effective coughing, with resultant constant and fatiguing efforts to clear the throat.
5. Nasal regurgitation of saliva and fluids caused by palatal paralysis, with an inability to separate the oropharynx from the nasopharynx during swallowing.
6. Deviation of the palate, uvula, or tongue.
7. Involvement of vital centers, as manifested by an irregularity in the rate, depth, and rhythm of respiration; by cardiovascular alterations that include changes in blood pressure (especially increased), alternate flushing and mottling of the skin, and cardiac arrhythmias; and by rapid changes in body temperature.
8. Paralysis of one or both vocal cords that causes hoarseness, aphonia, and, ultimately, asphyxia unless recognized by laryngoscopy and managed by immediate tracheostomy.
9. The "rope sign," an acute angulation between the chin and larynx caused by weakness of the hyoid muscles (the hyoid bone is pulled posteriorly, thus narrowing the hypopharyngeal inlet).

Myocardial failure sometimes develops secondary to pulmonary complications or as a result of acute myocarditis. The initial manifestation of poliovirus infection on occasion can resemble that of Guillain-Barré syndrome.[1201]

Congenital Infections

Abortion

Poliomyelitis is associated with an increased incidence of abortion. Horn[498] noted 43 abortions in 325 pregnancies complicated by maternal poliomyelitis. Abortion was related directly to the severity of the maternal illness, including the degree of fever during the acute phase of illness. However, abortion also has occurred in association with mild nonparalytic poliomyelitis. Greenberg and Siegel[428] noted that fetal death occurred in 14 of 30 instances (46.7%) of maternal poliomyelitis during the first trimester. Kaye and associates[603] reviewed the literature in 1953 and recorded 19 abortions in 101 cases of poliomyelitis in pregnancy. In a small study in Evanston Hospital in Illinois, the abortion rate in maternal poliomyelitis was little different from the expected rate.[111]

Congenital Malformations

Although isolated instances of congenital malformation and maternal poliomyelitis have been noted, little statistical evidence supports the suggestion that polioviruses are teratogens. In their review of the literature, Kaye and colleagues[603] noted 6 anomalies in 101 infants born to mothers with poliomyelitis during pregnancy. In the reviews of Horn,[498] Bates,[67] and Greenberg and Siegel,[428] no evidence of maternal polioviral infection–induced anomalies was found. Similarly, no evidence suggests that infection with poliovirus vaccine during pregnancy causes congenital malformations.[460]

Prematurity and Stillbirth

In Horn's study[498] of 325 pregnancies, nine infants died in utero. In each instance, the mother was critically ill with poliomyelitis. Horn[498] also noted that 45 infants weighed less than 6 pounds, and 17 of them had a birth weight less than 5 pounds. These low-birth-weight infants were born predominantly to mothers who had poliomyelitis early in pregnancy. In New York City, Greenberg and Siegel[428] also noted an increase in prematurity after maternal poliomyelitis infection. It was related specifically to maternal paralytic poliomyelitis.

Neonatal Infections

General Infections

In the excellent review by Bates[67] in 1955, 58 cases of poliomyelitis in infants younger than 1 month were described. Although complete data were not available on many of the cases, 51 had paralysis, died of their disease, or both. Of the total number of infants on whom these investigators had clinical data, only one infant had nonparalytic disease. More than one-half of the cases were secondary to maternal disease. Because other investigators have noted congenital infection without symptomatic maternal infection, infection in the mother probably was the source for an even greater percentage of the neonatal illnesses. The incubation period of neonatal poliomyelitis has not been established, and, therefore, determining how many of the babies were infected in utero is difficult. Probably, most illnesses that occurred within the first 5 days of life were congenital. Most of the neonates had symptoms of fever, anorexia or dysphagia, and listlessness. Almost one-half of the infants noted in this review died, and of those surviving, 48% had residual paralysis.

Infection Acquired in Utero

Elliott and associates[331] described an infant girl in whom "complete flaccidity" was noted at birth. This child's mother had mild paralytic poliomyelitis, with the onset of minor illness occurring 19 days before the infant's birth. Fetal movements had ceased 6 days before delivery, a finding suggesting that paralysis had occurred at this time. On examination, the baby was severely atonic; when supported under the back, she was passively opisthotonic. Respiratory efforts were abortive and were confined to the accessory muscles; laryngoscopy revealed complete flaccidity in the larynx.

Johnson and Stimson[575] reported a case in which the mother's probable abortive infection occurred 6 weeks before the birth of the baby. The baby initially was thought to be normal but apparently underwent no medical examination until the fourth day of life. At this time, the physician noted right hemiplegia. On the following day, a more complete examination revealed lateral bulging of the right side of the abdomen accompanied by crying and maintenance of the lower extremities in a frog leg position. Adduction and flexion at the hips were weak, and the knee and ankle jerks were absent. Laboratory studies were unremarkable except for examination of CSF. It revealed 20 lymphocytes and a protein level of 169 mg/dL. During a 6-month period, this child's paralysis gradually improved and resulted in only residual weakness of the left lower extremity.

Paresis of the left arm was noted shortly after birth in another child with apparent transplacentally acquired poliomyelitis.[724] At 2 days of age, the baby was quadriplegic, but patellar reflexes were present, and the child had no respiratory or swallowing difficulties. This child had pneumonia at 3 weeks of age, but otherwise, general neurologic improvement occurred. Examination at 8 weeks of age revealed bilateral atrophy of the shoulder girdle muscles. The CSF from this patient had 63 leukocytes/mm^3, 29% of them polymorphonuclear cells, and a protein concentration of 128 mg/dL.

All three of the infants just discussed apparently were infected in utero several days before birth. Their symptoms were exclusively neurologic; fever, irritability, and vomiting did not occur.

Postnatally Acquired Infection

In contrast to infections acquired in utero, those acquired postnatally are more typical of classic poliomyelitis. Shelokov and Weinstein[1025] described a child who was asymptomatic at birth. The onset of minor symptoms in the mother occurred 3 weeks before delivery, and the onset of major symptoms occurred 1 day before delivery. On the sixth day of life, the infant suddenly became ill with watery diarrhea. He looked grayish and pale. On the following day, he was irritable, lethargic, and limp and had a temperature of 38°C (100.4°F). Mild opisthotonos and weakness of both lower extremities developed. He was responsive to sound, light, and touch. The CSF had an elevated protein level and an increased number of leukocytes. His condition worsened during a total period of 3 days, and then gradual improvement began. At 1 year of age, he had severe residual paralysis of the right leg and moderate weakness in the left leg.

Baskin and associates[66] described two infants with neonatal poliomyelitis. The first child, whose mother had severe poliomyelitis at the time of delivery, was well for 3 days and then had a temperature of 38.3°C (100.9°F). On the fifth day of life, the boy became listless and cyanotic. Examination of CSF revealed a protein level of 300 mg/dL and 108 leukocytes/mm^3. His condition worsened, and extreme flaccidity, irregular respiration, and progressive cyanosis developed; he died on the seventh day of life. The second infant was a boy who was well until he was 8 days old but then became listless, with a temperature of 38.38°C (101.08°F). During the next 5 days, flaccid quadriplegia developed, as did irregular, rapid, and shallow respirations and an inability to swallow. The child died on the 14th day of life. Acute poliomyelitis had developed in his mother 6 days before the onset of his symptoms.

Abramson and colleagues[5] reported four children with neonatal poliomyelitis, two of whom died. In three of the children, the illnesses were typical of acute poliomyelitis in older children. The other child died at 13 days of age with generalized paralysis. The onset of his illness was difficult to define, and he was never febrile. Bates[67] described infants with acute poliomyelitis and clinical illnesses similar to those that occur in older persons.

DIAGNOSIS AND DIFFERENTIAL DIAGNOSIS

Clinical Diagnosis

Clinical differentiation of enteroviral disease frequently is thought to be impossible. Although treatable bacterial illnesses always should be considered and treated first, it is also true that when all the circumstances of a particular illness are considered, enteroviral diseases can be suspected on clinical grounds. The most important factors in clinical diagnosis are the season of the year, geographic location, exposure, incubation period, and clinical symptoms.

In temperate climates, the prevalence of EVs is distinctly seasonal, so disease usually is seen in the summer and fall. Enteroviral disease is less likely to occur in the winter. In the tropics, EVs are prevalent throughout the year, and the season therefore is not diagnostically helpful.

As with all infectious illnesses, knowledge of exposure and incubation time is important. A careful history of maternal illness is critical in neonatal disease. For example, nonspecific, mild febrile illness in a mother that occurs in the summer and fall should warn of the possibility of severe neonatal illness. Specific findings (i.e., aseptic meningitis, pleurodynia, herpangina, pericarditis, myocarditis) should alert the clinician to enteroviral illnesses. The short incubation period of enteroviral infections should be considered.

Laboratory Diagnosis

Virus Isolation and Detection Techniques

Most viral diagnostic laboratories have facilities for the recovery of most EVs that cause illness. A three-tissue culture system that includes primary monkey kidney, a diploid, human embryonic lung fibroblast cell strain, and the RD cell line will allow the isolation of virtually all group B coxsackieviruses and echoviruses and some coxsackieviruses A (e.g., coxsackieviruses A9 and A16). In a study in which Buffalo green monkey kidney cells and subpassage of primary human embryonic kidney cells were used in addition to primary monkey kidney and human diploid fibroblast (MRC-5) cells, the recovery rate of EVs was increased 11%.[210] For a complete diagnostic isolation spectrum, suckling mouse inoculation also should be performed.

Proper selection and handling of specimens are most important in the isolation of viruses. Enteroviral infections tend to be generalized, so collection of material from multiple sites is important; specimens should be collected from any or all of the following: nasopharynx, throat, stool, blood, urine, CSF, and any other body fluids that are available. Swabs from the nose, throat, and rectum should be placed in a carrying medium containing a small amount of protein. Hanks balanced salt solution with 2% agamma calf serum and antibiotics is satisfactory. Fluid specimens should be collected in sterile vials; specimens of postmortem material are collected best in vials that contain carrying medium. In general, specimens should be refrigerated immediately after collection and during transportation to the laboratory. The specimens must not be exposed to sunlight during transportation. If an extended period will elapse before a specimen is processed in the laboratory, shipping and storing it frozen are advisable.

Contrary to popular belief, tissue culture evidence of enteroviral growth takes only a few days in many cases and less than a week in most.[426] The use of spin amplification, the shell vial technique, and monoclonal antibodies has been shown to reduce the time of detection in enteroviral cultures significantly.[640,896,1023,1096] After an EV has been isolated, type identification is performed conventionally by neutralization, and this process, unfortunately, frequently takes a long time.

Nucleic acid techniques with cDNA and RNA probes have been shown to be useful for direct identification of EVs.[144,285,526,533,898,964,965,967] Most important, however, has been the development of numerous PCR techniques. Since 1990, many reports have described enteroviral, parechoviral, and SAFV PCR methods and their use in identifying viral RNA in clinical specimens.*

PCR has proved most useful for the direct identification of EVs and PeVs in the CSF of patients with meningitis.[34,526,970,996,1074,1086,1197] When compared with culture of CSF specimens, PCR is faster and more sensitive and the specificity is equal.

PCR also has proved useful in the identification of EVs and PeVs in blood, urine, and throat specimens.[10,24,133,835,838,1021,1053] Particularly impressive are the findings of Byington and associates[119,133] and Rittichier and associates.[952] Using PCR on specimens of blood and CSF, these investigators found that more than 25% of infants admitted to the hospital for suspected sepsis in 1997 had nonpolio enteroviral infections. On the basis of this study and the work of Andréoletti and coworkers,[24] we consider that the general workup for febrile children hospitalized for possible sepsis should include PCR for EVs and PeVs in both blood and CSF, if available. A shortcoming of PCR is that EV RNA is identified, but a specific enteroviral type is not. Because of this shortcoming, we recommend that conventional culture be performed in addition to PCR. However, in the research setting, further molecular study often can identify the genotype of a causative agent from the original sample submitted for PCR assay.[621]

EV RNA also has been identified in numerous tissue specimens from patients with chronic medical conditions such as idiopathic DCM. However, as discussed earlier in the section on cardiovascular manifestations, the possibility of a lack of specificity (false-positive results) is a concern. Polioviruses can be separated from other EVs, and poliovirus vaccine strains can be identified rapidly by PCR.[4,216,323,1194]

Serology

Except in special circumstances, the use of serologic techniques for establishing the primary diagnosis of suspected enteroviral infection is impractical. Standard serologic study depends on the demonstration of a rise in antibody titer to a specific virus as an indication of infection with that agent. Although enzyme-linked immunosorbent assay, hemagglutination inhibition, and complement fixation take only a short time to perform, these tests can be carried out only after a second, convalescent-phase blood specimen has been collected. These tests also are impractical in searching for the cause of a specific illness in a child because of the existence of so many antigenically different EVs. As noted previously in the discussion of antigenic characteristics, group antigens can be produced that allow one to establish a serologic diagnosis by IgM enzyme immunoassay and complement fixation, but these tests lack specificity.[989,1082,1083]

In the evaluation of a patient with a suspected enteroviral infection, serum should be collected as soon as possible after the onset of illness and then again 2 to 4 weeks later. This serum should be stored frozen. In most clinical situations, performing serologic tests on the collected serum is not necessary because demonstration of a rise in antibody

*References 4, 10, 24, 29, 50, 84, 133, 216, 246, 247, 251, 323, 364, 377, 423, 453, 534, 621, 660, 667, 699, 739, 765, 810, 835, 846, 849, 866, 928, 952, 956, 963, 966, 970, 993, 1001, 1020, 1021, 1026, 1034, 1052, 1064, 1073, 1074, 1086, 1102, 1126, 1129, 1134, 1182, 1194, 1197.

titer in the serum of an infant from whom a specific virus has been isolated from a body fluid obviously is superfluous. However, collected serum can be useful diagnostically if the prevalence of specific EVs in a community is known. In this situation, looking for antibody titer changes to a selected number of viral types is relatively easy. Faster diagnosis can be made with a single serum sample if a search for specific IgM enteroviral antibody is made.[175,227,390,408,409,420,1027,1101,1219]

Unfortunately, no EV IgM antibody tests are commercially available in the United States. Commercial laboratories offer enteroviral complement fixation antibody panels. However, these tests are expensive, and their results in the clinical setting almost always are meaningless unless acute-phase and convalescent-phase sera are analyzed.

Histology

Enteroviral infections have no specific histologic findings such as those seen in cytomegalovirus or HSV infection. However, tissues can be examined for specific enteroviral antigens by immunofluorescence and for RNA by PCR.[129,171,738]

Differential Diagnosis

The differential diagnosis of enteroviral infection depends on the clinical manifestations. In general, the most important considerations relate to bacterial diseases such as those commonly associated with pharyngitis, pneumonia, pericarditis, meningitis, and septicemia. Other viruses must be considered with upper respiratory tract illnesses, gastrointestinal infections, rashes, encephalitis, and neonatal illness.

Paralytic poliomyelitis usually presents no diagnostic problem in the presence of an outbreak, but sporadic cases are another matter, especially in countries such as the United States, where the disease (except for the vaccine-associated form) has disappeared and many pediatricians have never seen a case. Rarely, other EVs have been shown to cause paralytic syndromes that are indistinguishable from poliomyelitis.

Several other diseases must be considered in the differential diagnosis of sporadic cases of paralytic illness. Guillain-Barré syndrome is the most common and difficult differential diagnostic problem. Fever, headache, and meningeal signs usually occur less commonly in Guillain-Barré syndrome; the paralysis characteristically is symmetric, and sensory changes are common findings. Also in Guillain-Barré syndrome, the CSF contains few cells but a significant elevation in protein concentration. Other illnesses confused with paralytic poliomyelitis include peripheral neuritis (postinjection, toxic, herpes zoster), arboviral infection, rabies, tetanus, botulism, and tick paralysis.

TREATMENT

Specific Therapy

No specific therapy for any enteroviral infection is approved for use in the United States. In severe, catastrophic, and generalized neonatal infection, in all probability the baby received no specific antibody for the particular virus from the mother. In this situation, administering immunoglobulin to the infant is advisable because high titers of neutralizing antibody to most EVs and PeVs frequently are present in immunoglobulin.[16,235,274,1215] Little evidence supports the claim that this therapy is beneficial; however, it can be expected to stop further organ seeding secondary to continued viremia. Intravenous or intraventricular injection of immunoglobulin with IVIG and administration of hyperimmune plasma have been useful on some occasions and not others in the treatment of enteroviral infection in patients with agammaglobulinemia.*

Abzug and associates[8] performed a small but controlled study in which nine EV-infected neonates received IVIG and seven similarly infected infants received supportive care. In this study, no significant difference was found in clinical scores, antibody values, or the magnitude of viremia and viruria in those treated versus control infants. However, five infants received IVIG with a high neutralizing antibody titer (>1:800) to their individual viral isolates, and they experienced faster cessation of viremia and viruria. A neonate with disseminated echovirus 11 infection and hepatitis, pneumonitis, meningitis, DIC, decreased renal function, and anemia who survived after receiving a large dose of IVIG and supportive care was described.[577] Administering IVIG to older children with life-threatening enteroviral infection also seems reasonable. A specific recommended dosage is unknown, but 400 mg/kg per day for 4 days or 2 g/kg in one dose has been used.

Jantausch and associates[561] reported an infant with a disseminated echovirus 11 infection who survived after receiving maternal plasma transfusions. A neonate with fulminant echovirus 11 infection survived after undergoing orthotopic liver transplantation.[241]

The antiviral drug pleconaril offers promise for the treatment of enteroviral infections.* This drug is a novel compound that integrates into the capsid of EVs. It prevents virus attachment to cellular receptors and the uncoating and subsequent release of viral RNA into the host cell. In a double-blind, placebo-controlled study of 39 patients with enteroviral meningitis, a statistically significant shortening of duration of disease was noted—from 9.5 days in control subjects to 4.0 days in drug recipients.[969] Pleconaril also has been used on a compassionate-release basis for the treatment of patients with life-threatening infection.[69,125,971] The following categories of enteroviral illness have been treated: chronic meningoencephalitis in patients with agammaglobulinemia or hypogammaglobulinemia, neonatal sepsis, myocarditis, poliomyelitis (wild-type or vaccine associated), and encephalitis, as well as in bone marrow transplant recipients. Although these treatment studies did not have control arms, favorable clinical responses were observed in 26 of 50 treated patients, including 12 of 18 patients with chronic meningoencephalitis.

In subsequent randomized double-blind studies, 240 immunocompetent adolescents and adults with confirmed EV meningitis received pleconaril or placebo.[295] Post hoc analysis revealed that pleconaril-treated subjects reported headaches for a shorter period; no other differences in outcome were observed. The results of a lengthy double-blind placebo-controlled trial of pleconaril for the treatment of neonates with EV sepsis were published.[11,791] In intent-to-treat analysis, deaths were less common in pleconaril-treated infants than placebo recipients (10 of 43 [23%] vs. 8 of 18 [44%]; $P = .02$), but the differences in mortality rates of children with proven EV infection were not significantly different (7 of 31 [23%] vs. 5 of 12 [42%]; $P = .26$). The small study size of the study, low serum concentrations of pleconaril in the first 24 hours of treatment, and other factors make it difficult to assess the therapeutic potential of pleconaril in neonates. The investigators called for additional studies on the basis of evidence of viral suppression and other statistical signals suggesting drug efficacy.

The activity of pleconaril against EV D68 was evaluated using the reference Fermon strain and more recent 2014 isolates.[709,947] Although the reference strain was quite sensitive, the newer strains required much higher concentrations for inhibition.

Investigations of other antiviral agents are ongoing, driven both by the need for treatment options for nonpoliovirus EVs and by the proposal that antiviral agents may be needed to ensure eradication of poliovirus circulation.[253] Other capsid-binding agents exist, including pirodavir and vapendavir, and these exhibit activity against EV 71 and poliovirus strains.[7] However, clinical experience with these agents is very limited, and none had significant antiviral activity against the strains of EV D68 that circulated in 2014.[947] Other novel specific inhibitors of EV have been identified. However, progress toward the clinical studies has been impeded by limited antiviral activity, poor bioavailability, intrinsic resistance by some circulating strains, and pharmacoeconomic considerations.[7]

In severe illnesses such as neonatal myocarditis or encephalitis, a frequent temptation is to administer corticosteroids. Although some workers have thought that this therapy is beneficial in treating coxsackieviral myocarditis, we recommend that corticosteroids not be given during acute enteroviral infection. The deleterious effects of these agents in coxsackieviral infection of mice are particularly persuasive factors in this opinion.[106,629] Immunosuppressive therapy for myocarditis of unknown origin with prednisone and cyclosporine or azathioprine was

*References 12, 103, 264, 319, 335, 382, 448, 480, 751, 762, 766, 1120, 1153.

*References 11, 69, 125, 295, 604, 709, 718, 899, 947, 969, 971, 1150.

evaluated in a controlled trial of 111 adults, but no beneficial effect was observed.[741]

Because the possibility of bacterial sepsis cannot be ruled out in many instances of enteroviral infection, antibiotics frequently should be administered for the most likely potential pathogens. Care in the selection and administration of antibiotics is urged so that drug toxicity is not added to the problems of the patient.

Nonspecific Therapy

Mild, Nonspecific Febrile Illness

In patients in whom fever is the only symptom, careful observation is important. Many patients who eventually become severely ill initially have 2 to 3 days of fever without other localized findings. Care should be taken to administer adequate fluids to febrile infants, and excessive elevation of temperature should be prevented if possible.

Myocarditis

Myocarditis has no specific therapy. However, congestive heart failure and arrhythmias occur, and they should be treated by the usual methods. In administering digitalis to patients with enteroviral myocarditis, paying careful attention to the initial dosage is most important because the heart often is extremely sensitive; frequently, only small amounts of digoxin are necessary.

Meningoencephalitis

In patients with meningoencephalitis, seizures, cerebral edema, and disturbances in fluid and electrolyte balance all occur frequently and respond to treatment. Seizures are treated best with phenobarbital, phenytoin, or lorazepam. Cerebral edema can be treated with urea, mannitol, or large doses of corticosteroids. As noted, the use of corticosteroids in patients with active enteroviral infection seems unwise because the local benefit may be outweighed by the overall deleterious effects. Fluids should be monitored closely, and serum electrolyte levels should be determined frequently because inappropriate antidiuretic hormone secretion is a common occurrence.

Poliomyelitis

The broad principles of management are to allay fear, minimize the ensuing skeletal deformities, anticipate and meet complications in addition to the neuromusculoskeletal ones, and prepare the child and family for the prolonged treatment that may be required and for permanent disability when it seems likely. Patients with the nonparalytic and mildly paralytic forms of the disease may be treated at home.

Most patients with paralytic poliomyelitis require hospitalization. A calm atmosphere is desired. Suitable body alignment is necessary to avoid excessive skeletal deformity. A neutral position with the feet at a right angle, knees slightly flexed, and hips and spine straight is achieved by the use of boards, sandbags, and, occasionally, light splint shells. Active and passive motion is indicated as soon as the pain has disappeared. The orthopedist and physiatrist should see these patients as early in the illness as possible and should assume responsibility before fixed deformities develop.

Management of pure bulbar poliomyelitis consists essentially of maintaining the airway and avoiding all risks for inhalation of saliva, food, or vomitus. Gravity drainage of accumulated secretions is favored by the head-low (foot of the bed elevated 20 to 25 degrees), prone position with the face to one side. Aspirators with rigid or semirigid tips are preferred for direct oral and pharyngeal use, and soft flexible catheters may be used for nasopharyngeal aspiration. Fluid and electrolyte balance is maintained best by intravenous infusion because tube or oral feeding in the first few days may incite vomiting. After the initial few days, sips of sterile water may be given from a spoon, with increments as indicated by the child's ability to swallow. In addition to close observation for respiratory insufficiency, blood pressure should be recorded at least twice daily. Hypertension is not uncommon and occasionally leads to hypertensive encephalopathy. Patients with pure bulbar poliomyelitis may require tracheostomy because of paralysis of the vocal cords or constriction of the hypopharynx. Most patients with pure bulbar poliomyelitis who recover have little residual impairment; some patients exhibit mild dysphagia and occasional vocal fatigue with slurring of speech.

Impaired ventilation must be recognized early; mounting anxiety, restlessness, and fatigue are early indications for prompt intervention. Tracheostomy is indicated for some patients with pure bulbar poliomyelitis, spinal respiratory muscle paralysis, and bulbospinal paralysis. Unlike other patients on whom tracheostomy is performed, these patients generally are unable to cough, sometimes for many months. Frequent and swift endotracheal aspiration under aseptic conditions is necessary. Mechanical ventilation often is needed. Patients are fully conscious and aware; terrifying procedures are performed best with an outward atmosphere of calm. Explaining the procedure and having the parents on hand may be helpful. A reduction in thoracic compliance occurs early, and higher than expected pressure gradients may be required to achieve adequate ventilation. Weaning a patient from dependence on respiratory assistance is a torturous process, as is total musculoskeletal rehabilitation. Motivation of the patient and the team of personnel is paramount.

PROGNOSIS

The prognosis for nonpolio enteroviral infections is excellent in most instances. Virtually all morbidity and mortality are related to cardiac and neurologic diseases in older children and to these diseases in addition to general disseminated infection with hepatitis in neonates.

The prognosis for poliomyelitis varies with the degree of muscle involvement. In patients with mild muscle weakness, complete recovery is the rule. If paralysis is present, recovery of muscle function continues for a period of approximately 18 months to 2 years. By 3 months, approximately 60% of the ultimate improvement has been achieved, and by 6 months, 80%. The final result depends on the extent and localization of nerve cell damage.

Respiratory failure is responsible for most of the deaths in paralytic poliomyelitis. With the many improvements in techniques for handling this complication, the overall mortality rate has been reduced to approximately 4%; with the bulbar form and in adults, it still may be as high as 10%.

Occasionally, new neuromuscular symptoms develop later in life in patients who have had paralytic poliomyelitis.[145,276,277,568,929,1087,1175,1174] Although the cause of this late-onset weakness and muscle atrophy (postpolio syndrome) is not understood completely, it most likely is the result of routine attrition of anterior horn cells associated with aging rather than persistent neural infection with polioviruses. However, specific immunopathologic mechanisms possibly play a role in some instances.[405]

Leparc-Goffart and associates[681] presented data suggesting the presence of poliovirus-specific genomic sequences in the CSF of patients with postpolio syndrome. However, Muir and colleagues,[812] who performed similar studies, found no association of chronic neurologic disease with the presence of enteroviral RNA in CSF.

PREVENTION

Nonpolio Enteroviral Vaccines and Immune Globulin

Until recently no attenuated or live viral vaccines for EVs other than polioviruses were available. Because of its epidemic nature and disease severity, vaccines for EV 71 have been developed.[230,1217] The developed vaccines have been found to be safe and effective. In three different vaccine trials in children (6–60 months of age), an efficacy of greater than 90% against EV 71 hand-foot-and-mouth disease and greater than 80% against more serious diseases (CNS manifestations and hemorrhagic pulmonary edema) was observed.[230] Two of the vaccines have been approved for marketing in China.[1217]

Passive protection is IVIG may be useful in preventing disease. In practice, however, it would seem worthwhile only for sudden and virulent nursery outbreaks. For example, if several cases of myocarditis occurred in a nursery, administering IVIG to all babies in the nursery would seem reasonable. Pooled human immunoglobulin in most instances can be expected to contain antibodies against coxsackieviruses B1, B2, B3, B4, and B5, as well as several coxsackieviruses A, echoviruses, other

EVs, and PeVs 1,3, and 6.[16,274,1215] Therefore, this procedure would offer protection to infants without transplacentally acquired specific antibody who had not yet become infected. Immune serum was useful in the management of three nursery enteroviral outbreaks.[143,817,890]

Polioviral Vaccines

In the United States, the total annual number of paralytic cases fell from an average of 16,000 in the 5 years before the introduction of vaccine to approximately 10 cases per year between 1980 and 1984. The experience in 1979, however, when 26 paralytic cases were reported, served as a reminder that virulent polioviruses still could surface in susceptible persons.[152,151] Most of the 1979 cases occurred in Pennsylvania and several other states in Amish population groups who had not been immunized. A similar epidemic in Connecticut in 1972 involved a pocket of unimmunized students in a Christian Science school.[148] These outbreaks reflected the reality that poliomyelitis was still occurring in many parts of the world. The possibility of the introduction of virulent strains was ever present, and only through continued and extensive immunization programs could the disease be prevented from reappearing in epidemic form.[503]

The remarkable overall record of the decline in paralytic poliomyelitis in the United States was a result of the development and use of two effective vaccines.[503,1063,1130] IPV, the first to be licensed, was used extensively beginning in 1955 and considerably reduced the incidence of the disease, although epidemics continued to occur. Live-attenuated OPV, licensed in 1961 and 1962, subsequently was recommended as the method of choice in the United States on the basis of its superiority in terms of immunogenic capacity, ability to induce local IgA antibody in the oropharynx and intestinal tract and thus provide greater resistance to reinfection, and ease of administration. OPV gradually supplanted IPV, and between 1973 and 1978, it was the only vaccine available. Its extraordinary effectiveness at that time, despite reaching only 65% of children younger than 5 years of age with the recommended three doses, suggested that the capacity of the attenuated strains to spread contributed to a much higher immunization rate than was indicated by vaccination statistics. The potential impact of such spread on the immunity of the population was illustrated by the observations of Fox and Hall,[365] who conducted long-term virologic surveillance of middle-income families in Seattle, Washington. Polioviruses (vaccine strains) accounted for 50% of the 2937 viral isolates from healthy children, their parents, and others in the community. In an analysis of 611 of the poliovirus isolates, researchers found that 75.6% were from vaccinees, 10.5% were from vaccinee contacts, and 14% were from persons without recent known contact with vaccine or a vaccinee. These findings provided a vivid picture of the pervasiveness of the attenuated strains and their continuous circulation in the population. This feature also was supported by the almost invariable recovery of polioviruses from weekly samples of sewage that were collected throughout the year, in the early vaccine era, in urban communities.[504]

Despite its striking success, the oral vaccine had some problems. One was greatly reduced seroconversion rates when the vaccine was given to children living in the tropics: as few as 50% had satisfactory responses, in contrast to the more than 95% response rate in the United States and similar countries.[302,770] Viral interference from other EVs played some role, and the presence of an inhibitory substance in the oropharynx that prevented significant multiplication of the vaccine strains also was involved. The seroconversion problem was lessened by using pulse immunization programs.[567,980] For example, the strategy of national annual vaccination days twice per year, 2 months apart, has been successful in developing countries.

Another problem with OPV—and the major problem in the United States—was the occurrence of a small number of vaccine-associated cases of poliomyelitis.[503,770] The immunogenic effectiveness of the vaccine depends on multiplication of the attenuated strains in the intestinal tract. Because no poliovirus strain is completely stable, the progeny of vaccine strains underwent a certain degree of mutation, which rarely resulted in increased virulence and vaccine-associated cases in recipients and their contacts, most often their parents.

Since 1980, no indigenous cases of wild poliovirus disease have occurred in the United States.[158,1056] From 1980 to 1989, 80 cases of vaccine-associated paralytic poliomyelitis and five cases of imported disease were reported. The overall rate of vaccine-associated paralytic poliomyelitis was one case per 2.5 million doses of distributed vaccine; the risk for recipients was one case per 6.8 million doses, and for household contacts it was one case per 6.4 million doses. Of the 80 cases, 30 occurred in vaccinees, 32 occurred in household contacts, four were community acquired, and 14 occurred in immunologically abnormal persons.

Further analysis revealed that the risk associated with the first dose of vaccine was one case per 700,000 doses, but it was only one case per 6.9 million for subsequent doses; for vaccine recipients, the calculated risks were one case per 1.4 million initial doses and one case per 41.5 million subsequent doses. The calculated risks for contact cases were one case per 1.9 million initial doses of vaccine and one case per 13.8 million subsequent doses.

Immunodeficient children are at particular risk for acquiring vaccine-associated paralytic poliomyelitis.[149,1056] From 1969 through 1976, 11% of vaccine-associated cases occurred in immunodeficient patients; 10 of 11 of these patients were children younger than 1 year. From 1980 to 1989, 18% of vaccine-associated paralytic poliomyelitis cases occurred in immunodeficient patients.[1056]

Although the risks mentioned earlier were considered acceptable in view of the benefits provided, the question raised repeatedly since the 1970s was whether the United States should return to the use of IPV, which does not carry a risk for acquiring paralytic disease and has been highly successful in several small European countries in which more than 95% of the population is immunized.[363,378,490,583,601,815,884,983–986,1056]

The problem was reviewed in detail by a committee of the Institute of Medicine (IOM) of the National Academy of Sciences, which reported its recommendations in April of 1977.[840] The conclusion at the time was that given the situation in the United States, in which not more than 65% of susceptible children were vaccinated, OPV should continue to be the principal vaccine for routine immunization. IPV, conversely, should be provided for two groups: immunodeficient persons, because of their greatly enhanced risk for acquiring vaccine-associated disease after receiving the oral vaccine; and adults receiving primary immunization, because of their greater susceptibility to paralytic disease. Also suggested was that the inactivated vaccine be available as an alternative for those who prefer it. In addition, a single dose of trivalent OPV was suggested for all entrants into the seventh grade of school as a means of added protection for later years when they became parents.

In January of 1988, a panel appointed by the IOM again reviewed policy options for vaccination against poliomyelitis in the United States.[541] The IOM panel concluded that no change in policy should be recommended at that time. However, they did recommend that a new enhanced IPV replace the old vaccine when inactivated vaccine was indicated. They also suggested that when a new enhanced diphtheria-tetanus-pertussis IPV became available, a regimen of two or more doses of it followed by the oral vaccine be considered.

In 1996, the US poliovirus vaccine immunization program was evaluated extensively by both the Advisory Committee on Immunization Practices (ACIP) and the Committee on Infectious Diseases of the American Academy of Pediatrics (AAP). The ACIP recommended that sequential administration of IPV followed by OPV be the schedule of choice in the United States (W.A. Orenstein, personal communication, 1996). The schedule consisted of two doses of the inactivated vaccine at 2 and 4 months of age and two doses of the oral vaccine at 12 to 18 months and 4 to 6 years of age. Both committees indicated that schedules that include all the doses of each vaccine also were acceptable (R.E. Hanneman, personal communication, 1996; W.A. Orenstein, personal communication, 1996). At the present time, an all-IPV vaccination schedule is recommended in the United States.[23,784] It is a four-dose schedule with doses at 2 and 4 months, 6 to 18 months, and 4 to 6 years. The reader is advised to consult the recommendations of the ACIP and the AAP, as well as the manufacturers' literature, for full consideration of the contraindications and indications for poliovirus vaccines.

Routine primary poliovirus vaccination of adults older than 18 years is not conducted in the United States. However, adults at risk for exposure to wild polioviruses (i.e., laboratory workers, international travelers, health care workers) should be immunized. For the vaccination of adults, IPV is recommended. Patients with immunodeficiency diseases should not be given OPV; live virus also should not be used in households in which an immunodeficient person resides.

Global Eradication of Poliomyelitis

The WHO established the Expanded Program on Immunization (EPI) in 1974.[528,1145,1187] Subsequently, the use of OPV in developing countries vastly increased. In 1980 in Brazil, researchers demonstrated that mass administration with the oral vaccine on National Immunization Days (NIDs) led to a dramatic reduction in the incidence of poliomyelitis.[291] This demonstration led in 1985 to the targeted eradication of poliomyelitis from the Western Hemisphere by 1990. This campaign was successful in that the last confirmed case of paralytic poliomyelitis caused by wild poliovirus occurred in 1991 in Peru.[152] In September 1994, an international commission convened by the Pan American Health Organization certified that indigenous transmission of wild poliovirus had been interrupted in the Americas.[157]

In 1988, the World Health Assembly established the objective of global eradication of polio by 2000.[528] This program was based on four strategies recommended by the WHO: (1) maintenance of high vaccination coverage levels among children with at least three doses of OPV; (2) development of sensitive systems of epidemiologic and laboratory surveillance, including use of the standard WHO case definition (i.e., a confirmed case of poliomyelitis is defined as acute flaccid paralysis and at least one of the following: laboratory-confirmed wild poliovirus infection, residual paralysis of 60 days, death, or no follow-up investigation at 60 days); (3) administration of supplementary doses of OPV to all young children (usually those <5 years) during NIDs to interrupt the transmission of poliovirus rapidly; and (4) "mopping up" vaccination campaigns, which are localized campaigns targeted at high-risk areas where wild poliovirus transmission was most likely to persist at low levels. NIDs are mass campaigns conducted over the course of a short period (i.e., days to weeks) during which two doses of OPV are administered to all children in the target age group regardless of previous vaccination history, with an interval of 4 to 6 weeks between doses.

From 1985 through 1990, worldwide routine vaccination coverage levels increased from 47% to 85% and stabilized at 80% to 81% from 1991 to 1994.[158] From 1985 through 1994, the number of cases reported annually decreased 84%, from 39,361 to 6241. The number of countries reporting polio cases decreased steadily from 1985 (99 of 196 [51%]) to 1988 (88 of 196 [45%]) and 1994 (51 of 214 [24%]). In addition, the number of countries reporting zero polio cases increased from 1985 (84 [43%]) to 1988 (104 [53%]) and 1994 (145 [68%]). The number of countries with endemic polio that conducted NIDs each year increased from 15 in 1988 to 37 in April of 1995; 24 additional countries scheduled their first NIDs for later in 1995.

At the beginning of the 21st century, NIDs had been conducted in every country in the world with endemic polio. In 1999, 7141 cases of poliomyelitis were reported worldwide. These cases occurred in 30 countries, mainly in South Asia and Central Africa. By the end of 2000, fewer than 3500 cases occurred in endemic areas throughout the world, and wild-type 2 poliovirus has not been detected since October 1999.[988] At the close of 2001, the area of endemic poliomyelitis had been reduced to 10 countries, with fewer than 1000 cases reported.[827]

The global eradication program suffered a major setback in 2004 when OPV immunizations in northern Nigeria were suspended because of misinformation regarding vaccine safety.[481] After this suspension, epidemic disease caused by type 1 virus occurred throughout Nigeria and also spread directly or indirectly to 21 previously polio-free countries.[165] This epidemic, which had extensive spread, had a major negative impact on the Global Polio Eradication Initiative. During 2005, 1856 cases were reported globally, and 1000 of these cases occurred in countries with outbreaks caused by importation.

In 2011, there were four endemic countries (Afghanistan, India, Nigeria, and Pakistan).[169] In addition, reestablished transmission occurred in Angola, Chad, and the Democratic Republic of the Congo. In 2015 there were only 74 cases caused by wild polio virus found in Afghanistan and Pakistan.[800] As of May 2016 the only circulating wild-type virus is type 1. The last case caused by wild polio virus type 3 occurred in Nigeria in 2012.

Much attention is being paid to the end-game strategy for global polio eradication.[250,306,305,612,793,892,1063,1130] Of particular concern for the future after world eradication of wild poliovirus strains is vaccine-associated paralytic poliomyelitis.[250,297,298,614,615,799,1006] Other concerns are the long-term excretion of highly evolved vaccine-derived polioviruses in persons with primary immunodeficiencies and polio outbreaks associated with circulating vaccine-derived polioviruses in areas with low rates of OPV coverage. In 2014 to 2015 circulating vaccine-derived polio virus outbreaks occurred in five countries (Guinea, Laos, Madagascar, Myanmar, and Ukraine).[298,800] In 2015 vaccine-derived poliovirus infections were also noted in the Democratic Republic of the Congo, Nigeria, Pakistan, and South Sudan. Ideally, an end-game strategy would transition to the use of IPV, but this strategy is not realistic in much of the developing world. As of June 2015, 90 WHO member states were using IPV.[540] Twenty-two of these countries had introduced IPV after January 2013. Introduction of IPV in other member states is in progress. Currently in progress in countries using OPV is a switch from trivalent OPV to bivalent OPV (types 1 and 3).

Despite the substantial progress that has been made toward global eradication of polio, several challenges remain, including the following: (1) increasing vaccination levels in unvaccinated subpopulations; (2) preventing the reintroduction of wild poliovirus into polio-free areas by eliminating reservoirs in polio-endemic countries (particularly in the Indian subcontinent); (3) increasing the awareness of donor agencies and governments in industrialized countries of the substantial financial and humanitarian benefits of global eradication of polio, thus engendering support from unaffected countries beyond that already provided by organizations such as Rotary International; (4) encouraging all countries that remain polio endemic to make eradication of polio a high priority, including the implementation of NIDs and the initiation of acute flaccid paralysis surveillance; and (5) providing support to vaccination program managers for training to develop managerial skills for implementing and maintaining effective vaccination and surveillance programs in all countries.[158] The success of the Global Polio Eradication Initiative will depend on finding solutions to these financial, managerial, political, and technical challenges.

World events and new knowledge relating to reversion of poliovirus vaccine strains and recombination of poliovirus vaccine strains with nonpolio EVs led to the realization that decisions related to discontinuation of immunization after world eradication are exceedingly complex.[613,827,1080,1182]

NEW REFERENCES SINCE THE SEVENTH EDITION

3. Abedi GR, Watson JT, Pham H, et al. Enterovirus and human parechovirus surveillance—United States, 2009–2013. *MMWR Morb Mortal Wkly Rep.* 2015;64(34):940-943.
6. Abzug MJ. The enteroviruses: problems in need of treatments. *J Infect.* 2014;68(suppl 1):S108-S114.
11. Abzug MJ, Michaels MG, Wald E, et al. A randomized, double-blind, placebo-controlled trial of pleconaril for the treatment of neonates with enterovirus sepsis. *J Pediatric Infect Dis Soc.* 2016;5(1):53-62.
16. Aizawa Y, Watanabe K, Oishi T, et al. Role of maternal antibodies in infants with severe diseases related to human parechovirus type 3. *Emerg Infect Dis.* 2015;21(11):1966-1972.
20. Aliabadi N, Messacar K, Pastula DM, et al. Enterovirus D68 infection in children with acute flaccid myelitis, Colorado, USA, 2014. *Emerg Infect Dis.* 2016;22(8):1387-1394.
23. American Academy of Pediatrics. Infections. In: Kimberlin DW, Brady MT, Jackson MA, Long SS, eds. *Red Book 2015: Report of the Committee on Infectious Diseases.* Elk Grove, IL: American Academy of Pediatrics; 2015:644-650.
30. Aoki Y, Matoba Y, Tanaka S, et al. Isolation of Saffold virus type 2 from children with acute respiratory infections by using the RD-18S-Niigata cell line. *Jpn J Infect Dis.* 2015;68(5):438-441.
34. Archimbaud C, Chambon M, Bailly JL, et al. Impact of rapid enterovirus molecular diagnosis on the management of infants, children, and adults with aseptic meningitis. *J Med Virol.* 2009;81(1):42-48.
48. Ayscue P, Van Haren K, Sheriff H, et al. Acute flaccid paralysis with anterior myelitis—California, June 2012–June 2014. *MMWR Morb Mortal Wkly Rep.* 2014;63(40):903-906.

60. Banta J, Lenz B, Pawlak M, et al. Notes from the field: outbreak of hand, foot, and mouth disease caused by coxsackievirus A6 among basic military trainees—Texas, 2015. *MMWR Morb Mortal Wkly Rep*. 2016;65(26):678-680.
71. Begier EM, Oberste MS, Landry ML, et al. An outbreak of concurrent echovirus 30 and coxsackievirus A1 infections associated with sea swimming among a group of travelers to Mexico. *Clin Infect Dis*. 2008;47(5):616-623.
108. Bottcher S, Prifert C, Weissbrich B, et al. Detection of enterovirus D68 in patients hospitalised in three tertiary university hospitals in Germany, 2013 to 2014. *Euro Surveill*. 2016;21(19).
115. Branas P, Garcia M, Prieto C, et al. Saffold virus respiratory infection in children and immunocompromised patients in Spain. *J Infect*. 2015;70(6):679-680.
119. Britton PN, Dale RC, Nissen MD, et al. Parechovirus encephalitis and neurodevelopmental outcomes. *Pediatrics*. 2016;137(2):e20152848.
132. Buttery VW, Kenyon C, Grunewald S, et al. Atypical presentations of hand, foot, and mouth disease caused by coxsackievirus A6—Minnesota, 2014. *MMWR Morb Mortal Wkly Rep*. 2015;64(29):805.
138. Calvo C, Cuevas MT, Pozo F, et al. Respiratory infections by enterovirus D68 in outpatients and inpatients Spanish children. *Pediatr Infect Dis J*. 2016;35(1):45-49.
146. Centers for Disease Control and Prevention. Clusters of acute respiratory illness associated with human enterovirus 68—Asia, Europe, and United States, 2008–2010. *MMWR Morb Mortal Wkly Rep*. 2011;60(38):1301-1304.
147. Centers for Disease Control and Prevention. Notes from the field: severe hand, foot, and mouth disease associated with coxsackievirus A6—Alabama, Connecticut, California, and Nevada, November 2011–February 2012. *MMWR Morb Mortal Wkly Rep*. 2012;61(12):213-214.
178. Chang LY, Chang IS, Chen WJ, et al. HLA-A33 is associated with susceptibility to enterovirus 71 infection. *Pediatrics*. 2008;122(6):1271-1276.
201. Cherry JD. Enteroviruses. In: Remington JS, Klein JO, eds. *Infectious Diseases of the Fetus and Newborn Infant*. Philadelphia, PA: Saunders; 2016: 782-827.
207. Cherry JD, Krogstad P. Enteroviruses, parechoviruses, and Saffold viruses. In: Cherry JD, Harrison GJ, Kaplan SL, Steinbach WJ, Hotez PJ, eds. *Textbook of Pediatric Infectious Diseases*. 7th ed. Philadelphia, PA: Saunders; 2014:2051-2109.
225. Cho HK, Lee NY, Lee H, et al. Enterovirus 71-associated hand, foot and mouth diseases with neurologic symptoms, a university hospital experience in Korea, 2009. *Korean J Pediatr*. 2010;53(5):639-643.
226. Choi CS, Choi YJ, Choi UY, et al. Clinical manifestations of CNS infections caused by enterovirus type 71. *Korean J Pediatr*. 2011;54(1):11-16.
229. Chong JH, Aan MK. An atypical dermatologic presentation of a child with hand, foot and mouth disease caused by coxsackievirus A6. *Pediatr Infect Dis J*. 2014;33(8):889.
230. Chong P, Liu CC, Chow YH, et al. Review of enterovirus 71 vaccines. *Clin Infect Dis*. 2015;60(5):797-803.
240. Chua KB, Voon K, Yu M, et al. Saffold virus infection in children, Malaysia, 2009. *Emerg Infect Dis*. 2011;17(8):1562-1564.
242. Chung WH, Shih SR, Chang CF, et al. Clinicopathologic analysis of coxsackievirus a6 new variant induced widespread mucocutaneous bullous reactions mimicking severe cutaneous adverse reactions. *J Infect Dis*. 2013;208(12):1968-1978.
253. Collett MS, Neyts J, Modlin JF. A case for developing antiviral drugs against polio. *Antiviral Res*. 2008;79(3):179-187.
266. Crone M, Tellier R, Wei XC, et al. Polio-like illness associated with outbreak of upper respiratory tract infection in children. *J Child Neurol*. 2016;31(4):409-414.
284. Davis J, Fairley D, Christie S, et al. Human parechovirus infection in neonatal intensive care. *Pediatr Infect Dis J*. 2015;34(2):121-124.
298. Diop OM, Burns CC, Sutter RW, et al. Update on vaccine-derived polioviruses - worldwide, January 2014–March 2015. *MMWR Morb Mortal Wkly Rep*. 2015;64(23):640-646.
300. Division of Viral Diseases National Center for Immunization and Respiratory Diseases CDC, Division of Vector-Borne Diseases, Division of High-Consequence Pathogens and Pathology, National Center for Emerging and Zoonotic Infectious Diseases, CDC, et al. Notes from the field: acute flaccid myelitis among persons aged ≤21 years—United States, August 1–November 13, 2014. *MMWR Morb Mortal Wkly Rep*. 2015;63(53):1243-1244.
307. Drago F, Ciccarese G, Broccolo F, et al. Localized exanthem due to echovirus 9. *J Med Virol*. 2015;87(9):1447-1448.
329. El Houmami N, Minodier P, Dubourg G, et al. An outbreak of *Kingella kingae* infections associated with hand, foot and mouth disease/herpangina virus outbreak in Marseille, France, 2013. *Pediatr Infect Dis J*. 2015;34(3):246-250.
336. Esposito S, Lunghi G, Zampiero A, et al. Enterovirus-D68 in the cerebrospinal fluid of two children with aseptic meningitis. *Pediatr Infect Dis J*. 2016;35(5):589-591.
389. Gau SS, Chang LY, Huang LM, et al. Attention-deficit/hyperactivity-related symptoms among children with enterovirus 71 infection of the central nervous system. *Pediatrics*. 2008;122(2):e452-e458.
430. Greninger AL, Naccache SN, Messacar K, et al. A novel outbreak enterovirus D68 strain associated with acute flaccid myelitis cases in the USA (2012-14): a retrospective cohort study. *Lancet Infect Dis*. 2015;15(6):671-682.
431. Griffiths MJ, Ooi MH, Wong SC, et al. In enterovirus 71 encephalitis with cardio-respiratory compromise, elevated interleukin 1beta, interleukin 1 receptor antagonist, and granulocyte colony-stimulating factor levels are markers of poor prognosis. *J Infect Dis*. 2012;206(6):881-892.
465. Hayman R, Shepherd M, Tarring C, et al. Outbreak of variant hand-foot-and-mouth disease caused by coxsackievirus A6 in Auckland, New Zealand. *J Paediatr Child Health*. 2014;50(10):751-755.
495. Holm-Hansen CC, Midgley SE, Fischer TK. Global emergence of enterovirus D68: a systematic review. *Lancet Infect Dis*. 2016.
496. Hongyan G, Chengjie M, Qiaozhi Y, et al. Hand, foot and mouth disease caused by coxsackievirus A6, Beijing, 2013. *Pediatr Infect Dis J*. 2014;33(12):1302-1303.
500. Horner LM, Poulter MD, Brenton JN, et al. Acute flaccid paralysis associated with novel enterovirus C105. *Emerg Infect Dis*. 2015;21(10):1858-1860.
514. Hu YQ, Xie GC, Li DD, et al. Prevalence of coxsackievirus A6 and enterovirus 71 in hand, foot and mouth disease in Nanjing, China in 2013. *Pediatr Infect Dis J*. 2015;34(9):951-957.
520. Huang YC, Chu YH, Yen TY, et al. Clinical features and phylogenetic analysis of coxsackievirus A9 in northern Taiwan in 2011. *BMC Infect Dis*. 2013;13:33.
526. Huizing KM, Swanink CM, Landstra AM, et al. Rapid enterovirus molecular testing in cerebrospinal fluid reduces length of hospitalization and duration of antibiotic therapy in children with aseptic meningitis. *Pediatr Infect Dis J*. 2011;30(12):1107-1109.
537. Imamura T, Fuji N, Suzuki A, et al. Enterovirus 68 among children with severe acute respiratory infection, the Philippines. *Emerg Infect Dis*. 2011;17(8): 1430-1435.
538. Imamura T, Oshitani H. Global reemergence of enterovirus D68 as an important pathogen for acute respiratory infections. *Rev Med Virol*. 2015;25(2): 102-114.
539. Imamura T, Suzuki A, Lupisan S, et al. Detection of enterovirus 68 in serum from pediatric patients with pneumonia and their clinical outcomes. *Influenza Other Respir Viruses*. 2014;8(2):21-24.
552. Jaaskelainen AJ, Kolehmainen P, Kallio-Kokko H, et al. First two cases of neonatal human parechovirus 4 infection with manifestation of suspected sepsis, Finland. *J Clin Virol*. 2013;58(1):328-330.
556. Jacobson LM, Redd JT, Schneider E, et al. Outbreak of lower respiratory tract illness associated with human enterovirus 68 among American Indian children. *Pediatr Infect Dis J*. 2012;31(3):309-312.
579. Jones G, Muriello M, Patel A, et al. Enteroviral meningoencephalitis complicated by central diabetes insipidus in a neonate: a case report and review of the literature. *J Pediatric Infect Dis Soc*. 2015;4(2):155-158.
587. Kaida A, Kubo H, Sekiguchi J, et al. Enterovirus 68 in children with acute respiratory tract infections, Osaka, Japan. *Emerg Infect Dis*. 2011;17(8):1494-1497.
596. Karsch K, Obermeier P, Seeber L, et al. Human parechovirus infections associated with seizures and rash in infants and toddlers. *Pediatr Infect Dis J*. 2015;34(10):1049-1055.
617. Khamrin P, Thongprachum A, Kikuta H, et al. Three clusters of Saffold viruses circulating in children with diarrhea in Japan. *Infect Genet Evol*. 2013;13:339-343.
619. Khatami A, McMullan BJ, Webber M, et al. Sepsis-like disease in infants due to human parechovirus type 3 during an outbreak in Australia. *Clin Infect Dis*. 2015;60(2):228-236.
645. Kolehmainen P, Jaaskelainen A, Blomqvist S, et al. Human parechovirus type 3 and 4 associated with severe infections in young children. *Pediatr Infect Dis J*. 2014;33(11):1109-1113.
651. Kreuter JD, Barnes A, McCarthy JE, et al. A fatal central nervous system enterovirus 68 infection. *Arch Pathol Lab Med*. 2011;135(6):793-796.
664. Laitinen OH, Honkanen H, Pakkanen O, et al. Coxsackievirus B1 is associated with induction of beta-cell autoimmunity that portends type 1 diabetes. *Diabetes*. 2014;63(2):446-455.
695. Lewthwaite P, Perera D, Ooi MH, et al. Enterovirus 75 encephalitis in children, southern India. *Emerg Infect Dis*. 2010;16(11):1780-1782.
702. Lin TL, Lin TH, Chiu SC, et al. Molecular epidemiological analysis of Saffold cardiovirus genotype 3 from upper respiratory infection patients in Taiwan. *J Clin Virol*. 2015;70:7-13.
710. Liu Y, Sheng J, Fokine A, et al. Structure and inhibition of EV-D68, a virus that causes respiratory illness in children. *Science*. 2015;347(6217):71-74.
715. Lott JP, Liu K, Landry ML, et al. Atypical hand-foot-and-mouth disease associated with coxsackievirus A6 infection. *J Am Acad Dermatol*. 2013;69(5):736-741.
717. Lu QB, Wo Y, Wang HY, et al. Detection of enterovirus 68 as one of the commonest types of enterovirus found in patients with acute respiratory tract infection in China. *J Med Microbiol*. 2014;63:408-414.
718. Lugo D, Krogstad P. Enteroviruses in the early 21st century: new manifestations and challenges. *Curr Opin Pediatr*. 2016;28(1):107-113.
726. Lynch MD, Sears A, Cookson H, et al. Disseminated coxsackievirus A6 affecting children with atopic dermatitis. *Clin Exp Dermatol*. 2015;40(5):525-528.
742. Mathes EF, Oza V, Frieden IJ, et al. "Eczema coxsackium" and unusual cutaneous findings in an enterovirus outbreak. *Pediatrics*. 2013;132(1):e149-e157.
776. Merilahti P, Tauriainen S, Susi P. Human parechovirus 1 infection occurs via alphaVbeta1 integrin. *PLoS ONE*. 2016;11(4):e0154769.
778. Messacar K, Abzug MJ, Dominguez SR. 2014 outbreak of enterovirus D68 in North America. *J Med Virol*. 2016;88(5):739-745.

779. Messacar K, Schreiner TL, Maloney JA, et al. A cluster of acute flaccid paralysis and cranial nerve dysfunction temporally associated with an outbreak of enterovirus D68 in children in Colorado, USA. *Lancet*. 2015;385(9978):1662-1671.
780. Midgley CM, Jackson MA, Selvarangan R, et al. Severe respiratory illness associated with enterovirus D68 - Missouri and Illinois, 2014. *MMWR Morb Mortal Wkly Rep*. 2014;63(36):798-799.
781. Midgley CM, Watson JT, Nix WA, et al. Severe respiratory illness associated with a nationwide outbreak of enterovirus D68 in the USA (2014): a descriptive epidemiological investigation. *Lancet Respir Med*. 2015;3(11):879-887.
791. Modlin J. Treatment of neonatal enterovirus infections. *J Pediatric Infect Dis Soc*. 2016;5(1):63-64.
793. Modlin J, Wenger J. Achieving and maintaining polio eradication—new strategies. *N Engl J Med*. 2014;371(16):1476-1479.
799. Morales M, Nnadi CD, Tangermann RH, et al. Notes from the field: circulating vaccine-derived poliovirus outbreaks—five countries, 2014–2015. *MMWR Morb Mortal Wkly Rep*. 2016;65(5):128-129.
800. Morales M, Tangermann RH, Wassilak SG. Progress toward polio eradication—worldwide, 2015–2016. *MMWR Morb Mortal Wkly Rep*. 2016;65(18):470-473.
837. Nielsen AC, Gyhrs ML, Nielsen LP, et al. Gastroenteritis and the novel picornaviruses Aichi virus, cosavirus, Saffold virus, and salivirus in young children. *J Clin Virol*. 2013;57(3):239-242.
839. Nielsen TS, Nielsen AY, Banner J, et al. Saffold virus infection associated with human myocarditis. *J Clin Virol*. 2016;74:78-81.
844. Nilsson AL, Vaziri-Sani F, Andersson C, et al. Relationship between Ljungan virus antibodies, HLA-DQ8, and insulin autoantibodies in newly diagnosed type 1 diabetes children. *Viral Immunol*. 2013;26(3):207-215.
859. Obermeier PE, Karsch K, Hoppe C, et al. Acute disseminated encephalomyelitis after human parechovirus infection. *Pediatr Infect Dis J*. 2016;35(1):35-38.
864. Oberste MS, Maher K, Schnurr D, et al. Enterovirus 68 is associated with respiratory illness and shares biological features with both the enteroviruses and the rhinoviruses. *J Gen Virol*. 2004;85:2577-2584.
870. Oikarinen S, Martiskainen M, Tauriainen S, et al. Enterovirus RNA in blood is linked to the development of type 1 diabetes. *Diabetes*. 2011;60(1):276-279.
876. Orvedahl A, Padhye A, Barton K, et al. Clinical characterization of children presenting to the hospital with enterovirus D68 infection during the 2014 outbreak in St. Louis. *Pediatr Infect Dis J*. 2016;35(5):481-487.
880. Pallansch MA, Roos RP. Enteroviruses: polioviruses, coxsackieviruses, echoviruses, and newer enteroviruses. In: Knipe DM, Howley PM, eds. *Fields Virology*. Vol. 1. 6th ed. Philadelphia, PA: Lippincott Williams & Wilkins; 2013:490-530.
885. Pariani E, Pellegrinelli L, Pugni L, et al. Two cases of neonatal human parechovirus 3 encephalitis. *Pediatr Infect Dis J*. 2014;33(11):1191-1193.
891. Pastula DM, Aliabadi N, Haynes AK, et al. Acute neurologic illness of unknown etiology in children—Colorado, August-September 2014. *MMWR Morb Mortal Wkly Rep*. 2014;63(40):901-902.
892. Patel M, Orenstein W. A world free of polio—the final steps. *N Engl J Med*. 2016;374(6):501-503.
922. Principi N, Esposito S. Enterovirus D-68: an emerging cause of infection. *Expert Rev Respir Med*. 2015;9(6):711-719.
927. Racaniello VR. Picornaviridae: The viruses and their replication. In: Knipe DM, Howley PM, eds. *Fields Virology*. Vol. 1. 6th ed. Philadelphia, PA: Lippincott Williams & Wilkins; 2013:453-589.
947. Rhoden E, Zhang M, Nix WA, et al. In vitro efficacy of antiviral compounds against enterovirus D68. *Antimicrob Agents Chemother*. 2015;59(12):7779-7781.
998. Schieble JH, Fox VL, Lennette EH. A probable new human picornavirus associated with respiratory diseases. *Am J Epidemiol*. 1967;85(2):297-310.
1006. Schubert A, Bottcher S, Eis-Hubinger AM. Two cases of vaccine-derived poliovirus infection in an oncology ward. *N Engl J Med*. 2016;374(13):1296-1298.
1007. Schuffenecker I, Mirand A, Josset L, et al. Epidemiological and clinical characteristics of patients infected with enterovirus D68, France, July to December 2014. *Euro Surveill*. 2016;21(19).
1010. Schuster JE, Miller JO, Selvarangan R, et al. Severe enterovirus 68 respiratory illness in children requiring intensive care management. *J Clin Virol*. 2015;70:77-82.
1022. Sharp J, Harrison CJ, Puckett K, et al. Characteristics of young infants in whom human parechovirus, enterovirus or neither were detected in cerebrospinal fluid during sepsis evaluations. *Pediatr Infect Dis J*. 2013;32(3):213-216.
1032. Sinclair C, Gaunt E, Simmonds P, et al. Atypical hand, foot, and mouth disease associated with coxsackievirus A6 infection, Edinburgh, United Kingdom, January to February 2014. *Euro Surveill*. 2014;19(12):20745.
1037. Skowronski DM, Chambers C, Sabaiduc S, et al. Systematic community- and hospital-based surveillance for enterovirus-D68 in three Canadian provinces, August to December 2014. *Euro Surveill*. 2015;20(43).
1038. Skram MK, Skanke LH, Krokstad S, et al. Severe parechovirus infection in Norwegian infants. *Pediatr Infect Dis J*. 2014;33(12):1222-1225.
1053. Stellrecht KA, Lamson DM, Romero JR. Enteroviruses and parechoviruses. In: Jorgensen JH, Pfaller MA, Carroll KC, et al, eds. *Manual of Clinical Microbiology*. Washington, DC: ASM Press; 2015:1536-1550.
1063. Sutter RW, Kew OM, Cochi SL, et al. Poliovirus vaccine-live. In: Plotkin SA, Orenstein WA, Offit PA, eds. *Vaccines*. 6th ed. Philadelphia, PA: Saunders; 2012:598-645.
1081. Teoh HL, Mohammad SS, Britton PN, et al. Clinical characteristics and functional motor outcomes of enterovirus 71 neurological disease in children. *JAMA Neurol*. 2016;73(3):300-307.
1093. Torres JP, Farfan MJ, Izquierdo G, et al. Enterovirus D68 infection, Chile, spring 2014. *Emerg Infect Dis*. 2015;21(4):728-729.
1103. Tsou YA, Cheng YK, Chung HK, et al. Upper aerodigestive tract sequelae in severe enterovirus 71 infection: predictors and outcome. *Int J Pediatr Otorhinolaryngol*. 2008;72(1):41-47.
1109. Tyler KL. Rationale for the evaluation of fluoxetine in the treatment of enterovirus D68-associated acute flaccid myelitis. *JAMA Neurol*. 2015;72(5):493-494.
1118. Van Haren K, Ayscue P, Waubant E, et al. Acute flaccid myelitis of unknown etiology in California, 2012-2015. *JAMA*. 2015;314(24):2663-2671.
1130. Vidor E, Plotkin SA. Poliovirus vaccine-inactivated. In: Plotkin SA, Orenstein WA, Offit PA, eds. *Vaccines*. 6th ed. Philadelphia, PA: Saunders; 2012:573-597.
1170. Williams CJ, Thomas RH, Pickersgill TP, et al. Cluster of atypical adult Guillain-Barré syndrome temporally associated with neurological illness due to EV-D68 in children, South Wales, United Kingdom, October 2015 to January 2016. *Euro Surveill*. 2016;21(4).
1178. Wollersheim SK, Humphries RM, Cherry JD, et al. Serological misdiagnosis of acute liver failure associated with echovirus 25 due to immunological similarities to hepatitis A virus and prozone effect. *J Clin Microbiol*. 2015;53(1):309-310.
1199. Yip CC, Lau SK, Woo PC, et al. Recombinant coxsackievirus A2 and deaths of children, Hong Kong, 2012. *Emerg Infect Dis*. 2013;19(8):1285-1288.
1200. Yodmeeklin A, Khamrin P, Chuchaona W, et al. Saffold viruses in pediatric patients with diarrhea in Thailand. *J Med Virol*. 2015;87(4):702-707.
1214. Zhang XA, Lu QB, Wo Y, et al. Prevalence and genetic characteristics of Saffold cardiovirus in China from 2009 to 2012. *Sci Rep*. 2015;5:7704.
1215. Zhang Y, Moore DD, Nix WA, et al. Neutralization of enterovirus D68 isolated from the 2014 US outbreak by commercial intravenous immune globulin products. *J Clin Virol*. 2015;69:172-175.
1217. Zhou Y, Li JX, Jin PF, et al. Enterovirus 71: a whole virion inactivated enterovirus 71 vaccine. *Expert Rev Vaccines*. 2016;15(7):803-813.

The full reference list for this chapter is available at ExpertConsult.com.

167 Rhinoviruses

Robert L. Atmar • Janet A. Englund

Rhinoviruses (RVs) are one of the most common etiologies of infections in people, causing 25% to 30% of all acute respiratory illnesses.[104,116] RVs primarily lead to mild upper respiratory tract disease, but they also can cause bronchitis, sinusitis, and, on occasion, pneumonia in all age groups. These viruses are the most common precipitants of "infectious asthma" attacks, and they may also cause worsening of other lung diseases. Thus RVs constitute a significant health burden, particularly among children, children, hospitalized patients, and immunocompromised patients in both research and clinical practice.

HISTORY

The first recognized human RV (serotype 1A) was isolated in monkey kidney cell culture by Pelon and associates[232] in 1954 from a recruit at Great Lakes Naval Training Center in Chicago during an outbreak of afebrile common colds in his training company. Independently, Price and colleagues[243] reported the isolation of an antigenically identical virus from nurses and children with colds. In 1963, the RVs were so named because of their association with illnesses of the nasal passages.[292]

Before these actual virus isolations, evidence suggested that viruses cause the common cold. Despite indications that some coldlike illnesses could be complicated by bacterial infections,[80,304] bacteria-free nasal filtrates from persons with apparent symptomatic respiratory tract infections clearly were able to initiate these illnesses. Kruse,[184] in 1914, first demonstrated transmission with apparently sterile filtrates, and his results were confirmed in the late 1920s in a series of experiments in humans and chimpanzees by Dochez and associates.[80] In the 1930s, workers from this latter laboratory reported growth of the agent in tissue culture and embryonated eggs, but their results were not confirmed.[5] In the 1940s and 1950s, Andrewes and colleagues[6] at the Common Cold Unit in Salisbury, England, and Dingle and the members of the US Armed Forces Commission on Acute Respiratory Diseases were able to transmit colds from person to person with apparently sterile filtrates.[79] Jackson and colleagues[161] performed similar experiments in Chicago and also demonstrated immunity. In 1953, the Salisbury researchers reported isolation of an agent, DC, in serially passaged filtrates of tubed tissue cultures of human embryonic lungs; the virus was detected by its ability to produce colds in humans. Although these results could not be substantiated at the time, a virus *was* present; in 1968, the DC filtrates were found to contain RV serotype 9.[5,62]

The next major advance in growing common cold viruses took place in the late 1950s in Salisbury. Tyrrell and Parsons[293] inoculated human embryonic kidney cells with nasal filtrates and incubated the cultures under conditions simulating those of the nasal passages (e.g., 33°C, neutral pH, and in a roller drum for aeration). Six distinct types of RVs (serotypes 1B to 6) were isolated by observing cytopathic effects.[281] Shortly thereafter, Hamparian and coworkers[136,179] isolated 18 RVs (serotypes 7 to 12 and 18 to 29) by using a semicontinuous diploid cell strain obtained by Hayflick and Moorhead[144] from human fetal lung cultures. The use of Hayflick's cell lines greatly accelerated the isolation and characterization of "new" RVs, leading to the identification of 100 serotypes.[135]

The use of molecular methods for the sensitive detection of RVs, beginning in the 1990s, further revolutionized the field by enhanced detection and typing of RVs in the clinical setting.[187,197,233] In 2006, the detection of nonculturable RVs led to recognition of a wider diversity of recognized RVs associated with respiratory illness, including a new species (RV C).[10,34,187] Improvements in detection by polymerase chain reaction (PCR) and sequencing techniques have resulted in the identification of diverse new genotypes.[196,205] The application of molecular methods to viral diagnosis and improved methods of strain identification have led to a better understanding of the contribution of RVs to disease in children, hospitalized patients, and immunocompromised patients in both research and clinical practice.

ORGANISM

RVs are members of the *Enterovirus* genus in the family *Picornaviridae.*[182] Other members of the *Enterovirus* genus include polioviruses, Coxsackie viruses, and echoviruses. Like the other picornaviruses, the RVs are small (30 nm), nonenveloped (therefore resistant to lipid solvents such as ether and chloroform), and icosahedral (20-sided, hexagonal in cross section), with a genome consisting of single-stranded RNA (molecular weight, 2.5×10^6 Da) approximately 7200 nucleotides long.[182] A picornavirus can be thought of as an RNA genome surrounded by a 20-sided protein coat (the capsid) (Fig. 167.1). The RNA alone is infectious and can serve as a messenger.

RVs previously were distinguished from classical enteroviruses by being rendered noninfectious at an acidity lower than pH 5 and by their higher buoyant density in cesium chloride. RVs are subdivided based on various virus characteristics as follows: (1) into three species (RV A, RV B, and RV C) based on genomic sequence analysis; (2) into three groups based on receptor use (see later); (3) into two groups based on susceptibility to capsid-binding antiviral agents (groups 1 and 2); (4) into more than 100 serotypes, as described earlier; and (5) into more than 150 genotypes.[164,205] PCR assays or other molecular analyses are typically used to distinguish other enterovirus species from RVs.[164,196]

The genomes of the original 100 culturable serotypes and multiple nonculturable RV genotypes have been sequenced completely.[229] Classification is now based on phylogenetic analyses. Species and genotype can be assigned by analysis of the *VP1* or *VP4* genes. Within an RV species, there is no more that 12% to 13% nucleotide sequence divergence of the *VP1* gene within a genotype. The recognition of new genotypes requires the analysis of the complete *VP1* sequence.[205] With this classification system, RV genotypes are now identified by species and genotype; thus viruses belonging to the RV A species and genotype 100 are designated as A100.[115]

A virus previously classified as RV serotype 87 has greater sequence homology to the *Enterovirus D* species (EV-D68 and EV-D70) than to other RVs, leading to its reclassification into the *Enterovirus D* species.[30]

Structure of the Virion

The virion is composed of 60 copies of each of four structural proteins: VP1, VP2, VP3, and VP4. Knowledge of the structure of the RVs is based on the determination of the capsid structures in atomic detail for five types, A01, A02, A16, B03, and B14.[11,180,255,256,298,316] The thin (5-nm) protein capsid has an undulating exterior marked by 12 vertices (the icosahedral fivefold axis) equally spaced over the surface. Surrounding these vertices is a steep (2.5-nm deep), narrow canyon. VP1, VP2, and VP3 are exposed on the surface of the virion, whereas VP4 is buried within the capsid.

A pocket of unknown function whose walls are lined by 17 amino acids that vary with each RV type has been found at the base of the canyon.[7] Various organic molecules have been determined to bind in this pocket; when these molecules are bound, either the virus is prevented from uncoating (necessary to release viral RNA for its translation to viral protein) or the cell receptor is prevented from docking in the canyon.[105,236,258] Numerous drugs made by several different drug companies in the United States, Europe, and Japan have been developed to exploit the antipicornavirus potentialities of this pocket, and the sensitivity of the RVs to these drugs has been used as an additional means of classifying the RV A and RV B genotypes (into inhibitor groups 1 and 2).[8,7,115] One group

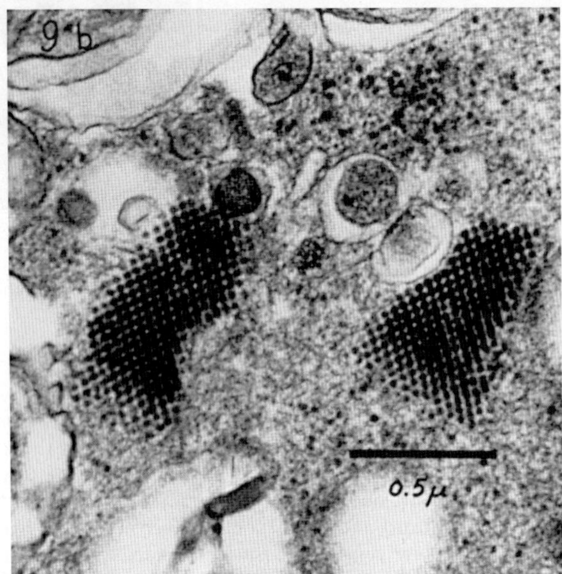

FIG. 167.1 Rhinovirus type 2 in human fetal lung cells. Note the hexagonal virus crystals closely packed in a rectangular lattice (×40,000). (From Kawana R, Matsumoto I. Electron microscopic study of rhinovirus replication in human fetal lung cells. *Jpn J Microbiol.* 1971;15:207-217.)

of these drugs, the WIN compounds synthesized by Sterling-Winthrop, has had wide scientific exposure; however, clinical trials have been discouraging.[284,286] One disadvantage of these compounds is that the various RV serotypes vary widely in sensitivity to these organic molecules.[7] Another problem has been failure to attain effective concentrations of drug at the site of infection.

Virus Life Cycle

The first step in the virus life cycle is binding to its cellular receptor. There are only two different receptor binding sites for the serotypes that belong to the RV A and B genotypes: 89 serotypes bind to intercellular adhesion molecule-1 (ICAM-1, the major receptor group), and 11 other serotypes (all from the RV A genotype) bind to members of the low-density lipoprotein receptor family (LDL-R, the minor receptor group).[1,115,122] The receptor(s) of RV C viruses have not been identified but are distinct from the two currently recognized receptors for RV A and RV B strains.[32]

ICAM-1 binds to the base of the canyon of RVs in the major receptor group.[257,295] Virus-neutralizing antibody prevents virus attachment to cells by adhering to serospecific sites and blocking the cell receptor from access to its binding site at the canyon base. These antibody sites may directly overlap ICAM-1–binding sites, or they may be separate from the ICAM-1–binding sites but at a point sufficiently close to allow the binding site to be blocked by steric hindrance.[50] Binding of the major receptor group RVs to ICAM-1 leads to destabilization of the virus capsid and uncoating of the viral RNA.[123] Some major group receptor viruses are also able to use heparan sulfate proteoglycans as an alternative receptor, either directly or following adaptation.[108]

The LDL-R family binds to a different site for the minor receptor group of RVs than that recognized by ICAM-1. The binding site for these RVs is the small, star-shaped dome above the canyon on the icosahedral fivefold axis. Multiple receptors are rapidly and sequentially bound.[251] Attachment of minor receptor group viruses to LDL-R does not lead to virus uncoating, in contrast to what is seen with binding of major receptor group RVs to ICAM-1. Instead, internalization into acidic endosomal compartments is required for uncoating of minor receptor group RVs.[150]

Replication of the RVs is similar to that of the enteroviruses.[249] After attachment to the cellular receptor and endocytosis of the virus, RNA is released into the cytoplasm. Genomic viral RNA functions as messenger RNA and attaches to ribosomes, which stimulates its translation by host enzymes into a single long polyprotein. This polyprotein is cleaved by viral proteases to yield viral RNA polymerase, capsid proteins, proteases, and proteins to halt the synthesis of host proteins and other products. Under laboratory conditions, infectious virus first is formed after approximately 2 hours and reaches a maximum of approximately 1000 infectious particles per cell at approximately 7 hours. Infectious virus, however, comprises a minority of the viruslike particles formed; only approximately one in 200 is a complete virus capable of replicating in cell culture. All viral replication occurs in the cytoplasm, and viruses are released by cell lysis in a process involving apoptosis.[71,249]

Host Range

Animals

RVs have been isolated from natural infections in only chimpanzees and humans. Chimpanzee infections are subclinical. A natural, subclinical outbreak of RV-31 in chimpanzees was reported in a primate center.[74,73]

Many attempts have been made to infect a wide variety of animals with RVs. In addition to the chimpanzee, the gibbon has been susceptible, although not reliably so.[74] Mice do not naturally express ICAM-1, the major receptor, and are not infected by these viruses. The block can be overcome by engineering mouse cells to express ICAM-1, a finding that led to the development of a transgenic mouse model for RV infection.[26,27,139] Mice also can be infected by RVs that express the minor receptor.[27,314] Mutations in viral nonstructural proteins can improve the replication efficiency of mouse-adapted RVs in both major and minor receptor groups.[139,314] Equine and bovine "rhinoviruses" have been described, but these viruses belong to different picornavirus genera.

Cell and Tissue Cultures

The spectrum of tissue culture cells infected by RVs also is narrow.[64,188] For initial isolation, human embryonic diploid cells generally are used for isolation of RV A and B strains (Fig. 167.2), although for some RV types, an especially sensitive strain[61] of a continuous cell line, HeLa, serves as well or better.[64,188] RV C strains are not cultivable in traditional cell lines. However, these viruses can be propagated in primary respiratory epithelium cultures and in three-dimensional human airway cultures.[138,279]

Antigenic Properties

A prominent characteristic of RV is its great antigenic diversity; more than 100 cultivable serotypes exist.[135] Genetic analyses suggest that close to 50 additional serotypes may exist among RV C strains.[206,267] The number of additional serotypes of cultivable strains may be limited.[104,135,218] There are conserved domains in the capsid to which cross-reactive cellular responses and heterosubtypic neutralizing antibody responses can be generated; these have been proposed as a potential target for future vaccine development efforts.[120] Certain serotypes cross-react, but there is little evidence to indicate that this cross-reaction can be exploited for vaccination.[63,102,215]

RVs often are poor antigens based on the immune responses observed after infection. Significant (fourfold or greater) increases in serum antibody may not develop in as many as 50% of patients from whom RVs are isolated, and the levels attained often are low.[102-104]

RVs may be undergoing continuous antigenic change.[215] Genetic analysis of the capsid genes of RV C strains found high substitution rates.[185] Another mechanism that may lead to the emergence of new strains is recombination. The sequencing of complete viral genomes has identified a number of probable recombination events between different virus serotypes, especially among RV A and C strains.[300] The recombinants then diverged further from the parental strains and became new serotypes.[229] Antigenic variation within serotypes RV-22 and RV-51 has been substantial enough to interfere with their typing.[262,275]

EPIDEMIOLOGY

RVs cause infection with a worldwide distribution, and large epidemiologic studies have consistently identified RVs as the most common cause of viral respiratory disease. For example, two population-based studies in Roehampton, England[154] and Tecumseh, Michigan[219] found RVs more frequently than other respiratory viruses, with RVs causing 26.3% and 38.1%, respectively, of all respiratory illnesses. More recent studies of acute respiratory illness in children also identified RVs most commonly.[39,202] Infection is more common in children than in adults. The annual incidence in children is approximately one infection per

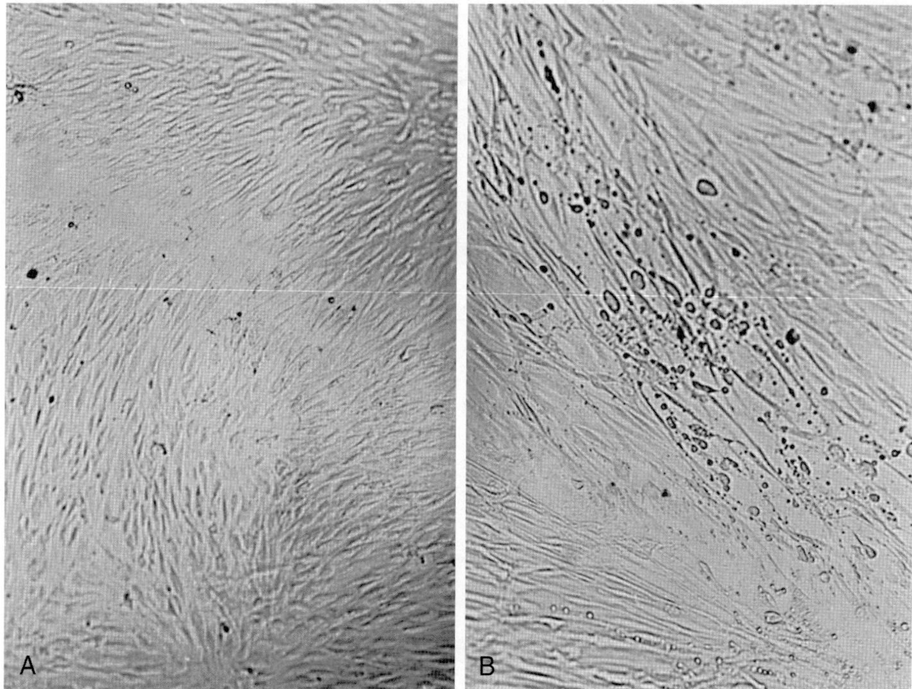

FIG. 167.2 Rhinovirus type 16 infection. (A) Normal human diploid (fetal tonsil) cell sheet. (B) Cell sheet infected for 2 days with rhinovirus type 16. The rounded and misshapen cells are characteristic. (Courtesy Dr. David M. Warshauer, University of Wisconsin, Madison, WI.)

year, although one study reported an incidence as high as six infections per year.[310]

Seasonal Distribution

RV causes infections year round, although there are seasonal peaks of occurrence.[217] During the usual September through May "cold season," RV infections often are predominant at both ends, early fall and middle to late spring (Fig. 167.3). They also are important causes of summer colds. In the Southern Hemisphere, a similar seasonal pattern occurs, but during opposing months.[170]

Cycling and Circulation of Individual Rhinovirus Types

Several RV serotypes usually circulate simultaneously within a community,[137] frequently coincident with other respiratory viruses.[72,154,219] For example, in a study of 24 neighboring families in Madison, Wisconsin (Eagle Heights Village), 14 different RV types, in addition to several nontypeable RVs, were found during the two academic years 1963 to 1965. Only a single type (RV-15) was found both years. The other common respiratory viruses also were present. In virus surveillance studies performed in families in Seattle and Tecumseh, a few "common" serotypes were found to be more prevalent in a given respiratory season and to be identified in subsequent respiratory seasons.[104,218] However, most individual RV types do not repeat within a population from year to year.

Although several RV types usually circulate concurrently, all types present are not equal in prevalence. In a Chicago nursery school study,[28] 14 different serotypes were isolated during the academic year 1962 to 1963, but 10 of the serotypes did not spread at all. Only 3 types disseminated widely, and they infected more than 40% of the children. Similarly, in the 1963 to 1965 Eagle Heights Village study, 14 RV types were isolated, but only 3 types (RV-43, RV-51, and RV-55) were "spreaders." Similar patterns of serologic prevalence were reported from laboratories in Tecumseh,[219] New York City, Seattle,[103,104] and Charlottesville, Virginia.[148]

Predominating Rhinovirus Types

Although the pattern of predominating RV types within a circumscribed population and a defined time frame seem to be well established, a predominance of serotypes over large geographic areas or over many years does not seem to occur. This phenomenon was studied exhaustively in widely separated locations and over many years: the Gulf South from 1962 to 1970, Tecumseh from 1966 to 1971 and from 1976 to 1981, and Seattle from 1965 to 1969 and from 1975 to 1979.[103,104,215,218,220] Although "common types" (usually the isolation of at least five to eight strains of a serotype during the period studied) occurred during each period and at each place, different types were "common" findings in different places and times. For example, Monto and colleagues,[218,220] during two 6-year study periods in Tecumseh, obtained 475 RV isolates covering 70 serotypes (of a possible 89 at that time), but only RV-1B, RV-10, RV-28, and RV-58 were isolated in both periods. However, these viruses were not particularly common because only 16, 22, 15, and 18 isolates, respectively, of these four types were found during the 12 years. In the neighboring state of Wisconsin from 1963 to 1965,[72] the common types were RV-43, RV-51, and RV-55, which were completely different from those in Michigan. Finally, the late John Fox sifted data from family populations surveyed by him and others in New York City, Seattle, and Tecumseh.[103,104] He found only 4 common serotypes (RV-1B, RV-12, RV-15, and RV-38) from among 802 isolates. Dominant RV serotypes often appear to occur locally over relatively short periods but do not extend for decades or over the nation, at least in the United States.

More recent studies using molecular assays indicate that the number of circulating strains in a given geographic area is even greater than previously appreciated using only cell culture methods. Investigators in the Netherlands identified 27 different genotypes of RV infection among a cohort of 18 healthy children 7 years of age and younger sampled at least every 2 weeks over a 6-month period.[297] Mackay and colleagues[197] identified 74 distinct RV genotypes from all 3 RV species circulating over a 1-year period in 234 children in Melbourne, Australia. Thus the diversity of RVs present in a community is greater than previously recognized.

Median Human Infectious Dose for Rhinovirus

As documented in RV challenge experiments with laboratory-grown virus administered by nose drops or aerosol, less than one median tissue culture infective dose ($TCID_{50}$) can initiate infection.[68,82] Much more (2000 times) is required when placed on the tongue or dried just outside the anterior nares (10,000 times).[68] How accurately these conditions approach the natural state is not known.

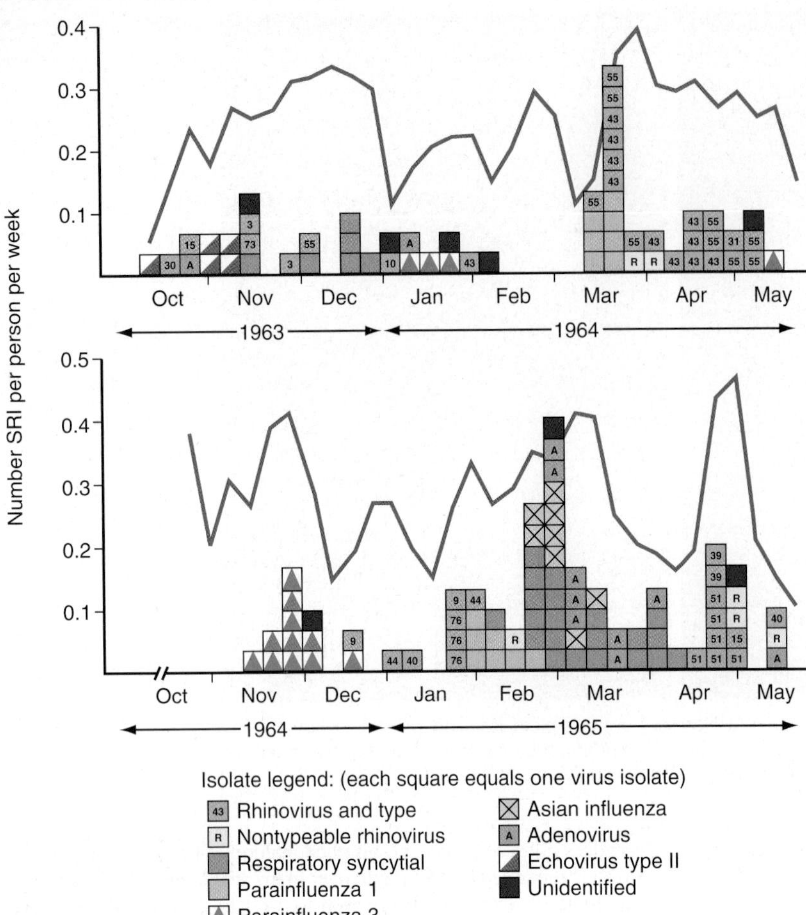

FIG. 167.3 Rhinoviruses and other respiratory viruses associated with symptomatic respiratory infection (SRI). This study included three neighboring apartment buildings in Eagle Heights, a University of Wisconsin housing village in Madison, Wisconsin (24–26 families, ≈100 persons), from 1963 to 1965.

PERSON-TO-PERSON TRANSMISSION

Epidemiologic Observations

Individual RV serotypes often disseminate with surprising difficulty, as noted in studies of Eagle Heights Village,[72] a Madison, Wisconsin, elementary school, and a Chicago nursery school.[28] At least within family populations, the most common finding was that a specific RV serotype did not spread from the index case. Hendley and associates,[148] in a study of 19 families in Charlottesville, found that RVs from 10 of 22 index cases did not spread at all, and dissemination to at least one other person occurred in only seven families. In only four of the 19 families did further sequential spread occur. Fox and associates,[103,104] in a surveillance of more than 200 Seattle families, found intrafamily secondary attack rates in susceptible individuals (no homotypic antibody) to be 44% from 1965 to 1969 and 28% from 1975 to 1979. In both periods, children younger than 5 years had the highest secondary attack rates of 60% and 30%, respectively. Monto and Johnson[216,221] reported similar findings in 48 Panamanian families: with five RV isolates used as antigens, the secondary attack rate varied from 10.5% to 56%.

In Madison, interfamily and intrafamily dissemination of the 3 "spreading" RV types, RV-43, RV-51, and RV-55, was examined in the 24 to 26 neighboring families living in fourplex apartments in Eagle Heights Village (Fig. 167.4).[72] These 3 serotypes were the only ones of 14 to spread beyond the index family. RV-51 attacked 23% of susceptible individuals, and many close contacts remained uninfected. RV-43 infected 34% of susceptible individuals; in one building, only the families in a single-end fourplex became infected. Conversely, RV-55 caused a mini-epidemic in two buildings. RV dissemination seemed to focus on the fourplex, probably because in the winter months the children played in the hallways and stairs connecting the apartments. Nonetheless, even the spreading RVs left many susceptible individuals in untouched families.

Determination of the reason for such erratic spreading patterns can be sought in well-controlled chain-of-infection experiments with human volunteers. RV transmission experiments from several laboratories are described next.

Person-to-Person Transmission to Human Volunteers

Early Experiments With Rhinovirus Colds

Early experiments with different RV serotypes showed that person-to-person transmission occurred infrequently. Couch and colleagues[67] attained no transmission after housing 15 donors (persons infected intranasally with laboratory-grown RV-15) with 12 antibody-negative recipients for 26 days. At approximately the same time, the Madison laboratory performed transmission trials with RV-55 and RV-16 in a series of experiments ranging in duration from a 1- to 1.5-minute kiss to a 3-day weekend in a dormitory room. In 26 donors and 33 recipients, only two transmissions occurred, one from a 1.5-minute kiss and the other from a weekend in a dormitory.[68] Only when young married student couples were used was a substantial rate attained; nine of 24 spouses infected their mates, for a transmission rate of 38%.[69]

Characteristics of a "Good" Rhinovirus Transmitter

In the experiments with married couples, "successful" donors shed enough virus to contaminate their environment, exhibited signs and symptoms of a moderate to severe cold, and spent many hours at home with their spouses.[69] As an example of the effect of high virus shedding, intracouple transmission rates were 71% for donors with nasopharyngeal RV titers of 5000 to more than 80,000 $TCID_{50}$, 33% for those with 1000 to 5000 $TCID_{50}$, and only 18% for those with less than 1000 $TCID_{50}$ ($P = .025$). Illustrative of both shedding and production of sufficient nasal secretions was contamination of the hands with RV: donors whose hands were assayed for virus and who transmitted infections to their spouses all had RV on their hands, whereas none of the nontransmitters did ($P = .03$). The amount of time spent together seemed important in transmission, although many infected spouses who spent hours of direct contact with their partners did not transmit the infection.

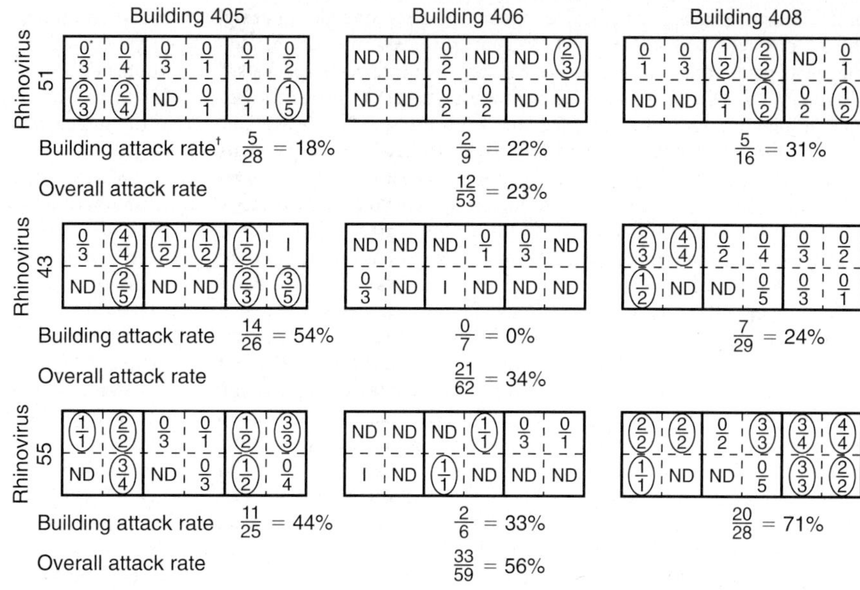

FIG. 167.4 Attack rates of three "spreading" rhinoviruses in three neighboring Eagle Heights apartment buildings in Madison, Wisconsin. *I*, all members immune; *ND*, not done; *O*, family with one or more infected members.

*No. diagnosed cases/no. susceptibles (no detectable antibody)
†As diagnosed by either virus isolation and/or a fourfold or greater serologic response

Some Early Conclusions

The preceding epidemiologic human volunteer studies suggest that attending a concert with persons who have even obvious signs of colds is unlikely to result in infection. Conversely, students who spend day after day in classrooms may have a higher chance of acquiring infection. In addition, a relatively short stay (a few hours) among friends or relatives with RV-caused colds is not likely to cause infection, even with brief embracing.

Route-of-Transmission Experiments

Because RVs often seem to spread with relative difficulty under many normal circumstances, the route of transmission becomes important because controlling respiratory virus transmission in habitats such as schoolrooms and families may be feasible by blocking transmission routes. Since the early 1970s, human volunteer experimental infection models have been used to explore RV transmission routes. These studies were performed primarily at the University of Virginia, England's Common Cold Unit, and the University of Wisconsin.

Gwaltney and Hendley[129] at the University of Virginia focused on the dissemination of RV colds by direct or indirect hand contact. Interest in this approach had been provoked by the inadvertent transmission of RVs from infected to noninfected persons through the vehicle of an ethanol-sterilized nasal speculum. Subsequently, the plausibility of direct hand transmission of RVs was supported by the observation that nose picking and eye rubbing were common among Department of Medicine Grand Rounds participants and Sunday school attendees,[149] following previous documentation of infection through conjunctival swabs.[40] These investigators then showed that RV-39 retained infectivity for several hours on various surfaces and could be found on the hands of persons infected with RV-39. In another study, infectious RV was isolated from the fingertips of 22% of persons who touched objects that had been contaminated with nasal mucus of adults with natural colds one hour earlier.[311] These experiments suggest that transmission of RV could occur through self-inoculation by environmentally contaminated hands and demonstrated RV-39 self-inoculation from an environmental source in human volunteers.[149]

The University of Virginia team in Charlottesville subsequently conducted a series of three experiments that identified direct inoculation as a route of RV transmission.[131] In two of the experiments, groups of recipients were exposed to aerosols generated by donors infected with an untypeable RV strain, HH, and the exposures occurred in separate closed rooms for large-particle (12 recipients) or small-particle (10 recipients) aerosols produced by donors during periods of 45 minutes (large particles) or 3 days (small particles). One of the large-particle aerosol recipients was infected, whereas no one exposed to small-particle aerosols was. These essentially negative transmission rates by aerosol exposure were not surprising.[129] Previously, Couch[65] had been unsuccessful in transmitting infection through the airborne route over a period of 26 days, and the Madison laboratory attained only a single RV transmission among 11 recipients after 3 days' exposure in a dormitory.[68] The third group of Charlottesville recipients was exposed to RV by inoculating themselves with the donor's nasal mucus. The donors blew their noses into their hands. The recipients then stroked the donors' contaminated hands for 10 seconds and then inoculated themselves by deliberately placing their fingers, two or three times, on their nasal and conjunctival mucosa on 3 successive days. Eleven of the 15 hand-contact recipients (73%) were infected with the donors' RV. The authors concluded that transmission by the hand-contact/self-inoculation route was much more efficient than the aerosol route and "may be an important natural route of RV transmission."[131]

One deficiency of this experiment was that donors and recipients shared the same air space over a measured, often brief, period during which fresh nasal mucus was transferred from the donor to the recipient. Nonetheless, Gwaltney did achieve a high rate of RV transmission with nasal secretions, something that had not been accomplished readily in more "natural" experiments.[68] Also in support of hand transmission was the observation in the aforementioned married-couple experiments that the ability to transmit RV was correlated significantly with the presence of the virus on the donors' hands.[69] As a result of this evidence, hand-to-hand or fomite transmission became the accepted route for RV contagion.[44,65] In later experiments, the Charlottesville group demonstrated approximately 50% transmission through fomites by using the same hand-contact/self-inoculation method with either a coffee-cup handle or a plastic tile interposed between donors' and recipients' hands.[130]

At England's Common Cold Unit, Reed[252] investigated the likelihood of natural hand-contact transmission among residents (roommates) of several housing units, 38 of whom had been infected with RV-2. Reed[252] found that 16 of the donors had RV on their fingers, but none of the virus was transmitted to the fingers of their 18 roommates, even though virus could be recovered from some (6 of 40) objects recently handled by RV-2–infected donors. Reed also found that none of 29 virus transfers from virus dried on the fingers could pass through a fomite to a recipient; the conclusion was that "spread of colds is unlikely to occur via objects contaminated by the hands of the virus shedder...."

Laboratory workers at the University of Wisconsin continued their attempts to devise a natural transmission model. Although the results of the transmission experiment with married couples were illuminating, the system itself had one great deficiency as an experimental model: the participants could not be observed during their interaction periods.[69] Ultimately, the scheme for such a system was suggested by two virologic-epidemiologic events in Antarctica, one from the summer seasons of 1975 to 1980 in which Dick and associates studied respiratory virus dissemination in an isolated Antarctic population, and the other from a human volunteer experiment conducted in an Antarctic field party by England's Common Cold Unit.[303] Both experiences suggested that high natural transmission rates after just a few days of exposure could be achieved only in an environment with a high donor-to-recipient ratio and population density. Accordingly, a model was devised in which donors (with the qualities of a "good" transmitter as described earlier) and recipients interacted during waking hours by playing cards and board and video games and engaging in communal studying. During the night, donors and recipients bunked together in the same or an adjoining room. With such an arrangement, graduate student monitors recorded activities and all clinical signs 24 hours a day. With eight donors and 12 to 16 recipients, a 50% recipient attack rate usually was attained over a 12-hour period and a 100% rate over the course of a week.[78,209] Informally, this model, a fully observed monotypic RV mini-epidemic, was named "Antarctic Hut," from its origins.[147]

Route-of-Transmission "Blocking" Experiments

With the use of the Antarctic Hut model, a series of four RV-16 route-of-transmission blocking experiments was conducted to determine whether the virus was spread by hand contact, aerosol, or both.[78] The first three experiments lasted 12 hours, with eight donors and 12 recipients; the donor-recipient interaction was through playing variants of stud and draw poker. This interaction mode facilitated both aerosol and fomite/hand-contact transmission. Half the recipients were blocked completely from any hand contact/self-inoculation by wearing arm restraints. Little transmission resulted from hand or fomite contact because the RV-16 infection rate in the restrained recipients was only slightly lower than in the unrestrained recipients, 56% versus 67%, an insignificant reduction ($P = .494$).

The fourth experiment, involving aerosol blocking, was begun immediately after the third. The poker game continued in the original room with eight donors alone, and all the equipment from the third experiment, including the cards (which literally were gummy from the previous 12-hour game), poker chips, pencils, and so forth, was moved to an identical room across the hall. The continuing eight-donor poker game in the room used for the third experiment was refurnished with poker implements. Subsequently, 12 new recipients entered the second room, began playing poker with the now heavily used cards and other paraphernalia, and made exaggerated hand-to-nose self-inoculation movements. Aerosol transmission was blocked effectively by the two brick walls between the rooms. Once each hour, the cards, poker chips, and other portables were exchanged between the donor and recipient rooms to maintain a freshly contaminated supply of fomites in the recipient room. The result was extremely surprising; not one of the 12 "fomite recipients" caught RV-16. Judging from the results of these Antarctic Hut experiments in which fomite/hand-contact and aerosol transmission were blocked alternately, aerosol transmission seemed the predominant route, at least for RV-16 among student poker players at the University of Wisconsin. A few months after the 1987 publication of these results, an editorial appeared in *The Lancet* titled "Splints Don't Stop Colds: Surprising!"[78,272] It concluded that "…it looks as though coughs and sneezes *do* spread these diseases more than sticky fingers."

Subsequently, a set of experiments was conducted to determine how RV-16 had disappeared along the five-step fomite transmission chain from nose to hand to fomite to hand to nose.[169] The same results that Reed[252] had observed previously were again noted. The virus seemed to disappear precipitously at each step in the chain; 10^6 $TCID_{50}$ of RV-16 in the donor's nose was reduced to 0 to 64 $TCID_{50}$ on the card-playing implements, and then the virus nearly disappeared on reaching the recipients' hands.

Additional studies examined other methods to interrupt transmission. The University of Virginia team performed a blocking experiment in the field in which mothers attempted to prevent hand contact/self-inoculation by dipping their fingers in iodine. The results of this 1979 to 1982 study were reported as part of a general review.[147] The illness rate during the 4 years was 40% lower in the mothers with iodinated fingers than in the placebo mothers ($P = .047$). However, the authors noted the difficulty of conducting and interpreting these investigations.[147] In another set of experimental human infection studies, the application of organic acids present in hand cleansers (e.g., salicylic acid, pyroglutamic acid) to the hands of volunteers decreased the likelihood of RV infection when volunteers subsequently touched their nasal or conjunctival mucosa 10 minutes after RV had been placed on their hands.[287]

The Madison group also examined transmission interruption methods to prevent spread from person to person. As part of an investigation of the epidemiology of respiratory viruses in an isolated (≈200 persons) Antarctic population at McMurdo Station in 1979, use of an iodinated facial tissue was successful in interrupting transmission.[75] Three days after all personnel began copious use of these tissues, the incidence of respiratory illness dropped rapidly and significantly ($P < .01$); in fact, respiratory illness nearly disappeared from the base.[77] Although this effect was striking, the trial could be controlled only historically. However, the apparent success was sufficient to interest the Kimberly-Clark Corporation in applying virucidal facial tissue technology to interrupt RV-16 transmission in the Antarctic Hut model. The Kimberly-Clark Corporation soon made available a nontoxic, highly virucidal facial tissue. The tissues completely stopped transmission of RV-16, in comparison to transmission rates of 42% and 75% in control recipients using ordinary cotton handkerchiefs ($P < .001$) (Table 167.1).[76] The corporation test-marketed these tissues under the brand name "Avert," but their sales were lower than expected. Subsequently, two field trials of Avert in families reduced viral transmission of 5% to 39%, respectively.[96,193] These results were disappointing but not unexpected. Changing established habits of personal nasal sanitation was not easy in the highly supervised, well-motivated adults in Antarctica; it may be impossible in unsupervised children.

Despite all the experimental studies to identify the principal route of virus transmission, no single route appears to be predominant. What is clear from these studies is that RV illnesses may be transmitted by both the hand-contact and aerosol routes.

TABLE 167.1 Apparent Complete Interruption by Virucidal Tissues of Rhinovirus Type 16 Transmission[a]

Study Group	Cotton Handkerchiefs Experiment A	Virucidal Tissues Experiment B	Virucidal Tissues Experiment C	Cotton Handkerchiefs Experiment D
Recipients who "caught" RV-16 colds/total (%)[b]	5/12 (42)	0/12	0/12	9/12 (75)

[a]In each of four experiments, eight volunteers with RV-16 colds played poker for 12 hours with 12 other volunteers (without RV-16 antibody) and for nasal sanitation used either ordinary cotton handkerchiefs (experiments A and D) or virucidal tissues (experiments B and C). Three-ply Kleenex tissues were treated, per 100 g, with 9.1 g citric acid, 4.5 g malic acid, and 1.8 g sodium lauryl sulfate. Cotton or paper handkerchiefs were used to clear nasal passages, to smother coughs and sneezes, and to wipe surfaces. Virucidal tissues were used carefully and copiously.

[b]Diagnosed by at least one isolation of RV-16 or a fourfold rise in antibody to RV-16 in the convalescent serum sample, or both.

RV-16, Rhinovirus type 16.

Modified from Dick EC, Hossain SU, Mink KA, et al. Interruption of transmission of rhinovirus colds among human volunteers using virucidal handkerchiefs. *J Infect Dis.* 1986;153:352-356.

PATHOGENESIS AND HOST FACTORS

General Course of Infection

Infection usually occurs through the respiratory route, although infection by the conjunctival route has been demonstrated.[40,149] When the virus is given intranasally by pipette, only one $TCID_{50}$ is needed to initiate infection.[68,82] The incubation period for a cold normally is 2 to 3 days, but a period of up to 7 days has been reported.[83,148] Ciliary dysfunction can predispose to respiratory tract infection.[31,43] RVs replicate well in both the upper and lower respiratory tracts.

RVs may be shed in large amounts (1000 to 1 million infectious particles per milliliter of nasal washing) during the first 2 to 3 days of a cold and may be produced for 2 to 3 weeks thereafter.[78,82,83,209] However, the effect on cells of the nasopharyngeal cavity seems benign despite much local reaction to the virus, which results in the usual signs and symptoms of a cold. Systematic studies of RV-inoculated human volunteers at the University of Virginia demonstrated that damage to the respiratory epithelium was slight, although a few sloughed ciliated epithelial cells did contain RV antigen.[288,307] RV was recovered only at focal sites in the nose and nasopharynx at the time of maximal symptoms, and in situ hybridization studies demonstrated evidence of RV infection in only a minority of epithelial cells.[16,24,309] Using primary monolayer cultures of ciliated and nonciliated epithelial cells, Winther and associates[308] demonstrated that RV, coronavirus, influenza A virus, and adenovirus all grew well in these cell cultures; however, RV and coronavirus produced no discernible cytopathic effect compared with the widespread destruction of the cell monolayer by influenza virus and adenovirus by 96 hours.

Innate Immune Response

Innate immunity is the initial host response to infection with RVs. Toll-like receptor 3 (TLR3) is activated during virus replication, is upregulated during RV infection, and is associated with decreased viral replication.[151] Signaling occurs through both retinoic acid inducible gene I (RIG-I) and melanoma differentiation associate gene 5 (MDA-5), and inhibition of these molecules leads to increased viral replication.[269] One mechanism of inhibition of intracellular signaling developed by the virus is cleavage of the signaling molecules (e.g., RIG-I, interferon-β [IFN-β] promoter stimulator 1 [IPS-1]) by the viral protease.[25,89] Toll-like receptor activation leads to the production of type 1 IFNs, which is likely the mechanism by which viral replication is inhibited. Impaired induction of IFN-β leads to increased viral replication and is a defect that has been identified in the respiratory epithelium of asthmatic patients.[231,302] Numerous other components of innate immunity are also induced by RV infection, including β-defensins, nitric oxide, and a variety of proinflammatory cytokines and chemokines (e.g., interleukin [IL]-1, IL-6, IL-8, RANTES [regulated on activation, normal T cell expressed and secreted]).[247,250]

Because RVs seem to cause only mild pathologic changes in cells of the respiratory tract, attention has focused on various immunologic or inflammatory substances as possible causes of symptomatic illness.[283] Researchers have long known that peripheral blood neutrophils increase in the first 2 to 3 days of illness in RV-infected volunteers.[45,283] Phagocytes (neutrophils and monocytes) also have been demonstrated in large numbers in the nasal secretions of RV-infected symptomatic human volunteers.[192] Although the microbe-killing ability of phagocytes is well known, these cells in themselves also can cause cold symptoms through the release of various toxic products, such as superoxide and hydrogen peroxide, during the respiratory burst.[280] In fact, increasing numbers of leukocytes in the peripheral blood correlate with increased symptoms and in infected human volunteers who are not ill the white blood cell count does not increase.[283] An association has been noted between the nasal levels of two proinflammatory mediators involved in granulocyte regulation, granulocyte colony-stimulating factor, and IL-8, and blood and nasal neutrophilia have been identified.[117,228] Nasal IL-8 levels also correlate with the severity of clinical symptoms.[124,290]

Increased nasal levels of other inflammatory mediators (e.g., IL-1β, IL-6, RANTES, kinins) have been associated with more severe clinical symptoms.[224,228,244,245,318] Furthermore, topical nasal administration of IL-6 or bradykinin leads to development of some of the symptoms of the common cold.[110,246] At least some of these inflammatory responses appear to depend on an activation pathway regulated by nuclear factor κB (NF-κB).[317,318] There may also be differential levels of cytokine induction by different RV species, with RV B strains inducing lower levels of chemokines and cytokines than RV A and RV C strains.[225] Resolution of clinical symptoms may be caused by the elaboration of inhibitors of inflammation, such as IL-1 receptor antagonist.[315] Transcriptome analysis of children with symptomatic RV infection has also shown upregulation of innate immune response genes, although there is little change in the expression of these genes in children with asymptomatic infection.[145] These inflammatory mediators may serve as a target for the development of drugs to relieve the symptoms of RV infection, although the use of a specific kinin inhibitor did not lead to clinical improvement.[127,153]

Immunity Associated With Serum Antibody

Serum antibody to the various RV types develops with age (presumably from repeated infections); and by adulthood, antibody may be detected against approximately 50% of RV types tested.[128] The presence of serum antibody correlates positively with immunity, and resistance to infection and the degree of disease expression are related to the amount of antibody present.[3,2,38] As examples, in the Eagle Heights Village families, 21 of 75 persons (28%) without antibody were infected with either RV-43 or RV-55, whereas only five of 35 (14%) with homologous antibody to either of these agents were infected.[72] No one was infected who had homologous serum antibody levels above 1:16. Similar results were observed in the Charlottesville and Seattle families.[103,104,148] However, large doses can overwhelm antibody. At the clinical center of the National Institute of Allergy and Infectious Diseases, where human volunteers were used, 1000 $TCID_{50}$ was found to infect persons with serum antibody titers up to 1:256.[46] Judging from the paucity of reports of natural infections in persons with serum antibody titers greater than 1:16, virus inocula in naturally contracted cases must be low.

Immunity Associated With Antibody in Nasal Secretions

Researchers at the National Institutes of Health found that the presence of antibody in nasal secretion is associated with protection from homologous RV infection and disease.[47] They found that intranasal administration of inactivated RV vaccine produced both serum and nasal antibody, whereas two intramuscular injections of this vaccine produced little, if any, nasal antibody.[235] When the volunteers given the vaccine intranasally were challenged with approximately 100 $TCID_{50}$ of homologous RV, they were protected significantly against both clinical illness and infection, whereas those administered the same vaccine intramuscularly remained susceptible.[235]

Conversely, when the same vaccine preparation was administered subcutaneously in three injections, nasal antibody responses were observed in 21 of 46 (45%) volunteers.[84,79] Challenge of these volunteers with 3 $TCID_{50}$ of virus produced significantly less virus shedding and reduced duration and severity of illness than were observed in unimmunized controls who had no RV-specific antibody. Possibly, this lower infectious dose more closely approximates a natural situation. This study also showed that protection against infection with the low virus challenge correlated with the magnitude of serum antibody and not with the presence of secretory antibody. The relative roles of serum and secretory antibody in RV infections are still unsettled.

Antibody Appearance Over the Course of Infection

There is a general pattern of the development of humoral (secretory and serum) antibody based on human studies.[38,86] Approximately 24 hours after infection, a sharp increase in nasal immunoglobulin (IgA) secretion occurs. At the time symptoms appear (approximately 48 hours after infection), rhinorrhea begins, and the transudate is composed of significant amounts of IgG. After approximately 1 week and after the actual episode of illness, virus-specific antibody, predominantly IgA, appears in the nasal passages, tears, and the parotid saliva. Serum antibody (usually IgG but occasionally IgM) also begins to be formed at 1 week and rises to peak levels at 1 month. Both serum and secretory antibodies appear sooner and rise more rapidly in persons with detectable neutralizing antibody in their preinfection serum specimens. Antibody has been detected in nasal secretions and serum approximately 1 year after infection and, judging from the high proportion of the adult population with antibody to many RV serotypes, probably lasts much longer.[36,128]

Cell-Mediated Immunity

Substantial evidence indicates that neutrophils increase both in the peripheral blood and in the nasopharynx during the first few days of an RV cold.[45,306] Peripheral blood lymphocytes actually decrease in the first 2 to 3 days of an RV cold, and migration of lymphocytes into the nasal secretions increases at this time.[45,192] Specific humoral antibody usually is not present in the serum or nasopharynx this early in the illness, a finding suggesting that these in situ nasopharyngeal lymphocytes, through cell-mediated immunity, play an important role in controlling RV proliferation. RV infection of primary epithelial cells cultured in vitro leads to increased expression of the T-cell attractant molecule CXCL10; and activated T cells cocultured with the epithelial cells produce IFN-γ and tumor necrosis factor (TNF) and activate the nitric oxide pathway, which can help inhibit viral replication.[172] Hsia and colleagues[156] examined the ability of peripheral blood lymphocytes to liberate various cytokines (IL-2 and IFN-γ) and participate in other cellular immune processes (cytotoxicity and antigen-stimulated blastogenesis) during the early days of RV colds in experimentally infected human volunteers. These investigators found that all these cell-mediated immunity activities during infection were increased significantly when compared with preinfection levels. Of special interest, the cellular ability to liberate higher levels of IL-2 correlated inversely and significantly ($P < .02$) with virus shedding and nasal mucus production. Cross-reactive T-cell epitopes are shared by RVs, and T cells isolated from peripheral blood and from tonsillar tissue proliferate and secrete a variety of cytokines (IFN-γ, IL-2, IL-4, IL-5, IL-13) after exposure to RV antigens.[113,140,273,305] Thus activation of T cells may contribute not only to virus clearance but also to airway inflammation.[113]

Interference Among Rhinoviruses

Interference in infection with heterotypic RV serotypes, which lasts between 5 and 16 weeks, has been reported in human volunteers.[97] Complete resistance to infection was observed after inoculation with as much as 2000 $TCID_{50}$ of RV-16 (administered by nasopharyngeal spray) in a subject with an unsuspected "wild" RV (not typed) infection present at the time of inoculation.[190] However, epidemiologic studies in a nursery school population,[28] a military population,[254] and a family population[214] showed sequential heterotypic RV infections occurring frequently, sometimes at intervals as short as 2 days. In the family population, one subject was infected by three different RVs within a 30-day period. The factor or factors responsible for the interference observed in the experimental human infection model have not been identified. Simultaneous infection with an RV and other respiratory viruses, including influenza A and B viruses, coronaviruses, parainfluenza type 1 virus, respiratory syncytial virus (RSV), adenoviruses, various enteroviruses, or other RV serotypes, also has been commonly reported, particularly in children.[90,104,202] However, coinfection with some other respiratory viruses (e.g., RSV) is less frequent than expected using molecular diagnostic assays, suggesting that these viruses may specifically suppress coinfection with each other.[175,202]

Influence of a Cold Environment on the Course of Infection

Exposure to cold temperatures has been thought either to initiate or to exacerbate respiratory tract infections. In fact, chilling animals was shown to increase the severity and frequency of viral infection.[299] However, investigation of the effects of chilling on humans infected with "common cold viruses" and with RV-15 did not demonstrate significant effects.[85] In the RV-15 experiments, the conditions were realistic. The subjects (men) were cooled sufficiently in air to cause shivering for approximately an hour or were immersed in water long enough to cause a decline in rectal temperature.

Effect of Age and Sex

A much higher prevalence of RV infection is found in infants and young children than in older persons. In Seattle,[103] the RV infection rate in children from birth to 5 years of age was nearly twice that of older children and adults (0.77 vs. 0.41 infections per person per year, respectively); in Tecumseh,[220] the isolation rate in the 1- to 4-year-old group was far higher than that in any other age bracket. The high attack rates in these young children were not unexpected because fewer than 10% of them would have been expected to have antibody to any of the 56 RV types,[128] and children ordinarily are subjected continuously to the family-like environment so conducive to transmission of RVs. Even higher prevalence rates among young children have been observed when molecular methods have been used for diagnosis; 34% of samples from children younger than 5 years were RV positive compared with 6% of samples from adults in a 1-year surveillance study of families in Utah.[39] In especially crowded populations, attack rates may be high. In an Alaskan Native village, 70% of 395 children were infected during a spring outbreak of RV-16 infection.[312]

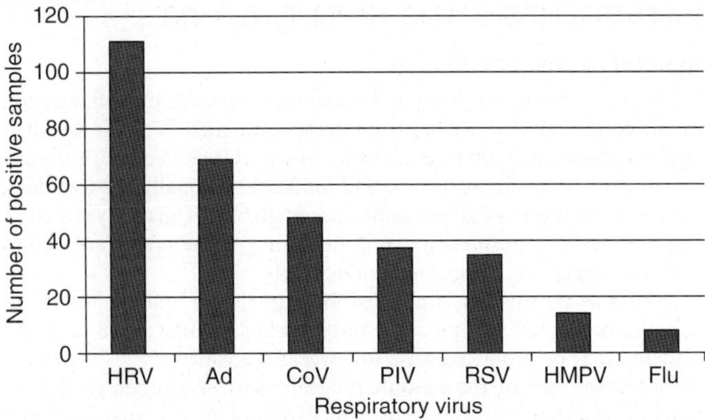

FIG. 167.5 Number of respiratory viruses identified using polymerase chain reaction from 318 respiratory tract illnesses in children attending a group child care center. *HRV*, Human rhinovirus; *Ad*, adenovirus; *CoV*, coronavirus; *PIV*, parainfluenza virus types 1 to 4; *RSV*, respiratory syncytial virus; *HMPV*, human metapneumovirus; *Flu*, influenza A and B. (Modified from Fairchok MP, Martin ET, Chambers S, et al. Epidemiology of viral respiratory tract infections in a prospective cohort of infants and toddlers attending daycare. *J Clin Virol.* 2010;49:16-20.)

The frequency of infection with RV generally declines throughout life. In a prospective study of children attending group child care where PCR methods were used to analyze samples collected weekly in symptomatic children, RVs were the most common respiratory virus identified (Fig. 167.5), and the incidence/child-year of RV infection was 1.3 per year for children enrolled in group child care at birth to 12 months of age versus 0.8 for children older than 12 to 24 months.[95] Beginning at the age of school attendance, the number of RV infections declines gradually from one to two per year to 0.25 per year in the age group older than 60 years.[128,222] Results from most laboratories have found that persons 20 to 30 years of age account for an exception to the general decline in incidence with age[103,148,219,222]; RV infections, as well as infections with other respiratory pathogens, increase during this period of life. Because the increase is especially marked in mothers,[103,148] it probably is the result of the transfer of respiratory illness in small children to parents.

In Tecumseh, the number of respiratory illnesses per year was consistently higher for female patients than for male patients (3 to >60 years of age).[222] If one assumed that RVs account for a similar proportion of disease in each gender, this finding would indicate that girls and women generally have more RV infections. As noted earlier, women with young children clearly seem to have more RV infections than do others in their age group. In Seattle,[103] mothers had 1.5 times more RV infections than fathers did, and in Charlottesville, women of childbearing age had approximately 1.2 times more RV illness than male study subjects did.[128]

The number of moderate to severe RV illnesses was higher in boys than girls during the first 3 years of life in a longitudinal birth cohort study examining factors associated with developing wheezing illness.[294] However, the number of RV-associated wheezing illnesses was similar between the two sexes.

Effect of Psychosocial Factors

Numerous psychosocial factors have been shown to influence susceptibility to RV infection, primarily in the experimental human infection model.

Increased psychological stress, as measured by numerous stress indices, and poorer sleep efficiency and sleep duration were associated with an increased susceptibility to infection and an increased likelihood of developing illness.[56,58,60,242] In contrast, having a more diverse societal network (increased number of social ties) and having a positive emotional style (i.e., sense of well-being, vigor, and calmness) were associated with resistance to infection and illness.[57,88] Antibody-negative (serum antibody levels <1:2) subjects were equally susceptible to infection regardless of the degree of stress or number of social ties, although these factors did influence the likelihood of clinical illness.[57,58] Increased stress in working adults also was associated with an increased risk for having a natural common cold.[278] Increased life stress also has been associated with glucocorticoid receptor resistance and an increased likelihood of illness following experimental RV challenge; the greater glucocorticoid receptor resistance also was associated with the production of higher levels of proinflammatory cytokines among RV-infected persons.[59]

CLINICAL MANIFESTATIONS

RV infections in any age group usually cause only mild upper respiratory tract illness or common colds. Investigators estimate that RVs cause 30% to 50% of common colds, at least in adults.[195] A variety of respiratory symptoms and signs can be present, and the relative frequency of such symptoms varies between children and adults (Table 167.2). The development of serious illness is also possible: RV-associated, radiograph-positive, atypical pneumonia has been described in military trainees[111] and in immunocompromised adults[119,158,166]; graft dysfunction has occurred in lung transplant recipients[174]; and exacerbation of underlying lung disease has been seen in adults with asthma and chronic obstructive pulmonary disease.[20,264] Severe respiratory disease, pneumonia, and death also have occurred in outbreaks of RV infection in geriatric patients residing in nursing homes.[152,194]

Children, particularly the very young, are subject to serious, sometimes fatal RV-caused illnesses. These include bronchiolitis and pneumonia. Viremia has been noted to occur in children with RV infection and respiratory disease.[94,313] Deaths of infants with rhinoviremia has also been observed, including one that occurred during a cold, and six "cot" deaths that were diagnosed as bronchiolitis/pneumonia and from which RVs were isolated.[253,296] At least in theory, generalized illness after viremia seems possible with RV infections; the RVs are a division of the larger picornavirus group, which contains many viruses capable of generalized and fatal infection and whose genomes have considerable homology with the RVs (see Structure of the Virion, earlier). RVs have also been isolated from patients with a variety of other respiratory clinical illnesses, including pharyngitis, epiglottitis, and laryngotracheobronchitis (croup) (Table 167.3). However, detection of RV may also occur in persons who are totally asymptomatic; up to 25% of infections detected by PCR assay in otherwise healthy children and adults are asymptomatic or subclinical,[159,268] and asymptomatic shedding for up to 3 months has been documented in immunocompromised hematopoietic stem cell transplant recipients.[210]

Rhinovirus Infections in Hospitalized Children

Many investigators have identified RV infections in children hospitalized with severe respiratory disease, and these studies continue to illustrate the high number of hospitalizations associated with RV in children overall. In 1971 in Bristol, England, before the widespread use of molecular diagnostic tools, 377 infants hospitalized for respiratory disease yielded 199 (53%) viral diagnoses.[165] RSV was the predominant virus, but RVs were second most common at 12% (23 patients). RV illnesses were comparable in severity to those caused by RSV.

At St. Anna Children's Hospital in Vienna, Kellner and colleagues[178] compared the clinical features of RV and RSV infection in 519 children aged 10 days to 3 years (median age, 6.6 months) from 1984 to 1986. Viral pathogens were detected in 227 (44%) of the children; and of these, 119 (23%) were RSV and 60 (12%) were RV. The physical findings (Table 167.4) and the clinical diagnosis (see Table 167.3) of the children with RV or RSV infection were the same, except RV infections were

TABLE 167.2 Signs and Symptoms of Respiratory Illness in 20 Adults and 15 Children With Rhinovirus Infections in Philadelphia and New Jersey, 1959–60[a]

Sign or Symptom	Adults	Children (Age 2 mo to 8 y)
Fever[b]	4 (20%)	9 (60%)
Eye, ear, nose, and throat		
Rhinorrhea	18 (90%)	10 (67%)
Purulent nasal discharge	4 (20%)	1 (7%)
Pharyngitis	10 (50%)	5 (33%)
Conjunctival infection	2 (10%)	1 (7%)
Anterior cervical lymphadenopathy	1 (5%)	8 (53%)
Hoarseness	4 (20%)	0
Croup	0	1 (7%)
Infection of the tympanic membrane	0	3 (20%)
Chest		
Cough	8 (40%)	15 (100%)
Dyspnea	0	4 (27%)
Refractions	0	3 (20%)
Rhonchi	0	7 (47%)
Rales	0	2 (13%)
Wheezing	0	4 (27%)

[a]The children were from outpatient clinics and wards of the Children's Hospital of Philadelphia, and the adults were employees of Merck and Company, Rahway, NJ.
[b]In adults, 37.2°C (99°F) or higher by mouth: the peak was 37.3°C (99.2°F). In children, 37.7°C (100°F) or higher by rectum; range, 37°C (98.6°F) to 39.1°C (102.4°F); mean, 37.9°C (100.4°F).
Modified from Reilly CM, Hoch SM, Stokes J Jr, et al. Clinical and laboratory findings in cases of respiratory illness caused by coryzaviruses. *Ann Intern Med.* 1962;57:515-525.

TABLE 167.3 Clinical Diagnosis of Respiratory Illnesses of Young Children[a] at St. Anna Children's Hospital, Vienna, from 1984–86: Comparison Between Rhinovirus and Respiratory Syncytial Virus Infections

Physical Findings	All Patients[b] (n = 519)	RSV (n = 119)	RV (n = 60)
Upper Respiratory Tract Infection			
Rhinitis	65 (12%)	4 (3%)	5 (9%)
Otitis media	10 (2%)	0	2 (3%)
Epiglottitis	6 (1%)	1 (1%)	2 (3%)
Pharyngitis	23 (4%)	3 (2%)	4 (6%)
Laryngitis	8 (2%)	1 (1%)	2 (3%)
Other diseases	25 (5%)	0	1 (2%)
Total	137 (26%)	9 (7%)	16 (26%)[b]
Lower Respiratory Tract Infection			
Croup	14 (3%)	4 (3%)	4 (6%)
Tracheobronchitis	100 (19%)	46 (39%)	16 (27%)
Bronchitis	24 (5%)	3 (2%)	0
Obstructive bronchitis[c]	78 (15%)	28 (24%)	8 (14%)
Pneumonia	126 (24%)	29 (25%)	15 (25%)
Other diseases	40 (8%)	0	1 (2%)
Total	382 (74%)	110 (93%)	44 (74%)

[a]Ten days to 3 years of age (median age, 6.6 months).
[b]Rhinoviruses were more likely to cause upper respiratory tract infection ($P < .01$).
[c]This diagnosis included children with expiratory wheeze and evidence of air trapping. In a later article, this same definition was used for wheezy bronchitis.
RV, Rhinovirus; *RSV,* respiratory syncytial virus.
Modified from Kellner G, Popow-Kraupp T, Kundi M, et al. Clinical manifestations of respiratory tract infections due to respiratory syncytial virus and rhinoviruses in hospitalized children. *Acta Paediatr Scand.* 1989;78:390-394.

TABLE 167.4 Physical Findings in Young Children[a] With Respiratory Illness at the Time of Admission to St. Anna Children's Hospital, Vienna, From 1984–86: Comparison Between Rhinovirus and Respiratory Syncytial Virus Infections

Physical Findings	All Patients[b] (n = 519)	RSV (n = 119)	RV (n = 60)
Stridor during expiration	67 (13%)	15 (13%)	10 (16%)
Cyanosis	18 (3%)	4 (3%)	2 (3%)
Swollen cervical glands	87 (17%)	17 (14%)	9 (15%)
Red throat	344 (66%)	75 (63%)	41 (68%)
Nasal flaring	75 (14%)	29 (16%)	11 (18%)
Crepitation	20 (4%)	7 (6%)	2 (3%)
Chest radiograph (positive)	260 (50%)	79 (66%)	35 (58%)
Wheezing	113 (22%)	30 (25%)	13 (22%)
Moist rales	174 (34%)	43 (36%)	22 (36%)
Dry rales	49 (9%)	13 (11%)	5 (8%)
Median respiratory rate/min (range)	43 (10–96)	40 (10–84)	36 (10–64)
Median body temperature (range)	38.4°C (36.4°C–41.8°C)	39.9°C (36.8°C–41.0°C)	38.5°C (36.9°C–41.0°C)
Median duration of illness (range)	11.6 days (2–45)	10.5 days (4–12)	12.8 days (3–31)

[a]Ten days to 3 years of age (median age, 6.6 months).
[b]One hundred twelve (21%) children had upper respiratory tract illnesses, and 342 (66%) children had lower respiratory tract illnesses: 471 (91%) were inpatients, and 48 (9%) were outpatients.
RV, Rhinovirus; *RSV,* respiratory syncytial virus.
Modified from Kellner G, Popow-Kraupp T, Kundi M, et al. Clinical manifestations of respiratory tract infections due to respiratory syncytial virus and rhinoviruses in hospitalized children. *Acta Paediatr Scand.* 1989;78:390-394.

more likely than were RSV infections to be associated with upper respiratory tract infection.

Glezen and colleagues[121] performed a prospective study to evaluate the occurrence of respiratory virus infection in subjects with respiratory or cardiac disorders in Houston, Texas, between 1991 and 1995. RV infections were identified by culture in 51 subjects from a total of 1198 evaluated illnesses; six were associated with a second respiratory virus infection.[93] In children younger than 5 years of age, exacerbation of asthma, bronchiolitis, and suspected sepsis were the most common clinical findings, whereas nearly all older children and young adults had an exacerbation of asthma. In older adults, a complication of an underlying disease (asthma, chronic obstructive lung disease, congestive heart failure) or pneumonia was diagnosed. In this prospective study, RV infections were an important cause of lower respiratory tract illness in all age groups.[93] When molecular methods were subsequently used to identify viral respiratory tract infections from specimens collected during this study, RVs were present in almost 25% of analyzed samples and in approximately half of children younger than 1 year of age.[21]

Studies of RV in hospitalized children with respiratory disease using molecular diagnostic techniques around the world document high rates of RV. In a large multicenter US study of children younger than 5 years, RV was detected in 17.4% of 1947 children hospitalized with acute respiratory illnesses compared with 12.5% of controls.[159] RV A viruses were significantly more common in hospitalized children 24 months and older compared with controls (8.1% vs. 2.2%), and RV C infection was significantly more frequent in hospitalized children 6 months and older (8.2% vs. 3.9%). RV B infection was uncommon in both groups (<1% each). RV has also been commonly detected at high rates in diverse geographic settings. Detection of RV was similar in hospitalized South African children infected or not infected with HIV with pneumonia (45.6 %) or bronchiolitis (52%).[9] RV was detected in 44% of Alaska Native children hospitalized in Alaska compared with 16% of healthy controls.[268]

Bronchiolitis is one of the more common reasons for young children to be hospitalized with respiratory illness. RVs have been identified in several studies as the second most common virus infection identified in association with bronchiolitis after RSV.[42,167,199,200] In some studies, the bronchiolitis associated with RV infection was less severe than that caused by RSV,[199,200,203,274] whereas in others the severity was similar.[42] In a large multicenter study reported by Mansbach and colleagues,[199] children younger than 2 years and coinfected with RSV and RV had significantly longer lengths of stay after adjustment for clinical and demographic parameters, whereas RV coinfections with other respiratory viruses were not associated with prolonged lengths of stay. Decreased severity of illness in hospitalized children who are coinfected with both RV and RSV or human metapneumovirus has also been documented.[33,203]

The contribution of RV to community-based illness has become both more sensitive and more practical with the advent of multiplex PCR. A prospective weekly sampling in 26 families with young children demonstrated that RV was the most common virus detected in any age group and represented 34% of the viral detection by week in children younger than 4 years.[39] Similarly, the burden of RV in children seeking care in a pediatric emergency department has been documented to be the most frequent respiratory virus detected in children younger than 3 years seeking acute care, with 59% of 425 children having lower respiratory tract disease, 52% requiring hospitalization, and 22% hospitalized for 3 or more days.[55] In this study, coinfection increased the risk for lower respiratory tract infection (odds ratio, 1.83; 95% confidence interval, 1.01–3.32).

Several studies have examined the prevalence of RV infection in pediatric patients presenting or hospitalized with community-acquired pneumonia. Juven and colleagues[173] found RV infection in 25% of 254 children hospitalized with community-acquired pneumonia; a concomitant bacterial copathogen was identified in half of the patients. Tsolia and associates[282] reported RV infection in 45% of 75 school-aged children hospitalized with community-acquired pneumonia, with a copathogen found in 58% of the RV-infected patients. García-García and colleagues[109] detected RV infection in approximately 20% of children hospitalized with pneumonia; RV was the most common viral pathogen identified in children older than 18 months of age and the sole virus identified in 55% of the RV-infected patients. Self and colleagues[265] performed a case-control study in Salt Lake City, Utah, and Nashville, Tennessee, to evaluate the importance of RV detection in pediatric patients with community-acquired pneumonia; RV infection was identified in 17% of controls compared with 22% of patients with community-acquired pneumonia, and its presence was not significantly associated with pneumonia. These indicate the need to account for background circulation of respiratory viruses among symptom-free subjects investigating the causes of pneumonia.

In summary, there is substantial evidence that RVs can cause serious lower respiratory tract illness, especially in young children. In some populations, RVs may be second to RSV in frequency and be associated with comparably severe signs and symptoms. However, the prevalence of asymptomatic virus shedding and the frequent identification of another viral respiratory tract infection make it difficult to determine the clinical significance of RV infection in the individual patient.

Asthma

RV infection is a risk factor both for the development of asthma and for exacerbations of wheezing in children with asthma. Having either an RSV or an RV infection that results in a wheezing illness during the first year of life is an independent risk factor for wheezing later in childhood.[183,186,191] Children who have a RV-associated wheezing illness in the first 3 years of life are more likely to be diagnosed with asthma at 6 years of age than are those who have an RSV-associated illness.[162] Sensitization to aeroallergens (atopy) in the first year of life also is an independent risk factor for the subsequent development of asthma, particularly after RV infection and precedes RV-induced wheezing.[160-162,186] Genetic factors also influence susceptibility to RV-induced wheezing.[41]

Viral respiratory tract infection is a common precipitant of wheezing in children with asthma.[37] RVs are the most frequent respiratory virus identified in children with acute wheezing exacerbation of asthma; however, not all RV infections in an asthmatic child will result in wheezing. Two investigative groups serotyped the RVs isolated from children with wheezy illness and found no types to be particularly "asthmagenic"; and a total of 30 different serotypes were associated with asthma exacerbations.[176,211-213] It is not clear whether RV strain differences are important factors in precipitating asthma attacks, although one small study found an increased risk for exacerbation with minor group RV A strains.[70] Strain differences in the level of cytokine and chemokine induction following infection of bronchial epithelial cells has also been reported.[301]

The mechanism of bronchospasm in virus-infected patients is an area of great research interest. RVs replicate in the lower respiratory tract.[114,230] RV infection induces the production of numerous proinflammatory cytokines in both the upper and lower airways, and an increased number of inflammatory cells has been demonstrated in the lower respiratory tract in association with RV infection.[99,107,112] The presence of activated cytotoxic T cells in the lower airways has been suggested to contribute to asthma-associated mortality.[226] Host factors also play a role, in that innate immune responses to RV are impaired. For example, bronchial epithelial cells from asthmatic individuals produce less IFN-β and have less apoptosis and greater viral replication after infection with RV than do cells from nonasthmatic subjects or in those with well-controlled asthma.[277,302] The timing of interferon expression during the course of RV infection may also be important.[263] Aeroallergen-sensitized asthmatic children have higher expression of the high-affinity IgE receptor FcεRI than nonallergic, nonasthmatic children, and this was associated with a decreased production of IFN-α and IFN-γ1 by plasma-derived dendritic cells after RV stimulation.[91] IFN production was further decreased after cross-linking of the FcεRI receptor. Animal models also suggest the possibility that reflex neurogenic pathways may be activated in association with viral respiratory tract infection and may lead to bronchoconstriction. The pathogenesis of respiratory virus–induced bronchospasm is an area of active research, with the hope that preventive or therapeutic intervention strategies can be developed.

Otitis Media

Although acute otitis media is chiefly a bacterial disease, with approximately two-thirds of middle ear fluid specimens yielding *Streptococcus pneumoniae, Haemophilus influenzae,* or both, and *Moraxella catarrhalis* and other bacteria playing lesser roles, otitic involvement often is preceded or accompanied by a putative viral upper respiratory tract illness.[12,14,181,260,251] Most bacterial pathogens found in middle ear fluid are colonizers of the nasopharynx, and bacterial infection of the middle ear is considered to be a direct extension from that area.[181] A history of a preceding viral upper respiratory tract illness is common, and clear and comprehensive evidence of viral extension from the nasopharynx to the middle ear has been established. Many different respiratory viruses have been identified in middle ear effusions from children with otitis media, and RVs are one of the most commonly identified when molecular methods of detection are used. Pitkaranta and colleagues[239] identified respiratory viruses from the middle ear effusions in 30% of 100 children who had otitis media with effusion. RVs constituted approximately two-thirds of the respiratory viruses identified. Bacterial pathogens were identified in 35% of the samples, and both bacteria and viruses were found in 11%. A criterion for selection was the absence of an upper respiratory tract illness within the preceding week; thus whether the presence of RV RNA represented evidence of ongoing or past infection is unclear. Blomqvist and colleagues[29] found RV RNA in middle ear effusions from 41% of children with otitis media in the first 2 years of life, and Chantzi and colleagues[49] found a similar prevalence of RV RNA in otitis media effusions.

The presence of both bacterial and viral pathogens in middle ear fluid does not, in general, interfere with the effectiveness of antibacterial therapy, although in those specific patients whose acute otitis media is refractory to treatment it may.[15] When measured against a comparison group of 66 "normal" acute otitis media cases (controls), 22 patients with refractory cases harbored significantly more viral pathogens than did controls (68% vs. 41%, respectively; $P < .05$). In addition, when only the middle ear fluid of these groups was examined for the presence of viruses, 32% of patients with refractory cases had virus versus 15% of controls. RVs were the dominant viruses in both groups. Bacterial pathogens were grown from the middle ear fluid of four of the 22 in the poor-responder group, and all harbored concomitant respiratory viruses, two of which were RVs; only one of the four bacteria was resistant to the antibacterial agent used in therapy. These investigators also examined patients in the 66-patient control group whose illnesses were refractory to treatment and found significantly more viruses ($P < .05$) in the middle ear fluid of this group than in those with a good response to therapy. These authors concluded that the presence of viruses in the middle ear fluid of children with acute otitis media can delay response to antibacterial therapy.

Chonmaitree and associates[53] in Galveston, Texas, also investigated the role of viruses in middle ear fluid as agents that may interfere with antibacterial therapy. In their initial report, viruses were cultured from the middle ear fluid of 11 of 58 children (19%); RSV and RV were the most frequent viruses isolated, at 3 each. Of the patients in whom therapy failed, significantly more ($P < .05$) harbored viruses as well, and of those whose bacteria were susceptible to the treatment antibiotic, significantly more had combined viral-bacterial infections. In two subsequent reports by these authors, the highest rate of poor bacteriologic outcome occurred when RV was isolated from middle ear fluid. Seven of nine instances of RV infection resulted in bacteriologic treatment failure.[276] Subsequent studies using molecular techniques by Chonmaitree and colleagues[52] found that acute otitis media does not occur after asymptomatic RV infection and that RV viral load in respiratory specimens is not a risk factor for the development of acute otitis media.

These studies suggest that viruses, including RVs, play a role in acute otitis media, especially in prolonging the response to antimicrobial treatment. McBride and associates[204] at the University of Pittsburgh and the University of Virginia used RV-infected human volunteers and found that the eustachian tube became occluded in 50% of the volunteers and that abnormal middle ear pressure was present for as long as 10 days. These studies were extended by Buchman and colleagues,[35] who inoculated 60 volunteers with RV-39. Middle ear pressures of less than −100 mm H_2O were noted in 22 subjects (37%). In two of the three subjects who had pressures less than −100 mm H_2O, upper respiratory tract illness with middle ear effusion developed. In this study, the otologic manifestations of experimental RV infection were extended to include otitis media.

Arola and colleagues[13] examined the role of viruses in 61 children (mean age, 3.2 years) with subacute or chronic asymptomatic otitis media with effusion. Five RVs and one adenovirus were found in the middle ear fluid. In addition, bacterial pathogens were isolated from the patient with adenovirus infection and from two of the patients with RV infection. None of these patients with otitis media and effusion were ill with an upper respiratory tract infection at the time the specimen was obtained, and the effusion had endured 30 to 60 days before myringotomy was performed.

Sinusitis

RVs can cause a clinical syndrome of rhinosinusitis similar to that caused by bacterial infection. Gwaltney and colleagues[132] performed computed tomography of the sinuses on adults with acute common colds of less than 4 days' duration in which RV infection was documented by culture in 27%. Radiographic abnormalities included mucosal thickening and air-fluid levels. Associated clinical signs and symptoms resolved without antibiotic therapy, a finding suggesting that the radiographic signs were caused by an acute viral infection. Few attempts have been made to recover viruses directly from the sinuses. Two reports from Virginia noted that 140 aspirates obtained by direct puncture of the maxillary sinuses yielded 86 positive specimens, and seven of 12 viruses were RVs.[133,134] Pitkaranta and associates[238,240] used real-time PCR analysis and in situ hybridization to identify RVs in 50% of adults with acute community-acquired sinusitis. A prospective, longitudinal pediatric study of acute bacterial sinusitis and viral respiratory infections in children younger than 3 years demonstrated that viruses were detected in 63% of children during the initial upper respiratory infection visit, and RV detection was positively correlated with the risk for acute sinusitis ($P = .01$).[201] Because the signs and symptoms of viral rhinosinusitis and bacterial sinusitis can be difficult to distinguish, the American Academy of Pediatrics developed clinical practice guidelines for the diagnosis and treatment of bacterial sinusitis, and these were updated in 2012 by the Infectious Diseases Society of America.[4,54]

Immunocompromised Patients

RV is the most common respiratory virus detected in immunocompromised patients. A cumulative 100-day incidence of 22.3% and 1-year incidence of 31% have been reported in hematopoietic stem cell transplant recipients in a prospective study conducted in Seattle.[210] Infections occurred year-round, and prolonged virus shedding for more than 12 weeks was noted. Clinical manifestations can range from mild upper respiratory tract symptoms to fatal pneumonia.[119,126,210] Fever, cough, sputum production, and dyspnea are the most common symptoms in hematopoietic stem cell transplant recipients with RV detected in the lower respiratory tract.[166]

When RV is identified as the sole pathogen in a transplant recipient with lower respiratory tract infection, it can cause severe pneumonia with a clinical picture similar to that of influenza virus–associated pneumonia.[51] A mortality rate of more than 40% was documented in a study of 87 patients with laboratory-proven RV detected in bronchoalveolar lavage fluid with symptomatic lower respiratory tract disease; risk factors for poor outcome included oxygen use at RV diagnosis (hazard ratio [HR] 2.6; $P = .04$), steroid use more than 1 mg/kg before diagnosis (HR, 5.5; $P = .002$), and bone marrow as a stem cell source (HR, 2.3; $P = .05$).[266] Many immunocompromised patients with fatal infections have been coinfected with other pathogens, making it difficult to determine the relative contribution of RV infection to the outcome.[119,158] Overall, higher viral loads in clinical samples correlated with more symptomatic and more severe disease.[118,210]

DIAGNOSIS OF INFECTION

RV infections cannot be diagnosed solely on the basis of clinical grounds because they cause such a wide spectrum of respiratory illness, particularly in infants, children, and immunocompromised hosts. However, because of the characteristic spring-summer-fall seasonal pattern of the RVs, tentatively assigning an RV origin in patients with mild to moderate respiratory illness during these months is reasonable.

Classical methods for diagnosis of RV have been based on culture, but culture of RV can be difficult. These viruses propagate unpredictably, even in relatively sensitive diploid cell cultures such as WI-38 and FT cells or in Ohio strain HeLa cells, and organ cultures or cultures of differentiated airway epithelial cells at an air-liquid interface are needed to propagate RV C strains in vitro.[19,32,66] Isolation of RV from children can also be hampered by the common practice of relying on a throat swab, which may contain only one tissue culture infectious virus particle or less (Table 167.5). Hendley and colleagues[148] found nasal specimens to be superior for RV diagnosis, with nasal aspirates successfully used worldwide.[155,177,208] If freezing is necessary and dry ice is used, great care must be taken to avoid contamination of the specimen with sublimed carbon dioxide because the resultant carbonic acid rapidly kills the virus. Cell cultures should be incubated and slowly rolled at 33°C. Evidence of viral growth usually is seen between 2 days and 2 weeks.

TABLE 167.5 Quantity of Virus Found in 87 Throat Swabs From Children Aged 3 to 11 Years: Madison, Wisconsin, 1971–72[a]

	Per 0.1 mL
$\leq$1 $TCID_{50}$	22
>1 to $\leq$50 $TCID_{50}$	46
$\geq$50 to <50 $TCID_{50}$	14
>50 to <500 $TCID_{50}$	5

[a]Fourteen rhinovirus types are represented.
$TCID_{50}$, Median tissue culture infective dose.

The availability of rapid, sensitive multiplex PCR assays in diagnostic laboratories has revolutionized the diagnosis of RV in the hospital and clinic. Because RVs have many nucleotide sequences in common among the RNA genomes of the various serotypes, especially in the noncoding region at the 5′ end, reverse transcriptase (RT)-PCR assays have been designed and widely used for the detection of RVs, often in panels with other respiratory viruses.[22,237] Some assays do not distinguish RVs from enteroviruses, whereas others are RV specific.[21,227] The superiority of RT-PCR techniques compared with cell culture methods first became evident in a clinical study of children with acute respiratory illnesses. Johnston and colleagues[171] detected RV by PCR in 146 of 292 samples (50%) that yielded RV in only 47 (16%) by standard culture. Many subsequent studies confirmed the superiority of RT-PCR assays over culture methods for the detection of RVs.[18,20,157] The increased sensitivity of molecular assays can make interpretation of a positive result problematic because many asymptomatic infections are identified. Viral quantitation may have a role in identifying clinically significant RV infections.[55,118]

PREVENTION AND TREATMENT

Prevention and treatment are addressed thoroughly in Chapter 7 and elsewhere, and only measures specific to the RVs are added here. Although some protection after the use of inactivated vaccines has been demonstrated,[84,234] the existence of more than 100 serotypes limits the prospect of vaccine development. However, based on the observation that cross-reacting neutralizing epitopes have been identified among the RVs, developing a vaccine that targets these epitopes may be possible.[92,120]

The most effective RV cold-preventive agent described to date that has been demonstrated to be effective for natural RV colds is IFN-α, a protein produced as part of the host's natural antiviral defense and now produced for experimentation by genetic recombinant methods.[87] Investigators administered this agent by nasal spray to other family members after symptoms appeared in the index case; 80% of the secondary RV colds were prevented. However, IFN given in this fashion does not seem to be effective against other respiratory viruses. For example, in a follow-up study in Seattle, IFN-α did not reduce the incidence of colds when administered in a protocol identical to that used in the previous family studies, chiefly because RV infections were not the majority of agents causing colds.[81,87,106] RVs often have a decided seasonality, so rapid diagnosis of the index case by PCR analysis might be helpful to determine when IFN-α could be used effectively to stop intrafamily spread. The disadvantage of IFN prophylaxis is that prolonged intranasal administration (>7 days) or repeated treatment produces an inflammatory response consisting of nasal stuffiness, ulceration, and blood-tinged discharge.[261]

Numerous antiviral agents with in vitro activity against RVs have been developed. The earlier section in this chapter on structure of the virion describes the development of some of these agents, which was made possible by taking advantage of current detailed knowledge of RV structure and specific cell receptors. Several of these preparations, including capsid-binding agents, soluble receptor (soluble ICAM-1), and antibody to the receptor (ICAM-1), have been tested in clinical trials, but development of most of these agents has not been pursued for a variety of reasons,[23,289] as reviewed by Arruda and Hayden.[17] Another capsid-binding agent, pleconaril, has in vitro antiviral activity against many enteroviruses and RVs, and phase III clinical trials on naturally acquired colds demonstrated some reduction in the severity and duration of several respiratory symptoms.[142] However, pleconaril induces the CYP3A4 enzyme that can lead to menstrual irregularities in women taking oral contraceptives.[98] This concern, along with the drug's modest efficacy, prevented pleconaril from being approved by the US Food and Drug Administration. Vapendavir is another capsid-binding agent in clinical trial; a phase 2 clinical trial in asthmatic adults demonstrated more rapid improvement in upper respiratory symptoms, better respiratory function, and decreased virus shedding compared with placebo.[141] However, early results of the SPIRITUS clinical trial conducted in adults with asthma did not demonstrate significant clinical improvement in asthma control compared with placebo based on questionnaire completion at study day 14. Whether to conduct further clinical studies of this agent is under consideration by its developer.

Rupintrivir, another class of antiviral drug for RVs, is a potent, irreversible inhibitor of viral 3C protease and has been administered as an intranasal drug; however, it had only moderate antiviral and clinical efficacy in a phase II clinical trial, and further development has been halted.[143]

Colds usually are treated symptomatically with mild nonsteroidal antiinflammatory drugs, sympathomimetics (e.g., phenylpropanolamine), and antihistamines; these agents are discussed in Chapter 7.[271] Anticholinergic agents (e.g., topical ipratropium bromide) and first-generation antihistamines reduce severity of rhinorrhea, whereas second-generation ("nonsedating") antihistamines have no effect. The efficacy of the first-generation antihistamines may result from the ability of these agents to block muscarinic as well as histaminic receptors and to cross the blood-brain barrier.[223] Sympathomimetics decrease nasal obstruction, although topical administration may lead to rebound nasal obstruction. Nonsteroidal antiinflammatory agents decrease the severity of some of the systemic symptoms associated with colds (e.g., malaise, headache).[284] A combination of antiviral and antimediator preparations may provide effective therapy. Various other treatments, including vitamin C,[48,146] *Echinacea*,[207,285] intranasal humidified air,[101,291] and zinc lozenges,[163,198,241] have been evaluated, and some studies have reported a clinical benefit, although other studies have failed to confirm such findings.[284] Almost all clinical evaluations of symptomatic and alternative therapies have been performed in adults; very few data exist on the utility of such therapy in children.[198,270] In 2007, the US Food and Drug Administration released a warning against using over-the-counter therapies including antihistamines, decongestants, and antitussives for the treatment of the common cold in children younger than 2 years because of potentially dangerous side effects linked to several deaths, in the absence of data demonstrating benefit in this age group.[100]

The use of oral or inhaled corticosteroids appears to enhance the shedding of viable virus.[125,248] One potential consequence of corticosteroid use, seen in a study of pediatric patients with a common cold syndrome, is a significant increase in the risk for developing acute otitis media in RV-infected subjects.[259] However, hospitalized children with a first episode of wheezing associated with RV infection were less likely to have recurrent wheezing over the following year if treated with prednisolone, and corticosteroid therapy can decrease the duration of symptoms associated with acute asthma exacerbations.[168,189] Available evidence indicates that corticosteroids do not have a role in the treatment of uncomplicated RV infections. Similarly, no role exists for the use of antibiotic therapy in uncomplicated RV infection.

Acknowledgment

We acknowledge the contributions of Elliot C. Dick, Stanley L. Inhorn, and W. Paul Glezen, who contributed to this chapter in previous editions of the text.

NEW REFERENCES SINCE THE SEVENTH EDITION

9. Annamalay AA, Abbott S, Sikazwe C, et al. Respiratory viruses in young South African children with acute lower respiratory infections and interactions with HIV. *J Clin Virol*. 2016;81:58-63.
19. Ashraf S, Brockman-Schneider R, Bochkov YA, et al. Biological characteristics and propagation of human rhinovirus-C in differentiated sinus epithelial cells. *Virology*. 2013;436(1):143-149.
26. Bartlett NW, Singanayagam A, Johnston SL. Mouse models of rhinovirus infection and airways disease. *Methods Mol Biol*. 2015;1221:181-188.
32. Bochkov YA, Palmenberg AC, Lee WM, et al. Molecular modeling, organ culture and reverse genetics for a newly identified human rhinovirus C. *Nat Med*. 2011;17(5):627-632.
39. Byington CL, Ampofo K, Stockmann C, et al. Community surveillance of respiratory viruses among families in the Utah Better Identification of Germs-Longitudinal Viral Epidemiology (BIG-LoVE) Study. *Clin Infect Dis*. 2015;61(8):1217-1224.
41. Caliskan M, Bochkov YA, Kreiner-Moller E, et al. Rhinovirus wheezing illness and genetic risk of childhood-onset asthma. *N Engl J Med*. 2013;368(15):1398-1407.
51. Choi SH, Huh JW, Hong SB, et al. Clinical characteristics and outcomes of severe rhinovirus-associated pneumonia identified by bronchoscopic bronchoalveolar lavage in adults: comparison with severe influenza virus-associated pneumonia. *J Clin Virol*. 2015;62:41-47.
52. Chonmaitree T, Alvarez-Fernandez P, Jennings K, et al. Symptomatic and asymptomatic respiratory viral infections in the first year of life: association with acute otitis media development. *Clin Infect Dis*. 2015;60(1):1-9.
55. Chu HY, Englund JA, Strelitz B, et al. Rhinovirus disease in children seeking care in a tertiary pediatric emergency department. *J Pediatric Infect Dis Soc*. 2016;5(1):29-38.
59. Cohen S, Janicki-Deverts D, Doyle WJ, et al. Chronic stress, glucocorticoid receptor resistance, inflammation, and disease risk. *Proc Natl Acad Sci USA*. 2012;109(16):5995-5999.
70. Denlinger LC, Sorkness RL, Lee WM, et al. Lower airway rhinovirus burden and the seasonal risk of asthma exacerbation. *Am J Respir Crit Care Med*. 2011;184(9):1007-1014.
92. Edlmayr J, Niespodziana K, Popow-Kraupp T, et al. Antibodies induced with recombinant VP1 from human rhinovirus exhibit cross-neutralisation. *Eur Respir J*. 2011;37(1):44-52.
94. Esposito S, Daleno C, Scala A, et al. Impact of rhinovirus nasopharyngeal viral load and viremia on severity of respiratory infections in children. *Eur J Clin Microbiol Infect Dis*. 2014;33(1):41-48.
108. Fuchs R, Blaas D. Productive entry pathways of human rhinoviruses. *Adv Virol*. 2012;2012:826301.
116. Gern JE, Pappas T, Visness CM, et al. Comparison of the etiology of viral respiratory illnesses in inner-city and suburban infants. *J Infect Dis*. 2012;206(9):1342-1349.
115. Gern JEP, Palmenberg AC. Rhinoviruses. In: Knipe DMH, Howley PM, eds. *Fields Virology*. 6th ed. New York: Lippincott Williams & Wilkins; 2013: 531-549.
120. Glanville N, McLean GR, Guy B, et al. Cross-serotype immunity induced by immunization with a conserved rhinovirus capsid protein. *PLoS Pathog*. 2013;9(9):e1003669.
138. Hao W, Bernard K, Patel N, et al. Infection and propagation of human rhinovirus C in human airway epithelial cells. *J Virol*. 2012;86(24):13524-13532.
141. Hayden FG. Advances in antivirals for non-influenza respiratory virus infections. *Influenza Other Respir Viruses*. 2013;7(suppl 3):36-43.
145. Heinonen S, Jartti T, Garcia C, et al. Rhinovirus detection in symptomatic and asymptomatic children: value of host transcriptome analysis. *Am J Respir Crit Care Med*. 2016;193(7):772-782.
164. Jacobs SE, Lamson DM, St George K, et al. Human rhinoviruses. *Clin Microbiol Rev*. 2013;26(1):135-162.
166. Jacobs SE, Soave R, Shore TB, et al. Human rhinovirus infections of the lower respiratory tract in hematopoietic stem cell transplant recipients. *Transpl Infect Dis*. 2013;15(5):474-486.
175. Karppinen S, Toivonen L, Schuez-Havupalo L, et al. Interference between respiratory syncytial virus and rhinovirus in respiratory tract infections in children. *Clin Microbiol Infect*. 2016;22(2):208 e201-208 e206.
185. Kuroda M, Niwa S, Sekizuka T, et al. Molecular evolution of the VP1, VP2, and VP3 genes in human rhinovirus species C. *Sci Rep*. 2015;5:8185.
201. Marom T, Alvarez-Fernandez PE, Jennings K, et al. Acute bacterial sinusitis complicating viral upper respiratory tract infection in young children. *Pediatr Infect Dis J*. 2014;33(8):803-808.
202. Martin ET, Fairchok MP, Stednick ZJ, et al. Epidemiology of multiple respiratory viruses in childcare attendees. *J Infect Dis*. 2013;207(6):982-989.
205. McIntyre CL, Knowles NJ, Simmonds P. Proposals for the classification of human rhinovirus species A, B and C into genotypically assigned types. *J Gen Virol*. 2013;94(Pt 8):1791-1806.
217. Monto AS. The seasonality of rhinovirus infections and its implications for clinical recognition. *Clin Ther*. 2002;24(12):1987-1997.

225. Nakagome K, Bochkov YA, Ashraf S, et al. Effects of rhinovirus species on viral replication and cytokine production. *J Allergy Clin Immunol.* 2014;134(2):332-341.
227. Osterback R, Tevaluoto T, Ylinen T, et al. Simultaneous detection and differentiation of human rhino- and enteroviruses in clinical specimens by real-time PCR with locked nucleic Acid probes. *J Clin Microbiol.* 2013;51(12):3960-3967.
231. Parsons KS, Hsu AC, Wark PA. TLR3 and MDA5 signalling, although not expression, is impaired in asthmatic epithelial cells in response to rhinovirus infection. *Clin Exp Allergy.* 2014;44(1):91-101.
242. Prather AA, Janicki-Deverts D, Hall MH, et al. Behaviorally assessed sleep and susceptibility to the common cold. *Sleep.* 2015;38(9):1353-1359.
249. Racaniello VR. Picornaviridae: The viruses and their replication. In: Knipe DMH, Howley PM, eds. *Fields Virology.* Vol. 1. 6th ed. Philadelphia: Lippincott, Williams & Wilkins; 2013:453-489.
250. Rajan D, McCracken CE, Kopleman HB, et al. Human rhinovirus induced cytokine/chemokine responses in human airway epithelial and immune cells. *PLoS ONE.* 2014;9(12):e114322.
251. Rankl C, Kienberger F, Wildling L, et al. Multiple receptors involved in human rhinovirus attachment to live cells. *Proc Natl Acad Sci USA.* 2008;105(46):17778-17783.
258. Roy A, Post CB. Long-distance correlations of rhinovirus capsid dynamics contribute to uncoating and antiviral activity. *Proc Natl Acad Sci USA.* 2012;109(14):5271-5276.
263. Schwantes EA, Denlinger LC, Evans MD, et al. Severity of virus-induced asthma symptoms is inversely related to resolution IFN-lambda expression. *J Allergy Clin Immunol.* 2015;135(6):1656-1659.
265. Self WH, Williams DJ, Zhu Y, et al. Respiratory viral detection in children and adults: comparing asymptomatic controls and patients with community-acquired pneumonia. *J Infect Dis.* 2016;213(4):584-591.
266. Seo SM E, Xie H, Kuypers JM, et al. Human rhinovirus RNA detection in the lower respiratory tract of hematopoietic cell transplant recipients: association with mortality. *Biol Blood Marrow Transplant.* 2013;19(2):S167-S168.
273. Steinke JW, Liu L, Turner RB, et al. Immune surveillance by rhinovirus-specific circulating CD4+ and CD8+ T lymphocytes. *PLoS ONE.* 2015;10(1):e0115271.
277. Sykes A, Macintyre J, Edwards MR, et al. Rhinovirus-induced interferon production is not deficient in well controlled asthma. *Thorax.* 2014;69(3):240-246.
279. Tapparel C, Sobo K, Constant S, et al. Growth and characterization of different human rhinovirus C types in three-dimensional human airway epithelia reconstituted in vitro. *Virology.* 2013;446(1-2):1-8.
300. Waman VP, Kolekar PS, Kale MM, et al. Population structure and evolution of Rhinoviruses. *PLoS ONE.* 2014;9(2):e88981.
301. Wark PA, Grissell T, Davies B, et al. Diversity in the bronchial epithelial cell response to infection with different rhinovirus strains. *Respirology.* 2009;14(2):180-186.

The full reference list for this chapter is available at ExpertConsult.com.

168 Hepatitis A Virus

Yen H. Pham • Daniel H. Leung

HISTORY

Hepatitis A has been recognized as a clinical entity for centuries, notably as large epidemics of jaundice among military camps in both ancient and modern times. During the past several decades, epidemiologic and clinical studies have defined the infectious nature of the disease, leading to the differentiation of "infectious hepatitis," now known as hepatitis A.[206] In the 1970s, isolation of hepatitis A virus (HAV) and identification by immune electron microscopy among stool samples of patients with HAV[133] led to understanding of the fecal-oral route of transmission, the clinical course of infection, and the efficacy of immunoglobulin in preventing disease.[206,207,423] This hastened the development of serologic tests that differentiate acute and resolved infections, definitions of pathogenic events during infection, and further epidemiologic study of HAV infection. Following propagation of HAV in cell culture,[88,304,404,406] the evolution and licensure of highly effective vaccines have dramatically changed the landscape of HAV infection, though certainly not eradicated it.[61,264,408]

PROPERTIES

Classification

HAV is a 27-nm, nonenveloped, positive-sense RNA virus belonging to the family Picornaviridae. Although HAV initially was classified in the genus *Enterovirus,* nucleotide analysis indicates that HAV is distinct from all other picornaviruses.[222,225,395,416] In contrast to other enteroviruses, HAV has essentially no nucleotide or amino acid homology, does not have an intestinal replication phase, replicates slowly in cell culture, rarely produces a cytopathic effect, and is relatively resistant to inactivation by heating.[87] For these reasons, HAV has been reclassified in a separate genus designated *Hepatovirus.*[257,416]

Genomic Organization and Genetic Variation

Hepatitis A is composed of an icosahedral capsid that contains a positive-sense, single-stranded RNA genome of approximately 7.5 kb in length with a single open reading frame flanked by 5′ and 3′ untranslated regions (UTR). The 5′ UTR is the most conserved region of the genome and contains an internal ribosome entry site. The open reading frame encodes a polyprotein organized into three functional regions: P1, P2, and P3. P1 is secondarily cleaved into four capsid proteins, VP1 to VP4, whereas P2 and P3 proteins encode nonstructural proteins associated with replication.[222,225,363,405,406,416]

HAV exists as a single serotype. The neutralization site appears to be conformational and derived from epitopes located on VP1 and VP3, as identified by neutralizing monoclonal antibodies.[268,299] A high degree of nucleotide conservation exists among geographically diverse human HAV isolates. However, enough genetic diversity exists to define several HAV genotypes and subgenotypes. The entire nucleic acid sequences of several HAV strains have been determined by molecular cloning, and a large number of HAV isolates have been characterized by sequencing of short genome segments.[270]

The genomic regions most commonly used to define HAV genotypes include (1) the C terminus of the VP3 region, (2) the N terminus of the VP1 region, (3) the junction of the VP1 and P2A regions, and (4) the VP1-P2B regions and the entire VP1 region (Fig. 168.1).[81,270]

Six genotypes (I to VI) are now defined based on analysis of the 900 nucleotides of the complete VP1 protein. Only genotypes I, II, and III, divided into subtypes A and B, infect humans. The other three (IV, V, and VI) appear to be restricted in their primary replication to Old World monkeys.[269,376]

The worldwide geographic distribution of HAV serotypes has been well described.[81,270,315] Genotype I is the most prevalent worldwide, particularly genotype IA, which dominates in North, Central, and South

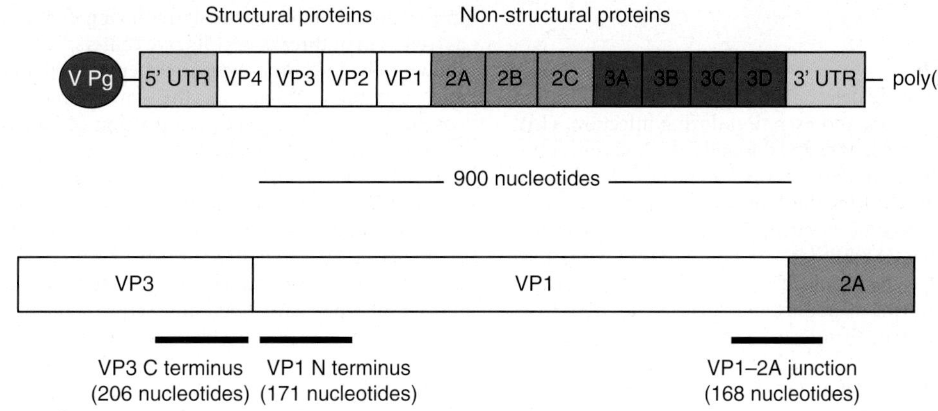

Fig. 168.1 Genomic organization of hepatitis A virus.

America; China; Japan; Thailand; and Europe.[48,177,184,315] Subgenotype IB is reported mainly from the Mediterranean region and South Africa and is the most prevalent in Turkey.[278] Subgenotype IIIA is the most prevalent in India, Nepal, and Korea.[170,348,421] In low-endemicity areas, such as the United States and Western Europe, subgenotype IA dominates, although all genotypes have been reported.[82,270] Of note, subgenotypes IIA, IIB, and IIIB rarely have been reported.[102]

The analysis of the other genomic regions (i.e., the N terminus of the VP1, VP1-2B regions, the entire VP, and the C terminus of VP3) allows better strain discrimination. Growing sequence databases allow for the identification of the geographic origin of a given subgenotype. This genetic variation has proved useful in identifying clusters and linking apparently sporadic cases.[10,101,167,172,267,313]

Genotype does not appear to influence the clinical presentation or outcome of infection,[2,144,170] although outbreaks in Korea suggest that genotypes might account for differences in disease severity. Report of a national hepatitis A outbreak in Korea from 2006 to 2008 indicated that genotype IIIA infection demonstrated significantly higher transaminase levels, prothrombin time, and leukocyte count, with more severe symptoms including fever and dark urine on admission compared to genotype IA infection.[421] Similarly, another Korean study found genotype IIIA to be associated with higher alanine transaminase (ALT) levels and longer hospitalization among adolescents and young adults in a multivariate logistic regression model.[419]

Virulence

HAV is known to produce disease in humans and nonhuman primates. HAV replicates more slowly in cell culture than other picornaviruses, and wild-type viruses may require many weeks of adaptation or serial passages before infectious foci or HAV antigen is detected.[33,219,222,284,342] With increasing passage in cell culture, the virus adapts to growth in vitro with more rapid production of viral antigen and increasing virus titers. HAV produces a high ratio of defective to complete (infectious) virus both in cell culture and during infection.[43,416] Cell culture adaptation is associated with mutations in nonstructural proteins and the 5′ nontranslated region.[121,123] Mutations in the VP1/2A and 2C genes are associated with loss of virulence, but virulence can be restored if genes from the wild-type virus are reintroduced.[122] Cell culture-adapted HAV rarely produces a cytopathic effect, although cytopathic strains have been isolated and serve as a useful model for laboratory studies.[88,272]

The HAV virion appears to be extremely stable, although the molecular determinants of this characteristic are not known. HAV is stable in the environment, with only a 100-fold decline in infectivity when it is stored for longer than 4 weeks at room temperature.[87,246,247,294] The virus retains infectivity even when treated with nonionic detergents, organic solvents, and low pH at 38°C (100.4°F) for 90 minutes.[87,256] HAV is more resistant than poliovirus to heat in that it is inactivated only partially at 60°C (140°F) for 1 hour.[87] Temperatures of 85° to 95°C (185°F–203°F) for 1 minute are required for complete inactivation of HAV in foods such as shellfish.[87,257] HAV is also completely inactivated by formalin (0.02% at 37°C [98.6°F] for 72 hours) but appears to be relatively resistant to free chlorine, especially when the virus is associated with organic matter.[235,339] For general-purpose disinfection, a 1 : 100 dilution of 5% sodium hypochlorite (i.e., household bleach) in tap water inactivates HAV in most situations.[61,130,131]

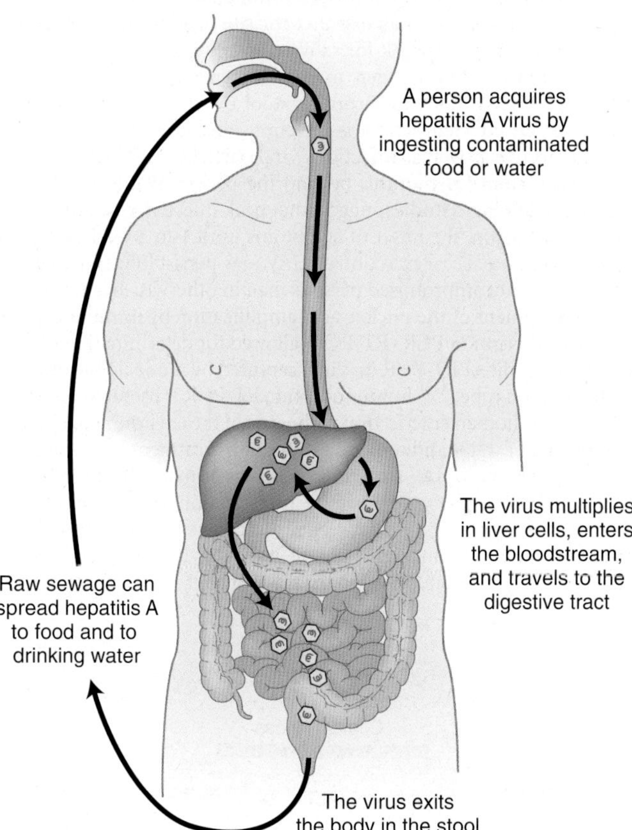

FIG. 168.2 Transmission of hepatitis A.

EPIDEMIOLOGY

Routes of Transmission

Routes of HAV transmission are determined by the timing and location of virus replication, circulation, and excretion during infection. HAV replicates in the liver, is excreted in bile, and is found in highest concentration in stool (up to 10^8 infectious particles per milliliter).[363] The highest concentration in stool occurs during the 2-week period before jaundice develops or liver enzymes become elevated, followed by a rapid decline after jaundice appears (Fig. 168.2).[133,346,363] Children and infants may shed HAV for longer periods than adults. Through the use of polymerase chain reaction (PCR) platforms to amplify viral nucleic acid, HAV RNA has been detected in the stool of infected neonates for as long as 6 months after infection, and some studies have shown excretion in older children and adults 1 to 3 months after the onset of clinical illness.[176,318,420] Chronic shedding of HAV does not occur, although virus may be detectable in stool during relapsing illness (see the section on relapsing hepatitis A).[345] Viremia occurs during the prodromal stage of infection and extends through the period of liver transaminase elevation (Fig. 168.3), with serum viral load several orders of magnitude lower than those in stool.[42,76,208,222,225] In experimentally infected animals, HAV can be detected in saliva during periods of peak excretion in stool.[76] HAV also has been detected in the saliva of infected humans with concurrent HAV viremia through HAV RNA with identical serum and saliva sequences.[233] This method is recommended for investigation of outbreaks.[6,7] The saliva as an extrahepatic site of early HAV replication could create a potential risk for saliva-transmitted infection.[5]

Detection of HAV antigen in stool by enzyme immunoassay or detection of HAV RNA in serum or stool by PCR does not demonstrate that an infected person is infectious, because these assays may detect defective as well as infectious viral particles. HAV RNA may be detected in stool for months, beyond the period of infectivity. Data from epidemiologic studies suggest that peak infectivity occurs during the 2 weeks before the onset of symptoms until 1 to 2 weeks after the onset of jaundice. Fecal excretion of HAV may persist longer in children and in immunocompromised persons than in otherwise healthy adults. The development of the nucleic acid amplification by immunocapture reverse transcription PCR (RT-PCR) allowed for determination of viral infectivity by direct RT-PCR on virus captured by monoclonal antibody in the reaction tube.[45,191] Immunocapture RT-PCR is useful to assess the infectivity of human enteric viral pathogens in the environment to aid in monitoring of water and food quality and for treatment processes.[184,316]

Not surprisingly, HAV transmission occurs primarily by the fecal-oral route, usually by person-to-person transmission in households and extended-family settings and between sexual contacts.[352] Person-to-person transmission results in high rates of infection in young children in developing countries and has been the predominant mode of transmission in the United States, particularly during community-wide outbreaks, as well as in outbreaks in childcare centers.[25,27,37] HAV in feces has been shown to be infectious even after being dried and stored for 1 month, and extremely stable in the environment as previously discussed.[247,87,246,247,294] Fecal contamination of food or water can result in common-source outbreaks. HAV has been transmitted by transfusion, but such transmission occurs rarely because the blood donation must occur during the early prodromal stage of the disease or from an asymptomatic person who is viremic.[221,224] In the United States, PCR is applied to screening of source plasma used for the manufacture of plasma-derived products. These assays are sufficiently sensitive to remove most units that have HAV, and serosurveillance for HAV infections among recipients receiving blood products in the United States indicates that HAV infections are now rare.[50,57]

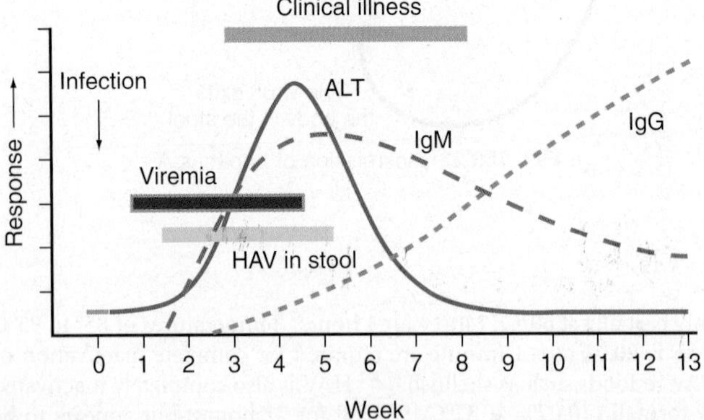

FIG. 168.3 Immunologic, virologic, and biochemical events during the course of a typical hepatitis A virus *(HAV)* infection. *ALT,* Alanine transaminase; *IgG,* immunoglobulin G; *IgM,* immunoglobulin M.

The risk for transmission to newborns by pregnant women with HAV appears to be low, although data are scarce.[71,310,] Most infants born to mothers with HAV infection were not affected and had normal antibody and transaminase levels.[262,327,371] A couple case reports have described vertical HAV transmission associated with jaundice and raised liver enzymes during the first weeks of life with uneventful improvement.[124,310] Newborns who acquire HAV infection perinatally or from a transfusion usually are asymptomatic, and the infection is detected by the development of hepatitis A in hospital staff or other persons having contact with the infant.[318,400] Two published case reports have described intrauterine transmission of HAV during the first trimester that resulted in fetal meconium peritonitis.[218,248] After delivery, both infants were found to have a perforated ileum. Another study in Korea of 12 pregnant women with HAV included 1 case of fetal ascites and intraabdominal calcification suggestive of meconium peritonitis which spontaneously resolved in serial sonographic imaging, and 1 case of confirmed vertical transmission in 2009.[71]

Although mothers infected with HAV can have anti-HAV immunoglobulin (Ig)M and IgG antibodies and HAV RNA in their breast milk,[90,96] transmission by breast milk has not been demonstrated.[96]

Patterns of Disease Worldwide

Worldwide, the endemicity of HAV infection differs markedly among and within countries (Fig. 168.4).[182] Patterns of HAV infection can be differentiated, each being characterized by distinct age-specific profiles of prevalence of antibody to HAV (anti-HAV), incidence of hepatitis A, and prevailing environmental (hygienic and sanitary) and socioeconomic conditions.[23,27,157,159,181,182]

In areas with a high endemic pattern of infection, represented by the least developed countries (i.e., parts of Africa, Asia, and Central and South America), poor socioeconomic conditions allow HAV to spread readily (see Fig. 168.4). Most persons are infected as young children, and essentially the entire population is infected before reaching adolescence, as demonstrated by the age-specific prevalence of anti-HAV (Fig. 168.5).[22,84,181,333,377] Because virtually all HAV infections occur in age groups in which asymptomatic infection predominates, reported disease rates may be low and outbreaks rare.

In areas of intermediate endemicity, HAV is not transmitted as readily because of better sanitary and living conditions, and the predominant age at infection is older than that in highly endemic areas.[73,181] Paradoxically, the overall incidence and average age of reported cases often increase because high levels of virus circulate in a population that includes many susceptible older children, adolescents, and young adults, in whom symptoms are likely to develop with HAV infection.[155] Large common-source outbreaks also can occur because of the relatively high rate of virus transmission and the large number of susceptible persons, especially among those of higher socioeconomic levels. Such an outbreak occurred in Shanghai in the late 1980s, with more than 300,000 cases associated with the consumption of contaminated clams.[160] Nonetheless, person-to-person transmission in community-wide epidemics continues to account for much of the disease in these countries.[391]

Considerable hepatitis A-related morbidity and associated costs can occur. A study at a tertiary care referral hospital in Karachi, Pakistan, identified 2735 patients younger than 15 years with confirmed hepatitis A during a 9-year period (1991–98). Of the 2735 patients, 232 were

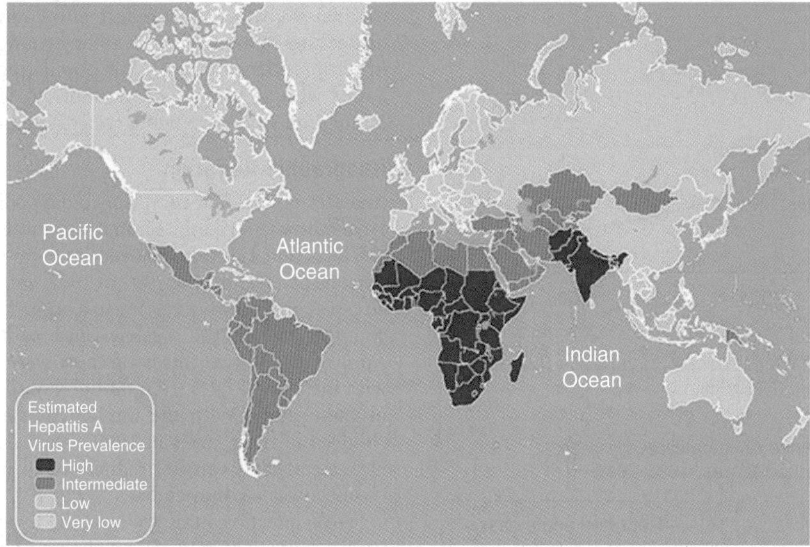

FIG. 168.4 Estimated geographic distribution of patterns of endemicity of hepatitis A virus infection.

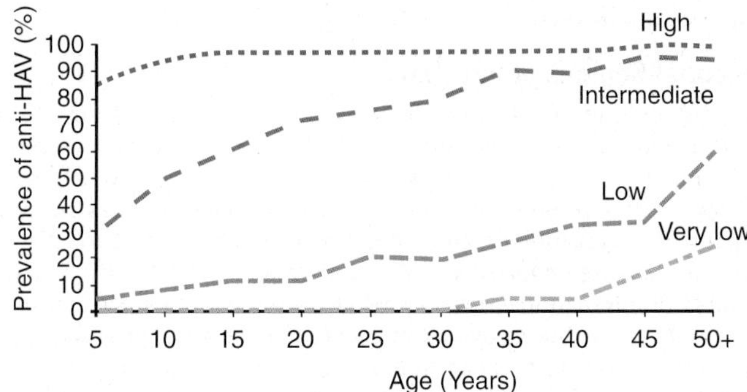

FIG. 168.5 Distinct age-specific profiles of prevalence of antibody to hepatitis A virus (anti-HAV).

admitted to the hospital, and 30 patients (1%) developed progressive hepatic dysfunction and liver failure.[329] In one Korean hospital, 304 patients older than 18 years were admitted from 2009 to 2011 with acute hepatitis A. Of those 304 patients, 18 (5.9%) progressed to acute liver failure, eight (2.6%) of whom died or underwent liver transplantation.[340]

In most areas of North America and Western Europe, sanitary and hygienic conditions are such that the endemicity of HAV infection is low. Relatively fewer children are infected, and disease often occurs in the context of community-wide and childcare-center outbreaks and occasionally as common-source outbreaks.[26,27,149,302,330,331,366] In some regions (e.g., Scandinavia), the endemicity of HAV infection is very low and disease occurs almost exclusively in defined risk groups, such as travelers returning from areas where HAV infection is endemic or illicit drug users.[40]

Changes have occurred in the epidemiologic trends and patterns of hepatitis A infection around the world related to vaccine A implementation, socioeconomic progress, and improvement in hygiene measures.[182,196,210,216,214,260,378]

Systematic review and meta-analysis of published data using IgG anti-HAV seroprevalence data between 1990 and 2005 from different world regions indicated that high-income regions (i.e., Western Europe, Australia, New Zealand, Canada, the United States, Japan, the Republic of Korea, and Singapore) remain as having very low HAV endemicity levels and a high proportion of susceptible adults. The low-income regions (i.e., sub-Saharan Africa and parts of South Asia) still present high endemicity levels and almost no susceptible adolescents and adults, and most middle-income regions (i.e., Asia, Latina America, Eastern Europe, and the Middle East) demonstrated a mix of intermediate and low endemicity levels.[182]

Patterns of Disease in the United States

The epidemiology of hepatitis A in the United States has been altered profoundly by the introduction of hepatitis A vaccines, with a significant reduction as a vaccine-preventable infectious disease (Fig. 168.6A). Rates have declined sharply since the mid-1990s. The rate of HAV disease was less than one case per 100,000 population in all age groups starting in 2009.[264] In 2010, 1670 cases were reported to the Centers for Disease Control and Prevention (CDC), representing a 94% decline in contrast to rates from 1990 to 1997 and significantly lower than previous incidence nadirs.[64,65,67,68] Numbers of acute cases reported to CDC further decreased to 1239 in 2014. However, national surveillance systems collect data on symptomatic cases, and incidence models indicate that most infections are not symptomatic. One such analysis estimated that an average of 271,000 infections occurred per year during 1980 to 1999—10.4 times the reported number of symptomatic cases.[12] With use of similar modeling methodology, an estimated 17,000 infections occurred in 2010 (see Fig. 168.6B).[55,66]

Variation by Age and Race or Ethnicity

Historically, the highest hepatitis A rates were reported among children 5 to 14 years of age, with approximately one third of cases occurring in children younger than 15 years.[62] Because many young children have unrecognized or asymptomatic infection, they also are likely to represent a major reservoir for HAV transmission. Incidence models indicated that during the 1980s and 1990s, more than half of HAV infections occurred among children younger than 10 years, most of whom were younger than 4 years.[12] Since the mid-1990s, decreases in rates among children have been greater than among adults, and the proportion of cases among children dropped from 35% in the prevaccine era to 19% in 2003.[399]

From 2002 to 2010, rates were similar and low among persons in all age groups (<1.0 cases/100,000 population). In 2010, the range was from 0.23 to 0.74 cases per 100,000 population.[64,65,67,68] The highest rates were for persons 15 to 24 years of age (0.74 cases per 100,000 population) and the lowest rates were among children younger than 9 years (0.3 cases/100,000 population).[64,67] Since then, the percentage of patients with acute hepatitis A in the United States who were 0 to 19 years of age has steadily decreased to 11.10% in 2013, with the highest percentage continuing to be the 20- to 59-year age group (65.26%).[230,231]

Before the use of hepatitis A vaccine, rates among Native Americans and Alaska Natives were more than 10 times higher than other racial and ethnic groups, and rates among Hispanics were approximately three

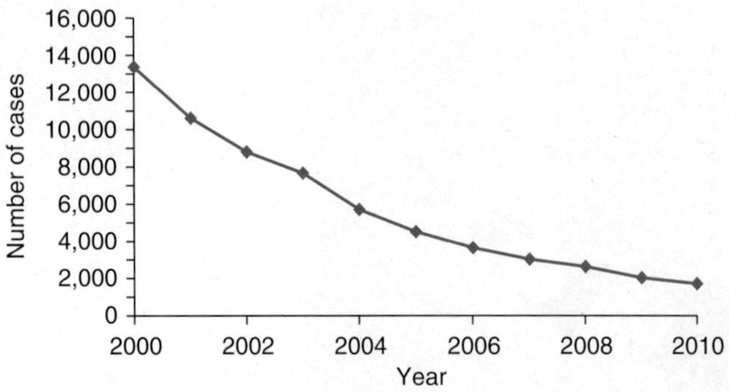

A Source: National Notifiable Diseases Surveillance System (NNDSS)

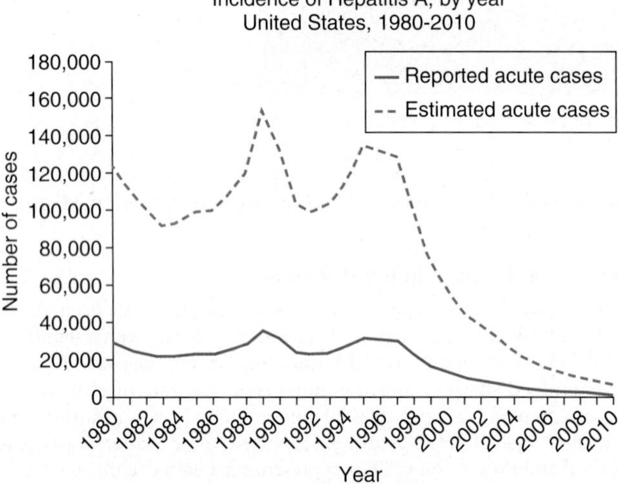

B Source: http://www.cdc.gov/hepatitis/HAV/HAVfaq.htm

FIG. 168.6 (A) Reported number of hepatitis A cases, United States, 2000–10. (B) Hepatitis A incidence rates (per 100,000 population) based on cases reported to the Centers for Disease Control and Prevention (1980–2010). (A, Courtesy National Notifiable Diseases Surveillance System (NNDSS) of the Centers for Disease Control and Prevention. Available at: https://www.cdc.gov/hepatitis/statistics/2010surveillance/slide2.1.htm.)

times higher than among non-Hispanics. These disparities have lessened or disappeared in the era of routine childhood vaccination, with rates among Hispanics in 2003 dropping to approximately twice those among non-Hispanics (86% decline in contrast to 1990–97); rates among Native Americans and Alaska Natives were the same as or lower than those among other ethnic groups.[399] In 2010, the rate for hepatitis A among Hispanics was 0.7 cases per 100,000 population, the lowest rate ever reported for this group.[264] Rates among Native Americans and Alaska Natives in 2010 were the lowest ever recorded (0.2/100,000 population) and the same as or lower than other ethnic groups.[64,67]

Seroprevalence of antibody to HAV (anti-HAV) in the population reflects immunity to either previous infection or vaccination. As determined by the National Health and Nutrition Examination Survey (NHANES), the overall seroprevalence of anti-HAV in the United States was 34.9% from 1999 to 2006.[199,201] HAV seroprevalence among children has increased from 8% in 1988–94 to 35.3% in 2007–08, reflecting increased immunization of children and others.[253] For US-born children 6 to 19 years of age, the strongest factor associated with seroprevalence was residence in vaccinating states. Among US-born adults aged older than 19 years, the overall age-adjusted seroprevalence of anti-HAV was 29.9% during 1999–2006, which was not significantly different from the seroprevalence during 1988–94.[199,201] Among US-born adults 40 years of age and older, HAV antibody prevalence decreased from 1988–94 to 2003–06, which may reflect lower rates of infection secondary to higher rates of immunization among younger age groups.[253] The decrease in seroprevalence in the adult population reflects the replacement of adults who were exposed naturally to HAV in the past by an adult population who were neither vaccinated nor previously exposed.[167]

Geographic Variation

Analyses of national surveillance data collected during the 1980s and 1990s showed striking regional variation in the incidence of hepatitis A. The national average incidence was approximately 10 cases per 100,000 persons per year during 1987 to 1997, with the highest rates and almost all cases consistently occurring in a limited number of states and counties concentrated in the western and southwestern United States.[54,63] Approximately two thirds of cases were reported from the 17 states with the highest rates, even though only one third of US residents lived in these states. With the implementation of routine vaccination of children in these states in 1999, rates equalized across the country,[399] with significantly greater reductions in incidence in areas where vaccination was recommended.[264,105,322,399]

HAV infection rates are now the lowest ever reported and similar in all regions. The rate of acute hepatitis A declined from 1.5 cases per 100,000 population to 0.54 per 100,000 population from 2005 to 2010.[64,67]

In 2010, the case rate ranged from 0.1 case per 100,000 population (Arkansas, Mississippi, and South Dakota) to 1.0 case per 100,000 population (Arizona).[65,68]

Potential Sources of Infection

The distribution of potential HAV exposures among cases for which information regarding exposures is available has changed in the vaccination era. The proportion of cases attributable to household or sexual contact with a person who has hepatitis A has declined as routine hepatitis A vaccination of children has increased, from 15% to 25% to 5.6% to 7.3% of reported cases in 2009 and 2010.[56-58,60,64,65,67,68] The number of international travel–associated cases has remained approximately the same, but as overall incidence declined, the proportion of cases attributable to this exposure has risen to 14% to 15% reported in 2009–10.[64,65,67,68] In sites conducting enhanced hepatitis surveillance during 2005–07 as part of the Emerging Infection Program of the CDC, the most frequent (46%) potential source of infection among persons reported with HAV disease was travel outside of the United States and Canada. These cases mostly reflected persons who traveled, but also included some who were exposed to a traveler but did not travel themselves.[200] As in previous years, most travel-related cases (85%) were associated with travel to Mexico, Central America, and South America.[200,333]

Recognized foodborne outbreaks account for a small proportion of cases in most years (3–5%), but large outbreaks such as those associated with contaminated green onions in 2003 have increased the proportion of cases associated with food in some years to as high as 16%.[10,56-58,60,404,406] In 2010, the linkage to an outbreak could be determined in only 10% of the reported cases for which this information was available.[65,68]

Cyclic outbreaks occur among men who have sex with men (MSM) and users of injecting and noninjecting drugs; during outbreak years, this exposure can account for 10% to 15% of nationally reported cases.[58,60,83,142,162,171,323]

In 2010, only 5% of the case reports with information available about sexual practices indicated sex with another man and only 2% reported use of injection drugs.[65,68] Nearly 50% of patients with hepatitis A do not have a recognized source of infection.[57,58,60,64,65,67,68]

Community-Wide Epidemic

Historically, most cases of hepatitis A in the United States occurred in the context of community-wide epidemics, during which infection is transmitted from person to person in households and extended-family settings.[26] Once initiated, these epidemics often persisted for several years and proved difficult to control[289,336,337] even when attempts were made to vaccinate some portion of the population rapidly.[16,86] Children played an important role in HAV transmission during these epidemics. During community-wide outbreaks, serologic studies of members of households with an adult case and no identified source found that 25% to 40% of contacts younger than 6 years had serologic evidence of having had recent HAV infection.[313,352] In one of these studies, 52% of households of adults without an identified source of infection included a child younger than 6 years, and the presence of a young child was associated with household transmission of HAV.[352] In this study, transmission chains were identified involving as many as six generations and more than 20 cases. With the advent of routine vaccination of children, community-wide outbreaks have largely ceased. Community-wide outbreaks that have been sustained by transmission among adults in high-risk groups continue to be identified, and novel strategies to provide vaccination in settings such as jails have had some success.[56,58,267,279,368,395]

Epidemiology of Hepatitis A in Specific Settings

Childcare Centers

The role of children with asymptomatic infection has been recognized in outbreaks in childcare centers since the 1970s.[330-332] Because infection in children usually is mild or asymptomatic, these outbreaks often are not recognized until adult contacts (usually parents) become ill.[158,159] Outbreaks rarely occur in centers that do not have children in diapers and occur more commonly in larger centers.[158,159] Both poor hygiene in these children and the need for staff to handle and change diapers contribute to spread. Despite the occurrence of outbreaks when HAV is introduced into a childcare center, studies of childcare center employees do not show a significantly increased prevalence of HAV infection in contrast to control populations.[140,180] On occasion, outbreaks in childcare centers can be the source of more extensive transmission within a community.[104,157,158,387] Hepatitis A outbreaks within childcare centers have become unusual events in recent years, as routine vaccination of all young children is the standard.

Other Groups and Settings

Hepatitis A cases in school-age children usually reflect disease that has been acquired in the community. However, multiple cases among children within a school may indicate a common-source outbreak.[172] Historically, HAV infection was endemic in institutions for the developmentally disabled; however, with smaller facilities and improved conditions, the incidence and prevalence of infection have decreased, and outbreaks rarely are reported in the United States.[357]

During the past 2 decades, outbreaks have been reported with increasing frequency in illicit drug users in North America, Australia, and Europe.[52,162,171,173,279,323,337,368,395] In the United States, these frequently involve users of injected and noninjected methamphetamine, who may account for as many as 30% of reported cases in these communities during outbreaks.[26,171,173,267,395] Cross-sectional serologic surveys have demonstrated that injection drug users have a higher prevalence of anti-HAV than the general US population.[178,393] More recent survey of 520 injection drug users age 18 to 40 years in San Diego from 2009 to 2010 found that 63% had no detectable anti-HAV antibodies,[78] suggesting that more aggressive implementation of the hepatitis A vaccine program is needed in this high-risk group.

Transmission among injection drug users probably occurs through both percutaneous and fecal-oral routes.[173]

Hepatitis A outbreaks in MSM have been reported frequently, most recently in urban areas in the United States, Canada, Europe, and Australia.[38,50,83,142,328,355,373,374] These outbreaks may occur in the context of an outbreak in the larger community.[26] Some studies conducted during outbreaks and seroprevalence surveys among MSM identified specific sex practices associated with illness, whereas others have not demonstrated such associations.[30,83,85,165,192,393]

Transfusion-related hepatitis A rarely occurs because HAV does not result in chronic infection and blood donors are screened for elevated transaminase levels. Currently, nucleic acid amplification tests also are used to screen source plasma used in the manufacture of plasma-derived products. However, during the mid-1990s, outbreaks were reported in Europe and the United States in patients who received factor VIII and factor IX concentrates prepared by solvent-detergent treatment to inactivate lipid-containing viruses.[238,349] HAV is resistant to solvent-detergent treatment, and contamination presumably occurred from plasma donors with hepatitis A who donated during the incubation period. The risk for acquiring infection in patients with hemophilia is not known, although data from one serologic survey of hemophiliac patients suggested that they might be at increased risk for acquisition of HAV infection.[234] However, no HAV infections attributed to blood products were identified in an analysis of serosurveillance data collected from 140 hemophilia treatment centers in the United States between 1998 and 2002, suggesting that improved viral inactivation procedures, donor screening, and increased hepatitis A vaccine coverage among clotting factor recipients can reduce the risk for transmission of HAV to recipients of clotting factors.[50,57] Transmission related to blood transfusions has resulted in nosocomial outbreaks in neonatal intensive care units.[198,277,318] Hepatitis A has been reported in adult cancer patients treated with lymphocytes that apparently were incubated in serum from a donor with HAV infection, although the patient source was not identified.[402]

Nosocomial transmission from adult patients to health care workers has often been associated with fecal incontinence of the patient.[153,287,288] Such transmission is a rare event, however, because most patients with hepatitis A are hospitalized after the onset of jaundice, when infectivity is low.[130,131,346] Health care workers have not been found to have an increased prevalence of anti-HAV in contrast to control populations in serologic surveys conducted in the United States.[148]

Persons from developed countries who travel to developing countries with a high, transitional, or intermediate endemicity of HAV infection are at substantial risk for acquiring hepatitis A (see Fig. 168.4).[182,333,354]

Hepatitis A infection is one of the most common vaccine-preventable infections acquired during travel.[333] A more recent study of Swiss travelers estimated the risk to be six to 30 cases per 100,000 person-months of stay in developing countries among persons who did not receive immunoglobulin or vaccine before departure.[266] The risk is higher among travelers staying in areas with poor hygienic conditions,[211] it varies according to the region and the length of stay, and it appears to be increased even among travelers who reported staying in urban areas or luxury hotels.[333,354] In some European countries, returning international travelers with hepatitis A account for a substantial proportion of reported cases (16–40%).[72,410] In the United States, the proportion of cases attributed to recent international travel has increased from 5% to 15%.[64,65,67,68]

The potential for new foodborne outbreaks around the world has been enhanced with the world globalization by importation of food products from countries where hepatitis A remains endemic to countries with low endemicity. This has been nicely demonstrated during recent outbreak investigations of hepatitis A infection, including the multistate outbreak associated with semidried tomatoes in Australia during 2009[113] and similar outbreaks in the Netherlands[296,297] and France during 2010.[146]

Foodborne hepatitis A outbreaks are now recognized relatively infrequently in the United States and are associated most commonly with contamination of food during preparation by a food handler with HAV infection. However, persons who work as food handlers are not at increased risk for acquiring hepatitis A because of their occupation. Food contaminated before retail distribution, such as lettuce or fruits contaminated at the growing or processing stage, has been recognized as the source of hepatitis A outbreaks.[10,101,103,172,275,309,317,406] Outbreaks related to contaminated shellfish, commonly noted in the past,[103,108,282,301] have become increasingly uncommon.[31] After the large multistate outbreaks linked to oysters in 2005,[31,101,404,406] another large outbreak of occurred United States in 2013 associated with frozen pomegranate arils imported from Turkey. A total of 165 people from 10 states became ill with hepatitis A genotype IB, 69 (42%) of whom required hospitalization, but no deaths were reported.[79] Waterborne transmission of HAV is now rare in the United States; earlier outbreaks were linked to sewage contamination or inadequate treatment of water.[29,36,41,46,98,143,235,398] In 2014, 13 (2.6%) of 500 case reports linked to an outbreak indicated exposure that may have been linked to a common-source foodborne or waterborne outbreak.[66,69,264]

Control of food outbreaks usually requires intensive public health effort.[93] HAV foodborne disease investigation with direct food testing through HAV RNA molecular techniques has made the recovery of implicated food faster and more efficient.[31] Molecular epidemiology through sequencing of outbreak strains has been demonstrated to be an excellent tool for the investigation of HAV infection outbreaks within the United States and European countries.[31,113,146,167,296,374]

PATHOLOGY AND PATHOGENESIS

Pathology

The light microscopic findings in acute hepatitis A, which include inflammatory cell infiltration, hepatocellular necrosis, and liver cell regeneration, are common to all forms of acute viral hepatitis. These histologic findings vary with the stage and severity of hepatitis. Early biopsy specimens generally show portal infiltration by lymphocytes, plasma cells, and macrophages positive for periodic acid–Schiff.[109,365] Spotty or focal necrosis, as evidenced by balloon degeneration, shrinkage, and fragmentation of hepatocytes, is seen commonly.[109] HAV antigen is found primarily in the cytoplasm of hepatocytes, but it also can be found in liver macrophages. However, because HAV infection is self-limited and does not result in chronic liver disease, liver biopsy rarely is indicated (see the discussion on treatment).

Differences have been noted in light microscopic findings of hepatitis A and other forms of viral hepatitis, particularly hepatitis B. In addition to degeneration of hepatocytes in the perivenular area, periportal inflammation and destruction of hepatocytes adjacent to the portal area may be more pronounced than in hepatitis B.[1,283,365] Findings in some patients, including extension of the inflammatory infiltration from the periportal area into the hepatic parenchyma and disruption of the limiting plate, may be difficult to distinguish from those of chronic hepatitis.[1,109] Cholestasis can be more prominent than in hepatitis B.[324]

The histologic findings in fulminant hepatitis A are indistinguishable from those in other forms of fulminant viral hepatitis. Examination of pathologic specimens shows massive hepatic necrosis, abnormal architecture of surviving hepatocytes, and a diffuse inflammatory response.[203,204] Viral antigen can be found in pathologic specimens.

Pathogenesis

The mechanism by which HAV crosses gastrointestinal epithelium and infects liver cells has not been completely established. Previous studies have shown that HAV-IgA complex can translocate across epithelial cells and that HAV-IgA complexes are taken up by hepatocytes through the asialoglycoprotein receptor.[114,115] In this model of HAV infection, virus would first infect gastrointestinal cells and then be transported into the enterohepatic circulation as part of an HAV-IgA complex, with subsequent selective uptake by hepatocytes. HAV is able to bind to human cells through a specific cellular receptor inserted into the plasma membrane, and DNA that encodes this receptor (huhavcr-1) has been identified in many human tissues.[132] HAVCR-1 was first discovered as the cellular receptor for HAV (HAVcr-1) in African green monkeys in 1996.[190] This cellular receptor is a member of the T-cell immunoglobulin mucin (TIM, also known as TIM-1) gene family. It appears to regulate the size and effector functions of T cells and also might play a role in the development of atopy.[249] The relationship of TIM1 and atopy with HAV exposure is important, and various epidemiologic studies around the world have shown lower prevalence of allergy and asthma among the HAV-seropositive individuals in contrast to HAV-seronegative individuals.[244,245] Immunoglobulin (Ig)A is a natural ligand of HAVCR-1, and the association of IgA with HAVCR1 enhances virus receptor activity with synergistic effect in virus-receptor interactions.[361]

HOST INNATE AND ADAPTIVE IMMUNE RESPONSES

Cellular Immune Response

Unlike other picornaviruses, infection of cultured cells with wild-type HAV has no cytopathic effect.[396] The general assumption is that HAV infection also is noncytopathic in vivo, and therefore the cytopathic changes in the liver associated with hepatitis A are immune mediated. HAV is able to suppress interferon (IFN)-β gene expression in the initial stages of infection, which might facilitate prolonged viral production and infection of neighboring cells.[134] This could be explained in part by a disruption in the signaling through the toll-like receptor 3 pathway.[242,306] A recent research study demonstrated that the interaction between HAV and its receptor HAVCR1 inhibits CD4 T-cell regulatory cell function, resulting in an immune imbalance allowing viral expansion with limited hepatocellular damage during the early phase of infection, which is characteristic of HAV infection.[237] Symptoms and biochemical evidence of liver injury do not occur at the time of maximum virus replication and fecal shedding (during the late incubation period). Rather, liver injury is associated closely with viral clearance. $CD8^+$, class 1-dependent, cytotoxic, and virus-specific T cells that are capable of producing IFN-γ are present in the circulation and the liver.[139,380] Additional inflammatory cells, recruited to the site of infection by IFN-γ and other cytokines secreted by $CD8^+$ cells, may be responsible for much of the liver injury. Complement has been shown to bind to HAV capsid proteins, and serum complement levels drop during infection, but whether complement-mediated cellular injury occurs is unclear.[241] The mechanism by which infection is resolved remains uncertain.

Humoral Immune Response

Unlike hepatitis C, the adaptive immune response to HAV is robust and extremely effective in eliminating the virus. Neutralizing antibodies to the virus (anti-HAV) generally appear in the serum concurrent with the earliest evidence of serum transaminase elevation and hepatocellular injury.

Antibodies directed against conformational epitopes displayed on intact virions as well as empty viral capsids are produced during the later stages of infection (see the earlier section on genomic organization and genetic variation). Virus-specific IgM and IgG and IgA antibodies are present in serum; IgM anti-HAV generally can be detected at the onset of symptoms (see Fig. 168.3).[242]

CLINICAL MANIFESTATIONS

Similar to other forms of viral hepatitis, the clinical manifestations of HAV infection are variable and range from asymptomatic anicteric infection to symptoms of acute hepatitis, including fever, malaise, anorexia, nausea, vomiting, right upper quadrant pain, and jaundice. The likelihood of having symptomatic HAV infection and the severity of the illness are related to the age of the patient. In early childhood, infection usually is asymptomatic, whereas infection in adulthood generally is accompanied by symptoms. The diagnosis of hepatitis A must be confirmed by serologic testing because no constellation of symptoms is pathognomonic of the disease.

Incubation Period

The average incubation period is 28 to 30 days but can range from 15 to 50 days.[206] The average incubation period has been reported to be shorter in patients who acquired HAV infection by parenteral transmission from contaminated blood products and in chimpanzees infected parenterally than in those infected orogastrically.[241,338]

Spectrum of Illness

HAV infection, confirmed by the detection of IgM anti-HAV in serum, can be inapparent (asymptomatic, with no elevation in serum transaminase levels), subclinical (asymptomatic, with elevation of serum transaminase levels), or clinically evident (with symptoms). Specific symptoms of liver dysfunction include jaundice and dark urine caused by hyperbilirubinemia. However, symptomatic hepatitis A without jaundice (anicteric) does occur. Nonspecific symptoms of acute hepatitis A can include fever, myalgia, anorexia, nausea, right upper quadrant pain or discomfort, diarrhea, and pruritus.

Many acute HAV infections, particularly subclinical and anicteric infection, are not recognized[352,418] The frequency of symptoms with acute infection is influenced strongly by age. Children are less likely than adults to have symptomatic infection, and jaundice rarely occurs in children younger than 6 years.[151] In one report describing outbreaks in several daycare centers, the proportion of infected children without symptoms was 84% in children younger than 3 years, 50% in children 3 to 4 years of age, and 20% in children 5 years or older.[158,159] Symptoms develop in most adults with acute infection. In a study of two outbreaks among young adult US military personnel, symptoms developed in 76% to 97% of infected persons, and approximately 55% were icteric.[213]

CLINICAL SIGNS AND SYMPTOMS

In an individual patient, the clinical symptoms of acute hepatitis A are indistinguishable from those caused by other forms of viral hepatitis. Particularly in older children and adults, the onset of illness often is quite abrupt and may consist of fever, myalgia, anorexia, malaise, nausea, intermittent dull abdominal pain, and vomiting. Fever (temperature rarely higher than 38.9°C [102°F]) and headache occur more frequently than in other forms of acute viral hepatitis.[358] Pediatric patients may have diarrhea or, less commonly, upper respiratory tract symptoms such as cough, sore throat, and runny nose, and the diagnosis of hepatitis A might not be considered in children with predominantly respiratory or gastrointestinal symptoms and transient fever without the typical malaise, fatigue, and anorexia.[138,219,225] Dark urine followed by jaundice and light-colored stool, if present, will appear within a few days to a week after onset of the prodromal symptoms.[28,156,213,219,225] When this icteric phase begins, symptoms often resolve and appetite returns in young children, but older children and adult patients may experience a transient worsening in the prodromal symptoms of anorexia, malaise, and weakness.[205,263]

In addition to jaundice and scleral icterus, physical findings may include mild hepatomegaly and tenderness, but severe tenderness suggests other diagnoses. The spleen may be palpable in 10% to 20% of patients, and posterior cervical adenopathy may be present.[75,213,372] Pleural effusions have been reported to occur, do not appear to be associated with more severe disease, and resolve spontaneously.[4] Ascites, peripheral edema, and findings indicative of hepatic encephalopathy suggest the presence of a more severe form of hepatitis but are rare (see the discussion on atypical clinical manifestations and complications of hepatitis A). Ultrasonographic findings in children with uncomplicated hepatitis A have included edema or thickening of the gallbladder wall, abdominal lymphadenopathy, and, less commonly, transient ascites and pancreatic abnormalities.[75,197]

The symptoms of hepatitis A last for several weeks on average and usually not longer than 2 months.[203,204] Prolonged or relapsing hepatitis A can occur (see the discussion on relapsing hepatitis A) and, in the case of prolonged hepatitis A, may be associated with genetic markers for autoimmune hepatitis.[128]

Laboratory Abnormalities

As in other forms of viral hepatitis, during HAV infection, inflammation of the liver is accompanied by abnormalities in serum hepatic enzymes, with increases in serum aspartate transaminase (AST), alkaline phosphatase, and γ-glutamyltranspeptidase (GGTP) levels. Elevations of serum ALT and AST occur most consistently and may precede the appearance of symptoms by a week or more (see Fig. 168.3). Peak levels generally occur 3 to 10 days after the onset of symptoms and are between 200 and 5000 IU but can reach as high as 20,000 IU. The level of ALT usually is higher than that of AST because the inflammatory response is destructive, particularly to the plasma membrane, in acute viral hepatitis. ALT is found in the cytosol of the plasma membrane, whereas AST is located mainly in cell mitochondria.[156]

Serum bilirubin levels, although frequently elevated, usually remain below 10 mg/dL and peak 1 to 2 weeks after illness begins. Higher levels can be seen in some patients, especially when HAV infection is complicated by cholestasis (see the section on cholestatic hepatitis A). Alkaline phosphatase is usually only mildly elevated, rarely reaching more than 2 or 3 times the normal level. GGTP levels generally are 3 to 10 times the upper limit of normal. Serum immunoglobulin levels often are elevated, and IgM levels frequently are higher than those in acute hepatitis B and non-A, non-B hepatitis, but not diagnostic.[422] Coagulopathy or elevated prothrombin time (PT)/ international normalized ratio (INR) are rare. A prolongation of these labs are generally associated with severe liver damage and a prognostic indicator for the development of fulminant hepatitis.[414]

Patients with acute HAV infection usually have a mild lymphocytosis with occasional atypical mononuclear cells.[263]

Apart from patients who have relapsing or cholestatic hepatitis A (see the section on atypical clinical manifestations and complications of hepatitis A), serum bilirubin and transaminase levels usually return to normal by 2 to 3 months after the onset of illness in most patients.[203,204]

Diagnostic Tests

Because the pattern and magnitude of symptoms and the hepatic enzyme abnormalities of hepatitis A are not distinctive for hepatitis A, the diagnosis requires serologic detection of IgM anti-HAV along with demonstration of an acute onset of signs and symptoms of hepatitis and jaundice or elevated transaminase levels. Persons with signs and symptoms of hepatitis and an epidemiologic link to other confirmed cases are likely to have hepatitis A, even if no laboratory confirmation is available. Sensitive and specific radioimmunoassays or enzyme immunoassays show that virtually all patients have detectable IgM anti-HAV during the acute or early convalescent phase of HAV infection (see Fig. 168.3).[227] A small proportion (3%) of patients tested within 3 days of the onset of symptoms may be IgM anti-HAV negative but become IgM anti-HAV positive within the initial 2 weeks of illness.[227] During the first 4 to 8 weeks after the onset of symptoms, the titer of IgM anti-HAV in serum is high.[163] Antibody generally disappears within 6 months, although rarely it can be detected for 2 years or longer.[111,163,202,227]

False-positive IgM anti-HAV test results among persons who have no other evidence of recent infection have been reported, suggesting a low positive predictive value when it is used to test asymptomatic persons with no known recent HAV exposures.[54,58,59,63] IgM anti-HAV may be detectable for a longer time in patients with symptomatic illness than in those with asymptomatic infection.[163,189,347]

IgG anti-HAV is present in low titer at or shortly after the onset of acute HAV infection, and the titer rises during the course of several weeks as the IgM anti-HAV titer falls (see Fig. 168.3). IgG anti-HAV remains detectable in serum for the lifetime of the individual and confers lasting protection against disease. Secretory IgA antibodies are detected in a minority of humans or primates with acute HAV infection but are unlikely to provide any significant protection against HAV infection.[353] IgG anti-HAV is transferred passively across the placenta and declines to undetectable levels in most infants by the time they reach 12 to 15 months of age.[25,26,228,229]

Commercially available enzyme immunoassays either detect total (IgG and IgM) antibody against HAV capsid proteins by using a competitive inhibition (blocking) format or detect IgM antibody to capsid proteins by using an IgM capture format.[220,223] These assays do not measure the neutralizing antibodies responsible for biologic activity against HAV, but detection of total anti-HAV by conventional assays is correlated with the appearance of neutralizing antibodies.[205,220,223] Neutralizing antibody can be detected by assays that measure inhibition of HAV in cell culture (i.e., radioimmunofocus inhibition test or plaque assay).[11,88,220,223] Neutralizing antibodies elicited against one strain of HAV have been shown to have biologic activity against other HAV strains.[220,223]

When tested in parallel with a World Health Organization anti-HAV reference reagent, the lower limit of detection of most commercially available assays is approximately 100 mIU/mL of anti-HAV.[147,220,223] Although antibody concentrations achieved by passive or active immunization are known to provide protection against HAV infection, they are generally 10- to 100-fold lower than those produced after natural infection.[220,223]

The lower limit of antibody necessary to provide protection against HAV infection is unknown. In vitro studies with cell culture–derived virus suggest that low levels of antibody (e.g., <20 mIU/mL) are neutralizing.[220,223] Clinical trials that evaluated vaccine efficacy have not provided an estimate of the minimum protective antibody level because vaccine-induced levels of antibody have been very high and few infections have occurred in vaccines. Experimental studies in chimpanzees indicate that very low levels of passively transferred antibody (<10 mIU/mL) obtained from immunized individuals do not protect against infection but prevent clinical hepatitis and shedding of virus.[305]

PCR techniques using serum specimens have been useful in some clinical, epidemiologic, or environmental studies. Although HAV concentrations in stool decline quickly after illness onset, HAV RNA can be detected in most serum specimens that are collected within 4 to 6 weeks after onset of illness.[42]

BOX 168.1 Atypical Clinical Manifestations and Complications of Hepatitis A Virus Infection

Relapsing hepatitis A[152,325,370]
Fulminant hepatitis A[243,280,308,369]
Cholestatic hepatitis A[154,370]
Hepatitis A triggering autoimmune hepatitis[370,388]
Extrahepatic manifestations
Transient rash or arthralgias[150,370]
Papular acrodermatitis of childhood[305]
Cutaneous vasculitis[94,174,175]
Cryoglobulinemia[174,175,325]
Guillain-Barré acute syndrome[359]
Other neurologic syndromes (e.g., myeloradiculopathy, mononeuritis, vertigo, meningoencephalitis)[19,39,359]
Renal syndromes (acute renal failure, nephritic syndrome, acute glomerulonephritis)[17,100,183]
Pancreatitis[259]
Aplastic anemia and thrombocytopenia[125,236]

Atypical Clinical Manifestations and Complications of Hepatitis A

Box 168.1 lists the atypical clinical manifestations and complications of hepatitis A.

Relapsing Hepatitis A

Relapsing hepatitis is a relatively common manifestation of hepatitis A that occurs in approximately 10% of patients.[325] One to 4 months after having the initial episode of acute hepatitis, these patients have a second episode; more than one relapse rarely occurs.[152,325,370] Patients with relapsing hepatitis A have no distinctive clinical features of their first disease episode. After the first episode, most patients experience a significant improvement in symptoms and biochemical abnormalities. However, the frequency with which serum transaminase levels completely normalize during this period has been variable; in one report, normalization occurred in only one of seven patients with relapsing hepatitis A.[370] The relapse episode of hepatitis rarely is more severe than the initial episode and is accompanied by elevated serum transaminase levels (typically to >1000 U/L) and persistence of IgM anti-HAV. Molecular studies have demonstrated the presence of HAV in stool and HAV RNA in serum during relapse, but whether patients are infectious is unknown.[152] The illness usually lasts a total of 16 to 40 weeks and results in full recovery.[152,325] Although the pathogenesis of relapsing hepatitis is unknown, it probably is immunologically mediated.[325] Persistent HAV infection with a relapsing clinical course has been reported in patients after they have undergone liver transplantation for fulminant hepatitis A; HAV-specific genomic sequences have been identified in the grafts of these patients.[127,414]

The IgA has been postulated as a carrier supporting hepatotropic transport of HAV, which may contribute to different clinical outcomes.[116] Over a period of several weeks after infection, anti-HAV IgA is able to promote an enterohepatic cycling of HAV, resulting in continuous endogenous reinfection of the liver. A mouse model demonstrated that highly avid IgG antibodies, which are present in later times of the infection, can terminate the reinfection. The endogenous reinfections in the presence of a developing neutralizing immunity might contribute to prolonged, as well as relapsing, courses of HAV infections, and the IgA may act as a protracting factor.[116]

Fulminant Hepatitis A

In the United States, a relatively small proportion of all fulminant hepatitis is caused by hepatitis A.[243,285,308,326,369] A prospective multicenter study conducted among 348 children with acute liver failure in the United States, Canada, and the United Kingdom found that only three cases (1%) could be attributed to hepatitis A.[351] However, 26% to 60% of children with acute liver failure had hepatitis A in tertiary care center–based studies conducted in Turkey, India, Argentina, and Pakistan.[15,18,21,329] In one Korean hospital, 304 patients more than 18 years of age were admitted from 2009 to 2011 with acute hepatitis A. Of those 304 patients, 18 (5.9%) progressed to liver failure, and of these, eight (2.6%) died or underwent liver transplantation.[340] Between 1998 and 2005, 29 adults with HAV IgM-positive acute liver failure were enrolled in the Acute Liver Failure Study Group (ALFSG) in the United States. Acute HAV accounted for 3.1% of the patients enrolled. At 3 weeks of follow-up, 16 had spontaneously recovered (55%), nine underwent transplantation (31%), and four had died (14%). The proportion of HAV cases enrolled in the ALFSG significantly decreased from 5% to 0.8% between 1988 and 2005 ($P < .007$).[364]

Among patients hospitalized with hepatitis A, the case-fatality rate has been estimated to be 0.14%.[252] In the 1988 Shanghai epidemic that involved primarily adolescents and young adults, 47 deaths (0.015%) were recorded among the 310,746 diagnosed cases.[80] A national cohort study in Taiwan looking at hospital admissions related to HAV from 1997 to 2011 showed an overall mortality rate of 16.8 per 1000 hospitalizations. Male sex, age over 40 years, cirrhotic liver, and long length of stay are significant factors associated with death in HAV-hospitalized cases.[70] On the basis of national surveillance data in the United States, death occurs in 0.3% to 0.6% of persons with symptomatic hepatitis A, reaching 1.8% among those over 50 years of age.[333] In 2013, nine (0.9%) cases of deaths related to HAV were reported to the CDC. None were reported in 2014.[65,68,69]

Host factors reported to be associated with an increased risk for development of fulminant hepatitis include older age[44,209,252,394,417] and underlying chronic liver disease.[3,95,193,224,389,394,415,417] Reported findings among persons with fulminant disease include nucleotide or amino acid substitutions in the 5′ untranslated region,[145] P2 region, and P3 region of the HAV genome.[270] Viral factors such as substitution rate in the entire genome were not associated with acute liver failure in the 29 patients identified with HAV liver failure in the adult ALFSG from 1998 to 2004; however, a negative PCR (undetectable or very low viral load) was the single factor that correlated more significantly with more severity and worse outcomes.[2] This finding has been previously described in the literature and suggests that the excessive host response maybe a determining factor in the development of fulminant hepatitis A.[311] An in-depth analysis conducted in India for a 5-year period concluded that higher CD8 T cells and coinfection with other viral hepatitis infections were more commonly associated with fulminant hepatitis; and, contrary to previous findings, higher viral load was also an important contributing factor.[170]

Fulminant hepatitis A has no distinctive clinical features that distinguish it from fulminant hepatic failure of other causes. Within approximately 8 weeks of the onset of illness, symptoms of hepatic encephalopathy and marked prolongation of PT are noted in patients with no history of previous liver disease.[281] Complications can include cerebral edema, sepsis, gastrointestinal bleeding, and hypoglycemia. The prognosis of fulminant hepatitis A without transplantation is better than that of fulminant disease related to other viral causes, and 40% to 70% of patients can be expected to recover.[150,280,326,369] In one hospital series, more rapid onset to liver failure after onset of jaundice was associated with improved outcome, and higher bilirubin concentration and more prolonged prothrombin time were associated with poor outcomes.[99]

Extrahepatic Manifestations

During acute hepatitis A, transient rash and arthralgias occur in as many as 14% and 19% of patients, respectively, particularly during the prodromal period.[150,370] Urticaria has been reported but occurs less frequently than in acute hepatitis B.[110] Papular acrodermatitis of childhood, the Gianotti-Crosti syndrome, rarely occurs in the United States but has been reported elsewhere in association with HAV infection.[320] The cutaneous lesions, which consist of nonpruritic, symmetric flat papules on the face, extremities, and buttocks, may persist for several weeks before spontaneously resolving.[117]

Other extrahepatic manifestations that occur chiefly in association with cholestatic or relapsing hepatitis A include cutaneous vasculitis and cryoglobulinemia.[94,174,175] The vasculitis, manifested as erythematous maculopapular lesions often affecting the lower extremities and buttocks and typically associated with purpura, appears as leukocytoclastic vasculitis and granular deposits of IgM anti-HAV and complement in blood vessel walls in skin biopsy specimens. Cryoglobulinemia includes cryoglobulins composed of IgG and IgM and IgM anti-HAV antibodies.[94,174,175,325] These manifestations resolve spontaneously with resolution of the hepatitis.

In the absence of fulminant disease, neurologic syndromes have been observed only rarely in association with hepatitis A. Guillain-Barré syndrome has been reported to occur 3 days to 2 weeks after the onset of hepatitis A, as have myeloradiculopathy, vertigo, mononeuritis (cranial or peripheral nerve), meningoencephalitis, and exacerbation of multiple sclerosis.[19,39,291,292,359] Renal complications, including acute renal failure, nephrotic syndrome, and acute glomerulonephritis, also rarely have been reported in children who did not have fulminant disease.[17,100,183] Self-limited, mild pancreatitis likewise appears to occur.[259] Reported hematologic complications include aplastic anemia and severe thrombocytopenia.[125,236] Gestational complications, including premature rupture of membranes and placental separation, have been reported among pregnant women with acute hepatitis A, but infants born to these women were healthy otherwise.[119,319]

Cholestatic Hepatitis A

Cholestatic hepatitis occurs in a small percentage of patients with hepatitis A. These patients are deeply icteric and may have pruritus, fatigue, fever, loose stools, anorexia, dark urine, and weight loss. In two reports of 10 patients with cholestatic hepatitis A, peak serum bilirubin levels generally were higher than 10 mg/dL, with some as high as 38 mg/dL, and remained elevated for 12 to 16 weeks.[154,370] Serum transaminase levels declined but remained elevated during the period of cholestasis. In one of these reports, five patients had prolonged prothrombin times that normalized with the administration of vitamin K.[154]

Cholestatic hepatitis A can be distinguished from obstructive jaundice by normal abdominal ultrasound findings. Conducting further invasive diagnostic procedures, such as liver biopsy or endoscopic retrograde cholangiopancreatography (ERCP), is not necessary in most cases.[325]

Hepatitis A Triggering Autoimmune Hepatitis

Several reports have described patients in whom hepatitis A is followed by type 1 autoimmune chronic hepatitis.[307,370,388] Laboratory studies demonstrated a T-cell defect in these patients, suggesting a genetic predisposition to the development of autoimmune hepatitis that is "triggered" by HAV infection. These patients have required corticosteroid therapy, sometimes for long periods.

TREATMENT

Hepatitis A has no specific therapy, and because HAV infection is self limited and does not result in chronic infection or chronic liver disease, treatment generally is supportive with hydration and good nutrition. Hospitalization may be necessary for patients who are dehydrated from nausea and vomiting or who have fulminant hepatic failure. Because no conclusive data indicate that bed rest or inactivity influences the course of illness, no restriction of activity is necessary. Similarly, no specific diet is indicated, although many patients may have an intolerance to fatty foods during their illness. Medications, particularly those that have the potential to cause hepatic damage and those that are metabolized by the liver, including acetaminophen, should be used with caution. The half-life of these medications may be prolonged.

No evidence exists that exchange transfusions, plasmapheresis, or corticosteroids are effective.[126,156] Liver transplantation is successful in the few who require it.[164,343,369,393] Persistent HAV infection has been demonstrated in some transplant recipients, but whether it affects survival is unknown.[118,127] Because survival rates of adult and pediatric patients are relatively high without transplantation and no single factor is predictive of a poor outcome, establishment of criteria for choosing candidates for transplantation has been difficult.[150,281,369,386] Reported survival rates after transplantation in patients with fulminant hepatitis from all viral causes range from 40% to 89%, depending on the severity of liver failure and other factors.[215,217,369]

Investigators are exploring direct-acting antivirals (DAAs) as a treatment option for the treatment of acute hepatitis infections, including HAV 3C cysteine protease inhibitors and HAV-specific siRNAs. HAV 3C proteinases play an important role in the processing of the HAV polyprotein, and inhibitors of HAV 3C can result in the suppression of HAV replication.[188] Studies revealed that siRNAs against the HAV 2C- and 3D-coding regions inhibited HAV 2C and HAV 3D expression and that the combination of 2C-siRNAs and 3D-siRNAs strongly inhibited HAV replication.[187,186] Exploration of DAAs for the treatment of HAV remains in the early stages of investigation in vitro and cell cultures. Human studies have yet to be performed.

PREVENTION

In addition to general measures of good personal hygiene, particularly handwashing; provision of safe drinking water; and proper disposal of sanitary waste, preexposure or postexposure immunization primarily with hepatitis A vaccine or with immunoglobulin can prevent the acquisition of hepatitis A.

Immunoglobulin

Immunoglobulin is a sterile solution of antibodies prepared by a serial cold ethanol precipitation procedure from pooled human plasma that has tested negative for hepatitis B surface antigen, antibody to human immunodeficiency virus (HIV), and antibody to hepatitis C virus.[77] When it is administered before exposure or within 2 weeks after exposure, immunoglobulin is more than 85% effective in preventing hepatitis A by passive transfer of anti-HAV.[202,261,355] Whether immunoglobulin completely prevents infection or leads to asymptomatic infection and the development of persistent anti-HAV (passive-active immunity) probably is related to the amount of time that has elapsed between exposure and administration of immunoglobulin.[219,225,355] Although in recent years immunoglobulin lots have had slightly lower titers of anti-HAV, probably because of a decreasing prevalence of previous HAV infection in plasma donors, no clinical or epidemiologic evidence of decreased efficacy has been reported.[362]

Hepatitis A immunoglobulin (IG) may be given instead of or in addition to hepatitis A vaccine to certain groups who are traveling to countries with high, transitional, or intermediate endemicity of HAV infection (see Fig. 168.4).[54,63] Travelers who are at increased risk of severe or fatal hepatitis A infection, including adults older than 40 years of age (particularly adults 75 years and older), persons with chronic liver disease, those who are immunocompromised, and those who are planning to depart in 2 weeks or less should receive IG (0.02 mL/kg) at a separate anatomic injection site in addition to the standard initial dose of vaccine. IG is also indicated for travelers who are allergic to a vaccine component or who elect not to receive the vaccine, as well as for travelers younger than 12 months, as hepatitis A vaccine is not licensed in the United States for children in this age group (see the section on vaccines).[54,63] Although hepatitis A often is asymptomatic in infants and young children, preexposure prophylaxis is indicated to prevent the rare severe cases and transmission to others after return from abroad.

For preexposure prophylaxis of travelers, the dose of IG is 0.02 mL/kg body weight if travel will be for less than 3 months. Because of the decay of passive immunity during the course of time, a dose of 0.06 mL/kg is necessary for persons who will be abroad for 3 to 5 months, and readministration every 5 months is necessary for extended trips. Hepatitis A vaccine, if it is not contraindicated, is a better choice for such persons and can be administered at any time prior to departure in healthy persons.

Aggressive use of vaccine immunoprophylaxis is indicated to control hepatitis A outbreaks[409,300] in childcare centers in which hepatitis A is diagnosed in a child or employee[54,61,63,330,331] and in other settings (e.g., hospitals and facilities for developmentally disabled persons) when outbreaks occur.[55,60] When a food handler is identified with hepatitis A, postexposure prophylaxis should be administered to other food handlers at the establishment and, under limited circumstances, to patrons.[49,54,63,135,136] Once cases are identified that are associated with a food service establishment, it generally is too late to administer postexposure prophylaxis to patrons because the 2-week postexposure period during which prophylaxis is effective will have passed.

Previously unvaccinated household or sexual contacts of patients with hepatitis A should receive postexposure prophylaxis. In the absence of postexposure prophylaxis, secondary attack rates of 15% to 30% have been reported in households, with higher rates of transmission occurring from infected young children than from infected adolescents and adults. Attack rates in food handlers are generally lower.[201]

IG is usually used for postexposure prophylaxis in susceptible persons who are either children younger than 12 months or persons older than 40 years, immunocompromised persons, and persons with chronic liver disease.[201]

For postexposure prophylaxis, 0.02 mL/kg body weight of IG is administered intramuscularly. For infants and young children, the injection can be administered in the anterolateral aspect of the thigh or the deltoid muscles; for older children and adolescents, the injection should be administered in the deltoid or gluteus muscles, into which a large volume of IG can be injected.[51,56] If the IG is administered in the gluteus, the injection should be given in the superolateral aspect to avoid injury to the sciatic nerve.[51,56]

Vaccine is recommended as postexposure prophylaxis in healthy persons 12 months through 40 years of age as of 2007, because it induces active immunity providing longer protection, has higher acceptability and availability, and is easy to administer.[54,55,63,66,201]

IG does not interfere with the immune response to oral poliovirus vaccine, to yellow fever vaccine, or, in general, to inactivated vaccines. However, IG can interfere with the immune response to some live attenuated vaccines (e.g., measles-mumps-rubella vaccine [MMR] and varicella vaccine). Administration of MMR and varicella vaccines should be delayed for at least 3 months and at least 5 months, respectively, after the administration of immunoglobulin. Immunoglobulin should not be given within 2 weeks after the administration of MMR or within 3 weeks of the administration of varicella vaccine, unless the benefits of immunoglobulin administration are greater than the benefits of vaccination.[51,56] For travelers younger than 1 year of age in whom the use of immunoglobulin may interfere with the administration of other needed vaccines (e.g., MMR and varicella), the use of inactivated hepatitis A vaccine could be considered (see the discussion on inactivated vaccines).

Serious adverse events from IG rarely occur. Because anaphylaxis has been reported after repeated administration to persons with IgA deficiency, these persons should not receive IG.[120] Pregnancy or lactation is not a contraindication to the administration of IG. For infants and pregnant women, a preparation that does not include thimerosal is preferable.

Hepatitis A Vaccine

The ability to propagate HAV in cell culture allowed the development of hepatitis A vaccines. Both inactivated and live attenuated hepatitis A vaccines have been developed by use of defined isolates from infected cell lines.[106,239,240,255,303,344] Available data indicate that both inactivated and live attenuated hepatitis vaccine are capable of providing long-term protection, but only inactivated vaccines are licensed in the United States.[232,286,176,403]

Vaccine Preparation and Performance

Inactivated hepatitis A vaccines are prepared by a method similar to that used to prepare inactivated poliovirus vaccine, by propagation of cell culture–adapted virus in human fibroblasts, purification by ultrafiltration or other methods, formalin inactivation, and adsorption to an aluminum hydroxide adjuvant.[14,74] Inactivated vaccines using the HM175 strain (HAVRIX, GlaxoSmithKline) and the CR326F′ strain (VAQTA, Merck) have been licensed in pediatric and adult formulations for intramuscular administration and are available in the United States for persons 12 months of age and older (Table 168.1). One of these vaccines (HM175 strain) is formulated with 2-phenoxyethanol as a preservative, whereas the other is formulated without a preservative.[290] The antigen content of one vaccine (CR326F′ strain) is expressed as units of HAV antigen as defined by a standard; the antigen content of the other vaccine

TABLE 168.1 Recommended Doses and Schedules for Inactivated Hepatitis A Vaccines Available in the United States

Age (y)	Vaccine[a]	Dose	Volume (mL)	No. of Doses	Schedule[b] (mo)
1–18	HAVRIX	720 ELU	0.5	2	0, 6–12
	VAQTA	25 U	0.5	2	0, 6–18
≥19	HAVRIX	1440 ELU	1.0	2	0, 6–12
	VAQTA	50 U	1.0	2	0, 6–18
>18	TWINRIX	720 ELU	1.0	3	0, 1, 6[c]

ELU, Enzyme-linked immunosorbent assay units.

[a]HAVRIX is manufactured from HAV strain HM175 by GlaxoSmithKline; VAQTA is manufactured from HAV strain CR326F′ by Merck & Co, Inc.; TWINRIX is a combined hepatitis A and hepatitis B vaccine that also contains 20 μg per dose recombinant hepatitis B surface antigen protein.

[b]Zero months indicates initial dose; subsequent numbers represent months after the initial dose.

[c]An alternative four-dose schedule, given on days 0, 7, 21–30, followed by a dose at month 12, also is licensed in the United States. This schedule is used prior to planned exposure with short notice.

From Centers for Disease Control and Prevention. Prevention of hepatitis A through active or passive immunization: recommendation from the advisory Committee on Immunization Practices (ACIP). *MMWR Morb Mortal Wkly Rep.* 2006;55(RR-7):1–23.

(HM175 strain) is determined by reactivity in a quantitative immunoassay for HAV antigen and is expressed as enzyme-linked immunosorbent assay units (ELU).

Two other inactivated hepatitis A vaccines are manufactured and available in Europe and other parts of the world.[175,212,293,392] In addition, a combination inactivated hepatitis A and recombinant hepatitis B vaccine is available in the United States for persons 18 years and older,[61] and a pediatric formulation is available in Europe, Canada, and other parts of the world.[107]

In extensive studies in children and adults, the inactivated hepatitis A vaccines available in the United States have been found to be highly immunogenic. In general, after one dose of vaccine, 95% to 100% of children 1 year or older and adults respond with concentrations of antibody considered to be protective; a second dose given 6 to 18 months later results in a boost in antibody concentration and probably is important for long-term protection.[20,25,74,169,251,271] Persons whose second dose is delayed as long as 3 to 8 years after the first dose have responses to vaccination similar to the responses of those who receive the vaccine on licensed schedules.[24,179,413] Studies conducted among infants and children younger than 18 months have demonstrated that simultaneous administration of hepatitis A vaccine with diphtheria-tetanus-acellular pertussis (DTaP), *Haemophilus influenzae* type b, hepatitis B, MMR, and inactivated poliovirus vaccines does not affect the immunogenicity and reactogenicity of these vaccines.[25,26,34,91,254,295,379] IgM anti-HAV occasionally can be detected by standard assays, primarily if it is measured soon (i.e., 2 to 3 weeks) after vaccination.[341,390]

Conditions that may result in reduced immunogenicity include HIV infection, chronic liver disease, and older age. Among adults with HIV infection, 61% to 87% had protective antibody concentrations after completing the vaccination series.[166,195,274,397] Higher $CD4^+$ T-lymphocyte count at baseline was associated with response to vaccination.[13,166,195,312,397] However, HIV-infected persons with normal or near-normal $CD4^+$ T-lymphocyte counts have response rates that exceed 95%.[401] A retrospective study in adult patients with HIV who received two doses of HAV vaccine demonstrated a durable seropositive response for up to 6 to 10 years after HAV vaccination. Suppressed HIV RNA levels were associated with durable HAV responses.[89] Awareness of hepatitis susceptibility and hepatitis coinfection status in HIV-infected patients is essential for optimal clinical management. Despite recommendations for hepatitis screening and vaccination of HIV-infected MSM, rates for screening and vaccination remained suboptimal in the United States from 2004 to 2007.[168] HIV-infected patients have an elevated risk for HAV coinfection, which is significant considering the elevated prevalence of liver disease in this population. Furthermore, HIV-infected persons may experience prolonged HAV viremia, which has important public health implications for transmission within the community.[89] Among persons with chronic liver disease, seroprotection rates were similar to those observed among healthy adults, but the final antibody concentrations were substantially lower.[193,194,215,217]

Most infants born to anti-HAV–positive mothers have lost detectable antibody by the time they reach 12 to 15 months of age, and both pediatric hepatitis A vaccines are now licensed for use in children as young as 12 months.[141,230,231] Studies in children younger than 1 year of age indicate that the vaccine is safe and immunogenic for those who do not have passively transferred antibody from previous maternal HAV infection.[26,226,298,375] However, there are concerns that the presence of passively acquired maternal anti-HAV may substantially reduce hepatitis A vaccine immuogenicity. A study following 183 children over a 15-year period showed a 90% to 100% seropositivity at 10 years of age. However, there was a decrease through ages 15 to 16 years in children in whom vaccination began at age 6 months (50–75%) when compared to infants in whom vaccination began at 12 to 15 months of age.[350] In studies of infants who received hepatitis A vaccine according to several different schedules, those with passively transferred maternal antibody at the time of vaccination responded, but final antibody concentrations were approximately one third to one tenth those of infants who did not have passively transferred antibody and were vaccinated according to the same schedule.[26,92,226,228,298,375]

The clinical significance, if any, of these lower antibody concentrations is unknown. One study found that all infants vaccinated in the presence of passively transferred maternal antibody responded to a booster dose given 6 months later with an anamnestic response, suggesting that they had been primed by the primary series.[92] However, in another small study, two of six children who had lost detectable antibody did not have an anamnestic response to a booster dose administered approximately 6 years after they had received the primary vaccine series in infancy in the presence of passively transferred antibody.[135,136]

Inactivated hepatitis A vaccine has been shown to be highly efficacious in preventing clinically apparent disease. In a study of approximately 40,000 Thai children 1 to 16 years of age, the efficacy of inactivated vaccine (HM175 strain) was 94% (95% confidence interval [CI], 79%, 99%) after two doses (360 ELU per dose) administered 1 month apart.[176] In a study of another inactivated vaccine (CR326F strain) involving approximately 1000 children 2 to 16 years of age in a New York community with high hepatitis A rates, efficacy was 100% (lower bound of the 95% CI, 87%) starting 17 days after the administration of one dose (25 U).[403]

Since hepatitis A vaccines became available in the United States in 1995, studies, demonstration projects, and surveillance data have evaluated their effectiveness in controlling and preventing the development of hepatitis A in communities. In areas with the highest hepatitis A rates, such as Native American and Alaska Native communities, vaccination of the majority of children—and in some cases adolescents and young adults—resulted in a rapid decline in the incidence of disease, and with ongoing routine vaccination of children, the reduction in incidence of disease has been sustained.[32,52,54,250] In larger, more heterogeneous communities with lower but consistently elevated hepatitis A rates, interruption of ongoing community-wide epidemics by vaccination of children proved more difficult.[86] In contrast, sustained routine vaccination of children can reduce hepatitis A incidence markedly during the course of time (see discussion on vaccine recommendations and use).[16,91,112] Examination of time trends of hospitalization for hepatitis A at a tertiary pediatric hospital in Athens in 1999 to 2013 shows that hospitalization rates significantly decreased after implementation of the universal vaccination program in 2008 (from 50.5 to 20.8 per 1000 hospitalizations).[287,288]

Hepatitis A vaccine also is effective when it is used to prevent infection after exposure. Hepatitis A vaccine administered soon after exposure prevented infection in a chimpanzee model.[314] Hepatitis A vaccine was found to be 79% efficacious in preventing infection in contrast to no treatment in a small randomized trial conducted in Italy.[321] In a randomized controlled trial conducted in Kazakhstan, among persons aged 2 to 40 years who were contacts of hepatitis A cases, the efficacy of hepatitis A vaccine administered within 14 days after exposure to HAV was shown to be similar to that of IG in healthy children and adults younger than 40 years of age.[390] Based on their results and because the vaccine offers advantages over IG, the Advisory Committee on Immunization Practices (ACIP) of the US Public Health Service currently recommends the hepatitis A vaccine in preference to IG for postexposure prophylaxis of healthy persons from the ages of 12 months to 40 years.[54,63] Advisory groups or expert panels in some other countries also have recommended that hepatitis A vaccine be used as the primary means of preventing hepatitis A after exposure.[273,360]

Experience to date indicates that the incidence of adverse events after vaccination is comparable to that after the administration of other widely used vaccines. In prelicensure clinical studies in children, the side effects reported most frequently included soreness, tenderness, warmth, or induration at the injection site (4–19%); feeding problems (8%); and headache (4%).[34,61,254] Through 2005, more than 188 million doses have been sold worldwide, including more than 50 million doses in the United States.[61] No serious adverse events in children or adults have been identified that could be definitively ascribed to hepatitis A vaccine.[35,61] The Vaccine Adverse Events Reporting System (maintained by the US Food and Drug Administration and the CDC) has received approximately 6000 reports of adverse events occurring after receipt of hepatitis A vaccine. The most common events were minor and of brief duration, such as fever, injection-site reactions, rash, and headache. The 871 serious adverse events included Guillain-Barré syndrome, elevated transaminases, idiopathic thrombocytopenic purpura, and seizures among children.[61,276] Rare adverse events reported after marketing include syncope, jaundice, erythema multiforme, anaphylaxis, brachial plexus neuropathy, transverse myelitis, encephalopathy, and others. For events for which incidence rates are available, such as Guillain-Barré syndrome, reported rates were not higher than reported background rates.[61]

Anti-HAV persists at protective levels in vaccinated adults for at least 10 to 12 years after vaccination,[381,385,384] and more recent publications have demonstrated protective levels up to 15 and 17 years after vaccination[383,382] and in children for at least 5 to 10 years after vaccination.[129,161,381] Available data indicate that both inactivated and live attenuated hepatitis A vaccine are capable of providing long-term protection for up to 15 years in both children and adults.[286] Recent studies using mathematical models predict that 84% to 95% of children and adults who receive the hepatitis A vaccination would remain seropositive for 30 years.[350,367]

In one follow-up study, two thirds of infants who did not have passively transferred maternal antibody at the time of vaccination had detectable anti-HAV 6 years later, and all who had lost antibody had an anamnestic response to a booster dose.[135,136] Estimates based on kinetic models of decline in antibody suggest that the duration of protection could be 15 to 25 years or longer.[381,411,412] A study randomized by maternal anti-HAV status included 197 children younger than 2 years of age who received different schedules of HAV vaccine and demonstrated that the seropositivity induced by hepatitis A vaccine can persists for at least 10 years regardless of presence of maternal anti-HAV.[334]

In some settings, performing prevaccination serologic testing may be considered in an attempt to reduce cost by not vaccinating persons with previous immunity.[47] Testing of children is not indicated because of their expected low prevalence of infection and the lower cost of vaccine for this age group. Testing may be considered for older adolescents and adults in certain population groups with a high prevalence of infection (e.g., Native Americans and Alaska Natives), persons who either were born in or lived for extensive periods in geographic areas that have high endemicity of HAV infection (e.g., Central and South America, Africa, and Asia), and adults 40 years of age and older. However, the cost of testing, the vaccine cost, and the likelihood that the person will return for vaccination should be taken into account. Postvaccination testing is not indicated because of the high rate of response to the vaccine. Furthermore, most anti-HAV testing methods licensed for use in the United States cannot reliably detect the low anti-HAV concentrations generated by immunization.[55,66]

TABLE 168.2 Advisory Committee on Immunization Practices Recommendations for Routine Preexposure Use of Hepatitis A Vaccine

Group	Comments
All children at age 12–23 months[a]	Integrate into routine childhood vaccination schedule; children who are not vaccinated by age 2 years can be vaccinated at subsequent visits
Children age 2–18 years	Maintain existing program[b]; can be considered in areas without existing programs
International travelers	Except persons traveling to Canada, Western Europe, Japan, Australia, or New Zealand, who are at no greater risk than in the United States Infants <12 months of age traveling to endemic area should receive immunoglobulin prophylaxis
Men who have sex with men	Includes adolescents
Illicit drug users	Includes adolescents
Persons with chronic liver disease	Increased risk of fulminant hepatitis A with HAV infection
Persons receiving clotting factor concentrates	
Persons who work with HAV in research settings	
Anyone wishing to obtain immunity	

HAV, Hepatitis A virus.

[a]Hepatitis A vaccine is not licensed for children younger than 12 months.

[b]States covered by 1999 ACIP recommendations (Alabama, Alaska, Arizona, California, Colorado, Idaho, Minnesota, Missouri, Nevada, New Mexico, Oklahoma, Oregon, South Dakota, Texas, Utah, Washington, Wyoming, and selected areas in other states).[55,60]

From Centers for Disease Control and Prevention: Prevention of hepatitis A through active or passive immunization. Recommendations of the Advisory Committee on Immunization Practices (ACIP). *MMWR Recomm Rep.* 2006;55(RR-7):1–23.

Vaccine Recommendations and Use

Recommendations for the use of hepatitis A vaccine were issued first by the ACIP (Table 168.2), the American Academy of Pediatrics, and other groups in 1996 and updated in 1999 and 2006.[8,51,55,59-61] As part of an incremental strategy aimed at achieving widespread routine vaccination, the 1999 recommendations called for routine vaccination of children living in areas where rates of hepatitis A consistently had been elevated. Various vaccination strategies that were suggested included vaccinating one or more single-age cohorts of children or adolescents, vaccinating children in selected settings (e.g., daycare), and vaccinating children and adolescents over a wide range of ages in a variety of settings, such as when they seek health care for other purposes. The final step in this incremental strategy, routine vaccination of children older than 12 months nationwide, was recommended by the ACIP in 2006.[61]

The impact of routine vaccination of children initially was shown in areas that historically have had the highest hepatitis A rates (e.g., Native American communities), where this strategy had been recommended since 1996. Surveys conducted in 1999 to 2000 indicated vaccination coverage of 50% to 80% of preschool- and school-age Native American and Alaska Native children, thus suggesting that the recommendation for routine vaccination was being implemented.[32] By 2000, the incidence of hepatitis A in Native Americans and Alaska Natives had declined by 97% in contrast to the beginning of the preceding decade and was the same as the overall US rate.[32]

National surveillance data indicate that routine vaccination of children living in areas with consistently elevated rates, which was recommended in 1999, has had an impact on the overall incidence of hepatitis A in the United States. Rates declined most dramatically among children in parts of the country where routine vaccination of children was recommended and where the estimated coverage was highest.[399]

Since 2001, incidence rates in each successive year have been historic lows, with the 2010 rate of 0.54 cases per 100,000 population demonstrating a 94% decline in contrast to previous lows observed in the early 1990s.[64,67]

Vaccine coverage data are limited but indicate that declines in incidence have occurred with modest levels of coverage, suggesting a strong herd immunity effect.[9,94,105,322,] Modeling studies suggested that 39% of potential cases were averted in 2001 because of the direct effects of immunization and herd immunity.[322] Similar observations have been made in Israel and Spain. The incidence of hepatitis A declined by 95% in Israel within 3 years after initiation of an immunization program among children 18 to 24 months old, even though no catch-up vaccination of other age groups was attempted.[92] Routine vaccination of 12-year-old children in Catalonia, Spain, was followed by a 58% reduction in overall incidence.[112] Hepatitis A incidence is cyclic, and data from additional years are needed to verify that low rates are sustained and attributable to vaccination and to provide a definitive determination of the overall impact of this strategy of routine childhood vaccination. However, the consistency and strength of these data render alternative explanations unlikely.

Vaccination of successive cohorts of children eventually should result in a sustained reduction in the incidence of disease nationwide and thus provide the opportunity to eliminate HAV transmission. To achieve this goal, implementation of recent ACIP recommendations for vaccination of young children nationwide will be needed. Pediatric combination vaccines that include hepatitis A vaccine would facilitate this effort.

Vaccination of persons at increased risk for acquiring hepatitis A, including travelers to countries where hepatitis A is endemic, adolescent and adult MSM, persons who use illegal drugs, those who work with HAV in research settings, and persons who have clotting factor disorders, also is recommended.[61,271,258] Persons with chronic liver disease who acquire hepatitis A have been reported to have a high case-fatality rate and are also recommended for vaccination.[61]

In 2009, ACIP recommended hepatitis A vaccination for all previously unvaccinated persons who anticipate close personal contact (e.g., household contact or regular babysitting) with an international adoptee from a country of high or intermediate endemicity during the first 60 days after arrival of the adoptee in the United States. The first dose of the two-dose hepatitis A vaccine series should be administered as soon as adoption is planned, ideally within 2 weeks before the arrival of the adoptee.[63,65]

ACIP considered the likelihood that a child adopted by parents in the United States may be actively infected with hepatitis A and shedding virus at the time of the adoption. During 1998 to 2008, approximately 18,000 children were adopted from foreign countries by families in the United States each year. Of these, 99.8% came from countries where hepatitis A is considered of high or intermediate endemicity and approximately 85% were younger than 5 years.

ACIP also considered reports of HAV infection among persons in close contact with new adoptees from countries of high or intermediate endemicity. In 2007, the CDC was notified of a case of fulminant hepatitis A in a non-traveling household contact of an asymptomatic Ethiopian adoptee confirmed to have acute hepatitis A (IgM HAV positive). This case prompted an investigation that led to an identification of 20 additional cases of acute hepatitis A among persons who had close contact with newly arriving international adopted children and no history of traveling abroad.[137,291,292] HAV infection in international adoptees and their contacts between 2007 and 2009 was also reported in Minnesota.[356]

HAV infection during pregnancy may be associated with a risk for gestational complications. HAV serology and vaccination for pregnant women should be considered in areas of high prevalence of acute hepatitis A.[319]

Hepatitis A vaccination is not routinely recommended for health care personnel, persons attending or working in childcare centers, or persons who work in liquid or solid waste management (e.g., sewer workers or plumbers). ACIP does not recommend routine hepatitis A vaccination for food service workers, but vaccination may be considered based on local epidemiology.[55,66,335]

NEW REFERENCES SINCE THE SEVENTH EDITION

68. Centers for Disease Control and Prevention. Viral Hepatitis Surveillance, United States. Atlanta: CDC; 2013.
69. Centers for Disease Control and Prevention. Viral Hepatitis Surveillance, United States. Atlanta: CDC; 2014.
70. Chen CM, Chen SC, Yang HY, et al. Hospitalization and mortality due to hepatitis A in Taiwan: a 15-year nationwide cohort study. *J Viral Hepat*. 2016;23(11):940-945.
71. Cho GJ, Kim YB, Kim SM. Hepatitis A virus infection during pregnancy in Korea: hepatitis A infection on pregnant women. *Obstet Gynecol Sci*. 2013;56(6):368-374.
78. Collier MG, Drobeniuc J, Cuevas-Mota J, et al. Hepatitis A and B among young persons who inject drugs—vaccination, past, and present infection. *Vaccine*. 2015;33(24):2808-2812.
79. Collier MG, Khudyakov YE, Selvage D, et al. Outbreak of hepatitis A in the USA associated with frozen pomegranate arils imported from Turkey: an epidemiological case study. *Lancet Infect Dis*. 2014;14(10):976-981.
97. Daudi N, Shouval D, Stein-Zamir C, Ackerman Z. Breastmilk hepatitis A virus RNA in nursing mothers with acute hepatitis A virus infection. *Breastfeed Med*. 2012;7:313-315.
105. Dhankhar P, Nwankwo C, Pillsbury M, et al. Public health impact and cost-effectiveness of hepatitis A vaccination in the United States: a disease transmission dynamic modeling approach. *Value Health*. 2015;18:358-367.
184. Jansen RW, Siegl G, Lemon SM. Molecular epidemiology of human hepatitis A virus defined by an antigen-capture polymerase chain reaction method. *Proc Natl Acad Sci USA*. 1990;87(8):2867-2871.
186. Jiang X, Kanda T, Wu S, et al. Suppression of La antigen exerts potential antiviral effects against hepatitis A virus. *PLoS ONE*. 2014;9(7):e101993.
187. Kanda T, Kusov Y, Yokosuka O, et al. Interference of hepatitis A virus replication by small interfering RNAs. *Biochem Biophys Res Commun*. 2004;318:341-345.
188. Kanda T, Nakamoto S, Wu S, et al. Direct-acting antivirals and host-targeting agents against the hepatitis A virus. *J Clin Transl Hepatol*. 2015;3:205-210.
230. Ly KN, Klevens RM. Trends in disease and complications of hepatitis A virus infection in the United States, 1999-2011: a new concern for adults. *J Infect Dis*. 2015;212(2):176-182.
231. Ly KN, Klevens RM, Jiles RB. Letter to the Editor in response to the editorial commentary by Dr Kenrad E. Nelson entitled, "The changing epidemiology of hepatitis A virus infections in the United States.". *J Infect Dis*. 2015;212(6):1009-1010.
232. Ma F, Yang J, Kang G. Comparison of the safety and immunogenicity of live attenuated and inactivated hepatitis A vaccine in healthy Chinese children aged 18 months to 16 years: results from a randomized, parallel controlled, phase IV study. *Clin Microbiol Infect*. 2016;22(9):811.e9-811.e811.
258. Mirzaei J, Ziaee M, Farsad SA. Vaccination against Hepatitis A for hemophilic patients: Is it necessary? *Hepat Mon*. 2016;16(4):e37447.
261. Murphy TV, Denniston MM, Hill HA. Progress toward eliminating hepatitis A disease in the United States. *MMWR Suppl*. 2016;65(1):29-41.
264. Murphy TV, Denniston MM, Hill HM, et al. Progress toward eliminating hepatitis A disease in the United States. *MMWR Suppl*. 2016;65(1):29-41.
270. Nainan OV, Xia G, Vaughan G, et al. Diagnosis of hepatitis A virus infection: a molecular approach. *Clin Microbiol Rev*. 2006;19(1):63-79.
287. Papaevangelou V, Alexopoulou Z, Hadjichristodoulou C. Time trends in pediatric hospitalizations for hepatitis A in Greece (1999-2013): assessment of the impact of universal infant immunization in 2008. *Hum Vaccin Immunother*. 2016;12(7):1852-1856.
295. Petrecz M, Ramsey KP, Stek JE. Concomitant use of VAQTA with PedvaxHIB and Infanrix in 12 to 17 month old children. *Hum Vaccin Immunother*. 2016;12(2):503-511.
300. Poovorawan K, Chattakul P, Chattakul S, et al. The important role of early diagnosis and preventive management during a large-scale outbreak of hepatitis A in Thailand. *Pathog Glob Health*. 2013;107(7):367-372.
316. Rodríguez RA, Pepper IL, Gerba CP. Application of PCR-based methods to assess the infectivity of enteric viruses in environmental samples. *Appl Environ Microbiol*. 2009;75(2):297-307.
335. Sharapov UM, Kentenyants K, Groeger J. Hepatitis A infections among food handlers in the United States, 1993-2011. *Public Health Rep*. 2016;131(1):26-29.
340. Shin HS, Kim SP, Han SH. Prognostic indicators for acute liver failure development and mortality in patients with hepatitis A: consecutive case analysis. *Yonsei Med J*. 2014;55(4):953-959.
350. Spradling PR, Bulkow LR, Negus SE. Persistence of seropositivity among persons vaccinated for hepatitis A during infancy by maternal antibody status: 15-year follow-up. *Hepatology*. 2016;63(3):703-711.
367. Theeten H, Van Herck K, Van Der Meeren O, et al. Long-term antibody persistence after vaccination with a 2-dose Havrix (inactivated hepatitis A vaccine): 20 years of observed data, and long-term model-based predictions. *Vaccine*. 2015;33:5723-5727.
396. Walker CM, Feng Z, Lemon SM. Reassessing immune control of hepatitis A virus. *Curr Opin Virol*. 2015;11:7-13.
398. Wallender EK, Ailes EC, Yoder JS, et al. Contributing factors to disease outbreaks associated with untreated groundwater. *Ground Water*. 2014;52:886-897.
408. WHO position paper on hepatitis A vaccines. *Wkly Epidemiol Rec*. 2012;87:261-276.
409. WHO position paper on hepatitis A vaccines: June 2012—recommendations. *Vaccine*. 2013;31:285-286.

The full reference list for this chapter is available at ExpertConsult.com.

SUBSECTION II RNA—Caliciviridae

Calicivirus (*Norovirus, Sapovirus, Vesivirus, Lagovirus, Nebovirus*) 169

Yalda C. Lucero • Miguel L. O'Ryan

Caliciviridae is a genetically diverse RNA virus family that currently includes five genera, *Norovirus, Sapovirus, Vesivirus, Lagovirus,* and *Nebovirus.*[182] In addition, six unclassified caliciviruses have been described (Atlantic salmon calicivirus, Bavovirus, Nacovirus, Recovirus, Valovirus, and Secalivirus).[87,128,165]

The first calicivirus-associated disease was described in animals in 1932, when outbreaks of a vesicular exanthema restricted to domestic pigs occurred in California and spread through the United States (vesicular exanthema of swine virus [VESV], prototype of the *Vesivirus* genus).[159,160] Although diagnostic tools were not available to identify the causative agent, epidemiologic observations suggested an infective origin that was probably transmitted through contaminated food. Extensive programs of sterilization and restriction of consumption of food products for the pigs finally stopped the outbreaks in the 1950s. In the 1970s, VESV strains were first visualized by electron microscopy; distinctive and unique features led to the name *calicivirus* (from "chalice," due to the virion's surface cup-shaped appearance).[27,87]

Caliciviruses in humans were first recognized in 1972, when viral particles were isolated from stool samples of gastroenteritis patients involved in an outbreak affecting schoolchildren, teachers, and their household contacts in Norwalk, Ohio.[1,97] Volunteer challenge studies proved the causal role of these round and rough-surfaced particles visualized by immune electron microscopy, which were named the Norwalk agent (prototype of the *Norovirus* genus). Many similar small, round-structured viruses (SRSVs) were described subsequently from outbreaks of gastroenteritis around the world. In parallel, investigators using electron microscopy to survey stool specimens from children with sporadic gastroenteritis visualized particles that did not have the appearance of SRSVs but instead were similar to the animal caliciviruses previously identified.[6,125] These "typical" caliciviruses occurred in a small percentage of sporadic diarrhea stool specimens and in a few outbreaks of gastroenteritis, including an outbreak in an orphanage in Sapporo, Japan (prototype of the *Sapovirus* genus). Biochemical and genomic sequencing analysis confirmed subsequently that the SRSVs (noroviruses) and human viruses with typical calicivirus morphologic features (sapoviruses) both belong to the Caliciviridae family.[91,123]

In 1984, a highly fatal, highly contagious hepatitis syndrome was observed in European rabbits bred in China.[54] This syndrome spread some 7000 miles across Asia into Europe and reached Spain within 4 years, a dispersal rate of approximately 8 km/day. European rabbit populations experienced mortality rates exceeding 90% within 3 days of exposure. Typical calicivirus particles were visualized in infected rabbit livers, hence the term rabbit hemorrhagic disease virus was accrued (RHDV; prototype of the *Lagovirus* genus).[137]

More recently, calicivirus isolates associated with gastroenteritis in bovines were recognized as a new genus, *Nebovirus*.[80,98]

This summary illustrates the diversity of the ecologic relationships, whether animals and humans can be infected by a particular virus, and the broad spectrum of illness (from mild gastroenteritis to fatal hepatitis) associated with members of the Caliciviridae family. Next, we discuss the virologic, epidemiologic, pathogenic, and clinical features of caliciviruses, with emphasis on human infection.

VIROLOGIC FEATURES

The Caliciviridae family includes a heterogeneous group of nonenveloped, icosahedral viruses with a positive-sense, polyadenylated, single-stranded RNA genome approximately 7500 nucleotides in length. Cryoelectron microscopy and x-ray crystallography have resolved the three-dimensional structure of representative members of four of the five genera.[36,147,183]

Typical calicivirus virion particles are 40 nm in diameter and have a T = 3 icosahedral symmetry, conformed by 90 dimers of the main structural protein, VP1 (Fig. 169.1).[36] VP1 is a 60-kDa protein that has two domains (S and P) linked by a hinge. The S domain is responsible for the shell structure of the capsid, and the P domain protrudes from the shell, generating spikes that denote the characteristic cuplike depressions that give name to this family.[36,147] The genomic RNA is covered by the capsid and remains covalently attached by its 5′ end to the viral genome-linked protein (VPg).[46]

The genomic organization among the calicivirus genera differ in the number and size of open-reading frames (ORFs), the presence of certain genes, and the need for posttranslational cleavage for gene product function (Fig. 169.2).[30,51,91,127] The genomes of noroviruses and vesiviruses have three ORFs. ORF1 encodes a polyprotein cleaved by a viral protease during replication into a set of nonstructural proteins, including the RNA-dependent RNA polymerase (RdRp), the nucleoside triphosphatase, the protease, and the VPg; ORF2 encodes the main capsid protein; and ORF3 encodes a protein that appears to be a minor structural protein.[79,91] Some vesivirus strains differ from noroviruses in harboring a longer genome (e.g., Pan-1),[150] although this is not universal (e.g., feline calicivirus).[30] ORF2 and ORF3 genes of these genera are included in a subgenomic RNA that can be transcribed independently of the genomic RNA.[91,150]

Sapoviruses, lagoviruses, and neboviruses have two ORFs. ORF1 is a fusion of the corresponding ORF1 and ORF2 of noroviruses and vesiviruses, whereas ORF2 encodes for a minor structural protein.[138,139] An additional ORF, in another frame, at the 5′ end of the capsid gene is present in some strains of sapoviruses.[138]

Calicivirus genomes have a highly conserved nontranscribed nucleotide sequence at the 5′ end of the whole genome and at the 5′ end of the capsid gene.[105] In addition, many caliciviruses have an overlap between the 3′ end of ORF1 and the 5′ end of the ORF2. Both features of genomic organization eventually favor recombination.[25]

The description of distinct phylogenetic clades within Caliciviridae genera, and discrepancies of genotyping of some strains when RdRp and capsid sequences were analyzed independently, encouraged studies aimed at recognizing strains that might be natural recombinants within caliciviruses. Multiple naturally recombinant noroviruses, sapoviruses, and lagoviruses have been identified worldwide.[7,56,78,118,145,180] Although this phenomenon has also been described in vesiviruses and neboviruses, it seems to be much more infrequent in these genera.[50,83] Other than recognizing a recombinant genomic structure, the recombinants themselves seem unremarkable in terms of clinical consequences. Recombination may be a mechanism by which caliciviruses quickly escape host immunity, analogous to antigenic shifts among influenza viruses but by a different molecular mechanism. The recombination event could be recent or could have occurred in the remote past.

Generation of recombinants within caliciviruses requires certain biologic and molecular attributes. First, single cells are infected simultaneously by two calicivirus strains, in the absence of immune or molecular interference.

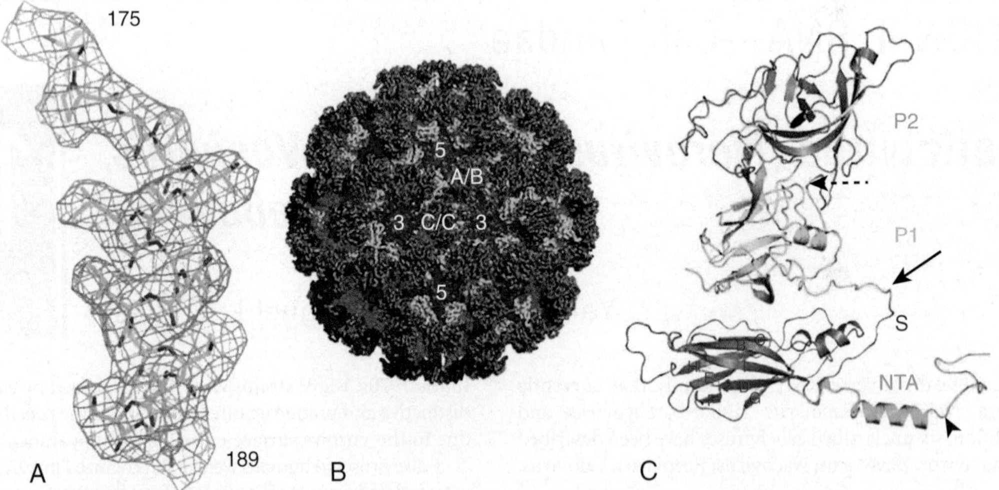

FIG. 169.1. X-ray structure of San Miguel sea lion virus (SMSV). (A) A sample region in the electron density map with modeled amino acid residues 175-189 (APAPTALATLATAST). (B) The x-ray structure of SMSV viewed along the icosahedral twofold axis (capsid protein subunits are shown as Cα trace). Locations of a set of A/B and C/C dimers and icosahedral fivefold and threefold axes are denoted. The NTA (internal, not visible in this view), S domain, and P1 and P2 subdomains of the subunits are colored in green, blue, yellow, and orange, respectively. (C) A ribbon representation of the B subunit structure. The NTA (residues 163-200, *green*), S domain (residues 201-361, *blue*), and P1 (residues 362-413 and 590-703, *yellow*) and P2 (residues 414-589, *orange*) subdomains are indicated. (From Chen R, Neill JD, Estes MK, et al. X-ray structure of a native calicivirus: structural insights into antigenic diversity and host specificity. *Proc Natl Acad Sci U S A.* 2006;103[21]:8048-8053.)

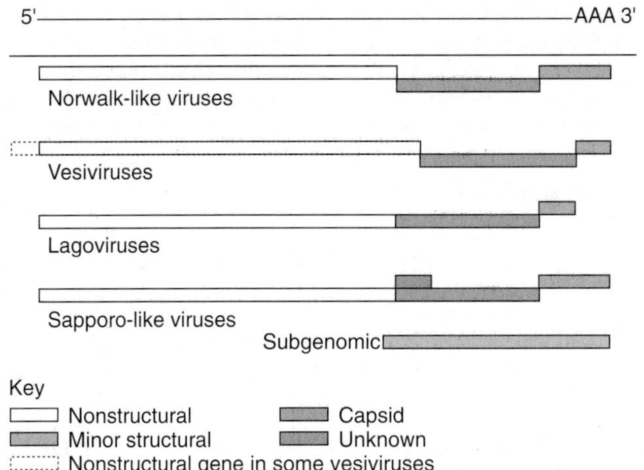

FIG. 169.2. Genomic organization of calicivirus genera. The genome of *Norovirus* has three open-reading frames (ORFs) that in the 5′ to 3′ direction include a nonstructural polypeptide, the virion capsid gene, and a minor structural protein. The genomes of the other three genera differ from that of noroviruses in the length of the ORFs, including a unique gene at the 5′ end of ORF1 in some vesiviruses and a post-translationally cleaved N terminus of the capsid protein in vesiviruses and sapoviruses. A subgenomic RNA beginning just 5′ of ORF2 and continuing to the poly-A tail is synthesized during replication. Some sequence comparisons suggest that the longer ORF3 of *Norovirus* (and the comparable gene of *Sapovirus*) arose by intragenic recombination.

Outbreaks caused by multiple *Norovirus* strains and coinfection with different *Norovirus* strains occur.[62,184,185] Second, the genomic structure of caliciviruses favors recombination, owing to overlapping regions between ORFs, conserved regions at the 5′ end of the ORFs, and independent transcription with a high copy number of the subgenomic region. Finally, the calicivirus RdRp can recognize and process the highly conserved 5′ end sequence of both ORF1 (for whole-genome transcription) and ORF2 (for subgenomic transcription) and can eventually switch from one RNA molecule to another.[25] The recognized recombinants may be a viable subset, among a larger set of recombination events occurring during replication.

Circulating caliciviruses are highly diverse.[5,77,78] This diversity is explained not only by recombination, but also by frequent mutations, as for other RNA viruses, mostly by the high error rate in genomic transcription performed by the viral RdRp, which has no proofreading activity. According to sequence analysis of whole-genome and capsid regions, multiple genogroups, denoted by "G" plus a Roman numeral (e.g., genogroup II is denoted as GII), and genetic clades, named by Arabic numbers following the genogroup name (e.g., GII.4 for genotype 4 of genogroup II), of uncertain immunologic/biologic significance have been identified within each genus.

Even though no human calicivirus (*Norovirus* or *Sapovirus*) has been successfully cultivated to date, reverse genetic systems and recombinant technology developed to express capsid protein in different cell lines have allowed studies of virus assembly and characterization of antigenic properties of viral capsids.[68,92,148,189,191] Enzyme-linked immunosorbent assays have been developed to detect viral antigens and antiviral antibodies directed against specific strains.[88,90,92] An intense, clear reaction is usually evidenced for the specific strain, but frequent cross reactivity between genotypes and genogroups has also been reported.[77] Neutralization assays have not been performed for human calicivirus because of culture limitations; however, innovative receptor (histo–blood group antigen [HBGA]) blocking assays, and hemagglutination inhibition assays have demonstrated a high correlation between blocking/inhibiting antibody titers and protection against a specific strain.[42,110,149]

EPIDEMIOLOGY

Human caliciviruses have worldwide distribution, and serologic studies indicate that infections by these agents occur commonly and early in life, with virtually all individuals having antibodies at 5 years of age.[3,68,135,142]

Human caliciviruses are described as causing acute gastroenteritis mainly in two distinct situations: sporadic endemic cases affecting children younger than 5 years of age and elderly people, and outbreaks affecting individuals of all ages. *Norovirus* is the second leading cause of endemic acute diarrhea in children after rotavirus, with an increasing proportion after rotavirus vaccine introduction, causing 10% to 20% of overall cases and nearly 15% to 20% of diarrhea-associated hospitalizations.[3,10,39,81,190,195] *Sapovirus* is comparatively less frequent, accounting for 1% to 12% of endemic gastroenteritis.[113,126,157,168]

Noroviruses are the main cause of gastroenteritis outbreaks, associated mostly with contaminated water and food, particularly shellfish.[75,76,174,186] Noroviruses account for approximately 50% of all outbreaks in countries with adequate sanitation and more than 90% of outbreaks for which no bacterial or parasitic cause can be found.[76,174,186] Unlike noroviruses, sapoviruses are known primarily from sporadic cases of diarrhea in children, although outbreaks in closed populations do occur.[106,174] Most human calicivirus outbreaks are recognized in close settings where common exposure occurs, such as nurseries, childcare centers, schools, hospitals, camps, hotels, and ships.[10,76] In these outbreaks, in addition to the primary source (contaminated water or food), person-to-person spread also plays a significant role in prolonging outbreak duration. Long persistence of *Norovirus* gastroenteritis outbreaks has been described and has been associated with persistent asymptomatic excretion in food handlers, continual surface contamination, and reexposure to the same strain from contaminated foods.[16,53] Primary attack rates in outbreaks frequently are high, near 30%, and secondary attack rates range from 5% to 30%.[66]

Although high genetic and antigenic diversity have been described for human caliciviruses, mainly for *Norovirus*,[60,77] a clear predominance of specific genotypes has been described and large changes in the relative prevalence of these genotypes have occurred during the past 40 years.[10] For example, Norwalk virus, the prototype of GI.1 strains, and closely related strains appear to have been the predominant noroviruses in the 1970s in several regions studied.[69] Thereafter, Snow Mountain virus (the prototype of GII.2 strains) and related strains predominated, whereas strains within the clade that contains the prototype Norwalk virus (GI) were found infrequently (<5%).[10,96,122] Beginning in the mid-1990s, GII.4 strains emerged and spread globally, currently representing more than 80% of noroviruses identified.[45,60,108] Distribution of GII.4 lineages differs remarkably from region to region and/or over time, which could be at least partially explained by selective pressure due to population-acquired immunity.[26,109,158] In the past 2 years the frequency of GII.17 genotype has markedly increased in some regions.[44,158]

Both sporadic and outbreak-associated *Norovirus* infections are more frequent in autumn and winter, at least in regions with temperate climate.[4,124,133] Exceptions to this trend are observed for particular transmission sources. Infections related to certain foods will occur when the foods are harvested and eaten fresh (fruit, salads, shellfish) or processed, shipped, and consumed later (frozen fruits, ice).[12,116,155] Infections from exposure associated with recreation facilities, such as swimming pools, tend to have a summer seasonal predominance.[154,194] In addition, contamination of water supplies occurs more frequently in a flooding situation resulting in the mixing of clear water and sewage and in situations associated with shellfish harvesting.[13,29,102]

A distinct seasonal prevalence of *Sapovirus*-associated illness is not as apparent, but winter predominance is suggested based on several studies.[49,143]

Vesiviruses include a large number of serotypes isolated from many different animal hosts, including pigs, cows, cats, dogs, sea lions, sea otters, walruses, whales, several snakes, pygmy chimpanzees, and gorillas, as well as a few isolates from humans.[55,64,107,121,161,164] These viruses have a worldwide distribution in terrestrial and marine environments. Vesiviruses include at least 40 neutralization types (serotypes). The prevalence of these serotypes in different regions has had little study.

The prototype *Lagovirus* is the rabbit RHDV. Rabbits also are infected with *Vesivirus* strains, which may lead to confusion.[121] RHDV has been epidemic in Asia and Europe since it was first recognized in China in 1984, and outbreaks in America and Australia have also been described.[28,70] Disease spreads rapidly and appears to "leap" large distances in a short time. The ability of the virus to spread rapidly across large bodies of water (e.g., the English Channel) suggests that arthropods or other flying vectors have a role in transmission. Accidental and deliberate importation and release have also been suspected.[35] RHDV infection is rabbit specific, and although this virus can bind HBGAs antigens, human disease has not been demonstrated.[136] In a food-associated outbreak in Mexico, antibody developed in one asymptomatic human.[70] Importantly, subclinical infection also occurred in some persons exposed to rabbits in Australia.[43] Zoo workers, rabbit breeders, and foresters have the largest occupational risk of RHDV exposure.

Nebovirus and its prototype strain Newbury-1 virus are bovine pathogens, causing acute gastroenteritis mainly in calves.[98,139] Although the first report of these bovine pathogens was in the mid-1970s, they were not recognized as a different Caliciviridae genus until recently. Neboviruses have been detected in 3% to 10% of calves with diarrhea[80,98] and have not yet been isolated in humans.

PATHOGENESIS

Human caliciviruses have not been successfully cultivated in cell lines to date, and animal models are still under development, a situation that has hindered elucidation of pathogenesis. Most of the information in this area comes from human volunteer studies, in vitro assays with virus-like proteins (VLPs), and animal models infected with murine, bovine norovirus, or porcine enteric calicivirus.[73] More recently, a probable breakthrough from Jones and colleagues is the development of an in vitro human *Norovirus* culture model using B cells in the presence of a commensal bacterium, *Enterobacter cloacae*.[94]

Human volunteer studies performed in the 1970s suggested that some individuals seemed resistant to Norwalk virus infection after challenge even with high viral loads.[10,144] The mechanism proposed for this differential risk was the absence or presence of HBGAs on digestive mucosa that could act as a host receptor. HBGAs are oligosaccharides present in human secretions and epithelia and are part of the innate immune system. The expression of HBGAs on mucosa is controlled by the activity of a fucosyl transferase-2 (FUT2), which is responsible for the synthesis of H antigen, the precursor of the A and B antigens. Individuals carrying an inactivating mutation of FUT2 do not express HBGAs on their epithelia, are eventually resistant to *Norovirus*, and are termed nonsecretors, whereas subjects with normal active FUT2 express these oligosaccharides and are called secretors. More recently, volunteer challenge studies, epidemiologic surveys, and in vitro assays have supported the role of these sugar structures in *Norovirus* virion attachment.[23,37,84,119] A genogroup-specific HBGA-attachment pattern has been described in vitro that could be related to strain-specific susceptibility.[84]

Secretor status does not completely explain the differences seen among infected and uninfected individuals for all *Norovirus* strains. Additional mechanisms are likely involved and remain an ongoing field of research.

The precise human calicivirus cell tropism is still under study, but evidence suggests infection of both immune cells (macrophages, dendritic cells, and B cells) and enterocytes.[99] According to current information, after ingestion, noroviruses reach the small intestine, where M cells can internalize viral particles and release them on lamina propria. From here, *Norovirus* may infect immune cells, triggering local inflammation and eventually translocation to mesenteric lymph nodes, leading to persistence.[99] Commensal bacteria, specifically those expressing HBGAs, are required for an efficient infection process.

Norovirus can be shed for up to 60 days in immunocompetent patients and for months to years in immunocompromised patients. Mechanisms of persistence are being researched. Evidence suggests that the ability of the strain to suppress CD8 T-cell response, antigenic changes to avoid recognition by antibodies, and suppression of IFN-γ by commensal bacteria may all contribute to *Norovirus* persistence.[99]

Small bowel biopsy specimens obtained from *Norovirus*-infected volunteers in challenge studies mainly evaluating the prototype Norwalk virus have given some pathologic clues.[8] Villous atrophy, epithelia disarrangement, crypt hyperplasia, cytoplasmic vacuolization, and lamina propria inflammatory infiltrate have been described in duodenal/jejunal biopsy specimens obtained from Norwalk virus–infected individuals. These morphologic changes have been evidenced both in symptomatic and asymptomatic infected subjects and as early as a few hours before the onset of clinical manifestations. No viral particle or specific cytopathic effects in enterocytes have been described. Histologic changes resolve after 2 weeks in immunocompetent individuals but could take months in immunosuppressed patients.[10,130] Sucrase, trehalase, and alkaline phosphatase activities from the intestinal brush border of symptomatic patients are decreased, inducing a transient malabsorptive state.[2]

The pathogenic features of *Sapovirus* infection in humans have not been determined and are presumed to be the same as those for *Norovirus*.

IMMUNOLOGY

The first barrier against human calicivirus is innate immunity, mainly represented by HBGA on the enterocyte surface, which acts as a virus receptor (see earlier discussion). Nonsecretor individuals lacking HBGA on their epithelia have a lower risk of *Norovirus* infection and *Norovirus*-associated gastroenteritis.[10,23,112] HBGAs present in human breast milk can inhibit binding of noroviral virus-like particles (VLPs) to saliva and synthetic oligosaccharides in vitro; breast-fed infants from secretor mothers have a lower risk of gastroenteritis caused by *Norovirus* compared with other enteric pathogens.[89,131]

Although human calicivirus infection triggers both humoral and cellular immune-acquired responses, infection by these agents can occur many times in the same individual and at any age. Protective acquired immunity to *Norovirus* seems to be complex and remains incompletely understood. Volunteer and clinical studies have demonstrated that 2 to 3 weeks after *Norovirus* infection, serum-specific antibodies can be detected and persist for many months.[41,112] Adult individuals rechallenged by the same strain seems to be protected shortly after (6–14 weeks) the initial exposure but can be infected again when the exposure occurs 24 to 72 months after the first challenge.[10,144] Cross reactivity has been described, but it seems to be restricted to strains of the same genogroups.[111] It has not been possible to correlate specific antibody titers with protection, and individuals with high serum and duodenal titers challenged with the same strain of *Norovirus* can be more susceptible than subjects who have lower titers or are seronegative.[20,93] However, the viral infectious dose given to volunteers in these challenge studies was several times greater than naturally occurring infective doses and thus may not actually represent the phenomenon of natural immunity. Importantly, in children, there is evidence suggesting that repeated infections is common, but that a previous infection with a given genogroup confers protection against symptomatic reinfection when a child is reexposed to a virus from the same genogroup, as discussed later.[140]

Viral neutralization assays have not been possible, owing to the lack of an adequate cell culture system. HBGA blocking assays and hemagglutination inhibition assays strongly suggest that natural infections are followed by the production of strain-specific protective antibodies.[42,110]

Phase II trials with a virus-like particles vaccine have demonstrated modest protection against severe disease.[9]

CLINICAL MANIFESTATIONS

The incubation period after exposure to *Norovirus* ranges from 12 to 60 hours, with a mean of 24 hours.[11,67] Stool excretion of *Norovirus* begins as early as 15 hours after the development of infection, peaks during the second day, and persists at least 7 days and up to 2 months.[11] Noroviruses also have been detected in vomitus, thus suggesting the possibility of spread by aerosol or dispersion of vomitus particles.[33,120] Illness is usually characterized by a self-limited episode of nonbloody diarrhea, nausea, vomiting, and low fever, lasting 1 to 2 days in outbreak settings and 5 to 6 days in endemic cases.[86,151] In children older than 1 year, vomiting predominates, whereas in infants and adults, diarrhea tends to predominate.[10,66] This clinical presentation is indistinguishable from those of other enteric pathogens.

A wide disease spectrum ranging from asymptomatic excretion to severe gastroenteritis with dehydration requiring hospital admission can occur for human caliciviruses as for all enteric viruses; death from *Norovirus* illness rarely occurs.[10,24,66,140] In general, human calicivirus gastroenteritis cases are milder than rotavirus cases, even though these agents may represent up to 20% of diarrhea-associated hospital admissions in children younger than 5 years of age.[132,141] Chronic symptomatic infections have been described in immunocompromised individuals.[59,153] Although the predominant feature of human calicivirus infections is by far gastrointestinal, some researchers have described viral RNA in serum samples, suggesting the possibility of occasional systemic infections.[85,170] Febrile and nonfebrile seizures during *Norovirus* gastroenteritis have been described.[34,38] Specific factors associated with clinical severity have not been clearly identified; GII.4 *Norovirus* strains were associated with more severe cases in one study.[24]

Sapovirus illnesses are also indistinguishable from those caused by other gastroenteritis pathogens, with a wide spectrum of severity, although most gastroenteritis cases are mild.[48,63,126]

Vesiviruses cause a variety of severe illnesses in animals and are not currently considered a relevant human pathogen, with rare cases reported mainly in people with close exposure to animals. Nevertheless, a role in human disease cannot be excluded because anti-*Vesivirus* antibodies have been detected in blood donors and patients with asymptomatic elevation of aminotransferases.[107,161] Smith and colleagues detected anti-*Vesivirus* antibodies in 12% of normal blood donors, at higher prevalence (21%) among otherwise normal donors with elevated serum levels of liver aminotransferases, and at highest prevalence (47%) among patients with hepatitis associated with blood exposures.[161] Some individuals in the groups with normal and elevated aminotransferase levels also had *Vesivirus* RNA circulating in the blood. The exact clinical significance of this finding is still unclear.

One laboratory worker was infected with San Miguel sea lion virus (SMSV)-5 and experienced an influenza-like illness, followed during the next several days by viremia and a vesicular exanthem similar to that observed in the original pinniped host.[160] SMSV-5 was visualized in vesicular fluid by electron microscopy and was cultured from the lesions; the genome was amplified and sequenced. The worker also mounted a greater than fourfold serum neutralizing antibody response to SMSV-5. Biologists working with marine mammals had similar illnesses but were studied less intensively than was the laboratory worker.[163]

Lagoviruses and neboviruses are not currently considered human pathogens.

DIFFERENTIAL DIAGNOSIS

Clinical presentations of acute sporadic gastroenteritis cases caused by human caliciviruses are indistinguishable from those of other viral and toxic causes of gastroenteritis. Individuals with calicivirus-associated infections tend to have less fever and more vomiting than those infected with other agents.[10,141] Characteristic human calicivirus outbreaks are associated with a rapid onset of symptoms after contaminated water or food ingestion (24–48 hours of incubation), high primary and secondary attack rate, and a broad age range of affected individuals. The pattern of symptoms is a fairly good marker for calicivirus-associated outbreaks: a brief duration of illness, 2 to 3 days; vomiting as a prominent symptom in more than 50% of the outbreak cases; and cultures of freshly processed stool specimens negative for bacterial, parasitic, or fungal pathogens.[13,66,74,92] When outbreaks have such characteristics, noroviruses will be detected in more than 80%.

DIAGNOSIS

Molecular and immunologically based techniques have been developed for human calicivirus detection in both clinical and environmental samples.

Real-time quantitative reverse transcription–polymerase chain reaction (RT-PCR) assays directed against a small region in the 5′ end of ORF2 (a highly conserved region) are currently the most sensitive test for *Norovirus* and *Sapovirus* detection in both stool and environmental samples,[95,177,179,178] and can be applied in endemic and outbreak gastroenteritis cases. Cautious interpretation has to be given to detection of very low viral loads, because asymptomatic excretion is common.[24,140] This assay discriminates between genogroups (GI and GII) but not between subtypes, which may make epidemiologic studies and tracking of a potential infectious source in outbreaks difficult.[178] Technical modifications have been developed for simultaneous screening of a high number of samples and simultaneous detection of multiple enteric pathogens.[58,82,166]

Conventional RT-PCR was the main diagnostic technique until the mid-2000s, after which it was largely replaced by the highly sensitive and faster real-time assay; currently its main application is for nucleic acid amplification for DNA sequencing and genotyping.[179,178] The gold standard for *Norovirus* genotyping is full-capsid sequencing; however, this procedure is very time consuming and technically difficult, making it impractical in clinical and epidemiologic settings.[193] In addition, recombination in the ORF1-ORF2 junction region is common. Currently a dual-nomenclature system has been proposed using small fragment sequences of both the RdRp region in ORF1 and a segment of VP1 in ORF2.[104,181] This system allows better discrimination between strains, with only slightly less differentiation when compared with full-capsid sequencing and detection of recombinant variants, which is the reason why it is more practical for clinical sample analysis.

To date, nine genotypes in GI, 22 in GII, two in GIII, two in GIV, one in GV, two in GVI, and one in the tentative new GVII have been recognized for *Norovirus*.[181] Human infection can be produced by GI, GII, and GIV *Norovirus*.

Enzyme immunoassays (EIAs) for stool antigen detection have been developed, and commercial kits are currently available.[31] Among the advantages of these methods are their high specificity, lower cost, and lower requirements for skilled personnel and complex instruments[32]; the disadvantage is their lower sensitivity due to a high antigenic diversity of human caliciviruses and a low stool viral load that can be under the threshold of detection. Compared with RT-PCR, the sensitivity of new-generation commercial EIA kits ranged from 61% to 80%, and specificity has ranged from 92% to 100%.[65,100] Because of the modest sensitivity of these commercial kits, they are not currently recommended for *Norovirus* detection in sporadic gastroenteritis cases. However, given their ease of use and rapid results, these methods have been recommended for screening of multiple stool samples obtained from gastroenteritis outbreaks; negative results do not exclude *Norovirus* etiology, and molecular tests should be performed in outbreak situations if *Norovirus* is highly probable.

Immunochromatographic rapid tests have also been developed. The advantages of these methods are their potential use as point-of-care tests to provide rapid results. However, their low sensitivity (near 70%) currently limits their clinical application.[65]

TREATMENT AND PREVENTION

Nonspecific Measures

Children with diarrhea are more likely than children without diarrhea to be excreting enteric viruses, including caliciviruses. Infection with noroviruses requires a very small inoculum, on the order of 100 particles, which favors transmission in closed settings and through fomites.[32,52,115] For children in care settings as well as for hospitalized children, a few infection control measures are likely to reduce the spread of infection. Such measures include personnel training in hygiene and isolation procedures, cleanliness of surfaces (with sodium hypochlorite solution or 70% ethanol) and in food preparation, exclusion of ill care providers, adequate hand washing, and exclusion or cohorting of ill children.[32,52] Laboratory workers exposed to caliciviruses should be aware of the risk for acquiring infection.

Specific Measures

No specific treatment for calicivirus infection has been established. Feline interferon and ribavirin inhibit the replication of feline calicivirus (a *Vesivirus*) in feline cell lines.[129,146] Morpholino antisense oligomers blocked production of *Vesivirus* and murine *Norovirus* virions cultivated in cell lines and inhibited the protein expression of Norwalk virus in replicon-bearing cells.[22,167] These antisense compounds have potential for prophylaxis and treatment of illness, although their potential future clinical use in humans seems highly unlikely.[162] More recently, a nucleoside analogue, 2′-C-MeC, showed significant in vitro activity against a GII *Norovirus* prototype and could be further explored for human use.[40] Use of HBGA receptor blocking molecules has also been postulated as a possible therapeutic strategy for the future.[134] Improved understanding of the pathobiology and life cycle of *Norovirus*, and advances in the identification of targets related with viral and host factors, in a new replicon system, in a small animal model for preclinical evaluation, and in high-resolution x-ray crystal structures provide some optimism regarding novel therapeutic and prophylactic molecules for *Norovirus*.[61]

Vaccines for feline calicivirus and RHDV indicated that this prevention method could work for other caliciviruses. The development of human vaccine candidates has focused on noroviruses, with substantial advances during the past decade. *Norovirus* vaccines incorporating an immunogen-expressed capsid protein that self-assembles into VLPs have been the candidates most extensively studied.[8,14,15,71,169] More recently, viral particles formed specifically by the P domain of the capsid protein (P particles) and viral vectors incorporating *Norovirus* capsid genes have been studied

TABLE 169.1 **Vaccine Candidates Against Norovirus**

Antigens in the Vaccine	Stage of Development	Comments	References
Norovirus VLPs GI.1 and GII.4	Clinical: phase I and II in adults completed, advancing to phase III trials in adults and children	Baculovirus expression system of VLPs. First delivered by intranasal route and currently developed for intramuscular administration. Immunogenic, well tolerated, moderate protection against severe disease after challenge.	18, 176, 196
Norovirus VLPs GI.1	Clinical: phase I in adults completed (data not published)	Recombinant vaccine using a replication-defective adenovirus 5 vector expressing GI.1 VP1 for oral administration.	197
Norovirus VLPs GI.1, GI.3, GII.4, and GII.12	Preclinical: in vitro and BALB/c mouse model	Baculovirus expression system, intramuscular administration. Triggers serum HBGA blocking antibodies.	198
Norovirus VLPs GI.3 and GII.4 and rotavirus rVP6	Preclinical: immunogenic in BALB/c mouse model	Baculovirus expression system, intramuscular administration. Norovirus VLPs associated with rVP6 rotavirus nanotubes elicited higher titers of anti-norovirus antibodies with higher blocking activity against binding to HBGAs than free VLPs alone.	199, 200
Norovirus VLPs GII.4 and enterovirus 71	Preclinical: immunogenic in BALB/c mouse model	Baculovirus expression system, intraperitoneal administration. Elicits production of HBGA blocking antibodies against GII.4 norovirus and neutralizing antibodies against enterovirus 71.	201
Norovirus P-particles	Preclinical: immunogenic in BALB/c mouse model and gnotobiotic pigs	High expression yield in *E. coli* system. Intranasal administration.	57, 103, 173
Norovirus GII.4 P-particle enhanced by adjuvant FlaB	Preclinical: immunogenic in BALB/c mice model	Expression in *E. coli* system. Administered by intranasal and sublingual route. Higher levels of response by intranasal administration. FlaB induces systemic and mucosal Th1 and Th2 responses.	202
Norovirus, hepatitis E, and astrovirus P-particles	Preclinical: immunogenic in a BALB/c mouse model	Expression of recombinant fusion protein including P domain of the three viruses. Intranasal administration. Elicits a significant increase in titers of antibodies against the three viruses. High blocking activity against norovirus binding to HBGAs.	203
Virus replicon particles including norovirus P domain	Preclinical: replication in vitro model and immunogenic in BALB/c mouse model	Replication in eukaryotic cell lines and inoculation in mice by intranasal administration. Elicits a Th1 predominant response. Higher levels of seric IgG than baculovirus-expressed VLPs.	101, 114, 204

HBGA, Histo–blood group antigen; *VLP*, virus-like particle.
Modified from Lucero Y, Vidal R, O'Ryan GM. Norovirus vaccines under development. *Vaccine.* 2017. Epub ahead of print.

as potential vaccine candidates. Candidate vaccines in different stages of development are shown in Table 169.1.

A safe and effective *Norovirus* vaccine could play a significant role in reducing the impact of large gastroenteritis outbreaks occurring in specific settings in which large groups of individuals are compromised. Army personnel (especially those allocated to large ships), foreign aid workers, cruise ship workers, and residents of elder care facilities are examples of populations that could benefit from *Norovirus* disease prevention.[52] More importantly, a vaccine targeted for infants, following the age strategy used for rotavirus, could have a significant impact in further reducing the toll from death, hospitalization, and medical visits associated with childhood endemic gastroenteritis. Current epidemiologic data indicate that an effective vaccine could reduce emergency department visits or hospitalizations associated with gastroenteritis by up to 20%.[141]

Barriers to *Norovirus* vaccine development have been to with the perception that immunity is short term and strain specific and that the significant genetic/antigenic variability may impair the effectiveness of a vaccine including a limited number of antigenic variants. The concept of short-term immunity was obtained from challenge studies in adults[144,187]; the situation in children may be different. A cohort study in infants from Chile indicates that *Norovirus* infections and reinfections are very common and caused largely by GII strains, but that symptomatic reinfections are uncommon during the first 3 years of life. Not a single case of a symptomatic GII infection was detected.[140] Thus, similar to rotavirus, it is possible that a GII *Norovirus* vaccine would be protective against symptomatic disease during the first critical 3 years of life and probably less protective against asymptomatic and mild infections. This vaccine outcome would be of unquestionable epidemiologic benefit worldwide.

The proof of concept for *Norovirus* vaccines came from a *Norovirus* VLP formulated in a powder form, adjuvanted with monophosphoryl lipid A (MPL) and chitosan, for intranasal use.[8] In a placebo-controlled trial including 90 adults receiving two doses of a Norwalk virus G1.1, VLP or placebo demonstrated a 70% immunoglobulin A antibody response in vaccine recipients. A Norwalk virus challenge caused gastroenteritis in 69% of placebo recipients and in 37% of vaccinated individuals ($P = .006$), whereas infection occurred in 82% and 61%, respectively ($P = .05$). Local and systemic side effects were similar among vaccinees and placebo recipients at about 70% each. Corporate decisions led to a change in vaccine strategy, moving to an intramuscular formulation that includes two VLPs, GI.1 and GII.4, because of the epidemiologic significance of both *Norovirus* types and the low level of cross reactogenicity between them. A first study concluded that 50 µg per antigen dose seemed optimal when administered with MPL in terms of an adequate balance between immunogenicity and side effects.[175] A GII.4 challenge study in adults using this candidate, although not optimal because of a low induction of disease in placebo recipients, suggested protective efficacy ranging from 47% to 100% with increasing disease severity.[18] This vaccine candidate is in rapid stage of development and intended to move to phase III trials in adults, children, and infants during 2017–18.

P-particle–based vaccines that include the protruding P domain of the VP1 protein induce both humoral and cellular immune responses in mice.[57] The advantages of this approach are lower cost of production, higher yield, and the possibility of combining different antigens such as rotavirus, influenza virus, hepatitis A, astrovirus, and HIV[171,188,192] in a parenteral vaccination strategy, although antigen combination also seems feasible for VLPs, at least with rotavirus VP6 antigen.[21]

Viral vectors incorporating *Norovirus* capsid genes have included[17] vesicular stomatitis virus,[117] avian paramyxovirus, avian "Newcastle virus,"[101] adenovirus,[72] and Venezuelan equine encephalitis virus.[17] The adenovirus recombinant candidate has moved to phase I clinical trials but the others are still in the preclinical development stage.

PROGNOSIS

Understanding of the features of calicivirus infection in humans has increased rapidly since 1990, when molecular tools for studying the viruses became available. The availability of refined diagnostic techniques has significantly increased our understanding of calicivirus-associated disease. Gastroenteritis that is mostly mild to moderate, but also can be severe, is the sole recognized disease associated with these viruses in humans. Severe cases have been reported mostly in infants, older adults, young healthy men under physical stress (e.g., military personnel), and immunocompromised patients.[47,59,140,153] Disease is usually short-lived, with the exception of infection in immunocompromised individuals, including children with solid-organ transplants, in whom it can cause prolonged diarrhea and viral shedding for months.[59,152,153] Severe chronic diarrhea can also occur in children with stem cell transplantation.[153] Deaths associated with *Norovirus* infections have been reported in adults with hematopoietic stem cell transplantation.[156] Nevertheless, these complications are rare, and most infected individuals fully recover within 1 week.

NEW REFERENCES SINCE THE SEVENTH EDITION

3. Ahmed SM, Hall AJ, Robinson AE, et al. Global prevalence of norovirus in cases of gastroenteritis: a systematic review and meta-analysis. *Lancet Infect Dis.* 2014;14(8):725-730.
4. Ahmed SM, Lopman BA, Levy K. A systematic review and meta-analysis of the global seasonality of norovirus. *PLoS ONE.* 2013;8(10):e75922.
7. Arana A, Cilla G, Montes M, et al. Genotypes, recombinant forms, and variants of norovirus GII.4 in Gipuzkoa (Basque Country, Spain), 2009-2012. *PLoS ONE.* 2014;9(6):e98875.
9. Atmar RL, Bernstein DI, Lyon GM, et al. Serological correlates of protection against a GII.4 norovirus. *Clin Vaccine Immunol.* 2015;22(8):923-929.
16. Barclay L, Park GW, Vega E, et al. Infection control for norovirus. *Clin Microbiol Infect.* 2014;20(8):731-740.
18. Bernstein DI, Atmar RL, Lyon GM, et al. Norovirus vaccine against experimental human GII.4 virus illness: a challenge study in healthy adults. *J Infect Dis.* 2015;211(6):870-878.
29. Campos CJ, Lees DN. Environmental transmission of human noroviruses in shellfish waters. *Appl Environ Microbiol.* 2014;80(12):3552-3561.
32. Centers for Disease Control and Prevention (CDC). Surveillance for foodborne disease outbreaks—United States, 2009-2010. *MMWR Morb Mortal Wkly Rep.* 2013;62(3):41-47.
42. Czakó R, Atmar RL, Opekun AR, et al. Experimental human infection with Norwalk virus elicits a surrogate neutralizing antibody response with cross-genogroup activity. *Clin Vaccine Immunol.* 2015;22(2):221-228.
44. Dang Thanh H, Than VT, Nguyen TH, et al. Emergence of norovirus GII.17 variants among children with acute gastroenteritis in South Korea. *PLoS ONE.* 2016;11(5):e0154284.
45. da Silva Poló T, Peiró JR, et al. Human norovirus infection in Latin America. *J Clin Virol.* 2016;78:111-119.
56. Fajardo Á, Tort FL, Victoria M, et al. Phylogenetic analyses of *Norovirus* strains detected in Uruguay reveal the circulation of the novel GII.P7/GII.6 recombinant variant. *Infect Genet Evol.* 2014;28:328-332.
57. Fang H, Tan M, Xia M, et al. Norovirus P particle efficiently elicits innate, humoral and cellular immunity. *PLoS ONE.* 2013;8(4):e63269.
60. Fu JG, Ai J, Zhang J, et al. Molecular epidemiology of genogroup II norovirus infection among hospitalized children with acute gastroenteritis in Suzhou (Jiangsu, China) from 2010 to 2013. *J Med Virol.* 2016;88(6):954-960.
61. Galasiti Kankanamalage AC, Weerawarna PM, Kim Y, et al. Anti-norovirus therapeutics: a patent review (2010-2015). *Expert Opin Ther Pat.* 2016;26(3):297-308.
73. Ha S, Choi IS, Choi C, Myoung J. Infection models of human norovirus: challenges and recent progress. *Arch Virol.* 2016;161(4):779-788.
75. Hall AJ, Lopman BA, Payne DC, et al. Norovirus disease in the United States. *Emerg Infect Dis.* 2013;19(8):1198-1205.
76. Hall AJ, Wikswo ME, Pringle K, et al. Vital signs: foodborne norovirus outbreaks—United States, 2009-2012. *MMWR Morb Mortal Wkly Rep.* 2014;63(22):491-495.
80. Hassine-Zaafrane M, Kaplon J, Sdiri-Loulizi K, et al. Molecular prevalence of bovine noroviruses and neboviruses detected in central-eastern Tunisia. *Arch Virol.* 2012;157(8):1599-1604.
81. Hemming M, Räsänen S, Huhti L, et al. Major reduction of rotavirus, but not norovirus, gastroenteritis in children seen in hospital after the introduction of RotaTeq vaccine into the National Immunization Programme in Finland. *Eur J Pediatr.* 2013;172(6):739-746.
83. Hou J, Sánchez-Vizcaíno F, McGahie D, et al. European molecular epidemiology and strain diversity of feline calicivirus. *Vet Rec.* 2016;178(5):114-115.
85. Huhti L, Hemming-Harlo M, Vesikari T. Norovirus detection from sera of young children with acute norovirus gastroenteritis. *J Clin Virol.* 2016;79:6-9.
98. Kaplon J, Guenau E, Asdrubal P, et al. Possible novel nebovirus genotype in cattle, France. *Emerg Infect Dis.* 2011;17(6):1120-1123.
99. Karst SM, Tibbetts SA. Recent advances in understanding norovirus pathogenesis. *J Med Virol.* 2016;88(11):1837-1843.
101. Kim SH, Chen S, Jiang X, et al. Immunogenicity of Newcastle disease virus vectors expressing Norwalk virus capsid protein in the presence or absence of VP2 protein. *Virology.* 2015;484:163-169.
102. Kittigul L, Thamjaroen A, Chiawchan S, et al. Prevalence and molecular genotyping of noroviruses in market oysters, mussels, and cockles in Bangkok, Thailand. *Food Environ Virol.* 2016;8(2):133-140.
103. Kocher J, Bui T, Giri-Rachman E, et al. Intranasal P particle vaccine provided partial cross-variant protection against human GII.4 norovirus diarrhea in gnotobiotic pigs. *J Virol.* 2014;88(17):9728-9743.
104. Kroneman A, Vega E, Vennema H, et al. Proposal for a unified norovirus nomenclature and genotyping. *Arch Virol.* 2013;158(10):2059-2068.
108. Lim KL, Hewitt J, Sitabkhan A, et al. A multi-site study of norovirus molecular epidemiology in Australia and New Zealand, 2013-2014. *PLoS ONE.* 2016;11(4):e0145254.
110. Lindesmith LC, Ferris MT, Mullan CW, et al. Broad blockade antibody responses in human volunteers after immunization with a multivalent norovirus VLP candidate vaccine: immunological analyses from a phase I clinical trial. *PLoS Med.* 2015;12(3):e1001807.
113. Liu X, Jahuira H, Gilman RH, et al. Etiological role and repeated infections of Sapovirus among children aged less than two years in a cohort study in a peri-urban community of Peru. *J Clin Microbiol.* 2016;54(6):1598-1604.
116. Loutreul J, Cazeaux C, Levert D, et al. Prevalence of human noroviruses in frozen marketed shellfish, red fruits and fresh vegetables. *Food Environ Virol.* 2014;6(3):157-168.
118. Mans J, Murray TY, Taylor MB. Novel norovirus recombinants detected in South Africa. *Virol J.* 2014;11:168.
128. Mikalsen AB, Nilsen P, Frøystad-Saugen M, et al. Characterization of a novel calicivirus causing systemic infection in Atlantic salmon (*Salmo salar* L.): proposal for a new genus of Caliciviridae. *PLoS ONE.* 2014;9(9):e107132.
132. Morton VK, Thomas MK, McEwen SA. Estimated hospitalizations attributed to norovirus and rotavirus infection in Canada, 2006-2010. *Epidemiol Infect.* 2015;143(16):3528-3537.
145. Phumpholsup T, Chieochansin T, Vongpunsawad S, et al. Human norovirus genogroup II recombinants in Thailand, 2009-2014. *Arch Virol.* 2015;160(10):2603-2609.
157. Shioda K, Cosmas L, Audi A, et al. Population-based incidence rates of diarrheal disease associated with Norovirus, Sapovirus, and Astrovirus in Kenya. *PLoS ONE.* 2016;11(4):e0145943.
166. Spina A, Kerr KG, Cormican M, et al. Spectrum of enteropathogens detected by the FilmArray GI Panel in a multicentre study of community-acquired gastroenteritis. *Clin Microbiol Infect.* 2015;21(8):719-728.
172. Tamminen K, Lappalainen S, Huhti L, et al. Trivalent combination vaccine induces broad heterologous immune responses to norovirus and rotavirus in mice. *PLoS ONE.* 2013;8(7):e70409.
173. Tan M, Jiang X. Vaccine against norovirus. *Hum Vaccin Immunother.* 2014;10(6):1449-1456.
174. Torner N, Martinez A, Broner S, et al. Epidemiology of acute gastroenteritis outbreaks caused by human calicivirus (norovirus and sapovirus) in Catalonia: A two year prospective study, 2010-2011. *PLoS ONE.* 2016;11(4):e0152503.
175. Treanor JJ, Atmar RL, Frey SE, et al. A novel intramuscular bivalent norovirus virus-like particle vaccine candidate—reactogenicity, safety, and immunogenicity in a Phase 1 trial in healthy adults. *J Infect Dis.* 2014;210(11):1763-1771.
179. Vega E, Barclay L, Gregoricus N, et al. Genotypic and epidemiologic trends of norovirus outbreaks in the United States, 2009 to 2013. *J Clin Microbiol.* 2014;52(1):147-155.
181. Vinjé J. Advances in laboratory methods for detection and typing of norovirus. *J Clin Microbiol.* 2015;53(2):373-381.
182. Virus Taxonomy: 2014 Release. 2015. http://www.ictvonline.org/virusTaxonomy.asp.
183. Wang X, Xu F, Liu J, et al. Atomic model of rabbit hemorrhagic disease virus by cryo-electron microscopy and crystallography. *PLoS Pathog.* 2013;9(1):e1003132.
184. Wang X, Yong W, Shi L, et al. An outbreak of multiple norovirus strains on a cruise ship in China, 2014. *J Appl Microbiol.* 2016;120(1):226-233.
185. Wang Y, Zhang J, Shen Z. The impact of calicivirus mixed infection in an oyster-associated outbreak during a food festival. *J Clin Virol.* 2015;73:55-63.
186. Wikswo ME, Kambhampati A, Shioda K, et al. Outbreaks of acute gastroenteritis transmitted by person-to-person contact, environmental contamination, and unknown modes of transmission—United States, 2009-2013. *MMWR Surveill Summ.* 2015;64(12):1-16.
188. Xia M, Wei C, Wang L, et al. A trivalent vaccine candidate against hepatitis E virus, norovirus, and astrovirus. *Vaccine.* 2016;34(7):905-913.
190. Yu J, Jing H, Lai S, et al. Etiology of diarrhea among children under the age five in China: Results from a five-year surveillance. *J Infect.* 2015;71(1):19-27.
192. Zang Y, Bi J, Du D, et al. Development of a Norovirus P particle platform for eliciting neutralizing antibody responses to the membrane proximal external region of human immunodeficiency virus type 1 envelope. *Protein Pept Lett.* 2014;21(12):1230-1239.
194. Zlot A, Simckes M, Vines J, et al. Norovirus outbreak associated with a natural lake used for recreation—Oregon, 2014. *MMWR Morb Mortal Wkly Rep.* 2015;64(18):485-590.

The full reference list for this chapter is available at ExpertConsult.com.

170 Hepatitis E Virus

Ravi Jhaveri

Hepatitis E virus (HEV) is a virus that was characterized just 20 years ago but has likely been infecting humans for hundreds of years. New information about its animal reservoirs, epidemiology, and molecular biology is constantly becoming available. Natural disasters and regional warfare constantly highlight HEV as an agent that causes epidemics in areas where sanitation and public health systems have broken down. New developments offer hope that protection using vaccine will soon become a reality. This chapter is a summary of the discoveries so far with emphasis on the impact of children infected with HEV.

HISTORY AND DISCOVERY OF VIRUS

As methods to detect hepatitis A and B virus as the major causes of fecal-oral and blood-borne hepatitis, respectively, became more reliable in the 1970s, more cases were being classified as "non-A, non-B hepatitis." Investigations in regions of South Asia looked at epidemic and endemic cases of acute hepatitis.[48,86,184] Case patients all had a clinical course that was very similar to hepatitis A virus (HAV) despite a remote history of HAV, and testing for other causes of viral hepatitis was negative. Many believed that a distinct enteric viral agent was the cause of these cases.

The first evidence of this came when Balayan and colleagues used stool extracts from infected humans orally administered to a human volunteer known to be HAV immune.[18] Classic hepatitis symptoms ensued, and stool from the infected volunteer was used to reinfect cynomolgus macaques. Electron microscopy of stool samples from the asymptomatic and early symptomatic phase showed virus-like particles (VLP) approximately 30 nm in diameter that banded at 1.35 g/cm^3 on a CsCl gradient.[28,29] The VLPs showed no cytopathic effect when passaged in tissue culture, and mice inoculated with the VLPs showed no signs of disease.[18]

The field experienced a major advance after the reverse transcription–polymerase chain reaction (RT-PCR) identification of hepatitis C virus in 1989.[34] Similar methods were used to determine the nature of the non-A, non-B enteric virus.[141] Reyes and colleagues constructed cDNA clones from infected bile that subsequently hybridized with RNA from infected animal and human liver, as well as isolates from five distinct geographic outbreaks. Sequence analysis revealed the presence of an RNA-dependent RNA polymerase, a common feature of plus-strand RNA viruses. Northern blot hybridization identified a 7.4-kB molecule present only in homogenates from infected liver samples. The agent was pronounced "hepatitis E virus," and further efforts by the same group cloned and sequenced HEV during the subsequent year.[159]

MICROBIOLOGY AND GENOME ORGANIZATION

HEV is a plus-sense RNA virus with a genome size of approximately 7200 base pairs.[159,186] Initial cloning of the Burma strain revealed the presence of three overlapping open-reading frames (ORFs).[159,172] ORF1 is approximately 5000 base pairs in length and encodes for the nonstructural proteins.[93,159] ORF2 begins 37 base pairs downstream from the ORF1 stop codon and codes for the viral capsid.[159] ORF3 is only 369 base pairs and overlaps both ORF1 and ORF2. The viral RNA contains a short 5′ untranslated region (UTR) of approximately 27 base pairs and a 3′ UTR of approximately 65 base pairs.[159] The genome has a 7-methyl cap at the 5′ UTR and a poly-A tail of approximately 150 to 200 bases.[76] The organization of the genome is represented in Fig. 170.1.

Initial comparative genomic analysis deduced the likely functions of the ORF1 nonstructural regions.[93] They include the methyltransferase "capping" motif (~amino acids 56–240), papain-like cysteine protease (~amino acids 433–592), RNA helicase (~amino acids 960–1204), and the RNA-dependent RNA polymerase (RdRp) (~amino acids 1207–1693). Details of ORF1 processing are limited, but recent data examining ORF1 using a baculovirus system showed extensive cysteine protease processing.[9,128,146] The enzymatic activities of the methyltransferase and RdRp have been demonstrated in independent studies.[7,105]

ORF2 codes for the viral capsid protein.[159] Specific studies of the ORF2 have shown a membrane export signal sequence (amino acids 1–36) at its extreme N terminus, several glycosylation sites, and multiple smaller processed forms.[72,142,159,193] ORF2 has dimerization sites and can assemble into VLPs when the first 110 amino acids are deleted.[100,101,189] Studies have shown that ORF2 dimers can encapsidate and deliver exogenous HEV RNA to naïve cells.[129]

The role of ORF3 appears to be multifaceted. A key function of the protein appears to be in mediating viral egress from cells.[190] ORF3 deletion mutant viruses can replicate RNA, but this RNA is almost entirely intracellular. Specific studies have shown that a specific proline-containing motif within ORF3 is responsible for interacting with cellular Tsg101, which has also been shown to interact with several other viruses.[47,84,122] Other effects include interaction with the MAPK/ERK pathway, ORF2, binding and self-association.[83,94,177,178] Recent studies have shown that ORF3 also mediates the evasion of interferon responses in A549 cells.[44]

Viral Structure and Stability

Electron micrographs from fecal samples of patients and animals infected with HEV show the virus to be approximately 27 to 30 nm in diameter.[18,28,29]

Ultrastructural studies of HEV have involved ORF2 expression, and the empty VLPs produced are slightly smaller than the infectious HEV virus.[101,189] The VLPs assemble from 30 dimers to form a spiky hollow sphere.[189] Although the empty VLP shares much similarity with the native virion in appearance, further confirmation is lacking until a tissue culture system is available. Similar to hepatitis A virus, HEV appears to exist in both an enveloped and nonenveloped form, depending on the setting of isolation.[137,192]

Several strains of HEV are almost completely heat inactivated by 60°C, compared to 66°C for HAV,[46] with some interstrain variability. Virus containing stocks have been stable at extreme cold temperatures with several freeze-thaw cycles.[46] Based on persistent HEV infections during an outbreak from water containing chlorine concentrations of 0.3 to 0.6 mg/L, HEV may be resistant to chlorine inactivation.[60]

Viral Life Cycle

For many years, HEV did not grow in tissue culture conditions, so detailed information regarding viral structure and life cycle were limited.[48] Studies have now shown evidence of HEV replication in primary macaque hepatocyte cultures and cell lines for many species known to become infected with HEV.[149,160,161] When in vitro transcribed RNA from a full-length cDNA clone was transfected into liver cell lines, viral proteins could be detected and the culture supernatant could be used to infect a rhesus monkey.[128] The cross-species cell-culture experiments discussed earlier discovered that a recombinant strain replicated in tissue culture to high levels and formed the basis of a subgenomic replicon.[148] Studies with this system have demonstrated that sofosbuvir, ribavirin, and mycophenolate can inhibit replication, whereas cyclosporine can promote replication.[41,181] HEV clinical strains isolated from feces and blood can replicate to high titers in the PLC/PRF/5 liver cell line and the A549 lung cell line.[162] Antibodies from patient serum, whether it was IgM, long after convalescence, or against heterotypic stains, were able to

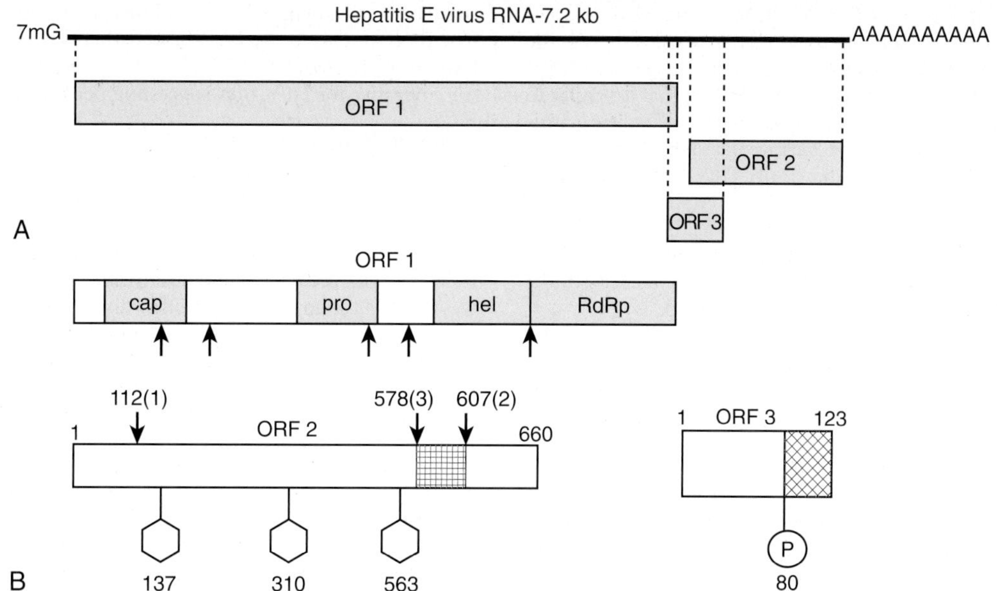

FIG. 170.1 Hepatitis E virus (HEV) genome and open-reading frames. (A) HEV genome overview. The HEV RNA is single stranded and features three overlapping reading frames: ORF1, ORF2, and ORF3. (B) Individual features of the HEV ORFs. ORF1 contains the nonstructural protein domains *(shaded)*, which include the methyltransferase *(cap)*, cysteine protease *(pro)*, helicase *(hel)*, and RNA-dependent RNA polymerase *(RdRp)*. Proposed cleavage sites are illustrated with the *bold arrows* at their approximate locations. ORF2 is the structural capsid protein, which is 660 amino acids in length. Cleavage sites are indicated by the *bold arrows* at their determined amino acid positions. Glycosylation sites are represented with *polygons* at their determined amino acid positions. The domain of ORF2 that has been determined to be the neutralization epitope is represented by the *cross-hatched box*. ORF3 is the smallest protein, and its phosphorylation site is represented by the *circle labeled P*. The domain responsible for dimerization is represented by the *diagonal hatched box*.

neutralize HEV in cell culture, demonstrating the validity and utility of the system.

Although the specific receptor for HEV is still unclear, much progress has been made in recent years. HEV VLPs enter the cell via clathrin-mediated endocytosis in a process that also involves dynamin-2, cholesterol, and asialoglycoprotein receptor.[66,81,196] After the virus gains access to the cell, it uncoats and translates its RNA in order to produce enough nonstructural proteins to begin the transcription/replication process.[128] A genomic and 2-kb subgenomic RNA are produced, as well as a negative-strand replication template.[56,161] Studies using real-time PCR coupled with live cell imaging demonstrated a peak of negative-strand RNA at 8 hours postinfection, followed by a decline.[180] Positive strand RNA peaked at 14 hours postinfection. With the accumulation of transcripts, structural proteins begin to accumulate, as well as more plus-sense daughter RNA. ORF2 gets cleaved, dimerizes, and associates with the HEV RNA to form new virions.[156] These accumulated virions are subsequently released by a mechanism that involves the endosomal secretory pathways and TSG101.[85,122]

Viral Genetics

There are four main genotypes of HEV.[186] Genotype 1 is distributed throughout the world from South Asia to North Africa. Genotype 2 is most common in Mexico but has been isolated in certain countries in Africa. Genotypes 3 and 4 are the zoonotic strains of HEV that are found in swine and humans from developed western countries and China, respectively. Genotypes 1 and 2 are approximately 70% to 80% homologous, whereas genotype 3 strains are more removed from genotype 2 strains (25–50% homology).[114] Generally, genotypes 1 and 2 are closer to each other and genotypes 3 and 4 are closer to each other.[104] This makes sense because genotypes 1 and 2 are responsible for endemic and epidemic diseases, whereas genotypes 3 and 4 are responsible for zoonotic disease and sporadic human cases.

There is only one serotype of HEV.[112,115,145,186] There is some evidence that HEV develops quasispecies during epidemics that allow for adaptation within individual hosts.[57]

Taxonomy and Classification

Prior to the characterization of HEV, it was proposed to be closely aligned with the calicivirus family based on physical characteristics.[18,159] After the full cloning of the virus and the identification of the three ORFs, the virus was formally classified with the caliciviruses.

Subsequent work showed that HEV shared several characteristics with rubella virus and other "alpha-like" viruses.[93] An analysis performed comparing the helicase and polymerase regions of HEV with members from the Caliciviridae, Picornaviridae, and Togaviridae families showed significant divergence.[22] The ICTV decided to separate HEV from the Caliciviridae family based on these findings and leave it unclassified.[58]

In 2014, after incorporating new genomic sequences of the new Hepeviridae family, two new genera were created: *Piscihepevirus* (which include those isolates that infect fish) and *Orthohepevirus* (which include those isolates that infect birds and mammals).[136] Within the *Orthohepevirus* are four types, and type A is the one containing HEV isolates that infect humans, swine, boar, and camels.

EPIDEMIOLOGY

Endemic Hepatitis E Virus

HEV is endemic in areas of the developing world where sanitation and clean water are not readily available. South/Southeast Asia and North Africa experience endemic disease, as well as regions of Mexico and South America. Large epidemics of HEV occur in these endemic countries related to widespread contamination of water after natural disasters. Cases of HEV outside these areas were inevitably traced back to some travel to one of these areas. Global estimates of the burden of HEV in endemic countries arrived at 20 million incident infections in 2005, with more than 3 million symptomatic cases and 70,000 deaths.[140] Sixty percent of these cases occur in South and East Asia, with another 14% in North Africa.

Most of the seroprevalence studies performed in endemic countries have shown that unlike HAV, children are not universally infected with

HEV early in life. Children in the first decade have anti-HEV+ rates of approximately 3% to 4%,[10,15] and the peak of HEV seropositivity is the second and third decades of life. However, studies from regions of Egypt and northern regions of India demonstrate a pattern that is similar to that of HAV, with 60% to 70% of children under 10 years being anti-HEV+.[6,50,111] Egypt has much higher prevalence than neighboring Israel, whereas southern and central India have anti–HEV rates much lower than the northern regions just described.[10,82,119] A study of children from Moscow had HEV seroprevalence rates that fell in between those of most other studies.[1] Explanations for these regional differences are lacking. Table 170.1 is a summary of HEV seroprevalence studies performed in children from different parts of the world.*

One of the Egyptian seroprevalence research groups performed a follow-up study to examine seroconversion and estimated the incidence of HEV.[154] Of the 919 villagers who were anti-HEV-negative at the beginning of the study, 34 seroconverted over 10 months, or an incidence of 41.6/1000PY for this group.

Studies of sporadic acute hepatitis in endemic areas indicate the burden of HEV disease in those countries. Studies examining children presenting with acute hepatitis symptoms in Egypt and Sudan show that HEV is either the leading cause or second leading cause in children.[45,69,70] A similar study from India showed that, although HEV was the second leading cause after HAV of acute hepatitis requiring admission to a children's hospital, it caused a slightly higher percentage of acute liver failure.[133] One study found that HAV/HEV infections led to worse outcomes in acute liver failure, but others have not substantiated those findings.[16,107]

There have also been several studies from endemic areas specifically designed to examine the differences in HAV and HEV infections.[31,144] The results of these studies have shown that HAV disease peaks earlier in life than HEV, and that although the clinical symptoms of acute hepatitis are very similar, the hepatic dysfunction from HEV tends to peak earlier in the illness and may take longer to resolve. Because the peaks of HAV and HEV seroprevalence and disease in endemic countries do not overlap, some believe that HAV disease somehow either protects against or interferes with HEV infection.[157] No specific proof of this hypothesis is available currently.

Although the reservoir for HEV is not known, the detection of HEV from various sewage samples combined with patients with prolonged viremia make it likely that the virus can exist in these environments to sustain its transmission cycle.[124,131,179]

Epidemic Hepatitis E Virus

HEV epidemics are often related to events that cause disruption of sanitary conditions (war, earthquakes, flooding, etc.). War-associated epidemics among the refugees from the Darfur region of Sudan and Iraq in 2004 illustrate the nature of HEV epidemic circulation.[25,54,60,182]

In a refugee camp in Western Sudan, there were more than 2600 reported cases of HEV among the estimated 78,000 residents in the second half of 2004.[25,60] Of the total cases, almost 10% required hospitalization, and of the hospitalized cases, 45 (17.8%) died.[25] The bulk of the mortality was among pregnant women, 19 of 45 (42.2%), and in fact, the sentinel cases for the HEV epidemic were two pregnant women who died in July 2004. The overall mortality for the epidemic was 1.7%. There were a total of 1133 pregnant women in the refugee camp, of whom 220 reported jaundice (19.4% attack rate), and the mortality rate was 8.2%.

The main source of water for the camp was unchlorinated groundwater pumped in through pipelines or surface water with chlorine added that refugees could access.[60] In the analysis of those patients with symptomatic HEV infection and those with asymptomatic infection, patients aged 15 to 45 years had a higher attack rate and more symptomatic infections (4.3% and 71% respectively) compared to the group aged less than 15 years (2.4% and 22%). Intrafamilial spread of HEV previously did not appear to play a significant role during epidemic conditions.[5,12] However, a large outbreak in northern Uganda with more than 3000 cases demonstrated in households with two or more cases that they were more likely to have had contact with people likely to have been infected with HEV.[165] All tested water and zoonotic sources were negative for HEV, thus suggesting person-to-person spread.

Zoonotic Hepatitis E Virus

As more widespread serologic studies were performed to assess rates of anti-HEV seropositivity, cases with no identifiable travel risks were discovered in developed countries with no known endemic HEV activity.[53,110,167] Many of the cases had heavy animal exposures, most commonly to swine. This led researchers to investigate the possibility that HEV was in fact a zoonosis, and that either direct animal contact or ingestion of raw or undercooked meat could produce HEV infection. Meng and colleagues conducted a multiphase study to determine if swine were infected with HEV and to isolate the virus.[116] They performed ELISAs on multiple swine herds and found the majority to be anti-HEV+ and that the seroprevalence increased with age. They followed newborn piglets, monitored for seroconversion, and demonstrated concurrent histologic hepatitis and viremia by RT-PCR. In a follow-up study, serum from the infected piglets was used to successfully infect pathogen-free experimental pigs.[113] Pigs could not be infected with human strains of HEV. Rhesus monkeys and chimpanzees, both human surrogates, were successfully infected with the swine HEV.[114] An isolate of HEV from the United States that was genetically similar to the swine HEV successfully infected pathogen-free pigs, thus proving that swine HEV could infect both pigs and humans and was the likely cause of sporadic cases of HEV in the United States and other developed countries. It has now been established that HEV genotypes 3 and 4 are the strains most frequently isolated from animals that are found in nonendemic HEV cases from industrialized countries.[38]

There are many animal species likely infected with HEV. Among those described are swine, deer, chickens, camels, rodents, and cats.[64,65,67,75,126,185] Of note, avian HEV, which has been demonstrated as the cause of hepatosplenomegaly syndrome in chickens, shares only 50% to 60% homology with human and swine HEV and has not been shown to be able to infect nonhuman primates.[65,68]

Vertical and Breast Milk Transmission

Studies done on pregnant women with HEV have also shown that vertical transmission does occur. The small studies performed show that HEV is likely transmitted at high rates, and the infants can be severely affected or die before or soon after birth.[89,90,151] Recent studies have shown that HEV RNA and protein can be identified in placental tissue from symptomatic mother-infant pairs.[26] This high mortality during pregnancy with HEV infection and vertical transmission has been recapitulated in a rabbit model.[188] Offering some insight into a possible mechanism for this severe illness, HEV infected A549 cells supplemented with serum from pregnant patients produced higher levels of OR2 and secreted lower levels of IFN-β.[24]

There have been limited studies on breast milk transmission. HEV RNA and anti-HEV antibody have been detected in colostrum components, but at significantly lower titers compared to serum.[33] No cases of HEV transmission in the infants were definitively linked to breast milk; however, mothers with advanced liver disease were not allowed or able to breast-feed in this study. In short, no recommendations exist to contraindicate breast-feeding in this population aside from those mothers with severe disease.

Other Modes of Transmission

Cases have been reported of HEV linked with transfusion of contaminated blood. Donors were in the presymptomatic viremic phase, and recipients of those blood products developed symptoms of acute hepatitis with a shorter incubation period than patients infected via the usual fecal-oral route.[13,14,27,91]

Consumption of undercooked wild game meat has been implicated in HEV infections. Several cases have been reported of acute HEV after consumption of uncooked or undercooked deer, wild boar meat, camel meat, and camel milk.[96,97,163,164] An outbreak in France was traced to consumption of uncooked pig liver sausage.[37] Comparison of HEV RNA sequences from index cases and sausages revealed 99.4% identity,

*References 1, 6, 8, 10, 19, 20, 23, 36, 40, 50, 51, 71, 82, 95, 102, 110, 111, 119, 134, 138, 150, 166.

TABLE 170.1 **Seroprevalence Studies of Hepatitis E in Children**

Country/Region	Age Group	% Positive	No. Positive/Tested	Reference
India: south Chennai	0–2 y	5.3	1/19	Mohanavalli 2003[119]
	2–4 y	9.0	2/22	
	4–6 y	7.3	4/55	
	6–8 y	7.9	3/37	
	8–10 y	16.7	3/15	
	10–12 y	9.0	3/33	
India: south Vellore	1–5 y	0.5	1/200	Daniel 2004[40]
	6–15 y	1.0	2/200	
	16–40 y	8.0	8/100	
India: central Pune	6–10 y	3.9	50/1302	Arankalle 2001[10]
India: north New Delhi	11–15 y	6.3	83/1349	
	6–12 mo	11.0	23/210	Mathur 2001[111]
	13–24 mo	9.3	19/203	
	25–48 mo	23.7	96/405	
	49–72 mo	29.5	126/426	
	73–96 mo	31.3	129/412	
	97–120 mo	35.8	152/424	
India: north Lucknow	0–5 y	64	18/28	Aggarwal 1997[6]
	6–10 y	59	13/22	
	11–18 y	64	16/25	
Bangladesh: southern	1–5 y	0.7	Not stated	Labrique 2009[95]
	6–10 y	1.8		
	11–15 y	11.7		
	16–20 y	28.2		
Nepal: Kathmandu	12–19 y	16	10/64	Clayson 1997[36]
Japan: Nagoya	1–11 y	2.6	8/309	Goto 2006[199]
Taiwan: central	3 y	3.1	6/196	Lin 2004[102]
	4 y	3.4	22/652	
	5 y	3.4	42/1247	
	6 y	3.4	15/443	
Russia: Moscow	0–3 y	11.8	2/17	Abe 2004[1]
	4–6 y	7.7	3/39	
	7–9 y	23.2	19/82	
	10–12 y	20	18/90	
	12–15 y	17.7	20/113	
Turkey: Istanbul	0.5–4 y	3.7	12/321	Sidal 2001[150]
	5–9 y	2.1	7/318	
	10–16	0.3	1/270	
Turkey: varied	<19 y	0	0/105	Thomas 1993[166]
Morocco: Melilla	Mean 9.2 y (±4.03)	0	0/321	Bernal 1995[23]
Israel: varied	1–5 y	1.1	1/93	Karetnyi 1995[82]
	6–10 y	0	0/30	
	11–15 yr	1.6	2/124	
	16–20 y	3.8	4/105	
Egypt: Nile delta + upper	0–4 y	36.2	130/359	Fix 2000[50]
	5–9 y	64.7	1600/2473	
	10–14 y	75.6	1944/2571	
	15–19 y	75.5	1438/1905	
Yemen	0–18	7.7	17/220	Bawazir 2010[20]
Spain: Madrid	2–10 y	1	7/724	Fogeda 2012[51]
	11–20 y	1.8	12/685	
United States: Northern California	<20 y	0.4–0.7	Not stated	Mast 1997[110]
Cuba: Havana	5–15 y	0	0/22	Quintana 2005[138]
Mexico: national sample	1–4 y	1.1	1/91	Alvarez-Munoz 1999[8]
	5–14 y	4.4	27/619	
	15–19 y	9.6	109/1138	
Chile: Valdivia	Not stated	36	60/166	Ibarra 1994[71]
Bolivia: Chaco region	1–5 y	3.9	2/51	Bartoloni 1999[19]
	6–10 y	3.8	4/105	
	11–20 y	5.5	5/90	
Venezuela: rural villages	4 y	1.3	1/75	Pujol 1994[134]
	5–9 y	2.7	2/75	
	10–15 y	5.8	4/69	

leading to a new package label recommending the sausage be cooked prior to eating.

PATHOGENESIS AND IMMUNITY

Pathogenesis

The details of pathogenesis in HEV infection are largely unknown. After an individual consumes HEV-contaminated water or food, it is unknown how the virus infects enterocytes and spreads from the intestine to the liver. Studies in swine show replicative HEV RNA present in colon, small intestine, lymph nodes, tonsils, and liver as early as 3 days postinfection.[183]

Evidence of HEV replication within the liver as detected by HEV antigen is apparent by 7 days postinfection. At its peak, HEV antigens can be detected in 70% to 90% of hepatocytes before the onset of symptoms and then drops off rapidly.[4] Viremia is detectable in serum, stool, and bile prior to the onset of symptoms.[32,103,169] Anti-HEV appears at the same time as the histologic signs of inflammation.[35] Similar to HAV, disease is likely caused by the immune response to the virus and not the virus itself.[4]

The majority of the information regarding progression and pathogenesis comes from HEV inoculation of animals.[18,103,169,173] These studies usually involved intravenous administration, with an incubation period from administration to viremia of approximately 3 weeks, approximately 1 week less on average than humans. HEV RNA can be detected in serum, stool, and bile 1 week before clinical symptoms become apparent.

In the HEV volunteer studies, the patients developed constitutional symptoms at approximately 4 weeks after administration.[18,32] Specific symptoms and the biochemical abnormalities of hepatitis developed 1 week later. Early studies showed that viral particles appeared in stool with the onset of symptoms and continued through the peak hepatitis symptoms, and antibody was present at the only time they tested, 1 week after the peak hepatitis symptoms.[18] Subsequent studies using RT-PCR showed that HEV RNA was present in serum earlier than in stool samples and was present from 1 week prior to 2 weeks after symptoms had begun.[32] Peak alanine aminotransferase (ALT) elevations corresponded with peak symptoms, and symptoms lasted between 30 and 80 days. HEV IgG persisted well beyond the study endpoint.[32]

The presence of HEV RNA in stool and serum can vary significantly from patient to patient.[3] In 20 patients diagnosed with sporadic HEV, HEV RNA appeared in serum at days 4 to 7 after the onset of symptoms in 89% of patients tested and persisted beyond day 22 in 21%. HEV RNA in stool samples was present in 73% of patients at days 8 to 14 after symptoms, peaking slightly later than serum HEV RNA, and persisted beyond day 22 in 13%. A subset of patients will have HEV RNA in serum and stool for up to 120 days.[124] It is possible that these patients with prolonged shedding may serve as a reservoir for spread of HEV to the environment.

A summary of the clinical progression of HEV infection is graphically represented in Fig. 170.2.

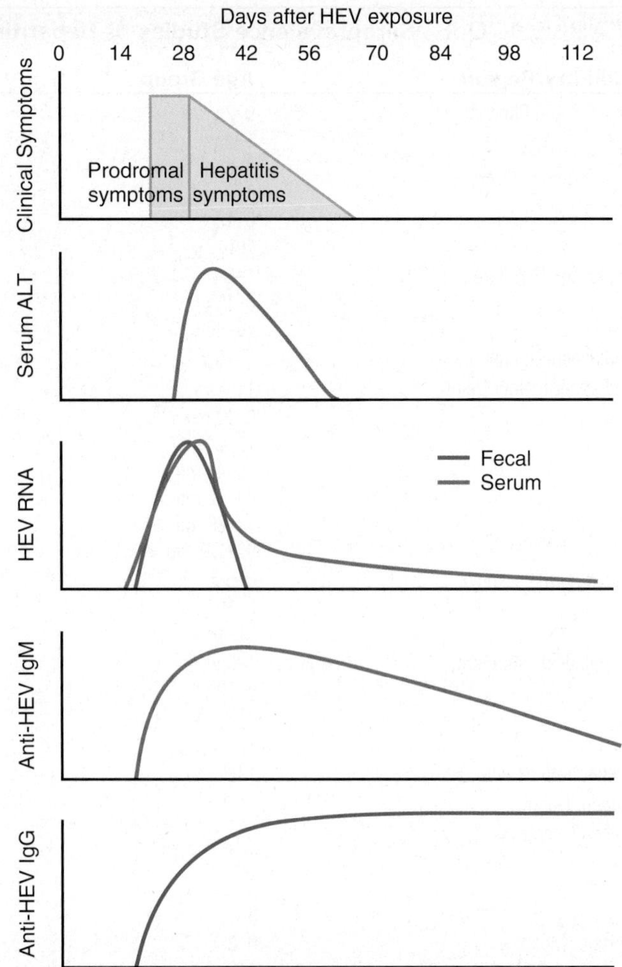

FIG. 170.2 Course of hepatitis E virus (HEV) infection with approximate times after HEV exposure. In volunteer and animal experiments, prodromal symptoms will appear approximately 3 weeks after infection, which precedes the symptoms of hepatitis by about 1 week. The hepatitis symptoms can last 4 to 6 weeks on average, with significant variation. Serum alanine aminotransferase (ALT) peaks with the onset of hepatitis symptoms. HEV RNA can be detected in either stool or serum approximately 3 weeks after infection with the onset of the prodrome and can be detected for a 1- to 3-week duration, with some patients experiencing prolonged viremia. HEV immunoglobulin (Ig)M and IgG appear in concert with the onset of symptoms and after the peak of HEV RNA. IgM peaks slightly earlier than IgG and can taper quickly, with some disappearing by 3 months. IgG peaks later and lasts for several months after infection.

Immunity

HEV antibody appears with the onset of symptoms and after the peak of viremia. IgM appears just ahead of IgG (see Fig. 170.2). HEV IgA appears at the same time as IgM and appears to persist slightly about 1 month longer after infection than IgM.[158,168] ORF2 is the dominant immunogen across all types of HEV, although antibodies to ORF3 can be detected in patients.[59,69,70,109,191] A more detailed discussion of neutralizing antibodies can be found in the vaccine subsection.

Some studies of patients after infection have shown that HEV IgG responses wane quickly after infection, whereas others show a more durable antibody response.[55] The waning of IgG levels observed forms the basis for the theory that susceptible adults accumulate to form the vulnerable population during HEV outbreaks.

Cellular immunity to HEV plays a role in eradication of infection and persistence of viral immunity.[123] Specific studies comparing patients with resolved acute HEV and transplant patients with resolved and chronic HEV have demonstrated a role for broad polyspecific T-cell responses against the virus.[155] Regulatory T cells appear to increase in number during acute HEV infection.[171]

CLINICAL MANIFESTATIONS

The signs and symptoms of acute HEV infection are indistinguishable from those seen with HAV.[4,31,70,144] A prodromal illness consisting of malaise, anorexia, nausea, abdominal pain, fever, myalgia, and headache precedes the findings of jaundice, hepatomegaly, and serum transaminase elevations.

One study examining children after a common source exposure provides insight into the manifestations of HEV in this group. Twenty students from a private school in urban North India were exposed to HEV while on a camping trip.[17] The exact source was never identified, but investigators were able to monitor the children for signs and symptoms of HEV infection as well as serologic and virologic confirmation of infection. The clinical symptoms are summarized in Fig. 170.3. Seventeen of the 20 children developed clinical illness (85%), but only

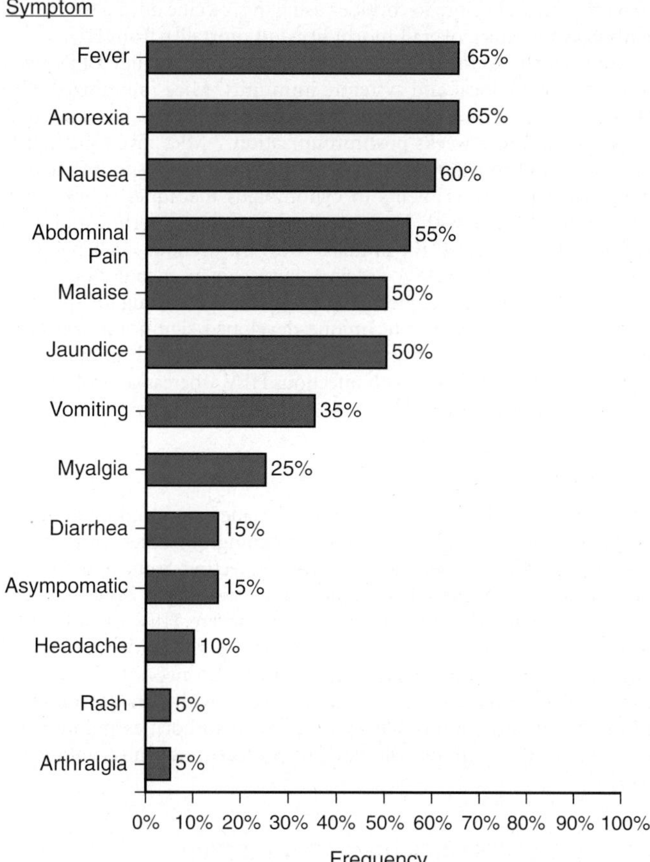

FIG. 170.3 Symptoms observed in children after a common-source exposure to hepatitis E virus. Jaundice was seen in only 50% of patients overall, and 15% were completely asymptomatic. (From Arora NK, Panda SK, Nanda SK, et al. Hepatitis E infection in children: study of an outbreak. *J Gastroenterol Hepatol.* 1999;14:572–577.)

10 children developed symptoms of acute hepatitis. The other seven remained anicteric, with symptoms of malaise, nausea, abdominal pain, and headache. The children with jaundice had a different incubation period (25–38 days; median, 33 days) compared to the children without jaundice (22–95 days; median, 27 days). HEV IgM was found in all patients. HEV RNA was found in 11 children, including one of the children who never developed any symptoms. Because this study is one of the few to have a point source of exposure, it is difficult to know if the very high rate of infection is due to the younger age of the patients, the strain of the virus, or the nature of the exposure.

Rates of fulminant hepatic failure and mortality from HEV are estimated to be approximately 1% to 4%. Studies from endemic areas suggest that the rate may be higher in children, but those data have not been widely substantiated.[132] The rate is closer to 15% to 50% in patients with preexisting liver diseases and compensated cirrhosis, whether due to chronic hepatitis B or C or other metabolic liver disease.[139]

Although it was previously thought that HEV only caused acute disease, many studies have demonstrated that chronic HEV can occur in immunocompromised and/or transplant patients.[61,79,118] This has been observed in children, with outcomes including cirrhosis and death.[62,63]

Pregnant women are highly vulnerable to HEV infection.[39,88] It was recognized before HEV was fully characterized that infected pregnant women had high rates of fulminant liver failure and mortality rates of 20% or higher.[92] One study from India of pregnant women with acute hepatitis demonstrated not only that HEV caused fulminant hepatitis and death more frequently, but also that it was associated with many obstetric complications (antepartum and postpartum hemorrhage, premature rupture of membranes, intrauterine fetal death) and poor fetal outcomes (preterm delivery, stillbirths) when compared with other forms of viral hepatitis.[130] This feature of HEV is not restricted to a particular region or genotype, as illustrated by the Darfur outbreaks. The mechanism for severe disease in these women is unknown, although one study showed an increased Th2 cytokine bias in peripheral blood mononuclear cells (PBMCs) from pregnant HEV-infected patients that could allow for a dysregulated inflammatory response.[25,127] Pregnant women with HEV have significantly longer periods of viremia than nonpregnant counterparts, also supporting the idea of a muted or dysfunctional immune response.[21]

Extrahepatic manifestations of HEV have been reported, but they are uncommon. Pancreatitis can occur shortly after the onset of acute hepatitis symptoms.[73,106,117] Several reports have described patients with significant hemolysis with glucose-6-phosphate dehydrogenase (G6PD) deficiency associated with acute HEV infection.[2,194] Neurologic manifestations described include transverse myelitis, Bell palsy, and Guillain-Barré syndrome.[42,43,77,108,152] All of these manifestations resolve spontaneously in conjunction with the hepatitis. It is not clear whether these are a result of direct viral effects or an immune-mediated phenomenon. It is interesting that most of the extrahepatic manifestations been reported in children.

DIAGNOSTIC TESTING

Serology

Antibody confirmation is the most widely available method used to diagnose HEV infection. Enzyme-linked immunosorbent assay (ELISA) for both IgG and IgM can be obtained at many reference laboratories. The ORF2 capsid protein is the most common antigen used to detect antibody.[174] Some studies have shown that inclusion of the other ORFs can increase the specificity and positive predictive value of the test. A few studies have shown that HEV IgA may perform better than IgM-based testing.[158,168] This needs to be confirmed in larger studies.

A comparison of different HEV ELISA kits during an epidemic in Indonesia found that the sensitivity of the tests was much better in symptomatic patients than in asymptomatic ones (72–91% vs. 39–51%, respectively).[120] Also, the Walter Reed kits for IgG and IgM performed better than the GeneLabs and Abbott IgG tests. Testing of normal healthy controls that were HEV PCR negative showed that the serologic testing had high specificity, again with the Walter Reed tests performing best. The caveat of the study is that the GeneLabs IgM kit was an older version of the test, and the limitations of the assay may not apply to the newer kit.

A new rapid immunochromatographic assay showed promising results when it was evaluated for use in resource poor countries to diagnose acute HEV.[121] Using 25 μL of serum or 35 μL of whole blood applied to the test strip and a 15-minute incubation period, the kit had a sensitivity of 93% and a specificity of 99.7%.

Polymerase Chain Reaction

RT-PCR for HEV RNA can be performed within the first month of illness on either serum or stool.[3] The testing is less available commercially and is likely conducted in research or select public health labs. Several recent studies have shown that real-time PCR testing may allow more rapid and sensitive detection of HEV RNA with the additional benefits of detecting multiple HEV genotypes and the ability to test environmental samples in addition to clinical samples.[49,74]

Electron Microscopy

HEV has also been visualized in stool samples from patients using electron microscopy.[18,153] In general, these methods incorporate HEV antibody to adsorb intact virus to increase the likelihood of detection. Again, this testing is not generally available.

DISEASE PREVENTION AND VACCINE CANDIDATES

Disease Avoidance

Practical measures can be taken to reduce the risk of HEV infection when traveling to endemic regions.[30] Consumption of only boiled or bottled water, avoidance of ice, eating fruits that can be peeled, and eating only well-cooked foods are all recommended measures.

Specific consideration should be made for pregnant women and patients with chronic liver disease to avoid travel to areas endemic for HEV or regions experiencing HEV outbreaks.

Antibody Preparations

There are no available antibody preparations that can be used as pre- or postexposure prophylaxis for HEV. There have been small studies showing successful passive immunization in animals.[175] There have also been studies with immune serum globulin in endemic areas with mixed effects.[11,87] These studies are all small, and the antibody preparations were of varying amounts given at varying times, so definitive conclusions about the role of antibody cannot be made.

Therapies

Most patients do not need therapy for acute HEV infection. Development of therapies for HEV is not likely to be effective for the simple reason that the peak of viral activity is usually prior to and along with the onset of symptoms. The patients with prolonged viremia are not necessarily the sickest patients; they are often asymptomatic. However, patients with less common manifestations might benefit if therapies existed. Ribavirin has been used with success in patients with fulminant infection, although it is not clear if the drug was critical in the recovery of the patient.[52] Ribavirin has also emerged as the primary option for immunocompromised patients with chronic HEV and appears to function by inducing lethal mutagenesis in the viral genome.[78,170]

Vaccine Candidates and Future Therapies

Early vaccine studies used cynomolgus monkeys actively immunized with a recombinant ORF2 protein. Subjects were protected after challenge with homologous virus compared to passively immunized or control animals.[175]

Work to identify neutralizing antibody showed that the epitopes recognized were in the terminal region of ORF2, amino acids 578 to 607.[145] These antibodies were protective of HEV infection when incubated with HEV prior to administration to monkeys. This epitope is present within the 56-kDa form of the capsid protein.

A recombinant 56-kDa ORF2 vaccine protected rhesus monkeys challenged with HEV 1 month after a two-dose series was complete.[135,176] Repeat challenge at 6 months and 1 year showed protection against hepatitis in 75%, which increased to 100% in animals given a third dose of vaccine 1 month prior to challenge.[195] Postexposure vaccination did not prevent HEV infection.

Subsequent phase I testing in humans induced anti-HEV titers ≥40 U/mL in 88% of vaccinees after three doses.[143] There were only few minor local reactions and no significant adverse events. Based on these early trials, a large human field trial was completed in Nepal in 2001. Two thousand seronegative soldiers were randomized to receive three doses over 6 months of the recombinant HEV vaccine or placebo.[147] The subjects were followed for signs and symptoms of acute hepatitis for 2.5 years. There were 69 total cases of acute HEV, 66 in the placebo group and three in the vaccine group, an efficacy of 95.5% in subjects receiving three doses of vaccine. The intent to treat analysis showed an efficacy of 88.5%. The vaccine was well tolerated, with local pain at the injection site being the most frequent complaint.

Another version of recombinant vaccine against hepatitis E produced in bacterial cells has moved through preclinical testing with promising results. A large phase III trial in China with more than 90,000 subjects showed that the vaccine was highly protective, with rates between 95% and 100%.[198] Only one case of HEV was observed in a subject who received only one dose of vaccine, compared to 22 in the placebo group. Follow-up studies have demonstrated durable vaccine-induced protection after almost 5 years.[197] A subsequent analysis of women in the study who became pregnant after enrollment demonstrated no associated pregnancy complications or fetal morbidity/mortality.[187] Antibody levels among those women who received study vaccine were comparable to those of nonpregnant counterparts in the study. These findings certainly raise the possibility that an HEV vaccine may become available to protect pregnant women in endemic areas. There have been some calls for public health authorities to consider using this vaccine during worldwide outbreaks to reduce overall morbidity and mortality from HEV.[125]

Alternative vaccine strategies being investigated include VLPs given orally to induce local and systemic immunity. Mice immunized with HEV VLPs in increasing amounts developed serum IgG and IgM responses at 2 to 4 weeks postimmunization.[99] Mice given the higher inoculums (50 and 100 μg) also developed fecal IgA responses. Subsequent challenge experiments in cynomolgus macaques showed that oral immunization with VLPs not only produced serum and fecal antibody but protected the animals from intravenous challenge with native HEV strains.[98] DNA vaccines have shown encouraging initial results as well. Macaques given a DNA plasmid encoding for the HEV ORF2 using the gene gun technique developed significant anti-HEV IgG within 4 months of vaccination, and vaccinated animals were protected against challenge with infectious HEV, whereas control animals developed clinical disease.[80]

SUMMARY

Many important developments have been made in our understanding of HEV, including the ability to conduct meaningful studies with in vitro systems and effective therapies for chronic infection. Some fundamental questions of virus entry and pathogenesis still linger, as well as why certain patients are highly susceptible to severe HEV disease while others are not. The nature of the differences in the epidemiology and clinical manifestations of HEV in children also needs to be studied further. The existence of an efficacious vaccine with durable immunity raises the question of how hard public health authorities and nongovernmental organizations will work to protect those most vulnerable to HEV.

NEW REFERENCES SINCE THE SEVENTH EDITION

24. Bi Y, Yang C, Yu W, et al. Pregnancy serum facilitates hepatitis E virus replication in vitro. *J Gen Virol*. 2015;96(Pt 5):1055-1061.
26. Bose PD, Das BC, Hazam RK, et al. Evidence of extrahepatic replication of hepatitis E virus in human placenta. *J Gen Virol*. 2014;95(Pt 6):1266-1271.
41. Dao Thi VL, Debing Y, Wu X, et al. Sofosbuvir inhibits hepatitis E virus replication in vitro and results in an additive effect when combined with ribavirin. *Gastroenterology*. 2016;150(1):82-85.e84.
66. Holla P, Ahmad I, Ahmed Z, et al. Hepatitis E virus enters liver cells through a dynamin-2, clathrin and membrane cholesterol-dependent pathway. *Traffic*. 2015;16(4):398-416.
78. Kamar N, Izopet J, Tripon S, et al. Ribavirin for chronic hepatitis E virus infection in transplant recipients. *N Engl J Med*. 2014;370(12):1111-1120.
81. Kapur N, Thakral D, Durgapal H, et al. Hepatitis E virus enters liver cells through receptor-dependent clathrin-mediated endocytosis. *J Viral Hepat*. 2012;19(6):436-448.
85. Kenney SP, Wentworth JL, Heffron CL, et al. Replacement of the hepatitis E virus ORF3 protein PxxP motif with heterologous late domain motifs affects virus release via interaction with TSG101. *Virology*. 2015;486:198-208.
96. Lee GH, Tan BH, Chi-Yuan Teo E, et al. Chronic infection with camelid hepatitis E virus in a liver transplant recipient who regularly consumes camel meat and milk. *Gastroenterology*. 2016;150(2):355-357.e353.
118. Moal V, Legris T, Burtey S, et al. Infection with hepatitis E virus in kidney transplant recipients in southeastern France. *J Med Virol*. 2013;85(3):462-471.
122. Nagashima S, Takahashi M, Jirintai, et al. A PSAP motif in the ORF3 protein of hepatitis E virus is necessary for virion release from infected cells. *J Gen Virol*. 2011;92(Pt 2):269-278.
125. Nelson KE, Shih JW, Zhang J, et al. Hepatitis e vaccine to prevent morbidity and mortality during epidemics. *Open Forum Infect Dis*. 2014;1(3):ofu098.
136. Purdy MA, Smith DB, Simmonds P, et al. New Classification Scheme for Hepeviridae; 2014. http://www.ictvonline.org/proposals/2014.008a-hV.A.v6.Hepeviridae.pdf.
137. Qi Y, Zhang F, Zhang L, et al. Hepatitis E virus produced from cell culture has a lipid envelope. *PLoS ONE*. 2015;10(7):e0132503.
148. Shukla P, Nguyen HT, Faulk K, et al. Adaptation of a genotype 3 hepatitis E virus to efficient growth in cell culture depends on an inserted human gene segment acquired by recombination. *J Virol*. 2012;86(10):5697-5707.
149. Shukla P, Nguyen HT, Torian U, et al. Cross-species infections of cultured cells by hepatitis E virus and discovery of an infectious virus-host recombinant. *Proc Natl Acad Sci USA*. 2011;108(6):2438-2443.
170. Todt D, Gisa A, Radonic A, et al. In vivo evidence for ribavirin-induced mutagenesis of the hepatitis E virus genome. *Gut*. 2016;65(10):1733-1743.

181. Wang Y, Zhou X, Debing Y, et al. Calcineurin inhibitors stimulate and mycophenolic acid inhibits replication of hepatitis E virus. *Gastroenterology*. 2014;146(7):1775-1783.
188. Xia J, Liu L, Wang L, et al. Experimental infection of pregnant rabbits with hepatitis E virus demonstrating high mortality and vertical transmission. *J Viral Hepat*. 2015;22(10):850-857.
192. Yin X, Ambardekar C, Lu Y, et al. Distinct entry mechanisms for nonenveloped and quasi-enveloped hepatitis E viruses. *J Virol*. 2016;90(8):4232-4242.
195. Zhang J, Zhang XF, Huang SJ, et al. Long-term efficacy of a hepatitis E vaccine. *N Engl J Med*. 2015;372(10):914-922.
196. Zhang L, Tian Y, Wen Z, et al. Asialoglycoprotein receptor facilitates infection of PLC/PRF/5 cells by HEV through interaction with ORF2. *J Med Virol*. 2016.

The full reference list for this chapter is available at ExpertConsult.com.

SUBSECTION III RNA—Reoviridae

171 Reoviruses

James D. Cherry

Reoviruses are ubiquitous in nature, but their role in human disease is vague. After reoviruses were classified in 1959, numerous reports noted their association with human disease.[46,75,79,86] Since that time, these viruses have been evaluated extensively in laboratory animal studies, but few cases of human disease have been reported during the last 5 decades.

HISTORY

On the basis of its cytopathic effect in monkey kidney tissue culture and its recovery from stool specimens at a time of enterovirus surveillance, the first recovered reovirus was designated ECHO virus type 10.[18,103] This virus and four similar strains were recovered in 1954 from the stools of healthy children in Cincinnati and Mexico.[68-70] By 1959, researchers were aware that ECHO 10 viral strains appeared to have many characteristics that were different from those of enteroviruses, such as large size and unique cytopathic effect, and they were withdrawn from this grouping. The term *reovirus* was chosen to stress the association of these agents with both the respiratory *(r)* and enteric *(e)* tracts. The *o* for orphan was retained in the designation. In the early 1960s, reoviral infections were noted in association with human illness.[16,31,36,46,75,76,79,80,113]

PROPERTIES

Reoviruses are members of the family Reoviridae.[19,13,60] This family has numerous double-stranded RNA viruses that infect mammals, birds, reptiles, fish, mollusks, insects, plants, and arthropods. The family Reoviridae contain 15 genera, which are divided into two groups based on their particle morphology. One subfamily (Sedoreovirinae) contains six genera, and three of these (*Orbivirus*, *Rotavirus*, and *Seadornavirus*) are presented in Chapters 172 and 173. The other subfamily (Spinareovirinae) contains nine genera, one of which (*Orthoreovirus*) is discussed in this chapter. Orthoreoviruses have a turtle-like protein that projects from the innermost capsid layer. Sedoreovirinae do not have this turtle-like protein. Orthoreoviruses commonly are called simply reoviruses. Historically, three serotypes of orthoreoviruses were noted to cause infection in humans. All mammalian reoviruses are related by a common group-specific, complement-fixing antigen.[13,82] Three distinct human serotypes can be identified by neutralization or hemagglutination inhibition.[73,80]

Reovirus particles are composed of an inner protein shell (core) with a diameter of 60 nm that is surrounded by an outer protein shell (outer capsid) measuring 81 nm in diameter.[13] The outer capsid has icosahedral symmetry and is composed of 92 to 180 hexagonal and pentagonal subunits (capsomers). The genome of orthoreoviruses has a total size of approximately 23,500 base pairs with 10 gene segments: three large (L1, L2, L3), three medium (M1, M2, M3), and four small (S1, S2, S3, S4). These genes encode 12 proteins. The outer capsid comprises four proteins: σ-1, σ-3, λ-2, and μ-1. The σ-1 protein is the reovirus cell-attachment protein against which serotype-specific neutralizing antibodies are developed. This protein also is the hemagglutinin. The reovirus receptor is the junctional adhesion molecule 1 (JAM1).[20,99] The σ-3 protein binds double-stranded RNA and is sensitive to protease degradation. It is a zinc metalloprotein that has effects on translation. The λ-2 protein is important in particle assembly and μ-1 in cell penetration.

The inner capsid is composed of four proteins: λ-3, λ-1, μ-2, and σ-2. The λ-3 protein is an RNA-dependent RNA polymerase. The λ-1 protein is a zinc metalloprotein that binds RNA. The μ-2 protein binds RNA, and σ-2 binds double-stranded RNA.

The four nonstructural proteins are μ-NS, μ-NSC, σ-1s, and σ-NS. The μ-NS protein is a core-binding protein, and σ-NS binds single-stranded RNA. The roles of μ-NSC and σ-1s are unknown.

Reoviruses are moderately heat stable. The half-life at 56°C (132.8°F) of a type 3 strain is 1.6 minutes; at 37°C (98.6°F), it is approximately 2.5 hours. Reoviruses are inactivated by visible light in the presence of heterocyclic dyes. They are inactivated by ultraviolet light but are more resistant to this treatment than are RNA viruses with single-stranded nucleic acid. Reoviruses are stable through a wide pH range and also as aerosols, particularly when the relative humidity is high. They are relatively resistant to 3% formaldehyde solution, 1% hydrogen peroxide, and 1% phenol but are inactivated completely by 70% ethyl alcohol at room temperature for 1 hour. Brief exposure to 70% ethanol is ineffective in disinfecting reoviruses, but brief exposure to 95% ethanol or sodium hypochlorite is effective.

Reoviruses replicate with a cytopathic effect in a large number of tissue culture systems of both primate and other animal origins. For recovery from clinical material, monkey kidney tissue culture is satisfactory. Cytopathic effect is enhanced in rolled in contrast to stationary cultures.[45] Infected cells develop characteristic cytoplasmic inclusions that contain double-stranded RNA, virus-specific proteins, and complete and incomplete viral particles. All three serotypes agglutinate human erythrocytes, and this virus-cell interaction is stable in a wide temperature and pH range.

Of all viruses that naturally infect humans, reoviruses have the broadest host range. They have been recovered from natural infections in cattle, chimpanzees, monkeys, mice, dogs, turkeys, sheep, pigs, chickens, and cats.[11,26,28,51,53,54,73,77,83,108,109] In addition, hemagglutination-inhibiting and neutralizing antibodies to one or more of the three reoviral serotypes have been found in the serum of rabbits, horses, trout, guinea pigs, antelopes, zebras, warthogs, bats, wallabies, quokkas, kangaroos, and several genera of New World monkeys.[59,73,74,77,80,82,93,95]

Because of their widespread prevalence in nature and the ease of causing infection in laboratory animals, reoviruses have been used widely in pathogenicity studies. The following unique illnesses have been observed: diabetes mellitus in mice; hydrocephalus in hamsters, ferrets, rats, and mice; encephalitis in mice; chronic infection with runting in mice; myocarditis in mice; chronic obstructive jaundice associated with choledochal obliteration in mice; and lymphomas in mice with chronic infection.[13,33,39,49,50,62,63,67,88,92,94]

EPIDEMIOLOGY

The serologic data presented in the preceding section of this chapter demonstrate that reoviruses are prevalent infectious agents in the animal world. Similarly, surveys of sera collected from humans indicate worldwide human infection.[4,5,6,22,37,44,46,47,66,81,85,100,101,105] The occurrence in nature of identical viruses in many different animals and humans leads to consideration of possible transmission from species to species. Chua and associates[8-10] and other investigators[21,89,90,110] present data suggesting that reoviruses associated with human respiratory infections were of fruit bat origin. In addition, Ouattara and colleagues[64] have noted a reovirus type 2 swine reovirus reassortant associated with encephalitis.

Reoviruses are recovered frequently from sewage.[17,35,42,48,52,61] In San Diego prior to 1972, reoviruses were recovered more consistently than has any other virus throughout the year from sewage.[17] This finding suggests that reoviral infection was endemic in humans in the San Diego area.

The type 2 hemagglutination-inhibiting antibody prevalence pattern by age in sera collected in Boston from 1959 to 1962 is presented in Table 171.1. Antibody is transmitted transplacentally to the newborn. During the first year of life, this acquired antibody wanes, after which antibody prevalence increases with increasing age. Approximately 50% of school-aged children have hemagglutination-inhibiting antibody titers to type 2 reovirus of 1:20 or greater; approximately 80% of adults have similar titers. Two more recent studies have shown a similar prevalence of antibody to reovirus type 3.[87,100]

The method of transmission of reoviruses is unknown. However, because they are recovered most frequently from the feces, the primary spread probably from person to person is by the fecal-oral route, similar to that of enteroviruses. Because the reoviruses are stable in aerosols and because respiratory illness has been associated with reovirus infections, the respiratory route is an additional possibility. The method of spread of fruit bat (flying foxes) reoviruses to humans is not known.

CLINICAL MANIFESTATIONS

The role of reoviral infections in human disease is far from clear. In most instances, virologic or serologic evidence of reoviral infection has been a sporadic finding in human illness, so that cause and effect are difficult to establish. However, in volunteer studies in young adults, infection resulted in clinical illness.[31,74,78]

The prevalence of antibody to all three reoviral types in humans and the frequency of reovirus isolation from human sewage indicate that human infection is a common occurrence, but the relative paucity of virus recovered during studies of community disease suggests that most infections are inapparent or associated with trivial illness.

Upper Respiratory Tract Illness

In the winter of 1957, Rosen and colleagues[75,79] noted an outbreak of infection with reovirus type 1 in nursery children in a welfare institution. Illness was noted in 16 of 22 infected children and was characterized by low-grade fever (rectal temperatures from 38.1°C to 38.6°C [100.6°F to 101.5°F]), rhinorrhea, and pharyngitis. The average duration of fever was 2.2 days; in nine children, the duration was only 1 day. Three children had diarrhea, and three had mild otitis media. In another study conducted at the same institution during the winter of 1955 to 1956, four children with reovirus type 3 infection and illness were noted.[76,80] One child had a temperature of 38.9°C (102°F), coryza, and tonsillitis; another child had fever (temperature of 38.2°C [100.8°F]), cough, and diarrhea; and two children had only coryza. During another reovirus type 3 outbreak in the fall of 1957, all six infected infants had symptoms. Five children had mild fever, five had coryza, and four had diarrhea. Pharyngitis was not observed in any of the infected children.

Other sporadic instances of similar mild upper respiratory tract illnesses have been described.[12,27,31,96,97] In volunteer trials in young adults, reovirus type 1 infection was associated with malaise, rhinorrhea, cough, sneezing, pharyngitis, and headache in some subjects in one study,[74,78] and coldlike illness was observed in 37% of subjects in another trial.[31] In both volunteer studies and natural infection, mild diarrhea occurred with the upper respiratory tract illness.

In three separate investigations, Chua and coworkers[8-10] noted acute influenza-like illnesses in four adult patients. The reoviruses in these four cases were of fruit bat origin, and in one instance evidence of human-to-human transmission was found.

Pneumonia

Tillotson and Lerner[104] described a 5-year-old girl who had extensive pneumonia and died after 15 days of illness. This child initially had fever, cough, rhinorrhea, and a generalized maculopapular rash. When admitted to the hospital on the tenth day of illness, the child was cyanotic and in marked respiratory distress; rash was no longer present, but mild pharyngitis and conjunctivitis were. A chest radiograph revealed diffuse confluent pneumonia, and reovirus type 3 was recovered from the lungs, adrenals, liver, spleen, kidney, a lymph node, heart, brain, and blood.

Joske and associates[36] described a 10-month-old girl who died after having a respiratory illness of 4 days' duration. A reovirus type 1 was recovered from the stool and brain of this child, and postmortem study revealed interstitial pneumonia, myocarditis, hepatitis, and encephalitis. El-Rai and Evans[16] reported the case of an 18-year-old man who had fever (temperature of 39.4°C [103°F]), nausea, vomiting, cough, and patchy pneumonia. He had serologic evidence of infection with reovirus type 1. Pneumonia has been noted in another child with reovirus type 3 infection.[96]

Gastrointestinal Manifestations

Mild diarrhea has been noted both in association with upper respiratory tract illness and as an isolated event.[69,70,74-76,78-80,83] Because reovirus type 3 consistently produces steatorrhea in mice, this clinical manifestation has been sought in illnesses of children and noted in six.[36,96] Three patients with hepatitis and encephalitis have been described.[36] Zalan and associates[113] have noted two patients in whom abdominal pain and cramps were prominent.

In 1980, Bangaru and associates[1] reported the similarity of induced hepatobiliary injury caused by reovirus type 3 infection in mice and biliary atresia in human infants. Subsequent to this observation, Glaser and associates[23] and Morecki and colleagues[23,57,58] looked for an association

TABLE 171.1 Hemagglutination-Inhibiting (H1) Antibodies to Reovirus Type 2 in 253 Serum Specimens Collected in Boston, Massachusetts, 1959–62

Age Group	% With H1 Titer ≥1:20
Premature newborn	68
0–6 mo	25
7–12 mo	9
13–24 mo	27
2–5 y	37
6–10 y	52
11–20 y	54
21–40 y	34
41–60 y	83
>60 y	73

From Lerner AM, Cherry JD, Klein JO, et al. Infections with reoviruses. *N Engl J Med.* 1962;267:947–952.

between reovirus type 3 infection and biliary atresia in humans. In their first report, they found that 17 of 25 patients (68%) with biliary atresia had antibodies (indirect immunofluorescent antibody technique) to reovirus type 3, whereas similar antibodies were recovered in only three of 37 control sera.[57] In a second study, they found that 62% of babies with extrahepatic biliary atresia and 52% of infants with idiopathic neonatal hepatitis had antibodies to reovirus type 3; only 12% of control children had similar antibodies.[23] In an ultrastructural and immunocytochemical study, they found evidence of reovirus type 3 in the porta hepatis of an infant with extrahepatic biliary atresia.[58]

Using similar serologic techniques, Dussaix and associates[14] were unable to find any relationship between reovirus type 3 antibody and either biliary atresia or neonatal hepatitis. They found reovirus type 3 antibody in sera from 45% of infants with biliary atresia, 50% of infants with neonatal hepatitis, and 50% of control infants. Minuk and colleagues[56] found no association between reovirus type 3 infection and idiopathic cholestatic liver disease in adults. Brown and colleagues[7] reported a relatively large study of reovirus type 3 infection and extrahepatic biliary atresia and neonatal hepatitis. They interpreted their data as demonstrating no correlation between the virus and the illnesses studied. However, the geometric mean antibody value in the combined biliary atresia and neonatal hepatitis groups was significantly higher than that of the control group. Richardson and associates[72] reported a study in which they examined the percentage of immunoglobulin (Ig)G, IgA, and IgM serum antibodies to reovirus type 3 in 40 infants with extrahepatic biliary atresia, 59 infants with neonatal hepatitis, 61 infants with cholestatic liver disease with causes other than extrahepatic biliary atresia or neonatal hepatitis, and 138 control infants with no liver disease. They found no difference in the prevalence of IgG and IgA antibodies between the groups with liver disease and the control subjects. They did, however, note a greater prevalence of IgM antibody in each of the groups with liver disease, in contrast to the rate in the control group. However, this increased prevalence of IgM antibody could be the result of false-positive titers as a result of the liver disease rather than evidence of recent or ongoing infection. Steele and associates,[98] using a reverse transcriptase-mediated polymerase chain reaction (RT-PCR), found no evidence of reovirus type 3 in preserved tissues from infants with cholestatic liver disease. Saito and associates,[84] using RT-PCR, could find no amplification product in tissue or stool specimens from patients with biliary atresia, infantile obstructive cholangiopathy, or congenital dilation of the bile duct.

In 2009, Rauschenfels and colleagues[71] did an extensive study on the incidence of hepatotropic viruses in biliary atresia. They obtained liver biopsies from 64 infants with biliary atresia at the time of the Kasai procedure. They identified reovirus type 3 RNA by RT-PCR in 21 (33%) biopsies. They noted that the 21 patients who were reovirus-positive were older (mean age 60 days) than those who were virus-negative (mean age, 54 days). This finding led them to suggest that the viral infection was a secondary phenomenon and not the cause of the biliary atresia.

Exanthem

Exanthem has been a common manifestation of clinically apparent reoviral infections.[16,36,46,104] Lerner and associates[46] noted exanthem in six of seven children infected with reovirus type 2. Predominant symptoms in these patients included fever, malaise, anorexia, and pharyngitis. Two children had adenopathy, and one had diarrhea. The rash was maculopapular in five patients and vesicular in one child. One child had a measles-like illness with photophobia, conjunctivitis, cervical lymphadenopathy, and a confluent maculopapular rash that lasted approximately 1 week.

Exanthem has been noted in a 5-year-old girl with pneumonia and type 3 reovirus infection, a 28-month-old girl with encephalitis and type 2 infection, and an 18-year-old adolescent male with pharyngitis and cervical and posterior occipital lymph node enlargement and type 2 infection.[16,36,104]

Neurologic Disease

Joske and colleagues[36] described three cases of hepatitis-encephalitis syndrome with reoviral infections. All of these cases had abnormal liver function test results and clinical and laboratory evidence of meningeal and cerebral involvement. One child died, one had mild neurologic residua at the 6-week follow-up, and one recovered without difficulty. Two patients were infected with reovirus type 2 and one with reovirus type 3.

El-Rai and Evans[16] found serologic evidence of reovirus type 2 infection in two children with aseptic meningitis, and Zalan and colleagues[113] described two children with reovirus type 2 infections associated with leg weakness and pain. Johansson and colleagues[34] noted a 3-month-old girl with meningitis, diarrhea, vomiting, and fever. Reovirus type 1 was isolated from this child's cerebrospinal fluid (CSF), and the child had a fourfold rise in neutralizing antibody to the isolated virus. Krainer and Aronson[43] described a 29-year-old woman who died of disseminated demyelinating encephalomyelitis in which a reovirus was recovered from the CSF and brain. Tyler and associates[106] isolated a type 3 reovirus from the CSF of a 6.5-week-old child with meningitis. This child recovered without obvious neurologic sequelae.

Ouattara and associates[64] reported a 6-year-old boy and his 2-month-old girl cousin with acute encephalitis associated with a reovirus type 2 infection. The boy had a febrile prodrome and then vomiting and impaired consciousness. On examination, he had a palsy of the left facial nerve. His CSF had a mildly elevated protein without pleocytosis. Magnetic resonance imaging (MRI) showed multiple symmetric lesions. He recovered completely in a few weeks. The cousin had fever, asthenia, and rhinorrhea. She also had a mildly elevated CSF protein and MRI findings similar to those of her older cousin. At hospital discharge at 18 days, she had marked hypotonia and the absence of language. At 1-year follow-up, she had uncoordinated movements. A similar virus was isolated from the urine of both children. This virus was thought to be a reassortant between human and swine strains.[43]

Other Manifestations

A 25-year-old man with Hodgkin disease had persistent reovirus type 1 viruria for a 5-week period, but no associated clinical illness was demonstrated.[15] Reoviruses have been recovered from biopsy material from patients with Burkitt lymphoma.[2,3] One child with hemorrhagic bullous myringitis was infected with reovirus type 2.[113] Terheggen and colleagues[102] noted a 28-year-old man with mild myocarditis in whom a reovirus was isolated from the stool sample.

Reoviruses as Potential Anti-Cancer Agents

Studies during the present and previous decades indicate the potential of reoviruses to selectively destroy many different types of neoplastic cells.[24,25,29,30,38,40,41,55,91,107,111,112] Many malignant cells have an activated Ras pathway that results in a deficient ability to mount an antireovirus response that is mediated by the cellular protein PKR. Organ culture and animal model systems have shown promising results with reovirus type 3 in numerous different malignant neoplasms. At present, many phase I and phase II trials are in progress or have been completed.[25,40,41,65] Also completed is one phase III head and neck cancer trial.[40,41]

DIAGNOSIS

Because no specific clinical features suggest reoviral infection, virologic and serologic studies are necessary for establishing the diagnosis. Reoviruses can be recovered from clinical material in primary monkey kidney tissue culture.[76,78] Care must be taken in interpreting results, however, because reoviruses can be contaminants of monkey tissue cultures. Cytopathic effect in tissue culture is enhanced by rolling during incubation.[45] Identification of virus is made by neutralization; the distinctive cytopathic effect should be helpful in selecting strains for study with reovirus antisera. In research laboratories, reoviruses also can be detected by molecular techniques such as in situ and dot-blot hybridization and PCR.[13,71] Paired serum specimens can be examined for antibody titer rise to reoviruses by neutralization, indirect immunofluorescent antibody technique, enzyme-linked immunosorbent assay (ELISA), or hemagglutination inhibition. Recent infection can also be identified by the demonstration of specific IgM antibody by ELISA.

With the exception of recent clinical illnesses associated with fruit bat orthoreoviruses,[8-10,89,90,110] the vast majority of clinical associations with reoviral infections occurred more than 45 years ago. This seems surprising because recent antibody studies in sera from children indicate that infections are still common.[100] I believe there are several reasons for the present lack of descriptions of clinical reovirus infections. The first reason is the fact that rolling of tissue cultures in virus laboratories is rarely done today. More importantly, many diagnostic laboratories have switched from studying specimens from patients in tissue culture systems to molecular diagnostic platforms. These platforms do not include reoviruses.

In regard to clinical illness, orthoreoviruses are the forgotten viruses of the 21st century. In the 11th edition of the *ASM Manual of Clinical Microbiology*, orthoreoviruses are not mentioned at all.[32]

NEW REFERENCES SINCE THE SEVENTH EDITION

40. Kim M. Naturally occurring reoviruses for human cancer therapy. *BMB Rep.* 2015;48(8):454-460.
89. Shi Z. Emerging infectious diseases associated with bat viruses. *Sci China Life Sci.* 2013;56(8):678-682.
90. Singh H, Shimojima M, Ngoc TC, et al. Serological evidence of human infection with Pteropine orthoreovirus in Central Vietnam. *J Med Virol.* 2015.
110. Yamanaka A, Iwakiri A, Yoshikawa T, et al. Imported case of acute respiratory tract infection associated with a member of species Nelson Bay orthoreovirus. *PLoS ONE.* 2014;9(3):e92777.

The full reference list for this chapter is available at ExpertConsult.com.

172 Orbiviruses, Coltiviruses, and Seadornaviruses

Gail J. Harrison • Theodore F. Tsai

Viruses in the genera *Orbivirus, Coltivirus,* and *Seadornavirus* differ from others in the family Reoviridae structurally, in physicochemical properties, and by their arthropod mode of transmission.[2,3] More than 100 orbiviruses are classified into serogroups by relationships in complement fixation, agar gel precipitation, and immunofluorescent assays. Additional serocomplex relationships are recognized, whereas individual viruses are differentiated by neutralization tests. Orbiviruses are principally animal pathogens (e.g., the bluetongue viruses); only viruses in the Kemerovo, Orungo, Lebombo, and Changuinola serogroups have been shown to cause human illness. Colorado tick fever (CTF) virus is the only *Coltivirus* recognized to cause human illness, and among the seadornaviruses, only Banna virus (BAV) is a confirmed human pathogen.[2-4,50,54]

The orbiviruses are spherical nonenveloped viruses with two protein shells: an outer shell (capsid) approximately 86 nm in diameter and an inner shell (core) 69 nm in diameter. The inner core VP7 protein, arranged in trimers, contains group-reactive antigens, and the outer capsid VP2 or VP5 proteins bear serotype-specific antigens. The viruses are acid labile, and some exhibit sensitivity to lipid solvents. The double-stranded RNA viral genome comprises 10 segments associated with viral structural and nonstructural proteins. Their complete nucleotide sequences and coding assignments have been determined for a bluetongue virus, and partial information is available for others. In general, reassortments of genomic segments among viruses within serogroups are viable, but not between groups, thus validating the broad serogroup classification. The genetic relationships (e.g., RNA hybridization) among viruses within serogroups diverge from the antigenic relationships in some instances, providing an additional basis for taxonomic classification.

The coltiviruses and seadornaviruses resemble the orbiviruses in size and in having two capsids but possess genomes organized into 12 RNA segments.[3] The morphologic features and structural protein similarities of seadornaviruses and rotaviruses suggest an evolutionary relationship.[40]

COLORADO TICK FEVER VIRUS

CTF virus is an acute tick-borne febrile illness caused by the eponymous *Coltivirus.*[5,13,18,19,30,48,51] Eyach virus, isolated from *Ixodes* ticks in France and Germany; S6-1403, isolated in California from a gray squirrel; and mosquito strains from Indonesia are related to but distinct from CTF virus and have not been confirmed to cause human illness.[3,29-31] RNA hybridization studies of CTF viral strains from a 33-year interval found minor heterogeneity, thus suggesting that a single gene pool has been maintained by mixing of viral strains and by constraints on viral replication within tick vectors and vertebrate hosts. Molecular characterization of the virus also continues by basic scientists.[43] A wide variety of small and large mammals are infected naturally with the virus, but clinical illness develops only in humans. Experimental infection of rhesus monkeys, hamsters, and mice produces hematologic changes similar to those occurring in human infections.[22]

Epidemiology

Cases occur sporadically in association with the habitats of the wood tick *Dermacentor andersoni.*[55] Most cases occur in May and June, when adult ticks are most active, but infections from March to November have been reported. Infections are acquired principally in the western part of the United States, especially Wyoming and Utah; Canada in the known geographic distribution of the vector; and at elevations between 4000 and 10,000 feet (Figs. 172.1 and 172.2).[8,11,12,13,46,47,55] In one study in Wyoming, 99% of the ticks reported were *D. andersoni*, found in areas with sagebrush at elevations higher than 7000 feet.[21] In rare cases, CTF has occurred in persons who had not traveled to areas of known risk, such as those exposed to ticks brought home on the clothing of family members and, in one case, by transfusion.[7,39,45,46,54] The annual incidence of disease in the Rocky Mountain region, approximately three per 1 million residents, is declining, possibly a result of a larger elk population that has reduced habitats of small vertebrate hosts.[4]

CTF virus is maintained in a 2- to 3-year cycle among small mammals, principally rodents, and *D. andersoni* ticks (Fig. 172.3).[5,13,19] Once infected in the larval stage, ticks remain infected through the nymphal and adult stages (transstadial transmission). Larvae are infected by viremic rodents. After molting, they carry the virus through the winter, and as nymphs, they infect other rodents and renew the cycle of transmission the following spring. Humans become infected incidentally by the bite of infected adult ticks (Fig. 172.4).

The least chipmunk *(Eutamias minimus)*, the golden-mantled ground squirrel *(Spermophilus lateralis)*, and the porcupine *(Erethizon dorsatum)* appear to be the primary hosts for larval, nymphal, and adult *D. andersoni;* secondary hosts include rock mice *(Peromyscus maniculatus)*, meadow voles *(Microtus pennsylvanicus)*, and pine squirrels *(Tamiasciurus hudsonicus)*.[6]

D. andersoni is found exclusively in the high plains and in mountainous terrain between 4000 and 10,000 feet in altitude in the geographic distribution previously mentioned. The specific microhabitats where

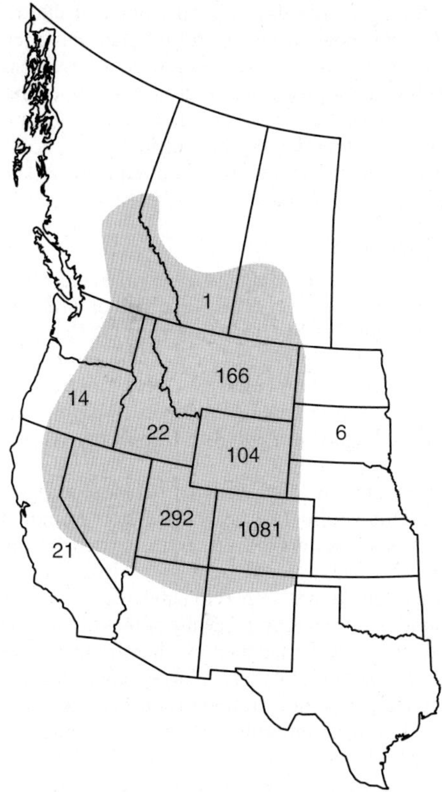

FIG. 172.1 Geographic distribution of *Dermacentor andersoni* ticks and reported cases of Colorado tick fever, 1980–91.

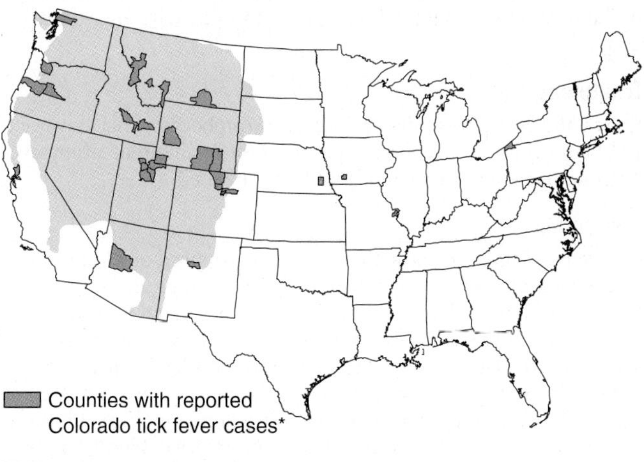

FIG. 172.2 Approximate geographic distribution of *Dermacentor andersoni* ticks and counties of residence for confirmed and probable Colorado tick fever virus disease cases, United States, 2002–12. (Courtesy Centers for Disease Control and Prevention. Available at: https://www.cdc.gov/coloradotickfever/statistics.html.)

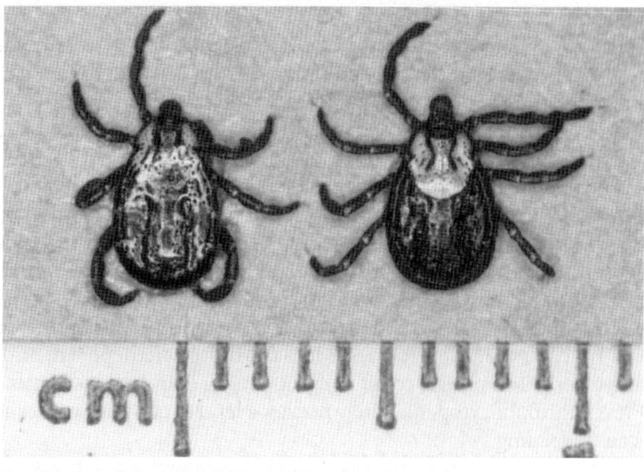

FIG. 172.3 Adult male *(left)* and female *(right) Dermacentor andersoni* ticks. Both can transmit Colorado tick fever virus.

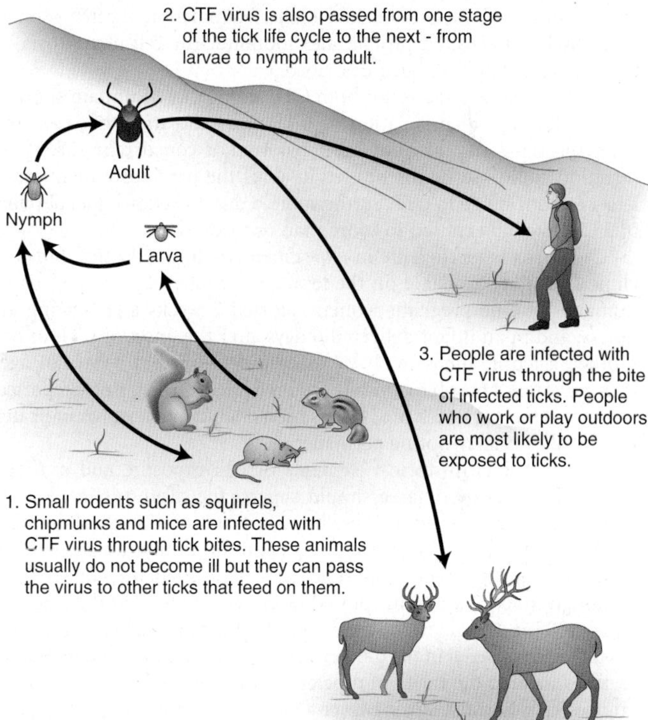

Ecology of Colorado Tick Fever Virus
Colorado tick fever (CTF) virus is spread by Rocky Mountain wood ticks (*Dermacentor andersoni*). Rocky mountain wood ticks are found in the western United States and Canda at 4,000–10,000 feet above sea level. Here are the steps in how the virus is spread:
2. CTF virus is also passed from one stage of the tick life cycle to the next - from larvae to nymph to adult.
Adult
Nymph
Larva
3. People are infected with CTF virus through the bite of infected ticks. People who work or play outdoors are most likely to be exposed to ticks.
1. Small rodents such as squirrels, chipmunks and mice are infected with CTF virus through tick bites. These animals usually do not become ill but they can pass the virus to other ticks that feed on them.
4. Other animals such as elk, marmots and deer also can be infected with CTF virus through tick bites. However, these animals probably do not play an important role in passing the virus to other ticks.

FIG. 172.4 Colorado tick fever virus ecology. (Courtesy Centers for Disease Control and Prevention. Available at https://www.cdc.gov/coloradotickfever/transmission.html.)

infected ticks are most prevalent are south-facing slopes with open stands of ponderosa pine, moderate shrubs, and rocky surfaces that provide favorable habitats for the intermediate rodent hosts.[6,38] Both male and female adult ticks can transmit infection to humans, and the period of attachment required for transmission of the virus may be very brief.

Clinical Manifestations

A history of a tick bite or tick exposure is given by more than 90% of patients.[23] The incubation period usually is 3 to 4 days, with a range of 0 to 14 days after known exposure to a tick.[4,23] The onset typically is abrupt, with fever, chills, malaise, headache, retroorbital pain, myalgia, lumbar pain, and hyperesthesia. Nausea, vomiting, and abdominal pain occur less frequently. Upper respiratory tract symptoms usually are absent, although conjunctival injection may develop. Lymphadenopathy and hepatosplenomegaly are found in some patients. Maculopapular and petechial eruptions have been observed in 5% to 12% of cases.[49]

The disease classically is biphasic; an initial attack lasting 2 to 3 days is followed by an equal interval of defervescence and a second and, rarely, a third recurrence. However, this saddleback pattern is absent in more than 50% of cases. Symptoms resolve several days after the second bout of fever, but prolonged asthenia lasting for several weeks is a typical finding, especially in adults.[23]

Leukopenia is a hallmark of the illness. The mean initial leukocyte count is 3900/mm^3, which diminishes to a nadir 5 to 6 days after the onset of illness, often during the period of remission. A left shift with an absolute neutropenia and relative lymphocytosis is a usual finding. Examination of bone marrow aspirates shows maturational arrest in the granulocytic series, with absent mature forms and numerous metamyelocytes and myelocytes. Megakaryocytes are depleted, and a reduced peripheral platelet count (<150,000/m^3) is found in most patients; however, thrombocytopenia rarely reaches a level of clinical significance to cause bleeding.[28,36]

Uncomplicated recovery is the rule. Epididymo-orchitis, pneumonitis, hepatitis, and pericarditis have been reported as complications, but the most serious complications are encephalitis and hemorrhage,[16,20,23,25,37] which have been reported nearly exclusively in children younger than 10 years.[11,23,50] Three deaths have been reported, all in children who exhibited signs of generalized bleeding accompanied by a reduced platelet count.[23,28] Examination of the bone marrow in one child disclosed a generalized depression of myeloid and erythroid elements and a marked reduction in megakaryocytes. Central nervous system signs consistent with meningitis and encephalitis, sometimes associated with coma, have been reported in both children and adults. Examination of cerebrospinal fluid disclosed elevated protein and mononuclear cell pleocytosis in the few cases that have been described.

D. andersoni is a vector for both CTF and Rocky Mountain spotted fever.[3] Although dual isolation of CTF virus and *Rickettsia rickettsii* from the same tick has not been reported, a concurrent rickettsial infection could not be discounted in all of the previously mentioned fatal cases attributed to CTF. Furthermore, a dual infection could develop in an individual exposed to more than one tick.

CTF virus is teratogenic in experimentally infected mice, but few clinical data are available on the teratogenic potential of the virus in humans.[24,27] One pregnant woman aborted 2 weeks after having an illness; and in an infant delivered 6 days after the onset of CTF in the mother, a febrile illness with leukopenia developed at 3 days of age, thus indicating a possible vertically acquired infection. In a single reported instance, a second attack of CTF has been documented, which indicates that immunity may not be permanent.[23,24]

The combined historical elements of tick exposure and outdoor activity in an enzootic area should suggest the diagnosis in patients with a spring-summer grippe-like illness. In a controlled study, abdominal pain, pharyngitis, and rash were less common symptoms in patients with CTF than in patients with other acute illnesses in the same season. Although Rocky Mountain spotted fever occurs rarely in the states in which CTF is prevalent, the possibility of this potentially fatal disease should be considered in the differential diagnosis. Helpful differentiating features include the rarity of a petechial rash in CTF and its biphasic course. Tick-borne relapsing fever also follows a remitting course, but it has a more acute and toxic onset; splenomegaly occurs commonly, and remission is by crisis. The geographic distribution of the diseases overlaps; however, human encounters with the argasid (soft) tick vectors of relapsing fever (*Ornithodoros* ticks) are likely to occur in cabins and other protected areas.

Eyach virus has been implicated in central nervous system infections and polyradiculitis in Europe. However, its tick-borne transmission from *Ixodes ricinus* that also transmits *Borrelia, Anaplasma,* and Kemerovo group viruses has prevented establishment of a clear interpretation.

Pathophysiology

Experimental infection of rhesus monkeys, rodents, and human marrow cells in vitro has shown that CTF virus infects the erythropoietic elements (erythroblasts to reticulocytes) at an early stage of infection.[13,14,22,28,45,47] After the infected cells mature and are released into the peripheral circulation, the virus persists intracellularly, where it has been identified by electron microscopy.[15,44,45] CTF virus has been cultured from circulating erythrocytes for up to 120 days after the onset of illness.[27] Red cell survival evidently is not shortened, and infected cells circulate in the presence of neutralizing antibody. Prolonged viremia has not been associated with either a protracted or a more severe course of illness. Infected CD34+ progenitor cells and impaired mononuclear cell production of colony-stimulating factors may contribute to the acute aregenerative cytopenia.[44,45] High levels of serum interferon-γ correlate with fever during the acute phase of illness.[1]

Laboratory Diagnosis

The most readily available diagnostic test is reverse transcriptase-polymerase chain reaction (RT-PCR) detection of viral RNA or virus-specific immunoglobulin M (IgM) in serum.[31,44] Cerebrospinal fluid may also be tested. Testing is available in some commercial and state health laboratories and at the Centers for Disease Control and Prevention Division of Vector-Borne Diseases Arbovirus Diagnostic Laboratory (https://www.cdc.gov/ncezid/dvbd/specimensub/arboviral-shipping.html).

RT-PCR may be positive on the first day of illness, and IgG seroconversion usually occurs within 14 to 21 days. Direct immunofluorescent examination of blood smears for intraerythrocytic viral antigen is also a rapid approach to laboratory diagnosis.[14,31] Isolation of virus from acute or convalescent blood samples in baby mice or Vero or BHK cells also can be done.[10,14] Freezing and thawing of the clot should be avoided, and it should instead be refrigerated for short-term storage. Virus has been isolated from a blood clot that had been refrigerated for 14 months. Serologic diagnosis by demonstration of fourfold rises in neutralizing, complement fixation, immunofluorescent, or enzyme-linked immunosorbent assay (ELISA) antibody is confirmatory. ELISAs that distinguish between CTF and Eyach virus antibodies are available. Neutralizing antibody rises slowly; only one-third of patients had detectable neutralizing antibody 10 days after onset, but fourfold rises appeared within 30 days of onset in 92%. Therefore acute serum should be collected 3 to 10 days after onset of symptoms, and convalescent serum for IgG antibody testing should be done at least 14 to 21 days after the acute serum.

Treatment

No specific therapy is available. Because thrombocytopenia may occur and hemorrhage is a reported complication in children, antipyretics that interfere with coagulation should not be used.

Prevention

Repellents containing permethrin should be sprayed on clothing, and repellents containing diethyltoluamide (DEET) or picaridin should be applied to exposed skin. Long pants should be tucked into socks and shirts tucked into slacks. Clothing, gear, and skin should be inspected frequently for unattached and attached ticks, especially if walking through sagebrush or spending time at elevations higher than 7000 feet.[21,22] Light-colored clothing facilitates such inspections. One case of human-to-human transmission by transfusion of infected blood has been reported.[7] Persons with documented CTF should be prohibited from donating blood until the often prolonged viremia has cleared.[46,47]

BANNA VIRUS

BAV is the prototype species of *Seadornavirus* within the family Reoviridae. It is a segmented double-stranded RNA virus with 12 segments in its genome.[34,35] It was originally isolated in patients with encephalitis in Xishuangbanna, Yunnan Province, People's Republic of China, from which it received its name. It is also found in mosquitoes in China, Vietnam, and Indonesia, and likely is distributed from the tropics of Southeast Asia to the northern temperate regions of China (Fig. 172.5).

BAV has been isolated from patients with febrile illness and encephalitis in China and is believed to be a major contributor to cases of viral encephalitis in China and, possibly, within a broader region of East and Southeast Asia.[2,32,35,50] It has been isolated from 10 different mosquito species from two genera (*Culex tritaeniorhynchus, Culex pipiens pallens, Culex annulus, Culex pseudovishnui, Culex modestus, Anopheles sinensis, Aedes vagus, Aedes albopictus, Aedes vexans,* and *Aedes dorsalis*), which

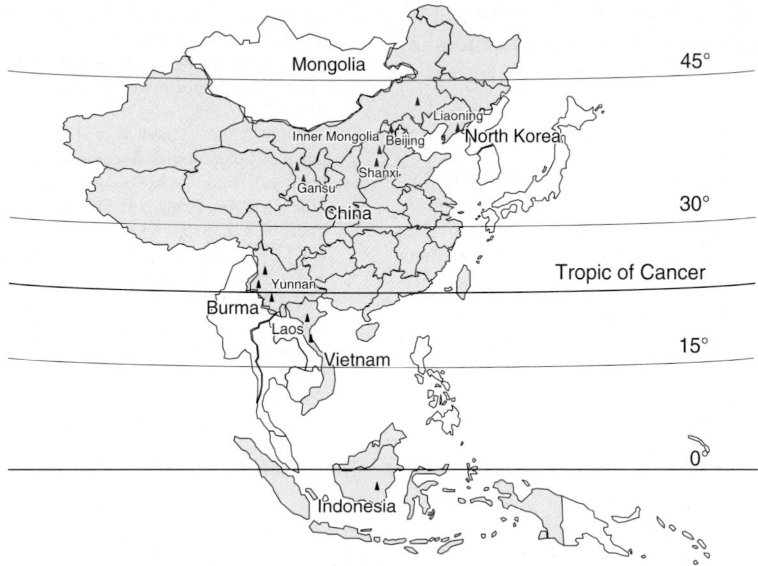

FIG. 172.5 Location of Banna viruses in China and southeast Asia countries of Vietnam and Indonesia *(shaded areas)*. Distinct areas of virus isolation from mosquitoes are shown *(triangles)*. (Courtesy Centers for Disease Control and Prevention. Available at: https://wwwnc.cdc.gov/eid/article/16/3/09-1160-f1.)

are widely distributed in China and other areas of the world.[26] A common ancestry and taxonomic link to rotaviruses have been indicated by similarities in the viruses' gene organization and certain gene segment sequences (e.g., for VP9), as well as their morphology.[41] Two genotypes/serotypes (A and B) have been defined with broadly overlapping geographic distributions. The virus has been isolated from far-northern China, Mongolia, southern China, Vietnam, and Indonesia and from *C. tritaeniorhynchus, C. pipiens pallens,* and other mosquito vectors that also transmit Japanese encephalitis virus (JEV), and, in one study, the virus was implicated as the cause of 14% of cases in a nominal JEV outbreak.[33,35,42] In addition, although the transmission dynamics of BAV are not well known, it is possible the virus may spread by infected mosquitoes caught by prevailing winds that move from South East Asia to East Asia, or associated with bird migration through East Asia–Australasia flyways.

Clinical symptoms in confirmed cases have included fever, arthralgia, and encephalitis, but few details have been published.

BAV appears to be an emerging virus with possible spread into nonendemic areas.

The potential public health impact of BAV infection could be substantial in the near future.[34,35] The diagnostic tests to confirm a specific diagnosis are not widely available; broader application of real-time PCR assays that have been developed and field studies are needed to define the burden of disease and need for public health intervention. In addition, several seadornaviruses related to BAV that have been described in China (e.g., mosquito-borne Liao ning virus, Balaton virus, and Mangshi virus) are suspected to cause human illness but currently remain orphan agents.[37,54]

KEMEROVO AND RELATED VIRUSES

The Kemerovo serogroup comprises tick-borne Kemerovo, Tribec, and Lipovnik viruses, which may have descended from ancestral mosquito-borne orbiviruses.[9] Kemerovo virus, a double-stranded RNA virus, was isolated from the cerebrospinal fluid of two patients with encephalitis and from ticks in the Kemerovo region of Russia; seroconversion was demonstrated in 10 other patients with meningoencephalitis with tick bites and in whom Russian spring-summer encephalitis was excluded.[8,33] The virus is transmitted in an *Ixodes persulcatus*–rodent cycle. Lipovnik virus has been reported in neurologic infections in the former Czechoslovakia, where flaviviral tick-borne encephalitis is endemic; one study showed seroconversion to Lipovnik virus in half of the patients with encephalitis who were studied, including some with suspected dual infection with tick-borne encephalitis virus.[32] This finding seems plausible because both viruses are transmitted by *I. ricinus* ticks, and multiple exposure to singly infected ticks or infection with a dually infected tick may be possible. In addition, serologic evidence of Lipovnik or Tribec infection was reported in patients with chronic polyradiculoneuritis; however, spirochetal infection was not ruled out in these cases. The increasing geographic range of *I. ricinus* ticks in Europe to more northerly latitudes and higher elevations, attributed to global warming, could lead to increased transmission of these orbiviruses, as has been observed with tick-borne encephalitis virus.

On the basis of serologic rises in patients with acute febrile illness diagnosed clinically as Rocky Mountain spotted fever, a Kemerovo-related virus is suspected to occur in the southwestern region of the United States. Patients with a history of a tick bite or tick exposure, whose sera were negative for *R. rickettsii,* demonstrated fourfold or greater changes in immunofluorescent titers to Lipovnik and Six Gun City viruses (Kemerovo group).[52,53] Rises in immunofluorescent antibody titers to 128 to 512 suggested recent infection with a Kemerovo-related virus, possibly a novel agent or related to rabbit syncytium virus, which is enzootic in the United States. The patients had acute febrile illnesses with myalgia, vomiting, and severe abdominal pain, along with leukopenia, thrombocytopenia, and anemia, similar to Rocky Mountain spotted fever. No agent was isolated from the patients, but neither was the possibility of *Ehrlichia* infection excluded. Quantitative PCR assays are also being developed to detect Kemerovo virus in mosquitoes and clinical specimens from humans.[52,53]

ORUNGO VIRUS

Orungo virus is unrelated antigenically to the other orbiviruses. Infection is prevalent in western, central, and eastern Africa and apparently is transmitted in a sylvatic monkey, with an *Aedes* mosquito cycle similar to that of yellow fever. Human-to-human transmission by *Anopheles* mosquitoes is speculated to occur. The virus is primarily a zoonotic infection of livestock and wildlife. However, it has been isolated from patients with fever and headache, and serologic evidence of infection has been reported in outbreaks of illness characterized by fever, headache, myalgia, nausea, and vomiting. Seroconversion has been observed in patients studied during yellow fever outbreaks, presumably because of concurrent transmission of the viruses. The virus also was isolated from the blood of a child with seizures and flaccid paralysis.[17,42]

LEBOMBO VIRUS

Lebombo virus is not grouped antigenically. The virus was isolated first from *Aedes circumluteolus* mosquitoes in South Africa. Subsequently, the virus was recovered from a Nigerian child with nonspecific febrile illness; the virus also was isolated from rodents and mosquitoes in Nigeria.[42]

CHANGUINOLA VIRUS

Changuinola virus belongs to an antigenic complex of 12 principally phlebotomine-borne orbiviruses. The virus is transmitted in Panama among forest mammals and *Phlebotomus* flies. Only one human case has been reported—a nonspecific febrile illness in a mosquito catcher.

NEW REFERENCES SINCE THE SEVENTH EDITION

21. Geissler A, Thorp E, Van Houten C, et al. Infection with Colorado tick fever virus among humans and ticks in a national park and forest, Wyoming, 2010. *Vector Borne Zoonotic Dis.* 2014;14(9):675-680.
26. Hong L, Ming-Hua L, You-Gang Z, et al. Banna Virus, China, 1987–2007. *Emerg Infect Dis.* 2010;16(3):514-517.
30. Klasco R. Colorado tick fever. *Med Clin North Am.* 2002;86(2):435-440.
34. Liu H, Gao X, Fu S, et al. Molecular evolution of emerging Banna virus. *Infect Genet Evol.* 2016;45:250-255.
37. Lv X, Jaafar M, Belhouchet M, et al. Isolates of Liao Ning virus from wild-caught mosquitoes in the XinJiang province of China in 2005. *PLoS ONE.* 2012;7(5):e37732.
44. Napthine S, Yek C, Powell M, et al. Characterization of the stop codon readthrough signal of Colorado tick fever virus segment 9 RNA. *RNA.* 2012;18(2):241-252.
48. Romero J, Simonsen K. Powassan encephalitis and Colorado tick fever. *Infect Dis Clin North Am.* 2008;22(3):545-559.
53. Varizhuk A, Zatsepin T, Golovin A, et al. Synthesis of oligonucleotides containing novel G-clamp analogue with C8-tethered group in phenoxazine ring: implication to qPCR detection of the low-copy Kemerovo virus ds RNA. *Bioorg Med Chem.* 2017;25(14):3597-3605.
54. Wang J, Li H, He Y, et al. Isolation and genetic characterization of Mangshi virus: a newly discovered Seadornavirus of the Reoviridae family found in Yunnan Province, China. *PLoS ONE.* 2015;10(12):e0143601.
55. Yendell SJ, Fischer M, Staples J. Colorado tick fever in the United States, 2002–2012. *Vector Borne Zoonotic Dis.* 2015;15(5):311-316.

The full reference list for this chapter is available at ExpertConsult.com.

173 Rotavirus

Timo Vesikari • Maria Hemming-Harlo • Suvi Heinimäki

Before universal rotavirus vaccinations, rotaviruses were the single most important cause of severe gastroenteritis of young children worldwide.[187,234] In the United States, rotaviruses were estimated to cause 55,000 to 70,000 hospitalizations (one in 72 children before the age of 5 years) and 20 to 60 deaths in young children annually before rotavirus vaccination.[83,84,188] In Europe, the number of hospitalizations was estimated at 87,000 (one in 54) per year.[228] Globally rotaviruses were estimated to be responsible each year for 453,000 deaths in children younger than 5 years at the time rotavirus vaccination was being introduced.[234] A more recent, and realistic, estimate puts the number at 197,000.[134] The latter is in line with the recent estimate of 0.6 million for total childhood mortality from acute diarrhea.[143] Deaths from acute diarrhea have greatly decreased in the past two decades because of better case management and improved sanitation and hygiene.

Rotavirus disease consists of diarrhea and vomiting accompanied by fever, a combination that may produce severe dehydration in infants and young children. Most deaths are due to dehydration and can be prevented by active rehydration therapy. Rotavirus infection is also associated with viremia (more often antigenemia) and may also cause extraintestinal symptoms.

Even though effective case management and "nonspecific" prevention have decreased rotavirus mortality over the past 25 years, rotavirus remains an important target for vaccination. Successful use of rotavirus vaccine has shown that rotavirus gastroenteritis (RVGE) is a vaccine-preventable disease. Since the introduction of rotavirus vaccines in 2006, RVGE has been drastically reduced in countries that have implemented universal vaccination, including the United States, Latin America, and many European countries. From Latin America, there is evidence that universal rotavirus vaccination has significantly reduced deaths from all-cause diarrhea.[193,213]

Human rotaviruses were discovered in 1973 by Bishop and colleagues based on electron microscopy (EM) of duodenal mucosa specimens from children with acute gastroenteritis.[21] At almost the same time, Flewett and coworkers demonstrated rotaviruses in stools by EM,[66] and EM of stools became the preferred diagnostic method for several years. Cultivation of human rotaviruses became possible when it was discovered that the viruses should be treated with trypsin to cleave the surface protein VP4.[37,54] This paved way for the development of human rotavirus vaccines.[236] Even earlier, animal (bovine and rhesus monkey) rotaviruses had been propagated in tissue culture to produce live (naturally) attenuated rotavirus vaccines that cross-protected against human rotavirus disease by sharing the common group A VP6 antigen, which is a major immunogenic protein of the rotavirus particle.[232]

ROTAVIRUSES

Rotaviruses are nonenveloped viruses with a segmented double-stranded RNA (dsRNA) genome. The name *Rotavirus* (Latin *rota*, meaning "wheel") originates from the distinctive wheel-like appearance of the complete virus particles visualized under electron microscope.[65] The mature infectious rotavirus particles consist of three concentric protein layers, therefore also called triple-layered particles (TLPs; Fig. 173.1A).

The innermost layer of the virion comprises 60 dimers of a VP2 protein (see Fig. 173.1B) enclosing the genome.[224] Complexes of two minor structural proteins, one copy of the viral RNA-dependent RNA polymerase VP1 and the viral capping enzyme VP3, are anchored to the inner surface of VP2 core shell (see Fig. 173.1B).[137,202] A middle layer consisting of 260 trimers of the VP6 protein surrounds the core (see Fig. 173.1B), forming a noninfectious but transcriptionally active double-layered particle (DLP).[160,167] The inner capsid protein VP6 is highly immunogenic and is the most abundant rotavirus protein.[110,232] VP6 is in direct contact with the core and external layers of the virus (see Fig. 173.1C). The outer layer is formed by 260 trimers of the VP7 glycoprotein, each trimer anchored to the underlying VP6 layer, and 60 spikes of VP4 trimers projecting from the VP7 shell (see Figs. 173.1B–C).[203,224] The VP7 and VP4 proteins serve as viral attachment proteins and neutralization antigens.[147,221] Proteolytic cleavage of VP4 protein into VP8* and VP5* fragments (see Fig. 173.1C) leads to the fully infectious TLP.[37,54]

A distinctive characteristic of the structure of rotavirus virion is the presence of 132 large channels of three types, which penetrate through the VP6 and VP7 layers.[203] These channels include 12 type I channels located at the fivefold axes, 60 type II channels surrounding the type I channels, and 60 type III channels around the threefold axes.

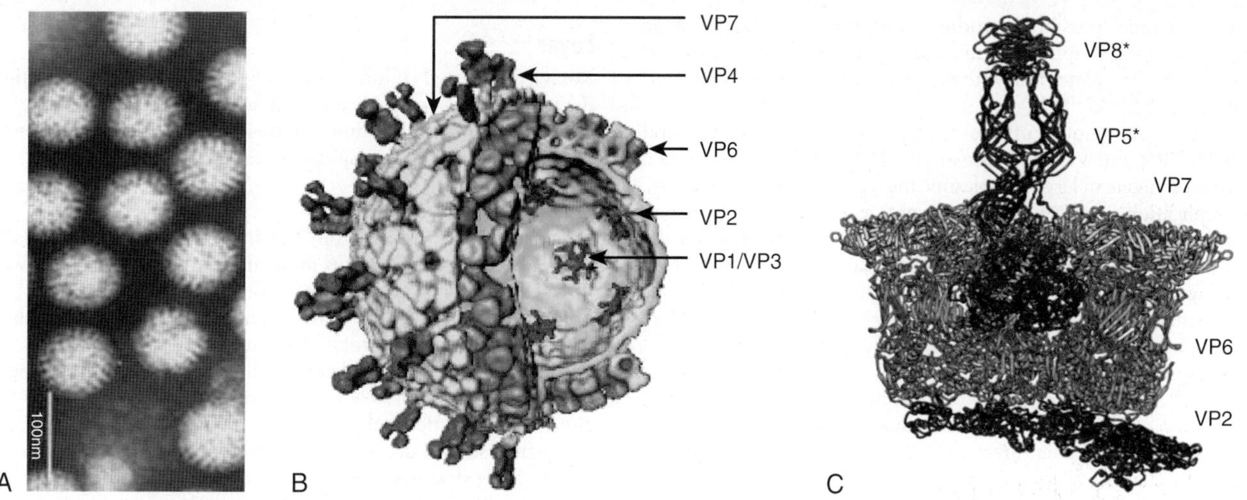

FIG. 173.1 Structure of rotavirus triple-layered particle (TLP) consisting of a VP2 core, a VP6 inner capsid and an outer capsid of VP7 with VP4 (VP5* + VP8*) spikes. (A) Electron microscopy image of TLPs. (B) Cutaway view of TLP demonstrating the VP7 layer with VP4 spikes, VP6 layer, VP2 core, and the transcriptional enzyme complex of VP1 and VP3 anchored to the inner surface of VP2. (C) Interactions of structural proteins. (B, Modified from Jayaram H, Estes MK, Prasad BV. Emerging themes in rotavirus cell entry, genome organization, transcription and replication. *Virus Res.* 2004;101:67-81. C, From Settembre EC, Chen JZ, Dormitzer PR, Grigorieff N, Harrison SC. Atomic model of an infectious rotavirus particle. *EMBO J.* 2011;30:408-416.)

The rotavirus genome consists of 11 dsRNA segments encoding six structural viral proteins (VP1–VP4, VP6, and VP7) and six nonstructural proteins (NSP1-NSP6). Each segment encodes one protein with the exception of segment 11, which codes for two proteins (NSP5/NSP6) because of overlapping open reading frames.[166] The nonstructural proteins are involved in replication, virus particle assembly, regulation of the host immune responses, and stimulation of viral gene expression.[12,15,55,235]

Classification and Strain Diversity

Rotaviruses can be classified into five groups (A–E) and three tentative groups (F–H) according to their antigenic properties or, more recently, the amino acid sequences of the VP6 protein. Group A rotaviruses cause more than 90% of human infections. Rotaviruses of groups B and C have been occasionally associated with diarrheal disease, primarily in older children and adults.

Within group A, rotaviruses are further divided into four subgroups (SGs) referred to as SGI, II, I+II, and non-I/II, based on the presence or absence of two SG-specific epitopes on VP6.[91] Human strains belong predominantly to either SGI or SGII.[113,201,238] Rotaviruses of group A have also been designated G- and P-serotypes according to the reactivity of VP7 (G for glycoprotein) and VP4 (P for protease-sensitive) antigens with reference antisera in neutralization assays.[105] At present, the rotavirus strains are classified into G- and P-genotypes based on the sequences of the VP7 and VP4 gene segments.[77,88] G-serotypes correspond one-to-one with G-genotypes, whereas part of P-serotypes comprise several P-genotypes. To date, 27 G-genotypes (G1-G27) and 37 P-genotypes (P[1]-P[37]) have been identified for rotaviruses.[164,241] In contrast, 14 P-serotypes, of which serotypes 1, 2, and 5 are further divided into subtypes with letter designations, have currently been discriminated. This has led to a double nomenclature for P-types in which the P-genotype is enclosed in square brackets after the P-serotype designation together with a possible subtype letter (e.g., P1A[8]). In practice, P-types are commonly denoted by their genotypes only.

The gene segments of rotaviruses can occasionally reassort during coinfections with different genotypes, leading to reassortant strains with segments originating from the two parent strains. More than 70 distinct G-P genotype combinations of human rotavirus strains belonging to the 12 G-types and 15 P-types have been identified, but only 5 G-types (G1, G2, G3, G4, and G9) and 3 P-types (P[4], P[6] and P[8]) are frequently associated with human diseases.[79] Still, the majority of rotavirus infections are associated with only five globally circulating genotype combinations: G1P[8], G2P[4], G3P[8], G4P[8], and G9P[8], of which G1P[8] strains are most common.[49] In developing countries, the incidence of strains with unusual genotypes (e.g., G8 and G12) as well as unusual genotype combinations (e.g., G1P[4], G2P[8] and G4P[6]) is higher.[13,223]

A novel comprehensive nucleotide-sequence–based classification system taking into account the complete genome of the virus was recently introduced as an extension to the binary G-and P-typing classification.[163,164] In the full genome classification system, the abbreviations Gx-P[x]-Ix-Rx-Cx-Mx-Ax-Nx-Tx-Ex-Hx represent genotypes of the gene segments respectively encoding VP7-VP4-VP6-VP1-VP2-VP3-NSP1-NSP2-NSP3-NSP4-NSP5/6. Currently, at least 27 G, 37 P, 17 I, 9 R, 9 C, 8 M, 18 A, 10 N, 12 T, 15 E, and 11 H genotypes have been differentiated according to cutoff points of nucleotide sequence identities. Regardless of the wide diversity rotaviruses exhibit, the majority of human rotaviruses appear to belong to two major genotype constellations sharing most of the genotypes of the internal non-G and non-P genes. Genotypes 1 (I1-R1-C1-M1-A1-N1-T1-E1-H1) are commonly encountered in combination with P[8] and various G-genotypes, and genotypes 2 (I2-R2-C2-M2-A2-N2-T2-E2-H2) with G2[P4].[165]

ROTAVIRUS INFECTION

Reproductive Cycle of Rotavirus

Rotaviruses infect nondividing mature enterocytes at the tips of the villi of the small intestine. Rotavirus infection depends on activation of the TLPs, involving cleavage of the VP4 into VP8* and VP5* (see Fig. 173.1C) by trypsin-like proteases in the intestinal lumen. VP8* domains located at the activated spike tips of the infectious TLPs can bind to sialic acids in the cellular glycans.[52,62] Recently, histo-blood group antigens (HBGAs) present on the surface of mucosal epithelial cells have also been described as receptors for certain rotavirus strains via binding of VP8*.[106,107] Other cell proteins implicated in rotavirus entry as probable coreceptors in a postattachment step include various cellular integrins and heat shock cognate protein 70 (hsc70) interacting with VP5* or VP7.[42,90,96,278] Following binding, the virus is internalized by receptor-mediated endocytosis, or direct membrane penetration and removal of the outer-layer proteins during entry leads to the release of transcriptionally active DLPs into the cytoplasm.[144,148,224,273,275]

Transcription complexes consisting of VP1 and VP3, localized at the inferior side of the VP2 core,[202] initiate the transcription of the 11 dsRNA gene segments. The synthesized capped plus-strand RNAs are extruded via type I channels passing through the layers of VP2 and

VP6, each channel possibly extruding transcripts of a specific gene segment.[198] The transcription products serve as mRNAs for viral protein synthesis and as templates for synthesis of the minus-strand RNAs and formation of dsRNAs.[118,194]

- Once a critical amount of viral proteins is synthesized, structural VP1, VP2, VP3, and VP6 and nonstructural NSP2, NSP5 and NSP6 proteins accumulate in large cytoplasmic inclusion bodies, "viroplasms," where replication, packing of genome, and assembly of DLPs occur. The presence of NSP2 and NSP5 has been found to be essential for the formation of viroplasms.[55] Viroplasm-associated plus-strand RNAs interacting with core proteins are packed into assembling VP2 cores and thereafter replicated into the dsRNAs by VP1 polymerase.[226] Core particles are coated with VP6 trimers, resulting in the formation of DLPs that bud into the endoplasmic reticulum via NSP4 transmembrane protein.[235,236] Subsequent assembly of VP4 and VP7 proteins completes the formation of TLPs, and release of the mature progeny virions from the infected cell occurs via direct cell lysis or a nonclassical vesicular transport mechanism.[121,172]

Transmission

Rotaviruses are highly infectious and transmitted via the fecal-oral route, in respiratory droplets or via fecally contaminated water.[4,68] Infected children start shedding rotaviruses in their stools before the onset of symptoms[200] and may excrete more than 10^{10} or 10^{11} rotavirus particles per gram of feces; fewer than 100 particles are required to infect new contacts.[64,124,265] The peak viral shedding in stools occurs on the third day of illness, and half of rotavirus-infected children shed for 10 days.[261] Prolonged shedding has been reported in immunocompromised children.[212]

ROTAVIRUS DISEASE

Pathogenesis

The clinical symptoms of primary rotavirus infection commonly start after a 48-hour incubation period, with forceful vomiting followed by fever and diarrhea. The symptoms usually last from 4 to 7 days.[242] Rotavirus infection may potentially cause elevation of transaminase levels and, in complicated diseases, seizures and encephalitis.[38,128,185,237] In several studies, the rotavirus viremia and/or antigenemia has been found to contribute to the clinical manifestations of rotavirus infections, as children detected with rotavirus RNA in serum are likely to have more severe vomiting and higher fever than those with rotavirus only in stools.[46,60,100] However, the antigen level has also been found to be associated with the probability of convulsions and level of interleukin 8 and 10 in rotavirus-infected children.[32,60,74,231]

Diarrhea

The most typical sign of rotavirus infection, diarrhea, may be caused by several mechanisms; it may be osmotic, secretory, and/or exudative.[59,151] Rotavirus diarrhea has been explained by damage to the epithelial cell line and by changes in the intracellular Ca^{2+} concentrations. After infection of mature enterocytes at the tip of the villi, the intracellular Ca^{2+} concentration increases, leading to inhibition of Na^{+} cotransporters, which reduces the absorptive capacity of the intestinal epithelium. The unabsorbed organic molecules increase the osmolality of the intestinal contents and absorb water from the epithelium, causing osmotic diarrhea. The increase of intracellular Ca^{2+} concentration is caused by NSP4, which also may stimulate the release of serotonin 5-hydroxytryptamine (5-HT) from the enterochromaffin cells, activating the enteric nervous system. In addition, NSP4 results in disruption of tight junctions of enterocytes while stimulating secretion in crypt cells.[97,108,109,150,176]

Vomiting

Rotavirus infection causes delay in gastric emptying, which changes the pressure between stomach and duodenum.[14] The pathology of gastric delay includes stimulation of vagal nerves and gastrointestinal hormones, mediated by the 5-HT3 receptors and sodium glucose co-transporter (SGLT-1).[174,208] During rotavirus infection intestinal enterochromaffin cells release 5-HT, which interacts with 5-HT3 receptors and stimulates the vagal afferent nerve projecting to the vomiting center of the brain.[97]

Fever

Rotavirus-infected children often have fever, as the infection stimulates the release of several pyrogens, such as prostaglandins and interleukin, from infected cells. In addition to their temperature-modulating effect, prostaglandins (PGE_2) may stimulate water secretion.[274]

Extraintestinal Spread

Rotaviruses may spread from the intestines into the circulation, as rotavirus RNA and rotavirus antigen have been detected in serum of infected children. The presence of rotavirus RNA or antigens in sera is not genotype specific.[23,24,116] In several studies, antigenemia has been found to correlate with rotavirus load in stools.[46]

Rotavirus RNAemia and antigenemia are common events, occurring in 58% to 72% and 33% to 90%, respectively, of rotavirus-infected children. Extraintestinal spread of rotavirus into cerebrospinal fluid has been described in case reports, and rotavirus RNA has been detected in multiple extraintestinal organs, such as heart, kidney, spleen, testes, bladder, and liver.[140,152,177,179,237] Even though the presence of rotavirus RNA and antigen in serum implies the presence of infectious rotavirus particles in blood, the isolation and culture of such infectious particles from human serum has been largely unsuccessful, apart from one study in which the infectious rotavirus particles were detected in HT-29 cells.[24] In the same study, the detection of antigenemia was found to be directly related to the presence of viral particles in serum. However, the presence of rotavirus RNA might be fully explainable by excess production of free viral proteins or release of noninfectious rotavirus particles (DLPs) from the intestines into the serum without any extraintestinal replication. It is plausible that previous rotavirus infections may reduce the extraintestinal spread of the virus and restrict the infection to the intestines, as an inverse association between baseline serum IgG titers and levels of serum antigen and serum RNA has been found.[207]

EPIDEMIOLOGY

Seasonality

In regions with a temperate climate, such as Europe or the United States, rotavirus has a clear seasonal distribution, the most active months being in the winter and/or early spring.[84,131] In subtropical and tropical climates, the distribution of rotavirus disease is not as clear as in Europe; the most active months are during the cool and dry season, but sporadic infections may be detected during the whole year.[99]

Genotype Distribution

Around the world, the most common circulating genotype before rotavirus vaccination was G1P[8] followed by G4P[8].[29,78] The most common genotypes—G1P[8], G2P[4], G3P[8], G4P[8], and G9P[8]—accounted for 86% to 99% of rotavirus infections in European countries.[49]

Fluctuations in the predominant genotypes are relatively frequent (such as shifts from G1P[8] to G4P[8]), but the shift commonly occurs within those genotypes. G1P[8] accounted for 78.5% of all rotavirus infections in the United States between 1996 and 2005, followed by G2P[4], G9P[8], and G3P[8] (9.2%, 3.6%, and 1.7%, respectively).[78] Similarly in Europe, for example in Finland, the most common rotavirus genotypes were G1P[8] (62%) and G9P[8] (12%), and other common genotypes, G4P[8], G2P[4], and G3P[8], were observed to a lesser extent.[205]

In Latin America, the same common genotypes account for the majority of the infections, but the annual genotype distribution is broader (Fig. 173.2). In developing area countries of Africa and Asia, more uncommon genotypes (such as G12 and G8) and different G- and P-type constellations (such as G12P[6] or G2P[8]) were and still are detected often.[29,43,129,175]

The implementation of rotavirus vaccination has changed the natural seasonality and genotype distribution of rotavirus disease. In the United States, a biennial pattern of rotavirus activity and delay in the most active months has been observed after mass vaccinations.[195] Altogether more variety in genotypes has been seen in countries that have implemented universal rotavirus vaccination, such as the United States and Finland (see later discussion).

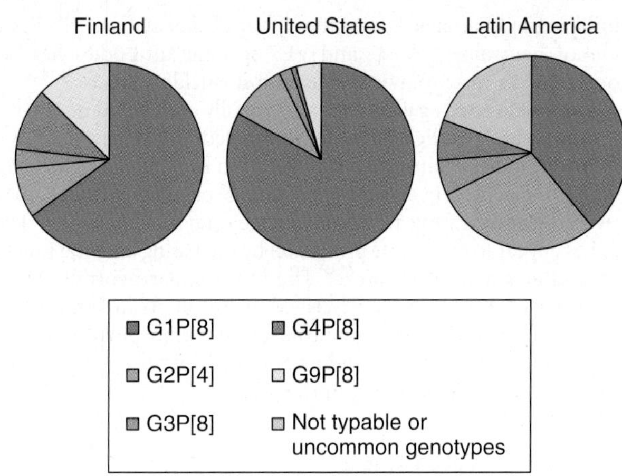

FIG. 173.2 Rotavirus genotypes in Finland, the United States, and Latin America before universal mass vaccination.

Age

Before the introduction of rotavirus vaccines, rotaviruses were the single most important cause of severe gastroenteritis of young children worldwide. Each child is infected at least once before the age of 5, the majority before their second birthday.[84] The occurrence of primary rotavirus infection is earlier in developing countries, possibly due to year-round exposure to rotavirus and high environmental viral loads. Generally, rotavirus causes the most severe gastroenteritis in infants and young children between the ages of 6 and 24 months.[157,242] Neonatal and adult rotavirus infections are less common and often asymptomatic; however, rotavirus may cause outbreaks in places such as retirement homes and neonatal units.[3,20,132] In a recent Finnish study of rotavirus epidemiology in adults, severe gastroenteritis due to rotavirus infection was detected mainly in the elderly (median age, 80 years); however, the burden of disease in elderly is small compared to that in young children.[159]

LABORATORY DIAGNOSIS

The first diagnostic method was demonstration of rotavirus particles by electron microscopy (EM) in stools.[66] An enzyme-linked immunosorbent assay (ELISA) detection method was developed soon after discovery,[276] and today ELISAs are the principal diagnostic test for rotavirus in stools. ELISAs recognize the rotavirus middle-layer protein VP6 antigen. Reverse transcription polymerase chain reaction (RT-PCR) is more sensitive than ELISA,[272] but the extra sensitivity is not usually needed because of the abundance of rotavirus antigen in stools. Usually RT-PCR targets gene segments encoding for VP7 and VP4, the outer capsid proteins applied as the results can also be used for classification.[78,88] Both ELISA and RT-PCR can be used for detection of rotavirus in serum and whole blood.[27] Rotaviruses may still be detected by EM and also by polyacrylamide gel electrophoresis.[103]

TREATMENT

Acute dehydration is the main clinical problem associated with RVGE. A 20-point score (Vesikari score) is commonly used for assessment of clinical severity of RVGE (Table 173.1). A score of 11 of 20 roughly correlates with severity that requires active rehydration therapy. The principles of treatment, oral rehydration, continued feeding, and possibly probiotics, as well as avoidance of drugs, are similar in all forms of gastroenteritis, rotavirus or not.

Reduced-osmolarity oral rehydration solution (224 mOsm/L) (ORS) has been shown to be more effective in RVGE than full-strength (iso-osmolar) ORS as measured by stool output, reduced vomiting, and reduced need for supplemental intravenous therapy[206]; consequently, ORS with sodium concentration of 50 to 60 mmol/L is recommended as first-line therapy.

TABLE 173.1 Numerical Scoring (1–2+ Points) for Severity of Rotavirus Diarrhea

Duration of Diarrhea (Days)	
1–4	1
5	2
≥6	3
Max No. Diarrheal Stools/24 h	
1–3	1
4–5	2
≥6	3
Duration of Vomiting (Days)	
1	1
2	2
≥3	3
Max No. Vomiting Episodes/24 h	
1	1
2–4	2
≥5	3
Fever	
37.1–38.4°C	1
38.5–38.9°C	2
≥39°C	3
Dehydration	
1–5%	2
≥6%	3
Treatment	
Clinic (oral) rehydration	1
Hospitalization	2
Total	**20**

From Ruuska T, Vesikari T. Rotavirus disease in Finnish children: use of numerical scores for clinical severity of diarrhoeal episodes. *Scand J Infect Dis.* 1990;22:259-267.

If oral rehydration is not successful, enteral rehydration by the nasogastric route is the next preferred rehydration method even in children with severe dehydration. Enteral rehydration, whether given orally or by nasogastric tube, is associated with significantly fewer major adverse events and a shorter hospital stay than intravenous rehydration. All guidelines state that if the child is breast-fed during the infection, breastfeeding should be continued throughout rehydration.

Probiotics, *Lactobacillus rhamnosus GG*[155] and *Lactobacillus reuteri*,[225] have been shown to significantly shorten the duration of rotavirus diarrhea.

ROTAVIRUS IMMUNITY

Individuals can experience multiple rotavirus infections during their lifetime, but natural rotavirus infection, whether symptomatic or asymptomatic, provides a protective effect against subsequent disease. The severity of rotavirus infections decreases with increasing number of infections, each reinfection broadening and boosting natural immunity.[17,20,61,184,244,245] The second infection provides practically complete protection against moderate-to-severe disease. Both humoral and cell-mediated immunity contribute to the resolution of ongoing rotavirus infection and protection from subsequent infection.

Immune Responses in Rotavirus-Infected Individuals

Rotavirus infection induces both systemic and mucosal antibody responses. Humoral anti-rotavirus responses include an early IgM response followed by the production of IgG and IgA.[47,92,214] Local response is considered to be important against rotavirus, as higher titers of intestinal IgA have correlated with protection from rotavirus infection and disease.[41,161] Of the serum antibody responses, IgA levels have been associated with protection against moderate-to-severe disease.[85,104,184,245]

Natural rotavirus infection generates antibodies directed against structural as well as nonstructural proteins.[210,211,232] Only VP4 and VP7 surface proteins are able to elicit classical neutralizing antibodies with type-specific and cross-reactive serotype responses.[5,31,211] The first rotavirus exposure is believed to induce a primarily homotypic antibody response, which is broadened to heterotypic responses upon recurrent exposure.[184] However, the occurrence of sequential infections even with the same serotype, although less frequent than with different serotypes, indicates that neutralizing antibodies are not sufficient for protective rotavirus immunity.[82,266,244] VP6 protein plays a role in protective immunity, because the strongest antibody response to rotavirus infection seems to be developed against this inner capsid protein.[210,211,232] VP6-specific antibodies have been identified as the dominant B-cell response following rotavirus infection in infants and adults.[267,268]

Cell-mediated immune responses have also been demonstrated after natural rotavirus infection. Because of the difficulty of studying intestinal antigen-specific T cells in situ in humans, characterization of T-cell responses has been concentrated on identification of the presence of rotavirus-specific T cells in circulation.[156,180] Rotavirus-specific $CD4^+$ and $CD8^+$ T cells have been detected in the circulation of rotavirus-infected and healthy adults,[115] but the induced responses appear to be lower or even undetectable in children with RVGE.[115,216] Chronic rotavirus infection in B- and/or T-cell immunodeficient children[81] indicates the importance of both the cellular and humoral arms of the immune system in the clearance of rotavirus infection.

According to the knockout mouse models, rotavirus-primed memory B cells, and hence rotavirus-specific antibodies, seem to provide more long-term protection against subsequent rotavirus infection, whereas rotavirus-specific T cells help to limit the course of infection.[71,69,171,169] According to these models, rotavirus-specific $CD8^+$ T lymphocytes are efficient in resolution of a primary rotavirus infection.[50,70,217] These murine cytotoxic T lymphocytes also mediate nearly complete short-term and partial long-term protection against reinfection.[72] Moreover, the development of protective anti-rotavirus intestinal IgA response is, at least partially, $CD4^+$ T-cell dependent.[70,171,243]

Mechanisms of Protection

Because of the replication site of rotaviruses in intestinal enterocytes, effector mechanisms are assumed to be active at the intestinal mucosa. The majority of circulating rotavirus-specific B cells and $CD4^+$ T cells express intestinal homing receptors, indicating trafficking of primed cells to the intestine for local action.[86,216,268]

The most evident effector is secretory IgA (SIgA), which is produced following polymeric immunoglobulin receptor–mediated transcellular transport of polymeric IgA (pIgA) across the epithelial cells into the gut lumen. As in humans, evidence of the role of SIgA is supported by the correlation of protection against rotavirus infection in mice and piglets with the levels of rotavirus-specific intestinal and serum IgA.[57,170,239] However, it has been shown that rotavirus-specific IgG or IgM in the gut or in sufficient amounts in serum can reach the intestine and mediate protection in IgA-deficient individuals.[112,183]

The protective nature of antibodies directed to VP4 and VP7 is based on the ability of these antibodies to neutralize rotavirus classically by inhibiting viral attachment to the cell or decapsidation.[63,149] Passive transfer of neutralizing VP4- and VP7-specific antibodies has been demonstrated to clear rotavirus infection in suckling mice.[162,181]

Antibodies directed against VP6 are generally considered nonneutralizing, but several studies have demonstrated inhibitory activity of anti-VP6 antibodies against rotavirus infection in vitro.[1,2,75,135] Moreover, certain VP6-specific pIgA antibodies have been shown to be capable of preventing and clearing a chronic murine rotavirus infection.[28] These antibodies appear to contribute protection by mediating antiviral function via intracellular neutralization.[40,58] The intracellular neutralization of rotavirus have recently been described to result from inhibition of rotavirus transcription during the transcellular transport of anti-VP6 pIgA antibodies via binding of these antibodies into the type I channel, thus blocking egress of RNA from the DLP.[1]

ROTAVIRUS VACCINES

Live attenuated rotavirus vaccines are given orally to multiply in the intestines and induce immunity mimicking that after natural rotavirus infection. The two major licensed rotavirus vaccines in the free market are a human rotavirus G1P[8] "monotypic" vaccine (Rotarix) and bovine-human reassortant "pentavalent" rotavirus vaccine (RotaTeq). These generic names are misleading and do not reflect their protective efficacy across human group A rotavirus types, whether included in the vaccine or not.

Other rotavirus vaccines are licensed in China,[73] India, and Indonesia (Table 173.2), and still others are being developed. Historically important are bovine rotavirus (heterologous) vaccine and rhesus rotavirus vaccine with its reassortants (RotaShield), which became the first licensed rotavirus vaccine but was withdrawn because of association with intussusception (IS). IS is still casting a shadow on all live oral rotavirus vaccines.

Bovine rotavirus strain RIT4237 (G6P[5]) was the first rotavirus vaccine tested in humans. The vaccine is highly attenuated with a history of 154 cell culture passages, much more than any other rotavirus vaccine strain. The adaptation to cell culture resulted in growth to a high titer over 10^8 $TCID_{50}$ /mL,[48] which is higher than in the present oral vaccines and may explain the good efficacy of this vaccine in the early trials in Finland. In its first efficacy trials in 1983, a single dose of RIT4237 vaccine induced 50% protection against any and 88% protection against severe ("clinically significant") rotavirus disease,[248] a result that remains a benchmark for other vaccines and trials. Two doses of the same did not improve efficacy.[249] In Peru the efficacy was 40% against any and 75% against severe RVGE,[133] and in Gambia the efficacy was 33% but severity of RVGE was not measured.[98] Thus, a gradient of efficacy between developed and developing countries was observed, as has later been seen with other rotavirus vaccines.

The higher efficacy of rotavirus vaccine against severe rotavirus disease was also documented using the 20-point score (see Table 173.1).[220,219] The same score has since been applied to measure efficacy of the other rotavirus vaccines; an example for RRV-TV is shown in Fig. 173.3.

TABLE 173.2 Licensed Live Oral Rotavirus Vaccines

Vaccine	Strain(s)	Developer/Manufacturer	Status in Development
Single-Strain Human Rotavirus Vaccines			
Rotarix	Human strain G1P1A[8]	GlaxoSmithKline (Belgium)	Licensed worldwide
Rotavac	Human neonatal strain 116E G9P[11]	Bharat Biotech International Limited (India)	Licensed in India
Rotavin-M1	Human strain G1P1A[8]	Polyvan (Vietnam)	Licensed in Vietnam
RV3-BB	Human neonatal strain G3P2A[6]	Murdoch Childrens Research Institute (Australia) and Biofarma (Indonesia)	Phase III trial
Animal-Human Reassortant Vaccines			
RotaShield	Tetravalent human-rhesus reassortant G1-G4 + P7[5]	Wyeth (US)	Withdrawn 1999, Phase II trials of neonatal administration in Ghana
RotaTeq	Pentavalent human-bovine reassortant G1-G4 + P7[5]; G6 + P1A[8]	Merck (US)	Licensed worldwide
LLR	Lamb rotavirus strain G12P[10][141]	Lanzhou Institute of Biological Products (China)	Licensed in China

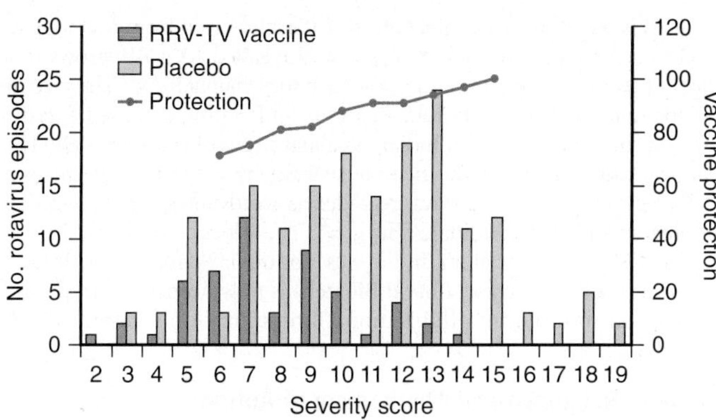

FIG. 173.3 Efficacy of RRV-TV (RotaShield) against rotavirus gastroenteritis of different severity as assessed using the Vesikari score. (From Joensuu J, Koskenniemi E, Pang XL, et al. Randomised placebo-controlled trial of rhesus-human reassortment rotavirus vaccine for prevention of severe rotavirus gastroenteritis. *Lancet.* 1997;350:1205-1209.)

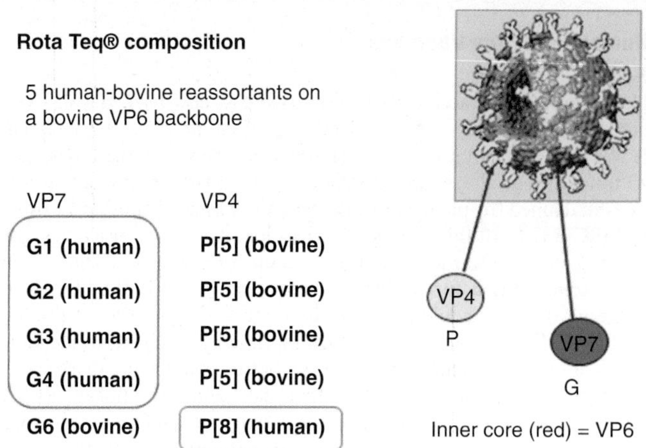

FIG. 173.4 RotaTeq composition.

The RIT4237 vaccine was withdrawn from further development for a combination of reasons. However, the series of studies of this bovine rotavirus vaccine established many general principles that were largely confirmed later for other oral rotavirus vaccines: (1) a higher titer of oral inoculum resulted in greater immune response[259]; (2) rotavirus vaccine virus was sensitive to gastric acidity, and buffering of the vaccine or milk feeding was needed for successful vaccine uptake[250]; and (3) breast milk or breastfeeding did not suppress the uptake to any significant degree, especially if the titer of vaccine was high.[259,260] Early studies also showed that concurrent administration of oral polio vaccine (OPV) suppresses the uptake of bovine rotavirus vaccine, whereas rotavirus vaccine had only minimal inhibitory effect (interference) on OPV.[80,264]

WC-3 Bovine Rotavirus Vaccine

WC-3 stands for Wistar Calf according to the Wistar Institute, where the vaccine was developed.[35] This bovine G6P[7] rotavirus strain is less adapted to cell culture (about 20 passages) and therefore grows only to a titer of approximately 10^7 PFU/mL. In the main US efficacy trial, the WC3 vaccine yielded only 20% protection against RVGE and was not developed further.[18] However, the strain is the backbone for bovine-human reassortants that are included in the current "pentavalent" (RV5) bovine-human reassortant rotavirus vaccine.

Rhesus Rotavirus (RRV) Vaccine

Rhesus (monkey) rotavirus strain (G3P[5]) was grown 9 times in monkey kidney and 7 times in fetal rhesus lung cells and adopted as human vaccine.[123] Unlike bovine rotavirus vaccine, RRV is clearly virulent in humans by causing fever, though not diarrhea.[252] At a high titer level of 10^5 PFU/dose the RRV vaccine was efficacious but reactogenic.[67,87] Importantly, however, RRV served as a backbone for the development of the rhesus-human reassortant vaccines,[173] of which the tetravalent composition (RRV-TV) became the first licensed rotavirus vaccine in 1998.

Rhesus-Human Reassortant Vaccine

Rhesus-human reassortant tetravalent (RRV-TV) vaccine (RotaShield, Wyeth) is the prototype of reassortant vaccines and contains four viruses expressing human G1, G2, and G4 VP7 antigens on the rhesus G3P[5] rotavirus genetic backbone plus the RRV itself. RRV-TV retained the high reactogenicity for fever of RRV. RotaShield vaccine was in use in the United States in 1998–99, but was withdrawn because of association with IS.[178,227]

RRV-TV is a more efficacious vaccine than the parent rhesus rotavirus vaccine.[209] In the pivotal efficacy trials before licensure of RotaShield, the RRV-TV vaccine showed an efficacy of 100% against hospitalization for RVGE and 68% against any RVGE in Finland[120] and 75% and 48%, respectively, in Venezuela.[197] These results were instrumental for wider acceptance of protection against severe RVGE as the primary endpoint of rotavirus vaccine efficacy. Lower vaccine efficacy in developing countries was also accepted with the understanding that rotavirus vaccination could still prevent a large number of severe RVGE cases.

RotaShield vaccine was withdrawn in 1999 in the United States because of association with IS, before it was launched in Europe or tested in developing countries. Recently, RRV-TV, given to neonates to minimize risk of IS, was tested in Ghana with promising results, and the possibility of reintroduction in developing countries remains viable.[6]

Bovine-Human Reassortant Vaccine

The "pentavalent" bovine-human reassortant rotavirus vaccine (RotaTeq, Merck; also termed RV5) was licensed in 2006 and is one of the two major rotavirus vaccines used globally. The vaccine is a combination of four G-type reassortants (for G1-G4) and one P-type (P[8]) reassortant on the WC-3 bovine rotavirus genetic backbone (see Fig. 173.3).[36] The terms pentavalent or RV5 refer to the five mono-reassortants present in the vaccine. However, it is now well established that the protection induced by the vaccine is not limited to the G or P types contained in the product. The vaccine is given in three doses. This was determined early on to accommodate the US childhood immunization program, but was also based on the demonstration of incremental immunogenicity up to the third dose.[33,34,247]

The efficacy and safety of RotaTeq vaccine were established in a large trial (70,000 infants) known as REST (Rotavirus Efficacy and Safety Trial). The overall efficacy against health care utilization (combined endpoint of hospital admission and outpatient clinic treatment) was about 95% with a narrow confidence interval.[251,258] An extension study of REST in Finland of 21,000 children confirmed that RotaTeq was efficacious not only against G1, G3, and G4, all P[8], and the heterologous P-type G2P[4], but also against G9P[8], which is not among the G-types in the vaccine.[253] In Japan the efficacy of RotaTeq was similar to that in the United States.[114] In Ghana and Kenya, the efficacy of RotaTeq was lower (64% and 83%, respectively) than in the United States or Europe.[7] In Asian developing countries, a point estimate of 45% was found.[277]

The G1 and P[8] reassortants included in RotaTeq vaccine (Fig. 173.4) may re-reassort with each other and form vaccine-derived (vd) double reassortants on the bovine rotavirus VP6 core.[51,102] vdG1P[8] viruses may be more virulent than the original single reassortant vaccine viruses, and they may be responsible for the low rate (about 1%) of diarrhea seen after vaccination. They may also be capable of transmission.[196] If transmitted to immunocompromised subjects, the vaccine viruses may cause prolonged infection.[190] Shedding of live infectious virus after the first dose of vaccination was found in about 9% in the REST study, but using RT-PCR shedding may be found in about 50% of the recipients, with G1 reassortants being the most common.[158]

UK-bovine rotavirus strain is another platform for reassortment.[256] However, development of UK-bovine tetravalent (G1-G4) reassortant vaccine was discontinued by Wyeth at the same time as the RotaShield vaccine was withdrawn. The technology has been licensed (by the US National Institutes of Health) to several manufacturers in India, China, and Brazil, but none of the vaccines have yet been licensed.

Human Rotavirus Vaccines

Rotarix

Human rotavirus vaccine RV1 (Rotarix, GSK, also termed RV1) was licensed in 2006 and is the most extensively used rotavirus vaccine today. It was derived from a G1P[8] rotavirus isolate in Cincinnati, passaged 33 times in cell culture, and designated 89-12.[16] The strain was acquired by GSK, cloned (by plaque purification), and passaged another 12 times in MRC-5 cells. In this process the virus lost its residual reactogenicity and is generally regarded as nonreactogenic for humans.[255] The titer of the vaccine chosen for the final formulation is about 10^5 PFU/dose, although the virus could be grown to a one-log higher titer.[222] Rotarix multiplies effectively in humans, as characterized by a high rate of shedding (60% or even more) after the first dose, but does not cause diarrhea.[255]

Rotarix is given in two doses. The uptake and immunogenicity are excellent (90%) even after the first dose when given in the presence of a low level of maternal antibody. The second dose under such circumstances does not add much, but the uptake is prevented by the immunity induced after the first dose, as indicated by the lack of shedding and lack of booster.[255] The pivotal safety and efficacy trial for licensure was carried out in 60,000 children in Latin America[218] and efficacy determined in a subset of 20,000 infants. Two endpoints were used: need for (oral) rehydration and score of 11 out of 20. Both yielded approximately 85% efficacy in 1-year follow-up.[218] In addition, before licensure in Europe, the vaccine was tested in five European countries and later in Japan[127] with similar results. In Europe, the follow-up was for two rotavirus seasons and the primary endpoint was severe RVGE as defined by a score of 11/20. Against this endpoint, efficacy for 2 years was 91%, with 96% efficacy in the first season and 86% in the second season, suggesting some decline over time. Against any RVGE, efficacy was 78% and 68% in the first and second year, respectively, for a total of 72% over 2 years. Furthermore, against severe RVGE on 2 years of follow-up, the efficacy for various G-types was similar, ranging from 96% for G1P[8] to 86% for G2P[4]; the differences were not statistically significant.[257] Evidence from Asia indicates that protection is sustained into the third year of life.[199]

Rotarix and RotaTeq have not been tested head-to-head for efficacy in any trial. On the other hand, both vaccines have been tested for efficacy in different environments, from developed to "intermediate" to developing countries, and the results of such studies can be compared with each other (Fig. 173.5A). In South Africa and Malawi, the efficacy of two doses of Rotarix against severe RVGE (score of 11 out of 20) was 61.2% and 49.4%, respectively, in 1-year follow-up.[153] Also in these African countries, there was no difference in vaccine efficacy against G1 and non-G1 (G2, G8, G12) rotaviruses.[154]

Other Human Rotavirus Vaccine Strains

(See Table 173.2.) Another human rotavirus vaccine has been prepared from a G1P[8] rotavirus isolate in Vietnam and designated as "Rotavin."[146] This vaccine is licensed in Vietnam.

RV3 is based on a neonatal G3P[6] rotavirus strain from Melbourne. A Vero cell adapted derivative of the strain, called RV3-BB, grows to a higher titer and is more immunogenic than the original RV3.[44] The vaccine will be manufactured in Indonesia and is undergoing a phase III trial.

The rotavirus 116E is an Indian neonatal strain of genotype G9P[11]. Natural attenuation of the neonatal strain by a modified P-antigen (VP4 gene of bovine origin) was regarded as an advantage in the selection of this strain as a candidate vaccine.[45] The efficacy of 116E against severe RVGE in a trial in India was about 55% for three doses,[19] and the vaccine (Rotavac, Bharat Biotech) is now licensed in India and is being introduced into the National Immunization Program (NIP) of India.

Immune Response and Mechanism of Action

Total rotavirus serum IgA antibody has been the most widely used immunologic marker for uptake of rotavirus vaccine. From studies on consecutive wild-type rotavirus infections, it is known that a high titer of serum rotavirus IgA antibody correlates with protection.[266,245] This can be applied to vaccine-induced immunity as well. High serum IgA responses are consistently induced by efficacious rotavirus vaccines such as Rotarix and RotaTeq, and it is logical to assume that serum IgA–mediated immunity is not only a surrogate marker[189] but also an actual mechanism of rotavirus vaccine-induced protection against severe rotavirus disease.

Wild-type rotavirus infections induce neutralizing antibodies against the rotavirus surface antigens VP7 and VP4, which protect against subsequent infections by the same serotype. Such antibodies are also induced after vaccinations, but the responses are inconsistent and the antibody levels often low.[246] Rotavirus vaccines do not induce much protection against rotavirus infection, and it is unlikely that these neutralizing antibodies are a major mechanism of action that reduces the severity of RVGE, although they may play some role in vaccine-induced protection. For both Rotarix and RotaTeq, G1-specific neutralizing antibody response and protection against G1 strains may be dominant.

G-type specific immunity induced by the vaccines may also "protect" against the homologous vaccine virus, that is, the subsequent dose of the vaccine itself. This is clearly seen by the lack of a booster effect to a monospecific human G1P[8] vaccine[255] and RRV.[209] The second dose of RV1 only "takes" if the first dose has not taken. Giving three or even five doses of monovalent human rotavirus vaccine does not much improve the uptake of this vaccine in developing countries.[130] In contrast, the reassortant vaccines may have an advantage of multiple doses "taking," as it is unlikely that all reassortants succeed in taking upon the first dose. A second and third dose of the "multivalent" vaccine may have a better opportunity of taking and inducing a booster effect, that is, an increase of rotavirus IgA serum antibody level.

In a recent study of mixed administration schedules of rotavirus vaccines in the United States, three doses of RotaTeq was clearly more immunogenic overall (rotavirus IgA response) than two doses of

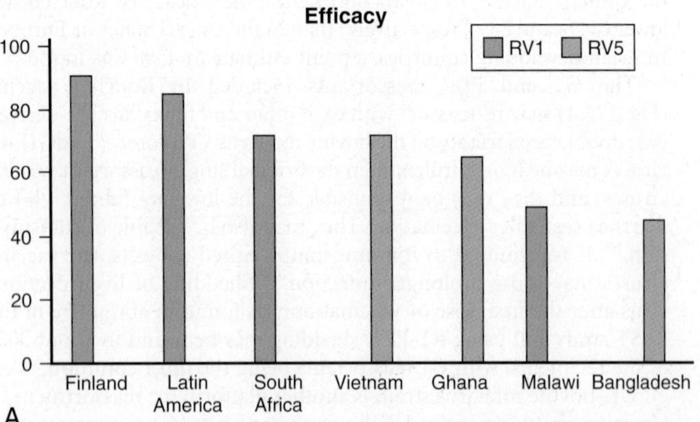

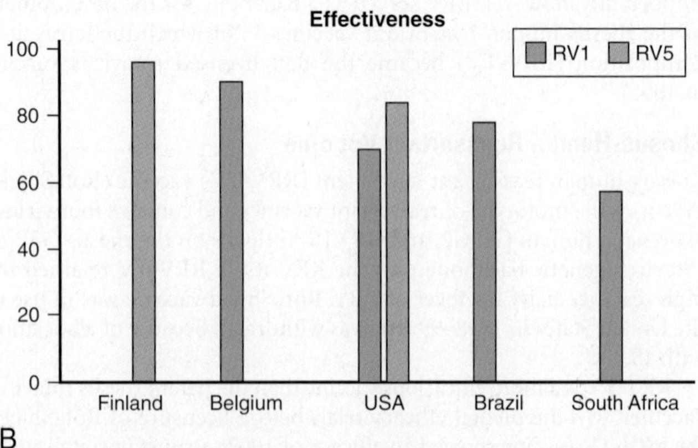

FIG. 173.5 Representative efficacy point estimates against severe RVGE with score of 11 out of 20 of RV5 and RV1 in (A) prelicensure trials and (B) postlicensure real-life effectiveness studies for RVGE hospitalizations in different geographic areas.

Rotarix.[142] All neutralizing antibody responses were broader after RotaTeq. The same study showed that replacing one dose of RotaTeq with Rotarix may actually be advantageous. The strongest rotavirus IgA response occurred when one dose of Rotarix was followed by two doses of RotaTeq.

The target antigen of serum rotavirus IgA is largely the rotavirus inner core protein VP6. VP6 is a strong immunogen, and immune responses to it overshadow those to other structural rotavirus antigens.[232,233] Anti-VP6 antibodies are "nonneutralizing" in the sense that they do not prevent rotavirus infection in vitro or in vivo (see earlier discussion). However, intracellularly acting anti-VP6 IgA antibodies block the infection at a later stage and, conceivably, may protect against rotavirus disease.[40] A plausible mechanism of the intracellular action may be that the anti-VP6 antibodies stabilize the VP6 inner core particle and prevent it from releasing rotavirus RNA.[1] An intracellular mechanism of effect is also consistent with the concept of rotavirus vaccines protecting against disease rather than infection.

Comparative Efficacy

In general, the overall and serotype-specific efficacies against severe RVGE of the two vaccines are remarkably similar, but depend on the environment.

Real Life Effectiveness

A recent review has addressed both the difference between developed (high-income) and middle-income countries as well as the lack of serotype specificity in protection against severe RVGE in postlicensure effectiveness studies.[139] The gradient between developed and developing countries that was found in prelicensure studies is seen also in postlicensure real-life effectiveness studies. Some representative examples of the point estimates are shown in Fig. 173.5B.

In Europe, the examples of Finland and Belgium are well representative, showing over 90% effectiveness for hospitalization with RVGE over some period of time in countries that have reached a high coverage with RV5 (Finland) and RV1 (Belgium), respectively.[26] In the United States, the 4-year follow-up of Payne et al reported 84% effectiveness for RotaTeq.[195] In Brazil, representing Latin America, the point estimate of effectiveness is of the order of magnitude 80%.[39,122] In South Africa, effectiveness of 57% was reported.[94]

Serotype (Genotype) Specific Effectiveness

The postvaccination experience confirms the finding in prelicensure studies that rotavirus vaccine effectiveness against severe RVGE is not strain specific and the terms "monovalent" for RV1 and "pentavalent" for RV5 are not functionally appropriate. Instead, these acronyms should only be used to refer to the number of constituents in each vaccine.

Although some serotype replacement of circulating rotaviruses has happened, new rotavirus serotypes have not permanently replaced old ones, and rotavirus vaccines have remained effective against severe RVGE associated with all circulating rotavirus strains. Soon after introduction of Rotarix vaccine in Latin America the G2P[4] rotaviruses became dominant among the RVGE cases, but Rotarix G1P[8] vaccine remained effective against severe RVGE caused by this G type.[39,122] Rotavirus G type G3P[8] has possibly become more common after introduction of RV5 vaccine in Finland and the United States, but it has never gained predominance.[101,195] G12P[8] has emerged in the United States and elsewhere, but has not remained predominant either. Recently, even more diversity of rotavirus genotypes has been observed in Finland, but total rotavirus activity has remained low.[159]

Impact of Rotavirus Vaccination: Direct and Indirect

The US experience shows that RVGE cannot be eliminated at a vaccine coverage of 75% to 80%, but rotavirus epidemics have occurred biannually instead of every year.[195] More generally, the impact of universal rotavirus vaccination cannot be reliably measured by short-term follow-up only. The first large-scale introduction of rotavirus vaccination will likely break the transmission chain of the wild-type rotavirus with resulting short-term direct and indirect impact, but rotavirus disease activity will resurge later.

The impact of rotavirus vaccination in early introducing European countries was recently reviewed by Karafillakis et al.[125] In Austria, with coverage of 72% to 74%, the reduction of RVGE hospitalizations in the target age group was 81% to 84% and remained sustained up to 3 years. However, while there was initially an indirect effect on unvaccinated children as well, after 3 years this was followed by an increase of RVGE hospitalizations in 5- to 14-year-old children. In Belgium, with a coverage rate of 90%, the direct impact on RVGE hospitalization in the target group has been about 80% and the 3-year indirect effect in older children 20% to 64%. In Finland, with rotavirus vaccination coverage of 95% to 97%, the reduction in cases of RVGE seen in hospitals was 94% in a period of 4 years after vaccination, but specifically in age group 5 to 14 years, no significant reduction has been seen over this period. Actually, the direct impact in the target age group of rotavirus vaccination has shifted the occurrence of RVGE to older unvaccinated children[101] and adults.[159]

It may be concluded that although higher coverage results in greater impact of rotavirus vaccination on severe RVGE, even very high coverage does not lead to elimination of RVGE through herd protection. Rotavirus vaccination has had a clear impact on rotavirus disease in all age groups, as reported from the United States,[76,145] but it remains to be seen whether this effect is durable over time.

Introduction of Universal Rotavirus Vaccination

The first country to introduce universal rotavirus vaccination was Brazil in March 2006, followed soon by Venezuela and Mexico, and about 20 more Latin American countries using Rotarix vaccine. Universal recommendation for RotaTeq vaccine was issued in the United States soon after licensure in 2006.[186] Other early introducers were Australia (both vaccines) and South Africa (Rotarix) since 2009.

In Europe, Austria (both vaccines) and Belgium (Rotarix) were the first introducers in 2007, followed by Finland (RotaTeq exclusively) in 2009. After that, there was a gap of a couple of years until Germany started vaccinations state by state. The most significant step forward is perhaps the UK introduction, and effective implementation, in 2014.[8]

Globally, the most significant recent progress has been introduction of rotavirus vaccination in Africa since 2013, made possible by support from GAVI. The true impact of these programs can only be assessed after several years, although the first results appear promising. With the exception of Rwanda, all African countries have introduced Rotarix vaccine.

Eight of the 10 countries with the highest mortality from RVGE are in Asia,[126,234] and none of these countries have yet implemented universal rotavirus vaccination. India has announced a program using the locally produced Rotavac, and the Philippines has a government program for the poorest section of the population.

Rotavirus Vaccine Recommendations

Before rotavirus vaccine introduction and also apart from universal vaccination programs, national recommendations for rotavirus vaccination have been issued in many countries. A crucial one was the US Advisory Committee on Immunization Practices (ACIP) recommendation that was issued immediately after licensure of RotaTeq.[186] Globally, the most important one is the World Health Organization (WHO) position and universal recommendation.[271] In Europe, there is no formal recommendation-issuing body, but the pediatric societies ESPID and ESPGHAN issued recommendations in 2008 that were updated as ESPID recommendations in 2015.[262]

All major recommendations have held that rotavirus vaccination should be given to all children, simply because no special "risk groups" for RVGE can be reliably identified. Vaccination of special groups is a separate issue discussed next.

Special Target Groups and Issues

Prelicensure efficacy trials of rotavirus vaccine were conducted in healthy infants and had many exclusion criteria. Therefore, knowledge on safety and efficacy of rotavirus vaccine in many special groups has accumulated slowly.

Premature Infants

Both RotaTeq and Rotarix, as well as RotaShield,[254] vaccines can be given to prematurely born infants regardless of gestational age, but following the recommendations according to calendar age.[89,182,230] If the infant is still in the hospital, a possible risk of local transmission of vaccine virus must be considered.

HIV-Infected Children

Asymptomatic HIV-infected infants can be vaccinated normally according to calendar age without any safety issues using either Rotarix[229] or RotaTeq.[136] Screening for maternally acquired HIV infection can often be done by the time of rotavirus vaccination at 6 to 8 weeks of age, but the result is not needed for decision making on rotavirus vaccination.[262]

Immunodeficiency

Rotavirus vaccine causes symptomatic disease (prolonged diarrhea and viral shedding) in children with severe combined immunodeficiency.[11,270] Vaccination is therefore contraindicated, and exposure to rotavirus vaccine shedders should be avoided in such children. Other immunodeficiencies may be regarded similarly. Selective IgA deficiency may result in prolonged shedding of rotavirus vaccine, but does not constitute a safety problem and, in any case, is usually not diagnosed by the time of rotavirus vaccination.[262]

Short Gut Syndrome and Intestinal Failure

Young children with intestinal failure are at risk for complications from RVGE and should therefore be considered for rotavirus vaccination. Two recent studies have shown that rotavirus vaccine may cause substantial symptoms in such children, but given the severity of wild-type rotavirus infection, they should nevertheless be vaccinated under close observation.[56,117]

Breastfeeding

Early studies with bovine and rhesus rotavirus vaccines showed little or no reduction of vaccine uptake in breast-fed infants compared with bottle-fed infants.[30,260] The question of possible suppressive effect of breastfeeding is largely theoretical, as there is no question of recommending against breastfeeding for the uptake of rotavirus vaccination. Specifically, it has been shown that a break in breastfeeding at the time of rotavirus vaccine administration does not increase uptake.[93]

Influence of Oral Polio Vaccine

The early studies of bovine rotavirus vaccine administered with OPV showed that OPV suppressed the uptake of rotavirus vaccine but not vice cersa.[80,264] The subject was recently reviewed by Patel et al with the same conclusion.[191] Rotavirus vaccines do not adversely affect OPV immunogenicity, but OPV does interfere with the uptake of (at least) the first dose of rotavirus vaccine. Also, rotavirus IgA antibody levels remain lower after a course of two doses of Rotarix or three doses of RotaTeq when administered concomitantly with OPV.[191]

To avoid interference, spacing of OPV and rotavirus vaccine (at least for the first dose) would be desirable.[262] This must be balanced against programmatic needs. In Latin America, Rotarix was coadministered with OPV and showed high efficacy.[240]

If OPV suppresses/prevents the uptake of the first dose of Rotarix, the second dose 2 months later may become effectively the first dose. This could explain why a small risk of IS after the second dose of Rotarix was identified in Brazil but not in Mexico.[192]

Intestinal Microflora

Composition of microflora may reduce the uptake of rotavirus vaccine in developing countries. It would be important to find ways to modulate the microflora for more optimal conditions for rotavirus vaccination, but no such intervention (e.g., probiotics) is proven as yet.

Intussusception

IS is the most important adverse effect of rotavirus vaccination and has already caused the withdrawal of the first licensed rotavirus vaccine, RotaShield, from the market. IS occurred mostly 3 to 7 days after the first dose of RotaShield, and the attributable risk was estimated at 1:10,000.[178] This rate was later challenged and a rate of 1:32,000 was proposed instead.[227] Furthermore, the risk of IS was shown to be age dependent, as most of the cases occurred in the catchup vaccination program in infants who were over 90 days of age at the time of the first dose.[227]

It is now well established that both of the leading licensed rotavirus vaccines, Rotarix and RotaTeq (and most likely other live rotavirus vaccines as well) are also associated with IS. This could not be detected in prelicensure trials that were designed to rule out a risk of IS of similar magnitude as that of RotaShield. Later, in prospective surveillance studies after the launch, the risk estimates of IS for both vaccines are between 1:50,000 and 1:80,000, and the relative risks over background of both vaccines in the 7-day period after dose 1 are about 5.[95]

The small risk of IS is often weighed against the benefits of rotavirus vaccination, and this comparison comes out in favor of vaccination in most settings.[271]

Although it is not currently known whether the risk of IS associated with the currently licensed rotavirus vaccines follows the same age-related pattern as that of RotaShield, it seems logical to assume that this is the case. It may be prudent to follow the current ESPID recommendation and give the first dose of rotavirus vaccine as early as possible, that is, at 6 to 8 weeks of age.

Porcine Circovirus

In 2010 both licensed rotavirus vaccines were found to have porcine circovirus (PCV) as contaminants.[168,263] This created some concern, although PCV is not known to infect humans, and the WHO and European Medicines Agency held that rotavirus vaccines may continue to be used. In Rotarix, PCV contamination was traced to virus seed, and the manufacturer is committed to provide a PCV-free vaccine in the future. In RotaTeq, the source of contamination was traced to batches of trypsin used in the manufacturing process,[204] and with changes in the process, PCV-free vaccine should be available.

Nonlive Rotavirus Vaccines

The need and rationale for the development of nonlive rotavirus vaccines as alternatives for live oral rotavirus vaccines are based on efficacy and safety concerns. All live rotavirus vaccines have shown a relatively (in comparison with developed countries) low efficacy in developing countries for reasons that may not be easily remedied, and repeated parenteral (or possibly intranasal) immunization might induce a high level of protection bypassing the intestinal obstacles. IS remains a serious safety concern, although the magnitude of the problem is regarded as tolerable. This may, however, change. Also, the possibility of contamination by adventitious agents such as PCV is limited to live vaccines.

Nonlive rotavirus vaccines might be administered mucosally or parenterally. The types of vaccines under consideration include three main categories:

1. Inactivated whole rotaviruses[119]
2. Rotavirus virus-like particles (VLPs) of double-layered (VP2/VP6) or triple-layered (2/6/7 or 2/4/6/7) composition[9,10,25,53,111,215]
3. Recombinant rotavirus proteins such as VP8[269] or VP6[22]

The only nonlive rotavirus vaccine that has reached human trials is the P-2 VP8* subunit vaccine in which VP8* from G1P[8] virus has been expressed in *Escherichia coli* and fused with P2 T-cell epitope of tetanus toxin to enhance immunogenicity.[269]

Under appropriate conditions,[138] rotavirus VP6 alone forms large tubular structures that are strong immunogens. VP6 is also the simplest possible rotavirus candidate vaccine, consisting of only a single protein, which is a group antigen common to and largely conserved among all group A rotaviruses. Rotavirus VP6 vaccine has been shown to protect against live rotavirus challenge in a mouse model.[135]

SELECTED READINGS

1. Aiyegbo MS, Sapparapu G, Spiller BW, et al. Human rotavirus VP6-specific antibodies mediate intracellular neutralization by binding to a quaternary structure in the transcriptional pore. *PLoS ONE*. 2013;8:e61101.

6. Armah GE, Kapikian AZ, Vesikari T, et al. Efficacy, immunogenicity, and safety of two doses of a tetravalent rotavirus vaccine RRV-TV in Ghana with the first dose administered during the neonatal period. *J Infect Dis*. 2013;208:423-431.

16. Bernstein DI, Sack DA, Rothstein E, et al. Efficacy of live, attenuated, human rotavirus vaccine 89-12 in infants: a randomised placebo-controlled trial. *Lancet.* 1999;354:287-290.
21. Bishop RF, Davidson GP, Holmes IH, et al. Virus particles in epithelial cells of duodenal mucosa from children with acute non-bacterial gastroenteritis. *Lancet.* 1973;2:1281-1283.
22. Blazevic V, Lappalainen S, Nurminen K, et al. Norovirus VLPs and rotavirus VP6 protein as combined vaccine for childhood gastroenteritis. *Vaccine.* 2011;29:8126-8133.
23. Blutt SE, Kirkwood CD, Parreno V, et al. Rotavirus antigenaemia and viraemia: a common event? *Lancet.* 2003;362:1445-1449.
44. Danchin M, Kirkwood CD, Lee KJ, et al. Phase I trial of RV3-BB rotavirus vaccine: a human neonatal rotavirus vaccine. *Vaccine.* 2013;31:2610-2616.
88. Gouvea V, Glass RI, Woods P, et al. Polymerase chain reaction amplification and typing of rotavirus nucleic acid from stool specimens. *J Clin Microbiol.* 1990;28:276-282.
120. Joensuu J, Koskenniemi E, Pang XL, et al. Randomised placebo-controlled trial of rhesus-human reassortant rotavirus vaccine for prevention of severe rotavirus gastroenteritis. *Lancet.* 1997;350:1205-1209.
142. Libster R, McNeal M, Walter EB, et al. Safety and immunogenicity of sequential rotavirus vaccine schedules. *Pediatrics.* 2016;137(2):20152603.
153. Madhi SA, Cunliffe NA, Steele D, et al. Effect of human rotavirus vaccine on severe diarrhea in African infants. *N Engl J Med.* 2010;362:289-298.
164. Matthijnssens J, Ciarlet M, McDonald SM, et al. Uniformity of rotavirus strain nomenclature proposed by the Rotavirus Classification Working Group (RCWG). *Arch Virol.* 2011;156:1397-1413.
195. Payne DC, Boom JA, Staat MA, et al. Effectiveness of pentavalent and monovalent rotavirus vaccines in concurrent use among US children <5 years of age, 2009-2011. *Clin Infect Dis.* 2013;57:13-20.
218. Ruiz-Palacios GM, Pérez-Schael I, Velázquez FR, et al. Safety and efficacy of an attenuated vaccine against severe rotavirus gastroenteritis. *N Engl J Med.* 2006;354:11-22.
220. Ruuska T, Vesikari T. Rotavirus disease in Finnish children: use of numerical scores for clinical severity of diarrhoeal episodes. *Scand J Infect Dis.* 1990;22:259-267.
227. Simonsen L, Viboud C, Elixhauser A, et al. More on RotaShield and intussusception: the role of age at the time of vaccination. *J Infect Dis.* 2005;192(suppl 1):S36-S43.
233. Svensson L, Sheshberadaran H, Vesikari T, et al. Immune response to rotavirus polypeptides after vaccination with heterologous rotavirus vaccines (RIT 4237, RRV-1). *J Gen Virol.* 1987b;68(Pt 7):1993-1999.
244. Velazquez FR, Matson DO, Calva JJ, et al. Rotavirus infections in infants as protection against subsequent infections. *N Engl J Med.* 1996;335:1022-1028.
246. Vesikari T. Rotavirus vaccination: a concise review. *Clin Microbiol Infect.* 2012;18(suppl 5):57-63.
248. Vesikari T, Isolauri E, D'Hondt E, et al. Protection of infants against rotavirus diarrhoea by RIT 4237 attenuated bovine rotavirus strain vaccine. *Lancet.* 1984;1:977-981.
258. Vesikari T, Matson DO, Dennehy P, et al. Safety and efficacy of a pentavalent human-bovine (WC3) reassortant rotavirus vaccine. *N Engl J Med.* 2006;354:23-33.

The full reference list for this chapter is available at ExpertConsult.com.

SUBSECTION **IV** RNA—Togaviridae

Rubella Virus 174

James D. Cherry • Amira Baker

Rubella (i.e., German measles) is a generally mild, exanthematous, infectious illness that usually causes minimal morbidity and mortality in children. However, infection during pregnancy can result in fetal infection, which usually is associated with considerable adversity for the developing infant. The rubella virus has only one known type.

HISTORY

In ancient history, rubella as a disease is lost among the other prominent exanthematous diseases such as scarlet fever, measles, and smallpox. In an extensive review, Griffith[234] suggested that rubella was known to the early Arabian physicians under the name *al-hamikah,* but they considered rubella a form of measles. Two German physicians, de Bergen in 1752 and Orlow in 1758, usually are credited with providing the first clinical descriptions of rubella as a specific entity.[234,623] In early writings, rubella was called *Röteln.*[187,623] However, because of the great interest of German physicians in the disease during the period from the mid-18th to the mid-19th centuries, the name *German measles* frequently was used in other countries.

In 1866, a Scottish physician named Veale[600] described 30 cases of German measles. In his paper, he gave the illness its present name, *rubella.* His opinion was that the German name Röteln was too harsh and foreign and that other possible names—*rubeola notha* and *rosalia idiopathica*—were too long for general use and could be confused with measles.[187] Other historical synonyms for rubella are rubeola, rubeola sine catarrho, rubeola epidemica, rubeola morbillosa, rubeola scarlatinosa, rosania, roseola, roseola epidemica, rosalia, scarlatina morbillosa, scarlatina hybrida, morbilli scarlatinosi, feuer masern, roséole, roséole idiopathique, rubéole, rougéole fausse, French measles, false measles, bastard measles, hybrid measles, and bastard scarlatina.[234]

In 1881, at the International Congress of Medicine in London, a consensus was reached that rubella was a distinct disease. Rubella was thought to be similar in some respects but not identical to measles or scarlatina. By the beginning of the 20th century, the clinical description of rubella was complete, except that joint manifestations had received curiously little description.[16,130,187,234,384,499,584]

Rubella gained its current importance in 1941, when Gregg,[233] an Australian ophthalmologist, reported congenital defects in infants of mothers who had rubella during early pregnancy. Despite considerable skepticism, Gregg's observations were confirmed quickly by Swan and colleagues[563,564] in Australia and other investigators in the United States and the United Kingdom.[168,473,480,623] By 1947, 28 communications describing 500 children with severe congenital defects associated with maternal rubella had appeared in the literature.[623]

In 1938, Hiro and Tasaka[274] demonstrated that rubella was caused by a virus transmitted to humans through the subcutaneous injection of filtered nasal washings. In 1942, Habel[242] infected monkeys with nasal washings and blood from human cases. In 1962, the rubella virus was propagated in the laboratory by two investigative teams, Weller and Neva[622] and Parkman and colleagues,[434] who used different techniques and reported the growth of rubella virus in tissue culture.

The isolation of rubella virus in 1962 paved the way for definitive study of the 1964 rubella pandemic.[358,422,606] The results of extensive virologic, serologic, and epidemiologic investigation were presented at a Rubella Symposium in May 1965.[326] After the rubella virus was isolated in tissue culture, an intensive worldwide effort to develop vaccines was mounted. The accumulation of these experiences resulted in an extensive body of knowledge related to rubella and rubella immunization that was presented at the International Conference on Rubella Immunization in February 1969.[327] Live attenuated rubella virus vaccines were licensed for use in mid-1969 in the United States.[328,383,470] In the 46-year period since vaccine licensure and its universal use in the United States occurred, the yearly occurrence of rubella fell from 40,000 cases to 11 cases in 2005.[79,80,78,84,82,84,457,469,629] During the next decade, the number of cases remained low.[86,89,334,431] Sustained transmission of rubella no longer occurs in the United States.[83,468]

PROPERTIES

Classification

Rubella virus is placed in the *Rubivirus* genus of the family Togaviridae.[178,275,330] It is the only species in this genus. The virus is similar physiochemically to the other member of its family (i.e., alphavirus) but is unrelated serologically. Rubella virus has no invertebrate host, which is a characteristic of all alphaviruses, and humans are the only known vertebrate host.

In 2005, the World Health Organization (WHO) adopted a systematic nomenclature to categorize the distinct genetic variants of rubella virus. Rubella virus genotypes were divided into two phylogenetic groups, clade 1 and clade 2, which have an 8% to 10% difference at the nucleotide level. This was updated in 2013 to upgrade three provisional genotypes, with 1a as the last remaining provisional genotype. Clade 1 includes 10 genotypes (i.e., 1a, 1B, 1C, 1D, 1E, 1F, 1G, 1H, 1I, and 1J), and clade 2 includes 3 genotypes (i.e., 2A, 2B, and 2C). Recognized genotypes are denoted with uppercase letters, in contrast to provisional genotypes that are designated with lowercase letters. Of these 13 genotypes, only 4 (i.e., 1E, 1G, 1J, and 2B) are repeated frequently in global distribution.[641] This classification has been especially important in the WHO's virologic surveillance and has greatly aided elimination efforts.[1,429,431,639]

Physical Properties

The rubella virion is spherical, with a diameter of 60 to 70 nm. It consists of a capsid protein (C) and two glycoproteins (E1 and E2).[96,275,346,366,443] E1 has a relative molecular weight of 58,000 daltons, and E2 has a relative molecular weight of 42,000 to 47,000 daltons. They are glycosylated and located on the viral surface membrane. E1 is the viral hemagglutinin that is found on 5- to 6-nm surface projections.[278,443] The nucleocapsid has a diameter of 30 to 40 nm and is composed of a polypeptide (i.e., C protein) and the genomic RNA. The nucleic acid of rubella virus is single-stranded RNA with a molecular weight of 3.2 to 3.8×10^7 daltons and a genome of 9762 nucleotides.[517] Its genome encodes five protein products, including two nonstructural proteins (i.e., P90 and P150) and three virion proteins (i.e., C, E1, and E2). The outer coat of the virus (i.e., envelope) is lipoprotein with host cell lipid and virus-specified polypeptides.

Rubella virus is relatively sensitive to heat; it can lose infectivity within 30 minutes at 56°C (132.8°F).[174,435,448] However, Kistler and Sapatino[317] observed that some infectivity persists even after heating for 60 minutes at 70°C (158°F). At 37°C (98.6°F) in the presence of 2% serum, 90% of virus is inactivated in 3 hours.[435] At 4°C (39.2°F) with protein stabilization, viral titers are maintained for 7 or more days. The virus is stable indefinitely at −60°C (−76°F) and below but labile at normal (−10°C to −20°C [14°F to −4°F]) refrigeration temperatures. When it is stabilized with protein, the virus can survive several rapid freeze-thaw cycles without significant loss of titer.[502]

Rubella virus is sensitive to ultraviolet light. In 1 hour, a high-titer, cell-free virus suspension was inactivated by an intensity of 1350 $\mu W/cm^2$; however, a tissue culture suspension of virus was not inactivated completely when it was exposed to a similar intensity of radiation.[317] Rubella virus is sensitive to visible light, and photosensitivity can be potentiated by the basic dye proflavine.[49]

The virus also is sensitive to pH extremes of less than 6.8 and greater than 8.1.[93] Several chemicals rapidly inactivate rubella virus: ether, acetone, chloroform, deoxycholate, formalin, β-propiolactone, ethylene oxide, free chlorine, and 70% alcohol.[448] It is resistant to thimerosal.

Antigenic Composition

Rubella virus infection of tissue culture cells results in the production of infectious virus that can be neutralized by specific antiserum. Specific viral antibodies can be identified by hemagglutination inhibition (HI), complement fixation (CF), precipitation in gel, platelet aggregation, passive hemagglutination, single radial hemolysis, latex agglutination, enzyme-linked immunosorbent assay (ELISA), and immunofluorescence.* Neutralization and HI identify antibodies that inhibit specific biologic functions of the virus, whereas the other assays identify only the formation of antigen-antibody complexes. The E1 glycoprotein is the predominant erythrocyte-binding and neutralization site of the virus.[586,617] Weak neuraminidase activity also has been associated with purified rubella virus.[25]

In 1967, Stewart and associates[553] reported that tissue culture–grown rubella virus produced hemagglutination of erythrocytes from chickens that were younger than 1 day old and from one goose and one lamb, but no hemagglutination was observed with adult chicken, guinea pig, and other red cell preparations commonly used. Subsequently, techniques involving careful control of test system diluents revealed that red cells from many different animals were agglutinated by rubella virus.[352,510] Viral hemagglutinin is stable at −20°C (−4°F) for months and at 4°C (39.2°F) for several weeks, but it is destroyed rapidly by heat.[206,246]

Sever and colleagues[524] first demonstrated that supernatant fluid from primary African green monkey kidney (AGMK) and rabbit kidney epithelial cell (RK-13) tissue cultures contained useful complement-fixing antigens. Two distinct rubella complement-fixing antigens exist.[512] One of the antigens is similar in size and weight to the hemagglutinin and infectious virus; the other soluble antigen is smaller, with a buoyant density of 1.08 g/mL. The soluble antigen is noninfectious and does not contain nucleic acid.[448] Rubella complement-fixing antigens retain their antigenicity after either treatment.

Two major small-particle antigens have been identified in the medium of tissue culture–infected cells by immunodiffusion.[341,345,513] The two soluble antigens are structural components of the virion, and natural infection with rubella virus results in the formation of serum-precipitating antibodies. The antigens have been designated *theta* and *iota*. Their importance lies in the fact that antibody to the iota antigen rarely is observed in the serum of recipients of some rubella vaccines; therefore, they may be of value in studying vaccine-induced immunity.[68,342]

The E1 glycoprotein is the dominant surface molecule of rubella virus.[97] It is the main target of the humoral antibody response for detection and elimination of the virus. HI and neutralization sites have been localized to a small segment of the E1 glycoprotein (i.e., $E1_{245}$ to $E1_{285}$). A study identified the myelin oligodendrocyte glycoprotein (MOG) as the host cell receptor for the rubella virus that interacts with the E1 glycoprotein. Blocking this MOG attachment site of rubella virus may be a way to prevent rubella virus infection of cells.[119]

Molecular analysis of rubella virus epidemiology from 1961 to 1997 in North America, Europe, and Asia found no major antigenic variations.[199] Further phylogenetic analysis of a collection of 103 E1 gene sequences from rubella viruses isolated from 17 countries from 1961 to 2000 found the existence of at least two genotypes.[647] Previous work identified rubella genotype 1 isolates predominantly in Europe, Japan, and the Western Hemisphere, whereas genotype 2 isolates were limited to Asia and Europe. In 2013, the WHO adopted a new nomenclature to categorize all of the genetic variants of rubella found.[641]

Tissue Culture Growth

Rubella virus grows in many different tissue cultures, including cell strains, cell lines, and primary cells.[137,370,371,435,448,634] Cell sources include mature and embryonic tissue from humans and other primates, rabbits, swine, dogs, birds, hamsters, and cattle. In tissue culture, growth of rubella virus can be identified by its cytopathic effect or its ability to interfere with the growth of another tissue culture–susceptible virus.

The method used most commonly for primary isolation of rubella virus from clinical material is the interference technique with primary AGMK cells.[434] In this system, nonadapted rubella virus grows readily but does not produce a cytopathic effect. Infection is demonstrated in AGMK tissue culture by the failure of a typical enterovirus cytopathic effect to occur after the culture is challenged with echovirus 11 or another suitable enterovirus. A common alternative to the

*References 33, 42, 95, 99, 100, 166, 167, 180, 196, 270, 341, 342, 367, 439, 448, 496, 495, 597, 648.

AGMK–echovirus 11 interference system for primary isolation of rubella virus is use of the RK-13 cell line, in which infection can be identified by a cytopathic effect. For laboratory study and determination of neutralizing antibody, many different cell lines (e.g., RK-13, baby hamster kidney cell [BHK]-21, rhesus monkey kidney epithelial cells [LLC-MK2]) can be used. The highest titers of rubella virus are produced in the BHK-21 and Vero cell lines.

Kinetic studies in tissue culture indicate that virus adsorption is complete within 90 minutes and that the eclipse period lasts approximately 12 hours. The first new virus observed is cell associated; it is followed in 2 to 4 hours by extracellular virus. In primary cell culture, titers of cell-associated and free virus reach 10^3 tissue culture infectious dose $(TCID)_{50}$/mL by the fourth day; peak titers are not attained until approximately the 17th day. In all cell systems, chronic infection occurs but is limited in some cultures by the cytopathic effect. Rubella virus induces the formation of plaques in several cell lines.

Animal Susceptibility

Although natural infection occurs only in humans, several other primates have been infected experimentally.[370,435,448] In addition to primates, rabbits, hamsters, ferrets, guinea pigs, and suckling mice have been infected with rubella virus.

EPIDEMIOLOGY

In contrast to measles and other diseases with apparent dramatic cycles, knowledge of rubella epidemiology has been acquired primarily during the past 85 years. Major events during this period that stimulated interest in its epidemiology were the observation of teratogenicity in 1941,[233] the isolation of the virus in the early 1960s,[434,622] and the pandemic of 1964. Because rubella was not a reportable disease in the United States until 1966, considerable gaps exist in the available information. We are in a new epidemiologic era because of the widespread use of rubella vaccine. Predicting the incidence of rubella must take into account the extent and method of vaccine use in the population under surveillance.

Incidence and Prevalence

Epidemic Behavior

The epidemic pattern of rubella in selected areas of the United States in the prevaccine and early vaccine eras is shown in Fig. 174.1. The rubella epidemic cycle was usually described as one of 6- to 9-year intervals, with each cycle consisting of a buildup and fall in incidence during the course of a 3- to 4-year period.[285,286] However, a close look at Fig. 174.1 suggests that the basic pattern in the prevaccine era was a 3.6-year cycle. Of the 11 peaks from 1928 to 1968, all but two occurred in a 2- to 4-year span, with a median of 3 years. Beyond the 3-year cycle is the better-known 6- to 9-year cycle of major disease. Pandemics occurred in the periods of 1941 to 1944 and 1963 to 1965.

The US rubella pandemic of 1964 to 1965, which initially began in Europe in 1963, exemplifies the extent of morbidity that rubella has the potential to cause.[449] At that time, there were an estimated 12.5 million cases of rubella, including more than 2000 cases of encephalitis, 11,250 fetal deaths, 20,000 cases of congenital rubella syndrome (CRS), 3580 deaf-blind children, and 1800 children with mental retardation.[639]

Since the introduction and widespread use of rubella vaccine in the United States, epidemic rubella has occurred only once on a national scale (Fig. 174.2).[82,81,467] In 1991, 1401 cases of rubella and 47 cases of CRS were reported.[84] During the next decade, 76 cases of rubella (yearly median of 8 cases) and six cases of CRS were reported (see Fig. 174.2). Rubella virus is no longer circulating in the United States, and the cases that have occurred in recent years have been importations.[83,468] On October 29, 2004, an expert review panel from the Centers for Disease Control and Prevention (CDC) declared that the rubella virus had not been an endemic threat since 2001 in the United States.

Another remarkable achievement has been rubella eradication from the Americas, especially because as many as 135,947 cases were confirmed in the Americas in 1998.[69,85] In 2003, the Pan American Health Organization strengthened efforts to eliminate rubella and CRS from the Americas by 2010. They accomplished this goal with high immunization coverage through programs targeting more than 450 million people, including mass vaccination of adolescents and adults, and increased surveillance for rubella and CRS that was integrated into existing measles surveillance programs. As a result of these comprehensive efforts, the last endemic rubella case documented in the Americas was reported in Argentina in February 2009, and the region was declared free of endemic rubella transmission in April 2015.[69,86,85,228,431]

In countries in which effective universal childhood immunization had not been achieved, epidemics continue to occur. Although the number of rubella cases on a global scale continues to decrease, rubella remains a problem in many areas of the world. Based on data from 2014 collected by the WHO, 33,068 rubella cases from 161 countries were reported, which is a 95% decrease from the 670,894 cases reported in 2000 from 102 countries.[228,558,638] There was also an increase in the number of countries reporting rubella cases and CRS cases during this time.

From 2002 to 2014, there were decreased numbers of cases in the Americas, European, and Eastern Mediterranean regions. In the Americas region, there was a decrease from 39,228 cases in 2000 to no new cases since 2009, a 1000-fold decrease in the European region (i.e., 621,039 cases in 41 countries in 2000 to 640 cases in 37 countries in 2014), and a 6% decrease in the Eastern Mediterranean region (i.e., 3122 cases to 2945 cases).[475]

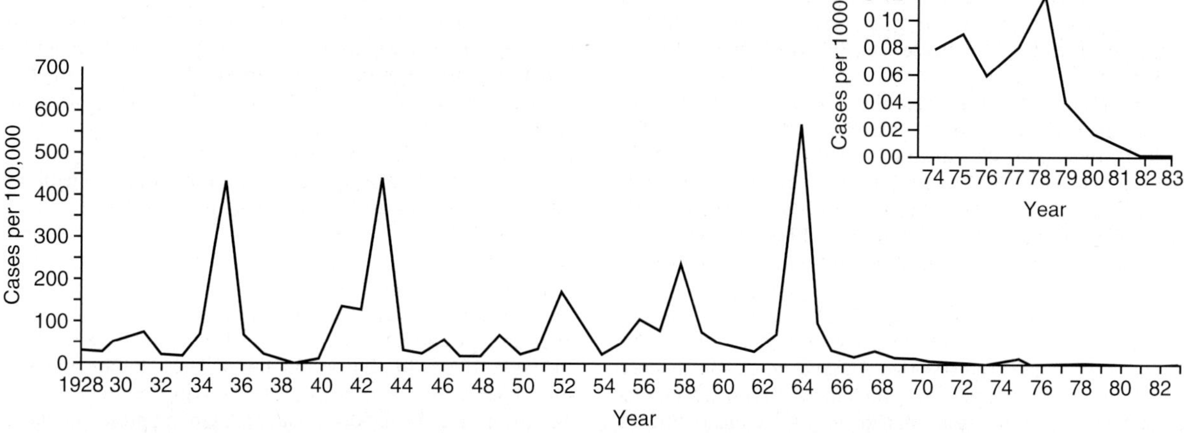

FIG. 174.1 Rubella incidence for 1928–83 in 10 selected US areas: Maine, Rhode Island, Connecticut, New York City, Ohio, Illinois, Wisconsin, Maryland, Washington, and Massachusetts. (From Williams NM, Preblud SR. Rubella and congenital rubella surveillance, 1983. *MMWR Surveill Summ.* 1984;33: 1SS–10SS.)

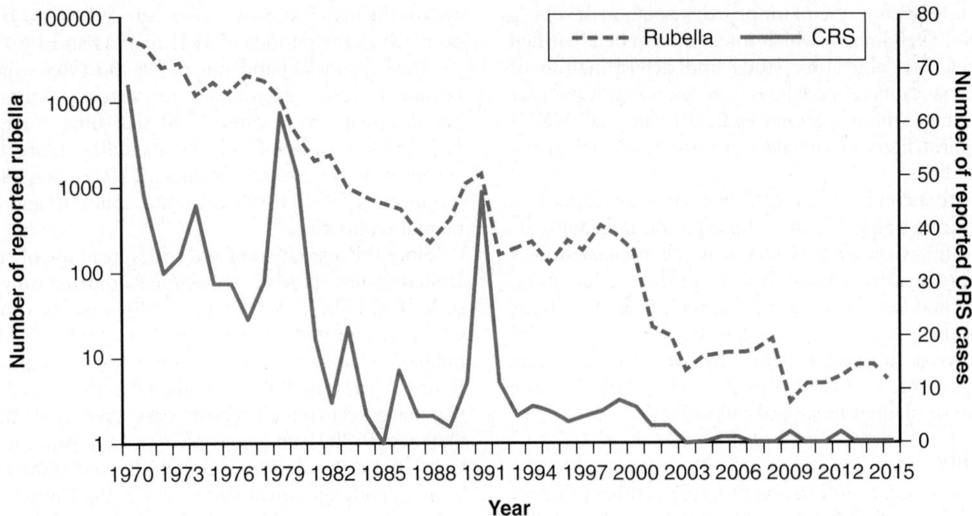

FIG. 174.2 Number of reported cases of rubella and congenital rubella syndrome (CRS) in the United States from 1970–2015. (Data from CDC yearly reports of selected notifiable diseases and Reef SE, Frey TK, Theal K, et al. The changing epidemiology of rubella in the 1990s: on the verge of elimination and new challenges for control and prevention. *JAMA.* 2002;287:464–72.)

TABLE 174.1 Age Distribution of Reported Rubella Cases and Estimated Incidence Rates[a] for Illinois, Massachusetts, and New York City, 1966–68,[b] and Total United States, 1985–87[b]

	1966–68 AVERAGE[c]		1985–87 AVERAGE[d]		1966–87
Age Group (y)	**%**	**Rate**	**%**	**Rate**	**Rate Change[e] (%)**
<5	21.6	63.3	24.8	0.6	−99.1
5–9	38.5	101.3	11.8	0.3	−99.7
10–14	17.0	44.0	5.2	0.1	−99.7
15–19	12.7	35.7	8.0	0.2	−99.5
≤20	10.2	3.7	50.2	0.1	−96.5
Total	100.0	24.3	100.0	0.2	−99.2

[a]Reported cases per 100,000 people. Patients with unknown age are excluded.
[b]Average annual figures during a 3-year period.
[c]Represents prevaccine years. National age data were not available before 1975 and were not reported consistently (i.e., >75% of cases) until 1980.
[d]Total United States data (i.e., 1986 population projections) are used for 1985–87; because the overall number of reported rubella cases currently is small, fluctuations (e.g., epidemic in New York City in 1985) in only these three reporting areas skewed the data for this period.
[e]Based on actual rates.
From Centers for Disease Control and Prevention: Rubella and congenital rubella syndrome: United States 1985–1988. *MMWR Morb Mortal Wkly Rep.* 1989;38:173–8.

In contrast, reported rubella cases increased in the Western Pacific, Southeast Asian, and African regions during this period. There was a twofold increase (i.e., 5475 to 12,814 cases) in the Western Pacific region, an eightfold increase (i.e., 1165 to 9263 cases) in the Southeast Asian region, and an eightfold increase (i.e., 865 to 7402 cases) in the African region.[228,472]

Epidemic rubella was documented in the former Czechoslovakia in 1972; in Greece in 1993 and 1999; in Australia in 1969 to 1970, 1975 to 1976, 1993 to 1996, and 2003; in Israel in 1972, 1979, and 1983; in Japan in 1975 to 1977, and 2012 to 2013; in Vietnam in 2010 to 2011, and 1982 to 1998; in Brazil in 1981 and 1997 to 2001; in Argentina in 2008; in the United Kingdom in 1971 to 1973, 1978, and 1983; and recently in some European countries.* A notable outbreak occurred in the Netherlands from 2004 to 2005, which primarily affected individuals unvaccinated due to religious beliefs. Three hundred eighty-seven cases of rubella were reported in the Netherlands and then spread to Canada, where an additional 309 cases were reported. An unfortunate consequence of vaccine refusal in these populations included 14 reported infants with congenital rubella infection and two fetal deaths.[243] Other outbreaks were also reported in Georgia in 2004 to 2005, northeastern Italy in 2008, Austria in 2008 to 2009, and Bosnia and Herzegovina in 2009, which were thought to be the result of vaccination failure rates during the war period in the early 1990s.[138,158,292,308,415,509]

*References 175, 186, 191, 211, 222, 244, 254, 284, 301, 309, 336, 337, 378, 432, 475, 500, 541, 561, 565, 566, 581, 599.

The incidence of rubella varies with the epidemic cycle, the number of susceptible people in a population group, and the level of intrapersonal contact within the group. In closed populations such as military training centers and institutions for the mentally handicapped, the attack rate after the disease is introduced approaches 100% among susceptible individuals.[288,289,347] Introduction of disease in the family also affects virtually all susceptible people.[208,209] In community epidemics, estimated attack rates for susceptible people are 50% to 90%.

Age Groups

The age distribution of reported rubella cases and estimated incidence rates in Illinois, Massachusetts, and New York City for 1966 through 1968 and the entire United States for 1985 through 1987[81] are presented in Table 174.1. In the period immediately before the vaccine was introduced (1966–68), the attack rate was highest in the 5- to 9-year-old age group, and the incidence was high among preschool-aged children. The overall reduction in the rate of rubella from the prevaccine era to 1987 was 99.2%. However, 50.2% of the cases reported between 1985 and 1988 were people older than 19 years; in the prevaccine period (1966–68), the percentage for this age group was 10.2%. In 1999, 75%

TABLE 174.2 Age-Specific Attack Rates in Two Communities During Rubella Epidemic in 1964

	DORAVILLE, GA			KINGSTON, TN		
Age Group (y)	**Total Population**	**Cases**	**Attack Rate (%)**	**Total Population**	**Cases**	**Attack Rate (%)**
0–4	87	32	36.8	69	30	43.5
5–9	206	104	50.5	127	90	70.9
10–14	208	59	28.4	127	68	53.5
15–19	78	9	11.5	90	25	27.8
20+	427	11	2.6	487	19	3.9
Unknown	8			—		
Total	1014	215	21.2	900	232	25.8 (average)

From Communicable Disease Center. Rubella surveillance—1964. *Morb Mortal Wkly Rep* 1964;13:349–60.

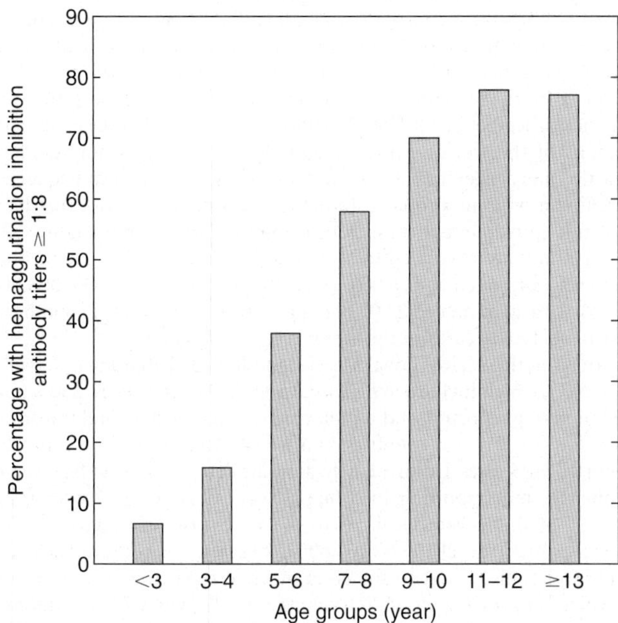

FIG. 174.3 Percentage of children with rubella hemagglutination inhibition antibody titers of 1:8 or greater in a St. Louis, Missouri, study in 1969. (From Cherry JD. Rubella: past, present, and future. *Volta Rev.* 1974;76:461–5.)

of the reported cases were people older than 19 years.[469] From 1980 to 2002, outbreaks of rubella occurred in prisons,[77] in colleges and universities,[75] in hospitals,[74,456,555] at work sites,[76,223,469] in communities with high concentrations of foreign-born people,[469] and among the Amish in six areas of the United States.[80]

Because rubella was not a reportable disease in the United States until 1966, few age-specific incidence or prevalence data on epidemic disease are available. In Table 174.2, age-specific attack rates are presented for two communities during epidemic rubella in 1964.[117] The attack rate curves during the 1964 rubella epidemic are similar to the curve for the prevaccine nonepidemic period from 1966 to 1968 (see Table 174.1). The overall attack rate during the 1964 epidemic in the two communities was 23%. Children younger than 15 years of age accounted for 86% of the cases. In 1999, 272 cases of rubella were reported in the United States, and of the 269 patients with known ages, children younger than 15 years of age accounted for only 14%.[469]

Data on antibody prevalence by age group in the prevaccine era in the St. Louis, Missouri, area are presented in Fig. 174.3.[103] The rubella HI antibody prevalence went from less than 10% among children younger than 3 years of age to almost 80% among preadolescents. Surveys of adolescents and young women of childbearing age conducted before 1969 typically indicated an immunity rate (i.e., HI antibody titer ≥1:8) of 75% to 85%.[118]

Immunity to rubella as indicated by the curve in Fig. 174.3 is affected by epidemic periods. With epidemic disease, the curve probably maintains the same slope, but it moves to the left; the prevalence of antibody in each age group of children increases significantly (10–30%). However, studies in the prevaccine era on sera from young adults indicate that the percentage of susceptible people in this age group is affected only slightly by epidemic disease.[118,186,522,527,634] In a survey of sera from 600 pregnant women in 1962, Sever and associates[527] found that 17.5% had no detectable antibody. In a similar study in 1966 in which the mean age was slightly less (23.6 vs. 25.6 years), 7.8% had no detectable antibody. Other surveys of rubella antibody in the sera of young adults acquired after the 1964 pandemic indicate a susceptibility rate in the 15% to 20% range, similar to pre-1964 data.[118,520,527]

Effect of Vaccination

Rubella vaccine was licensed for use in the United States and many other countries in 1969, and it has been used extensively for more than 50 years.[90,118,457,470,469,520,527,616] However, before the 1990s, rubella-containing vaccines were primarily limited to developed countries.[472] Significant progress has been made in increasing the number of countries that vaccinate routinely against rubella since 1996. As of 2014, the WHO estimated that 140 of 194 member states used rubella-containing vaccines in their national immunization schedules.[228,639]

As a result of successful rubella vaccination efforts, endemic rubella elimination has been achieved in the United States since 2001 and in many other developed countries. The success of elimination of rubella from the region of the Americas, with the last reported case in 2009, provided hope that rubella could be eradicated globally. However, the risk for importation of rubella into the United States remains high because rubella continues to be endemic in many parts of the world.[39] It is imperative to maintain rubella vaccination coverage greater than 90% in the United States. It was estimated by the National Immunization Survey (NIS) in the United States that vaccination coverage for children 19 to 35 months of age was greater than 90% during 2010 to 2014, and data from school surveys of kindergarten children estimated median vaccine coverage of 94% for two doses of measles-mumps-rubella (MMR) vaccine.[91,92,471]

It has been estimated by mathematical models that when vaccine coverage is low through suboptimal childhood-only immunization efforts, viral circulation may be decreased such that children normally infected during childhood may remain susceptible until adolescence and adulthood. The paradoxical effect of sustained low levels of rubella immunization in childhood can increase the risk of CRS more than without vaccine introduction. The WHO recommends rubella immunization coverage of 80% or greater, with at least one dose of rubella vaccine, because the effectiveness of one dose of vaccine is 95% or greater.[639]

The immunization effort in the United States initially focused on children.[146,324,328] A secondary goal was to immunize seronegative postpubertal girls and women of childbearing age, but little effort was extended in this area until 1978. The overall effect of the immunization effort in the United States on the young adult population is difficult to interpret. As shown in Table 174.1 and by subsequent data, the reported number of cases and the incidence of rubella decreased significantly from the prevaccine period until the present.[86,82,84,431,469,616] A marked reduction in the number of reported cases of congenital rubella also has occurred since 1969 (see Fig. 174.2). However, the actual number of cases and the incidence of rubella among adolescents and young adults did not decrease until 1981, and 58.2% of all patients from 1985 through 1987 were 15 years of age (see Table 174.1). The marked upswing in the number of congenital rubella cases in 1990 and 1991 was also alarming.[75,469] Antibody survey data reported between 1981 and 1993 indicate that 5% to 25% of the adolescent and young adult populations in the United States were susceptible to rubella.*

In four studies in which the prevalence of rubella antibody was analyzed by the vaccination status of the participants, differences were significant.[339,389,421,478] Between 87% and 96% of vaccinated people had rubella antibody, whereas only 70% to 80% of nonvaccinated people had antibody.

US serosurvey data for the period 1988 to 1994 found the following seropositive rates by age group: 6 to 11 years, 91.8%; 12 to 19 years, 82.6%; 20 to 29 years, 84.6%; 30 to 39 years, 88.7%; 40 to 49 years, 92.5%; 50 to 59 years, 93.7%; and 60 years or older, 95.7%.[164] In this survey, people born from 1970 to 1974 were found to have the lowest rate of seropositivity (78%). For the period 1999 to 2004, the overall US seropositivity level was 91.3%. Selected age-related rates for children 6 to 11 years of age and adolescents 12 to 19 years of age were 96.2% and 93.7%, respectively.[294] The seropositivity rate was 91.5% among women and 88.0% among men. Among air force recruits in Texas from 2013 to 2014, the rubella seropositivity rate was 82.1%.[351]

In contrast to the immunization program in the United States, which focused on children and elimination of epidemic rubella, immunization efforts in the United Kingdom and many other countries initially were aimed at girls 11 to 14 years of age, with selective immunization of women of childbearing age. This approach would not be expected to disrupt the epidemic pattern of rubella but only to decrease disease in young adult women. Serologic surveys in the United Kingdom indicated a significant reduction in the number of seronegative people in the target population.[112,247,389,390,392,484,580] In one study in which 10,000 serum samples were analyzed, 93% to 96% of girls born after 1956 (who would have been offered rubella vaccine in school) were found to have antibody, whereas only 80% to 89% of those born before 1954 were found to have antibody.[112]

Despite the high level of antibody prevalence among women of childbearing age, rubella infection in pregnancy and congenital rubella continued to be a major problem in the United Kingdom.[392,580] From 1971 to 1982, 625 cases of congenital rubella were reported, and from 1974 to 1981, 3273 women had their pregnancies terminated because they were infected with rubella or had been in contact with a person with rubella in England and Wales.[580]

In Finland, where initial immunization in 1975 involved 11- to 13-year-old girls and after 1982 involved a two-dose program for all children, the susceptibility rate in 1992 for 16- to 19-year-old girls was 3% to 5%, whereas it was 30% for boys.[593]

In Sweden, the initial immunization program, which began in 1973, targeted school girls, susceptible women after pregnancy, and women at special risk. Their second program, which began in 1982, was a universal two-dose schedule at 18 months and 12 years.[52] The rate of susceptibility among pregnant women in Sweden decreased from 12% in 1975 to below 2% in 1994.

Serosurveys from around the world have found various rates of seropositivity for adults.[115,143,155,302,587] In Jordan, 90.9% of women of childbearing age were immune, but only 83% of females 15 to 19 years of age were immune.[302] In Catalonia, Spain, 98.1% of adults had antibody to rubella.[155] In Israel, approximately 95% of women of childbearing age were immune to rubella, whereas only approximately 85% of men of similar age were immune.[115] In this serosurvey, as many as 40% of male adolescents were rubella nonimmune, but only approximately 5% of similarly aged girls were nonimmune.

In Taiwan, the prevalence of rubella antibody among women varied markedly by birth cohort.[587] Rubella antibody was undetectable in 19.9% to 29.2%, 7.1% to 7.3%, and 8.3% to 10.4% of cohorts born before 1971, between 1971 and 1976, and after 1976, respectively.[354] In Argentina in 2002, 91.2% of women of childbearing age had antibody to rubella.[143] A survey of 17 European countries and Australia from 1996 to 2003 showed seronegativity among women of children-bearing age without protective immunity to rubella ranging from 1.4% to 13.4%, lowest among the population of the Czech Republic and highest in Belgium.[410]

Data from pregnant women in Canada from 2002 to 2005 found that 8.8% of those tested were seronegative for rubella and that younger women were more likely to be seronegative.[310] A study from 2000 looking at women of childbearing age in Morocco found that 16.6% were seronegative for rubella immunoglobulin G (IgG) antibodies.[65] Seroprevalence data from Nepal in 2008 demonstrated that 90.8% of women of childbearing age were seropositive for rubella.[595]

*References 139, 157, 196, 312, 339, 421, 422, 478, 515, 551, 556, 608.

Congenital Rubella

Rubella infection during pregnancy, especially during the first 12 weeks of gestation, can lead to miscarriage, intrauterine fetal death, and a variety of birth defects associated with CRS.[162,530] As a result of rubella vaccine implementation, the number of cases of congenital rubella has decreased dramatically, especially in developed countries (see Fig. 174.2). As of 2015, rubella-containing vaccines were introduced into the vaccination schedules of 140 WHO member countries.[228] However, in many regions of the world, immunization against rubella is not standard practice, and congenital rubella infection and its devastating consequences remain an ongoing problem. In many developing countries that have still not implemented mass rubella immunization campaigns, CRS annual rates are estimated to be similar to those in 1996. CRS at that time was estimated at 110,000 cases annually (range, 14,000–308,000 cases), with an estimated 22,000 cases in Africa; 46,000 cases in Southeast Asia; and 12,634 cases in the Western Pacific Regions.[558,639]

In 2011, the WHO Global Measles and Rubella Laboratory Network (LabNet), which includes 690 laboratories in 183 countries, had a goal of improving reporting and monitoring vaccination and viral transmission.[640] As of 2014, 161 countries reported rubella cases and 114 countries reported CRS cases. Unfortunately, accurate data continue to be severely limited by underreporting. In 2014, only 141 cases of CRS were reported, and 86 of them were localized to the Southeast Asia region.[228] The global estimate for 2010 was 103,000 CRS cases.[558] Seroprevalence data and models also attest to the issue of underreporting. These models predicted approximately 46,621 infants annually with CRS in Southeast Asia, although only 86 cases were reported in 2014 in this region.[228,638,640]

Because congenital rubella was not a reportable disease in the United States until 1966, good data on incidence and prevalence during epidemics of rubella are not available. In the 1964 to 1965 rubella epidemic in the United States, 20,000 cases of congenital rubella occurred, 5000 therapeutic abortions were performed, fetal wastage in excess of 6250 was reported, and more than 2100 neonatal deaths occurred.[118] The estimated risk of acquiring congenital rubella after maternal infection vary considerably across studies. Studies performed before 1964, which included nonepidemic periods, tended to underestimate the risk, whereas early retrospective studies after epidemics resulted in high incidence values.[187]

The individual risk of acquiring congenital rubella depends on the month of pregnancy in which maternal infection occurs. Sallomi[494] analyzed eight published studies that met his rigid criteria and found the following rates of anomalies by gestational age when maternal infection occurred: weeks 1 to 4, 61%; weeks 5 to 8, 26%; and weeks 9 to 12, 8%. In pregnancies complicated by rubella in weeks 1 to 8, only 36% ended in normal live births, 39% ended in abortion or stillbirth, and 25% produced gross fetal anomalies. Peckham[438] found that 85% of infants born to mothers infected during the first 8 weeks of pregnancy had detectable defects during the first 4 years of life. Infection at other times during pregnancy revealed the following rates of detectable defects: 9 to 12 weeks, 52%; 13 to 20 weeks, 16%; and after 20 weeks, no defect. Other studies indicate a risk for malformation of 3% and a risk for abortion and stillbirth of 4% when intervals from conception to acquisition of rubella are greater than 12 weeks.[114]

Infection with rubella virus confers lifelong immunity against clinical illness, but asymptomatic reinfection does occur. Asymptomatic reinfection is observed frequently in pregnant women, but it usually has not been considered a risk to the fetus. However, in rare instances, reinfection has resulted in severely damaged infants.[2,24,27,63,141,479,618]

Transmission

Rubella infection likely spreads by the respiratory route. Although definitive evidence supporting this assumption is not available, data from volunteer projects and studies of natural disease strongly support this view.[232,268,506] Infected people regularly shed large concentrations of virus in the nose and throat, and droplets of secretions are released into the environment, which allows respiratory-to-respiratory transmission. It is also possible that the initial hosts contaminate their own hands and then transmit the infectious agent to environmental surfaces or directly to contacts. In this circumstance, new hosts can acquire infection through the fomite-hand-respiratory or hand-hand-respiratory route.

In experimental transmission studies, Green and colleagues[232] found that efficient transmission of infection to susceptible people required prolonged, repeated contact; after a brief, single contact, only one of five children acquired disease, whereas all but one of 17 patients with prolonged, repeated contact were infected. Although the period of communicability has never been determined accurately, almost 100 years ago, the period of infectivity was observed to precede the eruptive phase of illness.[234] Volunteer studies indicate that virus is present in nasopharyngeal secretions from 7 days before to 14 days after the onset of rash.[232,268] Maximal shedding and presumably maximal transmissibility occur for an 11-day period of 5 days before to 6 days after the appearance of rash. Infants with congenital rubella shed virus from the nose and throat for many months and have been responsible for the spread of virus to susceptible contacts.[287,504]

Seasonal Patterns

Rubella is a disease of winter and spring, with the largest number of cases in the United States occurring in March, April, and May.[118,117] This seasonal pattern occurs in years with a high or a low incidence of rubella. Presumably, some transmission and sporadic illness occur throughout the year in large urban areas.

Geographic Distribution

Rubella has been recognized in many countries throughout the world. In recent years, more information about circulating wild-type rubella viruses has been uncovered largely because of global virologic surveillance efforts for measles, which also incorporates surveillance for rubella. The WHO Global Measles and Rubella Network, which was developed in 2000, serves more than 183 countries and includes more than 690 laboratories, which helps confirm suspected cases of rubella and monitors rubella transmission patterns.[176,487] Nine of the 13 viral genotypes were identified during surveillance efforts from 2005 to 2010. Viruses 1E, 1G, 1J, and 2B have the widest geographic distribution and are the most frequently identified.[641] 1E Rubella viruses were found in the Middle East, Europe, Southeast Asia, Africa, and Western Pacific countries. This genotype is also the dominant one found in China. The 1G genotype viruses were found in Europe and Africa. The 2B genotype viruses were found in the Middle East, Europe, Southeast Asia, and South and Central America, Africa, and Western Pacific countries.[1]

In remote islands, rubella may not be endemic, and large segments of the population may be susceptible.[56,273] In these locales, the introduction of rubella results in epidemic infection that involves approximately 90% of the susceptible population. In populated areas of the world in the prevaccine era, rubella was endemic and epidemic, and between 80% and 90% of the adult population had serum rubella antibody.[114] In the prevaccine era in several well-populated large islands that were not remote (i.e., Jamaica, Taiwan, Barbados, Trinidad, Hawaii, and Japan), a smaller percentage of the total population had antibody, and rubella was not endemic.[114,173,209,229]

Other Factors

Sex

The incidence of clinical rubella is similar among boys and girls.[118,117] Among adults, more cases of rubella are reported for women than men.[118] This finding possibly is the result of interest and concern related to congenital rubella rather than a true difference on the basis of sex. In rubella vaccine trials, girls have had geometric mean convalescent-phase antibody titers higher than those of boys.[387,543]

Mitchell and associates[396] studied the IgG, IgM, and IgA antibody responses in men and women to rubella virus structural proteins (i.e., E1, E2, and C). IgA E2 antibodies did not develop in men, but they did in women. Men had lower IgG antibody levels to E2, an earlier onset of E1-specific IgG and IgM antibodies, and a greater proportion of total antibody against E1 than women did. In another study, Mitchell[393] reported that men had a more rapid cell-mediated immune response to whole, inactivated rubella virus and a panel of rubella virus peptides after reimmunization than women did.

Genetics

Hattis and associates[264] showed that individuals differ in their ability to transmit rubella. During a rubella epidemic, they identified a small number of people who had high potential for transmitting virus to susceptible people (i.e., spreaders). Most people demonstrated only minimal virus transmission (i.e., nonspreaders). Honeyman and colleagues[279,282] in 1975 suggested that the ability to spread rubella virus is favored by the cell surface human leukocyte antigen 1 (HLA-1) or the combination of HLA-1 and HLA-8. In a rubella vaccine trial in 1974, Spencer and associates[543] found that 44% of people with high rubella HI antibody titer (≥1:512) responses had HLA-W16. In this study, a high convalescent-phase geometric mean antibody titer was found in people with the AB blood type.

Ovsyannikova and associates[426] studied HLA haplotypes in the genetic control of the immune response to the MMR vaccine. They found that DRB1*04-DQB1*03-DPB1*03 was associated with high lymphoproliferative responses to rubella vaccine virus. They found that specific class II HLA haplotypes (i.e., DRB1*04-DQB1*03-DPB1*03 and DRB1*13/14-DQB1*06-DPB1*03) were associated with higher lymphoproliferative responses to rubella virus vaccine and that the haplotype DRB1*07-DQB1*02-DPB1*11 was associated with lower lymphoproliferative responses.[427]

Kennedy and associates[313] found that homozygosity within HLA DPB1 locus was associated with increased levels of rubella-specific IgG antibody. Haralambieva and colleagues[255] found associations between polymorphisms within the 2′-5′-oligoadenylate synthetase gene *(OAS)* cluster and rubella virus–specific cytokine secretion (i.e., IL-2, IL-10, and IL-6) and antibody levels.

PATHOLOGY AND PATHOGENESIS

Viral Infection

The sequence of events in uncomplicated, postnatally acquired rubella is presented in Table 174.3. Although much is known about rubella infection in humans, considerable gaps regarding specific events exist.[232,266-268,506] Estimates for the timing of events in rubella infection (see Table 174.3) have come from volunteer inoculation studies. In many instances, artificial inoculation has resulted in a reduction in the length of the incubation period of clinical disease. This finding suggests that the size of inoculum is important in the initial generation of human infection. It also helps explain the wide boundaries of the incubation period reported in many clinical studies.[234,384,499]

The primary site of infection is the respiratory epithelium of the nasopharynx. Initial infection of the respiratory epithelium apparently is minor; a more important event is early spread of virus to the regional lymphatics. In volunteers given 100 $TCID_{50}$ of rubella virus intranasally, viral multiplication at the respiratory site was found on the third day.[506] After viremia develops, extensive nasopharyngeal infection occurs. In people who have received attenuated or unattenuated virus by the subcutaneous route, nasopharyngeal shedding in various concentrations always occurs.[105,106,232,506] Concentrations of virus typically are greater in specimens collected from the nose than in those from the throat.

Viremia peaks just before the onset of exanthem and disappears shortly thereafter. In contrast, virus continues to be present consistently in the nasopharynx for a 6-day period after the onset of rash and occasionally for an additional week thereafter.[232] In addition to the blood and nasopharynx, other sites from which rubella virus has been

TABLE 174.3 **Sequence of Rubella Viral Infection in Uncomplicated Primary Disease**

Day	Event
0	Rubella virus from the respiratory secretions of an infected person comes in contact with the epithelial surface of the nasopharynx of a susceptible person. Localized infection in the respiratory epithelium is established, and virus spreads through lymphatics and possibly spreads by transient viremia to regional lymph nodes
1–22	Viral replication in localized areas of the nasopharynx and regional lymph nodes
3–8	First evidence of nasopharyngeal viral shedding
6–20	Viremia (i.e., virus free in serum and associated with leukocytes)
8–14	Establishment of infection in the skin and other viremic sites, including generalized nasopharyngeal involvement
10–17	Maximal viremia and viruria
10–24	Maximal nasopharyngeal viral shedding
17–19	Viremia decreases and then ceases. Viral content at viremic sites rapidly diminishes

Data from references 232, 266–268, 506.

recovered are the lymph nodes,[205] urine,[506] cerebrospinal fluid,[547] conjunctival sac,[267] breast milk,[60] synovial fluid,[271] and lungs.[531] In patients with rubella, the virus was recovered from the skin at sites with rash or without rash.[266,267]

Immunologic Events

Antibody

After having natural or vaccine rubella viral infection, patients regularly have an antibody response. Serum antibodies to different rubella viral antigens can be measured by HI, CF, neutralization, immunofluorescence, precipitation, radioimmunoassay, ELISA, single radial hemolysis, passive hemagglutination, latex agglutination, and platelet aggregation.*

In natural postnatal rubella infection, HI and neutralizing antibodies appear 14 to 18 days after exposure, at the time of the rash. HI antibody titers usually peak approximately 2 weeks after the onset of clinical illness, stay at a high level for several weeks, decrease about fourfold during the next year, and then generally persist for life. Immunofluorescence, ELISA, radioimmunoassay, and latex agglutination reveal antibody patterns similar to those determined by HI.[270] Antibody detected by passive hemagglutination does not appear until 3 to 4 weeks after the onset of illness, and that detected by single radial hemolysis is delayed until 1 to 2 weeks after onset. In an Amazon Indian tribe, the geometric mean rubella HI antibody titer 12 years after infection, with no intercurrent rubella exposure, was 1:33.[43] The pattern of the neutralizing antibody response is similar to the HI antibody response, except that the peak is delayed slightly. Brody and colleagues[56] found that all but 10% of an island population had rubella neutralizing antibody 22 years after the time of epidemic illness.

CF antibody first appears approximately a week after HI and neutralizing antibody, peaks approximately 1 month after illness, and usually does not persist as long as HI or neutralizing antibody. Occasionally, the CF antibody response is delayed and appears 1 month after the exanthem, with peak titers occurring 2 to 5 months later. Sever and colleagues[525] identified CF antibodies in only 44% of people with neutralizing antibody who were studied 10 to 20 years after illness. The use of an antigen prepared by alkaline extraction has increased the sensitivity of CF, but low levels of antibody are best identified by HI, ELISA, or neutralization.[448,511]

After natural infection occurs, precipitating antibodies develop to the theta and iota antigens.[341] Antibody to theta antigen appears early, parallels HI antibody, and is persistent. In contrast, the response to iota antigen is delayed, with a slow rise in concentration during a 2- to 3-month period. Five years after infection has occurred, anti-iota antibody cannot be detected.

After immunization has been administered, the antibody response pattern varies according to the type of vaccine used.[44,342,420,451,452,505,611] With RA 27/3 vaccine, the serum antibody response is similar to that after natural disease, except that the peak HI and neutralizing antibody titers attained usually are lower. Serum antibody responses found after HPV-77 and Cendehill vaccine viral infection are different from those found after natural infection in that CF and anti-iota antibodies are observed only irregularly and then in minimal concentrations.

Primary rubella virus infection that is naturally acquired or vaccine induced is characterized by the initial appearance of antibody in the IgM and IgG serum components.[30,41,132,151,241,436,437,548] The IgM-specific response is short lived and not detectable more than 8 weeks after the onset of infection. Occasionally, it has been detected in the serum for extended periods.

IgA nasal HI, ELISA, and neutralizing antibodies occur regularly after natural viral infection. After immunization, the nasal antibody response varies with the type of vaccine and the route of administration.[6,7,131,135,420,448] After subcutaneous immunization with HPV-77 vaccine is given, rubella-specific nasal IgA antibody is a rare finding; it occurs in most subjects who receive RA 27/3 vaccine administered intranasally and in approximately one half of those given this vaccine subcutaneously.

Specific Cell-Mediated Responses

Rubella-specific, cell-mediated lymphocyte responses regularly occur after infection with rubella virus.* Using an in vitro lymphocyte-mediated cytotoxicity assay, Steele and associates[550] found that lymphocytes from people who previously had rubella caused cell destruction in a tissue culture chronically infected with rubella virus. Rubella antigen–specific, cell-mediated immunity also has been demonstrated in lymphocyte cultures by blast transformation, production of migration-inhibition factor, and production of interferon (IFN).[62,280,403,540,573,603,604] With vaccination, rubella-specific, cell-mediated immunity begins 7 days after immunization, with peak responses at 3 weeks.[603,604] Honeyman and associates[280] observed that the rubella antigen-specific, cell-mediated response commenced 1 week before the humoral immune response occurred in natural and vaccine-induced rubella viral infection. They also found that the cell-mediated response was of greater magnitude and duration after natural disease than after immunization. Rossier and associates[486] studied cloistered nuns and found that specific cell-mediated immunity to rubella virus persisted until they reached 79 years of age in the probable absence of reinfection.

Morag and colleagues[403] demonstrated the specific appearance of cell-mediated immunity in tonsillar lymphoid tissue after natural infection or intranasal immunization with rubella vaccine. This responsiveness was conspicuously low after vaccination was administered by the subcutaneous route. In most instances, cell-mediated responsiveness correlates with the presence of antibody; however, specific rubella lymphocyte transformation has occurred in the absence of antibody.[540] The magnitude of the rubella-specific, cell-mediated response is suppressed during pregnancy.[573] Seventeen T-call epitopes have been identified with the lymphoproliferation assay.[97,394] They involve the capsid protein and E2 and E2 glycoproteins.

McCarthy and colleagues[369] identified potential determinants of human cellular immunity to rubella virus by using synthetic peptides

*References 15, 42, 129, 152, 179, 216, 226, 248, 270, 277, 342, 349, 367, 381–383, 407, 439, 448, 523, 524, 578, 601, 605, 630, 648.

*References 97, 269, 280, 307, 358, 361, 369, 393-396, 403, 425, 426, 485, 540, 550, 603, 604.

representing well-defined sequences of rubella virus structural proteins. They used two capsid domains (i.e., C_1 to C_{29} and C_{64} to C_{97}), a glycoprotein E1 domain (i.e., $E1_{202}$ to $E1_{283}$), and a glycoprotein E2 domain (i.e., $E2_{31}$ to $E2_{105}$). All but the C_{64} to C_{97} subsequences stimulated specific lymphoproliferative responses in peripheral blood mononuclear cells in 25% to 50% of immune subjects. The immunodominant T-proliferative epitope (i.e., C_{14} to C_{29}) was recognized by only 50% of the peripheral blood mononuclear cells of the study population. Relatively immunodominant T-cell epitopes vary among different people.

Using a lymphocyte proliferation assay, Mitchell and associates[395] reported positive cell-mediated immune responses to 16 peptides, including six that contained antibody neutralization domains after revaccination.

Nonspecific Responses

A large number of nonspecific, immunologically related responses can be demonstrated during rubella virus infections. Niwa and Kanoh[412] performed a comprehensive study of these responses in 85 children and adults during an epidemic of rubella. They found decreased numbers of neutrophils, T cells, and total leukocytes initially, which returned to normal values within 1 week. Some patients had slightly elevated levels of serum IgM, and total hemolytic complement was elevated in 12 of 30 patients. Marked increases in C4 and C9 were found, and they also observed a marked insensitivity to dinitrochlorobenzene and purified protein derivatives in many patients.

Atypical lymphocytes, autoantibodies, and reduced blastogenesis as measured by phytohemagglutinin (PHA) stimulation were detected in some patients. Other studies consistently have demonstrated a reduction in the lymphocyte response to PHA.[59,67,210,297,333,361,373,412] This reduction typically lasts less than 1 month, and infections with attenuated strains of rubella vaccine virus are less immunosuppressive than are infections with unattenuated rubella virus.

Hyypiä and colleagues[297] reported that during rubella virus infection, the proportion of suppressor-cytotoxic T cells was increased and the proportion of helper-inducer T cells was decreased. Polyclonal activation of B cells was associated with these findings.[298]

Zaknun and coworkers[645] noticed a marked increase in urine neopterin levels in two children with acute rubella. Their levels increased dramatically 4 days before the onset of exanthem.

Fetal Events

Viral Infection

A considerable amount of information about fetal infection became available from extensive studies during the 1964 epidemic of rubella,* and further information was obtained from natural and vaccine viral infections.[46,153,165,338,445,519,598,642] Despite the number and extent of investigations performed, little is known about transmission of the virus to the fetus in maternal infections during the latter half of pregnancy.

With maternal infection during the first trimester, placental infection regularly occurs and often persists throughout the remainder of the pregnancy. In the therapeutic abortion studies of Alford and associates,[10] fetal infection occurred in approximately 50% of placental infections. However, other studies have revealed almost identical isolation rates from placental and fetal tissue.[466,572] Persistent infection is the usual outcome of first-trimester fetal infection. Fetal infection usually involves multiple organs, and virus can be isolated at birth regularly from the throat, rectum, and urine.[287,446]

Little is known about events in second- and third-trimester maternal rubella infection. Most probably, placental infection is a regular occurrence, and transmission of virus to the infant in utero also may occur regularly. Because few infants have defects when they are born after maternal rubella infection in the second and third trimesters, a careful search for rubella infection in these infants by virologic or serologic methods rarely has been conducted. Random studies seem to indicate that rubella virus often infects the fetus after the first trimester and occasionally the infection becomes persistent.[134,153,257,287,399,606,626] Other studies have failed to show virologic or serologic evidence of infection in infants in whom maternal rubella occurred in the second and third trimesters.[107,400,554]

With maternal rubella infection, the cervix also is involved, and fetal infection can occur by the ascending route as well as by primary placental infection.[107,400,519,554,598] Fetal infection has resulted from maternal disease that occurred before conception.[185,627,642]

Rubella virus can be recovered regularly after birth from infants with congenital rubella. The percentage of infants with persistent infection decreases during the course of the first year of life; by their first birthdays; between 10% and 20% of children still shed virus in nasopharyngeal secretions.[124,466] Rawls and colleagues[466] were unable to isolate virus from the throats of 15 congenitally infected infants after they reached 18 months of age, and Sever and Monif[526] and Cooper and Krugman[124] were unable to demonstrate persistence of nasopharyngeal virus in older children. A 4.5-year-old boy with congenital rubella was found on one occasion to be shedding rubella virus in the throat.[532]

Immunologic Findings

Specific antibody. Humoral antibody in a congenitally infected fetus is acquired transplacentally from the mother and is produced actively by the fetus. In a normal maternal-fetal relationship, transport of antibody to the fetus is minimal until the midpoint of the second trimester (16–20 weeks).[8,9] With first-trimester maternal infection (i.e., transplacentally acquired), rubella antibody titers in serum amount to only approximately 5% of maternal values. The fetal immune system becomes functional during the second trimester,[340] and small amounts of specific rubella fetal IgM antibody can be detected. From the midpoint of pregnancy, antibody levels in the developing fetus rise, and at birth, the maternal and infant values are similar. Although the values of total antibody are similar, the composition is different. Maternal antibody at the time of delivery usually is composed entirely of IgG. In contrast, the infant titer consists of fetal IgM, presumably fetal IgG, and occasionally fetal IgA and transplacentally derived maternal IgG.

Long-term rubella antibody patterns in congenitally infected infants after birth are different from those of their mothers or from those of a group of children with acquired disease.[122,256,315,590] Cooper and colleagues[122] monitored a group of 223 mothers of children with congenital rubella and noticed that at the end of 5 years, all still had detectable HI antibody and that the geometric mean titer for the group had undergone a fourfold reduction. In contrast, 5-year follow-up of the congenitally infected infants revealed a 16-fold decline in geometric mean titer; eight of 29 infants had serum HI antibody titers less than 1:8 when they were examined at 5 years of age. Other investigators observed similar declines in rubella antibody titers of congenitally infected infants.[256,315,590]

Another unique aspect of rubella antibody in congenitally infected infants is the persistence of specific IgM. Cradock-Watson and colleagues[133] studied 40 infants with congenital rubella and found that IgM antibody persisted for approximately 6 months in most cases and for up to 2 years in a few children. De Mazancourt and colleagues[144] studied the antibody response to rubella virus structural proteins in infants with CRS and found that the immunoprecipitation patterns were different from those in sera from postnatally infected adults. The sera from congenitally infected infants had little or no C-specific antibody, occasionally only antibody to E1 was precipitated or E1 protein was precipitated in relative excess compared with E2 protein, and the relative amount of E2 antibody was greater than antibody to E1.

Specific cell-mediated immunity. Rubella-specific, cell-mediated immune responses have been studied in children with congenital rubella by the following assays: lymphocyte-mediated cytotoxicity, lymphocyte transformation, lymphocyte IFN production, and leukocyte migration-inhibition factor production.[61,204] By all methods of study, infants with congenital rubella have decreased rubella-specific, cell-mediated responses in contrast to people who had acquired rubella postnatally. Buimovici-Klein and associates[61] found that the degree of suppression correlated with the time of in utero infection; the earlier in pregnancy the maternal infection, the greater is the depression of specific cell-mediated responses. In the study of an infant with late-onset CRS, Verder and associates[602] observed decreased activity of killer and natural killer cells and alloreactive direct cytotoxic cells. Their data indicated that defective cytotoxic effector

*References 10, 72, 107, 124, 125, 126, 160, 253, 256–260, 287, 293, 398, 399, 401, 400, 446, 466, 504, 507, 554, 627.

cell function was the primary cause for failure to eliminate virus in the illness.

Nonspecific responses. Desmyter and colleagues[149] found that infants with congenital rubella produced normal amounts of IFN after receiving measles immunization. They also found that the clinical response and antibody development in these measles-vaccinated children were similar to those in normal children. Lebon and associates[343] observed that sera collected from rubella-infected fetuses and infants with congenital rubella contained an acid-labile IFN. Michaels[385] found that infants with congenital rubella who still were shedding virus in their throat or urine had depressed antibody responses to diphtheria and tetanus toxoids.

White and colleagues[625] reported decreased in vitro lymphocyte blast transformation responses to vaccinia and diphtheria toxoid antigens in children with congenital rubella in contrast to normal children. They also found depressed skin reactivity to intradermal *Candida* antigen in the congenital rubella group. Buimovici-Klein and associates[61] observed a marked reduction in lymphocyte transformation after PHA stimulation in their congenital rubella group. The most marked defect was seen in children in whom maternal rubella occurred during the first 8 weeks of pregnancy.

Pukhalsky and associates[459] reported that rubella immunization resulted in defective lymphocyte response to a mitogen (i.e., PHA). After immunization, serum IFN-α was slightly increased at day 7 and then fell significantly so that it was not measurable at day 30 in several subjects. The IFN-α to interleukin-10 ratio significantly decreased after immunization.

Pathology

Postnatally Acquired Disease

Almost no data on the histologic findings in uncomplicated rubella are available, but occasionally, postmortem tissue has been studied from patients with encephalitis. Giuliani and associates[220] studied lymph nodes from patients with rubella and reported edema, reticulum cell hyperplasia, and loss of the usual follicular morphologic features. Sherman and associates[531] reported six cases of rubella encephalitis and the autopsy findings in three cases. They specifically searched all organs for inclusion bodies, syncytial giant cells, focal cellular necrosis, and unusual proliferative changes, but none was found. Only mild, nonspecific, follicular hyperplasia in the spleen and lymph nodes was seen. Histologic examination of the brain of a 7-year-old girl who died of encephalitis revealed diffuse swelling, nonspecific degeneration, and a sparse, mononuclear perivascular and meningeal exudate.

A synovial biopsy specimen from a woman with rubella arthritis revealed scattered areas of fibrinopurulent exudate and synovial cell hyperplasia. Inflammatory cell infiltration composed mainly of lymphocytic cells was identified, and vascularity was increased.[643]

Congenital Infection

In contrast to postnatal rubella, the pathologic process of congenital infection has been studied extensively.* Table 174.4 summarizes the main pathologic findings of congenital rubella by anatomic location or system. Defects in congenital rubella result from specific cell damage and cellular deficiency. Although specific cellular necrosis is important in certain early lesions such as in the inner ear, the secondary effects of generalized vascular damage are of greater overall importance. The noncytolytic cellular infection characteristic of rubella virus is also important because it results in mitotic arrest and a reduction in the total number of cells in many organs.

CLINICAL MANIFESTATIONS

Postnatal Illness

Although clinical rubella is a distinctive exanthematous disease, its features are not as clearly discernible as those of measles or chickenpox.† The exanthematous illnesses caused by enteroviruses, adenoviruses, and other common respiratory viruses often are clinically similar or identical to those of rubella (see Chapter 58). Because of these other viral illnesses that simulate rubella, descriptions of clinical rubella made before modern virologic diagnostic techniques became available are not always accurate, particularly when rubella in infants and young children is described because exanthems caused by other viruses occur most commonly in these age groups. Despite the availability of a vast amount of clinical material collected during the rubella epidemic of 1964, most clinical knowledge about postnatally acquired rubella was formulated before the current virologic era.

Incubation Period

Although prodromal complaints and lymphadenopathy frequently precede the development of exanthem in rubella, the incubation period in most studies has been calculated as being from the time of exposure to the onset of rash. Almost a century ago, Michael[384] reviewed the incubation periods in 59 different reports and identified a variation of 5 days to 4 weeks. However, in most reports, the minimal incubation time was at least 14 days, and the maximum was 17 to 21 days. The mean incubation period from modern reviews is considered to be 18 ± 3 days.

In carefully controlled studies, Green and colleagues[232] found an incubation time of 13 to 15 days to the onset of rash after the intramuscular inoculation of serum from rubella-infected patients and a longer incubation time (16–21 days) in cases acquired by contact with ill patients. In similar volunteer studies in young adults, Schiff and colleagues[506] reported that the onset of rash occurred 11 to 12 days after the administration of 100 $TCID_{50}$ of tissue culture–grown rubella virus. The investigators attributed this shorter incubation period to a larger inoculum than that occurring in natural transmission.

Prodromal Period

Symptoms reported before the onset of rash in rubella vary with age. In young children, the first evidence of disease usually is the appearance of rash. Mild coryza and diarrhea sometimes precede the development of exanthem in younger patients. In contrast to the lack of prodrome in children, adolescents and adults usually have symptoms before the onset of rash (J. Cherry, unpublished data, 1963–73).[184,236] In one study, 94% of college students with rubella had prodromal symptoms. In decreasing order of frequency, the reported symptoms were eye pain, sore throat, headache, swollen glands, fever, aches, chills, anorexia, and nausea.[184] Gross and associates[236] reported prodromal upper respiratory tract complaints, including malaise, cough, sore throat, red eyes, and runny nose, in 65% of an infected adolescent study group.

Prodromal symptoms usually precede the onset of rash by 1 to 5 days. In the studies of Green and associates[232] involving volunteers, the onset of lymphadenopathy typically occurred 5 to 7 days before the onset of rash. In contrast, Schiff and colleagues[506] observed the appearance of lymphadenopathy only 1 day before the rash appeared; fever occurred 1 to 4 days before the onset of rash, and most of the volunteers also had malaise and sore throat. Pain on lateral and upward eye movement occurs frequently and is sometimes distressing (J. Cherry, unpublished data, 1963–76).[184]

Exanthem Period

The rubella exanthem appears first on the face. The rash spreads centrifugally from the head toward the hands and feet. The progression, extent, and duration of the exanthem vary considerably. In a typical case, the rash involves the entire body during the first 24 hours, begins to fade on the face during the second day, and has disappeared from the body by the end of the third day. The characteristic rash is erythematous, maculopapular, and discrete (Fig. 174.4). Its appearance on an adolescent's face occasionally is confused initially with an exacerbation of acne. Frequently, the rash is only macular with a scarlatiniform appearance. In some patients, the rash is present for less than a day, although sometimes it persists for 5 days or longer. Particularly in adults, the exanthem frequently is pruritic. This complaint is troublesome because it often leads the patient and the physician to attribute the rash to an allergic cause rather than rubella virus infection.

*References 5, 9, 31, 57, 71, 111, 125, 159, 171, 170, 169, 172, 193, 200, 201, 237, 251–253, 311, 319, 321, 322, 355, 398, 401, 408, 423, 444, 453, 454, 465, 467, 476, 481, 482, 489, 518, 536, 537, 544, 552, 557, 574, 583, 614, 617, 624, 637.

†References 101, 184, 187, 232, 234, 327, 335, 384, 499, 506, 588, 623.

TABLE 174.4 **Pathologic Findings in Congenital Rubella Cases**

Anatomic Location or System	Gross and Microscopic Findings	References
Placenta	Perivascular mononuclear cellular infiltration in the deciduas Edema, fibrosis, and necrosis of villi; cytoplasm inclusion bodies observed in swollen Hofbauer cells in villous stroma	423
Generalized growth retardation	Subnormal number of cells in many organs	408
Nervous system	Chronic meningitis with infiltrates of large mononuclear cells, lymphocytes, and plasma cells in the leptomeninges Vascular degeneration, ischemic lesions, and retardation of myelinization throughout brain	481, 482, 536, 574
Eye	Lens: cataract, cortical liquefaction, and spherophakia Iris and ciliary body: necrosis of ciliary body, iridocyclitis, iris atrophy, and pigmentation defects Retina: posterior pigmentary disturbances Cornea: usually normal; occasional endothelial degeneration Optic nerve: posterior bowing	48
Ear	Hemorrhage in fetal cochlea resulting in epithelial necrosis Inflammatory cells in stria vascularis Adhesions between the Reissner membrane and tectorial membrane Sacculocochlear degeneration of Scheibe (i.e., strial atrophy, collapse of the Reissner membrane, atrophy of organ of Corti, rolled-up tectorial membranes, and collapse and degeneration of sacculus) observed after birth	200, 201, 614
Cardiovascular system	Common heart defects in order of frequency: patent ductus arteriosus, pulmonary artery stenosis, ventricular septal defect, and atrial septal defect (these rubella-induced lesions are not different from similar non–rubella-induced lesions) Myocarditis with swelling of muscle fibers and loss of striations; necrosis Intimal proliferation of major arteries	5, 169, 193, 321, 322, 617
Pulmonary system	Chronic interstitial pneumonia with large mononuclear cells, lymphocytes, and plasma cells within interstitial spaces and alveoli	322, 444, 536
Liver	Hyalinization and swelling of hepatocytes, hematopoiesis, and multinucleated giant cells	171, 172, 552, 557
Skin	Purpuric lesion: focal areas of erythropoiesis in dermis and upper subcutaneous adipose tissue Chronic reticulated rash: acute and chronic inflammatory cells and histiocytes in dermis Edema in dermal papillae	71, 319
Bone	Thinning of metaphyseal trabeculae and decrease in number of osteoblasts and osteoclasts Many plasma cells in metaphyses and cartilaginous epiphyses and around vessels Occasional giant cells with cytoplasmic inclusions Thinning of cartilage	467, 489, 518, 624
Muscle	Focal abnormalities: very small fibers with darkly staining nuclei and muscle bundles containing empty connective tissue tubes	543
Teeth	Necrosis of enamel-forming epithelial cells	237, 583
Hematologic system	Transient thrombocytopenia with decreased megakaryocytes in bone marrow; increased platelet adhesiveness and platelet agglutinins Lymph nodes consistent with histiocytosis; unorganized cell mass made up of mononuclear cells with dense round nuclei and irregularly shaped cytoplasm	31, 111, 454, 465
Immunologic system	Spleen: fibrosis Loss of normal architecture and absence of germinal centers in spleen and lymph nodes Dysgammaglobulinemia usually with decreased IgG and IgA and elevated IgM levels	111, 250, 453, 476

The exanthem occasionally progresses to confluence with a morbilliform appearance. In these cases, the rash usually is less coppery and pinker than that in measles, and it heals without desquamation or brownish discoloration. The typical picture of erythema infectiosum (i.e., slapped-cheek appearance and reticular rash) has been observed in rubella-infected patients. Balfour and associates[22] described eight children with erythema infectiosum from whom rubella virus was recovered concurrently and two additional children with serologic evidence of rubella infection. The preliminary results of volunteer studies with a virus recovered from one of the patients in this study produced a slapped-cheek appearance but a nonreticulated rash in four of five men. One 3-year-old child from whom the investigator recovered rubella virus had typical erythema infectiosum (J. Cherry, unpublished data, 1972). A 14-month-old girl had a roseola-like illness and arthritis.[271]

In the volunteer studies of Schiff and associates,[506] the pink-red rash was maculopapular. It appeared initially on the face, chest, upper part of the arms, and shoulders and then spread rapidly over the abdomen, back, and thighs. It developed into an erythematous blush on the face and abdomen. The median duration was 3 days, with extremes of 2 and 5 days. Patients had no pruritus.

Rubella infection without rash is a common occurrence. In some patients, the infection occurs without symptoms; in other people, careful questioning reveals prodromal symptoms, and lymphadenopathy is found on examination. Green and associates[232] reported that approximately 25% of exposed children who became infected had subclinical infection. In an intensive study of 46 susceptible children and adults, all but one person had clinical symptoms with infection[521]; 60% of the group had rash and characteristic posterior auricular or suboccipital lymphadenopathy, and 40% had lymphadenopathy without rash. In another study of rubella in an institution for intellectually challenged children, Horstmann and associates[289] observed that only about one half of the children who became infected had a rash. Of nine children without rash, significant posterior auricular lymph node enlargement

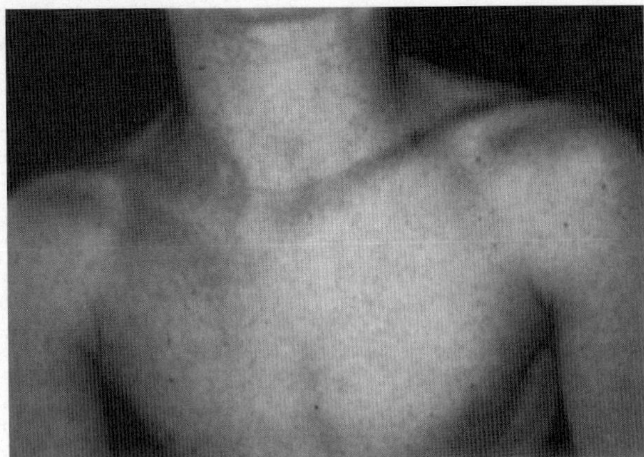

FIG. 174.4 Rubella exanthem. The rash is erythematous, maculopapular, and discrete. (From Cherry JD. Newer viral exanthems. *Adv Pediatr.* 1969;16:233–86.)

developed in five. Buescher[58] reported a subclinical-to-clinical infection ratio in a military recruit population of 6.5:1.

Lymphadenopathy is a major clinical manifestation of rubella. The most characteristic enlargement occurs in the suboccipital and posterior auricular nodes, but generalized involvement also occurs. In the volunteer studies of Schiff and colleagues,[506] the lymph node enlargement usually lasted 5 to 8 days. In two outbreak studies involving adolescents and young adults, posterior auricular and suboccipital lymphadenopathy occurred in all patients with rash.[184,236] In contrast to these findings, Landrigan and associates[335] reported that only 47% of children and 58% of adolescents had similar lymph node enlargement during epidemic rubella illness.

The frequent suggestion that the finding of exanthem and suboccipital lymphadenopathy is pathognomonic for rubella is incorrect. In young children, similar involvement is seen frequently with enteroviral and adenoviral infections. In adolescents and young adults, the association more strongly indicates rubella, but infectious mononucleosis, *Mycoplasma pneumoniae* infection, acquired toxoplasmosis, and other possibilities must be considered.

When fever develops in rubella, the temperature usually is elevated only minimally. For children with experimentally induced rubella, Krugman and Ward[329] reported that five of 13 had temperatures of 38°C (100.4°F) or higher. Two children had maximal temperatures of 38.5°C (101.6°F). Schiff and colleagues[506] found that all nine infected volunteers had fever with a median duration of 5 days. Landrigan and associates[335] found fever in 74% of children and only 47% of adolescents. Gross and coworkers[236] observed fever in only six of 17 adolescents. Children with apparent rubella occasionally have markedly elevated temperatures.

Because few of these cases have undergone virologic study, some doubt remains about whether the illnesses were induced by rubella virus or were caused by other viral agents more commonly associated with marked febrile responses, such as enteroviruses and adenoviruses. We have seen an 8-year-old boy with virologically and serologically confirmed rubella with a temperature of 40°C (104°F) on the day before the appearance of his rash. The 14-month-old girl with arthritis described by Hildebrandt and Maassab[271] had a temperature as high as 40.5°C (105°F).

In 1898, Forchheimer[188] described what he thought was the enanthem of German measles. He described pinhead-sized macular lesions with a rose-red color on the soft palate and uvula that appeared at approximately the time of the exanthem and lasted less than 24 hours. This exanthem has not been identified in children we have examined; however, petechial lesions on the soft palate and uvula have been seen occasionally. Mild pharyngitis is not an uncommon occurrence. Other signs and symptoms in rubella include mild conjunctivitis, sore throat, coryza, cough, and headache.

The duration of illness in uncomplicated rubella varies considerably. Most patients would continue normal activity if the rash were not present. Full return to normal activity usually occurs within 3 days. A few adults are bothered by persistent headache, eye pain, and pruritus for 7 to 10 days.

The white blood cell count in rubella tends to be low. Schiff and colleagues[506] found leukopenia in all nine volunteers. Their leukopenia paralleled the pattern of fever, with onset occurring 24 hours before the rash manifested and persisting for 4 to 5 days. Before rubella could be confirmed by specific serologic and virologic methods, many experts thought that rubella could be confirmed accurately by characteristics of the white blood cell count.[272,297] Leukopenia was found at the onset of disease; the total count rose to a high-normal value during a 10-day period. Relative neutropenia was reported by Hynes[296] in many patients; one patient had a neutrophil count of 868 cells/mm^3 on the first day of illness.

Plasma cells or Türk cells, or both, were seen in all cases of acute rubella studied by Hynes[296] and Hillenbrand.[272] A Türk cell is a developing plasma cell that is 25 to 40 µm in diameter and contains a 15- to 30-µm nucleus. The nucleus has two to five prominent nucleoli and a well-defined, light reticulum. The cytoplasm often is vacuolated. Twenty-five percent of the patients studied by Hynes[297] had elevated erythrocyte sedimentation rates during the first week of illness.

Complications

Joint involvement. The incidences of reported cases of arthritis and arthralgia vary considerably across studies.[37,94,212,236,306,335,534,592,623] Arthralgia and arthritis occur more commonly in adults than in prepubertal children. Women are afflicted more often than are men. In a large outbreak in Bermuda in 1971, 42% of 125 patients studied complained of joint pain or discomfort.[306] Three patients had swelling of the joints. The prevalence of joint symptoms increased from 18% in the 0- to 9-year-old age group by approximately 20% increments per decade; 73% of those older than 30 years had symptoms. Joint complaints were more common in females than in males older than 10 years of age. This difference was most marked in the 10- to 20-year-old age group. Landrigan and associates[335] studied the location of joint symptoms in adolescents and found that the fingers were involved most often; the knees and wrists were also commonly implicated.

Yanez and associates[643] studied 11 patients with rubella arthritis. In all instances, multiple joints were involved. The onset of arthritis occurred 1 to 6 days after the beginning of the exanthem and lasted 3 to 28 days (mean, 9 days). The erythrocyte sedimentation rate was elevated in three of seven cases, and one patient had markedly positive latex test results. The white blood cell count was below 5000 cells/mm^3 in five of seven patients. One woman had bilateral carpal tunnel syndrome. Four children with transient carpal tunnel syndrome accompanying rubella virus infection have been described.[45] Panush[430] identified serum hypocomplementemia with rubella arthritis in a 25-year-old woman.

The possibility that rubella viral infection is related to rheumatoid arthritis has been studied on several occasions.[51,146,365,418,426] Martenis and colleagues[365] described a 21-year-old woman in whom rheumatoid arthritis developed after typical rubella with arthritis. Deinard and associates[146] found that all serum specimens from 80 patients with rheumatoid arthritis contained rubella HI antibody. In contrast, only 86% of an equal number of nonarthritic controls and a group of people with other forms of arthritis had measurable rubella antibody titers. Ogra and associates[418] found that patients with juvenile rheumatoid arthritis had IgM and IgG serum rubella antibody levels that were four to six times higher than those observed in controls during rubella infection. They also found specific staining for rubella virus antigen in the synovial fluid of 33% of these patients with juvenile rheumatoid arthritis. Grahame and associates[225] repeatedly recovered rubella virus from the synovial fluid of six patients with inflammatory oligoarthritis or polyarthritis during a 2-year period.

Neurologic manifestations. Encephalitis is a rare complication of rubella.* Sherman and colleagues[531] reported six cases of encephalitis in an epidemic during the spring of 1964 that involved approximately 30,000 children. This rate of encephalitis (one of 5000 cases) is similar

*References 4, 29, 53, 110, 120, 142, 163, 364, 380, 403, 483, 531, 547, 610, 632.

to the rate of one of 6000 reported in Detroit in 1942.[364] Rubella encephalitis is clinically similar to encephalitis from measles virus infection but is thought to be less severe. Overall, the estimated mortality rate for rubella encephalitis is approximately 20%.[183] However, mortality and morbidity rates have varied considerably.

Although rubella encephalitis is a rare complication of rubella infection, rubella should still be considered in the differential diagnosis of encephalitis in unvaccinated individuals. Sherman and colleagues[531] reported that three of six children studied in Pittsburgh died of this complication during the spring of 1964, whereas in Atlanta during the same epidemic period, six patients recovered uneventfully. Rubella encephalitis typically is a self-limited illness with a favorable prognosis. Eighty percent of survivors tend to recover without any permanent sequelae.[238]

Guler and colleagues[238] reported a case of rubella encephalitis from Turkey. A 9-year-old, unvaccinated boy was admitted with headache, fever, and loss of consciousness. He had bilateral retroauricular lymphadenopathy but never developed a rash. Serum and cerebrospinal fluid (CSF) were positive for rubella IgM antibodies, and serum IgG was detected 3 weeks later.[238]

Figueiredo and associates[183] reported a case of rubella encephalitis from Brazil. An 18-year-old, unvaccinated man had fever, nausea, severe headache, confusion, aggression, and a generalized tonic-clonic seizure. Eight days earlier, he had a rash and fever. Serum and CSF tested positive for rubella virus IgM and IgG antibodies. Rubella virus was also isolated and confirmed with polymerase chain reaction (PCR) positivity from CSF and peripheral blood mononuclear cells. Phylogenetic analysis showed that it was rubella virus of the 1a genotype.[183]

The onset of encephalitis usually occurs 2 to 4 days after the rash appears, but occasionally, rash and neurologic symptoms occur at the same time. In other instances, the appearance of encephalitis is delayed as much as 1 week after the onset of illness. Examination of CSF usually reveals mild pleocytosis (20–100 cells/mm^3); most cells are lymphocytes. The protein content is normal or slightly elevated, and the glucose concentration is normal.

Kenny and associates[314] studied seven survivors of rubella encephalitis 1 year after their illnesses and could find no significant loss of intellectual function. Five of the seven had abnormalities on electroencephalography, and two patients had minor neurologic abnormalities. Gibbs and colleagues[215] found abnormal electroencephalographic tracings for six of 45 children with uncomplicated rubella.

Other neurologic complications associated with rubella include progressive panencephalitis, carotid artery thrombosis, myelitis, optic neuritis, Guillain-Barré syndrome, and peripheral neuritis.* Figueiredo and colleagues[182] also reported a case of Guillain-Barré syndrome associated with rubella from Brazil. An 18-year-old woman had fever, emesis, headache, neck pain, arthralgias, paresthesias, progressive weakness of her lower limbs, and left-sided facial paralysis. Six days earlier, she had rash, fever, cervical lymphadenopathy, and hepatomegaly. Rubella virus (genotype 1a) was isolated from CSF and peripheral blood mononuclear cells. Test results for serum IgM and IgG and CSF IgG antibodies against rubella were positive.[182]

Numbness, tingling, and other symptoms consistent with neuritis commonly occur during rubella infection. Cuetter and John[136] studied 20 patients with complaints of neuritis accompanying rubella and could find no objective sensory deficits or nerve conduction abnormalities.

Wolinsky and colleagues,[635] Lebon and Lyon,[344] and others described a slowly progressive and fatal nervous system disorder associated with rubella infection that was similar to subacute sclerosing panencephalitis. This illness has occurred as a late manifestation of congenital rubella and has occurred in children who acquired their initial infection in childhood.[54]

Thrombocytopenia. Thrombocytopenic purpura occurs in rubella at an incidence of one of 3000 cases.[31] Children are afflicted more frequently than adults, and girls are affected more often than boys.[22,31,240,303,357,404,428,549,615] The median interval between the onset of exanthem and the occurrence of purpura is approximately 4 days. Rash and purpura can develop simultaneously, but the hemorrhagic manifestations often do not become apparent until 2 weeks after the exanthem develops. The illness usually is self-limited, but its duration varies from a few days to several months. Although deaths caused by hemorrhagic complications have occurred, recovery is the general rule.

Other complications. Myocarditis and pericarditis are rare complications of rubella.[205] A 30-year-old woman had erythema multiforme exudativum and arthritis with apparent clinical rubella.[202] In an outbreak that involved 46 military recruits, testicular pain was a complaint of 25%.[508]

During a rubella epidemic in Japan in 1976 in which 79 patients were studied, 71% had mild catarrhal or follicular conjunctivitis.[254] Six patients had epithelial keratitis that persisted for 2 to 7 days. Seventeen patients had preauricular lymph node swelling associated with their eye findings. During the same epidemic, 13 cases of hemolytic anemia (including two cases of hemolytic uremic syndrome) occurred after the patients had rubella virus infections.[591] During an epidemic of rubella in Japan, Sugaya and colleagues[560] found that 7.5% of 241 patients had liver involvement.

Hepatitis has occurred in congenital rubella infections and acute infections in children and adults. Previously, severe hepatitis due to rubella had developed only in neonatal rubella infections. However, Figueiredo and colleagues[181] reported for the first time a case of acute liver failure necessitating liver transplantation that was associated with rubella virus infection in a child. Test results for serum IgM and IgG antibodies against rubella were positive, and peripheral blood mononuclear cells showed cytopathic effects characteristic of rubella. The rubella virus genome was also detected in liver fragments, and rubella virus antigen was found in the cytoplasm of hepatic cells, which suggests that the virus was replicating in hepatic tissue. Rubella virus genotype 1a was identified. This case report suggested that rubella could be an unrecognized cause of acute liver failure in children and should be included in the differential diagnosis even if there is no prior exanthem history.

Rubella virus also has been reported to cause uveitis. De Visser and associate[145] reported that rubella virus could cause a clinical spectrum of ocular symptoms similar to those of Fuchs heterochromic uveitis (FHU) and might be involved in the pathogenesis of FHU. Ruokonen and colleagues[491] and Suzuki and associates[562] showed a strong association between FHC and intraocular antibody synthesis against rubella virus.

Congenital Rubella

From Gregg's original observation in 1941 of congenital defects in infants born to mothers who had rubella during early pregnancy until the pandemic of 1964, CRS was considered to include only some combination of abnormalities involving the eyes, ears, brain, and heart. However, observations in 1964, supported by new virologic and serologic techniques, revealed a far more complex CRS picture, and rubella syndrome was expanded to include many new anatomic findings and to acknowledge the reality of chronic, persistent infection.

Congenital rubella is the result of in utero fetal infection, which usually occurs during the first 12 weeks of pregnancy. The fetal infection usually is subacute or chronic and can result in abortion, stillbirth, congenital malformations, active processes at birth (e.g., thrombocytopenia, encephalitis, hepatitis), and rarely, infected infants without defects. Table 174.5 summarizes the clinical findings in congenital rubella, an estimation of their frequency, and their main characteristics.

Infant Death and Growth Restriction

The most common manifestation of congenital rubella, which is readily apparent at birth, is generalized restriction of growth.* Between 50% and 85% of these infants weigh less than 2500 g, although gestational age is normal. Infants with intrauterine growth restriction have one or more other stigmata of congenital rubella. After birth, those with intrauterine growth restriction often demonstrate continued growth restriction. In some instances, the failure to thrive is severe. Others have a normal growth pattern, but the child is proportionally small.

The mortality rate for children with congenital rubella is high during the first year of life. Death is related to congenital pneumonia, heart

*References 4, 20, 66, 94, 120, 203, 261, 265, 276, 493, 582, 633, 635, 636.

*18, 124, 195, 230, 256, 287, 321, 348, 359, 376, 386, 436, 447, 490, 492, 494, 507, 523, 537, 574.

TABLE 174.5 **Clinical Findings and Characteristics of Congenital Rubella Virus Infection**

Clinical Findings	Frequency (%)	Main Characteristics	Selected References
Death and Growth Restriction			
In utero death	10–30	Spontaneous abortion; stillbirth	230, 256, 494
Intrauterine growth restriction	50–85	Generalized effects	109, 193, 195, 256, 258, 287, 321, 348, 359, 376, 454, 489, 490, 507, 537, 574
Extrauterine growth restriction	10	Failure to thrive	258, 348, 376, 386, 436, 574
Neonatal and infant deaths	10	Resulting from pneumonia, heart disease, hepatitis, thrombocytopenia, failure to thrive, immune deficiency, encephalitis	126, 230, 256, 321, 490, 507, 574
Ocular Effects			
Cataracts	35	Present at birth	18, 34, 48, 126, 195, 214, 230, 256, 258, 287, 321, 322, 376, 406, 490, 501, 507, 536, 574, 588, 589
Retinopathy	35	Present at birth; usually does not cause problems with vision	48, 116, 125, 214, 230, 256, 287, 324, 325, 376, 588, 589
Microphthalmos	5	Usually associated with cataract	48, 170, 214, 287, 321, 490, 516, 574
Glaucoma	5	Usually present at birth	48, 125, 256, 258, 287, 321, 490, 516, 523
Cloudy cornea	Rare	Usually present at birth; resolves spontaneously	48, 258
Severe myopia	Rare	Usually present at birth; defect may progress	121
Hypoplasia of the iris	Rare	Present at birth	48, 488
Strabismus	5	Associated with other eye defects	257, 376, 417
Iridocyclitis	Rare	Transient; associated with other eye defects	536
Auditory Effects			
Nerve deafness	80–90	May be bilateral or unilateral; moderate or severe; often not recognized early	18, 50, 147, 170, 195, 230, 239, 256, 258, 332, 376, 392, 442, 447, 507, 523, 582, 589, 594
Central deafness	5	Often associated with other central nervous system defects	253
Middle ear damage	5	Usually associated with nerve deafness	477
Intraoral, Nasal, and Facial Effects			
Cleft palate or lip	Rare	—	170, 230, 507
Dental abnormalities	Rare		71, 237, 376
Micrognathia	Rare	—	285, 507
Chronic rhinitis	Rare	Transitory finding	447
High-arched palate	Rare	—	256
Neurologic Effects			
Motor defects	10	Associated with mental and other neurologic defects	376, 523, 646
Hyperirritability (tremors)	Rare	Transitory finding	482
Microcephaly	Rare	—	18, 258, 287, 376, 523, 574, 613, 628
Mental disabilities	10–20	Associated with other stigmata	121, 230, 253, 256, 374, 523, 559
Full anterior fontanelle	10	Transitory finding related to meningoencephalitis	123, 490
Meningoencephalitis	10–20	Transitory finding but may last for 1 year	148, 258, 321, 322, 447, 490, 536, 574
Spastic diplegia and quadriparesis	Rare	Associated with other stigmata	123, 148
Seizures	Rare	Frequently transitory and related to meningoencephalitis	148, 259, 376, 447
Hypotonia	Rare	Transitory defect	147, 148
Brain calcification	Rare	—	442, 444, 536, 574
Cerebral arterial stenosis	Rare	—	253
Anencephaly	Rare	—	507
Encephalocele	Rare	—	507
Meningomyelocele	Rare	—	559
Behavior disorders	10–20	Frequently related to deafness	121, 147
Central language disorders	5	—	177, 230, 621
Autism	5	—	121, 177, 253
Aqueductal occlusion or hydrocephalus	Rare	—	230, 497
Poor balance	Rare	—	147, 646
Progressive panencephalitis	Rare	Has onset during adolescence	585, 620

TABLE 174.5 Clinical Findings and Characteristics of Congenital Rubella Virus Infection—cont'd

Clinical Findings	Frequency (%)	Main Characteristics	Selected References
Cardiovascular Effects			
Patent ductus arteriosus	30	Frequently associated with other defects	18, 34, 171, 195, 256, 258, 263, 304, 322, 399, 523, 536, 574, 589, 617
Pulmonary arterial hypoplasia, supravalvular stenosis, valvular stenosis, and peripheral branch stenosis	25	Frequently associated with other defects	195, 256, 258, 263, 304, 523, 535, 589, 617
Aortic stenosis	2–5		193, 263, 533, 607, 617
Ventricular and atrial septal defects	2–5		34, 523, 589, 617
Tetralogy of Fallot	2–5		170, 258
Myocarditis and myocardial necrosis	10		5, 15, 321, 399, 574, 617
Intimal fibromuscular proliferation of many arteries	5		169
Ventricular aneurysm	Rare		224
Pulmonary Effects			
Interstitial pneumonitis	5–10	May be acute, subacute, or chronic	47, 170, 258, 321, 322, 399, 442, 444, 447, 507, 536, 574, 628
Tracheoesophageal fistula	Rare		507
Respiratory distress	Rare	Secondary to acute pneumonia	376
Gastrointestinal Effects			
Esophageal atresia	Rare	—	507
Hepatitis	5–10	Associated with other evidence of disseminated disease	18, 170, 172, 258, 398, 552, 574
Obstructive jaundice	5	—	321, 322, 399, 482, 536
Chronic diarrhea	Rare	Related to failure to thrive and immune deficiency	447, 574
Pancreatitis	Rare	May lead to diabetes in later life	64, 156
Duodenal stenosis	Rare	—	150
Jejunal or rectal atresia	Rare	—	170
Genitourinary Effects			
Undescended testicle	Rare	Cause-and-effect relationship with rubella infection in doubt	376, 536
Polycystic kidney, ectopic kidney, renal agenesis, or bilobed kidney	Rare	Cause-and-effect relationship with rubella infection in doubt	170, 169, 379
Hypospadias	Rare	Cause-and-effect relationship with rubella infection in doubt	48, 195, 536
Duplication of ureter	Rare	Cause-and-effect relationship with rubella infection in doubt	34
Renal artery stenosis	Rare	—	375
Hydroureter and hydronephrosis	Rare	Cause-and-effect relationship with rubella in doubt	259, 442, 523, 536
Inguinal hernia	Rare	Cause-and-effect relationship with rubella in doubt	259, 442, 523, 536
Nephritis and nephrocalcinosis	Rare	—	536, 574
Testicular agenesis	Rare	Cause-and-effect relationship with rubella in doubt	170
Orthopedic Effects			
Bone radiolucencies	10–20	Radiolucencies in metaphyses of long bones	258, 376, 442, 454, 464, 467, 489, 490, 518, 613, 624, 628
Pathologic fractures	Rare	—	489[a]
Bone deformities	Rare	—	104, 230, 356
Clubfoot	Rare	—	507
Myositis	Rare	Transitory defect	544

Continued

TABLE 174.5 Clinical Findings and Characteristics of Congenital Rubella Virus Infection—cont'd

Clinical Findings	Frequency (%)	Main Characteristics	Selected References
Skin Effects			
Dermal erythropoiesis (blueberry muffin syndrome)	5	Transitory defect; usually associated with severe disease	319
Chronic rash	Rare	—	71, 251
Dermatoglyphic abnormalities	5	—	3, 11, 460
Dimples	Rare	—	249
Endocrine Effects			
Diabetes mellitus	Rare	—	192, 305, 377
Thyroid disorder	Rare	—	121
Precocious puberty	Rare	—	121
Growth hormone deficiency	Rare	—	458
Hematologic Effects			
Thrombocytopenic purpura	5–10	Usually associated with severe disease with high death rate; transitory	18, 31, 34, 38, 125, 195, 258, 287, 321, 331, 376, 442, 447, 454, 464, 465, 489, 507, 523, 609
Hemophagocytic syndrome	Rare	—	32
Hemolytic anemia	Rare	Transitory	397, 442, 465
Hypoplastic anemia	Rare	Transitory	123, 331
Extramedullary hematopoiesis	5–10	Usually associated with severe disease	574
Immunologic Effects			
Thymic hypoplasia	Rare	—	253
Dysgammaglobulinemia	Rare	—	114, 250, 453, 476, 537
Asplenia	Rare	—	286
Reticuloendothelial effects			
Generalized lymphadenopathy	10	—	123, 195, 251, 574
Hepatosplenomegaly	10–20	Usually associated with severe disease; transitory	34, 321, 454, 490, 507, 523
Genetic effects			
Chromosomal abnormalities	Rare	Cause-and-effect relationship with rubella not established	14, 416

[a]Cherry JD, unpublished data.

defects and myocarditis, hepatitis, thrombocytopenia, encephalitis, immune deficiency, and failure to thrive.

Eye Effects

Approximately one third of infants with congenital rubella have cataracts.* Cataracts may be bilateral or unilateral and are centrally located with a surrounding clear zone or diffuse. In most instances, cataracts are present at birth, but occasionally they are not observed until later in infancy. Retinopathy consisting of pigmentary defects occurs commonly in congenital rubella and is useful diagnostically, but it rarely adversely affects visual acuity. Microphthalmos occurs relatively frequently and usually is unilateral. Cataracts frequently are associated with microphthalmos.

Congenital glaucoma occurs in approximately 5% of congenitally infected infants. This defect usually is present at birth, but it often is overlooked. The diagnosis must be established early if sight is to be preserved.

Auditory Effects

Sensorineural deafness is the most common manifestation of congenital rubella, and most patients have some degree of hearing impairment.† The hearing loss usually is bilateral but may be unilateral. Frequently, the only manifestation of congenital infection is deafness. Deafness is frequently overlooked in infancy, and children incorrectly are considered to be developmentally delayed. All children born to mothers who had rubella during the first half of pregnancy should undergo evaluation of their hearing several times during the first 5 years of life, regardless of whether they have other manifestations of congenital infection.

Neurologic Effects

Between 10% and 20% of all infants with congenital rubella have active meningoencephalitis at birth.* Manifestations of this infection include one or more of the following: a full anterior fontanelle, irritability, hypotonia, seizures, lethargy, and head retraction and arching of the back. Examination of the CSF reveals elevated protein and mild pleocytosis. Later neurologic disease, such as intellectual disabilities and motor retardation, can be related to the severity and persistence of the initial meningoencephalitis. Active central nervous system infection has been demonstrated for a year or more.

Behavior disorders occur commonly in children with deafness and often cannot be associated with apparent meningoencephalitis. Children with congenital rubella who have generalized retardation of growth and a proportionally small head often have normal intelligence. In

*References 18, 34, 48, 116, 121, 124, 170, 195, 214, 221, 230, 256–258, 287, 321-325, 374, 406, 417, 488–490, 501, 507, 516, 523, 537, 574, 583, 588, 589,631.

†References 18, 50, 147, 170, 195, 230, 239, 253, 256, 258, 332, 376, 391, 442, 447, 477, 507, 523, 588, 589, 594.

*References 18, 20, 121, 123, 147, 148, 177, 230, 253, 256, 258, 287, 321, 322, 376, 442, 444, 446, 482, 483, 488, 490, 494, 497, 507, 523, 529, 536, 559, 574, 585, 613, 620, 621, 628, 632.

contrast, the prognosis for mental development of a child with true microcephaly is poor.

Chronic progressive panencephalitis has developed in a small number of adolescents with congenital rubella, similar to measles-related subacute sclerosing panencephalitis.

Cardiovascular Effects

In severe congenital rubella with multisystem involvement, myocarditis occurs and often is a cause of death.* Of the structural defects of the heart, patent ductus arteriosus (PDA) has been previously reported to be the most common. Although PDA may be the only lesion seen, two thirds of patients have other lesions. Historically, pulmonary artery stenosis has been considered the next most common defect and may involve the main pulmonary artery or its branches.

Pulmonary valvular stenosis is the third most common defect. Pulmonic valvular or arterial stenosis and PDA commonly occur together. However, a study by Oster and associates[424] that reviewed studies from 1941 to 2008 that used cardiac catheterization or echocardiography to evaluate cardiovascular malformations in CRS reported different patterns. They found that branch pulmonary artery stenosis was more common (78%) than PDA (62%) in patients who had been evaluated by catheterization. The combination of branch pulmonary artery stenosis and PDA (49%) was more frequently found than branch pulmonary artery stenosis (29%) or PDA (13%) alone.

Other Manifestations

The other manifestations of congenital rubella can be separated into three categories: those related to active, persistent infection; structural defects; and delayed manifestations of congenital rubella.†

Manifestations related to active, persistent infection. Manifestations related to active, persistent infection encompass a broad constellation of clinical events that largely were unknown before the pandemic of 1964. Collectively, they frequently are called the *expanded CRS* and include interstitial pneumonitis, hepatitis, nephritis, bone radiolucencies, myositis, dermal erythropoiesis, chronic rash, thrombocytopenic purpura, hemolytic and hypoplastic anemia, immunologic deficiency, generalized lymphadenopathy, hepatosplenomegaly, meningoencephalitis, and myocarditis. Most infants with the expanded CRS have low birth weight, exanthem caused by thrombocytopenia or dermal erythropoiesis (or both), hepatosplenomegaly, and jaundice. Radiographs usually reveal long-bone radiolucencies. Respiratory distress caused by diffuse pulmonary disease and myocarditis occurs commonly, and meningoencephalitis usually is evident.

The duration of chronic infection in these infants varies. Approximately 20% of survivors still are shedding virus at 1 year of age. Between 10% and 20% of those with hepatosplenomegaly and thrombocytopenia die during the first year of life.

Structural defects. Other than deafness, eye defects, and cardiac anomalies (discussed earlier), the association of other malformations with congenital rubella infection is less well established. Malformations such as tracheoesophageal fistula, jejunal atresia, inguinal hernia, and others recorded in Table 174.5 occur frequently without evidence of in utero infection. Because they are seen only sporadically in infants born after maternal rubella infection, they may be chance associations rather than cause-and-effect relationships.

Delayed manifestations. Important delayed manifestations of congenital rubella that were not seen in early life are deafness, ocular damage, progressive rubella panencephalitis, and vascular effects such as hypertension.[528] Endocrine delayed manifestations associated with congenital rubella include diabetes, thyroid disorders, early menopause, osteoporosis, and possible growth hormone deficiency.[140] Of particular importance is the association between endocrine abnormalities and autoimmunity.[113]

*References 5, 18, 170, 169, 193, 195, 256, 258, 263, 288, 304, 321, 322, 399, 523, 533, 535, 536, 574, 589, 607, 617.

†References 5, 11, 14, 18, 31, 34, 38, 47, 48, 64, 71, 104, 113, 114, 121, 123, 126, 156, 170–172, 192, 195, 218, 230, 249–251, 253, 258, 259, 287, 305, 319, 321, 322, 331, 356, 377, 397–399, 401, 416, 442, 444, 447, 453, 454, 458, 465, 467, 476, 482, 489, 490, 492, 507, 518, 523, 528, 536, 537, 544, 552, 557, 574, 609, 613, 624, 628.

In one study of 201 deaf adolescents with congenital rubella, 23.3% had positive thyroid microsomal or thyroglobulin antibodies, and of these patients, 19.6% had thyroid gland dysfunction.

Patients with congenital rubella have an increased incidence of insulin-dependent diabetes mellitus.[218] In a 40-year observational study of 280 Japanese patients with CRS, only three of the patients developed insulin-dependent diabetes.[568] HLA associations with diabetes in CRS have been reported. HLA A1-B8, which has been associated with insulin-dependent diabetes, has been found in many patients with congenital rubella who have diabetes (44%).[281] A review of literature by Gale[207] supports prior reports that CRS predisposes to diabetes. However, Gale's review suggests that only 1% of patients with congenital rubella instead of 20% will eventually develop diabetes.[207]

Psychiatric disorders are also often found in patients with CRS and may be seen in up to one half of patients. Rates of intellectual disability have been reported to be as high as 42%, and 4.12% to 7.3% of patients with CRS also may have autism. Higher rates of psychosis have been found along with increased rates of behavioral problems, including impulsivity, self-injury, and aggression.[293]

DIAGNOSIS

Differential Diagnosis

Postnatally Acquired Disease

Because no pathognomonic finding exists for rubella, the clinical diagnosis in an individual case often is difficult to establish (see Chapter 58). However, as with other exanthematous diseases, the key to establishing a diagnosis is careful elicitation of historical data. Rubella is an epidemic disease with a high clinical rate of expression of exanthem. When proper investigation is performed, it is unusual not to find the contact case or other cases in the community. Season also is an important consideration. Rubella typically occurs in the winter and spring, whereas enteroviral exanthems, which are the greatest masqueraders in young children, occur mainly in the summer and fall.

The incubation period also is important in separating rubella from exanthems caused by common enteroviruses or respiratory viruses. In rubella, the incubation period is long (18 ± 3 days), whereas the period in the other illnesses usually is much shorter (3–7 days). Age also is important. Today, rubella mainly is an illness of adolescents and young adults, and enteroviral exanthems are uncommon findings in patients at these ages.

The nature of fever also is useful in establishing the diagnosis of rubella. Temperature higher than 38.5°C (101.5°F) is an unusual occurrence in rubella but common with enteroviral exanthems, measles, and *M. pneumoniae* infection. A history of rubella infection is not particularly reliable, but if a past illness can be documented by year, season, and symptoms, accurate information can be obtained. Useful characteristics of the rubella exanthem are its mild, erythematous, maculopapular, and discrete nature; marked pruritus in adolescents and adults; and an acneiform appearance on the face in adolescents.

Although suboccipital and posterior auricular lymphadenopathy is thought by some investigators to be pathognomonic, its presence in nonrubella exanthems often leads to undue concern. In a young child, suboccipital and posterior auricular lymphadenopathy occurs as commonly with enteroviral illnesses as with rubella. In young adults, however, lymphadenopathy is much more useful because the enteroviral differential consideration is less of a problem. Similar lymphadenopathy does occur with acquired toxoplasmosis, infectious mononucleosis, and *M. pneumoniae* infection.

A major problem in the differential diagnosis for adults is allergy. However, fever (even low grade), lymphadenopathy, headache, and eye pain, which are common events in rubella, occur rarely in contact or other simple allergies.

Congenital Rubella

Establishing the diagnosis of congenital rubella in infants with known maternal exposure usually is not difficult. However, examining an apparently normal child at periodic intervals during the first few years of life is important so that deafness and subtle neurologic defects are not missed. The diagnosis of congenital rubella after an uneventful pregnancy is more difficult to make. All infants with evidence of intrauterine growth restriction or stigmata suggesting congenital infection should undergo virologic and serologic study for rubella and other infectious agents.

Determination of the amount of serum IgM can be useful in the study of infants with intrauterine growth restriction or those born to mothers in whom rubella or other infection was suspected to have occurred during pregnancy.[554] Values greater than 21 mg/dL during the first week of life strongly indicate congenital infection, but normal values do not rule out congenital infection.

Specific Diagnosis

Postnatally Acquired Disease

Rubella viral infection can be diagnosed specifically by isolation of virus from nasal or throat specimens in AGMK or other sensitive tissue culture systems or by PCR[36,128,129]; by the observation of a significant change in value of HI, ELISA, immunofluorescence, CF, or neutralizing antibody in two sequential serum samples; or by the demonstration of specific rubella IgM antibody in a single serum sample. The diagnosis of rubella usually is attempted by using a single serum test for identifying rubella IgM antibody.*

Commercial rubella IgM immunoassays are available, and their sensitivity and specificity ranges vary from 75% to 95% and from 85% to 100%, respectively.[152,578] Determination of rubella-specific IgM antibody in saliva 7 to 42 days after the onset of illness also is sensitive and specific.[463]

Although these tests are practical, the specificity and sensitivity of all routinely used tests are not 100% accurate. False-positive results often occur and commonly lead to unnecessary interventions. When the diagnosis is critical, such as with suspected rubella in pregnancy, a wise approach is to study IgG antibody in paired sera collected 1 to 2 weeks apart in addition to determining IgM antibody levels. One of the problems encountered with diagnosing rubella infection with serum IgM antibodies is that only 50% of serum samples from rubella cases collected on the day of rash onset are positive for the virus. Work by Abernathy and associates[1] compared detection of rubella IgM from sera and oral fluids with detection of rubella RNA from oral fluids by real-time PCR (RT-PCR) taken within 4 days after rash onset from suspected rubella cases during a rubella outbreak in Peru in 2004 to 2005. They found that RT-PCR testing of oral fluid confirmed more rubella cases than IgM testing of serum or oral fluid during days 1 and 2 after rash onset. However, the methods confirmed approximately the same number of cases on days 3 and 4 after rash onset.

Unfortunately, a rise in IgG antibody titer and an IgM-positive test result can occur in reinfection and in primary infection. Because reinfection in a pregnant woman is not likely to lead to damage of the in utero fetus, distinguishing primary infection from reinfection is important and can be done by measuring the avidity of rubella IgG antibody.[248,277,461] Rubella IgG avidity assays focus on the strength of the antigen-antibody interaction, which is different for first exposure to an antigen (e.g., primary infection) compared with a previous infection. In primary infection, the antigen-antibody interaction is low (i.e., low avidity), whereas in reinfection or prior infections, the antigen-antibody interaction is stronger (i.e., high avidity).[579]

Congenital Rubella

The best method for establishing a definitive diagnosis of congenital rubella is viral isolation or PCR. Specimens for viral culture or PCR should be obtained from the nose, throat, urine, buffy coat of blood, and CSF. Because of transplacental passage of maternal IgG, establishment of the diagnosis of congenital rubella in the neonatal period by serologic methods is fraught with difficulty. Usually, specific rubella IgM antibody can be demonstrated with currently available techniques. In questionable cases, follow-up studies comparing infant and maternal antibody values often establish the diagnosis. If the infant's value is the result solely of transplacentally acquired antibody, it should drop fourfold to eightfold by the time the infant reaches 3 months of age and continue to fall to nondetectable values by 6 to 8 months of age. Because the antibody value in some congenital infections also may fall, disappearance of antibody in serum does not rule out in utero infection completely. In questionable cases, the study of IgG rubella antibody avidity may be useful.[269,461]

The retrospective diagnosis of congenital rubella in late infancy and the second year of life has been difficult to make. However, researchers have shown that affected children have low avidity of specific IgG antibody, and a retrospective diagnosis of congenital rubella can be made by specific avidity assays.[269] Rubella IgG peptide–based enzyme immunoassay and rubella immunoblot assay also are useful for the serologic diagnosis of congenital rubella during the prenatal and newborn periods.[374] Newborns who were infected during the first 12 weeks of gestation have reduced levels of antibodies directed at the linear E1 epitope (SP15) and the topographic E2 epitope.

CDC investigators have identified serologic markers in school-aged children with CRS.[295] The children had more rubella virus–specific IgG antibody and stronger C protein and E2 signals than children without CRS. Fetal rubella also can be diagnosed in amniotic fluid samples by RT-PCR.[474,569]

Qualitative Demonstration of Rubella Antibody

The original screening method for rubella antibody was HI, which has been replaced by more rapid and easier tests involving enzyme immunoassay, erythrocyte agglutination, and latex agglutination. All are highly sensitive and specific.[99,179]

TREATMENT

Postnatally Acquired Disease

Uncomplicated Rubella

No specific therapy is necessary or indicated for uncomplicated rubella. Starch baths may be useful for adults with troublesome pruritus. Affected patients should understand that they are contagious and that transmission of infection to a pregnant woman could have serious consequences.

Complications of Rubella

Arthritis sometimes can be severe in adults. When weight-bearing joints are affected, rest is encouraged. Symptoms readily respond to aspirin therapy; corticosteroids are not indicated. For patients with rubella encephalitis, care is supportive, employing adequate maintenance of fluids and electrolytes.

Thrombocytopenia usually is self-limited. However, severe bleeding has occurred on occasion. Splenectomy is not indicated. Corticosteroid therapy often is used, but with little evidence of specific benefit in rubella-infected patients. In patients who do not recover rapidly and in those with severe bleeding, treatment with intravenous immunoglobulin should be considered.

Care of Exposed Pregnant Women

Ideally, all pregnant women should have received rubella vaccine previously or been shown to have rubella antibody by an appropriate serologic test. If a pregnant woman is exposed to a person with rubella and the history of previous immunization or antibody status is unknown, an immediate blood specimen should be obtained and a rubella antibody test performed. If antibody to rubella is demonstrated, no action is necessary.

If IgG antibody is not detectable in a pregnant woman exposed to rubella, she is not rubella immune. A second blood specimen should be obtained 2 to 3 weeks later and tested for rubella antibody concurrently with the first specimen. If the second test result is negative, a third blood specimen should be obtained 6 weeks after exposure and tested again for antibody concurrently with the first specimen. A negative result for the second and third specimens indicates that infection has not occurred. However, a positive test result for the second or third specimen but not the first indicates seroconversion and provides evidence for recent rubella infection.[12]

Susceptible rubella-exposed women should undergo careful clinical observation for fever, lymphadenopathy, or exanthem for a 4-week period. If illness occurs, a nasal specimen should be cultured for rubella

*References 13, 23, 33, 35, 36, 73, 87, 95, 100, 131, 152, 167, 180, 190, 219, 283, 362, 382, 405, 437, 514, 538, 578, 601.

virus, and serum should be examined for rubella IgM antibody. A second serum specimen should be submitted for rubella antibody examination. If rubella antibody seroconversion is identified or specific IgM antibody is demonstrated, the risk of fetal infection and malformation is considerable. Because false-positive rubella IgM antibody test results are not rare occurrences, all tests that yield positive results should be repeated for confirmation (by another assay and in another laboratory if possible). Because IgM antibody can occur in reinfections and fetal risk is then minimal, determining the avidity of IgG antibody also may be useful.[248,277,461] The patient should be advised, and therapeutic abortion should be discussed.

In situations of known exposure of a susceptible pregnant woman in which therapeutic abortion is not a consideration and exposure can be documented to have taken place within 72 hours, we think that 20 mL of immunoglobulin should be administered immediately. The use of immunoglobulin is controversial, but in certain controlled situations, it has been effective in preventing disease.[56,388,503,596,644]

Care of Pregnant Women With an Exanthem Thought to Be Rubella

Previous rubella serologic study results for a pregnant woman with an exanthem thought to be rubella are extremely useful. If previous serum antibody has been confirmed, the mother should be reassured that the current illness is not likely to be rubella. However, because false-positive rubella screening results do occur, a wise approach is to carry out rubella serologic study and, when possible, viral culture. An acute-phase serum sample should be examined for rubella-specific IgM antibody. A second serum specimen should be collected 1 to 2 weeks after the disappearance of the rash. If rubella antibody has risen significantly or IgM antibody is demonstrated, it is highly likely that congenital infection has occurred and that anomalies may result. A wise approach is to confirm IgM positive test results and, if available, do IgG rubella antibody avidity study. In this circumstance, the woman should be counseled about therapeutic abortion.

If a previous serum rubella antibody value is not available, a serum sample should be collected immediately and another collected 2 to 3 weeks later. These sera should be examined as paired specimens for rubella antibody and analyzed for specific rubella IgM antibody. If a rubella antibody increase is demonstrated or rubella IgM is confirmed, rubella viral infection can be assumed, and the patient should be advised about the risk for congenital infection and the possibility of therapeutic abortion.

Care of Children With Congenital Rubella

Isolation Procedures

Most infants with congenital rubella remain actively infected at the time of birth, are contagious, and therefore should be placed in isolation. Room isolation and urine precautions are the major necessities. The isolated baby should be cared for only by people known to be seropositive for rubella. Because rubella viral shedding can occur for a year or more from some infants, isolation of infants with congenital rubella should be continued for this duration unless repeated viral cultures have proved negative. Recommendations from the 2015 *Red Book* indicate that contact isolation of hospitalized children with proved or suspected congenital rubella is indicated until they are at least 1 year of age, unless two cultures of clinical specimens obtained 1 month apart after 3 months of age are negative for rubella virus.[12]

After the child is discharged from the hospital, no special precautions are necessary in the household setting. However, the parents should be advised of the potential risk to pregnant visitors.

Neonatal Period

The clinical manifestations of congenital rubella are varied, and many infants exhibit no symptoms during the first few months of life. In these apparently asymptomatic infants, no particular management problems are encountered. In other neonates, symptoms of continued viral infection are readily apparent and frequently are severe. Pneumonia, thrombocytopenia, eye findings, heart defects, hyperbilirubinemia, and hepatosplenomegaly are important findings in these infants.

Although purpura and petechiae due to thrombocytopenia may be impressively severe in these infants, true hemorrhagic difficulties have not been a major problem. Corticosteroid therapy does not seem to be indicated, but considering treatment with intravenous immunoglobulin may be worthwhile. Careful evaluation of the eyes is important. Of immediate concern is the search for corneal clouding because it probably indicates infantile glaucoma. Cataracts and retinopathy also should be sought carefully. Infants with glaucoma should be referred immediately for ophthalmologic evaluation and therapy. Children with cataracts or retinopathy also should be referred, but therapy for cataracts is best delayed until the child reaches a later age.

Respiratory distress due to extensive viral involvement should be managed similar to other neonatal respiratory disease: assisted ventilation and careful attention to arterial blood gas values and pH. Although jaundice due to congenital rubella infection rarely is severe, standard criteria for the treatment of hyperbilirubinemia should be followed. Newborns with pulmonary hypertension may respond to nitric oxide therapy.[462] Hepatosplenomegaly can be marked in some instances but is of no therapeutic concern.

Cardiac evaluation should be the same as for affected infants without rubella. Congestive cardiac failure should be treated vigorously. In malignant conditions (e.g., patent ductus arteriosus, coarctation of the aorta), lifesaving surgery should be contemplated.

Long-Term Problems

Deafness. Hearing disability is the most common abnormality after infection with congenital rubella; more than 80% of infected infants have some degree of hearing disability. In many instances, deafness is the only clinical manifestation of congenital rubella, and because the establishment of this diagnosis in early infancy is difficult, the diagnosis often is delayed. However, early diagnosis of deafness and institution of proper educational programs are the most productive measures in the long-term management of children with congenital rubella.

Poor medical advice often has been responsible for the delay in making an appropriate diagnosis and providing therapy. Any time that a mother suspects that her child is deaf, specific audiometric testing should be performed. Many general practitioners, pediatricians, and otolaryngologists think that hearing cannot be tested in infants. This concept must be discouraged vigorously. At proper centers, a severely deaf child can be recognized in virtually all instances.

If deafness is diagnosed, the child should be referred immediately to a training program. Information about training programs can be obtained from the Alexander Graham Bell Association for the Deaf (http://www.agbell.org) and the John Tracy Clinic (http://jtc.org). In virtually all instances, severely deaf children should be enrolled in an education program before or during the second year of life, and the child should be fitted with a proper auditory amplification device. Although deafness in congenital rubella is sensorineural, a surprising finding is that conduction defects also occur in many older children, for whom other aspects of otolaryngologic care may be indicated.

Eye problems. All children with eye problems (i.e., cloudy cornea, glaucoma, cataracts, retinitis, or strabismus) should be referred at an early age for ophthalmologic evaluation. Glaucoma requires immediate attention. Decisions about cataract surgery should be left to the discretion of the ophthalmologist, but they usually can be deferred until after the end of the first year. Retinopathy, although frequently impressive on ophthalmoscopic examination, rarely causes much visual defect. Strabismus is managed as it is in children without rubella. Advice on eye problems in congenital rubella can be obtained from the American Foundation for the Blind (https://www.afb.org/default.aspx).

Heart problems. Congenital heart disease due to in utero rubella infection should be managed as heart disease is in children without rubella. The children should be referred to cardiac centers where sophisticated diagnostic techniques and cardiac surgery facilities are available for correctable lesions.

Musculoskeletal problems. Isolated musculoskeletal defects are relatively uncommon findings in congenital rubella. However, when the symptoms indicate, referral to a cerebral palsy clinic is useful for specific therapeutic modalities and for the camaraderie of group therapy for the children and parents.

Central nervous system problems. Careful analysis of the available data suggests that many infants who have been labeled intellectually disabled are instead children with auditory or visual defects who have not had proper diagnosis and training for their handicaps. No child with congenital rubella should be labeled mentally subnormal until extensive audiologic and ophthalmologic investigations and perhaps specific therapy have been performed.

Immunologic defects. A few children with congenital rubella have specifically low levels of serum IgG. These infants have continued, systemic viral infection and fare poorly. Although outcome studies are not available, administration of immune serum globulin (i.e., intramuscular or intravenous immunoglobulin) to these infants periodically seems prudent.

Multiple handicaps. Children infected in utero with rubella virus often suffer from one or more of the handicaps mentioned. Care of these infants and children requires many different resources and modalities of therapy. Frequently, the physician is the one who must coordinate the diagnostic and long-term educational efforts that are necessary for optimal progress of an affected child.

In addition to the Alexander Graham Bell Association for the Deaf, the John Tracy Clinic, and the American Foundation for the Blind, several agencies can help physicians or the parents of congenital rubella children: United Cerebral Palsy Research and Educational Foundation (http://www.ucp.org), Easter Seal Research Foundation (http://www.easterseals.com), The Arc of the United States (http://www.thearc.org), and Maternal and Child Health Division, Department of Health and Human Services (http://mchb.hrsa.gov).

PREVENTION

Active Immunization Using Live Attenuated Rubella Virus Vaccine

In 1969, three rubella vaccines were licensed for use in the United States: HPV-77:DE-5 (i.e., duck embryo), HPV-77:DK-12 (i.e., dog kidney), and GMK-3:RK33 Cendevax (i.e., rabbit kidney) strains.[470,622] Use of the HPV-77:DK-12 vaccine was later discontinued because a higher rate of joint complaints was reported after vaccination with this strain.

In 1979, the RA 27/3 (i.e., human diploid fibroblast) strain, Meruvax-II, was licensed for use in the United States. The RA 27/3 rubella virus vaccine is the only vaccine currently licensed for use in the United States. The RA 27/3 rubella vaccine is a live attenuated virus vaccine. The virus used was first isolated from a rubella-infected aborted fetus from the Wistar Institute in 1965. Attenuation of the virus was achieved by 25 to 30 passages in tissue culture, using human diploid fibroblasts. This vaccine does not contain any duck, chicken, or egg protein. The rubella vaccine is available in combination with measles and mumps vaccines as MMR or combined mumps, measles, and varicella vaccine as MMRV (ProQuad). The single-antigen rubella vaccine is not available for use in the United States.

The MMR and MMRV vaccines are distributed as a lyophilized (freeze-dried) powder and require reconstitution with sterile, preservative-free water. These vaccines contain trace amounts of human albumin, neomycin, sorbitol, and gelatin.[88] Vaccination can be expected to produce antibodies in more than 95% of those immunized.[21,353,450,505,543,611,616,619] Antibody titers after RA 27/3 vaccination are slightly lower than those after natural infection, but they have been demonstrated to persist for an 11- to 15-year period with a pattern similar to that occurring after natural infection, even in the absence of reexposure to rubella virus.[43,290,450]

Because of universal immunization practices, indigenous rubella has been eliminated in the United States and from the Americas.[69,85,89,468,471] Finland's vigorous two-dose immunization program also resulted in the elimination of indigenous rubella.[440,441]

Recommendations for Use

Complete information about rubella immunization is available in the most recent recommendations of the Immunization Practices Advisory Committee of the US Public Health Service,[90,82] the recommendations of the Committee on Infectious Diseases of the American Academy of Pediatrics,[12] and the vaccine manufacturer's product information.

Rubella vaccine is recommended for all children 12 months of age or older, adolescents, and adults, particularly women, unless otherwise contraindicated. Vaccination of children protects them from rubella and prevents them from subsequently spreading it. Vaccination of susceptible postpubertal women confers individual protection from rubella-induced fetal injury. Vaccination of adolescents or adults in population groups such as those in colleges, places of employment, or military bases protects them from rubella and reduces the chance of epidemics occurring among partially immune groups.

Rubella vaccine should not be administered to infants younger than 1 year because persisting maternal antibodies may interfere with seroconversion. When rubella vaccine is part of a combination vaccine that includes measles antigen, it should be administered to children approximately 12 to 15 months of age. A second dose of rubella-containing vaccine is recommended at school entry, typically at age 4 through 6 years.[88] Children who have not received rubella vaccine at the optimal age should be vaccinated promptly. Because a history of rubella is not a reliable indicator of immunity, all children for whom vaccine is not contraindicated should be vaccinated.

Vaccination of all unimmunized prepubertal children, adolescents, and adult women of childbearing age must be emphasized. Because of the theoretical risk to the fetus, women of childbearing age should receive vaccine only if they are not pregnant and understand that they should not become pregnant for 28 days after receiving the vaccination.[12,88]

Special attention should be focused on targeted immunization of at-risk postpubertal males and females, especially college students, military recruits, recent immigrants, health care professionals, teachers, and child care providers. People born in 1957 or after who have not received at least one dose of vaccine or who have no serologic evidence of immunity to rubella should be immunized against rubella.[14] Educational and training institutions such as colleges, universities, and military bases should seek proof of rubella immunity (i.e., a positive serologic test result or documentation of previous rubella vaccination) from all students and employees of childbearing age. Nonpregnant women who lack proof of immunity should be vaccinated unless contraindications exist.

For the protection of susceptible female patients and female employees, people working in hospitals and clinics who may contract rubella from infected patients or who, if infected, could transmit rubella to pregnant patients should have serologically demonstrated immunity to rubella or should receive the vaccine.

Routine premarital serologic testing for rubella immunity could enhance efforts to identify susceptible women before pregnancy. Prenatal or antepartum screening for rubella susceptibility should be undertaken and vaccine administered in the immediate postpartum period—before hospital discharge. Previous administration of anti-Rh0(D) immunoglobulin (human) or blood products is not a contraindication to vaccination; however, 6- to 8-week postvaccination serologic testing should be performed for confirmation of seroconversion in those few who have received the globulin or blood products. Obtaining laboratory evidence of seroconversion in other vaccines is not necessary. The 2015 *Red Book* provides updated guidelines for the minimum recommended interval for rubella vaccination after receiving immunoglobulin.

No evidence has shown that live rubella virus vaccine given after exposure prevents illness or that vaccination of a person incubating rubella is harmful. Because postexposure vaccination can theoretically prevent illness if administered within 3 days of exposure and protect a person in the event of future exposure, postexposure vaccination is usually recommended unless otherwise contraindicated.[12]

Adverse Reactions

Vaccination of young children rarely is associated with symptoms. However, mild fever, rash, lymphadenopathy, and upper respiratory tract symptoms occasionally have been observed. Fever develops 6 to 12 days after immunization in approximately 5% to 15%of children receiving the MMR or MMRV vaccines. Rash may occur in approximately 5% of those immunized, and mild lymphadenopathy has been frequently observed. A twofold increase in febrile seizure risk has been observed among children vaccinated with the combined MMRV vaccine 5 to 12 days after immunization. In children 12 through 23 months of age, febrile seizures occur more frequently after administration of the MMRV vaccine (seven to nine of 10,000) than the MMR and varicella vaccines (three to four of 10,000) given separately. One additional febrile seizure may be expected to occur per 2300 to 2600 of the children immunized with the MMRV vaccine.[12,300,318]

More severe reactions have occurred rarely in children but have been an occasional problem for adults. Most of these complications were associated with the previously available vaccines, but complications with the RA 27/3 vaccine also have been reported.[21,161] Particularly troublesome are arthralgia and arthritis.* These symptoms occur most commonly in adults and have been seen more often in women than men.[88]

Joint pain, which is typically localized to smaller, peripheral joints, has been found in approximately 0.5% of young children. Joint involvement typically begins 7 to 21 days after immunization and is considered to be a transient reaction.[12,88] Arthralgia develops in approximately 25% of susceptible postpubertal females after they have received the RA 27/3 vaccination, and approximately 10% have had arthritis-like signs and symptoms.[40,235,455] Infrequently, chronic or recurrent arthralgia, sometimes with arthritis or neurologic symptoms, including paresthesias, carpal tunnel syndrome, and blurred vision, have developed in susceptible vaccinees, primarily adult women.[90,291] One group of investigators reported the frequency of chronic joint symptoms and signs among adult women to be as high as 5% to 11%[575–577]; however, some data from the United States and other countries suggest that these complications caused by RA 27/3 vaccine are rare or perhaps nonexistent.[127,189,198,262,414,539,545]

Patients with juvenile idiopathic arthritis (JIA) have been safely vaccinated with the rubella vaccine. However, a case report from Korematsu and colleagues[320] describes an 11-year-old girl with systemic JIA, previously in remission for 4 years, who then developed an abrupt and severe relapse with congestive heart failure 5 days after receiving the rubella vaccine. The study authors suggested that the exacerbation of the patient's systemic JIA might have resulted from molecular mimicry between the rubella virus and her JIA.

Other complications, mainly with vaccines other than RA 27/3, include polyneuropathies (i.e., catcher's crouch, carpal tunnel syndrome, neuritis, and myeloradiculoneuritis),[102,108,217,245,316,413,498] marked lymphadenopathy (J. Cherry, unpublished data, 1967–1976), vasculitis, and myositis.[252]

Geiger and associates[213] reported a persistent rubella virus infection in a 16-year-old boy with acute lymphoblastic leukemia in remission who was vaccinated. The virus was identified in the patient's peripheral blood mononuclear cells 8 months after immunization. In contrast, persistent infection could not be demonstrated in 10 children with symptomatic human immunodeficiency virus type 1 (HIV-1) infection.[197]

Cheong and colleagues[98] reported a fatal case of disseminated tuberculosis in a 14-year-old girl, which occurred immediately after a measles-rubella vaccination. Previously, the exacerbation of tuberculosis infection related to measles-rubella vaccine was reported only for severely immunocompromised patients. Although natural measles infection has been known to potentiate other infections such as tuberculosis, no evidence has shown that measles-rubella vaccinations may accelerate the progression of tuberculosis.

Other adverse reactions that occur after immunization with MMR or MMRV have been primarily associated with the measles, mumps, and varicella components of the vaccine. Particular focus has been placed on the risk of immune thrombocytopenia purpura after MMR immunization.[194,363] Chapter 245 offers details on other adverse reactions associated with the MMR and MMRV vaccines.

Contraindications

Administration of live rubella virus vaccine is contraindicated in women who are pregnant; in individuals with altered immune states, such as immunodeficiency, leukemia, lymphoma, and generalized malignant disease; and in patients treated with high doses of corticosteroids (≥2 mg/kg per day or >20 mg/day for 14 days or more), alkylating drugs, antimetabolites, and radiation.

Fever is not a contraindication to immunization, and children with mild illnesses such as upper respiratory tract infections can receive immunizations. However, immunization should be delayed until recovery in cases of moderate to severe acute illnesses.[12,88] A personal or family (i.e., sibling or parent) history of seizures of any cause is a precaution for MMRV vaccination because these children may have an increased risk of febrile seizures. This caveat does not apply for children vaccinated with MMR and varicella vaccines administered separately.[88] Rubella immunization in most instances should be deferred after the administration of blood products, including immune serum globulin (see Chapters 245 and 246).

Inadvertent Rubella Immunization in Pregnancy

From January 1971 to April 1989, the CDC observed to term 321 known rubella-susceptible pregnant women who had been vaccinated with rubella vaccine within 3 months before or 3 months after conception.[90] Ninety-four women received HPV-77 or Cendehill vaccine, one received a vaccine of unknown strain, and 226 received RA 27/3 vaccine. None of the 324 infants born to these women had malformations compatible with congenital rubella, but five of the infants (<2%) had serologic evidence of subclinical infection. From these data, the CDC estimated a 1.3% maximal theoretical risk of congenital rubella among women vaccinated with the RA 27/3 rubella virus vaccine within 1 to 2 weeks before and 4 to 6 weeks after conception.[12] Women who might have been inadvertently immunized with rubella during pregnancy should be counseled extensively regarding the potential risks to the fetus. However, these observations of outcomes do not necessitate pregnancy termination as a result of rubella vaccine receipt during pregnancy.[12]

Many other studies have investigated the risk of congenital rubella among women who have received the rubella vaccine during pregnancy and have confirmed its safety. Castillo-Solorzano and associates[70] collected data from 2001 to 2008 from more than six countries and 30,139 women who were pregnant or became pregnant within 1 month after receiving the rubella vaccine. Seventy infants (3.5%) showed positive rubella serology results, but none of the infants had features of CRS. The study authors concluded that the maximal theoretical risk for CRS after rubella vaccination of susceptible pregnant women was 0.2%.

A large study by Soares and colleagues[542] covering several states in Brazil investigated 22,708 women vaccinated during pregnancy and found 67 newborns (4.1%) showed evidence of congenital infection but none with CRS. Da Silva e Sa and associates,[136] Sato and associates,[484] and Minussi and associates[383] reviewed cases from Brazil and found low rates of congenital rubella infection (2%, 4.7%, and 6.7%) but no cases of vaccine-associated CRS. A smaller study from 2006 in Argentina by Pardon and associates[433] also did not show evidence of CRS in infants born to women unknowingly pregnant during their mass rubella vaccine campaign. Nasiri and colleagues[411] and Namaei and associates[409] looked at pregnant women inadvertently vaccinated with rubella during pregnancy during Iran's 2003 mass vaccination campaign and found no cases of CRS.[299]

In conjunction with a nationwide measles-rubella vaccination campaign in 2001, the fetal risk associated with rubella vaccination during pregnancy was studied in Costa Rica.[19] The study involved 1191 mother and child pairs, and no adverse pregnancy outcomes or cases of CRS occurred.

Passive Immunization

The use of immunoglobulin for the prevention of rubella has been controversial for many years.[26,55,154,231,360,368,372,388,503,596] However, I believe that its use is indicated in certain circumstances. The specific indication for immune serum globulin is for the prevention of rubella in a woman thought to be susceptible to rubella who is in the first 20 weeks of pregnancy. If the exposure can be documented clearly as one to a specific person with rubella and immunoglobulin is given within 72 hours of that exposure, maternal disease and congenital infection likely can be prevented. However, if the exposure was more general (e.g., schoolteacher exposed to children in the school setting), the woman probably was exposed for a considerable time before she realized the exposure. Because immunoglobulin probably will be administered too late—well into the incubation period of her disease and after viremia—congenital infection is not likely to be prevented. The dose of immunoglobulin for the prevention of rubella during pregnancy is 20 mL given intramuscularly.

*References 17, 28, 108, 127, 227, 350, 402, 419, 455, 546, 567, 570, 571, 575–577, 612.

Quarantine and Disease Containment

Patients with rubella should not have contact with susceptible people until the rash has disappeared. Containment of rubella is a vital part of the prevention policy in the United States. Rubella is a reportable disease, and compliance is the obligation of all physicians and other health care professionals. Reporting cases of rubella enables public health workers to organize vaccination programs so that small outbreaks of disease can be prevented from developing into major epidemics. During an outbreak, those without evidence of immunity should be immunized or excluded from school or child care attendance.

NEW REFERENCES SINCE THE SEVENTH EDITION

12. American Academy of Pediatrics. Rubella. In: *Red Book: 2015 Report of the Committee on Infectious Diseases*. Elk Grove Village, IL: American Academy of Pediatrics; 2015.
36. Bellini W, Icenogle J. Measles and rubella viruses. In: Jorgensen J, Pfaller M, Carroll K, et al, eds. *Manual of Clinical Microbiology*. 11th ed. Washington, DC: ASM Press; 2015:1519-1535.
74. Centers for Disease Control and Preventon. Documentation and verifcation of measles, rubella and congenital rubella syndrome elimiation in the region of the Americas. In: United States National Report, March 28, 2012. https://www.cdc.gov/measles/downloads/report-elimination-measles-rubella-crs.pdf.
89. Centers for Disease Control and Preventon. Nationwide rubella epidemic—Japan, 2013. *MMWR Morb Mortal Wkly Rep*. 2013;62:457-462.
91. Centers for Disease Control and Preventon. National, state, and selected local area vaccination coverage among children aged 19-35 months—United States 2014. *MMWR Morb Mortal Wkly Rep*. 2015;64:889-896.
228. Grant GB, Reef S, Dabbagh A, et al. Global progress toward rubella and congenital rubella syndrome control and elimination—2000-2014. *MMWR Morb Mortal Wkly Rep*. 2014;64:1052-1055.
275. Hobman TC. Rubella virus. In: Knipe DM, Howley PM, eds. *Field's Virology*. Vol 1. 5th ed. Philadelphia: Lippincott Williams & Wilkins; 2013:687-710.
295. Hyde TB, Sato HK, Hao L, et al. Identification of serologic markers for school-aged children with congenital rubella syndrome. *J Infect Dis*. 2015;212:57-66.
301. Janta D, Stanescu A, Lupulescu E, et al. Ongoing rubella outbreak among adolescents in Salaj, Romania, September 2011–January 2012. *Euro Surveill*. 2012;17:pii: 20089.
323. Kreps EO, Derveaux T, De Keyser F, et al. Fuchs' uveitis syndrome: no longer a syndrome? *Ocul Immunol Inflamm*. 2016;24:348-357.
330. Kuhn RJ. Togaviridae. In: Knipe DM, Howley PM, eds. *Field's Virology*. Vol 1. 5th ed. Philadelphia: Lippincott Williams & Wilkins; 2013:629-650.
334. Lambert N, Strebel P, Orenstein W, et al. Rubella. *Lancet*. 2015;385: 2297-2307.
351. Lewis PE, Burnett DG, Costello AA, et al. Measles, mumps, and rubella titers in Air Force recruits: below herd immunity thresholds? *Am J Prev Med*. 2015;49: 757-760.
429. Padhi A, Ma L. Molecular evolutionary and epidemiological dynamics of genotypes 1G and 2B of rubella virus. *PLoS ONE*. 2014;9:e110082.
431. Papania MJ, Wallace GS, Rota PA, et al. Elimination of endemic measles, rubella, and congenital rubella syndrome from the Western hemisphere: the US experience. *JAMA Pediatr*. 2014;168:148-155.
432. Paradowska-Stankiewicz I, Czarkowski MP, Derrough T, et al. Ongoing outbreak of rubella among young male adults in Poland: increased risk of congenital rubella infections. *Euro Surveill*. 2013;18:pii: 20485.
462. Raimondi F, Migliaro F, Di Pietro E, et al. Nitric oxide-sensitive pulmonary hypertension in congenital rubella syndrome. *Case Rep Crit Care*. 2015;2015: 198570.
470. Reef S, Plotkin SA. Rubella vaccine. In: Plotkin SA, Orenstein WA, Offit PA, eds. *Vaccines*. 6th ed. Philadelphia: Elsevier; 2013.
529. Severino M, Zerem A, Biancheri R, et al. Spontaneously regressing leukoencephalopathy with bilateral temporal cysts in congenital rubella infection. *Pediatr Infect Dis J*. 2014;33:422-424.
561. Sugishita Y, Shimatani N, Katow S, et al. Epidemiological characteristics of rubella and congenital rubella syndrome in the 2012-2013 epidemics in Tokyo, Japan. *Jpn J Infect Dis*. 2015;68:159-165.
581. Toda K, Reef S, Tsuruoka M, et al. Congenital rubella syndrome (CRS) in Vietnam 2011-2012—CRS epidemic after rubella epidemic in 2010-2011. *Vaccine*. 2015;33:3673-3677.
631. Winchester SA, Varga Z, Parmar D, et al. Persistent intraocular rubella infection in a patient with Fuchs' uveitis and congenital rubella syndrome. *J Clin Microbol*. 2013;51:1622-1624.
641. World Health Organization. Rubella virus nomenclature update: 2013. *Wkly Epidemiol Rec*. 2013;32:337-348.

The full reference list for this chapter is available at ExpertConsult.com.

175 Alphaviruses

175A ■ Eastern Equine Encephalitis

Gail J. Harrison • Theodore F. Tsai

Eastern equine encephalitis (EEE) is a highly pathogenic mosquito-borne viral zoonosis infection of humans, horses, and other vertebrates that occurs in North and South America and the Caribbean. It causes outbreaks of severe diseases in both humans and horses, with high mortality or neurologic impairment in survivors.

The disease EEE was first recognized in Massachusetts in 1831 when 75 horses died of viral encephalitis. The causative agent was isolated from infected horse brains in 1933, and in 1938 the first human case was identified when 30 children died of viral encephalitis in the northeastern United States. The vector and mode of transmission of EEE virus discovery was made by Dr. Charles William Lacaillade.[36]

In North America, infections recur in highly focal, primarily coastal locations in association with the habitat of the ornithophagic mosquito *Culiseta melanura,* the enzootic vector. In the United States, most cases are along the East coast and Gulf coast states. Florida continues to have the highest occurrence of human cases.[38] It is also endemic in the northeastern United States.[58] Birds are the amplifying hosts, and humans and horses are infected incidentally. Because it is a highly pathogenic virus in humans that may be disseminated in the population, it is considered a possible biologic agent, category B threat, that could be used against civilian populations.[59,68]

ETIOLOGIC AGENT

EEE virus is an antigenically distinct member of the *Alphavirus* genus in the Togaviridae family. On the basis of nucleotide differences, it has been inferred that EEE and Venezuelan equine encephalitis diverged 1000 to 2000 years ago, with a subsequent division of EEE virus into North American and South American varieties.[8,55,57] South American strains can be differentiated by monoclonal antibodies and by short-incubation hemagglutination-inhibition tests.

North American strains collected over a broad geographic and temporal span demonstrate remarkable genetic stability in one or two major lineages, with minor local divergences occurring within isolated geographic loci. South American strains are genetically heterogeneous. They have been isolated in northward-migrating birds captured in the United States, but they have never been shown to become established.

ECOLOGY

Equine cases have been reported as far north as Quebec, Ontario, and Alberta provinces; in South America, EEE viral activity has been reported from the Caribbean, Mexico, Guatemala, Honduras, Panama, Colombia, Venezuela, Peru, Guyana, and Brazil and as far south as Argentina.[5,9,25,67] The viral transmission cycles in the Caribbean and South America are not well characterized but apparently involve small mammals, birds, and *Culex (Melanoconion)* mosquitoes.[1,25,48,49]

In North America, the distribution of virus activity closely follows the distribution of freshwater swamps on the Eastern Seaboard, Gulf Coast, and other inland areas. Florida, with abundant fresh-water wetlands, is the state in the United States with the most cases in humans.[38] The distribution of virus corresponds to the distribution of the principal enzootic vector, *C. melanura*.[11,22,25] *C. melanura* feeds nearly exclusively on birds, so various epizootic (bridging) vectors are responsible for infecting humans and horses.[21,22,29–31,38,40,43,44,65] Numerous species may be involved, including *Coquillettidia perturbans, Aedes sollicitans, Aedes vexans,* and *Aedes canadensis.*

In 2011, expansion of EEE virus to northern New England was observed. Bites from mosquito *C. perturbans,* as well as *C. melanura,* feeding on both avian and mammalian hosts including humans, may both be important in the epidemic/epizootic transmission of EEE virus, according to recent insights of the recent emergence and expansion of the virus into northern New England.[48,49]

The bird species most commonly associated with *C. melanura* feedings and potentially responsible for this spread include the American robin, tufted titmouse, common grackle, wood thrush, chipping sparrow, black-capped chickadee, northern cardinal, and warbling vireo. The wood thrush and American robin especially may play a dominant role in supporting EEE virus amplification and have been termed *superspreaders* of EEE virus in North America.[48,49] Infection and viremia are subclinical in most native birds, whereas whooping cranes and exotic birds such as emus, house sparrows, ring-necked pheasants, Pekin ducks, and chukar partridges may become ill and die of infection.[4,13,15,44,66,72] Outbreaks resulting in thousands of deaths have occurred in commercial pheasant flocks, in some instances perpetuated by cannibalistic pecking or preening of persistently infected quills.[4] Illness and deaths in pigs, goats, calves, rodents, and other mammals also have been reported.[26,47]

C. melanura is found in and near freshwater swamps, where larval stages breed in acidic waters associated with mucky peat soils. These foci (from north to south) are found in upland red maple, coastal white cedar, and southern loblolly bay biotypes.[11,25]

The viral overwintering mechanism has not been elucidated, but the remarkable permanence of endemic foci is a strong argument for overwintering in local reservoirs, such as reptiles and amphibians.[11,34,35,40,47] Serosurveillance in amphibians and reptiles has shown that snakes, including garter snakes, have high seropositive rates and support viremia with EEE virus, whereas frogs, turtles, and lizards have little or low rates of infection.[30]

EPIDEMIOLOGY

EEE is a rare sporadic infection; historically, a median of three cases occurred annually in the United States[42] (Fig. 175A.1). More recently, a mean of eight cases per year (range, 3–21) have been reported to the ArboNET, Arboviral Diseases Branch, of the Centers for Disease Control and Prevention (Fig. 175A.2).

The states with the highest rates of infection show an average annual incidence of less than one per 10 million (Fig. 175A.3). EEE has been reported to occur in at least 17 states in the United States and is most commonly reported from Massachusetts, New Hampshire, and Florida (Fig. 175A.4).

However, these estimates obscure the remarkably consistent and focal distribution of cases on the Atlantic and Gulf Coasts, from Ontario to Texas, and in isolated pockets of activity inland.[5,9,20] For example, until 1995, all human cases in Massachusetts had occurred east of Highway 495 in Essex, Norfolk, Plymouth, Bristol, and Middlesex counties; the six southernmost counties account for most of the epizootic activity in New Jersey; and foci of EEE viral activity recur in upstate

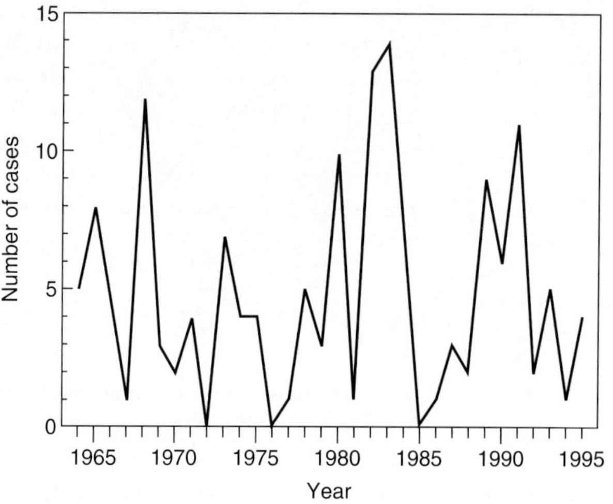

FIG. 175A.1 Reported cases of eastern equine encephalitis by year, 1964–95.

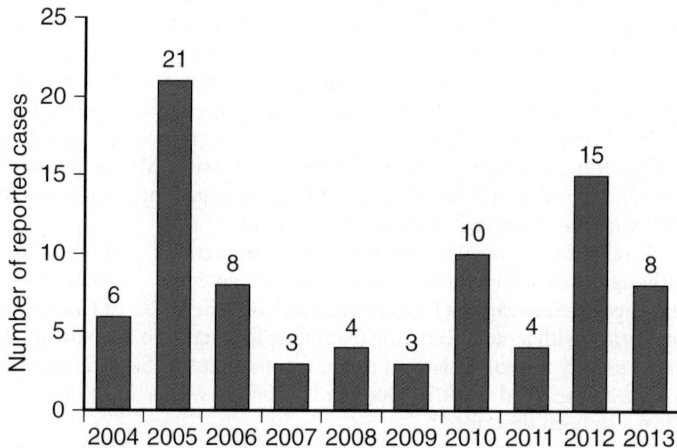

FIG. 175A.2 Eastern equine encephalitis virus neuroinvasive disease cases reported to the ArboNET, Arboviral Diseases Branch, Centers for Disease Control and Prevention, by year, 2004–13, showing an average of eight cases annually (range, 3–21) in the United States. (Courtesy Centers for Disease Control and Prevention. Available at: https://www.cdc.gov/easternequineencephalitis/tech/epi.html.)

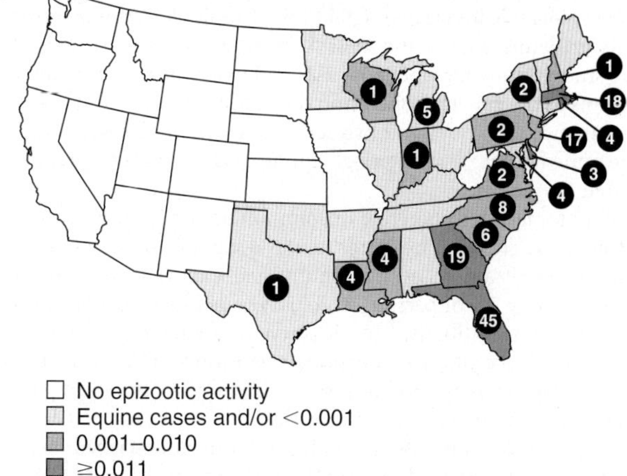

FIG. 175A.3 Reported cases and average annual incidence (per 100,000) of eastern equine encephalitis by state, 1964–95.

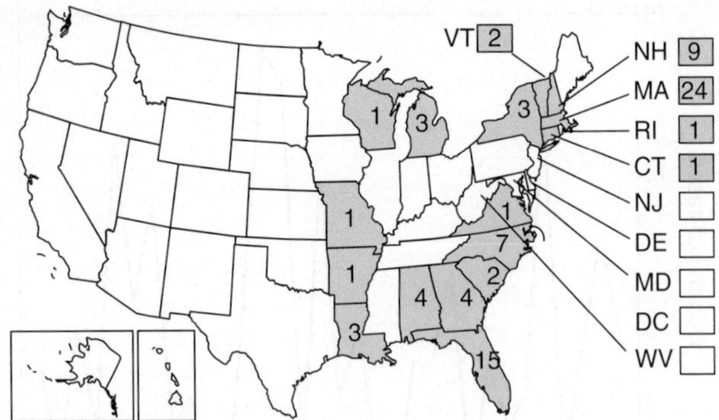

FIG. 175A.4 Eastern equine encephalitis (EEE) virus neuroinvasive disease cases reported by state, 2004–13. EEE cases have been reported in 17 states, with Massachusetts, New Hampshire, and Florida reporting the most cases. (Courtesy Centers for Disease Control and Prevention. Available at: https://www.cdc.gov/easternequineencephalitis/tech/epi.html.)

New York counties near Syracuse, southwestern Michigan, northeastern Indiana, and northeastern Florida.[12,20,29,31,35] Outbreaks of human cases caused by North American viral strains have been reported from Jamaica, Trinidad, and the Dominican Republic.[6,17,18] Isolated epizootics with sporadic human cases have occurred in South America.[67] The unpredictability of risk for EEE is underscored by the occurrence of a case in a United Kingdom tourist who had a brief itinerary in Massachusetts.[32] Therefore history of travel should be obtained in patients with possible EEE who are diagnosed in nonendemic areas.

Viral transmission, reflected in equine cases, occurs all year in Florida, although the peak incidence is from May to September.[7] Human cases have appeared as early as February and as late as in winter in December in Florida, with a peak occurring from June to August. In the Northeast, cases usually appear in late summer, from August to September, and as late as the third week in October.[42] Cases in winter in other areas have also been described.[61]

Cases occur chiefly at the extremes of age. However, serologic studies performed during a New Jersey outbreak disclosed that infection occurs with equal frequency in all age groups, thus indicating that biologic responses to infection rather than factors associated with exposure were responsible for the lower attack rates in young and middle-aged adults.[27] The ratio of inapparent infections to cases was highest in the middle years of life (29:1) and lowest in children younger than 4 years (8:1) and adults older than 55 years (16:1).[27] Immune-compromised hosts also are vulnerable to severe or fatal EEE.[62] Family clusters were observed in this epidemic and in the 1947 Louisiana outbreak.[33] In the New Jersey study, family members of cases had twice the rate of inapparent infections as the general population did; and in the southern Louisiana outbreak, two fatal cases and two seropositive members were observed in the same family.[27,33] Clusters of equine cases on a single premise are reported frequently.

Asymptomatic infections are uncommon occurrences, and long-term residence in an enzootic area leads to only a slight increase in population immunity. For example, even in an unusually active focus in southern New Jersey, only 7% of persons who had resided there 45 years or more had neutralizing antibody.[27] In serosurveys of endemic foci in Massachusetts, evidence of past infections was found in 0.5% to 0.7% of residents,[56] and a postepizootic serosurvey of at-risk Connecticut pheasant farmers showed no evidence of infection.[45]

Specific behavioral risk factors have not been described; however, residence, travel, and outdoor activity near swampy habitats have been reported anecdotally as possible contributing factors.

PATHOLOGY

Pathologic changes in the brain are consistent with severe meningoencephalitis with marked, diffuse cerebral edema and acute and chronic perivascular inflammation, and are characterized by lesions in the cortex, thalamus, basal ganglia, and brainstem, with cortical and deep gray matter neuronal loss from mild to extensive focal necrosis.[14,51] The areas on postmortem pathology correspond to lesions seen on neuroimaging, providing support that magnetic resonance imaging (MRI) findings represent virus-induced inflammatory and necrotic changes. Viral antigen is found predominantly in neurons and only occasionally in astrocytes.[23] Rare viral particles have been identified by electron microscopy in principally extracellular locations.[3,39] Neutrophils predominate in cellular infiltrates in the meninges, vascular cuffs, and foci of tissue damage in the cortex and brain nuclei of patients dying acutely; at later stages, neutrophilic infiltrates are replaced by mononuclear cells.[3,14,23,51] Immunohistochemical examination of one patient disclosed a predominance of helper T cells in perivascular infiltrates, with some B lymphocytes. The most intense inflammatory reaction occurred in areas where antigen-positive neurons were absent, presumably where cell lysis already had occurred. Perivascular macrophages contained cleared viral antigen, but antigen could not be demonstrated in vascular endothelial cells.[23]

PATHOGENESIS

After peripheral inoculation of experimental animals, local viral replication occurs at a low level or may be undetectable. Viremia develops after this eclipse period, with disseminated infection of the spleen, liver, and kidneys noted in monkeys and guinea pigs and infection of the spleen, heart, and lungs observed in mice. Infectivity can be demonstrated in the brain only after viremia and infection in the viscera are established, thus suggesting that invasion of the central nervous system occurs by hematogenous spread.[51] Neurologic injury is associated with vasogenic edema in the earliest stages and subsequently with virus-induced cytolysis and host inflammatory responses.[28]

The immune response in humans presumably is similar to that observed in experimental alphavirus infections in mice, in which host resistance depends on rapid elaboration of a humoral immune response. Infection with EEE virus confers lifelong immunity, but does not confer significant cross-immunity against other alphaviruses, such as western equine encephalitis virus; flaviviruses, such as West Nile virus; or bunyaviruses, such as LaCrosse virus.

CLINICAL MANIFESTATIONS

EEE is a fulminant encephalitis with rapid progression to coma and death in one-third of patients. Fever appears to be an almost universal presenting sign. In infants and children, an abrupt onset of fever, irritability, stiff neck, and headache is followed within 1 to 3 days by lethargy, confusion, seizures, and coma.[62] The often desperately ill infants may have a bulging fontanel, meningismus, high temperature, and generalized flaccid or spastic paralysis.[2,19,24,71,73] Seizures are often present, with complex partial seizures, generalized tonic-clonic seizures, or both types reported, and some patients present with status epilepticus.[62] The prodrome in adults and older children usually is brief, with nonspecific symptoms of fever, headache, and dizziness followed by clouding of the sensorium and rapid deterioration to coma. Remarkably, some patients have a prolonged prodrome lasting longer than a week, with a waxing and waning course of nonspecific symptoms, which may be associated with a better prognosis.[54,56,62,71] Various neurologic deficits have been described; in some cases, unilateral seizures, hemiparesis, hemiplegia, and aphasia have indicated focal areas of involvement.[16,50,54]

The peripheral leukocyte count usually is elevated with a shift to the left. White blood cell counts of 20,000/μL are typical, ranging as high as 60,000 with 55% to 89% neutrophils.[56] Cerebrospinal fluid (CSF) usually shows a polymorphonuclear pleocytosis with a total leukocyte count ranging from 500 to 2000/μL. The initial neutrophilic pleocytosis of 60% to 100% may persist into the second week before shifting to a predominance of mononuclear cells.[57] CSF protein level is elevated and glucose concentration is reduced in most cases.[62] Erythrocyte counts higher than 500/μL are found in some cases.

Imaging studies disclose only cerebral edema in three-fourths of patients. However, focal rim-enhancing lesions and areas of low alteration with mass effect have been observed on computed tomography (CT) scans in the frontal cortex, thalami, midbrain, and lentiform nuclei.[16,50,54]

CT of the brain may be abnormal as early as the first or second day of illness, with subtle attenuation abnormalities in the basal ganglia, cerebral cortex, and thalamus.[62] MRI will also show evidence of brain abnormalities, which correlate with pathologic viral inflammation on autopsy, early in the illness. Isointense diffusion-weighted images and hyperintensity on apparent diffusion coefficient images early in the course of illness in one case suggested vasogenic edema in the T2-weighted hyperintense areas.[28] In one small case series, T2-weighted fluid-attenuated inversion recovery (FLAIR) hyperintensities, with linear areas of hyperintensity in the external and internal capsule and sparing of the lentiform nuclei, were described as a so-called parenthesis sign that may be suggestive of EEE.[52] MRI also shows focal lesions in basal ganglia and thalami in patients with EEE.[18] Electroencephalographic tracings with focal or background slowing have been associated with a favorable outcome, whereas disorganized background activity, a burst-suppression pattern, and high-voltage delta slowing have been associated with a poor prognosis.[56] EEG may also show epileptiform activity or subclinical status epilepticus.[62] Mild nonencephalitic illnesses usually are not diagnosed. However, in the 1959 outbreak in New Jersey, fever, headache, nausea, vomiting, and sore throat were common symptoms in 19 patients who had serologic evidence of infection. One-third of the patients had illnesses sufficiently severe to motivate them to consult their physicians.[27] Other patients with bladder dysfunction, dysesthesias, weakness, and signs of myelitis have been described.[10,41] One case of infection during pregnancy has been reported. The third-trimester infection was severe, but the woman recovered from encephalitis and coma and was delivered of an apparently normal neonate. Serologic studies of the neonate's blood were not performed. Infection with EEE also was reported to trigger fatal hemophagocytic lymphohistiocytosis in an infant.[45]

PROGNOSIS AND SEQUELAE

The case-fatality rate is 33% among reported cases and is highest in elderly people; outcome is best in adults aged 20 to 59 years, in whom the case-fatality rate is 24%.[35] Patients with a long prodromal illness (>4 days) have a better prognosis, which is consistent with the protective effect of a peripheral antibody response in the preneuroinvasive phase.[46]

Residual neurologic damage is observed more often in young children. In a Florida series, serious sequelae were seen in four of seven survivors younger than 5 years and in one of 10 survivors in other age groups.[7] Similar findings were reported in a follow-up of epidemic cases in Massachusetts: seven of eight survivors younger than 3 years of age had neurologic sequelae, and only one of four surviving adults had residua.[2,21] Neurologic impairment ranged from mild unilateral spasticity to profound mental retardation, seizure disorders, and quadriplegia. A report published in 2013 of children with EEE from Massachusetts and New Hampshire showed that most survivors with severe neurologic impairment at the time of acute recovery were able to regain substantial cognitive and motor skills with appropriate rehabilitation therapy.[62]

DIAGNOSIS

A specific laboratory diagnosis usually is made from serologic studies. Isolation of virus from CSF is unusual. The virus should be sought from brain biopsy tissue or autopsy material. EEE virus grows rapidly in a variety of cell lines, including Vero A549 and MRC-5 cells, and causes widespread cytopathic effect in several days.[64] Specific identification of viral isolates can be accomplished rapidly by immunofluorescent or immunoperoxidase techniques. EEE virus has been identified by immunofluorescence and by electron microscopy in brain tissue.[3,23,39] Viral antigen in viremic bird blood, infected mosquito pools, and infected equine brains can be detected directly by antigen capture enzyme-linked immunosorbent assay (ELISA). Polymerase chain reaction analysis of CSF has been reported but has not been evaluated extensively for routine clinical diagnosis.[57,60] Testing of CSF for EEE is most often done at a state public health laboratory or the Division of Vector-Borne Diseases (DVBD) Laboratory at the Centers for Disease Control and Prevention (CDC).

Serologic testing is also available in many state and reference laboratories and is currently the preferred method for diagnosis in patients. It also may be done at the DVBD laboratory at the CDC. Virus-specific IgM usually can be detected in acute serum and CSF samples, using antibody-capture ELISA.[46,62] Indirect immunofluorescence, neutralization, and hemagglutination inhibition also are sensitive procedures. Confirmatory virus-specific neutralizing antibodies by plaque-reduction neutralization assay is a serologic test available at health department laboratories. Antibodies often are present in the first week of illness. Neutralizing antibody appears 3 to 4 days after the onset of illness, and hemagglutination-inhibition (HI) antibody appears with almost equal rapidity.[27] Both HI and neutralizing antibodies appear to be long lived.[27] Complement-fixing (CF) antibody is slower to rise and can be noted 11 days after onset, with diagnostic fourfold rises often appearing only in the third week after onset.[27] The peaks of both HI and CF titers are observed 3 to 4 weeks after onset.[28] CF antibody declines more rapidly. Measurable CF antibodies were found in approximately 50% of persons infected 8 years earlier in one study, although the effects of reexposure could not be ruled out in this endemic area.[27] Research and development of an ELISA-array platform that detects five different encephalitis viruses (Japanese encephalitis virus, tick-borne encephalitis virus, equine encephalitis virus, Sindbis virus, and dengue virus) has shown it to be easy to use, sensitive and specific, and accurate and potentially will be widely available for clinical use in areas where these viruses cause disease.[37] Immune-compromised patients may not have an immunoglobulin M (IgM) or IgG antibody response to EEE, and diagnosis may require direct detection of the agent in CSF or brain tissue.[63]

The low prevalence of EEE antibody in the general population suggests that detection of EEE viral antibody in the acute serum of a patient with encephalitis indicates a high probability of that diagnosis. Applying the Bayes theorem, if the "rate" of EEE is 1 in every 2000 cases of encephalitis, if HI antibody to EEE is present in 100% of cases in the first week of illness, and if the prevalence of HI antibody in the general population is 0.05%, the presence of EEE in a patient with encephalitis who has demonstrable EEE antibody in a single serum specimen is a certainty.[68] Thus the probability of the diagnosis is high when specific antibody is found in any (i.e., acute) serum specimen.

All EEE disease cases are reportable to the local public health department in order to recognize potential outbreaks and institute control measures.

DIFFERENTIAL DIAGNOSIS

The fulminant clinical course of EEE, the laboratory findings of neutrophilic leukocytosis and polymorphonuclear pleocytosis in the CSF, and focal findings on brain imaging may suggest bacterial cerebritis or meningitis as a working primary diagnosis until it is excluded with bacterial cultures. Because no specific antiviral therapy is available, EEE should be a diagnosis of exclusion, confirmed eventually with serologic and virologic testing, which may take several weeks or more to finalize. This should be done after every feasible effort has been made to diagnose and to treat empirically against bacterial meningitis and herpes simplex virus encephalitis, as well as after excluding other herpesvirus and arbovirus infections, influenza virus, enterovirus, rabies virus, and other infectious and noninfectious causes of encephalitis in humans. If exposure history is positive for endemic regions, Japanese encephalitis virus, tick-borne encephalitis, Sindbis virus, and dengue virus can all cause a similar clinical picture to EEE and should also be considered in the differential diagnosis.

TREATMENT

Specific antiviral treatment for EEE is unavailable. Therapy aimed at supporting cardiorespiratory function, homeostasis of fluid, electrolyte balance, and control of cerebral edema and seizures is indicated and may be lifesaving. Antiviral research and development initiatives have focused on agents with activity against EEE, but no specific antiviral agent is licensed for treatment of EEE in humans.[59] In case reports, intravenous immune globulin and glucocorticoids, as well as cyclophosphamide and interferon-α, were given for their potential immunomodulatory effects and were associated with survival.[28,70]

PREVENTION

An effective killed vaccine is licensed for horses, but no human vaccine is licensed. An investigational killed vaccine, available under investigatory permit, is used to protect laboratory personnel.[57] Other vaccine candidates, such as a Sindbis/EEE virus chimeric vaccine and a recombinant EEE virus attenuated by internal ribosomal entry site control, have been tested in vitro and in animal models.[53,69] Vaccination of the general public is not feasible as a public health measure because of the low incidence of disease.

Climatologic studies have shown a correlation between outbreaks and heavy rainfall in the summer of an epidemic year and in the preceding fall.[34,40,42] Although such predictors would have considerable utility in guiding control measures, outbreaks of EEE have been too few for their validity to be tested. Isolation of Highlands J virus, which shares a common enzootic cycle with EEE virus, often peaks 2 to 3 weeks before the appearance of EEE virus in *C. melanura.*

Surveillance and public health interventions to prevent EEE in endemic areas have been shown to be economical when they are balanced against the direct and indirect costs of even one human case.[69] Infection rates in *C. melanura* of 0.39 per 1000 population have been highly predictive of risk for human cases in areas of Massachusetts surveyed during a 26-year interval.[32] Larviciding of swampland to control *C. melanura* is difficult because of the large areas involved, the potential toxic effects in fish and other wildlife, and the relative inaccessibility of the larvae. Emergency application of adulticides to control epizootic vectors is indicated when viral, mosquito, and animal surveillance suggests a risk for epizootic transmission.

For the individual, public health advisories to avoid outdoor activity near enzootic foci and closure of campgrounds and parks in these locations may be necessary when viral transmission indices suggest a high level of risk. The use of repellents containing DEET, picaridin, IR3535, or oil of lemon eucalyptus on exposed skin or on clothing is recommended, and permethrin can be used on clothing as well. In addition, wearing long sleeves and long pants outdoors is recommended. Also, installation and repair of screens on windows and doors to keep out mosquitoes should be done. To keep mosquitoes from breeding and laying eggs near habitats, removal of even small amounts of standing water is an important preventive measure. Also, avoidance of outdoor activity 1 to 2 hours after sunset, when many mosquitoes are most active, may reduce the risk for exposure from *Culex* mosquitoes; however, some vector *Aedes* species are daytime biters. "Avoid bites day or night" is a popular public health slogan to help prevent all mosquito-borne illnesses.

NEW REFERENCES SINCE THE SEVENTH EDITION

36. Imperato P. Charles William Lacaillade. Biologist, parasitologist, educator, mentor. *J Community Health.* 2017;43(1):179-212.
37. Kang X, Li Y, Fan L, et al. Development of an ELISA-array for simultaneous detection of five encephalitis viruses. *Virol J.* 2012;9:56-60.
48. Molaei G, Armstrong P, Abadam C, et al. Vector-host interactions of *Culiseta melanura* in a focus of Eastern equine encephalitis virus activity in southeastern Virginia. *PLoS ONE.* 2015;10(9):e0136743.
49. Molaei G, Thomas C, Muller T, et al. Dynamics of vector-host interactions in avian communities in four eastern equine encephalitis virus foci in the northeastern U.S. *PLoS Negl Trop Dis.* 2016;10(1):e0004347.
52. Nickerson J, Kannabiran S, Burbank H. MRI findings in eastern equine encephalitis: the "parenthesis" sign. *Clin Imaging.* 2016;40(2):222-Oct 9; 8: 516.
58. Rocheleau J, Arenault J, Ogden N, et al. Characterization areas of potential human exposure to eastern equine encephalitis virus using serological and clinical data from horses. *Epidemiol Infect.* 2017;145(4):667-677.
61. Sha K, Cherabuddi K. Case of eastern equine encephalitis presenting in winter. *BMJ Case Rep.* 2016;2016.
62. Silverman M, Misasi J, Smole S, et al. Eastern equine encephalitis in children, Massachusetts and New Hampshire, USA, 1970–2010. *Emerg Infect Dis.* 2013;19(2):194-201.
63. Solomon I, Clarini P, Santagata S, et al. Fatal eastern equine encephalitis in a patient on maintenance rituximab: a case report. *Open Forum Infect Dis.* 2017;4(1): ofx021.
70. Wendell L, Potter N, Roth J, et al. Successful management of severe neuroinvasive eastern equine encephalitis. *Neurocrit Care.* 2013;19(1):111-115.

The full reference list for this chapter is available at ExpertConsult.com.

175B ■ Western Equine Encephalitis

Gail J. Harrison • Theodore F. Tsai

Western equine encephalitis (WEE) is an endemic and enzootic acute central nervous system (CNS) infection of humans, including children, and horses in the western part of the United States, Canada, Mexico, and parts of South America. In North America, *Culex tarsalis,* the principal mosquito vector, also maintains the virus in an avian enzootic cycle.[5,81] WEE virus is currently classified as a Biological Safety Level 3 (BSL-3) agent because it is highly infectious and potentially may be transmitted via aerosol, and a Category B bioterrorism agent based on its moderate ability to disseminate in the population and produce serious disease in humans.[67]

ETIOLOGIC AGENT

WEE and other alphaviruses (group A arboviruses) form a genus of principally mosquito-borne viruses in the family Togaviridae.[50,71] Three of the eight viruses constituting the WEE antigenic complex are found in North America: Highlands J, Fort Morgan, and WEE viruses. Among these, only WEE virus is a human pathogen. Much of what is known about the molecular biology of alphaviruses has been inferred from studies of the Sindbis (the type species and a member of the WEE complex) and Semliki Forest viruses.

Alphaviruses are small, enveloped, positive-stranded RNA viruses. Virions are spherical and 69 nm in diameter (including the length of their glycoprotein spikes), with a lipid bilayer enveloping a nucleocapsid core containing the 11.7-kb RNA viral genome.[67] Glycoprotein spikes embedded in the viral envelope bind to cell membrane receptors and initiate infection by endocytotic fusion. The viral and lysosomal membranes fuse in a pH-dependent step, and the viral nucleocapsid is released into the cell cytoplasm, where RNA and protein synthesis occurs. The 5′ terminal two thirds of the RNA genome encodes four nonstructural proteins, and the 3′ terminal third of the RNA genome encodes the three structural proteins. The 30-kDa nucleocapsid and two 50-kDa glycoproteins—E1 and E2—are translated as a polyprotein from subgenomic 26S RNA. The envelope proteins—E1 and E2—are assembled in trimers of a single E2 protein and an E1 dimer. Eighty such trimer spikes are arranged in an icosahedral lattice on the virion surface.[12] Capsid proteins assemble with the viral genome in the cytoplasm and then bud through the virally modified cell membrane and acquire an envelope.

The E1 glycoprotein possesses a group-reactive hemagglutinin and group-reactive epitopes linked to cross-protection and cell-mediated cytotoxic effects. E1 also mediates viral cellular membrane fusion and has been explored as a vaccine target.[72] Epitopes on E2 are linked to cell receptor recognition, viral neutralization and clearance, and neurovirulence and cellular apoptosis.[76]

Molecular genetic studies indicate that WEE virus arose more than 1000 years ago as a recombinant of eastern equine virus and an ancestral, now extinct, Sindbis-like virus, with the recombinant having acquired the neurotropic potential of eastern equine encephalitis (EEE) virus while retaining the antigenic and nucleocapsid characteristics of the nonneurotropic Sindbis virus.[23,50,63,67,73,74]

Alphaviruses are thought to have originated in the New World with separate introductions, presumably by birds, to the Old World, resulting in establishment of the present-day Sindbis-like viruses and Semliki

Forest–related viruses. A slow rate of evolution, circa 10^{-4} nucleotide changes per year (vs. 10^{-2}/year for other RNA viruses), probably reflects the natural pressure on viruses constrained to replicate in both insect and vertebrate cells.[74]

ECOLOGY

WEE virus is transmitted in an enzootic cycle to mosquitoes, birds, and other vertebrate hosts.[54,53,59] Surveillance is usually accomplished by public health department vector control programs by collection of mosquitoes from endemic areas and testing for vector-borne viruses, such as WEE, using reverse transcription loop-mediated isothermal amplification (LAMP), or single or multiplex quantitative reverse transcription polymerase chain reaction (qRT-PCR) assays.[9,77]

Horses and humans are dead-end hosts, but severe CNS infection may develop. Although WEE has been a public health and veterinary problem primarily in the western United States and Canada, the geographic range of the virus includes Mexico, Guyana, Brazil, Uruguay, and Argentina. Epizootics in horses, accompanied by small numbers of human cases, were reported in 1972 and 1983 in Argentina, where the virus apparently is transmitted by *Aedes albifasciatus* to introduced European hares and possibly birds. In addition, a distinct sylvatic subtype of WEE virus is transmitted in the subtropical Chaco province.[4,8]

In the United States, the geographic distribution of the virus and *C. tarsalis,* its principal vector, includes the western and central United States, southern Canada, and Mexico. A related virus—Highlands J virus, isolated from *Culiseta melanura* in the eastern United States—overlaps in its range in the east central part of the United States. Highlands J virus causes encephalitis in horses and possibly in humans.[40]

In the western region of the United States, *C. tarsalis* breeds in ground pools found on pasture lands; in irrigation wastewater; and at the margins of lakes, ponds, marshes, and flooded riversides. Some of these aquatic habitats are shared by birds that participate in the amplification of virus in nature.[54,53,59]

The female mosquito becomes infected after feeding on a viremic bird (or mammal or possibly reptile). After an extrinsic incubation period of 7 to 9 days, when the virus propagates in the mosquito and the salivary glands become infected, the mosquito can transmit virus to other birds or mammals or reptiles (amplifying hosts) or to humans and horses (dead-end hosts).

Passerine (perching) birds, especially sparrows and finches, have proved to be particularly important in amplification of the virus. In midsummer, the mosquito shifts its host-seeking activity to mammals. The shift may be influenced by an increase in the defensive behavior of nestling birds, which are its preferred host. The shift corresponds temporally to the appearance of cases in horses and people and appears to be a critical element enabling *C. tarsalis* to function as both an enzootic and an epizootic vector. In California, an auxiliary *Aedes melanimon*-jackrabbit *(Lepus californicus)* cycle has been demonstrated.

The overwintering mechanism for WEE virus has not been elucidated. However, virus has been recovered from adult *Aedes dorsalis* mosquitoes collected as larvae from a coastal area of California, thus indicating a possible role for vertical transmission of the virus in mosquitoes in some locations. Arguments also have been advanced for viral overwintering in adult mosquitoes and in persistently infected mammals, birds, and poikilotherms (snakes, frogs, and turtles). Experimental infection of snakes (garter snakes) and tortoises show them to be susceptible to chronic infection with WEE virus.[3] Seroepidemiology studies in the field show high prevalence of WEE virus antibody in reptile hosts, including snakes, lizards, turtles, and crocodiles. Reptiles, because of their low metabolic rate, may function as a reservoir host over the winter and transmit WEE virus to humans via an arthropod vector.[3] In Canada, *Aedes* spp. and *Culiseta inornata,* which emerge in the spring before *Culex tarsalis,* have been proposed as early amplifying vectors.[39]

Numerous climatologic and biologic indices with various degrees of predictive value have been shown to correlate with the occurrence of WEE outbreaks; these indices include vector population size, mosquito infection rates, and virus transmission rates to sentinel chickens or wild-caught sparrows. Such transmission indices are monitored in surveillance activities by public health agencies; however, their sensitivity, specificity, and predictive value for forecasting epidemics have been difficult to evaluate because of the sporadic nature of outbreaks.[75] A retrospective analysis of a 21-year experience in California showed correlation between average daily numbers of *C. tarsalis* females and the occurrence of human encephalitis.[46] In a Texas study, house sparrow infection and antibody rates were the best predictors of human disease, and *C. tarsalis* light trap indices were of borderline significance.[29]

Physical measures associated with the incidence of disease in humans or transmission of virus to sentinel species include the ambient air temperature, the snow pack in mountains providing runoff water, the river flow rate, the soil temperature inversion date (the date that the surface soil temperature exceeds the subsurface soil temperature), and the date when 50 or more days of 21°C (70°F) temperature have accumulated. Snow pack and river flow rate are associated with an abundance of irrigation water and flooding, which in turn are associated with the availability of breeding habitats and mosquito population size.[10,28,54,55,53]

Longitudinal and intraseasonal observations show that high temperatures are associated with a reduced risk for human disease. High ambient air temperature (32°F [>89.6°F]) decreases mosquito survival, adversely affects the competence of *C. tarsalis* to become infected with and to transmit WEE virus, and limits host-seeking activity.[58] In a model of global warming, higher temperatures are predicted to move the range of WEE viral transmission northward.[54,55]

EPIDEMIOLOGY

WEE occurs sporadically and in epidemic form, principally in Canadian provinces and states west of the Mississippi River (Figs. 175B.1 and 175B.2). Infections occur mainly in rural areas, where water impoundments, irrigated farmland, and naturally flooded sites provide breeding habitats for *C. tarsalis;* however, the increasingly rare interface between vector mosquitoes and humans has resulted in a point seroprevalence of 1% to 2% even in locations where the virus is transmitted in an enzootic cycle.[58] The annual median number of cases between 1964 and 1995 was only four, and only four cases were reported between 1988 and 1997, a lower incidence than that for EEE. Historically, however, periodic outbreaks have led to scores or hundreds of cases (Fig. 175B.3).

Recurrent endemic and epidemic transmission was recorded in the Yakima Valley, Washington (1939–42); California's Central Valley (1939–52); the north central states and Canadian provinces, including Minnesota, North and South Dakota, Alberta, Manitoba, and Saskatchewan (1941 and 1975); and the high plains panhandle of Texas (1963–66).[17,24,30,52,57] The largest outbreak on record, in 1941, resulted in more than 3400 human cases in Minnesota, North and South Dakota,

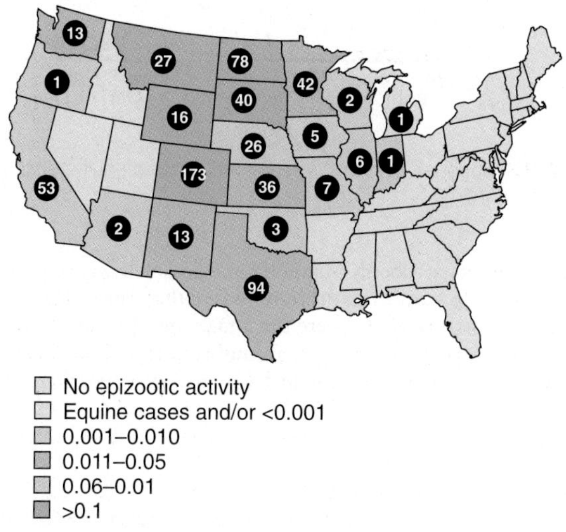

FIG. 175B.1 Reported cases and average annual incidence (per 100,000) of western equine encephalitis by state, 1964–95.

TABLE 175B.1 Western Equine Encephalitis Epidemic Attack Rates by Population Density[a]

Population Area	Minnesota, 1941	Kern County, CA, 1952	Hale County, TX, 1963–66	Manitoba, 1975
Rural	15.8–22.0	149.2	2.62	10.8
Small town	2.3–5.6			2.4
Urban		28.5	1.0	0.9

[a]Per 100,000 population.

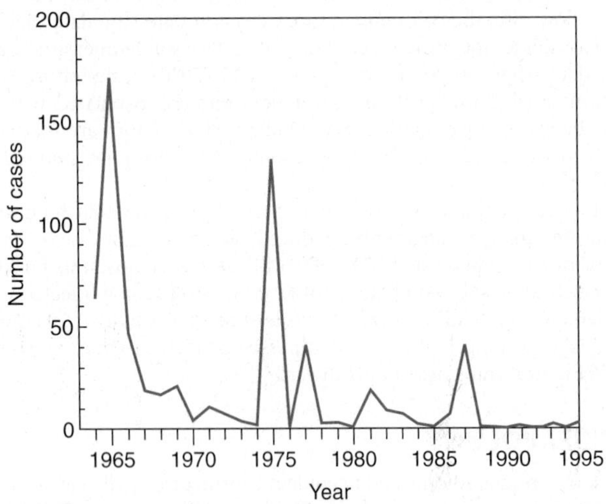

FIG. 175B.2 Reported cases of western equine encephalitis by year, 1964–95.

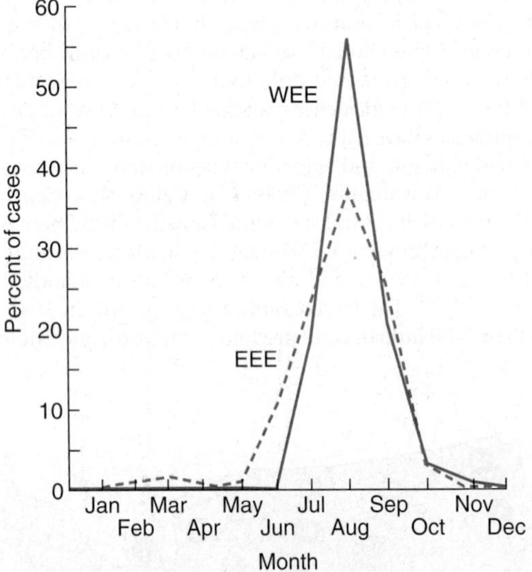

FIG. 175B.3 Reported cases of western and eastern equine encephalitis by month, 1972–89.

Nebraska, Montana, Alberta, Manitoba, and Saskatchewan; equine cases were estimated to number in the hundreds of thousands. The outbreak centered in North Dakota, where the attack rate for cases in the state was 167 per 100,000.[17,34] In 1952, an outbreak in California's Central Valley led to 348 reported cases, an incidence of 36 per 100,000 residents.[30] More recent outbreaks resulted in 277 cases in the central United States and Manitoba in 1975 and 40 cases in the central and mountain states in 1987.[15,35,39]

Most cases occur between June and September (see Fig. 175B.3), often preceded by cases occurring in horses several weeks earlier. Surveillance of equine cases is a widely used approach to assess the risk for epidemic transmission. However, the low frequency of laboratory-confirmed diagnoses, vaccination, and underreporting limit the precision of equine surveillance as a predictive marker.[49]

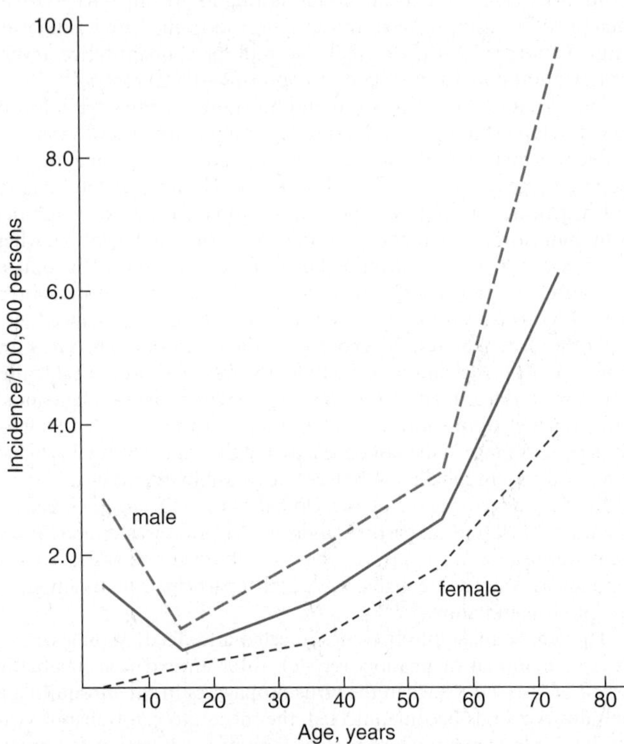

FIG. 175B.4 Age- and sex-specific incidence of western equine encephalitis, Colorado, 1987.

Several risk factors for acquiring WEE have been identified:

1. Attack rates usually are highest at the extremes of age[2] (Fig. 175B.4). The experience from the 1952 California outbreak showed that a third of cases occurred in infants younger than 1 year.[30,54] Other reports confirm the bimodal pattern of an elevated risk in infants, a declining risk in children and young adults, and a gradual increase in risk in the elderly.
2. Attack rates in males are twofold higher than those in females in every age group[2] (see Fig. 175B.2). Biologic differences in susceptibility to infection may account for the observed disparity in infancy, and greater occupational and recreational exposure outdoors might be responsible for the differences in adults. In the 1981 outbreak in Manitoba, 21 of 25 cases were in males; the four affected women were widows who maintained their premises alone.[15]
3. Rural residence is associated with attack rates 1.5 to 5 times higher than those for urban residence (Table 175B.1). Counties lying in major river drainage areas and with more irrigated acreage have had the highest incidence of equine and human disease[2] (Fig. 175B.5).
4. Agricultural occupation has been suggested as a risk factor in several studies.
5. Length of residence in areas where WEE is endemic is associated inversely with a risk for developing illness. Acquired immunity, through asymptomatic or mild infection, accumulates with length of residence; in endemic areas, the point prevalence of specific antibody previously approached 20% by adulthood.[54,53]

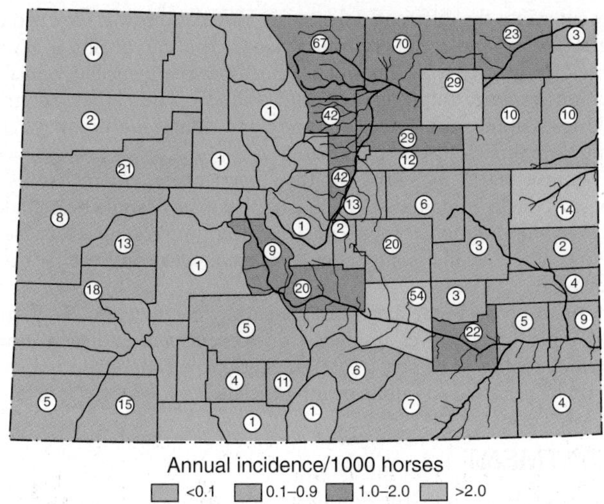

FIG. 175B.5 Reported equine cases and incidence of western equine encephalitis by county, Colorado, 1975–88.

CLINICAL MANIFESTATIONS

The clinical illness ranges from a nonspecific syndrome of headache and fever to aseptic meningitis, meningoencephalitis, and encephalitis with fatal outcome. The estimated case-infection ratio is 1:58 in children 1 to 4 years of age, but it declines to 1:1150 in adults.[14,20,54,59]

The onset of illness typically is abrupt, with sudden fever, headache, malaise, chills, and nausea and vomiting,[6,17,27,52] occasionally preceded by signs of an upper respiratory tract infection. Signs of CNS infection gradually become evident as dizziness, drowsiness, increasing headache, stiff neck, and disorientation develop during the course of hours or days. Infants typically have a sudden cessation of feeding, fussiness, fever, and protracted vomiting. The prodromal interval is abbreviated, and seizures and a lethargic unresponsive state develop rapidly.

On examination, patients appear somnolent and may have signs of meningeal irritation. The sensorium is depressed, and patients may alternate between agitation and somnolence. Generalized muscle weakness is present, and deep tendon reflexes are diminished. Focal neurologic signs suggesting herpes encephalitis have been reported in anecdotal cases[1,7]; however, in the 1941 Minnesota outbreak, only three of 226 cases reported had unilateral weakness.[17]

In infants, the fontanelle may be tense or bulging, often accompanied by spastic paresis and generalized seizures. The frequency of seizures is related inversely to age; they occur with greatest frequency in infants younger than 3 months (75% to 80% of cases), whereas in 2- to 4-year-old children, seizures have been reported in 15% of cases.[38]

The peripheral leukocyte count is unremarkable. Cerebrospinal fluid (CSF) obtained at an early stage in the illness generally exhibits normal glucose concentration, elevated protein level, and a leukocyte count between 10 and 300/mm^3.[35] Mononuclear cells usually predominate.

Five instances of late third-trimester infection in pregnant women have been reported to result in perinatal illness or encephalitis.[13,14,38] The women's illnesses had an onset 0 to 10 days before delivery, and the infants became ill on the fifth and sixth postpartum days. Teratogenic effects of infection occurring earlier in gestation have not been reported for WEE virus but are suspected for other group A arboviruses.[41]

PATHOLOGY

Specific pathologic changes are confined to the CNS.[6,35,44] On gross examination, the brain appears normal or may be congested and swollen, with minimal changes observed in the meninges. Microscopic lesions affecting gray and white matter appear throughout the brain but predominate in the basal ganglia. Disseminated small focal abscesses infiltrated with neutrophils are a distinctive feature. The vessels appear congested, and small focal hemorrhages or diffuse extravasations of erythrocytes are present along with neutrophilic infiltration of the vascular wall and endarteritis. Vascular lumina may be occluded by endothelial proliferation and swelling.

Extensive patchy areas of demyelination are found throughout the brain. Older lesions appear as sharply circumscribed, punched-out plaques. Secondary microglial reaction in demyelinated areas is minimal.

The spinal cord is affected in the same fashion, with focal, perivascular, and diffuse lesions attracting both polymorphonuclear and mononuclear cells. Lesions predominate in the central gray matter.

PATHOGENESIS

Peripheral inoculation of experimental animals with WEE virus is followed by viral replication in various extraneural sites before invasion of the CNS (including the peripheral site of inoculation, viscera, muscle, and perhaps vascular endothelial cells) occurs, usually at areas where the blood-brain barrier is weak or absent.[31,36,45,48,80]

Host resistance and recovery from infection depend chiefly on an effective antibody response. Antibody contributes to recovery by a variety of means, including viral neutralization and antibody-mediated restriction of viral gene expression.[22,76] Interferon may contribute to containment of local viral spread in the CNS. Antibodies are protective and may be cross-protective to other alphaviruses. Antibodies to the E2 glycoprotein typically are virus specific and associated with neutralization and protection. Antibodies to E1 exhibit greater cross-reactivity with other alphaviruses.[71] Immune serum given to monkeys prophylactically protects them from challenge with WEE virus, and passive protection has been demonstrated in monkeys inoculated with WEE virus and treated with immune serum within 24 hours.[80] However, immunotherapy in monkeys is uniformly unsuccessful in preventing death once signs of CNS infection have appeared. In guinea pigs peripherally inoculated with WEE virus, immunotherapy given within 24 to 48 hours of inoculation leads to survival of some animals and delayed death in others.[45] In one human case, passive immunization led to a delayed antibody response and was followed by the development of parkinsonism.[21]

The age-dependent virulence of specific Sindbis virus strains has been linked to the immaturity of the suckling mouse T- and B-cell repertoire. Fibroblasts from newborn but not weanling mice are susceptible to Sindbis virus infection, and viral infection of immature mouse neurons leads to apoptotic cell death. Mature neurons are protected against apoptosis by induction of the *bcl-2* oncogene, whose products convert the infection to a persistent nonlytic infection. Viral persistence in the brain of recovered mice is modulated by antibody.[22]

PROGNOSIS

Major neurologic sequelae of WEE, including quadriplegia, hemiplegia, spasticity, intracerebral calcifications, developmental delay in children, and epilepsy, have been reported in approximately 13% of cases.[16,18,27,82] The risk for development of serious neurologic sequelae in infants is triple that of other age groups, and 30% of recovered infants younger than 1 year remain seriously impaired.[18,20,70] In infants younger than 1 year, seizures during the acute phase of illness were associated with a greater risk for poor long-term outcome, including continued seizures. Multiple intracranial calcifications were observed in one recovered infant with persistent seizures.[69] Minor psychiatric or neurologic deficits remained in approximately one fourth of children and adults monitored for 18 months after infection.[18] Central apnea has been reported as a complication of encephalitis in two adult cases.[78]

Parkinson syndrome has been a residual effect in at least 15 cases of adults surviving WEE.[21,43,65,66] Its onset may be immediate or delayed for several years after recovery from the illness. Two retrospective investigations of patients with idiopathic Parkinson disease found no difference between cases and controls in seroprevalence to several arboviruses, including WEE virus.

The case-fatality rate in reported cases in the United States from 1955 to 1978 was 3% to 4%. In outbreaks in the central portion of the United States and Canada in 1941, 1975, and 1981, approximately 7% to 9% of patients died, with higher fatality rates in the elderly.

DIAGNOSIS

Virus rarely can be recovered from blood or CSF, but it can be isolated readily from the brains of patients who died of WEE. In a few attempts, WEE virus has been isolated from brain biopsy material; in principle, rapid diagnosis can be made by immunofluorescent identification of WEE viral antigen in brain biopsy tissue. The virus can be isolated readily, under BSL-3 containment precautions, in Vero cell culture or in suckling mice.[66] Nucleic acid–based sequence amplification and real-time reverse transcription polymerase chain reaction (RT-PCR) assays of CSF appear to be sensitive and specific. Duplex real-time RT-PCR assays that not only detect but also discern among alphaviruses have recently been developed.[32]

Immunoglobulin (Ig) M capture enzyme-linked immunosorbent assay (ELISA) is the preferred serologic procedure and is available from public health laboratories and commercial reference laboratories.[37] IgM antibody usually is present in acute serum within a week after the onset of illness, and its presence is presumptive evidence of recent infection. IgM often can be detected in CSF before it can be identified in serum, and its presence, which indicates intrathecal production of antibody, confirms a recent CNS infection.[37] Identification of virus-specific IgM in serum and CSF by immunofluorescence also is possible; however, this approach is somewhat less sensitive than IgM capture ELISA and may be confounded by the effects of rheumatoid factor.

Hemagglutination-inhibition and neutralizing antibodies are elevated in the first week of illness in most cases, and a diagnostic fourfold rise in titer usually is observed in the second week. Complement-fixing antibody is slower to rise, with fourfold changes delayed until the third to fifth week after onset. The complement-fixation response may be blunted in older patients.[70]

Neutralizing and hemagglutination-inhibition antibody titers have considerable longevity, with minimal decay noted 30 months after onset. In contrast, complement-fixing antibody is relatively short-lived, and its presence is a useful indicator of recent infection, particularly in endemic areas where long-term residents may have neutralizing and hemagglutination-inhibition antibody from previous exposure. Only two thirds of patients are estimated to show complement-fixing antibody 2 years after onset, and fewer than 15% have residual complement-fixing antibody after 5 years.[70]

DIFFERENTIAL DIAGNOSIS

The clinical findings in patients with encephalitis seldom are sufficiently characteristic that a specific diagnosis can be made on clinical grounds alone. Fever, vomiting, signs of meningeal irritation, and confusion are nonspecific features of encephalitis and cerebral edema. Early symptoms in infants, such as fever, lethargy, and vomiting, may be even less specific.[33]

Furthermore, the peak occurrence of arboviral infection in midsummer to late summer temporally overlaps the seasonal occurrence of other CNS infections by enteroviruses (e.g., echovirus 13, which recently has become epidemic in the United States), leptospires, free-living amoebae, and mosquito-borne Eastern equine encephalitis, Venezuelan equine encephalitis, and West Nile and St. Louis encephalitis.[57] CNS signs may be prominent in other summertime diseases, such as Rocky Mountain spotted fever, heat stroke, shigellosis, and lead encephalopathy. High priority should be given to establishing a specific diagnosis of treatable conditions, such as herpes simplex virus and enteroviral infection, while bearing in mind that dual arboviral and enteroviral infection has been reported.[7]

Other causes of CNS infection without an established summertime seasonality that also should be considered in the differential diagnosis include fungal, mycobacterial, and partially treated bacterial meningitis; brain abscess and infected subdural collections; bacterial endocarditis; toxoplasmosis; cat-scratch disease; and infections with rabies virus, mumps virus, herpes simplex virus, Epstein-Barr virus, human herpesvirus 6, adenovirus, lymphocytic choriomeningitis virus, and human immunodeficiency virus. Parainfectious disorders such as postinfectious viral encephalitis, acute cerebellar ataxia of childhood, mycoplasmal infection, neuroblastoma with opsoclonus, and Reye syndrome also may enter into the differential diagnosis. Vascular disorders formed the largest single group of disorders mimicking herpes encephalitis in several studies. Drugs (e.g., trimethoprim-sulfamethoxazole, penicillin, isoniazid, phenazopyridine, ibuprofen, tolmetin, sulindac, and carbamazepine), high doses of bismuth, OKT3 antibody, and vidarabine also may cause aseptic meningitis or encephalopathy.

Because of the potential for their overlapping circumstances of exposure, diethyltoluamide (DEET) encephalopathy should be excluded. DEET-containing insect repellents have been implicated as a cause of seizures and encephalopathy after brief cutaneous exposure (see later discussion).

Valuable clues to the diagnosis of an arbovirus infection are gleaned from a history of travel, residence, or occupational and recreational activities within the appropriate incubation period. Suspected cases should be reported to public health officials.

TREATMENT

Specific US Food and Drug Administration–approved antiviral therapy is not available for WEE. However, novel small-molecule inhibitors of neurotropic alphaviruses, including WEE virus, are in preclinical development.[47,56,68] Supportive treatment of acutely ill patients includes monitoring of cardiorespiratory function, fluid and electrolyte balance, and intracranial pressure. A case of laboratory infection treated with immune equine serum resulted in recovery; however, acute Parkinson syndrome developed in this patient and coincided temporally with serum sickness resulting from immunotherapy.[21]

PREVENTION

Killed vaccine prepared in chick embryo fibroblast culture is available in the United States under an investigatory permit for laboratory and field personnel who are at risk for occupational exposure. Effective killed vaccines are available for horses and usually are administered in bivalent or multivalent formulations (i.e., with EEE, Venezuelan equine encephalitis, and influenza viruses). Potential vaccine targets for WEE are under investigation and include E1 envelope protein targets and adenovirus vectored vaccines.[72,79] Vaccination of the general public, even in endemic areas, is not a practical consideration because of the low risk for disease.

Personal protective measures are encouraged when travel or living in endemic areas, and include avoidance of outdoor activity during the hours of peak mosquito activity at dusk and use of repellents.

The Centers for Disease Control and Prevention (CDC) recommends repellents containing DEET or picaridin (KBR 3023) as active ingredients.[10,11,19,25,51] DEET is absorbed readily through the skin, and its absorption and absorption of oxybenzone, a common sunscreen preparation, are increased when they are used in combination. Some authorities recommend that sunscreens be applied first and more liberally, followed by insect repellent applied sparingly because of concerns about the potential neurotoxicity of DEET.[10,61,62] Three cases were fatal. In one recovered child, encephalopathy and seizures developed after only two applications. In an additional child, seizures and encephalopathy occurred after the child had cutaneous and respiratory exposure to DEET in an automobile with closed windows. Additional cases of seizures in patients who used small quantities of DEET have been reported, but whether these events were coincidental in populations in which the prevalence of DEET use is high is unclear.[11] DEET may have an effect on ammonia metabolism; in one case, encephalopathy occurred in a patient with partial ornithine carbamoyltransferase deficiency.[26] DEET is a proved neurotoxin when it is ingested; however, the incidence of neurologic side effects after cutaneous exposure is unknown. Nonetheless, avoiding formulations containing DEET in high concentration is prudent; when it is applied simultaneously with sunscreen, DEET repellency is unhampered but ultraviolet protection may be reduced. Precautions for the prudent use of repellents as recommended by the CDC and US Environmental Protection Agency (EPA) are listed in Box 175B.1.

Repellents containing oil of lemon eucalyptus (but not "pure" oil of lemon eucalyptus) and registered with the EPA as repellents also may provide a similar level of protection.

BOX 175B.1 Precautions to Reduce Potential Adverse Reactions From Repellents

- DEET is approved for use on children older than 2 months. Read and follow label instructions.
- Repellents should be applied only to exposed skin and clothing (as directed on the product label). Do not use under clothing.
- Never use repellents over cuts, wounds, or irritated skin.
- Avoid mucosal contact—do not apply to the eyes and mouth, and apply sparingly around the ears. When using sprays, do not spray directly onto the face; spray on the hands first and then apply to the face.
- Do not allow children to handle the product, and do not apply to children's hands. When using on children, apply to your own hands and then put it on the child.
- Do not spray in enclosed areas. Avoid breathing a repellent spray.
- Avoid ingestion, and do not use the product near food.
- Use just enough repellent to cover exposed skin and clothing.
- Heavy application and saturation are unnecessary for effectiveness; if biting insects do not respond to a thin film of repellent, apply a bit more.
- After returning indoors, wash treated skin with soap and water or bathe. This precaution is particularly important when repellents are used repeatedly in a day or on consecutive days. Also, wash treated clothing before wearing it again.
- Pregnant and nursing women should minimize the use of repellents.
- If you suspect that you or your child is reacting to an insect repellent, discontinue use, wash treated skin, and then call your local poison control center. If you go to a physician, take the repellent with you.
- Specific medical information about the active ingredients in repellents and other pesticides is available at the National Pesticide Information Center at 800-858-7378.

Modified from US Environmental Protection Agency recommendations. Available at: http://www.epa.gov/pesticides/factsheets/chemicals/deet/htm.

Permethrin, a synthetic pyrethroid available as a 0.5% aerosol (Permanone), is both insecticidal and a repellent.[11,19,64] Permethrin is extremely effective in reducing the incidence of mosquito and tick bites when sprayed on clothing and shoes, and it also can be applied to tents, mosquito nets, and other gear.[19,63] Its use on the skin is not approved, except as treatment of scabies and head lice.

Prevention is focused primarily on interruption of the transmission of virus from mosquitoes to humans. In many localities where WEE is endemic, mosquito abatement districts monitor mosquito populations, virus infection rates in the vector population, or evidence of transmission of virus to wild or sentinel birds and chickens to provide a basis for predicting epidemic transmission and for emergency mosquito control.[42,60]

As a general rule, *C. tarsalis* densities exceeding 10 to 15 females per trap night and mosquito infection rates greater than five to 10 per 1000 signal a risk for epizootic transmission. Evidence of seroconversion in sentinel chickens and observations of equine cases are further indications that human cases may occur.

NEW REFERENCES SINCE THE SEVENTH EDITION

5. Bagdure D, Custer J, Rao S, et al. Hospitalized children with encephalitis in the United States: a pediatric health information system database study. *Pediatr Neurol.* 2016;61:58-62.
9. Brault A, Fang Y, Reisen W. Multiplex qRT-PCR for the detection of western equine encephalomyelitis, St. Louis encephalitis, and West Nile viral RNA min mosquito pools (Diptera: Culicidae). *J Entomol.* 2015;52(3):491-499.
48. Phillips AT, Rico A, Stauft C, et al. Entry sites of Venezuelan and Western equine encephalitis virus in the mouse central nervous system following peripheral infection. *J Virol.* 2016;90(12):5785-5796.
77. Wheeler S, Ball C, Langevin S, et al. Surveillance for western equine encephalitis, St. Louis encephalitis, and West Nile viruses using reverse transcription loop-mediated isothermal amplification. *PLoS ONE.* 2016;11(1):e0147962.

The full reference list for this chapter is available at ExpertConsult.com.

175C ■ Venezuelan Equine Encephalitis

Gail J. Harrison • Theodore F. Tsai

Mosquito-borne Venezuelan equine encephalitis (VEE) arguably is the most important viral zoonosis in Latin America. The disease, known locally as *peste loca,* has occurred in combined epizootics and epidemics at regular intervals since the 1920s, sometimes leading to hundreds of thousands of human and equine cases. Between 1935 and 1961, 11 outbreaks were reported, and from 1962 to 1973, epizootics recurred in every year except 1965.[1,4,20,44] The virus was isolated from horse brain in 1938 during an outbreak in Venezuela. Although outbreaks have arisen principally in northern South America, especially from Colombia and Venezuela, in a remarkable period between 1969 and 1971, epizootics and epidemics were reported from Colombia, Venezuela, Ecuador, Peru, all the countries of Central America (except Panama), Mexico, and the state of Texas.[1,4,14,30,44] Subsequently, no major epizootics or epidemics were recognized until a large outbreak emerged in Venezuela and Colombia in 1995.[7,8,35,48] Molecular phylogenetic analyses performed in the wake of that outbreak suggested that epizootic strains arise spontaneously from sylvatic viral strains circulating silently in nature.[3,6,25,48] VEE virus is classified as a Category B bioterrorism agent and a Biosafety Level 3 (BSL-3) agent, based on its ability to cause disease in humans, ease of production and stability, and potential for aerosol dissemination in the population.[51]

ETIOLOGIC AGENT

VEE virus is antigenically distinct from other alphaviruses in the Togaviridae family but is a complex of antigenically and ecologically distinct viral subtypes (Table 175C.1).[33,39,45,47,50] Epizootic subtypes IAB and IC are so named because they have been associated with major outbreaks in horses. Sylvatic viral subtypes circulate in silent cycles of rodent-mosquito or bird-mosquito transmission and in general do not cause encephalitis in equines. Both epizootic and sylvatic viral strains cause human illness. VEE virus is an enveloped virus with a nonsegmented, positive-sense RNA genome approximately 11 kilobases in length.

VEE virus is thought to have evolved about 1400 years ago from a now extinct ancestral alphavirus in one of two extant lineages of New World alphaviruses represented by eastern equine encephalomyelitis and VEE viruses.[33] Because epizootic VEE viral strains had never been isolated from nature except during epizootics, their reservoirs and the mechanisms by which they emerge to cause outbreaks had remained a puzzle. However, recent molecular phylogenetic analyses have found a close genetic relationship between the epizootic IC and the sylvatic ID strains, thus suggesting that these epizootic strains might arise spontaneously by mutation from naturally circulating ID virus.[1,3,6,47] Other outbreaks have had an iatrogenic source from improperly inactivated equine vaccine.[21,22,33,36,47,48]

Comparisons of the attenuated TC-83 vaccine strain of VEE virus and the epizootic IAB parent virus and mutations of virulent infectious clones have shown that changes associated with attenuation occur principally in genes encoding the E2 and E1 glycoproteins but also in the 5′ nontranslated region.[3,6,21,39] Attenuation is associated with reduced neuroinvasiveness (i.e., faster clearance from blood and lower viremia levels) and reduced neurovirulence (i.e., minimal histopathologic changes after intracerebral inoculation of horses).

TABLE 175C.1 **Viruses in the Venezuelan Equine Encephalomyelitis Complex**

Subtype	Variety	Pattern of Transmission	Location	Transmission Cycle
I	AB	Epizootic	South, Central, and North America	Various mosquitoes and biting insects: equines
	C	Epizootic	Northern South America	Various mosquitoes and biting insects: equines
	D	Enzootic	Ecuador, Panama, Colombia, and Venezuela	*Culex (Melanoconion) ocossa* and *panocossa:* rodents, aquatic birds
	E	Enzootic	Central America	*Culex (Melanoconion) taeniopus:* rodents
	F	Enzootic	Brazil	Unknown
II (Everglades)		Enzootic	Southern Florida	*Culex (Melanoconion) cedecei:* rodents
III	A (Mucambo)	Enzootic	South America	*Culex (Melanoconion) portesi:* rodents
	B (Tonate)	Enzootic	South America	Unknown
	Bijou Bridge	Unknown	Western North America	*Oeciacus vicarius:* birds
	C	Enzootic	Peru	Unknown
	D	Enzootic	Peru	*Culex (Melanoconion): Proechimys* spp.
IV (Pixuna)		Enzootic	Brazil	Unknown
V (Cabassou)		Enzootic	French Guiana	Unknown
VI		Enzootic	Argentina	Unknown

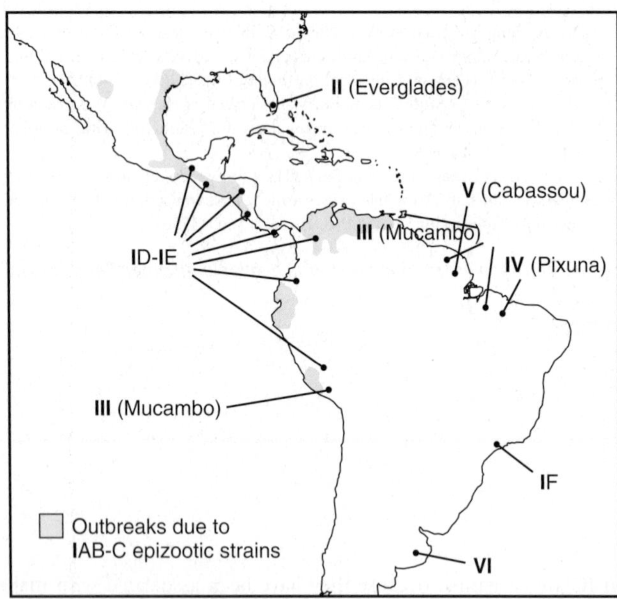

FIG. 175C.1 Locations of Venezuelan equine encephalitis (VEE) outbreaks caused by types IAB and IC epizootic strains and locations where VEE sylvatic subtypes have been recognized.

VEE virus rapidly produces cytopathic effects in a variety of cell cultures, including Vero, LLC-MK2, and BHK-21, and in primary chicken and duck embryo cells. Epizootic strains cause lethal infections in horses, donkeys, mules, rabbits, and dogs. In certain guinea pig strains, pathogenicity is correlated with equine virulence.

EPIDEMIOLOGY AND ECOLOGY

Epizootics and concurrent epidemics of VEE caused by the IAB and IC strains typically have led to thousands and, on at least one occasion, hundreds of thousands of cases in humans and equines. Surveillance for these mosquito-transmitted viruses are performed by public health laboratories using multiplex, reverse transcriptase polymerase chain reaction (RT-PCR), which can now detect multiple encephalomyelitis viruses in one reaction.[46] Most such outbreaks have occurred in Venezuela and Colombia and have been caused by IC viruses (see earlier discussion) (Fig. 175C.1).[35,38,47,48] The circumstances leading to the emergence of outbreaks are poorly understood, but outbreaks often have occurred in arid areas during years of heavy rainfall and flooding, especially during the dry season.[44] The importance of a nonimmune horse population to amplify the virus was underscored in the most recent outbreak in 1995, which occurred in areas of Colombia and Venezuela where equine immunizations had lapsed.[7,35,48] Equines are the most important vertebrate amplifying host because high levels of viremia develop and are sustained in equines, and they provide a large surface area for biting mosquitoes. Numerous species of mosquitoes and other blood-feeding insects, among them *Aedes taeniorhynchus,* a salt marsh mosquito, and *Psorophora confinnis,* found in ground pools, can transmit the virus from horse to horse and from horse to human.[41]

Infections are transmitted rapidly among animals and to people such that outbreaks can disseminate at rates of several miles per day. The epidemic curve of human cases usually follows the equine epizootic by several weeks, and epidemic transmission ceases when the number of susceptible horses has been exhausted by immunization or natural infection.[17,44]

The role of other animals, including humans, in sustaining epidemic viral transmission has been investigated in urban outbreaks, during which household clustering of cases has been observed, and in recent outbreaks, during which few horses were kept in the community. VEE virus levels in human blood are sufficiently high to infect mosquitoes, and virus also has been isolated from the pharynx of ill persons, indicating the possibility of person-to-person transmission by mosquitoes such as *Aedes aegypti* or by direct close contact.[3,40] Although such transmission mechanisms may account for some cases, a household survey found that rates of apparent secondary transmission were no higher than the underlying community attack rate.[7,35] Community attack rates of 20% to 50% have been recorded, and the brief course of epidemics in intervals as short as 1 month underscores the considerable force of epidemic transmission.

The series of epizootics beginning in Guatemala in 1969 and reaching Texas in 1971 was caused by an IAB virus that is almost genetically identical to the 1943 Trinidad donkey (epizootic IAB) virus used in inactivated vaccines, thus leading to the conclusion that these outbreaks were iatrogenic and caused by the use of inadequately inactivated equine vaccine.[4,22,47] Another outbreak in Argentina was traced to a similar cause. Serologic serosurveillance in the Gulf Coast region of Mexico conducted between 2003 and 2010 showed that the Gulf Coast lineage of VEE virus continues to actively circulate and be responsible for infection of animals and humans in this region.[35]

In contrast to the epizootic strains, sylvatic VEE viruses are avirulent in horses and cause a low level of viremia after infection, subclinical or mild illness, and minimal inflammatory change after direct intracerebral inoculation.[43] However, outbreaks of enzootic IE-like viruses rarely have caused outbreaks and deaths in horses (e.g., in Chiapas, Mexico, in 1993). The viruses are maintained in mosquitoes—principally *Culex (Melanoconion) taeniopus* in marshy coastal lowlands, in rodents—and in aquatic birds. In coastal lagoons in Panama, white ibises *(Endocinus albus)* and boat-billed heron *(Cochlearius cochlearius)* appear to serve as intermediate hosts.[2] VEE subtype II virus, the Everglades virus, is enzootic among cotton rats and other small mammals in the Everglades swamp and probably over a much larger area of Florida but rarely has caused human illness.[9,12] The other VEE virus found in the United States, Bijou Bridge virus, is a nonpathogenic virus thought to have evolved from South American subtype III virus transferred as recently as 40 years ago, probably by a migrating bird.

VEE infections caused by sylvatic strains can be considered "diseases of place" that occur sporadically in persons who enter sylvatic habitats where the viruses are maintained.[2,9] Sporadic cases and rare outbreaks among soldiers in field bivouacs have been reported, but seroprevalence rates in local populations range as high as 75% in some locations (e.g., Chiapas, Mexico).[18,37] Many infections are undoubtedly undiagnosed. Bridge vectors, mosquitoes that feed on mammals in the enzootic transmission cycle and subsequently on humans, usually are responsible for these infections.

Numerous cases and outbreaks of VEE have occurred in laboratories when infective aerosols were generated in laboratory procedures.[23] It also has been developed as a biologic weapon in the United States and the former Soviet Union.[51] Laboratory manipulations should be undertaken only in BL-3 laboratories and by immunized personnel.

Travelers to Central or South America may return to nonendemic areas with signs and symptoms of VEE. Careful travel history is therefore important in patients who seek medical care with signs and symptoms of encephalitis.[27]

CLINICAL MANIFESTATIONS

The incubation period is brief—2 to 5 days—and in many accounts, the onset of illness was so sudden that it was timed to an exact hour.[23] Fever, chills, headache, myalgia, and malaise are the earliest symptoms, and illness quickly leads to prostration. Photophobia, neck stiffness, backache, conjunctivitis, and sore throat are also common symptoms that occur in approximately one-fourth or more of cases. Gastrointestinal complaints, especially nausea and vomiting, and, to a lesser degree, loose stools or diarrhea, are reported frequently.[5] The case-fatality rate of VEE is estimated at 1%, but approximately 15% of survivors may experience severe neurologic sequelae. Asymptomatic infections also occur.

Physical examination discloses severe prostration and few specific findings. The face may appear hyperemic; inflammation of the pharynx is common; and, occasionally, tonsillitis, palatal ulcers, or petechiae are observed. The cervical lymph nodes may be enlarged and tender. Conjunctivitis and conjunctival suffusion are noted frequently. Nuchal rigidity can be elicited in 10% of cases, more often in children. Despite the disease's name, the symptoms of confusion, agitation, and mild disturbances in consciousness suggesting encephalitis are present in only 5% to 10% of cases, and patients with significant neurologic findings, such as cranial nerve palsy, motor weakness and paralysis, seizures, and coma, usually account for fewer than 5% of all cases.[5,35,36] In epidemics, neurologic findings and encephalitis occurred more commonly in children; however, sporadic cases, including encephalitis caused by VEE subtype II (Everglades) and III (Tonate) viruses, have occurred in middle-aged or elderly adults.[12,18] The fatality rate among patients with encephalitis is 10% to 25%, or about 0.5% of all cases.[35,36]

In many patients, the illness has an apparently biphasic course; seizures, projectile vomiting, and ataxia occur several days after the onset of fever, followed rapidly by a complete resolution of symptoms. Sequelae such as nervousness, forgetfulness, recurrent headache, and easy fatigability are common occurrences and may persist for months or even up to 1 year. Motor abnormalities usually resolve without residual deficit; however, rarely, sensory and motor abnormalities may persist. Long-term effects on psychometric examination have been reported.[24]

Experimental observations in animals suggest that congenital infection may lead to central nervous system (CNS) anomalies such as porencephaly, microcephaly, and hydrocephalus.[25] A similar pattern of structural brain abnormalities has been observed in virus culture–positive fetuses aborted during outbreaks.[48,49] Pancreatic β-cell infection occurs in experimentally infected animals and has led to speculation that VEE may be followed by diabetes, but epidemiologic studies have failed to find an association.[24]

The principal clinical laboratory finding is leukopenia (<4500/mm^3), the nadir of which occurs on the fourth day of illness.[5,11] After the onset of illness, the absolute neutrophil count declines from normal values to 500 to 2000; total lymphocytes are depressed at the onset of illness and gradually recover after 1 week. The platelet count may be diminished below 100,000 mm^3, and lactate dehydrogenase and hepatic transaminases may be elevated moderately. Cerebrospinal fluid (CSF) shows a lymphocytic pleocytosis of up to several hundred cells, moderately elevated protein level, and normal or slightly depressed glucose concentration.

PATHOLOGY AND PATHOGENESIS

VEE virus is both lymphotropic and neurotropic.[10,42] Pathologic changes are observed consistently in the lymph nodes, spleen, lungs, liver, gastrointestinal lymphoid tissue, and brain, with inflammatory infiltrates of mononuclear and polymorphonuclear cells. The lymph nodes and spleen show pronounced lymphoid depletion and necrosis of the germinal centers, along with neutrophilic infiltration and lymphophagocytosis. The selective depletion of lymphoid follicles, with sparing of the paracortical areas and the thymus, suggests that VEE virus principally destroys B cells. These histopathologic changes are reflected in the early lymphopenia seen in the peripheral blood. The liver shows patchy hepatocellular degeneration typical of viral hepatitis. A diffuse interstitial pneumonia with a mixed intraseptal inflammatory cell infiltrate is a consistent finding, and some cases also exhibit intraalveolar hemorrhage, secondary bronchopneumonia, or both. The brain shows only congestion and edema in most cases. Mild, often focal meningitis and changes associated with encephalitis, perivascular inflammatory infiltrates, and neuronal degeneration are found in a large number of cases.[10] The consistent presence of congestion and edema in various organs and the necrotizing vasculitis seen in some cases suggest that vascular endothelial cells may be a target of infection. This speculation is supported by the observation of VEE viral antigen in the vascular endothelial cells of experimentally infected animals. Secondary immune-mediated destruction of infected vascular endothelia and lymphoid cells may account for delayed clinical manifestations.

LABORATORY DIAGNOSIS

VEE virus can be recovered and grown in cell culture from blood during the first 3 days of illness in at least 75% of cases, although isolates have been made after 6 days.[3,4] Virus also has been recovered from throat swabs in approximately 25% of cases.[24] Specimens should be inoculated onto Vero or other susceptible cell cultures, but only in a laboratory with BL-3 level containment because of the risk for laboratory aerosol-associated infection. Virus in samples collected and transported in commercial transport media may not support the growth of VEE but will preserve the nucleic acid and protein integrity of the virus.[19] As an alternative to viral isolation, genomic sequences in acute viremic blood and other samples can be detected rapidly and with high sensitivity by PCR in reference laboratories and genotyped using nested RT-PCR assay.[31] Establishing the subtype of VEE viral isolates is vital because subtypes IAB and IC have a potential for epidemic spread. Isolates can be identified rapidly with subtype-specific monoclonal antibodies.

Immunoglobulin M (IgM) capture enzyme-linked immunosorbent assay is the recommended serologic procedure. Both serum and CSF specimens can be tested by this means. Elevated virus-specific IgM in a single serum or CSF specimen is diagnostic and often obviates the need for a second paired serum. An epitope-blocking assay can differentiate antibody responses among serotypes.[45]

DIFFERENTIAL DIAGNOSIS

The self-limited acute febrile illness that characterizes most VEE cases resembles infection caused by dengue, Oropouche, Mayaro, group C bunyaviruses, and various other arboviruses. The epidemic occurrence of cases may suggest dengue or Oropouche fever; however, the absence of rash and hemorrhagic manifestations and an association with equine deaths strongly indicate VEE until it is disproved. Eastern and western equine encephalitis infections overlap with VEE in some areas of Latin America, but only sporadic human cases have been recognized. Clinical recognition of sporadic VEE caused by sylvatic viruses is difficult; the diagnosis should be entertained in patients with CNS infection and an appropriate exposure history.

TREATMENT

No specific US Food and Drug Administration–approved antiviral treatment is available for VEE. Symptomatic treatment with antipyretics and fluids alone is sufficient in most cases. In patients with encephalitis, anticonvulsants may be needed, and intensive supportive care, especially early recognition and treatment of secondary pneumonia, may improve the outcome. Combinations of short interfering RNAs and passive immunization with humanized monoclonal antibodies are under preclinical development and investigation as therapeutic interventions.[16,28,34]

Development of VEE antibody preparations from human transchromosomic cows, a new therapeutic platform, may eventually reach clinical trials in humans.[15]

PREVENTION

Immunization with experimental live attenuated TC-83 vaccine is indicated for laboratory and field personnel with a high risk for exposure to VEE virus.[32] However, the vaccine is immunogenic in only 85% of vaccinees, and significant side effects consisting of fever, stiff neck, malaise, and myalgia develop in approximately 20% of vaccinees.[13] Previous vaccination with alphaviral vaccines may interfere with response to TC-83, but after immunization with experimental inactivated TC-84 vaccine, antibody will develop in approximately 75% of persons who failed to respond to TC-83.[13,26] Safer candidate vaccines that may provide better protection against respiratory infection are being investigated.

Immunization of equines with TC-83 vaccine is the best approach to preventing the emergence of outbreaks. Inadequately inactivated vaccine prepared from epizootic IAB strains poses a danger of producing iatrogenic outbreaks and should be used only if appropriate safety and quality assurance standards of vaccine production have been met. The original TC-83 vaccine virus also may be transmitted by mosquito vectors, and efforts have been made to improve its safety by preventing its ability to infect insects; this was done through manipulation of structural protein gene expression to produce further attenuation and render the vaccine virus incapable of replicating in insects.[29] Because the live vaccine provides rapid immunity after a single dose, it is the most effective approach in combating outbreaks. Attenuated vaccine is available commercially in certain Latin American countries, but in the United States, only inactivated vaccine formulated with western and eastern equine encephalitis and equine influenza and tetanus antigens is licensed. An improved candidate vaccine, V3526, has been shown to be efficacious in horses.[13] Preclinical development of new, novel VEE vaccines includes Sindbis virus and VEE chimeric viruses, alphavirus replicon particles, DNA vaccines, and adenovirus vector vaccines.[29]

Mosquito control with a combination of larvicides and adulticides may be indicated to mitigate large outbreaks. Taking precautions against mosquito bites, such as using repellents, staying in well-screened or air-conditioned areas when possible, and wearing long-sleeved shirts and long pants, is advised for persons who cannot avoid traveling to areas experiencing epidemics.

NEW REFERENCES SINCE THE SEVENTH EDITION

15. Gardner C, Sun C, Luke T, et al. Antibody preparations from human transchromosomic cows exhibit prophylactic and therapeutic efficacy versus Venezuelan equine encephalitis virus. *J Virol.* 2017;91(14):e00226-27.
46. Wang Y, Ostilund E, Jun Y, et al. Combining reverse-transcription multiplex PCR and microfluidic electrophoresis to simultaneously detect seven mosquito-transmitted zoonotic encephalomyelitis viruses. *Vet J.* 2016;212:27-35.

The full reference list for this chapter is available at ExpertConsult.com.

175D ■ Chikungunya

Scott B. Halstead

Chikungunya is a benign short-duration dengue-like febrile syndrome in children that in the very young carries a high risk for complicated outcomes. Infections of neonates may result in an elevated risk for neurologic complications and in a pantropic disease with a significant fatality rate. In adults, chikungunya produces fever followed by leukopenia, maculopapular rash, and arthralgia that may persist for months as polyarthritis. In the Makonde language *chikungunya* means "that which bends up," referring to the characteristic symptom of arthralgia.[80] In historical times, the terms *knokkel koorts, abu rokab, mal de genoux, dengue, dyenga,* and *3-day fever* have been given to epidemics probably caused by chikungunya virus.[14,35]

ETIOLOGIC AGENT

Chikungunya virus was isolated in 1952 by inoculating suckling mice with infected mosquitoes and blood from cases during an explosive dengue-like epidemic in the Makonde district on the border between Tanganyika and Mozambique.[52,59,80,82] Chikungunya genome consists of a capped 11.8-kilobase positive-sense single-stranded RNA with a poly(A) tail. The genome is composed of two open reading frames (ORFs) between nontranslated regions. The ORF located at the 5′ end of the genome encodes a polyprotein precursor of nonstructural proteins with replicative and proteolytic activities. The second ORF encodes the polyprotein precursor of the structural proteins.[70]

Chikungunya virus is an alphavirus in the Togavirus family and a member of the Semliki Forest complex related to Ross River, o'nyong-nyong, and Semliki Forest viruses.[70] Phylogenetic analysis of the E1 envelope glycoprotein divides chikungunya virus into two distinct geographic genotypes.[71,101] One genotype consists of viruses from Senegal and Nigeria and is named the *West Africa genotype.* These viruses have only 78% to 85% nucleotide sequence identity to viruses of East, Central, and South Africa (ECSA) and the closely related Asian viruses. The phyletic grouping is consistent with the introduction during 1879 to 1956 of East African strains into Asia, where it continues to circulate.[71,101]

Chikungunya virus produces death in infant mice, rats, and hamsters after intracerebral inoculation. Serial passage of the virus in mice has resulted in selection of a strain with a short incubation period that is lethal to weanling mice.[82] Virus grows to titers of 10^8 to 10^9 infectious doses per milliliter. Low-passage material is highly infectious for humans during routine laboratory handling, and therefore appropriate precautions should be taken by laboratory workers. If a mouse brain seed suspension of low-passage virus is prepared and inoculated into other mice at a 1:5 or 1:10 final concentration, death may be delayed significantly, may be sporadic, or may not occur at all. This difference is due to autointerference caused by an Asian strain that also produced hemorrhagic enteritis in rats and hamsters.[36]

Chikungunya virus produces a cytopathic effect in primary hamster kidney cells and in BHK-21, BSC-1, Vero, FL, HeLa, and rhesus kidney cells.[45] Virus multiplies in *Aedes albopictus, Aedes aegypti, Aedes vittatus, Anopheles stephensi,* and *Culex fatigans* continuous cell lines and in a cell line derived from *Drosophila.* Plaque assays have been described in LLC-MK2, Vero, and BHK-21 cells and in duck and chick embryo cell cultures.[45]

ZOONOTIC CYCLES

Chikungunya virus has been recovered from wild *A. aegypti* in Tanzania, Nigeria, India, and Thailand; from *Aedes africanus* in Uganda and Bangui; from *Aedes furcifer-taylori* in South Africa and Senegal; and from *Aedes luteocephalus* and *Aedes dalzieli* in Senegal.[3,20,26,44,59,61] Occasional isolates have been recovered from *Mansonia fuscopennata* in Uganda and from *C. fatigans* in Thailand and Tanzania. Transmission to humans has been demonstrated with the *A. furcifer-taylori* group; transmission to monkeys or mice has been demonstrated with *A. aegypti, A. albopictus, Aedes calceatus, Aedes triseriatus, Aedes togoi, Aedes pseudoscutellaris, Aedes polynesiensis, Anopheles albinanus, Mansonia africana,* and *Aedes apicoargenteus.*[45,57,67,87]

Chikungunya antibodies have been found in vervet monkeys, baboons, chimpanzees, and red-tailed monkeys in Zimbabwe, South Africa, and Uganda.[56] In Africa, zoonotic transmission to subhuman primates is surmised to take place in a wide variety of habitats, with transmission occurring in the forest canopy, at ground level, or both.[58] Chikungunya appears to be enzootic throughout much of eastern, central, southern, and western Africa.[45] Subhuman primate populations are affected in epizootics, which involve critical numbers of the susceptible population, followed by disappearance of the virus. Thus chikungunya may maintain itself in wildlife populations by constantly moving epizootic activity, in much the same fashion as respiratory tract and enteric virus infections are maintained in humans. A series of outbreaks originating from Central-South African lineage strains caused outbreaks in Cameroon and Gabon in 2007.[98]

Based on human outbreaks, chikungunya virus has emerged to cause Asian pandemics from its East African zoonotic cycle at roughly 50-year intervals since 1770. The factors that control this phenomenon are unidentified.

EPIDEMIOLOGY

History

The classical account, widely thought to be the initial description of "dengue fever," is a report by David Bylon, who was *staads chirurgyn* ("city surgeon") to the Batavia (capital of the Dutch East Indies, now Jakarta) in the year 1779.[12] Dr. Bylon, who himself contracted the illness, wrote the following:

> It was last May 25, in the afternoon at 5:00 when I noted while talking with two good friends of mine, a growing pain in my right hand, and the joints of the lower arm, which step by step proceeded upward to the shoulder and then continued onto all my limbs; so much so that at 9:00 that same evening I was already in my bed with a high fever....
>
> It's now been three weeks since I ... was stricken by the illness, and because of that had to stay home for 5 days; but even until today I have continuously pain and stiffness in the joints of both feet, with swelling of both ankles; so much so, that when I get up in the morning, or have sat up for a while and start to move again, I cannot do so very well and going up and down stairs is very painful.

This account of a febrile illness of acute onset with prominent involvement of the joints clearly suggests that this was chikungunya (see Clinical Manifestations). In the same year in Cairo and Alexandria, Egypt, a large outbreak occurred of a disease with these same features.[14,18,19,88] An important pandemic of a febrile exanthem occurred in the years 1870 to 1873 appearing first on the East African coast and then on the coasts of Arabia, Port Said, and Egypt. From there it was carried to Bombay and Calcutta, India, and Java. The 1870 outbreak led to the recognition that the Swahili words for this disease were *ki-dinga pepo*.[18] The term *denga* or *dyenga* had been used to designate this same disease in Africa during an earlier outbreak in 1823. In that pandemic, *denga* had spread with the slave trade to the Caribbean, where in 1827 the virus was introduced on St. Thomas then throughout the Caribbean and the Atlantic coastal cities of North and South America.[19,35] In Cuba, the Spanish homonym of *dyenga, dengue*, was introduced.

In 2005–06 a notable epidemic occurred on Reunion, Mauritius, Madagascar, Mayotte, and Seychelles.[76] This soon spread to India and to Southeast Asia.[48,73] The Reunion virus was brought by tourists to Europe, where modest autochthonous outbreaks occurred in southeastern France and northeastern Italy.[33,69] In 2013, the older ECSA-Asian genotype virus reached the American hemisphere after an absence of almost 200 years. As in 1827, chikungunya was first identified on an island adjacent to St. Thomas. As of April 2016, the Pan American Health Organization had reported that autochthonous transmission of the disease, first recognized in December 2013, was reported from 52 countries or territories in the Caribbean and Central, South, and North America. A total of 1,851,157 suspected and 65,066 laboratory-confirmed cases and 211 deaths had been attributed to chikungunya. During 2017, more than 150,000 cases and 88 deaths from suspected or confirmed chikungunya were reported to the Pan American Health Organization as of September 17, 2017.[104] Chikungunya virus completed the circumnavigation of the globe when Caribbean virus was introduced into Europe and Africa.[25]

Geographic Distribution

When susceptible human and *A. aegypti* or *A. albopictus* populations are above the threshold level required for chikungunya transmission, a person-mosquito-person cycle is established. This cycle probably is responsible for most of the large urban outbreaks of chikungunya studied during the past 40 years. Characteristically, chikungunya pandemics transmitted by *A. aegypti* are explosive. Studying *A. aegypti* in laboratory mice, Rao and colleagues documented mechanical transmission.[75] Viremia in humans may be as high as 10^8 infectious doses per milliliter.[75] Because the extrinsic incubation period in *A. aegypti* is relatively long, the explosive nature of chikungunya outbreaks was thought to be best explained by mechanical transmission, possibly complemented by biting *Culex* species. During the introduction of chikungunya on Reunion in 2005, an amino acid substitution in position 224 of the E1 protein resulted in enhanced transmissibility by *A. albopictus*. Subsequently, a further mutation occurred in E2-L210Q that enhanced fitness in *A. albopictus*. The new ECSA variants produced the huge Asian pandemic that followed the Reunion outbreak.[99,100] On Reunion the *A. albopictus*–borne outbreak, with a duration of about 4 months, affected an estimated 35% of a population of 800,000.[77] Ironically, it was the older ECSA-Asian strain that, when introduced into the Americas in 2013, produced the hemispheric pandemic.[103]

Serologic studies have demonstrated repeatedly the presence of antibodies in humans throughout the moist forests and semiarid savannas of East and West Africa.[1,26,61,84] In Africa, chikungunya outbreaks have been reported from Uganda, Tanzania, Zimbabwe, South Africa, Angola, Zaire, Nigeria, Senegal, Madagascar, and Reunion.[45] This distribution best fits the present location of virus research laboratories. A reasonable assumption is that chikungunya is endemic throughout sub-Saharan Africa. According to historical reports, pandemics swept into India in 1824, 1871, 1902, 1923, and during the modern virologic era in 1963 and 2006, extending into the Indonesian archipelago in the 18th and 19th centuries.[14,19,88]

At some point in time, the ECSA chikungunya virus became established in South East Asia. An extensive neutralizing antibody survey suggested chikungunya activity during World War II in Kalimantan and Sulawesi, Indonesia.[91] In the late 1950s and early 1960s, chikungunya was found to be transmitted continuously in urban and rural Thailand, Cambodia, and South Vietnam.[16,38,39,102] Involvement of urban populations in Burma appears to have been intermittent, with outbreaks recorded in 1963 and from 1970 to 1973.[60] A large chikungunya epidemic affected much of Indonesia in 1983 and 1984 and Burma in 1984 and 1985.[94] Chikungunya virus was isolated in Australia in 1989.[40] Serologic evidence of chikungunya virus infection has been found throughout the Philippines, possibly during World War II. Since then, localized outbreaks have occurred in Manila, Philippines, in 1967 and Negros, Philippines, in 1968,[5,13,53,85] and as recently as 2012–13.[85] After having disappeared in the 1970s, chikungunya was found again at low-level transmission in Thailand, Myanmar (formerly Burma), and Indonesia in 1990.[93] Little or no chikungunya virus activity was reported in the 20th century in Papua New Guinea, the Solomon Islands, Vanuatu (formerly New Hebrides), the Caroline Islands, the Pacific Islands, or any of the American tropics.[92]

A pertinent question to ask is why chikungunya and dengue viruses, both transmitted by *A. aegypti*, do not have an identical geographic distribution. This may be due partially to differences in the transmissability of chikungunya and dengue by vector mosquitoes. The threshold for infection of chikungunya virus in *A. aegypti* is relatively high, approximately 10^6 mouse infectious doses are required to infect 50% of adult female mosquitoes.[92] The infection threshold of female *A. aegypti* for dengue virus is rather similar. However, *A. aegypti* mosquitoes infected with chikungunya virus transmit virus to vertebrates poorly, whereas dengue-infected mosquitoes transmit with great regularity.[34] Thus transmission of chikungunya virus is expected in areas with high human susceptibility rates and high densities of *A. aegypti*.

CLINICAL MANIFESTATIONS

The global pandemic of chikungunya that followed the escape of virus from East Africa in 2005 has added substantially to our understanding of the clinical and pathophysiologic attributes of human infection. Infections in young children are predominantly inapparent.[4] The incubation period of chikungunya fever is usually 2 to 4 days. In infants, the disease typically begins with the abrupt onset of fever, followed by flushing of the skin. Febrile convulsions may occur in as many as one-third of patients. After 3 to 5 days of fever, a generalized maculopapular rash and lymphadenopathy are noted. Conjunctival injection, swelling of the eyelids, pharyngitis, and signs and symptoms of upper respiratory tract disease are common. No enanthem occurs. Some infants have a biphasic fever curve, and arthralgia may be quite severe, although it is not seen frequently. In Nicaragua, 2.9% of children older than 9 years had arthritis.[4,9,15,37,43,65]

Chikungunya infections early in pregnancy may infect the fetus rarely and result in a miscarriage.[30] Vertical transmission is rare. Of 678 women with antepartum or peripartum chikungunya who delivered live babies, none circulated chikungunya immunoglobulin M (IgM) antibodies. Perinatal infections of neonates were reported on Reunion, rising to nearly 50% when mothers were viremic in the week just preceding delivery.[74] Of 39 babies born to mothers experiencing chikungunya infections at the time of delivery, all developed a febrile illness beginning on day 4. Caesarean delivery of infants did not prevent chikungunya infections. Nine of these infants developed encephalopathy. Lymphopenia and thrombocytopenia were common, in some cases profound, but without severe bleeding. Most infants with chikungunya infections developed erythematous skin lesions and evidence of joint involvement. During the chikungunya outbreak on Reunion, 25% of young children developed neurologic symptoms, whereas in India 14% of all children presenting with suspected central nervous system infection had chikungunya.[51,78] Sequelae were studied in 35 Reunion babies infected perinatally. At 21 months, infected children exhibit poorer neurocognitive skills than uninfected peers as evidenced by lower global developmental quotient scores and diminished specific neurocognitive skills, even reaching abnormal ranges for coordination and language. The incidence of the global developmental delay in infected children was just more than 50%.[32] Rarely, infants younger than 6 months with chikungunya may exhibit extensive bullous skin lesions with blistering covering up to 35% of the body surface area.[79]

In older children, fever is accompanied by headache, myalgia, and arthralgia involving various joints. Residual arthralgia has been described but is uncommon.[41] Joint pain is typically polyarticular, bilateral, and symmetric and affects mainly the extremities (ankles, wrists, phalanges) but also larger joints (shoulders, elbows, knees).[55,89,95] Joint symptoms can fluctuate in intensity, but do not usually vary in their anatomic location. Swelling may also occur in the interphalangeal joints, wrists, and ankles, as well as pain along ligament insertions, notably in children. An early macular blush is followed by a maculopapular rash that accompanies or immediately precedes defervescence. At the same time, marked lymphadenopathy occurs. Febrile convulsions are observed commonly in younger children. Hemorrhagic findings, including a positive tourniquet test, are rare.[9,15,37,43,65] Chikungunya viruses were recovered from saliva obtained during acute illness in 10 of 13 children, some of whom had bleeding gums.[29] As further evidence that chikungunya replicates in oral and nasal mucosa, three adult Venezuelan patients with virologically confirmed disease developed extensive acute nasal skin necrosis early in the course of a life-threatening illness characterized by shock and organ dysfunction.[97] There is evidence of direct person-to-person spread of chikungunya, presumably through infected mucosal secretions.[81]

Although dengue and chikungunya illnesses are similar, important distinguishing features are summarized in Tables 175D.1 TO 175D.4 from clinical data obtained from children in Thailand.[37,65]

Table 175D.1 shows the abrupt onset and early severity of chikungunya versus dengue illnesses, many of which came to medical attention only several days after the onset of fever.

Chikungunya virus infections are shorter in duration than dengue virus infections (see Table 175D.2). Almost half of children with chikungunya had a fever that ended within 72 hours after onset, whereas the median duration of dengue fever was 2 days longer.

Many constitutional signs and symptoms occur with similar frequency in chikungunya and dengue viral infections and cannot be used to differentiate the illnesses clinically (see Table 175D.3). However, a terminal maculopapular rash, arthralgia or arthritis, and conjunctival injection were more common symptoms in chikungunya than in dengue (see Table 175D.4). Shock has been reported infrequently in chikungunya.[15,86,96] It was not observed in Thai cases.[65] Changes in taste perception and bradycardia, depression, or asthenia after illness are found rarely in

TABLE 175D.1 Chikungunya and Dengue in Children[a]: Comparison of Onset of Illness

	HOSPITALIZED				OUTPATIENT			
	Chikungunya (32 Cases)		Dengue (523 Cases)[b]		Chikungunya (17 Cases)		Primary Dengue (29 Cases)	
Day of Illness	No.	%	No.	%	No.	%	No.	%
0	8	25	2	0.4	0	0	0	0
1	15	47	44	8	11	65	8	27
2	5	16	67	13	1	6	5	17
3	2	6	145	28	2	12	3	10
4	1	3	148	28	0	0	7	24
5	1	3	84	16	3	17	4	14
6			20	4			2	
7			11	2			7	
≥8			3	0.6				

[a]Patients with simultaneous dengue and chikungunya are excluded from analysis.
[b]Includes primary and secondary infections.
Data from Nimmannitya S, Halstead SB, Cohen SN, et al. Dengue and chikungunya virus infection in man in Thailand, 1962–1964. I. Observations on hospitalized patients with hemorrhagic fever. *Am J Trop Med Hyg*. 1969;18:954–971; and Halstead SB, Nimmannitya S, Margiota MR. Dengue and chikungunya virus infection in man in Thailand, 1962–1964. II. Observations on disease in outpatients. *Am J Trop Med Hyg*. 1969;18:972–83.

chikungunya; these manifestations are distinctive findings in patients with dengue.

The frequencies of hemorrhagic findings in chikungunya and primary and secondary dengue viral infections in Thai children are compared in Table 175D.5. The frequency of minor hemorrhagic manifestations in outpatient and inpatient dengue did not differ significantly from that in chikungunya cases. However, petechial rash and spontaneous hematemesis or melena developed in only hospitalized dengue cases.

TABLE 175D.2 Chikungunya and Dengue in Children: Comparison of Duration of Illness

Duration of Fever (days)	CHIKUNGUNYA (32 CASES) No.	%	DENGUE (241 CASES)[a] No.	%
2	11	34.4	8	3.3
3	4	12.5	16	6.6
4	5	15.6	33	13.7
5	5	15.6	53	21.6
6	2	6.3	53	21.6
7	3	9.4	38	15.8
≥8	2	6.3	42	17.4
	Mean, 4 days		Mean, 5.85 days	

[a]Includes primary and secondary dengue infections.
Modified from Nimmannitya S, Halstead SB, Cohen SN, et al. Dengue and chikungunya virus infection in man in Thailand, 1962–1964. I. Observations on hospitalized patients with hemorrhagic fever. *Am J Trop Med Hyg.* 1969;18:954–971.

PATHOGENESIS AND PATHOLOGY

The pathophysiology of chikungunya chronic disease remains poorly understood, and to date, no animal model fully reproduces the chronic joint syndrome associated with many cases. In humans, patients with chronic chikungunya-induced arthralgia often have persistent virus-specific IgM that could result from continued exposure to chikungunya antigen.[7,50,54] A C57BL/6J mouse model results in arthritis, tenosynovitis, and myositis [62] Chikungunya infection in nonhuman primates (NHPs) results in acute fever, rash, viremia, and production of interferon type 1. NHPs develop CHIKV-specific B and T cells, generating neutralizing antibodies and specific $CD4^+$ and $CD8^+$ T cells.[11] In a cynomolgus monkey model with long-duration chikungunya, spleen, liver, muscle, and joint infection have been described.[47] Chikungunya antigens have been detected by immunohistochemistry in muscle satellite cells of muscle biopsy specimens from two patients with a myositic syndrome[66] and in fibroblasts of the joint capsule, skeletal muscle, and dermis from a fatal neonatal case.[22,23] Chikungunya virus infects and persists in human cornea tissue, and viral infection has been transmitted surgically.[21] In vitro studies have shown that other cell types, such as human epithelial and endothelial cells, primary fibroblasts, and to a lesser extent, monocyte-derived macrophages, are also able to sustain productive chikungunya infections.[22,23,47] Wild-type chikungunya strains produce a hemorrhagic enteritis in mice and hamsters.[36] NHPs are useful for

TABLE 175D.3 Chikungunya and Dengue in Children: Comparison of Frequency of Clinical Findings

	HOSPITALIZED				OUTPATIENT			
	Chikungunya (32 Cases)		Dengue (142 Cases)[a]		Chikungunya (17 Cases)		Primary Dengue (27 Cases)[a]	
Day of Illness	**No.**	**%**	**No.[b]**	**%**	**No.**	**%**	**No.**	**%**
Headache	13/19	68	37/83	45	2	12	4	15
Injected pharynx	28/31	90	121/125	97	12	71	27	100
Enanthem	3/27	11	7/84	8	0	24	0	22
Rhinitis	3/31	6	6/47	13	4	6	6	41
Cough	7/30	22	17/79	22	1	35	11	56
Vomiting	19/32	59	73/126	58	6	6	15	15
Constipation	12/30	40	16/30	53	0	18	4	4
Diarrhea	5/32	16	5/78	6	1		1	7
Abdominal pain	6/19	32	38/76	50	3		2	
Lymphadenopathy	8/26	31	32/79	41				
Restlessness	10/30	33	17/79	22				

[a]Includes primary and secondary dengue infections.
[b]Number with finding/number with observations recorded.
Data from Nimmannitya S, Halstead SB, Cohen SN, et al. Dengue and chikungunya virus infection in man in Thailand, 1962–1964. I. Observations on hospitalized patients with hemorrhagic fever. *Am J Trop Med Hyg.* 1969;18:954–971; and Halstead SB, Nimmannitya S, Margiota MR. Dengue and chikungunya virus infection in man in Thailand, 1962–1964. II. Observations on disease in outpatients. *Am J Trop Med Hyg.* 1969;18:972–983.

TABLE 175D.4 Chikungunya and Dengue in Children: Clinical Findings Occurring With Different Frequency

Manifestation	CHIKUNGUNYA (32 CASES) No.[b]	%	DENGUE[a] (32 CASES) No.[b]	%	Significance
Maculopapular rash	19/32	59.4	16/132	12.1	$P<.001$
Conjunctival injection	15/27	55.6	20/61	32.8	$.05 > P<.01$
Myalgias, arthralgias	8/20	40.0	9/75	12.0	$.05 > P<.01$

[a]Includes primary and secondary dengue infections.
[b]Number positive/number of observations.
From Nimmannitya S, Halstead SB, Cohen SN, et al. Dengue and chikungunya virus infection in man in Thailand, 1962–1964. I. Observations on hospitalized patients with hemorrhagic fever. *Am J Trop Med Hyg.* 1969;18:954–971.

TABLE 175D.5 **Chikungunya and Dengue in Children: Comparison of Frequency of Clinical Findings**

	CHIKUNGUNYA				PRIMARY DENGUE		SECONDARY DENGUE	
	Outpatients (17 Cases)		**Inpatients (32 Cases)**		**Outpatients (27 Cases)**		**Inpatients (135 Cases)**	
Day of Illness	***No.***[a]	***%***	***No.***	***%***	***No.***	***%***	***No.***	***%***
Positive tourniquet test result	3/17	18.0	24/31	77.4	4/27	14.8	94/112	83.9
Petechiae, scattered	0/17	0	10/32	31.2	4/27	7.4	60/129	46.5
Petechial rash	0/17	0	0/32	0	2/27	7.4	13/129	10.1
Maculopapular rash	0/17	0	19/32	59.4	1/27	3.7	16/132	12.1
Epistaxis	0/17	0	4/32	12.5	0/27	0	20/106	18.9
Gum bleeding			0/32	0			2/135	1.5
Melena, hematemesis			0/32	0			14/119	11.8

[a]Number positive/number of observations.
From Nimmannitya S, Halstead SB, Cohen SN, et al. Dengue and chikungunya virus infection in man in Thailand, 1962–1964. I. Observations on hospitalized patients with hemorrhagic fever. *Am J Trop Med Hyg.* 1969;18:954–971; and Halstead SB, Nimmannitya S, Margiota MR. Dengue and chikungunya virus infection in man in Thailand, 1962–1964. II. Observations on disease in outpatients. *Am J Trop Med Hyg.* 1969;18:972–983.

preclinical testing of vaccines and therapeutics and uncovering the details of pathogenesis.

DIAGNOSIS

The differential diagnosis includes the viral causes of dengue fever syndrome.[49] In Australia and the western Pacific area, Ross River fever is a frequent cause of epidemic, arthropod-borne, viral arthralgia.

Laboratory diagnosis depends on demonstrating chikungunya virus or viral RNA during the first 5 days after onset of fever or detection of IgM chikungunya antibodies 5 or more days after onset of fever.[42,72] Commercially, these are detected using the IgM-capture enzyme-linked immunosorbent assay. The assays currently on the market perform well, although they are unable to distinguish chikungunya from viruses in the Semliki Forest virus group.[6,46,64,72] Virus may be isolated by inoculating acute-phase serum or other suspect materials intracerebrally in 1- to 2-day-old mice or in tissue cultures. On initial passage, death may occur within 2 to 5 days after inoculation. An autointerference phenomenon is noted if low-dilution passages of infected mouse brain are performed. Passage at a 10^{-3} dilution or higher avoids this effect. Vero cells and suckling mice are equally effective for primary isolation. To differentiate infections caused by other members of the Semliki Forest viral group, neutralizing antibodies can be measured on convalescent sera.

TREATMENT

Treatment is supportive. Antirheumatoid drugs may be effective for management of chronic arthritis; however, chloroquine phosphate 250 mg/day, once touted for management of acute arthritic pain, had no effect in a double-blinded trial.[24] Analgesics or mild sedation may be required to control pain. Arthritis after illness may require continued treatment with antiinflammatory agents and graduated physiotherapy. Salicylates, because of their hemorrhagic potential, are contraindicated. Bed rest is advised during the febrile period. Antipyretics or cold sponging should be used to keep the body temperature below 40°C (104°F).

Seizures may be benign febrile seizures or may be a sign of encephalitis and may be treated with anticonvulsant medications. Children who have lost excessive fluid because of vomiting, fasting, or thirsting and who cannot take oral fluids may require intravenous rehydration. Individuals with severe hemorrhagic phenomena should be evaluated for underlying clotting disorders.

Human neutralizing monoclonal antibodies directed against E2 or E1 significantly delay lethality of chikungunya-infected mice, in both prophylactic and therapeutic settings.[27,28] It has been suggested that administration of chikungunya antibodies might protect infants exposed to infection perinatally.[22,23]

PROGNOSIS

In some instances, isolation or serologic evidence of recent infection has been obtained in persons with severe hemorrhagic findings and in individuals dying during an acute febrile illness.[15,43,63,76,86] In addition to hemorrhage, neurologic and myocardial involvement has been reported during chikungunya infection in adults.[15,17,22] In adults, arthralgia may persist for weeks, and exercise may prolong this symptom. Typically, pain shifts from joint to joint and is worse in the morning and on first use of the joint. Swelling of ankles, wrists, and fingers occurs frequently. In older patients, the sequelae may resemble rheumatoid arthritis.[8] In the Reunion Island outbreak, 57% of adult patients experienced long-duration symptoms, half of which impaired daily activities.[90] Chronic rheumatic manifestations were associated with age, severity of initial acute illness pain, and presence of osteoarthritis.[90] A destructive arthropathy after illness has been reported.[10,55] Chikungunya virus infection might coincide with other pathologic processes and result in death of the individual. Carefully studied, virologically documented cases have shown neither thrombocytopenia nor severe neutropenia.[43,55] Until more is known of the pathogenesis of chikungunya virus infection, estimating the frequency with which death can be attributed directly to chikungunya fever will be difficult.

Infants with chikungunya may experience residual neurologic deficits after recovery from encephalitis.[22,23,31]

PREVENTION

A very large number of chikungunya vaccine constructs have been developed and subjected to preclinical testing since the 1960s. These range from formalin inactivate whole virus and tissue culture passaged attenuated virus, to various chimeric, DNA, subunit and virus-like particle vaccines.[2] A measles chikungunya vaccine developed by the Institut Pasteur is projected to enter clinical trials by Themis Inc.[2] A vaccine engineered to carry an internal response sequence element between the nonstructural and the structural genes produced a successfully attenuated virus that prevented virus replication in vector mosquitoes. Further, in subhuman primates this vaccine was immunogenic and protective.[68,83] Whether and when safe and protective chikungunya vaccines will come on to the market is an open question.

At present, prevention consists of avoiding mosquito bites. For urban outbreaks in most of the Asian and African tropics, the regimen for individual protection and for chronic and emergency control is the same as has been described for dengue. When other vectors are involved, measures designed to combat *A. aegypti* may fail. In such outbreaks, expert entomologic advice will be needed to design appropriate preventive measures.

NEW REFERENCES SINCE THE SEVENTH EDITION

2. Ahola T, Courderc T, Ng LF, et al. Therapeutics and vaccines against chikungunya virus. *Vector Borne Zoonotic Dis*. 2015;15(4):250-257.
4. Balmaseda A, Gordon A, Gresh L, et al. Clinical attack rate of chikungunya in a cohort of Nicaraguan children. *Am J Trop Med Hyg*. 2016;94(2):397-399.
11. Broeckel R, Haese N, Messaoudi I, et al. Nonhuman primate models of chikungunya virus infection and disease (CHIKV NHP model). *Pathogens*. 2015;4(3):662-681.
23. Couderc T, Lecuit M. Chikungunya virus pathogenesis: from bedside to bench. *Antiviral Res*. 2015;121:120-131.
25. Delisle E, Rousseau C, Broche B, et al. Chikungunya outbreak in Montpellier, France, September to October 2014. *Euro Surveill*. 2015;20(17).
27. Fong RH, Banik SS, Mattia K, et al. Exposure of epitope residues on the outer face of the chikungunya virus envelope trimer determines antibody neutralizing efficacy. *J Virol*. 2014;88(24):14364-14379.
28. Fric J, Bertin-Maghit S, Wang CI, et al. Use of human monoclonal antibodies to treat chikungunya virus infection. *J Infect Dis*. 2013;207(2):319-322.
29. Gardner J, Rudd PA, Prow NA, et al. Infectious chikungunya virus in the saliva of mice, monkeys and humans. *PLoS ONE*. 2015;10(10):e0139481.
31. Gerardin P, Couderc T, Bintner M, et al. Chikungunya virus-associated encephalitis: a cohort study on La Reunion Island, 2005–2009. *Neurology*. 2016;86(1):94-102.
32. Gerardin P, Samperiz S, Ramful D, et al. Neurocognitive outcome of children exposed to perinatal mother-to-child Chikungunya virus infection: the CHIMERE cohort study on Reunion Island. *PLoS Negl Trop Dis*. 2014;8(7):e2996.
35. Halstead SB. Reappearance of chikungunya, formerly called dengue, in the Americas. *Emerg Infect Dis*. 2015;21(4):557-561.
41. Hawman DW, Stoermer KA, Montgomery SA, et al. Chronic joint disease caused by persistent chikungunya virus infection is controlled by the adaptive immune response. *J Virol*. 2013;87(24):13878-13888.
42. Jacobsen S, Patel P, Schmidt-Chanasit J, et al. External quality assessment studies for laboratory performance of molecular and serological diagnosis of chikungunya virus infection. *J Clin Virol*. 2016;76:55-65.
46. Kosasih H, Widjaja S, Surya E, et al. Evaluation of two IgM rapid immunochromatographic tests during circulation of Asian lineage chikungunya virus. *Southeast Asian J Trop Med Public Health*. 2012;43(1):55-61.
64. Niedrig M, Zeller H, Schuffenecker I, et al. International diagnostic accuracy study for the serological detection of chikungunya virus infection. *Clin Microbiol Infect*. 2009;15(9):880-884.
68. Plante KS, Rossi SL, Bergren NA, et al. Extended preclinical safety, efficacy and stability testing of a live-attenuated chikungunya vaccine candidate. *Plos Negl Trop Dis*. 2015;9(9):e0004007.
72. Prat CM, Flusin O, Panella A, et al. Evaluation of commercially available serologic diagnostic tests for chikungunya virus. *Emerg Infect Dis*. 2014;20(12): 2129-2132.
81. Rolph MS, Zaid A, Mahalingam S. Salivary transmission of the chikungunya arbovirus. *Trends Microbiol*. 2016;24(2):86-87.
83. Roy CJ, Adams AP, Wang E, et al. Chikungunya vaccine candidate is highly attenuated and protects nonhuman primates against telemetrically monitored disease following a single dose. *J Infect Dis*. 2014;209(12):1891-1899.
85. Salje H, Cauchemez S, Alera MT, et al. Reconstruction of 60 years of chikungunya epidemiology in the Philippines demonstrates episodic and focal transmission. *J Infect Dis*. 2016;213(4):604-610.
95. Thiberville SD, Boisson V, Gaudart J, et al. Chikungunya fever: a clinical and virological investigation of outpatients on Reunion Island, South-West Indian Ocean. *PLoS Negl Trop Dis*. 2013;7(1):e2004.
97. Torres JR, Cordova LG, Saravia V, et al. Nasal skin necrosis: an unexpected new finding in severe chikungunya fever. *Clin Infect Dis*. 2016;62(1):78-81.
103. Weaver SC, Forrester NL. Chikungunya: evolutionary history and recent epidemic spread. *Antiviral Res*. 2015;120:32-39.
104. Pan American Health Association. *Chikungunya*. Available at: http://www.paho.org/hq/index.php?Itemid=40931.

The full reference list for this chapter is available at ExpertConsult.com.

175E ▪ Ross River Virus Arthritis

John G. Aaskov • Roy A. Hall

Epidemics of a benign disease that caused polyarthralgia and rash were first described in Australia in 1927[69] and subsequently in 1943.[44] After recovery of the causative agent and the advent of serologic tests for diagnosing Ross River virus infection, epidemic polyarthritis was recognized as endemic in Australia. It has occurred as epidemics in numerous Pacific nations.

Approximately 4000 cases of epidemic polyarthritis are reported in Australia each year, with a peak of more than 9000 cases in 2015. In 2002, the median direct and indirect cost of a case of epidemic polyarthritis was estimated to be AUD\$2000. Approximately 50% of this amount resulted from disability and 30% from health care costs.[75]

Some confusion has been generated by use of the term *Ross River fever* to describe clinical Ross River virus infections because fever does not develop in more than one half of those with clinical disease.[65] Additional confusion resulted from efforts to describe polyarthritis caused by any Australian arbovirus as epidemic polyarthritis. The term *epidemic polyarthritis* should be used to describe only clinical disease caused by Ross River virus.

ETIOLOGIC AGENT

Investigations of an epidemic of polyarthritis in southern Australia in 1956[14,83] suggested that an alphavirus was the causative agent. This was confirmed when Ross River virus was isolated from *Aedes vigilax* mosquitoes collected beside the Ross River near Townsville in northern Australia, and serologic evidence showed it to be the causative agent of epidemic polyarthritis.[26,29] Although the first isolation of virus from a human was from a febrile child without arthritis,[25] subsequent use of mosquito cell lines enabled Ross River virus to be recovered regularly from epidemic polyarthritis patients.[11,30,86]

Ross River virus is related serologically to Getah and Bebaru viruses in the Semliki Forest virus subgroup.[23] Nucleotide sequencing has confirmed the close relationship among Ross River, Getah, and Semliki Forest viruses.[74] Phylogenetic analyses have identified four lineages of Ross River virus, three of which appear to have become extinct.[50] The appearance of the current lineage was associated with major genetic arrangements in the *nsP3* gene of Ross River virus.[7] No association has been observed between any particular virus genotype and disease in humans, but this may be because most studies employ consensus nucleotide sequences for what, genetically, are very diverse viral populations.[59]

Cryoelectron microscopic studies[19,72,90] suggest that the nucleocapsid of Ross River virus is approximately 400 Å in diameter and has a triangulation (T) = 4 quaternary structure. It is surrounded by a membrane bilayer that is penetrated by 80 spikes that are also arranged in a T = 4 lattice. Each spike is a trimer of heterodimers of the envelope glycoproteins E1 and E2. The E2 protein makes contact with heparin on the surface of host cells, and antibodies that combine with this protein neutralize infection in vitro.[5,84,87]

The virus can be adapted to grow to high titer in the muscle and brain of 1-day-old mice, in which it causes paralysis and death.[62,66] Ross River virus also grows to high titer in vertebrate and mosquito cell lines.[11]

TRANSMISSION AND EPIDEMIOLOGY

Ross River virus is endemic in all mainland states of Australia and in Papua New Guinea. The incidence of epidemic polyarthritis is highest in the Australian states of Queensland, Northern Territory, and Western Australia, with other states experiencing outbreaks of infection against a background of low incidence (http://www.health.gov.au/internet/main/publishing.nsf/Content/cda-surveil-nndss-nndssintro.htm).

No transmission of Ross River virus had been reported from the Pacific island states involved in the 1979 to 1980 epidemic (Fiji, Samoa, Tonga, and Cook Islands)[8,30,54,76,86] until 2003, when cases of epidemic polyarthritis began to be detected in travelers who had visited Fiji,[55,56] suggesting that Ross River virus may have become endemic in that country. Sporadic cases without local virus transmission have occurred in Europe, the United States and countries in Southeast Asia that included tourists and military personnel returning from Australia.

Isolation of Ross River virus from more than 20 species of mosquitoes,[77] particularly *A. vigilax*[29,42] and *Culex annulirostris*,[28,42] and the presence of antibody to the virus in almost as many species of animals, particularly mammals,[26,27,73] suggested a mammal-mosquito cycle with humans as an incidental host. However, improved laboratory diagnostic services have shown that clinical infection in humans occurs throughout the year, although most cases are seen in the late summer and in autumn, and most patients are city dwellers.[10,65] Taken together with the explosive spread of disease during the 1979 to 1980 epidemic of Ross River virus infection in the Pacific,[8,30,76,86] this virus appears to be maintained in either of two cycles, mammal-mosquito-mammal or human-mosquito-human, with movement of virus between the two. Evidence also has been obtained of transovarial transmission of Ross River virus in *Aedes* mosquitoes.[53,58]

Patients may be viremic for up to 7 days after the onset of symptoms.[10,76] The incubation time from infection to the onset of symptoms may vary from 1 to 27 days; an interval of 7 to 9 days is usual endemic areas.[35]

In endemic areas, the ratio of subclinical to clinical infection may be as high as 50 : 1,[10] but during outbreaks, the ratio can be reduced to 4 : 1 or less.[8,45] Approximately 1.5% of humans living in northern Australia are infected with Ross River virus each year,[10] but the rates are much higher in some areas.[21,22]

Infection rates are the same for both sexes, and early reports that clinical disease was more common in females than in males[24,65] are not supported by Australian national data for the past decade. An association between human leukocyte antigen DR7 (HLA-DR7) and clinical disease also has been observed.[41]

Ross River virus crosses the placenta in mice[4] and humans.[9] In mice, the result is extensive postpartum mortality,[4] but in humans, no evidence of morbidity or mortality for children infected in utero has been found.

Although there was evidence of subclinical infection in blood donors[2] and the risk of transmission in blood transfusions had been identified,[88] the first recorded transmission of Ross River virus in a blood donation occurred in 2014, prompting the risk of transfusion-transmitted Ross River virus infection to be reevaluated in 2016.[49,81]

CLINICAL MANIFESTATIONS

Epidemic polyarthritis occurs as a mild to severe illness characterized by joint pain, particularly in the knees and the small joints of the hands and feet. Frequently, the joint pain is accompanied by a maculopapular or vesicular rash on the trunk and limbs and sometimes by fever or chills, or both. Sore throat, lymphadenopathy, paresthesia, tenderness of the palms and soles, exanthems, and petechiae (rare) have been observed. Most patients experience several weeks of painful arthritis followed by a slow decrease in the severity of symptoms during the 30 to 40 weeks required by most for recovery.[3,67] Infrequently, symptoms may persist for a year or more,[33] and some patients may experience episodes of severe arthritis during convalescence. One study linked Ross River virus infection to a chronic fatigue syndrome.[48]

In less than 0.1% patients, clinical disease may develop without arthritis.[25] Rare cases of glomerulonephritis,[38] hematuria,[15] and central nervous system symptoms[1,60,71,78] accompanying Ross River virus infection in humans have been reported.

The severity and duration of symptoms are age related. Most clinical disease occurs in adults, who also have the most severe and prolonged symptoms. Teenagers may be incapacitated for only a few days and asymptomatic after only a few weeks.[25,31] Equines are the only other species known to develop clinical disease (i.e., musculoskeletal symptoms) after a natural infection with Ross River virus.[16]

PATHOLOGY

The pathogenesis of Ross River virus disease in humans is not understood. The literature describing the pathologic process of Ross River virus infection in mice is extensive,[47,57,63,64,66,79,80] but almost invariably, clinical symptoms are observed only in mice infected when younger than 4 weeks of age, which have key immunologic genes silenced, or which are infected by routes that could not occur in nature and with strains of virus that have been passaged extensively in cell culture.

Synovial tissue from patients with epidemic polyarthritis may show a marked mononuclear leukocyte infiltrate with small amounts of fibrin deposition and synovial cell hyperplasia.[46,85] No virus or viral antigen has been detected in synovial tissue from patients with epidemic polyarthritis, but a 250-nucleotide fragment of the viral genome was detected by reverse transcriptase polymerase chain reaction (RT-PCR) in synovium from 2 of 12 patients 5 weeks after the onset of symptoms.[85] Ross River virus can replicate for a similar period in human synovial cells maintained at 35°C (95°F) in vitro.[51] Whether virus persists in joints as long as symptoms are present remains unclear, and ethical and technical constraints prevent this issue being explored in a systematic manner.

Fluid from affected joints consists almost entirely of mononuclear leukocytes at all stages of disease.[20,34,36] Human synovial fibroblasts infected with Ross River virus in vitro produce elevated levels of messenger RNA (mRNA) coding for chemoattractants and other mediators, such as monocyte chemoattractant protein 1, interleukin-8 (IL-8), granulocyte-macrophage colony-stimulating factor, and tumor necrosis factor-α, but elevated levels of the proteins for which they code have not been demonstrated.[61] Viral antigen can be detected (in macrophages in synovial fluid) for only 5 to 7 days after the onset of symptoms, despite the persistence of arthritis for 30 to 40 weeks.[37] No evidence of immune complexes or complement activation in arthritic joints has been found.

No significant levels of anti-collagen antibodies were detected in serum from epidemic polyarthritis patients.[40] The significance of elevated levels of the pattern recognition molecule long pentraxin 3 (PTX3), which has a role in all three complement pathways, in serum from epidemic polyarthritis patients remains to be elucidated.[32] Neither anti–Ross River virus antibody levels nor a primary, virus-specific, cell-mediated immune response to Ross River virus infection correlated with the presence or absence of arthritis in human infections.[6] In patients with epidemic polyarthritis, a nonspecific immunologic response (i.e., natural killer cells) correlated well with the presence or absence of arthritic symptoms.[6,3] Functional natural killer cells have been recovered from the knee of a patient with epidemic polyarthritis,[46] and natural killer cells kill autologous synovial tissue in vitro.[3]

Infection of primary human osteoblasts with Ross River virus in vitro results in production of IL-6, chemokine (C-C motif) ligand 2 (CCL2), and IL-1β and an increased ratio of receptor activator of nuclear factor-κB (RANKL) to osteoprotegerin (OPG). Levels of RANKL proteins in synovial fluid from patients are elevated, and levels of OPG are lower than in healthy controls.[18] Chen and colleagues suggested that monocytes were recruited to the site of Ross River virus infection by the chemoattractant cytokines and chemokines where they are differentiated into bone-resorbing osteoclasts.

A rash develops in approximately 30% of patients with epidemic polyarthritis.[65] The dermis underlying these lesions contains a perivascular infiltrate of $CD8^+$ T cells and some monocytes and macrophages.[39] No immunoglobulin or complement deposition has been observed in these lesions, although Ross River virus antigen was detected in basal epidermal and eccrine duct epithelial cells.[39]

DIAGNOSIS

The signs and symptoms of a Ross River virus infection are too nonspecific to permit establishment of a diagnosis on clinical grounds alone.[43] Most clinical diagnoses of epidemic polyarthritis are confirmed by use of an indirect enzyme-linked immunosorbent assay (ELISA)[70] to detect Ross River virus–specific IgM antibodies in serum collected 7 to 10 days after the onset of symptoms. Various forms of this assay are available from commercial suppliers. Immunoglobulin M (IgM) can be detected for approximately 3 months after the onset of disease.[10]

In less than 1 of 5000) cases, anti–Ross River virus IgM antibody production may persist for years. Assays for serum anti–Ross River virus IgA may be an alternative to IgM assays because the duration of IgA production is shorter than that for IgM.[17] However, IgA assays have not been routinely adopted by diagnostic laboratories. Indirect ELISA assays that measure the avidity of anti–Ross River virus antibody can discriminate between recent and old infections with this virus.[52]

Although virus sometimes can be isolated from seronegative, acute-phase sera,[7,11,30,76,86] this procedure is not performed in most diagnostic laboratories. RT-PCR protocols,[82] mostly unpublished, have been developed for the detection of Ross River virus RNA, but they are less sensitive than is virus isolation for detection of the virus and are used routinely for the diagnosis of human disease only in large, central laboratories.

Because epidemic polyarthritis is an arthritic disease, care must be taken to avoid false-positive results caused by the presence of rheumatoid factor when indirect ELISA is used to detect anti–Ross River virus IgM antibodies. Precautions include removal of IgG or rheumatoid factor before testing sera and performing tests for rheumatoid factor in parallel with ELISA.

Another source of false-positive diagnoses is the production of anti–Ross River virus IgM antibody caused by polyclonal B-cell activation after infection of a Ross River virus–immune host with Epstein-Barr virus, cytomegalovirus, *Coxiella burnetii*, or *Plasmodium* spp. Other viral infections to be considered when an Australian patient or traveler is suspected of having epidemic polyarthritis include infections with Barmah Forest, Sindbis, Kunjin, Kokobera, or rubella viruses.

TREATMENT AND PROGNOSIS

No specific antiviral therapy is available, although experimental evidence suggests that interferon-γ may ameliorate acute disease.[80] Nonsteroidal antiinflammatory medication or steroids have been used to treat patients with severe disease or prolonged symptoms, but the therapeutic efficacy has not been evaluated in a systematic manner. A small study found that patients taking corticosteroids recovered more quickly than those using nonsteroidal antiinflammatory medication.[68] Rest while maintaining mobility and muscle tone appears to provide significant relief. Epidemic polyarthritis does not progress to chronic joint disease.

PREVENTION

A killed virus vaccine[12] was found to be safe and immunogenic in clinical trials.[13,89] In urban areas, public health mosquito control programs reduce mosquito numbers, but prevention of mosquito exposure for those with outdoor occupations and pastimes is impossible. Personal protection (i.e., insect screening of houses, wearing of protective clothing, and application of insect repellents) is the only reliable way to avoid the risk for being infected.

NEW REFERENCES SINCE THE SEVENTH EDITION

32. Foo SS, Chen W, Taylor A, et al. Role of pentaxin 3 in shaping arthritogenic alphaviral disease: from enhanced viral replication to immunomodulation. *PLoS Pathog*. 2015;11:e1004649.
49. Hoad VC, Speers DJ, Keller AJ, et al. First reported case of transfusion-transmitted Ross River virus infection. *Med J Aust*. 2015;202:267-269.
73. Potter A, Johansen CA, Fenwick S, et al. The seroprevalence and factors associated with Ross River virus infection in western grey kangaroos *(Macropus fuliginosus)* in Western Australia. *Vector Borne Zoonotic Dis*. 2014;14:740-745.
81. Seed CR, Hoad VC, Faddy HM, et al. Re-evaluating the residual risk of transfusion-transmitted Ross River virus infection. *Vox Sang*. 2016;110:317-323.

The full reference list for this chapter is available at ExpertConsult.com.

175F ■ Other Alphaviral Infections

Gail J Harrison • Theodore F. Tsai

O'NYONG-NYONG

The virus name *o'nyong-nyong* is derived from the Acholi dialect of the Southern Luo language of the people of East Africa. The term means "very painful and weak," which describes the acute constitutional symptoms and polyarthritis associated with the disease of the same name.[20] The o'nyong-nyong virus (ONNV) is a mosquito-borne RNA virus of the Togaviridae family, genus *Alphavirus*. It is genetically and serologically related closely to chikungunya virus and is seen in Africa. Unlike most arboviruses, ONNV is transmitted by anopheline mosquitoes in an interhuman cycle analogous to that of malaria in rural Africa. Apart from the human-to-human epidemic cycle, the natural transmission cycle and involvement of other vertebrate hosts are largely unknown. There is also a suggestion that *Aedes aegypti*, a mosquito found in some parts of Europe, may be a competent vector ONNV, indicating the virus may spread outside of Africa at some point.

The virus was first isolated in June 1959 in Gulu, Uganda, when ONNV disease first came to attention in the largest arboviral epidemic ever recorded. After emerging in Uganda in 1959, the epidemic spread to South and West Africa and produced an estimated 2 million cases before the outbreak died out spontaneously 3 years later. The disease apparently had disappeared from East Africa, although the virus was isolated sporadically from mosquitoes until 1996, when the second recognized outbreak of ONNV appeared in Uganda.[20] It has been responsible for several outbreaks in East Africa (Kenya, Uganda, Tanzania, Malawi, and Mozambique). In October 2013, a laboratory-confirmed imported case of ONNV infection was documented in a 60-year old woman from Germany who had returned home from a vacation to Uganda, Kenya, Rwanda, and Tanzania. She developed a recurring febrile illness with malaise, arthralgias of small joints, rash, edema, lymphadenopathy, arthralgia, and nausea, and a fourfold rise in anti-ONNV immunoglobulin G (IgG) titer was documented along with ONNV-specific neutralizing antibodies.[41]

In 2015 through 2016, there was a minor outbreak of 51 cases of ONNV infection reported in Uganda. The ONNV is considered endemic in coastal East Africa, similar to chikungunya virus.[22]

Clinically, the disease caused by ONNV is similar to chikungunya and should be considered in the differential diagnosis of acute febrile illness associated with travel to East Africa. It is also considered one of the tropical arthritogenic alphaviruses, along with chikungunya, Sindbis, Ross River, Mayaro, and Barmah Forest viruses, which have specific tropism for bones and joint tissue and can cause chronic rheumatic disease.[28] ONNV causes self-limited febrile illness with headache, rash, and joint pain. Lymphadenopathy is more pronounced in ONNV disease than in chikungunya and in some cases mimics the enlarged cervical lymph nodes of sleeping sickness.[6] The joint involvement is characteristically acute polyarthritis and polyarthralgia that is symmetric and involves the small peripheral joints. It may become chronic and cause painful arthropathy.[40]

The ONNV virus can be isolated from acute-phase blood samples performed in specialist public health laboratories. Detection of viral RNA by real-time reverse transcriptase polymerase chain reaction (RT-PCR) is also performed in reference public health laboratories.[5,24] The diagnosis can be confirmed serologically by detection of ONNV-specific immunoglobulin M (IgM) and a fourfold increase in ONNV-specific IgG by immunofluorescence assay. A virus neutralization test can also be done to confirm infection. There is a serologic cross-reaction with chikungunya virus, and interpretation of serologic testing should be done in this context. Serologic cross-reactivity has led public health officials to wonder how many true ONNV infections have been misdiagnosed as chikungunya infections.

There is no specific antiviral treatment available for ONNV infection. It is a self-limited illness. The arthralgias and arthropathy may respond to analgesics and nonsteroidal antiinflammatory drugs (NSAIDs).[40] There is no vaccine for prevention of ONNV infection. Personal protective measures against malaria (e.g., bed nets, mosquito repellants, protective clothing) should be effective against acquiring ONNV infection.

IGBO-ORA FEVER

Igbo-ora virus, first detected in Igbo-Ora, a community in western Nigeria, in 1967, has been determined genetically to be a subtype of ONNV. It is transmitted by anopheline mosquitoes and (without adaptation) is nonpathogenic in suckling mice.[33] The viral transmission cycle has not been defined. Sporadic cases and small outbreaks have been reported from Igbo-Ora and Ibadan, Nigeria; the Ivory Coast; and the Central African Republic. It has been detected in humans and anopheline mosquitoes in the Central African Republic, Nigeria, and the Ivory Coast. Based on a single case description, the illness consists of fever, polyarthritis, and pharyngitis.

BARMAH FOREST FEVER

Barmah Forest virus (BFV) is an RNA virus in the Togaviridae family, *Alphavirus* genus. It is named after the location in Northern Victoria, Australia, where it was first isolated in 1974. It occurs commonly in Australia, is the second most common arbovirus infection in Australia (after Ross River virus), and infects thousands annually.[30] BFV causes a sporadic and occasionally hyperendemic infection leading to a febrile, polyarthropathy-rash illness that is indistinguishable from Ross River fever.[12,23,35] It was first detected in Western Australia in 1989.

The mosquito-borne viral transmission cycle of BFV shares some features with that of the Ross River virus. However, independent outbreaks have occurred in all Australian locations where both viruses are enzootic, indicating differences in their transmission cycles or human susceptibility. BFV is hosted by marsupials, especially possums, kangaroos, and wallabies. It is transmitted to humans by bites of infected mosquitoes, including *Aedes* (especially *A. vigilax*) and *Culex* (especially *C. annulirostris*). Seroprevalence for BFV usually is lower than for Ross Valley virus.

Clinically, most BFV infections are subclinical or asymptomatic. When BFV causes disease, it is similar to chikungunya and ONNV and should be considered in the differential diagnosis of acute febrile illness associated with travel to Australia. It is also considered one of the tropical polyarthritis viruses, along with ONNV, chikungunya, Sindbis, Ross River, and Mayaro viruses, which have specific tropism for bones and joint tissue and can cause chronic rheumatic disease.[28]

BFV illness is self-limited and includes fever, malaise, rash, arthralgia, and muscle tenderness that lasts a few days to a week. The joint pain, however, may continue for 6 months in about 10% of patients infected with BFV. Anecdotal cases complicated by central nervous system signs and glomerulonephritis have been reported.[19,35] Serologic diagnosis using detection of BFV IgG and IgM enzyme-linked immunosorbent assays (ELISAs) and microneutralization assays for acute and convalescent sera to document seroconversion is straightforward in most cases, with little cross-reaction between the viruses.[8]

There is no specific antiviral treatment available for BFV infection. It is a self-limited illness.[30] The arthralgias and arthropathy may respond to analgesics and NSAIDs. There is no vaccine for prevention of BFV infection. Personal protective measures against malaria (e.g., bednets, mosquito repellants, protective clothing) should be effective against acquiring BFV infection.

SINDBIS FEVER

Sindbis virus (SINV) is an enveloped RNA virus of the family Togaviridae, genus *Alphavirus*. The virus was named after a district in the Nile River delta north of Cairo, Egypt, where it was isolated in 1952 from *Culex* mosquitoes.[42] It is the prototype of an antigenic complex that also includes western equine encephalitis virus and several Sindbis viral subtypes, including Ockelbo and related strains isolated from Scandinavia and the Babanki strain from West Africa.

Two SINV genotypes consisting of the South African and Scandinavian strains and the Australian and Asian strains have been defined. The close genetic relationship of the South African and Scandinavian strains indicates a recent introduction to Europe, possibly by a migrating bird.

The virus is distributed widely over four continents, although only sporadic cases have been reported from Asia and Australia. Transmission is endemic and occasionally hyperendemic in Africa and Scandinavia.[1] The virus is transmitted to birds by various species of *Culex* mosquitoes, and humans are infected when virus transmission spills out of the enzootic cycle by the intervention of bridging vectors that feed on viremic birds and later on humans.

Endemic infections occur with various intensities in areas of Africa.[18,27] Seroprevalence rates range from a few percent to 20% in some areas. Outbreaks producing hundreds to thousands of cases have been described. Concurrent transmission with West Nile virus, transmitted in the same avian cycle, is common. In South Africa, transmission occurs during the austral summer from December to April. Infections rarely are acquired during travel.[10]

An endemic focus in Scandinavia (i.e., between 60 and 63 degrees latitude in Sweden) was recognized after a series of outbreaks in 1981 led to several hundred cases in Sweden, Norway, Finland, and adjacent areas of western Russia and were locally called Ockelbo fever, Pogosta disease, or Karelian fever.[11,25,40] The seroprevalence rate is about 5% to 10%. By estimation from seroprevalence rates, 600 to 1200 clinical cases may occur annually in Sweden alone. Serosurveys indicate a wider distribution of unrecognized infection in Northern and Central Europe. Most cases occur from July to September, affecting middle-aged adults exposed to forested areas while picking berries or mushrooms or during other recreational activities. SINV outbreaks in Finland and other parts of northern Europe seem to peak at 7-year intervals and are associated with the size of grouse populations.[17]

Acute arthralgia and rash are the principal features of the illness.[1] They may be preceded by mild fever, headache, and myalgia, but patients can have arthralgia alone, and children can exhibit fever and nonspecific symptoms alone. The joints, especially the ankles, wrists, knees, fingers, and toes and less often the hips, shoulders, elbows, neck, and back, are involved symmetrically. The joints appear swollen, and movement is limited. The Achilles and wrist tendons can be inflamed, sometimes causing nerve entrapment and paresthesias. Some patients are confined to bed and unable to walk, but the joint pain and stiffness typically lead to a lesser degree of discomfort and compromised function.

A fine papular and sometimes pruritic rash appears on the trunk and extremities (including the palms and soles) but usually spares the face and head. After a few days, the rash develops a stained appearance and disappears. Lesions on the hands and feet may vesiculate. Joint symptoms resolve within 3 to 4 months in approximately 60% of cases; in the remainder of patients with SINV infection, symptoms may persist for 3 to 4 years.[21,32,36,38]

A higher prevalence of HLA-DRB1*01 and autoantibodies has been reported in patients with continued joint symptoms 3 years after the initial illness in contrast to a reference population.[38] Muscle biopsy from a patient with prolonged weakness and in vitro experiments suggest that the virus can infect and destroy myotubes and myoblasts.[36] Serologic evidence of infection in patients with central nervous system signs has been reported from China.[14]

The illness of SINV is not differentiated easily from West Nile fever, which is transmitted under similar epidemiologic circumstances, and has been mistaken for rubella.

The laboratory diagnosis is confirmed serologically by detection of SINV-specific IgM in acute-phase serum samples. IgM is detectable for months in some patients. The virus can be isolated, although not reliably, from acute-phase capillary blood specimens and skin lesions. Viral genomic products can be detected in skin biopsy samples.[16] A real-time RT-PCR assay for SINV has been used to screen for SINV in wildlife. However PCR application to the diagnosis of human SINV disease is limited because the viremia associated with SINV infection in humans is low and short lived.[24,37]

There is no specific antiviral treatment available for SINV infection. Symptomatic treatment with NSAIDs is sufficient in most patients with a self-limited illness. Anti–tumor necrosis factor antibodies have exacerbated alphaviral infection in experimental animals and should be avoided. There is no vaccine available to prevent SINV infection. However, personal protective measures used against malaria (e.g., bed nets, mosquito repellants, protective clothing) should be effective against acquiring SINV infection. Control of water areas infected by mosquito populations should be done to reduce SINV mosquito reservoirs.[17]

MAYARO FEVER

Mayaro virus (MAYV) is a member of the family Togaviridae, genus *Alphavirus*. The virus is placed in the Semliki Forest antigenic complex; its Una subtype causes arthritis in horses.

The virus was isolated first from sporadic fever cases on Trinidad and named after the island's Mayaro district.[3] It is another neglected tropical arbovirus infection that primarily affects people who live in forested areas in tropical South America, especially during the rainy season. Endemic infections with MAYV are highly prevalent in the forested areas of South and Central America, where MAYV is transmitted by *Haemagogus* spp. mosquitoes to marsupials and small mammals (e.g., monkeys), somewhat analogous to the jungle cycle of yellow fever.[4,13,43] Seroprevalence rates increase with age to higher than 50% among native populations in some locations.

Outbreaks have occurred in Bolivia, Pará (a state in Brazil), and Surinam, principally among men occupationally exposed to forested sites, residents of adjoining villages, and travelers returning from Central America.[9,34,39] Cases also have been reported among travelers returning to the United States, Switzerland, Netherlands, France, and Germany and should be included in the differential diagnosis of febrile illness in travelers returning from South America.[31] Epidemic transmission was reported in the city of Manaus, Brazil, and is a risk in other *Aedes aegypti*–infested cities.[29] Studies from 2017 suggest MAYV infection may occur more frequently in central Brazil than previously described and may be spreading to urbanized areas, similar to the Zika virus urbanization spread in 2015.[7]

The illness associated with MAYV may be mild, with acute febrile illness and an uneventful recovery. It may also be severe and dengue-like, with fever and severe, acute polyarthritis and rash.[34] Joint swelling, pain, and stiffness principally involve the hands, wrists, ankles, toes, elbows, and knees. The hands may be so swollen that they cannot be closed, and joints of the lower extremities may be so painful that patients limp or are unable to walk. Milder cases can occur.

The morbilliform rash is difficult to distinguish from rubella, with individual or coalescent papular lesions occurring on the trunk and extremities and usually sparing the face. Rash occurs more often in children than in adults. Mild fever, pharyngitis, conjunctivitis, headache, retrobulbar pain, lymphadenitis, and minor mucosal and petechial bleeding occur in some patients. The constitutional symptoms resolve rapidly, but the joint symptoms may wax and wane for several weeks or months, and they may be severe and debilitating. Pneumonitis and renal dysfunction that were described in rare cases might have been caused by concurrent infections. Transient leukopenia usually develops; some patients have had mild elevations in liver enzyme activities and bilirubin concentrations. A fatal case of yellow fever was described in a patient recovering from MAYV fever.

The illness is differentiated from other tropical febrile illnesses with rash and musculoskeletal pain by the specific involvement of the joints and the sylvatic setting of exposure. Some patients have features resembling those of rubella, human herpesvirus type 6 (HHV-6), parvovirus, Epstein-Barr virus (EBV) mononucleosis, malaria, chikungunya, Zika virus, or yellow fever.

Infection with MAYV may be laboratory confirmed by isolation from acute-phase blood specimens, but laboratory confirmation by MAYV-specific IgM ELISA serology is sensitive, specific, and more practical than culture.[7] IgG antibody may also be detected through indirect immunofluorescence assay or virus neutralization assay to document MAYV-specific seroconversion. There is no specific antiviral treatment for MAYV infection. However, thienopyridine-derivative antiviral compounds have shown promise in decreasing MAYV replication in vitro, suggesting the potential application of this class of compounds against MAYV and all alphaviruses.[2]

The illness is self-limited for most patients, and symptoms are treated with analgesics, antipyretics, NSAIDs, and rest. There is no vaccine to prevent MAYV infection or disease. However, personal protective measures used against malaria (e.g., bed nets, mosquito repellants, protective clothing) should be effective against acquiring MAYV infection when traveling to endemic areas.

SEMLIKI FOREST VIRUS FEVER

Semliki Forest virus (SFV) is an RNA virus in the Togaviridae family, *Alphavirus* genus. It was first isolated from mosquitoes in the Semliki Frost in Uganda in 1942. It causes infection and illness in humans and animals, including wild birds, rodents, domestic animals, and nonhuman primates. SFV is found in Central and West Africa, parts of Asia, and possibly in central and southern Europe, where it is transmitted principally by forest *Aedes* mosquitoes.[26] A rare case of inhalation transmission was reported. The virus appears to be a common cause of infection in horses and humans. The Me-Tri subtype has been implicated serologically in encephalitis cases in Vietnam; its transmission cycle has not been described.

Infection with SFV is thought to be subclinical or asymptomatic for most individuals, or it can cause a mild, self-limited flu-like illness with fever, severe and persistent headache, myalgia, and arthralgia. Fatal cases associated with meningoencephalitis have been reported.[44] It also may be severe in immunocompromised patients.[26] Several laboratory-acquired infections and at least one fatal case of SFV encephalitis in a laboratory worker have been reported.[15]

There is no known antiviral treatment for SFV infection, and no vaccine against SFV is available. However, because SFV has a broad host range and efficient viral replication, it has been developed as a vaccine vector for anticancer treatment agents and as a tool in gene therapy against glioblastoma brain tumors. Personal protective measures used against malaria and mosquito-borne arboviral infections (e.g., bed nets, mosquito repellants, protective clothing) should be effective against acquiring SFV infection when traveling to endemic areas. Laboratory workers working with SFV should take appropriate precautions to avoid skin contact or contact with aerosols from the virus.

NEW REFERENCES SINCE THE SEVENTH EDITION

1. Adouchief S, Smura T, Sane J, et al. Sindbis virus as a human pathogen-epidemiology, clinical picture and pathogenesis. *Rev Med Virol*. 2016;26:221-241.
2. Amorim R, de Meneses M, Borges J, et al. Thieno[2,3-b]pyridine derivatives: a new class of antiviral drugs against Mayaro virus. *Arch Virol*. 2017;162: 1577-1587.
4. Azevedo R, Silva E, Carvalho V, et al. Mayaro fever virus, Brazilian Amazon. *Emerg Infect Dis*. 2009;15:1830-1832.
5. Bessaud M, Peyrefitte C, Pastorino B, et al. O'nyong-nyong virus, Chad. *Emerg Infect Dis*. 2006;12:1248-1250.
7. Brunini S, Franca DD, Silva J, et al. High frequency of Mayaro virus IgM among febrile patients, Central Brazil. *Emerg Infect Dis*. 2017;23:1025-1026.
8. Cashman P, Hueston L, Duirrheim D, et al. Barmah Forest virus serology: implications or diagnosis and public health action. *Commun Dis Intell Q Rep*. 2008;32:263-266.
17. Jalava K, Sane J, Ollgren J, et al. Climatic, ecological and socioeconomic factors as predictors of Sindbis virus infections in Finland. *Epidemiol Infect*. 2013;141:1857-1866.
22. LeBeaud A, Banda T, Brichard J, et al. High rates of o'nyong nyong and Chikungunya virus transmission in coastal Kenya. *PloS Negl Trop Dis*. 2015;9:e0003436.
24. Liu J, Oschieng C, Wiersma S, et al. Development of a TaqMan array card for acute-febrile-illness outbreak investigation and surveillance of emerging pathogens, including Ebola virus. *J Clin Microbiol*. 2016;54:49-58.
28. Mejia C, Lopez-Velez R. Tropical arthritogenic alphaviruses. *Rheumatol Clin*. 2017;Mar 29:pii: S1699-258X(17)30025-6.
30. Naish S, Hu W, Mengersen K, Tong S. Spatio-temporal patterns of Barmah Forest Virus disease in Queensland, Australia. *PLoS ONE*. 2011;6:e25688.
31. Neumayr A, Gabriel M, Fritz J, et al. Mayaro virus infection in traveler returning from Amazon Basin, Northern Peru. *Emerg Infect Dis*. 2012;18:695-697.
37. Sane J, Kurkela S, Levanov L, et al. Development and evaluation of a real-time RT-PCR assay for Sindbis virus detection. *J Virol Methods*. 2012;179:185-188.
41. Tappe D, Kapaun A, Emmerich P, et al. O'nyong-nyong virus infection imported to Europe from Kenya by a traveler. *Emerg Infect Dis*. 2014;20:1766-1767.
42. Taylor R, Hurlbut H, Work T, et al. Sindbis virus: a newly recognized arthropod transmitted virus. *Am J Trop Med Hyg*. 1955;4:844-862.
44. Willems W, Kaluza G, Boschek C, et al. Semliki forest virus: cause of a fatal case of human encephalitis. *Science*. 1979;203:1127-1129.

The full reference list for this chapter is available at ExpertConsult.com.

176 Flaviviruses

176A ■ St. Louis Encephalitis

Kimberly C. Martin • José R. Romero

St. Louis encephalitis (SLE) virus was first identified in 1933 after an epidemic of encephalitis in St. Louis, Missouri, during August 1933.[87] Before the 1999 introduction of West Nile virus (WNV), SLE was the most important arboviral infection in the United States because of its leading role as a cause of widespread epidemics. Encephalitis is the principal clinical manifestation, although milder central nervous system (CNS) syndromes do occur, especially in children. The virus is transmitted between birds and *Culex* mosquitoes, with humans serving only as incidental, dead-end hosts.

ETIOLOGIC AGENT

The SLE virus is a member of the genus *Flavivirus* within the Flaviviridae family of viruses. SLE belongs to the Japanese encephalitis virus antigenic complex, which also includes important human pathogens such as Japanese encephalitis virus, WNV, and Murray Valley encephalitis virus.

Phylogenetic analysis of the E glycoprotein sequences from 62 strains from the United States and Central and South America identified seven genotypes corresponding to origins in the United States and South America.[36] A later analysis of 133 strains, including 30 novel strains from Brazil, identified an eighth genotype.[72] Individual clades exist within each genotype.

Genotype II is more prevalent in North America, and genotypes I and III through VIII are distributed throughout the Americas.[72] The most genetically diverse strains have only a 10.1% nucleotide divergence (i.e., 2.8% amino acid variation) in the total E gene nucleotide sequence, whereas strains within each lineage show less than a 5.5% nucleotide divergence, indicating a highly constrained viral adaptation to vector and vertebrate hosts.[49] The nucleotide diversity exhibited by SLE is substantially less than that seen for other members of the Japanese encephalitis virus antigenic complex. Strains from the three principal genotypes in the United States (I, II, and V) have different biologic characteristics. Epidemic-associated strains from the Ohio and Mississippi river basins and Florida display greater virulence in mice than do strains from the western United States associated with an endemic pattern of transmission.[17,51] Multiple viral genotypes with distinct biologic characteristics may be transmitted in relatively delimited areas within a region as small as a county in some years and more widely in others.[17,35]

ECOLOGY

SLE virus is transmitted in an enzootic cycle among birds and *Culex* mosquitoes in three distinct cycles associated with its four principal vector species: *Culex tarsalis* in the western and central United States, *C. pipiens* in the eastern and western United States, *C. quinquefasciatus* in the east central and Atlantic states, and *C. nigripalpus* in Florida. *C. salinarius* and *C. restuans* may have accessory roles in viral amplification and transmission (Fig. 176A.1).[13,40,43,50,82]

In the western United States, *C. tarsalis* serves as an enzootic and epizootic vector. This species feeds chiefly on birds early in the summer and switches to mammalian hosts, including humans, in midsummer. The transmission cycles of SLE virus and WNV overlap throughout the United States. Sparrows, finches, and other small birds and especially their nestlings are the principal amplifying hosts.[48] In the West, human infections result from encounters with the vector along natural and artificial waterways, irrigated farmland, and other breeding sites found chiefly in rural agricultural areas.

The introduction of WNV into an overlapping transmission cycle appears to have an effect of modulating SLE virus transmission because WNV-infected birds are more refractory to development of infection and viremia with SLE virus than the reverse.[27] In the Ohio and Mississippi valleys and on the Gulf Coast, infections are acquired in the peridomestic environment, where *C. pipiens* and *C. quinquefasciatus* are, respectively, the enzootic vectors in northern and southern states.

The mechanism by which the virus overwinters is unknown, but SLE virus has been shown to persist in overwintering *C. tarsalis* and *C. pipiens* for more than a month.[3] Vertical or transovarial transmission has been detected under laboratory conditions in *Culex* species.[3,30,46]

The intermittent occurrence of urban SLE outbreaks has been associated with climatic factors, such as a severe winter freeze in the 1 to 2 years before an outbreak or an antecedent mild winter, wet spring, and dry, hot summer.[21,50] Snowpack and the resultant availability of irrigation water and an area supportive of mosquito breeding appear to be highly predictive of viral transmission in southern California.[80] In a model of global warming, SLE transmission is predicted to move to northern latitudes and, in existing endemic areas, to become seasonal in the spring and fall.[66] Periods of drought followed by a briefer wet interval have been associated with viral transmission in Florida.[20,76]

EPIDEMIOLOGY

The epidemiologic patterns of SLE virus transmission reflect human interactions with reservoirs of the virus and its principal mosquito vectors.[39,41,50,82] In western states (Figs. 176A.2 and 176A.3), perennial transmission of SLE virus leads to an endemic pattern of transmission, but epidemics are limited by a high level of immunity in the population.[68,81] Infections occur chiefly in rural areas in association with the habitat of the vector. SLE outbreaks typically have taken place in rural agricultural areas and their small towns.[38] Studies in Texas indicated that an overlap of urban and rural cycles contributed to an urban outbreak in Dallas after introduction of the virus to the urban *C. quinquefasciatus* cycle from rural *C. tarsalis*.[33,39,40]

Epidemics frequently have occurred in urban locations or their peripheries. In 1975, a nationwide epidemic led to outbreaks in Houston, Chicago, Memphis, and Detroit and to smaller outbreaks in rural towns throughout the South and Midwest, resulting in more than 2000 cases (Fig. 176A.4). Outbreaks in large urban centers usually have been associated with attack rates of fewer than 40 cases per 100,000 residents and often have clustered in low socioeconomic status areas.[19,33,50,53,62,84,82,90] The US SLE outbreak in 2015 occurred concurrently with WNV in the Phoenix, Arizona, area and resulted in 19 cases.[11,14,23]

In modern urban outbreaks, homelessness and infection with human immunodeficiency virus (HIV) have been the principal risk factors for acquiring SLE.[59,86] However, in the 1933 St. Louis outbreak, attack rates were highest in wealthy areas where open sewers, streams, ponds, and weeds were prevalent. In other outbreaks, lush vegetation around houses, which provides shelter for *C. nigripalpus,* and closed sewer systems clogged with grass clippings were factors associated with high attack rates in upper socioeconomic areas.[20,49]

In outbreaks of disease from *C. pipiens* and *C. quinquefasciatus,* epidemic attack rates are 1.2 to 3 times higher among females than males, possibly reflecting increased exposure of females to these peridomestic vectors,[45,50,83] In western *C. tarsalis*–borne outbreaks, attack rates are usually higher among males.[38,68] A similar observation has been made in Florida, where SLE attack rates are highest among working-age men.[22,49,57] *C. nigripalpus* and *C. tarsalis* are most active in the twilight hours, and outdoor activity during these periods is associated with a greater risk of exposure.

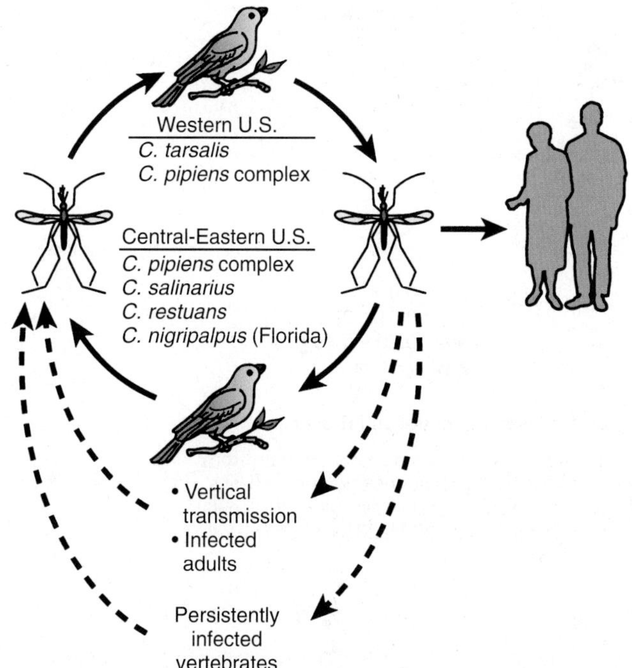

FIGURE 176A.1 Transmission cycles of St. Louis encephalitis virus in North America. *Culex* mosquito vectors cover different geographic areas: *C. tarsalis* in the West, *C. pipiens* and *C. quinquefasciatus* in the Ohio and Mississippi River Valleys, and *C. nigripalpus* in Florida. Epidemics occur when intense viral transmission in the enzootic cycle spills over and results in human infections. The viral overwintering mechanism, possibly in mosquitoes or persistently infected vertebrates, has not been proved *(dashed lines).*

Most cases (>80%) occur during the months of July through September.[67] However, in Florida, epidemics have continued through mid-December.[49,75] In the 1975 nationwide epidemic, outbreaks appeared first in the southeastern states in June, followed by an appearance in northern foci later in the summer and fall.[50]

From 2004 to 2013, 92 cases of SLE were reported to the Centers for Disease Control and Prevention (CDC). This included 25 cases of nonneuroinvasive and 67 cases of neuroinvasive disease, with an average of 7 neuroinvasive cases reported annually. Six states accounted for almost 80% of neuroinvasive cases during this period (in decreasing number): Arkansas, Texas, Louisiana, Mississippi, Arizona, and Michigan.[12] Within states reporting infections, cases were geographically restricted (see Fig. 176A.3).[12] Outbreaks occurring in 2014 and 2015 resulted in 10 and 19 cases, respectively.[11,14] In the latter, 17 were neuroinvasive. SLE has reemerged in areas where it had been absent for decades. In 2010, the District of Columbia reported two cases of nonneuroinvasive SLE. They were the first case reports from this jurisdiction since 1975.[10]

Although a case of neuroinvasive SLE in an infant as young as 19 days has been reported, the most important risk factor for acquiring neuroinvasive disease is advanced age.[41,50,89] Age-specific attack rates are lowest for children and rise steadily throughout adulthood, with attack rates 5 to 40 times higher in people older than 60 years than in those younger than 10 years of age. During outbreaks, infections occur uniformly in all age groups, with as many as 300 asymptomatic infections for each clinically apparent case. The higher clinical attack rates among the elderly are a function of susceptibility, not exposure.[41,50] The clinical expression of illness is more severe and the case-fatality rate is also highest among the elderly. The biologic basis for this age-related risk probably reflects aging of the immune system and comorbidities compromising cerebrovascular integrity.[9]

In the West, where SLE infections are endemic, an increasing level of immunity associated with length of residence leads to an adult population with lower susceptibility (i.e., 11% in the most recent serosurvey).[68] Consequently, cases often are seen in children and young adults. In a Florida outbreak, immunity to other flaviviruses (mainly from previous dengue infection) was shown to protect against the acquisition of SLE.[6]

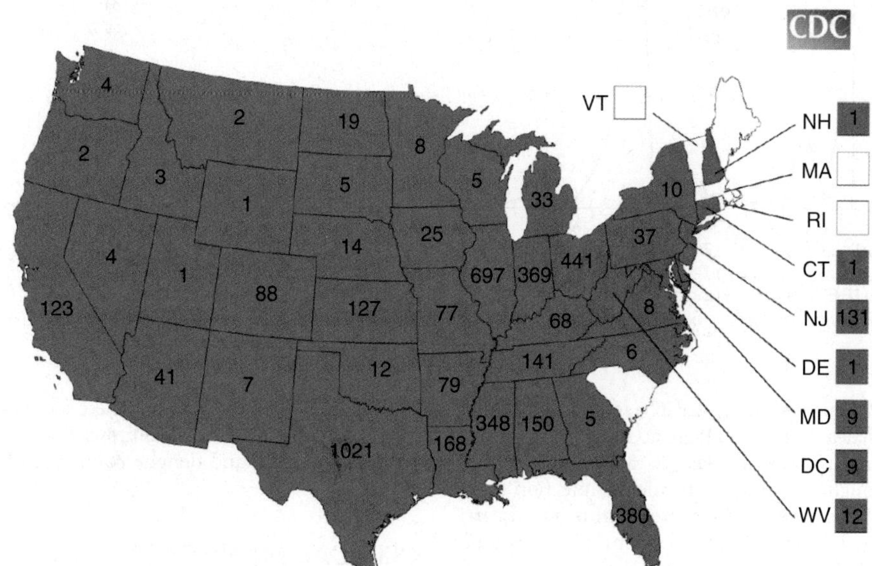

FIGURE 176A.2 Reported cases of St. Louis encephalitis virus neuroinvasive disease by state, 1964–2010. Cases were reported by state of residence. Neuroinvasive disease includes encephalitis, meningoencephalitis, or meningitis.

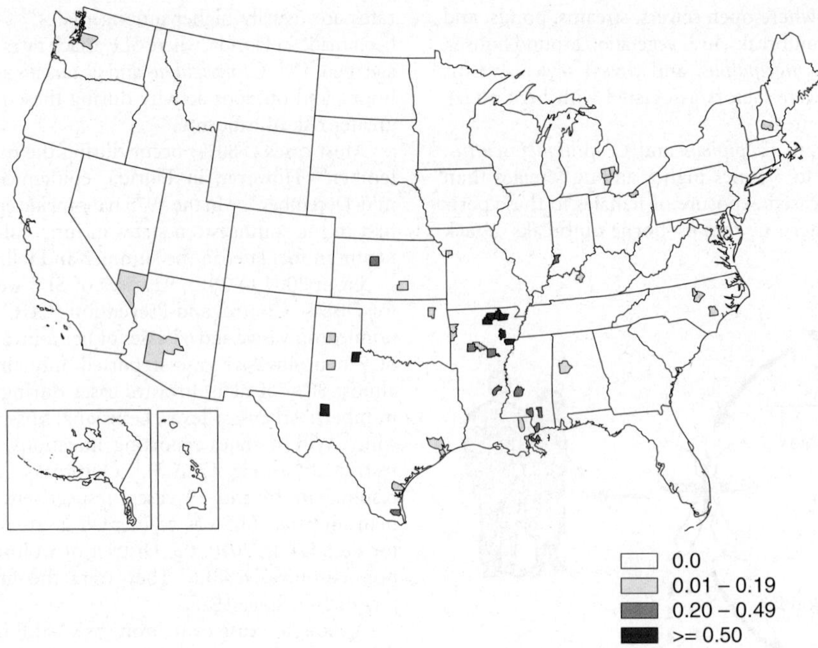

FIGURE 176A.3 Reported cases of St. Louis encephalitis virus neuroinvasive disease by state from 2004–13. Cases were reported by county of residence. Neuroinvasive disease includes encephalitis, meningoencephalitis, or meningitis. (From Centers for Disease Control and Prevention. St. Louis encephalitis virus neuroinvasive disease average annual incidence by county, 2004–2013. https://www.cdc.gov/sle/pdf/sle_county_map-04-13.pdf.)

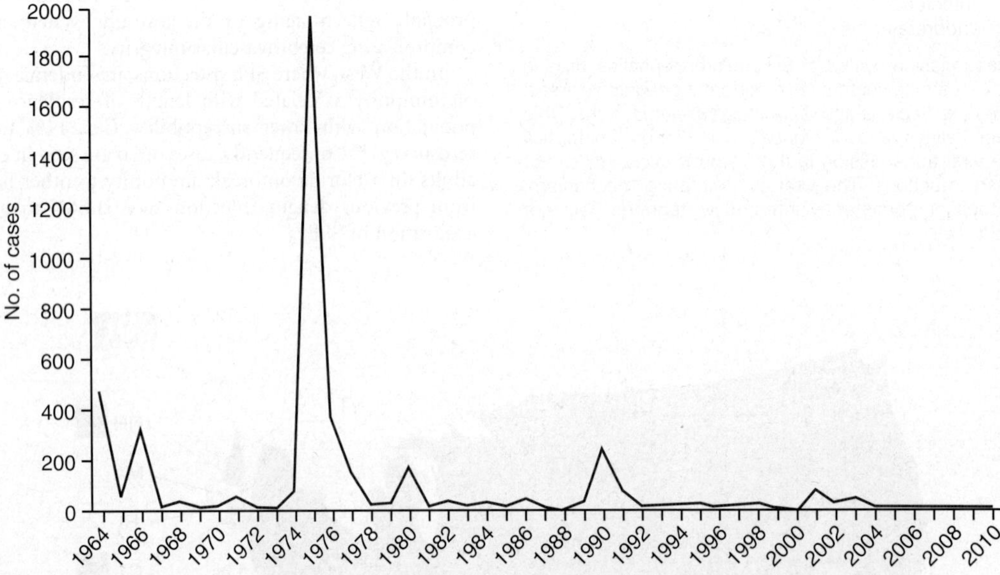

FIGURE 176A.4 Reported St. Louis encephalitis cases by year in the United States, 1964–2010. A nationwide epidemic in 1975 produced more than 2000 cases.

Cases of SLE have been reported in the Caribbean and South and Central America (i.e., Jamaica, Suriname, French Guiana, Argentina, Brazil, and Peru).[1,22,28,78] Increasing seroprevalence rates observed with increasing age indicates a higher frequency of endemic infection than is clinically apparent.[1,79] SLE is an emerging cause of arboviral disease in South America and has been responsible for sporadic cases and several outbreaks.[22,54,78] In 2005, the largest outbreak reported occurred in Cordoba, Argentina, resulting in 47 laboratory-confirmed or probable cases; 11 of the infections occurred in children. Nine adults died in this outbreak.[79] A smaller outbreak in Buenos Aires, Argentina, in 2010 resulted in 13 confirmed cases.[74] These sporadic SLE outbreaks principally have resulted in mild febrile illnesses that have been clinically confused with dengue. SLE and dengue coinfection has been demonstrated in Brazil.[32]

CLINICAL MANIFESTATIONS

Clinical manifestations range from a mild influenza-like illness to fatal encephalitis.[7,64,71,90] A case definition that stratifies cases into clinical syndromes of encephalitis, aseptic meningitis, and febrile headache[7]

BOX 176A.1 Definitions of Clinical Syndromes Caused by St. Louis Encephalitis

Encephalitis[a,b]
Acute febrile illness (oral temperature ≥37.8°C (≥100°F)
One or more signs in either of the following categories:
 Altered level of consciousness (i.e., confusion, disorientation, delirium, lethargy, stupor, or coma)
 Objective signs of neurologic dysfunction (i.e., seizure, cranial nerve palsy, dysarthria, rigidity, paresis, paralysis, abnormal reflexes, or tremor)

Aseptic meningitis[a]
Acute febrile illness
Signs of meningeal irritation (i.e., stiff neck with or without Kernig or Brudzinski sign)
No objective signs of neurologic dysfunction

Febrile headache[a]
Acute febrile illness
Headache (may have other systemic symptoms such as nausea or vomiting)
No signs of meningeal irritation or neurologic dysfunction

[a]Cerebrospinal fluid pleocytosis is seen in patients with encephalitis and aseptic meningitis; it also may be found in patients with the syndrome of febrile headache.
[b]Including meningoencephalitis and encephalomyelitis.
Modified from Brinker KR, Monath TP. The acute disease. In: Monath TP, ed. *St. Louis encephalitis.* Washington, DC: American Public Health Association; 1980:503–34.

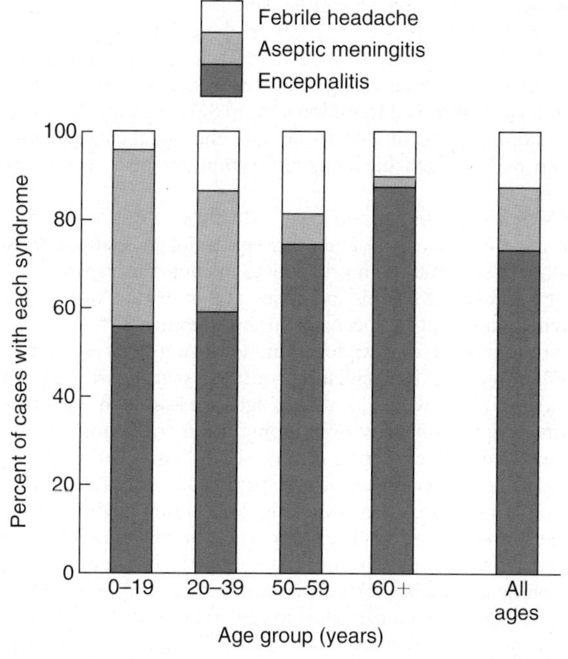

FIGURE 176A.5 Distribution of St. Louis encephalitis cases by clinical syndrome and age. Although mortality rates and disease severity increase with age, most pediatric cases are clinical encephalitis. (Data from Zweighaft RM, Rasmussen C, Brolnitsky O, et al. St. Louis encephalitis: the Chicago experience. *Am J Trop Med Hyg.* 1979;28:114–8.)

(Box 176A.1) has proved useful in surveillance (Fig. 176A.5). Although children as a group exhibit milder symptoms, encephalitis develops in more than one half of confirmed and presumptive pediatric cases, and 95% have objective clinical signs of CNS infection.[4,5,79,90]

SLE cannot be easily differentiated from other viral CNS infections on the basis of clinical features. Photophobia, headache, fever, nausea, vomiting, malaise, and neck stiffness are typical early symptoms. In approximately one half of reported cases, an abrupt onset of weakness, incoordination, disturbed sensorium, or other neurologic signs may occur, but equally often, patients have nonspecific symptoms with subtle changes in coordination or mentation during a prodromal phase lasting several days to more than a week. Seizures have been reported in a third of adult cases.[86]

In addition to fever of abrupt onset and signs of meningeal irritation, patients almost uniformly exhibit alterations in state of consciousness such as restlessness, confusion, lethargy, delirium, or coma. Neurologic examination usually reveals general weakness, hyperreflexia, and tremulousness, but focal deficits are unusual findings. Cranial nerve palsies, especially those involving nerves VII, IX, and X, occur in 10% to 25% of cases.[7] Clinical signs of increased intracranial pressure have been reported in a few patients.

Unusual localizing neurologic signs have been described in patients with involvement of the midbrain, thalamus, or brain stem. In a 4-year-old girl, paralysis of upward gaze was associated with a brain stem infection.[35] A 14-year-old boy with acquired parkinsonism attributed to SLE infection has been reported.[63] Ataxia has been observed in a fourth of the cases involving children, and several cases of opsoclonus have been reported for young adults.[25,26,86] In a series of 26 children with SLE, seizures were observed in eight patients, six of whom had focal seizures; however, enteroviruses were isolated concurrently from the stool in five of the eight patients.[4,61] It is not known whether they had enteroviral CNS infection. A confirmed case of SLE causing a seizure has been reported in a neonate.[89] In most cases, the fever abates 4 to 7 days after onset, and clinical improvement is evident early in the second week of illness. Polyradiculopathy and transverse myelitis have been reported.[5,73]

The peripheral leukocyte count is elevated modestly, with a shift to the left for most patients. Cerebrospinal fluid (CSF) usually contains fewer than 100 leukocytes/mm^3, but may, in some cases, contain fewer than 10 cells/mm^3. Occasionally no cells are discovered in the CSF. An increasing ratio of mononuclear to polymorphonuclear cells is observed on successive examinations. The CSF protein level rarely exceeds 200 mg/dL, and hypoglycorrhachia is unusual.[7]

In one series, elevated serum aldolase levels suggested a myopathic process, and muscle biopsy and electromyography disclosed lower motor neuron dysfunction, possibly from spinal root involvement. Moderate transaminase elevations have been reported in 19% to 48% of adult patients. Decreased serum osmolality attributed to inappropriate secretion of antidiuretic hormone was observed in one fourth to one third of cases in two series.[7,8]

Urinary incontinence, frequency, or retention and pyuria or proteinuria have been reported for adult patients, and viral antigen was detected on cells in the urinary sediment by immunofluorescence in one report.[42] Lower motor neuron lesions might have been the mechanism for bladder symptoms in some patients.

Electroencephalographic abnormalities have included focal discharges, including periodic lateralized epileptiform discharges, but they more consistently show diffuse generalized slowing.[4,8,86] Computed tomography scans may be normal, but magnetic resonance images have disclosed T2-weighted hyperintense abnormalities in the substantia nigra, consistent with edema.[16]

PATHOLOGY

Pathologic changes are found predominantly in the midbrain, thalamus, and brain stem but are also seen in the cerebral cortex and cerebellum. Lesions are observed in the spinal cord in some cases.[70,77,80] The leptomeninges are affected to some degree by edema, small hemorrhages, and round cell infiltration.

Perivascular and parenchymal inflammation is prevalent in the brain nuclei and scattered in the white matter of the brain stem and spinal cord and in subcortical and deep cerebral areas. Nodular collections of inflammatory cells composed of lymphocytes, microglial cells, and monocytes are found near to or surrounding degenerating neurons characterized by eccentric nuclear displacement, nuclear pyknosis, and cellular contraction. Vascular infiltrations and thrombosis have not been described as they have in cases of western equine encephalitis (WEE) and eastern equine encephalomyelitis (EEE). Focal demyelination, which is observed in WEE, has not been characteristic of SLE. Transmission electron microscopy may provide a pathologic diagnosis using tiny tissue fragments.[18]

PATHOGENESIS

After infection, viral replication occurs locally and in regional lymph nodes. After this eclipse phase, blood-borne (viremic) dissemination ensues, with secondary sites of replication occurring in muscle, endocrine, lymphoreticular, and other tissues, and in less than 1% of infections, replication occurs in the CNS. Vascular endothelial cells may have a role in actively transporting virus from the capillary lumen to the brain and in supporting secondary viral replication.[24] Conditions that compromise cerebrovascular integrity and disrupt the blood-brain barrier may predispose to neuroinvasion. For example, concurrent CNS cysticercosis can be a risk factor for acquiring Japanese encephalitis, a related flaviviral infection. Although some experimental studies suggest that CNS invasion occurs through the olfactory epithelium, pathologic studies of Japanese encephalitis cases indicate widespread involvement of the brain stem, deep nuclei, and cortex, which is most consistent with hematogenous infection.

Recovery from flaviviral encephalitis depends on early intrathecal synthesis of antibodies and viral clearance by macrophages. The inflammatory response in related CNS infections consists of helper-inducer T cells and, to a lesser degree, B lymphocytes infiltrating the perivascular space and parenchyma from the blood. Macrophages and activated microglial cells in the perivascular space and parenchyma, respectively, are responsible for viral clearance.

Outcome is determined by the comparative rates of viral spread and neuronal infection, the migration of inflammatory cells into the CNS, and the rapidity of the antibody response. Production of interferon is elicited in the brain of human SLE patients, but its role in limiting the spread of virus in the CNS is unclear.[43] The clinical course of SLE in HIV-infected persons has not been significantly different from that of other cases; however, few patients have been studied.[85]

Resistance and susceptibility to some flaviviral infections in mice have been linked to genes associated with permissiveness to infection and the immune response. Environmental factors that influence susceptibility to flaviviral infection in experimental models include stress from cold or isolation, reticuloendothelial cell blockade, and heavy metal intoxication.

DIAGNOSIS

A laboratory diagnosis of SLE usually is made serologically, although virus rarely has been recovered from blood in the acute phase of illness.[39] Virus can be sought from brain and other organs obtained by biopsy or at autopsy by inoculation of Vero cell cultures and suckling mice intracerebrally.[37] Viral antigen has been demonstrated in brain sections and in urinary cell sediment.[37,69] The clinical sensitivity of nucleic acid amplification tests (NAATs) is greater than that of antigen detection and viral culture using cell culture or suckling mouse inoculation,[37] although the ultimate sensitivity of NAATs depends on the dynamics of viral replication and host tropism.

Serologic studies comparing antibody titers in paired specimens collected during the first week of illness and 2 to 3 weeks later are considered the most appropriate for establishing the diagnosis.[37] Hemagglutination inhibition, complement fixation, and neutralizing antibody assays are used primarily in reference laboratories. A single immunoglobulin M (IgM) assay may be sufficient to establish the diagnosis in many cases. SLE-specific IgM capture enzyme-linked immunosorbent assay (ELISA) is the preferred serologic screening procedure.[37,52] Serum and CSF samples should be tested.

Intrathecal production of virus-specific IgM reflects recent infection because virus-specific IgM can be detected in serum or CSF in 75% or more of specimens obtained within 4 days of onset. In most patients, IgM levels decline in the convalescent sample and disappear approximately 4 months after onset, although IgM persisted at high titer in a few patients for 6 months.[84] In areas where SLE is endemic, virus-specific IgM carried over from the previous transmission season can lead to an erroneous diagnosis. The indirect immunofluorescent antibody procedure offers a similar capacity for rapid diagnosis, but it is less sensitive than ELISA, and IgM rheumatoid factor can lead to a false-positive result. Differentiation of antibody responses to WNV, particularly during simultaneous outbreaks of the infections, has been aided by development of a duplex immunoassay.[34,45]

The serologic response in a primary flavivirus infection is usually type specific, but repeated infections lead to broad heterologous responses that are often difficult to interpret. Human infections with indigenous flaviviruses (e.g., Rio Bravo, Powassan) other than SLE are rare occurrences. However, in patients with antecedent yellow fever immunization or infection with dengue virus acquired in areas of the United States where dengue was previously endemic and recently reemergent (e.g., Texas, Florida) or acquired during travel or residence abroad, a broadly reactive flavivirus antibody response may obfuscate the diagnosis. Recent immigrants with preexisting dengue antibodies are the most common source of flaviviral antibodies in most areas of the United States.

DIFFERENTIAL DIAGNOSIS

In an endemic setting, clinicians should consider SLE principally in the differential diagnosis of patients with aseptic meningitis or acute encephalitis. However, in the context of an outbreak, the diagnostic threshold should be lowered to include patients with less specific findings, especially acute febrile illnesses with headache and patients who exhibit confusion or are encephalopathic without fever. Increased suspicion of SLE in mildly ill patients should be directed particularly at children and young adults, in whom the infection often manifests without meningoencephalitis. In South America, SLE is a sporadic cause of acute febrile illness that as a syndrome has many non–vector-borne and vector-borne causes, including dengue.[44,81]

The clinical findings of SLE cannot be easily distinguished from those of other CNS infections, but focal neurologic deficits are less characteristic of SLE and suggest other diagnoses.[55] The combination of global confusion and tremulousness in SLE can suggest a metabolic encephalopathy, and in elderly patients, the initial manifestations of SLE can overlap with the signs and symptoms of a cerebrovascular accident.

WNV encephalitis and SLE have virtually identical clinical findings, predilection for the elderly, and other epidemiologic features, including late summer seasonality, an urban locus of epidemic transmission, and similar *Culex*-bird transmission cycles, and individual cases cannot be differentiated except by specific laboratory testing.[34,45,47]

The progression of symptoms and localizing signs associated with herpes simplex viral encephalitis contrasts sharply with the clinical findings in SLE, in which localizing signs are less often demonstrated. Enteroviral infections have overlapping summer seasonality but often are associated with clustering of illnesses in families and other epidemiologic clues of person-to-person spread. Skin eruptions, respiratory symptoms, pericarditis, myocarditis, and conjunctivitis are helpful distinguishing characteristics. Concurrent enterovirus infection and SLE can be associated with an increased risk of seizures during the acute phase of illness.[4,61] Enteroviral infections can be confirmed by detecting viral genomic sequences in CSF or blood by polymerase chain reaction or by recovery of virus from CSF or blood. Primary HIV, human herpesvirus 6, and mumps virus infections are other common infections that should be entertained in the differential diagnosis. One third of patients with mumps encephalitis do not have associated parotid gland swelling.

Adenoviral encephalitis is a rare infection in children, more severe than SLE, and sometimes associated with hepatic and other extraneural sites of infection. Lymphoreticular involvement and typical hematologic features suggest the clinical diagnosis of Epstein-Barr virus infection. Rabies virus encephalitis should be considered if the clinical picture is one of a progressive encephalitis.

Partially treated bacterial meningitis and parameningeal pyogenic infections are the principal bacterial causes to exclude. Cat-scratch disease can manifest as fever and encephalopathy mimicking arboviral encephalitis.[58] Seizures associated with *Shigella* enteritis and ataxia associated with typhoid fever can be interpreted as a primary CNS infection. Tuberculous meningitis is typically a subacute illness; evidence of active extraneural sites of infection should be sought. A low CSF glucose level is a clue to the diagnosis.

In urban areas or where parental occupational exposure may occur, lead intoxication remains an important potential cause of encephalopathy. Hyperthermia associated with sustained exposure to elevated environmental temperature likewise may lead to encephalopathy with seizures, signs of raised intracranial pressure, and evidence of hepatic dysfunction. This constellation of symptoms also can suggest Reye syndrome, although this disease typically occurs in the winter and spring after a respiratory viral infection, particularly influenza virus, and is characterized by hypoglycemia and an elevated blood ammonia level. Patients with salicylism exhibit similar clinical findings, but a history of salicylate ingestion, an elevated anion gap early in the course of illness, and an elevated blood salicylate level should suggest that diagnosis.

TREATMENT

Supportive therapy is aimed at maintaining cardiorespiratory function, ensuring fluid and electrolyte balance, controlling seizures, and monitoring and maintaining normal intracranial pressure.[47] No specific antiviral therapy is available.

PROGNOSIS

The principal risk factor for a fatal outcome is advanced age (see Fig. 176A.5).[19,33,50,53,62,84,82,90] Among all cases reported to the CDC from 1955 to 1971, 8% of the patients died, but the age-specific mortality rate for people 60 years of age or older was 19.5%. In the decade from 2004 to 2013, the mortality rate was only 2.2% for SLE-infected subjects.[15] Fatality rates as high as 38% to 80% were recorded in the 1933 St. Louis outbreak for patients who were 60 to 89 years of age. Mortality rates for children have ranged from 2% to 5%, with the highest risk for children younger than 5 years of age. The overall case-fatality rate in an outbreak in Hermosillo, Mexico, that involved principally children was 20%.[19] The high fatality rate in this instance is anomalous because fatality rates are usually lower in *C. tarsalis*–borne SLE outbreaks in the West.

Coma, a low CSF leukocyte count (<100 cells/mm^3), and underlying hypertensive vascular disease have been factors associated with fatal outcomes for adults.[6] For children, the risk factors for death have not been described.

Recovery from SLE usually is complete or associated with sequelae such as emotional disturbances, dizziness, headache, memory impairment, and tremor.[2,29,31,56] In one study of 193 cases, 25% of children who were 1 to 4 years of age at the time of infection had serious neurologic sequelae, which was the highest rate for any age group.[60] The incidence of sequelae was 10% for children 5 to 9 years of age. Children who were younger than 1 year at the time of infection appeared to be spared serious sequelae.

Deficits in motor and intellectual function were reported in some cases. Seizures were not a significant residual abnormality. The same cohort monitored at intervals of 6 months to 14 years had no perceptible residual differences in intelligence quotient in contrast to the normal population. In a case report, persistent ataxia of the extremities and trunk and dysarthria were reported as residual findings for a 54-year-old patient due to postinfectious encephalomyelitis temporally associated with SLE.[34,75]

No deleterious effects of SLE on the outcome of pregnancy have been reported. However, infection with Japanese encephalitis virus in the second trimester resulted in transplacental viral transmission and abortion, whereas infection in the third trimester was not associated with fetal damage. Prenatal Zika virus infection, another member of the family Flaviviridae, has been casually linked to microcephaly and other severe brain anomalies.[65]

PREVENTION

Preventive public health efforts have focused on surveillance of viral activity in the enzootic cycle to predict epidemic activity. In many east-central states, weekly serologic surveys of captured wild birds and sentinel chickens are conducted to detect rising seroprevalence rates that reflect viral amplification[53] and an increased risk for human infection. The abundance of female vector mosquitoes and increased viral infection rates in vectors have been correlated with the risk of epidemic transmission.[88]

When viral activity is elevated, ground and aerial application of insecticides is aimed at reducing the infected adult vector population. If insecticides are applied early enough, viral amplification can be potentially attenuated and epidemic transmission aborted.

Avoidance of outdoor activity during the twilight and evening hours, use of repellents appropriately, and repair of screens or installation of air conditioners in residences are simple but effective measures that reduce exposure to adult mosquitoes. Improvement of drainage and removal of containers that can serve as mosquito breeding sites are important steps in preventing the disease.

A vaccine is not available. Vaccination of the general public is not a realistic preventive measure because of low attack rates and the intermittent and focal nature of outbreaks.

NEW REFERENCES SINCE THE SEVENTH EDITION

11. Centers for Disease Control and Prevention. Concurrent outbreaks of St. Louis encephalitis virus and West Nile virus disease–Arizona, 2015. *MMWR Morb Mortal Wkly Rep*. 2015;64:1349-1350.
12. Centers for Disease Control and Prevention. Saint Louis Encephalitis. http://www.cdc.gov/sle/technical/epi.html#casesbyyear.
14. Centers for Disease Control and Prevention. Saint Louis encephalitis. http://diseasemaps.usgs.gov/mapviewer.
15. Centers for Disease Control and Prevention. Saint Louis encephalitis. http://www.cdc.gov/sle/resources/SLEbyYear_2004-2013.pdf.
65. Rasmussen SA, Jamieson DJ, Honein MA, Petersen LR. Zika virus and birth defects—reviewing the evidence for causality. *N Engl J Med*. 2016;374:1981-1987.
74. Seijo A, Morales A, Poustis G, et al. Outbreak of St. Louis encephalitis in the metropolitan Buenos Aires area. *Medicina (B Aires)*. 2011;71:211-217.
85. Viloria G, Kundro M, Toibaro J, et al. Two cases of Saint Louis encephalitis in HIV-1 infected patients in Buenos Aires. *Braz J Infect Dis*. 2011;15:607-608.

The full reference list for this chapter is available at ExpertConsult.com.

176B ■ West Nile Virus

José R. Romero

HISTORY

West Nile virus (WNV) was isolated first from the blood of a 37-year-old African woman in December 1937 in Omongo, West Nile district, in the Northern Province of Uganda while researchers were attempting to isolate yellow fever virus.[200] In the same report, these investigators demonstrated that sera from patients recovering from Japanese encephalitis virus could neutralize WNV. Shortly thereafter, this finding was confirmed and expanded to document that WNV was antigenically related not only to Japanese encephalitis virus but also to St. Louis encephalitis virus.[199]

In 1950, Melnick and coworkers[141] isolated WNV from the blood of three healthy children in Egypt, thereby demonstrating that WNV was not confined to a single geographic location. Before 1999, WNV was known to be endemic to Africa, the Middle East, Europe, west and central Asia, and Oceania. With its incursion into the United States in 1999[9,156] and subsequent spread throughout North America, Central America, and the Caribbean,[114,174] WNV has established a worldwide distribution.

The first reports of WNV as a cause of outbreaks of febrile illness came from Israel in the early 1950s and ultimately led to its being associated with a clinical entity coined West Nile fever.[19,77] Studies performed by Taylor and colleagues[206] at the US Naval Medical Research Unit in Egypt in the early 1950s provided information about the epidemiology of WNV infection and clinical picture of West Nile fever in children. This information was augmented by the seminal report by Marberg and colleagues[136] describing the clinical characteristics of serologically and virologically confirmed cases of West Nile fever among adolescent and young adult military personnel during a 1953 epidemic in Israel. Sporadic reports of central nervous system (CNS) complications associated with WNV infection followed closely after the early clinical descriptions of West Nile fever and pointed to the neuropathogenic potential of WNV.[18,87,202-204] Further characterization of West Nile neuroinvasive disease (encephalitis, meningitis, acute flaccid paralysis) followed as additional outbreaks of WNV were reported.

Outbreaks of WNV have occurred worldwide. Notable human outbreaks include Israel, 1951 to 1954, 1957, and 2000; France, 1962; South Africa, 1974; Algeria, 1994; Tunisia, 1997; Romania, 1996; and Russia, 1999.[19,49,60,65,87,168,209] Two of the largest epidemics recorded occurred in South Africa in 1974 and the United States in 2003. During the former, an estimated 18,000 cases of West Nile fever occurred.[87]

After the introduction of WNV into the North American continent in 1999, cases of West Nile fever and neuroinvasive disease remained at relatively low levels through 2001 and exploded in 2002 and 2003 when 4156 and 9862 cases, respectively, of WNV infection were reported to the Centers for Disease Control and Prevention (CDC) (Table 176B.1).[46] The 2002 epidemic of WNV in the United States resulted in the largest epidemic of neuroinvasive West Nile disease ever recorded, with nearly 3000 cases reported.[46] Currently, WNV has superseded all autochthonous North American arboviruses as the single most important cause of arboviral disease in the United States.[130] The magnitude of the cumulative number of WNV infections that occurred in the United States from 1999 to 2014 can be estimated from the studies suggesting that there are 30 to 70 nonneuroinvasive WNV disease cases for every case of neuroinvasive disease. Extrapolating from a total of 18,810 neuroinvasive disease cases reported to the CDC during the 16-year period,[46] an estimated 564,300 to 1,316,700 cases of nonneuroinvasive disease might have occurred.

VIROLOGY

WNV is a member of the Flaviviridae family of RNA viruses.[127] The viral family is composed of three genera: *Flavivirus, Pestivirus,* and *Hepacivirus*. WNV is a member of the *Flavivirus* genus and falls within the Japanese encephalitis virus serocomplex, along with Cacipacore, Japanese encephalitis, Kunjin, Murray Valley encephalitis, St. Louis encephalitis, Usutu, and Yaoundé viruses. Kunjin virus, which is endemic to Australia and Asia, is a subtype of WNV. Members within the Japanese encephalitis virus serogroup are antigenically related to each other.

WNV is a spherical, enveloped virus measuring approximately 50 nm in diameter. The viral envelope is derived from the lipid bilayer of the host cell and surrounds the approximately 25-nm nucleocapsid core of the virion. The host cell–derived envelope is modified by the insertion of two viral proteins: E (envelope protein) and M (membrane protein).

The genome of WNV is a single-stranded, positive-sense (messenger sense) RNA molecule measuring 11,029 nucleotides in length (Fig. 176B.1).[120,127,132] Two noncoding regions (5′ NCR and 3′ NCR) flank the 10,302-nucleotide viral single open reading frame and measure 96 and 631 nucleotides, respectively. The 5′ and 3′ NCRs contain conserved RNA secondary structures that play important roles in

TABLE 176B.1 West Nile Virus Infections in the United States, 1999–2014

Year	Total Cases	Total Deaths	Neuroinvasive Disease	Nonneuroinvasive Disease
1999	62	7	59	3
2000	21	2	19	2
2001	66	10	64	2
2002	4156	284	2946	1210
2003	9862	264	2866	6996
2004	2539	100	1148	1391
2005	3000	119	1309	1691
2006	4269	177	1459	2774
2007	3630	124	1227	2403
2008	1356	44	689	666
2009	720	32	386	334
2010	1021	57	629	392
2011	712	43	486	226
2012	5674	286	2873	2801
2013	2469	119	1267	1202
2014	2205	97	1347	858
Total	41,762	1,765 (4%)[a]	18,810 (45%)	22,952 (55%)

[a]Percentage of total cases.
From Centers for Disease Control and Prevention. West Nile virus disease cases and deaths reported to the CDC by year and clinical presentation. www.cdc.gov/westnile/statsmaps/cumMapsData.html#seven.

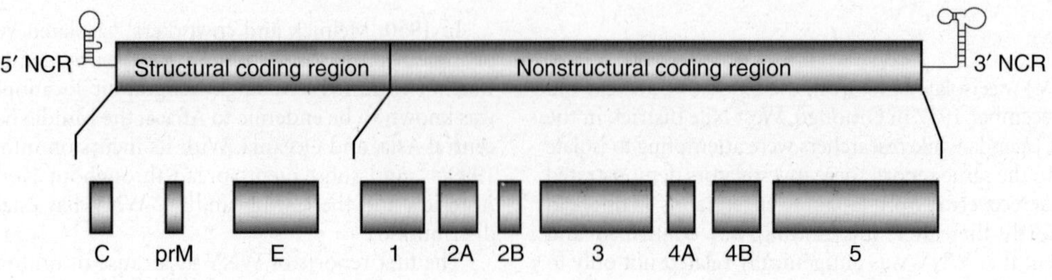

FIGURE 176B.1 Organization and protein products of the West Nile genome.

translation and replication. The open reading frame is organized as 5′-C-prM-E-NS1-NS2A-NS3-NS4A-NS4B-NS5-3′ and is transcribed into a single polyprotein of 3434 amino acids encoding three structural and seven nonstructural proteins.[120,127] The N-terminal portion of the polyprotein consists of viral structural proteins, whereas the remainder of the protein contains the nonstructural (NS) proteins. The viral polyprotein is cotranslationally and posttranslationally processed by host proteases and the viral protease NS2B-NS3 to yield three structural (i.e., E, premembrane [prM], and C) and seven NS (i.e., 1, 2A, 2B, 3, 4A, 4B, and 5) proteins.

Viral attachment, endocytosis, membrane fusion, and viral assembly are mediated by the E protein. The search for the cellular receptors of WNV has identified the integrin $\alpha_v\beta_3$ (vitronectin receptor) as the primary cellular receptor for lineage 2 WNVs.[50] The lectins DC-SIGNR and DC-SIGN are capable of binding WNV and promoting infection in vitro.[57] In addition, WNV has been shown to interact with several other cell surface proteins, but the whether they are physiologically relevant in vivo remains to be determined.[166] When bound to its receptor, WNV gains entry into the cell through endocytosis; after a pH-dependent change occurs in the conformation of the E protein, the viral and host endosomal membranes fuse. The viral nucleocapsid is then released into the cytoplasm of the cell. Viral replication is thought to occur on the membrane of the rough endoplasmic reticulum. The C or capsid protein binds to the viral RNA genome and forms a ribonucleoprotein complex required for packaging of the genome.[150] The immature virions are assembled, accumulate in vesicles, and bud into the endoplasmic reticulum. The immature virions are processed as they traverse the secretory pathway. Immature viral particles contain a prM protein that blocks premature viral fusion by the E protein. The prM protein is cleaved to the M protein by the trans-Golgi protein furin during the egress of the mature virion from the secretory pathway. Virions are transported to the cell membrane in vesicles and ultimately released through exocytosis or budding.

The NS proteins regulate viral transcription and translation, as well as attenuate host immune responses to WNV.[127,185] The NS1 protein serves as a cofactor for the viral replicase and modulates the host innate immune response by inhibition of TLR3 signal transduction.[222] NS1 can also bind complement factor H, thereby disrupting alternate complement pathway.[132] Host interferon (IFN) responses are inhibited by NS2A through inhibition of IFN-β promoter activity. This protein also may play a role in viral assembly. The NS3 protein is a serine protease and requires NS2B as a cofactor for activity. It also possesses NTPase and helicase activities. NS proteins 4A and 4B modulate IFN signaling. The NS5 functions as the RNA-dependent RNA polymerase and a methyltransferase. The NS5 protein from the virulent WNV strain NY99 is an antagonist of type 1 IFN-mediated JAK-STAT signal transduction.[121]

Phylogenetic analysis of WNV isolates from around the world has demonstrated the existence of up to six lineages.[120,135,167] Lineages 1 and 2 constitute the major lineages. Strains that make up lineage 2 were originally thought to be found exclusively in sub-Saharan Africa and Madagascar. However, isolates from this lineage have been found in recent outbreaks of human disease in Russia, Greece, Italy, Romania, and South Africa. Lineage 1 strains are found in geographically dispersed regions around the world and can be subdivided into two clades.[120] The clade can be further subdivided into six clusters (1–6). WNV strains from Africa, Europe, the United States, the Middle East, and Russia cluster within clade 1a. Kunjin virus and India WNV strains form clades 1b and 1c, respectively. WNV strains isolated from birds and a human during the 1999 outbreak in the United States and a WNV strain isolated in 1998 from a dead goose in Israel have been shown to be closely related.[119] Phylogenetic analysis of the prM protein and E glycoprotein demonstrated that they share more than 99.8% nucleotide homology, indicating that the North American strain of WNV almost certainly originated in the Middle East. Analysis of US WNV isolates has demonstrated a slowly evolving nucleotide divergence. The initial WNV strain in the United States, NY99, was displaced in less than 4 years by the current dominant genotype WN02.

Genetic correlations appear to exist between genotype/lineage and virulence/fitness phenotype.[95,120,135,167] Neurovirulence data by use of a murine model indicates that lineage 1 strains of WNV are more neuroinvasive than are those of lineage 2.[15] Nucleotide changes in the 3′ noncoding region and amino acid substitutions in the nonstructural and envelope proteins have been associated with increased morbidity and viral load in American crows, decreased incubation time for infection until transmission of WNV by *Culex pipiens* mosquitos, and modification of the host IFN signaling cascade. These changes have given rise to attenuated genotypes of WNV as it has spread across the United States.

EPIDEMIOLOGY

In temperate climates, WNV infections occur seasonally during the summer months, coinciding with periods of increased activity of its mosquito vectors. The peak period of activity for transmission of WNV to humans in the United States generally is from July through September.[130,45] As WNV has spread southward in the United States, the period of reported transmissions has increased, with human cases being reported as early as April and as late as December.[89] Year-round transmission may be possible in tropical climates.

Infections of humans (i.e., epizootic infection) by WNV are incidental to its enzootic life cycle and, with rare exception, result in a "dead-end" infection without subsequent human-to-human transmission. Epizootic transmission of WNV occurs when sufficient numbers of mosquitoes that bite both birds and humans become infected to allow transmission to humans. Important risk factors for the acquisition of human WNV infection are the amount of time spent outdoors when mosquitoes are biting; the presence of dead birds in the neighborhood; the exposure to mosquitoes; and the land cover, water, and soil suitable for harboring potentially infected mosquitoes.[26,51,84,149]

Climate and rainfall can influence the distribution and timing of WNV outbreaks. The competence of *Culex* mosquitoes as vectors increases at higher temperatures. Drought brings mosquito vectors and their hosts in closer contact.[21] Elevated environmental temperature accelerates viral replication within mosquito vectors and decreases the time span of the reproductive feeding cycle of *Culex* mosquitos.[62,85,109,177] Increases in WNV infections have been associated with economic factors, such as the downturn in the housing market and delinquent mortgages, which has led to large numbers of neglected residential swimming pools in some areas.[178]

The enzootic cycle of WNV requires replicative phases in its mosquito vectors and avian (or other) hosts. After WNV-infected blood meal has been ingested, the virus penetrates the mosquito's gut.[74] Viral replication then takes place in the salivary glands and nervous system of the mosquito. In mosquito tissues, WNV is nonlytic and results in persistent infection for the lifetime of the vector.

Mosquitoes play an important role in transgenerational and trans-seasonal maintenance of the WNV enzootic cycle. Female *C. pipiens* mosquitoes can transmit WNV vertically to F1 progeny.[63,212] In addition, WNV can survive the winter by overwintering in hibernating female mosquitoes, as documented with *C. pipiens,* which thereby serve as a source of WNV to initiate the enzootic cycle the following spring.[155]

Although numerous mosquito species have been found to be infected with WNV, ornithophilic members in the *Culex* genus are the principal vectors for the transmission of WNV around the world. These include *Culex pipiens* and *Culex quinquefasciatus* in Europe, *Culex perexiguus* in North Africa and the Middle East, *Culex univittatus* in sub-Saharan Africa, *Culex tritaeniorhynchus* in south Asia, *Culex annulirostris* in Australia, and species of the *Culex vishnui* complex in India.[113]

Although WNV has been found in 59 of the 172 North American species of mosquitoes, only about a half-dozen are considered to be important vectors for transmission to humans.[89] As in other regions of the world, *Culex* spp. of mosquitoes are important vectors[89]; *C. pipiens* (the northern house mosquito) and *C. quinquefasciatus* (the southern house mosquito) are considered to be the predominant vectors in the northeastern, southern, and southwestern United States, respectively. *Culex tarsalis* is a predominant vector west of the Mississippi River. *Culex nigripalpus* and *Culex salinarius* may be important vectors in regions where they are abundant. Last, *Culex restuans* also has been found to be a significant contributor to WNV-positive mosquito pools. Although arthropods can be infected with WNV, they are not thought to be important in transmission of WNV.

Birds are thought to be the principal amplifying hosts for WNV. Nearly 200 species of North American birds are susceptible to infection by WNV.[113] However, only birds capable of sustaining high-titer viremia for significant periods are capable of infecting the mosquitoes that feed on them. In vivo experiments using *C. tarsalis* have shown that 74% to 100% of mosquitoes consuming blood meals containing $10^{7.1}$ plaque-forming units (PFUs) per milliliter become infected. In contrast, 36% or fewer mosquitoes become infected after the consumption of blood containing $10^{4.9}$ PFUs/mL.[75] As a point of comparison, on the basis of blood tested from viremic blood donors, the maximum viral load in human blood is approximately $10^{3.2}$ PFUs/mL.[89] This finding indicates that humans fail to produce viremia titers of sufficient magnitude to infect mosquitoes. Most mammals also fail to have sufficient levels of viremia to permit transmission to mosquitoes.

Songbirds (Passeriformes), shorebirds (Charadriiformes), owls (Strigiformes), and falcons (Falconiformes) develop adequate viremia to infect mosquitoes feeding on them (pigeons and ducks do not). House finches, house sparrows, common grackles, and, in particular, corvids such as crows, magpies, and jays have been shown to be highly infectious to mosquitoes.[89,113] In addition, they have a high mortality rate after acquiring infection with WNV. Die-offs of avian species serve as epidemiologic markers for WNV activity in the environment.[79,149]

Unlike mammals, some amphibians appear to be capable of sustaining levels of viremia that potentially could be sufficient to infect mosquitoes and may serve as competent reservoirs for their infection. In the United States, alligators *(Alligator mississippiensis)* infected with WNV produced sufficient viral loads to infect mosquitoes.[112] Detection of WNV RNA in mosquitoes, alligators, and alligator-derived blood meals collected at alligator farms in Louisiana support the role of alligators as competent hosts for WNV amplification and transmission.[211] In Russia, the marsh frog *(Rana ridibunda)* may be a host for WNV.[89,115]

In areas where WNV traditionally has been endemic, seroprevalence studies document that most individuals acquire WNV infection during childhood. Such early acquisition of WNV infection results in large portions of the adult population with serologic evidence of immunity to WNV and may attenuate the occurrence of large outbreaks of WNV infection. Studies conducted in the 1950s in Egypt documented that a rapid rise in the presence of antibodies occurred in children 1 to 4 years of age such that by the time children were 4 years of age, 50% to 80% had neutralizing or complement-fixing antibodies to WNV.[141,206] Similar patterns of acquisition of WNV-specific antibodies have been documented in the Sudan, Central Africa, and Nigeria.[200,206] Interestingly, more recent studies conducted in Egypt indicate that the seroprevalence rates in children and young adults, although still high, may be decreasing.[53,56] One can speculate that mosquito abatement programs and, possibly, changes in lifestyle have resulted in decreasing numbers of infections in children.

Seroepidemiologic studies conducted in areas where initial WNV has resulted in large outbreaks of West Nile fever and neuroinvasive disease document low seroprevalence rates among the general population.[134,148,151,209] Investigation of the seroprevalence of WNV infection after an outbreak of WNV in Romania after the first major WNV epidemic in Europe found it to be 4.6%.[209] After the initial North American outbreak of West Nile encephalitis in New York in 1999, the seroprevalence at the outbreak's epicenter was found to be approximately 2.6%.[148] Based on data derived from the screening of the United States blood supply, the estimated prevalence of past WNV infection among the United States population is approximately 1%.[171] In areas where postepidemic seroprevalence has been conducted, it has been found to range from 1.9% to 14%—too low to protect against future large-scale outbreaks of WNV disease.[47,151,171]

Multiple non–vector-borne modes of WNV transmission have been identified. Transfusion-associated transmission of WNV was reported for the first time in 2002, when 23 cases were confirmed.[145,165] WNV virus infection has resulted from the transfusion of red blood cells, platelets, fresh frozen plasma, and granulocytes.[42-44,142,144,165,170] Of the 32 cases, five (16%) occurred in children younger than 18 years.[42,144,165] Three of the children had immunocompromising conditions (i.e., acute myeloid leukemia, rhabdomyosarcoma, stem cell transplant). The three children received platelet infusions and developed West Nile meningoencephalitis; all survived. The sole adolescent was a victim of a motor vehicle collision and received a transfusion of red blood cells. This patient subsequently became an organ donor and was implicated in four cases of transplantation-associated transmission of WNV.[36,100] A sole case of acquisition of WNV through granulocyte transfusion has been reported.[142]

National screening of blood donations for the presence of WNV by nucleic acid amplification–based testing was initiated in June 2003. However, rare cases of transfusion-associated transmission have continued to occur. Since then, 13 probable or confirmed cases of transfusion-acquired WNV infection occurred through 2012 (none of which occurred in children); they most likely were attributable to donations containing very low levels of virus.[40,44,46,129,142,144]

Transmission through organ transplantation has also been documented.[36,41,43,100,157,179] However, no cases in pediatric transplant recipients have been reported.[129] From 2002 to 2013, six clusters of organ transplant–associated WNV transmission were reported to the CDC.[12] WNV infection developed in 12 of 16 transplant recipients, nine of whom developed encephalitis and four of whom died. The risk for acquiring West Nile neuroinvasive disease is approximately 40 times greater in organ transplant recipients than in the general population.[116] Organ donations are not required to be screened by nucleic acid amplification for WNV infection, nor is it performed routinely.

Confirmed or suspected maternal-fetal and maternal-infant vertical transmission of WNV has been reported[3,34,35,90,161] but seems to be an unusual occurrence.[172] In a report of the outcomes of a small cohort of newborns whose mothers were infected with WNV during pregnancy, more than half occurring in the first and second trimesters, no infant was found to have evidence of WNV-specific immunoglobulin M (IgM) in cord blood.[172] In the most rigorously documented case of maternal-infant transmission,[3,34,90] confirmed maternal WNV infection occurred during the twenty-seventh week of gestation. The infant, delivered at 38 weeks of gestation, was found to have bilateral chorioretinitis, severe bilateral white-matter loss in the temporal and occipital lobes, and tissue destruction in a temporal lobe. The presence of WNV-specific IgM was confirmed in cord blood, infant serum, and cerebrospinal fluid (CSF), although the CSF contained red blood cells. Maternal serum also contained WNV-specific IgM at the time of birth. The WNV genome was detected in the umbilical cord tissue and placenta by reverse transcriptase polymerase chain reaction (RT-PCR). No WNV genome was detected in the infant's CSF.

Evaluation of 70 pregnancies reported to the CDC WNV pregnancy registry failed to identify any confirmed cases of congenital WNV infection.[161] However, three infants who lacked evidence of anti-WNV IgM in cord blood or infant serum at the time of delivery subsequently were found to have serologic evidence of infection that may have been acquired congenitally. A breast-fed term infant, whose mother had onset of West Nile neuroinvasive disease 6 days before delivery, developed West Nile meningitis at 10 days of age. Another breast-fed infant, born to a woman with acute West Nile fever at the time of delivery, was noted to have a transient rash at birth. No serum or cord blood was available for testing. However, at 1 month of age, the infant was found to have WNV-specific IgM antibodies. In the final case, the infant's mother had a febrile illness 3 weeks before delivery. The infant appeared to be healthy at birth, but at 7 days of age developed seizures. Evaluation of the infant at 17 days of age found lissencephaly and West Nile encephalitis with WNV-specific IgM antibodies detectable in the CSF. Because two of the infants were breast-fed, the possibility exists that WNV was transmitted in that manner. In addition, in none of the cases could the possibility of mosquito-borne transmission of WNV be excluded conclusively. This report also failed to link WNV infection during pregnancy with an increased frequency of spontaneous abortion, premature birth, or low birth weight.

The outcome of children born to mothers with West Nile illness during pregnancy appears to be good.[172,195] Two small studies have not identified developmental delays, neurologic defects, increased fetal loss, or an increased frequency of birth defects among infants born to women with confirmed WNV infection during pregnancy. However, it should be noted that both studies enrolled a small number of maternal-infant pairs. Larger studies are needed to confirm these findings.

WNV has been detected in the breast milk of infected women.[35,161] At least one case of possible transmission of WNV associated with breastfeeding has been reported.[35,88,161] The mother received packed red blood cell transfusions on the first 2 postpartum days. Ten days postpartum, the mother developed headache followed by fever. On evaluation, she was found to have CSF pleocytosis and the presence of WNV-specific IgM in the CSF. The infant was breast-fed for the first 17 days of life, and although the infant was clinically asymptomatic, a serum sample obtained at 25 days of age was found to have WNV-specific IgM. Because of the paucity of additional case reports, it appears that the risk for WNV transmission from mother to infant through breastfeeding is low. The current state of knowledge about transmission of WNV through breast milk does not warrant a change in breastfeeding recommendations.

Additional nontraditional modes of confirmed or possible transmission of WNV has been reported through laboratory exposure, animal autopsies, percutaneous injury, conjunctival inoculation, aerosol inhalation, and dialysis.[37-39,67,83,213,214]

With the exceptions of Alaska and Hawaii, every state in the United States has reported human, mosquito, avian, or animal WNV. From 1999 to 2014, 41,762 cases of WNV infection were reported to the CDC (see Table 176B.1).[46] Neuroinvasive syndromes accounted for 18,810 cases (45%), and nonneuroinvasive syndromes were reported in 22,952 cases (55%). During the same period, 1765 deaths (4%) were reported.[46]

Pediatric-specific epidemiologic and clinical data regarding WNV infections has become available but is most likely incomplete because of underreporting of cases.[88-90,129] After an Ohio outbreak of WNV, the county-wide seroprevalence rate was found to be 1.9%. However, among children younger than 17 years, the seroprevalence rate was nearly 3.5 times higher: 6.4%.[134] From 2003 to 2012, 13,108 cases of West Nile neuroinvasive disease were reported to the CDC (see Table 176B.1).[46] Children accounted for 505 cases (4%). The median number of pediatric cases per year was 49 (range, 7–137).[70] For that period, the median annual incidence of West Nile neuroinvasive disease was 0.68 cases per 1 million children and ranged from 0.09 to 1.85 cases per 1 million children. By way of comparison, for the same period the median annual incidence for adults was eightfold higher. States in the North Central and Mountain regions had the highest annual incidence. The four states with the highest annual pediatric incidences were South Dakota (10.36 per 1 million children), Wyoming (5.91 per 1 million children), North Dakota (5.34 per 1 million children), and Nebraska (5.23 per 1 million children). Seven states accounted for greater than half of all reported cases: Texas (77 cases), California (49), Louisiana (34), Colorado (32) Arizona (29), Nebraska (24), and South Dakota (21). Boys accounted for 61% of cases.

The distribution of WNV syndromes among children has been difficult to define because of underreporting of pediatric cases of West Nile infection.[88] Lindsey and colleagues reported cases of West Nile infection in children from 1999 through 2007 and noted that 1478 (5%) occurred in children younger than 18 years.[129] It is the only large study that has reported on the percentage of pediatric infections that result in nonneuroinvasive (68%) versus neuroinvasive (30%) disease.[129] In that report the median age of children with West Nile fever in one report spanning a decade was 14 years (range, 1 day to 17 years).[129] Children accounted for 4% of all neuroinvasive cases of West Nile infection from 1999 to 2013.[71,129] The median age of children with West Nile neuroinvasive disease was 12 years.[71,129] Of the children with neuroinvasive disease, 50% had meningitis, 40% encephalitis, and 3% acute flaccid paralysis.[70] Half of those with acute flaccid paralysis also had meningitis or encephalitis.

Three deaths have been reported—a 1-month-old boy, a 14-year-old boy, and a 16-year-old girl. Two of the children who died of neuroinvasive disease had underlying medical conditions; one had an immunodeficiency and the other lissencephaly.[90,129,159]

Available information indicates that WNV infection in children is typically mild, resulting in West Nile fever in more than two-thirds of children with symptomatic infection. The distribution of West Nile neuroinvasive disease in children indicates that the predominant West Nile neuroinvasive syndrome is meningitis, followed by encephalitis.

PATHOGENESIS

The pathogenesis of West Nile encephalitis has been explored in animal model systems. Subcutaneous inoculation of WNV is thought to result in WNV infection and replication in Langerhans dendritic cells.[27] Domain III of the WNV envelope (E) protein is believed to interact with DC-SIGN or DC-SIGNR to mediate cellular attachment. Under control of interleukin-1β, activated Langerhans cells migrate to regional lymph nodes and result in a primary viremia that develops after the virus reaches the systemic circulation through the thoracic duct.[27] In mice, peak viremia occurs by the second day after infection and clears by the sixth day. Virus subsequently can be detected in spleen, brain, and spinal cord. Because of the simultaneous appearance of virus in the brain and spinal cord, a hematogenous route for the CNS infection has been postulated. In humans, WNV can be detected in the neurons of the cerebral cortex, thalamus, brainstem, basal ganglia, cerebellum, and spinal cord, primarily in the anterior horn. Similar locations have been seen in mice and hamsters. Infection of the neurons in these sites results in meningoencephalitis and acute flaccid paralysis. Several mechanisms have been postulated for the neuronal injury seen in WNV infection[194]: viral injury to infected neurons through apoptosis, targeting of infected neurons by cytotoxic T lymphocytes, and neuronal death as a result of bystander injury. Cell death of WNV-infected neurons has been shown to be caspase-3 dependent.

The mechanism by which WNV gains access to the CNS is not fully understood. WNV binding to toll-like receptor-3 (TLR3) has been shown to result in TLR3 receptor–dependent inflammatory response with resultant production of tumor necrosis factor-α (TNF-α) and interleukin-6.[217] TNF-α may modulate the ability of WNV to invade the CNS, inducing breakdown of the blood-brain barrier. Macrophage migration inhibition factor, induced endothelial cell adhesion molecule-1 and matrix metalloproteinase-9 also have been shown to play roles in increased brain capillary epithelial permeability.[6,55,216] Additional postulated mechanisms through which WNV may breach the blood-brain barrier include infection or passive transport through the choroid plexus epithelial cells or the endothelium, infection of olfactory neurons, transport within infected immune cells that traffic into the CNS (Trojan horse mechanism), and retrograde axonal transport in infected peripheral neurons.[185]

Cessation of the viremia occurs by the sixth day in mice and is coincident with the appearance of type-specific antibody response. Viral clearance from all tissues is complete by 2 to 3 weeks after infection. Humoral immunity is essential to the recovery from WNV infection, as demonstrated by the uniform death of B-cell–deficient mice.[61] B-cell–deficient mice could be protected from lethal infection by the passive transfer of serum from infected and immune wild-type mice. Mice deficient in $CD4^+$ T cells exhibited prolonged detection of WNV in the CNS, lower WNV-specific levels of IgM and IgG, and uniform lethality, indicating that the principal protective role of these cells is to assist in antibody responses. γ/δ T cells that secrete IFN-γ may control viral replication through direct antiviral mechanisms and contribute to adaptive immune responses.[185]

Although clearance of WNV from the CNS and other tissues depends primarily on humoral immunity, cytotoxic T cells also play a role.[126,210] Increased mortality rates in association with higher and sustained WNV loads in the CNS and spleen were observed in mice deficient in $CD8^+$ T cells or class I major histocompatibility complex molecules.[193] In addition, control of WNV infection in the CNS requires IFN-α/β. IFN-α/β also may help increase the survival of neurons. Finally, chemokines such as CXCL10 and CCL5 and their ligands CXCR3 and CCR5 aid in the recruitment of $CD4^+$ and $CD8^+$ T cells and monocytes to the CNS.[185]

CLINICAL MANIFESTATIONS

Most WNV infections in children and adults result in subclinical disease. In general, WNV infection in children more frequently results in asymptomatic infection or milder disease than that in adults.[49,77,129,156,187,204] One report documented that children were 4.5 times more likely to become infected with WNV during an epidemic but 110 times less likely to develop neuroinvasive disease.[134] In another, the estimated incidence of neuroinvasive disease was 1.4 per 100,000 children aged 5 to 17 years in contrast to 14.3 per 100,000 individuals aged 18 years or older.[117] In adults, multiple reports have identified increasing age as the single most significant risk factor for the development of neuroinvasive disease, as well as adverse outcome.[129,152,168] The incidence of severe neurologic disease is 10 times higher in individuals aged 50 to 59 years and 43 times higher in persons aged 80 years or older in contrast to those 20 years or younger. Chronic illnesses, such as hypertension, diabetes mellitus, cardiovascular disease, and alcohol abuse, also have been identified as risk factors for severe disease.[22,152,156,168] These factors have not been linked to an increased risk for the development of severe disease in children.

In the early 1950s, therapeutic inoculation of WNV into patients with malignant neoplasms in advanced stages resulted in a high incidence of development of encephalitis among recipients and pointed to the role of immunosuppression as a risk factor for West Nile neuroinvasive disease.[203] This finding was substantiated by the recognition that transplant recipients were 40 times more likely to develop West Nile neuroinvasive disease.[116] Reports of West Nile neuroinvasive disease in immunocompromised children also are consistent with immunosuppression as a risk factor in this population.[7,68,94,176,201] Reports also have indicated that the use of immunomodulating agents such as infliximab, rituximab, methotrexate, and fludarabine may predispose to the development of severe WNV infection.[13,48,124,139]

Approximately 20% of infected adults develop West Nile fever. Because of the fever's mild nature, only about half of individuals with West Nile fever ever seek medical attention. WNV neuroinvasive syndromes (e.g., encephalitis, meningitis, meningoencephalitis, and acute flaccid paralysis) develop in less than 1% of adults (one in 140–320) infected with WNV.[148,156,168,209] The occurrence of West Nile neuroinvasive disease in children is significantly less.[117,134] In one study, it was calculated to occur in approximately one in 4200 infected children.[134]

The incubation period of WNV infection ranges from 2 to 14 days but usually is 2 to 6 days.[28,77,113,136] Viremia may be present from approximately 2 days before to approximately 4 days after the onset of the illness.[76] In immunosuppressed individuals, incubation periods up to 3 weeks have been reported and may exhibit prolonged periods of viremia.[100,165]

In children[52,68,77,90,98,136,223] and adults, West Nile fever is an influenza-like febrile illness characterized by an abrupt onset of fever that typically ranges from 38°C to 40°C (100.4°F–104°F). It is accompanied by fatigue, malaise, anorexia, headache, myalgias, and weakness.[28,77,136,168,218] Ocular pain on eye movement has been reported.[77,136] A diffuse, nonpruritic, macular, papular, maculopapular, or morbilliform exanthem and diffuse lymphadenopathy also may be seen. On occasion, it has been described as petechial.[24,52,181] The rash spares the palms and soles and generally involves the chest, back, and arms.[181] The exanthem may be present more frequently in children than in adults, regardless of the WNV syndrome, occurring in 50%.[25,52,181] The exanthem generally is present for less than a week. Neck pain and photosensitivity often are reported. Gastrointestinal complaints such as nausea, vomiting, abdominal pain, and diarrhea may occur. Sore throat and cough also have been reported. The illness generally is short-lived, lasting only 3 to 6 days.[77,98,136] Convalescence, however, may take many weeks and is characterized by fatigue.[77,136,218]

Other nonneurologic WNV syndromes that have been reported in adults include cardiac dysrhythmias, myocarditis, pancreatitis, hepatitis, rhabdomyolysis, myositis, and orchitis.[9,24,91,93,140,145,156,223] Myocarditis and hepatitis have been reported in children with West Nile infection.

Although cases of West Nile neuroinvasive disease have been reported in children,* most of the information about these clinical syndromes has been derived from reports that have involved predominantly adults.† However, on the basis of a limited number of pediatric cases and series, the clinical presentation in children appears to parallel that of adults.[187] Although discussion of each of the neuroinvasive syndromes individually (i.e., meningitis, encephalitis, and acute flaccid paralysis) is convenient, one should recognize that patients may have components of each in their clinical presentation. Finally, the clinical findings in West Nile neuroinvasive disease in children and adults are not sufficiently distinct to distinguish them from those of other viral meningitides or encephalitides.

*References 7, 24, 30, 52, 59, 60, 66, 68, 73, 88, 92,94, 96, 117, 146, 158, 159, 164, 173, 176, 180, 198, 201, 207, 215, 220, 223.

†References 9, 22, 28, 31, 48, 49, 102, 110, 125, 156, 168, 183, 189-191, 221.

In adults, the onset of West Nile meningitis tends to be abrupt, with fever, headache, and neck stiffness and meningeal signs (Kernig and Brudzinski signs).* Photophobia and phonophobia may be present. The headache pain may be severe enough to warrant the use of opioid analgesics. Weakness frequently is reported.[52,68] Additional associated symptoms may include those seen with West Nile fever: gastrointestinal and respiratory symptoms (i.e., nausea, vomiting, diarrhea, sore throat, and cough), rash, and lymphadenopathy. Dyskinesias in the form of tremors, myoclonus, or parkinsonism also may occur.

The reported clinical findings of West Nile encephalitis in children† are similar to those described in adults.[22,28,49,156,168,187] The onset of frank encephalitis may be preceded by a brief period, or prodrome, of fever, headache, rash, and malaise consistent with West Nile fever. In some cases, the appearance of fever is coincident with the onset of mental status changes. The mental status changes may range from a mild confusional state to severe encephalopathy and coma. Generalized weakness is a common component of the clinical spectrum of encephalitis. Paresis or palsies may be present. Ataxia, dysmetria, tremors, myoclonus, and parkinsonism may be seen.[52,146,158] Signs of bulbar dysfunction, such as dysarthria, dysphagia, and respiratory failure, have been reported. If a component of meningitis is present (i.e., meningoencephalitis), signs and symptoms described previously for meningitis also may be present. Seizures have been reported in children[7,30,68,159,180,201] and may be focal with associated neurologic signs similar to those of herpes simplex virus encephalitis.[180,215]

Acute flaccid paralysis in association with WNV infection was reported first in 1979[70] and may occur in the absence of meningitis or encephalitis. Several reports of acute flaccid paralysis, alone or in association with encephalitis, developing after the occurrence of WNV infection in children have been published.[24,68,80,92,183,198,207]

The onset of the paralysis occurs early in the illness, usually within the first 72 hours.[189] Pain or paresthesia in the affected limb preceding the onset of weakness is reported in most cases.[80,189] Patients exhibit asymmetric weakness, hypotonia, and absent or diminished deep tendon reflexes. Pain or sensory function in the affected limbs remains intact.[9,102,110,125,183,189] However, at least one report has documented electrophysiologic evidence of sensory fiber loss in association with severe spinal cord involvement.[64] It is postulated that this finding could be explained by damage to neurons in the dorsal root ganglia. Tremor, myoclonus, and parkinsonism are common findings.[190,191] In severe cases, changes in bowel and bladder function or quadriplegia may occur. Involvement of the brainstem motor nuclei of the vagus and glossopharyngeal nerves can result in dysphagia, dysarthria, and acute respiratory failure requiring assisted mechanical ventilation.[24] Patients with dysphagia and dysarthria are at greater risk for the development of respiratory failure.[189]

Ocular manifestations of WNV infection include chorioretinitis/retinitis, vitritis, and uveitis.[10,93,187] Chorioretinitis has been described in congenital and postnatal WNV infections[3,10,187] and may be more common than is realized.[91] Postnatal cases of West Nile chorioretinitis have been reported solely in adults. A recent study found that 24% of adults with a history of WNV infection had evidence of WNV-associated retinopathy. The finding of was even more frequently observed in those who presented with encephalitis, in whom it approached 50%.[86]

In the sole reported case of congenital WNV infection, the infant had a large chorioretinal scar involving the retina of the right eye. Mild chorioretinal scarring was observed in the far temporal periphery.[3,10] Vitritis also has been reported in children and can lead to blurring and loss of vision.[223]

*References 2, 22, 28, 49, 52, 57, 68, 88, 90, 96, 110, 117, 156, 168, 187, 191, 209, 221.

†References 7, 24, 30, 52, 59, 60, 68, 88, 90, 94, 108, 146, 159, 176, 180, 201, 215.

Other rarely reported neurologic manifestations of West Nile neuroinvasive disease in adults include optic neuritis, myelitis, Guillain-Barré syndrome,[2] and polyradiculitis.[164]

Recently, the possibility of long-term persistence of West Nile virus infection has been raised.[154] WNV genome was detected by RT-PCR in the urine in 20% of a cohort of patients with neuroinvasive disease 1.6 to 6.7 years after initial infection. All patients reported persistence of neurologic symptoms or signs. This finding is consistent with findings in the hamster model WNV infection and suggests ongoing replication in renal tissue. However, attempts to isolate virus from the urine were unsuccessful. In addition, a higher than expected prevalence of chronic kidney disease associated with proteinuria and hematuria has been documented in a cohort of patients with a history of neuroinvasive WNV.[160]

OUTCOME

Based on cases reported to the CDC from 1999 to 2012, the mortality rate in children is less than 1%.[70,129] Although reports of death in children as a result of WNV infection are rare,[32,73,88,94] WNV outbreaks associated with significant pediatric mortality rates (12.9%) have been documented.[60,122] From 2002 to 2011, the case-fatality rates in adults ranged from 2.6% to 6.8% (mean, 4.6%).[37] Hospitalized persons 75 years or older are nine times more likely to die than are younger patients. Other reported independent risk factors for death in adults are change in level of consciousness and anemia at presentation.[49] In addition to early mortality, delayed mortality, occurring years after infection, has been reported.[131]

Although complete recovery from West Nile fever is expected, it may take several weeks before children and adults return to preillness levels of health.[77,164] Watson and colleagues[219] found that the median time to complete recovery in adults was 60 days. Postillness fatigue was reported in 98%, and the median duration of fatigue was 36 days. Sixty-one percent of patients reported muscle weakness of a median duration of 28 days. Other symptoms that persisted for longer than 7 days were reported in more than half of the subjects and included headache, muscle pain and aches, difficulty concentrating, joint pain and aches, and sensitivity to light. Of those who worked or attended school, nearly 60% reported absenteeism of more than 7 days.

Neurologic outcome of children after West Nile neuroinvasive disease has not been assessed systematically. The published case reports of West Nile neuroinvasive disease in children are most likely biased by the disease severity or outcome and limited by a lack of long-term follow-up of patients. As such, reliable information about the outcome of West Nile encephalitis and acute flaccid paralysis is lacking. However, on the basis of the review of 47 reported cases of West Nile neuroinvasive disease in children and adolescents for whom clinical and outcome information was provided,* recovery from meningitis appears to be complete in children (n = 20). Among cases of encephalitis, meningoencephalitis, and acute flaccid paralysis (n = 27), approximately 50% of children were reported to have neurologic sequelae at the time of last medical encounter or at the time the report was submitted. The reported sequelae among children include seizures, weakness, paralysis, gait disturbances, motor difficulties, language and speech deficits, dysphagia, behavior problems, cognitive deficits, mental retardation, difficulty concentrating, difficulties with memory and comprehension, facial palsy, hypertonicity, and persistent vegetative state.[7,24,68,92,96,159,201,215,220,223]

Children and adults recovering from West Nile acute flaccid paralysis exhibited persistent associated neurologic signs, poor physical recovery, and atrophy of affected limbs.[103,190] Although the degree of initial paralysis was not correlated with long-term outcome in an early report,[29] a more recent publication indicates that the degree of initial paralysis may be an important indicator of long-term outcome.[190] The greatest recovery in strength occurred during the first 4 months after paralysis.[190]

LABORATORY FINDINGS

As is the case with the clinical findings of WNV infections, routine laboratory studies are nonspecific and do not provide conclusive evidence about the etiologic agent. Similar to those in adults, hematologic findings in children include leukocytosis, leukopenia, normal total white cell count, and lymphopenia.[7,52,59,117,180,201,215,220,223] Pediatric and adult cases of encephalitis hyponatremia have been reported.[24,49,221] Elevations of transaminases and creatine kinase may be seen in children with hepatitis and myositis.[24,223]

Cytochemical evaluation of the CSF generally reveals an abnormal white cell count and protein concentration.* A predominantly lymphocytic pleocytosis with, generally, fewer than 200 cells/mm³ is a frequent finding. Cell counts of more than 2000 cells/mm³ have been reported. Early in the infection, the CSF may show a polymorphonuclear cellular predominance that later shifts to a lymphocytic pleocytosis.[54] A mildly increased protein concentration of less than 100 mg/dL generally is seen. However, considerable variation in CSF protein concentration has been reported in patients with West Nile encephalitis. A normal CSF glucose concentration generally is observed.

*References 7, 24, 30, 49, 59, 68, 92, 94, 117, 159, 198, 201, 207, 215, 220, 223.

ELECTRODIAGNOSTIC STUDIES

Electrodiagnostic study findings are abnormal in most patients with West Nile encephalitis.† Electroencephalographic abnormalities have included diffuse irregular slow waves, focal sharp waves, and subclinical electrographic seizures. An anterior preponderance of slow waves has been suggested as characteristic of West Nile encephalitis.[72] Reports of focal electroencephalographic findings suggestive of herpes simplex virus encephalitis have been reported in children.[180,215]

In patients with acute flaccid paralysis, electromyography, and nerve conduction studies document normal nerve conduction velocities, normal or reduced compound muscle action potentials, and normal sensory nerve action potentials consistent with anterior horn cell disease.[4,33,64,80,92,110,123,125,156,191,192] Electrophysiologic documentation of severe loss of sensory fibers exists.[64]

NEUROIMAGING

Magnetic resonance imaging (MRI) is more sensitive than computed tomography in identifying CNS abnormalities in patients with West Nile neuroinvasive disease. However, even in cases of severe encephalopathy, MRI may fail to find any abnormalities.[25] Reported MRI findings in cases of West Nile neuroinvasive disease appear as hyperintense signal on T2-weighted and fluid-attenuated inversion recovery images and are nonenhancing and of normal intensity on T1 weighting.[102,169] In children and adults, lesions tend to be seen more frequently in the deep gray matter of the brain and, in particular, the basal ganglia, posterior thalami, and substantia nigra.[7,23,25,68,156,168,191,221] Leptomeningeal and paraventricular enhancement may also be seen.[24,176] Focal abnormalities occasionally may be seen, as noted in two cases of children with encephalitis in whom focal enhancement of the right temporal lobe was noted.[59,69,215]

In cases of acute flaccid paralysis, abnormal T2-weighted signals may be seen in the spinal cord gray matter.[4,92,102,125] In a case of a child with acute flaccid paralysis, MRI of the spine documented edema of the anterior horns of the cervical spinal cord.[92]

VIRAL CULTURE AND NUCLEIC ACID AMPLIFICATION DETECTION OF WEST NILE VIRUS

Multiple reports have documented that WNV can be detected from the blood and brain of infected individuals by use of mouse inoculation or cell culture.[19,73,76,77,83,97,141,200,203] However, this approach to establishing the diagnosis of WNV infections is of limited utility because of lack of sensitivity resulting from the brevity of the viremia, which begins approximately 2 days before and persists until approximately 4 days after the onset of the illness.[77,168,203] In addition, because of the potential

*References 7, 9, 25, 26, 30, 52, 54, 59, 68, 92, 94, 99, 110, 117, 156, 158, 159, 168, 176, 180, 191, 192, 196, 201, 215, 220, 221, 223.

†References 4, 7, 25, 33, 59, 92, 94, 102, 110, 123, 124, 156, 159, 180, 191, 192, 201, 215.

risk to laboratory personnel, attempts to isolate WNV from human specimens should be undertaken only in an appropriate biocontainment environment (i.e., biosafety level 3 containment).

Numerous nucleic amplification assays (i.e., RT-PCR, RT loop-mediated isothermal amplification) for the detection of WNV have been developed.[118,163] Diagnosis of acute WNV infections by nucleic acid amplification–based detection of WNV genome from blood and CSF clinical specimens also has limitations because of the short period of viremia.[118,168] Although genome could be detected in all brain tissue specimens tested, only 57% of CSF specimens and 14% of sera from patients with serologically confirmed infection were positive by a real-time RT-PCR assay.[118] Nucleic acid amplification–based detection of WNV has not been proved to be useful for the clinical diagnosis of WNV infections, but it has been extremely valuable in the screening and detection of asymptomatic viremia in blood donors.[144]

DETECTION OF WEST NILE VIRUS–SPECIFIC ANTIBODIES

Given the limitations of virologic and nucleic acid amplification–based diagnostic assays, detection of virus-specific antibodies forms the mainstay for establishing the diagnosis of WNV infections. In cases of neuroinvasive disease, the presence of WNV-specific IgM in serum and CSF increases by 10% per day the first week of illness such that it is usually detectable in 70% to 80% of patients by 8 days after onset of illness.[91,205] Interestingly, WNV-specific IgM may persist for long periods in serum and CSF of acutely infected individuals.[170] Fifty-eight percent of serum samples obtained approximately 500 or more days from onset of West Nile encephalitis were in the positive or equivocal range for WNV-specific IgM.[182] In a more recent study, serum anti-WNV IgM was detected in 23% of individuals up to 8 years after acute infection.[154] Similarly, WNV-specific IgM has been detected in the CSF for up to 199 days after onset of illness.[106]

The interflavivirus cross-reactivity of antiflaviviral IgG antibodies is well recognized. Traditionally, confirmation of antiflaviviral antibody specificity requires the use of a functional antibody assay such as the plaque reduction neutralization test.[128] Although multiple reports have documented greater specificity of antiflaviviral IgM antibodies and, in particular, those of WNV-specific IgM antibodies,[137,138,205] cross-reactions may still occur. On the basis of cross-reactivity with related flaviviruses (i.e., Japanese encephalitis virus and St. Louis encephalitis virus), an algorithm for the use of CDC-developed IgM capture enzyme-linked immunosorbent assay (MAC-ELISA) has been developed to differentiate human WNV and St. Louis encephalitis virus infections.[138] This algorithm has not been validated for commercial MAC-ELISA kits. In the absence of use of the CDC MAC-ELISA, confirmation of WNV infection may require documentation of presence of WNV functional (i.e., neutralizing or hemagglutination inhibition) antibodies.

The diagnosis of WNV infection currently relies on the detection of WNV-specific antibodies in CSF or paired serum samples.[91,187] The MAC-ELISA is the most sensitive and commonly used diagnostic assay. It is capable of detecting IgM antibodies in CSF 3 to 5 days into the clinical illness and 3 or more days earlier than detectable serum antibody.[205] The finding of WNV-specific IgM in the CSF of a child with a clinically compatible CNS syndrome generally is considered diagnostic of acute neuroinvasive infection. However, as discussed previously, persistence of WNV-specific IgM antibodies for as long as 199 days in the CSF has been reported.[106]

Detection of WNV-specific IgM antibodies in serum from a single specimen may not be diagnostic of WNV infection because of its prolonged persistence in serum.[153,182,187] When only serum is used for establishing a diagnosis, a second serum sample should be obtained at least 2 weeks later to document a fourfold increase in specific antibody titers with use of a functional assay such as neutralization or hemagglutination inhibition.[192] Serologic cross-reactions among St. Louis encephalitis virus, WNV, and Powassan virus may occur[208] and can confound the diagnosis in regions where multiple viruses are endemic. Serologic testing ideally should include a battery of region-specific arboviral antigens. Confirmatory assays, such as viral neutralization with the plaque reduction neutralization test, are available from the CDC Division of Vector-Borne Infectious Diseases, but only a limited number of commercial diagnostic laboratories and state public health laboratories have the capacity to perform the test.[101] The sensitivities and specificities of commercially available tests for the detection of WNV-specific antibodies may vary. An attenuated immune response may occur in immunocompromised hosts and result in a delayed antibody response.[165] Therefore serologic assays should be interpreted with caution in this population, and adjuncts such as nucleic acid amplification should be used to establish the diagnosis.

NEUROPATHOLOGY

Gross examination of the brain, spinal cord, and meninges generally is unremarkable but may demonstrate evidence of edema. In severe cases, the leptomeninges may show a perivascular monocytic infiltrate on microscopic examination.[209] Although the parenchymal findings of West Nile encephalitis can be seen distributed in nearly all areas of the CNS, the deep nuclei (i.e., thalamus, caudate, and lentiform nuclei), the substantia nigra, and other regions of the brainstem (in particular the pons and medulla), cerebellum, and spinal cord[28,78,107,156,162,184,209] may be more severely involved.

The CNS pathologic changes are the result of direct viral replication in neuronal and, less so, glial cells as well as the cytotoxic immune response to infected cells.[28,126] WNV demonstrates a penchant for infecting neurons. Viral antigen is detectable in neurons of fatal cases.[9,28,78,201] Neuronal pyknosis or neuronophagia is seen. Features in fatal cases of West Nile encephalitis include perivascular mononuclear inflammatory infiltrates composed predominantly of B lymphocytes, $CD8^+$ T-lymphocyte–dominant microglial nodules in the brain parenchyma, and focal mononuclear inflammation along the cranial nerve roots of the medulla.[9,12,23,69,78,111,156,184] In the cerebellum, the Purkinje cell layer demonstrates inflammation, neuronal loss, and gliosis.

In cases of acute flaccid paralysis, WNV demonstrates a penchant for infection of the anterior motor neurons. The anterior horns of cervical and lumbar regions are the most severely involved areas.[23,69,78] Evidence of neuronophagia, neuronal loss, and perivascular monocytic infiltrates has been found.[23] Loss of ganglionic neurons, nodules of Nageotte, and perivascular lymphocytic aggregates have been seen in the dorsal roots and sympathetic ganglia.[22,69]

TREATMENT

Treatment of West Nile fever and neuroinvasive syndromes is primarily supportive. In the case of West Nile encephalitis and meningoencephalitis, close monitoring of respiratory status is essential. Patients with severe muscle weakness, paralysis, dysphagia, or dysarthria may require mechanical ventilation.

No effective antiviral therapy currently is available for the treatment of WNV syndromes. Ribavirin, a broadly active antiviral, has been shown to be active against WNV in vitro and may have as its mechanism of action error-prone replication.[58,104] In the sole pediatric case report, ribavirin was administered orally to a 14-year-old with Hodgkin lymphoma and West Nile meningoencephalitis who recovered completely.[204] Although encouraging, a report of ribavirin in an unblinded, uncontrolled manner for the treatment of WNV infection in 37 patients during an outbreak in Israel in 2000[49] associated its use with a higher mortality rate. Bivariate analysis indicated that its use was associated with a greater likelihood of death (odds ratio, 6.7; 95% confidence interval, 3.0–15.2). Because this was an uncontrolled trial, selection bias for its use in more severely ill patients cannot be excluded. However, in a hamster model of WNV infection, ribavirin treatment alone increased the mortality rate.[147] These reports indicate that the use of ribavirin for the treatment of WNV infections appears to be unwarranted and unsupported at this time.

In cell culture, animal models, and a pilot study, IFN-α has been shown to be beneficial against some flavivirues.[147,175] Although anecdotal reports[105,186] in humans suggest that the use of interferon-α2b may improve recovery from West Nile encephalitis, an open-label, nonblinded trial did not indicate benefit.[187]

Anecdotal reports of the use of an intravenous immunoglobulin preparation containing a high neutralizing titer of anti-WNV antibodies (Omr-IgG-am) for the treatment of West Nile neuroinvasive disease in adults[17,81,82,124,133,179,188] and children[24,94] have been published. The limited information suggests a benefit from their use in some cases. Case reports and a case series suggest that use of hyperimmune gammaglobulin as early as possible in the course of encephalitis and acute flaccid paralysis may be associated with better outcome.[133,207]

A report of the treatment of macular edema associated with WNV chorioretinitis with bevacizumab has been published.[1] Bevacizumab is a humanized monoclonal antibody that inhibits angiogenesis by inhibition of vascular endothelial growth factor A.

In a phase I study a monoclonal antibody to WNV was demonstrated to have mild adverse effects and be well tolerated in healthy adults.[16] However, further clinical trials have not been reported.

PREVENTION

Prevention of WNV infections requires both community-based public health programs and personal measures. Mosquito abatement through elimination of mosquito breeding sites, use of larvicides to breeding areas, and application of pesticides targeted to adult mosquitoes are approaches used to reduce the abundance of mosquitoes in the environment.

The use and maintenance of door and window screens as physical barriers to prevent mosquitoes gaining access to homes can limit exposure to mosquitoes. Similarly, during engagement in outdoor activities where mosquitoes are prevalent, the use of mosquito netting in sleeping quarters also may decrease exposure to mosquito bites. Individuals should use insect repellent on skin and clothes when exposure to mosquitoes is probable or possible. Repellents such as N,N-diethyl-meta-toluamide (DEET), picaridin, and lemon eucalyptus oil have been shown to be effective and provide long-lasting protection.[11] Permethrin and DEET have been shown to be effective protection against mosquitoes when applied to clothing.

Finally, avoidance of environments where mosquitoes are found to be in high concentrations and avoidance of outdoor activities during dusk and dawn, when mosquito activity is the highest, should be encouraged. Efforts to prevent transmission of WNV through blood transfusions have led to the use of nucleic acid amplification–based tests for the screening of donated blood. At this time, screening of organ donors for the possible presence of West Nile infection has not been recommended.[108]

The development of WNV vaccines for use in humans has taken various approaches: live, attenuated virus, inactivated virus, viral subunits, DNA, and chimeric/recombinant viruses.[5] To date, eight phase I or II vaccine trials have been completed using a DNA vaccine containing the prM and E coding sequences (NIAID), soluble E protein lacking the C-terminal transmembrane domains (Hawaii Biotech), and two chimeric vaccines derived from dengue 4 virus (NIAID) and yellow fever virus (Sanofi-Aventis).

Only the latter has progressed to phase II trials. An infectious clone of yellow fever 17D virus was used as the background for the homologous exchange and insertion of the WNV prM and E genes.[143] The WNV E gene was mutated at three sites to reduce neurovirulence.[8] A phase I chimeric WNV–yellow fever virus vaccine was well tolerated, and the incidences of adverse events were similar in both the vaccine and the placebo groups.[143,197] A transient viremia was observed in 93% of recipients of chimeric vaccine. High levels of neutralizing antibodies were detected in 100% of the recipients. $CD8^+$ responses were induced in 93% to 100% of vaccine recipients. The phase II study[14,20] used a small plaque variant of the vaccine strain, which exhibited reduced viremia in a hamster model. It contained an additional amino acid mutation in the membrane protein. In part one of the study a short-lived viremia was observed but was lower than that seen in the phase I study, regardless of dose of given. Dose-ranging studies demonstrated that more than 96% of all vaccine recipients developed neutralizing antibodies. The highest dose (3.7×10^5 PFUs) was used for the second part of the study. The mean peak titer of the viremia and its duration were greater in the cohort 65 years and older than in the 41- to 64-year-old cohort. Older patients exhibited higher neutralizing titers. Both cohorts had detectable neutralizing antibodies at 12 months and were higher in the 65 years and older cohort.

NEW REFERENCES SINCE THE SEVENTH EDITION

5. Amanna IJ, Slifka MK. Current trends in West Nile virus vaccine development. *Expert Rev Vaccines.* 2014;13:589-608.
12. Basavaraju SV, Kuehnert MJ, Zaki SR, et al. Encephalitis caused by pathogens transmitted through organ transplants, United States, 2002–2013. *Emerg Infect Dis.* 2014;20:1443-1451.
21. Blitvich BJ. Transmission dynamics and changing epidemiology of West Nile virus. *Anim Health Res Rev.* 2008;9:71-86.
44. Centers for Disease Control and Prevention. Fatal West Nile virus infection after probable transfusion-associated transmission—Colorado, 2012. *MMWR Morb Mortal Wkly Rep.* 2013;62:622-624.
45. Centers for Disease Control and Prevention. West Nile virus disease cases reported to CDC by week of illness onset, 1999–2014. http://www.cdc.gov/westnile/resources/pdfs/data/4-wnv-week-onset_1999-2014_06042015.pdf.
46. Centers for Disease Control and Prevention. West Nile virus disease cases and deaths reported to CDC by year and clinical presentation, 1999–2014. http://www.cdc.gov/westnile/resources/pdfs/data/1-wnv-disease-cases-by-year_1999-2014_06042015.pdf.
47. Cervantes DT, Chen S, Sutor LJ, et al. West Nile virus infection incidence based on donated blood samples and neuroinvasive disease reports, Northern Texas, USA, 2012. *Emerg Infect Dis.* 2015;21:681-683.
62. Dohm DJ, O'Guinn ML, Turell MJ. Effect of environmental temperature on the ability of *Culex pipiens* (Diptera: Culicidae) to transmit West Nile virus. *J Med Entomol.* 2002;39:221-225.
71. Gaensbauer JT, Lindsey NP, Messacar K, et al. Neuroinvasive arboviral disease in the United States: 2003 to 2012. *Pediatrics.* 2014;134:e642-e650.
85. Hartley DM, Barker CM, Le Menach A, et al. Effects of temperature on emergence and seasonality of West Nile virus in California. *Am J Trop Med Hyg.* 2012;86:884-894.
86. Hasbun R, Garcia MN, Kellaway J, et al. West Nile Virus Retinopathy and Associations with Long Term Neurological and Neurocognitive Sequelae. *PLoS ONE.* 2016;11(3):e0148898.
109. Kilpatrick AM, Meola MA, Moudy RM, Kramer LD. Temperature, viral genetics, and the transmission of West Nile virus by Culex pipiens mosquitoes. *PLoS Pathog.* 2008;27:e1000092.
111. Kleinschmidt-DeMasters BK, Beckham JD. West Nile virus encephalitis 16 years later. *Brain Pathol.* 2015;25:625-633.
130. Lindsey NP, Lehman JA, Staples JE, et al. West Nile virus and other nationally notifiable arboviral diseases—United States, 2014. *MMWR Morb Mortal Wkly Rep.* 2015;64:929-934.
132. Londono-Renteria B, Colpitts TM. Brief review of West Nile virus biology. *Methods Mol Biol.* 2016;1435:1-13.
135. Mann BR, McMullen AR, Swetnam DM, et al. Molecular epidemiology and evolution of West Nile virus in North America. *Int J Environ Res Public Health.* 2013;10:5111-5129.
153. Murray KO, Garcia MN, Yan C, et al. Persistence of detectable immunoglobulin M antibodies up to 8 years after infection with West Nile virus. *Am J Trop Med Hyg.* 2013;89:996-1000.
157. Nett RJ, Kuehnert MJ, Ison MG, et al. Current practices and evaluation of screening solid organ donors for West Nile virus. *Transpl Infect Dis.* 2012;14:268-277.
166. Perera-Lecoin M, Meertens L, Carnec X, et al. Flavivirus entry receptors: an update. *Viruses.* 2014;6:69-88.
168. Petersen LR, Busch MP. Transfusion-transmitted arboviruses. *Vox Sang.* 2010;98:495-503.
172. Pridjian G, Sirois PA, McRae S, et al. Prospective study of pregnancy and newborn outcomes in mothers with West Nile illness during pregnancy. *Birth Defects Res A Clin Mol Teratol.* 2016;106(8):716-723.
177. Reisen WK, Fang Y, Martinez VM. Effects of temperature on the transmission of West Nile virus by *Culex tarsalis* (Diptera: Culicidae). *J Med Entomol.* 2006;43:309-317.
195. Sirois PA, Pridjian G, McRae S, et al. Developmental outcomes in young children born to mothers with West Nile illness during pregnancy. *Birth Defects Res A Clin Mol Teratol.* 2014;100:792-796.
200. Soldatou A, Vartzelis G, Vorre S, et al. A toddler with acute flaccid paralysis due to West Nile virus infection. *Pediatr Infect Dis J.* 2013;32:1023-1024.
207. Thabet FI, Servinsky SE, Naz F, et al. Unusual case of West Nile Virus flaccid paralysis in a 10-year-old child. *Pediatr Neurol.* 2013;48:393-396.

The full reference list for this chapter is available at ExpertConsult.com.

176C ■ Yellow Fever

Duane J. Gubler • Gail J. Harrison

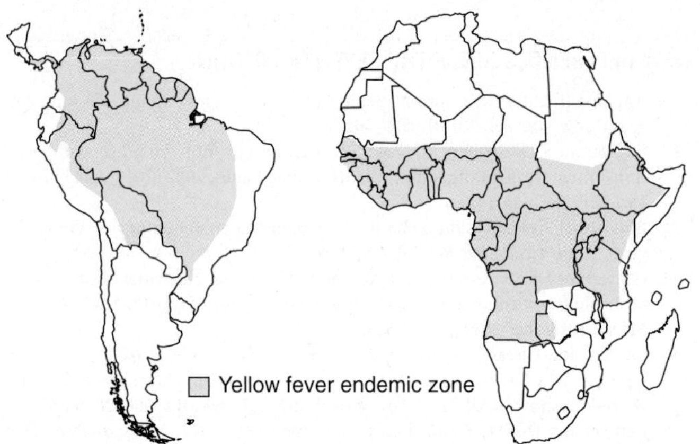

FIGURE 176C.1 Geographic distribution of yellow fever in Africa and the Americas.

Yellow fever is a mosquito-borne viral disease of humans and lower primates that occurs naturally in tropical Africa and the Americas (Fig. 176C.1). Epidemics, which can occur in both urban and rural areas, often are associated with severe hemorrhagic disease and high fatality rates. It is considered a reemerging disease, with increased incidence documented since the 1980s[2] Globally, yellow fever virus infects more than 200,000 people every year and causes approximately 30,000 deaths annually.

HISTORY

Yellow fever was described as a disease entity first in 1648 in the Yucatan, Mexico. It apparently was part of a larger regional epidemic that affected the Caribbean islands and Central America from Barbados to Mexico from 1647 to 1649.[22,23] Although it was first described in the Americas, yellow fever virus, along with its principal urban epidemic mosquito vector, *Aedes aegypti*, most likely originated in Africa and was introduced to the New World by the slave trade. During the 17th, 18th, 19th, and early 20th centuries, epidemic yellow fever was a major public health problem in the Western Hemisphere. Large epidemics occurred in tropical America, as well as in the United States (as far north as Boston) and Europe (as far north as England).[33] Epidemics occurred primarily in port cities as a result of spread by sailing vessels and commerce.

After transmission by mosquitoes was documented by Reed and the Yellow Fever Commission in Cuba,[30] major efforts were undertaken to keep the disease in check by mosquito control. The first yellow fever virus was isolated in 1927 from a patient in Ghana, West Africa. By 1938, an effective live, attenuated virus vaccine had been developed. Yellow fever was controlled in the Americas by eradication of the mosquito vector of urban disease, *A. aegypti*, from most Central and South American countries. In Francophone countries of West Africa, yellow fever was controlled by mass vaccination programs. The result was the disappearance of major urban epidemics of yellow fever in both Africa and the Americas during the 1950s, 1960s, and 1970s. In the mid-1980s, however, the urban form of disease reemerged in West Africa, with major epidemics in Nigeria and increased transmission in other countries.[22] Kenya experienced its first epidemic in history in 1993. Yellow fever outbreaks continue to occur in Africa. For example, Uganda experienced its largest yellow fever outbreak in 2010–11, related to occupational activities of males working in and around forests.[37] In 2015 Angola experienced a yellow fever outbreak; and 2016, the Democratic Republic of Congo Ministry of Health declared a yellow fever outbreak.[29] Previously, yellow fever was not seen in Asia. During the Angola outbreak, 11 unvaccinated Chinese workers were infected in Angola and imported yellow fever to China in 2016. At least one of these workers died.[5] This recent importation of yellow fever to China from unvaccinated workers and travelers exposed a low vaccination rate in Chinese travelers and workers in Angola and also exposed a potential threat of yellow fever spread to Asia.[36,40] Imported cases of severe, fatal yellow fever have also been reported from other areas of the world, such as Europe (Germany and Belgium).[1] In the Americas, *A. aegypti* has reinfested most Central and South American countries from which it had been eradicated, and urban centers of the American tropics are at their highest risk for epidemic urban yellow fever in more than 60 years.[13] Thus the disease continues to be an important public health problem in both Africa and the Americas. Yellow fever transmission has never been recognized in Asia or the Pacific, but the recent importation of yellow fever into China from unvaccinated travelers returning from an area with a yellow fever outbreak makes this occurrence a distinct possibility in the future.[36,40]

ETIOLOGIC AGENT

Yellow fever is caused by the yellow fever virus, the prototype of the genus *Flavivirus*, family Flaviviridae. The genus *Flavivirus* contains 53 viruses, which are small (40–50 nm in diameter), spherical, and enveloped, with single-stranded RNA approximately 11 kilobases in length.[9] The genome produces 10 proteins but has complex host interaction. Many of the flaviviruses are very closely related antigenically, which has resulted in extensive cross-reactivity in most serologic tests, so a laboratory diagnosis is difficult to make. Yellow fever virus has seven genotypes that are geographically separated, and outbreaks of disease are often associated with specific genotypes.[2] The virus is part of an antigenic complex that is different from other members of the family Flaviviridae.[14]

EPIDEMIOLOGY

Yellow fever viruses are maintained in natural zoonotic cycles involving lower primates and canopy-dwelling mosquitoes that breed in tree holes in the rain forests of both Africa and the Americas, called the *jungle* or *sylvatic cycle* of yellow fever.[22,24,33] Humans become involved accidentally when they encroach on this forest cycle. Humans thus infected may transport the virus back to a village or city during the incubation period of 2 to 14 days. If infected persons are fed on by urban *A. aegypti*, the virus then can be transmitted to other humans by mosquito bite after an extrinsic incubation of 8 to 10 days. Major urban epidemics are transmitted by this highly domesticated mosquito, which lives in close association with humans in most tropical cities of the world.[2,13]

Yellow fever occurs throughout much of sub-Saharan Africa and tropical America in the sylvatic cycle (see Fig. 176C.1). In Africa, cercopithecoid and celobid monkeys are the main vertebrate hosts; infection rarely causes illness and death in these species. Year-round enzootic transmission by *Aedes africanus* occurs in the rain forests. In wet savanna areas bordering the rain forests of western and central Africa, transmission increases during the rainy season and decreases during the dry season. *Aedes furcifer*, *A. africanus*, and *Aedes leuteocephalus* are the main mosquito vectors in this zone of emergence, and the virus is transmitted from monkey to monkey, monkey to human, and human to human. In the dry savanna zones, yellow fever activity is intermittent and takes place mainly during the rainy season, but it also occurs in major epidemics in urban areas, where stored water provides the ideal larval habitat for *A. aegypti*. In East Africa, *Aedes simpsoni (Aedes bromeliae)* provides the link between the *A. africanus* sylvatic cycle and humans in areas bordering gallery forests.

In tropical America, howler, spider, squirrel, owl, capuchin, and wooly monkeys all act as vertebrate hosts for yellow fever virus. Mosquitoes of the genus *Haemagogus* are the principal vectors in tropical American rain forests, where they feed in the canopy as well as at ground level. Other mosquito species, such as *Sabethes chloropterus*, *Aedes leucocelaenus*, and *Aedes fulvus*, may play secondary roles. Although most cases of yellow fever have been reported from Bolivia, Brazil, Venezuela, and Peru in recent years, the enzootic zone probably includes the rain forests of at least 10 countries (i.e., Colombia, Ecuador, Peru, Bolivia, Brazil, Venezuela, Guyana, Suriname, French Guiana, and Trinidad[41]) and involves "wandering" enzootic transmission among the monkey populations. The humans involved are mainly adult men who work in the forest.

Vertical transmission of yellow fever virus from an infected female mosquito through the eggs to her offspring plays an important role in survival and maintenance of yellow fever virus in enzootic cycles and has been demonstrated in nature in West Africa by isolation of the virus from male *A. furcifer* mosquitoes. Experimentally, *Haemagogus* and *A. aegypti* mosquitoes have been shown to be capable of vertical transmission. This mechanism is thought to be of major importance in survival of the virus during prolonged dry periods in both enzootic regions.

Urban epidemics of yellow fever have reappeared in West Africa in the past 17 years.[28] Unfortunately, surveillance is very poor, and the actual number of cases reported is thought to be grossly underestimated. For example, in Nigeria in 1986 and 1987, the numbers of reported cases and deaths during epidemics were 2612 and 973, respectively. Seroepidemiologic studies, however, estimated that the actual numbers of cases and deaths were 130,000 and 29,000, respectively.[28]

In the Americas, the last urban yellow fever epidemic occurred in 1942. Reinvasion of American tropical urban centers by *A. aegypti*, however, has placed more than 300 million susceptible individuals at risk. As might be expected, urban transmission has been reported recently. In 1998, urban transmission of yellow fever was documented in Santa Cruz, Bolivia.[35] Although not comprising a large number of cases, this outbreak underscores the high risk that many tropical urban centers have at the beginning of the 21st century. In addition, six fatal cases of yellow fever in travelers who visited South America (four cases) or Africa (two cases) in recent years have been confirmed. Three of these cases were US citizens, and three were European. Why contemporary yellow fever epidemics have not occurred in the Americas, despite the high risk, is not known. The dramatic increase in transmission of dengue in urban centers of the American tropics in recent years possibly has resulted in a high prevalence of heterotypic flavivirus antibody that protects against severe yellow fever clinical illness. Another possibility is that the enzootic virus strains are not well adapted to urban transmission by *A. aegypti*.

Epidemic yellow fever has never been reported in Asia or the Pacific, although imported yellow fever from unvaccinated travelers recently has occurred in 2016.[36,40] The reason is not known, but both variation in mosquito vector competence and partial protection by heterotypic flavivirus antibody have been suggested as reasons that this virus has never become established in that part of the world. If urban epidemics do occur in the American tropics, however, the virus is expected to move very quickly to this and other permissive areas where urban *A. aegypti* mosquitoes are found; this movement of yellow fever virus undoubtedly would cause a major international public health emergency.

CLINICAL MANIFESTATIONS

Infection with yellow fever virus causes a spectrum of illness ranging from inapparent infection to severe yellow fever with the classic triad of jaundice, hemorrhage, and albuminuria, which is associated with a high case-fatality rate. Most yellow fever infections are manifested clinically as a mild to severe viral syndrome without symptoms of intoxication; 10% to 20% of infections may result in classic yellow fever.[21,24,25]

The incubation period may be as long as 13 days but generally is 3 to 6 days.[24] The onset of illness is abrupt, with fever, headache, backache, myalgia, nausea, and other nonspecific signs and symptoms. In mild cases, the illness will last for several days, after which recovery is uneventful and complete. In severe cases, prostration occurs commonly, and examination reveals congestion of the skin, conjunctivae, and mucous membranes. The pulse rate usually increases early in the illness, and blood pressure is normal. Leukopenia is a frequent finding, and mild albuminuria may be noted. The temperature generally ranges between 38.5°C and 40°C (101.3°C and 104°F). Nausea and vomiting are common manifestations. Minor hemorrhagic manifestations such as epistaxis and bleeding gums may be observed. This period of infection may last for approximately 3 days, at which time the congestion declines and a relative bradycardia may occur despite the elevated temperature (Faget sign). The temperature falls to or below normal, and the patient feels better.

In most patients, this period of remission signals the beginning of convalescence; but in severe cases, it may last only a few hours, after which the patient enters a "period of intoxication" characterized by venous congestion and extreme bradycardia, despite a secondary rise in temperature.[10] Nausea and vomiting are severe and associated with epigastric pain. Prostration and jaundice from liver failure, and marked albuminuria and anuria from renal failure are present. Hemorrhagic manifestations include hematemesis ("black vomit") and melena.

The jaundice in some patients is not striking; it is difficult to detect in early disease and often is not detected until after death. The severity of hemorrhagic manifestations also varies greatly, but some hemorrhage can be found in most cases. As indicated earlier, minor hemorrhagic manifestations may be observed in the early stage of illness; severe hemorrhage usually develops late in the illness, although it may occur in fulminant cases as early as the second or third day. Hemorrhage may be so severe that it causes shock and death from blood loss. Albuminuria is one of the most common findings in yellow fever, and it occurs in all but very mild cases. It is present early in the illness and may increase rapidly. The albuminuria probably is related to renal involvement during the period of infection. Anuria, on the other hand, appears to be related to hepatic involvement and never is seen in the absence of other signs of liver infection. These terminal events may be related to "cytokine storm." Involvement of the brain with viral encephalitis is rare in yellow fever, although the brain may exhibit edema and hemorrhages in fatal cases.

Death may ensue as early as 2 to 4 days after onset but occurs after 7 to 10 days of illness in 20% to 50% of severe cases. In patients in whom death occurs later, autopsy generally reveals a cause other than yellow fever. Patients with severe infection often have lowered resistance to secondary infection, which may develop at the time of convalescence. Other complications include kidney abscess, pneumonia, suppurative parotitis, and skin infection. Viral encephalitis is rare. Convalescence usually is rapid and complete except for a general weakness that may last for several weeks. Permanent damage to the liver or kidneys does not apparently occur in survivors.

PATHOLOGY

The gross pathologic findings in fatal cases of yellow fever are not striking.[25] The skin, sclerae, serosa, some internal organs, and subcutaneous fat usually have moderate icterus. Serous effusions, edema, and hemorrhages, including petechiae and purpuric lesions on the skin, conjunctivae, mucous membranes, stomach, duodenum, and bladder, often are present. Gastrointestinal hemorrhage may be prominent.[15]

The most characteristic lesions caused by yellow fever virus are seen in the liver, although liver failure is not generally the cause of death. The liver may have a yellowish color and be enlarged and fatty in consistency. In typical cases, marked necrosis of the midzone of the lobule is present. The necrosis extends both centrally and peripherally and on average involves 80% of the lobule in fatal cases.[21,25] The cells bordering the central vein and portal areas usually are spared. Councilman and Torres bodies can be observed in hepatocytes and are characteristic of yellow fever. Little or no inflammatory response occurs, and the reticulin framework is preserved.

The kidneys generally are tense and swollen. Glomerular changes are minor, but acute tubular necrosis and fatty metamorphosis may be significant. Cloudy swelling, degeneration, and fatty infiltration may occur in the myocardial fibers. The spleen and lymph nodes are depleted of lymphocytes, and mononucleocytes or histiocytes accumulate in the follicles of the spleen. Edema and petechiae may be observed in the brain.

LABORATORY FINDINGS

Leukopenia and albuminuria are common findings in early stages of the disease.[10] In severe cases, prolonged prothrombin and partial thromboplastin times, thrombocytopenia, fibrin split products, and elevated liver enzymes are observed. Total and conjugated serum bilirubin levels are elevated. Albumin levels in urine usually are less than 5 g/L, but in rare cases they may reach 40 g/L. The urine contains bile. Cerebrospinal fluid usually is normal but may be under increased pressure. Patients who are suspected of having or are diagnosed with yellow fever should have complete blood counts with platelet counts to detect leukopenia and thrombocytopenia; hemoconcentration with hemoglobuin and hematocrit measurements, coagulation studies, and metabolic panel with electrolytes to detect elevated creatinine, metabolic acidosis, and hypoglycemia from liver failure; liver function tests to detect transaminitis and elevated direct bilirubin levels; and urinalysis to detect proteinuria and urobilinogen. Imaging studies include chest radiograph to detect cardiomegaly or pulmonary edema or pneumonia, electrocardiogram and cardiac monitoring for arrhythmias, and brain imaging to detect hemorrhages.

DIFFERENTIAL DIAGNOSIS

Yellow fever should be considered in patients living or traveling from endemic areas.[10] Clinically, yellow fever is difficult to differentiate from many other viral, bacterial, and parasitic infections, including other viral hemorrhagic fevers such as Lassa, Ebola, Marburg, and Rift Valley in Africa; the illnesses caused by arenaviruses in the Americas; and dengue hemorrhagic fever in both continents. Other diseases that cause fever and jaundice, such as typhus, louse-borne relapsing fever, typhoid fever, viral hepatitis, hepatitis A, B, C, or E virus, leptospirosis, falciparum malaria, tick-borne relapsing fever, and Q fever, as well as other flavivirus infections with mild to moderate illness, such as Zika virus, West Nile virus, Chikungunya fever, and dengue virus, also should be considered in the differential diagnosis. Noninfectious causes of liver dysfunction including toxins and Reye syndrome should also be considered.

A definitive diagnosis of yellow fever can be made only by use of the appropriate laboratory test.

LABORATORY DIAGNOSIS

Specific laboratory diagnosis requires isolation of the virus or serologic, nucleic acid amplification, or immunohistochemical tests. Virus can be isolated most easily from acute-phase serum taken during the first 4 days of illness, but it has been isolated as long as 14 days after the onset of illness and from the liver after death.[25] The most sensitive method of virus isolation is inoculation of mosquitoes followed by AP-61 cell culture from *Aedes pseudoscutellaris* mosquitoes. Vero cells and inoculation of suckling mice also can be used but are less sensitive. Polymerase chain reaction (PCR) is highly sensitive, and yellow fever RNA can be amplified from these same tissues with a sensitivity higher than that of virus isolation.[13,18] Viral antigen can be demonstrated in the liver by immunohistochemical methods.[15] Either fresh or formalin-fixed tissue can be used with these techniques, which may be performed to establish a virologic diagnosis after virus has been cleared from the blood.

Serologic diagnosis depends on the collection of properly timed acute- and convalescent-phase serum samples to demonstrate a rise in specific antibody. Serologic tests commonly used to diagnose yellow fever include hemagglutination inhibition, complement fixation, and the plaque reduction neutralization test (PRNT), as well as newer tests, such as enzyme-linked immunosorbent assay (ELISA) for both immunoglobulin G (IgG) and IgM antibodies.[14] The immunofluorescent assay is used in some laboratories.

Antibodies detected by hemagglutination inhibition, PRNT, immunofluorescent assay, and IgM capture ELISA appear within 5 to 7 days after the onset of illness.[12] The presence of a positive IgM test is diagnostic of recent yellow fever virus infection, as long as the patient has not had a recent yellow fever vaccine, which also may induce IgM antibodies. The complement fixation antibodies appear later than the other tests, usually after 10 to 14 days. Hemagglutination inhibition and PRNT antibodies persist at detectable levels for many years (>50) in most patients, whereas the duration of complement fixation and IgM antibodies is uncertain, but they probably wane to undetectable levels after 12 to 18 months.

PRNT is the most sensitive and specific of the serologic tests.[32] In patients who have had no previous flavivirus infection, this test can be used to make a specific diagnosis of yellow fever, as can IgM capture ELISA. Cross-reaction between yellow fever antigen and antibodies to other related flaviviruses complicates the serodiagnosis of this and other flavivirus diseases. Hemagglutination inhibition, immunofluorescent assay, and IgG ELISA are nonspecific tests in which considerable cross-reactivity with heterologous flavivirus antibodies occurs. Therefore positive results should be interpreted in clinical and epidemiological context.

The use of yellow fever 17D vaccine in disease-endemic areas also may complicate serologic diagnosis. Vaccination induces low-titer (1:10 to 1:40) hemagglutination inhibition and neutralizing antibodies but no detectable immunofluorescent or complement fixation antibodies. Vaccination also induces IgM antibody, which may remain at detectable levels for as long as 3 to 4 years.[12,31] Vaccination of individuals who have had a previous flavivirus infection induces an anamnestic response of heterotypic flavivirus antibodies at high titer (≥1:1280).[19]

Yellow fever virus genome also may be detected by molecular methods such as quantitative real-time PCR and isothermal protocols that have been simplified and used in reference laboratories and point-of-care field situations.[8,18,23]

TREATMENT

Treatment of yellow fever is primarily supportive. Patients with severe disease requiring hospitalization should have complete bed rest with good nursing care and close monitoring of vital organ functions. Salicylates should be avoided, but mild sedatives may be helpful. Maintenance of fluid and electrolyte balance is critical. Guidelines for intensive care of severe yellow fever cases have not been established. Secondary bacterial infections may occur and should be treated with appropriate antibiotics.

No specific antiviral therapy is licensed for treatment of yellow fever.[10,21,23] However, ribavirin has activity against yellow fever virus and has been used to treat other *Flavivirus* infections.[26] In addition, investigations on the use of compounds such as T-705 and T-1106, as well as derivatives of the antibiotics doxorubicin and teicoplanin, as inhibitors of yellow fever virus replication are reported.[7,16] Research and development for antiviral compounds effective against yellow fever virus continues, in novel areas such as lipid metabolism and carbohydrate-based inhibitors.[17,20]

PROGNOSIS

Mortality in all yellow fever infections is low (<5%), but in severe cases requiring hospitalization, it may be 20% to 50%.[21,25] The prognosis is poor for patients who enter a period of deterioration of clinical status with rapidly increasing albuminuria, jaundice, fever, and severe hemorrhage. Patients in the terminal stage of illness usually are somnolent, have below-normal temperatures, and may have intractable hiccups.

PREVENTION AND CONTROL

The most practical and cost-effective method of preventing yellow fever is vaccination.[6,10]

A single dose of 17D-based live, attenuated yellow fever vaccine provides effective, long-term (10 years to life) protection and used in the World Health Organization (WHO) Expanded Program of Immunization in enzootic countries of Africa and the Americas.[3,41] Two substrains of 17D strain of yellow fever virus (17D-204 and 17DD) are included in a live, attenuated vaccine dose of 10^5 plaque-forming units, which is manufactured in four countries in the world.[11] Yellow fever is the only disease where an international certificate of vaccination is required under International Health Regulations for travelers to endemic areas. In addition, yellow fever vaccination is recommended by the WHO to be included in routine infant immunization programs for infants older than 9 months in countries with endemic yellow fever. The vaccine is given every 10 years, although recently, the WHO stated that only one yellow fever vaccination per lifetime is probably all that is necessary.[29] It is one of the most effective vaccines ever created, promoting well-characterized humoral neutralizing antibody and robust T-cell $CD4^+$ and $CD8^+$ cellular immunity responses.[38,39] Also, $CD4^+$ cells may be particularly important in preventing severe disease after wild-type yellow fever virus challenge in vaccinated animal models.[39] Detection of yellow fever IgG antibody persists for at least 10 years and possibly for life in some populations, and detection of yellow fever IgM antibodies may persist up to 3 to 4 years after vaccination, confounding serologic diagnosis of yellow fever in vaccinated travelers.[12]

The live, attenuated 17D vaccine was introduced in the 1930s and remains the mainstay of control of yellow fever in endemic zones of Central and South America and sub-Saharan Africa. The vaccine is prepared from infected chicken embryos and produces effective immunity in more than 95% of recipients.[4,25] The same seed-lot system of vaccine production developed in 1945 is still used and contributes to limited vaccine availability. The vaccine is administered routinely to infants in endemic areas and also is used to provide protection for travelers to and residents of endemic areas of tropical South America, South Africa, and Africa. Traditionally, the vaccine is given every 10 years. However, in 2016, the WHO modified its guidance from a 10-year booster dosing schedule to a recommendation that one dose gives lifelong protection in most populations.[5]

The decision to administer yellow fever vaccine should include the geographic destination, season of the year, local evidence for yellow fever transmission, likelihood of exposure to vector mosquitoes, and individual risk factors for adverse events.[4,27,25] Up to 25% of vaccines will have mild side effects, including injection site pain or redness, headache, malaise, and myalgia. Moderate to severe adverse reactions rarely occur and are categorized as neurotropic ("postvaccinal encephalitis") or viscerotropic. Neurotropic complications occur at a rate of 1 per 5 million doses and with a case-fatality rate of 5%.[10,11] Viscerotropic reactions are systemic illnesses that occur at a frequency of 4 million doses with a case-fatality rate of more than 50%. Severe adverse events occur more often in elderly persons, infants, and pregnant women.[4,19,25,27] Elderly people appear to have a delayed antibody response and a prolonged viremia after vaccination, possibly leading to the higher incidence of adverse events in this group.[19,31] Infants younger than 4 months have a high risk for development of encephalitis and should not be vaccinated with the live, attenuated 17D vaccine until they are 9 months of age. Pregnant women also should avoid being vaccinated because vaccine virus may infect the developing fetus, although the risk for adverse events associated with congenital infection is unknown. The live, attenuated 17D vaccine should not be given to persons who are allergic to eggs or to those who are immunodeficient or receiving immunosuppressive drugs.

In 2016, a yellow fever vaccine shortage occurred in Angola and the Democratic Republic of Congo.[3,42] In response to this shortage, temporary fractional dosing of the vaccine was approved to meet the vaccine demands.[42] In 2017, because of a manufacturing problem, a yellow fever vaccine shortage occurred in the United States, affecting immunization of US travelers.[11] The importation of an alternative yellow fever vaccine manufactured in France with safety and efficacy characteristics similar to the US licensed yellow fever vaccine may help address the US shortage.

The other method of preventing yellow fever is mosquito control, especially during epidemic activity. The principal mosquito vector of urban yellow fever, *A. aegypti,* is a highly domesticated species that lives in and around the houses of humans.[2,13] It breeds primarily in artificial containers that collect rainwater or in domestic water storage containers and is notoriously difficult to control. The most sustainable and effective prevention, therefore, is to control, discard, or chemically treat larval habitats in the domestic environment.[2,13] This process is labor intensive but can be done with the help of the citizens in the community.

Some authorities recommend adult mosquito control with insecticide space sprays, primarily ultra-low-volume sprays. Recent field trials, however, have shown this approach to be ineffective unless portable sprayers are used to treat the inside of each dwelling. Because of the excessive cost and lack of efficacy of ultra-low-volume application of insecticides, this method is not recommended. Recently, the ability of the intracellular bacterium *Wolbachia* to reduce the replication of yellow fever virus in the mosquito vector *A. aegypti* shows promise for a novel biocontrol strategy for yellow fever.[34]

Using mosquito repellants, wearing protective clothing (long sleeves, long pants, and mosquito netting), and using screened windows and doors in habitats and sleeping areas also will decrease exposure to mosquitoes bearing yellow fever virus.

Patients in whom yellow fever is suspected or proved should also be protected from mosquitoes to reduce spread of the virus. The most effective protection is to use a mosquito net on the bed during the acute febrile period of illness. Alternatively, patients can be kept in screened rooms. Effective repellents are available to treat clothing and exposed skin.

NEW REFERENCES SINCE THE SEVENTH EDITION

1. Bae H, Drosten C, Emmerich P, et al. Analysis of two imported cases of yellow fever infection from Ivory Coast and The Gambia to Germany and Belgium. *J Clin Virol.* 2005;33(4):274-280.
3. Barrett A. Yellow fever live attenuated vaccine: a very successful live attenuated vaccine but still we have problems controlling the disease. *Vaccine.* 2017;[Epub ahead of print].
5. Chen Z, Liu L, Lv Y, et al. A fatal yellow fever virus infection in China: description and lessons. *Emerg Microbes Infect.* 2016;5(7):369.
6. Collins N, Barrett A. Live attenuated yellow fever 17D vaccine: a legacy vaccine still controlling outbreaks in modern day. *Curr Infect Dis Rep.* 2017;19(3):14.
10. Gardner C, Ryman K. Yellow Fever: a re-emerging threat. *Clin Lab Med.* 2010;30(1):237-260.
11. Gershman M, Angelo K, Ritchey J, et al. Addressing a Yellow Fever vaccine shortage-United States, 2016–2017. *MMWR Morb Mortal Wkly Rep.* 2017;66(17):457-459.
17. Kim S, Li B, Linhardt R. Pathogenesis and inhibition of Flaviviruses from a carbohydrate perspective. *Pharmaceuticals (Basel).* 2017;10(2):E 44.
20. Martin-Acebes M, Vazquez-Calvo A, Saiz J. Lipids and flaviviruses, present and future perspectives for the control of dengue, Zika and West Nile viruses. *Prog Lipid Res.* 2016;64:123-137.
29. Otshudiema J, Ndakala N, Mawanda E, et al. Yellow fever outbreak—Kongo Central Province, Democratic Republic of the Congo, August 2016. *MMWR Morb Mortal Wkly Rep.* 2017;66(12):335-338.
36. Wamala J, Malimbo M, Okot C, et al. Epidemiological and laboratory characterization of a yellow fever outbreak in northern Uganda, October 2010–January 2011. *Int J Infect Dis.* 2012;16(7):e536-e542.
37. Wasserman S, Tambyah P, Lim P. Yellow fever cases in Asia: primed for an epidemic. *Int J Infect Dis.* 2016;48:98-103.
38. Watson A, Kilmstra W. T cell-mediated immunity towards yellow fever virus and useful animal models. *Viruses.* 2017;9(4):E77.
39. Watson A, Metthew-Lam L, Kilmstra W, Ryman K. The 17D-204 vaccine strain-induced protection against virulent yellow fever virus is mediated by humoral immunity and $CD4^+$ but not $CD8^+$ T cells. *PLoS Pathog.* 2016;12(7):e1005786.
40. Wilder-Smith A, Leong W. Importation of yellow fever into China: assessing travel patterns. *J Travel Med.* 2017;24(4).
42. Wu J, Peak C, Leung G, Lipsitch M. Fractional dosing of yellow fever vaccine to extend supply: a modeling study. *Lancet.* 2016;388(10062):2904-2911.

The full reference list for this chapter is available at ExpertConsult.com.

176D ▪ Dengue, Dengue Hemorrhagic Fever, and Severe Dengue

Scott B. Halstead

Dengue fever is an acute febrile illness syndrome caused by several arthropod-borne viruses and characterized by biphasic fever, myalgia or arthralgia, rash, leukopenia, and lymphadenopathy. Synonyms are *dengue* and *breakbone fever*. Dengue hemorrhagic fever (DHF), a febrile disease syndrome caused by dengue viruses, is characterized by abnormalities in hemostasis and leakage of fluid and protein from capillaries, which in severe cases result in shock (dengue shock syndrome [DSS]) (Box 176D.1). Both are manifestations of the dengue vascular permeability syndrome, an immune-complex mediated immunopathology.[107] Synonyms are *hemorrhagic dengue, acute infectious*

BOX 176D.1 World Health Organization 1997 Case Definition[a] for Dengue Hemorrhagic Fever and Dengue Shock Syndrome

Dengue Hemorrhagic Fever

- Fever, or history of acute fever, lasting 2 to 7 days, occasionally biphasic
- Hemorrhagic tendencies, evidenced by at least one of the following:
  - A positive tourniquet test
  - Petechiae, ecchymosis, or purpura
  - Bleeding from the mucosa, gastrointestinal tract, injection sites, or other locations
  - Hematemesis or melena
  - Thrombocytopenia (100,000 cells per mm^3 or less)
- Evidence of plasma leakage due to increased vascular permeability, manifested by at least one of the following:
  - A rise in the hematocrit equal to or greater than 20% above average for age, sex, and population
  - A drop in the hematocrit following volume replacement treatment equal to or greater than 20% of baseline
  - Signs of plasma leakage such as pleural effusion, ascites, and hypoproteinemia

Dengue Shock Syndrome

All of the above criteria for dengue hemorrhagic fever must be present, along with evidence of circulatory failure, manifested by the following:

- Rapid and weak pulse
- Cold, clammy skin and restlessness
- Narrow pulse pressure (<20 mm Hg)
- Hypotension for age

[a]No. 10693.

thrombocytopenic purpura, and *Philippine, Thai, Singapore hemorrhagic fever.* The 2009 World Health Organization (WHO) case definitions of *dengue, dengue with warning signs,* and *severe dengue* are provided in Box 176D.2. Useful general reviews are available.[85,102,231]

The dengue subgroup is composed of four antigenically distinct members. In the first decade of the 21st century, based on records of dengue occurrences and modeling frameworks, dengue viruses were epidemic or endemic in 128 tropical countries, placing nearly 4 billion people at risk for infection and resulting in an estimated 390 million dengue infections. Of these infected people, 96 million developed clinical symptoms, 26.6 million sought medical care, and 2.5 million were hospitalized, with case-fatality rates in some countries of 5%.[28,36,225,226,242] In tropical Asian countries, dengue is among the 10 leading causes of death in children 1 to 15 years of age.[100] Small indigenous outbreaks of dengue 1 occurred in Hawaii in 2001 and 2015–16 and in Key West, Florida, in 2009 to 2011[68,195] (http://health.hawaii.gov/docd/dengue-outbreak-2015/). Dengue infections are major causes of febrile illnesses in tourists to tropical destinations, some of whom develop life-threatening disease.[267-269]

The term *dengue,* of Spanish origin, came into use in 1828 during a Cuban outbreak that undoubtedly was chikungunya.[44,108] The Swahili term for chikungunya, *ki denga pepo,* had been used to describe an 1823 outbreak on Zanzibar.[52] The first outbreak that resembled a disease now recognized clinically and epidemiologically as dengue fever was described by Benjamin Rush in Philadelphia in 1780.[214] Epidemics probably caused by dengue viruses were common from the 18th century onward in inhabitants of the Atlantic coastal areas of the United States and South America, the Caribbean islands, and the Mississippi basin.[229] Dengue viruses almost certainly were the cause of the 5- and 7-day fevers that occurred in European colonists in tropical Asia. Similar epidemics occurred commonly in settlers in tropical Australia, where in 1905 *Aedes aegypti* was identified as a dengue vector by Bancroft.[21] Ashburn and Craig first found the etiologic agent in human blood and showed that it could pass through a diatomaceous earth filter.[16] An intrinsic incubation period of 3 to 8 days in humans, an extrinsic incubation period of 8 to 11 days in mosquitoes, immunity in humans and monkeys, and the nonsusceptibility of most domestic animals were demonstrated in the classic studies of Siler and associates[229] and Simmons and coworkers[232] in the Philippines between 1924 and 1930. When dengue viruses were isolated in laboratory mice in 1943 and 1944, the modern era of dengue research began.[147,217] Two strains from Hawaii and Papua New Guinea failed to cross-protect humans. From this experiment, researchers recognized the existence of at least two different dengue viruses; they were named *dengue viruses type 1 and type 2.*[216,217,235]

During most of the previrologic era, dengue viruses were thought to be the cause of a generally benign, self-limited febrile exanthem. However, death, shock, and severe hemorrhagic manifestations

BOX 176D.2 World Health Organization 2009 Case Definition[a] for Dengue

Probable Dengue

The patient lives in or travels to dengue-endemic area and has a fever and two of the following:

- Nausea, vomiting
- Rash
- Aches and pains
- Positive tourniquet test
- Leukopenia
- Any "warning sign"

Dengue With Warning Signs

- Abdominal pain or tenderness
- Persistent vomiting
- Clinical fluid accumulation
- Mucosal bleed
- Lethargy, restlessness
- Liver enlargement >2 cm
- Laboratory increase in HCT concurrent with rapid decrease in platelet count

Severe Dengue (Short Form)

- Severe plasma leakage
- Shock (DSS)
- Fluid accumulation with respiratory distress
- Severe bleeding (as evaluated by clinician)
- Severe organ involvement
- Liver AST or ALT ≥1000
- CNS-impaired consciousness
- Heart and other organs

Severe Dengue (Long Form)

- Evidence of plasma leakage, such as the following
  - High or progressively rising HCT
  - Pleural effusions or ascites
  - Circulatory compromise or shock (tachycardia, cold and clammy extremities, capillary refill time >3 seconds, weak or undetectable pulse, narrow pulse pressure, or, in late shock, unrecordable blood pressure)
- Significant bleeding
- An altered level of consciousness (lethargy or restlessness, coma, convulsions)
- Severe gastrointestinal involvement (persistent vomiting, increasing or intense abdominal pain, jaundice)
- Severe organ impairment (acute liver failure, acute renal failure, encephalopathy or encephalitis, cardiomyopathy) or other unusual manifestations

[a]No. 13630.

ALT, Alanine aminotransferase; *AST,* aspartate aminotransferase; *CNS,* central nervous system; *DSS,* dengue shock syndrome; *HCT,* hematocrit.

accompanied classic dengue fever outbreaks in Australia in 1897 and thereafter for 15 years. Similar phenomena were recorded in Greece in 1928 and in Formosa in 1931.[91] This "new" syndrome was recognized again in Manila in 1954. It was called *Philippine hemorrhagic fever* because of a resemblance to the epidemic hemorrhagic fever then occurring in United Nations troops on the Korean Peninsula.[194] In 1956, Philippine hemorrhagic fever was associated with dengue when types 3 and 4 were recovered.[118] All four dengue viruses are now endemic in tropical countries throughout the globe.[28] In 1966, the terms *dengue hemorrhagic fever* and *dengue shock syndrome* came into general use.[110] In 2009, a WHO committee advised that these terms be subsumed under the diagnostic categories of "dengue with warning signs" and "severe dengue."[277]

By epidemiologic criteria, dengue viruses are arthropod-borne (arboviruses) because they are transmitted biologically by various members of the genus *Stegomyia*.[167] Gene structure, replicative strategy, and antigenic relatedness place the dengue viruses in the family Flaviviridae.[143,262] At present, 68 members of the flavivirus family have been identified; 29 of them are established as human pathogens.[143] Cross-comparisons by plaque-reduction neutralization tests have shown dengue viruses to be an antigenic subgroup.[60] In addition to their antigenic relatedness and their ability to be transmitted by *Stegomyia,* each type of dengue virus produces a closely similar clinical syndrome in susceptible humans.[93,140,182,216,229,232]

Dengue is an enveloped, positive-strand RNA virus that produces a spherical particle with a diameter of approximately 500A. Dengue RNA consists of approximately 11,000 nucleotides coding from the 5′ end for core, premembrane, envelope, and five nonstructural proteins.[48,90] The crystal structures of the E protein of several dengue viruses have been solved.[171,170,172] The viral envelope contains two membrane proteins, envelope (E) and premembrane (prM). Individual subunits of E protein consist of three β-barrel domains designated domains I (EDI), II (EDII), and III (EDIII). These proteins form head-to-tail homodimers. Each virus particle has 180 monomers of E that are organized into 90 tightly packed dimers that lie flat on the surface of the viral membrane. Individual E subunits are organized in twofold, threefold, and fivefold axes of the T-3 icosahedral structure of the virion. E protein subunits are not placed in identical environments on the viral surface. The hydrophobic viral fusion peptide is located at the tip of domain II and is shielded by domain III of the adjacent subunit. Steric and other considerations can result in preferential interactions of some E subunits over others with receptors and antibodies. The E proteins, the main target of neutralizing antibodies, bind to cellular receptors and mediate fusion of viral and cellular membranes during viral entry into cells. Domain III appears to be responsible for binding to cellular receptors. The structural arrangement of viral surface proteins plays an important role in dictating how antibodies neutralize viruses.

When the virion is assembled the envelope protein bears quaternary epitopes unique to serotypes. These quaternary epitope pockets are bounded variously by domains II, III, and I.[58,71,76,260] Antibodies directed to these epitopes neutralize by hindering viral attachment to cell receptors or fusion entry into cells.[192,260] Other structural epitopes are shared between dengue viruses (dengue subgroup antigens) and other flaviviruses (group antigens).

Four clearly defined types exist, as determined by plaque-reduction neutralization tests using antibodies raised by infection of monkeys or fluorescent antibody tests using monoclonal antibodies raised in mice.[215] The four types have distinctive genetic structures and antigenic structures separable by homotypic antibodies.[60,120,144,266] Phylogenetic studies suggest that human dengue viruses diverged from four zoonotic dengue types relatively recently, whereas the four zoonotic types evolved in subhuman primates from a common viral ancestor in the more remote past, most likely in Indonesia.[122,257,262] Sylvatic dengue viruses retain the capacity to infect and cause disease in humans.[42,254,255] Different dengue strains cluster in groups that differ genetically (genotypes).[53,54,200,201,249] Genotypes consist of viruses of similar genetic structure that usually circulate within one geographic area.[249] Genotyping can be used to trace the movement of dengue viruses between persons over short and long distances.[137] Of particular interest, a strain of dengue type 2 isolated in Jamaica in 1981 and the dengue 2 viruses recovered from 1981 Cuban DHF patients belong to a Southeast Asian genotype.[200,218] The most sharply divergent genetic differences are among human viruses and strains from Asian and African zoonotic cycles.[200,257,262]

Dengue virus can be grown in 1- to 2-day-old mice or hamsters by intracerebral inoculation or in various mosquitoes by oral or parenteral inoculation. High mouse-passaged virus grows and produces deaths in weanling mice. Various tissue cultures of vertebrate and invertebrate origin support dengue virus growth in vitro, as reviewed in the following section.

TRANSMISSION

A. aegypti, a crepuscular daytime-biting mosquito, is the principal vector. All four virus types have been recovered from naturally infected *A. aegypti.*[91] In most tropical areas, *A. aegypti* is highly domesticated and breeds in water stored for drinking, washing, or bathing or in any container collecting fresh water. Dengue viruses also have been recovered from naturally infected *Aedes albopictus,* which breeds outdoors in vegetation.[68,91] Outbreaks in the Pacific area have been attributed to *Aedes scutellaris* and *Aedes polynesiensis*.[210]

Transmission of dengue by *A. aegypti* may be explosive and involve as much as 70% to 80% of the population.[229] Because *A. aegypti* has a limited flight range, spread of virus is mainly by mobile viremic humans.[197,234,280] Transmission of dengue viruses by *A. albopictus* results in indolent, long-duration small outbreaks, as exemplified by the introduction of dengue virus type 1 into Hawaii in 2001.[68]

Dengue viruses replicate in the gut, brain, and salivary glands of infected mosquitoes without apparent harm to adult mosquitoes.[207] Mosquitoes are infectious for a lifetime and for as long as 70 days in experimental circumstances.[232] Because female mosquitoes take repeated blood meals, long-lived female mosquitoes have great potency as vectors.[113] Several species of *Stegomyia* are infected readily by intrathoracic inoculation, although the threshold for infection by oral feeding is higher.[207,206] *A. aegypti* and *Culex quinquefasciatus* can transmit dengue mechanically by interrupted feeding.[232] The contribution of mechanical feeding to the spread of dengue virus during epidemics has never been measured. Because of the "skittishness" of *A. aegypti* and its habit of feeding during the day when its intended victim is awake and often moving, interrupted feeding with simultaneous transmission to multiple hosts within a household must be a common occurrence.

A. aegypti preferentially feeds on people and hence is most abundant in and around human habitations. The mosquito breeds in clean water. Biting activity is reduced at temperatures below a wet bulb temperature of 14°C (57.2°F).[37,38,63] Transmission of dengue in temperate countries is interrupted during winter weather, and dengue has not established itself endemically at latitudes above 25 degrees north or south. Breeding sites may be provided by humans through living habits, as in Thailand, where water is stored in and around homes in large earthenware jars.[91,98] In contrast, *A. aegypti* is not abundant in some parts of India because only small amounts of water are brought to homes from village wells for immediate use. Water in flower vases, household offerings, ant traps, coconut husks, tin cans, and rubber tires may supply breeding sites for *A. aegypti*.[81]

In the tropics, outbreaks of dengue generally coincide with the monsoon season. Eggs, which resist desiccation, are deposited inside water containers above the water line.[81] With the beginning of monsoon rains, a large number of eggs laid outdoors are hatched.[103,223] Indoor populations do not show seasonal change. Temperature is important in controlling viral transmission. Evidence indicates that the extrinsic incubation period shortens with increasing mean temperatures; mosquito biting rates increase with increased temperature and relative humidity.[227]

In sylvan settings, dengue virus has been isolated from three subgenera of *Aedes,* namely, *Stegomyia, Diceromyia,* and *Finlaya,* some in circumstances suggesting the occurrence of transovarial transmission. This phenomenon has been demonstrated experimentally, but its contribution to maintenance of virus in a habitat is unknown.[211]

EPIDEMIOLOGY

Host Range

Inoculation of strains of dengue with known human pathogenicity does not produce demonstrable infection in adult chickens, lizards, guinea pigs, rabbits, hamsters, or cotton rats.[221,232] Subhuman primates generally are susceptible to infection by dengue viruses. Numerous species belonging to *Macaca, Cercopithecus, Cercocebus, Papio, Hylobates,* and *Pan* can be infected by the bite of virus-infected mosquitoes or by injection of infectious virus preparations.[109,219,220,232] Infection is essentially asymptomatic. Viremia occurs at levels sufficient to infect mosquitoes. Simmons and colleagues were the first to note that wild-caught *Macaca philippinensis* resisted dengue infection, whereas *Macaca fuscatus* (Japanese macaque) was susceptible.[232] Work by Rudnick in Malaysia has revealed a jungle cycle of dengue transmission involving canopy-feeding monkeys and *Aedes niveus,* a species that feeds on both monkeys and humans.[213] Although the existence of a jungle dengue cycle in the Malaysian rain forest has been documented, the full geographic range of the subhuman primate zoonotic reservoir in Asia is not known.[255] In the 1980s and 1990s, extensive epizootics of dengue virus type 2 involved subhuman primates over wide areas of West Africa.[204,256] Genetic and epidemiologic studies have shown that urban human dengue and jungle monkey dengue are only relatively compartmentalized.[200,254,255,262] Urban dengue is vectored by anthropophilic mosquitoes, and the virus travels with people along routes of transportation.[159,234] *A. aegypti* and susceptible humans are so abundant and so widespread that should dengue viruses be exchanged between humans and monkeys, detection would be extremely difficult. If, in the future, urban dengue is eliminated but vector mosquito populations are unabated, dengue viruses may once again be introduced from jungle cycles.

Geographic Distribution

Outbreaks of dengue fever have been documented on every continent except Antarctica.[28,36,38] Evidence suggests that human dengue may have originated from enzootic subhuman primate foci in tropical Asia.[255,262,264] *A. aegypti* originated in Africa where its ancestral form was a tree hole–breeding mosquito named *A. aegypti* formosus.[39] This mosquito evolved into a domestic form in Africa.[40] The spread of *A. aegypti* during historical times from Africa throughout the world provided an ecologic niche quickly occupied by several human viral pathogens: yellow fever, chikungunya, Zika, and the dengue viruses.[39] During the 18th and 19th centuries, epidemics occurred in newly settled lands, largely because of the necessity for storage of domestic water in frontier areas. Isolated shipboard or garrison outbreaks often confined to nonindigenous settlers or visitors were reported in Africa, the Indian subcontinent, and Southeast Asia.[44,43,162,229] During World War II, dengue virus infections occurred commonly in combatants of the Pacific War and spread to staging areas not normally infected—Japan, Hawaii, and Polynesia.[104,100,216] DHF-like disease was described clinically in Thailand beginning in 1950 and in the Philippines from 1953; cases were confirmed etiologically as dengue in 1958 and 1956, respectively.[110,117,118] DHF was described in Singapore and Malaysia in 1962, Vietnam in 1963, India in 1963, Ceylon (Sri Lanka) in 1965, Indonesia in 1969, Burma (Myanmar) in 1970, China in 1985, and Kampuchea and Laos from about 1985; major outbreaks have occurred in Sri Lanka and India since 1988, in French Polynesia since 1990, in Pakistan since 1998, and in Bangladesh since 1999.[96,104,100] DHF has occurred at consistently high endemicity in Thailand, Burma, Vietnam, Cambodia, Laos, Philippines, India, and Indonesia.[104] Since 2008, repeated outbreaks have occurred in Pakistan.[129] In Thailand, DHF is the third ranking cause of hospitalization and death in children. Intermittent epidemics have involved the Maldives, Singapore, and Bangladesh.

During the past 20 years, major epidemics of all four dengue serotypes have occurred on several Pacific islands, with repeated severe epidemics on Tahiti, and in 2001, with a subsequent introduction into Hawaii.[54,68,83,100,127]

American genotype dengue 2 virus circulated in the American hemisphere for hundreds of years and was the only virus to survive an intensive period of control of *A. aegypti* designed to eradicate urban yellow fever.[6,81] In 1963, an Asian strain dengue 3 was introduced into the Caribbean and died out in the 1980s. Dengue viruses became fully established in the hemisphere after the introduction of a Southeast Asian dengue 1 in 1977.[62,101] Dengue 1 spread rapidly and now is endemic on the larger Caribbean islands and in Mexico, coastal Central America, and the tropical areas of Guyana, Venezuela, Colombia, Ecuador, Peru, Bolivia, and Brazil.[101] A sharp dengue virus type 2 epidemic in Cuba in 1981 involving 116,000 hospitalizations in a 3-month period led to apparent eradication of *A. aegypti,* but reintroduction of dengue type 2 into Santiago de Cuba in 1997 and type 3 in Havana in 2001 resulted in particularly severe outbreaks of DHF.[3,88,153] In 1981, an Asian dengue 4 was introduced into the Caribbean, spread widely, and now is endemic throughout the Caribbean basin. In 1986 and 1987, dengue virus type 1 spread through most of coastal Brazil and from there to Paraguay, Peru, and Ecuador.[196] In 1990, more than 9000 dengue cases were reported from Venezuela; 2600 of them were classified as DHF, and 74 deaths were associated with the epidemic.[196] Dengue virus types 1, 2, and 4 were isolated.[196] Shortly thereafter, DHF/DSS caused by dengue type 2 was reported from Brazil and French Guiana.[184,198] In 1994, dengue virus 3 was introduced into the region, and dengue 4 in 2010.[70,101] All four dengue virus types are now endemic in most of Brazil. Initially, in the Americas, because the population was dengue naïve owing to decades of mosquito control, most dengue infections produced disease in adults, and occasionally severe disease in older individuals with preexisting chronic diseases but with low mortality. As two or more dengue viruses became endemically established, classic DHF was recognized throughout most of South and Central America, with severe disease increasingly involving children.[101,205]

In the 1960s, dengue viruses 1 and 2 were recovered from humans with mild clinical illnesses in Nigeria in the absence of epidemic disease.[45] In 1983, dengue virus type 3 was isolated in Mozambique.[4] Since then, all four dengue virus types have been recovered from individuals with febrile diseases in much of Africa or in nonindigenous persons living in or returning from Africa.[4] Dengue virus type 3 infections were notable in the past decade with a sharp outbreak of classic dengue fever observed in adults on the Cape Verde islands, and cases and deaths resulting from classic DHF/DSS in Kassala, Sudan, and Port Sudan on the Gulf of Aden.[61,1,163] In sub-Saharan Africa, DHF/DSS have not been reported and even dengue fever outbreaks are rare, although a substantial outbreak was reported in Angola in 2013.[187,222] In this respect, sub-Saharan Africa resembles the situation in Haiti, where multiple dengue serotypes are transmitted at high rates among a predominantly black population but severe disease is not recognized.[115,136,202]

CLINICAL MANIFESTATIONS

Dengue Fever

In children, clinical manifestations of both primary and secondary dengue infections are varied and often mild. Duration and degree of fever are highly variable. When brought to the attention of health care workers, the disease often presents with upper respiratory tract symptoms and signs and/or gastrointestinal disturbances. Patients often have leukopenia, positive tourniquet test, cough, and pharyngeal injection. Maculopapular rash, petechiae, facial flush, liver enlargement, and cool extremities are observed infrequently but at similar frequency in children with primary or secondary dengue infections.[77,112,142,174]

When studied in the open population, primary infections with dengue virus types 2 and 4 are largely inapparent.[73,88,258] By contrast, primary infections with dengue virus types 1 and 3 in children somewhat more often result in mild to moderate febrile disease, sometimes accompanied by low-grade vascular permeability. Epistaxis, petechiae, and purpuric lesions are uncommon manifestations but may occur at any stage of the disease. Swallowed blood from epistaxis may be passed per rectum or be vomited and could be interpreted as bleeding of gastrointestinal origin.

Because chikungunya and the dengue viruses are transmitted by the same vector mosquitoes, the diseases frequently are observed in the same patient populations. Chikungunya virus, now distributed globally in the tropics, produces a dengue fever–like syndrome. Chikungunya illnesses begin more abruptly than dengue illnesses and are of shorter duration. Maculopapular rash, conjunctival injection, and myalgia or arthralgia occur more frequently in chikungunya than in dengue illnesses, but other features associated with both viruses are remarkably similar.[44,112,182] Similarities and differences in mild dengue syndromes, hospitalized dengue cases (predominantly during secondary dengue virus infections), and chikungunya illnesses are illustrated in the Chapter 175D.

In classic dengue fever (seen most frequently in adults), after an incubation period of 2 to 7 days, patients experience a sudden onset of fever, which rapidly rises to 39.5°C to 41.4°C (103°F–106°F) and usually is accompanied by frontal or retroorbital headache. On occasion, back pain precedes the fever. A transient, macular, generalized rash that blanches under pressure may be seen during the first 24 to 48 hours of fever. The pulse rate may be slow in proportion to the degree of fever. Myalgia or bone pain occurs soon after onset and increases in severity. During the second to sixth day of fever, nausea and vomiting are likely to occur, and generalized lymphadenopathy, cutaneous hyperesthesia or hyperalgesia, aberrations in taste, and pronounced anorexia may develop. One or 2 days after defervescence, a generalized morbilliform, maculopapular rash appears, with sparing of the palms and soles. It disappears in 1 to 5 days. In some cases, edema of the palms and soles may be noted, and desquamation may occur. About the time of appearance of this second rash, the body temperature, which has fallen to normal, may become elevated slightly and establish the biphasic temperature curve.

A dengue 2 strain circulating in Cuba in 1997 produced predominantly silent primary infections in adults and children.[88] Primary infections with dengue 1 and 3 viruses in adults are often overt with biphasic fever, rash, myalgia, anorexia, and gastrointestinal disturbances as characteristic features.[72,73,232] In Taiwan, primary dengue 1 infections in individuals with peptic ulcer resulted in gastrointestinal hemorrhage, in some cases severe.[253] This syndrome may be confused with DSS (see later discussion) and contribute to a misunderstanding of its pathogenesis. Gastrointestinal bleeding, menorrhagia, and bleeding from other organs have been observed in many outbreaks of dengue fever.[199,253,265] The mechanism of the hemorrhagic diathesis that commonly occurs with primary dengue virus infections is not known. In some cases, dengue infections, whether primary or secondary, in adults or elderly people, particularly those with diabetes, asthma, or hypertension, are serious and pose a risk for death.[157,186,191,248]

Dengue Hemorrhagic Fever, Dengue Shock Syndrome, and Severe Dengue

The dengue vascular permeability syndrome (DVPS) is the core pathophysiologic phenomenon in DHF/DSS and severe dengue (Box 176D.3).[12,107,241] The incubation period of DVPS is unknown but is presumed to be the same as that of dengue fever. In infants and children, progression of the illness is characteristic.[56,155,182,250-252,272] A relatively mild first phase with an abrupt onset of fever, malaise, vomiting, headache, anorexia, and cough may be followed after 2 to 5 days by acute midepigastric abdominal pain, lassitude, then rapid deterioration and physical collapse. In Thailand, the median day of admission to the hospital after the onset of fever is day 4. In this second phase, the patient usually has cold and clammy extremities, a warm trunk, flushed face, diaphoresis, and anuria. Patients are lethargic or restless and irritable and complain of midepigastric pain. Frequently, scattered petechiae appear on the forehead and extremities, spontaneous ecchymoses may develop, and easy bruisability and bleeding at sites of venipuncture are common findings. Circumoral and peripheral cyanosis may occur. There is slow venous filling time. Respirations are rapid and often labored. The pulse is weak, rapid, and thready, and the heart sounds are faint. Systolic pressure may remain normal or even elevated, and the patient appears deceptively well, retaining full consciousness. When hypotension ensues, the pulse pressure becomes narrow (<20 mm Hg) and systolic and diastolic pressures fall rapidly and may become unobtainable. The liver may become palpable two or three fingerbreadths below the costal margin and usually is firm and nontender. Chest radiographs may show unilateral (right) or bilateral pleural effusions. Ultrasonographic evidence of plasma leakage may be detected in some cases within 3 days after fever onset. Pleural effusion is the most common ultrasonographic sign of plasma leakage (62% of DHF cases 1 day after defervescence). Thickening of the gallbladder wall, postvesicular edema, and ascites are detected less frequently and resolve more rapidly than pleural effusions.[238,239] Up to 10% of patients may have gross ecchymosis or gastrointestinal bleeding. During the transition from the febrile to the critical phase, it is crucial for the clinician to be aware of warning signs of impending vascular permeability: persistent vomiting, increasingly severe abdominal pain, rising hematocrit, and falling platelet count. After a 24- or 36-hour period of crisis, convalescence is fairly rapid in children who recover. The temperature may return to normal before or during the stage of shock.

It should be noted that DVPS occurs regularly in infants in countries where multiple dengue viruses are hyperendemic.[111,130,131,179] These babies are born to mothers with two or more lifetime dengue infections but do not occur when mothers have experienced only a single dengue infection before pregnancy.[46,50,149] Infants, predominantly aged 5 to 10 months, experience physiologically the same dengue vascular permeability syndrome as older children, except that they are more difficult to diagnose and treat and their case-fatality rates are higher.[130,131,141,179]

BOX 176D.3 Dengue Vascular Permeability Syndrome

A dengue syndrome that occurs late in the course (on or near defervescence) of an acute dengue illness consisting of:

- Thrombocytopenia
- Altered hemostasis: most commonly prolonged bleeding time and/or elevated activated partial thromboplastin time and/or elevated prothrombin time
- Activated complement, by classical and alternative pathways
- Elevated liver transaminase enzymes
- Vascular permeability: clinically significant loss of fluid and small macromolecules (e.g., albumin) into interstitial spaces, most commonly to serosal cavities

Case Definitions

Dengue Fever, Dengue Hemorrhagic Fever, and Dengue Shock Syndrome

Case definitions were introduced in Thailand in the 1960s to assist pediatricians in outpatient settings to identify patients with acute dengue infections and to initiate triage.[110] A positive tourniquet test, thrombocytopenia, and enlarged liver were regarded as a case of "dengue," whereas an elevated hematocrit suggested vascular leakage (see Box 176D.1). These diagnostic criteria were applied successfully over 30 years in several Southeast Asian countries, successfully reducing mortality rates.[9,52,181] In retrospect, this success could be attributed to the widespread availability of microhematocrit centrifuges in outpatient facilities and the stationing of centrifuges on hospital wards where they were widely used by staff. Frequent microhematocrit determinations made possible the rapid and responsive management regimen as described in WHO case management recommendations.[9] Defining DHF/DSS proved difficult because estimates of 20% hemoconcentration could only be made in retrospect, comparing convalescent hematocrit values with those obtained during acute illness. Except during formal research studies, this requirement was seldom satisfied. Accordingly, DHF was a clinically based diagnosis without a "hard" diagnostic end point.

Dengue Fever Warning Signs and Severe Dengue

When multiple dengue viruses of Southeast Asian origin successfully invaded the American hemisphere beginning in 1977, DVPS gradually emerged throughout the region. Two major epidemiologic differences were noted between dengue in the Americas and in Asia: disease was common in susceptible adults and was predominantly the dengue fever syndrome.[101] A few severe cases occurred in adults, but over time more severe cases including classic shock syndrome and deaths were observed. In the Americas, the predominant hospital management system specified that hematocrit centrifuges be located in pathology laboratories. Thus inexpensive and easy access to multiple microhematocrit determinations was not available. This obstacle generated a movement to bypass the quantitative, laboratory-based 1997 WHO case definitions in favor of the qualitative descriptors of the 2009 WHO Technical Guideline (see Box 176D.2). The rationale for developing and the experience with these case definitions have been extensively documented.[22,123-126]

A useful focus of the 2009 WHO case definitions is the effort to alert clinicians through clinical signs to anticipate onset of dengue vascular permeability (dengue with warning signs). But the suggestion that all patients with a warning sign be hospitalized has resulted in vast overhospitalization as in, for example, the 2011 classical dengue fever epidemic in Pakistan. In addition, the diagnosis of severe dengue includes a broader range of pathologic responses to dengue infections than did the earlier DHF, which included cases classified as "unusual dengue." These cases include altered levels of consciousness, severe liver disease, acute renal failure, cardiomyopathy, respiratory distress, and severe bleeding. Many of these are end-stage syndromes that may follow prolonged shock or are due to comorbidities. More problematic is identifying those patients who are in respiratory distress because of fluid overload as having severe dengue. This labels as severe dengue an all too frequent iatrogenic complication caused by administration of excess intravenous fluid. In this way inadequate patient management may be confused diagnostically and epidemiologically as an instance of the vascular permeability shock syndrome.

PATHOLOGY AND PATHOGENESIS

Using relatively insensitive virus recovery systems, tissue cultures and suckling mice, recovery of dengue virus is difficult and usually absent in tissues at the time of death.[183,208] If patients experienced a second dengue infection, their tissue suspensions contain large quantities of dengue-neutralizing antibodies. The use of mosquito inoculation techniques improves viral isolation rates.[207,206,209] Genetic probes increase viral detection sensitivity still further.[18,128,208] In humans, dengue viruses infect and replicate efficiently in intracutaneous Langerhans cells in vitro and in tissue explants.[278] Virus ultimately targets liver parenchymal cells, where infection produces apoptosis, but hepatocytes may not serve as replicative hosts.[18,57,128,165] Late in infection, virus is found associated in circulating monocytes.[66] Fluorescent antibody, virus isolation, electron microscopic, and in situ hybridization studies suggest that tissue mononuclear phagocytes are major hosts for dengue infection.[18,19,27,29,34,35,279]

On pathologic examination, usually no gross or microscopic lesions are found that might account for death.[27] In rare instances, death may be caused by gastrointestinal or intracranial hemorrhage. Minimal to moderate hemorrhage is seen in the upper gastrointestinal tract, and petechial hemorrhage occurs frequently in the intraventricular septum of the heart, on the pericardium, and on the subserosal surfaces of major viscera. Focal hemorrhaging is seen occasionally in the lungs, liver, adrenals, and subarachnoid space. The liver usually is enlarged, often with fatty changes. Yellow, watery, at times blood-tinged effusions are present in serous cavities in approximately three-fourths of patients. Retroperitoneal tissues are markedly edematous. On microscopic examination, perivascular edema in soft tissues and widespread diapedesis of red blood cells can be seen. Maturational arrest of megakaryocytes may be noted in the bone marrow,[30,175,177] and increased numbers of such megakaryocytes are seen in the capillaries of the lungs, in the renal glomeruli, and in the sinusoids of the liver and spleen. Proliferation of lymphocytoid and plasmacytoid cells, lymphocytolysis, and lymphophagocytosis occur in the spleen and lymph nodes.[27] In the spleen, evidence shows infected tissue macrophages, and malpighian corpuscle germinal centers are necrotic.[18,176] Depletion of lymphocytes occurs in the thymus. In the liver, widespread evidence of infection with varying degrees of fatty metamorphosis, focal midzonal necrosis, and hyperplasia of Kupffer cells is present. [18,19,27,138,176] Dengue infection of hepatocytes may result in apoptosis, with evidence of assembled virions lacking.[18,57,138,166] Nonnucleated cells with vacuolated acidophilic cytoplasm resembling Councilman bodies (apoptotic hepatocytes) are seen in the sinusoids.[18,26,128] A mild, proliferative glomerulonephritis is present. Biopsy specimens of the rash reveal swelling and minimal necrosis of endothelial cells, subcutaneous deposits of fibrinogen, and, in a few cases, dengue antigen in extravascular mononuclear cells and on blood vessel walls.[35]

Epidemiologic, clinical, and virologic studies of DHF/DSS in humans have shown a significant association between the dengue vascular permeability syndrome and dengue virus infection in the presence of circulating dengue antibody, whether it is passively acquired from the mother or actively acquired from previous infection. Risk for developing vascular permeability syndrome is inversely correlated with age; the youngest children are at highest intrinsic risk.[5,87] In humans, circulating antibody appears to have two biologic activities: neutralization of virus and enhancement of infection.[99,97] In Thailand and Vietnam, DHF/DSS developed in infants during dengue virus type 2 infection only when maternal neutralizing antibody had catabolized to low titer and infection-enhancing antibodies were left in circulation.[49,111,149,178,230] Similarly, in a prospective study of dengue virus infection in Thai children, DHF/DSS occurred in children who had circulating enhancing antibodies from a previous single dengue virus infection, but it did not occur in children whose first infection left them with low levels of cross-reactive dengue virus type 2 neutralizing antibody at the time of the second dengue virus infection.[150] It is now known that heterotypic protective immunity spaces clinically second severe dengue infections to at least 2 or more years after first infections.[7] Cross-protective immunity may also explain the failure of secondary infections to produce DHF/DSS with the American genotype dengue type 2.[263] American genotype dengue 2 viruses are significantly neutralized by human anti–dengue 1, whereas Southeast Asian dengue 2 viruses are not.[151,152]

In rhesus monkeys experimentally infected with dengue virus by subcutaneous inoculation, virus replicates initially in the skin. Virus disseminates rapidly to regional lymph nodes and then to lymphatic tissue throughout the body.[164] Early in the viremic period, virus can be recovered only from the skin inoculation site and lymph nodes, whereas 2 to 3 days later, evidence of general dissemination to skin and other tissues is found. Virus is recovered from the skin, lymph nodes, and several leukocyte-rich tissues for up to 3 days after termination of viremia. Virus can be recovered from circulating leukocytes and from the skin only at the end of the viremic period. The number of sites from which virus can be recovered increases as the infection progresses. Intracellular infection is terminated abruptly 2 to 3 days after viremia ceases.

Monkeys infected initially with dengue viruses 1, 3, or 4 and then with dengue virus 2 had higher viremia than when the same virus was inoculated into susceptible animals.[95,114] A similar phenomenon was observed in monkeys given diluted human polyclonal dengue antibodies and then challenged with dengue 2 virus.[94] This phenomenon, in vivo antibody-dependent enhancement of dengue infection, provides an explanatory hypothesis of the immunopathogenesis of dengue in humans.[99,105,106]

Dengue pathogenesis models have been developed in mice that lack interferon receptors. Dengue virus dose-dependent early infection events result in severe vascular permeability.[19,228] Of importance, dengue antibody concentrations modulate infection in Fc receptor–bearing cells across a range of responses from protection to enhancement.[20,228,282,283] To date, mutant dengue virus 2 is required to produce DHF-like disease in immunocompromised mice after peripheral or intravenous infection. These mutations affect efficiency of viral replication or cell entry. A single amino acid change in NS4B modulates replicative efficiency, and two amino acid changes in the envelope protein affect interactions with heparan receptors for dengue infection.[78,193,283] The operative correlate of vascular permeability is the inoculum dose of mouse-adapted dengue viruses. Using nonlethal virus concentrations, enhancing antibodies increase viremia, thrombocytopenia, liver disease, and vascular permeability. Recent studies tie these pathologic changes directly to cellular infection dynamics.

Epidemiologic evidence suggests the existence of a human dengue resistance gene. Epidemiologic studies of the 1981 Cuban outbreak demonstrated a higher risk for DHF/DSS in white than in black individuals.[86,153] A search for DHF/DSS in black children in Haiti revealed no cases, despite the presence of high rates of dengue types 1, 2, and 4 infections and circulation of the Southeast Asian genotype dengue 2 viruses.[115] Human leukocyte antigens and other genetic factors have shown differing frequencies in DHF/DSS cases and controls.[51,231,243,244]

Early in the acute stage of secondary dengue virus infection, rapid activation of the complement system occurs.[33,168] During shock, blood levels of C1q, C3, C4, C5, C6, C7, C8, and C3 proactivators are depressed and C3 catabolic rates are elevated. The blood clotting and fibrinolytic systems are activated.[237,271,272] Studies find high levels of tumor necrosis factor, interleukin-2, interleukin-10, and interferon-γ sometimes attributed to activated T lymphocytes or original antigenic sin, a phenomenon thought to direct pathogenic T-cell responses to cells infected with a second heterotypic dengue virus.[154,173,212,224]

Two groups have shown that nonstructural protein 1 (NS1) of the dengue viruses are viral toxins that contribute to dengue pathogenesis by mechanisms analogous to those of bacterial endotoxins in the toxic shock syndrome.[24,169] DENV NS1 activates the toll-like receptor 4 (TLR4) on primary human myeloid cells, resulting in increased production of proinflammatory cytokines and chemokines as a byproduct of this interaction. In both in vitro and in vivo models, DENV NS1 activates TLR4 on human and mouse endothelial cells, resulting in loss of endothelial integrity and vascular permeability. In early work, NS1 was shown to activate complement by the alternative pathway and to target liver cells promoting intracellular DENV infection, and it was detected as a complex with thrombin in acute-phase blood of dengue patients.[2,17,160] The direct toxicity of DENV NS1 provides a single causal mechanism for the dengue vascular permeability syndrome, reconciling severe disease in infants born to dengue-immune mothers to that of older individuals experiencing a second dengue infection. It is still not understood why peak vascular permeability is delayed until defervescence rather correlating with peak NS1 blood levels observed earlier in disease.[158] It has long been suggested that the cellular immune response targeting dengue-infected cells triggers DVPS.[92] But the failure of cortisone to prevent DVPS argues against a direct cytopathic role for cytokines and chemokines.[246] It has been suggested that as dengue-infected target cells are disrupted by cytotoxic T cells, a final pathogenic bolus of DENV NS1 is released.

DIAGNOSIS

Dengue Fever

Activities of the patient during the period preceding the onset of illness may give important clues to the possibility of infection. The differential diagnosis includes many viral, respiratory, and influenza-like diseases and the early stages of malaria, typhoid fever, scrub typhus, hepatitis, and leptospirosis. Abortive forms of these diseases may never evolve beyond a DHF-like stage. At least five arbovirus diseases are similar to dengue: chikungunya and o'nyong-nyong fever (togaviruses), West Nile fever (flavivirus), Oropouche (bunyavirus), and Zika (flavivirus). Four other diseases are DHF-like but without rash: Colorado tick fever, sandfly fever, Ross River fever, and the mild form of Rift Valley fever. Many nonviral acute infectious diseases are DHF-like, malaria being number one. Because of the variation in clinical findings and the multiplicity of possible causative agents, the descriptive term *denguelike disease* should be used until a specific etiologic diagnosis is provided by the laboratory.

Dengue Hemorrhagic Fever, Dengue Shock Syndrome, and Severe Dengue

Children presenting with any warning sign should be hospitalized or placed under observation to initiate fluid resuscitation.[12] Using the DHF diagnostic algorithm, patients presenting with an acute fever plus complaints suggesting early cardiovascular collapse, thrombocytopenia (<100,000 mm^3), liver enlargement, hemorrhagic manifestations, or a positive tourniquet test and suggestive hemoconcentration are hospitalized or placed under observation with fluid resuscitation.[56,238] No matter which admission criteria are used, patients should be monitored to detect and quantitate vascular permeability. A research tool, strain-gauge plethysmography, was able to document microvascular permeability early and differentiate cases from controls.[25] However, repeated measurements of hematocrits are most frequently used to estimate hypovolemia by recording changes in hemoconcentration. Pleural or peritoneal effusions may be observed and fluid loss estimated using ultrasonography or radiography.[238-240] New noninvasive diagnostic modalities are being investigated. Near-infrared spectroscopy has been used to measure muscle oxygen saturation as a correlate of vascular permeability.[236] DSS is diagnosed when these manifestations are accompanied by hypotension or narrow pulse pressure (<20 mm Hg).

In areas endemic for dengue, DHF/DSS or severe dengue should be suspected in children with a febrile illness who exhibit shock and hemoconcentration with thrombocytopenia, hypoproteinemia, hemorrhagic manifestations, and hepatic enlargement. Because leptospirosis, many rickettsial diseases, meningococcemia, and other severe illnesses caused by a variety of agents may produce a similar clinical picture, the diagnosis should be made only when epidemiologic or serologic evidence suggests the possibility of dengue. Hemorrhagic manifestations have been described in other diseases of viral origin, including the arenavirus hemorrhagic fevers of Argentina, Bolivia, and West Africa (Lassa fever); the tick-borne hemorrhagic fevers of India and the former Soviet Union; hemorrhagic fever with renal syndrome, which occurs across northern Eurasia, specifically from Scandinavia to Korea; and Marburg and Ebola virus infections in Central and West Africa.[59,139]

LABORATORY STUDIES

An etiologic diagnosis can be made by serologic study of properly collected serum samples, by isolation of the virus, and by identification of viral RNA or the nonstructural protein NS1 in acute-phase sera.[85,277] The acute-phase serum or plasma collected for isolation of virus should be stored optimally at less than 65°C (149°F). Serologic diagnosis depends on a fourfold or greater increase in antibody titer by hemagglutination inhibition, complement fixation, radioimmunoassay, enzyme-linked immunosorbent assay (ELISA), or neutralization. Immunoglobulin M (IgM)-capture ELISA has revolutionized dengue serology, and commercial kits are available.[31,32,132-135] Primary and sequential (secondary) dengue virus infections result in the production of dengue-reactive IgM antibodies, which appear during the acute phase and disappear within 60 days of infection.[135,277] Secondary or primary dengue virus infections can be confirmed in a single serum specimen by quantitating IgM/IgG antibody ratios. IgG antibody concentrations are abundant in secondary but minimal in primary dengue virus infection. Dengue NS1 proteins can be detected in blood during the acute illness phase by dengue group–specific antibodies, and these have been formatted into commercial ELISA or rapid immunochromatographic tests.[31,74,158,281] By combining IgM-capture ELISA and NS1 detection, point-of-care tests are available to diagnose acute dengue infections. Accurate use of diagnostic tests requires an understanding of the kinetics of primary and secondary dengue virus infections. Dengue IgM antibodies are seldom detected until 5 or more days after onset of fever. By contrast, dengue NS1 protein circulates in blood during and shortly after the febrile period, with higher detection in primary and secondary dengue infections.[31,32]

Numerous techniques are available for the recovery and identification of dengue viruses.[277] Recommendations for general use have been made by a WHO expert committee.[277] Diagnostic testing for dengue virus infection is available through commercial reference laboratories, selected public health laboratories, and the Dengue Branch of the Centers for Disease Control and Prevention (http://www.cdc.gov/dengue). Acute-phase serum, mosquito suspensions, or other materials thought to contain dengue virus may be inoculated into suckling mice, which may be examined for sickness or subtle neurologic signs or challenged at 14 days with a neurovirulent dengue virus. Repeated subpassage markedly increases the neurovirulence of dengue virus. Alternatively, materials may be inoculated into any of several tissue cultures of mammalian or mosquito origin and examined for plaques under agar or methylcellulose overlay, for cytopathic effect, resistance to a challenge cytopathic virus by use of a fluid overlay, or fluorescence or other markers with the use of an appropriate detection system. Intrathoracic inoculation of *A. albopictus, A. aegypti,* or *Toxorhynchites* spp. is a highly sensitive dengue virus recovery system.[206,209]

TREATMENT

Dengue Fever

Treatment is supportive. Bed rest is advised during the febrile period. Antipyretics or tepid sponging should be used to keep the body temperature below 40°C (104°F). Paracetamol (10–15 mg/kg every 4–6 hours), or acetaminophen, is the preferred antipyretic agent. Analgesics or mild sedation may be required to control pain. Fluid and electrolyte replacement therapy is required when deficits caused by sweating, fasting, thirsting, vomiting, or diarrhea are present. Because of the potential for Reye syndrome and the dengue hemorrhagic diathesis, aspirin or other nonsteroidal antiinflammatory (NSAIDs) medications should not be given to reduce fever or to control pain. During dengue fever without detectable hypovolemia, adult patients may develop severe menorrhagia or gastrointestinal bleeding. Bleeding may be severe and require blood transfusions.

Outpatients With Mild Dengue Hemorrhagic Fever or Warning Signs

The Southeast Regional Office of the WHO has issued a special guideline for the diagnosis and management of dengue patients in small clinical facilities.[10] In the absence of increased vascular permeability, clinically significant hemoconcentration may result from thirst, dehydration, fever, anorexia, and vomiting. Fluid intake by mouth should be as ample as tolerated. Electrolyte and dextrose solution (as used in diarrheal disease), fruit juice, or both are preferable to plain water. With high fever, a risk for seizures exists, so antipyretic drugs may be indicated. Salicylates should be avoided because they are known to cause bleeding and acidosis. Acetaminophen is preferable at the following doses: younger than 1 year, 60 mg per dose; 1 to 3 years, 60 to 120 mg per dose; 3 to 6 years, 120 mg per dose; and 6 to 12 years, 240 mg per dose.

Dengue Hemorrhagic Fever (Compensated Shock) and Dengue Shock Syndrome

Explicit recommendations for management of DHF (compensated shock), DSS, and severe dengue have been made by a number of international and national authorities.[10,12-14] The 2009 WHO case definitions are widely accepted in the American hemisphere, whereas the 1997 WHO case definitions are still used in most of Asia. Despite these diagnostic differences, treatment in all cases focuses on the recognition and management of acute vascular permeability and is based on research observations.[56,65,140,270]

Inpatients

Treatment of patients with Nonshock Dengue hemorrhagic fever (compensated shock). Critical care management of dengue vascular permeability syndrome is a major challenge to pediatricians because more than half of the world's children are at risk. Because dengue is a major disease of travelers, children experiencing dengue illnesses may present to any clinical care facility in the world. These children require that all pediatricians have access to detailed diagnostic and treatment guidelines and develop the skills to recognize and manage dengue shock, hemorrhage, and fluid overload (an all too frequent complication and cause of death). Basic treatment guidelines are given in this section. The reader is referred to authoritative texts, the most comprehensive being the 2012 WHO *Handbook for Clinical Management of Dengue.*[12]

A baseline hematocrit should be obtained. Immediate administration of intravenous fluid to expand plasma volume is essential. In children, shock may develop or subside during the course of a 48-hour period, so close observation 24 hours per day is imperative. Patients with similar degrees of severity should be grouped together. Those with shock require intensive 24-hour care by nurses and physicians. Paramedical workers or parents can assist in provision of oral fluid therapy or in surveillance of the rate of intravenous fluid administration and general status of the patient.

Treatment for patients with nonshock dengue hemorrhagic fever is as follows:

- Start intravenous fluid resuscitation with isotonic crystalloid solution at 5 to 10 mL/kg per hour over 1 hour. Then reassess the patient's condition (i.e., vital signs, capillary refill time, hematocrit, urine output).
- If the patient's condition improves, intravenous fluids should be gradually reduced to 5 to 7 mL/kg per hour for 1 to 2 hours, then to 3 to 5 mL/kg per hour for 2 to 4 hours, and then to 2 to 3 mL/kg per hour and then further depending on hemodynamic status.
- If vital signs are still unstable, check hematocrit after first bolus. If the hematocrit increases or is still high (>50%), administer a second bolus of crystalloid solution at 10 to 20 mL/kg per hour for 1 hour. After the second bolus, if there is improvement, reduce the rate to 7 to 10 mL/kg per hour for 1 to 2 hours. If the hematocrit decreases from the initial reference hematocrit, this indicates bleeding. Immediately obtain cross-match and transfuse blood.
- Further boluses of crystalloid solutions may be necessary for the next 1 to 2 days.

Treatment of patients with shock. Treatment for patients with shock is as follows:

- For patients with narrow pulse pressure or systolic hypotension, initiate intravenous fluid resuscitation with crystalloid or colloid (gelatin has the least effect on blood coagulation, dextran 40 and 70 are in wide use) solution at 20 mL/kg as a bolus over 15 minutes to bring the patient out of shock as quickly as possible.
- If the patient's condition improves, give a crystalloid/colloid infusion of 10 mL/kg per hour for 1 hour. Then continue with crystalloid infusion and gradually reduce to 5 to 7 mL/kg per hour for 1 to 2 hours, then to 3 to 5 mL/kg per hour for 2 to 4 hours, and then to 2 to 3 mL/kg per hour or less, which can be maintained for up to 24 to 48 hours.
- If vital signs are still unstable, review the hematocrit obtained before the first bolus. If the hematocrit is low, this indicates bleeding and the need for blood transfusion.
- If the hematocrit was high in contrast to the baseline value, change intravenous fluids to colloid solutions at 10 to 20 mL/kg per hour as a second bolus given over 30 minutes to 1 hour. After the second bolus, reassess the patient. If the condition improves, reduce the rate to 7 to 10 mL/kg per hour for 1 to 2 hours, then change back to crystalloid solution and reduce the rate of infusion as mentioned earlier. If the condition is still unstable, repeat the hematocrit after the second bolus.
- If the hematocrit decreases from the previous value, this indicates bleeding and the need for blood transfusion. If the hematocrit increases from the previous value or remains very high, continue colloid solutions at 10 to 20 mL/kg per hour as a third bolus over 1 hour. After this dose, reduce the rate to 7 to 10 mL/kg per hour for 1 to 2 hours, then change back to crystalloid solution and reduce the rate of infusion as mentioned earlier.
- Further boluses may need to be given during the next 24 hours. The rate and volume of each bolus infusion should be titrated to the clinical response.

General management. If resources permit, patients with severe shock syndrome should have an arterial catheter placed. The reason for this is that in shock states, estimation of blood pressure using a cuff is commonly inaccurate. An indwelling arterial catheter allows for continuous and reproducible blood pressure measurements and frequent blood sampling on which decisions regarding therapy can be made. Monitoring of electrocardiogram and pulse oximetry should be available. Urine output should be checked regularly (i.e., hourly until patient is out of shock, then every 1 to 2 hours). Hematocrit should be monitored before and after fluid boluses until stable and then every 4 to 6 hours. In addition, there should be monitoring of arterial or venous blood gases, lactate, total carbon dioxide/bicarbonate every 30 minutes to 1 hour until stable, and blood glucose before fluid resuscitation and afterward as indicated.

Treatment of hemorrhagic complications.

- Patients in danger of bleeding are those with prolonged or refractory shock, hypotensive shock, and renal or liver failure or persistent metabolic acidosis; those who were given nonsteroidal antiinflammatory agents; those with preexisting peptic ulcer disease; those who are on anticoagulant therapy; and those who have any form of trauma, including intramuscular injections. Patients with hemolytic conditions are at risk for acute hemolysis with hemoglobinuria and will require blood transfusion.
- Severe bleeding can be recognized by refractory shock that fails to respond to consecutive fluid resuscitation of 40 to 60 mL/kg, hypotensive shock with low or normal hematocrit before fluid resuscitation, or persistent or worsening metabolic acidosis despite well-maintained systolic blood pressure, especially if accompanied by severe abdominal tenderness and distention.
- Give 5 to 10 mL/kg of fresh-packed red cells or 10 to 20 mL/kg of fresh whole blood at an appropriate rate and observe the clinical response.

- Consider repeating the blood transfusion if there is further blood loss or no appropriate rise in hematocrit after blood transfusion.
- There are no evidence-based data supporting the use of platelet concentrates or fresh-frozen plasma as a treatment for profound thrombocytopenia or severe bleeding. This treatment option is widely practiced in dengue-endemic countries and may contribute to fluid overload.

Recognizing fluid overload begins with knowing when to decrease or stop intravenous fluids. Intravenous fluids should be discontinued or reduced when there are signs of cessation of plasma leakage; stable blood pressure, pulse, and peripheral perfusion; hematocrit decreases in the presence of good pulse volume; no fever for more than 24 to 48 hours; resolving bowel and abdominal symptoms, and improving urine output.

Causes of fluid overload are excessive or too rapid intravenous fluids; incorrect use of hypotonic rather than isotonic crystalloid solutions; inappropriate use of large volumes of intravenous fluids in patients with unrecognized severe bleeding; inappropriate transfusion of fresh-frozen plasma, platelet concentrates, or cryoprecipitates; continuation of intravenous fluids after plasma leakage has stopped; and comorbid conditions, such as congenital or ischemic heart disease and chronic lung or renal disease.

Early clinical features of fluid overload are respiratory distress, difficulty in breathing, rapid breathing, chest wall retractions, wheezing (rather than crepitations), large pleural effusions, tense abdominal ascites, and increased jugular venous pressure.

Late clinical features are pulmonary edema (cough with pink or frothy sputum with or without crepitations; irreversible shock (i.e., heart failure with ongoing hypovolemia); the chest radiograph shows cardiomegaly, pleural effusion, upward displacement of the diaphragm by the ascites, and varying degrees of "bat wings" appearance with or without Kerley B lines suggestive of fluid overload and pulmonary edema.

Action plan for treatment of fluid overload. Treatment of fluid overload is as follows:

- Begin oxygen therapy immediately.
- Stop intravenous fluids.
- Check physiologic status: electrocardiogram to exclude ischemic changes and arrhythmia; arterial blood gases; echocardiogram for assessment of left ventricular function and regional wall dyskinesia that may suggest underlying ischemic heart disease; and cardiac enzymes.
- If necessary, give oral or intravenous furosemide 0.1 to 0.5 mg/kg per dose once or twice daily, or a continuous infusion of furosemide 0.1 mg/kg per hour. Monitor serum potassium and correct the ensuing hypokalemia.
- Patients who are in shock with low or normal hematocrit levels but who show signs of fluid overload may have occult hemorrhage. Further infusion of large volumes of intravenous fluids will lead only to a poor outcome. Careful transfusion of fresh whole blood should be initiated as soon as possible. Repeated small boluses of colloid solution may be helpful.

REGULATORY MEASURES

Dengue diseases are not subject to international quarantine or surveillance regulations. Dengue is a nationally notifiable disease in the United States, and suspected cases should be reported to the local health department. An intensive and effective voluntary reporting system has been devised by the regional offices of the WHO. People traveling to areas where dengue is endemic should assess the risk (http://www.healthmap.org/dengue/) and take necessary precautions to protect themselves against mosquito exposure.

PROGNOSIS

Not all patients suspected of having DHF need to be hospitalized because circulatory failure and shock may develop in only approximately one-third of patients. Mild and moderate cases may be treated on an outpatient basis. For the purpose of early recognition of shock, parents should be advised to bring the patient back if evidence of clinical deterioration is noted or such warning signs as restlessness with or without lethargy, severe abdominal pain, cold extremities, and skin congestion occur on or after the third day after the onset of fever.

In most cases, early and effective replacement of lost plasma with plasma, plasma expanders, or fluid and electrolyte solutions (or any combination of these products) results in a favorable outcome. The acute onset of shock and the rapid, often dramatic clinical recovery, together with the fact that no destructive or inflammatory vascular lesions are observed, suggest that the disease is produced by transient functional vascular changes caused by short-acting pharmacologic mediators.

Sequelae in dengue and DHF have not been studied systematically. Common sequelae of mild and uncomplicated dengue virus infection include bradycardia and ventricular extrasystoles during the convalescent stage, often persisting for several weeks. Profound asthenia with or without mental depression has been described. In patients with DHF/DSS, great care must be taken to reduce use of invasive procedures for managing shock. Nosocomial infections such as gram-negative sepsis can masquerade as DHF/DSS. Overhydration during the shock resuscitation phase may lead to heart failure and a complicated, stormy postshock stage. Infrequently, residual brain damage occurs, apparently as a result of either prolonged shock or, occasionally, intracranial hemorrhage. Children in whom profound shock develops rapidly with no detectable diastolic pressure or with unobtainable blood pressure, children in shock with delayed admission to the hospital, or children in shock with gastrointestinal hemorrhage have a poor prognosis. Mortality rates may exceed 50% in these groups.

PREVENTION

Three immunogenic tissue culture–based vaccines containing antigens for dengue virus types 1, 2, 3, and 4 are in phase III human clinical trials. A vaccine now licensed in 16 countries, manufactured by Sanofi Pasteur, is a chimera of the nonstructural genes of yellow fever 17D vaccine spliced with structural genes of the four dengue viruses.[84] It is designed as a two-dose vaccine to be given at months 0, 6, and 12 to individuals 9 to 45 years of age who have overall prevalence of dengue antibodies of 70%. This vaccine has received endorsement from the WHO.[15,89,116] This vaccine is not designed for, nor available for use by, tourists to protect against dengue infection. Another vaccine, comprising one chimeric and three mutagenized dengue viruses, was designed by the US National Institutes of Health and licensed to Merck, as well to several dengue endemic country vaccine manufacturers. [67] In human challenge studies, this vaccine has been shown to be highly protective.[148] A final vaccine, developed by the Centers for Disease Control and Prevention, was licensed to Takeda Pharmaceuticals and comprises chimeras of dengue 2 virus. [189,190]

Today, for most at-risk countries, prophylaxis depends on killing vector mosquitoes or avoiding mosquito bites. This involves the use of insecticides, repellents, protective body clothing, and screens on houses to avoid mosquito bites. Destruction of *A. aegypti* breeding sites also is effective. The WHO issues definitive guidelines with technical information and advice on organizing national vector control programs.[11,14,277] If water storage is mandatory, a tight-fitting lid or a thin layer of oil may prevent eggs from being deposited or hatching. A larvicide such as temefos (Abate), which is available as a 1% sand granule formulation and effective at a concentration of 1 ppm, may be added safely to drinking water.

Epidemic Measures

The WHO recommends integrated vector management, which requires training, preparation, and application of appropriate technologies.[277] Control of *A. aegypti* is mainly achieved by eliminating container habitats that are favorable oviposition sites, permitting development of aquatic stages. In emergencies, space sprays can be applied either as thermal fogs at 10 to 50 L/hectare or as ultra-low-volume applications of undiluted or slightly diluted technical-grade insecticide in the form of a cold aerosol or droplets of controlled size (15–25 μm) at a rate of 0.5 to 2 L/hectare . Portable or vehicle-mounted thermal or cold-fog generators can be used for ground application. If the target area exceeds

1000 hectares or cannot be covered for ground equipment within 10 days, aerial cold fog application is sometimes used. Applications vary with the susceptibility of the target species and environmental conditions, such as wind speed. Cold-fog applications from large fixed-wing aircraft are made at approximately 240 km/h and 60 m above the ground.

Eradication and Control

A. aegypti was eradicated successfully from countries and whole continents with use of the techniques pioneered by the Rockefeller Foundation in its worldwide program to control urban yellow fever.[82,245] An eradication campaign in the United States was abandoned and replaced by a program of disease surveillance and containment of introduced virus. After 1970, the species successfully reestablished itself in much of its former range. Mosquito control or eradication programs require the simultaneous use of two approaches: a reduction in breeding sites and the application of larvicides. Alternatively, a significant reduction in population may be effected by closely spaced applications of adulticide.[79,80] Vehicle-mounted or portable ultra-low-volume aerosol generators or mist blowers can be used to apply technical-grade malathion or fenitrothion at 438 mL/hectare. Three applications made at 1-week intervals can suppress *A. aegypti* populations for approximately 2 months.

Source reduction requires public support by either legal sanctions or voluntary actions (see the following section). Source reduction campaigns should be well organized, supervised, and evaluated. Proper disposal of discarded cans, bottles, tires, and other potential breeding sites not used for storage of drinking or bathing water should be performed. Sides of water storage containers should be scrubbed to remove eggs when the water level is low. Water storage containers for drinking and bathing and flower vases should be emptied completely once weekly. Water containers that cannot be emptied should be treated with Abate 1% sand granules at a dosage of 1 ppm (e.g., 10 g of sand to 100 L of water). Treatments should be repeated at intervals of 2 to 3 months.

In dengue-endemic countries, little effort has been made to adopt building codes or waste collection methods to reduce the number of mosquito breeding sites.[156] Furthermore, almost no way has been found to use the resources and skills of the private sector to implement vector control despite ample evidence of long-term successful vector mosquito abatement programs in the United States.[47,55]

New generations of vector control methods are under active development and testing. *Mesocyclops,* an antilarval insect predator, has been introduced into water storage containers in rural Vietnam with near eradication of *A. aegypti* larvae.[145,146,233,259] Infection of *A. aegypti* by *Wolbachia,* a species of rickettsial-like organism, blocks replication of dengue virus and vectoral capacity of the mosquito.[121,185,261] *Wolbachia* has been successfully introduced into wild populations of *A. aegypti* with sufficient spread to prevent dengue transmission.[41,180,203,247] Various methods of achieving and spreading sterile *A. aegypti* males or flightless females are being tested in the field.[69,75,119,275,276] Autocidal mosquito traps may be effective in areas of recent mosquito introduction or low, dispersed populations.[23]

Health Education

Control of *A. aegypti* has been maintained effectively in some tropical areas through the simple expedient of emptying water containers once per week. During the yellow fever campaigns, strong sanitary laws made the breeding of mosquitoes on premises a crime punishable by fine or jail.[245] In the modern era, Singapore and Cuba have adopted these measures with moderate degrees of success.[188] Health education through mass media and schools has been attempted in Myanmar, Thailand, Malaysia, and Indonesia, but without spectacular success.[64] The goals of health education and community participation approaches are to make the population aware of the identity of the vector of DHF, to describe its biting habits (daytime feeding) and its breeding habits (containers holding clean water), and to motivate people to reduce breeding sources by emptying water from containers on a regular basis.[8,273,274] The use of piped water rather than water storage should be encouraged. Studies in Malaysia after the 1973 epidemic of DHF indicated a very low level of functional knowledge among the inhabitants of Kuala Lumpur, Malaysia, about the vector of DHF.[64] Discouragingly, persons who were informed correctly, in most instances, took no action to protect themselves against mosquito breeding in their homes. Extensive effort is being made to apply social science methods to gain the voluntary participation of the population in sustained mosquito control programs.[8,161]

NEW REFERENCES SINCE THE SEVENTH EDITION

7. Anderson KB, Gibbons RV, Cummings DA, et al. A Shorter Time Interval Between First and Second Dengue Infections Is Associated With Protection From Clinical Illness in a School-based Cohort in Thailand. *J Infect Dis.* 2013;209(3):360-368.
8. Andersson N, Nava-Aguilera E, Arostegui J, et al. Evidence based community mobilization for dengue prevention in Nicaragua and Mexico (Camino Verde, the Green Way): cluster randomized controlled trial. *BMJ.* 2015;351:h3267.
11. Dengue: Guias para la atencion de enfermos en la region de las Americas; 2016. http://iris.paho.org/xmlui/bitstream/handle/123456789/31207/9789275118900-eng.pdf?sequence=1&isAllowed=y.
13. *Handbook for clinical management of dengue.* Geneva: World Health Organization; 2012. http://www.who.int/tdr/publications/handbook_dengue/en/.
15. Summary of the April 2016 Meeting of the Strategic Advisory Group of Experts on Immunization (SAGE). Available at: http://www.who.int/immunization/sage/meetings/2016/april/SAGE_April_2016_Meeting_Web_summary.pdf?ua=1.
15. National Guidelines for Clinical Management of Dengue Fever; 2015. New Delhi, India: Southeast Asia Office of the World Health Organization National Vector Borne Disease Control Program. http://www.searo.who.int/india/publications/national_guidelines_clinical_management_dengue1.pdf?ua=1.
18. Aye KS, Charngkaew K, Win N, et al. Pathologic highlights of dengue hemorrhagic fever in 13 autopsy cases from Myanmar. *Hum Pathol.* 2014;45(6):1221-1233.
23. Barrera R, Amador M, Acevedo V, et al. Use of the CDC autocidal gravid ovitrap to control and prevent outbreaks of *Aedes aegypti* (Diptera: Culicidae). *J Med Entomol.* 2014;51(1):145-154.
24. Beatty RP, Puerta-Guardo H, Killingbeck S, et al. Dengue virus non-structural protein 1 triggers endothelial permeability and vascular leak that can be inhibited by anti-NS1 antibodies. *Sci Transl Med.* 2015;7(304):304-141.
28. Bhatt S, Gething PW, Brady OJ, et al. The global distribution and burden of dengue. *Nature.* 2013;496(7446):504-507.
32. Blacksell SD, Jarman RG, Gibbons RV, et al. Comparison of seven commercial antigen and antibody enzyme-linked immunosorbent assays for detection of acute dengue infection. *Clin Vaccine Immunol.* 2012;19(5):804-810.
37. Brady OJ, Golding N, Pigott DM, et al. Global temperature constraints on *Aedes aegypti* and *Ae. albopictus* persistence and competence for dengue virus transmission. *Parasit Vectors.* 2014;7:338.
38. Brady OJ, Johansson MA, Guerra CA, et al. Modelling adult *Aedes aegypti* and *Aedes albopictus* survival at different temperatures in laboratory and field settings. *Parasit Vectors.* 2013;6:351.
39. Brown JE, Evans BR, Zheng W, et al. Human impacts have shaped historical and recent evolution in *Aedes aegypti,* the dengue and yellow fever mosquito. *Evolution.* 2014;68(2):514-525.
41. Caragata EP, Dutra HL, Moreira LA. Exploiting Intimate Relationships: Controlling Mosquito-Transmitted Disease with *Wolbachia. Trends Parasitol.* 2016;32(3):207-218.
46. Castanha PM, Braga C, Cordeiro MT, et al. Placental transfer of dengue-specific antibodies and kinetics of dengue infection enhancing-activity in Brazilian infants. *J Infect Dis.* 2016;214(2):265-272.
58. de Alwis R, Smith SA, Olivarez NP, et al. Identification of human neutralizing antibodies that bind to complex epitopes on dengue virions. *Proc Natl Acad Sci USA.* 2012;109(19):7439-7444.
59. DeBiasi RL, Song X, Cato K, et al. Preparedness, Evaluation, and Care of Pediatric Patients Under Investigation for Ebola Virus Disease: Experience From a Pediatric Designated Care Facility. *J Pediatric Infect Dis Soc.* 2016;5(1):68-75.
69. Ernst KC, Haenchen S, Dickinson K, et al. Awareness and support of release of genetically modified "sterile" mosquitoes, Key West, Florida, USA. *Emerg Infect Dis.* 2015;21(2):320-324.
70. Fares RC, Souza KP, Anez G, et al. Epidemiological Scenario of Dengue in Brazil. *Biomed Res Int.* 2015;2015:321873.
71. Fibriansah G, Tan JL, Smith SA, et al. A potent anti-dengue human antibody preferentially recognizes the conformation of E protein monomers assembled on the virus surface. *EMBO Mol Med.* 2014;6(3):358-371.
76. Gallichotte EN, Widman DG, Yount BL, et al. A new quaternary structure epitope on dengue virus serotype 2 is the target of durable type-specific neutralizing antibodies. *MBio.* 2015;6(5):e01461-15.
77. Gordon A, Kuan G, Mercado JC, et al. The Nicaraguan pediatric dengue cohort study: incidence of inapparent and symptomatic dengue virus infections, 2004–2010. *PLoS Negl Trop Dis.* 2013;7(9):e2462.
84. Guy B, Briand O, Lang J, et al. Development of the Sanofi Pasteur tetravalent dengue vaccine: One more step forward. *Vaccine.* 2015;33(50):7100-7111.
85. Guzman MG, Harris E. Dengue. *Lancet.* 2015;385(9966):453-465.
89. Hadinegoro SR, Arredondo-Garcia JL, Capeding MR, et al. Efficacy and Long-Term Safety of a Dengue Vaccine in Regions of Endemic Disease. *N Engl J Med.* 2015;373(13):1195-1206.

92. Halstead SB, Cohen SN. Dengue Hemorrhagic Fever at 60 Years: Early Evolution of Concepts of Causation and Treatment. *Microbiol Mol Biol Rev*. 2015;79(3):281-291.
98. Halstead SB, Thomas SJ. Dengue Vaccines. In: Plotkin SA, Orenstein W, Offit PA, eds. *Vaccines*. Vol 2. 7th ed. Philadelphia: Elsevier; 2017.
112. Halstead SB. Pathogenesis of Dengue: Dawn of a New Era. *F1000Res*. 2015;4.
115. Halstead SB. Reappearance of chikungunya, formerly called dengue, in the Americas. *Emerg Infect Dis*. 2015;21(4):557-561.
124. Horstick O, Jaenisch T, Martinez E, et al. Comparing the usefulness of the 1997 and 2009 WHO dengue case classification: a systematic literature review. *Am J Trop Med Hyg*. 2014;91(3):621-634.
125. Horstick O, Martinez E, Guzman MG, et al. WHO dengue case classification 2009 and its usefulness in practice: an expert consensus in the Americas. *Pathog Glob Health*. 2015;109(1):19-25.
126. Horstick O, Ranzinger SR. Reporting progress on the use of the WHO 2009 dengue case classification: A review. *Southeast Asian J Trop Med Public Health*. 2015;46(suppl 1):49-54.
132. Hunsperger EA, Munoz-Jordan J, Beltran M, et al. Performance of Dengue Diagnostic Tests in a Single-Specimen Diagnostic Algorithm. *J Infect Dis*. 2016;214(6):836-844.
134. Hunsperger EA, Yoksan S, Buchy P, et al. Evaluation of commercially available diagnostic tests for the detection of dengue virus NS1 antigen and anti-dengue virus IgM antibody. *PLoS Negl Trop Dis*. 2014;8(10):e3171.
136. Jaenisch T, Junghanss T, Wills B, et al. Dengue expansion in Africa—not recognized or not happening? *Emerg Infect Dis*. 2014;20(10).
144. Katzelnick LC, Fonville JM, Gromowski GD, et al. Dengue viruses cluster antigenically but not as discrete serotypes. *Science*. 2015;349(6254):1338-1343.
148. Kirkpatrick BD, Whitehead SS, Pierce KK, et al. The live attenuated dengue vaccine TV003 elicits complete protection against dengue in a human challenge model. *Sci Transl Med*. 2016;8(330):330-336.
155. Lam PK, Tam DT, Diet TV, et al. Clinical characteristics of dengue shock syndrome in Vietnamese children: a 10-year prospective study in a single hospital. *Clin Infect Dis*. 2013;57(11):1577-1586.
159. Liebman KA, Stoddard ST, Morrison AC, et al. Spatial dimensions of dengue virus transmission across interepidemic and epidemic periods in Iquitos, Peru (1999–2003). *PLoS Negl Trop Dis*. 2012;6(2):e1472.
160. Lin SW, Chuang YC, Lin YS, et al. Dengue virus nonstructural protein NS1 binds to prothrombin/thrombin and inhibits prothrombin activation. *J Infect*. 2012;64(3):325-334.
169. Modhiran N, Watterson D, Panetta AK, et al. Dengue virus NS1 is a viral toxin that activates cells via TLR4 and disrupts endothelial cell monolayer integrity. *Sci Transl Med*. 2015;7(304):304-142.
174. Montoya M, Gresh L, Mercado JC, et al. Symptomatic versus inapparent outcome in repeat dengue virus infections is influenced by the time interval between infections and study year. *PLoS Negl Trop Dis*. 2013;7(8):e2357.
179. Nguyen TH, Nguyen HL, Nguyen TY, et al. Field evaluation of the establishment potential of wMelPop *Wolbachia* in Australia and Vietnam for dengue control. *Parasit Vectors*. 2015;8:563.
187. Ongoing dengue epidemic—Angola, June 2013. *MMWR Morb Mortal Wkly Rep*. 2013;62(24):504-507.
189. Osorio JE, Partidos CD, Wallace D, et al. Development of a recombinant, chimeric tetravalent dengue vaccine candidate. *Vaccine*. 2015;33(50):7112-7120.
190. Osorio JE, Wallace D, Stinchcomb DT. A recombinant, chimeric tetravalent dengue vaccine candidate based on a dengue virus serotype 2 backbone. *Expert Rev Vaccines*. 2016;15(4):497-508.
195. Radke EG, Gregory CJ, Kintziger KW, et al. Dengue outbreak in key west, Florida, USA, 2009. *Emerg Infect Dis*. 2012;18(1):135-137.
197. Reiner RC Jr, Stoddard ST, Scott TW. Socially structured human movement shapes dengue transmission despite the diffusive effect of mosquito dispersal. *Epidemics*. 2014;6:30-36.
203. Ritchie SA, Townsend M, Paton CJ, et al. Application of wMelPop *Wolbachia* Strain to Crash Local Populations of Aedes aegypti. *PLoS Negl Trop Dis*. 2015;9(7):e0003930.
222. Schwartz E, Meltzer E, Mendelson M, et al. Detection on four continents of dengue fever cases related to an ongoing outbreak in Luanda, Angola, March to May 2013. *Euro Surveill*. 2013;18(21).
224. Screaton G, Mongkolsapaya J, Yacoub S, et al. New insights into the immunopathology and control of dengue virus infection. *Nat Rev Immunol*. 2015;15(12):745-759.
225. Selck FW, Adalja AA, Boddie CR. An estimate of the global health care and lost productivity costs of dengue. *Vector Borne Zoonotic Dis*. 2014;14(11):824-826.
226. Shepard DS, Undurraga EA, Halasa YA, et al. The global economic burden of dengue: a systematic analysis. *Lancet Infect Dis*. 2016;16(8):935-941.
233. Sinh Nam V, Thi Yen N, Minh Duc H, et al. Community-based control of *Aedes aegypti* by using *Mesocyclops* in southern Vietnam. *Am J Trop Med Hyg*. 2012;86(5):850-859.
234. Smith DL, Perkins TA, Reiner RC Jr, et al. Recasting the theory of mosquito-borne pathogen transmission dynamics and control. *Trans R Soc Trop Med Hyg*. 2014;108(4):185-197.
235. Snow GE, Haaland B, Ooi EE, et al. Review article: Research on dengue during World War II revisited. *Am J Trop Med Hyg*. 2014;91(6):1203-1217.
236. Soller B, Srikiatkachorn A, Zou F, et al. Preliminary evaluation of near infrared spectroscopy as a method to detect plasma leakage in children with dengue hemorrhagic fever. *BMC Infect Dis*. 2014;14:396.
239. Srikiatkhachorn A, Kelley JF. Endothelial cells in dengue hemorrhagic fever. *Antiviral Res*. 2014;109:160-170.
240. Srikiatkhachorn A, Krautrachue A, Ratanaprakarn W, et al. Natural history of plasma leakage in dengue hemorrhagic fever: a serial ultrasonographic study. *Pediatr Infect Dis J*. 2007;26(4):283-290, discussion 291-282.
242. Stanaway JD, Shepard DS, Undurraga EA, et al. The global burden of dengue: an analysis from the Global Burden of Disease Study 2013. *Lancet Infect Dis*. 2016;16(6):712-723.
246. Tam DT, Ngoc TV, Tien NT, et al. Effects of Short-Course Oral Corticosteroid Therapy in Early Dengue Infection in Vietnamese Patients: A Randomized, Placebo-Controlled Trial. *Clin Infect Dis*. 2012;55(9):1216-1224.
247. Tantowijoyo W, Arguni E, Johnson P, et al. Spatial and Temporal Variation in Aedes aegypti and *Aedes albopictus* (Diptera: Culicidae) Numbers in the Yogyakarta Area of Java, Indonesia, With Implications for *Wolbachia* Releases. *J Med Entomol*. 2016;53(1):188-198.
248. Thein TL, Leo YS, Fisher DA, et al. Risk factors for fatality among confirmed adult dengue inpatients in Singapore: a matched case-control study. *PLoS ONE*. 2013;8(11):e81060.
250. Trung DT, Thao le TT, Dung NM, et al. Clinical features of dengue in a large Vietnamese cohort: intrinsically lower platelet counts and greater risk for bleeding in adults than children. *PLoS Negl Trop Dis*. 2012;6(6):e1679.
275. Winskill P, Carvalho DO, Capurro ML, et al. Dispersal of Engineered Male *Aedes aegypti* Mosquitoes. *PLoS Negl Trop Dis*. 2015;9(11):e0004156.
280. Yoon IK, Getis A, Aldstadt J, et al. Fine scale spatiotemporal clustering of dengue virus transmission in children and *Aedes aegypti* in rural Thai villages. *PLoS Negl Trop Dis*. 2012;6(7):e1730.
283. Zellweger RM, Shresta S. Mouse models to study dengue virus immunology and pathogenesis. *Front Immunol*. 2014;5:151.

The full reference list for this chapter is available at ExpertConsult.com.

176E ■ Japanese Encephalitis

Theresa Barton

Japanese encephalitis (JE), a mosquito-borne flavivirus infection, is the leading vaccine-preventable viral encephalitis in Asia.

HISTORY

JE first was recognized after an outbreak in Japan in 1924 led to an alarming 6125 cases of encephalitis. In retrospect, similar summer and autumn outbreaks were recognized as early as 1871 to 1873.[28,43] In 1933, Hayashi recovered the virus from monkeys and the brain of a patient, and in 1938, Mitamura confirmed its mosquito-borne mode of transmission by isolating the virus from *Culex tritaeniorhynchus*.[43] An inactivated vaccine was licensed in Japan in 1956, and its use successfully controlled the disease in Asian countries where it was deployed. New inactivated cell culture–derived and live, attenuated vaccines are now displacing the efficacious but reactogenic 50-year-old mouse brain–derived product.[33] Despite preventative measures, JE causes 15,000 deaths per year and continues to evolve in new geographic regions.[11] It is considered a neglected tropical disease despite its impact.

ETIOLOGIC AGENT

JE virus is a member of the flavivirus antigenic complex that includes St. Louis encephalitis, Murray Valley encephalitis, and West Nile viruses. Five viral genotypes have been described. Since the 1980s, viruses in genotype I have displaced previously predominant genotype III strains, and genotype V viruses also may be emerging.[16,17,58,79,113] Because humans are incidental to the viral transmission cycle, the changing distribution of viral genotypes indicates evolving viral adaptation to vertebrate hosts and mosquito vectors responsible for viral maintenance. However, the virus exists as a single serotype, and all vaccines are made from genotype III strains, with no evidence that they fail to prevent disease caused by viruses in other genotypes. Genotypic strains were previously associated with distinct geographic distribution, but subsequent observations have shown shifts in genotype presence within areas.[87,97]

As with other flaviviruses, important biologic functions, including attenuation and viral neutralization, are associated with the E glycoprotein. With repeated cell culture passage, biologically derived neuroattenuated strains have been produced for use as vaccines.[111] Combinations of mutations in genes of the E protein, nonstructural proteins, and noncoding regions have been associated with attenuation of the live vaccine strain SA 14-14-2 and so have been selectively incorporated with others into a chimeric JE vaccine using nonstructural proteins from the itself attenuated yellow fever 17D vaccine strain.[33]

JE virus is perpetuated in both wild, or sylvatic, and domestic cycles. JE mosquito vectors are largely opportunistic, feeding on numerous available hosts.[105] JE virus is transmitted between birds and *Culex* mosquitoes; however, pigs, when present, are the most important source of viral amplification (Fig. 176E.1).[3,5,93,94] This domestic cycle of JE is the most important source for human disease. Domestic pigs maintain high sustained viremias and may be hosts to thousands of mosquitoes in a single night, thereby serving as prolific sources of infected vectors capable of transmitting the virus onward. In rural Asia, the onset of human cases each summer occurs shortly after pigs become infected, following which the epidemic curves of human and pig infections evolve in parallel.[82] However, outbreaks of JE have occurred in areas devoid of pigs, where birds, including ducklings, pigeons, sparrows, and possibly other small birds found near human residences, have served as amplifying hosts.[3,5,29,93]

In the sylvatic cycle vectors transmit to mammalian reservoirs, with bats and peridomestic wild mammals such as wild boar and raccoons playing an integral role.[55,75] The bird-associated sylvatic cycle is crucial to viral persistence in the environment as well as spread of the virus to new geographic areas.[5] More than 90 bird species can amplify and serve as viral reservoirs. Wading birds such as egrets and herons are particularly effective reservoirs with high viremia and ability to infect vector mosquitos.[105]

C. tritaeniorhynchus is the major mosquito vector in most areas of Asia, and distribution in niches below 1000-m elevation (valleys in Tibet and Kathmandu are conspicuous exceptions), along with other environmental and climatic features, corresponds well to the distribution of human cases.[70,94] That distribution also overlaps the land cover used for rice paddies. *C. tritaeniorhynchus* exploits ground pools and especially rice paddies in its preadult stages, emerging in immense numbers from the flooded rice paddies responsible for 80% of the land cover in some areas and that frequently surround individual residences and villages. The vector is zoophilic and prefers to feed on large animals such as pigs and less so on humans, but with the custom of keeping pigs near or inside houses in rural Asia, residents live in the midst of the viral transmission cycle and are at high risk for exposure to infected mosquitoes, starting at an early age. Living in proximity to a rice field and pig ownership understandably are risk factors for acquiring the illness.[64] Although *C. tritaeniorhynchus* is most active in the evening and night, because adults feed outdoors, bed nets are not entirely protective.

In various regions, other species *(Culex pseudovishnui, Culex vishnui, Culex gelidus, Culex fuscocephalus, Culex annulirostris,* and *Culex bitaeniorhynchus)* with different habitats may also serve as vectors.[3,94] Anopheline mosquitoes may contribute to transmission in northeastern India. The viral overwintering mechanism for JE virus has been a matter of speculation; however, vertical infection of mosquito eggs has been demonstrated as a means by which transmission is reestablished.[25,94]

Ecologic factors have been modeled to describe the seasonality of infection and to predict the occurrence and severity of outbreaks; surveillance tools include monitoring infections in pigs, birds, dogs, and horses, as well as precipitation and temperature. The potential impact of global climate on JE seasonality has been speculated because warmer environmental temperature shortens the extrinsic incubation period of related flaviviruses, thereby speeding the transmission cycle. In support of this hypothesis, a secular trend toward an earlier onset of JE transmission in Taiwan has been noted, from June to May, whereas

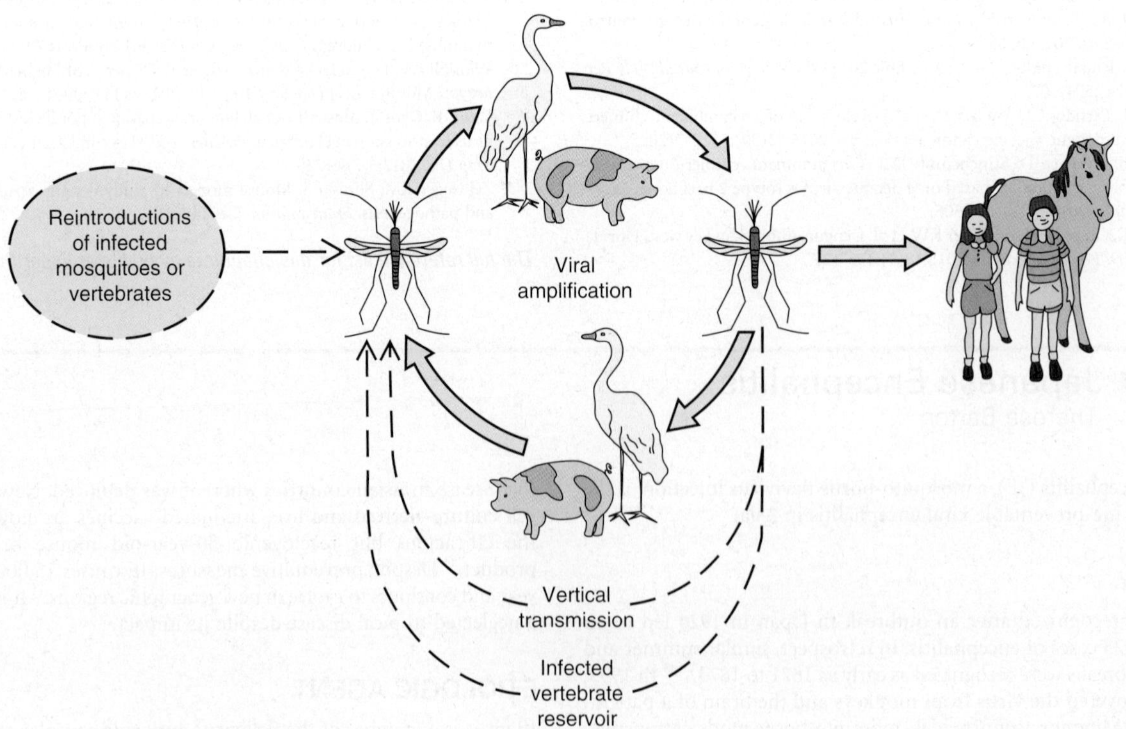

FIGURE 176E.1 Transmission cycle of Japanese encephalitis virus. Speculative portions of the cycle are shown in *broken lines.*

high summertime temperatures have been associated with the occurrence and severity of West Nile and St. Louis encephalitis outbreaks.

EPIDEMIOLOGY

JE is the largest worldwide cause of epidemic viral encephalitis.[10] Approximately 68,000 JE cases occur annually, causing about 10,000 to 15,000 deaths across Asia and the Australian continent. In areas where children are not routinely vaccinated, cases occur mainly in children after the first year of life, with a slight preponderance in boys. More than 99% of infections are subclinical, and cumulative exposure with age leads to seroprevalence rates of 80% or more by adulthood.[31] In Japan and other developed Asian countries, where children are protected by routine vaccination, adult cases now predominate.[2,50,57] A majority of cases occur in adults older than 45 years, because of immunosenescence and age-related chronic diseases that may be risk factors. Waning protection from remote childhood vaccination may also be shifting epidemiology to adult disease.[42]

Transmission is seasonal, during late summer and early fall in temperate regions (July to October) and over a longer interval in tropical and subtropical regions, such as southern China and Southeast Asia (April to November).[113] Mosquitoes proliferate after monsoon rains, and multiple epidemic seasons or year-round transmission is possible in some tropical locations. In many locations, vector populations now follow irrigation-controlled schedules of rice field flooding and other patterns dictated by mechanized rice production rather than the traditional rainy season.[78]

JE transmission is endemic in nearly every country in Asia (Fig. 176E.2).[11] Annual incidence rates range widely from less than 0.01 to 5 per 100,000, depending on vaccine coverage and environmental conditions, and epidemic attack rates as high as 100 per 100,000 have been described.[106] Incidence is underestimated because the unavailability of laboratory confirmation limits specific diagnosis and surveillance. In addition to seasonal epidemics, self-limited outbreaks can occur after the virus is introduced by migrating birds or other mechanisms, coupled with unusual conditions of human activity or weather patterns, but transmission is usually not sustained after the exhaustion of susceptible hosts.[35,80] Few cases are reported from countries where vaccination rates are high (e.g., Japan, Korea, and Taiwan) and where development through urbanization, decreased agricultural land use, and improved standards of living have reduced human exposure. The use of agricultural pesticides and centralized pig rearing also may have contributed to lowering risk. Although the number of human cases has decreased in some areas, enzootic animal transmission persists. Horses can develop encephalitis, and outbreaks and economically significant loss of prize horses have led to routine use of equine vaccines in China, Mongolia, and Japan. Sows also are vaccinated, not to prevent illness in the animals, which remain asymptomatic after infection, but to prevent congenital infection of piglets, which may die in utero or may be born with lethal neurologic malformations. For example, in Japan, more than 80% of pigs and 2.6% of the human population still are infected each year.[2,51] Domestic animals such as dogs and cattle can be infected, but their viremias are insufficient to support further transmission. Because they are attractive hosts to JE vectors, they may divert mosquitoes from humans, thereby protecting them from infection (zooprophylaxis).

Although economic development has paralleled a decline in JE, in some areas, development in the form of deforestation, construction of dams, and irrigation schemes has led to increases in transmission of JE virus or its emergence in areas where the disease had not occurred previously. Examples include development projects in the Terai in southern Nepal and the Mahaweli Valley in Sri Lanka, where JE and malaria have become hyperendemic after large-scale programs of deforestation and agricultural development.

Travelers to areas where JE is endemic may be at risk for acquiring the illness.[37] Updated information can be obtained from the Centers for Disease Control and Prevention (CDC) at the website http://www.cdc.gov/travel/. Approximately 80 cases have been reported in travelers and expatriates (including military personnel and their family members) from North America, Europe, Russia, and Australia in the past 20 years, but the number undoubtedly is larger because of underreporting.[37] The risk for acquiring the disease can best be described as serendipitous—cases have been reported in travelers who were infected within days of arriving in Asia, who never visited a rural area, and who had none of the risk issues cited in recommendations. The generally low but difficult-to-predict risk can be understood by factoring the probability of development of an illness after a single mosquito bite—only certain vector species transmit the virus, typically less than 3% of vector mosquitoes are infected, and only one in several hundred infections leads to clinical illness. Other factors entering into the risk for acquiring infection and illness are described in Table 176E.1.

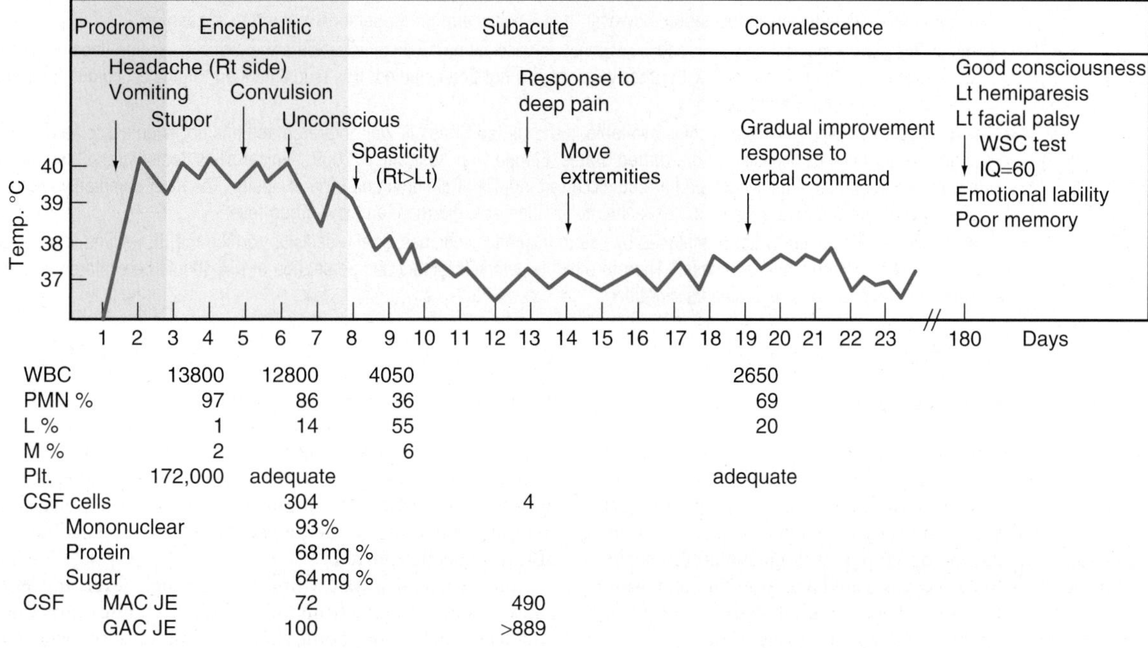

FIGURE 176E.2 Clinical stages of a typical Japanese encephalitis case.

TABLE 176E.1 Factors to Consider in Recommending Japanese Encephalitis (JE) Vaccine for Travelers to Asia

Factor	Comment
Expatriates	During extended assignments, expatriates likely will make unanticipated trips within the region, including to areas where the risk for acquiring JE is high or unknown.
Visiting friends or relatives	Returning families may be more likely to visit ancestral villages or other locations that pose a greater risk for viral transmission. Parents may have been vaccinated or have acquired natural infections before they emigrated and may not realize that their own children are unprotected.
Travelers with open itineraries	"Year abroad" and other travelers who have open itineraries may journey to locations where risk for disease is higher, including rural areas.
Frequent travelers	Travelers who have second homes in the region or who travel frequently to Asia, even if individual trips are brief, have a cumulative risk for exposure.
Season	In East Asia, which has a temperate or subtropical climate, transmission usually is described as extending from April to October, but within individual countries even the size of Thailand, transmission periods may differ by several months from north to south, or, as in China, from West to East. In the tropical zone, the virus may be transmitted year-round with superimposed patterns of higher risk. In many locations, seasonal monsoons dictate the periods when mosquito vectors are prevalent, and those patterns can differ within surprisingly delimited geographic bounds, such as for Southeastern versus Southwestern India. Historical seasonal patterns may not be predictive in any given year. As rice cultivation has become more industrialized, the timing of rice field flooding and resulting blooms of vector mosquitoes may not correspond only to natural patterns of rainfall.
Activity out of doors	Persons with extensive occupational or recreational outdoor activities, especially at twilight and evening, are more likely to be exposed to the principal JE mosquito vectors. Even brief episodes outdoors (e.g., an elephant ride) have been reported in case histories of travel-associated JE.
Exposure to vector mosquito habitat	Most recommendations cite "rural exposure" as a risk factor for acquiring JE. However, "rural" is used in this context as a proxy for exposure to rice paddies that are highly productive habitats for JE vectors. Rice paddies, however, are found at the edges or even within major Asian cities (e.g., in Denpasar, Indonesia, the city greenbelts are rice fields). Moreover, other pools of water (e.g., flooded ditches) can support species capable of transmitting JE virus; thus infected mosquitoes and seroconverting sentinel animals have been detected in urban or suburban surveillance sites.
Exposure to pigs	Pigs are highly important in amplifying JE virus in the usual transmission cycle. Although locations with few or no pigs may pose a lower risk for encountering virus-infected mosquitoes, birds, ducks, and potentially other vertebrates also can amplify the virus and have been implicated in outbreaks.
Age	Infants and older adults are at an increased risk for developing neurologic disease after infection, in contrast to young adults.
Chronic disease	Immunocompromising conditions, including HIV infection, increase risk for illness. Other chronic diseases, including cardiovascular disease, hypertension, and metabolic conditions, have been associated with risk for illness or increased severity of illness for other flaviviruses. Because observational and experimental data indicate that certain underlying neurologic diseases (e.g., neurocysticercosis and other concurrent neurologic infections) can facilitate neuroinvasion, it seems possible that CSF shunts, cochlear implants, baclofen pumps, and other implanted devices, as well as other neurologic disorders, could pose a similar risk.
Pregnancy	JE acquired in pregnancy has been associated with miscarriage and fetal death. However, no safety or immunogenicity data in pregnant women are available on use of the only available JE vaccine in the United States, an inactivated cell culture–derived vaccine (Pregnancy Category B). Pregnancy is a precaution for vaccination, and vaccination in pregnant women should only be done when there is a clear risk for infection.
Genetic factors	Several studies suggest that persons homozygous for *CCR5*Δ32 are at increased risk for clinical illness from the flaviviruses, West Nile virus and tick-borne encephalitis virus. This deletion is so uncommon in Asia that it is unlikely to be unimportant as a risk factor among the indigenous population; however, it is a consideration for persons with other ancestries.
Concurrent medication	Immunosuppressant medications may reduce response to vaccination. Coadministration of hepatitis A vaccine does not reduce immunogenicity. Coadministration with other vaccines has not been studied. It is recommended to give concomitant vaccines at different sites using different syringes.
Vaccine safety	The inactivated Vero cell–derived vaccine available in the United States is well tolerated and has not been associated with any safety issues since its licensure in the United States, Europe, and Australia in 2009. Clinical trials demonstrated serious adverse events in 1% of recipients. Minor side effects occurred in 40% of children and 59% of adults. The most commonly reported side effects were injection site reactions, headache, flulike illnesses, diarrhea, and low-grade fever.
Vaccine cost	Travel vaccines are generally not reimbursed by health insurance schemes, so the decision to take the JE vaccine is a decision for an out-of-pocket discretionary "purchase." Therefore highly personal factors and perception of risk should be explored and respected when advising travelers regarding vaccination.

CLINICAL MANIFESTATIONS

The majority of JE infections are asymptomatic or manifest as mild self-limited illnesses. Occasional cases of JE viremia are identified in serologic studies of children with undifferentiated fever, which might otherwise have been diagnosed clinically as dengue or another viral syndrome. However, patients who develop neurologic infection usually are profoundly ill, and 5% to 25% of cases are fatal. After an incubation period of 4 to 14 days, the illness begins with lethargy, nausea or abdominal pain and vomiting, headache, and fever (Fig. 176E.3).[4,52,53,61,92] The prodrome is followed by increasing lethargy or changes in behavior and motor disturbances over several days, leading eventually to impaired consciousness and coma. The initial presentation varies, however; in some cases, it may be a sudden seizure, whereas in others, there may be a long prodrome of a week or more, with periods of confusion or agitation and unsteadiness of gait and other motor abnormalities. Unusual manifestations, such as acute psychosis and Guillain-Barré syndrome, also have been reported.[90]

The principal physical findings are high fever and alterations in consciousness, ranging from mild mental clouding, frank disorientation, and delirium, to coma. Some children exhibit bizarre behavior, including mutism, shouting, spitting, and personality changes. Signs of meningeal

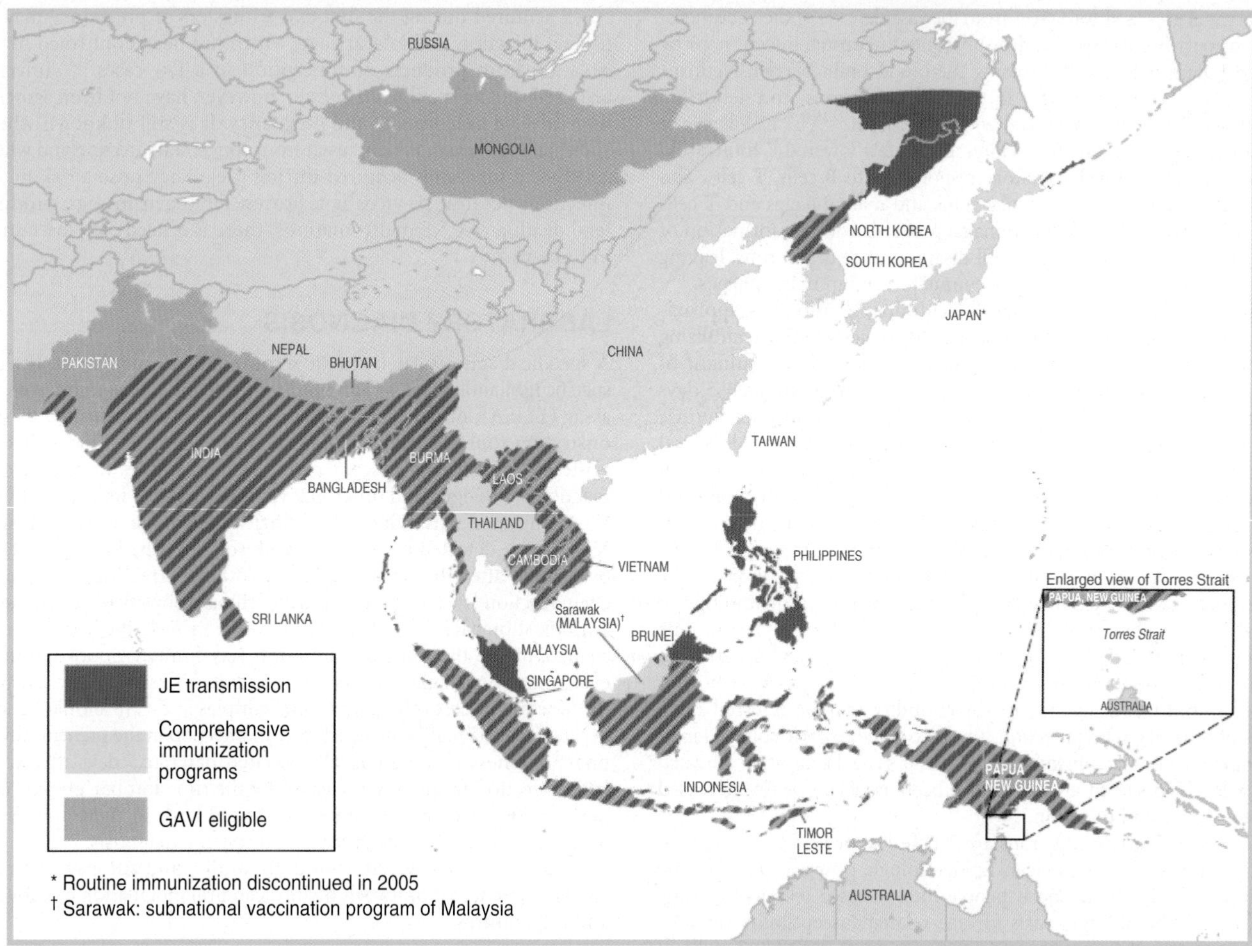

FIGURE 176E.3 Locations where Japanese encephalitis (JE) is prevalent.

irritation are present. Cranial nerve palsies, mainly disconjugate gaze and central facial paralysis, are observed in one-third of cases, and generalized or focal motor weakness can usually be demonstrated, presenting with either flaccid or spastic paralysis. Some patients exhibit erratic flailing movements, tremor, rigidity, expressionless facies, or thick slurred speech; frequently, choreoathetosis and other extrapyramidal signs become evident only in the second week of illness. Focal or generalized seizures develop in 50% to 75% of patients. Papilledema is seen in 10% of cases, along with hypertension, indicating increased intracranial pressure. In more than one third of patients, coma and respiratory failure necessitate ventilatory support. Patients with fulminant infections may die within the first 5 days of illness.

Recovery is slow, with defervescence of fever followed by gradual improvement of neurologic function over several weeks. During convalescence, stasis ulcers, urinary tract infections, pneumonia, and bacteremia may complicate the course. In anecdotal cases, a biphasic pattern of illness has been described, with a recurrence of motor and behavioral abnormalities 2 to 5 weeks after initial improvement, accompanied by larger and more numerous associated lesions on magnetic resonance imaging (MRI).[69] Recovery of motor function and adaptation to sequelae may progress over a period of months to years.

Routine laboratory studies initially show a peripheral leukocytosis, often with bandemia. Opening pressures on lumbar puncture usually are normal or slightly elevated. Cerebrospinal fluid (CSF) pleocytosis ranges from fewer than 10 cells to several thousand, with a median of several hundred per cubic millimeter, potentially leading to a misdiagnosis of bacterial meningitis. Lymphocytic pleocytosis follows, and CSF glucose and protein levels frequently are normal (80% of cases); when elevated, protein levels rarely exceed 100 mg/dL.

Electroencephalograms typically show diffuse theta to delta wave slowing, whereas spike and wave discharges are relatively uncommon. MRI is more sensitive using T2-weighted and fluid attenuation inversion recovery (FLAIR) sequences in early stages of illness, with a relatively lower sensitivity from diffusion-weighted signals.[34,69] A distinct pattern of hyperintensity in the thalamus, basal ganglia, and brainstem has been noted, although cortical, cerebellar, and spinal cord involvement is are seen. Electromyograms show a neurogenic pattern consistent with anterior horn cell involvement.[101] Central motor conduction times are prolonged, indicative of diffuse subcortical damage.

PATHOLOGY

Although JE presents clinically as a central nervous system (CNS) infection, often overlooked is that the infection is pantropic, with pathologic changes found in the lungs and viscera, in addition to the brain.[23,24,39,44,59,99,114] On gross examination, the brain appears swollen and the meninges may be congested with macroscopically visible punctate hemorrhages. Microscopic examination discloses a moderate inflammatory response in the meninges. The parenchyma shows foci of neuronal degeneration and parenchymal and perivascular inflammatory responses principally in the thalamus and brainstem, but also more widely, in the hippocampus, temporal cortex, cerebellum, and spinal cord. Areas of neuronophagia may be surrounded by microglial nodules, but sharply defined round areas of softening or necrolysis without an inflammatory response also are seen. Purkinje cells and cerebellar glial shrubs also may be lost.[114]

PATHOPHYSIOLOGY

After virus is introduced by a mosquito bite, replication within regional lymphatic tissue leads to a secondary amplified viremia and disseminated infection that includes the CNS. Neuroinvasion is thought to occur through cerebral capillaries as virions cross from the vascular side of the endothelial cell to the perivascular space, with subsequent neuronal infection, or by infected inflammatory cells crossing the blood-brain barrier. Neurons show evidence of viral antigen in the cell body, axons, and dendrites, indicating cell-to-cell viral spread within the brain.[22,23,48,58] CSF levels of catecholamines and their metabolites are acutely lowered.[39] Infiltrating T cells elicit a broad inflammatory response, with B cells, T cells, and macrophages found in perivascular cuffs and macrophages and T cells in the parenchyma.[48,109] Neuronophagia proceeds with the formation of microglial nodules and the eventual disappearance of neurons, leaving ghostlike remnants with antigen accumulated within macrophages.

Relatively low levels of circulating neutralizing antibodies, approximately 1 : 10, correlate with protection, and the rapidity of the neutralizing antibody response in naïve individuals is a principal determinant of outcome.[8,9,48,74] Most fatal cases occurring within approximately 5 days after the onset of illness have no detectable CSF antibody response while virus is recoverable from the CSF, indicating unimpeded viral replication.[8,9] In experimentally infected animals, passive immunization reduces mortality, even when it is given 4 to 5 days after inoculation.[74] However, the persistence of viral antigen in neurons for extended periods in the presence of intrathecal antibody and immune complexes in some cases, and development of antineurofilament antibodies, indicate the importance of viral clearance and potential for immunopathology in delayed or incomplete resolution of illness.[22-24] The role of innate immune responses is not well characterized, but they may contribute to both control of infection and immunopathology.[104,109] The contribution of interferon and CCR5 ligands in susceptibility may be inferred from studies of other flaviviral infections that associated risk with oligoadenylate synthetase polymorphisms and *CCR5*Δ32 gene deletions.[9,60] Elevated CXCL8 levels in serum and CSF have been associated with increased disease severity and duration.

Why most JE virus infections are subclinical or lead to no signs of infection in the CNS is unclear. Epidemiologic observations indicate an elevated risk for JE in elderly people and increased severity in young children, but the biologic basis for age-related susceptibility remains poorly understood. Tumor necrosis factor-α promoter polymorphism also has been suggested as a specific risk factor.[86] Pathologic observations have shown a higher prevalence of neurocysticercosis in fatal JE cases than in deaths from other causes, which suggests that physical or physiologic disruption of the brain architecture by infection or other mechanisms could facilitate neuroinvasion [20,63,101] Experimental dual infection of animals with JE virus and other agents supports this hypothesis. In experimental animals, other host factors associated with a risk for acquiring illness and poor outcome include flavivirus-specific susceptibility genes, age, levels of sex hormones, and cold and stress responses. Because dengue infections are prevalent across much of the JE-endemic region, the role of cross-reactive flavivirus immunity in the clinical outcome of JE is of considerable interest; unfortunately, no clear pattern of protection or increased risk has been confirmed.[1,27]

COMPLICATIONS

The principal risk is secondary bacterial infection occurring in the acute and subacute phases of illness. In addition, concurrent malaria and other parasitic or bacterial infections that are endemic in Asia may complicate management. Although JE occurs in areas of Asia where human immunodeficiency virus (HIV) infection is prevalent, data are insufficient to conclude differences in outcome in coinfected patients. Hyponatremia caused by inappropriate antidiuretic hormone secretion also can complicate treatment.

Cases of clinical relapse with seizures, coma, and weakness, several occurring 6 to 9 months after recovery from the acute illness, have been reported.[85,89] These and other patients experiencing relapse had evidence of persistent JE virus infection in peripheral blood mononuclear cells.[100] A study of 253 patients found laboratory evidence of subacute CNS infection in 5% of cases, with persistent intrathecal production of JE virus–specific immunoglobulin M (IgM) beyond 50 to 180 days or CSF containing JE virus antigen or virus more than 3 weeks after recovery.[89] These observations suggest that some infections may be followed by viral persistence, but additional confirmatory studies are needed.

JE acquired during the first two trimesters of pregnancy may lead to fetal infection and miscarriage, which has been confirmed by viral isolation from products of conception in a few cases.[15,67] Infections acquired during the third trimester, however, have not been associated with adverse outcomes to the pregnancy. It is still unknown whether sublethal malformations can result from congenital infection and whether subclinical infections acquired during pregnancy pose a risk for fetal infection. Because JE virus is a proven teratogen in pigs, producing fetal death and CNS malformations, there is a need for closer studies in humans.[2,3,10]

LABORATORY DIAGNOSIS

A specific diagnosis can be made serologically by identifying JE virus–specific IgM antibody in serum or CSF by enzyme-linked immunosorbent assay (ELISA); often, however, results need to be confirmed by demonstrating fourfold titer changes in neutralizing antibodies between acute-phase and convalescent-phase serum samples to resolve cross-reactions to dengue and other flaviviruses.[66] Several IgM detection kits exhibiting good sensitivity and specificity are commercially available.[71,88] IgM can be detected in serum or CSF (or in both) in nearly all cases by 1 week after the onset of illness. Although real-time polymerase chain reaction (PCR) and reverse transcriptase loop-mediated isothermal amplification (RT-LAMP) assays have been described, their limited availability in the endemic situation has limited opportunities for evaluation.[21] Available reports indicate that as a result of the sensitivity of these methods, both acute serum samples and CSF should be tested because viremia may be detected early in infection in the preneuroinvasive phase of illness, although usually no later than 6 to 7 days after onset.[40] Viral infection frequently is cleared by the time lumbar punctures are performed; therefore CSF should be tested both for IgM and by PCR to maximize the chances of making a specific diagnosis.

Virus can be recovered from brain biopsy and autopsy material in special reference laboratories, by intracerebral inoculation of baby mice and cell cultures.

DIFFERENTIAL DIAGNOSIS

Other mosquito-borne arboviruses also cause encephalitis—West Nile, Banna, and Chandipura viruses—and may be responsible for occasional or epidemic encephalitis in the same regions where JE occurs.[32] Because specific diagnostic assays are even less accessible for these infections than for JE virus itself, they may be responsible for some of the cases currently attributed to JE. Infections caused by West Nile virus, and also dengue virus, which frequently produces encephalopathy, are particularly difficult to differentiate by routine serologic methods because of the antigenic relatedness of the viruses.[66] JE often cannot be differentiated clinically from other causes of viral encephalitis and has also been misdiagnosed as tubercular or pyogenic meningitis.[56,77] Enterovirus 71, Nipah virus, and hepatitis E virus—the latter two also associated with pig contact—are transmitted in Asia and can present with CNS signs and symptoms. Other infections that may enter the differential diagnosis include typhoid fever, which can present with tremor and lethargy similar to the prodrome of JE. Acute encephalitis with seizures is encountered in two-thirds of patients with neurocysticercosis, a prevalent chronic condition in some areas of Asia that may increase the risk for acquiring JE (see Pathophysiology). Where poliomyelitis still has not been confirmed to be eradicated, JE should be included among the possible causes of acute flaccid paralysis.

Noninfectious causes of acute encephalopathy can be considered, as well, including heat stroke, autoimmune encephalitis, vascular occlusion and intracranial hemorrhage, acute electrolyte disturbances, Reye syndrome, lead encephalopathy and other poisonings (including insect repellent toxicity), and inherited metabolic disorders.[102]

TREATMENT

No specific antiviral therapy is available. Supportive care and control of increased intracranial pressure are critical for a good outcome. Mannitol or hypertonic saline is used routinely to control raised intracranial pressure, and early high-dose dexamethasone therapy was shown to have no clinical efficacy in a prospective controlled clinical trial.[41] Other supportive measures, including control of fever and seizures, attention to fluid balance, respiratory support, and prevention and treatment of secondary infections, have contributed to increased survival and improved outcomes. A small randomized double-blind placebo controlled trial of intravenous immunoglobulin in children with JE demonstrated higher levels of neutralizing antibodies in the treatment group, but no difference in outcome measures.[91] A few patients have been treated with interferon-α, but its efficacy has not been evaluated in wider trials.[36] Small interfering and hairpin RNA molecules, and minocycline, administered as an immunomodulator, are being investigated as therapeutic agents.

PROGNOSIS

The case-fatality ratio varies from 5% to 35%, depending on the accessibility and quality of supportive care.[11] Younger children (<10 years) are more likely to die of the infection and to have more serious neurologic complications acutely and as sequelae. Gross neurologic impairment, such as paralysis, weakness, abnormal muscle tone, seizures, ataxia, and extrapyramidal movement disorders, are found in approximately one-third to one-half of recovered patients several months to a year after onset.[38,65,72,96] Electroencephalographic abnormalities have been detected in more than 50% of surviving children 1 year after recovery. The graver clinical consequences of JE, in contrast to other forms of encephalitis necessitating hospitalization, were clearly shown in a follow-up study 6 to 27 years after hospitalization that disclosed neurologic deficits on examination in 22% versus 2% of the subjects and subnormal intelligent quotients in 28% versus 2%, respectively.[25] Thus, in areas where the disease is prevalent, JE may account for substantial disability in the resident population. Optic atrophy and chronic seizures have been reported to have a delayed onset of 3 to 17 years after hospital discharge, indicating the need for long-term follow-up.[25,95]

PREVENTION

JE vaccine is administered routinely under the World Health Organization Expanded Programme on Immunization and national schedules in most Asian countries (see Fig. 176E.3). Vaccination effectively reduces the incidence of JE disease.[108,116] Several JE vaccines are used in humans: (1) mouse brain–derived killed, inactivated; (2) cell culture–derived live, attenuated; (3) Vero cell–derived killed, inactivated; and (4) genetically engineered live, attenuated chimeric vaccine.[33,108,112] Availability of these products varies by country. Only the Vero cell–derived vaccine is licensed in the United States.

The first JE vaccine was the mouse brain–derived inactivated vaccine (JE-VAX) and was the only vaccine available for decades. Although highly immunogenic, JE-VAX had a considerable incidence of adverse side effects, including rare allergic and neurologic effects.[83,84] Its use has been replaced with the cell-derived vaccines, and worldwide production of JE-VAX was halted in 2006.

The cell-derived live, attenuated vaccine made from the SA14-14-2 strain was first licensed in China in 1988 and is now the most widely used vaccine in JE-endemic areas, also licensed in India, South Korea, Nepal, Sri Lanka, Cambodia, Laos, Myanmar, and Thailand. The SA14-14-2 vaccine is highly immunogenic, achieving high levels of neutralizing antibodies after one dose in 80% to 99% of children, and almost complete protection after two doses.[18,54,76] Previously given at 1, 2, and 6 years of age, the 2015 WHO position statement for JE vaccine recommends a single dose at 8 months or older.[107] Although the strain is highly attenuated, with low reactogenicity, safety studies are limited. A report of four JE cases occurring in temporal relationship to vaccination could not distinguish vaccine failure from vaccine-associated encephalitis, indicating a need for additional safety surveillance.[47] No data are available on its use in HIV-infected or other immunocompromised patients.

The inactivated Vero cell–derived JE vaccine, also made from the SA14-14-2 strain, is licensed in the United States for children older than 2 months and adults, and internationally for use in travelers.[12,13,45,112] Two intramuscular doses separated by 28 days produces seroconversion to protective neutralizing antibody titers in 96% of adult subjects with few local and systemic reactions.[49] After primary immunization, seroprotection rates were 83%, 58%, and 48% at month 6, month 12, and month 24, respectively.[26] When subjects were vaccinated 15 months after primary immunization, all responded to the booster dose with persistence of a high geometric mean titer (GMT) at 1 year later.[13] Trials in children indicate 100% seroconversion after two 3-μg (children <3 years) or 6-μg doses (children 3–18 years), with protection in 88% of children 2 years and younger and 95% of children 3 years and older at 6 months after the two-dose series.[14] Reactogenicity was similar to that of the PCV7 control vaccine, and no safety signals have emerged in postmarketing surveillance.[98]

The live chimeric vaccine leads to seroconversion in 97% of adults 6 months after a single dose, with 93% retaining protective antibody levels at 5 years.[103] Antibody persistence was modeled to show that 90% of subjects would remain seroprotected at 8 years.[22,24] Well-tolerated, compatible, or sequential administration with yellow fever 17D vaccine was shown.[73] In 12- to 19-month-old toddlers, more than 92% seroconverted, with persistence of antibodies in more than 84% after 2 years.[19,30] Cautions associated with the use of the live vaccine in immunocompromised persons, at the extremes of age, and in other populations have not been specifically defined.

The WHO recommends the following dosing schedule for JEV in endemic areas:

- Inactivated Vero cell–derived vaccine: primary series according to manufacturer's recommendations (these vary by product), generally two doses at 4-week intervals starting the primary series at 6 months and older in endemic settings.
- Live, attenuated vaccine: single dose administered at 8 months and older.
- Live, recombinant vaccine: single dose administered at 9 months and older.[107]

The duration of protection of these vaccines is not known, although protection of childhood vaccination extends into adulthood and likely confers long-lasting immunity. A surveillance of birth cohorts in Taiwan, where a vaccination program has been in place for more than 40 years using mostly the inactivated mouse brain–derived vaccine, demonstrated neutralizing antibodies in 54% of people whose last JE virus vaccine was more than 20 years earlier.[42] Antibodies did appear to wane in older individuals. Long-term follow-up of subjects receiving the inactivated Vero cell–derived SA14-14-2 vaccine showed persistence of protective levels of antibodies in 96%, and modeling predicted duration of approximately 14 years.[81]

More than 100 JE cases have been reported in travelers; therefore, vaccination of certain travelers is recommended.[6] Current US recommendations specify vaccination for expatriates, for travelers spending 30 days or more in an endemic area during the transmission season, and for persons with briefer itineraries if they have a high risk for exposure (see Table 176E.1).[12,37] The course of immunization should be completed 7 to 10 days before the onset of travel. These recommendations are highly conservative, however, because cases in travelers have been reported in individuals with briefer itineraries and without the cited risk factors, who later died or survived with serious neurologic damage. The narrow criteria defined in the recommendation are a legacy of committee efforts to limit use of the highly reactogenic mouse brain–derived vaccine, which was the only licensed vaccine when recommendations initially were formulated.[12] With the availability of a safer inactivated vaccine, the changed risk-to-benefit ratio of vaccination has prompted reconsideration of these recommendations.[6,7,68,108] Because the illness has such a high clinical impact and the risk for acquiring the infection is serendipitous—although low—thoughtful counseling is needed while discussing the risks for the disease, vaccine cost, and other factors so that travelers can make an informed decision (see Table 176E.1). From a public health perspective, routine childhood vaccination with the live SA14-14-2 vaccine has been shown to be highly cost effective.[62,110] Pig vaccination is ineffective and impractical, although keeping pigs sties and pig production facilities at a distance from the human population can reduce disease risk.

Another avenue for JE prevention could be vector control. Mosquito control is impractical in most areas where JE is endemic, but agricultural practices, such as schedules of rice production and changes in water levels, and nontargeted effects of agricultural pesticides have had secondary effects in reducing the vector population and cannot be excluded to have reduced human infections. A growing area of study is the use of the bacterial endosymbiont *Wolbachia* to reduce viral proliferation, a strategy that has shown reduced replication of yellow fever, West Nile, and Chikungunya viruses and potentially JE.[46]

Although vaccination is recommended to prevent infection and illness, avoidance of outdoor activities during the evening hours, staying in screened or air-conditioned quarters, and sleeping under a bed net also will lower the risk for acquiring the illness by reducing exposures to vector mosquitoes. Wearing long-sleeved shirts and long pants and using mosquito repellents on clothing and exposed skin are recommended for outdoor activities.

NEW REFERENCES SINCE THE SEVENTH EDITION

10. Burns KF. Congenital Japanese B encephalitis infection of swine. *Proc Soc Exp Biol Med.* 1950;75(2):621-625.
14. Centers for Disease Control and Prevention. Use of Japanese Encephalitis Vaccine in Children: Recommendations of the Advisory Committee on Immunization Practices, 2013. *MMWR Morb Mortal Wkly Rep.* 2013;62(45):898-900.
21. Deng J, Pei J, Gou H, et al. Rapid and simple detection of Japanese encephalitis virus by reverse transcription loop-mediated isothermal amplification combined with a lateral flow dipstick. *J Virol Methods.* 2015;213:98-105.
26. Dubischar-Kastner K, Eder S, Buerger V, et al. Long-term immunity and immune response to a booster dose following vaccination with the inactivated Japanese encephalitis vaccine IXIARO, IC51. *Vaccine.* 2010;28(32):5197-5202.
28. Erlanger TE, Weiss S, Keiser J, Utzinger J, Wiedenmayer K. Past, present, and future of Japanese encephalitis. *Emerg Infect Dis.* 2009;15(1):1-7.
40. Hobson-Peters J. Approaches for the development of rapid serological assays for surveillance and diagnosis of infections caused by zoonotic flaviviruses of the Japanese encephalitis virus serocomplex. *J Biomed Biotechnol.* 2012;2012:379738.
42. Hsu LC, Chen YJ, Hsu FK, et al. The incidence of Japanese encephalitis in Taiwan—a population-based study. *PLoS Negl Trop Dis.* 2014;8(7):e3030.
46. Jeffries CL, Walker T. The potential use of Wolbachia-based mosquito biocontrol strategies for Japanese encephalitis. *PLoS Negl Trop Dis.* 2015;9(6).
54. Kwon HJ, Lee SY, Kim KH, et al. The immunogenicity and safety of the live-attenuated SA 14-14-2 Japanese encephalitis vaccine given with a two-dose primary schedule in children. *J Korean Med Sci.* 2015;30(5):612-616.
55. Le Flohic G, Porphyre V, Barbazan P, Gonzalez JP. Review of climate, landscape, and viral genetics as drivers of the Japanese encephalitis virus ecology. *PLoS Negl Trop Dis.* 2013;7(9):e2208.
66. Mansfield KL, Horton DL, Johnson N, et al. Flavivirus-induced antibody cross-reactivity. *J Gen Virol.* 2011;92(Pt 12):2821-2829.
75. Ohno Y, Sato H, Suzuki K, et al. Detection of antibodies against Japanese encephalitis virus in raccoons, raccoon dogs and wild boars in Japan. *J Vet Med Sci.* 2009;71(8):1035-1039.
81. Paulke-Korinek M, Kollaritsch H, Kundi M, et al. Persistence of antibodies six years after booster vaccination with inactivated vaccine against Japanese encephalitis. *Vaccine.* 2015;33(30):3600-3604.
87. Pyke AT, Williams DT, Nisbet DJ, et al. The appearance of a second genotype of Japanese encephalitis virus in the Australasian region. *Am J Trop Med Hyg.* 2001;65(6):747-753.
91. Rayamajhi A, Nightingale S, Bhatta NK, et al. Correction: a preliminary randomized double blind placebo-controlled trial of intravenous immunoglobulin for Japanese encephalitis in Nepal. *PLoS ONE.* 2015;10(8).
97. Schuh AJ, Tesh RB, Barrett AD. Genetic characterization of Japanese encephalitis virus genotype II strains isolated from 1951 to 1978. *J Gen Virol.* 2011;92(Pt 3):516-527.
102. Swale DR, Sun B, Tong F, Bloomquist JR. Neurotoxicity and mode of action of N, N-diethyl-meta-toluamide (DEET). *PLoS ONE.* 2014;9(8):e103713.
106. Wang H, Liang G. Epidemiology of Japanese encephalitis: past, present, and future prospects. *Ther Clin Risk Manag.* 2015;11:435-448.
107. WHO. Japanese Encephalitis Vaccines: WHO position paper, February 2015—Recommendations. *Vaccine.* 2016;34(3):302-303.
112. Yun SI, Lee YM. Japanese encephalitis: the virus and vaccines. *Hum Vaccin Immunother.* 2014;10(2):263-279.

The full reference list for this chapter is available at ExpertConsult.com.

176F ■ Murray Valley Encephalitis

Roy A. Hall • John Aaskov

Outbreaks of an acute, severe, encephalitic illness, clinically similar to Japanese and St. Louis encephalitis, occurred in rural areas of southeastern Australia in 1917, 1918, 1922, 1925, 1951, and 1974.[1,10,15-17] and in north and northwestern Australia in 1981, 1993, 2000, and 2011.[9,13,44,45] Approximately 437 cases were reported in these 10 outbreaks.[44] They are thought to represent a single entity for which various names (Australian X disease, Murray Valley encephalitis, Australian encephalitis) have been used.

Case-fatality rates, as high as 70% in the early years,[10,12] declined to 20% in the 1974 outbreak and have remained at about this level since then.[4-6,11,13] However, significant residual neurologic disability occurs in as many as 50% of survivors.[11,13]

The presence of this disease in Papua New Guinea was confirmed in 1956.[21] The causative virus was transmitted to experimental animals as early as 1918,[7,12] although those strains could not be maintained. The definitive isolation and characterization of Murray Valley encephalitis virus in 1951[20] led to epidemiologic studies that suggested its survival in bird-mosquito cycles in northern Australia but not in the area of epidemic occurrence in southern Australia.[1]

Murray Valley encephalitis is caused by Murray Valley encephalitis virus. In an effort to dissociate a disease from a specific locality, the term *Australian encephalitis* was proposed by residents of the Murray Valley region for the disease caused by Murray Valley encephalitis virus. Some researchers subsequently have attempted to expand the term *Australian encephalitis* to include encephalitis caused by any Australian arbovirus. Because the term *Australian encephalitis* has no scientific validity and is ambiguous, it should not be used.

ETIOLOGIC AGENT

Murray Valley encephalitis virus was isolated postmortem from the brain of patients in 1951 and 1974 and shown to be a flavivirus, related antigenically to Japanese encephalitis virus.[20,29]

A partial nucleotide sequence of Murray Valley encephalitis virus[14] confirmed the previous classification of this virus, on serologic grounds, as being a member of the Japanese encephalitis, St. Louis encephalitis, West Nile fever subgroup of flaviviruses.[39] Four genotypes of Murray Valley encephalitis have been identified, two exclusively from Papua New Guinea.[25,30] However, more recent isolates from Papua New Guinea cluster with Australian strains in genotype 1.[50]

TRANSMISSION AND EPIDEMIOLOGY

The mosquito *Culex annulirostris* is thought to be the major vector of Murray Valley encephalitis virus,[17,18,33] although other mosquitoes, such as *Aedes normanensis, Aedes tremulus,* and *Culex quinquefasciatus,* also may play a significant role in transmission of the virus.[8]

Murray Valley encephalitis virus is thought to survive in cycles of infection between birds and mosquitoes in northern Australia and Papua New Guinea,[1] where regular infection of humans and other animals is indicated by seroconversion in the summer-autumn "wet" season,[17] as well as by clinical disease.[8,44] Studies also suggest that the virus might survive, after vertical transmission, in desiccation-resistant eggs of *A. tremulus* mosquitoes.[8] Epidemics that occurred in more populous areas of southeastern Australia are thought to have followed the introduction of virus when abnormal spring rainfall allowed chains of bird-mosquito transmission to occur through northern Australia.[2] However, several studies have also suggested that interepidemic survival of virus occurs in southern Australia.[22]

Although disease occurs most commonly in children, clinical infection occurs in individuals of all ages (see Clinical Manifestations). Data are insufficient to determine whether the lower incidence of disease in adults is due to immunity acquired from previous subclinical infections.

Recent reports of sporadic clinical Murray Valley encephalitis virus infection in horses, with pathologic changes in the brain and spinal cord similar to those seen in humans,[5,24] confirm a previous, unconfirmed report of possible Murray Valley encephalitis virus infections in horses[23] and raise the possibility that both wild and domestic horses could play a role in the transmission and dissemination of this virus. The association of Murray Valley encephalitis virus infection with neurologic disease in horses also was observed in a large outbreak of equine encephalitis in southeastern Australia in 2011. Although a virulent strain of the Kunjin subtype of West Nile virus was responsible for most cases, Murray Valley encephalitis virus RNA was detected in the brain of several diseased animals.[43]

CLINICAL MANIFESTATIONS

An initial period of nonspecific, fluctuating, prodromal symptoms and signs, with fever, headache, nausea, vomiting, muscle pain, and photophobia, is followed within 2 to 5 days by drowsiness, mental obtundation, confusion, disorientation, incongruous behavior, ataxia, speech disturbance, or seizures.[32] Bennett[6] recognized three groups of patients according to eventual clinical outcome:

1. Patients with mild disease commonly had disturbed mentation short of coma, incoherent or slurred speech, aphasia, speech perseveration, incontinence, neck stiffness, intention tremor, and limb hypertonicity but rarely required assisted ventilation. The neurologic changes stabilized in 5 to 10 days, and the patients' clinical condition improved.
2. Patients with severe disease showed more profound central nervous system (CNS) involvement consisting of impairment of consciousness to coma, more marked signs of upper motor neuron involvement, and pharyngeal or respiratory paralysis requiring assisted ventilation.
3. In fatal cases, patients had either spastic quadriplegia progressing to almost complete loss of nervous function or severe disease with superimposed infection.

There also may be a fourth group with even milder signs and symptoms than Bennett's group 1. These are patients with mild or no encephalitis whose principal features are fever and headache.[42]

PATHOLOGY

A period of viremia probably precedes infection of the CNS, during the 1- to 3-week incubation period,[1] but it has not been demonstrated. Pathologic changes in fatal cases were restricted to the CNS and included extensive perivascular cuffing (especially in the cortex), lymphocytic infiltration of the meninges, neuron degeneration and neuronophagia in the cerebellum and spinal cord, and thalamic necrosis. Evidence of repair, including calcification, was described in patients who died late in the course of the disease.[7,11,12,38,41] These pathologic changes do not distinguish Murray Valley encephalitis from other arthropod-borne encephalitides.

In rodents infected peripherally with Murray Valley encephalitis virus, the virus enters the CNS through the olfactory pathway after replicating in regional lymph nodes. From the olfactory lobe, it spreads through interconnected neural circuits to the cortex, hippocampus, thalamus, cerebellum, medulla oblongata, and spinal cord. Extensive neuronal necrosis was observed in the olfactory bulb and hippocampus. The severity of the subsequent encephalitis correlated with the magnitude of mononuclear and polymorphonuclear cell infiltrates. Infiltration of neutrophils was preceded by increased expression of tumor necrosis factor-α and the chemokine N51/KC in the CNS. Previous depletion of neutrophils or inhibition of inducible nitric oxide synthetase resulted in prolonged survival and decreased incidence of mortality in mice infected with Murray Valley encephalitis virus.[3,34] However, the pronounced mononuclear cell content of cerebrospinal fluid in some patients with Murray Valley encephalitis[11,21] contrasts with the picture in rodents.[34] However, a recent study of the pathogenesis of Murray Valley encephalitis virus in weanling New Zealand white rabbits suggests this animal model more closely mimics human infection with this virus. Rabbits infected through the footpad developed low-titer viremias with dissemination of virus to the lymph nodes and spleen. As with humans, most infections in the rabbits were asymptomatic and were associated with no, or mild, pathology in the CNS.[48]

DIAGNOSIS

Clinical and epidemiologic features may suggest the diagnosis of Murray Valley encephalitis, especially during recognized epidemics, but individual cases may be difficult to distinguish from cases of encephalitis or encephalopathy of other cause (e.g., herpesvirus or Japanese encephalitis or Kunjin viruses).[6,36,51] A differential diagnosis of Murray Valley encephalitis may be assisted by observing signs attributable to spinal cord involvement and cranial nerve palsies, tremor, and frequency of seizures (seizures rarely develop in adults with Murray Valley encephalitis, whereas they may occur in up to 90% of children). Although computed tomographic scans in these patients may be normal and electroencephalograms may not show focal features,[11] magnetic resonance imaging (MRI) reveals changes within a week of symptoms, similar to those reported in the brain of patients with Japanese encephalitis[26]—thalamic edema, hypointensity on T1-weighted images, and hyperintensity on T2-weighted images.[19,27,28] Changes also were noted in the reticular formation, the substantia nigra, and the cervical spinal cord.[19] In the absence of serology, MRI findings might be regarded as diagnostic of an infection with herpes simplex virus rather than with Murray Valley encephalitis virus.[51]

Establishment of a specific diagnosis depends on serologic evidence of infection concurrent with disease. Detection of IgM antibody that reacts with Murray Valley encephalitis virus in enzyme-linked immunosorbent assays is the most useful indication of recent infection. Other flaviviruses, especially Kunjin virus, may cause encephalitis, subclinical infection, or minor illness during epidemics of Murray Valley encephalitis,[44] and interpretation of serologic cross-reactions between Kunjin and Murray Valley encephalitis viruses may require specific tests (e.g., neutralization) with several viruses.[17] Serologic tests for the laboratory diagnosis of Murray Valley encephalitis are not available commercially and so are performed only at larger regional laboratories. Isolation of virus has not been successful for antemortem diagnosis. Reports[19,35] document the detection of Murray Valley encephalitis viral RNA in serum or cerebrospinal fluid from patients by use of reverse transcriptase polymerase chain reaction (RT-PCR), and some laboratories use in-house RT-PCR assays as part of routine diagnosis.[35,40]

TREATMENT AND PROGNOSIS

No specific antiviral therapy is available. Administration of corticosteroids has been recommended during the acute phase of the illness to reduce brain edema. Artificial respiration has been lifesaving, and all patients should be transported to base hospitals with facilities for the management of patients with respiratory paralysis.[6] Most patients also require parenteral nutrition or nasogastric feeding.[11]

The early epidemics left some patients with neurologic and psychiatric sequelae, but the lower case-fatality rate in recent outbreaks, presumably because of use of modern intensive care techniques, has been associated with a high rate of residual disability.[11,13] Bennett[6] observed 18 patients up to 16 months after they experienced infection. Four of 11 patients with mild disease had emotional problems and mild degrees of impaired motor coordination and mental acuity. All 7 patients with severe disease had serious defects, including paraplegia or quadriplegia and mental disturbance. This pattern of high residual disability has continued to the present.[11,13,47]

PREVENTION

Because of the irregularity of outbreaks and the large areas over which they occur, implementation of cost-effective measures to prevent Murray

Valley encephalitis is difficult. There is no evidence that mosquito control measures, even during outbreaks, have had any effect on transmission of Murray Valley encephalitis virus. Several Australian states have established surveillance programs for Murray Valley encephalitis virus employing flocks of sentinel chickens to provide warning of transmission of this virus. In combination with observing rainfall patterns, this information appears to have predictive value and serves to alert public health authorities and local residents to the need of enhanced mosquito management and avoidance measures.[46]

A more recent technology to detect Murray valley encephalitis virus RNA in mosquito saliva expectorated during feeding on sugar-baited, nucleic acid preservation cards has the potential for use in surveillance programs over much wider areas than the sentinel chicken flocks but has yet to be evaluated as an early warning tool.[49]

There is no vaccine to prevent infection with Murray Valley encephalitis virus; however, studies in animal models have shown that cross protective immunity can be generated against the virus with an inactivated Japanese encephalitis vaccine in the presence of a suitable adjuvant.[31] Although these data suggest that the recently licensed Japanese encephalitis virus vaccine (IMOJEV)[37] might protect against infection with Murray Valley encephalitis, the cost of the human clinical trials to confirm this renders the use of the vaccine for this purpose unlikely.

NEW REFERENCES SINCE THE SEVENTH EDITION

5. Barton AJ, Prow NA, Hall RA, et al. A case of Murray Valley encephalitis in a 2-year-old Australian Stock Horse in south-east Queensland. *Aust Vet J*. 2015;93:53-57.
43. Roche SE, Wicks R, Garner MG, et al. Descriptive overview of the 2011 epidemic of arboviral disease in horses in Australia. *Aust Vet J*. 2013;91:5-13.
45. Selvey LA, Dailey L, Lindsay M, et al. The changing epidemiology of Murray Valley encephalitis in Australia: the 2011 outbreak and a review of the literature. *PLoS Negl Trop Dis*. 2014;8:e2656.
46. Selvey LA, Johansen CA, Broom AK, et al. Rainfall and sentinel chicken seroconversions predict human cases of Murray Valley encephalitis in the north of Western Australia. *BMC Infect Dis*. 2014;14:672.
47. Selvey LA, Speers DJ, Smith DW. Long-term outcomes of Murray Valley encephalitis cases in Western Australia: what have we learnt? *Intern Med J*. 2016;46:193-201.
48. Suen WW, Uddin MJ, Wang W, et al. Experimental West Nile Virus Infection in Rabbits: An Alternative Model for Studying Induction of Disease and Virus Control. *Pathogens*. 2015;4:529-558.
49. van den Hurk AF, Hall-Mendelin S, Townsend M, et al. Applications of a sugar-based surveillance system to track arboviruses in wild mosquito populations. *Vector Borne Zoonotic Dis*. 2014;14:66-73.
50. Williams DT, Diviney SM, Niazi AU, et al. The molecular epidemiology and evolution of Murray Valley encephalitis virus: recent emergence of distinct sub-lineages of the dominant genotype 1. *PLoS Negl Trop Dis*. 2015;9:e0004240.

The full reference list for this chapter is available at ExpertConsult.com.

176G ▪ Tick-Borne Encephalitis

Gail J. Harrison • Andrea Duppenthaler • Christoph Aebi • Theodore F. Tsai

Tick-borne encephalitis (TBE) refers to the neurotropic hard tick–transmitted flaviviral infection caused by tick-borne encephalitis virus (TBEV), which occurs across the Eurasian landmass from the Far East to western Europe. TBE is usually divided into European, Far Eastern, and Siberian subtypes, and it infects thousands of people each year in these regions. It has been a growing public health problem in Europe and other parts of the world since 1999.[87] The Far Eastern form of the disease frequently is called *Russian spring-summer encephalitis* (RSSE); in Europe, where the disease is distinctly milder and often biphasic, it is called *tick-borne encephalitis, spring-summer meningoencephalitis, central European encephalitis,* or, because sometimes it is transmitted by raw infected milk, *biphasic milk fever.*[31,43,82,124] The presence of TBEV in ticks and the Roe deer, in the Netherlands, has recently been reported.[61]

HISTORY

After an outbreak of encephalitis in the Far Eastern region of Russia in 1932, Zilber isolated the virus from viremic humans and from *Ixodes persulcatus* ticks.[167] A milder form of the disease with a similar seasonality was described previously in Sweden and Austria, but its etiology was not defined until 1948, when the virus was isolated in the Czech Republic and Slovakia. Milk-borne transmission of TBEV from infected livestock first was recognized in an outbreak in 1951 and 1952.

ETIOLOGIC AGENT

TBEV and the closely related viruses of RSSE and Powassan encephalitis are flaviviruses placed antigenically within a complex of tick-borne flaviviruses that also includes the agents of Kyasanur Forest disease, Omsk hemorrhagic fever, and an encephalomyelitis syndrome in sheep variously called *louping ill* in the British Isles and *Spanish, Greek,* or *Turkish sheep encephalomyelitis* in their respective countries.[51] Molecular taxonomic studies based on nucleotide sequence differences in the E glycoprotein gene of the virus show the early divergence of a mammal-associated clade from seabird-associated agents. Viruses in the mammal-associated clade exhibit a continuous east-to-west cline consistent with an evolutionary origin of TBEV in the Far East and dispersion westward to Europe and the British Isles (Fig. 176G.1).[39,103]

ECOLOGY

The viruses of RSSE and TBE are transmitted principally by hard ticks in the *Ixodes ricinus* complex—*I. ricinus* in Europe and *I. persulcatus* in the Far East.[43,82,124] Other tick vectors include *Ixodes arboricola, Ixodes hexagonus, Haemaphysalis punctata, Haemaphysalis concinna, Dermacentor marginatus,* and *Dermacentor reticulatus.* Viral circulation is maintained by continuous horizontal infection between ticks and animals and through the winter by vertical transmission in vector ticks and by latent infection in hibernating animals. The viruses are transmitted transstadially from larval to nymphal to adult tick stages and also transovarially. All stages of the tick and both male and female ticks transmit infection to animals and humans. Ixodid ticks feed on three hosts, one for each of the stages, during the typical 3-year life cycle. Larval and nymphal ticks feed preferentially on birds and small mammals, such as wild mice, voles, and dormice; adult ticks feed on larger mammals, such as roe deer, hedgehogs, foxes, hares, badgers, deer, domestic livestock (pigs, goats, sheep, and cows), dogs, cats, and humans. RNA sequence heterogeneity of the 5′ noncoding region in different TBEV isolates recovered from the same biotope suggest that virus populations consist of subtypes with specificities for individual vertebrate hosts.[15] Infections in animals, except occasionally in dogs, are asymptomatic, and the viremia is of brief duration. Therefore a large population of susceptible vertebrate hosts is needed to maintain viral transmission. Human infections are incidental to the natural cycle of transmission. Birds and large mammals contribute to the spread of vector ticks and viral foci.[94]

Ticks in the *I. ricinus* complex require high soil and ambient humidity (>80–90% relative humidity) and moderate temperature, within the 8°C (46.4°F) isotherm. They typically are found in the transitional vegetation zone from the forest edge to fields or meadows or in areas where dense brush or ground vegetation provides a sheltered microenvironment. Vector ticks are absent from mountainous areas with an elevation above 1200 to 1500 m. Foci of TBE transmission are restricted geographically and ecologically to these biotopes and have tended to be highly stable over years. However, global warming has been speculated to underlie the changes, both expansion and contraction of transmission foci, in northern and central-southern Europe, respectively.[93,124] New data also suggest a shift of tick activity to higher altitudes in recent years, potentially allowing vertical expansions of TBE foci.[26]

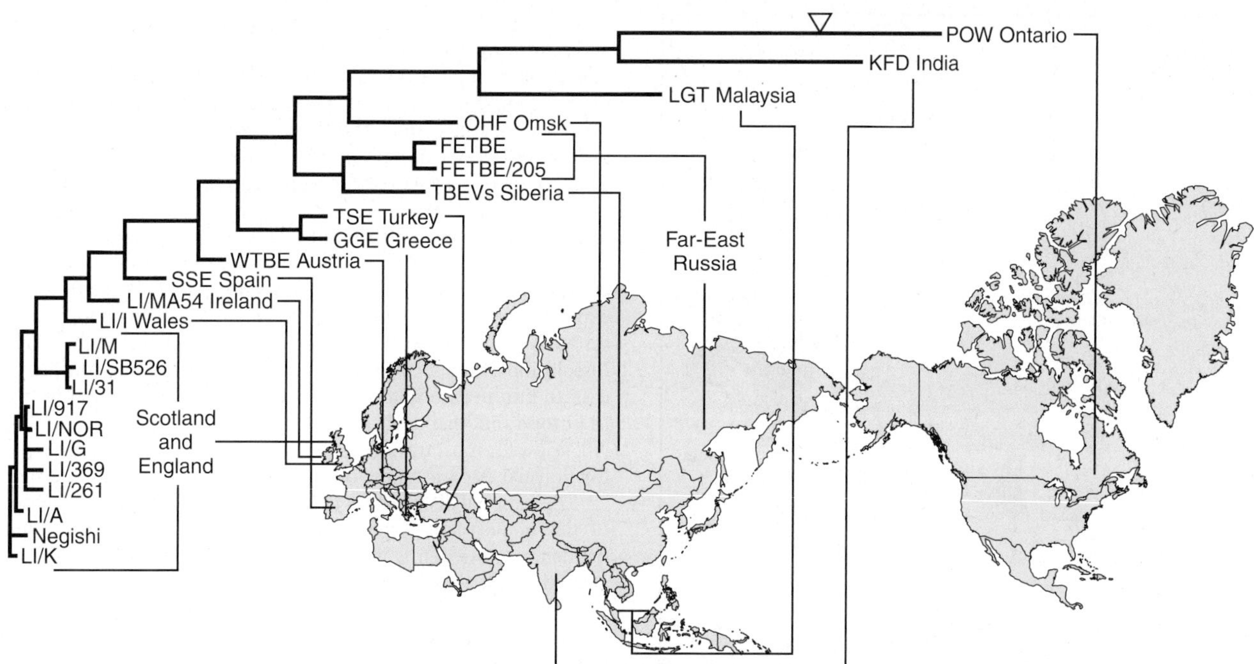

FIGURE 176G.1 Cladogram of tick-borne encephalitis complex viruses based on E gene sequences presented from west to east with respect to louping ill *(LI)* virus. *FETBE,* Far Eastern tick-borne encephalitis; *GGE,* Greek goat encephalitis; *KFD,* Kyasanur Forest disease; *LGT,* Langat; *OHF,* Omsk hemorrhagic fever; *POW,* Powassan encephalitis; *SSE,* Spanish sheep encephalitis; *TSE,* Turkish sheep encephalitis; *WTBE,* Western tick-borne encephalitis. The phylogenetics of these and other mosquito-borne flaviviruses are rooted in the Powassan branch indicated by the triangle. (From Zanotto PM, Gao GF, Gritsun T, et al. An arbovirus cline across the Northern Hemisphere. *Virology.* 1995;210: 152-159.)

Tick activity varies with seasonal temperature and humidity. In central Europe, activity begins in March and April, reaches a peak in May, and declines during the summer in July and August. With the return of cooler temperatures, a second peak of activity occurs in September. In temperate regions, tick activity begins later and is greatest in the summer months. In Mediterranean climates, ticks are most active from November to January.

In foci with hyperendemic transmission, tick density may exceed 1/mm^2. Viral infection rates in ticks generally are in the range of 0.1% to 5%.[18] These rates typically are 10-fold lower than *Borrelia burgdorferi* (sensu lato) infection rates in *I. ricinus* in the same areas, although *I. persulcatus* infection rates greater than 10% have been reported.[75] The mechanisms underlying this difference are unclear but may include the following[115]:

- The variable infectiousness of the agents and their interactions with modulatory factors in tick saliva
- The relatively brief duration of TBE viremia in animals, which lasts only a few days and thus results in a reduced chance of transmission of virus to feeding ticks, as opposed to the persistent *B. burgdorferi* infections in rodents, with tick feeding more likely to result in infection
- The potential differences in the principal reservoir hosts for the respective infectious agents, with a more limited and focal distribution of important hosts for TBEV, such as goats.

The two agents evidently do not interfere with each other in their infection of *I. persulcatus* ticks; dually infected ticks and singly TBE-infected and *Borrelia*-infected ticks stand in a ratio of approximately 1:4:14.[75] *I. ricinus* also can be infected with and transmit *Francisella tularensis* and *Anaplasma phagocytophilum,* the agent of human granulocytic ehrlichiosis.[159]

The geographic distributions of RSSE and European TBE correspond to the ranges of their principal tick vectors; however, transmission is highly focal within this range because of the locations of biotopes that support viral circulation (Fig. 176G.2). New foci are reported periodically as a result of better recognition of the disease, its natural spread, human modifications of the landscape, and environmental and climate changes (e.g., global warming).[36,65,93,124]

EPIDEMIOLOGY

TBE is transmitted through hard tick bites or through ingestion of unpasteurized diary products. TBE has been recognized in all countries of Europe except Portugal and the Benelux countries, but endemic transmission is most intense in central Europe.[82,124] Slovenia currently has one of the highest notified incidences of TBE in Europe.[35] TBE also has been detected in Japan and northern mainland China, in areas of forests, presence of *I. persulcatus* ticks, and appropriate altitude and climate.[149] Human TBE has increased since the 1990s in all endemic European countries except Austria, where a well-organized vaccination campaign was initiated.[6,62,93] The incidence of TBE previously ranged as high as 50 per 100,000 population in Austria, Poland, Hungary, Russia, Czech Republic, Slovakia, Bulgaria, and former Yugoslavia; in certain areas, similar levels of transmission still may prevail. TBEV also has been reported recently in the Netherlands in 2% of the ticks and Roe deer population of the areas, and there is increasing evidence of TBEV transmission in the Netherlands.[20,53,61,158]

Vaccination has reduced the incidence of disease regionally, especially in Austria, where a national program of immunization since 1981 has reduced the incidence to less than 1 per 100,000 population.[165] However, breakthrough illnesses, and rarely even fatal breakthrough cases of TBE, have been reported in vaccinated children and adults and in elderly individuals.[14,145] Currently, isolated cases are reported from Norway, Denmark,[146] France,[47] Greece, and Liechtenstein, and fewer than 200 cases are reported annually in Sweden, Germany, and Italy. The Swedish Institute for Communicable Disease Control recently reported the highest annual incidence of human TBE in 2011 and 2012.[62] Switzerland reported a threefold increase in human TBE cases between 2004 and 2006,[166] which resulted both from more infections in endemic areas and from infections in newly recognized foci. Since then, the number of newly diagnosed cases in Switzerland has decreased again but has remained

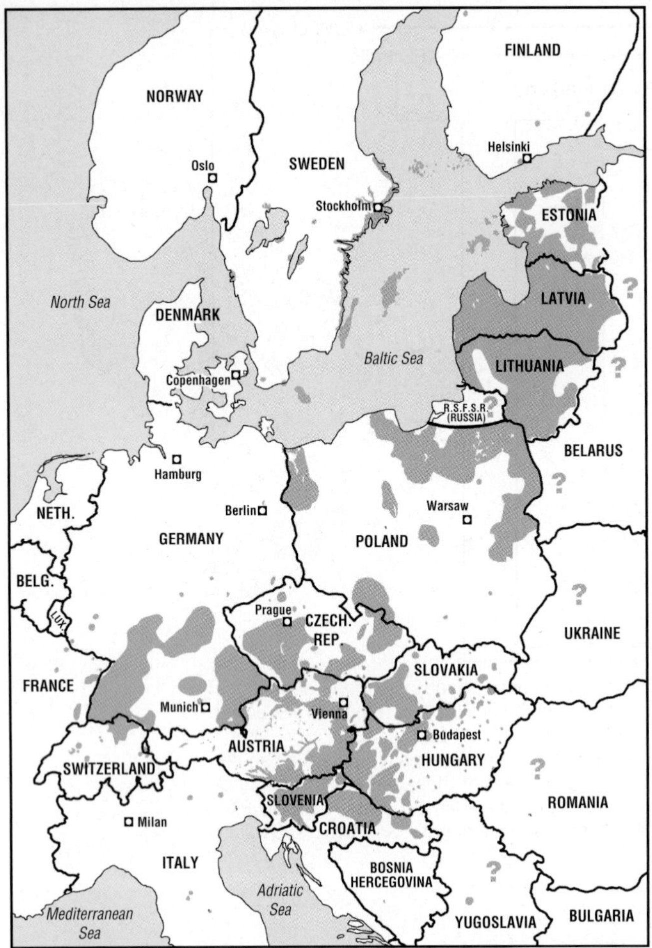

FIGURE 176G.2 The geographic distributions of Russian spring-summer encephalitis and European tick-borne encephalitis correspond to the ranges of their principal tick vectors; however, transmission is highly focal within this range because of the locations of biotopes that support viral circulation.

higher than before 2004. In the Far East, cases of RSSE occur principally in forest workers. The disease is recognized in Russia and China, and the first cases acquired in Japan (transmitted by *Ixodes ovatus*) were reported recently.

Within each country, the distribution of cases is highly focal in certain areas and may vary with each year. Local seroprevalence may exceed 20%, but the general seroprevalence usually is less than one per 100,000 population. Frequent exposure during long-term residence leads to a general trend of increasing seroprevalence with age. Seroprevalence rates as high as 50% have been observed in groups at high risk for exposure, such as farmers and forestry workers. Although, in general, rates are lower (1–5%) and in certain groups are similar to the seroprevalence of hantaviruses, lymphocytic choriomeningitis virus, and *Anaplasma* spp., *B. burgdorferi* seroprevalence rates are 10-fold higher or more.[107,113] The frequency of clinical cases of TBE, borreliosis, and dual infection closely approximates the relative frequency of tick infection, singly and dually. Adults 20 to 50 years of age characteristically accounted for most of the cases. In some studies, cases in males (adults and children) predominate by a ratio of 2 : 1.[32,48,92]

Cases have occurred in children as young as 3 weeks,[59,66] but generally, risk in children increases with age as a result of their increased mobility and activity in the sylvatic environment.[92] These epidemiologic patterns are changing in areas with high immunization coverage.[165] Vaccination effort has focused principally on hyperendemic areas and on high-risk occupational groups such as forestry workers. The low number of cases currently reported from areas where vaccination coverage is high belies the continued transmission of virus in these locations.

Cases may be acquired during outdoor activities, such as berry picking and mushroom gathering, and infection occasionally has been acquired from ticks brought from endemic areas on Christmas trees and other objects. One study found that the seroprevalence in Swedish orienteers (1%) was not substantially different from the general seroprevalence in residents of Stockholm County (5%), an area where TBE is endemic. The absence of a higher risk for acquiring TBE in persons with occasional sylvatic exposure reflects the low infection rate of ticks and the generally low risk to persons with sporadic or short-term exposure. Neither of two studies of American soldiers stationed in central Europe found a clinical case, although one seroconversion in 3297 person-months of exposure, an infection rate of 0.9 per 1000 person-months and four seroconversions in 959 persons (0.4%) were detected.[105,134] With the dissolution of the former Soviet Union and increasing commerce with eastern Europe, interest in the risk for TBE being acquired by travelers to Europe and Russia has increased. The available data suggest that the risk is low for most travelers and that vaccination is not indicated except for unusual circumstances of prolonged stay in an endemic area.

The seasonal distribution of cases lags roughly 1 month behind that of tick activity and extends from April until November. The peak incidence in Sweden is in August; in Austria, the peak occurs in June and July, with a secondary rise in October.

Milk-borne TBE previously accounted for 10% to 20% of all cases in central Europe. Infections frequently were acquired from consuming unpasteurized milk or cheese from infected goats, sheep, and cows, and outbreaks resulting in thousands of cases have been reported. Transmission from infected milk now is a rare occurrence, but as recently as 1994, an outbreak in Slovakia led to 7 cases in a group that regularly drank raw milk from a family goat.[75] Also, an outbreak of 21 human cases caused by contaminated cheese produced from unpasteurized sheep milk has been reported.[162] Contact infection, acquired during slaughter of an infected goat, also has been observed.

Recently, transmission of TBE to three patients who received solid organ transplants from a single donor occurred. They developed fatal encephalitis within 17 to 49 days after transplantation, and the illness was confirmed to be TBE by RT-PCR of brain tissue and cerebrospinal fluid. The high fatality rate in these patients was most likely related to their immunosuppression. These cases raise the awareness that organ donors from TBE endemic areas should be screened for TBEV infection.[159]

CLINICAL MANIFESTATIONS

Seroepidemiologic studies indicate that as many as 90% of human infections with TBEV remain asymptomatic or result in a nonspecific illness.[2,7,46,70] The classic manifestation of the European form of TBE is an acute febrile illness characterized by a biphasic course consisting of a nonspecific prodromal syndrome followed by central nervous system (CNS) disease (Fig. 176G.3).[42,156] Infection with TBEV may occur solely as the primary, nonspecific phase without the secondary CNS phase.[31,98] Infection with Far Eastern strains of TBEV results in a more severe, monophasic illness that progresses directly to neurologic involvement with a poorer prognosis for survival and full recovery. TBE has been observed in all age groups. The median age in pediatric case series is 8 to 10 years (range, 0–17 years).[22,48,92,96,153] The youngest patient with serologically and virologically documented TBE described in the literature was a 17-day-old infant.[66] Congenital infection has not been reported. Fatal TBE disease has been described in immunocompetent individuals and immune-compromised transplant recipients.[159]

The clinical features of TBE in children are summarized in Table 176G.1. The clinical spectrum ranges from nonfocal mild aseptic meningitis to severe meningoencephalitis, without paralysis, or meningoencepahloradiculitis, associated with paralysis. Patients may also have a cranial nerve palsy or cerebellar signs of ataxia on presentation, as well as aphasia and autonomic dysfunction.[13,158] A rare abortive form of TBE may also occur, as well as a chronic progressive form of TBE. There is also a postencephalitis syndrome. The diagnosis of TBE should be considered in all acutely ill patients with fever, CNS abnormalities, and a history of potential tick exposure or ingestion of raw milk in an area endemic for TBE, especially if the patient presents during peak

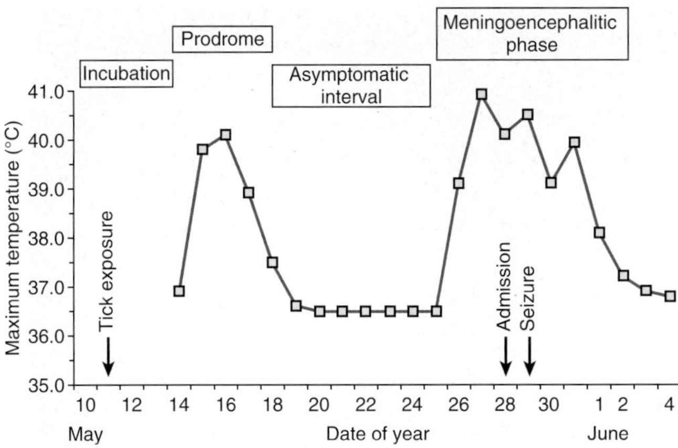

FIGURE 176G.3 Clinical course of tick-borne encephalitis (TBE) in a 5-year-old boy exposed to a tick bite in a known endemic area for TBE in the pre-alpine region of central Switzerland. Lumbar puncture on admission revealed mild cerebrospinal fluid (CSF) pleocytosis (14×10^6/L, 50% polymorphonuclear cells). Serum anti-TBE virus immunoglobulin (Ig) M and IgG were present; serum and CSF antibodies against *Borrelia burgdorferi* were absent. CSF enteroviral polymerase chain reaction was negative. Recovery was uneventful.

TABLE 176G.1 Clinical Features of Serologically Documented Tick-Borne Encephalitis in Five Pediatric Case Series (333 Children)

Clinical Features	Rate (%)
History	
Tick exposure	47–78
Biphasic illness	77–90
Major Symptoms at Presentation	
Fever >38.0°C (100.4°F)	100
Headache	90–100
Vomiting	60–90
Central Nervous System Signs	
Nuchal rigidity	74–90
Photophobia	10–25
Impaired consciousness	9–11
Ataxia or tremor	5–26
Seizures	0–5
Paresis	0–5
Extent of Central Nervous System Involvement	
Meningitis alone	49–89
Meningoencephalitis	9–48
Meningoencephalomyelitis	0–5
Fatal outcome	0
Cerebrospinal Fluid Parameters	
Pleocytosis >15 × 10⁶/L	98–100
Glucose normal	100
Protein elevated	9–55
Abnormal electroencephalogram	80–87

Data from references 21, 44, 62, 82, 89, 144.

tick season April to November.[13] A high degree of diagnostic awareness is required because the clinical presentation of TBE is nonspecific. After an incubation period of 2 to 28 days, in most cases 7 to 14 days,[32,48,92,96,156] the patient may have a prodromal illness consisting of fever, malaise, nausea and vomiting, headache, myalgia, and, occasionally, upper respiratory tract symptoms.[32,48,77,156] Defervescence occurs after 2 to 7 days, and the patient subsequently remains asymptomatic for 1 to 20 days, usually 2 to 10 days.[32,48,77,92,153] This prodromal illness may be absent. In various case series, a biphasic course was reported in 30% to 90% of children with TBE.[48,68,92,96,153] An abrupt onset of fever, headache, emesis, and symptoms of meningeal irritation heralds the beginning of the second phase of disease.[96] In adults, no association exists between the length of the incubation period and the severity of clinical illness.[68] The typical evolution of fever in a child with TBE is shown in Fig. 176G.4.

In this second phase of illness, most affected children (50–90%) have meningitis without clinical evidence of parenchymal CNS involvement.[48,76,80,96,110,128,153] In adult patients, by contrast, meningitis without encephalitis or myelitis occurs only in 20% to 60% of cases.[2,68,77,125,144] On physical examination, fever, signs of meningeal irritation, and photophobia are the most common features.[96,153] In uncomplicated cases, patients defervesce within 5 to 10 days.[48,92,96,153] Meningoencephalitis, meningoencephalomyelitis, or both manifested by impaired consciousness, seizures, and focal neurologic signs, including limb paresis, associated with meningoencephaloradiculitis, occurs in 0% to 34% of children.[22,48,70,92,96,153] In a large series of 139 pediatric patients with TBE meningoencephalitis, Lesnicar and coworkers[92] observed tremor in all patients, impaired consciousness in 27 (7%), ataxia in 18 (5%), behavioral changes in 16 (4%), cranial nerve paresis in 14 (4%), and limb paresis in 11 (3%). In a series of 13 children, Harasek[48] observed ataxia in 10 patients, somnolence in four, paresthesias and seizures in two each, and central facial palsy and nystagmus in one each. In two of these patients, transient unilateral shoulder girdle weakness that occurred during the second week of CNS disease suggested involvement of the cervical anterior horn or radiculitis. Overall, limb or cranial nerve paresis occurs in 0% to 5% of children with TBE (see Table 176G.1). In a series of 133 children with TBE, Cizman and colleagues[22] reported transient paresis in five patients and irreversible hemiparesis in one.

In large case series of predominantly adult patients, a paralytic course secondary to bulbar, spinal, or radicular injury was observed in 5% to 25% of cases.[70,72,105,144,150,156] Unilateral, flaccid paresis of an upper extremity is the most common manifestation of lower motor neuron disease complicating adult TBE.[105,150,156] Involvement of the cranial nerves occurs somewhat less frequently and is revealed most commonly by external ocular muscle paralysis (usually cranial nerve VI), peripheral facial palsy (VII), otovestibular manifestations (VIII), or involvement of the pharyngeal muscles (IX, X, and XI).[32,68,105,147] Lower extremity weakness and, occasionally, autonomic nervous system affliction manifested as bladder dysfunction also may occur.[32,69,147] Whereas most manifestations of parenchymal CNS involvement evolve during the acute stage of TBE, paralysis resulting from radiculitis may develop up to 14 days after the onset of CNS disease.[48,82]

As many as 5% of children with TBE experience seizures during the acute stage of TBE.[22,48,153] Because most patients are older than 6 years and thus are unlikely to suffer from febrile seizures, these episodes probably reflect encephalitis. In adults, seizures have been observed in less than 2% of patients.[32,68]

Extracerebral manifestations of TBE seldom are reported and are of minor clinical relevance. Mild hepatitis[54,68] and electrocardiographic abnormalities have been described in adults.[151] A single case of myopericarditis in a child with TBE has been reported.[33]

The peripheral white blood cell (WBC) count is not altered in a characteristic way. Although it is usually in the normal range, both leukopenia and moderate leukocytosis may be found.[48,96,147] In adult patients, several investigators observed leukopenia during the viremic prodrome and normal or moderately elevated WBC counts during the second phase of illness.[68,77,96,99] In a report describing hematologic values during the prodromal phase of TBE, 23 of 28 (82%) patients had mild to moderate thrombocytopenia ($60–130 \times 10^9$/L), with values returning to normal during the second phase of illness.[99] Cerebrospinal fluid (CSF) analysis in children with serologically proven TBE reveals predominantly mononuclear pleocytosis in all patients. However, as with enteroviral meningitis, neutrophils may predominate during the first 1 to 3 days of illness.[64] Typically, the CSF WBC count is 100 to 1000×10^6/L.[48,79,92,96,147,153] On occasion, lower values occur, as reported by Krausler and associates,[76] who found less than 100×10^6/L in 24 of 75 (32%) pediatric cases. Wahlberg and colleagues[156] reported an absence of pleocytosis in 18% of 94 adult patients examined. Harasek[48] could not

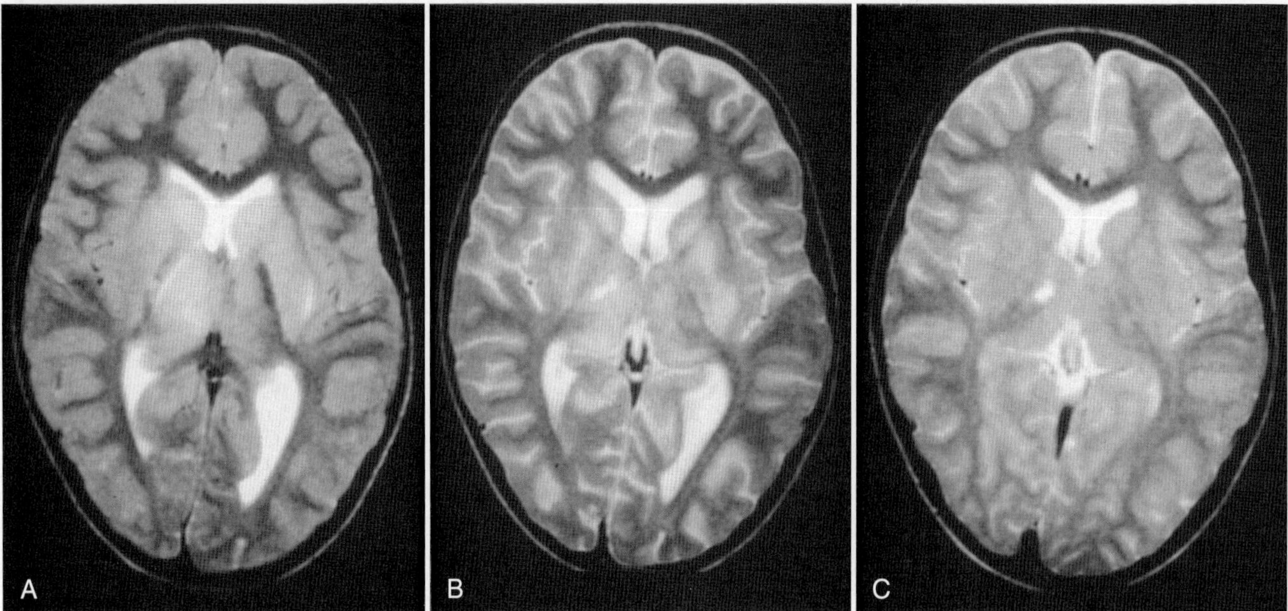

FIGURE 176G.4 T2-weighted magnetic resonance imaging series of a 5-year-old girl with a severe course of tick-borne encephalitis. (A) Acute phase. Note the T2 hyperintensity in the right side of the thalamus, basal ganglia, and diencephalon. (B) One month later, partial recovery of T2 hyperintensity and enlargement of cerebrospinal fluid spaces can be seen. (C) Three months later, normal T2 intensity and a cerebrospinal fluid–filled cavity in the right side of the thalamus are apparent. (Courtesy David Nadal, MD, University Children's Hospital, Zurich, Switzerland.)

find any correlation between the CSF leukocyte count and the severity of clinical disease. In contrast, some investigators[69,68,72] reported that adult patients with a high CSF white blood cell count (>300 × 10^6/L) were more likely to experience a severe course of TBE and persistent neurologic sequelae. CSF pleocytosis disappears within 4 to 5 weeks of the onset of acute CNS disease. The CSF glucose concentration is normal,[96] and the protein concentration is normal or moderately elevated (<1000 mg/L),[48,77,96,147] with evidence of dysfunction of the blood-brain barrier in most patients.[69] Electroencephalographic examination findings during acute TBE usually are abnormal and characterized by a nonspecific reduction in rhythmic background activity, bilateral periodic slowing, and, rarely, focal abnormalities.[48,67,68] Attenuation of background activity with periodic delta groups has been shown to correlate with parenchymal CNS involvement in adult TBE patients.[67] Reorganization of electroencephalographic activity commonly lags behind clinical improvement, and abnormalities may persist for months to years.[48,67,153]

The limited information available on magnetic resonance imaging (MRI) in children with severe TBE indicates that parenchymal lesions characteristically are located in the thalamus (see Fig. 176G.4).[22,68,71,91,157] The diagnostic and prognostic value of neuroimaging studies in pediatric TBE has not been established as well as in adults. In adults, MRI studies may detect abnormality in approximately 20% of patients.[68] Focal lesions are more likely to be found in those with severe neurologic abnormalities[68] and are located mainly in the thalamus.[5,10,70,97,121,154,157] Less frequently, lesions are located in the basal ganglia,[5,68,97,121] cerebellum,[10,68] brainstem,[11,22,68] and anterior portions of the cervical spine.[10,22] Available case series suggest that brain lesions visible on MRI in TBE do not appear to correlate with disease severity.[122] However, in patients with paralysis associated with meningoencephaloradiculitis, high-resolution MRI is helpful in determining alpha motor neuron injury.[91]

PATHOLOGY

CNS findings are mainly those of acute meningeal inflammation and focal gray-matter encephalomyelitis. The white matter rarely is involved. Macroscopic findings include congestion of the leptomeninges and swelling and hyperemia of the cerebral parenchyma, particularly in the brainstem and cervical region of the spinal cord.[43,112] Petechial hemorrhages are seen in the brainstem, the anterior horns of the spinal cord, and, less consistently, the cerebellum and the anterior central region of the cortex. Histologic changes are dominated by infiltration and ganglion cell damage in the gray matter of these same areas. Changes are particularly pronounced in the anterior horns of the cervical spine (consistent with the poliomyelitis-like manifestations of paralytic courses of TBE),[138] the medulla oblongata, the cranial nerve nuclei of the pons, and the Purkinje cell layer of the cerebellum.[43] Inflammatory foci are characterized by lymphocytic perivascular infiltration and various stages of degenerative changes in neuronal cells. Areas of neuronal necrosis are characterized by perifocal edema, lymphocytic and neutrophilic infiltration, and, at a later stage, nodular microglial proliferation at sites of complete neuronophagia. The presence of granzyme, B-expressing, cytotoxic T cells in close contact with TBE-expressing neurons indicates that immune mechanisms contribute to tissue injury in these areas.[40] Rarely, the spinal nerve roots, spinal ganglia, and peripheral nerves are involved. Spongiform changes, particularly after protracted illness, appear as sharply defined areas of softening with minimal inflammatory reaction. In the Far Eastern form of the disease, extensive poliomyelitis of the spinal cord with destruction of anterior horn cells, particularly in the upper cervical and lower lumbar areas, and poliomyelitis of the brainstem are noted.

PATHOGENESIS

Tick-mediated inoculation of TBEV and viral replication within local dermal cells are followed by lymphatic spread to regional lymph nodes, where further replication occurs.[69] Subsequently, viremia leads to generalized infection, especially of reticuloendothelial cells, followed by secondary rounds of viremia that result in neuroinvasion. Viral penetration of the CNS occurs through microvascular capillary endothelial cells and by TBEV-infected, infiltrating mononuclear cells, without compromising the integrity of the blood-brain barrier.[119] Envelope glycoprotein E, the immunodominant TBEV-encoded surface protein, mediates attachment to and fusion with the host cellular membrane.[102] The molecular mechanisms of neural invasion by TBEV have not been elucidated in detail. Current knowledge of the molecular pathogenesis of TBEV has been reviewed elsewhere.[51,50,49]

LABORATORY DIAGNOSIS

Because neither clinical nor CSF findings differentiate TBE from other causes of meningitis or meningoencephalitis, the diagnosis of TBE rests on demonstration of specific antibody by serologic testing. The presence of specific serum immunoglobulin M (IgM) or a significant rise in titer of specific IgG antibody in paired sera (or both) is diagnostic of TBE,[57,58,69] unless the patient previously received TBE vaccine doses. Enzyme-linked immunosorbent assay (ELISA) has replaced complement fixation, hemagglutination inhibition, and neutralization assays in the routine laboratory diagnosis of TBE.[56,58] ELISA technology offers increased sensitivity, reliably differentiates between IgM and IgG antibodies, and, in contrast to neutralization, uses nonviable viral antigens.[52,129] For the detection of specific anti-TBEV IgM, an IgM-capture ELISA system has proved to be more sensitive and specific than the conventional three-layer ELISA system because high titers of specific IgG and rheumatoid factor do not interfere with IgM binding.[52,129] With this method, specific IgM virtually always can be demonstrated during the acute illness and thereafter may persist for as long as 9 months.[57,69,129] The highly sensitive capture ELISA format allows a determination of anti-TBEV IgM, even in serum samples obtained late during the acute illness, when high titers of specific IgG already are present. A potential problem of TBEV IgG ELISA systems is cross-reactivity with other flaviviruses, notably yellow fever virus, dengue virus, and Japanese encephalitis virus.[29,30,114] This limitation should be considered in the interpretation of seroprevalence studies and in patients with a relevant travel or immunization history.

Specific IgM and IgG to TBEV also can be measured in CSF.[52,129] Detection of TBEV-specific intrathecal antibody production by ELISA is highly specific for the diagnosis of TBE but somewhat less sensitive than is determination of serum IgM during the first several days of CNS disease.[58,69] Up to 16% of patients with TBE will not have intrathecal TBEV-specific IgM detectable; therefore absence of intrathecal antibody does not exclude the diagnosis of TBE.[53] Intrathecal TBEV antibody assays are less widely used in clinical practice, but they may be useful if serum antibody titers fail to differentiate between infection- and vaccine-induced immunity.

Detection of virus by culture is technically feasible, but it is not used routinely in clinical practice. TBEV can be recovered from blood by viral culture, but because detectable viremia occurs during the prodromal stage (when the diagnosis of TBE seldom is considered), culture is not useful in clinical practice. TBEV may be recovered from the brain tissue of patients who died at an early stage of disease.[23] Amplification of TBEV-specific RNA by reverse transcriptase polymerase chain reaction (RT-PCR) has been established for detection of TBEV in ticks, in tick surveys as part of national surveillance systems,[38,123] and, in humans, for individual patient diagnosis.[143] Primers that amplify the highly conserved 5′ noncoding region of the TBEV genome have been shown to be sensitive and specific.[142] Successful amplification of TBEV-specific RNA from blood, CSF, or brain tissue has been reported.[24,143,152,157] However, like culture, RT-PCR usually is positive only during the prodromal stage and thus generally is not useful in clinical practice.[66]

DIFFERENTIAL DIAGNOSIS

The clinical course of TBE is nonspecific in most cases, and a history of exposure to ticks in an endemic area can be elicited in 40% to 75% of pediatric patients.[48,70,92,96,110,140,153] Because serologic confirmation of the diagnosis is not available immediately in most cases, the differential diagnosis includes a wide spectrum of diseases causing fever and CNS manifestations.

Enteroviruses are the most common cause of symptomatic CNS infection in children during the warm seasons in regions where TBE is prevalent. Fever in enteroviral infection may occasionally be biphasic,[108] although the durations of both the first phase and the asymptomatic interval usually are shorter than those noted in TBE.[19] Routine tests of CSF do not differentiate between the two entities. Skin and mucosal manifestations are indicative of enteroviral infection rather than TBE, whereas encephalitis and myelitis can occur in both. Enteroviral meningitis is diagnosed most readily by PCR of CSF[135] or by culture of virus from CSF and mucosal surfaces. Mumps meningitis is to be considered in the differential diagnosis in cases without parotid enlargement, particularly in areas with low rates of mumps immunization.[148] The diagnosis of mumps meningitis is made by viral culture of CSF or detection of specific serum IgM antibody. Although it is a rare occurrence in childhood, herpes simplex virus (HSV) encephalitis always should be considered in the differential diagnosis. Because the case-fatality rate of HSV encephalitis is greater than 90% if it is left untreated, therapy with intravenous acyclovir should be initiated without delay, if that diagnosis is thought possible. The combination of fever, which may be biphasic,[130] and localizing signs observed by neurologic examination, electroencephalographic studies, or MRI[60] suggests HSV encephalitis and rarely occurs in pediatric TBE, particularly if the temporal lobe or the orbital portion of the frontal lobe is affected. Meningeal irritation usually is absent in HSV encephalitis. The diagnosis of HSV encephalitis is confirmed by PCR of CSF.[9,89] Epstein-Barr virus encephalitis can occur in immunocompetent children, and Epstein-Barr virus shares with TBEV a preference for causing thalamic and basal ganglia lesions.[68,117] Other viral causes include common respiratory tract viruses such as influenza, parainfluenza, and adenovirus.

Among bacterial infections, partially treated pyogenic meningitis, encephalitis in association with *Mycoplasma pneumoniae* infection,[132] and encephalopathy caused by *Bartonella henselae* may resemble TBE. Tuberculous meningitis runs a subacute course, and although near-normal CSF chemistry may be recorded very early in the disease, hypoglycorrhachia invariably develops and CSF protein rises to high levels. CNS infection by *B. burgdorferi* is particularly important in the differential diagnosis because in Europe this pathogen and TBEV are transmitted by the same tick vectors—*I. ricinus* and *I. persulcatus*—and because one of the most prevalent European genospecies, *Borrelia garinii,* is more neurotropic than *B. burgdorferi* sensu stricto.[131] In contrast to TBE, the incubation period for early neuroborreliosis in children generally is 4 to 10 weeks, high-grade fever is unusual, and most patients have cranial nerve paresis. However, several cases of concomitant infection with TBEV and *B. burgdorferi* have been reported in the literature,[1,21,78,116] and coexistence of TBEV and *B. burgdorferi* in ticks has been documented.[75] In some cases of TBE, persistent or late-appearing limb paralysis has been suggested to be attributed to concomitant, but undiagnosed, borrelial radiculoneuritis rather than TBE-related myelitis with anterior horn involvement.[78] In this situation, diagnostic evidence of Lyme borreliosis coinfection with TBEV-associated TBE should be sought because this condition requires antimicrobial therapy.[16] Seroepidemiologic and clinical evidence indicates that concomitant infection with TBEV and *Anaplasma phagocytophilum,* the agent of human granulocytic ehrlichiosis, also may occur.[75,100]

TREATMENT

No specific antiviral therapy is available to treat TBE. However, recent studies suggest TBEV is inhibited by LCTA-949, an analog of the antibiotic teicoplanin, and the anthelminthic compound ivermectin.[27,104] In severe cases, supportive therapy is aimed at preventing the development of sequelae related to increased intracranial pressure, seizures, and bulbar dysfunction. After the acute stage, neurorehabilitation may be necessary for patients with motor, cognitive, or emotional disturbances. Because TBE rarely causes a chronic seizure disorder, prolonged anticonvulsive therapy seldom is indicated in patients who had convulsions during acute disease.

PROGNOSIS

Approximately 4% of patients will die during the acute illness of TBE. The main risk factor for neurologic residua and a fatal outcome of TBE is advanced age.[2,68,144] Also, patients with meningoencephaloradiculitis are more likely to have more severe and fatal illness.[91]

Substantial sequelae also may occur in two-thirds of children,[48,70,80,96,139,153] and according to long-term follow-up studies of pediatric TBE patients, a variety of neurocognitive and motor sequelae may occur, including issues with short- and long-term memory, learning, executive functions, and physical impairments of gross and fine motor skills, balance problems, and coordination problems. Children also may experience chronic headaches, fatigue, and irritability.[34,37,151,155]

Individual cases of children, presenting more likely with meningoencephalitis in the acute phase, show persistent neurologic damage, including hemiparesis,[22,66,71,157] unilateral arm paresis,[156] epilepsy,[66,71,128] and extrapyramidal movement disorder.[71] Recent evidence, however, indicates that subtle abnormalities in attention and psychomotor skills may persist in many children for prolonged periods.[139] In adult patients, long-term neurologic defects are observed in 2% to 10% of patients with clinical evidence of parenchymal CNS involvement during the acute illness.[2,42,68,72,156]

Risk factors for persistent sequelae have been assessed by Kaiser[68] and, by univariate analysis, include impaired consciousness (i.e., Glasgow Coma Scale score <7), ataxia, paresis, abnormal findings on MRI, CSF pleocytosis greater than 300 × 10^6/L, and CSF protein concentration of more than 600 mg/L. Gunther and colleagues[45] reported that encephalitic symptoms were associated with low levels of intrathecal IgM in early stages of TBE. Paresis of the extremities and ataxia are the most common persistent findings on neurologic examination.[2,32,70,72,101,144] Much more common, however, are ill-defined manifestations such as chronic fatigue, headache, sleep disorders, memory dysfunction, and emotional disturbances, which are reported by most adults recovering from TBE and persist for months to years.[32,90,144] In some patients, electroencephalographic findings may remain abnormal for prolonged periods, with seizure activity occasionally demonstrated.[48,139] Most of these patients are symptom free, although epilepsy secondary to TBE has been described infrequently.[48,111] For these reasons, children who recover from TBE should have their neurologic, cognitive, and developmental status assessed on a regular basis.

The reported case-fatality rate in adult TBE patients is approximately 1% in large series,[2,32,42,70,72,101] with most deaths being attributed to severe bulbar encephalitis or related to underlying cardiovascular disease in elderly patients.[32] Fatal outcome of TBE in children is exceedingly rare.[106] Fatal outcomes from TBE have been reported in transplant recipients.[95]

PREVENTION

General preventive principles include avoidance of known endemic areas of TBE, use of protective clothing, and rapid removal of ticks attached to the skin. The topical repellent *N,N*-diethyl-*m*-toluamide (DEET) has a definite, albeit moderate, effect against ticks.[133] Because of its potential neurotoxicity, the content of DEET in products used for children should not exceed 15%.[15,118] These measures are effective in reducing tick exposure and transmission of TBEV to some degree. Pasteurization of raw milk prevents enteric transmission of TBEV.[4,73] Travelers should assess their risk for TBE by knowing whether the countries and regions to be visited are endemic with TBE illness, whether they will be traveling during peak (April to November) season, whether they will travel at an altitude less than 1500 m above sea level, whether the travel stay will be of long duration, whether the travel will involve tick exposure–associated activities in forests or other tick-infested areas, and whether the travelers are of advanced age or have comorbidities of illness that may put them at higher risk for severe or fatal illness with TBE.

Reliable protection, however, requires active immunization against TBE. Inactivated whole-virus vaccines are produced in Austria (Baxter), Germany (Chiron), and Russia. These vaccines are made from different central European TBEV strains; they are produced by concentrating and purifying cell culture fluid from infected chick embryo cells and consist of a three-injection immunization schedule.[63] Adjuvants (aluminum hydroxide) are added to the formalin-inactivated cell culture fluid. The Russian vaccine is an inactivated, unconcentrated cell culture fluid from infected African green monkey kidney cells. An inactivated, purified whole-virus vaccine produced in primary hamster kidney cell lines is now produced in China and is effective against the Far Eastern TBEV strain seen in that country.[161] TBE vaccine is also available in the United States under investigational drug exemption to military personnel deployed in endemic areas.[12,25]

Currently approved TBE vaccines are approved for children 12 months and older. Basic immunization consists of three doses given at 0, 1 to 3, and 5 to 12 months. Rapid immunization schedules also are available. The vaccines are immunogenic and safe.[28,41,42,44,120,140] Seroconversion rates for neutralizing antibodies after the first, second, and third dose are 70%, 95%, and 99%, respectively.[81,85] Reliable protection is achieved 2 weeks after administration of the second dose.[164] Data on the kinetics of vaccine-induced serum antibodies led to the first recommendation for booster doses every 3 years.[81,83] Recent data on the decay of neutralizing antibodies, however, indicate that protection may last at least 5 years in children and 10 years in adults.[74,126,127,160] Therefore booster doses are recommended only every 5 to 10 years in some European countries. Minor adverse events (i.e., fever and local reactions) are reported by 4% to 15% of vaccinees after receiving the first dose and less frequently after receiving subsequent doses.[83,120,163] Mostly transient neurologic adverse events temporally associated with the administration of TBE vaccine have been reported rarely.[41,42,136,137,141] Their true incidence has not been established. Based on passive notification of adverse events, an incidence of one neurologic illness in 1 million doses of TBE vaccine has been calculated.[55] Placebo-controlled trials of vaccine efficacy have not been conducted. Observational studies in Austria using historical controls indicate that the effectiveness of the vaccine is greater than 90%.[84,88]

In Austria, the TBE vaccine is recommended for mass immunization of all potentially exposed individuals. Since the beginning of the vaccination campaign in 1981, a dramatic reduction in nationally notified cases has been observed (Fig. 176G.5).[88,165] Mass immunization is the probable cause of this decrease because neighboring countries (e.g., Switzerland, southern Germany, and Slovenia) reported stable or increasing numbers of cases of TBE during the same time. In these and other endemic countries of central and eastern Europe, authorities recommend immunization of school-aged children and adults who live in endemic areas and have a risk for exposure to ticks.[22,113] In younger children, TBE vaccination is not recommended routinely because neurologic complications are exceedingly rare.[22,92]

Specific IgG against TBEV has been used historically for passive immunization within 96 hours of exposure to ticks in endemic regions. Because of reports from some patients[3,86] who developed a severe form of

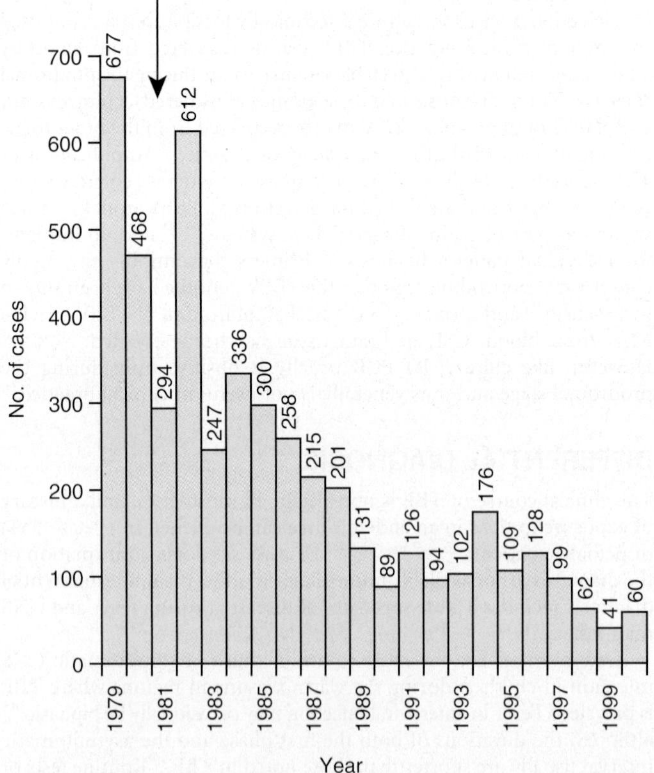

FIGURE 176G.5 Annual number of cases of tick-borne encephalitis in Austria before and after the introduction of mass immunization in 1981 *(arrow)*. (Data from the International Scientific Working Group on Tick-Borne-Encephalitis, http://www.tbe-info.com/report.)

TBE disease after immunoglobulin administration, these products have been withdrawn in many countries and are no longer recommended. These severe cases raised concern about a causative role of TBE immunoglobulin in enhancement of disease.[8,70,71,97,154,157] Also, postexposure vaccine administration is not recommended, because of similar concern about antibody-dependent enhancement.[17] Antibody-dependent enhancement, a mechanism of pathogenicity proposed in dengue hemorrhagic fever,[109] is a possible explanation for both phenomena,[71] and although plausible, experimental data in support of this hypothesis in TBE are lacking.[71]

NEW REFERENCES SINCE THE SEVENTH EDITION

13. Bogovic P, Strie F. Tick-borne encephalitis: a review of epidemiology, clinical characteristics, and management. *World J Clin Cases.* 2015;3(5):430-441.
14. Brauhli Y, Gittermann M, Michot M, et al. A fatal tick bite occurring during the course of tick-borne encephalitis vaccination. *Pediatr Infect Dis J.* 2008;27(4):363-365.
16. Broker M. Following a tick bite: double infections by tick-borne encephalitis and the spirochete Borrelia and other potential multiple infections. *Zoonoses Public Health.* 2012;59(3):176-180.
17. Broker M, Kollaritsch H. After a tick bite in a tick-borne encephalitis virus endemic area: current positions about post-exposure treatment. *Vaccine.* 2008;26(7):863-868.
20. Christova I, Panayotova E, Tchakarova S, et al. A nationwide seroprevalence screening for West Nile virus and Tick-borne encephalitis virus in the population of Bulgaria. *J Med Virol.* 2017;89(10):1875-1878.
34. Engman M, Lindsrom K, Sallamamba M, et al. One-year followup of tick-borne central nervous system infections in childhood. *Pediatr Infect Dis J.* 2012;32(6):570-574.
35. Fafangel M, Cassini A, Colzani E, et al. Estimating the annual burden of tick-borne encephalitis to inform vaccination policy, Slovenia, 2009–2013. *Euro Surveill.* 2017;22(16):30509.
37. Fowler A, Forsman L, Eriksson M, Wickstrom R. Tick-borne encephalitis carries a high risk of incomplete recovery in children. *J Pediatr.* 2013;163(20):555-560.
53. Hira V, Rockx B. Human tick-borne encephalitis, the Netherlands. *Emerg Infect Dis.* 2017;23(1):169.
61. Jacob L, Kostev K. Compliance with vaccination against tick-borne encephalitis virus in Germany. *Clin Microbiol Infect.* 2017;23(7):460-463.
63. Jahfari S, de Vries A, Rijks M, et al. Tick-borne encephalitis virus in ticks and Roe deer, the Netherlands. *Emerg Infect Dis.* 2017;23(6):1028-1030.
74. Konior R, Brzistej J, Poellabauer E, et al. Seropersistence of TBE virus antibodies 10 years after first booster vaccination and response to a second booster vaccination with FSME-IMMUN 0.5 mL in adults. *Vaccine.* 2017;5(8):551-556.
88. Kunze U. The International Scientific Working Group on Tick-Borne Encephalitis (ISW-TBE): review of 17 years of activity and commitment. *Ticks Tick Borne Dis.* 2016;7(3):399-404.
91. Lenhard T, Ott D, Jakob N, et al. Predictors, neuroimaging characteristics and long-term outcome of severe European tick-borne encephalitis: a prospective cohort study. *PLoS ONE.* 2016;111(4):e0154143.
95. Lipowski D, Popiel M, Perlejewski K, et al. A cluster of fatal tick-borne encephalitis virus infection in organ transplant setting. *J Infect Dis.* 2017;215(6):896-901.
119. Palus M, Vancova M, Simarova J, et al. Tick-borne encephalitis virus infects human brain microvascular endothelial cells without compromising blood-brain barrier integrity. *Virology.* 2017;507:110-122.
122. Pichler A, Sellner J, Harutyunyan G, et al. Magnetic resonance imaging and clinical findings in adults with tick-borne encephalitis. *J Neurol Sci.* 2017;375:266-269.
145. Sendi P, Hirzel C, Pfister S, et al. Fatal outcome of European tick-borne encephalitis after vaccine failure. *Front Neurol.* 2017;8:119.
149. Sun R, Lai S, Yang Y, et al. Mapping and distribution of tick-borne encephalitis in mainland China. *Ticks Tick Borne Dis.* 2017;8(4):631-639.
155. Veje M, Nolskog P, Petzoid M, et al. Tick-borne encephalitis sequelae at long-term followup: a self-reported case-control study. *Acta Neurol Scand.* 2016;134(6):434-441.
158. Weststrate A, Knapen D, Laveman G, et al. Increasing evidence of tick-borne encephalitis (TBE) virus transmission, the Netherlands, June 2016. *Euro Surveill.* 2017;22(11):30492.
160. Witteman C, Izu A, Petri E, et al. Five year follow-up after primary vaccination against tick-borne encephalitis in children. *Vaccine.* 2015;33(15):1824-1829.
161. Xing Y, Schmitt H, Arguendas A, Yang J. Tick-borne encephalitis in China: a review of epidemiology and vaccines. *Vaccine.* 2017;35(9):1227-1237.
167. Zlobin V, Pogodina V, Kahl O. A brief history of the discovery of tick-borne encephalitis virus in the late 1930s (based on reminiscences of members of the expeditions, their colleagues, and relatives). *Ticks Tick Borne Dis.* 2017. [Epub ahead of print].

The full reference list for this chapter is available at ExpertConsult.com.

176H ■ Zika Virus Infections*

Kristina Adachi • Claudia Raja Gabaglia • Patricia Brasil • Karin Nielsen-Saines

Zika virus (also known as ZIKV) is a mosquito-borne flavivirus that was discovered in 1947 in a yellow fever sentinel rhesus monkey stationed in Uganda's Zika forest, from which it takes its name.[111,193,299] (Figs. 176H.1 and 176H.2). Although ZIKV's history since discovery spans nearly seven decades, it was only in 2016 that ZIKV rose from obscurity and received global, household recognition as an emerging infectious disease of cataclysmic proportions. During those early years, ZIKV had only caused sporadic, denguelike infections with smaller human epidemics, most notably those reported in 2007 in Micronesia and in 2013–14 in French Polynesia and other South Pacific Islands.[65,121,193,298,299,303]

ZIKV has emerged as a formidable opponent, posing a major threat to global health security, particularly for pregnant women and their infants.[326] Some have even drawn parallels between ZIKV's potential to cause human devastation worldwide and the HIV pandemic.[173,199] From February to November 2016, the World Health Organization (WHO) declared ZIKV a "Public Health Emergency" owing to concerns that infection in pregnancy may lead to congenital anomalies such as microcephaly and other neurologic complications.[180,427,467] Leaders at the WHO and Centers for Disease Control and Prevention (CDC) now consider ZIKV to be the first major infectious disease associated with congenital birth defects to be discovered in more than half a century, joining a pantheon of infections such as rubella, cytomegalovirus, lymphocytic choriomeningitic virus, toxoplasmosis, syphilis, and others.[73,88,322,332,352]

FIGURE 176H.1 Zika forest in Uganda, where Zika virus was first isolated in 1947. (Courtesy Dr. Andrew D. Haddow, USAMRIID, Fort Detrick, MD.)

EPIDEMIOLOGY

History of ZIKV as an Emerging Infection From 1947 to the Present

Discovery of ZIKV

The known history of ZIKV[222,257,329] begins in 1947 with three scientists: G.W.A. Dick, S.F. Kitchen, and A.J. Haddow from the Medicine, Public Health, and International Health Divisions of the Rockefeller Foundation,

*Our understanding of Zika infections has changed dramatically over the past several years. This chapter is based on the authors' review of the literature in May 2016 and again in December 2016. We highly recommend that readers refer to key reference sources (WHO, CDC, PAHO, etc.) listed at the end of this chapter for the most up-to-date information, especially with regard to epidemiology and clinical care, which are constantly changing.

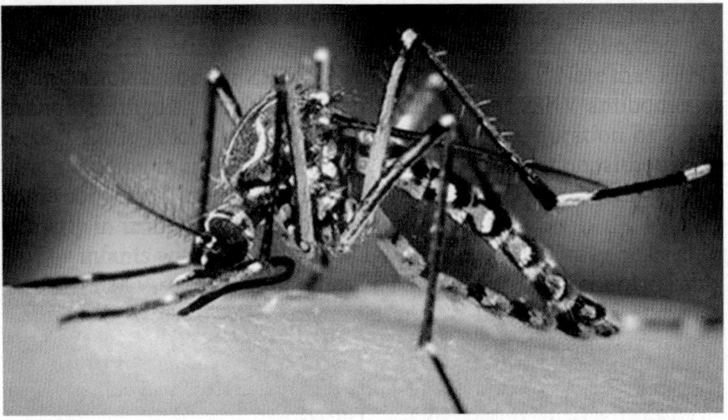

FIGURE 176H.2 *Aedes* mosquito. The *Aedes* species of mosquito have been primarily responsible for the spread of Zika virus around the world. (From the World Health Organization, http://www.portal.pmnch.org/emergencies/zika-virus/history/en/.)

the National Institute for Medical Research in London, and the Virus Research Institute in Entebbe, Uganda.[111] They were studying yellow fever in the Zika forest, which neighbors Lake Victoria and the Entebbe-Kampala road in Uganda[111] (see Fig. 176H.1). From one of their captive, sentinel rhesus monkeys (#766) that developed a low-grade fever, they were able to isolate a new virus.[111] With serum obtained from this rhesus monkey, they inoculated adult and infant mice intracerebrally, which triggered illness after 1.5 weeks and ultimately led to recovery of a filterable virus, which we now know as *Zika virus.*[111] The following year, in 1948, the same researchers were able to demonstrate that ZIKV could also be recovered from captured, wild *Aedes africanus* mosquitoes in the same forest.[110,111]

A few years later, in 1952, during additional investigations of yellow fever in the East African countries of Uganda and Tanzania, the first reported cases of human infection were incidentally discovered during serologic surveys of 297 residents for antibodies to multiple viruses (Zika and others such as West Nile, Bwamba fever, Semliki Forest, Bunyamwera, Ntaya, Mengo, and Uganda S viruses).[416] Researchers were evaluating whether antibodies to those viruses could potentially be used to neutralize yellow fever virus.[416] Subsequently during an investigation of jaundice and yellow fever in Eastern Nigeria, ZIKV was isolated from one patient, a 10-year-old girl with fever and headache, who was coinfected with malaria.[249] Serologic antibody response to ZIKV was also detected in two other patients during that investigation.[249]

After this period of fortuitous early discovery, the presence of ZIKV was acknowledged only in a few case reports and was primarily documented through serologic surveys, albeit without reports of hospitalization for severe infection or deaths. Yet, it is now apparent that unbeknownst to many, a smoldering level of human ZIKV infection was well maintained across diverse populations spanning half a century. Some have speculated that cocirculating arboviruses such as dengue and chikungunya, as well as ZIKV's propensity to cause primarily mild illness, were the primary factors that allowed it to persist and hide unnoticed for decades. Given the lack of human ZIKV outbreaks reported during this time and a handful of isolated human cases reported, it is only through retrospective phylogenetic mapping of ZIKV that has allowed researchers to trace ZIKV's temporal and geographical path from its early origins to the present. From Uganda, ZIKV appeared to have traveled across the African continent and later to Asia during the latter part of the 20th century. Evidence of ZIKV has been found in multiple additional countries, including Senegal, Sierra Leone, Ivory Coast, Burkina Faso, Nigeria, Cameroon, Central African Republic, Gabon, Ethiopia, Egypt, Kenya, Tanzania, Somalia, Pakistan, India, Thailand, Vietnam, Malaysia, Indonesia, and the Philippines, among others.* A detailed report of ZIKV human serologic surveys by year and country is available in the literature.[206,222,301]

*References 10, 96, 111, 137, 144, 187, 206, 208, 222, 254, 257, 268, 286, 301, 319, 320, 329, 388, 398, 412, 471.

First ZIKV Epidemics: The 2007 Federated States of Micronesia (Yap Island) and the 2013–14 French Polynesia, New Caledonia, and Cook Island ZIKV Epidemics

It was not until 2007 that the first major human ZIKV outbreak was identified in one of the Pacific Islands known as Yap Island in the Federated States of Micronesia.[121] It was estimated that 73% of the population older than 3 years of age had been infected with ZIKV, and approximately 900 or more Yap residents had illness from ZIKV infection.[121] Yet, the majority of those infected with ZIKV did not appear to develop clinical disease.[121] In one study of 185 suspected ZIKV cases, ZIKV was confirmed in 49 (26%) cases, whereas the other 59 (32%) were considered probable cases.[121]

The following year, in 2008, the first case of suspected sexual transmission of ZIKV was noted and subsequently reported in 2011.[156] An American researcher contracted ZIKV in Senegal and transmitted the infection to his wife upon return to the United States.[156] This was the first time evidence existed suggesting an arbovirus could be acquired by sexual transmission.[156]

In 2012, researchers discovered that there were two distinct Zika viruses: the African and the Asian lineages. The Asian lineage was first documented in the Yap Island ZIKV epidemic.[182,389] In the following years from 2013 to 2014, additional outbreaks of Asian lineage ZIKV were reported in other Pacific Islands, most notably in French Polynesia but also in New Caledonia and the Cook Islands, with later spread to other islands in the region including Vanuatu, Solomon Islands, and Easter Island.[329,389] Phylogenetic analysis demonstrated that the French Polynesia ZIKV strain was closely related to ZIKV strains recovered from the Yap Island outbreak in 2007 and Cambodian cases seen in 2010.[28,303]

These cases of ZIKV in the Pacific were first identified by the French Polynesia public health authorities during investigations of a major dengue outbreak. French Polynesia, best known for its most populated island, Tahiti, is a country comprising five archipelagos with 67 inhabited islands. During that time, French Polynesia and other surrounding Pacific islands reported approximately 28 new outbreaks of cocirculating arboviruses (dengue, chikungunya, and ZIKV), with reports of more than 120,000 people infected with at least one of those three arboviruses.[389] The largest ZIKV outbreak occurred in French Polynesia, where it was estimated that 11% of the population was infected, with 8746 suspected ZIKV cases and an estimated 30,000 seeking medical attention due to ZIKV concerns.[105,227,380,389] It also included 1400 confirmed cases in New Caledonia and 932 cases in the Cook Islands.[389] This epidemic in the Pacific exported ZIKV cases to other countries: from Tahiti to Norway, from French Polynesia to Japan, from Thailand to Germany and Canada, and from Indonesia to Australia.[152,231,232,433,457]

The resulting investigations of the Pacific region ZIKV outbreaks, particularly the outbreak in French Polynesia, formed the basis of our early understanding of clinical aspects of ZIKV infection, including its potential to be transmitted from mother to child (perinatal transmission) as well as its potential to cause clinical complications.[33,64,65,314] Before these investigations, cases of ZIKV infections had been described as primarily self-limited, nonspecific viral infections characterized by mild symptoms. However, during the French Polynesia ZIKV outbreak, 42 cases of Guillain-Barré syndrome (GBS) were reported, which was the first time concerns were raised about ZIKV's potential to cause neurologic complications.[64,314,389] In addition, recently conducted retrospective analyses revealed that congenital anomalies such as microcephaly and other cerebral malformations also occurred with increased frequency during the ZIKV outbreak in French Polynesia, strengthening evidence of ZIKV as a cause of congenital anomalies.[32,68] The outbreak was also significant because it increased awareness about the potential for ZIKV infection to be asymptomatic and the possibility of ZIKV blood-borne transmission. More than 42 (3%) of the 1505 asymptomatic blood donors were found to be positive for ZIKV, and only one-fourth of these donors later developed symptomatic ZIKV infection.[34,301,302]

ZIKV's Rapid Global Expansion: Epidemics in Brazil, Other Latin American Countries, and Beyond

The first case of autochthonous circulation of ZIKV in the Americas was actually reported in February 2014 by Chile with regard to ZIKV transmission on Easter Island, an island located in the southeastern region of the Pacific.[331,337] The following year in March 2015, the Brazilian Ministry of Health gave its first notification to the WHO about clusters of an unknown acute, exanthematic, denguelike illness that was occurring in the northeastern region of the country since late 2014.[66,482] From February to April 2015, they reported more than 7000 cases of a clinically mild infection, of which only 13% were positive for dengue virus; and tests for other infections in the differential diagnosis, including chikungunya, measles, rubella, parvovirus B19, and enterovirus, were all negative.[222,257,329] A few months later, in May 2015, the Brazilian National Reference Laboratory identified that this mysterious infection being transmitted in the state of Bahia in Brazil was, in fact, ZIKV.[63,257,334,482] Brazilian public health authorities promptly notified the Pan American Health Organization (PAHO) and the WHO. The PAHO then released an epidemiologic alert to its member states about the potential for additional ZIKV outbreaks in regions where *Aedes* mosquitoes were present.[134,257,329]

Subsequently, the ZIKV strain in Brazil was shown to be of the Asian lineage and appeared to have originated from French Polynesia.[92,141,168] Some have speculated that it may have been introduced by tourists from the Pacific Island regions attending the World Cup Soccer Event in Brazil from June to July 2014 or the Va'a World Sprint Championship Canoe Race in Rio de Janeiro, Brazil in August 2014, where the four Pacific region countries of French Polynesia, New Caledonia, Cook Islands, and Easter Island competed.[141,297] Another study suggested that the virus might actually have reached Brazil a year earlier, being introduced in mid-2013 during a prequalifying soccer World Cup event, the 2013 Fédération Internationale de Football Association (FIFA) Confederations Cup.[141]

By mid-July 2015, the ZIKV situation in Brazil had become more worrisome, with reports suggesting that increased neurologic disorders such as GBS were being seen in patients following a recent history of ZIKV infection.[15,45] Apart from Brazil, by October 2015, additional reports of ZIKV were surfacing from Colombia and Cabo Verde, an island on the northwest coast of Africa also known as Cape Verde.[257,271,329,334] By October 2015, the ZIKV epidemic had grown substantially in Brazil, with 14 states reporting autochthonous ZIKV transmission, which coincided with new concerns about the discovery of a substantial increase in microcephaly cases identified at birth, particularly in the state of Pernambuco.[42,257,277,329,331,334] In the months following, Brazil declared a national public health emergency over growing concerns about an association of ZIKV and microcephaly with 1248 reported cases, more than 20 times greater than expected.[42,257,276,281,329,337,361]

Shortly after this announcement, progress was made in establishing evidence linking the ZIKV epidemic with congenital anomalies such as microcephaly in Brazil.[42,361,406] ZIKV was recovered from the amniotic fluid of two pregnant women whose fetuses were found to have microcephaly on prenatal ultrasound; the ZIKV genome was also recovered from tissue and serum samples of an infant with microcephaly.[59,150,204,224] An official investigation by the PAHO and the WHO response team was also launched.[336] Other alerts were issued in the Americas about ZIKV's potential to cause both congenital anomalies such as microcephaly and neurologic complications such as GBS. By the end of 2015, it was estimated that there were nearly 210,000 suspected and confirmed ZIKV cases in Brazil, but numbers may have been as high as 440,000 to 1.3 million cases.[128,193,335,405]

Subsequently, further additional evidence from Brazil strengthened links of ZIKV with congenital anomalies.[406] Microcephaly of four fetuses/infants (two miscarriages and two early neonatal deaths) was described among four women with rash and fever during pregnancy and placenta and fetal/infant brain tissue testing positive for ZIKV RNA and immunohistochemistry.[127] Reports from ophthalmologists in Brazil also described severe ocular anomalies, including macular atrophy, accompanying microcephaly in three infants.[448,450] By the end of January 2016, the consequences of ZIKV in Brazil were astounding, with more than 3893 suspected cases of microcephaly and 1708 cases of GBS reported.[257] On February 1, 2016, in response to the concerns of the emerging ZIKV epidemic in Brazil and its complications, the WHO Director General issued a declaration that ZIKV constituted a "Public Health Emergency of International Concern" in an effort to mobilize governments, public health, and scientific community into action worldwide.[180,467]

TABLE 176H.1 Countries and Territories in the Americas With Reported Congenital Syndrome Associated With Zika Virus

Country	No. of Confirmed Cases
Argentina	1
Brazil	2289
Bolivia	14
Colombia	72
Paraguay	2
Dominican Republic	22
French Guiana	16
Grenada	1
Guadeloupe	6
Haiti	1
Martinique	18
Puerto Rico	10
Suriname	2
Trinidad and Tobago	1
Costa Rica	2
El Salvador	4
Guatemala	15
Honduras	2
Nicaragua	2
Panama	5
United States	39
Canada	1
TOTAL	2525

From Word Health Organization and Pan American Health Organization. Regional Zika Epidemiological Update (Americas). 2016. http://www.paho.org/hq/index.php?option=com_content&view=article&id=12390&Itemid=42090&lang=en.

As of December 29, 2016, there were 2289 confirmed cases of ZIKV congenital syndrome in Brazil, which includes cases of microcephaly and other congenital malformations, with most (approximately 90%) having occurred in the northeast region of the country.[335,338] Interestingly, this exponential increase in microcephaly cases in northeastern Brazil contrasts to the lower numbers of potential ZIKV congenital syndrome cases in other countries of the Americas[335,338] (Table 176H.1).

After establishing itself in the *Aedes* mosquito populations in Brazil, ZIKV transmission rapidly spread.[193,326] Some have cited two major factors behind ZIKV's "explosive spread" throughout Latin America, the Caribbean, and other regions: namely the unmatched ability of *Aedes aegypti* to flourish in urban settings, and the lack of preexisting immunity to ZIKV among resident populations.[326] Outside of Brazil, locally acquired ZIKV infection was being reported in many other Central and South American countries, including Suriname, El Salvador, Guatemala,[107] Mexico,[179] Paraguay, and Venezuela.[257,329] During the end of 2015 to early 2016, ZIKV spread to additional countries, including Panama,[16] Honduras, French Guiana, Martinique, Puerto Rico, Maldives, Guyana, Ecuador,[480] Barbados, Bolivia, Haiti, Saint Martin, the Dominican Republic, Saint Croix (US Virgin Islands), Nicaragua, Curaçao, and Jamaica.[257,329] The list of affected countries further expanded by February 2016 to include Samoa, Bonaire, Aruba, Trinidad and Tobago, Saint Vincent, Grenadines, and Argentina, as well as Kosrae and other Federated States of Micronesia, Dominica, and Cuba by March 2016.[257,329] In addition, during that time, reports of increasing cases of GBS in conjunction with ZIKV transmission were also surfacing first from El Salvador and then from Venezuela, Suriname, and Honduras.[257,329] By November 2016, more than 18 countries and territories in the Americas had reported cases of GBS following confirmed ZIKV infection.[468] Furthermore, other global regions, including Africa (Guinea-Bissau) in July 2016, as well as Southeast Asia, began reported locally acquired ZIKV cases, with two confirmed cases reported in Vietnam in April 2016.[469] In September 2016, additional countries apart from Vietnam in the Western Pacific

Region reported ZIKV cases, including Singapore, Philippines, Malaysia, and Thailand.[469]

Based on WHO surveillance as of December 2016, the level of global ZIKV transmission is staggering. Recent ZIKV transmission has been reported in more than 75 countries, which include at least 48 countries in the Americas with new ZIKV circulation since 2015.[141,328,339,352,470] (Figs. 176H.3 and 176H.4). In light of the ZIKV epidemic in Brazil and the rest of the Americas, the decision to continue to hold the August 2016 Rio de Janeiro Olympic Games was also a source of considerable controversy.[177,267] However, ZIKV had declined considerably by that

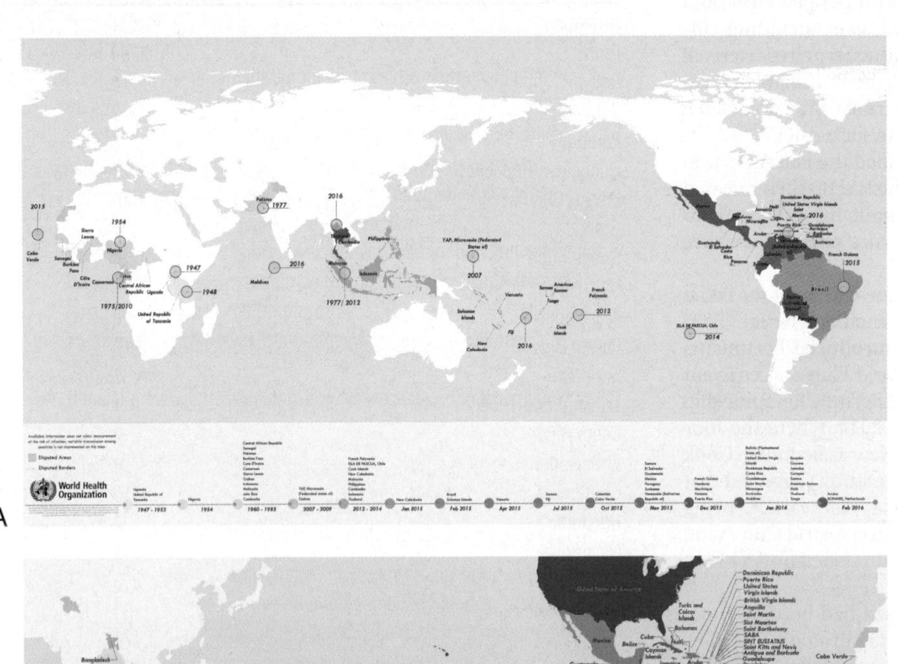

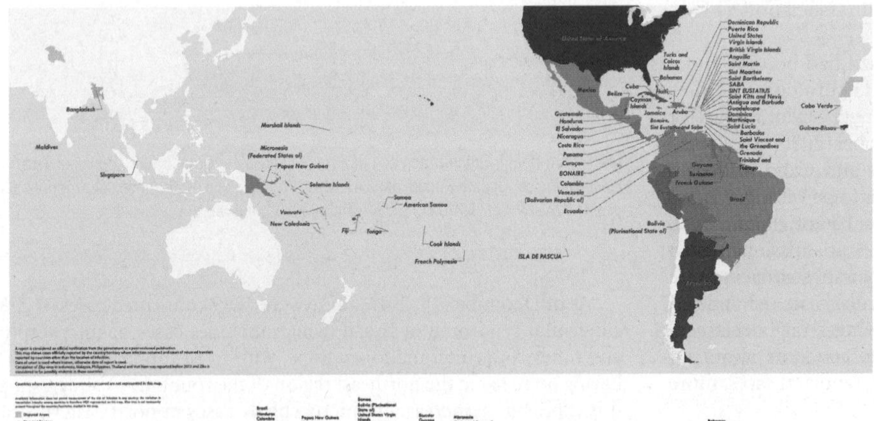

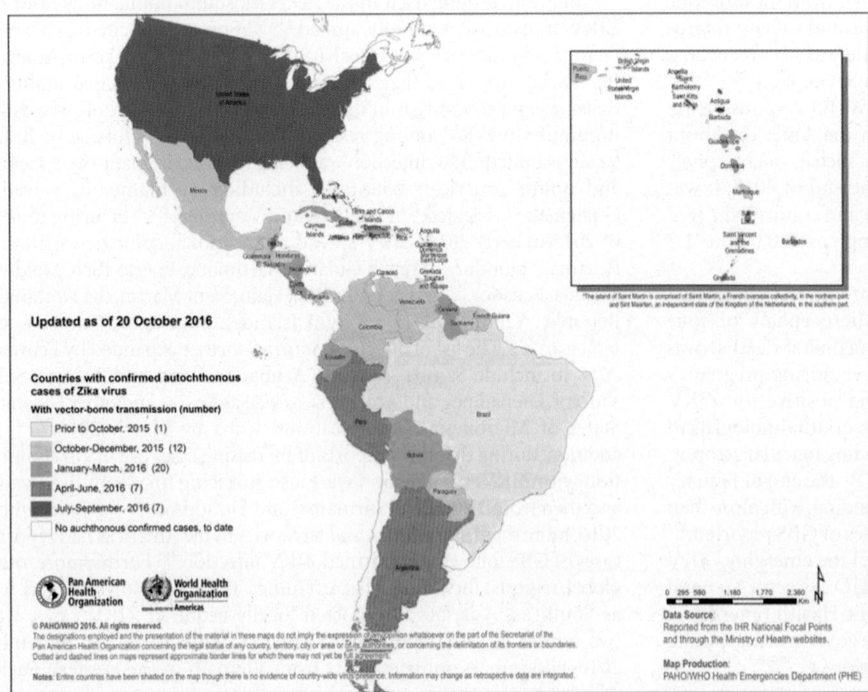

FIGURE 176H.3 (A) The figure is a timeline from the WHO that shows ZIKV global distribution from 1947 to early 2016. (B) The figure shows more recent ZIKV transmission from 2013 to August 2016. (C) The figure focuses on countries with demonstrated autochthonous (vector-borne) ZIKV transmission in the Americas from 2015 until November 2016. (A, From http://www.portal.pmnch.org/emergencies/zika-virus/zika-historical-distribution.pdf; and Kindhauser MK, Allen T, Frank V, Santhana RS, Dye C. Zika: the origin and spread of a mosquito-borne virus. *Bull World Health Organ.* 2016;94[9]:675-686. B, From WHO, http://www.who.int/emergencies/zika-virus/situation-report/10-november-2016/en/. C, From WHO, http://www.paho.org/hq/index.php?option=com_docman&task=doc_view&Itemid=270&gid=36623&lang=en.)

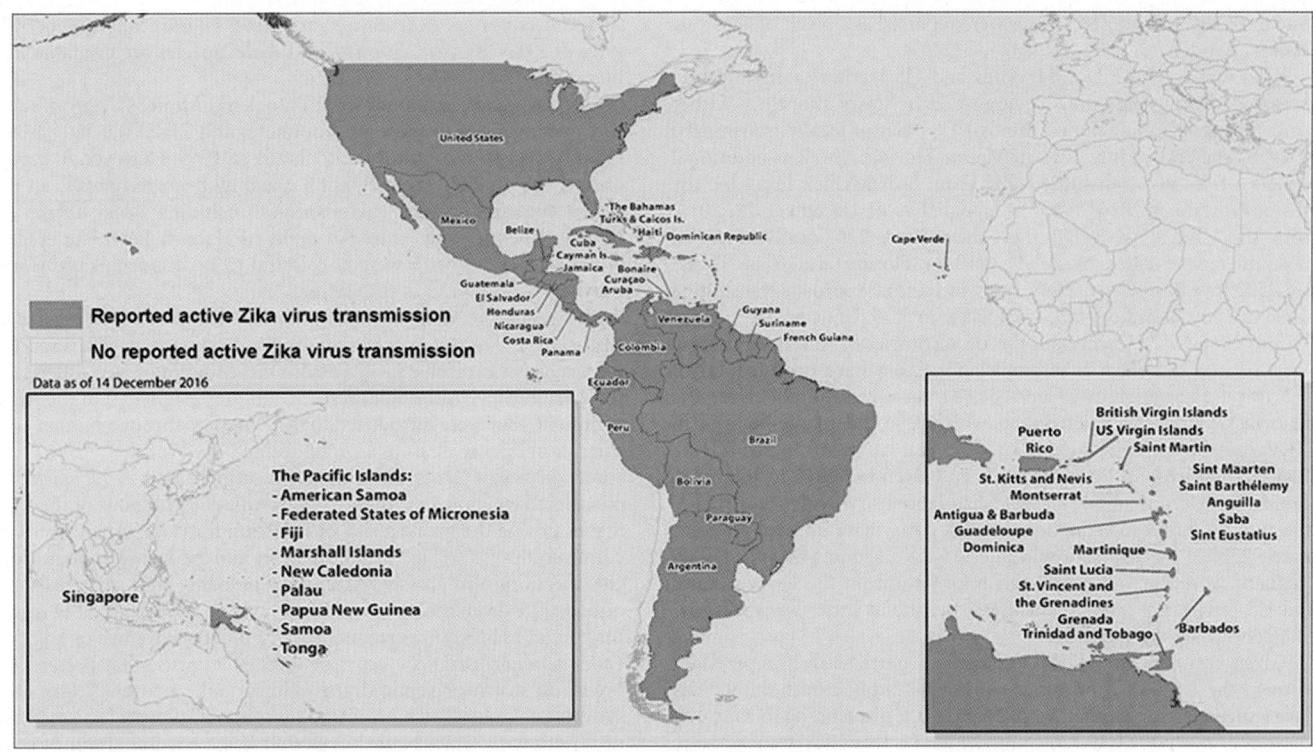

A

Americas

- Anguilla
- Antigua and Barbuda
- Argentina
- Aruba
- The Bahamas
- Barbados
- Belize
- Bolivia
- Bonaire
- Brazi
- British Virgin Islands
- Cayman Islands
- Colombia
- Commonwealth of Puerto Rico, US territory
- Costa Rica
- Cuba
- Curacao
- Dominica
- Dominican Republic
- Ecuador
- El Salvador
- French Guiana
- Grenada
- Guadeloupe
- Guatemala
- Guyana
- Haiti
- Honduras
- Jamaica
- Martinique
- Mexico
- Montserrat
- Nicaragua
- Palau
- Panama
- Paraguay
- Peru
- Saba
- Saint Barthélemy
- Saint Lucia
- Saint Martin
- Saint Vincent and the Grenadines
- Sint Eustatius
- Sint Maarten
- St. Kitts and Nevis
- Suriname
- Trinidad and Tobago
- Turks and Caicos
- United States
- U.S. Virgin Island
- Venezuela

Asia, Oceania/Pacific Islands

- American Samoa
- Fiji
- Kosrae
- Federated States of Micronesia
- Marshall Islands
- New Caledonia
- Palau
- Papua New Guinea
- Samoa
- Singapore
- Tonga

Africa

- Cape Verde

B

FIGURE 176H.4 All countries and territories with active Zika virus (ZIKV) transmission as of December 16, 2016. The figure shows countries and territories with active ZIKV transmission according to the CDC. (From http://www.cdc.gov/zika/geo/index.html; Centers for Disease Control and Prevention. Zika virus: all countries and territories with active Zika virus transmission. 2016. http://www.cdc.gov/zika/geo/active-countries.html.)

time in Brazil, and no ZIKV cases were reported as a result of Olympic Games attendance.

ZIKV cases in the United States and US territories significantly increased during the June to August 2016 travel months.[97] Other contributing factors included the first US cases of locally transmitted ZIKV by the end of July 2016 in Miami, Florida as well as additional reports of locally transmitted ZIKV in Brownsville, Texas by the end of November 2016.[74,246,262,264] Updated as of December 28, 2016, from the CDC's ArboNET, there have been 216 locally acquired mosquito-borne cases of ZIKV (210 in Florida and 6 in Texas) and 4592 travel-associated ZIKV cases, including 38 sexually transmitted cases and 1 laboratory-acquired case in the United States from 2015 to 2016.[375,378] However, in the US territories of American Samoa, Puerto Rico, and the US Virgin Islands, there have been a total of 132 travel-associated cases and 34,841 locally acquired cases, the majority occurring in Puerto Rico, which reported a large increase in ZIKV cases starting in July 2016.[375,378] Evaluation of 16,522 ZIKV-suspected patients in Puerto Rico from November 2015 to July 2016 found that more than 5351 (32%) had laboratory evidence of ZIKV infection.[5] It has been estimated that ZIKV may have infected approximately 25% of the population in Puerto Rico, including 6000 to 11,000 pregnant women.[161] (For updated information on the United States and US territories, refer to the CDC website at http://www.cdc.gov/zika/geo/united-states.html.)

Given concerns about ZIKV infection, particularly for pregnant women, the US CDC and other worldwide public health authorities have issued alerts to women who are pregnant or planning to conceive, to avoid or postpone travel to countries with active ZIKV transmission. Travel warnings were issued for South Florida and Brownsville, Texas in the United States and for the majority of countries and territories in Latin America, the Caribbean, Cape Verde in Africa, Oceania, and the Pacific Islands, as well as Singapore, where a cluster of locally transmitted cases was noted at the end of August 2016[74,260,327,362] (see Fig. 176H.4). Since September 2016, the CDC and WHO also acknowledged Southeast Asia (including Cambodia, Laos, Malaysia, Maldives, Philippines, Thailand, Vietnam) as another region with active ZIKV transmission, but the risk for transmission is thought to be lower given prior population immunity.[252,275,376,456,471] After the Americas, the Asia-Pacific region ranks second in countries affected by ZIKV, with 19 countries reporting ZIKV cases.[126] The WHO has also issued warnings regarding the likely increasing spread of ZIKV to Australia,[184] China,[488] Japan,[410] other Pacific Islands, and Southeast Asian countries.[126,436] Epidemic levels of ZIKV transmission in resource-limited countries in Asia-Pacific and Africa may be of particular concern given the 2.6 billion people living there, as well as socioeconomic and environmental conditions that may facilitate ZIKV spread.[37,400]

Areas with active ZIKV transmission are being continually updated on the CDC website (http://wwwnc.cdc.gov/travel/page/zika-travel-information; http://www.cdc.gov/zika/geo/active-countries.html) (see Fig. 176H.4).

Transmission of ZIKV

Arbovectors: Aedes *Mosquitoes*

The *Aedes* species of mosquitoes are primarily responsible for the rapid global spread of ZIKV because the mosquito bite is considered the predominant mode of ZIKV transmission to humans (see Fig. 176H.2). The mosquito acquires the virus during its blood meal from a viremic person or animal, and the virus replicates in the salivary glands of the mosquito.[301] Then, during a subsequent blood meal, the mosquito introduces saliva infected with ZIKV into a new host.[301] Mosquito saliva not only is important in transmitting the virus but also may be relevant in the establishment of viral infection. Recent work in experimental mice infected with Semliki Forest virus, a mosquito-borne alphavirus relative of the chikungunya virus, has shown that the *A. aegypti* saliva potentiates viremia 10-fold compared with viral infection alone, by causing inflammation attracting neutrophils and myeloid cells to the mosquito biting site.[357] Since ZIKV was isolated from the *A. africanus* mosquito back in 1948 in the forests of Uganda,[110,111] it has been subsequently detected in several other sylvatic (forest-dwelling) *Aedes* mosquito species, including the *Aedes apicoargenteus, Aedes furcifer, Aedes luteocephalus, Aedes taylori,* and *Aedes vitattus,* among others.[142,301] Lists of ZIKV by year, country, and *Aedes* species are available in the literature.[142,301]

An early laboratory study from 1956 demonstrated *A. aegypti's* ability to transmit ZIKV to mice and monkeys, and ZIKV was later isolated from *A. aegypti* mosquitoes in Malaysia in 1969. However, *A. aegypti's* critical role in ZIKV transmission has only been recognized in more recent epidemics. Other *Aedes* species, including *Aedes hensilli* (Yap Island epidemic) and *Aedes polynesiensis* (French Polynesia epidemic along with *A. aegypti*), were also found to be important transmitters during the outbreaks in the Pacific.[142,176,187,190,240,244,254,464,473]

Currently, the "citified" *Aedes* species, *A. aegypti* and *Aedes albopictus* (Asian tiger mosquito), appear to be the dominant players responsible for the recent explosive spread of ZIKV throughout Latin America and the Caribbean.[326] Although these mosquitoes originated in the African continent, they were introduced to the Americas through human (slave) migration by way of ships coming to the New World.[294,360] As a result, some species of *Aedes* mosquitoes (*A. aegypti* and *A. albopictus*) are considered endemic in southern and southeastern regions of the United States, posing the greatest risk of infection for poor urban Gulf Coast communities[199,460] (Fig. 176H.5). It should be noted that mosquito classifications also grossly reflect their breeding sites, and *Aedes* mosquitoes differ from other mosquitoes such as *Anopheles* (vector of malaria) that prefer to breed in permanent water sources (swamps or lakes) and *Culex quinquefasciatus* (vector of West Nile virus) that preferentially breeds in storm or septic drains with organic matter.[169] Termed the "gothic cockroach" of mosquitoes by some, *A. aegypti* is a small black mosquito with white banded legs that has a natural affinity for dark colors and spaces along with an uncanny ability to thrive in close proximity to humans.[169,326] Flourishing in densely populated urban environments, they attack in the day (morning and afternoon) and even prefer to breed in artificial containers with water, which may be as small and as seemingly innocuous as discarded bottle caps or plastic wrappers.[169,187,326,364]

A recent study of mosquitoes in Mexico has provided additional evidence confirming suspicions that *A. aegypti* has been the primary species of mosquito linked with ZIKV transmission in the Americas because they were unable to detect ZIKV in other frequently encountered tropical, urban-dwelling mosquitoes (i.e., *Culex* species such as *C. quinquefasciatus*).[179] Similar findings were also reported in other studies in the United States and Brazil.[147,463]

The true, definitive natural hosts and reservoirs of ZIKV still remain under investigation, but nonhuman primates and humans are believed to be the main reservoirs, with anthropocentric (human-to-vector-to-human) transmission characterizing outbreaks.[187,364] ZIKV antibodies have been detected in many primates in Africa and Asia, and ZIKV epizootic (nonhuman animal) transmission cycles, which included monkeys, were reported in Uganda and Senegal.[301] ZIKV has also been isolated from two species of monkeys, *Cercopithecus aethiops* and *Erythrocebus patas.*[86,142] However, other studies have detected ZIKV antibodies in several animals, including rodents, goats, bats, sheep, and others.[96,182,301,460] Although some have even suggested that bats may play a role in sylvatic ZIKV transmission cycles,[214] uncertainty still exists about whether other, nonprimate animal species can serve as ZIKV reservoirs.[86,142,183,187,190]

Nevertheless, it is clear that ZIKV appears to have a remarkable ability to adapt and persist in new ecological environments. In April 2016, researchers reported detection of ZIKV in monkeys in Northeastern Brazil and Ecuador.[326] Furthermore, ZIKV has been detected in wild *A. albopictus* mosquitoes in Mexico, which is worrisome because of its ability to survive in even cooler climates than other *Aedes* species.[326] A more recent study has also suggested that vertical transmission of ZIKV in *A. aegypti* mosquitoes may occur, which may further facilitate ZIKV's survival during adverse environmental conditions.[435] The incubation period of ZIKV in the mosquito host is 10 days, whereas the mosquito itself has a lifespan of 30 days. Therefore, hypothetically, the mosquito would have two-thirds of its lifetime at best to successfully transmit the infection.

Refer to Fig. 176H.4 and the CDC website for updated information about all countries and territories with active ZIKV transmission[75] (http://www.cdc.gov/zika/geo/index.html).

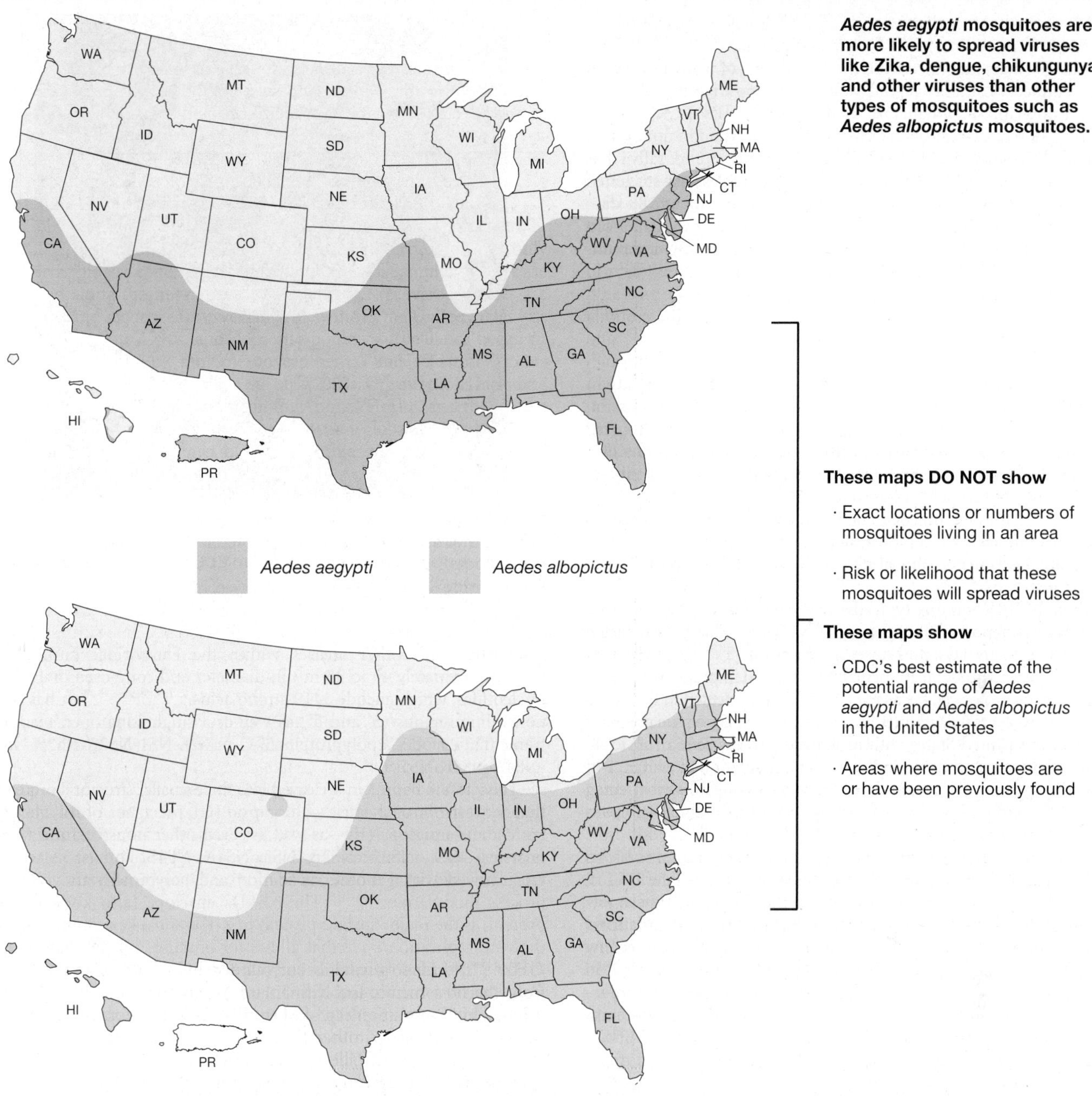
Aedes aegypti mosquitoes are more likely to spread viruses like Zika, dengue, chikungunya and other viruses than other types of mosquitoes such as Aedes albopictus mosquitoes.
These maps DO NOT show
· Exact locations or numbers of mosquitoes living in an area
· Risk or likelihood that these mosquitoes will spread viruses
These maps show
· CDC's best estimate of the potential range of Aedes aegypti and Aedes albopictus in the United States
· Areas where mosquitoes are or have been previously found
Aedes aegypti
Aedes albopictus
WA
OR
CA
NV
ID
MT
WY
UT
CO
AZ
NM
ND
SD
NE
KS
OK
TX
MN
IA
MO
AR
LA
WI
IL
MI
IN
OH
KY
TN
MS
AL
GA
FL
SC
NC
VA
WV
PA
NY
VT
ME
NH
MA
RI
CT
NJ
DE
MD
HI
PR

FIGURE 176H.5 Estimated range of *Aedes aegypti* and *Aedes albopictus* mosquitoes in the United States and the potential for Zika virus spread. Maps have been updated from a variety of sources. These maps represent the Centers for Disease Control and Prevention's best estimate of the potential range of *A. aegypti* and *A. albopictus* in the United States. Maps are not meant to represent risk for spread of disease. (From http://www.cdc.gov/zika/pdfs/zika-mosquito-maps.pdf. Last updated by the CDC on August 2, 2016.)

Other Modes of Transmission

Apart from mosquito-vector transmission, other modes of transmission of ZIKV have been documented, including case reports of sexual transmission, transfusion-associated transmission (which includes at least four cases of probable transfusion-related ZIKV transmission in Brazil),[27,209,290,302,307,447] and perinatal transmission.[32,33,44,59,68,450]

Suspected cases of ZIKV sexual transmission (including male-to-female, male-to-male, and female-to-male sexual transmission) were reported from French Polynesia, as well as at least 12 other countries, including France, Germany, Italy, New Zealand, and the United States, in returning travelers.* Updates from the CDC as of December 28, 2016, have now documented more than 38 cases of ZIKV from sexual transmission in the United States.[196,378] ZIKV may be transmitted sexually before, during, or after symptom onset, and in known cases from unprotected sexual activity (vaginal, anal, or oral).[363] At least one case and possibly another case (male-to-female sexual transmission) have also suggested the potential for ZIKV to be sexually transmitted from an asymptomatic carrier.[49,160] There are no studies evaluating the relevance of sexual transmission in the human population, but based on mathematical modeling studies, sexual transmission may account for a small portion of ZIKV transmission (3%), although it may be a significant contributor to prolonging the ZIKV epidemic and serving as an additional risk factor for ZIKV transmission.[164] Likewise, some sexually transmitted infection (STI) experts have suggested that sustained sexual transmission of ZIKV in the population seems unlikely given the relatively short infectious duration of ZIKV compared with other STIs.[13,477]

*References 13, 98, 100, 115, 156, 158, 160, 189, 196, 266, 288, 306, 309, 340, 341, 442, 451.

ZIKV has been detected in semen[22,251,309,390,442] as well as spermatozoa,[253] breast milk,[123] urine,[35,38,174,205,309,391,410,486] and saliva.[30,35,38,247,305,309,413,434,472] ZIKV has also been identified from the genital tract of women (cervical mucus, endocervical, and genital swabs tested positive for ZIKV by reverse transcriptase polymerase chain reaction [RT-PCR]).[98,308,379] Similarly, ZIKV has also been detected from vaginal fluid in nonhuman primates.[120] Prolonged ZIKV shedding in the urine and saliva has also been reported for 29 to 91 days.[155,259,309] Some studies have suggested even more prolonged virus detection in semen for up to 188 days after symptom onset.[22,189,251-253,259,309,353,363,372] Interestingly, ZIKV was detected in the semen for up to 39 days in a man, who was asymptomatically infected.[160] ZIKV has also been detected in semen for 69 days in a vasectomized man.[18]

The epidemiologic relevance of detection of ZIKV in these bodily fluids, apart from semen and the female genital tract,[22,98,251,379,390,442] and the risks for transmission have not been yet determined, although replication-competent (infective) virus has been isolated from patient urine and saliva.[38] A case of secondary nonsexual ZIKV transmission (presumably through unprotected contact with sweat or tears) occurred after visiting a hospitalized patient with extremely high levels of ZIKV viremia and has raised new and unanswered questions about the infectious risks of contact with bodily fluids in those with severe ZIKV infection.[48,428] Although mucocutaneous transmission of flaviviruses is rare, animal models have demonstrated its possibility, and nosocomial mucocutaneous transmission of dengue has also been reported in at least one instance.[79,80,428]

Although ZIKV viremia typically may range from a few days to 1 week, some case reports did suggest that ZIKV viremia has been detected in patients 10 to 16 days after onset of symptoms.[30,155,480] However, in pregnant women with fetal abnormalities detected in pregnancy, ZIKV viremia may be prolonged because ZIKV has been detected in the blood as long as 10 weeks (70 days) after infection.[119,444] A study of five pregnant women in the United States with prolonged ZIKV viremia (up to 46 days after symptom onset) found that only one infant had evidence of fetal ZIKV infection.[269] In another report of a congenitally infected infant, ZIKV viremia was noted 67 days after birth, and ZIKV was detected from urine and saliva on his 54th day of life.[316]

Importantly, ZIKV has been detected in as many as 1.1% blood donors in regions with active ZIKV transmission, such as Puerto Rico, which has led to subsequent efforts to protect the blood donation supply through US Food and Drug Administration (FDA) recommendations, which include deferral of donations from high-risk individuals, screening of blood donors, and special management of blood products.[228,353] In addition, given modes of ZIKV transmission, organ and tissue transplantation, fertility treatment, and breast-feeding may all pose theoretical risks for ZIKV transmission.[363] (Refer to the later section on ZIKV Prevention for further details about prevention efforts from vector and nonvector transmission standpoints.)

VIROLOGY AND PATHOGENESIS

Virology of ZIKV

Viral Classification and Structure

ZIKV is classified within the mosquito-borne clade X and *Flavivirus* cluster within the *Flavivirus* genus and Flaviviridae family[178,230,301] (Fig. 176H.6). It is one of 73 viruses and includes 53 distinct species within the *Flavivirus* genus, which have been classified based on molecular-based taxonomy into appropriate clusters, clades, and species.[85,178,301,356] However, only one other virus, Spondweni virus, is in ZIKV's clade, with which it shares about 70% of its nucleotides.[125] Other closely related viruses are Ilheus, Rocio, and St. Louis encephalitis viruses.[85,190,230] Other well-known viruses within the *Flaviviridae* family are yellow fever, Japanese encephalitis, West Nile, dengue, and hepatitis C viruses. Of these, ZIKV shares approximately 60% of its nucleotides with Japanese encephalitis, West Nile, and dengue virus.[125]

Similar in structure to other viruses in the Flaviviridae family, ZIKV is an icosahedral-shaped, enveloped single-stranded positive-sense RNA virus (+ssRNA). In fact, with almost atomic resolution (3.7 Å), the three-dimensional cryo–electron microscopy (cryo-EM) structure of ZIKV has now been demonstrated and has highlighted structural similarities with other viruses within the Flaviviridae family.[26,226] It is approximately 40 to 45 nm in diameter and composed of 10,794 nucleotides, which encode 3419 amino acids.[85,109,190,229,230,397] It has two noncoding regions (5′ and 3′) as well as a single long open reading frame that encodes a polyprotein: 5′-C-prM-E-NS1-NS2A-NS2B-NS3-NS4A-NS4B-NS5-3′.[144,355]

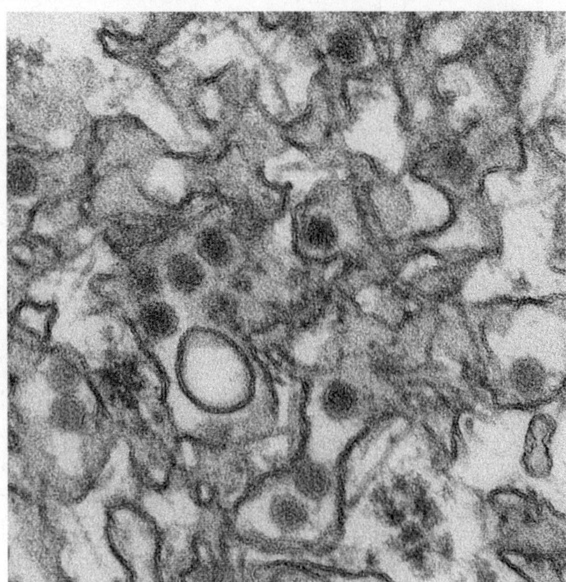

FIGURE 176H.6 Colorized electron micrograph depicting Zika virus (ZIKV) particles in red. The ZIKV particles are 40 nm in diameter with an outer envelope and an inner dense core. (From CDC/Cynthia Goldsmith, http://phil.cdc.gov/phil/details.asp.)

This ZIKV polyprotein is cleaved into three smaller structural proteins that form the virus particle—the capsid (C), precursor of membrane (prM), and envelope (E)—as well as seven other nonstructural (NS) proteins—NS1, NS2A, NS2B, NS3, NS4A, NS4B, and NS5—which are involved with genome replication and polyprotein and cellular process modulation.[52,144,355] The 53-kDa envelope (also known as E protein) is the major surface protein of ZIKV and a key component in the viral replication cycle that allows for binding and cell membrane fusion.[144] Its nucleocapsid is surrounded by a lipid bilayer derived from the host membrane with E and M envelope proteins. As seen through high-resolution cryo-EM studies, the ZIKV E envelope protein shows resemblance to other flavivirus E proteins, such as Japanese encephalitis and West Nile viruses, which are also known to exhibit neurotropism.[226] The E protein is the most common target for neutralizing antibodies, and antibody responses to the envelope protein are often protective.[422]

NS1 is a nonstructural protein seen in ZIKV and other flaviviruses and functions as a virulence factor that is important for viral replication and also has immune-modulatory roles, including immune evasion. Although the overall ZIKV NS1 structure is similar to other flaviviruses, crystallographic studies of the ZIKV NS1 have shown an extended hydrophobic and polar surface different from West Nile and dengue serotype 2 that may affect cellular membrane attachment.[52,476] NS5, which is the largest ZIKV protein, has dual functions with RNA-dependent RNA polymerase (C-terminal) activity and RNA capping owing to its methyltransferase (N-terminal) activity.[144] The 3′-noncoding region may also have roles in translation, genome stabilization, RNA packaging, cyclization, and cellular/viral factor recognition functions.[144] The ZIKV helicase is considered an important component in viral replication, and some hypothesized that it may be a target for an antiviral drug after recent determination of the crystal structure of the ZIKV helicase was reported.[207,438] Other studies have also suggested that polyamines (small, positively charged ornithine-derived molecules) are important for ZIKV replication.[292]

Flaviviruses are known to be inactivated by high temperatures (>56°C for at least 30 minutes), pH ≤6, ultraviolet-light and gamma radiation and are susceptible to 30 minutes of contact with disinfectants like 1% sodium hypochlorite, 2% glutaraldehyde, 70% ethanol, 3% to 6% hydrogen peroxide and 3% to 8% formaldehyde, TRIzol, and Buffer AVL.[23,36,55,139,171,304] Subsequent preliminary studies on ZIKV inactivation have also determined that certain types of disinfectants used in laboratories typically will inactivate ZIKV.[295] Loss of ZIKV infectivity was observed after exposure to all types of alcohols, 1% hypochlorite (typically used to inactivate viruses in BSL-2/3 laboratory liquid waste), 2% paraformaldehyde, 2% glutaraldehyde, ultraviolet-light radiation, temperatures of 60°C or higher, and pH ≥12 or pH ≤4.[295] These studies also observed that dried ZIKV could remain infectious for more than 3 days and that standard contact barriers such as intact nitrile and latex gloves are protective.[295]

ZIKV Phylogeny and Genetics

Although ZIKV's origins can be traced back to East Africa, evolutionary patterns in ZIKV sequencing have been described.[233,352] The full genome of the original ZIKV from Uganda (MR 766 prototype) was sequenced in 2007, as were genomes of ZIKV strains from other outbreaks in Brazil, Cambodia, Central African Republic, French Polynesia, Guatemala, Malaysia, Nigeria, Puerto Rico, Senegal, Thailand, and Yap, which are available in GenBank.[229,301]

The initial phylogenetic analyses done after the Yap Island outbreak in 2007[233] identified several ZIKV lineages, including two African lineages (eastern and western) and one Asian lineage, which are referred to as the East African (Uganda prototype), West African (Senegal), and Asian (Yap) strains.[144,233,301,352] Subsequently, full genome sequencing identified two primary ZIKV lineages, the African lineage (including Nigeria, Senegal, and Uganda strains) and the Asian lineage (including Malaysia, Yap, and Cambodia strains); the study suggested that ZIKV likely arrived in the Yap Islands by way of Southeast Asia.[182,301] An additional phylogenetic analysis of 43 ZIKV strains from 1947 to 2007 confirmed earlier findings of African (MR-766 prototype Uganda and Nigeria clusters) and Asian (Yap and Malaysian) ZIKV strains.[144,301] It was suggested that ZIKV likely appeared in East Africa in the 1920s, traveled to West Africa, and then dispersed to Asia in the 1940s.[144,301] Sequencing of ZIKV in Brazil has suggested that it is of the Asian lineage, likely originating from French Polynesia.[41,92,141,168] Although African strains were typically responsible for asymptomatic or mild infection, the Asian strain, which may also cause asymptomatic or mild infection, has been largely responsible for the reported congenital anomalies. Some have speculated that recombination events of ZIKV may have contributed to changes in its pathogenicity.[144,301,344,462]

Other unresolved questions involve the pathogenicity, particularly neuropathogenicity, of different ZIKV strains. A recent study has reported a shared mutation of amino acids at NS5, a nonstructural ZIKV protein, in isolates from Colombia, Mexico, Panama, and Martinique.[8] It has been suggested that this NS5 mutation may form a "Latin American" clade of ZIKV that appears to be distinct from the virus isolated from Brazil and has been speculated that it may affect ZIKV's neutropism.[8] In addition, one study comparing African (strain from Central African Republic) and Asian lineages has demonstrated higher infectivity of human astrocytes and neural stem cells, cell death, and antiviral response of the Central Republic African strain; the researchers hypothesized that the older African MR-766 original strain used in the experiments may have lost its neurovirulence because of serial in vitro passages compared with other African ZIKV lineage strains.[411]

Of note, the WHO has recently developed a ZIKV candidate reference strain (ZIKV strain PF13/251013-18) for the development of nucleic acid amplification tests (NAATs).[441] The reference strain was isolated from serum from a French Polynesian patient with ZIKV in 2013 and related to ZIKV strains recently detected in Central and South America, the Caribbean, and the Pacific regions.[441]

Viral Pathogenesis

Current understanding about ZIKV's pathogenesis is limited, although rapidly evolving. As with other mosquito-transmitted flaviviruses, it is believed that after ZIKV is transmitted through the mosquito's bite. The virus initially sustains itself by replicating locally in dendritic cells at the site of inoculation before spreading to lymph nodes and more distant sites of the body.[108,190] Because dendritic cells, dermal fibroblasts, and epidermal keratinocytes may be infected with ZIKV, these cells in humans are thought to be important in ZIKV's pathogenesis.[186,301] One study from the 1980s has suggested that ZIKV may also be able to replicate in the host cell nucleus because its antigens have been detected in cell nuclei; this finding is unusual for flaviviruses, which are known to replicate in the cellular cytoplasm.[54,190]

Early animal studies provided some basic insight into ZIKV's pathogenesis in humans. Apart from the initial rhesus monkey (#766) that developed mild fever from ZIKV infection and thereby enabled ZIKV's discovery, other rhesus monkeys did not develop symptoms of acute infection after being inoculated with the virus, even after demonstrating viremia.[109,111] Interestingly enough, other small animals inoculated intracerebrally with ZIKV, including cotton rats, guinea pigs, and rabbits, also did not demonstrate apparent symptoms of ZIKV infection.[109] However, both rhesus monkeys and rabbits were able to demonstrate an antibody response to ZIKV.[109,111] More contemporary studies of rhesus monkeys inoculated with a recent 2016 ZIKV clinical isolate demonstrated that monkeys did develop fever and viremia.[120,243,342] ZIKV was excreted in multiple bodily secretions, including urine, saliva, tears, semen, and vaginal secretions, and evidence of ZIKV was detected in the central nervous system (CNS) (brain and spinal cord) and other organs (lymph nodes, parotids, stomach, liver, kidney, bladder, spleen, intestines, testes and other male and female reproductive tissue, and heart).[120,243,342] Detection in saliva and urine was prolonged for approximately 4 weeks, and repeat challenge with ZIKV after primary infection resulted in protection from subsequent infections.[342]

Other fascinating observations in early animal studies included reports that ZIKV was highly neurotropic in mice and was only recovered from brain tissues of infected mice.[109,111] Upon autopsy of ZIKV-infected mice, these early studies observed neuronal degeneration, cellular infiltration, Cowdry type A inclusion bodies, and "softening" of brain tissue, with young mice demonstrating the most extensive brain lesions.[109] In addition, although mice of all ages were found to be susceptible to infection when inoculated intracerebrally, only mice younger than 2 weeks of age became sick when infected intraperitoneally with ZIKV.[111] Of note, one study in mice also reported lesions in tissues other than the CNS induced by ZIKV, including skeletal myositis, myocarditis, and lung edema.[464] In contrast to these findings in mice, other early animal studies of rhesus monkeys, cotton rats, guinea pigs, and rabbits did not demonstrate ZIKV's neurotropism.[109,111,301]

Additional in vitro studies have investigated nonhuman cell lines that support ZIKV infection. Nonhuman cell lines, including nonhuman primate (Vero and LLC-MK2), pig (PK-15), rabbit (RK-13), hamster (BHK21), and chicken (DF-1) cell lines, supported productive ZIKV replication.[78]

Human in Vitro Cellular Studies and Histopathology From Neonatal Autopsies

ZIKV replication and its cytopathic effects have also been observed in several human cell lines, including placental (JEG-3), neuronal (SF268), muscle (RD), retinal (ARPE19), pulmonary (Hep-2 and HFL), colonic (Caco-2), and hepatic (Huh-7) cell lines.[78] In addition, several other human cell lines, including prostatic (LNCaP), testicular (833KE), and renal (HEK) cell lines, have also shown increased ZIKV viral load without cytopathic effects.[78]

Further in vitro studies have also suggested that ZIKV may exhibit a wide range of maternal and fetal tissue and cell tropism and have helped elucidate potential mechanisms of ZIKV maternal-fetal intrauterine transmission.[130,383,430] ZIKV has the capability of infecting various umbilical cord (mesenchymal stem cells), human placental cell, and chorionic villus cell types (cytotrophoblasts, endothelial cells, fibroblasts, Hofbauer cells [also known as primary human placental macrophages]) in chorionic villi, amniotic epithelial cells and trophoblast progenitors in amniochorionic membranes, which express the ZIKV cofactor (TIM1).[130,213,383,430] One study demonstrated that ZIKV had particular affinity for replication in placental macrophages (Hofbauer cells) and that ZIKV viral replication coincided with induction of type I interferon (IFN), proinflammatory cytokines, and antiviral gene expression, but with minimal cell death.[383] Overall, these results suggest that ZIKV may cause fetal infection by initially infecting placental cells, which disrupts the placental barrier.[383] ZIKV can infect these cells from early, mid, and late gestation, suggesting not only placental but paraplacental transmission.[430] Target inhibitors of TIM1 may also have the potential to inhibit ZIKV infection at the uterine-placental interface.[430]

One study also found that serially passaged ZIKV strain (MR-766) was able to infect human neural progenitor cells and increase cellular death.[279,431] Likewise, the Asian/Brazilian ZIKV strain has also been shown to infect human cortical progenitor cells and lead to increased cell death with disruption of proliferative zones and cortical brain layers.[89,245,321] ZIKV may also damage cranial neural crest cells, which are important precursors of skull bone and cartilage, which leads to increased cytokine production and abnormal in vitro neurodevelopment.[31] Furthermore, others have suggested that high AXL expression, which may serve as a ZIKV cellular entry receptor in neural stem cells, may be one of the factors contributing to ZIKV's observed neurotropism.[279,312] A link between ZIKV neural progenitor cells and the upregulation of toll-like receptor 3 (TLR3) has been suggested and may lead to cell death and abnormal regulation of neurogenesis, axon guidance, and cell differentiation.[95]

Pathologic evaluation of fetuses and infants with congenital ZIKV infection has also confirmed findings of direct ZIKV cytopathic effects primarily localized to the brain.[407] Histopathology of congenital ZIKV syndrome from spontaneous abortions and neonatal autopsies has demonstrated microcalcifications, scattered microglial nodules, cell degeneration, and necrosis of brain tissue, along with identification of ZIKV antigens in neurons and glial cells.[255] Placental pathology has shown villous edema, increased Hofbauer cells, and ZIKV antigens in Hofbauer cells in the chorionic villi.[255] The lack of significant inflammatory response in the fetal or infant brain, along with distinguishing viral cytopathic features, appear to be more characteristic of ZIKV (as well as congenital rubella infection) as opposed to other congenital infections such as cytomegalovirus and herpes simplex virus.[255]

Recent Insight Into ZIKV's Pathology, Including Experimental Animal Model Studies (Mice and Nonhuman Primates)

One important discovery has been the development of ZIKV mouse models because immunocompetent mice are typically resistant to ZIKV challenge. However, mice lacking type 1 IFN receptors, either knockouts (genetically deficient) or treated with antibodies that block these receptors, are susceptible to ZIKV infection.[197] One study has reported that type I IFN signaling–deficient mice infected with ZIKV early in pregnancy can lead to infection of placental trophoblasts, and hence to placental damage and fetal demise,[278] a finding previously reported in human observational studies.[44] Researchers have also demonstrated that the Brazilian ZIKV strain can infect murine fetuses and lead to intrauterine growth restriction, including signs of microcephaly, mimicking what was previously described in humans.[44,89] Other studies of pregnant mice have shown that ZIKV can replicate in the vaginal tract, and pregnant mice infected vaginally with ZIKV during early pregnancy can lead to fetal growth restriction and fetal brain infection.[478]

Another study investigated the effect of ZIKV infection in several types of knockout mice, with differences in IFN receptors and abilities to produce IFN-α and IFN-β. Neurologic disease was observed and high ZIKV viral loads were detected in the brain, spinal cord, and even the testes, which appears to have relevance to both neurodevelopmental defects seen in human fetuses and ZIKV's ability to be transmitted sexually.[237] A recent study reported that ZIKV (Asian strain SZ01) was able to replicate efficiently in the mice embryonic brain by targeting neuronal progenitor cells, which led to cell cycle arrest, apoptosis, and inhibition of neuronal progenitor cell differentiation.[245] Similar findings in other murine studies and human cells have also suggested that undifferentiated neurons are very susceptible to ZIKV infection,[47,202] especially during periods of rapid brain growth.[200] Furthermore, ZIKV-infected mice brains were smaller, had larger ventricles, and had a thinner cortex, which appears to be consistent with the microcephalic phenotype observed in ZIKV-infected human fetuses and infants.[245] Apart from reproducing fetal brain pathology in mice models and human in vitro cell studies, ZIKV inoculation of pregnant nonhuman primates (pigtail macaque) has also produced ZIKV-associated fetal brain pathology with periventricular lesions in occipital and parietal lobes, cerebral white-matter hypoplasia, periventricular white-matter gliosis, and axonal and ependymal damage.[6]

Mouse studies have also demonstrated that ZIKV infection in adult mice can infect multiple parts of the eye (iris, retina, optic nerve) and can lead to conjunctivitis, panuveitis, and neuroretinitis, with high levels of ZIKV detected in the eye, lacrimal glands, and tears.[280] ZIKV studies in mice have demonstrated that ZIKV may persist in the testes, preferring to infect spermatogonia, primary spermatocytes, and Sertoli cells, and epididymis of male mice and resulting injury including inducement of cell death may lead to decreased testosterone and sperm production.[175]

Other Studies Providing Insight Into ZIKV's Pathogenesis (ZIKV and Dengue Antibodies)

Researchers have also been interested in investigating whether prior exposure to dengue may affect ZIKV's pathogenesis given similarities of ZIKV to dengue (differences of 41% to 46% in the amino acid sequence of envelope proteins of dengue and ZIKV, whereas differences of 30% to 35% have been noted between dengue serotypes).[102] A theory that has been used to explain dengue hemorrhagic complications that may occur after secondary infections with different dengue serotypes is antibody-dependent enhancement (ADE), which can lead to higher viral loads.[102] This occurs because cross-reactive but nonneutralizing antibodies may bind to other dengue serotypes and facilitate entry through Fc-γ receptors present on monocytes and macrophages (primary viral replication sites) and thereby lead to increased viral replication.[125,185] Some preliminary in vitro studies have also suggested that plasma immune to dengue may also lead to ADE and enhance ZIKV replication.[102,219] However, at this time epidemiologic studies have not suggested dengue antibody enhancement of ZIKV infection.[125]

Although little is known about the protective antibody responses to ZIKV, antibodies to other flaviviruses have been known to result in lasting, lifelong immunity to subsequent infection with the same virus.[429] Some studies have suggested that convalescent ZIKV-immune sera has the potential to neutralize various ZIKV strains (South American, Asian, and early African ZIKV strains).[117,487] Other studies have even demonstrated conserved epitopes between ZIKV and dengue that are targets for cross-neutralizing antibodies.[26,429] Specifically, human monoclonal antibodies (reactive to the envelope dimer epitope 1) from dengue patients can neutralize all four dengue serotypes as well as ZIKV in cell cultures and can even be protective in murine models.[429] In contrast, another interesting study characterizing the antigenic specificity of antibodies generated from patients that had been infected by ZIKV only, or coinfected with dengue virus, found that antibodies to NS1 were typically ZIKV specific, whereas those reactive to the E protein domain I/II (ED I/II) did not neutralize ZIKV and dengue and instead strongly enhanced ZIKV and dengue infection, whereas EDIII or quaternary epitope ZIKV antibodies provided the best ZIKV protection.[424]

CLINICAL MANIFESTATIONS AND COMPLICATIONS

Acute ZIKV Infection

As with many other infections, ZIKV may cause an acute febrile, exanthematous illness that is typically clinically indistinguishable from many other infections, especially other arboviral infections such as dengue and chikungunya, which are transmitted by the same *Aedes* mosquito species.[44,58,121,148,460] The exact incubation period has not been conclusively established for ZIKV but has been generally considered to be anywhere from 3 days to 2 weeks, which has its basis in other flaviviruses and mosquito studies.[151,187,352,354,363,394]

The WHO has developed interim case definitions for any person infected with ZIKV.[330] A suspected case is considered to be "a person presenting with rash and/or fever and at least one of the following signs or symptoms: (1) arthralgia or (2) arthritis or (3) conjunctivitis (nonpurulent/hyperemic)."[330] The CDC suspected case definition includes an epidemiologic linkage and clinical criteria with one or more of the following, not explained by another diagnostic etiology: (1) acute onset of fever,

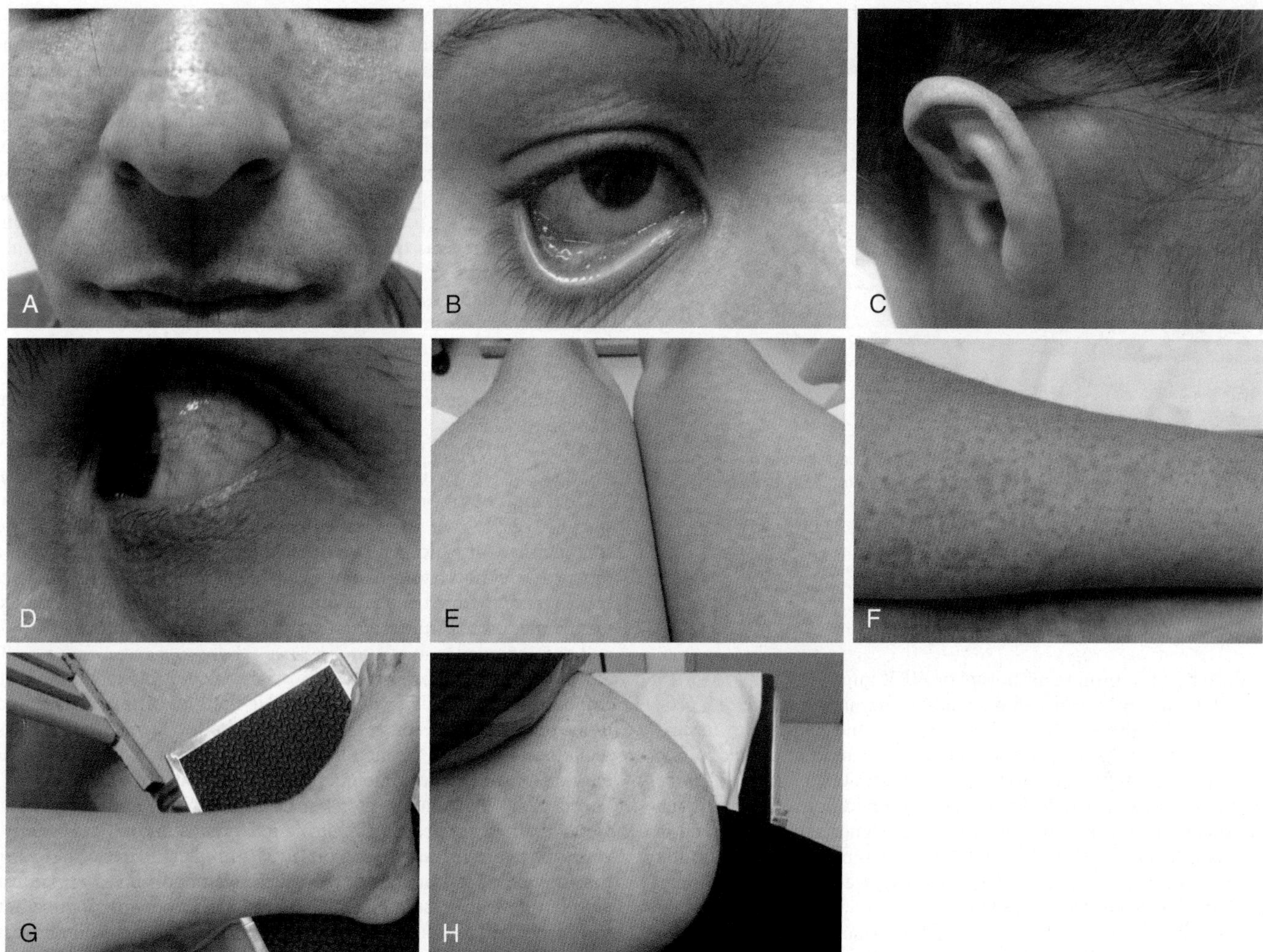

FIGURE 176H.7 Clinical manifestations of Zika virus in pregnant women in Rio de Janeiro, Brazil. (A) Maculopapular rash on the face. (B) Conjunctival and palpebral erythema. (C) Retroauricular lymphadenopathy. (D) Conjunctival injection with prominence of vasculature. (E) Rash on the legs, with a lacy reticular pattern. (F) Maculopapular rash on the inner arm. (G) Edema of the foot, which the patient reported was painful. (H) Blanching macular rash on the gravid abdomen. (From Brasil P, Pereira JP Jr, Moreira ME, et al. Zika virus infection in pregnant women in Rio de Janeiro. *N Engl J Med.* 2016;375[24]:2321-2334.)

(2) maculopapular rash, (3) conjunctivitis, (4) arthralgia, (5) complications of pregnancy (fetal loss or fetus or neonate with congenital microcephaly, intracranial calcifications, other structural brain or eye abnormalities, other congenital CNS-related abnormalities such as clubfoot or joint contractures), or (6) GBS or other neurologic manifestations.[373,374]

As highlighted by the WHO and CDC suspected case definitions of ZIKV, the most commonly reported symptoms in adults include rash, transient fever, arthralgia, and conjunctivitis[97,332,374] (Fig. 176H.7). From what has been learned from studies of patients from the Pacific Island region (Yap Island, French Polynesia, and others) as well as from Brazil and other countries in Latin America, acute ZIKV infection is typically considered mild.[44,179,332] Fever is present in less than one-third of cases and is low grade and short lived, and the infection tends to subsist for about 2 to 7 days.[332,44]

The exanthem of ZIKV is typically described as a nonspecific, diffuse, macular or maculopapular eruption appearing 3 days to 2 weeks after initial infection[140] (see Fig. 176H.7). The rash often starts on the trunk and descends to include the lower extremities, usually sparing palms and soles.[44,106] Of note, other reports have emphasized variability in rash presentation, which may be more morbilliform or scarlatiniform, may begin on the face before spreading to the extremities, and may include the palms and soles in rare cases.[140] One case report described a patient with a ZIKV exanthem of the abdomen, trunk, and face, marked by erythema and edema of the malar region of the face.[41,44] Pruritus generally accompanies the exanthema, and desquamation may be seen after the rash subsides.[44,49,140] Occasionally, gum bleeding and petechiae, including palatal petechiae, and oral blisters or ulcers have been observed in some patients.[24,41,44,65,106,140,152,156,428] Skin biopsies have shown mild and focally moderate perivascular lymphocytic infiltrate in the upper dermis.[106]

Profuse tearing has also been described in one patient with ZIKV conjunctivitis.[428] Other symptoms, such as abdominal pain, diarrhea, emesis, and pharyngitis, are less common on presentation but have been reported.[24,189,428] Lymphopenia, neutropenia, thrombocytopenia, and elevation in liver enzymes also appear less frequently but have been reported in the literature.[24,155,189,275,428] Respiratory findings are generally not part of ZIKV's clinical presentation.

Definitive diagnosis of ZIKV is difficult based on clinical features alone, especially given considerable overlap in presenting features and transmission regions for other arbovirus such as chikungunya and dengue[16,58,91,138,146] (Table 176H.2). Some have even coined the term *ChikDenMaZika syndrome* to describe the diagnostic conundrum of predominant arboviral infections in Latin America (chikungunya, dengue, Mayaro virus [a togavirus], and ZIKV) with similar presenting symptoms.[241,346] Yet, some symptoms may be more or less common features of ZIKV compared with dengue and chikungunya. For instance, fever

TABLE 176H.2 Clinical Features of Zika Virus Compared With Dengue and Chikungunya[a]

Features	Zika	Dengue	Chikungunya
Fever	+ to ++	+++	+++
Maculopapular rash	+++	+	++
Pruritus	++	−/+	−/+
Conjunctivitis	++	−	+/−
Arthralgia	++	+	+++
Myalgia	+	++	+
Headache	+	++	++
Facial edema	+/−	++	+
Palatal petechiae	+/−	++	+
Hemorrhage	−	++	−
Shock	−	+	−

[a]Note that one study of all three viruses of patients in Nicaragua suggested more similarities among the three viruses with regard to fever, conjunctivitis, arthralgia, and headache.[459]

Primarily adapted from a Centers for Disease Control and Prevention Presentation by Ingrid Rabe,[363] "Zika Virus: What Clinicians Need to Know," a Clinician Outreach and Communication Activity (COCA), Call, Atlanta, GA, January 26, 2016. With similar tables also noted in references 21 and 138.

tends to be a less prominent feature of ZIKV infection compared with the other two, with which fever tends to be higher and more prolonged.[138,363] Arthralgia is a much more prominent symptom in chikungunya, in which it occurs more frequently, affects multiple joints, and tends to be more severe, long lived, and debilitating than in ZIKV.[138] Thrombocytopenia with facial edema or complications of hemorrhage and shock often has been suggestive of a diagnosis of dengue and is not characteristic of ZIKV.[363] In addition, rash is much more frequently observed with ZIKV; conjunctivitis is not typically seen with dengue, unless hemorrhagic, and is less frequently seen with chikungunya than with ZIKV.[363] (See Table 176H.2 for further detail on a comparison of clinical features of ZIKV, dengue, and chikungunya.)

It should also be noted that some studies have also indicated the potential for other arboviral coinfections in as many as 13.3% to 20.5% of patients,[459] including ZIKV with dengue [58,124,453] and ZIKV with chikungunya.[58,401,480] There have even been reports from Colombia and Nicaragua of patients infected simultaneously with all three arboviruses: ZIKV, chikungunya, and dengue.[453,459]

ZIKV Presentation From the Yap Island Case Series

In 2007, one of the earliest and largest case series of ZIKV infection was performed from 49 laboratory-confirmed and 59 probable cases from Yap Island in the Federated States of Micronesia.[121] The symptomatic attack rate from Yap Island among those infected with ZIKV was estimated to be 18% (95% confidence interval [CI], 10–27%).[121,363] The most common symptoms reported were rash (90%) with a median duration of 6 days, subjective fever (65%), arthralgia (65%) with a mean duration of 3.5 days, and nonpurulent conjunctivitis (55%).[121] Other frequently reported symptoms were headache (45%), retroorbital pain (39%), myalgia (48%), edema (19%), and vomiting (10%).[121] All of the ZIKV infections were considered mild; none of the patients required hospitalization, had serious complications such as hemorrhagic symptoms, or died[121] (Table 176H.3).

ZIKV Presentation From Several Case Series From Brazil and Other Countries

A study from Rio de Janeiro, Brazil of 119 PCR-proven adult cases of ZIKV in 2015 corroborated the early findings from Yap Island that ZIKV is primarily a self-limited, viral illness.[41] Early in the infection, the most commonly reported symptoms were rash (97%), primarily maculopapular with a mean duration of 5.5 days; pruritus (79%); prostration (73%); headache (66%); and arthralgia (63%) with a mean duration 9 days. Interestingly, fever was only observed in 36% of patients and was often transient (≤1 day).[41] Other, less common findings included low back pain (51%), retroorbital pain (45%), and lymph node enlargement (41%), particularly in cervical and retroauricular areas,[181] but generalized lymphadenopathy was also observed.[41] Less than one-fourth of patients (21%) reported mild hemorrhagic symptoms such as petechiae or mild bleeding from mucosal sites.[41] Median leukocyte count (4590 cells/mm^3), hematocrit (41.2%), and platelets (201,000 cells/mm^3) were not significantly impaired in this cohort[41] (see Table 176H.3). These presenting ZIKV symptoms corresponded to those seen in another Rio de Janeiro cohort of patients by the same group of investigators, but the second report was exclusive to pregnant women,[44] as well as another smaller retrospective review of ZIKV cases in 2015 in Rio de Janeiro by another group[76] (see Table 176H.3 and Fig. 176H.7).

These studies from Brazil, as well another study from Puerto Rico, underscore that the use of the term *Zika fever* may be a misnomer because many patients infected with ZIKV do not have fever.[41,44,76,330,437] This finding was probably best exemplified in the case study of pregnant women from Rio de Janeiro, Brazil, in which fever was only seen in 28% of women and, if present, was typically low grade and transient.[44] Another important clinical feature highlighted by these studies in Brazil is the frequency of pruritus in ZIKV infections, which may help distinguish ZIKV from other arboviral infections such as dengue and chikungunya, in which pruritus appears less frequently,[41] although a case of severe protracted pruritus for 3 weeks secondary to chikungunya has been reported in the literature.[93] In the case series of ZIKV-infected pregnant women, pruritus was observed in nearly all women (90–96%) and accompanied rash.[43,44]

Although the largest case series of acute ZIKV infection are from Yap Island and Brazil,[121,41,44,121,485] similar findings of this nonspecific, mild viral clinical presentation have been reported in other countries, including Mexico,[210] Thailand,[53] and Nicaragua,[459] as well as in the majority of other case reports of travelers returning from Colombia,[291] Puerto Rico,[106] Thailand,[152,201,410,433] Maldives,[225] French Polynesia,[231,481] Dominican Republic,[122] and Suriname.[122] In addition, most ZIKV-confirmed cases in Americans acquired from travel abroad have also been either asymptomatic or have demonstrated only mild clinical disease.[97] Smaller case series of patients presenting with acute ZIKV infection have also been published from Mexico, Panama, and Brazil (Sao Paulo).[16,146,179] A summary table of some of the presenting features of smaller case series since the discovery of ZIKV is available in the literature.[146]

Acute ZIKV Infection in Children

Similar to the WHO definition of a ZIKV infection in any person, the CDC has also released recommendations specific to pediatric patients regarding when to suspect acute ZIKV disease in an infant or child younger than 18 years. This includes having at least two or more clinical manifestations of fever, rash, conjunctivitis, or arthralgia and meeting criteria for ZIKV exposure.[151] Similarly, because maternal-to-child transmission of ZIKV in pregnancy or at delivery is also possible, acute ZIKV disease should also be considered during the first 2 weeks of an infant's life among those with mothers meeting ZIKV exposure and clinical criteria.[151] (ZIKV exposure criteria are discussed further in the ZIKV evaluation and management section).

Apart from those with in utero ZIKV exposure, relatively few reports of children with ZIKV have been published.[12,19,124,151,192,249,318,320] Based on clinical information collected in 2007 from the Yap Islands, which included children, it has been suggested that children have similar symptoms as adults (fever, macular or maculopapular rash, arthralgia, and conjunctivitis) but generally experience more mild ZIKV infection and have lower reported attack rates than adults.[121,151] In sentinel studies of ZIKV surveillance in Rio de Janeiro, very few nonadolescent children with symptomatic ZIKV infection were identified compared with adults (P. Brasil, personal communication, 2016). It is likely that in prepubertal children, ZIKV may be more frequently asymptomatic than in adults.

One brief review of six publications of 10 children with ZIKV infection from various regions of the world, including Cambodia, Colombia, Indonesia, New Caledonia, Nigeria, and the Philippines, also described clinical features of children with ZIKV in the literature from 1954 to 2016.[12,19,124,151,192,217,249,318,320,354] The children ranged in age from 3 to 16 years, but the illness duration was less than 1 week and consisted

TABLE 176H.3 **Clinical Characteristics of Zika Virus–Infected Patients From Studies in Micronesia, Brazil, and Mexico**

	Yap Island, Federated States of Micronesia	Rio de Janeiro, Brazil	Rio de Janeiro, Brazil	Rio de Janeiro, Brazil	Multiple States, Mexico
Reference(s)	121	41	76	43, 44	210
Time period	April–July 2007	January–July 2015	April–June 2015	September 2015–June 2016	November 2015–February 2016
Total no. of cases	49 laboratory confirmed	119 laboratory confirmed	57 laboratory confirmed	134 laboratory confirmed	93 laboratory confirmed
Method of laboratory confirmation	Zika RNA RT-PCR blood or Zika IgM and Zika PRNT90 ≥20 and Zika virus/dengue virus PRNT90 ratio ≥4	Zika RNA RT-PCR blood	Zika RNA RT-PCR blood	Zika RNA RT-PCR blood or urine	
No. of cases surveyed	31	119	57	134	93
Cohort characteristics age	Various ages of children and adults ≥3 y	Adults 37 y (median age)	34 y (median age)	Pregnant women 31 y (median age)	Various ages of children and adults; mean age, 35 y; range, 6–90 y
Sign or symptom	No. of patients (%)	No. of patients (%)	No. of patients (%)	No. of patients (%)[a]	No. of patients (%)[b]
Rash	28 (90%)	115 (97%)	56 (98%)	134 (100%)[c]	(93)%
Rash median or mean duration	6 days	5.5 days	—	5 days	—
Pruritus	—	94 (79%)	32 (56%)	116 (90%)	(81%)
Fever	20 (65%)	43 (36%)	38 (67%)	34 (2.%)	(97%)
Fever median duration	—	≤1 day	—	50% <1 days, 50% <3 days	—
Arthritis or arthralgia	20 (65%)	75 (63%)	33 (58%)	81 (62%)	(72%)/(17%)
Arthritis/arthralgia median duration	3.5 days	9 days	—	—	—
Nonpurulent conjunctivitis	17 (55%)	66 (56%)	22 (39%)	73 (58%)	(89%)
Back pain	—	61 (51%)	—	—	(16%)
Myalgia	15 (48%)	73 (61%)	28 (49%)	53 (41%)	(84%)
Headache	14 (45%)	78 (66%)	38 (67%)	69 (54%)	(85%)
Retroorbital Pain	12 (39%)	53 (45%)	23 (40%)	53 (41%)	(47%)
Lymphadenopathy	—	49 (41%)	—	48 (38%)	(7%)
Edema	6 (19%)	34 (29%)	23% joint swelling	54 (55%)	—
Vomiting	3 (10%)	5 (4%)	—	41 (31%)[d]	(9%)
Hemorrhagic symptoms (mild mucosal bleeding or petechiae)	None	25 (21%)	—	12 (9%)	—
Median CBC values Leukocytes Hematocrit Platelets	—	4590 cells/mm^3 41.2% 201,000 cells/mm^3	—	—	—

[a]Note that denominator for calculating symptom percentages varied and is not necessarily 134.
[b]Only percentages were listed in the original article.
[c]Rash was one of the enrollment criteria for this study.
[d]Includes both nausea and vomiting.
PRNT90, 90% endpoint of the plaque reduction neutralization test; *RT-PCR,* reverse transcriptase polymerase chain reaction.
Data from references 41, 44, 76, 121, 210.

of some of the common nonspecific findings of ZIKV, such as fever, malaise, headache, and myalgia, that have been reported.[217] However, in that brief review, gastrointestinal complaints (abdominal pain, nausea, vomiting, diarrhea) were more frequently reported (seven of 10 children), and rash was not seen.[151,217] Three fatalities in children (all female teenagers from Brazil and Colombia) have also been reported[19,24,191] (for further details, see the later section on Potential Complications Following ZIKV Infection) (Table 176H.4).

Similar findings were noted in the initial unpublished data collected by the CDC in 2016 for eight children and the more recent updated version that now includes 158 cases of travel-acquired ZIKV among children younger than 18 years (range, 1 month to 17 years of age).[151,172] Almost all of the children with ZIKV had rash (82%), about one-half had fever (55%), and more than one-fourth had conjunctivitis (29%) and/or arthralgia (28%).[172]

Other reported symptoms included myalgia, abdominal symptoms (vomiting and diarrhea), retroorbital pain, and sore throat.[172] No complications such as meningitis, encephalitis, septic shock, GBS, or death were noted. However, two children (aged 1 and 4 years) were hospitalized for what appears to be more minor concerns, such as cough, fever, and poor oral intake[172] (see Table 176H.4).

The presentation of ZIKV disease in neonates acquired from perinatal transmission near or at the time of delivery is also unclear apart from what is known from two reported cases.[33,151] In these cases, the mothers

TABLE 176H.4 Pediatric ZIKV Cases in the Literature

Study	Year	Country	No. of Pediatric Cases	Age of Patient (s)	Signs/Symptoms	Other Comorbidities	Outcome	Other Comments
Macnamara et al.[249]	1952	Eastern Nigeria	1	10	Fever, headache	Malaria coinfection	Complete recovery	—
Olson et al.[320]	1977, 1978	Central Java, Indonesia	5	12	Fever (high), malaise, dizziness, GI complaints (abdominal pain, constipation)	—	Unknown	Zika virus cases in this study differ from in others because of high fever, no rash, and GI complaints reported in all patients
				12	Fever (high), malaise, dizziness, GI complaints (anorexia, abdominal pain, constipation), hypotension	—	Unknown	
				13	Fever (high), malaise, GI complaints (anorexia, abdominal pain, constipation), hypotension	—	Unknown	
				14	Fever (high), conjunctivitis, dizziness, arthralgia, myalgia, GI complaints (diarrhea), hematuria	—	Unknown	
				16	Fever (high), malaise, chills, dizziness, GI complaints (anorexia, abdominal pain vomiting, diarrhea), leg pain	—	Unknown	
Duffy et al.[121]	2007	Yap Island, Micronesia	Not specified	Included some children ≥3 y, number not specified	For cohort that included children and adults: fever, rash, conjunctivitis, arthralgia most common; also reports of myalgia, headache, retroorbital pain, edema, vomiting	—	Unknown	Infection generally more mild than in adults and lower attack rates than in adults, although specific comparisons of presentation of children and adults not available
Heang et al.[192]	2010	Kampong Speu Province, Cambodia	1	3	Fever, headache, sore throat, cough	—	Complete recovery	—
Alera et al.[12]	2012	Cebu City, Philippines	1	15	Fever, conjunctivitis, headache, myalgia, GI complaints (abdominal pain, anorexia, nausea, vomiting), sore throat	—	Complete recovery	—
Besnard et al.[33]	2013, 2014	French Polynesia	2	Infant	Asymptomatic	—	Complete recovery	Zika virus perinatal transmission. Infants born to women with Zika had symptoms shortly before (2 days) or after (3 days) delivery
				Infant	Rash, thrombocytopenia	Pregnancy complicated by gestational diabetes and IUGR noted in second trimester, caesarean delivery. Infant with hypotrophy and hypoglycemia, neonatal jaundice, and low birth weight	Complete recovery	

Dupont-Rouzeyrol et al.[124]	2014	New Caledonia and French Polynesia	1	14	Fever, headache, arthralgia, myalgia, asthenia, mild thrombocytopenia and leukopenia	Dengue coinfection	Complete recovery	—
Arzuza-Ortega et al.[19]	2015	Malambo, Northern Colombia	1	15	Fever, malaise, headache, arthralgia, myalgia, GI complaints (abdominal pain and jaundice)	Sickle cell disease (Hb SC)	ICU for ARDS, hemothorax, hepatic necrosis, splenic sequestration, and death	Suspected that ZIKV triggered vasoocclusion crises given history of sickle cell disease
Sarmiento-Ospina et al.[402]	2015	Tolima, Central Colombia	1	2	Fever, altered mental status, jaundice, hepatomegaly, splenomegaly, severe abdominal pain, thrombocytopenia, mucosal hemorrhage, anemia, dehydration	Autopsy revealed probable acute leukemia (lymphoblastic)	ICU for DIC, respiratory distress, shock, and death	
Brazil Ministry of Health[191]	2015	Brazil	1	16	Headache, nausea, petechiae	—	Likely encephalitis and death	—
Azevedo et al.[24]	2016	Brazil	1	16	Headache, fever, malaise, myalagia, rash, and later hemorrhagic findings of petechiae, epistaxis, hematuria, vaginal bleeding, ecchymoses, mild hepatosplenomegaly, thrombocytopenia, anemia	—	Hypovolemic shock and death	—
Mecharles et al.[270]	2016	Guadeloupe	1	15	Headache, conjunctivitis 7 days followed by left hemiparesis, paresthesia, urinary retention, T4 sensory bilateral level	—	Lesions cervical and thoracic spinal cord consistent with acute myelitis; able to walk unassisted after methylprednisolone for 5 days	Zika virus detected serum, urine, and CSF
Fleming-Dutra et al.[151]	2016	US (travel acquired)	8	Not specified	All with rash and ≥1 other sign/symptom such as fever, arthralgia, or conjunctivitis	—	—	—
Goodman et al.[172]	2015–2016	US (travel acquired)	158	Median age 14 y	82% had rash, 55% with fever, 29% conjunctivitis, 28% arthralgias	—	2 hospitalized; no cases of meningitis/encephalitis, GBS, and no fatalities	
Meltzer et al.[274]	2015–16	Israel (travel acquired)	1	2	Not specified but had first occurrence of febrile seizures with normal CSF, neurologic exam, and brain MRI	—	Developed recurrent seizures 3 mo later	

ARDS, Acute respiratory distress syndrome; *CSF,* cerebrospinal fluid; *DIC,* disseminated intravascular coagulation; *GBS,* Guillain-Barré syndrome; *GI,* gastrointestinal; *ICU,* intensive care unit; *IUGR,* intrauterine growth restriction.
Data from Karwowski MP, Nelson JM, Staples JE, et al. Zika virus disease: A CDC update for pediatric health care providers. *Pediatrics.* 2016;137(5):e20160621.

developed ZIKV symptoms either near delivery (2 days prior) or immediately after delivery (3 days after).[33] One infant was symptom free, and the other had a rash and thrombocytopenia, but both made full recoveries without any issues[33,151] (see Table 176H.4). It is known from reports of perinatal transmission of other arboviruses that infection during this period may range from asymptomatic infection to severe infection that may include a neonatal sepsislike presentation with fever, thrombocytopenia, and hemorrhagic complications in those with dengue and chikungunya, as well as reports of rash, meningitis, or encephalitis in those with West Nile virus infection.[151,162,166,315,359] Of note, the CHIMERE study of infants with perinatal chikungunya exposure (in utero exposure) on the French Reunion Island in the Indian Ocean also found high rates of neonatal encephalopathy and global developmental delay, as well as some cases of microcephaly.[167]

Potential Complications Following ZIKV Infection

Excluding the special circumstance of ZIKV infection in pregnancy, the prognosis following ZIKV infection is generally considered favorable, with most of those infected making a full recovery without any lasting sequelae. In fact, a review of 2382 confirmed or probable ZIKV cases in the United States found that only 65 (3%) required hospitalization.[461] However, some reported complications have been observed in patients following acute ZIKV infection.[57] Unusual but reported symptoms that have been seen after acute infection include short-term impairments in hearing, described as having a "dull and metallic" quality, dysgeusia (abnormal taste), recurrent nightmares, seizure disorder, hypertensive iridocyclitis, uveitis, unilateral acute maculopathy, and rare genitourinary symptoms, including hematospermia and prostatitis.[152,153,156,163,274,297,348,432,465] A positive antinuclear antibody test was also reported in a ZIKV-infected patient with exacerbation of severe immune thrombocytopenia, but whether it can lead to other autoimmune diseases such as lupus is for the present time unknown.[484]

In contrast to the hemorrhagic complications that may follow infection with dengue virus, hemorrhagic complications such as hematomas and severe thrombocytopenia (including immune thrombocytopenic purpura with mucosal [palate and vaginal], subcutaneous bleeding, and gross hematuria) after infection with ZIKV are considered rare.[5,61,82,206,215,300,402,409,426,481,484] In a case report of two ZIKV patients in Puerto Rico, both presented with bloody buccal mucosal lesions, which developed the day after resolution of their fever and rash.[409] Both were found to have severe thrombocytopenia (1000 and 2000 platelets/μL).[409] One recovered after receiving intravenous immunoglobulin, whereas the other died after complications from multiple hemorrhages.[409] Based on these recent observations, some have hypothesized that the rare cases of thrombocytopenia seen in patients with acute ZIKV appear to be different than those that complicate dengue infections.[409]

At least 10 cases of death have been reported in adult patients with ZIKV without GBS.[428] Cases of reported death from ZIKV included a patient from the United States,[428,461] four patients from Brazil,[24,191,419] one from Puerto Rico,[5,409] and four from Colombia. Of these was a 2-year-old Colombian child with altered mental status, hepatomegaly, and thrombocytopenia, which evolved to disseminated intravascular coagulation, respiratory distress, and shock.[402,409] Another was a 30-year-old Colombian woman with ZIKV infection that was complicated by severe thrombocytopenia, leukopenia, and later intracerebral and subarachnoid hemorrhages, sepsis, acute respiratory distress, seizures, and shock.[402] Autopsy revealed probable leukemias in the child and woman.[402] Another fatality was reported in a 15-year-old teenager with underlying sickle cell disease (hemoglobin SC disease), who was infected with ZIKV and presented with fever, abdominal pain, myalgia, and jaundice; her infection likely triggered vasoocclusion crises that then caused severe acute respiratory distress, hemothorax, hepatic necrosis, and severe splenic sequestration, which ultimately led to her death.[19] Regarding the Brazilian females who died from ZIKV, two were teenagers, including one that presented with thrombocytopenia, anemia, and hemorrhagic manifestations and died of hypovolemic shock, whereas the other was believed to have encephalitis; another was a young woman with thrombocytopenia, hemorrhages, and pneumonia.[24,191,419] The other fatal case was a Brazilian man with rheumatoid arthritis and lupus, which is described in the next section on Special Populations With Acute ZIKV.[24] The patient from the United States was a 73-year old man who had recently completed radiation therapy for prostate cancer; he died from septic shock with multiple-organ failure from ZIKV after presenting with tachypnea, tachycardia, abdominal pain, pharyngitis, conjunctivitis, diarrhea, fever, and myalgias after a trip to Mexico.[428,461] ZIKV serum testing showed extremely high levels of viremia with 2×10^8 genome copies per milliliter.[428]

Special Populations With Acute ZIKV Infection (HIV-Infected and Other Immunosuppressed Patients)

It is currently unknown whether people with HIV infection or other immunocompromised conditions have a higher risk for acquiring ZIKV infection, are more likely to have symptomatic infection, or suffer from more severe or complicated infection.[369] For other arboviruses such as dengue virus, yellow fever virus, or West Nile virus, the risk for an HIV-infected person acquiring one of these viruses is the same as the general population, but there have been some reports that indicate that HIV-infected adults with severe immunosuppression may have more complications from dengue virus.[194,216,345,369,439] Three cases of ZIKV infection have been reported in HIV-infected adults in Brazil, and all had mild infection.[60,369]

A fatal ZIKV case was reported in a 36-year-old Brazilian man with rheumatoid arthritis and lupus on chronic daily prednisone, who presented with severe denguelike symptoms and respiratory distress.[24] A small series of four patients in Brazil with renal and liver transplants that acquired acute ZIKV infection noted that none of these patients presented with rash or conjunctivitis, but they demonstrated various constellations of symptoms ranging from fever, myalgia, headache, and abdominal symptoms to thrombocytopenia, anemia, and acute graft dysfunction.[311] Although all the patients eventually recovered, complications included bacterial superinfections, and one patient even required repeat liver transplantation from hepatic artery thrombosis and biliary stenosis 3 months after ZIKV infection.[311]

Neurologic Complications Including Guillain-Barré Syndrome

Early animal experiments of ZIKV in the 1950s discovered that ZIKV appeared to be neurotropic, a finding that has corresponded to more recent studies that have demonstrated ZIKV's ability to cause neuron cell death.[51,89,109,237,245] Reported neurologic complications following acute ZIKV infection include encephalopathy, meningoencephalitis (including a case of fatal encephalitis secondary to severe cerebral edema),[419] seizures, acute sensory polyneuropathy, myelitis (including acute disseminated encephalomyelitis), and GBS.*

ZIKV and Guillain-Barré Syndrome

Although GBS may be a rare complication of other bacterial and viral infections, including other arboviral triggers such as Japanese encephalitis virus, West Nile virus, dengue virus, and chikungunya, considerable concern has been expressed over the increased incidence of GBS seen with or following ZIKV infection. GBS, a form of acute or subacute immune-mediated progressive flaccid paralysis, is considered a medical emergency requiring hospitalization and may also pose a risk for death.[64,170,415,479] The scientific community has recently come to the consensus that ZIKV is, indeed, a cause of GBS.[332]

Early observations of the ZIKV epidemic in Brazil appeared to coincide with an increased incidence of GBS and other neurologic complications seen since May 2015, with some having estimated that the incidence of GBS increased fivefold since 2015.[15,45,154] Approximately 49 cases of GBS in patients with a history of recent infection consistent with ZIKV were identified in Bahia, Brazil in July 2015.[469] In Rio de Janeiro, Brazil, the RIO GBS-ZIKV Research Network reported that 17 of 20 patients with GBS seen from December 2015 to March 2016 were suspected to have had a ZIKV infection that preceded the development of GBS symptoms.[149] A study investigating temporal relationships between ZIKV and GBS in Salvador, one of the main epicenters of the ZIKV epidemic in Brazil, determined that the number of GBS cases peaked

*References 15, 17, 20, 45, 64, 67, 113, 114, 116, 136, 154, 218, 270, 272, 296, 308, 314, 349, 391, 392, 408, 414, 461, 480.

5 to 9 weeks after outbreaks of a new acute exanthematous illness were observed in Salvador, Brazil in 2015.[347] The study provided additional support for an association between ZIKV and the development of complications such as GBS.[347] Following these observations in Brazil, in June 2016, the WHO reported that 11 additional countries and territories (Colombia, Dominican Republic, El Salvador, French Guiana, Honduras, Martinique, Suriname, Venezuela, Haiti, Panama, Puerto Rico) demonstrated an increased incidence of GBS cases or reported cases of GBS in the context of ZIKV infection.[218,339,391] Five GBS cases were also identified in returning US travelers with ZIKV infection.[375,461] More recently, a multicountry review of GBS cases in Brazil, Colombia, Dominican Republic, El Salvador, Honduras, Suriname, and Venezuela has suggested a twofold to nearly 10-fold increase in GBS cases above baseline.[116]

GBS case series from French Polynesia, Brazil, Colombia, and Puerto Rico. Before the French Polynesia outbreak, ZIKV was largely believed to be a mild, febrile illness without serious complications.[64] However, during the 2013–14 outbreak in French Polynesia, significant rates of neurologic complications were observed, including GBS, that were not observed in earlier outbreaks such as the one on the Yap Islands.[64,314] To date, the largest study documenting GBS after ZIKV infection was a case-control study during the French Polynesia outbreak, which included 42 GBS cases and provides the strongest evidence, thus far, that ZIKV is a cause of GBS (odds ratio [OR], >34).[64,352] Of these patients, rapid deterioration was frequently noted, with 16 (38%) requiring intensive care admission and 12 (29%) requiring mechanical ventilation.[250,323] Some have estimated that the incidence of GBS in French Polynesia was 0.24 to 0.41 per 1000 ZIKV infections, which would have constituted as high as a 21-fold increase in GBS incidence.[64,479] Of note, none of the cases of GBS in the French Polynesia study were in children.[151]

Three additional case series of GBS patients from Colombia (two series) and Puerto Rico (one series) have also been reported. One included 68 patients with GBS, most of whom had the acute inflammatory demyelinating polyneuropathy GBS subtype. Almost all presented with limb weakness (97%), many reported paresthesias (76%) and facial palsy (32%), and about one-half (50%) had bilateral facial paralysis on examination.[349] Nearly one-third (31%) required mechanical ventilation, and three patients died from respiratory failure and sepsis.[349] Prolonged ZIKV viruria was also noted in patients with GBS and was reported in another case series.[391] Another case series of 19 patients with GBS from Colombia with a mean age of 44 years has also provided important information.[17] The majority required respiratory ventilation (79%) and received intravenous immunoglobulin treatment (84%), with a few (16%) requiring plasmapheresis; severe disability (Hughes scale 4–5: chair-bound or bedridden and/or requiring ventilation assistance for at least part of the day) was noted in most (80%) on discharge.[17] In both studies the mean time to development of GBS after ZIKV symptoms was 7 to 10 days.[17,349] Both studies also found that the majority (80–82%) had albuminocytologic dissociation of the cerebrospinal fluid (CSF) (i.e., increased protein levels without pleocytosis).[17,349] Another review of 56 patients with GBS from Puerto Rico, of whom 76% had confirmed or presumed ZIKV infection, reported that the majority had acute illness 5 days before development of GBS symptoms and 35% required ventilation (35%).[113] All required hospitalization and were treated with standard GBS treatment of intravenous immunoglobulin G, but one patient died from complications of septic shock.[113]

ZIKV in Pregnancy and Congenital ZIKV Syndrome (Microcephaly and Other Congenital Complications)

Although it is believed that pregnant and nonpregnant women present similarly with acute ZIKV infection in terms of infectious symptoms, ZIKV infection in pregnancy presents unique challenges because it may have devastating consequences on the developing fetus.[133] In 2015, based on novel observations of infants exposed to ZIKV infection during pregnancy in Brazil, unprecedented global alarm was raised about the potential of ZIKV to cause congenital anomalies, including microcephaly.[284,352,393,399] The PAHO subsequently issued alerts to its member states based on the troubling observations in Brazil. Additional evidence, including subsequent detection of ZIKV RNA from fetal brain and amniotic fluid specimens from fetuses and infants with microcephaly, ultimately led to involvement of the European Centre for Disease Prevention and Control and the US CDC.[406] By February 2016, the WHO declared ZIKV a "Public Health Emergency of International Concern."[467,406]

Since then, leaders at the WHO and CDC have come to the scientific consensus that ZIKV infection is a cause of microcephaly, and ZIKV is now considered to be the first major infectious disease associated with congenital birth defects to be discovered in more than half a century.[73,322,332,352,385] As summarized in a special review published in the *New England Journal of Medicine* employing Shepard's Criteria for Proof of Human Teratogenicity to ZIKV, the causal relationship between in utero ZIKV infection and microcephaly and other brain anomalies was substantiated by several factors: temporal relationship of ZIKV infection in pregnancy and anomalies observed; the otherwise rare phenotypic condition of microcephaly and other brain anomalies seen in fetuses and/or infants with congenital ZIKV infection; and detection of virus from brain tissue of ZIKV-infected fetuses and/or infants suggesting "biologic plausibility."[385] It has been suggested that ZIKV infection in pregnancy and sequelae may be due to direct infection of the trophoblast, viral invasion across the placenta, movement of infected cells leading to embryonic infection, or resulting effects of inflammatory cytokines released from infected placenta as well as ZIKV activation of neural cells' TLR3 paths that then lead to neural cell death and thus fetal pathology seen in ZIKV-exposed infants.[223]

Per CDC definitions, congenital ZIKV is confirmed by a positive serum or urine ZIKV PCR collected ideally within the first 2 days of life.[395] Whereas, a diagnosis of "probable congenital ZIKV infection" is based on a positive infant ZIKV immunoglobulin M (IgM) test with a negative ZIKV PCR.[395] Although complete understanding of the complete spectrum of congenital anomalies that may be caused by ZIKV is still in evolution, reports of infants with congenital ZIKV have begun to describe a wide array of potential anomalies associated with in utero ZIKV infection. Lessons can be learned from other well-known viral congenital infections such as cytomegalovirus (CMV) and rubella, which have demonstrated the adverse effects these infections may have on the developing fetus, including the ability to affect hearing, vision, cognition, and motor development among others.[88,223] It is believed that congenital ZIKV infection may also have the potential to cause widespread effects on the developing fetus with the most detrimental effects occurring during exposure in the first two trimesters of pregnancy.[44,224,352]

Although early reports of ZIKV's effects in pregnancy had primarily focused on microcephaly, later reports have described a host of other significant congenital anomalies; in fact, microcephaly appears to be just the tip of the iceberg.[317] In response to these observations of distinctive congenital anomalies observed in infants with in utero ZIKV exposure, the term *congenital Zika syndrome* was introduced. Based on preliminary studies, classic findings of congenital ZIKV syndrome now include fetal brain disruption sequence phenotype (severe microcephaly, craniofacial disproportion including collapse of skull and overriding cranial sutures, biparietal depression, prominent occiput, excess nuchal or scalp skin, and neurologic impairment), intracranial calcifications, eye abnormalities as well as sequelae of fetal akinesia deformation syndrome, including arthrogryposis (congenital contractures) and clubfoot.[59,77,87,255,273,283,385,406] It is important to note that these brain anomalies may be observed in infants with or without microcephaly at birth. Many fetuses are also noted to have intrauterine growth restriction (IUGR).[43,455] In addition, other adverse pregnancy outcomes, including miscarriage, stillbirth, and hydrops fetalis (with hydrothorax, ascites, and subcutaneous edema) have also been reported.[44,255,256,404,444]

Specifically, the other congenital brain anomalies described with ZIKV include cerebral calcifications, gyral pattern anomalies, cerebellar and brainstem hypoplasia, absence of the corpus callosum, ventricular dilation, and hydranencephaly.* Reviews of literature and neuroimaging cases have suggested the most common brain abnormalities seen with congenital ZIKV syndrome apart from microcephaly include (1) diffuse intraparenchymal calcifications (often punctate, at the corticomedullary junction of the frontal/parietal lobes but may also be in the basal ganglia

*References 44, 90, 101, 104, 212, 238, 273, 284, 289, 317, 351, 352, 403, 448, 450, 466.

and cerebellum), (2) ventriculomegaly, and (3) cortical development malformations (abnormal gyration patterns).[287,455,483]

These congenital neurologic abnormalities observed with in utero ZIKV infection, primarily characterized by severe fetal brain destruction, is most reminiscent of other congenital infections such as CMV, lymphocytic choriomeningitis virus, and toxoplasmosis, although to a lesser degree.[455] Nevertheless, the presence of certain features of congenital ZIKV syndrome appear to help distinguish it from these other congenital infections.[287] These findings include the severe microcephaly with partial skull collapse, the thin cerebral cortex with calcifications, dysgenesis of the corpus callosum, congenital contractures (including arthrogryposis along with early and severe hypertonia with extrapyramidal symptoms), macular scarring, and focal pigmentary retinal mottling.[287]

Arthrogryposis, which has been reported in 5.7% to 11% of congenital ZIKV cases, is thought to be due to the damage to upper and lower motor neurons.[287,445] It may involve upper or lower limbs (proximal or distal) and may vary in severity.[287,445] In extreme cases, bilateral congenital hip dislocation and even partial or full knee dislocation have been reported.[287,445] Apart from arthrogryposis, other findings of fetal akinesia disruption sequence include isolated clubfoot, which has been seen in 3.8% to 14% of cases of congenital ZIKV.[287] Other neurologic problems observed in these infants include seizures, tremors, posturing, hypertonia with spasticity, severe irritability, and dysphagia.[43,287,446]

Sensorineural hearing loss (in 6% of cases of congenital ZIKV infants with microcephaly), including severe bilateral hearing loss, has also been described.[238,239] In addition, ocular abnormalities in infants with congenital ZIKV also appear to be common, ranging from 35% to 46% of infants with microcephaly and intracerebral calcifications to as many as 100% of these infants in some small case series.[104,443,448,449] One study suggested that infants with ocular findings were more likely to have smaller cephalic perimeters and have been born to women who had ZIKV symptoms during the first trimester of pregnancy.[449] ZIKV ocular abnormalities described include focal retinal pigment mottling, chorioretinal atrophy, optic nerve changes, lens subluxation, loss of foveal reflex, iris colobomas, microophthalmia, cataracts, intraocular calcifications, and myopia, among others.[104,282,287,443,448-450] Interestingly enough, active chorioretinitis, a classic finding in congenital infections, has not yet been reported with congenital ZIKV, and pathology of the posterior eye has been more commonly seen.[287]

Microcephaly and Other Congenital Cerebral Abnormalities

Although ZIKV is now considered to be a cause of microcephaly, the condition itself can be due to a variety of etiologies, including other congenital infections (rubella, toxoplasmosis, CMV), severe malnutrition, fetal ischemia during development, chromosomal changes, craniosynostosis, metabolic disorders, and in utero exposure to drugs, alcohol, and other environmental toxins.[84,367,386,406,454] Historically, in the general population microcephaly is considered a rare clinical finding; it is characterized by a small head and typically reflects brain growth disturbances during development that often lead to developmental delay, vision and hearing impairment, and other neurologic problems such as seizures. Specifically, it is believed that disruption to the fetal brain growth sequence can lead to fetal skull collapse, which ultimately can give rise to microcephaly.[352] Microcephaly prevalence was previously reported to be 0.5 to 2 per 10,000 live births in Brazil and 1.9 to 2 per 10,000 live births in the United States and Europe.[57,68,129,352,367,420] (See Figs. 176H.8 and 176H.9E for depictions of microcephaly.)

The definitions of microcephaly have varied by country and have been one challenging aspect impeding accurate monitoring of microcephaly incidence in the setting of ZIKV.[217] Some have defined microcephaly as head circumference (occipitofrontal) less than the 3rd percentile or less than 2 standard deviations (SD) for gestational age and sex, with severe microcephaly being defined as less than 3 SD for gestational age and sex.[217,352,452] The working microcephaly case definition used by the CDC is head circumference less than the 3rd percentile adjusted for gestational age and sex.[71,151,354,363] (In Brazil, since December 2015, the Ministry of Health has been using a case definition of microcephaly as a head circumference ≤32 cm in any full-term newborn or <2 SD for gestational age and sex for premature infants in their surveillance, but had previously used the definition of ≥3 SD below the mean for gestational age and sex, which is more restrictive and would correspond to 30.3 cm for females and 30.7 cm for males; this was followed by a temporary change in ad hoc surveillance definitions in November 2015 to ≤33 cm before the new case definition was being used.[224,452])

Another important consideration regarding the characterization of microcephaly is whether it is proportional or disproportional. It should be noted that microcephaly is generally a postnatal diagnosis that cannot be clearly ascertained by fetal ultrasound. IUGR will render an infant who is universally small for gestational age (SGA), a finding that has been reported in ZIKV congenital infection.[43,44,455] For gestational age, these SGA infants may be considered microcephalic; however, microcephaly in this instance would be proportional to the infant's overall size. In contrast, most reports of microcephaly in ZIKV-infected infants describe disproportionate microcephaly, in which the head circumference

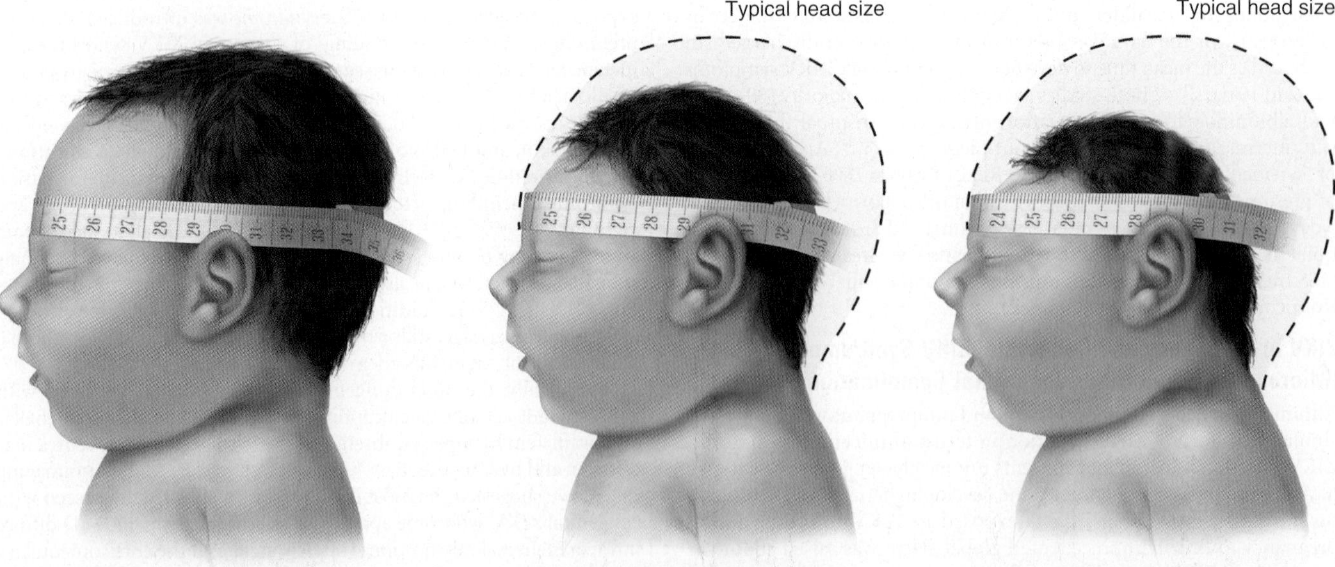

FIGURE 176H.8 Depiction of measurements of typical infant head size, microcephaly, and severe microcephaly. (From Centers for Disease Control and Prevention. Zika virus: information for clinicians. June 13, 2016. https://www.cdc.gov/zika/hc-providers/qa-pediatrician.html.)

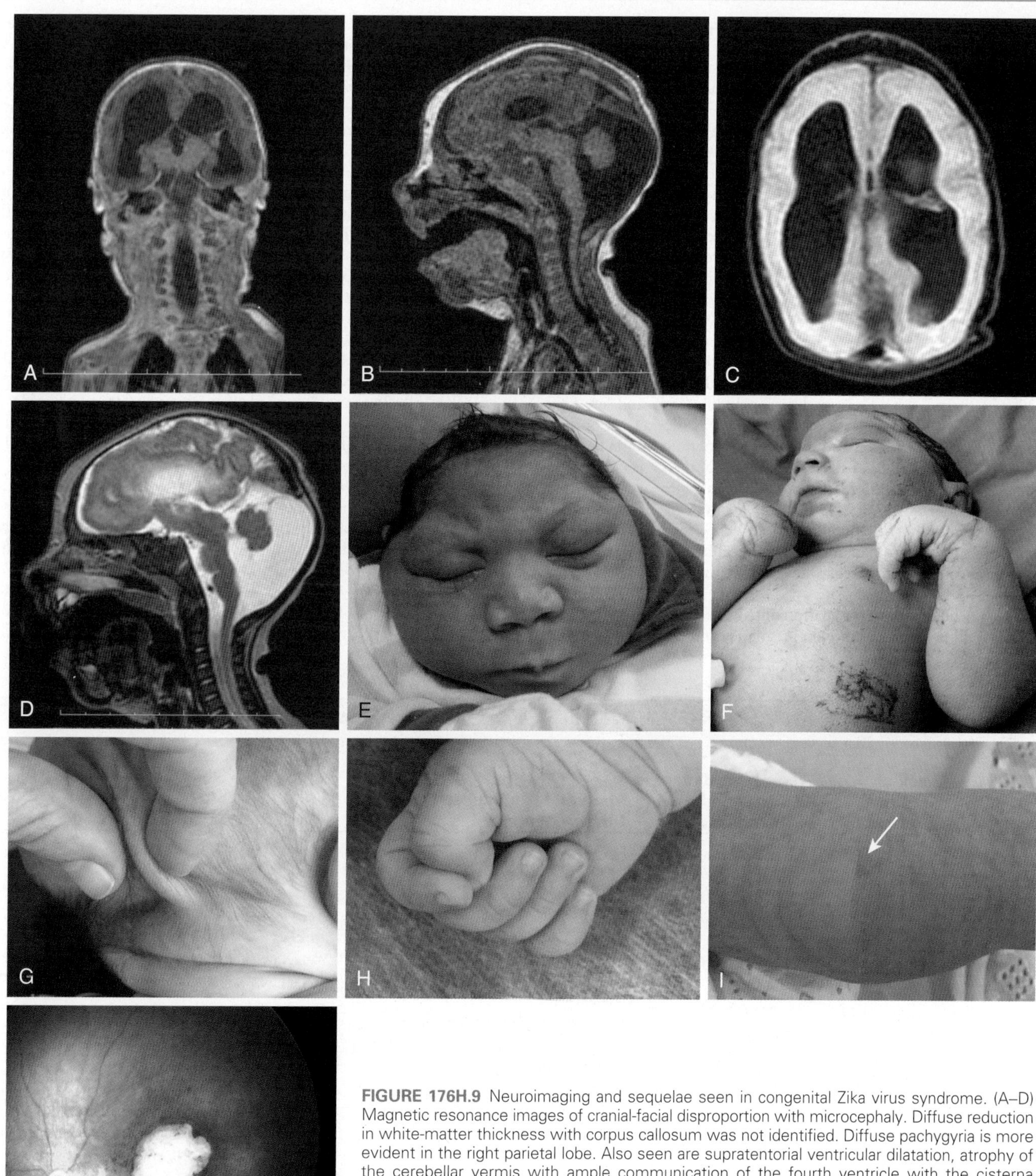

FIGURE 176H.9 Neuroimaging and sequelae seen in congenital Zika virus syndrome. (A–D) Magnetic resonance images of cranial-facial disproportion with microcephaly. Diffuse reduction in white-matter thickness with corpus callosum was not identified. Diffuse pachygyria is more evident in the right parietal lobe. Also seen are supratentorial ventricular dilatation, atrophy of the cerebellar vermis with ample communication of the fourth ventricle with the cisterna magna, and widening of the perivascular spaces of the cerebellar hemispheres with surrounding gliosis. (E–J) Clinical features of Zika virus infection in infants. (E) Disproportionate microcephaly. (F) Arthrogryposis at birth. (G) Redundant scalp. (H) Cortical thumb. (I) Knee fovea. (J) Left infant retina demonstrating optic disc hypoplasia, peripapillary atrophy, and macular chorioretinal atrophy with a colobomatous-like aspect with hyperpigmented halo and pigmentary mottling. (From Brasil P, Pereira JP Jr, Moreira ME, et al. Zika virus infection in pregnant women in Rio de Janeiro. *N Engl J Med.* 2016;375[24]:2321-2334.)

does not correspond to other anthropometric measures, including weight and length.[165]

ZIKV Cases in Pregnant Women in Brazil, French Polynesia, Other Latin American Countries, and the United States

ZIKV cases in pregnant women in Brazil. After recognition of clusters of a febrile rash illness observed in Northeastern Brazil since late 2014, which was later attributed to ZIKV transmission, with confirmed subsequent transmission in all five regions of the country, a substantial increase in cases of microcephaly was reported to the Ministry of Health in Brazil in October 2015.[224] By January 2016, a total of 3530 suspected microcephaly cases had been reported, which was a significant increase over the 0.5 to 0.6 cases per 10,000 live births previously reported.[224,406] A Brazilian Zika Embryopathy Task Force was then established to review cases of microcephaly born to mothers with suspected ZIKV infection during pregnancy.[406] One study analyzing data on microcephaly and ZIKV-infected pregnant women from the Bahia state in northeast Brazil has estimated that the risk for microcephaly following ZIKV infection during pregnancy ranges from 0.88% to 13.2%.[211,263]

Because the majority of cases of global ZIKV-associated microcephaly have occurred in Brazil, many of the early reports from Brazil were critical in supplying evidence linking ZIKV infection with microcephaly and other cerebral anomalies (see Table 176H.1). Reports from Brazil also continue to provide important information that has helped define the range of sequelae resulting from the congenital ZIKV epidemic. One of the two major epidemiologic studies providing evidence for a causal relationship between ZIKV and congenital anomalies such as microcephaly and other cerebral anomalies seen on fetal ultrasound was a preliminary report of 72 pregnant women in Rio de Janeiro enrolled with PCR-confirmed ZIKV from September 2015 to February 2016 at various gestational ages (5–38 weeks).[44] Although clinical infection in these women was mild, fetal anomalies were detected by ultrasound in 29% of them.[44] Fetal abnormalities, including early and late fetal death, IUGR with and without microcephaly, CNS lesions, abnormal amniotic fluid, and cerebral and umbilical artery flow anomalies were observed[44] (Table 176H.5). A subsequent report of the same prospective cohort revealed that in 125 ZIKV-affected pregnancies, overall adverse outcomes occurred in 46%, including fetal death in 7% of pregnancies. In addition, among 117 live infants born to PCR-proven ZIKV-infected women, 42% of infants had abnormal clinical or neuroimaging, with adverse outcomes noted regardless of the trimester of maternal infection.[43]

Early Brazilian case reports also contributed to the accumulating evidence linking ZIKV infection in pregnancy and congenital sequelae such as microcephaly. One was a case study of two pregnant women with fetal microcephaly and clinical manifestations of acute ZIKV infection (fever, myalgia, and rash).[59] ZIKV was recovered from the amniotic fluid in both women, and the full ZIKV genome was sequenced from one of them.[59] The study demonstrated that ZIKV had the capability to breech placental barriers, and sequencing of the virus' genome revealed that the ZIKV strain circulating in Brazil likely originated from the outbreak in French Polynesia.[59] Similarly, another case report detailed the evaluation of brain and placental tissue from two miscarriages and two newborns born to mothers from Rio Grande do Norte with symptomatic ZIKV infection in pregnancy.[256] Histopathologic changes in the neonates' brains showed parenchymal calcification, microglial nodules, gliosis, cell degeneration, and necrosis but did not show other organ tissue abnormalities.[256] Placental tissue from one of the miscarriages showed heterogeneous chorionic villi with calcification, fibrosis, perivillous fibrin deposition, and patchy intervillositis and focal villisitis.[256] The ZIKV RT-PCR assay was also positive, and the complete ZIKV genome was again recovered.[256] In addition, compatible findings with ZIKV infection were also noted on autopsy of a fetus of a European woman with a history of suspected ZIKV infection while living in Brazil during the end of her first trimester.[284] The fetus had microcephaly, agyria, hydrocephalus, and calcifications of the brain and placenta.[284] Electron microscopy of fetal brain tissue appeared to demonstrate viral replication in the brain.[284] Investigators noted that ZIKV also appeared to be able to damage the placenta based on placental pathology, but ZIKV was not detected in other fetal organs apart from the brain, which reinforced findings of other studies suggesting ZIKV's neurotropism.[284]

Preliminary results from the first case-control study of microcephaly and congenital ZIKV from Recife, one of the epicenters of microcephaly

TABLE 176H.5 Preliminary Prenatal Ultrasound Findings From Pregnant Women With Zika Virus Infection in Rio de Janeiro, Brazil

No. of Fetuses	Week of Gestation at Infection	Week of Gestation at Ultrasound Examination	Abnormal Findings on Doppler Ultrasonography	Findings at Birth
19	8	35	Microcephaly, cerebral calcifications, abnormal middle cerebral artery, intrauterine growth restriction	Microcephaly, cerebral calcifications on CT, global cerebral atrophy, macular lesions
40	8	20	Choroid plexus cyst, cerebellar atrophy (transverse diameter <5th percentile)	Still in utero
24	12	29	Microcephaly, cerebral calcification, Blake's cyst, agenesis vermis, club foot, intrauterine growth restriction	Still in utero
41	12	24	Mega cisterna magna (>95th percentile)	Still in utero
39	21	30	Cerebellar and cerebral right periventricular calcifications	Still in utero
17	22	26	Middle cerebral artery flow <5th percentile	Still in utero
12	22	27	Microcephaly, placental insufficiency as assessed by Doppler study, oligohydramnios, intrauterine growth restriction	Small for gestational age, head circumference proportional to body size, macular lesions
10	25	30	Normal first ultrasonogram, fetal death detected at 36 weeks on repeat ultrasonogram	Stillbirth
36	26	35	Microcephaly, abnormal umbilical artery flow (>95th percentile on the pulsatile index), intrauterine growth restriction	Small for gestational age, head circumference proportional to body size
38	27	35	Cerebral calcifications, ventriculomegaly, brachycephaly	Still in utero
2	30	34	None	Normal at birth
3	31	33	None	Normal at birth
53	32	38	Fetal death	Stillbirth
23	35	40	Anhydramnios, intrauterine growth restriction	Normal growth measure, poor sucking reflex, EEG abnormalities

CT, Computed tomography; *EEG*, electroencephalogram.

From Brasil P, Pereira JP Jr, Raja Gabaglia C, et al. Zika virus infection in pregnant women in Rio de Janeiro: preliminary report. *N Engl J Med*. 2016;375(24):2321-2334.

cases in Brazil, also reported a strong association between congenital ZIKV and microcephaly (OR, 55.5; 95% CI, 8.6–∞), which was even higher for those cases of microcephaly with other brain abnormalities identified by imaging (OR, 113.3; 95% CI, 14.5–∞); 41% of microcephaly cases and none of controls had laboratory-confirmed ZIKV.[42,99] Although these preliminary results from the 32 infant cases with microcephaly and 62 controls provide additional evidence supporting ZIKV as a cause of microcephaly, the results of the complete study (200 cases and 400 controls anticipated) will be reported when available.[261]

Other studies from the Bahia State have also found ecologic evidence of a temporal relationship between maternal ZIKV infection during pregnancy and microcephaly.[347,387] In 2015, it was noted that suspected cases of microcephaly in Salvador, Brazil peaked 30 to 33 weeks after the emergence of acute exanthematous illness outbreaks.[347] Similar conclusions were drawn from another study of 574 microcephaly cases in Brazil that established both temporal and geospatial evidence linking ZIKV disease in the first trimester of pregnancy with increased prevalence of microcephaly.[224] However, findings of one study and a case report have suggested that even ZIKV infection in the third trimester of pregnancy may lead to serious neurologic damage in the developing fetus.[43,421]

The studies from Brazil on microcephaly, congenital brain anomalies, and ZIKV have demonstrated that our knowledge about ZIKV congenital syndrome is quickly evolving. Of the 20 Brazilian states reporting cases of microcephaly, the state of Pernambuco initially reported the most, with 874 reported cases.[277,406] A preliminary analysis of 104 microcephaly cases (defined as head circumference <3% for gestational age and sex) in Pernambuco was conducted by the CDC and published in June 2016 and demonstrates the frequency and extent of neurologic damage seen in congenital ZIKV cases.[277] Approximately 67% of these infants had severe microcephaly with a head circumference of <30 cm^3. Of the 58 infants who underwent radiographic imaging, nearly all (93%) had calcifications, which were primarily localized to the cortical and subcortical junctions, although some were also seen in the periventricular region, basal ganglia, thalamus, midbrain, and cerebellum.[276] Many infants (69%) also had cortical development malformations, including neuronal cell migration abnormalities such as lissencephaly ("smooth brain"), pachygyria (malformed cortical folds with "thick gyri"), and agyria (lack of cortical folds).[276] Many infants (66%) also had ventriculomegaly due to cortical or subcortical atrophy.[276] Similar findings were seen in other, smaller series of infants with congenital ZIKV infection, in whom calcifications, cortical development malformations, decreased brain volume, ventriculomegaly, and hypoplasia of the brainstem or cerebellum were extremely common.[101,293,406] Redundant scalp skin and arthrogryposis resulting from central and peripheral nervous system damage following in utero cerebral growth arrest were also common findings, and some had detectable IgM antibodies to ZIKV in their CSF[101,406] (see Fig. 176H.9).

Yet, it may be also important to keep in mind that although microcephaly is one potential marker of the ZIKV congenital syndrome, focusing on microcephaly alone may underestimate the true magnitude of this major epidemic.[157] This idea is underscored by recent findings of a report evaluating 13 Brazilian infants from the states of Pernambuco and Ceará with prenatal ZIKV exposure who developed microcephaly after birth.[446] At birth these infants were not microcephalic, but they had abnormal findings on neuroimaging, with nearly all having decreased brain volume (92%), ventriculomegaly (85%), calcifications (100%), or cortical malformations (100%).[446] In addition, all infants had decreases in their rate of head circumference growth after birth, and 11 of 13 (85%) were ultimately given a diagnosis of postnatal or secondary microcephaly.[446] Other common findings included hypertonia (100%), pyramidal and extrapyramidal signs (92%), dysphagia (77%), no voluntary hand movement (69%), epilepsy (54%), irritability (39%), arthrogryposis or hip dysplasia (23%), and chorioretinal abnormalities of the eye (23%).[446]

Although long-term outcomes of infants with congenital ZIKV syndrome are still under investigation, one study of 48 Brazilian infants with probable congenital ZIKV syndrome (all with abnormal neuroimaging) evaluated over the first 1 to 8 months of life has provided some early insight into some of their long-term health issues.[293] Common chronic issues included irritability (85%); pyramidal/extrapyramidal syndrome (56%), including hypertonia, clonus, and hyperreflexia; epileptic seizures (50%); dysphagia (15%); and orthopedic morbidities associated with congenital clubfoot (10%) and arthrogryposis (10%).[293] Similar to the previously mentioned study, three infants with abnormal neuroimaging but without microcephaly at birth were later noted to have microcephaly postnatally, which underscores the importance of close monitoring of postnatal growth parameters, particularly head circumference.[293]

Reports from the Brazilian Ministry of Health at the end of July 2016 have also begun to question whether other factors apart from ZIKV may have contributed to the number of ZIKV-related microcephaly cases in Brazil because the majority of cases of microcephaly (90%) were from only a small region of the country (Northeast Brazil) and primarily were among poor, young, single, black pregnant women. These findings have prompted questions about the possibility of other biologic and socioeconomic factors, including coinfections with dengue and chikungunya, low yellow fever vaccination rates, and even the bovine viral diarrhea virus, of which proteins have been recovered from three fetuses with microcephaly.[56] Another hypothesis for contributing factors for the microcephaly epidemic, particularly in Northeast Brazil, focused on the use of the larvicide pyriproxyfen in potable water tanks, but ecological studies have not supported any association.[11] Thus far, no contributing factors to the ZIKV-associated microcephaly and congenital cerebral anomalies epidemic in Brazil have been identified. An alternative explanation is that ZIKV attack rate in Northeastern Brazil was exceedingly high, with most of the population becoming infected.

ZIKV cases in pregnant women in French Polynesia. After the announcement of observations of congenital anomalies such as microcephaly observed in Brazil during the 2015 ZIKV outbreak, researchers recently retrospectively reviewed 19 cases of infants with congenital cerebral malformations and dysfunction born from pregnancies during the 2013–14 French Polynesia ZIKV epidemic.[32] From 2014 to 2015, in the year following the French Polynesia ZIKV epidemic, an increase in congenital brain malformations was observed there, which included cerebral malformations (2-fold), brainstem dysfunction (31-fold), and severe microcephaly (14-fold) increases in fetuses and newborn infants.[32] Cerebral lesions included septal and callosal disruption, ventriculomegaly, abnormal neuronal migration, cerebellar hypoplasia, occipital pseudocysts, and brain calcifications.[32] ZIKV RNA was also isolated retrospectively from amniotic fluid in four of seven cases with severe neurologic impairment, demonstrating in utero ZIKV infection.[32]

An additional retrospective modeling study of microcephaly cases from 2013 to 2015 in French Polynesia by the same group of researchers suggested that the cluster of cases of microcephaly could best be explained by ZIKV infection in the first trimester of pregnancy, and the risk for microcephaly was 95 cases (95% CI, 34–191) per 10,000 pregnant women infected in the first trimester (or 0.95%),[211] which greatly exceeded the baseline microcephaly prevalence of 2 cases (95% CI, 0–8) per 10,000 neonates in that region.[68]

ZIKV cases in pregnant women in Colombia and other Latin American countries. After recognition of the Brazilian ZIKV outbreak, monitoring quickly became established in other Latin American countries, including Colombia in August 2015, where the first laboratory-confirmed cases of ZIKV were reported in October 2015. Initially, there were 50 reported cases of microcephaly, of which 20 were determined to be due to causes other than ZIKV.[343] As of December 29, 2016, there have been approximately 72 infants born with congenital ZIKV syndrome in Colombia.[335,338,343] In addition, early findings from some of the studies in Brazil,[44] as well as from French Polynesia,[69] have also prompted hypotheses, including whether symptomatic ZIKV infection may be a predictor of ZIKV complications such as fetal abnormalities in pregnant women.[70,159] However, four cases of infants in Colombia with congenital ZIKV were born to women with asymptomatic ZIKV infection in pregnancy, and additional analyses evaluating the severity of ZIKV infection in pregnancy with infant outcomes have failed to substantiate those earlier hypotheses.[265,343]

Two case reports of pregnant European women traveling to Latin American countries have provided additional insight into the timing and pathogenesis of ZIKV-induced complications in pregnancy. One case was a woman traveling to several Latin American countries (Mexico,

Guatemala, and Belize) during 11 weeks' gestation, who became symptomatic after contracting ZIKV infection.[119] Seven weeks after resolution of her symptoms, her sequential fetal ultrasounds at 19 and 20 weeks showed fetal intracranial anomalies with diffuse cerebral cortical thinning and significant decrease in head circumference.[119] Maternal viremia (ZIKV RNA RT-PCR) was still detected at 4 and 10 weeks after clinical ZIKV infection, which was hypothesized to be due to high levels of fetal or placental viral replication.[119] Postmortem fetal autopsy revealed high ZIKV loads from fetal brain, membranes, umbilical cord, and placenta; histopathology demonstrated significant apoptosis of intermediately differentiated postmigratory neurons and isolation of ZIKV from fetal brain tissue.[119] The other case was a woman visiting Suriname at 6 to 7 weeks' gestation whose pregnancy was complicated by ZIKV infection and miscarriage at 11 weeks' gestation.[444] Histopathologic analysis determined evidence of ZIKV infecting amniotic epithelial and fetal mesenchymal cells, particularly the perichondrium.[444] These findings suggested ZIKV replication in pluripotent amniotic stem cells, which are critical in early embryonic development.[444]

ZIKV Cases in Pregnant Women in the United States and US Territories

A summary report released by the CDC noted that by March 2016, 3335 pregnant women in the United States had received ZIKV testing, with only 28 (0.8%) having confirmed ZIKV infection.[97] Overall, the percentage of symptom-free pregnant women tested for ZIKV, who had the infection, was very low (0.3%).[97] In fact, more than 99% of these symptom-free pregnant women tested for ZIKV did not have the infection, whereas 64% of pregnant women with confirmed ZIKV had at least one of the typical ZIKV-associated symptoms.[97] Current aggregate data from the CDC's US Zika Pregnancy Registry, updated on December 13, 2016, revealed that there are more than 1246 pregnant women with laboratory evidence of possible ZIKV infection and another 2701 women in the US Territories (American Samoa, Puerto Rico, and the US Virgin Islands).[371] Of these women with outcomes available in the United States as of December 29, 2016, there have been 39 cases of congenital ZIKV syndrome.[370] Some have estimated that as many as 100 to 270 cases of congenital microcephaly from ZIKV will follow the epidemic in Puerto Rico.[132] A preliminary report of 442 completed pregnancies found that ZIKV-related birth defects were observed in 6% of pregnancies, with no difference for pregnant women with symptomatic versus asymptomatic infection.[198] ZIKV-related birth defects were as high as 11% when ZIKV infection occurred in the first trimester, and the rate of microcephaly for completed pregnancies was 4% (18 cases).[198] (Refer to the CDC webpage for the most recent released data at http://www.cdc.gov/zika/geo/pregwomen-uscases.html.)

The full extent of problems that ZIKV may cause in pregnancy is an evolving story and currently under intense investigation by researchers around the world. At the present time, there is no evidence that prior infection with ZIKV will negatively affect future pregnancies.[363] However, the true impact of ZIKV infection in women of childbearing age and the degree of chronic morbidities faced by infants with congenital ZIKV infection remain to be seen.

ZIKV DIAGNOSIS, MANAGEMENT, TREATMENT, AND PREVENTION

ZIKV Diagnostics

Accurate diagnosis of acute ZIKV infection is difficult to make based on clinical presentation because of significant overlap in symptoms of ZIKV with dengue virus and chikungunya as well as a broad differential of other infections with a rash that may be considered. Infections in the differential diagnosis of ZIKV include other flavivirus infections (dengue, West Nile virus, yellow fever), malaria, leptospirosis, rickettsia, other alpha viruses (chikungunya, Mayaro, Ross River, Barmah Forest, O'nyong-nyong, and Sindbis viruses), other viral illnesses associated with exanthems such as parvovirus B19, enterovirus, rubella, measles, adenovirus, herpesviruses (CMV, Epstein-Barr virus, human herpesvirus type 6), and acute HIV infection.[346,364,460]

Historical Methods for ZIKV Evaluation

Historically, viral cultures have been used for ZIKV research, but these are not available for routine clinical use.[460] ZIKV can be cultured in several cell lines, including African green monkey (Vero), rhesus monkey kidney (LL-MK2), *Aedes pseudoscutellaris* (MOS61 or AP61), and *Aedes albopictus* (C6/36).[460] (See also earlier section on Viral Pathogenesis.) In early animal studies, for successful isolation of the virus, intracerebral mouse inoculation was required.[111,112,182,232,460] Early studies of ZIKV infection in humans were based on seroepidemiologic studies of ZIKV neutralizing antibodies detected in serum, which even then observed some cross-reactivity of ZIKV antibodies with those of dengue and yellow fever virus.* Since 2008, RT-PCR has been used to detect ZIKV RNA in a variety of specimens, including serum, plasma, urine, saliva, amniotic fluid, breast milk, and tissues.[25,143,458,460] Recently, whole blood was also included as a specimen option for RT-PCR per CDC guidelines.[14] Specific ZIKV RT-PCR assays that were used from 2008 to 2014, including the type of RT-PCR, source, primer/probe, sequence, and position, are available in the literature.[460]

Current Methods for ZIKV Evaluation

At present, the primary methods available for diagnostic testing of ZIKV include RT-PCR, serology (IgM) including neutralizing antibodies by plaque reduction neutralization test (PRNT), and immunohistochemical staining.[362,363] In the United States, testing is primarily done at the CDC. Some state health departments and commercial laboratories have efforts underway to expand diagnostic capabilities in several states. It is recommended that clinicians contact their state health departments to facilitate any ZIKV diagnostic testing.[362,363]

Acute Phase ZIKV Testing Using RT-PCR–Based Methods

During the acute phase of the illness, ZIKV RT-PCR may be used to detect virus RNA from clinical specimens, depending on the time of presentation after the onset of clinical symptoms.[205,362] It was previously recommended that ZIKV RT-PCR from serum only be used early in the illness (<7 days after clinical illness onset), whereas urine (<14 days after illness onset) may be used for a longer period after the onset of symptoms.[205,363] However, based on newer CDC guidelines from November 2016, it is now recommended that *both* serum and urine be collected from all patients with symptoms who present less than 14 days after onset of their symptoms in order to test using ZIKV RNA RT-PCR.[72] Whole blood may also be collected along with serum because ZIKV RNA may be detected for longer periods in whole blood than in serum.[72] If these ZIKV RT-PCR results are negative, then serology (serum ZIKV IgM testing) should be done as well as testing for dengue, particularly if there are exposures or if the patient is pregnant.[72] (See more information later regarding ZIKV serology considerations) (Fig. 176H.10).

Of note, a recent study conducted by the Florida Department of Health in 70 patients with suspected ZIKV disease highlights the differences in diagnostic yield using ZIKV RT-PCR on different bodily fluid specimens.[35] In this study, 95% of urine specimens collected within 5 days of symptom onset tested positive for ZIKV RNA RT-PCR, as opposed to only 56% of serum specimens.[35] The study also demonstrated that ZIKV RNA detection in saliva within the first 5 days of symptoms was better than that in serum, with the percentage of detection in saliva approaching that of urine specimens.[35] However, despite this study's findings, it should be noted that because of issues with processing saliva samples for ZIKV RT-PCR, saliva is not currently recommended as part of routine specimen collection in the evaluation of ZIKV infection.[234]

Note that various NAATs have been approved by the FDA through Emergency Use Authorization (EAU), and a list of all of these ZIKV EUAs are available on the FDA website (http://www.fda.gov/MedicalDevices/Safety/EmergencySituations/ucm161496.htm).[72,234] Apart from CDC Trioplex RT-PCR, this includes other tests by Focus Diagnostics, Altona Diagnostics, Hologic, Viracor-IBT, Siemens Healthcare Diagnostics, Luminex, and Roche Molecular Systems.[234]

*References 7, 111, 137, 181, 188, 248, 319, 358, 416–418, 460.

Beyond the Period of ZIKV Acute-Phase Testing (Serology and PRNT Testing)

Beyond the acute phase of the illness after 2 weeks (≥14 days), it is recommended that serology for ZIKV IgM (typically the IgM antibody capture enzyme-linked immunosorbent assay [MAC-ELISA]) from collected serum be used to diagnose infection up to 12 weeks after illness onset.[72,205,363] This also includes the use of the PRNT to evaluate for virus-specific neutralizing antibodies in paired serum samples for any test result on MAC-ELISA indicating anti-ZIKV IgM antibodies (which includes a positive, equivocal, or presumptive/possible ZIKV-positive result)[72,205,363] (Fig. 176H.11).

Anti-ZIKV IgM antibodies will be detectable in serum within the first week after symptom onset (possibly as early as 4–5 days) and be present for 8 to 12 weeks after.[72,384] It should also be noted that in some patients RT-PCR testing may be positive (particularly for urine and whole blood) for longer than 2 weeks after onset of ZIKV symptoms.[72] Thus it may be of benefit to send serum as well as whole blood and urine for ZIKV RNA NAATs even beyond the acute phase of illness of 2 weeks.[72]

Note that testing recommendations for pregnant women are somewhat different and include testing using ZIKV RT-PCR on all available specimens (serum, urine, whole blood), even if presenting more than 2 weeks beyond symptom onset, as well as dengue IgM testing.[72] For symptom-free pregnant women, repeat testing should be done 2 to 12 weeks after exposure, even if the first test results were negative.[72]

Because ZIKV serology (IgM) may cross-react with antibodies to other flavivirus infections such as dengue and yellow fever viruses, neutralizing antibody testing (PRNT) can be used to help differentiate between these cross-reacting antibodies that may occur in patients with primary flavivirus infections and those occurring in previously infected patients or patients vaccinated against flaviviruses.[363] PRNT evaluates for neutralizing antibodies to ZIKV as well as other flaviviruses that can cross-react with ZIKV serology.[72] For instance, cases of acute ZIKV infection in travelers returning from the Pacific Islands and Southeast Asia have been reported to have false-positive testing results for dengue virus IgM[152,232,410,425,433,481] (Box 176H.1). In the United States, PRNT is typically done either at the CDC or at another CDC-qualified laboratory.[72] However, the use of PRNT for ZIKV and dengue in Puerto Rico is an exception to these CDC guidelines and is not routinely recommended given high rates of cross-reactivity.[72]

Guidelines from the CDC and from local and state health departments can assist providers in interpreting serology results.[384] Further details regarding interpretation of ZIKV testing results and ZIKV laboratory testing protocols are available on the CDC website (http://www.cdc.gov/zika/state-labs/index.html) and in Box 176H.1.

It should also be noted that both MAC-ELISA and PRNT are labor-intensive methods for ZIKV infection diagnosis, and there is a great need for the development of more specific, user-friendly, rapid ZIKV diagnostic tests.[234] A potential future diagnostic method is the ultrasensitive electrogenerated chemiluminescence-based immunoassay for ZIKV detection in bodily fluids.[4]

Other Specimen-Testing Methods

ZIKV testing can also be done on other bodily fluids, although these are not considered primary diagnostic specimens. Cerebral CSF can be tested using ZIKV RNA RT-PCR and ZIKV IgM.[72] Amniotic fluid may also be tested for ZIKV RNA using RT-PCR.[72] At present, there are no FDA-authorized tests that accept use of saliva or semen for ZIKV testing.[72]

In addition, if tissue samples are available for testing, immunohistochemical staining can be done to look for ZIKV antigens, and RT-PCR can also be done on fixed tissues.[363] Of note, ZIKV testing that can be used in formalin-fixed, paraffin-embedded (FFPE) tissue samples has

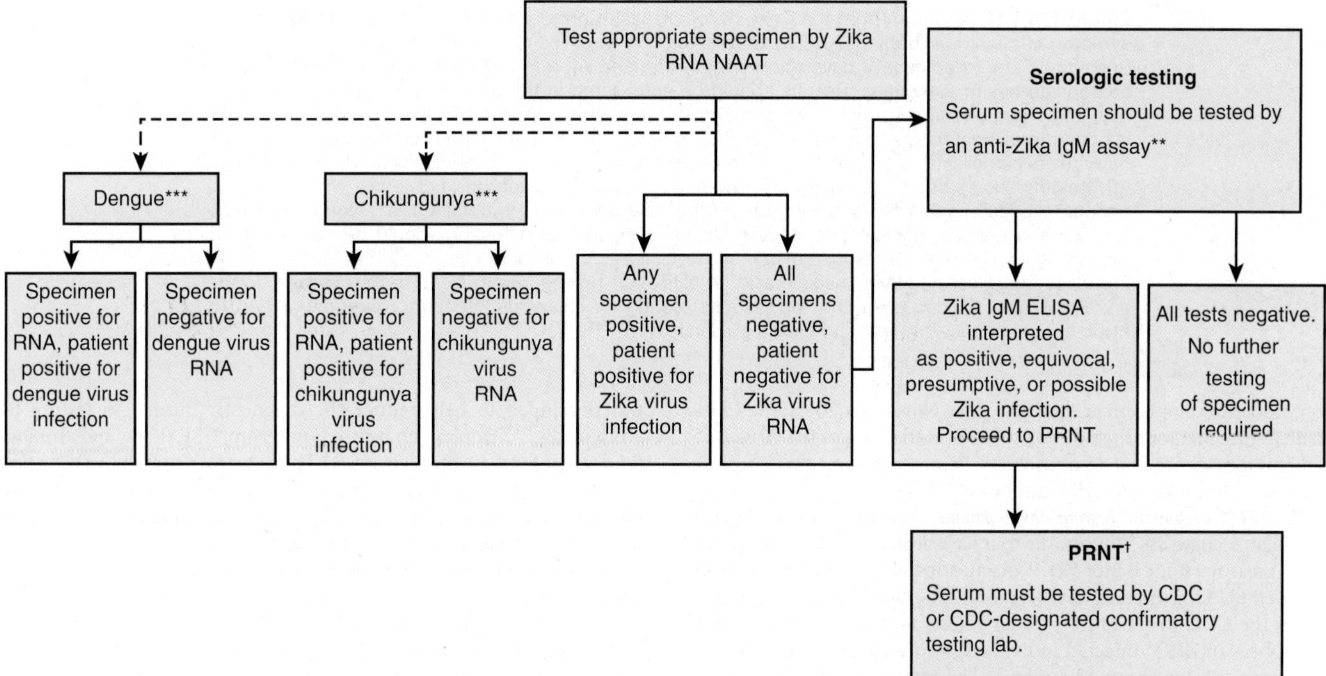

FIGURE 176H.10 Algorithm created by the Centers for Disease Control and Prevention (CDC) to help guide testing of individuals in the United States with symptomatic acute Zika virus infection. Specimens are collected <14 days after symptom onset. All test results should be reported. Results should be considered in the context of symptoms, exposure risk, and time point of specimen collection. *Pregnant and nonpregnant symptomatic individuals. **Note that antibody cross-reactivity to other flaviviruses (e.g., dengue) complicates interpretation of the current anti-Zika immunoglobulin M (IgM) tests. Dengue IgM testing should be conducted for symptomatic pregnant women, for individuals with a potential dengue exposure, and when a presumptive other flavivirus result is obtained. ***Testing and interpretation for the CDC Trioplex assay. Note that when testing urine and amniotic fluid with the CDC Trioplex assay, only report the Zika result. †Plaque reduction neutralization test (PRNT) confirmation is not currently routinely recommended in Puerto Rico. NAAT, nucleic acid amplification testing. (From Centers for Disease Control and Prevention. Guidance for U.S. laboratories testing for Zika virus infection. November 16, 2016. https://www.cdc.gov/zika/images/laboratories/zikaalgorithm-1.jpg. https://www.cdc.gov/zika/hc-providers/testing-guidance.html.)

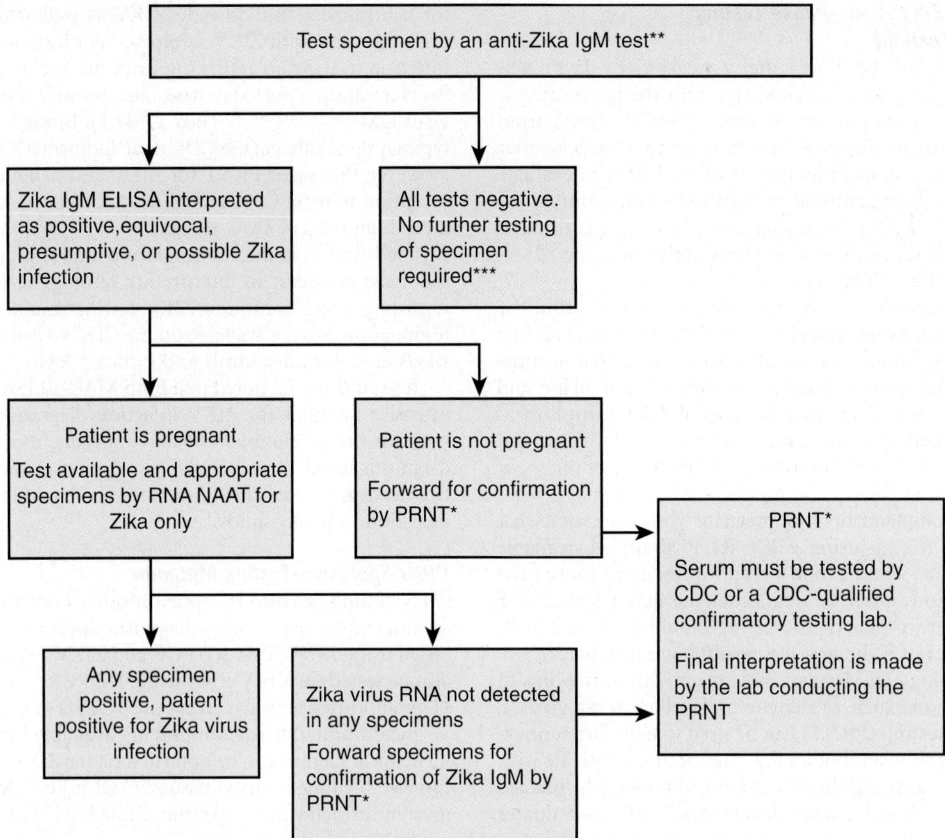

Figure 176H.11 Algorithm from the Centers for Disease Control and Prevention (CDC) for testing of symptomatic individuals in the United States for Zika virus beyond the acute period of infection. Specimens are collected ≥14 days after symptom onset. All test results should be reported to the appropriate health authorities. Results should be considered in the context of symptoms, exposure risk, and time point of specimen collection. *Plaque reduction neutralization test (PRNT) confirmation is not currently routinely recommended for Puerto Rico. **Note that antibody cross-reactivity to other flaviviruses complicates interpretation of the current anti-Zika immunoglobulin M (IgM) tests. Dengue IgM testing should be conducted for symptomatic pregnant women, for individuals with a potential dengue exposure, and when a presumptive other flavivirus result is obtained. ***Note that if tests for Zika and dengue IgM are not reactive, anti-chikungunya IgM testing should be performed for persons with chikungunya exposure risk and a clinically compatible illness. ELISA, enzyme-linked immunosorbent assay; NAAT, nucleic acid amplification testing. (From Centers for Disease Control and Prevention. Guidance for U.S. laboratories testing for Zika virus infection. November 16, 2016. https://www.cdc.gov/zika/laboratories/lab-guidance.html.)

been under development at the CDC since November 2015. The FFPE tissue testing methods include ZIKV RT-PCR that targets the virus NS5 and envelope genes and immunohistochemistry testing that employs a mouse polyclonal anti-ZIKV antibody.[256,460]

New ZIKV diagnostic testing developments. According to the WHO, more than 55 new ZIKV diagnostic tests have been developed in response to the great need for better ZIKV diagnostics.[469] In addition, the FDA approved EUA for several ZIKV diagnostic kits. One of the most popular tests is the CDC MAC-ELISA, which detects IgM antibodies to ZIKV that appear in ZIKV-infected individuals 4 to 5 days after the start of illness and last for about 12 weeks.[384] The test is intended to be used on blood from individuals with a history of symptoms associated with ZIKV or recent travel to an area with active ZIKV transmission.[384] Furthermore, a recent novel ZIKV ELISA based on the ZIKV NS1 antigen was also developed and evaluated in European patients for cross-reacting serum antibodies to dengue, yellow fever, hepatitis C, and also tick-borne encephalitis (TBE).[203] The test has particular relevance in Europe, where TBE vaccination coverage is more widespread in certain countries, such as South Germany and Austria, and the test has shown early promise as highly specific and reliable.[203]

Another new test has also received FDA EUA.[366] The Trioplex real-time RT-PCR assay, which was developed by the CDC, is a single-reaction multiplex RT-PCR used to detect ZIKV, chikungunya, and dengue and was developed to help reduce the diagnostic burden in testing for arboviruses.[458] Trioplex can be used on serum, CSF, urine, and amniotic fluid to test for these three viruses.[366] The test strives to improve detection, workflow, and testing costs associated with ZIKV and other arboviral testing; the test also shows initial promise in being able to simplify diagnostic workload for these three arboviruses and was designed to minimize cross-reactivity of testing results between the three viruses.[366,458] Others have also developed nested, multiplex RT-PCR tests for simultaneous detection of ZIKV, chikungunya, and dengue.[62] In addition, the US Department of Health and Human Services assisted in funding the development of a rapid ZIKV serologic test (ZIKV *Detect* IgM Capture ELISA from InBios International) that can diagnose ZIKV in 4 hours, which is much faster than the current serologic test used by the CDC, which takes 2 to 3 days.[2,195] This rapid serologic test received FDA EUA. However, recent FDA warnings have been issued about high false-positive rates observed.[145,489]

ZIKV Diagnostic Definitions and Testing Guidelines

Note that CDC interim guidelines for ZIKV testing may change. Therefore it is highly recommended that the most updated guidelines be reviewed to guide any clinical evaluation of patients with suspected ZIKV infection. See http://www.cdc.gov/zika/hc-providers/index.html.

BOX 176H.1 Possible Results of Plaque Reduction Neutralization Antibody Testing

The following result interpretations from plaque reduction neutralization antibody testing (PRNT) testing are possible for Zika and dengue based on the detection of immunoglobulin M (IgM) by enzyme-linked immunosorbent assay (ELISA) and the levels of neutralizing antibody titers identified in the PRNT. The results given here will be determined by the laboratories performing PRNT.

Interpretation of Antibody Testing[a,b]

Recent Zika virus infection[c]
Recent dengue virus infection[c]
Recent flavivirus infection; specific virus cannot be identified[c]
No evidence of Zika virus or dengue virus infection
Evidence of Zika virus infection; timing cannot be determined[d]
Evidence of dengue virus infection; timing cannot be determined[d]
Evidence of flavivirus infection; specific virus and timing cannot be determined[d]
Presumptive recent Zika virus infection[c,d]
Presumptive recent dengue virus infection[c,d]
Presumptive recent flavivirus infection[c,d]
Equivocal results[d]
Inconclusive results[d]
No evidence of recent Zika virus or dengue virus infection

Report any positive or equivocal IgM Zika or dengue results to state or local health department. PRNT is not currently routinely recommended in Puerto Rico for specimens that have "positive, presumptive, equivocal or possible" Zika interpretations based on testing with current Emergency Use Authorization Zika IGM tests.

[a]For persons with suspected Zika virus disease, Zika virus RNA nucleic acid amplification tests should be performed on specimens collected <14 days after onset of symptoms.

[b]To resolve false-positive results that might be caused by cross-reactivity or nonspecific reactivity, presumptive positive Zika IgM results should be confirmed with PRNT titers against Zika, dengue, and other flaviviruses to which the person might have been exposed.

[c]In the absence of RNA nucleic acid amplification testing, negative IgM or neutralizing antibody testing in specimens collected <7 days after illness onset might reflect collection before development of detectable antibodies and does not rule out infection with the virus for which testing was conducted.

[d]Zika IgM positive result is reported as "presumptive positive" to denote the need to perform confirmatory PRNT.

Modified from Rabe IB, Staples JE, Villanueva J, et al. Interim guidance for interpretation of Zika virus antibody test results. *MMWR Morb Mortal Wkly Rep.* 2016;65(21):543-546.

Diagnostic Definitions of ZIKV Cases

According to the 2016 WHO interim ZIKV disease definitions, a probable case is a suspected case (signs and symptoms as described earlier) with the presence of IgM antibody against ZIKV and an epidemiologic link (e.g., contact with a confirmed case, or a history of residing in or traveling to an area with local transmission of ZIKV within 2 weeks before the onset of symptoms).[330] A confirmed case is defined as the presence of ZIKV RNA or antigen in serum or other samples (e.g., saliva, tissues, urine, whole blood), or a positive IgM antibody against ZIKV and $PRNT_{90}$ for ZIKV with a titer of 20 or higher and ZIKV $PRNT_{90}$ titer ratio of 4 or higher compared with other flaviviruses, and the exclusion of other flaviviruses.[330]

Similarly, according to CDC guidelines, laboratory evidence of ZIKV infection includes the following: (1) detectable ZIKV, ZIKV RNA, or ZIKV antigen in any clinical specimen; and (2) positive ZIKV IgM with confirmatory antibody titers that are fourfold or more higher than dengue virus neutralizing antibody titers in serum or cerebrospinal fluid. Testing is considered inconclusive if titer criteria are not met.[151] Negative results from a molecular ZIKV test (i.e., ZIKV PCR) does not exclude a diagnosis of ZIKV infection, and ZIKV serology (ZIKV IgM) testing should also be done.[72]

For congenital ZIKV cases, the CDC considers a positive infant serum *or* urine ZIKV RT-PCR result as confirmatory for the diagnosis of congenital ZIKV,[395] whereas a positive ZIKV IgM result with a negative ZIKV RT-PCR is suggestive of "probable" congenital ZIKV infection.[395] As discussed previously, congenital ZIKV infection is a cause of microcephaly along with other anomalies, including intracranial calcifications and other brain or eye abnormalities, but the full clinical spectrum of ZIKV effects in pregnancy is still under determination.[395] (See earlier descriptions of findings that may be seen in congenital ZIKV syndrome.) In addition, it should again be noted that a negative PCR test result may confirm infection but does not necessarily rule out congenital ZIKV infection.[395]

General Guidelines for ZIKV Testing

The CDC recommends ZIKV testing for any *symptomatic* person who meets one of the following criteria: (1) currently lives in an area identified as having active ZIKV transmission, or (2) has recently returned from travel to an area identified as having active ZIKV transmission, or (3) has had unprotected sex with a partner with confirmed ZIKV infection.[363] With regard to sexual transmission of ZIKV, it is currently not recommended to test blood, semen, female genital tract, or urine as a means to risk-stratify a male or female's likelihood of transmitting ZIKV through sexual intercourse given the current limited knowledge regarding ZIKV's sexual transmission.[341,363]

ZIKV testing in pregnancy was previously recommended for both symptomatic and asymptomatic women with possible exposure to ZIKV (a history of recent travel to an area with active transmission, residing in an area with active ZIKV transmission, or having had unprotected sexual activity with a partner with confirmed ZIKV infection). Further details of testing and management of ZIKV in pregnancy are beyond the scope of this chapter and are consistently changing.[313,354] Refer to specific CDC guidelines and testing algorithms for further details on testing during pregnancy. There are different algorithms available for pregnant women traveling to or residing in regions with local ZIKV transmission along with accompanying recommendations for repeat testing and serial fetal ultrasounds during pregnancy.

ZIKV Testing for Infants and Children for Suspected Acute ZIKV Infection

For infants or children younger than 18 years, postnatal ZIKV infection should be suspected in the following situations per the CDC: (1) recent travel or residing in areas with active ZIKV transmission in the past 2 weeks or other possible ZIKV exposure (i.e., adolescent with sexual contact with a partner with exposure risk factors); and (2) two or more symptoms of ZIKV infection (i.e., fever, rash, conjunctivitis, or arthralgia).[365]

Because vertical transmission of ZIKV from mother to child at the time of delivery is also possible, perinatal ZIKV infection should be suspected in infants in the first 2 weeks of life in the following situations: (1) mother with a history of traveling or residing in a region with active ZIKV transmission 2 weeks or less before delivery or exposure through sexual transmission; and (2) infant with at least two or more symptoms consistent with ZIKV infection (fever, rash, conjunctivitis, arthralgia).[365]

According to the CDC guidelines for testing of children for acute ZIKV infection, if symptoms have been present for less than 2 weeks (14 days), it is recommended to test for ZIKV RNA by RT-PCR on serum and urine.[151] A positive ZIKV RT-PCR test confirms infection, but a negative result does not rule out ZIKV infection. If RT-PCR testing is negative or if it is beyond the 2-week period at presentation, serologic testing is recommended, as discussed earlier[365,377] (see Figs. 176H.10 and 176H.11).

Infant ZIKV Testing for Suspected ZIKV Congenital Infection

The CDC recommends workup for congenital ZIKV infection for the following groups of infants: (1) infants of mothers with laboratory-confirmed ZIKV infection in pregnancy or (2) infants with abnormal examinations or neuroimaging consistent with congenital ZIKV syndrome whose mothers had ZIKV exposure in pregnancy, regardless of maternal ZIKV laboratory results.[395]

Infant evaluation for congenital ZIKV infection includes both RT-PCR for ZIKV RNA (serum and urine) and serologic ZIKV IgM testing, ideally from infant specimens collected within the first 2 days of life.[151,395] Although cord blood was initially recommended to be collected along with serum, most updated CDC guidelines from the end of August 2016 *no longer recommend testing* for ZIKV via cord blood given the false-positive results from maternal blood contamination.[395] In addition to serum, newer guidelines also recommend collecting urine for ZIKV RNA RT-PCR testing, as well as consideration for also collecting and testing whole blood for ZIKV RNA RT-PCR testing.[72] Note that PRNT cannot distinguish between maternal and infant ZIKV antibodies at birth.[72] Little is known at this time regarding the duration of ZIKV viral shedding in infants with congenital ZIKV infection, although in some congenital infections such as CMV and rubella, shedding (particularly in urine) may be prolonged.[395]

For infants with positive ZIKV IgM testing, PRNT may be used to confirm ZIKV-specific antibodies.[395] However, PRNT cannot reliably distinguish between ZIKV maternal and infant antibodies and may need to be repeated after the child is 18 months or older, at which time maternal antibodies are expected to have waned.[395] For children whose initial ZIKV RNA RT-PCR and IgM testing results were negative at birth, PRNT testing may be useful to evaluate for ZIKV congenital infection.[72] In that situation, PRNT may be used to evaluate for congenital infection in children 18 months or older.[14]

In addition, if CSF is collected for other reasons and is available for testing, it is recommended to test CSF for both ZIKV RNA and ZIKV IgM.[151,395]

Histopathologic evaluation of placenta and umbilical cord with ZIKV immunohistochemical staining on fixed tissue and ZIKV RT-PCR on fixed and frozen tissue (umbilical cord and placenta) are also recommended for infants born to women with confirmed ZIKV infection and should be considered for those born to women with presumptive ZIKV infection.[151,313] It should be noted as well that a positive result for ZIKV RNA from placenta can confirm maternal ZIKV infection but cannot reliably determine whether congenital infection has also occurred.[72] If testing of the mother was not performed during pregnancy, it should also be done and should include testing serum for ZIKV IgM and neutralizing antibodies and for dengue virus IgM and neutralizing antibodies.[151]

In addition, ZIKV testing (RT-PCR and immunohistochemical staining of fixed tissues) should be offered to pregnant women with confirmed or possible ZIKV infection that suffer from fetal loss or stillbirth.[313] Further details about laboratory testing protocols are given later, and interpretation of ZIKV testing results are available on the CDC website (http://www.cdc.gov/zika/state-labs/index.html).

EVALUATION AND MANAGEMENT OF PEDIATRIC PATIENTS WITH ZIKV

Recommendations for Evaluation and Management of Possible Pediatric ZIKV Cases

In February 2016, the CDC released interim guidelines for the evaluation and management of infants and children with possible ZIKV infection.[151,423] Subsequent updates (last in August 2016) have been made to these guidelines released for the evaluation and testing of infants with possible congenital ZIKV infection.[151,395,423] Remember that ZIKV disease is considered a nationally notifiable condition that warrants reporting all confirmed cases to state health departments.[363,151]

Evaluation of Children for Acute ZIKV Disease

Recommendations for laboratory evaluation were discussed previously in the section ZIKV Testing for Infants and Children for Suspected Acute ZIKV Infection.

Evaluation for Congenital ZIKV Infection

Recommendations for laboratory evaluation were discussed previously in the section Infant ZIKV Testing for Suspected ZIKV Congenital Infection. However, it is important to note that the need for additional evaluation (other tests and evaluation by subspecialists) is based on whether (1) the infant has any findings consistent with congenital ZIKV syndrome or (2) the infant has laboratory-confirmed congenital ZIKV infection (Fig. 176H.12 and Table 176H.6). Note that recommendations for evaluation have been changed from previous CDC guidelines issued before August 2016 and now include a broader definition of possible congenital ZIKV infection beyond that of just microcephaly or intracranial calcifications.[151,313]

TABLE 176H.6 Interpretation of Results of Laboratory Testing of Infant's Blood, Urine, and Cerebrospinal Fluid for Evidence of Congenital Zika Virus Infection

rRT-PCR	IgM	Interpretation
Positive	Positive or negative	Confirmed congenital Zika virus infection
Negative	Positive	Probable congenital Zika virus infection[a]
Negative	Negative	Negative for congenital Zika virus infection[a]

IgM, Immunoglobulin M; *rRT-PCR,* real-time reverse transcriptase polymerase chain reaction.

[a]Laboratory results should be interpreted in the context of timing of infection during pregnancy, maternal serology results, clinical findings consistent with congenital Zika syndrome, and any confirmatory testing with plaque reduction neutralization testing.

From Russell K, Oliver SE, Lewis L, et al. Update: interim guidance for the evaluation and management of infants with possible congenital zika virus infection—United States, August 2016. *MMWR. Morb Mortal Wkly Rep.* 2016;65(33):870-878.

For infants born to women with laboratory-confirmed ZIKV infection, a comprehensive physical examination at birth is essential, which includes measurement of head circumference, length, and weight; gestational age assessment; and evaluation for dysmorphic features and neurologic abnormalities.[395] They should also have a postnatal head ultrasound and a hearing screen. Infants with laboratory evidence of ZIKV infection but no abnormalities consistent with congenital ZIKV infection should also undergo an ophthalmologic examination and auditory brainstem response hearing evaluation before 1 month of age.[395] In contrast, infants with negative ZIKV testing results and no abnormalities consistent with congenital ZIKV infection should continue their routine newborn care[395] (Table 176H.7).

In contrast, infants with abnormalities consistent with congenital ZIKV syndrome will need a comprehensive evaluation at birth and may require access to a facility with pediatric subspecialties.[395] Before discharge from the hospital at birth, the recommended evaluation includes a complete blood count and a metabolic panel including liver function tests, an ophthalmologist examination, an ABR hearing evaluation, and consideration for additional neuroimaging, as well as evaluation for other genetic conditions and congenital infections. (Refer to Table 176H.7 and Box 176H.2 for more details.) Specifically, for infants with abnormalities and laboratory results consistent with congenital ZIKV infection, additional evaluation by subspecialists, including infectious disease specialist (for other congenital infections), geneticist (for other causes of microcephaly or other abnormalities), neurologist (for additional neurologic evaluation), and endocrinologist (for hypothalamic or pituitary dysfunction), is also recommended in the early newborn period. (See Box 176H.2 for further detail.)

Infants with congenital ZIKV syndrome will require a medical home with access to multiple subspecialists for regular outpatient care and monthly visits for at least the first 6 months of life. (See further details in Box 176H.2.[395]) Infants should be evaluated for feeding difficulties and may require assistance with lactation, occupational therapy, speech therapy, and nutrition, and they should be evaluated by a gastroenterologist regarding reflux, aspiration, poor suck, and swallowing dysfunction.[395] In particular, issues with swallowing dysfunction may be evident as the infant grows.[395] Neurologic examinations should be done at 1 and 2 months of age and may require referrals for additional neurologic issues such as sleeping problems and excessive irritability.[395] Repeat ophthalmology examination should be done at 3 months of age if earlier results were normal.[395] If the ABR before 1 month of age was normal, repeat examination should be done at 4 to 6 months of age.[395] Given the risks for hypothalamic dysfunction and pituitary insufficiency, thyroid screening, including thyroid-stimulating hormone and thyroxine (either free T_4 or both total T_4 and estimated free T_4) should also be conducted at 2 weeks of age and 3 months of age.[40] In addition, growth and development parameters should be monitored at each visit and may require referral to developmental specialists.

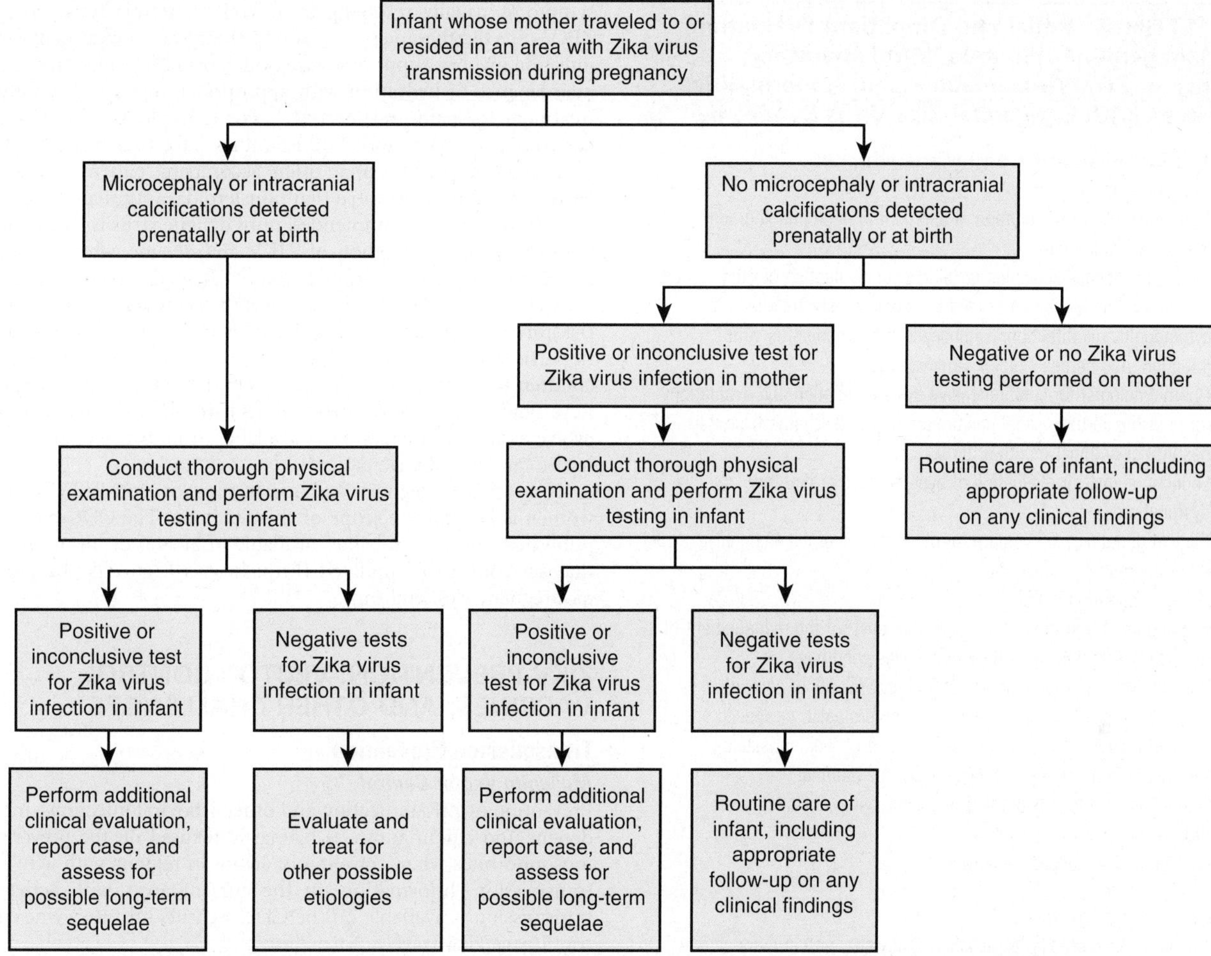

FIGURE 176H.12 Algorithm from the Centers for Disease Control and Prevention (CDC) for Zika virus evaluation of infants born to mothers with Zika virus exposure in pregnancy. Areas with Zika virus transmission are listed on the CDC website at http://wwwnc.cdc.gov/travel/page/zika-travel-information. Microcephaly is defined as occipitofrontal circumference less than the 3rd percentile for gestational age and sex based on standard growth curves, not explained by other etiologies. Laboratory evidence of Zika virus infection includes (1) detectable Zika virus, Zika virus RNA, or Zika virus antigen in any clinical specimen; or (2) positive Zika virus immunoglobulin M (IgM) with confirmatory neutralizing antibody titers more than fourfold higher or greater than dengue virus neutralizing antibody titers in serum or cerebrospinal fluid. Testing is considered inconclusive if Zika virus neutralizing antibody titers are less than fourfold higher than dengue virus neutralizing antibody titers. For infants, perform reverse transcriptase polymerase chain reaction (RT-PCR) testing for Zika virus RNA and Zika virus and dengue virus IgM and neutralizing antibodies on serum collected from the umbilical cord or directly from infant within 2 days of birth, if possible. If cerebrospinal fluid is obtained for other reasons, test for Zika virus RNA, Zika virus IgM and neutralizing antibodies, and dengue virus IgM and neutralizing antibodies. Consider histopathologic evaluation of the placenta and umbilical cord with Zika virus immunohistochemical staining on fixed tissue and Zika virus RT-PCR on fixed and frozen tissue. More information on laboratory testing for Zika virus infection is available at http://www.cdc.gov/zika/state-labs/index.html. (From Russell K, Oliver SE, Lewis L, et al. Update: interim guidance for the evaluation and management of infants with possible congenital Zika virus infection–United States, August 2016. *MMWR Morb Mortal Wkly Rep.* 2016;65[33]:870-878. Modified from Staples JE, Dziuban EJ, Fischer M, et al. Interim guidelines for the evaluation and testing of infants with possible congenital Zika virus infection—United States, 2016. *MMWR Morb Mortal Wkly Rep.* 2016;65:63-67.)

In addition, infants with laboratory evidence of congenital ZIKV syndrome but no abnormalities consistent with congenital ZIKV infection should also have close outpatient follow-up. They should be monitored for neurologic issues (e.g., seizures and cognitive delay) and for vision and hearing abnormalities.[395] Refer to Table 176H.7 and Box 176H.3 for detailed recommendations regarding follow-up for development, ophthalmology, and hearing evaluations during infancy for this particular group of infants.[395]

Any confirmed or suspected ZIKV cases should be relayed to local, state, or territorial health departments, which will assist in the coordination of laboratory testing and in the prevention of potential risks for local transmission of ZIKV in regions where *Aedes* spp. mosquitoes are found.[151,423] To help facilitate better understanding of ZIKV infection, the CDC has established a US Zika Pregnancy Registry to collect information about pregnancy and outcomes for women and their infants with laboratory diagnosis of ZIKV infection.

Health care providers who suspect congenital ZIKV infection in an infant should contact their state, tribal, local, or territorial health department if the infant meets the clinical criteria for testing as outlined in the CDC guidelines. The state, tribal, local, or territorial health department can facilitate laboratory testing for ZIKV infection in infants who meet these clinical criteria. A similar system (Zika Active Pregnancy Surveillance System) has also been established by the CDC in Puerto Rico.[363] In addition, health care providers can contact the CDC Zika

BOX 176H.2 Initial and Outpatient Evaluation and Management of Infants With Laboratory Evidence of Zika Virus infection and Abnormalities Consistent With Congenital Zika Virus Syndrome

Initial Clinical Evaluation and Management

- Consultation with:
  - Neurologist for determination of appropriate neuroimaging and additional evaluation.
  - Infectious disease specialist for diagnostic evaluation of other congenital infections (e.g., syphilis, toxoplasmosis, rubella, cytomegalovirus infection, lymphocytic choriomeningitis virus infection, and herpes simplex virus infection)
  - Ophthalmologist for comprehensive eye examination and evaluation for possible cortical visual impairment before discharge from the hospital or within 1 month of birth
  - Endocrinologist for evaluation of hypothalamic or pituitary dysfunction
  - Clinical geneticist to evaluate for other causes of microcephaly or other anomalies if present
- Consider consultation with:
  - Orthopedist, physiatrist, or physical therapist for the management of hypertonia, clubfoot, or arthrogrypotic-like conditions
  - Pulmonologist or otolaryngologist for concerns about aspiration
  - Lactation specialist, nutritionist, gastroenterologist, or speech or occupational therapist for the management of feeding issues
- Perform auditory brainstem response to assess hearing.
- Perform complete blood count and metabolic panel, including liver function tests.
- Provide family and supportive services.

Outpatient Management

- A medical home should be established, and visits with primary care provider should occur monthly for at least the first 6 months of life.
  - Follow growth parameters; monitor development; provide routine immunizations, anticipatory guidance, and psychosocial support; and ensure infants receive necessary testing and consultations.
- Neurologic examination by the primary care provider at 1 and 2 months of age. Refer to neurology for any abnormalities, or for any parental or provider concerns.
- Refer to developmental specialist and early intervention services.
- Repeat comprehensive ophthalmologic examination at age 3 months, and refer to ophthalmology for any abnormal findings, or for any parental or provider concerns.
- Repeat auditory brainstem response testing at age 4 to 6 months, and refer to audiology for any abnormal findings or for any parental or provider concerns.
- Repeat testing for hypothyroidism at age 2 weeks and age 3 months, even if the initial testing results were normal. Refer to endocrinology for any abnormal findings.
- Provide family and supportive services.

From Russell K, Oliver SE, Lewis L, et al. Update: interim guidance for the evaluation and management of infants with possible congenital Zika virus infection—United States, August 2016. *MMWR Morb Mortal Wkly Rep*. 2016;65(33):870-878.

Pregnancy Hotline (previously available through CDC's Emergency Operations Center watch desk at 770-488-7100, ZikaMCH@cdc.gov or ZikaPregnancy@cdc.gov) to discuss information on infants suspected of having congenital ZIKV infection.

Management of Pediatric Patients Infected With Acute ZIKV

Although a few isolated case reports of fatalities have been reported in the literature, acute ZIKV infection in children is typically mild, with symptoms usually resolving in 1 week.[151] At this time, no specific ZIKV-directed therapies exist, and the mainstay of treatment for acute infection involves supportive care, which primarily constitutes bed rest, maintenance of hydration with appropriate fluids, and symptomatic treatment for pain and fever.[151,217] For example, acetaminophen has been used for fever and antihistamines have been used to alleviate symptoms of pruritus that often accompany patients with rash.[217] However, it should be noted that nonsteroidal antiinflammatory drugs (NSAIDs) are not recommended until dengue virus is ruled out given the overlap in presentation of ZIKV and dengue, which may pose a risk for hemorrhagic complications.[151] It is also recommended that NSAIDs be avoided in children younger than 6 months given the potential risk for nephrotoxicity, particularly for children with dehydration.[217] In particular, use of aspirin and other salicylates should be avoided in children with acute viral illnesses given the potential association with Reye syndrome.[151] Recommendations from the CDC will continue to evolve as more information is available to inform recommendations in the care of pediatric patients.[151]

Note that the diagnosis and management of acute ZIKV in pregnant women is beyond the scope of this textbook. The CDC has multiple published interim guidelines available in greater detail on its website that are continually updated (http://www.cdc.gov/zika/hc-providers/qa-pregnant-women.html).

ZIKV PREVENTION: VECTOR CONTROL, VACCINES, AND OTHER CHALLENGES

Transmission Prevention

Mosquito Vector Control

Prevention of ZIKV infection and other arboviral infections, including dengue and chikungunya, is primarily focused on the prevention of mosquito bites when traveling or living in regions with active ZIKV transmission. Information on the current areas with active ZIKV transmission is available on the CDC website, http://wwwnc.cdc.gov/travel/page/zika-travel-information.

Appropriate mosquito protection is especially critical during the daytime because *Aedes* species are typically daytime feeders but differ from others such as *Culex* species, which are carriers of West Nile virus and are primarily active evening to morning, and *Anopheles* species, which may transmit malaria and primarily bite from dusk to dawn.[236] Recommended means of mosquito bite prevention include barrier methods to cover exposed skin, such as wearing long-sleeved shirts, pants, and hats, and the use of permethrin-treated clothing and insect repellents.[151] Substances such as DEET (*N,N*-diethyl-*m*-toluamide), picaridin (which is a long-acting repellent), oil of lemon eucalyptus, or ethyl butylacetylaminopropionate (IR3535) provide protection against mosquito bites.[151,217] Of these, DEET appears to have the best track record (longest history and most studied) of providing the most long-acting and effective protection.[236,474] DEET is considered safe to use in pregnant women and children, and its use in these groups was reviewed by the US Environmental Protection Agency (EPA) in 1998 and again in 2014.[474] Local reactions involving the skin are the primary adverse effects reported with DEET use.[474] After DEET, picaridin comes in second with regard to the strength of evidence supporting its use as an effective mosquito repellent.[350]

Most insect repellents that can protect against mosquito bites and meet registration criteria with the EPA can be safely used in children 2 months and older.[151] As such, products with DEET should not be used in children younger than 2 months.[151] The maximum permissible concentration for DEET for use on infants and children is 30%, and efforts should be made to avoid contact of the product with children's hands, eyes, mouth, and areas of open skin.[151,217] The CDC recommends against the use of oil of lemon eucalyptus on children younger than 3 years.[151,217] Screening on windows and doors to prevent mosquitoes from entering residencies and mosquito netting for bedding in rooms while sleeping with lack of adequate window and door screening methods or air-conditioning can also be used to prevent mosquito contact and thereby transmission of infections.[151,217]

In addition, prevention of additional mosquito bites in infants, children, and any persons already infected with ZIKV is especially

TABLE 176H.7 CDC Updated Initial Evaluation and Recommended Outpatient Management in First Year of Life for Infants With Possible Congenital Zika Virus

Mother	Infant Clinical Exam	Before Hospital Discharge	Infant Testing	2 wk	1 mo	2 mo	3 mo	4–6 mo	9 mo	12 mo
Laboratory evidence of Zika virus infection[a]	No evidence of abnormalities	Routine newborn care: PE, HC, weight/length, and neurologic exam Hearing screen Head ultrasound Infant Zika virus testing	Negative for Zika virus infection	Routine care, including monitoring of OFC and development at every well-child visit and age-appropriate developmental screening						
			Laboratory evidence of Zika virus infection[a]	Ophthalmology exam ABR				Consider ABR repeat	Behavioral audiology if ABR not done at 4–6 mo	
				Monitoring of OFC and development at every visit and age-appropriate developmental screening						
	Abnormalities consistent with congenital Zika syndrome	As above plus: Consider transfer to hospital with subspecialty care CBC, metabolic panel, LFTs, ophthalmology exam ABR Consider advanced neuroimaging	Negative for Zika virus infection Laboratory evidence of Zika virus infection[a]	Evaluate for other causes of congenital anomalies Further management as clinically indicated						
				Thyroid screen	Neurologic exam	Neurologic exam	Thyroid screen, ophthalmology exam		Repeat ABR	
				Routine preventive health care including monitoring of feeding and growth Routine and congenital infection-specific anticipatory guidance Referral to specialists, including evaluation of other causes of congenital anomalies as needed						
Not tested, or tested outside of appropriate window	No evidence of abnormalities	Maternal Zika virus testing[b] Consider Zika virus placental testing Routine newborn care: PE, HC, weight/length and neurologic exam Hearing screen Head ultrasound	Perform infant Zika virus testing of evidence of Zika virus infection on maternal testing[a,b]	Outpatient management for appropriate infant clinical exam and test results						
	Abnormalities consistent with congenital Zika syndrome	As above, plus: Consider transfer to hospital with subspecialty care CBC, metabolic panel, LFTs, ophthalmology exam ABR Consider advanced neuroimaging Infant Zika virus testing	Negative for Zika virus infection Laboratory evidence of Zika virus infection[a]	Evaluate for other causes of congenital anomalies Further management as clinically indicated Refer to outpatient management for infant with abnormalities consistent with congenital Zika syndrome						

[a]Laboratory evidence of maternal Zika virus infection includes (1) Zika virus RNA detected by real-time reverse transcriptase polymerase chain reaction (rRT-PCR) in any clinical specimen; or (2) positive Zika virus immunoglobulin M (IgM) with confirmatory neutralizing antibody titers. Confirmatory neutralizing antibody titers are needed in addition to IgM for maternal Zika virus infection.

[b]Mothers should be tested by rRT-PCR within 2 weeks of exposure or symptom onset, or by IgM within 2–12 weeks of exposure or symptom onset. Because of the decline in IgM antibody titers and viral RNA levels over time, negative maternal testing 12 weeks after exposure does not rule out maternal infection.

ABR, Auditory brainstem response; *CBC,* complete blood count; *CDC,* Centers for Disease Control and Prevention; *LFTs,* liver function tests; *HC,* head (occipitofrontal) circumference; *PE,* physical examination.

From Oduyebo T, Igbinosa I, Peterson EE, et al. Update: interim guidance for health care providers caring for pregnant women with possible Zika virus exposure—United States, July 2016. *MMWR Morb Mortal Wkly Rep.* 2016;65:739-744; Russell K, Oliver SE, Lewis L, et al. Update: interim guidance for the evaluation and management of infants with possible congenital Zika virus infection—United States, August 2016. *MMWR Morb Mortal Wkly Rep.* 2016;65(33):870-878.

BOX 176H.3 Outpatient Management of Infants With Laboratory Evidence of Zika Virus infection but No Abnormalities Consistent With Congenital Zika Virus Syndrome

- A medical home should be established.
  - Follow growth parameters and perform developmental screening at each well-child visit.
  - Emphasize anticipatory guidance for families regarding developmental milestones, feeding and growth, sleep and irritability, and abnormal movements.
- Use a standardized, validated developmental screening tool at 9 months as currently recommended, or earlier for any parental or provider concerns.
- Referral to ophthalmology for comprehensive eye examination within 1 month of birth. Perform vision screening and assess visual regard at every well-child visit and refer to ophthalmology for any abnormal findings or for any parental or provider concerns.
- Perform auditory brainstem response within 1 month of birth. Consider repeat auditory brainstem response at age 4 to 6 months or perform behavioral diagnostic testing at age 9 months and refer to audiology for any abnormal findings or for any parental or provider concerns.
- Provide family and supportive services.

From Russell K, Oliver SE, Lewis L, et al. Update: interim guidance for the evaluation and management of infants with possible congenital Zika virus infection—United States, August 2016. *MMWR Morb Mortal Wkly Rep*. 2016;65(33):870-878.

important during the first week of illness.[151] During this time, infected individuals are more likely to be viremic, and any mosquito bites during this period are more likely to perpetuate the human-mosquito-human cycle of ZIKV transmission, which has allowed ZIKV to flourish in many densely populated urban areas around the world.[151] This also applies to returning travelers from ZIKV endemic regions because most ZIKV infections appear to be asymptomatic.[236]

Additional guidance on mosquito bite prevention is also available on the following EPA and CDC websites:

- http://www.cdc.gov/zika/prevention
- http://wwwnc.cdc.gov/travel/yellowbook/2016/the-pre-travel-consultation/protection-against-mosquitoes-ticks-other-arthropods
- http://www.epa.gov/insect-repellents/using-insect-repellents-safely-and-effectively

Another critical part of vector control includes efforts to remove potential sources of mosquito breeding in endemic areas. In fact, some experts believe that clearing mosquito breeding sites around the home is the most crucial component in effective mosquito control for ZIKV, more efficacious than mass-spraying towns or cities because of *Aedes* spp. mosquitoes' tendency to prefer breeding in artificial containers.[169] Unfortunately, *Aedes* spp. mosquitoes are extremely well adapted to coexist near human habitation; they breed well in the artificial containers with even minimal amounts of water that often surround homes.[332] Instructions regarding mosquito control at home are available on the CDC website (http://www.cdc.gov/zika/prevention/controlling-mosquitoes-at-home.html) but primarily include removing any sources collecting standing water.[236]

Mosquito control at the city level is also important. After the discovery of the first locally acquired ZIKV cases in the United States (Florida), the CDC implemented a combination of the strategies listed previously in an effort to limit the spread of ZIKV. Mosquito control strategies deployed included use of larvicides and insecticides to remove larval and adult mosquitoes, aerial spraying with Naled and larvicide, and removal of standing water.[161]

Other ZIKV Transmission Considerations

Breast milk transmission: interim guidelines for breast-feeding mothers with ZIKV. The CDC has published preliminary guidelines based on available data with regard to the safety of breast-feeding for mothers with ZIKV infection.[151,423] It has been acknowledged that ZIKV RNA and infective viral particles have been recovered from breast milk in mothers with ZIKV infection.[33,123,151] However, at this time, no cases of infant ZIKV acquired through breast-feeding have been reported.[151,423] It is believed that, based on available evidence, the benefits that come with breast-feeding are greater than theoretical risks for ZIKV transmission to infants through breast milk.[151] As such, the CDC continues to support breast-feeding for ZIKV-infected mothers currently living in regions with active ZIKV transmission.[151]

Other ZIKV transmission risks: sexual transmission, blood transfusion, and travel. ZIKV has been detected in semen and female genital fluid,[98,353,379] and most sexual transmission has been reported from symptomatic ZIKV cases, including male-to-female or male partners and from female-to-male partners.[22,251,390,442] However, two cases have suggested the potential for ZIKV to be transmitted sexually from an asymptomatic carrier.[49,160,353] It is not known at this time whether detection of ZIKV in semen reflects any adverse effects on spermatozoids or negatively impacts future semen quality and fertility.[381]

To reduce the risk for sexual ZIKV transmission to pregnant partners, it is recommended that males who live in or have recently traveled to an area with ZIKV transmission, abstain from sexual activity or use condoms with pregnant partners throughout the duration of pregnancy, particularly in regions where local ZIKV transmission is actively occurring.[217,340,353,354] This is particularly important because sexual transmission may occur even in the absence of symptoms. The CDC and WHO recommend that men both with and without symptoms who are returning from regions with local ZIKV transmission use condoms or abstain from sexual activity for at least 6 months after return from travel or after symptom onset to prevent ZIKV transmission to partners.[50,332,353] Infected females should abstain from sexual activity or use condoms for at least 8 weeks from symptom onset to prevent ZIKV sexual transmission to others.[50,332,340,354] It should be noted that the 6-month guideline for prevention of ZIKV sexual transmission from men was based on the initial finding that ZIKV was detected in semen up to 62 days multiplied by a factor of 3.[259] However, given more recent reports that ZIKV has been detected in semen 80 to 188 days after symptom onset, some experts question whether this may warrant extending this interval to at least 9 months.[252,253,259,309]

Women who have recently traveled to regions with ZIKV local transmission and do not have symptoms are advised to wait at least 8 weeks before planning a pregnancy.[332,340,354] Men, regardless of symptoms, should wait at least 6 months.[353] If one of the partners has ZIKV clinical illness or confirmed ZIKV infection, the WHO recommends waiting at least 6 months before attempting conception; similar recommendations have been made by the CDC, but with differences in the duration of waiting before attempts at conception for men (at least 6 months) and women (at least 8 weeks) with ZIKV infection.[332,340,354]

Additional details and updates are available on the CDC and WHO website (http://www.cdc.gov/zika/transmission/sexual-transmission.html).

It is also recommended by the CDC that pregnant women avoid travel to areas with continued ZIKV transmission.[217] Updated travel notices from the CDC are available on their website (http://wwwnc.cdc.gov/travel/notices).

Deferral of blood donations is also recommended for individuals that have recently traveled to regions with ZIKV transmission with or without confirmed ZIKV infections.[217]

As with many other infections, standard precautions should be taken in the care of patients and family members with ZIKV infection.[368] Of note, an unusual case of secondary nonsexual ZIKV transmission, possibly through mucocutaneous contact with sweat or tears of a ZIKV-infected patient with high levels of ZIKV viremia, also underscores the importance for health care workers to adhere to standard precaution procedures in the care of ZIKV patients.[48,428] Refer to the CDC for more detailed guidance on this matter (https://www.cdc.gov/zika/hc-providers/infection-control.html).

Vaccine Development

The ability of effective antiviral vaccines to combat devastating congenital viral infections is best exemplified with the successes of the rubella vaccine, which has virtually eliminated congenital rubella syndrome in countries with a high level of vaccine coverage.[344] A similar strategy could be employed with ZIKV after an effective vaccine is available.[344] However, at present, no approved vaccines against ZIKV exist.

Yet, after declaration by the WHO that ZIKV was a global public health emergency, multiple organizations have joined efforts, and creating a ZIKV vaccine is now considered a leading research priority around the world.[333,440] This ZIKV vaccine collaborative includes 18 active programs comprising five academic groups and 15 commercial groups that are researching different strategies to create a successful ZIKV vaccine (purified inactivated virus vaccine; nucleic acid–based [RNA, DNA] vaccine; live, vectored vaccine; subunit vaccine; viruslike particles [VLP] vaccine; and live, recombinant vaccine) that build on existing flavivirus knowledge and technology.[83,221,333,333,382,440]

Some vaccine experts believe that developing an effective ZIKV vaccine is foreseeable given that vaccines exist for several other flaviviruses, including yellow fever, Japanese encephalitis, and dengue, which are all live, attenuated vaccines.[83,440] Yet, important questions that will help guide this process include determining whether infection will lead to lifelong immunity, whether other related flaviviruses may have the potential to provide any cross-protection against ZIKV, and whether an appropriate primate model or other animal models to evaluate ZIKV vaccines can be developed.[46,83] Other potential hurdles include ZIKV's ability to cause neurologic complications such as GBS and the potential for complications related to antibody-dependent enhancement seen with its close relative, dengue,[220] which will require exercising prudence and caution during the development and testing of any successful vaccine candidates.[344] This will also need to be balanced with the importance of providing protection in special populations such as pregnant women. Other challenges include the possibility that ZIKV spread has already peaked in countries such as Brazil and Colombia, resulting in herd immunity that may make it more difficult to perform vaccine clinical trials to evaluate vaccine efficacy.[83]

The first human trials (phase I study) of a ZIKV vaccine (Inovio Pharmaceuticals), a DNA vaccine, began in the end of July 2016.[83] Other vaccines (three, including another ZIKV DNA vaccine, which has a genetically engineered plasmid that encodes premembrane [prM] and envelope [E] ZIKV structural proteins that then allow release of viruslike subviral particles that can trigger an immune response) created in collaboration with NIAID, Walter Reed, Sanofi Pasteur, and Butantan Institute in Brazil are also in development.[2,83,118] Among these, the NIAID ZIKV DNA vaccine has already begun phase I clinical trials with testing in at least 80 volunteers for immune response and vaccine safety and plans to enter phase II clinical trials in 2017.[2,310] The vaccine was designed after previously developed NIAID investigational West Nile virus vaccines.[310] Another whole-particle inactivated ZIKV vaccine will also begin phase I clinical trials.[2]

In addition, in August and September 2016, it was reported that another research group, which had developed several ZIKV vaccines (three different platforms) used in rhesus monkeys, had demonstrated protection against ZIKV.[3,83] These ZIKV vaccines showing preliminary success by producing ZIKV neutralizing antibodies included (1) an inactivated ZIKV vaccine, (2) a plasmid DNA vaccine, and (3) a recombinant rhesus adenovirus serotype 52 vector vaccine.[3] Earlier studies had also demonstrated protection using these vaccines (purified inactivated ZIKV vaccine and plasmid DNA vaccine) in mice model challenges.[3,235] Vaccine-induced antibodies against ZIKV also provided protection against ZIKV in ZIKV challenge studies.[3] A list of candidate vaccines, including institution, vaccine category, and stage of development, are available from the WHO and other reviews.[333,382]

Future Therapeutics, Vector Control, and Other Interventions to Address ZIKV

Therapeutics

Although considerable efforts have already jump-started the development of vaccines against ZIKV, the role of developing new antiviral therapeutics, although theoretically important, has been deemed less of a priority by the WHO given current limitations in understanding the virus, clinical progression of disease, and pathogenesis of the infection.[333] However, some therapeutic agents that may be further evaluated in the future or are under development and have variable activity against some flaviviruses include amodiaquine, chloroquine, ribavirin, interferon-α, BCX4430 (Biocryst), GS-5734 (Gilead), and NITD008.[333]

In addition, because the development of new drugs is time-consuming and expensive, one strategy used to expedite drug discovery in ZIKV has included repurposing drugs by screening other FDA-approved drugs for ZIKV activity.[81] One research group did this by screening 774 FDA-approved drugs to determine whether they had activity in vitro against ZIKV and found that more than 20 of these drugs had some activity against ZIKV.[29] These included anti-flavivirus drugs (bortezomib, mycophenolic acid, ivermectin), as well as others (daptomycin, micafungin, clofazimine, mebendazole, mefloquine, pyrimethamine) whose antiviral activity was not previously known.[29] Of these, mycophenolic acid and daptomycin had high activity against ZIKV.[29] Some of the drugs had activity against ZIKV in several human cell types (placental, cervical, and neural stem cells).[29,81] ZIKV's role in cell cycle and proapoptotic paths may be one reason that drugs used in cancer treatment have also shown in vitro activity against ZIKV.[81] A similar study was performed by another group that screened 6000 compounds for potential to inhibit ZIKV or protect ZIKV-infected cells from death (by inhibiting caspase-3 activity) in neural cells. This group identified 116 compounds and confirmed that 35 showed potential to inhibit ZIKV replication or cellular death, with notable ones including niclosamide (antihelminth drug) and emricasan (caspase inhibitor); combined treatment with compounds from both categories also enhanced protection.[1,94,475] However, issues with many of these compounds in both studies include having antiviral activity that may also be accompanied by cell death, belonging to known classes of pregnancy teratogens (category D drugs), having immunosuppressive effects that may encourage virus persistence, and even having concentration-dependent antiviral effects that may enhance the virus at higher concentration, which was seen with daptomycin.[29,94,475]

Others have also begun to investigate the effects of hepatitis C (member of the flavivirus family) drugs on the ZIKV polymerase (NS5, a RNA-dependent RNA polymerase) with nucleotide inhibitors (sofosbuvir, ribavirin, and IDX-184 and MK0608 as nucleotide inhibitors against HCV polymerase), which have shown some preliminary promise in activity against ZIKV.[131,396] Similar studies have evaluated other nucleoside analogs for in vitro activity against ZIKV's RNA-dependent RNA polymerase that are currently in use to treat other types of infection such as HIV, hepatitis B, CMV, and herpes simplex virus, with 2′-*C*-methylated nucleosides showing some preliminary promise.[135] Bithionol, which inhibits host caspases, has also shown broad activity against a variety of bacterial toxin pathogenic effects as well as ZIKV.[242]

Given the difficulties of testing new therapeutic drugs in pregnant women, the WHO early on had anticipated that therapeutics for use in pregnancy will not be a research and development priority, apart from the potential development of prophylactic interventions or passive immunization therapies.[333] Possibilities for such immunotherapies include the use of pooled immunoglobulin from heterologous serum or monoclonal antibodies to aid in ZIKV neutralization at the blood-placenta barrier.[333] These approaches have been employed for other viral in utero infections such as CMV and HIV.[344] A list of several potential drug therapy candidates currently under investigation are available from several reviews.[333,382]

Vector Control

ZIKV is one of the many vector-borne diseases that have been estimated to account for 22% of the communicable global disease burden.[333] Vector control efforts have demonstrated their ability to reduce and halt disease transmission in endemic regions.[333] Novel tools that aid in mosquito control to employ in the battle against ZIKV include several different strategies: (1) mechanical approaches (e.g., ovitraps, which mimic preferred *Aedes* spp. breeding sites); (2) chemical approaches (e.g., development of chemical agents with adulticidal and larvicidal properties, including investigation of plant-based secondary metabolites with insecticide properties such as alkaloids derived from Amaryllidaceae plants, novel approaches to outdoor spraying, and others); (3) biologic approaches (e.g., use of bacteria such as *Bacillus thuringiensis, Bacillus israelensis,* and *Wolbachia* species that can reduce transmission of arboviruses in mosquitoes), fungal control (e.g., *Metarhizium anisopliae* and *Beauveria bassiana* biocontrol activity against *Aedes* species), copepod predators (e.g., fish that feed on mosquito larvae), or Sterile Insect Technique through irradiation of male mosquitoes; and (4) genetic approaches (e.g., Sterile Insect Technique, creation of insects with dominant lethal genes [RIDL], RNAi-boosted insect immune responses that lead to sterility and inhibit female insect development, and homing endonuclease genes (gene drives to limit ability to transmit pathogens).[258,325,333] A WHO Vector Control Advisory Group has also been convened to review new tools and strategies that may be relevant to addressing the ZIKV global public health crisis.[333]

CONCLUSION

Although ZIKV represents a formidable global health challenge, it was initially met by an impressive and early response from public health and scientific leaders around the world. To catalyze and strengthen global commitment to fighting ZIKV, the WHO had created the Zika Strategic Response Framework. The goals included defining and prioritizing research into ZIKV by bringing experts and partners together, enhancing surveillance and potential complications, strengthening capacity to engage communities to increase understanding of ZIKV risks, improving laboratory capacity to detect ZIKV effectively, supporting health authorities to implement vector control to reduce *Aedes* mosquitoes, and creating recommendations for clinical management and follow-up of those with ZIKV complications.[332,490] As a major step in this direction, the WHO, along with multiple international organizations, convened an International ZIKV Summit at the Institute Pasteur in Paris, France in April 2016. Scientists and public health professionals from around the world came together to discuss key issues surrounding this ZIKV Public Health Emergency, which included topics such as epidemiology and clinical cohorts, neurologic complications, vaccine development, diagnostics, animal models, and vector control.[324]

By October 2016, the WHO had effectively convened four Emergency Committee meetings on ZIKV and microcephaly and had received nearly $24 million dollars in contributions from 13 major global donors to combat ZIKV. The rapid response of the scientific community has also been laudatory. Nearly 1 year since declaring ZIKV a public health emergency, a flurry of scientific reports has been generated with more than 2000 ZIKV publications available on the US National Library of Medicine Pubmed.gov website alone. By November 2016, the WHO announced that it no longer considered ZIKV a global health emergency.[427] Instead, ZIKV would be considered a "significant and enduring public health challenge" requiring a sustained focus of resources and activities within the WHO.[427] The WHO's ZIKV strategic response is estimated to cost more than $122 million.[173] Yet, although WHO experts argue that the change in status is actually an escalation in ZIKV's standing as a global health priority, some critics worry that it may lead to international government and funding apathy.[427]

Nevertheless, it is clear that the societal and economic costs that the ZIKV epidemic leaves in its wake are tremendous and will continue to grow. Estimates of caring for even one child with microcephaly have been estimated to be as high as $10 million dollars. By the end of August 2016, in the United States alone, the CDC had already spent $194 million of the $222 million dollars received from Congress to respond to the ZIKV threat.[103,173] The World Bank has estimated that the ZIKV economic losses in 2016 in just Latin America will total more than $3.5 billion dollars.[173] To effectively combat ZIKV, it is clear that a sustained, dedicated, and multifaceted approach to prevention, diagnosis, and management will be needed to halt further morbidity and mortality from this emerging pathogen. Issues of economic, gender, and racial/ethnic inequality will all be pushed to the forefront and will need to be addressed effectively as we deal with ZIKV's global societal ramifications.[173] As with many other infections, it is women and children, particularly from poor urban regions around the world, that will continue to pay the highest price from ZIKV.[9,199]

See Fig. 176H.13 and Box 176H.4 for other Zika resources.

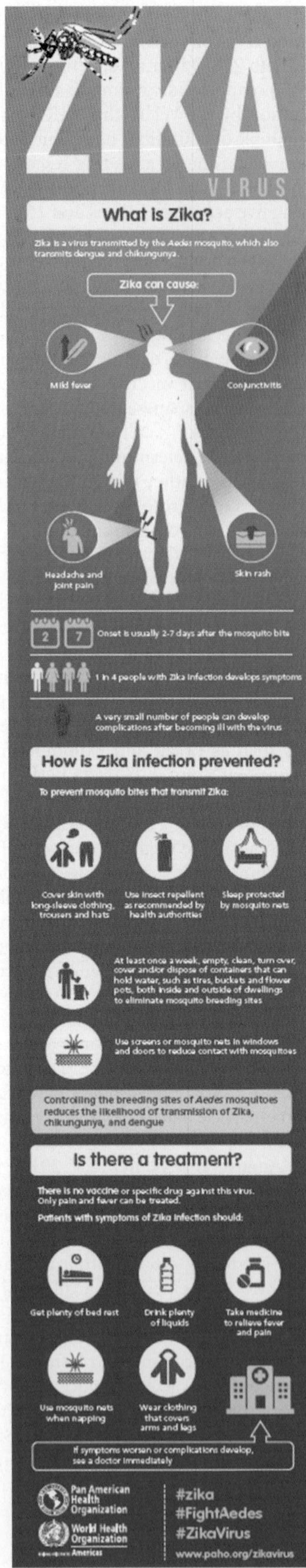

Figure 176H.13 Zika patient infographics from the Centers for Disease Control and Prevention.

BOX 176H.4 **Other Zika Resources**

General

Centers for Disease Control and Prevention: www.cdc.gov/zika

For Health Care Providers

For healthcare providers: https://www.cdc.gov/zika/hc-providers/index.html

Includes clinical guidance on:

- Pregnant women and women of reproductive age
- Infants and children

Clinical guidance for healthcare providers caring for infants and children: https://www.cdc.gov/zika/hc-providers/qa-pediatrician.html

Sexual transmission: https://www.cdc.gov/zika/hc-providers/qa-sexual-transmission.html

Additional Publications

Countries and regions with active Zika transmission: http://www.cdc.gov/zika/geo/index.html

Zika virus disease statistics in the United States and US Territories: http://www.cdc.gov/zika/geo/united-states.html

Pregnant women with any laboratory evidence of possible Zika infection in the United States and US Territories: http://www.cdc.gov/zika/geo/pregwomen-uscases.html

Other Scientific Resources

Morbidity and Mortality Weekly Report—Zika: http://www.cdc.gov/mmwr/zika_reports.html

Emerging Infectious Diseases (EID) Zika Spotlight: http://wwwnc.cdc.gov/eid/page/zika-spotlight

Zika Compiled Resources and Collections by Publisher: http://www.cdc.gov/zika/resources/index.html

Zika Video Resources: http://www.cdc.gov/zika/comm-resources/video.html

World Health Organization (WHO): www.who.int/csr/disease/zika/en

WHO Zika App: http://www.who.int/risk-communication/zika-virus/app/en/

Pan American Health Organization (PAHO): www.paho.org/zikavirus

American Academy of Pediatrics: https://www.aap.org/en-us/advocacy-and-policy/aap-health-initiatives/Children-and-Disasters/Pages/ZikaVirus.aspx

SELECTED REFERENCES

32. Besnard M, Eyrolle-Guignot D, Guillemette-Artur P, et al. Congenital cerebral malformations and dysfunction in fetuses and newborns following the 2013 to 2014 Zika virus epidemic in French Polynesia. *Euro Surveill.* 2016;21(13).
41. Brasil P, Calvet GA, Siqueira AM, et al. Zika virus outbreak in Rio de Janeiro, Brazil: clinical characterization, epidemiological and virological aspects. *PLoS Negl Trop Dis.* 2016;10(4):e0004636.
44. Brasil P, Pereira JP Jr, Raja Gabaglia C, et al. Zika virus infection in pregnant women in Rio de Janeiro: preliminary report. *N Engl J Med.* 2016;37(24):2321-2334.
59. Calvet G, Aguiar RS, Melo AS, et al. Detection and sequencing of Zika virus from amniotic fluid of fetuses with microcephaly in Brazil: a case study. *Lancet Infect Dis.* 2016;16(6):653-660.
64. Cao-Lormeau VM, Blake A, Mons S, et al. Guillain-Barre Syndrome outbreak associated with Zika virus infection in French Polynesia: a case-control study. *Lancet.* 2016;387(10027):1531-1539.
69. Cauchemez S, Besnard M, Bompard P, et al. Association between Zika virus and microcephaly in French Polynesia, 2013–15: a retrospective study. *Lancet.* 2016;387(10033):2125-2132.
76. Cerbino-Neto J, Mesquita EC, Souza TM, et al. Clinical manifestations of Zika virus infection, Rio de Janeiro, Brazil, 2015. *Emerg Infect Dis.* 2016;22(7):1318-1320.
89. Cugola FR, Fernandes IR, Russo FB, et al. The Brazilian Zika virus strain causes birth defects in experimental models. *Nature.* 2016;534(7606):267-271.
93. Cunha MS, Esposito DL, Rocco IM, et al. First complete genome sequence of Zika virus (Flaviviridae, Flavivirus) from an autochthonous transmission in Brazil. *Genome Announc.* 2016;4(2).
111. Dick GW. Zika virus. II. Pathogenicity and physical properties. *Trans R Soc Trop Med Hyg.* 1952;46(5):521-534.
109. Dick GW, Kitchen SF, Haddow AJ. Zika virus. I. Isolations and serological specificity. *Trans R Soc Trop Med Hyg.* 1952;46(5):509-520.
121. Duffy MR, Chen TH, Hancock WT, et al. Zika virus outbreak on Yap Island, Federated States of Micronesia. *N Engl J Med.* 2009;360(24):2536-2543.
144. Faye O, Freire CC, Iamarino A, et al. Molecular evolution of Zika virus during its emergence in the 20th century. *PLoS Negl Trop Dis.* 2014;8(1):e2636.
151. Fleming-Dutra KE, Nelson JM, Fischer M, et al. Update: interim guidelines for health care providers caring for infants and children with possible Zika virus infection—United States, February 2016. *MMWR Morb Mortal Wkly Rep.* 2016;65(7):182-187.
182. Haddow AD, Schuh AJ, Yasuda CY, et al. Genetic characterization of Zika virus strains: geographic expansion of the Asian lineage. *PLoS Negl Trop Dis.* 2012;6(2):e1477.
190. Hayes EB. Zika virus outside Africa. *Emerg Infect Dis.* 2009;15(9):1347-1350.
217. Karwowski MP, Nelson JM, Staples JE, et al. Zika Virus Disease: A CDC Update for pediatric health care providers. *Pediatrics.* 2016;137(5).
224. Kleber de Oliveira W, Cortez-Escalante J, De Oliveira WT, et al. Increase in reported prevalence of microcephaly in infants born to women living in areas with confirmed Zika virus transmission during the first trimester of pregnancy—Brazil, 2015. *MMWR Morb Mortal Wkly Rep.* 2016;65(9):242-247.
243. Li C, Xu D, Ye Q, et al. Zika virus disrupts neural progenitor development and leads to microcephaly in mice. *Cell Stem Cell.* 2016;19(5):672.
278. Miner JJ, Cao B, Govero J, et al. Zika virus infection during pregnancy in mice causes placental damage and fetal demise. *Cell.* 2016;165(5):1081-1091.
300. Musso D, Gubler DJ. Zika Virus. *Clin Microbiol Rev.* 2016;29(3):487-524.
341. Oster AM, Russell K, Stryker JE, et al. Update: Interim guidance for prevention of sexual transmission of Zika virus—United States, 2016. *MMWR Morb Mortal Wkly Rep.* 2016;65(12):323-325.
354. Petersen LR, Jamieson DJ, Powers AM, et al. Zika virus. *N Engl J Med.* 2016;374(16):1552-1563.
385. Rasmussen SA, Jamieson DJ, Honein MA, et al. Zika virus and birth defects: reviewing the evidence for causality. *N Engl J Med.* 2016;374(20):1981-1987.
406. Schuler-Faccini L, Ribeiro EM, Feitosa IM, et al. Possible association between Zika virus infection and microcephaly—Brazil, 2015. *MMWR Morb Mortal Wkly Rep.* 2016;65(3):59-62.
460. Waggoner JJ, Pinsky BA. Zika Virus: Diagnostics for an emerging pandemic threat. *J Clin Microbiol.* 2016;54(4):860-867.

The full reference list for this chapter is available at ExpertConsult.com.

176I ■ Other Less Commonly Recognized Flaviviruses

Theodore F. Tsai • Gail J. Harrison

The less medically recognized flaviviruses include dozens of arthropod-borne pathogens that may cause life-threatening illness and may potentially become emerging pathogens causing public health problems worldwide. The well-known flaviviruses, such as dengue, West Nile, yellow fever, tick-borne encephalitis, and Japanese encephalitis virus infections, as well as the recently emerged Zika virus, are discussed under their own chapters.[10,16,21]

POWASSAN VIRAL ENCEPHALITIS

Powassan viral encephalitis is the only zoonotic tick-borne flavivirus detected in North America. Powassan virus was isolated from a fatally infected patient and named after the patient's Ontario town of residence.[9] The virus is classified within the antigenic complex of tick-borne flaviviruses, with North American viruses circulating in two genetic lineages in distinct enzootic cycles.[11,12] More than half of surviving cases suffer from residual neurologic deficits, frequently associated with upper cervical damage leading to upper extremity muscle weakness and wasting. Powassan encephalitis should be considered in the differential of acute childhood encephalitis.

Epidemiology, Ecology, and Pathogenesis

Fewer than 50 sporadic cases of naturally acquired Powassan encephalitis have been reported from North America and others from Russia, as well as two laboratory-acquired cases. Approximately one fourth of the cases from North America have occurred in children younger than 15 years, and the preponderance of cases have been in males. Most cases have occurred in the summer or early fall, and one patient had an onset in December.[17,37]

Reported cases have been acquired chiefly in eastern and upper Midwestern US states and Canadian provinces; however, the geographic distribution of the virus is far wider, with strains recorded from West Virginia, Colorado, South Dakota, and California, and serologic evidence of infection in humans or animals reported from Wyoming, Minnesota, North Dakota, British Columbia, Alberta, and Sonora, Mexico.[4,11,24,41] Since 2008, the number of confirmed cases has increased.[4] Viral isolates also have been recovered from ticks, mosquitoes, and birds from southeastern Russia, and evidence of viral transmission in China and Southeast Asia has been reported.[33]

In North America, viruses in lineage 1 are transmitted to small mammals by *Ixodes cookei* ticks, chiefly to groundhogs, skunks, and weasels; by *Ixodes marxi* ticks mainly to red squirrels; and by *Dermacentor andersoni* ticks to chipmunks.[11,12] The virus is transmitted transstadially in *D. andersoni* and *Ixodes pacificus*, and transovarial transmission has been shown in other species. Lineage 2 viruses (deer tick virus) are transmitted by *Ixodes scapularis;* however, although infections have been demonstrated in *Peromyscus* mice, details of the viral transmission cycle are poorly defined. Because *I. scapularis* also is the vector of *Borrelia burgdorferi*, *Babesia microti*, and *Anaplasma phagocytophilum*, it is of interest that in a collection of adult ticks from Long Island and Westchester County, New York, 2% were infected with Powassan virus, whereas infection rates for the other pathogens were 64%, 20%, and 20%, respectively.[50] The absence of a Powassan epidemic paralleling that of Lyme disease suggests differences in the agents' transmission cycles. Because the deer tick virus has been implicated in two fatal Powassan encephalitis cases, it seems unlikely that the strain is less virulent to humans than lineage 1 strains.[17,49] Russian strains of the virus are identical to lineage 1 viruses, suggesting an introduction from North America within the last century, possibly with the importation of farmed minks.[30] *Ixodes persulcatus* and various *Haemaphysalis* ticks are the principal vectors, and *Apodemus* mice and *Microtus* voles are the main vertebrate hosts.

Seroprevalence in humans is low, from less than 1% to 3%. Human infections probably are rare because *I. cookei* ticks usually confine themselves to animal host burrows, limiting opportunities for human exposure. Patients usually give a history of outdoor exposure but, in one case involving a 13-month-old infant, an infected tick was brought into the home by a domestic cat.[53] Animal serosurveys indicate that infections occur in dogs, and exposure to ticks on domestic animals may be an alternative source of infection. In a survey of New York goats, 2% had serologic evidence of past Powassan virus infection, which indicates the possibility of raw milk-borne Powassan virus infection in the United States, similar to the alimentary transmission of tick-borne encephalitis from infected raw milk products in Europe.[55] Although no such cases of Powassan cases infection have been reported, experimental studies have shown that domestic goats can be infected with Powassan virus and can shed the virus into milk.

Clinical and pathologic signs of encephalitis have been produced in experimentally infected horses and mouse models.[45] In one mouse model, the disease progresses rapidly, with a poliomyelitis-like syndrome with a high level of POWV antigen in the ventral horn of the spinal cord, as well as marked infection of the spleen, suggesting that the lymphoid organs may play an important role in pathogensis.[45] Also, unlike Lyme disease and some rickettsial infections, Powassan virus infection can be transmitted after only a brief period of tick attachment.[11,12]

Clinical Manifestations

The incubation period may be several weeks after known exposure to a tick. Early symptoms of fever, headache, lethargy, vomiting, retro-orbital pain, and photophobia are followed by changes in sensorium, confusion, generalized or focal seizures, progressive weakness, difficulty ambulating and moving limbs, paresis, and paralysis, that may lead to coma and require ventilator support and intensive care.* Magnetic resonance imaging has shown restricted diffusion and abnormal enhancement in parietal and temporal lobes and thalamic hemorrhage, which is often seen in other forms of flaviviral encephalitis. Approximately 10% of cases have been fatal; however, significant neurologic sequelae follow in the majority of survivors, including hemiplegia, quadriplegia, aphasia, and cognitive impairment. Residual shoulder girdle atrophy and weakness, analogous to sequelae that occur after European and Far Eastern tick-borne encephalitis, are common.[7] In another patient, wasting and weakness of a leg consistent with lumbosacral poliomyelitis were reported.[9,25] On the other hand, a laboratory-confirmed case was reported in a febrile patient without neurologic signs.[24]

Clinical and experimental observations of tick-borne encephalitis suggest that chronic central nervous system infection characterized by a seizure disorder (i.e., epilepsia partialis continua), weakness, and dementia may occur after recovery from the acute phase of illness. A retrospective study of 22 Canadian patients with a similar clinical syndrome and in whom histologic changes in the brain resembled those of chronic tick-borne encephalitis showed no evidence of Powassan virus infection. However, none of these patients had a history of acute encephalitis.

Laboratory Diagnosis

Virus has been recovered from the brains of patients with fatal cases of the disease. A serologic diagnosis can be achieved more rapidly by detecting specific immunoglobulin (Ig)M antibody by IgM antibody capture-enzyme immunosorbent assay (MAC-EIA) in acute-phase serum or spinal fluid. Confirmatory testing using dilution plaque reduction neutralization test (PRNT) can be performed by the Centers for Disease Control and Prevention. Early in the illness, IgM MAC-EIA serologic studies on serum and cerebrospinal fluid (CSF) may be negative.[29] Heterologous antibodies from other flavivirus infections (e.g., dengue and West Nile and St. Louis encephalitis and Zika virus) or vaccinations (e.g., tick-borne encephalitis and yellow fever) may interfere with interpretation.

Differential Diagnosis

Powassan encephalitis should be considered in the differential diagnosis of acute childhood encephalitis. The clinical findings of encephalitis in a patient with a history of a tick bite acquired in an endemic area should suggest the possibility of Powassan encephalitis. However, because ixodid tick bites may be inconspicuous, a negative history does not exclude the diagnosis. Other viral agents of encephalitis, especially eastern equine encephalitis virus and California group viruses, which are prevalent in New York State and eastern Canada, should be considered in the differential diagnosis. Lyme disease, because of its known geographic distribution and association with a tick vector, also may be associated with neurologic complications; however, a history of having a typical rash and arthritis should differentiate the conditions. In a series of 145 clinical encephalitis cases at a Canadian tertiary pediatric hospital, one was attributed to Powassan virus.[28] Imported travel-associated cases of tick-borne encephalitis acquired in Europe have been reported, underscoring the value of obtaining a travel history.

Treatment and Prevention

No specific therapy for Powassan encephalitis is available. Personal protective measures to avoid tick bites are advised. Consumption of unpasteurized goat milk should be avoided because of the theoretical risk for contracting Powassan virus infection and the well-documented risk for acquiring other infections associated with raw milk. Inactivated tick-borne encephalitis vaccines licensed in Europe do not cross protect against Powassan virus infection.

ROCIO VIRAL ENCEPHALITIS

Rocio viral encephalitis should be considered in the differential diagnosis of viral encephalitis in endemic people or travelers from South America.

*References 4, 6, 7, 9, 11, 13, 14, 16, 17, 19-21, 23-25, 30, 34, 36, 37, 41, 42, 48, 49, 53.

Rocio encephalitis virus is a flavivirus and was isolated from the brain of a fatal case of encephalitis in a patient during an outbreak in 1975 in São Paulo State, Brazil.[14,31] The virus is antigenically to viruses in the Japanese encephalitis virus complex. The disease has been reported exclusively in São Paulo State and adjacent Paraná State, Brazil, principally in the Ribiera Valley and Santista lowlands. More than 1000 cases were documented in outbreaks between 1975 and 1977; only one symptomatic case (in an infant) has been recognized subsequently, although recent infections (IgM in asymptomatic individuals) were documented in later serosurveys in northeastern and southeastern Brazil. Thus, the virus may be transmitted undetected in an area beyond the Ribiera Valley. Because of deforestation and global and geographic changes, as well as the competency of a wide variety of mosquito species for transmitting Rocio virus, it may emerge, like other previously obscure flaviviruses such as Zika virus, to become a more widely distributed pathogenic flavivirus. The viral transmission cycle has not been elucidated; however, field and laboratory observations suggest transmission between birds and *Psorophora* or *Aedes* mosquitoes. Seroprevalence studies in healthy Brazilian horses showed 6% were seropositive for Rocio virus, yet were entirely asymptomatic.[47] Humans are dead-end hosts. Human cases have occurred principally in men with outdoor occupations, especially fishermen.

The incubation period is estimated to be 7 to 14 days. Prodromal symptoms of fever, headache, malaise, vomiting, and conjunctivitis are followed by mental status changes, meningismus, and motor impairment. Cerebellar signs occur commonly. Signs of bulbar involvement also are seen. Coma and a fatal outcome occur most commonly in children (30%) and in older people; overall, 10% of cases are fatal, and 20% of patients have had neuropsychiatric sequelae. Pathologic findings of encephalitis principally involve the thalamus, cerebellar dentate nucleus, brain nuclei, brain stem, and spinal cord.

The diagnosis should be suspected in patients with acute encephalitis acquired in South America. The presence of virus-specific IgM in CSF or a fourfold change in serum antibody titer confirms a case, but cross reactions with St. Louis encephalitis, dengue, and other flaviviruses should be ruled out using virus specific PRNT serologic studies. There is no specific antiviral therapy effective for Rocio viral encephalitis, and treatment is therefore supportive.[29] Emergency application of adulticide and larvicide pesticides has been used to control epidemics.

LOUPING ILL VIRUS

Louping ill virus encephalitis should be considered in the differential of viral encephalitis in endemic individuals and travelers from the British Isles, especially in individuals with occupational or household exposure to sheep, cattle, and economically valuable game birds such as the red grouse.[18,26] Louping ill virus derives its name from an old Scottish term describing the leaping motions of encephalitic sheep. Historical accounts of the disease in sheep date from 1795, and the virus was isolated in 1931. The virus is a member of the antigenic complex of tick-borne flaviviruses and is transmitted by *Ixodes ricinus* ticks.[8,18,19,35] Sheep, deer, mountain hares, and grouse are the principal amplifying hosts. Grouse may become infected by tick bites or by ingesting infected ticks. The disease is enzootic in pasturelands of Scotland, England, Wales, and Ireland, where human infections have occurred mainly in sheep farmers, veterinarians, and slaughterhouse workers or butchers who had direct contact with animals or their meat. Antibody prevalence is 10% in slaughterhouse workers in enzootic areas. Laboratory-acquired infections are common and account for half of all reported human cases. These observations suggest that infections are transmitted easily by direct mucous membrane or respiratory infection. Hospital surveillance in an enzootic area found louping ill virus to be a rare occurrence that was responsible for fewer than 0.5% of encephalitis cases. Related tick-borne viruses in Spain, Greece, Norway, and Turkey have not been associated with human disease. The virus is shed in sheep and goat milk, but unlike tick-borne encephalitis, milk-transmitted cases have not been reported. Sheep in the United Kingdom are routinely vaccinated with a crude inactivated vaccine.

The incubation period can be as short as 3 days. Four distinct clinical syndromes have been described.[8] These syndromes are influenza-like illness, biphasic encephalitis illness, poliomyelitis-like illness, and hemorrhagic fever. Approximately a third of patients have a self-limited influenza-like illness with fever, headache, dizziness, and myalgias. The febrile illness is followed by clinical improvement and a second encephalitic phase in more than half of cases. Neurologic symptoms include meningismus, severe headache, vomiting, drowsiness, and tremor; one fatal case was reported. A poliomyelitis syndrome with muscle weakness or paralysis has been described in a few cases; the final presentation is hemorrhagic fever, which was reported in one atypical laboratory-acquired case.

The diagnosis should be suspected in febrile patients with occupational or other exposure, especially if central nervous system symptoms are present. The diagnosis can be confirmed by polymerase chain reaction or, serologically, by demonstrating virus-specific IgM in CSF or serum or by a fourfold rise in antibody titer. Treatment is symptomatic. Consumption of unpasteurized milk products should be avoided. Persons with outdoor exposure in enzootic areas are advised to use repellents and other protective measures against tick bites. Treatment of the disease is supportive, there is no specific antiviral therapy available for louping ill disease.[15,29] Protective vaccination against louping ill virus infection in sheep is effective.[26] Licensed human vaccines against other tick-borne encephalitis virus are likely to be protective against louping ill virus infection, because of cross-protective antibodies.

KYASANUR FOREST DISEASE

Kyasanur Forest disease (KFD), also known as "monkey fever," is a tick-borne arboviral fever in the Russian spring-summer encephalitis complex of flaviviruses. It infects humans with a severe biphasic course of illness, characterized by a hemorrhagic fever presentation in the first phase, and an encephalitis presentation in the second phase of illness, with an endemic geographical distribution in southern Karnataka, India.[3] The disease is, however, emerging in other areas of India, despite surveillance and the availability of a vaccine. An outbreak occurred in 2016 in the Wayanad and Malappuram districts of Kerala, India, emphasizing that tick-borne diseases may emerge in new areas.[44] Exposure of the 2016 epidemic included indigenous tribes that depended on the forest for their livelihood and likely had high exposures to infected ticks in the forest.[44,46] Kyasanur Forest virus was isolated in 1957 after an outbreak of hemorrhagic fever, initially suspected to be the first outbreak of yellow fever in Asia, appeared in India in the Kyasanur Forest of Mysore (now Karnataka).[2,38-40] The virus subsequently was identified as a member of the tick-borne flaviviral antigenic complex and shown to be transmitted by *Haemaphysalis spinigera* (among numerous other ixodid ticks). Forest rodents, insectivores, and possibly bats, participate in the transmission cycle, and langur monkeys sicken in epizootics and die of the infection. Human cases occur in dry-season epidemics, chiefly in persons who have contact with tick-infested forests. The disease has spread geographically as villagers clear forests for pastureland. Between 1982 and 1988, 1847 cases were reported, 254 of which were fatal.[38] Hyperendemic transmission in Karnataka State continues despite the introduction of mass vaccination with a locally produced, inactivated chick embryo fibroblast-derived vaccine.[38] The geographic distribution of the virus is now known to be much broader, with virologic or serologic evidence of infection throughout China and on the Andaman and Nicobar Islands.[52]

Additionally, a viral variant of the virus that has caused outbreaks of hemorrhagic fever in Saudi Arabia, Alkhumra virus, was transmitted to Italian tourists visiting the Egypt-Sudan border, indicating a distribution possibly encompassing a broad swath of Northern Africa, the Middle East, and into Central, South, and East Asia.[6,34] Molecular epidemiologic studies support the ancestral eastward spread of tick-borne flaviviruses, possibly along camel trade routes or by migrating birds carrying infected ticks.[22] Alkhumra virus has been acquired principally by persons who had close contact with livestock animals or their meat during or after slaughter, although mosquito-borne transmission from infected animals also has been suspected.[34] Tick-borne transmission was strongly suspected in the case of the Italian tourists.[6]

After an incubation period of 3 to 8 days, illness begins abruptly with fever, headache, myalgias, chills, and gastrointestinal symptoms.[2,39,40]

Patients are seriously ill with facial hyperemia, conjunctival suffusion, lymphadenopathy, and hepatomegaly, and they may be bradycardic and hypotensive. A papulovesicular enanthem and petechiae are seen, and mucosal bleeding from the gums, epistaxis, hemoptysis, and gastrointestinal and vaginal bleeding may be prominent. Bronchopneumonia and hemorrhagic pulmonary edema complicate the illness in 40% of cases. Renal failure may develop. After the resolution of symptoms and an afebrile interval of 1 to 3 weeks, fever, recurrence of symptoms, and meningoencephalitis develop in 15% to 50% of cases, as occurs in tick-borne encephalitis. Although biphasic febrile illness also occurs in patients infected with Alkhumra virus, encephalitis, which complicates one fourth of cases, usually is a component of the primary illness.[34] Ocular findings may also occur. Leukopenia with a left shift, thrombocytopenia, and an elevated hematocrit reflecting hemoconcentration are seen, and, in some cases, evidence of disseminated intravascular coagulation. Elevations in liver enzymes are present in the majority of cases. The case-fatality rate is 3% to 15%. Keratitis and iritis have been reported to occur as sequelae. The virus frequently can be isolated from acute-phase blood specimens (<12 days after onset), or the diagnosis can be confirmed serologically. There is no specific antiviral treatment for tick-borne flavivirus infection associated with KFD, so treatment is supportive.[15,29] Prevention is possible through an available vaccine with a formalin-inactivated tissue-culture vaccine available in India. Two doses administered 1 month apart confer temporary immunity for 6 to 12 months, and annual booster doses are recommended if outbreaks occur. However, because of vaccine side effects and the need for multiple doses and boosters, vaccine coverage is low, even in high-risk groups.[27]

OMSK HEMORRHAGIC FEVER

Omsk hemorrhagic fever (OHF) virus was isolated from a viremic human during a series of outbreaks in the Omsk region of western Siberia, Russia, from 1945 to 1949.[32,43] Omsk hemorrhagic fever is a tick-borne infection that occurs in the western Siberia regions of Omsk, Novosibirsk, Kurgan, and Tyumen. Between 1945 and 1958, approximately 1500 cases were reported in the forest-steppe zones within the Omsk, Novosibirsk, Kurgan, and Tyumen regions; however, the distribution of enzootic and human infections has shrunk considerably, and human cases now are reported sporadically only from Novosibirsk. The virus is related antigenically to other tick-borne flaviviruses and is spread by *Dermacentor marginatus, D. reticulatus,* and *Ixodes persulcatus* ticks that may be dually infected with tick-borne encephalitis virus. Numerous small mammals, especially *Microtus* voles, are infected in the transmission cycle, but it was the introduction of muskrats *(Ondatra zibethicus)* into the region from Canada in the early 20th century that resulted in an expansion of viral transmission and large outbreaks in trappers, despite high mortality in the infected muskrats. Seasonal peaks of infection are in May to June and August to September, but recent cases, occurring principally among hunters and trappers, occur through the end of the year. Infections are transmitted by tick bites, directly from infected muskrats during skinning, and potentially from streams where the virus survives for months after being shed by infected animals. Alimentary infection from consumption of infected goat milk is possible but has not been reported. Laboratory-associated cases frequently have occurred.

The incubation period may be as brief as 2 to 4 days. The illness is similar to Kyasanur Forest disease from India and Alkhumra hemorrhagic fever from Saudi Arabia, but with an earlier onset of hemorrhagic phenomena (e.g., epistaxis). Hemorrhages tend to be less severe, and the overall mortality rate is lower (<3%). A second phase of illness develops after an asymptomatic period of 1 to 2 weeks in 30% to 50% of cases and frequently is dominated by neurologic symptoms and encephalitis. Laboratory diagnosis of OHF is by detection of the virus in blood samples by virus isolation or molecular techniques such as polymerase chain reaction (PCR) to detect the viral genome in blood or CSF during the acute first phase of illness. Treatment is supportive, and there is no specific antiviral therapy available for OHF.[15,29] Antibody production may also be detected in serum and CSF later in the second phase of illness. Vaccine produced against tick-borne encephalitis virus is reported to provide some degree of cross protection for OHF.

OTHER FLAVIVIRAL INFECTIONS

Flaviviral infections of lesser public health importance or that are recognized less frequently are listed in Table 176I.1.[1,5,33,36,54] Several of the viruses are known to cause human illness only after laboratory exposure, and others, such as Usutu virus, have been reported to cause illness only in highly immunocompromised patients.[51] Alkhumra virus infection emerged in Saudi Arabia in 2001, as a serious zoonotic hemorrhagic fever, causing acute viral hemorrhagic fever in humans, and appeared to be transmitted from sheep or goats to humans by mosquito bites or direct contact with these animals.[34] The clinical

TABLE 176I.1 Less Commonly Recognized Flaviviral Infections

Virus	Clinical Syndrome	Geographic Distribution	Transmission Cycle	Mode of Transmission
Alfuy	Fever	Australia	Unknown	V
Alkhumra virus	Hemorrhagic fever	Saudi Arabia	Mosquito: sheep, goat	V
Apoi	Encephalitis	Japan	Rodent: ?	L
Banzi	Nonspecific febrile illness	South, East Africa	*Culex rubinotus:* Rodent	V
Bussuquara	Fever, arthralgias	Brazil, Colombia, Panama	*Culex melaconion:* Rodent	V
Edge Hill	Fever, polyarthritis	Australia	*Aedes vigilax:* Marsupial	V
Ilheus	Fever, myalgia, encephalitis	Argentina, Brazil, Colombia, Guatemala, Panama, Trinidad	*Psorophora ferox:* Bird	V, E
Karshi	Nonspecific febrile illness	Uzbekistan	Various ticks: Rodent	V
Kokobera	Fever, polyarthralgia	Australia, Papua New Guinea	*Culex annulirostris:* ? Marsupial	V
Koutango	Fever, rash, arthralgia	Western and central Africa	Tick: Rodent	L
Langat	Fever, encephalitis	Malaysia, Thailand, Russia	*Ixodes* tick: Rodent	L
Modoc	Aseptic meningitis	Western United States, Canada	Rodent: Rodent	Z
Negishi	Encephalitis	Japan, China, Russia	Tick: Unknown	L, V
Rio Bravo	Nonspecific febrile illness, meningitis	Western United States, Canada	Bat: Bat	Z, L
Sepik	Nonspecific febrile illness	Papua New Guinea	*Mansonia* spp.: ?	V
Spondweni	Fever, arthralgia, rash	Southern and western Africa	*Aedes* spp.: ?	L, V
Usutu	Fever, rash, encephalitis	Southern and central Africa, Europe	*Culex* spp.: Bird	V
Wesselsbron	Fever, arthralgia, rash, encephalitis	Sub-Saharan Africa, Thailand	*Aedes* spp.: ?	V, L, DC?

DC, Direct contact with infected sheep; *E,* experimental infection; *L,* laboratory-acquired infection; *V,* vector-borne infection; *Z,* zoonotic infection.

manifestations of these infections may differ from naturally acquired infection because of their mode of transmission by respiratory, mucosal, or other routes of infection. Other viruses that cause nonspecific syndromes of febrile illness were discovered through fever surveys; although few cases may have been reported, their prevalence may be underestimated because few cases are recognized.[1,5,33,36,54] Because immune responses to repeated flaviviral infections lead to broadly cross-reactive responses, serologic diagnosis may be misleading unless extensive cross-neutralization assays are undertaken. Of the zoonotic flaviviruses (transmitted from animal to animal without an arthropod vector), only Rio Bravo and Modoc viruses are known to cause human illness.

NEW REFERENCES SINCE THE SEVENTH EDITION

3. Awate P, Yadav P, Patil D, et al. Outbreak of Kyasanur Forest disease (monkey fever) in Sindhudurg, Maharashtra State, India, 2016. *J Infect.* 2016;72(6):759-761.
4. Birge J, Sonnesyn S. Powassan virus encephalitis, Minnesota, USA. *Emerg Infect Dis.* 2012;18(10):1669.
15. Flint M, McMullan L, Dodd K, et al. Inhibitors of the tick-borne, hemorrhagic fever-associated flaviviruses. *Antimicrob Agents Chemother.* 2014;58(6):3206-3216.
18. Gilbert L. Louping ill virus in the UK: a review of the hosts, transmission, and ecological consequences of control. *Exp Appl Acarol.* 2016;68(3):363-374.
26. Jeffires C, Mansfield K, Phipps L, et al. Louping Ill virus: an endemic tick-borne disease of Great Britain. *J Gen Virol.* 2014;95(Pt5):1005-1014.
27. Kiran S, Pasai A, Kumar S, et al. Kyasanur Forest disease outbreak and vaccination strategy, Shimoga District, India, 2013-12014. *Emerg Infect Dis.* 2015;21(1):146-149.
29. Lani R, Moghaddam E, Haghani A, et al. Tick-borne viruses: a review from the perspective of therapeutic approaches. *Ticks Tick Borne Dis.* 2014;5(5):457-465.
41. Raval M, Singhai M, Guererro D, Alonto A. Powassan virus infection: case series and literature review from a single institution. *BMC Res Notes.* 2012;5:594.
44. Sadanandane C, Elango A, Marja N, et al. An outbreak of Kyasanur forest disease in the Wayand and Malappuram districts of Kerala, India. *Ticks Tick Borne Dis.* 2017;8(1):25-30.
45. Santos R, Hermance M, Geiman B, Thangamani S. Spinal cord ventral horns and lymphoid organ involvement in Powassan virus infection in a mouse model. *Viruses.* 2016;8(6):E220.
46. Shiji P, Viswanath V, Sreekumar S, et al. Kyasanur Forest disease—first reported case in Kerala. *J Assoc Physicians India.* 2016;64(3):90-91.
47. Silva J, Romeiro M, Souza V, et al. A Saint Louis encephalitis and Rocio virus serosurvey in Brazilian horses. *Rev Soc Bras Med Trop.* 2014;47(4):414-417.

The full reference list for this chapter is available at ExpertConsult.com.

Hepatitis C Virus 177

Ravi Jhaveri • Samer S. El-Kamary

Hepatitis C virus (HCV) is a major cause of chronic liver disease in both adults and children. HCV was officially discovered only 27 years ago, but progress in understanding the viral life cycle and developing therapies has been very rapid over the past decade. In the last few years alone, the rate of drug discovery has been breathtaking, with a major shift in HCV prognosis from a chronic and difficult-to-treat disease, to an illness that is readily curable using a combination of oral drugs. For children, the challenge will continue to be which patients require therapy and when is the right time to initiate treatment. This chapter attempts to summarize what is known about the HCV life cycle, how HCV presents in children, and how HCV treatment will change in the next decade.

HISTORY

After reliable testing for both hepatitis A and B was developed, it became clear that a significant number of bloodborne, transfusion-related cases of hepatitis existed. These patients appeared to be infected with an agent that tested negative for both hepatitis A and B and thus was deemed "non-A, non-B hepatitis." The agent was suspected to be viral because transfer of blood from affected patients into naïve chimpanzees resulted in hepatitis. After a great deal of effort, the virus was finally identified in 1989.[26] A group at Chiron Corporation used molecular methods to identify RNA sequences from infected chimpanzees that were distinct from any known virus. HCV was the first pathogen to be described using only molecular methods, a practice that has now become the standard form of pathogen discovery. After a great deal of validation work, they named the virus hepatitis C virus.[68]

VIROLOGY

HCV is classified in its own *Hepacivirus* genus within the Flaviviridae family.[74,104] It is an enveloped, single-stranded, plus-sense RNA virus organized into one long open reading frame of approximately 9500 nucleotides.[75] It has the structural protein genes at its 5′ end and its nonstructural proteins toward the 3′ end.[36,97] Fig. 177.1 illustrates how the HCV genome is organized and lists the names of individual proteins and their main role during infection. The details of the molecular and structural biology of HCV are reviewed elsewhere,[36,75,97] but several unique features of the HCV genome are worth noting here. The HCV RNA 5′ untranslated region (5′UTR) contains an internal ribosomal entry site (IRES), a feature that no other flavivirus contains.[28] The IRES allows for direct binding of host ribosomes to the viral RNA using a set of proteins different from those required for conventional capP-dependent translation. The 3′UTR does not feature a poly-A tail as many flaviviruses do.[36] The HCV E2 protein contains a hypervariable region that responds to immune-mediated pressure with hypermutation.[36] The viral RNA polymerase lacks proofreading ability and, with a replication rate of approximately 10^8 virions per day,[12] has the potential to generate a mutation in every single position of the genome in one infected host every 24 hours. Whereas many of these are "lethal mutants" and do not survive, enough are generated that allow for one or more viable viruses that are able to rapidly escape antibody neutralization in a fashion very similar to that observed with human immunodeficiency virus (HIV). Each infected individual may harbor innumerable HCV variants that constitute a "quasispecies," which often overwhelms the immune response and makes vaccine development highly complicated.[50,51] The HCV NS3 is a multifunctional protein, with both helicase and protease domains.[74,75] The HCV NS5A protein is an important cofactor for many viral processes, including RNA replication and viral assembly, and the HCV NS5B is the RNA-dependent RNA polymerase.[74,75]

In vitro systems used to study HCV include subgenomic replicons, which are RNA constructs containing only the nonstructural region of the virus that can replicate themselves but produce no functional virus.[16,76] Pseudoviruses using a retrovirus or Semliki Forest virus as a backbone have been used to study virus-receptor interaction.[15,51] In 2005, a one-of-a-kind isolate of HCV was discovered in Japan, deemed "JFH1," which was found to replicate in vitro and produce infectious virus in several liver cell lines.[132] This discovery has since allowed for incredibly rapid progress in understanding the HCV viral life cycle.

HCV exists in the bloodstream in several different forms: naked virus, which would be the enveloped virus alone; HCV bound to antibody in higher density fractions; and HCV bound to low-density lipoproteins (LDL) and very-low-density lipoproteins (VLDL).[6,9,10] These last two

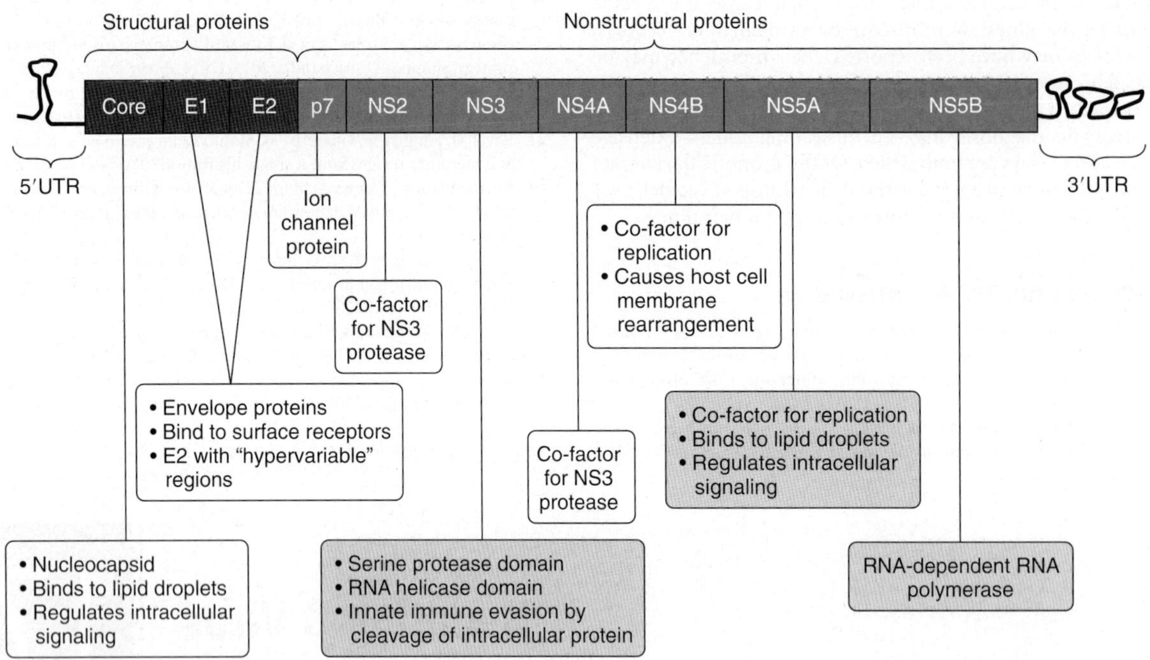

FIG. 177.1 Genomic organization of hepatitis C virus (HCV). HCV is organized as a single open reading frame coding for one polyprotein that is subsequently cleaved into multiple individual proteins. Structural proteins are shaded in *dark gray,* nonstructural proteins in *light gray.* The name and most important functions of each protein are provided. Proteins that are current or near-future direct antiviral targets are indicated by a *shaded* function box. *UTR,* Untranslated region.

fractions are deemed lipo-viro particles (LVPs) and have been shown to be the most infectious form of HCV.[6,10,14,41]

PATHOGENESIS

After gaining access to the bloodstream, the virus enters the liver through the sinusoidal blood, after which viral cell entry is a complex multistep process, requiring several cellular factors that trigger virus uptake into the hepatocytes. The virus replicates within the infected cell but does not cause cytolysis.[74,75] HCV replicates to very high levels within liver cells, and a significant proportion of the virus is released into the bloodstream. The exact levels of virus in the liver vary considerably from patient to patient based on age, genetics, and other host factors, with the interaction between virus, host liver cells, and host immune cells resulting in either resolution of infection or progression to chronic infection.[25,29] Resolved acute HCV has no long-term consequences. During chronic infection, inflammatory signals are released from the infected cells that, over time, contribute to the fibrosis and necrosis that is observed with long-standing infection.[114]

VIRAL LIFE CYCLE

HCV has been shown to interact with several proteins that serve as primary receptors or coreceptors depending on whether it is the initial infection or whether cell-to-cell spread has occurred within an already infected liver.[99] Viral entry occurs in three main steps, by poorly understood mechanisms: (1) viral attachment to the hepatocyte; (2) receptor-mediated viral particle endocytosis; and (3) endosomal fusion.[141] The first interaction appears to be when LVPs interact with the scavenger-receptor B1 (SR-B1) protein.[21] This interaction is not required, and other lipid-related proteins such as the low-density lipoprotein receptor (LDLR) may substitute for SR-B1.[87] Given the enrichment of these proteins on liver cells, this step likely provides much of the tissue specificity for the virus. After this initial binding step, a more specific interaction takes place between the HCV E2 protein and the CD81 molecule.[62,140] This interaction is thought to be a critical one for initial infections. This E2-CD81 complex then traffics to the tight junction of the cell, where interactions with both tight junction proteins claudin-1 and occludin-1 mediate the final steps in viral entry.[34,47,100] It has been shown that for direct cell-to-cell spread, the tight junction proteins can mediate infection alone, bypassing the need for CD81 or SR-B1.[126] After cell entry, HCV relies on a specific interaction with a liver-specific microRNA, miR-122, as a necessary cofactor.[60] The HCV RNA has two sites in the 5′UTR that are complementary to miR-122.[59] This is the first instance of a microRNA enhancing the function of an RNA, because in almost every other circumstance, microRNAs serve to silence gene expression by causing degradation of mRNA.

Another key step in the HCV life cycle is the association of the core protein with lipid droplets as part of viral assembly and release.[18,85] When first discovered, this was unique among flaviviruses, although it is now understood that dengue virus also associates with lipid droplets.[110] When bound to lipid droplets, the core protein recruits other viral proteins and newly synthesized RNA to form new virions.[85] Disruption of this association prevents the release of infectious virus.[18] HCV has evolved to co-opt many host lipid synthesis and trafficking pathways—binding to lipid droplets, requiring several apolipoproteins for assembly, and using VLDL export pathways for viral release.[10,14,54,63,85,109,115,117]

EPIDEMIOLOGY

The epidemiology of HCV varies significantly based on age and geography. In the general US population, approximately 4 million have HCV antibody-positive status and approximately two thirds of those have chronic infection.[8,12] In children, between 0.1% and 0.4% have evidence of HCV antibody.[8,32] In recent years, cases of HCV have been rising in teenagers and young adults due to widespread opioid abuse.[142]

Certain countries are known to have exceedingly high rates of HCV seroprevalence, largely as a result of unsafe injection practices and a contaminated blood supply. Pakistan is known to have HCV seroprevalence rates of 4% to 10%.[65,129] In Egypt, 10% to 15% of the general population, including children, have HCV antibody-positive status.[46,61,116]

This the highest rate in the world and is largely due to widespread inoculation of many individuals during a 20-year public health intervention to control schistosomiasis.[37,40] After screening for the parasite in the stool and urine, patients were treated with an intravenous tartar preparation.[119] While this was a well-intentioned public health intervention by the Ministry of Health, there were no disposable syringes available and, unknown to them at the time, boiling of glass syringes and needles in water was not sufficient to kill the virus. Once oral praziquantel replaced the intravenous treatment, the rates of HCV infection from this intervention were reduced significantly. However, the seroprevalence in the population was already high, and other modes of transmission serve to perpetuate the epidemic.[2,33,86,98]

VIRAL GENETICS

HCV has six major genotypes of HCV that vary in their geographic distribution.[36,84,118] Genotypes 1a and 1b are the most prevalent genotypes in the United States and Western Europe. Genotypes 2 and 3 are minority genotypes in this region, but are more frequently observed in Asia and Australia. Genotype 4 is frequently observed in Africa, particularly in Egypt. Genotypes 5 and 6 are minority genotypes, mostly in Africa.

The different genotypes are associated with important clinical phenotypes. Response to interferon (IFN)-based therapy varies widely based on genotype.[39] Genotypes 2 and 3 are exceedingly responsive to IFN, with sustained response rates between 80% and 90%. Genotypes 1a, 1b, and 4 all respond to IFN at much lower rates, closer to 40% to 50%. Genotype 3 is associated with more frequent and more severe steatosis (fatty liver) in contrast to other genotypes.[53,95]

TRANSMISSION

HCV is transmitted efficiently by exposure to blood and blood-containing solutions, tissue, and equipment.[74,139] Before the advent of effective tests for screening blood and blood products in the early 1990s, virtually all patients dependent on regular transfusions, such as hemophiliacs and patients with hemoglobinopathies, became chronically infected with HCV.[7,134] In the current era, in which blood supplies are rigorously screened, the primary route of blood-borne transmission is among injection drug users. Nosocomial transmission from medical and dental equipment is a constant issue that manifests when intentional and unintentional breaches of sterile techniques occur.[4,48,22,105,122]

For children, the major route of transmission is mother to infant (vertical transmission).[13] It is clear that only mothers with active viremia will transmit HCV, but beyond that, no clear risk factors for transmission have been defined.[131,79,103,116] Although higher viral loads increase risk, no threshold level has been defined. Cesarean section has not been demonstrated to be protective against transmission.[31,22,79,83] Studies from countries with different prevailing genotypes demonstrate comparable rates of transmission.[131,79,116] Overall transmission rates vary between 5% and 10%, depending on the study. In the era before highly active antiretroviral therapy (HAART), HIV coinfection raised the vertical transmission rate to 20% to 25%.[92,103,125] However, in the current HAART era, if a woman's HIV disease is suppressed or well controlled, the risk for HCV vertical transmission is comparable to that with HCV monoinfection.[23] For reasons that are not entirely clear, a significant rate of spontaneous resolution of HCV infection occurs among young children such that up to 50% of those with an initial transmission resolve their HCV viremia, leaving a rate of chronic infection after vertical transmission of 3% to 5%.[22,116]

Other, less frequent modes of transmission deserve some discussion. Sexual transmission is an inefficient and uncommon route of transmission.[78,89,123] This has been demonstrated largely in long-term studies of serodiscordant couples, in whom the infection rate was only 1% to 2%, and many of those who seroconverted had independent risk factors for HCV infection. The exception to this is for men who have sex with men, which is a high-risk exposure.[69] Tattooing is not considered a high-risk exposure, particularly in the current era when sterile techniques are commonplace.[127] This may not be true for a war veteran or prisoner, or community "tattoo parties" where sterile techniques may not be used. Breast-feeding has never been documented as a source of infection and is not contraindicated in new mothers who have HCV infection.[31,67,72] Other microscopic blood exposures from razors and toothbrushes are possible and are targets for prevention measures.[131] In a fraction of patients, no obvious risk factor for HCV exists. It is presumed that some of these microscopic exposures may have been the cause in these cases or that patients either may not recall their high-risk exposure or may not be entirely forthcoming.

CLINICAL MANIFESTATIONS

HCV in most cases is an asymptomatic infection.[7,58] Patients are often diagnosed when seeking medical attention for other reasons and are found to have elevated liver enzymes. In the minority of cases, patients will have acute signs of hepatitis, including malaise, jaundice, abdominal pain, and discomfort.[133] This is often the sign of a robust immune response that may portend clearance of the acute infection. In most patients, there are no acute symptoms and the infection quietly progresses from acute to chronic over the course of several months.

For children infected with HCV, these same observations largely hold true.[58] Infants infected at birth manifest no symptoms for many years.[128] They are often diagnosed only because the mother is known to be infected or has several high-risk factors that warrant screening. Some infants may have elevated transaminases early in life, but most do not. HCV does not alter physical growth or cognitive development. This is an important point to emphasize with parents in counseling during early visits.

Children are also frequently diagnosed during their teenage years during screening for other reasons. Commonly encountered scenarios include testing of those who were preterm infants born in the late 1980s or early 1990s, especially those who needed blood transfusions, or teenagers who were screened as part of a school blood donation drive and tested positive for HCV antibody.

The major risk for chronic HCV infection is the progression to chronic liver disease, which includes both cirrhosis and subsequent hepatocellular carcinoma (HCC).[114] The rate of these complications in children is low, approximately 5% of the time, but it increases with duration of infection. A European study demonstrated that cirrhosis was observed only in children infected for more than 10 years.[57] A large US study demonstrated that many infected children who underwent biopsy had either mild or no fibrosis.[45] Teenagers can have HCV-associated cirrhosis or HCC requiring transplant.[108]

HCV has a variety of extrahepatic manifestations that are primarily observed in adults, but may be possible in children.[20,55] These are skin and joint manifestations such as porphyria cutanea tarda, mixed cryoglobulinemia, and vasculitis that are due to immune complex deposition in small vessels. HCV has also been associated with insulin resistance and resulting diabetes.[91] Although the specific mechanism of this is unknown, it is likely due to effects of the HCV core protein on regulation of glucose metabolism at multiple levels within liver cells.[90,96] HCV also has been associated with extreme levels of fatigue and altered mood and concentration.[111] It has recently been demonstrated that HCV can infect brain endothelial cells in vitro, and immunohistochemistry has shown HCV to be present in the brain tissue of chronically infected patients.[35] This raises the possibility that HCV may have some direct effect on the brain.

IMMUNITY

HCV infection is associated with both a cellular and humoral immune response.[19] Responses can be detected after approximately 6 to 8 weeks of infection. Patients with acute infection have evidence of a robust cell-mediated response, with readily detected HCV-specific $CD8^+$ T cells.[133] This response mediates clearance of acute infection in these patients. Most patients, however, have specific T cells detected, but the response is weak and ineffective. These patients progress to chronic infection, and over time their T cells display an exhausted phenotype that has little impact on the course of infection.[102]

HCV antibodies are detectable throughout the course of infection, but their role in preventing infection is unclear.[19] As mentioned earlier, neutralizing antibodies to HCV are not observed because of the hypermutation observed in the HCV E2 protein generating many "quasispecies" of HCV that escape neutralization. However, the presence of antibody may alter progression of infection over time in ways not yet understood. HCV also interacts with the innate immune system to subvert host response to viral infection.[49] Multiple proteins have been demonstrated to directly cleave IFN-induced mediators of host protection.[121] A more specific discussion of these effects can be found in several in-depth reviews.[40,49]

DIAGNOSIS

HCV infection can be diagnosed by demonstration of HCV-specific antibody, the presence of HCV RNA from serum or blood samples, or direct demonstration of HCV proteins in serum or blood samples.[56] First-pass screening of at-risk children is usually done with enzyme-linked immunosorbent assay (ELISA)-based testing. If positive, patients can be tested using a highly specific recombinant immunoblot assay, which detects the presence of antibodies to several HCV proteins. However, this is very rarely necessary. Most practitioners would move immediately to testing for HCV RNA, because the presence of RNA demonstrates chronic infection, which is the most important biomarker of infection. HCV RNA is now done using a real-time polymerase chain reaction (PCR)-based assay that offers the advantages of both reliability for presence of viral RNA and a broad dynamic range for quantitation.[24] If HCV RNA is detected, a frequent next step is determination of HCV genotype, which is done by characterizing the sequence of the HCV polymerase gene.[118] As has been discussed previously, knowledge of genotype can have a major impact on the choice of how and when to treat a patient. Liver biopsy is now rarely performed in favor of noninvasive methods of fibrosis assessment. An algorithm for the evaluation of a child with HCV-positive antibody testing is outlined in Fig. 177.2.

The testing of those infants who are vertically exposed is an altogether different matter. Because of the persistence of maternal antibody and the significant potential for spontaneous resolution of infection in young children, simple ELISA or single-point HCV RNA can be misleading.[131,116] There is no consensus on the best time to test these infants. The approach of this author is outlined in Fig. 177.3. Because no treatment is initiated during infancy, testing is not recommended in the first year. The possible exception to this is if a parent has considerable anxiety over the possibility of infection or if there is a concern about possible loss of follow-up. In that case, performing an HCV RNA test in the first 2 to 6 months of life can be considered. If the test is negative, it is very reassuring, although not absolute that the child is not infected. A positive result indicates infection but still leaves open the possibility that the infant may spontaneously resolve the infection over the next 1 to 2 years. Preferred timing for testing would be after the first birthday and should include both an HCV antibody and HCV RNA PCR. A repeat result several months later confirming a negative test should be performed before declaring a child uninfected. If the initial test result is positive, a repeat in 6 to 12 months should be performed, and, if the result is still positive, an annual monitoring plan that includes a careful history and physical, liver function testing, and HCV RNA testing should be initiated.

Assessment for Severity of Disease

In addition to a careful physical examination to determine if signs of chronic liver disease are present, assessment of laboratory, radiologic, and pathologic specimens should be performed. The severity of transaminase elevation, if any, should be determined. These tests are notoriously insensitive for disease of mild and moderate severity but are helpful when normal or significantly elevated.[101] Other laboratory tests should be performed to assess the synthetic function of the liver (albumin, prothrombin time, partial thromboplastin time, etc.).[77]

Routine radiologic studies are not necessary for all HCV-infected patients. Ultrasound of the liver can be used at an initial visit for an assessment of any anatomic factors that may complicate future assessments.[77] Unlike hepatitis B virus, with which the risk for HCC is independent of liver damage, with rare exception, HCC with HCV occurs only after cirrhosis is present.[52] If a patient is known to have HCV-induced cirrhosis, annual ultrasounds are justified. If not, periodic testing every 5 years or so may be more appropriate.

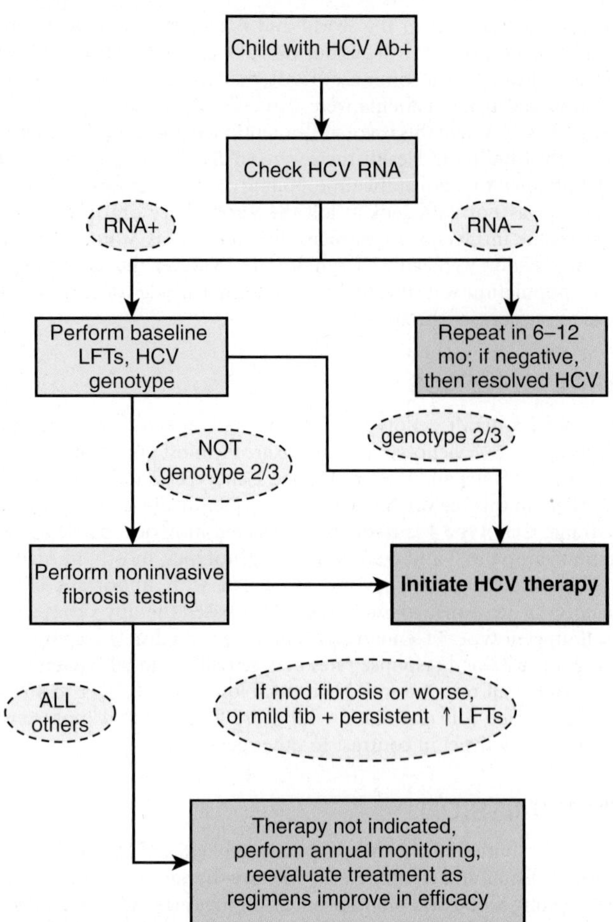

FIG. 177.2 Suggested algorithm for evaluation of a child with evidence of hepatitis C virus (HCV) antibody. Endpoints are highlighted by a *shaded box,* while key result branch points in the decision tree are highlighted in the *ovals* with *dashed borders. Ab+,* Positive for antibodies; *LFTs,* liver function tests.

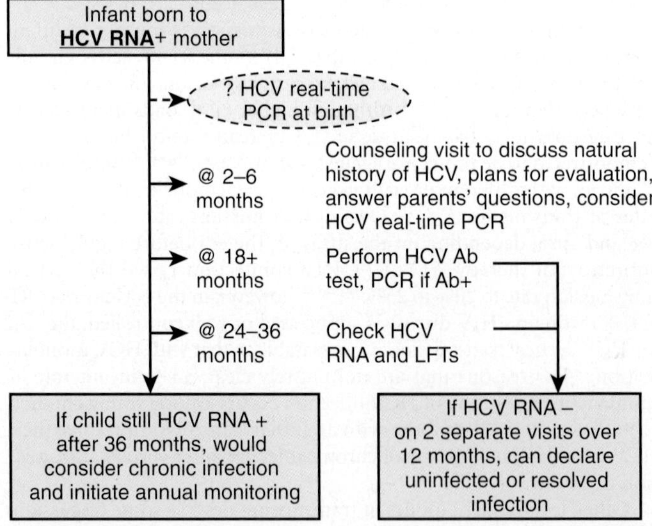

FIG. 177.3 Suggested algorithm for evaluation of the infant vertically exposed to hepatitis C virus (HCV). Endpoints are highlighted by a *shaded box,* while testing that has not yet been studied are highlighted with *dashed borders. Ab,* Antibody; *LFTs,* liver function tests; *PCR,* polymerase chain reaction.

Definitive assessment of HCV-induced liver damage is done using a liver biopsy, but this is rarely performed in the current era unless there is concern for other causes of liver disease.[77] More recently, sensitive ultrasound-based methods have been approved that are used to evaluate liver stiffness and fibrosis.[30,94] These are now being increasingly used to follow liver fibrosis and cirrhosis in HCV-infected adults and children in lieu of liver biopsy. Many studies have been performed to determine if combinations of laboratory or radiologic tests can be used to assess for liver fibrosis in the absence of a liver biopsy. These so-called noninvasive markers of fibrosis consist of a variety of blood tests that are used to create a score or index that allows for subsequent selection of those more likely to have severe liver damage. Most of these tests perform reasonably well at the ends of the disease severity spectrum, but very poorly in the middle.[93] This is true in children as well.[80]

Host Genetics

Studies performed in the past several years have now demonstrated that host genetics plays a significant role in the course of HCV disease. As part of a genome-wide associated study, polymorphisms within the *IL28b* gene were initially shown to have an exceedingly high correlation to response to treatment with IFN-based therapy.[42] In examination of the rates of the favorable polymorphisms in different ethnic groups, these polymorphisms potentially accounted for most of the racial and ethnic differences seen using IFN-based therapy. Further studies demonstrated that these polymorphisms also correlated very highly with patients resolving acute HCV in contrast to those whose disease progressed to chronic infection.[124] The mechanism underlying these significant differences has yet to be determined, but because *IL28b* encodes for a lambda-IFN that then regulates subsequent host antiviral responses, studies are being conducted to closely examine the initial lambda-IFN dynamics. No studies have thus far been performed in children, but because these are genetic differences, they likely will have the same impact there. One study searched for a potential role of this polymorphism in predicting and determining vertical transmission, but no correlation was found.[107] It is important to emphasize that although this polymorphism on a population level is an exceedingly powerful predictor of HCV clearance and response to therapy, it is still unclear how to use this information for the individual patient. Although this polymorphism is not absolutely predictive of response, it was used as a general guide for counseling patients in the era of interferon-based therapy.[27]

However, with the advent of oral direct-acting antiviral therapies that are not affected by the patient's IL28B status, it is no longer taken into consideration when planning an adult patient's therapeutic regimen.[1] A similar management approach is expected for children once these therapies are approved for younger age groups.

TREATMENT

The issue of when to initiate therapy for a child infected with HCV is still under contention.[77] There is no controversy in the case of a child who has clear evidence of liver compromise from long-standing HCV infection, but these cases are the minority. Because natural history studies of children with HCV do indicate that many of them will do well with only minimal progression of liver fibrosis, treatment initiation remains a controversial issue. Proponents of therapy argue the many potential benefits of treating children: the cost advantage of using less of an expensive drug when treating a smaller person; the number of years of "virus-free" life still ahead for a child; the absence of comorbidities in a child that may complicate treatment; eradicating virus before entering adolescence, when high-risk behavior that can potentially transmit the virus traditionally begins; and for girls, eliminating the potential for vertical transmission. At this point, the decision about when to treat is one that should be individualized on a case-by-case basis.

HCV treatment recommendations are rapidly changing, so the AASLD/IDSA have partnered to form a guidelines panel to maintain an up-to-date website with the most current information that now includes children.[1] The reader is referred there for a detailed discussion of drug doses, adjustments, and side effects. HCV therapy is undergoing a significant transition as more agents against specific viral proteins emerge from preclinical studies. This section attempts to cover currently approved information for HCV as well as what is anticipated in the next several years. Specific attention is focused on the existing data for treating children. The goal of HCV treatment is the eradication from the bloodstream of viral RNA that persists after the discontinuation of therapy. This is in stark contrast to HIV therapy, which is suppressive only while the medications are continued. It is thought that treatment for HCV reduces the burden of virus in the liver such that either HCV is completely eradicated from the system or the immune system is able to control the virus to such low levels as to be undetectable in the bloodstream. Rare cases have been reported of viral reemergence long after treatment response when immunosuppression is initiated for an unrelated reason, supporting the latter as a likely scenario.[73] For interferon-based therapy, the endpoint of HCV therapy is the sustained viral response (SVR), which was defined as the absence of detectable HCV RNA at 6 months after completion of therapy.[39,82] However, in the current era of direct-acting antiviral (DAA) therapy in adults, SVR is now defined as the absence of HCV RNA at 12 weeks after completion of therapy[1] and will presumably be the same after the new therapies are approved for children younger than 18 years of age. If patients do not achieve SVR, they are categorized as nonresponders (i.e., patients who never suppressed virus during treatment), partial responders (i.e., patients who partially suppressed virus early but then had recrudescence), or relapsers (i.e., patients who completely suppressed virus for some amount of time but then had recrudescence at some point later). Knowledge of this terminology is helpful in interpreting the HCV treatment literature and important because each group has a different prognosis if new treatment regimens are attempted later.

IFN-α and its chemically modified derivatives have long been the backbone for HCV therapy. Old preparations given subcutaneously three times per week offered SVR rates of only 15% to 20%.[29] In an attempt to improve the poor pharmacokinetics of traditional IFN, a polyethylene glycol (PEG-IFN) moiety was added to allow for much higher serum concentrations combined with less frequent weekly subcutaneous dosing. The use of PEG-IFN improved SVR rates by almost 20%.[39] It is interesting to note that studies examining patients with the favorable and unfavorable IL28b polymorphisms have shown that HCV patients who achieve SVR are those with low levels of IFN-induced gene expression that are readily enhanced with IFN administration, whereas patients who do not respond to treatment have high IFN-induced gene expression that is ineffective in counteracting the virus and incapable of being augmented with exogenous IFN.[3,130] It has long been known that significant racial and ethnic differences exist in rates of response to IFN therapy. African-American and Hispanic/Latino patients achieve SVR at rates significantly lower than those of Caucasian or Asian patients.[82,88] Much of this may be due to differences in IL28b status, but not entirely.

Ribavirin was mainstay of HCV therapy in children and can still be used in combination for certain genotypes. When traditional IFN was still being used with very low SVR rates, other agents were sought to boost its effects. With the addition of orally administered ribavirin, SVR rates increased to almost 40% for patients infected with genotypes 1a or 1b.[81] When PEG-IFN was developed, the combination of PEG-IFN and ribavirin resulted in SVR rates of 40% to 50% for genotype 1a and 1b patients and 80 to 90 for genotype 2 and 3 patients.[39] The mechanism of action of ribavirin is still unknown, but it is thought to inhibit viral replication efficiency enough to make the virus more susceptible to other agents. Ribavirin monotherapy has no effect on HCV RNA levels and does not lead to SVR.[17]

Although no longer the standard of care, PEG-IFN and ribavirin have been studied and approved for use in children at reduced doses.[56,112,113,135] Small pharmacokinetic studies determined that dosing of PEG-IFN based on either weight or body surface area led to serum drug levels comparable to those in adult administration.[113] Ribavirin is given on a weight-based dose for both children and adults.[44] The largest single study of HCV treatment in children was the Pediatric Study of Hepatitis C (PEDS-C) trial, which compared PEG-IFN alone to PEG-IFN plus ribavirin.[112] The rationale for this design was that many thought that PEG-IFN alone may be sufficient in younger children with the absence of many other adverse risk factors. The PEDS-C trial demonstrated that children had overall SVR rates comparable to their adult counterparts (53%) when treated with both drugs, significantly better in contrast to when PEG-IFN was used alone (37%). Several factors must be considered when treating children with these agents.[77,112] Side effects of PEG-IFN include flulike symptoms and malaise. For children attending school who require maximal function during the school week, PEG-IFN administration on Friday with coadministration of a nonsteroidal antiinflammatory agent has been effective in alleviating these effects. IFN can also cause neutropenia and hemolytic anemia, both of which can be managed with dose reduction. PEG-IFN has been shown to cause depression and suicidal ideation, dangerous at any age but particularly worrisome during the usually emotionally turbulent adolescent years. A side effect unique to children is the associated arrest of linear growth during PEG-IFN treatment. Although children do experience catch-up growth once the drug is discontinued, long-term follow-up is still being conducted to determine whether children actually attain their predicted midparental height.[64]

Starting in 2009, several directly acting antiviral drugs were approved by the FDA for adults. In 2009, two oral protease inhibitors were approved, boceprevir and telaprevir, which when combined with pegylated interferon and ribavirin increased the cure rate to 70% to 75% but had increased side-effects.[10,50,94,128] Two additional oral drugs were approved by the FDA in 2013, sofosbuvir (nucleotide analogue NS5B polymerase inhibitor) and simeprevir (protease inhibitor) which improved the cure rate to 90% when individually combined with pegylated interferon and ribavirin.[38,66] In July 2014, the first all-oral HCV-treatment regimen without interferon or ribavirin was approved by the FDA: a combination of ledipasvir (NS5A inhibitor) and sofosbuvir.[5] Later in 2014 (November), simeprevir and sofosbuvir were approved as another interferon-free all-oral treatment.[71] In December 2014, another all-oral regimen consisting of a combination of four drugs was approved by the FDA: ombitasvir (NS5A inhibitor), paritaprevir (NS3/4A protease inhibitor), ritonavir (CYP3A inhibitor), and dasabuvir (nonnucleoside NS5B polymerase inhibitor).[11] In 2015, another oral medication was approved, daclatasvir (NS5A inhibitor), for use with sofosbuvir to treat HCV genotype 3 infections without the need for coadministration of interferon or ribavirin.[120] In January 2016, the FDA approved elbasvir (NS5A replication complex inhibitor) and grazoprevir (NS3/4A protease inhibitor) with or without ribavirin for the treatment of chronic HCV genotypes 1 and 4 infections in adult patients.[70,106] In April 2017, sofosbuvir/ledipasvir was approved for use in children ages 12 to 17 years.[143] Clinical trials are currently ongoing with several DAA regimens in children down to 3 years of age.[136-138]

What also becomes possible in the future is interruption of vertical transmission using these specific antiviral agents in and around the time of delivery in a manner similar to treatment of HIV.[13] Given the much lower risk for transmission and lower morbidity and mortality in contrast to HIV, further studies into understanding better which mothers transmit HCV and when they transmit the virus would allow more selective drug use.

PREVENTION AND COUNSELING

No specific prevention measures are currently available against HCV infection. Attempts to create a vaccine have been frustrated by the heterogeneity of the virus and an incomplete understanding of immune correlates of protection that can reliably predict protection against the virus. Prevention largely rests on avoiding high-risk behaviors, rigorous sterile technique to avoid nosocomial transmission, and screening to identify HCV-infected adults and children so patients can be evaluated and treated. Counsel for the child who is already infected with HCV should include prompt care of bloody injuries, vaccination against other forms of viral hepatitis (hepatitis A and B) to avoid potentiated injury to the liver, being aware of prescription and nonprescription drugs that cause liver toxicity, and being aware of the risks of alcohol use when chronically infected with HCV and that no known safe level of alcohol consumption exists for HCV-infected patients.[77] It is also important to reiterate to parents that HCV-infected children grow and develop normally and do not present a risk to classmates. It is also important to advocate for HCV-infected children because some schools and other agencies needlessly continue to try to restrict the attendance and activities of HCV-infected children.

SUMMARY

Children with HCV infection often do very well with few or no long-term effects, but a few children do develop significant liver disease. A working knowledge of how to monitor and manage these patients can assist in mitigating the severity of disease. The treatment of HCV is in the midst of major changes that will revolutionize the field. Although multiple new oral anti-HCV direct-acting antiviral agents have been approved in adults,[1,43] they are still not ready to be used for children. Nevertheless, familiarity with what will ultimately become available will assist providers in discussions with their patients.

NEW REFERENCES SINCE THE SEVENTH EDITION

1. AASLD-IDSA. Recommendations for testing, managing, and treating hepatitis C. Available at: http://www.hcvguidelines.org.
2. Abdelwahab S, Rewisha E, Hashem M, et al. Risk factors for hepatitis C virus infection among Egyptian healthcare workers in a national liver diseases referral centre. *Trans R Soc Trop Med Hyg*. 2012;106(2):98-103.
5. Afdhal N, Zeuzem S, Kwo P, et al. Ledipasvir and sofosbuvir for untreated HCV genotype 1 infection. *N Engl J Med*. 2014;370(20):1889-1898.
11. Andreone P, Colombo MG, Enejosa JV, et al. ABT-450, ritonavir, ombitasvir, and dasabuvir achieves 97% and 100% sustained virologic response with or without ribavirin in treatment-experienced patients with HCV genotype 1b infection. *Gastroenterology*. 2014;147(2):359-365.e1.
33. Esmat G, Hashem M, El-Raziky M, et al. Risk factors for hepatitis C virus acquisition and predictors of persistence among Egyptian children. *Liver Int*. 2012;32(3):449-456.
37. Frank C, Mohamed MK, Strickland GT, et al. The role of parenteral antischistosomal therapy in the spread of hepatitis C virus in Egypt. *Lancet*. 2000;355(9207):887-891.
38. Fried MW, Buti M, Dore GJ, et al. Once-daily simeprevir (TMC435) with pegylated interferon and ribavirin in treatment-naive genotype 1 hepatitis C: the randomized PILLAR study. *Hepatology*. 2013;58(6):1918-1929.
43. World Health Organization. *World Health Organization Guidelines for the Screening Care and Treatment of Persons with Chronic Hepatitis C Infection: Updated Version*. Geneva: 2016.
46. Guerra J, Garenne M, Mohamed MK, et al. HCV burden of infection in Egypt: results from a nationwide survey. *J Viral Hepat*. 2012;19(8):560-567.
61. Kandeel A, Genedy M, El-Refai S, et al. The prevalence of HCV infection in Egypt 2015: implications for future policy on prevention and treatment. *Liver Int*. 2016.
66. Kowdley KV, Lawitz E, Crespo I, et al. Sofosbuvir with pegylated interferon alfa-2a and ribavirin for treatment-naive patients with hepatitis C genotype-1 infection (ATOMIC): an open-label, randomised, multicentre phase 2 trial. *Lancet*. 2013;381(9883):2100-2107.
71. Lawitz E, Gane E, Pearlman B, et al. Efficacy and safety of 12 weeks versus 18 weeks of treatment with grazoprevir (MK-5172) and elbasvir (MK-8742) with or without ribavirin for hepatitis C virus genotype 1 infection in previously untreated patients with cirrhosis and patients with previous null response with or without cirrhosis (C-WORTHY): a randomised, open-label phase 2 trial. *Lancet*. 2015;385(9973):1075-1086.
72. Lawitz E, Sulkowski MS, Ghalib R, et al. Simeprevir plus sofosbuvir, with or without ribavirin, to treat chronic infection with hepatitis C virus genotype 1 in non-responders to pegylated interferon and ribavirin and treatment-naive patients: the COSMOS randomised study. *Lancet*. 2014;384(9956):1756-1765.
100. Ploss A, Evans MJ. Hepatitis C virus host cell entry. *Curr Opin Virol*. 2012;2(1):14-19.
102. Radziewicz H, Ibegbu CC, Fernandez ML, et al. Liver-infiltrating lymphocytes in chronic human hepatitis C virus infection display an exhausted phenotype with high levels of PD-1 and low levels of CD127 expression. *J Virol*. 2007;81(6):2545-2553.
106. Roth D, Nelson DR, Bruchfeld A, et al. Grazoprevir plus elbasvir in treatment-naive and treatment-experienced patients with hepatitis C virus genotype 1 infection and stage 4-5 chronic kidney disease (the C-SURFER study): a combination phase 3 study. *Lancet*. 2015;386(10003):1537-1545.
120. Sulkowski MS, Gardiner DF, Rodriguez-Torres M, et al. Daclatasvir plus sofosbuvir for previously treated or untreated chronic HCV infection. *N Engl J Med*. 2014;370(3):211-221.
123. Terrault NA, Dodge JL, Murphy EL, et al. Sexual transmission of hepatitis C virus among monogamous heterosexual couples: the HCV partners study. *Hepatology*. 2013;57(3):881-889.
136. www.clinicaltrials.gov. Safety and Efficacy of Ledipasvir/Sofosbuvir Fixed Dose Combination +/- Ribavirin in Adolescents and Children with Chronic HCV-Infection. NCT02249182. https://clinicaltrials.gov/ct2/show/NCT02249182?term=harvoni+children&rank=1.
137. www.clinicaltrials.gov. Safety and Efficacy of Sofosbuvir + Ribavirin in Adolescents and Children with Genotype 2 or 3 Chronic HCV Infection. NCT02175758. https://clinicaltrials.gov/ct2/show/NCT02175758?term=sofosbuvir+children&rank=1.
138. www.clinicaltrials.gov. A Study to Evaluate the Pharmacokinetics, Safety, and Efficacy of Glecaprevir/Pibrentasvir in Pediatric Subjects With Genotypes 1-6 Chronic Hepatitis C Virus (HCV) Infection. Available at: https://clinicaltrials.gov/ct2/show/NCT03067129?term=NCT03067129&rank=1.
141. Zhu YZ, Qian XJ, Zhao P, et al. How hepatitis C virus invades hepatocytes: the mystery of viral entry. *World J Gastroenterol*. 2014;20(13):3457-3467.
142. Suryaprasad AG, White JZ, Xu F, et al. Emerging epidemic of hepatitis C virus infections among young nonurban persons who inject drugs in the United States, 2006-2012. *Clin Infect Dis*. 2014;59(10):1411-1419.
143. Balistreri WF, Murray KF, Rosenthal P, et al. The safety and effectiveness of ledipasvir-sofosbuvir in adolescents 12-17 years old with hepatitis C virus genotype 1 infection. *Hepatology*. 2017;66(2):371-378.

The full reference list for this chapter is available at ExpertConsult.com.

Influenza Viruses 178

Jonathan A. McCullers

Influenza is an acute respiratory disease caused by influenza viruses. Children are the main amplifiers of the virus, because of their naïve immune systems, and the main vectors for transmission, because of their high social contact rate. The clinical attack rate and hospitalization rate are also highest in young children. Evolutionarily, all influenza viruses are zoonoses, arising in the animal reservoir and spilling over into the human population. Children are often the first hosts in which infections are detected following cross-species transmission events, which are typically with swine or avian influenza A viruses. Several times a century, one of these zoonotic events results in a new influenza virus lineage becoming established in humans and circulating for years or decades as an endemic strain. The worldwide pandemic that occurs shortly after the nascent virus becomes established can have a profound impact on morbidity and mortality in children and young adults, with high rates of severe disease requiring intensive care and a higher case fatality rate in children than is typical with seasonal influenza. Because influenza viruses continually evolve and the illness they engender can vary considerably based on characteristics of the strain, the weather, and other circulating or endemic pathogens, as well as the number of susceptible hosts, the impact of each season on human health is unpredictable. To remain abreast of the latest information, clinicians are therefore referred to sources such as the Centers for Disease Control and Prevention (CDC)[58] and the World Health Organization (WHO)[503] for updated guidance on epidemiology, treatment, prevention, and control of influenza.

HISTORY

The origin of the term influenza has several possible derivations; the most likely is from the Latin *influentia* in the astrological sense of believing the stars have influence on disease. The first application of the word influenza to actual influenzal disease was probably during the 1743 pandemic, which started in Italy and spread worldwide,[15] but the term had been used since at least 1357 to describe various disease outbreaks, some of which were clearly not influenza.[192] Descriptions of epidemic respiratory disease that were likely to be influenza date back to as early as 412 BCE in an account by Hippocrates.[192] Numerous accounts of similar outbreaks can be found throughout the next two millennia.[440] The first description of an outbreak from multiple continents widespread enough to represent a pandemic occurred in 1580. Sporadic observations from autopsies document likely secondary bacterial pneumonia associated with an influenza epidemic as far back as the early 1700s.[328] René T.H. Laennec, the inventor of the stethoscope and the technique of auscultation, was the first to fully appreciate this association between epidemic influenza and bacterial pneumonia. During an 1803 epidemic of "la grippe" in Paris, he described several autopsies on patients who developed fatal lobar pneumonia shortly after an influenza-like illness.[249] This association of secondary bacterial infections with mortality came into sharper focus during the 1918 pandemic, which killed an estimated 50 million persons worldwide. More than 95% of all deaths from the 1918 influenza virus were associated with a secondary bacterial infection[329]; Louis Cruveilhier succinctly summed this up with the phrase, "if grippe condemns, the secondary infections execute."[85] The first influenza virus isolate came from an experimental infection of swine by Richard Shope in 1930.[411] Pigs only exhibited disease from *Haemophilus influenzae suis* when they were coinfected with a second agent, which turned out to be swine influenza virus upon isolation.[411,412] The first human isolation was in 1933 when scientist Wilson Smith, working with experimental infection models in ferrets, contracted influenza from one of the animals and developed secondary pneumococcal pneumonia.[12] Identification of influenza B viruses followed in 1936.[122] The discovery of the wild bird reservoir of influenza did not occur until the early 1970s when avian influenza viruses were isolated from wild birds,[419] allowing the ecology of these viruses to be elucidated through a series of field studies.[480]

BIOLOGY

Properties and Life Cycle

The hemagglutinin (HA) of influenza A and B viruses is the primary attachment protein. Structurally, the HA is a glycoprotein that exists in the virus as a trimer, with a globular head positioned as a spike through the captured cell membrane, and a fusion domain that protrudes through the membrane toward the virus's protein shell.[128,490] The nascent HA (termed HA0) must be proteolytically activated through a cleavage step mediated by a furin-like protease, resulting in HA1 and HA2 subunits that are capable of significant structural changes during membrane fusion.[38,128] Binding of the HA's evolutionarily conserved receptor binding domain to cell surface sialic acids allows internalization of virions by endocytosis into the acidic endosome (Fig. 178.1). The M2 protein, which is an ion channel spanning the virus's captured cell membrane, then acidifies the interior of the virion, triggering HA-mediated fusion of the virus envelope with the endosome through a "spring-action" extension of the fusion domain through the membranes that results in merging of these membranes and creation of an opening between the cytoplasm and the virion interior.[49,133] This merger allows release of viral ribonucleic acids and the proteins that make up the RNA polymerase complex (PB2, PB1, and PA) into the cytoplasm.

The vRNAs and polymerase complex proteins move to the nucleus, where transcription of (−) sense gene segments using a (+) strand copy-RNA intermediate (cRNA) takes place, together with production of (+) sense mRNAs.[238,406] Nascent (−) strand viral RNAs (vRNAs) are incorporated with NP into vRNPs and exported from the nucleus via the nuclear export protein NS-2 and the matrix protein 1 (M1).[96] mRNA leave the nucleus and act as template for synthesis of accessory, structural, and glycoproteins. Structural proteins, primarily M1, congregate at the cell membrane, initiating assembly and preparing for budding.[327] The glycoproteins, HA and the neuraminidase (NA), are shunted through the endoplasmic reticulum (ER) and Golgi network for folding and posttranslational modification, including addition of glycans, prior to shuttling to the assembly site where they are inserted into the cell membrane.[88,386,407] Budding of mature virions is facilitated by the sialidase activity of the NA (Fig. 178.2), which clears cell surface sialic acids from the HAs on the nascent virion[155,450] (see Fig. 178.1).

Nonstructural and accessory proteins are typically not incorporated into the virus[212,492,493] (Fig. 178.3). The nonstructural protein NS-1 has multiple functions within the cell, primarily in countering the antiviral response.[167] The influenza A and B virus NS-1 proteins differ in the specific interferon stimulatory genes that they target, and in other cellular binding partners, but perform a similar role in the life cycle.[239] The accessory protein PB1-F2, which is expressed from an alternate start codon in the +1 reading frame of the PB1 gene segment, is variably present in the genome and is variable in length.[7,65,421] When present as the full-length version, PB1-F2 targets mitochondria inducing cell death and triggering an inflammatory response.[5,6,79,295] The functions of multiple other accessory proteins are only now being elucidated, but many appear to impact viral and cellular gene regulation (Table 178.1).[212,462,492,494]

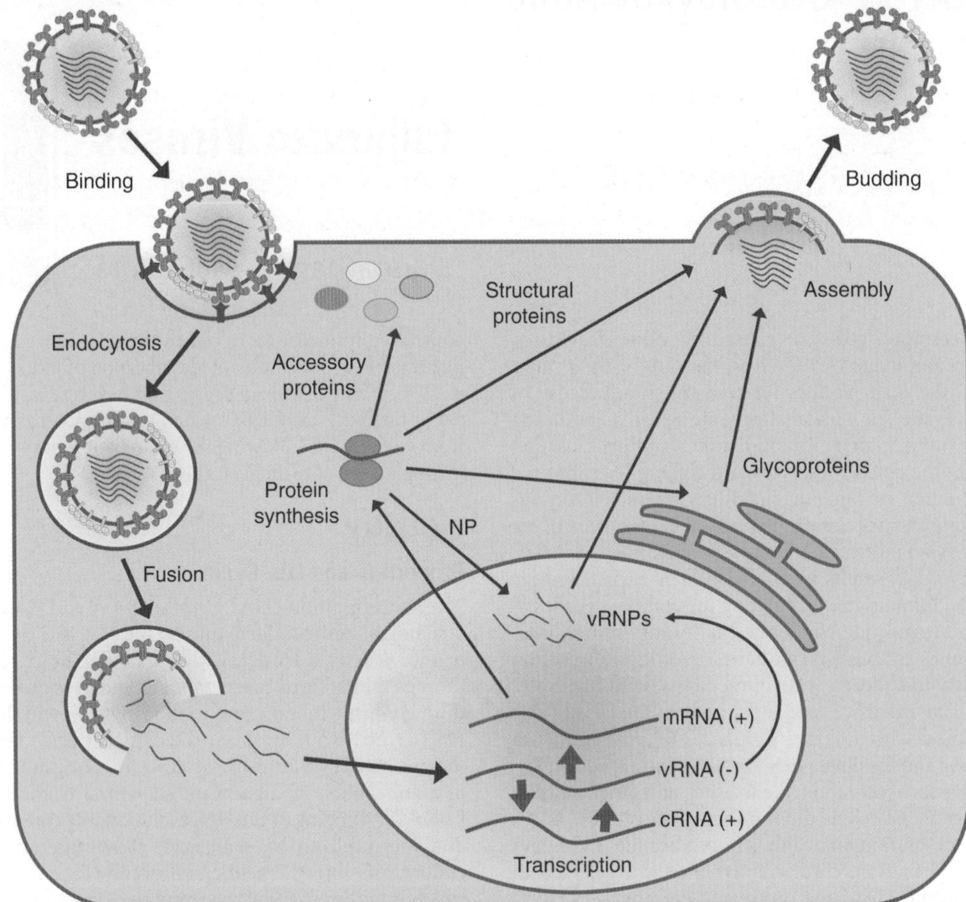

FIG. 178.1 Influenza A virus life cycle in cells. (Modified from McCullers JA. The role of punctuated evolution in the pathogenicity of influenza viruses. In: Scheld WM, Hughes JM, Whitley RJ, eds. *Emerging Infections*. Washington, DC: ASM Press; 2016.)

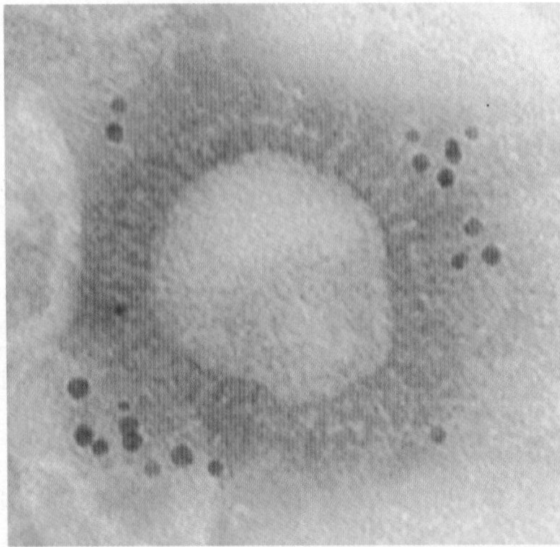

FIG. 178.2 Electron micrograph of an influenza virion with gold particle labeling of neuraminidase molecules to highlight their polar distribution. The other visible spikes are hemagglutinin glycoproteins. (Modified from Peltola VT, Murti KG, McCullers JA. Influenza virus neuraminidase contributes to secondary bacterial pneumonia. *J Infect Dis*. 2005;192:249-257.)

Classification

Influenza viruses are segmented, negative strand, RNA viruses (see Fig. 178.3). They are divided based on divergence of nucleotide sequences and by functional coding strategies into four types, termed A, B, C, and D. Influenza B viruses diverged evolutionarily from influenza A viruses between 100 and 350 years ago and are stably adapted to humans.[349] Influenza B viruses share a functional organizational strategy with influenza A viruses, having homologous versions of 10 proteins important for the life cycle encoded on 8 RNA gene segments (see Table 178.1). A number of accessory proteins with varying functions differ between the types. Influenza C viruses are thought to have diverged from influenza A viruses much further in antiquity, and have a slightly different organization with seven gene segments encoding nine proteins.[468] The hemagglutination and sialidase functions of influenza C viruses are combined in a hemagglutinin-esterase-fusion protein; evolutionary remnants of the esterase domain can be found in the influenza A virus HA. Influenza C viruses are very stably adapted to humans and undergo much less evolutionary change over time than the other types. Influenza D viruses have to this point been found only in cattle and swine and are distantly related to influenza C viruses.[173]

Influenza A viruses are zoonoses that are constantly crossing over from animal reservoirs into humans, causing individual infections and occasionally restricted epidemics.[147] Several times a century one of these zoonotic strains will establish endemicity and circulate for, typically, several decades before being replaced by a new incursion. Human influenza A virus lineages do not fully diverge over this evolutionarily short time period and frequently cross back over into animals such as swine.[464] Although rare interspecies transmission events have been documented with influenza B viruses (e.g., from humans to harbor seals),[356] influenza B and C viruses are predominantly restricted to humans as a "dead-end" adaptation. Influenza D viruses have not been detected in humans,[420] although few studies have been performed because of the relatively recent discovery of this type. Individual gene segments of the different influenza virus types have diverged enough evolutionarily that they cannot functionally coexist in a reassortant virus without significant alterations to the noncoding sequences at the termini of the individual gene segments.

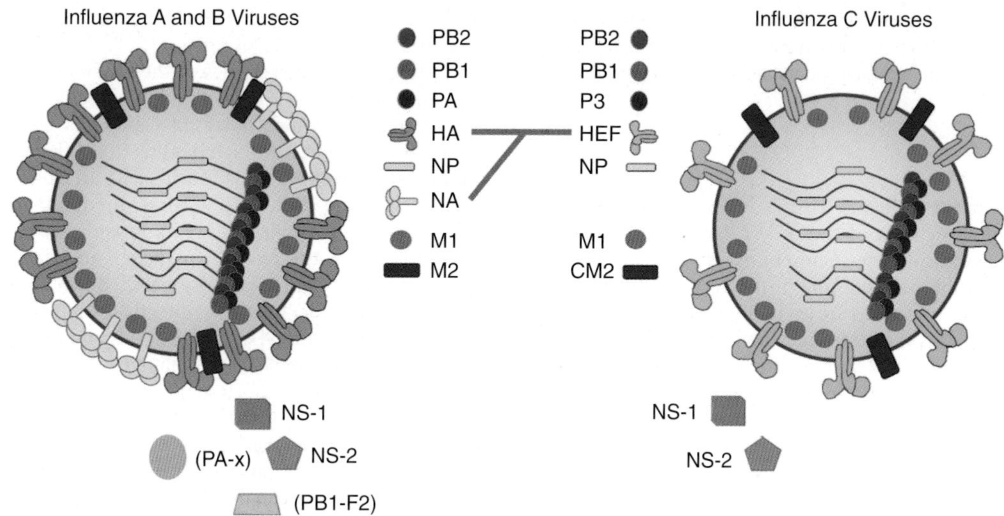

FIG. 178.3 Comparison of influenza A, B, and C virus proteins. Influenza C viruses encode nine known proteins on seven gene segments, two of which are accessory proteins (NS-1 and NS-2). Influenza A and B viruses encode at least 10 proteins on eight gene segments, including many homologous proteins with structures and functions similar to those in influenza C viruses, but also encode a neuraminidase (NA) on an eighth gene segment. In addition, influenza A viruses encode several other accessory proteins including PA-X and PB1-F2 that are not found in influenza B and C viruses (indicated by parentheses), and influenza B viruses encode an accessory protein termed NB on the NA gene segment. The hemagglutinin-esterase-fusion (HEF) protein of influenza C viruses performs similar functions in the life cycle, as do the hemagglutinin (HA) and NA of influenza A and B viruses. Nomenclature for the three types of virus differs somewhat; the third polymerase of influenza C viruses is termed P3, whereas the M2 of influenza B viruses is termed BM2 (see Table 178.1). (Modified from Wang M, Veit M. Hemagglutinin-esterase-fusion [HEF] protein of influenza C virus. *Protein Cell.* 2016;7:28-45.)

TABLE 178.1 Influenza A, B, and C Virus Proteins

Segment	Type	Gene/Product	Function
1. PB2	A, B, C	Basic polymerase 2	Part of transcription and replication complex
2. PB1	A, B, C	Basic polymerase 1	Part of transcription and replication complex
	A	PB1-F2	Cell death via mitochondrial targeting
	B	PB1-N40	Unknown
3. PA	A, B	Acid polymerase	Part of transcription and replication complex
P3	C	Polymerase	Part of transcription and replication complex
	A	PA-X	Host shutoff endonuclease
	A	PA-N155	Unknown
	A	PA-N182	Unknown
4. HA	A, B	Hemagglutinin	Attachment and fusion
HEF	C	Hemagglutinin-esterase-fusion	Attachment, fusion, and esterase activity
5. NP	A, B, C	Nucleoprotein	Scaffolding for viral ribonucleoproteins
6. NA	A, B	Neuraminidase	Sialidase facilitating budding
		NB	Ion channel?
7. M	A, B, C	Matrix protein 1	Primary structural protein of virions
	A	Matrix protein 2	Ion channel
	B	BM2	Ion channel
	C	CM2	Ion channel
	A	M42	Alternate form of matrix protein 2?
8. NS	A, B, C	Nonstructural gene 1	Multifunctional including interferon inhibition
	A, B, C	Nonstructural gene 2	Nuclear export
	A	Nonstructural gene 3	Unknown

Influenza A viruses are subtyped by serologic characterization of the two surface glycoproteins, HA and NA. Historically, this nomenclature was adopted because HA and NA are the major antigens of the virus. Thus far, 18 HA subtypes and 11 NA subtypes have been identified in nature.[446] The majority of these subtypes and many of their various possible combinations of HA and NA pairs are found in the wild bird reservoirs of the world.[513] Only H1, H2, and H3 and N1 and N2 have been demonstrated to form endemic lineages in humans, with the major caveat that virologic data are only available for the past century. Thus, it is presently unclear whether there are difficult or insurmountable restrictions on other subtypes crossing over into humans and circulating widely, or if this limited sample is a recency bias. However, there have been numerous instances of interspecies transmission from birds or swine with other subtypes that have not, to this point, established endemicity.[147,218,259,367] A variety of these subtypes can cause epidemics in domestic poultry, such as chickens, ducks, turkey, and quail, whereas a more restricted set have been found in mammals such as swine, horses, cats, and dogs.[7,170,313,513] Subtypes containing the H17, H18, N10, and N11 glycoproteins have been exclusively detected in bats to this point.[446]

ECOLOGY

Animal Reservoirs

The primary reservoir for influenza viruses is migratory waterfowl, including ducks and shorebirds of the orders Anseriformes (ducks, geese, swans) and Charadriiformes (shorebirds, gulls, alcids).[152,480,513] Sixteen of the 18 HA subtypes and nine of the 11 NA subtypes have been found in wild birds. Infections are asymptomatic, and the natural site of replication in birds is the gastrointestinal tract. Virus is shed in the feces into the environment and transmission between wild waterfowl is by the fecal-oral route. Free virus can be isolated from bird droppings on the shore and from the water of lakes where the birds congregate for breeding prior to migration.[237] There are multiple north-south migratory flyways for these birds, some of which span thousands of miles.[340] It is likely that young waterfowl are infected by contaminated water in the lakes prior to migration, and then carry the viruses with them, leaving it behind in their feces along the route.[21]

A number of domestic species, primarily poultry such as chickens, turkeys, quail, and domesticated ducks, come into direct contact with infected waterfowl during their migration.[131,365,512] Viruses may cross over into these populations intact, or may reassort with existing lineages in the domestic poultry to form new viruses. Some of these viruses can cause severe respiratory disease in species such as chicken and turkeys, causing epizootics with high mortality rates. Symptomatic disease will often result in large-scale culling of birds to prevent further spread, with resulting economic losses.[1,154,418] Inapparent infections also occur, and viruses can be maintained for prolonged periods of time in farms or in live bird markets, where they may come into contact with other species of birds or with mammals such as swine. Avian strains are typically classified as highly pathogenic avian influenza viruses (HPAI) or low pathogenicity avian influenza viruses (LPAI) based on the presence or absence of a multibasic cleavage site in the HA (a cleavage site containing the amino acid motif RX(R/K)R↓G or R(R/K) XR↓G, where X is any amino acid and the downward arrow indicates the site of cleavage).[38,331] With a typical cleavage site, LPAI are restricted to the respiratory tract, where furin-like proteases are available, and may cause inapparent, mild, or moderate disease.[38,128,331] The HA of HPAI with a multibasic cleavage site, however, can be cleaved by a wide variety of host proteases, allowing systemic spread and high mortality. Most avian influenza viruses are LPAI; HPAI are currently limited to a subset of H5 and H7 strains.

Infections in domestic ducks are typically gastrointestinal and asymptomatic, as is seen in their wild counterparts.[237,435] Swine have been considered somewhat unusual for many years, as they are susceptible to both avian influenza viruses and to human strains, raising the possibility of reassortment and generation of novel strains capable of establishing lineages in mammals.[259,464] Pigs were therefore proposed to be a "mixing vessel" that could act as an intermediate host in the creation of new pandemic strains.[396] Indeed, the 2009 H1N1 pandemic appears to have arisen in just such a manner.[366] However, other viruses with pandemic potential have arisen through adaptation and reassortment in birds, indicating that this mechanism is not universal.

Reassortment and Establishment of New Lineages

Influenza viruses reassort frequently in nature in humans and in animals.[268,314,507] There appear to be functional limitations on what specific pairings are possible, but a wide variety of HA and NA combinations are seen.[222,391] Structurally, HAs can be placed into several related groups and share similarities in function.[428,429] Individual gene segments can form evolutionary lineages that may or may not match well with other gene products following reassortment, resulting in low-fitness or high-fitness viruses. There also appear to be functional limitations on which gene constellations can be tolerated in which species, since, outside of waterfowl, a restricted set of viruses is typically found in any one species. For example, H3N8 viruses have established endemicity in dogs, while both H3N8 and H7N7 have formed lineages in horses.[77,426] Cats can be infected with human H1N1 and H3N2 strains, but also are susceptible to HPAI H5N1 viruses.[170,241,313,361] Swine may be the most interesting mammalian species, as they are more permissive of multiple subtypes.[131,204,259,464,465] This is thought to be due to the frequency and distribution of the major forms of sialic acids, which serve as receptors for the influenza virus through binding to HA. Birds including waterfowl typically display terminal sialic acids with an alpha-2,3 galactose linker, and most avian influenza viruses predominantly recognize this moiety.[180,291] Human viruses predominantly recognize alpha-2,6 sialic acids because of the relative frequency and distribution of the two versions in the human respiratory tract, a difference that creates a species barrier to zoonotic infection directly from wild waterfowl.[289] Pigs, however, display both types of sialic acids and can be infected by viruses with either receptor preference, facilitating dual infections and potentially avian-human virus reassortment events.[277,396,397]

Swine viruses have an evolutionary history that in some ways parallels that of humans. The "classic" H1N1 linage is believed to have entered swine in 1918 at the same time that it emerged in humans.[328] This lineage remained stable in the United States for many decades, maintained in an endemic cycle in swine and causing only mild disease. Multiple lineages circulated in Europe in the 1970s and 1980s, including a variant of the classic swine strain, H3N2 strains descended from the 1968 pandemic strain, and a novel avian H1N1 strain.[464] In 1998 the classic H1N1 strain began to evolve in the United States through acquisition of new gene segments via reassortment. The first event led to the emergence of a new strain termed the "double reassortant" H3N2, composed of classic swine genes and human genes from an H3N2 strain. This was quickly replaced by a novel "triple reassortant" that took two new avian genes from the wild bird population.[477] This variant not only spread widely throughout the world in the ensuing decade, but was a very promiscuous strain, reassorting frequently with circulating human viruses to generate new lineages.[464]

Zoonoses

Many of these novel viruses generated by reassortment between wild birds and domestic species have the potential to infect humans. Incursions of multiple subtypes have occurred in diverse areas of the world, typically through close association of humans with domestic animals. Bird markets, where poultry can be bought live for later consumption, have been shown to be a source of many of these outbreaks in regions where this practice is common, such as Southeast Asia and North Africa.[418] An outbreak with an HPAI H5N1 strain in Hong Kong in 1997 infected 18 persons, resulting in six deaths and was halted only by closing the markets and culling all birds on the island.[154,365,482] This virus reemerged in 2003 in mainland China[154] and has since spread to poultry across the world, with zoonotic infections of more than 850 humans and a 53% case fatality rate.[501] A similarly concerning HPAI H7N9 strain emerged in 2013 in China and has infected more than 790 persons[119] with a 41% case fatality rate. H9N2, H7N7, and H5N6 avian influenza viruses have also caused limited outbreaks in humans.[126,125,263,262,469] In the United States, zoonotic infections have most frequently come from contact with swine, often affecting children who visited state fairs and came into close contact with pigs.[147,464,496] More than 350 infections and one death have been detected during outbreaks from swine variant subtypes including H1N2, H1N2, and H3N2 viruses.[337] Asymptomatic infections are probably also common, as poultry workers, workers in swine abattoirs, and others with close contact with species that harbor endemic lineages frequently have serologic evidence of past infection without a clinically apparent illness.[70,280]

SURVEILLANCE

Animals

Because of the frequency of zoonotic infections and the pandemic potential of many of these strains, surveillance of influenza viruses in animals is essential both to improve our understanding of the ecology and evolution of these pathogens, and to provide an early warning of possible strains of special significance, such as newly emerging HPAI. These strains have the potential to cause huge economic losses through epidemic spread and through the culling of animals that is necessary to halt disease progression in a population and to reassure the public of the safety of the food supply. Some of these strains are likely to also possess pandemic potential. A set of molecular signatures of virulence in humans is being established that should allow improved pandemic planning through surveillance and genetic analysis of these emerging strains.[304,305,421]

Surveillance of wild aquatic birds was established by the WHO Collaborating Center for Studies of the Ecology of Influenza Viruses at St. Jude Children's Research Hospital in Memphis in 1976. There are six Collaborating Centers at present, including Centers in Atlanta at the CDC, in London, Tokyo, Beijing, and in Melbourne. However, only the Memphis site concentrates on animal viruses. Samples of feces are collected along the migratory flyways, and the recovered viruses are subtyped and sequenced. Surveillance of swine in the United States was added in the late 1990s, and domestic poultry surveillance began in multiple locations by multiple governmental and scientific groups following the H5N1 outbreaks in the early 2000s. Organizations including the WHO, the World Organization for Animal Health, and the United Nations Food and Agricultural Organization global networks report outbreaks in member states of animal influenza viruses, particularly HPAI H5 and H7 strains.

Humans

Virologic surveillance in humans is coordinated globally by the WHO Collaborating Centers and the WHO Global Influenza Response and Surveillance System,[502] which was established in 1952. Approximately 143 national centers in 113 member states participate by performing influenza virus testing, isolation, typing, and subtyping. Health care facilities participating in surveillance send samples from patients with influenza-like illness to these national centers for testing; viral isolates are then forwarded to the WHO Collaborating Centers for further investigation, including antigenic characterization, genetic sequencing, and antiviral susceptibility testing. The WHO Collaborating Centers share these data for decisions on annual vaccine composition and pre-pandemic vaccine development. In the United States, approximately 140 state, governmental, and hospital laboratories conduct surveillance, perform testing, and collect viral specimens that are ultimately sent to CDC for more detailed characterization. CDC generates a weekly surveillance report that can be accessed at http://www.cdc.gov/flu/weekly/.

Disease

Influenza disease surveillance is also coordinated globally by the WHO, although the degree of surveillance in individual countries varies widely. The WHO Global Influenza Programme publishes standards for estimating disease burden and publishes biweekly summaries of national data from about 100 countries.[502] Disease surveillance for influenza began in the 19th century as an outgrowth of the desire to better measure causes of mortality in populations. In 1847, the eminent London epidemiologist William Farr, remembered chiefly for his assistance to John Snow in determining that cholera was a waterborne disease, coined the term "excess mortality" to describe the increase in deaths that occurred during the influenza season that were attributed on medical certificates to causes other than influenza itself. Using this concept, he developed in detail the methodology used today to quantitate mortality in influenza epidemics.[115,252] Selwyn Collins of the US Public Health Service then further refined the terms by which we classify outcomes after influenza in a series of thorough and detailed reports on epidemic mortality in the early part of the 20th century.[73-76] Today, data are collected from 122 cities, covering about one third of the US population, on deaths from pneumonia and influenza (P&I) and reported weekly by CDC. P&I mortality includes deaths from the primary viral infection as well as from secondary bacterial pneumonia and are considered together because they are difficult to distinguish using mortality data. This measure does not include deaths attributed to other causes such as exacerbation of an underlying condition by the viral infection. This provides a proxy for the severity of any given influenza season, by comparing the level of excess mortality to the seasonal baseline. Influenza-associated pediatric mortality surveillance began in 2003 and is now reported separately from excess mortality.

Surveillance for influenza-associated hospitalizations began in the United States in 2003 in children and in 2005 in adults through the Influenza Hospitalization Surveillance Network (FluSurv-NET) at the CDC.[64] Currently, hospitals in 13 states participate by collecting data on age and clinical characteristics of persons with severe influenza. This allows estimation of age-specific hospitalization rates, description of disease presentation, and determination of comorbid conditions for weekly reporting. Surveillance for influenza-like illness in outpatients is performed at more than 2900 health care providers, which report more than 36 million outpatient visits annually through the Outpatient Influenza-like Illness Surveillance Network (ILINet). This allows estimation of the percentage of clinician visits attributable to influenza-like illness as a proxy for the prevalence of influenza in each state or US territory.

EVOLUTION AND ADAPTATION

Pandemics

Pandemics of influenza occur several times a century when a novel influenza A virus enters humans and spreads worldwide. According to Edwin Kilbourne's framework,[227,302] a virus must meet three criteria to be considered pandemic: (1) a novel HA protein to which most of the population is immunologically naïve, allowing a high clinical attack rate, (2) ease of transmission enabling worldwide spread, and (3) the ability to cause severe disease. Four pandemics have taken place in the past 100 years. In 1918, an H1N1 subtype virus entered humans from the animal reservoir, causing severe disease and killing more than 40 million people worldwide. This virus adapted to humans and circulated until 1957, when it was replaced by an H2N2 subtype virus that took part of its gene constellation from the circulating H1N1 strain, and the remainder from an avian source (Fig. 178.4). The 1957 pandemic was severe, killing several million persons, but not on the same scale as that of 1918. In 1968 another novel strain emerged, again by reassortment. This H3N2 virus had a novel HA, but retained the NA and several other genes from the 1957 strain. Disease and mortality were milder than in previous pandemics, perhaps because of the retention of the NA antigen from the previously circulating strain. Adapted versions of this virus continue to circulate today. This virus was joined in circulation in humans in 1977 when a 1950 version of the previously circulating H1N1 strain was released from a frozen source. Although this virus achieved worldwide circulation and continues to be endemic in humans today, cocirculating with H3N2 strains, this event was not considered to be a pandemic because much of the population was immune and little disease ensued.

In 2009, the most recent pandemic strain emerged as a complex mixture of genes of avian, human, and swine derivation.[366] It was again of the H1N1 subtype, but was most antigenically similar to the 1918 strain among viruses that circulated in the 20th century. Because of this, only older persons who experienced influenza in the 1930s and 1940s and persons who had received the 1976 "swine flu" vaccine had any cross-reactive immunity.[312,382] Sero-archaeologic evidence suggests that as far back as the mid-1850s, H1, H2, and H3 subtype viruses have successively replaced each other as pandemic strains. It is not known whether this recycling phenomenon is limited to these subtypes because of factors presently not understood, or whether other subtypes are also capable of causing pandemics.[328,440] The repeated incursions of highly pathogenic avian influenza viruses of the H5N1 subtype into humans since 1997 have created significant concern that a truly novel pandemic strain could arise, but as yet these viruses seem incapable of sustaining chains of transmission in humans.[154,260]

Adaptation

Common characteristics of RNA viruses such as influenza virus are use of a low-fidelity polymerase coupled with lack of proofreading mechanisms to correct base-pair mismatches.[406] This results in a high mutation rate and the opportunity for significant variation between influenza viruses to arise under specific conditions. The rapid cycle time and high mutation rate generate a large pool of "quasi-species" variants that interact together, complementing each other by providing flexibility as environmental conditions change.[300] As a result of this quasi–species-driven diversity, influenza viruses undergo not only positive selection for traits that aid

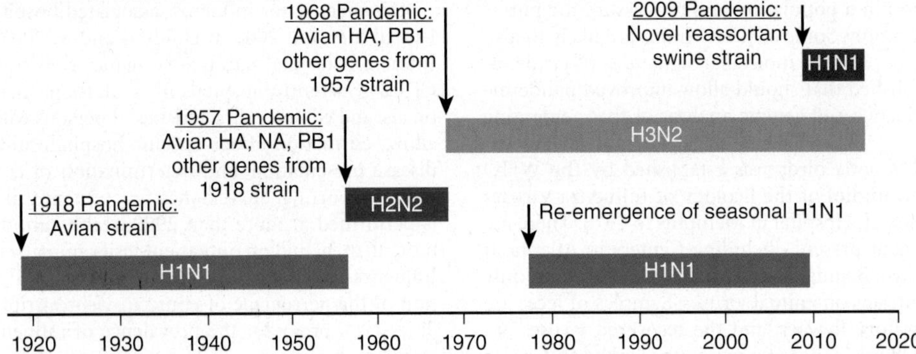

FIG. 178.4 Pandemic timeline. Four major lineages of influenza A virus have established endemicity in humans in the past 100 years. The 1957 and 1968 pandemic viruses were reassortants that included genes from the previously circulating viruses that they replaced. The 1918 and 2009 pandemic strains came directly from animal reservoirs. The seasonal H1N1 lineage, which circulated early in the 20th century, was replaced in 1957 but reemerged in 1976 and co-circulated for 32 years with seasonal H3N2 strains. (From McCullers JA. The role of punctuated evolution in the pathogenicity of influenza viruses. In: Scheld WM, Hughes JM, Whitley RJ, eds. *Emerging Infections.* Washington, DC: ASM Press; 2016.)

in adaptation, but also negative (purifying) selection for disadvantageous traits.[305] These selection events can be at the level of mutation of individual gene segments, or via reassortment to acquire completely new gene segments that are a better fit for the evolutionary pressure being applied to the quasi-species pool. Because small RNA viruses have limited genome sizes to facilitate rapid replication and easier packaging, they typically have complex coding strategies with multiple gene products capable of being expressed from any individual gene or gene segment.[194,492-494] Mutations of nonessential gene products may result in expression, deletion, truncation, or other alterations to these accessory proteins changing their function and role in the life cycle.[5,7,421] Influenza viruses tend to adapt very rapidly (on a scale of years) to positive selection pressure and more slowly (on a scale of decades) to lose or modify undesirable traits through negative selection.[46,156,495]

Rapid Evolution

Several common scenarios are known to drive evolution of influenza A viruses through positive selection. The most striking is establishing a lineage in a new host through a cross-species jump.[222,391] In humans this occurs immediately following the introduction of a new pandemic strain. The virus evolves rapidly for several years, then slows, and eventually (after decades) reaches an equilibrium such that, in the absence of other sources of positive selection, most genes are not changing except through gradual negative selection for improved fitness in the host.[495] The most common positive selection pressure is from antibodies induced either by natural infection or by vaccination. This typically results in mutations in the HA and NA, since they are the primary targets of the immune system. These events, termed antigenic drift, occur seasonally and are a combination of mutations around the receptor binding site of the HA that alter antigenicity and bystander or compensatory structural changes. Antiviral drug use is another commonly encountered selective pressure. Rapid evolution of the NA can be seen in sites related to NA activity following introduction of neuraminidase inhibitor antivirals into a population.[506] Finally, reassortment is a common event, both within human virus populations and between human and animal strains. The presence of gene products from different influenza A virus lineages in a newly reassorted virus causes functional mismatches that drive selection of genes coding for variants of proteins that work better together. A classic example is the need for a balance of HA binding to sialic acids to enable entry and NA sialidase activity to facilitate budding.[222,223] Reassortment-induced mismatches are corrected by evolutionary change.[472]

EPIDEMIOLOGY

Seasonality and Transmission

Seasonal influenza is primarily a disease of children, with clinical attack rates of 20% to 30% during some epidemics. In addition to having the largest burden of infection, children exhibit a high social contact rate,[158,278] facilitating transmission.[415] They also possess a relative lack of cross-reactive immunity, allowing unrestricted replication and shedding of large quantities of the virus. However, most deaths are in persons with chronic comorbidities, so mortality is concentrated in older persons. The excess mortality rate for influenza A viruses varies significantly by strain and season, based on both the degree of preexisting immunity in the population, the potency of viral virulence factors, and how well the circulating viruses support secondary bacterial infections from regionally endemic bacterial strains. Because influenza B viruses do not have an animal reservoir and are well adapted to humans, the epidemiology of these viruses resembles that of well-adapted seasonal strains with a high clinical attack rate in children and little mortality outside of those with underlying chronic illnesses. The epidemiology of influenza C viruses is poorly understood at present, but it may cause epidemics related to antigenic drift and emergence of new strains similar to the other influenza virus types.[293]

Human-to-human transmission of influenza viruses can occur by contact, large droplet, and aerosol routes.[8,60,478] Since most viruses are expelled during coughing and sneezing, direct contact with infected secretions or contaminated objects is thought to dominate in most settings. Transmission is affected by both temperature and humidity and is favored in cold conditions and significantly diminished in the setting of high humidity.[274,275] It has been suggested that aerosol transmission is more efficient in cool, dry environments, facilitating epidemic spread when optimal conditions are met. Most outbreaks in temperate regions therefore occur in the winter months when the aerosol transmission route is favored. However, a low level of infection can be detected year-round when testing is employed. In tropical parts of the world, circulation of viruses can occur in any season, with the timing of peaks of disease being associated with poorly understood climatic changes.[67]

Herd immunity plays some role in the seasonality of influenza. Antigenic drift can lead to larger epidemics, and conversely lack of significant drift can restrict disease mostly to naïve subjects such as children or to those with comorbidities and increased susceptibility. Pandemic strains appear to transmit efficiently in the summer in temperate climes, likely because of elimination of the contribution of herd immunity; the increased availability of susceptible hosts may overcome the temperature and humidity barriers to transmission. For example, the largest peaks of disease during the 2009 H1N1 pandemic occurred in the summer in many parts of the world.[225,243] The relative ability of influenza viruses to transmit is expressed by a term called the reproductive number R_0, which represents the average number of persons an infected individual will themselves infect.[124] Any value over 1.0 suggests that sustained transmission is possible and therefore an outbreak can occur. Seasonal strains of influenza virus have an R_0 in the range of 1.3 to 1.7, which is much lower than comparable viruses such as measles, which may have an R_0 of 10 to 15. The R_0 of the 2009 pandemic strain varied between 1.1 and 2.0, depending on the population studied.[247] Most zoonotic infections, such as with the recent incursions of HPAI H5N1 viruses in Southeast Asia, have an R_0 below 1.0, a factor in these viruses failing to achieve endemicity.[240]

Global Disease Burden

Until recently, comprehensive surveillance had been conducted predominantly in high-income, developed countries. Data from recent decades suggested that the rate of hospitalization was highest in children younger than 1 year and adults older than 65 years. The great majority of deaths are in persons older than 65 years. Hospitalization rates by age for children have been estimated in the United States at approximately 130 to 150 per 100,000 for age less than 1 year, 36 to 39 per 100,000 for ages 1 to 4 years, and 11 per 100,000 for ages 5 to 17 years.[144,515] However, these are likely underestimates by a factor of about 2, because only a proportion of patients are tested for influenza, many testing methods have poor sensitivity and specificity, and hospitalizations for influenza are often coded as something else.[144,381,413,515] Adjusting for this systematic bias, it was estimated that during three influenza seasons from 2010 to 2013, the total number of hospitalizations in US children (<18 years) varied from approximately 10,000 to 42,000, the number of ICU admissions from 1900 to 7600, and the number of deaths from 50 to 840 annually.[381] Because only about 0.5% of children with symptomatic influenza are hospitalized,[413] it can be further extrapolated that about 2.2 to 9.3 million illnesses occur in children annually in the United States. The severity of any particular influenza season varies considerably based on the predominant type or subtype circulating, the overall burden of disease, and the hospitalization rate of children in different age groups.[57]

Globally, few systematically collected data have been available until very recently. A recent meta-analysis of studies using polymerase chain reaction (PCR) diagnostic testing suggests that the rate of hospitalization is about threefold higher in developing compared to industrialized countries[250] and is highest in Africa and Southeast Asia.[132,191,250,316,416] On average, an estimated 900,000 children are hospitalized for influenza annually, with 96.3% of these hospital stays occurring in the developing world. In a different meta-analysis, it was recently estimated that in 2008 more than 90 million influenza-associated illnesses occurred in children younger than 5 years, with more than 20 million cases of influenza-associated acute lower respiratory tract infections (ALRI) and 1 million cases of severe ALRI.[334] In this study, 93% to 97% of all ALRI and severe ALRI were in the developing world. These numbers are probably also underestimates, as in many developing parts of the world passive surveillance fails to detect many persons who for cultural preferences or because of financial constraints do not seek health care,[379] or use alternative forms of health care such as private clinics where surveillance is not taking place.[266] Prospective community- or household-based surveillance may better capture the true incidence of disease.[81,149,341,353]

Coinfections

The epidemiology of influenza-associated coinfections remains difficult to assess with any accuracy because it is difficult to attribute disease or death to influenza instead of its complications,[73,473] and because most of the burden of disease occurs in outpatient settings, where few studies have comprehensively assessed coinfections.[304] It is also difficult to assign an etiology for clinical syndromes such as otitis media and pneumonia; it is particularly difficult to define precisely the contribution to the pathogenesis of disease of the various pathogens that can be co-detected in infected individuals when sensitive methodologies are used.[214] Current testing paradigms for identifying bacterial pathogens within the lung suffer from a lack of both sensitivity and specificity.[348] Recent advances in use of PCR-based assays for detection of viral pathogens help in identifying viral causes of pneumonia,[213] but positive tests from the upper respiratory tract do not always correlate with the etiology of deep lung infections. Direct examination of the middle ear is possible through otoscopy and tympanocentesis, such that etiology is better established for otitis media, where viruses are the predominant pathogens in the conjugate vaccine era and coinfections are common.[347] An issue specific to coinfections is that sequential infections may be more difficult to accurately diagnose if the preceding pathogen (e.g., influenza) has resolved by the time the patient presents for medical attention due to secondary bacterial pneumonia.[484] Because viruses other than influenza are also found in coinfections, specific attribution of etiology is difficult in this "hit and run" scenario. Despite these challenges, there is an increasing appreciation that most episodes of otitis media and community-acquired pneumonia, particularly when associated with influenza, result from coinfections.[303]

The 1918 pandemic was comprehensively studied by leading microbiologists and pathologists of the era, and many of these early studies have been reanalyzed in recent years.[43,68] Estimates from clinical and autopsy series suggest that more than 95% of all severe illnesses and deaths were complicated by bacterial pathogens.[329] Many of the victims of this pandemic were children and healthy young adults.[44] This contrasts sharply with seasonal influenza, in which mortality is most often seen in persons with chronic medical conditions, a propensity that shifts the age distribution toward an older population. Respiratory pathogens such as *Streptococcus pneumoniae*, *Staphylococcus aureus*, *Haemophilus influenzae*, and *Streptococcus pyogenes* (group A streptococcus) were all identified as common pathogens in various studies.[44] The overall picture that is evident from these data is that severe disease and mortality were linked to the presence of secondary invaders, with factors such as variations in which strains were endemic, modified by personal immunity, dictating the epidemiology in a particular region.[44,219,303]

Beginning in the antibiotic age,[216] the overall pattern of mortality in the subsequent 1957 and 1968 pandemics was closer in character to seasonal influenza than that seen in the pandemic of 1918. Pneumonia accounted for a higher proportion of deaths in 1957–58 and 1968–69[33,45,399,405,449] than during most of the preceding interpandemic years,[76,89] but did not approach the 95% seen in 1918.[329] Similar to seasonal influenza, the highest incidence of disease was in healthy children and young adults of school and working age, with an attack rate that averaged about 40%.[441] In contrast to 1918, however, most excess deaths were linked to cardiopulmonary conditions and thus occurred primarily in older persons.[89,187,449] When pneumonia was associated with mortality in 1957–58, *S. aureus* was the most frequent secondary invader.[185,186,287,355,387] The clinical course was often fulminant, with death occurring in less than 7 days, and severe pulmonary edema and hemorrhage were commonly found on autopsy.[187] The higher incidence of *S. aureus* was a striking departure from previous pandemics and seasonal epidemics and was initially blamed on the use of antibiotics that were effective against *S. pneumoniae*, *S. pyogenes*, and many strains of *H. influenzae*, but not against the emerging antibiotic-resistant strains of *S. aureus* prevalent in hospitals at the time.[216,387] However, in 1968–69, the clinical attack rate and incidence of pneumonia were comparable to rates in 1957, but *S. pneumoniae* was once again the predominant pathogen. *S. aureus* was diagnosed more frequently during the 1968 pandemic than in the immediately preceding interpandemic years,[399] but was not the dominant etiologic agent as it had been in 1957–58 despite similar availability of antibiotics.

Although *S. pneumoniae* was considered the most common cause of secondary pneumonia in the decades after the 1968 pandemic, in the past two decades *S. aureus* has emerged as a cause of fulminant pneumonia in association with influenza in many parts of the world, particularly in children.[117,142] The USA300 and USA400 clonotypes of *S. aureus* seem to be particularly likely to cause secondary pneumonia with influenza compared to other circulating strains, for unclear reasons. *H. influenzae* has become less prominent as a cause of secondary bacterial pneumonia with the introduction of the type B conjugate vaccine, although it remains important in regions of the world with poor vaccine coverage.[476] Group A streptococcus is entirely absent from many series describing community-acquired pneumonia in association with viruses and is typically third in incidence when it does appear.[63]

During the 2009 H1N1 pandemic,[93] in a departure from the previous two pandemics, mortality rates were similar to recent seasonal epidemics. However, most deaths occurred in older children and young adults, often with no underlying chronic conditions, and morbidity rates were high.[92,113] Respiratory deaths associated with an aberrant response to the virus accounted for most of this mortality in previously healthy persons.[92,325,382] It remains unclear what the precise impact of secondary bacterial disease was; some estimates put excess mortality from influenza and pneumonia as low as 10%,[62] a rate lower than many seasonal epidemics.[417] In careful studies of severely ill or fatal cases, bacterial pneumonia was found to complicate around one third of infections.[51,103,113,141,294,408] *S. pneumoniae* and *S. aureus* were the most common etiologies of secondary bacterial pneumonia, with regional variation in which was more prominent.[51,141,294,342,385] It is unclear whether the prominence of *S. aureus* in 2009–10 was due to the strain-specific features of the recently emerged USA300 clonotype, or was a reflection of increased penetrance of pneumococcal vaccination in the last decade.[336] *S. pyogenes* was absent as a secondary pathogen from many series, but was surprisingly frequent in others, suggesting further differences in regional endemicity of the most common co-pathogens.[9,51] In some carefully conducted studies, few serious bacterial superinfections were identified despite extensive sampling to detect them.[243] When present, however, it was clear that bacterial superinfections from *S. pneumoniae* or *S. aureus* resulted in worse outcomes.[99,342,359,385]

Economic Impact

Influenza has a tremendous economic impact from direct costs (outpatient visits, testing, medications, travel costs, hospital stays), intervention costs (vaccines, school closures), and indirect costs (missed days of work for parents or guardians). This impact varies based on the severity of the season, cultural and infrastructure factors that vary by country, and the characteristics of the patient population. Estimates of economic impact for a mild pandemic in the developed world range from $81 million in a mid-sized North American city[10] to $330 million in Hong Kong, a city of 7 million persons.[497] In this latter study, outpatient costs for children with influenza ranged from $236 for an illness not requiring medical attention, to $542 for an illness requiring an outpatient visit, to $1926 for a hospitalization, and cost $352,284 for each death.[319,497] Using 2003 data, the overall impact of seasonal influenza in the United States has been estimated at $87.1 billion per year, based on 31.4 million outpatient visits, 3.1 million hospitalization days, and 610,660 life-years lost.[324] Economic impact is lower in low-to-middle-income countries, primarily because the direct costs are lower for treatment and hospitalization,[95] and patients may not choose to seek health care as often for cultural reasons.[379] However, indirect costs reflected in productivity losses are higher in low-to-middle-income countries, and these are the countries least able to sustain such an impact.[95] In children, the economic impact is highest in young children under 5 years, especially under 2 years, and in those with chronic medical conditions.[319] Interestingly, public health interventions such as school closings, although effective at reducing the burden of disease, are estimated to increase costs due to loss of productivity,[497] whereas use of antivirals and vaccines can both reduce the burden and reduce costs.[10]

High-Risk Pediatric Groups

Age and chronic medical conditions are the predominant risk factors for increased severity of influenza. Hospitalization rates for influenza by age presents as a U-shaped curve, with rates in children highest in infants younger than 1 year, but still higher in the 1- to 2-year range and 2- to 5-year range than in school-age children.[211,338,350,443] Children with chronic medical conditions have a higher rate of outpatient and emergency department use and higher rate of hospitalization in all groups compared to children without such conditions. Children with chronic respiratory diseases, such as cystic fibrosis, are at risk for hospitalization and worse outcomes from influenza.[8,378,474] Because asthma is such a common chronic disease of children, affecting about 8% of children in the United States,[59] co-occurrence of asthma in children hospitalized for influenza is common and asthma has long also been considered a risk factor for hospitalization.[8,55] However, recent retrospective studies have found that asthmatics were less likely to have complications from influenza, including pneumonia and intensive care admission, and were less likely to die compared to nonasthmatics.[94,139,273,315,459] It has been proposed that the immune profile of the lungs in asthmatics, in contrast to the situation in cystic fibrosis,[378] may diminish replication of influenza viruses and ameliorate disease.[395] Other common chronic conditions of children associated with increased rates of hospitalization include cardiovascular (except hypertension alone), renal, hepatic, hematologic (including sickle cell disease), neurologic or neurodevelopmental (including cerebral palsy, epilepsy, stroke, and intellectual disability), and metabolic (including diabetes mellitus) disorders.[8] Children with cancer or other forms of immunosuppression are at a particularly[256] high risk for complications and poor outcomes from influenza, including prolonged shedding, pneumonia, delay in chemotherapy, and death.[129,165]

Mortality in Children

Despite high rates of morbidity, influenza-associated mortality is uncommon in children in the developed world. Since pediatric influenza-associated deaths became a nationally notifiable occurrence in the United States in 2004,[364] an annual average of 93 deaths (range, 37 to 171) have been attributed to seasonal influenza in children.[57] Surprisingly, up to 43% of these influenza-associated fatalities were in healthy children without comorbidities.[498] Of those with one or more comorbidities, neurologic and developmental disorders (33%) were most common, followed by respiratory disorders (26%), chromosomal or genetic disorders (12%), and congenital heart or other cardiac disease (11%). In the group of children without preexisting chronic medical problems, 55% had bacterial pneumonia as a complication, and 46% died before being admitted to a hospital.[498] *S. aureus* was the most common bacterial pathogen complicating influenza in these cases, accounting for about half of diagnoses.[117,498] It is likely that these are underestimates of the actual number of deaths, because mandatory reporting does not capture all patients for a variety of reasons, including lack of testing and categorization of deaths as attributable to other processes, such as complications of comorbidities. Outside the United States, the case fatality rate is thought to be much higher, with the total burden worldwide attributable to influenza estimated in one study as between 28,000 and 111,500 deaths in children under 5 years.[334]

Avian Influenza

Humans who have close contact with avian species such as chickens, ducks, quail, geese, or turkeys are frequently exposed to avian influenza viruses.[198,335] However, because of barriers to cross-species transmission, symptomatic infections are rare. Infections resulting in respiratory illness have been identified for multiple subtypes, both LPAI and HPAI strains.[125,246,260,365,501] Many of the reported LPAI H9N2 infections have occurred in children.[47,367] Person-to-person transmission of LPAI has not been reported.[457] LPAI virus infections commonly cause uncomplicated illness with fever, myalgias, and upper respiratory tract symptoms such as cough, sore throat, rhinorrhea, and nasal congestion.[47,457] Both LPAI and HPAI can cause conjunctivitis, either with or without accompanying respiratory tract disease.[121,343,377] H7 subtype viruses seem to have particular tropism for the eye.[121,343,377,451]

The first case of HPAI H5N1 infection was reported in a child in Hong Kong in 1997.[72] Eighteen cases, including 11 children, were identified in Hong Kong in 1997 prior to the closing of all live bird markets and slaughter of all poultry on the island.[514] The spectrum of disease in children ranged from uncomplicated influenza-like illness to acute respiratory distress syndrome (ARDS), multiorgan failure, and death. This virus reemerged in 2003 in mainland China and, since that time, has continued to circulate throughout Southeast Asia and parts of the Middle East and Africa in wild birds, with outbreaks in domestic poultry and occasional transmission to humans.[154,217,335,458] Limited chains of human-to-human transmission have been identified, but in most cases direct contact with poultry has been implicated.[1,26,365,402] However, studies on transmission in ferrets suggest that relatively few mutations are needed to achieve respiratory droplet transmission,[184,205,392] which could presage improved spread and trigger a pandemic. As of spring 2016, 850 human cases had been confirmed in 15 countries, with 449 deaths (52.8% case fatality ratio).[501] Clinical disease from HPAI H5N1 is often severe or fatal in adults, but can present as a mild upper respiratory tract infection in children.[41,354] The case fatality ratio is lowest in children, perhaps because they present to medical attention and are hospitalized earlier in the course of illness than with adults.[354] Atypical presentations such as gastroenteritis or encephalitis have been seen,[17] and cases have been misdiagnosed as other common febrile diseases such as dengue and typhoid.[1]

Other HPAI outbreaks have ranged from conjunctivitis with or without mild respiratory tract illness (H7N3 and H7N7 strains)[377,451] to more severe disease including ARDS and death (H7N7, H7N9).[121,126] The current H7N9 outbreak began in 2013 in China, and cases have occurred in Malaysia and Taiwan. To date 778 cases have been identified,[119] although very few have been children. Severe disease including ARDS is common, occurring in more than 70% of patients.[126,263] Diagnosis of avian influenza virus infections including HPAI viruses is made by testing respiratory specimens by reverse transcription (RT)-PCR, targeting persons with a history of travel to an endemic area and contact with poultry. Clinical management is by early initiation of antiviral treatment with an NA inhibitor, and supportive therapy for complications such as respiratory failure, shock, and multiorgan system failure.[456,487] Nosocomial infection with H5N1 has been reported, and adherence to infection control measures including standard, droplet, and contact precautions with eye protection and enhanced respiratory protection with N95 or equivalent respirators is important to prevent acquisition by health care workers.[456]

Swine Influenza

Swine influenza was first described in association with the 1918 pandemic[480] and was first isolated in 1930 by Richard E. Shope.[411] Experimentally infected swine could be demonstrated to have respiratory disease when coinfected with *H. influenzae suis*. Most human strains of influenza and some avian strains can infect pigs, and human viruses often cross the species barrier, reassort in pigs, and establish lineages. Swine influenza can cause viral pneumonia in pigs, typically in the setting of bacterial coinfection.[301] Sporadic zoonotic infections occur from direct contact with swine, often in children.[148] An outbreak at Fort Dix in 1976 caused great national concern in the United States over the possibility of a new H1N1 pandemic when 13 soldiers were infected and one died.[130] This fear became reality in 2009 when a reassortant H1N1 strain emerged in swine and started the first pandemic since 1968.[93] Fortunately, this virus did not cause high mortality, likely because it was missing several virulence factors associated with virulence and support for secondary bacterial infections.[162] However, multiple other strains currently circulating in swine do possess these virulence factors and do support secondary bacterial infections well, creating the worry that a new, more pathogenic pandemic strain will emerge from this reservoir.[483] In recent years, multiple cases of swine influenza acquisition have been documented at state fairs and other agricultural exhibitions where direct contact with pigs is common.[56]

CLINICAL MANIFESTATIONS

Primary Influenza

Influenza has a short, 2- to 3-day incubation period, after which both respiratory and systemic symptoms appear together. After the first several days of illness when systemic symptoms dominate the clinical course, a transition takes place and systemic symptoms subside and cough and other respiratory tract–related symptoms become more prominent. Systemic symptoms include fever, chills, malaise, headache, dizziness, gastrointestinal disturbances, and myalgias.[83,253,258] An erythematous maculopapular rash may be present briefly but is not a common or prominent sign of infection. Common respiratory symptoms include cough, sore throat, rhinitis, nasal congestion, and eye irritation. Cough may be productive or nonproductive and may persist for weeks or longer. Disease in adolescents and older children is similar to that of adults and is dominated by the triad of fever, cough, and myalgias (Table 178.2). Cough is less prominent in younger children and is sometimes absent entirely in infants. Myalgias are much less frequent in children than in adults. Gastrointestinal symptoms are frequent in young children and can manifest as vomiting, diarrhea, or abdominal pain. Infants may have fever and diarrhea as their sole presenting signs. Gastrointestinal symptomatology was more common during the 2009 H1N1 pandemic than is typically observed in seasonal influenza, and commonly affected older children and adults.[352,413] Apnea and a sepsis-like syndrome can also occur in neonates and infants. In 5% to 30% of cases, infection is asymptomatic; this rate varies somewhat by strain.[207,363]

TABLE 178.2 Clinical Manifestations of Influenza

Symptoms	Infants	Children	Adults
Fever	++	+++	+++
Cough	+	++	+++
Myalgias	–	+	++
Sore throat	–	+	++
Headache	–	++	++
Conjunctivitis	++	++	++
Cervical adenopathy	+	+	–
Anorexia	++	++	+
Diarrhea	++	+[a]	–[a]
Vomiting	++	+[a]	–[a]
Rhinitis	++	+	+
Malaise/lethargy	++	+	+
Neurological symptoms	+	–[a]	–

– rare, + uncommon, ++ common, +++ very common.
[a]Common (++) with 2009 pandemic influenza.
Modified from McCullers JA. Influenza. In: Elzouki AY, Harfi HA, Nazer H, et al, eds. *Textbook of Clinical Pediatrics*. 2nd ed. New York: Springer; 2012.

Most children with influenza have a normal white blood cell count, but both leukopenia and leukocytosis can be seen. Leukocytosis with a predominance of neutrophils can be a sign of secondary bacterial infection, but can also occur with uncomplicated influenza. Blood chemistries are typically normal unless dehydration or complications are present. Influenza A and influenza B are indistinguishable clinically, although specific strains may have a predilection for certain clinical syndromes, and influenza B is more likely to cause clinical disease in younger children than in adults.[371] Influenza C viruses are more likely to be asymptomatic or pauci-symptomatic, but when symptomatic disease is present it can be severe, resulting in hospitalization and complications.[292]

Complications

Both viral and bacterial complications are common during childhood influenza. Otitis media, sinusitis, and pneumonia all can be due either to the primary viral infection or to manifestations of coinfecting bacteria.[160,183,243,303,369] Laryngotracheobronchitis (croup) can be a manifestation of acute influenza in young children. Viral pneumonia was more common with the 2009 pandemic H1N1 strain than in recent seasons with other influenza A or B virus strains and was particularly prevalent in older children and young adults.[91-93,113] This appears to be due both to unique characteristics of this virus and to an aberrant immune response causing immunopathology in the lung. Lack of surface glycosylation on the HA coupled with a polymorphism at amino acid 222 of the HA allows deeper penetration into the lung and diminished clearance by surfactant protein D.[141,193,384,463,510] Enhanced inflammation triggered by aberrant antibody and T-cell memory responses and innate recognition of the poorly glycosylated HA during transit through the Golgi contribute to acute lung injury.[197,325,471] Bacterial pneumonia was relatively uncommon during the 2009 pandemic compared to previous pandemics, but when superinfections were present, outcomes were worse and hospitalization was prolonged.[90,342,344,359,385,459] Otitis media associated with influenza may present as a mild, serous exudate if it is solely due to the virus, but in young children, mixed viral-bacterial infections are common and a painful, purulent exudate may result. Symptoms of sinusitis are common during acute influenza, and opacification of the sinuses can be seen on computed tomography in a significant proportion of affected persons. Bacterial sinusitis may result as a secondary complication, manifest as increased pain and a return of fever after an initial period of recovery.[160]

Mild elevations of hepatic transaminases occur commonly during acute influenza. Severe elevations, accompanied by steatosis, may be seen in Reye syndrome in the setting of salicylate exposure.[27,168,434] Reye syndrome appears to be more common with influenza B virus, and encephalopathy, hepatic failure, and death may result. The incidence of this complication has decreased markedly since warnings to avoid aspirin in febrile children were issued, but occasional cases still occur[27,168,346] An acute myositis manifest by severe pain and tenderness of both calves may occur during the early convalescence stage. This syndrome may have a rapid onset and is accompanied by elevations of serum creatine kinase and aspartate transaminase and, occasionally, rhabdomyolysis in severe cases.[475] Cardiac complications including myocarditis and pericarditis are associated rarely with influenza.[210,452] The pathogenesis of these complications is unclear, as virus is rarely identified in affected tissues.

Severe neurologic symptoms can be associated with influenza.[404] These complications are confined almost exclusively to young children who are naïve to the virus and have never received the influenza vaccine.[143,330] Mild neurologic complications, such as exacerbation of a seizure disorder, occur more frequently in patients with preexisting neurologic disorders.[376] Febrile seizures are relatively common and uncomplicated in young children with or without a previous diagnosis of seizure disorder, and up to 30% of all febrile seizures of childhood are due to influenza.[110,489] Encephalopathy during influenza can present with a variety of symptoms and signs, but mental status changes ranging from delirium to behavioral disturbances to coma are most prominent.[307,339] Cranial nerve pareses are unusual, as are meningitic presentations. Cerebrospinal fluid (CSF) examination is typically normal or reveals a mild pleocytosis, and virus can be detected in CSF by PCR or in biopsy or autopsy material from affected brains in about 15% of cases. Diagnosis is made on a clinical basis, with supporting information from electroencephalography (EEG) and magnetic resonance imaging (MRI) to rule out other causes. Computed tomography (CT) scans and MRI either are normal or demonstrate diffuse edema and are generally unhelpful in establishing a definitive diagnosis or prognosis.[209] EEG typically shows a general slowing without an acute focus. A subset of patients present with a more fulminant course and have findings on CT or MRI suggestive of necrosis in the subthalamic regions, a syndrome termed acute necrotizing encephalopathy.[203,209] Influenza-associated encephalopathy is uncommon in much of the world during circulation of seasonal strains, but was relatively common in Japan in the late 1990s and early 2000s for reasons that remain unclear. During the 2009 H1N1 pandemic, neurologic complications were more common than in preceding years, and older children were affected more commonly than is typically seen with seasonal influenza.[376]

PATHOLOGY

The hallmark of pandemic influenza is pneumonitis with diffuse alveolar damage, since these viruses typically penetrate well into the lower respiratory tract.[141,186,242,294,329,408,439] Hemorrhage, fibrin deposition, edema, and formation of hyaline membranes are common in the alveolar spaces. Submucosal congestion, hemorrhage, inflammation, and necrosis are common in the trachea and bronchi. In severe cases typical features of ARDS are seen. Myocarditis can be seen on autopsy in fatal cases.[242,358] Findings suggestive of bacterial pneumonia, primarily manifest as a neutrophilic infiltrate with consolidation, may be superimposed on this pathologic picture.[51,68,141,141,329,439] Antigen testing for bacteria in autopsy cases has been useful in recent studies to define the differences between primary viral and secondary bacterial pneumonia.[51] Seasonal influenza rarely presents as severe, primary viral lower respiratory tract disease; a mild to moderate tracheobronchitis is a more common presentation. Infiltration of lymphocytes in a peribronchial and perivascular distribution is typical.[140,242,439] The epithelial lining of the major airways is predominantly affected, with cell death and sloughing of epithelial cells exposing basement membrane elements, upon which extracellular matrix material is deposited. Ciliated cells may also be killed during infection, or may merely be functionally disrupted so that beat frequency and coordination of beat direction are altered, reducing clearance of mucus secretions.[362] Pathologic alterations in other affected organs (e.g., heart, brain), are most commonly nonspecific, with edema and inflammatory changes present.[358,432]

PATHOGENESIS

Virulence Factors

Hemagglutinin

The surface glycoprotein HA contributes to virulence both by facilitating efficient infection and by triggering inflammatory immune responses. HAs that have recently emerged from the avian reservoirs (including many pandemic strains) demonstrate enhanced virulence by both of these mechanisms. Avian origin HAs will typically have residual specificity for α-2,3-sialic acids, the predominant form in birds, while gaining specificity for α-2,6-sialic acids,[111,508] which are the predominant receptor for influenza A viruses in the human respiratory tract. It has been suggested that this residual α-2,3 recognition facilitates lower respiratory tract invasion by H5N1 viruses due to the deep lung distribution of α-2,3-sialic acids in humans.[71,460] Recently, a role for glycosylation in modulation of innate immune surveillance has been recognized. Influenza virus glycoproteins are flagged in the ER as "nonself" when they are poorly glycosylated, triggering the unfolded protein response and ER stress.[197] Mediated by IRE1α, signal transduction downstream of the c-Jun N-terminal kinase (JNK) drives inflammatory responses in the respiratory tract leading to acute lung injury. This contributes substantially to the pathology during influenza virus infections, particularly pandemic strains.

Neuraminidase

The role of NA in virulence is as a complement to HA, facilitating budding by cleaving sialic acids and disrupting sialic acid–HA binding. This requires maintenance of a balance between HA binding affinity and NA activity; viruses with NA activity that is too high relative to HA affinity have difficulty binding and establishing an infection, whereas viruses with too little relative NA activity have difficulty budding. The NA also contributes substantially to support for bacterial coinfections.[369] Sialic acid cleavage uncovers receptors for bacteria[306] and releases sialic acids into the extracellular medium where they can be used as a carbon source, facilitating bacterial growth.[414] The strength of the cleavage activity of the NA correlates broadly with the severity of epidemic influenza; circulating viruses with high NA activity map to some of the most severe seasons of the last century, and pandemic strains tend to have high NA activity.[369]

Polymerase Genes and PB1-F2

Much like the HA, the polymerase complex of genes (PB1, PA, PB2) are essential to infection, and viruses with high-efficiency polymerases replicate faster and can cause more pathology by outpacing the immune responses. This contributes to the high virulence of recent HPAI H5N1 and H7N9 strains.[436,509] The PA and PB1 proteins from certain virulent viruses also contribute to pathogenesis by interfering with RIG-I-mediated recognition of viral RNPs during the first stages of replication, which blocks early interferon signaling preventing cellular control of the infection.[264,265] PB1-F2 is a small, multifunctional accessory protein of influenza A viruses that is evolutionarily conserved in avian strains, including the pandemic strains from 1918, 1957, and 1968.[421] It contributes to pathogenicity by triggering cell death through mitochondrial interactions and through support of secondary bacterial infections.[295,296]

Nonstructural Protein 1

NS-1 is another nonstructural protein with several functions.[167] Its main role is as an antagonist of interferon and the antiviral response; artificial viruses without canonical NS-1 activity are severely attenuated.[127] The influenza A virus NS-1 also contains three potential src homology binding domains, one SH2bm and two SH3bm, which are conserved in many avian lineages. Most avian strains excluding H5N1 and H9N2 variants share a consensus sequence from amino acids 212 to 217 defining an SH3(II)bm.[195] This domain allows binding of NS-1 to c-Abl and subsequent inhibition of its functions in lung homeostasis. The end result of this blockade is acute lung injury and greatly increased pathogenicity of viruses that carry the motif.[196]

Evolution of Virulence

Because influenza A viruses are all zoonoses from the wild bird reservoirs of the world, newly emergent pandemic strains of avian origin must adapt to their new hosts. Many of the virulence factors just described are found in pandemic strains or other HPAI capable of infecting humans, but are lost during subsequent evolution.[304,305] The binding affinity of HA for α-2,3-sialic acids tends to weaken or disappear over time during adaptation. Over several decades, the HAs of strains that achieve endemicity in humans gain additional glycans on the head region of the protein, abrogating innate sensing in the ER and diminishing the resulting inflammatory response in the lung.[197,463] Considerably less lung pathology then occurs during the infection with seasonal strains.[197] These heavily glycosylated viruses are also more easily neutralized by collagenous lectins such as surfactant protein D and are cleared from the lower respiratory tract more efficiently.[380,463]

Reassortant strains with mismatched HA/NA pairs, such as the 1968 pandemic virus, undergo rapid adaptation, with the NA often evolving to match HA and regain the balance between HA affinity and NA cleavage.[472] Changes in NA activity either to match HA affinity changes during adaptation or in response to neuraminidase inhibitors[156] have a downstream impact on pathogenicity through change in support for secondary bacterial infections. Loss of NA activity as a compensatory mechanism to escape these drugs in a population with frequent treatment[157] should diminish pathogenicity in this manner.

Because its role in the life cycle of the virus is dispensable in mammalian hosts, nonfunctional forms of PB1-F2 are negatively selected over decades during adaptation in both humans and swine. These pathogenic functions are lost through truncation to shorter forms that lack the active sites in the C-terminal portion of the protein (typically to 11 or 56 amino acids, reduced from the full length of 87 to 90 amino acids[421]), or through loss of the start codon itself or mutation of the active site amino acids to a neutral or even antibacterial configuration.[5] Strains lacking the cytotoxic functions supported by the C-terminal domain do not support secondary bacterial infections very efficiently, and in the human H3N2 lineage, the antibacterial effect appears to be a form of viral-bacterial warfare supporting the virus in its host niche.[5,297] The 1918 pandemic strain expressed an avian NS-1 that contained the SH3(II)bm domain that inhibits c-Abl; however, the motif was mutated during adaptation of the H1N1 lineage to humans to a form that could not bind c-Abl and did not enhance acute lung injury.[196] The overall pattern for changes in virulence is a gradual decrease in pathogenicity of viruses during adaptation to the mammalian host after emerging from birds.[305] Evolutionarily, this is likely to benefit the virus by helping it avoid immune surveillance, facilitating transmission and a continuation of the adapted lineage.

Animal Models

The earliest examples of modeling influenza infections in animals came during the 1918 pandemic prior to the discovery of viruses. Wherry and Butterfield passed unfiltered sputum from ill patients by aerosol into a variety of animal species, including guinea pigs, mice, and rats.[486] Approximately a third of the exposed animals developed pneumonia and died, likely from a combination of the virus and coinfecting bacteria. Although a number of attempts had been made to prove influenza was caused by a filterable agent both before and after the 1918 pandemic, it was not until the 1926 demonstration, by Dunkin and Laidlaw using dogs and ferrets, that canine distemper was caused by a virus[106-108] that similar experiments in pigs were successfully conducted for influenza virus by Richard Shope.[411] Pigs remain a viable model for study of both human and swine viruses,[516] although size and husbandry requirements limit their use to specialized facilities.

The first well-controlled study of secondary bacterial pneumonia in mice using an influenza virus was conducted by Thomas Francis and Mercedes V. de Torregosa in 1945.[123] They reported that *H. influenzae*, *S. pneumoniae*, and *S. aureus* could all cause a fatal pneumonia in an intranasal coinfection model with the mouse-adapted influenza virus A/Puerto Rico/8/34 (PR8). Today, most laboratory models of viral-bacterial coinfection are derived from a similar sequential infection model that uses influenza virus PR8 followed by a laboratory strain of *S. pneumoniae*, which faithfully recapitulates many of the hallmarks of the clinical syndrome of severe secondary bacterial pneumonia.[309] Because mouse models are limited to a select set of mouse-adapted viruses, however, ferrets are commonly used as a second animal model to study human viruses. Early studies of influenza infectivity, transmission, and isolation of viruses were done in ferrets[11] in the 1930s and 1940s, and ferrets remain the favorite model for study or respiratory droplet transmission.[184,205] Mice, ferrets, and chinchillas have all been used in vaccine studies,[200,202,389] and chinchillas are particularly useful in studies of influenza-associated otitis media because of the ease of access to their middle ear space by tympanocentesis.[137,368] Guinea pigs are also used as an alternative model for transmission.[275,427]

Research and Modeling

Unraveling the relationships between pathogen replication and the resulting airway alterations and inflammatory responses that are driving host pathology and disease is complicated. Animal models have limitations in terms of both what can be studied and the ethics of using animals when alternatives are available. Kinetic mathematical models are a robust means of analyzing experimental results and explaining biologic phenomena without testing every scenario experimentally. A growing body of work modeling in vivo influenza virus infections has led to improved knowledge about the viral life cycle, viral control by the host, pathogenic differences in strains, and efficacy of antiviral treatment (reviewed in references 24, 422, and 424). These models have characterized the spread of virus during early infection and yielded estimates of strain-specific viral infection and production rates, infected cell life spans, and infectious virus half-life, all of which are not amenable to experimental investigation. It is likely that this field will continue to advance rapidly in the coming years and will be useful both to aid experimental interpretation of findings in animal models, and in some cases to replace animal studies altogether.

Dual Use Research

A significant controversy arose when two papers were published in 2012[184,205] that demonstrated that HPAI H5N1 viruses could be adapted to transmit between ferrets by the airborne route with only a few amino acid changes using reverse genetics systems.[190] This was a critically important discovery, as it not only serves as a warning that such viruses could evolve in nature, perhaps relatively easily,[392] but also allows targeted surveillance in H5N1 strains for these amino acid changes as a part of pandemic planning. Two concerns arose following the announcement of this discovery: the possibility that accidental release of these pathogens might cause a pandemic, and the fear that terrorists would either acquire such a virus or create it themselves for intentional release.[270] This led to unprecedented steps by the Dutch government to censor one of the publications by making it subject to "export laws,"[112] and by the US government to halt all research and research funding on "gain of function" studies for influenza viruses. It has been argued by prominent scientists who study influenza that, while the risks related to failures of biocontainment and biosecurity are real, albeit minuscule, the true threat is nature.[479] Influenza viruses evolve and adapt easily and in unpredictable ways, and if such a virus is possible (as shown by the published studies), nature is likely to produce it. Deliberately eschewing research and open scientific discourse that might prevent another pandemic on the scale of 1918, which killed more than 50 million persons worldwide, is near-sighted and dangerous to the public health.[479] Four years after publication of the original papers, the National Science Advisory Board on Biosecurity in the United States continues to debate the appropriate regulatory framework for balancing the ethical concerns about dual-use research with the scientific gains that are needed to prevent the next pandemic, and research remains in a hiatus.[351]

DIAGNOSIS

Differential Diagnosis

Because influenza can manifest as a variety of clinical syndromes, the differential diagnosis is broad. This is particularly true in infants, who may not have common signs of infection such as cough. Depending on the particular disease manifestations, many other pathogens can be either the primary cause or a co-pathogen. Other respiratory viruses such as parainfluenzaviruses, respiratory syncytial virus, human metapneumovirus, rhinoviruses, and coronaviruses should be considered in the differential diagnosis for upper respiratory tract infections, otitis media, and croup, particularly if they are circulating in the community in the same time frame. Accuracy of clinical diagnoses of specific respiratory viruses is very poor, with a sensitivity for diagnosing influenza as low as 38% and a positive predictive value of only 32%.[370] Influenza A and B viruses cannot be distinguished clinically by signs and symptoms of the presentation.[87] In general, testing for influenza is valuable to understand when influenza is circulating in a community, but testing is not necessary to establish the diagnosis in every patient once an epidemic is underway.

Bacterial causes of epiglottitis such as *H. influenzae*, *S. aureus*, and *S. pneumoniae* must also be considered in the child with croup, particularly if acutely ill. *S. pneumoniae*, *S. aureus*, and *S. pyogenes* are common lower respiratory tract co-pathogens with influenza, but must also be considered in the differential diagnosis as primary agents of disease along with other common causes of community-acquired pneumonia such as *Mycoplasma pneumoniae* and *Chlamydophila pneumoniae*. Numerous viral and bacterial pathogens can also present with fever and diarrhea, although gastrointestinal symptomatology with influenza is generally mild and the diarrhea nonbloody. The encephalopathy syndrome associated with influenza can mimic either bacterial meningitis or a viral encephalitis, so multiple causes must be considered. Finally, neonates with influenza can present with lethargy, poor circulation, and apnea without other typical signs of influenza, so other causes of sepsis must be considered.

Diagnostic Testing

Classically, influenza has been diagnosed on the basis of a compatible clinical presentation in the setting of supportive epidemiology, with testing being used to establish circulation. Local or regional data suggesting increased presentation to primary care centers coupled with an increased rate of laboratory diagnosis of influenza can usually be relied on to indicate the start of wintertime epidemics in temperate climes. Sentinel programs to track influenza are in place in many countries (e.g., through the CDC in the United States[64]) and internationally through the WHO. As an important epidemiologic clue, influenza will more frequently affect both adults and children together than other causes of similar clinical syndromes. In this context, an age-appropriate clinical presentation can usually be assumed to be influenza and appropriate measures taken without specific diagnostic testing. Testing is generally most useful to inform treatment decisions. A positive test may be useful to prompt antiviral treatment and avoid unnecessary use of antibiotics, whereas a negative test may reduce the cost of treatment by avoiding antiviral treatment. In the hospital setting, testing may also help to guide the need for or type of isolation and personal protective equipment to be employed. Chest radiographs may be helpful in some cases to confirm lower respiratory tract involvement or define a complicating bacterial pneumonia, which may need antibacterial therapy.

Three methods of diagnosis of influenza are in widespread use at present. Point-of-care testing in outpatient settings is typically limited to antigen-based testing. This is accomplished through the use of inexpensive kits that use colorimetric changes upon antibody recognition of virus in nasal swab material to rapidly demonstrate the presence of antigen.[244] Some tests can distinguish type A from type B influenza, but none can currently subtype influenza A strains or distinguish specific strains within an influenza A subtype or between the two major influenza B lineages. These kits typically have a low sensitivity but reasonable specificity compared to PCR, so although a positive result is useful for directing care, a negative result does not rule out influenza.[322] Use in the proper setting when influenza is likely to be circulating is important, as the pretest probability of influenza being present can have a dramatic impact on positive predictive value with tests with poor sensitivity.[150] Rapid antigen testing is also commonly employed in hospitals as a point-of-care diagnostic in acute care settings such as emergency rooms, but typically with a more sensitive and specific test as a backup, performed in a central laboratory.[2] Two methods are commonly employed in tertiary care settings. A fluorescent antibody test where clinical material from a nasal swab or nasal wash is used as the sample, and the presence of virus is determined by microscopy to detect fluorescence of dyes bound to those antibodies which recognize the virus, has been in common use for decades. This method is more sensitive and specific than rapid antigen tests, but may take several hours to achieve a result and requires special training and experience. This has been replaced in many centers by the use of PCR-based testing, particularly using rapid and sensitive real-time PCR assays. These assays have the advantages of quick turnaround times, improved sensitivity and specificity compared to all other methods, and can be designed to differentiate viruses by type, subtype, and even strain.[25,244] In parallel, similar methods are now available to rapidly sequence portions of the viral genome to provide indicators of the most common resistance mutations.[98,438] Other potential methods to diagnose influenza, such as virus isolation or acute and convalescent serology, are now confined to research settings.

MANAGEMENT

Antiviral Therapy

Several antiviral compounds have been developed against influenza virus to interfere with specific events in the replication cycle.[299] Among these, two classes of drugs are currently approved as antiviral agents by the Food and Drug Administration (FDA) of the United States. The adamantanes (amantadine, rimantadine) are inhibitors of viral uncoating, while the NA inhibitors (zanamivir, oseltamivir) interfere with the viral budding process.

Adamantanes

The adamantanes have been shown to be efficacious in the treatment of influenza A virus infection caused by different subtypes (H1N1, H2N2, and H3N2) but are ineffective against influenza B viruses.[104,177,461,491] Defervescence, improvement in symptoms, resolution of symptoms, and return to normal activity all occurred about 1 day earlier in treated subjects than in those receiving placebo. Although no studies of sufficient size have been performed to convincingly address whether adamantane treatment prevents complications of influenza, animal data[298] and a challenge trial in adult volunteers[104] suggest that there is a lack of effect. Efficacy in populations other than healthy adults or when administration is delayed beyond 48 hours has not been studied thoroughly. Prophylaxis of healthy adults during influenza outbreaks showed 71% to 91% efficacy compared to placebo in preventing laboratory-confirmed influenza virus infection in two trials using amantadine,[102,326] and 85% efficacy using rimantadine in a single trial.[102] A meta-analysis of published clinical data concluded that the major effects of amantadine and rimantadine treatment were to shorten the duration of fever by about 1 day in treated, infected individuals, and prevent about 60% to 70% of influenza cases when used as prophylaxis.[215]

Adamantanes possess two concentration-dependent mechanisms of antiviral action.[374] At micromolar concentrations (0.1-5 μM), adamantanes selectively inhibit two different steps in the replication cycle in a strain-specific manner.[18] Prior to membrane fusion, the low pH of the endosome activates the M2 channel to conduct protons across the viral envelope, which results in the acidification of the viral interior. Adamantanes block the ion channel activity of the M2 protein of influenza A virus, and viral replication is inhibited by the blockade of hydrogen ion flow into the virus particle, principally at the stage of virus entry and uncoating.[467] Amantadine also acts at a late stage of replication by preventing virus release of certain influenza strains that possess intracellularly cleavable hemagglutinin (HA), in particular the H5 and H7 subtypes. This effect is proposed to result from irreversible conversion of the HA to its low-pH conformation form within the trans-Golgi network in the absence of M2 function.[32,146]

Rapid development of fully pathogenic and transmissible resistant variants after amantadine or rimantadine treatment and their ineffectiveness against influenza B virus infection are the main drawbacks of M2 blockers.[175] The markers of resistance to adamantanes are well established and include substitution of one of five amino acids (positions 26, 27, 30, 31, and 34) within the transmembrane domain of M2 protein; each change confers resistance to both amantadine and rimantadine.[31,174,374] Amantadine-resistant influenza A viruses are found among 30% to 80% of isolates after only a few days of drug therapy in both immunocompetent and immunocompromised patients.[410]

The incidence of naturally occurring amantadine-resistant variants has increased dramatically since 2003, and these resistant influenza A

(H1N1) and A (H3N2) viruses have spread widely and reached nearly 100% even in countries without substantial amantadine use.[40,50] For this reason, the US CDC discourages use of M2 inhibitors[50] except in specific instances with susceptible strains as a part of combination therapy.[505]

Neuraminidase Inhibitors

Development of the NA inhibitors was a significant milestone in antiviral development, as this was the first example of synthesis of such a drug based on the crystal structure of a target enzyme.[20,230,466] The NA inhibitors zanamivir and oseltamivir were approved by FDA for the treatment and prevention of influenza in 1999. Oseltamivir is not thought to distribute into the brain,[431] although central nervous system toxicity in juvenile rats with an immature blood-brain barrier led to cautionary warnings about the use of this agent in children under 1 year of age.[231] A subsequent study demonstrated that the incidence of neurologic side effects in infants was no greater with oseltamivir than with amantadine,[231] suggesting an acceptable safety profile. Reports of neuropsychiatric events in patients taking oseltamivir, particularly in Japan where use is heavy, have prompted many countries to add cautionary warnings to the drug's label. However, it is unclear whether these effects are due to the drug or to influenza itself, which has well-known neurologic side effects.[376] In general, adverse events after oral administration of oseltamivir are considered to be mild and include nausea and vomiting. Inhalation of zanamivir is generally well tolerated but may cause bronchospasm in some patients with underlying lung disease.[155]

Both oseltamivir and zanamivir are effective and well tolerated in adults treated for natural influenza infection, including hospitalized patients.[178,345,448] Reduced effectiveness for influenza B viruses as compared to influenza A viruses has been reported for oseltamivir.[224] The therapeutic benefits of NA inhibitors have been reported to include reductions of about 1 day in the time to alleviation of illness, resumption of usual activities, and duration of fever, as well as decreases in illness severity, ancillary medication use, viral titers, and the frequency of antibiotic prescriptions for lower respiratory complications.[178,345,448] Oseltamivir both decreases the incidence of secondary bacterial pneumonia and reduces the severity of complications in an animal model.[298] Similar data are not available from a single, well-powered trial in humans, although a meta-analysis of data from multiple trials suggests that these results can be extrapolated at least to healthy adults.[220] In children, however, oseltamivir was shown to reduce the occurrence of otitis media by 44% compared to placebo.[488] Retrospective reviews of insurance claims databases suggest that NA inhibitors reduce the risk of otitis media, pneumonia, respiratory illnesses other than pneumonia, and hospitalization in both adults and children.[159,373]

Both zanamivir and oseltamivir have demonstrated the ability to interrupt household transmission.[176,485] A meta-analysis of 78 trials during the 2009 pandemic showed a reduced risk of mortality; earlier treatment was associated with a further reduction in risk.[332] Early administration of oseltamivir increases the benefit seen in healthy adults relative to treatment at 48 hours,[16] but no randomized, controlled trials have been conducted studying treatment outside of the first 48 hours, so no data are available to examine the effects of late treatment on prevention of complications. Because persons with chronic illness, who might be more likely to benefit from late treatment as viral control might be established later in such individuals, have typically been excluded from antiviral studies, this question is currently unanswered. Intravenous zanamivir has been used under an emergency investigational new drug program in several hundred hospitalized children and adults with severe illness for whom oral or inhaled therapy was impractical, but efficacy and safety information will require prospective study.[61] Higher doses and longer durations of therapy with oseltamivir (150 mg twice daily for 10 days) have been attempted anecdotally for severe infections with H5N1 subtype viruses or in immunocompromised subjects,[26,254,321] but no data from randomized trials are available to assess the effectiveness of these measures.

The NA inhibitors were designed based on the knowledge of the three-dimensional structure of the NA complex with sialic acid[466] and act as competitive inhibitors by binding within the enzyme's active site. The primary function of the NA enzyme in the life cycle of influenza viruses is to remove sialic acid residues from the surface of the infected cell and from mucins in the respiratory tract, facilitating the release of newly synthesized virus particles and allowing the virus to spread.[290] Blockade of this activity prevents virion budding and leads to aggregation of viruses on the cell surface and within the mucosal layer, preventing subsequent infection of new cells.[145]

Two mechanisms of resistance to NA inhibitors have been described. The first is mutations within the NA enzyme catalytic site that disrupt a direct interaction with the drug. The second is mutations in the HA that reduce affinity for its receptor, thus compensating for the effect of the drug on NA activity.[155] The most frequently observed mutations for NA inhibitor-resistant variants for influenza A viruses of N1 NA subtype are H275Y and N295S (N1 numbering); for influenza A viruses of N2 NA subtype are R292K and E119V (N2 numbering), and for influenza B viruses are R152K and D198N. Prior to the 2007-08 influenza season, oseltamivir-resistant variants were found in only a small proportion of patients (approximately 4%-8% of children and <1% of adults) after treatment with the NA inhibitor.[430] However, rigorous detection techniques identified resistant mutants in 9 of 50 (18%) Japanese children during treatment with oseltamivir.[234] A high level of oseltamivir resistance among influenza H1N1 viruses was reported in many European countries starting in the 2007-08 influenza season.[100,248]

During the 2009 H1N1 influenza pandemic, almost all tested viruses remained susceptible to oseltamivir and zanamivir. Oseltamivir-resistant variants with H275Y NA mutation were isolated from individuals receiving prophylaxis[23] and from immunocompromised patients[52] under drug selection pressure. Oseltamivir-resistant variants also have been isolated from untreated patients[257,517] and from a few community clusters.[255] The reasons for the relative paucity of resistant strains and the lack of widespread transmission are not yet clear. However, experimental evidence suggests that the oseltamivir-resistant H275Y mutant of the pandemic 2009 H1N1 virus retained efficient transmission through direct contact in a ferret model, but respiratory droplet transmission was decreased as compared to an oseltamivir-sensitive virus.[105] This suggests that transmission efficiency of the mutants may be decreased, limiting spread between humans.

Steroids

Corticosteroids have been widely used to treat many inflammatory and immune diseases including severe pulmonary infections such as ARDS.[317] Clinical use of corticosteroids as an adjunctive therapy for treating pneumonia or to reduce cytokine loads during ARDS has been controversial.[323,401] Most data on their use derives from studies in adults, and data are lacking in children. Despite controversy, the use of steroids in severe influenza, particularly in the setting of ARDS, is common in both adults and children. In a recent prospective case registry analysis in Japan, 33% of children mechanically ventilated for pandemic H1N1 influenza received corticosteroids as part of their therapy.[445] A similar study in France showed that 40% of children with ARDS from influenza received corticosteroids.[42] Some randomized controlled clinical trials suggest beneficial activity in treating pneumonia with a significant reduction in the length of hospital stay[80,318] or a decrease in mortality of patients with septic shock.[14] Based on these studies in severe pneumonia, some have advocated for use in influenza as well.[13] However, other studies of pneumonia have shown no benefit or harmful outcomes from corticosteroids.[286,425] Similar findings, including increased secondary bacterial infections and mortality, have also been demonstrated in clinical trials in influenza, although most studies are in adults.[42,101,229] Animal data suggest that the primary detrimental effect of steroids during influenza treatment is prolongation of viral replication due to suppression of T-cell responses.[134] Based on these data and expert opinion, the WHO discouraged corticosteroid treatment during the 2009 influenza pandemic.[500] Generally, consensus expert opinion suggests that the data are insufficient to recommend use of corticosteroids in children for treatment of influenza or ARDS.[437] However, children receiving corticosteroids for chronic pulmonary, rheumatologic, or other disorders should not have these drugs withheld.

INFECTION CONTROL

Clinical management of influenza in both the outpatient and inpatient settings requires an infection control plan for prevention of nosocomial influenza in health care workers and transmission of influenza virus to other patients. All health care workers should receive influenza vaccination.[153] Influenza vaccine coverage among health care personnel in the United States has increased dramatically from the early 2000s (rates typically ranged from 34–49%[172]) to the mid-2010s (rates of 75–77%).[34] Coverage is highest in hospitals, likely because of required reporting instituted in 2013 by the Centers for Medicare & Medicaid Services.[267] Educational programs have only a modest impact on vaccination rates.[311,388] Requiring vaccination as a condition of employment (with few exceptions allowed) improves rates markedly, and hospitals mandating vaccination achieve rates as high as 96%.[34,267,279] Instituting a policy that requires unvaccinated health care personnel to wear a mask throughout the influenza season when working in patient care areas increases the acceptance rate and may close some of the gaps that persist despite mandates from employers.[109] Unfortunately, vaccination rates among health care workers remain low in many countries other than the United States.[19,135,388]

Patients with confirmed or suspected influenza should be isolated in single patient rooms, or cohorted with other patients with confirmed infection if this is not possible. Because influenza can transmit by both droplet and aerosol routes, standard, contact, and droplet precautions are recommended, including a gown, gloves, and surgical mask as personal protective equipment (PPE).[60] Hand hygiene should be employed after removal of PPE. Both soap and water and alcohol-based gels are effective at neutralizing influenza viruses. Enhanced respiratory protection (e.g., fit-tested N95 respirator and goggles or a face shield) should be used during aerosol-generating procedures and when providing care to patients with confirmed or suspected HPAI influenza viruses such as H5N1 or H7N9 strains.[60,478] Negative-pressure rooms, when available, should be used for isolation of confirmed or suspected cases of HPAI influenza. Antiviral treatment of ill patients and postexposure prophylaxis with an NA inhibitor is effective at reducing infection after exposure of unvaccinated health care personnel and other household contacts.[171] In particular, pregnant health care workers should be vaccinated and included in postexposure prophylaxis programs, because the mother and the fetus are at high risk for adverse events from influenza, including primary viral pneumonia and fetal loss.[444]

VACCINES

History

About a decade after the first isolation of influenza viruses, a monovalent, inactivated, whole virus influenza A vaccine was developed by the US military.[308] It entered widespread use in the Armed Forces in 1943 and was licensed commercially shortly thereafter in 1945 as a bivalent product with the addition of influenza B antigen. A trivalent vaccine with two type A H1N1 antigens was introduced in 1947.[235] During the 1960s, inactivated, split antigen and subunit vaccines were introduced in an attempt to reduce reactogenicity of whole-virus preparations, a particular concern in children due to side effects such as intense local reactions, fever, and febrile seizures.[199] The development of the master donor virus backbones for the live, attenuated influenza vaccines (LAIV) that were first licensed for human use in 2003 was also accomplished in this decade.[281] Trivalent influenza vaccines (TIV) containing a type B antigen, and both H1N1 and H3N2 type A antigens have been in use since 1978 following the reemergence of H1N1 strains in 1977. The divergence of influenza B into two antigenically distinct lineages in the 1980s created a problem with vaccine matching, as there was reduced immunogenicity when the "wrong" strain was chosen for inclusion in the vaccine and the circulating strains did not match.[310] Quadrivalent influenza vaccines (QIV) containing two influenza A antigens and two influenza B antigens were approved in the United States in both LAIV and inactivated forms in 2012 to address this problem through inclusion of both circulating influenza B virus strains.[251]

Strain Selection

A strain selection committee, organized by the WHO, meets twice a year in February (for the Northern Hemisphere) and September (for the Southern Hemisphere). The Committee reviews data on the characteristics of strains circulating in different parts of the world as collected by the WHO Collaborating Centers.[499] Characteristics include type and subtype, associated disease and epidemiology data (e.g., severity by outcomes), antigenicity compared to prior vaccine strains as determined by hemagglutination-inhibition assays using ferret sera, and genetic analyses to understand evolution of virulence factors and other markers in strains over time. Taking all of these factors into account, the panel of experts appointed to the committee chooses vaccine strains for the upcoming influenza season, prioritizing those that are likely to be in wide circulation, grow well in eggs to facilitate large-scale production, have the possibility of antigenic drift with reduced population immunity, and are predicted to cause more severe disease. The WHO Collaborating Centers then develop vaccine seed strains through reverse genetics techniques, creating viruses that should grow well in eggs or tissue culture by virtue of internal genes adapted to the planned growth medium, but which have the desired antigenicity due to use of the chosen HA and NA glycoproteins. Individual countries then make a decision on whether to use these seed strains or closely matched alternative strains during production and distribution. In the United States, this decision is made by the FDA's Vaccines and Related Biological Products Advisory Committee shortly after the WHO's February strain selection meeting for the upcoming fall and winter season. In about 7 of 10 years the vaccine is well matched to the circulating strains the following season; in other years significant drift occurs in the intervening months or a minor variant unexpectedly emerges, leading to reduced vaccine efficacy. The process of producing vaccine takes 5 to 8 months for egg-grown viruses and may be limited by the growth properties of individual viruses and production capacity. A 5- to 10-fold reduction in replication capacity of one of the viruses leads to a need for 5 to 10 times as many eggs, with associated increased costs and increased lag time until vaccine is available.[453] Many countries outside of the developed world do not have the capacity to produce vaccines and rely on either purchase at reduced cost from manufacturers in developed countries or on vaccine donation programs.[245]

Immunogenicity

Currently, influenza immunization focuses on induction of immunity to the exposed globular head of the HA glycoprotein.[118] For the purpose of vaccine licensure, the serum hemagglutination-inhibition (HI) titer is considered the gold standard correlate of anti-influenza immunity by both the US FDA and the European Agency for the Evaluation of Medicinal Products.[78,455] This assay indirectly measures the ability of antibodies from sera to disrupt binding of HA to sialic acids on red blood cells, which serves as a correlate for the ability of these antibodies to prevent attachment of the virus to sialic acids on respiratory tract epithelial cells. The initial association between a specific HI titer and protection from clinical illness was made by Thomas Francis Jr,[228] who cited unpublished data when he suggested that an HI titer of 1:32 or better was protective in early clinical trials in the military and in mental institutions.[320,393] This spurred the use of HI titer as a threshold for protection for licensure purposes, and currently a serum HI titer of 1:40 or greater is defined as a protective response by the FDA and the European Agency for the Evaluation of Medicinal Products.[78,455] Human vaccination-challenge studies later showed that protection from infection could be conferred in many subjects by a titer between 1:30 and 1:40, but protection was not absolute even over 1:40.[189,375]

Additional assays that can detect specific immune responses (e.g., microneutralization, enzyme-linked immunosorbent assays [ELISA]) are being tested in laboratory settings and in clinical trials of influenza vaccines and offer additional information about the degree of responsiveness to a vaccine and functional quality of the response.[308] However, these assays are not yet useful as stand-alone correlates of protection. Because the mucosa is the site of replication of influenza viruses, there is interest in the development of mucosal correlates of immunity to guide improved vaccine design. IgA antibodies can be detected in the nasal wash of humans after influenza, and they are induced by LAIV vaccines.[29] A contribution of IgA antibodies to protective immunity to pulmonary infections can be demonstrated in murine models, but IgA is not required for protection in mice.[360] The contribution of IgA to protection in humans is unclear because of the difficulty in obtaining appropriate mucosal samples in humans, compared to the ease with which secretions from the entire lung surface can be assayed in mice. This lack of appropriate correlates of mucosal immunity makes immunogenicity assessments of mucosal vaccines, such as the licensed LAIV product, difficult. LAIV shows better relative efficacy in some patient populations compared to TIV,[28] but generally is accompanied by a modest serum antibody response as measured by HI, so better correlates of immunity are needed. In addition to antibodies toward the HA protein, antibodies to alternative antigens on influenza (e.g., NA, M2) can also be measured and are used in clinical trials to understand the contribution of other forms of immunity to protection, but there are not enough data available in humans to demonstrate utility as correlates of protection.

Pediatric Vaccination

Universal vaccination of all children is recommended in the United States.[153] In children, influenza vaccines are typically poorly immunogenic in the first several years of life, and prior infection or repeated vaccination is required to boost responses to the vaccine above thresholds predicted to be effective. Current recommendations are for children 6 months to 8 years to be given two doses of vaccine during their first season of vaccination to optimize responses.[153] Two doses are also required if a child received only one dose in prior seasons, but children with two prior lifetime doses need only one dose each year. Some children with chronic diseases have reduced responses to influenza vaccines, particularly those with immunosuppressive states such as human immunodeficiency virus (HIV) infection or after cancer chemotherapy.[48,163,164,166] In other chronic conditions, such as sickle cell, responses are not blunted.[163] Children with cancer or HIV may benefit from two doses of vaccine regardless of past history of vaccine uptake.[163,164,236] Because no influenza vaccines are licensed for children under 6 months of age, household contacts should be vaccinated to prevent transmission to the infant, and pregnant women should be vaccinated.[372] Inactivated influenza vaccine is safe and effective in pregnant women.[208,442] Because 10% to 20% of all pregnancies end in spontaneous abortion and influenza is one of the causes of early termination of pregnancies, vaccination is protective against spontaneous abortion by preventing an infection that may trigger fetal demise.[39] Influenza vaccine is also safe in breastfeeding mothers and provides protection for infants through the breast milk.[283]

In the United States, several formulations of inactivated vaccine are available from several different manufacturers, and many have different age ranges for use. In the 2015–16 season, different vaccine products were licensed for use in children, with the lower bound for age set for various preparations at greater than 6 months, 3 years, 4 years, 9 years, or for use only in adults greater than 18 years.[153] These differing age ranges do not stem from different anticipated safety or efficacy profiles of the vaccines, but from the need to conduct a small clinical trial of immunogenicity in the specific age groups prior to release of each vaccine, leading each company to make a decision on target ages based on cost and timing of their specific trial versus anticipated use and profit margin. A larger age range means a larger, more expensive trial and perhaps a longer time to market. Both trivalent (H1, H3, and B) and quadrivalent (H1, H3, and two strains of B) preparations were available in 2015–16. Preparations were available in multiuse vials, containing trace amounts of thimerosal as a preservative, and as single-dose syringes or vials with or without thimerosal. LAIV was available as a quadrivalent preparation and is indicated for children older than 2 years, excluding immunocompromised patients and children younger than 4 years with asthma or wheezing. Multiple additional preparations are available for adults, including vaccine delivered by needleless intradermal microinjection systems, cell-culture–based vaccines that do not trigger allergic reactions to eggs, and a recombinant protein vaccine.[153]

Influenza vaccines are considered to be safe and well tolerated in children. Common side effects of inactivated vaccines include fever as well as mild and transient pain, tenderness, and/or swelling at the injection site, each generally noted in 10% to 20% of vaccinees.[161,169,261] Other side effects are extremely rare, and in some cases are linked to specific batches of vaccine. Whole-virus vaccines were associated with higher rates of fever and a clear association with febrile seizures in children, prompting replacement by split-virus and subunit vaccines in the 1970s.[199,261,308] Although febrile seizures are still reported with influenza vaccines, and at a somewhat higher incidence during first exposure to the 2009 pandemic vaccine, they are not more common than is seen in the unvaccinated population unless the influenza vaccine is coadministered with pneumococcal conjugate vaccine.[22,161,169,261] More severe skin reactions resembling cellulitis occur at a rate of about 1 in 10,000 and typically resolve in 2 or 3 days without antibiotics.[169] Other rare side effects linked to specific vaccine products include anaphylaxis (one per million exposures); Guillain-Barré syndrome (one per 100,000 exposures), predominantly during the 1976 "swine flu" vaccine program[403]; narcolepsy (one to six per 100,000 exposures), limited to a set of European countries using an adjuvanted H1N1 pandemic vaccine in 2009[3,4]; and Bell palsy (odds ratio of 84, 1–2 months after receipt of vaccine, compared to controls), limited to persons receiving a specific vaccine in Switzerland in the 2000–01 season.[333] Subsequent population-based studies from large databases suggest that none of these rare side effects are clearly linked to inactivated influenza vaccines in general, but either can be attributed to specific products through unclear mechanisms or are spurious associations because they do not occur at a rate above that of the unvaccinated population.[161,169,261,390] Because Guillain-Barré syndrome and Bell palsy can be caused by influenza itself, the vaccine is considered protective against these conditions outside of the epidemics cited. LAIV is also safe and well tolerated. About half of children receiving LAIV report nasal congestion; other side effects including fever, sore throat, and headache are mild and transient and occur in less than 5% of recipients.[28,30,35,233]

EFFICACY AND EFFECTIVENESS

Vaccine efficacy is defined as the ability of a vaccine to prevent laboratory-diagnosed infection in the context of a clinical trial.[116] By contrast, effectiveness is a broader term indicating the ability of a vaccine to provide a benefit to the vaccinee; this benefit may be by preventing various manifestations of disease, ameliorating symptoms, abrogating subsequent transmission, facilitating a return to normal activities sooner, or providing cost savings for a person, business, or society. Both inactivated influenza vaccines and LAIV are efficacious when compared to placebo.[28,30,84,232,233] Generally, inactivated influenza vaccine and LAIV have similar efficacy when compared head-to-head in children of all ages as a group, although LAIV is typically superior in young children when immunity to the live virus contained in the vaccine is lowest and immunogenicity of inactivated vaccines is poorest.[28] Although it has not been well studied in older adults, it is likely that decreased replication of the vaccine virus in individuals with significant lifetime exposure to influenza may lead to decreased efficacy of LAIV in this population. There are strong data suggesting that inactivated vaccines are not as immunogenic or efficacious in older people as they are in healthy younger adults, which has led to the development of high-dose inactivated vaccines for this age group.[54,114] Several generalizations can be made on vaccine efficacy from data accumulated over the past several decades. First, there are age gradients of efficacy for each vaccine type. LAIV is most efficacious in very young children, with decreasing efficacy seen with increasing age and immune experience. Inactivated influenza vaccines are most efficacious in healthy older children and young adults and have much less efficacy in young children, particularly under 2 years of age, and in older persons. Second, there is great variability in efficacy based on underlying comorbidities in an individual and season, subtype, and vaccine strain such that efficacy of the vaccine in particular patient groups and from year to year is very difficult to predict.

Influenza vaccines provide a variety of benefits beyond direct prevention of infection in the individual vaccinated. Influenza vaccines are generally effective at preventing most medically attended illnesses due to influenza, as well as severe influenza requiring hospitalization.[36,69,82,221,470] Estimates generally range from 60% to 70% for prevention of influenza-like illness for well-matched strains. Despite concerns about immunogenicity, effectiveness against hospitalization in children with chronic medical conditions is typically very good, around 70%.[37] Both inactivated influenza vaccines and LAIV are effective at reducing the incidence of acute otitis media and otitis media with effusion.[86,181,182,357] Effectiveness against influenza-related pneumonia is between 50% and 60%.[151,284] Both LAIV and inactivated vaccines are cost saving or cost effective in children and show a higher cost benefit in children who are at increased risk for complications of influenza.[188,276,285,394,409,423] The value of cost savings varies considerably by severity of the influenza season and match of the vaccine to the circulating strains, but is typically estimated between $5 and $150 per child immunized. However, these are probably low estimates for vaccine programs in children, as most analyses do not consider the impact of herd immunity and decreased transmission from children into other groups, including older persons and other vulnerable populations.[120,136,138,383,433]

PANDEMIC PREPAREDNESS

Careful planning and several critical advances are needed in order for the world to be prepared for the inevitable next influenza pandemic (Table 178.3). At the most basic level, the magnitude and nature of the threat must be understood and monitored with thorough and structured surveillance. Currently, continuous surveillance in birds takes place at a limited number of sites relative to the scope of wild bird ecology and is often confined to specific countries or regions with artificial borders.[21,152,513] Targeted surveillance takes place during outbreaks,[66,262] and more than 80 countries have some sort of surveillance program,[282] but these are poorly coordinated and do not share standards or reporting measures. There are even fewer structured, continuous programs for monitoring swine influenza,[204,259,464] so it is unsurprising that the emergence of the 2009 pandemic strain went undetected until multiple human cases had occurred and transmission of the virus could not be constrained.[53] Programs should be aimed at understanding the patterns of circulation of influenza viruses in their natural hosts, aquatic waterfowl, and incidental hosts at the human-avian interface such as domestic poultry and swine.[269,481] In addition to surveillance, further research is required.[303,305] Answers to many basic questions are needed, such as, "Why are HPAI strains so lethal? What will allow transmission to humans from birds, or between humans? Can H5N1, H7N9, or other pandemic precursors reassort with currently circulating human strains? What patient groups or age ranges will be most affected? Will mortality stem from our immune response to the virus, from comorbid conditions, or from secondary bacterial infections?" We know very little at present about most of these critically important questions.

In the United States and at the WHO, significant progress in pandemic planning has been made at the level of strategic planning. In a sea change from the situation that existed prior to the 2009 pandemic, comprehensive websites including detailed information for health care workers and businesses, risk assessment tools, and guidelines for entities ranging from individuals to businesses to entire countries are now available.[454,504] The US strategy takes three parts: preparedness and communication, surveillance and detection, and response and containment. Much of the governmental focus in the United States in the area of response and containment has been on stockpiling antivirals.[511] This is appropriate as a stopgap measure to control the pace of viral spread[271] or protect key individuals, but is insufficient as a total solution because of cost, distribution, and effectiveness concerns.[206] Unfortunately, the least expensive and most widely available agents, the adamantanes, are not effective against most H5N1 strains.[179,299] The most popular choice for stockpiling, the NA inhibitor oseltamivir, has not been highly effective thus far in laboratory-confirmed cases of H5N1 infection,[398] and resistance has been shown to develop in select treated cases.[254] Strategies based on prophylaxis of contacts at the start of a pandemic to slow or limit the spread of the pandemic, buying time for development of a vaccine, may be the best option available.[272,272] However, this strategy was ineffective during the 2009 pandemic because of delayed recognition of early cases.

Numerous pandemic or universal vaccine candidates are in pre-clinical or clinical development at present.[97,201,400] Perhaps the most difficult obstacle to developing such a vaccine is that we will not know what strain or even subtype to make a vaccine against until the pandemic starts. Because of the long production timeline for influenza vaccines (6–10 months), it is unlikely that an effective, well-matched vaccine can be prepared before the first wave of the pandemic virus has circumnavigated the world. Thus, most of the emphasis for planning has to be on mitigation strategies such as antiviral use, or implementation of other measures broadly dubbed "nonpharmaceutical interventions."[226,288,447] This includes strategies to prevent or decrease the likelihood of both transmission and acquisition of virus by maintaining personal spacing and decreasing contact between individuals, practicing good hand hygiene, using masks when close contact cannot be avoided, and intervening at the community level by closing schools and discouraging gatherings.

TABLE 178.3 Priorities for Pandemic Planning

Surveillance	Wild birds, human-avian and human-swine interface, human-to-human transmission
Research	Virulence determinants, capacity to reassort with human strains, requirements for transmission, interactions with the immune system
Stockpiling antivirals	Capacity for early intervention before vaccine is available
Pandemic vaccines	Pre- and postpandemic vaccine strategies
Nonpharmaceutical interventions	Utility of hand hygiene, masks, social distancing strategies, and community-based interventions

Modified from McCullers JA. Preparing for the next influenza pandemic. *Pediatr Infect Dis J* 2008;27:S57-S59.

NEW REFERENCES SINCE THE SEVENTH EDITION

2. Abraham MK, Perkins J, Vilke GM, et al. Influenza in the emergency department: vaccination, diagnosis, and treatment: clinical practice paper approved by American Academy of Emergency Medicine Clinical Guidelines Committee. *J Emerg Med.* 2016;50:536-542.
81. Cowling BJ, Chan KH, Fang VJ, et al. Comparative epidemiology of pandemic and seasonal influenza A in households. *N Engl J Med.* 2010;362:2175-2184.
117. Finelli L, Fiore A, Dhara R, et al. Influenza-associated pediatric mortality in the United States: increase of *Staphylococcus aureus* coinfection. *Pediatrics.* 2008;122:805-811.
167. Hale BG, Randall RE, Ortin J, et al. The multifunctional NS1 protein of influenza A viruses. *J Gen Virol.* 2008;89:2359-2376.
169. Halsey NA, Talaat KR, Greenbaum A, et al. The safety of influenza vaccines in children: An Institute for Vaccine Safety white paper. *Vaccine.* 2015;33(suppl 5):F1-F67.
197. Hrincius ER, Liedmann S, Finkelstein D, et al. Acute lung injury results from innate sensing of viruses by an ER stress pathway. *Cell Rep.* 2015;11:1591-1603.
206. Infectious Diseases Society of America. Pandemic and Seasonal Influenza—Principles for U.S. Action; 2012. Available at: http://www.idsociety.org/influenzaprinciples/.
214. Jain S, Williams DJ, Arnold SR, et al. Community-acquired pneumonia requiring hospitalization among U.S. children. *N Engl J Med.* 2015;372:835-845.
244. Kumar S, Henrickson KJ. Update on influenza diagnostics: lessons from the novel H1N1 influenza A pandemic. *Clin Microbiol Rev.* 2012;25:344-361.
250. Lafond KE, Nair H, Rasooly MH, et al. Global role and burden of influenza in pediatric respiratory hospitalizations, 1982-2012: a systematic analysis. *PLoS Med.* 2016;13:e1001977.
253. Lau LL, Cowling BJ, Fang VJ, et al. Viral shedding and clinical illness in naturally acquired influenza virus infections. *J Infect Dis.* 2010;201:1509-1516.
263. Li Q, Zhou L, Zhou M, et al. Epidemiology of human infections with avian influenza A(H7N9) virus in China. *N Engl J Med.* 2014;370:520-532.
275. Lowen AC, Steel J. Roles of humidity and temperature in shaping influenza seasonality. *J Virol.* 2014;88:7692-7695.
294. Mauad T, Hajjar LA, Callegari GD, et al. Lung pathology in fatal novel human influenza A (H1N1) infection. *Am J Respir Crit Care Med.* 2010;181:72-79.
304. McCullers JA. The co-pathogenesis of influenza viruses with bacteria in the lung. *Nat Rev Microbiol.* 2014;12:252-262.
308. McCullers JA, Huber VC. Correlates of vaccine protection from influenza and its complications. *Hum Vaccine Immunother.* 2012;8:1-12.
329. Morens DM, Taubenberger JK, Fauci AS. Predominant role of bacterial pneumonia as a cause of death in pandemic influenza: implications for pandemic influenza preparedness. *J Infect Dis.* 2008;198:962-970.

392. Russell CA, Fonville JM, Brown AE, et al. The potential for respiratory droplet-transmissible A/H5N1 influenza virus to evolve in a mammalian host. *Science.* 2012;336:1541-1547.
433. Sugaya N. A review of the indirect protection of younger children and the elderly through a mass influenza vaccination program in Japan. *Expert Rev Vaccines.* 2014;13:1563-1570.
442. Thompson MG, Li DK, Shifflett P, et al. Effectiveness of seasonal trivalent influenza vaccine for preventing influenza virus illness among pregnant women: a population-based case-control study during the 2010-2011 and 2011-2012 influenza seasons. *Clin Infect Dis.* 2014;58:449-457.
513. Yoon SW, Webby RJ, Webster RG. Evolution and ecology of influenza A viruses. *Curr Top Microbiol Immunol.* 2014;385:359-375.

The full reference list for this chapter is available at ExpertConsult.com.

SUBSECTION **VII** Paramyxoviridae

179 Parainfluenza Viruses

Robert C. Welliver Sr

The human parainfluenza viruses (hPIVs) are ubiquitous agents with well-earned recognition as being among the most important viral respiratory pathogens of humans. The three major hPIVs (1 to 3) have been estimated to be among the three most frequent causes of hospitalizations for young children with respiratory tract illnesses.[91,92,101] The impact of these three hPIVs on health care resources is demonstrated by the 16,000 to 100,000 hospitalizations each year they are estimated to cause among children younger than 5 years.[48] Hospitalizations from hPIV-3 alone are estimated to range from about 9000 to 52,000 each year. The rates of outpatient visits for hPIV infections among young children are even higher, estimated to be 10 times the hospitalization rates.[62] One study estimated that the cost of emergency visits and hospitalization from croup resulting from parainfluenza alone was $20 to $56 million.[92] The costs imposed by the burden of all the hPIVs, types 1 to 4, and at all ages have not been estimated.

Respiratory tract illnesses from the hPIVs may occur and recur throughout life, and they are subordinate only to respiratory syncytial virus (RSV) in the morbidity caused by acute lower respiratory tract disease in infants and young children.[216] Among the causative agents of acute laryngotracheitis or "croup," the hPIVs are second to none.[175] The epidemic nature of hPIV types 1 and 2, the prolonged seasonal occurrence of type 3, and the ability of all types to cause repeated infections throughout life indicate why they continue to be important despite the technological advances that have been made toward control of viral diseases.

HISTORY

The historical delineation of the parainfluenza viral family is intertwined with the discovery of the related animal viruses and marked by the colorful names descriptive of their origin (Table 179.1). The first strain of PIV was discovered in Japan and named *Sendai,* or the hemagglutinating virus of Japan (HVJ).[120] This agent was recovered from mice that had been inoculated with postmortem lung tissue of infants with pneumonia (some confusion may have existed, as mouse Sendai virus essentially does not infect humans). The first PIV from human sources was recovered several years later by Chanock[36] from infants with croup, and thus it became known as the croup-associated (CA) virus. Subsequently, three additional hPIVs that were distinct antigenically were isolated from children with acute respiratory illness.[38,105] In contrast to the CA virus, which was recognized by its ability to produce syncytia in tissue culture, the strains of the next two types of PIVs produced few or no cytopathic effects but were recognized by their ability to cause hemadsorption of guinea pig erythrocytes to infected tissue culture. These viruses thus were called hemadsorption type 1 (HA-1) and hemadsorption type 2 (HA-2) viruses.

Once the similarity of the familial characteristics of the CA virus to those of the other three viruses was recognized, the viruses were renamed the hPIVs, type 1 (HA-2), type 2 (CA), and type 3 (HA-1).[6] The fourth hPIV, discovered subsequent to this reclassification, is without a sobriquet and simply is termed hPIV-4, with two subtypes, A and B. The first type 4 strain was recovered in monkey kidney cell culture from a college student afflicted with a common cold.[105]

Several animal species appear to be natural hosts to the PIVs (see Table 179.1), with the exception of hPIV-4, which has been found only in humans. In animals, PIVs may be important pathogens. Bovine PIV (bPIV), similar to hPIV-3, often in combination with infection by *Pasteurella* organisms, causes an illness of considerable morbidity and cost in cattle termed *shipping fever.* Naturally acquired antibodies to the PIVs are found not only in cows but also in rodents, monkeys, rabbits, and other mammals. Various rodents, along with ferrets, dogs, and lambs, have been used for experimental infection.[208] The virus previously named *equine Morbillivirus* has been demonstrated to be in the Paramyxoviridae family and named *Hendra virus.* This virus, which causes lethal illness in horses, was recognized to cause illness in humans also. Individuals in close contact with horses in Australia contracted the virus, and two died.[162] Subsequently, in 1998, an outbreak of severe, often fatal encephalitis occurred in Malaysia and Singapore in individuals who had close contact with pigs.[43,72] The agent of this outbreak, Nipah virus, is phenotypically and antigenically similar to Hendra virus (80% genomic homology).

CHARACTERIZATION OF PARAINFLUENZA VIRUSES

Classification and Structure

The five hPIVs, hPIV serotypes 1, 2, 3, 4A, and 4B, are members of the Paramyxoviridae family, belonging to the *Respirovirus* and *Rubulavirus* genera (Fig. 179.1). The Paramyxoviridae family also includes other human viral pathogens transmitted via the respiratory route, such as RSV, measles, mumps, and metapneumovirus. The PIVs are distinguishable from the orthomyxoviruses (i.e., influenza viruses) in their size, nucleocapsid structure, antigenic composition, and laboratory growth characteristics.

hPIVs are nonsegmented, single-stranded, negative-sense, enveloped RNA viruses appearing as pleomorphic particles of medium size, with an average diameter of 150 to 200 nm.[111,195] The genomes of all the hPIVs, consisting of an average of approximately 15,000 nucleotides, code for at least six structural proteins (3′-N-P-M-F-HN-L-5′) and one or more nonstructural proteins (C, V, D) (Fig. 179.2). The viral ribonucleoprotein (RNP) is the viral RNA, tightly encapsulated by the nucleoprotein (NP). It is surrounded by the envelope, derived from the

TABLE 179.1 Parainfluenza Viruses

Parainfluenza Virus Type/ Related Animal Virus	Natural Host	Experimental Infection	Preferred Tissue Culture for Initial Isolation	CYTOPATHIC EFFECT	
				Initial Isolation	Passage
Parainfluenza type 1, hemadsorption type 2 (HA-2)	Human, guinea pig, rabbit, monkey, marmoset	Hamster, ferret	Monkey kidney, human diploid, human embryonic kidney	±	Rounding, cell destruction
Sendai, hemagglutinating virus of Japan (HVJ)	Mouse, pig				
Parainfluenza type 2	Human, monkey, rabbit, guinea pig	Hamster, dog	Monkey kidney, human embryonic kidney	+ (syncytial on monkey and human cells)	Syncytial, "Swiss cheese"
Simian virus 5 (SV 5)	Monkey				
Simian virus 41 (SV 41)	Monkey				
Parainfluenza type 3, hemadsorption type 1 (HA-1)	Human, guinea pig, monkey	Hamster, ferret, cotton rat, mouse, lamb	Monkey kidney, human embryonic kidney	±	In monkey cells: elongated, detachment of cell sheet In human cells: syncytial
Shipping fever (SF-4) Parainfluenza type 4	Cow, human	Hamster, guinea pig	Monkey kidney	±	Rounding granular, vacuolated

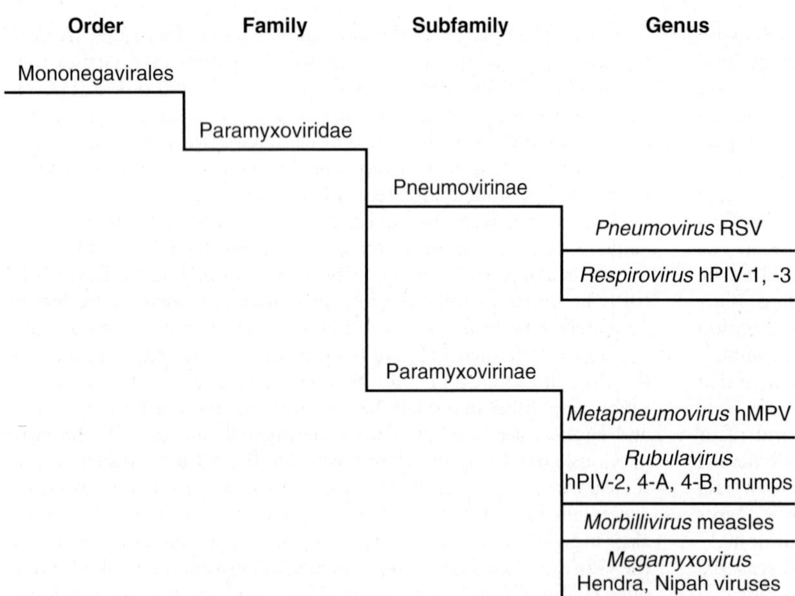

FIG. 179.1 Classification of parainfluenza viruses that cause human infection.

host cell, which is studded with spikes of surface glycoproteins, the hemagglutinin-neuraminidase (HN) and fusion (F) proteins, which are the major protective antigens. The large polymerase (L) protein and the phosphorylated nucleocapsid-associated (P) protein also form clusters within the nucleocapsid structure. The sixth structural protein is the nonglycosylated matrix (M) protein, located between the nucleocapsid and the envelope.

Replication and assembly of the virus occur solely in the cytoplasm of the host cell.[111,197] The NP, along with the P and L proteins, is responsible for the primary transcription that occurs sequentially, beginning from the 3′ end of the genome, producing predominately nonoverlapping subgenomic messenger RNAs from which the viral proteins are translated. The genome also is replicated from the formation of a full-length antigenome with positive-sense RNA. The NP and the genomic RNA make up the helical structure, and with the subsequent addition of the P and L protein complexes, the nucleocapsid is formed. The envelope proteins are assembled at the cell surface. The M protein is the smallest of the major structural proteins and is the most abundant of the virion's proteins. The M protein facilitates the interaction between the nucleocapsid and the surface glycoprotein by the attachment and insertion of the surface glycoproteins to the host cell and recruitment of the completed NP to the budding site of new virions, which are released from the cell surface by evagination of the plasma membrane. Like the M protein of RSV and paramyxoviruses, the PIV M is responsible for reassembly of viral proteins newly synthesized in the infected cell.[222]

The HN protein is a dimer of two polypeptide portions held together by a disulfide link in the hydrophilic region and at the bases by hydrophobic bonds. The HN is the major immunogenic and type-specific determinant. It is important in multiple viral functions, including mediating the attachment of the virus to the host cell by binding to sialic acid (*N*-acetylneuraminic acid), a terminal saccharide receptor present on the cell glycans. The hemagglutination component of the HN protein mediates the hemagglutination of mammalian erythrocytes. The neuraminidase component of the HN protein functions during late infection to release progeny virions by dislodging the cellular bond by cleaving the sialic acid residues and prevents reattachment of the viral particles to the cell surface.

The F protein effects entry of virus by fusing the host and viral cellular membranes. Once adsorption of the virus occurs, the F protein precursor, F0, is cleaved by host proteases into the active F1 and F2 protein fragments, which mediate penetration of the virus into the cell, with subsequent fusion of the viral and cell membranes and hemolysis. The N-terminal residues of the F1 protein (the fusion peptide) promote the penetration and fusion of the virus with the cellular membrane. In

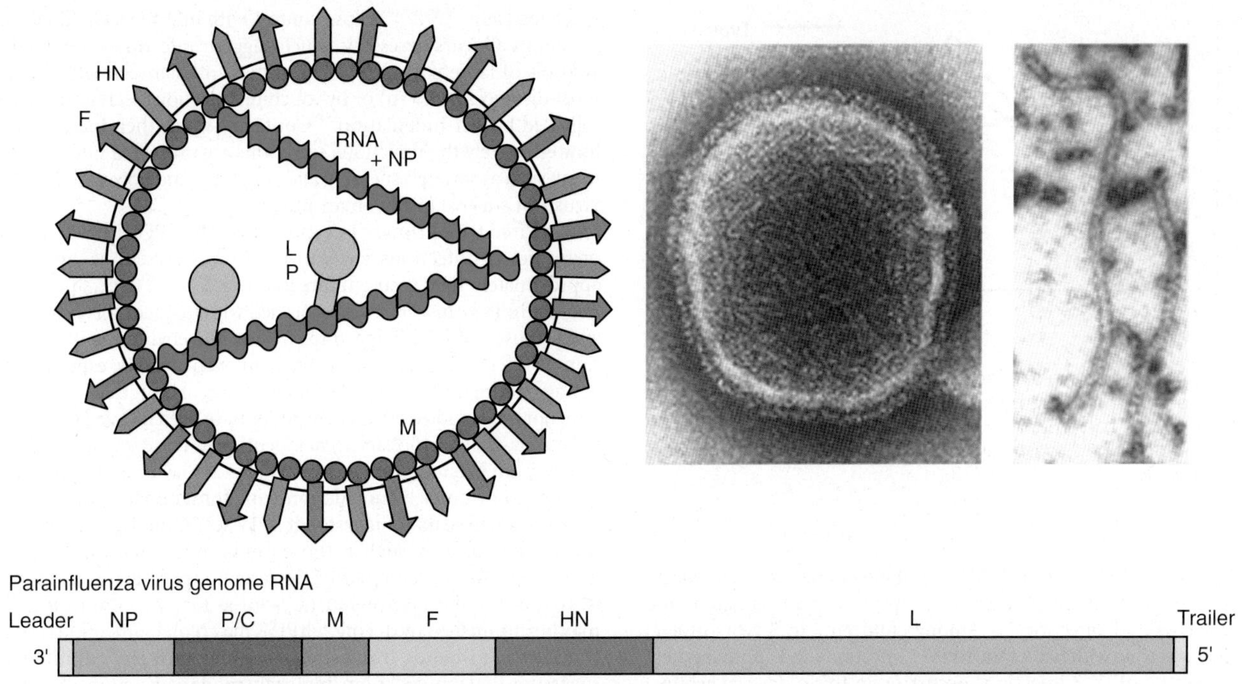

FIG. 179.2 Structure of parainfluenza virus (Sendai virus, *top left*) and its genomic RNA *(bottom)*. Electron micrograph of Sendai virus *(top middle)* and its helical nucleocapsid *(top right)*. (From Takimoto T. Parainfluenza viruses. In: Harper D, editor. *Encyclopedia of Life Sciences*. Chichester, UK: John Wiley & Sons; 2006:678-684.)

contrast to the foregoing proteins, the nonstructural C, V, and D proteins are not encoded by all the hPIVs but are produced variably by the different hPIV types and appear to have roles in transcription, replication, production, and pathogenicity of the virions. At least with hPIV-3, the C protein has been shown to inhibit viral transcription.[50,89,111,134] Recent structural studies led to a better understanding of the various mechanisms by which hPIVs and other Paramyxovirinae attachment glycoproteins use cell-surface receptors to facilitate viral entry[26] and form particles that assemble and bud from the cellular membranes.[86]

hPIVs share common antigens but also may be differentiated into two antigenic groups. hPIV-1 and hPIV-3 are within the Paramyxovirinae genus *Respirovirus*, and hPIV-2 and hPIV-4A and hPIV-4B are within the Paramyxovirinae genus *Rubulavirus*[111] (see Fig. 179.1). Their common antigenicity is illustrated by serologic heterotypic antibody responses to infection with hPIV-1, hPIV-2, and hPIV-3 and mumps viruses. Although the hPIVs do not undergo major antigenic alterations in their surface antigens similar to influenza virus, genetic and antigenic variations within all four types have been detected, and their evolution can be determined by analyses of strains obtained over time.[89,111,220]

Isolation and Identification

The hPIVs are inactivated rapidly by acid at a pH of 3.0 and by exposure to lipid solvents, such as ether and chloroform, which destroy the envelope of the virus. They also are relatively labile to temperatures higher than 37°C (98.6°F).[52,53] Media containing protein, however, tend to protect against loss of infectivity when the virus is exposed to heat and when it is frozen at −70°C (−94°F).[52,98]

Isolation of the hPIVs occurs in permissive cell cultures after an incubation period of 3 to 7 days at 35° to 37°C (95° to 98.6°F). The preferred cell cultures for the isolation of the hPIVs are primary or continuous monkey kidney cells, such as LLC-MK and human embryonic kidney cells, along with a continuous line of mucoepidermoid human lung carcinoma cells, NCI-H292.[63,89,111] The production and characteristic type of cytopathic effect in tissue culture vary according to the hPIV strain (see Table 179.1).[166] hPIV-1 and hPIV-3 on initial isolation are unlikely to demonstrate distinctive cytopathic effects, but, depending on the cell line, they may on passage. hPIV-4 is the most difficult hPIV to grow and identify in tissue culture because the cytopathic effect is not evident, and 2 to 4 weeks may be required before identification by hemadsorption is possible. Identification of hPIVs in tissue culture traditionally has relied on the ability of the hPIVs to hemadsorb erythrocytes, most commonly guinea pig, human group O, or chicken erythrocytes, at 4°C or 25°C (39.2°F or 77°F). However, the sensitivity of this method is variable, especially for the rubulaviruses hPIV2 and hPIV4.[89]

EPIDEMIOLOGY

Geographic Distribution

The ubiquitous nature of the hPIVs has been illustrated among diverse populations, in many parts of the world, and in differing climates.[68,139,144,156,193,211] Despite these wide variations, experience with the hPIVs is similar in most countries.

Prevalence and Age at Infection

The frequency and impact of hPIV infections are greatest among preschool-aged children and are estimated to account for approximately one third of the lower respiratory tract infections in this age group.[68,89,92,119,173] Among the hPIVs, the type most commonly isolated is hPIV3, which usually is acquired first, followed by hPIV-1 and hPIV-2 (Fig. 179.3).

Like RSV infection, hPIV-3 infection is a common occurrence during the first few months of life. Half to two thirds of infants have acquired infection by the time they reach 12 months of age.[68,144,148] Experience with hPIV-1 and hPIV-2 usually occurs later, most commonly during the preschool years.[68,69,144,173] In a study in Tecumseh, Michigan, the annual isolation rate of hPIV per 1000 person-years was 53.8 for children birth to 4 years of age, 14.3 for those 5 to 19 years of age, 3.9 for adults 20 to 39 years of age, and 2.3 for those 40 years of age or older.[143]

The frequency of hPIV infection among young children was well illustrated by the Houston Family Studies, in which infections were detected by both viral isolation and serology among children observed from birth.[68,69] By the time they reached 2 years of age, 92% of the children had experienced at least one infection with hPIV-3 and 32% had been infected more than once. hPIV-3 is the most frequent cause of hospitalizations associated with hPIV infections. hPIV-1 and hPIV-2 are associated primarily with hospitalizations of children 2 to 6 years old. The age distribution of children with hPIV-1 and hPIV-3 viral infections cared for in private pediatric practices, however, may overlap substantially (see Fig. 179.3). Among outpatients in Rochester, New

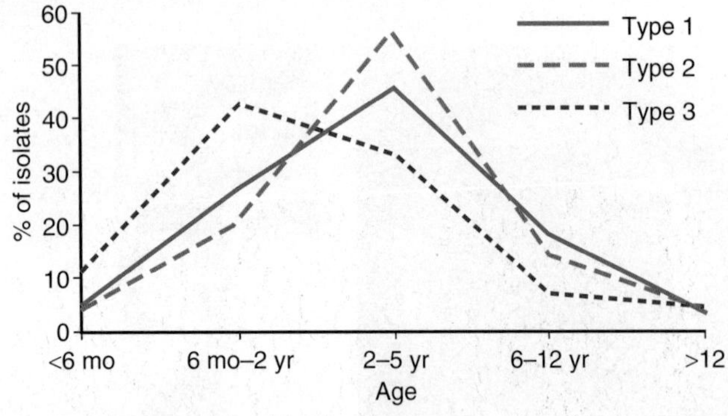

FIG. 179.3 Age distribution of infections with human parainfluenza virus types 1, 2, and 3 in outpatient children in Rochester, New York, from 1976–1992. (From Knott A, Long CE, Hall CB. Parainfluenza viral infections in pediatric outpatients: seasonal patterns and clinical characteristics. *Pediatr Infect Dis J.* 1994;13:269-273.)

York, approximately half of the hPIV-3 viral infections occurred among children younger than 24 months, in contrast to approximately one third of the hPIV-1 infections.[119] Among children 2 to 5 years of age, the reverse was true, with half of the hPIV-1 infections and approximately one third of the hPIV-3 infections occurring in this older age group.

Until recently, the epidemiology of hPIV-4 was less well described, in part because the clinical disease is mild and its recovery from cell cultures is inherently low, and thus its prevalence was underestimated.[122,123,178] More recent studies using sensitive reverse transcription polymerase chain reaction (RT-PCR) methods show that hPIV-4 infection is more frequent and sometimes can cause more serious illnesses than previously recognized.[31,60,210] Serologic studies have suggested that infection with hPIV-4 is particularly frequent during the preschool years, with between 50% and 90% of 5-year-old children possessing antibodies.[117,123,124]

Seasonal Occurrence

The seasonal patterns of the hPIVs vary according to location and year. In temperate regions, the incidence of parainfluenza viral infections appears to correlate with seasonal weather conditions, but in tropical regions it is less well defined. Different hPIV strains have different seasonal activities.[64] hPIV-1 tends to occur in the fall and commonly causes outbreaks of croup every other year.[68,114,173] The behavior of hPIV-2 has been more erratic.[68,89,119,173] During 20 years of surveillance in Rochester, New York, hPIV-2 appeared sporadically and in low numbers of cases, usually at the end of the fall outbreaks of hPIV-1 in the odd-numbered years.[80,119] hPIV-3 may be present in a community in case numbers for many months, but swells of more epidemic activity occur in the spring to fall.[68,80,119] During long-term surveillance, approximately 75% of hPIV-3 isolates were recovered in the spring and summer and most of the remainder were obtained in the autumns of the even-numbered years, when hPIV-1 was absent.[119] hPIV-4 usually occurs during late fall and winter in temperate countries,[123,124] but in China it is more prevalent during the spring and summer.[174] Studies from a more diverse geographic range are needed to better understand the global seasonal patterns of hPIV-4.

PATHOGENESIS

Transmission

Experimental studies using Sendai viruses have shown that even a low inoculum (70 plaque-forming units) to the upper respiratory tract resulted in robust growth and efficient contact transmission.[29] Of note, the efficiency and timing of transmission were independent of clinical symptoms and severity, which is consistent with data from animal models and with the epidemiology of hPIV outbreaks.[80,89] Furthermore, more severe infection involving the lower respiratory tract was a poor predictor of transmission.[29] Several clinical and experimental observations also have indicated that the hPIVs are able to spread readily and effectively.[7,47,84,107,148] Close contact with infected individuals or their secretions appears necessary, which suggests infection is spread through aerosols of large particles (>10 μm mass median diameter) that travel short distances (<0.9 m) or by touching infectious secretions on fomites followed by self-inoculation.[81] Contagiousness, therefore, is related to how effectively the infectious secretions are propelled into the environment, such as through sneezing and coughing, and how well the infectious virus can survive in the environment.[27]

Children with primary infection caused by hPIV-1 have considerable quantities of infectious virus in their nasal secretions, an average of approximately 1000 tissue culture infective doses ($TCID_{50}$) per milliliter.[84] Because hPIVs cause illnesses associated with frequent sneezing, coughing, and profuse nasal discharge, transmission and environmental contamination of infectious secretions is likely to occur readily, especially among young children. Although the routes of inoculation that occur naturally have not been studied adequately, adults have been infected experimentally by intranasal and oropharyngeal inoculation. The eye as a site of inoculation has not been examined similarly, but it may be an important portal of infection from self-inoculation with contaminated hands.

Experimental data suggest that hPIV secretions survive well on hard, nonporous surfaces, such as those found in hospitals, workplaces, and homes. The hPIVs remain infectious on nonporous surfaces for as long as 10 hours and on porous surfaces for as long as 4 hours, but survival may be diminished by drying.[27] hPIVs may remain infectious after being transferred to hands from environmental surfaces, a finding further suggesting that fomites are an important mode of dissemination. A curious conundrum is the survival and persistence of hPIV-1 and hPIV-3 infections among a group of individuals isolated in the frigid environs of the South Pole for 8.5 months.[147,161] Despite no outside contacts, infection with hPIV-1 and hPIV-3 occurred repetitively in the quarantined individuals. This phenomenon raised the possibility that persistent infection may be engendered not only in tissue culture but also in humans under such circumstances as extreme environmental conditions.

Pathology

Inoculation of the hPIVs into the upper respiratory tract results in infection of the nasal epithelium and nasopharynx and the appearance of clinical signs after an incubation period of 2 to 4 days. The hPIVs appear to replicate preferentially in the superficial ciliated epithelial cells lining the airways of the upper and lower respiratory tract. The factors determining the tropism and severity of the viral infection are incompletely understood. Such factors may include host genetics, age, and immunity; the protease activity of various tissues; and virus-specific determinants, such as the cleavage phenotype of the F_0 protein.[111,145]

The magnitude of viral replication appears important in the pathogenesis, as evidenced by the correlation of viral loads with severity of disease.[24,78,81] This has been confirmed by the development of live attenuated PIV vaccines using reverse genetics, which demonstrated precise viral mutations correlated with clinical attenuation.[18,55,108,155] Viral shedding is most abundant and prolonged in young children with primary and severe disease and may begin several days to a week before the onset of symptoms.[84] Children with hPIV-1 infections shed the virus for an average of 4 to 7 days, but may shed for as long as 12 days. With hPIV-3 infections, shedding tends to be longer, occasionally for 2 to 3 weeks, and in adults with chronic lung disease, shedding may be both prolonged and intermittent.[77,87]

The pathophysiology of hPIVs has been explored in animal models.[111,159,170] Inoculation of rodents with hPIV-3 produced histologically evident, but usually asymptomatic, interstitial pneumonitis or bronchiolitis. Ferrets also can be silently infected, but in newborn ferrets, PIV infection may be progressive and fatal.[142] Chimpanzees and several species of monkeys may be infected, but clinical manifestations generally are lacking, except with hPIV-3 infection of chimpanzees and African green monkeys.[201] Inoculation of hPIV-2 into the respiratory tract of a canine model produced clinical signs of cough and rhinitis accompanied by histologic changes in the airways.[111]

Pathologic studies of children with hPIV infections are limited. The few cases of confirmed hPIV infection examined have shown that in the young child with primary infection, inflammation, marked primarily by necrosis of the epithelium, is evident throughout the respiratory tract. The subglottic tissues in croup appear particularly involved, but with primary infection, the conducting airways at all levels and the alveoli may be affected.[37,224] Lung tissue samples from 200 young children who died from severe respiratory disease, which were examined for hPIV types 1, 2, and 3, RSV, influenza, and adenoviruses, showed no distinctive histologic changes that would allow identification of a specific virus.[54] hPIV was identified as the sole pathogen in 4% of the 200 samples tested and was the sole pathogen in 10% of virus-positive samples. Of the hPIVs identified, hPIV-3 was the most common serotype. hPIV infections caused bronchopneumonia and interstitial pneumonitis, which had infiltrates consisting mainly of mononuclear inflammatory cells in the bronchial lumen. Most of the children with bronchopneumonia had cellular necrosis and destruction of the bronchial pseudostratified columnar epithelium and diffuse alveolar damage. Immunohistochemical assessment on tissue microarray slides showed the virus in bronchial and bronchiole epithelial cells and in alveolar cells.[54]

IMMUNE RESPONSE: ROLE IN PATHOGENESIS AND PROTECTION

Innate immunity's role in controlling PIV infection and how it is elicited are of increasing interest, but data are currently of limited clarity. Better understanding of the pathogenesis of the innate response and its effect on the transition to adaptive immunity may lead to novel and better means of controlling the ubiquitous hPIV infections that occur during infancy and thereafter.

The innate antiviral responses to infection of viruses of the Paramyxoviridae family have been studied in experimental models. The response is elicited within the respiratory tract once the viral genome enters and replicates in the cytoplasm of the host cell and is characterized by the production of a cascade of immunomodulatory mediators, chemokines, and proinflammatory cytokines.[49,67,111,157,158] Toll-like receptors (TLRs), a class of pattern-recognition receptors, appear to be important early in the innate antiviral defense.[49,140] The products of viral replication trigger and activate specific TLRs that allow the binding of the virus to the host cell and the expression of the genes associated with the host immune response. TLRs may help mediate the immune response, both by their interaction with infected respiratory epithelial cells and by the induction of dendritic cell maturation that is integral in the subsequent development of adaptive immunity with the production of effector and memory T cell and B cells.[128,180] Although TLRs appear to have a pivotal place in innate antiviral defense, experimental evidence suggests that replicating infection of paramyxoviruses and other respiratory viruses may induce and enhance the innate immune response by other pathways that are not dependent on TLR-mediated signaling.[126,128,130]

The major components of the adaptive immune response to hPIV infection that play important and independent roles in primary infection and reinfection are both humoral and cellular. Rodent models using Sendai virus have shown that $CD8^+$ cytotoxic T lymphocytes are necessary for clearing the virus from the lung.[96,115] The viral antigen is carried by dendritic cells and macrophages to the draining lymph nodes, and activated cytotoxic T lymphocytes subsequently migrate to the site of pulmonary inflammation, resulting in viral clearance. The cellular immune response of memory T cells, which was established during the primary infection, persists in high titers in the spleen and rapidly responds to a repeated infection. In addition, virus-specific interferon (IFN)-γ–producing $CD4^+$ T cells have been shown to increase in the airways of infected mice during viral clearance, and IFN-α and IFN-β may be produced by experimental PIV infection.[74,83,111] IFN production also has been demonstrated during natural parainfluenza infection in young children.[87,219] However, some hPIVs may be able to evade this protective response by inhibiting IFN production through accessory proteins (C and V) expressed from the P gene.[25,74,111,116]

In contrast to infection with hPIV-1 and hPIV-2, the most serious illness caused by hPIV-3 infection usually occurs during the first year of life, when infants possess maternally derived specific antibody. This finding has raised the question of whether interactions of maternal antibody and virus may be detrimental.[139] In animal models, however, passively administered PIV antibody and monoclonal antibodies against the F and HN proteins appeared protective. Furthermore, the trials with an inactivated trivalent hPIV vaccine in the 1960s did not suggest a pathogenic role for antibody.[66] Although not protective, the vaccine was immunogenic and produced serum antibody in the vaccinees. Subsequently, the vaccinees did not experience augmented disease, as observed with the simultaneously tested formalin-inactivated RSV vaccine.

In animal models the specific antibody response is generated only during the later phase of the primary infection and does not play an important role in clearing the infection.[223] However, specific antibodies are protective against secondary challenge with the same parainfluenza virus. Clinical observations also show that the more severe infections involving the lower respiratory tract occur during initial infection in young, seronegative children, but recurrent infections usually are mild. Naturally acquired immunity, therefore, although not complete, and of variable durability, does provide protection against more severe disease.[69,111] Antigenic variation in the hPIVs is not sufficient to explain the lack of complete or durable immunity. The cause is more likely the waning of both humoral and cellular immune responses that occurs during the intervals between exposures to one of the hPIVs.

Serum hemagglutination-inhibition antibody and neutralizing antibody are detectable within 1 to 2 weeks.[114] Neutralizing antibody is directed primarily to epitopes on the HN and F proteins. The importance of neutralizing antibody in providing protection against infection of the lower respiratory tract, and to some extent of the upper respiratory tract, has been well established in animal models. Infants with primary hPIV infection usually produce a greater antibody response toward HN than F, and the response is relatively specific to the PIV serotype. With repeated infections, an anamnestic and broader humoral antibody response occurs, producing antibodies with cross reactivity against the different hPIV serotypes. In young children with primary hPIV-3 infection, the antibody response to the HN protein has been shown to be directed at multiple neutralizing antigenic sites.[202] The response to the F protein, whether with primary or recurrent infection, appears to be more variable in magnitude and restricted in terms of antigenic sites. The presence of maternal antibody, however, inhibits the infant's ability to produce specific humoral antibody.

Primary and secondary infections result in secretory immunoglobulin (Ig)G, IgM, and IgA antibodies that peak at 2 weeks after onset of symptoms.[49,219] Infection induces relatively incomplete protection in infants because of the lower titer of antibodies and the different IgG subclasses produced.[49] IgG_1 and IgG_3 antibodies are the predominant subclasses, contrary to the IgG_2 antibodies generated in older children and adults. Protection of the upper respiratory tract is mediated by secretory IgA and that of the lower tract by local IgG antibodies.[49] The transient nature of the induced secretory IgA antibodies may partially explain the common occurrence of reinfections throughout life.

Understanding the cell-mediated immune response to hPIV infection is important for vaccine development, and observations about the functions of $CD4^+$ and $CD8^+$ T cells in the recall response to PIV infection suggest that this system plays a major role in protection from primary and recurrent infections.[189,217] The increased severity and prolonged period of viral shedding in immunocompromised hosts, such as those receiving organ transplants, indicate the importance of intact cellular immunity in the control of disease and recovery from hPIV infection.[39,58,203]

CLINICAL MANIFESTATIONS

Primary Infection

The types of illnesses caused by hPIV infections have characteristic associations with the age of the child, the season, and the hPIV serotype (see Figs. 179.3 and 179.4).[69,71,100,119,124,173,211,218] Most primary infections are symptomatic, and many affect the tracheobronchial and lower respiratory tract. Of the primary infections that involve only the upper respiratory tract, fever and laryngeal or tracheal signs are common occurrences. Even an influenza-like illness with sudden onset of high fever, chills, cough, headache, myalgia, or fatigue has been reported to occur with hPIV infection.[168,184] Reinfections occur frequently at all ages and usually are mild and limited to the upper respiratory tract, or sometimes they are asymptomatic.[69]

The hPIVs cause a greater proportion of acute respiratory tract illnesses among outpatients than among hospitalized children.[119,124] Of

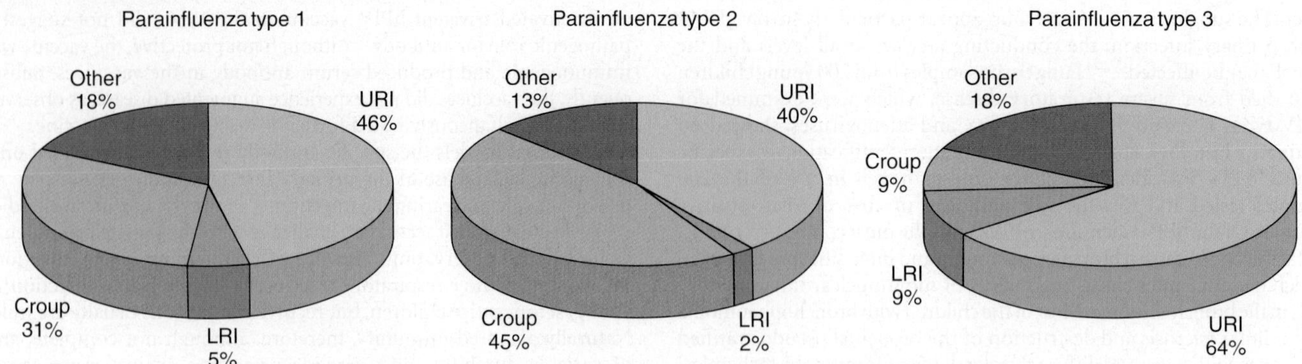

FIG. 179.4 Clinical manifestations of parainfluenza virus infections according to serotype in pediatric outpatients in Rochester, New York (1976–92). *LRI,* Lower respiratory tract infection other than croup; *URI,* upper respiratory tract infection (including otitis, colds, and pharyngitis). (From Knott A, Long CE, Hall CB. Parainfluenza viral infections in pediatric outpatients: seasonal patterns and clinical characteristics. *Pediatr Infect Dis J.* 1994;13:269-273.)

all viral respiratory illnesses examined in a pediatric practice, the hPIVs caused approximately two thirds of the croup cases, one fourth of the tracheobronchitis cases, and approximately half of the upper respiratory tract illnesses, including colds, laryngitis, pharyngitis, and otitis media.

hPIV infections account for almost 7% of all hospitalizations for respiratory illnesses with or without fever among children younger than 5 years of age.[211] The proportion of children with hPIV infection who require hospitalization, mainly those with croup, has markedly diminished in recent years, primarily because of better outpatient management and therapy of croup (see discussion of management and therapy).[185,218] Currently, most children hospitalized with hPIV infections are infants with pneumonia and bronchiolitis from hPIV-3, who are most likely to be admitted during the spring. hPIV infections may cause 11% of admissions for virus-induced asthma attacks; fatalities are uncommon, but may occur.[4] Pneumonia has been described with hPIV infections in previously healthy adults, such as among military recruits, but has been considered to be uncommon in normal, healthy populations of adults and school-aged children.[59,212] However, hPIV types 1 through 3 account for 4% to 6% of community-acquired pneumonias among adolescents and adults.[171] As many as 20% of pneumonias occurring in children in lower socioeconomic circumstances are caused by hPIV.[102] In contrast, hPIV infections in children are asymptomatic in less than 2.2% of cases.[97]

The onset of the typical primary hPIV infection generally is acute and associated with mild fever and upper respiratory tract signs of the common cold, such as rhinitis, sore throat, and cough. Laryngeal involvement manifesting as hoarseness is apt to be more prominent than with other viruses that commonly produce colds in young children. After 3 to 4 days, these upper respiratory tract symptoms may progress, primarily in infants with hPIV-3 infection, to involve the lower respiratory tract. The characteristic manifestations of pneumonia or bronchiolitis, including dyspnea, crackles, wheezing, and hyperaeration, follow. Children with hPIV-1 or hPIV-2 infection, who usually are 2 years of age or older, also have acute onset of fever and upper respiratory tract signs, but if the infection progresses in this age group, it is more likely to evolve into croup. Children with hPIV-1 infections who were seen in a private pediatric practice during a community outbreak of hPIV-1 predominantly had fever, upper respiratory tract signs, and tracheobronchial or tracheolaryngeal signs of croup.[84]

In children with croup, upper respiratory tract illness is generally present for 2 to 3 days before the patient abruptly (and usually at night) develops markedly increased work of breathing. The classical "croup triad" (barking cough, stridor, and laryngitis) distinguishes croup from other illnesses. Patients may also exhibit nasal flaring, retractions of the chest wall, and dyspnea.[192] The course of croup varies, with lessening in the intensity of the stridor and dyspnea during the day, with return of symptoms (usually of lesser severity) in the ensuing evenings. The acute symptoms usually last for 3 to 4 days, although cough may continue for longer.[23] Fewer than 10% of children with croup have hypoxemia from viral involvement of the lung parenchyma, which, although important in management, may not be recognized because of the focus on the apparent major site of inflammation, the subglottic area. Because obstruction occurs in the subglottic area, marked CO_2 retention may occur in the absence of significant hypoxia. The most reliable findings to assess illness severity are the severity of stridor and the degree of retractions.[35,40] Very few patients need intubation in the era of high-dose dexamethasone therapy, and the mortality is low.[177] Recurrent (spasmodic) croup usually occurs without fever or other respiratory tract symptoms. It has a viral etiology similar to that of acute laryngotracheobronchitis,[209] but allergic reactions or gastroesophageal reflux may cause a somewhat similar syndrome.[40]

Otitis media may complicate hPIV upper respiratory tract infection among young infants and older children.[42,88,119,146,172,213] hPIVs are commonly isolated from children with and without a history of otitis media, and thus their role in acute and recurrent otitis media is unclear. However, of the otitis media cases that have been associated with hPIV, the serotypes most frequently identified were hPIV-1 and hPIV-3. hPIVs have also been detected in middle ear aspirates as the sole agent or with a bacterial agent, suggesting that hPIVs may play both primary and secondary roles in predisposing children to middle ear infection.

The association of acute hPIV infection with a nonrespiratory illness or the isolation of hPIV from sites other than the respiratory tract occurs rarely. Case reports have associated hPIV infections with a variety of diseases, including adult respiratory distress syndrome, pertussis-like disease, parotitis, myopericarditis, and diseases of the central nervous system.[9,50,95,101,121,206,215] Anecdotal reports also have associated hPIV infection with collagen vascular diseases and sporadic severe hepatitis, characterized histologically by syncytial giant hepatocytes.[164,165]

The clinical manifestations associated with hPIV-4 are less well described, which may be explained partially by the technical difficulty of isolating hPIV-4.[31,60,93,123,127,210] Most have been associated with a mild, usually afebrile upper respiratory tract infection, but more severe disease and lower respiratory tract illness also have been reported.[127]

Reinfection

Immunity to PIV infection is transient and incomplete; therefore, reinfections commonly develop among healthy older children and adults. hPIV reinfections usually are mild, with symptoms of the common cold. In adults, hPIV-1, hPIV-2, and hPIV-3 cause approximately 2% to 5% of the upper respiratory tract infections, but one fifth or more of these infections may be asymptomatic.[24,93] Of those with clinical illness, approximately 30% to 92% develop fever, which is often associated with malaise, sore throat, and cough. Rhinorrhea occurs in fewer than 25% of infections among adults and usually less among children.

hPIV infection may cause more severe disease in elderly persons and also may exacerbate symptoms in both children and adults with chronic lung disease, including chronic bronchitis, asthma, and cystic fibrosis.[46,70,106,153,199,200]

Infection in Immunocompromised Patients

As demonstrated by multiple reports of outbreaks of hPIV infections occurring on transplant units, children and adults with compromised immunity, especially those with deficient cellular immunity, are at high risk for development of severe, and sometimes fatal, hPIV disease.[22,39,58,125-137,167,203,205] Some of these hPIV outbreaks are not associated with a concurrent increase in hPIV infections in the community, which suggests that many hPIV infections are nosocomial.[125,152] Most of the hPIV infections occur more than 1 year after transplantation. Close to half of the hPIV infections involve the lower respiratory tract, and approximately 15% to 40% of these infections are fatal.[15,204] Improved survival may accompany better supportive care, and better screening for hPIV infection.[196] In some studies, hPIV infection is as common as RSV infection in causing pneumonia in these patients.[32] Corticosteroid administration for graft-versus-host disease (GVHD) increases the risk for developing lower respiratory tract infection.[151] Recipients of nonmyeloablative conditioning regimens appear to have a lower risk for developing lower respiratory tract disease.[182]

Very high viral loads have been found in bone marrow transplant patients with pneumonia,[32] and the duration of shedding of hPIV is prolonged. These two features significantly augment the risk for an outbreak of infection among patients and personnel in transplant units. Furthermore, hPIV infection often is not considered among the opportunistic infections that plague these patients, and the diagnosis is confounded by the observation that hPIV infection may lead to bacterial and fungal pneumonia.[56,151] In addition, the sensitivity of detecting the virus in specimens from the upper respiratory tract is poor.

The incidence of hPIV infections among lung transplant recipients has been estimated to be 1.6% to 11.9% and is most often associated with hPIV-3.[203,205] Among these patients the initial manifestations of hPIV infections are usually nondistinctive upper respiratory tract symptoms, such as cough and sore throat, and, less commonly, rhinorrhea and fever.[203] Progression to involvement of the lower respiratory tract or rejection of the transplant follows in approximately 10% to 70% of cases, depending on multiple host factors, including being a child, presence of GVHD, degree of immunosuppression, and corticosteroid or antilymphocyte therapy.[99,198] The risk for developing lower airway disease in transplant recipients is further enhanced because of mechanical factors present in transplanted lungs and because of altered or absent mucosal immunity.[203] The bronchus-associated lymphoid tissue in the lung, which is integral to the protective immune response against pulmonary infections, is injured during transplantation, thus resulting in diminished control and clearance of the viral infection.

Therefore, the high rate of symptomatic infection (95%) with hPIV infections among lung transplant recipients is not surprising.[203] Cough has been reported as present in 70%, dyspnea in 66%, fever in 16%, and lower respiratory tract disease, which is diagnosed as viral pneumonia, in 16%. hPIV and other viral infections may lead not only to graft rejection but also to severe long-term complications. Thirty-two percent of lung transplant recipients have developed acute bronchiolitis obliterans, which has occurred an average of 6 months (range, 1 to 14 months) after their hPIV infection.[58,203,204] hPIV infection occasionally has been reported also to be complicated by pancytopenia, Guillain-Barré syndrome, parotitis, and acute disseminated encephalitis.[10,121,176]

Among children with immunodeficiency syndromes who have diminished cellular immunity, especially children with severe combined immunodeficiency syndrome, hPIV has been notably severe and frequently fatal.[104] Complicated disease and lower respiratory tract involvement are observed less frequently with hPIV infection among children with less severely compromised cellular immunity, such as patients with human immunodeficiency virus (HIV) infection.[109,132,141] The clinical severity of hPIV infection among patients with HIV infection is variable, but even among those with mild disease, the shedding of hPIV usually is prolonged and may persist beyond the period of clinical symptoms.

DIAGNOSIS

The diagnosis of hPIV infections may be surmised on clinical and epidemiologic grounds, such as the patient's age, the type of illness, and the seasonal patterns of hPIV in the community. However, the nonspecific clinical presentation of many other viral respiratory infections makes the specific laboratory diagnosis of hPIV necessary. During the acute phase of the illness, hPIV may be diagnosed in specimens of nasal secretions by the following methods:

1. Detection of viral RNA using RT-PCR in single or multiplex assays.[2,16,214] RT-PCR has markedly increased the detection and specific identification of the hPIVs in patient specimens.[28,89,91,211] RT-PCR assays can detect a single respiratory virus or multiple viruses simultaneously and provide sensitive, specific, and rapidly available identification of hPIVs from clinical specimens.[30,160,214,]
2. Isolation of the virus by culture or enhanced by shell viral culture techniques.[166]
3. Serologic assays during the patient's convalescence (see discussion of isolation and identification).

Numerous serologic assays exist, including complement fixation, hemagglutination-inhibition, hemadsorption inhibition, neutralizing, enzyme immunoassay, and immunofluorescence.[61,90] However, serologic diagnosis is confounded by heterotypic antibody responses (see discussion of immune response). During reinfection, both homotypic and heterotypic antibody rises may occur, or sometimes little antibody response is detected, despite shedding of the virus from the nasopharynx.[111] Less is known about the antibody response to hPIV-4 infection, but during primary infection, a homotypic response usually occurs.[117] Detection of specific IgM antibodies, which usually persist for 2 to 11 weeks after infection, has been of limited success as a diagnostic technique.[207]

PCR-based methods should be the preferred diagnostic tool for hPIV infection over culture or serologic assays because they have a sensitivity of 95% to 100% and a specificity of 97% to 100% in contrast to viral isolation.[8,89] Although most hPIV infections do not require specific diagnosis, among more severely ill and hospitalized patients the diagnosis using these newer molecular techniques, if rapidly available, offers several advantages in addition to their high sensitivity and specificity. Among these are giving the health care provider a known specific viral diagnosis, diminished use of unnecessary antibiotics, and the implementation of effective infection control procedures, potentially reducing the risk for nosocomial infection with a different virus from patients with the same clinical presentation.

Differential Diagnosis

Most of the other major respiratory viral pathogens can mimic the illnesses produced by hPIV infections. Clinical differentiation rarely is possible. More helpful are such epidemiologic clues as the differing seasonal patterns and age-related attack rates of the common viral agents of respiratory illnesses in children.[82]

Croup from hPIVs or any other virus must be differentiated from bacterial tracheitis, retropharyngeal abscess, and epiglottitis, which have rapidly progressive courses and a potentially fatal outcome. With the widespread use of the *Haemophilus influenzae* type b vaccine, epiglottitis now occurs very rarely. Reports of epiglottitis have not been published in the past 10 years. Retropharyngeal abscess is also less common because of the widespread use of antibiotics for upper respiratory tract infections. However, bacterial tracheitis has been occasionally observed, usually as a complication of refractory hPIV croup, in which the patient is being intubated for respiratory failure.[94]

Children with croup associated with hPIV infection usually have peripheral white blood cell counts that are normal or initially slightly elevated, with a mild left shift. In contrast, among children with stridor from epiglottitis, retropharyngeal abscess, or bacterial tracheitis, the left shift usually is marked.

In countries that continue to have diphtheria, laryngeal diphtheria may be a consideration in an unimmunized child. However, laryngeal diphtheria usually is gradual in onset and manifests with characteristic membranous pharyngitis. Stridor and other signs of croup also may be present in children with congenital or acquired conditions that obstruct the laryngeal airflow, such as aspiration of a foreign body, tracheomalacia, stenosis, and acute angioneurotic edema.

MANAGEMENT AND THERAPY

Most hPIV infections are self-limited and require no treatment. Specific therapy currently is not available for hPIV infections. In vitro studies have shown that ribavirin inhibits hPIV, but clinical studies produced mixed results. A few small studies showed some benefit in controlling hPIV infections among a limited number of immunocompromised patients,[34,45,57,138,194] but larger studies have not shown such an effect, and the duration of viral shedding was not shortened.[56,151] Controlled trials, however, are lacking. Thus, until more data are available, aerosolized ribavirin currently should be considered only for high-risk patients with severe lower respiratory tract disease. Among potential therapies being explored are sialic acid inhibitors, such as those used for treating influenza, which inhibit hPIV F and HN activities.[2,76,150,169] Other therapeutic approaches include interference with viral attachment and replication with the use of inhibitors of protein and nucleic acid synthesis, synthetic peptides, and antivirals inhibiting *S*-adenosyl-L-homocysteine hydrolase[19,89,111,197] or protein kinase B (AKT), which is critical for viral replication.[65]

Management of croup in the home is primarily supportive.[218] The armamentarium used during the past century has been varied and usually anecdotal, ranging from cold night air to humidification or putting the child in a comfortable position. No such home therapies have proved beneficial. Simply holding the child may relax them, lessening the degree of dyspnea.

Children who are more severely affected require outpatient evaluation, usually in an emergency department. With the current management offered in emergency departments, few children's symptoms progress such that hospitalization is required.[48,185,218] Intravenous immunoglobulin (IVIG) is not recommended; a retrospective analysis of its administration did not find any benefit.[151] The current consensus and recommendations for the management of acute viral laryngotracheitis have afforded a more consistent beneficial outcome.[3,40,218] Administration of 0.05 mL/kg (maximum, 5 mL) nebulized 2.25% racemic epinephrine (a 1:1 mixture of D-and L-isomers of epinephrine) has been demonstrated to provide rapid relief for the airway obstruction. The relief from nebulized epinephrine is transient, usually lasting no longer than 2 to 3 hours; however, this is often long enough to allow for the onset of activity of corticosteroids. Patients who improve after receiving racemic epinephrine should be observed for at least 3 hours after the last racemic epinephrine dose, to be sure that illness does not return as the effect of the aerosol wears off. Furthermore, hypoxemia, if present, and the outcome are not affected by treatment with nebulized epinephrine.[188,218]

Administration of corticosteroids has become the cornerstone of management for the more severely affected child who fails to improve with the usual supportive care. Corticosteroids administered intramuscularly, intravenously, or orally have been shown to provide significant and lasting benefit on the clinical course and outcome, in contrast to placebo or other therapies, and also decreased the need for nebulized epinephrine.[3,5,179] Although studies have shown that any dexamethasone dose between 0.15 mg/kg and 0.6 mg/kg (with a maximum of 10 mg/day) will be effective in relieving the symptoms and diminishing the severity of disease and need for hospitalization,[44,103] the recommended dose most commonly used is a single dose of dexamethasone 0.6 mg/kg given intramuscularly or intravenously.[179,218] Prednisolone 1 mg/kg is less effective than dexamethasone 0.15 mg/kg, probably because of its shorter half-life (36 hours vs. 54 hours, respectively).[195] Although nebulized steroids (e.g., budesonide) have been shown to be effective, they are expensive and less effective than oral dexamethasone.[33] The treatment of croup is discussed more thoroughly in Chapter 18. Antibiotic therapy should be reserved for documented episodes of secondary bacterial tracheitis.

PROGNOSIS

Most previously healthy children recover from hPIV infections completely and without complication. Follow-up studies of normal children with hPIV infections support the generally good prognosis. Some children who have had croup have pulmonary function abnormalities detected subsequently, but proof that these abnormalities were caused by their hPIV infection is lacking.[79,129]

The potential for development of acute complications, morbidity, and mortality is related to the presence of a comorbid condition such as immunodeficiency and diseases that affect cardiopulmonary function, including congenital malformations and acquired conditions obstructing the airway.[218] Of children hospitalized with hPIV infections who were studied during a 4-year period, 35% had preexisting pulmonary or cardiac abnormalities, prematurity, or asthma.[87] In contrast to the children who previously were normal, the children with underlying conditions had significantly more severe disease and more complicated courses requiring longer hospitalization. Immunodeficient patients, as described previously, have particular difficulty in controlling and clearing hPIV infections; thus, these children have complicated, prolonged, and recurrent respiratory tract infections. Prolonged or persistent infection with hPIVs, especially with hPIV-3, has been noted to occur in some patients with chronic bronchitis, possibly related to the lack of a sufficient specific antibody response in the sputum.[77] The possibility that hPIV may cause central nervous system involvement has been suggested by the occasional detection of such viruses in the central nervous system in patients with previous transplantation, but there is little evidence for an hPIV encephalitis in otherwise healthy subjects.[10,176]

Short interfering RNA (si-RNAs) that bind to messenger RNA of the virus-infected host cell are logically attractive candidates for therapy of infections caused by hPIV and other viruses, but their use is largely theoretical at this time.[12]

PREVENTION

Infection control measures to prevent the spread of hPIV through direct contact with fomites or other infected objects are integral in preventing infection. Hand washing and droplet precautions should be implemented as soon as hPIV infection is suspected and continued throughout the period of shedding, which in immunocompromised patients may be for extended periods (>100 days).[56] Nonetheless, infection control measures may fail because many hPIV infections are mild, and prolonged asymptomatic shedding may occur among immunocompromised patients[163] and adults with chronic bronchitis.

For decades, attempts to prevent hPIV infections have focused on the development of effective vaccines. The current lack of a licensed vaccine for hPIV infections attests to the problematic nature of infection with hPIVs and of the response of the human host at different ages. Many of the hurdles encountered in the development of an effective vaccine for hPIV are similar to those for RSV. The vaccine, at least for hPIV-3, would have to be administered during the first few months of life when the infant's immunologic system is not fully developed[51,221] and when the potential inhibitory effect of passive maternal antibody exists. Furthermore, to elicit durable protection, the vaccine would have to produce an immunologic response superior to that derived from natural infection, because recurrent infections occur throughout life.

Hence, the goals of immunization for hPIVs, like those for RSV, currently may need to be modified toward prevention of more serious disease and attenuating disease associated with primary infection and reinfections by restricting viral replication. Because the greatest clinical and economic burdens have been estimated to occur with hPIV-3 infection among infants, compromised patients, and elderly individuals, many of the candidate vaccines have been aimed at providing protection against hPIV-3 infection.[5,55,149,197]

Initially formalin-inactivated, parenteral hPIV vaccines, along with formalin-inactivated vaccines for RSV, were developed and evaluated in clinical trials.[41,66,118,191] In general, these vaccines, whether monovalent, trivalent, or combined with other respiratory vaccines, were immunogenic, inducing a variable humoral and mucosal antibody response, but they were not protective.[41,66] In many cases the serum antibody titers were insufficient, and nasal neutralizing antibodies were not induced.[191]

Development of candidate vaccines currently focuses primarily on live-attenuated and subunit vaccines.[55,75,190] Live-attenuated vaccines, in contrast to inactivated or subunit vaccines, have the potential advantages of inducing immunity by more closely mimicking natural infection by eliciting both humoral and mucosal immunity and a longer duration of protection. Furthermore, because significant yearly antigenic change, as observed with the influenza viruses, does not occur with hPIVs, a single monovalent or polyvalent vaccine may suffice, although later booster doses may be required. The potential disadvantages of a live vaccine are more adverse or symptomatic reactions, the possible transmission of the vaccine virus, and insufficient genetic stability to prevent reversion to the more virulent virus from which it was derived.

Cold-passage hPIV-3 mutant strains derived from a wild-type hPIV-3 strain produced in cell culture (by 45 passages at low temperature; cold passages *[cp]*) were demonstrated to be stable and to grow well at the lower temperatures of the nasal passages, but not at the higher temperatures of the lower respiratory tract, and they were attenuated clinically.[55] The *cp*45 mutant strain was developed into a candidate hPIV-3 vaccine (hPIV-3 *cp*45) containing 20-point mutation with the desired characteristics of cold adaptation *(ca)*, temperature sensitivity *(ts)*, attenuation *(att)*, and genetic stability.[17,18,186,187] A second candidate hPIV-3 vaccine was developed from a closely related bovine hPIV-3 (bPIV-3). The protective surface glycoproteins, HN and F, of bPIV-3 and hPIV-3 share amino acid identities of 75% and 78%, respectively.[202] In contrast to hPIV, the bPIV-3 has restricted replication in humans and thus is attenuated. The hPIV-3 *cp*45 was evaluated in phase I and II clinical trials in adults, seropositive children, and seronegative infants as young as 1 month of age. In seropositive children and adults, the vaccines were not sufficiently immunogenic or protective.[108] In some trials of seronegative infants, the hPIV3 *cp*45 vaccine was too reactogenic and was associated with otitis media.[55,108] Nonetheless, the vaccine readily produced infection and was immunogenic. Most toddlers and infants developed both humoral IgG and IgA anti-HN antibody responses, and the presence of maternal antibodies did not affect vaccine virus replication in the upper airway. Low titers of the attenuated virus were shed for 2 to 3 weeks after vaccination. The observation that a higher percentage of infants shed the virus after receiving the second dose 3 months after the first dose (62%), in contrast to those receiving the second dose 1 month after the first dose (24%), suggests a rapid waning of protective immunity.[108] In a subsequent trial of hPIV3 *cp*45 vaccine involving seronegative children 6 to 18 months old, the vaccine was found to be well tolerated, safe, and immunogenic.[18] No significant difference was observed in frequency of side effects (including otitis media) between the vaccine and placebo. An attempt to combine the hPIV3 *cp*45 with live-attenuated RSV (*cpts* 248/404) found that replication of the attenuated RSV interfered with that of the attenuated hPIV-3.[17]

When a bovine PIV-3 (bPIV-3) vaccine was evaluated as a live-attenuated vaccine against hPIV-3, it was demonstrated to be safe and immunogenic against bPIV-3, but because of its antigenic differences from hPIV-3, it induced only a modest immune response against hPIV-3 in seronegative infants and children.[75,112]

The use of reverse genetics is particularly applicable and beneficial in advancing the development of hPIV vaccines because the molecular virology of the PIVs has been relatively well deciphered.[149] This technology has allowed the development of such PIV candidate vaccines as those produced by recovering infectious hPIV and bPIV from cDNA. The systematic introduction of desired mutations into the viral genome with a well-defined passage history and with minimal risk for biologic contamination resulted in recombinant and chimeric vaccines with more precise and promising profiles. In a phase I trial with the recombinant virus (9r) hPIV-3 *cp*45 in seronegative infants 6 to less than 12 months of age, the vaccine appeared safe, well tolerated, and immunogenic.[20] After three vaccine doses administered at 2-month intervals, 76.9% of the infants had over a fourfold increase in hemagglutination inhibition antibody. Shedding of the vaccine virus was restricted in titer and in duration after the second and third doses, suggesting that an immune response was elicited. The cDNA-derived virus was also shown to be comparable to previously observed results with the biologically derived hPIV-3 *cp*45 vaccine.[110] In an attempt to improve the immunogenicity, cDNA-derived chimeric human-bovine vaccines for PIV-3 were constructed by replacing the HN and F glycoproteins of bPIV-3 with those of hPIV-3, and substituting the N of hPIV-3 with that of bPIV-3.[11,85,111] The chimeric vaccine was evaluated in adults and in hPIV-3 seropositive and seronegative children. Although the vaccine's viral replication was highly restricted in both adults and seropositive children, it remained infectious in seronegative children, and antibody was produced after a single dose.[113] However, the titer was lower than that observed among children with natural hPIV-3 infection, suggesting that a series of vaccinations, such as three injections 2 months apart, may improve the antibody response.

The need to protect against both hPIV and RSV early in life led to further modifications of the chimeric rB/hPIV3 that also allowed the expression of the G and/or F proteins of RSV.[183] The vaccine, when administered to seropositive children 1 to 9 years of age, appeared to be safe, but with restricted replication, and was minimally immunogenic.[73] Further investigation among seronegative infants (6 to 24 months of age) showed that seroconversion occurred for RSV in 67% and for hPIV-3 in 100% of the infants.[21] Subunit vaccines containing HN and F proteins from hPIV-1 in hPIV-3 have not been encouraging, but the introduction of amino acid substitutions in various hPIV-1 genes was successful in creating an attenuated virus. A vaccine containing three attenuating elements that protected against hPIV-1 infection of both the upper and lower respiratory tract of African green monkeys[14] has been tested in seronegative children, but immunogenicity was limited.[131] Another Sendai-based hPIV1 vaccine has been only mildly immunogenic in 3- to 6-year-old children.[1] Although the need for a vaccine against hPIV-2 is less because of its lower prevalence and clinical significance in the first 6 months of life, several candidate hPIV-2 live-attenuated vaccines have been developed. Mutations in the L protein produced strains that were both temperature sensitive and attenuated. One of these mutant strains was found to be attenuated in an in vitro model of human ciliated airway epithelium and to provide significant protection against wild-type hPIV-2 challenge in African green monkeys.[154,181]

Multiple other approaches to develop candidate hPIV vaccines through recombinant DNA technology are being explored and include chimeric PIV vaccines with heterologous paramyxoviruses and with viruses for which concurrent immunization would be desirable, such as RSV and influenza.[13,133] Approaches combined with these creative techniques, such as novel adjuvants, immunomodulators, and vehicles for incorporation and administration of the vaccine, are evolving and may further enhance the protective immune response from PIV immunization.

NEW REFERENCES SINCE THE SEVENTH EDITION

1. Adderson E, Branum K, Sealy RE, et al. Safety and immunogenicity of an intranasal Sendai virus-based human parainfluenza virus type 1 vaccine in 3- to 6-year-old children. *Clin Vaccine Immunol.* 2015;22(3):298-303.
4. Amina NM, El Bashaa NR, El Rifala NM, et al. Viral causes of acute respiratory infection among Egyptian children hospitalized with severe asthma exacerbation. *J Egypt Public Health Assoc.* 2013;88:52-56.
12. Barik S, Lu P. Therapy of respiratory viral infections with intranasal sRNAs. *Methods Mol Biol.* 2015;1218:251-262.
96. Howard LM, Johnson M, Williams JV, et al. Respiratory viral dete4ctions during symptomatic and asymptomatic periods in young Andean children. *Pediatr Infect Dis J.* 2015;34(10):1074-1080.
104. Johnson AWBR, Osinusi K, Andrele WI, et al. Etiologic agents and outcome determinants of community-acquired pneumonia in urban children: a hospital-based study. *J Natl Med Assoc.* 2008;100(4):370-385.
130. Mackow N, Amaro-Carambol E, Liang B, et al. Attenuated human parainfluenza virus type 1 (HPIV-1) expressing the fusion glycoprotein of human respiratory syncytial virus (RSV) as a bivalent HPIV/RSV vaccine. *J Virol.* 2015;89(20):10319-10332.
159. Parker J, Fowler N, Walmsley ML, et al. Analytical sensitivity comparison between Singleplex real-time PCR and a Multiplex PCR platform for detecting respiratory viruses. *PLoS ONE.* 2015;10(11):e0143164.
170. Qu JX, Gu L, Pu ZH, et al. Viral etiology of community-acquired pneumonia among adolescents and adults with mild or moderate severity and its relation to age and severity. *BMC Infect Dis.* 2015;15:89-98.
195. Srinivasin A, Gu Z, Smith T, et al. Prospective detection of respiratory pathogens in symptomatic children with cancer. *Pediatr Infect Dis J.* 2013;32:e99-e104.
197. Tamaki K, Kinjo T, Aoyama H, et al. Fatal pneumonia and viremia due human parainfluenza virus type 1 in a patient with adult T-cell leukemia-lymphoma treated with mogamulizumab. *J Infect Chemother.* 2015;21(11):820-823.
221. Zhang G, Zhong Y, Qin Y, Chen M. Interaction of human parainfluenza virus type 3 nucleoprotein with matrix protein mediates internal viral protein assembly. *J Virol.* 2016;90(5):2306-2315.

The full reference list for this chapter is available at ExpertConsult.com.

180 Measles Virus

James D. Cherry • Debra Lugo

Measles virus is a singular agent that causes a relatively distinct, exanthematous disease characterized by fever, cough, coryza, conjunctivitis, an erythematous maculopapular confluent rash, and a pathognomonic enanthem. Clinical measles is an epidemic disease, the incidence of which in the United States was reduced by the use of attenuated vaccines from 315 reported cases per 100,000 persons in the prevaccine era to fewer than 1 per 100,000 persons in 1992.[86] At present, measles no longer is an endemic disease in the United States.[380] However, measles is still a major problem because of its worldwide prevalence, associated morbidity and mortality, and changing epidemiologic patterns in countries where vaccine use has been less than optimal.[78,80,173,379]

HISTORY

In antiquity, measles and smallpox frequently were confused with each other, as well as with other exanthematous diseases.[26,371] Major epidemics of both measles and smallpox occurred 1800 years ago in the Roman Empire and China.[48,319] The first written record of measles generally is credited to Rhazes, a 10th century Persian physician.[26,48,248,494,495] However, Rhazes quoted writers, including El Yahudi, a famous Hebrew physician, who lived 300 years earlier.[48] Rhazes identified measles as an entity distinct from smallpox.

During the Middle Ages in Europe, smallpox and measles continued to be confused. By the beginning of the 17th century, however, differentiation between the two diseases was relatively clear; death reports by London parish clerks in 1629 listed measles and smallpox separately.[494,495] Repeated epidemics of measles were described in the English medical literature during the 17th and 18th centuries.[248]

The first account of measles in America was given by John Hall, who described epidemic disease in Boston in the fall of 1657.[70] The next epidemic in colonial America was reported in 1687. During the next 150 years, the interval between epidemics in Boston gradually decreased from 30 years to approximately 3 years. Epidemics during the 17th and 18th centuries involved persons of all ages, including neonates; coincident with a reduction in the interval between epidemics was a reduction in the age-specific incidence of measles. The reduction in time between epidemics can be attributed to the increased incidence of importation of measles that occurred as more and faster ships crossed the Atlantic and the population density in North America gradually increased. By the turn of the 19th century, both Boston and Philadelphia had sufficient populations for measles to propagate itself.

The first recognition of the contagiousness of measles is unclear. Shakespeare in *Coriolanus* was aware of its human-to-human transmission.[494,495] Home,[219] in 1758, attempted to immunize against measles by applying a technique similar to the variolation used in smallpox.[399] In 1911, Goldberger and Anderson[180] produced clinical measles in monkeys by injecting filtered material from acute cases of human disease.

The classic epidemiologic study of measles is the account described by Panum[385] of the 1846 epidemic in the Faroe Islands. In this study, Panum confirmed that spread occurred solely through human-to-human contagion by the respiratory route, the incubation period was 14 days, and infection conveyed lifelong immunity.

The enanthem of measles, which is pathognomonic, was described carefully and presented by Koplik[267-269] in 1896, 1898, and 1899.[55] However, Koplik spots clearly were recognized specifically about a century earlier by John Quier, a physician in Jamaica,[55,178] as well as by Richard Hazeltine, a general practitioner in rural Maine.[70] Although Plotz[400] reported cultivation of measles virus in 1938 and Rake and Shaffer[405] noted similar findings in 1940, reliable tissue culture methods were not available until approximately 10 years later. In 1954, Enders and Peebles[142] isolated eight strains (from cases of measles) in human or simian renal cell cultures. These investigators also demonstrated the ability of convalescent-phase serum from a patient with measles to neutralize the viral cytopathogenic effect. The stage for vaccine development was set by recovery in tissue culture of the virus,[142] adaptation of viral growth in chicken embryos,[327] and, finally, cultivation of the virus in chicken embryo tissue culture cells.[250]

After extensive trials were conducted from 1958 through 1962, tissue culture–grown, inactivated ("killed"), and attenuated ("live") measles viral vaccines became available for general use in 1963.[100,247,274,275] In the United States, a nationwide immunization effort instituted in 1965 and 1966 led to a dramatic reduction in the incidence of epidemic measles for several years. Epidemic measles recurred in 1971, 1977, and 1989, but at overall levels less than those in the prevaccine era.[21,76,77,81,84,91,100,273] After initiation of the Childhood Immunization Initiative in 1977 and the Measles Elimination Program in 1978, the incidence of measles in the United States fell in 1981 to fewer than 1.5 cases per 100,000 population and remained at this low level until 1986.[21,82,83,90] In 1990, the rate was 11.2 cases per 100,000 population, which was the highest it had been since 1977. After 1990, a substantial decline in the incidence of measles occurred in the United States, to a low of 86 confirmed cases in 2000.[85]

PROPERTIES

Classification

Measles virus is a relatively large virus with helical capsid symmetry and an RNA genome.[36,144,145,192,283] It is a singular virus, but phylogenetically it is most closely related to rinderpest virus, a pathogen of cattle. Genetic relationships suggest both viruses also share common ancestry with canine distemper.[170,192] These agents, as well as peste des petits ruminants virus, dolphin morbillivirus, phocine distemper virus, and rinderpest virus, currently are included in the genus *Morbillivirus;* they are members of the Paramyxoviridae family.[283] Formation of intranuclear inclusion bodies differentiates *Morbillivirus* species from other Paramyxoviridae.[293,353] Measles virus differs from the other paramyxoviruses in that it does not possess specific neuraminidase activity and does not adsorb to neuraminic acid–containing cellular receptors.[339,362,394,484] Measles virus hemagglutinates, whereas the other members of its genus do not.

Physical Properties

Measles virus is a roughly spherical but pleomorphic virus that ranges from 100 to 300 nm in diameter.[36,144,145,192,353,371,484,485] The virion is composed of an outer lipoprotein envelope and an internal helical ribonucleocapsid. The virion contains eight proteins. The outer viral envelope is 10 to 22 nm thick, has short surface projections (peplomers), and contains three virus-coded proteins (F, H, and M).[104,339,371]

Fusion (F) protein is a dumbbell-shaped transmembrane peplomer that causes membrane fusion of the virus and host cell and enables penetration of the virus into the host cell. The presence of both the H protein and the F protein is required for fusion. Syncytia formation requires basolateral targeting of F and H proteins, overcoming the epithelial barrier and increasing cell-to-cell spread.[337]

Hemagglutinin (H) protein is the receptor binding and hemagglutinating protein and is a conical transmembrane peplomer. In infection, H protein reacts with a host cellular receptor and triggers major conformational changes in F protein, ultimately resulting in insertion of the F protein into target membrane. More than one F trimer may interact with each H tetramer.[398]

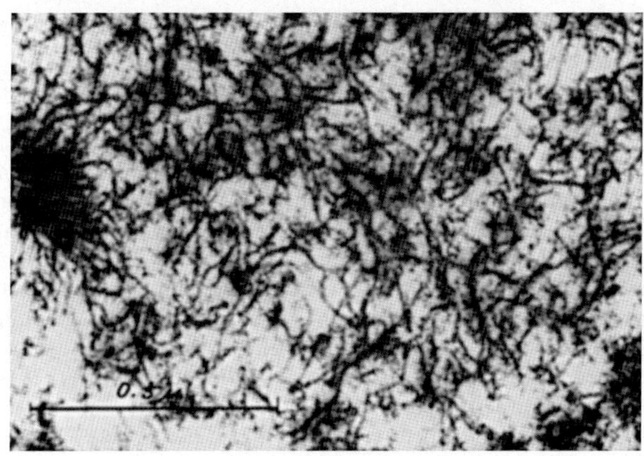

FIG. 180.1 Electron micrograph of nucleocapsid fragments. (Courtesy Dr. John M. Adams.)

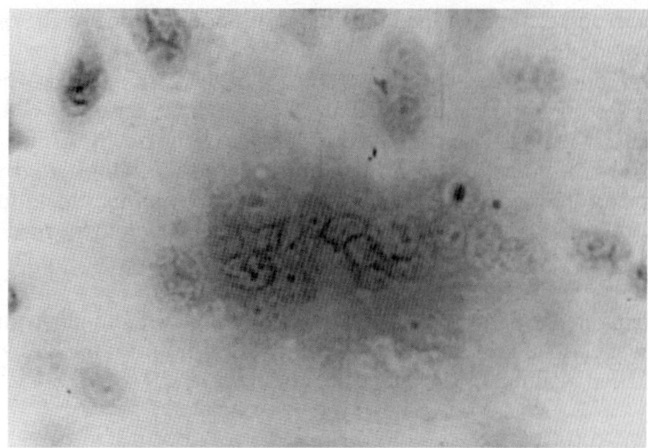

FIG. 180.2 Giant cell with approximately 20 nuclei showing measles virus cytopathogenic effect in monkey kidney tissue culture.

Matrix (M) protein is nonglycosylated and associated with the inner lipid bilayer of the envelope. It plays an important role in the maturation of the virus. In infected cells M protein interacts with the nucleocapsid and regulates MeV RNA synthesis and assembly.[232] Matrix protein interacts with the transmembrane proteins, modulates fusogenic capacity, and directs release of the virus from the apical surface, and F actin also interacts with these proteins, further modulating cell-to-cell fusion and virus assembly.[49,352,478]

The nucleocapsid (N) protein (Fig. 180.1) wraps the 16-kilobase viral genomic RNA to form the helical ribonucleocapsid, a coiled rod with a diameter of 18 nm and a length of 1 μm.[366,369-371,482,484] N protein has a molecular weight of approximately 60 kDa. Approximately 5% of the nucleocapsid is RNA.[204,471,483] The phosphoprotein (P) and the large polymerase (L) proteins are attached to the helical ribonucleocapsid. The other internal proteins of the virus are the C, and V proteins.

The phospho (P), C, and V proteins are all encoded by the P gene and alter innate response to infection. P protein forms the replicase complex along with L and N, and is a polymerase cofactor bonding to the nucleoside capsid and forming a dynamic protein interaction.[58] Both C and V proteins interact with cellular proteins and regulate response to infection. C regulates viral RNA synthesis, suppressing interferon (IFN) induction and cellular protein kinases and interfering with the innate immune response.[354]

The virus genome has a molecular weight of 4.5×10^6 daltons. It is a linear, single strand of RNA that contains approximately 15,900 nucleotides.

Cellular Receptors

Measles virus uses varying receptors for infection, depending on cell type, including CD46, signaling lymphocyte activation molecule (SLAM)/CD150, and nectin 4. CD46 appears to be the cellular receptor for attenuated measles vaccine strains but not wild-type viral strains.[59,133,303,304,356,377] More recent data suggest that SLAM is the cellular receptor for wild-type virus.[131,377,504] Nectin 4 allows measles virus entry in airway epithelial cells, sustains lateral spread, and is downregulated in infected cells.[344] It appears that measles virus also uses other receptors for entry into central nervous system (CNS) cells and endothelial cells. Measles virus also interacts with cell surface molecules to enhance infection and to increase viral spread and pathogenicity, including toll-like receptor 2 (TLR2), intercellular adhesion molecule 3 (ICAM-3), and nonintegrin (DC-SIGN), and interacts with the cyclophilin ligand CD147/EMMPRIN.[40,107,124,322,323]

Measles virus is labile.[248,249,347] It is inactivated rapidly by heat, ultraviolet light, lipid solvents such as ether and chloroform, and extreme degrees of acidity and alkalinity (i.e., pH <5 and >10). Longevity is prolonged when protein is present in the virus-suspending medium and when the virus is lyophilized with a protein stabilizer. Protein specifically protects against the adverse effects of heat and light. Protein-stabilized measles virus can be stored at −70°C for 5 or more years without significant loss of infectivity. At room temperature, a 60% loss in titer occurs in 3 to 5 days; at 56°C, the virus is inactivated within 30 minutes.[42,43,259,347]

Antigenic Composition

Clinical and epidemiologic data and early laboratory study suggested antigenic homogeneity of all measles strains.[249] More recent nucleotide sequence analysis identified distinct lineages among wild-type measles virus isolates, with most variation in H, N, and P genes.[36,346,347,419,420,463] There are eight clades (A to H) that contain at least 24 genotypes. The global distribution of measles genotypes and measles molecular epidemiology has been extensively studied since the early 1990s by Rota and colleagues at the Centers for Disease Control and Prevention (CDC).[419-421] Their work has been extremely useful for tracking global measles transmission patterns and for documenting the interruption of measles transmission in some countries.

The following properties have been associated with measles virus: a hemagglutinin (for simian cells), complement-fixing antigens, hemolytic activity, and a giant-cell–inducing factor.[61,205,248,249,364,365,369,370,394,431,433] Human measles virus infection results in serum antibodies that are capable of neutralizing viral infectivity, fixing complement with viral antigen, and inhibiting viral hemagglutination and hemolysis.

Cross-seroreactivity occurs among members of the genus *Morbillivirus* but not with other members of the Paramyxoviridae family.[45,65,229] Measles virus serum antibody in humans reacts with distemper virus, but canine serum after a case of distemper does not react with measles virus. A two-way cross between measles and rinderpest viruses has been demonstrated.

Tissue Culture Growth

Measles virus can be propagated in many different primary and cell line tissue cultures.[44,231,288] However, for isolation of virus from patient specimens, primary human and monkey kidney cultures have been most successful over the years. Recently, isolation of wild-type strains of measles virus has been more successful in other cell lines, including an Epstein-Barr virus–transformed B-lymphocyte line, continuous monkey kidney cell lines (Vero) engineered to express measles virus receptor SLAM, or a human T-cell line from cord blood (COBL-a).[262,270] In one study, an Epstein-Barr virus–transformed marmoset lymphocytic line (B95-8) was found to be superior to primary monkey kidney cell culture for isolation of virus from nasopharyngeal specimens.[263]

In tissue culture, measles virus has two distinct cytopathogenic effects. With initial isolation, syncytial formation occurs as a result of cell fusion, and the resulting giant cells may contain 10 to 50 or more nuclei (Fig. 180.2). On stained preparations, both the nuclei and cytoplasm contain eosinophilic inclusions. The second type of cytopathogenic effect is characterized by the alteration of single cells into spindle shapes or stellate forms. In general, tissue culture–adapted measles viral strains are more likely to cause this cytopathogenic effect than is giant-cell formation. In most cultures, both forms of cytopathogenic effect are evident, and changes in medium composition render one or the other type predominant.

Infection in tissue culture is associated with an attachment-adsorption phase lasting approximately 1 hour and an eclipse period of 6 to 12 hours.[313,339] Antigen first is noted in the perinuclear cytoplasm by 12 hours; by 24 hours, it is distributed throughout the cytoplasm. By 30 hours, most antigen is detected at the cell surface. In mature cultures, more cell-associated virus is present than is found free within the medium.

Animal Susceptibility

Humans are the natural hosts of measles virus, but, with human contact, monkeys also are infected easily.[324] Laboratory strains of measles virus have been adapted to suckling mice and hamsters.[60,64,230,479]

EPIDEMIOLOGY

Prevalence

The prevalence of measles throughout history has been affected markedly by population density and, since the 1960s, by the use of measles vaccine. Reported cases of measles in the United States from 1963 to 2015, analyzed by year, are presented in Fig. 180.3. After the universal use of measles vaccine began in 1965, the number of cases in the United States decreased to 22,231 in 1968.[84,91] In 1971 to 1972 and 1976 to 1977, epidemics occurred; then, after a national commitment to measles immunization, the number of cases of measles fell to an all-time low of 1497 cases reported in 1983. Beginning in 1986, the number of measles cases again increased, with 27,786 cases reported in 1990.

From 1995 through 2015, there have been 3250 cases of measles reported in the United States.[72,73,75] The mean number of reported cases during this period was 155 cases per year, with a range between 37 cases in 2004 and 667 cases in 2014 (see Fig. 180.3). Since 1998, the endemic transmission of measles in the United States has been eliminated.[380] In 2005, 66 cases were reported in the United States, and 95% of these were linked to importations.[86] Half of all the cases in 2005 were traced to one unvaccinated traveler who was infected in Europe. All but two of the contact cases in this outbreak were unvaccinated because their parents had declined immunization. In 2011, there were 220 measles cases in the United States with 17 different outbreaks.[79,91] Two hundred (90%) of these cases were associated with importations from other countries; this included United States residents returning from abroad and foreign visitors. Most patients (86%) were unvaccinated or had unknown vaccination status.

Between January 4 and April 2, 2015, a total of 159 measles cases (155 US residents and four foreign visitors) from 18 states and the District of Columbia were reported to the CDC.[71,74,512] At least 111 of these cases were directly related to exposures in December 2014 at Disney theme parks in Orange County, California. Of the 110 California patients linked to the Disneyland outbreak, 45% were unvaccinated, 5% had one dose of measles-containing vaccine, 7% had two or more doses of vaccine, 43% had unknown or undocumented vaccination status, and one patient was found to have measles immunoglobulin G (IgG) antibody indicating previous vaccination or infection.[512] Of the unvaccinated, 12 were infants too young to be vaccinated and 28 were intentionally unvaccinated.

In the 20th century, before the widespread use of measles vaccine, between 200,000 and 600,000 cases of measles were reported annually in the United States.[112,285] Careful survey suggested that in the past, reported cases accounted for only approximately 15% of the actual number of cases of measles.[100]

In the prevaccine era in the United States and other concentrated populations throughout the world, measles epidemics occurred regularly. In the United States, urban-centered measles epidemics took place every 2 to 5 years, with each epidemic lasting 3 to 4 months.[26,48,201,213,295,490,506] In general, the larger the community, the shorter the interval between epidemics. In the vaccine era, the epidemic pattern has been changed. As noted in Fig. 180.3, the total number of cases has been reduced, and the cycle between peaks has lengthened.

Age Incidence and Prevalence

In modern times in populous areas, measles has been a disease of children. The age-specific incidence in the United States for selected years is presented in Table 180.1. In the prevaccine era during the 20th century, the highest measles attack rate occurred in children aged 5 to 9 years.[26,48,213,494,495] In the period 1960 to 1964, data from five reporting areas showed that more than half of all measles cases occurred in this age group.[207] Before the present vaccine era, infections and epidemic loci centered in elementary schools. Younger children acquired measles as secondary cases from their older siblings who were attending school. In rural areas, the interval between measles epidemics tended to be greater; therefore, a broader spread in ages occurred in the percentage

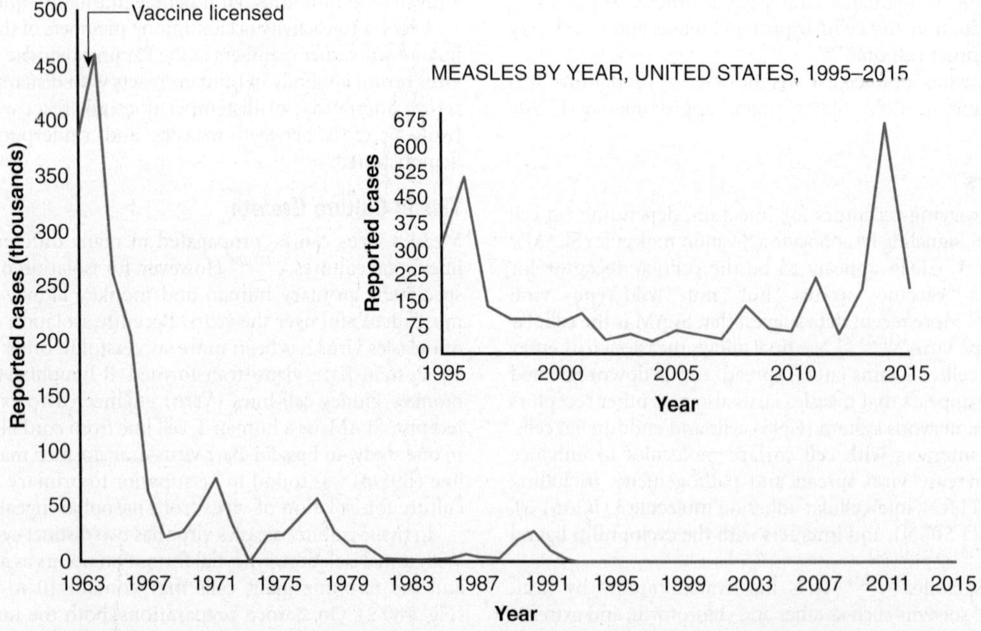

FIG. 180.3 Reported measles cases by year in the United States (From Centers for Disease Control and Prevention. Summary of notifiable diseases—United States, 1998. *MMWR Morb Mortal Wkly Rep.* 1999;47:48.) Supplement to Centers for Disease Control and Prevention. Summary of Notifiable Diseases—United States, 2010. *MMWR Morb Mortal Wkly Rep.* 2012;59:96. Centers for Disease Control and Prevention. Measles Cases and Outbreaks. http://www.cdc.gov/measles/cases-outbreaks.html.

TABLE 180.1 **Incidence and Percent Distribution of Reported Measles Cases by Age Group in Selected Years, United States**

	1960–64[a]			1974			1979			1991		
Age Group	***Cases***	**%**	***Incidence***[b]	***Cases***	**%**	***Incidence***[b]	***Cases***	**%**	***Incidence***[b]	***Cases***	**%**	***Incidence***[b]
<1–4	93,653	37.2	766	5899	26.7	36	2331	20.7	18.0	4756	49.3	24.7
5–9	132,956	52.8	1237	5391	24.4	30	2473	21.9	18.1	991	10.2	5.5
10–14	16,403	6.5	169	7799	35.3	38	3054	27.1	20.4	905	9.4	5.3
15–19	8,635	3.4	10	2475	11.2	12	2633	23.3	15.2	1102	11.4	6.2
20+				552	2.5	>1	786	7.0	0.6	1890	19.6	1.8
Totals	251,647			22,094			11,277			9643		

[a]Data from four reporting areas: Washington, DC, New York City, Illinois (including Chicago), and Massachusetts.[21,76,80,83,88,207]
[b]Incidence, cases per 100,000 population, extrapolated from the age distribution of known cases.

of measles cases. In a nationwide serum survey of US military recruits in 1962, Black[44] found that 99% had measles antibody.

As noted in Table 180.1, the age-related incidence and percentage of measles cases by age group have changed markedly since 1964. In 1991, more than 40% of measles cases occurred in persons older than 10 years; in the period from 1960 to 1964, fewer than 10% of the patients were older than 10 years. Approximately one-third of the cases in 1991 were in adolescents and young adults. Evidence also indicates high primary measles attack rates in neonates to 4-year-old children in areas of suboptimal vaccine utilization.[21,85,100,158,210] Because there has been no endemic sustained transmission of measles in the United States since 1998, cases today relate to international travel by US residents and importations.[71,74,79,86,91,419,422] Of the 159 cases between January 4 and April 2, 2015 in the United States, 26 (16%) were younger than 12 months, 18 (12%) were aged 1 to 4 years, 27 (17%) were aged 5 to 19 years, 58 (36%) were aged 20 to 39 years, and 30 (19%) were 40 years or older.[71,74] Measles in heavily populated but developing countries has its greatest incidence in children younger than 2 years.[109,151,212,340,341,372]

Geographic Distribution

In the 20th century, measles occurred regularly throughout the world in all but the most remote areas.[26,48] In island and other isolated populations, intervals between epidemics can be 10 years or more, and the occurrence of disease depends on its introduction from outside the area.

Seasonal Patterns

Epidemic measles is a winter-spring disease in temperate climates, with peak activity in the Northern Hemisphere occurring in March or April. In equatorial regions, epidemics of measles are less marked but tend to occur in the hot, dry seasons.[26,340,342,414,460]

Host and Social Factors

No difference is found in the incidence of measles in males and females. One suggestion, however, is that complication rates are higher in boys or men than in girls or women. Tidstrom[465] found that acute laryngitis occurred more than twice as frequently in male patients compared with female patients. In other studies, otitis media, pneumonia, and death occurred slightly more often in male patients.[26,373] Miller,[325,326] in a large survey in England in 1963, found no difference in the incidence of complications in male and female patients. Christensen and associates,[105] in studies of an epidemic in Greenland, noted a greater number of complications in female patients older than 15 years, attributable primarily to an increased incidence of pneumonia. In a review of 375 confirmed cases of subacute sclerosing panencephalitis (SSPE), the male-to-female ratio was 2.4 : 1.[335] In one study,[48] antibody titers were slightly higher in women than in men. The studies by one of us (JDC) involving young adults in 1976 failed to reveal a similar sex-associated difference in antibody levels, however.[446] Garenne and Aaby[172] noted that a group of women had a higher postimmunization geometric mean antibody titer than did vaccinated men.

It had been observed in the 18th and 19th centuries that importation of measles into isolated populations resulted in devastating epidemics.[319,440] The reason for this is not totally clear. However, McNeil[319] thought that, in populations where measles had been circulating for long periods of time, a pattern of mutual adaption had occurred. This allowed both the virus and people to survive.

Although the severity of disease in certain populations in more recent times appears to suggest differences based on race, this difference may be the result of nutritional and other environmental factors. Deseda-Tous and associates[128] were unable to demonstrate any differences in measles antibody by human leukocyte antigen (HLA) or by ABO blood types. In a more recent study, the findings of Ovsyannikova and coworkers[382] suggested that HLA alleles relate to antibody responses after immunization. The following alleles were positively associated with hyperseropositivity: HLA-B*7, HLA-DQA1*0104, and HLA-DPA1*0202. In contrast, HLA-B*44, HLA-DRB1*01, HLA-DRB1*08, HLA-DQB1*0301, and HLA-DPD1*0401 alleles were negatively associated with hyperseropositivity. In another study, the same group looked for associations between HLA homozygosity and measles antibody levels.[447] They found a negative correlation between homozygosity (=1/loci) and antibody value. More recently, the same group of investigators found significant associations with class I HLA-B, as well as class II HLA-DPBI and HLA-DPA1 genes for measles vaccine–induced antibody values after the second vaccine dose.[234] This group also noted associations between single nucleotide polymorphisms and haplotypes in cytokine and cytokine receptor genes and immunity after measles immunization.[209]

In the prevaccine era, the age of patients at the time of acquiring measles infection was related inversely to the number of siblings in the family.[26,48,501] In general, measles occurred at an earlier age in city dwellers and those of lower socioeconomic classes than in rural families and well-educated, upper-income groups.

In the present era of antibiotics and other medical modalities, the greatest factors in measles-related morbidity and mortality are age and nutritional status. The mortality rates for measles are highest in children younger than 2 years and in adults.[26,48] The severity of measles and rates of mortality correlate in general with the severity of malnutrition.[44,337] However, extensive investigations by Aaby and others[3,4,172] since the 1980s suggest that overcrowding and intensive exposure may be more important determinants of measles-related mortality than is nutritional status alone.

Studies of measles conducted early in the 20th century and in developing countries indicated that secondary cases in households were likely to be more severe than were primary cases.[2-4,172] However, more recent studies in the United States found no difference in severity between primary and secondary cases in families.[457]

Spread of Infection

Measles is a highly contagious disease in nonimmune persons. It is spread from an infected ill person to a new host by the respiratory route.[26,48,411,412,415] Although monkeys can acquire measles from humans, practically speaking, no animal reservoir exists.[324] Available evidence suggests that infection is spread by persons ill with measles. Asymptomatic contagious carriers are unknown, and persons with acute asymptomatic infection probably are not contagious.[289] Recent California data indicate that secondary vaccine failure cases are less contagious than cases with primary measles. (J.D. Cherry and J. Zipprich, unpublished data).

However, a small number of secondary vaccine failure cases did transmit to contacts after prolonged contact. The period of greatest contagion occurs during the prodromal period.[180]

Transmission of measles is thought to occur mainly by aerosolized droplets of respiratory secretions. Acquisition of infection by a new host is by the nose and possibly the conjunctivae.[386] Infection can be initiated by small-droplet nuclei, which stay suspended in air for considerable periods of time, or by direct hits of large droplets at close range.[50,409] Also possible is that spread involves close person-to-person contact in young children, with large virus-containing droplets of nasal secretions being picked up on the hands of the future host and then applied to the nose.

PATHOGENESIS AND PATHOLOGY

Viral Infection

The sequence of viral events in uncomplicated measles is presented in Table 180.2. Although much is known about measles virus infection in humans, considerable gaps exist regarding specific events. Experimental studies in other primates have been performed in an attempt to fill in the gaps and thereby provide a more complete picture.[245,314,361,376,435,503] The primary site of infection appears to be the respiratory epithelium of the nasopharynx. Measles vaccine virus instilled into the nose or by aerosol results in infection.[46,47,272] Papp[386] reported studies suggesting that infection resulted from conjunctival contact and proposed that this means was the primary portal of entry. However, experiments with vaccine virus generally have been unsuccessful when conjunctival inoculation has been performed.[46,47] Initial infection of the respiratory epithelium appears to be minimal; a more important event is the early spread of virus to regional lymphatics. A presumption based on data derived from Fenner's ectromelia-mouse experimental model[144,145] is that after such spread, primary viremia occurs, followed by extensive multiplication of virus in the reticuloendothelial system at both regional and distant sites. Multiplication of virus also continues at the site of initial infection.

During the fifth to seventh days of infection, extensive secondary viremia takes place and results in the establishment of generalized measles viral infection. The skin, conjunctivae, and respiratory tract are obvious sites of infection, but other organs may be involved as well. From the 11th to the 14th days, the viral content of the blood, respiratory tract, and other organs peaks and then rapidly diminishes over the ensuing 2- to 3-day period.

In immunologically compromised patients with defects in cell-mediated factors, measles virus is not cleared from the secondary infection sites, and progressive, frequently fatal illnesses occur.[8,141,329,331,343] During infection, measles virus replicates in endothelial cells, epithelial cells, and monocytes and macrophages.[195,336]

TABLE 180.2 Sequence of Measles Virus Infection in Uncomplicated Primary Disease

Day	Event
0	Measles virus in droplet nuclei or large droplet comes in contact with the epithelial surface of the nasopharynx or possibly the conjunctiva Infection of epithelial cells and virus multiplication
1–2	Extension of infection to regional lymphoid tissue
2–3	Primary viremia
3–5	Multiplication of measles virus in respiratory epithelium at the site of initial infection and in the reticuloendothelial system regionally and at distant sites
5–7	Secondary viremia
7–11	Establishment of infection in the skin and other viremic sites, including the respiratory tract
11–14	Virus in blood, respiratory tract, skin, and other organs
15–17	Viremia decreases and then ceases Viral content in organs rapidly diminishes

Data from references 190–192,195, 199, 245, 251, 257, 290, 361, 376, 393, 415, 424, 435, 503.

Pathology

The characteristic pathologic feature of measles is the widespread distribution of multinucleated giant cells, which are the result of cell fusion.[45,245,248,290,313,361,376,416,435,503] Two main types of giant cells occur in measles: (1) Warthin-Finkeldey cells, which are found in the reticuloendothelium; and (2) epithelial giant cells (Fig. 180.4), which occur principally in the respiratory epithelium but also on other epithelial surfaces.[290]

Warthin-Finkeldey giant cells are found throughout the reticuloendothelial system in the adenoids, tonsils, Peyer patches, appendix, lymph nodes, spleen, and thymus. They vary in size and contain as many as 100 or more nuclei. The cells contain both cytoplasmic and intranuclear eosinophilic inclusions, with cytoplasmic inclusions more common than intranuclear lesions. During the prodromal stage of measles, epithelial giant cells regularly are present on respiratory surfaces and frequently are sloughed free (see Fig. 180.4).

Measles Exanthem

Hematoxylin and eosin–stained sections of skin biopsy specimens have revealed typical epithelial syncytial giant cells with nuclear and cytoplasmic inclusions.[257,456] The giant cells contain three to 26 nuclei. Other findings include the following: focal parakeratosis, dyskeratosis, spongiosis, and intracellular edema. The superficial blood vessels are dilated, with a sparse, surrounding lymphohistiocytic infiltrate.

Koplik Spots

Suringa and colleagues[456] observed that the histopathologic features of Koplik spots were similar to those of the rash. These investigators noted more giant cells with more nuclei, a greater degree of edema, and a lessened inflammatory response in the enanthem biopsy sample, however.

Respiratory Tract

The extent of respiratory involvement in uncomplicated measles is not known. However, clinical symptoms and the extensive radiographic studies of Kohn and Koiransky[265] suggested that pharyngitis, tracheitis, bronchitis, and pulmonary infiltration are the rule rather than the exception. Unfortunately, the human pathologic data available have been obtained mainly from complicated cases, so the findings cannot be considered representative.[126,416] In a study in monkeys, Nii and colleagues[361] noted giant cells in the mucosal epithelium of the trachea,

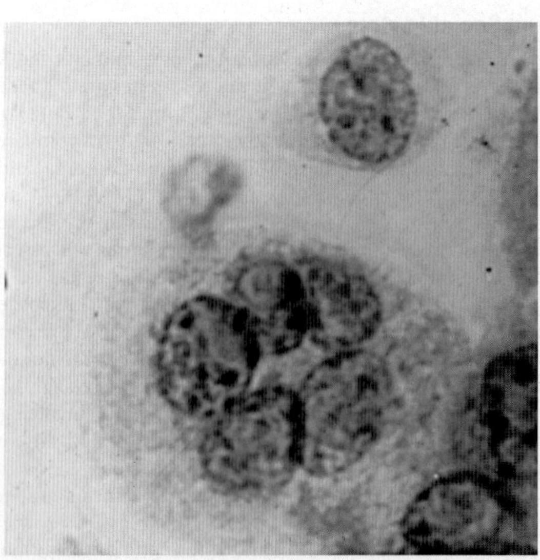

FIG. 180.4 Pharyngeal smear of epithelial giant cell with five nuclei. (Courtesy Dr. John M. Adams.)

bronchi, and bronchioli. The lumina of these airways contained sloughed syncytial cells. Warthin-Finkeldey cells were found in the adjacent lymphatics.

In the lungs of experimentally infected monkeys, interstitial pneumonitis was observed with giant-cell formation.[361] Infiltration of neutrophils, eosinophils, and mononuclear cells also was noted.

Immunologic Events

After natural or attenuated measles virus infection develops, large numbers of specific and nonspecific immunologic responses occur. Many questions relating to immunity in measles remain unanswered, although a considerable body of knowledge has been gathered since the 1950s.

Antibody

After measles viral infection develops, an antibody response regularly occurs. Serum antibodies to the N, F, H, and M proteins of measles virus can be demonstrated by hemagglutination inhibition (HI), complement fixation (CF), neutralization, immune precipitation, hemolysin inhibition, enzyme-linked immunosorbent assay (ELISA), and fluorescent antibody (FA) methods.[118,168,169,186,258,275,276,357,363,364,473] Antibody-dependent cellular cytotoxicity and antibody-dependent complement-mediated lysis also have been demonstrated.[156,157,254] In natural infection, HI and neutralizing antibodies appear at approximately the 14th day, peak at around 4 to 6 weeks, and decrease approximately fourfold from the peak over the course of a year. Most naturally infected persons have demonstrable HI and neutralizing antibodies for life. Krugman[273,274] noted an average 16-fold reduction in HI antibody titer 15 years after natural infection in a group of children who had no measles exposure during the observation period.

After measles vaccine has been administered, both HI and neutralizing antibodies are present by the 14th day.[168,169,275,276] CF antibody appears slightly later than does HI antibody and in general does not persist as long as either HI or neutralizing antibody. Primary infection is characterized by the initial appearance of antibody in the IgM and IgG serum components.[154,214,431-433,468] The IgM-specific response is short-lived, and rarely can measles antibody in this fraction be demonstrated more than 9 weeks after infection. IgA secretory antibody also occurs regularly after vaccine viral infection and after natural infection.[34,163]

IgG antibody appearing after infection is primarily subclasses IgG1 and IgG4.[311] Antibody detected by neutralization and by HI is mainly to H protein and correlates with clinical protection against illness.[123,195,364] Antibody to N protein is the main antibody detected by CF.[364] Antibody to F protein is demonstrated by inhibition of hemolysis of monkey erythrocytes by measles virus or by immunoprecipitation.[363,365] Antibody to F protein may contribute to neutralization by disrupting the fusion of virus membrane with host cell membranes. Only small amounts of antibody to M protein are elicited after infection with wild virus or vaccine virus.[186]

Specific Cell-Mediated Responses

Investigators recognized in the 1960s that patients with defective cellular resistance factors frequently died of progressive measles virus infections.[351] In the 1970s, techniques became available that demonstrated measles-specific lymphocyte sensitization.[171,187,188,271,282,423] Graziano and colleagues[187] found that lymphocytes from persons who previously had measles had a blastogenic response in vitro when these cells were incubated with measles antigen. Labowskie and associates,[282] using an in vitro lymphocyte-mediated cytotoxicity assay, noted that lymphocytes from persons who previously had measles caused cell destruction in a tissue culture chronically infected with measles virus. Ruckdeschel and colleagues[423] observed that two physicians without detectable measles antibody who had experienced repeated recent exposure to measles without developing illness had strong in vitro cellular responsiveness to measles virus. T cells are appreciated to be important both in B-cell antiviral antibody responses and as effector cells for the clearance of virus-infected cells from tissues.[195] Both helper ($CD4^+$) and suppressor ($CD8^+$) cells participate in the cellular response.[481] During infection, $CD8^+$ T cells eliminate virus-infected cells by major histocompatibility complex (MHC) class I–restricted cytotoxic mechanisms.[195] $CD4^+$ T cells respond to measles virus infection by the secretion of cytokines. After initial exposure to virus occurs, $CD4^+$ T cells mount a helper T-cell subtype 1 (Th1) response. Before the rash develops, levels of plasma IFN-γ are increased, and, with the rash, interleukin-2 (IL-2) appears. With clinical recovery, plasma levels of IL-4 increase (a Th2 response) and stay elevated for several weeks, whereas the initial Th1 response subsides.

On reexposure, Th1 and Th2 responses occur as indicated by the production of IFN-γ, IL-2, tumor necrosis factor-β (TNF-β), IL-4, IL-5, and IL-10. The Th1 cytokine response is important for macrophage activation (through the action of IFN-γ), lymphocyte proliferation (through IL-2), and MHC class II–restricted cytotoxicity (through TNF-β). The Th2 cytokine response is important for macrophage deactivation (through the action of IL-4 and IL-10) and B-cell help (through IL-4, IL-5, and IL-10). In studies in rhesus monkeys, researchers found that humoral immunity had only a limited role in the control of measles virus replication in primary infection.[395]

Ovsyannikova and colleagues[383] found a predominant Th1 cytokine pattern after measles vaccine viral infection. This pattern occurred after both primary immunization and revaccination. In this study, no relationship was found between any specific cytokine level and serum measles antibody values. In another study, the same research group found a subset of vaccinees in whom the cytokine responses were skewed toward the Th2 type.[132] These investigators suggested that this response in this subset may not be sufficient for long-term immunity.

Other Responses

Listed in Table 180.3 are nonspecific, immunologically related responses that can be demonstrated during natural or vaccine measles virus infection. Anderson and colleagues[15] demonstrated a temporary defect in neutrophil motility during acute measles that resolved by the 11th day after the onset of rash. Leukopenia has been observed in natural measles[37] and after immunization.[46,47] With immunization, the numbers of both neutrophils and lymphocytes are reduced; this reduction lasts approximately 1 week, with an onset occurring approximately 7 days after vaccination. Coovadia and colleagues[114,115] showed that the numbers of T, B, and null cells in the lymphocyte population are reduced. With a reduction in the number of T lymphocytes, no change occurs in the ratio of helper and suppressor cytotoxic cell phenotypes.[10,18,239]

Thrombocytopenia occasionally has been associated with natural measles[225] and vaccination.[11,492] Oski and Naiman[381] noted a mild reduction in the peripheral platelet count during routine measles immunization. Transitory complement defects vary in measles; Charlesworth and associates[94] found evidence of pathologic complement activation in 20 of 50 patents studied. Coovadia and colleagues[115] noted slight but significant reductions in serum IgA levels and elevated IgM values in acute measles virus infections. These investigators found the IgG concentrations to be normal. Increased levels of serum or plasma IgE were noted in two studies.[193,436] Delayed hypersensitivity responses in skin are suppressed in both natural and vaccine measles virus infection.[148,448,449] Similarly, in vitro lymphocyte blastogenic responses to common antigens are suppressed.[491]

Mechanisms in Recovery From Measles Viral Infection

Acute clinical measles is characterized by viral multiplication in many organs of the body and then rapid subsidence of the infection by the 17th day. As noted earlier, measles virus infection is associated with both serum and secretory antibody responses and specific cell-mediated responses that coincide with clinical recovery. All three factors would seem to be important in recovery from acute measles virus infection, but confusing information clouds the issue. For example, researchers have noted that children with simple agammaglobulinemia in whom measurable measles antibodies do not develop after measles virus infection recover from the disease normally.[182] This finding suggests that development of measles antibody is not important for recovery from acute infection. However, by using a sensitive plaque-reduction measles neutralizing antibody technique, Black[42,43] found small amounts of antibody in the sera of three agammaglobulinemic patients.

In contrast to antibody data, data on patients with defects in the cell-mediated immune system show that they clearly do poorly with

TABLE 180.3 Nonspecific, Immunologically Related Responses During Measles Virus Infection

Category	Findings	Reference
Leukocytes	Defective neutrophil motility	15
	Leukopenia (both lymphocytes and neutrophils)	37, 48
	Decreased T, B, and null lymphocytes	10, 18, 114, 115, 239
	Decreased natural killer cell activity	198
	Decreased helper T cells	119, 255
	Prolonged suppression of interleukin-12 production	20
	Prolonged depression of virus-specific interferon-α production	355
Interferon-α	Elevated plasma levels	196, 197
Neopterin	Elevated plasma levels	196, 197
Interleukin-2 receptor (soluble)	Elevated plasma levels	196, 197
Platelets	Reduction in peripheral count	381
Complement	Frequent pathologic activation of the complement system; reduction of C1q, C4, C3, and C5	94
Serum immunoglobulins	IgA reduced and IgE and IgM elevated	115, 193, 436
In vitro lymphocyte response to phytohemagglutinin	Suppressed in presence of autologous serum; normal in presence of calf serum	491
In vitro lymphocyte response to *Candida*	Suppressed	491
Cutaneous delayed hypersensitivity	Depressed	148
C-reactive protein	Elevated at onset of rash	194
Circulating immune complexes	Noted in 25% of patients 7 to 13 days after rash onset	511

measles virus infection and frequently succumb to progressive infection despite the administration of large doses of measles antibody-containing immunoglobulin. T cells (both $CD4^+$ and $CD8^+$) clear virus-infected cells from tissues by cytotoxicity. IFN-α, which is released by a variety of cells, including T cells, inhibits the spread of virus infection.

In studies in a transgenic mouse model system, Tishon and associates[467] showed that CD4, CD8, or B cells alone controlled measles virus infection. However, combinations of CD4 T cells and B cells or CD4 and CD8 T cells were essential in clearing infection. In contrast, the combination of CD5 T cells and B cells was ineffective.

Mechanisms in Prevention of Repeat Illness in Persons Previously Infected With Measles Virus

In contrast to mechanisms of recovery in acute measles, the role of serum antibody in protection against recurrent disease is solid. Before the present vaccine era, researchers repeatedly demonstrated that the administration of measles antibody-containing immunoglobulin could prevent clinical measles.[235,453] Similarly, infants with transplacentally acquired measles antibody are immune.[275,276] Whether other factors also are important in protection against reinfection is not clear. Often cited is that patients with agammaglobulinemia do not have repeated measles virus infections, so other factors must be involved.[182]

Of interest is that patients have been described in whom antibody did not prevent acquisition of atypical measles after immunization with killed measles vaccine.[292] The data of Krause and associates[271] suggested that persons in whom the capacity for exaggerated measles-specific lymphocyte activity (when tested with formalin inactivated measles virus) persists (some previous killed vaccine recipients) may be subject to illness despite the presence of antibody. However, the antibody produced after receipt of killed measles vaccine was incomplete; it lacked specific antibody to F protein.[42,43,104] Black noted one child with a low measles neutralizing antibody titer, presumably from natural measles virus infection, in whom measles later developed. Chen and coworkers[96] found that some students with measurable but low neutralizing antibody titers were not protected from clinical measles on exposure.

CLINICAL MANIFESTATIONS

Before the present vaccine era, measles was an inevitable disease of childhood that was recognized readily by parents and other laypersons, as well as by physicians. Despite the occasional confusion with other exanthematous diseases,[98] the epidemic character of measles usually resulted in an accurate diagnosis. Currently in North America, few of the new generation of parents, physicians, and other medical personnel have seen measles; therefore, the illness can be misdiagnosed.

Typical Illness

Incubation Period

The incubation period[26,99,100,248,278,415,452] of measles is approximately 10 days (range, 8–12 days). Although extensive virologic and immunologic events occur during this period, the individual has virtually no outward sign of illness. Goodall[183] suggested (and Partington and Quinton[388] presented supporting data) that some patients have mild transient respiratory symptoms and fever shortly after initial acquisition of the virus.

Prodromal Period

The prodrome of measles lasts approximately 3 days (range, 2–4 days). Initial symptoms are respiratory and suggest the possibility of a cold, except that fever is an early sign. In fact, in situations of close observation, slight temperature elevation has occurred and then subsided for a day or so before the appearance of typical respiratory symptoms.[452]

The onset of clinical measles is characterized by general malaise, fever, coryza, conjunctivitis, and cough. These symptoms worsen during a 2- to 4-day period. Early in the prodromal phase, a transitory rash occasionally has been observed. It has been urticarial or macular, has occurred with the initial onset of fever, and has disappeared before onset of the typical exanthem.

During the prodromal period, the temperature increases gradually to a value of 39.5° ± 1.1°C (103° ± 2°F) over the course of a 4-day period. The nasal symptoms resemble those of other viral respiratory tract infections and are similar to those of the common cold or acute nasopharyngitis. Sneezing, rhinitis, and congestion are common symptoms. The degree of prodromal conjunctivitis varies considerably. Initially, the conjunctival infection is divided by a transverse marginal line across the lower lids.[451] The conjunctivitis is associated with considerable lacrimation, and older patients in particular are bothered by photophobia, which frequently is severe. Slit-lamp examination reveals both corneal and conjunctival lesions.[25,150]

The cough in prodromal measles frequently is troublesome. It worsens throughout the period and often has a brassy quality suggesting laryngeal and tracheal involvement. On day 10 ± 1, Koplik spots, the pathognomonic enanthem of measles, first appear (Fig. 180.5). Koplik[267-269] originally described the lesions as bluish-white specks on a bright-red mucosal surface. In the experience of one of us (J.D.C.), the lesions always have appeared white, and a blue component was not observed. Koplik spots

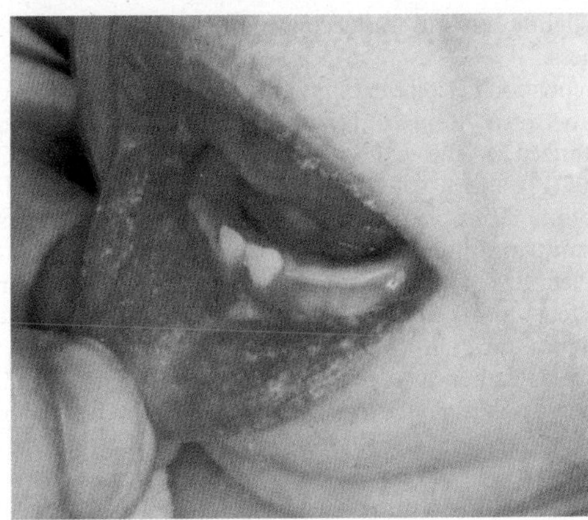

FIG. 180.5 Koplik spots with involvement of the buccal and lower labial mucosa.

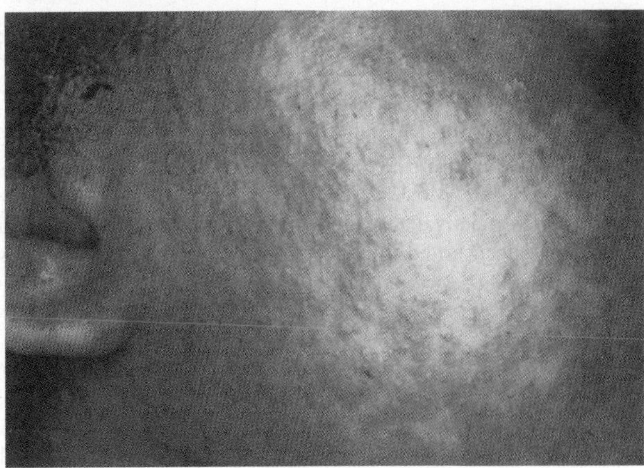

FIG. 180.6 Measles exanthem. Note the generalized erythematous confluent base supporting small papular and microvesicular lesions.

first arise on the buccal mucosa opposite the lower molars but usually spread quickly to involve most of the buccal and lower labial mucosa. The lesions are approximately 1 mm at first but occasionally seem to coalesce into larger lesions. Initially, only a few lesions appear, but within 12 hours the number usually is uncountable. Of equal importance in establishing the diagnosis is the appearance of the background mucosal surface, which is always bright red and granular. Frequently, 1-mm lesions (Fordyce aphthae), which commonly occur normally in adolescents and adults, are confused with Koplik spots.[97] These lesions, however, can be differentiated easily because they appear on a normal pale mucosal surface rather than the bright-red background of measles.

During the prodromal period, erythematous maculopapular lesions also are observed occasionally on the palate. At the end of the prodromal period, the posterior pharyngeal wall usually is erythematous, and the patient may complain of a sore throat.

Exanthem Period

In typical measles, the exanthem appears on approximately the 14th day after exposure. The exanthem occurs at approximately the peak of the respiratory symptoms and when the temperature usually is approximately 39.5°C (103°F). At this time, the manifestation of Koplik spots has peaked, and during the next 3 days the spots disappear. However, after the specific white spots have disappeared, the red, sandpapery mucosal background remains for a day or so.

The measles exanthem first appears behind the ears and on the forehead at the hairline. Spread of the rash is centrifugal from the head to the feet. By the third day, the rash has involved the face, neck, trunk, upper extremities, buttocks, and lower extremities sequentially. The rash initially is erythematous and maculopapular but progresses to confluence in the same centrifugal manner as it is spread. Confluence always is more prominent on the face; frequently, the lesions on the lower extremities remain discrete. At the height of the rash, the appearance suggests microvesicles on top of a generalized erythematous confluent base (Fig. 180.6).

The exanthem begins to clear on the third to fourth day, again following the centrifugal course of progression. During the initial stages of the rash, its color is red and it readily blanches on pressure. As the rash fades, it takes on a coppery appearance, after which a brownish discoloration is seen that does not clear with pressure. With healing, a fine desquamation frequently occurs in confluent areas with brownish discoloration. The duration of the exanthem usually is 6 to 7 days.

During the exanthem period, the fever generally peaks on approximately the second or third day of the rash and then falls by lysis during a 24-hour period. Fever that persists after the third or fourth day of exanthem usually is an indication of a complication. Conjunctivitis and nasal symptoms generally subside at about the time of defervescence. Continued nasal discharge, whether purulent or not, suggests bacterial secondary infection. With the appearance of the rash, the cough loosens up, and in older persons it frequently becomes productive. The cough may persist for 10 days or more.

Pharyngitis is a common development during the exanthem period, as is enlargement of cervical lymph nodes. Generalized lymphadenopathy with suboccipital and postauricular involvement is not an uncommon finding, nor is splenomegaly. Young children occasionally have diarrhea, vomiting, laryngitis, and croup. Abdominal pain also can be troublesome.

Laboratory Findings

Laboratory studies rarely are indicated for acute uncomplicated typical measles because the diagnosis can be established on a clinical and epidemiologic basis, and the results of studies rarely affect management of the patient. During the periods of prodrome and rash, the total leukocyte count is low. Numbers of neutrophils and lymphocytes are reduced, but the most marked reduction, when absolute counts are considered, is in the number of lymphocytes.[37] As noted in Table 180.3, there may be a reduction in the platelet count and an elevation in C-reactive protein value, and skin test (such as the tuberculin) reactions may be suppressed.

Modified Illness

Modified measles* is an infection that occurs in a partially immune person. It is characterized by a generally mild illness that usually follows the regular sequence of events in measles. The prodromal period is shorter; cough, coryza, and fever are minimal. Koplik spots are few and transient, and they frequently do not occur. The exanthem follows the progression pattern of regular measles, but confluence of the lesions does not occur. Because serologic studies reveal some children with measles antibody who have never had clinical disease suggestive of measles, some modified infections probably occur without exanthem and perhaps without overt symptoms at all.[42,43,276,277]

Modified measles develops under a variety of circumstances, the most important of which historically was the result of intentional alteration of disease by the administration of immune serum globulin to an exposed susceptible child. Naturally occurring modified measles is seen occasionally in infants younger than 9 months because of the presence of transplacentally acquired maternal measles antibody.

Today the main cause of modified measles is secondary vaccine failure. In this instance, patients have had modified illness but demonstrated a secondary measles serum antibody response (only IgG antibody).[100,103,444] With increasing time from immunization, this response will occur more frequently.[24,96,127,139]

Recurrent measles also rarely results in modified illness. The frequency of recurrent measles is unknown. In general, most authorities have discounted the existence of recurrent measles and suggested that the recorded experiences were the result of confusion with infection by other exanthem-producing agents.[98,274,275] However, Cherry and colleagues,[100] Schaffner and associates,[429] and Schluederberg[432,433] have

*References 26, 30, 96, 100, 103, 139, 168, 169, 216, 235, 278, 390, 410, 429.

described children with modified illnesses, secondary immunologic responses, and well-documented instances of previous cases of measles.

Atypical Measles

Atypical measles is a clearly defined clinical syndrome that occurs in some previously immunized persons after they have been exposed to natural measles. Most cases have occurred in persons who initially received inactivated (killed) measles viral vaccines, but some cases also have been noted in children who received only live measles vaccines.[101,292,358]

Historical Aspects

The initial studies with inactivated measles vaccines in the early 1960s demonstrated that multiple doses were necessary to stimulate an antibody response and that measurable serum antibody levels were short-lived.[168,169,200,246,275,276,496] In the initial trials, it soon became apparent that some study participants who had received killed vaccine were still susceptible to measles. On being exposed to natural measles, some children developed typical measles, and others developed a mild, modified illness.[168,169] As a result, regimens were developed in which children were immunized with two or three doses of killed vaccine at monthly intervals, followed in a month or more by a single dose of Edmonston B live measles vaccine (KKL or KKKL). Studies at the time demonstrated that good antibody levels were achieved after administration of both regimens. After measles vaccine was licensed in 1963, killed-live measles vaccine regimens enjoyed modest popularity in the United States (as well as in other countries) because live Edmonston B strain vaccine frequently was associated with alarming febrile responses and occasional febrile convulsions.

In 1965, Rauh and Schmidt[407] reported an unusual illness after exposure to natural measles in some children who had received killed vaccine 2 years previously. The significance of their findings became more apparent during the following 2 years when Fulginiti and colleagues[166] and Nader and coworkers[349] noted many instances of "atypical measles" in previous recipients of KKK and KKL vaccination regimens. In these two instances, original immunization had taken place 4 to 6 years before the occurrence of atypical illness.

In 1968, killed measles vaccine was taken off the market in the United States after the distribution of approximately 1.8 million doses in the period from 1963 to 1968.[378] During the 12-year period from 1968 to 1980, atypical measles was reported frequently.* We are unaware of reports since 1980 of further cases of atypical measles. However, one of us (J.D.C.) observed one 26-year-old physician and a 28-year-old nurse with the syndrome in the 1980s. Sporadic cases in adults may still be occurring but are misdiagnosed because physicians caring for adults are unaware of the syndrome; therefore, the history of killed measles vaccine is not uncovered and specific antibody studies are not performed.

In 1971, during study of an extensive measles epidemic, Cherry and colleagues[101] observed six children who had relatively mild, atypical measles-like illnesses but had received only live measles vaccine. Linnemann and colleagues[292] similarly noted two children with atypical measles-like illnesses who had received only live measles vaccine. Nichols[358] and St. Geme and associates[174] also have reported bizarre measles illnesses in patients who formerly received live vaccine.

Clinical Characteristics

Atypical measles was a common illness from 1967 to 1978. Because killed measles vaccines have not been available in the United States since 1968, two obvious facts need to be mentioned: with each passing year, potential patients and actual patients with atypical measles will be 1 year older and also 1 year farther from the time of receiving the primary killed measles vaccine immunization series. Both these aspects raise concern about whether the clinical manifestations of the syndrome will remain the same today as when the illness first was described. It was the opinion of one of us (JDC) in 1981 that the syndrome had changed slightly but still was recognizable from original descriptions of the illness.[99]

The incubation period of atypical measles is similar to that of typical measles—between 7 and 14 days in duration. The prodromal period is characterized by the sudden onset of high fever (39.5°C–40.6°C [103°F–105°F]) and usually headache. Abdominal pain and myalgia also are common complaints. Dry, nonproductive cough occurs in most patients, and vomiting is noted in approximately one-third of those afflicted. Pleuritic chest pain and weakness also are common complaints. Although few reports to the contrary exist, Koplik spots appear to be rare in atypical measles.

Two to 3 days after onset of the illness, the rash appears. It is unique in that it first develops on the distal ends of the extremities and progresses in a cephalad direction. Usually, the rash initially is erythematous and maculopapular. One of us (J.D.C.) has been impressed by a slight yellowish hue of the exanthem when compared with that of typical measles. The rash is particularly prominent on the wrists and ankles; it involves the palms and soles. Spread of the rash varies considerably. In some patients, only the wrists and ankles are involved, whereas in others, the entire extremities and the lower part of the trunk are affected. In a peculiar fashion, the rash frequently seems to end its cephalad progression in a line at the level of the nipples. Occasionally, a few erythematous, maculopapular but discrete lesions are found on the face. In some cases, the rash becomes vesicular, with the lesions 2 to 3 mm in diameter; they do not proceed to scab formation as in varicella, but occasionally pruritus is a problem, and excoriation occurs from scratching. The exanthem often has a petechial or purpuric component, and urticaria also occurs frequently. Edema of the extremities has been a common finding.

Although coryza has been noted in a few reports, it is not a prominent feature, nor is conjunctivitis. Respiratory distress with dyspnea and rales occurs commonly, and radiographic examination reveals pulmonary involvement in virtually all cases. Most patients have hilar adenopathy and pneumonia. Pleural effusion also occurs frequently. The pneumonia in atypical measles usually is lobular or segmental, and the lesions often appear nodular (Fig. 180.7). Although initial descriptions of the syndrome suggested an illness of approximately 1 week's duration, later observations indicated illnesses of 2 weeks or more. In one case, fatigue and other symptoms persisted for more than 1.5 years.

In the original description by Rauh and Schmidt,[407] one patient had an exanthem that was biphasic; initially, a transitory rash suggested modified measles. Two weeks later, the more characteristic atypical exanthem developed. The same observers also noted a second case with a biphasic exanthem in which the first lesions were vesicular and occurred when the child had little fever. The second exanthem was maculopapular

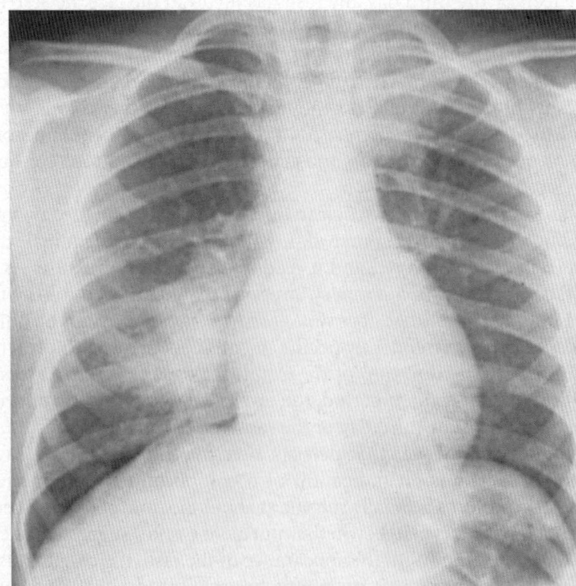

FIG. 180.7 Nodular pulmonary infiltrates in a child with atypical measles.

*References 17, 57, 95, 101, 167, 179, 203, 217, 223, 286, 317, 328, 358, 360, 367, 368, 488, 489, 507–509.

and associated with a febrile response. Zahradnik and colleagues[509] also noted a similar sequence in two young adults. Two patients who had received killed measles vaccine in the past had radiographic evidence of characteristic pulmonary findings, but the typical exanthem did not develop.[367,368,507,508]

Other findings in atypical measles include marked hepatosplenomegaly,[407] marked hyperesthesia,[349] weakness,[286] and numbness and paresthesia.[317] Personal observations by one of us (J.D.C.) of cases in adolescents and young adults suggest that the exanthem is less prominent than in past cases, and the fever and overall morbidity are of greater duration. Follow-up radiographic studies demonstrated the persistence of nodular pulmonary lesions for longer than 1 year in several patients and up to 6 years in one patient.[286,328,507,508]

Measles antibody studies in atypical measles are remarkably diagnostic. If an initial serum sample is obtained before or at onset of the exanthem, CF and HI titers usually are less than 1:5. By the 10th day of illness, both titers are elevated markedly, and most are 1:1280 or greater. In contrast, in typical natural measles at the 10th day of illness, the titer rarely is greater than 1:160.

Measles virus was not recovered from any patients with atypical measles, but only a few adequately performed studies were performed. The epidemiologic data currently available suggest that patients with atypical measles are not contagious. Other laboratory studies are not particularly useful in atypical measles. The erythrocyte sedimentation rate is elevated. When serial blood cell counts have been performed, slight early leukopenia and late eosinophilia have been noted.[166]

The pathogenesis of atypical measles was studied by several investigators, and several possible mechanisms were suggested,[401] including a generalized Arthus reaction, induction of abnormal measles virus–specific, delayed-type hypersensitivity, and an imbalance in antibody responses to H and F proteins caused by denaturation of F protein during formalin inactivation of the vaccine virus. In a study in monkeys, Polack and associates[401] found that atypical measles resulted from previous priming for a nonproductive type 2 $CD4^+$ T-cell response and not from the lack of functional antibody against F protein. In revaccination studies performed by Cherry and colleagues in the 1970s, it was found that vaccinees with severe local reactions had marked lymphocyte reactivity to formalin inactivated measles virus and absent or minimal HI antibody.[271]

Unusual Manifestations and Complications of Measles

In addition to typical measles, modified measles, and atypical measles, many other clinical manifestations and complications occur at a broad range of frequency. By definition, unusual manifestations are a direct result of the primary viral infection, whereas complications are a result of damage by a secondary infection with another microorganism. In many instances, determining whether a particular manifestation is just viral or involves a second agent is difficult. Combinations of infections are common occurrences.

In general, complications resulting from secondary infection are not as common today as they were before the antibiotic era; however, no evidence suggests that unusual manifestations of illness occur less frequently today than formerly. To demonstrate the magnitude of the problem today, the findings in a 1970 to 1971 hospital survey in St. Louis are revealing.[100,102] In this period, an extensive epidemic occurred, with 10,000 cases of measles. In eight area hospitals, 130 children (1.3%) were admitted; 66 cases of pneumonia and six fatalities occurred, and six children had encephalitis.

The records of measles patients in three hospitals were reviewed carefully. Of this group of 71 patients, 53 had pneumonia; 37 of the patients with pneumonia had either previous cardiorespiratory or other chronic systemic disorders. Two children had mediastinal and subcutaneous emphysema. All six deaths were caused by fulminant pneumonia. Of the six children with encephalitis, severe residual neurologic damage developed in three. One child had acute measles appendicitis with perforation and peritonitis, and another patient had mesenteric lymphadenitis.

Pneumonia

Pulmonary involvement in measles, as a result of the viral infection, is probably the rule rather than the exception. Kohn and Koiransky[265] performed careful radiographic studies in 130 children with measles and noted that 55% had pneumonic infiltration and 74% had hilar adenopathy. In most instances, the pneumonia was observed early in the course of the illness, a finding that suggested primary viral involvement rather than secondary bacterial infection. In the 1970 to 1971 St. Louis measles epidemic, approximately one in every 150 patients with measles was hospitalized because of pneumonia.

Pneumonia in measles has varied radiographic manifestations.[6,102,189,265,294,302,310,373,458] Clearly, viral pneumonia is characterized by bilateral hyperinflation with diffuse fluffy infiltrates that are more confluent at the hilum. Unilateral, segmental, and lobar pneumonias also are observed. Gremillion and Crawford[189] reviewed 106 cases of pneumonia that occurred in 3220 Air Force recruits with measles between 1976 and 1979. Illnesses were severe, but no deaths occurred. Bacterial superinfection was documented in 30.3% of the cases; bronchospasm occurred in 17% of the recruits with pneumonia. In one study, seven children with massive and bilateral lung consolidation had clinical findings consistent with adult respiratory distress syndrome.[6]

Clinically, young infants have a picture of bronchiolitis with expiratory distress. In severe cases at all ages, a marked ventilation-perfusion deficit is noted.[294,389] Patients with defects in the cell-mediated immune system are particularly prone to progressive fatal bilateral infection.[141,264,329,331,442,445]

Secondary bacterial pneumonia is the result of common respiratory pathogens, particularly *Streptococcus pneumoniae, Haemophilus influenzae, Streptococcus pyogenes,* and *Staphylococcus aureus.* Coinfection with other viruses also was noted in an extensive study of measles-associated pneumonia in the Philippines.[404] In this study, parainfluenza virus and adenoviruses were isolated most frequently.

Other Respiratory Manifestations

Otitis media is the most common complication and is age related. In the immediate prevaccine era in the United States, otitis media developed in 5% to 15% of patients with measles. It now is less of a problem because of the change in the age-related incidence of measles. The bacterial pathogens in otitis media associated with measles are similar to those in otitis media in children without measles. Mastoiditis was a common complication of measles in the era before antibiotics, but fortunately today it is rare.

Laryngitis and mild laryngotracheitis occur commonly. Occasionally, frank, severe laryngotracheobronchitis occurs and may require tracheotomy.[417,418] Measles-associated bacterial tracheitis is not an uncommon finding.[110] Secondary bacterial infection of the cervical lymph nodes and secondary bacterial pharyngitis also are rather frequent complications of measles. Field[146] attributed 3.2% of cases of childhood bronchiectasis to former infection with measles virus.[146] Measles also has a deleterious effect on the course of tuberculosis.[448,449]

Cardiac Manifestations

Myocarditis and pericarditis occasionally occur in cases of measles.[126,147] Nonspecific, transient electrocardiographic abnormalities were noted in more than half of 71 children with measles in one study.[417,418] In another study, 19% of patients had transient but clear-cut abnormalities, including T-wave changes, atrioventricular conduction defects, and premature auricular contractions.[181] Although cardiac involvement appears to occur frequently in measles, clinical consequences from such involvement are rare developments.

Neurologic Manifestations

Neurologic involvement is not an uncommon finding in patients with measles.* Gibbs and associates noted that 51% of 680 patients with measles who had no clinical evidence of encephalitis had abnormal electroencephalographic results during acute or immediate postacute illness. Although the incidence varies, clinically evident encephalitis occurs in 0.5 to 1 of every 1000 measles cases.[25,78,80,100,140,247] From 1962 to 1979, the average measles encephalitis-to-case ratio was 0.73:1000.[78,80] Both mortality and the incidence of sequelae have varied in the reports available. LaBoccetta and Tornay[281] noted a mortality rate of 32% in

*References 5, 26, 38, 140, 143, 177, 185, 281, 297, 316, 384, 402, 470, 510.

50 patients in a group seen before 1947 and a rate of 11.5% in a group seen between 1947 and 1957. Ziegra[510] reported only two deaths in a group of 38 cases. Long-term morbidity data also vary considerably. In general, between 20% and 40% of patients who recover from measles encephalitis have manifestations of brain damage. Douglas[134] could find no evidence of later subnormal school performance in a group of children who had uncomplicated measles.

Symptoms of encephalitis usually develop during the period of measles exanthem and within 8 days of the onset of illness.[5,281,416] Occasionally, the onset of CNS signs and symptoms occurs during the prodromal period. LaBoccetta and Tornay[281] noted the following frequencies of signs and symptoms at the onset of measles encephalitis: convulsions, 56%; lethargy, 46%; coma, 28%; and irritability, 26%. Patients with encephalitis frequently have multiple findings: headache, abnormalities in respiratory rate and rhythm, twitching and other involuntary movements, and disorientation. Cerebellar ataxia, myelitis, retrobulbar neuritis, transient mental disorders, and hemiplegia are findings noted during the subacute stages of illness. Long-term sequelae include various degrees of retardation and selective brain damage, recurrent seizures, deafness, and hemiplegia and paraplegia. An 8-year-old girl developed pseudotumor cerebri 3 weeks after having a case of measles.[461]

Examination of cerebrospinal fluid (CSF) in measles encephalitis usually reveals mild pleocytosis with a predominance of mononuclear cells, mildly elevated protein values, and a normal glucose level.[281,316,374,470] In one study, in 15% of the cases, CSF pleocytosis was not found.[281]

Considerable controversy relates to the mechanisms in measles encephalitis.* Some investigators failed to isolate measles virus or to demonstrate measles virus RNA or other viral antigens in the brain of affected patients.[175,243,252,336] These findings led to the widespread consensus that the illness is autoimmune (acute disseminated encephalomyelitis [ADEM]) and that viral invasion of the CSF is unnecessary. However, other investigators have recovered measles virus from the CSF and brain of affected patients, a finding indicating that the virus is involved directly in the process.[143,153,316,464] In the hamster model of measles virus encephalitis, virus can be cultured directly from the brain.[387]

Other Manifestations

Measles has been associated with many other manifestations and complications. Of historical interest was the occurrence of a severe, often fatal, form of measles called *black measles* that was characterized by a confluent hemorrhagic skin eruption.[278] Patients with this illness had signs of both encephalitis or encephalopathy and pneumonia. Extensive bleeding from the mouth, nose, and bowel frequently occurred. Severe hemorrhagic measles rarely is seen today, and little is known about its pathogenesis. Disseminated intravascular coagulation would appear to play a role.

Another complication of measles involving bleeding is thrombocytopenic purpura.[6,225] It is a postinfectious illness and different from hemorrhagic measles. Although bleeding is extensive on occasion, the ultimate prognosis usually is good. Stevens-Johnson syndrome has been noted occasionally in measles.[305] Other manifestations include pneumomediastinum, subcutaneous emphysema, hepatitis, appendicitis, ileocolitis, mesenteric lymphadenitis, cervicitis, acute glomerulonephritis, corneal ulceration, and gangrene of the extremities.[159,215,247,253,278,291,318,338,359,441,466,502] Measles in pregnancy results in significant maternal and fetal morbidity and mortality.[23,138,238,343,450] Jespersen and associates[238] retrospectively reviewed 10 epidemics of measles in Greenland; these investigators obtained adequate data on 327 women infected during pregnancy, and they also were able to examine 252 of the offspring. Thirty-two percent of women infected during the first trimester had spontaneous abortions, and 9% of these pregnancies that continued to term resulted in stillbirths. Congenital malformations occurred in 8 of 300 live-born infants.[238] Pneumonia is a frequent maternal complication of measles during pregnancy.[23,138]

Clinical measles shortly before birth in the mother-to-be has resulted in congenital infection and illness in the neonate.[176] Congenital measles is often severe, with death occurring in approximately 32%.

*References 7, 149, 153, 175, 195, 196, 241–243, 252, 316, 336, 350, 391, 397, 464.

Subacute Sclerosing Panencephalitis

SSPE is an uncommon, slowly progressive disease of the CNS, with an almost invariably fatal outcome. The disease was recognized by a number of investigators early in the 20th century.[53,120,425] Several early accounts, especially those published by Dawson in 1933,[120] suggested a viral origin of this disease; however, not until the mid-1960s was measles virus clearly demonstrated to be the causative agent.[42,43,94,111,221,391,463] Today, SSPE is extremely rare in countries, such as the United States, where measles is no longer epidemic. However, in countries where measles is still endemic, it is still a relatively common occurrence.[24,202,211,227,228,256]

Epidemiology

The estimated incidence of SSPE after wild-type measles virus infection in the prevaccine era was approximately one case per 100,000 population. The incidence of SSPE in the prevaccine era in some developing nations greatly exceeded that of developed nations. In southern India the incidence of SSPE was as high as 21 per 100,000 population,[426] and in Pakistan the rate was estimated to be 100 per 100,000.[266] A report from Papua New Guinea suggested a similarly high incidence of SSPE.[296] Several characteristics of natural measles virus infection in developing countries in the prevaccine era were associated with the development of SSPE and included the high incidence of measles and the frequent occurrence of measles in children younger than 2 years. Both these risk factors for SSPE are modifiable, if not preventable, by vaccination.

The disease has been reported in all countries of the world, and although no outbreaks have been reported, clustering of cases prompted suggestions that environmental factors or unique strains of viruses may contribute to the development of SSPE after measles. The epidemiologic study of SSPE in the Netherlands described four cases of SSPE that occurred in 1 year in one city of 120,000 people, a number that calculated to four cases of SSPE per 6000 cases of measles, a rate 10-fold greater than that for the rest of the country.[33]

The incidence of SSPE in the prevaccine era was approximately five times higher in the southeastern United States than that in other regions of the country,[206,233,334] also suggesting the possibility of environmental cofactors. In addition, in the prevaccine era, a preponderance of cases of SSPE occurred in the United States, as well as in other developed and developing countries, in children from rural areas, independent of the incidence of measles in these areas.[63,64,206,299,333] SSPE appears to have no racial predilection, although the largest number of cases occur in whites.[231,334] The incidence of SSPE consistently is two to three times more common in male than in female patients.[33,231] No relationship between any HLA genotype and the development of SSPE has been demonstrated, and cases of SSPE in only one member of identical twins have been reported.[106,130,224] The usual age at presentation in the prevaccine era was between 6 and 10 years, with ranges of 2 to 35 years reported.[33,164,165,206] The youngest case reported was in a 10-month-old child, and the oldest was in a 52-year-old man with depressed cellular immunity.[39,459] In most cases, symptoms attributable to SSPE begin 4 to 8 years after measles virus infection; however, in some series, older patients (>10 years) appeared to have experienced a prolonged interval between measles virus infection and the development of SSPE.[33,231,334]

Although several risk factors for the development of SSPE have been demonstrated repeatedly, the most consistent is the acquisition of measles before reaching the second birthday.[33,129,206,334,426] An estimated minimum of 50% of those with SSPE have had early measles.[206] In India, an estimated 60% of measles infections occurred before the patients reached 2 years of age, a factor possibly contributing to the high incidence of SSPE in the United States.[426] Other risk factors have included exposure to animals.[206]

The decreased incidence of SSPE after institution of an effective measles vaccine program was demonstrated in several countries.[33,51,89,91,326,375,486] The incidence of SSPE in the Netherlands decreased 10-fold after universal vaccination was initiated.[33] The incidence in Japan decreased at least 10-fold and possibly more.[375] Development of SSPE after receipt of measles vaccination has been noted to occur. In a case-control study of patients with SSPE in the United States, 17 of 52 patients (32.7%) with SSPE had received measles vaccine before they developed disease.[206] Similarly, SSPE occurring after measles immunization was noted in the Netherlands, but the incidence of vaccine-related SSPE was less than one case per 2.5 million immunizations.[33] In Japan, the estimated incidence of measles vaccine–related SSPE was 0.9 cases per million doses of vaccine.[375] An inherent problem common to all of these studies was the inability to identify patients with subclinical, wild-type measles virus infection before they received vaccination. Subclinical measles virus infections are thought to be common in developing countries, as illustrated by studies from India that suggested that as many as 20% to 40% of patients with measles may have had a subclinical or unrecognized infection.[426]

In the United States, the success of measles immunization clearly resulted in a profound reduction in the incidence of SSPE.[51,89,91,486] In the earlier years of the immunization program in the United States, rare cases of SSPE developed in vaccinees. Some of these children and perhaps all of them had unrecognized measles infection before they were vaccinated, and the SSPE was caused by the natural measles virus infection and not the vaccine virus.[486] We are unaware of any cases of SSPE in the United States since the year 2000 that can be attributed to measles vaccine virus.

Bellini and associates[35] studied brain samples from 11 patients with SSPE during the period 1992 to 2003. Nine of the patients in this group had a history of measles immunization. Nonetheless, in all 11 cases, the measles virus genotype identified was that of wild measles and was not consistent with vaccine virus. These researchers attributed the measles infections to the epidemic that occurred in the United States from 1989 through 1991.

In the period 1989 through 1997, 55,622 measles cases were reported. From these data, a rate of 22 cases of SSPE per 100,000 reported cases of measles was calculated. This rate is approximately 10 times higher than previous estimates in the United States and similar to those noted in developing countries in the prevaccine era.[266,296,426] In Germany, from 2003 to 2009, there were 39 SSPE cases. The rate of SSPE was calculated as one case per 1700 to 3300 measles cases in children less than 5 years of age.[434]

Pathogenesis and Pathology

Autopsy specimens from patients who died of SSPE reveal mild to striking changes in the gross appearance of the cerebral cortex, with ventriculomegaly in some cases. Histopathologic changes include minimal meningeal cellular infiltrate, with a perivascular accumulation of lymphocytes and plasma cells. Within involved areas of the brain, dense infiltrates of T lymphocytes and marked cellular expression of MHC class II antigens have been described.[56] A prominent microglial and astrocytic hyperplasia often is present. One of the characteristics of SSPE is the presence of intranuclear and cytoplasmic inclusion bodies.

The study of these structures by electron microscopy in 1965 led to the finding of paramyxovirus-like particles in autopsy material.[54,463] Subsequently, Connolly and colleagues[111] described the presence of measles virus antibody in the CSF of patients with SSPE, as well as the presence of measles virus antigens in brain tissue from autopsy specimens of patients who had SSPE. Shortly thereafter, several laboratories reported the recovery of defective measles virus in specimens of brain from patients with SSPE.[56,220,221] Virus was isolated only by cocultivation and not as cell-free material. Together, these findings suggested that SSPE was caused by a persistent infection of the brain by measles virus.

Several mechanisms, such as an abnormal host immune response to a common infection or a mutant virus, have elicited the most interest. Available data suggest that it may be a combination of these two possibilities. Several observations of the natural history of SSPE are consistent with an abnormal host immune response to a primary measles infection. They include the following: (1) the chronicity of measles virus infection in children with SSPE indicated a failure to eliminate the agent; (2) the importance of early acquisition of measles virus in the development of SSPE suggested that the immature immune system may predispose the host to a persistent infection; and (3) the onset of clinical disease long after a primary infection also suggested a failure of a previously protective immune response. Early on, the consensus was that patients with SSPE had subtle defects in cellular immune responses as measured by decreased cutaneous reactivity to common skin test antigens, decreased lymphocyte proliferative responses to mitogens and measles virus antigens, and reduced production of cytokines. Subsequent studies failed to confirm these conclusions, and most investigators now suggest that patients with SSPE can generate vigorous cellular immune responses after exposure to mitogen and measles-specific antigens. [56] Studies demonstrated the presence of several cytokines, including IL-1b, IL-2, IL-6, TNF, heat-labile toxin, and IFN-γ, as well as other markers of immune activation, in brain lesions from patients with SSPE.[56] Still, some debate continues about the immunocompetence of patients with SSPE. Finally, measles virus is associated with chronic progressive encephalitis in immunocompromised patients (measles inclusion body encephalitis); however, the clinical course and histologic findings of this disease clearly are different from those of SSPE.

In contrast to the questions that surround the cellular response to measles virus in patients with SSPE, antibody responses to measles virus–encoded proteins are well preserved. Antibodies of all isotypes are produced peripherally and within the CNS. Antibodies against all the proteins encoded by measles, including the M (matrix) protein, have been detected in the sera from patients with SSPE.[56] The paradox of elevated levels of circulating antimeasles antibody as well as CSF antimeasles antibody in the presence of persistent infection suggested a possible immune-mediated origin of this disease. Evidence was presented that antimeasles antibody could interfere with spread of the virus and syncytial formation. Fujinami and Oldstone[164] demonstrated that antimeasles antibody reversibly could modulate the intracellular expression of measles virus–encoded proteins, thereby providing a mechanism by which antiviral antibody could convert an acute productive infection into a chronic persistent infection. This decrease in expression of measles antigen also could shelter virus-infected cells from immunologic recognition. This hypothesis also is supported by observations suggesting that early acquisition of measles predisposes the individual to the development of SSPE because the limited quantity of passively acquired maternal antimeasles antibody may be insufficient to prevent development of infection and dissemination of measles virus but adequate to modulate expression of measles virus. This series of events then would predispose the patient to the development of a chronic persistent infection. Animal models consistent with this disease mechanism have been described.[56]

The second general mechanism for the development of SSPE is the generation of viral mutants during acute infection that then can establish a persistent infection. Persistence may result from antigenic variability or a viral mutation leading to decreased production of viral proteins below a level recognizable by the immune system or an extension of cell tropism. That measles viruses from the CNS of patients with SSPE are defective in replication is well documented. Analysis of these isolates does not define a virulence feature of SSPE strains but does suggest several mechanisms that could account for the generation of viral mutants. Much interest has been focused on the decreased expression of the M protein in explants of brain tissue from patients with SSPE.[56] This viral phenotype also was consistent with the decreased production of anti-M antibody in patients with SSPE, a finding suggesting the possibility of subthreshold production of antigen in these patients. Although the decreased expression of M protein was proposed originally as the mechanism for the persistence of mutant measles virus in patients with SSPE, subsequent studies showed that this is only one of many mutant phenotypes in strains of measles virus associated with SSPE.

Further studies of the replication of measles virus revealed several mechanisms that favor the production of mutant viruses. The RNA polymerase of measles viruses, like that of other RNA viruses, does not have proofreading functions and therefore frequently misincorporates nucleotides.[67] Thus mutant progeny virus arises regularly and can be selected either by host immune responses or because of its extended host-cell tropism. In addition to this general mechanism of genetic diversity in RNA viruses, measles virus also exhibits what has been described originally as biased hypermutation and more recently as A/I hypermutation.[68,69] This mutational event results in clusters of U (uridine) to C (cytidine) or A (adenosine) to G (guanosine) transitions, possibly as the result of novel host-derived enzymatic activity referred to as *double-stranded RNA unwindase.*[56] This activity results in the replacement of A residues with inosines in duplex RNA molecules formed between genomic RNA and mRNA. Replication of the inosine-modified genomic strand then results in the replacement of U by C. Evidence of this proposed mutational event has been found in the genomes of measles viruses from the brains of patients with SSPE, in which up to 132 of a possible 266 U residues in the M coding sequence were converted to C.[67]

Studies clearly demonstrated that the M gene is the most heavily mutated of measles virus genes, often with early stop codons. Researchers stressed that this mechanism of genetic change is operative during lytic as well as persistent infection, and mutants that persist must do so as the result of growth advantage, such as evasion of the host immune response. The frequent mutations found in the M gene suggest that the measles virus can tolerate extensive genetic change in the M protein yet still replicate within cells of the CNS. The finding of clonal spread of a hypermutated measles virus genome within the brain of a patient with SSPE is consistent with this hypothesis.[28] Kweder and associates[280] have noted that B3 genotype viral strains have not been associated with SSPE cases. These B3 strains do not have the PEA motif in their M protein. Other genes of the measles virus also exhibit mutations that alter function, including the gene encoding the hemagglutinin (H) protein. Mutations of this protein were shown to limit cell surface expression but not the function of hemagglutinin in the replicative cycle of measles virus.[41] Cells infected with this phenotype likely are poorly recognized by the immune system because of the limited cell surface expression of the H protein, yet enough functional activity remains to allow spread of the mutant virus within the CNS by a mechanism of cell-to-cell fusion. Thus the generation of measles viruses that can induce disease and establish persistent infections results from viral strategies of genetic diversity coupled with selective pressure of the host immune response.

Clinical Manifestations

The initial stage of the disease can be described best as a period of progressive psychointellectual disturbances.[202,413] These disturbances can include lability of mood, deterioration of school performance, hyperactivity or lethargy, depression, and occasionally altered states of consciousness. Although retrospective analysis often allows precise definition of the onset of SSPE to be established, many of these disturbances are so subtle that they escape parental or physician detection. Physical findings vary and often are nonspecific. A peculiar pigmented retinopathy has been observed in a small number of patients.[65] The duration in stage I varies, depending on the clinical staging system, but in larger series, this stage is relatively short, usually lasting fewer than 6 months.[413] The duration in stage I appeared to be prolonged in older patients compared with patients younger than 10 years in the series from the Netherlands.[33] Accelerated progression to stage II has been reported.[413]

Stage II is characterized best by a variety of convulsive and motor disorders. The motor disorders are striking, ranging from akinetic drop attacks to violent myoclonic jerks. The motor disturbances have been described consistently as stereotypic and rhythmic. Rigidity or spasticity may be present in the later part of this stage.[56] Extrapyramidal findings, such as choreoathetotic and ballistic movements, as well as parkinsonism with abnormalities in the basal ganglia, have been reported. Intellectual functions continue to deteriorate, but patients may retain receptive function during this stage. In one series of patients, as many as 50% with stage II disease had abnormal retinal findings, including optic atrophy. The duration of this stage is quite protracted; as many as 50% of patients remain in this stage for longer than 6 months, and as many as 20% remain so for more than 1 year.

Progression to stage III is suggested by increased frequency of myoclonic jerks, development of spasticity or rigidity, and decerebrate and decorticate posturing. Hypothalamic dysfunction becomes prominent, with hyperpyrexia, diaphoresis, and periods of pallor and flushing. Cortical activity rapidly decreases, and patients usually become comatose in this preterminal stage of disease. Duration of this stage is relatively short, lasting fewer than 6 months in most cases. Death usually is associated with complications that accompany the vegetative state, although destruction of essential structures within the brainstem or hypothalamus may result in death.

The previous descriptions account for most patients with SSPE; however, a significant number may exhibit a less predictable course. Some 5% to 10% of patients can be expected to have a prolonged survival measured in years. These patients may progress to stage II or III and then remain static without relapse, or they can experience a periodic and sometimes fatal relapse of disease. Conversely, some 10% of patients may have a fulminant, rapidly progressive course lasting less than 3 months.[184,300,416]

Laboratory Findings

The definitive diagnosis of SSPE relies on a combination of laboratory findings and a compatible clinical course. Before the association between measles and SSPE was made, the electroencephalogram (EEG) was extremely helpful in establishing the diagnosis.[160,161,306,413] The classic pattern of the EEG in SSPE is described as periodic, synchronous, bilateral discharges with a frequency of 3 to 20 seconds.[108] The discharge contains high-amplitude polyphasic slow-wave complexes, often consisting of two or more delta waves.[306] Frequently, the background of the EEG is suppressed, thus creating the familiar burst suppression pattern. The EEG provides little help in predicting progression of SSPE. Also of note is that the absence of the classic findings, as well as other abnormalities on the EEG, has been reported in patients with SSPE.[160,161,227,228,240] Alternatively, the finding of periodic generalized bursts of fast waves should prompt consideration of SSPE.[309]

More recent advances in imaging technology have aided greatly in the diagnosis of SSPE. Computed tomographic (CT) scans are abnormal in more than 50% of patients with SSPE, but the findings often are nonspecific.[56,114,125,135,345] In the later stages of the disease, cortical atrophy often is a prominent finding on CT scan. Magnetic resonance imaging (MRI) of patients with SSPE has revealed the presence of focal lesions consistent with inflammation, often in the white matter, in multiple areas of the brain.[125] In some cases the location of abnormalities detected by MRI closely reflects the clinical symptoms of the patient, whereas in others the MRI findings do not correlate with clinical findings.[462] Finally, brain biopsy has been used as an important means of establishing the diagnosis in the past and still is of considerable value in atypical cases.

Perhaps the most useful laboratory examination of the patient with suspected SSPE is the examination of the CSF. Normal to slightly increased levels of protein with an absolute increase in the γ-globulin fraction are a consistent finding in patients with SSPE.[240] Furthermore, the increase in the γ-globulin fraction is caused almost exclusively by elevation of immunoglobulin.[443,480] Additional studies showed that 20% to 40% of the CSF IgG was oligoclonal and that the oligoclonal fraction contained antimeasles antibodies.[474,475] This finding almost is pathognomonic for SSPE in patients with compatible clinical presentations. All isotypes of antibodies have been found in the CSF, although the finding of IgM antimeasles antibody remains controversial.[56,141,222,482] Because the levels of antimeasles antibodies within the CSF are elevated, as well as oligoclonal, most investigators contend that these antibodies are produced locally within the CNS, apparently in response to ongoing measles virus replication. Other CSF findings include normal levels of glucose and slight pleocytosis consisting primarily of lymphocytes. Patients with SSPE have normal to elevated levels of circulating antimeasles antibody; in some cases, this antibody response also appears clonally restricted.[56]

Treatment

In the past, 5-bromo-2-deoxyuridine, transfer factor, ribavirin, and amantadine proved to be of little value.[56] In the 1970s, the antiviral agent inosiplex was introduced and was thought to have antiviral activity in vivo and in vitro, although this claim remains controversial. Some studies suggested that treatment with inosiplex may result in stabilization, prolongation of survival, or actual clinical improvement in as many as 50% to 60% of patients. In a large study, 98 patients with SSPE were treated continuously, and their actuarial survival was compared with that of 500 historical controls.[244] The results of this study showed that median survival for the treated patients was 3.2 years compared with 1.2 years for the historical controls. The use of historical controls, however, raised a number of questions about the validity of the results. The results of this trial also suggested a greater benefit of treatment with inosiplex in patients with more slowly progressive SSPE. Other studies did not demonstrate any efficacy of inosiplex.[56] Inosiplex and intrathecal IFN-α seem to elicit transient improvement in some patients.[136,137,279,301,332] IFN-β combined with inosiplex also may offer benefit in patients with SSPE.[16] Other treatment approaches that may have shown some benefit in children include levetiracetam, ribavirin, amantadine, cimetidine, corticosteroids, plasmapheresis, and intravenous immunoglobulin.[31]

Measles in Developing Countries

Measles has been and continues to be a staggering problem in developing countries. The mortality rate in much of Africa was approximately 10%,[372] and a reasonable assumption is that the rates are similar in some regions of Asia.[121,396,414,460] In developing countries, measles is a disease of young children. For example, in Kenya in the prevaccine era, 25% to 30% of children contracted measles before reaching their first birthday, and 55% to 60% did so before they were 2 years of age; virtually all children had measles by the time they were 4 years old.[212] In Kenyan children, mortality peaked in the 17- to 20-month age group, and the median age for hospital admission was 14 months.

Although many factors, such as the age at infection, suboptimal medical facilities, and failure to seek medical care, contribute to the excessive morbidity and mortality in children of developing countries, the single overriding factor generally has been thought to be the nutritional status of the infected children.[340-342,372] The data of O'Donovan[372] clearly indicate a direct relationship between malnutrition and hospital admissions for measles and deaths. Studies by Coovadia and colleagues[113] and by Carney and associates[66] indicated both humoral and cell-mediated defects in protein-calorie malnutrition. The clinical picture of measles in children with malnutrition is frequently similar to that in patients with known defects in cell-mediated functions.

Low serum retinol concentrations nearly always are present in children with measles in developing countries.[29,116,226,231,307,408,476] Low retinol levels correlate directly with measles mortality, and treatment with vitamin A reduces this mortality rate.[29,226,307] Studies performed since the 1980s indicate that the intensive exposure that occurs in children in developing countries is a major factor in measles mortality.[1,3,172]

Clinical Manifestations

Measles in children in developing countries is characterized by two different types of severe disease. One type of illness is a fulminant, toxic illness without apparent localizing complications. The other is a more prolonged illness with obvious complications; the complications may be caused by infection with secondary bacterial or other infectious agents, persistent measles virus infection, or a combination of both.

In a group of 507 hospitalized children, O'Donovan[372] noted that 301 had pneumonia, 96 had gastroenteritis, 36 had croup, 11 had convulsions, 67 had two or more complications, and 140 had nonlocalized systemic toxic effects. The measles rash in malnourished children tends to result in greater confluence and progresses to dark red and then violet.[340,342] Desquamation is marked and occurs in large scales.[430] After desquamation, patchy depigmentation lasts for some weeks. Other common problems are stomatitis and the resultant sore mouth, which leads to further loss of nutritional intake. Acute corneal ulceration, which occurs after measles in malnourished children, is a common cause of blindness.[427] Multiple skin abscesses and noma (cancrum oris) are rare secondary infectious problems.[247]

Measles in Immunocompromised Hosts

Today, because of the extensive use of immunosuppressive therapeutic modalities and greater duration of survival in certain rapidly fatal diseases, a sizable population of children and adults is immunologically compromised. Measles virus infection in a patient with disease-induced or iatrogenically caused immune deficiency usually is severe and protracted and frequently is fatal.

The most common severe measles virus infection in an immunocompromised host is giant-cell pneumonia.[141,264,320,329,330,406,442] The mode of manifestation of this illness varies. Some patients initially have severe but otherwise typical measles after a normal incubation period. Clinical findings at the time of the exanthem indicate pulmonary involvement and respiratory distress, and radiographic findings become rapidly worse over a period of about a week or less. Other patients initially have rather vague illness, frequently without rash. In these cases, the pulmonary process may progress over the course of a month or longer. Siegel and associates[442] reported a child with leukemia who recovered from typical measles and then died the following year of diffuse interstitial pneumonia in which characteristic measles giant cells were seen.

A unique form of measles encephalitis also is manifested in immunosuppressed patients.[8,160,161,208,321,345,348,403,469,497] Although the symptoms in different described cases varied, the illness appears to be intermediate between the acute encephalitis occurring in patients without known immune defects and the chronic picture of SSPE. The incubation period has varied between 5 weeks and 6 months.[8] Convulsions frequently are the initial symptom, and they are a prominent aspect of the illness. The seizures have been focal, unilateral, or permanent localized twitching. Other findings include hemiplegia, stupor, coma, hypertonia, and slurred speech. Most cases have been fatal, and the duration of illness has been from 1 week to 2 months. It should be noted that successfully treated children with leukemia, solid tumors, and Hodgkin disease lose humoral immunity to measles and thus should all be revaccinated.[52]

DIFFERENTIAL DIAGNOSIS

The differential diagnosis of typical measles must include all illnesses in which an erythematous maculopapular rash occurs (see Chapter 58). The following are most important in establishing the diagnosis of measles: a consideration of possible exposure; the duration of the incubation period; the presence of Koplik spots; the presence of the typical febrile prodrome with cough, coryza, and conjunctivitis; and progression of the rash in a caudal direction. The brown discoloration and the intensity of the measles rash are such that the illness usually should not be confused with rubella, erythema infectiosum, roseola infantum, or enteroviral infection. Of greatest differential difficulty are the exanthems of infectious mononucleosis, *Mycoplasma pneumoniae* infection, and drug eruptions.

In the past, atypical measles was extremely difficult to diagnose. Today for children born in the United States, this disease will occur only in adults aged 50 years or older. The key to diagnosing this illness is careful elicitation of an accurate vaccination history. Even if it is not known whether the vaccination that the patient received as a child was live or killed vaccine, it usually can be determined by the number of doses given; if a child received more than one dose of vaccine in a short interval, killed vaccine almost certainly was administered. Differential considerations in atypical measles include Rocky Mountain spotted fever, anaphylactoid purpura, *M. pneumoniae* infection, and drug eruptions.

DIAGNOSIS

Measles virus infection can be diagnosed specifically by the following methods: isolation of virus in an appropriate tissue culture system; demonstration of measles antigen in exfoliated cells and tissues by FA techniques or polymerase chain reaction (PCR)[312]; or the demonstration of a rise in HI, CF, ELISA, FA, or neutralizing antibody titer in two sequential serum samples or specific measles IgM antibody in a single serum sample (see Chapter 253).

In the recent past, measles was usually diagnosed by the demonstration of specific IgM antibody in an acute-phase serum specimen. False-positive IgM enzyme immunoassay results may occur.[71,73,76,90,237,472] Perhaps more importantly, false-negative results may occur in secondary vaccine failure cases. These patients may have vigorous IgG measles antibody response but no IgM response. Therefore, today, the preferred diagnostic method is the detection of measles RNA by reverse transcriptase PCR or by culture.[72,74] Virus can be detected in samples from the throat, nasopharynx, and urine.

TREATMENT

Uncomplicated Measles

No specific therapy for uncomplicated measles exists. During the febrile period of illness, activity should be discouraged, and fluid status should be maintained by the liberal provision of soft drinks and ice. Fever may be controlled with acetaminophen. Coughing frequently is distressing and can be managed by the judicious use of common antitussive agents. Room humidification also is useful in controlling the cough and generally can be expected to make the patient more comfortable. As the fever disappears, a gradual return to normal activity is indicated. However, measles virus infection is associated with considerable damage to the ciliated epithelium of the respiratory tract; therefore, resumption of normal activities too soon and exposure to other children and their bacterial pathogens can be associated with severe secondary infection.

Children in developing countries frequently have vitamin A deficiency. Measles morbidity correlates with this deficiency, and treatment with vitamin A is beneficial.[29,116,226,231,307,408,476] Studies in the United States indicate that vitamin A levels are low in a substantial number of measles cases and that morbidity is increased in these deficient children.[12,19,62,162] Vitamin A supplementation also has been shown to enhance IgG antibody levels and total lymphocyte numbers.[117] In 1993, the Committee on Infectious Diseases of the American Academy of Pediatrics recommended providing vitamin A supplementation for children with measles in selected circumstances.[12,14] Vitamin A was recommended for children aged 6 months to 2 years who require hospitalization and all patients 6 months or older with immune deficiencies or possible vitamin A deficiency. The World Health Organization now recommends vitamin A for all children with measles in all countries.[12,13] The doses are: 200,000 IU for children 12 months or older; 100,000 IU for infants 6 through 11 months of age; and 50,000 IU for infants younger than 6 months of age. Following this, an additional age-specific dose should be given 2 through 4 weeks later in children with clinical signs and symptoms of vitamin A deficiency.

Atypical Measles

The most important aspect of therapy for atypical measles is proper diagnosis. In patients with atypical measles, Rocky Mountain spotted fever, other septic conditions, lymphoma, or collagen vascular disease frequently is diagnosed erroneously, and their workup is associated with extensive blood cultures, other diagnostic procedures, and vigorous antibiotic therapy. Careful attention given to a history of previous administration of killed measles vaccine should clarify the diagnosis and preclude the unnecessary trauma associated with extensive diagnostic and therapeutic procedures.

In atypical measles, chest radiographs always should be obtained because the pneumonia that usually develops in these patients frequently is much more extensive than the clinical findings would indicate. Activity should be discouraged in acutely ill patients, and follow-up chest radiographs should be used as a guide to resumption of normal activity. In some patients, pulmonary abnormalities have persisted for a considerable period.

Complications of Measles

Otitis Media

Otitis media is the most frequent complication of measles. The infectious agent of otitis media in measles is no different from that in other children without measles of comparable age, so conventional antibiotic therapy is all that is necessary (see Chapter 16).

Laryngotracheitis

Management of the laryngotracheitis caused by measles virus infection is similar to that in other patients with croup caused by other viral etiologic agents. Administration of corticosteroids is contraindicated in measles, and antibiotics are indicated only in patients with laboratory or clinical evidence of secondary bacterial infection (see Chapter 18).

Pneumonia

Pneumonia is a common complication of measles, and it is the leading cause of death. Pneumonia may be a manifestation of primary viral infection, or it may result from a superimposed bacterial infection. The differential diagnosis between primary viral and superimposed bacterial disease cannot be made with certainty. Because the diagnosis of viral pneumonia often is uncertain, most patients should be treated with antibiotics. In primary measles pneumonia, treatment with aerosolized ribavirin should be considered.

In one uncontrolled study in adult patients, intravenous ribavirin was found to be well tolerated, and its use was associated with clinical improvement.[155] In a study in pregnant women, Atmar and associates[23] were unable to demonstrate clear clinical benefit with the administration of aerosolized ribavirin.

Encephalitis

The course of measles encephalitis is unpredictable, and treatment is symptomatic and supportive. Trained nursing care is essential. Careful attention given to fluid and electrolyte balance is necessary. In prolonged states of coma, parenteral hyperalimentation is indicated. Status epilepticus should be treated vigorously with the use of a structured protocol for ensuring optimal control (see Chapter 36).

Numerous review articles indicate that measles encephalitis is a postinfectious encephalitis and is predominantly a disease of white matter (ADEM).[192,241,242] This concept resulted from a study of 19 patients with measles encephalitis that was published in 1984 by Johnson and associates.[243] I am aware of only two patients subsequent to this article who had ADEM associated with measles virus infection. Clinical evidence supports the finding that ADEM not related to measles virus infection is responsive to corticosteroid therapy.[152,315]

Considerable evidence indicates that measles encephalitis usually is not ADEM and that active direct CNS infection is involved in the process.[143,153,316,392,464] A controlled trial of 32 children with measles encephalitis failed to find benefit in the corticosteroid-treated group.[510] These data suggest to us that corticosteroids should not be used to treat measles encephalitis unless evidence of ADEM is clear and active measles virus infection has subsided. In patients with severe intractable seizures or other evidence of cerebral edema, the use of intravenous mannitol therapy (0.25–1 g/kg of a 20% solution administered over the course of a 30- to 60-minute period) is indicated. In occasional circumstances, respiratory arrest is a problem, and artificial ventilators should be used to tide patients over until respiration becomes normal. Mustafa and coworkers[348] noted improvement in an immunocompromised child with subacute measles encephalitis who was treated with intravenously administered ribavirin.

Appendicitis

Acute abdominal pain occurs occasionally in primary measles, and it can be caused by generalized mesenteric adenitis secondary to measles virus appendicitis. In appendicitis, evidence of measles virus involvement of the appendix is present. However, therapy should be similar to that in other cases of appendicitis; removal of the appendix is indicated because measles appendicitis perforates with a frequency equal to that in non–measles virus infection.

Prophylactic Antibiotics

In the developing world, secondary bacterial infections in measles are a major cause of mortality. Accordingly, interest has arisen in the use of antibiotics prophylactically.[93,437] A meta-analysis in 1997 of studies involving the use of prophylactic antibiotics noted that the available data were poor and provided only weak evidence for giving antibiotics to all children with measles.[437] The recommendation from this study was that antibiotics should be given only if a child has clinical signs of pneumonia or other evidence of sepsis. Chalmers[93] pointed out the necessity and urgency for performing controlled prophylactic trials.

PREVENTION

Active Immunization: Live, Attenuated Measles Virus Vaccine

The original attenuated measles vaccine was developed from the Edmonston strain of measles virus by passage in human kidney and human amnion tissue cultures, then in chicken embryos, and finally in chicken embryo fibroblast tissue culture.[455] Today in the United States, measles vaccines are prepared in chicken embryo fibroblast tissue culture. Vaccines available in other countries are prepared in chicken embryo fibroblast tissue culture, Japanese quail tissue culture, chicken embryo, and WI-38 tissue culture. Vaccination produces a mild or inapparent noncommunicable infection that induces active immunity in more than 95% of recipients. Following two doses of a measles-containing vaccine,

99% of vaccinees will be immune, and this immunity is long-lasting.[273,277,278] However, the decay in antibody values over time with the present measles vaccine used in the United States is greater than that following natural infection. It was noted by Chen and associates[96,308] that low levels of measles antibody (values <120 IU) were not protective against infection and illness. Today, there is a large population of previous two-dose vaccine recipients who have not had natural antibody boosts from wild virus exposure. Many of these people will get measles when exposed. One of us (J.D.C.) with colleagues at the California Department of Public Health has analyzed measles cases between 2000 and 2015 in California (J.D. Cherry and J Zipprich, unpublished data). In this study, 29 instances of secondary vaccine failure were noted. Illness in these patients was less severe than primary infections. and the patients were less contagious. Similar findings were noted in Canada in an epidemic in 2011.[122]

Symptoms associated with measles immunization are minimal and are limited to fever, mild malaise, and occasionally a faint rash occurring approximately 1 week after immunization. For complete information and recommendations related to measles immunization, refer to Chapter 245 and the most recent recommendations of the Advisory Committee on Immunization Practices,[22] the CDC "Pink Book,"[78,92] the Committee on Infectious Diseases of the American Academy of Pediatrics,[12,13] and the manufacturer's package insert. The vaccines in routine use in the United States today are measles-mumps-rubella (MMR) or measles-mumps-rubella-varicella (MMRV). Only a summary of recommendations is presented here.

Recommendations for Use

The widespread epidemics of measles in the United States in 1989 to 1991 were the result of a failure to immunize children at the appropriate age and the increased number of susceptible older children and adults because of vaccine failure.[21,82,83,90,287,308] Therefore continued eradication of measles in the United States depends on ongoing programs that (1) enroll all children of initial vaccination age and (2) allow revaccination of all persons whose primary vaccine failed. Because routine immunity testing is not a viable public health option, revaccination of primary vaccine failures can be accomplished only by universal reimmunization.

Currently, live measles vaccine is recommended in a two-dose schedule.[12,13,82,486] In general, live measles vaccine is recommended to be administered at 12 to 15 months of age and the second dose at entry into school.[9,12,13,22,79,84,273,277,438,486,493,505] However, the second dose can be given after any interval longer than 1 month after administration of the first dose.[29,78,92] Because of numerous importation cases in the United States in recent years, it is our opinion that the second dose of measles-containing vaccine should be given in the second year of life. The rationale for this suggestion is based on the fact that the one dose vaccine failure rate is 5%. Therefore, in the age group of 1 to 4 years, there are presently about 800,000 young children in the United States who are susceptible. Children who have not received vaccine during infancy may be immunized at any age, and adults who have not had natural measles also should be immunized. When measles is endemic or epidemic in a community, all children aged 6 months or older should be immunized. In children who initially were vaccinated before they were 12 months of age, a second vaccination should be administered at 12 to 15 months of age, and a third dose at entry into school is necessary to complete the schedule.

It should also be noted that persons born between 1962 and 1981 usually had received just one dose of vaccine. Many of the vaccine failures in this group will have been protected by herd immunity. In our opinion, persons in this group should be offered a second dose of a measles-contained vaccine or have their serum tested for measles IgG antibody.

Precautions

Measles vaccination should be deferred at times of febrile illness or when interference from another viral infection could cause failure of measles vaccine. Measles immunization also should be postponed for 3 to 11 months in persons who have received whole blood, blood plasma, or immunoglobulin because these products may contain sufficient measles antibody to neutralize the vaccine virus. The duration of postponement depends on the product administered and the dose.[12,13,22] Children treated with intravenous immunoglobulin for Kawasaki disease should not receive measles vaccine until 11 months after receiving the immunoglobulin, whereas 3 months' time is adequate for children given immunoglobulin for hepatitis A prophylaxis.

Contraindications

Live measles vaccine should not be administered to pregnant women or to some persons with diseases or therapeutic programs associated with impaired cell-mediated immunity. These conditions in general include the following: leukemia, lymphoma, or other generalized malignant diseases; primary and secondary immunologic disorders; and therapy with corticosteroids, radiation, antimetabolites, or alkylating agents. Measles immunization is recommended for children and adults with asymptomatic human immunodeficiency infection and for symptomatic patients who are not severely immunocompromised.[12-14]

Complications

Serious complications associated with administration of measles vaccine are exceedingly rare. Serious neurologic disease (encephalitis, Reye syndrome, cranial nerve palsy, cerebellar ataxia, and Guillain-Barré syndrome) within 30 days of immunization occurs at a rate of approximately one case per million doses of vaccine administered.[76,83,284] This rate is lower than the rate of occurrence of encephalitis of unknown cause in children for any 30-day period. However, the clustering of cases on days 8 and 9 after immunization noted from claims submitted to the National Vaccine Injury Compensation Program suggests that a causal relationship between measles vaccine and encephalopathy may be a rare complication of immunization.[487] In addition, recovery of measles virus from the CSF of a vaccinated child with encephalitis also suggests that rare vaccine-induced neurologic disease may occur.[153] In a large population-based study in Denmark between 1991 and 1998 it was found that MMR immunization was associated with a transient increased rate of febrile seizures.[477] However, the long-term rate of epilepsy was not increased in children who had febrile seizures after receiving vaccination compared with children who had febrile seizures related to other causative events. Studies in the United States and Canada also noted an increased risk for febrile seizures during the first 2 weeks after the first dose of MMR.[88,92] Further study noted that the risk for febrile seizures was significantly greater after MMRV than after MMR.[260,280,298] In a recent study, Klein and associates[260] found no increased risk for febrile seizures after the second dose of measles-containing vaccines in children 4 to 6 years of age. Thrombocytopenic purpura, anaphylaxis, hearing loss, and toxic epidermal necrolysis also have been associated with measles immunization.[11,27,32,236,428,439,454,492]

In developing countries, high-titer measles vaccines were used to induce seroconversion at a young age.[498] However, follow-up studies in some countries noted that the mortality rate was increased in female recipients of these high-titer vaccines over the course of a 3-year period compared with children who received conventional doses of vaccine.[218,261] Nonetheless, follow-up studies in other countries showed no increased mortality rates in recipients of high-titer measles vaccine.[3,288]

Global Progress Toward Measles Eradication

Measles has been a major cause of death in the developing world, with 750,000 deaths in 2000.[87] A World Health Organization (WHO) global immunization vision meeting in 2005 established a commitment to achieve a 90% reduction in measles mortality by 2010 compared with 2000.[499] This commitment focused on 47 priority countries in the developing world. The components of the strategy included achieving and maintaining high coverage (>90%) with routinely scheduled first dose of measles-containing vaccine among children aged 1 year and ensuring that all children receive a second opportunity for measles immunization. In 2007, 82% of the target population was vaccinated, but the coverage varied substantially by geographic region. During the period 2000 through 2007, the global measles mortality rate was reduced by 74% (from 750,000 deaths in 2000 to 197,000 deaths in 2007).

Endemic measles has been eliminated in North America, Sweden, Finland, and selected other countries in the world. In the WHO

European Region (EUR), substantial progress was made between 2003 and 2009 in eliminating measles.[77,89] However, since late 2009, measles outbreaks have become widespread. In 2010, 30,639 measles cases were reported in the EUR, and up to October 26, 2011, an additional 26,074 cases were reported. Most of the cases occurred in the western European subregion.

In 2011 in the EUR, 49.4% of the cases occurred in persons 15 years or older, 25% occurred in children younger than 5 years, and 24.7% occurred in children 5 to 14 years of age.[77,89] Of the reported cases in 2011, 54% occurred in France and 11% in Spain. Nine deaths occurred (six in France), and seven of these occurred in persons older than 10 years. In 2011, 90% of the cases occurred in unvaccinated persons or in persons with an unknown vaccination status.

In the EUR, the overall coverage with at least one dose of a measles-containing vaccine is below the target of 95%.[77,89] This is a particular problem in the western European subregion.

There are multiple reasons for the underuse of vaccines in the EUR.[77,89,346] In contrast to North America, compulsory school immunization laws do not exist in Western Europe. Some degree of herd immunity has allowed unvaccinated children to become susceptible adolescents and adults. Important and serious barriers to increasing population immunity in the EUR and, in particular, the western European subregion, are religious or philosophical objections to vaccination.[346]

Perry and associates[396] reviewed the progress toward regional measles elimination worldwide from 2000 to 2014. During the observation period, there was an increase in worldwide coverage with both first dose and second dose of measles-contained vaccines. There was a 73% decrease in reported measles incidence and a 79% reduction in estimated measles mortality. However, it was also noted that the 2015 goals of the WHO global vaccine action plan for 2011 to 2020 will not be met.[499,500]

Quarantine and Disease Containment

Before the use of measles vaccines became widespread, quarantine measures were practiced widely but were largely ineffective in preventing the spread of measles. However, containment of disease is practical today because the widespread use of measles vaccine has reduced the general number of susceptible young children and thus has decreased the rapidity of epidemic development. Epidemic measles now generally involves a greater age range of the population (cases in adolescents and young adults occur frequently), and progression of disease from one age group to another is slower than in epidemics that involve one uniform, largely susceptible population.

Containment is a vital part of the measles prevention policy in the United States. Measles is a reportable disease throughout the United States, and compliance is the obligation of all physicians. After receiving early reports of sporadic measles, health department workers can organize local immunization clinics so that the disease often can be contained in a small geographic area rather than developing into a widespread epidemic.

Passive Immunization: Immunoglobulin

In the present vaccine era, there should be little need for passive immunization. However, as seen in California in 2014 and 2015, there were a significant number of exposed personal-belief, nonvaccinated children and also exposed infants too young to have been vaccinated. Passive immunization is highly effective when given 7 days of exposure.[507,508] When a known susceptible child has had definite exposure to measles, immunoglobulin should be administered in a dose of 0.25 mg/kg (maximal dose, 15 mL). If this treatment is administered within 5 days of exposure, prevention of infection and disease can be expected. Administration of immunoglobulin later in the incubation period may modify the illness but does not prevent it. The use of immunoglobulin is particularly important in children who have not been immunized because of the contraindications to vaccination mentioned previously. In these children, immunoglobulin (0.5 mL/kg; maximal dose, 15 mL) should be administered when measles is epidemic in the community in which they reside. The dosage should be repeated every 4 weeks until the epidemic subsides. Intravenous immunoglobulin in a dose of 400 mg/kg may be used (also see Chapter 246).

NEW REFERENCES SINCE THE SEVENTH EDITION

12. American Academy of Pediatrics. Measles. In: Kimberlin DW, Brady MT, Jackson MA, Long SS, eds. *2015 Red Book: Report of the Committee on Infectious Diseases*. 30th ed. Elk Grove Village, IL: American Academy of Pediatrics; 2015:535.
24. Aulakh R, Tiwari A. Subacute sclerosing panencephalitis in a toddler: changing epidemiological trends. *Case Rep Pediatr*. 2013;2013:341462.
52. Bochennek K, Allwinn R, Langer R, et al. Differential loss of humoral immunity against measles, mumps, rubella and varicella-zoster virus in children treated for cancer.
71. Centers for Disease Control and Prevention. False-positive measles test: Maine, February 2012. *MMWR Morb Mortal Wkly Rep*. 2012;61:396.
72. Centers for Disease Control and Prevention. *Specimens for Detection of Measles RNA by RT-PCR or Virus Isolation*. Available at: http://www.cdc.gov/measles/lab-tools/rt-pcr.html.
73. Centers for Disease Control and Prevention. Summary of Notifiable Diseases—United States, 2010. *MMWR Morb Mortal Wkly Rep*. 2012;59(53):96-98.
74. Centers for Disease Control and Prevention. Measles—United States, January 4–April 2, 2015. *MMWR Morb Mortal Wkly Rep*. 2015;64(14):373-376.
75. Centers for Disease Control and Prevention. Measles Cases and Outbreaks. *MMWR Morb Mortal Wkly Rep*. 2015. Available at: http://www.cdc.gov/measles/cases-outbreaks.html.
92. Centers for Disease Control and Prevention. Measles. In: Hamborsky J, Kroger A, Wolfe S, eds. *Epidemiology and Prevention of Vaccine-Preventable Diseases*. 13th ed. Washington DC: Public Health Foundation; 2015.
122. De Serres G, Markowski F, Toth E, et al. Largest measles epidemic in North America in a decade—Quebec, Canada, 2011: contribution of susceptibility, serendipity, and superspreading events. *J Infect Dis*. 2013;207(6):990-998.
192. Griffin DE. Measles virus. In: Knipe DM, Howley PM, eds. *Fields Virology*. 6th ed. Philadelphia: Lippincott Williams & Wilkins; 2013.
202. Gutierrez J, Issacson RS, Koppel BS. Subacute sclerosing panencephalitis: an update. *Dev Med Child Neurol*. 2010;52(10):901-907.
211. Hausler M, Aksoy A, Alber M, et al. A Multinational Survey on Actual Diagnostics and Treatment of Subacute Sclerosing Panencephalitis. *Neuropediatrics*. 2015;46(6):377-384.
228. Ibrahim SH, Amjad N, Saleem AF, et al. The upsurge of SSPE: a reflection of national measles immunization status in Pakistan. *J Trop Pediatr*. 2014;60(6):449-453.
256. Kija E, Ndondo A, Spittal G, et al. Subacute sclerosing panencephalitis in South African children following the measles outbreak between 2009 and 2011. *S Afr Med J*. 2015;105(9):713-718.
260. Klein NP, Lewis E, Fireman B, et al. Safety of measles-containing vaccines in 1-year-old children. *Pediatrics*. 2015;135(2):e321-e329.
280. Kweder H, Ainouze M, Brunel J, et al. Measles Virus: Identification in the M Protein Primary Sequence of a Potential Molecular Marker for Subacute Sclerosing Panencephalitis. *Adv Virol*. 2015;2015:769837.
283. Lamb RA, Kolakofsky D. Paramyxoviridae: The viruses and their replication. In: Knipe DM, Howley PM, eds. *Fields Virology*. 6th ed. Philadelphia: Lippincott Williams & Wilkins; 2013.
289. Lievano FA, Papania MJ, Helfand RF, et al. Lack of evidence of measles virus shedding in people with inapparent measles virus infections. *J Infect Dis*. 2004;189(suppl 1):S165-S170.
298. MacDonald SE, Dover DC, Simmonds KA, et al. Risk of febrile seizures after first dose of measles-mumps-rubella-varicella vaccine: a population-based cohort study. *CMAJ*. 2014;186(11):824-829.
396. Perry RT, Murray JS, Gacic-Dobo M, et al. Progress Toward Regional Measles Elimination—Worldwide, 2000–2014. *MMWR Morb Mortal Wkly Rep*. 2015;64(44):1246-1251.
421. Rota PA, Brown K, Mankertz A, et al. Global distribution of measles genotypes and measles molecular epidemiology. *J Infect Dis*. 2011;204(suppl 1):S514-S523.
434. Schonberger K, Ludwig MS, Wildner M, et al. Epidemiology of subacute sclerosing panencephalitis (SSPE) in Germany from 2003 to 2009: a risk estimation. *PLoS ONE*. 2013;8(7):e68909.
440. Shulman ST, Shulman DL, Sims RH. The tragic 1824 journey of the Hawaiian king and queen to London: history of measles in Hawaii. *Pediatr Infect Dis J*. 2009;28(8):728-733.
454. Strebel PM, Papania MJ, Dayan GH, et al. Measles vaccine. In: Plotkin SA, Orenstein WA, Offit PA, eds. *Vaccines*. 5th ed. Saunders; 2008.
500. World Health Organization. Meeting report of the Strategic Advisory Group of Experts (SAGE) on Immunization. Geneva: WHO; 2015.
508. Young MK, Cripps AW, Nimmo GR, et al. Post-exposure passive immunisation for preventing rubella and congenital rubella syndrome. *Cochrane Database Syst Rev*. 2015;(9):CD010586.
512. Zipprich J, Winter K, Hacker J, et al. Measles outbreak—California, December 2014–February 2015. *MMWR Morb Mortal Wkly Rep*. 2015;64(6):153-154.

The full reference list for this chapter is available at ExpertConsult.com.

Mumps Virus

181

James D. Cherry • Kevin K. Quinn

Mumps (epidemic parotitis) is an acute communicable disease caused by the mumps virus, a member of the genus *Rubulavirus*. As a result of universal immunization, mumps was an uncommon disease in children in the United States at the end of the 20th century; however, a 2006 epidemic and subsequent outbreaks indicate the need for renewed study of mumps. In addition, mumps continues to be an epidemic problem worldwide.

HISTORY

In the fifth century BCE, Hippocrates described an outbreak on the island of Thasos.[115,227] He noted that most patients had bilateral swelling near the ears and that the others had unilateral swelling. He also noted that some patients had bilateral or unilateral pain and swelling of the testes.

The origin of the name mumps is not known. It may be from the English noun *mump*, which means "a lump," or the English verb *mump*, one of whose definitions is "mumble." This latter possible origin is based on the mumbling speech that patients with significant parotitis may have.

In 1790, Robert Hamilton[85,86] presented an extensive study of mumps in which he noted orchitis, associated the illness with neurologic involvement, and described the neuropathology of a fatal case. In 1886, Hirsch[97] noted that mumps occurred throughout the world and that it was a major cause of morbidity in Confederate troops during the American Civil War. In the first half of the 20th century, investigators recognized that mumps virus infection involved multiple organs, and the causative agent was shown by Johnson and Goodpasture in 1934[59,108] to be a filterable virus.

The growth of mumps virus in embryonated eggs was reported in 1945, and 10 years later its propagation in tissue culture was noted.[83,90] This latter development led to the development and licensure in the United States of a live attenuated mumps vaccine in 1967.

CLASSIFICATION

Mumps virus is a member of the genus *Rubulavirus*, subfamily Paramyxovirinae, and family Paramyxoviridae.[133] It contains a single-stranded, nonsegmented, negative-sense RNA genome that is surrounded by a helical nucleocapsid and a surface envelope.

PROPERTIES

Physical Properties

The virus generally is spherical, but marked pleomorphism occurs.[117,132,183] Its size varies from 100 to 600 nm. The mumps viral genome is 15,384 nucleotides in length and encodes for 9 known viral proteins: a nucleocapsid-associated protein (NP), a phosphoprotein (P), a membrane or matrix protein (M), a fusion protein (F), a hydrophobic membrane-associated protein (SH), a hemagglutinin-neuraminidase (HN), a polymerase protein (L), and nonstructural proteins within the P protein (I and V, which counteracts the interferon [IFN]–induced host antiviral response).[228] The genes for these proteins have been sequenced, and the gene order is 3-NP-P-M-F-SH-HN-L-5. The viral envelope is studded with 12- to 15-nm projections that contain either of the two structural glycoproteins (HN or F).

The P structural protein is associated with the nucleocapsid, and an RNA-dependent RNA polymerase is located within the nucleocapsid structure. The envelope has a high lipid content, and it contains the M protein.

The SH protein gene is the most variable region of the genome and therefore can be used to differentiate viral strains.[5,122,163,202] Analysis of the variations in SH gene nucleotide sequences has been used to study outbreaks, identify vaccine viruses, study vaccine adverse events, and identify new viral strains. Antigenic differences among vaccine strains result in variable cross-neutralization of unknown significance.[151]

Mumps virus infectivity is destroyed by heat (56°C for 20 minutes), and its infectivity is reduced by ultraviolet light, Tween 80, ether, and formalin. The virus is stable at 4°C for several days; and when placed in a buffered salt solution (e.g., Hanks) with 1% to 2% inactivated fetal calf serum, the virus can be stored indefinitely at −70°C.

Antigenic Composition

The three major antigenic components of mumps virus are the two glycoproteins (HN or V antigen and F protein) and the nucleocapsid protein (NP or S antigen).[117] The glycoproteins that project from the viral surface are the antigenic target for specific antibodies. Host antibodies to HN and F proteins confer protective immunity against the virus. Mumps viral particles agglutinate erythrocytes of several mammalian and avian species (human, avian, rodent, and simian); at 37°C, the virus causes partial hemolysis of susceptible erythrocytes when it is attached to cellular surface receptors. Specific antibody blocks hemagglutination, hemadsorption, and hemolysis.

Mumps virus is considered to have a single immunotype. However, polyclonal antibodies to parainfluenza and Newcastle disease viral antigens cross react with antibodies to mumps virus in complement-fixation and hemagglutination-inhibition assays. With monoclonal antibodies, an antigenic relationship between the NH and NP proteins of Sendai virus (a murine parainfluenza type 1 virus) and mumps virus has been demonstrated.[164]

Although mumps is a monotypic virus, genetic variation among strains exists. A standardized nomenclature and an analysis protocol have been proposed for the genetic characterization of mumps strains to facilitate the expansion of molecular epidemiologic studies.[106,107] This nomenclature includes 12 genotypes assigned letters from A to N (excluding E and M) based on the nucleotide sequence of the hydrophobic (SH) gene. The 2004 to 2005 UK outbreak and the 2006 US outbreak were of serotype G,[37,178] whereas the F serotype is most prevalent in recent Chinese outbreaks.[139] Historically, C, D, G, and H predominate in the Western Hemisphere, and B, F, and I occur in Asia.[102] The Western Hemisphere tends to use vaccines to the A serotype.[228]

Tissue Culture Growth and Animal Susceptibility

Mumps virus can be propagated in many different primary and cell-line tissue cultures.[117,136] To isolate the virus, primary monkey kidney cells generally are used. Its cytopathic effect is similar to that of other paramyxoviruses. When the virus is stained, multinucleated giant cells and cytoplasmic eosinophilic inclusions may be observed. In culture, the addition of erythrocytes results in hemadsorption to surface virus.

Mumps virus infects monkeys, rabbits, dogs, cats, and rodents. The virus is isolated readily after inoculation of the amniotic sac of 7- to 8-day-old chicken embryos.

EPIDEMIOLOGY

Incidence

In the United States, mumps was a reportable disease from 1922 to 1950 and has been again since 1967. Between 1950 and 1967, incidence data were gathered from voluntary reporting by cooperating states. Incidence data from 1922 to 1982 are presented in Fig. 181.1, and

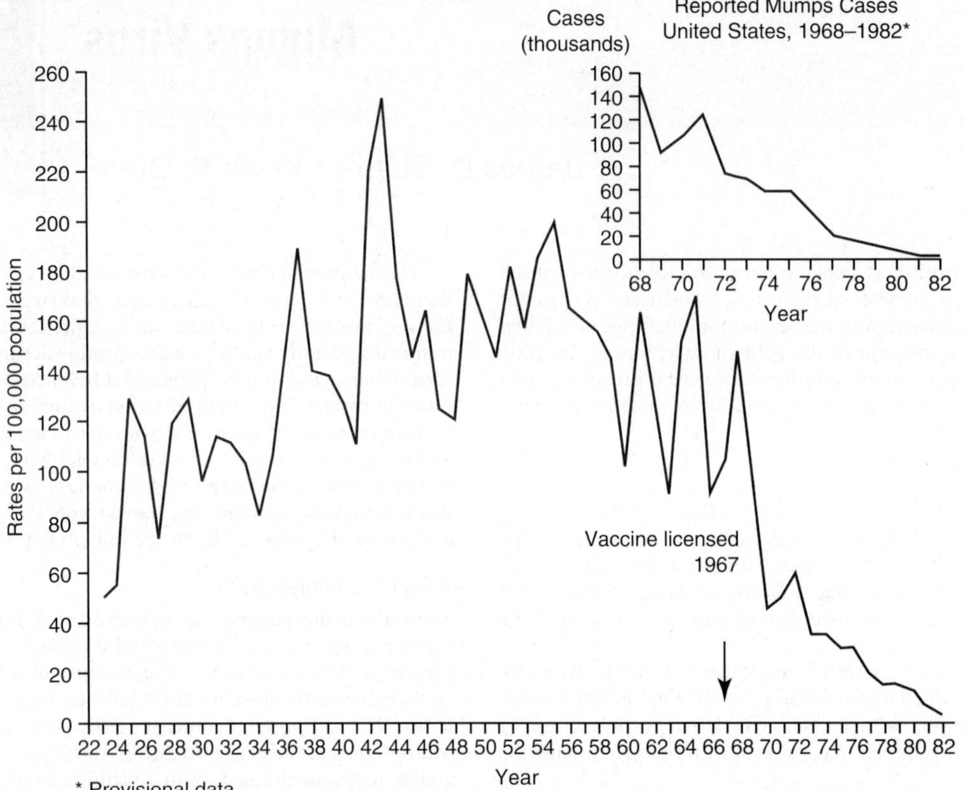

FIG. 181.1 Incidence of reported mumps in the United States from 1922 to 1982 and the number of reported cases from 1968 to 1982. (From Centers for Disease Control and Prevention. Mumps—United States, 1983–1984. *MMWR Morb Mortal Wkly Rep.* 1984;33:533–5.)

vaccine-era data are presented in Fig. 181.2.[30,41] In the prevaccine era, mumps was a yearly disease, with epidemic peaks occurring approximately every 4 years. The peak epidemic year was 1944, when the rate was 250 per 100,000 population.

In the prevaccine era, mumps was a disease predominantly of young children.[30] However, outbreaks of mumps were a significant problem in young adults in the military.[77,147] The age distribution of mumps in the United States during selected years is presented in Table 181.1. After the mumps vaccine was licensed in 1967, mumps remained a disease of predominantly young children from 1967 to 1971. However, by 1981, most reported patients were 10 years old or older. In 1987, 76% of the cases occurred in persons 10 years old or older (see Table 181.1). In 1994, 1537 cases were reported, and of those with age noted, 21.8% were in patients 20 years old or older. The increase in reported cases that occurred in 1987 (see Fig. 181.2 and Table 181.1) was the result of a marked increase in cases in nonimmunized persons 10 to 19 years of age. This group had been protected for a time by herd immunity because of the rapidly declining incidence of mumps as a result of routine vaccine use beginning in 1977.[47] In 1998, only 666 cases of mumps were reported in the United States.[34] Nineteen percent of the patients were younger than 5 years old, and 36% were 15 years old or older. In 2010, 54.6% of the reported cases were in persons 15 years of age or older (see Table 181.1).

In the prevaccine era, the peak incidence of mumps occurred in the winter and spring months, and this peak continued well into the vaccine era.[29,77,120] After licensure of the mumps vaccine, reported cases in the United States dropped from 152,209 cases (87.9 cases per 100,000 persons) in 1968 to less than 300 cases (<0.1 case per 100,000 persons) from 2001 through 2005.[36,28] However, a 2006 outbreak in primarily Midwestern college student populations revealed a dramatic resurgence of disease.[36,38,39] By March 28, 2006, a total of 219 mumps cases were reported in Iowa alone; this was a 44-fold increase in cases from the preceding decade. Of the 219 cases, the median patient age was 21 years (range, 3 to 85 years), with 48% of the patients 17 to 25 years old; 30% of the patients were known to be college students. This outbreak in Iowa in December 2005 was found to involve 10 additional states by May 2, 2006.[38] A total of 6584 cases were reported nationwide.[35,56] There were 85 hospitalizations, 85% of patients lived in eight contiguous Midwestern states, and 83% were college students. Sixty-three percent of the case patients with known vaccination status had received two doses of either mumps or mumps-measles-rubella (MMR) vaccine, and affected colleges reported 84% two-dose MMR vaccine coverage. The year 2006 represented a historical national two-dose coverage peak of 87% among adolescents.[16,51,56,144]

In 2004 to 2005, a mumps epidemic occurred in the United Kingdom.[37] There were 56,390 reported cases. In 2004, 79.1% of the confirmed cases were in persons 15 to 24 years of age, and two-thirds of all cases occurred in persons who had not been vaccinated. In many respects, this epidemic is similar to the one in the United States in 1987; herd immunity had protected this adolescent and young adult cohort for a number of years.*

A 2009 to 2012 mumps outbreak in the New York–New Jersey area had 3502 cases.[17] The index case in this outbreak was a twice-vaccinated 11-year-old boy who returned to the United States from the United Kingdom on June 17, 2009. At the time of this boy's visit to the United Kingdom, there was a continuing large outbreak of mumps in the region. After returning home, this boy attended a camp in Sullivan County, New York. At the camp, he developed mumps. At the camp, there were 400 Orthodox Jewish boys. Of this group, 22 campers developed mumps, as well as three adults. The 25 camp cases were the index cases for 1813 cases in New York City, 449 cases in Rockland County, 425 cases in Ocean County, NJ, and 790 cases in Orange County, NY.

Of the 3405 cases in the outbreak, 97% occurred among Orthodox Jewish persons. Seventy-one percent of the cases occurred among male patients. Twenty-seven percent of the cases occurred in adolescents 13

*References 14, 64, 64, 76, 96, 101, 105, 129, 150, 152, 167, 188, 199, 216, 217, 225, 226.

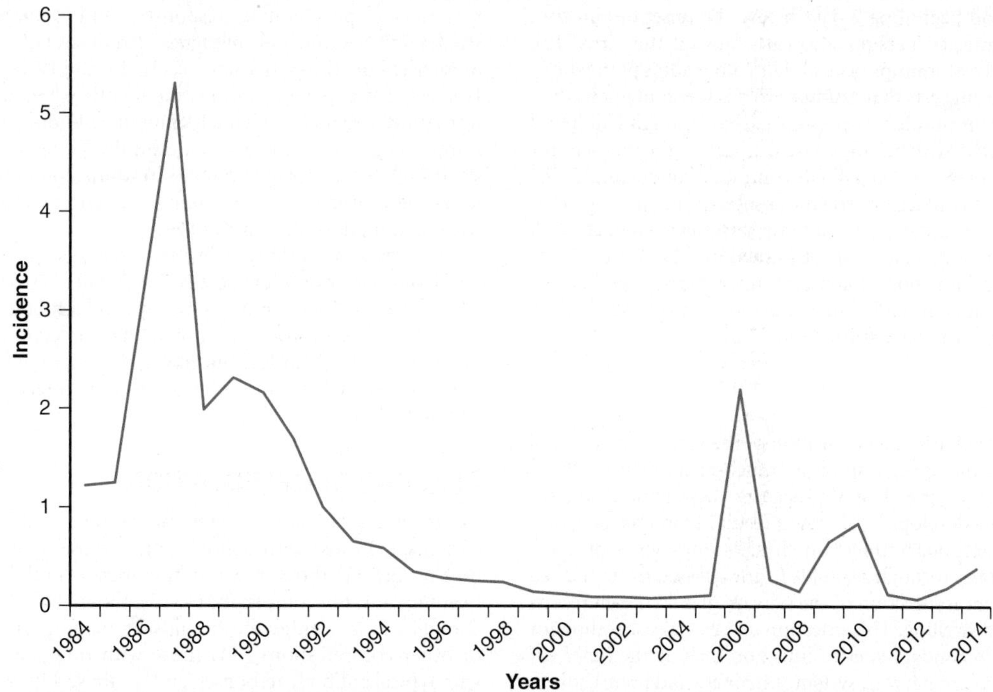

FIG. 181.2 Incidence of reported mumps in the United States from 1985 to 2014. (Modified from Centers for Disease Control and Prevention. Summary of notifiable diseases—United States, 2013. *MMWR Morb Mortal Wkly Rep.* 2013;62[53]:1–119.)

TABLE 181.1 Age Distribution of Mumps Cases in the United States During Selected Years

	1967–71[A]		1987		1994			2010	
Age Group (y)	**Cases**	**%**	**Cases**	**%**	**Cases**	**%**	**Age Group (y)**	**Cases**	**%**
<5	2932	17.1	804	6.5	250	17.4	<5	297	11.4
5–9	10,413	60.8	2196	17.9	473	33.0	5–14	884	33.8
10–14	2372	13.8	4567	37.3	271	18.9	15–24	767	29.4
15–19	1418[b]	8.3	3455	28.2	128	8.9	≥25	657	25.2
≥20			1235	10.1	312	20.8			

[a]Average annual reported cases for California, Massachusetts, and New York City.
[b]Includes all reported cases in patients age ≥15 years.Data from references 30, 41, and 214.

to 17 years of age. Of the 2317 patients (68%) in whom vaccinated status was verified, 10% were unvaccinated, 14% had received one dose of MMR, and 70% had received two doses of MMR vaccine.

A small outbreak of 29 cases on a university campus occurred in California in 2011. The presumed source patient was an unvaccinated student with a history of recent travel to Western Europe.[40]

Worldwide recent outbreaks have occurred in the United Kingdom (2013),[2] France (2013),[75] Belgium (2012–13),[22] the Czech republic (2011–12),[137] Bosnia and Herzegovina (2010–11[101] and 2010–12[100]), Germany (2010–11),[206] Guam (2009–10),[141] the Netherlands (2007–09[226] and 2009–12[64,80,131,186,225]), Canada (2007–09[226] and 2009–10[217]), Spain (2007–08),[76] Poland (2009),[167] Israel (2009–10),[152,199] Scotland (2010–11),[216] Moldova (2007–08),[188] Macedonia (2008–09),[129] Australia (2007–08),[14] the United Kingdom (2003–06),[105] Luxembourg (2008),[150] Palestinian refugee camps of the West Bank (2003–05),[96] Serbia (2012),[154] Portugal (2012–13),[50] and Denmark (2013).[200]

Morbidity and Mortality

The most common clinical manifestations of mumps virus infection are fever and parotitis. However, approximately 30% of infected persons do not have parotitis and therefore are not recognized.[119] Epididymo-orchitis occurs in 20% to 30% of clinical cases in postpubertal male patients. Approximately 60% of clinical mumps cases involve cerebrospinal fluid (CSF) pleocytosis, but only one-sixth of these patients have meningeal symptoms.[13] In 1966, 628 cases of encephalitis (0.5% of total reported cases) were reported, and of these, 10 (1.6%) had a fatal outcome.[31] Encephalitis occurs more frequently in male patients (61%) than in female patients (39%), and the rate of occurrence is greatest in adults. Deafness after a case of mumps has been estimated to occur in 0.5 to 5.0 per 100,000 cases.[63,215]

From 1966 to 1975, 200 mumps-associated deaths were reported in the United States.[31] Of these, 44 (22%) were in patients with encephalitis; in the others, the causes of death were not identified. Forty-one percent of the deaths occurred in adults 40 years old or older. During the 10-year period from 1988 through 1997, only eight deaths caused by mumps were reported.[34]

In the 2006 mumps outbreak in the United States there were 85 hospitalizations (2%), but no deaths were reported. Parotitis or other salivary gland inflammation was reported in 99%, nonspecific symptoms (headache, myalgia, or fatigue) in 57%, and fever in 29%. Overall complications were 5%, with orchitis most prevalent. Encephalitis and meningitis occurred in less than 1%.[56]

Spread of Infection

Mumps virus is contagious for nonimmune persons. It is spread from an infected person to a new host by the respiratory route. The virus can be isolated from the saliva of infected patients from 7 days before the onset of parotitis to 9 days after onset.[117] Transmission is greatest during a 7-day period beginning 2 days before the onset of parotitis. Asymptomatically infected persons also can transmit the virus. The finding that outbreaks of mumps occurred in young adult populations in the prevaccine era suggests that mumps virus is less contagious than is measles; a significant number of persons passed through childhood without being infected with mumps virus. In 2011, the Centers for Disease Control and Prevention (CDC) discontinued conducting airline flight–related mumps contact investigations after prior investigations failed to reveal any secondary cases among passenger contacts.[156] A serologic study reported by Black[20] in 1964 noted that 24% of US Army recruits lacked hemagglutination-inhibition antibody to mumps, whereas only 1% lacked measles antibody. The incubation period usually is 16 to 18 days, although it can vary from 12 to 25 days.[117]

PATHOGENESIS

After respiratory or perhaps oral acquisition of the virus, primary viral replication occurs in the upper respiratory mucosal epithelium.[65,117,227] Virus multiplies and is spread by drainage to local lymph nodes.[65] Subsequently, viremia develops.[112,166,211] As a result of viremia, infection occurs in multiple secondary infection sites. Mumps virus prevents macrophage chemotaxis through a soluble factor released from infected cells[23] Most prominent is infection of the salivary glands, which results in inflammation and swelling. This infection causes virus shedding for 1 to 2 weeks. Other secondary sites of infection include the inner ear (cochlea), pancreas, heart, nervous system (meninges and brain), joints, kidneys, liver, gonads, and thyroid.

PATHOLOGY

In the salivary glands, virus infects the ductal epithelium and causes periductal interstitial edema and a local inflammatory reaction involving lymphocytes and macrophages[180,224,227] Tissue damage ensues, and the involved cells desquamate. Virus enters the central nervous system (CNS) by the choroid plexus through infected mononuclear cells. Virus multiplies in choroid and ependymal cells on the ventricular surfaces, and these cells desquamate into the CSF and result in meningitis. In encephalitis, perivascular infiltration with mononuclear cells, scattered foci of neuronophagia, and microglial rod-cell proliferation occur.[25] Periventricular demyelination also takes place. In the male gonad, the primary site of viral replication is the seminiferous tubules, where infection results in lymphocytic infiltration and edema of interstitial tissue.

Immunologic Events

Infection gives rise to serum antibodies to the HN glycoprotein (V antigen), the F antigen, and the NP protein (S antigen).[117] Antibody to NP protein develops first, 3 to 7 days after the onset of symptoms. Antibodies to NP protein are short lived and usually are absent after 6 months; they cross react with parainfluenza viruses. Antibodies to HN glycoprotein develop 2 to 4 weeks after the onset of illness and persist for long periods after infection.

Immunoglobulin (Ig) G and IgM antibody responses (determined by enzyme-linked immunosorbent assay [ELISA]) regularly occur after infection.[210] IgG antibody levels measured by ELISA correlate best with those derived by complement-fixation and hemolysis-in-gel assays. ELISA results are less specific than are those achieved with the plaque-reduction neutralization assay because of the high rate of cross-reacting antibodies against parainfluenza viruses detected by ELISA.[145,172] IgM antibodies develop early in the course of infection (second day of illness), peak within the first week of illness, and usually are undetectable 3 months after the onset of illness; occasionally, mumps-specific IgM antibody persists for 5 to 6 months.[117,210] Mumps-specific IgG antibody appears at the end of the first week of illness, peaks 3 weeks later, and persists throughout life. The IgG response is mainly the IgG1 subclass; a minor IgG3 subclass response also occurs.[187] Salivary IgA antibodies to mumps virus regularly appear after infection.[70]

During infection with vaccine virus, the cell-mediated response to tuberculin is diminished for up to 4 weeks.[123] During the same period, a mumps-specific, cell-mediated immune response develops.[117,227] This response has been demonstrated by skin test hypersensitivity, in vitro lymphocyte proliferative responses, and cytotoxic T-lymphocyte studies.[24,26,118] Asano and colleagues[8] demonstrated a significant increase in interleukin (IL)–8, IL-10, IL-12, IL-13, and IFN-γ levels in sera from Japanese patients with mumps meningitis when compared with sera from other patients with viral meningitis, a finding suggesting a distinct immunologic response. More specifically, Wang and associates,[218] in a study of 960 patients with mumps in China, found that IL-6 and IFN-γ levels were predictive of meningitis or encephalitis when compared with uncomplicated mumps cases.

In general, immunity against recurrent disease has been thought to be lifelong. However, Gut and associates[82] noted 26 patients with mumps who had a previous history of mumps and antibody response patterns suggestive of reinfection and not primary infection. Specifically, these patients had a rise in IgG but not IgM titers. In a study of mumps in 281 children, reinfection after a previous infection was noted in 9 children.[184]

CLINICAL MANIFESTATIONS

In epidemics of mumps, cases can be separated into five groups of patients: (1) those with a short course whose signs and symptoms are nonspecific, (2) those in whom the disease is full blown with salivary swelling but no complications, (3) those with severe mumps and complications (epididymo-orchitis or meningoencephalitis, or both, or other complications), (4) those with no apparent symptoms but with typical antibody responses, and (5) those with meningoencephalitis or orchitis but without involvement of the salivary glands.[201] Approximately 75% of all cases of apparent mumps in children are of the full-blown type without complications. Involvement of the gonads rarely occurs before puberty.

Typical Mumps Without Complications

The average case in children has a prodromal period of 1 to 2 days that consists of fever, anorexia, headache, vomiting, and generalized aches and pains. The headache often is particularly marked and probably is caused by mild meningoencephalitis.[68] The temperature usually rises slowly to 38.9°C or 39.4°C (102°F or 103°F) as the disease becomes full blown, but at times fever is only slight or absent.[201]

After the prodromal period, one or both parotid glands will begin to enlarge (Fig. 181.3). Mumps is bilateral in 70% to 80% of cases. A few days to a week or more may intervene between the swellings of the

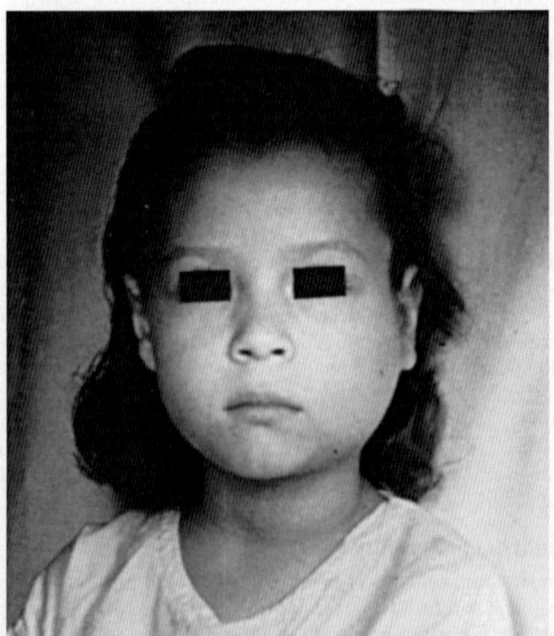

FIG. 181.3 Note the swelling on the left side of the face related to parotitis secondary to mumps virus infection. The left ear protrudes from the side of the head.

two sides. A distinctive "puckering" sensation is experienced at the angle of the jaw in the early stage, and it may be increased by the application of sour liquids, such as lemon juice or vinegar, to the tongue. This sign, when present, may be useful for early establishment of the diagnosis. The swelling of the gland also is distinctive in that a brawny type of edema occurs about the parotid gland, the borders of which are not discrete, in contrast to the discrete swelling typical of lymphadenitis, in which the node generally is outlined easily. The lobe of the ear is in the center of the swelling, which usually cannot be separated by palpation from the angle of the mandible. Pressure is painful, and opening the jaw often is difficult.

The swelling of an individual gland reaches its maximum in approximately 3 days, remains at its peak for approximately 2 days, and then slowly recedes. The extent of the swelling varies considerably but at times is sufficient to distort the outline of the face and head completely. The submaxillary and sublingual glands may be involved separately or with the parotids in any combination.

During the prodromal phase, slight redness of the orifices of the Stensen or Wharton ducts, when present, has diagnostic significance. The amount of saliva usually is unchanged, although the mouth may be dry or salivation may be extreme. Gellis and Peters[74] described a few cases with edema over the upper part of the sternum, apparently caused by pressure on the lymphatics in the neck.

In uncomplicated mumps, the white blood cell count usually is low, with slight relative lymphocytosis. The serum amylase value typically is elevated.

Meningitis, Meningoencephalitis, and Encephalitis

Meningitis and mild meningoencephalitis are the most frequent complications of mumps in children. Azimi and colleagues[11] reviewed 51 children with mumps meningoencephalitis who were admitted to Columbus Children's Hospital in Columbus, Ohio, between July 1964 and December 1967. Of this group of patients, fever occurred in 94%, vomiting in 84%, nuchal rigidity in 71%, lethargy in 69%, parotid swelling in 47%, headache in 47%, convulsions in 18%, abdominal pain in 14%, sore throat in 8%, diarrhea in 8%, and delirium in 6%.

Clinical findings in neurologic illness caused by mumps virus infection differ according to the age of the patient. Meningeal signs are recognized more readily in older children, adolescents, and adults, whereas nonspecific findings such as drowsiness and lethargy occur more frequently in young children.[227] Although seizures develop in 20% to 30% of hospitalized patients, electroencephalographic results usually are normal. Even in patients with severe obtundation, the electroencephalogram reveals only diffuse slowing with increased voltage. Focal findings are rare. The outlook in mumps meningoencephalitis generally is good and usually is better than in encephalitis of other viral causes (see Chapter 36). Even patients with profound obtundation generally recover without having residual damage. Rarely, deaths do occur, however.[34]

In the typical case, CSF has normal glucose and elevated protein levels and pleocytosis. Glucose levels are slightly low in approximately 20% of cases. At the onset of symptoms, modest mononuclear pleocytosis is present. The CSF cell count peaks on the third day of illness; counts average 250/mm^3, but counts greater than 1000/mm^3 are not uncommon. Mumps meningitis usually develops in patients with parotitis approximately 5 days after the onset of illness, but CNS findings can precede the parotid findings and can develop without any salivary gland involvement.

Herndon and colleagues[92] noted that ependymitis regularly occurs in cases of mumps meningitis. A rare complication of mumps appears to be acquired aqueductal stenosis, and researchers have suggested that it may be caused by the preceding ependymitis.[92,159,198,208] In one reported fatal case, hydrocephalus developed within 5 days of onset of disease.[162] More recently, acute hydrocephalus associated with mumps meningoencephalitis was noted in an 8.5-year-old boy.[6] This child received a ventriculoperitoneal shunt and at follow-up had no neurologic deficit.

A 3-year-old boy with mumps cerebellitis, nystagmus, and focal localization of brain lesions noted by electroencephalography was described.[142] Also reported were facial palsy in a 3-year-old Japanese boy and transverse myelitis in an adult.[60,213] A case in a girl 4 years and 3 months of age who had brainstem encephalitis and acute disseminated encephalomyelitis after mumps has been reported.[196] This child responded rather dramatically to treatment with glucocorticoids and intravenous immunoglobulin. Haginoya and associates[84] reported the case of a 14-year-old Japanese girl who had chronic progressive mumps virus encephalitis. This child had an illness similar to subacute sclerosing panencephalitis, and her antibody titers suggested that the infecting virus may have had a defect in the HN protein.

Gonadal Infection (Epididymo-Orchitis and Oophoritis)

Epididymo-orchitis and oophoritis almost never occur before puberty.[201] However, in adolescent boys and adult men, epididymo-orchitis is second only to parotitis as a manifestation of mumps virus infection.[119] Cases of orchitis have been reported in children as young as 3 years old.[176] In postpubertal male patients, orchitis develops in 30% to 38% with mumps.[18,171] The rate of orchitis is highest in those 15 to 29 years of age. The greatest numbers of cases occur during the second, third, and fourth decades of life. Approximately 80% of cases of epididymo-orchitis appear during the first 8 days of involvement of the salivary gland, but a few cases occur a considerable time after the parotitis has subsided.[201]

The onset of testicular involvement usually is manifested as chills, recurrence of fever, and swelling of the testes. Pain over the renal area or in the lower part of the abdomen, bilateral or unilateral, may precede or accompany the orchitis. Occasionally, this pain, if on the right side, may suggest appendicitis.

The orchitis usually is unilateral, but bilateral involvement has been reported in 17% to 38% of cases.[18,171] Although atrophy may develop after orchitis, in patients with unilateral involvement, sterility is not a concern. Sterility has resulted after some cases of bilateral orchitis, however. A 16-year-old adolescent with mumps epididymo-orchitis was found to have persistent mumps virus RNA in his semen for 40 days.[104] In follow-up studies, he was found to have antisperm antibodies. The development of malignant disease in affected testes also has been reported.[18,111]

Oophoritis occurs in approximately 7% of postpubertal female patients. Pelvic pain and tenderness are noted.[189]

Pancreatitis

In a retrospective survey of 2482 hospitalized patients with mumps, pancreatitis was noted in 75 (3%).[1] Cases occurred in children and adults, and pancreatitis was 1.6 times more common in male than in female patients. Severe involvement of the pancreas is a rare occurrence, but mild or subclinical infection may occur more frequently than recognized.[189] It may be unassociated with salivary gland manifestations and be misdiagnosed as gastroenteritis. Epigastric pain and tenderness are suggestive; they may be accompanied by fever, chills, vomiting, and prostration. A child with acute hemorrhagic pancreatitis and a pseudocyst caused by mumps virus infection has been reported.[66]

Diabetes Mellitus

Diabetes mellitus long has been suspected to be associated with antecedent mumps.[31,87] In experimental animals, mumps virus infection has been linked to hyperglycemia and histologic lesions of the pancreatic islets. Mumps virus can invade the human pancreas and can infect and destroy human and rhesus beta cells in vitro,[175] but pancreatic damage has not been documented in reported cases of diabetes that developed after mumps or mumps vaccination.[195]

In humans, many cases of temporal association have been described both in individuals and in siblings,[52,53,116,149,158] and outbreaks of diabetes mellitus a few months or years after outbreaks of mumps have been reported.[81,148,205] Although evidence has not established a causal association in these cases, a study in Surrey, England, suggested that a small proportion, if any, of diabetes cases that start in childhood (only 15 of the 1663 patients in the study [<1%]) may have resulted from a recent mumps virus infection.[72] Antibody studies have shown fewer positive titers for mumps in diabetic patients than in normal subjects, even in children.[185] Infection may contribute to the development of diabetes either by specifically damaging islet cells or by precipitating diabetes in patients whose disease is latent. Teng and colleagues[207] reported the case of an 11-year-old girl with mumps infection complicated by transient hyperinsulinemic hypoglycemia.

Nephritis

Viruria is a common occurrence in uncomplicated mumps, and mild abnormalities in renal function occur.[211] Severe and fatal nephritis was reported as a rare complication of mumps occurring 10 to 14 days after parotitis.[189] Fujieda and associates[71] reported the demonstration of mumps virus genomic RNA by polymerase chain reaction (PCR) in a renal biopsy specimen from a 5-year-old girl with IgA nephropathy. Baas and colleagues[12] reported a case of a 56-year-old renal transplant recipient who developed acute irreversible transplant failure secondary to interstitial nephritis with mumps RNA detected in urine and renal biopsy.

Deafness

Deafness is an important but rare complication of mumps virus infection.[29,77,120] Its incidence has been estimated at 0.5 to 5.0 per 100,000 cases of mumps.[47,187] However, the incidence rate of minor degrees of hearing impairment, such as high-tone hearing loss, is probably much higher.[44]

Mumps-associated deafness occurs with or without meningoencephalitis and may develop after asymptomatic infection.[31,63,157] The deafness usually is unilateral and often permanent. Twenty-two of 103 cases (21%) reviewed by Everberg[63] were bilateral. Mumps virus has been isolated from perilymph fluid in a case of sudden-onset, unilateral, complete deafness that began 2 days after the onset of mumps.[14,144] Vertigo also is noted occasionally in patients with mumps; it occurs most commonly in those in whom deafness develops.[103]

Mumps and Pregnancy[34]

The incidence of mumps during pregnancy was estimated at 0.8 to 10 cases per 10,000 pregnancies[190] before vaccine was licensed in the United States. No vaccine-era data are available for comparison. Maternal complications such as mastitis,[171] aseptic meningitis,[14] aseptic meningitis,[21] and fatal glomerulonephritis[58] have been reported. Mumps virus has been isolated from human breast milk.[113]

Increased rates of fetal mortality were reported in women who contracted mumps during the first trimester. In a large prospective case-control study, a 27.3% rate of fetal wastage was noted in women with mumps during the first trimester versus a 13.0% rate in matched, healthy controls during the first trimester.[194] No significant differences in birth weight were noted among the live births.[193] Because fetal loss usually occurs in such cases within 2 weeks of development of maternal infection, investigators postulated that factors related to maternal gonadal infection with resulting hormonal changes may be responsible. A histopathologic study of the products of conception in mothers with gestational mumps revealed severe proliferative necrotic villitis and vasculitis in the placenta and viral inclusions, as seen in mumps infection, in fetal tissues.[73] Mumps virus was isolated from a spontaneously aborted 10-week-old human fetus.[125]

No evidence has shown that gestational mumps in humans increases the risk of development of fetal malformations,[192] although a few cases of various congenital malformations with no consistent pattern have been reported.[98]

Other Manifestations

Other rare clinical manifestations include exanthem and enanthem,[43] arthritis,[78] myocarditis,[19] thrombocytopenia,[124,130,173] keratouveitus,[161] lower respiratory tract infection,[69] and other glandular involvement (thyroiditis, mastitis, dacryoadenitis, and bartholinitis).[119,169]

DIFFERENTIAL DIAGNOSIS

Not all patients with mumps have parotid swelling, and mumps virus is not the only cause of parotitis. Mumps virus infection must be considered in all children with aseptic meningitis, meningoencephalitis, and encephalitis (see Chapters 35 and 36). In addition to mumps virus infection, many other infectious agents and noninfectious conditions are associated with parotitis or parotid swelling (see Chapter 13). Other viruses that can cause parotitis include Epstein-Barr virus, coxsackieviruses and echoviruses, influenza A virus, parainfluenza viruses, cytomegalovirus, human herpesvirus-6, and lymphocytic choriomeningitis virus.[15,27,55] Purulent parotitis can be differentiated from mumps by the exquisite tenderness of the region, an elevated white blood cell count, and the observation of pus coming from the Stensen duct. Other viral causes of parotitis can be differentiated by the respective epidemiologic and clinical characteristics of specific agents and appropriate culture, serologic study, or both.

Enlargement of lymph nodes in proximity to the parotid gland must be differentiated from parotid enlargement (see Chapter 12). The cervical lymph nodes are below the ramus of the mandible. The preparotid nodes generally are anterior to the parotid, and their enlargement usually is associated with conjunctivitis. Occasionally, an enlarged lymph node within the parotid gland may cause some confusion. Lesions of the ramus of the mandible, such as osteomyelitis, occasionally have been mistaken for parotid enlargement. In this case, the enlargement usually is persistent.

DIAGNOSIS

In an epidemic situation, the diagnosis of mumps is clinically straightforward, and performing laboratory tests is unnecessary. The critical points are a history of exposure, an incubation period of 2 to 3 weeks, and a typical clinical picture consisting of fever and parotitis. In a sporadic case or in a previously vaccinated child, confirming the cause by laboratory study is important. Mumps virus, as well as most other viruses that cause parotitis, can be demonstrated readily by culture or nucleic acid detection from saliva, throat swabs, or mouth washings during acute illness. Oral fluid specimens can also be assayed for virus-specific IgM. In patients with meningoencephalitis, virus also can be recovered from CSF. Virus is isolated in primary monkey kidney tissue culture. In unusual cases in which the source of facial swelling is obscure, determination of a serum amylase level may be helpful; a high value indicates parotid involvement.

Mumps virus infection also can be confirmed by demonstrating a significant rise in antibody titer in paired serum specimens by complement fixation, hemagglutination inhibition, or ELISA. However, because mumps cross reacts with parainfluenza viruses, these methods are not ideal.[172] Mumps-specific IgM antibody determined by ELISA is the usual test performed; the presence of this antibody indicates a recent infection. Mumps-specific IgM antibodies determined by enzyme immunoassay in oral fluid also are useful for establishing the diagnosis.[219] Mumps virus RNA also can be detected directly from clinical samples by real-time PCR.[209] In outbreaks today, many cases occur in previously vaccinated individuals. Many of these vaccine failures are secondary and, therefore, there is less likely to be a mumps-specific serum IgM antibody response.[134,179] Therefore, greater diagnostic sensitivity will occur when using culture or PCR assay. In the 2009 to 2010 New York mumps outbreak, an increase in sensitivity with either method was noted after 2 to 3 days of symptoms.[177]

TREATMENT

Conservative therapy is indicated in the treatment of mumps. Adequate attention given to hydration and alimentation of patients is important. Patients may have difficulty with acidic foods such as orange juice. In addition, orange juice may cause vomiting in an already nauseated patient. The diet should be light, with a generous offering of fluids.

Occasionally, analgesics are necessary to treat severe headache or discomfort caused by parotitis. Stronger analgesics such as codeine or meperidine (Demerol) rarely are required for headache but may be useful for orchitis. Vomiting seldom is sufficiently severe to require intravenous fluids. In these instances, however, electrolytes lost by vomiting should be replaced.

Although lumbar puncture seldom is necessary for establishing a diagnosis in patients with meningoencephalitis accompanying mumps, patients often indicate that they have experienced relief of headache after undergoing this procedure. No antiviral agent is appropriate or indicated for the treatment of mumps, which is a self-limited illness. Systemic reviews of the literature failed to identify useful information regarding the utility of traditional Chinese medicine or acupuncture for the treatment of mumps.[89,191]

A potential new treatment for mumps orchitis specifically is IFN-α2b. In a small study of 12 patients, both symptom resolution and normospermia were improved versus results in untreated control subjects.[62,121]

PROGNOSIS

The overall prognosis in uncomplicated mumps is excellent. The outlook in meningoencephalitis also generally is favorable, but death and neurologic damage can occur. Deafness and sterility are rare complications.

PREVENTION

Immunization

Numerous different mumps vaccines are available in different countries throughout the world.[182] These vaccines have different effectiveness and reactogenicity profiles. In this chapter, recommendations relating to the vaccines available in the United States are presented.

A summary of the recommendations of the Advisory Committee on Immunization Practices (ACIP) and the Committee on Infectious Diseases of the American Academy of Pediatrics for the use of mumps vaccine follows.[7,40] For more complete information, the reader should consult the most recent ACIP statement or the Report of the Committee on Infectious Diseases of the American Academy of Pediatrics.

The mumps virus vaccine available in the United States (official name: mumps virus vaccine, live) is the Jeryl Lynn strain and is prepared in chick embryo cell culture. The vaccine produces a subclinical, noncommunicable infection with few side effects. Mumps vaccine is available in the following combinations: MMR and measles-mumps-rubella-varicella (MMRV) vaccines.

In initial trials, mumps vaccine had an approximately 95% effectiveness in preventing mumps disease[95,114,203]; and after vaccination, measurable antibody developed in more than 97% of persons known to be susceptible to mumps.[223] Vaccine-induced antibody was protective and long lasting,[221,222] although it was of considerably lower titer than antibody resulting from natural infection.[223] The duration of vaccine-induced immunity is unknown, but serologic and epidemiologic data collected during 35 years of use of live vaccine suggested both persistence of antibody and continuing protection against infection. The epidemic occurrence of mumps in 2006 in the United States and in other countries resulted in further evaluations of vaccine efficacy and waning immunity.[24,40,48,88,109,168,212] In a study in England, the effectiveness of vaccine after one dose declined from 96% in 2-year-old children to 66% in children 11 to 12 years old.[48] In the 2010 to 2001 outbreak in Germany, a very small sampling ($n = 20$) revealed poor (50%) vaccine effectiveness in young adults given one dose in childhood and good protection with no evidence of waning if two doses had been administered.[206] In those children who had received two doses, the effectiveness declined from 99% in children 5 to 6 years old to 86% in children 11 to 12 years old. These data suggest that waning immunity contributes to outbreaks of mumps in older, previously vaccinated populations. Studies in Belgium and Korea also demonstrated waning immunity as contributing to outbreaks of mumps.[42] However, a small study in Wisconsin compared the mumps antibody titers of children who received their second MMR shot at age 4 to 6 years (as is typical) with delaying until age 9 to 11 years. At age 17 years, both groups had similar titers.[135]

In Finland, a two-dose MMR vaccination program with the Jeryl Lynn mumps vaccine strain was launched in 1982.[170] This program was highly successful, and Finland was the first country documented to be free of indigenous mumps, as well as rubella and measles. In a study in Finland that was published in 2007, researchers found that previous vaccinees who were found to be seronegative nonetheless had mumps antigen-specific lymphoproliferative responses.[109]

In a review of 47 publications documenting the vaccination status of patients during 50 outbreaks from 1977 through 2008, Dayan and Rubin[57] calculated that the effectiveness of prior vaccination with one dose of vaccine ranged from 72.8% to 91% for the Jeryl Lynn strain, from 54.4% to 93% for the Urabe strain, and from 0% to 33% for the Rubini strain. Vaccine effectiveness after two doses of mumps vaccine was reported in three outbreaks and ranged from 91% to 94.6%.[181] In the 2009 to 2010 New York outbreak, two-dose effectiveness was 86.3%.[140]

Clinical isolates sequenced from recent outbreaks have revealed genotypes distinct from those of vaccine viruses, thus raising concern that certain mumps virus strains may escape vaccine-induced immunity. Rubin and colleagues[181] performed a study in which sera obtained from children 6 weeks after MMR vaccination were tested for the ability to neutralize genetically diverse mumps virus strains. Although antibody titers varied, all viruses were readily neutralized, arguing against immune escape.

An immunoinformatic analysis performed by a private laboratory in Wisconsin in 2014 revealed significant differences in the $CD4^+$ helper T cells elicited by wild-type and vaccine response, and the investigators postulated that vaccine efficacy with the original strains (including JL5) may have overemphasized vaccine efficacy as a result of frequent wild-type boosting that overcame a potential lack of appropriate T-helper stimulation from exposure to the JL5 vaccine strain.[99] These investigators concluded that serologic methods to evaluate vaccine efficacy and immunity may have overemphasized the conservation of one neutralizing epitope at the expense of others that could more accurately predict amnestic responses.

The vaccination rates in the United States in 1999 through 2004 were 90%, which is at the low end of the estimated population immunity (90–92%) needed for herd immunity.[126] It appears that outbreaks have occurred when vaccination rates drop below that required for herd immunity, and both vaccinated and unvaccinated individuals are at risk of infection. At present, the contribution of waning immunity to outbreaks is not well understood, and additional booster vaccinations are not routinely recommended in nonoutbreak settings. Notably, the 2006 Midwestern US outbreak and the 2009 to 2010 New York outbreak occurred in the setting of very high two-dose vaccine coverage, thereby leading to the suggestion that a more effective vaccine or an updated vaccination policy was needed.[56,128] Additional outbreak reports worldwide corroborate that high vaccination coverage is not necessarily protective.[22,75,80,131,141,143] Analysis of the seroepidemiology of mumps in 18 European countries between 1996 and 2008 suggests that in endemic-prone areas, repeating vaccination every 4 to 8 years is a potential strategy to prevent outbreaks.[61] Abrams and colleagues[4] described a computer-based mathematical model to estimate the risk of a mumps outbreak in highly vaccinated population by using spatial seroprevalence data.

A 2014 phase I clinical trial of a new F-genotype live attenuated mumps vaccine in China suggested adequate safety and effective immunogenicity.[138]

General Recommendations

Susceptible children, adolescents, and adults should be vaccinated against mumps unless vaccination is contraindicated. Mumps vaccine is of particular value for children approaching puberty and for adolescents and adults who have not had mumps. MMR and MMRV are the vaccines of choice for routine administration and should be used in all situations in which recipients also are likely to be susceptible to measles, rubella, or varicella. Persons should be considered susceptible to mumps unless they have documentation of (1) physician-diagnosed mumps, (2) two doses of live mumps virus vaccine with the first dose on or after their first birthday, or (3) laboratory evidence of immunity.

Persons who are unsure of their history of mumps disease or mumps vaccination should be vaccinated. No evidence has shown that persons who previously either received mumps vaccine or had mumps are at any increased risk for developing local or systemic reactions from receiving live mumps vaccine. Testing for susceptibility before administering vaccination, especially in adolescents and young adults, is not necessary.

Dosage

Two doses of MMR vaccine separated by at least 1 month in the volume specified by the manufacturer should be administered subcutaneously.

Age

Live mumps virus vaccine is recommended at any age on or after the first birthday for all susceptible persons, unless a contraindication exists. In routine circumstances, mumps vaccine should be given as MMR or MMRV, and the currently recommended schedule for administration of measles vaccine should be followed. It should generally not be administered to infants younger than 12 months old because persisting maternal antibody may interfere with seroconversion. To ensure that the patient has developed immunity, all persons vaccinated before their first birthday should be revaccinated on or after their first birthday.

Persons Exposed to Mumps

Use of Vaccine

When given after exposure to mumps, live mumps virus vaccine may not provide protection; although in a small cohort, it showed some promise when given as postexposure prophylaxis in the 2009 to 2010 New York outbreak.[67] However, if the exposure did not result in infection, vaccine should induce protection against infection from subsequent exposure. No evidence has indicated that the risk of vaccine-associated adverse events increases if vaccine is administered to persons incubating disease. In the 2009 to 2012 outbreak in New York, eligible 6th- to 12th-grade students were offered a third MMR vaccine, with a dramatic decline in incidence shortly after the intervention.[160] A lower rate of adverse events (with no serious events) was also observed, and it was concluded that a third dose of MMR vaccine may be effective in controlling future outbreaks.[3] In the 2009 to 2010 Guam outbreak in a cohort of 1068 students with two-dose coverage, there was a trend toward protection with a prophylactic third dose, and no serious adverse events were reported.[155]

Use of Immunoglobulin

Immunoglobulin has not been demonstrated to be of established value in postexposure prophylaxis and is not recommended.

Adverse Effects of Vaccine Use

In field trials in the United States before vaccine was licensed, illnesses did not occur more often in vaccinees than in unvaccinated control subjects.[94] Reports of illnesses occurring after receipt of mumps vaccination have been episodes mainly of parotitis and low-grade fever. Allergic reactions, including rash, pruritus, and purpura, have been associated temporally with mumps vaccination but are uncommon and usually mild and of brief duration. The reported development of encephalitis within 30 days of receiving a mumps-containing vaccine in the United States (0.4 per million doses) is not greater than the observed background incidence rate of CNS dysfunction in the normal population. Other manifestations of CNS involvement in the United States, such as febrile seizures and deafness, also have been reported infrequently. Complete recovery usually occurs. Reports of nervous system illness occurring after receipt of mumps vaccination do not necessarily denote an etiologic relationship between the illness and the vaccine. In parts of Europe, Canada, and Japan, where different mumps vaccines (Leningrad 3 strain and Urabe Am 9 strain) have been used, rates of vaccine-induced aseptic meningitis have been high.[45,49,146,153,204] Orchitis is a very rare complication of mumps vaccination.[46] Most cases have occurred in adolescents and adults, and five different vaccine strains have been associated with orchitis.

Contraindications to Vaccine Use

Pregnancy

Although mumps vaccine virus has been shown to infect the placenta and fetus,[229] no evidence has indicated that it causes congenital malformations in humans. However, because of the theoretic risk of fetal damage, a prudent approach is to avoid giving live virus vaccine to pregnant women. Women should avoid becoming pregnant for 3 months after receiving vaccination. Routine precautions for vaccinating postpubertal women include asking whether they are or may be pregnant, excluding those women who say that they are, and explaining the theoretic risk to those who plan to receive the vaccine. Being vaccinated during pregnancy should not be considered an indication for termination of pregnancy. However, the final decision about interruption of pregnancy must rest with the individual patient and her physician.

Severe Febrile Illness

Administration of vaccine should not be postponed because of minor or intercurrent febrile illnesses such as mild upper respiratory tract infections. However, vaccination of persons with severe febrile illnesses generally should be deferred until they have recovered.

Allergies

Because live mumps vaccine is produced in chick embryo cell culture, persons with a history of anaphylactic reactions (e.g., hives, swelling of the mouth and throat, difficulty breathing, hypotension, shock) after ingesting eggs should be vaccinated only with caution and according to published protocols.[79,91] Children known to be allergic should not leave the vaccination site for 20 minutes after being vaccinated. Evidence indicates that persons are not at increased risk if they have egg allergies that are not anaphylactic. Such persons may be vaccinated in the usual manner. No evidence has demonstrated that persons with allergies to chickens or feathers are at increased risk of having a reaction to the vaccine.

Because mumps vaccine contains trace amounts of neomycin (25 μg), persons who have experienced anaphylactic reactions to topically or systemically administered neomycin should not receive mumps vaccine. Most often, allergy to neomycin is manifested as contact dermatitis, which is a delayed-type (cell-mediated) immune response rather than anaphylaxis. In such persons, the adverse reaction, if any, to 25 μg of neomycin in the vaccine would be an erythematous, pruritic nodule or papule at 48 to 96 hours. A history of contact dermatitis to neomycin is not a contraindication to receiving mumps vaccine. Live mumps virus vaccine does not contain penicillin.

Recent Immunoglobulin Injection

Passively acquired antibody can interfere with the response to live attenuated virus vaccines. Therefore, mumps vaccine should be given at least 2 weeks before the administration of immunoglobulin or be deferred for 3 to 11 months after the administration of immunoglobulin. The duration of deferral depends on the dose of immunoglobulin administered.[220]

Altered Immunity

In theory, replication of the mumps vaccine virus may be potentiated in patients with immunodeficiency disease and by the suppressed immune responses that occur with leukemia, lymphoma, or generalized malignancy or with therapy with corticosteroids, alkylating drugs, antimetabolites, or radiation. In general, patients with such conditions should not be given live mumps virus vaccine. Because vaccinated persons in the United States do not transmit mumps vaccine virus, the risk of exposure to mumps in these patients may be reduced by vaccinating their close susceptible contacts. Interestingly, a handful of cases of horizontal transmission have been reported in Belarus and Croatia, all associated with the Leningrad-Zagreb or Leningrad-3 MuV virus strains.[9,10,110,165]

An exception to these general recommendations is in children infected with human immunodeficiency virus (HIV): all asymptomatic HIV-infected children should receive MMR vaccine at 12 months of age.[32,220] If measles vaccine is administered to symptomatic HIV-infected children, the combination MMR vaccine generally is preferred.[33]

Patients with leukemia in remission whose chemotherapy has been terminated for at least 3 months also may receive live mumps virus vaccine. Short-term (<2 weeks' duration) corticosteroid therapy, topical corticosteroid therapy (e.g., nasal, skin), and intraarticular, bursal, or tendon injections with corticosteroids are not contraindications to the administration of mumps vaccine. However, mumps vaccine should be avoided if systemic immunosuppressive levels are reached by prolonged, extensive, topical application.

Live vaccines have historically been avoided in patients who have received bone marrow, stem cell, and solid-organ transplantation. An international consensus conference recommends two doses of the MMR vaccine for allogeneic hematopoietic stem cell transplant recipients starting 24 months after transplant and once they are no longer receiving immunosuppressive therapy.[93] A review by Danerseau and Robinson in 2008[54] concluded that there were insufficient published data to determine the safety and/or efficacy of live viral vaccines in transplant recipients still receiving immunosuppressive therapy.

Containment of Disease

Containment is important in prevention of mumps in the United States. Mumps is a reportable disease, and compliance is the obligation of all physicians. After early reports of sporadic mumps cases, health department workers can organize local immunization clinics and exclude susceptible students from school so that disease can be contained in a small geographic area. Kutty and colleagues[127] published a discussion of containment strategies in wake of the 2006 US outbreak. Isolation of case patients was the primary outbreak control measure.

A 2008 CDC update recommended isolation of infected persons for 5 days after onset of parotitis and for contact and droplet precautions during this time.[40] These recommendations were based on data from the 2006 Iowa outbreaks, which yielded information on the duration of virus shedding after symptom onset,[174] as well as poor compliance with 9-day as compared with 5-day isolation regimens.[197]

NEW REFERENCES SINCE THE SEVENTH EDITION

2. Aasheim ET, Inns T, Trindall A, et al. Outbreak of mumps in a school setting, United Kingdom, 2013. *Hum Vaccin Immunother.* 2014;10(8):2446-2449.
3. Abedi GR, Mutuc JD, Lawler J, et al. Adverse events following a third dose of measles, mumps, and rubella vaccine in a mumps outbreak. *Vaccine.* 2012;30(49):7052-7058.
4. Abrams S, Beutels P, Hens N. Assessing mumps outbreak risk in highly vaccinated populations using spatial seroprevalence data. *Am J Epidemiol.* 2014;179(8): 1006-1017.
9. Atrasheuskaya A, Kulak M, Fisenko EG, et al. Horizontal transmission of the Leningrad-Zagreb mumps vaccine strain: a report of six symptomatic cases of parotitis and one case of meningitis. *Vaccine.* 2012;30(36):5324-5326.
10. Atrasheuskaya AV, Neverov AA, Rubin S, et al. Horizontal transmission of the Leningrad-3 live attenuated mumps vaccine virus. *Vaccine.* 2006;24(10):1530-1536.
15. Barrabeig I, Costa J, Rovira A, et al. Viral etiology of mumps-like illnesses in suspected mumps cases reported in Catalonia, Spain. *Hum Vaccin Immunother.* 2015;11(1):282-287.
17. Barskey AE, Schulte C, Rosen JB, et al. Mumps outbreak in Orthodox Jewish communities in the United States. *N Engl J Med.* 2012;367(18):1704-1713.
22. Braeye T, Linina I, De Roy R, et al. Mumps increase in Flanders, Belgium, 2012-2013: results from temporary mandatory notification and a cohort study among university students. *Vaccine.* 2014;32(35):4393-4398.
23. Briggs CM, Mayer AE, Parks GD. Mumps virus inhibits migration of primary human macrophages toward a chemokine gradient through a TNF-alpha dependent mechanism. *Virology.* 2012;433(1):245-252.
50. Cordeiro E, Ferreira M, Rodrigues F, et al. Mumps outbreak among highly vaccinated teenagers and children in the central region of Portugal, 2012-2013. *Acta Med Port.* 2015;28(4):435-441.
61. Eriksen J, Davidkin I, Kafatos G, et al. Seroepidemiology of mumps in Europe (1996-2008): why do outbreaks occur in highly vaccinated populations? *Epidemiol Infect.* 2013;141(3):651-666.
67. Fiebelkorn AP, Lawler J, Curns AT, et al. Mumps postexposure prophylaxis with a third dose of measles-mumps-rubella vaccine, Orange County, New York, USA. *Emerg Infect Dis.* 2013;19(9):1411-1417.
75. Gobet A, Mayet A, Journaux L, et al. Mumps among highly vaccinated people: investigation of an outbreak in a French military parachuting unit, 2013. *J Infect.* 2014;68(1):101-102.
80. Greenland K, Whelan J, Fanoy E, et al. Mumps outbreak among vaccinated university students associated with a large party, the Netherlands, 2010. *Vaccine.* 2012;30(31):4676-4680.
89. He J, Jia P, Zheng M, et al. Acupuncture for mumps in children. *Cochrane Database Syst Rev.* 2015;(2):CD008400.
99. Homan EJ, Bremel RD. Are cases of mumps in vaccinated patients attributable to mismatches in both vaccine T-cell and B-cell epitopes? An immunoinformatic analysis. *Hum Vaccin Immunother.* 2014;10(2):290-300.
100. Hukic M, Hajdarpasic A, Ravlija J, et al. Mumps outbreak in the Federation of Bosnia and Herzegovina with large cohorts of susceptibles and genetically diverse strains of genotype G, Bosnia and Herzegovina, December 2010 to September 2012. *Euro Surveill.* 2014;19(33):20879.
106. Jin L, Orvell C, Myers R, et al. Genomic diversity of mumps virus and global distribution of the 12 genotypes. *Rev Med Virol.* 2015;25(2):85-101.
110. Kaic B, Gjenero-Margan I, Aleraj B, et al. Transmission of the L-Zagreb mumps vaccine virus, Croatia, 2005-2008. *Euro Surveill.* 2008;13(16):18843.
128. Kutty PK, McLean HQ, Lawler J, et al. Risk factors for transmission of mumps in a highly vaccinated population in Orange County, NY, 2009-2010. *Pediatr Infect Dis J.* 2014;33(2):121-125.
131. Ladbury G, Ostendorf S, Waegemaekers T, et al. Smoking and older age associated with mumps in an outbreak in a group of highly-vaccinated individuals attending a youth club party, the Netherlands, 2012. *Euro Surveill.* 2014;19(16):20776.
133. Lamb RA, Parks GD. Paramyxoviridae. In: Knipe DM, Howley PM, eds. *Fields Virology.* Vol. 1. 6th ed. Philadelphia, PA: Lippincott Williams & Wilkins; 2013:957-995.
136. Leland DS. Parainfluenza and mumps viruses. In: Jorgensen JH, Pfaller MA, Carroll KC, et al, eds. *Manual of Clinical Microbiology.* Vol. 2. 11th ed. Washington, DC: ASM Press; 2015:1487-1497.
137. Lexova P, Limberkova R, Castkova J, et al. Increased incidence of mumps in the Czech Republic in the years 2011 and 2012. *Acta Virol.* 2013;57(3):347-351.
138. Liang Y, Ma J, Li C, et al. Safety and immunogenicity of a live attenuated mumps vaccine: a phase I clinical trial. *Hum Vaccin Immunother.* 2014;10(5):1382-1390.
140. Livingston KA, Rosen JB, Zucker JR, et al. Mumps vaccine effectiveness and risk factors for disease in households during an outbreak in New York City. *Vaccine.* 2014;32(3):369-374.
141. Mahamud A, Fiebelkorn AP, Nelson G, et al. Economic impact of the 2009-2010 Guam mumps outbreak on the public health sector and affected families. *Vaccine.* 2012;30(45):6444-6448.
143. Malaiyan J, Menon T. Low vaccine efficacy of mumps component among MMR vaccine recipients in Chennai, India. *Indian J Med Res.* 2014;139(5):773-775.
154. Nedeljkovic J, Kovacevic-Jovanovic V, Milosevic V, et al. A mumps outbreak in Vojvodina, Serbia, in 2012 underlines the need for additional vaccination opportunities for young adults. *PLoS ONE.* 2015;10(10):e0139815.
155. Nelson GE, Aguon A, Valencia E, et al. Epidemiology of a mumps outbreak in a highly vaccinated island population and use of a third dose of measles-mumps-rubella vaccine for outbreak control—Guam 2009 to 2010. *Pediatr Infect Dis J.* 2013;32(4):374-380.
156. Nelson KR, Marienau KJ, Barskey AE, et al. No evidence of mumps transmission during air travel, United States, November 1, 2006-October 31, 2010. *Travel Med Infect Dis.* 2012;10(4):165-171.
160. Ogbuanu IU, Kutty PK, Hudson JM, et al. Impact of a third dose of measles-mumps-rubella vaccine on a mumps outbreak. *Pediatrics.* 2012;130(6):e1567-e1574.
165. Otrashevskaia EV, Kulak MV, Otrashevskaia AV, et al. [Mumps vaccine virus transmission]. *Vopr Virusol.* 2013;58(6):42-45.
177. Rota JS, Rosen JB, Doll MK, et al. Comparison of the sensitivity of laboratory diagnostic methods from a well-characterized outbreak of mumps in New York City in 2009. *Clin Vaccine Immunol.* 2013;20(3):391-396.
180. Rubin S, Eckhaus M, Rennick LJ, et al. Molecular biology, pathogenesis and pathology of mumps virus. *J Pathol.* 2015;235(2):242-252.
181. Rubin S, Plotkin S. Mumps vaccine. In: Plotkin S, Orenstein W, Offit P, eds. *Vaccines.* Philadelphia, PA: Elsevier; 2013:419-446.
182. Rubin S, Sauder CJ, Carbone K. Mumps virus. In: Knipe DM, Howley PM, eds. *Fields Virology.* Vol. 1. 6th ed. Philadelphia, PA: Lippincott Williams & Wilkins; 2013:1024-1041.
184. Sakata R, Nagita A, Kidokoro M, et al. Virus genotypes and responses of serum-specific antibodies in children with primary mumps and mumps reinfection. *Pediatr Res.* 2015;78(5):580-584.
186. Sane J, Gouma S, Koopmans M, et al. Epidemic of mumps among vaccinated persons, the Netherlands, 2009-2012. *Emerg Infect Dis.* 2014;20(4):643-648.
191. Shu M, Zhang YQ, Li Z, et al. Chinese medicinal herbs for mumps. *Cochrane Database Syst Rev.* 2015;(4):CD008578.
199. St-Martin G, Knudsen LK, Engsig FN, et al. Mumps resurgence in Denmark. *J Clin Virol.* 2014;61(3):435-438.
206. Takla A, Bohmer MM, Klinc C, et al. Outbreak-related mumps vaccine effectiveness among a cohort of children and of young adults in Germany 2011. *Hum Vaccin Immunother.* 2014;10(1):140-145.
218. Wang W, Zhu Y, Wu H, et al. IL-6 and IFNgamma are elevated in severe mumps cases: a study of 960 mumps patients in China. *J Infect Dev Ctries.* 2014;8(2):208-214.

The full reference list for this chapter is available at ExpertConsult.com.

182 Respiratory Syncytial Virus

Robert C. Welliver Sr • Caroline B. Hall[†]

Respiratory syncytial virus (RSV) is the most important respiratory pathogen of infancy and early childhood and the major cause of hospitalization for bronchiolitis and pneumonia in infants globally.[39,101-103,152,225,228] In the United States, RSV has been estimated to be the leading cause of all hospitalizations for infants, resulting in an estimated 74,000 to 126,000 hospitalizations each year from 1994 to 1996.[175,250] More recent studies suggest that these figures are lower than the current number of infant hospitalizations associated with RSV infections and that the associated annual costs are approximately $2.6 billion.[131,133,145] Furthermore, the considerable burden of RSV infections among older children, adults, and outpatients has not been recognized. It is estimated that more than 2 million children younger than 5 years require outpatient management annually because of RSV infection, and 2% to 3% require hospitalization in the United States.[102,103,131] The situation is worse in developing countries, where it is estimated that RSV may cause 66,000 to 199,000 deaths annually.[25,208] In contrast, fewer than 100 deaths occur annually in the United States, and death rates are declining.[44] Overall, little doubt exists that the worldwide burden of lower respiratory tract disease attributable to RSV exceeds that of *Haemophilus influenzae* type b and *Streptococcus pneumoniae*.[215] The annual rate of hospitalizations caused by RSV, compared with that for influenza or the parainfluenza viruses, has been approximately three times greater for children aged 5 years and younger and six to eight times greater for children younger than 1 year. Adding to this burden of disease are emergency department and pediatric office visits, which occur at 5 to 10 times the rates of hospitalization.[71,72,91,112]

Among previously healthy working adults between 18 and 60 years of age, more than one-third require time away from work or school because of RSV infection. Among adults older than 65 years, RSV is a common cause of both upper and lower respiratory tract disease. Among elderly people, RSV-related deaths in the United States are estimated to exceed 10,000 annually; those with cardiopulmonary comorbidities are at greatest risk.[49,50,86,88]

RSV is marked by its contagiousness and by its propensity to cause the most severe disease during the first few months of life, despite the uniform presence of specific maternal antibody. Sizable outbreaks occur each year, with the result that most children become infected at least once in their first 2 years of life.[104,105,131] Nearly all first infections are symptomatic, and 20% to 30% involve the lower respiratory tract.[99,102,104,105] Reinfections occur throughout life despite an absence of major antigenic changes in viral surface proteins and commonly are sufficiently symptomatic to cause absence from work or school.[103,127]

HISTORY

In 1956, Morris and associates[202] noted an outbreak of colds with coryza in a colony of chimpanzees that had been under observation for the previous 3 to 24 weeks. A new virus was recovered from 1 of the 14 afflicted chimpanzees, and it was appropriately named chimpanzee coryza agent (CCA). Specific antibody to the CCA agent developed in the remaining 13 animals during convalescence; thus the attack rate was 100%. An upper respiratory tract infection and a serologic antibody response to CCA also developed in a person working with these chimpanzees, but the virus was not isolated from his secretions. However, further evidence of the pathogenicity of CCA was obtained subsequently when the CCA virus isolated from one chimpanzee was inoculated into susceptible chimpanzees and a coryzal illness developed after 3 days.

The suspected human origin of the chimpanzee coryza agent was confirmed a year later when Chanock and Finberg[54] recovered two agents indistinguishable from the CCA virus from the throat swabs of an infant with bronchopneumonia (Long strain) and from a child with laryngotracheobronchitis (Snyder strain). These investigators also observed an antibody response to these viruses in patients with respiratory disease and noted that by the time they reached 4 years of age, 80% of children had neutralizing antibody against the Long strain. Nonetheless, these investigators could not determine a definite etiologic association between the virus and lower respiratory tract disease in their young patients. They proposed naming this group of viruses (Long, Snyder, and CCA) respiratory syncytial virus because of their similar clinical manifestations and striking viral cytopathic effect of syncytial formation and multinucleated giant cells when the virus was grown in vitro. Confirmation of RSV as a major agent of respiratory disease soon accumulated from studies throughout the United States, and investigators from many countries subsequently documented and further delineated the importance of RSV.[25]

STRUCTURAL AND ANTIGENIC PROPERTIES

A tiny thistle—
of coiled spine
and outer quill...

—C.B.H.

Classification

The original classification of RSV with the Newcastle disease and parainfluenza group of viruses was based on their similar internal particle structure, eosinophilic inclusions, and syncytial appearance in tissue culture. However, RSV is antigenically distinct and does not hemagglutinate erythrocytes. Subsequently, the diameter of the nucleocapsid of RSV was determined to be between that of the larger paramyxoviruses and that of the smaller influenza viruses. Further study of the structure of RSV resulted in its current classification in the order Mononegavirales, family Paramyxoviridae, subfamily Pneumovirinae, and genus *Pneumovirus*.[64] RSV belongs, along with pneumonia virus of mice, bovine RSV, ovine RSV, caprine RSV, and turkey rhinotracheitis virus, to the subfamily Pneumovirinae, which consists of two genera, *Pneumovirus* and *Metapneumovirus* (MPV). The second genus, *Metapneumovirus*, contains human metapneumovirus (hMPV).[64]

Structural and Antigenic Properties

The virion of RSV consists of a nucleocapsid enclosed within an envelope consisting of a bilipid layer derived from the plasma membrane of host cells. Transmembrane glycoprotein spikes on its surface give the virus the appearance of a thistle on electron microscopy. The genome of RSV (strain A2) has been completely sequenced and is composed of 15,222 nucleotides. It is a nonsegmented, single-stranded, negative-sense RNA genome that encodes 11 proteins. Each of the major messenger RNAs (mRNAs) (Fig. 182.1) encodes for one of the major proteins, except for M2 mRNA, which possesses two overlapping open reading frames that encode for two separate proteins (M2-1 and M2-2).[64,295] Eight of these, including the seven largest (L, G, F, N, P, M, and SH), are structural proteins; two (NS1 and NS2) are nonstructural proteins that interfere with the interferon type I and type III response; M2-1 and M2-2 proteins are involved in RNA synthesis.[199]

Of the structural proteins, three form the viral capsid: N (nucleoprotein), P (phosphoprotein), and L (polymerase). Two are matrix

[†]Deceased.

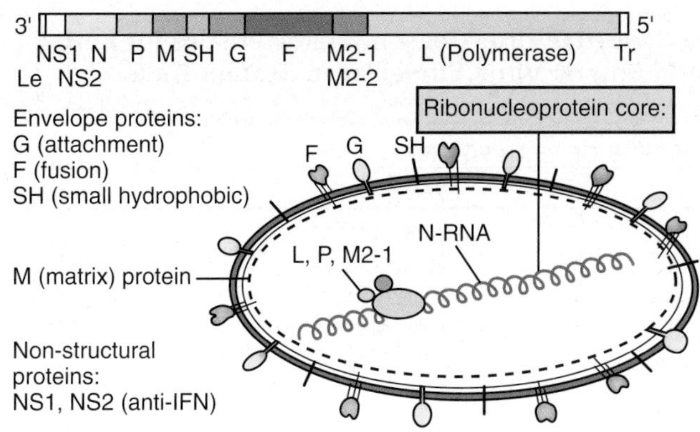

FIG. 182.1 The genome of respiratory syncytial virus (RSV) and a schematic diagram of an RSV virus particle. *Le*, leader; *Tr*, trailer.

membrane–associated proteins: the nonglycosylated M and M2 (the transcriptional antiterminator protein or transcriptase processivity factor, M2-1). The other three structural proteins, the glycosylated F (fusion) and G (attachment) proteins and the small, nonglycosylated hydrophobic SH protein, are transmembrane surface proteins.[64] The larger M protein is responsible for reassembly of the virus after it has entered a target cell and synthesized all of its proteins.[199] The F and G proteins are integral to RSV's infectivity and pathogenicity. The primary function of G, the largest glycoprotein, appears to be in the initial attachment of the virus to the host cell and is unusual compared with the attachment proteins of other paramyxoviruses because it has no hemagglutinin or neuraminidase. Initial penetration of the virus then is mediated by the F protein by fusing the viral and host cellular membranes, a process that allows cell-to-cell spread of the virus and results in the syncytia characteristic of RSV. However, all three of the surface glycoproteins, F, G, and SH, appear to act in concert to enhance the fusion process. Binding to a cellular receptor produces conformational changes in the F protein resulting in fusion of the virion envelope with the membrane of the cell.[196] Previously, G protein was identified as the major attachment protein, but more recently the F protein also has been recognized as having an important role in attachment of the virus.[263]

Significant strain variations among RSV isolates cause strains to be divided into two major groups.[13,295] These two major groups, A and B, have intergroup and intragroup variations in several proteins, including F, G, P, and N. The primary differences reside in the largest surface glycoprotein, the G protein. The amino acid sequence of the G protein varies by approximately 50% between the RSV A and RSV B strain groups. Intragroup strain variation also occurs mainly within the G protein. In contrast, within F protein, the amino acid sequence is conserved relatively well, and thus neutralizing antibody to F protein is cross-reactive between the two strain groups.[64] The F proteins of prototype strains from groups A and B have greater than 90% amino acid homology and a high degree of antigenic relatedness.

Laboratory Growth

RSV is relatively labile and is destroyed rapidly at 55°C. At 37°C, infectivity does not diminish for 1 hour, but by 24 hours, only 10% remains. RSV can grow in a variety of human and animal cell cultures. Human heteroploid cells, such as HEp-2, HeLa, and A549 cells, are used most frequently for primary isolation. Additional cell cultures that may be used, but generally are less sensitive, include diploid fibroblastic, monkey kidney, human kidney, and amnion cells. However, the sensitivity of these cell lines is variable, especially with passage, and must be monitored constantly. The characteristic cytopathic effect of RSV in continuous cell lines is syncytial formation with eosinophilic cytoplasmic inclusions. The syncytia usually are evident 2 to 7 days after inoculation and progress to complete degeneration within about 4 days.[64,120] The cytopathic effect, however, depends on the strain of virus, the medium, the sensitivity and thickness of the cell cultures, and the number of passages. Syncytia tend to be less evident in fibroblast cell lines; and in some primary cell cultures, RSV may produce rounded, refractile cells.

The growth cycle of RSV has been shown to consist of a period of adsorption, in which 50% of the inoculum is adsorbed in 2 hours, followed by an eclipse period of 12 hours. New virus appears shortly thereafter and enters a log phase of replication lasting approximately 10 hours. Viral antigen can be documented by fluorescent antibody staining 7 to 10 hours after inoculation. Shortly thereafter, cell-free virus may be demonstrated in the culture medium, but 50% to 90% of the virus remains associated with the cell surface at the time maximal titers are reached. Most of the cell-associated virus consists of incomplete noninfectious virions that may be released by agitation and sonication. With the laboratory Long strain (group A), peak titers usually are reached in 48 hours. For each infected cell, approximately 10 plaque-forming units generally result. Titers of virus are enhanced by inoculation of cell monolayers that are not yet confluent.[64]

Animal Susceptibility

An animal model of human RSV disease is a critical step in the search for effective antiviral therapy as well as for development of a vaccine. The natural hosts for symptomatic RSV infection are primarily humans and chimpanzees. Susceptible animals that could serve as a model for the lower respiratory tract disease of infants have been sought for some time.[20,82] Although RSV grows in the lung of a variety of animals, direct inoculation into their respiratory tract generally produces infection that is clinically and pathologically silent. Cattle are naturally infected with bovine, but not human, RSV.[82] RSV also has been recovered from asymptomatic goats and sheep. Other domestic animals, such as dogs and cats, have been found to possess antibody to RSV, the significance of which is unclear.

Chimpanzees resemble humans in some aspects in their clinical response to RSV, in that they develop rhinorrhea with natural RSV infection, and may transmit the virus to others of their species. Histologic pneumonia and some degree of clinical disease have been induced in many other adult primates, but the illness is mild in nature.[20,82] Infant baboons, however, develop tachypnea and reduced oxygenation following infection with RSV, with interstitial pneumonia, bronchiolitis, and obstruction of bronchiolar airways with inflammatory and sloughed epithelial cells similar to that observed in human infants. Fatal bronchiolitis can occur in infant baboons challenged with RSV. As in human infants, CD8 lymphocyte responses are absent with severe disease in infant baboons.[221] Infection in cattle can result in lung disease, but secondary bacterial infection may be required for symptoms to be evident. Marked lung pathology can be observed in sheep infected with RSV, but infection remains asymptomatic.[45] Infection in ferrets is age dependent, with limited histopathologic features developing in the nasal turbinates and trachea (but not lung) of adults. In infant ferrets, however, the virus replicates in the lung, although symptomatic respiratory disease is not apparent. RSV replicates in cotton rats better than in most animal models.[231] With intranasal inoculation, viral titers peak in the lung and nasal turbinates after 4 to 5 days. Illness is not apparent clinically, however. Histologic changes in the lung are present but are inconsistent, and immunologic reagents are limited compared with those for mice. Replication of RSV in other rodents generally is limited. BALB/c mice are among the most susceptible, and marked pulmonary disease may occur with high-titer inocula, which in older mice is accompanied by tachypnea and evidence of airway obstruction.[276] Disease in these mice, however, is mediated by aggressive CD4 and CD8 lymphocyte responses, which is the opposite of what occurs in humans, where CD8 responses are absent in infants with fatal disease.[113,292]

A human model of RSV infection has been reported in which healthy adult volunteers are infected intranasally with an attenuated strain of RSV and observed for viral load, immune markers, and clinical symptoms.[76-78] It is hoped that the availability of a safe and reproducible human model will permit more rapid testing of novel drugs and immunotherapies.

EPIDEMIOLOGY

What occult power pries loose the lid
to give you winter flight,
But with the lengthening light of spring
gives cloak and leaden wing?

—C.B.H.

TABLE 182.1 Summary of Median Values of Respiratory Syncytial Virus Season Characteristics for Entire Nation and US Census Regions From National Respiratory and Enteric Virus Surveillance System Data, 1990–2000

	MEDIAN WEEKS OF YEAR FOR RSV			
Location	***Onset***	***Peak***	***Offset***	***Duration***
Nation	51 (late December)[a]	5 (early February)	13 (end of March)	15
West	52 (late December)	6 (mid February)	13 (end of March)	14
Midwest	1[b] (early January)	7 (late February)	13 (end of March)	13[b]
South	47[c] (late November)	1 (early January)	10 (mid March)	16[b]
Northeast	49 (early December)	4 (end of January)	12 (late March)	15

[a]Numbers in parentheses, time of year.
[b]Statistically different from the rest of the nation, $P < .05$.
[c]Statistically different from the rest of the nation, $P < .01$.
From Mullins JA, LaMonte AC, Bresee JS, Anderson LJ. Substantial variability in community respiratory syncytial virus season timing. *Pediatr Infect Dis J.* 2003;22:857-862.

Geographic Distribution

Infection with RSV occurs worldwide, with its predominant pathogenicity occurring in the very young, in elderly people, and in those in each of those age groups who have underlying high-risk conditions, largely heart and lung disease. All geographic areas of the world experience RSV activity in every year. The timing, length, and intensity of RSV outbreaks, however, vary geographically.

Seasonal Patterns

In temperate locations, community outbreaks generally occur during the cold season. Outbreaks in warm and tropical climates tend to be more prolonged, with essentially continuous activity.[89,97] Within the United States, the inevitability of the RSV season is predictable, but the severity of the season, the time of onset, the peak of activity, and the end of the season cannot be predicted with precision (Table 182.1). The timing of RSV outbreaks often shows variation from year to year within the same community. This variation, however, occurs within the overall pattern of RSV seasonality in temperate climates, with epidemic activity generally beginning in November or December, peaking in January or February, and ending in March or April. Trends in RSV seasonality are monitored by the National Respiratory and Enteric Virus Surveillance System maintained by the Centers for Disease Control and Prevention.[49,50] Communities in the southern states tend to experience the earliest onset of RSV activity, and those in the upper Midwest tend to experience the latest onset. The duration of the season for the western and northeast regions typically occurs between that observed in the South and the Midwest. During the four RSV seasons of 2007 through 2011, the seasonal onset occurred from mid-November to early January, and the season's end occurred from mid-March to late April across all 10 Department of Health and Human Services regions. The median duration ranged from 13 to 23 weeks, and the peak of RSV activity occurred from mid-December to early February.[49,50] In regions where the season begins in November or December, the season ended by April or early May. In the few areas where the RSV season began in October, the season ended in March or early April. Florida is reported separately because, in some parts of the state, there is an earlier onset and earlier end to RSV circulation than the rest of the United States. Southeastern Florida (Miami area) has continuous RSV activity throughout the year.[49,183] Regional differences in RSV activity probably have a multifactorial explanation, including temperature, humidity, ultraviolet light exposure, social behavior, and probably other factors.[90,221,284] Areas near the equator and those in extremely cold climates have nearly continuous activity.[307] In contrast to data from the Western Hemisphere, where epidemic peaks occur annually in January and February, RSV activity in central Europe occurs in a biennial cycle, with peaks alternating between January and February in one year and between March and April in the following year.[151] The number of RSV infections causing hospitalization correlates with RSV activity in the community (Fig. 182.2).[49,183,250]

Specific groups of American Indian/Alaska Native children in certain geographic areas (particularly young children in southwestern Alaska) may experience more severe RSV disease and a longer RSV season than those in other parts of the United States.[254] Navajo and White Mountain Apache infants and young children may experience RSV hospitalization rates that are two to three times those of similar-aged children in other parts of the country.[43,215]

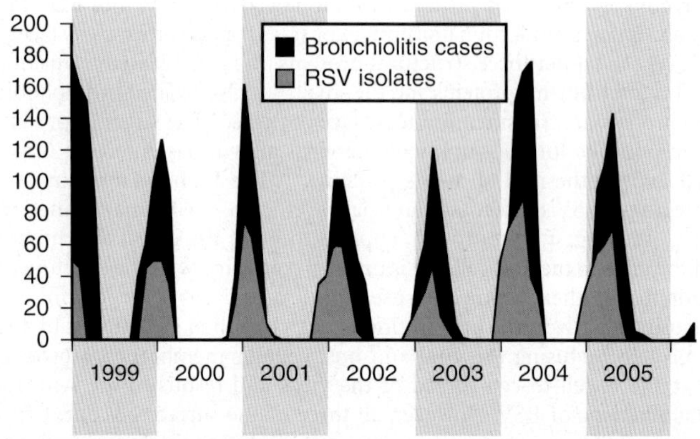

FIG. 182.2 The number of cases of bronchiolitis and the number of isolates of respiratory syncytial virus (RSV) from children younger than 5 years who were evaluated in private offices and outpatient facilities from 2000–05 identified by a community surveillance program in Monroe County, NY.

In geographic regions with temperate climates, including both the Northern and Southern Hemispheres, periods of RSV activity correlate with cold weather. In equatorial countries, RSV activity continues for much of the year. These patterns suggest the possibility that meterologic conditions influence the dissemination of virus. Efforts have been made to correlate RSV activity in different geographic locations with mean daily temperature, dew point, absolute humidity, ultraviolet B radiance, relative humidity, and precipitation. Results show a complex interaction between RSV circulation and environmental conditions that cannot be correlated easily.[92,288,291] In addition, weather conditions are likely to alter behavior, such that colder temperatures and rainy weather result in more time spent indoors, resulting in closer contact with other individuals and facilitating the spread of virus.

Results from several epidemiologic studies suggest that vitamin D may be protective against RSV lower respiratory tract infection. Vitamin D serum concentrations are lowest during winter months. Plasma concentrations of 25-hydroxyvitamin D concentrations are lower in infants hospitalized with RSV infections compared with healthy controls,[197,241] and a low 25-hydroxyvitamin D plasma concentration at birth correlates with a subsequent risk for RSV.[19] Whether vitamin D supplementation can reduce the frequency and severity of RSV infection has not been determined.

Strain Variation

Variation in circulating strains of RSV has been suggested as partly accounting for the fluctuating clinical impact of RSV epidemics.[13,221,245] The two major strain groups, A and B, differ mostly in the antigenic nature of the G and N proteins.[192,226] Importantly, A and B strains usually circulate simultaneously during an outbreak. The proportion of strains from each group may vary by season and geography, as does predominance of the subgroups of A and B strains.[13,192,226,245] In most areas, the usual dominant strains are in group A. In Rochester, New York, during a 20-year period, group A strains predominated in 11 of the years, group A and B strains were relatively equal in another 5 years, and in four seasons group B strains accounted for more than 75% of the year's isolates.[130] A study of strains from 14 cities across the United States demonstrated that the variability of strains occurs both seasonally and geographically.[13] Several distinct but varying genotypes within the A and B strain groups predominate each year in a community, a finding suggesting that local preexisting immunity to previously circulating RSV strains may engender a selective advantage for strains with genotypes most diverse from those recently present in a community.[192,226,295] Nevertheless, the relationship between the circulating strain group or subgroup and the size or clinical severity of an RSV outbreak has not been strong or consistent.[200,226] Further understanding of these relationships and the molecular mechanisms, pathogenesis, and clinical importance of differing genotypes may be integral to the development of effective vaccines and the control of RSV. A novel genotype, named ON1, originated in Toronto and spread rapidly across the world. Nevertheless, despite the penetrance of this genetically new strain in most global areas, the severity of disease has not increased.[84,261]

Acquisition and Ramifications of Infection

The availability of molecular-based detection techniques has allowed identification of a diverse group of viruses capable of causing lower respiratory tract disease.[265] Although the reported proportion of hospitalizations attributable to each virus differs depending on the geographic area and the year, the most common pathogen in these studies is uniformly RSV, followed by human rhinovirus. During the first year of life, 50% to 70% or more of infants acquire RSV infection, despite the presence of maternal-specific neutralizing antibody in the sera of all newborns. The level of antibody in a term newborn is similar to the maternal level, which gradually declines during the first 6 months of life. In patients older than 7 months of age, detectable specific serum antibody usually is the result of natural infection. Essentially all children possess specific serum antibody by 3 years of age.[104,225]

RSV accounts for 30% to 90% of bronchiolitis cases and up to 50% of pneumonia admissions during infancy. The major burden that RSV inflicts on the health care of children is illustrated by its ubiquity and the proportion of lower respiratory tract disease it causes in early childhood, especially among young infants. RSV accounts for 30% to 90% of bronchiolitis cases, up to 50% of pneumonia admissions during infancy, and 10% to 30% of cases of pediatric bronchitis.[39,131] In contrast, only relatively small proportions, less than 10%, of croup cases have been associated with RSV infection. RSV is isolated rarely from patients (<1%) without respiratory disease.[131] Fatal pediatric RSV cases are uncommon in industrialized countries. In the United States, the number of deaths associated with RSV infection each year among children younger than 5 years was estimated in 1985 to be 4500.[267] During 1979 to 1997, this number was reported to have declined to an estimated 510 or less each year in children younger than 5 years.[251] An analysis of mortality rates between 2004 and 2011 among children hospitalized because of RSV reported fewer than 100 deaths per year.[44] The deaths often occurred mostly in patients with congenital heart disease and after several weeks of hospitalization, suggesting that RSV infection alone was not the cause of death.

In the United States, inpatient hospital charges for hospitalized children were estimated to exceed $1.5 billion in 2009.[133] The economic and clinical costs related to RSV infections among young outpatient children have not been determined completely because costs from visits to emergency departments, clinics, and physicians' offices are difficult to quantify but are certainly quite substantial.[131]

Determination of the epidemiologic and clinical importance of coinfections in hospitalized children with bronchiolitis is an area of active research. Coinfection rates vary widely among studies and range from 6% to greater than 30%.[15,62] Studies of coinfections oddly have not established whether disease severity is enhanced, reduced, or unaffected by coinfection.[15]

Reports that use nuclear amplification assays suggest that one or more viral respiratory pathogens (particularly rhinoviruses) can be isolated from the upper respiratory tract of as many as 30% of symptom-free young children.[152,153] Whether viral genome detection in this setting represents prolonged shedding following a resolved infection, the incubation period for a pending infection, a persistent low-grade infection producing small amounts of virus, or infection by a serotype with limited ability to cause disease is not known.

The impact of RSV infections on communities around the world has been examined in numerous studies and varies depending on the geographic location, the population, and the methods of assessment. Nonetheless, several generalizations are evident: (1) RSV is highly contagious, resulting in ubiquitous infection by 2 to 3 years of age; (2) in this age group, RSV is the major cause of lower respiratory disease, predominantly bronchiolitis and pneumonia; (3) RSV infection of the lower respiratory tract in normal children almost always results from primary infection; (4) reinfections occur throughout life and tend to be milder and usually are upper respiratory tract infections; (5) the severity of illness from reinfections remains appreciable at any age in persons with comorbid conditions; and (6) medical visits by outpatients with RSV infection represent an appreciable portion of the burden to health care. Annual population-based hospitalization rates attributable to RSV from European countries are reported to be similar to those reported in the United States among children in different age groups.[93]

Risk Factors for Severe Disease

Most infants hospitalized with RSV lower respiratory infection are full-term infants with no known risk factors. Chronologic age is the single most important determinant for severe bronchiolitis based on the observation that approximately two-thirds of pediatric RSV hospitalizations occur in the first 5 months of life. Hospitalization rates are highest between 30 and 90 days after birth.[131] Infants with underlying chronic conditions are at high risk for requiring hospitalization for RSV illness, but numerous environmental and other host factors have been reported to augment the risk for a previously healthy infant's developing more severe RSV infection.[104,244,255] These factors include becoming infected within the first few months of life, living in crowded and lower socioeconomic circumstances, geographic location, and gender. Although the rate of infection among girls and boys is equal, boys are hospitalized more frequently than are girls.

In the United States, an estimated 55,000 to 125,000 RSV-associated hospitalizations occur each year.[156,198,294,292] The annual rate of hospitalizations caused by RSV compared with that from influenza or the parainfluenza viruses has been approximately three times greater for children aged 5 years and younger and six to eight times greater for children younger than 1 year.[131,152,213] Adding to this burden of disease are emergency department and pediatric office visits, which occur at 5 to 10 times the rates for hospitalization.[131]

The rate of admissions attributable to RSV is markedly higher among infants within the first year of life than among children aged 1 to 4 years. In infants, the estimated rates have varied from 5 to 41 per 1000 each year, depending on the area and the methods used.[36,176,189]

Population-based studies have reported annual hospitalization rates attributable to RSV in the United States of 3 to 3.5 per 1000 children younger than 5 years.[36,131,160] These rates were approximately six times greater than those associated with the influenza viruses and three times greater than those associated with the parainfluenza viruses. The rates of hospitalization for RSV among infants were even greater, 12.9 per 1000 children younger than 1 year, compared with 1.7 for influenza and 3.2 for the parainfluenza viruses. The youngest infants, those younger than 6 months, had the greatest risk for requiring admission for their RSV infection, with a yearly rate of 17 per 1000 children.[131]

In other developed countries, population-based studies demonstrated similarly high rates of hospitalizations related to RSV among infants and young children.[93,189,213] Annual population-based hospitalization rates attributable to RSV from European countries were reported per 1000 children to be 2.5 for those younger than 4 years of age, 11 for children younger than 3 years of age, and 4 to 7 for those younger than 2 years of age. Among children within the first 12 months of life, 19 to 22 per 1000 children were admitted each year with RSV infection.[93]

Children with certain comorbidities, including prematurity, chronic lung disease of prematurity, and congenital heart disease, may experience more severe RSV disease relative to children without such comorbidities.[10] Studies indicate a marked increase in risk for severe RSV disease among preterm infants born before 29 weeks' gestation and those born between 29 and 35 weeks' gestation, relative to infants born at or after 36 weeks' gestation.[36] Current controversy exists as to whether premature infants born relatively later in gestation (32 to 35 weeks) are at higher risk for severe RSV disease.[8,49]

Population-based data are not available on the incidence or severity of RSV disease among children who undergo solid organ transplantation or hematopoietic stem cell transplantation (HSCT), receive chemotherapy, or are immunocompromised because of other conditions. Progression of RSV infection from upper to lower respiratory tract disease depends on the virulence of the RSV strain as well as specific abnormalities in the immunocompromised host's immune response due to the underlying disease or to chemotherapy.[81,140,166,238]

The magnitude of ambulatory visits among children resulting from RSV infection has not been well quantified and generally has received less attention. Surveillance conducted in Nashville, Tennessee, and Rochester, New York for acute respiratory illness occurring among children aged up to 59 months showed that RSV was the agent most frequently identified among ambulatory children evaluated for respiratory illness.[131] RSV accounted for 18% of emergency department visits and 15% of pediatric practice visits from November to May. The estimated average rate of RSV-associated outpatient visits was 80 per 1000 children younger than 5 years and was estimated to be three times the rate of emergency department visits and 27 times the hospitalization rate for RSV. This appreciable impact of RSV outpatient visits on health care resources is further supported by a German study in which the annual incidence rate for RSV illness among outpatients was notably high at 77 per 1000 children younger than 3 years.[93]

The economic and clinical costs related to RSV infections among young outpatient children have been poorly characterized. In the United States, the cost for emergency department visits was estimated in 1997 to 2000 at more than $200 million per year for infants, and for all children younger than 5 years the cost for hospitalizations and other medical visits was $652 million in 2000. The contributions to this economic burden from office practices have not been estimated but are likely significant.[131,175]

Spread of Infection

RSV spreads effectively through exposed families, and introduction of the virus into the family appears to occur most commonly through a school-aged child. Serious disease in infancy is likely to follow a mild "cold" in an older sibling.[122] In a prospective study of families with an infant and one or more older siblings, 44% of the families became infected with RSV during a 3-month epidemic. In almost all these families, older siblings (2–16 years of age) introduced the virus into the family, and the infants became secondarily infected (Table 182.2).

These clinical observations and volunteer studies indicate that RSV is predominantly spread by two modes: (1) large particle droplet aerosols (>10–100 μm mass median diameter), which generally travel short distances (≤0.9 m) through sneezing, coughing, and even in some individuals by normal quiet breathing; and (2) self-inoculation of infectious secretions contaminating environmental surfaces.[117,113] Small particle aerosols (≤10 μm mass median diameter), which can produce distant spread, may also occur with RSV, but their clinical importance is controversial.

These modes of spread have been supported by volunteer and experimental studies. One study demonstrated that infection occurs in volunteers who touch surfaces contaminated by secretions and then their eyes or nasal mucosa.[117] In contrast, no infections developed in volunteers exposed to infected infants at a distance of greater than 6 feet, thus suggesting that small-particle aerosol spread of RSV was not a major mode of transmission. RSV infection therefore appears in most instances to require close contact with infected individuals or their secretions.

RSV in the nasal secretions of infants with acute infection remains infectious on countertops for longer than 6 hours and on cloth and tissue paper for approximately 30 minutes. These nasal secretions can remain infectious after transfer from objects or hands to the hands of another person, thus indicating that contact with clothing, furniture, or tissues contaminated by the secretions of infected children can result in spread.[120] Furthermore, the potential for RSV's transmission is augmented by the long duration of shedding and high viral loads commonly observed among young infants with RSV infection.[73,119,300]

TABLE 182.2 Attack Rate of Respiratory Syncytial Virus in Families According to Age

Age (y)	CRUDE RATE[a]		RATE IN RSV-POSITIVE FAMILIES		SECONDARY RATE	
	No.[b]	%	*No.*[b]	%	*No.*[b]	%
<1	10/34	29.4	10/16	62.5	5/11	45.4
1–<2	2/7	28.6	2/5	40.0	0/3	0.0
2–<5	9/34	26.4	9/19	47.0	2/12	16.6
5–<17	9/48	18.7	9/24	38.0	4/19	21.0
17–45	9/55	16.8	9/21	43.0	6/18	33.3
Total	39/178	21.9	39/85	45.9	17/63	27.0

[a]The crude attack rate according to age is shown for all family members studied and for members of RSV-positive families. The secondary attack rate is also shown for members of RSV-positive families, excluding all primary and co-primary cases.

[b]Number of persons infected with RSV per total number of persons exposed.

From Hall CB, Geiman JM, Biggar R, et al. Respiratory syncytial virus infection within families. *N Engl J Med.* 1976;294:414-419.

PATHOLOGY AND PATHOGENESIS

The incubation period of illness from RSV has been reported variably as being between 2 and 8 days, most frequently as 4 to 6 days. Experimental infection in adult volunteers produced an incubation period of 3 to 6 days, with an average of 5 days.[121,171] With primary infection, the incubation period may be shorter.[121,129] Inoculation is through the upper respiratory tract, followed by infection of the respiratory epithelium. Both the eye and the nose appear to be equally sensitive routes of inoculation.[121] In contrast, inoculation by mouth results in infection much less frequently. Spread along the respiratory tract may occur by cell-to-cell transfer of the virus along intracytoplasmic bridges and may involve the conducting airways at all levels. However, aspiration of secretions into the lung during sleep cannot be excluded as a means by which virus may reach the lower lung.

The major pathologic findings shown in the lungs of infants dying from RSV bronchiolitis are (1) peribronchiolar mononuclear infiltration; (2) necrosis of the epithelium of the small airways; (3) plugging of the lumina with necrotic epithelial cells, leukocytes, and fibrin; and (4) hyperinflation and atelectasis (Fig. 182.3).[6,154,292] The initial lesions in bronchiolitis occur in the small airways (75–300 μm).[278] Macrophage and neutrophil peribronchiolar infiltration develops, along with edema of the walls, the submucosa, and adventitial tissue. Lymphocytes, especially CD8 T cells, are notably absent in fatal RSV infections of infants[292] but are present in cases with milder outcomes.[154] Subsequently, the epithelium of the bronchioles undergoes striking necrosis, sometimes with proliferation of the epithelium into the lumen. Sloughing of necrotic material into the lumina of the small airways impedes the flow of air, which is aggravated by the presence of inflammatory debris.[278,292] Amorphous material plugging the lumen is negative in stains for mucus (periodic acid–Schiff and Alcian blue), therefore more likely representing fibrin.[292]

Peripheral to the sites of partial occlusion, air trapping occurs, similar to a ball-and-valve mechanism. During the negative intrapleural pressure of inspiration, air can flow past the site of partial obstruction, but with the positive pressure of expiration, the lumen narrows, resulting in more complete obstruction and the hyperinflation characteristic of bronchiolitis. The trapped air may be absorbed and result in multiple areas of focal atelectasis. Functionally, these pathologic changes translate into an increased lung volume (unless atelectasis is extensive) and higher expiratory resistance in the infant. Pneumonia may be present concurrently and is marked by infiltration of mononuclear cells into the alveolar interstitium. The lung parenchyma appears edematous, with areas of necrosis leading to alveolar filling, consolidation, and collapse.

Initial recovery from acute bronchiolitis may be evident in 3 to 4 days, with regeneration of the bronchiolar epithelium, but ciliated cells rarely are present before 2 weeks.[279] Complete histologic and functional recovery may require another 4 to 8 weeks.[123]

IMMUNE RESPONSE: IMMUNITY AND DISEASE PATHOGENESIS

Despite the recent rapid rise in our knowledge of the immune response to RSV infection, it remains unclear whether disease results primarily from the direct cytotoxic effect of viral replication or from the evoked immune response. Evidence for the direct viral replication being the prime cause has been long suggested by the observation of a correlation between increased RSV concentration in nasal secretions and disease severity seen in some studies,[73,119,188] but not in others.[187,300] Experimental studies in humans suggest that upper respiratory symptoms begin near the onset of viral shedding in nasal secretions, peak at the time of peak viral shedding, and begin to subside as viral load declines.[78] Nevertheless, because upper respiratory symptoms precede clinical signs of bronchiolitis and pneumonia by several days, it is unclear whether the degree of viral shedding will correlate with the time of development of severe forms of RSV illness in infants. More recent evidence showed that T-lymphocyte–derived cytokine concentrations in respiratory secretions of infants with RSV infection were lower than those in children with influenza infection.[292] In addition, lung tissue from infants with fatal RSV infection demonstrated abundant RSV antigen, but few $CD4^+$ and $CD8^+$ lymphocytes and few natural killer (NK) cells, leading to the conclusion that cytotoxic lymphocyte responses do not have an important role in the pathogenesis of RSV lower respiratory tract disease. Instead, severe RSV lower tract disease is characterized by abundant viral replication and an inadequate adaptive immune response.[290,292] These findings suggest that during acute illness the pathogenesis of RSV disease is related more to the infant's inability to develop an adaptive cytotoxic T-cell response to curb viral replication than to an aberrant immune response that enhances the disease process.

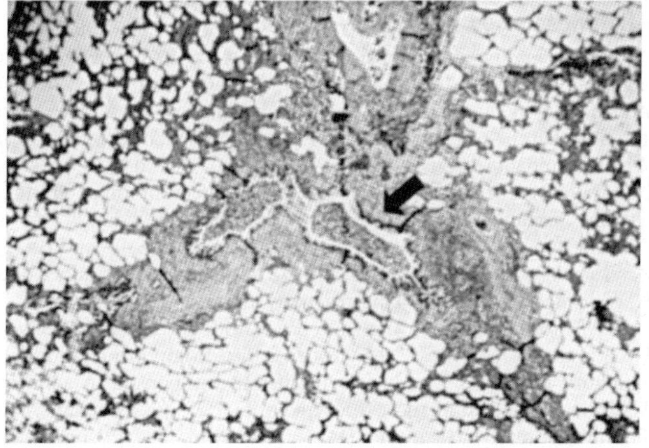

FIG. 182.3 Histologic examination of an infant dying of respiratory syncytial virus bronchiolitis. The *arrow* denotes a bronchiole filled with inflammatory exudate and comparatively normal alveoli.

Evidence supporting an immunopathic contribution comes from observations of enhanced disease among recipients of a formalin-inactivated RSV vaccine in the 1960s.[164] Current research also suggests that the innate and adaptive immune responses may participate in producing disease as well as limiting primary infection and immunizing against subsequent infection (Fig. 182.4). It is likely that both the direct effect of the virus and immune factors of the host are involved in causing disease following infection with RSV.[290]

Innate Immunity

RSV targets type I alveolar cells, airway epithelial cells, and alveolar macrophages, resulting in impairment of ciliary action and sloughing of infected epithelial cells.[275,278] Dendritic cells scavenge the lung for foreign antigen and are important in generating a viral-specific immune response against RSV. After ingesting viral antigen, dendritic cells migrate to lymph nodes where antigen is presented to cognate, naïve T cells.[100] Cytokines released from dendritic cells polarize the cytokine responses toward a helper T-cell subtype 1 (Th1) or Th2 profile. Although it has been attractive to attribute wheezing in association with RSV infection

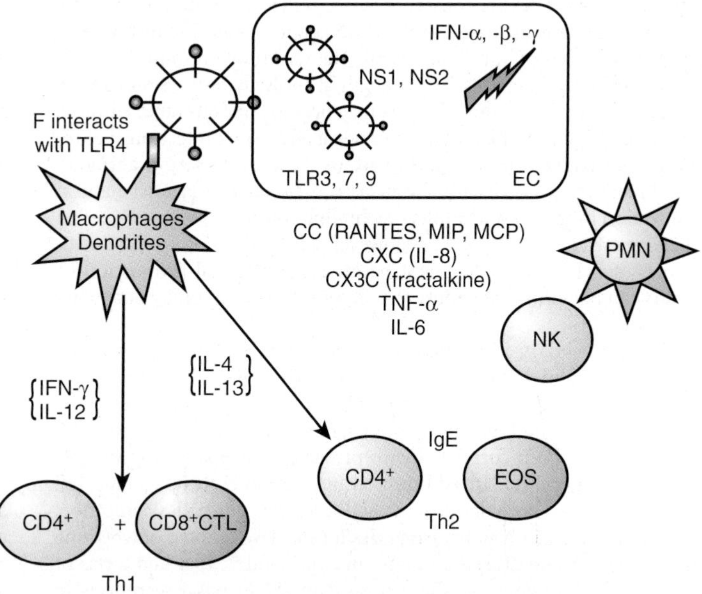

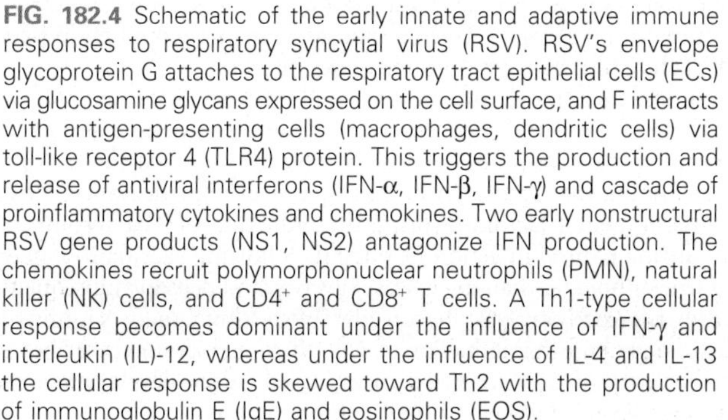

FIG. 182.4 Schematic of the early innate and adaptive immune responses to respiratory syncytial virus (RSV). RSV's envelope glycoprotein G attaches to the respiratory tract epithelial cells (ECs) via glucosamine glycans expressed on the cell surface, and F interacts with antigen-presenting cells (macrophages, dendritic cells) via toll-like receptor 4 (TLR4) protein. This triggers the production and release of antiviral interferons (IFN-α, IFN-β, IFN-γ) and cascade of proinflammatory cytokines and chemokines. Two early nonstructural RSV gene products (NS1, NS2) antagonize IFN production. The chemokines recruit polymorphonuclear neutrophils (PMN), natural killer (NK) cells, and $CD4^+$ and $CD8^+$ T cells. A Th1-type cellular response becomes dominant under the influence of IFN-γ and interleukin (IL)-12, whereas under the influence of IL-4 and IL-13 the cellular response is skewed toward Th2 with the production of immunoglobulin E (IgE) and eosinophils (EOS).

to the induction of a Th2 response, there is virtually no evidence to support this in humans.[98]

The infant's early innate immune response to the infection of these cells is characterized by the synthesis of chemokines and proinflammatory cytokines and the recruitment of inflammatory cells to the infected pulmonary tissues.[154,155,246,269] Among these are neutrophils, eosinophils, and interferon-γ (IFN-γ)–secreting NK cells. There is a suggestion that strong innate cytokine responses are necessary to limit the severity of RSV infection.[23]

Toll-like receptors (TLRs) have an important role in mediating and modulating the inflammatory cytokine and chemokine production during RSV infection. RSV's interaction with specific TLRs (TLR3, TLR4, TLR7, TLR8, TLR9) on mononuclear cells and alveolar macrophages results in production of antiviral and immunomodulatory mediators, including type I and III interferons; IFN-α, IFN-β, and IFN-γ; chemokines CXCL8 (interleukin-8 [IL-8]) and CCL5 (RANTES), and cytokines IL-6 and tumor necrosis factor-α (TNF-α) (see Fig. 182.4).[22,29,110,111,135,157,169,195,218,242] The outcome of RSV infection may vary according to the interaction of RSV with individual TLRs. This is illustrated in rodent models by TLR4-deficient mice having impaired viral clearance, whereas TLR3-deficient mice develop Th2-polarized responses but continue to eliminate virus with normal kinetics.[135,242] Some evidence currently supports the role of TLR4 signaling in modulating human RSV disease.[46]

Passively Acquired Antibody

During the neonatal period, protection against RSV infection is mediated in part by transplacentally acquired IgG. Glezen and coworkers showed that the age at the time of hospitalization for infants with primary RSV infection was directly correlated with the cord blood–neutralizing antibody titer.[104] Because maternally derived antibody has a half-life in the infant of approximately 21 days, the protective effect rapidly wanes. These observations, among others, led to the development and use of high-titered RSV intravenous immunoglobulin (RSV-IVIG) and, subsequently, of the monoclonal antibody palivizumab for RSV prophylaxis in high-risk infants.[109,149]

B-Cell Responses

After acquiring RSV infection, infants develop antibodies to several RSV-specified proteins, the most important of which are directed against the F and G proteins, which have viral neutralizing activity.[303] Serum-neutralizing and F and G protein–specific antibodies develop in most infants after RSV infection, regardless of the severity of their illness.[293] However, neutralizing and F antibody responses are diminished in those younger than 6 months, and high levels of preexisting maternal antibody inhibit antibody responses to the G protein. The antibody response to the F protein is broadly cross-reactive with both A and B strains because neutralizing epitopes are conserved between the two strain groups. This is in marked contrast to the group- and genotype-specific response to the highly variable G protein. Overall, the serum IgG response to RSV is relatively weak in infants. The strength of antibody responses increases with secondary infections.[293] Titers may become undetectable within a year after infection, thus requiring several additional infections before levels approximate those found in adults.[279] Levels of serum antibody are directly correlated with the degree of protection against natural reinfection in infants and adults,[283] a finding confirmed in experimental challenge studies in adults.[129,178] However, solid protection from reinfection is of brief duration at best because a substantial proportion of adults can be reinfected within several months of a naturally occurring infection.[129]

During primary RSV infection of mice and humans, RSV-specific immunoglobulin A (IgA) antibody is detectable in nasal secretions and coincides with the cessation of viral replication, as judged by culture.[129,257] Using a human adult challenge model, high levels of RSV-specific IgA antibody have been correlated with protection against symptoms following challenge.[17,129] In addition to IgA antibody, RSV-specific IgE antibody has also been detected in nasal secretions during RSV infection, which correlated with an increased risk for the development of wheezing both during acute disease and later in childhood.[294] Elevated levels of cysteinyl leukotrienes also have been detected in nasal secretions in infants with RSV infection, although quantities of leukotrienes detected are not clearly related to the severity of illness.[277] Mucosal antibody responses to nonreplicating RSV antigens are not strong but may be enhanced by the concurrent administration of ligands (TLR9/NOD2) before application.[248]

Efforts to develop a monoclonal antibody to be used for prophylaxis initially focused on the F protein because of its highly conserved amino acid sequence. By contrast, most portions of the RSV G protein are heavily glycosylated and highly variable, except for a short central motif that appears to be invariant. The G protein appears to induce neutralizing antibodies and protective immunity, but the G protein also has been implicated in disease pathogenesis, particularly modulation of the host immune response.[156,219] The conserved region of the G protein demonstrates molecular mimicry with the chemokine fractalkine, which induces leukocyte transit to the site of inflammation. Both membrane-bound and secreted forms of G protein can bind to the fractalkine receptor CX3CR1, thereby blocking the interaction of fractalkine with its receptor and potentially interfering with the recruitment of NK cells and $CD4^+$ and $CD8^+$ T cells to the site of inflammation.[42,272] Antibodies that block this motif of the G protein have been shown to reduce both viral replication and disease severity in animals.[134] However, there is tremendous duplication of chemokine functions in humans, and whether antibody to this G protein motif, or to the G protein itself, will modify disease in humans has not been established.

T-Cell Responses

Our understanding of cell-mediated immunity to RSV has been derived principally from studies in rodent models and from more limited information in humans. A hypothesis that has emerged from these studies is that the severity of disease is best controlled by the generation of Th1-dominant responses by IFN-γ–secreting $CD4^+$ and $CD8^+$ cytotoxic T lymphocytes, in concert with the combined effects of innate immune cytokines, serum neutralizing antibody, and mucosal antibody.[17,98,142,252,256] Conversely, a Th2-polarized response, which induces IL-4– and IL-13–secreting $CD4^+$ cells, eosinophils, and IgE antibody, theoretically would be associated with airway hyperreactivity and more severe disease.[61,193]

RSV infection has been shown to have a wide spectrum of effects on T-cell immune responses.[205] RSV, when added to in vitro cultures, has inhibitory effects on lymphocyte proliferative responses. In addition, dendritic cells, including those recovered from RSV-infected infants, have diminished capacity to activate $CD4^+$ T cells in vitro.[58,70,100,184] Nonetheless, RSV infection can induce a full range of T-cell responses in vivo, including Th1 $CD4^+$ and $CD8^+$ cytotoxic T lymphocytes as well as Th2 $CD4^+$ cells. These responses are, however, generally quite weak in human infants with RSV infection.[194] Human and murine $CD8^+$ cytotoxic T lymphocytes recognize F, M2, M, and NS2 epitopes in the context of class I antigens.[38,53,57,136] Both $CD4^+$ and $CD8^+$ T cells can clear virus from the lungs of infected animals. However, disease in mice is mediated by excessive T-cell responses; removal of CD4 or CD8 T cells permits greater virus replication, but illness is less severe.[106] The relevance of these studies to human disease, where illness seems related to inadequate cytotoxic lymphocyte responses,[292] is unclear. Also, although a predominance of Th2 lymphocytes has been hypothesized as a factor in severe forms of RSV infection, most studies have failed to detect the presence of Th2 cytokines in human infants with RSV disease.[3,98,252,271,292] In one report, RSV-specific lymphoproliferative responses were relatively short-lived after primary infection and were not boosted by reinfection.[33] RSV is a poor inducer of protective central memory T-cell responses, perhaps accounting in part for the failure of long-term immunity after infection.[53]

In summary, humoral and mucosal antibodies provide some protection from infection, although it is variable and transient. The innate and adaptive T-cell responses elicited by RSV infection may have a role in determining the disease pathogenesis and in viral clearance. Host and environmental factors favoring the induction of Th1 responses, either during natural infection or possibly following vaccination, may minimize pathologic changes, disease severity, and perhaps subsequent airway hyperreactivity. Despite considerable research, there is minimal evidence suggesting that induction of Th2 cytokine responses contributes to the severity of RSV infection or is linked to the development of wheezing episodes following infantile bronchiolitis.

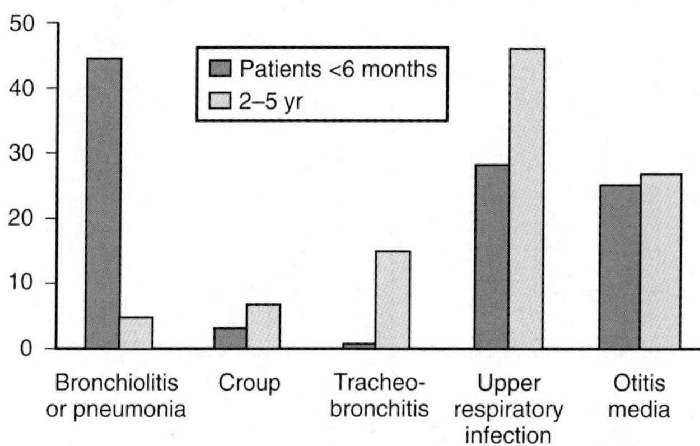

FIG. 182.5 Clinical diagnoses of children with respiratory syncytial virus (RSV) infection according to age. The proportion of children presenting with each respiratory syndrome who were younger than 6 months and had primary RSV infection is shown in comparison with those children aged 2 to 5 years who had a repeated RSV infection. Data were obtained from 415 outpatient infants and children evaluated in Rochester, NY. (Courtesy C.B. Hall, unpublished data.)

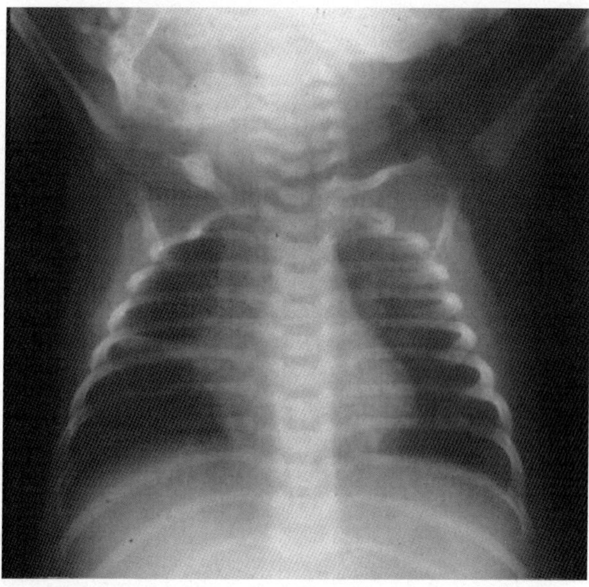

FIG. 182.6 Bronchiolitis from respiratory syncytial virus (RSV) infection. This chest radiograph of a 3-month-old infant with bronchiolitis from RSV infection shows hyperaeration of the lung and area of atelectasis in the right middle lobe.

CLINICAL MANIFESTATIONS

We view their chests ballooning, with the fears
that they're "pink puffers" of more tender years.

—C.B.H.

Primary Infection

An infant's first encounter with RSV almost always is apparent, but the symptoms may range from those of a mild cold to severe bronchiolitis or pneumonia. Various definitions of bronchiolitis have been proposed, but generally the term *bronchiolitis* is limited to infants less than 12 to 18 months of age with wheezing precipitated by a viral infection. An infant with bronchiolitis typically presents during the winter months after 2 to 4 days of low-grade fever, nasal congestion, and rhinorrhea with symptoms of lower respiratory tract illness, including cough, tachypnea, and increased respiratory effort as manifested by grunting, nasal flaring, and intercostal, subcostal, or supraclavicular retractions.[124] Rarely is a child's first encounter with RSV entirely asymptomatic. Among infants examined over the course of a 10-year period with known primary RSV infection who initially were younger than 6 months, 45% had the clinical manifestations of bronchiolitis or pneumonia, compared with 5% of children 2 to 5 years of age who had experienced two or more outbreaks of RSV infection (Fig. 182.5).[225] Higher rates of lower respiratory tract disease have been documented to occur in children with underlying cardiopulmonary disease, those in closed populations such as group child care centers, and those from certain geographic areas or with particular ethnic backgrounds.[139,186]

In the longitudinal Houston family studies,[105] 69% of children in their first year of life acquired RSV infection, and one-third of these infections were lower respiratory tract illnesses. By the time they were 24 months of age, essentially all children had been infected at least once and about half had experienced two infections, such that the rate of infections during the second year of life was 83%. The proportion of RSV infections involving the lower respiratory tract remained appreciable during the second, third, and fourth years of life, but the severity decreased. In general, lower respiratory tract illnesses associated with RSV after the second year of life most frequently are tracheobronchitis and reactive airway disease.[105]

Pneumonia and bronchiolitis, the most common forms of RSV lower respiratory tract disease in infants, generally coexist and are nearly impossible to differentiate clinically or radiographically. Children with hyperinflation and wheezing, the hallmarks of bronchiolitis, may have densities on a chest film that may appear similar to infiltrates from pneumonia (Fig. 182.6). However, in bronchiolitis, these shadows most likely result from atelectasis rather than from the interstitial inflammation and alveolar filling of pneumonia.

Upper respiratory tract symptoms usually precede lower respiratory tract involvement by several days. Low-grade fever is a common manifestation during this initial phase of the illness, but it may have disappeared by the time of hospitalization (Fig. 182.7). Among 565 children hospitalized with RSV infection, fewer than half had a temperature higher than 38°C (100.4°F) at the time of admission.[128] Among children undergoing their second, third, or fourth infections, 20% to 40% of children may be febrile.[139]

Increased coughing commonly heralds involvement of the lower respiratory tract, which subsequently may be indicated by an increased respiratory rate, dyspnea, and retractions of the chest wall (see Fig. 182.7). Auscultatory findings of crackles and wheezing may be present on initial examination but absent on reexamination shortly thereafter. Variability of the child's clinical findings within minutes to hours is characteristic of RSV lower respiratory tract disease. Ill children who elicit concern because they are lethargic and short of breath may have minimal audible wheezing and crackles because of limited air entry with inspiration. There is not a consistent correlation between the findings on auscultation or on the chest radiograph with severity of disease or with length of hospital stay. Respiratory rate and the degree of chest wall retraction are better predictors.

Radiographic Findings

The radiographic findings in infants hospitalized with RSV lower respiratory tract disease may be variable, but with bronchiolitis, hyperinflation with hyperlucency of the lung, flattened diaphragms, and peribronchiolar thickening usually are evident. Patchy areas of atelectasis also may be present, most often in the right middle and upper lobes. Areas of atelectasis may be large and are too often interpreted as representing bacterial pneumonia. Less frequently observed are interstitial infiltrates of pneumonitis, which tend to be present diffusely (see Fig. 182.6).

Current guidelines recommend that bronchiolitis should be diagnosed on the history and physical examination and that chest radiographs should not be obtained routinely. Infants with bronchiolitis will have abnormalities on a chest radiograph, but data do not indicate that the chest radiograph findings correlate well with disease severity. Routine radiography has been shown to increase the risk for receipt of antibiotics without any impact on outcome. Initial radiography should be reserved for cases in which respiratory effort is severe enough to warrant intensive care unit (ICU) admission or where signs of airway complication (such as pneumothorax) are present.[19]

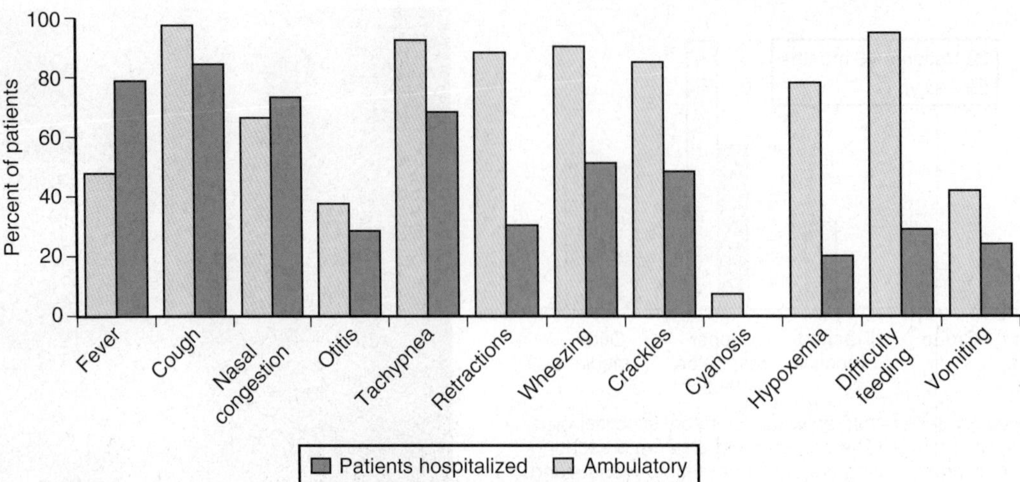

FIG. 182.7 Clinical manifestations in children with respiratory syncytial virus (RSV) infection who were evaluated in Rochester, NY. Shown are the proportions of 1132 hospitalized children compared with the proportions of 489 outpatient children with each clinical sign.

With tracheobronchitis and upper respiratory tract infections, the accompanying signs and symptoms tend to be more severe in RSV infection than in infections with other common respiratory agents. Coughing is often prolonged. Otitis media frequently is associated with both initial RSV and recurrent RSV infection.[137,230] Among children with RSV infection, the virus has been detected in 30% to 74% of middle ear aspirates. Among children presenting with otitis media, RSV is one of the most frequently identified viral pathogens and has been associated with prolonged symptoms and apparent failure of therapy. RSV may be detected as the sole pathogen or simultaneously with a bacterial agent, thus suggesting that RSV may play both a primary and a secondary role in the pathogenesis of otitis media.[297]

RSV infection has been associated occasionally with a variety of neurologic, cardiac, and other conditions.[18,210,260] However, in most of these reports, the causal role of RSV is arguable; alternatively, a simultaneous RSV infection may be occurring that is unrelated to the more unique clinical event.

Infection in Neonates

Symptoms of RSV infection are largely dependent on the age of the host at the time of infection. In Washington, DC, the incidence of RSV infection during the first month of life was noted to be only one-third of that during the second month of life.[225] The protected environment of newborns with diminished exposure to others, as well as the high levels of maternal antibody or other early immune factors, may explain the lower incidence of illness in the neonatal period. RSV infection in neonates may be variable and atypical. Apnea and hemodynamic instability may occur in the presence of only with minimal respiratory signs, resulting in an incorrect or delayed diagnosis.[125] Apnea usually develops at the beginning of the RSV infection before wheezing occurs, often as the first manifestation of illness, and is short-lived and nonobstructive.[12] Most infants do not have apnea subsequently, even with later respiratory tract infections.

In full-term infants, RSV infection in the neonatal period may manifest primarily as a mild, afebrile upper respiratory tract illness, often associated with atypical findings such as feeding difficulties, poor weight gain, periodic breathing, or apnea.[12] However, among premature infants, the morbidity may be more pronounced. During a community outbreak of RSV infection in Rochester, New York, 25% of infants kept in a neonatal ICU for more than 6 days acquired RSV infection. Infants older than 3 weeks of age tended to have lower respiratory tract disease characteristic of RSV infection and apnea, whereas infants in the first 3 weeks of life were more likely to have nonspecific findings without clinical evidence of lower respiratory tract disease. Fewer than half had upper respiratory tract signs; nonetheless, four (17%) of the infants died.[125]

Acute Complications

Apnea, a major complication of acute RSV infection in young infants, occurs in 1% to 20% of infants hospitalized with RSV infection.[12,124,234] Apnea is most likely to occur among infants born prematurely, in those with a young postnatal age, especially infants who have not yet reached a postconceptional age of 44 weeks, and in infants with a history of apnea of prematurity. The apnea usually develops at the beginning of the RSV infection, often as the first manifestation of illness, and is short-lived and nonobstructive.[12] Most infants do not have apnea subsequently, even with later respiratory tract infections.

Simultaneous or secondary bacterial infection appears to be a relatively frequent complication of RSV infection in some countries in the developing world.[208,270] In the United States and other developed countries, it is an unusual complication, and most clinical and pathologic studies indicate that RSV infection rarely predisposes to acquisition of a bacterial infection.[128,232]

In a 9-year prospective study of 565 children hospitalized with RSV lower respiratory tract disease, the rate of subsequent bacterial infection was 1.2% in the total group of children infected with RSV and 0.6% in the 352 children who received no antibiotics.[128] If a bacterial infection is present simultaneously, it most frequently involves the urinary tract. The diagnosis is made by a positive urine culture (using the criterion of 50,000 colonies/mL) in about 3% of infants.[180,198,232,236] Concurrent urinary tract infections, however, may be coincidental to RSV infection or may represent asymptomatic bacteriuria. Serious concurrent bacterial infections are unusual enough that evaluations for sepsis and meningitis, and the empiric use of antibiotics, are not recommended routinely.[9] Controlled studies with randomized antibiotic treatment of lower respiratory tract disease caused mostly by RSV have shown no difference in the severity or duration of illness or in the child's outcome.[9]

More frequently, coinfection with other respiratory viruses occurs.[146,179,190,191] Using real-time polymerase chain reaction (PCR) assays, infection with two or more viruses has been reported to occur in more than 15% of hospitalized children with acute respiratory tract infection.[34,146] Studies examining whether coexistent viral infections in normal children augment the severity of infection show mixed results.[19,146,190,191] Among the commonly found agents that are simultaneously detected in young children with RSV infection are adenoviruses, rhinoviruses, hMPV, bocavirus, enteroviruses, influenza viruses, and parainfluenza viruses.[191] Respiratory disease from bacterial coinfection is uncommon, but bacterial pathogens have been detected simultaneously in the respiratory secretions of children intubated for RSV infection, including *Staphylococcus aureus, Bordetella pertussis, Bordetella parapertussis, S. pneumoniae, Moraxella catarrhalis,* and *H. influenzae*.[214,258,264,282] These bacterial isolates likely represent colonization among infants with

RSV infection, often being found with approximately equal frequency in intubated, uninfected, control infants.

PROGNOSIS

Thus, if infected at this tender stage
will they become "blue bloaters" as they age?

—C.B.H.

Prediction at Time of Initial Evaluation

Determining whether an infant with RSV infection who initially presents as an outpatient is likely to require subsequent hospitalization has been problematic. Numerous clinical findings have been evaluated, but most have relatively poor predictive value for individual patients.[9] Among the more consistent and helpful findings at the time of evaluation are oxygen saturation and global assessment of the degree of illness. Fever does not correlate with the severity of disease.[40] Tachypnea (≥70 breaths/min) has been mildly correlated with the presence of lower respiratory tract infection in infants and progression to the need for intensive care.[9,40] Repetitive assessments are helpful because rapid fluctuations in clinical manifestations are characteristic of RSV lower respiratory tract disease.

Clinical scoring systems commonly are used, but their use is limited by variable design, rendering comparison and standardization difficult. The Respiratory Distress Assessment Instrument has been standardized, but it is not validated in predicting the severity or outcome of children with bronchiolitis.[9] Another report described a scoring system to predict which healthy, term newborns in the Netherlands are at increased risk for RSV lower respiratory tract infection during the first year of life.[143] Independent predictors for RSV lower respiratory tract disease were group child care attendance and/or having siblings, birth weight less than 4000 g, birth outside of the months of April to September, and a low level of parental education.

Pulse oximetry is a convenient method to assess the percentage of hemoglobin bound by oxygen in vivo. However, only a moderate correlation exists between respiratory distress and oxygen saturations among infants with viral lower respiratory tract infections, and the use of oximetry has been demonstrated occasionally to prolong hospitalizations unnecessarily.[247] The difficulty seems to center around the use of an oxygen saturation of 95% as a criterion for admission and discharge. Using a lower value, perhaps 92%, may improve the precision of oximetry in determining the need for admission or continued hospitalization.

Infants hospitalized on inpatient floors for RSV infection rarely require subsequent transfer to ICUs. The risk in one study was 1.2%, with young age and high respiratory rates providing the best predictive value.[40]

Infants hospitalized with RSV bronchiolitis or pneumonia usually show clinical improvement within 24 to 48 hours, and most previously normal infants are discharged within 1 to 7 days, most commonly after 2 to 3 days in the United States.[9,233] However, children with underlying conditions that increase their risk for developing more complicated illness may require a longer hospitalization. Among infants in the first year of life who present to the emergency department with bronchiolitis, the median duration of symptoms until complete recovery was 15 days, and this did not vary in regard to viral etiology.[229]

Patients at Risk for Complicated RSV Infection

The primary risk factors for hospitalization and increased severity of RSV infection are premature birth, underlying congenital heart disease, and particularly bronchopulmonary dysplasia. Infants with these conditions have rates of hospitalization that are many times that of the population without these factors.[7,37,149,285] Secondary factors reported to be associated with an increased risk for severe RSV disease include a greater number of older siblings, impaired neuromuscular function or certain congenital malformations, low socioeconomic status, crowded living conditions, birth during the first half of the RSV season, multiple births, exposure to indoor air pollution including secondhand smoke, malnutrition, living at an altitude greater than 2500 meters, Down syndrome, nonwhite race, and low antibody concentration in cord blood. Other chronic diseases, chromosomal abnormalities, and congenital malformations have been associated with an increased risk for RSV hospitalization.[43,61,72,92,168,233,239] However, these secondary risk factors either have been reported inconsistently or have been associated with only a slightly increased risk for hospitalization.[174]

Infants with hemodynamically compromising congenital heart disease, particularly conditions associated with pulmonary hypertension or cyanosis, have been shown to have a markedly elevated risk for fatal outcomes.[44] The mortality rate of children with certain functionally important cardiac conditions has declined from greater than 30% to approximately 3%.[44]

Deficits in innate and adaptive immunity have long been assumed to predispose a child to the development of more severe forms of RSV infection, but the nature of these defects remains mostly undefined. More recent studies show some correlation of genetic polymorphisms with primary RSV disease and severity. Variations within a number of genetic loci potentially associated with controlling immune function, such as the expression of IL-4 and other T-lymphocyte cytokines and chemokines associated with the production of IgE antibody and hyperactive airways, have been shown to be overrepresented in children with RSV lower respiratory tract disease and with disease that is more severe[61,141,147,172,217,262] (see Immune Response: Immunity and Disease Pathogenesis).

Immunocompromised Patients

RSV infection can occasionally become life-threatening in subjects with severe immune deficiencies, either from acute infection or by causing the long-term development of bronchiolitis obliterans.[62,83] The risk for RSV infection becomes more significant with increasing numbers of highly immunosuppressed patients, such as recipients of bone marrow and solid organ transplants.[212] Progression of RSV infection from upper to lower respiratory tract disease depends on the degree of specific vulnerabilities in the immunocompromised host's immune response because of the underlying disease or to chemotherapy.[81,140,166,238] Lymphopenia has been recognized as a risk factor for disease progression in several studies of immunocompromised patients. One study in adults noted that progression of RSV to lower tract disease did not occur in patients with a lymphocyte count greater than 1000 cells/mm^3 at time of onset of upper respiratory tract infection. An absolute lymphocyte count of 100 cells/mm^3 or less at the time of RSV upper tract infection was associated with nearly uniform progression to lower tract disease. In contrast to lymphopenia, analysis of antibody concentration in these adult HSCT patients indicated no correlation between preexisting anti-RSV antibody concentration and progression from upper to lower respiratory tract disease.[166]

Reported risk factors for a poor outcome due to RSV infection in an immunosuppressed child include age less than 2 years, presence of lower respiratory tract symptoms at presentation (particularly in the absence of symptoms of upper respiratory infection), and varying degrees of lymphopenia.[55]

RSV infection has been reported as occurring in approximately 50% of bone marrow transplant recipients and often is acquired nosocomially.[2] The morbidity and clinical manifestations associated with RSV in these patients are highly variable.[2,32,31,51,63] Risk factors for development of more severe disease in transplant recipients include not only the degree of immunosuppression but also allogeneic transplantation, acquisition of the RSV infection within 2 months of undergoing transplantation but before engraftment, and the presence of graft-versus-host disease. The associated mortality rate among transplant recipients with lower respiratory tract disease has been reported as 70% to 100%, but mortality has been reported more recently as ranging from 0% to 50%, depending on the patient population.[161,163,243] Findings on the chest radiograph include focal interstitial infiltrates, sometimes associated with lobar consolidation or with hyperinflation, or more severe involvement of generalized alveolar and interstitial infiltration, and marked hypoxemia. The major findings with high-resolution computed tomography (CT) are small centrilobular nodules, airspace consolidation, ground-glass opacities, and bronchial wall thickening. These abnormalities frequently are present in both the periphery and central areas of the lung, are bilateral, and are asymmetric in distribution.[31]

RSV infection in immune-compromised subjects may not be recognized or considered because it may occur when RSV is not circulating in the community, and the clinical picture may mimic that of other opportunistic agents that commonly infect immunocompromised patients. Furthermore, establishing the diagnosis is problematic because the most frequently available assays—rapid antigen assays applied to swabs of upper respiratory tract secretions—often lack sensitivity in these patients. Greater accuracy is achieved using quantitative PCR assays in specimens obtained through bronchopulmonary lavage specimens.[47]

Instituting therapy with ribavirin in RSV-infected patients while they still have only symptoms of upper respiratory tract infection has shown variable results in terms of survival.[55,249] Outcomes may be improved with the combined use of ribavirin and palivizumab,[55] but larger, controlled studies are needed to establish the optimal form of treatment. Because many RSV infections on a hematology-oncology ward are nosocomial, strict enforcement of infection control policies is critical.[246]

Patients With Human Immunodeficiency Virus Infection

RSV infection may be more severe among HIV-infected children. In a cohort of South African children observed for 5 years, the incidence of hospitalization from RSV lower respiratory tract disease in children with HIV infection was three to five times greater than that in those not infected with HIV, and RSV deaths were increased 31-fold.[203] Studies have not confirmed a similar risk in HIV-infected children in the United States or United Kingdom, perhaps related to better care for HIV-infected children in developed countries.[52,65,167]

Pulmonary Sequelae

RSV infection in infancy is associated with an increased risk for wheezing in childhood and perhaps longer. Abnormalities of lung function have been noted in later childhood following infantile bronchiolitis as well, although the risk is also associated with respiratory viruses other than RSV.[94,110,166,214,298,302] Variations on three basic theories have been proposed to explain the link between early RSV infection and subsequent asthma. One possibility, a causal relationship, is that changes induced by viral replication alter the pattern of normal lung development in such a way that the infant is predisposed to subsequent episodes of wheezing. A second possibility, a triggering relationship, is that certain infants have a preexisting aberration of either airway function or the immune response, and early viral infection serves as a triggering event to episodes of acute airway obstruction. For example, several polymorphisms in cytokine genes have been associated with RSV severity and asthma suggesting a shared predisposition.[94,148,215,257,268] A third possibility is that a preexisting abnormality of airway function (possibly airway hyperreactivity) predisposes to wheezing with viral bronchiolitis in infancy and again with allergen exposures in later life. Intervention studies with a vaccine or other preventive and therapeutic measures will determine the presence of a link between RSV bronchiolitis and subsequent wheezing illnesses.

Repeated Infection

Recurrent infections with RSV occur across the age span from toddlers to elderly persons, whether healthy or infirm. Reinfection occurs most frequently among those in close contact with young or school-aged children, as in group child care facilities and primary schools, or among those in confined settings, including military recruits.[105,127,112,139,220] Most of these infections are upper respiratory tract illnesses, which often are complicated by sinusitis and otitis media. Recurrent infections involving the lower respiratory tract usually are manifest as tracheobronchitis or as exacerbations of wheezing. Even among young, healthy adults without asthma or other chronic pulmonary conditions, acute RSV infection produces hyperreactivity of the airways that may persist for as long as 8 weeks.[123]

Among children observed longitudinally, as many as three-fourths can be reinfected each year. Among children in group child care, attack rates of 98%, 75%, and 65% have been reported for first, second, and third infections, respectively. Immunity resulting from a single infection appeared to have no ameliorating effect on illness associated with reinfection 1 year later. Not until the third infection was severity reduced appreciably.[139] Among preschool-aged children, 20% to 50% of the repeated RSV infections involved the lower respiratory tract, but the illness tended to be milder than that following primary RSV infection.[103] Most children had lower respiratory tract illness only once, and those with repetitive lower respiratory tract infections had other features suggesting the presence of asthma.

Healthy adults frequently are exposed to RSV in their workplace and as parents or members of families with preschool-aged and elementary school–aged children. Despite these repetitive exposures, most subjects remained susceptible to RSV infection during the subsequent outbreaks and, if infected, developed symptoms.[127,220,283] Very recent infection, however, may result in diminished symptoms. In one study, 15 previously well adults became naturally infected with an RSV A strain during a community outbreak and developed upper respiratory tract illnesses (Fig. 182.8). These individuals subsequently were inoculated intranasally with an RSV A strain at repetitive intervals over the course of 2 to 26 months. The number reinfected and the proportion manifesting any symptoms continually declined during the 26 months. The quantity and duration of virus shedding also diminished concurrently.[129]

Among 211 working adults observed over the course of multiple seasons, RSV reinfection was symptomatic in 84% and manifested as an upper respiratory tract illness in 74%.[127] The remaining fourth of the reinfections caused tracheobronchitis or wheezing. Some individuals became infected with RSV and, later, with both RSV and influenza virus simultaneously. Comparison of the two illness episodes revealed that symptoms associated with influenza and RSV were generally similar (Fig. 182.9), although influenza was accompanied more frequently by fever and absence from work, whereas RSV infection was associated significantly more often with sinusitis, otitis, and a longer duration of illness.

The clinical similarity of illness from RSV and from influenza among young adults and the difficulty of differentiating the two also were shown in university students and in military recruits.[185,220] Findings associated with RSV and influenza infections were similar, except that wheezing was associated more frequently with RSV infection. The proportion of patients requiring inpatient confinement was the same for those with RSV infection as for those with influenza.

The importance of RSV infection as a cause of morbidity and mortality in older adults, both those previously healthy and those with underlying conditions, is being recognized increasingly.[88,281,298] Between 2% and 9% of all lower respiratory tract hospitalizations in elderly persons have been estimated to be caused by RSV, with an estimated annual cost of more than $1 billion.[88] Additional hospitalizations and costs may be incurred from the exacerbations of underlying chronic conditions associated with unrecognized RSV infections.

The impact of RSV infection in elderly individuals was illustrated in a prospective, multiyear study of 608 healthy community-dwelling elderly patients and 504 adults with high-risk conditions. An additional 1388 individuals who were hospitalized with acute cardiopulmonary conditions also were studied.[88] The mean age of the individuals studied ranged from 70 to 75 years. Using viral isolation, reverse transcriptase polymerase chain reaction (RT-PCR), and serology, RSV infection was identified at an annual rate in 3% to 7% of the healthy cohort, in 4% to 10% of the high-risk group, and in 8% to 13% of the hospitalized patients. In comparison, influenza A infection was detected annually in 2% to 4% of the healthy elderly cohort, in 1% to 5% of the high-risk group, and in 1% to 20% of hospitalized patients. The illnesses from RSV and influenza A could not be distinguished clinically. Among the hospitalized patients, intensive care was required by 15% of those with RSV and by 12% of those with influenza A infection; 8% of the RSV and 7% of the influenza A infections were fatal. Although RSV infection generated fewer office visits than did influenza among the healthy, older age group, those with high-risk conditions used health care services similarly if they were infected with RSV or influenza. The impact on health care services and costs by RSV is underscored by the proportion of hospitalizations caused by RSV for pneumonia (10.6%), chronic obstructive pulmonary disease (11.4%), congestive heart failure (5.4%), and asthma (7.2%). The role of RSV in elderly patients with these diagnoses frequently is unrecognized.

Further evidence of the burden of RSV disease is provided by a prospective, three-season study evaluating patients 50 years or older

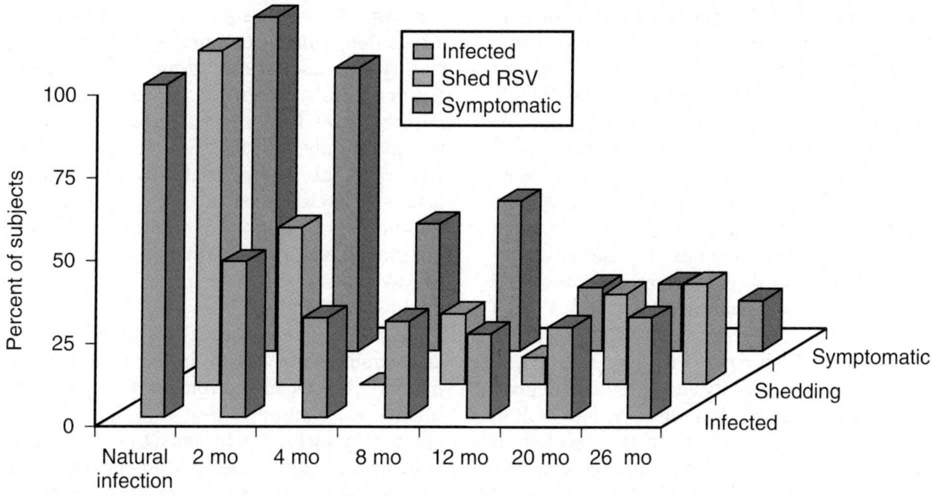

FIG. 182.8 Reinfection with respiratory syncytial virus (RSV). Proportion of young adults with natural RSV A infection who became reinfected, shed virus, and were symptomatic when they were subsequently rechallenged intranasally with RSV A after intervals of 2, 4, 8, 12, 20, and 26 months from time of their natural infection. (From Hall CB, Walsh EE, Long CE, Schnabel KC. Immunity to and frequency of reinfection with respiratory syncytial virus. *J Infect Dis.* 1991;163:693-698.)

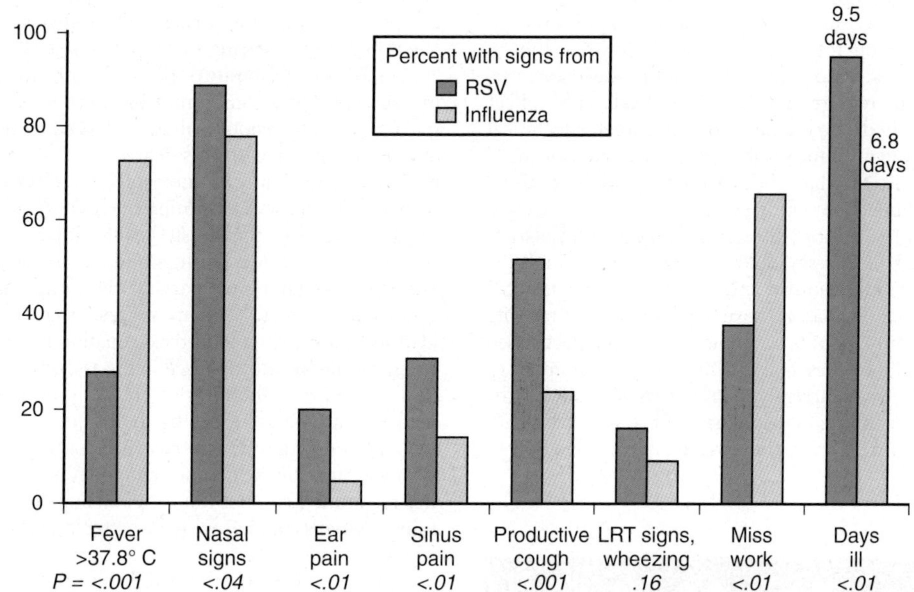

FIG. 182.9 Respiratory syncytial virus (RSV) infection and influenza. Comparison of clinical findings observed during RSV infection compared with influenza infection among 211 prospectively followed previously healthy adults who acquired both infections, RSV infection at one time and influenza infection at a separate time. (From Hall CB. Nosocomial respiratory syncytial virus infections: the "cold war" has not ended. *Clin Infect Dis.* 2000;31:590-596.)

admitted to the hospital with respiratory symptoms caused by infection attributable to RSV, hMPV, or influenza viruses.[296] The length of hospitalization, rate of admission to the ICU, number of days spent in the ICU, need for mechanical ventilation, and death were no different among patients infected with any of the three viruses. The rates of hospitalization during the 3-year period were 15.0, 9.8, and 11.8 per 10,000 residents for infection caused by RSV, hMPV, and influenza, respectively. For adults 65 years or older, rates of hospitalization were statistically higher for those with RSV and hMPV infections than for those with influenza. RSV accounted for 6.1% of hospitalizations for acute respiratory illness in these elderly individuals over the 3 years. In a separate study among high-risk adults 65 years or older, hospitalization rates were estimated at 23.4 per 10,000 for infections with both RSV and influenza.[204]

DIAGNOSIS

A presumptive diagnosis of RSV lower respiratory tract disease often is made on the basis of the age of the child, the presence of symptoms of bronchiolitis, and presentation within the usual period of peak RSV seasonal activity (if not monitored locally, nationwide data are available through the Centers for Disease Control and Prevention).[50] A marked increase in the number of outpatient visits and admissions for bronchiolitis and respiratory illness in children younger than 2 years usually is a strong indication that RSV is active within the community (see Fig. 182.2).[116]

However, PCR techniques have shown that an increasing number of viruses other than RSV may produce clinically similar illnesses, although the intensity of epidemic activity with these other viruses is still less than that caused by RSV.[126,289,299] Routine viral testing of outpatient or hospitalized young children with bronchiolitis is not recommended in the Clinical Practice Guidelines from the American Academy of Pediatrics.[9] However, viral testing may be useful for epidemiologic monitoring, for evaluating children with an atypical presentation, or for decisions regarding cohorting of particularly high-risk patients.[126]

A specific diagnosis of RSV infection alternatively may be made by viral isolation using standard cell culture or shell vials, direct and indirect fluorescent assays, and enzyme immunoassays, when PCR technology is not available. Nevertheless all of these methods lack the sensitivity and specificity of PCR.[206] Indirect and direct fluorescent assays and enzyme immunoassays applied to nasopharyngeal secretions from children, especially infants, have an average sensitivity and specificity of approximately 95% when these tests are performed by experienced personnel.[114] However, the ranges of sensitivity and specificity depend on the laboratory's expertise. These tests are less sensitive than PCR in older children and adults, who have preexisting antibody in secretions that may interfere with detection of RSV. False-positive results may occur when non-PCR tests are used during seasons of the year in which RSV activity is low.

The specimens employed for diagnosis usually are upper respiratory tract secretions from a nasopharyngeal swab or, less frequently, nasal aspirate. A flocked nasal swab is satisfactory for detection of RSV by PCR, but nasal washing or tracheal aspiration is more sensitive than is a nasopharyngeal swab specimen if the other diagnostic techniques are be used.[138] Nasal wash specimens may be obtained with a suction apparatus or by the use of a tapered rubber bulb (Fig. 182.10).

In the past, tissue culture isolation of the virus was the standard technique used for establishing the diagnosis of RSV. However, culture techniques now are used less frequently because of the added expense, the greater number of days required until a syncytial cytopathic effect appears (an average of 3–5 days), the need for considerable technical expertise and time, and the need for reliably sensitive tissue culture.[115]

PCR techniques consistently have been shown to be the optimal means for detecting viral infections among populations of children and adults, and they detect 30% or more infections than do viral isolation techniques.[87,185,288] Nested PCR assays add sensitivity, allow multiple viruses to be identified simultaneously, and help to differentiate RSV group A versus B strains. RT-PCR assays have the advantages of rapidity because of a diminished number of procedural steps and of a decreased chance of contamination, but they may be limited in the number of viruses that can be detected concurrently. Quantitative RT-PCR has the further advantage of determining the viral load, which correlates with viral quantitation by culture during the early phase of infection. In contrast, PCR signals persist well beyond the time when virus is no longer detectable by culture.[76,265,274] In addition, higher viral loads may predict a more severe clinical course,[73,144] although not all studies agree.[187] A considerable proportion of symptom-free children have specimens positive by PCR to various respiratory viruses, although this occurs less commonly with RSV than with other viruses, particularly rhinoviruses.[266] This may be related to the sensitivity of PCR techniques to detect low levels of shedding during the convalescent phase of a previously symptomatic infection, or indicate a concurrent asymptomatic viral infection. It is also possible that detection by PCR may indicate persistence of RSV infection somewhere in the epithelial or inflammatory cells of the lower airways.

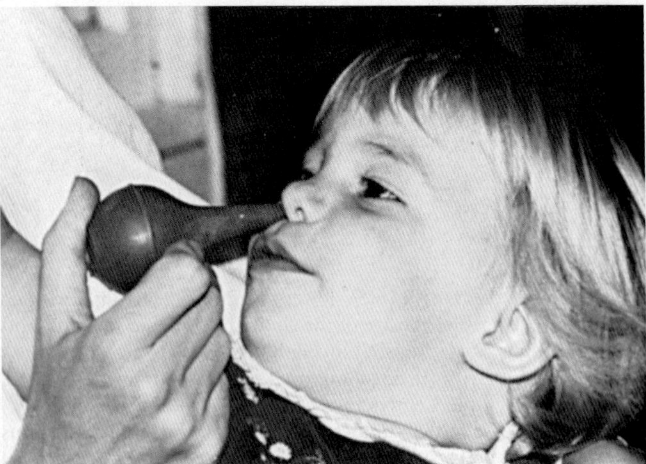

FIG. 182.10 Simple method for obtaining nasal wash specimens from young children. A 1-oz tapered rubber bulb is used to inject and collect 5 to 10 mL of saline with one squeeze. (From Hall CB, Douglas RG Jr. Clinically useful method for the isolation of respiratory syncytial virus. *J Infect Dis.* 1975;131:1-5.)

Serologic diagnosis usually is reserved for research purposes because it generally is not helpful in the acute diagnosis and management of patients. A detectable serologic response is inconsistently observed in infants, even among those with severe disease.[94,293] Serologic assays commonly include neutralizing antibody assays against whole virus, and enzyme immunoassays using purified F and G proteins of RSV to detect IgM and IgG responses. A number of other assays are used in research. Serologic diagnosis appears to be more sensitive among elderly than younger subjects.[280] Using the presence of a single high titer to identify infection has led to variable results and is not employed currently.

TREATMENT

For most children with RSV lower respiratory tract disease, supportive care is sufficient. Monitoring hydration status and oxygenation and, when necessary, clearing the nasal passages by gentle bulb suctioning are important. Respiratory rates of more than 60 to 70 breaths per minute are likely to compromise the infant's ability to take fluids, creating the need for intravenous hydration. The administration of supplemental oxygen to infants with this degree of tachypnea may be necessary to make the infant more comfortable and to prevent tiring.[312]

The criteria for determining the need for administration of supplemental oxygen to previously healthy infants are not well defined. A correlation of clinical findings and oxygen saturation (Spo_2) values is present, although it is not particularly strong, with an overall correlation coefficient of −0.4.[60,286] This suggests that the use of oximetry may identify infants with reduced oxygenation that is not apparent clinically, and it should be one tool used in the assessment of need for hospitalization. In contrast, the rates of hospitalization and length of stay may inadvertently be increased by the use of oximetry.[247] Current recommendations suggest that persistent measurements of Spo_2 of less than 90% may indicate the need for initiating supplemental oxygen.[9] However, this recommendation is not based on any direct studies; therefore other values perhaps could prove to be better indicators of the need for oxygen support.

A Cochrane report reviewed the results of nine controlled trials comparing chest physiotherapy (vibration and percussion techniques) to no intervention among hospitalized, nonintubated patients with acute bronchiolitis. No differences were detected between groups in respiratory rates, oxygen requirement, length of stay, or severe side effects.[211] In addition, deep pharyngeal or tracheal suctioning has not been shown to be beneficial.[9]

Conflicting results have come from trials evaluating the role of hypertonic saline inhalation for acute bronchiolitis. Results from some studies suggest a modest reduction in the length of hospitalization among patients treated with nebulized 3% saline versus those treated with 0.9% saline,[14,235] but studies in which predefined endpoints (as opposed to randomly determined discharge times) have not demonstrated any benefit of hypertonic saline.[85,253]

Several randomized trials have evaluated the usefulness of inhaled helium-oxygen therapy among children with bronchiolitis. This approach is based on the theory that helium-oxygen mixtures may improve gas flow through the high-resistance airways that characterize bronchiolitis.[165] A Cochrane review of published studies concluded that helium-oxygen therapy may have an early, transient benefit but does not result in a reduced rate of intubation, less mechanical ventilation, or shortened length of stay in a pediatric ICU.[182]

The use of bronchodilating agents in the management of infants with RSV lower respiratory tract illness has varied considerably among centers in the United States and other countries.[285] Bronchodilators have been administered to an average 75% to 80% of infants hospitalized with RSV infection.[312] Trials evaluating α-adrenergic or β-adrenergic bronchodilating agents have given inconsistent results.[162] The patients studied have varied in age, presence of underlying conditions, and history of previous episodes of wheezing, rendering comparisons somewhat difficult to make. A Cochrane review of bronchodilator therapy concluded that a limited transient improvement in assessment scores may be observed in one of every seven children treated, but the degree of improvement was minimal.[162] A second Cochrane review of bronchodilator therapy for hospitalized infants and young children with bronchiolitis found no effect on oxygen saturation or length of stay. Outpatient bronchodilator treatment did not reduce the rate of hospitalization or reduce time to resolution of illness at home.[96] The American Academy of Pediatrics Subcommittee on Diagnosis and Management of Bronchiolitis[9] recommended that for management of infants with a first episode of wheezing, bronchodilators should not be used routinely. The guidelines note that a carefully monitored trial of inhaled α-adrenergic and β-adrenergic agents was a possible option in some cases. However, bronchodilator administration should be continued only if benefit was documented by objective means of evaluation. Anticholinergic medications alone or in addition to bronchodilatory agents have not been shown to improve the course of viral bronchiolitis.[9]

Numerous publications evaluating the effects of corticosteroids in bronchiolitis have appeared, with variable results. More recently, a study involving 20 emergency departments over the course of three RSV seasons examined the outcomes of 608 children aged 2 to 12 months who presented with a first episode of bronchiolitis in a double-blind, placebo-controlled trial that administered one dose of oral dexamethasone of 1 mg/kg.[66] The rate of hospitalization and the Respiratory Assessment Change Score (RACS) of these groups did not differ significantly. Furthermore, no benefit was observed among the subgroup of children with asthma or with a family history of asthma. The results of other original studies and a meta-analysis are in agreement.[68] The American Academy of Pediatrics guidelines[9] concluded that current data do not support a recommendation for using corticosteroid therapy to prevent hospitalization, nor should corticosteroid medication be used routinely in the management of inpatient bronchiolitis. Some evidence exists that older children and those with prior episodes of wheezing and with asthma may potentially benefit from the administration of systemic glucocorticoid therapy.[227]

Montelukast is a selective leukotriene receptor antagonist that inhibits the cysteinyl leukotriene 1 receptor and is a modestly effective treatment for asthma and allergic rhinitis.[28,56] Because increased leukotriene levels are present in nasal secretions during many viral infections, including RSV,[69,277] montelukast was evaluated for its effectiveness in RSV lower respiratory tract disease. Although an initial controlled trial suggested a beneficial effect in infants with RSV bronchiolitis,[27] a large follow-up study randomizing 979 subjects failed to show a difference between the groups in the primary outcome (days with no cough, wheeze, or shortness of breath).[26]

In developed countries, pulmonary bacterial superinfection is an unusual occurrence among children with RSV lower respiratory tract disease, and the administration of antibiotics in placebo-controlled trials has not been associated with beneficial outcomes.[190,262] Moreover, prolonged administration of intravenous broad-spectrum antibiotics may augment the rate of secondary bacterial infection.[153] Antibiotics presumably should not be administered prophylactically to children with RSV infection or as therapy unless clear indications of the coexistence of a bacterial infection are present.

The only specific treatment currently approved for children hospitalized with RSV infection is ribavirin (1-β-D-ribofuranosyl-1H-1,2,4-triazole-3-carboxamide). This synthetic nucleoside has been administered as a small-particle aerosol for 12 to 22 hours per day until clinical improvement is evident, usually about 3 days. Much shorter, intermittent courses of higher doses also appear to be an acceptable mode of administration.[90] Although aerosolized ribavirin therapy has been associated with a small but statistically significant increase in oxygen saturation during the acute infection in several small studies, a consistent decrease in mortality, need for mechanical ventilation, decrease in length of stay in the pediatric ICU, or reduction in days of hospitalization among ribavirin recipients has not been demonstrated. The need for specialized nebulizers to deliver the drug, concern about potential toxic effects among exposed health care personnel, unconvincing results of efficacy trials, and extremely high cost have led to infrequent use of this drug.[9] Ribavirin is not recommended for routine use but may be considered for use in immunocompromised patients with documented, potentially life-threatening RSV infection, although it is not licensed for this indication.[249,273]

Other compounds continue to be investigated for their possible therapeutic benefit in RSV infection. Polyclonal neutralizing antibodies against RSV have been shown to have no therapeutic effect.[109] Palivizumab, a monoclonal antibody against the RSV fusion protein, has been demonstrated to have an antiviral effect when used therapeutically in infants with RSV infection, but no clinical benefit has been demonstrated.[188] A small randomized controlled trial of motavizumab, another monoclonal antibody, also failed to demonstrate any therapeutic benefit.[171] A complementary, antisense sequence of RNA (a short interfering RNA) that suppresses expression of the RSV nucleocapsid gene has been evaluated in adult volunteers who received the drug intranasally before RSV inoculation. No significant differences in the symptom scores between treatment and placebo groups were noted.[75] This compound was also investigated among lung transplant recipients for whom RSV lower respiratory disease may be fatal, but no positive effect was observed.[308] Another promising area of investigation is inhibitors of RSV fusion. Inhibition of enzymatic activity associated with several epitopes within the fusion (F) RSV glycoprotein prevents viral entry into the host cell as well as inhibition of cell-to-cell spread.[310] Two fusion-inhibiting drugs have been studied in adult volunteers experimentally challenged with RSV intranasally. Each compound was able to reduce the degree of viral replication and the magnitude of symptoms following RSV challenge.[76,77] It should be noted that, in each case, antiviral therapy was instituted before subjects developed symptoms following challenge. It remains possible that fusion inhibitors may have beneficial effects when started after symptoms appear, but this remains to be seen. Other small-molecule compounds that bind specific epitopes on viral-encoded proteins, including G, L, N, and P proteins, interfere with the viral replication cycle.[58] Clinical efficacy of these compounds has not yet been demonstrated.

PREVENTION

Breastfeeding

Most studies evaluating the protective effect of breastfeeding against RSV infection show a diminished likelihood of acquiring more severe infection.[16,223] Although colostrum and breast milk contain IgG and IgA antibodies and neutralizing activity against RSV, the exact mechanism of the protective effect is unknown. Other possibly protective factors include multifunctional components in human milk.[209] Longer term protection from breast milk against bronchiolitis may relate to human milk factors that modulate the infant's developing immune system.[41] The degree and duration of breastfeeding necessary to provide protection against RSV infection remain undefined.[170]

In a meta-analysis, infants who were exclusively breast-fed for 4 months were almost three times less likely to be hospitalized for lower respiratory tract disease (risk ratio, 0.28). It was estimated that 30% of hospitalizations of infants for infection would have been avoided for each additional month of full breastfeeding beyond 3 months.[223] The authors thus estimated that if all 4-month-old infants had been exclusively breast-fed, 56% of hospital admissions for infants in the first year of life would have been prevented. This number seems unrealistic, possibly because many breastfeeding studies do not control for other factors that can influence the rate of hospitalization for RSV.

Infection Control and Nosocomial Infection

Infection control procedures in the home should focus on interrupting the spread of RSV by using effective hand hygiene practices, including frequent hand washing or the use of hand sanitizers.[37] If hands are not visibly soiled, alcohol-based sanitizers are preferentially recommended.[37] Objects contaminated with respiratory secretions, which act as fomites, should be cleaned and used tissues discarded carefully.

Within medical settings, infection control procedures are the mainstay of controlling nosocomial infections from RSV.[37] More than 70 years ago, in 1941, Adams[4] described an epidemic of pneumonitis that occurred in January through February in the nurseries of two Minneapolis hospitals. Thirty-two infants, mostly in the second and third months of life, were affected, and 29% died. Cytoplasmic inclusions in the bronchial epithelium were observed in all fatal cases. The distinctive epidemiology, clinical syndrome, and pathology of these cases led Adams to propose a viral origin. Twenty years later, he and his colleagues described a markedly similar epidemic of respiratory illness in infants in whom they identified RSV as the cause.[6] RSV was thus implicated as the agent of the earlier, first-described nosocomial outbreak.

During community RSV epidemics, the risk for the nosocomial spread of RSV infection is high and, if not recognized, may result in prolonged hospitalization of infants and even increased mortality.[118] The risk for acquiring nosocomial infection is related to the child's age, underlying disease, and length of hospitalization.

Among immunocompromised children and adults, nosocomial RSV infections often are serious and difficult to control. Outbreaks in transplantation units in particular have been associated with a high mortality rate and prolonged and intermittent transmission.[35,91]

RSV infection frequently is introduced to the ward by hospital staff, families, and visitors who may have only a mild cold. Genetic analysis has demonstrated that nosocomial outbreaks may be caused by one or multiple strains of RSV during a single outbreak or season.[16,205,259] Infection rates may be high among staff members, who often require absence from work.

Various infection control procedures have been employed to prevent the nosocomial spread of RSV (Table 182.3). Integral to any effective infection control program are assiduous hand hygiene and education of health care personnel, as well as families and visitors, including frequent reminders to ensure compliance throughout the RSV season.[37] Careful and continued education regarding the importance of infection control practices has reduced the incidence of nosocomial RSV infection in many pediatric facilities. These practices generally include (1) early identification of RSV-infected patients through laboratory screening of symptomatic patients, (2) cohorting of infected patients and staff, (3) excluding visitors with current or recent respiratory tract infections, (4) excluding staff with respiratory tract illness from caring for susceptible infants, (5) emphasizing hand hygiene before and after direct patient contact or contact with objects in the vicinity of patients, and (6) limiting visitation by young siblings and other young children during the RSV season.[9] The efficacy of additional barrier precautions such as gowns, gloves, and masks has varied in different settings. In two controlled studies, the routine use of gowns and masks did not add further benefit to conscientious hand washing and other infection control procedures.[139,207] With widespread application of infection control practices, the occurrence of nosocomial RSV infection in neonatal ICUs has become an uncommon event.[24]

As many as 70% of RSV infections on hematology-oncology wards are nosocomial.[2,55] More severe RSV disease is recognized to occur early after transplantation and among patients with persistent lymphopenia, chronic graft-versus-host disease, and allogeneic stem cell transplantation.[11,55,79,150] Application of hand hygiene measures in conjunction with a private room, central HEPA-filtered air supply, and positive-pressure ventilation has been shown to significantly reduce RSV transmission on an oncology ward.[173]

TABLE 182.3 Infection Control Procedures, Both Standard Precautions and Contact Precautions for Prevention of Respiratory Syncytial Virus Infection, Recommended by the Centers for Disease Control and Prevention

Category I-B Recommendations[a]	Comment(s)
Hand washing	Water with soap or antibacterial agent or waterless antiseptic hand rub
Wearing gloves	Combined with hand washing before and after each glove change; may diminish self-inoculation
Wearing gowns	When direct contact with patient or patient secretions is likely
Wearing masks and eye protection	Eyes and nose are major sites for inoculation
Housing patient in private room or in a cohort isolated from other patients	Patients with documented infection can be grouped and isolated from other patients; beds should be separated by >0.9 m
Use of dedicated patient care equipment sometimes recommended with less or no supporting evidence	Equipment, including toys, assigned to specific patients
Staff assigned according to patient's RSV status	Specific staff care only for patients with RSV infection
Visitor restrictions during RSV season	Some qualify by restricting young children only
Screening visitors for illness during RSV season	Visitor assessed by trained personnel or advised by use of an educational patient information list

RSV, Respiratory syncytial virus.
[a]Centers for Disease Control and Prevention I-B recommendations based on "strong rationale and suggestive evidence" and strongly recommended for all hospitals and "reviewed as effective by experts in the field."
Modified from Hall CB. Nosocomial respiratory syncytial virus infections: the "cold war" has not ended. *Clin Infect Dis.* 2000;31:590-596.

Prophylaxis

Interest in immunoprophylaxis against RSV infection for high-risk infants came from the observation that although maternally derived RSV antibodies may not completely protect against RSV disease in young infants, the severity of RSV lower respiratory tract disease was inversely correlated with neutralizing antibody titers. Subsequent trials with an enriched RSV immune globulin preparation (RSV-IVIG) demonstrated statistically significant differences in hospitalization rates between RSV-IVIG recipients and control groups, and the compound was licensed for clinical use in infants with risk factors for severe RSV disease.[240] Standard IVIG preparations lacking high-titer RSV antibodies were less effective. Disadvantages associated with RSV-IVIG included the need for intravenous access, the risk for infectious disease transmission associated with plasma-derived products; supply issues; interference with live, attenuated vaccines; and most important, a significantly increased rate of adverse events when used in children with cyanotic congenital heart disease. These issues led to the development of monoclonal antibodies that can be administered in smaller volumes, and RSV-IVIG is no longer available.

In 1998, the US Food and Drug Administration (FDA) licensed a monoclonal anti-RSV antibody preparation, palivizumab, which targets a highly conserved epitope on the RSV F glycoprotein. Palivizumab was 50 to 100 times more effective than the polyclonal immunoglobulin, and the smaller volume administered circumvented many of the difficulties and adverse effects of use of a larger intravenous dose.[149,224] Palivizumab was modified from a mouse monoclonal antibody recognizing a protective epitope of the RSV fusion glycoprotein. Only the antigen-binding site from the mouse monoclonal antibody was inserted into the spine of a human antibody, thus diminishing the chance of allergic reactions to the mouse-raised antibody. A randomized, multicenter, double-blind, placebo-controlled trial involving 1502 premature infants with or without chronic lung disease demonstrated that monthly intramuscular injections of palivizumab reduce the overall incidence of RSV hospitalization by 55% compared with placebo recipients.[149] A second randomized, placebo-controlled trial involving 1287 infants with hemodynamically significant congenital heart disease published in 2003 confirmed the safety and efficacy of immunoprophylaxis in high-risk infants and young children.[89] The rate of hospitalization for RSV illness was reduced by approximately 50% among the infants who received prophylaxis in comparison with the placebo group. In different subgroups, the reduction of RSV hospitalization rates ranged from 39% to 78%, with the lower rates of protection observed among infants with chronic lung disease and congenital heart disease. Postlicensure studies suggested that reduction rates in the necessity for hospitalization with RSV infection may be even greater.[10]

A second-generation humanized IgG1 monoclonal antibody (motavizumab) derived by in vitro affinity maturation of the complementarity-determining regions of the heavy and light chains of palivizumab demonstrated approximately 18-fold greater neutralizing capacity than palivizumab.[1] Motavizumab was evaluated in a randomized, double-blind, noninferiority trial to palivizumab in 6635 infants with prematurity and/or chronic lung disease of prematurity. Motavizumab proved to be noninferior to palivizumab in terms of reduction in RSV hospitalization rates.[48] However, because of several concerns, including an increased incidence of hypersensitivity reactions among motavizumab recipients, motavizumab was not licensed by the FDA. Other monoclonal antibody preparations are now being studied in infants.

The mechanism by which RSV-neutralizing monoclonal antibodies interrupt the viral replicative cycle appears to be through inhibition of viral cellular fusion. Pretreatment of virus with either palivizumab or motavizumab does not inhibit the ability of the F protein to interact with the target cell receptor, but viral replication does not occur. This suggests these antibodies block virus-to-cell fusion, perhaps by preventing conformational changes in the F protein after attachment.[171]

RSV isolates resistant to palivizumab due to mutations in the palivizumab-binding site on the F protein initially were described in vitro during long-term incubation of infected cells in the presence of antibody.[74,309,311] Subsequent reports have isolated palivizumab-resistant RSV isolates from RSV infected children who were receiving palivizumab prophylaxis.[5] Palivizumab-resistant RSV isolates appear to account for only a subset of RSV cases occurring among infants receiving palivizumab. These escape mutants appear to have impaired growth characteristics relative to wild-type RSV. The importance of these escape mutants as a cause of breakthrough disease is poorly understood, but does not seem substantial.[275]

Current Guidelines for Immunoprophylaxis

Palivizumab is the only licensed product available to reduce the risk for RSV lower respiratory tract disease in infants and children, particularly those with underlying risk factors for more severe RSV disease. The American Academy of Pediatrics recommends prophylaxis for subgroups of high-risk children for different periods of time depending on their gestational and postnatal ages, the severity of their underlying conditions, their need for recent medical therapy, and the presence of other risk factors. Prophylaxis with palivizumab is recommended for otherwise healthy infants who were born at less than 29 weeks, 0 days of gestation. Palivizumab is also recommended for infants in their first year of life who have chronic lung disease (essentially bronchopulmonary dysplasia [BPD], using the definition of a requirement for supplemental oxygen through the first 28 days of life), and again in their second year of life if they continue to require medical therapy (largely oxygen) for BPD within 6 months of the onset of the RSV season.[10,9]

Palivizumab is administered intramuscularly at a dose of 15 mg/kg once every 30 days throughout the RSV season. For most areas of the United States, monthly prophylaxis should begin in November, but knowledge of local epidemiologic patterns can help in making a more informed decision.[10,9] After a child has qualified at the beginning of the season for the administration of prophylaxis, it should be continued until the epidemic season ends, but with no more than five monthly doses.[10] These guidelines have been contested, largely because they oppose the initial FDA guidelines established as a result of the initial clinical trials that led to the approval of palivizumab and because the changes are not based on newer, controlled trials.[304]

The use of palivizumab in itself remains controversial. Economic analyses, in general, have not demonstrated an overall savings in health care costs if all high-risk children receive prophylaxis.[80,237] Cost-benefit analyses have been difficult to complete because of considerable geographic variation in hospitalization costs for such infants. Most published cost-effectiveness analyses have found that the cost of immunoprophylaxis exceeds the economic benefit of avoiding an RSV hospitalization.[132,287,306] Palivizumab immunoprophylaxis has not reduced mortality for infants with RSV infection in any study, although this may be difficult to accomplish because the mortality rate from RSV currently is very low. An effect of palivizumab prophylaxis on short-term wheezing has been suggested in some studies,[30,305] but not longer-term studies,[216] and no firm conclusions on the strength of this effect can be drawn currently.

Vaccines

Control of RSV has long lured but eluded investigators. Although the outcome of infants with RSV infection has improved greatly in recent years, the burden on health care that RSV imposes yearly remains notable among both children and adults.[228] Immunoprophylaxis with palivizumab administration will lower the RSV hospitalization rate among high-risk infants and young children, but the vast majority of hospitalized young children do not have risk factors that justify the use of palivizumab. Thus immunoprophylaxis will have only a modest impact on the overall burden of RSV disease in the United States. Only effective immunization is likely to alleviate this burden. Certain characteristics of RSV infection, however, continue to pose barriers to the successful development of a vaccine.

The shroud of past experience with the formalin-inactivated vaccines has conferred caution and concern regarding the development of candidate vaccines. The initial RSV vaccine trials, with the alum-precipitated, formalin-inactivated vaccine (FI-RSV), were conducted in 1966 to 1967 among seronegative children 2 months or older with the administration of an inactivated and trivalent parainfluenza vaccine. When naturally infected during the subsequent RSV outbreak, the FI-RSV vaccinees experienced an unanticipated increased severity of disease. Almost 80% required hospitalization, and two died.[59,95,158] The unfortunate outcomes of these trials stimulated research that has been integral to the evolution of future vaccines. Subsequent examination of the vaccinees' immune response and experiments in rodent models with exaggerated disease indicated that the formalin-inactivated vaccine produced a poor and defective neutralizing antibody response and mild peripheral blood and pulmonary eosinophilia (not observed in human disease), perhaps suggesting an excessive Th2-type CD4 T-cell response.[95,158,164] These studies suggested that a successful vaccine should evoke a balanced immune response with both $CD4^+$ and $CD8^+$ cytotoxic lymphocytes (see Immune Response: Immunity and Disease Pathogenesis).[113,193]

An RSV vaccine should reflect the immune response of natural infection, yet improve its inconsistent and nondurable protection. In addition, an RSV vaccine would need to be administered in the first few weeks of life, when the most severe disease usually occurs. Little experience exists regarding immunization with live viruses during the neonatal period when the immune system is incompletely developed and interfering maternal antibody is present.[218] However, pregnant women respond well to vaccines with resulting placental transfer of maternal antibodies during the third trimester, which may be a potential approach to offer protection to infants early in life. Furthermore, the effect of the multiple antigens from other vaccines administered in the first few months of life must be considered.

Vaccine development subsequently has cautiously taken several approaches with production of live, attenuated, protein subunit, and vectored candidate vaccines. Protein subunit vaccines have raised concern for disease enhancement, particularly in the pediatric population, and thus trials have been largely restricted to older children and adults. Candidate subunit vaccines have used primarily the two major surface glycoproteins, F and G, which are the major targets for the production of neutralizing antibodies.[67] Clinical investigation has focused on vaccines of the F protein, which has greater cross-reactivity between RSV A and RSV B strains. Three generations of purified F protein vaccines, PFP-1, PFP-2, and PFP-3, which consist of immunoaffinity-purified, alum-absorbed F glycoprotein, have been evaluated in clinical trials. The initial PFP-1 vaccine contained small amounts of the G protein, which did induce an antibody response. PFP-1 and PFP-2 vaccines have been administered to normal adults, institutionalized adults, normal children, and individuals with chronic underlying conditions including chronic lung disease, cystic fibrosis, and asthma.[107,108,222]

The PFP vaccines generally were safe and modestly immunogenic. The PFP-2 vaccine, administered during the third trimester in a study of maternal immunization, showed no adverse effects on the infants. At delivery, only low levels of maternal neutralizing antibody were present in the infant. However, increased levels of IgG, but not IgA, antibody to the F protein did occur in breast milk. A meta-analysis of the PFP vaccine trials concluded that a significant relative risk of 0.55 (95% confidence interval, 0.35–0.88) in the overall number of RSV infections existed, but the heterogeneity of the studies cast doubt on the validity of this conclusion. Vaccination with PFP did not show any effect on reducing the incidence of RSV lower respiratory tract disease.[222]

Numerous nonreplicating vaccines, including other protein subunits of the G and F proteins and DNA vaccines have been developed, and some are in stages of development at the present time. DNA plasmid vaccines expressing F or G glycoproteins have shown limited immunogenicity.[21,181] Nanoparticle vaccines have interesting properties that may prove advantageous in vaccine development.[177] One of these vaccines is now in phase III trials in a maternal immunization protocol. Licensing of these vaccines is not likely for at least 5 years.

Live, attenuated vaccines have the advantage over subunit vaccines of producing an immune response that more closely mimics the natural route of inoculation into the upper respiratory tract, thus eliciting more balanced local and systemic humoral and cellular responses and offering potentially broader and more durable protection. The initial live, attenuated candidate vaccines were derived from cold-passaged mutants propagated from wild-type RSV (wt RSV) strains grown at progressively lower temperatures, and strains were selected by growth at low temperatures, similar to that of the upper respiratory tract. Subsequent passage in the presence of chemical mutagenic agents produced candidate strains that were temperature sensitive *(ts)* and unable to replicate at the higher body temperatures of the lower respiratory tract.[301] These candidate (*cp* and *ts*) vaccines were tested in adult volunteers and seropositive children without complication but proved to be unsuitable for infants and young, seronegative children.[159,160] These vaccines were associated with unacceptable degrees of illness, were overattenuated and not protective, or were genetically unstable; some were accompanied by prolonged shedding of wild-type virus, which most frequently was observed in infants and resulted in transmission of the shed virus to 20% to 25% of the unvaccinated contacts.[159]

More recent vaccine candidates have been derived from previously combined *cp* and *ts (cpts)* mutants, which contain mutations generated by reverse genetics that allow the precise desired enhancements of stability, attenuation, and immunogenicity. For example, one candidate, *cpts 248* strain, was further mutated and attenuated into *cpts 248/404*. Each of its mutations was introduced alone or in combination into wt RSV for evaluation in experimental animals of the mutations' immunogenic and attenuating effects. This candidate *cpts 248/404* vaccine was immunogenic in seropositive and seronegative children older than 6 months, but upper respiratory tract illness with appreciable nasal congestion developed in younger infants 1 and 2 months of age.[160] These vaccines are not being further developed presently.

Reverse genetics has produced a lineage of further "designer gene" candidate vaccines with one or combined deletions of *NS1, NS2, M2-2,* and *SH* genes.[159,256] Of these, the M2-2 is undergoing the most intensive investigation currently.[160]

Novel adjuvants also are being developed, some of which can shift the immune response evoked by subunit vaccines from a Th2- to a Th1-type response in experimental animals. Enhanced immunogenicity appears possible with enterically active adjuvants and carriers, such as liposomes and biodegradable microspheres, and with adjuvants in vesicles of immunostimulating complexes.[67]

A third approach to vaccine development involves engineered live viral vectors, including vaccinia virus, adenovirus, Sendai virus, and parainfluenza virus. Results from animal models indicate that these vaccines are immunogenic, but antibody responses in human children have been minimal.[201]

NEW REFERENCES SINCE THE SEVENTH EDITION

8. Ambrose CS, Anderson EJ, Simoes EA, et al. Respiratory syncytial virus disease in preterm infants in the U.S. born at 32-35 weeks gestation not receiving immunoprophylaxis. *Pediatr Infect Dis J.* 2014;33(6):576-582.
9. American Academy of Pediatrics. Clinical practice guideline: the diagnosis, management, and prevention of bronchiolitis. *Pediatrics.* 2014;134(5):e1474-e1502.
10. American Academy of Pediatrics Committee on Infectious D, American Academy of Pediatrics Bronchiolitis Guidelines C. Updated guidance for palivizumab prophylaxis among infants and young children at increased risk of hospitalization for respiratory syncytial virus infection. *Pediatrics.* 2014;134(2):e620-e638.
15. Asner SA, Science ME, Tran D, et al. Clinical disease severity of respiratory viral co-infection versus single viral infection: a systematic review and meta-analysis. *PLoS ONE.* 2014;9(6):e99392.
17. Bagga B, Cehelsky JE, Vaishnaw A, et al. Effect of Preexisting Serum and Mucosal Antibody on Experimental Respiratory Syncytial Virus (RSV) Challenge and Infection of Adults. *J Infect Dis.* 2015;212(11):1719-1725.
23. Bennett BL, Garofalo RP, Cron SG, et al. Immunopathogenesis of respiratory syncytial virus bronchiolitis. *J Infect Dis.* 2007;195(10):1532-1540.
30. Blanken MO, Rovers MM, Molenaar JM, et al. Respiratory syncytial virus and recurrent wheeze in healthy preterm infants. *N Engl J Med.* 2013;368(19):1791-1799.
44. Byington CL, Wilkes J, Korgenski K, et al. Respiratory syncytial virus-associated mortality in hospitalized infants and young children. *Pediatrics.* 2015;135(1):e24-e31.
46. Caballero MT, Serra ME, Acosta PL, et al. TLR4 genotype and environmental LPS mediate RSV bronchiolitis through Th2 polarization. *J Clin Invest.* 2015;125(2):571-582.
60. Chin HJ, Seng QB. Reliability and validity of the respiratory score in the assessment of acute bronchiolitis. *Malays J Med Sci.* 2004;11(2):34-40.
62. Chorazy ML, Lebeck MG, McCarthy TA, et al. Polymicrobial acute respiratory infections in a hospital-based pediatric population. *Pediatr Infect Dis J.* 2013;32(5):460-466.
76. DeVincenzo JP, McClure MW, Symons JA, et al. Activity of Oral ALS-008176 in a Respiratory Syncytial Virus Challenge Study. *N Engl J Med.* 2015;373(21):2048-2058.
77. DeVincenzo JP, Whitley RJ, Mackman RL, et al. Oral GS-5806 activity in a respiratory syncytial virus challenge study. *N Engl J Med.* 2014;371(8):711-722.
84. Eshaghi A, Duvvuri VR, Lai R, et al. Genetic variability of human respiratory syncytial virus A strains circulating in Ontario: a novel genotype with a 72 nucleotide G gene duplication. *PLoS ONE.* 2012;7(3):e32807.
85. Everard ML, Hind D, Ugonna K, et al. SABRE: a multicentre randomised control trial of nebulised hypertonic saline in infants hospitalised with acute bronchiolitis. *Thorax.* 2014;69(12):1105-1112.
89. Feltes TF, Cabalka AK, Meissner HC, et al. Palivizumab prophylaxis reduces hospitalization due to respiratory syncytial virus in young children with hemodynamically significant congenital heart disease. *J Pediatr.* 2003;143(4):532-540.
97. Gamba-Sanchez N, Rodriguez-Martinez CE, Sossa-Briceno MP. Epidemic activity of respiratory syncytial virus is related to temperature and rainfall in equatorial tropical countries. *Epidemiol Infect.* 2016;144(10):2057-2063.
100. Gill MA, Long K, Kwon T, et al. Differential recruitment of dendritic cells and monocytes to respiratory mucosal sites in children with influenza virus or respiratory syncytial virus infection. *J Infect Dis.* 2008;198(11):1667-1676.
124. Hall CB, Hall WJ, Speers DM. Clinical and physiological manifestations of bronchiolitis and pneumonia. Outcome of respiratory syncytial virus. *Am J Dis Child.* 1979;133(8):798-802.
133. Hasegawa K, Tsugawa Y, Brown DF, et al. Trends in bronchiolitis hospitalizations in the United States, 2000–2009. *Pediatrics.* 2013;132(1):28-36.
151. Ivancic-Jelecki J, Forcic D, Mlinaric-Galinovic G, et al. Early Evolution of Human Respiratory Syncytial Virus ON1 Strains: Analysis of the Diversity in the C-Terminal Hypervariable Region of Glycoprotein Gene within the First 3.5 Years since Their Detection. *Intervirology.* 2015;58(3):172-180.
153. Janssen R, Bont L, Siezen CL, et al. Genetic susceptibility to respiratory syncytial virus bronchiolitis is predominantly associated with innate immune genes. *J Infect Dis.* 2007;196(6):826-834.
177. Lee YT, Ko EJ, Hwang HS, et al. Respiratory syncytial virus-like nanoparticle vaccination induces long-term protection without pulmonary disease by modulating cytokines and T-cells partially through alveolar macrophages. *Int J Nanomedicine.* 2015;10:4491-4505.
187. Luchsinger V, Ampuero S, Palomino MA, et al. Comparison of virological profiles of respiratory syncytial virus and rhinovirus in acute lower tract respiratory infections in very young Chilean infants, according to their clinical outcome. *J Clin Virol.* 2014;61(1):138-144.
199. Mitra R, Baviskar P, Duncan-Decocq RR, et al. The human respiratory syncytial virus matrix protein is required for maturation of viral filaments. *J Virol.* 2012;86(8):4432-4443.
203. Moyes J, Cohen C, Pretorius M, et al. Epidemiology of respiratory syncytial virus-associated acute lower respiratory tract infection hospitalizations among HIV-infected and HIV-uninfected South African children, 2010–2011. *J Infect Dis.* 2013;208(suppl 3):S217-S226.

216. O'Brien KL, Chandran A, Weatherholtz R, et al. Efficacy of motavizumab for the prevention of respiratory syncytial virus disease in healthy Native American infants: a phase 3 randomised double-blind placebo-controlled trial. *Lancet Infect Dis*. 2015;15(12):1398-1408.
247. Schroeder AR, Marmor AK, Pantell RH, et al. Impact of pulse oximetry and oxygen therapy on length of stay in bronchiolitis hospitalizations. *Arch Pediatr Adolesc Med*. 2004;158(6):527-530.
249. Shah DP, Ghantoji SS, Shah JN, et al. Impact of aerosolized ribavirin on mortality in 280 allogeneic haematopoietic stem cell transplant recipients with respiratory syncytial virus infections. *J Antimicrob Chemother*. 2013;68(8):1872-1880.
253. Silver AH, Esteban-Cruciani N, Azzarone G, et al. 3% Hypertonic Saline Versus Normal Saline in Inpatient Bronchiolitis: A Randomized Controlled Trial. *Pediatrics*. 2015;136(6):1036-1043.
261. Tabatabai J, Prifert C, Pfeil J, et al. Novel respiratory syncytial virus (RSV) genotype ON1 predominates in Germany during winter season 2012–13. *PLoS ONE*. 2014;9(10):e109191.
265. Templeton KE, Scheltinga SA, Beersma MF, et al. Rapid and sensitive method using multiplex real-time PCR for diagnosis of infections by influenza a and influenza B viruses, respiratory syncytial virus, and parainfluenza viruses 1, 2, 3, and 4. *J Clin Microbiol*. 2004;42(4):1564-1569.
276. van Schaik SM, Enhorning G, Vargas I, et al. Respiratory syncytial virus affects pulmonary function in BALB/c mice. *J Infect Dis*. 1998;177(2):269-276.
277. van Schaik SM, Tristram DA, Nagpal IS, et al. Increased production of IFN-gamma and cysteinyl leukotrienes in virus-induced wheezing. *J Allergy Clin Immunol*. 1999;103(4):630-636.
304. Yogev R, Krilov LR, Fergie JE, et al. Re-evaluating the New Committee on Infectious Diseases Recommendations for Palivizumab Use in Premature Infants. *Pediatr Infect Dis J*. 2015;34(9):958-960.
305. Yoshihara S, Kusuda S, Mochizuki H, et al. Effect of palivizumab prophylaxis on subsequent recurrent wheezing in preterm infants. *Pediatrics*. 2013;132(5):811-818.

The full reference list for this chapter is available at ExpertConsult.com.

Human Metapneumovirus 183

Jennifer E. Schuster • John V. Williams

Human metapneumovirus (MPV, HMPV) is a paramyxovirus that is a ubiquitous respiratory tract pathogen with seropositivity demonstrated in virtually all adults around the world.* The spectrum of disease varies from minor upper respiratory tract illness to lower respiratory tract disease, with significant morbidity and mortality.[68,220,233,248] The clinical manifestations of MPV include bronchiolitis, croup, pneumonia, asthma exacerbations, and acute otitis media, similar to other common respiratory viruses. MPV can cause severe disease in children and adults with underlying medical conditions as well as in older adults.† Multiple epidemiologic studies have demonstrated that MPV is widely prevalent and is usually second to respiratory syncytial virus (RSV) in incidence.[67,68,165,167] Research groups have begun to elucidate the pathogenesis and immunity of MPV, thereby facilitating the development of preventive strategies and vaccines.

HISTORY

In 2001, van den Hoogen and colleagues[220] discovered a novel virus in respiratory specimens collected from 28 Dutch children with acute respiratory illness over a 20-year period. Clinical symptoms were similar to those of RSV, and disease severity ranged from mild respiratory infection to respiratory failure requiring mechanical ventilation. The unknown virus produced cytopathic effects, including syncytia, in monkey kidney cells. However, the polymerase chain reaction (PCR) result for known respiratory viruses was negative, and the virus did not adsorb red blood cells (hemagglutination). Elegant random reverse-transcriptase (RT)-PCR experiments provided sufficient genomic sequence data to place the virus in the Pneumovirinae subfamily of the Paramyxoviridae (*Pneumoviridae* have now been classified as a separate family within *Mononegavirales*). MPV, like avian metapneumovirus (AMPV), is a member of the *Metapneumovirus* genus, but it is the first described human pathogen in the genus. The virus most closely related genetically to MPV is avian metapneumovirus type C (AMPV-C); evolutionary analyses of viral genes estimate that MPV diverged from AMPV-C 200 to 300 years ago.[48,255] MPV-specific antibodies were present in human sera from 1958,[220] a finding confirming that the virus circulated before recent identification.

*References 55, 68, 94, 133, 135, 136, 138, 149, 151, 159, 220.
†References 19, 61, 68, 132, 141, 153, 168, 201, 203, 224, 233, 245.

PROPERTIES

Structural and Antigenic Properties

MPV contains a single-stranded, negative-sense RNA genome with a lipid envelope, as do all paramyxoviruses.[220] MPV lacks the two nonstructural proteins, NS1 and NS2, encoded by RSV (Fig. 183.1). The eight genes are nucleoprotein (N), phosphoprotein (P), matrix protein (M), fusion protein (F), second matrix protein (M2), small hydrophobic protein (SH), and polymerase protein (L). The M2 gene has two open reading frames, M2-1 and M2-2, for a total of nine viral proteins. The gene order in MPV (3′N-P-M-F-M2-SH-G-L-5′) demonstrates a different placement of the F and M2 genes compared with RSV (3′NS1-NS2 -N-P-M-SH-G-F-M2-L-5′). The absent nonstructural proteins and the different gene order characterize MPV as a member of the *Metapneumovirus* genus.[219,220] Like all pneumoviruses and paramyxoviruses, the fusion protein is synthesized as an active precursor cleaved by host proteases.[219] The fusion protein binds to integrins, which serve as entry receptors, as well as heparan sulfate.[29,39,41] Entry occurs by multiple mechanisms, including membrane fusion with endosomes.[40]

Electron microscopy demonstrates paramyxovirus-like pleomorphic spherical, and filamentous particles 150 to 600 nm in size, with short envelope projections of 13 to 17 nm representing glycoprotein spikes.[170,220] Nucleocapsid diameter averages 17 nm.[170] The genome is about 13.3 kb in size.[15,172,219] Sequence analysis demonstrates that MPV is most similar to AMPV-C, with six of the nine proteins having a 70% to 80% amino acid identity with AMPV-C.[172,219] The SH and G proteins are the most divergent between the two viruses, as well as among MPV genotypes.[15,219] The F protein is highly conserved with 93% to 97% amino acid identity among all strains of MPV.[15,20,222,255] Phylogenetic analysis of MPV genes identifies four distinct genetic lineages.[12,20,48,222,255] These lineages are classified into two groups (A and B), each with two subgroups (A1, A2, B1, and B2). Further subdivision of A2 into A2a and A2b has been proposed but not confirmed.[95] All four strains have been identified in different global regions over multiple years, a finding demonstrating that they are not exclusive to countries or seasons.

Most evidence suggests that the different genetic lineages of MPV do not represent distinct serotypes. Animal studies in rodents and nonhuman primates show a high degree of cross neutralization and cross protection among subgroups,[139,204,214] although one study in ferrets identified a 16-fold difference in serum neutralizing antibody titer.[222]

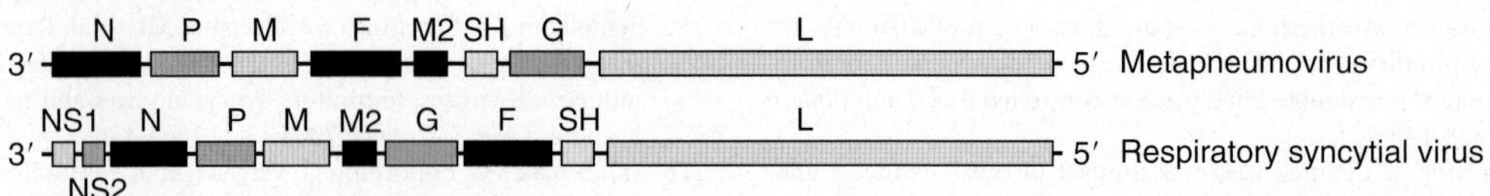

FIG. 183.1 Genomic map of human metapneumovirus compared with human respiratory syncytial virus. The putative open-reading frames and the approximate nucleotide positions within the genome are indicated.

Laboratory Growth

MPV requires trypsin for optimal replication in most cell types and is difficult to culture.[220] LLC-MK2 and Vero cells, two monkey kidney epithelial cell lines, are the most permissive, with viral replication enhanced by supplemental trypsin.[215] A low level of replication occurs in LLC-MK2 and MA-104 cells without trypsin, and some strains exhibit a reduced dependence on trypsin.[190] No growth is observed on MDCK or CEF cells even with exogenous trypsin.[170,220] In LLC-MK2 cells, plaques tend to be small and round with occasional syncytia.[17,170] Cytopathic effects are noted between 3 and 23 days (average, 17 days).[17] The subtle, late cytopathic effects in primary isolates and trypsin requirement likely account for the failure to detect MPV previously.

Animal Susceptibility

Van den Hoogen and colleagues[119,220] infected turkeys, chickens, and cynomolgus macaques with MPV. No overt clinical symptoms were observed in the birds, but one-half of the monkeys exhibited upper respiratory tract disease. Viral replication was not detected in poultry but was present in all macaques.[220] African green monkeys appear to be the most permissive nonhuman primate species.[204] Fatal MPV infections have occurred in wild chimpanzees and gorillas, as well as in zoologic facilities, likely transmitted from humans based on sequencing of the isolates.[107,118,162,206] Hamsters, ferrets, cotton rats, and several strains of inbred mice display viral replication in the upper and lower respiratory tract, thus allowing for small animal models.[139,246,253] Cotton rats displayed the highest lung viral titers, whereas Syrian golden hamsters had the highest nasal titers.[246] Ferrets and guinea pigs have been infected for generation of antisera but do not manifest clinical symptoms.[220]

EPIDEMIOLOGY

Geographic Distribution

Epidemiologic studies have verified the presence of MPV worldwide. The incidence of the virus varies among countries and years, but MPV circulates in every year.*

Seasonal Patterns

In temperate regions, MPV is present during most of the year but peaks in late winter-early spring, typically following peak RSV incidence.† In subtropical climates such as Hong Kong, a spring-summer season similar to that seen with RSV occurs.[167] Biannual peaks of seasonality have been described in some European studies.[1,85] In general, rates of MPV acute respiratory infection are lower than RSV and comparable to parainfluenza and influenza,[31,92,101,125,155,167,207] although MPV does on occasion surpass RSV in incidence.[110]

Strain Variation

The predominant subtype varies by site and year.[74,109,160,195,207,248] In Italy, the incidence of MPV varied from 8% to 20% over a 3-year period. All four subtypes were identified each season; however, the predominant subtype changed. In 2001 to 2002, A1 accounted for 59% of all strains, the following year B1 and B2 were present equally, and in 2003 to 2004, 72% of strains were A2.[74] Similar variation was observed in a 20-year prospective US study, with multiple genotypes present in most years.[248] In recent years, A1 has not been identified in multiyear studies in diverse regions.[137,156,164,195] Whether groups and subgroups differ in virulence remains unclear. Vicente and colleagues[231] reviewed MPV strains isolated in Spain and noted that children with group A infection had significantly more frequent pneumonia and higher disease severity. Similarly, Jordanian children with MPV A were more likely to require supplemental oxygen.[195] A Canadian study found that genotype B was associated with more severe disease in hospitalized patients.[165] In France, patients with group B strains were more likely to have abnormal chest radiographs, but they did not have significant differences in oxygen saturation, hospitalizations, or clinical severity scores.[171] Other studies have found no major distinctions in disease severity,[3,56,207] laboratory abnormalities,[149] or symptoms[109,234] among genotypes. Group A viruses replicate more efficiently in animal models, a finding suggesting some meaningful biologic differences among groups.[204,221]

*References 4, 31, 56, 58, 72, 101, 110, 125, 167, 177, 195, 207, 220, 244.

†References 56, 58, 66–68, 98, 101, 125, 160, 175, 195, 207, 220, 244, 248.

Viral Load

The relationship between viral load and disease severity is unclear. Roussy and colleagues[186] noted that an MPV viral load 1000 copies per 10^5 cells or larger was associated with hospitalization and use of adjunctive therapies, including corticosteroids and bronchodilators. Other studies have identified an association between higher viral load and fever, bronchodilator use, lower respiratory tract involvement, duration of oxygen therapy, need for hospitalization, and length of hospital stay.[23,146,183] However, an association with viral load and disease severity has not been confirmed in all studies. In a large cohort of Jordanian children, viral load was not associated with supplemental oxygen use.[195] Similarly, viral load was not associated with disease severity in Kenyan children[71] or with progression of disease in a hematopoietic stem cell transplant population.[199]

Incidence and Prevalence

Many epidemiologic studies of MPV include convenience samples collected in single-center clinical settings from patients with acute respiratory infection and report incidence rates of MPV between 5% and 25%.* Some prospective and multicenter studies exist.

A prospective study of all hospitalized children younger than 18 years over a single winter in Hong Kong detected HMPV in 32 of 587 (6%), slightly less than the rate of 8% for both RSV and influenza. The estimated incidence of HMPV-associated LRI requiring hospitalization was four in 1000.[167] A systematic study of all lower respiratory illnesses in Queensland, Australia over 4 years detected HMPV in 707 of 10,025 (7%), with seasonal peaks of 15%; the rates of RSV and influenza in this cohort were 9% and 4%, respectively.[207] A 25-year prospective study of children with acute lower respiratory illness in Tennessee identified MPV in 12% of all specimens.[244] A large, population-based, prospective surveillance study in 2 United States cities found that the incidence of hospitalization for MPV in children younger than 5 years old was 1.2 per 1000, lower than the rate of RSV-associated hospitalization in the same cohort (three in 1000) but similar to the rates for influenza (0.9 in 1000) and parainfluenza virus type 3 (PIV-3) (0.5 in 1000).[243] A prospective 1-year study of outpatient children with acute respiratory illness in Melbourne, Australia tested 543 specimens by RT-PCR and detected MPV in 6%, RSV in 7%, and influenza in 4%.[125] A prospective study that enrolled 878 hospitalized children during a winter in China detected HMPV in 26% and RSV in 36%.[30]

Hospitalization rates from MPV are similar to those from other viruses, including PIV, adenovirus, rhinovirus, and influenza.[92,144] Hospitalization rates vary annually similar to incidence rates. In a retrospective study of children in Utah, annual hospitalization rates varied from nine to 79 of 100,000 person-years.[44] Young infants typically

*References 4, 31, 56, 72, 101, 110, 125, 160, 167, 177, 207, 220, 244.

have the highest rates of hospitalization. In a prospective study of Jordanian children, hospitalization rates in children younger than 6 months exceeded seven per 1000 children in years with high MPV activity.[195] Over a 6-year prospective multicenter study in the United States, rates of MPV hospitalization in children younger than 5 years averaged one per 1000. Rates of outpatient clinic and emergency department visits in children younger than 5 years were 55 and 13 per 1000 children, respectively. In some years, outpatient visits in children 6 to 11 months of age exceeded 130 visits per 1000 children, a finding indicating a significant burden of outpatient disease.[58]

A South African study of children hospitalized with acute respiratory infection found that MPV was present in 126 of 1409 (9%) and was the most common virus after RSV; the incidence of MPV-associated hospitalization in human immunodeficiency virus (HIV)–negative children was 29 in 1000.[141] A Japanese 2-year, multicenter study of inpatient and outpatient children with acute respiratory infection identified MPV in 57 of 637 (9%), with many cases proven by serologic study to be primary infections.[56] A 5-year observational study of Korean children younger than 5 years found MPV in 24 of 515 (5%), similar to the rates for influenza and PIV-3.[31] In Argentina, MPV was isolated from 11% of previously negative specimens in children with respiratory illnesses.[72] In Jordanian[4] and Israeli children,[177] MPV without coinfection caused 6% and 10% of acute respiratory infections, respectively.

Children hospitalized with MPV infection tend to be older than those admitted with RSV.[18,31,101,153,160,167,220] In a prospective analysis of Chinese children with acute respiratory infection, MPV-infected children averaged 22 months of age compared with 10.5 months in children with RSV ($P < .001$).[101] A male predominance has been observed in some studies but is not always statistically significant.[31,66,101,167,243]

There are fewer studies of adults with MPV infection, but the rate of MPV in studies of adults with acute respiratory infection is 2% to 14%.[60,68,79,102,233,240] A 4-year prospective study detected MPV in 8.5% (range, 4.4–13.2%) of adults hospitalized with acute respiratory infection.[233] A population-based study found that the incidence of hospitalization with MPV in adults age 50 years or older was one per 1000, similar to the rates for influenza (1.2 in 1000) and RSV (1.5 in 1000).[60] In patients 18 to 49 years of age, hospitalization rates were about two per 100,000, although emergency department visits were 5 to 6 times more common.[238,239]

MPV has been implicated in outbreaks in hospitals and long-term care facilities for adults and children, thus leading to mortality with rates as high as 25% in oncology patients or extremely old adults.[19,91,97,124,148,157,216,256] Kim and colleagues[111] reported transmission of MPV to pediatric hematology-oncology patients during a nosocomial outbreak. Two children shared a room with an infected child. Standard, but not droplet, precautions, were used. The incubation period was between 7 and 9 days. In laboratory studies, virus has been isolated from metal and nonporous surfaces for up to 8 hours,[215] although another study suggests that drying of MPV resulted in loss of infective particles, whereas viral RNA could still be detected at day 7.[154] Because of the significant morbidity and mortality of MPV in high-risk children, isolation precautions are important.

Exposure to MPV is ubiquitous by adulthood. In one Dutch study, 100% of patients older than 5 years demonstrated a positive antibody response to MPV.[220] Serosurveys testing large sample collections in Canada, China, Croatia, Germany, Israel, Japan, Taiwan, Thailand, the United States, and Uruguay showed that 95% to 100% of children have antibodies against HMPV by the age of 5 years.[94,130,133,135,136,138,149,151,166,251] In many of these studies, 50% to 75% of children were seropositive by age 2 years, a finding suggesting that most children acquire primary HMPV infection early.

Hospitalizations from MPV have significant associated costs, varying widely by country.[144] The estimated median hospitalization cost exceeded $5513 per child from a cohort of MPV-positive children in the United States from 2007 to 2013, with a median length of stay of 2.8 days.[44] Children with chronic medical conditions had significantly higher costs.

PATHOGENESIS AND PATHOLOGY

The pathogenesis of MPV has been described in animals and humans, although human data are limited. In macaques, the incubation period was short, at about 2 days. Necropsy revealed mild erosive and inflammatory changes in the mucosa and submucosa of the airways. Alveolar macrophages were increased, and virus replicated in ciliated respiratory epithelial cells.[119] In a mouse model, inflammatory infiltrates with a lymphocytic and monocytic predominance and perivascular edema were seen in the peribronchial areas. Histopathologic features peaked between days 5 and 7 with evidence of abnormalities remaining on day 14.[116] Similar patterns of bronchiolitis were observed in the cotton rat model.[246] Sumino and colleagues[211] reviewed the lung pathologic features of five adults with MPV infection. Histopathologic findings in three patients demonstrated acute, organizing lung injury with diffuse alveolar membrane formation and the presence of smudge cells. The fourth patient had no evidence of lower respiratory tract infection, and the fifth patient had nonspecific acute and chronic inflammation. A similar study in children revealed chronic inflammatory changes of the airways with intra-alveolar macrophages.[226] In a mouse model, depletion of alveolar macrophages was associated with milder disease, suggesting an important role for host inflammation in MPV pathogenesis.[117] However, natural killer (NK) cells did not contribute to viral clearance or immunopathology in a murine model.[237] A major limitation of the reports of human pathology is that the patients had been mechanically ventilated for a prolonged period before death, and thus it is impossible to distinguish virus-induced pathologic features from barotrauma and nonspecific inflammation.

The interaction between MPV and the immune system has been studied in humans and animal models, but the relationship is poorly understood. Laham and colleagues[122] evaluated cytokines from nasal wash specimens of children with acute viral lower respiratory infections. Comparing MPV-infected with RSV-infected children, interleukin (IL)-12, tumor necrosis factor-α, IL-1β, IL-6, and IL-8 were lower, but IL-10 was not different. Cytokine profiles of hospitalized versus outpatient children with MPV were not significantly different. Another study evaluated cytokine production induced by MPV in the lungs of mice. Interferon (IFN)-α and IFN-γ were present at higher levels than RSV, as well as granulocyte-macrophage colony-stimulating factor.[78] In peripheral blood mononuclear cells, MPV produced more IL-6 compared with RSV but less IFN-γ.[54] Mice lacking type 1 IFN responses are able to clear the virus and have less lung inflammation, a finding suggesting that type 1 IFN may contribute to MPV pathogenesis.[83] MPV lacks the genes that mediate innate immune inhibition in other paramyxoviruses. Nonetheless, MPV is capable of blocking type 1 interferon responses by an unclear mechanism; studies have implicated the G, M2-1, P, and SH proteins.[11,50,76,82,115,117,129,179,180] MPV and other respiratory viruses induce functional impairment of lung $CD8^+$ T cells, which fail to secrete IFN-γ or exhibit cytotoxic degranulation in response to viral peptides. This lung $CD8^+$ T-cell impairment is primarily driven by programmed cell death-1 (PD-1) signaling and resembles $CD8^+$ T-cell exhaustion induced by cancer and chronic infections such as with HIV and hepatitis C virus.[62,63] These exhausted T cells remain impaired during challenge infection in an animal model, thereby suggesting a potential mechanism for the capacity of MPV to reinfect humans throughout life.[64]

Humans mount robust antibody responses to MPV, and antibodies alone can protect in animal models. However, immunity likely wanes over time and provides limited cross protection among genotypes because recurrent infections in children and adults are well described,[68,240] with genetically different strains,[56,109,168,170,244] as well as with strains from the same lineage.[248] In vitro, antisera show evidence of cross protection between A and B strains, with neutralization titer generally four-fold higher against homologous versus heterologous strains.[222] Using a mouse model, Kolli and colleagues[116] demonstrated that initial infection with MPV was protective against reinfection 6 weeks later with a homologous strain. Early protection was confirmed in macaques; however, when these animals were challenged 12 weeks after initial infection, virus replication was detectable despite the presence of serum antibodies. At 11 months, antibody levels and protection had waned further; all macaques infected with heterologous virus and two of three macaques reinfected with homologous virus had no evidence of protection.[221] These data suggest that in primates, and likely humans, antibody levels wane over time, facilitating reinfection. A prospective study in humans noted that baseline MPV antibodies were lower in patients who subsequently became infected versus those who did not become infected.[69] Thus, cross-protection and duration of antibody responses are important issues for vaccine development.

CLINICAL MANIFESTATIONS

MPV causes upper and lower respiratory tract disease, as well as systemic symptoms, although signs and symptoms vary in incidence among studies. Clinically, MPV causes symptoms similar to those of RSV and other respiratory viruses.[18,56,155,244,257] Fever is present in the majority of cases.[31,56,66,110,167,207,248] Transient maculopapular rash has been described in 8% to 12% of patients.[110,167,207] Gastrointestinal symptoms are described with low frequency.[56,167,244] Duration of hospitalization does not differ between children with RSV and MPV.[18,167] White blood cell count and C-reactive protein are not significantly different between RSV and MPV.[101,243] Similarly, abnormalities in transaminases are uncommon, although the previous study identified 27% of patients with alanine transaminase and aspartate transaminase values more than twice normal.[110]

MPV is rarely detected in asymptomatic persons,[10,27,58,67,93,161,197,223,244] although in otherwise healthy young adults, MPV infection can be subclinical.[68] The duration of shedding in healthy individuals is approximately 7 to 14 days.[56,121] However, symptomatic episodes with shedding in healthy persons for 3 weeks or longer have been reported,[27] and shedding in patients with hematologic malignant diseases is also prolonged.[184]

Upper Respiratory Tract Manifestations

Rates of upper respiratory tract disease are less than lower respiratory tract disease.[65,101,244,248] Hoarseness, laryngitis, sore throat, and croup are less common than pulmonary symptoms, although rhinorrhea is a frequent finding.[31,56,101,167,207,243] One study in Nashville, Tennessee, detected MPV in 5% of children with upper respiratory disease, an incidence similar to that of RSV, influenza, and PIV but lower than adenovirus and rhinovirus. In that cohort, fever was present in 54% of patients, coryza in 82%, cough in 66%, pharyngitis in 44%, hoarseness in 8%, and conjunctivitis in 3%.[248]

MPV is associated with acute otitis media and has been isolated by nasal wash and tympanocentesis.[158,191,212,244,247,248] Schildgen and colleagues[191] isolated MPV in NP specimens from 13% of children with acute otitis media. Nokso-Koivisto and colleagues[158] noted that 24% of children with MPV and upper respiratory infection had acute otitis media; the incidence of acute otitis media was lower in children with MPV than in those with adenovirus, coronavirus, RSV, influenza virus, PIV, and rhinovirus. In a study of 118 children with MPV and upper respiratory tract infection, 63% had an abnormal tympanic membrane, although this was not significantly different from children with RSV, PIV, or influenza.[248] Bacterial coinfection is common, but MPV has been isolated as the sole pathogen in middle ear fluid.[212] In another study, children with MPV had a more common history of acute otitis media necessitating tympanocentesis compared with RSV.[250] Peak MPV activity has been temporally associated with an increased number of visits and diagnoses of acute otitis media.[210] However, in a prospective study of 362 children, MPV was associated with symptomatic upper respiratory tract infection but not the development of acute otitis media compared with other viruses.[33]

Lower Respiratory Tract Manifestations

Lower respiratory tract signs and symptoms include cough, wheeze, and rhonchi. In a cohort of Bangladeshi children, MPV accounted for 14% of all early childhood wheezing episodes.[45] In a large study of Chinese children with acute respiratory infection, wheezing was more common in children with RSV, but MPV-infected children were diagnosed with pneumonia more than were RSV-infected children: 47% versus 31% ($P = .002$)[101] Conversely, a larger percentage of children with RSV were diagnosed with bronchiolitis compared with MPV: 62% versus 42% ($P < .001$). Other studies also note the trend toward a higher percentage of children with MPV and pneumonia compared with RSV,[243,244] although this is not always statistically significant.[167] Jroundi and colleagues[103] noted that in Moroccan children with World Health Organization–defined severe pneumonia, MPV was associated with more severity and a higher risk of intensive care need than RSV. MPV has been implicated as a cause of pediatric community-acquired pneumonia because it is detected significantly more frequently in children with community-acquired pneumonia than in healthy control subjects.[182,197] MPV-associated community-acquired pneumonia requiring hospitalization was significantly more common in children younger than 5 years than in other age groups.[98] Frequency ranges of signs and symptoms of MPV infections in young children are presented in Table 183.1. As can be seen, the ranges vary considerably by feature in the studies reviewed. Presented in Fig. 183.2 is the chest radiograph of a child with MPV pneumonia.

TABLE 183.1 Signs and Symptoms in Young Children With Human Metapneumovirus Acute Respiratory Tract Infections

Clinical Feature	Frequency Ranges (%)
Acute otitis media	11–26
Asthma exacerbation	9–47
Conjunctivitis	3–9
Coryza	82–88
Cough	67–100
Crackles, rales	4–89
Cyanosis	2–85
Dyspnea	5–91
Febrile seizures	4–16
Fever	36–97
Pharyngitis, sore throat	10–46
Rash	4–13
Rhinorrhea	18–91
Tachypnea	59–81
Vomiting and/or diarrhea	0–54
Wheezing	15–56

Data from references 5, 9, 22, 30, 46, 52, 56, 101, 109, 110, 143, 167, 223, 244, 248, 249, 257.

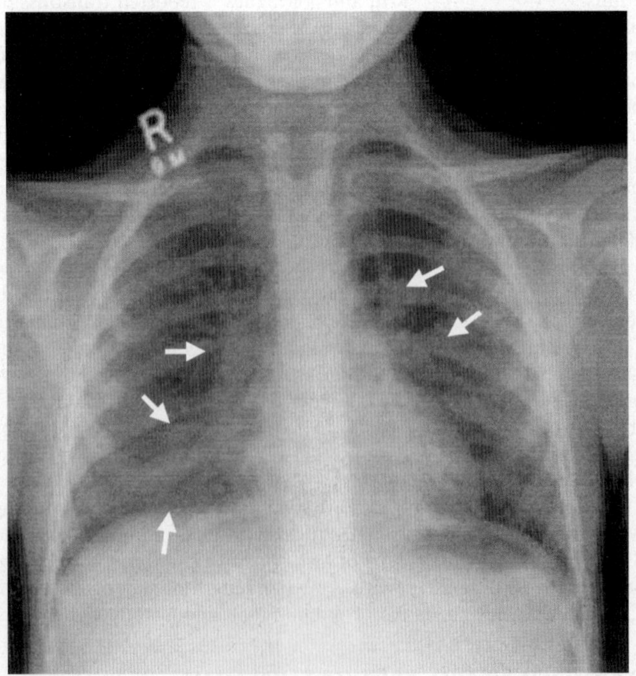

FIG. 183.2 Chest radiograph of a child infected with human metapneumovirus demonstrating bilateral pneumonic infiltrates *(arrows)* and hyperinflated lung fields.

In one study, 75% of children with MPV had no underlying medical conditions[18]; however, in some cohorts, the majority of hospitalized MPV-positive children had a complex medical condition.[44] Although death is most commonly described in immunocompromised patients and in patients with underlying conditions, healthy children do have fatal sequelae of MPV. Donoso and colleagues[53] reported a case of a previously healthy 2-year-old child with fatal pneumonia, hypotension, and acute respiratory distress syndrome secondary to MPV. A similar case was reported in a 20-month-old male child with acute respiratory distress syndrome who developed multiorgan system failure with hepatitis, cytopenia, coagulopathy, and renal failure requiring extracorporeal membrane oxygenation.[193] In a cohort of pediatric intensive care unit (ICU) patients, children with MPV required a longer duration of mechanical ventilation than those with RSV (11 days vs. 7 days).[59] Spaeder and colleagues[208] described a cohort of 111 MPV positive children requiring ICU care, and 9% did not survive to discharge. Female sex, chronic medical conditions, and hospital acquisition of the virus were associated with mortality. Severe symptoms have also been reported in healthy adults.

Viral coinfection has been described with MPV and is common in young children.[145] Dual infection with RSV and MPV increased the risk of pediatric ICU admission compared with RSV alone in one small study,[198] but this finding was not confirmed by subsequent larger reports.[127,202,225] Other studies demonstrated no significant clinical differences in children with coinfections, including adenovirus, bocavirus, coronavirus, influenza virus, PIVs, or RSV.[31,101,105,109,110,128,195,207] The increased sensitivity of molecular viral detection methods has uncovered high rates of codetection for many viruses, not just MPV; the clinical significance of this finding remains unclear.

Streptococcus pneumoniae acute otitis media is associated with MPV infection,[212,247] and it may be a cause of pneumonia. Verkaik and colleagues[229] noted that frequent carriage of *S. pneumoniae* in children increased seroconversion rates of MPV. Infection with both organisms may contribute to more severe disease.[196] Pneumococcal vaccination decreased the number of children with MPV who have severe pneumonia in both HIV and non-HIV infected children.[140] Secondary bacterial pneumonia following MPV infection has been reported, although the frequency of this complication is unknown.[6,196] Mice infected with MPV and subsequently challenged with sublethal doses of *S. pneumoniae* exhibited more severe lung disease than did mice infected with MPV or pneumococcus alone.[120] In vitro models suggest increased adherence of *S. pneumoniae* as a possible mechanism.[123]

Asthma

MPV has been linked to asthma exacerbations, although the incidence is lower than with RSV or human rhinovirus (HRV).[99,108,176] MPV was detected in 10 of 132 hospitalized Finnish children with acute wheezing.[100] Similarly, MPV was isolated from 7% of adults hospitalized for an acute asthma exacerbation.[242] As with RSV, infection with MPV within the first 2 years of life is a risk factor for later development of asthma.[73] Broughton and colleagues[24] prospectively followed premature infants who developed MPV bronchiolitis within the first year of life and noted that they had decreased lung function at 12 months of age.

Infections in Immunocompromised Persons

Severe and fatal MPV disease has been described in immunocompromised individuals, including solid-organ and stem cell transplant recipients, HIV-infected individuals, chemotherapy recipients, and persons with chronic cardiopulmonary disease. In a study of hospitalized South African children, children with underlying medical problems accounted for 88% of positive MPV specimens, not significantly different from findings with RSV.[153] MPV is a cause of death in children and adults with hematologic malignant disease,[34,245] as well as stem cell transplants.[51,96,199] MPV was detected in bronchoalveolar lavage specimens from 5 of 163 (3%) episodes of acute respiratory infection in stem cell transplant recipients, and 4 patients died.[61] In a retrospective study of hematopoietic stem cell transplant recipients with MPV-positive bronchoalveolar lavage specimens, mortality rates within the first 100 days were 43%, identical to those from RSV.[181] Chu and colleagues[34] noted that in their cohort of MPV-positive immunocompromised children, hematopoietic stem cell transplant recipients were more likely to require ICU care compared with patients with other conditions. One patient who tested positive for MPV before transplantation developed symptoms after transplantation and died.[28]

In a South African study, HIV-positive children with MPV were significantly more likely to receive a diagnosis of pneumonia and experience longer hospitalization, lower mean oxygen saturation, and bacteremia. Children with HIV infection were five-fold more likely to be infected with MPV than were HIV-negative children.[141] However, Groome and colleagues[77] noted that hospitalizations from MPV were increased only in HIV-positive children 5 to 17 years of age, whereas rates in younger children were similar between HIV-infected and HIV-uninfected children. HIV-exposed, uninfected children were more likely to have MPV lower respiratory tract infection than HIV-unexposed, uninfected children.[35]

MPV causes severe disease in children with underlying cardiac and respiratory disease or prematurity,[113,153,165,227] with some evidence suggesting that it is more common than RSV in these children, possibly related to the use of palivizumab.[257] Esper and colleagues[66] noted that 34% of patients with MPV had a history of prematurity, chronic lung disease, complex congenital heart disease, or immunodeficiency, findings emphasizing that these children are at risk for MPV disease. Ulloa-Gutierrez and colleagues[218] described a 3-month-old 27-week premature infant who required 10 days of extracorporeal membrane oxygenation. In a study of preschool children with MPV, 32.7% had a history of severe prematurity (<32 weeks), and they were more likely to have longer hospitalizations, need for supplemental oxygen, and higher severity scores.[163] Anderson and colleagues[7] noted that high-risk hospitalized children with MPV were more likely to be more premature and more commonly have chronic lung disease than children with RSV. MPV has been detected in 3% to 12% of adults hospitalized for exacerbations of chronic obstructive pulmonary disease.[147,185,230]

Encephalitis and Encephalopathy

MPV has been associated with neurologic complications including febrile seizures, status epilepticus, and altered mental status, but there is no conclusive evidence for direct central nervous system infection. Schildgen and colleagues[192] reported a case of one patient who died and had MPV isolated by RT-PCR from brain and lung tissue. Glaser and colleagues[75] detected MPV by RT-PCR in nasal specimens from four of 1570 patients with encephalitis of unknown etiology. Several other reports described the detection of MPV in a respiratory specimen from patients with encephalitis.[8,70,84,104,192,228] There are two case reports of detection of MPV RNA in brain or cerebrospinal fluid.[188,192]

MPV has been isolated from nasopharyngeal specimens in patients with myopericarditis, although the virus has not been directly associated with cardiac disease.[32,235]

DIFFERENTIAL DIAGNOSIS

Clinical illness caused by MPV cannot be reliably distinguished from disease caused by other common respiratory viruses, including RSV, PIVs, rhinoviruses, and influenza virus. Complications such as acute otitis media and supervening bacterial pneumonia may occur.

DIAGNOSIS

Because detection in tissue culture can require prolonged incubation for viral replication, other diagnostic tests have been used. Shell vial culture offers increased sensitivity over traditional culture.[126,178] Immunofluorescence assay has demonstrated a sensitivity of 73% and specificity of 97% with RT-PCR as the gold standard.[57] Direct fluorescent assay has shown similar results.[169] Commercial antibody reagents for immunofluorescent detection of MPV are available. RT-PCR is widely used for detection of the virus in epidemiologic studies; primers have been directed at the F, M, L, P, and N protein.[17,37,170,220] Real-time RT-PCR directed toward the N gene has a high sensitivity for virus detection and can detect the four subgroups.[114,142] Several commercial multiplex molecular assays that include MPV are available.[26,173]

TREATMENT

The mainstay of therapy for MPV infections is supportive care, including oral or intravenous hydration for infants unable to feed, monitoring of respiratory status and oxygen saturation, supplemental oxygen as needed, and mechanical ventilation for respiratory failure. Reports of pharmacologic treatment of MPV are limited to immunocompromised and severely ill patients. Ribavirin, an antiviral agent used in severe RSV infection, has been used in animal models and humans, although there are no controlled studies. Hamelin and colleagues[81] demonstrated that ribavirin reduced inflammation and viral replication in mice with MPV infection. Commercial intravenous immunoglobulin (IVIG), ribavirin, and $NMSO_3$ effectively inhibited MPV in vitro.[252,254] Spetch and colleagues[209] noted that in a mouse model, $NMSO_3$ decreased viral replication, weight loss associated with infection, and pulmonary inflammation. Ribavirin, with and without IVIG, has been used in immunocompromised adults.[106] Bonney and colleagues[21] reported successful treatment of an immunocompromised child with MPV by using intravenous ribavirin and IVIG. Subsequently, oral ribavirin and inhaled ribavirin with and without IVIG have been described as successful in several case reports.[34,112,200,201] However, ribavirin is not routinely recommended in patients with hematologic malignant diseases or in patients undergoing hematopoietic stem cell transplantation.[49,90,232] Alternate therapies studied in vitro and in animals include plant-derived compounds and short-interfering RNA.[43,47,150,174] Human and murine monoclonal antibodies exhibit therapeutic efficacy in animal models, with improvements in viral load and lung pathologic findings.[80,194,217,241]

PROGNOSIS

Most patients with MPV infection experience a full recovery. Fatalities are uncommon and occur primarily in severely immunocompromised persons (e.g., hematopoietic stem cell or solid-organ transplant recipients, patients receiving intensive chemotherapy, patients with HIV infection), persons with significant underlying conditions (e.g., severe chronic obstructive pulmonary disease), and adults older than 65 years who are in poor health ("frail" older adults). MPV may be associated with the subsequent development of asthma.

PREVENTION

Development of candidate MPV vaccines began shortly after identification of the virus. The F protein is highly immunogenic and is the only target of neutralizing antibodies; in contrast to RSV, the MPV G protein does not induce neutralizing antibodies and is not a protective antigen.[152,187,205] A recombinant PIV encoding the MPV F protein demonstrated protection against wild-type virus.[214] Soluble F protein vaccines have shown a reduction in viral titers in cotton rats and hamsters,[42,87] and addition of the M protein to F subunit vaccines may have an adjuvant effect.[2] Many of the candidate vaccines produced both homologous and heterologous viral protection.[87,131,134,204,236] Other candidate vaccines include a Venezuelan equine encephalitis virus–based viral replicon particle vaccine expressing the F protein, which was effective at controlling viral load and producing F-specific antibodies with neutralizing activity in mice, cotton rats, and African green monkeys.[13,152] Virus-like particles are also a promising vaccine candidate.[38,131,236] Monoclonal antibodies directed at the fusion protein are effective prophylactically at decreasing viral replication in mouse and cotton rat models.[36,80,174,194,217] Two different human monoclonal antibodies against the F protein have shown therapeutic efficacy against both MPV and RSV in small animal models.[36,194] Reverse genetics has been developed for MPV and has been used to develop recombinant strains for vaccine development.[16,86] Viruses lacking the G, M2-1, M2-2, or SH proteins or with point mutations are attenuated and immunogenic in rodent and primate models.[14,16,25,88,89,189] A human challenge model has been established, which will facilitate the development and testing of MPV vaccines.[213]

NEW REFERENCES SINCE THE SEVENTH EDITION

2. Aerts L, Rheaume C, Carbonneau J, et al. Adjuvant effect of the human metapneumovirus (HMPV) matrix protein in HMPV subunit vaccines. *J Gen Virol.* 2015;96(Pt 4):767-774.
7. Anderson EJ, Simoes EA, Buttery JP, et al. Prevalence and characteristics of human metapneumovirus infection among hospitalized children at high risk for severe lower respiratory tract infection. *J Pediatric Infect Dis Soc.* 2012;1(3):212-222.
13. Bates JT, Pickens JA, Schuster JE, et al. Immunogenicity and efficacy of alphavirus-derived replicon vaccines for respiratory syncytial virus and human metapneumovirus in nonhuman primates. *Vaccine.* 2016;34(7):950-956.
16. Biacchesi S, Skiadopoulos MH, Yang L, et al. Recombinant human metapneumovirus lacking the small hydrophobic SH and/or attachment G glycoprotein: deletion of G yields a promising vaccine candidate. *J Virol.* 2004;78(23):12877-12887.
23. Bosis S, Esposito S, Osterhaus AD, et al. Association between high nasopharyngeal viral load and disease severity in children with human metapneumovirus infection. *J Clin Virol.* 2008;42(3):286-290.
26. Butt SA, Maceira VP, McCallen ME, et al. Comparison of three commercial RT-PCR systems for the detection of respiratory viruses. *J Clin Virol.* 2014;61(3):406-410.
27. Byington CL, Ampofo K, Stockmann C, et al. Community surveillance of respiratory viruses among families in the Utah Better Identification of Germs-Longitudinal Viral Epidemiology (BIG-LoVE) study. *Clin Infect Dis.* 2015;61(8):1217-1224.
28. Campbell AP, Guthrie KA, Englund JA, et al. Clinical outcomes associated with respiratory virus detection before allogeneic hematopoietic stem cell transplant. *Clin Infect Dis.* 2015;61(2):192-202.
32. Choi MJ, Song JY, Yang TU, et al. acute myopericarditis caused by human metapneumovirus. *Infect Chemother.* 2016;48(1):36-40.
33. Chonmaitree T, Alvarez-Fernandez P, Jennings K, et al. Symptomatic and asymptomatic respiratory viral infections in the first year of life: association with acute otitis media development. *Clin Infect Dis.* 2015;60(1):1-9.
34. Chu HY, Renaud C, Ficken E, et al. Respiratory tract infections due to human metapneumovirus in immunocompromised children. *J Pediatric Infect Dis Soc.* 2014;3(4):286-293.
35. Cohen C, Moyes J, Tempia S, et al. Epidemiology of acute lower respiratory tract infection in HIV-exposed uninfected infants. *Pediatrics.* 2016;137:e20153272.
36. Corti D, Bianchi S, Vanzetta F, et al. Cross-neutralization of four paramyxoviruses by a human monoclonal antibody. *Nature.* 2013;501(7467):439-443.
37. Cote S, Abed Y, Boivin G. Comparative evaluation of real-time PCR assays for detection of the human metapneumovirus. *J Clin Microbiol.* 2003;41(8):3631-3635.
38. Cox RG, Erickson JJ, Hastings AK, et al. Human metapneumovirus virus-like particles induce protective B and T cell responses in a mouse model. *J Virol.* 2014;88(11):6368-6379.
39. Cox RG, Livesay SB, Johnson M, et al. The human metapneumovirus fusion protein mediates entry via an interaction with RGD-binding integrins. *J Virol.* 2012;86(22):12148-12160.
40. Cox RG, Mainou BA, Johnson M, et al. Human metapneumovirus is capable of entering cells by fusion with endosomal membranes. *PLoS Pathog.* 2015;11(12):e1005303.
44. Davis CR, Stockmann C, Pavia AT, et al. Incidence, morbidity, and costs of human metapneumovirus infection in hospitalized children. *J Pediatric Infect Dis Soc.* 2016;5(3):303-311.
45. Dawood FS, Fry AM, Goswami D, et al. Incidence and characteristics of early childhood wheezing, Dhaka, Bangladesh, 2004-2010. *Pediatr Pulmonol.* 2016;51(6):588-595.
49. Dignan FL, Clark A, Aitken C, et al. BCSH/BSBMT/UK Clinical Virology Network guideline: diagnosis and management of common respiratory viral infections in patients undergoing treatment for haematological malignancies or stem cell transplantation. *Br J Haematol.* 2016;173(3):380-393.
51. Dokos C, Masjosthusmann K, Rellensmann G, et al. Fatal human metapneumovirus infection following allogeneic hematopoietic stem cell transplantation. *Transpl Infect Dis.* 2013;15(3):E97-E101.
58. Edwards KM, Zhu Y, Griffin MR, et al. Burden of human metapneumovirus infection in young children. *N Engl J Med.* 2013;368(7):633-643.
59. Eggleston HA, Gunville CF, Miller JI, et al. A comparison of characteristics and outcomes in severe human metapneumovirus and respiratory syncytial virus infections in children treated in an intensive care unit. *Pediatr Infect Dis J.* 2013;32(12):1330-1334.
63. Erickson JJ, Lu P, Wen S, et al. Acute viral respiratory infection rapidly induces a CD8+ T cell exhaustion-like phenotype. *J Immunol.* 2015;195(9):4319-4330.
64. Erickson JJ, Rogers MC, Hastings AK, et al. Programmed death-1 impairs secondary effector lung CD8+ T cells during respiratory virus reinfection. *J Immunol.* 2014;193(10):5108-5117.
70. Fok A, Mateevici C, Lin B, et al. Encephalitis-associated human metapneumovirus pneumonia in adult, Australia. *Emerg Infect Dis.* 2015;21(11):2074-2076.
71. Fuller JA, Njenga MK, Bigogo G, et al. Association of the CT values of real-time PCR of viral upper respiratory tract infection with clinical severity, Kenya. *J Med Virol.* 2013;85(5):924-932.
76. Goutagny N, Jiang Z, Tian J, et al. Cell type-specific recognition of human metapneumoviruses (HMPVs) by retinoic acid-inducible gene I (RIG-I) and TLR7 and viral interference of RIG-I ligand recognition by HMPV-B1 phosphoprotein. *J Immunol.* 2010;184(3):1168-1179.

77. Groome MJ, Moyes J, Cohen C, et al. Human metapneumovirus-associated severe acute respiratory illness hospitalisation in HIV-infected and HIV-uninfected South African children and adults. *J Clin Virol.* 2015;69:125-132.
82. Hastings AK, Amato KR, Wen SC, et al. Human metapneumovirus small hydrophobic (SH) protein downregulates type I IFN pathway signaling by affecting STAT1 expression and phosphorylation. *Virology.* 2016;494:248-256.
83. Hastings AK, Erickson JJ, Schuster JE, et al. Role of type I interferon signaling in human metapneumovirus pathogenesis and control of viral replication. *J Virol.* 2015;89(8):4405-4420.
84. Hata M, Ito M, Kiyosawa S, et al. A fatal case of encephalopathy possibly associated with human metapneumovirus infection. *Jpn J Infect Dis.* 2007;60(5):328-329.
90. Hirsch HH, Martino R, Ward KN, et al. Fourth European Conference on Infections in Leukaemia (ECIL-4): guidelines for diagnosis and treatment of human respiratory syncytial virus, parainfluenza virus, metapneumovirus, rhinovirus, and coronavirus. *Clin Infect Dis.* 2013;56(2):258-266.
91. Hoellein A, Hecker J, Hoffmann D, et al. Serious outbreak of human metapneumovirus in patients with hematologic malignancies. *Leuk Lymphoma.* 2016;57(3):623-627.
92. Homaira N, Luby SP, Hossain K, et al. Respiratory viruses associated hospitalization among children aged <5 years in Bangladesh: 2010-2014. *PLoS ONE.* 2016;11(2):e0147982.
93. Howard LM, Johnson M, Williams JV, et al. Respiratory viral detections during symptomatic and asymptomatic periods in young Andean children. *Pediatr Infect Dis J.* 2015;34(10):1074-1080.
95. Huck B, Scharf G, Neumann-Haefelin D, et al. Novel human metapneumovirus sublineage. *Emerg Infect Dis.* 2006;12(1):147-150.
96. Hutspardol S, Essa M, Richardson S, et al. Significant transplantation-related mortality from respiratory virus infections within the first one hundred days in children after hematopoietic stem cell transplantation. *Biol Blood Marrow Transplant.* 2015;21(10):1802-1807.
97. Ibrahim S, Scott M, Bixler D, et al. Outbreaks of human metapneumovirus in two skilled nursing facilities—West Virginia and Idaho, 2011–2012. *MMWR Morb Mortal Wkly Rep.* 2013;62(46):909-913.
98. Jain S, Williams DJ, Arnold SR, et al. Community-acquired pneumonia requiring hospitalization among U.S. children. *N Engl J Med.* 2015;372(9):835-845.
103. Jroundi I, Mahraoui C, Benmessaoud R, et al. A comparison of human metapneumovirus and respiratory syncytial virus WHO-defined severe pneumonia in Moroccan children. *Epidemiol Infect.* 2016;144(3):516-526.
104. Kaida A, Iritani N, Kubo H, et al. Seasonal distribution and phylogenetic analysis of human metapneumovirus among children in Osaka City, Japan. *J Clin Virol.* 2006;35(4):394-399.
112. Kitanovski L, Kopriva S, Pokorn M, et al. Treatment of severe human metapneumovirus (hMPV) pneumonia in an immunocompromised child with oral ribavirin and IVIG. *J Pediatr Hematol Oncol.* 2013;35(7):e311-e313.
114. Klemenc J, Asad Ali S, Johnson M, et al. Real-time reverse transcriptase PCR assay for improved detection of human metapneumovirus. *J Clin Virol.* 2012;54(4):371-375.
115. Kolli D, Bao X, Liu T, et al. Human metapneumovirus glycoprotein G inhibits TLR4-dependent signaling in monocyte-derived dendritic cells. *J Immunol.* 2011;187(1):47-54.
117. Kolli D, Gupta MR, Sbrana E, et al. Alveolar macrophages contribute to the pathogenesis of human metapneumovirus infection while protecting against respiratory syncytial virus infection. *Am J Respir Cell Mol Biol.* 2014;51(4):502-515.
123. Lai SH, Liao SL, Wong KS, et al. Preceding human metapneumovirus infection increases adherence of *Streptococcus pneumoniae* and severity of murine pneumococcal pneumonia. *J Microbiol Immunol Infect.* 2016;49(2):216-224.
124. Laine O, Laine J, Saila P, et al. An outbreak of human metapneumovirus in a rehabilitation center for alcoholics in Tampere, Finland. *Infect Dis (Lond).* 2015;47(7):499-503.
128. Le Nouen C, Hillyer P, Brock LG, et al. Human metapneumovirus SH and G glycoproteins inhibit macropinocytosis-mediated entry into human dendritic cells and reduce CD4+ T cell activation. *J Virol.* 2014;88(11):6453-6469.
131. Levy C, Aerts L, Hamelin ME, et al. Virus-like particle vaccine induces cross-protection against human metapneumovirus infections in mice. *Vaccine.* 2013;31(25):2778-2785.
134. Liu P, Shu Z, Qin X, et al. A live attenuated human metapneumovirus vaccine strain provides complete protection against homologous viral infection and cross-protection against heterologous viral infection in BALB/c mice. *Clin Vaccine Immunol.* 2013;20(8):1246-1254.
137. Lu G, Li J, Xie Z, et al. Human metapneumovirus associated with community-acquired pneumonia in children in Beijing, China. *J Med Virol.* 2013;85(1):138-143.
144. Marcone DN, Durand LO, Azziz-Baumgartner E, et al. Incidence of viral respiratory infections in a prospective cohort of outpatient and hospitalized children aged ≤5 years and its associated cost in Buenos Aires, Argentina. *BMC Infect Dis.* 2015;15:447.
145. Martin ET, Fairchok MP, Stednick ZJ, et al. Epidemiology of multiple respiratory viruses in childcare attendees. *J Infect Dis.* 2013;207(6):982-989.
146. Martin ET, Kuypers J, Heugel J, et al. Clinical disease and viral load in children infected with respiratory syncytial virus or human metapneumovirus. *Diagn Microbiol Infect Dis.* 2008;62(4):382-388.
148. Matsuda S, Nakamura M, Hirano E, et al. Characteristics of human metapneumovirus infection prevailing in hospital wards housing patients with severe disabilities. *Jpn J Infect Dis.* 2013;66(3):195-200.
156. Neemuchwala A, Duvvuri VR, Marchand-Austin A, et al. Human metapneumovirus prevalence and molecular epidemiology in respiratory outbreaks in Ontario, Canada. *J Med Virol.* 2015;87(2):269-274.
157. Neu N, Plaskett T, Hutcheon G, et al. Epidemiology of human metapneumovirus in a pediatric long-term care facility. *Infect Control Hosp Epidemiol.* 2012;33(6):545-550.
163. Pancham K, Sami I, Perez GF, et al. Human metapneumovirus infection is associated with severe respiratory disease in preschool children with history of prematurity. *Pediatr Neonatol.* 2016;57(1):27-34.
164. Papenburg J, Carbonneau J, Isabel S, et al. Genetic diversity and molecular evolution of the major human metapneumovirus surface glycoproteins over a decade. *J Clin Virol.* 2013;58(3):541-547.
173. Popowitch EB, O'Neill SS, Miller MB. Comparison of the Biofire FilmArray RP, Genmark eSensor RVP, Luminex xTAG RVPv1, and Luminex xTAG RVP fast multiplex assays for detection of respiratory viruses. *J Clin Microbiol.* 2013;51(5):1528-1533.
175. Pretorius MA, Madhi SA, Cohen C, et al. Respiratory viral coinfections identified by a 10-plex real-time reverse-transcription polymerase chain reaction assay in patients hospitalized with severe acute respiratory illness—South Africa, 2009–2010. *J Infect Dis.* 2012;206(suppl 1):S159-S165.
179. Ren J, Kolli D, Liu T, et al. Human metapneumovirus inhibits IFN-beta signaling by downregulating Jak1 and Tyk2 cellular levels. *PLoS ONE.* 2011;6(9):e24496.
180. Ren J, Liu G, Go J, et al. Human metapneumovirus M2-2 protein inhibits innate immune response in monocyte-derived dendritic cells. *PLoS ONE.* 2014;9(3):e91865.
181. Renaud C, Xie H, Seo S, et al. Mortality rates of human metapneumovirus and respiratory syncytial virus lower respiratory tract infections in hematopoietic cell transplantation recipients. *Biol Blood Marrow Transplant.* 2013;19(8):1220-1226.
182. Rhedin S, Lindstrand A, Hjelmgren A, et al. Respiratory viruses associated with community-acquired pneumonia in children: matched case-control study. *Thorax.* 2015;70(9):847-853.
183. Ricart S, Garcia-Garcia JJ, Anton A, et al. Analysis of human metapneumovirus and human bocavirus viral load. *Pediatr Infect Dis J.* 2013;32(9):1032-1034.
184. Richardson L, Brite J, Del Castillo M, et al. Comparison of respiratory virus shedding by conventional and molecular testing methods in patients with haematological malignancy. *Clin Microbiol Infect.* 2016;22(4):380.e381-380.e387.
186. Roussy JF, Carbonneau J, Ouakki M, et al. Human metapneumovirus viral load is an important risk factor for disease severity in young children. *J Clin Virol.* 2014;60(2):133-140.
194. Schuster JE, Cox RG, Hastings AK, et al. A broadly neutralizing human monoclonal antibody exhibits in vivo efficacy against both human metapneumovirus and respiratory syncytial virus. *J Infect Dis.* 2015;211(2):216-225.
195. Schuster JE, Khuri-Bulos N, Faouri S, et al. Human metapneumovirus infection in Jordanian children: epidemiology and risk factors for severe disease. *Pediatr Infect Dis J.* 2015;34(12):1335-1341.
196. Seki M, Yoshida H, Gotoh K, et al. Severe respiratory failure due to co-infection with human metapneumovirus and *Streptococcus pneumoniae*. *Respir Med Case Rep.* 2014;12:13-15.
197. Self WH, Williams DJ, Zhu Y, et al. Respiratory viral detection in children and adults: comparing asymptomatic controls and patients with community-acquired pneumonia. *J Infect Dis.* 2016;213(4):584-591.
199. Seo S, Gooley TA, Kuypers JM, et al. Human metapneumovirus infections following hematopoietic cell transplantation: factors associated with disease progression. *Clin Infect Dis.* 2016;63(2):178-185.
206. Slater OM, Terio KA, Zhang Y, et al. Human metapneumovirus infection in chimpanzees, United States. *Emerg Infect Dis.* 2014;20(12):2115-2118.
208. Spaeder MC, Custer JW, Bembea MM, et al. A multicenter outcomes analysis of children with severe viral respiratory infection due to human metapneumovirus. *Pediatr Crit Care Med.* 2013;14(3):268-272.
210. Stockmann C, Ampofo K, Hersh AL, et al. Seasonality of acute otitis media and the role of respiratory viral activity in children. *Pediatr Infect Dis J.* 2013;32(4):314-319.
213. Talaat KR, Karron RA, Thumar B, et al. Experimental infection of adults with recombinant wild-type human metapneumovirus. *J Infect Dis.* 2013;208(10):1669-1678.
228. Vehapoglu A, Turel O, Uygur Sahin T, et al. Clinical significance of human metapneumovirus in refractory status epilepticus and encephalitis: case report and review of the literature. *Case Rep Neurol Med.* 2015;2015:131780.
230. Vicente D, Montes M, Cilla G, et al. Human metapneumovirus and chronic obstructive pulmonary disease. *Emerg Infect Dis.* 2004;10(7):1338-1339.
232. Waghmare A, Englund JA, Boeckh M. How I treat respiratory viral infections in the setting of intensive chemotherapy or hematopoietic cell transplantation. *Blood.* 2016;127(22):2682-2692.

234. Wei HY, Tsao KC, Huang CG, et al. Clinical features of different genotypes/genogroups of human metapneumovirus in hospitalized children. *J Microbiol Immunol Infect.* 2013;46(5):352-357.
235. Weinreich MA, Jabbar AY, Malguria N, et al. New-onset myocarditis in an immunocompetent adult with acute metapneumovirus infection. *Case Rep Med.* 2015;2015:814269.
236. Wen SC, Schuster JE, Gilchuk P, et al. Lung CD8+ T cell impairment occurs during human metapneumovirus infection despite virus-like particle induction of functional CD8+ T cells. *J Virol.* 2015;89(17):8713-8726.
237. Wen SC, Tollefson SJ, Johnson M, et al. acute clearance of human metapneumovirus occurs independently of natural killer cells. *J Virol.* 2014;88(18):10963-10969.
238. Widmer K, Griffin MR, Zhu Y, et al. Respiratory syncytial virus- and human metapneumovirus-associated emergency department and hospital burden in adults. *Influenza Other Respir Viruses.* 2014;8(3):347-352.
239. Widmer K, Zhu Y, Williams JV, et al. Rates of hospitalizations for respiratory syncytial virus, human metapneumovirus, and influenza virus in older adults. *J Infect Dis.* 2012;206(1):56-62.
256. Yang Z, Suzuki A, Watanabe O, et al. Outbreak of human metapneumovirus infection in a severe motor-and-intellectual disabilities ward in Japan. *Jpn J Infect Dis.* 2014;67(4):318-321.

The full reference list for this chapter is available at ExpertConsult.com.

SUBSECTION VIII Rhabdoviridae

184 Rabies Virus

Charles E. Rupprecht • Stephen J. Scholand

Rabies is an acute, progressive viral infectious disease of the central nervous system (CNS). It causes a devastating encephalitis, classically characterized by hydrophobia, hypersalivation, and certain death. Only warm-blooded vertebrates can be infected, and humans are considered a dead-end host. Sadly, children make up a more than one-half of the total annual deaths around the world.[312]

The disease occurs following the introduction of virus by a bite or scratch from an infected animal. Rarely, aerosol or mucosal exposure or transplanted tissue enables infection. In most cases, saliva from an infected animal serves as the transfecting medium. Laden with infectious virions, inoculation can occur through breaks in the skin or direct contact with mucous membranes. From there, the virus can attach to and migrate by peripheral nerves to the spinal cord and brain. Encephalomyelitis develops, with subsequent centrifugal dissemination of progeny virions. The clinical symptoms at first may be nonspecific, such as with headache, fever, and malaise. Neurologic symptoms then manifest, such as numbness or paresthesias relative to the inoculation site. Each presentation of human rabies, however, can be quite variable. Inevitably, the disease progresses to coma and almost always death. Recent experience indicates that in extremely rare cases, survival may be possible. The mainstay of medical intervention, however, remains prevention. Redoubled efforts around the world to control this zoonosis have begun, but enormous challenges remain. A thorough appreciation of viral epidemiology, transmission, pathophysiology, and prevention methods is of great value in the study of pediatric infectious diseases.

HISTORY

Rabies is an ancient disease that has plagued humankind throughout history. Frightful myths, admixed with astute observations of the disease, have been described by all major civilizations. For a detailed historical account of rabies throughout the ages, one may refer to a previous version of this chapter and other relevant publications.[223,264,308] More recently, in this 21st century, rabies remains a major public health problem throughout most of the developing world. Current estimations of the global burden of human rabies suggest that 60,000 or more victims may succumb each year,[312] with most deaths in Asia and Africa.[162] However, the actual number is unknown as a result of difficulties in reporting and surveillance.[273] Costs in disability-adjusted life years are estimated at more than 3.7 million USD (95% confidence interval, 1.6–10.4 million), with 8.6 billion USD (95% confidence interval, 2.9–21.5 billion) in annual losses.[118]

Canine rabies is the source for the majority of human cases in the developing world, but it has been eliminated in developed countries. The United States was declared free of canine rabies transmission in 2007,[288] and by 2008 most of Western Europe was "rabies free" (except for the disease in bats). However, even with the control of canine rabies in some regions, importation of infected dogs from rabies-endemic countries was responsible for sporadic reintroduction, such as in France and Italy in recent years.[25,86] Thus, it is important to remain vigilant for rabies reintroduction.[63] Whereas the Old World still has canine rabies as an important public health problem, within Latin America, significant progress was achieved, with a 95% decline in human rabies cases since 1983, when a large regional effort for animal rabies elimination was launched.[251]

In the United States, wildlife rabies reservoirs, such as raccoons, skunks, foxes, and bats, remained an important source of rabies at the end of the 20th century. Human and animal rabies prevention recommendations in the United States were adjusted to this reality, and a national oral rabies vaccination program targeted to free-ranging carnivores was launched to contain the spread of wildlife rabies.[257] Oral rabies vaccination programs for wildlife have increased in recent times, by using baits containing a vaccinia-rabies recombinant vaccine and, more recently, an adenovirus-rabies recombinant vaccine.[91] Although progress in the development of tools to control carnivore rabies was notable in the beginning of the 21st century, little progress has occurred regarding rabies transmitted by bats. This is because of an extensive global biodiversity of bats, and as such, these mammals and the rabies viruses circulating within those populations represent a new frontier for rabies management.[17,71,218]

Besides basic approaches focused on animals, advancement of human rabies biologics was also notable in the late 20th century. Both human rabies immune globulin (RIG) and rabies cell culture vaccines, to replace older nerve tissue vaccines (NTVs), were made available.[28,311] These more modern rabies biologics became the standard in many developing countries.[31,241] Historical NTVs are not recommended by health authorities and are in the process of being phased out worldwide. A few remaining countries in Africa and Asia, however, still permit their use.[56] Social determinants underlying basic health disparities, such as poverty, limited education, and geographic isolation, became relevant factors for more innovative strategies to control and prevent rabies at the local community level.[250] A global strategy for a transdisciplinary response to rabies is required, given increased movements of disenfranchised populations, illegal hunting and trade of animals, and overnight travel. In this regard, new stakeholders and partners were created in the 21st century.[211] These global academic, industrial, and nongovernmental organizations (NGOs) coordinate efforts for advocacy, education, awareness, and joint human and animal campaigns for improved disease prevention and control in the world. Coordinated efforts with leading rabies research groups, international philanthropic institutions, and global health agencies, such as the United Nations Food and Agriculture Organization, World Organization for Animal Health, Pan American Health Organization, World Health Organization (WHO), and many others have had a major impact.[179] For example, the first global rabies campaign was held in 2007, by recognizing World Rabies Day, and September 28 was established officially as a date for rabies outreach. Currently, more than 150 countries participate annually in World Rabies Day activities. Another important underlying element for global rabies mitigation in the 21st century was the adoption of a One Health approach, fostering collaborative work among animal, environmental, and human health sectors to accomplish management of zoonotic diseases. Such a basic strategy is a current mainframe for integrated public health actions, especially concentrated on diseases of nature.[154]

ETIOLOGY

As fundamental hosts, all mammals are believed to be susceptible to infection with the viruses that cause rabies. In fact, rabies virus proper (RABV) is only one of several related viruses that cause the disease.

The gross morphologic characteristics and biochemical composition of the etiologic agents of rabies place them within the family Rhabdoviridae, genus *Lyssavirus.* These viruses, however, share antigenic and genetic relationships that set them apart from other rhabdoviruses. They can be distinguished by fluorescent antibody and complement-fixation tests, reactions with monoclonal antibodies, and, importantly, sequencing studies.

The *Lyssavirus* genus contains at least 14 viruses recognized by the International Committee for the Taxonomy of Viruses (ICTV), and all of them cause rabies. The 14 species include RABV as the type species, Aravan virus, Australian bat lyssavirus (ABLV), Bokeloh bat virus, Duvenhage virus (DUV), European bat lyssavirus (EBLV, types 1 and 2), Ikoma virus (IKOV), Irkut virus (IRKV), Khujand virus, Lagos bat virus (LBV), Mokola virus (MOKV), Shimoni bat virus (SHIBV), and West Caucasian bat virus (WCBV).[39,148,169,170,188,242] Fig. 184.1 shows the known lyssaviruses and the three phylogenetic groups in which they are classified.[17] The lyssaviruses are antigenically variable, with IKOV, LBV, MOKV, SHIBV, and WCBV being the most distant from RABV.[136] Additionally, many more lyssaviruses will be discovered in the near future as scientists conduct pathogen discovery, especially in poorly studied animal populations. Besides RABV, cases of human disease have been described with ABLV,[101] DUV,[286] EBLV,[100] IRKV[29] and MOKV lyssaviruses.[87]

Electron microscopic studies reveal that these viruses are rod or bullet shaped. Viruses typically mature at cytoplasmic plasma membranes and intracellular membranes of the endoplasmic reticulum in infected cultured cells (Fig. 184.2).[137] Standard virions are approximately 75 nm in diameter and 160 to 180 nm in length. Regular arrays of standard-size virions maturing from plasma membranes are observed in infected salivary glands. Budding of virus from plasma membranes is much less pronounced in neurons of the CNS than in cell culture or salivary gland cells. However, meticulous electron microscopic examination of

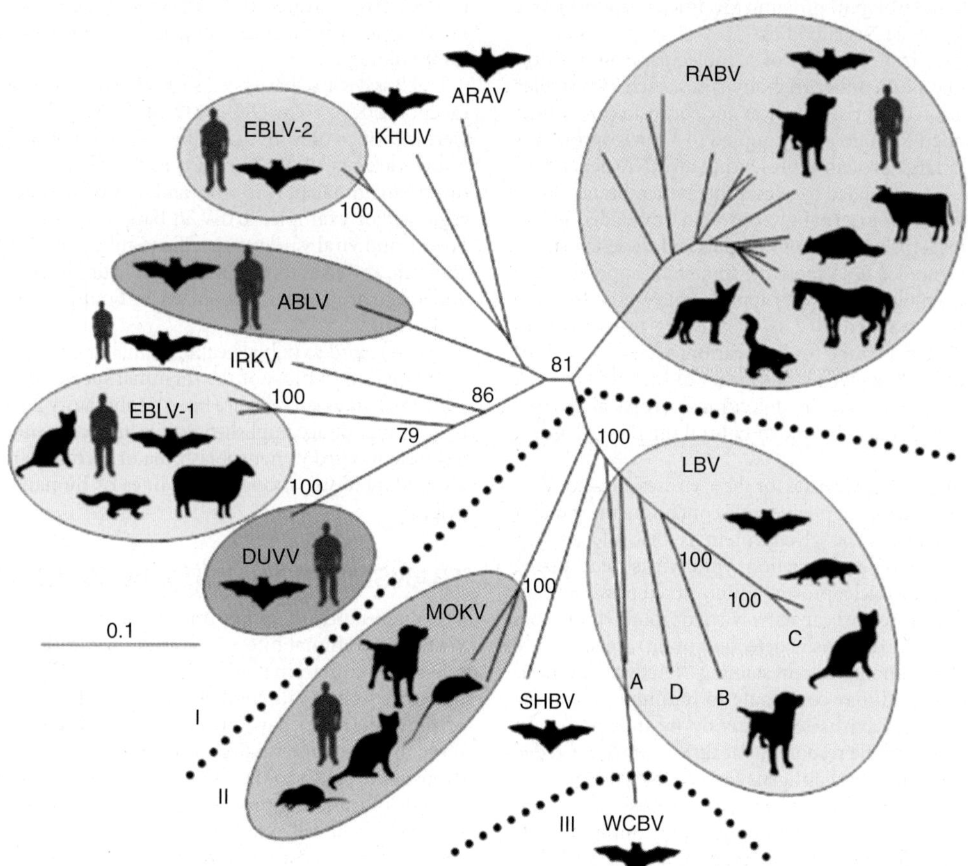

FIG. 184.1 Phylogenetic analysis of characterized *Lyssavirus* isolates based on 405 nucleotides of the nucleoprotein, grouped by phylogenetic groups I, II, and III and indicating main hosts and reservoirs identified. *ABLV,* Australian bat lyssavirus; *ARAV,* Aravan virus; *DUVV,* Duvenhage virus; *EBLV,* European bat lyssavirus; *IRKV,* Irkut virus; *KHUV,* Khujand virus; *LBV,* Lagos bat virus; *MOKV,* Mokola virus; *RABV,* rabies virus; *SHBV,* Shimoni bat virus; *WCBV,* West Caucasian bat virus. (From Banyard AC, Hayman D, Johnson N, et al. Bats and lyssaviruses. Adv Virus Res 2011;79:239–289. Available at: http://dx.doi.org/10.1016/B978-0-12-387040-7.00012-3.)

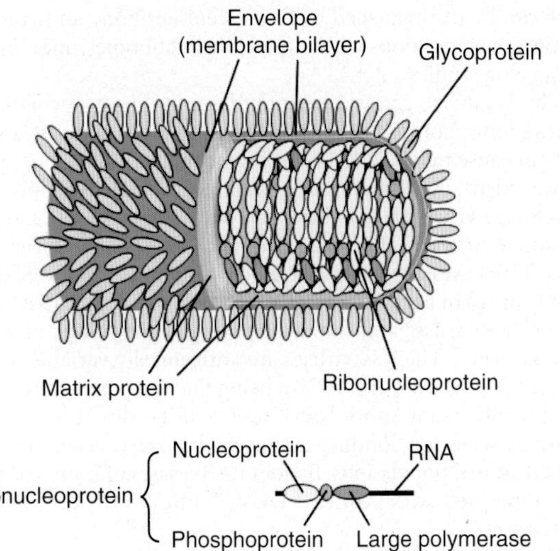

FIG. 184.2 **Structural diagram of a *Lyssavirus*.** (From Orciari LA, Rupprecht CE. Rabies. In Versalovic J, Carroll KC, Funke G, et al, editors. *Manual of clinical microbiology,* 10th ed. Washington, DC: ASM Press; 2011:1470–1478.)

experimentally and naturally infected tissues has revealed that budding from membranes of perikarya and dendrites, as well as the presence of virus in intracellular spaces of brain (especially at synaptic junctions), occurs regularly.[139] In addition, CNS neurons often exhibit both typical and bizarre morphologic forms of virus maturing in the cytoplasm. Cytoplasmic forms often develop in proximity to nucleocapsid matrix inclusions forming the classic Negri bodies.[190]

The basic *Lyssavirus* virion consists of a molecular composition somewhat similar to that of the other rhabdoviruses, such as vesicular stomatitis virus. The virion comprises a helical nucleocapsid core, which contains a single-stranded RNA genome coupled to a nucleoprotein, a phosphoprotein, and a large protein representing an RNA-dependent polymerase.[60] This core is surrounded by a lipoprotein membrane, which contains a matrix protein, an external glycoprotein embedded in the envelope, and several lipids (primarily phospholipids and cholesterol).[27,261] The genome is a single-stranded RNA molecule containing approximately 11,932 nucleotides with a molecular mass of approximately 4.0×10^6 Da.[23] The genome is negative stranded; that is, it must be transcribed to produce messenger RNA necessary for replication. Defective virions containing characteristic (for a given strain) sizes of incomplete RNA molecules have been demonstrated in cell culture–propagated virus populations, but their occurrence or role in natural infections has not been determined.

Important surface antigenic properties for these viruses are associated primarily with the glycoprotein,[261] a polypeptide containing three major oligosaccharide side chains.[72] The glycoprotein is the sole antigen responsible for induction of and reaction with virus-neutralizing antibodies. Antibodies to the nucleoprotein administered passively have no virus-neutralizing or protective capacity. Nucleoprotein antibodies are essential, however, for the diagnostic detection of intracellular viral antigens in the CNS by immunofluorescent staining.[314] Active immunization with rabies nucleocapsid may contribute to immune protection, especially to heterotropic lyssaviruses, apparently by induction of a *Lyssavirus*-specific T-cell immune response, but further work is needed to appreciate the role of other viral antigens for prophylaxis.[40,78]

Historically, viral specificity can be recognized on the basis of genomic sequence analysis[280] and differentiation by monoclonal antibodies. By these means, animal-specific variants and geographic distribution of viruses can be discerned, and isolates from human cases can be traced to the animal and place of origin.[260] Researchers have suggested that lyssaviruses, like several other RNA virus populations, may exist as a quasispecies. The presence of such viral subpopulations may permit rapid adaptation to new hosts.[160,202]

Antigenic differences between both strains of classic laboratory-fixed virus strains and variants of different field isolates of diverse origin have been detected with the use of monoclonal antibodies[316] directed against viral antigens, including the glycoprotein and nucleoprotein.[77] The use of monoclonal antibodies allowed rapid distinction of RABV from the other rabies-related lyssaviruses.[238] Studies with monoclonal antibodies have revealed that, worldwide, clustering of certain RABV antigenic subtypes is geographic and may be species specific.[225] Many genetic groups of RABV with relatively specific geographic localizations exist.[32,260] Within those areas, the viruses may be transmitted by different species, such as dogs or foxes. In the United States, readily distinguishable subtypes of RABV have been determined to circulate in each of the major mammalian reservoir species (primarily skunks and raccoons) and in bats.[26] In all well-studied rabies enzootic areas, researchers have determined that rabies circulates predominantly in a limited number of mammalian species characteristic of that area, and a major antigenic phenotype is characteristic of that transmission cycle.[77] However, distinct bat-adapted RABV may circulate independently in these areas or in areas where other animals (e.g., dogs) are free of rabies. Different geographic subtypes of RABV share varying proportions of the immunologically important glycoprotein epitopes with the vaccine strains of virus. Those RABV subtypes isolated from human cases in the United States have been shown to differ from vaccine strain viruses in their antigenic composition.[316] Despite intense investigation, however, no evidence supports the contention that cross protection between the RABV vaccine and antigenically distinguishable wild-type viruses is reduced to a degree justifying inclusion of new RABV strains in human vaccines. Physicians should have every reason to believe that present vaccines protect against all classic RABV and other members of the phylogenetic group I, provided the vaccine is sufficiently potent. The same degree of cross reactivity does not exist for the other lyssaviruses in phylogenetic groups II and III. Studies using virtual tridimensional models demonstrated that antigenic distances among the known lyssaviruses are the basis for antigenic variation and unequal response to rabies biologics.[136]

All lyssaviruses have been suspected or associated with bat reservoirs, except MOKV.[245] The DUV, IKOV, LBV, MOKV, and SHIBV lyssaviruses were identified only in Africa; the WCBV was isolated in Eurasia only.[84,299] Many variants of RABV exist, and such variants are adaptations to diverse mammalian reservoirs and may be specific to certain geographic regions. For example, RABV in bats is widely distributed in the New World, and viral variants specific to different bat species exist in North America, as well as to vampire bats in Latin America, and to insectivorous and frugivorous bats recognized in South America, such as in Chile and Brazil.[26,102,221,242,252]

With regard to public health, animal rabies reports include laboratory confirmation in most of the mammal species in contact with humans, with an obvious surveillance bias.[242] Laboratory isolation and propagation of virus may be accomplished readily in mice or other standard laboratory animals; in vitro in neuroblastoma or certain hamster cell cultures; or, after adaptation, in certain cell lines of human or other mammalian origin.[215]

TRANSMISSION AND EPIDEMIOLOGY

The main mode of rabies transmission is through inoculation of the virus by an animal bite. Once an injury to the skin occurs, infectious saliva may contaminate the wound. Thus, the virus may gain access to nerves as well as muscle tissue. Unlike skin, mucous membranes (e.g., of the eyes, nose) have no protective epithelial barrier and therefore serve as other potential entry points for the virus, such as a splash exposure of saliva to the mouth. A rabid animal's saliva contains virus capable of initiating productive infections. Importantly, however, viral shedding in the saliva can occur for several days before the classic clinical signs occur in most animals.[93,204] This makes capture and observation of the biting domestic animal very important; otherwise, a default pathway assuming an RABV exposure typically ensues. Animal scratches may become contaminated with saliva during an exposure and therefore are managed in the same way as bites.[79]

Other secretions from rabid animals, such as urine, feces, and milk, are considered at low or no risk for viral transmission[43]; however, exposure to those secretions can potentially allow transmission of other diseases.[187]

Consuming the meat of rabid animals is not recommended; however, in the developing world, rabid animals, especially livestock, may be killed and eaten, even animals with the onset of neurologic signs. Although eating cooked meat of a rabid animal is not considered a risk for viral transmission, the people handling the carcasses and in contact with the head, saliva, brains, nervous tissues, and other organs may be exposed.[293]

In very rare circumstances under special conditions, infection may occur by inhalation of virus. Experimental studies with animals left exposed in caves heavily colonized with bats indicate that this form of transmission is possible.[66] In contrast, bat "fly by" exposures are not considered exposures to rabies. Concentrated virus aerosols produced in the laboratory setting have caused human rabies cases.[149] Optimum biosafety practices and equipment will prevent this kind of exposure. Finally, transmission of rabies has occurred from human to human by corneal and other tissue transplants.[46,137,186,263,291] Because human rabies in the United States and Europe is very rare, occasionally a case will be missed, and screening may neglect the possibility of death from rabies. There are a number of well-known rabies cases transmitted by corneal transplant from fatal cases of undiagnosed encephalitis.[137,263] Several other human rabies cases caused by organs transplanted from donors with unrecognized rabies encephalitis have also occurred, thus raising concerns about proper diagnostics available for viral encephalitis in the modern health care setting.[186,263,291]

Domestic animals constitute the largest sources of human exposure in most parts of the world. Dogs are the primary reservoirs and vectors in Asian countries, such as India, Indonesia, China, and the Philippines. Cats are a distant second in terms of RABV transmission. The magnitude of the rabies problem is illustrated by the observation that approximately 12,000 to 20,000 deaths are attributed to rabies annually in India alone,[310] and as many as 50,000 to 100,000 deaths occur each year throughout the world.[162] The incidence of rabies deaths in India of 2 to 4 in 100,000 population may be exceeded only by that of Ethiopia, where the rate may approximate 18 in 100,000.[122] The total number of people given postexposure prophylaxis (PEP) is estimated to exceed 12 million or more annually. In contrast, many areas, including Japan, Singapore, many parts of the Caribbean, New Zealand, Pacific Oceania, and others, are considered "rabies free."[16,30] China has averaged about 1500 human cases per year, but in at least 1 year there were more than 3000 cases. Dogs were by far the most important sources of human rabies.[262]

The veterinary challenge has always been to vaccinate the local dog population adequately, a measure that would essentially resolve the majority of the problem in these developing countries. Given the severely constrained resources in some areas and the lack of adequate infrastructure, a cycle of neglect continues.

Indeed, the burden to people is directly related to the perpetuation of the disease in local animal populations. For example, in a single year of an urban epizootic of dog rabies in one city in Mexico, an estimated 2.5% of the human population received dog bites, and 2.7% were given rabies PEP.[85] In Africa, the dog still is the most important reservoir and vector, although in the southern portion of the continent, jackals and mongooses also are common sources of viral exposures.[22,62,155,331,332] In much of Africa, the incidence of rabies in humans and dogs has increased in recent years because of social and political disruptions.[310,311] Hence, rabies is a significant tropical disease. Resources directed toward vaccinating dogs against rabies would follow a One Health paradigm and yield great dividends to animals and humans alike.[211]

Rabies in Central and South America is related predominantly to dogs, but vampire bats also have considerable importance.[147] Although humans sometimes are bitten, they are also exposed to rabid cattle infected by these bats. Fortunately, despite these relatively common exposures, viral transmission from livestock to humans is an extremely rare event.[69]

In the United States and Canada, foxes and skunks once were the primary rabid wild animals that most commonly attacked humans. In more recent years, the raccoon has replaced these carnivores as the most important potential source of infection. The reason is because of an outbreak of rabies in these animals stemming from the introduction of infected animals into the mid-Atlantic states from Florida and southeastern Georgia. Subsequently, a rapid expansion of raccoon rabies moved northward and southward in North America, in a range now continuous from Canada to Florida and west to Ohio.[44,80] This massive spread of raccoon rabies continues to incur large costs in human prevention related to PEP, domestic animal care, and efforts at wildlife control. Fortunately, human cases of rabies attributable to raccoons have remained very rare.[35,45,200,291]

The significance of bats to rabies epidemiology varies globally. In the United States, bats serve as a reservoir in every state except Hawaii. Bats are responsible for a high proportion of all North American cases, including those in persons with no antecedent history of animal bite.[24] For example, between 2003 and 2015, an average of three human rabies cases occurred per year,[200] of which almost three-fourths were bat RABV variants, discounting imported and transplant cases. A review from 1990 to 2005 showed that more than 90% of domestic cases (42 of 45 cases, excluding four transplant-transmitted infections)[263] were caused by bat RABV, predominantly from the silver-haired *(Lasionycteris noctivagans)* and eastern tricolored bats *(Perimyotis subflavus)*.[24,90,187]

Viruses isolated from silver-haired bats may be better able to grow in non-neuronal cells, and although prophylactic vaccination is effective when exposure is recognized, the infectiousness of these viruses apparently appears high.[202] In Colorado, 15% of laboratory-tested bats were found rabid.[215] The most recent national data from the Centers for Disease Control and Prevention (CDC) indicate that approximately 6% of submitted bats were rabid from biased surveillance of ill animals and those in contact with humans.[200] As with other animals, clinical signs may not be apparent immediately, even though the animal is infected.[231] However, certain behaviors raise suspicion, and bats found paralyzed on the ground have a high likelihood of being rabid, compared with healthy, wild-caught individuals, in which the prevalence is typically much less than a fraction of 1%.[65] Problems regarding human exposure to bats that are potentially rabid may arise. In particular, a child sleeping in a room may not be able to report a scratch or a bite, and there may be little physical evidence of such an exposure.[166,297] Ideally, capture of the bat with laboratory analysis of the brain would help guide therapeutic decisions. Vaccination may be indicated if the bat is confirmed to be rabid. Finally, decisions may favor vaccination if a bat entered a room but escaped, and there is a reasonable probability of bite exposure. In Europe, bats have been responsible for transmission of other rabies-related lyssaviruses.[100] Despite the rarity of such an event, bats and vampirism were linked inextricably in legend with Dracula, the 15th-century despot who lived in current-day Romania.[124] In contrast, true vampire bats (subfamily Desmodontinae) in Central and South America are responsible for considerable losses of domestic animals and for human rabies cases.[147,178]

On average, about two to three cases of human rabies are reported in the United States each year, but thousands of animals are diagnosed as rabid by laboratory analysis. All reservoirs are within wildlife hosts, with spillover infection to other mammals. The distribution of infection among animals is shown in Table 184.1.[24,200] The cat continues to be a more important host of domestic rabies than the dog in the United States. In Puerto Rico, the mongoose is the major reservoir, and almost all the mongooses that bite people may be expected to be rabid.[209]

True canine RABV transmission has been eliminated in the United States. The most recent data from the CDC reports that only 59 dogs were found rabid in 2014, in contrast to the thousands of rabid dogs during the 1940s. True vaccine failure is rare. Of those rabid dogs for which immunization records were available, none had been immunized or had proper immunization.[200] Interestingly, the RABV variants found in dogs were largely from skunk variants ($n = 17$), with raccoon rabies second ($n = 7$); however, the majority of rabies variants were not typed ($n = 33$). Thus, public health authorities advocate RABV variant testing for all dogs as surveillance against reintroduction of canine rabies by imported dogs.

Vaccination has reduced the overall prevalence of rabies in cats in the United States, yet these animals remain the most common rabid domestic animal, comprising almost two-thirds of the total.[200] Although only about one-fourth of the rabid cats had RABV variant typing, data showed that primarily skunk (59%) and raccoon variants (40%) were implicated. Clearly, more public health emphasis on immunizing cats is needed.

TABLE 184.1 Cases of Animal Rabies in the United States, 2014, and 5-Year Average

Animal	Number	Percent	Number 2009–2013	Percent 2009–2013
Wild				
Raccoons	1822	30	2101	34
Skunks	1588	26	1536	25
Bats	1756	29	1547	25
Foxes	311	5	409	7
Rodents/lagomorphs	45	<1	NA	NA
Other	66	1	NA	NA
Total	5588	93	5717	92
Domestic				
Cats	272	5	283	5
Dogs	59	<1	79	1
Cattle	78	1	82	1
Horses/mules	25	<1	40	<1
Sheep/goats	10	<1	10	<1
Swine	0	0	NA	NA
Other	1	<1	NA	NA
Total	445	7	6213	8

NA, Not available.
From Monroe BP, Yager P, Blanton J, et al. Rabies surveillance in the United States during 2014. *J Am Vet Med Assoc.* 2016;248(7):777–788.

Wildlife rabies continues to be a major concern, with more than 6000 rabies-positive animals reported during 2014. Most rabid animals were raccoons (30%), bats (29%), and skunks (26%). Table 184.1 summarizes the data for wildlife in more detail.

Rabies host shifts were recognized during the last decade for multiple species. Virologists refer to this as spillover, as a virus from one primary reservoir that may transmit to other species of animals. This transmission could be a dead end (as in humans) or may allow for adaptation, differentiation, and circulation of the virus in a new reservoir. Thus, a host shift could occur, as described in Arizona where rabies virus jumped species from bats to foxes and skunks.[171] This important phenomenon highlights the potential dangers of uncontrolled wildlife rabies and supports the need for continued surveillance and research. For example, there could be significant public health and veterinary impacts should a new rabies outbreak occur.

PATHOGENESIS

The initial stages of RABV and other lyssavirus infection are perhaps the least understood. Disease certainly depends on the entry of the virus into peripheral nerves, after which centripetal spread occurs rapidly toward the CNS. Replication of virus in muscle cells at a peripheral inoculation site has been demonstrated experimentally, and the virus has been suggested to persist in myocytes for many days after inoculation,[52] but this has not been proven to occur in nonexperimental situations.[53,207] Nonetheless, replication at a low level in myocytes, followed by subsequent infection of nerve cells, would help to explain the occasionally extended incubation periods of disease. Entry of virus into the peripheral nerve endings is mediated by attachment to various receptors, such as the nicotinic acetylcholine receptor (nAChR) and other ganglioside receptors, such as neural cell adhesion molecule (NCAM or CD56).[172,253] Once the virus is in nervous tissue, spread can occur by cell-to-cell contact.[51,281] In any case, virus is thought to enter peripheral nerves at an extremely variable time after exposure, presumably at the site of neuromuscular or neurotendinal spindles, at motor end plates, or (in the case of aerosol exposure) at olfactory end organs.[208] Viremia is of no known importance in the dissemination of infection.

Historically, amputation or cauterization of the bite site was used as a means of intervention even before pathobiologic insights. More recently, the finding that virus transits along nervous pathways has been demonstrated directly by repeated experimental observations, such that the progress of infection may be interrupted by surgical excision or chemical destruction of nerves at sites distal to the inoculation site.[12] Central progression of virus along neuronal pathways has been demonstrated by electron microscopic, immunofluorescent, and serial infectivity studies. Virus appears to be sequestered within neuronal cells during transmission (by axoplasmic flow) through peripheral nerves, and the virus can therefore be used experimentally to trace synaptic circuits.[156] Intra-axonal retrograde transport appears to be aided by interaction of the viral phosphoprotein (P protein) with the cytoplasmic protein dynein light chains.[143,230] Minimal numbers of virions are observed within neurons, and connective tissue elements of nerve sheaths are not involved. Given viral tropic stealth, little maturation or release of virus from nerve plasma membranes occurs during transit, and scant or no virus is presented to the immune system. This feature explains in part the absence of detectable humoral antibody until late in the disease that is characteristic of even prolonged incubation periods with rabies. Nonetheless, neutralizing antibody may enter the neuronal cytosol by endocytosis and block viral transcription.[76] One study described an immunoevasive strategy triggered by RABV to infect the CNS. Moreover, LGP2, a protein that regulates retinoic acid–inducible gene I (RIG-I), mediates immune responses and reacts with negative immune signals in the presence of negative-stranded RNA viruses, thereby preventing the elimination of T cells infiltrated by virus.[55]

Entry from the periphery to brain occurs through the spinal cord or cranial nerves. Early selective infection of the limbic system in the brain may cause disease characterized by extreme excitability and agitation (furious rabies), whereas the encephalitic depressive symptoms are associated with early, widespread infection in the brain.[198] In either case, infection rapidly spreads to affect nearly all brain neurons within a few days of the onset of brain entry and acute CNS symptoms. Brain infection leads rapidly to death by respiratory or cardiac failure. Fatal cases of encephalitis reveal little damage of neuronal cells, despite the ubiquitous neuronal infection.[104] Alternatively, persons kept alive by vigorous supportive therapy for lengthy periods after onset of disease may develop severe histopathologic encephalitic lesions. Studies in mice have shown that apoptotic mechanisms may be induced by laboratory strains of RABV,[141,284] but other virulent street RABV variants induce little if any apoptosis by expressing less G protein in neurons.[203] RABV G protein expression may contribute to pathogenesis by downregulating apoptosis.[203] Although ascending infection is specific to neurons, once the CNS is infected, virus spreads centrifugally to peripheral nerve plexuses, the salivary glands, muscle fibers, hair follicles, and other innervated sites.[142]

The entire manner of progression of the infecting virus, particularly those points in its transit vulnerable to immune intervention, remains to be fully determined. Clearly, preexisting humoral antibody protects by inactivating virus before it gains entry into the nervous system. After an RABV-naïve person is exposed to RABV, disease can be delayed or prevented by passive antibody, interferon (IFN) treatment, or both,[146] but protection becomes efficient only when active immunization with potent vaccine accompanies such PEP.

The presence of neutralizing antibodies after exposure but before illness is a key facet of protection against rabies. However, studies have demonstrated the complexity of the immune response after infection.[103,210] Although some experimental evidence argues for the importance of cytotoxic T lymphocytes in protection against rabies, Hooper and colleagues[134] infected mice that were unable to mount a cellular response and found no difference in disease with respect to normal mice. Nonetheless, early inflammatory responses, as well as rapid production of antibody, correlated with recovery from rabies. Thus, IFN and other mediators may supplement antibody in the prevention of disease. Interestingly, virus-specific cytotoxic T lymphocytes do not usually develop during infection, and street RABV may act as an immunosuppressor. Moreover, chemical immunosuppression enhances the development of experimental rabies. IFN[13] and interleukin-2,[213] both important immunomodulators produced by cells, enhance protection against rabies. More sophisticated understanding of rabies pathogenesis is required before ideal combinations of immunotherapeutic procedures, possibly including IFN, can be applied.

The reverse side of the infection-immunity coin is reflected by the "early death" phenomenon, in which exposed animals or humans develop earlier onset of rabies if previously they received incomplete immunization. Sugamata and associates[267] demonstrated that early death depends on the presence of T cells, a finding indicating that it is mediated by an immunopathologic cellular response. In addition, some investigators have argued that cytotoxic T lymphocytes actually may contribute to rabies neuritic paralysis.[267,309]

CLINICAL MANIFESTATIONS

Animal Rabies

Rabies encephalitis in animals is expressed as either a paralytic (dumb) or encephalitic (furious) syndrome. Typical infections are characterized by behavioral changes and a rapid clinical course leading to paralysis, coma, and death. Rarely encephalitis can be nonfatal, and the animal recovers.[10] Because literally millions of animal bites of humans occur annually in the United States, the identification of aberrant behavior and whether animal attacks can be considered provoked or unprovoked are critical factors in many decisions to administer prophylaxis against rabies.[113]

The prodromal stage of disease is marked by nonspecific signs, such as restlessness and malaise. Subsequently, placid dogs, cats, cattle, or horses may become vicious. Wild animals may lose their fear of humans and of periurban areas. Thus, rabid foxes, normally nocturnal, may be seen wandering aimlessly in the daylight. Similarly, rabid bats often have been encountered flying oddly in daytime hours. Early behavioral changes are not accompanied by paralysis.

The clinical course progresses rapidly to either dumb or furious disease. Dumb rabies typically is a depressed ascending neurologic type disease. In addition to lethargy, selectively severe paralysis of throat muscles may be observed, which causes drooling of saliva because of difficulty in swallowing. Hydrophobia is not noted in animals. Furious rabies is characterized by an unusual state of alertness in which any visual or sound stimulation may incite an attack. Animals may roam, indiscriminately biting at inanimate objects. Caged animals have been observed biting furiously at traps without obvious pain. Companion animals, such as dogs and cats, may exhibit unusually affectionate and playful behavior and then suddenly bite those playing with them. Very aggressive biting behavior may occur in herbivores such as horses, mules, and cattle, which may produce outright fatal injuries.

Both dumb rabies and furious rabies have a rapid clinical course in domestic and wild animals. The period between onset of prodromal signs and death caused by respiratory paralysis rarely exceeds 7 to 10 days.[274] Although 10 days usually is given as the limit of virus excretion in the saliva of dogs before death supervenes, rare exceptions involving longer excretion have been reported experimentally and in animals observed in both Africa and Asia.[92,287]

The diagnosis of rabies in an animal depends on the demonstration of postmortem viral antigens in the brain by fluorescent antibody tests or of viral RNA by reverse transcriptase polymerase chain reaction (RT-PCR) followed by sequencing.

Management of Animal Rabies

Aside from the historical ineffective large-scale removal of potentially rabid animal species, such as community dogs, most modern control methods focus on the induction of herd immunity by vaccination. In domestic animals, immunization is accomplished readily by a variety of veterinary vaccines, although boosters must be given annually or after other stated intervals, depending on the product.[35]

In wild animals, primarily raccoons in the United States and foxes in Europe, oral vaccination with baits containing recombinant-vectored RABV glycoprotein or attenuated live virus has been successful,[80,217] with the more recent addition of a rabies-adenovirus recombinant vaccine.[133,257,279]

Human Rabies

The incubation period in human rabies has been observed to be quite variable. Most cases develop within 3 weeks to 3 months following an exposure (20–90 days). About 14% of cases occurred after 1 year in a large case series of patients with rabies.[79] Some well-documented cases have occurred as long as 6 to 8 years after the bite.[26,296] The longer incubation times, reputed even up to 27 years, may result from unrecognized exposures.[79] In contrast, the shortest incubation periods reported range from 4 to 7 days. These cases may occur with direct viral inoculation into the brain, such as a dog bite puncturing a child's skull.

Incubation periods are longer after bites on the legs than after bites on the face. The reason for this appears to be related not to the length of the nerve that the virus must traverse, because it travels rapidly even from the farthest site, but to the extent of innervation of different parts of the body. Bites on the tips of the fingers or on the genitalia have relatively short incubation periods for this reason. Children in general tend to have shorter incubation periods than adults.

Hemachudha[126] published a comprehensive review of human rabies. The first symptoms of rabies usually are vague and insidious. The patient simply may feel unwell or have anxiety or depression. Some fever or nausea may be present. A striking prodromal symptom is itching, pain, or tingling at the site of the bite. This paresthesia is not present always and may take various forms, but its localization is a definite harbinger of rabies. The prodrome lasts 2 to 10 days, when the acute neurologic phase begins. The symptoms of this second phase are divided into furious versus paralytic rabies, with most cases being in the furious category. The signs and symptoms as reported from human rabies cases in the literature over the last 50 years (1958–2011) are listed in Table 184.2.

In furious rabies, the emphasis is on agitation, hyperactivity, fluctuating consciousness, bizarre behavior, and perhaps nuchal rigidity. Sore throat and hypersalivation are prominent complaints, and laryngospasm may cause hoarseness. A high percentage of human cases exhibit hydrophobia.[224] In fact, in many clinical settings where advanced diagnostics are lacking, the presence of a dog bite history and the sign of hydrophobia are considered sufficient to make the diagnosis.[312] The disease of rabies itself, in older literature, was sometimes referred to as "hydrophobe." Such a dramatic presentation is a startling sign and is considered pathognomonic of furious rabies. Initial attempts to swallow liquid result in painful spasms of the pharyngeal and laryngeal muscles, with aspiration into the trachea. A conditioned response appears to be created, in which fear exacerbates the actual spasms. Warrell and associates[302] hypothesized that brainstem encephalitis leads to destruction of inhibitors of inspiratory motor neurons. Respiratory tract instant reflexes are exaggerated, leading to inspiratory spasms. Hydrophobia has an important psychological element. At times, the sound of rushing water or the sight of water can induce the terrible reaction.[305] Interestingly, hydrophobia has been reported in only about one-third of the human cases in the United States,[220] and with even less frequency among children affected with a vampire bat rabies variant (Table 184.3). Whether this may have to do with the infecting virus variant (bat vs. dog rabies)[285] or clinical familiarity with rabies remains unknown. Also frequently present is aerophobia, in which spasms occur when a current of air is fanned across the face. Priapism, spontaneous ejaculation, and increased libido also have been reported.

The neurologic examination findings in rabies are not uniform. In fact, virtually any neurologic finding can occur. Meningismus is somewhat common. Cranial nerve abnormalities can be seen, especially paralysis of the palate and vocal cords. Deep tendon reflexes may vary from hyperactive to absent, and involuntary movements are prominent.[79,285,305] Table 184.2 also examines clinical differences in dog-associated versus bat-associated cases. Patients with dog-acquired cases tended to have greater incidence of hydrophobia, aerophobia, and encephalopathy. Patients with bat-acquired cases, in contrast, exhibited more cranial nerve abnormalities and motor and sensory symptoms. These data certainly have limitations related to the heterogeneity of reporting, including the lack of detailed assessments and nonstandardization. These differences could, however, relate to viral pathogenicity, viral tropism, route of inoculation, or other factors that are worthy of further study.[285]

A distinct pattern of neurologic involvement is shown by approximately 20% to 30% of patients with rabies, particularly those bitten by vampire bats. Flaccid paralysis may start in the limb that was bitten originally and spread to other limbs. The cranial nerves become involved, and the face, rather than showing agitation, becomes expressionless.

TABLE 184.2 Select Clinical Aspects of Human Rabies: Dog vs. Bat Cases, A Review From the Published Literature, 1958–2011[a]

Clinical Feature Rabies Specific	Naturally Acquired N (%)	Dog Acquired N (%)	Bat Acquired N (%)	Dog vs. Bat Difference
Headache	31 (100)	12 (100)	12 (100)	0
Malaise	80 (100)	29 (100)	36 (100)	0
Hallucinations	23 (100)	8 (100)	13 (100)	0
Sore throat	33 (100)	9 (100)	17 (100)	0
Slurred speech	14 (100)	2 (100)	8 (100)	0
Late-onset encephalopathy	19 (100)	6 (100)	10 (100)	0
Hyperarousal	74 (98.6)	28 (100)	37 (97.3)	2.7
Fever	84 (97.6)	32 (96.9)	39 (97.4)	−0.6
Larynx or facial spasms	13 (92.3)	6 (83.3)	5 (100)	−16.7
Meningismus	10 (80)	3 (66.7)	3 (66.7)	0
Hydrophobia	53 (77.4)	27 (81.5)	18 (72.2)	9.3
Aerophobia	22 (72.7)	15 (80)	6 (50)	30
Encephalopathy	106 (50.9)	42 (64.3)	52 (46.2)	18.1
Bite Site				
Any local sensory symptoms	79 (88.6)	29 (79.3)	40 (97.5)	−18.2
Pain	58 (84.5)	21 (71.4)	30 (96.7)	−25.2
Paresthesias	38 (73.7)	15 (60)	18 (88.9)	−28.9
Numbness	34 (67.6)	13 (46.2)	17 (88.2)	−42.1
Other				
Autonomic dysfunction	18 (100)	5 (100)	11 (100)	0
Convulsive seizures	25 (96)	11 (100)	7 (100)	0
Hypersalivation	35 (94.3)	14 (85.7)	18 (100)	−14.3
Motor-Sensory Examination				
Fasciculations	6 (100)	3 (100)	2 (100)	0
Ascending flaccid weakness	49 (71.4)	21 (76.2)	18 (72.2)	4
Dysphagia	65 (90.8)	25 (84)	31 (93.5)	−9.5
Cranial nerve abnormality	37 (67.6)	14 (57.1)	16 (68.8)	−11.6
Abnormal deep tendon reflexes	38 (50)	17 (47.1)	17 (58.8)	−11.8
Late Complications				
Coma	89 (100)	31 (100)	42 (100)	0
Cardiovascular	55 (100)	28 (100)	20 (100)	0
Respiratory	44 (100)	17 (100)	22 (100)	0

[a]Lack of uniform reporting accounted for variance in each characteristic. A positive difference in dog to bat comparisons indicated a higher percentage of cases favored dog-transmitted rabies, whereas a negative value favored bat cases. Naturally acquired cases were those acquired (or presumed acquired) from an animal vector, whereas transplant cases were excluded. Modified from Udow SJ, Marrie RA, Jackson AC. Clinical features of dog- and bat-acquired rabies in humans. *Clin Infect Dis.* 2013;57(5):689–696.

Hydrophobia is not a common feature. Paralytic rabies is confused easily with Guillain-Barré syndrome. Hemachudha and colleagues[130,132] emphasized the importance of fever, intact sensation, urinary incontinence, and percussion myoedema in paralytic rabies.

The cerebrospinal fluid (CSF) is abnormal in a minority of patients, particularly those with clinical meningitis. When abnormal, the CSF shows mild pleocytosis, mainly mononuclear. The peripheral white blood cell count shows increased polymorphonuclear cells.

Magnetic resonance imaging shows involvement of gray matter in the hippocampus, hypothalamus, and brainstem.[128,189] Advanced magnetic resonance imaging techniques such as diffusion-weighted imaging and diffusion tensor imaging can provide finer imaging about microstructural and macrostructural damage from rabies encephalitis.[177] Brain imaging is, of course, only adjunctive because findings maybe absent or otherwise nonspecific.

The acute neurologic phase lasts 2 to 10 days, with eventual deterioration of the patient's mental status into coma. The patient may survive in this state for 2 weeks or more, particularly in dumb rabies. Before the final deterioration, the patient may have alternating periods of wild agitation and alert cooperation. During the alert state, patients may be able to discuss their illnesses and express fear of impending death. However, most often, death rapidly follows onset of coma unless intubation and ventilatory assistance are offered, in which case survival may be prolonged for weeks to even months. During the comatose state, a variety of problems may manifest, including cerebral edema, inappropriate antidiuretic hormone secretion, diabetes insipidus, and other manifestations of hypothalamic dysfunction; hypotension or arrhythmia; and pneumonia. Death caused by rabies in the acute stage occurs because of cardiac or respiratory problems. Cardiac arrhythmias with circulatory collapse commonly occur, and virus may be recovered at autopsy from cardiac tissue that shows pathologic evidence of myocarditis. Respiration becomes increasingly labored, and death may occur during a laryngeal spasm or from aspiration.

However, cases of spontaneous recovery and survival have been documented, thus challenging conventional opinion of absolute rabies mortality.[1,48,49] Additionally, published evidence of survival after bites from rabid vampire bats without clinical rabies among indigenous Amazon communities challenges the paradigm of certain fatality from viral exposures.[109] Survival also has been documented in a small number of individuals who had been vaccinated,[2,41,121,227] as well as in an unvaccinated 15-year-old girl who was treated with coma induction, midazolam, ribavirin, ketamine, and amantadine.[325] The last two drugs may have rabies receptor–blocking ability. This experimental rabies treatment has been termed the Milwaukee Protocol, and its original version has been modified by dropping ribavirin because of its effect delaying immune response, adding tetrahydrobiopterin to cover the deficiency observed in CSF, and including calcium channel blockers to prevent vasospasm.[323] Using the Milwaukee Protocol, a 15-year-old boy survived

TABLE 184.3 Symptoms and Signs Reported in 17 Children From a Vampire Bat Rabies Outbreak: Peru, 2011

Signs, Symptoms, or Factor	Frequency	%
Mean age, y (range)	5.7(1–14)	
Female sex	14	82.3
Fever	17	100
Somnolence	12	70.6
Dysphagia with solids	12	70.6
Dyspnea	11	64.7
Dysphagia with liquids	10	58.8
Headache	10	58.8
Paralysis	9	52.9
Fatigue	9	52.9
Hypersalivation	9	47.1
Sore throat	8	41.2
Abdominal pain	7	41.2
Vomiting	7	41.2
Spasm, chorea, seizures	6	35.3
Anorexia	5	29.4
Cough	5	29.4
Stridor	5	29.4
Hallucinations	5	29.4
Weakness	4	23.5
Muscle pain	4	23.5
Anxiety	3	17.6
Otalgia	3	17.6
Hydrophobia	3	17.6
Gaze palsy	2	11.8
Diarrhea	2	11.8
Photophobia	2	11.8
Back pain	2	11.8
Paresthesia	2	11.8
Arthralgia	2	11.8
Neck pain	2	5.9
Chest pain	1	5.9
Tachycardia	1	5.9
Tachypnea	1	5.9
Aerophobia	1	5.9
Restlessness	1	5.9
Polydipsia	1	5.9
Delirium	1	5.9
Altered sensorium	1	5.9
Priapism	1	5.9

From Dirección General de Epidemiología, Ministerio de Salud del Perú, and US Centers for Disease Control and Prevention. Unpublished data, 2011.

rabies in Recife, Brazil, but this patient received rabies vaccine and developed the disease anyway.[214] Additional attempts for the use of the Milwaukee Protocol were not successful for survival but resulted in extended survival, thus allowing an increased understanding of the complex pathophysiology of rabies, its complications, and viral clearance.[8,138,234,324] Many failures of the Milwaukee Protocol have been recorded, and the requirement for a high level of intensive care and laboratory handling of cases may not be possible to fulfill in small hospitals or health care systems with limited budgets, such as in the developing world, where the greatest impact can be achieved with rabies prevention activities.[140]

DIAGNOSIS

The diagnosis of rabies in humans begins with its discovery in the implicated animal. Hopefully, the animal remains available for testing, and euthanasia with analysis of brain tissue can be undertaken. Traditional testing requires fluorescein-labeled antibody to detect viral antigens. More recently, enzyme-coupled antibodies have been introduced, allowing colored neuronal inclusions to be observed under the light microscope.[180] RABV RNA also can be detected by dot hybridization or by RT-PCR amplification.[152] Virus isolation may be used for confirmation, either through intracerebral inoculation in mice or by inoculation of neuroblastoma cells with subsequent fluorescent antibody staining for viral antigens. When the animal is unavailable for rabies testing, such as if a bat in a room flies away, or the biting dog is never captured, more involved assessments are required. This is particularly true if the clinical presentation leaves any doubts. The classic clinical expression of rabies in humans is made clear with a history of animal bite exposure, paresthesia at the wound site, and hydrophobia. In fact, in developing countries where advanced laboratory testing is not available, the presence of hydrophobia and aerophobia is considered diagnostic of rabies.[79,312] The differential diagnosis includes other viral-borne causes of encephalitis, such as from arboviruses, enteroviruses, and herpes simplex virus (Box 184.1). Occasionally cerebral malaria, acute demyelinating encephalomyelitis (ADEM), or other limbic forms of encephalitis may demonstrate significant clinical overlap.[246] However, further testing, such as isolation of malaria parasites in the blood, or finding a space-occupying lesion on head imaging, should yield an alternative diagnosis.

BOX 184.1 Differential Diagnosis of Rabies

- Viral-borne encephalitis
- Herpes simplex virus (HSV-1)
- Arboviruses (e.g., Eastern equine encephalitis, Western equine encephalitis, West Nile, Japanese encephalitis, California encephalitis, Rift Valley fever)
- Enterovirus: Enterovirus 71
- Cerebral malaria
- Acute disseminated encephalomyelitis (ADEM)
- Limbic encephalitis
- Guillain-Barré syndrome
- Poliomyelitis
- Post–rabies vaccine encephalomyelitis
- Tetanus
- Botulism
- Drugs
  - Direct toxicity: drug-induced psychosis (e.g., phencyclidine [PCP])
  - Drug syndromes: serotonin syndrome, neuroleptic malignant syndrome
  - Drug withdrawal: severe alcohol withdrawal
- Florid mental illness
- Rabies hysteria

Paralytic rabies, conversely, may present special diagnostic challenges. Important differential diagnosis includes Guillain-Barré syndrome, poliomyelitis, or post–rabies vaccine encephalomyelitis. Tetanus is sometimes considered as well, particularly because animal bites and penetrating injuries are tetanus-prone wounds by definition. However, tetanus examination findings, such as sustained muscle spasm and trismus, are not found in rabies.

Botulism (either from a wound or from ingestion) may be more difficult to rule out because drooling may be found with oropharyngeal paralysis, but the absence of sensory changes should exclude rabies. Other important differential considerations include psychosis from drug effects or florid mental illness. In one tragic human case,[88] a 16-year-old boy was tested repeatedly for drugs, and even went to a psychiatric facility, before hydrophobia was noted and the diagnosis of rabies was finally made.

Relatively new research on encephalitis has shed light on some of the specific causes of this disease.[19,106,112] This is important because of clinical overlap with rabies encephalitic symptoms, such as in anti–*N*-methyl-D-aspartate (anti-NMDA) receptor encephalitis. In these

TABLE 184.4 Antemortem Diagnostic Test Results for 62 Human Patients With Rabies: United States, 1960–2010

Test	No. of Patients Positive for Rabies Virus/ Total No. Tested (%)	Earliest Positive (Day of Test Illness)
RT-PCR of saliva for rabies virus RNA	27/32 (84)	2
Brain biopsy for rabies virus antigen	4/6 (67)	7
Nuchal skin biopsy for rabies virus antigen	24/41 (59)	2
Virus isolation from saliva	11/23 (48)	3
Antibody to rabies virus in serum	38/53 (72)	4
Rabies virus antigen in touch impression from cornea	9/19 (47)	2
Antibody to rabies virus in cerebrospinal fluid	17/41 (5)	5

RT-PCR, Reverse transcriptase polymerase chain reaction.
Modified from Petersen B, Rupprecht C. Human rabies epidemiology and diagnosis. In: Tkachev S, ed. *Non-flavivirus Encephalitis.* New York: InTech; 2011.

patients, symptoms include agitation, psychosis, autonomic dysfunction, and other neurologic symptoms. In-depth workup and evaluation are often necessary to identify potential causes. In fact, in up to two-thirds of encephalitis cases in the United States, an underlying cause is never discovered.[19] In the past, postvaccination encephalitis with NTVs was a diagnostic dilemma, yet this is a vanishing disease entity because NTVs are phasing out globally. In addition, rabies hysteria is largely a syndrome of the past, when rabies threats were much more palpable. In this disease, similar to conversion disorder, patients complain of rabies-like symptoms such as hydrophobia, but the examiner's insights supported by normal laboratory testing can eliminate that diagnostic consideration. Thus, the differential diagnosis of encephalitis may include rabies, and the astute clinician needs to remain vigilant for that possibility. Indeed, nearly one-half of rabies cases are diagnosed post mortem,[47] a finding suggesting that cases may be missed every year, even in highly developed countries. Multiple transplant-associated rabies cases[46,137,186,263,291] support such a hypothesis. Thorough history taking, including that from extended family members and friends, careful neurologic examination, and appropriate laboratory analysis (especially of the CSF) are of critical importance, especially in the pediatric patient.

Laboratory diagnosis is possible before death through rabies antemortem rule-out testing. Antemortem rabies diagnosis has increased relevance with the improvement of intensive care and potential new treatment for rabid patients. Such antemortem testing requires a set of four samples: saliva, skin biopsy from the nape of the neck, CSF, and serum.[131] Viral antigens may be demonstrated by fluorescent antibody staining of smears of corneal epithelial cells[163,249] or sections of skin from the neck at the hairline.[36,259] Corneal impressions are not routinely used in the presence of modern diagnostic techniques. These test results become positive once virus migrates down the nerves from the brain because both the cornea and hair follicles are richly innervated.

Serologic diagnosis also can be obtained if the patient survives beyond the acute period. In persons not given PEP, only low levels of antibodies appear.[131,130] In contrast, patients who have received vaccine show a rapid rise in titer of virus-neutralizing antibodies between 6 and 10 days after the onset of symptoms.[119] Such antibodies are detected by an in vitro method, such as the rapid fluorescent focus inhibition test (RFFIT) or historically by mouse neutralization tests. Rabies may be diagnosed in immunized persons by a rise in titer after the onset of clinical symptoms and is suggested by any antibody titer 1:5000 or greater, a level not usually achieved by routine vaccination. High antibody levels in CSF are characteristic late in the course of rabies encephalitis; CSF antibody is not induced efficiently by vaccination.[119,304]

Virus has been isolated from human saliva between days 2 and 24 after onset of disease.[119,220] Virus also may be isolated in some rare cases from CSF or from concentrated urine sediment during the first 2 weeks of illness. In persons surviving longer than 2 weeks, isolation of virus from body tissues or fluids (or from postmortem brain) may be more difficult, presumably because of virus neutralization by humoral antibody.

Postmortem diagnosis can be confirmed by the presence of pathognomonic cytoplasmic inclusions (Negri bodies) in brain tissue, but they are present in fewer than 80% of cases. RABV antigens may be detected by fluorescent antibody examination, with higher frequency in brain tissues of persons dying after a brief, acute course of disease. In postmortem tissues, histochemical staining with monoclonal antibody to viral internal antigens especially may be useful because ribonucleoprotein possesses epitopes resistant to the formalin fixation and the paraffin-embedding process.[194] In studies of paraffin-embedded brain tissues (samples up to 40 years old), digestion of sections with proteinase K followed by immunofluorescence or RT-PCR testing gave 100% (300 of 300) positive results.[295] TaqMan real-time RT PCR is particularly useful.[292]

However, as in the case of virus isolation attempts, identification of viral antigens in brains of persons kept alive for prolonged periods after onset of disease may be extremely difficult.

Petersen and Rupprecht[220] summarized the results of antemortem attempts to diagnose rabies in humans. Their data are summarized in Table 184.4,[220] which shows that RT-PCR analysis of saliva and brain biopsy is the most accurate method of diagnosis; results can be positive as early as the second day after onset. Because of the different times in which antemortem test results can be negative in any of the four required samples (i.e., skin, saliva, serum, and CSF), ruling out of rabies can occur definitively only when all samples taken at the same time test negative. Serial sampling may be required if other etiologic explanations fail.

PROPHYLAXIS

Local Wound Management

Human rabies is virtually 100% preventable after an exposure. The immediate washing of a wound after an animal bite or scratch is a crucial part of PEP. These wounds are contaminated with saliva that contains virus and should be flushed copiously with soap and water, for no less than 10 to 15 minutes. This immediate lavage helps to reduce viral load, thus leading to increased survival after exposure in 50% of patients, and this inexpensive but effective intervention is especially useful in medically underserved health care settings.[153,298] Some investigators suggest an additional local application of povidone-iodine or ethanol. The concentration of ethanol is important: 43% (86 proof) or higher gave the best results.[315]

Experimental data suggest that regardless of the solutions used, thorough irrigation and flushing are important, particularly in deep puncture wounds. Catheters should be inserted into puncture wounds and fluid instilled by means of an attached syringe.[67,256] If this procedure proves to be too painful, the area may be anesthetized safely with local procaine-type anesthetic agents.[153,315] Suturing should be done only in line with good surgical practice and limited as much as possible to minimize the opportunity for driving virus deeper into surrounding tissues.[322]

Passive Immunity

The administration of rabies immune globulin (RIG) is an essential component of PEP in a previously unimmunized patient. The delivery of antibodies enables immediate virus neutralization at the site of injury while the active immune response from rabies vaccination starts to mature. The production of endogenous antibodies induced by rabies vaccination may take at least 7 days or more to reach adequate levels. Thus, RIG should be used only up to 1 week after the first rabies vaccine is given. RIG is never used in patients previously vaccinated against rabies because this may mute the body's normal immune response. Instead, for those patients previously vaccinated, booster doses of vaccine on days 0 and 3 are given per Advisory Committee on Immunization Practices (ACIP) and WHO guidelines.[28,114]

The role of passive immunity in saving lives after exposures had been demonstrated under field conditions, and it is more relevant when a short rabies incubation period is presumed, such as in head and neck exposures.[97,115] Despite the WHO recommendation of RIG use as part of routine PEP, it is still rarely used in most of the developing world. Delayed initiation of PEP because of limited health care access may allow progression of viral infection. In these cases, the use of RIG should not be ignored because of the increased risk for prophylaxis failure. In other words, there could still be a significant benefit from RIG, regardless of the time between exposure and presentation for PEP.[298]

Two major formulations of RIG are available: human (HRIG) and equine (ERIG). The former is more expensive to produce and is available mostly in the developed world, whereas ERIG is certainly less costly and is found in the developing world where available.[320] Often, however, even ERIG is unavailable in resource-constrained countries.

As an alternative to RIG, virus-specific monoclonal antibodies (MAbs) have been developed that would provide an economical and more readily available product.[74] Clinical studies are ongoing in animals and humans.[15,68,254] Such MAb formulations would likely improve access to passive immunity.[15,28,68,206]

Equine Rabies Immune Globulin

Animal rabies serum is no longer available in the United States and most developed countries. Previous versions of this chapter go into more detail regarding the use and history of ERIG.[174,223,247,321,318,319]

Human Rabies Immune Globulin

HRIG is prepared from the fractionation of gamma globulin (immunoglobulin G [IgG]) from the plasma of volunteers hyperimmunized with rabies vaccine. HRIG is currently the standard in the United States for immediate passive immunity in rabies PEP.[187] Because the gamma globulin is homologous in humans, HRIG persists for longer in the circulation compared with ERIG, which obviously is an animal protein. For this reason, HRIG may have a greater dampening effect on active immunization compared with ERIG. This factor may not be relevant, however, given the excellent quality and potency of modern-day rabies vaccines.

Dosing of HRIG derives from pharmacokinetic measurements,[120,125,185,193,236] such that 20 IU of HRIG per kilogram should be administered immediately, with as much as possible being injected locally. The remainder can be injected at a distal site intramuscularly, away from the vaccine administration site. Local HRIG injection is extremely important (Fig. 184.3) because serum levels of antibody after intramuscular injection are not high.[54] Although intravenous administration of HRIG produces higher serum titers,[5] local injection is still preferred. No further dose is necessary or desirable because excessive antibody diminishes the active response to vaccine. Two equivalent preparations of HRIG are available in the United States, one produced by Sanofi Pasteur (Imogam Rabies-HT, Sanofi Pasteur) and the other by Grifols (HyperRAB S/D, Grifols). If HRIG is unavailable, vaccination should be started immediately, followed by administration of HRIG if it arrives within a week.[158]

Nerve Tissue Vaccines

NTVs revolutionized rabies prevention after the introduction of the original Pasteur vaccine. However, NTVs have been replaced by cell culture vaccines in developing countries. NTVs produced in sheep or goat brain were widely used throughout Asia and Africa but were associated with a high incidence of postvaccine encephalitis.[7] The previous version of this chapter goes into greater detail regarding NTVs[105,222] and duck embryo vaccines,[157,235,248] which were designed as a replacement yet are now considered obsolete in the developed world.[223]

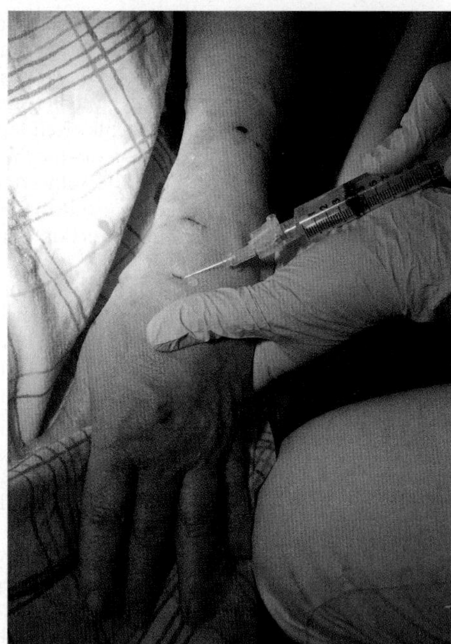

FIG. 184.3 Injection of human rabies immunoglobulin after a savage attack by a stray cat.

Cell Culture Vaccines

Rabies immunization evolved further with the development of safe and potent cell culture vaccines. RABV grown in cell culture is by definition free of neural tissue. Choosing a human cell line for growth avoids issues with foreign host proteins that could cause serious adverse events. The first widely used cell culture vaccine was the human diploid cell vaccine (HDCV). A human fibroblast cell line (WI-38) was developed,[123] and the Pitman-Moore strain of RABV was grown in these cells by Wiktor and associates.[313] Subsequently, the virus was harvested and concentrated by ultrafiltration to increase antigen content. Inactivation was performed with β-propiolactone. After various schedules of HDCV were compared, researchers found that three properly spaced intramuscular doses consistently produced a robust immune response.[14] A similar schedule of duck embryo vaccine resulted in antibody titers 10 to 20 times lower. The excellent immunogenicity of HDCV was confirmed,[6,37,64,108,187,226,283,317] and it became a gold standard against which other vaccines were measured.

A crucial test of any rabies vaccine is protection of those actually exposed to the virus. In Europe, the HDCV was used to vaccinate thousands of people exposed to rabies. However, those situations in which rabies was confirmed in the biting animal were particularly important to consider. Kuwert and associates[167,168] in Essen, Germany, vaccinated 68 persons after exposure to dogs, cats, cows, or wild animals with laboratory-confirmed RABV infection or exposed as a result of a laboratory accident. The schedule used was 1 mL intramuscularly on days 0, 3, 7, 14, 30, and 90. These investigators had no failures of protection, no significant reactions, and excellent neutralizing and complement-fixing antibody responses.

Bahmanyar and associates[14] in Iran conducted another test of HDCV. Forty-five persons who were bitten by rabid wolves or dogs were given rabies antiserum, followed by the same schedule of vaccine used in Germany. Once again, no rabies cases developed in vaccinees, despite an estimated 40% risk of disease if they had remained unvaccinated. Antibody measurements showed mean titers as follows: 7 days, 1.1 IU; 14 days, 10.7 IU; 30 days, 49 IU; and 100 days, 312 IU.

Later, the CDC distributed HDCV of US manufacture for persons whose exposure to rabies was established.[3] No vaccine failures occurred, and all healthy persons who received the full schedule of five 1-mL doses intramuscularly responded with antibodies, to date.

Although a few vaccine failures have been reported in other countries after administration of HDCV, ancillary prophylaxis recommendations were not followed scrupulously in each case.[4] The failure rate is estimated to be at most 1 in 12,000 courses of vaccination given in countries with a high risk for rabies.[212] General anesthetic agents given locally while the wound is repaired may increase the risk for vaccine failure.[95] The exact mechanism of protection afforded by PEP is uncertain. It may be blockage by antibodies of virus passage from subcutaneous tissue to the CNS, or it may actually be through the induction of innate and adaptive immune responses in parts of the CNS.[135,181]

An effort has been made to produce vaccines with the desirable properties of HDCV at a lower cost that would make them broadly available in developing nations, where the risk for human rabies is most severe. For example, purified Vero cell rabies vaccine (PVRV) is the Pasteur strain of RABV (as used in HDCV) grown in a Vero cell line in industrial fermenters. The virus is concentrated, inactivated, and purified. The PVRV has an immunogenic potency similar to that of HDCV. Successful PEP experiences have been reported in multiple countries, including Tunisia,[50] China,[294] and Thailand, even after severe exposure.[144,268,304] The PVRV has been purified further by chromatography.[175]

Purified chick embryo cell (PCEC) rabies vaccine is produced in primary chick embryo cell culture with use of the Flury low egg passage strain of RABV. It is inactivated, concentrated, and purified, yielding a vaccine preparation of antigenic potency similar to that of PVRV and HDCV.[18] The PCEC rabies vaccine was uniformly successful in preventing rabies in PEP trials in the former Yugoslavia, including subjects who were exposed by wolf bite.[61,289] The PCEC rabies vaccine also was shown to be equivalent to HDCV for PEP,[229] for boosting previously immunized subjects,[33] and in animal models for protection against bat rabies virus variants.[75]

Two types of rabies vaccine are now licensed and available in the United States: HDCV and PCEC. A tissue culture vaccine made in fetal rhesus diploid cells previously by the Michigan State Department of Health (and later Bioport), termed rabies vaccine adsorbed (RVA), is no longer distributed.[20] Either HDCV or PCEC rabies vaccine is recommended for PEP when given by the intramuscular route according to the regimens listed in Table 184.5. In 2011, the PEP regimen in the United States was reduced from five to four intramuscular doses in those with a normal immune system, in recognition of the high immunogenicity of the vaccines. Immunosuppressed patients should continue to receive five doses.[237] Decreased immune responses have been noted in vaccinees given injections in the gluteal area,[98] and therefore all intramuscular injections of rabies vaccine should be given in the deltoid muscles. In the event of repeat exposure of persons with a prior history of vaccination, two intramuscular booster doses should be given (see Table 184.5). Virtually 100% of these patients will have an anamnestic response.[270]

Numerous regimens have been developed for rapid immunization of exposed patients in developing countries who may seek medical help late or who may not return for subsequent doses.[269,290,304] To reduce costs, intradermal administration is often used because of the smaller volume required, which enables cost sharing of a standard dose among vaccinees. Moreover, because appropriate follow-up of patients for subsequent doses is more erratic in developing countries, the intradermal schedules generally are relatively short.[116,255,300,301] Some workers propose a 1-week schedule.[196,266] These regimens are listed in Table 184.5 and have the advantage of being less expensive. Note that if the 2-1-1 regimen is chosen, RIG may interfere with the body's native response to the vaccine.[312]

No intradermal rabies vaccine schedule is licensed in the United States,[187] partly because of the scarcity of mass exposures, the lack of bite clinics, and a relative inexperience with such delivery. Indeed, there is a small risk of failure with improper administration because intradermal vaccination requires some skill, given the millimeter depth of the dermis.

The effectiveness of current rabies vaccines to protect against most rabies-related lyssaviruses appears to be adequate; however, for those viruses in phylogroups II or III, there may be no protection afforded.[111,205]

Clinical Considerations

Decisions to Immunize

A physician must weigh numerous factors in deciding when to immunize a patient against rabies (Table 184.6). Some important considerations include the type of animal involved, the biting or exposure incident, the geographic area, patient-related factors such as immunosuppressive medications, or pregnancy. Costs, potential adverse events, pain, and inconvenience also need to be balanced against risk. With rabies, clinicians tend to favor overt vaccination, given the fatal nature of the disease. In fact, a study in the United States[201] revealed that rabies prophylaxis was inappropriately administered in 40% of cases. However, the study also showed that 6% of those not receiving prophylaxis should have received it. Thus, physician education regarding rabies certainly needs improvement.[233]

Pregnancy

The modern cell culture rabies vaccines are considered safe in pregnant women.[58,265] In the developing world, the issue of saving the unborn child of an expectant mother with rabies has occurred, and healthy infant delivery has been reported. Because rabies viremia is not known to occur, and a maternal-fetal barrier exists (the placenta), experts favor urgent cesarean section to save the child if feasible. The infant usually would not require rabies prophylaxis to ensure survival. However, data and evidence-based medicine available to provide guidance in such a rare clinical circumstance are not available, and each case should be

TABLE 184.5 Regimen Examples for Preexposure and Postexposure Vaccination With Rabies Vaccines

Vaccination	Route	Days on Which Doses Are Given	Remarks
Preexposure	IM[a]	0, 7, 21, or 28	Standard US and WHO three-dose regimen
	ID[b]	0, 7, 21, or 28	Economical, but not to be used in those taking antimalarial medications; unlicensed route in United States; WHO recommended
Postexposure[c]	IM[a]	0, 3, 7, 14	Standard US four-dose recommendation
	IM[a]	0 (2 doses), 7, 21	Used in some countries when RIG is not indicated; so-called 2-1-1 schedule
	ID[b]	0, 3, 7 (2 doses each), 28	Used in Thailand with PVRV, PCECV; so-called 2-2-2-0-1 schedule
	ID[b,d]	0 (8 doses), 7 (4 doses), 28, 90	Used in developing countries with HDCV, PCECV, or PVRV cell culture vaccines; so-called 8-0-4-0-1-1
Booster (for reexposure)	IM[a]	0, 3	Only after documented vaccination with cell culture vaccine[e]
	ID[b]	0, 3	Only after documented vaccination with cell culture vaccine[e]

HDCV, Human diploid cell vaccine; *ID,* intradermal; *IM,* intramuscular; *PCECV,* purified chick embryo cell vaccine; *PVRV,* purified Vero cell rabies vaccine; *RIG,* rabies immune globulin; *WHO,* World Health Organization.

[a]Together with rabies immunoglobulin.

[b]Give 0.1 mL, over the deltoids.

[c]Give 0.5 mL (PVRV) or 1 mL, depending on the vaccine, into the deltoid.

[d]Give 0.1 mL at multiple sites (see text).

[e]Or demonstrated presence of virus-neutralizing antibodies after other vaccines.

TABLE 184.6 Rabies Postexposure Prophylaxis Guide: United States

Animal Type	Evaluation and Disposition of Animal	Postexposure Prophylaxis Recommendations
Dogs, cats, and ferrets	Healthy and available for 10 days of observation	Persons should not begin prophylaxis unless animal develops clinical signs of rabies[a]
	Rabid or suspected rabid	Immediately vaccinate
	Unknown (e.g., escaped)	Consult public health officials
Skunks, raccoons, foxes, and most other carnivores; bats[b]	Regarded as rabid unless animal proven negative by laboratory tests[c]	Consider immediate vaccination
Livestock, small rodents, lagomorphs (rabbits and hares), large rodents (woodchucks and beavers), and other mammals	Consider individually	Consult public health officials. Bites of squirrels, hamsters, guinea pigs, gerbils, chipmunks, rats, mice, other small rodents, rabbits, and hares almost never require antirabies postexposure prophylaxis.

[a]During the 10-day observation period, begin postexposure prophylaxis at the first sign of rabies in a dog, cat, or ferret that has bitten someone. If the animal exhibits clinical signs of rabies, it should be euthanized immediately and tested.

[b]Postexposure prophylaxis should be initiated as soon as possible after exposure to such wildlife unless the animal is available for testing and public health authorities are facilitating expeditious laboratory testing or it is already known that brain material from the animal has tested negative. Other factors that may influence the urgency of decision making regarding initiation of postexposure prophylaxis before diagnostic results are known include the species of the animal, the general appearance and behavior of the animal, whether the encounter was provoked by the presence of a human, and the severity and location of bites. Discontinue vaccine if the result of an appropriate laboratory diagnostic test (i.e., the direct fluorescent antibody test) is negative.

[c]The animal should be euthanized and tested as soon as possible. Holding for observation is not recommended.

From Manning SE, Rupprecht CE, Fishbein D, et al; Advisory Committee on Immunization Practices Centers for Disease Control and Prevention (CDC). Human rabies prevention—United States, 2008: recommendations of the Advisory Committee on Immunization Practices. *MMWR Recomm Rep*. 2008;57:1–28.

individualized when the need for rabies prophylaxis in the newborn exposed to maternal rabies is considered.

Exposures to Bats, Wildlife, and Domestic Animals

In the United States, significant rabies reservoirs are found in multiple species of wildlife.[200] Bats and rabies are a special problem, as earlier discussion in this chapter has highlighted. When in doubt, bat testing in the setting of possible human exposures is the best way to rule out any risk of RABV transmission.[187]

Wild carnivores such as raccoons, skunks, and foxes involved in exposures must be considered rabid until proven otherwise. Rodents, with the exception of woodchucks and possibly beavers, are unlikely to be rabid.[200] Cat bites and cat scratches need important consideration, especially because rabid cats have consistently outnumbered dogs over the years by several factors. Cat immunization rates are lower compared with dogs, and cats may engage in more free-roaming activity wherein they may acquire infection. Cats always are suspect if they go out of their way to bite. Dog exposures, conversely, are less worrisome, given the successes of public health measures in recent times. This concept may not apply, however, for dogs residing close to the US-Mexican border, where circulating wildlife (gray fox) strains present a potential for reintroduction in nonimmunized animals.[187]

Circumstances of Bite

Clinical consideration of a provoked versus an unprovoked animal attack deserves some attention. For example, an attempt to feed an undomesticated animal is considered provocative behavior. Invasion of an animal's space or territory may be seen as a threat. This normal behavior for the animal is therefore less concerning for rabies compared with a spontaneous attack by an animal in a human environment. In rabies-enzootic areas, however, this concept of a provoked versus unprovoked attack is poorly predictive of rabies.[165]

If an animal appears clinically rabid, it should be euthanized immediately for confirmation of rabies by brain examination. If a dog, cat, or ferret appears normal, it may be kept for 10 days to see whether it develops rabies.[197] Clinical judgment about whether to start rabies prophylaxis depends on factors including the prevalence of rabies in the particular region, the species of animal, and the circumstances of the incident.

Rabies is extremely rare in properly vaccinated animals, yet it can occur.[200] Thus, prophylaxis may be administered if clinical or epidemiologic data suggest rabies, even in a vaccinated animal.

Table 184.6 summarizes recommendations by the ACIP on vaccination against rabies.[187] Advice can be sought from state and local health departments (particularly with regard to the occurrence of rabies in animals) and from the CDC directly.

Failure of Rabies Prophylaxis

The most common causes of human rabies are that no prophylaxis was given, a delay in PEP occurred, or there was a deviation from protocol such as the improper use of RIG.[70,107,322] Active immunization with vaccine does not regularly produce antibodies until 7 to 14 days after the first dose is given, hence the need for RIG for immediate passive protection. RIG is best given locally around the wound. If a large area is needed, the product can be diluted with saline.[322] Additionally, certain diseases and drugs such as chloroquine may exert an immunosuppressive effect and may account for other failures. The presence of B-cell immunodeficiency in a patient requires measurement of antibodies (titers) after vaccination. Patients infected with human immunodeficiency virus (HIV) are likely to respond if their $CD4^+$ lymphocytes are higher than 300/μL. If not, their postvaccination antibodies also should be measured.[144] In HIV-infected children, a standard PEP course of HDCV had no effect on the level of $CD4^+$ lymphocytes or the HIV-1 viral load.[275] However, even with correct prophylaxis, failures may occur, perhaps because in severe exposures, virus is deposited directly onto nerve endings.[129] Failures of the health care system such as inadequate monitoring of vaccine and RIG potency in developing countries may also be implicated.[11]

PREEXPOSURE IMMUNIZATION

Human rabies is 100% preventable with appropriate preexposure immunization. Modern vaccines are highly effective in persons at risk of exposure. Veterinarians, animal handlers, laboratory workers, and spelunkers should receive preexposure immunization (Table 184.7). Large numbers of veterinary students have been vaccinated under a three-dose schedule at 0, 7, and 21 or 28 days. Rabies virus antibody titers were determined on the serum of each veterinary student. Nearly 100% developed antibodies, with geometric mean titers of 10 IU or greater, which is equivalent to a neutralizing antibody titer of at least 1 : 200.[232] The three-dose regimen listed in Table 184.5 induces antibodies in 100% of healthy recipients. Preexposure immunization may be given with the use of HDCV and PCEC rabies vaccines by intramuscular administration. Outside the United States, any of the alternative cell culture vaccines on the WHO preapproved list can be used on the same schedule.[244] In addition, economic considerations may lead to immunization by the intradermal route, according to the same schedule.[305]

TABLE 184.7 **Rabies Preexposure Prophylaxis Guide: United States**

Risk Category	Nature of Risk	Typical Populations	Preexposure Recommendations
Continuous	Virus present continuously, often in high concentrations Specific exposure likely to go unrecognized Bite, nonbite, or aerosol exposure	Rabies research laboratory workers[a] Rabies biologics production workers	Primary course Serologic testing every 6 months; booster vaccination if antibody titer is below acceptable level[b]
Frequent	Exposure usually episodic with source recognized, but exposure also could be unrecognized Bite, nonbite, or aerosol exposure	Rabies diagnostic laboratory workers,[a] cavers, veterinarians and staff, and animal-control and wildlife workers in areas where rabies is enzootic All persons who frequently handle bats	Primary course; serologic testing every 2 y; booster vaccination if antibody titer is below acceptable level[b]
Infrequent (greater than in population at large)	Exposure nearly always episodic with source recognized Bite or nonbite exposure	Veterinarians and animal-control and wildlife workers in areas with low rabies rates Veterinary students Travelers visiting areas where rabies is enzootic and immediate access to appropriate medical care, including biologics, is limited	Primary course No serologic testing or booster vaccination
Rare (population at large)	Exposure always episodic with source recognized Bite or nonbite exposure	US population at large, including persons in rabies-epizootic areas	No vaccination necessary

[a]Judgment of relative risk and extra monitoring of vaccination status of laboratory workers are the responsibilities of the laboratory supervisor.
[b]Minimum acceptable antibody level is complete virus neutralization at a 1:5 serum dilution by the rapid fluorescent focus inhibition test, equivalent to ~0.1 IU/mL. A booster dose should be administered if the titer falls below this level.
From Manning SE, Rupprecht CE, Fishbein D, et al; Advisory Committee on Immunization Practices Centers for Disease Control and Prevention (CDC). Human rabies prevention—United States, 2008: recommendations of the Advisory Committee on Immunization Practices. *MMWR Recomm Rep* 2008;57:1–28.

Because rabies in developing countries is primarily a disease of children, exploratory studies have been performed to determine whether preexposure vaccination could be incorporated into routine pediatric schedules. Preliminary results from Vietnam show that routine rabies vaccination in infancy is feasible,[176] and it could even be performed by low-dose intradermal administration.[83] In areas enzootic for canine rabies, universal vaccination of children could be cost effective if the incidence of dog bite is high.[57] Children at routine risk for vampire bat exposures throughout Amazonia should be considered as well for preexposure vaccination. Children infected with HIV can be immunized successfully if their $CD4^+$ cells exceed 15% of lymphocytes. Those children with fewer $CD4^+$ cells may need at least double doses of rabies vaccine.[275] Missionaries and Peace Corps personnel operating in rabies-endemic countries should receive preexposure vaccination.[9]

Intradermal Vaccination

For preexposure use, the intradermal route is considered an acceptable alternative to intramuscular injection, with the important proviso that persons receiving antimalarial or other immunosuppressive agents and perhaps older persons should have their titers checked after vaccination or receive the injections by the intramuscular route. The success of intradermal vaccination depends on a technique that ensures intradermal rather than subcutaneous injection, but a margin of error exists.[21,97]

Today, essentially all intradermal vaccinations abroad are done with PVRV and PCEC rabies vaccine. To reduce the costs of vaccination, intradermal vaccination for postexposure use has become popular in developing countries, but it is no longer approved in the United States. Although single-dose preparations are not available for the intradermal administration of the 0.1-mL dose, extensive experience in Thailand and elsewhere has validated the successful prevention of rabies with vaccine extracted from vials intended for intramuscular use.[83,282,303,306,] However, attention must be paid to the correct administration of the dose into the skin, the sterility of unused portions of the vial for only a few hours while maintaining the cold chain, the volume of vaccine in the ampule, and the antigenic content of the vaccine used. The antigenic content should be at least 0.25 IU/0.1 mL. A popular intradermal schedule is one developed by the Thai Red Cross, consisting of inoculations on days 0, 3, 7, and 28 days, with double doses given in the first three administrations. A former recommendation for a 90-day dose has been abandoned.[159] Poor responses to intradermal vaccine have been noted in those concurrently receiving chloroquine or immunosuppressive agents, such as corticosteroids.[187,216] Therefore, persons who must be vaccinated while they are taking chloroquine or related antimalarial agents should be given injections into the deltoid muscle, and postvaccination rabies serologic studies should be obtained on those patients and others who are immunosuppressed.

Alternative Schedules

Although the WHO schedules are firmly established for the induction of optimal immune responses, other schedules have been tested extensively to reduce the number of vaccination visits, particularly in the developing world. One of the most popular of these is the 2-1-1 schedule, in which a double dose is given intramuscularly at day 0, followed by single doses on days 7 and 21,[59,195] and the regimen developed by Warrell and associates,[303] consisting of eight intradermal doses on day 0, four intradermal doses on day 7, and single doses on days 28 and 90.

The 2-1-1 schedule may not be as reliable if immunoglobulin (RIG) is administered.[173,176]

Booster Doses

Even with administration of cell culture vaccine, antibodies fall off rapidly after initial immunization, although most vaccine recipients have some detectable antibody decades after initial vaccination.[89,151] Nonetheless, once an immune response to rabies vaccine has developed, revaccination is almost certain to evoke a rapid response.[270] One booster of cell culture vaccine given to previously vaccinated persons results in a dramatic anamnestic response, with titers in one study rising from 2.8 to 94 IU at 14 days and more than 100 IU in 35 days.[225] As mentioned, with exposure to rabies in a previously vaccinated person, two intramuscular booster doses are recommended to provide a margin of safety. Single intramuscular or intradermal boosters are given to maintain immunity in individuals chronically exposed to rabies, according to the recommendations made by the ACIP and WHO in Table 184.7 if serologic testing suggests a waning titer.

In persons who have received preexposure immunization to rabies, the necessity of boosters is an important issue. Persons who definitely were exposed to a rabid animal should receive two booster doses of vaccine by the intramuscular route. Individuals who are likely to be exposed to actual virus, such as rabies laboratory workers, should be bled every 6 months and receive booster injections as needed to maintain their antibody titers above 0.5 IU (or complete neutralization at a dilution of 1:5, equal to ~0.1 IU/mL). A follow-up study by Briggs and Schwenke[34] found maintenance of an adequate titer (>0.5 IU) at 1.5 to 2 years after vaccination in 99% of subjects who received vaccine by the intramuscular route and in 93% who received vaccine by the intradermal route. In Thailand, researchers demonstrated that persons who received preexposure rabies vaccination by the intradermal route mounted a slow response to boosters, and the investigators suggested that in severe exposures, rabies RIG should be given despite the prior immunization.[144] However, the intradermal route can be used successfully to boost prior immunity.[272] Thraenhart and associates[277] observed 100% of antibodies induced in 18 subjects studied between 2 and 14 years after they received vaccination. Thus, if a person is properly vaccinated with modern cell culture vaccines, subsequent administration of RIG is not indicated in PEP.

Adverse Events

The available tissue culture vaccines are well tolerated. In more than 1770 human volunteers receiving preexposure immunization with HDCV administered intramuscularly, a sore arm was noted in approximately 20%, headache in about 8%, malaise in 5%, and allergic edema in 0.1%.[225] During incidents involving mass PEP, pain, swelling, and other local symptoms occurred in 30% to 74% of individuals.[187] Pregnancy is not a contraindication to receiving modern rabies vaccines.[59] Guillain-Barré syndrome and other neurologic problems have been rare occurrences, and their relationship with HDCV is uncertain.[161] Guillain-Barré syndrome that occurs after administration of NTV is associated with antibodies to myelin basic protein.[127]

In contrast, booster vaccinations with HDCV have been associated with allergic reactions in approximately 6% of subjects.[42] Those reactions were believed to be caused by the presence in the vaccine of human albumin that has been altered by the β-propiolactone used to inactivate the virus.[3,271,307] The reactions are of the immune complex type (type III), with urticaria, edema, joint manifestations, fever, and malaise. CDC data suggest that when primary vaccination is given intramuscularly and booster intradermally, or vice versa, reactions are more common than if all vaccination is by the same route.[99] Because the reaction is associated with the particular formulation of HDCV rather than with the virus antigen itself, additional boosters may be given if necessary with PCEC rabies vaccine, PVRV, or HDCV manufactured in Canada (Sanofi Pasteur).[96] Reactions to PVRV and PCEC cell culture vaccines generally have been mild.[81] A comparative study of PVRV with HDCV showed lower or equivalent rates of local and systemic reactions, with no serious adverse events.[150] Because PCEC rabies vaccine is manufactured in chicken cells, egg allergy is a possible problem, and anaphylactic events as well as some rare and perhaps unrelated neurologic complications have been reported.

FUTURE DEVELOPMENTS

Rabies, both the disease and progress in its prevention, is far from static. For example, Table 184.8 shows the progress of rabies vaccine development for humans. Perhaps the most dramatic future prospect is the development of vaccines in which the gene for RABV glycoprotein has been inserted into a viral vector, such as a poxvirus or adenovirus, or the use of rabies virus as a cloning and expression vector system by reverse genetics.[38,243] These vaccines already have been used extensively in a large variety of animal species, in which they have been found to be safe and highly immunogenic.[239] In field studies, raccoons and other wild animals have been immunized successfully by the oral route with baits containing rabies recombinant vaccines. Such vaccination has eliminated fox rabies from large areas of Western Europe[30] and has reduced raccoon rabies in the eastern United States.[240,257,258] Other avenues being pursued include the use of potent adjuvants to enhance the immunogenicity of subunit vaccine,[94] the addition of the internal ribonucleoprotein to enhance protection through induction of cellular immune responses and higher antibody responses,[278] synthetic peptides constructed from epitopes of the single glycoprotein and nucleoprotein,[73] and plasmid vectors containing cDNA of the glycoprotein (G protein) gene.[328]

TABLE 184.8 Examples of Rabies Vaccines Tested in Humans

Vaccine Types	Remarks
Pasteur: dried rabbit spinal cord	Residual live virus; NLU
Fermi: phenolized sheep or goat brain	Residual live virus; NLU
Semple: phenol-inactivated sheep or goat brain	Contains nerve tissue; NLU
Fuenzalida-Palacios: phenol-inactivated suckling mouse brain	Contains less myelin; once used extensively throughout Latin America
Duck embryo: BPL inactivated	Allergy to duck proteins
Human diploid cell (HDCV): BPL-inactivated fetal human cell culture vaccine	First tissue-culture standard; booster allergic reactions
Rabies vaccine adsorbed (RVA): fetal rhesus cell culture, BPL inactivated	Fewer allergic reactions; no longer marketed in United States
Vero cell (PVRV): BPL-inactivated virus	Purified by density gradient centrifugation; grown in Vero monkey kidney cell line
Chick embryo cell (PCEC rabies vaccine): inactivated virus grown in chick embryo cells	Purification similar to PVRV
Avipox recombinant-glycoprotein (V-RG): genetic construct expressing rabies virus glycoprotein	Limited clinical trials

BPL, β-Propiolactone; *NLU,* no longer used.

Particular effort has been directed toward the development of DNA vaccines. They are alleged to be potentially inexpensive and particularly thermostable, but to date most have required an unsatisfactory interval to produce virus-neutralizing antibodies or to have induced virus-neutralizing antibodies of inadequate titer.[182,183,184] Dogs given two doses of Pasteur strain G protein DNA, administered intramuscularly, were shown to develop virus-neutralizing antibodies to rabies and to European bat lyssaviruses 1 and 2 and to have protection against virus challenge.[219] Jallet and colleagues[145] produced chimeric G DNAs of rabies and EBLV1, or rabies and Mokola virus, to generate vaccines designed to induce virus-neutralizing antibodies in dogs to either all European lyssaviruses or all African lyssaviruses, respectively. In primates, rabies G DNA induced virus-neutralizing antibodies only if it was administered by gene gun.[181]

Other approaches have included efforts to express rabies G protein in yeast cells, which failed,[276] and in baculovirus in insect cells, which was successful. Although it is less glycosylated than the virion G protein, the baculovirus-expressed G-protein–induced virus-neutralizing antibodies efficiently in mice; its immunogenicity was not improved by adding baculovirus-expressed rabies nucleoprotein (N protein).[82] In approaches using the rabies G protein cloned into adenovirus, researchers have shown that a replication-defective recombinant elicited enzyme-linked immunosorbent assay antibodies in mice inoculated onto mucosal surfaces,[327] and an adenovirus incorporating a special promoted-intron expression cassette efficiently induced rabies G protein in cell culture that induced virus-neutralizing antibodies in intraperitoneally inoculated mice.[191] The rabies G-protein gene was cloned into canine herpesvirus; this recombinant induced virus-neutralizing antibodies efficiently in dogs inoculated by the intranasal route, a finding suggesting that it may be useful as an oral product to control canine rabies.[329] Similar hopes are offered by a new recombinant canine adenovirus vaccine, but widespread infection by canine adenoviruses may preclude such a possibility.

Molecular biologic approaches have not yet produced an ideal vaccine, especially for human use. In the near future, the most cost-effective and protective vaccines may be virion products propagated to high titer in an easily managed cell culture system (e.g., a suitable BHK-21 continuous cell line or transgenic plants).[199] In addition, MAbs may offer effective alternatives to HRIG.[110,117,228]

More recent work has shown potential for a broadly acting antiviral compound, favipiravir (T-705), to make an impact in rabies PEP.[330] A significant 3- to 4-$\log_{10}$ reduction in viral multiplication in a mouse model was shown. The agent reduced viral positivity in the brain but was thought to be most effective before neuroinvasion occurred, at about an effect equal to ERIG in PEP. Dr. Hilary Koprowski, considered by many as a leading authority on rabies, envisaged possible human rabies treatment in the 21st century, although acknowledging the great challenges.[164]

Regardless of developments in human medicine, the key to future progress is a focus on elimination of canine rabies, with greater global partnerships from a One Health perspective.[192,326]

NEW REFERENCES SINCE THE SEVENTH EDITION

19. Beattie GC, Glaser CA, Sheriff H, et al. Encephalitis with thalamic and basal ganglia abnormalities: etiologies, neuroimaging, and potential role of respiratory viruses. *Clin Infect Dis.* 2013;56(6):825-832.
29. Botvinkin AD, Poleschuk EM, Kuzmin IV, et al. Novel lyssaviruses isolated from bats in Russia. *Emerg Infect Dis.* 2003;9:1623-1625.
41. Centers for Disease Control and Prevention. First human death associated with raccoon rabies—Virginia 2003. *MMWR Morb Mortal Wkly Rep.* 2003;52(45):1102-1103.
42. Centers for Disease Control and Prevention. Human rabies—Kentucky/Indiana, 2009. *MMWR Morb Mortal Wkly Rep.* 2010;59(13):393-396.
56. Chowdhury FR, Basher A, Amin MR, et al. Rabies in South Asia: fighting for elimination. *Recent Pat Antiinfect Drug Discov.* 2015;10(1):30-34.
63. Cliquet F, Picard-Meyer E, Robardet E. Rabies in Europe: what are the risks? *Expert Rev Anti Infect Ther.* 2014;12(8):905-908.
65. Davis A, Gordy P, Rudd R, et al. Naturally acquired rabies virus infections in wild-caught bats. *Vector Borne Zoonotic Dis.* 2012;12(1):55-60.
66. Davis AD, Rudd RJ, Bowen RA. Effects of aerosolized rabies virus exposure on bats and mice. *J Infect Dis.* 2007;195(8):1144-1150.
68. de Thoisy B, Bourhy H, Delaval M, et al. Bioecological drivers of rabies virus circulation in a neotropical bat community. *PLoS Negl Trop Dis.* 2016;10(1):e0004378.
79. Dimaano EM, Scholand SJ, Alera MT, et al. Clinical and epidemiological features of human rabies cases in the Philippines: a review from 1987 to 2006. *Int J Infect Dis.* 2011;15(7):e495-e499.
87. Familusi JB, Osunkoya BO, Moore D, et al. A fatal human infection with Mokola virus. *Am J Trop Med Hyg.* 1972;21(6):959-963.
88. Faulkner R. We lost our son to rabies. The Guardian. September 29, 2009. http://www.theguardian.com/society/2009/sep/28/health-usa.
92. Fekadu M, Shaddock JH, Baer GM. Excretion of rabies virus in the saliva of a dog two and six months after it had recovered from experimental rabies. *Am J Trop Med Hyg.* 1981;30(5):1113-1115.
100. Fooks AR, McElhinney LM, Pounder DJ, et al. Case report: isolation of a European bat lyssavirus type 2a from a fatal human case of rabies encephalitis. *J Med Virol.* 2003;71(2):281-289.
101. Francis JR, Nourse C, Vaska VL, et al. Australian bat lyssavirus in a child: the first reported case. *Pediatrics.* 2014;133:e1063-e1067.
106. Gable MS, Gavali S, Radner A, et al. Anti-NMDA receptor encephalitis: report of ten cases and comparison with viral encephalitis. *Eur J Clin Microbiol Infect Dis.* 2009;28:1421-1429.
112. Graus F, Titulaer MJ, Balu R, et al. A clinical approach to diagnosis of autoimmune encephalitis. *Lancet Neurol.* 2016;15(4):391-404.
118. Hapson K, Coudeville L, Lembo T, et al. on behalf of the Global Alliance for Rabies Control Partners for Rabies Prevention. Estimating the global burden of endemic canine rabies. *PLoS Negl Trop Dis.* 2015;9(4):1-20.
147. Johnson N, Arechiga-Ceballos N, Aguilar-Setien A. Vampire bat rabies: ecology, epidemiology and control. *Viruses.* 2014;6:1911-1928.
164. Koprowski H. Rabies in the face of the 21st century. *Zoonoses Public Health.* 2009;56(6-7):258-261.
180. Lembo T, Niezgoda M, Velasco-Villa A, et al. Evaluation of a direct, rapid immuno- histochemical test for rabies diagnosis. *Emerg Infect Dis.* 2006;12(2):310-313.
200. Monroe BP, Yager P, Blanton J, et al. Rabies surveillance in the United States during 2014. *J Am Vet Med Assoc.* 2016;248(7):777-788.
204. Mshelbwala PP, Ogunkoya AB, Maikai BV. Detection of rabies antigen in the saliva and brains of apparently healthy dogs slaughtered for human consumption and its Public Health implications in Abia State, Nigeria. *ISRN Vet Sci.* 2013;2013:468043.
211. Nel LH, Taylor LH, Balaram D, et al. Global partnerships are critical to advance the control of neglected zoonotic diseases: the case of the Global Alliance for Rabies Control. *Acta Trop.* 2017;165:274-279.
241. Rupprecht CE, Nagarajan T, Ertl H. Current status and development of vaccines and other biologics for human rabies prevention. *Expert Rev Vaccines.* 2016;15(6):731-749.
246. Santhoshkumar A, Kalpana D, Sowrabha R. Rabies encephalomyelitis vs. ADEM: usefulness of MR imaging in differential diagnosis. *J Pediatr Neurosci.* 2012;7(2):133-135.
273. Taylor LH, Hampson K, Fahrion A, et al. Difficulties in estimating the human burden of canine rabies. *Acta Trop.* 2017;165:133-140.
285. Udow SJ, Marrie RA, Jackson AC. Clinical features of dog- and bat-acquired rabies in humans. *Clin Infect Dis.* 2013;57(5):689-696.
286. Van Thiel PAM, de Bie RMA, Eftimov F, et al. Fatal human rabies due to Duvenhage virus from a bat in Kenya: failure of treatment with coma-induction, ketamine, and antiviral drugs. *PLoS Negl Trop Dis.* 2009;3(7):e428.
288. Velasco-Villa A, Reeder SA, Orciari LA, et al. Enzootic rabies elimination from dogs and reemergence in wild terrestrial carnivores, United States. *Emerg Infect Dis.* 2008;14(12):1849-1854.
291. Vora NM, Basavarju SV, Feldman KA, et al. Raccoon rabies virus variant transmission through solid organ transplantation. *JAMA.* 2013;310(4):398-407.
302. Warrell MJ, Warrell DA. Rabies: the clinical features, management and prevention of the classic zoonosis. *Clin Med.* 2015;15(1):78-81.
311. WHO. WHO expert consultation on rabies: second report. World Health Organization technical report series no. 982. Geneva: World Health Organization; 2013, p 139.
330. Yamada K, Noguchi K, Komeno T, et al. Efficacy of favipiravir (T-705) in rabies postexposure prophylaxis. *J Infect Dis.* 2016;213(8):1253-1261.

The full reference list for this chapter is available at ExpertConsult.com.

SUBSECTION IX Arenaviridae and Filoviridae

185 Lymphocytic Choriomeningitis Virus

Rémi N. Charrel • Xavier de Lamballerie

Lymphocytic choriomeningitis virus (LCMV) is maintained in nature through persistent infection of its reservoir host, the common house mouse (*Mus musculus*). Human infection occurs through direct contact with infected rodents or by inhaling infectious rodent excreta or secreta. Although infection with LCMV usually is asymptomatic or mild and self-limiting, it can be severe and manifest as meningitis and encephalitis. Infection during pregnancy may cause fetal loss or congenital malformations.

HISTORY

In the 1930s, LCMV was discovered, at about the same time and independently, in three different localities in the United States. Armstrong and Lillie encountered the agent in a monkey when they passaged a recent isolate of St. Louis encephalitis virus.[6-9] In 1935, Rivers and Scott[63] described the first two cases of human infection with LCMV. Both these patients developed febrile illnesses characterized by headache, vomiting, and stiff neck; lumbar puncture revealed 720 and 1700 cells/mm^3, nearly all of which were lymphocytes. These investigators subsequently isolated five strains from patients with meningitis.[63] Traub[71] revealed the virus in a colony of albino mice. Mice were incriminated in these first isolations, and later observations proved beyond a doubt that *M. musculus* is the principal reservoir of LCMV in nature. However, not until 2007 was definitive evidence presented that LCMV-infected rodents caused disease in humans, as established by genetic comparative analysis.[32] For some time after its discovery, LCMV was regarded as the sole etiologic agent of Wallgren acute aseptic meningitis. However, it became clear that Wallgren syndrome had a multitude of viral causes, among which LCMV was of little relevance. In the years after other etiologic agents of acute aseptic meningitis were identified, such as enteroviruses, mumps, or herpesviruses, LCMV progressively disappeared from the sight of virologists and general practitioners. This situation is exemplified by the low numbers of human cases or outbreaks of LCMV infection reported in the medical literature (<80 articles). Meanwhile, LCMV was used as an excellent model for the study of a variety of phenomena of biologic and medical relevance, such as immunologic tolerance, viral immunopathology, slow viral diseases, and latent viral infections, the last demonstrated by the large number of scientific articles on that topic (>3700 references in the PubMed bibliographic database found using "lymphocytic choriomeningitis" as the search criterion).

EPIDEMIOLOGY

LCMV belongs to the genus *Arenavirus*, family Arenaviridae. *M. musculus* (the common house mouse) constitutes the reservoir of LCMV in nature, but hamsters also can carry the virus. Humans usually become infected through direct contact with infected rodents or by inhaling infectious rodent excreta or secreta during occupational exposure (laboratory workers, rodent sellers) or household exposure (pet owners). The epidemiologic features vary when animals other than *M. musculus* are involved. Thus, LCMV transmitted from Syrian hamsters has occurred in areas where infected mice are not found. Altogether, 47 human cases have been traced to these pets and may have caused family outbreaks but no epidemics.

Human infection with LCMV is a rare occurrence. Specific tests conducted with diagnostic materials from several large hospitals revealed an incidence seldom exceeding one case per year.[64] Because *M. musculus* is the reservoir from which most human infections can be traced, efforts were made to clarify the geographic distribution of LCMV-carrying mice. Of 1795 house mice trapped in Germany, 65 carried the virus.[1] In 44 of 376 trapping areas, infected mice were found; these 44 positive sites were unevenly distributed, with a majority located in northern and northwestern Germany. Recently 2 of 37 *Mus musculus* juveniles trapped in French Guinea were found to be infected with LCMV.[44] In 2015, LCMV RNA was detected for the first time in Africa from *Mus musculus*.[57] Together, all these results indicate sustained worldwide presence of LCMV.

In a serologic survey, the proportion of people with LCMV-specific antibodies was significantly higher in rural areas where infected mice were known to live as compared with zoonosis-free districts. In areas where LCMV-carrier mice are frequently found, 9.1% of the rural population had neutralizing antibodies. In contrast, only 1.2% of the people residing in southern Germany, which is essentially free of LCMV-carrying mice, had neutralizing antibodies. Extrapolating from these statistics, approximately 1000 persons are newly infected each year in Germany. Thus, researchers estimate that in western Germany, at least 72,000 persons must have had an infection with LCMV, based on an average life expectancy of 70 years and an approximate rate of new cases of 1000 per year. If this estimation is correct, most infections are not diagnosed and many remain unapparent.

The occurrence of LCMV infection in persons from homes where mice have been proved to be carriers of the virus is well known.[7] Researchers have suggested that small, persistent zoonotic foci of infection exist, on the basis of the known natural history of the disease in mice and the circumscribed range of activity of mice. The percentage of infected house mice apparently varies in different communities, and it has been recorded at 21.5% in Washington, DC,[5,8] and at 4% in Boston and New York.[41,76] However, because infected mouse colonies are dispersed unevenly, the proportion of infected animals in a given infected colony can be high, up to 95%.[32,35]

Many human cases have been reported in the context of occupational exposure to rodent colonies.[7,16,18,19,29,31,37–39,46,51,72] Outbreaks and isolated cases of LCMV infections were reported in laboratory personnel having contact with hamsters, not mice.[16,22,47,48] Recently a case acquired through occupational exposure presented initially as an influenza-like syndrome, complicated by pericarditis and meningoencephalitis.[3]

A study by real-time polymerase chain reaction (RT-PCR) assay of 130 samples of cerebrospinal fluid (CSF) from patients with acute aseptic meningitis in Switzerland showed no cases of acute infection with LCMV.[26] This suggests that LCMV infections are extremely rare in hospitalized patients. Until 2005, no case of person-to-person transmission had been documented, and the general consensus was that LCMV could infect humans only after direct or indirect contact with an infected rodent. The more recent evidence that LCMV can be transmitted through organ donation should lead physicians to evoke LCMV as a possible cause of infection in the absence of established close contact with mice or hamsters.[20,21,34] In a report of LCMV infection developing after organ transplantation, the fatality rate was much higher (seven deaths in eight cases) than previously noted, perhaps a reflection of the immunosuppressive regimens required by these transplant recipients.[34] Another, similar episode occurred in Australia, where three patients died after receiving an organ transplant from the same donor. Next-generation sequencing provided clues about possible involvement of an arenavirus related to LCMV.[45,61]

On April 15, 2008, an organ procurement organization notified the Centers for Disease Control and Prevention (CDC) of severe illness in two kidney transplant recipients from a common donor; at the time of notification, one of the recipients had died. Samples from the donor and both recipients were tested at the CDC; on April 22, test results revealed evidence of acute LCMV infection in the donor and both recipients. This report summarizes the results of the subsequent public health investigation.[20,21]

Serologic studies conducted in healthy populations of large cities by either immunofluorescence assay (IFA) or enzyme-linked immunosorbent assay (ELISA) found immunoglobulin G (IgG) antibody prevalence varying between 0.3% and 4.7%: 0.3% in Marseille, France[27]; 1.7% in Spain by IFA[49]; 3.3% in Argentina[62]; and 4.7% in Baltimore.[25] A study conducted in a region where murine typhus is endemic in Croatia reported an unexpectedly high prevalence, 36%, through IFA.[30]

Serologic evidence of four acute LCMV infections was retrospectively reported in Spain in serum and CSF samples from 341 patients.[28]

CLINICAL MANIFESTATIONS

In most cases, LCMV infection is minimally symptomatic or asymptomatic and consists of an influenza-like illness with fever, headache, myalgia, fatigue, and general malaise. These symptoms are self-limited and resolve after a few days. These mild illnesses, which usually do not motivate patients to see a physician, most likely represent most LCMV infections, but the exact proportion is unknown. Historical articles reported that respiratory symptoms occur in LCMV infections. In a certain (but unknown) proportion of cases, a second phase is observed during which neurologic manifestations, such as meningitis, encephalitis, or even acquired hydrocephalus, can be recorded.

In 1942, Farmer and Janeway[33] proposed the following classification of LCM into four clinical categories:

1. *Inapparent and subclinical infections:* Immunologic studies suggested that these forms are quite common: 11% of 2000 sera tested contained neutralizing antibodies against LCMV.[9]
2. *Nonmeningeal form, non–central nervous system (CNS) infection, systemic infection, influenza-like infection:* This form consists of two stages: systemic illness, then convalescence. The incidence probably is underestimated because of the lack of laboratory documentation and the absence of specific or suggestive signs. Only vague assumptions can be made concerning the number of underdiagnosed cases. The diagnosis of LCMV usually is not suspected unless attention is

directed to signs and symptoms suggestive of meningoencephalitis, although researchers have shown that generalized systemic infection may occur without any evidence of involvement of the CNS.[67] How often the disease manifests in this form or how often apparently asymptomatic infection occurs is not known. The demonstration of neutralizing antibodies in the blood of as many as 10% of the adult population suggests that infection with LCMV may occur more frequently than is suspected.[74]

3. *Lymphocytic choriomeningitis, meningeal form:* This form usually consists of three stages: systemic illness, meningitis (possibly delayed up to 2–3 weeks), and convalescence.[10] A striking example was recently reported: a 37-year old woman was admitted for meningitis 3 weeks after being bitten (and probably infected through this pathway) by a mouse at home.[73]
4. *Lymphocytic choriomeningitis, encephalomyelitic form:* This form has three stages: systemic illness, encephalitis (possibly delayed), and convalescence. A recent case perfectly illustrates this form: a 15-year old girl was admitted to the emergency department for fever, myalgia, headache, and photophobia, and was released after a negative initial investigations; 1 week later, she was admitted again with neuroinvasive febrile manifestations.[68]

Other CNS manifestations such as transverse myelitis, Guillain-Barré–type syndrome, and transient or permanent acquired hydrocephalus can be associated with LCMV infection.[12,13] LCMV-associated acquired hydrocephalus has been described only five times since the virus was discovered.[11,23,43,70] In all cases, the clinical picture was severe and patients required ventriculostomy.

A fifth category (congenital LCMV) should be added to the previous classification, corresponding to fetal consequences of LCMV infection during pregnancy. LCMV is a fetal teratogen. It can cause hydrocephalus, microcephaly or macrocephaly, intracranial calcifications, chorioretinitis, and nonimmune hydrops. More than 50 cases of congenital LCMV infection have been documented since 1955, with more than two thirds of these cases diagnosed since 1993. Chorioretinitis and hydrocephalus are the predominant characteristics among children diagnosed with congenital LCMV infection.[40] LCMV was isolated for the first time in the CSF of a congenitally infected infant, who had congenital hydrocephalus caused by LCMV infection with severe neurologic sequelae, including, in addition to hydrocephalus, chorioretinitis, blindness, and developmental delay.[65] The differential diagnosis of congenital LCMV infection includes toxoplasmosis, rubella, cytomegalovirus infection, herpes simplex, enteroviral infection, human parvovirus B19 infection, and syphilis.[13,14,56,75]

Last, immunosuppressed patients, such as organ transplant recipients, can develop fatal hemorrhagic fever–like disease. Several occurrences of transmission of LCMV via organ transplantation have been documented recently.[20,21,34] Of 11 recipients described in those clusters, 10 died of multisystem organ failure, with LCMV-associated hepatitis as a prominent feature. The surviving patient was treated with ribavirin (an antiviral agent with in vitro activity against LCMV) and reduction of immunosuppressive therapy.[20,21] During 2002–13, the US CDC investigated several clusters of LCMV cases in patients who had received solid organ transplantation in the preceding weeks.[4,12,14,15,59] Such events indicate that diagnosis of LCMV in the donor was undetected because of the lack of obvious manifestations and that enforcing measures for preventing similar cases is likely to be challenging.[15]

DIAGNOSIS

As in other viral diseases, direct diagnosis can be established by virus isolation using cell culture; Vero and L929 cells have proved effective for LCMV isolation, but other mammalian cells also can be used. Usually, either no effect or a mild cytopathic effect is noted. Routine clinical laboratories, however, may not offer isolation of LCMV in culture. Several molecular techniques using PCR technology have been described.[17,24,32,54,60] An RT-PCR assay has recently been described.[26,52] The main problem with all these techniques is that the genetic diversity of LCMV is poorly understood and clinical laboratories may not offer PCR assays for LCMV detection. Sequence data acquired from newer LCMV strains indicate that the genetic heterogeneity could be greater than 20% between two strains.[32] Therefore, a diagnostic assay able to amplify recognized LCMV strains may provide false-negative results with a new, uncharacterized strain. Further genetic analysis of newly discovered strains therefore will be key to developing better diagnostic tools in the future.

Several serologic techniques have been described for establishing the diagnosis of LCMV infection in patients. Among these techniques, the one that was used commonly in the past, complement fixation assay, has been demonstrated to have poor sensitivity.[47] IFA and ELISA techniques are equivalent in terms of specificity and sensitivity, although home-made ELISA may display higher sensitivity.[42] However, because of broad cross reactivity among members of the genus *Arenavirus*, confirmation should rely on neutralization assays to discriminate between LCMV and other arenaviruses.

Serologic study can be performed with serum or CSF samples. As in other viral diseases, a fourfold difference in titers indicates a recent infection. In a single sample, detection of specific IgM suggests a recent infection. Molecular detection of LCMV genomic RNA, as well as virus isolation, can be performed from CSF during CNS manifestations and possibly from serum or plasma.

TREATMENT

No treatment exists for LCMV infection. Ribavirin has been shown to be efficient for Lassa fever,[53] a viral hemorrhagic fever caused by another arenavirus related to LCMV. Ribavirin was used once in a kidney transplant recipient whose immunosuppressive medications were discontinued and who received intravenous immunoglobulin when the diagnosis was established; the issue was favorable, with complete recovery.[20,21] T-705 (favipiravir) was shown to interfere with LCMV minigenome transcription and/or replication.[55] Interestingly, this molecule is FDA approved for influenza virus infection treatment, has been recently used in clinical trials in humans during the West African Ebola virus outbreak, and has been successfully tested against a large variety of RNA viruses severely affecting humans such as Lassa virus, CCHFV, and SFTSV.[50,58,66,69]

CONCLUSION

Since 2000, several reports have shown that LCMV has not disappeared and that it still can cause severe or fatal cases. Renewed attention was drawn to LCMV after seven recipients of solid-organ transplants died of LCMV infection.[34] Historically, this virus was a major cause of aseptic meningitis in the United States; LCMV ranked first during the World War II era and second during the 1947 to 1952 period.[2] At that time, other major causes were mumps, herpes simplex virus, and leptospirosis. The focus on LCMV declined over the intervening decades, even though the rate of unrecognized causes of CNS infections still remains high, at more than 50%.[36] The reason for the diminishing interest in LCMV is not clear, but it may be related to the historical prevalence of the disease in rural rather than urban populations of developed countries. However, the growing proportion of urban people living below the poverty level may lead to conditions compatible with contact with mice and, therefore, may boost the incidence of rodent-associated diseases.

In addition, the capacity to diagnose LCMV has declined dramatically since the 1980s. Hence, the decreasing number of reported cases may reflect the decrease in clinical interest and the lack of diagnostic tests, rather than a genuine modification of the epidemiology of the disease. Standard techniques, such as IFA or virus isolation, have been virtually abandoned in clinical microbiology laboratories. In Europe, the situation has been critical since 2000; barely a handful of laboratories are capable of performing recognized serologic or molecular diagnostic tests. LCMV infection still exists, and cases are reported when physicians include LCMV in the differential diagnosis and when appropriate diagnostic tests are conducted. Efforts are essential to determine the epidemiologic landscape of the disease and to implement etiologic investigations of neonates with congenital malformations who have CNS infections. The combination of poor diagnostic testing capacity and a lack of awareness of the virus among physicians may contribute directly to an underestimation of the current role of LCMV in medicine.

NEW REFERENCES SINCE THE SEVENTH EDITION

3. Aebischer O, Meylan P, Kunz S, Lazor-Blanchet C. Lymphocytic choriomeningitis virus infection induced by percutaneous exposure. *Occup Med (Lond)*. 2016;66(2):171-173.
4. Al-Zein N, Boyce TG, Correa AG, Rodriguez V. Meningitis caused by lymphocytic choriomeningitis virus in a patient with leukemia. *J Pediatr Hematol Oncol*. 2008;30:781-784.
12. Barton LL. LCMV transmission by organ transplantation. *N Engl J Med*. 2006;355:1737.
15. Basavaraju SV, Kuehnert MJ, Zaki SR, Sejvar JJ. Encephalitis caused by pathogens transmitted through organ transplants, United States, 2002-2013. *Emerg Infect Dis*. 2014;20(9):1443-1451.
21. Centers for Disease Control and Prevention. Brief report: lymphocytic choriomeningitis virus transmitted through solid organ transplantation—Massachusetts, 2008. *MMWR Morb Mortal Wkly Rep*. 2008;57:799-801.
22. Centers for Disease Control and Prevention. Notes from the field: lymphocytic choriomeningitis virus infections in employees of a rodent breeding facility-Indiana, May-June 2012. *MMWR Morb Mortal Wkly Rep*. 2012;61:622-623.
26. Cordey S, Sahli R, Moraz ML, et al. Analytical validation of a lymphocyticchoriomeningitis virus real-time RT-PCR assay. *J Virol Methods*. 2011;177:118-122.
28. De Ory F, Gegúndez MI, Fedele CG, et al. Toscana virus, West Nile virus and lymphochoriomeningitis virus as causing agents of aseptic meningitis in Spain. *Med Clin (Barc)*. 2009;132:587-590.
42. Lapošová K, Lukáčiková Ľ, Ovečková I, et al. Development and application of ELISA for the detection of IgG antibodies to lymphocytic choriomeningitis virus. *Acta Virol*. 2016;60(2):143-150.
44. Lavergne A, de Thoisy B, Tirera S, et al. Identification of lymphocytic choriomeningitis mammarenavirus in house mouse (*Mus musculus*, Rodentia) in French Guiana. *Infect Genet Evol*. 2016;37:225-230.
50. Madelain V, Guedj J, Mentré F, et al. Favipiravir pharmacokinetics in non-human primates and insights for future efficacy studies of hemorrhagic fever viruses. *Antimicrob Agents Chemother*. 2016;61(1).
52. McCausland MM, Crotty S. Quantitative PCR technique for detecting lymphocytic choriomeningitis virus in vivo. *J Virol Methods*. 2008;147:167-176.
55. Mendenhall M, Russell A, Juelich T, et al. T-705 (favipiravir) inhibition of arenavirus replication in cell culture. *Antimicrob Agents Chemother*. 2011;55(2):782-787.
57. N' Dilimabaka N, Berthet N, Rougeron V, et al. Evidence of lymphocytic choriomeningitis virus (LCMV) in domestic mice in Gabon: risk of emergence of LCMV encephalitis in Central Africa. *J Virol*. 2015;89(2):1456-1460.
58. Oestereich L, Rieger T, Lüdtke A, et al. Efficacy of favipiravir alone and in combination with ribavirin in a lethal, immunocompetent mouse model of Lassa fever. *J Infect Dis*. 2016;213(6):934-938.
59. Palacios G, Druce J, Du L, et al. A new arenavirus in a cluster of fatal transplant-associated diseases. *N Engl J Med*. 2008;358:991-998.
66. Sissoko D, Laouenan C, Folkesson E, et al. Experimental treatment with favipiravir for Ebola virus disease (the JIKI Trial): a historically controlled, single-arm proof-of-concept trial in Guinea. *PLoS Med*. 2016;13(3):e1001967. Erratum in: PLoS Med. 2016;13(6):e1002066.
68. Talley P, Holzbauer S, Smith K, Pomputius W. Notes from the field: lymphocytic choriomeningitis virus meningoencephalitis from a household rodent infestation—Minnesota, 2015. *MMWR Morb Mortal Wkly Rep*. 2016;65(9):248-249.
69. Tani H, Fukuma A, Fukushi S, et al. Efficacy of T-705 (favipiravir) in the treatment of infections with lethal severe fever with thrombocytopenia syndrome virus. *mSphere*. 2016;1(1).
73. Verhaegh EM, Moudrous W, Buiting AG, et al. [Meningitis after a mouse bite]. *Ned Tijdschr Geneeskd*. 2014;158:A7033.

The full reference list for this chapter is available at ExpertConsult.com.

186 Arenaviral Hemorrhagic Fevers

Remi N. Charrel • Priya R. Soni • James D. Cherry

The Arenaviridae family of viruses consists of 38 distinct viral species, some of which cause disease in humans characterized by hemorrhagic fever syndromes. The majority of these viruses are associated with rodent-transmitted disease to humans and in one case, transmission by phyllostomid bats to humans. Arenaviruses have been classified into one of two groups based on the virus's ability to infect rodents in different geographic areas—Old World (Eastern Hemisphere) versus New World (Western Hemisphere). The New World Arenaviruses are further divided into three distinct lineages. In 1933, the original arenavirus, lymphocytic choriomeningitis virus (LCMV), was isolated by chance when a researcher was studying the St. Louis encephalitis epidemic.[149] Although the etiology of the outbreak was later identified as St. Louis encephalitis virus, LCMV was found to be a cause of aseptic meningitis. By the early 1950s, several other similar viruses were isolated and discovered and added to the family. Since the late 1950s it has been thought that a new Arenavirus species was discovered about every one to three years. (Lymphocytic choriomeningitis virus is discussed in Chapter 185.)

HISTORY

In the 1950s, a new disease emerged in the Buenos Aires province of Argentina, a rich farming region. The causative agent of the Argentine hemorrhagic fever (AHF), named Junín virus, was isolated in 1958.[113] Junín virus is hosted by rodents widely distributed in the region, and human infection occurs through contact with infected excreta, usually by a respiratory pathway. AHF is a severe disease that is fatal in approximately 20% of cases in the absence of specific treatment. Intensive deforestation and extensive agricultural practices in this region have increased considerably the number of contacts between humans and rodents and thereby fueled the emergence of severe annual outbreaks. Cases were expanding progressively into north-central Argentina until they finally were controlled by the availability of a live attenuated vaccine (Candid #1) developed in the early 1980s, which is licensed for use for endemic areas in Argentina.[2] Junín virus is estimated to have caused approximately 30,000 cases of symptomatic disease since its discovery.

Bolivian hemorrhagic fever (BHF) was described first in 1959 in the El Beni department of eastern Bolivia. The causative agent, named Machupo virus, was isolated in 1963 and was found to be antigenically and genetically distinct from but related to Junín virus.[75] Machupo virus was responsible for large outbreaks with high incidence (up to 21% of the population) and a case-fatality rate of approximately 20% during the 1960s. Effective rodent-control efforts interrupted these epidemics, and after the mid-1970s, no cases of BHF were reported. After 20 years of silence, however, 19 additional cases were reported in the same region from 1993 to 1999.[8]

An outbreak of severe hemorrhagic fever began in the state of Portuguesa, located in the central plains of Venezuela, in 1989. Initially thought to be dengue hemorrhagic fever, the causative agent was isolated in 1990, identified as a new arenavirus species, and named Guanarito after the municipality where the first epidemic occurred.[125] Venezuelan hemorrhagic fever (VHF) presents a seasonal occurrence clearly related to intense agricultural activity and to human contact with the soil and the rodents hosting Guanarito virus.

Little is known about Sabiá virus, which was responsible for one fatal case of hemorrhagic fever near São Paulo (Brazil) in 1994.[83] Subsequently, two other cases were reported in laboratory workers. The epidemiology and the natural reservoir of Sabiá virus remain unknown.

In 1999 and 2000, three fatal cases of illness were reported in female patients aged 14, 30, and 52 years; two resided in northern California and one in southern California.[24,25] These cases were associated with Whitewater Arroyo virus infections, a recently described arenavirus indigenous to the southwestern United States and hosted by *Neotoma* rodents.[54]

In the Old World, Lassa fever was described initially in Nigeria in 1969 when two missionary nurses died in the town of Lassa, and the causative virus was identified during that same year.[17] The disease occurs also in Sierra Leone, Guinea, and Liberia and several neighboring countries in the West African region, including Mali and Ghana.

ETIOLOGIC AGENTS

Arenaviruses are enveloped single-stranded negative sense RNA viruses with a genome consisting of two RNA segments, designated large (L) and small (S). The L genomic segment (~7.2 kb) encodes the viral RNA-dependent RNA polymerase and a zinc-binding protein (matrix protein Z). The S genomic segment (~3.5 kb) encodes the nucleocapsid protein (N) and glycoprotein precursor (GPC; secondarily cleaved into the G1 and G2 envelope glycoproteins) in nonoverlapping open reading frames of opposite polarities.[132] Nucleocapsid antigens are shared by most arenaviruses, and quantitative relationships show a basic split between viruses of Africa and viruses of the Western Hemisphere. Individual viruses are distinguished immunologically by neutralization test, which depends on the specificity of epitopes contained in the envelope glycoproteins.[115]

At present, 38 arenaviruses are recognized (Table 186.1). They have been classified according to their immunologic characteristics. Two groups are recognized (Fig. 186.1): the Tacaribe serocomplex, including the New World viruses; and the Lassa–lymphocytic choriomeningitis (LCM) serocomplex, including the ubiquitous LCM virus and all recognized Old World viruses. Genetic studies are congruent with serologic analyses.[40] They also indicate that the 38 arenaviruses represent four phylogenetic lineages. The Old World (Lassa-LCM serocomplex) lineage comprises 14 viruses (LCM, Lassa, Mopeia, Mobala, Ippy, Merino Walk, Menekre, Gbagroube, Morogoro, Kodoko, Lujo, Lemniscomys, Mus minutoides, and Luna). The three New World (Tacaribe serocomplex) lineages are designated A, B, and C (see Fig. 186.1). The lineage A includes eight North American viruses (Whitewater Arroyo, Tamiami, Bear Canyon, Real de Catorce, Tonto Creek, Skinner Tank, Big Brushy Tank, and Catarina) and five South American viruses (Pirital, Pichindé, Flexal, Paraná, and Allpahuayo). The lineage B includes nine South American viruses (Sabiá, Junín, Machupo, Guanarito, Amapari, Tacaribe, Cupixi, Ocozocoautla de

TABLE 186.1 List of Arenaviruses That Have Caused Illness in Humans

Virus	Acronym	Lineage	Country	(Possible) Host	Reference
Allpahuayo	ALLV	NW-A	Peru	*Oecomys bicolor, Oecomys paricola*	114
Amapari	AMAV	NW-B	Brazil	*Oryzomys goeldi, Neacomys guianae*	28
Bear Canyon	BCNV	NW-Rec	USA	*Peromyscus californicus, Neotoma macrotis*	56
Big Brushy Tank	BBTV	NW-Rec	Arizona, USA	*Neotoma albigula*	110
Catarina	CTNV	NW-Rec	USA	*Neotoma micropus*	16
Chapare	CHPV	NW-B	Bolivia	Unknown	38
Cupixi	CPXV	NW-B	Brazil	*Oryzomys capito*	28
Flexal	FLEV	NW-A	Brazil	*Oryzomys* spp.	28
Gbagroube		OW	Ivory Coast	*Mus (Nannomys) setulosus*	33
Guanarito	GTOV	NW-B	Venezuela	*Zygodontomys brevicauda, Sigmodon alstoni*	145
Ippy	IPPYV	OW	Central African Republic	*Arvicanthus* spp.	141
Junín	JUNV	NW-B	Argentina	*Callomys musculinus*	123
Kodoko		OW	Guinea	*Mus (Nannomys) minutoides*	
Lassa	LASV	OW	West Africa	*Mastomys natalensis*	14
Latino	LATV	NW-C	Bolivia	*Callomys callosus*	158
Lymphocytic choriomeningitis	LCMV	OW	Ubiquitous	*Mus musculus, Mus domesticus*	119, 131
Lujo	LUJV	OW	South Africa	Unknown	124
Luna	LUNV	OW	Zambia	*Mastomys natalensis*	75, 76
Lunk	LNKV	OW	Zambia	*Mus minutoides*	75, 76
Machupo	MACV	NW-B	Bolivia	*Callomys callosus*	159
Menekre		OW	Ivory Coast	*Hylomyscus* spp.	33
Merino Walk	MWV	OW	South Africa	*Myotomys unisulcatus*	120
Mobala	MOBV	OW	Central African Republic	*Praomys* spp.	108
Mopeia	MOPV	OW	Mozambique, Zimbabwe	*Mastomys natalensis*	
Morogoro	MORV	OW	Tanzania	*Mastomys* spp.	67
Ocozocoautla de Espinosa	OCEV	NW-B	Southern Mexico	*Peromyscus mexicanus*	17
Oliveros	OLVV	NW-C	Argentina	*Bolomys* spp.	8
Pampa		NW-C	Argentina	*Bolomys* spp.	
Paraná	PARV	NW-A	Paraguay	*Oryzomys buccinatus*	157
Pichindé	PICV	NW-A	Colombia	*Oryzomys albigularis*	109, 147
Pirital	PIRV	NW-A	Venezuela	*Sigmodon alstoni*	53
Real de Catorce	RCTV	NW-Rec	Mexico	*Neotoma leucodon*	74
Sabiá	SABV	NW-B	Brazil	Unknown	87
Skinner Tank	SKTV	NW-Rec	USA	*Neotoma mexicana*	15
Tonto Creek	TTCV	NW-Rec	USA	*Neotoma* spp.	110
Tacaribe	TCRV	NW-B	Trinidad	*Artibeus* bat	41
Tamiami	TAMV	NW-Rec	USA	*Sigmodon hispidus*	19
Whitewater Arroyo	WWAV	NW-Rec	New Mexico, USA	*Neotoma* spp.	52

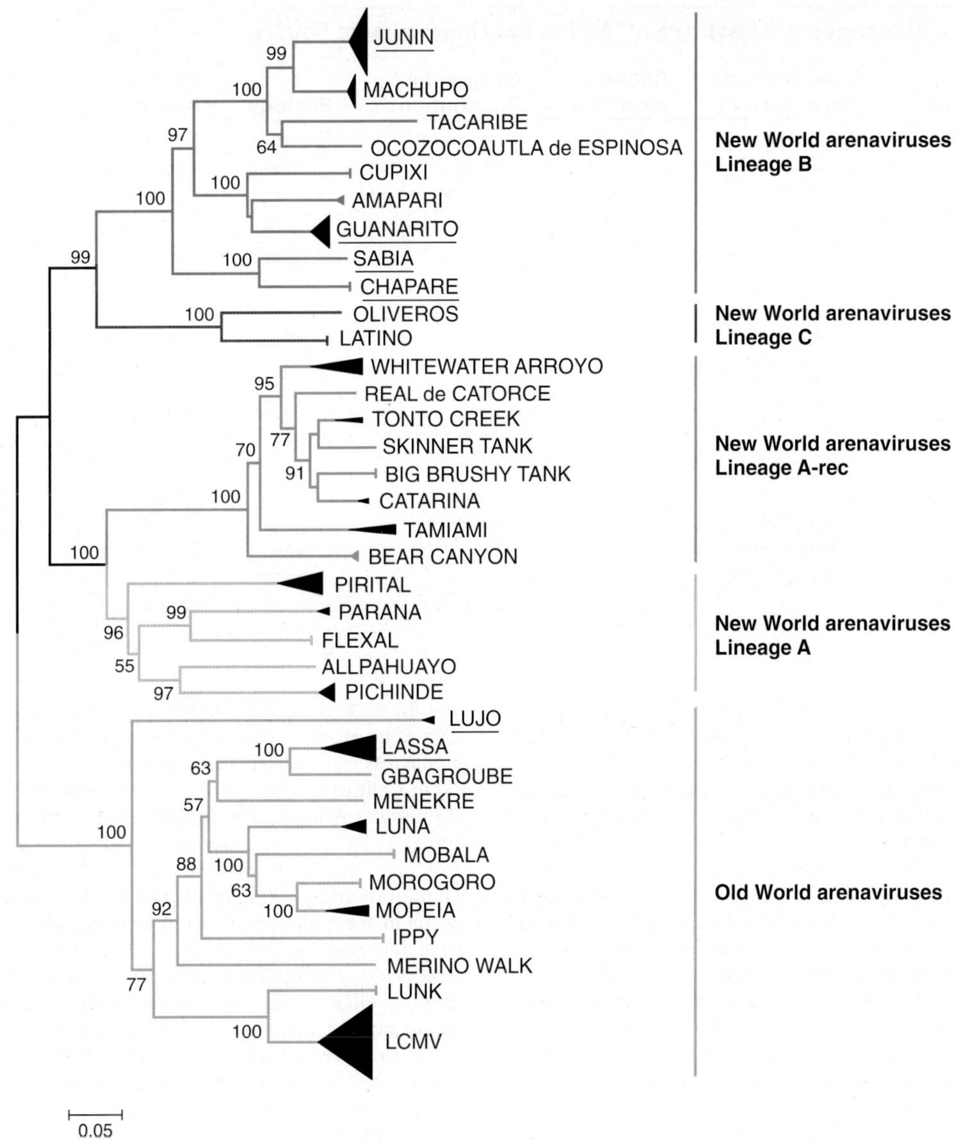

FIG. 186.1 Phylogeny of arenaviruses based on the analysis of complete sequences of the NP gene. A, B, and C show the three evolutionary lineages of New World arenaviruses. A-Rec denotes the recombinant lineage including the North American viruses. Bootstrap values above 75% are indicated and correspond to 500 replications.

Espinoza, and Chapare). The lineage C comprises three South American viruses (Oliveros, Latino, and Pampa). Phylogenies reconstructed from each of the four genes independently demonstrated that the eight North American arenaviruses possess a chimeric genome, with the glycoprotein gene inherited from a clade B ancestor and the nucleoprotein gene inherited from a clade A ancestor; this mechanism could not be identified within the large genomic segment, with both polymerase and matrix genes more closely related to those of clade A viruses.[27-29]

Lassa and Lujo viruses are the only Old World arenaviruses that cause human hemorrhagic fever, whereas five New World members of the lineage B (Junín, Machupo, Guanarito, Sabiá, and Chapare) have been associated with hemorrhagic fever in South America. Although Whitewater Arroyo virus has been associated with three fatal human cases in North America in 1999-2000, other cases of infection have not been reported since.

During the past decade, novel arenaviruses were discovered in snakes (in the families Boidae and Pythonidae, i.e., boas and pythons), in which they cause an illness called inclusion body disease that is characterized by behavioral abnormalities, wasting, and secondary infections.[121,134] The three new viruses were provisionally named California Academy of Sciences virus (CASV), Golden Gate virus (GGV), and Collierville virus (CVV). These viruses have a typical arenavirus genome organization but are highly divergent, belonging to a lineage separate from that of the Old and New World arenaviruses. Interestingly, these viruses encode envelope glycoproteins that are more similar to those of filoviruses than to those of other arenaviruses.[134]

Specific rodents (usually one or two closely related species) are the principal hosts of the arenaviruses for which natural host relationships have been characterized (Table 186.2); the only exception is Tacaribe virus, which was first isolated during a rabies surveillance survey from bats and mosquitoes in the late 1950s.[127]

The consensus is that the diversity of arenaviruses is the result of a long-term, shared evolutionary relationship (termed co-evolution or co-speciation) between the virus members of the family Arenaviridae and the rodents of the family Muridae.[11,12] Chronic infections of the host appear to be crucial to the long-term persistence of arenaviruses in nature. The infection in rodents is accompanied by a chronic viremia or viruria. Because of this specific association, the geographic area where each arenaviral disease is diagnosed is limited by the geographic distribution of the corresponding rodent host.

The rodent host of Junín virus is *Calomys musculinus*, a small field rodent. Since it was first isolated in 1959, the endemic area has expanded

TABLE 186.2 Epidemiologic Features of Arenaviral Hemorrhagic Fevers

Fever	Virus	Case, Season, Place, Pattern	Annual Incidence	Geographic Distribution	Ecology	Rodent Reservoir	Comment
Argentine hemorrhagic fever	Junín	Males; corn harvest; March-June	20-200	North-central Argentina	Temperate pampa	*Calomys musculinus*	3- to 4-year rodent-disease cycle
Bolivian hemorrhagic fever	Machupo	All ages, both sexes; villages; February-July	<10	Northeast Bolivia	Tropical savanna	*Calomys callosus*	Rodent control successful
Venezuelan hemorrhagic fever	Guanarito	All ages, both sexes equally; house, gardens; no seasonality	0–100	Central Venezuela	Tropical mixed savanna	*Zygodontomys brevicauda* *Sigmodon alstoni*	Recently described
Brazilian hemorrhagic fever	Sabiá			Brazil		Unknown	
	Chapare			Bolivia		Unknown	Recently described
Lassa fever	Lassa	All ages, both sexes; villages; no seasonality	10,000	West Africa	Tropical forest savanna	*Mastomys natalensis*	No long-term cycle; nosocomial infections
	Lujo			South Africa		Unknown	Recently described

from a region of 16,000 km^2 in the north of Buenos Aires Province to a region that is now 150,000 km^2 (reaching north of Buenos Aires, south of Santa Fé, southeast of Córdoba, and northeast of La Pampa provinces). The human population at risk now is estimated to be almost 5 million.[42,44] AHF caused by Junín virus is typically a seasonal disease, with a peak frequency in the corn harvesting season from March to June; during this period, 75% of the infected people are male agricultural workers who are contaminated by inhalation of infected aerosols produced from rodent excreta or from rodents caught in mechanical harvesters.[90] Since 1958, cases have been recorded annually, with a variation ranging from several hundred to 3500. The mortality rate for patients with confirmed AHF was 14% to 17% before immune plasma was used routinely.[91] Evidence indicates that the number of human cases reflects the proportion of infected *C. musculinus* in a particular area.[106] Since vaccination has been started with Candid #1 vaccine, there has been even a significant reduction in the incidence of AHF.[15,16]

Machupo virus, the causative agent of Bolivian hemorrhagic fever (BHF), is hosted by *Calomys laucha* rodents. As for Junín virus, the dynamics of the rodent population determine the epidemiologic features in humans.[101] By contrast to *Calomys callosus*, *C. laucha* invades houses during inundation at the rainy season; this invasion results in human cases occurring with an attack rate identical in men, women, and children. The disease has been recorded only from a sparsely populated region in northeast Bolivia, the El Beni Province. From 1962 to 1964, a series of outbreaks involved more than 1000 patients, 180 of whom died. Nosocomial transmission of Machupo virus was clearly demonstrated,[116] although most of the recorded infections were acquired by direct contact with *C. laucha* or by aerosol contact through infected excreta.

In 1990, new cases of hemorrhagic fever were investigated in Venezuela; the culprit was found to be a new arenavirus, designated Guanarito virus after the region where the outbreak occurred.[125] Natural and experimental data suggest that two different rodent species are involved in the transmission cycle of Guanarito virus in nature: the cane rat, *Zygodontomys brevicauda*; and the cotton rat, *Sigmodon alstoni*.[55,57,137] Since its discovery, Guanarito virus has been responsible for at least 200 cases of VHF. For unknown reasons, the number of reported human cases has dropped spontaneously since 1992, although rodent infection can still be demonstrated easily inside and even outside the original endemic zone.[146]

In December 2003 and January 2004, a small number of hemorrhagic fever cases were reported in rural Bolivia, outside of the known Machupo hemorrhagic fever endemic zone. The patients had symptoms similar to those seen with other arenaviral hemorrhagic fever cases—acute febrile illness beginning with headache, joint and muscle pain, and vomiting—and rapidly progressed to shock, bleeding, and death at 14 days after onset of illness. In the serum from one fatal case, a novel arenavirus was isolated and sequenced.[36]

In California, three fatal cases in 1999–2000 were associated with Whitewater Arroyo virus, initially isolated from a wood rat (*Neotoma* spp.).[24,25,54] The present-day geographic range of rodents of the genus *Neotoma* extends from western Canada southward to Guatemala, Honduras, and Nicaragua. Of the 20 recognized *Neotoma* spp., nine occur in the United States, and evidence of arenavirus infection has been reported for five of them. Field studies have provided strong evidence that Whitewater Arroyo virus circulates in the states of New Mexico, Utah, Texas, Oklahoma, Arizona, and Colorado.[18,56] The abundance and habits of wood rats suggest that potential contact between *Neotoma* rodents and humans is limited. Recent data support the fact that Whitewater Arroyo virus can infect humans.[103]

Lassa virus (LASV) is associated with a primary reservoir species, which is the natal multimammate mouse of the *Mastomys* genus. These mice are widely distributed in sub-Saharan Africa. However, it seems that the virus's range is restricted to West Africa. Documented cases of Lassa fever have been reported in several West African countries, such as Nigeria, Liberia, Sierra Leone, Burkina Faso, Guinea, Ivory Coast, Ghana, Senegal, Gambia, and Mali.[19,50,52,69,98,126,138] It is important to note that in some countries, including Guinea-Bissau, Senegal, Togo, Niger and Cameroon, fewer cases of Lassa fever are reported because of their low level of health care infrastructure.[119] Between 1985 and 1987, three of 5000 (0.06%) randomly selected persons living in six central African countries (Cameroon, Central African Republic, Chad, Congo, Equatorial Guinea, and Gabon) tested for serologic evidence of LASV infection were found to have antibody.[61] In contrast, a second study conducted with individuals living in different parts of Nigeria found that 21.3% of the 1677 tested antibody positive.[138] Lassa fever is a disease of major public health importance in West Africa because it causes an estimated 5000 to 10,000 deaths and as many as 300,000 infections annually in endemic areas.[65] The first epidemic was described in 1969 in Nigeria when two missionary nurses died[17] and soon was followed by several other epidemics in nearby countries. Among hospitalized patients, the mortality rate is estimated at 15% to 20%.[147] In hospitals located within the endemic area, 10% to 17% of admissions are caused by Lassa fever. However, serologic surveys suggest that subclinical cases occur and result in a lower overall mortality (<1%).[98] The overall incidence of Lassa fever in West Africa may be tens of thousands to hundreds of thousands annually. An important characteristic of Lassa fever is that there is a risk of secondary transmission of the virus from human to human through direct contact with blood or secretions from infected

TABLE 186.3 **Laboratory Findings in Arenaviral Hemorrhagic Fevers**

Disease	Viremia	RBC Increase	WBC	Urine Protein	AST/ALT
Argentine hemorrhagic fever	+	++	↓↓	+	N-200
Bolivian hemorrhagic fever	+/–	++	↓↓	+	N-200
Venezuelan hemorrhagic fever	++	++	↓↓	+	??
Lassa fever	++++	++	N-↑	++	100-1500

ALT, Alanine aminotransferase; *AST*, aspartate aminotransferase; *N*, normal; *RBC*, red blood cell; *WBC*, white blood cell.

patients and by aerosol exposure.[77] Many nosocomial outbreaks have been described. Another characteristic of Lassa fever is that a number of cases are acquired by local residents who seek out rodents for consumption.[136] Because of the prevalence of virus transmission, Lassa fever is a prominent threat of imported hemorrhagic fever cases; such cases have been reported in England,[31] Germany,[64] Japan,[70] the Netherlands,[143] Israel,[129] and the United States.[71] A comprehensive report of imported Lassa fever recorded 24 cases occurring from 1969 to 2004, with a fatality rate of 29%.[88] Currently it is observed that the overall case-fatality rate is 1%, with overall case-fatality among patients hospitalized with severe cases up to 15%.[148]

In fall 2008, five cases of hemorrhagic fever were reported in South Africa after air transfer of a critically ill index case from Zambia. Four of them were fatal; the fifth case received ribavirin and recovered. Next-generation sequencing from serum and tissue samples detected a novel arenavirus that was subsequently completely sequenced. Lujo virus (LUJV) was named after its geographic origin (Lusaka, Zambia, and Johannesburg, South Africa).[14]

PERSON-TO-PERSON TRANSMISSION

Although human-to-human transmission of BHF has been seen only rarely and then only after intimate contact, Machupo virus clearly was responsible for severe nosocomial outbreaks in which all cases were associated with a single index case who had returned from the endemic region. The only recognized hospital-based outbreak resulted in four secondary cases followed by a tertiary case acquired from a necropsy incident; all but one died. An epidemic was reported in which seven members of the same family were infected, with a fatal outcome for six.[23]

Nosocomial transmission is a common feature of Lassa fever, and many nosocomial outbreaks have been described.[48,77] However, it is apparent that this aspect of Lassa fever has been overestimated in reports based on infections in hospitals. The additional risk to hospital workers within the endemic zone is not great as judged by serosurveys, provided that basic hygiene measures are respected in hospitals in dealing with suspected cases.[68] Good barrier nursing and protection of personnel by use of gloves, gowns, and eye shields have reduced the incidence of such infection in recent years. Broader surveys of community infections have revealed Lassa fever to be an important community-acquired disease, with a wide spectrum of clinical manifestations. Because LASV has been isolated from breast milk, there is a risk to nursing children.

Concerning Lujo virus (LUJV) infection, an index patient was airlifted from Zambia to a clinic in South Africa, after infection from an unidentified source. Secondary infections were recognized in a paramedic (case 2) who attended the index case during air transfer from Zambia, in a nurse (case 3) who attended the index case in the intensive care unit in South Africa, and in a member of the hospital staff (case 4) who cleaned the room after the index case died. One case of tertiary infection was recorded in a nurse (case 5) who attended case 2 after his transfer from Zambia.[114] The distribution of this newly described arenavirus is still not fully known.

In conclusion, the data demonstrating nosocomial and human-to-human transmission of several arenaviral diseases highlight the necessity for implementing biocontainment precautions in dealing with arenavirus-infected patients and materials. LASV is classified as a Biosafety Level 4 (BSL4) and NIAID Biodefense category A agent, because of high case-fatality rates, ability to spread quickly through secondary human-to-human transmission, and the potential for aerosolized release.

It is important to note that agricultural workers and those in rural communities are at highest risk. It is thought that transmission to humans in these settings results from the virus being carried on dust particles or by direct ingestion of contaminated food products. Overall the majority of human infections occur primarily by aerosol or close contact with rodent excreta or contamination of food or through skin abrasions.[106]

CLINICAL MANIFESTATIONS

The clinical pictures of the South American arenaviral hemorrhagic fevers are almost identical, regardless of the virus responsible for the disease. The incubation period usually is 10 to 14 days, with an extreme incubation time extending from 5 to 21 days. Infection secondary to high-load inoculum may result in the reduction of the incubation period to 2 days. The onset is gradual with fever and malaise, secondarily joined by myalgia, back pain, headache, and dizziness. Hyperesthesia of the skin is a common manifestation. Petechiae of the skin and hemorrhages from the gums, vagina, and gastrointestinal tract beginning about the fourth day of illness herald the advent of hypovolemic clinical shock. Blood loss usually is minor, so the hematocrit generally increases as capillary leak syndrome, a hallmark of the disease, becomes more severe (Table 186.3). Bleeding and prothrombin time may be prolonged, and reductions of factors II and VII of the coagulation cascade have been noted. Renal function is generally preserved until shock occurs, but urinary protein concentration may be high. Neurologic manifestations are prominent and include intention tremor of the hands, and inability to swallow or to speak clearly may develop. These symptoms can progress to grand mal convulsions, coma, and death in the absence of significant capillary leak or hemorrhagic signs. Death usually occurs 7 to 12 days after onset of disease. Those who survive generally recover completely without permanent sequelae, although transient loss of scalp hair and Beau lines in digital nails are a common consequence of the high and sustained fever.

Symptoms that appear to be more specifically associated with one or another of the viruses have been reported.[142] Although the frequency of clinical and laboratory findings is identical for Junín and Machupo virus infections, clear differences exist with Guanarito virus infections. Pharyngitis, vomiting, and diarrhea are observed more frequently with Guanarito virus; in contrast, petechiae, erythema, facial edema, hyperesthesia of the skin, and shock are observed more frequently in the case of Junín or Machupo infection. There seems to be little difference, if any, between clinical manifestations caused by these three viruses and the recently isolated Chapare virus; the patient, a 22-year-old man, had lived for the last 4 years in the same region. He was a tailor and also a farmer. He had no history of travel and no contact with any case with compatible illness for at least 4 weeks before his disease onset. In addition, no members of the case household or other close contacts were affected. His clinical course included fever, headache, arthralgia, myalgia, and vomiting, with subsequent deterioration and multiple hemorrhagic signs and death 14 days after onset.[36]

Fatal outcome of Junín virus infection is observed more frequently in pregnant women in the third trimester, and a high fetal mortality is associated with Junín and Machupo virus infections.[15,16,38,73]

The symptoms of Argentine hemorrhagic fever (Junín virus), Bolivian hemorrhagic fever (Machupo virus), and Venezuelan hemorrhagic fever (Guanarito virus) are distinct from those of Lassa fever in that hepatitis rarely occurs, whereas it occurs frequently in severe Lassa fever. Overall, hemorrhaging, neurological signs and symptoms, leukopenia, and thrombocytopenia are more common in the three Latin American hemorrhagic fevers in comparison to Lassa fever. The increased urinary protein and increased hemoconcentration seen in these three viral infections are associated with a higher rate of mortality.[118] In severe episodes, patients with these viral infections develop hemorrhagic fever, leukopenia, thrombocytopenia, leukopenia, hematuria, tremors, pulmonary edema, respiratory distress, coma, and shock.[131]

The patients infected with Whitewater Arroyo virus were healthy before acquiring the virus infection. In one case, the patient probably acquired the virus by aerosol pathway while cleaning rodent droppings at home. In all cases, no history of travel outside California was found during the 4 weeks preceding the illness. The onset was characterized by nonspecific febrile symptoms including fever, headache, and myalgia. All patients presented with acute respiratory distress syndrome, and two developed liver failure and hemorrhagic manifestations. Death occurred within 8 weeks after the onset.[24,25]

Concerning Lassa fever, the clinical description is based on signs observed in hospitalized patients.[51,76,115] After an incubation period that ranges from 7 to 14 days, patients suffer an insidious onset characterized by progressive fever, malaise, and generalized myalgia. Retrosternal pain frequently is associated with this phase. In these earlier stages, Lassa fever is often misdiagnosed as influenza, typhoid, or malaria. The symptoms, however, increase in severity during the following week and are accompanied by nausea, vomiting, diarrhea, chest pain, abdominal pain, headache, sore throat, cough, and dizziness. Patients complain of sore throat, pharyngeal inflammation, and chest pain. As the disease progresses, vomiting, diarrhea, hemorrhagic manifestations, encephalopathy, and evidence of vascular permeability may be noted. During the second week, recovery may begin or the disease progressively worsens until harbingers of a fatal outcome are evident: severe edema, mucosal hemorrhages, pulmonary involvement, encephalopathy (with seizures and coma), or shock; at this stage, pleural and pericardial effusions and ascites are not rare findings. Liver involvement is frequent, but icterus is not usual. Death occurs in 15% to 20% of the hospitalized patients, usually in the second or third week of the course, and is associated with sudden cardiovascular collapse caused by hepatic, pulmonary, and myocardial damage. Few patients develop severe central nervous system (CNS) signs, and disturbances in consciousness and convulsions are markers of a poor prognosis. Deafness is an important sequela of Lassa fever; it may be unilateral or bilateral and is a consequence of eighth cranial nerve dysfunction. It can be observed in as many as 30% of patients.

Clinical disease among children generally is similar to that in adults. Systematic data are available only for Lassa fever patients.[105,147] Fever, vomiting, diarrhea, and cough are common presenting symptoms. Pulmonary signs, including rales and pleural effusion, are seen more commonly in children than in adults. Among very young children, especially those infected antepartum, an unusual condition called swollen baby syndrome has been described. It is marked by abdominal distention, widespread edema, and spontaneous bleeding. In a small review of cases from Liberia, it seemed that the absence of this clinical presentation was a good prognostic indicator in children.[105]

LASV replicates at a very high level in the placenta of pregnant women, which might account for the high mortality rate observed in these patients. The risk for death in pregnant women is estimated to vary from 7% in the first two trimesters to 30% in the third trimester, compared with the 13% mortality in nonpregnant women. A high fetal mortality rate varying from 92% in early pregnancy to 75% in the last trimester has been observed.[102,104,120]

Although few cases of LUJV infection have been reported, it appears that the clinical manifestations are not drastically different from those observed with other arenaviruses. The putative incubation period ranged from 7 to 13 days, and the period of illness varied from 10 to 13 days. All patients presented with nonspecific febrile illness with headache and myalgia. The severity increased for 7 days with diarrhea and pharyngitis. A morbilliform rash was observed on the face and trunk of white patients but was lacking in African patients. Transient subjective improvement after approximately 1 week of illness was reported; afterward, the patients endured a rapid deterioration with respiratory distress, neurologic signs, and circulatory collapse, the terminal features in patients who died. Bleeding was not a prominent feature. However, petechial rash, gingival bleeding, and oozing of blood from venipuncture sites were observed. Chest pain was a prominent symptom for two patients. All patients had thrombocytopenia on admission to the hospital (platelet count range, 20 to 104×10^9 cells/L). Three patients had leukocyte counts in the normal range, and two had leukopenia on admission, whereas leukocytosis developed in four patients during the illness. The highest aspartate transaminase values recorded in the patients who died ranged from 549 to 2486 U/L, compared with 240 U/L in the survivor who was treated with ribavirin.[114]

Very little is known about the health consequences of infection with the other arenaviruses. Aerosol infections are common in those who work in laboratories where arenaviruses are manipulated. Pichindé virus has resulted in several seroconversions without any notable clinical significance.[13] Flexal virus has resulted in two severe laboratory infections and should be regarded as potentially dangerous (F. Pinheiro, personal communication). Tacaribe virus has resulted in a single case of febrile disease with mild CNS symptoms (J. Casals, personal communication).

PATHOGENESIS AND PATHOLOGY

Human and nonhuman primate infection initially involves virus replication at the site of infection, usually in the lung after infected aerosol deposition in the terminal respiratory bronchioles. Replication occurs in the hilar lymph nodes, and despite interstitial infiltration, pneumonic foci usually are not observed. Regardless of the route of infection, the macrophage is a site of important viral replication. With the exception of the hepatitis peculiar to Lassa fever, the pathologic process of arenaviral hemorrhagic fever is notable for the general lack of parenchymal histologic damage. Edema of tissues and focal hemorrhages in mucosal surfaces and fascia of many organs are common events. Rarely, blood clots are found that are large enough to be of clinical significance. Thus, the crucial and life-threatening lesion in these diseases appears to be the capillary leak. How capillary leak, in which plasma protein and fluid escape the circulation at a much higher rate than erythrocytes do, occurs is not clear.[115]

Hemorrhages are common findings with New World arenaviruses causing hemorrhagic fever. The prominent thrombocytopenia seen has a central origin possibly linked to high levels of interferon observed in these patients.[82] Minor foci of necrosis with acidophilic inclusions (Councilman bodies) have been reported in patients with BHF,[30] and erythroid hypoplasia of bone marrow as well as lymphoid depletion of nodes and spleen may be present. Histologic evidence of disseminated intravascular coagulation generally is absent. Inflammatory lesions of the CNS are lacking. Mild inflammation of the myocardium has been noted in patients with BHF. The Argentine and Bolivian fevers may be marked by encephalopathy. Virus is not recovered from cerebrospinal fluid of patients presenting such CNS symptoms with the South American agents. Macrophages and lymphocytes or their precursors are targets for infection, and an activation of the complex cytokine cascade occurs, which can cause endothelial cells of small capillaries to lose the tight continuity that keeps proteins and red cells inside the circulation. As part of this cascade, levels of interferon are elevated. Analysis of the serum levels of hematopoietic growth factors suggested a link between granulocyte colony-stimulating factor serum levels and the severity of the illness in humans.[93] Similarly, interleukin-8 is thought to play an essential role in neutrophil activation.[94] Specific antibodies may not appear until 3 to 4 weeks after the onset of the disease. However, New World arenaviruses that cause hemorrhagic fever are neutralized more readily, and immune serum–based therapy has been successful in humans. Preliminary studies of VHF suggest that this disease resembles those caused by other South American relatives.[35,125] Genetic analysis of Junín and Guanarito virus sequences amplified from human cases in Argentina and Venezuela, respectively, failed to identify any genetic marker correlating with human pathogenicity or with the severity of clinical forms.[58,146]

Although only three cases have been reported to date, Whitewater Arroyo virus infection seems to be associated with profound lymphopenia and thrombocytopenia.[24,25] To date, no studies have been performed to investigate the pathogenesis of Whitewater Arroyo virus infection. An interesting note is that Whitewater Arroyo virus belongs to lineage A (based on genetic analysis performed in the nucleocapsid gene), in which no other members have been recognized so far as human pathogens. However, the small genomic segment of Whitewater Arroyo virus has been shown to have a dual origin: the gene encoding the nucleocapsid is inherited from an ancestor belonging to lineage A, whereas the glycoprotein precursor gene is inherited from an ancestor belonging to lineage B.[27] Further investigations are needed to clarify whether the lineage B–inherited GPC gene is responsible for the putative human pathogenicity of Whitewater Arroyo virus.

The model for LASV pathogenesis has been carefully studied. Macrophages and dendritic cells represent the targets of early infection in humans, as in many of the other virus infections as mentioned earlier. In LASV, instead of the virus then being recognized and presented as a foreign antigen, the virus establishes an infection that evades the immune system and therefore does not stimulate T cells. This contributes to immunosuppression. It is also known that LASV infection in macrophages does not result in the production of excessive cytokines, but the cells release high amounts of infectious virus. In the hepatocytes, the infection leads to elevation in transaminases and hepatocellular necrosis. The virus is also known to replicate heavily in the adrenal cortex. The high viral load there may contribute to alterations in mineralocorticoids leading to fluid imbalance. LASV is also known to infect vascular endothelial cells without causing the overt cytopathology seen in other viruses.[106]

The hepatitis of Lassa fever is represented by different stages successively characterized by hepatocellular injury, necrosis, and regeneration, any of which may be present at death. In no instance is the degree of hepatic damage sufficient to be responsible for hepatic failure; consequently, the hepatitis of Lassa fever is not the primary cause of death.[74,97] For the cases characterized by encephalopathy, correlation could not be established with the presence of LASV in the cerebrospinal fluid or with virus antibodies in cerebrospinal fluid or serum; no evidence shows that the encephalopathy observed in Lassa fever is the consequence of either direct cytopathic or immune-mediated mechanisms.[32] Direct damage to circulating leukocytes is not demonstrated, and profound thrombocytopenia does not occur.

In human cases of Lassa fever, no correlation exists between antibody levels and outcome of the disease.[46] More than one third of patients have antibodies to the nucleocapsid of the virus on admission to the hospital. These antibodies do not neutralize the virus, which is found in blood in concentrations much higher in severe infection than in any of the other arenaviral diseases. During convalescence, viral neutralizing antibodies evolve for months and rarely reach levels even one tenth of those that develop after infection with the other viruses in this group. Recovery from LASV infection usually precedes the appearance of neutralizing antibodies, indicating that cellular immunity plays a primary role in viral clearance. Thus, it seems reasonable to speculate that compromise of cell-mediated immunity is responsible for uncontrolled virus replication and functional capillary collapse. Primates challenged with LASV or naturally infected patients who recovered from acute Lassa fever usually do not exhibit a measurable neutralizing antibody response. Individuals who are seropositive exhibit a strong memory CD4+ T-cell response against the nucleocapsid protein of LASV.[135] Experiments based on inactivated vaccines have shown that in spite of the resulting synthesis of high titers of antibodies, vaccination did not prevent virus replication and death in nonhuman primates.[46] It therefore seems obvious that control of human Lassa fever involves mostly T cells through a Th1-type immune response. In addition, immune response requires epitopes located on both GP1 and GP2 glycoproteins to protect efficiently primates challenged with Lassa virus.[46]

Furthermore, α-dystroglycan has been identified as a major receptor for LCM and Lassa viruses. In New World arenaviruses, only clade C viruses (Oliveros and Latino) use α-dystroglycan as a major receptor, whereas clade A and clade B arenaviruses use distinct and widely expressed receptors.[123,133] Functional receptors for South American hemorrhagic fever arenaviruses (Guanarito, Junín, and Machupo) were found on most human cell types and cells derived from nonhuman primates and rodents.[124]

Last, it is important to note that several animals have provided reasonable models for the clinical disease seen in humans. Junín virus causes fatal hemorrhagic disease in guinea pigs; rhesus monkeys are good models for Lassa[72] and Machupo virus infections; and marmosets (*Callithrix jacchus*) reproduce the pathogenesis of Junín virus. Indeed, rhesus monkeys were used to predict the effectiveness of the antiviral drug ribavirin to treat Lassa fever, and guinea pigs were instrumental in the development of an attenuated vaccine for AHF. The paired Syrian golden hamster and Pirital virus (a nonpathogenic clade A arenavirus) has been shown to be a model to mimic clinical virologic and pathologic changes observed with Lassa fever in humans.[128]

DIAGNOSIS

Differential Diagnosis

Differential diagnosis of Lassa fever should include malaria, typhoid, shigellosis, dengue, and yellow fever. For South American viruses causing hemorrhagic fever, the differential diagnosis includes yellow fever, dengue hemorrhagic fever, hepatitis, leptospirosis, hemorrhagic fever with renal syndrome (caused by hantaviruses), rickettsial diseases, typhoid, sepsis with disseminated intravascular coagulation, and, in the case of CNS involvement, viral encephalitis.

For biosafety reasons, suspected cases must be reported to national laboratories having the expertise and capacity for molecular diagnostics of viral hemorrhagic fevers together with a procedure for handling and transportation of specimens. Isolation of virus must be attempted in biosafety level 4 laboratory facilities.

Predictive Value

In West Africa, the association of fever, pharyngitis, retrosternal pain, and proteinuria presented a predictive value of 81%. In the endemic area of Argentina, the constellation of asthenia and dizziness accompanied by petechiae and conjunctival congestion has been shown to be indicative for the diagnosis of AHF; the presence of leukopenia, thrombocytopenia, and proteinuria further reinforces the diagnostic suspicion based on clinical findings. The association of a platelet count of less than 100,000/mm^3 and a white blood cell count of less than 2500/mm^3 or less than 4000/mm^3 was reported to have a sensitivity of 87% and 100%, respectively, and a specificity of 88% and 71%, respectively.[66]

Direct Diagnosis

Serum or heparinized plasma should be collected during the acute febrile stages of the disease. The samples should be frozen on dry ice or in liquid nitrogen. Storage at temperatures higher than −40°C will result in the progressive loss of infectivity. Classically achieved by virus isolation, direct diagnosis now may be performed by reverse transcription polymerase chain reaction (RT-PCR) assay, more specifically through real-time RT-PCR. Isolation of the virus is achieved readily in cell culture; Vero cells are a sensitive substrate for such direct diagnosis. Because cytopathic effect is not always observed, arenavirus-infected cells are detected by an immunofluorescence test.

For South American arenaviruses causing hemorrhagic fevers, the delay for isolation on Vero cells is 1 to 5 days, much faster than animal inoculation, which requires 7 to 20 days before illness develops. Serum and throat washings collected 3 to 10 days after onset usually yield virus. Virus is isolated less frequently from urine. Specifically, Machupo virus is recovered from only 20% of acute-phase sera and even less frequently from throat washings or urine. When serum or throat samples are collected within 2 weeks of clinical onset, the level of success in isolating LASV is very high.

Currently there are no commercially available diagnostic assays for LASV, and the limitation of research laboratories in endemic areas makes laboratory diagnosis more difficult. However, when possible, viral RNA can be purified from serum, plasma, urine, throat washings, and tissues and can be used as a target for cDNA synthesis with use of a reverse transcriptase. This cDNA can be amplified by a PCR assay with consensus primers or specific primers. The amplified region finally is sequenced for diagnostic confirmation. RT-PCR–based diagnosis offers the advantages of reducing the delay of response and possessing a greater sensitivity compared with cell culture. Specifically, several protocols using conserved primers have been used. These target the 5′ region of S-RNA. These techniques have been applied successfully to Lassa fever diagnosis, and several of these methods have been validated with large numbers in field isolates of LASV strains.[78] Molecular tests based on the RT-PCR methodology are being developed increasingly for the diagnosis of arenaviral infections.[87] For Junín and Machupo virus infection specifically, this technique is the only one that is early and sensitive enough to detect low viremia encountered during the period in which immune plasma therapy can be used effectively.[85] At the time of admission to the hospital, RT-PCR detected LASV RNA in 79% of patients; for comparison, in these patients, immunofluorescence assay detected antibodies in only 21%. By the third day of admission, 100% of the patients tested positive by RT-PCR analysis, whereas only 52% tested positive by the immunofluorescence assay.[37] The drawbacks of molecular methods consist mostly of the need for sophisticated equipment to be fully applicable in the field conditions when an outbreak occurs. Although considerable progress has been recently made, and equipment for RNA extraction and real-time PCR is accessible more easily, the Ebola outbreak in West Africa has underlined that the situation is far from optimal.

Additional techniques for direct detection of virus in tissues are being actively developed; they include in situ nucleic acid hybridization techniques. Antigen-detection enzyme-linked immunosorbent assay (ELISA) has been a sensitive tool in a number of patients.

More recently, molecular assays taking advantage of the real-time PCR technology have been reported for the detection of the four South American arenaviruses causing VHF. Apart from assays specific for one virus, a universal clade B PCR assay proved able to detect 5 to 500 $TCID_{50}$ per reaction for Junín, Machupo, Guanarito, and Sabiá viruses and also for Tacaribe, Cupixi, and Amapari viruses.[144] These tests have application to laboratory diagnosis on human specimens but also can be used to detect arenaviruses in rodent tissues. Real-time RT-PCR assays have been recently developed and published.[5,33,45,53,110-112,139,145]

The first quality assurance study on the rapid detection of LASV RNA included 24 participant laboratories from 17 countries; 10-fold dilutions of LASV-inactivated genetic material were detected with success varying from 21% to 85%, depending on the concentration in the sample.[108] Of interest is that specimens containing high concentration of viral RNA may lead to false-negative results by the inhibition of enzymatic reaction, suggesting that clinical specimens should be either spiked with internal control to monitor enzymatic reaction efficacy or tested after dilution.[39,108] A second EQA for LASV detection was organized and showed that molecular diagnosis remains challenging, and that none of the participants used probe-based real-time RT-PCR assay because of the lack of a suitable protocol.[109]

Indirect Diagnosis

Serologic diagnosis is made by demonstration of a fourfold rise in the titer of specific antibody. A high IgG antibody titer or the presence of specific IgM is indicative of a probable case. Nucleocapsid antigens are shared by most of these viruses, and quantitative relationships show the basic split between the viruses of Africa and the Western Hemisphere. Individual viruses immunologically are distinct by neutralization test, which depends on the specificity of epitopes contained in the envelope glycoproteins G1 and G2. Samples collected for serologic diagnosis can be kept at −20°C. Blood obtained in early convalescence may be infectious despite the presence of antibodies and should be handled accordingly. Antibodies often are detected by indirect immunofluorescence because it is an inexpensive, rapid, and sensitive test. An alternative is ELISA, the specificity of which is greater than and the sensitivity of which is on the level of the neutralization test. ELISA is therefore the test of choice for differentiation of viral strains of arenaviruses, for confirmation of unexpected results, and for detection of infection from the distant past. All these tests have been tested in the conditions of an outbreak and shown to be effective.

Antibodies specific to South American arenaviruses appear 12 to 30 days after onset, which often correlates with clinical improvement.[117] Traditionally, Lassa fever has been diagnosed using antibody detection assays, including indirect immunofluorescence (IIF) and ELISA. IIF, however, has many false-positive results, especially for IgM antibodies, which in addition to being false positive, are known to persist for months to years in these settings and are therefore not of much value.[78]

In the case of Lassa fever, antibodies detectable by immunofluorescence appear early and often are present during the acute illness with no apparent relation to viremia or clinical status; 50% of patients with Lassa fever develop IgM or IgG antibody during the first week, and more than 66% do so during the next week. Antigen-detection ELISA in conjunction with IgM-capture ELISA has shown promise for rapid and sensitive diagnosis of Lassa fever. Neutralizing antibodies usually develop only after 4 to 6 months of convalescence.

PROGNOSIS AND TREATMENT

Prognosis

The case-fatality ratio of AHF, which is greater than 15% without specific treatment, drops spectacularly to less than 1% when specific treatment is available.[66] Granulocyte colony-stimulating factor serum level seems to be a marker of severity of the illness.[93]

For Lassa fever, no correlation exists between antibody levels and outcome. Viremia levels in Lassa fever are important in terms of prognostic value; the higher the viral concentration, the higher the mortality rate. The serum aspartate transaminase level also is an accurate prognostic marker; values above 150 U/mL are associated with a 55% mortality rate, whereas the overall mortality rate is approximately 15%.[74]

Treatment

Arenaviral hemorrhagic fever should be managed by monitoring and correction of fluid, electrolyte, and osmotic imbalances and of metabolic acidosis. Hydration should be administered cautiously because of generalized capillary leak and the possibility of precipitating pulmonary edema. If possible, bleeding should be treated with clotting factor and platelet replacement as guided by laboratory test results.

For Junín virus infection, immune serum therapy is effective in reducing the incidence of mortality when it is given within the first 8 days of illness.[42,43,91] Experimental evidence suggests that the plasma may work through attacking infected cells as well as viral neutralization. In approximately 10% of patients with AHF due to Junín virus who are treated with immune plasma develop an entity called "late neurologic syndrome," with symptoms that include fever, cerebellar signs, and cranial nerve palsies. These clinical signs are transient; they are thought to be related to immunopathologic mechanisms induced by the treatment with convalescent plasma. Surprisingly, this late neurologic syndrome has not been noted in patients with AHF who recover without administration of immune plasma therapy.[78]

Despite the recognized efficacy of convalescent plasma for treatment of Machupo virus infection, the paucity of survivors and the lack of programs for collection and storage of BHF immune plasma anticipate the problem of shortage in case of a new outbreak. In recent cases, ribavirin was offered to two patients presenting with life-threatening infection; both recovered without sequelae. These promising results suggest the need for performing more extensive clinical studies to assess the usefulness of ribavirin for treatment of BHF.[79]

Junín and Guanarito viruses showed very high in vitro sensitivity to ribavirin, which also showed antiviral effect in patients.[43,44] One of the laboratory-acquired Sabiá virus infections was treated successfully with ribavirin; the treatment was started early after onset, and there was no production of neutralizing antibodies.

The late evolution and low titers of LASV neutralizing antibodies render immune serum–based therapy less efficient than in treatment of South American arenaviral fevers.[95] In contrast, clinical studies have shown ribavirin to be of benefit in severe cases and that it therefore should be used as early as possible in the course of the disease. Ribavirin, a guanosine analogue, has broad-spectrum antiviral activity and, if given within the first 6 days of onset of symptoms, has been shown to decrease the mortality of severe Lassa fever from 55% to 5%. Oral ribavirin has also been used but is less effective than the intravenous form because it can take 2 to 4 weeks of administration to achieve steady-state levels.[6] The intravenous regimen that is recommended for treatment of LASV is as follows:

- A loading dose of 30 mg/kg, then
- 15 mg/kg every 6 hours for 4 days, then
- 7.5 mg/kg every 8 hours for 6 days.

A well-recognized side effect of ribavirin is hemolytic anemia, which is reversible when drug administration is interrupted. It is also important to note that the half-life of ribavirin is about 24 hours. The large volume of distribution indicates that the drug will still have an effect long after cessation. The mechanism of action of ribavirin consists of interference of RNA capping, RNA polymerase inhibition, and lethal mutagenesis.[6]

Postexposure prophylaxis (PEP) with oral ribavirin has also been discussed. Patients who had a definitive high-risk exposure—including (1) penetration of skin by a contaminated sharp instrument, (2) contamination of mucous membranes or broken skin with blood or bodily secretions, (3) participation in emergency procedures, or (4) prolonged and continuous contact in an enclosed space without appropriate use of personal protective equipment—may all be examples of when ribavirin PEP is indicated. The following oral regimen for adults has been proposed:

- Ribavirin 35 mg/kg loading dose (max: 2.5 g), followed by
- Ribavirin 15 mg/kg by mouth 3 times per day for 10 days.[6]

There are many other experimental antiviral drugs that have been tested in vitro or even in small animal models for activity against LASV, but none have progressed into clinical trials for Lassa fever. One particular drug is favipiravir (T-705), which is an RNA polymerase inhibitor that has also been studied for its effectiveness in the recent Ebola epidemic.[78]

The Future of Antivirals in the Domain of Arenaviruses

In the past 5 years, basic research has used reverse genetics to develop replicons and infectious clones that are used to investigate virus replication mechanisms, to test antivirals in vitro, and to better understand arenavirus cycles. The development of reverse genetic systems allows detailed molecular characterization of the viral *cis*-acting signals and *trans*-acting factors that control each of the steps of the virus cycle, including RNA synthesis, packaging, and budding. Likewise, the ability to generate predetermined specific mutations in the genome and to analyze their phenotypic expression will contribute to elucidation of the arenavirus-host interactions as well as the mechanisms leading to severe hemorrhagic disease in humans. The development of a mini-replicon system for LASV will help the investigation of replication and transcription and may facilitate the testing of antivirals outside biosafety level 4 laboratories.[67]

Infectious LCM virus has been recovered entirely from cDNA. Intracellular transcription from polymerase I–driven vectors and co-expression of the minimal viral *trans*-acting factors NP and L from polymerase II–driven plasmids resulted in the efficient formation of infectious virus with genetic tags in both genome segments; this cDNA-derived virus behaves identically to wild-type virus in both cell culture and infected mice.[49]

High-throughput screening of molecules for their antiviral effects is being performed increasingly by both public laboratories and private companies. From 2003 to 2006, seven articles reporting testing of molecules with antiviral efficacy on arenaviruses were published.[1,4,8,19,21,63,140] In recent years research activity in antivirals against these viruses has accelerated.[20,26,81,99,100,107,122,130,141] Unique small molecules have been identified as inhibitors of arenavirus infection. They prevent arenavirus entry and protect against risk of lethal infection in animal models.[78]

PREVENTION AND CONTROL

Prevention of arenavirus disease consists of preventing transmission from rodents to humans, from humans to humans, and from infected specimens to laboratory personnel. It seems that patients pose minimal risk of contagion in early stages of disease. However, as the process continues and viremia increases, the opportunities for spread rise as well. Strategies for avoiding contact between rodents and humans have been effective in BHF.[89] Simple trapping of *C. callosus* in towns was successful in reducing human contact and thus reducing the disease to essentially zero. This is more difficult in AHF because conditions under which human exposure occurs are different from those in BHF. *C. musculinus* (reservoir of Junín virus and AHF) distribution is much wider than that of *C. callosus* (reservoir of Machupo virus and BHF), and Argentine agricultural practices continue to place workers at risk for exposure to reservoir hosts.

A collaborative effort conducted by the United States and Argentine governments led to the production of a live attenuated Junín virus vaccine named Candid #1, which has passed safety and immunogenicity tests in U.S. volunteers. Its efficacy was established in a double-blind trial in 15,000 agricultural workers at risk for natural infection in Argentina. Subsequently, more than 100,000 persons were immunized with Junín virus vaccine in Argentina. Currently the vaccine is approved in Argentina for adults older than 15 years of age.[78] Animal protection studies suggest that the Junín vaccine could be protective against Machupo virus infections as well. A prospective study conducted during two epidemic seasons among 6500 male agricultural workers in Argentina showed that Candid #1 vaccine efficacy was 84% or higher and that no serious adverse effects could be expected.[92]

Neutralizing antibody titers to Candid #1 vaccine against AHF were studied for 2 years after vaccination in 330 volunteers. Of a total of 160 volunteers who received Candid #1, 54 had no detectable preinfection with arenaviruses, 55 had preexisting antibodies to Junín virus, and 51 had preexisting antibodies to LCM virus; the remaining 170 individuals received placebo. Levels of anti-Junín virus antibodies displayed a trend in which titers increased with the virulence of the infecting strain, from Candid #1 through subclinical Junín virus infection, vaccination after subclinical infection, and Junín virus symptomatic infection. The study also demonstrated that the mean titer of neutralizing antibodies to Candid #1 did not vary significantly during the 2 years, was significantly lower than that elicited by wild strains of Junín virus, significantly increased the titers of preexisting anti-Junín antibodies, and was not modified by preexisting anti-LCM virus antibodies.[3]

Comparative sequence analysis of the L RNA segment of Candid 1 strain and the more virulent ancestors (XJ 44 and XJ 13) revealed 12 point mutations in the L polypeptide that are unique to the vaccine strain.[60] Whether these changes are associated with the attenuated phenotype remains to be investigated by the use of reverse genetic systems.

For VHF, no preventive measures have been developed. Attenuated Junín virus strains do not protect experimental animals against challenge with Guanarito virus. In VHF, the evidence suggests that transmission occurs around houses and in fields as in BHF, so measures to avoid contact between rodents and humans should be effective, as shown for BHF.

For Lassa fever, reducing the contact with *Mastomys natalensis* is a formidable task in West Africa, and this option does not seem to have a promising future. Because person-to-person transmission has been reported in Lassa fever, precautions should be taken to place patients in single rooms. The health care team should be small and adequately trained; they should wear appropriate personal protective equipment including gloves, gowns, and filter masks.[22,24,25] All secretions should be decontaminated.[84] Laboratory procedures should be performed with care by use of inactivating methods of heat, chemicals, or irradiation.

In rhesus monkeys (*Cercopithecus aethiops*), the humoral antibody response measured after they were challenged with purified inactivated LASV, although as high as in humans who recovered from Lassa fever, was insufficient to protect the animals from a fatal outcome.[96] A naturally attenuated strain (Mopeia virus, from Mozambique) protects rhesus monkeys against challenge with LASV, but field studies are required to establish the extent and nature of natural human infection with this virus before it can be considered seriously as a candidate for human vaccine development. Alternative approaches, including the use of vaccinia virus vectors bearing the LASV GPC or N gene, are being investigated actively and show promising preliminary results.[46,47] Two peptides encoded by the glycoprotein precursor were shown to display high-affinity binding to human leukocyte antigen (HLA)-A*0201 transgenic mice; mice immunized with these peptides were protected against challenge with a recombinant vaccinia virus that expressed LASV glycoproteins. These two epitopes represent candidates for inclusion in epitope-based vaccine constructs.[9]

The Future of Vaccine Research

Although there is currently no licensed vaccine against LASV, in recent years tremendous advances have been made toward vaccine development.[10,34,41,59,62,80] Many different approaches were used. Reverse genetic exchange of the viral glycoprotein for foreign glycoproteins created attenuated vaccine strains that remained viable although unable to cause disease in infected mice; this phenotype remained stable even after extensive propagation in immunodeficient hosts. The engineered viruses induced T-cell–mediated immunity, protecting against systemic infection and severe liver disease on wild-type virus challenge.[7] The yellow fever vaccine 17D has been used as a vector for the LASV glycoprotein precursor, resulting in construction of recombinant virus, which was replication competent and processed LASV glycoprotein in cell culture. The recombinant virus replicated poorly in guinea pigs but still elicited specific antibodies against Lassa and yellow fever antigens, and single subcutaneous injection protected guinea pigs against fatal Lassa fever.[13] Clone ML29 is a reassortant virus that encodes the nucleocapsid protein and glycoproteins from LASV and the RNA polymerase and matrix protein of Mopeia virus; replication of ML29 was attenuated in guinea pigs and nonhuman primates. Guinea pigs vaccinated with ML29 survived after challenge with LASV without developing either signs of disease or histologic lesions. Rhesus macaques inoculated with clone ML29 developed primary virus-specific T cells capable of secreting interferon in response to homologous and heterologous challenge (the latter with Mopeia virus and LCM virus). Vaccinated monkeys did not present any histologic lesions or signs of disease.[86] Future strategies should focus on continuing the development of human monoclonal antibodies for passive immune therapy for the South American hemorrhagic fevers and to develop antivirals for Lassa fever and Argentine hemorrhagic fever as well. There should also be follow-through with several advanced Lassa fever vaccine candidates.

NEW REFERENCES SINCE THE SEVENTH EDITION

2. Ambrosio A, Saavedra M, Mariani M, et al. Argentine hemorrhagic fever vaccines. *Hum Vaccin.* 2011;7(6):694-700.
5. Atkinson B, Chamberlain J, Dowall SD, et al. Rapid molecular detection of Lujo virus RNA. *J Virol Methods.* 2014;195:170-173.
6. Bausch DG, Hadi CM, Khan SH, et al. Review of the literature and proposed guidelines for the use of oral ribavirin as postexposure prophylaxis for Lassa fever. *Clin Infect Dis.* 2010;51(12):1435-1441.
15. Briggiler A, Sinchi A, Coronel F, et al. [New transmission scenarios of the Argentine hemorrhagic fever since the introduction of the live attenuated Junín virus vaccine (Candid #1): an experience in migrant workers]. *Rev Peru Med Exp Salud Publica.* 2015;32(1):165-171.
33. Das S, Rundell MS, Mirza AH, et al. A multiplex PCR/LDR assay for the simultaneous identification of category A infectious pathogens: Agents of viral hemorrhagic fever and variola virus. *PLoS ONE.* 2015;10(9):e0138484.
45. Fajfr M, Neubauerova V, Pajer P, et al. Detection panel for identification of twelve hemorrhagic viruses using real-time RT-PCR. *Epidemiol Mikrobiol Imunol.* 2014;63(3):238-244.
53. Fukuma A, Kurosaki Y, Morikawa Y, et al. Rapid detection of Lassa virus by reverse transcription-loop-mediated isothermal amplification. *Microbiol Immunol.* 2011;55(1):44-50.
65. Gunther S, Lenz O. Lassa virus. *Crit Rev Clin Lab Sci.* 2004;41(4):339-390.
78. Kerber R, Reindl S, Romanowski V, et al. Research efforts to control highly pathogenic arenaviruses: a summary of the progress and gaps. *J Clin Virol.* 2015;64:120-127.
106. Moraz ML, Kunz S. Pathogenesis of arenavirus hemorrhagic fevers. *Expert Rev Anti Infect Ther.* 2011;9(1):49-59.
109. Nikisins S, Rieger T, Patel P, et al. International external quality assessment study for molecular detection of Lassa virus. *PLoS Negl Trop Dis.* 2015;9(5):e0003793.
111. Olschlager S, Lelke M, Emmerich P, et al. Improved detection of Lassa virus by reverse transcription-PCR targeting the 5′ region of S RNA. *J Clin Microbiol.* 2010;48(6):2009-2013.
118. Pfau C. Arenaviruses. In: Baron S, ed. *Medical Microbiology.* 4th ed. Galveston: University of Texas Medical Branch at Galveston; 1996.
119. Pigott DM, Golding N, Mylne A, et al. Mapping the zoonotic niche of Marburg virus disease in Africa. *Trans R Soc Trop Med Hyg.* 2015;109(6):366-378.
121. Radoshitzky SR, Bao Y, Buchmeier MJ, et al. Past, present, and future of arenavirus taxonomy. *Arch Virol.* 2015;160(7):1851-1874.
127. Sayler KA, Barbet AF, Chamberlain C, et al. Isolation of Tacaribe virus, a Caribbean arenavirus, from host-seeking Amblyomma americanum ticks in Florida. *PLoS ONE.* 2014;9(12):e115769.
131. Shao J, Liang Y, Ly H. Human hemorrhagic fever causing arenaviruses: molecular mechanisms contributing to virus virulence and disease pathogenesis. *Pathogens.* 2015;4(2):283-306.
148. World Health Organization. Lassa Fever Fact Sheet. http://www.who.int/mediacentre/factsheets/fs179/en/.
149. Zhou X, Ramachandran S, Mann M, et al. Role of lymphocytic choriomeningitis virus (LCMV) in understanding viral immunology: past, present and future. *Viruses.* 2012;4(11):2650-2669.

The full reference list for this chapter is available at ExpertConsult.com.

187 Filoviral Hemorrhagic Fever: Marburg and Ebola Virus Fevers

Amy S. Arrington • David Hilmers • Judith R. Campbell • Gail J. Harrison

I came to understand firsthand what my own patients had suffered.... I was isolated from my family and I was unsure if I would ever see them again. Even though I knew most of my caretakers, I could see nothing but their eyes through their protective goggles.

Dr. Kent Brantly, medical missionary, Ebola survivor, Senate Hearing on Ebola Outbreak, September 16, 2014

Hemorrhagic fevers due to Marburg and Ebola viruses, are among the most virulent infections known to mankind.[47] Ebola virus disease (EVD) and outbreaks are associated with high attack rates and substantial mortality and until recently were only encountered by those in remote, rural areas of sub-Saharan Africa or maximum security infectious disease laboratories such as the US Army Medical Research Institute of Infectious Diseases (USAMRIID). For decades these pathogens were studied at institutions such as USAMRIID because of the biohazard of Marburg and Ebola viruses and their potential use as biologic weapons.[21,135] On the other extreme, the public, mostly unaware of this exotic disease, became familiar with this rare infection through novels such as Richard Preston's *The Hot Zone*, which vividly described the devastating effects of this disease.[140] In 2014, this drastically changed. The impact of viral hemorrhagic fever, specifically due to Ebola virus, became known to people worldwide. Scientists, health care workers, public health officials, politicians, and the general public became familiar with this rare but devastating infection. Viral hemorrhagic fever is actually caused by viruses from four diverse viral families: Arenaviridae, Bunyaviridae, Flaviviridae, and Filoviridae. *Ebolavirus* and *Marburgvirus* are the only genera of the family Filoviridae, which belongs to the order Mononegavirales.[44] Human outbreaks of acute hemorrhagic fever caused by these viruses are associated with case fatality rates of up to 88%. The outbreak of 2014 demonstrated the high potential for large-scale dissemination, high rates of mortality, potential for major public health effects, public panic, social disruption, and necessity for special preparedness globally. Furthermore, this most recent Ebola outbreak exposed gaps in infrastructure and processes for global public health emergencies.[55] *Ebolavirus* and *Marburgvirus* are classified as Biohazard Level 4 and Biothreat Category A agents; thus, they should be manipulated only in maximum-security facilities. Research performed decades earlier at such facilities provided the scientific foundation for diagnostic assays, therapeutic options, and candidate vaccines employed during the 2014 outbreak.[107,60] This established scientific evidence then contributed to an unprecedented rapid review and FDA approval of candidate vaccines and therapeutic agents.[202]

ETIOLOGIC AGENTS

The *filovirus* family consists of three different genera, *Ebolavirus, Marburgvirus,* and *Cuevavirus.* Although all members of this family cause highly lethal viral hemorrhagic fevers, Ebola virus has proven to be a pathogen capable of large-scale human morbidity and mortality, with mortality rates ranging from 30% to 90%. The most recent Ebola virus epidemic in 2014–15 affecting West Africa and beyond has reminded us of the virulence of these agents, as well as provided new knowledge regarding the pathogenesis and potential treatments for this biologic threat.

Members of the Filoviridae all have similar morphologic features. The viral particles are filamentary and often form bizarre configurations, such as "6"-shaped forms and hairpins (Fig. 187.1), and may be up to 14,000 nm in length.[44,148] In contrast, the filaments are always 80 nm wide. The capsid contains a single negative-stranded RNA genome that encodes seven structural proteins and one nonstructural protein, the soluble glycoprotein.[149,184,183] Members of the Filoviridae family are enveloped, nonsegmented, single-stranded negative-sense long (~19 kb) RNA genomes with a uniform 80-nm diameter. They contain seven sequentially arranged genes and are distinguished by virions that are a characteristically filamentous shape (see Fig. 187.1). Filoviruses replicate readily in Vero, MA-104, or SW-13 cell cultures, all of which are derived from primates. These viruses are highly pathogenic for macaques. To date, there are seven designated species within the three genera in the Filoviridae family, with eight identified viruses (Table 187.1). Of these eight viruses, six are known to cause disease in humans, with Zaire Ebola virus being the virus responsible for the largest outbreak yet in the world, with more than 28,000 cases and more than 11,000 deaths to date (Centers for Disease Control and Prevention [CDC] case count, 2016). The evolutionary profile of Filoviridae suggests that Marburg virus and Ebola virus represent distinct filovirus lineages. Within the species of Ebola virus, there is a high degree of genetic stability, indicating a high level of fitness adapted to their respective niches.

Lloviu virus, obtained from bats in Spain (2002), is the only known virus in the Cuevavirus family, and its potential to cause human infections remains undetermined as no virus has yet been isolated.[128] This review is therefore limited to Ebola virus and Marburg virus.

Virtually no antigenic relationship exists between Marburg virus and any of the Ebola virus species. Virus neutralization has been virtually impossible to measure for any of the filoviruses, which has hindered epidemiologic and ecologic studies of these agents. Only the three African Ebola virus species appear to be pathogenic for humans. Interestingly, these strains are also the only Ebola species originating and circulating in Africa. Unlike these three Ebola species, *Reston Ebola virus* is found only in the Philippines among nonhuman primates, and although antibodies to Reston Ebola virus has been detected in those exposed, it has not been found to cause disease in humans.[72] These four Ebola virus species exhibit extensive cross reactivity in immunofluorescence methods and enzyme-linked immunosorbent assays (ELISAs). Filoviruses are classified as biosafety level 4 agents (BSL-4), based on their easy person-to-person transmission, high mortality rate, and lack of approved vaccine or drug therapies (www.cdc.gov/ncezid/dhcpp/vspb/).[80,208]

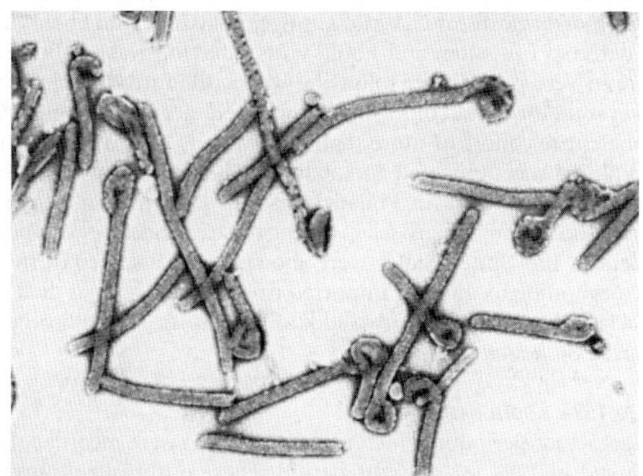

FIG. 187.1 Electron micrograph of Ebola virus (magnification ×38,750). (Courtesy T.W. Geisbert.)

HISTORY AND EPIDEMIOLOGY

Marburg Virus

Marburg hemorrhagic fever was first described after concurrent outbreaks of this unusual, severe infection among laboratory workers in Marburg and Frankfurt, Germany, and Belgrade, Yugoslavia, in 1967 (see Table 187.1).[117,115,160,199] Seven of 31 patients died, and the source was determined to be African green monkeys (*Cercopithecus aethiops*) that had been exported from Uganda and shipped to laboratories in all three locations. The etiologic agent was isolated, characterized, and identified by scientists in Marburg and Hamburg and later named *Marburg virus* after the city with the most cases.[1,2] For decades sporadic outbreaks of Marburg occurred in rural villages in several African countries including Kenya, Democratic Republic of the Congo (formerly known as Zaire), and Angola. Civil war and political unrest hindered detailed characterization of these outbreaks other than the notably high case fatality rates.[57,156]

A lengthy outbreak occurred between 1998 and 2000 in Durba (eastern Democratic Republic of the Congo), affecting 154 people and killing 83% of victims (Fig. 187.2).[13] Most patients (94%) worked in underground gold mines. Because of the civil war raging in 1997, the cause of the outbreak was not identified until 1999, a year after the first cases occurred. The Durba outbreak was characterized by the circulation of multiple viral strains, pointing to several independent introductions from the unknown natural reservoir.[12,13] The largest recorded Marburg outbreak occurred in Uige Province of northern Angola. It was the first recorded outbreak in the west side of Africa and lasted from October 2004 to July 2005, causing 252 cases and 227 deaths (fatality rate, 90%).[26,199] Complete genomic characterization showed that the culprit strain, named *Angola marburgvirus,* was closely related to previous East African isolates.[171,172,176,183-186,196-198] In 2007, a small outbreak of Marburg hemorrhagic fever among mine workers in Kamwenge District of Uganda was reported. In 2008, two cases of Marburg hemorrhagic fever occurred in tourists who visited the Python Cave, a bat cave in Queen Elizabeth National Park in western Uganda.[199] One of these had a rapidly fatal disease. The last reported outbreak of Marburg occurred in Uganda in 2012 during which there were 26 confirmed or probable cases and 15 (58%) fatalities. In November 2014 there was a single confirmed, fatal case of Marburg hemorrhagic fever in Kampala, Uganda. Investigation of 197 contacts and testing of 8 suspect cases were all negative.[190] The Viral Special Pathogens Branch of the CDC hosts a web page with archived and current outbreak postings, case counts, and location lists of viral hemorrhagic fevers (www.cdc.gov/vhf/marburg/outbreaks/index.html) reported from around the world.

Confirmed cases of Marburg hemorrhagic fever have been sporadically reported in Uganda, Zimbabwe, the Democratic Republic of the Congo, Kenya, and Angola. It characteristically occurs in outbreaks. However, cases of Marburg hemorrhagic fever outside of Africa have been reported infrequently, in laboratory workers and travelers. The emergence of the other filoviral cause of hemorrhagic fever, *Ebola virus,* has surpassed Marburg in the regional and global impact.

Ebola Virus

1976 to 1979: First Recorded Ebola Outbreaks

Ebola first emerged in the form of two nearly simultaneous outbreaks in 1976, one caused by *Sudan ebolavirus* and the other by *Zaire ebolavirus.* The first outbreak was due to *Sudan ebolavirus* and occurred in Sudan, near the border with the Democratic Republic of the Congo, mainly affecting the towns of Nzara and Maridi.[126,157] The first cases were reported among cotton factory workers, but spread to household contacts and

TABLE 187.1 Year and Location of Filoviral Hemorrhagic Fever Cases and Outbreaks

Year	Virus Species	Country	No. of Human Cases	Fatality Rate (%)
1967	Marburg	Germany and Serbia	31	23
1975	Marburg	South Africa	3	33
1976	Zaire Ebola	Zaire	318	88
1976	Sudan Ebola	Sudan	284	53
1976	Sudan Ebola	England	1	0
1979	Sudan Ebola	Sudan	34	65
1980	Marburg	Kenya	2	50
1987	Marburg	Kenya	1	100
1989	Reston Ebola[a]	United States	0	0
1990	Reston Ebola[a]	United States	0	0
1992	Reston Ebola[a]	Italy	0	0
1994	Marburg	DRC[b]	11	Unknown
1994	Zaire Ebola	Gabon	52	60
1994	Tai Forest Ebola	Ivory Coast	1	0
1995	Zaire Ebola	DRC[b]	315	82
1996	Zaire Ebola	Gabon	37	57
1996	Zaire Ebola	Gabon	60	75
1996	Zaire Ebola	South Africa	1	100
1996	Reston Ebola[a]	United States	0	0
1996	Reston Ebola[a]	Philippines	0	0
1998-2000	Marburg	DRC[b]	154	83
2000	Sudan Ebola	Uganda	425	53
2004-2005	Marburg	Angola	374	80
2007	Marburg	Uganda	4	20
2008	Marburg	Netherlands by way of Uganda	2	50
2008	Marburg	United States by way of Uganda	1	0
2008	Ebola-Reston[†]	Philippines	6	0
2011	Ebola	Uganda	1	1
2012	Ebola	Uganda	24	17
2012	Marburg	Uganda	23	65
2012	Ebola	DRC[b]	35	12
2014- 2016	Zaire Ebola	Sierra Leone, Liberia, Nigeria, Senegal, Spain, United States, Mali, United Kingdom, Italy	28, 652	40
2017	Zaire Ebola	DRC	29	10[c]

DRC, Democratic Republic of Congo, formerly was known as Zaire.
[a]Symptomatic infections and fatal cases were observed in nonhuman primates only.
[b]New strain detected in swine with asymptomatic transmission to humans.
[c]As of May 2017.

health workers who cared for them during their illness. The outbreak spread from Nzara to Maridi through exposed persons who were incubating this infection and were later hospitalized in Maridi. Hospitalization of these cases resulted in transmission within the hospital in Maridi and then throughout the township among close contacts of those sick and dying of Ebola. The disease in Maridi was particularly amplified because of transmission in the very large and busy hospital due to use of nonsterile needles and syringes.[90] The outbreak had 284 cases, and the mortality rate was 53%, a proportion characteristic of *Sudan ebolavirus* infection. The outbreak due to *Zaire ebolavirus* occurred in the Democratic Republic of the Congo, near the border with Sudan, 2 months later.[90] The epicenter was Yambuku, about 800 km from Nzara. This previously unknown disease was named for the river Ebola, which flows past Yambuku. The initial cases were people who had received recent injections at an outpatient clinic; many were women attending prenatal and outpatient clinics. In this outbreak the majority of cases were thought to be due to reuse of nonsterile needles and syringes, although close contact with those dying of Ebola was also associated with secondary cases. There were 318 cases, and the mortality rate was 89%, characteristic of *Zaire ebolavirus* infection. Later, an unconfirmed lethal case was reported involving a 9-year-old girl living in Tandala, Democratic Republic of Congo,[61,76] followed by another *Sudan ebolavirus* outbreak in 1979, again in Nzara, with 34 cases and 22 deaths.[9]

Reston Ebolavirus

In 1989, it became apparent that Ebola virus is not restricted to Africa. A group of cynomolgus monkeys *(Macaca fascicularis)* from the Philippines, quarantined in a laboratory in Reston, Virginia, developed a lethal hemorrhagic disease.[87] Virions antigenically similar to Ebola virions were detected in tissues, and Ebola virus infection was confirmed by culture in Vero cells. In the following weeks, the introduction of new monkeys and the spread of the infection to several animal rooms meant that the entire cohort of more than 400 animals had to be destroyed. The building was fumigated and abandoned. The virus was recovered from another macaque in Philadelphia and later in a laboratory in Italy.[134] Although no humans fell ill during these episodes, several monkey handlers in the United States were shown to have seroconverted. In 1996, a cynomolgus monkey imported from the Philippines died in an animal facility in Texas, where two additional cases subsequently occurred, all caused by *Reston ebolavirus.*[145]

1994 to 1997: Ebola Resurgence

After a 15-year period in which no human cases were recorded, Ebola reemerged in 1994 for a 3-year period. These outbreaks occurred in more populated areas of Gabon and Zaire and for the first time in West Africa. This new phase was marked by the identification of a new species, *Ivory Coast,* and by four *Zaire ebolavirus* outbreaks. The only case caused

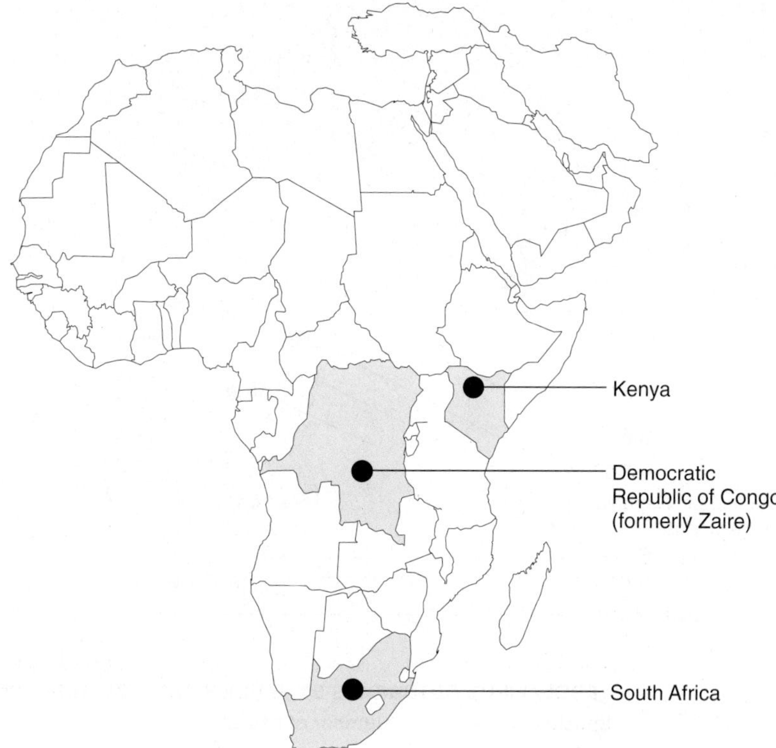

FIG. 187.2 Geographic distribution of human outbreaks of Marburg virus fever in Africa.

by *Ivory Coast ebolavirus* occurred in 1994, when an ethnologist was sickened a few days after performing an autopsy on a chimpanzee found dead in Tai National Park in Ivory Coast.[51,105,106] A large outbreak then occurred in 1995, in and around the town of Kikwit in the southern Democratic Republic of Congo,[133] with 315 cases and a mortality rate of 81%. Despite the deployment of more sophisticated scientific and medical resources than were available in 1976, this outbreak was as large as the 1976 one, probably because it affected a town of several hundred thousand inhabitants and person-to-person transmission occurred mainly in two hospitals. Three other outbreaks, all from *Zaire ebolavirus,* struck northeast Gabon between 1996 and 1997.[68] The first occurred in northeastern Gabon, close to the border with Cameroon,[3] in three gold-digger camps located in the heart of the forest. Some of the victims left the camps for the nearest hospital, located in Makokou, where they infected other patients and caused a second wave of virus dissemination. In total, 49 clinical cases and 29 deaths were recorded. The second outbreak hit the village of Mayibout, located south of Mekouka.[68] The first victims were 18 children who had helped carry and butcher a chimpanzee carcass found in the forest. These 18 children infected their families and friends, who in turn transmitted the disease to neighboring villages. In total, this outbreak involved 31 people and caused 21 deaths. The third outbreak in this region occurred between October 1996 and March 1997.[68] It started among hunters, who infected a traditional healer, his assistant, and some of his patients, who in turn transmitted the disease to several towns and villages in Gabon. Fifteen cases and 11 deaths were recorded in Libreville, and a South African nurse was infected by a Gabonese physician who had traveled to Johannesburg. This outbreak, with 60 cases and 45 deaths occurring in a 6-month period, was noteworthy for its wide geographic range. Although sporadic, these outbreaks in the 20th century provided a basic understanding about the epidemiology, pathogenesis, treatment, and complications of this rare and deadly infection.[151]

2000 to 2004: Geographic Pattern of Zaire Ebolavirus and Sudan Ebolavirus Resurgence

Zaire ebolavirus outbreaks. The first outbreak during this period occurred in northeast Gabon and northwest Democratic Republic of Congo between October 2001 and May 2002.[111] It spread along the main road between Mekambo (Gabon) and Mbomo (Democratic Republic of Congo) and, in fact, involved several independent epidemic chains of human-human transmission with different source animals.[110] These epidemic chains started when local hunters found and manipulated the carcasses of an antelope, chimpanzees, and gorillas. Simultaneously, a second outbreak occurred in the Democratic Republic of Congo, in villages close to the Gabonese border, 200 km south of Mbomo. It then spread to the town of Kelle, about 65 km away. The origin of this outbreak is unknown. The third outbreak also affected the region of Mbomo, between 2002 and 2003.[54] It had two independent sources resulting in two separate chains, one in Mbomo and the other in Kelle. This outbreak involved 143 cases and caused 128 deaths. The fourth outbreak again affected the region of Mbomo, in late 2003; the first cases occurred in Mbanza, a village located about 30 km north of Mbomo. In this outbreak, 35 cases and 29 deaths were recorded.[196] Two years later, in 2005, an outbreak occurred in Etoumbi, 60 km south of Mbomo, where 12 cases and 9 deaths were reported. Simultaneously with the human outbreaks, *Zaire ebolavirus* also infected animals belonging to several species, including gorillas, chimpanzees, and duiker antelopes, probably accounting for the sharp declines in animal populations observed in these regions between 2001 and 2005.[81,110,186]

Sudan ebolavirus outbreaks. Two outbreaks of *Sudan ebolavirus* also occurred during this period (Fig. 187.3). One occurred in Uganda in 2000, causing 173 deaths among its 425 victims (mortality rate, 41%).[196] It was the largest of all recorded *Sudan ebolavirus* outbreaks and comprised three foci, one in the immediate area of Gulu, one in the town of Masindi, and one in Mbarara; of note, the index patient in the Mbarara focus was a soldier. A second *Sudan ebolavirus* outbreak occurred in Sudan in 2004 in the town of Yambio, located only a few dozen kilometers from Nzara and Maridi, which had been sites of Ebola virus outbreaks in 1976 and 1979. In this outbreak, 17 cases and seven deaths occurred.[197]

2007 to 2012: Ebola Outbreaks

In 2007, an outbreak of 264 cases of Ebola hemorrhagic fever caused by *Zaire ebolavirus* species was reported in the Democratic Republic of Congo. In this outbreak, 187 deaths occurred and the mortality rate was 71%. In Uganda in late 2007 and early 2008, 149 cases of Ebola hemorrhagic fever, caused by a new strain, *Ebola Bundibugyo,* was reported from the Bundibugyo District. In this outbreak, 37 deaths occurred, with a mortality rate of 25%. In November 2008, the first known occurrence of *Reston ebolavirus* strain in pigs was reported from the Philippines, with asymptomatic transmission to six human workers (no fatalities) in contact with the pigs.[94,114] In December 2008 through

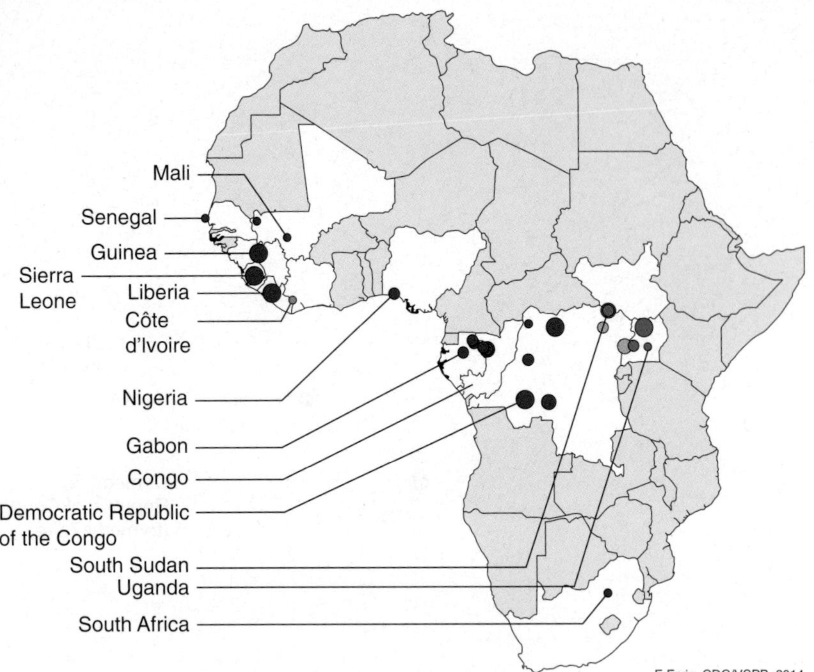

FIG. 187.3 Cases of Ebola Virus Disease in Africa, 1976–2016. (Courtesy Elizabeth Ervin, Centers for Disease Control and Prevention, Viral Special Pathogens Branch, 2014.)

February 2009, 32 human cases of Ebola hemorrhagic fever caused by the *Zaire ebolavirus* strain, resulting in 15 deaths (47% mortality rate), were reported from the Democratic Republic of Congo. In 2011, one case of Ebola hemorrhagic fever was reported from Uganda and quickly contained, with no other known cases from that incident reported. In 2012, Uganda reported an outbreak of Ebola hemorrhagic fever in the Kibaale District with 24 human cases and 17 fatalities, and Democratic Republic of Congo reported 35 confirmed cases of Ebola hemorrhagic fever, 12 of them fatal. The Viral Special Pathogens Branch of the CDC hosts a webpage with archived and current outbreak postings, case counts, and location lists of viral hemorrhagic fevers (www.cdc.gov/vhf/Ebola/outbreaks/2014-west-africa/index.html) reported from around the world.

Largest Ebola Outbreak in History (2014–15)

Previously recorded Ebola outbreaks consisted of seven to 425 cases each and were limited to one or two countries. Even in these resource limited settings transmission was contained. The Ebola epidemic of 2014–15 was unprecedented in several ways. The number of cases in this single epidemic surpassed the total of all previous Ebola epidemics combined (see Table 187.1). Within 6 months of the index case, there were more cases of Ebola than all previous Ebola outbreaks combined, and for the first time in history, the Ebola outbreak was in a capital city.[89] The rapidity with which infection spread through villages, communities, and even to other countries was unprecedented and exposed deficiencies in national health care infrastructures and organizations globally. Although the majority of cases occurred in West Africa, this epidemic had global impact and implications, as cases were diagnosed or treated in seven countries outside of West Africa. Detailed interviews and investigation of events conducted by the World Health Organization (WHO) and other international agencies and institutions significantly expanded our understanding of the epidemiology and pathophysiology of what was previously considered a rare and obscure infection. The rapid spread from Guinea to two other West African countries, Liberia and Sierre Leone, and infections in travelers presented unique challenges yet served as an opportunity to prospectively study this disease. Furthermore, this unprecedented outbreak served as an impetus for global preparedness for responding to highly virulent pathogens. Despite heightened awareness and scientific advances as a result of this epidemic, other aspects of Ebola virus, such as the natural reservoir, best therapeutic interventions, and optimal postexposure prophylaxis, remain uncertain.

Guinea. The index case was a 2-year-old child in the remote Guinean village of Meliandou, Guéckédou. In December 2013, the child had fever, black stools, and vomiting and died 4 days later.[34,167] Several family members, health workers, and those who attended his funeral developed similar symptoms and a rapidly fatal illness. Detailed case tracing in Guinea revealed that family and village caregivers, as well as health care workers in hospitals in Guéckédou and Macenta, were sources for additional cases before the outbreak was recognized. Complete genome sequences from three of these patients early in the epidemic had a high degree of similarity, suggesting a single introduction of the virus into this population.[167] When these sequences were compared to 48 sequences of filoviruses available from GenBank, the Guinean *Zaire ebolavirus* strain was closely related, yet a distinct clade, to strains from DRC and Gabon, and that evolution of the Guinean strain of Ebola virus emerged in parallel with strains from the DRC.[167,70] Potential sources of Ebola virus in the epicenter of the 2014–15 epidemic include fruit bats (*Hypsignathus monstrosus, Epomops franqueti, and Myonycteris torquata)* which are prevalent in this part of West Africa. Studies conducted by Leroy et al sought to identify the source or reservoir of Ebola through trapping primates, bats, birds and small terrestrial vertebrates that were tested for evidence of infection by Ebola virus. Three different bat species had evidence of immunoglobulin G (IgG) specific for Ebola virus detected in serum. Furthermore, viral nucleotide sequences were detected in the liver and spleens of bats and clustered phylogenetically with the Zaire clade.[109] The child thought to be the index case lived near a hollowed-out tree which was a roosting place for fruit bats. Unfortunately, when the epidemiologist investigated this village, the tree had been burned down.[146] Factors that contributed to the unusual rapidity of the spread of this Ebola epidemic included: delay in early recognition and reporting of the outbreak, the crowded, urban setting at the epicenter, villages and cities connected by roads and limited public health resources and facilities in this poverty stricken area of West Africa. By March 2014 Ebola virus was reported for the first time in a West African capital city,

Conakry. From there a large number of transmission of cases occurred in Guinea and throughout the southeastern part of the country. From December, 2013 to December, 2015 there were 3814 suspected, probable or confirmed cases of EVD and 2544 deaths in Guinea. Once Ebola reached Conakry there was a large nosocomial outbreak affecting health care workers at the Hôpital de l'Amitié Sino-Guinéenne. One third of the initial cases at that Ebola treatment unit were health care workers. The other groups most often infected were household members of confirmed cases and burial workers. The observed mortality in Conakry was reported to be 43%.[5] On December 29, 2015, WHO declared Guinea free of Ebola virus transmission after 42 days (two incubation periods) had passed since the last Ebola patient tested negative.[27,200] Unfortunately, recent cases have been reported in Guinea. In this report sexual exposure to an EVD survivor was the only epidemiologic link to the new case. At the time, there were no other EVD cases in Guinea. Ebola virus RNA was detected in seminal fluid of the survivor 531 days after onset of disease and was genetically identical to that of the new case, his sexual partner. This report highlights the fact that Ebola virus remains viable and infectious during the long-term persistence.[17]

Ebola spread rapidly to other countries within 3 months of the index case. Transmission to neighboring countries was fueled in part by interconnection of these communities and villages with access across open borders via roads and pathways in even the most rural areas. In addition, within these communities some who had been exposed to Ebola in Guinea sought medical care in Liberia and Sierra Leone. People in these three countries often travel across the borders to visit family or seek care from traditional healers. Some had attended funerals in Guinea and then returned to Liberia and Sierra Leone incubating Ebola. It was not until March 2014 that the Ministry of Health of Guinea notified WHO of a rapidly evolving outbreak of Ebola virus disease in Guekedou, Macenta, Nzerekore, and Kissidougou districts, forested areas south of eastern Guinea and the capital Conakry. After this notification, neighboring countries were alerted, but the virus had already been introduced into the populations of Liberia and Sierra Leone.[34,192]

Liberia. In March 2014, Liberia was alerted of the EVD outbreak in neighboring country of Guinea. The first cases of EVD in Liberia occurred 1 week after reports of EVD in Guinea.[170] There were 20 suspected cases reported and thought to be contained in Lofa and Margivi counties. Months later in May 2014, cases reemerged and rapidly spread to the capital city, Monrovia, by June 2014 and throughout the country by September 2014. Between March 2014 and January 2016, when Liberia was declared Ebola free, there were 10,678 suspected, probable, or confirmed cases of EVD and 4810 deaths. Core interventions from local government and international entities included the building of treatment centers, implementation of local communication and social mobilization, case management and surveillance, and hygienic measures. The decline in the number of cases coincided with community leadership in control efforts and changing of beliefs and burial practices in the population.[93]

Sierra Leone. The coastal country of Sierra Leone shares national borders with Guinea to the north and east and Liberia to the south and is connected to Monrovia by roads and rivers. The first case of EVD in Sierra Leone was on May 25, 2014.[34,200] These initial cases were detected soon after introduction into the country because of a clinical research program on Lassa hemorrhagic fever at the Kenema Government Hospital. This hospital, being in close proximity to the epicenter of the Ebola outbreak in Guinea, had mobilized and established surveillance and diagnostic capabilities given the existing hemorrhagic fever program. Investigation of the first case in Sierra Leone revealed an epidemiologic link between this cases and the burial of a traditional healer who had treated several EVD patients from Guinea. Genomic sequencing of 78 cases in Sierra Leone was compared with that of three Guinean samples and suggested that two genetically distinct viruses from Guinea had been introduced into Sierra Leone.[70] The Lassa fever research program at Kenema Government Hospital provided infrastructure for clinical and laboratory evaluation for EVD for cases early in the epidemic in Sierra Leone.[151] Observations from this site described clinical features and complications associated with the 2014 outbreak. Sierra Leone was initially declared free of Ebola in November 2015. However, two new confirmed cases were reported in January 2016.

Ebola outside West Africa. Another unprecedented feature of the Ebola epidemic of 2014 was the introduction of Ebola into seven countries outside of West Africa from travelers or expatriate health care workers who had exposure to EVD while working in Ebola treatment units. Although most cases of EVD occurred within three countries in West Africa (Guinea, Liberia, and Sierra Leone), 36 cases and 15 deaths occurred in other African countries (Nigeria, Senegal, and Mali), Europe (Italy, Spain, and the United Kingdom) and the United States.[200]

The Nigeria EVD outbreak began on July 20, 2014, when a traveler from Liberia arrived in Lagos, Nigeria, and sought care for fever and body weakness. Although he denied exposure to a known EVD case or funeral attendance, his condition worsened, and on the third hospital day EVD was suspected and confirmed by PCR testing 2 days later. This index case transmitted Ebola to 13 first-generation contacts. Disease was spread to another large city, Port Hartcourt, by one of these contacts, who traveled against medical advice and subsequently exposed three other individuals.[49,129] From July to September 2014, there were 20 cases (eight fatal) in Nigeria. Although Lagos is the most populous city in Africa, the rapid deployment of epidemiologists, existing laboratory capacity, an established health care system led to an effective containment. Through aggressive tracing of first, second and third generation contacts of their index case, health officials in Nigeria were able to avoid widespread disease in this populous country.[49,129]

The first laboratory-confirmed case of Ebola in the United States was diagnosed on September 30, 2014, in a Liberian traveler who was incubating the disease when he departed Liberia. He developed symptoms 5 days after arrival in the United States and sought care at a hospital in Dallas, Texas. Investigation by the CDC and local health authorities identified 48 contacts. Of these, 17 were persons with exposure to the patient in the community, 10 were persons who had been transported in the same ambulance that had transported the patient before it was completely cleaned and disinfected, and 21 were health care workers. All underwent direct active monitoring for 21 days. Although none of the community contacts developed disease, two nurses who provided direct patient care to the index case each developed fever and symptoms during this observation period. No secondary cases occurred in the contacts of these two health care workers.[28] These cases prompted detailed review of Ebola preparedness throughout the nation and multifaceted efforts on the local, state, federal, and global level.[56,75] The fourth case of EVD diagnosed in the United States was in late October 2014, when a physician who had worked in an Ebola center in Ebola center in Guéckédou, Guinea, returned to New York City. This case required monitoring of three close contacts and 114 health care personnel, none of whom developed disease.[204]

Additional cases of EVD outside of Africa occurred in Europe. Single cases occurred in Spain, Italy, and the United Kingdom in humanitarian health care workers who had worked in Ebola treatment centers in West Africa and returned to their home country. Given active monitoring for fever and symptoms, all were diagnosed early and isolated. There were no secondary cases reported in Europe.[200]

Latest Outbreak, 2017: Democratic Republic of the Congo

The most recent outbreak of EVD is in the Democratic Republic of the Congo (DRC). Initially, a small cluster of cases was first recognized on April 22, 2017, in the province of Bas Uélé, a remote forested area of the DRC, close to the border with the Central African Republic and some 1400 km northeast of the capital, Kinshasa. On May 9, WHO was first alerted of potential new EVD cases in this region, consisting of patients experiencing symptoms including hematuria, epistaxis, bloody diarrhea, and hematemesis. Rapid reverse-transcription polymerase chain reaction (RT-PCR) testing of samples conducted by the Institut National de Recherche Biomédicale (INRB) in Kinshasa confirmed Ebola Zaire virus. As of May 22, 2017, 29 cases had been confirmed, with three deaths, and more than 400 contacts were being actively monitored. To date, the outbreak is limited to a remote, geographically limited area of the DRC. This is the eighth Ebola outbreak in the DRC since 1976, where the virus was first isolated. The last outbreak of Ebola in the DRC's Boende region was in 2014, resulting in 49 fatalities.[25,195]

Ebola and Marburg Virus Transmission

Animal to Human

The sources of most human outbreaks of viral hemorrhagic fever, including most Marburg outbreaks, the *Zaire ebolavirus* outbreaks that occurred between 1976 and 1997, and all outbreaks of *Sudan ebolavirus,* have not been identified. Prior to 2014, there were 13 recorded outbreaks and two isolated cases of Ebola, totaling about 1850 human cases, and 1300 deaths had struck countries spanning the equatorial forest regions of Africa.[198] In the 2014–15 Ebola epidemic, there were 28,616 human cases and 11,232 deaths that occurred primarily in West Africa. A review of the epidemiologic surveillance during Ebola and Marburg hemorrhagic fever epidemics in Africa over a 15-year period delineated several factors that affected transmission.[1] During rural epidemics, multiple introductions of the virus into the human population through wildlife were observed. In contrast, during epidemics in more urban settings, the introduction of a single case in the community was responsible for epidemics.

Several outbreaks have been firmly linked to infected animal carcasses. The 1967 outbreak of Marburg virus infection in Marburg and Belgrade was linked to the handling of organs and tissues from vervet monkeys imported from Uganda.[115,160] As mentioned before, an ethnologist became infected by *Ivory Coast ebolavirus* in 1994 while performing an autopsy on a chimpanzee.[106] Similarly, the 1996 Mayibout outbreak in Gabon started among children who found and butchered a chimpanzee carcass in the forest.[68] Likewise, the sources of the *Zaire ebolavirus* outbreaks that occurred in the border region of Gabon and Democratic Republic of Congo between 2001 and 2003 are well documented; they all occurred after people handled animal carcasses they had found in the forest (mainly gorillas, chimpanzees, and duikers).[110]

Ebola hemorrhagic fever is thus a zoonotic disease that often is transmitted to humans by direct contact with infected animal carcasses, which are themselves probably infected from the reservoir animal species that harbor the virus, symptomatically or asymptomatically. Since the first recorded human outbreak occurred, many field and laboratory studies have been conducted in attempts to identify Ebola virus reservoir species. Wild animals (vertebrates and invertebrates) were captured in the field, and blood and tissues were used to inoculate Ebola virus-permissive Vero cells. Six field studies, conducted from 1976 to 1995, examined a total of 7000 vertebrates and 30,000 invertebrates, but none was found to harbor Ebola virus.[90,125] Although small Ebola virus nucleotide sequences and Ebola virus-like nucleocapsids were detected in organs of six mice (*Mus musculus* and *Praomys* spp.) and a shrew (*Sylvisorex ollula*) caught in Central African Republic in 1999,[125] no conclusions could be drawn as to their reservoir status.

All attempts at experimental inoculation of rodents, bats, birds, reptiles, mollusks, arthropods, and plants have failed, although some bat species belonging to the genera *Epomophorus* and *Tadarida* developed transient viremia lasting nearly 4 weeks.[166,176] These results did not provide conclusive evidence that bats serve as an Ebola virus reservoir.

Other field collections were conducted during 2002 and 2003 in Gabon and the Republic of Congo, in areas hit by the different outbreaks. A total of 1030 animals were captured, necropsied, and analyzed. The captures and laboratory analyses spanned a period of 4 years. The results showed that three species of fruit bat (*Hypsignathus monstrosus, Epomops franqueti,* and *Myonycteris torquata*) were asymptomatically infected by Ebola virus.[46,109] Indeed, anti-Ebola virus immunoglobulin (Ig)G was detected in the serum of 16 bats (four *Hypsignathus,* eight *Epomops,* and four *Myonycteris*), but no other animal species, including other bat species, were positive. Likewise, Ebola virus nucleotide sequences were detected in the organs of 13 bats (three *Hypsignathus,* five *Epomops,* and five *Myonycteris*). Sequencing of the amplified fragments confirmed they were specific to Ebola virus. Phylogenetic analysis of the sequences by the Bayesian and maximum parsimony methods showed they belonged to the species *Zaire.* Although the virus itself was not isolated, this work provided the first biologic evidence that some fruit bat species harbor Ebola virus. In addition, these findings were in keeping with certain epidemiologic clues from previous outbreaks and with the transient viremia observed in some bat species after experimental challenge. The distribution of the bat species also matched that of the outbreaks. Recent studies implicate the Egyptian fruit bat (*Rousettus aegyptiacus*) as the reservoir host for Marburg virus. This Egyptian fruit bat is a cave-dwelling species widely distributed across Africa and carries the virus asymptomatically.

The most recent Ebola epidemic has added further evidence of the potential role of fruit bats in the transmission of Ebola virus. In Guinea, the epicenter of the 2014–15 epidemic, large fruit bat colonies (*Eidolon helvum, Hypsignathus monstrosus, Mops condylurus*) inhabit the Ziama Biosphere Reserve. Bats were commonly found under roofs of houses in the villages. The house where the index case in the 2014–15 epidemic lived was in one of these villages and was very close to a hollow tree that was inhabited by bats. A field mission in southeastern Guinea in April, 2014 investigated human exposure to bats, bushmeat, and captured local wildlife and bats in the village and neighboring forest. Bat hunting in this village was common practice as a food source. Children often caught bats, and the index case reportedly frequently played in the hollow tree inhabited by a bats. The hollow tree had been burned prior to arrival of the investigation team, and no Ebola virus RNA was detected at the site or in trapped animals in the area.[146]

In 2009, domestic pigs in the Philippines were discovered to host *Reston ebolavirus,* meaning that they might pose a transmission risk to farm, veterinary, and slaughterhouse workers exposed to infected pigs.[10,114] In 2011, domestic pigs in China had evidence of *Reston ebolavirus,* and strains were closely related to the *Reston ebolavirus* variant discovered in domestic pigs the Philippines.[131] Pigs have also been experimentally infected with *Zaire ebolavirus* via respiratory exposure and shown to develop lower respiratory tract disease and shed high titers of Ebola virus. In this animal model it was unclear if spread to naïve animals was from virus contaminating the environment with oronasal secretions or via an aerosol route.[94]

Human to Human

Although the first case of human infection in the 2014 epidemic was probably acquired from an animal, all subsequent cases are likely to have arisen from human-to-human transmission. The main route of transmission in this and in previous outbreaks was direct personal contact with blood or body fluids of a person with symptomatic EVD. In contrast to outbreaks occurring in remote rural villages in Africa, epidemics in more urban settings are due to the introduction of a single case in the community, as was the case in the largest Ebola epidemic ever recorded. In the 2014-2015 Ebola epidemic, phylogenetic analyses of Ebola virus from early cases in Guinea were indistinguishable, yet they were distinctly different from an emerging clade of Ebola virus in DRC during the same time period.[8] Later genetic sequencing from Ebola virus from Conakry suggested three related lineages. Historic outbreaks as well as the most recent outbreak have shown that household exposure is a significant risk factor, especially for those caring for someone ill with Ebola. Of interest, household exposure for children is not as great a risk. This might be because although they lived within the household, young children did not have responsibility for caring for ill family members.[18,35,73,96]

Cultural practices. Cultural practices played a significant role in the ongoing transmission of Ebola in the 2014 Ebola epidemic. Through contact tracing and exposure risks assessment, it was determined that many individuals' only contact with Ebola was attending a funeral of someone who died of the disease. Titers of Ebola virus are very high at time of death, and risk of transmission is great with direct physical contact with an infected person or their body fluids during the later stages of illness or after death. Contact with the bodies and fluids of persons who have died of Ebola is especially common in West Africa, where family and community members often touch and wash the body of the deceased in preparation for funerals. These cultural practices were shown to be a route of Ebola transmission in the 2014 epidemic. As an example, an investigation of a cluster of cases in a remote village of Guinea, the investigation found that 85 confirmed Ebola cases were linked to one traditional funeral ceremony.[31,182]

Health care–Associated. Prior to the 2014 Ebola epidemic Ebola transmission to health care workers was rare.[1] Health care workers are especially at risk for acquiring EVD if proper personal protective equipment (PPE) is not available or is not used appropriately. The most recent epidemic impacted health care workers significantly, with many health care workers dying of the disease.[182] Nosocomial transmission to two health care workers at a hospital in the United States highlighted that the potential for transmission is not limited to resource-limited settings.[28]

Although it was suspected sexual transmission of Ebola virus occurred in cases in the Democratic Republic of the Congo in 1995, the 2014–15 outbreak provided convincing evidence of sexually acquired EVD. Ebola virus is detected in the semen of survivors up to 7 to 9 months after resolution of the acute illness.[181;33] Cases have been reported of EVD in sexual contacts of survivors who had negative blood Ebola virus PCR and after transmission in the community had been eradicated.[29;119]

CLINICAL MANIFESTATIONS

Marburg virus and the four Ebola virus species all cause severe, usually fatal hemorrhagic fever, but they differ in terms of the incubation period, clinical severity, and case fatality rate.[116]

Among the four species of Ebola virus that cause *human* infections, the clinical syndrome may vary significantly, though the majority of all outbreaks in humans are secondary to Zaire Ebola virus, including the 2014–15 outbreak in West Africa. After infection occurs, there is an incubation period ranging from 2 to 21 days (mean, 4-10 days), followed by the onset of fever, malaise, and myalgias. With the abrupt onset of fever, the patient now becomes infectious and capable of spreading the virus. The clinical course then progresses rapidly, followed by multisystem involvement, with severe gastrointestinal symptoms including abdominal pain, nausea, vomiting, and diarrhea leading to severe electrolyte disturbances. Other symptoms include headaches, sore throat, persistent hiccups, and a maculopapular rash. Symptoms rapidly progress to septic shock and resultant multiorgan failure, including renal failure, delirium, severe liver failure, and, in 50% of cases, disseminated intravascular coagulation followed by hemorrhage. Although massive hemorrhage occurs infrequently, it is usually manifested by significant GI bleeding and is typically not the cause of death. Defects in blood coagulation more commonly include mucosal bleeding, bleeding from peripheral IV sites, petechiae, and ecchymoses.[11,120] In the 2014 outbreak, only 19% of patients reported symptoms of unexplained bleeding as compared to previous reports of 50%.[43;151]

The incubation period of Marburg virus fever is almost identical to that of Ebola virus fever; clinical onset also is abrupt, starting with fever, chills, headache, and muscle pain. A week later, some patients develop a maculopapular rash, nausea, vomiting, chest pain, abdominal pain, diarrhea, and sore throat. Clinical status deteriorates gradually, with jaundice, delirium, shock, liver failure, massive hemorrhaging, and multiorgan dysfunction.[23,83,137,159] Although the virus disappears quickly from the bloodstream of survivors, it can persist in the eyes and testicles.[38,117] Marburg virus was recovered from the semen of one patient some weeks after clinical recovery.

Pediatric Patients and 2014 Outbreak

Pediatric patients have typically represented a minority of all patients presenting with suspected or confirmed Ebola virus. The incubation time is usually reduced relative to adults, and the progression of the disease appears to be faster.[193] The case fatality rate in children, especially those younger than 5 years, is quite high, though mortality rates for neonates are reportedly 100%.[96] Major risk factors for infections during the 2014 outbreak in West Africa, such as washing of bodies during ritual burials and direct care of sick relatives, were less likely to occur in children and may partially account for the lower overall incidence of infection in pediatric patients. In some reports children accounted for 10% to 33% of the patients being treated in Ebola Treatment Units (ETUs) (Fig. 187.4).[175] Other authors suggest that there might be underreporting of Ebola virus cases in children as a result of faster progression to death, lower rates of attribution of fever to Ebola, and a lower likelihood of being reported as a contact.[73]

Similar to adults, there is a wide range of symptoms that occur in children infected with Ebola virus. After an incubation of 2 to 21 days, patients usually develop fever, chills, anorexia, headache, and myalgia. A rash is commonly seen. In contrast to adults, children more often present with fever and are less likely to report specific complaints of pain, dyspnea, dysphagia, and hiccups. Although Ebola is designated as a hemorrhagic virus, significant bleeding or bloody diarrhea is seen in a minority of patients. Gastrointestinal involvement predominates after the initial symptomatology, which may include significant diarrhea, emesis, and abdominal pain. It has been suggested that young children are less likely to be able to report such symptoms, which may distort these differences.[40]

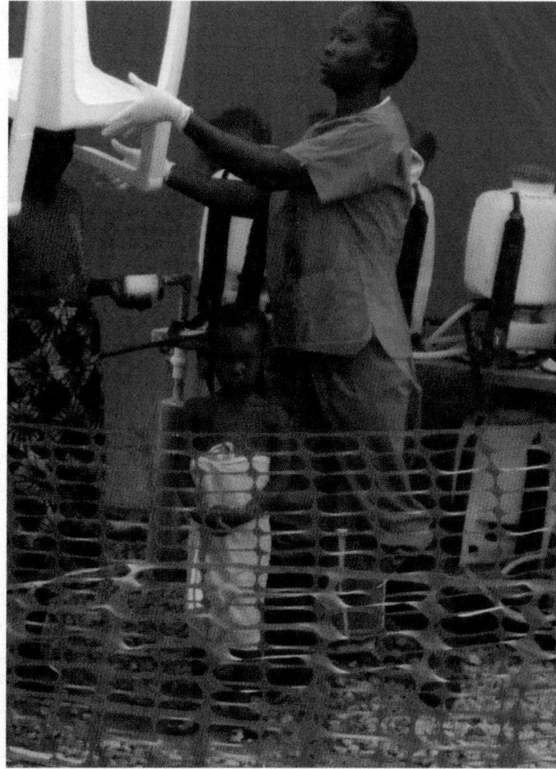

FIG. 187.4 An unidentified little boy, standing outside an Ebola Treatment Unit in Liberia, who was the sole survivor from a family of 12 who died during the Ebola outbreak of 2013–16 in Liberia, Africa. (Photo courtesy Dr. Majid Sidigh.)

Post Ebola Sequelae

Little is understood about how survivors of Ebola virus fare, particularly in regard to long-term sequelae. A "post-Ebola syndrome" has been described and includes prolonged abdominal pain, ocular disease and vision loss, neuropsychiatric issues, significant fatigue, and arthralgias.[191,152] In a recent study evaluating 166 survivors in Sierra Leone, the most common complaints and diagnoses included arthralgia (77%), fatigue (70%), abdominal pain (54%), headache (52%), anemia (50%), and skin disorders (48%). Ocular complications were noted in 56% of survivors, including uveitis.[169] The psychiatric affects are also significant. Survivors are prone to depression and anxiety, posttraumatic stress disorder, and survivor guilt. Mental health facilities and support in West Africa after the 2014–15 outbreak were limited if available at all. Survivors with mental health issues are shunned and rejected from families.[22] The PREVAIL III study in Liberia is an ongoing clinical study that will track more than 1500 Ebola survivors for up to 5 years in an effort to better elucidate the long-term consequences of surviving with Ebola virus.[22] The reports of relapses of disease in patients weeks to months after discharge is concerning not only in regard to patient care, but because of the serious implications that prolonged viral persistence may have for transmission and reinfection. Two significant cases include a 43-year-old physician who recovered from EVD and was subsequently found to have severe unilateral uveitis during convalescence. Ebola virus was detected in the patient's aqueous humor using quantitative RT-PCR, 9 weeks after the clearance of viremia.[179] The second patient was a 39-year-old nurse who had recovered from Ebola virus and had been discharged from the hospital with undetectable Ebola virus RNA in peripheral blood. Nine months after discharge, she developed rapid-onset severe headache, neck pain, photophobia, fever, and vomiting. She was readmitted to the hospital, and lumbar puncture showed high levels of Ebola virus RNA in her cerebrospinal fluid (CSF). The patient was isolated appropriately, and treated with early supportive therapy, as well as antiepileptics, appropriate antibiotics, and GS-5734 (see treatment section, nucleoside analogue). The patient slowly improved and was eventually discharged from the hospital after 52 days of treatment, with only residual weakness of her left leg as well as left-sided deafness.[84] Although the cause of post-Ebola syndrome is likely multifactorial, further research and adequate funding is needed to further elucidate the true scope and improved therapies to offer patients.

PATHOLOGY

With the unprecedented 2014–15 Ebola virus outbreak, more information than ever is now available regarding the pathology of Ebola virus infections in humans. In the past, the largest body of data had existed in experimentally infected rodents and nonhuman primates. Still, why some people recover from filovirus fevers and others die remains unclear.

No major difference exists in the pathogenesis of the different filovirus diseases. Studies of *Zaire ebolavirus* show that dendritic cells and macrophages are the initial host targets at the entry site.[42,63,66] These infected cells then disseminate through the bloodstream and lymphatics to all organs, where they release virions that infect monocytic cells in lymph nodes, spleen, liver, and other organs and tissues.[2] In the later stages of the disease, the virus also infects other cell types, such as hepatocytes, adrenal cortical cells, and endothelial cells, causing lysis and necrosis.[65] Lymphocytes do not seem to be infected, but they nonetheless undergo bystander apoptotic lysis.[61]

The pathogenetic mechanisms of filovirus infection involve both direct damage to infected cells[50,130,164,185] and indirect insults through interactions between the virus and the adaptive immune system.[20,124] By contrast with other viruses, filoviruses can infect and kill a wide variety of cells throughout the body. This apparent lack of target cell specificity may be due to the binding of the viral surface glycoprotein to widely distributed cell surface lectins.[154] Infection of macrophages and dendritic cells can suppress various cellular functions, including the production of proinflammatory mediators such as interferon (IFN)-α, interleukin-1β, and tumor necrosis factor-α (TNF-α),[6,16,71] contributing to the suppression of innate antiviral responses and weakening adaptive immune responses. Studies of serial samples from infected nonhuman primates have shown that lymphocytes undergo apoptosis in vivo, probably through the TNF-related apoptosis-inducing ligand (TRAIL) and FAS pathways.[46,63,61] These findings are compatible with the massive intravascular apoptosis of peripheral monocytic cells observed in patients who died (but not in those who survived) during the 1996 outbreaks in Gabon.[7] This bystander lymphocyte destruction has been suggested to play a major role both in immunosuppression and in the onset of septic shock observed in nonsurvivors.[50] Various studies have shown that filovirus infection of endothelial cells causes their lysis and a loss of vascular integrity, leading to disseminated intravascular coagulation, vascular dysfunction, and finally shock.

DIFFERENTIAL DIAGNOSIS

In the clinical setting, Marburg and Ebola virus fevers must be distinguished from other viral hemorrhagic diseases occurring likely simultaneously in Africa, including Lassa fever and yellow fever, as well as from the many bacterial, rickettsial, and protozoal diseases that can cause similar initial signs and symptoms. The absence of jaundice helps eliminate yellow fever and Rift Valley fever. Because of their prevalence in the population in African countries in particular, it is important to rule out and treat malaria and typhoid fever, but it is still important to realize these may be coinfections. For patients seen outside Africa, the travel history is the most important diagnostic sign available to physicians. Imported cases in travelers have occurred, resulting in significant public health consequences,[15] and the increase in global air travel, the rise of tourism in Africa, and the greater dispersion of military troops increases the possibility for importation of filoviruses to non-endemic areas.[12]

DIAGNOSIS

Early laboratory diagnoses of Ebola virus and Marburg virus infection are based on antigen-capture ELISA, RT-PCR, real-time PCR, and virus isolation.[100,99,101,108,172] These tests are the most accurate tools for diagnosis of acute Ebola virus fever. Later in the course of the disease, or after recovery, diagnosis relies on IgM-capture ELISA or IgG antibody detection. Interestingly, however, in a significant proportion of patients in whom the disease is fatal, specific antibodies do not develop. These diagnostic tools also may be used for oral fluid specimens obtained from clinical patients.[52] Quantitative PCR and viral load of Ebola virus has also been used to monitor patients during the recovery phase of and as a predictor of outcome.[173,30,32,104] During the 2014-2015 Ebola epidemic, the CDC Viral Special Pathogens Branch set up a molecular diagnostic laboratory in Sierra Leone and tested paired blood and oral swab specimens obtained from living patients in the Médecins Sans Frontières Ebola treatment center in Bo, Sierra Leone's second largest city. Testing of the oral swab specimens was consistently less sensitive. As in previous outbreaks, swab specimens for detection of Ebola virus was of limited utility except in severely ill patients or corpses.[139,52] These recent field laboratories studies also demonstrated that neither delay from collection to testing nor settings without temperature or humidity controls impaired the sensitivity of the RT-PCR assay. The disadvantage of these RT-PCR assays is the requirement for electrical power, laboratory expertise, and training to perform the assays.[39] Lateral flow immunoassays are point-of-care assays that are designed for use outside of a formal laboratory setting. These assays are activated when a liquid sample is applied to a membrane that contains a specific antibody and then a second antibody with a colored or fluorescent detector creates a visible change when the target antigen is present. During the 2014 outbreak lateral flow immunoassays were studied at several sites. One that was previously developed by the Naval Medical Research Center for Ebola virus detection was studied at the Liberian Institute for Biomedical Research using clinical samples from patients with suspected Ebola virus infection or oral swabs from deceased individuals as part of the Ebola outbreak response. Ebola virus by RT-PCR and laminar flow immunoassay were compared on 527 samples from patients in Liberia. The Ebola virus laminar flow assay results had greater than 95% accuracy for both plasma and oral swabs when compared with RT-PCR.[136] Because large quantities of Ebola virus are present in dermal tissue, skin necropsy with immunohistochemical analysis was previously proposed for postmortem diagnostic confirmation; however, in the most recent outbreak, use of oral swabs and testing by RT-PCR or laminar flow assay was implemented.[206] These specimens are easy to collect, and formalin fixation renders them safe for transport. Skin biopsy testing is not sufficiently sensitive for early diagnosis, however, and thus should be reserved for dead or dying patients.

Cases have been classified depending on epidemiologic risk category and the patient's clinical manifestations. The first consideration of risk is if the exposure occurred in a country with high rates of transmission, as was the case in West Africa in 2014–15. Next the type of exposure is considered, with the greatest risk being exposure to a patient in the severe stage of the infection or someone who has died of Ebola. Listed next are categories developed by the CDC for exposure risk assessment outside the high-transmission areas:

High risk includes any of the following:

- Percutaneous (e.g., needle stick) or mucous membrane exposure to blood or body fluids (including but not limited to feces, saliva, sweat, urine, vomit, and semen) from a person with Ebola who has symptoms
- Direct contact with a person with Ebola who has symptoms, or the person's body fluids, while not wearing appropriate PPE
- Laboratory processing of blood or body fluids from a person with Ebola who has symptoms while not wearing appropriate PPE or without using standard biosafety precautions
- Providing direct care to a person showing symptoms of Ebola in a household setting

Some risk includes any of the following:

- Being in close contact with a person with Ebola who has symptoms while not wearing appropriate PPE (for example, in households, health care facilities, or community settings)

Low (but not zero) risk includes any of the following:

- Brief direct contact (such as shaking hands) with a person in the early stages of Ebola, while not wearing appropriate PPE. Early signs can include fever, fatigue, or headache
- Brief proximity with a person with Ebola who has symptoms (such as being in the same room, but not in close contact) while not wearing appropriate PPE

- Laboratory processing of blood or body fluids from a person with Ebola who has symptoms while wearing appropriate PPE and using standard biosafety precautions
- Traveling on an airplane with a person with Ebola who has symptoms and having had no identified some-risk or high-risk exposures
- Direct contact with a person with Ebola who has symptoms, or the person's body fluids, while wearing appropriate PPE
- Being in the patient-care area of an Ebola treatment unit

No identifiable risk includes any of the following:

- Laboratory processing of Ebola-containing specimens in a Biosafety Level 4 facility
- Any contact with a person who is not showing symptoms of Ebola, even if the person had potential exposure to Ebola virus
- Contact with a person with Ebola before the person developed symptoms
- Any potential exposure to Ebola virus that occurred more than 21 days previously
- Having been in a country with Ebola cases, but *without* widespread transmission, cases in urban settings with uncertain control measures, or former widespread transmission and now established control measures, and not having had any other exposures
- Having stayed on or very close to an airplane or ship (for example, to inspect the outside of the ship or plane or to load or unload supplies) during the entire time that the airplane or ship was in a country with widespread transmission or a country with cases in urban settings with uncertain control measures, and having had no direct contact with anyone from the community
- Having had laboratory-confirmed Ebola and subsequently been determined by public health authorities to no longer be infectious (i.e., Ebola survivors)

A patient under investigation is defined as the following:

- A person with fever and a history of contact with a confirmed or suspected case (i.e., a person with fever, headache, vomiting, loss of appetite, diarrhea, weakness or severe fatigue, abdominal pain, body aches or joint pains, difficulty swallowing, difficulty breathing, and hiccups; and any person having died of unknown causes in a country with high transmission rate).

Laboratory-confirmed cases are defined as the following:

- A case that meets the surveillance case definitions, and the patient has positive test results for Ebola virus antigens, Ebola virus IgG antibodies, or Ebola virus genomic sequences (RT-PCR).

INFECTION CONTROL AND PREVENTION

In the United States, the first step in managing suspected patients was first identifying those patients at risk for infection based on travel and symptom screening. Next, patients were to be placed in isolation until a full assessment and diagnostic testing, if indicated, could be performed. In the United States a tiered approach was developed for hospitals: Tier 1 hospitals identify and isolate patient under investigation. Tier 2 hospitals are Ebola assessment facilities that have the capacity to care for the patient until confirmatory testing is performed. Tier 3 are Ebola treatment centers to care for confirmed cases for the duration of illness. In each of these settings standard, contact, and droplet precautions should be employed. Additional infection control and prevention measures when evaluating patients under investigation or patient confirmed as having Ebola virus disease include the following key components: (1) patient placement in a single room (with a bathroom) with log maintained of all persons entering the room, (2) PPE to be used by health care workers, (3) dedicated or disposable medical equipment, (4) hand hygiene, (5) active monitoring of all personnel for exposure, signs and symptoms, and (6) environmental cleaning and management of waste. The specific type of PPE varies, but the proficiency of use and specific training and practice in donning and doffing PPE is what has been shown to be most important. Active training, including computer simulation and spoken instructions, led to fewer errors with guidance on which PPE to use and how to remove it among health care staff compared to passive training.[180]

In countries with high rates of Ebola virus transmission, infection control measures included identifying and isolating patients under investigation for Ebola virus disease, prioritizing protection of both patients and health care workers, cleaning up safely after caring for patients under investigation, and safe and compassionate care and burials. In these settings PPE may be limited to PVC or rubber boots, gloves, impermeable gown or coveralls, apron to provide maximal protection to the front of the body against contaminated body fluids, face mask to protect nose and mouth, goggles or face shield to protect eyes, and a head cover to protect the head from contamination when removing mask or face shields, but this proved to be effective when used properly.

Management of Filoviruses

Ebola Treatment Unit in Resource-Limited Settings

ETUs became the central point for the diagnosis, isolation, and management of patients suspected or confirmed to have Ebola virus. Although no two ETUs are exactly alike, they all share certain features (Fig. 187.5). Access to the unit is restricted by some sort of barrier, usually a large, gated fence. The ETUs are divided into two large areas, the "hot" or "red" zone and the "cold" or "green" zone. In the cold zone workers can work without any special protection, and office spaces, electrical generating equipment, laundry facilities, chlorinated water production, structures for supplies, laboratory, and pharmacy can be found here. The cold and hot zones are separated by a double fence with sufficient separation to provide protection from contamination, typically 3 meters. In the hot zone there are patient wards and lavatory facilities. The patient wards are usually divided into "suspect" and "confirmed," with the suspect wards sometimes further divided into "wet" (patients with vomiting and diarrhea) and "dry" (few gastrointestinal symptoms). Some facilities have had special wards for pregnant women and pediatric patients.[174] An isolation fence with a gate separates the suspect and confirmed wards. Within the hot zone there exists provisions for the disposal of contaminated waste, as well as a morgue for deceased patients (Fig. 187.6). A gate near the morgue allows for ambulances and a specially trained team to remove bodies for safe burial. The triage area where patients enter the ETU can reside within the cold zone, but must have an entryway for patients to enter the hot zone directly without passing through, and therefore contaminating, the cold zone. In the triage area there exists a barrier between the health care worker and the patient. Workers don their PPE in the "donning station" which is located in the green zone. PPE is not standardized but usually consists of a body suit, gloves (two or three pair), a hood, goggles, boots, masks, and an apron (Fig. 187.7). Once the PPE has been donned, the worker can enter the hot zone through a gate near the donning station. Once the hot zone is accessed, the workers must use a unidirectional path. First they enter the suspect wards, next the confirmed wards, and then they must remove their PPE, which by this point can be highly contaminated. A "doffing station," which is partly located in the hot zone and partly in the cold zone, allows the worker to carefully remove the components of the PPE

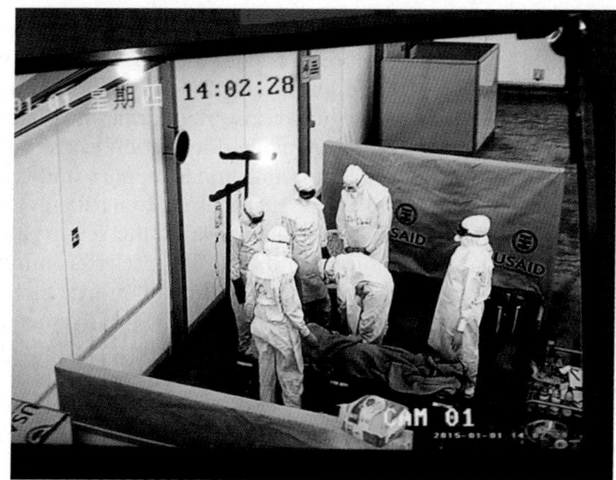

FIG. 187.5 A video surveillance photo from inside the "hot zone" of an Ebola Treatment Unit in Liberia, Africa, during the 2013–16 Ebola outbreak. Dr. David Hilmers (one of the chapter authors) and colleagues care for a dying woman with suspected Ebola hemorrhagic fever. (Courtesy Dr. Kenneth Marx.)

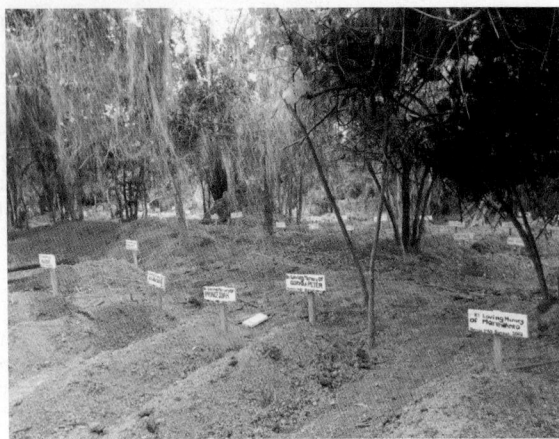

FIG. 187.6 A graveyard outside an Ebola Treatment Unit in Liberia, Africa, during the 2013–16 Ebola outbreak. (Courtesy Dr. Majid Sadigh.)

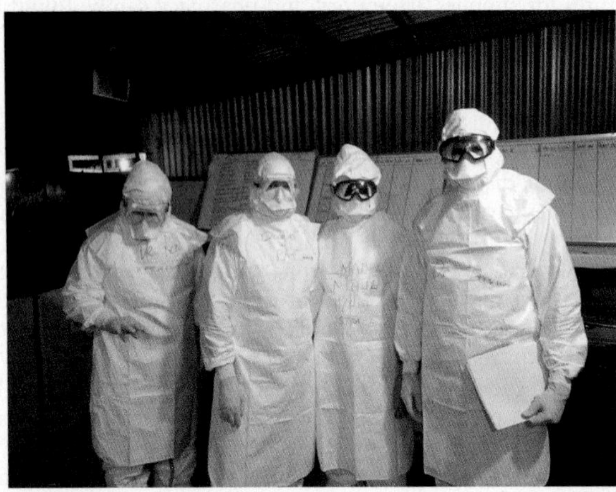

FIG. 187.7 Dr. David Hilmers (far right) (one of the chapter authors) and colleagues in personal protective equipment in an Ebola Treatment Unit in Liberia, Africa, during the 2013–16 Ebola outbreak. (Courtesy Dr. David Hilmers.)

in a standardized and highly choreographed manner. This is done in coordination with another worker standing in the cold zone, who directs the doffing process and sprays the person exiting the hot zone with chlorinated water as the PPE is taken off. Once the PPE has been removed, the now decontaminated worker will step across into the cold zone.

Biocontainment Units in Developed Countries

With the 2014-2015 Ebola outbreak, a total of 27 cases of EVD were treated in the United States and Europe, in 15 different hospitals in 9 different countries. All patients required close monitoring and aggressive supportive care, including intravenous fluid hydration, correction of significant electrolyte abnormalities, nutritional support, and critical care management for respiratory and renal failure. Seven patients (26%) received invasive mechanical ventilation. Five of the seven patients who received invasive mechanical ventilation also received continuous renal replacement therapy. Five patients died, with an overall 18.5% mortality rate after 28 days of illness.[177] This public health emergency highlighted the need for increased overall preparedness, including the ability to provide high-level care for critically ill patients with serious communicable diseases such as Ebola virus in biocontainment units where staff were not only safe, but trained in the concepts of biocontainment, PPE, and the equipment needed to care for these complex patients.[90] In resource-rich settings, it may be feasible to build true biocontainment facilities in the hospital setting, as exemplified at the University of Nebraska Medical Center (Omaha), Emory University (Atlanta) and Texas Children's Hospital (Houston). This requires advance planning, adequate space, and institutional support. Key concepts to such a unit include negative air pressure ventilation systems, disinfectant pass-through boxes, restricted access, cleanable surfaces, laboratory facilities, and the ability to handle and process biohazardous waste[158] (Figs. 187.8 to 187.13). Last, purposeful recruitment of staff is crucial to the success of such a unit, and staff should be a mix with different skill sets. A varied group of nurses and physicians is helpful to have on a team, but having a majority with critical care skills is helpful. Ongoing, quarterly training is required to maintain competency in special skills, including training in PPE, procedures, and unit protocols to ensure the safety of the staff, as well as build the team dynamic, helping them to work together in a high-risk, unfamiliar environment (Figs. 187.14 to 187.16).

Supportive Care

No specific antiviral treatment for filoviral hemorrhagic fevers is licensed.[14,45] Standard medical treatment relies on symptomatic measures aimed at maintaining hydration, managing severe electrolyte disturbances, reversing cytokine storm and disseminated intravascular coagulation, treating hemorrhage with transfusions, and managing organ failure. In addition, maintaining nutritional status and preventing or curing bacterial and parasitic superinfections are important for management. Appropriate control measures for health care workers and family members to prevent secondary transmission are important to follow. Barrier techniques to prevent direct physical contact with the patient and the patient's secretions and blood, including wearing of protective gowns, gloves, and masks; placing the infected patient in strict isolation; and sterilization or incineration of needles, equipment, and patient excretions are recommended. A manual prepared collaboratively by the CDC and WHO is available and addresses early provisional diagnosis, medical response, and measures to prevent spread of filovirus disease and other viral hemorrhagic fevers within a limited infrastructure that is likely in the African health care setting[79] (http://cdc.gov/ncidod/dvrd/spb/mnpages/vhfmanual.htm).

Treatment of Ebola in Children and Pregnant Women

In developing countries, there is a lack of comprehensive guidelines for care of pregnant women and pediatric patients infected with Ebola virus. One ETU reported the creation of a pediatric ward within the confirmed and suspect zones.[145,175] Parents who were also patients were allowed to stay with their children in these wards until a discordancy in their status was confirmed, with subsequent separation of the dyad. As for all patients, treatment is mainly supportive. The majority of children are given a full course of malaria treatment, even if testing negative, as most treatment units are located in areas where malaria is endemic. Likewise, broad-spectrum antibiotics are often administered empirically, given the difficulty in distinguishing between the symptoms of Ebola virus and a bacterial process as well as possible translocation of bacteria through the intestinal mucosa while infected with Ebola virus. Zinc is given to those patients with significant diarrhea. Patients are allowed to drink oral rehydration solutions liberally if able. If unable to tolerate oral therapy, intravenous fluids are administered to replace gastrointestinal losses. However, care must be taken not to be overly aggressive with rapid fluid resuscitation, as increased mortality rates have been reported with large fluid boluses in recent studies in children with children in Africa with severe infections, as compared to children in the United Kingdom and United States.[113,194] Some possible approaches include vital signs, signs of dehydration on physical exam, direct measurement of input and output, and measurement of electrolytes. The use of bedside ultrasound to measure the inferior vena cava diameter has been reported. In the developing world, many children may have underlying malnutrition that predates infection with Ebola virus, and this can affect the immunologic response. Therefore, moderate and severe malnutrition must be addressed early and aggressively. Ready-to-use therapeutic foods (RUTF) and available formulas should be used to treat malnourished patients.

The care of EVD in pregnancy is particularly difficult. There is a high rate of spontaneous abortions, high mortality rate for the mother, and elevated risk of preterm complications, as well as a high risk of transmission to health care workers who are attending a delivery[77,127] (http://apps.who.int/iris/bitstream/10665/184163/1/WHO_EVD_HSE_PED_15.1_eng.pdf) For women who give birth with active EVD, there are no reports of survival beyond the neonatal period. Intrauterine contents appear to be PCR positive for Ebola virus. As a result, the WHO issued guidelines for the diagnosis and management of Ebola virus in pregnant women[77] (http://apps.who.int/iris/bitstream/10665/184163/1/WHO_EVD_HSE_PED_15.1_eng.pdf).

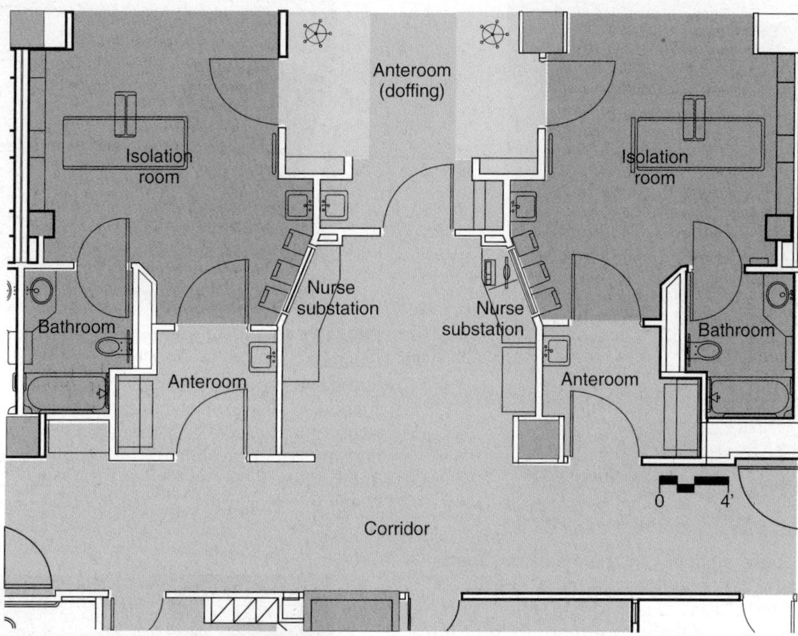

FIG. 187.8 Typical floor plan of a set of two rooms in the eight-bed Pediatric Special Isolation Unit at Texas Children's Hospital West Campus, Houston. It is designed for pediatric biocontainment of fluid-borne and air-borne contagious pathogens, such as Ebola and Marburg viruses, Lassa fever virus, smallpox, monkeypox, Middle East respiratory syndrome, severe acute respiratory syndrome, avian influenza, measles, pneumonic tularemia, and multidrug-resistant tuberculosis. It provides for containment at the level of the room, not at the level of the entire unit. The floor plan includes a safe or "cold" "green zone" secured corridor where parents and other visitors and health care professionals may walk, and a "green" "cold" anteroom for passing of needed materials and supplies and observation. The "yellow zone" is the separate anteroom with specialized negative air flow, for donning and doffing of personal protective equipment and preparation of contaminated trash for exit from the isolation room. The "red zone" or "hot" zone is the isolation room and bathroom for the patient and contains all potentially infectious materials. In addition, each room has a designated nurse substation with large glass window and electronic communications. (Courtesy Dr. Amy Arrington and Texas Children's Hospital.)

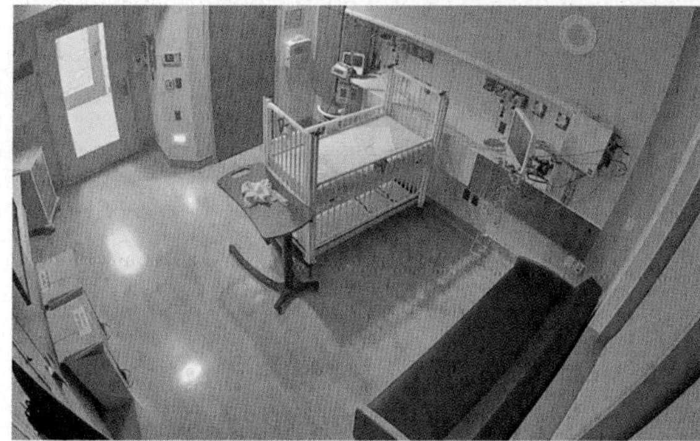

FIG. 187.9 The patient room area in the Pediatric Special Isolation Unit at Texas Children's Hospital, Houston. To the far left is the nurse substation patient window with specialized communication technology to limit staff exposure and to facilitate patient care. The top left is the "yellow zone" anteroom doffing-donning glass entry door for easy visibility, and to the right the door to the patient bathroom and the patient care area. All floor surfaces and counter surfaces are smooth, impermeable, and designed for easy cleanup and decontamination. To reduce the stress associated with isolation, age-appropriate toys and distractions are available, and patients are able to communicate with their family via video chat using a special tablet computer. These flexible, dual-purpose patient rooms, when not "activated" and secured for special isolation, may be used for routine pediatric inpatient care. (Courtesy Dr. Amy Arrington and Texas Children's Hospital.)

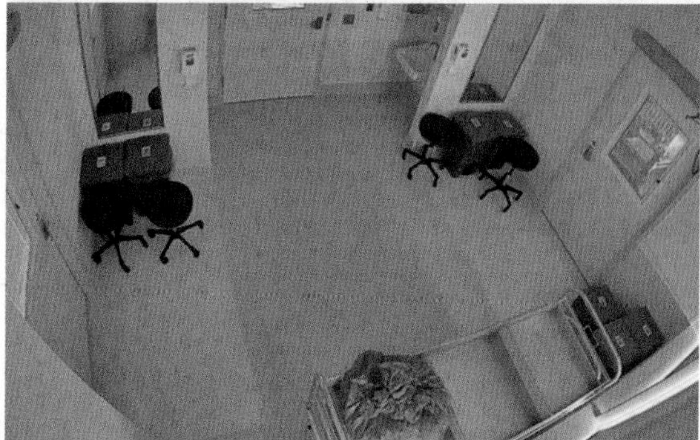

FIG. 187.10 "Yellow zone" anteroom doffing-donning area, shared by two patient rooms in the Pediatric Special Isolation Unit at Texas Children's Hospital, Houston. The anteroom has three doors, two providing entrance to each of the patient rooms, and one for entry to and from "green zone" to "yellow zone." In the donning and doffing anteroom, members of the Special Response Team put on or remove personal protective equipment according to a standard procedure. In addition, in the "yellow zone" anteroom waste and trash will be appropriately bagged and sealed prior to removal and transfer to the on-site, in-unit autoclaves. (Courtesy Dr. Amy Arrington and Texas Children's Hospital.)

Because pregnancy may mask some of the symptoms of early Ebola virus, a heightened awareness must be maintained. Pregnant women in endemic areas should be admitted to facilities that have obstetric facilities with proper infection control.[36] For those assisting with delivery, full PPE with double gloving and elbow-length gloves is recommended.[4]

Experimental Therapies

Phosphorodiamidate Morpholino Oligomers

Administration of positively charged phosphorodiamidate morpholino oligomers (PMOs), delivered with various dosing strategies, protected more than 60% of rhesus monkeys against lethal Zaire Ebola virus challenge and 100% of cynomolgus monkeys against Lake Victoria Marburg virus infection, suggesting PMOs may be useful for treatment.[14,67] AVI 6002 is a combination of positively charged phosphorodiamidate morpholino

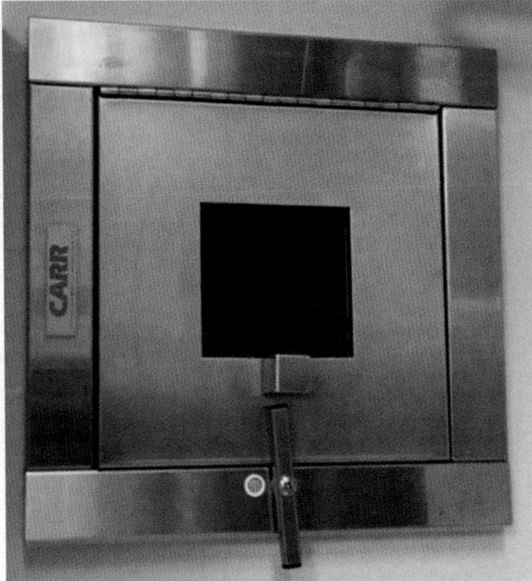

FIG. 187.11 Secure "pass-through window" in the Pediatric Special Isolation Unit allows for safe transfer of needed supplies, small equipment, and patient samples back and forth from clean "green zone" nurse substation to contaminated "red zone" patient care room. Use of the pass-through window reduces the need for patient caregivers to repeatedly don and doff personal protective equipment when transfer of equipment, supplies, or samples is needed. (Courtesy Dr. Amy Arrington and Texas Children's Hospital.)

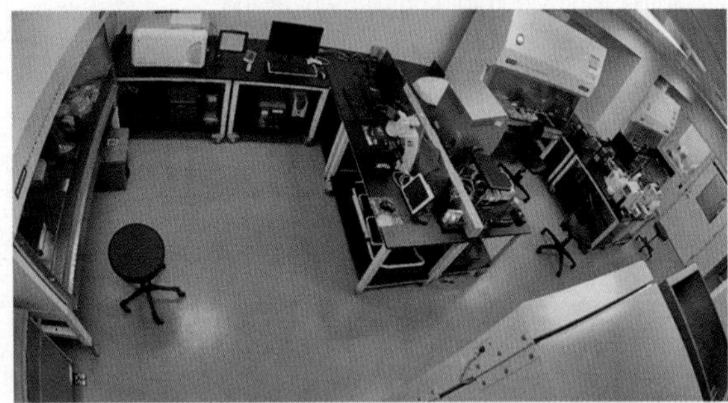

FIG. 187.12 On-site, unit-based Biosafety Level 3 Laboratory in the Pediatric Special Isolation Unit at Texas Children's Hospital, Houston. This laboratory is designed for rapid detection of unusual and usual pathogens that may be needed to diagnose patient illness and also may perform other laboratory monitoring tests. It contains a biosafety hood, specialized air flow, and laboratory autoclave and is staffed by trained laboratory technicians. (Courtesy Dr. Amy Arrington and Texas Children's Hospital.)

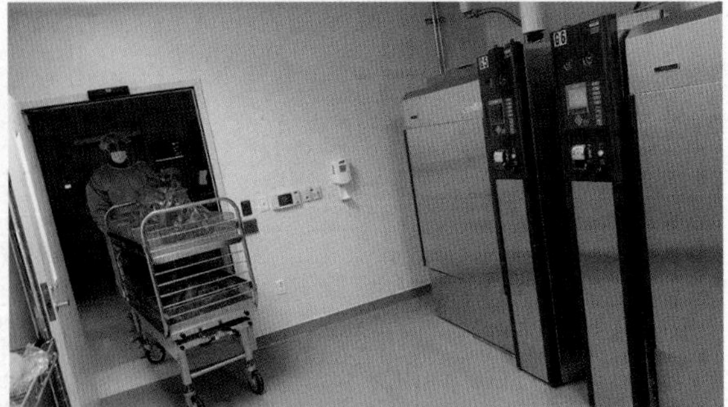

FIG. 187.13 On-site, unit-based autoclave room located in the Special Isolation Unit at Texas Children's Hospital, Houston. It contains two autoclaves and is staffed by environmental service technicians specially trained in disposal of contaminated waste products. Disposal of the large quantity of contaminated waste and trash produced during care of patients with Ebola hemorrhagic fever is critical to maintain appropriate biocontainment. (Courtesy Dr. Amy Arrington and Texas Children's Hospital.)

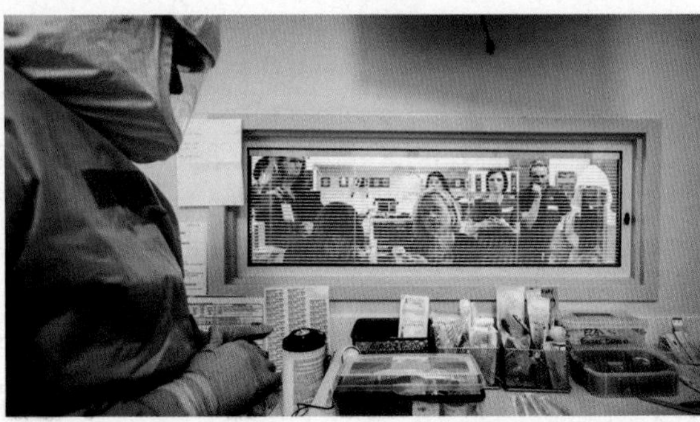

FIG. 187.14 The Special Isolation Unit (SIU) of Texas Children's Hospital is staffed by a Special Response Team (SRT) consisting of doctors, nurses, respiratory therapists, medical technicians, and environmental services technicians. The SRT members are all trained in biocontainment and management of patients with Ebola hemorrhagic fever and other airborne and fluid-borne contagious diseases. The SRT has quarterly in-service didactic sessions, review of donning and doffing procedures, review of laboratory procedures, and simulation sessions of patient care scenarios. Shown here is one such simulation in the SIU. A health care worker, in full personal protective equipment, is performing a laboratory test in the patient care area during a patient simulation session, while Dr. Amy Arrington, Pediatric SIU Medical Director, and other SRT members provide oversight of the simulation session through the observational window in the nurses' anteroom area. (Courtesy Dr. Amy Arrington and Texas Children's Hospital.)

oligomers designed to target mRNA sequences of VP24 and VP35 in Ebola virus. AVI-6002 was administered intravenously to rhesus macaques 30 to 60 minutes after Ebola virus exposure at varying doses for up to 14 days. Results of this study demonstrated that 60% of macaques given doses of 28 mg/kg and 40 mg/kg survived with 100 times greater suppression of mean viral load at the peak of plasma viremia compared to control animals.[188] Phase I safety trials have shown AVI 6002 to be well tolerated in healthy adult subjects.

Nucleoside/Nucleotide Viral Polymerase Inhibitors

Brincidofovir is a nucleotide analogue and conjugate of cidofovir originally studied as a treatment for double-stranded DNA viruses. Its mechanism of action in RNA viruses such as Ebola virus is not well understood, but it has been found to inhibit in vitro infection of Ebola virus in multiple human cell lines.[121] Oral brincidofovir was administered to four patients in Liberia with laboratory-confirmed EVD in a single-arm, phase 2 trial; all four patients died.[37]

Favipiravir is a RNA polymerase inhibitor that has shown strong antiviral efficacy against lethal doses of Ebola virus in mice.[161] From a clinical research standpoint, favipiravir is currently the most advanced of the small molecules and is currently in phase 3 clinical trials.[155]

BCX4430 is an adenosine nucleoside analogue, designed to inhibit viral RNA polymerase activity indirectly through non-obligate RNA chain termination, and has been shown to provide complete protection to cynomolgus macaques from Marburg virus infection when administered as late as 48 hours after infection.[189] Phase 1 clinical trials of this drug are currently ongoing in healthy subjects.

GS-5734 is the newest small molecule to be developed against filoviruses and has shown several important findings. In a macaque monkey model, a 10 mg/kg loading dose of GS-5734 was administered 3 days after infection with Ebola virus followed by daily maintenance dosing for 12 days with 3 mg/kg, resulting in a 100% survival rate. Additionally, intravenous administration of GS-5734 to nonhuman primates resulted in persistent GS-5734 levels in peripheral blood mononuclear cells and distribution to sanctuary sites for viral replication including testes, eyes, and brain, suggesting that the drug may be usefully for postexposure prophylaxis as well as post-Ebola syndrome.[187] The drug has been used in an individual suffering from postexposure relapse resulting in meningoencephalitis 9 months after discharge from the initial hospital stay.[84]

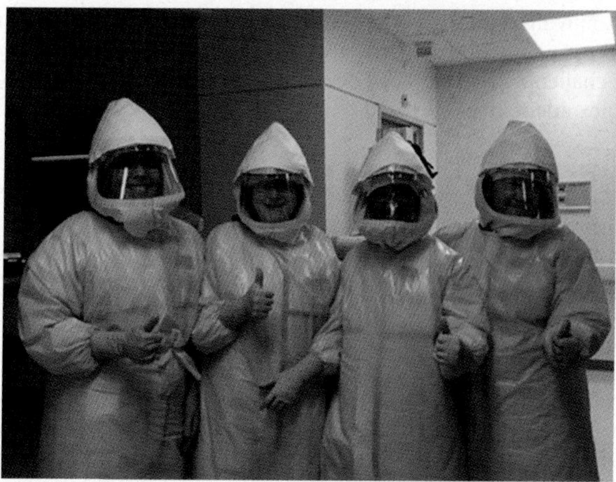

FIG. 187.15 Personal protective equipment (PPE) is an important part of staff safety when caring for patients with Ebola hemorrhagic fever or other highly contagious diseases. Shown here are doctors on the Special Response Team for the Pediatric Special Isolation Unitat Texas Children's Hospital, Houston, during a donning and doffing practice session. The PPE includes first layer as hospital scrubs for clothing and plastic crocks as shoes, a battery-powered air purifying respirator with face mask on the head and neck, hooded liquid-repellent one-piece coverall that zips in the front, isolation gown/apron over coverall that ties in the back, hospital shoe covers over Crocs, which are then covered by water-resistant plastic booties, and three pairs of gloves. PPE is donned and doffed according to a specific checklist of instructions in the anteroom area before entering and after leaving the patient care isolation room. Shown here in the photo are two of the chapter authors, Dr. Judith Campbell (second from right) and Dr. Gail Harrison (far right), and Dr. Maria Carolina Gazzaneo (far left) and Dr. Regina Okhuysen-Crawley (second from left), who are all members of the Special Isolation Unit Special Response Team. (Courtesy Dr. Amy Arrington.)

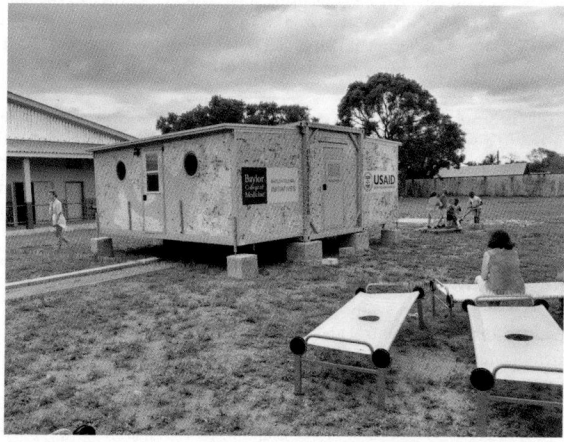

FIG. 187.16 The United States Agency for International Development (USAID) Emergency Isolation Smart Pod set up at EWA Hospital, Monrovia, Liberia, in September 2017. These modular, deployable, portable isolation pods are used as a mobile hospital unit for physicians and technicians to evaluate and care for Ebola patients during their acute illness and after recovery for evaluation of complications. They contain a water sanitation system, drug and supply tracking system, laboratory, and patient isolation beds. They can be shipped by air, land, or sea directly to remote destinations and can be assembled in 5 to 10 minutes by a team of four. (Courtesy Dr. David Hilmers; www.bcm.edu/global-initiatives/innovation-center/emergency-smart-pod.)

Immunotherapeutics

Convalescent plasma has been used for treatment of filovirus infection, but its efficacy has not been proved in randomized clinical trials. In a study conducted during the 1995 Kikwit Ebola epidemic, seven of eight patients who received blood collected from convalescent donors recovered, warranting a thorough evaluation of passive immune therapy.[88,126] One person infected by *Sudan ebolavirus* after a laboratory accident survived after receiving plasma from *Zaire ebolavirus* survivors. In the 2014–15 EVD outbreak, several clinical trials evaluating convalescent plasma were conducted in three separate studies.[178] Only the Ebola-Tx trial in Guinea enrolled a sufficient number of patients ($n = 102$); the Ebola-CP trial in Sierra Leone and theEVD001 trial in Liberia both enrolled a small number of subjects ($n = 4$ and $n = 5$, respectively). Data available from these studies showed no severe adverse reactions to convalescent plasma, with no efficacy data yet available. Two patients in the 2014–15 EVD outbreak who were cared for in the United States (Nebraska Biocontainment Unit and Emory University Hospital Serious Communicable Diseases Unit) both received convalescent plasma in addition to an investigational therapeutic drug, TKM-100802, and supportive care. Both critically ill patients recovered completely,[98] although the role convalescent plasma played in their recovery is unknown. In past studies using convalescent plasma as a treatment in other viral infections including avian influenza, Middle East respiratory syndrome, and hemorrhagic fevers including Lassa and Marburg, results have been conflicting.[98,178,147]

Hyperimmunoglobulin from horses protected baboons in experimental studies.[122] Goat immunoglobulin has been tested in laboratory animals and also was given to laboratory researchers suspected of being infected by Ebola virus[102]; one researcher with highly probable infection made a full recovery. Studies have investigated the potential therapeutic utility of a variety of monoclonal antibody preparations for treatment and postexposure prophylaxis of Ebola virus infection.[24,168] Mouse and human chimeric monoclonal antibodies active against Ebola virus and produced in Chinese hamster ovary and in whole plant cells have been shown to successfully protect rhesus monkeys against lethal viral challenge. Fucose-free monoclonal antibody against Ebola virus has also been found effective in preclinical trials.[207]

In addition to antibody-based strategies, preclinical development of a variety of antiviral drug strategies for treatment of filovirus infection is in progress. Compound library screening in vitro, with small molecules, and in silicon structure-based drug design are being explored to treat filovirus infection.[67,132,153] Administration of recombinant nematode anticoagulant protein c2 (rNAPc2), a potent inhibitor of tissue factor–initiated blood coagulation, attenuated proinflammatory and coagulopathic responses and prolonged the survival of macaques that had received a lethal inoculum of Ebola virus.[62]

ZMapp is an experimental drug composed of three different chimeric humanized monoclonal antibodies that bind specifically to the Ebola surface glycoprotein. In a rhesus macaque model, 100% of these animals survived when ZMapp was administered up to 5 days post-challenge with Ebola virus. Additionally, after ZMapp administration, advanced disease including elevated liver enzymes, mucosal hemorrhages, and generalized petechiae could be reversed, leading to full recovery in these animals.[143] The recent Partnership for Research on Ebola Virus in Liberia II (PREVAIL II) study was a randomized, controlled trial evaluating ZMapp in patients who had been diagnosed with Zaire Ebola virus during the 2014–15 outbreak in in Liberia, Sierra Leone, or Guinea. The study enrolled 72 patients and compared ZMapp to the standard of care: providing fluids, balancing electrolytes, and maintaining blood pressure and oxygen support. Twenty-one of the 72 patients died, a case fatality rate of 29%. Thirteen of the 35 patients (37%) who received only standard care died, while eight of the 36 people (22%) who received ZMapp plus standard care died. The study found ZMapp to be safe and well tolerated; however, because of lack of power due to the small sample size, the study was unable to show statistical significance and determine definitively whether it is a better treatment for Ebola virus disease (EVD) than the best available standard of care alone.[141]

Vaccine Therapies for Ebola Virus

A variety of vaccine platforms, including DNA vaccines, recombinant replication-deficient adenovirus serotype 5 vector vaccines, recombinant human parainfluenza virus 3, vesicular stomatitis virus-based vaccines, and virus-like particle vaccines, have been investigated and shown to be effective against filovirus infection in animal models.[20,41,58,92,138,150,163] Successful preclinical developments suggest that studies on the safety and efficacy of a filovirus vaccine for human use may be possible.[92,150]

Several candidate vaccines against Ebola virus are effective in guinea pigs but less so in macaques.[64,163] Experimental vaccines in the past had been based on viral particles inactivated by heat, formalin, or γ-irradiation[112]; plasmids coding for the Ebola virus glycoprotein (GP) or nucleoprotein (NP),[203] recombinant GP-expressing Venezuelan equine encephalitis virus,[142] or variola virus; and Ebola virus particles encapsulated in liposomes.[144] In contrast, a vaccine candidate based on three injections of GP-encoding DNA given 4 weeks apart, followed by a booster with recombinant inactivated GP expressing adenovirus, protected macaques from infectious challenge 1 week later.[165] However, the small inoculum used to challenge the macaques (six plaque-forming units [PFU]), together with the lengthy immunization protocol, renders this candidate vaccine impractical.

With the 2014 Ebola virus outbreak in West Africa leading to an unprecedented loss of human lives, heightened awareness on vaccine development led to new advances, including several potential candidate vaccines showing protection against Ebola virus in both animal and human subjects. The first of these is vesicular stomatitis virus (VSV)-EBOV, also known as rVSV-ZEBOV, a recombinant live-attenuated VSV-based vaccine developed against Ebola virus and currently is the first vaccine with reported efficacy against Ebola virus infections in humans in phase 3 clinical trials. This vaccine was shown to completely protect macaques against lethal challenge with the West African Ebola virus-Makona strain with a single dose.[118] This vaccine as been used as postexposure prophylaxis as well following a needle-stick injury in a US physician caring for patients in an Ebola treatment center in Sierra Leone. Forty-three hours postexposure, rVSV-ZEBOV was administered to the patient evacuated to the US for treatment.[103] This patient developed a postvaccine febrile syndrome beginning 12 hours after vaccination, which was self-limited and associated with the brief detection of recombinant vesicular stomatitis vaccine virus in the blood. Strong innate and Ebola-specific adaptive immune responses were detected postvaccination, with no evidence of Ebola virus infection.[103]

A large study was conducted in Guinea using the viral stomatitis vaccine (rVSV-ZEBOV) that included 7651 people who had either been in contact with a patient with known Ebola virus or were a contact of a direct contact.[82] However, children and pregnant or lactating women were excluded. The patients were divided into two groups; one group received the vaccination immediately after randomization, and the other was given the vaccination 21 days after randomization. None of the 2014 patients in the first group became infected with Ebola, and 16 of the second group of 1930 became infected. Thus, the vaccine was considered 100% effective in those immediately vaccinated and 75.1% overall in this trial. Two other vaccines are currently in phase 3 development. The durability of these vaccines remains to be studied, and there is an urgent need for a vaccine that can be administered to children and pregnant or lactating women.[48]

Other vaccine candidates with promising results include a recombinant adenovirus of various serotypes. A study in 2016 evaluated the reactogenicity and immunogenicity of immunization schedules using two novel candidate Ebola vaccines—an adenovirus type 26 vector vaccine encoding Ebola glycoprotein (Ad26.ZEBOV), and a modified vaccinia Ankara (MVA) vector vaccine, which is an attenuated vaccine of a poxvirus. This vector vaccine encodes glycoproteins from Ebola virus, Sudan virus, Marburg virus, and Tai Forest virus nucleoprotein (MVA-BN-Filo). Vaccines were administered to healthy adult volunteers in the United Kingdom in a Phase I trial. In the randomized groups, 28 of 29 Ad26.ZEBOV recipients and 7 of 30 MVA-BN-Filo recipients had detectable Ebola glycoprotein-specific IgG 28 days after primary immunization. All vaccine recipients had specific IgG detectable at 8-month follow-up. Within randomized groups, at least 86% of vaccine recipients showed Ebola-specific T-cell responses.[123] These vaccines are now being further evaluated in Phase II and III studies. In recent studies, recombinant adenovirus (Ad5)-vectored vaccine expressing the Makona Ebola virus glycoprotein (MakGP) was shown to elicit specific B- and T-cell immunity in cynomolgus macaques and conferred 100% protection when these animals were challenged 4 weeks after immunization.[201]

Virus-like particles have shown promise and protect small laboratory animals and nonhuman primates against lethal challenge by Ebola or Marburg viruses.[205] Also, a vaccine system based on recombinant vesicular stomatitis virus that expresses filovirus glycoprotein in place of the vesicular stomatitis virus glycoprotein has shown protection against infection with Marburg and Ebola virus.[58,59,69,163] Protection of nonhuman primates against Ebola virus infection by both parenteral and aerosol route challenges also has been documented by vaccination with a single complex adenovirus vector vaccine.[19,138]

CONCLUSION

Filoviruses remain a threat to mankind, but important advances were made following the 2014–15 Ebola outbreak in West Africa. Advances included vaccine development and novel drug therapies, and several Phase III drug trials are underway. We have yet to truly understand the effects of Ebola on long-term survivors, but data showing Ebola virus RNA present in semen and CSF samples of survivors up to 9 months after infection is concerning.[84,162] Perhaps one of the most important lessons learned from the 2014–15 Ebola outbreak was how to be more prepared both locally and globally for the next one. It is critical to strengthen the medical infrastructure in developing countries where outbreaks are most likely to occur. This includes improvement in staffing and training of medical personnel at the local and national level, reporting of suspected cases, and public education. Critical lessons were learned in how we respond to public health emergencies and the need for improved infection control, isolation of highly infectious patients, and the ability to care for them in specialized units. Being prepared for the next outbreak is critical for preventing a catastrophic epidemic, both locally and abroad. The world is vulnerable to global epidemics as never before, and constant surveillance and preparedness are required on all of our parts.

NEW REFERENCES SINCE THE SEVENTH EDITION

4. Baggi FM, Taybi A, Kurth A, et al. Management of pregnant women infected with Ebola virus in a treatment centre in Guinea, 2014. *Euro Surveill.* 2014;19(49).
5. Bah EI, Lamah MC, Fletcher T, et al. Clinical presentation of patients with Ebola virus disease in Conakry, Guinea. *N Engl J Med.* 2015;372(1):40-47.
8. Baize S, Pannetier D, Oestereich L, et al. Emergence of Zaire Ebola virus disease in Guinea. *N Engl J Med.* 2014;371(15):1418-1425.
11. Baseler L, Chertow DS, Johnson KM, et al. The pathogenesis of Ebola virus disease. *Annu Rev Pathol.* 2017;12:387-418.
15. Bell BP, Damon IK, Jernigan DB, et al. Overview, control strategies, and lessons learned in the CDC response to the 2014-2016 Ebola epidemic. *MMWR Suppl.* 2016;65(3):4-11.
17. Diallo B, Sissoko D, Loman NJ, et al. Resurgence of Ebola virus disease in Guinea linked to a survivor with virus persistence in seminal fluid for more than 500 days. *Clin Infect Dis.* 2016;63(10):1353-1356.
18. Bower H, Johnson S, Bangura MS, et al. Exposure-specific and age-specific attack rates for Ebola virus disease in Ebola-affected households, Sierra Leone. *Emerg Infect Dis.* 2016;22(8):1403-1411.
21. Bray M. Defense against filoviruses used as biological weapons. *Antiviral Res.* 2003;57(1-2):53-60.
22. Burki TK. Post-Ebola syndrome. *Lancet Infect Dis.* 2016;16(7):780-781.
25. Centers for Disease Control and Prevention. Ebola (Ebola Virus Disease). 2017 Democratic Republic of the Congo, Bas Uélé District: Outbreak Update. https://www.cdc.gov/vhf/Ebola/outbreaks/drc/2017-may.html.
27. Centers for Disease Control and Prevention. 2014-2016 Ebola Outbreak in West Africa. https://www.cdc.gov/vhf/Ebola/outbreaks/2014-west-africa/index.html.
28. Chevalier MS, Chung W, Smith J, et al. Ebola virus disease cluster in the United States—Dallas County, Texas, 2014. *MMWR Morb Mortal Wkly Rep.* 2014;63(46):1087-1088.
29. Christie A, Davies-Wayne GJ, Cordier-Lassalle T, et al. Possible sexual transmission of Ebola virus—Liberia, 2015. *MMWR Morb Mortal Wkly Rep.* 2015;64(17):479-481.
30. Cnops L, van Griensven J, Honko AN, et al. Essentials of filoviral load quantification. *Lancet Infect Dis.* 2016;16(7):e134-e138.
31. Curran KG, Gibson JJ, Marke D, et al. Cluster of Ebola virus disease linked to a single funeral—Moyamba District, Sierra Leone, 2014. *MMWR Morb Mortal Wkly Rep.* 2016;65(8):202-205.
32. de La Vega MA, Caleo G, Audet J, et al. Ebola viral load at diagnosis associates with patient outcome and outbreak evolution. *J Clin Invest.* 2015;125(12):4421-4428.
33. Deen GF, Knust B, Broutet N, et al. Ebola RNA persistence in semen of Ebola virus disease survivors—preliminary report. *N Engl J Med.* 2015;Epub before print.
34. Dixon MG, Schafer IJ. Ebola viral disease outbreak—West Africa, 2014. *MMWR Morb Mortal Wkly Rep.* 2014;63(25):548-551.
35. Dowell SF. Ebola hemorrhagic fever: why were children spared? *Pediatr Infect Dis J.* 1996;15(3):189-191.
36. Dunn AC, Walker TA, Redd J, et al. Nosocomial transmission of Ebola virus disease on pediatric and maternity wards: Bombali and Tonkolili, Sierra Leone, 2014. *Am J Infect Control.* 2016;44(3):269-272.

37. Dunning J, Kennedy SB, Antierens A, et al. RAPIDE-BCV trial team. Experimental treatment of Ebola virus disease with brincidofovir. *PLoS ONE.* 2016;11(9):e0162199.
39. Erickson BR, Sealy TK, Flietstra T, et al. Ebola virus disease diagnostics, Sierra Leone: Analysis of real-time reverse transcription-polymerase chain reaction values for clinical blood and oral swab specimens. *J Infect Dis.* 2016;214(suppl 3):S258-S262.
40. Eriksson CO, Uyeki TM, Christian MD, et al. Care of the child with Ebola virus disease. *Pediatr Crit Care Med.* 2015;16(2):97-103.
43. Feldmann H, Geisbert TW. Ebola haemorrhagic fever. *Lancet.* 2011;377(9768):849-862.
48. Fitzgerald F, Yeung S, Gibb DM, et al. Ebola vaccination. *Lancet.* 2015;386(10012):2478.
49. Folarin OA, Ehichioya D, Schaffner SF, et al. Ebola virus epidemiology and evolution in Nigeria. *J Infect Dis.* 2016;214:S102-S1029.
52. Formenty P, Leroy EM, Epelboin A, et al. Detection of Ebola virus in oral fluid specimens during outbreaks of Ebola virus hemorrhagic fever in the Republic of Congo. *Clin Infect Dis.* 2006;42(11):1521-1526.
55. Forum on Microbial Threats (US), Board on Global Health (US), Health and Medicine Division (US), National Academies of Sciences, Engineering, and Medicine (US). *The Ebola Epidemic in West Africa: Proceedings of a Workshop.* Washington, DC: National Academies Press; 2016.
56. Frieden TR, Damon IK. Ebola in West Africa—CDC's Role in epidemic detection, control and prevention. *Emerg Infect Dis.* 2015;21:1897-1905.
60. Geisbert TW, et al. Single-injection vaccine protects nonhuman primates against infection with Marburg virus and three species of Ebola virus. *J Virol.* 2009;83(14):7296-7304.
70. Gire SK, Goba A, Andersen KG, et al. Genomic surveillance elucidates Ebola virus origin and transmission during the 2014 outbreak. *Science.* 2014;345(6202):1369-1372.
73. Helleringer S, Noymer A, Clark SJ, McCormick T. Did Ebola relatively spare children? *Lancet.* 2015;386(10002):1442-1443.
75. Herstein JJ, Biddinger PD, Kraft CS, et al. Current capabilities and capacity of Ebola treatment centers in the United States. *Infect Control Hosp Epidemiol.* 2016;37(3):313-318.
77. World Health Organization. *Interim Guidance: Ebola Virus Disease in Preegnancy: Screening and Management of Ebola Cases, Contacts, and Survivors.* Available at: https://www.cdc.gov/vhf/abroad/pdf/african-healthcare-setting-vhf.pdf.
79. Centers for Disease Control and Prevention. *Viral Hemorrhagic Fevers: Information for Healthcare Workers.* Available at: https://www.cdc.gov/vhf/abroad/healthcare-workers.html.
80. Centers for Disease Control and Prevention. Viral Special Pathogens Branch (VSPB). https://www.cdc.gov/ncezid/dhcpp/vspb/.
82. Huttner A, Dayer JA, Yerly S, et al. The effect of dose on the safety and immunogenicity of the VSV Ebola candidate vaccine: a randomised double-blind, placebo-controlled phase 1/2 trial. *Lancet Infect Dis.* 2015;15(10):1156-1166.
84. Jacobs M, Rodger A, Bell DJ, et al. Late Ebola virus relapse causing meningoencephalitis: a case report. *Lancet.* 2016;388(10043):498-503.
89. Jezek Z, Szczeniowski MY, Muyembe-Tamfum JJ, et al. Ebola between outbreaks: intensified Ebola hemorrhagic fever surveillance in the Democratic Republic of the Congo, 1981-1985. *J Infect Dis.* 1999;179(suppl 1):S60 S64.
90. Johnson DW, Sullivan JN, Piquette CA, et al. Lessons learned: critical care management of patients with Ebola in the United States. *Crit Care Med.* 2015;43(6):1157-1164.
93. Kirsch TD, Moseson H, Massaquoi M, et al. Impact of interventions and the incidence of Ebola virus disease in Liberia—implications for future epidemics. *Health Policy Plan.* 2016;29:1-10.
94. Kobinger GP1, Leung A, Neufeld J, et al. Replication, pathogenicity, shedding, and transmission of Zaire ebolavirus in pigs. *J Infect Dis.* 2011;204(2):200-208.
96. Kourtis AP, Appelgren K, Chevalier MS, McElroy A. Ebola virus disease: focus on children. *Pediatr Infect Dis J.* 2015;34(8):893-897.
98. Kraft CS, Hewlett AL, Koepsell S, et al. The use of TKM-100802 and convalescent plasma in 2 patients with Ebola virus disease in the United States. *Clin Infect Dis.* 2015;61(4):496-502.
103. Lai L, Davey R, Beck A, et al. Emergency postexposure vaccination with vesicular stomatitis virus-vectored Ebola vaccine after needlestick. *JAMA.* 2015;313(12):1249-1255.
104. Lanini S, Portella G, Vairo F, et al. Blood kinetics of Ebola virus in survivors and nonsurvivors. *J Clin Invest.* 2015;125(12):4692-4698.
107. Ledgerwood JE, Costner P, Desai N, et al. A replication defective recombinant Ad5 vaccine expressing Ebola virus GP is safe and immunogenic in healthy adults. *Vaccine.* 2010;29:304-313.
113. Maitland K, Kiguli S, Opoka RO, et al. FEAST Trial Group. Mortality after fluid bolus in African children with severe infection. *N Engl J Med.* 2011;364(26):2483-2495.
118. Marzi A, Robertson SJ, Haddock E, et al. Ebola vaccine. VSV-EBOV rapidly protects macaques against infection with the 2014/15 Ebola virus outbreak strain. *Science.* 2015;349:739-742.
119. Mate SE, Kugelman JR, Nyenswah TG, et al. Molecular evidence of sexual transmission of Ebola virus. *N Engl J Med.* 2015;373(25):2448-2454.
120. Mattia JG, Vandy MJ, Chang JC, et al. Early clinical sequelae of Ebola virus disease in Sierra Leone: a cross-sectional study. *Lancet Infect Dis.* 2016;16(3):331-338.
121. McMullan LK, Flint M, Dyall J, et al. The lipid moiety of brincidofovir is required for in vitro antiviral activity against Ebola virus. *Antiviral Res.* 2016;125:71-78.
123. Milligan ID, Gibani MM, Sewell R, et al. Safety and immunogenicity of novel adenovirus type 26- and modified vaccinia Ankara-vectored Ebola vaccines: a randomized clinical trial. *JAMA.* 2016;315(15):1610-1623.
127. Mupapa K, Mukundu W, Bwaka MA, et al. Ebola hemorrhagic fever and pregnancy. *J Infect Dis.* 1999;179(suppl 1):S11-S12.
128. Negredo A, Palacios G, Vázquez-Morón S, et al. Discovery of an ebolavirus-like filovirus in Europe. *PLoS Pathog.* 2011;7(10):e1002304.
129. Ohuabunwo C, Ameh C, Oduyebo O, et al. clinical profile and containment of Ebola virus disease outbreak in two large West African cities, Nigeria, July-September 2014. *Int J Infect Dis.* 2016;53:23-29.
131. Pan Y1, Zhang W, Cui L, et al. Reston virus in domestic pigs in China. *Arch Virol.* 2014;159(5):1129-1132.
135. Peters CJ. Marburg and Ebola—arming ourselves against the deadly filoviruses. *N Engl J Med.* 2005;352(25):2571-2573.
136. Phan JC, Pettitt J, George JS, et al. Lateral flow immunoassays for Ebola virus disease detection in Liberia. *J Infect Dis.* 2016;214(suppl 3):S222-S228.
139. Prescott J, Bushmaker T, Fischer R, et al. Postmortem stability of Ebola virus. *Emerg Infect Dis.* 2015;21(5):856-859.
140. Preston R. *The Hot Zone: The Terrifying True Story of the Origins of the Ebola Virus.* New York: Anchor; 1995.
141. PREVAIL II Writing Group; Multi-National PREVAIL II Study Team, Davey RT Jr, Dodd L, et al. A randomized, controlled trial of ZMapp for Ebola virus infection. *N Engl J Med.* 2016;375(15):1448-1456.
143. Qiu X, Wong G, Audet J, et al. Reversion of advanced Ebola virus disease in nonhuman primates with ZMapp. *Nature.* 2014;514(7520):47-53.
146. Saez AM, Weiss S, Nowak K, et al. Investigating the zoonotic origin of the West African Ebola epidemic. *EMBO Mol Med.* 2015;7:17-23.
147. Sahr F, Ansumana R, Massaquoi TA, et al. Evaluation of convalescent whole blood for treating Ebola virus disease in Freetown, Sierra Leone. *J Infect.* 2017;74(3):302-309.
151. Schieffelin JS, Shaffer JG, Goba A, et al. Clinical illness and outcomes in patients with Ebola in Sierra Leone. *N Engl J Med.* 2014;371(22):2092-2100.
152. Scott JT, Sesay FR, Massaquoi TA, et al. Post-Ebola syndrome, Sierra Leone. *Emerg Infect Dis.* 2016;22(4):641-646.
155. Sissoko D, Laouenan C, Folkesson E, et al. JIKI Study Group. Experimental treatment with favipiravir for Ebola virus disease (the JIKI Trial): a historically controlled, single-arm proof-of-concept trial in Guinea. *PLoS Med.* 2016;13(3):e1001967.
158. Smith PW, Anderson AO, Christopher GW, et al. Designing a biocontainment unit to care for patients with serious communicable diseases: a consensus statement. *Biosecur Bioterror.* 2006;4(4):351-365.
161. Smither SJ, Eastaugh LS, Steward JA, et al. Post-exposure efficacy of oral T-705 (Favipiravir) against inhalational Ebola virus infection in a mouse model. *Antiviral Res.* 2014;104:153-155.
162. Sow MS, Etard JF, Baize S, et al. Postebogui Study Group. New evidence of long-lasting persistence of Ebola virus genetic material in semen of survivors. *J Infect Dis.* 2016;214(10):1475-1476.
167. Baize S, Pannetier D, Oestereich L, et al. Emergence of Zaire Ebola virus disease in Guinea. *N Engl J Med.* 2014;371:1418-1425.
169. Tiffany A, Vetter P, Mattia J, et al. Ebola virus disease complications as experienced by survivors in Sierra Leone. *Clin Infect Dis.* 2016;62(11):1360-1366.
170. Nyenswah TG, Kateh F, Bawo L, et al. Ebola and its control in Liberia, 2014-2015. *Emerg Infect Dis.* 2016;22(2):169-177.
172. Towner JS, Rollin PE, Bausch DG, et al. Rapid diagnosis of Ebola hemorrhagic fever by reverse transcription-PCR in an outbreak setting and assessment of patient viral load as a predictor of outcome. *J Virol.* 2004;78(8):4330-4341.
174. Trehan I, Kelly T, Marsh RH, et al. Moving towards a more aggressive and comprehensive model of care for children with Ebola. *J Pediatr.* 2016;170:28-33, e27.
175. Trehan I, Kelly P, Shaikh N, Manary MJ. New insights into environmental enteric dysfunction. *Arch Dis Child.* 2016;101(8):741-744.
177. Uyeki TM, Mehta AK, Davey RT Jr, et al. Clinical management of Ebola virus disease in the United States and Europe. *N Engl J Med.* 2016;374(7):636-646.
178. Van Griensven J, De Weiggheleire A, Delamou A, et al. The use of Ebola convalescent plasma to treat Ebola virus disease in resource-constrained settings: a perspective from the field. *Clin Infect Dis.* 2016;62(1):69-74.
179. Varkey JB, Shantha JG, Crozier I, et al. Persistence of Ebola virus in ocular fluid during convalescence. *N Engl J Med.* 2015;372(25):2423-2427.
180. Verbeek JH, Ijaz S, Mischke C, et al. Personal protective equipment for preventing highly infectious diseases due to exposure to contaminated body fluids in health care staff. *Cochrane Database Syst Rev.* 2016;(4):CD011621.

181. Vetter P, Fischer WA, Schibler M, et al. Ebola virus shedding and transmission: review of current evidence. *J Infect Dis*. 2016;214(suppl 3):S177-S184.
182. Victory KR, Coronado F, Ifono SO, et al. Ebola transmission linked to a single traditional funeral ceremony—Kissidougou, Guinea, December, 2014–January 2015. *MMWR Morb Mortal Wkly Rep*. 2015;64(14):386-388.
187. Warren TK, Jordan R, Lo MK, et al. Therapeutic efficacy of the small molecule GS-5734 against Ebola virus in rhesus monkeys. *Nature*. 2016;531(7594):381-385.
188. Warren TK, Warfield KL, Wells J, et al. Advanced antisense therapies for postexposure protection against lethal filovirus infections. *Nat Med*. 2010;16(9):991-994.
189. Warren TK, Wells J, Panchal RG, et al. Protection against filovirus diseases by a novel broad-spectrum nucleoside analogue BCX4430. *Nature*. 2014;508(7496):402-405.
190. Wasswa H. International agencies help fight Marburg disease outbreak in Uganda. *BMJ*. 2014;349:g6185.
191. Wendo C. Caring for the survivors of Uganda's Ebola epidemic one year on. *Lancet*. 2001;358(9290):1350.
192. WHO Ebola Response Team. Ebola virus disease in West Africa—the first 9 months of the epidemic and forward projections. *N Engl J Med*. 2014;371(16):1481-1495.
193. WHO Ebola Response Team, Agua-Agum J, Ariyarajah A, et al. Ebola virus disease among children in West Africa. *N Engl J Med*. 2015;372(13):1274-1277.
195. *WHO: Statement on Ebola in the Democratic Republic of the Congo*. Available at: http://www.who.int/mediacentre/news/statements/2017/ebola-drc/en/.
201. Wu S, Kroeker A, Wong G, et al. An adenovirus vaccine expressing Ebola virus variant Makona glycoprotein is efficacious in guinea pigs and nonhuman primates. *J Infect Dis*. 2016;214(suppl 3):S326-S332.
202. US Food and Drug Administration. *Ebola Response Updates From FDA*. Available at: https://www.fda.gov/EmergencyPreparedness/Counterterrorism/MedicalCountermeasures/MCMIssues/ucm410308.htm.
204. Yacisin K, Balter S, Fine A, et al. Ebola virus disease in a humanitarian aid worker—New York City, October 2014. *MMWR Morb Mortal Wkly Rep*. 2015;64(12):321-323.

The full reference list for this chapter is available at ExpertConsult.com.

SUBSECTION X Coronaviridae and Toroviridae

188 Human Coronaviruses, Including Middle East Respiratory Syndrome Coronavirus

Janet A. Englund • Yae-Jean Kim • Kenneth McIntosh

The family Coronaviridae contains two subfamilies, Coronavirinae and Torovirinae. The subfamily Coronavirinae is currently divided into four genera, the alpha-, beta-, gamma-, and deltacoronaviruses; the human coronaviruses (HCoVs) belong in the first two of these. Until recently, HCoVs were considered to cause upper respiratory tract illness and possibly also some undetermined fraction of viral diarrhea. In 2002, a new coronavirus, the SARS coronavirus (SARS-CoV), was found to be the cause of an acute, severe, frequently fatal respiratory disease with prominent systemic symptoms: severe acute respiratory syndrome, or SARS. In 2012, another highly pathogenic coronavirus, the Middle East Respiratory Syndrome coronavirus (MERS-CoV), appeared in Saudi Arabia and neighboring countries.[41,198] This virus, with a high case-fatality rate and the ability to spread in families and among patients and caregivers in hospitals, is in at least some instances contracted from camels with respiratory disease.[10] The origin of this virus, as with SARS-CoV, may also have been in bats.[5] In retrospect, the emergence of SARS and MERS-CoV is consistent with what was already known about coronaviruses: these viruses are widespread pathogens in the animal kingdom, evolving rapidly through mutation and recombination, and with a capacity for jumping species barriers.[87] Coronaviruses cause a wide variety of important diseases in animals, including infectious bronchitis and nephrosis in chickens; gastroenteritis and encephalitis in young piglets; enteritis in turkeys, dogs, and calves; hepatitis and encephalitis in mice; pneumonitis and sialodacryoadenitis in rats; infectious peritonitis in cats; and pneumonia and hepatitis in whales. Multiple strains of unknown pathogenicity have been recovered from numerous species of bats.[189]

BACKGROUND

Since the first report of HCoV isolation in 1965,[170] the HCoV group has been repeatedly confirmed to be an important and frequent cause of the common cold and a likely cause of more serious respiratory tract infections in the elderly.[52,53,64,183] They also have been implicated as contributors to lower respiratory tract infections in children and adults. The first HCoV was cultivated by Tyrrell and Bynoe at the Common Cold Unit in Salisbury, England, with the use of human embryonic tracheal and nasal epithelial mucosal organ cultures.[170] These investigators were able to produce colds regularly in volunteers inoculated with organ culture fluid from the first and later passages of an agent, B814, obtained from a boy with a cold.[16] Working independently, Hamre and Procknow in 1966 described the isolation of five viruses, including the prototype strain HCoV-229E, in primary human embryonic kidney cell cultures.[68] Four of these agents were obtained from medical students with upper respiratory tract illnesses and one from a healthy student. The growth of six additional HCoVs, including the second human prototype HCoV-OC43, was reported in 1967 by McIntosh and associates, who used human embryonic tracheal organ cultures inoculated with secretions from adults with upper respiratory tract infections.[105,107]

The relationship of HCoVs to similar agents known to infect animals soon became evident. By electron microscopy, 229E and B814 were demonstrated to be morphologically identical to each other as well as to avian infectious bronchitis virus.[2] Subsequently, mouse hepatitis virus was demonstrated to be very similar morphologically and to be antigenically related to HCoV-OC43.[105,109] Shortly thereafter, these and similar agents were given the name "coronaviruses" owing to the crownlike appearance of their surface projections on electron microscopy.[169]

Poor growth and a lack of cytopathic effect in cell culture were, until recently, major deterrents to research on HCoV. With the development of molecular diagnostic techniques including the polymerase chain reaction (PCR), and following the emergence of SARS-CoV[45,84,135] and, in 2012, MERS-CoV,[10,41] the field of coronavirology has developed widely and rapidly. Two additional community-acquired respiratory coronaviruses were discovered in the wake of the SARS epidemic: HCoV-NL63 in 2004,[49,55,175] and HCoV-HKU1 in 2005.[90,188] These two virus species joined HCoV-229E and HCoV-OC43 as common, endemic respiratory viruses with worldwide distribution and similar, although probably not identical, mild-to-moderate pathogenicity in normal human hosts. In this chapter, these four HCoVs are referred to as "community-acquired respiratory coronaviruses" to distinguish them from SARS-CoV and MERS-CoV.

VIROLOGY

Coronaviruses are medium to large (80–220 nm), pleomorphic, spherical or elliptical enveloped RNA viruses with widely spaced, petal-shaped,

20-nm–long surface projections giving the virus the appearance of a solar corona[104] (Fig. 188.1). They are labile to heat, lipid solvents, and acid pH. The genomes of multiple coronaviruses have been sequenced completely, including those of HCoVs 229E, OC43, NL63, HKU1, MERS-CoV, and multiple strains of the SARS-CoV.[38,55,65,71,144,175,181,182,188] The genome and its surrounding capsid are arranged in helical symmetry and enclosed within a lipoprotein envelope.

Within the coronavirus particle, a nucleoprotein (N) surrounds the RNA genome, and together they appear as a coiled tubular helix within the bilayer lipid-containing envelope. The envelope contains two or three glycoproteins: (1) a matrix protein M, which is embedded in the envelope; (2) a surface component S, which is the structural protein of the petal-shaped spikes and the target of neutralizing antibody; and (3) a hemagglutinin esterase HE, which is found in several of the betacoronaviruses, including OC43 and HKU1, and contains sequences closely related to influenza C hemagglutinin. The four respiratory HCoV species plus the SARS-CoV and MERS-CoV, along with several other mammalian coronaviruses, have been placed in the alphacoronavirus genus (229E and NL63) or the betacoronavirus genus (OC43, HKU1, SARS-CoV, and MERS-CoV) (Box 188.1); avian infectious bronchitis virus and several other coronaviruses have been placed in the gammacoronavirus genus, and several recently discovered avian coronaviruses in the deltacoronavirus genus.[187]

Coronaviruses contain a positive-sense, single-stranded RNA genome of molecular weight 26 to 31 kilobases, the largest of any RNA virus group.[87] In coronavirus replication, all processes take place in the cytoplasm. In the first step, the virus attaches to the cell membrane by using its HE or S protein in the petal-shaped spike. HCoV-229E uses aminopeptidase N (CD-13) as a cellular receptor,[195] both the SARS-CoV and NL63 use angiotensin-converting enzyme 2,[72,93] and MERS-CoV uses dipeptidyl-peptidase 4 (CD26),[145] whereas the receptor for HCoV-OC43 still has not been identified definitively. Penetration occurs as a result of S protein–mediated fusion of the viral envelope with the plasma membrane. The large viral replicase gene, which occupies two-thirds of the genome, then codes for a large polyprotein. This polyprotein is cleaved into 15 or 16 nonstructural proteins by two or three virally encoded proteases, and a replication complex is formed. Within this complex, an RNA-dependent RNA polymerase initiates the transcription of subgenomic mRNAs through negative-stranded intermediaries. The mRNA molecules, as in other members of the virus order Nidovirales, form a nested set, with the sequences of the first open reading frame at the 5′ end (after a leader sequence) containing the coding region and subsequent sequences through to the polyadenylated 3′ end being untranslated.[132] Virions then are assembled by budding into cytoplasmic vesicles in the rough endoplasmic reticulum and Golgi region. Virus particles are released by cell lysis or fusion of post-Golgi, virion-containing vesicles with the plasma membrane.

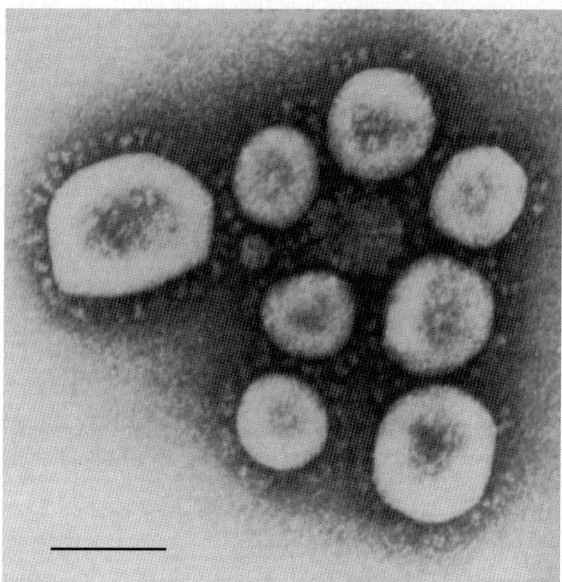

FIG. 188.1 Human coronavirus. Electron micrograph of one of the earliest coronaviruses found from an adult with a cold (OC16), negatively stained with phosphotungstic acid. The bar is 100 nm.

BOX 188.1 Taxonomy of Selected Coronavirus Species

- Alpha coronavirus
  - HCoV-229E
  - HCoV-NL63 (new)
  - SARS-CoV (new)
  - MERS-CoV (new)
- Beta coronavirus
  - HCoV-OC43
  - HCoV-HKU1 (new)
- Gamma coronavirus
  - Avian infectious bronchitis virus
- Delta coronavirus
- Porcine coronavirus HKU15

EPIDEMIOLOGY OF COMMUNITY-ACQUIRED RESPIRATORY CORONAVIRUSES

Early epidemiologic surveys of HCoV infections were carried out by serologic methods of complement fixation, hemagglutination inhibition, and enzyme immunoassays, with 229E or OC43 viruses as antigens.[24,43,83,99,110] More recently, epidemiologic surveys of 229E, OC43, NL63, and/or HKU1 infection have been based on PCR of respiratory tract samples.[50,86,95,96,102,127,162,172,190]

Recent epidemiologic studies of enteric HCoVs have been based on PCR detection in stool and respiratory samples obtained simultaneously and are described in the section on clinical manifestations of enteric HCoVs. The epidemiology of SARS-CoV and MERS-CoV is described in the following sections.

Geographic Prevalence

Community-acquired respiratory coronavirus infections occur worldwide. Seroprevalence studies using 229E and OC43 antigens have been conducted in the United States, Europe, Brazil, and Iraq.[17,25,69,70,80,81,110] With enzyme-linked immunosorbent assay (ELISA), antibody prevalence in adults from all areas where they have been examined approaches 90% to 100%. All four of the community-acquired human coronaviruses have been identified frequently using PCR analysis wherever they have been sought.[50,86,95,96,102,127,162,172,190]

Seasonal Incidence and Annual Recycling Pattern

Although HCoV infection may occur at any time of the year (Fig. 188.2), the highest rates in temperate climates are seen in midwinter to early spring. The irregular year-to-year pattern described for OC43 and 229E, namely, that individual species predominate for 1 or more years, followed by 1 or more years of lower activity,[80,81,117,118] appears also to hold for NL63 and HKU1.[39,142,167,174] More sensitive molecular assays using multiplex PCR have provided more insight into these patterns, confirming earlier reports that one of the four known HCoV species may be the predominant HCoV in a particular area during a particular season, with all four types circulating simultaneously in many years.[86] Evaluation of community-acquired respiratory coronavirus epidemiology must include tests that are sensitive for all four species.[86] Because of unpredictable variability, studies carried out over relatively short periods, such as 6 months or even 1 year, are likely to yield misleading results regarding prevalence and incidence. The experience of one laboratory over 4 successive years where symptomatic children were sampled in outpatient and hospital settings is shown in Fig. 188.2.

During outbreaks, specific coronavirus types may be responsible for a large fraction of respiratory tract infections. At the University of Chicago in 1966 and 1967, 229E was associated with a significant outbreak in medical students; 66 (35%) of 191 sampled students were infected.[67]

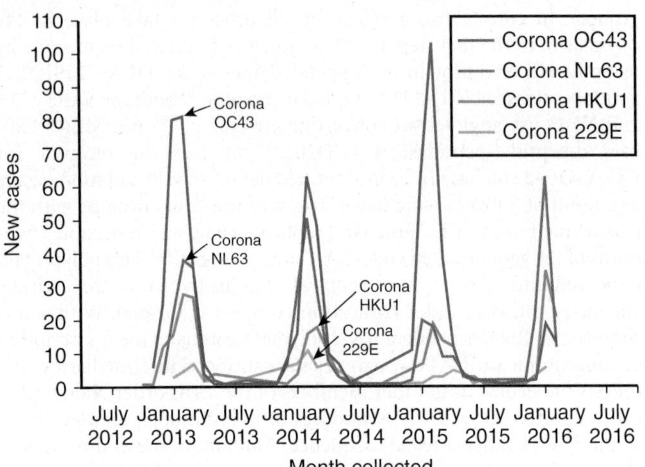

FIG. 188.2 Distribution of human coronavirus types in respiratory specimens from symptomatic inpatient and outpatient pediatric patients over 4 years at Seattle Children's Hospital using a commercial rapid multiplex polymerase chain reaction (FilmArray, Biofire Diagnostics). This demonstrates concurrent circulation of all four types of human coronavirus (HCoV) during winter months, with predominance of HCoV-OC43 in three seasons and HCoV-229E in another. (Unpublished data courtesy J. Stapp, Seattle Children's Hospital Microbiology Laboratory.)

In Tecumseh, Michigan, a large 229E outbreak in 1967 affected 68% of 38 families and 34% of 159 individuals tested. Distinct outbreaks also can occur in hospitalized infants; at National Jewish Hospital in Denver, 16 of 20 hospitalized asthmatic infants were infected with HCoV-OC43 in December 1968,[108] and smaller outbreaks have been seen in neonatal intensive care units with OC43,[161] 229E,[58] and NL63.[49]

Ratio of Clinical to Subclinical Illness

Although B814, 229E and OC43 clearly caused symptomatic upper respiratory tract disease in adult volunteers, asymptomatic infections were also seen in these volunteer studies. Early surveys of 229E and OC43 that identified infection in infants and children by a rise in antibody indicated that at least 50% of infections were subclinical.[80,81,110] In contrast, in the Denver children hospitalized with atopic asthma, 19 were infected with either 229E or OC43 and 17 were symptomatic.[108] A 2-year prospective PCR-based study of respiratory illness in more than 600 rural Alaskan children demonstrated similar rates of coronavirus infection in hospitalized children and community controls.[159] Other surveys of HCoVs in both symptomatic and asymptomatic children using detection by PCR have shown almost identical rates of positivity, indicating that in otherwise normal children, community-acquired respiratory coronaviruses may be of low pathogenicity or are shed for prolonged periods.[15,39,85,142]

The importance of coronavirus in severely immunocompromised patients, such as hematopoietic stem cell transplant (HSCT) patients, has been investigated. In a 2-year prospective study conducted in HSCT recipients of all ages who were sampled weekly before and for 100 days after transplantation, the rates of detection of any of the four species of community-acquired respiratory HCoV in symptomatic versus asymptomatic patients were similar.[116] Of note, the duration of shedding of coronaviruses in immunocompromised patients varied from less than 2 weeks (35%) to more than 10 weeks (17%).

Age Specificity of Infection

The first infection with all four HCoVs takes place during childhood, probably during the first 6 years of life.[200] Antibody to the HCoVs appears in early childhood, with a tendency for antibody to OC43 and NL63 to appear earlier and more frequently than antibody to 229E and HKU1.[43] Prevalence increases rapidly with age. Asymptomatic and symptomatic infection occurs at all ages, including in the elderly. In the Tecumseh families studied during a community-wide 229E epidemic in 1967, only 3 of 54 infections occurred in children younger than 4 years. The attack rate then rose to a peak of 14% in individuals 15 to 29 years of age and subsequently fell with increasing age.[25] The results were different in an outbreak of HCoV-OC43 infection. With this virus, the highest rate, 29%, occurred in children 4 years of age or younger, and rates decreased very little even into adult years, when the incidence was 22%.[118]

Prospective studies during the first year of life of viruses found by PCR in nasopharyngeal samples obtained during acute respiratory symptoms have found coronaviruses, including OC43, 229E, NL63, and HKU1, in 6% to 16% of episodes.[85,91,148,177] In a birth cohort study that included samples obtained from asymptomatic as well as symptomatic infants, the proportions in the two groups were not significantly different (4.4% in asymptomatic infants vs. 5.5% in symptomatic infants).[85] In a prospective study of symptomatic children younger than 2 years attending daycare, coronavirus was detected as a sole pathogen in only 4% of upper respiratory tract illnesses but in an additional 11% of illnesses when more than one virus was present.[51] In the same study, the incidence of coronavirus detection by age cohort decreased from a rate of 0.6 infection per child-year for children observed beginning at 0 to 6 months of age to 0.5 infection per child-year for those observed from 7 to 12 months of age and further to 0.2 for those observed from 1 to 2 years of age. Similarly, a longitudinal study among 26 households with children in Utah demonstrated higher (although not necessarily significantly higher) rates of symptomatic disease associated with all four types of HCoV in children ages 0 to 4 years, with relatively similar rates in older children and adults.[22] Several studies have emphasized the importance of coronavirus infection in the elderly, particularly in individuals in chronic care facilities and those with underlying cardiopulmonary disease.[53,60,126]

Transmission

Human volunteers can be infected readily by nose drops containing OC43 or 229E, and a typical cold develops 2 to 3 days later. Natural infections are therefore assumed to occur through the respiratory route. Nosocomial transmission of coronavirus respiratory tract infection has been reported. One study took place in a neonatal intensive care unit, where prospective surveillance by immunofluorescence testing of nasal aspirates performed for 15 months detected 10 infections with coronavirus OC43, all of them nosocomially acquired.[161] All infants had apnea, bradycardia, or abdominal distention, or a combination of these pathologic effects, at the time of infection. Another study using PCR analysis for HCoV-229E found three outbreaks occurred in 1 year involving 28% of neonates (43 of 152, most of whom were symptomatic) and 52% of staff members (most of whom were asymptomatic).[59] The mode of transmission was not demonstrated in either study.

INFECTION AND IMMUNITY

Pathogenesis, Incubation Period, and Serologic Response

In healthy adults, community-acquired respiratory HCoVs seem to replicate only in the upper respiratory tract and to produce little direct cytopathologic effect. In immunocompromised adults, HCoV has been detected in bronchoalveolar lavage fluid,[60,116] indicating potential replication in the lower airway. In human embryonic tracheal organ culture, a decline in ciliary activity after serial passage was the only cytopathic effect observed.[107,170] Very similar events appear to take place in vivo. Electron microscopy of nasal epithelial biopsy specimens from a young girl with chronic rhinitis and bronchitis showed preservation of cellular structures and cilia despite replication of coronavirus particles.[1]

OC43 and 229E have been detected in nasopharyngeal cells,[111] and 229E virus titers from 10 to more than 1000 $TCID_{50}$ (median tissue culture infective dose) were found for a week or more in nasopharyngeal washings.[122] Bende and associates studied the course of 229E colds in 24 volunteers and delineated the typical signs, symptoms, and virus shedding patterns; eight volunteers were asymptomatic.[13] The incubation period of HCoV colds is, on average, 2 days, and they usually last approximately 1 week.[16] In small infants, virus may be detectable in respiratory secretions for 3 weeks and longer.[148] Recovery is likely to be dependent on cell-mediated immunity. Infections in immunocompromised subjects may be associated with severe and prolonged disease,[7,54,136] although prospective studies have identified asymptomatic infections and prolonged shedding in severely immunocompromised hosts such as bone marrow transplant patients.[116] More studies have been devoted to the pathogenesis of SARS[137] and MERS.

Reinfection

Evidence from human volunteer experiments demonstrates that postinfection immunity can be strain specific. Reed infected volunteers with one of several 229E-like viruses. She found that immunity to homotypic challenge endured for at least 1 year but that immunity to heterotypic HCoV-229E strains in these same volunteers was much lower.[147] IgA antibody may play an important protective role.[23]

CLINICAL MANIFESTATIONS OF RESPIRATORY TRACT INFECTIONS

Common Cold and Other Upper Respiratory Tract Illnesses

A significant association of HCoVs 229E and OC43 with respiratory tract illnesses—most of them coldlike—was demonstrated in early prospective serologic studies of adolescents and young adults. In the Chicago medical students described earlier, HCoV-229E attack rates were 31% during "illness periods" and only 9% in matched "wellness periods" ($P < .001$); the illnesses did not differ significantly from undifferentiated acute respiratory tract infections caused by respiratory syncytial virus, parainfluenza viruses, or rhinoviruses.[67] Similarly, respiratory disease, including pneumonia, was significantly associated with OC43 seroconversion by complement fixation in military recruits at Parris Island and Camp Lejeune in 1971.[184]

Symptoms in the adolescents and adults in the two investigations cited earlier were much like those in human volunteers inoculated with HCoV.[13,16,23,24,147] Infected volunteers contracted typical common colds, with perhaps more rhinorrhea than in rhinovirus colds. Sore throat, cough, malaise, and headache were noted in approximately 50% of volunteers; 20% had fever.

The proportion of total respiratory tract disease or colds attributable to community-acquired respiratory HCoVs varies by season, from year to year, as well as the methodology used. Most serologic surveys have concluded that approximately 8% to 10% of all colds are associated with coronavirus infection.[101] A well-controlled study in the Netherlands used PCR for 229E and OC43 to estimate the contribution of coronaviruses to illness at all ages leading to a visit to general practitioners. Coronaviruses were found in 8.0% of subjects with acute respiratory tract infection, in comparison to 5.5% of nonrespiratory controls. Rhinoviruses were found most commonly in this group (24.7% vs. 16.6% of controls).[178] A survey of first respiratory tract illnesses in the first year of life using PCR with primers for 229E, OC43, and NL63 found coronaviruses in 13 of 82 (16%) infants.[148] As more studies are performed that span longer periods, sample properly matched asymptomatic controls, and include all four known respiratory HCoV strains, the true incidence is likely to become clearer.

The possible role of coronaviruses in the etiology of otitis media with effusion has been the subject of several studies that used PCR for 229E and OC43 in both nasal secretions and middle ear fluid. In one study, 92 children with acute otitis media were investigated. Coronavirus sequences were found in 16 children (17%), in the nasopharynx in 14 children, and in middle ear fluid in seven. This prevalence was less than that of both respiratory syncytial virus (26%) and rhinoviruses (32%).[138] Another 3-year survey of viral upper respiratory tract infections with or without otitis media in the United States used PCR for OC43, NL63, and 229E as well as for other respiratory viruses. Otitis complicated approximately 50% of upper respiratory tract infections in which respiratory syncytial virus, HCoVs, and adenoviruses were found and a smaller proportion in which other viruses (influenza, rhinovirus, metapneumovirus, and parainfluenza viruses) were detected.[36]

Lower Respiratory Tract Disease

Pneumonia and Other Severe Lower Respiratory Tract Infections

The first evidence of a possible causative role of coronaviruses in lower respiratory tract disease was found in a serologic study of hospitalized infants during 1967 to 1970.[106] Infections with both HCoV-229E and HCoV-OC43 were noted, and HCoV was the third most frequently occurring virus (behind respiratory syncytial virus and parainfluenza virus type 3), both in incidence and specifically associated with pneumonia and bronchiolitis. Many of these infants required oxygen. HCoV-229E was grown in tissue culture from oropharyngeal swabs obtained from two of the infants with pneumonia and rises in antibody.

With the increasing availability of PCR for detection of coronaviruses and the addition of two new HCoV strains, NL63 and HKU1, information about the presence of these viruses in children with serious respiratory tract disease has expanded greatly. A large number of studies have demonstrated that HCoVs can be found in the respiratory tract of 4% to 8% of children hospitalized with acute respiratory infection, often accompanied by coinfection with other respiratory tract viruses.[32,35,61,86,96,127,146,156,167,180] A much smaller number of surveys have included age- and season-matched control children without respiratory symptoms. When these controls are properly chosen and studied, however, HCoV detection rates in well and ill children have been similar.[39,142,159] It appears likely that coronaviruses are pathogenic in some instances whereas in others they are not, or persistent shedding of these viruses may occur, and it is difficult to assign an etiologic role in individual cases.[103]

In newborns, apnea, bradycardia, and increased demand for oxygen have been described during coronavirus infection.[39,59,160,161] One prospective nursery study, with sampling at regular intervals regardless of symptoms, associated HCoV-229E infection with symptomatic disease in high-risk neonates.[57] Another outbreak study in a neonatal intensive care setting implicated NL63 in acute symptomatic disease.[49]

There is a suggestion that NL63 is seen particularly in croup.[35,166,176] Carefully conducted epidemiologic studies do not link coronavirus infection or disease with Kawasaki syndrome.[12]

Infections in Children With Underlying Respiratory Disease or Immunodeficiency

Substantial evidence indicates that HCoVs can precipitate asthma attacks,[73,77,108,114,133] although their role in this regard is clearly secondary to that of rhinoviruses and respiratory syncytial virus.[74] In a 2-year surveillance (1967–69) of 32 mostly atopic children aged 1 to 5 years hospitalized in Denver for severe, recurrent bouts of wheezing, 19 HCoV infections were diagnosed.[108] Six children were infected simultaneously with either parainfluenza virus or respiratory syncytial virus. Of the remaining 13 patients, all were symptomatic: three had mild wheezing, and seven had acute asthma attacks, two of which required intravenous therapy.

Several studies of HCoVs in children with cystic fibrosis have identified all four species by PCR.[21,40] In a study from Brazil, HCoVs were found in 19 of 408 samples, with a correlation of NL63 infection with exacerbations of respiratory symptoms, although this did not hold up in a logistic regression model for independent association.[40] In a 2-year prospective Seattle study in 44 participants, HCoVs were detected in only three subjects, but in both upper airway and sputum samples.[21]

Coronavirus has been detected as the sole respiratory pathogen in upper and lower respiratory tract samples in immunocompromised children with pneumonia receiving chemotherapy or having received a solid-organ transplant as well as in adults undergoing HSCT.[86,171] Respiratory disease in six immunocompromised children with coronavirus and no other viral, bacterial, or fungal pathogen detected by sensitive testing began as fever and rhinorrhea; only two children had cough at the time of first medical encounter.[86] Only one of three children had evidence of abnormalities on chest radiographs, although all six children required hospitalization for coronavirus-linked illness for 2 to 12 days. A prospective study with weekly sampling in 215 asymptomatic and symptomatic HSCT recipients of all ages during the first 100 days after transplantation demonstrated prolonged coronavirus shedding (frequently for 6 weeks, occasionally up to 12 weeks). Moreover, coronavirus was not found as a sole pathogen associated with pneumonia, demonstrating that coronavirus-associated pneumonia is relatively infrequent in immunocompromised patients and that the detection of coronavirus is probably insufficient evidence to assess causality.[116]

Severe Acute Respiratory Syndrome

SARS emerged in 2002 as a new infectious disease that originated in Guangdong Province, China, in November 2002. After a few sporadic cases, the virus spread at first within China and then, through Hong Kong, to Vietnam, Singapore, Europe, Canada, and the United States. By the time the epidemic ended in the summer of 2003, there were 8096 probable cases in 29 countries and areas with 774 deaths (9.6% mortality).[192] The total number of health care workers affected was 1706 (21.1% of all probable cases). Globally, children younger than 18 years likely accounted for only about 5% of cases. The severity of the syndrome appears to have been greater in adults and adolescents than in young children, and there was no reported mortality in children.[193] Further detail is provided in the sixth edition of this book.

Etiology

The etiologic agent of SARS is a novel coronavirus, the SARS-CoV, identified independently and collaboratively by multiple investigators.[45,84,135,141] The virus was classified as a betacoronavirus, lineage B (HCoV-OC43 and HKU1 are in lineage A). The virus undoubtedly originated in animals, probably bats, and then spread to exotic animals kept for human consumption in southeastern China, and then to humans.[31,65,78,89,94] The genome of the SARS-CoV is about 29,700 nucleotides in length and has a genetic organization similar to that of other coronaviruses. The SARS-CoV uses angiotensin-converting enzyme 2 as a key functional cellular receptor. The virus also binds to the C-type lectin CD209L (also known as L-SIGN) and DC-SIGN.[72,88,93]

Epidemiology

Through case identification and rigorous implementation of barrier methods, the SARS epidemic was quenched after only about 8 months of activity despite the fact that the virus could potentially spread widely through aerosols. One well-described airplane cluster and several explosive community epidemics were well documented.[129,197] Children with SARS are apparently less infectious than their adult counterparts.

Clinical Presentation

There are two large series of serologically proven pediatric cases of SARS.[33,92] In Leung's series (median age, 12 years) the disease had many features similar to that in adults: onset with fever and systemic, influenza-like symptoms, followed by cough in 64% and diarrhea in 20%; progressive pneumonia, common in adults, appeared in only a small minority of children and mostly in adolescents.[92]

Chest radiography and high-resolution computed tomography findings were similar to those found in adults, showing peripheral consolidations and ground-glass opacities, with pleural effusions being rare.[11] In spite of the apparent universality of viremia, no evidence of perinatal transmission to infants was documented.[123,124,154,158,186,199] However, maternal SARS-CoV infection was associated with both maternal and fetal morbidity and mortality.[123,124,158,185,186]

Specific Diagnosis, Treatment and Prevention

The World Health Organization and the Centers for Disease Control and Prevention developed case definitions for SARS.[26,191] Laboratory diagnosis depended on antibody titer during illness or detection of virus in plasma or respiratory tract secretions using specific reverse transcriptase (RT)-PCR platforms.[125,140] No specific treatment other than careful supportive care is recommended.

The mainstay of prevention of SARS was effective and enforced hospital infection control practices and quarantine procedures outside hospitals: isolation at triage in negative air-pressure rooms, use of appropriate masks and goggles or face shields while tending patients, and handwashing before and after contact with patients.[37]

Middle East Respiratory Syndrome

The first report of Middle East respiratory syndrome (MERS) was in a man hospitalized in Jeddah, Saudi Arabia, in June 2012, who died of severe pneumonia and renal failure and from whose sputum a novel coronavirus was isolated.[198] This new betacoronavirus was initially called human coronavirus Erasmus Medical Center (HCoV-EMC).[173] In September 2012, a similar virus was identified from a patient with severe pneumonia who had been transferred from the Gulf region of the Middle East to London, United Kingdom, and was named human coronavirus England 1.[14] Later, this novel coronavirus was renamed MERS-CoV by global consensus.[41] Multiple studies have reported outbreaks associated with health care facilities and with transmission in household contacts.[9,46,128] As of March 2016, WHO had reported 1698 laboratory-confirmed cases of MERS-CoV infection in 26 countries with 609 deaths globally, an approximate 36% mortality rate (http://www.who.int/emergencies/mers-cov/en/). Most cases have been in adults living or traveling in the Arabian peninsula and with underlying chronic diseases or immunosuppression.

Etiology

MERS-CoV is a betacoronavirus, belongs to lineage C, and is closely related to *Tylonycteris* bat coronavirus HKU4 (Ty-BatCoV HKU4) and *Pipistrellus* bat coronavirus HKU5 (Pi-BatCoV HKU5).[41] The widely expressed cell-surface protease dipeptidyl-peptidase 4 (DPP4, also known as CD26) was identified as a functional receptor for host cell entry.[145]

Epidemiology

The epidemiology of MERS-CoV infection has not been well described. The role of bats has been investigated. In four countries in Europe and Ghana, Africa, viruses related to MERS-CoV were identified from 24.9% of *Nycteris* bats and 14.7% of *Pipistrellus* bats.[5] In Saudi Arabia virus from one bat contained a 190-base-pair sequence in the large replicase gene identical to the analogous sequence from the human index case virus.[113]

The first definitive isolation of MERS-CoV in nonhuman animal species was reported from dromedary camels in an outbreak investigation in Qatar.[66] An analysis of a 4β2-kb partial viral sequence collected from one animal showed that the camel virus was almost identical to isolates collected from two human cases who had been working on the affected farm. In addition, neutralizing antibodies to MERS-CoV in persons with and without dromedary contact were detected only in those with contact.[150]

A study from United Arab Emirates showed that dromedaries had antibodies against MERS-CoV in sera obtained in both 2003 and 2013,[115] and positive antibody responses were also detected among dromedary in several countries in Africa, such as Nigeria, Tunisia, and Ethiopia.[151] MERS-CoV thus circulated among camels long before human cases were identified, and MERS may also have been underdiagnosed in humans outside the Arabian Peninsula. In a serosurveillance of domestic animals, no evidence of infections in cows, goats, or sheep has been found.[151]

All known MERS-CoV infections can be traced to countries in the Middle East, primarily Saudi Arabia. In early reports, limited person-to-person spread in families and health care settings was demonstrated. Calculations from these early data suggested a reproductive coefficient less than 1, indicating a likely low pandemic potential.[18] However, in the large, predominantly nosocomial 2015 outbreak in the Republic of Korea, a potential episode of "superspreading" was described in which a single patient infected more than 80 other individuals in an emergency department setting.[82]

Clinical Presentation

The incubation period for MERS has been reported to be from 2 to over 14 days with a mean of 5 days from exposure to symptom development.[9] Patients with MERS often develop symptoms with fever, chills, cough, sore throat, myalgia, and arthralgia followed by dyspnea and rapid progression to pneumonia requiring ventilatory and other organ support within the first week.[3,8,9] Of note, some patients with fever, myalgia, and arthralgia have severe disease prior to or without the development of pneumonia. Other common symptoms have included nausea, vomiting, diarrhea, sore throat, myalgia, and headache. Some of those infected, including children and adolescents, have been asymptomatic or only mildly affected.

Many clinical features are similar among patients with MERS and SARS. However, it appears that patients with MERS have higher respiratory tract viral loads during the first week of the illness, a shorter time from illness onset to clinical presentation and requirement for ventilatory support, and a higher overall case-fatality rate than do patients with SARS.[201]

There has been only one summary of proven MERS-CoV infections in children.[112] Of 11 pediatric cases reported, nine were asymptomatic. A 14-year-old morbidly obese girl with Down syndrome was hospitalized with pneumonia but recovered uneventfully. A 2-year-old with cystic fibrosis died after a prolonged hospital course with respiratory and multiorgan failure. In one further report from the World Health Organization, a 14-month-old child in Italy exposed to an adult relative who had returned from Amman, Jordan, with proven MERS developed a mild respiratory illness with PCR-proven MERS-CoV infection and made a full recovery.[194]

Diagnosis

The World Health Organization and the US Centers for Disease Control and Prevention have published case definitions and urge the early submission of respiratory samples, preferably from the lower respiratory tract, for PCR diagnosis, using laboratories with approved protocols and reagents. Serologic diagnosis has not been standardized[27,193] but has been important in outbreak investigations.

Treatment

Multiple experimental treatment modalities have been attempted, including ribavirin, interferon, lopinavir/ritonavir, and convalescent plasma, but data are lacking on the benefits of these therapies.[4,100,143,157,164]

Prevention

In the absence of specific information about the mode of MERS-CoV spread and because of the high lethality of infection, full barrier precautions are recommended for all contacts, with details very similar to the precautions that were used in the SARS epidemic.[28] Strict adherence to good infection control practices is essential because of the potential for nosocomial spread (Fig. 188.3).[34]

Enteric Human Coronavirus

Coronaviruses are important causes of diarrhea in young calves and pigs, and therefore attempts have been made to find human coronaviruses in the stool and to associate them with enteric disease. Most early studies used electron microscopy to detect coronavirus-like particles (CVLPs), but because such particles have, in many studies, appeared as frequently in well subjects as in those with diarrhea, their relevance or authenticity has been questioned.[44,98,119,134] Isolated reports of coronavirus growth in vitro from cases of diarrhea[97,199] have similarly not been confirmed.

The firmest link of CVLPs to human enteric disease may be with gastroenteritis in the very young, especially neonatal necrotizing enterocolitis (NEC). An epidemiologic investigation of NEC was conducted in two hospitals in France, one with and one without an NEC outbreak.[29] Within each hospital, newborns with "no pathologic

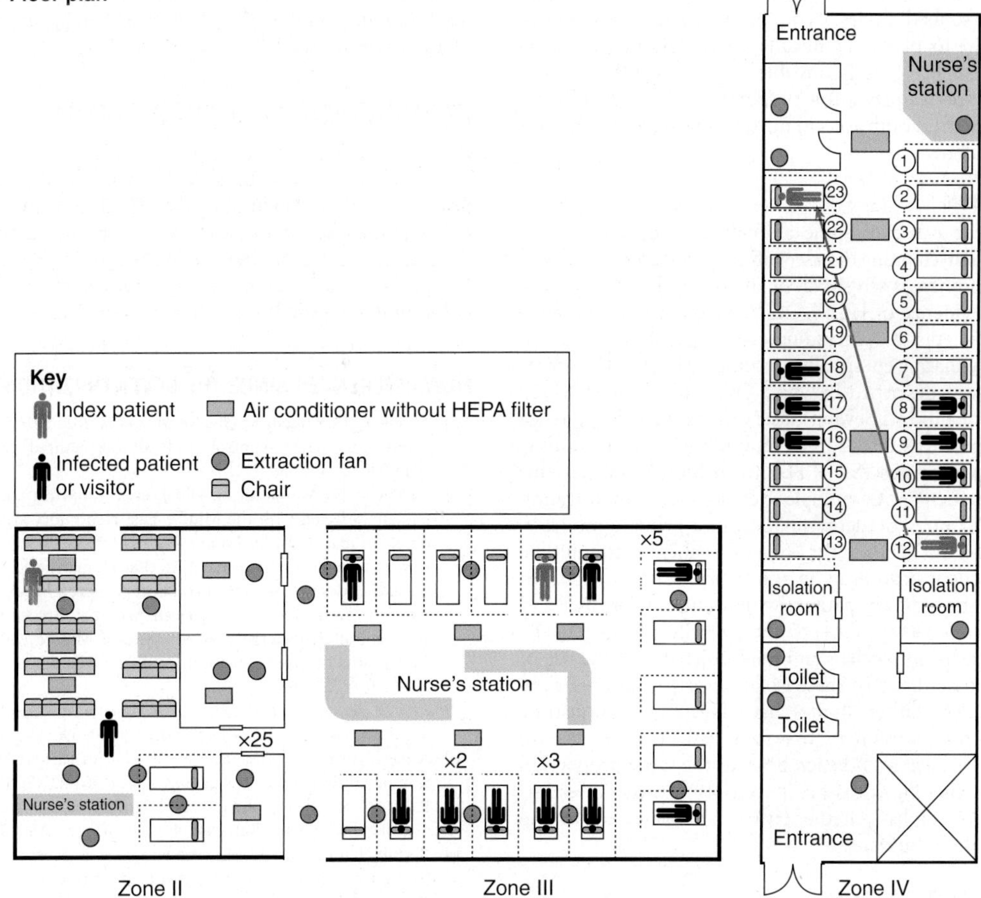

FIG. 188.3 Transmission of Middle East respiratory syndrome coronavirus (MERS-CoV) within a hospital setting. The index patient is shown in red and infected patients and visitors in black in various zones in an emergency room (ER). Over 3 days, the index patient moved from the sitting area (left) to a bed in the central zone of ER (middle), to a preadmission zone of ER (right), and from bed 12 to bed 23 in that zone. MERS-CoV transmission occurred despite the fact that the distance from the index patient's bed to beds of other patients was as great as 6 meters; "×2" indicates two infected MERS cases, successively, in patients or visitors occupying or visiting that bed or that zone. Average ventilation rate in the ER was maintained at three air changes per hour, and all zones in the ER were covered by the same air handling unit. (From Cho SY, Kang J, Ha YE, et al. MERS-CoV outbreak following a single patient exposure in an emergency room in South Korea: an epidemiological outbreak study. *Lancet.* 2016;388[10048]:994-1001.)

occurrence" were used as controls. In the NEC-free hospital, no CVLPs were found in the stools of 21 controls, but two patients with mild diarrhea had CVLPs. In the NEC hospital, 23 of the 32 (72%) NEC patients had fecal CVLPs compared to 3 of 26 (11.5%) controls ($P < .02$). Similar nursery outbreaks of severe diarrhea or NEC in Italy and the United States have been studied by electron microscopy, with similar significant association of CVLPs with disease.[179,62,149]

More recently, clinical studies have used RT-PCR directed at the four community-acquired respiratory coronavirus species in simultaneously collected stool samples and nasopharyngeal swabs from children in the community and the hospital who have acute gastroenteritis (AGE).[48,76,130,131,153] These studies have been conducted in the United States, Finland, and Slovenia and have failed to identify HCoV as an important cause of AGE. One large study, which included asymptomatic control samples, evaluated 878 samples from children with gastrointestinal complaints during 2 years, and detected one of the four HCoV species in 22 children.[153] However, in all but four cases, either rotavirus or norovirus was also found. About half the children had respiratory as well as gastrointestinal symptoms. A prospective study in Finland studied HCoV in hospitalized children with AGE ($n = 172$), acute respiratory tract infection ($n = 545$), or both ($n = 238$) using RT-PCR.[131] As in Risku's previous study, HCoVs were detected in the stools of children with AGE, but usually in the presence of other well-known gastroenteritis viruses, and concomitantly in the respiratory tract. To date, most symptomatic children with HCoV RNA in the stool also have evidence of coinfection by viruses with known gastrointestinal pathogenicity. Thus, the currently described species of community-acquired respiratory HCoV do not appear to play a significant causal role in childhood gastrointestinal illness.[76,131,153] It is possible that some other, as yet undescribed, HCoV species play a role in diarrhea. Controlled longitudinal studies of diarrheal outbreaks in nurseries using PCR have not been published to date.

Neurologic Diseases

Coronaviruses are the cause of some animal neurologic disorders, including a murine demyelinating disease with some features resembling multiple sclerosis. In humans, a serosurvey of HCoV infection in southern Finland discovered evidence of HCoV-OC43 infection in six patients with acute neurologic episodes, including one with polyradiculitis.[152] A case of acute demyelinating encephalitis accompanying OC43 respiratory tract infection was described in which OC43 RNA was detected by PCR in the spinal fluid.[196] Several observations have suggested a possible role of coronavirus infection in multiple sclerosis including: (1) isolation of coronaviruses (SK + SD) from the central nervous system tissue of two patients with multiple sclerosis,[20] (2) demonstration that coronavirus SD can cause demyelination in a primate model,[121] (3) direct visualization of CVLPs in the brain of a patient with multiple sclerosis,[168] and (4) identification by in situ hybridization or PCR of coronavirus RNA in the brains of patients with multiple sclerosis.[6,120,165] However, coronaviruses SK and SD are antigenically and genetically very similar to mouse hepatitis virus and were isolated with the use of mouse tissues; the possibility that these isolates were of mouse origin has not been excluded. Other studies have failed to demonstrate coronavirus RNA in the central nervous system tissue of patients with multiple sclerosis[163] or have found such RNA in the same proportion of patients with demyelinating diseases as in controls.[42] Further investigation will be needed to establish whether HCoVs are related causally to any neurologic disease in humans.

LABORATORY DIAGNOSIS

Virus Isolation

Community-Acquired Respiratory Coronaviruses

Human embryo tracheal or nasal mucosal organ cultures were first used for primary isolation of multiple community-acquired respiratory HCoV strains, including B814, OC43, and several less well characterized strains.[107,170] OC43 was subsequently adapted to growth in monkey kidney, BSC-1, and rhabdomyoma cells.[19,155] The 229E-type strains were shown to replicate and produce a cytopathic effect in secondary human embryo kidney[68] or certain diploid cell lines: WI-38, MRC-5, and MA-177.[67,79] There has been a report of the growth and cytopathic effect of OC43-like and HKU1 strains in the HuH7 hepatocarcinoma cell line.[56,172] NL63 strains grow directly from clinical samples in tertiary monkey kidney cells, with subsequent growth in LLC or Vero cells.[55,175]

Virus Detection Techniques

Community-Acquired Respiratory Coronaviruses

Respiratory coronaviruses can be found in clinical samples by direct antigen detection techniques or by nucleic acid detection. Immunofluorescence[75,111,161] and antigen-detecting ELISA have been used successfully for the diagnosis of HCoV infection,[73,99,114] but nucleic acid detection using PCR techniques has opened up the field of coronavirus diagnosis. Not only is this method the most sensitive for all the known strains of HCoV, but it can also be designed to detect new strains.[49] Attempts to design a set of "pan-coronavirus" primers have, however, always led to suboptimal sensitivity.[49,61] The exact design of the tests greatly influences their sensitivity and specificity.

Serodiagnosis

A rise in antibody titer after day 28 of onset of symptoms is the gold standard for diagnosis of SARS-CoV and MERS-CoV infection, most commonly by ELISA or immunofluorescence assay in Vero-E6 cells. The finding of antibody in convalescent serum is highly specific, although there are one-way cross-reactivities with both 229E and, notably, OC43 for SARS-CoV.[30] For respiratory coronaviruses, complement fixation,[25,106,110,118,152] hemagglutination inhibition (for HCoV-OC43 only),[81] neutralization,[47] ELISA,[24,43,63,83,99] indirect hemagglutination,[80] and Western blot have been used.[139]

PREVENTION AND TREATMENT

Barrier methods with attention to infection control practices were extraordinarily successful in the limitation and final elimination of the SARS epidemic and in limiting the MERS epidemic. The high reinfection rate with the respiratory HCoVs as well as the number of related strains suggests that a vaccine may be ineffective in preventing HCoV-caused respiratory illness. There are no known effective antivirals for the community-acquired respiratory coronaviruses.

NEW REFERENCES SINCE THE SEVENTH EDITION

3. Al-Tawfiq JA, Hinedi K, Ghandour J, et al. Middle East respiratory syndrome coronavirus: a case-control study of hospitalized patients. *Clin Infect Dis.* 2014;59(2):160-165.
4. Al-Tawfiq JA, Momattin H, Dib J, et al. Ribavirin and interferon therapy in patients infected with the Middle East respiratory syndrome coronavirus: an observational study. *Int J Infect Dis.* 2014;20:42-46.
5. Annan A, Baldwin HJ, Corman VM, et al. Human betacoronavirus 2c EMC/2012-related viruses in bats, Ghana and Europe. *Emerg Infect Dis.* 2013;19(3):456-459.
8. Assiri A, Al-Tawfiq JA, Al-Rabeeah AA, et al. Epidemiological, demographic, and clinical characteristics of 47 cases of Middle East respiratory syndrome coronavirus disease from Saudi Arabia: a descriptive study. *Lancet Infect Dis.* 2013;13(9):752-761.
9. Assiri A, McGeer A, Perl TM, et al. Hospital outbreak of Middle East respiratory syndrome coronavirus. *N Engl J Med.* 2013;369(5):407-416.
10. Azhar EI, El-Kafrawy SA, Farraj SA, et al. Evidence for camel-to-human transmission of MERS coronavirus. *N Engl J Med.* 2014;370(26):2499-2505.
12. Baker SC, Shimizu C, Shike H, et al. Human coronavirus-NL63 infection is not associated with acute Kawasaki disease. *Adv Exp Med Biol.* 2006;581:523-526.
14. Bermingham A, Chand MA, Brown CS, et al. Severe respiratory illness caused by a novel coronavirus, in a patient transferred to the United Kingdom from the Middle East, September 2012. *Euro Surveill.* 2012;17(40):20290.
18. Breban R, Riou J, Fontanet A. Interhuman transmissibility of Middle East respiratory syndrome coronavirus: estimation of pandemic risk. *Lancet.* 2013;382(9893):694-699.
21. Burns JL, Emerson J, Kuypers J, et al. Respiratory viruses in children with cystic fibrosis: viral detection and clinical findings. *Influenza Other Respir Viruses.* 2012;6(3):218-223.
27. Centers for Disease Control and Prevention. MERS—Interim Patient under Investigation (PUI) Guidance and Case Definitions; http://www.cdc.gov/coronavirus/mers/interim-guidance.html.
28. Centers for Disease Control and Prevention. Interim Infection Prevention and Control Recommendations for Hospitalized Patients with Middle East Respiratory

Syndrome Coronavirus (MERS-CoV); 2015. http://www.cdc.gov/coronavirus/mers/infection-prevention-control.html.

34. Cho SY, Kang J, Ha YE, et al. MERS-CoV outbreak following a single patient exposure in an emergency room in South Korea: an epidemiological outbreak study. *Lancet*. 2016;388(10048):994-1001.
36. Chonmaitree T, Revai K, Grady JJ, et al. Viral upper respiratory tract infection and otitis media complication in young children. *Clin Infect Dis*. 2008;46(6):815-823.
38. Cotten M, Lam TT, Watson SJ, et al. Full-genome deep sequencing and phylogenetic analysis of novel human betacoronavirus. *Emerg Infect Dis*. 2013;19(5):736-742B.
40. da Silva Filho LV, Zerbinati RM, Tateno AF, et al. The differential clinical impact of human coronavirus species in children with cystic fibrosis. *J Infect Dis*. 2012;206(3):384-388.
39. Dare RK, Fry AM, Chittaganpitch M, et al. Human coronavirus infections in rural Thailand: a comprehensive study using real-time reverse-transcription polymerase chain reaction assays. *J Infect Dis*. 2007;196(9):1321-1328.
41. de Groot RJ, Baker SC, Baric RS, et al. Middle East respiratory syndrome coronavirus (MERS-CoV): announcement of the Coronavirus Study Group. *J Virol*. 2013;87(14):7790-7792.
43. Dijkman R, Jebbink MF, Gaunt E, et al. The dominance of human coronavirus OC43 and NL63 infections in infants. *J Clin Virol*. 2012;53(2):135-139.
46. Drosten C, Meyer B, Muller MA, et al. Transmission of MERS-coronavirus in household contacts. *N Engl J Med*. 2014;371(9):828-835.
48. Esper F, Ou Z, Huang YT. Human coronaviruses are uncommon in patients with gastrointestinal illness. *J Clin Virol*. 2010;48(2):131-133.
49. Esper F, Weibel C, Ferguson D, et al. Evidence of a novel human coronavirus that is associated with respiratory tract disease in infants and young children. *J Infect Dis*. 2005;191(4):492-498.
51. Fairchok MP, Martin ET, Chambers S, et al. Epidemiology of viral respiratory tract infections in a prospective cohort of infants and toddlers attending daycare. *J Clin Virol*. 2010;49(1):16-20.
53. Falsey AR, McElhaney JE, Beran J, et al. Respiratory syncytial virus and other respiratory viral infections in older adults with moderate to severe influenza-like illness. *J Infect Dis*. 2014;209(12):1873-1881.
57. Gagneur A, Dirson E, Audebert S, et al. Materno-fetal transmission of human coronaviruses: a prospective pilot study. *Eur J Clin Microbiol Infect Dis*. 2008;27(9):863-866.
59. Gagneur A, Vallet S, Talbot PJ, et al. Outbreaks of human coronavirus in a pediatric and neonatal intensive care unit. *Eur J Pediatr*. 2008;167(12):1427-1434.
64. Graat JM, Schouten EG, Heijnen ML, et al. A prospective, community-based study on virologic assessment among elderly people with and without symptoms of acute respiratory infection. *J Clin Epidemiol*. 2003;56(12):1218-1223.
66. Haagmans BL, Al Dhahiry SH, Reusken CB, et al. Middle East respiratory syndrome coronavirus in dromedary camels: an outbreak investigation. *Lancet Infect Dis*. 2014;14(2):140-145.
68. Hamre D, Procknow JJ. A new virus isolated from the human respiratory tract. *Proc Soc Exp Biol Med*. 1966;121(1):190-193.
76. Jevsnik M, Steyer A, Zrim T, et al. Detection of human coronaviruses in simultaneously collected stool samples and nasopharyngeal swabs from hospitalized children with acute gastroenteritis. *Virol J*. 2013;10:46.
82. Korea Centers for Disease Control and Prevention. Middle East respiratory syndrome coronavirus outbreak in the Republic of Korea, 2015. *Osong Public Health Res Perspect*. 2015;6(4):269-278.
86. Kuypers J, Martin ET, Heugel J, et al. Clinical disease in children associated with newly described coronavirus subtypes. *Pediatrics*. 2007;119(1):e70-e76.
87. Lai MM, Holmes KV. Coronaviridae: the viruses and their replication. In: Knipe DH, PM, ed. *Fields Virology*. 5th ed. Philadelphia, PA: Lippincott-Raven; 2007.
95. Liao X, Hu Z, Liu W, et al. New epidemiological and clinical signatures of 18 pathogens from respiratory tract infections based on a 5-year study. *PLoS ONE*. 2015;10(9):e0138684.
100. Mair-Jenkins J, Saavedra-Campos M, Baillie JK, et al. The effectiveness of convalescent plasma and hyperimmune immunoglobulin for the treatment of severe acute respiratory infections of viral etiology: a systematic review and exploratory meta-analysis. *J Infect Dis*. 2015;211(1):80-90.
102. Matoba Y, Abiko C, Ikeda T, et al. Detection of the human coronavirus 229E, HKU1, NL63, and OC43 between 2010 and 2013 in Yamagata, Japan. *Jpn J Infect Dis*. 2015;68(2):138-141.
103. McIntosh K. Proving etiologic relationships to disease: the particular problem of human coronaviruses. *Pediatr Infect Dis J*. 2012;31(3):241-242.
112. Memish ZA, Al-Tawfiq JA, Assiri A, et al. Middle East respiratory syndrome coronavirus disease in children. *Pediatr Infect Dis J*. 2014;33(9):904-906.
113. Memish ZA, Mishra N, Olival KJ, et al. Middle East respiratory syndrome coronavirus in bats, Saudi Arabia. *Emerg Infect Dis*. 2013;19(11):1819-1823.
115. Meyer B, Muller MA, Corman VM, et al. Antibodies against MERS coronavirus in dromedary camels, United Arab Emirates, 2003 and 2013. *Emerg Infect Dis*. 2014;20(4):552-559.
116. Milano F, Campbell AP, Guthrie KA, et al. Human rhinovirus and coronavirus detection among allogeneic hematopoietic stem cell transplantation recipients. *Blood*. 2010;115(10):2088-2094.
127. Nunes MC, Kuschner Z, Rabede Z, et al. Clinical epidemiology of bocavirus, rhinovirus, two polyomaviruses and four coronaviruses in HIV-infected and HIV-uninfected South African children. *PLoS ONE*. 2014;9(2):e86448.
128. Oboho IK, Tomczyk SM, Al-Asmari AM, et al. 2014 MERS-CoV outbreak in Jeddah—a link to health care facilities. *N Engl J Med*. 2015;372(9):846-854.
130. Osborne CM, Montano AC, Robinson CC, et al. Viral gastroenteritis in children in Colorado 2006-2009. *J Med Virol*. 2015;87(6):931-939.
131. Paloniemi M, Lappalainen S, Vesikari T. Commonly circulating human coronaviruses do not have a significant role in the etiology of gastrointestinal infections in hospitalized children. *J Clin Virol*. 2015;62:114-117.
142. Prill MM, Iwane MK, Edwards KM, et al. Human coronavirus in young children hospitalized for acute respiratory illness and asymptomatic controls. *Pediatr Infect Dis J*. 2012;31(3):235-240.
143. Public Health England. Treatment of MERS-CoV: Information for Clinicians. Clinical decision-making support for treatment of MERS-CoV patients; 2015. https://www.gov.uk/government/uploads/system/uploads/attachment_data/file/459835/merscov_for_clinicians_sept2015.pdf.
144. Pyrc K, Berkhout B, van der Hoek L. The novel human coronaviruses NL63 and HKU1. *J Virol*. 2007;81(7):3051-3057.
145. Raj VS, Mou H, Smits SL, et al. Dipeptidyl peptidase 4 is a functional receptor for the emerging human coronavirus-EMC. *Nature*. 2013;495(7440):251-254.
146. Raymond F, Carbonneau J, Boucher N, et al. Comparison of automated microarray detection with real-time PCR assays for detection of respiratory viruses in specimens obtained from children. *J Clin Microbiol*. 2009;47(3):743-750.
148. Regamey N, Kaiser L, Roiha HL, et al. Viral etiology of acute respiratory infections with cough in infancy: a community-based birth cohort study. *Pediatr Infect Dis J*. 2008;27(2):100-105.
150. Reusken CB, Farag EA, Haagmans BL, et al. Occupational exposure to dromedaries and risk for MERS-CoV infection, Qatar, 2013-2014. *Emerg Infect Dis*. 2015;21(8):1422-1425.
151. Reusken CB, Messadi L, Feyisa A, et al. Geographic distribution of MERS coronavirus among dromedary camels, Africa. *Emerg Infect Dis*. 2014;20(8):1370-1374.
153. Risku M, Lappalainen S, Rasanen S, et al. Detection of human coronaviruses in children with acute gastroenteritis. *J Clin Virol*. 2010;48(1):27-30.
156. Self WH, Williams DJ, Zhu Y, et al. Respiratory viral detection in children and adults: comparing asymptomatic controls and patients with community-acquired pneumonia. *J Infect Dis*. 2016;213(4):584-591.
157. Shalhoub S, Farahat F, Al-Jiffri A, et al. IFN-alpha2a or IFN-beta1a in combination with ribavirin to treat Middle East respiratory syndrome coronavirus pneumonia: a retrospective study. *J Antimicrob Chemother*. 2015;70(7):2129-2132.
159. Singleton RJ, Bulkow LR, Miernyk K, et al. Viral respiratory infections in hospitalized and community control children in Alaska. *J Med Virol*. 2010;82(7):1282-1290.
164. Spanakis N, Tsiodras S, Haagmans BL, et al. Virological and serological analysis of a recent Middle East respiratory syndrome coronavirus infection case on a triple combination antiviral regimen. *Int J Antimicrob Agents*. 2014;44(6):528-532.
166. Sung JY, Lee HJ, Eun BW, et al. Role of human coronavirus NL63 in hospitalized children with croup. *Pediatr Infect Dis J*. 2010;29(9):822-826.
167. Talbot HK, Shepherd BE, Crowe JE Jr, et al. The pediatric burden of human coronaviruses evaluated for twenty years. *Pediatr Infect Dis J*. 2009;28(8):682-687.
171. Uhlenhaut C, Cohen JI, Pavletic S, et al. Use of a novel virus detection assay to identify coronavirus HKU1 in the lungs of a hematopoietic stem cell transplant recipient with fatal pneumonia. *Transpl Infect Dis*. 2012;14(1):79-85.
173. van Boheemen S, de Graaf M, Lauber C, et al. Genomic characterization of a newly discovered coronavirus associated with acute respiratory distress syndrome in humans. *MBio*. 2012;3(6).
174. van der Hoek L, Ihorst G, Sure K, et al. Burden of disease due to human coronavirus NL63 infections and periodicity of infection. *J Clin Virol*. 2010;48(2):104-108.
177. van der Zalm MM, Uiterwaal CS, Wilbrink B, et al. Respiratory pathogens in respiratory tract illnesses during the first year of life: a birth cohort study. *Pediatr Infect Dis J*. 2009;28(6):472-476.
180. Venter M, Lassauniere R, Kresfelder TL, et al. Contribution of common and recently described respiratory viruses to annual hospitalizations in children in South Africa. *J Med Virol*. 2011;83(8):1458-1468.
184. Wenzel RP, Hendley JO, Davies JA, et al. Coronavirus infections in military recruits. Three-year study with coronavirus strains OC43 and 229E. *Am Rev Respir Dis*. 1974;109(6):621-624.
187. Woo PC, Huang Y, Lau SK, et al. Coronavirus genomics and bioinformatics analysis. *Viruses*. 2010;2(8):1804-1820.
193. World Health Organization. Interim surveillance recommendations for human infection with Middle east respiratory syndrome coronavirus; 2013. http://www.who.int/csr/disease/coronavirus_infections/update_20130709/en/.
194. World Health Organization. MERS-CoV summary and literature update - as of 20 June 2013; 2013. http://www.who.int/csr/disease/coronavirus_infections/update_20130620/en/.
192. World Health Organization. Summary of probable SARS cases with onset of illness from 1 November 2002 to 31 July 2004; 2004. http://www.who.int/csr/sars/country/table2004_04_21/en/.

198. Zaki AM, van Boheemen S, Bestebroer TM, et al. Isolation of a novel coronavirus from a man with pneumonia in Saudi Arabia. *N Engl J Med.* 2012;367(19):1814-1820.

200. Zhou W, Wang W, Wang H, et al. First infection by all four non-severe acute respiratory syndrome human coronaviruses takes place during childhood. *BMC Infect Dis.* 2013;13:433.

201. Zumla A, Hui DS, Perlman S. Middle East respiratory syndrome. *Lancet.* 2015;386(9997):995-1007.

The full reference list for this chapter is available at ExpertConsult.com.

SUBSECTION XI Bunyaviridae

189 Hantaviruses

Louisa E. Chapman† • C.J. Peters • James N. Mills • Kelly T. McKee Jr

HISTORICAL PERSPECTIVE

Hantaviruses are the etiologic agents of a diverse group of rodent-borne hemorrhagic fevers that are responsible for considerable morbidity and mortality worldwide. Although recognized by Western Hemisphere medical practitioners relatively recently, clinical syndromes now known to be associated with these viruses have been described by traditional practitioners across the globe from antiquity.[31,127] Russian scientists documented sporadic outbreaks of febrile renal failure with hemorrhage in the eastern Soviet Union between 1913 and 1930,[21] and Japanese and Soviet scientists recognized annual outbreaks of a similar syndrome in Manchuria and Siberia between 1932 and 1935.[52,62,63,100,133,153,154,204]

In 1934, Swedish scientists described a novel disorder, characterized by fever, abdominal and back pain, and renal abnormalities.[75,161,210,246] Epidemic disease with these features occurred among German and Finnish troops stationed in Lapland during World War II.[94,210] Physicians called this syndrome nephropathia epidemica (NE). North American medical practitioners initially became acquainted with a similar syndrome in the early 1950s when a previously unrecognized febrile illness characterized by shock, hemorrhage, and renal failure developed in thousands of soldiers serving with United Nations forces during the Korean War. Physicians called this syndrome, which had a case-fatality rate of 5% to 15%, epidemic hemorrhagic fever.[52,154]

In 1953, Gajdusek[62] noted similarities among epidemic hemorrhagic fever, the severe and frequently fatal Far Eastern diseases described by Soviet and Japanese scientists, and the Scandinavian disorder and proposed a common origin. Subsequent validation of this hypothesis (see Organism) ultimately prompted adoption of the collective term hemorrhagic fever with renal syndrome (HFRS) to describe this clinical entity characterized by varying degrees of renal dysfunction and hemorrhage with fever.

In June 1993, investigation of a cluster of unexplained respiratory deaths in previously healthy young adult residents of rural areas in the southwestern United States led to recognition of a "new" febrile disorder in North America. Application of sophisticated serologic and virologic tools to diagnostic specimens from patients with this disease quickly pointed to a hantavirus related to, but distinct from, those causing HFRS.[120,164] This disorder, now called hantavirus pulmonary syndrome (HPS) or hantavirus cardiopulmonary syndrome (HCPS), appeared to be different clinically from classic HFRS; however, as virologic and epidemiologic studies of the etiologic agent and its reservoirs were completed, similarities to other hantaviruses became apparent. Subsequent studies searching for hantaviruses associated with febrile pulmonary rather than renal disease established HPS as endemic throughout the Western hemisphere and identified a large number of unique hantaviruses associated with rodents indigenous to the Americas, not all of which have been associated with human disease[31,50,147] (Fig. 189.1).

†Deceased.

Twenty-four hantavirus species were recognized by the International Committee on Taxonomy of Viruses (ICTV) in its 2015 release.[1] Molecular analyses of these and more recent isolates or sequences have revealed three to four or more phylogenetic clusters, thus reflecting the complex evolutionary history and diverse range of mammalian hosts harboring these agents.[11,78,222]

ORGANISM

Classification and Antigenic Composition

The genus *Hantavirus* of the family *Bunyaviridae* was defined in 1985.[191–194] Members of the genus *Hantavirus* are classified among the bunyaviruses because of their shared morphologic, physicochemical, and molecular properties. Like other members of the *Bunyaviridae* family, hantaviruses are negative-stranded, lipid-enveloped RNA viruses with tripartite genomes; genomic segments are designated as large (L, approximately 6500 nucleotides, encodes the virus L protein, an RNA-dependent RNA polymerase), medium (M, approximately 3600 nucleotides long, encodes the envelope glycoprotein precursor [GPC], which is processed into two transmembrane glycoproteins: mature Gn and Gc glycoproteins), and small (S, 1600–2004 nucleotides long, encodes an RNA-binding nucleocapsid protein, the N protein).[90,147,195] Puumala virus and some other hantaviruses also encode a nonstructural protein NS that can function as a weak interferon inhibitor.[161]

Also like other bunyaviruses, hantaviruses display Golgi-associated morphogenesis and usually acquire their envelopes by budding into intracytoplasmic vacuoles.[194] However, they are serologically distinct from other family members and possess unique terminal genomic sequences.[192,195] The genus *Hantavirus* contains the only members of *Bunyaviridae* that lack arthropod vectors. As a general rule, each of the hantaviruses associated with human disease is adapted to a specific rodent host species and depends on persistent infection in wild rodents for maintenance in nature.

Physical Properties

Morphologically, hantaviruses are spherical or pleomorphic, 70 to 210 nm in diameter, and have a surface glycoprotein complex consisting of Gn interconnected with Gc embedded in a lipid bilayer envelope.[222] These Gn and Gc tetramers form spikes that protrude approximately 10 nm from the membrane, creating a fourfold symmetry that is apparently unique among enveloped viruses (Fig. 189.2).[222]

Integrins have been implicated as primary host cell surface receptors for hantaviruses, with α5β3 integrin serving as a receptor of pathogenic hantaviruses and α5β1 integrin as a receptor for nonpathogenic hantaviruses in vitro.[42,68,222] The viral surface glycoproteins (Gn and Gc) mediate virus attachment to cells. The virus appears to use a variety of pathways for entry (e.g., both clathrin-dependent and clathrin–independent endocytosis).[222] After internalization, virions migrate to

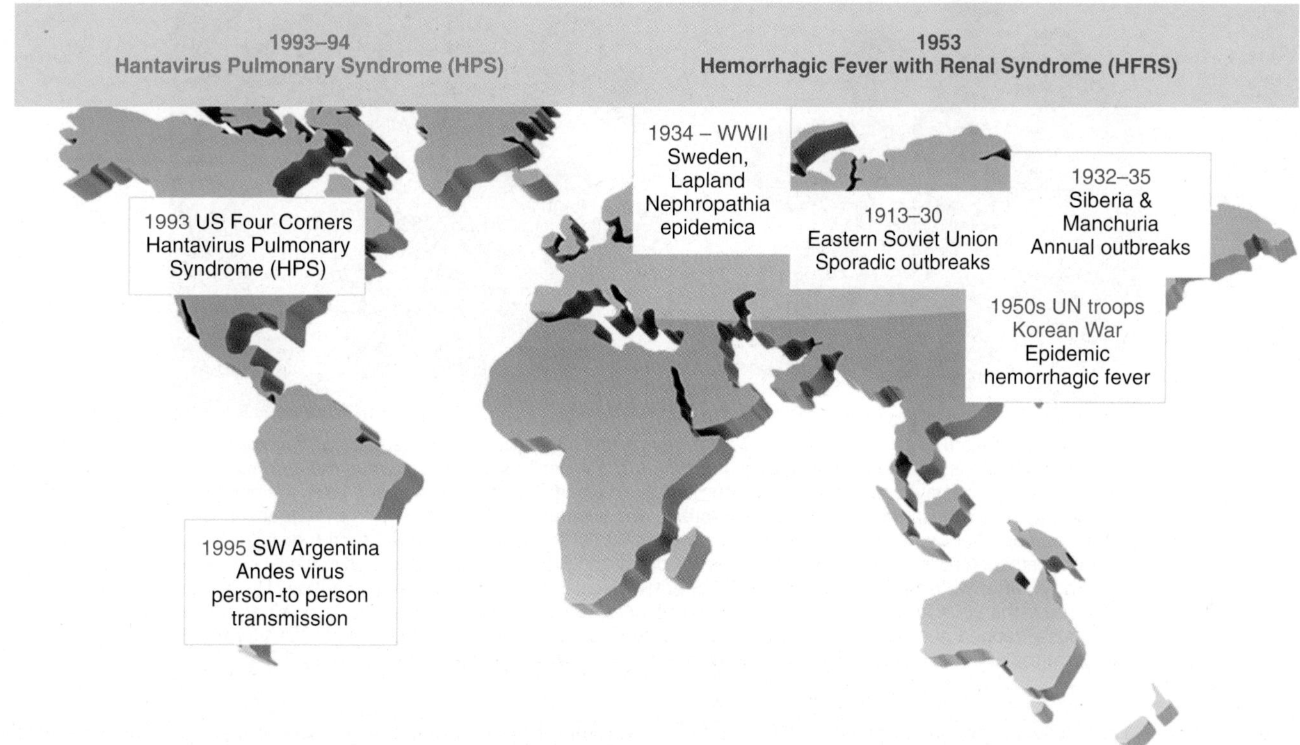

FIG. 189.1 Map demonstrating the temporal and geographic recognition of human diseases associated with hantavirus infections. *UN,* United Nations; *WWII,* World War II.

endosomes, where low pH triggers conformational changes resulting in fusion of the virus and endosomal membranes and release of virion ribonucleocapsid (RNP) cores into the cell cytoplasm. The virion-associated RNA-dependent RNA polymerase transcribes its negative-sense RNA segments to produce messenger RNAs (mRNAs) encoding the viral proteins (N protein, L polymerase protein, and the GPC).[90,222] Details of transcription are still unclear, but the polymerase appears to be involved in so-called 5′-cap snatching (similar to that for other negative-sense RNA viruses), as well as transcriptase, replicase, and endonuclease functions critical for mRNA transcription, as well as for subsequent translation and replication activities.[147,222] The GPC mRNA is translated by membrane-bound ribosomes and by analogy with other *Bunyaviridae*, presumably in the Golgi complex and endoplasmic reticulum. The N and L mRNAs are translated by free ribosomes.[147] The multifunctional N protein protects the virus genomic RNA (vRNA) from nuclease degradation by limiting access of RNA to host nucleases and is involved in encapsidation of vRNA and antigenomic RNA (cRNA), but not viral mRNA. The N protein plays an active role in virus RNA transcription, interacts with ribosomal protein RPS19 to facilitate the loading of the 40S ribosomal subunit onto the virus mRNA, and plays an active role in virus assembly.[147] N protein activities are linked not only to fundamental requirements of viral replication but also to interference with intracellular processes of the host cell, including inflammatory processes.[90,113]

Hantavirus assembly involves the RNP core (containing the vRNA and N and L proteins) and the acquired host cell membrane containing the embedded virus Gn and Gc glycoproteins. Direct interaction of the virus Gn or its cytoplasmic tail with N protein and RNA is believed to facilitate virus assembly.[147] Virus glycoproteins are believed to determine the site of virus assembly and budding. The Gn and Gc proteins of so-called New World (endemic to the Western Hemisphere) hantaviruses accumulate in the Golgi, but the process by which virions make their way to the cell surface remains poorly defined.[147,222] Two sites of New World hantaviral maturation have been described. During infection in polarized epithelial cells, Black Creek Canal virus was released from the apical membrane,[185] but Andes virus was released from both apical and basolateral sites in primary hamster epithelium.[186]

Susceptibility

Hantavirus transmission may occur through indirect contact with contaminated environmental surfaces. Puumala virus excreted by experimentally infected bank voles into bedding maintained infectivity to recipient voles at room temperature for 12 to 15 days.[102] Knowledge about the survival time in the environment in the absence of disinfection is limited, but survival appears to be temperature dependent. Infectivity persists in dried cell culture medium for as long as 2 days and in neutral solutions for several hours at 37°C or several days at lower temperatures.[23] Infectious Hantaan virus was detected after 96 days under "wet" conditions at 4°C, and it remained viable for 2 minutes in 30% ethanol.[81] Cell culture supernatants of Puumala and Tula hantaviruses remained infectious for 5 to 11 days at room temperature and for as long as 18 days at 4°C but were inactivated after 24 hours at 37°C.[191]

However, hantaviruses are inactivated readily by lipid solvents and most disinfectants, including dilute hypochlorite solutions, detergents, ethyl alcohol (70%), most general-purpose household disinfectants, and β-propiolactone (0.1% at 4°C for 3 days).[75,116,181] Limited studies with Hantaan virus have shown sensitivity to a pH of 5 or less and to temperatures of 56°C or higher.[75]

Laboratory Propagation and Tissue Culture Growth

Hantaviruses are fastidious but can be grown in culture through serial blind passage. They routinely establish persistent, noncytolytic infections and generally do not replicate to high titer.[75,192,194] The prototype hantavirus, Hantaan virus, was isolated in 1978,[135] and it was propagated in cell culture in the A-549 cell line in 1981.[60] Vero E-6 cells subsequently were found to be a better cell culture system for this and other hantaviruses.[75] Hantaviruses have been isolated and propagated through direct inoculation of homogenates of infected tissue from wild-caught rodent hosts onto cell lines or after amplification through serially infected, colonized rodent hosts.[53,60,73,75,135,166,196,239] Recovery of hantaviruses from human specimens has been difficult and infrequent. Some hantaviruses have been isolated in cell culture, but many are known only from genetic material amplified from human or rodent tissue. Laboratory infection of persons working with cell culture–adapted Hantaan virus has occurred occasionally, but laboratory transmission of hantaviruses from infected

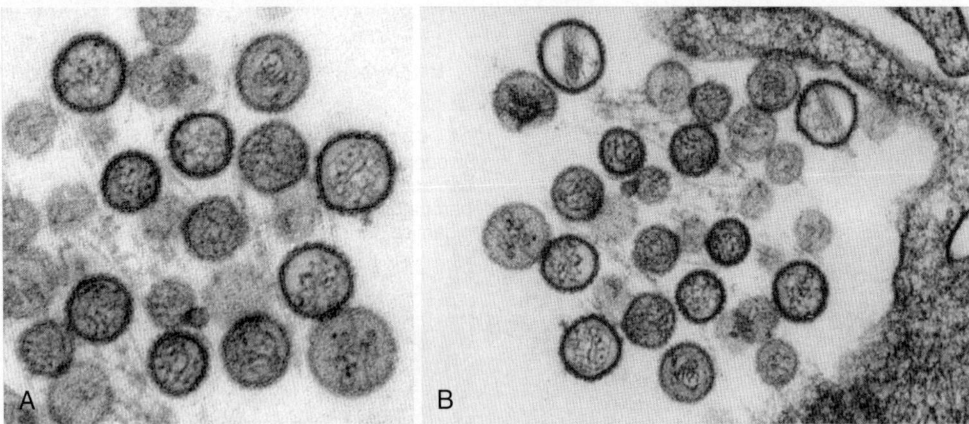

FIG. 189.2 Transmission electron micrographs reveal the ultrastructural appearance of several virus particles, or virions, of a hantavirus known as Sin Nombre virus. This is the hantavirus most commonly responsible for hantavirus pulmonary syndrome in the United States. In November 1993 the specific hantavirus that caused the Four Corners outbreak was isolated. (A) Using tissue from a deer mouse that had been trapped near the New Mexico home of a person who had contracted the disease, the Special Pathogens Branch at Centers for Disease Control and Prevention grew the virus in the laboratory. (B) Shortly afterward, and independently, the US Army Medical Research Institute of Infectious Diseases also grew the virus from a person in New Mexico who had contracted the disease, as well as from a mouse trapped in California. (Courtesy Centers for Disease Control and Prevention[CDC]/Cynthia Goldsmith, Luanne H. Elliott, Brian W. Mahy, and the CDC Viral Special Pathogens Branch.)

rodents to humans is a particularly common occurrence.[44,49,104,130,132,142,221] Consequently, attempts to propagate the virus in cell culture or rodents should be performed only when using biosafety level 3 or 4 facilities and practices.[23,27]

Transmission

Hantaviruses are zoonotic; with few exceptions, each of the hantaviruses that are pathogenic for humans is naturally associated with a distinct rodent species or subspecies in which it establishes chronic infection (Table 189.1). Hantavirus infection of rodents produces brief viremia that results in dissemination of virus to the lungs, salivary glands, and kidneys. The infected rodent sheds virus in urine, saliva, and (to a lesser extent) feces persistently or occasionally throughout its life, despite the development of neutralizing antibodies.[134] In contrast to early laboratory data suggesting that infection does not adversely affect host longevity or reproduction, field evidence is accumulating that deer mice infected with Sin Nombre virus have reduced survivorship in nature.[3,47,48,144] Vertical transmission has not been demonstrated, and pups born to infected dams appear to be protected by maternal antibody.[46,103,159] Enzootic infection appears to be maintained by exposure to nesting materials contaminated with infectious secretions, by grooming, and by intraspecies biting.[48,130,134]

Humans typically become infected with hantaviruses after contact with saliva or excreta from infected rodents (or material contaminated by these), by inhalation of small-particle aerosols, by direct contact of infectious materials with broken skin or mucous membranes, or by percutaneous inoculation of infectious materials (e.g., rodent bite). The primacy of respiratory droplets or airborne particles as the mode of transmission to humans is supported by evidence from outbreaks of disease among laboratory workers and sporadic cases resulting from brief exposure to rodent-infested habitats.

The risk of human hantavirus infection is a function of the density of the local rodent reservoir population, the prevalence of infection among rodents, and the frequency of activities that result in contact between humans and rodents or rodent excreta. Individual hantavirus infections usually occur when humans disturb rodent habitats or rodents enter human housing.[245] The risk for contracting disease after rodent exposure remains unquantified; however, one serosurvey suggested that persons in North America whose occupation entails close physical contact with rodents have a low risk for acquiring hantavirus infection.[61] Epidemics generally are associated with changes in the behavior of human populations that result in large-scale exposure of persons to rodent-infested areas (e.g., military maneuvers, agricultural or forestry activities) or environmental changes that result in rapid increases in the abundance of certain rodent host species (e.g., increased availability of food or preferred habitat).[158,241]

Person-to-person transmission of hantaviruses associated with HFRS has not been demonstrated. The experience with HPS has been similar in North and Central America.[233] However, interpersonal spread clearly occurred during a 1996 HPS outbreak in southern Argentina.[56,235] Subsequent independent investigations support this observation by having identified clusters in Argentina and Chile that suggest person-to-person transmission associated with Andes virus.[125,151,231] Interpersonal transmission thus appears to be an infrequent but clear feature peculiar to Andes virus[29,150] (see Fig. 189.1).

EPIDEMIOLOGY

Geographic Distribution

Approximately 28 hantavirus genotypes are currently recognized as causing human disease, although many of them have not been fully characterized, and the reservoirs of a few have not been clearly determined. Only 15 of the known pathogenic genotypes are currently recognized as distinct species by the ICTV (see Table 189.1). Nevertheless, several other hantavirus genotypes are associated with distinct host species, occur in disjunct geographic areas, and are individually studied and commonly referred to in the literature. Therefore, we believe that listing those names is important (Table 189.1). In addition, there are at least 58 named hantavirus genotypes with no known association with human disease. This list will continue to grow and be modified as surveillance increases our knowledge of genetic relatedness among viruses and hosts improves.

Hantaviruses have been found on every continent except Antarctica. All rodent-borne hantaviruses are associated with four subfamilies of rodents in the large superfamily Muroidea. These are the Old World rats and mice (subfamily Murinae), the New World rats and mice (subfamilies Sigmodontinae and Neotominae), and the voles and lemmings (subfamily Arvicolinae). With the exception of HFRS caused by Seoul virus, hantavirus diseases occur almost exclusively in rural areas. Hantaan virus, the cause of classic HFRS, is carried by the striped field mouse, *Apodemus agrarius manchuricus*, which is distributed across eastern Russia, China, and the Korean peninsula.[135] The principal reservoir for Puumala virus, the etiologic agent of the milder HFRS variant (NE) found in Scandinavia, northern Europe, and Russia west of the Ural Mountains, is the bank vole, *Myodes glareolus.*[198] Puumala is the sole cause of HFRS in Nordic countries.[162] Finland has the highest recognized annual incidence of NE (case-fatality rate, <0.4%).[162]

TABLE 189.1 **Named Genotypes of Hantaviruses Known to Be Pathogenic for Humans**

Virus	Principal Reservoir	Known Distribution of Virus	Disease Association[a]
Old World Rodent-Borne			
Hantaan[b]	*Apodemus agrarius manchuricus*	Far East Northern Asia	HFRS (severe)
Seoul[b]	*Rattus norvegicus*	Worldwide	HFRS (mild/moderate)
Dobrava[b]	*Apodemus flavicollis*	Balkans	HFRS (severe)
Puumala[b]	*Myodes (Clethrionomys) glareolus*	Scandinavia, Northern Europe, Balkans	HFRS (mild; nephropathia epidemica)
Tula[b]	*Microtus arvalis/Microtus levis*	Western Russia, eastern Europe	HFRS
Saaremaa[b]	*Apodemus agrarius agrarius*	Europe	HFRS (mild)
Amur	*Apodemus peninsulae*	Far eastern Russia, Korea, China	HFRS
Muju	*Myodes regulus*	South Korea	HFRS
Thailand[b]	*Bandicota indica*	Thailand	HFRS
Sangassou[b]	*Hylomyscus alleni*	West Africa	Febrile syndrome
New World Rodent-Borne			
Sin Nombre[b]	*Peromyscus maniculatus*	North America	HPS
New York[b]	*Peromyscus leucopus*	Eastern United States	HPS
Monongahela	*Peromyscus maniculatus nubiterrae*	Eastern United States	HPS
Black Creek Canal[b]	*Sigmodon hispidus spadicipygus*	Florida	HPS
Bayou[b]	*Oryzomys palustris*	Southeastern United States	HPS
Andes[b]	*Oligoryzomys longicaudatus*	Southern Chile, Argentina	HPS
Oran	*Oligoryzomys chacoensis*	Northern Argentina	HPS
Laguna Negra[b]	*Calomys laucha*	Central South America	HPS
Choclo	*Oligoryzomys fulvescens costaricensis*	Panama	HPS
Juquitiba	*Oligoryzomys nigripes*	Southeastern Brazil	HPS
Araraquara	*Necromys lasiurus*	Southeastern Brazil	HPS
Castelo dos Sonhos	Unknown	Northern Brazil	HPS
Lechiguanas	*Oligoryzomys flavescens*[c]	Central Argentina, Southwest Uruguay	HPS
Central Plata	*Oligoryzomys flavescens*[c]	Southern Uruguay	HPS
Hu39694	*Oligoryzomys flavescens*[c]	Central Argentina	HPS
Bermejo	*Oligoryzomys chacoensis*	Northwestern Argentina, Central Brazil	HPS
Anajatuba	*Oligoryzomys fornesi*	Northeastern Brazil	HPS
Río Mamoré[b]	*Oligoryzomys microtis*	Bolivia, Peru, Brazil, French Guiana	HPS

[a]An additional 58 hantavirus genotypes not known to be associated with human disease are not listed here.
[b]Virus species recognized by the International Committee on the Taxonomy of Viruses.
[c]The taxonomy of the genus *Oligoryzomys* in general and *O. flavescens* in particular is still unresolved. The uniqueness of the viruses these rodents carry is also debated.
HFRS, Hemorrhagic fever with renal syndrome; *HPS,* hantavirus pulmonary syndrome.

In Europe, at least four viruses have been linked etiologically with HFRS: Puumala, Tula, Saaremaa, and Dobrava; Tula virus is associated with voles (*Microtus* spp.); Saaremaa virus is hosted by a subspecies of the striped field mouse *(Apodemus agrarius agrarius);* Dobrava virus is associated with *Apodemus flavicollis,* the yellow-necked field mouse.[4,7,9,10,73,178,179] *Rattus* spp. (primarily the brown rat, *Rattus norvegicus*) serve as reservoirs for the Seoul-like viruses identified worldwide; human infections have been seen most frequently in eastern Asia. Outbreaks of severe, and occasionally fatal, HFRS among animal handlers and laboratory scientists have been caused by exposure to laboratory rats with inapparent infection with Seoul-like viruses.[132] Although infections with Dobrava and Saaremaa viruses are more likely to be fatal, Puumala virus remains the most common cause of HFRS in Europe.[162]

Genome sequences of a novel hantavirus species have been detected in an African wood mouse *(Hylomyscus alleni)* in Guinea.[112] This agent, Sangassou virus, was more similar to Eurasian hantaviruses than to those causing HPS in the Western Hemisphere. Neutralizing antibodies to Sangassou virus were subsequently (and retrospectively) detected in sera from two human patients with fever of unknown origin in Sangassou Village.[114] The virus is sufficiently distinct to represent a separate clade.

Numerous hantaviruses associated with native muroid rodents are known in the Americas (see Table 189.1). Several, all associated with New World rats and mice, are of medical importance in the United States.[175] The deer mouse, *Peromyscus maniculatus,* is the reservoir for Sin Nombre virus, the agent associated most frequently with HPS in the United States and Canada (Fig. 189.3).[34,54,146] This rodent is distributed widely over the United States, Canada, and parts of Mexico. In addition, HPS cases in the eastern United States have been associated with New York virus (hosted by the white-footed mouse, *Peromyscus leucopus*) and Monongahela viruses (also hosted by the deer mouse), which are closely related to Sin Nombre virus.[88,207] Rare cases of HPS also have been associated with Black Creek Canal virus, which is associated with the hispid cotton rat *(Sigmodon hispidus)* and Bayou virus, hosted by the marsh rice rat *(Oryzomys palustris).*[86,106,109,163,185,217] Several hantaviruses associated with voles (Arvicolinae) in North America are not associated with human disease: Prospect Hill virus has been recovered from meadow voles *(Microtus pennsylvanicus)* in Maryland,[238] and related but distinct hantaviruses (Bloodland Lake and Isla Vista) have been shown in other voles by detection of genetic sequences by reverse transcriptase-polymerase chain reaction (RT-PCR).[87,208] The Old World, murine-borne Seoul virus, introduced by the brown rat, has been associated with human infections in several large cities throughout the Americas, but acute (HFRS-like) disease has been recognized and confirmed only in Recife, Brazil.[37,71,72,126]

South America clearly has surpassed North America in numbers of human HPS cases and numbers of hantaviruses and host species identified.[13,91,232,234] All HPS-causing hantaviruses in South America are associated with sigmodontine rodents. Some of the most important viruses include the following: Andes virus in southern Argentina and Chile; Lechiguanas virus in central Argentina; Laguna Negra virus in northern Argentina, Paraguay, and Bolivia; Juquitiba virus in Brazil and eastern Paraguay; and Choclo virus in Panama. Numerous other hantaviruses, both pathogenic and not known to be pathogenic, occur throughout South America (see Table 189.1). Although HPS is clearly a panhemispheric disease, all HPS agents identified or suspected to date

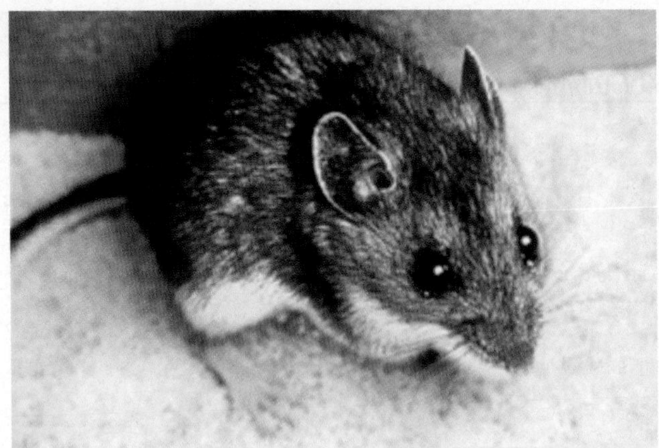

FIG. 189.3 The deer mouse, *Peromyscus maniculatus,* the carrier of Sin Nombre virus, the most common agent of hantavirus pulmonary syndrome in North America. (Courtesy Centers for Disease Control and Prevention Special Pathogens Branch.)

belong to a single genetic group of hantaviruses and are associated with two subfamilies of rodents, the Neotominae (North America) and the Sigmodontinae (primarily Central and South America). These rodent species are restricted to the Americas, in accordance with findings that HPS is an exclusively Western Hemisphere disease.[157]

One finding has been the apparently widespread occurrence of a divergent clade of hantaviruses associated with a group of small mammals unrelated to rodents, the insectivores (shrews and moles, order Soricomorpha).[240] Although Thottapalayam virus and its association with the common house shrew *(Suncus murinus)* have been recognized since 1971,[20] this association was thought to be a unique exception. At least 27 newer insectivore-borne hantaviruses have been described from North America, Asia, Europe, and Africa.[240]

Finally, and most recently, approximately five hantaviruses have been reported in association with bats (order Chiroptera).[240] Clearly, the association of hantaviruses with insectivores and bats is ancient, and understanding their distribution and evolution will be a challenge. Nevertheless, none of these bat, shrew, or mole viruses has so far been associated with human disease.

Seasonal Patterns

The natural population cycles of rodents and the seasonal nature of certain human behaviors result in a pattern of human hantavirus disease that varies seasonally and annually.[21,31,63,127,219] Although incidence varies by season, cases of hantavirus-associated human disease are recognized year round in all disease-endemic areas.[24,107,128,198] In eastern Asia and Russia east of the Ural Mountains, HFRS occurs primarily during late fall and early winter, with smaller peaks in spring and summer. Most Scandinavian HFRS occurs between late summer and early spring, whereas European HFRS in warmer regions (e.g., France, Belgium) tends to peak in spring. In the Balkans, the presence of multiple hantavirus-host combinations results in a more diffuse seasonal distribution of human disease.

Persons whose occupations or avocations bring them to rural settings, such as agricultural workers, foresters, biologists, hunters, campers, and soldiers stationed in the field, are at greatest risk for contracting HFRS. HFRS caused by Seoul virus tends to occur throughout the year, but there are conflicting descriptions of a seasonal occurrence of Seoul virus infection as well.[33,129] Presumably because of the peridomestic nature of the reservoir, cases of Seoul virus disease are also less likely to have a skewed age and sex distribution than are rural hantavirus infections.

The temporal distribution of HPS cases in the United States displays strong seasonality. Maximum numbers of cases occur in May, June, and July, whereas minimum case numbers are seen during December, January, and February.[146] However, environmental and geographic factors influence this pattern[157]; HPS cases have been identified throughout the winter and early spring.[24,25,54,70,241] Seasonal patterns vary by region in the United States; in the midwestern and northwestern regions the highest proportion of cases occur in May, whereas cases peak in July in the southwestern region.[146]

Prevalence and Incidence

Worldwide, human hantavirus infections may number in the hundreds of thousands of cases annually.[241] Because of the predominantly rural nature of the disease and its prevalence in developing regions of the Eurasian land mass (e.g., rural China), accurate case reporting (and statistical data) for HFRS is challenging. Researchers have estimated that 100,000 or more cases of HFRS may occur each year in China.[205] One report suggested an incidence of 1.6 to 29.6 per 100,000 population during 1980.[100] In the former Soviet Union, more than 4000 cases per year were recorded between 1978 and 1989, 96% of which occurred in "European" republics. Rates in western regions near the Ural Mountains were higher (20–40 per 100,000 population) than were those in eastern districts (2–5 per 100,000 population).[216] In Korea, approximately 500 persons with HFRS, approximately half of whom are soldiers, are hospitalized annually.[216] In central and northern Sweden, a mean annual incidence of 4.3 per 100,000 population has been reported, although northern locales have rates of more than 20 per 100,000 population.[198] In Finland between 1995 and 2008, the average annual incidence of Puumala virus infection was 31 per 100,000 population.[148]

As of January 2016, 692 cases of HPS had been laboratory confirmed in the United States. Although 30 cases were identified retrospectively, most recognized cases have occurred since 1993.[28] HPS is rare in the United States; the annual incidence is estimated to range from 0.04 to 0.19 cases per million persons.[146] Case counts were relatively stable across a 17-year period in the northwestern and midwestern regions of the United States, but greater variability in the southwestern part of the country drove fluctuations in the national HPS case counts.[146] Updated US surveillance data can be found on the Centers for Disease Control and Prevention (CDC) website.[28] HPS is less common in Canada, with between 2 and 8 reported cases per year, but more common in South America. More than 4800 cases were documented in South America between 1993 and 2015, with Brazil, Argentina, and Chile reporting most of the cases.

Demographic and Geographic Features

Hantavirus infections are recognized relatively infrequently in the pediatric age group.[2,5,8,64,107,108,198,216,242] The disease occurs principally in adults, with a significant minority (≤15%) of cases diagnosed in children. Reports from Argentina, China, Sweden, and the United States confirm a male predominance in reported incidence of disease,[92,111,146,147,150] despite serologic evidence that similar proportions of men and women are infected with Puumala virus in Sweden.[4] In a survey from Finland, 85% of patients were 20 to 64 years old; 62% were male; 52% were hospitalized; 3% were registered as having occupational diseases; and the case-fatality proportion was 0.08%.[148] Case-fatality rates appear to be higher among female patients with HRFS in China (Hantaan and Seoul viruses),[111] women infected with Andes-associated HPS in Argentina,[150] and women with Puumala virus–associated NE in Sweden.[92] In all studies, these sex-based differences were most marked among populations at peak reproductive ages (20s and 30s) and older than 50 years.[92,111,147,147,150] Analysis of US data did not support a similar sex-based difference in case-fatality rates.[147] Interpretations conflict regarding the likelihood that these differences are biologically based. The peak incidence of HFRS in Europe, the Balkans, and the Far East and of HPS in the United States occurs in persons who are 20 to 50 years of age.[122,128,146,173,219] Few cases have been reported in children younger than 10 years of age. Both HFRS and HPS cases in young children often are recognized in association with cases in other family members.[8,64,122,161,173,171]

A male predominance has been observed for both the severe (Korean) and milder (European) forms of HFRS in children.[2,5,115,161,242] Although this pattern, also seen in adults with HFRS and with HPS in the United States, suggests differential susceptibility or risk for exposure by sex, the number of recorded cases, particularly in the youngest age groups, is too small to be used to draw firm conclusions.

In the United States, fewer than 7% of reported HPS cases occur in children younger than 17 years [146]; in South America, the proportion of cases in the pediatric age group may be somewhat higher.[59] The underrepresentation of children recognized to have HFRS and HPS may not be explained by age-related avoidance of activities resulting in exposure. The limited data available (see Clinical Manifestations below) suggest that hantavirus infections in children may induce milder HFRS and NE syndromes than those seen in adults. In contrast, typical HPS has been repeatedly described in children, particularly teenagers. Comprehensive population-based serosurveys are sparse and have been inadequate to define age-associated infection rates. The apparently immune-mediated pathologic process of hantavirus diseases (see Pathogenesis and Pathology below) is possibly more evident in persons experiencing infection in adulthood.

CLINICAL MANIFESTATIONS

Hemorrhagic Fever With Renal Syndrome

Two major clinical variants of HFRS have been recognized traditionally. Severe disease associated with high morbidity and mortality rates occurs primarily in areas of the world where Hantaan, Dobrava, Saaremaa, and Tula viruses are endemic: across the northern half of Asia, China, the Korean Peninsula, and the Balkan nations. Milder illness with little mortality occurs in areas where Puumala and related viruses have been recovered; this latter disease, a milder variant of HFRS known as NE, is found throughout northern Europe, Scandinavia, and western areas of the former Soviet Union.[122,123] In the Balkans, the coexistence of Puumala virus–like strains with viruses causing more serious disease has resulted in a mixture of clinical findings in the former Yugoslavia and neighboring countries. Benign manifestations of HFRS are well recognized in many regions where Hantaan virus is found, however, and clinically severe disease occasionally results from Puumala virus infection.[133,176] Hence, it is important to appreciate the protean nature of this disorder and to recognize the potential for disease of any severity whenever and wherever human infection with hantavirus occurs.

Severe HFRS, such as that associated with Hantaan or Dobrava virus, is a complex, multiphasic disorder that presents substantial challenges to patient management. The clinical course of HFRS caused by Hantaan virus in adults spans a wide spectrum from mildly symptomatic disease to severe hemorrhagic fever and death. Subclinical infections probably occur infrequently.[242,180] In most cases, the clinical course is relatively benign; severe disease develops in 20% to 30% of patients. Modern-day case-fatality rates range from 2% to 7%. In Korea, approximately one-third of recognized Hantaan virus infections follow a clinical course consisting of progression through five clinically and pathophysiologically defined stages: febrile, hypotensive, oliguric, diuretic, and convalescent.[129,199] Phases often blur, however, and in milder cases, one or more phases may not be discernible.

After an incubation period of 2 to 3 weeks (range, 4–42 days), most patients report the abrupt onset of high fever, headache, chills, dizziness, myalgia, anorexia, and backache. Approximately one-third of patients experience prodromal mild respiratory or gastrointestinal symptoms. Nausea, vomiting, abdominal pain, and intense thirst may be evident at initial evaluation but increase in severity in succeeding days. Photophobia, blurred vision, and eyeball pain are reported frequently. Physical examination reveals a restless, acutely ill patient with flushing of the face, neck, and upper thoracic region. Relative bradycardia is present. Conjunctival and pharyngeal injection, together with facial puffiness, is characteristic. In more than 90% of patients, petechiae develop on the soft palate, axillae, lateral aspect of the thorax, conjunctivae, or face, generally between the third and sixth days of illness. Tenderness occurs commonly over the costovertebral angles and diffusely throughout the abdomen.

Hematologic studies in the first 3 to 4 days of illness reveal leukocytosis with a left shift in more than 90% of patients, as well as almost universal thrombocytopenia; the hematocrit at this stage generally is normal or slightly increased. Proteinuria develops by the third to fourth day, and microscopic hematuria, hyposthenuria, and mild pyuria are reported in most patients; fibrin clots in urine are characteristic findings.

This febrile phase generally lasts approximately 1 week, followed by abrupt defervescence. Approximately 40% of patients then become hypotensive; in most cases, the drop in blood pressure is mild and brief, but in severely ill persons (30–50% of hypotensive patients), clinical shock develops. Tachycardia replaces bradycardia, the pulse pressure narrows, and cyanosis and mental confusion may be seen. The hypotensive phase may last from a few hours to 3 days, and 30% to 40% of deaths occur during this period.

As patients recover from hypotension, they enter a period of oliguria. This phase occurs in approximately 60% of patients and generally lasts for several days. Anuria develops in approximately 10% of patients. Blood pressure normalizes, and hypertension often develops. Clinical manifestations of uremia, including protracted vomiting and hiccups, may be seen. More extensive hemorrhagic manifestations such as ecchymoses, hemoptysis, hematemesis, melena, gross hematuria, and, rarely, bleeding in the central nervous system (CNS) become evident during the oliguric phase. Striking elevations in blood urea nitrogen and creatinine levels are common findings. Biochemical disturbances (electrolyte derangements, metabolic acidosis, uremia) may be severe, and, in such cases, dialysis may be lifesaving. Approximately one-half of fatalities occur during the oliguric phase.

Between 10 and 14 days into the illness, renal function is restored spontaneously in most patients, and a period of diuresis follows. Polyuria may be substantial, and urine output frequently exceeds 3 to 6 L/day. With the onset of diuresis, clinical recovery is initiated; however, the rapid change in fluid status may precipitate further electrolyte disturbances, so close monitoring remains necessary.

Convalescence typically lasts from 3 to 6 weeks, but in many cases a longer period passes before health is restored completely. Body weight and strength are recovered slowly. Proteinuria resolves, but hyposthenuria persists for months. Most patients recover completely, although permanent sequelae may result from such complications as anterior pituitary or other CNS hemorrhage.

The disease has been reported infrequently in children.[64,115,242] The data available indicate that clinical manifestations are similar to and perhaps somewhat less severe than those observed in adults. In a series of 63 children identified retrospectively over a 15-year period in Korea, fever was universal, whereas abdominal pain, headache, and vomiting were present in 73% or more of patients (Table 189.2).[242] Proteinuria (100%), leukocytosis (71%), thrombocytopenia (80%), hypocholesterolemia (87%), and elevations in creatinine (94%), blood urea nitrogen (94%), and alanine aminotransferase (80%) were the laboratory abnormalities found most commonly. Petechiae and hypotension occurred infrequently (38% and 11%, respectively), and frank hemorrhage occurred rarely. Eleven patients (18%) required dialysis. The mortality rate was 5%, and the remaining patients recovered without sequelae.[242]

HFRS occurring in adults after they are infected with Seoul virus resembles that described for Hantaan virus infection, but the clinical manifestations generally are milder.[129] Fever and constitutional symptoms are similar in the two types of infection, but hypotension occurs infrequently in persons infected with Seoul virus (10% of cases), and clinical shock is a rare event. The frequency and severity of thrombocytopenia are less with Seoul virus infection, whereas elevations of aminotransferases occur commonly (>60% of cases). The mortality rate for HFRS caused by Seoul virus is 1% or less.

Nephropathia Epidemica

The Scandinavian or European form of HFRS (NE) generally is a more benign disease than that attributed to Hantaan virus; fatal outcomes are observed, but the case-fatality rate is less than 1%.[98] In contrast to the findings with Hantaan virus, subclinical infection apparently occurs commonly with Puumala virus; one report suggested a case-to-infection ratio of 1:10.[167] Host related factors influence severity of disease. In Finland, the most severe disease is more likely to occur in persons with human leukocyte antigen (HLA) alleles B8, C4A·Q0, and DRB1·0301. HLA-B27 predicted a more benign course. In Slovenia, Puumala-infected persons with severe disease were more likely than Dobrava-infected persons with severe disease to have HLA-DRB1·13 haplotype. HLA-B·07 appeared possibly to protect against severe disease following Puumala virus infection. HLA-B·35 was significantly more frequent among Dobrava virus–infected patients than among Puumala virus–infected persons.[162]

In adults, NE is typically described as a biphasic disease of 1 to 3 weeks' duration.[38,173,228] However, NE resulting from Puumala virus infection has been further divided by some investigators into five phases (febrile, hypotensive, oliguric, polyuric, and convalescent) analogous to prototypical Hantaan infection.[162] The onset of the febrile phase usually is abrupt, with no apparent prodrome. High fever is the initial symptom in 95% of patients. On examination, a facial flush is a usual

TABLE 189.2 **Prominent Clinical and Laboratory Features of Hemorrhagic Fever With Renal Syndrome in Children**

Features	Korea[242] (%)	Sweden[5] (%)	Finland[124,161] (%)	Austria[2] (%)
Fever	100	100	100/NR	89
Headache	76	100	62/59	58
Anorexia	33	100	NR/NR	NR
Nausea	62	86	NR/81	89
Vomiting	73	91	NR/72	84
Abdominal pain	91	93	100/59	100
Back/costovertebral angle pain	35	76	92/63	NR
Dizziness	21	73	NR/9	NR
Thirst	NR	75	NR/NR	NR
Polyuria	NR	57	100/NR	NR
Diarrhea	NR	57	NR/9	NR
Petechiae	38	NR	0/NR	NR
Conjunctival hemorrhage	35	NR	0/3	NR
Proteinuria	100	100	100/97	100
Hematuria	67	80	NR/73	100
Pyuria	8	43	NR/44	NR
Glucosuria	NR	26	NR/12	NR
Casts	NR	33	NR/NR	NR
Leukocytosis	71	22	NR/41	NR
Thrombocytopenia	80	68	100/87	84
Elevated hemoglobin	39	NR	NR/28	NR
Elevated C-reactive protein	NR	28	100/89	100
Elevated erythrocyte sedimentation rate	NR	58	NR/74	NR
Elevated alanine aminotransferase	80	NR	83/53	63
Elevated creatinine	94	76	92/84	95

NR, Not recorded.

finding. This febrile phase lasts from 3 to 6 days. Typical acute febrile phase laboratory abnormalities are anemia, leukocytosis, thrombocytosis, elevated liver function test results and serum creatinine levels, and proteinuria and hematuria.[162]

The development of nausea, vomiting, abdominal pain, back pain, somnolence, and, occasionally, joint pain heralds the onset of the second, or renal, phase. The abdominal pain may be of such severity and character that an acute abdomen is suspected, and many patients have undergone surgical intervention for suspected appendicitis before NE was diagnosed. Visual disturbances are common manifestations (≈43%).[82–84,98] In one prospective study, 70% of patients hospitalized in Finland with acute Puumala infection reported ocular symptoms. Examinations identified decreased intraocular pressure (88%), reduced visual acuity and chemosis (87%), thickening of the lens (82%), myopic shift (78%), and shallowing of the anterior chamber (64%) and of the vitreous length (52%) during the acute phase compared with measurements taken after clinical recovery. That myopic shift was less common than diminished visual acuity suggested that multiple mechanisms, possibly including extraocular CNS involvement, contribute to visual disturbances during acute NE.[82]

Hypotension, if it develops, usually is mild. Petechiae are seen relatively infrequently (11%).[98] Severe internal bleeding is rare, seen almost exclusively in adults, and frequently associated with a fatal outcome.[98] The severity of acute kidney injury does not correlate with hypotension.[162]

The renal stage generally lasts 1 to 2 weeks and is characterized by the subsequent development of an oliguric phase with proteinuria, hematuria, and hyposthenuria. Among hospitalized patients, the decline in glomerular filtration rate can be precipitous.[162] Proteinuria begins abruptly, can be massive, and is nonselective, indicating contributions from both a defective glomerular barrier and from tubular injury.[162] Modest elevations in blood urea nitrogen and creatinine accompany the oliguria, which typically lasts for no more than a few days before diuresis begins (polyuric phase). Mild leukocytosis and thrombocytopenia occur during the renal phase. Electrolyte disturbances sufficient to require dialysis are infrequent events but occur in up to 6% of hospitalized patients.[162] Renal biopsy results reveal histopathologic findings characteristic of acute tubulointerstitial nephritis that correlate with the clinical severity of acute kidney injury but not with the severity of proteinuria.[162]

As with other forms of HFRS, the convalescent phase may be prolonged, and hyposthenuria may persist for many months. With Puumala infection, viremia can last 3 to 4 weeks.[162] Recovery typically is complete, although minor abnormalities in renal function and blood pressure have been described.[122,165] Hypertension, hypopituitarism, and cardiovascular disease are the most commonly described long-term consequences.[162]

As with Hantaan virus–associated HFRS, NE in children is recognized relatively infrequently. Clinically, the disease also appears to be similar to, although milder than, that seen in adults. Abdominal pain and vomiting are more frequently observed among children than adults, and children are more often hypertensive, thrombocytopenic, and oliguric.[98] Arthralgias, myalgias, and visual disturbances are more commonly reported in adults, as are epistaxis, leukocytosis, polyuria, and proteinuria.[98] Results of chest radiographs are more frequently abnormal in pediatric patients.[98] Among 32 Swedish cases reported (18 identified retrospectively and 14 prospectively), fever (100%), headache (100%), anorexia (100%), abdominal pain (93%), vomiting (91%), nausea (86%), and back pain (76%) were the most prevalent symptoms (see Table 189.2).[5] Proteinuria (100%), microscopic hematuria (80%), elevated serum creatinine concentration (76%), and thrombocytopenia (68%) were the laboratory abnormalities most frequently found. Leukocytosis was a relatively uncommon finding (22%) in this series. Six children (19%) had hemorrhagic manifestations, and one complained of blurred vision. In a 32-patient series from Finland, fever (100%), nausea (81%), vomiting (72%), and back pain (63%) again were prevalent, but headache and abdominal pain (59%) were reported less frequently.[161] Proteinuria (97%), hematuria (73%), and elevated serum creatinine level (84%) were common findings. In a separate 13-patient retrospective series from the same country, abdominal pain was universal as a presenting symptom, with temperature elevation, oliguria, polyuria, proteinuria, thrombocytopenia, and elevated serum creatinine level ultimately reported in all (see Table 189.2).[124]

Among 19 Austrian children 6 to 18 years old who were identified retrospectively, abdominal pain (100%), fever (89%), nausea (89%), vomiting (84%), and headache (58%) were the most frequent signs and symptoms reported.[25] Ninety-five percent of these children developed acute renal failure, but all appeared to recover fully while under clinical observation. No long-term follow up is available. Thrombocytopenia was reported more prominently among Austrian and Finnish than Swedish children. Up to one-fourth of Austrian and Finnish children displayed hemorrhagic manifestations. The proportion of transient visual blurring was identical to that seen in adults (25%). Some disease manifestations (e.g., thrombocytopenia, renal function abnormalities) may be absent, however, and the disease should be considered in the differential diagnosis of "fever of unknown origin" in endemic areas.[225] Three children with Puumala virus nephropathy in the Czech Republic were admitted with interstitial nephritis after a flulike prodrome. All were mildly febrile and had the following findings: anemia; elevated C-reactive protein values, erythrocyte sedimentation rates, and serum creatinine levels; and proteinuria. Biopsy-confirmed renal abnormalities returned to normal within 4 weeks after corticosteroid treatment.[51] No children in any of these series required dialysis.

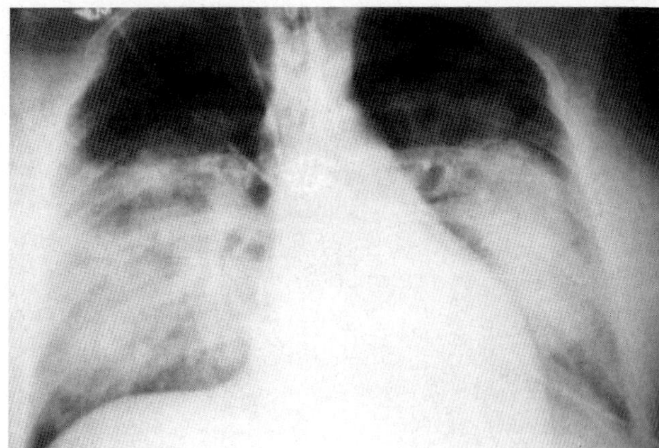

FIG. 189.4 Anteroposterior chest radiograph reveals the midstaged bilateral pulmonary effusion caused by hantavirus pulmonary syndrome. The radiologic evolution begins with minimal changes of interstitial pulmonary edema and progresses to alveolar edema with severe bilateral involvement. Pleural effusions are common and are often large enough to be evident radiographically. (Courtesy Centers for Disease Control and Prevention and D. Loren Ketai, MD.)

Hantavirus Pulmonary Syndrome

Classic HPS in adults is a biphasic illness that challenges the diagnostic acumen and clinical management skills of physicians.[22,169–171,175] The incubation period was 7 to 39 days (median, 18 days) for 20 people with defined exposure to Andes virus in a high-risk area,[231] an observation consistent with the incubation period of 9 to 33 days (median, 14–17 days) for 11 patients with HPS and well-defined exposure in the United States,[243] as well as the 3-week incubation period observed in two boys with HPS who were bitten by the same mouse.[203]

The clinical features of the prodrome phase are not pathognomonic; the diagnosis is rarely suspected before abrupt clinical deterioration heralds the onset of the cardiopulmonary phase. HPS characteristically begins with a prodrome that lasts 3 to 4 days but may extend as long as a week or more.[30,50,138,175,230] This phase is typified by fever and myalgia, particularly of the back or lower extremities. Although a cough may develop as the prodrome progresses, illnesses initially characterized predominantly by upper respiratory tract symptoms, such as cough and coryza, are unlikely to be HPS.[30,138,151,160] More than one-half of patients with HPS also have gastrointestinal symptoms (e.g., nausea, vomiting, diarrhea) that usually are mild.[30,50] Occasionally, HPS-associated gastrointestinal symptoms have been mistaken for an acute surgical abdomen or another intraabdominal process. The presence of thrombocytopenia in the context of a compatible prodrome is highly suggestive of HPS.[30,50,117,160,202]

The onset of the cardiopulmonary phase is abrupt and often life threatening. Patients usually are hospitalized within 12 to 24 hours of initial medical evaluation, and most deaths occur during the first 24 to 48 hours in the hospital.[30,32,50,138] Among fatal HPS cases identified in the United States between 1993 and 2009, the mean time from onset of symptoms to death was 6.4 days (median, 5 days) and the 35% case-fatality rate was similar across demographic characteristics and geographic regions.[146] Clear lungs shown by radiography have progressed to diffuse bilateral pulmonary involvement during the course of several hours. Interstitial edema, present in only 5% of patients with adult respiratory distress syndrome, is present in most patients with HPS on initial radiography, and alveolar flooding that is usually indistinguishable from the peripheral pattern seen in the acute phase of adult respiratory distress syndrome develops in most patients (Fig. 189.4).[105] This noncardiogenic pulmonary edema, resulting from a diffuse pulmonary capillary leak, can be differentiated from cardiac (hydrostatic) pulmonary edema by the presence of low pulmonary artery occlusion pressure and an increased protein content in edema fluid.[80] Secretions recovered when patients with HPS are intubated generally are acellular, resemble plasma or pulmonary edema fluid, and have been observed to clot in severe cases.[50,80] The presence of significant numbers of polymorphonuclear leukocytes in pulmonary secretions suggests an alternative cause.

The pulmonary decline usually is accompanied by the onset of shock caused by myocardial dysfunction and relative hypovolemia.[30,80,138] In severe cases, hemodynamic measurements show high systemic vascular resistance combined with low cardiac and stroke volume indices. Progression to death is associated with worsening cardiac dysfunction unresponsive to treatment, despite provision of adequate oxygenation.[80] Increased hematocrit, creatinine levels, and leukocyte counts; requirement for supplemental oxygen; and necessity for intubation are all associated with fatal outcome, and thrombocytopenia, although common, is more pronounced among patients who die compared with survivors.[30,146] At autopsy, the myocardium of patients who died of Araraquara virus–associated HPS contained endothelial cells and interstitial macrophage-type cells harboring hantavirus antigen and viral particles accompanied by a mononuclear cell inflammatory interstitial infiltrate that met the international consensus criteria for infectious inflammatory myocarditis. These findings were absent from the autopsy myocardium of persons who died after having either necrotizing pancreatitis associated with acute lung injury or nonthoracic trauma.[183,188] This infectious inflammatory form of cardiomyopathy may be responsible for HPS-associated myocardial depression and shock. In one South American study, the absence of clinical and laboratory signs of circulatory shock on admission was associated with a favorable outcome.[189]

Thrombocytopenia may be present in the late prodrome and almost always is found during the cardiopulmonary phase. Additional laboratory abnormalities in hospitalized patients include hemoconcentration, prolonged prothrombin and partial thromboplastin times, elevated serum lactate and serum lactate dehydrogenase concentrations, decreased serum protein concentration, mild leukocytosis with a marked left shift, and the frequent presence of myeloid precursors on the peripheral smear (Fig. 189.5).[30,50,117,138,175] The left shift and leukocytosis can, on occasion, be so marked as to represent a leukemoid reaction. Proteinuria is a common occurrence. The serum creatinine value often is elevated modestly in severe cases, although renal failure is not characteristic of infection with Sin Nombre virus, despite episodes of hypotension and other predisposing conditions that are present in many patients. Renal failure was more prominent in two reported North American cases of HPS caused by infection with Black Creek Canal virus and Bayou virus.[86,106,109,185]

Patients who survive enter a diuretic phase after recovery from cardiovascular collapse and improve rapidly thereafter. Surviving patients may be extubated within 3 to 7 days after admission to the intensive care unit and may be discharged from the hospital within 2 weeks.[30,32,175,188]

Subclinical or mild disease is rarely recognized after Sin Nombre virus infection.[202] However, although initial case-fatality rates of 70% to 80% were reported in 1993, a wider clinical spectrum became recognized once clinicians developed heightened suspicion and diagnostic assays

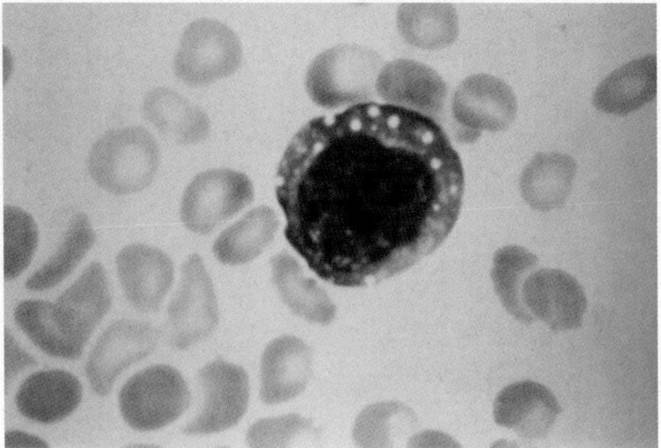

FIG. 189.5 Micrograph shows an atypical enlarged lymphocyte found in the blood smear from a patient with hantavirus pulmonary syndrome. The large atypical lymphocyte shown here is an example of one of the laboratory findings that, when combined with bandemia and a dropping platelet count, is characteristic of hantavirus pulmonary syndrome. (Courtesy Centers for Disease Control and Prevention.)

became more readily available. As of 2011, the overall case-fatality rate for HPS cases in the United States was 35%[146,147]; case-fatality rates are similar throughout the Americas.[147] This apparent decline in the incidence of mortality compared with initial reports in the early 1990s may reflect improvements in survival attributed to improved clinical management. However, it undoubtedly also reflects a decrease in the tendency to suspect this diagnosis only with the fatal and nearly fatal disease that existed early in the clinical understanding of this syndrome.

The hantavirus disease pulmonary manifestations associated with Andes virus[143] in Argentina and Chile and those from other related virus infections in Brazil[163] and Paraguay[236] closely resemble Sin Nombre virus disease. However, hemorrhagic and renal symptoms are more often associated with HPS in South America.[22,170,184,218,236] Renal failure accompanied some cases in a focus in northern Argentina,[171] and both viral antigen and infectious virus have been isolated from urine of Andes virus–infected patients with HPS.[74] The association of person-to-person transmission with Andes and a few other South American hantavirus infections suggests the need for increased infection control, although some transmission occurs before hospitalization.

HPS is relatively uncommon (7–15% of reported cases) in children younger than 17 years of age. Several case reports and reviews of North American pediatric patients with HPS have indicated that the geographic distribution, clinical course, and mortality rates in children and adolescents are similar to those described for adults.[8,19,26,108,131,168,182] In South America (predominantly Chile and Argentina), clinical manifestations of HPS in children appear to be similar to those described in North America.[59,125] Fever, headache, dyspnea or cough, gastrointestinal disturbances, and myalgia are common manifestations in the prodromal phase. Tachypnea and fever are frequent on hospital admission; in one case series, however, hypotension at presentation was an uncommon finding (33%).[182] In one patient, dizziness with an apparent vestibular component was described.[108] Thrombocytopenia, a left shift in the leukocyte differential count, elevated levels of hepatic aminotransferases and lactate dehydrogenase, and hypoalbuminemia typically are noted on admission. Although leukocytosis and hemoconcentration are generally not found early, they may appear later in the course of illness. Investigators suggested that the mortality rate among prepubertal children may be somewhat lower than that seen in older persons,[19] but as patients' numbers have accumulated over time, overall case-fatality rates in pediatric and adolescent patients seem to be similar to those seen in adults (30–40%). In one series, hypotension and the absence of fever at admission were found to be predictive of respiratory failure, whereas elevated prothrombin time (≥14 seconds) at admission was predictive of mortality.[182]

The overall mortality rate among 82 children with HPS contracted in Chile was 37%[59]; in one small case series from Argentina, however, the case-fatality rate for HPS in 5- to 11-year-old children was higher (60%).[177] In the same report the investigators noted evidence of passive hantavirus antibody transfer from a pregnant woman to her fetus, without subsequent illness in the infant. Additionally, a woman who nursed a 7-month-old infant contracted HPS and subsequently died. Hantavirus antibodies were detected to high titer (>1:6400) 8 and 15 months later in the infant (who remained healthy), a finding suggesting possible asymptomatic mother-to-child transmission of the infection through breastfeeding.[177]

One report suggests that one or more hantaviruses may be infecting children on the Caribbean island of Barbados. Among 272 children younger than 15 years of age who were hospitalized with suspected dengue and who tested negative for dengue but were also tested for hantavirus over a 2-year period, 22% had positive anti–hantavirus immunoglobulin M (IgM) antibody when a commercially available enzyme-linked immunosorbent assay was used. All these children had nonspecific febrile illnesses, with and without accompanying respiratory or gastrointestinal symptoms; four had mild bleeding, but none required intensive care, and there were no fatalities.[121]

COMPLICATIONS

In general, human infection with HFRS-associated hantaviruses results in an acute illness with prolonged incapacitation followed by complete recovery. Unless the illness is complicated by organ hemorrhage (e.g., CNS bleeding), long-term sequelae generally have not been observed.

In a Finnish study of 58 hospitalized Puumala virus–infected patients, 87% of these patients had symptoms suggestive of CNS involvement (headache, light sensitivity, nausea or vomiting, or dizziness). Two patients experienced symptoms indicative of encephalitis (vomiting, headache, somnolence, confusion). Two patients experienced an abrupt, complete loss of vision with spontaneous recovery, associated with severe headache, vomiting, dizziness, and pituitary hemorrhage demonstrated by magnetic resonance imaging.[84] One of the two patients with demonstrated pituitary hemorrhage recovered spontaneously within 3 months.[84] Young male patients may be at increased risk of developing serious CNS complications during acute Puumala virus infections.[83] Epidemiologic associations between previous infections with Seoul virus in the United States and hypertensive renal disease have been reported.[71,72] In one study, 5 years after recovery, 50% of patients who had HFRS were hypertensive, with a higher glomerular filtration rate and urinary protein excretion compared with 21% of control subjects. These differences resolved by 10 years.[156] These data require further study to determine their significance.

Although prolonged prothrombin and partial thromboplastin times occur commonly among Sin Nombre–infected patients hospitalized in North America, overt disseminated intravascular coagulation and overt hemorrhage are infrequent.[30,244] Patients with established disseminated intravascular coagulation rarely survive longer than 48 hours. One patient who did survive a cardiopulmonary phase accompanied by overt disseminated intravascular coagulation died 3 weeks later of gangrenous complications.

One 5-year follow-up study of 30 North American HPS survivors (29 infected with Sin Nombre and 1 with Bayou virus) identified proteinuria of more than 150 mg total protein by 24-hour urine collection in more than one-half of the cohort; 17% also had decreased creatinine clearance. Proteinuria prevalence appeared to increase over time and to be associated with increased severity of HPS disease, although treatment by extracorporeal membrane oxygenation (ECMO) may have lowered the risk.[174]

The South American HPS-associated viruses have been associated with more extrapulmonary manifestations than have the Sin Nombre infections in the United States. Evidence of disseminated intravascular coagulation, bleeding, and renal manifestations are reported with greater frequency among Andes virus–infected patients.[22]

PATHOGENESIS AND PATHOLOGY

In humans, hantaviruses infect alveolar macrophages and follicular dendritic cells, but they primarily target and replicate in endothelium, without apparent cytopathic effect.[244] Signs and symptoms of hantavirus disease are likely the result of both direct effects of the virus on endothelium and the innate and adaptive immune response to infection.[222] Hantaviruses infect human kidney tubular epithelial cells, glomerular endothelial cells, and podocytes, thereby disrupting cell-to-cell contacts, decreasing barrier functions, and causing proteinuria.[162] Barrier breakdown appears to be caused directly by infection and release of cytokines and is not the result of endothelial cell death.[162]

Early clinical events are presumed, and with Andes virus demonstrated, to be accompanied by viremia[58]; however, significant signs and symptoms develop in temporal association with the onset of a measurable antibody response.

In HPS, Andes viral RNA (detected by RT-PCR) has been observed up to 2 weeks before symptom onset.[58] A statistically significant association has been demonstrated between plasma viral RNA levels at hospital admission and the severity of HPS disease.[237] Survivors rapidly clear virus.[214]

Increased capillary permeability is a hallmark of hantavirus infection, and it appears to be responsible for most of the clinical stigmata observed (e.g., hypotension, extravascular fluid extravasation, pulmonary edema, abdominal pain). Although endothelial cells of small vessels are the primary targets for hantavirus infection, the absence of cytopathic effects suggests that host immune or inflammatory mechanisms are likely principal contributors to capillary leakage.[162] Increased monolayer permeability and loss of integrity of the endothelial cell barrier in association with early increase in secreted vascular endothelial growth factor (VEGF) and concomitant decreased vascular endothelial (VE)-cadherin have been demonstrated during HPS-associated hantavirus infection of human primary lung endothelial cells.[67,200] VEGF is a potent vascular permeability agent and when present, it binds to vascular endothelial growth factor receptor-2 (VEGFR2), thus initiating the internalization and degradation of VE-cadherin and the disruption of the adherens junctions of the endothelial cell barrier.[68,200] Virus-induced inactivation of β3 integrins and subsequent deregulation of this VEGF/VEGFR2/VE-cadherin cascade is thought to be central to the increase in vascular permeability observed in hantavirus-infected endothelial cells.[68,76,77,200]

Thrombocytopenia with a nadir of approximately 100×10^8/L occurs in most patients with NE approximately 4 to 5 days after the onset of fever and usually resolves within 1 week, although severe thrombocytopenia can predict a severe course of acute kidney failure.[162] The mechanisms underlying thrombocytopenia observed in both HFRS and HPS are not well understood. Decreased platelet count without evidence of decreased function or production is the most common coagulation profile abnormality. Bone marrow biopsy specimens have demonstrated increased megakaryocytes and active platelet function during hantavirus infections. Thus thrombocytopenia may result from increased platelet consumption, and endothelial injury likely contributes to enhanced coagulation, fibrinolysis, and platelet consumption.[162] Cell-associated pathogenic hantaviruses demonstrate direct binding and inactivation of platelets to endothelial cell surfaces by interaction with platelet integrin αIIβ3, perhaps contributing to pathogenesis.[42,68,222] The differential use of β3 integrins as receptors by pathogenic hantaviruses is therefore likely relevant to pathogenesis because β3 integrins are present on platelets and endothelial cells, and interaction with these proteins can regulate vascular permeability, platelet activation, and adhesion.[147] Bleeding in NE is characteristically mild with petechiae and epistaxis, although hemorrhage has been identified by magnetic resonance imaging and at autopsy and bleeding into multiple organs documented in some cases.[162] Less than 30% of Scandinavian patients with Puumala virus infection have met strict criteria for overt disseminated intravascular coagulation.[162]

Pathologic studies of fatal HFRS cases indicated that multiple organ systems are involved, but a triad of lesions consisting of hemorrhagic necrosis of the renal medulla, anterior pituitary, and cardiac right atrium is described as characteristic.[97] Magnetic resonance imaging has demonstrated clearly enlarged spleens during acute NE, but the degree of splenic enlargement did not correlate with the degree of thrombocytopenia.[162] Among hospitalized patients with NE, 16% to 35% have abnormal chest radiographs, with pleural effusions, atelectasis, and interstitial infiltrates that correlate with the degree of renal failure, fluid overload, leukocytosis, and thrombocytosis as the most common findings.[162] Endobronchial mucosal biopsy specimens show increased CD8 T cells in epithelium and submucosa, and increased submucosal CD4 T cells, demonstrating a local immune response.[162] Puumala virus antigens are present in lung capillary vascular endothelium of patients with NE as well as in bronchoalveolar lavage fluid.[162] Patients with NE occasionally have myocarditis with nonspecific electrocardiographic changes that may be attributed to acute kidney injury with altered plasma electrolytes and cytokine release, sometimes associated with impaired cardiovascular contraction observed with echocardiograpy.[162] CNS symptoms are common in Puumala virus infection and include headache, insomnia, somnolence, dizziness, anxiety, and amnesia. About one-half of infected persons who undergo lumbar puncture have elevated IgM, increased protein, or increased leukocytes counts in spinal fluid.[162] Pituitary hemorrhage has been reported during acute HFRS, but recovered patients remain at increased risk of hypopituitarism for reasons unrelated to the severity of HFRS and for which the underlying pathophysiology remains unclear.[162]

In HPS, multiple organ involvement with variable degrees of vascular congestion is noted in all fatal cases. However, the predominant findings at autopsy have involved the lungs, with pulmonary edema and serous effusions seen grossly and interstitial pneumonitis with a mononuclear cell infiltrate, intraalveolar edema, and focal hyaline membrane formation described microscopically (Fig. 189.6). Immunohistochemical studies demonstrated the widespread presence of hantavirus antigens in endothelial cells of the microvasculature, particularly in the lungs, but also in the kidneys, heart, spleen, pancreas, lymph nodes, skeletal muscle, intestine, adrenal gland, adipose tissue, urinary bladder, and brain. However, few histologic changes have been noted in autopsy examination of the kidney, brain, and heart of patients who died of HPS.[244]

Endothelial cell mRNA responses to infection by pathogenic and nonpathogenic hantaviruses, observed by DNA array analyses, showed differential patterns of gene activation.[69] Pathogenic Hantaan and New York viruses appeared to suppress early interferon (IFN) responses that were activated by nonpathogenic Prospect Hill virus. Hantaan virus uniquely induced multiple chemokines (interleukin-8 [IL-8], IL-6, growth-regulated oncogene-β [GRO-β]), cell adhesion molecules (intercellular cell adhesion molecule [ICAM]), and complement cascade–associated factors that could play a role in HFRS immunopathogenesis. Although New York virus failed to induce most of the cellular chemokines activated by Hantaan virus, it uniquely induced β3 integrin–linked potassium channels, an action that could be important to HPS-induced vascular permeability.[69,147] Evidence exists that hantaviruses work to subvert host innate immune responses.[65,211] Hantaviruses use a transcription mechanism that avoids activation of the IFN pathway.[66,79] Hantavirus Gn and Gc glycoproteins can downregulate the host IFN response and contribute, along with the nucleocapsid protein, to inhibition of the IFN signaling pathway.[6,137,209] Pathogenic and nonpathogenic hantaviruses both downregulate the IFN induction, but pathogenic hantaviruses do not induce the early IFN responses activated by nonpathogenic hantaviruses described earlier.[69,147] This difference in innate immune activation has been speculated to contribute to differences in pathogenicity.

Whereas the mechanisms underlying the observed pathologic lesions are incompletely understood, both cellular and humoral immune-mediated mechanisms have been implicated.[15,39,97,220] Serum antibodies develop within 3 to 7 days of the onset of illness in patients infected with hantaviruses. In patients with HPS, N protein–reactive antibodies are present in serum soon after onset of disease; neutralizing antibodies directed against Gn and Gc glycoproteins follow.[99,224] High-titer neutralizing antibodies in serum correlate with milder disease, and higher hantavirus-specific IgG levels early in disease are associated with survival.[12,145]

The abrupt onset of noncardiogenic pulmonary edema in HPS occurs after the development of an immune response directed against viral antigen present throughout the endothelial cells lining the pulmonary capillaries. This temporal association suggests an immune-mediated capillary leak syndrome in addition to direct effects of virus replication and indirect effects of increased VEGF and decreased VE-cadherin on the permeability and integrity of the endothelial cell barrier.[67,76,77,200]

Virus-specific cytotoxic T lymphocytes have been observed during acute phases of HFRS,[95] and elevated levels of inflammatory cytokines (IFN-γ, tumor necrosis factor [TNF]-α, TNF-β, IL-6, and IL-10) have been found in sera and renal biopsy specimens of patients.[95,118,140,212] Animal

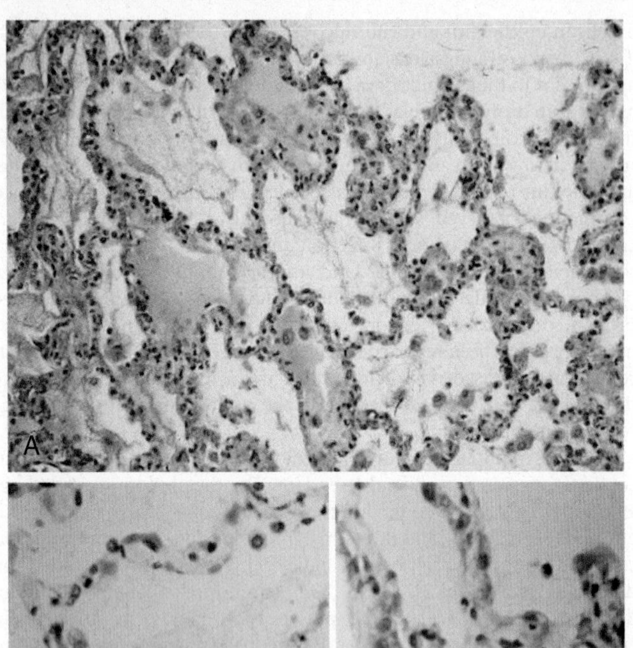

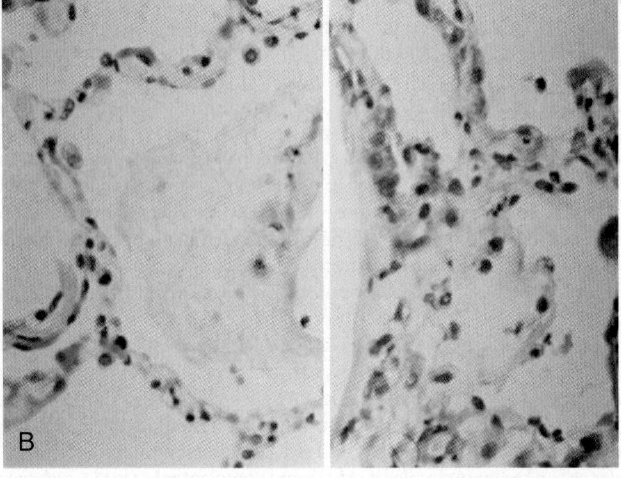

FIG. 189.6 (A) Histopathologic features of the lung in hantavirus pulmonary syndrome (HPS), with interstitial pneumonitis and intraalveolar edema. (B) Histopathologic comparison between HPS *(right)* and acute respiratory distress syndrome *(left)*. HPS is characterized by interstitial lymphocytic infiltrates and alveolar edema, whereas acute respiratory distress syndrome is characterized by neutrophilic presence and damage to pneumocytes. (Courtesy Centers for Disease Control and Prevention and Dr. Sherif R. Zaki.)

studies have also suggested a role for T-helper cells and antibodies.[43] $CD4^+$ and $CD8^+$ T-cell clones that recognize Hantaan virus N, Gn, and Gc proteins are present in acute and convalescent patient blood samples.[55,110,215,226,227] Several studies suggest that cytotoxic T lymphocytes play a major role in induction of HPS. Patients with more severe HPS had higher frequencies of Sin Nombre virus–specific $CD8^+$ T cells compared with patients with milder disease, and the presence of Sin Nombre virus–specific $CD8^+$ T cells has been shown to increase permeability of infected HLA-matched human endothelial cells in vitro.[85,213]

DIAGNOSIS AND DIFFERENTIAL DIAGNOSIS

A high index of suspicion is essential for recognition of hantavirus infection in persons living or traveling in disease-endemic areas and participating in activities that could provide appropriate exposures. The protean nature of the disease in children is such that almost any ill-defined febrile disease (or fever of unknown origin) associated with abdominal or back pain in an appropriate geographic setting should stimulate consideration of the diagnosis, particularly if the clinical syndrome is accompanied by myalgia, if thrombocytopenia or proteinuria is present, or if a history of exposure to rodents or rural environments in disease-endemic areas is elicited.[201]

The differential diagnosis of HFRS includes rickettsial disease, leptospirosis, meningococcemia, other viral diseases, poststreptococcal syndromes, pyelonephritis, leukemia, and hemolytic uremic syndrome. Differentiating from an acute intraabdominal or pelvic process, such as appendicitis, may be extremely difficult on clinical grounds.

The differential diagnosis of HPS includes rickettsial diseases, leptospirosis, influenza, streptococcal pneumonia, legionellosis, *Yersinia pestis* infection (plague), meningococcemia, brucellosis, mycoplasmal and fungal pneumonias (including *Coccidioides immitis* and *Histoplasma* pneumonias), tularemia, psittacosis, pancreatitis accompanied by adult respiratory distress syndrome, inhalation anthrax, and autoimmune disorders (including thrombotic thrombocytopenia purpura). A prominent cough or sore throat or a localized infiltrate on a chest radiograph that does not generalize within hours argues for a cause other than hantaviral.[30,32,117,160] A constellation of the absence of a cough in the presence of dizziness, nausea or vomiting, a low platelet count, a low serum bicarbonate level, and an elevated hematocrit discriminated HPS from similar patients with unexplained adult respiratory distress syndrome in two studies.[30,160] Thrombocytopenia or a falling platelet count provides a valuable clue late in the prodrome. After the onset of pulmonary edema, the presence of four of five findings (thrombocytopenia, myelocytosis, hemoconcentration, lack of significant toxic granulations in neutrophils, and more than 10% of lymphocytes with immunoblastic morphologic findings) has a sensitivity for HPS of 96% and a specificity of 99%.[117]

Laboratory Studies

Serologic testing remains the mainstay of clinical diagnosis and is widely available through commercial laboratories or, in the United States, state public health laboratories and the CDC. IgM antibodies to nucleocapsid antigen are universally present in symptomatic patients with HPS and almost universally in patients with HFRS; seroconversion takes place up to 5 days after the onset of disease in 2% to 5% of Puumala virus–infected patients with NE.[90,101,202,223] The extent of viremia, and therefore the utility of testing for viral RNA, varies depending on the infecting hantavirus. Plasma viral RNA correlates with disease severity for both HFRS and HPS, and a high viral load is generally identifiable in the blood circulation of patients with severe HFRS and HPS disease (i.e., infections with Hantaan, Dobrava, Sin Nombre, or Andes viruses).[90,223] Prospective surveillance of household contact of Andes virus–infected patients with HPS detected hantaviral RNA 5 to 15 days before symptom onset or detection of IgM antibodies.[223] Although the viremia level is lower in Puumala virus–associated NE cases, viral RNA detection may be successful on blood samples collected within the first 7 days after symptom onset.[223] Detection of viral RNA in urine or cerebrospinal fluid of hantavirus-infected patients helps describe pathophysiology but has little diagnostic utility, although detection of hantavirus RNA in saliva may prove useful for diagnostic applications.[223] Kidney biopsies were used for diagnosis of HFRS in earlier years, but findings were generally nonspecific; interstitial hemorrhage was found in only 25% of HFRS cases, and identification of viral markers was rare.[223]

Routine immunohistologic methods can detect hantavirus antigens in autopsy samples.[223] Laboratory diagnosis of HFRS or HPS is made by demonstrating specific anti-hantavirus IgM antibodies in acute-phase serum by enzyme immunoassay in the IgM capture format. A fourfold or greater rise in specific IgG antibodies by enzyme immunoassay or immunofluorescence[120,136] in sequential sera (ideally obtained ≥2 weeks apart) also is useful. The availability of purified recombinant hantavirus antigens has enhanced diagnostic specificity in both the enzyme immunoassay and the Western blot assay systems.[57,99,101,223,248] Enzyme-linked immunosorbent assay and indirect fluorescent antibody tests are broadly cross reactive, particularly among viruses from rodents of the same subfamily.[35,36] For example, a recombinant Sin Nombre virus antigen detects antibodies against Bayou, Black Creek Canal, Andes, and several other viruses from sigmodontine and neotomine rodents, and it maintains reactivity with antibodies directed against arvicoline rodent–associated viruses (e.g., Puumala and Prospect Hill viruses). Neutralizing antibody assays are more specific, but technical requirements preclude their routine use.[101,223] Immunohistochemical techniques have been applied to tissue samples from patients infected with hantaviruses.[244,223] Nucleic acid primers from several hantavirus strains have been generated, and they have enabled nucleotide sequences from fresh or frozen tissues to be amplified by RT-PCR. RT-PCR usually is successful on whole blood or blood clots obtained within the first 7 to 10 days of illness. However, the expense and effort of performing the method are not justified unless the resulting genetic sequence information is needed for definition of the viral strain or for epidemiologic studies.[7,164] Attempts to isolate hantaviruses from human specimens are generally unrewarding.

TREATMENT

Cautious fluid management and hemodynamic management in an intensive care unit setting are the most important aspects of the clinical management of any hantavirus disease.[138,80] Early hospitalization and avoidance of even minor trauma are essential to maintain the integrity of damaged vascular beds in these patients. Transport of patients should be minimized; the barotrauma associated with transport in underpressurized aircraft may be particularly hazardous.[18] Attention to fluid management and metabolic status is especially critical.

In patients with HFRS, restriction of fluids may be necessary early in the course of disease as renal function diminishes, but large input may be required later during diuresis to correct massive losses. Electrolyte abnormalities and metabolic acidosis occur commonly. Peritoneal dialysis or hemodialysis may be lifesaving in severe cases.[18]

In patients with HPS, the nature of the pulmonary disease predisposes to iatrogenic pulmonary edema; careful attention must be paid to maintaining appropriate central venous and pulmonary arterial pressure to avoid such complications. Tissue perfusion and adequate oxygenation are the goals of supportive therapy with this syndrome. Oxygen supplementation and mechanical ventilation are nearly always required. Inotropic agents may be necessary to maintain tissue perfusion.[80,138] ECMO has been used in severe HPS cases; some studies suggest that this procedure may improve survival.[41,45] One study suggested that ECMO may also be associated with a lower risk of proteinuria after acute disease.[74]

Studies have suggested that cytotoxic T-lymphocyte activity and other aspects of the inflammatory response contribute to the capillary leakage observed in patients with HFRS or HPS, and case reports have attributed clinical improvement to treatment with corticosteroids and venovenous hemodiafiltration.[85,197] Immunotherapeutic approaches that may inhibit the vascular permeability induced by hantavirus infection were under clinical investigation in 2011.[147]

Hantaan, Sin Nombre, and several Old and New World hantaviruses exhibit similar in vitro sensitivity to ribavirin. One prospective, placebo-controlled trial suggested that intravenous ribavirin was effective in reducing the mortality and morbidity rates associated with HFRS in China.[96] In contrast, although 30 patients with HPS who received investigational, open-label intravenous ribavirin generally tolerated it well, treatment was accompanied by a low frequency of early drug-associated adverse events, most significantly anemia and resulting transfusion, and no clear evidence of benefit was obtained.[30,32] A subsequent randomized placebo-controlled trial was stopped short of a definitive end point because of small enrollment without trends supporting either efficacy or adverse events.[155] However, the study sample size was insufficient to exclude adverse events that occurred at a rate of less than 27%.[149] Similar doses of intravenous ribavirin resulted in hemolysis in 76%, a 2 g/dL hemoglobin level decrease in 49%, and discontinuation because of toxicity in 18% of 126 patients treated for severe acute respiratory syndrome, findings consistent with observations during the open-label trial.[14,30,32,149] This contrast in clinical experience is not explained by differences in dosing schedules; patients in all three protocols received identical doses.[14,32,96] Because all hantaviruses have been sensitive to the antiviral effects of ribavirin in vitro, the lack of any dramatic effect by intravenous ribavirin in HPS is probably the result of the rapid progression of the disease; HPS-associated deaths usually occur within the first 48 hours after admission and therapeutic intervention.[30–32,50,80,96,138] Although ribavirin administered at 3 days after infection provided complete protection from disease in a hamster animal model,[187] the 2- to 3-week incubation period associated with Andes and Sin Nombre–virus infections leading to HPS precludes administration of ribavirin comparably early in human infection.

Administration of 5000 or more neutralizing antibody units (NAU) of human polyclonal antibody obtained from fresh frozen plasma of an HPS survivor per kilogram or of 12,000 NAU/kg of a despeciated (Fc removed) polyclonal immunoglobulin-based product purified from the eggs of ducks vaccinated with a DNA vaccine protected against lethal disease when given up to 8 days after intranasal Andes virus challenge in the same hamster model.[16] Therapeutic approaches attempting to combine ribavirin with other therapeutic agents, including immune modulators, may be more efficacious. Ribavirin is not licensed for intravenous use in the United States. Teratogenic concerns mandate careful informed consent if the use of this drug is considered in children, pregnant women, or nursing mothers. A single case report of a patient with severe NE suggested that treatment with a synthetic polypeptide licensed for treatment of hereditary angioedema, icatibant, may have improved survival.[162]

PREVENTION

Primary Prevention

The most effective preventive measure available for hantavirus infection is the avoidance of rodents and their habitats. However, eradication of rodent reservoir hosts in disease-endemic areas is not feasible. Prevention efforts are directed more appropriately toward reducing the frequency of rodent-human interactions through environmental hygiene practices that minimize rodent abundance in home and work environments and avoidance of known rodent-infested areas and activities that increase the risk of human exposure to aerosolized infectious rodent excreta. Such avoidance may be particularly important during times of high rodent populations in specific localities.

In the United States hantavirus infection is a nationally notifiable condition reported to state health departments, who notify the federal public health agency, the CDC.[40] In the southwestern United States remote sensing patterns from the year before have predicted local areas of increased risk for HPS, thus allowing precisely targeted public health messages and interventions.[70]

Detailed guidelines on measures appropriate to eliminate rodents from homes in disease-endemic areas, to clean rodent-contaminated areas safely, and to minimize the risk for workers occupationally exposed to rodents and participants in outdoor recreational activities have been published.[158] Although rodent ectoparasites do not transmit hantaviruses, in the southwestern United States, several rodent species are also hosts to fleas that transmit *Yersinia pestis*. In such areas, insecticides should be used in conjunction with rodent extermination measures because eradication of rodents without concurrent control of the associated fleas may increase the risk of human plague.[158]

One study[229] reported a strong association between smoking and infection with Puumala virus, but more study is needed to demonstrate cause and effect. As these authors hypothesized, one potential mechanism would be that smoking impairs respiratory ciliary action, thereby increasing the likelihood that Puumala virus in an aerosol exposure would reach the alveoli and remain long enough to cause an infection.

Vaccine Prospects

Both rodent brain–derived and cell culture–derived inactivated vaccines to Hantaan and Seoul viruses have been developed in South Korea and China. Some of these vaccines induce neutralizing antibody responses in humans and are being tested in field studies, but none has been approved in the United States.[172,190,205,206] A commercial suckling mouse brain–derived vaccine marketed in Korea, Hantavax, has no reported safety issues but placebo-controlled trials have not been conducted, and a case-control study did not have sufficient statistical power to demonstrate efficacy.[189] Monovalent and bivalent cell culture–based Hantaan virus– and Seoul virus–inactivated vaccines produced in China elicited neutralizing antibodies in more than 90% of persons tested who received three doses.[190]

A recombinant vaccinia strain expressing Hantaan virus antigens has been tested in human volunteers in the United States and has been shown to induce a serum neutralizing antibody response.[193] However, because only 26% of vaccinia virus–immune volunteers developed neutralizing antibodies, this vaccine has not been pursued.[190] A plasmid DNA platform vaccine delivered by gene gun was developed because the platform allows ready construction of combination vaccines and because the absence of a protein component means that preexisting vector immunity is not a problem. DNA vaccines for Hantaan and Puumala viruses have been developed, tested in animals, and moved into phase I clinical trials.[190] Various other approaches to vaccine development against hantaviruses across the globe are under way,[17,119,139,141,152,247] but none have progressed to clinically relevant interventions. An immediate need exists for a vaccine to Hantaan virus and perhaps other hantaviruses, but until recently a lack of realistic animal models of human disease hampered efforts to perform full preclinical evaluation of candidates. This is particularly important because the diseases are immunopathologic, and some monoclonal antibodies can enhance macrophage infection in vitro. The discovery that hamsters infected with Andes virus provide a reproducible model for HPS that mimics the human disease very closely[93] provides an avenue to explore mechanisms of disease and also vastly improves preclinical evaluation of hantavirus vaccine candidates. Nonetheless, even more than with other viral vaccines, double-blind, placebo-controlled trials are needed to provide definitive evidence of protection and to exclude adverse effects.

Hospital Infection Control

The use of universal precautions in handling the blood and body fluids of all patients is prudent practice. In addition, a certified biologic safety cabinet should be used for all handling of human body fluids in situations in which splatter or aerosolization is possible.[23,27] Viral antigens can be detected in necropsy specimens, and RT-PCR readily detects viral genetic material in necropsy tissue and in blood and plasma obtained from hantavirus-infected persons early in the course of the disease.[89,244] However, secondary transmission of hantaviruses associated with HFRS has not been documented after contact with acutely ill persons or exposure to their clinical laboratory specimens.[221] The experience with North American hantaviruses linked to HPS has been similar.[233]

In contrast, a well-documented episode of person-to-person spread during an Andes virus outbreak in South America and subsequent molecular and epidemiologic studies have demonstrated numerous occurrences of person-to-person transmission of Andes virus. Person-to-person spread has been reported to result in secondary cases among up to 3.4% of household contacts of primary HPS cases, with sexual partners at greatest risk.[56,58,125,151,170,218,235] With the possible exception of Andes virus infections, the many years of experience with HFRS and HPS indicate that once the diagnosis has been confirmed, isolation of hospitalized patients to prevent nosocomial transmission generally is not required. In plague-endemic areas, respiratory isolation pending confirmation of hantavirus infection may be a wise precaution. Sera and other specimens from hantavirus-infected persons can be handled safely by using biosafety level 2 facilities and practices. Higher biosafety levels are recommended for attempts to propagate hantaviruses.[27]

NEW REFERENCES SINCE THE SEVENTH EDITION

1. Virus taxonomy: 2015 release. International Committee on Taxonomy of Viruses (ICTV). 2016. http://www.ictvonline.org/virusTaxonomy.asp.
11. Bennett SN, Gu SH, Kang HJ, Arai S, Yanagihara R. Reconstructing the evolutionary origins and phylogeography of hantaviruses. *Trends Microbiol.* 2014;22:473-482.
40. Nationally notifiable conditions. Council of State and Territorial Epidemiologist (CSTE). 2013. https://c.ymcdn.com/sites/cste.site-ym.com/resource/resmgr/CSTENotifiableConditionListA.pdf.
42. Dalrymple NA, Mackow ER. Virus interactions with endothelial cell receptors: implications for viral pathogenesis. *Curr Opin Virol.* 2014;7:134-140.
68. Gavrilovskaya I, Gorbunova E, Matthys V, Dalrymple N, Mackow E. The role of the endothelium in HPS pathogenesis and potential therapeutic approaches. *Adv Virol.* 2012;2012:467059.
78. Guo WP, Lin XD, Wang W, et al. Phylogeny and origins of hantaviruses harbored by bats, insectivores, and rodents. *PLoS Pathog.* 2013;9:e1003159.
114. Klempa K, Koivogui L, Sylla O, et al. Serological evidence of human hantavirus infections in Guinea, West Africa. *J Infect Dis.* 2010;201:1031-1034.
121. Kumar A, Krishnamurthy K, Nielsen AL. Hantavirus infection among children hospitalized for febrile illness suspected to be dengue in Barbados. *J Infect Public Health.* 2016;9:81-87.
162. Mustonen J, Mäkelä S, Outinen T, et al. The pathogenesis of nephropathia epidemica: new knowledge and unanswered questions. *Antiviral Res.* 2013;100:589-604.
222. Vaheri A, Strandin T, Hepojoki J, et al. Uncovering the mysteries of hantavirus infections. *Nat Rev Microbiol.* 2013;11:539-550.
240. Yanagihara R, Gu SH, Arai S, Kang HJ, Song J-W. Hantaviruses: rediscovery and new beginnings. *Virus Res.* 2016;187:6-14.

The full reference list for this chapter is available at ExpertConsult.com.

190 La Crosse Encephalitis and Other California Serogroup Viruses

W. Garrett Hunt • James E. McJunkin

La Crosse virus (LACV) is a member of the California serogroup viruses within the family Bunyaviridae and the genus *Orthobunyavirus*. The term *California serogroup* does not describe the widespread geographic distribution of viruses in the serogroup but simply reflects the name of the prototype virus, California encephalitis virus (CEV), initially discovered in California in 1943.[67] LACV, the most prevalent and pathogenic member of the serogroup, causes disease in the upper Midwestern, mid-Atlantic, and southeastern United States, particularly in Appalachia in more recent reports, but not on the West Coast (Figs. 190.1 and 190.2).[20,55,59,64,93,99,124,144,145] LACV is estimated to cause 8% to 30% of all cases of encephalitis in the United States annually, and in 2011, LACV was the most common arboviral infection of children in North America, a finding consistent with previous reports.[26,27,126] In 2014, there were 80 cases of LACV disease reported from 9 states, with 72 cases in persons younger than 18 years old and 76 cases of neuroinvasive disease.[95] From 2003 to 2012, LACV neuroinvasive disease was reported from 204 counties in 21 states. The average annual incidence in children was 0.090 cases per 100,000 children (range, 0.053–0.151 cases), compared with the rate in adults, 0.004 per 100,000 adults.[49] In a separate analysis, the average annual reported incidence of neuroinvasive disease (meningitis, encephalitis, and meningoencephalitis) caused by the California serogroup viruses as a whole from 1999 to 2007 was 0.035 case per 100,000 population per year (all those patients in whom the etiology was tested had confirmed or probable California serogroup–associated disease).[124]

The medical, psychosocial, and economic costs to affected persons in endemic areas are significant. Acute morbidity includes seizures in roughly 50% to 60% of hospitalized cases, mental status changes in one- to two-thirds, cerebral edema in 16%, and cerebral herniation in 2% to 3%. Approximately 9% to 25% of all hospitalized patients require mechanical ventilation.[101,106] Long-term morbidity after severe disease may include cognitive delays in up to one-third and attention-deficit/hyperactivity disorder in up to two-thirds of all patients.[101] The mortality rate of LACV encephalitis (LACVE) is relatively low compared with that of certain other arboviral illnesses, such as West Nile virus (WNV) infection or eastern equine encephalitis. However, the first risk assessment mapping of LACVE cases, reported to the Centers for Disease Control and Prevention (CDC) from 2003 to 2007, found a mortality rate

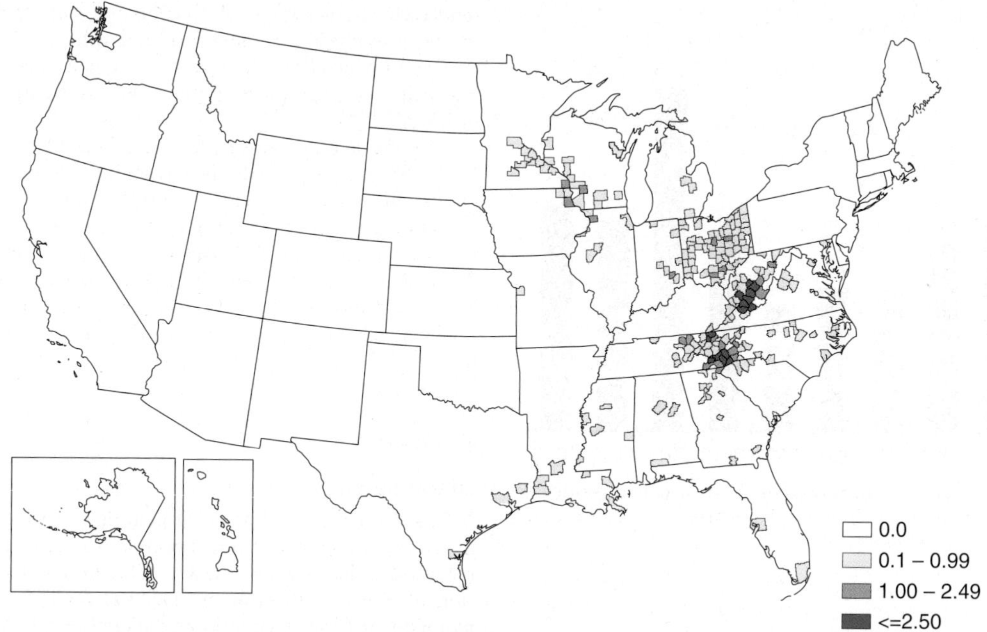

FIG. 190.1 La Crosse virus neuroinvasive disease average annual incidence by county, 2004–13. (Modified from ArboNET, Arboviral Diseases Branch, Centers for Disease Control and Prevention.)

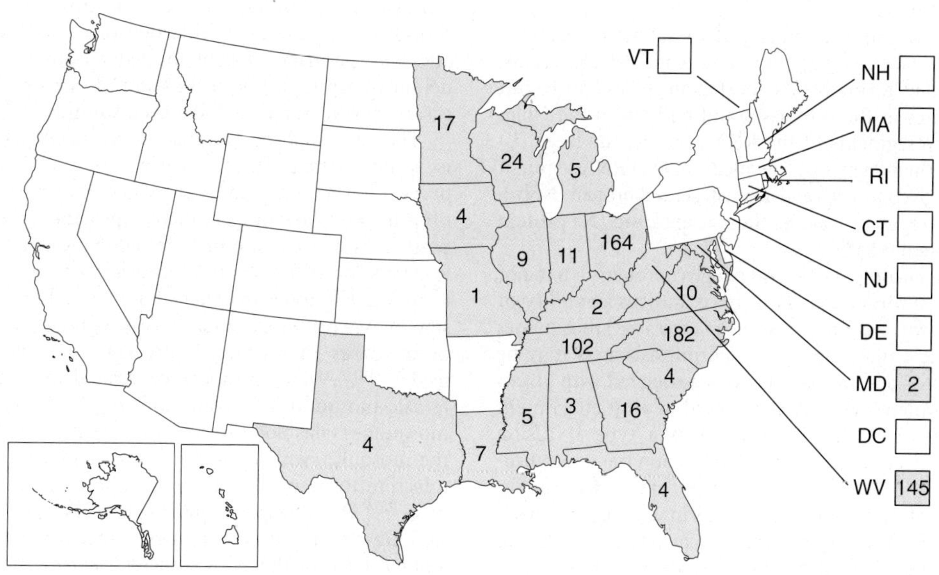

FIG. 190.2 La Crosse virus neuroinvasive disease cases reported by state, 2004–13. (From ArboNET, Arboviral Diseases Branch, Centers for Disease Control and Prevention.)

of 1.9% among confirmed cases, higher than previously reported (0.3%).[64,124,126] In a study of the economic and social impact of LACVE in an endemic region of western North Carolina, the average direct and indirect medical costs per patient (from a group of 24 patients studied over 89.6 life-years) were roughly $33,000 (≤$35,000). The projected cost for five patients with neurologic sequelae ranged from approximately $50,000 to $3 million per patient.[147] Although the number of confirmed cases of LACV-associated neuroinvasive disease in the United States is usually 80 to 100 per year, with an approximate range of 30 to 170 per year from 1964 to 2014, underrecognition and underreporting within a voluntary national reporting system are common problems (Fig. 190.3).[93,95] Because LACV is the most clinically significant member of the California serogroup viruses, it is the focus of this chapter, but other members of the serogroup are addressed briefly.

ETIOLOGIC AGENT

In 1960, a 4-year-old girl died of "rural encephalitis" in a hospital in La Crosse County, Wisconsin. In 1965, Thompson and colleagues[141,143] reported the isolation of a novel virus from frozen homogenates of the child's brain by intracerebral inoculation of suckling mice. Soon after its discovery, LACV was identified as a member of the California serogroup viruses on the basis of complement fixation and virus neutralization tests; it is one of five such viruses causing human disease in North America.

The prototype, CEV, is 1 of 16 viruses in the *Orthobunyavirus* genus. CEV was discovered in mosquitoes from Kern County in the San Joaquin Valley of California in 1943 and linked to human cases of encephalitis in the same region in 1945.[66,67] The other four viruses of this serogroup

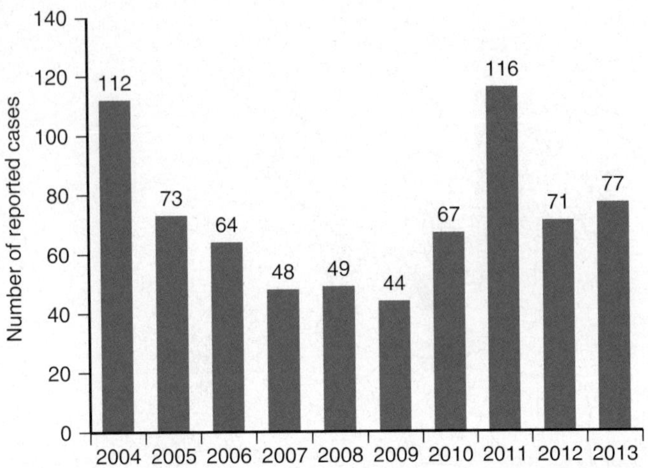

FIG. 190.3 La Crosse virus neuroinvasive disease cases reported by year, 2004–13. (From ArboNET, Arboviral Diseases Branch, Centers for Disease Control and Prevention.)

in North America include LACV, snowshoe hare virus (SSHV), Jamestown Canyon virus (JCV), and trivittatus virus (TV). Inkoo virus (INKV) and Tahyna virus (TAHV) are members of the California serogroup viruses distributed in Europe.

The LACV virion is pleomorphic, roughly 90 to 100 nm in diameter, and has a host-derived viral envelope with virus-encoded glycoproteins, Gc (formerly G1) and Gn (formerly G2), located on spikes 5 to 10 nm long. The virus replicates in the cytoplasm and buds from the Golgi apparatus. Of the three segments of the RNA genome, the large (L) RNA segment encodes the polymerase, the medium (M) RNA segment encodes the Gc and Gn glycoproteins and a nonstructural protein (NSm), and the small (S) RNA segment encodes the nucleocapsid (N) protein and nonstructural protein NSs.[15,121]

The M segment that encodes the Gc and Gn glycoproteins is a major determinant of viral neuroinvasiveness in mice and susceptibility of *Ochlerotatus triseriatus* (formerly known as *Aedes triseriatus*) mosquitoes to oral and intrathoracic infection.[53,55,128] Neuroinvasiveness may be linked to the cell receptor and fusion functions associated with glycoproteins.[53,54] The Gc protein of LACV is involved in viral attachment to mammalian cell receptors, by functioning as a type II fusion protein,[120,121] and is involved in hemagglutination and viral neutralization.[53,55,86,87,128] Group- and LACV-specific epitopes are present on Gc. Gc is also required for infection of mosquito cells in vitro and in vivo.[63] The Gn glycoprotein mediates viral attachment to insect cells.[96] Whereas the M segment genome has been defined in great detail in terms of its neuroinvasiveness, that is, the ability to invade the central nervous system (CNS) from an extraneural site, through its glycoprotein products Gc and Gn, viral reassortants have implicated the L segment as a major factor in determining neurovirulence, which is the ability to cause CNS disease after direct cerebral injection.[38,132] Furthermore, studies of Gc fusion peptide mutants have shown significantly reduced replication but a persisting ability to cause neuronal death in culture, findings implicating the native Gc fusion protein as important in neuroinvasion but not necessarily in neurovirulence.[132] Finally, a viral component encoded by the S segment also seems to serve a role in pathogenesis. NSs was shown in insect and mammalian cells to inhibit the RNA interference pathway, thus interfering with a mechanism of innate immune response to viral infection. NSs has also been shown to be involved in apoptosis, the main mechanism by which LACV causes cell death.[15,131] Investigators have shown that a truncated Gc protein preparation induces a protective immune response in suckling mice through neutralizing antibody (see Prevention).[116] Apparently, neutralizing antibody can prevent neuroinvasion by interruption of transient viremia, which occurs just after virus inoculation. A study by Taylor and colleagues[139] found that the myeloid dendritic cell, an early response cell type, was critical to protect adult animals and that this cell type was reduced in young animals. Activation of the myeloid dendritic cell line during virus infection or after treatment with type 1 interferon in young animals provided protection from LACV neuroinvasion.[139] This finding may help to explain the preponderance of pediatric versus adult cases of LACVE.[138,139]

Oligonucleotide maps of LACV isolates from various areas of the United States have grouped the viruses into three types. Upper Midwest viral strains are of two types, A and B, and type C varieties are found in scattered areas of the eastern part of the United States.[45,89] Variations in strains indicate that changes in the viral genome occur by genetic drift. Genetic reassortment through exchange of RNA segments also has been demonstrated in nature; one proposed mechanism involves dually infected mosquitoes, particularly those mosquitoes with initial transovarial infection preceding superinfection with a second closely related virus.[16]

ECOLOGY

La Crosse Virus

Borucki and coworkers[17] provided an in-depth review of LACV replication in vertebrate and invertebrate hosts. *O. triseriatus*, the eastern tree hole mosquito, is the reservoir of LACV in nature and the vector for transmission of infection to humans (Fig. 190.4).[59,101,149,150] Humans do not maintain prolonged viremia and therefore are dead-end hosts. The mosquito is distributed principally in eastern hardwood deciduous forests, where it breeds in tree holes; however, it also is adapted to breeding in small artificial containers that hold rainwater, such as discarded cans, bottles, and tires. The mosquito is diurnal (i.e., it feeds actively during the day). Although these insects disperse over a wide area, fairly permanent foci of infected mosquitoes are observed in sharply delimited areas, and both isolation of virus and detection of human cases recur in established foci each summer.[9,59,88,136]

The most important mechanism for maintenance of LACV in nature is vertical (transovarial) transmission in *O. triseriatus*. The virus overwinters in infected eggs, which give rise to infected mosquito progeny the following year, thereby providing the mechanism of recurrent disease each summer in endemic areas.[107,135,150] Transovarial transmission of LACV in *O. triseriatus* is controlled by a single gene locus.[57] LACV also is maintained in nature through horizontal transmission by venereal propagation in *O. triseriatus* and through amplification of the virus in the vertebrate hosts on which vector mosquitoes feed.[107,149,150] Vector competence, related in part to the ability of the female mosquito to become infected in the first place (only female mosquitoes take blood meals), may be associated with malnutrition of the mosquito, which compromises its mesenteric barrier and allows infection to occur after the mosquito takes an LACV-infected blood meal.[57,114] The principal amplifying hosts involved in horizontal transmission are chipmunks and squirrels, specifically the eastern chipmunk, *Tamias striatus*, the gray squirrel, *Sciurus carolinensis*, and the fox squirrel, *Sciurus niger*.[91,110,156] Other wild vertebrates, such as foxes and woodchucks, may contribute to amplification. Although domestic livestock and pets are thought not to contribute to horizontal amplification of the virus, certain species do show seroconversion to California serogroup viruses, and these species may prove to be useful markers of viral presence in a given area.[52] Concern that *Aedes albopictus*, the Asian tiger mosquito, has entered the transmission cycle for LACV was heightened in 2001 when LACV-infected *A. albopictus* mosquitoes were isolated in nature in areas proximate to human cases.[7,8,34,35,51,60,75] In addition, an elevated burden of *A. albopictus* near the residence of patients with LACVE was associated significantly with LACV infection in cases versus controls.[47] This mosquito species, which was first discovered in the United States in 1985 in Houston, Texas, has since dispersed widely throughout the southeastern United States. The presence of LACV in *A. albopictus* mosquitoes in Dallas County, Texas, in the late summer of 2009 signified the possible expansion of the geographic range of LACV within this invasive mosquito species in Texas.[93] *A. albopictus* has significant further potential to expand the geographic range and frequency of transmission of LACV and possibly other California serogroup viruses. Most recently, another mosquito vector, *Aedes japonicas*, has been identified.[69,151]

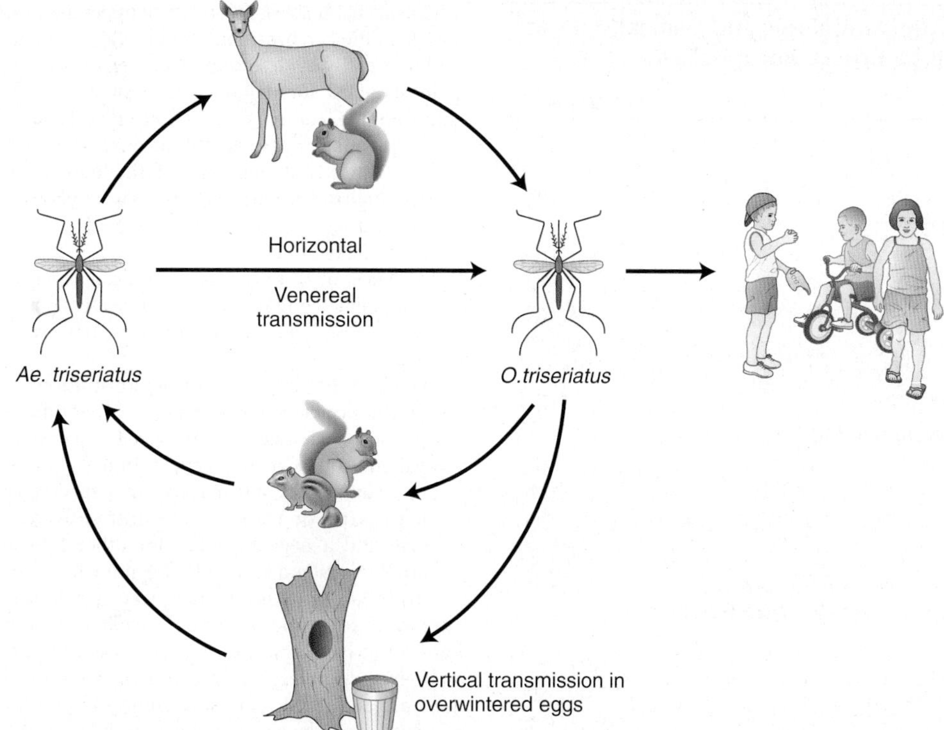

FIG. 190.4 La Crosse virus transmission cycle. The virus is maintained by vertical transmission in *Ochlerotatus triseriatus* mosquitoes; the virus overwinters in infected eggs that usually are deposited in tree holes or in artificial containers holding rainwater. Horizontal transmission by viral amplification in small vertebrates, such as squirrels and chipmunks, or by the venereal route, among adult mosquitoes, is required to supplement vertical transmission. The role of deer in viral amplification is uncertain. Human infections are incidental to the transmission cycle. (From McJunkin JE, Khan RR, Tsai TF. California–La Crosse encephalitis. *Infect Dis Clin North Am.* 1998;12:83–93.)

Other California Serogroup Viruses

A brief discussion of the ecology of other California serogroup viruses follows. Although JCV was isolated first in Colorado and is distributed widely in the West and Midwest, most cases of human illness have been reported in New York, New England, Ontario, and the upper Midwest. Seroconversion to JCV also has been found frequently (18%) in native Alaskans.[148] Various *Aedes* mosquitoes, including *Aedes communis* in the West, *Aedes stimulans* in the upper Midwest, and *Aedes abserratus* in Connecticut, function as vectors.[37,59,60,61] As opposed to LACV, for which large mammals do not play a role in viral propagation in nature, the horizontal amplification of JCV includes deer as the primary amplifying host, with up to 80% seroconversion found in adult deer populations in endemic areas.[112,113,157] The overwintering mechanism of JCV has not been elucidated, although transovarial transmission in *Aedes provocans* has been demonstrated.[14]

SSHV is distributed throughout Canada, including the Yukon and Northwest Territories, and in Russia and China. *Culiseta inornata* and various *Aedes* spp. transmit the virus to snowshoe hares *(Lepus americanus)*, ground squirrels *(Citellus undulatus)*, and other mammals. Transovarial transmission in vector mosquitoes has been demonstrated.[70]

TV is transmitted and maintained through vertical transmission by *Aedes trivittatus* in the Midwest and by *Aedes infirmatus* in the South. CEV is distributed in the western part of the United States, where *Aedes melanimon* and *Aedes dorsalis* are the principal vectors.[57,66,122,142]

INKV and TAHV cause a febrile illness typified by CNS or respiratory tract symptoms, respectively, within the same regions: Scandinavia, central Europe, and western Russia. INKV also has been found in native Alaskans,[148] whereas TAHV has additional endemicity in Asia and Africa.[58,65] Viral recombinants of these viruses have been demonstrated.[38]

EPIDEMIOLOGY

LACV-associated neuroinvasive disease occurs principally in children. From 2003 to 2012, 754 cases of neuroinvasive disease caused by LACV were reported from 204 counties in 21 states within the United States, and 88% (665, including five reported as unspecified California serogroup virus) of all cases occurred in persons younger than 18 years of age.[49] Of the 665 pediatric cases, 412 (62%) occurred in boys. The median age of patients was 7 years (range, 1 month–17 years), and 309 (46%) were 5 to 9 years of age. The average annual incidence in children (persons <18 years) reported to the CDC was 0.09 per 100,000 children per year (range, 0.053–0.151 cases).[49] LACV infections are endemic in the United States, typically occurring from July through October and mainly in rural areas of the east-central states.[84,144] In CDC data from 2003 to 2012, 544 cases (82%) of LACV-associated neuroinvasive disease in children occurred from July through September, but 8% occurred in June and October, respectively.[49] The medical and economic burden to affected persons and society in endemic areas is significant.[147] Table 190.1 summarizes demographic data and clinical characteristics for a large series of hospitalized children.[101]

The geographic distribution of LACV infection corresponds to natural divisions in which beech, oak, and maple woodlots are prevalent.[59] Although LACVE has been considered a disease of the Midwestern and mid-Atlantic states (with highly endemic zones along the upper Mississippi River Valley, specifically in Minnesota, Wisconsin, Illinois, and Iowa, and in Appalachia, particularly in Ohio and West Virginia), cases were reported in 21 states from 2004 to 2013, mostly east of the Mississippi River (see Fig. 190.2). From 2003 to 2012, the four states with the highest average annual incidence rates of LACV-associated neuroinvasive disease and 81% of cases were the following: (1) West Virginia (3.769 per 100,000 children and 146 cases); (2) Tennessee (0.628 per 100,000 children and 94 cases); (3) North Carolina (0.622 per 100,000 children and 142 cases); and (4) Ohio (0.586 per 100,000 children and 160 cases).[49] One highly endemic focus has been recognized in western North Carolina for many years,[135] and sporadic cases have been found as far south as Louisiana and as far east as Connecticut (see Fig. 190.2). Although certain foci of infection appear to remain well localized,[108,135] investigations in eastern Tennessee showed a low seroprevalence in the

TABLE 190.1 Epidemiologic and Clinical Data of 127 Children With La Crosse Encephalitis[a]

Variable	Value
Sex: No. (%)	
Male	90 (71)
Female	37 (29)
Age in Years: No. (%)	
0.5–2	9 (7)
3–5	30 (24)
6–8	42 (33)
9–11	26 (20)
12–14	19 (15)
15	1 (1)
Month of Presentation: No. (%)	
June	3 (2)
July	31 (24)
August	38 (30)
September	44 (35)
October	11 (9)
Symptoms on Presentation: No. With Findings/ Total No. (%)[b]	
Headache	105/126 (83)
Fever	107/125 (86)
Vomiting	89/127 (70)
Disorientation	50/119 (42)
Seizures[c]	58/127 (46)
Signs on Admission: No. With Finding/Total No. (%)	
Nuchal rigidity	31/120 (26)
Glasgow Coma Scale score ≤12	42/127 (33)
Focal neurologic signs	23/126 (18)

[a]For symptoms on presentation and signs on admission, data were missing for some patients. Because of rounding, not all percentages total 100.
[b]Typically, the patients with headache or fever were admitted 3 or 4 days after presentation; those with vomiting were admitted 1 or 2 days after presentation; and those with disorientation or seizures were admitted on the day of presentation.
[c]Seizures were generalized in 22 patients, partial in 24, and partial with secondary generalization in 22.
Data from McJunkin JE, de los Reyes EC, Irazuzta JE, et al. La Crosse encephalitis in children. *N Engl J Med.* 2001;344:801–807.

general population (only 0.5%) despite a recent marked increase in the number of pediatric cases in that region, a finding suggesting that true increases in the incidence of LACV infection (indicating a newly established endemic focus) do occur in some areas.[81,82] For true increases of case incidence to be detected, it may be necessary to track cases at a county level as opposed to a state level. The variability of case incidence within a state is apparent in CDC county incidence data, for which the county incidence varied from 0.2 to 228.7 cases per 100,000 persons, with both confirmed and probable cases combined (see Fig. 190.1). Therefore a wide variation results from the focal nature of the virus among counties reporting LACV infections, and this phenomenon highlights the need to report the range of incidence risk in relatively smaller zones (e.g., county) rather than only the mean incidence risk (e.g., state), which may not provide an accurate assessment of risk within focal areas.[64]

Most LACV infections are asymptomatic. Clinical disease ranges from mild illness with or without fever to severe encephalitis. For the purposes of surveillance and reporting, cases of LACV-associated clinical disease, like all cases of arboviral disease, are often categorized as either neuroinvasive (meningitis, encephalitis, or meningoencephalitis) or nonneuroinvasive. Signs of central and peripheral neurologic function are included in the clinical criteria for neuroinvasive disease. Although lower motor neuron disease such as acute flaccid paralysis is included as a part of the clinical criteria, this finding is much more pathognomonic of disease caused by WNV than LACV. LACVE is, however, associated with acute hemiparesis secondary to upper motor neuron disease. Because LACV in the cerebrospinal fluid (CSF) is difficult to isolate by culture and to identify by detection of antigen or nucleic acid, the most typical gold standard for diagnosis is serology. Confirmed cases of LACV infections are required to meet both clinical and laboratory requirements set by the CDC's case definition for arboviral disease.[21] A confirmed neuroinvasive case must meet all the following criteria:

1. Meningitis, encephalitis, acute flaccid paralysis, or other acute signs of central or peripheral neurologic dysfunction, as documented by a physician, *and*
2. Absence of a more likely clinical explanation. Other clinically compatible symptoms of arbovirus diseases include headache, myalgia, rash, arthralgia, vertigo, vomiting, paresis, and/or nuchal rigidity, *and*
3. Isolation of virus from or demonstration of specific viral antigen or nucleic acid in tissue, blood, CSF, or other body fluid; *or* fourfold or greater change in virus-specific quantitative antibody titers in paired sera; *or* virus-specific immunoglobulin M (IgM) antibodies in serum with confirmatory virus-specific neutralizing antibodies in the same or a later specimen; *or* virus-specific IgM antibodies in CSF and a negative result for other IgM antibodies in CSF for arboviruses endemic to the region where exposure occurred.[21]

A probable case is one that meets the clinical definition for neuroinvasive disease and has LACV-specific IgM antibodies in the CSF or serum but lacks convalescent titers, neutralization titers, or testing to help exclude other endemic arboviruses. The clinical case definition for nonneuroinvasive disease requires fever (chills) as reported by the patient or health care provider, as well as the absence of neuroinvasive disease and any more likely clinical explanation; the laboratory criteria are the same as for neuroinvasive disease, excluding those criteria involving the CSF or other CNS fluids or tissues. A change in the 2014 and 2015 clinical case definitions for arboviral disease from the 2011 clinical case definition is that documented fever is not required, whether for neuroinvasive or nonneuroinvasive disease, and fever is not required at all for neuroinvasive disease (reported fever or chills required for nonneuroinvasive disease).[21] It has been appreciated for some time that the absence of documented fever does not exclude LACV-associated clinical disease, and now this is formally recognized in the epidemiologic definitions of disease.

Active surveillance efforts can increase case findings markedly, as seen in West Virginia,[85] where after a child died of LACVE in 1987, more than 150 cases were diagnosed during the next 8 years (vs. only 15 cases ever previously reported in West Virginia).[103] The CDC records from 1987 to 1997 reveal that West Virginia became the most highly endemic state in the United States.[25] This trend has continued, with West Virginia highest among the states with 235 (26%) of the 895 suspected or confirmed cases of neuroinvasive California serogroup–associated neuroinvasive disease from 1999 to 2007 (see Fig. 190.1 for relative case rates by county and Fig. 190.2 for total cases of neuroinvasive disease by state, 2004–13).[124] Knowledge of the public health importance of LACVE is not complete because the virus is distributed discontinuously in the eastern part of the United States, where the disease could be endemic but underrecognized. Nevertheless, more recent use of spatial mapping techniques has increased the understanding of regional transmission patterns.[12,64,76,124,153] In addition, the high ratio of inapparent to apparent infections (see Clinical Manifestations) implies that most persons who are infected will not come to medical attention, and thus the infection will not be reported.[82] Even the presentation of symptomatic patients occurs along a continuum from fever and headache to alteration of consciousness and seizures. To improve case diagnosis and reporting to state health departments, clinicians need to cultivate an appreciation for the epidemiology of LACV, the range of clinical presentations of LACVE, and the appropriate diagnostic tests. The virus typically is not recoverable on culture of CSF and therefore requires specific serologic testing (see Laboratory and Radiologic Diagnosis).

Seroprevalence rises with age in endemic areas.[135,136] Serosurveys have shown that point prevalence rates vary in endemic locations from 30% in rural areas to 15% in urban locations.[109] Although risk appears to be highest in rural areas, many cases occur in suburban residential locations. Some patients with clinical disease have reported travel to forested recreational areas in endemic regions.[38,76,142] A case-control study performed in a highly endemic county found several characteristics of the peridomestic environment to be associated with a risk of acquiring LACVE: tree holes on the residential premise, proximity of the house to the forest edge, and the presence of artificial containers and large numbers of discarded tires.[153] A case-control study in eastern Tennessee also showed an association of LACVE with proximity (within 100 m) of tree holes to the residence, increased time that patients spent outdoors, and increased burden of *A. albopictus* in the peridomestic environment.[47] A more recent noncontrolled study in West Virginia that investigated the residences of patients with LACVE found the presence of a wooded area in 92.0% and outside containers in 70.5%.[65] The presence of standing water was observed at almost one-half of the case residences (49.4%), and most case residences (76.7%) were located within 45.6 m (149.0 feet) of a wooded area. In general, these epidemiologic data support the use of public health and spatial mapping techniques to identify hyperendemic areas where preventive efforts should be focused. National and state maps (including county-level data) from the United States Geological Survey (USGS) from 2004 to the present can be found at http://diseasemaps.usgs.gov/mapviewer/.

With regard to California serogroup viruses in the United States other than LACV, JCV seroprevalence rates of 5% to 40% have been found in the upper Midwest. In 2014, there were 11 cases of JCV disease reported from 4 states (Massachusetts, Minnesota, Tennessee, and Wisconsin), including the first case reported from Tennessee.[95] Dates of illness onset occurred from May to September, and the age distribution of patients was bimodal, with four patients younger than 18 years old and six older than 60 years. Seven patients were hospitalized, and none died. Six of the 11 patients were female. In contrast, most of the previously reported cases (21 of 29 in one series) occurred in male patients.[133] In contrast to LACV, JCV infections occur earlier, in May or June, and continue through the end of the summer. In addition, JCV is more likely to cause illness in adults than in children.[38,65] As for SSHV, human infections have been documented by serosurveys in Alaska and throughout Canada.[59] In these serosurveys, antibody prevalence rates were more than 30% in some areas; seroprevalence in the male population was twice the rate in the female population. Sporadic infection with California serogroup viruses other than LACV is likely to occur frequently in the western part of the United States.[122] However, symptomatic cases of infection with CEV occur rarely.[44]

PATHOGENESIS

LACV, which infects the salivary glands of the mosquito vector, is introduced into the host's skin and subcutaneous tissue during feeding. Probing alone is sufficient for infection. Completion of a blood meal is not necessary for transmission to occur. Local viral replication in adjacent muscle tissue leads to systemic viremia that seeds the reticuloendothelial system, muscle, and chondrocytes. This seeding results in further amplification of viremia and allows infection of vascular endothelial cells abutting the CNS.[54,55,77,79] Entrance into the CNS probably is initiated by infection of these vascular endothelial cells, which provide a route for infection of neurons and glial cells.[77,79] In a murine model, LACV probably gained direct access to the CNS through the bloodstream or olfactory neurons, or both.[13] The ability to infect mice efficiently by the intranasal route raises the possibility that LACV could use this route to infect its natural hosts. Case reports suggest that vascular involvement in human LACVE may be important in the pathogenesis of focal deficits (from stroke) and more generalized cerebral edema (possibly from vasogenic edema).[94,104] Polymerase chain reaction (PCR) studies of the location of LACV within the CNS found viral RNA within the cortex but not in other CNS tissues.[29] This finding is consistent with the results of magnetic resonance imaging (MRI) in one study that showed evidence of lesions predominantly in cortical areas.[101]

Most studies indicate that the extraneural phases of viral replication and neuroinvasiveness are mediated largely by the M segment of the genome, primarily through Gc glycoprotein, which appears to promote binding to and entry into cells.[53,54,55,120,128] A study in adult mice indicated that once the virus has gained access to the CNS, replication in CNS tissue (i.e., neurovirulence) is mediated largely by the L RNA segment, probably through the viral polymerase.[46,55] Previous work implicated the M segment in neurovirulence, but in that study neurovirulence was defined as time to death after intracutaneous inoculation.[128] The host immune response involves neutralizing antibody, which mediates viral aggregation, inhibition of viral attachment to cells, and inhibition of viral penetration and uncoating.[87] Other aspects of the immune response shown to play a role in protection against LACV infection of the CNS in animal models include $CD4^+$ T cells and MxA protein, which is induced by the interferon-α/γ system.[70,90,123,127] Susceptibility to and complications of LACVE may have an immunogenic component, as indicated by an association of illness and seizures with certain human leukocyte antigens.[22] Neuronal cell death may be mediated largely by apoptosis (programmed cell death), as determined by studies in mice,[117] and the nonstructural protein NSs has been found to promote apoptosis and to interrupt the RNAi pathway.[15,131] It is interesting that bcl-2 expression can inhibit apoptosis in certain cell lines.[117]

CLINICAL MANIFESTATIONS

The clinical spectrum of illness in LACV infections ranges from inapparent infection or mild febrile illness to aseptic meningitis and fatal encephalitis.[5,6,30,31,33,62,71,101,137,155] The ratio of inapparent to clinically apparent infection ranges from 26:1 to 322:1.[84] Most clinically apparent infections in children are associated with signs and symptoms of meningoencephalitis and occur within an average incubation period of 5 to 15 days after inoculation. Severe cases tend to mimic herpes simplex virus encephalitis (HSVE) at initial evaluation, whereas mild cases may manifest similarly to enterovirus-associated aseptic meningitis. Of the 665 cases reported from 2004 to 2012, 521 (78%) were classified as encephalitis, 134 (20%) as meningitis, and 10 (2%) as acute flaccid paralysis (see case definition in Epidemiology). All the patients with acute flaccid paralysis also had meningitis or encephalitis. Nine patients (1%) died. Of the patients with the 562 cases with available data, 543 (97%) were hospitalized.[49] In largest series of hospitalized children published in 2001, three children had the nearly lethal complication of cerebral herniation.[115] In addition, nearly one-half of all patients required admission to intensive care, and one-fourth required mechanical ventilation.[64,101,124,137]

Children typically have a 3- to 4-day prodrome of fever, headache, and vomiting; diarrhea is usually absent. The illness often progresses such that disorientation (42%) or seizures (46%) may be seen on the day of admission. Most seizures are partial or partial with secondary generalization (58%), and the remaining seizures are generalized. Status epilepticus develops in approximately one-fourth of children with seizures. Rarely, patients may have sudden onset of seizures with little or no preceding fever or headache.[101] In a more recent retrospective analysis of 47 patients younger than 18 years of age with LACV infection in western North Carolina, admission signs and symptoms included fever (43%), headache (94%), vomiting (78%), altered mental status (58%), seizures (61%), and hyponatremia (15%).[106] Three more patients (6%) developed hyponatremia during their hospital stay. A case series of LACVE in 10 adults ranging from 20 to 80 years of age found that fever, headache, and hyponatremia were common, as they are for children. Mental status changes occurred in about one-half of adults, but seizures may occur less frequently in adults (20%) than in children.[140] Neuroinvasive disease in adults is probably underrecognized and is not trivial in terms of morbidity, with prolonged acute hospital stays (average stay longer than 1 week) and nearly one-half of patients requiring discharge to rehabilitation facilities. Symptoms or diagnosis of LACV-associated disease in adults may be a sentinel to cases in children and vice versa.

On examination, signs of meningeal irritation and changes in mental status are found in approximately one-fifth to one-fourth and one- to two-thirds of patients, respectively.[101,106] Focal neurologic signs, principally focal seizures, paresis, aphasia, and abnormal reflexes, are seen in 16% to 25% of patients with LACVE. Focal and generalized seizures occur in 42% to 62% of cases, and status epilepticus develops in 10% to 15%.[30,100,101,151] Focal neurologic signs, whether found on physical examination, electroencephalographic (EEG) examination, or imaging studies, should be taken as evidence of presumptive HSVE, thus indicating the need to start empiric acyclovir until diagnostic studies have been completed.[154] Table 190.1 summarizes the clinical characteristics and demographic data of a large series of hospitalized children with LACVE.[101]

From the same study, the hospital course was complicated by the following: hyponatremia (21%), a finding generally consistent with the syndrome of inappropriate antidiuretic hormone secretion; recurrent or de novo seizures (13%); signs of increased intracranial pressure (ICP; 13%); and, rarely, cerebral herniation (2.3%).[115] Approximately one in 10 patients (including the three with herniation and 10 others with recurrent seizures, coma, or both) experienced neurologic deterioration after hospital admission, usually between 36 and 72 hours after admission. Risk factors associated with deterioration were the presence of disorientation or vomiting at admission and a trend toward seizures at admission. Neurologic deterioration appeared to be related temporally to a decrease in serum sodium concentration or an increase in body temperature, findings suggesting that these conditions may also be risk factors for in-hospital deterioration. The tendency for one in 10 hospitalized children with LACVE to deteriorate neurologically after admission represents a significant challenge for clinicians (see Treatment).

Clinical findings in patients infected with other members of the California serogroup viruses deserve brief mention. JCV infections often are associated with prodromal respiratory symptoms in conjunction with aseptic meningitis or clinical encephalitis. Among 39 patients with proven or suspected CNS infection with JCV, 10 had encephalitis, and seven reported upper respiratory symptoms or pneumonia.[59,133]

The few patients described with SSHV infection have had manifestations ranging from an influenza-like illness to aseptic meningitis or fatal encephalitis. One fatality was reported in a 14-year-old girl who had symptoms and signs that suggested Reye syndrome.[42] In a 59-year-old man, radiologic and EEG findings showed a temporal lobe focus, which led to performance of a brain biopsy and a clinical and pathologic diagnosis of herpes encephalitis, even though herpes virus was not isolated. Serologic examination later confirmed the diagnosis of SSHV infection. Mild febrile illness attributed to infection with TV has been described in some patients, and CNS infections with TV have been identified in others.[109] Three cases of symptomatic infection caused by CEV have been reported. All three patients had signs and symptoms of encephalitis.[66]

LABORATORY AND RADIOLOGIC DIAGNOSIS

Despite the lack of an effective antiviral agent for the treatment of LACV, early diagnosis of LACVE is important in guiding triage and management decisions. Initially, such a diagnosis is often probable or presumptive rather than definitive because at best a single elevated IgM or IgG antibody titer is available in the acute phase of illness, meaning that clinicians should continue to be vigilant for alternative diagnoses. In addition, when choosing diagnostic tests for encephalitis, clinicians should communicate with virology laboratory colleagues so that the limitations of these tests are understood. For example, results of viral culture of CSF is usually negative. There have been only two reports of successful growth of LACV from CSF.[98] Isolation from brain tissue has occurred on four occasions.[83,102] Improvements in the detection of LACV RNA,[28,72,92] including nucleic acid–based amplification and reverse transcription PCR, have been tested in mosquitoes and human brain tissue,[93] but clinical diagnostic capabilities with blood or CSF samples remain experimental. Therefore, at this time, serologic methods to detect LACV antibody continue to be the best method for diagnosis, with a fourfold rise between acute and convalescent titers remaining the gold standard. IgM-specific antibody to LACV can be detected reliably in serum and CSF by two methods: (1) indirect immunofluorescent antibody (IFA), which is a Food and Drug Administration (FDA)–approved test with rapid turnaround available for use by clinical laboratories; and (2) enzyme immunoassay (EIA), which is available only through the CDC and some state laboratories. The IFA assay is a two-stage "sandwich" procedure. In the first stage, the patient's serum is diluted, added to appropriate slide wells bearing the antigen, and incubated. After incubation, unbound antibodies are washed away, and then each antigen well is overlaid with fluorescein-labeled antihuman goat antibody to IgG or IgM. The slide is incubated a second time, to allow complexes of antigen and either LACV IgM or LACV IgG antibody to react with the fluorescein-labeled anti-IgG. After the slide is washed, dried, and mounted, it is examined by fluorescence microscopy. Positive reactions appear as cells exhibiting bright apple-green cytoplasmic fluorescence against a background of red negative control cells (Fig. 190.5). The cutoff for a positive IgM or IgG IFA is a titer of 1:16 or higher. One study used the standard fourfold rise in antibody titer as the gold standard for comparison to diagnosis by single acute-phase LACV titers and reported that a single elevated acute LACV IgM or LACV IgG titer by IFA has a sensitivity of 75% and a specificity of 98%.[111] The available IFA kit also provides tests for St. Louis encephalitis virus (SLEV), eastern equine encephalitis virus (EEEV), and western equine encephalitis virus (WEEV).[3] The IFA test for LACV IgM has the advantage of providing a rapid diagnosis within 24 to 48 hours, but a single titer defines only a probable case under the CDC case definition. For a probable case to become a confirmed case, it is necessary to obtain positive serum convalescent titers by either IFA or EIA (i.e., a fourfold rise) or confirmatory neutralization titers performed at the CDC, done either on a serum sample (acute or convalescent) or CSF (see Epidemiology).

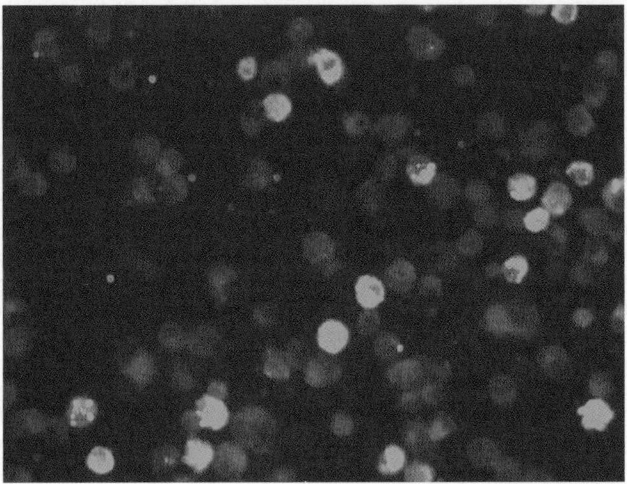

FIG. 190.5 California serogroup viruses immunofluorescent antibody. The indirect immunofluorescent antibody assay is a two-stage "sandwich" procedure. In the first stage, the patient's serum is diluted, added to appropriate slide wells bearing the La Crosse virus antigen, and incubated. After incubation, unbound antibodies are washed away, and then each antigen well is overlaid with fluorescein-labeled antibody to immunoglobulin G (IgG). The slide is incubated a second time, to allow complexes of antigen and antibody to react with the fluorescein-labeled anti-IgG. After the slide is washed, dried, and mounted, it is examined by fluorescence microscopy. Positive reactions appear as cells exhibiting bright apple-green cytoplasmic fluorescence against a background of red negative control cells. The so-called starry night pattern of stippling along the cell membrane and cytoplasm is a finding unique to the California serogroup viruses. Semiquantitative end-point titers are obtained by testing serial dilutions of positive specimens.[3,18]

IgM capture EIA is used by the CDC as a sensitive serologic test that detects virus-specific IgM in 83% to 100% of cases (see Fig. 190.5).[3,10,11,18,19,41,43] An IgG capture EIA method has been developed as well, but preliminary work suggests that it lacks reliability at this time.[80,97] The main advantage of IgM capture is that it is less operator dependent than the IFA method, which requires careful observance of visual reading criteria by experienced personnel. For this reason, IgM capture EIA is the method used by the CDC for detection of LACV IgM. Sometime in the future, the CDC may replace the EIA capture method with a microsphere immunofluorescence assay (MIA) for the concurrent detection of either IgM or IgG antibody to LACV, WNV, SLEV, WEEV, EEEV, and Powassan virus (a tick-transmitted flavivirus) (A.J. Basile, personal communication). An MIA is similar to an EIA, except that viral antigens are either directly attached to beads instead of a plate or attached indirectly by an intermediate antibody. Results are read by use of a modified flow cytometer. Relative advantages of the MIA in comparison with EIA include decreased time to test completion, improved technical ease, and decreased sample volume. Confirmatory testing of patients with a positive IgM result by IFA or EIA involves the detection of LACV-specific neutralizing antibodies by plaque reduction assay, performed by the CDC. Despite the current CDC recommendations that a probable case should be confirmed with additional testing, more recent work suggests that a single acute serologic sample tested by IFA may eventually be considered sufficient for clinical purposes if not also epidemiologic uses.[111] For more on surveillance and reporting of cases, see also the CDC case definition of arboviral disease in the Epidemiology section. Instructions for sending diagnostic specimens to the CDC Division of Vector-Borne Diseases Arbovirus Diagnostic Laboratory can be found at http://www.cdc.gov/ncezid/dvbd/specimensub/index.html. In fatal cases, nucleic acid amplification, histopathologic examination with immunohistochemistry, and virus culture of autopsy tissues can also be useful. Only a few state laboratories or other specialized laboratories, including those at CDC, are capable of doing this specialized testing.

In all diagnostic tests for LACVE, even a minimal decrease in specificity (a false-positive result) can present a key clinical dilemma, with the potential to distract clinicians from diagnosis of treatable conditions. Unfortunately, neither currently available serologic method for LACV IgM detection can guarantee 100% specificity, especially because in rare instances LACV IgM reportedly has remained elevated in serum for more than 1 year. Therefore, even in the context of positive acute titers for LACV, it may be prudent to consider continuation of empiric therapy for HSVE with intravenous acyclovir until a negative CSF PCR assay result for herpes simplex virus is obtained. Although the occurrence of false-positive test results for LACV is the major concern clinically, false-negative results may occur as well, particularly within the context of a rapidly progressive acute infection. IgM antibodies are generally first detectable at 3 to 8 days after onset of illness and usually persist for 30 to 90 days. Serum collected within 8 days of illness onset may not have detectable IgM.[21] In patients with a negative result for IgM and a clinical syndrome compatible with LACVE, it may be helpful to obtain convalescent-phase IgM and IgG titers in 1 to 2 weeks and in some cases in as little as 3 or 4 days from initial testing at clinical presentation.

Ancillary laboratory examinations for LACV infection were well outlined in one series (Table 190.2).[101] The total CSF leukocyte count was elevated only moderately (the median white blood cell [WBC] count in the CSF was 75 cells/mm^3), with a predominance of lymphocytes, and 25% of patients had sparsely elevated red blood cells in the CSF.[101] In a more recent retrospective analysis of 47 patients with probable or confirmed LACVE, the median CSF WBC count was 160/mm^3 (range, 10–1063/mm^3), with a median lymphocyte percentage of 44% (0–98%).[151] In the classic study, the 75th percentile for the CSF protein level was 45 mg/dL (normal range, 5–40 mg/dL), consistent with numerous reports in which elevated protein levels were observed in less than one-third of cases.[5,30,33,71,101] Approximately 10% of children had negative or equivocal findings on initial CSF analysis, only to have numerous WBCs in the CSF within 24 to 48 hours on repeated lumbar puncture. The peripheral WBC count was elevated (≥15,000 WBCs/mm^3) in half of the cases at admission and was frequently associated with neutrophilia, which in general may raise suspicion for bacterial meningitis or partially treated bacterial meningitis. Serum electrolyte values should be monitored for hyponatremia, which occurs frequently and has been associated with worsening clinical status in LACVE.[101]

Even though the Infectious Diseases Society of America recommends that all children and adolescents with encephalitis should have brain MRI with and without contrast enhancement, optimally with diffusion-weighted imaging, at this time most available data in children with LACVE are from computed tomography (CT) scans (see Treatment for basic recommendations on obtaining imaging in this clinical setting).[146] In 127 hospitalized children with LACVE, 92 had non–contrast-enhanced CT scans. Only 11 of these scans had abnormal findings; eight showed generalized edema, and three showed focal findings, all in supratentorial locations.[115] In three children whose courses were complicated by cerebral herniation, CT scans detected an abnormality only after the herniation event (i.e., CT scans on admission were normal). From this same series, each of 10 children had MRI of the brain; four of these children had abnormal MRI findings that showed focal areas of gadolinium enhancement, predominantly in cortical areas (Fig. 190.6).[101] Case reports of LACVE suggest that MRI may reveal lesions not detected by CT. In a 20-month-old infant with right hemiparesis, CT findings on admission were normal, but MRI on day 1 showed evidence of acute infarction of the left basal ganglia.[94] In a 12-month-old child with clinical evidence of worsening neurologic status, MRI showed areas of increased signal intensity in the periventricular white matter, even though the initial CT scan had been normal.[50]

EEG abnormalities have been found in 71% to 90% of patients tested. Focal EEG findings, usually slowing, may appear in as many as 44% of abnormal EEG tracings.[30,100,101] Periodic lateralizing epileptiform discharges (PLEDs), previously thought to be virtually pathognomonic for HSVE, also occur in LACVE. In a case series of LACVE, 8 of 90 EEG tracings were positive for PLEDs[39,101]; in four of these eight cases, patients required continuous EEG surveillance to monitor treatment of nonconvulsive status epilepticus.[101] Patients with PLEDs represent a worrisome subgroup of all patients with LACVE because they have longer, more complicated hospitalizations and are likely to have worse long-term outcomes.[40]

DIFFERENTIAL DIAGNOSIS

The principal consideration in the differential diagnosis of LACVE is HSVE.[101,130] Clinical descriptions of LACVE consistently disclose a high rate of focal neurologic findings or focal seizures, or both (~30%). The frontal and temporal lobe locations of abnormalities detected by EEG examinations (including PLEDs) and by brain imaging studies in some

TABLE 190.2 Laboratory Values at Admission in Patients With La Crosse Encephalitis

Variable	Mean Value ± SD	Range	PERCENTILE 10th	25th	50th	75th	90th	Remarks
Cerebrospinal Fluid								
White blood cell count (per mm^3)	130 ± 151	2–867	10	26	75	184	316	<200/mm^3 in most cases
Differential count (% lymphocytes)	—	2–100	10	27	62	77	90	Predominance of lymphocytes
Red blood cell count (per mm^3)	71 ± 213	0–1,500	0	1	5	20	177	Elevated (≥20/mm^3) in 25%
Glucose (mg/dL)a	75 ± 20	37–149	56	62	71	83	105	Normal
Protein (mg/dL)	37 ±± 15	10–85	20	27	34	45	56	Rarely elevated
Peripheral Blood								
White blood cell count (per mm^3)	15,700 ± 5,900	6,800–49,700	8,900	11,500	14,800	19,000	22,600	Usually elevated (>15,000/mm^3)
Differential count (% polymorphonuclear leukocytes)	—	17–94	58	66	76	82	86	Predominance of polymorphonuclear leukocytes

[a]To convert values for glucose to millimoles per liter, multiply by 0.05551.
SD, Standard deviation.
Data from McJunkin JE, de los Reyes EC, Irazuzta JE, et al. La Crosse encephalitis in children. *N Engl J Med.* 2001;344:801–807.

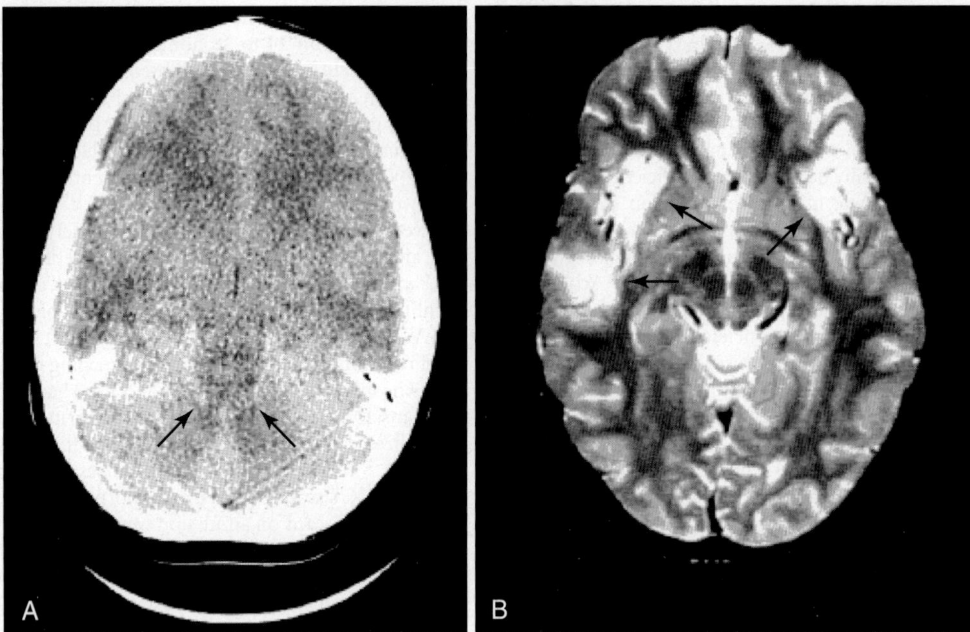

FIG. 190.6 Radiographic studies in patients with severe La Crosse encephalitis. (A) Computed tomography (CT) scan (obtained on the second hospital day) of an 8-year-old boy with severe La Crosse encephalitis complicated by uncal herniation reveals brain edema with associated obliteration of perimesencephalic cisterns *(arrows)*. (B) T2-weighted magnetic resonance image obtained in a 7-year-old boy with severe La Crosse encephalitis shows focal areas of increased signal intensity in the right temporoparietal and left frontotemporal regions *(arrows)*. A CT scan obtained at the time of uncal herniation 7 days earlier showed hypodensity in the same areas. (From McJunkin JE, de los Reyes EC, Irazuzta JE, et al. La Crosse encephalitis in children. *N Engl J Med.* 2001;344:801–807.)

cases of LACVE initially may suggest a presumptive diagnosis of HSVE.[5,101] Hemorrhagic pleocytosis, which can occur in both HSVE and LACVE, also may favor a presumptive diagnosis of and therapy for HSVE. Because delay of therapy for HSVE is associated with a poor outcome, a reasonable approach in cases of encephalitis with focal findings or severe encephalitis is to treat empirically for HSVE with intravenous acyclovir pending definitive diagnosis.[146,152]

In patients with less fulminant signs of CNS infection, enteroviral aseptic meningitis is a common consideration, especially because it often occurs with similar seasonality, in summer and early fall. The presence of rash, pharyngitis, conjunctivitis, or myocarditis is a clue to enterovirus and is not characteristic of LACV infection. In a study comparing enteroviral CNS infection with LACVE, patients with LACVE were significantly more likely to have aphasia, loss of consciousness, seizure, and admission to the pediatric intensive care unit than were patients with enteroviral CNS infection.[68]

For undervaccinated or unvaccinated persons and communities, poliomyelitis remains an important diagnostic consideration. In September 2005, a 7-month-old Amish child from Minnesota with failure to thrive, diarrhea, and recurrent infections was diagnosed with type 1 vaccine-derived poliovirus (VDPV) in the context of newly diagnosed severe combined immunodeficiency.[24] Although 8 of 23 children (including the infant) in the index community tested positive for VDPV, none had paralytic disease.[1] Mumps encephalitis is another consideration, even in the absence of parotid swelling, and low or low-normal CSF glucose levels may be a clue to this diagnosis.[93]

Patients with Rocky Mountain spotted fever may exhibit signs of CNS disturbance, and one should remember that rash may be absent in 20% of patients. *Bartonella henselae* infection (cat-scratch disease) or *Mycoplasma pneumoniae*–associated encephalopathy may be valid considerations in the differential diagnosis. Certainly, other Arboviridae should be considered, and many laboratories now test simultaneously for Arboviridae known to occur in the United States (WNV, SLEV, EEEV, and WEEV) in patients with severe seasonal (summer or fall) encephalitis. A rare and tragic consideration in a child presenting with encephalitis is rabies, which may occur in the absence of a known animal bite. Certainly, a wide array of viruses, bacteria, and even amebas and parasites can cause CNS disease. These etiologic agents are reviewed in other chapters of this text as well as in the Infectious Diseases Society of America practice guidelines for the management of encephalitis.[146]

TREATMENT

Because no specific FDA-approved antiviral treatment of LACVE is currently available, careful supportive care is the mainstay of therapy. A reasonable general supportive strategy is to assess these patients as one would assess children with closed head injury. In both instances, (1) changes in the level of consciousness cannot be assumed to be caused by a normal need to sleep and therefore require serial monitoring, and (2) changes in the level of consciousness generally are the best and earliest indicators of evolving intracranial disease, as opposed to later brainstem signs such as pupillary abnormalities or bradycardia with hypertension. Therefore, serial monitoring of the level of consciousness is the most important aspect of neurologic monitoring (i.e., use of the Glasgow Coma Scale [GCS]), even if the child has minimal changes in level of consciousness at the time of admission.

Three particularly important decision points in management depend on the presence or absence of (1) disorientation, (2) further deterioration in GCS scores, and (3) focal findings. Once the child becomes disoriented (GCS score typically <13), as shown by changes in mental status in an older child or perhaps by lack of recognition of parents in an infant, the child is monitored best in an intensive care setting. Children presenting with seizures on admission or children documented to have elevated opening pressure on lumbar puncture also deserve consideration for admission to intensive care, as do those with unremitting vomiting or headache or both despite appropriate medical care on the general pediatric ward.[101] Further deterioration in the GCS score to 8 or lower generally indicates that the patient no longer is able to protect the airway adequately, and appropriate intervention is needed. Cases suggesting HSVE because of focal findings or coma or both warrant presumptive treatment with intravenous acyclovir pending definitive diagnosis.

Many of the same strategies that apply in treating children at risk for increased ICP are used in treating children with LACVE. A reasonable approach is to perform funduscopy and to consider a non–contrast CT scan of the brain to evaluate for a mass lesion or other cause of increased ICP that would be a contraindication to lumbar puncture. When performing lumbar puncture, measure the opening pressure whenever possible. In patients with encephalitis, brain MRI with and without gadolinium contrast and with diffusion-weighted imaging is the recommended imaging modality, and this should be performed as soon as feasible. Nevertheless, practical considerations (e.g., the need to perform lumbar puncture with minimal delay and the lack of the patient's cooperation because of young age or disorientation) still often favor CT over MRI in the early phase of illness. General treatment strategies in patients at risk for increased ICP include the following: airway and (if necessary) ventilatory management designed to avoid hypercapnia; hemodynamic management to optimize mean arterial pressure (and presumably cerebral perfusion pressure); neurologic strategies to optimize control of seizures; and strategies designed to avoid hypoosmolality, hyperthermia, and other factors that may exacerbate intracranial hypertension or avoidable increases in the cerebral metabolic rate. Intubated patients should be sedated adequately and may need additional analgesia or sedation before noxious procedures such as endotracheal suctioning are performed.

In a large series of hospitalized patients with LACVE, the condition of 1 in 10 patients with LACVE deteriorated neurologically after admission. Risk factors identified to occur more often before in-hospital deterioration were the occurrence of disorientation (consistent with a GCS score ≤13), vomiting, and seizures.[101] In addition, hyponatremia and hyperthermia may be related temporally to clinical deterioration in patients with LACVE.[101] Regarding therapeutic implications of the risk for development of hyponatremia, isotonic fluids (normal saline or 5% dextrose in normal saline) should be used at maintenance rates, in addition to deficit replacement, to minimize the tendency for the development of hyponatremia while maintaining intravascular volume.[101] Serum sodium concentration should be monitored approximately every 8 hours during the acute phase of the illness. If evidence of the syndrome of inappropriate antidiuretic hormone secretion is documented and cerebral salt wasting is ruled out by careful monitoring of fluid status as well as sodium level and osmolality of the urine and serum, careful restriction of fluids may be considered. Because hyperthermia may be associated with neurologic deterioration in some patients, a low threshold for prevention or treatment of fever with antipyretics is recommended. In critically ill patients with evidence of increased ICP, methods other than antipyretics (e.g., cooling blankets) may be considered to address persistent hyperthermia, provided shivering and discomfort are controlled.

Patients with neurologic deterioration may need to have repeated EEG or brain imaging studies or both because nonconvulsive status epilepticus can occur and because the initial brain imaging results may be normal, but later imaging may show evidence of cerebral edema. Some experience has been gained in the monitoring of ICP in LACVE.[83] In one particular study, high ICP was documented in three of six patients in whom monitors were placed, and such monitoring was considered by clinicians to be a useful adjunct in these cases.[101] Establishment of clinical and imaging criteria to determine which patients could benefit from insertion of an ICP monitoring device remains a dilemma, particularly because ictal and postictal events in LACVE can confound the neurologic examination regarding possible signs of increased ICP.

No specific antiviral therapy is approved by the FDA for the treatment of LACV infection or LACVE. Although previous laboratory studies suggested the potential of ribavirin (RBV) as a therapeutic agent,[23,32,73,74,104,119,129,134] a report summarizing the largest study of antiviral treatment of LACVE documented overall poor clinical efficacy and a narrow therapeutic index.[105] This report summarized three studies of children treated with intravenous RBV during a 10-year period from 1994 to 2003, each study exploring a different phase (I, IIA, and IIB) of clinical trial development. In a group of 15 children treated in phase I and phase IIA, RBV appeared safe at moderate dosing, but on the basis of steady-state RBV levels of 9.3 μM, estimated CSF levels were less than 20% of the half-maximal effective concentration of RBV for LACV. No trends to suggest efficacy of intravenous RBV could be detected in the statistically underpowered phase IIA randomized controlled trial. At the escalated dose used in phase IIB, each of the first two enrollees experienced adverse effects (elevated serum ammonia and elevated serum pancreatic enzymes, respectively) considered likely to be related to RBV, and therefore the trial was discontinued. In view of the limitations of RBV for LACVE, it is encouraging to note a group of novel broad-spectrum RNA virus inhibitors known as the pyrazinecarboxamide derivatives: T-705 (favipiravir), T-1105, and T-1106.[48] These compounds have demonstrated good activity in treating laboratory animals with viral infections caused by various RNA viruses, including influenza virus, arenaviruses, bunyaviruses, and others. Whether these agents will prove capable of treating viral infection in the CNS, however, remains to be investigated. Most recently, research on inhibition of certain cellular enzymes called deubiquitinases, important for cellular processes such as the response to unfolded proteins in the endoplasmic reticulum, implicates this pathway as a possible target for the inhibition of replication of certain RNA viruses, including LACV.[118] Even though this finding is certainly interesting, the mechanism of inhibition of viral replication has not been elucidated. In summary, the search for antiviral treatment of LACVE remains important because of the high morbidity caused by this virus as well as its potential to increase in prevalence and severity.[51,101]

OUTCOME

LACV infections are associated with a case-fatality rate of up to 1.9%.[64] A series of hospitalized patients ($n = 127$) showed nearly lethal disease from cerebral herniation in three cases. Furthermore, in this study many patients required mechanical ventilation (25%) or intensive care (50%).[101]

In the 1960s and 1970s, psychometric evaluation of patients who had recovered from their acute LACV–associated encephalitis failed to show significant differences in standard tests of cognitive ability compared with control subjects or normative data in the general population.[100,125] In 2001, however, a study of 28 recovered patients, most of whom had severe LACVE (e.g., associated with seizures or coma, including three patients with cerebral herniation), showed a mean full-scale intelligence quotient (IQ) of 87.8 (95% confidence interval, 82.2–93.2). Thirty-five percent of these patients had an IQ lower than 80, and 46% demonstrated significant disparities between verbal and performance IQ scores. In addition, 60% of this group had test results indicative of attention deficit–hyperactivity disorder.[101] This study lacked a contemporaneous, matched control group, but certainly compared with normative data, these findings strongly suggest that neurocognitive and behavioral deficits do occur after LACVE, particularly in patients with severe disease. In addition, previous data indicating changes in performance on tests administered before and after illness suggested effects in children who were more seriously ill.[100] In another small series, visual-motor function abnormalities and intellectual impairment were observed more often in patients who had focal abnormalities during the acute illness.[100]

Of the patients who recover from LACVE, 6% to 15% have recurrent seizures.[30,36] The risk of having a recurrent convulsive disorder is approximately 25% in patients who experienced a seizure during the acute phase of illness.[36,56] The interval between the onset of recurrent seizures and recovery from acute infection ranges from a few days to years (mean, 4 years).[36] Persistent hemiparesis was a residual abnormality in two of 151 patients monitored for up to 6 years after recovery from LACVE, but one patient had a brain biopsy performed, which may have accounted for some of his neurologic deficit.[30] Unilateral infarction of the basal ganglia and hemiparesis were described in the case of an infant.[94] Another infant with a presumed LACV infection initially had an apparent neurodegenerative disease secondary to acute disseminated encephalomyelitis.[50] See the description at the beginning of this chapter for a discussion of the economic costs of LACVE.

PATHOLOGY

The original model of LACV disease in LACVE proposed that the virus first replicates in muscle cells, thus leading to viremia with subsequent hematogenous spread to the vascular endothelium and ultimately to access in the CNS.[13,78] In a more recent study, weanling mice inoculated intraperitoneally with 100 median lethal doses of LACV/human/1960 had histopathologic lesions on day 6 after inoculation in the following: (1) the brain, including olfactory bulb, cerebral cortex, thalamus, hippocampus, and medulla oblongata; and (2) the spinal cord, including perivascular cuffing, neuronal degeneration, necrosis (either single cell or small foci), and apoptosis.[13] Histopathologic changes were minimal outside the CNS. Viral antigens were not observed in the nasal turbinates, muscle, spleen, or pancreas. However, viral antigen was detected in the olfactory bulb of the brain, thalamus, cerebrum, medulla oblongata, and spinal cord. Therefore this more recent study suggests that LACV can enter the CNS through the olfactory neurons from nasal olfactory epithelium, although the virus may alternatively or additionally enter through the bloodstream and vascular endothelium.

Pathologic descriptions of two fatal cases in humans have been reported.[83] In gross appearance, the brain was swollen, and the meninges were congested. The principal brain lesions were neuronal degeneration, patchy inflammatory lesions, and vasculitis. The cerebrum and basal ganglia were the principal sites of involvement, but petechial hemorrhages and edema were noted in the spinal cord of one patient. In both cases, lesions in the cerebrum were confined to the frontal, parietal, and temporal lobes, and the cerebellum was not involved. Focal inflammatory lesions and perivascular reactions were composed primarily of mononuclear cells. Neuronolysis and neuronophagia were observed in foci of inflammation and necrosis, along with reactive polymorphonuclear, mononuclear, and microglial responses. Small extravasations of erythrocytes were seen, as were lymphocytic perivascular cuffs, but inclusion bodies were not. In one case, a focal area of necrosis, hemorrhage, and formation of a hematoma was present in the temporal lobe, a finding corresponding to a mass lesion seen on CT. From a patient in a separate case report, brain biopsy material examined by indirect immunofluorescence demonstrated LACV antigen in neurons and perhaps in endothelial cells. The same biopsy material from this patient showed minimal necrosis and perivascular cuffing on light microscopy.[102] The finding of minimal necrosis despite abnormal CT findings and deep coma is interesting in view of the relatively benign outcome of LACVE in most patients, even in those who experience deep coma or exhibit CT abnormalities. This finding is in marked contradistinction to HSVE, in which the presence of either coma or CT lesions is a poor prognostic factor, consistent with the extensive necrosis seen on pathologic examination.[152]

PREVENTION

Reduction of exposure to mosquito bites is the best method for prevention of infection by LACV or other mosquito-borne viruses. To accomplish this goal, community campaigns have emphasized using repellent, using barriers (mosquito nets, screens, or protective clothing), avoiding peak biting hours (dawn until dusk), and eliminating mosquito breeding sites. Large-scale spraying of insecticides is not an effective intervention for elimination of *O. triseriatus* because this tree-dwelling mosquito tends to be protected by the leaf canopy of its habitat. Public health prevention has focused on common-sense methods of elimination of breeding sites of *O. triseriatus*. Such efforts in endemic areas have included removal of used tires and other containers that hold small pools of water and (less commonly) sealing of tree holes with cement or gypsum wool insulation.[142] Other methods of minimizing standing water include drilling holes in tire swings so that water drains out; emptying standing water from flower pots, buckets, and barrels; replacing water in bird baths weekly; and emptying children's wading pools and storing the pools on their side after use.[93] Home public health or mosquito control program visits to patients with new cases of LACVE may identify risk factors around the home or in neighboring areas, with implications for uninfected siblings of the index case and possibly for other children in the community. Counties identified with cases may be targeted during the subsequent spring for educational town meetings or television coverage or interventions such as tire removal campaigns. Such targeted interventions have been tracked in highly endemic areas of West Virginia in recent years. The proper use of insect repellents and avoidance of tree-shaded areas during the vector's active feeding period (from dawn until dusk) may confer a reduction in risk by minimizing exposure to the vector.

Repellents are synthetic compounds or derivatives of plant oils that can be used during outdoor activities when mosquitoes are present to discourage mosquitoes from biting. The most active insect repellents for use on skin contain either *N,N*-diethyl-*m*-toluamide or *N,N*-diethyl-3-methyl-benzamide (DEET), picaridin (KBR 3023), IR3535 (3-[*N*-butyl-*N*-acetyl]-aminopropionic acid, ethyl ester), or the plant-based oil of lemon eucalyptus and its synthetic equivalent, *p*-menthane-3,8-diol.[2] Insect repellents acceptable for children may contain up to 30% DEET per recommendation of the American Academy of Pediatrics (and up to 50% DEET per recommendation of the CDC), but DEET-containing products should not be used on infants younger than 2 months. As of 2005, the American Academy of Pediatrics and the CDC revised recommendations such that repellents containing picaridin are considered an acceptable alternative to DEET.[2] Oil of lemon eucalyptus should not be used in children younger than 3 years, according to specifications of the Environmental Protection Agency. A possible advantage of DEET and permethrin is that each has been proven to repel ticks (and to kill ticks in the case of permethrin). DEET is an effective solvent and should be used with caution next to clothing because it may dissolve some plastics, rayon, spandex, or other synthetic fibers. In contrast, permethrin is a repellent and insecticide registered by the Environmental Protection Agency for use on clothing and will provide excellent protection through multiple washes. It should not be applied to skin. All products should be used as directed by the manufacturer.

The potential for development of a vaccine comes from work with a truncated Gc protein preparation that induces a protective immune response in suckling mice through generation of neutralizing antibodies.[116] Protection against neuroinvasion was achieved by interruption of transient viremia, which occurred just after inoculation of the virus. A DNA-based vaccine that encodes viral glycoproteins (Gc and Gn) also induced a protective neutralizing antibody response in mice.[115,127] Should ecologic preventive measures fail to lower disease rates in endemic areas, development of a vaccine for use in persons living in these areas may prove worthwhile.

Acknowledgments

Regarding the interpretation of diagnostic studies for LACV, the authors recognize the valuable input of Kathy Mack, Supervisor of the Virology and Immunoserology Laboratories at Nationwide Children's Hospital, and Linda Minnich, Virology Supervisor at Charleston Area Medical Center Memorial–Charleston. We also thank Marc Fischer, MD, MPH, medical officer at the CDC Division of Vector-Borne Diseases and liaison to the American Academy of Pediatrics Committee on Infectious Diseases from 2010 to 2012, for his insight into the epidemiologic investigation of arboviruses.

NEW REFERENCES SINCE THE SEVENTH EDITION

21. Centers for Disease Control and Prevention. *Case Definitions: Nationally Notifiable Conditions Infectious and Non-Infectious Case.* Atlanta: Centers for Disease Control and Prevention; 2012.
49. Gaensbauer JT, Lindsey NP, Messacar K, et al. Neuroinvasive arboviral disease in the United States: 2003 to 2012. *Pediatrics.* 2014;134:e642-e649.
69. Harris MC, Dotseth EJ, Jackson BT, et al. La Crosse virus in *Aedes japonicas japonicas* mosquitoes in the Appalachian region, United States. *Emerg Infect Dis.* 2015;21(4):646-649.
95. Lindsey NP, Lehman JA, Staples E, et al. West Nile virus and other nationally notifiable arboviral diseases—United States, 2014. *MMWR Morb Mortal Wkly Rep.* 2015;64(34):929-934.
106. Miller A, Carchman R, Long R, et al. La Crosse viral infection in hospitalized pediatric patients in western North Carolina. *Hosp Pediatr.* 2012;2:235-242.
138. Taylor KG, Peterson KE. Innate immune response to La Crosse virus infection. *J Neurovirol.* 2014;20:150-156.
139. Taylor KG, Woods TA, Winkler CW, et al. Age-dependent myeloid dendritic cell responses mediate resistance to La Crosse virus-induced neurological disease. *J Virol.* 2014;88(19):11070-11079.
140. Teleron ALA, Rose BK, Williams DM, et al. La Crosse encephalitis: an adult case series. *Am J Med.* 2016;129:881-884.
151. Westby KM, Fritzen C, Paulsen D, et al. La Crosse encephalitis virus infection in field-collected *Aedes albopictus, Aedes japonicas,* and *Aeses triseriatus* in Tennessee. *J Am Mosq Control Assoc.* 2015;31:233-241.

The full reference list for this chapter is available at ExpertConsult.com.

Other Bunyaviridae 191

191A ■ Rift Valley Fever

Gail J. Harrison

Rift Valley fever (RVF) is a severe, mosquito-borne disease that is caused by a phlebovirus of the family Bunyaviridae and affects both domestic ruminant animals and humans. Outbreaks usually occur during years of heavy rainfall. RVF is caused by a virus with selective affinity for the parenchymal cells of the liver, which undergo characteristic eosinophilic degeneration. Infection with RVF virus causes a short but severe disease in sheep and cattle and other domestic mammals. Most pregnant ewes and cows abort, and more than 90% of newborn lambs die. Case-fatality rates in older sheep and cattle are lower but nonetheless significant. People usually acquire the infection from direct contact or aerosols generated from the body fluids and tissues of animals dying of the disease and from bites of infected mosquitoes, especially during epidemics.[7,14,27] In humans, Rift Valley virus causes hepatitis, encephalitis, retinitis, and hemorrhagic fever. The public health importance of this disease in humans is emerging because outbreaks in Africa, sub-Saharan Africa, Madagascar, Saudi Arabia, Yemen, and Egypt have resulted in an increase in human fatalities, including neonatal deaths, along with miscarriages and fetal deaths in pregnant women.[1,3,5] (Fig. 191A.1). With the presence of the competent mosquito vectors in currently RVF-free countries, the wide range of animal susceptible to infection with RVF virus around the world, global changes in climate and geography, and increased animal trade and human travel, RVF may emerge as a global pathogen in the near future, potentially threatening Europe and the Americas.[12,26,29] In addition, RVF virus has been classified as a potential bioterrorist agent.[7,14]

HISTORY

RVF probably has occurred for many years in Africa and was recognized first at the beginning of the 20th century with the introduction of intensive livestock husbandry. In 1912 large numbers of newborn lambs died of an unknown disease in the Rift Valley of Kenya, and in the following year the clinical features were described. Daubney and associates[9] proved that the causal agent was a filterable virus that they suspected was transmitted by mosquitoes because animals protected by screens did not contract the disease. In 1944 the virus was isolated from mosquitoes caught in the Semliki Forest in western Uganda, and it was proved later that *Erethmapodites chrysogaster* was able to transmit the infection under experimental conditions. Between 1950 and 1974 at least 15 major epizootics of RVF occurred in livestock in various areas of sub-Saharan Africa. During 1975 an extensive epizootic of RVF took place in South Africa, with many human cases and several deaths documented.[11,12]

An extensive epizootic of RVF also occurred in lower Egypt in 1977. Hundreds of thousands of domestic animals, including cattle, buffaloes, goats, and sheep, were lost. Associated with this epizootic was the largest human epidemic of the disease ever known, in which 200,000 humans were infected and 600 died.[17] This outbreak emphasized the increasing threat of RVF to humans and domestic animals and showed that RVF virus was an important cause of hemorrhagic fever in Africa. In 1987, an epidemic of RVF occurred in Mauritania after flooding of the Senegal River basin following completion of the Diama Dam; at least 1200 human cases and 200 deaths occurred in one affected area alone. Epidemics and epizootics were reported in Madagascar in 1990,[19] in Egypt in 1993,[4] in eastern Africa in 1997 to 1998,[2] and in Yemen and Saudi Arabia in 2000. In November 2006 through January 2007 Kenya experienced an outbreak of RVF, with a total of 404 cases, 118 deaths, and a case-fatality rate of 29%. Similar to previous outbreaks, this more recent outbreak was associated with a heavy rainfall, and most cases occurred in young men, who herded and slaughtered livestock, and in young women, who likely handled uncooked animal products as they prepared meals for the family.[8] The cases in the Arabian peninsula are the first outside Africa and demonstrate the potential of RVF to spread. Based on isolation of the virus, RVF probably occurs sporadically throughout most of sub-Saharan Africa. Zinga virus, previously described as a cause of sporadic human disease in central Africa, has been shown to be a strain of RVF virus. With increase in international trade and tourist travel, as well as climate changes affecting northern Africa and southern Europe, it is likely that future outbreaks of RVF may soon affect the agricultural industry and humans in Europe, Asia, and the Americas.[7,22,25,28]

ETIOLOGIC AGENT

RVF virus is a member of the genus *Phlebovirus,* belonging to the *Bunyaviridae* family of viruses. It is a negative-stranded RNA virus, with tripartite S, M, and L segments of its RNA. It is a biosafety level 4 pathogen that is easily cultivated in Vero cells or in mice from blood and tissue specimens of infected animals and human patients. It also is classified as a category A overlap select agent by the Centers for Disease Control and Prevention.[7] The virus is destroyed by solvents such as ether and is inactivated readily by formalin; it is destroyed by heating at 56°C for 40 minutes. When stored at 4°C or −10°C, the virus loses its infectivity in approximately 3 months. The virus can be preserved indefinitely on dry ice at −70°C or in lyophilized form.

Fully formed virions are spherical and approximately 94 nm in diameter. They mature in the cytoplasm, although intranuclear inclusions occur in vivo and in cell culture. The virus multiplies readily in a variety of cell lines of animal and human origin. The virus is highly pathogenic for mice, young rats, and hamsters, and death occurs in 95% to 100% of these animals 36 to 96 hours after inoculation.

VECTORS AND EPIDEMIOLOGY

In studies in South Africa, the virus has been transmitted experimentally by a variety of mosquitoes, including *Culex theileri, Culex zombaensis, Culex neavei, Aedes juppi, Anopheles,* and *Erethmapodites quinquevittatus.* Epizootics of RVF have occurred in years of unusually heavy rains that filled natural depressions in the land (pans or dambos), thereby favoring the proliferation of flood-water mosquitoes. Studies in Kenya have shown that transovarial transmission of the virus in pan-breeding *Aedes* of the subgenus *Neomelanoconion* is the probable mechanism of virus maintenance and periodic recrudescence. Seroprevalence in humans in Kenya ranges from 2% in children to 30% in older men and women, with young men and women with reported seroprevalence of seropositivity of 13% to 18%. Risk factors for seropositivity included contact with dead animals and slaughterhouses.[22,26] *Culex pipiens* was implicated as a vector in Egypt during the 1977 to 1978 epidemic. During epizootics, domestic livestock serve as viremic, amplifying hosts in the transmission cycle. Although currently the virus is limited to Africa and the Middle East, regions in Europe and North America have mosquito genera capable of transmitting RVF virus. One seroepidemiologic study in Saudi Arabia indicated that 5% of children and adolescents were seropositive for

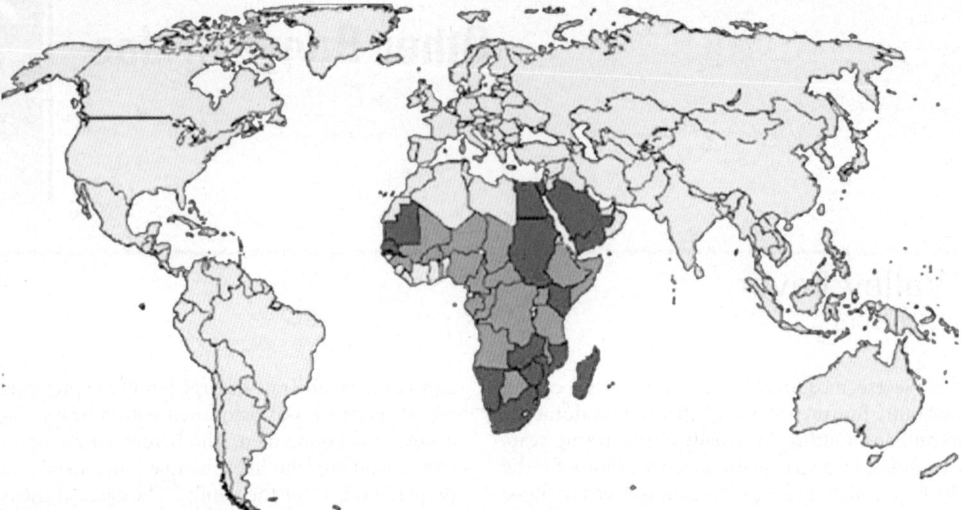

FIG. 191A.1 Rift Valley fever world distribution map. (From Centers for Disease Control and Prevention Special Pathogens Branch. Available at: http://www.cdc.gov/ncidod/dvrd/spb/mnpages/dispages/rvf/rvfmap.htm.)

RVF virus.[26] Prolonged periods of rainfall, which allow mosquito eggs to hatch, may increase chances for RVF outbreaks, and "early warning systems" using satellite measurements of sea surface temperature, rainfall, and vegetation have been used to predict human and livestock outbreaks of RVF in Africa.[7,14] In addition to arthropod-borne transmission from domestic livestock to humans by mosquitoes, RVF virus also is transmitted by aerosol and by direct contact with infected tissues from aborted livestock or carcasses of freshly slaughtered animals infected with RVF virus. Therefore persons who herd, care for, or slaughter livestock, as well as persons who prepare raw meats for cooking and consumption, are at greatest risk for RVF. Laboratory worker–acquired cases also occur. The person-to-person transmission of RVF has not been documented, but infected travelers may spread the virus to nonendemic countries, with potentially global implications for severe disease in livestock and humans.[7,14]

CLINICAL MANIFESTATIONS

Humans are very susceptible to RVF virus. During the epizootics in South Africa, most veterinarians and many farmers engaged in work with sick sheep and cattle became infected. In most cases infection was linked to direct contact with the carcasses, tissues, and organs of animals that died of RVF. Transmission probably occurred by the aerosolized body fluids of the animals. Some patients gave no history of such contact; in these cases the infection was transmitted by mosquitoes or possibly acquired by drinking infected milk. The virus can be transmitted readily to laboratory personnel by direct contact with infected animals or by the respiratory route from aerosol droplet infection. Travelers from endemic areas may also acquire RVF, so a careful travel history should be ascertained.[7,14]

The incubation period of RVF is 3 to 7 days. Infection may be asymptomatic or cause a febrile illness or fever of undetermined origin. Illness with RVF onset is sudden, with chills, myalgia, joint pain, dizziness, headache, and an influenza-like illness. A biphasic fever that lasts approximately 1 week may occur. Patients often feel nauseated and may vomit or complain of abdominal fullness and pain. The face is flushed, the conjunctivae are injected, and the tongue is furred. Icterus may develop. Bradycardia is present, and slight tenderness over the liver, which may be enlarged, can be present. Many patients become delirious, and some have hallucinations. In a small proportion (1% to 10%) of patients the infection is complicated by retinitis.[20] Late in the course of the illness or early in convalescence, unclear vision may be noted, and the patient may have a central blind spot. This visual defect is associated with a cotton-wool exudate on the macula, with permanent vision loss. Both eyes are involved occasionally, and the loss of vision from retinal lesions is a severe handicap. These lesions gradually resolve, and the patient's vision may return to normal; however, some people are left with permanent retinal scars and vision loss. Some investigators have suggested that possible immune or autoimmune factors are involved in the pathogenesis and contribute to the severity of RFV retinitis.[20]

Meningoencephalitis manifested as intense headache, confusion, and stupor may occur as a complication in less than 1% of patients during or after the second wave of fever. Lumbar puncture relieves the headache. Cerebrospinal fluid shows slight pleocytosis, mostly of lymphocytes, a normal glucose level, and a slightly increased protein content. Antibody to RVF virus also may be demonstrated in the cerebrospinal fluid. Few patients with encephalitis die. Recovery usually is complete, but convalescence may be prolonged. Occasionally, the patient is left with permanent neurologic sequelae or vision loss. Hemorrhagic fever, a complication with a case-fatality rate of 15%, develops in approximately 1% of patients with RVF. The mortality rate was disproportionately lower in children than in adults during the 1977 Egyptian epidemic. In cases of severe illness, a hemorrhagic diathesis may develop that includes epistaxis, hematemesis, melena, and, sometimes, cerebral hemorrhage. Profuse gastrointestinal hemorrhage may be fatal. Jaundice may be evident.

Infection with RVF virus in pregnant women is also associated with miscarriages and fetal deaths.[5] In addition fatal disease in the newborn associated with vertical transmission from the mother has been reported.[1,3]

The human genes *TLR3, TLR7, TLR8, MyD88, TRIF, MAVS,* and *RIG-1* have been associated with severe symptoms of RVF in humans, and this finding suggests that certain genetic polymorphisms may contribute to the severity of disease.[16]

LABORATORY FINDINGS

The patient has initial leukocytosis that is followed by leukopenia. Profound thrombocytopenia and other defects in coagulation may be observed. Disturbance in liver and kidney function also may be documented. The diagnosis of RVF is clinically suggested when humans have an acute, severe, but short febrile illness at the same time that an epizootic with high mortality is occurring in sheep.

The laboratory diagnosis usually can be confirmed by isolation of the virus in mice or cell culture from blood during the early days of illness and, in fatal cases, from the liver. Immunohistochemical study of tissues from necropsy or biopsy samples also may provide the diagnosis. Because the virus is a biosafety level 4 pathogen, virus cultivation should be attempted only in restricted laboratories. Detection using polymerase chain reaction assays also may be performed under appropriate safety precautions in specialized laboratories. Quantitative real-time polymerase chain reaction detection and quantification of RVF virus in serum appear sensitive and useful as routine diagnostic tests for identifying the virus in the early stage of the disease in individual humans, for identification of cases during outbreaks, and for follow-up of antiviral therapy.[10,24] The development of serum antibodies can be demonstrated by immunofluorescence, immunoglobulin (Ig) M enzyme-linked immunosorbent assay, hemagglutination inhibition, complement fixation, and neutralization. In patients with encephalitis, RVF virus–specific IgM and IgG antibodies are detectable in cerebrospinal fluid.

TREATMENT

Treatment is symptomatic and supportive, with appropriate isolation precautions. When a hemorrhagic diathesis develops, treatment should be directed toward controlling bleeding. Transfusions of fresh frozen plasma and platelets may be beneficial for bleeding. Convalescent-phase plasma from survivors of RVF may also provide benefit and improve survival. There is no licensed specific antiviral therapy for RVF, but effective therapeutic agents are needed because of the serious human and veterinary threat of this virus.[6] Ribavirin has activity against Bunyaviridae and is used to treat disease caused by hemorrhagic fever viruses.[7,14] In addition, treatment with amantadine, rifampicin, and dexamethasone in a patient with encephalitis was reported.[7,14]

PREVENTION

RVF is mainly a disease of adults and is usually acquired occupationally. It is a serious hazard faced by veterinarians, ranchers, and laboratory personnel in the course of their work. Because RVF usually is acquired by direct contact with the tissues of infected sheep and cattle, the risk for acquiring infection can be reduced by wearing gloves, protective masks, and goggles when postmortem examinations are carried out on animals that have died of unknown causes. Because of the value of domestic animals in many economically depressed areas of Africa, sheep and cattle often are housed within family compounds. Sick or dying animals usually are killed to salvage their meat. In this peridomestic environment, children also can be exposed to virus aerosols and readily become infected. Infection from a mosquito bite is also a mode of transmission for RVF, and for this reason the use of mosquito repellents and mosquito bed nets is recommended.

The primary strategy for preventing RVF in both humans and animals relies on vaccination of sheep and cattle, which are the amplifying hosts, and vaccination of humans in high-risk situations. Humoral immunity appears protective against RVF virus infection, but the role of cellular immunity is not clearly understood.[21] Attenuated strains of the virus have been developed and used successfully on a mass scale to immunize livestock. These attenuated vaccines are associated with some abortions in pregnant ewes and cows. An inactivated vaccine for livestock is safe and is in widespread use in Africa.[23]

A live attenuated vaccine designated MP-12 was developed by passage of RVF virus in the presence of the mutagen 5-fluorouracil.[18] The vaccine has proved safe for use in domestic livestock, does not produce abortions, and offers considerable promise as a veterinary and human vaccine. It is conditionally licensed for veterinary use in the United States.[21] More recently an attenuated strain, designated clone 13, has been investigated and shown effective in protecting sheep without any noticeable adverse effects. Another strain, designated R566, derived from both clone 13 and MP-12 through reassortment, is also under investigation.[7,13,15] Formalin-inactivated vaccine RVFV TSI-GSD-200 is being used to vaccinate military and laboratory personnel who are in contact with RVF virus.[7,8,13,15] Virus-like particles generated by reverse genetics or expression vectors, as well as DNA vaccines, are in development.

NEW REFERENCES SINCE THE SEVENTH EDITION

1. Adam I, Karsany M. Case report: Rift Valley fever with vertical transmission in a pregnant Sudanese woman. *J Med Virol.* 2008;80(5):929.
3. Arishi H, Aqeel A, Al Hazmi M. Vertical transmission of fatal Rift Valley fever in a newborn. *Ann Trop Paediatr.* 2006;26(3):251.
5. Baudin M, Jumaa A, Jomma H, et al. Association of Rift Valley fever virus infection with miscarriage in Sudanese women: a cross sectional study. *Lancet Glob Health.* 2016;4(11):e864.
6. Bird B, McElroy A. Rift Valley fever virus: unanswered questions. *Antiviral Res.* 2016;132:274.
12. Goinar A, Turell M, LeBeaurd A, et al. Predicting the mosquito species and vertebrate species involved in the theoretical transmission of Rift Valley fever virus in the United States. *PLoS Negl Trop Dis.* 2014;8(9):e3163.
16. LaBeaud A, Pfell S, Muiruri S, et al. Factors associated with severe human Rift Valley fever in Sangailu, Garissa County, Kenya. *PLoS Negl Trop Dis.* 2015;9(3):e0003548.
20. Newman-Gerhardt S, Muiruri S, Muchiri E, et al. Potential for autoimmune pathogenesis of Rift Valley fever retinitis. *Am J Trop Med Hyg.* 2013;89(3):495.
21. Nishliyama S, Lokugamage N, Ikegami T. The L, M, and S segments of Rift Valley fever virus MP-12 vaccine independently contribute to a temperature-sensitive phenotype. *J Virol.* 2016;90(7):3735.
22. Paweska J. Rift Valley fever. *Rev - Off Int Epizoot.* 2015;34(2):375.
25. Sindato C, Pfeiffer D, Karimuribo E, et al. A spatial analysis of Rift Valley fever virus seropositivity in domestic ruminants in Tanzania. *PLoS ONE.* 2015;10(7):e0131873.
26. Sow A, Faye O, Ba Y, et al. Widespread Rift Valley fever emergence in Senegal in 2013-2014. *Open Forum Infect Dis.* 2016;3(3):ofw149.
28. Tran A, Ippoliti C, Balenghien T, et al. A geographical information system-based multicriteria evaluation to map areas at risk for Rift Valley fever vector-borne transmission in Italy. *Transbound Emerg Dis.* 2013;60(suppl 2):14.
29. Xue L, Cohnstaedt L, Scott H, Scooglio C. A hierarchical network approach for modeling Rift Valley fever epidemics with applications in North America. *PLoS ONE.* 2013;8(5):e62049.

The full reference list for this chapter is available at ExpertConsult.com.

191B ■ Crimean-Congo Hemorrhagic Fever

Gail J. Harrison

Crimean-Congo hemorrhagic fever (CCHF) is a serious and potentially fatal viral illness that often has hemorrhagic manifestations.[3,32] The clinical entity as a tick-borne hemorrhagic fever and its viral origin were described first in Russia in the Crimean Peninsula by Chumakov in 1945. The agent was not propagated or available for study until 1967 and was further studied in 1969 in the Congo.[35,38,39] Since then, CCHF virus has been reported from many countries in Eastern Europe, Central Asia, and Africa.[9,35,38] The virus currently can be found in Africa, Asia, the Middle East, and Eastern Europe. During 2001, CCHF was diagnosed in patients in Kosovo, Albania, Iran, Pakistan, and South Africa. In the 21st century, outbreaks have become more frequent in the region of the former Yugoslavia, Turkey, and Iran.[24,29] In 2010, an outbreak in India was reported.[1] Exposure to ticks and contact with the blood of infected livestock or people are the usual sources of human infection. Travelers also should be evaluated for CCHF if they traveled to areas where CCHF transmission has occurred.[24]

ETIOLOGIC AGENT

CCHF virus, the etiologic agent, is a member of the genus *Nairovirus* in the family Bunyaviridae. It is lethal to newborn mice after intracerebral inoculation. CCHF virus replicates in some vertebrate cell lines, but isolation in mice is more sensitive because the virus usually does not cause any discernible cytopathic effect under fluid overlay. Thus indirect methods such as immunofluorescence or reverse-transcriptase polymerase chain reaction must be used to detect CCHF viral antigen or nucleic acid in the cells. The complete genome of CCHF viruses isolated from geographically and climate diverse areas indicates that distinct geographic lineages exist but also that these viruses are highly variable within lineages.[5,11,27,31,39]

A relatively high level of viremia develops in persons with CCHF and persists for 6 to 8 days after onset of the illness.[35] Blood from acutely ill patients with CCHF is quite infectious, and numerous nosocomial infections have occurred in hospital personnel caring for patients with this disease.[4,9,20] CCHF virus is relatively stable in blood and serum and has been recovered from specimens stored as long as 2 or 3 weeks at 4°C.

EPIDEMIOLOGY

CCHF virus is known to occur over a wide geographic area, including Eastern Europe, southern Europe, Central Asia, western China, the Middle East, India, and Africa (Fig. 191B.1).[1,5,9,11,27,39] The global distribution of CHFF virus appears to be migrating and expanding. Because it is expected that future outbreaks may extend to new areas, increased surveillance and geographic mapping of this potentially lethal viral infection are needed. Most cases of the disease probably are unrecognized because of its sporadic occurrence and largely rural distribution or its occurrence in developing countries. It is often considered an occupational disease of health care workers and persons who work with or around animals. Travelers also may acquire CCHF and are at risk to import the infection.[24] It also is considered a possible bioterrorism agent.[39,40]

The epidemiology of CCHF is complex and not fully understood because of the variety of tick and mammalian species that have been found to be naturally infected with the virus.[38] The *Hyalomma* spp. ticks have been incriminated in transmission of CCHF virus in the field, but the role of other ticks in transmission is also possible.[5] The basic transmission cycle of CCHF virus varies from region to region, depending on the developmental stage and species of ticks involved and their preferred mammalian hosts.[38] In addition, transovarial and transstadial transmissions of CCHF virus also have been demonstrated in some tick vectors. In general, human cases of CCHF usually are associated with periods of tick abundance and feeding activity.[9] For example, in Eastern Europe, cases of CCHF typically occur between May and August, when the tick population is active. Models of global warming climate scenarios project that the northern limit of the tick range may increase and change the distribution of the disease.[5,11] Humans usually acquire CCHF from a tick bite or from contact with blood or other tissues of infected livestock.[9,35,38] Most patients have a history of contact with large domestic animals (farmers, abattoir workers, and veterinarians). Health care workers are another high-risk group.

Numerous CCHF health care–associated outbreaks have occurred in hospital workers and laboratory technicians.[4,9,20,39] These persons usually have had direct contact with the blood of patients with CCHF. The mortality rate reported in secondary cases has been high, particularly in persons with needle-stick injury or those involved in management of patients with gastrointestinal bleeding.[9]

PATHOGENESIS

The pathogenesis of CCHF is not well understood, but the available evidence suggests that endothelial damage and dysfunction play important roles in the hemostatic failure.[9,20,36] Excessive proinflammatory cytokine production, cytokine storm, and dysfunction of the innate immune response also appear to contribute to the disease process. Lymphocyte depletion also seems to occur.[2] CCHF sometimes leads to reactive hemophagocytic histiocytosis in children.[7,26] Fluorescent antibody studies on organs in fatal cases of CCHF show a concentration of viral antigen in the reticuloendothelial cells of the liver and spleen, a finding suggesting that these cells are major sites of virus replication.[36] Other pathologic

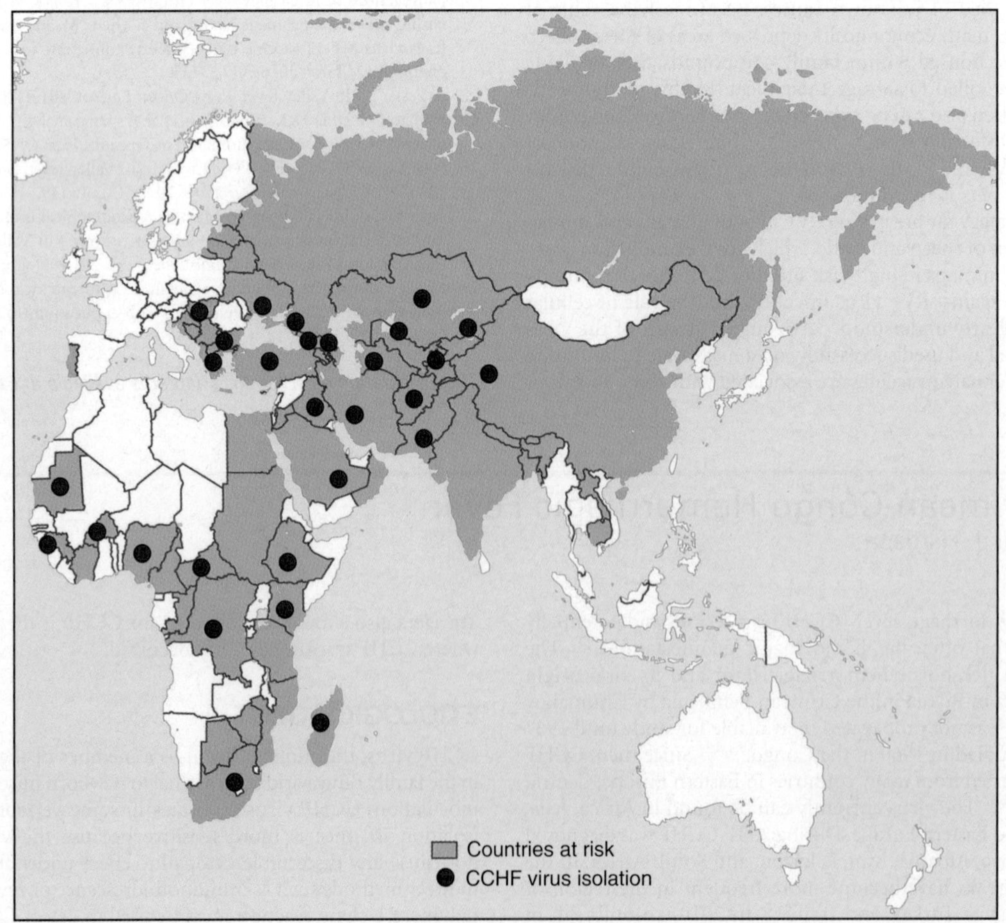

FIG. 191B.1 Known distribution of Crimean-Congo hemorrhagic fever *(CCHF)* virus in the world. (From Ergonul O. Crimean-Congo hemorrhagic fever. *Lancet Infect Dis.* 2006;6:203–14.)

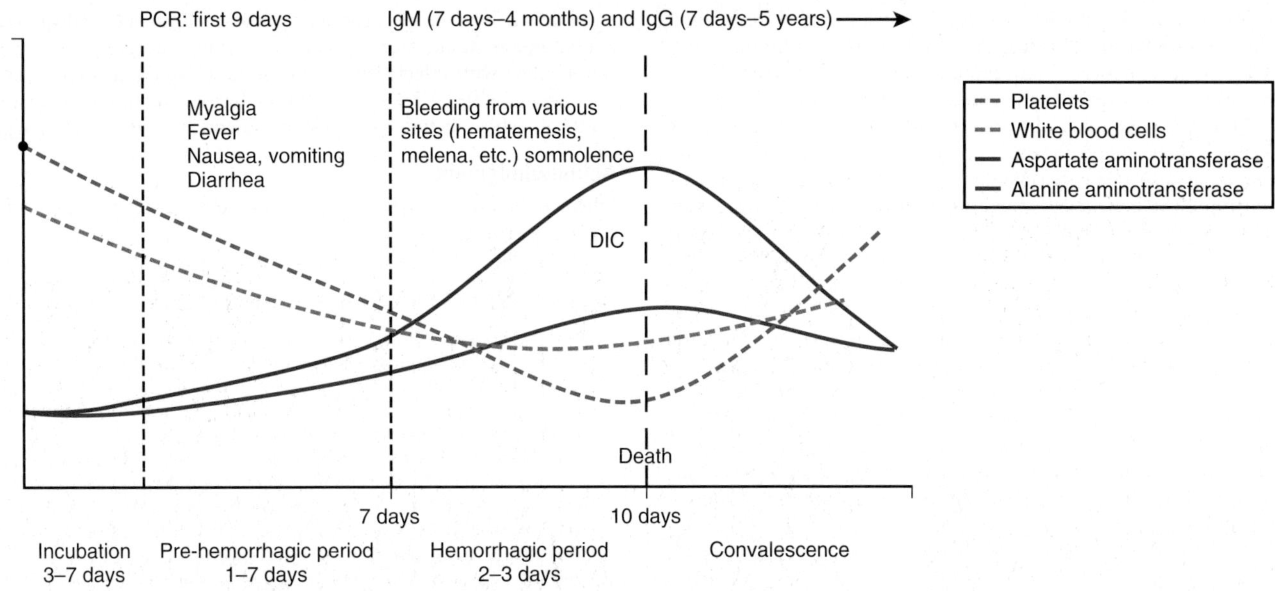

FIG. 191B.2 Clinical and laboratory course of Crimean-Congo hemorrhagic fever. *DIC,* Disseminated intravascular coagulation; *IgM,* immunoglobulin M; *PCR,* polymerase chain reaction. (From Ergonul O. Crimean-Congo hemorrhagic fever. *Lancet Infect Dis.* 2006;6:203–14.)

changes observed at autopsy include generalized vascular lesions with endothelial damage that give rise to scattered focal hemorrhage and edema in most organs.[9] In severe cases, dysfunction of the coagulation system and disseminated intravascular coagulation appear to be prominent features of the disease.

CLINICAL MANIFESTATIONS

The course of CCHF infection typically has four distinct phases: incubation, prehemorrhagic, hemorrhagic, and convalescent (Fig. 191B.2).[9,8,36] The incubation period generally is 3 to 7 days. The prehemorrhagic phase begins suddenly with fever (39–41°C [102.2–105.8°F]), nausea, diarrhea, vomiting, myalgia, rash, and general toxemia. Patients usually are flushed, with red eyes associated with conjunctival and scleral injection. Children commonly have pharyngitis and tonsillitis as presenting signs.[37] Hepatosplenomegaly with hepatitis commonly occurs in as many as 30% of cases. Thrombocytopenia also occurs. This second phase lasts approximately 3 days (range, 1–7 days). The hemorrhagic phase usually begins between the third and fifth days of the disease and lasts only 2 to 3 days. The appearance is sudden and can vary from petechiae to large hematomas on the skin and mucous membranes. Profuse bleeding from the nose, gums, gastrointestinal and genitourinary tracts, and lungs can occur at this stage, resulting in tachycardia, shock, and, sometimes, death. Not infrequently, intraabdominal bleeding occurs during this third phase and causes acute pain; some of these patients are subjected to surgery because of suspected appendicitis or intestinal perforation. Hemorrhagic pleural effusions and cardiac manifestations may occur.[14,16,33] Bradycardia may also occur and often is reversible.[14,16,30] Fatality is higher in patients with diarrhea, melena, hematemesis, hematuria, and confusion at presentation.[18] If the patient survives the hemorrhagic phase, convalescence begins about the 10th day, with a slow convalescent period lasting 2 to 6 weeks.[9] Viremia is intense and prolonged in CCHF, especially in fatal cases, so blood from these patients should be treated with extreme care.

Pregnant women who acquire CCHF may transmit the infection to their fetus. Infection in the first trimester may result in miscarriage. Infections in pregnancy later in gestation may result in normal newborn delivery.[6,13]

Leukopenia and thrombocytopenia are consistent features of CCHF and occur early in the disease.[9,8,18] Other abnormal laboratory findings usually include elevated levels of serum aspartate and alanine aminotransferase, lactate dehydrogenase, bilirubin, creatinine, and urea. Fatality is associated with higher levels of aspartate aminotransferase, alanine aminotransferase, and C-reactive protein levels and with prolonged coagulation tests such as prothrombin time and activated prothrombin time.[18] Fibrinogen may be decreased, and fibrin degradation products may be increased. These laboratory values generally return to normal levels with the onset of convalescence.

DIAGNOSIS

A clinical diagnosis of CCHF is difficult to establish before the onset of hemorrhagic manifestations because the initial symptoms are nonspecific, and cases usually occur sporadically. The differential diagnosis of CCHF in children includes viral upper respiratory tract infections, brucellosis, periodic fever syndrome, and cellulitis associated with the tick bite.[21] As a result of the frequency and severity of the abdominal pain associated with the prehemorrhagic and hemorrhagic phases of CCHF, the disease sometimes is misdiagnosed as appendicitis or gastric ulcer. Such patients may be subjected to unnecessary surgery, which can be fatal to both the patient and the attending medical personnel.[4,9,35] Once hemorrhagic manifestations appear, the differential diagnosis should include erythema multiforme (Stevens-Johnson syndrome), leptospirosis, hemorrhagic fever with renal syndrome, Ebola virus infection, Lassa fever, Rift Valley fever, Q fever, and yellow fever, depending on the region of the world where the patient was exposed. Unusual complications of CCHF include hemorrhagic pleural effusions, and myocarditis.[30]

A definitive diagnosis of CCHF can be made by isolating the virus from the patient's serum or by detecting viral nucleic acids by polymerase chain reaction during the first week of illness[34] Molecular methods for diagnosis are being applied by many laboratories in endemic areas for accurate and timely diagnosis. However, performance of these molecular methods may vary depending on method used, type of CCHF virus strain tested, and the concentration of the virus in the sample.[10] Immunoglobulin (Ig) G and IgM antibodies do not appear until 7 to 10 days after the onset of symptoms in nonfatal cases.[35,36] Establishing the diagnosis early is critical for proper management of the patient and prevention of potential transmission to health care workers caring for the patient.

TREATMENT

Treatment of CCHF is largely supportive and should include immediate hospitalization and strict bed rest.[9,35] High mortality rates (average, 30%) have been reported. Because death usually results from acute blood loss and shock, patients may require transfusions of fresh blood, platelets, or plasma (or all three). Administration of immune plasma or CCHF-negative hyperimmune globulin obtained from convalescent donors can be used early in the course of the illness or for persons, such as hospital personnel, who are exposed to the virus inadvertently, especially if they reside in endemic areas.[7,26,39] Therapeutic plasma exchange has also been successfully performed in selected patients. Ribavirin may be beneficial for treatment of CCHF, even in pregnant women, and especially if treatment is begun within the first 4 days of illness, and it is recommended by the World Health Organization.[6,9,8,12,13] The mechanism of action is unknown. Ribavirin also has been shown to protect mice from lethal CCHF virus challenge.[19,25,26] A World Health Organization report recommended intravenous ribavirin treatment for 10 days, with 30 mg/kg as an initial loading dose, then 15 mg/kg every 6 hours for 4 days, and then 7.5 mg/kg every 8 hours for 6 days.[9,12,19,25] Oral ribavirin also has been reported to have potential benefit.[12,19,25] In patients with CCHF associated with reactive hemophagocytic histiocytosis, administration of high-dose methylprednisolone, 5 to 30 mg/kg per day, fresh frozen plasma, and intravenous immunoglobulin has been shown possibly to be effective.[7]

PROGNOSIS

The mortality rate for CCHF has been estimated at 30%, but estimates have varied from 15% to 70%.[9,35,38] These figures may be high because milder cases of the disease may not be recognized or reported. The illness associated with CCHF in children may be milder and less often fatal than the illness in adults. Factors predictive of fatality include clinical signs of melena, hemorrhage, and confusion, and laboratory findings of elevated transferase levels, elevated C-reactive protein value, elevated procalcitonin levels, CCHF viral load in serum, and high concentrations of interkeukin-6 and tumor necrosis factor-α, as well as lack of virus-specific IgG humoral response and the presence of prolonged coagulation factors.[17,18,22] These factors may help clinicians in countries with limited resources decide which patients may benefit from care in a tertiary care center. If the patient survives the hemorrhagic phase of the disease, recovery is complete, and permanent immunity results. Survivors may experience posttraumatic stress disorder, especially if they were critically ill and required care in an intensive care unit.[15]

PREVENTION

No vaccine of proven safety or efficacy for prevention of CCHF is licensed. However, an inactivated, suckling mouse brain–derived Bulgarian CCHF vaccine has been shown to produce anti–CCHF-specific T-cell activity and high levels of CCHF-specific antibodies.[23,28] Personal protective measures, including insect repellents containing diethyltoluamide (DEET), are recommended for people living or working in heavily tick-infested areas. People exposed occupationally to potentially infected animal blood should wear protective clothing and gloves to prevent skin contact with infected tissue or blood. Hospital personnel caring for patients with CCHF should follow barrier nursing and isolation protocols, which include use of gloves, gowns, face shields, and goggles.

Acknowledgment

I thank Robert B. Tesh for his contributions to this chapter in the previous editions of this text.

NEW REFERENCES SINCE THE SEVENTH EDITION

3. Bente D, Forrester N, Watts D, et al. Crimean-Congo hemorrhagic fever: history, epidemiology, pathogenesis, clinical syndrome and genetic diversity. *Antiviral Res*. 2013;100(1):159.
6. Dizbay M, Aktas F, Gaygisiz U, et al. Crimean-Congo hemorrhagic fever treated with ribavirin in a pregnant woman. *J Infect*. 2009;59(4):281.
13. Gozel M, Eladi N, Engin A, et al. Favorable outcomes for both mother and baby are possible in pregnant women with Crimean-Congo hemorrhagic fever disease: a case series and literature review. *Gynecol Obstet Invest*. 2014;77(4):266.
14. Guihan B, Kanik-Yuksek S, Cetin I, et al. Myocarditis in a child with Crimean-Congo hemorrhagic fever. *Vector Borne Zoonotic Dis*. 2015;15(9):565.
15. Gul I, Kaya A, Guven A, et al. Cardiac findings in children with Crimean Congo hemorrhagic fever. *Med Sci Monit*. 2011;17(8):CR457.
16. Gul S, Ozturk D, Kisa U, et al. Procalcitonin level and its predictive effect on mortality in Crimean-Congo hemorrhagic fever patients. *Jpn J Infect Dis*. 2015;68(6):511.
21. Kara S, Kara D, Fettah A. Various clinical conditions can mimic Crimean-Congo hemorrhagic fever in pediatric patients in endemic regions. *J Infect Public Health*. 2016;9(5):626.
22. Kaya S, Eladi N, Kubar A, et al. Sequential determination of serum viral titers, virus-specific IgG antibodies, and TNF-alpha, IL-6, IL-10, and INF-gamma levels in patients with Crimean-Congo hemorrhagic fever. *BMC Infect Dis*. 2014;14:416.
24. Leblebicioglu H, Ozaras R, Fletcher T, et al. Crimean-Congo haemorrhagic fever in travellers: A systematic review. *Travel Med Infect Dis*. 2016;14(2):73.
29. Nurmakhanov T, Sansyzbaev Y, Atshabar B, et al. Crimean-Congo haemorrhagic fever virus in Kazakhstan (1948-2013). *In J Infect Dis*. 2015;38:19.
30. Oflaz M, Kucukdurmaz Z, Guven A, et al. Bradycardia seen in children with Crimean-Congo hemorrhagic fever. *Vector Borne Zoonotic Dis*. 2013; 13(11):807.
32. Peyrefitte C, Marianneau P, Tordo N, Bouloy M. Crimean-Congo haemorrhagic fever. *Rev - Off Int Epizoot*. 2015;34(2):391.
33. Sahin I, Guven A, Kaya A, et al. A child with an unusual complication of Crimean-Congo hemorrhagic fever: hemorrhagic pleural effusion. *J Vector Borne Dis*. 2016;53(1):87.
34. Shayan S, Bokaean M, Shahrivar M, Chinikar S. Crimean-Congo hemorrhagic fever. *Lab Med*. 2015;46(3):180.
37. Tezer H, Sucakil I, Sayli T, et al. Crimean Congo hemorrhagic fever in children. *J Clin Virol*. 2010;48(3):184.
40. Yadav P, Patil D, Shete A, et al. Nosocomial infection of CCHF among health care workers in Rajasthan, India. *BMC Infect Dis*. 2016;16(1):624.

The full reference list for this chapter is available at ExpertConsult.com.

191C ▪ Phlebotomus Fever (Sandfly Fever)

Gail J. Harrison

Phlebotomus fever is an acute, self-limited febrile illness of 2 to 4 days' duration that usually is acquired from the bite of infected phlebotomine sandflies. Phlebotomus fever also is known as sandfly fever, pappataci fever, and 3-day fever. Sandflies have sporadically been in Central Europe since the Holocene climate optima (c. 4500 BC). The disease is currently endemic in many areas of Central Asia, northern Africa, and southern Europe. Global warming is predicted to extend the distribution of sandfly fever into Central Europe.[1,14] Both historically and currently, phlebotomus fever has been largely of military interest because the introduction of large numbers of susceptible troops into endemic areas often has resulted in epidemics of the disease.[5,11] More recently, the disease has been reported with increasing frequency in civilian populations and in tourists visiting endemic areas. An outbreak of sandfly fever virus has been reported in Turkey.[12] Sandfly fever virus infection imported from Malta into Switzerland by travelers also has been reported.[20]

In 1909, Doerr and associates first demonstrated that the causative agent of the illness was a virus transmitted by *Phlebotomus papatasi*. In 1954, Sabin successfully adapted the agent to mice and described two distinct serologic types, designated the Naples and Sicilian strains.[22,23] Subsequently, 44 additional serotypes were isolated from various regions of the world; all these agents are included in the genus *Phlebovirus*, family Bunyaviridae. Although most of the phleboviruses probably are capable of producing human illness, the discussion here is limited to the three (Naples, Sicilian, and Toscana) that are associated most commonly with human illness. Rift Valley fever virus, which causes a severe disease acquired from the bite of infected mosquitoes or aerosol, and Toscana virus, a phlebovirus that causes meningoencephalitis, also are members of this genus and frequently cause a phlebotomus fever–like illness in infected persons. In addition, Saddaguia virus and sandfly fever Sicilian virus and Utique virus also are phleboviruses found in association with sand flies.[9,13] Some of these diseases are covered in more detail in other chapters.[4,7,17,21]

ETIOLOGIC AGENT

The phleboviruses are RNA-containing viruses, spherical, and 90 to 100 nm in diameter.[22] The Naples, Sicilian, and Toscana viruses produce a cytopathic effect, as well as plaques in Vero cells. A novel sandfly fever virus variant of the Sicilian virus, termed sandfly fever Turkey virus, has been identified by consensus polymerase chain reaction and sequencing methodology.[12] Most laboratory animals are not susceptible to infection with these viruses, although the viruses usually can be adapted to newborn mice by serial passage intracerebrally. For this reason, tissue culture is recommended for primary isolation of these agents, and molecular detection using real-time reverse-transcriptase polymerase chain reaction is useful for rapid detection and characterization.[12,16]

EPIDEMIOLOGY

The geographic distribution of the Naples and Sicilian virus types in the Old World closely parallels that of their presumed vector, *P. papatasi* (Fig. 191C.1).[22] Toscana virus has been isolated in Portugal, Spain, France, Italy, Greece, Croatia, Turkey, Corsica, Malta, and Cyprus and has been associated with two other peridomestic sandfly species, *Phlebotomus perniciosus* and *Phlebotomus perfiliewi*.[3,7,6,13,22]

These phlebotomine species are tiny, sand-colored, biting flies that are 2 to 3 mm long. Because of their small size, they have little difficulty squeezing through ordinary screens and mosquito netting. They usually are nocturnal, and only the female bites. Sandflies move in short hops and usually do not travel more than a few hundred meters from their resting and breeding sites. During the day, peridomestic species such as *P. papatasi* and *P. perniciosus* rest in dark corners and crevices, often within houses. The larvae develop in loose soil and organic debris in stone walls, animal sheds, privies, open wells, and gardens. Because of their indoor habits, these peridomestic species are quite vulnerable to residual insecticides.

In Central Asia and the Mediterranean region, sandflies are active during the late spring and summer. The incidence of phlebotomus fever follows the same seasonal pattern. Global warming patterns are predicted to alter the epidemiology of sandfly fever in the future.[1,14]

Many phlebotomus fever viruses appear to be maintained in the sandfly population by transovarial (vertical) transmission.[22] Thus sandflies appear to serve as both vectors and reservoirs of these viruses. Unlike most other arboviruses, whose activity depends on the presence of susceptible and viremic vertebrate hosts, phlebotomus fever viruses are probably active continuously during each sandfly season, regardless of the immune status of the local human population. Serologic studies of persons living in endemic areas of the disease indicate that most of the residents are infected early in life.[22,23] In these communities, sporadic cases of phlebotomus fever occur in children because most of the adult population is already immune. However, because of the benign nature of the disease, its sporadic occurrence, and its similarity to many other viral diseases of childhood, most cases are unrecognized. When large numbers of susceptible persons (e.g., soldiers, tourists, refugees) enter an area where phlebotomus fever is endemic, however, bite transmission occurs, and an epidemic of the disease quickly ensues.[10,22]

CLINICAL MANIFESTATIONS

The incubation period for phlebotomus fever averages 3 to 5 days.[2,22] The influenza-like illness begins suddenly with fever, severe frontal headache, retroorbital pain, red eyes from conjunctival injection, photophobia, malaise, anorexia, nausea, vomiting, myalgia, and lower back pain.[18] The face may be flushed, but a true rash is absent. The disease is self-limited, and symptoms usually disappear within 1 to 3 days; however, a general feeling of weakness and depression often occurs for a week or more after the illness.[18,19]

Meningitis and meningoencephalitis with Toscana virus infection have been described with increasing frequency in southern Europe.[2,4,7,6] In addition to the classic symptoms of phlebotomus fever, these patients exhibit nuchal rigidity, a positive Kernig sign, a clouded sensorium, and, occasionally, nystagmus and tremor. To date, no deaths have been recorded. Childhood cases of the meningoencephalitic form of Toscana virus infection have been reported,[2] but this form of the infection occurs more commonly in adults.

One attack of phlebotomus fever usually confers lifelong immunity against the infecting virus type but not against heterologous serotypes.[11] For this reason, second cases of the disease have been reported in the same person in areas where two or more virus serotypes are active.

Marked leukopenia usually is observed in patients with phlebotomus fever.[1] It is characterized by initial lymphopenia, followed by protracted neutropenia (Fig. 191C.2). In patients with central nervous system involvement, pleocytosis and an elevated protein content are observed in the cerebrospinal fluid.

PATHOLOGY

Fatalities caused by phlebotomus fever have not been reported, and little is known of the pathologic changes produced by these viruses.

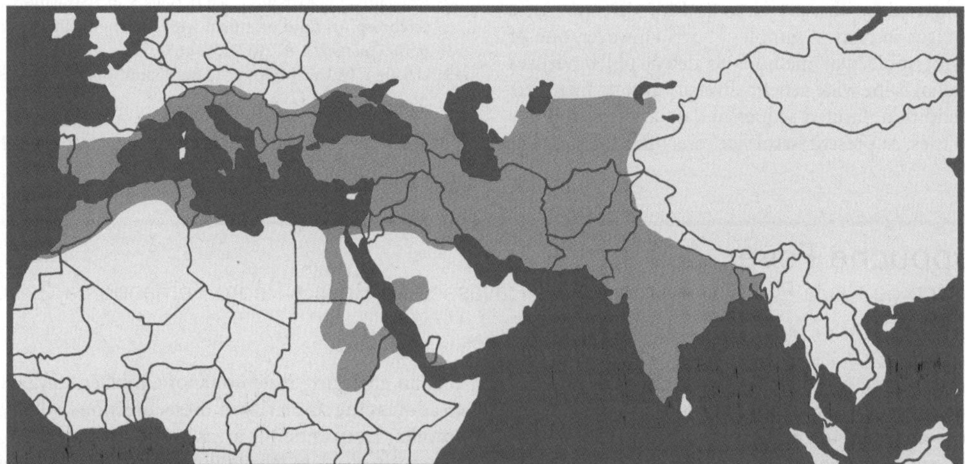

FIG. 191C.1 **The known geographic distribution of *Phlebotomus papatasi*, the presumed vector of sandfly fever (Naples and Sicilian types), in Central Asia, the Mediterranean region, and adjacent areas of Africa.** (Modified from Tesh RB, Saidi S, Gajdamovic SJ, et al. Serological studies on the epidemiology of sandfly fever in the Old World. *Bull World Health Organ.* 1976;54:663–674.)

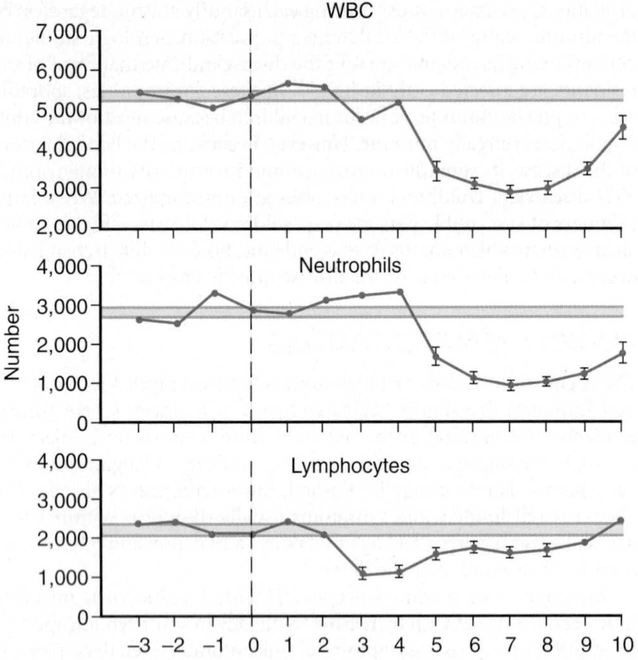

FIG. 191C.2 Mean total white blood cell *(WBC)* count as well as absolute neutrophil and lymphocyte counts in 11 adult volunteers inoculated (day 0) with the Sicilian strain of sandfly fever virus. The average incubation period in the subjects was approximately 70 hours. (Modified from Bartelloni PJ, Tesh RB. Clinical and serologic responses of volunteers infected with phlebotomus fever virus [Sicilian type]. *Am J Trop Med Hyg.* 1976;25:456–462.)

DIAGNOSIS

The diagnosis of phlebotomus fever often can be made on the basis of clinical and epidemiologic evidence. A sudden outbreak during the summer months of a short febrile illness with severe headache and marked leukopenia in visitors or other newcomers to an endemic area where sandflies are abundant should suggest the disease. Depending on the region, the differential diagnosis may include dengue, West Nile fever, malaria, influenza, and numerous other respiratory tract and enteroviral infections.

Transient (24–36 hours), low-level viremia occurs during this illness; therefore, isolation of the virus from blood is unusual. In a few instances, Toscana virus has been isolated directly from the cerebrospinal fluid of persons with central nervous system symptoms.[4] Molecular techniques (reverse-transcriptase polymerase chain reaction) have been described for direct detection of Toscana and Sicilian virus and clinical diagnosis of aseptic meningitis caused by Toscana virus and for detection of a novel Turkey variant virus in clinical samples.[7,12,16,18] However, one of the problems with using molecular methods to detect phleboviruses directly in clinical material is the wide genetic diversity among members of each serotype. In addition, limited sequence data are available for many of the phleboviruses. At present, serologic tests offer the simplest method for establishing a specific diagnosis of phlebotomus fever. Antibodies are present in serum 7 to 14 days after infection and can be demonstrated by immunofluorescence,[2] enzyme immunoassay,[11] or neutralization testing.[2] A fourfold rise in antibody titer from acute to convalescent sera or the presence of specific immunoglobulin M antibodies provides presumptive evidence of a recent phlebotomus fever virus infection. At present, these serologic tests are not generally available and usually are performed in only a few arbovirus laboratories.

TREATMENT

There is no licensed specific antiviral treatment available for sandfly fever. However, ribavirin inhibits a late step of the virus replicative cycle and, when combined with interferon-α, has shown a synergistic antiviral effect.[8] In addition, the pyrazine carboxamide derivatives T-705 (favipiravir), T-1105, and T-1106, which are compounds with broad activity against RNA viruses, for treatment of phlebovirus infections, have been evaluated.[15] Treatment is symptomatic, currently, and hospitalization usually is not necessary, except in patients with more severe cases of Toscana virus infection. Occasionally, pain relievers are required to relieve the severe headache associated with the disease.

PROGNOSIS

Phlebotomus fever is a self-limited, nonfatal illness. Recovery is complete.

PREVENTION

Control measures are directed primarily against the vector. Household spraying with residual insecticides is quite effective in reducing peridomestic sandfly vectors and controlling the disease. The use of personal insect repellents (e.g., diethyltoluamide) and fine-mesh bed nets is also effective in avoiding sandfly bites.

Acknowledgment

I thank Robert B. Tesh for his contributions to this chapter in the previous editions of this text.

NEW REFERENCES SINCE THE SEVENTH EDITION

3. Bichaud L, Izri A, de Lamballerie X, et al. First detection of Toscana virus in Corsica, France. *Clin Microbiol Infect.* 2014;20(2):O0101.
6. Charrel R, Bichaud L, de Lamballerie X. Emerence of Toscana virus in the Mediterranean area. *World J Virol.* 2012;1(5):135.
9. Dachaoul K, Fares W, Bichaud L, et al. Phleboviruses associated with sandflies in arid bio-geographical areas of Central Tunisia. *Acta Trop.* 2016;158:13.
13. Fares W, Charrel R, Dachraoui K, et al. Infection of sandflies collected from different bio-geographical areas of Tunisia with phleboviruses. *Acta Trop.* 2015;14:1.
18. Nougairede A, Bichaud L, Thiberville S, et al. Isolation of Toscana virus from the cerebrospinal fluid of a man with meningitis in Marseille, France, 2010. *Vector Borne Zoonotic Dis.* 2013;13(9):685.
19. Ozkale Y, Ozkale M, Kiper P, et al. Sandfly fever: two case reports. *Turk Paediatri Ars.* 2016;51(2):110.

The full reference list for this chapter is available at ExpertConsult.com.

191D ■ Oropouche Fever

Francisco de Paula Pinheiro • Amelia P.A. Travassos da Rosa • Pedro Fernando da C. Vasconcelos • Gail J. Harrison

Oropouche (ORO) fever is currently only in Central or South America and is one of the most important arbvoviral infections in the Brazilian Amazon. ORO fever is an emerging arbovirus infection that causes sporadic outbreaks in Central and South America that are characterized by an acute febrile illness accompanied by headache, myalgia, arthralgia, and other systemic symptoms.[13,23,35] The symptoms of ORO fever overlap with several other emerging arboviral-like illnesses, such as dengue, chikungunya, West Nile virus, and Mayaro virus, a finding suggesting that an emerging mnemonic of ChikDenMayZikOrov should be used to address the similarity of these infections, which may infect returning travelers from endemic areas, and to include them all in the differential diagnosis of acute febrile illness with headache, arthralgia, and rash.[23]

The initial symptoms of ORO fever usually recur a few days after the end of the first febrile episode, at which time they generally are less severe. Aseptic meningitis may develop in some patients. Patients make a full recovery, without any apparent aftereffects, even in the most serious cases. No fatalities have been confirmed as being attributable to ORO fever. One of the most striking characteristics of ORO virus (OROV) is its ability to produce epidemics in urban population centers, most of which reportedly have occurred in the Brazilian Amazon region, although some have occurred in other countries in northern South America, Central America (Panama), and the Caribbean region (Trinidad and Tobago). Many of these outbreaks have had a major impact on the stricken cities.

The first case of the disease was described in 1955 in a resident of Vega de Oropouche, Trinidad, from whose blood the agent was isolated.[2] The disease was detected again in 1961, this time in the city of Belém, in northern Brazil, where it caused an epidemic that affected at least 11,000 people.[26] This epidemic was followed by many other epidemics, several of an explosive nature, in urban population centers throughout the Brazilian states of Pará, Amapá, Amazonas, Tocantins, Maranhão, Rondônia, and Acre.[12,17,26,30,31,32,38,41] Outside Brazil, epidemics of ORO fever were reported in Panama in 1989 (E. Quiroz and associates, Panama, unpublished data, 1989) and in the Amazon region of Peru in 1992[5] and in 1994 (Ministry of Health, Peru, and US Naval Medical Research Institute Detachment [NAMRID], Lima, unpublished data, 1994) (Fig. 191D.1). On June 22, 2010, the Pan American Health Organization reported an outbreak of OROV infection in the northern Amazonian region of Peru. As of mid-June 2010 the Peruvian Ministry of Health reported a total of 282 cases, of which 41 cases were confirmed and

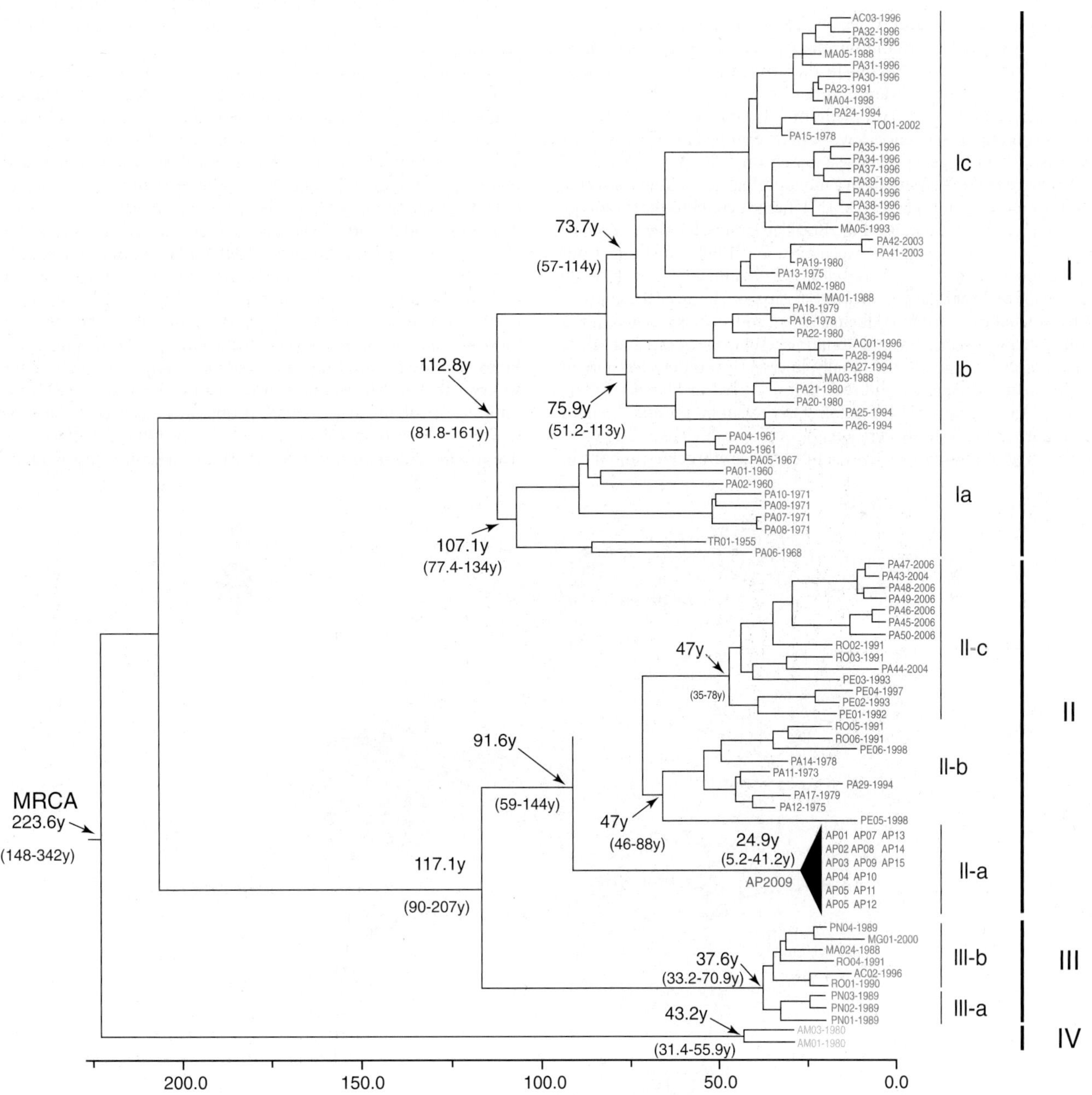

FIG. 191D.1 Phylogenetic tree based on the complete nucleotide sequence of the N gene (693 nt) of 96 OROV strains isolated from different hosts, locations, and periods. The main phylogenetic groups are represented by the genotypes I *(red),* II *(dark blue),* III *(green),* and IV *(light blue).* The values above the main nodes represent the dates of emergence of common ancestors expressed in years from 2009. *Arrows* indicate the probable date of emergence of genotypes I, II, III, and IV. ***MRCA,*** Most recent common ancestor. The numbers inside the parentheses are its value for high population density (HPD) 95%. The numerical data in the bar represent the time scale of molecular dating. (From Vasconcelos HB, Nunes MRT, Casseb LMN, et al. Oropouche fever virus: molecular epidemiology and evolution. *Emerg Infect Dis.* 2011;17:800–806.)

241 were probable. The outbreak has centered on Bagazán, in the district of Pachiza in the department of San Martín, and was the first outbreak to be reported in the region.[22] In January through March 2016, an outbreak of 57 confirmed cases of ORO fever occurred in towns in the northern part of the Cusco Region, in the Amazon Rainforest.[45] In February 2016, a mixed outbreak of dengue fever and ORO fever occurred in Peru. Because the competent vector for OROV has a broad geographic distribution, the risk of cases being identified in other countries is now significant, and the World Health Organization and the Centers for Disease Control and Prevention will monitor the status of OROV infection globally.

ETIOLOGIC AGENT

ORO fever is caused by OROV, which belongs to the genus *Orthobunyavirus* of the family Peribunyaviridae.[32,37] The virus has enveloped spherical particles 90 to 100 nm in diameter; the capsid has helical symmetry; and the single-stranded, negative-sense RNA contains three segments, designated large (L), medium (M), and small (S) RNA.[18,32] Complete nucleotide sequences have been determined for all three RNA segments.[3,36,42] Phylogenetic analysis based on S RNA (N gene) has revealed that all OROV strains form a monophylogenetic group consisting of four distinct lineages (Fig. 191D.2).[40] Lineage I contains the prototype strain from Trinidad and most of the Brazilian strains; lineage II contains the Peruvian strains isolated between 1992 and 1998 and strains from western Brazil isolated in 1991, as well as isolates obtained more recently from Amapá and Pará states in the eastern Amazon; lineage III comprises strains isolated from Panama during 1989[36] and strains isolated in the Brazilian states of Acre, Pará, and Rondônia (Amazon region) and Minas Gerais (Southeast region); and, finally, lineage IV was detected only in a strain isolated during an outbreak that occurred in Manaus, Brazil, in 1981.[40] Antigenically, OROV belongs to the Simbu group, which, in turn, is part of the Bunyamwera supergroup of arboviruses. The virus has a hemagglutinin that is active against geese erythrocytes, and it can be recovered from infected hamster serum treated with acetone (A. P. A. Travassos da Rosa, Belém, unpublished data, 1969). Intracerebral and intraperitoneal inoculation of OROV into baby mice and intracerebral, intraperitoneal, and subcutaneous inoculation of the virus into adult hamsters produce lethal infections. The virus replicates in numerous cell cultures, including Vero, BHK-21, and primary chicken embryo fibroblast, and it causes a cytopathic effect.[32] The agent is sensitive to the action of sodium deoxycholate.[16]

EPIDEMIOLOGY

Geographic Distribution

Thus far the only reported cases of ORO fever have occurred in Argentina, Brazil, Panama, Peru, and Trinidad (see Fig. 191D.2). However, most cases have been limited to the Brazilian Amazon region, with none reported in other areas of Brazil.

With a few exceptions, all episodes of ORO fever have been in the form of urban epidemics, including those in Belém and Manaus, the largest cities in the Brazilian Amazon region. The city of Belém, capital of Pará, was struck by three major epidemics during a 20-year period. The city of Santarém and surrounding villages also were affected by a major epidemic in 1974 and 1975.[30] The first epidemics that occurred outside Pará, those striking the cities of Manaus and Barcelos in Amazonas[8] and the city of Mazagão in what was then the Amapá Territory, were reported early in the 1980s.[24] After a period of quiescence lasting until 1988, new outbreaks of the disease struck the cities of Porto Franco and Tocantinópolis in the states of Maranhão and Tocantins, respectively.[41] The next reported epidemics occurred in 1991, this time in more distant locations, namely, in the cities of Ariquemes and Ouro Preto D'Oeste in Rondônia; the epidemic's impact on these cities was so great that it was reported in the national press. In 1994, another outbreak involving at least 6000 people was recorded in Serra Pelada in Pará.[38] Other outbreaks were recorded in 1996 and affected at least five urban centers in the states of Pará, Amazonas, and Acre.[31] Thus,

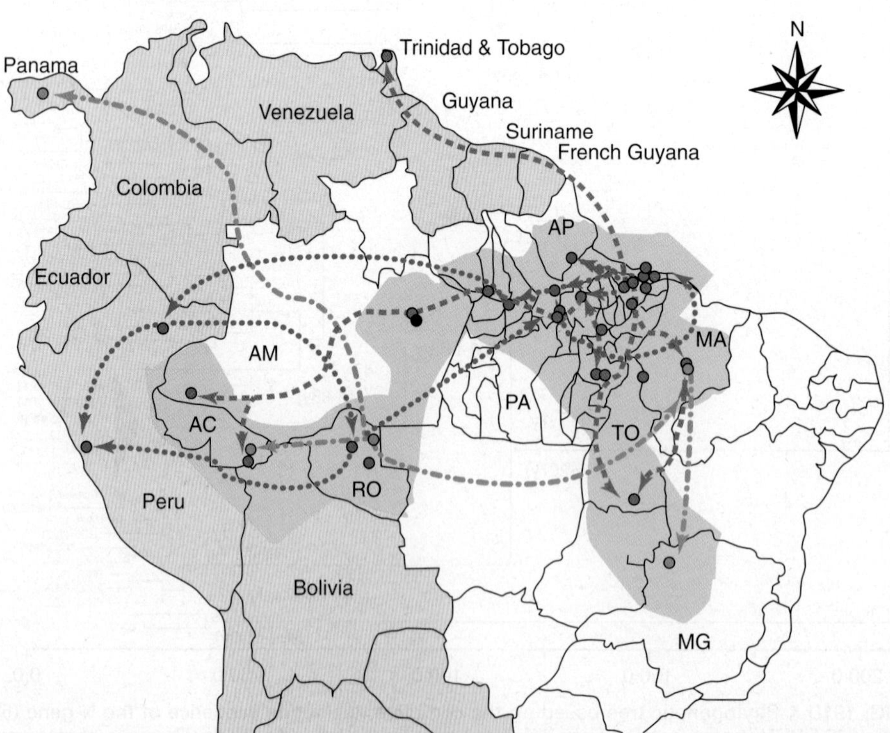

FIG. 191D.2 Geographic dispersion of OROV genotypes in the Americas between 1955 and 2009 based on the N gene genetic data. *Red line,* dispersion route for genotype I; *blue line,* dispersion route for genotype II; *green line,* dispersion route for genotype III; *black dot,* genotype IV. Coverage area of the OROV in Brazil: *AC,* Acre; *AP,* Amapá; *AM,* Amazonas; *MA,* Maranhão; *MG,* Minas Gerais; *PA,* Pará; *RO,* Rondônia; *TO,* Tocantins. (From Vasconcelos HB, Nunes MRT, Casseb LMN, et al. Oropouche fever virus: molecular epidemiology and evolution. *Emerg Infect Dis.* 2011; 17:800–806.)

during 1961 to 1996, more than 30 epidemics of ORO fever were recorded in Brazil. Several small outbreaks also were recognized in Canãa dos Carajás in 2003 and in Tapará Village at Porto de Moz in 2004, both municipalities in Pará.[4,21] In April of 2006, a large epidemic of ORO fever occurred in northeastern Pará that affected several municipalities. Autochthonous cases of ORO fever also were diagnosed in the municipalities of Magalhães Barata, Maracanã, Marapanim, Igarapé-Açu, São Francisco do Pará, and Viseu. A retrospective serologic study conducted among inhabitants of urban and rural communities of the municipality of Magalhães Barata showed that 320 of 631 persons had immunoglobulin (Ig) M OROV antibodies detected by enzyme-linked immunosorbent assay, thus suggesting that approximately half of the 8000 inhabitants had been infected. In this episode, several isolates were obtained and sequenced, and the OROV genotype II was recognized.[39] The last recorded epidemic in those municipalities occurred in 1980.[12] In 2016, The Ministry of Health of Peru reported 57 nonfatal cases of ORO fever in towns in the northern part of the Cusco Region, in the Amazon rainforest.[45]

Serologic surveys[12,24,28,31] estimated that more than 360,000 people were infected during this period (P.F.C. Vasconcelos, M.R.T. Nunes, unpublished data, 2006). However, this estimate actually is quite conservative because the incidence of this viral disease was not computed in many major outbreaks (Belém, 1968; Porto Franco and Tocantinópolis, 1988). In 2009 a large epidemic of ORO fever was reported in Mazagão, Amapá, and was caused by genotype III (P.F.C. Vasconcelos, unpublished data, 2009); the last report of ORO fever in the municipality occurred in 1980. Possibly more than a half million people in the Brazilian Amazon region may have been infected with OROV since the beginning of the 1960s.

In addition to the aforementioned epidemic areas, countless small villages scattered throughout virtually the entire Amazon region have residents who show hemagglutination-inhibition antibodies against OROV. In general, the prevalence of these antibodies is less than 3%, with the exception of Ilha de Gurupá, where it is 10.7%.[31] An OROV strain was isolated from a novel primate host (*Callithrix* spp.) in Arinos in Minas Gerais in southeastern Brazil,[20] thus extending the enzootic area farther to southern Brazil.

Outside Brazil, outbreaks were reported in Panama and Peru. The outbreak in Panama occurred in 1989 in the village of Bejuco, which is located approximately 50 km west of the capital (E. Quiroz and associates, Panama, unpublished data, 1989). The first epidemic in Peru was reported in 1992 in the city of Iquitos in the Peruvian Amazon region.[9] Subsequently, an outbreak occurred in Puerto Maldonado, Madre de Dios, also in the Peruvian Amazon region (Ministry of Health, Peru, and NAMRID, Lima, unpublished data, 1994). Studies performed in Peru suggested that transmission of OROV occurs continuously in the population of the city of Iquitos and surrounding villages.[43] Evidence of immunity to OROV was detected in nonhuman primates in Colombia, a finding suggesting the presence of OROV in that country as well.[16] OROV has been detected by reverse-transcriptase polymerase chain reaction assay from febrile persons in Jujuy, northern Argentina (P. F. C. Vasconcelos, unpublished data, 2009). The nucleotide sequencing of S RNA showed that the Argentinian strains belonged to genotype IV.

Incidence

A significant characteristic of ORO fever is the exceptionally high attack rates seen during several outbreaks. Although incidence rates varied in different outbreaks, a rate of 30% was quite common. The proportion of those infected who had overt disease is not known with certainty, but in one epidemic clinical disease developed in 63% of those infected.[12]

Sex-specific attack rates vary. Rates in female patients were slightly higher than those in male patients in villages in the Bragantina area, in eastern Pará, which was struck by the virus in 1979,[12] and the opposite was true in the outbreak in Belém that same year. However, in the reported epidemics in Santarém, the infection struck female patients twice as often as male patients.[11] ORO fever affects all age groups, although in certain outbreaks the incidence was higher in children and young adults.

Diffusion of Epidemics

As indicated earlier, ORO fever epidemics have struck different locations at varying intervals. However, many outbreaks have been marked by bona fide epidemic sweeps, with countless numbers of villages within a particular geographic area affected by the virus. This diffusion phenomenon was observed in Bragança in 1967, in Santarém in 1974 and 1975, and even more dramatically in Belém and in the Bragantina area from 1978 to 1980 (where at least 10 towns were stricken), as well as in Rondônia in 1991. Spread of the virus most likely is attributable to the movement of viremic persons throughout areas in which the virus vector is present.

Seasonal Fluctuation

Most epidemics of ORO fever typically occur during the rainy season, which, in the case of Pará in Brazil, corresponds to the period between January and June. However, many epidemics have extended into the dry season, although with less intensity. The seasonal nature of ORO fever most likely is linked to the higher density of populations of *Culicoides paraensis,* commonly known as the biting midge, the urban virus vector, in months with higher levels of rainfall, combined with a higher concentration of exposed individuals. Downward trends in epidemics of ORO fever generally are associated with the arrival of the dry season and the resulting lower density of biting midge populations and smaller numbers of exposed persons.[18,33]

Endemic Transmission

During interepidemic periods, isolated cases of ORO fever undoubtedly occur in Brazil but remain undiagnosed. Although no systematic studies have been conducted to investigate endemic transmission of OROV in Brazil, seroepidemiologic investigations have indicated that the prevalence of anti-OROV antibodies in humans is 0% to 2% in areas where endemic transmission has not been reported,[31] but it increases to 17% to 44% after outbreaks.[11,18,32] These data suggest that endemic transmission of OROV is quite low in Brazil.

Transmission Mechanism

Laboratory studies and broad-based surveys conducted by the Evandro Chagas Institute of Belém during the course of epidemics point to the importance of the insect *C. paraensis* in the Ceratopogonidae as the urban vector for OROV.[25,29] These tiny insects, commonly known as maruins (biting midges) in the Amazon region, are active during the day, particularly in the late afternoon hours. They crave human blood and bite people inside as well as outside their homes.[15,20,34] The disease is transmitted by inoculation of the virus into exposed individuals by bites of infected midges.

Transmission Cycles

Studies conducted by the Evandro Chagas Institute[31] suggest that OROV is perpetuated in nature through two different cycles, namely, an urban cycle and a wild cycle. In the urban or epidemic cycle, the virus is transmitted from person to person by the bite of *C. paraensis.* One of the most conclusive pieces of evidence attesting to this assertion lies in demonstration of the ability of *C. paraensis,* after feeding on the blood of viremic patients, to transmit the virus to hamsters bitten by the midges 5 or more days later.[29] Moreover, these midges typically are found in high densities during periods of epidemics. They breed mostly in the decomposing trunks of felled banana trees, in rotting husks of cocoa beans,[14] and in piles of detritus formed in tree hollows.[19] They are scattered throughout tropical and subtropical areas of the Americas.[19]

Attempts to transmit the virus from one hamster to another through the bite of the *Culex quinquefasciatus* mosquito (a species commonly found in urban areas throughout the Amazon region) demonstrated that the virus was transmitted only in the presence of extremely high levels of viremia, which rarely occurs in infected humans.[25] Thus this finding virtually rules out all likelihood that the epidemic vector is *C. quinquefasciatus.* Curiously, the virus isolation rate from *C. paraensis* during periods of epidemics is only one in 12,500,[18] a finding suggesting that it is a low-efficiency vector. Apparently, humans are the only vertebrates in the urban cycle of OROV because studies of domestic animals conducted during the course of numerous outbreaks ruled out the possibility that these animals play an amplifying role.

As far as the wild, silent cycle of the virus is concerned, evidence suggests that among vertebrates, the *Edentata* (sloth), nonhuman primates, and possibly certain species of wild birds serve as hosts. Although to date OROV has been isolated from mosquitoes (from a single pool of *Aedes serratus* in Brazil and once from *Coquillettidia venezuelensis* in Trinidad[2,27]), the possible involvement of biting midges in the wild cycle of the virus nonetheless should be investigated.

The link between the two cycles most likely is humans themselves, who, after contracting the infection in enzootic forested areas and then returning to an urban setting during the viremic phase, become a source of infection for biting midges. The virus replicates in the tissues of biting midges, which, after the extrinsic incubation period, bite and infect exposed individuals. These individuals, in turn, serve as a source of infection for other midges, thereby forming a chain of transmission resulting in the unleashing of an epidemic.

Incubation Period

Observations conducted during numerous epidemics suggest that the incubation period ranges from 4 to 8 days. A laboratory worker who accidentally was infected orally exhibited symptoms of the viral disease 3 days later, and another technician fell ill 4 days after being infected, probably through the respiratory route.[31]

Transmissibility Period

The blood of infected patients is infectious to *C. paraensis* for the first 3 or 4 days after the onset of symptoms, when the level of viremia is high enough to infect the midges. Experimental studies have shown the length of the extrinsic incubation period to be 5 days or more.[29] The virus is not transmitted directly from one person to another.

Ratio of Symptomatic Cases

A prospective study conducted in the city of Santa Izabel in Pará in Brazil during the course of the epidemic of 1979 showed the ratio of symptomatic to asymptomatic cases to be roughly 2 : 1.[12] The study was performed during the period from March through June of that year. It involved 274 persons exposed to the virus who were monitored by clinical examination and laboratory testing on a weekly basis throughout the study. By the end of the study period, 78 (28.5%) of these persons had serologic evidence of OROV infection, with clinical manifestations of the disease developing in 49 (63%) of the 78.

CLINICAL MANIFESTATIONS

In most cases of ORO fever, the infection takes the form of an acute febrile episode, which runs its course. However, certain patients may show typical signs and symptoms of aseptic meningitis, which also runs its course without complications.

Classic Febrile Form

This form of the disease is characterized by the sudden onset of symptoms after an incubation period ranging from 4 to 8 days. The first symptoms to appear are fever, headache, chills, dizziness, muscular pain, arthralgia, and photophobia. Retroocular pain and conjunctival congestion also may be present. In addition, some patients have nausea, which may be accompanied by episodes of vomiting. Not uncommonly, patients have severe anorexia and insomnia. At times, cough and coryza are present as well, although these manifestations may be attributable to intercurrent infections. Certain patients complain of fleeting burning or stinging sensations in different parts of their body. The presence of an exanthem is a rare finding. Two laboratory workers who were infected accidentally reported a longer and heavier menstrual flow than usual.[30,31] The fever can be quite high, 39°C or 40°C (102.2°F–104°F), and in some cases it may be higher than 40°C. The headache usually is localized in the front or back part of the head, although it also may be diffuse. It generally is severe and, in some cases, may not respond readily to common analgesics. Generalized myalgia is present and sharpest in the neck, along the vertebral column, and in the area of the sacrum. The pain may be extremely severe. Patients generally describe feeling as though their body had been crushed or they had been beaten. Usually, generalized arthralgia also is present. Certain patients have dizzy spells so severe that in some cases they collapse. Any epigastric pain generally is mild. Patients have no sign of jaundice, hepatomegaly, or splenomegaly. Occasionally, swollen lymph nodes are detected in the submaxillary and occipital regions, and these findings could be totally unrelated to the viral infection.

The intensity of the clinical symptoms varies. In some cases, the symptoms are quite severe and even may cause prostration, whereas in others, they can be rather mild. Many patients are bedridden and, during epidemics, flood area hospitals, thus causing serious overcrowding.

The acute phase of the disease generally lasts 2 to 5 days but can be as long as a week. The myalgia, conversely, may persist for 3 to 5 days after the fever has disappeared. Some patients report having prolonged asthenia for as long as a month. Certain patients complain of a persistent headache lasting up to several weeks. No human deaths have been attributed to OROV infection.[18]

Nearly 60% of all patients have one or more recurrences in the first or second week after disappearance of the manifestations of the acute phase of the disease.[12,24,31] Relapses may take the form of reappearance of all the acute-phase symptoms of the disease, or they may be limited strictly to fever, asthenia, and dizziness. In some reported patients, relapses were accompanied by a urinary tract infection of bacterial origin. An abscess, most likely bacterial, developed in the oropharynx of one particular patient approximately 10 days after recovery from the original febrile condition. In some cases, patients may have a series of relapses during a period of 2 to 3 weeks.[31] All attempts to isolate OROV during relapses have failed.

Observations made during the course of the 1980 outbreak in Belém revealed that an exanthem developed in approximately 5% of all laboratory-confirmed cases.[24] The exanthem appeared between the third and sixth day after onset of the fever, disappeared 2 or 3 days later, and mainly involved the thorax, back, arms, and legs.[24,28] During the outbreak in Manaus, many patients exhibited a maculopapular exanthem beginning on the torso and spreading to the upper and lower extremities.[5] In another rare case, a 4-year-old child whose infection was confirmed by serodiagnosis experienced nystagmus, generalized tremors, and somnolence.[12] These symptoms lasted approximately 8 days, and the child apparently made a full recovery.

The effects of ORO fever on pregnancy are unknown. The only available data in this regard come from studies conducted in Manaus of nine pregnant patients, two of whom, both in the second month of pregnancy at the time, had miscarriages.[5]

Aseptic Meningitis

At first, patients exhibit manifestations typical of the initial acute phase of the infection. As the illness progresses, a few days later the headache and dizziness become increasingly severe, and some patients begin to experience other neurologic symptoms, generally during the second week of the illness, that lead them to seek medical care. The main complaints cited by patients are fever, extremely severe headache in the back of the head, and dizziness. Approximately one-third of all patients complain of nausea and vomiting. Some patients have moderate lethargy. They also may have trouble holding themselves upright. Some patients complain of double vision or diplopia. They generally try to keep from moving their heads to avoid aggravating their pain. In most cases, physical examination of these patients reveals varying degrees of stiffness of the neck but no signs of paresis or paralysis. Some patients experience nystagmus. Despite the seriousness of these neurologic symptoms, patients make a full recovery. Electroencephalograms taken of four patients showed no abnormalities. The incidence of meningitis in patients who seek medical care is less than 5%.[27]

PATHOGENESIS

Little is known about the pathogenesis of ORO fever. The viral agent produces a systemic infection in humans that induces viremia during the first 2 days of illness.[10]

By the third day, the rate of viremia drops to 72%, and it falls to 44% and 23% by the fourth and fifth days, respectively. Viremia titers generally are higher than 3.0 $\log_{10}$ median lethal dose/0.02 mL in mice, with approximately 10% of patients exhibiting virus titers as high as 5.0 to 5.3 during the course of the first 2 days of their illness. By the third day, virus titers are 1 log lower than in the first 2 days, and titers plummet by the fourth day.[29]

Similarly, little is known about the pathogenesis of relapses, which occur commonly. That no sign of viremia could be detected in any of the countless patients examined during relapses is noteworthy.

The finding that OROV is capable of causing aseptic meningitis, combined with isolation of the virus from the cerebrospinal fluid (CSF) in one patient with meningitis,[27] suggests that the virus has the ability to penetrate the blood-brain barrier. With no known confirmed fatalities attributable to OROV, no data are available on the possible organic lesions caused by this agent in humans.

Laboratory tests on young hamsters inoculated with OROV showed that the virus has essentially hepatoviscerotropic properties, with isolated necrosis of hepatocytes or focal necrosis and the involvement of Kupffer cells exhibiting reactive hyperplasia; animals invariably succumb to the infection. In newborn mice the virus exhibits marked neurotropism, and animals show signs of focal encephalitis within 24 to 48 hours after being inoculated.[4]

LABORATORY FINDINGS

Leukopenia associated with neutropenia is found commonly, although in certain cases moderate leukocytosis may be present. The leukopenia can be severe, with reports of leukocyte counts as low as $2000/mm^3$. No signs of cell abnormalities are present. Aspartate and alanine aminotransferase levels are normal or may show a moderate increase, but in no case do they exceed 135 units/mL of serum. Platelet counts usually are normal but occasionally may be slightly low. The erythrocyte sedimentation rate and levels of urea, creatinine, and glucose in blood are normal, as are urine test results.[29]

The CSF of patients with aseptic meningitis shows pleocytosis and an increased concentration of protein.[27] The cell count varies from 7 to 310 $cells/mm^3$ of CSF; both segmented and mononuclear cells are present, with a predominance of segmented cells. In one case the cell count in CSF fell from 130 to 30 $cells/mm^3$ in a 1-week period, and another patient's cell count fell from 70 to 10 $cells/mm^3$ over a 3-week interval. In general, a moderate increase in protein levels occurs in the CSF, although one patient's protein level was more than 100 mg/mL. Glucose levels remain normal. The viral RNA from the causative agent has been detected in the CSF of patients with meningoencephalitis associated with ORO fever, as well as OROV-specific IgG and IgM antibodies.[6]

DIAGNOSIS

Specific confirmation of the infection is made by isolating the virus from a patient's blood or by performing OROV-specific serologic assays.[7,32] To isolate the virus, blood samples need to be taken during the first 5 days of the illness, preferably in the first 2 days, when viremia is present in virtually all cases. The virus can be isolated by intracerebral or intraperitoneal inoculation of serum from infected patients into baby mice or young hamsters (in this case, subcutaneous inoculation can be used as well). Viral isolates also can be recovered in different cell cultures, such as Vero and BHK-21. The virus is identified by complement fixation or neutralization using OROV-specific ascitic fluid or antisera. Serodiagnosis is accomplished by the demonstration of an increase in antibody in paired serum samples taken during the acute and convalescent phases of the disease by hemagglutination inhibition, complement fixation, or neutralization. A positive IgM antibody capture enzyme-linked immunosorbent assay (MAC-ELISA) on a single serum sample provides a presumptive diagnosis of recent infection, particularly in the presence of a clinical picture consistent with the disease; the test result usually is positive after the fifth day of illness. A rapid and highly sensitive one-step TaqMan reverse-transcriptase polymerase chain reaction assay has been described for detection of OROV and certain other orthobunyaviruses; it was found to be more sensitive than the established nested polymerase chain reaction system.[44] A recent real-time RT-PCR was developed and has been used to diagnosis OROV and IQUV.[46]

A comprehensive and large molecular study performed with OROV isolates focused on phylogenetic analysis, as well as on dispersal and evolutionary aspects (see Figs. 191D.1 and 191D.2).[41] The conclusions of the study were that OROV emerged in the Brazilian Amazon approximately 223 years ago and that, based on N gene (S RNA) data, the genotype I was the first genetic lineage to emerge and was responsible for the emergence of the other genetic lineages, as well as for virus dispersal in northern South America.[41]

DIFFERENTIAL DIAGNOSIS

Because of the nonspecific nature of the symptoms, a clinical diagnosis of ORO fever is difficult to make, and often the disease is mistaken for other febrile illnesses such as dengue fever, Zika virus infection, yellow fever, chikungunya, and malaria. In fact, malaria and dengue fever initially were suspected as the cause of numerous epidemics of ORO fever. Detailed clinical records combined with epidemiologic data can help establish a differential diagnosis, the certainty of which hinges on the absence of plasmodia in blood samples and the lack of laboratory evidence of dengue infection. Other viral and bacterial febrile diseases must be considered in the differential diagnosis. Accordingly, clinical and epidemiologic data and nonspecific tests will need to be taken into account, although establishing an accurate diagnosis requires specific tests.

Febrile forms of the disease accompanied by an exanthem need to be distinguished from other exanthematous febrile symptoms caused by dengue, measles, parvovirus B19 infection, infection with human herpesvirus type 6 or 5, enteroviral infections, and allergies to medication. A potential problem in differentiating ORO fever was observed in Peru after the emergence of a new orthobunyavirus named Iquitos virus (IQTV), a reassortant virus containing the S and L segments of OROV and the M segment of an unknown Simbu serogroup virus.[1] Clinically the febrile disease caused by IQTV is identical to ORO fever.[1] Finally, differentiating cases of aseptic meningitis associated with OROV infection from cases of aseptic meningitis associated with other causative agents requires a specific etiologic diagnosis.

TREATMENT

Because ORO fever has no specific treatment, management is symptomatic. Rest is important and should be continued for several days after disappearance of the initial acute manifestations because relapses are thought to occur more often in patients who prematurely resume regular activities, particularly strenuous activities. Aspirin or another antipyretic should be taken to lower the fever, and the use of ordinary analgesics is recommended for headache, myalgia, and arthralgia. However, certain reported patients whose headaches failed to respond to this treatment were treated with morphine derivatives. Also recommended are fruit juices or glucose solutions. Severely dehydrated patients may be treated with intravenous fluids.

PREVENTION AND CONTROL

The most effective way to prevent, avert, or curb the impact of epidemics of ORO fever is to combat its vector, *C. paraensis.* To be effective, vector control effort needs to focus on the midge's adult and larval forms. Given that *C. paraensis* is habitually active during the day, application of insecticides to its habitats by thermonebulization or ultra-low-volume aerosolization may help to reduce populations of adult biting midges. Because this *Culicoides* species is most active during the late afternoon hours,[34] ultra-low-volume spraying may be more effective during this period. However, carefully planned studies are needed to assess how to maximize the effectiveness of spraying by determining the type and concentration of insecticide to be used, the necessary volume of insecticide per treatment area, the size of the droplets, the frequency and timing of applications, and other factors. At the same time, making an effort to control the larvae by applying larvicides to corresponding habitats or, better yet, by conducting drives to eliminate or burn breeding sites such as rotting cocoa bean husks and the decomposing trunks of felled banana trees is essential.[14] Obviously, the success of these measures will depend largely on community involvement. Providing proper community education is important. People can protect themselves by applying insect repellent directly to the skin. However, these types of products provide only temporary action, and they may be unaffordable to the poor.

No vaccine against ORO fever exists at this time. In light of the relatively benign nature of this viral disease, developing a general-purpose vaccine for at-risk populations living in areas where they are exposed to the disease is difficult to justify.

NEW REFERENCES SINCE THE SEVENTH EDITION

6. Bastos M, Lessa N, Nvec F, et al. Detection of herpesvirus, enterovirus, and arbovirus infection in patients with suspected central nervous system viral infection in the western Brazilian Amazon. *J Med Virol.* 2014;86(9):1522.
7. Belgath F, Otacillia P, de Vilva Heinen, et al. Detection of Oropouche virus segment S in patients and in *Culex quinquefasciatus* in the state of Mato Grosso, Brazil. *Mem Inst Oswald.* 2015;110(6):745.
10. De Souza Luna L, Rodrigues A, Dos Santos R, et al. Oropouche virus is detected in peripheral blood leukocytes from patients. *J Med Virol.* 2017;89:1108-1111.
13. Ginier M, Neumayr A, Gunther S, et al. Zika without symptoms in returning travellers: what are the implications? *Travel Med Infect Dis.* 2016;14(1):16.
23. Paniz-Mondolfi A, Rodrigue-Morales A, Blohm G, et al. ChikDenMaZika syndrome: the challenge of diagnosing arboviral infections in the midst of concurrent epidemics. *Ann Clin Microbiol Antimicrob.* 2016;15(1):42.
35. Rodriguez-Morales A, Paniz-Mondolfi A, Villamil-Gomez W, Navarro J. Mayaro, Oropouche and Venezuelan equine encephalitis viruses: following in the footsteps of Zika? *Travel Med Infect Dis.* 2017;15:72-73.
37. Tilston-Lunel N, Hughes J, Acrani G, et al. Genetic analysis of members of the species Oropouche virus and identification of a novel M segment sequence. *J Gen Virol.* 2015;96(7):1636.
45. World Health Organization. Oropouche Virus Disease: Peru. http://www.who.int/csr/don/03-june-2016-oropouche-peru/en/.

The full reference list for this chapter is available at ExpertConsult.com.

191E ■ Toscana Virus

Rémi N. Charrel • Xavier de Lamballerie

HISTORY

Toscana virus (TOSV) was discovered in 1971 in phlebotomines in Italy. Three strains were isolated from female *Phlebotomus perniciosus* collected in Monte Argentario (Grosseto Province, central Italy).[86–88] The first evidence that TOSV was causing disease in humans was provided 14 year later.[36] Subsequent clinical and epidemiologic studies performed in Italy confirmed its role in aseptic acute meningitis.[14,15] Then studies from other Mediterranean countries confirmed the medical importance of TOSV as one of the major causes of aseptic acute meningitis and encephalitis during the summer in regions where phlebotomine vectors are present.[50,60,71,76] A bibliographic search using "Toscana virus" as key words in the PubMed database retrieved 273 research and review articles, of which less than 30% reported clinical cases of infection in southern Europe and the islands of the Mediterranean.[26,42,74] More recently, TOSV was isolated in northern Africa, thus demonstrating its presence on the southern shore of the Mediterranean.[3,13] Despite increasing evidence of its major role in human disease, TOSV remains poorly studied, and most physicians have little awareness of its potential to cause central nervous system (CNS) infections.

ETIOLOGIC AGENT

Phleboviruses are arthropod-borne viruses that contain a negative-sense, single-stranded RNA genome that consists of three segments, designated large, medium, and small, that encode the RNA-dependent RNA polymerase,[40] the envelope glycoproteins, and the nucleoprotein, respectively. Phylogenetic analyses performed using the medium segment identified three major lineages separate from Rift Valley fever virus and Uukuniemi virus. Given that cross-reactivity among phleboviruses when using serologic techniques is not uncommon, the identification of these viruses has increasingly involved incorporating genetic approaches to characterize these virus isolates. According to the ninth report of the International Committee on Taxonomy of Viruses, TOSV is a serotype of the species *Sandfly fever Naples virus* within the genus *Phlebovirus* in the Bunyaviridae family.[72] Serologic cross-reactions are observed among the viruses included in the Sandfly fever Naples virus antigenic group by using indirect immunofluorescence assay (indirect IFA), hemagglutination inhibition, complement fixation, or enzyme-linked immunosorbent assay (ELISA), thus distinguishing TOSV antibody from antibody directed to Naples, Tehran, Massilia, Punique, Granada, Zerdali viruses is not possible.[22,24,91] Therefore studies based on ELISA or IFA techniques must be interpreted carefully because of possible misinterpretations as a result of antigenic cross-reactivity among distinct viruses. Only neutralization assays can discriminate viruses that belong to the same antigenic complex or species.

EPIDEMIOLOGY

Sandfly-borne phleboviruses have been isolated from phlebotomines in southern Europe, Africa, central Asia, and the Americas. Data indicate that the same may apply to TOSV and *P. perniciosus* (or *Phlebotomus perfiliewi*). Until recently *P. perniciosus* and *P. perfiliewi* were the only recognized vectors of TOSV. Evidence if TOSV in regions where these two species are either absent or rarely found suggests that other species of phlebotomines that belong to the *Larroussius* subgenus are possible vectors (*P. ariasi, P. neglectus, P. tobbi*). The geographic distribution of TOSV covers southern Europe and northern Africa, the Balkans, and Turkey (Fig. 191E.1); additional studies are needed to assess whether it expands beyond this area.[35,39,50,57,71]

Italy

Preliminary clues pointing to the role of TOSV in CNS infections in Italy were provided by case reports of imported cases diagnosed in the United States[18,36] and Germany.[80] A large study carried out between 1977 and 1988 showed that the virus was the cause of meningitis in two different regions of Italy, Tuscany and Marche, with a seasonal peak occurring in August, corresponding to the peak of sandfly activity.[63] Striking evidence that TOSV was the most prominent viral cause of summertime meningitis was reported in the late 1990s.[81,84] A study of children living in rural or suburban areas of Siena (central Italy) showed that 40% of meningitis or encephalitis cases could be linked to infection with TOSV.[15] A 7-year study (1990–96) performed in Siena showed that 52% of aseptic meningitis cases in adults were associated with TOSV.[14] All studies are in agreement regarding the monthly distribution of human cases of TOSV infections—the highest risk for acquiring TOSV is in August, then July and September, and finally June and October. Many reports describe TOSV cases in other regions of Italy, such as northern Italy, Emilia Romagna, Naples, Sicily, and Sardinia.[19,25,32,48,54,55,66,73,85,89] Seroprevalence studies report rates that vary between 9% and 25%, indicating different levels of exposure according to regional and local environmental conditions; however, most of these serologic studies are based on ELISA or indirect IFA and should be considered with caution because of cross-reactions with other phleboviruses related with TOSV. The same comment applies to other countries but is not repeated, to avoid redundancy.

Spain

The first case of TOSV infection reported from Spain occurred in the late 1980s in a Swedish tourist after visiting Catalonia and was documented by plaque reduction neutralization test.[37] Subsequently, Spanish researchers and physicians reported many cases of TOSV infection and conducted several comprehensive epidemiologic studies demonstrating that TOSV was a major cause of meningitis in Spain.[60] A total of 15 strains of TOSV were isolated between 1988 and 1996 from the cerebrospinal fluid (CSF) of patients with acute aseptic meningitis in Granada, Spain.[57] A total of 724 CSF samples from patients with suspected aseptic meningitis were tested through viral isolation in cell culture. TOSV was isolated from the CSF of 17 patients (7% of all viral isolates), 15 of whom were previously reported in the foregoing reference. TOSV was ranked as the third most common cause of aseptic meningitis after

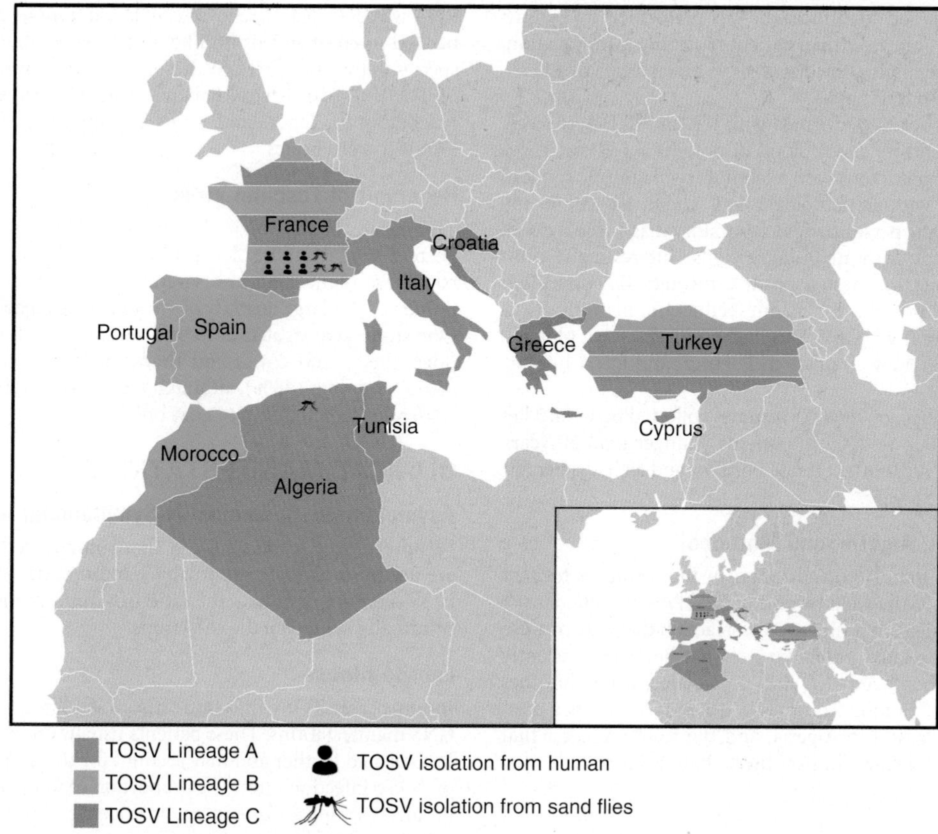

FIG. 191E.1 Geographic distribution of Toscana virus *(TOSV)* in the Mediterranean Area.

enteroviruses and mumps virus, a finding suggesting that its etiologic role in CNS infections in Spain is not as high as observed in central Italy. These data suggest that the situation in Spain is similar to that observed in France, with lower prevalence of CNS infections in contrast to those observed in central Italy. The testing of clinical samples with these assays confirmed the role of TOSV as a causative agent of acute aseptic meningitis in the central region of Spain.[75] In a collection of 88 serum and 53 CSF samples taken from 81 patients with acute aseptic meningitis of unknown origin who were living in Madrid or on the southern Mediterranean coast of Spain, seven patients were found to have acute TOSV infection (3 residents from the Mediterranean region and four from the Madrid region).[35] A large study conducted in different regions of Spain showed the presence of immunoglobulin (Ig) G antibodies to TOSV (26.2%), and Sandfly fever Naples virus (2.2%) in 1181 adults and 87 children.[57] A total of 457 serum samples taken from healthy persons, 2 to 60 years of age, from the south of the Madrid region was investigated for anti-TOSV IgG. The overall prevalence of anti-TOSV was 5%.[35]

In the Granada region, the overall seroprevalence rate was 24.9%. A statistically significant increase in the seroprevalence rate was observed with age (9.4% in persons younger than 15 years in contrast to 60.4% in persons older than 65 years). In addition, several cases of TOSV infection were documented in numerous geographic areas of Spain (Badajoz, Málaga, Granada, Almería, Murcia, Alicante, Valencia, Madrid, and Barcelona), mostly in the southern, central, and Mediterranean areas of the country (EVITAR network, A. Tenorio, personal communication, 2003).

France

The first reported case of TOSV infection acquired in France was in a German traveler returning from southern France.[33] Five of 205 CSF samples retrospectively tested for TOSV RNA were positive, and they corresponded to patients living in the city of Marseille in southeastern France with no history of travel abroad. Sequence analysis indicated that these strains were most closely related to TOSV circulating in Italy.[21] A total of 13 of 72 serum samples collected from April to September of 2003 in patients admitted for meningitis contained specific IgM by using an ELISA test.[28] Twelve percent (n = 11) of 92 healthy blood donors from Marseille tested positive for specific IgG.[28] Similar prevalence rates were reported later.[16]

During the national surveillance for West Nile virus in southern France, many cases of acute TOSV infections were diagnosed by the National Reference center for Arboviruses and the virology laboratory of the Public Hospitals of Marseille.[34,58,64] Together these findings indicate that strains of TOSV belonging to both the Italian and Spanish genotypes are co-circulating in the region, and both cause human infections.[9,21,50,71]

Together, these data confirm that TOSV circulates in southwestern and southeastern France, as well as in Corsica island,[12,27] and it ranks third as an etiologic agent of aseptic meningitis.

Cyprus

Several studies were conducted in Swedish United Nations soldiers based in Cyprus in 1985. Blood samples were obtained from the 362-soldier battalion just before and immediately after their 6-month tour of duty. Of 298 serum pairs available, seroconversion for TOSV was observed in a single case without any clinical manifestations.[39] Seroprevalence studies showed that 20% (96 of 479) of the healthy population of the island had TOSV IgG.[38]

Greece

Studies of populations living on two Ionian Islands and in northern Greece showed a seroprevalence of 11% and 48%, respectively.[5,68]

The first direct evidence for the presence of TOSV in Greece was described in 2014 with a case of encephalitis caused by a strain belonging to the lineage C (also reported in Croatia).[67] Seroprevalence studies (using IFA) demonstrated that TOSV and antigenically related viruses were actively circulating in the islands of Aegean Sea, in northern Greece and in the Ionian islands.[5,6,68]

Portugal

One imported case of TOSV was reported in Portugal, in a man who presented with severe headache and fever without neck stiffness. Viral isolation was successful, and identification was performed by plaque neutralization.[36] In addition, a German patient returning from vacation in Portugal developed meningitis; the diagnosis was established by ELISA and confirmed by immunoblot assay.[79]

A seroepidemiologic study, performed with IFA and ELISA, showed that TOSV IgG was found in 2% of blood donors (n = 150), in 1.3% of sera from symptomatic persons with a laboratory diagnostic request for vector-borne viruses without neurologic signs, and in 4.2% of serum samples from symptomatic persons with a laboratory diagnostic request for vector-borne viruses with neurologic signs. Interestingly, only five of 29 serum samples that tested positive through IFA or ELISA were confirmed to be positive by plaque reduction neutralization assay with the Italian strain of TOSV. This finding suggests that phleboviruses other than TOSV may circulate in Portugal and infect human populations.[4]

In the north of Portugal, of 106 CSF samples collected between May and September from 2002 to 2005 in patients younger than 30 years who were tested for TOSV RNA, six tested positive, and all had a benign course and self-limited disease.[76]

North Africa (Tunisia, Algeria, and Morocco)

Several studies suggest that TOSV circulates in the countries located on the southern shore of the Mediterranean Sea. Present data consist of serologic studies,[8] which are prone to cross-reaction that may confuse TOSV with genetically related phleboviruses that have been recently discovered.[59,91] TOSV has been detected or isolated from sandflies collected in Morocco [45,46] and in Tunisia.[13] Human infection has been demonstrated in Tunisia and in Algeria, and the results suggest that TOSV may have a much greater impact there than in Europe.[2,47]

Turkey

TOSV is present in Turkey, where it causes human infections.[42,44] Human cases were described in Aegean Turkey, in eastern Thrace, and in central Anatolia. Molecular evidence indicates that strains belonging to the lineages A and B are present in Turkey.[30,41,42,65] To date, lineage A TOSV RNA has been described in phlebotomies in dogs and in humans, whereas lineage B TOSV RNA has been reported in dogs only.[30] A comprehensive review is available for details of TOSV in Turkey.[43]

Other Countries

TOSV neutralizing antibodies were detected in humans populations living in Djibouti (East Africa).[7] Patients presenting with neurologic manifestations or with fever of unknown origin should be tested for TOSV using polymerase chain reaction (PCR) assay or cell culture to assess the medical importance suggested by serologic findings.

CYCLE IN NATURE

Vectors of Toscana Virus

TOSV was isolated first from *P. perniciosus*. Other strains have been isolated from *P. perfiliewi* but never from *P. papatasi*. TOSV also has been isolated from the brains of the bat *Pipistrellus kuhlii* trapped in areas where *P. perniciosus* and *P. perfiliewi* were present.[86–88] Isolation from bats has been reported for a large number of mosquito-borne arboviruses, including flaviviruses such as yellow fever virus, dengue virus, West Nile virus, and St. Louis encephalitis virus, with no clear information on implications for the ecologic cycle of these viruses. Transovarial transmission of TOSV in sandflies has been demonstrated in the laboratory and by viral isolation from male *Phlebotomus* species. Venereal transmission from infected males to uninfected females also has been demonstrated. *P. perniciosus* is distributed throughout the Mediterranean region as two races. The typical *P. perniciosus* race occurs in Italy, as well as in Malta, Tunisia, and Morocco. It is replaced in southern Spain by the Iberian race (with the pni mitochondrial DNA sublineage).[70] TOSV was detected in both male and female pools of phlebotomine sandflies captured during the summer seasons of 2003 and 2004 in Granada. The most probable transmission vector for TOSV in Spain is *P. perniciosus,* because approximately 70% of captured individuals corresponded to this species. Detection in pools of males suggests vertical or sexual transmission of TOSV among sandflies. TOSV RNA was detected once in *Sergentomyia minuta*; additional studies are needed to confirm this finding and to assess the potential role of this species in the cycle of TOSV. Results showing a much larger distribution of TOSV (North Africa, Balkans, Turkey) raise the question whether phlebotomines other that *P. perniciosus* and *P. perfiliewi* can also transmit TOSV to vertebrates.

Reservoir of Toscana Virus

The nature of the reservoir remains highly controversial. TOSV has been isolated from the blood of humans, dogs, and the *Pipistrellus kuhlii* bat.[88] Transient and low viremia occurs after TOSV infection in humans.[11,82] A large quantity of virus must be ingested to infect sandflies.[23] One study investigated domestic animals (i.e., horses, goats, pigs, cats, dogs, sheep, and cows) and found high seroprevalence rates in cats (60%) and dogs (48%), although no virus could be isolated, and TOSV RNA was detected in one goat only.[61]

CLINICAL MANIFESTATIONS

Asymptomatic or Minimally Symptomatic Infection

Seroprevalence studies suggest that some infections caused by TOSV are asymptomatic or minimally symptomatic. Additional studies will be necessary to evaluate the ratio of symptomatic to asymptomatic or minimally symptomatic infections.

Febrile Illness

In some cases, TOSV infection causes a self-limiting febrile illness without CNS manifestations. These patients usually are neither hospitalized nor investigated further and may account for the probable underestimation of TOSV infection rates. The proportion of this clinical form is unknown because of the lack of systematic documentation of fever of unknown origin in regions where TOSV is present.

Meningitis

After an incubation period ranging from a few days to a maximum of 2 weeks, the onset of disease is brutal (70%), with headache (100%, 1–5 days), fever (76–97%), nausea and vomiting (67–88%), photophobia (86%), malaise (62%), and myalgias (18%). On physical examination, stiff neck (53–95%), Kernig signs (87%), encephalitis (44%), focal neurologic defect (21%), seizures (12%), poor levels of consciousness (12%), paresis (1.7%), and nystagmus (5.2%) are apparent.[34,52,63,89] In most cases reported thus far, CSF samples have contained more than 5 to 10 cells, with normal levels of glucose and protein. Leukocytosis (29%) or leukopenia (6%) may be observed in the blood. The mean duration of the disease is 7 days, and the outcome usually is favorable.[34,56,64]

Other Central Nervous System Manifestations

Although TOSV infection in most cases is a mild disease with a favorable outcome, a few severe cases have been reported in the literature. Meningoencephalitis and pure encephalitis are not so infrequent, as shown in several series.[10,25,31,34,52,56] One case of meningitis complicated by abducens nerve palsy was reported in a German tourist returning from Italy.[77]

Other Disease Manifestations Not Involving the Central Nervous System

Other manifestations should also be considered during the warm season, such as myositis and fasciitis.[58]

DIAGNOSIS AND DIFFERENTIAL DIAGNOSIS

For diagnosis of suspected cases of TOSV, it is important to follow the clinical criteria and laboratory tests as recommended for the detection of arboviral infections.[20] A clinically compatible case of TOSV infection is defined as follows:

- Fever (≥38°C [≥100.4°F]) as reported by the patient or a health care provider, *and* absence of neuroinvasive disease, *or*
- Fever (≥38°C [≥100.4°F]) as reported by the patient or a health care provider, *and*

- Meningitis, encephalitis, acute flaccid paralysis, or other acute signs of central or peripheral neurologic dysfunction, as documented by a physician, *and*
- Absence of a more likely clinical explanation.

The laboratory tests necessary for virologic documentation are as follows:

1. *For confirmed cases:* A case that meets the foregoing clinical criteria and one or more of the following laboratory criteria for a confirmed case:
   - Isolation of virus from, or demonstration of specific viral antigen or nucleic acid in, tissue, blood, CSF, or other body fluid, *or*
   - Fourfold or greater change in virus-specific quantitative antibody titers in paired sera, *or*
   - Virus-specific IgM antibodies in serum with confirmatory virus-specific neutralizing antibodies in the same or a later specimen, *or*
   - Virus-specific IgM antibodies in CSF and a negative result for other IgM antibodies in CSF for arboviruses endemic to the region where exposure occurred.
2. *For probable cases:* A case that meets the foregoing clinical criteria for neuroinvasive disease and the following laboratory criteria:
   - Virus-specific IgM antibodies in CSF or serum but with no other testing.

Serology

Techniques such as indirect IFA, ELISA, complement fixation, and hemagglutination inhibition are broadly reactive (i.e., they can identify antibodies against virus strains within the Sandfly fever Naples antigenic complex). However, they cannot discriminate among the different strains. In other words, these techniques can hardly distinguish antibodies elicited by virus belonging to this serocomplex: TOSV versus other viruses such as Naples virus, another demonstrated human pathogen, but also Tehran, Massilia, Punique, Granada, Zerdali. Although some of these viruses are not demonstrated human pathogens, most of them can infect vertebrates; because sympatric distribution of several of these viruses is established (Massilia and TOSV, Punique and TOSV, Naples and TOSV), serologic cross-reactions can overestimate the prevalence of TOSV.[22,91]

Immunofluorescence Assay

Seroconversion and the detection of IgG or IgM can be achieved in cells infected with TOSV. Apart from homemade assays, Euroimmun AG (Lübeck) is commercializing a mosaic test that incorporate TOSV, Naples, Sandfly fever Sicilian virus, and Cyprus virus. This assay can more or less easily discriminate between Naples and TOSV antibodies and between Sicilian and Cyprus antibodies.

Enzyme-Linked Immunosorbent Assay

ELISA tests have been developed with crude antigens, purified virus, or recombinant nucleoprotein. One ELISA test detecting IgG and IgM is commercially available (DIESSE Diagnostica Senese).[35,57]

Rapid Immunochromatographic Test

An immunochromatographic assay has been developed for human anti-TOSV IgG or IgM detection, with performance similar to that observed with the commercial ELISA test.[51]

Neutralization Test

Techniques detecting neutralizing antibodies (plaque reduction neutralization test, virus neutralization test, microneutralization) are the tests of choice for definitive identification or confirmation of the results observed with broadly reactive assays. Although seroconversion remains the serology gold standard for establishing the diagnosis of viral diseases, the presence of specific IgM in a single serum sample is indicative of a recent infection.

Viral Isolation

Isolation from clinical samples can be achieved by using CSF or serum. TOSV replicates in a variety of animals; intracerebral, intraperitoneal, and subcutaneous routes lead to death in the newborn mouse; intracerebral and intraperitoneal routes lead to death in the weanling mouse; in the guinea pig and rabbit, intracerebral inoculation results in paralysis and irregular death, whereas intraperitoneal inoculation is not fatal and results in antibody synthesis. *Macaca fascicularis* succumbs after intracerebral inoculation but recovers with antibody production after intraperitoneal inoculation.[53] TOSV replicates in Vero, BHK-21, CV-1, and SW13 cells with cytopathic effect but not in C6/36 cells.[53,86]

Genome Amplification by Reverse Transcriptase Polymerase Chain Reaction Assays

Molecular diagnosis of TOSV can be achieved using three different real-time reverse transcriptase PCR assays that can be used to detect viral RNA in either CSF or serum of suspect cases.[17,69,90] Over time, this technology has progressively supplanted classic PCR and nested PCR assays.[75,78,83]

GENETIC DIVERSITY OF TOSCANA VIRUS

TOSV has been isolated from sandflies of two different species, *P. perniciosus* and *P. perfiliewi;* from humans; and once from a bat *(P. kuhlii).* Viral TOSV RNA was detected in dog sera, but no virus isolation was obtained.[30,92] The prototype TOSV strain, ISS Phl.3, isolated from *P. perniciosus* in 1971, has been sequenced completely and is used as reference for further genetic studies.[1,29,49]

Many strains from Italy have been partially sequenced, and only minor differences in nucleoprotein sequences were found among strains isolated in the early 1980s from both species of sandflies, from the bat, and from humans, with no more than one amino acid substitution.[62] Studies conducted with partial sequences in the polymerase gene indicate that a distinct genotype of TOSV is present in Spain.[75] This finding suggests the presence of at least two topotypes of TOSV, commonly designated lineage A and lineage B. Interestingly, strains from both lineages are co-circulating only in France and in Turkey.[30] A third lineage (lineage C) was identified in Croatia and in Greece.[67,74] Distribution of the topotypes or lineages is presented in Fig. 191E.1.

NEW REFERENCES SINCE THE SEVENTH EDITION

2. Alkan C, Allal-Ikhlef AB, Alwassouf S, et al. Virus isolation, genetic characterization and seroprevalence of Toscana virus in Algeria. *Clin Microbiol Infect.* 2015;21(11):1040.e1-1040.e9.
6. Anagnostou V, Papa A. Seroprevalence of Toscana virus among residents of Aegean Sea islands, Greece. *Travel Med Infect Dis.* 2013;11(2):98-102.
7. Andayi F, Charrel RN, Kieffer A, et al. A sero-epidemiological study of arboviral fevers in Djibouti, Horn of Africa. *PLoS Negl Trop Dis.* 2014;8(12):e3299.
9. Baklouti A, Leparc-Goffart I, Piorkowski G, et al. Complete coding sequences of six Toscana virus strains isolated from human patients in France. *Genome Announc.* 2016;4(3).
12. Bichaud L, Izri A, de Lamballerie X, Moureau G, Charrel RN. First detection of Toscana virus in Corsica, France. *Clin Microbiol Infect.* 2014;20(2):O101-O104.
17. Brisbarre N, Plumet S, Cotteaux-Lautard C, et al. A rapid and specific real time RT-PCR assay for diagnosis of Toscana virus infection. *J Clin Virol.* 2015;66:107-111.
19. Calzolari M, Angelini P, Finarelli AC, et al. Human and entomological surveillance of Toscana virus in the Emilia-Romagna region, Italy, 2010 to 2012. *Euro Surveill.* 2014;19(48):20978.
27. Dahmani M, Alwassouf S, Grech-Angelini S, et al. Seroprevalence of Toscana virus in dogs from Corsica, France. *Parasit Vectors.* 2016;9(1):381.
30. Dincer E, Gargari S, Ozkul A, Ergunay K. Potential animal reservoirs of Toscana virus and coinfections with *Leishmania infantum* in Turkey. *Am J Trop Med Hyg.* 2015;92(4):690-697.
31. Dincer E, Karapinar Z, Oktem M, et al. Canine Infections and Partial S Segment sequence analysis of Toscana virus in Turkey. *Vector Borne Zoonotic Dis.* 2016;16:611-618.
35. Dupouey J, Bichaud L, Ninove L, et al. Toscana virus infections: a case series from France. *J Infect.* 2014;68(3):290-295.
42. Erdem H, Ergunay K, Yilmaz A, et al. Emergence and co-infections of West Nile virus and Toscana virus in Eastern Thrace, Turkey. *Clin Microbiol Infect.* 2014;20(4):319-325.
44. Ergunay K, Ayhan N, Charrel RN. Novel and emergent sandfly-borne phleboviruses in Asia Minor: a systematic review. *Rev Med Virol.* 2017;27(2).
46. Es-Sette N, Ajaoud M, Anga L, Mellouki F, Lemrani M. Toscana virus isolated from sandflies, Morocco. *Parasit Vectors.* 2015;8:205.

48. Fezaa O, M'ghirbi Y, Savellini GG, et al. Serological and molecular detection of Toscana and other Phleboviruses in patients and sandflies in Tunisia. *BMC Infect Dis*. 2014;14:598.
56. Magurano F, Baggieri M, Gattuso G, et al. Toscana virus genome stability: data from a meningoencephalitis case in Mantua, Italy. *Vector Borne Zoonotic Dis*. 2014;14(12):866-869.
57. Marlinge M, Crespy L, Zandotti C, et al. Afebrile meningoencephalitis with transient central facial paralysis due to Toscana virus infection, southeastern France, 2014 [corrected]. *Euro Surveill*. 2014;19(48):20974.
59. Mosnier E, Charrel R, Vidal B, et al. Toscana virus myositis and fasciitis. *Med Mal Infect*. 2013;43(5):208-210.
65. Nougairede A, Bichaud L, Thiberville SD, et al. Isolation of Toscana virus from the cerebrospinal fluid of a man with meningitis in Marseille, France, 2010. *Vector Borne Zoonotic Dis*. 2013;13(9):685-688.
66. Ocal M, Orsten S, Inkaya AC, et al. Ongoing activity of Toscana virus genotype A and West Nile virus lineage 1 strains in Turkey: a clinical and field survey. *Zoonoses Public Health*. 2014;61(7):480-491.
67. Osborne JC, Khatamzas E, Misbahuddin A, et al. Toscana virus encephalitis following a holiday in Sicily. *Pract Neurol*. 2016;16(2):139-141.
69. Papa A, Paraforou T, Papakonstantinou I, et al. Severe encephalitis caused by Toscana virus, Greece. *Emerg Infect Dis*. 2014;20(8):1417-1419.

The full reference list for this chapter is available at ExpertConsult.com.

SUBSECTION XII Retroviridae

192 Human Retroviruses

192A ▪ Oncoviruses (Human T-Cell Lymphotropic Viruses) and Lentiviruses (Human Immunodeficiency Virus Type 2)

Michael A. Tolle • Susan L. Gillespie

In the 1980s retroviral infections were identified to be the cause of significant disease in humans, namely, human immunodeficiency virus (HIV) and human T-lymphotropic virus (HTLV) infections. Since that time, approximately 78 million people have been infected with HIV and 10 to 15 million with HTLV. Human retroviruses have a zoonotic origin. It is now well established that HIV and HTLV originated from simian retroviruses in nonhuman primates (NHPs) that crossed the species barrier to humans on several occasions, leading to the HIV and HTLV epidemics.[418]

The discovery of human T-cell lymphotropic virus type 1 (HTLV-1) in 1980 demonstrated for the first time that humans could be infected by retroviruses, which previously were known as animal pathogens that could cause malignant disease.[426] HTLV-1 subsequently was found to cause adult T-cell leukemia/lymphoma (ATLL) and now is recognized to be associated with the following spectrum of disease manifestations: a chronic degenerative neurologic disease (HTLV-1–associated myelopathy [HAM]/tropical spastic paraparesis [TSP]); relapsing, severe generalized dermatitis in children (infective dermatitis); and numerous inflammatory or autoimmune conditions, or both, such as uveitis, arthropathy, polymyositis, bronchoalveolitis, and Sjögren syndrome.[440] In 1982, a second antigenically related retrovirus of the oncovirus subfamily, HTLV-2, was identified from a patient with a T-cell variant of hairy cell leukemia.[250] The pathogenicity of this virus has become more clear over the years, being associated with other lymphoproliferative diseases and neuromyopathies, including diseases similar to HAM/TSP.[52,86,458,487] The subsequent discovery of HTLV-3 and HTLV-4 demonstrated that diversity among these viruses is greater than previously understood.

HIV-1 was identified as the cause of acquired immunodeficiency syndrome (AIDS) in 1983. HIV-2, a related but antigenically distinct virus, was isolated for the first time in 1986 from two West African patients.[101] HIV-1 and HIV-2 are lentiviruses.

CLASSIFICATION

Retroviruses form a large and diverse family of single-stranded RNA viruses that are unusual because they contain a diploid RNA genome that replicates by flow of genetic information through a DNA intermediate, a process known as reverse transcription. The name retrovirus is derived from this characteristic. This unique capability results from the presence of a virally encoded RNA-dependent DNA polymerase, reverse transcriptase, which catalyzes transcription of viral RNA into a double-stranded DNA copy. This viral DNA intermediary becomes integrated into host-cell DNA, where it then resides as a provirus; this process occurs by a specialized recombination mechanism requiring another viral protein, integrase. This capacity for genomic integration correlates with the capability of retroviruses to cause lifelong infection, evade the usual mechanisms of immune clearance, and produce chronic diseases in the host that manifest only after a long asymptomatic period that may last years to decades. Retroviruses infect both animals and humans.

Retroviruses can be categorized as being either exogenous or endogenous. Exogenous retroviruses such as HIV and HTLV are transmitted between individuals and across species, whereas endogenous retroviruses have become part of the genetic material of their host species through the chromosomal integration of viral DNA in the host germ cells, which then allows for vertical transmission of viral genetic material and fixation in the host population. Through whole-genome sequencing, it is estimated that 1% of the human genome consists of human endogenous retrovirus sequences resulting from infections millions of years ago.

The classification of retroviruses has been complicated by the ongoing discovery of new viruses and elucidation of their genetic organization and replication. At one time, retroviruses were divided historically into three subfamilies on the basis of nucleotide sequences and genetic organization. The subfamilies were the Oncovirinae (oncogenic or transforming viruses, which include HTLV), the Lentivirinae (slow viruses with cytopathic effects, which include human immunodeficiency virus types 1 [HIV-1] and 2 [HIV-2]), and the Spumavirinae (foamy viruses). Retroviruses have been also classified according to morphologic and biologic criteria based on the observance of retroviral particles in infected cells. Currently, human retroviruses have been broadly classified in to five groups, three of which include only endogenous viruses

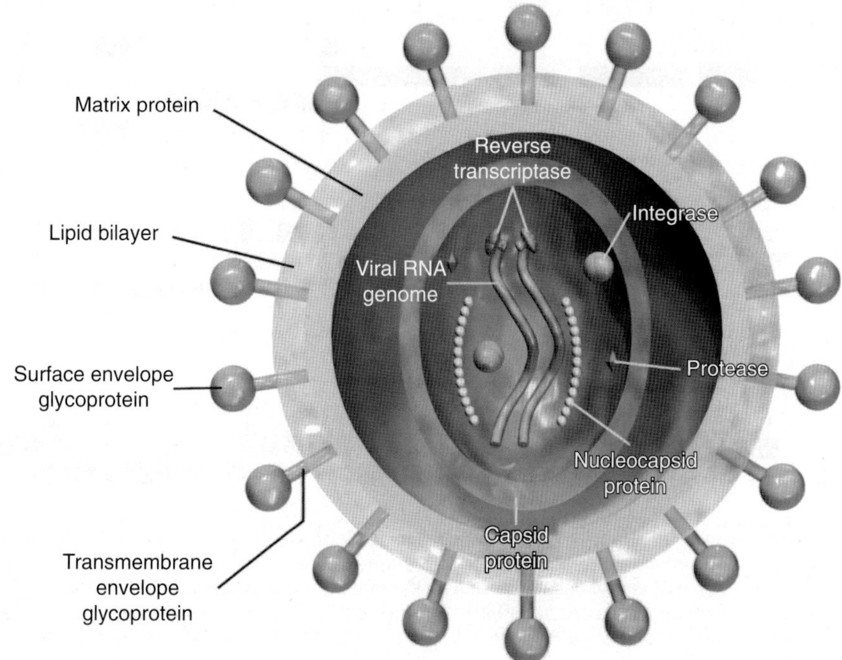

FIG. 192A.1 Retroviral structure. The mature retroviral virion is spherical; the central viral core is spherical in human T-cell lymphotropic virus oncoviruses and cylindric in human immunodeficiency virus lentiviruses. The core is surrounded by a lipid bilayer envelope derived from the host-cell membrane during bussing, the surface projections consisting of the viral surface and transmembrane envelope proteins. The viral matrix protein surrounds the virion core and is associated with the viral transmembrane envelope glycoproteins. The virion core is a structural shell composed of the viral capsid proteins. Within the shell are two copies of single-stranded viral RNA and multiple copies of the virally encoded reverse transcriptase, protease, and integrase enzymes. The viral nucleocapsid protein is bound to the RNA copies and may serve to condense the viral RNA into the capsid shell during virion assembly.

(betaretroviruses, spumaviruses, and gammaretroviruses) and two groups for exogenous viruses (lentiviruses [e.g., HIV] and deltaretroviruses [e.g., HTLV]).

Morphology and Genomic Structure

Retroviruses have a distinct morphology. They are enveloped RNA viruses that have a diameter of 80 to 120 nm; a thin, electron-dense outer envelope; and an electron-dense core that is either spherical (HTLV) or cylindrical (HIV). The envelope of all retroviruses comprises a lipid bilayer derived from the host-cell plasma membrane during budding of the virus from the cell surface, with surface projections consisting of the viral envelope proteins (Fig. 192A.1). The retroviral core protein encloses a ribonucleoprotein of genomic RNA complexed with viral reverse transcriptase and integrase.[102] The genome is a messenger-sense, linear, single-stranded RNA comprising two identical subunits held together by hydrogen bonds at their 5′ ends. The 5′ and 3′ ends of the RNA contain repeated sequences that give rise to elements in viral DNA called *long terminal repeats* (LTRs).

The LTRs are composed of nucleic acid sequences that provide signals critical for structural transformation of the viral genome, including initiation and progression of reverse transcription of viral RNA into DNA, integration of viral DNA into the host genome by viral integrase, and initiation of viral messenger RNA (mRNA) transcription from the integrated provirus and binding sites for viral and cellular proteins, and that positively and negatively influence mRNA transcription.[445,515,541,581] Between the LTRs are the genes that encode the major structural proteins of the virus, the enzymes found in the viral particles, and additional proteins with specialized intracellular functions.

As noted earlier, all retroviruses contain a minimum of three genes: *gag, pol,* and *env.* They are arranged in a 5′ to 3′ order, with LTRs at each end (Fig. 192A.2). The *gag* gene encodes the structural protein products that form the core particle of the virus, including nucleocapsid, capsid, and matrix proteins. The *pol* gene products include the enzymes required for genome replication (viral RNA–dependent DNA polymerase and ribonuclease H), proviral integration (integrase), and polyprotein processing (protease). The *env* gene encodes the major components of the viral coat, the surface, and transmembrane glycoproteins. Retroviral genes generally are expressed first as large, overlapping polyproteins that undergo processing into functional peptide products by viral or cellular proteases.

Oncoviral Regulatory and Accessory Genes

In addition to the standard retroviral genes, the oncoviruses HTLV-1 and HTLV-2 contain several regulatory and accessory genes important for viral replication and activation of host genes that are encoded in open reading frames (ORFs) in a unique region at the 3′ end of the genome called the pX region.[5,230] The HTLV-1 pX region contains four ORFs, whereas HTLV-2 contains five ORFs. Two of these ORFs common to both viruses (ORF III and ORF IV) encode the regulatory proteins Rex and Tax.

The regulator of expression of virion proteins gene *(rex)* encodes a nucleolus-localizing phosphoprotein that affects mRNA splicing and export from the nucleus to the cytoplasm. For cellular genes, mRNA splicing and export are tightly coupled. After cellular genes are transcribed into mRNA, splicing occurs in the cell nucleus before mRNA can be exported into the cytoplasm for translation into proteins. Incompletely spliced mRNA molecules are retained in the nucleus.[343,344,515] However, for retroviral reproduction, the export of full-length, unspliced viral RNA into the cytoplasm is required to serve as genomic RNA for integration into progeny virions and mRNA for the production of viral structural proteins. Thus retroviruses had to develop a mechanism to bypass the cellular regulatory process; for HTLV, the Rex protein serves this function. This protein is expressed predominantly at an early stage of viral gene expression and enhances the transport of single-spliced and unspliced viral mRNA coding for structural proteins, as well as transport of the viral genome from the nucleus to the cytoplasm. The Rex protein also

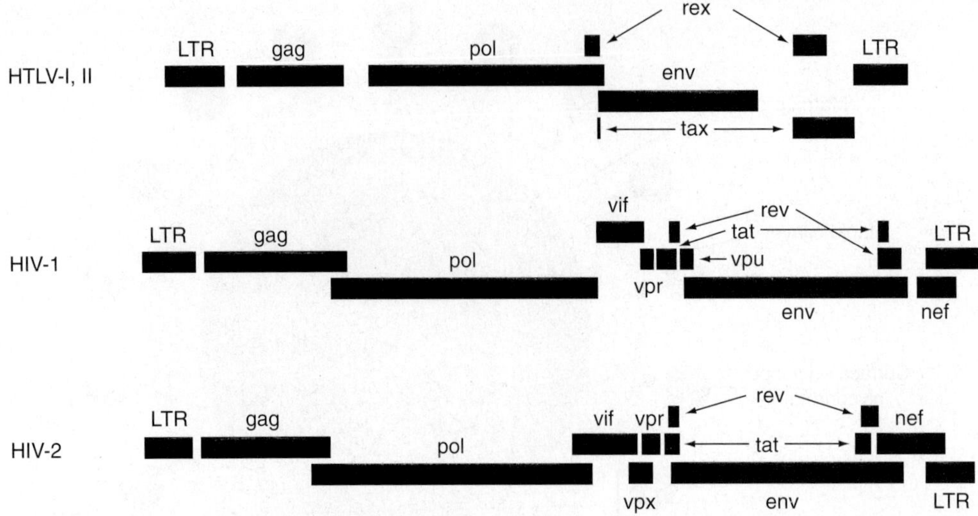

FIG. 192A.2 Retroviral genome. This schematic depiction of the human T-cell lymphotropic virus (HTLV) and human immunodeficiency virus (HIV) genomes shows that HTLV has a more complex genome than most animal retroviruses do and that HIV, in turn, has additional regulatory genes. Details of the functions of these genes are summarized in the text. *LTR,* Long terminal repeat. (From Gallo RC, Wong-Staal F, Montagnier L, et al. HIV/HTLV gene nomenclature. *Nature.* 1988;333:504.)

exerts a negative effect on the transport of multiply spliced viral mRNA to the cytoplasm. These multiply spliced mRNA molecules code for regulatory proteins, including Rex and Tax.[541]

The transactivator gene *(tax)* encodes a nuclear protein that plays a critical role in the regulation of viral replication and also stimulates a large number of cellular genes involved in activation and proliferation of T cells, including lymphokines, lymphokine receptors, and nuclear protooncogenes.[595,596] The Tax protein does not bind directly to DNA but rather interacts with host-cell transcriptional factors to produce a multifaceted array of molecular effects.[46] The Tax protein activates mRNA transcription by binding to several different host-cell transcription-enhancing factors, including those of the nuclear factor (NF)-κB family. In addition to activating transcription of the HTLV genome, the Tax transcription factor complex stimulates transcription of many cellular genes, including those encoding interleukin-2 (IL-2), IL-2 receptor-α, tumor necrosis factor (TNF), cyclooxygenase 2 (a prostaglandin synthetase), and some nuclear oncogenes.[358,595,596] Tax also represses transcription of tumor suppression genes and the expression of cellular DNA polymerase-β, a key enzyme for repair of damaged DNA. Additionally, Tax can bind directly to and inhibit some cell cycle regulation and tumor suppressor proteins, thereby interfering with cell cycle regulation and resulting in abnormal promotion of the cell cycle and enhancement of cellular proliferation.[596] Finally, Tax increases the genetic instability of the cell by impairing cellular DNA repair mechanisms, a process that leads to an accumulation of mutations and an increase in chromosomal anomalies. In vitro, Tax protein can immortalize human T cells and induce tumors in transgenic mice. However, in vivo, malignant disease develops in fewer than 5% of HTLV-1–infected individuals. Thus, although the *tax* gene probably is involved in malignant transformation of infected T cells, this is not sufficient by itself to explain the final development of malignancy.[7,546,595,596]

Less is known about the function of the HTLV accessory proteins that are encoded by the remaining ORFs in the pX region (e.g., p12, p13, and p30 in HTLV-1; p10, p11, p22/20, and p28 in HTLV-2). The best characterized accessory protein is HTLV-1 p12 from ORF I, which is a conserved, hydrophobic protein localized to the internal cell plasma membrane and perinuclear regions of the cell.[92] The p12 protein contains amino acid motifs commonly found in proteins involved in intracellular signaling pathways and probably interacts with cellular proteins, perhaps cellular kinases, to modulate intracellular signaling in infected cells. The protein also interacts with the β and γ chains of the IL-2 receptor. This protein may be required for activation of host cells during the early stages of infection, for cellular transformation, and for efficient viral infectivity, similar to the function of the *nef* gene of the lentivirus HIV-1.[3] The corresponding ORF I protein in HTLV-2, p10, does not bind the IL-2 receptor and is not associated with the constitutive activation of the IL-2 signaling pathway that is seen with HTLV-1–transformed cells.[92] These differences may be associated with differences in pathogenicity between the two oncoviruses.

Lentiviral Regulatory and Accessory Genes

More detailed data are available on the function of lentiviral genes.[144] The lentiviruses HIV-1 and HIV-2 have more complex genomes containing at least six regulatory genes in addition to *env, gag,* and *pol.* The lentiviral genes corresponding to the oncoviral *tax* and *rex* are called *tat* and *rev*; these genes are found in all known human and animal lentiviruses and appear to be essential for replication.[343,344]

Like the oncoviral *rex* gene, *rev* is expressed early in the viral replication cycle and undergoes splicing in the nucleus; multiply spliced *rev* mRNA transcripts then are exported to produce Rev protein in the cytoplasm. This protein contains a nuclear localization signal that facilitates entry of the protein back into the nucleus. Rev then binds to unspliced viral mRNA at a *cis*-acting Rev response element (RRE) located on the mRNA. A nuclear export signal sequence on the carboxy-terminal domain of Rev next targets the unspliced viral mRNA for export to the cytoplasm by binding to the cellular protein CRM1 (exportin 1) and exiting the nucleus through the host-cell export pathway.[108] The full-length unspliced viral mRNA then serves as a translational template for expression of the Gag and Pol proteins and also serves as genomic RNA for incorporation into new virions.

In contrast to the oncoviral Tax protein, which binds to host-cell proteins and has multiple effects in addition to promoting initiation of HTLV gene transcription, the lentiviral Tat protein binds to an RNA target, the Tat activation region (TAR), located immediately 3′ to the LTR transcription start site, and plays a primary role in the expression of HIV viral transcripts by enhancing mRNA elongation. At least two host-cell cofactors are involved in this process.[599] Cellular cyclin T binds to the activation domain of Tat, which increases both the affinity and specificity of the resulting complex for TAR. A host-cell encoded kinase then is recruited to the Tat-cyclin T-TAR complex and phosphorylates the carboxyl-terminal domain of the host-cell RNA polymerase II, which in turn enhances mRNA transcript elongation.

The remaining lentiviral accessory regulatory genes *nef, vpr,* and *vif* provide fine-tuning by enhancing or, less commonly, by diminishing viral replication. Another accessory gene, *vpu,* is found only in HIV-1, whereas HIV-2 and simian immunodeficiency virus lack the *vpu* gene but contain a gene called *vpx*. The *nef* gene, like *tat* and *rev*, is expressed early in the replication cycle. Similar to the HTLV-1 p12 protein, *nef* encodes a hydrophobic, membrane-associated protein that probably interacts with and modulates cellular signaling pathways and is required for optimal infectivity in vivo and for activation of infected host cells. Nef protein significantly enhances the cytoplasmic delivery of viral particles entering the cell through fusion at the plasma membrane, possibly by enhancing phosphorylation of the viral matrix protein and thereby allowing dissociation of the matrix and associated preintegration nucleoprotein complex from the virion capsid proteins.[470,515] Nef also downregulates cell surface expression of CD4+ by accelerating $CD4^+$ receptor endocytosis through interaction with the cytoplasmic tail of $CD4^+$ and a protein complex (i.e., AP-2 adaptor complex) responsible for recruiting membrane-associated proteins to clathrin-coated pits for endocytosis.[144] This process reduces the potential interference of membrane-associated $CD4^+$ with the release of budding virions. Major histocompatibility complex (MHC) class I receptor expression also is downregulated by Nef.

The Vpr protein is present in the virion itself, may act to regulate cellular events after penetration and uncoating of the virus to facilitate viral replication, and is involved in efficient localization of the nucleoprotein preintegration complex into the nucleus.[102,214] Vpr appears to interact with a specific site on nucleoporins in the nuclear pore complex to facilitate nuclear entry.[515] Similar to the Vpr protein, the HIV-2 Vpx protein is found in the virion and appears to affect the efficiency of early replication events, but the precise mechanism is unknown.[102,290]

The virion infectivity factor *(vif)* accessory gene is expressed late, along with structural and enzymatic proteins. The Vif protein is predominantly cytoplasmic but also exists in a membrane-associated form.[343,344] Vif protein is phosphorylated by a host-cell protein kinase, which seems to be important for viral growth in primary cells.[201] Vif appears to stabilize the preintegration provirus; viral particles that are produced in the absence of Vif are incapable of incorporating the provirus into host-cell chromosomes.[343,344] Vif also may function to prevent premature processing of Gag precursor proteins by viral protease in the cytoplasm, thereby ensuring that the Gag-derived peptides that form the viral nucleoprotein core are available at the plasma membrane for assembly with other viral components.

The HIV-1 *vpu* gene also is expressed late. The Vpu protein is associated with the endoplasmic reticulum in infected cells, where it binds the $CD4^+$ molecule and prevents it from translocating to the plasma membrane; instead, the $CD4^+$ molecule is targeted for proteolysis through the cytoplasmic ubiquitin-proteasome pathway.[144,515] This process prevents trapping and subsequent degradation of HIV envelope proteins by $CD4^+$ in the cytoplasm, thus increasing the ability of the viral envelope proteins to reach the cell membrane. Vpu, like Nef, also downregulates MHC class I receptor expression. In addition, Vpu may be important in virion assembly and release of particles.[95,177,564]

Viral Replication

The lentiviruses can infect and replicate in nondividing, terminally differentiated cells, and transmission can occur by cell-free or cell-associated virus. HIV-1 has high replication rates in vivo, with an average of 10^9 to 10^{10} viral particles produced each day. Free viral particles are estimated to have a half-life of less than 6 hours, and productively infected cells have a half-life of approximately 1 day.[228,387,570] The relentless rounds of reverse transcription rapidly generate extensive viral genetic variation within a single individual that results in a genetically related "swarm," or quasi-species, of viruses and provides the ability to escape the host immune response rapidly.

In contrast, the oncoviruses require that host cells undergo division for productive infection to be established, and they replicate in vivo largely by mitosis rather than by reverse transcription.[320] In addition, transmission is predominantly, if not solely, accomplished by means of cell-to-cell contact.[126] The events that occur during primary HTLV infection are reverse transcription of the viral genome, integration of the provirus into DNA, transcription of mRNA, synthesis of viral proteins, and a burst of viral expression. However, after a period of active replication, viral persistence is facilitated by a prolonged phase of clonal proviral expansion produced by transactivation of host-cell genes by Tax, which results in cellular DNA replication and the production of new cells containing the HTLV proviral genome.[361] Unlike viral nucleic acid replication by the error-prone viral reverse transcriptase, cellular mitosis is much less prone to mutation and generates little viral genetic variation. Moreover, the provirus remains hidden from immune surveillance. Thus oncoviruses have extraordinary genetic stability, in contrast to lentiviruses. The genetic variability of the HIV-1 envelope protein that exists within the viral quasi-species in a single individual 5 years after infection is greater than the genetic variability found in all HTLV-1 proteins identified worldwide to date.[569]

These differences are related to divergence among the retroviral subfamilies in genetic organization, transcription, and function of the major regulatory genes (*tax* and *rex* for the HTLVs and *tat* and *rev* for HIVs). The Tax and Tat proteins both are transactivating enhancer proteins. However, the HTLV Tax protein interacts with cellular proteins and activates cellular genes, thereby resulting in disruption of the cell cycle and induction of cell proliferation. In contrast, the HIV Tat protein has more focal effects; it recognizes a small RNA domain in the HIV LTR and serves primarily to transactivate HIV replication. The Rex and Rev proteins have similar functions; both interact with genomic mRNA structures (the Rex-responsive element and Rev-responsive element) to enhance transport of the unspliced and partly spliced viral mRNA molecules from the nucleus to the cytoplasm, and both also downregulate the transport of multiply spliced mRNA transcripts that encode for early regulatory proteins, including the mRNA molecules coding for themselves. In the oncoviruses, Tax and Rex are derived from the same mRNA; therefore downregulation of Rex mRNA transport results in decreased Tax mRNA transport and protein production. This process leads to diminished transactivation of HTLV genome transcription and prevents massive viral production. In contrast, the HIV Tat protein comes in two functionally equivalent forms, a 72- and an 86-residue protein. The 72-residue Tat protein is derived from a joint Rev/Tat mRNA, but the 86-residue Tat protein comes from a small Rev-independent mRNA. Although Rev, like Rex, has a negative effect on its own expression, as well as that of Tat, this effect is mitigated by the expression of a Tat mRNA that is not dependent on expression of Rev mRNA, thereby resulting in continued production of the Tat transactivating protein and constant and massive transcription of the HIV genome.

Retroviral Life Cycle

All retroviruses have two phases in their life cycle: an infection phase (including viral attachment, entry, reverse transcription, and proviral integration) and an expression phase (including transcription, translation, assembly, and budding of the virion) (Fig. 192A.3).[102] In general, more detail is known about replication in lentiviruses than in oncoviruses.

Infection phase of retroviral replication. Retroviruses attach to cells through recognition and binding of viral outer surface envelope proteins to specific proteins on the surface of the host cell; such cell surface receptor specificity probably accounts for the species and cellular tropism of retroviruses.[246,383] The surface glycoprotein of the retroviral envelope has three structural and functional domains separated by conserved hinges and is noncovalently linked to the transmembrane protein by disulfide bonds. The envelope transmembrane protein anchors the entire envelope glycoprotein complex on the virion surface and is responsible for the fusogenic capacity of the viral envelope. The transmembrane protein of all retroviruses has several conserved motifs, including a "leucine zipper" coiled motif followed by the N-terminal hydrophobic "fusion peptide" responsible for fusion with the host-cell membrane. After binding of the viral surface protein to the host-cell receptor occurs, conformational changes permit correct exposure of the transmembrane fusion peptide to the host-cell membrane. The interaction of several fusion peptides may serve to destabilize the lipid bilayer of the target-cell membrane by forming a "fusion pore" between the two bilayers[82] to facilitate fusion of the viral and cellular membranes and release of the viral RNA–protein complex into the cytoplasm.[198,500,546]

The cell surface receptor for HTLV-1 and HTLV-2 has not been characterized completely. Oncoviruses transmit infection primarily by fusion of infected cells with uninfected cells and the subsequent formation of syncytia. In HTLV-1, fusion is thought to be mediated by the HTLV envelope proteins expressed on the surface of infected cells and by cell

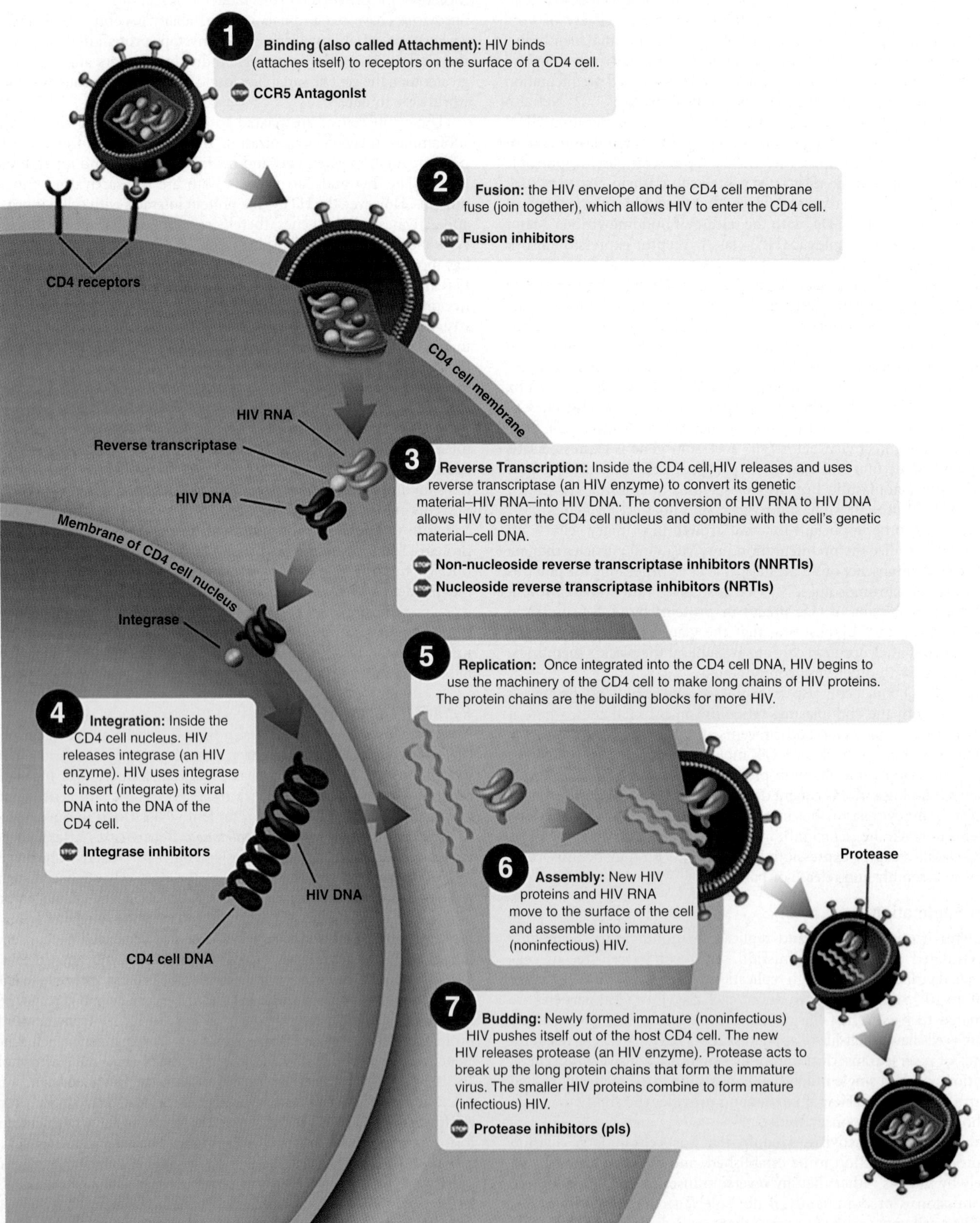

The HIV Life Cycle
HIV medicines in six drug classes stop HIV at different stages in the HIV life cycle.
1
Binding (also called Attachment): HIV binds (attaches itself) to receptors on the surface of a CD4 cell.
CCR5 Antagonist
2
Fusion: the HIV envelope and the CD4 cell membrane fuse (join together), which allows HIV to enter the CD4 cell.
Fusion inhibitors
CD4 receptors
CD4 cell membrane
HIV RNA
Reverse transcriptase
HIV DNA
3
Reverse Transcription: Inside the CD4 cell,HIV releases and uses reverse transcriptase (an HIV enzyme) to convert its genetic material–HIV RNA–into HIV DNA. The conversion of HIV RNA to HIV DNA allows HIV to enter the CD4 cell nucleus and combine with the cell's genetic material–cell DNA.
Non-nucleoside reverse transcriptase inhibitors (NNRTIs)
Nucleoside reverse transcriptase inhibitors (NRTIs)
Membrane of CD4 cell nucleus
Integrase
5
Replication: Once integrated into the CD4 cell DNA, HIV begins to use the machinery of the CD4 cell to make long chains of HIV proteins. The protein chains are the building blocks for more HIV.
4
Integration: Inside the CD4 cell nucleus. HIV releases integrase (an HIV enzyme). HIV uses integrase to insert (integrate) its viral DNA into the DNA of the CD4 cell.
Integrase inhibitors
HIV DNA
CD4 cell DNA
6
Assembly: New HIV proteins and HIV RNA move to the surface of the cell and assemble into immature (noninfectious) HIV.
Protease
7
Budding: Newly formed immature (noninfectious) HIV pushes itself out of the host CD4 cell. The new HIV releases protease (an HIV enzyme). Protease acts to break up the long protein chains that form the immature virus. The smaller HIV proteins combine to form mature (infectious) HIV.
Protease inhibitors (pls)

FIG. 192A.3 Life cycle of retroviruses. Details of viral replication are discussed in the text. (From AIDSinfo: The HIV Life Cycle. https://aidsinfo.nih.gov/education-materials/fact-sheets/19/73/the-hiv-life-cycle. Last updated 9/13/16.)

adhesion molecules, such as vascular cell adhesion molecule type 1 (VCAM-1), intracellular adhesion molecule type 1 (ICAM-1), ICAM-3, and the membrane permease CD98, on target-cell surfaces.[46] Although HTLV-1 envelope–expressing infected cells can form syncytia with cells from most cell lines, in vivo, HTLV-1 is found only in CD4$^+$ lymphocytes.[126] In contrast, HTLV-2 displays a preferential tropism for cells of the CD8$^+$ T-lymphocyte phenotype.[240,282]

The lentiviruses HIV-1 and HIV-2 infect cells that express CD4$^+$, the human leukocyte antigen (HLA) class II receptor, on their cell surface.[383] These cells include CD4$^+$ T lymphocytes, cells of the monocyte and macrophage lineage, and microglia in the brain. A high-affinity interaction between the surface glycoprotein and the CD4$^+$ receptor produces a conformational change that results in exposure of another site with high affinity for a secondary coreceptor required for the entry of HIV-1 and some HIV-2 isolates into the cell. The chemokine receptor CCR5 is the coreceptor used by monocyte-tropic and macrophage-tropic HIV-1, whereas the CXCR4 chemokine receptor is used by T-lymphocyte–tropic HIV-1; although most HIV-1 strains use only one receptor, some strains of HIV-1 are dually tropic and can use both receptors.[126] Additional coreceptors may support the entry of more restricted types of HIV isolates. For example, the chemokine receptor CCR3 is used by some macrophage-tropic HIV-1 strains and mediates entry of the virus into microglia; CCR2b, CR8, STLR/STRL-22, GPR15, GPR1, and the cytomegalovirus protein US28 also support entry by various HIV-1 and HIV-2 strains.[206,515] Whereas nearly all strains of HIV-2 can use CD4$^+$ together with the chemokine receptor CCR5 or CXCR4 (or both), most HIV-2 isolates also can interact with multiple other coreceptors.[206,515] Additionally, some HIV-2 isolates can use CXCR4 or other receptors, such as CCR3, as a primary receptor and infect cells lacking the CD4$^+$ molecule.[145]

Early postentry events include uncoating of the virus, which appears to require interaction of viral structural proteins with host-cell components that may have been incorporated into the virion during viral assembly. In HIV-1, interaction of the viral capsid protein with the host-cell cyclophilin A that is associated with the virion core during viral assembly may destabilize the multimeric capsid complex.[298,515] Additionally, a virion-associated host-cell protein kinase phosphorylates the viral matrix protein and thereby allows dissociation of the capsid and nucleocapsid proteins from the rest of the virus at the cell membrane. The HIV-1 Vif protein, which colocalizes with the Gag-derived proteins, is thought to confer enhanced stability to the remaining cytoplasmic viral nucleoprotein complex.

Retroviral RNA-to-DNA transcriptional events are initiated in the cytoplasm through the action of the viral enzymes reverse transcriptase (RNA-directed DNA polymerase) and ribonuclease. Viral single-stranded RNA is transcribed into a viral RNA/DNA hybrid complex by the DNA polymerase; the ribonuclease then destroys the original RNA and permits the DNA polymerase to complete transcription of a second DNA strand to form a linear double-stranded DNA copy of the original viral RNA.[198] Retroviral integration is mediated by a large nucleoprotein complex that forms in the cytoplasm and is called the preintegration complex. This complex includes the viral nucleic acids and a subset of viral proteins, including the matrix protein, reverse transcriptase, integrase, and, in the lentiviruses, Vpr.[515] The viral integrase enzyme component of this complex recognizes specific sequences within the viral LTR and cleaves two nucleotides from the 3′ ends as an initial processing step for integration; this process occurs while the preintegration complex is still in the cytoplasm.[19] Integrase appears to be the principal viral determinant of integration specificity.[292] In the lentiviruses, which can infect nondividing cells, the preintegration complex is imported actively into the nucleus during interphase. Nuclear transport is mediated by nuclear localization sequences on the matrix protein and on integrase and by interactions of Vpr with nucleoporins in the nuclear pore complex.

After nuclear entry has been gained, the integrase joins the recessed 3′ ends to phosphates in the host DNA for insertion of the DNA duplex into the host genome.[19,103] A final step in integration is thought to involve cellular factors that participate in DNA repair, in particular, a DNA-dependent protein kinase. This kinase is hypothesized to repair gaps left by the integrase around the sequence inserted into the host DNA; the result is a fully integrated provirus.[111]

Expression phase of retroviral replication. After viral DNA is integrated into the host cell, the proviral genome resembles other cellular genes and becomes highly dependent on the host cell for further replication, with the host-cell machinery used for replication, expression, and production of protein. Regulation of transcription is a complex process requiring interaction among the integrated proviral LTRs, host-cell DNA transcription factors, and the lentiviral Tat protein or oncoviral Tax protein.

The early phase of viral gene expression is characterized by the presence of spliced and unspliced viral mRNA in the nucleus, but only multiply spliced mRNA in the cytoplasm. In HTLVs, these mRNA molecules serve to direct production of the Tax and Rex regulatory proteins; in HIVs, they direct production of the Tat, Rev, and Nef proteins. The transition from early regulatory to late structural gene expression is characterized by the selective transport of unspliced and partially spliced mRNA into the cytoplasm. As discussed previously, in lentiviruses, this process depends on sufficient amounts of the Rev protein and, in oncoviruses, the Rex protein.[102,546] The unspliced or partially spiced mRNA transcripts that enter the cytoplasm encode for structural proteins and are first expressed as large, overlapping polyproteins. These polyproteins undergo processing into functional peptide viral structural components by the action of virally encoded and host-cell protease enzymes.

The retroviral Env protein is synthesized as a large precursor protein; it undergoes initial glycosylation in the endoplasmic reticulum, with subsequent disulfide bonding, folding, and oligomerization, and then is transported to the Golgi complex, where it is cleaved by a host-cell protease into surface and transmembrane proteins, which undergo further glycosylation.[126] The two mature glycoproteins are noncovalently associated through disulfide bonds. After cleavage occurs, the complexed proteins are transported and inserted into the plasma cell membrane by the cellular secretory pathway.[158,159]

The retroviral *gag* and *pol* genes are transcribed into a single mRNA transcript, which subsequently is translated into two separate polyprotein precursors, the Gag and Gag-Pol precursor proteins; the Gag-Pol polyprotein is translated by a ribosomal frame shift between the Gag and Pol mRNA reading frames. The Pol component of the Gag-Pol precursor protein is cleaved to form the viral enzymes reverse transcriptase, ribonuclease, and protease. The Gag precursor encodes the major structural proteins of the virion core, which do not undergo proteolytic processing into mature proteins until after assembly of the immature virion at the plasma membrane occurs.

Virion assembly and budding occur through targeting, accumulation, and association of different domains of the Gag and Gag-Pol precursor proteins at the inner face of the plasma membrane where the envelope proteins are being expressed.[158,159,562] The M domain, an amino acid sequence contained in the N-terminal area of the matrix portion of the Gag protein, has a membrane-targeting sequence that directs the Gag and Gag-Pol polyproteins to the cytoplasmic face of the plasma membrane. Myristylation of the N-terminal portion of some (lentiviruses) or all (oncoviruses) of the Gag precursor protein matrix domain is required for membrane targeting to occur and to allow Gag protein assembly at the membrane. In lentiviruses, the matrix domain interacts with the long cytoplasmic tail of the viral envelope transmembrane protein inserted into the membrane of the cell.[158,159] The I domain, an amino acid sequence contained in the nucleocapsid portion of the Gag polyprotein, participates in the Gag–Gag interactions to promote protein polymerization and also appears to be required for incorporation of the Gag-Pol precursor into virions.[158,159] The nucleocapsid domain of the Gag polyprotein interacts with viral genomic RNA through specific (sequence-specific nucleic acid binding) and nonspecific (interaction of basic residues with RNA) mechanisms and plays an important role in RNA binding, dimerization, and encapsidation and in facilitating Gag protein interactions and packaging into tight complexes.[98,158,159]

The interactions of these three domains in the precursor protein thus lead to assembly and emergence (but not release) of the viral "bud" from the cell surface.[413] On electron microscopy, large, electron-dense patches of Gag multimers, visualized under the plasma membrane, deform the membrane outward as they grow. More advanced intermediates appear as spheres connected to the cell by a thin stalk. During the process of budding, substantial amounts of cellular surface antigens, such as β_2-microglobulin and HLA-DR, are incorporated into the viral envelope. Additionally, during the process of virion assembly, host-cell proteins may be incorporated into the virion. For example, in HIV-1, a host-cell protein, cyclophilin A, interacts with the Gag polyprotein to form a complex in the virion core.[157,521] This host factor appears to be required for the formation of infectious virions, and it may play a role in early events after viral entry, as discussed earlier.[515]

In addition to the capsid, nucleocapsid, and matrix protein domains, other polypeptide segments that are required during the late stages of viral assembly are contained in the Gag polyprotein. They are referred to collectively as "late assembly" or "L" domains, and they are found in both lentiviruses and oncoviruses. In lentiviruses, the C-terminal portion of Gag (p6) includes a highly conserved amino acid motif that is needed to recruit the cellular machinery required for efficient release of budding virus from the cell membrane.[413,475,495,562] The Gag protein of oncoviruses also contains a late domain, although it is located in the N-terminal region of the protein.[495] Some investigators have suggested that these domains engage in interactions with host proteins that are located at the plasma membrane and that facilitate final release of the budding virus from the cell.

In HIV-1, the late domain is thought to interact with the cellular protein ubiquitin. Ubiquitin is a small protein present in cells that, together with cellular proteasomes, is involved in collecting or destroying cellular proteins that are damaged or no longer needed; it exists in cells as a free molecule or is covalently attached to lysines in a variety of proteins. When a protein is linked to multiple ubiquitin molecules (polyubiquitination), the protein becomes targeted for degradation by cellular proteasomes. However, when a protein is linked to a single ubiquitin molecule (mono-ubiquitination), instead of degradation, protein function is modulated; for example, mono-ubiquitination of plasma membrane receptor proteins promotes internalization and downregulation of the receptor through endocytosis in a nonproteolytic process that has some similarities to virus budding. After protein degradation occurs, the ubiquitin molecule is recycled as a free molecule. HIV-1 particles have been shown to contain ubiquitin, predominantly as a free molecule, but 2% to 5% of the Gag-derived, L domain protein p6 is mono-ubiquitinated.[495] One hypothesis is that the late domain of Gag contains an amino acid sequence that binds to residues on the ubiquitin ligase enzyme and thereby results in mono-ubiquitination of the Gag protein. The Gag-ubiquitin conjugate then may attract undefined cellular factors, perhaps those normally involved in endocytosis, that trigger release of the retrovirus from the cell membrane.[413] In the absence of the late domain, an infected cell becomes covered with virus that remains tethered to the plasma membrane by narrow stalks.

Maturation of the virion requires cleavage of the Gag precursor by the virally encoded protease and triggers structural changes that produce mature virions with the characteristic spherical oncoviral or cylindric lentiviral capsid. The Gag polyprotein gives rise to the following: the matrix protein, which lines the inner face of the viral membrane; the capsid protein, which forms a core shell surrounding the viral RNA genome and its associated proteins; and the nucleocapsid protein, which coats and condenses the RNA genome. This step occurs concomitantly with or immediately after the external budding process.

Diagnosis

Detection of retroviral antibody has been the test most widely used to diagnose infection in older children and adults. However, because of transplacental passage of maternal antibody, antibody testing during infancy (children <18 months) is not diagnostic of infection, and direct viral detection methods are necessary for establishing the diagnosis. Additionally, during primary infection, a window period exists during which ongoing viral replication is detectable by virologic tests, but antibody tests will be negative or indeterminant because a detectable antibody response has not yet developed.

Antibody testing for retroviruses most frequently involves the use of an initial screening test followed by performance of a more specific confirmatory test. Initial screening generally involves the detection of viral antigens from disrupted whole virus or synthetic or recombinant viral antigens in an enzyme-linked immunosorbent assay (ELISA). A positive ELISA is confirmed by the more specific immunoblot (or Western blot), which measures the presence of antibodies to various virus-associated proteins, both structural and nonstructural. Viral antigens (from disrupted whole virus or synthetic or recombinant antigens) undergo electrophoresis through polyacrylamide gel to separate the antigens by size. The separated antigens then are transferred to nitrocellulose paper, incubated with the patient's serum, and subsequently incubated with enzyme-linked antihuman antibody and chromogenic substrate, which results in visible bands where patient antibodies are bound by antigens. Analysis of band patterns permits more specific identification of the virus. Other techniques used to measure antibodies to retroviruses include indirect immunofluorescence assay (IFA), radioimmunoprecipitation assay (RIPA), and biologic assays for antibody to envelope glycoproteins (neutralization or syncytium inhibition assays).

Because antigenic differences exist between HIV-1 and HIV-2, HIV-1 screening tests are not reliable for the detection of HIV-2. Commercial HIV-1 and HIV-2 combination assays are available that have high sensitivity for detection of both viruses; a supplemental immunoblot assay is used to confirm the viral subtype.[91,325] Serologic diagnosis of HTLV infection is similar to that of HIV and involves the use of a screening enzyme immunoassay (EIA) and confirmatory immunoblot or RIPA. However, these tests do not distinguish between antibodies directed at HTLV-1 or HTLV-2.[90] In patients with positive serology, virologic detection tests, such as proviral amplification by polymerase chain reaction (PCR) or viral isolation, have been used.[115] Assays containing several synthetic peptides and recombinant proteins have been developed and appear to be capable of differentiating between HTLV-1 and HTLV-2.[65,454]

Direct detection of virus by culture is intensive, expensive, and time-consuming; several weeks often are required for results. The ability to isolate HTLV and HIV depends on the patient's disease state, immune status, and viral load. The ability to culture retroviruses has been improved by cocultivation of patient cells with human peripheral blood mononuclear cells that have been stimulated in vitro with mitogens (e.g., phytohemagglutinin) and growth factors (e.g., IL-2), as well as by removal of patient CD8+ (suppressor) cells from the coculture. In infants and children, the small volume of blood available for culture and the low virus load in some cases may render virus isolation challenging.

Other methods used for detecting virus include (1) antigen capture assays to detect free circulating viral antigens (e.g., p24 HIV-1 core antigen), (2) IFA and immunohistochemistry to detect viral antigens in tissue, (3) detection of viral nucleic acids by Southern blot analysis, (4) in situ hybridization or dot blots, (5) PCR to detect proviral DNA in leukocytes or tissue, and (6) assays to detect viral RNA in plasma or other fluids. DNA PCR can be used to quantitate virus and is highly sensitive because it is capable of amplifying tiny quantities of viral nucleic acids enzymatically to detectable levels with a system of specific nucleotide primers and probes. This technique can be modified to detect viral RNA by using reverse transcription to convert viral RNA to DNA and by performing PCR on the DNA product or by using other techniques such as branched-chain amplification or nucleic acid sequence-based amplification.[75,406,488]

ONCOVIRUSES: HUMAN T-CELL LYMPHOTROPIC VIRUS TYPES

Human T-Cell Lymphotropic Virus Type I

In 1980, HTLV-1 was reported as having been isolated from lymphocytes from a patient with cutaneous T-cell lymphoma, becoming the first oncoretrovirus to be described as infecting and causing disease in humans.[426] HTLV-1 is now recognized as the causative agent of not only ATLL but also HTLV-associated HAM/TSP and uveitis and is strongly associated with a variety of inflammatory and infectious disorders[577] (Table 192A.1), including autoimmune disorders, pneumonitis, tuberculosis, bronchiectasis, and, particularly in children, a severe infectious dermatitis. Unlike HTLV-2, in which coinfection with HIV-1 is associated with a survival benefit, HIV-1 and HTLV-1 coinfections are associated with reduced survival and possible increased risk for malignancies, HAM/TSP, and other neurologic disease.[39,41]

TABLE 192A.1 Basis for and Lifetime Risk for Diseases Associated With Human T-Cell Lymphotropic Virus Type 1

	EPIDEMIOLOGIC EVIDENCE			BIOLOGIC EVIDENCE		
	Case Reports or Case Series	**Case-Control Studies**	**Cohort Studies**	**HTLV-1 Present in Lesions**	**Animal Model**	**Lifetime Risk for Developing (for HTLV-1 Carriers) (%)**
Malignant Diseases						
ATLL	+	+	+	+	+	1–5[a]
Cutaneous T-cell lymphoma	+			+		
Inflammatory Syndromes						
HAM/TSP	+	+	+	+	+	0.3–4[a]
Uveitis	+	+		+	+	
Pulmonary disease	+					
Arthritis/arthropathy	+	+		+	+	
Polymyositis	+			+	+	
Sjögren syndrome	+			+	+	
Infectious Complications						
Infective dermatitis	+					
Tuberculosis	+	+				
Strongyloides stercoralis	+	+	+			
Crusted scabies	+					

[a]For HTLV-1–associated diseases in general, including ATLL, HAM/TSP, uveitis, arthritis/arthropathy, and polymyositis, lifetime risk approaches 10%.
ATLL, Adult T-cell leukemia/lymphoma; *HAM/TSP,* HTLV-1–associated myelopathy/tropical spastic paraparesis; *HTLV-1,* human T-cell lymphotropic virus type 1.
Modified from Verdonck K, Gonzalez E, Van Dooren S, et al. Human T-lymphotropic virus 1: recent knowledge about an ancient infection. *Lancet Infect Dis.* 2007;7:266-281.

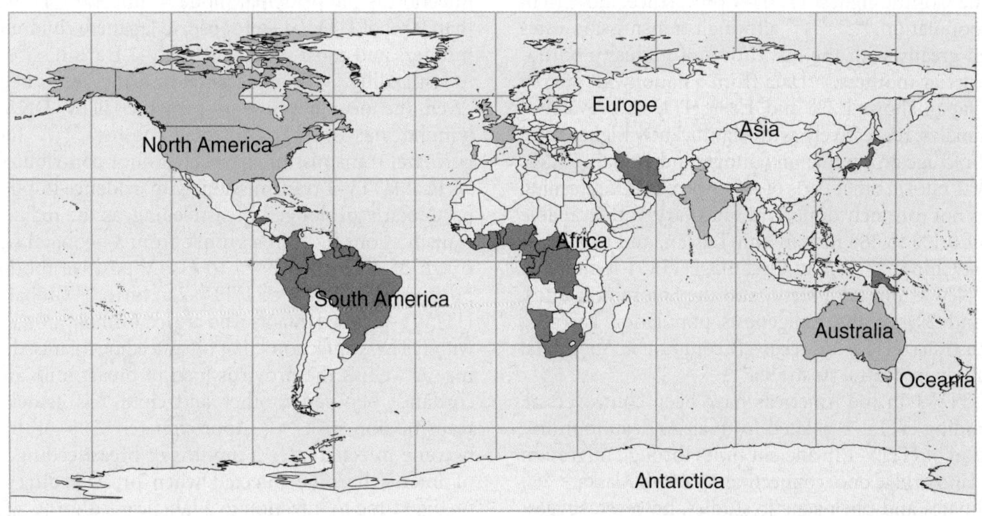

FIG. 192A.4 HTLV-1 epidemiology map. (From Proietti FA, Carneiro-Proietti AB, Catalan-Soares BC, Murphy EL. Global epidemiology of HTLV-I infection and associated diseases. *Oncogene.* 2005;24[39]: 6058-6068.)

Epidemiology

Although its disease implications are clear, most HTLV-1 infections are asymptomatic. It is estimated that 15 to 20 million persons are infected globally.[399] HTLV-1 is found in human populations around the world; however, its distribution is highly clustered, with highest prevalence in Japan, the Caribbean, and parts of tropical Africa and South America.[440] (Fig. 192A.4). Southwestern Japan, in particular, has the world's highest HTLV-1 prevalence, with rates as high as 37% in some communities,[364,586] whereas in much of Europe and North America, HTLV-1 rates are very low (<1%).[527]

Seven subtypes of HTLV-1 have been identified[550,551]: HTLV-1a is termed Cosmopolitan, and although its origins are in Africa, it is most widely distributed globally. Other subtypes include Australo-Melanesian subtype HTLV-1c and Central African subtypes HTLV-1b, HTLV-1d, HTLV-1e, HTLV-1f, and HTLV-1g.[550,551,558] The Cosmopolitan group has been divided further into five subtypes based on LTR sequencing: Transcontinental (A), Japanese (B), West African (C), North African (D), and Black Peruvian (E).[77,78] Transcontinental, subtype A, the most widespread, has been isolated from Japan, the Caribbean basin, South America, India, Iran, far-eastern Russia, and South Africa. Subtypes B and C are more restricted geographically, with subtype B found primarily in Japan and rarely in India and subtype C found in West Africa and the Caribbean basin. Subtype D has been identified in Morocco, Algeria, and elsewhere in North Africa. Subtype E, the most rare of the Cosmopolitan subtypes, was characterized from two Peruvians of African heritage.[77,78]

Phylogenetic data indicate substantial similarity between all HTLV-1 subtypes, with the exception of the Australo-Melanesian subtype HTLV-1c, which appears to have undergone a lengthy independent evolution separate from the other strains.[550,551] Molecular clock studies suggest that HTLV-1a, HTLV-1b, HTLV-1d, and HTLV-1e appear to have diverged in Africa from precursor primate T-cell lymphotropic virus type 1 (PTLV-1) between approximately 21,100 and 5300 years ago, with HTLV-1f a more recent emergent approximately 3000 years ago.[550,551] Phylogenetic studies,[550,552,556] along with the fact that Africa is the only continent where all PTLVs have been found (HTLV types 1 to 4 and their simian counterparts simian T-lymphotropic viruses [STLV] types 1 to 3),[558] suggest PTLV originated in central Africa.[550,552,556,558]

Growing interest in the population impacts of HTLV-1 in Africa have yielded new epidemiologic data from the continent in recent years.[213] A recent meta-analysis of data from 25 African countries yielded HTLV-1 seroprevalence ranging from 0% to 17%, with highest rates in West and Central Africa and lowest rates (0%) in many North African countries.[156] Within a given locale, risk varies among groups of individuals; in a Cameroonian study, HTLV-1 prevalence in individuals who had been bitten by an NHP was 8.6%, whereas in matched controls the rate was 1.5%.[153] Data from equatorial Africa indicate that a north-south gradient exists for HTLV-1 prevalence, with rates of 0% to 2% in Chad, the northern Central African Republic, and northern Cameroon to 5% to 10% in forested areas of Gabon, Equatorial Guinea, southern Cameroon, and southern Central African Republic.[301] Indeed, a cross-sectional survey in southern Central African Republic yielded a 7.4% prevalence of HTLV-1,[419] as well as suggestions that HTLV-1 was likely transmitted in Central Africa during the 1940s and 1950s when prophylactic injections of pentamidine were used as chemoprophylaxis for African trypanosomiasis.[420,419]

The broad dissemination of HTLV-1 beyond Africa was likely driven by the slave trade, along with increased mobility among populations, with HTLV-1a being introduced to Japan, the Middle East, North Africa, and the Americas.[170,171,179,491,551,552,558] Japan's southern islands of Kyushu and Okinawa have the world's highest HTLV-1 prevalence, more than 10% in the general population,[268,336,360,505] although transmission rates to infants have fallen greatly with the institution of exclusive bottle-feeding by HTLV-1 carrier mothers.[505] Data from a nationwide survey of blood donors in Japan showed 2% and 1.8% HTLV-1 prevalence rates in females and males, respectively, with significantly higher rates in the 40- to 64-year-old age group than in younger individuals.[469] Less is known about HTLV-1 rates in other parts of Asia where HTLV screening of blood donations is not routinely done, and rates vary, with available data showing rates of 0.1% to 1% in Iran and Taiwan, and as high as 2.6% in large cities in China.[1,303,567,584] In Oceania, HTLV-1 is endemic to Irian Jaya, Papua New Guinea, Vanuatu, and the Solomon Islands, with between 1% and 2% of the indigenous population carrying HTLV-1c.[82,166,509] In Australia, HTLV-1 is relatively common in Aboriginal populations, particularly in central Australia.[137]

The origins of HTLV-1 in the Americas have been controversial, with some data, including HTLV-1 isolated from an Andean mummy, suggesting introduction of HTLV-1 in ancient times through migration of persons across the land bridge once connecting Asia with Alaska.[77,78,551] Molecular clock estimates and phylogenetic studies, however, suggest that HTLV-1 arrived in the Americas first with the slave trade, and then again with Japanese immigration in the early 1900s.[77,78,421] Indeed, where HTLV-1 is prevalent in the region, including Jamaica and Trinidad and Tobago (up to 6% in both),[77,78,366] Martinique, Guyana, French Guiana, Suriname, Colombia, and northern Brazil, HTLV-1 is especially frequent among descendants of African slaves.[57,435,526] Studies of blood donors in Argentina and Peru demonstrate HTLV-1 rates up to 2%,[174,262,286] with higher prevalence in indigenous peoples.[191,409,467,601] HTLV-1 is generally rare in Central and North America, although there, too, notable rates (1–3%) have been seen in some indigenous groups.[409,191,558]

In Western Europe, HTLV-1 infection is generally rare,[558] with infections clustered in specific risk groups. In a British sexual health clinic, 0.7% of an HIV-infected population was coinfected with HTLV-1, with 80% of HIV-1 or HITLV-1 coinfected persons being females born in either sub-Saharan Africa or the Caribbean.[105] In a comprehensive survey of individuals infected with HTLV-1 in England and Wales between 2002 and 2004, more than 50% were of Afro-Caribbean origin.[133] In some parts of Western Europe, HTLV-1 is nearly nonexistent; in a survey of young heroin users in Spain, no HTLV-1 infections were recorded.[119] Eastern European rates may be higher, between 0.5% and 1%,[414] with Romania considered an endemic area for HTLV-1 and its associated pathologies, particularly ATLL.[309] However, in Eastern Europe, too, rates vary, with a recent survey of HTLV rates in IVDU in Estonia yielding a 0% prevalence.[247]

Modes of Transmission

Unlike HIV, HTLV-1 is not produced by infected T cells in appreciable quantities. Plasma HTLV-1 viral loads are virtually undetectable,[232] and its efficiency of transmission is accordingly much lower than that of HIV. HTLV-1 is transmitted by cell-to-cell contact as a provirus.[232] Hence its modes of transmission are those in which T cells themselves are transmitted and cell-to-cell interactions possible[249]—most commonly from mother-to-child during breastfeeding; parenterally through transfusion of infected cellular blood products or reuse of needles and syringes; and, much less efficiently,[399] through sexual intercourse. In areas endemic for HTLV-1, infection generally clusters in communities. This, along with the observation that seroprevalence declines in subsequent generations of people migrating from endemic to nonendemic areas,[343,344] suggest that biologic or social cofactors exist that affect HTLV-1 transmission.[316]

Mother-to-child transmission. Occurring in 4% to 22% of infants born to HTLV-1–positive women,[559] mother-to-child ("vertical") HTLV-1 transmission is the most important route of HTLV-1 acquisition[568] because, in addition to being the most common manner in which HTLV-1 is transmitted,[249] HTLV-1 infection in early life is associated with the development of adult T-cell leukemia/lymphoma (ATL), a key HTLV-I–associated pathology, later in life; indeed, approximately 1% to 5% of children infected through vertical transmission will develop ATL.[441,187,162] Vertical transmission rates as great as 31% have been seen in mothers coinfected with *Strongyloides* spp.[559] Vertical transmission of HTLV-1 infection is the principal mode of infection in children,[568] with more than 90% of HTLV-1–seropositive Japanese children having seropositive mothers and most perinatal HTLV-1 transmission occurring through breastfeeding.[372] Transplacental transmission is believed to be unlikely, given the near absence of proviral HTLV DNA in umbilical cord lymphocytes of HTLV-infected mothers.[465,545] Indeed, prenatal and perinatal transmission are likely minor contributors to the entirety of vertical HTLV-1 transmission, with evidence implicating breastfeeding, particularly prolonged breastfeeding, as the major source of perinatal transmissions.[372,512] In a sample from a neonatal screening program in Brazil of 42 infants born to HTLV-positive mothers, none was PCR positive for HTLV-1 or HTLV-2 at birth.[449] Globally, fewer than 3% of HTLV-1–exposed infants who are fed formula are subsequently diagnosed with HTLV-1 infection.[17] For breastfeeding infants, duration of breastfeeding, as well as the provirus load in breast milk and HLA class I concordance between mother and child,[50] is associated with increased transmission risk.[50,295] Approximately 5% of breastfeeding infants become infected after 3 months of breastfeeding, whereas up to 40% of infants become infected when breastfeeding is prolonged.[17] The median time to infection in a Jamaican cohort was 11.9 months,[163] and the passive transfer of maternal HTLV-1 is believed to be protective against infection.[17,449,512] Other associations with risk for vertical transmission of HTLV-1 include female gender of the child, older maternal age, long duration of membrane rupture (>4 hours), and lower maternal income.[220-222,257,506,545,574,575]

In some countries where HTLV-1 is endemic, including Japan, Brazil, and Martinique, HTLV-1 is screened for either in pregnancy or in neonates.[10,451,450,507] Policy in these countries and in other similarly well-resourced settings is for HTLV-infected mothers to completely avoid breastfeeding and for formula to be provided for HTLV-1–exposed infants. If breastfeeding is unavoidable, weaning before 6 months will prevent most HTLV-1 infections. Indeed, where this approach has been put into practice, HTLV prevalence has dropped sharply.[219,257]

Yet, although complete cessation or limiting breastfeeding has clear advantages for preventing perinatal transmission of HTLV-1, no international guidelines (World Health Organization, United Nations Children's Fund, Centers for Disease Control and Prevention [CDC], or similar) exist for breastfeeding and HTLV-1 prevention in resource-poor settings, which include most developing countries and most HTLV-1–endemic settings, particularly sub-Saharan Africa.[15] Although clear risks exist in HTLV-1 infection, including severe disease (e.g., ATL or HAM/TSP) in approximately 5% to 10% of infected persons and many other morbidities of variable impact, well-defined and substantial risks exist to both early weaning and formula-feeding,[553] particularly in resource-poor countries, yet high HTLV-1 prevalence is found in pregnancy in many settings.[17,148,553] Southeast Gabon, for example, has HTLV-1 prevalence in pregnancy in excess of 5%, one of the highest rates in the world,[148] whereas recent data from Malawi indicating maternal HTLV-1 prevalence of 2.6% demonstrate that mother-to-child transmission risks in Africa exist outside the previously recognized areas of West and Central Africa.[156]

Complicating issues for HTLV-1 transmission prevention in resource-poor settings is the recognition of breastfeeding as one of the most powerful child survival interventions, a cornerstone of efforts to reduce mortality worldwide in children younger than 5 years,[248] although African studies on prevention of perinatal HIV transmission have shown serious morbidity and mortality risks to be associated with formula-feeding. In Botswana's Mashi trial, cumulative mortality from all causes at 7 months was significantly higher (9.3% vs. 4.9%) in infants randomly assigned to formula-feeding versus those assigned to breastfeeding plus zidovudine (AZT). HIV-free survival at 18 months was equivalent between the two groups, showing that the early mortality increase seen with formula-feeding negates the benefits of reduced HIV transmission.[522] Work in Guinea-Bissau, where HTLV-1 prevalence is 5% and socioeconomic indicators are among the most austere in Africa, has shown increased risk for diarrheal diseases and mortality among children weaned before 12 months of age.[553,554] Additionally, during an outbreak of diarrhea in Botswana in early 2006, more than 22,000 Botswanan infants experienced diarrhea (in contrast to just more than 9000 over the same period in 2005), and the number of deaths in children younger than 5 years of age increased by 20-fold.[107] Virtually all deaths in the diarrheal cohort were in formula-fed infants, suggesting a lack of protective immunity in formula-fed versus breast-fed infants, a finding consistent with the long-appreciated immunologic benefits of breastfeeding. Malnutrition and growth failure are also more common in formula-fed than breast-fed HIV-exposed infants.[273]

It is unclear to what extent cesarean delivery or the use of antiretroviral drugs during and after delivery help prevent perinatal HTLV-1 transmission, as they have been shown to do with perinatal HIV transmission. Indeed, there have been no prospective studies of either antiretroviral therapy (ART) or delivery mode to evaluate the potential for augmenting perinatal HTLV-1 transmission efforts.[77,78] In a Brazilian study, none of the HTLV-1–exposed infants subsequently diagnosed with HTLV-1, including both those born vaginally and by cesarean delivery, were PCR positive for HTLV-1 shortly after birth, yet all had breast-fed, supporting perinatal HTLV-1 transmission as postnatal via breastfeeding.[449] Yet the finding that the duration of rupture of the membrane is associated with transmission of HTLV-1 suggests that some percentage of transmissions may occur intrapartum, and some HTLV-1–infected infants by maternal report did not breastfeed. The utility of cesarean delivery in preventing perinatal HIV transmission is chiefly in mothers with a detectable viral load at term, especially when viral load is high.[411] Currently, in most settings globally, HTLV-1 proviral load testing is not readily available for incorporation into decisions on mode of delivery, nor is formal guidance accessible on the use of either HTLV-1 proviral load testing or cesarean delivery in the management of perinatal HTLV-1 prevention.

Parenteral transmission. Parenteral transmission by transfusion and intravenous drug use is well documented and appears to be the most efficient mode of transmission, with an estimated 44% chance of infection occurring in those receiving HTLV-1–infected cellular products.[319] Comparative rates of transmission of HTLV-1, HTLV-2, and HIV-1 were evaluated retrospectively in a large repository of US blood donor serum from the Transfusion Safety Study.[130] Consistent with a requirement for cell-to-cell contact for transmission of HTLV and in contrast to HIV-1, transmission of HTLV-1 and HTLV-2 was observed only with the transfusion of cellular blood components. Infectivity appeared to decrease with an increasing period of blood storage; no apparent transmission occurred after the transfusion of components stored more than 10 days, a finding suggesting that the known decrease in the ability of donor lymphocytes to be activated or to proliferate with storage renders the cells noninfectious. In this study, rates of transfusion-related transmission of HTLV-1 and HTLV-2 were similar; approximately 27% of recipients of blood components from seropositive donors became infected. In contrast, 89% of the recipients of HIV-1–positive blood became infected, regardless of the blood product component type, and no effect of storage on transmission risk was seen. The median time to seroconversion after the transfusion of HTLV-1–contaminated blood products is 51 to 65 days.[440]

Over the past two decades in Japan, the United States, Canada, and much of South America and Western Europe, screening of blood donors for HTLV-1 and HTLV-2 has dramatically reduced the number of transfusion-associated HTLV infections and has contributed to reductions in HTLV prevalence in the general population.[120,133,440,558] Because many blood donors are repeat donors, exclusion of HTLV-infected donors from the eligible pool yields a resource-use benefit over time for blood banks, with fewer HTLV-positive tests seen year to year after instituting screening.[133] In the United Kingdom, where screening was instituted in 2002, by 2004 the number of HTLV-positive screens had fallen by more than 80%.[133]

However, in countries in which screening of blood for HTLV-1 and HTLV-2 is not performed, transfusions continue to provide an important source of infection. Patients with transfusion-dependent conditions, such as sickle cell disease, are especially at risk. In a study of hospitalized children in Gabon in Africa, multiple blood transfusions secondary to complications of sickle cell disease were as predominant a mode of transmission of HTLV-1 as perinatal transmission.[128] Similarly, in Martinique, HTLV-1 seroprevalence in patients with sickle cell anemia was 10% versus 1% to 3% in blood donors, and HTLV-1–seropositive patients had received more transfusions than had seronegative persons.[467]

Case reports detail multiple cases—in endemic countries or involving donors from endemic countries—of HTLV-1–associated disease after solid organ or bone marrow transplantation.[525] In all these cases, HTLV-1–associated disease occurred within a brief time (<2 years) after transplantation; it is likely that immunosuppressive treatment facilitates accelerated replication of HTLV-1.[525] In Japan, North America, and many European countries, organ donors are now screened for HTLV-1 infection.[18,331]

Intravenous drug use is a notable source of other parentally transmitted infections, such as HIV. Somewhat paradoxically, however, HTLV-1 is rarely detected in injection drug users,[119,440] especially younger cohorts.[119] A Spanish study of young injection heroin users showed no HTLV-1 in 981 injection drug users screened, whereas 27 individuals were HTLV-2 positive.[119] This study's HTLV-2 findings are not novel because HTLV-2 is considerably more commonly detected in injection drug users than HTLV-1,[440,558] and in Spain, almost all HTLV-2 infections are diagnosed in such users.[43,305,524] Some cohorts, however, defy this trend, with HTLV-1 prevalent among injection drug users in New York and Brazil,[149,558] and sharing needles is considered an effective transmission route for HTLV-1.[186]

Sexual transmission. Sexual transmission is a significant source for acquisition of HTLV-1 in adults. In serodiscordant couples, incident infection is low, with one cohort of 30 couples followed for 10 years yielding an HTLV-1 infection incidence estimate of 0.9 per 100 person-years.[460] Older cross-sectional studies suggested higher transmission efficiency from males to females,[284,371,440] but more recent cohort studies have shown no significant difference in male-to-female transmission compared with female-to-male transmission.[460] Nonetheless, HTLV-1 rates in settings worldwide are higher in females than in males, as are rates in older cohorts than in younger ones, suggesting a cumulative risk over time.[481,505] The infected individual's proviral load is likely an important factor in risk for transmission between discordant partners. In the Retrovirus Epidemiology Donation Study, which has enrolled volunteer blood donors from five participating blood centers since 1988, HTLV-transmitting men had proviral loads higher than those of nontransmitters.[256] Transmitting men also tended to have higher antibody titers against various viral proteins than did nontransmitters; in general, antibody titers correlated highly with proviral load.[256]

Similar to other sexually transmitted infections (STIs), HTLV-1 seropositivity is associated with higher numbers of lifetime sexual partners, presence of genital sores, paying for or receiving money for sex, and anoreceptive intercourse among men who have sex with men.[28,43,440,490,572] In studies from several different countries, prevalence of HTLV-1 has been found to be elevated in female sex workers.[127,192,576] In these studies, the lack of consistent use of condoms, the duration of prostitution, older age, infection with *Chlamydia trachomatis* or syphilis, antibody to herpes simplex virus type 1, and concomitant HIV-1 infection were associated with elevated HTLV-1 prevalence.[192,378] Among sex workers in Peru, condom use has been shown to protect against HTLV-1c infection.[192,531] An increased risk for HTLV-1 seropositivity has been observed in persons attending clinics that treat STIs.[152,264,378,572] In such clinics in the United States, HTLV seropositivity ranges from 0.18% to 2%; in the United Kingdom, rates in similar clinics were between 0.5% and 1%,[105,133] well higher than rates in the general population of less than 0.01% in both settings.

Descriptive studies have suggested that ecologic factors may influence the rate of seropositivity in a population; for example, residence in a lower altitude, tropical environment was associated with higher rates of seropositivity in some reports.[316,343,344] A role for insect vectors, such as mosquitoes, was postulated. However, no evidence has shown that retroviruses can replicate in arthropods, and any hypothesized insect-borne transmission would need to occur mechanically by the mouth parts of biting insects that were contaminated with a significant amount of infected and infectious lymphocytes; such transmission, if it occurred, would be expected to be very unusual.[154] However, a very strong epidemiologic association exists between infection with *Strongyloides* and HTLV.[185] A case-control study from Guadeloupe ties together *Strongyloides* infection and the socioeconomic and environmental risk factors (i.e., low socioeconomic status, low educational level, and agricultural activity) associated with many HTLV clusters noted in diverse tropical settings worldwide, suggesting that *Strongyloides* infection may increase susceptibility to HTLV infection and be responsible in some settings for both the notable clustering of HTLV within endemic areas and the decrease in HTLV prevalence noted in migrant communities from endemic areas over time.[106]

Disease Associations

In HTLV-1–infected individuals, persistent viral infection and antigen production elicit a strong humoral and cellular immune response that results in high antibody titers to HTLV-1 structural and regulatory proteins and increased circulating activated HTLV-1 Tax protein–specific cytotoxic T lymphocytes.[109,236] In addition, even in asymptomatic patients, spontaneous in vitro proliferation of lymphocytes is observed.[271]

Early in the course of primary infection, the HTLV-1 proviral load is high but becomes controlled rapidly. Within 90 days of primary infection, a narrow range of proviral load is observed in an individual that generally stays relatively constant over the course of time.[318,395,519] Antibody titer is highly correlated with proviral load after the initial set point is reached. The HTLV-1 proviral load in asymptomatic HTLV-1 carriers can be as high as 5% of all peripheral blood mononuclear cells, and it is particularly high in individuals with HAM/TSP, in whom as many as 20% of peripheral blood mononuclear cells can be infected.[318,361] A high peripheral blood proviral load appears to predate the development of neurologic and ophthalmologic HTLV-1–associated disease entities.

Although most individuals infected with HTLV-1 will remain symptom-free lifelong, regardless of age at time of infection or infection route, between 5% and 10% of infected individuals will develop HTLV-associated illness, which can be, especially in the case of ATL and HAM/TSP, extraordinarily severe.[381] Indeed, HTLV-1 may be a prototype for other retroviruses yet to be discovered that predispose to the development of active diseases with long latency after exposure at birth or early in life.

A variety of less intense clinical manifestations have been noted in HTLV-infected individuals, including uveitis, other rheumatic and neurologic conditions, pulmonary disease, other coinfections, and, especially in children, infective dermatitis.[25,81,425,440,558] Some manifestations of HTLV-associated disease are different in children and adolescents than in adults; HAM/TSP in children, for example, while rare, usually is associated with infective dermatitis and, unlike most cases in adults, is rapidly progressive.[25] Studies from Brazil of recently diagnosed individuals indicate that neurologic, ocular, and rheumatologic symptoms may be the first manifestations of HTLV-1 infection,[425] and in Brazilian cohorts with long-standing HTLV-1 infection, HTLV-1–infected individuals were more likely than controls to report extremity weakness or hand or foot numbness, arthralgia, nocturia, and oral findings such as gingivitis, periodontitis, or dry mouth.[81]

Adult T-Cell Leukemia and Other Malignancies

HTLV-1 is a truly oncogenic virus, with its prototype manifestation being ATLL.[381] First described in Japan by Takatsuki in 1977,[541] and the first disease to be causally linked to HTLV-1 infection, ATLL is a malignancy of mature peripheral T lymphocytes.[238] Approximately 3% of HTLV-I carriers will ultimately develop ATLL,[381] and ATLL is much more common in individuals who are thought to have acquired HTLV-1 infection perinatally.[542] After infection, HTLV-1 produces cell immortalization through Tax-1, which yields a clonal expansion of HTLV-1–infected T cells in a proportion of asymptomatic carriers who then manifest high proviral loads,[381,511,542] a risk factor for developing ATLL.[241,396] Other risk factors include increasing age (a mean of 57 years in Japan) and a family history of ATLL.[242]

The distribution of ATLL follows that of HTLV-1, with most cases in southwestern Japan, tropical Africa, the Caribbean, Middle East, Irian Jaya, Papua New Guinea, and parts of South America.[541] In hyperendemic southwestern Japan as many as 9.3% of patients newly diagnosed with hematologic disorders have ATLL,[238] and more broadly in Japan data suggests an incidence of approximately 0.37 per 100 HTLV-1 carrier years.[494] ATLL epidemiology is similar in endemic areas of the Caribbean such as Jamaica and French Guiana,[367] as well as in Brazil and Iran,[309] although average age of onset in Africa, Brazil, and the Caribbean is lower (42–49 years), and in both regions ATLL is more common in women than in Japan,[24,59,428,587,590] where the male-to-female ratio is 1.4 : 1.[309] One hypothesis for the younger age of ATLL onset in the tropics is the presence of *Strongyloides* coinfection. *Strongyloides stercoralis* stimulates clonal expansion of HTLV-1–infected cells in asymptomatic carriers, potentially serving as a cofactor for ATLL development.[169]

Outside endemic areas, ATLL is most commonly seen in immigrants from endemic areas, most of whom are assumed to have obtained their HTLV-1 infection perinatally.[337,339] In Great Britain and France, almost all ATLL cases are seen in first- or second-generation immigrants of African or Afro-Caribbean descent.[309,337,339] In the United States, the incidence of ATLL is low; cases are seen primarily in immigrants from HTLV-1–endemic areas or in blacks in the southeastern United States, in whom endemic HTLV-1 infection has been documented.[445] In a study in central Brooklyn, which has a large Caribbean migrant population, the annual incidence of ATLL in African Americans of all geographic backgrounds was approximately 3.1 per 100,000 person-years.[288]

Given the long incubation period generally associated with ATLL, the condition in children is quite rare. Most cases of ATLL in childhood occur in tropical countries; nearly half of those reported have been from Brazil.[59,103] Mean age of diagnosis in case reports in the literature is 15 years,[59,308,427,428] although cases have been diagnosed in children as young as 2 years.[427,428] In one case series, maternal HTLV-1 serology was positive in 16 of 19 cases where it was available,[59] with one of the three cases with maternal serology having received a blood transfusion and the other two having been breast-fed by women of unknown serologic status.[293,427,428] Most cases in children present similarly to cases in adults and, like adult cases, have poor outcomes.[59]

Given substantial diversity in how ATLL presents and evolves clinically, diagnostic criteria developed in Japan are used for classifying the malignancy into four major subtypes.[309,486] For diagnosis, histologically or cytologically proved lymphoid malignancy must be found, with expression of specific T-cell surface antigens; abnormal $CD4^+$ and $CD25^+$ T lymphocytes[37] with characteristic lobulated nuclei (so-called flower cells, containing monoclonal or oligoclonal HTLV-1 provirus integrated into the cell genome) in peripheral blood (except in the ATLL type), with many asymptomatic HTLV-1 carriers expressing a persistent leukocytosis; and positive serum antibodies against HTLV-1 at the time of diagnosis.[309] These criteria are summarized in Box 192A.1. Monoclonal expansion of HTLV-I–infected cells in carriers is directly associated with ATLL onset.[309] A method for detecting a persistently infected HTLV-1 monoclonal cell population could serve as a monitoring approach, especially for perinatally infected individuals at highest risk for developing ATLL.[309]

Why ATLL develops in only a small percentage of HTLV-1–infected individuals, including those infected perinatally and at greatest risk for ATLL, is not completely clear. Although ATLL is clearly linked to the integration of HTLV-1 into every malignant cell,[337,339] ex vivo studies of ATLL cells indicate lack of expression of viral proteins or RNA, and occasionally defective viral genomes are detected.[106,337] Because malignant transformation probably is a multistep process, intermediate factors such as the host immune response, oncogenic environmental stimuli, or both, may be involved.[230] Familial ATLL has been documented in several countries, including Japan, the United States, and the United Kingdom,[337,338,589,590] yet it is not known whether genetic predisposition is involved in the development of ATLL in such cases.[337,339]

Monoclonal HTLV-1 provirus is found integrated into the DNA of ATLL malignant cells. HTLV-1 is known to transform normal CD4+ lymphocytes in vitro and results in immortalization, high levels of IL-2 expression, and increased expression of the IL-2 α-chain receptor on the cell surface. The presence of excessive receptors for IL-2, a known growth factor for T cells, may be linked to development of the proliferative leukemic process of ATLL.[587,590] Additionally, the HTLV-1 Tax protein activates the promoters of many genes involved in cell growth and differentiation and interferes with DNA repair functions.[362] Indeed, studies of transgenic mice and human CD34+ stem cells suggest that Tax initiates ATLL because leukemia with ATLL features has been induced by Tax expression.[23,210,431]

One hypothesis is that the continuous proliferation observed in HTLV-1–infected cells may render them more susceptible to spontaneous mutagenesis, as well as to the effect of external carcinogens.[2] The finding that persistent clonal expansion of HTLV-1–infected cells precedes the development of ATLL suggests that tumor cells may originate in clonally expanding nonmalignant cells through a multistep process that may include the mutation or deletion of tumor suppressor genes such as *p53* or $p15^{INK4B}/p16^{INK4A}$, which are detected in 30% to 50% of ATLL cases and associated with clinical subtypes and prognosis.[42,168] Along with affecting tumor suppression genes and reducing DNA repair, Tax downregulates DNA polymerase B, affecting base excision repair[42] and suppressing nucleotide excision repair.[118,254] Tax also reduces the activity of telomerase, contributing to changes in chromosome number[42,168,254]; ATLL cells are usually aneuploid.[328] Accordingly, chromosomal fusions and shortened telomeres are also regularly detected in ATLL cells, perhaps reflecting this decreased human telomerase expression in early transformation stages.[42,168]

The host immune response also may be involved in malignant transformation because cells may escape immune surveillance by deleting Tax,[37] the major target of cytotoxic T cells in HTLV-1 infection.[224] Indeed, HTLV-1–infected patients with ATLL have poorly detectable Tax-specific cytotoxic T-cell activity,[253,393] which could permit more unrestrained proliferation of infected cells and lead to increased HTLV-1 viral load, higher HTLV-1 antibody levels to non-Tax viral proteins, and, eventually, malignant transformation. HTLV-1 bZIP *(HBZ)* factor gene has growth-promoting activity and is expressed in all ATLL cells,[464] suggesting *HBZ* also may play a role in cellular transformation and leukemogenisis.[37,335] *HBZ* expression correlates with provirus load,[37] which itself correlates with risk for developing ATLL.[259]

The Japanese Lymphoma Study Group has defined ATLL in four major subtypes, based on how the condition presents[486] and for which there are clinical and laboratory criteria (Table 192A.2). The distribution of clinical ATLL subtypes varies geographically. In Japan, most cases are acute ATLL with leukemic manifestations; however, in the Caribbean, most cases are initially of the lymphoma subtype.[288,289] ATLL frequently presents aggressively, either as a leukemia or with lymph node enlargement without peripheral blood involvement (<1% leukemic cells in peripheral blood).[37] Most commonly globally (about 60% of cases),[37] ATLL presents acutely as leukemia along with systemic symptoms, organomegaly, and prominent lymphadenopathy.[337,339] The lymphoma subtype represents 20% of global ATLL cases.[37] In both aggressive subtypes, massive lymphadenopathy usually is present, although sparing the mediastinum,[37] as are hepatosplenomegaly and multiple visceral lesions, including skin, lung, and gastrointestinal infiltration.[37] ATLL cells in vitro express receptor activator of NFκ-β ligand on their surface and, along with

BOX 192A.1 Requirements for Diagnosis of Adult T-Cell Leukemia/Lymphoma

1. HTLV-1 seropositivity
2. Histologically or cytologically proven lymphoid malignancy with T-cell surface antigens present
3. Abnormal T lymphocytes ("flower cells") consistently present in peripheral blood (except for lymphoma subtype of ATLL)
4. Demonstration of clonality of proviral DNA as well as clonal integration of proviral DNA

ATLL, Adult T-cell leukemia/lymphoma; *HTLV-1,* human T-cell lymphotropic virus type 1.

TABLE 192A.2 Clinical Subtypes of Adult T-Cell Leukemia/Lymphoma: Clinical and Laboratory Findings

	ADULT T-CELL LEUKEMIA/LYMPHOMA CLINICAL SUBTYPE			
	Acute	**Chronic**	**Lymphoma**	**Smoldering**
Percentage With Subtype (%)	***55***	***20***	***20***	***5***
Survival				
Median	6 mo	24 mo	10 mo	>24 mo
Four-year survival rate (%)	5	27	6	66
Clinical Findings				
Lymphadenopathy	±	±	Yes	No
Hepatomegaly/splenomegaly	±	±	±	No
Skin involvement	±	±	±	±
Bone lesions	±	No	±	No
Bone marrow involvement	±	No	±	No
Laboratory Findings				
Absolute lymphocyte count (×10[9])	Not definitive	≥4	<4	<4
Abnormal circulating lymphocytes (%)	≥5[a]	≥5[a]	≤1	≥5[a]
Polylobulated lymphocytes ("flower cells")	Yes	Occasionally	No	Occasionally
Calcium	Normal or elevated	Normal	Normal or elevated	Normal
Lactate dehydrogenase	Normal or elevated	<2 times normal	Normal or elevated	<1.5 times normal

[a]If <5% of circulating abnormal lymphocytes are present, at least one histologically proved tumor lesion from the lungs, skin, or elsewhere is required for diagnosis.
Modified from Verdonck K, Gonzalez E, Van Dooren S, et al. Human T-lymphotropic virus 1: recent knowledge about an ancient infection. *Lancet Infect Dis* 2007;7:266-281.

elevated levels of mononuclear phagocyte colony-stimulating factor, induce the differentiation of hematopoietic precursor cells to osteoclasts.[309] The resultant acceleration in bone resorption leads to lytic bone lesions in some cases,[309,337,339] and, with or without lytic bone lesions, to the prominent hypercalcemia characteristic of acute ATLL.[309] Of acute ATLL cases, 20% to 30% present with hypercalcemia at diagnosis and more than 70% manifest hypercalcemia at some point in the illness course.[309,337,517] ATLL cells also have been found to secrete excessive amounts of parathyroid hormone–related peptide, probably because of Tax-mediated transactivation of the gene for this protein, which also contributes to hypercalcemia.[139] Skin lesions also are common in acute ATLL,[337,339] caused by dense skin infiltration by clonal HTLV-1 tumoral cells.[337,339,588,589] Multiple types of skin lesions have been described, from papules and nodules to erythroderma and ulcerative lesions.[309] In some acute ATLL presentations, cutaneous findings dominate the clinical picture; so-called cutaneous ATLL can be challenging to differentiate from mycosis fungoides and Sézary syndrome.[123,309]

The chronic form of ATLL manifests as lymphocytosis with ATLL cells, often stable for months to years, skin findings, low-grade lymphadenopathy and hepatosplenomegaly, occasional lung involvement and the absence of systemic symptoms, hypercalcemia, and lactate dehydrogenase (LDH) either normal or only slightly raised.[37,106,108,109,337,487] The central nervous system (CNS) is not involved in chronic ATLL,[37] which is separated into favorable and unfavorable subgroups, with the worse prognosis defined by low serum albumin, high LDH or high urea levels, and an elevated expression of Ki-67 antigen.[586] In smoldering ATLL, the least common ATLL presentation, affected individuals usually do not have symptoms but may have skin rash pulmonary infiltrates, with absence of other visceral involvement.[37,237,337,339] Cutaneous manifestations of smoldering ATLL often respond to topical steroids, and pulmonary findings may be misdiagnosed as infectious or other processes.[337,339] Key to the diagnosis of smoldering ATLL versus the chronic form of ATLL is a normal leukocyte count,[337,339] of which abnormal lymphocytes make up 1% to 5%.[37] Although not common, cases have been reported of disease progression from chronic or smoldering ATLL to acute, leukemic manifestations.[337,339] Table 192A.3 details clinical findings in ATLL presentations.

Although the described classification scheme is used globally as the standard for describing ATLL and its prognosis and treatment, gaps exist in its definitions.[37] Given the definition of lymphoma subtype by the presence of fewer than 1% circulating abnormal lymphocytes, patients with aggressive presentations and more than 1% circulating abnormal lymphocytes are classified as having acute ATLL, even when bulky lymphadenopathy or visceral involvement is present. Current data indicate that such patients with substantial lymph node or organ involvement do not respond to antiviral therapy alone, as do leukemic ATLL patients with less prominent lymph node and organ involvement,[37] suggesting, from a treatment perspective, that a third aggressive category may exist and be in need of description. As well, debate is ongoing about how to classify patients with isolated circulating abnormal lymphocytes (>5%). In the current approach, they are classified as having smoldering ATLL, although data suggest that this group of patients has outstanding long-term survival,[229] in contrast to patients with smoldering ATLL with infiltration of skin or lung.[510]

Individuals with ATLL are immunosuppressed, with severely impaired T-cell–mediated immunity.[337,339,571] Opportunistic infections are common and are a common cause of mortality;[381] indeed, most deaths in ATLL patients are due to opportunistic infections and complications of opportunistic infections, such as hypercalcemia.[389] *S. stercoralis* infection is commonly present, and a hyperinfection syndrome may develop, accompanied by gram-negative sepsis, with a mortality rate of greater than 70%. As mentioned earlier, evidence suggests that *S. stercoralis* infection may be a cofactor for HTLV-1–induced leukemogenesis.[309] Other common opportunistic infections include bacterial infections, *Pneumocystis* pneumonia, and serious fungal infections. Findings indicative of poor survival include age older than 40 years, increased tumor bulk, poor performance status, high LDH level, hypercalcemia, and the presence of clones of cells containing multiple or defective copies of the HTLV-1 provirus.[11,449] The CNS, which is affected in 2.5% to 10% of patients, can act as a sanctuary and has been found to be an important site for relapse when chemotherapy is given to treat ATLL.[415]

The prognosis and treatment of ATLL depend on the subtype, and for prognosis purposes, ATLL is classified into low-, intermediate-, and high-risk groups based on age (high risk >70 years of age), stage, performance status and biochemical markers (serum albumin <3.5 g/dL, and serum IL-2 >20,000 U/mL[259]), and median survival times are estimated at 16.2, 7.3, and 3.6 months, respectively[260]). Survival rate varies markedly by subtype, with a 4-year survival of 66% for smoldering ATLL, 27% for the chronic form of ATLL, and 5% to 6% for acute and lymphoma types. Aggressive ATLL presentations (acute and lymphoma) are among the most severe lymphoproliferations known to medicine[33] and have very poor prognoses for multiple reasons, including large tumor burden, hypercalcemia, liver or kidney dysfunction, and substantial immunodeficiency resulting in frequent infectious complications.[33,37,309] Importantly, as well, ATLL cells possess intrinsic chemoresistance resulting from elevated expression of the multidrug resistance gene[285] and mutations in the *p53* gene.[466] Complete remission in ATLL is defined by normalization of the complete blood count and resolution of all tumor masses, lasting for at least 1 month,[37] although patients with these factors but maintaining fewer than 5% atypical lymphocytes are also considered to be in complete remission because this situation may be noted in HTLV-1 carriers without malignant disease ("pre-ATL," which may either disappear or progress to clinical ATLL).[37,569]

Given ATLL's intrinsic chemotherapy resistance, alternative treatment approaches have been explored. Antiviral therapy is an important aspect of ATLL treatment,[31,33,211,259,331,560] especially for acute ATLL,[34,37,216,263,338,339,571] and even more so for acute ATLL that has not been previously treated.[571] By a mechanism that remains unclear, treatment with AZT and interferon-α (IFN-α) has proved to increase survival rates in both chronic and acute forms of ATLL.[35,322] As well, it was recently reported that IFN-α induces a gene expression suppressive effect inducing an arrest of cell cycle in infected cells; by adding AZT, an added effect is observed wherein *p53* is induced and cell apoptosis takes place.[267] Previous reports of AZT effect were similar, showing inhibition of telomerase activity along with stabilization and reactivation of *p53, p21,* and *p27,* resulting in the induction of cell apoptosis.[114] The combination of IFN and arsenic has also been shown to cause cell apoptosis mediated by Tax degradation and has also been proposed as an alternative therapy.[112,311] A meta-analysis of ATL survival since 1995 compared different treatment strategies for ATLL—antiviral therapy alone, chemotherapy alone, and chemotherapy followed by maintenance antiviral therapy. The 5-year overall survival rates were 46% for 75 patients who received first-line antiviral therapy, 20% for 77 patients who received first-line chemotherapy, and 12% for patients who received first-line chemotherapy followed by antiviral therapy.[34] Patients with acute, chronic, and smoldering ATLL substantially benefitted from first-line antiviral therapy, and ATLL lymphoma patients did better with chemotherapy.[37] Acute ATLL patients achieved a 5-year survival rate of 28%, in contrast to

TABLE 192A.3 Clinical Findings in Adult T-Cell Leukemia/Lymphoma

Median age of onset	40–60 y
Gender	Caribbean, Africa: Females > males Japan: Males slightly > females (1.4 : 1)
Clinical and Laboratory Findings	
Generalized lymphadenopathy (%)	50–80
Hepatosplenomegaly (%)	25–67
Skin involvement (%)	40–60
Elevated white blood cell count (%)	60–66
Hypercalcemia (%)	32–63
Pulmonary involvement (%)	14
Lytic bone lesions (%)	2–10
Central nervous system involvement (%)	2–10

the 10% 5-year survival rate with chemotherapy with or without maintenance antiviral therapy.[37] Achievement of complete remission with antiviral therapy was important, with 82% of this subgroup surviving at 5 years.[37] Antiviral therapy resulted in 100% 5-year survival in chronic and smoldering forms, yet in ATLL lymphoma a survival disadvantage (median survival time of 7 months; 5-year survival of 0) was seen compared with first-line chemotherapy with or without maintenance antiviral therapy.[34] Other antiretroviral agents, including lamivudine (3TC), have been evaluated in ATLL, but without benefit being shown.[37]

Standard therapy for acute ATLL is now AZT/IFN, with patients possessing wild-type *p53* at substantial survival benefit over those with mutated *p53*.[113] Long-term therapy is required because relapse will occur if treatment is stopped, and eventually, even though survival is prolonged, patients with acute ATLL usually relapse eventually and die.[37] For young patients with acute ATLL and a matched donor, allo-hematopoeitic stem cell transplantation (allo-HSCT) is recommended.[37]

Arsenic trioxide synergizes with IFN to induce cell cycle arrest and apoptosis in HTLV-1–infected ATLL leukemia cells,[32] eradicating leukemia-initiating cell activity.[143] Trials are currently ongoing to assess the role of arsenic/IFN as consolidation therapy for patients achieving satisfactory responses to induction therapy.[37] Particularly with chronic and smoldering subtypes, suggestions have been made that arsenic may have a role in achieving cure by eliminating leukemia-initiating cell,[32,143] and arsenic/IFN maintenance therapy is being investigated in acute ATLL as well.[37]

Several other therapies are accepted as second- and subsequent-line treatments for ATLL, including multiagent chemotherapy, allo-HSCT, and newer agents, such as purine analogs, histone deacetylase inhibitors, and monoclonal antibodies.[533,534]

Different chemotherapy combinations and regimens have been investigated over the years,[37] particularly in Japan, where ATLL is common and the resources to intensively address it exist, unlike in most HTLV-1–endemic settings. First- and second-generation Japanese protocols with the regimen of cyclophosphamide, hydroxydaunomycin, vincristine (Oncovin), and prednisone (CHOP) and other combined chemotherapies obtained complete remission of up to 42%, but with early relapses and 4-year survival rates of less than 10% for aggressive subtypes.[37] Similar results were seen historically from outside Japan.[453] Intensive induction therapy supported by granulocyte colony-stimulating factor yielded complete remission rates as high as 67% for lymphoma subtype, but still poor long-term survival.[586] Newer cytotoxic agents, including deoxycoformycin (a nucleoside analog),[533,534] irinotecan (a topoisomerase I inhibitor),[532] and MST-16 (a topoisomerase II inhibitor), have been studied in relapsed ATLL patients,[513] but with poor outcomes, as with earlier chemotherapy approaches.[37]

In Japan, allo-HSCT has improved ATLL prognosis, with several studies showing that discontinuation of immunosuppressant therapy induces sustained remission in substantial numbers of posttransplantation relapsed patients, suggesting that ATLL may be susceptible to a graft-versus-leukemia effect.[251] In a large Japanese review, outcomes were evaluated for 386 patients who had undergone allo-HSCT.[225] At a median follow-up of 41 months, 3-year overall survival was 33%.[225] Donor lymphocyte infusions have been used in Japan for relapse after allo-HSCT, with sustained complete remission of more than 8 years in case reports.[251] Allo-HSCT, while promising in some cases, has limited utility for ATLL presenters as a whole, given limits to eligibility for allo-HSCT based on severe immunosuppression at presentation, older age, and poor overall health status.[37] Especially in acute ATLL, complete remission remains low even with allo-HSCT.[37]

Noting ATLL cells' ubiquitous surface expression of IL-2 receptors, monoclonal antibodies against the IL-2 receptor have been used in trial in patients with relapsed or refractory ATLL.[37,109] Good responses are uncommon.[37] Case reports indicate some initial success with alemtuzumab anti-CD52 antibody, but duration of response is short and substantial risk for opportunistic infections exists, especially cytomegalovirus reactivation.[351,447] Helper T cell type 2 and regulatory T cells express CC chemokine receptor 4 (CCR4), and a next-generation humanized anti-CCR4 antibody, KW-0761, has demonstrated possible benefit versus relapsed ATLL expressing the CCR4 phenotype.[592] In chronic and smoldering ATLL subtypes, monoclonal antibodies can be used as single agents, although clinical trials of monoclonal antibodies with chemotherapy in the lymphoma subtype and ART in the acute subtype are needed to better define their ultimate utility in treating ATLL.[37]

Supportive therapy is necessary in managing ATLL, including treatment of hypercalcemia and prophylaxis against *Pneumocystis jiroveci* pneumonia, viral infections, and fungal infections.[535] In patients with potential past or present *Strongyloides* exposure, prophylaxis with ivermectin or albendazole should be given.[37] Patients with aggressive ATLL should be considered for intrathecal prophylaxis because more than half of relapses at new sites after chemotherapy are in the CNS.[37]

Other malignant diseases have been associated with HTLV-1 infection, although the supporting evidence for these associations is less clear than that for ATLL. Cutaneous T-cell lymphomas, such as mycosis fungoides and Sézary syndrome, have been described in adults and a child with HTLV-1 infection.[36,204,565,599] In one small study of eight patients with Sézary syndrome, HTLV-1 mRNA expression was found in four patients,[183] and HTLV-1–like sequences have been found in patients with mycosis fungoides.[64] Multiple myeloma, B-cell chronic lymphocytic leukemia,[26] acute lymphoblastic leukemia (ALL), and acute myeloid leukemia (AML) also have been described in patients infected with HTLV-1.[26] These malignancies may arise as a result of chronic antigenic stimulation of B cells by HTLV-1–infected T cells, with such stimulation leading to uncontrolled B-cell expansion. In the Caribbean and Chile, HTLV-1 has been associated with the development of T-cell non-Hodgkin lymphoma.[26,317] Although some cases of adult HTLV-1–associated lymphomas are similar in character to anaplastic large cell lymphoma (ALCL), in a series of 33 cases of pediatric ALCL from Brazil, where HTLV-1 is endemic, no cases demonstrated proviral HTLV-1 DNA, suggesting no relationship between HTLV-1 and ALCL in children.[199] A case of primary brain T-cell lymphoma in a young HTLV-1–positive adult has been reported,[300] as has a case of small cell cancer of the lung with monoclonally integrated HTLV-1. A pulmonary infiltrative syndrome resembling lymphoid pulmonary hyperplasia seen in HIV-1–infected children has been reported in patients with HTLV-1–associated myelopathy.[497]

Human T-Cell Lymphotropic Virus Type 1–Associated Myelopathy

In the 1880s, a "multiple neuritis" syndrome with a predominantly ataxic motor neuropathy was reported in Jamaica. In subsequent years, similar syndromes of unknown origin were described in other geographic locales and given different names, including Strachan disease, central neuritis, Jamaican neuropathy, tropical spastic paraplegia, and tropical spastic paraparesis.[600] The identification of HTLV-1 in 1980, the development of antibody tests to diagnose HTLV-1 infection, and the recognition that HTLV-1 and TSP were endemic in the same geographic locations led to the hypothesis that these entities could be associated. In 1985, Gessain and colleagues[178] performed a case-control study in Martinique in which patients with TSP of unknown cause were compared with a control group of nurses and blood donors without neurologic disease. Sixty percent of the patients with TSP versus only 4% of controls had HTLV-1 serum antibodies detected.[161,178] In the same year, a report was published on the detection of HTLV-1 antibodies in the cerebrospinal fluid (CSF) and serum of individuals afflicted with TSP.[456] In 1986, a series of Japanese patients with a similar clinical syndrome who also had HTLV-1 antibodies in their CSF were described, and these investigators proposed that the syndrome be called *HTLV-1–associated myelopathy*.[402] At a 1988 meeting of the World Health Organization (WHO) Scientific Group on HTLV-1 Infections and Its Associated Disease, researchers proposed that HAM and HTLV-1–associated TSP were clinically and pathologically identical and recommended that the disorder be known by the acronym *HAM/TSP*.[582,583]

Diagnostic criteria developed at this meeting, and revised in 1989, base diagnoses of HAM/TSP on the presence of a variety of clinical and laboratory criteria,[196] including anti–HTLV-1 antibodies in serum and CSF.[59,439] With advances in diagnostic technology, particularly molecular techniques and HTLV-1 proviral load testing, in 2006 De Castro-Costa and colleagues proposed simplified diagnostic criteria for HAM/TSP that may allow diagnosis at earlier stages, when treatment may be more successful. Widely adopted in Brazil, the De Castro-Costa criteria[116] use myelopathic symptoms, serologic findings or detection of HTLV-1 DNA, the exclusion of other disorders, and the results of HTLV-1 proviral load testing to ascertain one of three categories of HAM/TSP: possible, probable, or definite. HTLV-1 proviral load progressively increases by De Castro-Costa ascertainment category,[13,196] with a level higher than 50,000 HTLV-1 copies/10^6 peripheral blood mononuclear cells (PBMCs) an additional criterion for differentiating definite from probable HAM/TSP cases (Box 192A.2).[196]

The disease usually occurs in HTLV-1–endemic areas, including the Caribbean, southern Japan, equatorial Africa, Central and South America, Melanesia, and southern Africa. Sporadic cases have been described in nonendemic areas, usually in immigrants from endemic areas or their sexual contacts or in recipients of blood transfusions (before the advent of HTLV blood screening). Incidence and prevalence estimates suggest that between 0.3% and 3% of asymptomatic carriers will develop HAM/TSP,[195] and women are more commonly affected than men.[314] Yet clinically recognized and diagnosed HAM/TSP is likely the tip of a neurologic iceberg in HTLV-1; a recent cohort study demonstrated that up to 30% of asymptomatic carriers presenting with mild neurologic symptoms did not fulfill HAM/TSP criteria.[514]

As with ATLL, the chief risk factor for developing HAM/TSP is a high HTLV-1 proviral load. Yet genetic factors appear to play a role as well, with gene polymorphisms, such as for IL28B, associated with disease development[20]; that cases aggregate in families has long been recognized.[388]

Case rates differ geographically. In HTLV-1–seropositive persons in Japan, the incidence of HAM/TSP is 3.1 per 100,000 HTLV-1–infected persons per year. In contrast, the annual incidence of HAM/TSP in HTLV-1–infected persons in Jamaica and Trinidad was 22.1 per 100,000 persons.[314] This difference in incidence is hypothesized to reflect an association between the time that HTLV-1 infection is acquired and the type of disease manifestation that occurs. In the Caribbean, most HTLV-1 infection being acquired sexually during adult life is more common than in Japan, and HAM/TSP is the most common clinical manifestation of the disease. In Japan, sexual transmission is less common, most infection is acquired by maternal-to-child transmission during infancy, and ATLL is the most common disease manifestation. Case reports of HAM/TSP occurring after receipt of blood transfusions and the finding in Japan and Martinique that 13% to 20% of patients with HAM/TSP had a history of receiving blood transfusions accelerated the decision of blood banks in the United States to screen for HTLV-1 antibodies. In Japan, a 16% decrease in the number of HAM/TSP cases occurred in the 2 years after initiation of blood screening.[170,171,401]

Although the mean onset of disease is in the fourth decade of life, incubation of this disease appears to be shorter than that of ATLL. In patients with HTLV-1 infection acquired by transfusion in whom HAM/TSP subsequently developed, the median time to development of symptoms after receiving a transfusion was 3.3 years, and in one report, HAM/TSP occurred 18 weeks after blood transfusion.[194,401] Onset of symptoms is uncommon in persons younger than 20 years or older than 70 years, and incidence increases from age 20 years through age 50 years and then declines.[189] However, HAM/TSP has been reported in children and adolescents, and the majority of cases are from Brazil,[59,121,205,439,443] with a predominance in girls.[59] Most pediatric and adolescent cases have been in vertically infected children,[205,439] although HAM/TSP has been described in a 6-year-old child after transfusion-acquired HTLV-1 infection.[401] Most HAM/TSP cases in children and adolescents occur in patients with active, or a history of, HTLV-1–associated infective dermatitis.[439] In one study from Brazil, 60% of pediatric and adolescent infective dermatitis cases had neurologic symptoms, and one-third had frank HAM/TSP.[59,439]

Clinical features of HAM/TSP in children and adolescents are similar to those in adults,[59] and it typically presents as a slowly progressive neurologic disease[180] involving the pyramidal tracts and including chronic progressive spastic paraparesis and weakness of the limbs, particularly the legs, that results in an insidious onset of gait disturbance (see Table 192A.5). Mild sensory loss and painful paresthesias may develop and result in complaints of extremity numbness or dysesthesia and low back pain. Vesical dysfunction generally presents later in the illness but is particularly characteristic of pediatric disease and is characterized by urinary urgency, difficulty emptying the bladder, and incontinence.[439] Urodynamic studies are important in children for diagnosis as well as for follow-up treatment of vesical dysfunction.[59] Bowel issues in adults include constipation and incontinence. Erectile dysfunction may be seen. Neurologic examination shows hyperactive deep tendon reflexes, clonus, extensor plantar reflexes, proximal muscle wasting, and a spastic paraparesis with a slow, scissoring gait; mild sensory changes may be observed. Cognitive function and the cranial nerves usually are spared. Systemic nonneurologic symptoms suggestive of an autoimmune process, such as pulmonary alveolitis, uveitis, arthropathy, Sjögren syndrome, and vasculitis, also may be noted.[230,233,498] Progression is variable, but, on the whole, prognosis is poor, with complete motor disability of the lower extremities in half of patients 10 years after onset, whereas 30% of patients become bedridden.[181,186]

In endemic areas, patients, particularly children and adolescents, without previously known HTLV-1 infection, with symptoms of myelopathy should be serologically screened for HTLV-1.[59,439] Even when HTLV-1 infection status is known, the differential diagnosis of the symptoms described earlier is broad. Of particular importance are CSF studies to rule out other infectious diseases that may involve the spinal cord, including tuberculosis, syphilis, and toxoplasmosis, and, in at-risk geographic areas, cysticercosis and schistosomiasis.[439]

BOX 192A.2 Diagnostic Criteria for Human T-Cell Lymphotropic Virus Type 1–Associated Myelopathy/Tropical Spastic Paraparesis: Levels of Ascertainment

Definite

1. A nonremitting progressive spastic paraparesis with sufficiently impaired gait to be perceived by the patient. Sensory symptoms or signs may or may not be present. When present, they remain subtle and without a clear-cut sensory level. Anal and urinary sphincter signs and symptoms may or may not be present.
2. Presence of HTLV-1 antibodies in serum and CSF confirmed by Western blot and/or a positive PCR for HTLV-1 in blood and/or CSF.
3. Exclusion of other disorders that can mimic HAM/TSP.[a]

Probable

1. Monosymptomatic presentation: Spasticity or hyperreflexia in the lower limbs or isolated Babinski sign with or without subtle sensory signs or symptoms, or neurogenic bladder only confirmed by urodynamic testing.
2. Presence of HTLV-1 antibodies in serum and/or CSF confirmed by Western blot and/or a positive PCR for HTLV-1 in blood and/or CSF.
3. Exclusion of other disorders that can mimic HAM/TSP.[a]

Possible

1. Complete or incomplete clinical presentation.
2. Presence of HTLV-1 antibodies in serum and/or CSF confirmed by Western blot and/or a positive PCR for HTLV-1 in blood and/or CSF.
3. Disorders that can mimic HAM/TSP have not been excluded.[a]

[a]The following conditions should be excluded by appropriate laboratory and clinical evaluation to minimize risk for misdiagnosis of HAM/TSP: multiple sclerosis; carcinomatous meningitis; familial spastic paraparesis; transverse myelitis; primary lateral sclerosis; paraneoplastic syndromes; syringomyelia; Lyme disease; vitamin B_{12} and folate deficiency; Behçet disease; neurosyphilis; neurotuberculosis; sarcoidosis; HIV vacuolar myelopathy; collagen vascular diseases; autoimmune myelopathies; Sjögren syndrome; toxic myelopathies; amyotrophic lateral sclerosis; fungal myelopathy; spinal arteriovenous fistula; hepatic myelopathy; parasitic myelopathy (visceral larva migrans of *Toxocara canis* and *Ascaris suum*); spinal cord compression (e.g., spinal tumor, cervical spondylosis, brain parasagittal tumor); endemic regional myelopathies with similar clinical manifestations (including schistosomiasis and neurocysticercosis).

CSF, Cerebrospinal fluid; *HAM/TSP,* HTLV-1–associated myelopathy/tropical spastic paraparesis; *HTLV,* human T-cell lymphotropic virus; *PCR,* polymerase chain reaction.

Modified from De Castro-Costa CM, Araujo AQ, Barreto MM, et al. Proposal for diagnostic criteria of tropical spastic paraparesis/HTLV-I-associated myelopathy (TSP/HAM). *AIDS Res Hum Retroviruses.* 2006;22:931-935.

Helminthic coinfections are common in HTLV-1–infected persons,[432,433,502] including helminths other than *Strongyloides,* such as *Ascaris* and *Schistosoma* spp.[502] HTLV-1 infection is associated with a high Th1 response, although helminthic infections have been shown in some studies to downregulate Th1 responses and attenuate chronic inflammatory diseases.[76,341,407] It has been suggested that treatment of helminths in HTLV-1–infected persons may raise the risk for subsequent development of HAM/TSP, yet data to date suggest that treatment of helminthic coinfections do not affect the risk for developing neurologic disease in HTLV-1 infection or otherwise adversely affect HTLV-1–infected persons.[502]

The pediatric form of HAM/TSP has been associated with multiple comorbidities, including short stature, hypocalcemia, and increases in urinary phosphorus and cyclic adenosine monophosphate after parathyroid hormone administration, raising the question of whether HTLV-1 may induce pseudohypoparathyroidism (PHP) in some children.[597] Current thinking is that HTLV-1 does not induce PHP, rather PHP may be a risk factor for developing HAM/TSP in HTLV-1 carriers.[304] Unlike in most adult cases, in which progression is insidious, pediatric HAM/TSP is generally rapidly progressive, in some cases with substantial disability within weeks to months of first symptoms.[439] Some adult populations, such as persons older than 60 years acquiring HTLV-1 through blood transfusion, are more likely to experience rapid progression.[297] Subacute HAM/TSP progression (requiring wheelchair use during first 2 years of symptoms[297]) is also uncommon (<10% of cases), with almost all cases in women, most of whom acquired their HTLV-1 infection through sexual contact.[297] Both rapidly progressive and subacute HAM/TSP may be more amenable to improvements with aggressive immunosuppressive treatment, and attempts to risk-stratify HAM/TSP presentations for projected chronicity of symptoms have been made.[297] Studies to date have not shown an association between HTLV-1 proviral load and risk for more rapid progression, suggesting that factors other than proviral load are involved in this determination.[297]

Nonspecific lesions of the brain are observed with magnetic resonance imaging (MRI) in as many as 75% of patients, but no clear correlation has been established between the lesions and symptoms. Atrophy of the spinal cord may occur, usually in the thoracic region, as may discrete lesions visible on MRI.[297] Multiple foci of increased T2 signal intensity are found in the periventricular white matter, similar to the findings observed in patients with multiple sclerosis. However, cognitive impairment may be noted in multiple sclerosis but is not found in HAM/TSP, and HTLV-1 sequences have not been detected in the peripheral blood or CNS of patients with multiple sclerosis.[397]

High HTLV-1 antibody levels are found in both peripheral blood and CSF. In CSF, mild to moderate pleocytosis, increased protein, oligoclonal immunoglobulin bands, or any combination of these findings may be observed. Elevated CSF neopterin, an indicator of cellular immune activation, may be present, and its CSF concentration correlates with disease severity.[464] In approximately 50% of patients, atypical flower lymphocytes are observed and account for approximately 1% to 15% of peripheral blood lymphocytes; these cells also may be seen in CSF.[233] Unlike the monoclonal integration observed in ATLL, polyclonal integration of HTLV-1 is noted in cells from patients with HAM/TSP.

Pathologically, HAM/TSP is characterized by perivascular demyelination and neuronal lesions. Macroscopic atrophy of the spinal cord occurs, with changes consistent with a chronic inflammatory process characterized by perivascular cuffing of mononuclear cells and lymphocytic infiltration of the brain and spinal cord. Early in the disease, these lymphocytes consist of both $CD8^+$ and $CD4^+$ T cells, along with B lymphocytes and macrophages in areas of parenchymal damage.[243] HTLV-1 proviral DNA can be demonstrated in $CD4^+$ cells in the infiltrates by in situ PCR. Evidence suggests that these HTLV-1–infected $CD4^+$ cells migrate from the peripheral blood and cross the blood-brain barrier to enter the nervous system.[13,88] Later in the disease process, the inflammatory cells are fewer in number and consist primarily of $CD8^+$ cytotoxic T cells.[13] Marked myelin and axonal destruction and astrocytic gliosis are prominent. The lower thoracic spinal cord is particularly affected, and parenchymal damage of both white and gray matter of the cord may be present. In the brain, although perivascular mononuclear cell infiltration may be seen, parenchymal damage is an unusual finding. However, rare patients may have white-matter lesions, cerebellar symptoms, amyotrophic lateral sclerosis–like symptoms, or neuropathy.[233]

The pathogenesis of HAM/TSP is not fully understood, but it is believed to be related to a high HTLV-1 provirus burden and an exaggerated proinflammatory cellular immune response,[13,563] with the risk for HAM/TSP increasing exponentially as proviral load exceeds $10{,}000/10^6$ peripheral blood mononuclear cells.[13] In a large Brazilian cohort, a proviral load cutoff of $11{,}400/10^6$ has a 78.2% sensitivity for identifying HAM/TSP diagnoses over a 14-year follow-up.[164] When compared with asymptomatic HTLV-1–seropositive individuals or those with ATLL, patients with HAM/TSP have higher HTLV-1 antibody titers, a higher proviral load, and elevated levels of spontaneous lymphocyte proliferation and proinflammatory cytokines, including IL-1, IFN-α, and TFN-α.[318,373,374]

One postulated mechanism for nervous system damage is direct infection of CNS glial cells by HTLV-1; a direct cytotoxic immune response to the glial cell is generated and results in demyelination.[230] However, HTLV-1 expression appears to be localized to infiltrating $CD4^+$ lymphocytes within the spinal cord lesions rather than nervous system parenchymal cells, and no clear evidence has established that HTLV-1 infects CNS cells.[375] Alternatively, the heightened HTLV-1–specific immune response in patients with HAM/TSP and neuropathologic findings suggests that immune-mediated mechanisms may have a role in the pathogenesis of disease.[287]

Tax has a role in inducing HAM/TSP.[464] HTLV-1 *tax* mRNA expression is significantly higher in HAM/TSP patients than in asymptomatic HTLV-1 carriers, and this correlates with HTLV-1 proviral load, Tax-specific $CD8^+$ T-cell frequency, and disease severity.[177,593] Mononuclear cells infiltrating the spinal cord overexpress several cytokines, chemokines, and matrix metalloproteinases (MMPs) that are transactivated by Tax protein[121,464] and that may induce demyelination, as well as increase the transmigration of additional HTLV-1–infected lymphocytes to the inflammatory lesion.[230,373,374] These include TNF-α,[543] monocyte chemoattractant protein-1 (MCP-1),[544] and MMP-9. Expression of the *HBZ* gene also correlates with CSF neopterin concentration and disease severity, as well as decreases after successful immunomodulatory treatment for HAM/TSP, suggesting a role for *HBZ* in HAM/TSP pathogenesis.[464] HTLV-1–specific $CD8^+$ cytotoxic T cells can be found in the CSF and in the peripheral blood of patients with HAM/TSP, and a significant reduction in the naïve T-cell population occurs with a concomitant increase in the memory/effector $CD8^+$ cell population.[244,245,373] Examination of the T-cell receptor repertoire shows significant expansion of the $CD8^+$ T-cell population in patients with HAM/TSP as opposed to asymptomatic carriers. Many of these $CD8^+$ cells correspond to cytotoxic T lymphocytes directed against epitopes of the immunodominant Tax protein of HTLV-1.[545]

Specific characteristics of the virus also may influence disease manifestations. In one study, a specific *tax* gene phylogenetic subgroup, *tax A,* was found to occur more commonly in patients with HAM/TSP than in healthy HTLV-1 carriers, suggesting that functional or immunogenic differences in the transactivating Tax protein among HTLV-1 viral types may play a role in causing disease.[165] Another hypothesized mechanism is more indirect and involves an HTLV-1–associated activation of autoreactive cells that could lead to an autoimmune process inducing myelin destruction. The finding that numerous autoimmune-like diseases may occur in HTLV-1–infected patients and may coexist with HAM/TSP is consistent with the latter hypothesis.[233]

Despite extensive effort over the more than 35 years since its definition, HAM/TSP still has no specific treatment,[330] and current approaches do not affect the natural history of HAM/TSP.[184,330] Mean survival after the onset of symptoms is 10 years, although prolonged survival may be seen, and the major causes of death are infection and cancer.[541] Many strategies, including corticosteroids, IFN-α and IFN-β, danazol, pentoxifylline tamibarotene,[145] and plasmapheresis, have had their efficacy evaluated, yet none of these has shown an effect on long-term prognosis and there is not, currently, enough evidence to inform recommendations on a standard treatment.[392]

Case reports suggest that, particularly in early phases of HAM/TSP when substantial parenchymal inflammation is present, responses to such therapies are more likely, whereas later in the disease course, degeneration of the white matter and glio-mesenchymal tissue reactions dampen the odds for success.[297] In Brazilian pediatric cases treated with intravenous methylprednisolone early in disease course, vesical status improved in most cases, but motor responses were generally poor.[440] In most reports, corticosteroids and IFN treatments are of only transient benefit and often associated with serious side effects.[330] Patients with HAM/TSP, particularly children and adolescents, are often highly affected by the psychological and social aspects of disability, and care is best provided by a multidisciplinary team including a psychologist, physical and occupational therapists, physicians, and nurses.[59] Depression and anxiety substantial enough to require specific treatment are common.[173] Symptomatic treatments with agents such as baclofen and anticonvulsants to relieve spasticity and neuropathic pain are of benefit in many patients,[59] as are oxybutynin for urinary incontinence and bethanechol for urinary retention, along with high doses of vitamin C (2 g/day) to acidify the urine and daily oral nitrofurantoin when recurrent urinary tract infection is an issue.[13] Valproic acid may prove dually useful, for both symptoms and disease activity, because it induces reductions in proviral load by activating viral gene expression and exposing HTLV-1–infected cells to the immune system.[294]

Several studies have evaluated antiretrovirals in the treatment of HAM/TSP, with and without myelopathy.[518] Specifically evaluated have been AZT, 3TC, and raltegravir, with different but consistently poor results.[518] This may not be surprising, considering the limited role intracellular viral replication plays in HTLV-1–associated disease compared with division of infected cells yielding high proviral levels. With its favorable safety profile, raltegravir has been proposed as an option for individuals with high HTLV-1 proviral loads to treat early or reduce the rate of development of HTLV-1–associated conditions[530]; a clinical trial initiated in 2013 evaluating this is ongoing.[444]

Given the implication of activated T cells and mononuclear phagocytes, along with their associated cytokines, in the pathogenesis of HAM/TSP, there is interest in assessing whether inhibition of T-cell and/or mononuclear phagocyte activation is of benefit in patients with early or clinically progressing HAM/TSP.[330] An open-label, proof-of-concept, 48-week pilot study enrolled onto cyclosporine A (an immunosuppressive inhibitor of activated T cells) therapy seven patients older than 16 years with early (<2 years) or progressive (>50% deterioration in timed walk during the preceding 3 months) HAM/TSP.[330] Five of the seven patients showed objective clinical improvement after 3 months of treatment with cyclosporine A, and the two who did not show improvement experienced clinical deterioration and stopped therapy.[330] Overall pain, mobility, spasticity, and bladder function improved by 48 weeks, and larger, randomized controlled studies are planned.[330] Minocycline is known to inhibit activated mononuclear phagocytes,[146] and recent in vitro work has shown minocycline's ability to inhibit TNF-α and IL-1β expression in cultured CD14$^+$ cells of patients with HAM/TSP, while also inhibiting IFN-γ expression in CD8$^+$ T cells of patients with HAM/TSP, and suggesting that minocycline may offer a novel treatment strategy directed at suppression of CD8$^+$ T-cell activation in patients with HAM/TSP and other HTLV-1–associated neurologic disease.[146]

Human T-Cell Lymphotropic Virus Type 1–Associated Uveitis

Defined as uveitis of unknown etiology in an HTLV-1–infected individual, HTLV-1 uveitis was first described in Japan in 1992 based on studies showing higher incidence of HTLV-1 seropositivity in individuals with uveitis of unknown etiology compared with to uveitis of known etiology.[72] In HTLV-1–endemic areas in Japan, 38% of patients with idiopathic uveitis were infected with HTLV-1, in contrast to 19% of patients with nonuveitic ocular disease and 10% with uveitis of known origin.[349] In the younger age group (20–49 years) with idiopathic uveitis, HTLV-1 seroprevalence was 49%. Similarly, in Brazil, an area of lower HTLV-1 endemicity, HTLV-1 seroprevalence was elevated in patients with idiopathic uveitis; 1.8% of patients with idiopathic uveitis were HTLV-1–seropositive versus none of those with uveitis of known origin.[591] Along with epidemiologic associations, the causality of HTLV-1 in HTLV-1 uveitis was suggested. HTLV-1 antibody was detected in the aqueous humor of patients with HTLV-1 uveitis,[349] as was the presence of HTLV-1 virus itself and HTLV-1–infected cells in ocular fluid from HTLV-1 uveitis cases,[347] including more than 50% of Japanese patients with HTLV-1 uveitis. In Japan, HTLV-1 uveitis prevalence in the general population is 0.112%[508]; in a survey of 105 asymptomatic Brazilian HTLV-1 carriers, uveitis was found in 2.8% of infected persons. Women are almost twice as likely to be affected as men in Japan, yet mean age of onset is earlier in men (34.8 years vs. 48.1 years).[377] As noted for HAM/TSP, genetic factors also may be associated with a susceptibility to, or the severity of, HTLV-1–associated uveitis.[478]

HTLV-1 uveitis is likely the result of HTLV-1–infected T cells infiltrating the eye and producing inflammatory cytokines.[345,349,463,478] The long-term follow-up of Japanese patients informs HTLV-1 uveitis presentation and clinical course.[377] Clinically, HTLV-1 uveitis presents as an acute, moderate to severe vitreitis, along with mild iritis and mild retinal vasculitis, in what typically are healthy, asymptomatic HTLV-1 carriers.[72,346,348,376,485] Uveitis is unilateral in 60% of cases, with blurred vision and floaters the most common symptoms. Onset is typically abrupt. Characteristic findings on examination are mild anterior segment inflammation, nongranulomatous in more than 80% of cases, as well as vitreitis with fine granular and lacework-like membranous vitreous opacities. Retinal vasculitis, exudative retinal lesions, and optic disc abnormalities are common, occurring in 60%, 25%, and 20% of cases, respectively. HTLV-1 uveitis anatomic characterization is intermediate in more than 75% of cases. Five percent of HTLV-1 uveitis cases have iritis alone.[349] The uveitis is generally mild to moderate, and visual acuity is only mildly affected in most patients. The disease usually responds to topical, periocular, or systemic steroids, with complete resolution in 4 to 8 weeks, although recurrence is seen in 40% to 50% of cases after steroid therapy is discontinued.[349,376] Approximately 33% of cases are associated with complications, including cataract, glaucoma, epiretinal membranes, persistent vitreous opacities, retinochoroidal degeneration, retinal vascular occlusion, and optic atrophy,[72,197] and poor visual outcomes may be seen in 4% to 10% of cases.[72] Clinical studies suggest that retinal vasculitis unresponsive to corticosteroid therapy may be a poor prognostic sign.[377] In Japanese patients, 15% to 20% are diagnosed with Graves disease before onset of HTLV-1 uveitis, and approximately 7% have concomitant HAM/TSP before or after onset of HTLV-1 uveitis.[72,197] A study of the association between Graves disease and HTLV-1 uveitis found that methimazole was administered in all cases before HTLV-1 uveitis onset.[468] ATLL has not been associated with HTLV-1 uveitis, although rare cases of ATLL can present with ocular findings that mimic severe HTLV-1 uveitis, principally a necrotizing retinal vasculitis.[291] A study of 105 asymptomatic Brazilian HTLV-1–seropositive adults found abnormal results in at least one lacrimal film evaluation test in 40% versus 23% of uninfected controls,[591] a finding suggesting that abnormal early ocular abnormalities may be present in asymptomatic HTLV-1 carriers.

Non-Japanese HTLV-1 uveitis cases may be associated with findings not typically described in Japan, such as corneal pathology in Brazilian patients and patients from the Caribbean.[72] HTLV-1 uveitis in children and adolescents is rare, with cases reported as young as 3 years; girls more commonly affected than boys; and presenting symptoms and ocular examination findings similar to those in adults.[258,266] As in adults, topical or systemic steroids are usually effective in pediatric HTLV-1 uveitis cases, and topical steroids may need to be continued as maintenance therapy to prevent relapses.[266] As in adults, the presence of retinal vasculitis predicts long-term visual compromise, usually with slow progression poorly responsive to corticosteroids and resulting in diffuse chorioretinal degeneration.[59]

Pediatric Manifestations

Infective dermatitis. A chronic recurrent eczema of childhood called *infective dermatitis* was first described in 1966 as a series of 17 cases in Jamaican children.[503] These cases were reported as presenting with severe, infected lesions involving the ears, face, scalp, shoulders, and neck, with onset of illness at approximately 2 years of age and rarely before 18 months of age.[122,503] In 1967, researchers observed that cultures of the nares or skin lesions in children with infective dermatitis often were positive for *Staphylococcus aureus* or β-hemolytic streptococci.[566] It is now recognized that infective dermatitis is always associated with either or both of these organisms, typically with nonvirulent strains.[56] Patients with these infections responded well to antibiotic therapy but relapsed after therapy was withdrawn. The refractory nature of the disorder with frequent exacerbations, infections with bacteria that usually were nonvirulent, and resistance to treatment suggested an association with immune dysfunction. After HTLV-1 was identified in 1980, epidemiologic studies demonstrated that HTLV-1 was endemic in Jamaica. Because HTLV-1 infection was known to be associated with immune dysfunction and enhanced susceptibility to infections,[329] an association between infective dermatitis and HTLV-1 infection was hypothesized. Approximately 10% of childhood eczema cases in Jamaica are infective dermatitis,[276,278] and the probability of developing infective dermatitis in Jamaican children after perinatal HTLV-1 infection is estimated at 2%.[315]

In 1990, La Grenade and colleagues[274,275] first linked infective dermatitis to HTLV-1 infection in Jamaican children, after observing that of 14 children with typical infective dermatitis and 11 with atopic dermatitis, all children with infective dermatitis were HTLV-1 seropositive compared with none of those with atopic dermatitis. A subsequent report described 50 children with infective dermatitis, all of whom were HTLV-1 seropositive, as opposed to only 14% of 35 children with atopic dermatitis.[271] Subsequently, cases of infective dermatitis were reported in HTLV-1–infected children in Brazil,[56,122,398] Trinidad and Tobago,[499] French Guiana,[379] Colombia, Peru,[12] Senegal,[12] and Japan.[62,536] In Japan, however, infective dermatitis is very rare,[59] despite high HTLV-1 prevalence, suggesting that genetic and environmental factors may be involved in its development.[279,312] In 1996, infective dermatitis began to be referred to as infective dermatitis associated with HTLV-1 (IDH),[274,277] and criteria for its diagnosis were established in 1998.[275,276] In 2010, revised criteria for the diagnosis of IDH were suggested,[56] and these are detailed in Box 192A.3. Given that the diagnosis of HTLV-1 is mandatory to the diagnosis of IDH, it is advised that in endemic areas serology for HTLV-1 be performed in all cases of severe eczema in children and adolescents.[56]

A recently reported study of 42 IDH cases from Bahia, Brazil details the epidemiologic and dermatologic characteristics of the condition.[122] In this series, approximately two-thirds of the patients are females, and all are of African descent and from underprivileged backgrounds. Of the 42 patients, 41 were perinatally infected with HTLV-1; one with an HTLV-1–seronegative mother had received a blood transfusion early in life. Mean age at onset of IDH was 2.6 years (range, 2 months to 11 years), and in 37% of children skin lesions first appeared before 12 months of life. All patients were symptomatic, with pruritus of mild to moderate intensity. Dermatologically, all patients had lesions on the scalp and retroauricular area; crusting of the nares was found in only 64% of children and in two children was seen only during relapses. Antecubital and popliteal fossae were involved in 57%, and 83% had disseminated IDH (i.e., simultaneous involvement of scalp, neck, trunk, and limbs). Lesions were generally severe and exudative, associated with erythematous scale, and grossly infected. Other lesions noted in fewer patients included erythematous scaly papules, follicular papules (always disseminated), retroauricular fissures, and blepharoconjunctivitis. *S. aureus* was isolated from the skin lesions of 97% of children evaluated bacteriologically; in fewer than 10%, *Streptococcus pyogenes* was detected.

BOX 192A.3 Major Criteria for Diagnosis of Infective Dermatitis Associated With Human T-Cell Lymphotropic Virus Type 1

1. Lesions of the scalp, ears, retroauricular areas, paranasal and perioral areas, neck, axillae, thorax, abdomen, groin, and other sites. Lesions may be erythematous/scaly, exudative, and/or crusted
2. Crusting of nostrils
3. Chronic, relapsing condition with prompt response to specific appropriate therapy, but recurrence promptly on discontinuation of antibiotics
4. Serologic or molecular evidence of HTLV-1 infection

Fulfillment of criterion 1 requires involvement of three or more areas, including scalp and retroauricular areas. Of the 4 major criteria, 3 are required for diagnosis; 1, 3, and 4 must be present.

Modified from Bittencourt AL, de Oliveira Mde F. Cutaneous manifestations associated with HTLV-1 infection. *Int J Dermatol.* 2010;49:1099-110.

Immunohistologic findings were similar to those from other studies,[58] in which inflammatory infiltrates in IDH comprise mostly $CD8^+$ T cells, as opposed to atopic dermatitis and seborrheic dermatitis, in which $CD4^+$ lymphocytes predominate.[58] The HTLV-1 genome has been detected by PCR in lymphocytes cultured from biopsy specimens of skin lesions in patients with infectious dermatitis, although cultured fibroblasts were negative, suggesting that HTLV-1–infected lymphocytes had infiltrated the skin.[277] Cultured keratinocytes from children with infectious dermatitis have been shown to exhibit overexpression of proinflammatory and antiinflammatory cytokines that could be induced directly or indirectly by HTLV-1 infection.[557] Secretion of cytokines by HTLV-1–infected cells may amplify or maintain a persistent inflammatory reaction in the skin and, when combined with the enhanced susceptibility to infection induced by HTLV-1–associated immunodysfunction, could result in the clinical manifestations of infective dermatitis. Although likely secreting cytokines that contribute to the disease process, in IDH infiltrating $CD8^+$ lymphocytes are typically not activated with cytotoxic granulations, whereas in atopic dermatitis lymphocytes are activated, expressing perforin and granzyme-B and contributing to the inflammatory process.[58] This distinction, along with the difference in $CD4^+$/$CD8^+$ ratios among infiltrating cells, may present a distinguishing feature in the differential diagnosis between atopic dermatitis and IDH.[56,58]

In the Bahia series, all patients responded to antibiotic treatment; trimethoprim-sulfamethoxazole is commonly used. Yet relapse was very common after discontinuation of antibiotics. Although active disease continues in approximately two-thirds of patients, persistent disseminated disease is rare (a single child), indicating long-term improvements over time with treatment. In this series, in which cases have been followed for up to 12 years, the mean age at which IDH disappeared (one-third of patients) was 15 years (range, 10–20 years).

Not infrequently, IDH progresses to HAM/TSP and rarely to ATLL.[56,122,379] In the Bahia case series, 47% of children with IDH progressed to HAM/TSP in childhood or adolescence, with more than 80% of HAM/TSP cases defined as definite. An association with development of HAM/TSP has been reported from other settings, as well.[56,379] IDH has similar virologic and immunologic features to HAM/TSP, with high proviral load and high levels of TNF-α and IFN-γ[379]; in a Brazilian study, no differences were found between IDH and HAM/TSP patients in the latter two markers. It is suggested, then, that IDH is a risk factor for the development of HAM/TSP.[379] IDH may also be a risk factor for progression to ATLL.[56,59] Progression to ATLL has been seen in the Bahia cohort and others, although much less commonly than progression to HAM/TSP.[56,122,379] Of 52 cases of ATLL with skin involvement observed in Bahia, 37% of patients reported a history of severe childhood eczema suggestive of IDH,[55] and flower cells were observed in 17% of a 30-patient IDH cohort in childhood or puberty, possibly representing a prodromal stage of ATLL.

In addition to the risk for subsequent TAM/HSP and ATLL in children with IDH, warranting periodic neurologic examinations as part of follow-up, IDH's other complications, occurring in 30% to 35% of patients, also should be appreciated. *Strongyloides* is a common coinfection in IDH cases. Given its putative role in the pathogenesis of ATLL through stimulating clonal expansion of lymphocytes and its generally asymptomatic nature, *Strongyloides* should be actively sought in all IDH cases and treated when present because appropriate *Strongyloides* treatment can reverse clonal expansion and may reduce the risk for ATLL developing.[167] Other reported complications include crusted (Norwegian) scabies, chronic bronchiectasis, lymphocytic interstitial pneumonitis, and glomerulonephritis, which reflect the systemic complications of HTLV-1 infection. Early death caused by severe bacterial infections with sepsis may occur, and rheumatic heart disease and kidney failure have been reported as causes of death in adolescents with IDH.[122]

Other Disorders in Adults and Children

Numerous autoimmune disorders have been associated with HTLV-1. In a study of 113 HTLV-1–infected patients in southern Florida, rheumatologic or autoimmune diseases were not uncommon manifestations.[209] In two settings, HTLV-1 infection is associated with arthritis[340]:

in patients with ATLL and in those who are HTLV-1 seropositive but do not have ATLL or HAM/TSP.[340,382] Polyarthritis is a common presenting feature of ATLL, with some patients manifesting arthritis for as much as 5 years before ATLL diagnosis. Most patients with ATLL-associated arthritis are negative for rheumatoid factor. In patients with HTLV-1–associated arthritis (HAA) without ATLL, onset is typically after 50 years of age, and presentation is a chronic oligoarthritis with large joints (shoulders, knees, and wrists) most commonly affected. As with HAA in ATLL, rheumatoid factor is typically negative. Strong suspicion exists that HAA represents another disease caused by HTLV-1, as opposed to simply HTLV-1 associated, because synovial fluid and tissue in HAA cases contain high proportions of ATLL-like cells, along with HTLV-1 proviral DNA. As well, HAA occurs in HTLV-1 *tax*-transgenic mice,[239] and there are suggestions that HTLV-1 Tax protein may be associated with proliferation of synovial cells, leading to erosion of cartilage and bone.

HTLV-1–associated polymyositis has been well described in patients with HAM/TSP.[353,354,405,587,590] Muscle biopsy is consistent with myositis with mononuclear interstitial infiltrates, necrosis, and regeneration. HTLV-1 provirus has been identified by in situ hybridization in CD4$^+$ cells in the inflammatory cell infiltrate.[217] The mechanism by which HTLV-1 produces disease is unknown. It is probably not a direct viral effect because HTLV-1 does not appear to infect muscle cells.[353,354] As hypothesized for HAM/TSP, the pathologic process could be the result of an autoimmune response, or it could be caused by the production of cytokines in focal inflammatory infiltrates in muscle by activated HTLV-1–infected CD4$^+$ cells and subsequent bystander damage to the myofibers. Cases complicating HAM/TSP may be severe, with diaphragmatic involvement and respiratory failure.[299] As well, non–HAM/TSP-associated polymyositis has been noted in HTLV-1–infected carriers without HAM/TSP, with predominance in children.[150] Muscular dystrophy–like presentations have been noted,[150] with onset of muscular weakness in early childhood, initially in the lower limbs and progressing to the upper limbs, in the absence of bladder dysfunction or signs of spinal cord or other CNS dysfunction, markedly elevated muscle enzymes, myopathic pattern on electroneuromyography, and diffuse muscular atrophy on MRI.[150] Polymyositis may be associated with uveitis.[265] In some HTLV-1–infected patients coinfected with HIV, inclusion-body myositis has been noted.[110] Therapy includes immunosuppressants and immunomodulators, particularly corticosteroids.[85,150]

Asymptomatic, subclinical lymphocytic pneumonitis has been described in patients with HAM/TSP, and radiologic studies have shown higher rates of pulmonary involvement in HTLV-1 carriers than in individuals not infected with HTLV-1.[394] HTLV-1 carriers have increased risk for pulmonary tuberculosis, cryptococcosis, and community-acquired pneumonia.[21,269,324] The innate immunosuppression induced by HTLV-1 infection contributes to this and can result in frankly immunosuppression-associated infections such as *P. jiroveci* pneumonia. Pulmonary manifestations vary in HTLV-1–associated lung disease, with bronchiolitis, including diffuse panbronchiolitis, alveolitis, and interstitial pneumonia having been noted.[261] HTLV-1 proviral load in peripheral blood mononuclear monocytes corresponds to the degree of bronchoalveolar lymphocytosis,[355] and HTLV-1 mRNA appears to be upregulated in bronchoalveolar lavage fluid cells, in contrast to peripheral blood mononuclear monocytes.[261] Bronchoalveolar lavage has shown the presence of a T-lymphocyte alveolitis, with highly soluble IL-2 receptor levels, increased mRNA levels of cytokines and chemokines, and high proportions of HTLV-1–specific CD8$^+$ cells also found in lavage fluid from these patients, suggesting that HTLV-1 induces pulmonary inflammation.[261,497,498,594] On lung biopsy, marked lymphocytic infiltration of the lung is seen.

Destructive lung disease associated with HTLV-1 has been noted in some populations. HTLV-1 has been shown to be a risk factor for the development of bronchiectasis in some endemic areas, especially in the indigenous central Australian population, where HTLV-1 is prevalent (7.2%–13.9%, although rare elsewhere in Australia) and where bronchiectasis exacts a heavy toll in morbidity and mortality[137]; specifically, higher HTLV-1 subtype c proviral loads have been associated with bronchiectasis and higher risk for lower respiratory infections in indigenous Australians.[136] Annually, 1.5% of indigenous children in central Australia require admission for bronchiectasis[93]; in a recent study, 13% of indigenous Australian adults with bronchiectasis died during a single year of follow-up.[493]

HTLV-1 also has been associated with Sjögren syndrome, a chronic exocrinopathy causing keratoconjunctivitis sicca, xerostomia, and sialadenitis and characterized by a lymphocytic infiltration of the lacrimal and salivary glands; the origin has been hypothesized to be autoimmune. In a study in Japan, HTLV-1 seroprevalence in patients with Sjögren syndrome was 23%, significantly higher than the 3% HTLV-1 seroprevalence in blood donors.[520] HTLV-1 antibody titers in HTLV-1–seropositive patients with Sjögren syndrome were significantly higher than those in asymptomatic HTLV-1 carriers and similar to those seen in patients with HAM/TSP. However, in contrast to that in patients with HAM/TSP, the HTLV-1 proviral load in peripheral blood was not consistently high. In a study of HTLV-1–infected patients from Guadeloupe, French West Indies, a sicca-like syndrome was found in almost 80% of patients, approximately half of whom also had neurologic findings.[38] HTLV-1 provirus has been identified by PCR in acini cells and inflammatory infiltrates in the labial salivary glands of patients with HAM/TSP, as well as in healthy HTLV-1 carriers with the sicca syndrome.[516] In addition, one of the symptoms of Sjögren syndrome is impaired sweating, and HTLV-1 pX sequences have been identified in samples of eccrine sweat gland epithelia from HTLV-1–infected individuals.[480] Transgenic animal models have indicated that HTLV-1 is tropic for ductal epithelium of the salivary and lacrimal glands.[197] Human studies also suggest this, and add to the suggestion that HTLV-1 may be causal in some patients with Sjögren syndrome, because expression of *tax* but not other HTLV-1 genes has been reported in the salivary glands of 29% of patients with Sjögren syndrome from areas of Japan endemic for HTLV-1[501] and in 23% of patients with Sjögren syndrome from French regions not endemic for HTLV-1.[323]

As mentioned earlier, the immunosuppression induced by HTLV-1 is associated with a variety of infectious complications in HTLV-1–infected patients, including higher rates of both leprosy cases and leprosy treatment failures in areas of Africa where both conditions are endemic, as well as a generally increased susceptibility to parasitic diseases. Although malaria is common in many HTLV-1–endemic areas, there does not appear to be an association between HTLV-1 and risk for severe malaria. The association between *Strongyloides* and HTLV-1 infection has been discussed previously, including the possible role of *Strongyloides* in the pathogenesis of HTLV-1–related disease.[79,80,446] As well, HTLV-1 infection is a strong risk factor for the development of *Strongyloides* hyperinfection,[79,80,223,352] which is often fatal,[79,80] as well as for refractory *Strongyloides* and the development of gastrointestinal lymphoma in coinfected patients.[97]

Dual Infection With Human Immunodeficiency Virus Type 1

HIV-1 coinfection in HTLV-1 and HTLV-2 carriers occurs with highest prevalence in large metropolitan areas in Europe, the Americas, and Africa and is probably more frequent than clinicians generally realize because HTLV-1 and HTLV-2 testing is not routine in most HIV programs.[90] Estimates are that HTLV-1 and HTLV-2 rates in HIV-1–infected persons are 100 to 500 times greater than in the general population.[39,41] In some endemic settings,[27,28,149] and in at-risk populations in nonendemic settings, such as intravenous drug users in the United States, 5% to 10% of HIV-1–infected persons may be coinfected with HTLV-1 or HTLV-2.[49,68] A recent study in Brazil showed almost 3% of HIV-positive patients also coinfected with HTLV (64% HTLV-1, 35% HTLV-2).[70]

The natural histories of HIV-1/HTLV-1 and HIV-1/HTLV-2 coinfections appear to be different; HTLV-1 appears to accelerate progression to AIDS[70] and is a risk factor for developing ATLL and HAM/TSP,[538] whereas HTLV-2 may produce an immunologic protection against HIV and delay the progression of immunocompromise.[31]

Indeed during the era before highly active antiretroviral therapy (HAART) (mid-1980s), in a cohort of HIV-1–infected men who have sex with men in Trinidad, progression to AIDS within 48 months of observation occurred in 50% of HTLV-1–coinfected men, in contrast to less than 10% of men without HTLV-1 coinfection.[27] Additional studies in the 1980s also observed accelerated progression to AIDS in

HTLV-1–coinfected individuals.[207,211,484] HTLV-2 coinfection, in contrast to that with HTLV-1, was rarely implicated with HIV-1 disease progression. Multiple studies in adults with HIV-1/HTLV-1 and HIV-1/HTLV-2 coinfections have been carried out since the advent of HAART in the 1990s,[30,71,69,218,540] with consistent findings that HIV-1/HTLV-1 coinfection is associated with shortened survival and a possible increase in risk for HAM/TSP and other neurologic conditions,[234] leukemia, and lymphoma,[39,40,71,83,84] including the otherwise unusual presentation of these conditions in patients with high CD4 counts. On the other hand, HIV-1/HTLV-2 coinfection is associated with delayed progression to both AIDS and death[39,41] and is associated in some cases with long-term nonprogression of HIV-1.[170,171] Pediatric data suggest that the findings in HIV-1/HTLV-1–coinfected adults are also seen in children, with HIV-1/HTLV-1–coinfected children more likely to present with HIV disease signs and symptoms, and to die, than HIV-1–monoinfected children, despite higher CD4 cell counts at presentation in the coinfected cohort.[416] In both adults and children, CD4 levels may be a less reliable predictor of immunodeficiency in HIV-1/HTLV-1–coinfected patients because HTLV-1 may induce elevated CD4 levels through enhancing lymphocyte proliferation, but the function of these cells may be abnormal.[83,84]

Why the clinical differences between HTLV-1 and HTLV-2 coinfection with HIV-1 exist is of substantial interest, and the answer likely lies with an interaction between the Tax-2 protein and several aspects of the HIV-1 replicative cycle along with the modification of several immunologic phenomena.[424]

Human T-Cell Lymphotropic Virus Type 2

First reported in 1982 in association with a T-cell variant of hairy cell leukemia,[250] HTLV-2 is closely related to HTLV-1,[30] with approximately 70% homology in nucleotide sequences[272] and sharing a tropism for T lymphocytes[170,171] and similar mechanisms of transmission.[30] Importantly, however, it has not been shown to be a true oncogenic virus like HTLV-1.[381]

HTLV-2 infection is endemic to indigenous central African (pygmies) and Amerindian populations[203,307] and is epidemic among users of intravenous drugs in urban North and South America, Asia, and Europe.[307,368] Whereas most HTLV-2 infections in urban North and South America, Asia, and Europe are associated with sharing of HTLV-2–infected needles among intravenous drug users, in central African and indigenous American populations, HTLV-2 is probably an ancient infection that has been maintained in the population by sexual transmission and mother-to-child transmission through breastfeeding.[197,281,283] As mentioned earlier, HTLV-2's role in disease causation is less clear than that of HTLV-1,[131] but a possible association with lymphoproliferative and neurologic disorders and increased rates of infectious diseases has been suggested.[52,86,487]

Viral Pathogenesis and Molecular Biology

Characterization at the molecular level of HTLV-2's envelope gene *(env)*, LTR genomic region, and *tax* gene have recognized three HTLV-2 subtypes: HTLV-2a, HTLV-2b, and HTLV-2d. A unique HTLV-2 subtype discovered in the Brazilian Amazon region originally was christened HTLV-2c,[235] but subsequent complete sequencing of this strain demonstrated it to be a molecular variant of HTLV-2a.[307]

Like HTLV-1, HTLV-2 can transform cells in vitro, with experimental evidence suggesting that Tax-2 is able to immortalize $CD4^+$ T lymphocytes in vitro by oncogenic activation, as well as by promoting autophagy, resulting in increased survival and proliferation of immortalized T cells.[448] However, in vivo, HTLV-2 displays a preferential tropism for and induces clonal expansion of cells of the CD8+ T-lymphocyte phenotype,[131] whereas HTLV-1 provirus is chiefly found in $CD4^+$ T lymphocytes. Whether the difference in cell tropism between HTLV-1 and HTLV-2 may explain the differential pathogenicity between the two viruses is unknown. Differences in the two viruses' *tax* gene expression and Tax protein itself have been explored. *Tax-1* possesses a PDZ binding motif in its sequence, a motif that is crucial for *tax-1's* cell-transforming activity and absent from *tax-2*.[96] The results of other gene expressions are also likely involved in the two viruses' divergent virulence. HTLV-1 and HTLV-2 encode accessory proteins p30 and p28, respectively, which possess some homology in amino acid sequence and are required for in vivo viral persistence.[131] Yet p30 and p28 have distinct host protein interaction profiles, resulting in differential expression of a variety of HTLV-1 and HTLV-2 viral genes.[131]

Some molecular differences exist between gene products of the various HTLV-2 subtypes, the clinical importance of which is not clear. Of note, Tax-2 protein appears to differ in length between the HTLV-2a and HTLV-2b subtypes, with the HTLV-2b Tax protein being 25 amino acids longer than the HTLV-2a Tax protein.[412] Functionally, the HTLV-2a Tax protein is a weaker inactivator of the *p53* tumor suppressor gene and a less potent transactivator of the viral LTR in vitro than is the Tax protein from HTLV-1 or HTLV-2b, and limited data suggest that the proviral load may be lower in HTLV-2a–infected than HTLV-2b–infected individuals.[138,312] To date, nonetheless, no indications suggest that disease associations differ in magnitude or effect between HTLV-2 subtypes.

Epidemiology

It is likely that HTLV-2's ancient origins were, like those of HTLV-1, in central Africa, where STLV-2 has been isolated alongside HTLV-2.[460] HTLV-2–infected migrants likely brought the virus to the Americas 15,000 to 35,000 years ago across the land bridge once connecting Asia and North America.[51,280] In the past several decades, HTLV-2 has passed from indigenous Americans to intravenous drug users by sharing of contaminated needles,[555] resulting in an urban HTLV-2 epidemic among this group in Europe, Asia, and the Americas that is well documented.[30,86,307,460]

HTLV-2 prevalence is highest among indigenous communities in the Americas, particularly in the Amazon region, where prevalence as high as 58% has been reported in some tribal groups. Rates of 8% to 10% have been noted among the Guaymi of Panama and Costa Rica[560]; in North American indigenous groups, fewer than 1% of Mayans in the Yucatan are HTLV-2 infected,[188] with higher rates in Pueblo, New Mexico (2–3%),[227] Seminole, Florida (13.2%),[302] and Nuu-chah-nulth Amerindians in British Columbia (1.6%).[422] HTLV-2 seroprevalence is much higher in Amerindian blood donors in New Mexico than non-Hispanic white donors (1–1.6% vs. 0.009–0.06%, respectively).[227] HTLV-2 prevalence in nonindigenous, non–intravenous drug user populations in South America is low, with 0.1% HTLV-2 prevalence noted in an urban Brazilian cohort of pregnant women[200] and less than 0.1% in Brazilian and Venezuelan blood donors.[104,286]

Although HTLV-2 is endemic in Africa, HTLV-2 seroprevalence appears to be relatively low, although in some settings, such as Malawi, HTLV-2 prevalence exceeds that of HTLV-1.[156] Cases are reported sporadically in West and Central Africa,[182,539] and serosurveys suggest low prevalence.[66,148] Only 1 in 907 Gabonese pregnant women screened for HTLV-1 and HTLV-2 was HTLV-2 positive, and HTLV-1 prevalence in the same cohort was 2.1%.[148] HTLV-2 prevalence of 0.8% has been noted in Ivory Coast, 0.05% in Guinea, and 0.02% in Senegal.[66] In higher risk groups in Africa, however, HTLV-2 prevalence may be higher; 2.1% of female sex workers in Eritrea were noted to be HTLV-2 seropositive.[9]

In the United States, Brazil, Europe, and Southeast Asia, HTLV-2 infection is epidemic among intravenous drug users. Globally, the highest rates among intravenous drug users are seen in southern Vietnam, where more than 60% are HTLV-2 infected,[163] with HTLV-2 most likely introduced during the Vietnam War by US military personnel.[460] High rates are also noted in intravenous drug users in south and southeast Brazil[307,356]; in the United States, rates as high as 20% have been noted in some urban populations.[460] In the United States, HTLV-2 accounts for most of the HTLV infections in intravenous drug users.[90] In a study of HTLV-2 and HIV seroprevalence in drug users from eight metropolitan areas in the United States, the overall prevalence of HTLV-2 alone was 15.1%, the prevalence of HIV-1 alone was 9.9%, and that of dual HIV-1/HTLV-2 infection was 3.3%. HTLV-2 prevalence was higher in the Southwest and Midwest than the Northeast, whereas HIV-1 prevalence was highest in the Northeast.[28] Rates of HTLV-2 infection in European intravenous drug users are also high, from 1.6% to 8% in Italy,[184] 0.4 to 11.5% in Spain,[119,459] and 15% in an Irish cohort.[135]

In a recent study of blood donors in North America, 14.7 cases per 100,000 individuals were noted.[94] Peak HTLV-2 prevalence has been previously noted among middle-aged donors, suggesting an age-cohort effect linked to an epidemic of intravenous drug use (including sex with an intravenous drug user) in the 1960s and 1970s.[460] Much lower HTLV-2 rates have been seen in Danish, Swiss, and French blood donors.[63,129,423]

The geographic distribution of HTLV-2 subtypes varies.[201,460] HTLV-2a is the predominant infection in intravenous drug users in North America, the British Isles, northern Europe, and southeast Asia,[135,460] while also being seen in Brazilian Amerindians and intravenous drug users.[6,307] HTLV-2b is endemic in Central and South American indigenous groups, as well as more common among intravenous drug users in southern Europe.[6,135,307,460] It is also the most common strain detected in Central and West Africa,[460] although HTLV-2d is also found in Central African pygmy populations.[460]

Modes of Transmission

HTLV-2, like HTLV-1, is transmitted by transfusion of contaminated cellular blood products, sharing of contaminated needles during injection drug use, from mother to child, and sexually; indeed, parenteral routes of transmission appear to be particularly effective for HTLV-2.[381]

Sexual transmission is also an important mode of HTLV-2 acquisition. Although data are more limited for HTLV-2 than for HTLV-1, sexual transmission of HTLV-2 appears to be an important infection route in multiple populations,[460] including prostitutes and patients attending STI clinics,[44,460] where two-thirds of HTLV infections diagnosed are HTLV-2.[264] This is especially the case for individuals with both an injection drug use history and a history of STIs.[68,476,562] High HTLV-2 prevalence is also noted in non–intravenous drug using patients who have STIs.[474] In Amerindian populations in whom HTLV-2 is common, and injection drug use rare,[460,560] HTLV-2 prevalence is high among both men and women, and there is a strong association of HTLV-2 infection between spouses.[313,560] Seropositivity in Guaymi women is associated with an early age at first sexual intercourse, the number of lifetime sexual partners, and the number of long-term sexual relationships; in men, sexual intercourse with prostitutes is associated with seropositivity.[313] Preferential male-to-female transmission has been suggested by cross-sectional data, as with HTLV-1; the female preponderance of HTLV-2 infection may indicate more efficient sexual transmission of HTLV-2 from men to women than vice versa, and higher HTLV-2 proviral loads in seropositive males are associated with higher rates of HTLV-2 transmission to their partners.[372] Prospective incidence data are sparse; the US study referenced earlier showed equivalent proportions of female-to-male and male-to-female transmissions.[462] In HTLV-2–positive blood donors, a history of sexual contact with an intravenous drug user or an HTLV-2–infected sexual partner was associated with increased risk for HTLV-2 seropositivity.[475]

Injecting drug use is the primary mode of HTLV-2 acquisition in North America, Europe, Asia, and parts of Brazil, where HTLV-2 is endemic among injection drug users.[86,460] In a study of HTLV-infected blood donors (the Retrovirus Epidemiology Donor Study), HTLV-2 infection was associated significantly with injection drug use or sexual contact with an injection drug user, whereas HTLV-1 infection was not.[475] Other risk factors, such as seven or more sexual partners, were common to both HTLV-1 and HTLV-2. Sex with an injection drug user was a particular risk factor for women; 65% of HTLV-2–infected women reported that they had a sexual partner who used injection drugs, and 20% of women reported that they also injected drugs themselves. HTLV-2 infection in drug users has been associated with nonwhite race, older age, markers of previous hepatitis B virus infection, the use of a specific needle-sharing practice called backloading, a history of herpes simplex virus type 2 infection, and a history of receiving money for sex.[76,477,561] In a Spanish study of young injection and noninjection heroin users, approximately 3% of the cohort was HTLV infected, with all HTLV infections being HTLV-2.[119] Indeed, almost all cases of HTLV-2 reported from Spain have been in injection drug users, and the prevalence in Spain in this group is one of the highest in Europe.[43,305,524] Among injection drug users in Spanish prisons, HTLV-2 prevalence is 18%, whereas outside prisons, HTLV-2 rates countrywide in Spain average 5%.[83,84] In an Italian study, seroprevalence among injection drug users for HTLV-2 was 8.2% versus 2.1% for HTLV-1.

HTLV-2 also has been detected in the breast milk of carrier mothers,[460] and mother-to-child transmission has been described in those who breastfeed.[215,274,275,277,278,546] High proviral load in the mother is a clear transmission risk factor.[461] Prolonged breastfeeding is common in Amerindian populations, and high prevalence rates (12–16%) have been documented in children younger than 15 years in several Central and South American indigenous populations.[61,151,560] Like HTLV-1, HTLV-2 appears to be transmitted infrequently in the absence of breastfeeding,[170,171,202,255] and breastfeeding interruption has been shown to prevent perinatal transmission of HTLV-2.[449] Passive immunization with HTLV-2 hyperimmunoglobulin in rabbits prevented blood-borne transmission of HTLV-2–infected cells.[357] Only HTLV-2, and not HTLV-1, immunoglobulin was effective in preventing HTLV-2 transmission, a finding suggesting that despite some cross-reactivity on conventional ELISAs, cross-neutralization between the viruses is minimal or nonexistent.[357]

Clinical Disease

As mentioned previously, HTLV-2 is less virulent than HTLV-1, its main associations being lymphocytosis, infections, and inflammatory manifestations.[29] Why this is is unclear. It has been suggested the reasons lie in higher expression of gene products inducing viral latency (p28 and tRex) as well as differences between Tax-1 and Tax-2 between the two viruses.[99]

Whereas HTLV-1 has been causally linked to diseases such as ATLL and HAM/TSP, as detailed earlier, to date HTLV-2 has not, although an association exists between HTLV-2 and HAM/TSP, especially in HIV-coinfected individuals.[434] In otherwise healthy individuals, HTLV-2 has been associated with increased mortality from a variety of causes.[54,400] In a prospective cohort study of non–HIV-infected American blood donors, controlling for intravenous drug use, all-causes mortality was increased among HTLV-2–infected patients, although no single cause of death could be identified as responsible for the effect.[400] Another prospective study noted a similar effect of HTLV-2 on all-causes mortality, tying the effect to an increase in cancer mortality.[54] Specific cancers noted in excess included lung, cervical, and colorectal cancer, as well as hepatocellular carcinoma, leukemia, lymphoma, and melanoma,[54] suggesting that HTLV-2 may have a facilitating role in cancer development similar to that in HIV, mediated by reduced immunosurveillance of malignant cells in emerging neoplasms.[54]

Although HTLV-2–infected patients commonly have hematologic abnormalities, and cases have been reported of hairy cell leukemia, large granulocytic leukemia, T-prolymphocytic leukemia, and cutaneous lymphoma, including mycosis fungoides, in larger studies HTLV-2 has not been proved to cause leukemia/lymphoma, as has HTLV-1.[280,460] Importantly, HTLV-2 integration in transformed cell or tumor samples has not been detected.[155,310] Yet, although HTLV-2 has not demonstrated a causal role in leukemia/lymphoma, HIV-coinfected individuals may be at higher risk for T-cell leukemia/lymphoma, suggesting that the expansion of HTLV-2–transformed lymphocytes may be prone to dysregulation in the presence of HIV-induced immune system dysfunction and highlighting the oncologic risks for HTLV-2/HIV–coinfected patients.[460]

Evidence suggests that HTLV-2 may be associated with neurologic disorders ranging from a spastic paraparesis-myelopathy similar to HAM/TSP to more widespread involvement of the CNS.[365,434] Myeloneuropathies indistinguishable from HAM/TSP have been reported in patients infected with HTLV-2 alone or coinfected with HIV-1.[45,226,365,370] In a prospective Brazilian cohort, 10% of HTLV-2/HIV–coinfected patients developed HAM/TSP over a 7-year observational period, whereas no patients infected with only HTLV-2 did, suggesting HIV coinfection is a substantial risk factor for developing neurologic disease when infected with HTLV-2.[434] In addition, sensory neuropathies have been noted in patients with HTLV-2 alone,[53] as well as with HIV coinfection,[598] and a chronic neurodegenerative disorder with ataxia as a prominent feature has been reported in HTLV-2–infected individuals.[208,483]

An increased risk for other infections in HTLV-2–infected patients has been suggested, including serious infections such as pneumonia and pyleonephritis.[460] An initial report from San Francisco described an association of HTLV-2 seropositivity and bacterial infections, particularly skin and soft tissue infections and bacterial pneumonia, but the results were confounded by intravenous drug use, which in itself could increase the risk for infections, in nearly all HTLV-2–seropositive patients.[350] In a case-control study of intravenous drug users from Baltimore with an overall HTLV-2 seroprevalence of 7%, no significant association between HTLV-2 seropositivity and the development of bacterial pneumonia, infective endocarditis, and skin abscess was found.[460] However, a prospective study of HIV-negative, HTLV-1–infected and HTLV-2–infected, and uninfected individuals from several large American cities found that HTLV-2–infected persons were more likely to develop asthma, acute bronchitis, bladder or kidney infection, arthritis, and pneumonia than HTLV-2–uninfected persons and that HTLV-1 infection was associated with only bladder or kidney infection or arthritis.[369] Although suggesting that HTLV-2 may inhibit immunologic responses to bacterial infections,[369] the natural history and clinical manifestations of HTLV-2 need further delineation in the context of ongoing prospective studies.

Given HTLV-2's unclear pathogenic role, treatment of HTLV-2 is not established and has not been evaluated systematically.[381]

Other Forms of Human T-Cell Lymphotropic Virus

Three new primate T-cell lymphotropic viruses have been discovered in recent decades. In East Africa in 1994, STLV-3 was described in a nonhuman primate.[193] In the mid-2000s, the identification of HTLV-3 and HTLV-4 among bushmeat hunters in Cameroon demonstrated greater HTLV diversity than was recognized previously. Preliminary data suggest that HTLV-3 comes from a simian origin, whereas HTLV-4 does not appear to have a known simian counterpart, despite extensive screening of monkeys in Cameroon.[310] It is predicted that HTLV-3 and HTLV-4 may be widespread in central Africa, although of low prevalence.[74,580]

Both of these newer forms of HTLV cross-react with current HTLV-1 and HTLV-2 assays, giving positive or indeterminate results and highlighting the need for more specific subtype testing. Currently PCR assays specific for PTLV-3 and PTLV-4 are required for HTLV-3 or HTLV-4 detection.[421] Although both HTLV-3 and HTLV-4 contain sequences encoding for some of the proteins believed to be involved in the pathogenesis of HTLV-associated T-cell malignancies,[421] no clinical maladies in either humans or simians have been attributed to HTLV-3 or HTLV-4 to date,[134,310,421,504] and concern exists about the spread of infection by blood donations from infected persons or by those who participate in primate hunting. A 2010 sample from New York State of more than 1000 HTLV-infected patients, HTLV-indeterminate blood donors, and other subjects with epidemiologic or clinical features suggesting risk for HTLV-associated disease was negative for HTLV-3 and HTLV-4.[421] Molecular studies have established that in terms of transcriptional activation, Tax-3 is a functional analogue of Tax-1 and is distinctly different from Tax-2, suggesting that HTLV-3 may have pathogenic features in common with HTLV-1.[96] HTLV-4's Tax protein has similarities to that of HTLV-2, missing the PDZ motif present in Tax-1 and Tax-3 important for cellular signal transduction and transformation, as is Tax-2.[504] Further study is required to understand more clearly what implications these newer forms of HTLV have on human disease.

Future Directions

Effective treatments for HTLV-1-associated disease are of great clinical interest, and trials are ongoing in pursuit of HTLV-1 therapies (Table 192A.4).

LENTIVIRUSES: HUMAN IMMUNODEFICIENCY VIRUS TYPE 2

First identified in 1986, HIV-2 has a morphology and life cycle similar to those of HIV-1 but with significant antigenic, biologic, epidemiologic, and clinical differences (Table 192A.5). The viruses have similar modes of transmission, and each can result in immune depletion and AIDS. However, whereas HIV-1 has a global distribution, HIV-2 is confined primarily to West Africa and is found only sporadically in Europe, the United States, and other countries. In all settings in recent decades, the incidence and prevalence of HIV-2 have declined and HIV-1 infection has become more likely. The clinical course of HIV-2 infection is generally more indolent than that of HIV-1; the clinical latency period is longer, progression to AIDS is less common, and rates of perinatal and sexual transmission are lower. The basis of such differences in natural history between these two lentiviruses is unknown and may result from characteristics of the virus, the host, or both.

Viral Genome and Pathogenesis

Like HIV-1, HIV-2 is thought to have entered human populations through cross-species transmission. HIV-2 is closely related to simian immunodeficiency virus from the sooty mangabey (SIV_{SM}) indigenous to West Africa. Nine genetic groups of HIV-2 have been identified. However, current data suggest that only HIV-2 groups A and B are established in significant amounts in the human population,[47] with the remaining groups being identified in single individuals. Intergroup recombinant forms of HIV-2 involving groups A and B have been identified.[231,587,588] No significant differences in transmission, pathogenicity, or disease progression have been observed between the HIV-2 groups A and B.

The genomes of HIV-1 and HIV-2 encode 16 viral proteins that play roles essential for HIV infection and replication. Three major genes, *gag*, *pol*, and *env*, encode structural proteins (capsid, matrix, nucleocapsid, and p6), viral enzymes (protease, reverse transcriptase, and integrase),

TABLE 192A.4 Registered Studies in Human T-Cell Lymphotropic Virus (2010–15)

Clinical Trial Identifier	Sponsor (Location)	Initiation Date	Objectives
NCT01867320	NINDS (USA)	May 2013	To evaluate the effect of raltegravir in decreasing viral load of patients with HAM/TSP
NCT01754311	Centre Hospitalier Universitaire de Fort-de-France (France	December 2012	To evaluate prevalence and influence of CT/TT genotype in HTLV-1 infection and HAM/TSP
NCT01712659	NCI (USA)	October 2012	To test safety and efficacy of ruxolitinib in treating HTLV-1–associated ATLL
NCT01472263	Hospital Universitario Professor Edgard Santos (Brazil)	November 2011	To evaluate the efficacy of pentoxifyline in HTLV-1 patients with neurologic diseases: HAM/TSP or neurogenic bladder
NCT01640002	Hospital Universitario Professor Edgard Santos (Brazil)	July 2011	To assess the efficacy of propantheline bromide to treat OAB in HTLV-1–infected patients
NCT01343355	St. Marianna University School of Medicine (Japan)	April 2011	To evaluate the efficacy of tamibarotene in motor and urination function, HTLV-1 proviral load, immunologic parameters, and markers in the spinal fluid in patients with HAM/TSP
NCT01274533	Columbia University (USA)	January 2011	To determine the efficacy of lenalidomide monotherapy in relapsed or refractory HTLV-1–associated ATLL

ATLL, Adult T-cell leukemia/lymphoma; *HAM/TSP*, HTLV-1–associated myelopathy/tropical spastic paraparesis; *HTLV-1*, human T-cell lymphotropic virus type 1; *OAB*, overactive bladder.
From Nicolas D, Ambrosioni J, Paredes R, et al. *Expert Rev Anti Infect Ther.* 2015;13(8):947-963.

TABLE 192A.5 **Comparison of Human Immunodeficiency Virus Types 1 and 2**

Characteristic	HIV-2	HIV-1
Viral genome	Genes encoding structural proteins: *gag, pol, env*	Genes encoding structural proteins: *gag, pol, env*
	Genes encoding regulatory proteins: *tat, rev*	Genes encoding regulatory proteins: *tat, rev*
	Genes encoding accessory proteins: *vif, vpr, vpx*	Genes encoding accessory proteins: *vif, vpr, vpu*
Co-receptor usage	CCR5, CXCR4, CCR3, CCR8, GPR1, GPR15, CXCR6, RDC1 and apj[359]	CCR5, CXCR4
Geographic distribution	West Africa: Guinea-Bissau, Burkina Faso, the Gambia, Senegal, Ivory Coast Outside of West Africa, primarily in countries with political and economic ties with West Africa: Portugal, France, Germany, Brazil	Global
Prevalence over time	Declining[109,352]	Increasing
Mode of transmission	Sexual, blood-borne, mother to child	Sexual, blood-borne, mother to child
Risk of mother-to-child transmission (without antiretroviral prophylaxis)	1.2–4%[4,391]	24.4–24.7%
Viral set point	2500 copies/mL (28-fold lower than HIV-1)[8]	70,000 copies/mL
Progression to AIDS (without antiretroviral treatment)	Infrequent (probability of remaining AIDS free at 1 and 3 years being 96.6% and 94.5%, respectively)[333]	Frequent
Increase in mortality above that of HIV-seronegative individuals	2-fold to 4-fold increase[48,436,452]	10-fold increase
Mortality rates	52 deaths/patient-years observed[332]	87 deaths/patient-years observed
Antiretroviral medication resistance	Intrinsically resistant to nonnucleoside reverse transcriptase inhibitors[579] and fusion inhibitors[437,578]	

AIDS, acquired immunodeficiency virus; *HIV*, human immunodeficiency virus; *LTR*, long terminal repeat.

and envelope proteins (GP120 and GP41). The remaining genes code for regulatory proteins (Tat and Rev) and accessory proteins (Vif, Vpu/Vpx, Vpr and Nef). Vpu is found exclusively in HIV-1, and Vpx is found in HIV-2. The function of and the interactions between the various HIV proteins in the viral lifecycle,[296] as well as how HIV accessory proteins interact with host cellular proteins to overcome host pathways and processes that act to limit viral infection and replication, are areas of active investigation.[496,334]

Both HIV-1 and HIV-2 bind to CD4 receptors on the surface of susceptible cells. In addition to CD4, binding to a chemokine coreceptor is required for effective infection of target cells. Chemokines act as potent chemoattractants of a large variety of mononuclear cells to sites of inflammation or secondary lymphoid organs by interacting with chemokine receptors. The seven-transmembrane G-protein–coupled chemokine receptors CCR5 and CXCR4 are the major coreceptors used for HIV-1 and HIV-2 infection in vivo. Binding of HIV to chemokine receptors together with CD4 molecules permits fusion of the virus and cell membranes to occur and ultimately viral entry into target cells. Cell tropism of HIV is determined by the expression of CD4$^+$ and these coreceptors.

The CCR5 receptor is used by the majority of HIV-1 isolates (R5 viruses), but some isolates from individuals with more advanced immunodeficiency use CXCR4 (X4 viruses) instead of or in addition to CCR5. CXCR4-binding viruses emerge late in disease in as many as 50% of patients with AIDS. The presence of X4 virus, as well as a switch from CCR5 to CXCR4 use, is associated with accelerated rate of disease progression, although it is not a prerequisite because not all infected individuals demonstrate this coreceptor switch.

Whereas both HIV-1 and HIV-2 infect CD4$^+$ T lymphocytes and use CXCR4 or CCR5 coreceptors for cell entry, primary HIV-2 isolates can use multiple additional coreceptors to infect indicator cell lines in vitro,[359] including CCR3, CCR8, GPR1, GPR15, CXCR6, RDC1, and apj.

The cytopathicity of HIV-2 appears similar to that of HIV-1 and is determined in part by the type of coreceptor used for cell entry. In an in vitro study comparing HIV-1 and HIV-2 coreceptor use and cytopathicity in human lymphoid cells, HIV-2 specificity for the CCR5 coreceptor alone or in combination with other coreceptors was associated with restricted cytopathicity, whereas specificity for CXCR4 was linked to a more virulent phenotype, as observed for HIV-1.[474] Coreceptor use of primary HIV variants isolated from individuals who had undetectable viral loads, preserved CD4$^+$ cell counts, and a nonprogressive clinical course was compared with those from individuals with more progressive disease. In this comparison, HIV-2 variants were found to use CCR5, GPR15, and CXCR6 with high efficiency regardless of the clinical course, but only HIV-2 variants isolated from individuals with viremia or overt progressive disease could use CXCR4. X4 variants were not observed in all individuals with progressive infection, a finding indicating that the capacity to use CXCR4 is not the only determinant of HIV-2 virulence. Studies have shown that the use of CCR1, CCR2b, and CCR3 coreceptors is rare.[60] Thus the lesser virulence of HIV-2, in contrast to that of HIV-1, does not appear to be the result of a restriction in coreceptor use or lower intrinsic cytopathic potential. In addition, the broadening of the coreceptor use did not necessarily increase the pathogenic potential of HIV-2 strains.[548]

Lentiviral envelope glycoproteins can induce production of cytokines and other immunologic disturbances; differences in the effect of the HIV-1 and HIV-2 envelope glycoprotein also could contribute to differences in the pathogenicity of the viruses. Recombinant HIV-2 envelope glycoprotein is superior to the HIV-1 envelope in stimulating the production of IFN-γ and IL-16, both of which inhibit viral replication, and less effective in producing expression of IL-4, which stimulates viral replication.[380,479] The HIV-2 envelope glycoprotein inhibits T-cell proliferation more than does the glycoprotein of HIV-1 in vitro and also was found to inhibit expression of cell surface activation markers.[87] The presence of an HIV-2 protein that reduces immune system stimulation may decrease replication, result in lower levels of HIV-2 viremia, and decrease CD4$^+$ cell apoptosis. The rate of total lymphocyte apoptosis has been found to be lower in HIV-2 than in HIV-1 infection.[342] In one study, 50% of peripheral blood mononuclear cells from HIV-2–infected commercial sex workers resisted in vitro challenge with CCR5-dependent HIV-1, but not CXCR4-dependent HIV-1.[270] Additionally, high levels of β-chemokines RANTES (regulated on activation, normal T-cell expressed and secreted), macrophage inflammatory protein (MIP)-1α, and MIP-1β, the natural ligands of the CCR5 receptor, were secreted when these resistant peripheral blood mononuclear cells from HIV-2–infected individuals underwent stimulation. These investigators hypothesized that β-chemokine–mediated resistance could play a role in the potential protection of some HIV-2–infected individuals from secondary HIV-1 infection.

Epidemiology

Although the global prevalence of HIV-2 infection has been far exceeded by that of HIV-1, HIV-2 remains endemic in former Portuguese and French colonies in West and South Central Africa, including Guinea-Bissau, Burkina Faso, the Gambia, Cape Verde, Senegal, and the Ivory Coast, as well as in Angola and Mozambique.[325]

In these settings, there has been diverging epidemiology between HIV-2 and HIV-1 infections, with the prevalence of HIV-2 declining while that of HIV-1 has increased. Guinea-Bissau, for example, had the highest recorded adult prevalence of 8.9% in 1987.[436] In the decade between 1996 and 2006, Guinea-Bissau had a reduction in the prevalence of HIV-2 from 7.4% in 1996 to 4.4% in 2006, particularly among men and women younger than 45 years. Over the same time period, the prevalence of HIV-1 increased from 2.3% to 4.6%.[109,321] Mathematical models predict a continued decline in HIV-2 acquisition and prevalence, with eventual extinction of HIV-2 in areas of West Africa.[160]

Outside of the countries in West and South Central Africa in which it is endemic, HIV-2 has been reported primarily in regions in Europe, South America, and India with historical socioeconomic ties to West Africa. In Europe, the greatest numbers of HIV-2 cases have been reported in Portugal, France, and Germany. The cultural and economic ties of Portugal to its former colonies in West Africa likely facilitated the spread of HIV-2 to Europe and possibly Brazil, also a former Portuguese colony. Portugal has experienced great changes in the epidemiology of HIV-2 infections over time. By the end of 2008, the cumulative number of HIV-2 infections in Portugal was 1813. Until 2000, the majority of HIV-2–infected individuals in Portugal were Portuguese-born males living in the north of the country, many with direct or indirect relationships with Africa. In contrast, from 2000 to 2007, most of the patients diagnosed with HIV-2 infection were females of West African origin living in the capital city of Lisbon.[79,80] These shifts in infection trends have been attributed to sociopolitical events in West African countries and population migration both to and within Portugal. Indigenous HIV-2 transmission also may occur, inasmuch as HIV-2 infections not directly linked to West Africa have been reported in Portugal, France, and Spain.

Sociopolitical pressures and international migration have resulted in the identification of individuals infected with HIV-2 in other countries as well. In England, Wales, and Northern Ireland, the prevalence of HIV-2 infection among clinic attendees with STIs was 0.006% (6 per 104,006) in 2002. Most of these patients likely were infected through heterosexual intercourse in West Africa. Of 1324 HIV-infected adults, 917 (69%) were HIV-1 infected and 52 (6%) were HIV-2 or HIV-1/HIV-2 coinfected; the HIV type was not reported in the remaining 355 (27%). The ratio of HIV-2 and HIV-1/HIV-2 dual infections to HIV-1 infections varied greatly by country of infection, with the Gambia (11.7–15.2%) and Ivory Coast (7.2–9.8%) having a high proportion of HIV-2 infections and Nigeria (0.7–1%) a low proportion.[132] From 1988 to June 2010 in the United States, 166 cases met the CDC working case definition for HIV-2 infection. Most cases (66%) were concentrated in the northeastern United States, particularly New York City, and 81% occurred among individuals born in West Africa.[523] Between 2000 and 2008 in New York City alone, 62 HIV-2–infected individuals were identified, of whom 82.7% (48 per 62) were born in West African countries.[523] It is important to note that in the past, HIV-2 infection has been difficult to diagnose, hampered by diagnostic algorithms that inadequately distinguished HIV-1 and HIV-2 monoinfections and HIV-1/HIV-2 dual infection. Now that better HIV-2 diagnostics are available, it may be found that although HIV-2 infections contribute only marginally to the overall global HIV burden, HIV-2 may be less geographically restricted than previously thought.

Dual Infections With Human Immunodeficiency Virus Types 1 and 2

Dual infection with HIV-1 and HIV-2 has been observed in areas that are endemic for both viruses.[125,176,417] In a cross-sectional survey of Guinea-Bissau households, the prevalence rates of HIV-1 and HIV-2 are similar (4.6% and 4.4%, respectively), but HIV-1/HIV-2 dual infections remained rare (0.5%).[124] In the United States, 11% (19 per 166) of HIV-2 cases were confirmed to be HIV-1/HIV-2 coinfections.[523]

Although some reports suggested that infection with HIV-2 may be protective against subsequent acquisition of HIV-1 infection, this was not confirmed in other studies.[16,384,528,529,573] In two studies, HIV-2–positive subjects actually had a tendency toward a higher risk for acquiring HIV-1 infection than did seronegative individuals.[385,576] Susceptibility to dual HIV-1 and HIV-2 infection was studied in a macaque model of HIV infection.[404,442] The timing of secondary virus exposure was found to be a critical factor in the risk for acquiring infection. Productive mixed infections were established with simultaneous exposure or when viral challenge occurred within 4 weeks after primary infection developed. However, animals exposed at 8 weeks or more after primary inoculation were resistant to secondary infection. The mechanism of protection is not known.[404,442]

A retrospective examination of data from the long-term follow-up of a cohort of members of the Guinea-Bissau police force suggests that the progression of HIV-1 infection may be inhibited by concomitant HIV-2 infection, particularly when HIV-2 infection occurred before HIV-1 infection. Differences were found in progression of infection, with the median time to developing AIDS being 68 months for those with HIV-1 infection alone and 104 months for individuals with HIV-1/HIV-2 dual infection. When those with dual infection were stratified by whether HIV-2 infection occurred before or simultaneously with HIV-1, the median times to development of AIDS were 129 months and 88 months, respectively.[147]

Mode of Transmission

The modes of acquisition of HIV-2 are identical to those of HIV-1: heterosexual and homosexual intercourse, intravenous drug use, receipt of contaminated blood products, and transmission from mother to child. The infectivity of HIV-2 is lower than that of HIV-1, and transmission of HIV-2 by sexual intercourse and from mother to child is much less frequent than that observed with HIV-1.[252]

Sexual Transmission

The likelihood of sexual transmission of HIV depends in part on the quantity of HIV in genital tract secretions, which correlates with plasma viral loads. Accordingly, because plasma viral loads are higher in those with HIV-1 infection compared with HIV-2, HIV-1 is detected in semen more commonly and at higher quantities. In one report, HIV-2–infected subjects had a 0.7 $\log_{10}$ lower HIV semen viral load than those with HIV-1, even after adjusting for plasma viral load.[190]

Female genital shedding of HIV is important in both heterosexual and mother-to-child transmission of the virus. In a cross-sectional sampling of HIV-infected women living in Dakar, Senegal, HIV-1 shedding occurred more commonly than did shedding of HIV-2. HIV-2 shedding was associated with older age, severe vitamin A deficiency, advanced HIV disease, and $CD4^+$ cell counts lower than 200 cells/mm^3. Viral shedding was not detected in any women with HIV-1/HIV-2 dual infection.[477] In a subsequent study of HIV-infected women in Senegal, again HIV-1–infected women were more likely to shed virus and to have high levels of virus in the genital tract than those infected with HIV-2: 78% versus 58%, respectively. Viral shedding correlated more with plasma viral load than HIV type or CD4 count. HIV-1 and HIV-2 shedding was always detected in women with genital or cervical ulcerative disease. Women with HIV-1/HIV-2 dual infections were not included in this study.[212]

Perinatal Transmission

Perinatal transmission of HIV-2 appears to be a rare occurrence, with vertical transmission from breastfeeding mothers with HIV-2 infection in the absence of ART being less than 4%.[4,390,408] In a large prospective study from the Ivory Coast, the risk for perinatal transmission from HIV-1–infected mothers was 21-fold greater than from HIV-2–infected mothers; transmission rates were 24.7% from HIV-1–infected mothers versus 1.2% from HIV-2–infected mothers.[4] In another large study in the Gambia, the estimated rate of mother-to-child transmission of HIV-2 was 4% compared with 24.4% for HIV-1. In this study, three of seven HIV-2–infected infants were infected after reaching 2 months of age, a finding suggesting that HIV-2, like HIV-1, can be transmitted postnatally through breast milk.[391]

In a large French cohort of 8660 HIV-infected mothers who delivered babies between 1994 and 2007, 2.6% of the women were HIV-2 monoinfected. The mother-to-child transmission rate was much lower for HIV-2–infected women than for those infected with HIV-1 (0.6% vs. 5.2%) and was most pronounced in those women not receiving ART and those receiving nucleoside reverse transcriptase inhibitor (NRTI) monotherapy. The mother-to-child transmission among women with CD4 cell counts greater than 350 cells/mm^3 was significantly lower in HIV-2–infected mothers than in HIV-1–infected mothers. For those women with severe immunosuppression (CD4 cell counts <200 cells/mm^3), however, the risks for transmission were more similar between the groups, 5.3% and 9%, respectively, for women infected with HIV-2 and HIV-1.[73] Maternal plasma viral load at delivery has been demonstrated to be a significant risk factor for perinatal transmission of both HIV-1 and HIV-2 infection. Among mothers in the Gambia, for every 1 $\log_{10}$ increase in plasma RNA, the odds of transmission were 2.7 for HIV-1 and 2.8 for HIV-2.[391] After adjusting for viral load, the odds for transmitting HIV-1 were similar to those for HIV-2; this finding suggests that the level of viremia, as opposed to the type of virus, is the major determinant of the difference in mother-to-child transmission rates between HIV-1 and HIV-2.

HIV transmission from women who are dually seropositive for HIV-1 and HIV-2 has been described; HIV-1 appears to be transmitted more efficiently than does HIV-2, and HIV-1 transmission rates from dually infected women are similar to those from women infected with HIV-1 alone. Transmission of dual infection to the infant, although a rare occurrence, has been described. In the Ivory Coast cohort, 19% of women with HIV-1/HIV-2 dual infection transmitted HIV to their infants; of 11 infected infants, 10 were infected with HIV-1 alone and 1 was dually infected.[4]

Diagnosis of Human Immunodeficiency Virus Type 2

The CDC and the US Preventive Services Task Force both recommend routine HIV screening for adolescent and adult patients unless the patient declines testing. This "opt-out" testing is offered regardless of whether the patient or the health care provider identifies a specific risk for acquisition of HIV infection. If risk factors are identified that place the patient at increased risk for HIV acquisition, annual or more frequent testing may be recommended.[67,363]

The current HIV testing algorithm (Fig. 192A.5) better detects HIV-2 monoinfection and HIV-1/HIV-2 dual infections. Testing begins with a US Food and Drug Administration (FDA)-approved antigen/antibody combination immunoassay that detects HIV-1 and HIV-2 antibodies and HIV-1 p24 antigen to screen for established infections with HIV-1 or HIV-2 and for acute HIV-1 infection. Because of the use of the antigen/antibody screening immunoassay, this algorithm identities HIV infection sooner after infection than previous immunoassays. For specimens that are nonreactive on this initial immunoassay, no further testing is required. Specimens reactive to the antigen/antibody combination immunoassay are then tested with an antibody assay that differentiates between HIV-1 antibodies and HIV-2 antibodies. The use of the HIV-1, HIV-2 antibody discriminating assay allows the more accurate diagnosis of HIV-2 monoinfection and HIV-1/HIV-2 dual infection. If the differentiation test is reactive, the result is positive for HIV-1, HIV-2, or both. Specimens reactive by antigen/antibody combination immunoassay but negative or indeterminate for antibody by the type-differentiating immunoassay would proceed to HIV-1 nucleic acid testing for resolution of HIV-1 infection status. Individuals with a positive HIV-1 nucleic acid test and a negative or indeterminate result on the HIV-1, HIV-2 differentiation test are considered to have acute HIV-1 infection. Specimens reactive for HIV-2 with or without reactivity to HIV-1 should be confirmed with a supplemental HIV-2 antibody test such as a HIV-2 Western blot. Ideally, to confirm HIV-2 infection, HIV-2 virus would be isolated by nucleic acid testing, particularly demonstrating HIV-2 proviral DNA in peripheral blood monocytes because HIV-2 viral loads may be low. Currently, there are no FDA-approved qualitative or quantitative HIV-2 nucleic acid assays, and such testing is available through the CDC.[89]

Natural History

Although HIV-2 is fully pathogenic in humans and may lead to AIDS that is indistinguishable from HIV-1–associated AIDS,[332,333] the clinical course of HIV-2 infection has been found to be more indolent, characterized by a longer asymptomatic phase with slower CD4 cell depletion and progression to AIDS than that of HIV-1 infection.[306,326,327,430] HIV-2 infection may resemble a slowly progressive or nonprogressive HIV-1 infection, with 86% to 95% of people infected with HIV-2 being long-term nonprogressors.[549] Compared with that of HIV uninfected

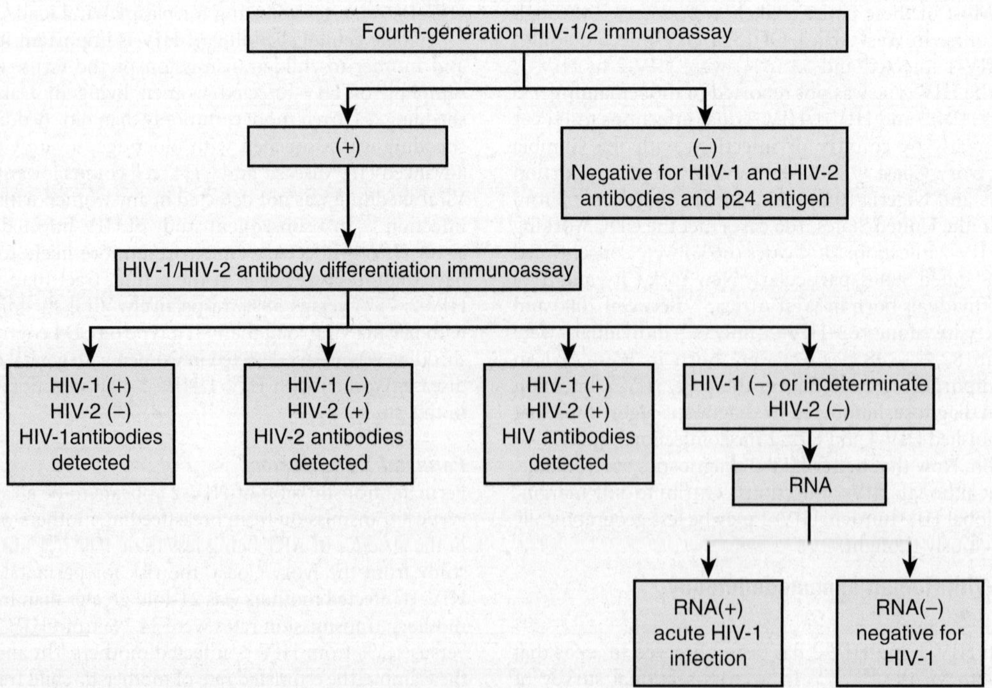

FIG. 192A.5 Recommended laboratory HIV testing algorithm for serum or plasma specimens. (From Centers for Disease Control and Prevention and Association of Public Health Laboratories. Laboratory testing for the diagnosis of HIV infection: updated recommendations. 2014. https://stacks.cdc.gov/view/cdc/23447.)

individuals, the HIV-2 mortality rate is increased by 2-fold to 4-fold, in contrast to a 10-fold increase with HIV-1 infection.[48,436,452]

Similar to those with HIV-1 infection, the clinical course for those infected with HIV-2 can be heterogeneous. But whereas most HIV-1–infected individuals experience disease progression to AIDS, most HIV-2–infected individuals experience little or no disease progression, with only a minority progressing to AIDS. For asymptomatic HIV-infected individuals, CD4 cell counts are higher in those infected with HIV-2 than in those infected with HIV-1 (946 cells/μL and 560 cells/μL, respectively).[306] Among individuals enrolled in the French HIV-2 cohort, immunosuppression as indicated by CD4 cell depletion was correlated with clinical progression of disease, with CD4 cell counts of 482 cells/μL, 293 cells/μL, and 81 cells/μL for individuals at CDC stages A, B, and C respectively.[333] In this cohort, disease progression occurred infrequently, with the probability of remaining AIDS-free at 1 and 3 years being 96.6% and 94.5%, respectively. Only 19 of the 152 (12.7%) patients classified as CDC group A or B at enrollment experienced at least one group B or C event. Only 9 of those who progressed developed AIDS. The most common AIDS-defining events were tuberculosis and wasting syndrome. Overall survival rates within the cohort were 97% and 93.4% at 1 and 3 years, respectively.[333]

In a clinic-based cohort of enrollees infected with HIV-1 and HIV-2 in Gambia, fewer individuals with HIV-2 than with HIV-1 developed AIDS (36.4% vs. 27.6%).[332] In this cohort, among those individuals with AIDS, CD4 cell counts were higher in those with HIV-2 in contrast to HIV-1 (176 cells/μL vs. 109 cells/μL). More individuals with HIV-2 than with HIV-1 had CD4 cell counts greater than 200 cells/μL (44% and 33%, respectively). Overall, similar to the French cohort, the most common AIDS-defining conditions included wasting syndrome and pulmonary tuberculosis. The pattern was similar between patients infected with HIV-1 and HIV-2, with two exceptions: compared with those infected with HIV-1, individuals with HIV-2 had significantly more wasting syndrome and significantly less Kaposi sarcoma.[332] After the diagnosis of AIDS, individuals with HIV-2 survived twice as long as those with HIV-1, with median lengths of survival after AIDS diagnosis of 6.3 months and 12.6 months, respectively. Mortality rates were 52/patient years observed (PYO) for HIV-2–infected individuals and 87/PYO for those with HIV-1. At the time of death, CD4 cell counts remained higher for those with HIV-2 than for those with HIV-1 (120 cells/μL and 62 cells/μL, respectively).[332]

Just as for HIV-1, HIV-2 plasma viral load correlates with progression of disease as measured by CD4 cell decline or mortality. The viral set point is significantly lower in HIV-2 infection than in HIV-1 infection. Recent HIV-2 seroconverters have plasma HIV RNA levels 28 times lower than those of recent HIV-1 seroconverters. For HIV-1, the viral set point has been demonstrated to be a very good predictor of outcome of disease. Differences in viral load throughout most of the natural history of HIV-1 and HIV-2 infection likely account for the differences in progression of disease and transmissibility reported between the two viruses.[8,15,430,492]

HIV-2 viremia has been associated with more pronounced immunosuppression, more rapid disease progression, and a greater likelihood for death. In a comparison of HIV-1–infected and HIV-2–infected persons with similar CD4 cell counts, the quantitative viral load was significantly lower in those infected with HIV-2.[482] Plasma viral load is inversely related to CD4 counts, with each decline in $CD4^+$ cell count by 100 cells/μL associated with an increase in plasma viral load of 0.07 $\log_{10}$ copies/mL.[333] In this study the risk for disease progression was higher in individuals with plasma viral loads of 1000 copies/mL or greater than in those with plasma viral loads less than 1000 copies/mL—26% versus 6%. In patients with no immunosuppression ($CD4^+$ cell count >500/mm^3), none of the HIV-2–infected individuals had a detectable plasma viral load, in contrast to 52% of HIV-1–infected persons. Individuals with HIV-2 had a significantly lower mortality rate than that of HIV-1–infected patients or those with HIV-1/HIV-2 dual infections.[472] Among HIV-infected patients with advanced disease ($CD4^+$ counts <200 cells/μL), all had a poor prognosis, and no difference in mortality rates occurred among HIV-1, HIV-2, or dually infected patients.[472] In fact, the mortality rates of HIV-2–infected patients with undetectable plasma viral loads was similar to that of uninfected individuals, whereas HIV-2–infected patients with plasma viral loads of 10,000 copies/mL or greater had mortality rates similar to those observed with HIV-1.[549]

The lower HIV-2 plasma viral load could possibly be due to lower viral replication, enhanced host immune control, or a combination of the two factors. HIV-2 and HIV-1 have comparable cytopathicity. It is clear, however, that the two viruses have different dynamics in vivo, with plasma viral loads set points and plasma RNA levels being approximately 30-fold lower than with HIV-1.[8,430] At corresponding levels of CD4 cell depletion, despite greatly disparate plasma viral loads, levels of integrated proviral HIV-2 DNA in peripheral blood mononuclear cells are similar to those in comparable groups of HIV-1–infected individuals,[14,240,430] indicating that HIV-2 is able to establish provirus. HIV-2 viral mRNA accumulates at much lower amount, indicating that HIV-2 has tighter transcriptional control.[306,490]

Autologous neutralizing antibodies more frequently are found in HIV-2–infected individuals than in HIV-1–infected individuals and also may contribute to the slower disease progression in HIV-2.

Similar to the clinical outcome of HIV-2 infection in adults, slower rates of disease progression and better survival rates have been observed in HIV-2–infected versus HIV-1–infected or dually infected children.[4,118,386,403,438] In a prospective study in the Gambia, the 18-month mortality rate of children born to HIV-2–infected mothers did not differ significantly from that of children born to HIV-seronegative women (7% vs. 6%, respectively). In contrast, the relative risks for death in children born to HIV-1–infected versus HIV-2–infected or seronegative mothers were increased by 2.3-fold and 2.6-fold, respectively.[403]

The excess number of deaths in children of HIV-1–infected mothers was caused primarily by HIV-1 infection in the child; the mortality rate was 35% in HIV-1–infected children, as opposed to 9% in uninfected children born to HIV-1–infected mothers. In contrast, no deaths occurred in HIV-2–infected children. In Guinea-Bissau, the overall child mortality rates were similar in children born to HIV-2–seropositive and HIV-seronegative women (16.3% vs. 14.6%, respectively).[386] However, despite generally slower progression in HIV-2–infected children, severe immunodeficiency and AIDS occurring early in life rarely have been reported with HIV-2 infection.[175,353,354] Mortality rates in infants born to HIV-1–infected or dually infected mothers were 2.6 to 4.2 times higher than those in infants born to HIV-2–infected mothers (mortality rates of 133, 82, and 32 per 1000, respectively).[117] This finding is similar to that observed in the Gambia, where the childhood mortality rate was 15% for children born to HIV-1–infected mothers compared with 7% for those born to HIV-2–positive mothers and 6% for those born to HIV-seronegative mothers.[403] In a small cohort study investigating the survival of children born to HIV-1–positive and HIV-2–positive mothers, the mortality rates for infected children were significantly higher than those for uninfected children.[471]

The mortality hazards ratio of HIV-1–infected children was 3.1 times that of HIV-2–infected children but was not statistically significant.

The overall mortality of HIV-uninfected children of HIV-1–seropositive and HIV-2–seropositive mothers was not significantly different from that in children of HIV-uninfected children.[473]

Treatment

Currently available antiretroviral medications (ARVs) have been specifically developed for treatment of HIV-1, and some ARVs are not active against HIV-2 virus. Combination ART is recommended for the treatment of HIV-2, as it is for HIV-1. Observational cohort studies have shown variable but largely poor outcomes for ART in HIV-2 infection.[100,140-142,189,333,455] Poorer outcomes of treatment of HIV-2 can be attributed to a number of operational, clinical, and public health challenges, including diagnostic tools that have not adequately differentiated between HIV-1, HIV-2, and HIV-1/HIV-2 dual infections. Failure to diagnose HIV-2 or dual infection may lead to treatment with inappropriate and ineffective ARV regimens, which can result in poor immunologic response and disease progression. Optimal disease monitoring is not possible because there are no commercially available viral load assays to identify virologic failure and no commercially available genotypic assays to identify drug-resistant virus. Lastly, there have been no randomized trials addressing the optimal time to start ART or the choice of first- or second-line therapy for HIV-2. US guidelines recommend initiating ART before there is clinical progression of the infection or severe immunosuppression.[410]

Significant differences exist in the effectiveness of specific ART medications in treatment of HIV types 1 and 2 that must be considered in establishing an effective therapeutic regimen. Nonnucleoside reverse transcriptase inhibitors (NNRTIs) generally show little to no inhibition of HIV-2 in vitro at nontoxic levels.[579] HIV-2 is intrinsically resistant to NNRTIs because of a naturally occurring polymorphism in all HIV-2 isolates.[537] NNRTIs inhibit HIV-2 but at effective concentrations at least 50 times higher than those that inhibit HIV-1. These concentrations limit the clinical utility of these agents against HIV-2. HIV-2 is also resistant to enfuvirtide, a fusion inhibitor.[437,578]

HIV-2 is sensitive to currently available nucleoside and NRTI drugs, although with a lower barrier to resistance than HIV-1.[489]

Clinical studies of HIV-2 clones taken from patients receiving NRTI-containing ART confirmed that phenotypic resistance is associated with genotypic changes. Amino acid changes associated with HIV-1 NRTI resistance at M184 and Q151M also seem to occur in HIV-2 and have been associated with NRTI treatment failure.[547] The significance of other mutations in the HIV-2 reverse transcriptase gene after exposure to NRTI is unknown; also not known is whether mutations in the NRTI gene accumulate in a stepwise fashion, conferring increasing resistance to NRTI therapy.

Protease inhibitors are effective against HIV-2 protease but have variable activity and accelerated genotypic resistance.[389] The ritonavir-boosted protease inhibitors darunavir (DRV) and lopinavir (LPV) are more active against HIV-2 than other approved protease inhibitors and are preferred agents for first-line treatment.

The integrase strand transfer inhibitors (INSTs) raltegravir (RAL), dolutegravir (DTG), and elvitegravir (EVG) have demonstrated activity against HIV-2 in vitro. Clinical response to raltegravir was reported in a patient with highly treatment-exposed HIV-2 infection.[172,585] The CCR5 coreceptor antagonist maraviroc (MVC) appears to be active against some HIV-2 isolates. Use of coreceptor antagonists is hampered by the lack of approved assays to determine HIV-2 coreceptor tropism and by the fact that HIV-2 is able use a broad range of coreceptors, including CXCR4, CCR5, CCT-5, GPR15, and CXCR6.[170,171,457,585]

Because there are current recommendations for universal treatment of HIV-infected individuals without regard for CD4 count or clinical stage,[582,583] more HIV-2 infected individuals will be started on ART. Until more definitive data are available, it is recommended that ART-naïve patients with HIV-2 monoinfection or HIV-1/HIV-2 dual infection be started on a regimen containing two NRTIs plus an HIV-2–active boosted protease inhibitor or INSTI before the individual has clinical disease progression.[410,582,583]

Disease Monitoring

Progression of HIV disease and response to ART are usually assessed by considering clinical, immunologic, and virologic criteria. Clinical assessment and measuring CD4 count are the most readily available means for monitoring disease progression in HIV-2 infection because no HIV-2 viral load assays are yet commercially available. In response to ART, CD4 counts do not increase in HIV-2 infection as dramatically as can be seen in HIV-1 infection,[22,140-142] further highlighting the need for access to HIV-2 viral loads and genotypic testing as key components of comprehensive care for HIV-2 infections.

NEW REFERENCES SINCE THE SEVENTH EDITION

10. Ando Y, Saito K, Nakano S, et al. Bottle-feeding can prevent transmission of HTLV-I from mothers to their babies. *J Infect.* 1989;19:25-29.
18. Armstrong MJ, Corbett C, Rowe IA, et al. HTLV-1 in solid-organ transplantation: current challenges and future management strategies. *Transplantation.* 2012;94(11):1075-1084.
20. Assone T, de Souza FV, Gaester KO, et al. IL28B gene polymorphism SNP rs8099917 genotype GG is associated with HTLV-1-associated myelopathy/tropical spastic paraparesis (HAM/TSP) in HTLV-1 carriers. *PLoS Negl Trop Dis.* 2014;8(9):e3199.
22. Balestre E, Ekouevi DK, Tchounga B, et al. Immunologic response in treatment-naive HIV-2-infected patients: the IeDEA West Africa cohort. *J Int AIDS Soc.* 2016;19(1):20044.
29. Bartman MT, Kaidarova Z, Hirschkorn D, et al. Long-term increases in lymphocytes and platelets in human T-lymphotropic virus type II infection. *Blood.* 2008;112(10):3995-4002.
30. Bassani S, Lopez M, Toro C, et al. Influence of human T cell lymphotropic virus type 2 coinfection on virological and immunological parameters in HIV type 1-infected patients. *Clin Infect Dis.* 2007;44(1):105-110.
35. Bazarbachi A, Plumelle Y, Carlos RJ, et al. Meta-analysis on the use of zidovudine and interferon-alfa in adult T-cell leukemia/ lymphoma showing improved survival in the leukemic subtypes. *J Clin Oncol.* 2010;28(27):4177-4183.
67. Branson BM, Handsfield HH, Lampe MA, et al. Revised recommendations for HIV testing of adults, adolescents, and pregnant women in health-care settings. *MMWR Recomm Rep.* 2006;55(RR-14):1-17. quiz CE11-14.
69. Brites C, Alencar R, Gusmao R, et al. Co-infection with HTLV-1 is associated with a shorter survival time for HIV-1-infected patients in Bahia. Brazil. *AIDS.* 2001;15(15):2053-2055.
74. Calattini S, Chevalier SA, Duprez R, et al. Discovery of a new human T-cell lymphotropic virus (HTLV-3) in Central Africa. *Retrovirology.* 2005;2:30.
77. Carneiro-Proietti ABF, Amaranto-Damasio MS, Leal-Horiguchi CF, et al. Mother-to-child transmission of human T-cell lymphotropic viruses-1/2: what we know, and what are the gaps in understanding and preventing this route of infection. *J Pediatr Infect Dis Soc.* 2014;3(suppl 1):S24-S29.
89. Centers for Disease Control and Prevention and Association of Public Health Laboratories. Laboratory Testing for the Diagnosis of HIV Infection: Updated Recommendations; 2014. https://stacks.cdc.gov/view/cdc/23447.
94. Chang YB, Kaidarova Z, Hindes D, et al. Seroprevalence and demographic determinants of human T-lymphotropic virus type 1 and 2 infections among first-time blood donors—United States, 2000(2009. *J Infect Dis.* 2014;209(4):523-531.
99. Ciminale V, Rende F, Bertazzoni U, Romanelli MG. HTLV-1 and HTLV-2: highly similar viruses with distinct oncogenic properties. *Front Microbiol.* 2014;5:398.
101. Clavel F, Guetard D, Brun-Vezinet F, et al. Isolation of a new human retrovirus from West African patients with AIDS. *Science.* 1986;233(4761):343-346.
112. Dassouki Z, Sahin U, El HH, et al. ATL response to arsenic/interferon therapy is triggered by SUMO/PML/RNF4-dependent Tax degradation. *Blood.* 2015;125(3):474-482.
113. Datta A, Bellon M, Sinha-Datta U, et al. Persistent inhibition of telomerase reprograms adult T-cell leukemia to p53-dependent senescence. *Blood.* 2006;108(3):1021-1029.
120. de Mendoza C, Caballero E, Aguilera A, et al. HIV-2 and HTLV-1 infections in Spain, a non-endemic region. *AIDS Rev.* 2014;16(3):152-159.
136. Einsiedel L, Cassar O, Goeman E, et al. Higher human T-lymphotropic virus type 1 subtype C proviral loads are associated with bronchiectasis in indigenous Australians: results of a case-control study. *Open Forum Infect Dis.* 2014;1(1):ofu023.
142. Ekouevi DK, Tchounga BK, Coffie PA, et al. Antiretroviral therapy response among HIV-2 infected patients: a systematic review. *BMC Infect Dis.* 2014;14:461.
141. Ekouevi DK, Balestre E, Coffie PA, et al. Characteristics of HIV-2 and HIV-1/HIV-2 dually seropositive adults in West Africa presenting for care and antiretroviral therapy: the IeDEA-West Africa HIV-2 cohort study. *PLoS ONE.* 2013;8(6):e66135.
140. Ekouevi DK, Avettand-Fenoel V, Tchounga BK, et al. Plasma HIV-2 RNA according to CD4 count strata among HIV-2-infected adults in the IeDEA West Africa Collaboration. *PLoS ONE.* 2015;10(6):e0129886.
153. Filippone C, Betsem E, Tortevoye P. A severe bite from a nonhuman primate is a major risk factor for HTLV-1 in hunters from Central Africa. *CID.* 2015;60:1667-1676.
156. Fox JM, Mutalima N, Molyneux E, et al. Seroprevalence of HTLV-1 and HTLV-2 amongst mothers and children in Malawi within the context of a systematic review and meta-analysis of HTLV seroprevalence in Africa. *Trop Med Int Health.* 2016;21(3):312-324.
160. Fryer HR, Van Tienen C, Van Der Loeff MS, et al. Predicting the extinction of HIV-2 in rural Guinea-Bissau. *AIDS.* 2015;29(18):2479-2486.
162. Fujino T, Nagata Y. HTLV-I transmission from mother to child. *J Reprod Immunol.* 2000;47:197-206.
180. Gessain A, Mahieux R. Tropical spastic paraparesis and HTLV-1 associated myelopathy: clinical, epidemiological, virological and therapeutic aspects. *Rev Neurol (Paris).* 2012;168(3):257-269.
181. Gessain A, Mahieux R. Tropical spastic paraparesis and HTLV-1 associated myelopathy: clinical, epidemiological, virological and therapeutic aspects. *Rev Neurol (Paris).* 2012;168(3):257-269.
185. Gillet NA, Cook L, Laydon DJ, et al. Strongyloidiasis and infective dermatitis alter human T lymphotropic virus-1 clonality in vivo. *PLoS Pathog.* 2013;9(4):e1003263.
186. Giuliani M, Rezza G, Lepri AC, et al. Risk factors for HTLV-I and II in individuals attending a clinic for sexually transmitted diseases. *Sex Transm Dis.* 2000;27(2):87-92.
187. Gonçalves DU, Proietti FA, Ribas JG, et al. Epidemiology, treatment and prevention of human T-cell leukemia virus type 1-associated diseases. *Clin Microbiol Rev.* 2010;23:577-589.
193. Goubau P, Van BM, Vandamme AM, et al. A primate T-lymphotropic virus, PTLV-L, different from human T-lymphotropic viruses types I and II, in a wild-caught baboon (Papio hamadryas). *Proc Natl Acad Sci USA.* 1994;91(7):2848-2852.
194. Gout O, Baulac M, Gessain A, et al. Rapid development of myelopathy after HTLV-I infection acquired by transfusion during cardiac transplantation. *N Engl J Med.* 1990;322(6):383-388.

202. Hall WW, Ishak R, Zhu SW, et al. Human T lymphotropic virus type II (HTLV-II): epidemiology, molecular properties, and clinical features of infection. *J Acquir Immune Defic Syndr Hum Retrovirol.* 1996;13(suppl 1):S204-S214.
213. He X, Maranga IO, Oliver AW, et al. Analysis of the prevalence of HTLV-1 proviral DNA in cervical smears and carcinomas from HIV positive and negative Kenyan women. *Viruses.* 2016;8(9):E245.
232. Igakura T, Stinchcombe JC, Goon PK, et al. Spread of HTLV-I between lymphocytes by virus-induced polarization of the cytoskeleton. *Science.* 2003;299(5613):1713-1716.
234. Isache C, Sands M, Guzman N, Figueroa D. HTLV-1 and HIV-1 co-infection: a case report and review of the literature. *ID Cases.* 2016;4:53-55.
242. Iwanaga M, Watanabe T, Yamaguchi K, Adult T. cell leukemia: a review of epidemiological evidence. *Front Microbiol.* 2012;3:322.
247. Jogeda EL, Avi R, Pauskar M, et al. Human T-lymphotropic virus types 1 and 2 are rare among intravenous drug users in Eastern Europe. *Infect Gent Evol.* 2016;43:83-85.
249. Jones KS, Petrow-Sadowski C, Huang YK, et al. Cell-free HTLV-1 infects dendritic cells leading to transmission and transformation of CD4(+) T cells. *Nat Med.* 2008;14(4):429-436.
259. Katsuya H, Yamanaka T, Ishitsuka K, et al. Prognostic index for acute- and lymphoma-type adult T-cell leukemia/ lymphoma. *J Clin Oncol.* 2012;30(14):1635-1640.
267. Kinpara S, Kijiyama M, Takamori A, et al. Interferon-alpha (IFN-alpha) suppresses HTLV-1 gene expression and cell cycling, while IFN-alpha combined with zidovudine induces p53 signaling and apoptosis in HTLV-1-infected cells. *Retrovirology.* 2013;10:52.
296. Li G, De Clercq E. HIV genome-wide protein associations: a review of 30 Years of Research. *Microbiol Mol Biol Rev.* 2016;80(3):679-731.
311. Mahieux R, Pise-Masison C, Gessain A, et al. Arsenic trioxide induces apoptosis in human T-cell leukemia virus type 1- and type 2-infected cells by a caspase-3-dependent mechanism involving Bcl-2 cleavage. *Blood.* 2001;98(13):3762-3769.
318. Manns A, Wilks RJ, Murphy EL, et al. A prospective study of transmission by transfusion of HTLV-I and risk factors associated with seroconversion. *Int J Cancer.* 1992;51(6):886-891.
321. Marcais A, Suarez F, Sibon D, et al. Therapeutic options for adult T-cell leukemia/ lymphoma. *Curr Oncol Rep.* 2013;15(5):457-464.
331. Martin-Davila P, Fortun J, Lopez-Velez R, et al. Transmission of tropical and geographically restricted infections during solid-organ.
334. Matheson NJ, Greenwood EJ, Lehner PJ. Manipulation of immunometabolism by HIV-accessories to the crime? *Curr Opin Virol.* 2016;19:65-70.
363. Moyer V. Screening for HIV: U.S. Preventive Services Task Force Recommendation Statement. *Ann Intern Med.* 2013;159(1):51-60.
381. Nicolas D, Ambrosioni J, Paredes R, et al. Infection with human retroviruses other than HIV-1: HIV-2, HTLV-1, HTLV-2, HTLV-3 and HTLV-4. *Expert Rev Anti Infect Ther.* 2015;13(8):947-963.
388. Nozuma S, Matsuura E, Matsuzaki T, et al. Familial clusters of HTLV-1-associated myelopathy/tropical spastic paraparesis. *PLoS ONE.* 2014;9(5):e86144.
391. Oh U, Jacobson S. Treatment of HTLV-I-associated myelopathy/tropical spastic paraparesis: toward rational targeted therapy. *Neurol Clin.* 2008;26(3):781-797.
392. Oh U, Jacobson S. Treatment of HTLV-I-associated myelopathy/tropical spastic paraparesis: toward rational targeted therapy. *Neurol Clin.* 2008;26(3):781-797.
399. Oo Z, Barrios CS, Castillo L, Beilke MA. High levels of CC-chemokine expression and downregulated levels of CCR5 during HIV-1/HTLV-1 and HIV-1/HTLV-2 coinfections. *J Med Virol.* 2015;87:790-797.
409. Paiva A, Casseb J. Origin and prevalence of human T-lymphotropic virus type 1 (HTLV-1) and type 2 (HTLV-2) among indigenous populations in the Americas. *Rev Inst Med Trop Sao Paulo.* 2015;57(1):1-13.
410. Department of Health and Human Services. Panel on Antiretroviral Guidelines for Adults and Adolescents. *Guidelines for the Use of Antiretroviral Agents in Adults and Adolescents Living with HIV.* Available at: http://www.aidsinfo.nih.gov/ContentFiles/AdultandAdolescentGL.pdf.
418. Peeters M, Arc MD, Delaporte E. Origin and diversity of human retroviruses. *AIDS Rev.* 2014;16(1):23-34.
424. Pilotti E, Bianchi MV, De MA, et al. HTLV-1/-2 and HIV-1 co-infections: retroviral interference on host immune status. *Front Microbiol.* 2013;4:372.
440. Proietti FA, Carneiro-Proietti AB, Catalan-Soares BC, Murphy EL. Global epidemiology of HTLV-I infection and associated diseases. *Oncogene.* 2005;24:6058-6068.
444. Raltegravir for HAM/TSP. https://clinicaltrials.gov/ct2/show/NCT01867320.
450. Ribeiro MA, Martins ML, Teixeira C, et al. Blocking vertical transmission of human T cell lymphotropic virus type 1 and 2 through breastfeeding interruption. *Pediatr Infect Dis J.* 2012;31:1139-1143.
451. Ribeiro MA, Proietti FA, Martins ML, et al. Geographic distribution of human T-lymphotropic virus types 1 and 2 among mothers of newborns tested during neonatal screening, Minas Gerais, Brazil. *Rev Panam Salud Publica.* 2010;27:330-337.
458. Rossheim AE, Cunningham TD, Troy SB. Human T-lymphotropic virus co-infections in adults infected with human immunodeficiency virus. *Am J Med Sci.* 2016;352(3):258-260.
460. Roucoux DF, Wang B, Smith D, et al. A prospective study of sexual transmission of human T lymphotropic virus (HTLV)-I and HTLV-II. *J Infect Dis.* 2005;191(9):1490-1497.
469. Satake M, Yamada Y, Atogami S, Yamaguchi K. The incidence of adult T-cell leukemia/lymphoma among human T-lymphotropic virus type 1 carriers in Japan. *Leuk Lymphoma.* 2015;56(6):1806-1812.
489. Smith RA, Anderson DJ, Pyrak CL, Preston BD, Gottlieb GS. Antiretroviral drug resistance in HIV-2: three amino acid changes are sufficient for classwide nucleoside analogue resistance. *J Infect Dis.* 2009;199(9):1323-1326.
494. Stienlauf S, Yahalom V, Shinar E, et al. Malignant diseases and mortality in blood donors infected with human T-lymphotropic virus type 1 in Israel. *Int J Infect Dis.* 2013;17(11):e1022-e1024.
496. Strebel K. HIV accessory proteins versus host restriction factors. *Curr Opin Virol.* 2013;3(6):692-699.
507. Takahashi K, Takezaki T, Oki T, et al. The Mother-to-Child Transmission Study Group. Inhibitory effect of maternal antibody on mother-to-child transmission of human T-lymphotropic virus type I. *Int J Cancer.* 1991;49:673-677.
514. Tanajura D, Castro N, Oliveira P, et al. Neurological manifestations in human T-cell lymphotropic virus type 1 (HTLV-1)-infected individuals without HTLV-1-associated myelopathy/tropical spastic paraparesis: a longitudinal cohort study. *Clin Infect Dis.* 2015;61(1):49-56.
518. Taylor GP, Goon P, Furukawa Y, et al. Zidovudine plus lamivudine in human T-lymphotropic virus type-I-associated myelopathy: a randomised trial. *Retrovirology.* 2006;3:63.
525. Toro C, Rodes B, Poveda E, Soriano V. Rapid development of subacute myelopathy in three organ transplant recipients after transmission of human T-cell lymphotropic virus type I from a single donor. *Transplantation.* 2003;75(1):102-104.
527. Murphy EL. Infection with human T-lymphotrophic virus types-1 and -2 (HTLV-1 and -2): implications for blood transfusion safety. *Transfus Clin Biol.* 2016;23(1):13-19.
530. Trevino A, Parra P, Bar-Magen T, et al. Antiviral effect of raltegravir on HTLV-1 carriers. *J Antimicrob Chemother.* 2012;67(1):218-221.
533. Tsukasaki K, Tobinai K. Biology and treatment of HTLV-1 associated T-cell lymphomas. *Best Pract Res Clin Haematol.* 2013;26(1):3-14.
538. Tulius SM, de Melo EO, Bezerra Leite AC, Araujo A. Neurological aspects of HIV/human T lymphotropic virus coinfection. *AIDS Rev.* 2009;11(2):71-78.
559. Villaverde JA, Romani FR, Montano Torres S, Zunt JR. Transmisión vertical de HTLV-1 en el Perú. *Rev Peru Med Exp Salud Publica.* 2011;28:101-108.
568. Watanabe T. Current status of HTLV-1 infection. *Int J Hematol.* 2011;94(5):430-434.
577. Willems L, Hasegawa H, Accolla R, et al. Reducing the global burden of HTLV-1 infection: An agenda for research and action. *Antiviral Res.* 2016;137:41-48.
580. Wolfe ND, Heneine W, Carr JK, et al. Emergence of unique primate T-lymphotropic viruses among central African bushmeat hunters. *Proc Natl Acad Sci USA.* 2005;102(22):7994-7999.
583. World Health Organization. Consolidated Guidelines on the Use of Antiretroviral Drugs for Treating and Preventing HIV Infection: Recommendations for a Public Health Approach. 2nd ed; 2016. http://apps.who.int/iris/bitstream/10665/208825/1/9789241549684_eng.pdf.
584. Xie J, Ge S, Zhang Y, et al. The prevalence of human T-lymphotropic virus infection among blood donors in Southeast China, 2004(2013. *PLoS Neg Trop Dis.* 2015;9(4):e0003685.

The full reference list for this chapter is available at ExpertConsult.com.

192B ■ Human Immunodeficiency Virus and Acquired Immunodeficiency Syndrome

Karin Nielsen-Saines • Mary E. Paul • William T. Shearer

In the absence of treatment, infection with human immunodeficiency virus type 1 (HIV-1), a retrovirus, causes a chronic, eventually fatal illness. Human retroviruses include human T-cell lymphotropic viruses (i.e., HTLV-I, HTLV-II, HTLV-III, and HTLV-VI), also known as oncoviruses, and lentiviruses (i.e., HIV-1 and HIV-2). Retroviruses are RNA viruses capable of transforming themselves into DNA viruses and integrating into the host cell genome. Before 1980, retroviruses were known to cause disease only in animals, but shortly thereafter, HTLV-I and HTLV-II were shown to be associated with human disease.

In 1983, the virus responsible for the newly identified human acquired immunodeficiency syndrome (AIDS) was described by several investigators worldwide. It was initially called human lymphotropic virus III or lymphadenopathy-associated virus, but further identification revealed the syndrome was caused by a single novel virus renamed HIV. Two species of HIV (i.e., HIV-1 and HIV-2) were later identified. Both are lentiviruses responsible for the development of AIDS, but transmission patterns, demographics, and disease progression are different. HIV-2 is closely related to simian immunodeficiency virus (SIV) and is not responsible for pediatric HIV disease because it has lower rates of mother-to-child transmission (MTCT) and a very protracted disease course. HIV-1 is responsible for pediatric disease.

HIV infection continues to be one of the world's most serious health and development challenges. An estimated 36.7 million people worldwide are living with HIV/AIDS.[269] Of these, 1.8 million are children younger than 15 years.[269] Every year, approximately 2.1 million people acquire HIV infection, including 150,000 children, most of whom were infected perinatally and live in sub-Saharan Africa[269] (Fig. 192B.1).

Despite significant advances in prevention, diagnosis, and treatment of HIV infection, most of those living with or at risk for HIV infection

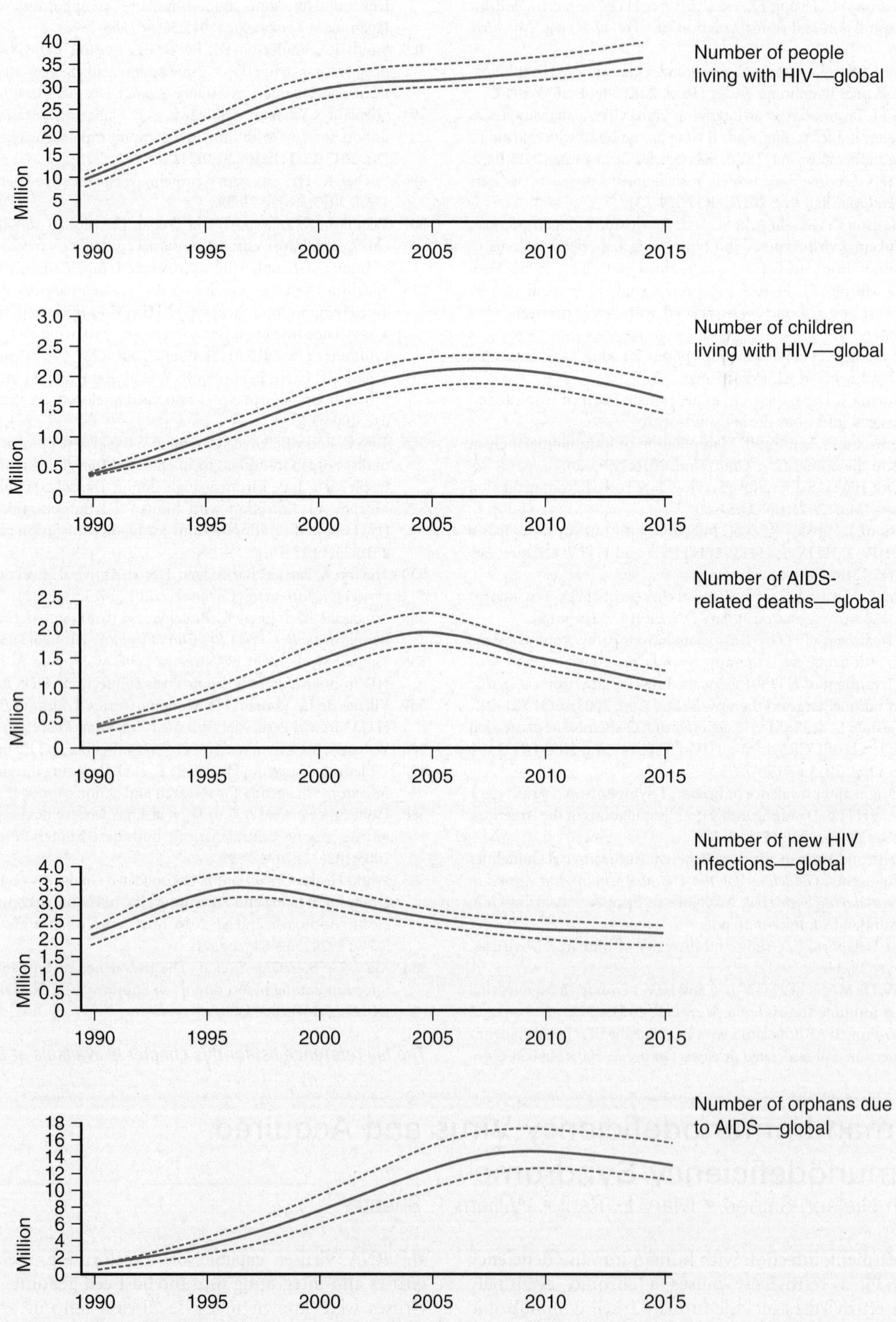

FIG. 192B.1 Global statistics for HIV infection. (From UNAIDS. AIDS by the numbers—AIDS is not over, but it can be. http://www.unaids.org/en/resources/documents/2016/AIDS-by-the-numbers.)

do not have access to prevention and appropriate treatment. It is estimated that only 54% of people with HIV infection are aware of their HIV infection status.[288] Sub-Saharan Africa has almost two thirds of the global total of incident HIV infections, for an estimated total of 25.6 million infected people in the region.[288] An estimated 35 million people have died of AIDS since the start of the epidemic, including 1.1 million in 2015.[288]

Despite the sobering statistics, global efforts in the past decade have been successful in reducing HIV prevalence rates worldwide, and the number of incident infections has declined. The number of people with HIV receiving treatment globally increased, from 7.5 million in 2010 to 17 million by the end of 2015.[270] In the absence of a successful vaccine, the recognition that treatment of infected individuals significantly reduces sexual transmission of the virus[59] has created the treatment for prevention paradigm. Observational and modeling studies have demonstrated the dramatic impact global antiretroviral treatment can have on curtailing the epidemic.[108,210] The use of preexposure prophylaxis (PREP) has been highly beneficial in protecting against new infections,[45,110] and much progress has been made in preventing MTCT. An estimated 77% of pregnant women with HIV worldwide had access to antiretroviral treatment to prevent infection of their babies in 2015, and perinatal infections have declined by more than 50% since 2010.[271]

Renewed optimism that a functional cure for HIV may be obtainable followed reports such as the successful transplantation of CCR5-Δ32/Δ32–deleted stem cells to suppress viremia in an individual with HIV infection,[127] the Mississippi baby who had a prolonged period of HIV aviremia while off antiretrovirals after very early initiation of antiretroviral therapy,[161] or the Visconti trial participants who remained aviremic off antiretroviral therapy after early treatment initiation.[237] Despite some progress, much work still needs to be done to reduce basic health disparities that favor HIV spread even in developed countries such as the United States.[271]

Research continues to demonstrate that racial and ethnic disparities in health are often a marker of a range of broader social and economic challenges. Eradicating racial disparities and preventing HIV infections in the changing face of the US and global epidemic will be the medical and public health challenges for this century.[36]

DEFINITION AND STAGING OF PEDIATRIC HIV INFECTION

The natural history of pediatric HIV-1 infection is bimodal.[243] Studies conducted in developed countries before the availability of antiretrovirals demonstrate that approximately 20% of children exhibit very rapid disease progression with rapid loss of $CD4^+$ cell counts and development of AIDS-defining conditions before 2 years of age.[203] Approximately 60% to 65% of HIV-infected children have intermediate disease progression, with the appearance of AIDS-defining events by 7 to 8 years of age in the absence of treatment. As in adults, there is a small subset of children (≈5%) who have very slow to no disease progression by 8 years of age. These children enter adolescence with minimal or no symptoms of HIV disease. Studies conducted in Africa demonstrated a faster pace of disease progression, with most pediatric patients having AIDS-defining conditions by 5 years of age.[201] This may reflect the higher overall burden of disease and multiple coinfections.

Antiretroviral treatment makes it possible to alter the natural history of HIV disease and transform disease progressors into nonprogressors. This translates into improvements in the quality of life and reduction in HIV-associated disease morbidity and mortality. In this context, current staging of HIV disease does not carry the same implications as in the early 1990s because immune preservation and immune reconstitution supported by continuous antiretroviral treatment allow children with advanced immunodeficiency to regenerate their immune system and revert from full-blown AIDS to an asymptomatic disease presentation.

From a historical perspective, pediatric AIDS was first reported to the Centers for Disease Control and Prevention (CDC) in 1982; AIDS was first reported in adults in 1981.[35] The first definitions of pediatric AIDS were published in 1985. In 1994 and again in 2008, the classification system was revised to include more advanced viral diagnostic technology and a system for staging pediatric HIV disease that involved clinical and immunologic axes.[40,187]

Table 192B.1 outlines the clinical axis of the staging system, which is composed of four clinical categories: N, A, B, and C.[187] The clinical axis was originally intended for unidirectional use for an individual child. Severity of disease proceeds from category N (i.e., asymptomatic), to A (i.e., mildly symptomatic), to B (i.e., moderately symptomatic), to C (i.e., severely symptomatic), and then to HIV-associated death. Clinical category C describes children with AIDS-defining characteristics (i.e., wasting, encephalopathy, opportunistic infections, and malignancies), but it excludes lymphoid interstitial pneumonitis or pulmonary lymphoid hyperplasia (LIP/PLH). Clinical category B describes children with other specific HIV-associated illnesses (e.g., single episodes of bacteremia, leiomyosarcomas, lymphoproliferative lung disorders, anemia, thrombocytopenia) and excludes children with a clinical category C event. Clinical category A describes children with two or more specific HIV-associated illnesses (i.e., lymphadenopathy; hepatomegaly; splenomegaly; upper respiratory tract infections, sinusitis, or otitis media; parotitis; and dermatitis) and excludes children with a clinical category C or B event. Clinical category N describes children without clinical category C, B, or A events; these children may or may not be completely asymptomatic (i.e., single category A events such as lymphadenopathy may exist).

Tables 192B.2 and 192B.3 provide expanded descriptions of the immunologic axis of the staging system. They include categories 1 (no evidence of immune suppression), 2 (moderate immunosuppression), and 3 (severe immunosuppression).[187]

In resource-limited settings, the World Health Organization (WHO) staging system has been implemented as a guide to describe the severity of HIV-related symptoms in children with disease classifications ranging from 1 to 4, with 1 being asymptomatic and 4 corresponding to AIDS.[290]

EPIDEMIOLOGY AND TRANSMISSION AND PREVENTION

Transmission by Blood Products

Documented spread of pediatric HIV infection has occurred through blood and blood products, perinatal transfer from mothers with identified risk factors, breast milk,[79] and sexual transmission to children and adolescents.[99] Most adolescents are infected through sexual exposure and frequently are unaware of their HIV status, which renders them good candidates for early intervention studies.[3] Since HIV screening techniques, including nucleic acid amplification testing of pooled blood products, were adapted and recombinant factor products were increasingly used, transmission of HIV by blood products has been rare in the United States.[72]

TABLE 192B.1 Factors Affecting Intrapartum and In Utero Transmission of HIV

Viral Transmission	Immune Transmission	Maternal Transmission	Fetal Transmission
Virus load	Decreased $CD4^+$ count	Advanced disease	Prematurity
Virus phenotype/ tropism	Maternal neutralizing antibodies	Primary infection during pregnancy	Chorioamnionitis
Virus genotype	Cell-mediated immunity	Coinfection	Infant immune response
	Mucosal immunity	Twins: higher risk for first born	
		Timing of infection	
		Obstetric events	

TABLE 192B.2 Clinical Categories of Pediatric HIV Classification

	CLINICAL CATEGORIES			
Immunologic Category	**N: No Signs or Symptoms**	**A: Mild Signs or Symptoms**	**B: Moderate Signs or Symptoms**	**C: Severe Signs or Symptoms**
1. No evidence of suppression	N1	A1	B1	C1
2. Evidence of moderate suppression	N2	A2	B2	C2
3. Severe suppression	N3	A3	B3	C3

Modified from Mofenson LM, Brady MT, Danner SP, et al. Guidelines for the prevention and treatment of opportunistic infections among HIV-exposed and HIV-infected children: recommendations from CDC, the National Institutes of Health, the HIV Medicine Association of the Infectious Diseases Society of America, the Pediatric Infectious Diseases Society, and the American Academy of Pediatrics. *MMWR Recomm Rep.* 2009;58(RR-11):1–166.

TABLE 192B.3 Immunologic Categories Based on Age-Specific CD4⁺ T-Lymphocyte Counts and Percentage of Total Lymphocytes

	AGE OF CHILD					
	<12 mo		**1–5 y**		**6–12 y**	
Immunologic Category	***μL***	**%**	***μL***	**%**	***μL***	**%**
1. No evidence of suppression	≥1500	≥25	≥1000	≥25	≥500	≥25
2. Evidence of moderate suppression	750–1499	15–24	500–999	15–24	200–499	15–24
3. Severe suppression	<750	<15	<500	<15	<200	<15

Modified from Mofenson LM, Brady MT, Danner SP, et al. Guidelines for the prevention and treatment of opportunistic infections among HIV-exposed and HIV-infected children: recommendations from CDC, the National Institutes of Health, the HIV Medicine Association of the Infectious Diseases Society of America, the Pediatric Infectious Diseases Society, and the American Academy of Pediatrics. *MMWR Recomm Rep.* 2009;58(RR-11):1–166.

Perinatal Transmission

In the absence of interventions to curtail MTCT of HIV-1, HIV-1 infection among children parallels that of women of childbearing age. Perinatal transmission of HIV-1 accounts for most worldwide cases of pediatric HIV-1 infection, with the exception of adolescent acquisition of HIV-1 via adult risk behaviors. HIV-1 transmission from mother to child occurs in 25% to 30% of cases when there is no maternal antiretroviral treatment,[200,244] and if breastfeeding until 12 months of age is included, the transmission risk can be as high as 40%. Infection can be transmitted during pregnancy, at the time of labor and delivery, and through breastfeeding.

Worldwide, approximately 2000 HIV-exposed infants are born daily, with 90% of cases occurring in sub-Saharan Africa.[174] Breastfeeding transmission contributes another 240,000 infant infections per year.[273] Although combination antiretroviral therapy (cART) can reduce MTCT transmission to less than 1% in developed countries,[75] failure to recognize HIV-1 infection in women and unavailability of treatment contribute to continuing MTCT of HIV worldwide. Management of HIV-1 infection must consider early diagnosis of infection, the natural history of HIV-1 infection in children and surrogate markers of disease, suitable pediatric drug formulations, drug metabolism and pharmacokinetics of antiretrovirals in children, and the paucity of pediatric treatment data compared with that for adults.

Acquisition of HIV infection can occur in utero, during the intrapartum period, or through breastfeeding. Even before antiretroviral treatment was recommended to pregnant women, two thirds of HIV-exposed infants escaped HIV infection. Perinatal HIV infection rates have declined substantially in the developed world since 1994, following publication of the landmark PACTG 076 study, which demonstrated reduction of perinatal HIV transmission in women who used zidovudine in pregnancy compared with placebo.[61] Approximately 30% to 50% of infants who contract HIV infection acquire it in utero, and 50% to 70% acquire the infection during the intrapartum period.[32,71,178]

To characterize the timing of HIV infection, a working definition was created for acquisition of infection in utero and intrapartum.[26] An infant is considered to have in utero infection if virologic tests (i.e., HIV DNA or RNA polymerase chain reaction [PCR] assays) are positive within 48 hours of life. Due to the risk of contamination with maternal blood, cord blood samples should not be used for diagnostic evaluations. Infants are considered to have intrapartum HIV infection if diagnostic tests within the first 48 hours of life are negative but further virologic testing after 1 week of life is positive. There is evidence that most cases of HIV transmission occur late in pregnancy or at delivery.

Infants with in utero infection appear to have a more rapid disease course compared with infants with intrapartum HIV infection.[70] In utero infected infants have normal CD4⁺ cell values at birth and are usually born with a low virus load (as measured by DNA or RNA PCR).[177] Infants infected by HIV in utero are asymptomatic at birth. In utero HIV infection appears to result from transplacental passage of virus or ascending viral infection in patients with prolonged rupture of membranes.[183] In the animal model, researchers demonstrated that viral infection of the amniotic fluid with SIV resulted in infection of all offspring.[276]

Intrapartum transmission of HIV infection is responsible for most perinatal cases. In a prospective study of 271 HIV-infected infants using HIV DNA PCR, 38% of children were found to be positive for HIV within 48 hours of life, 93% were positive by 14 days of age, and 96% were positive by 4 weeks of age.[78] A few infants may not have detectable virus as late as 3 months after delivery. Untreated infants tend to maintain a very high virus burden throughout their first year of life, and immunologic patterns of primary viremia in infants have been described.[160] High-level viremia can persist for a longer period in infants than in adults with primary infection; untreated early infection is associated with a high risk of death.[279] Before the advent of combination antiretroviral therapy, discordant twin infections were reported, with the first-born twin having a higher risk of infection.[77]

Postpartum transmission of HIV through breastfeeding has been a continuing problem for the prevention of HIV MTCT efforts worldwide. HIV-1 can be transmitted as a cell-associated or cell-free virus in breast milk.[165] Mastitis, which triggers migration of inflammatory cells, is also a known risk factor for HIV transmission by breast milk,[248] as is nonexclusive breastfeeding[63] or oral thrush in the infant.[226] Longer duration of breastfeeding is another risk factor for transmission,[12] as is maternal primary infection during lactation.[192] However, in areas where safe alternatives to breastfeeding are not available, formula feeding is associated with higher morbidity and mortality rates.

Provision of combination antiretroviral therapy to lactating, HIV-infected mothers has significantly increased HIV-free survival of infants and produced improved infant outcomes in terms of growth and reduced rates of infections.[169–171] Successful screening of pregnant women with availability of antiretroviral treatment for HIV-infected pregnant and lactating women through the WHO B and B+ program[128] has decreased early and late postpartum HIV-transmission through breastfeeding in recent years.

Early diagnosis of HIV-1 infection is crucial for identification of at-risk infants and initiation of treatment. All HIV-1–exposed infants carry maternal HIV-1 antibodies until approximately 15 to 18 months of age. Early pediatric diagnosis relies on identification of the virus by HIV-1 DNA or RNA PCR techniques. The former technique measures integrated virus in the host genome, and the latter method measures circulating plasma virus. HIV-1 coculture is not routinely performed because of cost and time, although it is also a reliable diagnostic method. Infants infected in utero usually have positive PCR results within the first 48 hours of birth, whereas infants infected at the time of labor and delivery can have a negative HIV DNA or RNA PCR result at birth, followed by a positive result 1 week to 2 months after birth. Because breastfed infants have continuing HIV-1 exposure, they can develop a positive HIV DNA or RNA PCR result at any time. The risk of breastfeeding transmission by an HIV-1–positive mother is approximately 16%.[91] Repeat PCR testing in the first few months of life is required to determine the timing of infection, and the sensitivity of PCR results increase over time in the absence of breastfeeding.[79,202]

In the United States, the total annual number of AIDS cases resulting from perinatal transmission peaked in 1992, with slightly fewer than 1000 newly affected children reported.[21] Predominance of perinatal transmission is found worldwide, especially in countries where adult heterosexual transmission is uniquely prevalent (e.g., Africa).[44,236] Before the use of perinatal antiretroviral interventions, the reported transmission rate for perinatally acquired HIV infection was between 12% and 25% in the United States and Europe and higher in Africa.[61,263]

Maternal risk factors associated with enhanced perinatal HIV transmission and identified through national surveillance of reported AIDS cases include untreated HIV disease, seroconversion during pregnancy or breastfeeding, drug abuse, heterosexual infection by sexual partners with risk factors for acquiring HIV disease, and maternal transfusion before 1985. Prospective and retrospective evaluations of maternal predictors for perinatal HIV transmission have been the focus of many studies. Maternal transmission predictors identified include maternal viremia (i.e., measured by quantitative HIV RNA PCR or viral load),[93,166] maternal immunosuppression, an inadequate immune response (i.e., measured by the $CD4^+$ T-cell count and neutralizing antibody production),[166] and viral characteristics (e.g., chemokine receptor tropism, resistance patterns of maternal virus at delivery or infant virus at birth).[239]

Pregnancy and placental variables (e.g., delivery mode, duration of rupture of membranes, chorioamnionitis) can influence the risk of perinatal transmission of HIV.[196,257,262] Infant variables evaluated as predictors of transmission of HIV include specific human leukocyte antigen (HLA) markers and the infant cellular immune response (e.g., cytokine production, activated T-cell function).[83,162,166,220] Immunogenetic factors (e.g., chemokine coreceptor expression) may confer protection against progression of disease.[246]

Advances in perinatal primary antiretroviral therapy, such as antepartum, peripartum, and postpartum administration of zidovudine in nonbreastfeeding HIV-infected women without severe immunosuppression in the United States, led to a decrease in perinatal transmission rates. The CDC estimated that the number of infants born annually with HIV in the United States decreased from 1650 in 1991 to 100 to 200 in 2004, which remained the number reported in 2016.

The provision of antiretrovirals to infants born to HIV-infected mothers as prophylaxis has been standard of care in the Unites States since 1994, when results of the Pediatric AIDS Clinical Trials Group study 076 were published.[61] The study demonstrated that zidovudine administered to the mother starting at 16 weeks' gestation, accompanied by an intravenous zidovudine infusion during labor and delivery and followed by four times daily dosing of zidovudine to the infant from birth to 6 weeks of age, was highly effective in preventing HIV MTCT compared with placebo (8% vs. 25%, $P < .001$). In developed countries, infants are provided 4 to 6 weeks of zidovudine starting at birth and given at 2 mg/kg per dose four times daily or 4 mg/kg per dose twice daily as the standard of care.[214]

The major toxicities of zidovudine prophylaxis for infants include anemia and neutropenia, but the effects are dose dependent and self-limited, tend to occur toward the end of the course of treatment, and rarely require interruption of prophylaxis.[147] In resource-limited settings, single-dose nevirapine (2 mg/kg) given to the infant shortly after birth is the standard of care and has been implemented in multiple studies after publication of the HIVNET 012 results,[115] which documented the efficacy of this approach in reducing MTCT when associated with single-dose nevirapine given to the mother at the time of labor. Among HIV-infected infants whose mothers were not treated with antiretrovirals throughout the course of pregnancy and are therefore at higher risk for HIV acquisition, double antiretroviral prophylaxis initiated within 48 hours of birth with three doses of nevirapine in the first week of life concurrently with 6 weeks of zidovudine is more effective for the prevention of HIV intrapartum infection than zidovudine alone.[204]

An equally efficacious alternative regimen is the use of lamivudine and nelfinavir in the first 2 weeks of life concurrent with 6 weeks of zidovudine.[204] Due to the lack of availability of pediatric formulations of nelfinavir, the nevirapine plus zidovudine combination is preferable.[214] A lopinavir plus ritonavir suspension is not recommended by the US Food and Drug Administration (FDA) for use in infants younger than 2 weeks of age. In resource-limited settings, the use of daily nevirapine prophylaxis for HIV-exposed infants for the prevention of MTCT has been evaluated for those up to 6 months of age and shown to be effective and safe in the prevention of postpartum HIV acquisition.[62] However, most settings in sub-Saharan Africa have transitioned to the WHO program options B or B+, which recommend treatment with cART to all HIV-infected women during pregnancy and lactation or from pregnancy onward with no further treatment interruption.[289]

The selection of antiretroviral therapy to reduce perinatal HIV transmission must consider optimal treatment for infected pregnant women and the potential for fetal harm. Maternal factors include the mother's viral load, degree of immunosuppression, medications for use in treatment of comorbid conditions (e.g., tuberculosis, hepatitis C virus infection), and the potential for inducing viral resistance. Transmission of treatment-resistant HIV to infants has been described in the literature, but it occurs infrequently.

Other considerations to prevent perinatal transmission of HIV include scheduled delivery to minimize prolonged rupture of membranes, including a recommendation from the American College of Obstetrics and Gynecology for scheduled cesarean section for women with viral loads exceeding HIV RNA levels of 1000 copies/mL.[60] In a meta-analysis of 15 North American and European cohorts of HIV-infected pregnant women ($n = 100$ women), there was a 5% difference in vertical transmission rates for those with scheduled delivery by cesarean section (2% transmission rate) compared with those with other delivery modes (7.3% transmission rate).[262] Evaluation of the morbidity and mortality related to scheduled cesarean sections suggests that HIV-infected pregnant women may have a higher incidence of postpartum hemorrhage with resultant transfusion, sepsis, pneumonia, and death than their noninfected pregnant peers undergoing the same scheduled procedure (odds ratio, 1.6).[159] HIV-infected pregnant women without detectable viral loads should be informed preoperatively about the risk of morbidity related to cesarean section performed to prevent perinatal HIV transmission.

Sexual Transmission: Second Wave of Pediatric AIDS

In the adult, young adult, and adolescent populations, sexual acquisition of HIV infection is the predominant transmission pattern. The intersection of pediatric sexual abuse and transmission of HIV has been reported. Sexual abuse of young children and infants may be associated with the transmission of sexual disease (e.g., syphilis, gonorrhea, human papillomavirus). HIV infection should be considered in the differential diagnosis of sexually transmitted diseases in children assessed for sexual assault. In contrast to the infrequent reports of sexual transmission to infants and children younger than 13 years, adolescents are infected frequently by sexual transmission. In an inner-city urban US community, 41% of sexually active female youth described having vaginal intercourse and receptive anal intercourse in casual relationships.[124] Use of condoms was reported by 64% of youth, but receptive anal intercourse was used by some as a form of contraception, and condom use in this setting was reported in only 41% of these encounters.

The American Academy of Pediatrics (AAP) stressed the importance of preadolescent and adolescent care and encouraged performing examinations of patients who are 11 to 14 years of age. Health care providers can take advantage of these preteen and teen visits as an opportunity to explore sexual exposures of youth in their care and to educate sexually active youth on options for contraception.

Because the symptom-free period for clinical expression of HIV infection in adolescents may approach adult standards (>10 years), many young adults 20 to 29 years of age with AIDS probably became infected with HIV during adolescence. Adolescents with AIDS, like affected infants and children, are more likely to be poor and black or Hispanic. Reported risks of transmission to adolescents vary by age, sex, and race or ethnicity. Behavioral transmission (i.e., men who have sex with men and heterosexual contact) and transmission of unknown risk predominate as reported risk behaviors of US youth.[287] The category of heterosexual contact accounts for the largest proportional increase in the reported risk of transmission for female and male adolescent cases of AIDS. The nature of youth (e.g., experimentation, search for self and sexual identity, inability to access health care easily) places adolescents at risk for heterosexual transmission of HIV infection.[283]

Recommendations for postexposure prophylaxis for nonoccupational exposure to blood, genital, or other body fluids were updated by the CDC in 2016.[47] After exposure to these fluids from an HIV-infected individual and with determination of significant exposure risk, a 28-day regimen of combination antiretrovirals (many containing integrase inhibitors) is recommended if administration can begin within 72 hours of exposure.

Other Modes of Transmission

Less frequently reported transmission routes of HIV infection are important for pediatric health care providers to acknowledge and target. The risk of HIV transmission through breastfeeding is reported infrequently in the United States. In a study of HIV-infected, breastfeeding mothers and their exposed infants, Dunn and associates[79] documented a 14% risk of HIV transmission through breastfeeding above the established perinatal transmission risk. Study results prompted the adoption of guidelines for preventing transmission by this route by avoiding breastfeeding by HIV-seropositive mothers in the United States. Transmission of HIV to infants by breastfeeding represents approximately one half of all perinatal transmission worldwide, and the risk of transmission continues with prolonged breastfeeding after the first year of life.[143]

Children may be prone to needlestick or sharps injuries that occur in a nonhospital, nonmedical setting, such as needlestick injury associated with inappropriately discarded needles in public places such as public parks and bathrooms. Recommendations for psychological support, discussion of adherence to prescribed medications, and toxicity monitoring are provided by the AAP Committee on Pediatric AIDS.[119]

An estimated 13% of 159 diagnoses of HIV and AIDS among children younger than 13 years were attributed to modes other than perinatal transmission. In 2008, a study of three pediatric HIV cases concluded that premastication was the likely route of HIV transmission through blood in saliva.[98] A cross-sectional survey conducted by the CDC in nine pediatric HIV clinics in the United States indicated that among primary caregivers of children 6 months of age or older, 31% of the 154 reported the children received premasticated food from themselves or someone else. Although data on the risk of HIV transmission by premastication are limited, the CDC recommends that HIV-infected caregivers not premasticate food for HIV-uninfected children.[37] Health care providers should routinely inquire about premastication of foods fed to infants, instruct HIV-infected caregivers to avoid this practice, and advise patients about safer feeding options.

No data have suggested that HIV infection is transmitted casually from HIV-infected children to siblings, playmates, or caregivers.[255] Documentation of transmission routes and lack of casual transmission have prompted defining appropriate measures for mainstreaming of HIV-infected children and families.[74] This measure includes school, childcare, and foster care and adoption placement for HIV-infected children, and it promotes social incorporation of the children.

ETIOLOGY

Identification of the origin of AIDS followed closely behind the clinical description of this complex immunodeficiency. In 1983, investigators worldwide identified a viral cause for AIDS and described human lymphotropic virus III, lymphadenopathy-associated virus, and a virus associated with persistent generalized lymphadenopathy.[56,92] These viruses subsequently were identified as similar and were called HIV.[64] Two species of HIV are recognized: HIV-1 and HIV-2. HIV-1 has been the more prevalent pathogenic species and, especially in the United States, almost uniformly has been associated with reported AIDS cases.

Viral divergence is common, and HIV-1 can be divided into three groups: M, major; O, outliers; and N, non-M/non-O. The M group represents the major group, with subtypes (i.e., clades) showing significant symmetry.[116] The major subtypes have been identified, and data from the WHO HIV Vaccine Initiative identified clade C in 50% of global infections in 2004.[116] Clade B is identified most frequently in industrialized countries, including the United States. In 2004, recombinant subtypes were responsible for 18% of worldwide infections. Continued collection of data is important for the successful development of a vaccine that can be applied universally to stem transmission of HIV. A detailed description of these RNA viruses, their method of viral introduction into the affected host, and their impact on critical immune components is provided in Chapter 192A.

PATHOGENESIS

The Developing Immune System

HIV affects almost all immune cell types and alters their ability to produce important chemokines and interleukins that are integral to immunologic homeostasis.[53] Independent of cell damage, the host response can vary according to individual genetic HLA representation and predict probability of infection occurring after exposure or progression of disease.[85] $CD4^+$ T cells bear a receptor (i.e., the $CD4^+$ T-cell molecule itself) for the gp120 component of the HIV virion coat, and viral entry into the host cell takes place through this mechanism. Entry does not occur in isolation, and host expression of a chemokine receptor (i.e., CXCR4 for T-lymphotropic HIV strains and CCR5 for monocyte-tropic HIV strains) interacts in promoting viral particle binding to the host cell membrane and release of viral particles into the cytoplasm.[55] Heterozygous allele expression of these coreceptors affects expression and progression of HIV disease. Density expression of CCR5 molecules in infants has been correlated with progression of disease even in the presence of antiretroviral therapy and with the slope of $CD4^+$ T-cell decline from birth.[100]

After infection, the infant with perinatal transmission exhibits a quick rise in detectable HIV viral load that can exceed 750,000 copies/mL in the first weeks or months of life and that persists unchecked without institution of antiviral therapy through the first years of life.[2] The persistent and lengthy viremia in early perinatal HIV infection is different from acute HIV-1 infection in adults, in which viremia initially may be equally elevated but abates with host immunologic response (albeit without complete elimination) over the course of weeks to months. These distinctions in host response reflect the more ineffective infant immunologic host response to HIV infection.

Proposed mechanisms of immune dysfunction associated with continued viremia in infants include thymic damage with thymocyte depletion, disruption of thymic architecture, early $CD4^+$ T-cell depletion that affects the $CD8^+$ cell response to HIV antigens, early lymphocyte activation as measured by $CD8^+DR^+CD38^+$ T cells that impede effective host T-cell response, and genetic predisposition to allow enhanced HIV entry into host cells.[238,292] Most clinicians opt for early treatment of HIV-infected infants younger than 1 year of age, independent of the clinical or immunologic (i.e., $CD4^+$ T-cell count) presentation. Studies have documented that early therapy slows immune system destruction and preserves immune function, preventing clinical disease progression.[52]

Immune Dysfunction

Abnormalities in adult HIV infection include leukopenia, lymphopenia, and decreased CD4$^+$ helper-inducer T cells with an expanded CD8$^+$ T-cell population, which results in an inverted CD4/CD8 ratio, typically less than 1.0. Early in the course of infection, T-lymphocyte function is diminished (<50%), with decreased in vitro responses to soluble antigens preceding CD4$^+$ T-cell depletion. Proinflammatory cytokines appear to induce viral replication by activating the host cell.[58] HIV-infected CD4$^+$ T cells release soluble interleukin-2 (IL-2) receptors. The elevated serum IL-2 receptor levels block cell-bound IL-2 receptors by competition for IL-2. The CD8$^+$ T-cell response to HIV-specific antigens is impaired.[209]

Children with HIV infection seldom are lymphopenic in terms of the values observed in adults. If lymphopenia is observed in children with HIV infection, it usually is seen in older children or in children who have progressed to end-stage HIV disease. CD4$^+$ T-cell counts in HIV-infected children commonly exceed 400 cells/mm^3. In infants 12 to 24 months of age, a CD4$^+$ T-cell value of less than 1000 cells/mm^3 is significant for selective HIV-related CD4$^+$ T-cell depletion. In infants younger than 12 months, a value of less than 1500 cells/mm^3 similarly applies.

After administration of highly active antiretroviral therapy (HAART), T-cell function against specific HIV antigens continues to be imperfect. Despite lowering of viral load, CD4$^+$ T-cell depletion may not be completely restored for many weeks. Differential restoration of subpopulations of CD4$^+$ T cells (i.e., effector memory cells more commonly encountered than naïve cells) may occur. In 643 children with significant CD4$^+$ depletion (i.e., CD4$^+$ T cells <250 cells/mm^3) and viremia, HAART resulted in a median rise of the CD4$^+$ T-cell count of 100 cells/mm^3 over the course of 2 years, but anergy was reported in 80%, lack of proliferative response to the specific antigen of tetanus in 73%, and impaired serologic response to hepatitis A virus vaccination in 54%.[151] Despite administration of antiretroviral therapy, T-cell immune restoration may not be complete in all affected children.

B-cell dysfunction is similarly identified in HIV-infected adults and children and manifests as hypergammaglobulinemia. HIV-infected adults also demonstrate circulating immune complexes and production of autoantibodies due to polyclonal activation of B cells by HIV itself or concomitant viral infection with cytomegalovirus (CMV) or Epstein-Barr virus (EBV).[148] Immunoglobulin G (IgG) levels may rise to 2 to 3 standard deviations above the mean of normal values, and serum IgA, IgM, and IgE levels also may be elevated. This extreme hypergammaglobulinemia in children may be caused by polyclonal stimulation of B cells by HIV or coinfection with CMV or EBV, or it may be caused by the absence of normal CD4$^+$ T-cell immunoregulatory cells. Specific antibody functions measured as childhood vaccine responses often are abnormal and are not always completely restored in the most severely immunocompromised individuals after administration of HAART therapy.[151]

Other host defense cells affected by HIV infection include natural killer (NK) cells.[7,245] In adults with chronic HIV infection, reported NK cell abnormalities include differential representation of certain NK cell subpopulations, downregulation of NK ligand expression that affects cytotoxicity of HIV-infected cells, and NK cell–dendritic cell (DC) interactions. Human DCs have myeloid and plasmacytoid subsets. Both subsets have additional roles in HIV infection that lead to viral elimination or control.[6] Activated myeloid DCs produce cytokines such as IL-12, IL-15, and IL-18. IL-12 is critical for myeloid DCs to induce helper T-cell type 1 (Th1) responses, which promote the potent cytotoxic T-lymphocyte responses that are necessary for clearing virus-infected cells.[149] Plasmacytoid DCs produce more type I interferons (IFNs) in response to HIV than any other cell in the body; they stimulate myeloid DCs in a bystander fashion and directly activate NK cells.[231] The implications of these events underlie the need to develop vaccine strategies that enhance the ability of DCs to prime potent T-cell responses that can subvert the potential inhibitory effects of HIV on the immune system.

Monocytes and macrophages play important roles in the pathogenesis of HIV infection by serving as reservoirs of HIV. Defective chemotaxis and bacterial killing have been observed in HIV-infected monocytes and macrophages, as has defective induction of IL-1, which possibly accounts for the decreased IL-2 response in CD4$^+$ T cells.[291]

The immune system also seems to contribute directly to HIV-induced encephalopathy.[25,123] HIV-induced encephalopathy is particularly devastating in young infants, who fail to reach early motor milestones or, worse, regress from acquired early development. The incomplete state of myelination of central nervous system (CNS) tissue may account for susceptibility to the neurologic effects of HIV infection.

In adults with progression of disease, depletion of CD4$^+$ T cells has been linked to shifts in coreceptor use (from CXCR4 to CCR5), and individuals with more severe disease appear to harbor predominantly CCR5-dependent (R5) viral strains.[103] HIV-containing monocytes are thought to transport HIV into the CNS and infect microglial cells, including astrocytes.[56] Also implicated in HIV-associated neurologic complications are glial soluble factors that may have a direct neurotoxic effect.[146] Cytokines and reactive oxygen species released by HIV-infected lymphocytes and macrophages in the CNS may damage exposed nerve tissue.[280] The normal CNS immune defense system can attempt to enhance neuronal survival.

T-Cell Depletion

Loss of T cells in HIV infection occurs by direct lysis of T cells, apoptosis, and autophagy. Direct T-cell lysis is the result of massive destruction of T cells, as exemplified by the significant lysis of T cells in the gastrointestinal tract early in HIV infection. Almost all T cells are destroyed. The CD4$^+$ T-cell number drops precipitously at this time and frequently confirms the clinical suspicion of HIV infection, which is then diagnosed by laboratory testing. Activation of cytokine inflammatory cytokine pathways plays an important role in cell destruction.

Apoptosis is a well-known phenomenon of programmed cell death in HIV infection. Several hypotheses have been offered to explain the mechanism of apoptosis, including a viral cytopathic effect, bystander effect from HIV-infected neighbor cells, death of HIV effector cells migrating into HIV-infected tissue sites, activation of co-proapoptotic signaling on immune cells due to chronic immune activation, and destruction of HIV-infected cells by immune effector cells. Older HIV-infected patients exhibit syncytial formation by interaction on HIV viral proteins and their receptors on neighboring cells. These cells undergo apoptosis by a FAS-dependent pathway.[120]

Autophagy can be considered a form of autophagocytosis in which cytoplasmic organelles are lysed by lysosomes and histone deacetylase. Common regulating factors, such as tumor necrosis factor–related apoptosis-inducing-ligand (TRAIL), serve as stimuli for autophagy in uninfected CD4 T cells through the T-cell receptor for HIV gp120.[30]

Investigators hypothesize that HIV first depletes mucosal CCR5$^+$CD4$^+$ effector memory cells, leaving short-lived central memory or naïve CD4$^+$ T cells and other immunoregulatory cells in a chronic state of activation that leads to an ineffective host response.[69,113] Infection of CCR5$^+$CD4$^+$ effector memory cells also is associated with higher expression of cytotoxic T-lymphocyte-associated protein 4 (CTLA4 or CD152), a potent negative regulator for CD4$^+$ T cells.[294] High expression of CTLA4 can interrupt IL-2 production by CD4$^+$ T cells, impeding the ability of these cells to proliferate and depleting the population. The resultant chronic immune activation may lead to disorganization of the host immune response and further deplete CD4$^+$ T-cell regeneration. For patients with the most profound CD4$^+$ T-cell depletion, reduction of viral load with antiviral agents does not immediately result in correction of their immune defects.[103] The study of immune reconstitution with HAART may illuminate the immunopathogenesis of HIV infection.

CLINICAL MANIFESTATIONS

In children and adults, HIV infection causes a spectrum of clinical abnormalities that affect multiple organ systems and include the symptom constellation of AIDS. Box 192B.1 lists the pre-HAART frequency of AIDS-defining events per 100 child-years.[188]

Infection with HIV, independent of a diagnosis of AIDS, can be attended by nonspecific clinical findings, including mild failure to thrive, hepatosplenomegaly, acquired microcephaly, parotitis, generalized lymphadenopathy, nonspecific intermittent diarrhea, intermittent fever,

BOX 192B.1 Frequency of Opportunistic Infections in HIV-Infected Children Before Widespread Use of Highly Active Antiretroviral Therapy (HAART)

Pre-HAART Era (Event Rates >1/100 Child-Years)

Candidiasis
Disseminated *Mycobacterium avium* complex
Serious bacterial infections (e.g., pneumonia)
Herpes zoster
Pneumocystis jiroveci pneumonia
Serious bacterial infections (pneumonia)

Pre-HAART Era (Event Rates <1/100 Child-Years)

Cryptosporidiosis
Cytomegalovirus disease
Systemic fungal disease
Tuberculosis
Toxoplasmosis

Modified from Mofenson LM, Oleske J, Serchuck L, et al. Treating opportunistic infections among HIV-exposed and infected children: recommendations from CDC, the National Institutes of Health, and the Infectious Diseases Society of America. *MMWR Recomm Rep* 2004;53:1–92.

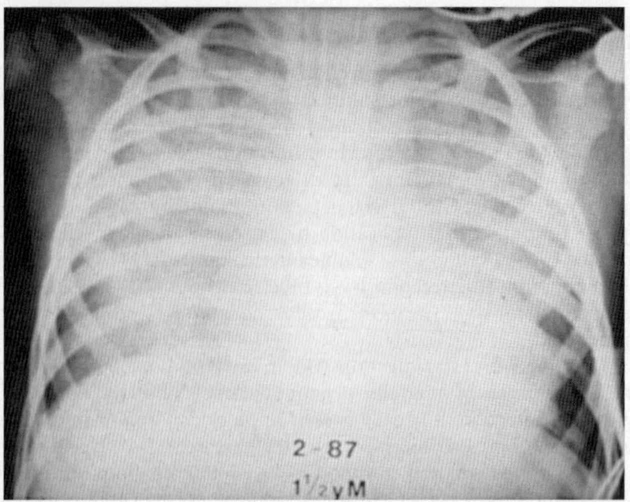

FIG. 192B.2 The classic, diffuse interstitial infiltrates of acute and fatal pneumonia due to infection with *Pneumocystis jiroveci* are seen in a 15-month-old child with perinatal acquired immunodeficiency syndrome. (From Hanson IC. Respiratory infections in HIV-infected children. *Immunol Allergy Clin North Am.* 1993;13:205–17.)

and chronic skin disease. These clinical symptoms are shared by other pediatric disease processes and can, when manifested singly in an HIV-infected host, delay establishing the diagnosis. However, a careful and detailed history should provide insight into potential HIV risk factors and prompt inclusion of HIV infection in the differential diagnosis. With the use of HAART, HIV infection has become a chronic disease and new clinical disease manifestations (e.g., lipodystrophy, hyperlipidemia) that are most closely related to chronic antiviral use have been described.

The health of HIV-infected children has improved during the past decade. Kourtis and associates reported a dramatic decrease (71%) in the number of hospitalizations of children with HIV infection who were 18 years of age or younger between 1994 (before HAART) and 2004 (after HAART).[142]

Opportunistic Infections

Opportunistic infections plague HIV-infected individuals and are the most prominent cause of morbidity and mortality in this cohort. Before the use of HAART, opportunistic infections in children usually were primary infections rather than the reactivation of infection seen in adults.[188] The introduction of effective HAART with associated host immune restoration significantly modified the expression of certain opportunistic infections in adults and children.[259] Among children, the overall incidence of these infections declined from 14.4 cases per 100 patient-years before 1997 to 1.1 cases per 100 patient-years.[199] In pre-HAART years, the age at clinical presentation was much younger, and an age younger than 3 years was associated with very rapid $CD4^+$ cell decline. Although the number of these opportunistic diseases has diminished, their prevalence appears to be unaffected. The administration of combination HIV therapy, including protease inhibitors (PIs) in adults and children, has improved the survival of perinatally infected children.[104]

Pneumocystis *Pneumonia*

P. jiroveci pneumonia (PJP) is the opportunistic infection most commonly reported for HIV-infected children. Declines in the incidence of PJP have been documented, with rates of 5.8 cases per 100 patient-years reported before 1997 and 0.3 cases per 100 patient-years reported after 1997.[199] PJP has a fulminant course in the pediatric population, with the highest mortality rates for affected children younger than 1 year of age. In a study of 172 children with perinatal HIV infection without HIV-specific intervention, 9% had PJP when they were younger than 1 year, with a median survival of 1 month.

Clinical expression of pediatric PJP often can be distinguished from other pulmonary diseases by the severity of the hypoxemia (i.e., higher alveolar-arterial oxygen gradients), elevated serum lactate dehydrogenase levels, the rapidity of progression of disease with tachypnea and fever, characteristic diffuse interstitial infiltrates on radiography, and the usual lack of digital clubbing.[117] The more insidious manifestations of PJP characteristic of HIV-infected adults, such as prolonged fever (>7 weeks), cough, and dyspnea (averaging 3 weeks), less commonly occur in infants and children.

Radiographically, pediatric PJP is associated with diffuse interstitial markings progressing to the white-out pattern of adult respiratory distress syndrome (Fig. 192B.2).[118] However, PJP can be seen initially as a unilateral streaky pneumonic infiltrate, as lobar consolidation, or with accompanying pleural effusions.

Aggressive diagnostic measures may be indicated to establish a diagnosis of PJP. Bronchoscopic alveolar lavage (BAL) is the preferred diagnostic tool for adults and children and should be considered a first choice for presumed PJP in children who cannot provide sputum specimens for evaluation. In older children and adults, evaluation of sputum for the presence of *Pneumocystis* with appropriate stains or monoclonal antibodies may preempt the need for using invasive diagnostic measures. PCR assays have been developed for diagnostic evaluation of PJP that are usually more sensitive but less specific than microscopic methods.[125] Lung biopsy carries the highest sensitivity for identifying the organism but has attendant morbidity related to thoracotomy or video-assisted thoracoscopy (VATS) and placement of a chest tube.

Acute PJP is treated with parenteral trimethoprim-sulfamethoxazole (TMP-SMX) or pentamidine or atovaquone for patients with TMP-SMX or pentamidine hypersensitivity. TMP-SMX treatment consists of 15 to 20 mg/kg per day of the TMP component delivered intravenously three to four times daily. Adjunctive corticosteroid therapy given early for moderate to severe PJP provides significant benefit with only limited evidence of concomitant immune suppression and attendant infectious complications.[95,256] Concomitant CMV and PJP has been documented in HIV-infected children. For the clinical situation of concomitant viral infection, no existing data recommend delay of corticosteroid use. Treatment of PJP should not be altered. Dosing regimens for corticosteroids are published and include options for use of oral prednisone or oral methylprednisolone or intravenous methylprednisolone.[42]

After the occurrence of PJP infection, secondary PJP prophylaxis (i.e., therapy initiated after acute disease treatment and resolution) is

TABLE 192B.4 Recommendations for *Pneumocystis* Pneumonia Prophylaxis and CD4+ Monitoring for Infants and Children Exposed to or Infected With HIV

Age, HIV Infection Status	Prophylaxis	CD4+ Monitoring
Birth to 4–6 wk, HIV exposed	No prophylaxis	—
4–6 wk to 12 mo, HIV exposed	No prophylaxis[a]	—
<12 mo, HIV infected or indeterminate	Prophylaxis	Every 3–4 mo
1–5 y, HIV infected	Prophylaxis if CD4+ count is <500 cells/μL or CD4+ percentage is <15%	Every 3–4 mo
6–12 y, HIV infected	Prophylaxis if CD4+ count is <200 cells/μL or CD4+ percentage is <15%	Every 3–4 mo

[a]Until HIV infection is presumptively excluded (i.e., documentation of two negative virologic test results, one at age ≥2 wk and one at age ≥4 wk) or definitively excluded (i.e., documentation of two negative virologic test results, one at age ≥1 mo and one at age ≥4 mo). For these definitions of HIV exclusion to be valid, the infant must not be breastfeeding.

Modified from Mofenson LM, Brady MT, Danner SP, et al. Guidelines for the prevention and treatment of opportunistic infections among HIV-exposed and HIV-infected children: recommendations from CDC, the National Institutes of Health, the HIV Medicine Association of the Infectious Diseases Society of America, the Pediatric Infectious Diseases Society, and the American Academy of Pediatrics. *MMWR Recomm Rep.* 2009;58(RR-11):1–166.

recommended (Table 192B.4). Proposed pediatric regimens include TMP-SMX at 150 mg/m^2 per day and 750 mg/m^2 per day, respectively, given in two divided doses on 3 consecutive days/week (alternative regimens include a single dose on 3 consecutive days/week, two divided doses on 3 alternate days/week, and two divided doses daily); dapsone for children 1 month of age or older at 2 mg/kg daily (single dosing not to exceed 100 mg/day) or 4 mg/kg weekly (single dosing not to exceed 200 mg); pentamidine (aerosolized [300 mg by Respirgard II inhaler monthly]) for children 5 years or older; and atovaquone (30 mg/kg daily for children 1–3 months and >24 months and 45 mg/kg daily for children 4–24 months).[187]

For adults and adolescents, recommendations to discontinue secondary PJP prophylaxis can be considered when there is documentation of immune restoration (i.e., CD4+ T-cell counts that have increased to >200 cells/mm^3 for ≥3 months as a result of HAART).[42] Data from the European PJP-Withdrawal Study Group suggest that with immunorestoration by HAART, the risk for PJP development is low and that withdrawal of PJP prophylaxis as recommended if the adult host appears to be a reasonable risk.[274] US guidelines continue to recommend lifelong primary PJP prophylaxis for individuals who acquired PJP before reaching 13 years of age.[188]

Primary PJP prophylaxis (i.e., therapy initiated to prevent primary infection) for adults and children is accepted as standard care.[42] Pediatric regimens and dosing for secondary PJP prophylaxis are not different from those outlined earlier. In 1993, the CDC published the first PJP prophylaxis guidelines for HIV-infected children. The guidelines linked the institution of therapy to the level of immunosuppression as measured by the CD4+ cell count or percentage.[38] Guidelines for PJP prophylaxis were modified in 2009.[187] The most significant change in the revised guidelines concerned diagnosing HIV infection and presumptively excluding HIV infection in infants, which affected the need for initiation of prophylaxis to prevent PJP in neonates.

Based on the revision, prophylaxis is not recommended for infants who meet criteria for being definitively or presumptively not HIV infected. For nonbreastfeeding infants with no positive HIV virologic test results, presumptive exclusion of HIV infection can be based on two negative virologic test results (i.e., one obtained at age ≥2 weeks and one obtained at 4 weeks of age), on one negative virologic test result obtained at 8 weeks of age or older, or on one negative HIV-antibody test result obtained at 6 months of age or older. Definitive exclusion of HIV infection is based on two negative virologic test results (one obtained at age ≥1 month and one obtained at age ≥4 months) or on two negative HIV-antibody test results from separate specimens obtained at 6 months of age or older. For presumptive and definitive exclusion of infection, the child should have no other laboratory or clinical evidence of HIV infection.

Infants born to HIV-infected mothers should be considered for prophylaxis beginning at 4 to 6 weeks of age. HIV-infected infants should be administered prophylaxis until 1 year of age, at which time they should be reassessed on the basis of the age-specific CD4+ T-cell count or percentage thresholds. Infants with indeterminate HIV infection status should receive prophylaxis until they are determined to be HIV uninfected or presumptively uninfected with HIV. Data from the Pediatric AIDS Clinical Trials Group protocol 1088 documented that primary PJP prophylaxis for HIV-infected children could be discontinued safely with immune restoration on stable antiretroviral therapy.[198]

Infection with Mycobacterium avium *Complex*

The incidence of *Mycobacterium avium* complex (MAC, formerly *Mycobacterium avium-intracellulare*), which caused disseminated infections in HIV-infected adults and children in the early 1980s and 1990s, waned significantly with the increasing and successful use of HAART. In a 1990 review of opportunistic infections in pediatric patients with AIDS, 43 (7.8%) of 552 children from birth to 9 years of age were found to have disseminated MAC infection.[117] The incidence of pediatric MAC infection among HIV-infected children dropped from 1.3 cases per 100 patient-years reported before 1997 to 0.2 cases per 100 patient-years after 1997.[199] Epidemiologically, MAC has been linked to significant immunosuppression (i.e., CD4+ T-cell counts <50 cells/mm^3) in adults.[42,189] Researchers observed that the development of MAC infection in children can be associated with CD4+ T-cell counts greater than 50 cells/mm^3, especially in children younger than 6 years.[235]

Symptoms of MAC infection include fever, malaise, weight loss, anorexia, and night sweats. Gastrointestinal manifestations have included abdominal pain, diarrhea, malabsorption, and intestinal perforation. Rarely, MAC has been reported with extrabiliary obstructive jaundice (presumably due to lymphadenopathy) and endobronchial masses. The diagnosis of disseminated MAC infection relies on identification of the microorganisms from the blood, lymph tissue, bone marrow, liver, lungs, and gastrointestinal tract.

Therapy for disseminated MAC infection in the pediatric population includes some combination of clarithromycin or azithromycin (maximal dosing of 500 mg and 250 mg, respectively) or rifabutin (maximal dosing of 300 mg), or both regimens. The epidemiologic link with severe immunosuppression and the advent of therapeutic prophylactic interventions (i.e., clarithromycin or azithromycin and/or rifabutin) prompted the implementation of MAC prophylaxis guidelines for adults, adolescents, and older children (≥6 years) with CD4+ T-cell counts lower than 50 cells/mm^3.[39] Primary MAC prophylaxis can be discontinued in HIV-infected children older than 2 years of age receiving stable HAART for 6 months or more and sustaining (>3 months) CD4+ T-cell recovery.[198]

An unusual immune reconstitution inflammatory syndrome (IRIS) has been described as a paradoxical event after immune recovery has been achieved in adults and adolescents receiving HAART.[258] IRIS is associated with reactivation of opportunistic infections such as MAC. Activation of other latent complications, including carcinoma and neurologic symptoms, has been described.[267] Data indicated that MAC prophylaxis with azithromycin did not prevent IRIS.[217] In children with IRIS, treatment of the reactivated opportunistic infection can include administration of antiinflammatory agents, including systemic corticosteroids.

Tuberculosis

Overall case rates of tuberculosis in the United States are declining, with 4.4 new cases per 100,000 people (total of 13,299 cases) reported in 2007. The percentage of patients with tuberculosis and known HIV infection also decreased from 15.0% in 2003 to 12.4% in 2006.[36] Primary disease accounts for one third or more of cases of tuberculosis in HIV-infected populations.[286] In a cohort of pregnant and nonpregnant HIV-infected women monitored in a multicenter longitudinal study, the prevalence of tuberculosis determined by medical history or positive skin tests was 14%.[188]

Children most commonly are infected with *Mycobacterium tuberculosis* from exposure in their immediate environment, usually the household. In a study of 60 HIV-infected families, the incidence of tuberculosis was approximately 6%, with HIV-infected and HIV-uninfected children affected. The vector for transmission was identified as an infected family member or caregiver.[11] Tuberculosis should be considered in the differential diagnosis of pulmonary disease in HIV-exposed children.

The principles for treating tuberculosis in the HIV-infected child are the same as for the HIV-uninfected child and should include at least a four-drug regimen. However, treating tuberculosis in an HIV-infected child is complicated by antiretroviral drug interactions with the rifamycins and overlapping toxicities caused by antiretroviral agents and tuberculosis medications. The duration of treatment is 9 to 12 months, with the longest duration for children with extrapulmonary disease.[34] Secondary prophylaxis is not recommended for children who have had a prior episode of tuberculosis.

Cytomegalovirus

In the pre-antiretroviral era, CMV caused 8% to 10% of pediatric AIDS-defining illness.[138] The adult spectrum of CMV disease, including retinitis, pneumonitis, esophagitis, gastritis, colitis, hepatitis, cholangitis, and encephalitis, is not reported uniformly in the pediatric AIDS literature. CMV can cause primary pneumonitis in children and can be associated with other pulmonary pathogens, especially *Pneumocystis*. Unusual gastrointestinal manifestations have included pyloric obstruction, enterocolitis, and oral and esophageal ulcers. CMV retinitis is the most frequent severe manifestation of CMV disease among HIV-infected children, accounting for approximately 25% of CMV AIDS-defining illnesses.[51] However, it appears to be decreasing in incidence with the wider use of HAART.[199] Annual CMV antibody testing is recommended beginning at 1 year of age for CMV-seronegative, HIV-infected infants and children who are severely immunosuppressed.

Treatment of CMV disease associated with HIV infection focuses on slowing progression of disease and not on a curative outcome. Therapeutic intervention includes the use of ganciclovir, valganciclovir, foscarnet, or cidofovir. These drugs have significant side effects, including bone marrow suppression and renal toxicity. Administration of these agents is divided into induction and maintenance dosing. The optimal interval for efficacy has not been determined and often is selected on an individual basis. Although many adults report experiencing subjective and objective improvement while receiving therapy, discontinuation of therapy is associated with high relapse rates, independent of the affected site.

Careful monitoring of children receiving treatment for CMV and antiretroviral therapy is imperative because the use of both classes of agents can depress bone marrow function. CMV end-organ disease is best prevented by antiretroviral therapy to maintain $CD4^+$ T-cell count greater than 100 cells/mm^3. If this is not possible, prophylaxis with valganciclovir can be considered for HIV-infected older children who are CMV seropositive and have severe immune suppression (i.e., $CD4^+$ T-cell count <50 cells/mm^3) at a dose of 15 mg/kg per dose every 12 hours and using a 50-mg/mL pediatric solution or using tablets if the child weighs enough to receive adult doses of valganciclovir.

Prevention of complications of CMV in HIV-infected children with severe immunosuppression includes careful and regular (i.e., every 4–6 months) retinal monitoring for evidence of eye disease. After secondary prophylaxis for disseminated CMV disease is initiated, its discontinuation should be considered on a case-by-case basis because current data to support discontinuation are limited.[281] As reported with MAC, reactivation of CMV disease in IRIS has been described.

Other Herpesvirus Infections

Infections with the herpesvirus family occur in HIV-infected children. In a US study during the HAART era, the incidence of systemic HSV infection was 0.9 case per 100 child-years. Infection was most common among children with a reduced $CD4^+$ T-cell percentage (<25%).[102] HSV infection in pediatric AIDS typically has been limited to mild to severe localized infections without reports of dissemination. Varicella-zoster virus (VZV) and herpes zoster virus (HZV) infections have contributed significant morbidity to HIV-infected people. Disseminated and chronic HZV infections are reported for pediatric patients with AIDS.

Because episodes of HSV disease can be treated successfully, chronic therapy with acyclovir is not required after lesions resolve. However, children who have frequent or severe recurrences can be administered daily suppressive therapy with oral acyclovir.[82] Prevention of herpes infections in school-aged children is especially important because exposure to varicella may be considerable. Administering varicella-zoster immune globulin (VariZIG) should be considered for susceptible HIV-infected children with exposure to VZV. Because the varicella vaccine is an attenuated live viral vaccine, its use in HIV-infected children is limited to children with asymptomatic or mildly symptomatic HIV disease and no evidence of immune suppression.[43]

Fungal Diseases

The most common fungal infections among HIV-infected children are caused by *Candida* spp. Oral thrush and diaper dermatitis occur among 50% to 85% of HIV-infected children.[102] Affected mucous membranes or skin often does not respond well to treatment with topical antifungal agents. Systemic therapy with one of the oral azoles, including fluconazole, ketoconazole, or itraconazole, is effective in oropharyngeal or esophageal candidiasis. In severe fungal infections, amphotericin B or other agents effective against the *Candida* spp. should be administered intravenously. Because of limited experience with children and no information about HIV-infected children, data are insufficient to recommend echinocandin class antifungal medications, including caspofungin, micafungin, and anidulafungin, as first-line agents for invasive candidiasis in children.[247] Prophylaxis for candidal infections is not recommended because of concern about development of resistance to azoles such as fluconazole, which could limit the use of these agents in the care of disseminated or mucosal disease.[42]

Other disseminated fungal diseases, such as histoplasmosis and cryptococcosis, less commonly affect pediatric patients with AIDS. Histoplasmosis may be prevalent among HIV-infected children who reside in parts of the United States where *Histoplasma capsulatum* is endemic. Symptoms of histoplasmosis include fever, rash, cough, lymphadenopathy, splenomegaly, thrombocytopenia, low-grade disseminated intravascular coagulopathy, acute respiratory distress syndrome, meningoencephalitis, and neurologic abnormalities consistent with intracranial mass lesions. Symptoms of cryptococcosis include fever, headache, pulmonary involvement, and subacute meningitis or meningoencephalitis.[185]

Because of the low incidence of histoplasmosis among pediatric HIV-infected patients, possibility of drug interactions, potential antifungal drug resistance, and cost, the routine use of antifungal medications for primary prophylaxis of *Histoplasma* infections in children is not recommended. However, primary prophylaxis for adults and adolescents is suggested for those with compromised immune systems. Fluconazole is suggested as primary cryptococcosis prophylaxis for adults and adolescents with $CD4^+$ T-cell counts of less than 50 cells/mm^3, and itraconazole is advised for histoplasmosis prophylaxis in adults and adolescents with $CD4^+$ T-cell counts of less than 150 cells/mm^3.

The safety of discontinuing secondary prophylaxis for cryptococcosis after immune reconstitution with HAART has not been studied in children, and decisions in this regard should be made on a case-by-case basis. Recommendations to discontinue prophylaxis as a result of HAART-related improved immune function have been developed for cryptococcosis and include sustained (>6 months) $CD4^+$ T-cell counts higher than 200 cells/mm^3.[137] No such recommendations exist for discontinuation of histoplasmosis prophylaxis in HIV-infected adults or adolescents with evidence of HAART-related reconstitution of immunity.

Bacterial Diseases

Pediatric patients have an increased incidence of severe bacterial infections, including infections with *Streptococcus pneumoniae, Staphylococcus aureus,* and various gram-negative organisms. One of the most common first-time infections in HIV-infected children is a bacterial infection (e.g., bacterial pneumonia).[102] In a study of 372 HIV-infected children monitored for a median of 17 months, 14% experienced one or more laboratory-proven serious bacterial infections. Later findings suggested that the rates of bacterial disease dropped from 4.7 cases per 100 patient-years before 1997 to 0.2 cases per 100 patient-years after 1997 (i.e., HAART era).[199]

Reported clinical infections included bacteremia, pneumonia, osteomyelitis, meningitis, and sinusitis. Therapy is directed against the specific isolated bacterial pathogen, and the dosing and duration of therapy depend on the affected site. Prophylaxis against bacterial infections initially should include vaccination with appropriate childhood vaccines, including *Haemophilus influenzae* type b (Hib) vaccine, pneumococcal conjugate vaccines, meningococcal conjugate vaccines, and influenza vaccine.[206] Other medications available for bacterial prophylaxis include intravenous immune globulin (IVIG), TMP-SMX, atovaquone, and azithromycin. IGIV is no longer recommended for primary prevention of serious bacterial infections in HIV-infected children unless hypogammaglobulinemia exists or functional antibody deficiency is demonstrated.

COMPLICATIONS

Pulmonary Complications

In addition to PJP and chronic sinopulmonary infection, noninfectious pulmonary complications of pediatric AIDS cause morbidity. Chronic lung disease is common in HIV-infected children with increasing age.[252] A longitudinal birth cohort study reported a cumulative incidence of chronic radiographic lung changes in HIV-infected children of 33% by 4 years of age.[205] The spectrum of chronic HIV-associated lung disease includes lymphocytic interstitial pneumonia (LIP) or pulmonary lymphoid hyperplasia (PLH), chronic infections, IRIS, bronchiectasis, and malignancies.[293] Lymphoid interstitial pneumonitis and *P. jiroveci* pneumonitis have largely disappeared in developed countries but remain a significant problem in developing countries.[293] The incidence of *P. jiroveci* pneumonitis (previously 1.3 per 100 child-years) is now 0.13 per 100 child-years. LIP is similarly affected by HAART. The rate of bacterial pneumonia remains relatively high (2.2 per 100 child-years), although it is markedly reduced from the period before HAART, when the incidence was fivefold higher.[293] Bronchiectasis may reappear as a serious complication of HIV infection if chronic inflammation of the lung (usually controlled by HAART) takes its toll over the years; the oldest surviving HIV-infected children are now approaching 30 years of age.

Histopathologically, LIP and PLH appear to be distinct entities, although whether these disorders represent a continuum of reactive hyperplasia of lymphoid tissue is somewhat controversial. In LIP, small lymphoid infiltrates are dispersed throughout parenchymal lung tissue and often are accompanied by alveolar epithelial hyperplasia and interstitial widening. PLH describes larger, dense nodular aggregates of lymphoid tissue in distal parenchymal tissue and the walls of bronchi and bronchioles (Fig. 192B.3B). Compression of blood and lymphatic vessels by these nodules may contribute to the accompanying clinical interstitial widening. The cause of LIP/PLH has not been defined. Simultaneous infection with EBV and HIV may amplify the risk of LIP. B lymphocytes infected with EBV are very susceptible to HIV infection in vitro and can enhance intrapulmonary replication of HIV.[264]

Clinically, LIP/PLH is characterized by a nonproductive cough and the insidious onset of progressive hypoxia. The hypoxemia may be subtle and best appreciated during febrile, upper respiratory tract illnesses. Digital clubbing, generalized lymphadenopathy, chronic parotitis, or failure to thrive may accompany LIP/PLH.[216,260] Radiographically, LIP/PLH often demonstrates characteristic interstitial infiltrates with a nodular pattern (see Fig. 192B.3A). This radiographic picture frequently mimics that of miliary tuberculosis and warrants exclusion of this pulmonary infection.

In an immunocompromised, anergic, HIV-positive child, simple delayed hypersensitivity skin testing for exclusion of tuberculosis may not suffice, and BAL or gastric aspiration for detection of acid-fast microorganisms may be necessary. Lung biopsy is the definitive diagnostic procedure for LIP/PLH. However, in HIV-infected children, a presumed diagnosis of LIP/PLH by the less invasive exclusion of infectious pathogens is preferred.

Therapy for LIP/PLH is not defined clearly because the clinical outcome varies. HIV-infected children with LIP/PLH have had spontaneous remissions without therapeutic intervention, whereas other affected children progress to respiratory insufficiency and failure. Therapeutic

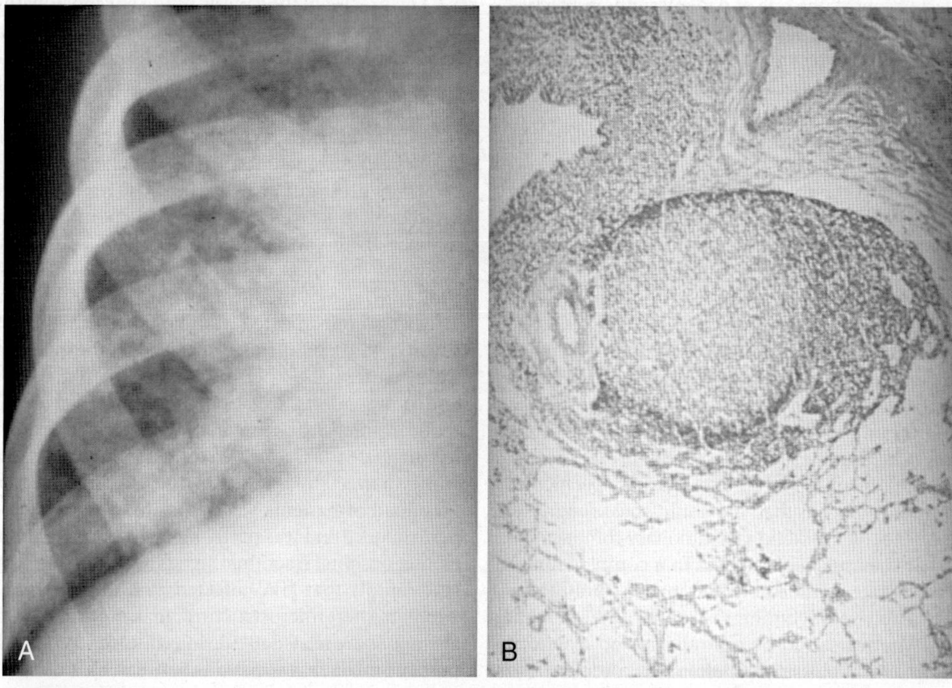

FIG. 192B.3 (A) Chest radiograph documents parenchymal nodularity in a 3-year-old child with perinatal AIDS. (B) Pulmonary lymphoid hyperplasia in the child produced histologic changes, including interstitial widening and prominent peribronchial lung nodes.

interventions have included IVIG supplementation, antiretroviral therapy, corticosteroids (i.e., daily or alternate-day dosing of 0.5–2.0 mg/kg per day), and observation. No significant associated infectious sequelae (e.g., bacteremia, fungemia) of corticosteroid use were reported for treated children. Supportive therapy consisting of oxygen supplementation, chest physical therapy, and adequate nutritional intake is helpful.[106,216]

Other noninfectious pulmonary complications have been reported less frequently for the pediatric HIV-infected population. Evidence of an increased incidence of asthma among HIV-infected children, adolescents, and young adults was shown in a series of peer-reviewed publications.[88–90,116,254] In the most recent of these, physician-diagnosed asthma and asthma medication use associated with at least a 30% increase in the asthma incidence (i.e., HIV-infected vs. HIV-exposed but not infected patients) and offered compelling evidence that patients had more than one manifestation of allergic disease.[254] The rate of atopic dermatitis also increased among HIV-infected patients, It appeared shortly after birth and before the asthmatic child was diagnosed, resembling the order that it appears in the general pediatric population.

Two mechanisms that may underlie the increased incidence of asthma among HIV-infected youth have been discovered. The first is genetic inheritance of HLA class I genes that are associated with new disease appearance after patients with HIV infection have had immune reconstitution with HAART.[88] The second mechanism that may be applicable to the appearance of new disease in immunoreconstituted patients infected with HIV is a sudden return of cellular immunity (i.e., measured by $CD4^+$ T-cell increases), which may precipitate a dysregulated attack on HIV in the airways, and commensal fungi that colonize or infect the airways of HIV-infected patients.[16] In experimental animal models, the sudden burst of immune stimulation precipitates an asthma attack.[222,223]

Studies of asthma and HIV infection have been extended in the Pediatric HIV/AIDS Cohort Study of a cohort of older children, adolescents, and young adults who were HIV infected ($n = 218$) and HIV exposed but uninfected ($n = 152$).[252] The stimulus for this ongoing research was the National Heart, Lung, and Blood Institute supplemental grant that enabled the performance of pulmonary function tests (PFTs) to augment the clinical information on asthma, asthma medications, and physician examination with objective evidence of abnormal pulmonary airflow recorded by a spirometer. A key outcome of PFTs is the rate (i.e., number of abnormal/total number of patients) with obstructive airflow (i.e., difficulty breathing). For the HIV-infected and HIV-exposed but uninfected cohort, the rate of patients with obstructive airflow is elevated at 17% to 20% (vs. 8.6% for US youth), but the rate of reversal of obstructive airflow after inhalation of a bronchodilator (i.e., criteria for asthma) was less for the HIV-infected group compared with the HIV-exposed but uninfected group of youth.

When only the obstructive subgroup was identified by PFTs, the rate of reversal of obstructive airflow for the HIV-infected group was only 50%, compared with 75% for the HIV-exposed but uninfected subgroup. The lack of reversibility of airflow obstruction in patients with asthma can be attributed to a complex mixture of asthma and chronic obstructive pulmonary disease (COPD), known as the asthma-COPD overlap syndrome. Immune dysregulation has been implicated in these disorders. Investigators looked for evidence of objective involvement of the immune system and showed reversibility by using time-honored methods: control of total nonspecific serum IgE levels by the $CD4^+$ T cells and. ability of both subgroups to produce specific IgE in response to common inhaled allergens, such as dust mites.

These approaches revealed that the HIV-infected subgroup showed no immune control of total serum IgE levels and had less specific IgE levels in response to common allergens than the noninfected subgroup. The tests indicated the presence of an additional pulmonary complication of HIV infection, one that coexisted with asthma in a complex illness that will most likely demonstrate considerable pulmonary comorbidity as patients grow older. The overall findings strongly indicate that perinatally HIV-infected youth need to be followed for an extended period in case they develop serious obstructive pulmonary complications of HIV infection and that additional control subgroups are essential for the demonstration of the specific destructive nature of the asthma-COPD overlap syndrome (e.g., HIV-unexposed, uninfected subjects).

Central Nervous System, Neurobehavioral, and Neurocognitive Complications of Pediatric HIV/AIDS

Neurologic abnormalities have been documented in people with HIV and can be attributed to opportunistic infections, adverse events of primary treatment, or primary infection with HIV, especially in light of HIV's described tropism for monocytes. Diverse neurologic and neurobehavioral deficits that occur in children with HIV-1 infection include abnormal neurologic examination findings (e.g., global pyramidal tract signs, hemiparesis, peripheral neuropathy, visual, hearing impairment), neurobehavioral problems, encephalopathy, and epilepsy.[13,105,131] Children with severe immunosuppression, those with immune activation not receiving antiretroviral therapy, and those who are growth impaired and younger than 1 year of age are at greatest risk for neurologic complications.[145,180] Antiretroviral treatment is associated with fewer severe CNS effects of HIV infection, such as encephalopathy. However, increases have been found in mental health and neurodevelopmental conditions. A study of two cohorts, P219C (2004–07) compared with P1074 (2008–14), showed the largest increases in substance or alcohol abuse, anxiety disorders, trauma- or stress-related disorders, impulse control and mood disorders, and learning and communication disorders.[184]

An encouraging study of early viral suppression improving neurocognitive function of HIV-infected children was made by Crowell and colleagues.[64] Measurements for almost 400 HIV-infected children from two US-based multisite studies in which IQ scores, perceptual receptive reasoning, and verbal comprehension were compared for HIV-infected patients with or without viral suppression. HIV-infected children with viral suppression scored significantly higher in several neurocognitive assessments than HIV-infected children not viral suppressed.

In 1994, HIV encephalopathy in children was adapted as a criterion for the diagnosis of AIDS. It consists of at least one of the following features persisting for at least 2 months: failure to attain or loss of developmental milestones or loss of intellectual ability, verified by a standard developmental scale or neuropsychological tests; impaired brain growth or acquired microcephaly demonstrated by head circumference measurements or brain atrophy identified by computed tomography (CT) or magnetic resonance imaging (MRI) (i.e., serial imaging is required for children <2 years); and acquired symmetric motor deficit manifested by two or more of the following: paresis, pathologic reflexes, ataxia, or gait disturbance.[40]

The precise pathogenesis of the encephalopathic changes associated with HIV infection remains elusive, although cellular tropism of HIV has been implicated.[141] Most children with involvement of the CNS show significant brain atrophy histopathologically. Inflammatory lesions usually are sparse and alone cannot account for the significant amount of atrophy observed. Other factors potentially contributing to diminished brain size have included the following: direct or indirect interference of HIV with brain growth (i.e. HIV toxic effect vs. competition with brain growth factors such as neuroleukin), severe malnutrition, severe hypoxia from cardiac and pulmonary compromise, and therapeutic regimens for infectious or noninfectious processes that mandate the prolonged use of medications that can inhibit brain growth.[157,242]

Using sophisticated radiologic scanning technology, Uban and coworkers[268] demonstrated alteration of the microstructure of the cerebral white matter cells in perinatally HIV-infected older children, adolescents, and young adults.[268] Patients with more severe HIV disease exhibited reduced fractional signaling of the right inferior frontal-occipital and left uncinate tracts, elevated diffusion in the F minor tract, and increased white matter streamlines in the left inferior bundle. Increased peak viral load of patients was associated with decreased working memory performance and was partly mediated by reductions in the right inferior frontal occipital fractional signaling node. Conclusions of this pediatric study imply that HIV-infected youth have a higher risk of changes in white matter microstructure than youth controls and that certain alterations are related to previous disease severity. White matter alterations possibly mediate associations between HIV disease severity and working memory.

A prospective study of a cohort of 319 perinatally HIV-infected children 6 to 17 years of age observed over a 2-year period indicated associations of past and current CDC class C designation with less severe attention-deficit/hyperactivity disorder (ADHD) inattention symptoms, older age at nadir CD4$^+$ T-cell percentage and lower CD4$^+$ T-cell percentage at study entry with more severe conduct disorder symptoms, higher RNA viral load at study entry with more severe depression symptoms, and lower CD4$^+$ T-cell percentage at study entry with less severe symptoms of depression. There was little evidence of an association between specific antiretroviral therapy and severity of psychiatric symptoms. A lower nadir CD4$^+$ T-cell percentage was associated with worse quality of life, worse Wechsler Intelligence Scale for Children Coding Recall scores, and worse social functioning.[197] In a cohort of perinatally HIV-infected children with severe disease, Kapetanovic and colleagues concluded that higher CD4$^+$CD38$^+$HLADR$^+$ percentage was associated with a neuroprotective effect and higher percentage of CD4$^+$CD38$^+$ but that HLADR$^-$ T cells may be deleterious.[132] ADHD, learning disability, and graphomotor weakness have been described in higher proportions among HIV-infected children with transfusion-acquired infection.

Behavioral, neurodevelopmental, and occasionally, imaging improvements have been documented with antiretroviral therapy. In a study of 146 perinatally HIV-infected children born between 1990 and 2003, the prevalence of encephalopathy (i.e., progressive or static) decreased from 40.7% before 1996 (i.e., limited combination antiviral therapy) to 18.2% after that year.[249] In this cohort, neurocognitive scores remained stable over the course of a 6-month period for children receiving combined antiviral therapy, and only a weak association with lowered viral load could be found. Antiviral therapy must achieve effective serum and plasma concentrations and must be able to cross the blood-brain barrier and affect HIV-infected CNS monocytes. On the contrary, a longitudinal cohort study involving HIV-infected and HIV-exposed but uninfected infants and children reported the effects of PI-based HAART and showed a positive but limited impact on neurodevelopmental trajectories and the rate of significant cognitive and motor impairment in HIV-infected infants and young children during the first 3 years of life.[155] In this study, infants with immune suppression (i.e., CD4$^+$ T-cell levels <25%) seemed to be most vulnerable with respect to neurodevelopmental functioning, demonstrating mental and motor scores lower than those of the HIV-negative infants and HIV-infected infants with less immune suppression.

Sleep disturbances, neurocognitive deficits, and abnormal psychosocial function are associated with abnormal cytokine levels in children with HIV infection.[18,207,241,285] A National Heart, Lung, and Blood Institute (NHLBI)–funded study attempted to discern a molecular pathway of these complications of pediatric HIV infection by assessing proinflammatory cytokine production in CD4$^+$ and CD8$^+$ T cells, disturbed sleep patterns, and results of neurodevelopmental testing in HIV-infected versus HIV-exposed children.[87] Compared with HIV-exposed children, there were significant associations for HIV-infected children for changes in intracellular proinflammatory cytokines (i.e., tumor necrosis factor-α, IFN-γ, IL-12), sleep patterns (particularly increased daytime sleep), and lower neurocognitive scores on socioemotional, behavioral, and executive function: working memory and mental fatigue; verbal memory; and sustained concentrations and vigilance. The authors of this sleep study of HIV-infected children proposed that therapies that reduced immune-mediated inflammation and prescribed sleeping habits could improve the neurocognitive and psychosocial problems.[87]

Gastrointestinal Complications

Gastrointestinal complications of HIV disease are encountered frequently in children and adults. In untreated children, malnutrition is one of the most frequent and devastating complications of pediatric HIV, and it predicts morbidity and mortality. Malnutrition in HIV-infected children has several causes, including reduced oral intake (i.e., HIV-induced primary cachexia, opportunistic infections of the upper gastrointestinal tract, and medication side effects), malabsorption (i.e., HIV alone or infections of the gastrointestinal tract), altered metabolic states (i.e., proinflammatory effects of chronic HIV infection), and socioeconomic factors.[135]

Although the prevalence of AIDS-associated wasting has declined in the developed world because of HAART, it is still a concern for children in rich and poor nations. HIV and its complications also have been associated with specific nutritional disorders. Higher HIV viral load, lower CD4$^+$ T-lymphocyte counts, infections, maternal drug use, and some antiretrovirals such as zidovudine and lopinavir plus ritonavir, have been associated with growth problems.[153,182] Wasting and weight loss in HIV-infected individuals appear to be independent predictors of death and are associated with lower CD4$^+$ T-cell counts.[86,168]

The intestine is a primary target organ for HIV and is important in the pathogenesis of HIV infection. Among untreated HIV-infected children, as many as 80% will have one or more intestinal abnormalities at a given time. The pattern of intestinal dysfunction may change with time and can occur without evident cause or change in clinical HIV stage or immunologic status.[66,114] The transactivator of transcription (Tat), a regulatory protein that drastically enhances the efficiency of HIV DNA transcription, may be involved in intestinal dysfunction (i.e., HIV enteropathy) because it can impair enterocyte proliferation by targeting its L-type calcium sodium-glucose symporter. This pathway may explain many features of intestinal dysfunction, such as intestinal atrophy, carbohydrate malabsorption, and diarrhea, that are frequently observed.[66] Associated protein and micronutrient (e.g., zinc, selenium) deficiencies have been documented in HIV-infected adults and children.[50] Despite use of HAART, gastrointestinal conditions, nutritional deficiencies, and fluid and electrolyte disorders continue to be the most frequently described diagnoses for hospitalized HIV-infected children.[144]

Specialized nutritional supplements such as nucleotides, polyamines, probiotics, and zinc can improve gastrointestinal absorption. Zinc may control diarrhea in HIV-infected children because it specifically counteracts Tat-induced intestinal ion secretion.[31] Polyamines such as spermine, spermidine, and putrescine can modulate intestinal maturation. Probiotics, including *Saccharomyces boulardii,* target the gastrointestinal tract and have antioxidant, antibacterial, enzymatic, antiinfective, metabolic, and antiinflammatory activity. However, their effectiveness in HIV care is not well established.[73,97]

The use of more potent antiretroviral therapy regimens, particularly those including PIs, has resulted in unwanted biochemical lipid abnormalities and changes in body composition for some HIV-infected adults and children. In a 2004 study of 94 infected children receiving long-term PI-containing antiviral regimens, 10% developed redistribution of fat, 52% developed dyslipidemia without associated somatic changes, and 38% had no associated findings.[261] In this cohort, changes in redistribution of fat and dyslipidemia were most likely to occur near ages consistent with the start of puberty (age 10–15 years).

In a multicenter US Perinatal AIDS Collaboration Transmission Study, 178 HIV-infected children were evaluated for hypercholesterolemia or hypertriglyceridemia, and 47% and 67%, respectively, met criteria for these diagnoses at least once during their follow-up.[33] In this cohort, hypercholesterolemia was associated with multiple PI-containing regimens and an undetectable HIV viral load as measured by RNA PCR. Hypertriglyceridemia was predicted by elevated body mass index and use of the PI ritonavir (RTV). These clinical findings of lipodystrophy and dyslipidemia have been treated with some success with diet, exercise, or lipid-lowering medications, although the lipid-lowering medications may result in drug-drug interactions when they are combined with antiviral agents. Antiretrovirals regimens with integrase inhibitors are less associated with lipodystrophy and dyslipidemia.

Nutritional goals for HIV-infected children should include preservation of normal growth and development, provision of adequate amounts of all nutrients, and prevention of malabsorption and deficiencies of nutrients that alter immunologic function while improving quality of life.[181]

Malignancy

HIV infection has been associated with an increased risk of AIDS-defining and non–AIDS-defining malignancies.[80] Initiation of HAART in the mid-1990s has resulted in a significant decrease in AIDS-defining neoplasms such as Kaposi sarcoma and certain lymphomas, particularly primary CNS lymphoma and high-grade B-cell non-Hodgkin lymphoma, but malignancies continue to be reported.[57,80,109,130] Most malignancies that affect HIV-infected children are non-Hodgkin lymphomas, although the leading cause of malignancy in youth in Africa is Kaposi sarcoma.[81,109,136,140]

In a retrospective study of 4954 children with AIDS in the United States (1978–96), approximately 2.5% had documented malignant diseases: non-Hodgkin lymphoma ($n = 100$), Kaposi sarcoma ($n = 8$), leiomyosarcoma ($n = 4$), and Hodgkin disease ($n = 2$); 10 others had unspecified cancers.[15] Associated in situ infection with HIV or EBV, or both, has been documented in pediatric malignancies, although the precise role in pathogenesis is not defined. In a case-control study, a high viral burden of EBV was associated with the development of malignancy, but only in children with CD4+ T-cell counts greater than 200/μL.[219] Early chemotherapeutic intervention has enhanced quality of life and longevity and often has been provided in conjunction with antiretroviral therapy.

The pathogenesis of HIV-related and non–HIV related Kaposi sarcoma has been elucidated, and human herpesvirus 8 has been documented in lesions.[121,150] Pathogenesis has been linked to oncogenesis and cytokine-induced growth. The clinical manifestations of Kaposi sarcoma associated with AIDS affect many organs. The skin, gastrointestinal tract, lungs, and heart are affected by Kaposi sarcoma.[8] Management of Kaposi sarcoma has improved with increasing use of HAART to restore immune function in HIV-infected individuals.[81,215]

Leiomyomas and leiomyosarcomas are among the common malignancies observed in HIV-infected children. Although these cancers are usually seen in the gastrointestinal tract, the lungs or spleen can also be involved. The pulmonary lesions are usually visible as nodules on chest CT, whereas the gastrointestinal tumors manifest as obstruction, abdominal pain, and bloody diarrhea.[109]

Since the advent of HAART, HIV-related malignant disease in the United States is reported less frequently. In a study of 2969 HIV-infected children observed in the Pediatric AIDS Clinical Trials Group 219/219C from 1993 to 2003, only 37 cases of malignant disease were reported, representing a prevalence of 0.6% malignancies and an incidence of 1.56 cases per 1000 person-years.[136] In this analysis, the standardized incidence cancer rate for infected children was 10.08 compared with uninfected but exposed controls. The incidence of cancer was highest among children with severe immunocompromise and those who had received HAART for less than 2 years.

Other Complications

Cardiac Abnormalities

The most direct way to study pediatric cardiovascular disease in HIV infection is to study adults with HIV-related cardiovascular disease. Adults with HIV infection are 50% to 100% more likely to have cardiovascular disease.[266] Studies at the Veterans Affairs Agency have found a less than 50% incidence of myocardial infarction among non–HIV-infected people compared with HIV-infected individuals.

Coronary artery plaque is the leading factor in the cause of myocardial infarction.[92] Scanning techniques have demonstrated that plaque is the culprit in the ensuing myocardial infarction.[158] Adherence to antiretroviral therapy by adults has produced a significant reduction in cardiovascular events.[186]

Cardiac manifestations of HIV infection in children include left ventricular dysfunction, increased left ventricular mass, myocarditis, and pericardial effusion.[277] HIV-infected children have been described with congestive heart failure and cardiomegaly, cardiac tamponade, nonbacterial thrombotic endocarditis, conduction disturbances, and sudden death, presumably due to primary ventricular arrhythmia associated with severe cardiomyopathy. In a postmortem analysis of 30 HIV-infected children followed longitudinally in the prospective P2C2 HIV Multicenter Study, 50% had cardiomegaly with associated clinical findings of increased heart rate, increased left ventricular mass, and chronic heart disease.[133]

Asymptomatic children with HIV infection can exhibit cardiac abnormalities. In a cross-sectional study of 49 HIV-infected children, carotid artery wall stiffness was larger and systolic-diastolic variations in diameter of the carotid artery were significantly lower compared with controls in the absence of cardiovascular risk factors.[17] Other investigators reported higher carotid intima-media thickness in HIV-infected subjects than in healthy controls, suggesting early atherosclerosis; duration of antiretroviral therapy and CD4+ T-cell percentage were associated with these changes.[233]

A prospective cohort study of HIV-exposed infants suggested associations of in utero antiretroviral therapy exposure with reduced left ventricular mass and dimension, reduced septal wall thickness Z-scores, and increased left ventricular fractional shortening and contractility up to 2 years of life.[152] In a later study of this problem by the same group of investigators but with a more contemporary cohort of HIV-exposed but uninfected children, there was no evidence of cardiac toxicity of perinatal antiretroviral therapy exposure.[156] There were some subclinical differences in cardiac structure and function with certain antiretroviral medications and first trimester of pregnancy medication. The study authors proposed long-term follow-up of patients to determine future harmful effects of prenatal and postnatal antiretroviral drugs.

The increasing use of HAART and specifically of PIs in the pediatric HIV-infected population prompted careful management of associated hypercholesterolemia and hyperlipidemia. In univariate analysis, hypercholesterolemia in children with HIV infection treated with a PI regimen was associated with elevated systolic blood pressure but not with body mass.[84] Careful follow-up of lipid profiles should be evaluated routinely for HIV-infected children receiving antiretroviral therapy.

Renal Dysfunction

Renal disease is a well-known complication of HIV infection. HIV-1–associated nephropathy (HIVAN) is a clinical and renal histologic disease characterized by heavy proteinuria and nephrotic syndrome leading to rapid progression to chronic renal failure. The renal abnormalities described in HIVAN include nephritis (i.e., focal and segmental glomerulosclerosis and mesangial hyperplasia) and nephrosis.[14] The immunopathologic characteristics of HIVAN include inflammatory infiltrations predominantly composed of activated T cells, with CD4+ T cells usually exceeding CD8+ T cells.[229]

Persistent metabolic acidosis associated with renal tubular disease and high anion gap acidosis has been reported for pediatric HIV infection.[229] Renal disease in HIV-infected children often appears in concert with profound immunodeficiency and end-stage HIV disease. Because most pediatric patients with AIDS and renal disease have perinatally acquired HIV infection, the importance of congenital or early concomitant infections (e.g., CMV) has been postulated to affect pathogenesis. Host genetic factors also play an essential role in HIVAN.[224]

The nephrosis of HIV disease can be particularly difficult to treat in an already malnourished, hypoproteinemic, HIV-infected child. HAART is considered the best treatment for HIVAN. Corticosteroids in combination with HAART can be attempted. However, the risks associated with their long-term use in HIV-infected children should be balanced against their potential benefits.[225] Many of the reported children with renal disease have associated growth failure. Nutritional supplementation and dietary restriction can offer supportive adjunctive therapy.

Bone Marrow Suppression

Hematologic abnormalities associated with HIV infection in children include leukopenia, anemia, and thrombocytopenia. The cause of neutropenia is often multifactorial in HIV-infected patients, representing the combined effects of systemic infection, medications, and the virus itself.[10] Neutropenia often has been associated with circulating anti-neutrophil antibodies and may respond to blockade therapy with IVIG. Granulocyte colony-stimulating factor has been used successfully in drug-induced and HIV-associated neutropenia.[111,112,195]

The anemia of HIV infection may be microcytic, hypochromic as seen in chronic infection, autoimmune with positive Coombs testing, or typical of nutritional deprivation (i.e., iron or vitamin B_{12} deficiency). Determining the origin of anemia in AIDS is confounded by multiple cofactors that affect red blood cell counts, such as poor nutritional status and concomitant use of toxic therapeutic agents (e.g., zidovudine).

In adults and children, recombinant erythropoietin has been beneficial in treating anemia associated with antiviral therapy.[195] In developing nations, infant anemia of HIV exposure or infection coupled with acute local parasitic infections (e.g., malaria) can significantly affect infant morbidity. The risk of developing severe and potentially fatal malarial anemia is increased for HIV-exposed or -infected children with concomitant acute parasitemia compared with HIV-negative controls.[208]

Immune thrombocytopenia has been reported for 13% of children with symptomatic HIV infection with an onset as early as the first year of life.[101,173] Thrombocytopenia in HIV-1–infected patients is multifactorial, including a direct effect of HIV-1 with a depressed platelet production due to HIV infection of megakaryocytes and peripheral destruction due to platelet-associated autoantibodies triggered by molecular mimicry between some HIV-1 peptides and membrane-associated platelet glycoproteins.[154] Therapy for thrombocytopenia in children and adults has included no intervention, platelet transfusions, systemic corticosteroids, IVIG, antiretroviral therapy, and in adults, IFN-α. Immune thrombocytopenia has resolved spontaneously in some children with simple supportive measures.

DIAGNOSIS OF HIV INFECTION IN INFANTS AND CHILDREN

Early Transmission to Fetuses

Human placenta plays a role in prenatal transmission of HIV infection from mother to fetus. Studies suggested that fetal infection can take place as early as 9 to 11 weeks' gestation.[24,176] Preliminary examination of birth placental tissue from HIV-infected mothers in another study indicated that HIV core antigens could be detected in approximately 50% (23 of 51) of the cases studied and HIV antigens were localized in the Hofbauer cells.[272] Investigators documented that placental trophoblasts could be infected by CD4-independent isolates of HIV-1 in vitro.[4] Placental cytokines and chemokines influence HIV replication in trophoblasts. Genetic analysis of HIV-1 sequences can verify the interaction of HIV-1 and placental tissue. The vertical transmission of HIV-1 is characterized by selection of genotype variants that escape the mother's immune system.[5]

An increase in the incidence of intrauterine fetal demise was demonstrated for HIV-infected pregnant women.[76] In HIV-negative fetuses, placental lesions associated with fetal demise were identified: abruption, infarction, and other infections (e.g., CMV). In HIV-positive fetuses, similar placental lesions could not be identified, and death was attributed to HIV infection of fetal tissue detected by in situ hybridization. Two hypotheses for transmission are proposed: direct cell-to-cell spread of HIV from infected maternal mononuclear cells through the placental cells and eventually to fetal tissue itself and infected maternal cells that gain access to the fetal circulation.

Methods for Diagnosing Infection in Children Older Than 18 Months

In children older than 18 months of age in whom maternal anti-HIV antibody no longer is a confounding variable, the conventional tests used to diagnose HIV infection in adults are applicable (Box 192B.2). Antibody detection tests, including the HIV rapid test, enzyme immunoassays (EIAs), Western blot analysis, indirect fluorescent antibody assay, and p24 HIV antigen (p24Ag) analysis, HIV culture, and HIV PCR assay, may be used.

The period between infection and detection of HIV antibody by a particular test is referred to as the *window period* for that assay. The window period for detection of HIV has been progressively shortened as EIA techniques have improved. Various generations of screening EIAs begin to detect anti-HIV antibody 2 to 6 weeks after HIV RNA is detected. EIAs that test for HIV-1 and HIV-2 are used for screening. Western blots, which have been used for confirmation of positive screening EIA results, become diagnostically reactive 5 to 6 weeks after infection. Aside from the HIV-1 Western blot, confirmation of HIV-1 infection can be achieved with qualitative or quantitative HIV RNA PCR or HIV DNA PCR analysis. Combined fourth-generation tests that detect HIV p24 antigen and HIV antibody have been used for initial screening, with confirmation of infection provided by HIV RNA PCR testing to reduce the window period for diagnosis with newer diagnostic algorithms.[20]

Methods for Diagnosing Infection in Children Younger Than 18 Months

The clinical manifestations of HIV infection in children are varied and nonspecific and include chronic pneumonitis, failure to thrive, hepatosplenomegaly, thrombocytopenia, and chronic diarrhea. For children younger than 18 months, a positive serologic determination of HIV is not accepted as indicative of HIV infection because of passive maternal antibody. Documentation of HIV infection in children younger than 18 months requires identification of viral components from blood. The most commonly used virologic assay in the United States is PCR for HIV DNA or RNA.[214]

Pediatric PJP prophylaxis guidelines suggest that infants with two negative virologic assay results, both performed at 1 month or older and at 4 months or older, are not infected with HIV and that interruption of the therapeutic intervention is warranted.[41] The early diagnosis of HIV-exposed infants has been improved for identification of HIV-infected children (as early as the first month of life) and for uninfected children labeled as seroreverters (as early as the fourth month of life). Schedules for testing of HIV-exposed infants vary nationally. However, advances in diagnostic technology allow for early testing of HIV-exposed infants, including shortly after birth through 14 days of life, at 1 to 2 months of age, and again at 3 to 6 months. Confirmation of negative virologic assay (e.g., HIV PCR) results can be performed with typical antibody testing when the child is 18 months of age.

The assays outlined earlier easily detect HIV-1 subtype B that is commonly found in developed nations. To detect non-B HIV infection in individuals from or in developing countries, HIV RNA PCR may be preferred because it has a lower rate of false-negative assay results compared with HIV DNA PCR. If non–subtype B HIV is suspected, use of HIV RNA testing that is sensitive for these subtypes (i.e., more sensitive RNA PCR assays or branched DNA assays that are commercially available in the United States) should be considered.

BOX 192B.2 Guidelines for the Diagnosis of HIV Infection in Infants Born to HIV-Infected Mothers

Diagnosis of infants age <18 months: Virologic assays that directly detect HIV, preferably HIV RNA assays or the HIV DNA polymerase chain reaction (PCR) assay, must be used to diagnose HIV infection in infants age <18 months. A positive virologic test result should be confirmed by a repeat virologic test on a second specimen.

Diagnosis of infants age ≥18 months: A positive HIV antibody test result with confirmatory Western blot or immunofluorescent antibody (IFA) assay or virologic assay is used for the diagnosis of infants age ≥18 months.

Exclusion of HIV infection in infants: Definitive exclusion of HIV infection in non-breastfed infants is based on two or more negative virologic test results, one obtained at age ≥1 months and one at age ≥4 months, or on two negative HIV antibody test results from separate specimens obtained at age ≥6 months.

Modified from Panel on Antiretroviral Therapy and Medical Management of HIV-Infected Children. Guidelines for the use of antiretroviral agents in pediatric HIV infection. http://aidsinfo.nih.gov/contentfiles/lvguidelines/pediatricguidelines.pdf; Department of Health and Human Services. Guidelines for the use of antiretroviral agents in pediatric HIV infection, 2012. https://aidsinfo.nih.gov/guidelines/html/2/pediatric-arv-guidelines/0.

IMMUNOLOGIC AND CLINICAL MONITORING OF HIV-INFECTED CHILDREN

Laboratory monitoring of HIV-infected children is linked to variables that predict morbidity and mortality: $CD4^+$ T-cell percentage and HIV RNA PCR assay results. Clinical evaluations should occur at a minimum of every 3 to 6 months or sooner if the patient has clinical signs or AIDS-defining events, and measures of $CD4^+$ T-cell and HIV RNA PCR values should be performed. Because of variations across commercially available RNA PCR assays that may be as great as twofold, the HIV-infected patient should be tested with a single assay type. Recommendations for changes in treatment based on changes in $CD4^+$ T-cell percentages or HIV RNA PCR should be undertaken in consultation with a specialist who routinely provides care to HIV-infected individuals.

Evaluation of the individual HIV-infected child for viral resistance can be accomplished with the use of commercially available phenotyping or genotyping assays. Studies should be performed in consultation with an HIV specialist. Depending on treatment regimens, most children also should have laboratory studies performed to assess their potential for developing treatment-induced toxicities, including bone marrow suppression, metabolic acidosis, dyslipidemia disorders, and pancreatitis. It is recommended that this cohort annually receive dental and ophthalmologic assessments and tuberculosis screening. Routine recommendations for childhood vaccine delivery are outlined later.

TREATMENT

Primary Anti-HIV Infection Treatment

Implementation of combination antiretroviral therapy consisting of at least three antiviral drugs has enhanced survival rates, improved immune status, and reduced opportunistic infections.[23,102,179,228] Increased survival of HIV-infected children brings challenges in selecting successive new antiretroviral therapy regimens, and specific issues to address include short-term and long-term toxicities related to therapy and development of drug resistance.

The principles of therapy are similar for all affected age groups. Treatment should be aggressive and use multiple drugs as early in the course of the infection as possible to suppress viral replication fully, reduce development of resistant viral strains, minimize drug-related toxicity, and preserve immune function. Considerations specific to the pediatric host include early clinical severity of HIV disease, viral load, and level of immune suppression; availability of appropriate drug formulations and dosing; unique pharmacokinetics (e.g., body composition, renal excretion, liver metabolism, enzyme maturation); regimen potency, complexity, short-term and long-term toxicity potential; impact of changing therapy; comorbidities that affect drug choice; drug interactions; and the ability of the parent or child to adhere to a prescribed regimen.

Guidelines for initiation of therapy are somewhat different for adults and children. Pediatric recommendations include initiation of therapy for all HIV-infected children, with the strongest support for the recommendation for symptomatic and immunosuppressed HIV-infected children and children younger than 12 months of age, regardless of clinical, immunologic, or virologic status. Current antiretroviral therapy is designed to target different steps in the replication cycle of HIV (Fig. 192B.4).[139]

The Working Group on Antiretroviral Therapy and Medical Management of HIV-Infected Children recommends aggressive combination of at least three medications from at least two drug classes for initial treatment of HIV-infected infants, children, and adolescents. With improvements in treatment formulations, dosing recommendations for antiviral agents can change over time. Updated information on specific antiretroviral medications, including dosing and drug-drug interactions of antiviral agents, is provided in the guidelines from the Panel on Antiretroviral Therapy and Medical Management of HIV-Infected Children.[213]

Inhibitors of HIV Cell Entry

Entry of HIV-1 into target cells begins with interactions of the viral envelope protein gp120 with CD4 and a chemokine coreceptor, usually CCR5 or CXCR4. The cellular receptors and structures in envelope proteins associated with membrane attachment and fusion are targets for therapeutic intervention.

Blockade of HIV by CD4-Receptor Inhibitors

CD4-based molecules can neutralize HIV by several mechanisms. Initial studies demonstrated the efficacy of soluble preparations of CD4 (sCD4) against HIV in vitro.[126,240,277] A chimeric molecule consisting of

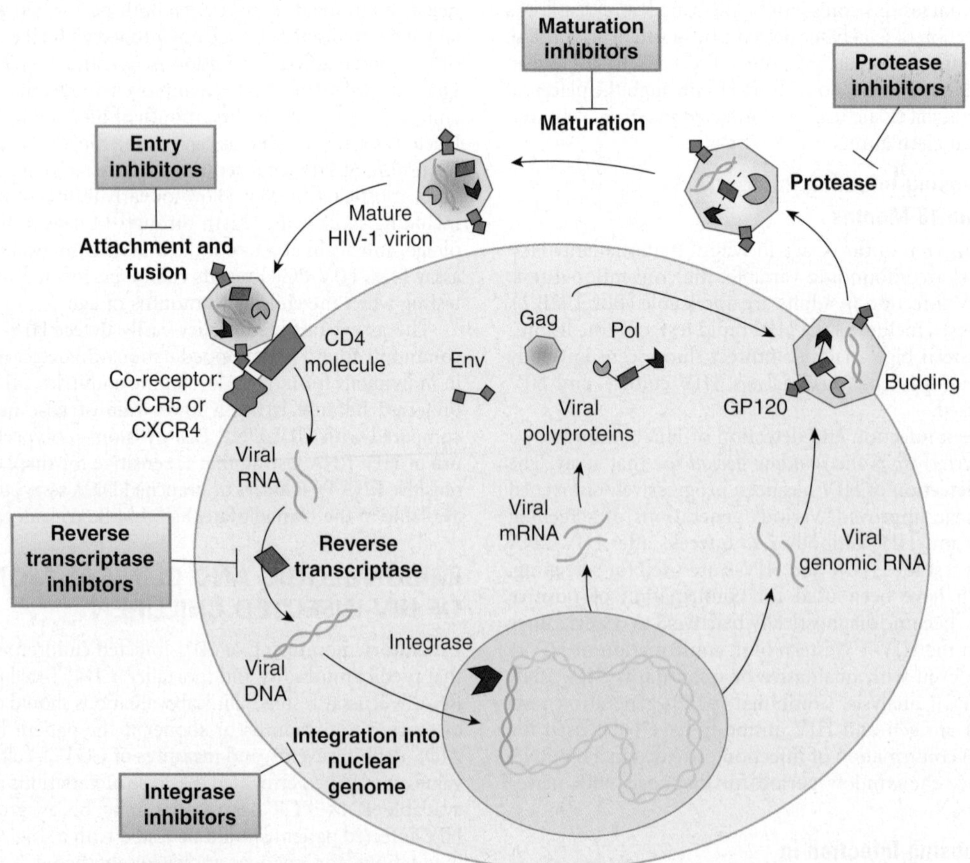

FIG. 192B.4 Inhibition of HIV-1 replication can be accomplished at different steps in the viral life cycle. (From Smith RL, de Boer R, Brul S, Budovskaya Y, van Spek H. Premature and accelerated aging: HIV or HAART? *Front Genet.* 2013;3:328.)

recombinant CD4 and immunoglobulin G (rCD4-IgG) was developed with an extended half-life and enhanced efficacy. Shearer and colleagues[253] documented safety, evidence of placental transfer, and appropriate elimination after intravenous administration of rCD4-IgG2 in pregnant women. In a phase I/II study, 18 children infected with HIV-1 received single or multiple intravenous doses of rCD4-IgG2 and demonstrated evidence of antiviral activity and tolerance.[251]

Certain small molecules may competitively inhibit viral entry by binding gp120, blocking the gp120-CD4 interaction. These small molecules in development as antiretroviral medications are thought to interfere with the gp120-CD4 interaction by altering the conformation of gp120 induced by CD4 instead of directly blocking CD4 binding.[65]

Blockade of HIV by Chemokine Inhibitors

Agents that block CXCR4 and CCR5 are being evaluated in clinical trials. Concerns about the use of chemokine (i.e., coreceptor) inhibitors include the potential for unintended immune modulation and for viral escape to occur from tropism selection, with resultant disease progression.[194] Maraviroc, a first-in-its-class selective CCR5 coreceptor antagonist, received approval by the FDA for use in adults in August 2007. It is recommended as adjunctive therapy for combination antiviral regimens and targets treatment of CCR5-tropic HIV-1 (i.e., R5 virus). The most common adverse effects are cough, fever, upper respiratory tract infections, rash, musculoskeletal symptoms, abdominal pain, and dizziness.

Blockade of HIV by Interference With gp120-CD4 Interactions

Polyanionic compounds such as dextran sulfate and heparin inhibit binding of HIV to the cell membrane, targeting the V3 loop of gp120.[193] Because of their systemic toxicity, most of these compounds have been evaluated in clinical trials as topical microbicides to prevent sexual transmission of HIV in humans. Unfortunately, clinical trials involving polyanion-containing microbicide formulations demonstrated that these products were ineffective, and in some circumstances, they might have increased the risk of HIV-1 infection.[218] An additional substance, the green tea flavonoid epigallocatechin gallate (EGCG), binds to the CD4 molecule at the gp120 binding site, inhibiting gp120-CD4 interaction in a dose-dependent manner.[282] These adjunctive mechanisms to restrict HIV infection remain under development.

Blockade of HIV by Fusion Inhibitors

Fusion of the HIV envelope (i.e., glycoprotein gp41) with the target cell membrane is an important step in host cell infection. During fusion, the gp41 fusion peptide inserts into the target cell membrane, and gp41 heptad repeats (i.e., HR1 and HR2) alter their conformations to form a six-helix bundle. This process produces a fusion pore through which the HIV capsid passes into the target cell.

Fusion inhibitors represent the first class of entry inhibitors for which there is a licensed drug. Enfuvirtide (T-20) is a synthetic peptide that binds to the HR1 domain of gp41, prevents six-helix formation, and inhibits fusion.[48,227] Enfuvirtide is approved for use in HIV-infected adults and children 6 years of age or older whose HIV infection has not been controlled by other anti-HIV drugs. Addition of enfuvirtide to an optimized background regimen of antiretroviral agents has demonstrated modest decreases of HIV viral load for long periods.[284]

Although enfuvirtide is FDA approved for use in children, it is not commonly used because of its high cost; need for twice-daily, subcutaneous injections; and high rate of injection-site reactions. The most common adverse effects include mild to moderate erythema, induration, pain, lymph node swelling, itching, and tenderness at the injection site. Other reported side effects are diarrhea, nausea, fatigue, headache, dizziness, peripheral neuropathy, and hypersensitivity reactions.[68] In the absence of a fully suppressive antiretroviral therapy regimen, mutations associated with resistance to enfuvirtide have been rapid.

Nucleoside Reverse Transcriptase Inhibitors

Nucleoside reverse transcriptase inhibitors (NRTIs) have no direct effect on HIV reverse transcriptase. After phosphorylation by the host cell kinases, they inhibit viral reverse transcriptase by competing with the natural substrate at the same binding site on the enzyme. With their incorporation into the newly forming proviral DNA, further viral transcription is prematurely terminated.

Six NRTIs are licensed in the United States: zidovudine (ZDV), didanosine (ddI), stavudine (d4T), lamivudine (3TC), abacavir (ABC), and emtricitabine (FTC). They are also available in combinations (e.g., zidovudine + lamivudine, abacavir + lamivudine, abacavir + zidovudine + lamivudine).

Nucleotide Reverse Transcriptase Inhibitors

Nucleotide reverse transcriptase inhibitors (NtRTIs) function like the previously described NRTIs, but they do not require phosphorylation. Tenofovir disoproxil fumarate (tenofovir DF [TDF]) and tenofovir alafinamide (TAF) are orally bioavailable prodrugs of tenofovir. TDF has good in vivo potency against HIV-1 and hepatitis B virus (HBV).[96] TDF has long serum and intracellular half-lives that allow once-daily dosing.

High-dose TDF treatment has been associated with skeletal abnormalities in young animals[275] and a significant decrease in absolute bone mineral density in HIV-infected children.[94] The changes in bone mineral density appeared to stabilize by 24 weeks of treatment, and none of the patients experienced fractures during the study period. US pediatric guidelines suggest judicious use in children and young adolescents because of unfavorable bone mineral density changes at a time when bone growth is so important. New-onset or worsening of renal impairment has been reported in adults and children receiving tenofovir and may be more common in those with higher tenofovir trough plasma concentrations.[230]

Oral-administration TDF is well absorbed and is so rapidly metabolized to TFV that TDF itself cannot be measured in blood, even when plasma is sampled within 5 minutes of administration.[213] TFV is the main compound measurable in plasma after TDF administration. From the bloodstream, TFV enters cells and is phosphorylated to the active agent tenofovir diphosphate (TFV-DP).

TAF also has good oral bioavailability.[9] Within the enterocyte and liver, TAF is not metabolized to TFV as quickly as TDF. The plasma TFV concentration is much lower with administration of TAF compared with TDF, and the main component in plasma is the prodrug itself, TAF.[234] Relative to TDF, TAF more effectively delivers TFV to cells throughout the body.[9] A lower dose of TAF results in equivalent or higher concentrations of TFV-DP inside cells compared with the much higher doses of TDF needed to attain a similar intracellular TFV-DP concentration.

The key pharmacokinetic difference between TDF and TAF is that TDF results in a higher plasma TFV concentration compared with TAF, but when administered at FDA-approved doses, both result in equivalent intracellular TFV-DP concentrations.[234] Because it is intracellular TFV-DP that suppresses viral replication, TAF should have antiviral efficacy equivalent to TDF, but it should avoid the toxicities that are specifically related to plasma TFV.

A combined product, Truvada, provides a preformed tablet formulation of FTC (200 mg) and TDF (300 mg) available for use once daily. Truvada is the recommended drug for HIV PREP.[46]

Nonnucleoside Reverse Transcriptase Inhibitors

Nonnucleoside reverse transcriptase inhibitors (NNRTIs) work by binding directly to the reverse transcriptase enzyme, rendering it nonfunctional. Five available drugs in this class are approved for use in the United States: nevirapine (NVP), delavirdine (which is not recommended in pediatrics), efavirenz (EFV), etravirine (ETR), and rilpivirine (RPV). The major disadvantage of the two drugs widely used in pediatrics in this category, NVP and EFV, is the rapid development of resistance with resultant cross-resistance between the two drugs. ETR, a newer NNRTI, retains activity against NVP- or EFV-resistant viruses when used in a regimen that also contains darunavir or ritonavir and if the number of NNRTI resistance-associated mutations is limited.[22] Additional NNRTIs are in development.[278]

Protease Inhibitors

PIs are relatively small peptides that share structural features with the substrates for viral protease. These molecules bind to and inhibit viral protease, preventing the virus from maturing into an infectious virion. These drugs are extremely potent in reducing plasma RNA viral loads. They exhibit a high barrier for development of drug resistance. As a class, they interact with the hepatic cytochrome P450 enzyme system, and many induce their own metabolism. As a result, the potential for significant drug-drug interactions is considerable. Examples of these interactions include those with oral contraceptives, antituberculous drugs, antiepileptic drugs, some antihistamines, and methadone.

Adverse events of PI use include previously described metabolic complications (e.g., dyslipidemia, lipodystrophy, insulin resistance, gastrointestinal effects of nausea or diarrhea), higher pill burden than with NRTI- or NNRTI-based regimens, and poor palatability of liquid preparations. PIs approved for the treatment of HIV infection include saquinavir, RTV, lopinavir (LPV) plus RTV, indinavir, nelfinavir (NFV), atazanavir (ATV), fosamprenavir (FPV), tipranavir (TPV), and darunavir (DRV). Previously used amprenavir is no longer manufactured in the United States. Saquinavir, which has a high pill burden, must be boosted with another PI due to low bioavailability, and limited pediatric pharmacokinetics data, and indinavir, which has an unfavorable toxicity profile and limited pediatric pharmacokinetics data, typically are not used in pediatrics.

Integrase Inhibitors

Joining of the viral genome and the host's chromosomal DNA is the hallmark of a retroviral infection. Integrase, the enzyme that catalyzes this step of the HIV life cycle, is an effective therapeutic target. On binding to specific sequences in viral DNA, HIV-1 integrase catalyzes two consecutive steps during integration: 3′ processing, endonucleolytic cleavage of the 3′ ends of the viral cDNA, and strand transfer, achieved by ligation of the viral 3′-OH cDNA ends to the 5′-DNA phosphate of an acceptor DNA (i.e., host chromosome).[221]

Several compounds have been developed to block integration at different steps. Compounds that inhibit integrase at its catalytic site with an effect on strand transfer, known as strand-transfer inhibitors (i.e., raltegravir [RAL], elvitegravir, and dolutegravir), are approved for use. Elvitegravir is available in a combination quad pill containing elvitegravir, a novel boosting agent with no antiviral activity (i.e., cobicistat), tenofovir DF, and emtricitabine. Dolutegravir is available in combination with abacavir and lamivudine.

Allosteric integrase inhibitors intended to interfere with the integrase-LEDGF/p75 interaction are being designed. These new inhibitors (i.e., LEDGINs) have an effect on 3′ processing and strand transfer.[167] Long-acting antiretroviral agents such as cabotegravir, a novel parenteral integrase inhibitor similar to dolutegravir, are under investigation.[172] In research studies, the agent has been packaged into nanoparticles, conferring an exceptionally long half-life of 21 to 50 days after a single dose.[19,265]

Antiretrovirals available for use in the United States are listed at https://aidsinfo.nih.gov/guidelines/html/2/pediatric-arv-guidelines/0. Optimal antiretroviral combinations for children may be slightly different from those for adults. For infants, particularly those younger than 1 year, there is often a need to use very potent antiretroviral regimens for reduction of persistently elevated virus loads.[163,211] In this scenario, four-drug combinations that include a protease inhibitor, two nucleoside analogues, and a nonnucleoside analogue such as nevirapine may be indicated.

The use of many antiretrovirals is limited in younger children (especially those younger than 4 years of age) because of the lack of liquid formulations. Prevalent combination antiretroviral regimens in pediatrics include one protease inhibitor drug such as ritonavir plus lopinavir or use of atazanavir or darunavir (in older children) in combination with a double NRTI backbone such as ZDV + 3TC, D4T + 3TC, ZDV + DDI, D4T + ABC, ABC + 3TC, or FTC or 3TC (in older children).

The PIs may be substituted by NNRTI drugs such as nevirapine or efavirenz (the latter in older children). In special circumstances, it may be necessary to boost the main PI with additional PIs such as ritonavir or saquinavir to achieve higher blood concentrations. For instance, this is the case of atazanavir when used with tenofovir. Additional boosting with 100 mg of ritonavir in the treatment of older children is often warranted.

Triple NRTI regimens may have a role in specific case scenarios, however they are less potent antiretroviral regimens. Specific antiretroviral regimens to be avoided include any type of single or dual therapy; efavirenz during pregnancy; atazanavir with tenofovir without ritonavir boosting; combinations of ZDV + D4T; DDC with 3TC, D4T or DDI; and D4T and DDI in pregnant patients.

US clinical trials are evaluating the pharmacokinetics of integrase inhibitors in children and the pharmacokinetics of R5 receptor blockers. Newer-generation NNRTI drugs such as etravirine or rilpivirine have not been evaluated in children, nor are there dosing recommendations for multiple antiretrovirals in children younger than 4 years of age. In resource-limited settings, treatment studies have demonstrated greater durability of virus load suppression in children treated with ritonavir plus lopinavir regimens compared with nevirapine-based regimens, although nevirapine has been associated with improved growth in this population.[49]

Change in Therapy

The decision to change antiretrovirals varies slightly according to the pediatric guidelines employed. The decision mostly depends on the surrogate markers used. Most experts agree that indicators of treatment failure include progression of HIV disease, growth failure, development of opportunistic infections while on established therapy, decline in CD4 percentiles, development or worsening HIV encephalopathy, and significant increases in virus load.

Toxicities and Adverse Effects

Specific antiretrovirals have many complications and side effects. The most frequent toxicities of ZDV are hematologic, particularly anemia, and neutropenia. They may resolve with dose reduction. All NRTIs can cause some degree of mitochondrial toxicity. ZDV can cause myopathy, and peripheral neuropathy is seen with this drug and with DDI, D4T, and rarely, 3TC. DDI is associated with pancreatitis. D4T is associated with lipoatrophy, and in combination with DDI, it may induce liver fatty acid syndrome, particularly during pregnancy. Abacavir is famous for a fatal hypersensitivity reaction, which occurs in 1% of pediatric patients. It manifests as flu-like symptoms with or without a rash, abdominal pain, sore throat, and myalgias. If the drug has been interrupted in this scenario, shock will ensue when it is restarted.

The NNRTIs most commonly cause rashes (≈40%) and have been associated with Stevens-Johnson syndrome. Efavirenz is teratogenic, and central nervous system findings such as dizziness, insomnia, and nightmares have been reported shortly after initiation of treatment with this drug. There is some concern about the prolonged use of nevirapine during pregnancy in patients with higher $CD4^+$ T-cell counts who developed hepatic failure,[122] but there is still controversy on the subject because additional studies have failed to demonstrate an association.[67]

Protease inhibitors have multiple drug-drug interactions because of their cytochrome P450 metabolism in the liver. Their most common side effects are gastrointestinal symptoms. Hepatitis and hyperbilirubinemia also occur. In adults, they have induced lipodystrophy, diabetes, and increased atherosclerosis because of lipid abnormalities. These findings are beginning to be recognized in children, although complications occur less often. Indinavir may induce renal stones by precipitation of the drug in the kidneys or tubules. There are also concerns about the potential in children for osteopenia and osteoporosis induced by combination antiretrovirals or HIV disease itself.[191]

One recognized complication of potent antiretroviral therapy is IRIS. It occurs most frequently in patients who initiate treatment with lower $CD4^+$ T-cell counts. It is attributed to a wide range of pathogens, and tuberculosis is a common underlying condition. The pathogenesis appears to be colonization with opportunistic pathogens when patients have moderate to severe immunosuppression. With the initiation of combination antiretroviral treatment and subsequent recovery of immunity to the organism, there is a paradoxical clinical deterioration due to a dysregulated immune response.

IRIS usually manifests in the first 6 weeks of antiretrovirals and may resolve with the use of steroids or temporary discontinuation of antiretroviral treatment. It is infrequently seen in pediatric HIV cases in developed countries, particularly because children are treated earlier. However, it is prevalent in the developing world and may produce high morbidity and mortality rates.

Benefits of Therapy

Despite the complications and controversies, the benefits of antiretroviral treatment of children with HIV are overwhelming. In the United States, the annual mortality rate for pediatric HIV patients decreased to less than 1% as of 1999 due to the availability of treatment.[104,129] HAART decreases the virus load, preserves and restores the immune function, decreases the risk of comorbidities, decreases hospitalizations, improves survival, improves quality of life, and restores hope to children and their families. Perinatally HIV-infected children who received antiretroviral treatment are now young adults attending college and preparing for an adult life.

Treatment very early in the perinatal period or in the acute stages of HIV infection has dramatically reduced viral reservoirs, a situation that may render the environment amenable to a functional cure. Pediatric studies of HIV perinatally infected infants treated very early with potent antiretroviral therapy[164] and studies of adult cohorts treated during acute infection[237] have shown that very early treatment of HIV is associated with control and decrease of the viral reservoir burden, which is likely a predictor of long-term HIV control. Although the early treatment approach has not been shown to induce a functional HIV cure, it has been associated with an extended period of complete viral quiescence, also known as HIV-free remission (i.e., no detectable plasma HIV RNA).

Antiretroviral treatment improves immune reconstitution and immune preservation of infected individuals. It also prevents HIV dissemination in susceptible or infected individuals, and it can potentially provide a functional cure.

Immune-Based Therapies

The cardinal immune manifestation of HIV infection is development of progressive CD4$^+$ T-cell lymphopenia with resultant clinical disease associated with severe immunodeficiency. Replacement of the CD4$^+$ T-lymphocyte pool is therefore a logical approach for immune-based therapies.[250]

Immune modulators have been assessed as single therapeutic agents and in combination regimens in adult clinical trials. An immune-based therapy (IL-2) demonstrated CD4$^+$ T-cell count increases but no clinical benefit in two large, randomized studies.[1] Other immune-based therapies (e.g., gene therapies, growth hormone, IL-7) are being studied and should be used in the treatment of HIV only in the context of a clinical trial. IFN-α initially was studied as a therapeutic agent for Kaposi sarcoma and had good response rates, but significant side effects limit its use in HIV infection. The utility of immune-based therapies in pediatric or adolescent HIV infection may include treatment of concomitant chronic hepatitis B and C virus infection and HIV-associated immune thrombocytopenia.[54]

Chronic immune activation has been associated with poor outcomes for AIDS-defining and non–AIDS-defining clinical events and for persistent CD4$^+$ T-cell depletion. The cause of chronic immune activation in well-controlled HIV infection in the era of combined antiretroviral therapy, aside from coinfecting pathogens, can include low-level viral replication and microbial translocation. Therapeutic interventions that target immune activation, including interfering directly with activation and inflammatory pathways, are being developed.[29] Long-acting, potent neutralizing monoclonal antibodies that have the potential to control HIV viremia in the absence of antiretrovirals are being studied.[27]

Vaccines

Goals for the development of an HIV vaccine include prevention of persistent HIV infection, prevention of severe clinical disease (i.e., AIDS), and therapeutic immunization to control HIV infection. The first candidate preventive vaccines tested in human trials in the late 1980s were based on the HIV-1 envelope glycoproteins gp120 and gp160, an approach aiming to induce neutralizing antibodies. The major limitations of this approach were lack of neutralizing antibody activity against a diversity of primary patient isolates of HIV-1 because of genetic variation and structural complexity of the HIV-1 envelope glycoproteins and absence of envelope-specific cytotoxic T-lymphocyte responses.[107,134,175]

More than 30 HIV vaccines have been tested in human trials.[233,242] The vaccines produced disappointing results until a HIV-1 vaccine efficacy trial completed in 2005 in Thailand (RV144) showed that priming with a recombinant canarypox vector (vCP1521) and boosting with this vector plus bivalent gp120 protein (AIDSVAX B/E) provided partial protection against HIV infection in heterosexual men and women.[232] A subsequent study showed that the peak neutralizing antibody response (Nab) in RV144 was substantially weaker than the peak Nab response in a study of AIDSVAX B/E in injection drug users that showed no efficacy.[190] The results suggest that weak neutralizing antibody responses can be partially protective against HIV in low-risk heterosexual populations or that the efficacy seen in RV144 was mediated by other immune responses, alone or in combination with neutralizing antibodies.

Antigenically diverse viruses, including HIV, contain highly conserved exposed sites, usually associated with function, that can be targeted by broadly neutralizing antibodies, and advances in the field have enabled increasing numbers to be identified.[28] Molecular characterizations of the antibodies and of the HIV antigens that they recognize offer hope for the discovery of new vaccines and drugs.

NEW REFERENCES SINCE THE SEVENTH EDITION

3. AIDSinfo, U.S. Department of Health and Human Services. Guidelines for the use of antiretroviral agents in HIV-1-infected adults and adolescents. https://aidsinfo.nih.gov/guidelines/html/1/adult-and-adolescent-treatment-guidelines/21/hiv-infected-adolescents-and-young-adults.
7. Altfeld M, Gale M Jr. Innate immunity against HIV-1 infection. *Nat Immunol.* 2015;16:554-562.
9. Babusis D, Phan TK, Lee WA, et al. Mechanism for effective lymphoid cell and tissue loading following oral administration of nucleotide prodrug GS-7340. *Mol Pharm.* 2013;10:459-466.
12. Becquet R, Ekouevi DK, Viho I, et al. Acceptability of exclusive breast-feeding with early cessation to prevent HIV transmission through breast milk, ANRS 1201/1202 Ditrame Plus, Abidjan, Côte d'Ivoire. *J Acquir Immune Defic Syndr.* 2005;40:600-608.
14. Bhimma R, Purswani MU, Kala U. Kidney disease in children and adolescents with perinatal HIV-1 infection. *J Int AIDS Soc.* 2013;16:18596.
26. Bryson YJ, Luzuriaga K, Sullivan JL, et al. Proposed definitions for in utero versus intrapartum transmission of HIV-1. *N Engl J Med.* 1992;327:1246-1247.
27. Burton DR, Hangartner L. Broadly neutralizing antibodies to HIV and their role in vaccine design. *Annu Rev Immunol.* 2016;34:635-659.
30. Campbell GR, Bruckman RS, Chu YL, et al. Autophagy induction by histone deacetylase inhibitors inhibits HIV type 1. *J Biol Chem.* 2015;290:5028-5040.
32. Cao Y, Krogstad P, Korber BT, et al. Maternal HIV-1 viral load and vertical transmission of infection: the Ariel Project for the prevention of HIV transmission from mother to infant. *Nat Med.* 1997;3:549-552.
45. Centers for Disease Control and Prevention. Pre-exposure prophylaxis (PrEP). http://www.cdc.gov/hiv/research/biomedicalresearch/prep/index.html.
46. Centers for Disease Control and Prevention. Preexposure prophylaxis for the prevention of HIV infection in the United States—2014: a clinical practice guideline. http://www.cdc.gov/hiv/pdf/prepguidelines2014.pdf.
47. Centers for Disease Control and prevention. Updated guidelines for antiretroviral postexposure prophylaxis after sexual, injection drug use, or other nonoccupational exposure to HIV—United States, 2016. http://www.cdc.gov/hiv/pdf/programresources/cdc-hiv-npep-guidelines.pdf.
53. Chevalier MF, Weiss L. The split personality of regulatory T cells in HIV infection. *Blood.* 2013;121:29-37.
59. Cohen MS, Chen YQ, McCauley M, et al. Antiretroviral therapy for the prevention of HIV-1 transmission. *N Engl J Med.* 2016;375:830-839.
61. Connor EM, Sperling RS, Gelber R, et al. Reduction of maternal-infant transmission of human immunodeficiency virus type 1 with zidovudine treatment. Pediatric AIDS Clinical Trials Group Protocol 076 Study Group. *N Engl J Med.* 1994;331:1173-1180.
62. Coovadia HM, Brown ER, Fowler MG, et al. Efficacy and safety of an extended nevirapine regimen in infant children of breastfeeding mothers with HIV-1 infection for prevention of postnatal HIV-1 transmission (HPTN 046): a randomised, double-blind, placebo-controlled trial. *Lancet.* 2012;379:221-228.
63. Coutsoudis A, Pillay K, Spooner E, et al. Influence of infant-feeding patterns on early mother-to-child transmission of HIV-1 in Durban, South Africa: a prospective cohort study. South African Vitamin A Study Group. *Lancet.* 1999;354:471-476.
64. Crowell CS, Huo Y, Tassiopoulos K, et al. Early viral suppression improves neurocognitive outcomes in HIV-infected children. *AIDS.* 2015;29:295-304.
67. De Lazzari E, Leon A, Arnaiz JA, et al. Hepatotoxicity of nevirapine in virologically suppressed patients according to gender and CD4 cell counts. *HIV Med.* 2008;9:221-226.

70. Dickover RE, Dillon M, Gillette SG, et al. Rapid increases in load of human immunodeficiency virus correlate with early disease progression and loss of CD4 cells in vertically infected infants. *J Infect Dis.* 1994;170:1279-1284.
71. Dickover RE, Garratty EM, Herman SA, et al. Identification of levels of maternal HIV-1 RNA associated with risk of perinatal transmission. Effect of maternal zidovudine treatment on viral load. *JAMA.* 1996;275:599-605.
75. Dorenbaum A, Cunningham CK, Gelber RD, et al. Two-dose intrapartum/newborn nevirapine and standard antiretroviral therapy to reduce perinatal HIV transmission: a randomized trial. *JAMA.* 2002;288:189-198.
77. Duliege AM, Amos CI, Felton S, et al. Birth order, delivery route, and concordance in the transmission of human immunodeficiency virus type 1 from mothers to twins. International Registry of HIV-Exposed Twins. *J Pediatr.* 1995;126:625-632.
78. Dunn DT, Brandt CD, Krivine A, et al. The sensitivity of HIV-1 DNA polymerase chain reaction in the neonatal period and the relative contributions of intra-uterine and intra-partum transmission. *AIDS.* 1995;9:F7-F11.
79. Dunn DT, Newell ML, Ades AE, et al. Risk of human immunodeficiency virus type 1 transmission through breastfeeding. *Lancet.* 1992;340:585-588.
81. El-Mallawany NK, Kamiyango W, Slone JS, et al. Clinical factors associated with long-term complete remission versus poor response to chemotherapy in HIV-infected children and adolescents with Kaposi sarcoma receiving bleomycin and vincristine: a retrospective observational study. *PLoS ONE.* 2016;11:e0153335.
91. Fowler MG, Newell ML. Breast-feeding and HIV-1 transmission in resource-limited settings. *J Acquir Immune Defic Syndr.* 2002;30:230-239.
92. Freiberg MS, Chang CC, Kuller LH, et al. HIV infection and the risk of acute myocardial infarction. *JAMA Intern Med.* 2013;173:614-622.
104. Gortmaker SL, Hughes M, Cervia J, et al. Effect of combination therapy including protease inhibitors on mortality among children and adolescents infected with HIV-1. *N Engl J Med.* 2001;345:1522-1528.
108. Granich RM, Gilks CF, Dye C, et al. Universal voluntary HIV testing with immediate antiretroviral therapy as a strategy for elimination of HIV transmission: a mathematical model. *Lancet.* 2009;373:48-57.
110. Grant RM, Lama JR, Anderson PL, et al. Preexposure chemoprophylaxis for HIV prevention in men who have sex with men. *N Engl J Med.* 2010;363:2587-2599.
115. Guay LA, Musoke P, Fleming T, et al. Intrapartum and neonatal single-dose nevirapine compared with zidovudine for prevention of mother-to-child transmission of HIV-1 in Kampala, Uganda: HIVNET 012 randomised trial. *Lancet.* 1999;354:795-802.
120. Heigele A, Joas S, Regensburger K, et al. Increased susceptibility of CD4+ T cells from elderly individuals to HIV-1 infection and apoptosis is associated with reduced CD4 and enhanced CXCR4 and FAS surface expression levels. *Retrovirology.* 2015;12:86.
122. Hitti J, Frenkel LM, Stek AM, et al. Maternal toxicity with continuous nevirapine in pregnancy: results from PACTG 1022. *J Acquir Immune Defic Syndr.* 2004;36:772-776.
127. Hutter G, Nowak D, Mossner M, et al. Long-term control of HIV by CCR5 Delta32/Delta32 stem-cell transplantation. *N Engl J Med.* 2009;360:692-698.
128. Inter-agency Task Team on the Prevention and Treatment of HIV Infection in Pregnant Women Mothers and Children (IATT), CDC, WHO, and UNICEF. Monitoring & evaluation framework for antiretroviral treatment for pregnant and breastfeeding women living with HIV and their infants, 2015. http://www.who.int/hiv/mtct/iatt-me-framework/en/.
129. Jeremy RJ, Kim S, Nozyce M, et al. Neuropsychological functioning and viral load in stable antiretroviral therapy-experienced HIV-infected children. *Pediatrics.* 2005;115:380-387.
135. Kelly P, Saloojee H, Chen JY, et al. Noncommunicable diseases in HIV infection in low- and middle-income countries: gastrointestinal, hepatic, and nutritional aspects. *J Acquir Immune Defic Syndr.* 2014;67(suppl 1):S79-S86.
147. Lahoz R, Noguera A, Rovira N, et al. Antiretroviral-related hematologic short-term toxicity in healthy infants: implications of the new neonatal 4-week zidovudine regimen. *Pediatr Infect Dis J.* 2010;29:376-379.
153. Lindsey JC, Hughes MD, Violari A, et al. Predictors of virologic and clinical response to nevirapine versus lopinavir/ritonavir-based antiretroviral therapy in young children with and without prior nevirapine exposure for the prevention of mother-to-child HIV transmission. *Pediatr Infect Dis J.* 2014;33:846-854.
156. Lipshultz SE, Williams PL, Zeldow B, et al. Cardiac effects of in-utero exposure to antiretroviral therapy in HIV-uninfected children born to HIV-infected mothers. *AIDS.* 2015;29:91-100.
158. Lo J, Abbara S, Shturman L, et al. Increased prevalence of subclinical coronary atherosclerosis detected by coronary computed tomography angiography in HIV-infected men. *AIDS.* 2010;24:243-253.
160. Luzuriaga K, Bryson Y, Krogstad P, et al. Combination treatment with zidovudine, didanosine, and nevirapine in infants with human immunodeficiency virus type 1 infection. *N Engl J Med.* 1997;336:1343-1349.
161. Luzuriaga K, Gay H, Ziemniak C, et al. Viremic relapse after HIV-1 remission in a perinatally infected child. *N Engl J Med.* 2015;372:786-788.
163. Luzuriaga K, McManus M, Mofenson L, et al. A trial of three antiretroviral regimens in HIV-1-infected children. *N Engl J Med.* 2004;350:2471-2480.
164. Luzuriaga K, Tabak B, Garber M, et al. HIV type 1 (HIV-1) proviral reservoirs decay continuously under sustained virologic control in HIV-1-infected children who received early treatment. *J Infect Dis.* 2014;210:1529-1538.
165. Lyimo MA, Mosi MN, Housman ML, et al. Breast milk from Tanzanian women has divergent effects on cell-free and cell-associated HIV-1 infection in vitro. *PLoS ONE.* 2012;7:e43815.
169. Marazzi CM, Germano P, Liotta G, et al. Implementing anti-retroviral triple therapy to prevent HIV mother-to-child transmission: a public health approach in resource-limited settings. *Eur J Pediatr.* 2007;166:1305-1307.
170. Marazzi MC, Liotta G, Nielsen-Saines K, et al. Extended antenatal antiretroviral use correlates with improved infant outcomes throughout the first year of life. *AIDS.* 2010;24:2819-2826.
171. Marazzi MC, Nielsen-Saines K, Buonomo E, et al. Increased infant human immunodeficiency virus-type one free survival at one year of age in sub-saharan Africa with maternal use of highly active antiretroviral therapy during breast-feeding. *Pediatr Infect Dis J.* 2009;28:483-487.
172. Margolis DA, Brinson CC, Smith GH, et al. Cabotegravir plus rilpivirine, once a day, after induction with cabotegravir plus nucleoside reverse transcriptase inhibitors in antiretroviral-naive adults with HIV-1 infection (LATTE): a randomised, phase 2b, dose-ranging trial. *Lancet Infect Dis.* 2015;15:1145-1155.
174. Marston M, Becquet R, Zaba B, et al. Net survival of perinatally and postnatally HIV-infected children: a pooled analysis of individual data from sub-Saharan Africa. *Int J Epidemiol.* 2011;40:385-396.
177. Mayaux MJ, Burgard M, Teglas JP, et al. Neonatal characteristics in rapidly progressive perinatally acquired HIV-1 disease. The French Pediatric HIV Infection Study Group. *JAMA.* 1996;275:606-610.
178. Mayaux MJ, Dussaix E, Isopet J, et al. Maternal virus load during pregnancy and mother-to-child transmission of human immunodeficiency virus type 1: the French perinatal cohort studies. SEROGEST Cohort Group. *J Infect Dis.* 1997;175:172-175.
183. Minkoff H, Burns DN, Landesman S, et al. The relationship of the duration of ruptured membranes to vertical transmission of human immunodeficiency virus. *Am J Obstet Gynecol.* 1995;173:585-589.
184. Mirani G, Williams PL, Chernoff M, et al. Changing trends in complications and mortality rates among US youth and young adults with HIV infection in the era of combination antiretroviral therapy. *Clin Infect Dis.* 2015;61:1850-1861.
186. Mitka M. Exploring statins to decrease HIV-related heart disease risk. *JAMA.* 2015;314:657-659.
191. Mora S, Zamproni I, Beccio S, et al. Longitudinal changes of bone mineral density and metabolism in antiretroviral-treated human immunodeficiency virus-infected children. *J Clin Endocrinol Metab.* 2004;89:24-28.
192. Morrison S, John-Stewart G, Egessa JJ, et al. Rapid antiretroviral therapy initiation for women in an HIV-1 prevention clinical trial experiencing primary HIV-1 infection during pregnancy or breastfeeding. *PLoS ONE.* 2015;10:e0140773.
200. Newell ML. The natural history of vertically acquired HIV infection. The European Collaborative Study. *J Perinat Med.* 1991;19(suppl 1):257-262.
201. Newell ML, Coovadia H, Cortina-Borja M, et al. Mortality of infected and uninfected infants born to HIV-infected mothers in Africa: a pooled analysis. *Lancet.* 2004;364:1236-1243.
202. Nielsen K, Bryson YJ. Diagnosis of HIV infection in children. *Pediatr Clin North Am.* 2000;47:39-63.
203. Nielsen K, McSherry G, Petru A, et al. A descriptive survey of pediatric human immunodeficiency virus-infected long-term survivors. *Pediatrics.* 1997;99:E4.
204. Nielsen-Saines K, Watts DH, Veloso VG, et al. Three postpartum antiretroviral regimens to prevent intrapartum HIV infection. *N Engl J Med.* 2012;366:2368-2379.
210. Palombi L, Bernava GM, Nucita A, et al. Predicting trends in HIV-1 sexual transmission in sub-Saharan Africa through the Drug Resource Enhancement Against AIDS and Malnutrition model: antiretrovirals for reduction of population infectivity, incidence and prevalence at the district level. *Clin Infect Dis.* 2012;55:268-275.
226. Read JS, Mwatha A, Richardson B, et al. Primary HIV-1 infection among infants in sub-Saharan Africa: HPTN 024. *J Acquir Immune Defic Syndr.* 2009;51:317-322.
234. Ruane PJ, DeJesus E, Berger D, et al. Antiviral activity, safety, and pharmacokinetics/pharmacodynamics of tenofovir alafenamide as 10-day monotherapy in HIV-1-positive adults. *J Acquir Immune Defic Syndr.* 2013;63:449-455.
237. Saez-Cirion A, Bacchus C, Hocqueloux L, et al. Post-treatment HIV-1 controllers with a long-term virological remission after the interruption of early initiated antiretroviral therapy ANRS VISCONTI Study. *PLoS Pathog.* 2013;9:e1003211.
243. Scott GB. HIV infection in children: clinical features and management. *J Acquir Immune Defic Syndr.* 1991;4:109-115.
244. Scott GB, Hutto C, Makuch RW, et al. Survival in children with perinatally acquired human immunodeficiency virus type 1 infection. *N Engl J Med.* 1989;321:1791-1796.
245. Scully E, Alter G. NK Cells in HIV Disease. *Curr HIV/AIDS Rep.* 2016;13:85-94.
248. Semrau K, Kuhn L, Brooks DR, et al. Dynamics of breast milk HIV-1 RNA with unilateral mastitis or abscess. *J Acquir Immune Defic Syndr.* 2013;62:348-355.

252. Shearer WT, Leister E, Siberry G, et al. Pulmonary complications of HIV-1 in youth: the PHACS AMP Study. Paper presented at the 22nd Conference on Retroviruses and Opportunistic Infections (CROI), 2015, Seattle, Washington.
265. Trezza C, Ford SL, Spreen W, et al. Formulation and pharmacology of long-acting cabotegravir. *Curr Opin HIV AIDS*. 2015;10:239-245.
266. Triant VA, Lee H, Hadigan C, et al. Increased acute myocardial infarction rates and cardiovascular risk factors among patients with human immunodeficiency virus disease. *J Clin Endocrinol Metab*. 2007;92:2506-2512.
268. Uban KA, Herting MM, Williams PL, et al. White matter microstructure among youth with perinatally acquired HIV is associated with disease severity. *AIDS*. 2015;29:1035-1044.
269. UNAIDS. AIDS by the numbers—AIDS is not over, but it can be. http://www.unaids.org/en/resources/documents/2016/AIDS-by-the-numbers.
270. UNAIDS. Fact sheet—latest statistics on the status of the AIDS epidemic. http://www.unaids.org/en/resources/fact-sheet.
271. UNAIDS. Global AIDS update, 2016. http://www.unaids.org/sites/default/files/media_asset/global-AIDS-update-2016_en.pdf.
273. UNICEF. 2014 Annual results report—HIV and AIDS, 2014. http://www.unicef.org/publicpartnerships/files/2014_Annual_Results_Report_HIV_and_AIDS.pdf.
276. Van Rompay KK, Otsyula MG, Marthas ML, et al. Immediate zidovudine treatment protects simian immunodeficiency virus-infected newborn macaques against rapid onset of AIDS. *Antimicrob Agents Chemother*. 1995;39:125-131.
279. Violari A, Cotton MF, Gibb DM, et al. Early antiretroviral therapy and mortality among HIV-infected infants. *N Engl J Med*. 2008;359:2233-2244.
288. World Health Organization. HIV/AIDS fact sheet, 2017. http://www.who.int/mediacentre/factsheets/fs360/en/.
289. World Health Organization. March 2014 supplement to the 2013 consolidated guidelines on the use of antiretroviral drugs for treating and preventing HIV infection: recommendations for a public health approach. http://apps.who.int/iris/bitstream/10665/104264/1/9789241506830_eng.pdf?ua=1.
290. World Health Organization. WHO case definitions of HIV for surveillance and revised clinical staging and immunological classification of HIV-related disease in adults and children, 2007. http://www.who.int/hiv/pub/guidelines/hivstaging/en/.

The full reference list for this chapter is available at ExpertConsult.com.

SUBSECTION XIII Prion-Related Diseases

193 Transmissible Spongiform Encephalopathies (Creutzfeldt-Jakob Disease, Gerstmann-Sträussler-Scheinker Disease, Kuru, Fatal Familial Insomnia, New Variant Creutzfeldt-Jakob Disease, Sporadic Fatal Insomnia)

Gail J. Harrison • William J. Britt

The prion-associated, neurodegenerative diseases classified as transmissible spongiform encephalopathies (TSE) are Creutzfeldt-Jakob disease (CJD), Gerstmann-Sträussler-Scheinker disease (GSS), kuru, fatal familial insomnia (FFI), and sporadic fatal insomnia (SFI).[150] They represent a subset within a group of diseases that also have been termed infectious amyloidoses or cerebral proteopathies.[80,175,224,283] The TSE diseases affect both humans and animals (Table 193.1). CJD is the TSE of most relevance to pediatrics at this moment, although kuru historically also affected children and adolescents and young adults at one time.[85] The other TSEs are known to affect only adults and the elderly (Table 193.2).

It has been shown that these neurodegenerative diseases are prion diseases, caused by disease-associated prion protein (PrPD or PrP^{Sc}), a self-propagating beta sheet–rich aberrant conformation of the normal cellular self prion protein (PrP^{C}) with neurotoxic and aggregation-prone properties that is capable of misfolding the PrP^{C} molecules and producing progressive neurodegenerative disorders. These disorders are characterized by progressive cortical dysfunction and are linked to the accumulation of insoluble, proteinaceous aggregates of PrP^{Sc} in the central nervous system (CNS).[98,106,204] (see Table 193.1). The abnormal PrP^{Sc} is the main component of the TSE agent, called the prion, and is responsible for the prion diseases.

HISTORY

TSE diseases were recognized only in domestic livestock in northern Europe until late in the 20th century. Scrapie, a disease of sheep, was described first in the mid-1700s.[40,248] Farmers soon realized early that the agent responsible for scrapie was communicable and instituted control measures that included isolation and destruction of affected animals and herds.[40] Evidence suggests that the scrapie agent can persist in contaminated soil for at least 16 years, a finding that explains the reported recurrences of this disease in flocks that had been culled decades earlier.[116] Although farmers were aware of the communicability of scrapie between herds of sheep and had documented its spread among sheep, its transmissibility was not formally demonstrated until 1936.[91] Shortly thereafter, scrapie developed in a flock of sheep that had been inoculated with a vaccine for louping that was ill prepared from CNS tissue derived from sheep that had been exposed to scrapie.[40,248] Together, these reports provided definitive evidence of the transmissible nature of scrapie. The term slow virus disease was initially coined by veterinarians to describe the natural history of this curious group of diseases in domestic animals, which includes a prolonged incubation period measured in years and a relentlessly progressive clinical deterioration once symptoms appear.[250] This term was used until the 1980s, when investigators began to consider that although the agent responsible for the spongiform changes in scrapie-infected mice was transmissible, it could not be classified as a conventional virus.

A decade earlier, the observational and laboratory studies of kuru, a progressive cerebellar ataxia and dementia occurring predominantly in adolescent and young adults of the Fore tribe in Papua New Guinea, provided an important piece of the puzzle of the etiology of this group of diseases.[3,120] The natural history of kuru was described initially by Vincent Zigas and Carleton Gajdusek, who noted that the disease was associated with the ritual cannibalism practiced by the Fore tribe.[85] In 1959, an astute veterinary neuropathologist, William Hadlow, observed a striking similarity of the spongiform changes in the brains of patients with kuru to the brains of sheep with scrapie and suggested that these two diseases could be caused by similar mechanisms, possibly a transmissible agent.[129] Gajdusek and coworkers[109–111] eventually demonstrated that the clinical and histopathologic findings of kuru can be transmitted to chimpanzees and other nonhuman primates by inoculation of brain tissue from patients with kuru. Interestingly, they initially thought that

TABLE 193.1 Naturally Occurring Transmissible Spongiform Encephalopathies in Humans and Animals

Host	Disease
Human	Kuru
	Creutzfeldt-Jakob disease
	Sporadic
	Familial
	Infectious or iatrogenic
	Variant Creutzfeldt-Jakob disease
	Gerstmann-Sträussler-Scheinker syndrome
	Fatal familial insomnia, sporadic fatal insomnia
Sheep, goats	Scrapie
Mink	Transmissible mink encephalopathy
Deer, elk	Chronic wasting disease
Cattle	Bovine spongiform encephalopathy, bovine amyloidotic spongiform encephalopathy
Cats, tigers, pumas, cheetahs	Feline spongiform encephalopathy

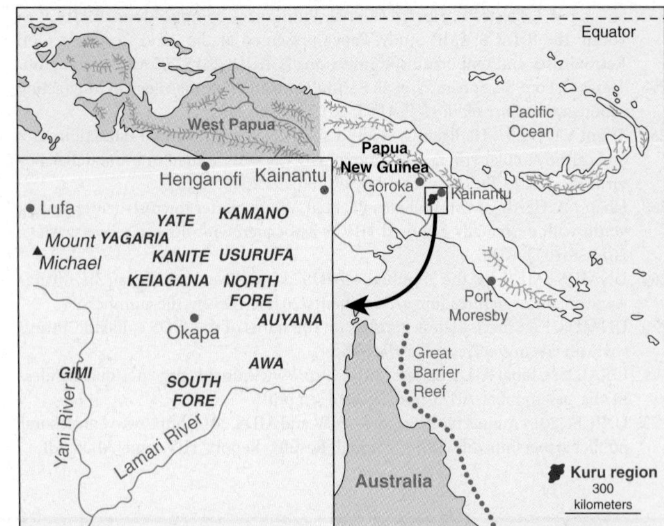

FIG. 193.1 Area and linguistic groups historically affected by kuru in the Eastern Highlands Province of Papua New Guinea. (From Whitfield JT, Pako WH, Collinge J, Alpers MP. Cultural factors that affected the spatial and temporal epidemiology of kuru. *R Soc Open Sci.* 2017;4:160789. Available at https://www.ncbi.nlm.nih.gov/core/lw/2.0/html/tileshop_pmc/tileshop_pmc_inline.html?title=Click%20on%20image%20to%20zoom&p=PMC3&id=5319347_rsos160789-g1.jpg.)

the experiment was a failure because the animals did not become symptomatic until 18 to 21 months after intracranial inoculation was performed, and later reports from this same laboratory indicated that almost 20 years elapsed between inoculation and the development of disease in some chimpanzees.[16,40,85] Subsequent studies by other investigators demonstrated that brain homogenates from patients with CJD, GSS disease, FFI, or, most recently, variant CJD (vCJD) can transmit spongiform changes to nonhuman primates.[24,30,222,260]

A variant of FFI, SFI, was identified in the 1990s and added to this group of transmissible neurodegenerative diseases.[194,215]

The hypothesis that transmissible neurodegenerative diseases are caused by a protein was suggested first by Griffith[128] in 1967 and later more extensively developed by Prusiner[222] and coworkers. The claim that the etiologic agent of scrapie is an isoform of a normal host protein, PrP^C (prion protein) that can transmit disease in the absence of nucleic acid was met initially with great skepticism and even today continues to evoke debate.[69,70,187,222] Over the next decade, the hypothesis that a protein can promote the formation of a polymeric fibrillary, insoluble plaque without the requirement of a nucleic acid–encoded a protein of an infectious agent was supported by studies from several laboratories. This hypothesis represented a paradigm shift in biology, and Stanley Prusiner was awarded the Nobel Prize in 1997 for his groundbreaking studies of prion diseases. Approximately 20 years earlier, Gajdusek had also been awarded a Nobel Prize for his description of the transmissible nature of kuru and similar diseases of the CNS.

An important chapter in the TSE saga was the appearance of "mad cow disease" (bovine spongiform encephalopathy [BSE]) in Great Britain in the mid-1980s; by the late 1990s, almost 200,000 diseased animals had been destroyed.[53] Mad cow disease was discovered in cattle in several European countries and later in the United States. Of greatest concern has been the transmission of BSE to more than 100 individuals in Great Britain and the report of at least 3 cases in France.[53] A significant increase in the incidence of TSE among elk and deer (i.e., chronic wasting disease) has been reported in wild deer herds in the midwestern United States and in wild game farms in the western states.[195,284] Because of the concern that large numbers of human cases could eventually result from contamination of food products and pharmaceutical reagents with BSE or contact with contaminated tissue from deer or elk, there has been substantial interest in the diagnosis, treatment, and prevention of TSE and in surveillance for BSE in livestock.

EPIDEMIOLOGY AND NATURAL HISTORY

The epidemiology and natural history of human TSE spans a variety of geographical, cultural, and medical exposures (see Table 193.2). Clues from molecular epidemiology and genetic mutations provide insight into disease origins, transmission, and expression.

Kuru

Although farmers and neuropathologists were well aware that scrapie is readily transmissible, the possibility that human TSEs also are transmissible was not demonstrated until Gajdusek and coworkers defined the natural history of kuru in the Fore tribe in Papua New Guinea[3,289] (Fig. 193.1). Kuru was originally named after the shivering noted early in the disease when the patients were cold. It was seen most commonly in children, adolescents, and young adults of both sexes, as well as older women, but rarely if ever in older men (Fig. 193.2). The disease was common in the specific area, with an incidence of 1% in the Fore tribe, and was a significant cause of death in this population.[3] Gajdusek carried out a detailed observational study of the Fore people, including their ritualistic endocannibalism or transumption of the bodies of the dead.[108,289] This ritual included eating of body parts and homogenization of the brains of dead relatives in bamboo cylinders with use of crude hand tools. The brain was reportedly ingested as well as smeared over the body by relatives and other members of the tribe.[288] During most of their childhood, the Fore children remained with their mothers and other women of the village, including the time spent preparing the brains of dead relatives for ritual endocannibalism or transumption. It is during this time that exposure to the agent responsible for kuru was thought to occur, either by ingestion of the contaminated brain material or through skin abrasions that were present secondary to the nearly universal scabies infestation. Those affected had cerebellar ataxia, tremors, and choreiform and athetoid movements. Kuru affected all ages of individuals, including children. Gajdusek observed three stages of kuru: the early ambulatory stage, in which the patient remained able to walk upright; the second sedentary stage, in which the patient was able only to sit; and the terminal immobile stage, in which the patient was unable to sit up independently.

Gajdusek and coworkers hypothesized that kuru is caused by an infectious agent and injected homogenates prepared from the brain of a deceased kuru patient into nonhuman primates; after an incubation period of more than 2 years, a disease similar to kuru was observed in the primates.[16] After the transmissibility of kuru was demonstrated in experimental animals, several other TSEs were shown to be transmissible in nonhuman primates and other animals.[16,48,83,264,266] Subsequent studies demonstrated that kuru could be transmitted to nonhuman primates by oral ingestion of contaminated tissue.[118] Although the origin of the TSE agent responsible for kuru in the Fore tribe is unknown, the most plausible explanation is that a spontaneous mutation in *PRNP*, the gene encoding the normal cellular PrP^C, resulted in a case of CJD with the abnormal isoform PrP^{Sc} in the Fore tribe that then was introduced and propagated in the population by ritual endocannibalism/transumption of their dead relatives.[282] After ritual endocannibalism/transumption was halted by the government of these districts in Papua New Guinea, new cases of the disease disappeared; the last case of kuru in an individual younger than 30 years of age was reported in 1985.[3] Cases of kuru have developed some 40 to 50 years after exposure to infectious material, illustrating the prolonged incubation period of these diseases.[84,85,164] The last recorded case of kuru was reported in 2009, and no one in the area born after 1959 has developed kuru.[85,87] The surveillance of kuru ceased in 2012, after 55 years of fieldwork started by Gajdusek and colleagues in 1957.

TABLE 193.2 Human Transmissible Spongiform Encephalopathies: Clinical and Diagnostic Criteria

Disease	Acquisition	Clinical Features
Kuru	Ingestion of or percutaneous inoculation with contaminated central nervous system tissue during ritual endocannibalism/transumption in the Fore tribe in Papua New Guinea First case reported in 1957 Last case reported in 2004 (last case identified was born before 1960 in Papua New Guinea)	Bimodal age distribution with disease in adolescents and in older adults Adolescents presented with ataxia and dementia with prominent cerebellar involvement Rapidly progressive disease
Creutzfeldt-Jakob disease (CJD)	85% are sporadic reported cases of CJD; first reported in 1921 5–10% are familial cases caused by a defined mutation in PrP^C protein; first reported in 1924 <5% are secondary to infection or iatrogenic sources from neurosurgical procedures, injection of cadaveric growth hormone or blood product, or clotting factor transfusions; first reported in 1974 **Sporadic CJD** **Definite** Brain biopsy or postmortem examination shows plaques on histopathology and/or immunohistochemistry, and/or Western blot confirmed protease-resistant PrP, and/or presence of scrapie-associated fibrils, and/or RT-QuIC prion PrP^{Sc} specific positive detection in cerebrospinal fluid (CSF), brain, or nasal olfactory mucosa **Probable** Progressive dementia, myoclonus, visual signs, cerebellar signs, pyramidal/extrapyramidal signs, akinetic mutism *plus* Electroencephalogram with periodic sharp wave complexes CSF positive for 14-3-3 protein assay Magnetic resonance imaging (MRI) high signal abnormalities in the caudate nucleus and/or putamen areas *plus* No alternative diagnosis found on routine evaluation **Possible** Progressive dementia with myoclonus, visual or cerebellar signs, pyramidal/extrapyramidal signs, akinetic mutism *plus* No alternative diagnosis found on routine evaluation **Infectious/Iatrogenic CJD** Progressive neurological/cerebellar syndrome *or* Criteria for definite or probable CJD met *plus* Recipient human cadaveric-derived pituitary hormone *or* Antecedent neurosurgery with a dura mater implantation **Familial CJD** Definite or probable criteria for CJD met Neuropsychiatric disorder *plus* Disease-specific PrP gene mutation *plus* First-degree relative with definite or probable CJD	Classic presentation of dementia and sensory abnormalities followed by loss of motor functions Rapid progression of symptoms with death usually occurring <6 mo to <1 y after onset Disease of late middle age except in cases acquired after iatrogenic transmission from neurosurgical procedures (strong) or possibly blood product transfusions (weak)
Variant Creutzfeldt-Jakob disease (vCJD)	First reported in 1996 Acquired through exposure to beef or beef byproducts contaminated with bovine spongiform encephalopathy (BSE); route of acquisition presumed to be oral (ingestion)	Presentation similar to CJD but disease progresses more slowly, with death occurring >12 mo after symptoms develop

Continued

TABLE 193.2 **Human Transmissible Spongiform Encephalopathies: Clinical and Diagnostic Criteria—cont'd**

Disease	Acquisition	Clinical Features
	vCJD Prominent neuropsychiatric symptoms, painful dysthesiasis *plus* EEG periodic sharp waves *plus* MRI pulvinar sign in brain *plus* Florid plaques on brain biopsy neuropathology *plus* Detection of agent in lymphoid tissue *plus* Accumulation of protease resistance prion protein in brain *plus* Positive RT-QuIC* for PrP^{Sc} in CSF or nasal olfactory brushings	Mean age of cases approximately 28 y, with documented cases in adolescents
Gerstmann-Sträussler-Scheinker syndrome (GSS)	First reported in 1936 Autosomal dominant inheritance with documented point mutations in PrP^{C} gene	Disease of middle age, with mean age at onset of 45 y; motor abnormalities and progressive dementia
Familial fatal insomnia (FFI)	First reported in 1986 Autosomal dominant inheritance with point mutations in PrP^{C} gene (missense mutation codon 178)	Disease of middle age; presentation includes insomnia, dysautonomia, and motor dysfunction
Sporadic fatal insomnia	First reported in 1999 No genetic mutations identified, but homozygosity at methionine 129 is characteristic	Presentation similar to FFI and neuropathologic changes similar

*RT-QuIC real-time quaking-induced conversion PrP^{Sc} prion–specific detection test.

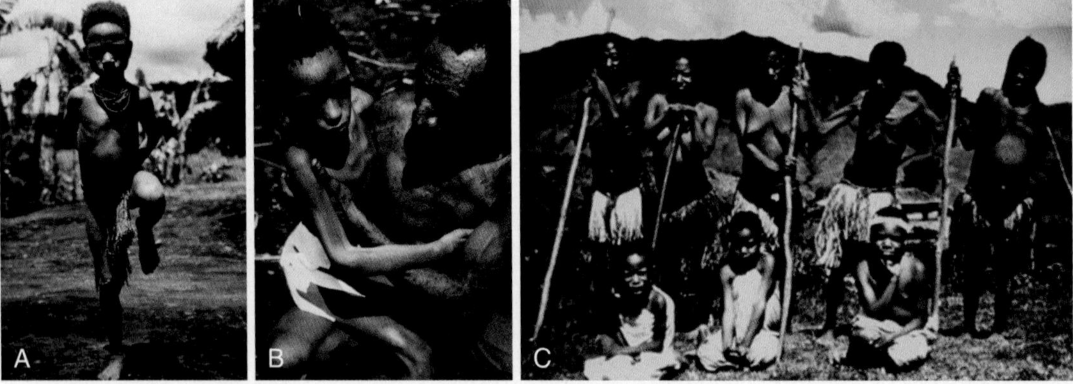

FIG. 193.2 (A) Little girl in Papua New Guinea in 1957 has the early signs of kuru in the ambulatory stage. (B) The same girl 2 years later has advanced kuru in the sedentary stage. She is unable to sit or walk and is held in the arms of a family member. (C) In this photograph, taken in Papua New Guinea in 1957, five women standing in back have advanced kuru and require long walking sticks to support them while standing and to help them walk. The three young girls sitting in front also have kuru. Young children, adolescents, and older women were affected by the kuru epidemic more than other demographic groups. (From Gajdursek DC. Early images of kuru and the people of Okapa. *Philos Trans R Soc Lond B Biol Sci.* 2008;363:3636–43.)

Creutzfeldt-Jakob Disease

Four different modes of acquisition of CJD have been described: (1) sporadic (sCJD), which occurs worldwide at a rate of 1 to 2 cases per million population per year and equally in men and women; (2) classic (cCJD), which results from inherited or familial mutations in the *PRNP* gene (>30 mutations found so far); (3) iatrogenic (iCJD), acquired or infectious, which occurs after exogenous exposure to prion-contaminated material (e.g., after neurologic procedures, injection of growth hormone, transfusion of blood products); and (4) variant (vCJD), which is acquired through oral ingestion of meat contaminated with BSE. Variant CJD is distinctly different from the other forms of CJD in presentation and diagnosis[92,93,303] (see Table 193.1).

Little is known about genetic or environmental factors that contribute to the development of sporadic forms of these diseases, although numerous epidemiologic studies have claimed associations ranging from ingestion of mutton to exposure to blood products after surgery or treatment for clotting disorders such as hemophilia.[4,44,89,92,93,193] The risk of cCJD after blood product transfusion is theoretical, but the risk of iCJD is estimated to be 14% in recipients of blood transfusions from individuals who died of iCJD. Two reports of sCJD have been published recently.[92,93,303] Common migratory scavenger birds, such as crows, may also play a role in the geographic spread of TSE diseases.[277]

Studies of CJD cases have revealed numerous genetic mutations in the *PRNP* gene associated with the development of disease, and they have been defined as genetic causes of CJD and other TSEs.[156]

Polymorphism in the methionine at position 129 in the coding sequence of PrP^C is the genetic variation most commonly recognized as being associated with sCJD.[213] Homozygosity at methionine 129 of PrP^C is seen in 64% to 81% of patients with sCJD but in only approximately 39% of the general population; it is thought to predispose an individual to both iCJD and sCJD.[2,213,295] Valine homozygosity at this position was associated more frequently with cases of CJD in which onset occurred before 40 years of age.[2] A retrospective analysis of a small number of patients with kuru revealed that all were homozygous for methionine at position 129 and all had more rapidly progressive disease with a shorter incubation period than did other patients with kuru from the same cohort.[173] In Papua New Guinea, Fore women who had survived exposure to contaminated material during the ritual cannibalistic feasts were shown to be more likely to be heterozygous at methionine 129 (76%) than similarly aged Fore women who had not been exposed to the cannibalistic feasts.[198] This result suggested that heterozygosity at methionine 129 provided a survival advantage.

Population geneticists have argued that haplotype diversity at codon 129 of *PRNP* (the gene that encodes the cellular prion protein) may have developed in response to an epidemic of prion disease. If so, this response would represent a recent balancing selection in humans.[199,200] The codon at position 129 also appears to modulate the clinical course of inherited TSEs such as FFI, and patients homozygous for methionine at position 129 have a more rapid clinical course than do patients who are heterozygous at this codon.[206] Polymorphisms in the PrP^C, including those that occur at position 129, have not been associated with the development of vCJD after exposure to BSE-contaminated material; in fact, all human cases in Great Britain have been homozygous for methionine at position 129.[151] Heterozygosity at methionine 129 is thought to confer resistance by inhibiting PrP^C protein-protein interactions.[213] Sequence analysis of the *PRNP* gene from populations throughout the world suggested that the observed increased frequency of heterozygosity at position 129 could be explained by widespread cannibalism among primitive humans and selection of methionine 129 heterozygotes secondary to increased disease penetrance associated with exposure of susceptible methionine 129 homozygotes to prion-contaminated tissue.[198] This conclusion has been challenged by other investigators.[252]

Sporadic CJD is the most common TSE in humans and accounts for approximately 85% of all cases of CJD (see Table 193.1).[44,156] It occurs worldwide at a rate of approximately 1 per million population.[44] CJD is a disease of late middle age, with a mean age at onset of 55 to 65 years. Cases of CJD range from 20 to 84 years, with the youngest patients being 16 to 18 years old.[43,102,205] Little evidence exists for case-to-case transmission of CJD, with the obvious exception of iatrogenic transmission of CJD.[67] Vertical transmission of CJD in humans has not been reported. Two cases of sCJD, in contrast to vCJD, in patients with clotting disorders who received blood product transfusions have been reported.[92,93,275] Anecdotal reports of occurrence of CJD in the spouses of individuals with CJD raise the possibility of horizontal transmission.[46] Alternatively, disease in spouses could result from shared environmental exposures. Sporadic cases of non-CJD TSE previously thought to be caused solely by genetic mutations have been reported, thus extending the spectrum of TSE in humans.[176,194] With the exception of cases that can be linked to an inherited genetic mutation, no epidemics of CJD have been reported. This an observation led British epidemiologists to suspect that a link exists between what was initially thought to be an increased frequency of CJD in young adults and the outbreak of BSE in the British Isles.[6,15,90,123,276,293]

Genetic mutations in *PRNP* can result in a variety of inherited TSEs and are likely to account for the reported outbreaks of TSE in isolated populations. Because of the relatively late onset of disease even in patients with well-characterized mutations in *PRNP*, the possibility that TSEs are inherited diseases of the CNS was not considered until more recent studies of the host cell origin of prions and the discovery that a cellular gene encoded the pathogenic protein associated with TSE. Estimates from various studies suggest that between 5% and 15% of cases of CJD may arise from mutations in *PRNP*.[43] Genetic linkage studies have demonstrated that TSEs are inherited in an autosomal dominant fashion, an observation consistent with several studies in families with FFI and GSS.[23,146,179,201] In addition, defined mutations in *PRNP* have been shown to account for the increased rate of TSE in geographically or ethnically isolated populations, such as Libyan-born Jews, an ethnic group with an incidence of TSE almost 40 times greater than that observed in other populations.[67,95,122,147,148,151,254] More than 20 mutations in *PRNP* have been described; they appear to be scattered throughout the gene. Reported mutations include both point mutations in the coding sequence changes, which result in amino acid substitutions, and octapeptide insertions.[61,67,120,148,219,227] Because mutations in *PRNP* by definition are not present in sCJD, mutations of this cellular gene are not thought to play a direct role in the development of sCJD. The mode of acquisition of the TSE agent in these individuals has not been defined. In sporadic cases of CJD, the proposal has been made that spontaneous generation of the TSE agent could be occurring extremely infrequently and resulting in CJD. However, since scrapie was eliminated in sheep in New Zealand and Australia by culling diseased herds, spontaneous development of scrapie has not been described in those herds, suggesting that spontaneous development of the agent of TSE leading to scrapie in sheep is almost nonexistent.[70] In most cases, disease secondary to a genetic mutation in *PRNP* develops in patients of middle age, suggesting that although these diseases exhibit an autosomal dominance inheritance, the genetic background of the host contributes significantly to the observed phenotypes.

Before the 1980s, cases of TSE occurring in children and adolescents, with the exception of kuru, were either extremely rare or not recognized. In the late 1980s, cases of TSE resembling CJD were reported in young adults who as young children had received injections of human growth hormone prepared from cadaveric pituitary glands.[39,48,50] The thought was that the practice of pooling pituitary glands from a large number of cadavers increased the risk of contamination of the preparation with prions from subclinical cases of TSE. More than 100 cases of TSE occurring after injection of contaminated growth hormone preparations have been reported.[66] Whether new cases of TSE will develop in adults who were given cadaveric growth hormone before the mid-1980s remains uncertain, but with a mean incubation period of 12 years in documented cases, it is unlikely that significant numbers of new cases will be reported.[41,50] Other sources of TSE have included dura grafts, corneal transplants, contaminated stereotaxic neurosurgical equipment, and, more recently, blood transfusions.[7,27,41,45,96,127,130,143,209,211,219,211] An alarming case of TSE occurred in a chimpanzee after the use of a stereotaxic electrode that 2 years previously had been used in a procedure involving a patient with CJD. Because this electrode had been decontaminated numerous times with conventional sterilization methods before its use in this experimental animal, this case illustrated the potential for the occurrence of iatrogenic transmission of TSE to humans undergoing neurosurgical procedures.[119] Two confirmed and two probable cases of CJD occurring after receipt of blood transfusions have been described in Great Britain.[130] Studies of experimental models of TSE, primarily scrapie in mice, have shown that the scrapie agent initially amplifies in titer in spleen and regional lymph nodes and enters the CNS by a bloodborne route or by infection of the peripheral nervous system.[1,158,160,163,172,188] In addition, studies in mice have demonstrated that brain tissue from animals injected with hamster scrapie can harbor the infectious agent for a prolonged time without evidence of disease.[138,230] Even during a period of inactive persistence and replication, the scrapie prion could be detected, suggesting that transmission of prion disease by contaminated blood products or surgical instruments may occur even if screening assays for the detection of prions are mandated.[216] To further cloud the issue, other investigators have postulated that less virulent strains of prions can attenuate the virulence of other strains of prions, which then can be transmitted readily during asymptomatic periods.[190,279] After transmission to a secondary host has occurred, the phenotype of the more virulent strain could be expressed. These findings are particularly worrisome because of the possibility that food products from cattle with subclinical BSE could continue to be consumed. Similarly, the possibility exists that the low incidence of vCJD in Great Britain, in spite of what most authorities consider was a much larger exposure to BSE before eradication of BSE-containing herds, can be explained by persistence of infectious agents in genetically resistant individuals or persistence in non-CNS organ systems.[33,138]

Such studies raised the possibility that TSE could be acquired by transfusion of blood and blood products obtained from infected hosts,[174] although considerable controversy existed about the importance of this transmission route.[92,93,135,303] Investigators argued that the risk was exceedingly small on the basis of experimental studies in rodents and epidemiologic studies involving patients receiving quantities of blood products, such as hemophiliacs. However, at least four patients are believed to have contracted CJD from blood transfusions and at least one from human plasma–derived clotting factor.[1,34,37,99,135,271,273,294] BSE has been transmitted to sheep by blood transfusions, and buffy coat preparations have been shown to transmit TSE to experimental primates.[29,145] The US Food and Drug Administration has recommended a very conservative policy for blood and blood products because of these theoretical concerns; more recently, this policy has been reinforced after reports of blood transfusion–acquired CJD.[134,177,299] In addition to the exclusion of donors with symptoms consistent with TSE, individuals who lived in or visited Great Britain or other countries with BSE for a cumulative period of 3 months during the interval 1980 to 1996 are also excluded as donors (http://www.redcross.org/services/biomed/0,1082,0_557_,00.html).

With the possible exception of kuru, little evidence was available previously to suggest that TSEs such as CJD could be acquired by ingestion of contaminated tissue.[44] This claim was challenged in the early 1990s by the reports of several young adults with CJD in Great Britain.[90,293] The rate of CJD in England was found to be approximately 15-fold higher than in surveillance studies from previous decades.[39] In the years preceding this startling increase in the rate of CJD, the cattle industry in Great Britain was devastated by a spreading epidemic of BSE, a disease ultimately shown to be a TSE.[132,251,291] A similar disease had been noted in domestic cats and in animals housed in zoos that had been fed British beef and beef byproducts.[30,84,251] The first case of human disease thought to be associated with BSE, termed vCJD, was described in 1995, about 10 years after the first cases of BSE were reported in cows. However, more careful analysis suggested that the first cases of BSE probably occurred in the 1970s.[251,293] During the ensuing years, investigators have closed the circle of evidence, showing that vCJD represents the transmission of BSE to humans, presumably by ingestion of contaminated beef or byproducts from BSE-infected cattle.[78,140,250,253] These byproducts include many common household and medical products, such as gelatin in food products and in pharmaceutical capsules, bouillon cubes used for food preparation, and a wide variety of foodstuffs containing beef.

Although the origin of BSE is far from settled, most investigators concur that changes in the rendering of beef and sheep carcasses to remove fat as part of the preparation of meat and bone meal protein supplements in animal feeds led to the epidemic. Before the late 1970s, beef carcasses were heated and extracted with hydrocarbons such as chloroform to delipidate the homogenate.[35,94,265,291,293] Omission of the hydrocarbon-extraction step apparently decreased inactivation of bovine prions, allowing introduction of this agent into the food products of British cattle. The epidemic began slowly in cattle, with the first case documented in 1986; by the mid-1990s, more than 3500 new cases of BSE were being reported each year. As a result of the BSE epidemic, 200,000 diseased cattle died from BSE and almost 4.5 million cattle were slaughtered preemptively, at a cost of approximately £4 billion, to curtail the epidemic.[5,53,251,298] BSE also has been documented in US herds, resulting in a ban on exportation of beef to several economically important markets.[234]

As noted earlier, transmission to humans was suggested first in 1995 after three cases of CJD in young adults were reported; by 1996, additional cases of CJD in young adults were thought to have be secondary to transmission from exposure to beef from BSE-infected cows.[78] Of the initial 20 human cases, only one individual was older than 40 years of age, and the mean age was 28 years.[6,223,276,279,301] Additional evidence from in vitro studies of the protein agents responsible for BSE and vCJD and from animal inoculation indicated that vCJD represented a human infection with the agent responsible for BSE.[56,83,139,170] Because the BSE epidemic was recognized first in 1985, researchers argued that the incubation period was approximately 10 years. On the basis of studies in kuru and experimental animal models of TSE, this estimate was determined to be dependent on exposure, genetic susceptibility, and other, as yet unrecognized risk factors.[66,178] For this and other reasons, mathematical projections of the extent of the human epidemic have been based on theoretical estimates of exposure rates, possible dose-dependent incubation periods, and undefined host genes that might alter susceptibility to TSE. Even though most of these variables cannot be quantified, arguments have been put forth that the epidemic in humans has peaked and that the approximately 120 cases of vCJD resulting from consumption of contaminated beef represents the extent of human disease associated with BSE.[117,279] In contrast, other models of the current data suggest that as many as 100,000 people may be affected. Perhaps the most compelling argument against such a large number of human cases has been the slowly evolving epidemic of vCJD in humans, with the number of new cases declining; however, several investigators have contested this hypothesis.[76,117,279,292]

Gerstmann-Sträussler-Scheinker Disease

GSS disease is a rare, sporadic, autosomal dominant, neurodegenerative disease caused by mutations within the *PRNP* gene (most commonly a codon 129 PrP102L mutation).[236] It is worldwide in distribution, with an incidence of one per 100 million (see Table 193.2). It was the first TSE for which a mutation in a gene encoding for the PrP was discovered. Originally reported by Gerstmann, Sträussler, and Scheinker in 1936, it was probably recognized earlier by Viennese psychiatrists. There can be marked phenotypic variability in presentation, even among families, but GSS often manifests with hereditary ataxia or dementia in older adults. Also, patients may exhibit ocular dysmetria, gait abnormalities, dysarthria, myoclonus, spastic paraparesis, parkinsonian signs, and hyporeflexia or areflexia in the legs.

Fatal Familial Insomnia

FFI is a rare autosomal dominant disease caused by a mutation in *PRNP* (most commonly in codon 178 at position 129M) (see Table 193.2). It occurs worldwide and causes insomnia, movement disorders, ataxia, dysarthria, dysphagia, autonomic hyperactivity, and dementia in older adults. It was originally called thalamic dementia until the term FFI was adopted in 1986. At least 100 affected families in Europe, the United States, Australia, Japan, China, and Morocco have been reported.[179]

Sporadic Fatal Insomnia

SFI, a rare disease originally reported in 1999, exhibits phenotypes similar to those of FFI but without the family history or the FFI genetic mutation (see Table 193.2). Fewer than two dozen cases have been studied in several countries around the world. All cases have shown 129 MM homozygosity and propagating PrP^{Sc}.

ETIOLOGIC AGENT AND PATHOGENESIS

The TSEs are now known to be caused by prion proteins associated with identified specific genetic mutations of the prion protein gene *PRNP*. Each of the TSE diseases is associated with a specific genetic mutation, with variants. Human PrP has a common polymorphism residue 129 (encoding methionine or valine), and homozygosity confers genetic susceptibility to CJD. Heterozygosity at codon129 confers survival advantage.

The protein aggregates characteristic of prion-associated TSE are composed of polymeric fibrils of a host-encoded protein that are deposited in several different regions of the CNS and within other organ systems, particularly in lymphoid organs. Amyloid may be present in TSEs, and its role in the pathogenesis of these diseases is uncertain. However, the symptoms associated with the spongiform encephalopathies arise from cellular and end-organ dysfunction associated with the abnormal deposition of an isoform of the normal cellular protein, PrP^C.[14,40,79,224] The physiologic function of PrP^C remains incompletely defined, and no null alleles of the *PRNP* gene have been identified, raising the possibility that some of the symptoms associated with these diseases are caused by a loss of normal PrP^C function.[198] Although the biologic determinants of the phenotypic expression and variation of CJD are not clear, prions may exist as multiple prion strains or genotypes that influence disease expression, and prion propagation may also be associated with production of toxic species that cause disease.[81,113,154] Six subgroups (MM1, MM2, MV1, MV2, W1, and VV), based on prion protein codon 129 genotype and biochemical characteristics of PrP, have been proposed to correlate with transmissibility and with the clinical and pathologic features of CJD.[22,121,240] The TSEs share several clinical features with other cerebral amyloidoses, and the insoluble protein aggregates exhibit biophysical properties similar to those of plaques found in Alzheimer disease, currently the most common cerebral proteopathy.[106] However, the TSEs can by definition be transmitted by parenteral inoculation or by other less efficient routes, such as ingestion of contaminated tissue from the nervous system. Therefore, prion diseases are believed to be unique infectious diseases.

The initial claim that TSE resulted from a transmissible protein was met with considerable skepticism, both because a paradigm of biology was challenged and because key elements of the supporting scientific data were incomplete. Most experimental studies have been performed with the agent responsible for scrapie in sheep, which was adapted for growth in mice and other small animals. Early studies arguing that the scrapie agent did not contain nucleic acid were based on studies in which the agent was inactivated with ultraviolet radiation. These studies did not exclude the possibility that the scrapie agent contained nucleic acid but instead suggested that if it did contain nucleic acid, the coding sequence was so limited that it could not encode any replicative functions.[18,19,222] Later calculations based on inactivation by gamma rays suggested that the scrapie agent could contain between 2- and 4-kilobase pairs of DNA.[237] Other experiments demonstrated that the infectivity of the scrapie agent could be eliminated or significantly reduced by treatment with agents that denatured proteins, such as guanidine hydrochloride, sodium hypochlorite (bleach), and proteases.[222]

Together, these data led several groups of investigators to postulate that the agent is an infectious protein.[26,128,225] Prusiner[222] isolated an infectious fraction from a scrapie-infected hamster brain homogenate and obtained a partial amino acid sequence. This fundamental finding led to identification of the prion protein (PrP^C) and eventually to the finding that a cellular gene on chromosome 20, *PRNP*, encoded the transmissible agent that was responsible for the development of scrapie in mice and hamsters.[15,72] Not all investigators have been convinced that the scrapie agent is an infectious protein, and some data have suggested that it is a small virus.[187,189] Once the protein encoded by the *PRNP* gene had been identified and definitively linked to scrapie and other TSEs, many investigators thought that the pathogenesis of these diseases would be elucidated quickly. However, the pathogenesis remains uncertain, perhaps because of the inability to assign a function to the normal protein product, PrP^C. The conformation of the normal cellular form of PrP^C is primarily α-helical and is susceptible to protease digestion. Various functions have been proposed for the normal, nonpathogenic isoform of the cellular PrP^C, yet transgenic mice lacking the *PRNP* gene have a normal lifespan and exhibit only minor variations in normal sleep patterns.[58,59,88,226] These mice are completely resistant to prion disease regardless of the source of exposure, a finding that is consistent with the hypothesis that PrP^C is necessary for the disease process associated with scrapie and other TSEs.[1,58]

In contrast to the normal cellular form of PrP^C, which is composed of four α-helical domains, the pathogenic form of PrP^{Sc} (scrapie prion protein) exists in an extended beta sheet, is insoluble, and is partially resistant to protease digestion, as indicated by the designation PrP^{res} (PrP protease resistant). The partial resistance of PrP^{res} to proteinase K digestion is a characteristic that allows pathogenic prions to be detected in tissue specimens and has been widely used to identify products of the conversion reaction of PrP^C to PrP^{res}.[197,242] The conversion of PrP^C to PrP^{res} represents a central paradigm of the prion hypothesis. It is thought to occur as the result of a process similar to crystal formation by nucleation (i.e., seeding the normal cellular pool of PrP^C with PrP^{res}) or, alternatively, by a template-directed misfolding of a normal cellular protein. Thus, PrP^{res} can be viewed as a transmissible, infectious agent that catalyzes the conversion of the normal cellular protein to a form associated with protein deposition in the CNS, cell death, and, eventually, clinical disease in the host.

The normal cellular protein, PrP^C, is a small membrane glycoprotein that is covalently linked to cellular membranes, including the plasma membrane, by a glycosyl phosphoinositol (GPI) linkage.[255–257] This cell surface form can be released by treating cellular membranes with phospholipases.[255] A secreted form of the protein also is expressed. Genetic mutations in *PRNP* appear to predispose the protein to assume other topologies, including a transmembrane form.[131,270] Membrane-associated forms are postulated to play an important role in the neurodegeneration associated with accumulation of the misfolded forms of PrP^C, and secreted forms can accelerate disease in a genetically susceptible animal.[131,228] Chesebro and coworkers[71,73,259] demonstrated that transgenic mice encoding a GPI-anchorless form of PrP^C generated an abnormal protease-resistant PrP^{res} that could be transmitted to other animals and induce formation of amyloid plaques but failed to cause clinical spongiform encephalopathy (scrapie equivalent in mice) in experimental animals. When the anchorless form was coexpressed with the wild-type form of PrP^C, accelerated disease was seen. Therefore, it appears that a cell surface–linked PrP^C is required for induction of disease, yet amyloid-like deposits can be formed from the secreted form of PrP^C, and disease can be induced when both secreted and wild-type PrP^C are expressed.[73] Consistent with this observation was the description of a transmissible PrP^C amyloid disease without spongiform encephalopathy after inoculation of tissue containing amyloid deposits from a patient with GSS without CNS spongiform degeneration.[221,228] Together, these studies argue that PrP^C misfolding, protease resistance, and amyloid formation are sufficient to confer transmissibility to the PrP^{res} but may not, by themselves, be directly responsible for transmissible disease.

The challenge to existing paradigms of molecular biology and genetics, including self-replication of a protein, were quickly noted by investigators in this field. Several investigators had previously demonstrated that distinctive strains of the scrapie agent exist and that these strains induce definable and reproducible phenotypes of disease in experimental animals.[20,32,54,55,159] These well-accepted and reproducible studies strongly argued for the presence of a genetic program in the scrapie agent that was most consistent with a nucleic acid–containing agent. More recently, several studies have suggested that the phenotypic behavior of scrapie strains may be entirely dependent on the pathogenic conformation assumed by the PrP^C when it is exposed to pathogenic forms of PrP^C, which in turn is dependent on its posttranslational modifications.[21,64,65,262,279,280,285] Researchers argued that the phenotypes of scrapie strains are entirely dependent on the protein structure of PrP^C and are independent of any nucleic acid–encoded genetic trait. A second characteristic of etiologic agents of TSE that was difficult to ascribe to an infectious protein was the species barrier for transmission of prions. This characteristic was noted when the scrapie agent from sheep was first adapted to mice and then to other species, including hamsters. Other examples of a species barrier include BSE: 1000 lethal doses (as defined in cattle) must be given to a mouse to induce disease.[286] The species barrier not only contributes to the absolute resistance of species to infection with prions derived from other species but also can lengthen the mean incubation period in a population. The species barrier often is invoked to explain the rarity of TSE, even in populations repeatedly exposed to TSE in other species (e.g., humans exposed to scrapie-infected sheep), and it may explain the relatively low number of human cases of vCJD that develop after exposure to beef contaminated with BSE.[78] A more worrisome aspect of the phenomenon of species barrier is that subclinical infections could result from exposure to BSE and subsequent transmission, leading to secondary cases with clinical symptoms.[138,279] A proposed unifying explanation for the restricted transmission of prion disease between species argues that species restriction is related to the efficiency with which exogenous prions interact with endogenous host-derived PrP^C to form PrP^{res}.[1,64,65,78,144,166,231,262,278]

Although considerable gaps in understanding of the infectious agent responsible for TSE persist and at times have contributed to the controversy that surrounds the infectious protein hypothesis, in vitro studies have shifted the view of the field toward the infectious protein hypothesis. For example, protease-resistant prions (PrP^{res}) that appear identical biochemically to PrP^{res} derived from infected brain can be produced in cell-free systems in vitro.[1,64,165] However, these preparations at first could not transmit disease to uninfected animals unless they were supplemented with brain tissue derived from diseased animals, presumably because their titer was too low.[136] A more recent study using a system to amplify prion production through sequential folding, sonication, and feeding of new substrate produced titers of in vitro–derived prions that could transmit TSE to susceptible animals and accelerate the development of symptoms in infected animals.[63] These results have provided compelling evidence for a mechanism of recruitment of cellular proteins by a misfolded protein and subsequent protein deposition as an etiology of diseases classified as TSE.

Although several mechanisms can be envisioned to explain how a misfolded host protein could lead to the recruitment and misfolding of additional copies of the protein, the process by which deposition of PrP^{res} might lead to disease remains unclear. Based on solid-state nuclear magnetic resonance and x-ray crystallography, the underlying structures of prion amyloids appear to share common structural features, and single molecular methods will continue to advance understanding of misfolding and aggregation.[169] There are several well-studied examples (e.g., cystic fibrosis) in which loss of normal protein function leads to the development of disease in humans.[126,296] These diseases are associated with loss of function of an essential cellular protein. The accumulation of cellular proteins (e.g., amyloid accumulation secondary to overproduction of a normal protein) also can lead to disease and usually is associated with deposition and loss of organ function. In the case of TSE, the proposed mechanism for the generation of pathogenic prions appears to be fundamentally different: the conformational change from a predominance of α-helical PrP^C to PrP^{res} molecules containing extensive amounts of an extended beta sheet results in the accumulation of insoluble, protease-resistant proteins that can recruit additional normal cellular proteins into this conformation. In vitro cell-free systems and studies from kindreds with inherited TSEs such as GSS and FFI have shown that exposure to the misfolded prion protein (e.g., PrP^{res}) can result in this conversion.[1,64,65,68,107,235] In genetic TSEs such as GSS and FFI, the genetic mutation is inherited as an autosomal dominant trait, and the PrP^{res} pathogenic form of the prion protein was shown to be derived from the mutant allele of an individual heterozygous for this allele.[1,64,68] The energetics required for the conversion in conformation of PrP^C to PrP^{res} are thought to be unfavorable and could require a mutant template or perhaps a chaperone protein (protein X).[64,157,164,267] Because the conversion reaction is essentially irreversible, this change in protein conformation results in accumulation of the insoluble and protease-resistant PrP^{res} protein. Arguments have been put forth that certain conformations of PrP^C favor the conversion to pathogenic forms of PrP^{res}; this would provide additional constraints on the expression of disease that could explain the non-PrP^C genetic contributions to disease susceptibility and provide a final common pathway for genetic and infectious forms of the disease.[1,270] Several studies have argued that the various protease fragments generated after PrP^{res} treatment with protease K may be associated with different patterns of disease in the CNS; this could account for additional diversity in disease phenotype attributed to this single, small protein.[216,217,279] Once the pathogenic PrP^{res} accumulates, additional newly synthesized molecules are converted into PrP^{res}, and clinical symptoms develop, depending on the site of cell loss in the CNS. Accumulation of the PrP^{res} isoform probably involves a combination of new synthesis of PrP^{res} and decreased clearance of the misfolded aggregate. Failure to clear the misfolded pathogenic isoform may ultimately be the major pathway leading to accumulation of PrP^{res} and disease.[1,241] Finally, studies have linked copper binding to PrP^C with oxidation of the prion protein.[1,38,232,245,297] Alternatively, a copper-containing prion complex localized to the synaptic junction could protect normal synapses from oxidants or perhaps play a direct role in copper metabolism or transport.[153,245] Loss of normal prion function by misfolding could then lead to neuronal loss. The importance of these newly described characteristics of PrP^C remains incompletely defined at this time.

Although inoculation of a susceptible host with prion-contaminated cadaveric growth hormone or the use of contaminated instruments during neurosurgical procedures clearly can transmit CJD, the route of infection leading to vCJD is only assumed to be oral ingestion of contaminated beef, based on studies in nonhuman primates.[27,30,279] As noted earlier, studies have demonstrated that other TSEs, including kuru, can be transmitted by oral ingestion of infectious material, but only with large inoculums and often requiring extended incubation periods.[118] Researchers have shown that 10 g of BSE-infected cow brain can infect and kill most mice.[13] Even though, extrapolating from these data, a comparable dose required for human infection would be difficult to achieve, these findings demonstrate that the BSE agent can be transmitted by oral ingestion.

The pathway leading from ingestion of PrP^{res} tissue to deposition in the CNS has been shown to require local replication in lymphoid tissue, which is thought to be followed by bloodborne dissemination to the CNS.[1,133,160,163] High titers of infectious prions can be found in liver and spleen as well as in the tonsils and other lymphoid tissue of the oropharynx and gut, suggesting that the titer of the infecting PrP^{res} is amplified in these tissues before spread to the CNS. In vCJD, PrP^{res} can be found in the tonsils at levels as high as 10% of the levels in infected brain.[136,281] However, these findings were reported to be restricted to vCJD; this may reflect a characteristic of the PrP^{res} of vCJD or possibly the route of inoculation. Studies in mice have shown that performing splenectomy before inoculation with the scrapie agent can prolong the disease course, and subsequent studies have demonstrated the importance of replication in cells derived from bone marrow for neuroinvasion.[75,155,167] Other studies have demonstrated that expression of PrP^{res} in the peripheral nervous system is sufficient to transmit disease, suggesting that direct hematogenous dissemination to the brain is not necessary for transmission of TSE.[229] Prions are thought to replicate in these tissues before spreading to the CNS, and one study documented the presence of PrP^{res} in an appendix that was removed 8 months before the onset of TSE in the patient.[136] Although the B lymphocytes were once thought to represent a likely candidate for the cell transmitting the PrP^{res} to the CNS, studies have provided data inconsistent with this mechanism of transmission.[11,52,82,163,207,208,247] There is evidence for the role of follicular dendritic cells in lymphoid tissue as sites of prion replication, and they may direct the prion to the CNS.[155,167] Other investigators have suggested that unidentified host cell molecules may provide the necessary interactions with the prion molecule to permit their trafficking with migratory myeloid cells and, ultimately, entry into the CNS.[181] Candidate molecules have included components of the complement system, based on the study of PrP^{res} in transgenic mice lacking specific complement components, perhaps secondary to the expression of Fcγ and complement receptors CD21/CD35 by follicular dendritic cells.[23,162,182]

PATHOLOGY

The pathologic findings of TSE include a hallmark triad of histologic findings: neuronal loss, proliferation of reactive astrocytes, and status spongiosis.[17] *Status spongiosis* is a descriptive term for degeneration of neurons and collapse of the cortical cytoarchitecture leading to vacuolation of the neuropil.[17] Amyloid plaques also are observed in some patients, and in some cases PrP^{res} is present in these plaques.[17,57,161] Whether the distribution of spongiform lesions is related to the pathogenesis of these disorders or merely reflects the duration of disease before the onset of clinical symptoms is unknown; however, some TSEs, such as FFI, exhibit a preponderance of histopathologic changes in specific locations (e.g., thalamus).[17,57,185,215,268] Descriptions of the neuropathologic process of vCJD have suggested distinctive histopathologic changes,[279] including a distinctive plaque containing a central amyloid core and fibrillary periphery with extensive spongiform changes in the immediate periphery of the plaque (Fig. 193.3).[103,151] The surrounding spongiform changes are proximal to the plaque, and the remaining neuropil is relatively intact.[57,151] These findings are unique to vCJD cases and have not been seen in sCJD cases from outside Great Britain.[56,152] Histopathologic lesions in the cerebral and cerebellar cortices, basal ganglia, thalamus, and brain stem also have been described.[152] Involvement of the cerebellum appears to be more common in vCJD than in reported cases of sCJD, but this finding may be related to the differences in age at onset of disease in these two populations; findings from young patients with sCJD have suggested that these patients have a syndrome more closely resembling vCJD than sCJD in older patients.[25] Extensive widespread CJD findings that included involvement of cerebellar white matter, corticospinal degeneration, and ballooned neurons were also reported in an 11-year-old child who died of CJD after

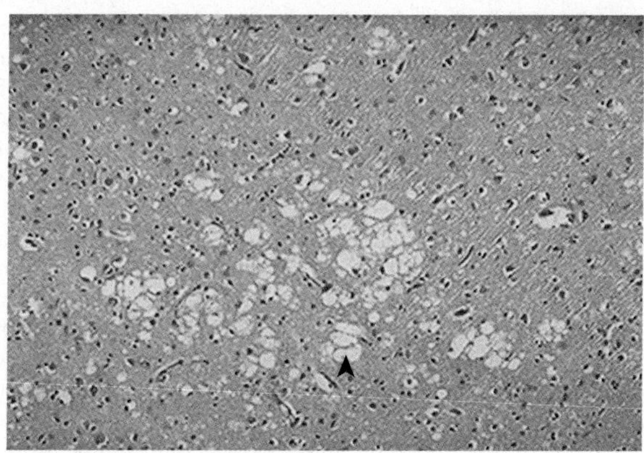

FIG. 193.3 Microscopic appearance of a specimen from a person with Creutzfeldt-Jakob disease (CJD), which produces rapidly progressive dementia. The vacuoles in the cerebral cortical gray matter *(arrowhead)* represent the spongiform encephalopathy that occurs with CJD. There is marked gliosis in response to the neuronal loss as CJD progresses. CJD has the potential for infectious spread, but cases appear sporadically. The agent of CJD is a prion protein (PrP), a neuronal cell surface sialoglycoprotein. Disease results when the normal prion protein (PrP^C) undergoes conformational change to an abnormal form (PrP^{Sc}), which is protease resistant (PrP^{res}) and can accumulate and cause loss of neuronal cell function, vacuolization, and death. (From Klatt EC, ed. *Robbins and Cotran Atlas of Pathology*. 2nd ed. Philadelphia: Saunders; 2010.)

treatment with native human growth hormone.[203] Finally, electron microscopic studies of plaques from vCJD brain tissue have suggested subtle but recognizable differences between plaques obtained from patients with vCJD and those from patients with CJD.[103,107]

CLINICAL MANIFESTATIONS

Only the clinical manifestations of sCJD and vCJD are discussed in this chapter. The other TSEs, such as GSS and FFI, are diseases that are unlikely to be encountered in children, and kuru, a horizontally transmitted form of CJD, is no longer reported to be occurring (see Table 193.2). The interested reader is referred to referenced discussions of these diseases in adults and in the Papua New Guinea unique population.[42,100,112,141,180,185]

Clinical signs and symptoms during the early stages of CJD are subtle and often complex and include both motor and sensory dysfunction.[141] Abnormalities in gait, ataxia, vision problems, and complaints of headache, dizziness, and paresthesias often are noted.[42,51,210,238] Intellectual dysfunction, including loss of memory, speech abnormalities, anxiety, and depression, also are often presenting complaints of patients with early stages of CJD.[25,42,51] Neurologic abnormalities may include corticospinal tract dysfunction as manifested by hyperreflexia, spasticity, and extensor plantar reflexes. Visual disturbances include visual field abnormalities and, in some cases, cortical blindness. Seizures are not a frequent clinical symptom of patients with CJD. Presentation mimicking a stroke syndrome has also been reported in elderly adult patients.[246] Other, less frequent findings include evidence of autonomic system dysfunction and, rarely, lower motor neuron disease.[210,243] Although death secondary to complications associated with the vegetative state usually occurs within 1 year after onset of symptoms, a small percentage of patients exhibit a prolonged disease course.[51]

The clinical symptoms of vCJD are distinct from those of sCJD. This disease has been reported in an 11-year old child with neonatal growth hormone deficiency who was treated from infancy with injections of native human growth hormone, as well as in an adolescent; therefore, CJD or vCJD could potentially be encountered by pediatricians.[203] The age range for reported cases of vCJD is 11 to 48 years, a distribution clearly outside that of sCJD. Symptoms included psychiatric and sensory disturbances such as dysesthesias and paresthesias with electromyographic evidence of denervation. Psychiatric symptoms included anxiety, depression, anorexia, social withdrawal, and other nonspecific complaints. As the disease progressed, more familiar findings of TSE, including pyramidal tract dysfunction, rigidity, cerebellar dysfunction, and myoclonus, developed. Visual disturbances also were noted late in the disease. The duration of illness has exceeded 1 year in most patients with vCJD and death follows complications associated with the vegetative state. As noted earlier, the clinical presentation of sCJD in young individuals more closely resembles that of vCJD than that of sCJD in older individuals.[25] In these young patients, prion-specific proteins are present in brain, cerebrospinal fluid (CSF), and nasal olfactory brushings.

DIAGNOSIS

The diagnosis of CJD or vCJD requires a high index of suspicion and, in the case of vCJD, a history compatible with exposure to contaminated beef or beef byproducts or, possibly, a previous blood product transfusion from a high-risk area, neurosurgical procedure, growth hormone injection, or corneal transplantation. Routine laboratory findings are nonspecific and not helpful.[92,93,274,303] No consistent reports demonstrate systemic or CNS inflammation. Therefore, routine laboratory analysis of CSF often is nondiagnostic. Laboratory tests, electroencephalography (EEG) and brain imaging can provide support for the diagnosis.

Laboratory Diagnosis

Assays for specific CSF protein biomarkers, such as the 14-3-3 protein, tau, or neuron-specific enolase, may provide helpful laboratory evidence of CJD or vCJD.[124,125,149,168,244,302] Definitive premortem diagnosis requires biopsy tissue, and histopathologic diagnosis can be facilitated by use of PrP^{res}-specific antibodies in both immunocytochemistry and Western blot assays.[8,57,279,281] The use of monoclonal antibodies specific for PrP^{res} has permitted a more thorough understanding of the distribution of prions in CNS and non-CNS tissue in patients with TSE. Hill and coworkers reported that tonsillar biopsy followed by detection of PrP^{res} by both Western blot and immunocytochemistry or *PRNP* sequencing is useful for establishing the diagnosis of vCJD disease.[105,137] This approach has been particularly valuable for defining the incidence of vCJD infection in populations, such as has been carried out in studies in Great Britain.[105,142] The National Prion Disease Pathology Surveillance Center (http://www.cjdsurveillance.com) offers diagnostic testing assays for 14-3-3 and tau proteins in CSF, *PRNP* sequencing, Western blot analysis to identify and characterize PrP, histologic processing of brain tissues, and expert neuropathologic consultation for patients with suspected CJD.[113] More recently, in vitro prion formation using CSF has been shown to be very sensitive and specific for the diagnosis of prion disease.[10,196,214]

A second-generation, highly sensitive real-time quaking–induced conversion (RT-QuIC) prion test has been developed and evaluated in more than 2000 patients to detect the specific target of prion protein PrP^{Sc}; this provides a more specific diagnostic test for CJD than surrogate biomarkers do. The RT-QuIC assay shows favorable diagnostic performance compared with surrogate biomarker tests for prion disease such as 14-3-3 and tau proteins; together with *PRNP* gene sequencing, it can be used to differentiate major prion subtypes, which can help predict the disease progression. This new test can provide an early and accurate diagnosis and may be used to diagnose CJD by testing CSF or olfactory nasal mucosa brushings from patients who present with clinical signs and symptoms consistent with CJD.[28,104,171,212,218,300]

Neuroimaging

Imaging of patients with suspected prion disease has been extremely helpful in establishing the diagnosis of these rare diseases.[114] Although computed tomography may reveal a variety of structural abnormalities, none is sufficiently specific to be considered diagnostic. In contrast, magnetic resonance imaging findings of increased T2 signals from the striatum and thalamus are specific for prion diseases, especially vCJD.[12,101] Abnormal signals originating from the pulvinar in the posterior thalamus (pulvinar sign) are distinctive for vCJD and should be considered highly predictive for the disease.[12,77,184] Other studies have shown lesions in the cortex and basal ganglia, without involvement of the thalamus, in patients with biopsy-confirmed CJD.[202,269] Therefore, cortical signal increases, as well as hyperintensities in the basal ganglia and the thalamus, may occur in patients with CJD.

Electroencephalography

EEG tracings from patients with CJD and vCJD are characteristic but not diagnostic. The classic findings are synchronous, bilateral biphasic or triphasic periodic sharp waves of 1 to 2 cycles per second on a background of generalized slowing. Repeat or serial tracings may be necessary to document these changes.[31,74,258]

TREATMENT

No known treatments of TSE are licensed for medical practice. In vitro models of PrP^C folding have suggested that a variety of agents may limit production of pathogenic forms of PrP^{res} in neuroblastoma cells in vitro. Comprehensive reviews of treatment modalities have been published, and the interested reader is referred to these publications.[62,272] Derivatives of Congo red, polyene antibiotics related to amphotericin B, branched polyamines, and phenothiazines all have been reported to exhibit some activity and to delay onset of disease in experimental animals.[272] To date, no evidence that any of these proposed therapies would be effective in human TSE has been reported. Small molecules that target protein misfolding are in preclinical development, as are adoptive immunotherapy techniques using transfer of $CD4^+$ T cells.[60,115,249]

Immunotherapy with antibody vaccines targeting prion disease–specific epitopes that are exposed in the misfolded PrP^{Sc} conformation, dendritic cell vaccines that use antigen-loaded dendritic cells with the ability to bypass immune tolerance, and adoptive transfer of physiologic prion protein–specific $CD4^+$ T cells are in early development for treatment of prion diseases.[60] At least two reports have suggested that anti-prion monoclonal antibodies may offer a therapeutic approach to TSE. These reports suggested that anti-prion antibodies directed at cell surface PrP^C prevented infection of susceptible cells and also eliminated infection in a chronically infected cell line.[97,220,287] These findings argue that impaired clearance of misfolded PrP^C contributed to disease in animals infected with PrP^{res} and that passive antibody therapy could potentially cure similar infections in vivo.[60] Treatment of mice with soluble lymphotoxin-β blocked follicular dendritic cell maturation and inhibited the development of scrapie in inoculated, susceptible mice, suggesting that interventions with agents that can block neuroinvasion may be efficacious.[183,208]

PREVENTION

Because effective treatments of TSE are still undefined, prevention of disease remains the goal of current medical practice. Iatrogenic transmission of CJD has been reported in more than 250 patients around the world. Infection occurs after exposure during neurosurgical procedures (including dural grafts and stereotaxic electrodes), after exposure to contaminated CNS tissue in the form of growth hormone or gonadotropic hormone preparations, and after corneal grafting. These forms of iCJD have declined due to awareness and appropriate interventions to avoid these exposures in patients. Because transmissions by blood and blood products have been reported, the American Red Cross has placed restrictions on donors to exclude those who may have been exposed to agents or geographical locations associated with TSE. Cases of TSE that follow exposure to human feces, urine, or mucosal secretions have not been reported; therefore, current universal precautions employed in health care settings should suffice to prevent health care–associated transmission during routine care of patients with TSE. Recent evidence has shown shedding of PrP in olfactory nasal washings of patients with CJD, but transmission to health care workers or close contacts by contact with nasal secretions of patients with CJD has not been documented.[28,212] The infectivity category of brain, spinal cord, and eye tissues is high, compared with CSF, kidney, liver, lung, lymph nodes, spleen and placenta, which are likely to be low. However, some experts think that lymphoid tissue may be in the moderate to high category in some patients. All other blood products, tissues, and body secretions are believed to be in a low or no infectivity category, based on limited data on actual infectivity titers.[290]

Inactivation of tissue and fluid suspected of being contaminated with prions is problematic because they exhibit unusual resistance to conventional chemical and physical decontamination methods.[290] Early studies indicated that subjecting prion-containing brain tissue to temperatures in excess of 360°C resulted in a reduction of only about 90% in infectivity.[36,49] In addition, formalin- and glutarldehyde-fixed tissue retains infectivity indefinitely, and CJD has been transmitted from paraffin-embedded tissue sections.[46,47] Several different approaches for decontamination of prion-contaminated tissue and instruments have been proposed.[186,233,239] Tissues such as brain, eyes, lymphoid tissue, and spinal cords from infected patients may have high levels of infectivity. Therefore, the tissues and instruments in contact with these tissues should be handled as highly biohazardous materials. Instruments should be cleaned with high concentrations of sodium hydroxide or undiluted sodium hypochlorite and then autoclaved at high temperatures for prolonged periods or, if practical, incinerated. The high concentration of prions in lymphoid and nervous tissue in these patients should be emphasized to anyone in contact with patients with TSE, and material that may be contaminated with prions should be handled in a rigorous manner to ensure safe disposal. There are also special procedures for autopsies and embalming and burial of patients with CJD. The World Health Organization (www.who.int) provides guidelines for infection control, including sterilization, disposal, and biocontamination for prevention of TSE in health care and surgical settings, in certain occupations, and after death. These guidelines are also endorsed by the US Centers for Disease Control and Prevention.[290]

No documented cases of TSE transmission after routine dental procedures have been reported in humans. However, invasive endodontic procedures involving contact with nerve rich dental pulp may theoretically transmit prions from affected individuals.[261] Universal precautions for dental procedures are currently recommended; however, if the patient in need of invasive dental procedures is suspected of having a TSE, then referral to a major medical center is advised for special precautions and single-use instruments.[290]

Genetic counseling may be helpful in familial disease in families with a *PRNP* mutation.[156]

There is no licensed vaccine available against prion disease. However, protocols are being considered to develop vaccines with disease-specific epitopes specifically targeting the misfolded prion conformation associated with TSE diseases.[192,191,263]

Prevention of prion-associated disease in individuals also may be genetic. A naturally occurring variant of the human prion protein that may completely prevent prion disease in exposed individuals has been discovered. This novel PrP variant has a single amino acid substitution of G to V at codon 127 (G127V, or PrP V127). It likely resulted from positive evolutionary selection during the kuru epidemic in Papua New Guinea. Studies in transgenic mice expressing different ratios of the variant and wild-type PrP indicate that presence of the PrP V127 variant is refractory to prion conversion and also acts as a dose-dependent inhibitor of wild-type prion propagation.[9]

NEW REFERENCES SINCE THE SEVENTH EDITION

9. Asante E, Smidak M, Grimshaw A, et al. A naturally occurring variant of the human prion protein completely prevents prion disease. *Nature.* 2015;522:478-481.
27. Bonda D, Manjila S, Mehnddiratta P, et al. Human prion disease: surgical lessons learned from iatrogenic prion transmission. *Neurosurg Focus.* 2016;41:E10.
28. Bongianni M, Orru C, Goveman B, et al. Diagnosis of human prion disease using real-time quaking-induced conversion testing of olfactory mucosa and cerebrospinal fluid samples. *JAMA Neurol.* 2017;74:155-162.
60. Burchell J, Panegyres P. Prion diseases: immunotargets and therapy. *Immunotargets Ther.* 2016;5-57.
80. Collinge J. Mammalian prions and their wider relevance in neurodegenerative diseases. *Nature.* 2016;539(7628):217-226.
85. Collinge J, Whitfield J, McKintosh E, et al. Kuru in the 21st century: an acquired human prion disease with very long incubation periods. *Lancet.* 2006;367:2068-2074.
87. Collinge J, Whitfield J, McKintosh E, et al. A clinical study of kuru patients with long incubation periods at the end of the epidemic in Papua New Guinea. *Philos Trans R Soc Lond B Biol Sci.* 2008;363:3725-3739.
92. Davidson L, Llewelyn C, Mackenzie J, et al. Variant CJD and blood transfusion: are there additional cases? *Vox Sang.* 2014;107:220-225.

93. Diack A, Head M, McCutcheon S, et al. Variant CJD: 18 years of research and surveillance. *Prion*. 2014;8:286-295.
98. Erana H, Benegas V, Morena J, Castilla J. Prion-like disorders and transmissible spongiform encephalopathies: an overview of the mechanistic features that are shared by the various disease-related misfolded proteins. *Biochem Biophys Res Commun*. 2017;483:1125-1136.
104. Foutz A, Appleby B, Hamlin C, et al. Diagnostic and prognostic value of human prion detection in cerebrospinal fluid. *Ann Neurol*. 2017;81:79-92.
114. Gaudino S, Gangemi E, Colantonio R, et al. Neuroradiology of human prion diseases, diagnosis and differential diagnosis. *Radiol Med*. 2017;122:369-385.
150. Imran M, Mahmood S. An overview of human prion diseases. *Virol J*. 2011;8:559-561.
171. Lattanzio F, Abu-Rumelleh S, Franceschini A, et al. Prion-specific and surrogate CSF biomarkers in Creutzfeldt-Jakob disease: diagnostic accuracy in relation to molecular subtypes and analysis of neuropathological correlates of p-tau and Abeta42 levels. *Acta Neuropathol*. 2017;133:559-578.
175. Liberski P. Gerstmann-Straussler-Scheinker disease. *Adv Exp Med Biol*. 2012;724:126-137.
179. Lu T, Pan Y, Peng L, et al. Fatal familial insomnia with abnormal signals on routine MRI: a case report and literature review. *BMC Neurol*. 2017;17:104.
191. Marciniuk K, Maattanen P, Taschuk R, et al. Development of a multivalent, PrP(Sc)-specific prion vaccine through rational optimization of three disease-specific epitopes. *Vaccine*. 2014;32:1988-1997.
192. Marciniuk K, Taschuk R, Napper S. Methods and protocols for developing prion vaccines. *Methods Mol Biol*. 2016;1403:657-680.
212. Orru C, Bongianni M, Tonoli G, et al. A test for Cretuzfeldt-Jakob disease using nasal brushings. *N Engl J Med*. 2014;371:519-529.
218. Park J, Choi Y, Lee Y, et al. Real-time quaking-induced conversion analysis for the diagnosis of sporadic Creutzfeldt-Jacob disease in Korea. *J Clin Neurol*. 2016;12:101-106.
236. Riudavets M, Sraka M, Schultz M, et al. Gerstmann-Straussler-Scheinker syndrome with variable genotype in a new kindred with PRNP-P102L mutation. *Brain Pathol*. 2014;24:142-147.
246. Shama D, Bogglid M, van Heuven A, White R. Creutzfeldt-Jakob disease presenting as stroke: a case report and systemic literature review. *Neurologist*. 2017;22:48-52.
260. Sun L, Li X, Lin X, et al. Familial fatal insomnia with atypical clinical features in a patient with D178N mutation and homozygosity for Met at codon 129 of the prion protein gene. *Prion*. 2015;9:228-235.
261. Sushma B, Gugwad S, Pavaskar R, Malik S. Prions in dentistry: a need to be concerned and known. *J Oral Maxillofac Pathol*. 2016;20:111-114.
263. Taschuk R, Marciniuk K, Maatanen P, et al. Safety, specificity and immunogenicity of a PrP(Sc)-specific prion vaccine based on the YYR disease specific epitope. *Prion*. 2014;8:51-59.
274. Urwin P, Mackenzie J, Llewelyn C, et al. Creutzfeldt-Jakob disease and blood transfusion: updated results of the UK Transfusion Medicine Epidemiology Review Study. *Vox Sang*. 2016;110:310-316.
282. Wadsworth J, Joiner S, LInehan J, et al. Kuru prions and sporadic Creutzfeld-Jakob disease prions have equivalent transmission properties in transgenic and wild-type mice. *Proc Natl Acad Sci USA*. 2008;105:3885-3890.
288. Whitfield J, Pako W, Collinge J, Alpers M. Mortuary rites of the South Fore and kuru. *Philos Trans R Soc Lond B Biol Sci*. 2008;3631:3721-3724.
289. Whitfield J, Pako W, Collinge J, Alpers M. Cultural factors that affected the spatial and temporal epidemiology of kuru. *R Soc Open Sci*. 2017;4:1607-1689.
290. WHO Infection Control Guidelines for Transmissible Spongiform Encephalopathies. Report of a WHO consultation; World Health Organization Communicable Disease Surveillance and Control. Geneva, Switzerland, 1999. www.who.int.
300. Zanusso G, Monaco S, Pocchiari M, Caughey B. Advanced tests for early and accurate diagnosis of Creutzfeld-Jacob disease. *Nat Rev Neurol*. 2016;12:325-333.
303. Zou S, Fang C, Schonberger L. Transfusion transmission of human prion diseases. *Transfus Med Rev*. 2008;22:58-69.

The full reference list for this chapter is available at ExpertConsult.com.

194 Chlamydia Infections

Margaret R. Hammerschlag • Stephan A. Kohlhoff

Chlamydiae are obligate intracellular pathogens that have established a unique niche within the host cell. They cause a variety of diseases in animal species at virtually all phylogenic levels. In 1999, Everett and colleagues[48,55] reported a taxonomic analysis involving the 16S and 23S rRNA genes that found that the order Chlamydiales contained at least four distinct groups at the family level and that within the family Chlamydiaceae there were two distinct lineages; they suggested splitting of the genus *Chlamydia* into two genera, *Chlamydia* and *Chlamydophila.* This classification was not universally accepted, and it was agreed that the family Chlamydiaceae contains a single genus, *Chlamydia.*[67,154] This position has been supported by additional data on *Chlamydia* genome sequences. The genus *Chlamydia* now contains 11 recognized species: *C. trachomatis, C. psittaci, C. pneumoniae, C. pecorum* (infects cattle, other ruminants, and koalas),[48,55,154] *C. muridarum* (formerly the agent of mouse pneumonitis), *C. suis* (an important pathogen of swine), *C. abortus* (causes abortion in cattle and sheep; rarely has caused abortion in humans), *C. caviae* (formerly *C. psittaci* guinea pig conjunctivitis strain), *C. felis* (causes epidemic keratoconjunctivitis in cats) and *C. avium* and *C. gallinacea* (two new species causing infection in wild and breeding birds).[67] *C. trachomatis* and *C. pneumoniae* are the most significant human pathogens, and *C. psittaci* is an important zoonosis.

Recently, several chlamydia-like organisms that are endosymbionts of free-living amoebae have been identified.[68] These organisms, which include *Parachlamydia acanthamoebae, Simkania negevensis, Waddlia chondrophilia,* and *Neochlamydia hartmannellae,* have been termed *environmental chlamydiae.*[68,112] Analyses of nearly full-length 16S rRNA gene sequences of these isolates showed that they clustered with other members of the order Chlamydiales but in a lineage separate from those of *Chlamydia* (16S rRNA sequence similarities of >88%). Data on the potential role of these organisms in human disease are limited. This bacteria-protozoa interaction might have been a driving force for the development of effective mechanisms by bacteria to survive phagocytosis by unicellular eukaryotes, which in turn may have been a first step in the evolution of intracellular bacterial pathogens of higher organisms.[36,137]

Chlamydiae are characterized by a unique developmental cycle with morphologically distinct infectious and reproductive forms: the elementary body and the reticulate body. They have a gram-negative envelope without detectable peptidoglycan, although recent genomic analysis has revealed that both *C. trachomatis* and *C. pneumoniae* encode proteins forming a nearly complete pathway for the synthesis of peptidoglycan, including penicillin-binding proteins.[93,136,138,151] This finding is the basis for the so-called chlamydial peptidoglycan paradox, given that it has been known for decades that chlamydial development is sensitive to β-lactam antibiotics.[136] An explanation for this has been recently described: Chlamydia species do produce a small amount of peptidoglycan during cell division that is necessary for proper localization of septal proteins.[97] Chlamydiae also share a group-specific lipopolysaccharide (LPS) antigen and use host adenosine triphosphate (ATP) for the synthesis of chlamydial protein.[151] Although chlamydiae are auxotrophic for three of four nucleoside triphosphates, they encode functional glucose-catabolizing enzymes that can be used for the generation of ATP. As with peptidoglycan synthesis, for some reason these genes are turned off.[151] All chlamydiae also encode an abundant protein, the major outer membrane protein (MOMP or OmpA), that is surface exposed in *C. trachomatis* and *C. psittaci* but apparently not in *C. pneumoniae.*[151] MOMP is the major determinant of the serologic classification of *C. trachomatis* and *C. psittaci* isolates.

After infection develops, the infectious elementary bodies, which are 200 to 400 μm in diameter, attach to the host cell by a process of electrostatic binding and are taken into the cell by endocytosis that does not depend on the microtubule system. Within the host cell, the elementary body remains within a membrane-lined phagosome. The phagosome does not fuse with the host cell lysosome. The inclusion membrane is devoid of host cell markers, but lipid markers traffic to the inclusion, which suggests functional interaction with the Golgi apparatus. The elementary bodies then differentiate into reticulate bodies that undergo binary fission. After approximately 36 hours, reticulate bodies differentiate into elementary bodies. At approximately 48 hours, release may occur by cytolysis or by a process of exocytosis or extrusion of the whole inclusion, with the host cell left intact. Chlamydiae also may enter a persistent state after treatment with certain cytokines such as interferon-γ, treatment with antibiotics, or restriction of certain nutrients. In the persistent state, metabolic activity is reduced. The ability to cause prolonged, often subclinical infection is one of the major characteristics of chlamydiae.[80]

INFECTIONS CAUSED BY *CHLAMYDIA TRACHOMATIS*

Epidemiology

C. trachomatis infection is the most prevalent sexually transmitted infection (STI) and infectious disease in the United States today.[28-30] In 2010, more than 1.3 million cases were reported to the Centers for Disease Control and Prevention (CDC).[29,30] The prevalence of chlamydial infection is associated less with socioeconomic status, urban or rural residence, and race or ethnicity than are gonorrhea and syphilis. Infection with *C. trachomatis* tends to be asymptomatic and of long duration. If a pregnant woman has active infection during delivery, the infant may acquire the infection and, as a consequence, either conjunctivitis or pneumonia.[28,53,74,76,157] Children also may acquire chlamydial infection as a result of sexual abuse.

Chlamydia trachomatis Infections in the Neonate

History

At the beginning of the 20th century, before expectant mothers were being screened for STIs, the term *ophthalmia neonatorum* was, for all practical purposes, synonymous with gonococcal conjunctivitis. As neonatal conjunctivitis came under control with silver nitrate prophylaxis, the importance of another form of ophthalmia neonatorum, *inclusion blennorrhea,* was noted. The relationship between maternal genital infection and conjunctivitis of the newborn associated with inclusion bodies within epithelial cells was established by Thygeson and Stone in 1942.[170] Respiratory infection in infants caused by *C. trachomatis* probably was reported first in 1941 by Botsztejn,[23] who described an entity that he called *pertussoid eosinophilic pneumonia.*

Epidemiology

The rate of cervical infection with *C. trachomatis* during pregnancy varies from 1% to 37%, with the highest rates occurring in women 25 years and younger. *C. trachomatis* infection is acquired by the infant from the mother during parturition, as demonstrated in multiple well-controlled prospective studies conducted in the 1970s and 1980s of maternal-infant infection in which infection occurred only in infants born to infected mothers.[28,53,74,72,157] No convincing evidence demonstrates

TABLE 194.1 **Selected Studies of Perinatal Chlamydial Infection**

	PREVALENCE OF MATERNAL GENITAL INFECTION		PROPORTION OF INFANTS WITH CHLAMYDIAL INFECTION BORN TO INFECTED MOTHERS				
Reference, City	**Total**	**No. Infected (%)**	**Total**	**Conjunctivitis (%)**	**Pneumonia (%)**	**NP (%)**	**Rectum/Vagina (%)**
Frommell et al., 1979, Denver[53]	340	30 (8.8)	67	39	11	6	NS
Schachter et al., 1986, San Francisco[157,158]	5531	262 (4.7)	131	17.6	16	11.5	14
Hammerschlag et al., 1989, Brooklyn[76]	4357	341 (7.8)	45	15	1	4	NS

NP, Nasopharynx; *NS*, not studied.

horizontal transmission from mother to infant, from other family members to the infant, or from infant to infant after delivery. Infection after cesarean delivery, usually associated with rupture of the membranes, or infection through intact membranes is a rare event but may occur.[13] The overall risk for an infant born to a mother with active chlamydial infection becoming infected at any anatomic site has been reported to be approximately 50% to 75% in various studies (Table 194.1).[53,76,157] Infants can be infected at more than one site, including the conjunctiva, nasopharynx, rectum, and vagina. The most frequent clinical manifestation of neonatal chlamydial infection, inclusion conjunctivitis, has been reported to occur in 15% to 37% of infants born to mothers with untreated cervical chlamydial infection.[53,76,157] The most frequent site of infection, however, is the nasopharynx, with 78% of infected infants having positive nasopharyngeal cultures in one study.[70] Approximately half of infants with inclusion conjunctivitis also will be infected in the nasopharynx. In only a minority of infants with nasopharyngeal infection does chlamydial pneumonia eventually develop; Hammerschlag and colleagues[74] found that pneumonia subsequently developed in only 4 of 12 infants (33%) with isolated nasopharyngeal infection. The overall risk for pneumonia developing in infants born to chlamydia-positive mothers has been reported to range from 1% to 22%.[53,76,157]

Data on the risk for acquiring rectal or vaginal infection are more limited. Bell and colleagues[14] demonstrated that perinatally acquired *C. trachomatis* infection may persist for months to more than 2 years. Twenty-two infants born to women with culture-documented chlamydial infection were monitored, and positive cultures from the nasopharynx and oropharynx in the infants were detected as late as 28.5 months after birth. Rectal and vaginal infections were asymptomatic and persisted for at least 1 year, which can become an important confounding variable when young children are tested for the presence of *C. trachomatis* during evaluation for suspected sexual abuse.

Conjunctivitis. *C. trachomatis* was the most frequent identifiable infectious cause of neonatal conjunctivitis, and conjunctivitis was the major clinical manifestation of neonatal chlamydial infection in the United States in the 1990s. The introduction of systematic screening and treatment of pregnant women has resulted in a dramatic decrease in the number of perinatal chlamydial infections, including conjunctivitis, in the United States.[2,71] However, in countries in which pregnant women are not screened routinely, including many developing countries, *C. trachomatis* remains the most frequent cause of neonatal conjunctivitis.[130,147,152,176,180,181] The incubation period of *C. trachomatis* conjunctivitis is 5 to 14 days after delivery or earlier if premature rupture of membranes has occurred. At least 50% of infants with chlamydial conjunctivitis also will have nasopharyngeal infection. The manifestation is extremely variable and ranges from mild conjunctivitis with scant mucoid discharge to severe conjunctivitis with copious purulent discharge, chemosis, and pseudomembrane formation. The conjunctiva can be very friable and may bleed when stroked with a swab. Eyelid erythema and edema frequently are present. A Gram-stained conjunctival smear initially may reveal a predominance of polymorphonuclear leukocytes. Chlamydial conjunctivitis needs to be differentiated from gonococcal ophthalmia in some infants, especially those born to mothers who did not receive any prenatal care, had gonorrhea during pregnancy, or abused drugs.

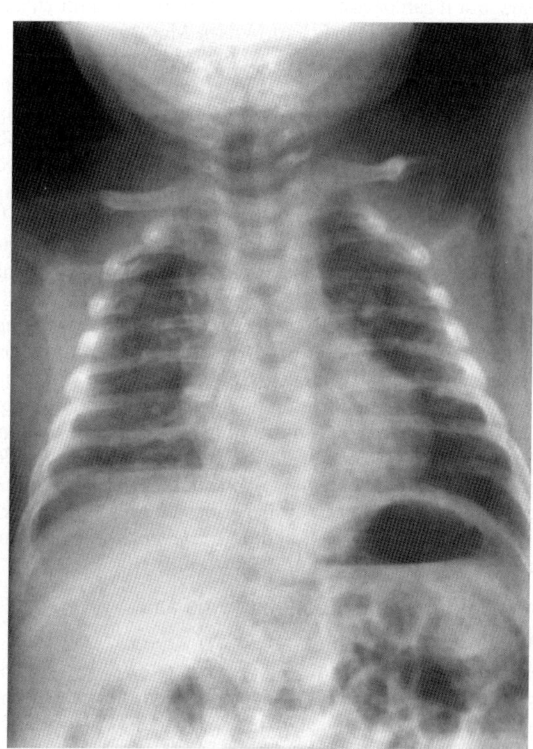

FIG. 194.1 Anteroposterior chest radiograph of a severely ill 1-month-old male infant with *Chlamydia trachomatis* pneumonitis. Diffuse interstitial infiltrates and hyperaeration with a flattened diaphragm are prominent.

An overlap in both incubation periods and clinical findings can occur. Bilateral infections are present in two-thirds of cases. A follicular reaction is not seen because infants younger than 3 months of age do not have the requisite lymphoid tissue present in the conjunctiva.

Pneumonia. As stated previously, approximately 70% of infected infants will have positive nasopharyngeal cultures, but most of these infections are asymptomatic.[74,153] Chlamydial pneumonia develops in only approximately 30% of infants with nasopharyngeal infection.[74] In infants in whom pneumonia does develop, the manifestations and clinical findings are very characteristic.[11,85,171] The children usually are seen initially when they are between the ages of 4 and 12 weeks. A few cases have been reported in infants as young as 2 weeks, but no cases have been seen in infants older than 4 months. The infants frequently have a history of cough and congestion, with an absence of fever. On physical examination, the infant is tachypneic, and rales are heard on auscultation of the chest; wheezing is a distinctly uncommon finding.[11,85,171] No specific radiographic findings except hyperinflation are found (Fig. 194.1). Significant laboratory findings include peripheral eosinophilia (>300 cells/cm^3) and elevated serum immunoglobulin levels. If cultures are performed, infants with *C. trachomatis* pneumonia may remain symptomatic and shed the organism from the nasopharynx for protracted periods.[14,71] Generally, infantile pneumonia caused by *C. trachomatis* appears to be self-limited. Most infants can be managed as outpatients, although a few cases of severe disease requiring hospitalization and assisted ventilation have been reported. *C. trachomatis* pneumonia in infants also appears to be associated with few sequelae, although data are limited. Rarely, infants with *C. trachomatis* pneumonia may have concomitant otitis media.[171]

Diagnosis of *Chlamydia trachomatis* Infection in Infants

The diagnosis of neonatal conjunctivitis cannot be made on clinical grounds alone. Significant overlap in both incubation period and clinical findings occurs with infections by other organisms, especially *Neisseria gonorrhoeae*. In a high-risk population, particularly infants born to women with no prenatal care, gonococcal ophthalmia must be considered seriously.[76] The incubation period for gonococcal conjunctivitis is usually 3 to 5 days, but it can be longer. The incubation period for chlamydial conjunctivitis is approximately 5 to 14 days. Most cases will be evident by the time the infant is 2 weeks of age, which is after the infant leaves the hospital. Epidemiologic clues can help the physician decide whether gonococcal ophthalmia needs to be considered. Hammerschlag and colleagues[72,76] noted that seven of the eight infants with gonococcal conjunctivitis in their studies were born to mothers who had not received prenatal care. Five of these women were abusers of crack cocaine. Another epidemiologic clue is a history of gonorrhea or other STI during pregnancy. The clinical manifestation of *C. trachomatis* pneumonitis in infants is fairly characteristic, and clinical diagnosis may be established with a degree of certainty.

The gold standard for diagnosis of *C. trachomatis* infection in infants and children remains isolation of *C. trachomatis* by culture from the conjunctiva, nasopharynx, vagina, or rectum. Seven commercially available nucleic acid amplification tests (NAATs) have been approved by the US Food and Drug Administration (FDA) for the diagnosis of *C. trachomatis* infection (described in detail in the discussion on infection in older children and adolescents).[31] None of these have been approved for use in children. However, available data suggest that NAATs are equivalent to culture for detection of *C. trachomatis* in the conjunctiva and nasopharynx of infants with conjunctivitis.[83,181]

Treatment of Chlamydial Conjunctivitis and Pneumonia in Infants

Oral erythromycin suspension (ethylsuccinate or stearate) 50 mg/kg per day for 14 days is the therapy of choice for the treatment of chlamydial conjunctivitis and pneumonia in infants.[12,28,71] Additional topical therapy is not needed. The efficacy of this regimen has been reported to range from 80% to 90%; however, as many as 20% of infants may require another course of therapy.[12,71] Erythromycin given at the same dose for 2 weeks is the treatment of choice for pneumonia and results in clinical improvement and elimination of the organism from the respiratory tract. One small study evaluated azithromycin and found that a short course of azithromycin suspension, 20 mg/kg per day given orally as one dose daily for 3 days, was as effective as 2 weeks of erythromycin for eradication of *C. trachomatis* from the conjunctivae and nasopharynx of infants with conjunctivitis.[107,78] The CDC included azithromycin as an alternative to erythromycin in the 2015 Sexually Transmitted Diseases Treatment Guidelines.[28]

Treatment with oral erythromycin has been associated with hypertrophic pyloric stenosis in infants younger than 6 weeks who were given the drug for prophylaxis after nursery exposure to pertussis.[37,89] Erythromycin is a motilin receptor agonist. However, a recent retrospective cohort study of children born between 2001 and 2012 performed using the military health system database found that infants prescribed azithromycin in the first 2 weeks of life were also at increased risk for development of pyloric stenosis.[44]

Prevention and Control Strategies

Because *C. trachomatis* infections are transmitted vertically from mother to infant during delivery, several possible options for intervention exist. Prospective studies of mother-to-infant transmission of *C. trachomatis* have demonstrated that neonatal ocular prophylaxis with silver nitrate, erythromycin, or tetracycline ophthalmic ointment does not prevent the development of chlamydial conjunctivitis.[32,76] The most effective method of control of perinatal *C. trachomatis* infection is screening and treatment of pregnant women.[71,79,128] In the 1980s, McMillan and colleagues[124] and Schachter and coworkers[158] reported that treatment of pregnant women infected with *C. trachomatis* with erythromycin resulted in a dramatic decrease in chlamydial infection (i.e., conjunctivitis and nasopharyngeal infection) in their infants in contrast to infants born to untreated infected women. The introduction of NAATs for diagnosis and the use of well-tolerated antibiotic regimens, including amoxicillin and single-dose azithromycin, have increased the efficacy of prenatal screening and treatment.[28] This approach has been validated by a dramatic decrease in perinatal chlamydial infection in the United States[71,75] and a persistence of these infections in countries in which screening and treatment of pregnant women are not standard practice, such as the Netherlands, Ireland, India, and China.[130,147,152,176,180] Rates of maternal chlamydia infections frequently exceed 20% in many nations in sub-Saharan Africa and Asia.[1] The Canadian Pediatric Society recently recommended that neonatal ocular prophylaxis for *C. trachomatis* and gonococcal infection be stopped and emphasized the importance prenatal screening and treatment; this program was implemented in 2016.[132] The American Academy of Pediatrics is considering similar recommendations.

Infections in Older Children

C. trachomatis has not been associated with any specific clinical syndrome in older infants and children. Most attention given to *C. trachomatis* infection in these children has concentrated on its relationship to sexual abuse. Isolation of *C. trachomatis* from a rectal or genital site in children without previous sexual activity may be a marker of sexual abuse; moreover, evidence for other modes of spread, such as through fomites, is lacking for this organism.[28,72,79,91-94] Perinatal maternal-to-infant transmission resulting in vaginal or rectal infection has been documented, with prolonged infection lasting for periods up to 3 years.[14,155,157] This duration can be an important confounding variable in evaluation of possible sexual abuse in a young child.

Four studies examining the epidemiology of STIs in children and adolescents being evaluated for suspected sexual abuse have been published since 2005. Three were retrospective chart reviews, including one each from Vienna, Austria,[103,106] Auckland, New Zealand,[100,102] and Miami, Florida.[161] Despite differences in populations and methodologies,[161,163] the results of the retrospective studies were fairly consistent. Charts were examined from a total of 4350 children, who were seen over periods ranging from 4 to 7 years. Their ages ranged from 0 to 17 years, and most were girls. The prevalence of STIs, specifically gonorrhea and *C. trachomatis*, was low, ranging from 0.4% to 1.8%. These findings are consistent with earlier published studies.[45,91-94] Because these were retrospective chart reviews, they had some major limitations. Inclusion criteria varied, and not every child or adolescent was tested for every STI. In the one prospective study, Girardet and colleagues[61,60] examined children 0 to 13 years of age being evaluated for suspected sexual abuse or assault at seven tertiary care centers in the United States (in Houston, Texas, Atlanta, Georgia, Harrisburg, Pennsylvania, and New York City). All children were tested at multiple sites for *N. gonorrhoeae* and *C. trachomatis* by culture. Vaginal and urethral swabs and urine were also tested using two NAATs. A total of 536 children were enrolled, and 485 (90.5%) were girls. None of the 51 boys enrolled were positive for an STI. Overall, 40 (8.2%) of the girls were found to have one or more STIs. *C. trachomatis* was detected by culture or NAAT in 15 of the girls (3.1%) enrolled. Sixty percent of the children who were positive for *C. trachomatis* gave a clear, credible, detailed description of molestation.

In the setting of repeated abuse by a family member over a long period, the development of infection would be difficult to demonstrate. The 2015 CDC Sexually Transmitted Diseases Treatment Guidelines do not recommend that samples for culture of *C. trachomatis* be obtained routinely from the pharynx and urethra in children who are suspected victims of sexual abuse.[28] The major reasons are the low yield from the urethra, the tendency for longer persistence of perinatally acquired pharyngeal infection, and the potential confusion with *C. pneumoniae*.[9]

Genital *Chlamydia trachomatis* Infections in Adolescents

As stated previously, *C. trachomatis* is the most prevalent STI and infectious disease in the United States. At least 70% (930,000) of cases were among men and women between 15 and 24 years of age, with the highest rates in women 15 to 19 years of age.[30,52] In sexually active adolescents, the prevalence commonly exceeds 10% and may exceed 20%.[52] The case rate of infection in females 15 to 19 years of age was 3378.2 per 100,000, more than 4 times the rate in males of the same age (774.3 per 100,000).[30] The reasons for this gender discrepancy, which is seen in almost every age bracket, are not clear but may include better screening of female adolescents and increased susceptibility to infection in women. More than 70% of infections in women are asymptomatic. Reinfection is very common, with as many as 40% of adolescent women being reinfected, usually from an untreated partner, within 9 months.[8] Women sustain a disproportionate share of the morbidity from these *C. trachomatis* infections through their well-known complications of pelvic inflammatory disease, ectopic pregnancy, and tubal factor infertility.[28] Although *C. trachomatis* infection can be treated effectively with antibiotics, infections may result in tissue damage even with appropriate antimicrobial therapy. Although most infections are asymptomatic, in men they can cause urethritis, and *C. trachomatis* infection is the most frequent cause of epididymitis in men younger than 30 years.[28] The symptoms of chlamydial genital tract infections are less acute than those of gonorrhea, consisting of a discharge that is usually mucoid rather than purulent.

Lymphogranuloma Venereum

Lymphogranuloma venereum (LGV) is an STD caused by the L1 to L3 serovars of *C. trachomatis* that are endemic in tropical and subtropical areas (e.g., parts of Southeast Asia, Africa, South America, India, and the Caribbean) but rare in the United States.[16,28] About 20 cases of LGV have been reported in children. Fewer than 1000 cases are reported in adults in the United States annually. Recently a resurgence of LGV infections has occurred among men who have sex with men (MSM) in Europe and the United States. Some common characteristics of these outbreaks are (1) it affected predominantly white MSM, (2) it presented mostly as proctocolitis (with no inguinal syndrome), (3) individuals affected had very high HIV coinfection rates (about 70%), (4) patients often reported multiple sexual contacts met at casual sex gatherings, (5) 71% met partners at sex-on-premises venues or sex parties, and (6) 23% met partners on the Internet.[6]

LGV is a disease of the lymphatic tissue that has acute and chronic manifestations. Unlike other anogenital *C. trachomatis* infections, in which replication is confined to mucosal epithelial cells, LGV can replicate in macrophages and produce chronic invasive infection. Progression follows several defined stages, similar to syphilitic infection. The primary lesion of LGV is a small, inconspicuous, asymptomatic genital papule or ulcer that heals without a scar. Days to weeks later, unilateral acute lymphadenitis with bubo formation occurs at the site of lymphatic drainage of the primary lesion; acute hemorrhagic proctitis develops after a rectal lesion. Systemic symptoms can include fever, myalgia, or headache. Approximately one-third of inguinal buboes become fluctuant and rupture; the remainder involute slowly. Although most patients recover from LGV after this secondary stage, a small number develop a chronic inflammatory response with fibrosis (as a result of the persistence of *Chlamydia* organisms in anogenital tissues) that can result in chronic genital ulcers or fistulas, rectal strictures, or genital elephantiasis. In females, the vulvar lymph drains to the retroperitoneal nodes; thus they may not have inguinal lymphadenopathy but rather the genitoanorectal syndrome with rectovaginal fistulas and rectal strictures.

To our knowledge, cases in the pediatric population have not been reported since the emergence of the new clusters of cases in 2003. We reported a case of a 16-year-old boy with LGV proctocolitis after having receptive unprotected anal intercourse with a 30-year-old man he met on the Internet.[6] This history was obtained after the boy was found to be HIV positive. The diagnosis of LGV, in particular when it presents with proctocolitis, relies on a high index of suspicion that would lead to emphasizing certain aspects of the history and ordering the pertinent diagnostic tests. Many pediatricians and pediatric gastroenterologists might not be familiar with the entity and might not entertain it as a diagnostic consideration in pediatric patients. The diagnosis can be further suggested by *C. trachomatis* testing that involves culturing the organism or, more commonly, by NAATs. Currently available NAATs will not differentiate LGV from other *C. trachomatis* serovars.[28] NAATs for *C. trachomatis* are also not cleared by the FDA for testing rectal specimens. Trying to ascertain the *C. trachomatis* serovar for confirmation of LGV has therapeutic implications because a single dose of azithromycin is unlikely to eradicate the infection and a 3-week course of doxycycline is the preferred treatment.[28]

Trachoma

Trachoma, the most important preventable cause of blindness in the world, is caused primarily by the A, B, Ba, and C serotypes of *C. trachomatis*.[17,116] It is endemic in sub-Saharan Africa and Southeast Asia. The disease is spread from eye to eye through infected secretions. Flies are frequent vectors.

Trachoma begins as a follicular conjunctivitis, usually in early childhood. The follicles heal, leading to conjunctival scarring that may result in entropion, in which the eyelid turns inward so that the lashes abrade the cornea. It is the corneal ulceration secondary to the constant trauma that leads to scarring and blindness. Bacterial superinfection also may contribute to scarring. Blindness occurs years after the active disease.

Trachoma can be diagnosed clinically. The World Health Organization (WHO) suggests that at least two of four criteria must be present for a diagnosis of trachoma: (1) lymphoid follicles on the upper tarsal conjunctivae, (2) typical conjunctival scarring, (3) vascular pannus, and (4) limbal follicles.[17] The diagnosis is confirmed by culture, microscopy, or NAAT for *C. trachomatis* performed during the active stage of disease. Serologic tests are not helpful clinically because of the long duration of the disease and the high seroprevalence in endemic populations.

Poverty and lack of sanitation are important factors in the spread of trachoma. As socioeconomic conditions improve, the incidence of the disease decreases substantially. The WHO recommends a single dose of azithromycin, 20 mg/kg (maximum, 1 g), for the treatment of trachoma in children. Numerous studies have demonstrated that mass community treatment with a single dose of azithromycin to all residents of a village dramatically reduced the prevalence and intensity of infection.[17,116] This effect continued for 2 years after treatment, probably by interrupting the transmission of ocular *C. trachomatis* infection. Other important interventions include fly control, through providing pit latrines, and face washing, either alone or with topical tetracyclines.[116]

Diagnosis of *Chlamydia trachomatis* Infections

Culture remains the gold standard of diagnosis for detection of *C. trachomatis* from the vagina or rectum in prepubertal children. *Chlamydia* culture has been defined further by the CDC as isolation of the organism in tissue culture and confirmation by microscopic identification of the characteristic inclusions by fluorescent antibody staining using a species-specific conjugated monoclonal antibody.[28]

The major advance in the diagnosis of *C. trachomatis* infection during the past decade has been the introduction of NAATs. These tests have high sensitivity, perhaps even detecting 10% to 20% more cases than is possible with culture, while retaining high specificity.[28] Three commercially available NAATs are approved by the FDA and available in the United States: polymerase chain reaction (PCR), transcription-mediated amplification (TMA), and strand displacement amplification (SDA).[77,83] PCR and SDA are DNA amplification tests; both use primers that target gene sequences on the cryptogenic *C. trachomatis* plasmid, which has approximately 10 copies per cell. TMA is an RNA amplification assay. NAATs that are commercially available have FDA approval for cervical and vaginal swabs from women, urethral swabs from men, and urine samples from men and women. Several studies have demonstrated that self-collected vaginal swabs also are suitable specimens.[28,77,83] *C. trachomatis* DNA and RNA may persist for 9 or more days after treatment.[56]

Even though culture is considered the gold standard for detection of *C. trachomatis* in children being evaluated for suspected sexual abuse, *C. trachomatis* culture is not standardized or regulated in any way. Sensitivity may vary significantly across laboratories. Enzyme immunoassays (EIAs) are not acceptable as confirmatory tests and have been associated with false-positive results, especially when used with vaginal and rectal specimens.[79,73,145] The methods used for culture confirmation became an issue when several large commercial laboratories started using an EIA instead of fluorescent antibody staining and visual identification of inclusions for culture confirmation. This has resulted in at least one "outbreak" of *C. trachomatis* infection in the evaluation of suspected sexual abuse among residents and staff of an institution for those with intellectual disabilities in Ohio in 1990.[79,74] All of the "positive" cultures, mostly rectal specimens, were subsequently determined to be false-positive cultures resulting from carryover of fecal material and bacteria in the culture specimens. The major advantage of culture is that it is 100% specific; however, because confirmation depends on visual identification of inclusions, a subjective component exists that could lead to misidentification of artifacts as chlamydial inclusions. This appears to have happened in two pseudo outbreaks in other states, one in a residential institution[69] and one among children being evaluated for suspected sexual abuse.[162] In the latter, specimens for culture were outsourced to a commercial laboratory.

NAATs are not currently approved for the detection of *C. trachomatis* in rectogenital specimens or urine from prepubertal children and in rectal specimens from adults.[28,77] Several studies, predominantly from MSM, found NAATs to be sensitive and specific for detection of rectal chlamydial infection. Data on the use of NAATs for vaginal specimens or urine from children are very limited.[28,77,80] To date, four studies have been published comparing NAATs to *C. trachomatis* culture in children being evaluated for suspected sexual abuse.[18,61,60,101,122] They include the recent multicenter study by Black and colleagues[18,19] that evaluated SDA and TMA. Girardet and colleagues[61] and Kellogg and associates[101] primarily evaluated girls, most of whom were postpubertal. Both studies used ligase chain reaction (LCR), which is no longer manufactured. Kellogg and associates[101] also evaluated PCR in addition to LCR. These studies had major limitations, including failure to use an independent reference standard in estimating test performance, failure to separately analyze test performance by age and gender, and the fact that most of the girls were postpubertal and many were sexually active. The ages of the children ranged from 1 month to 17 years, with a mean age of 8.6 years, and 82.4% were female. Anatomic sites tested included vagina, cervix, rectum, pharynx, male urethra, and urine. The overall prevalence of *C. trachomatis* infection in these studies ranged from 6.6% to 8.3% by LCR or PCR and 0.8% to 5.3% by culture. Many discrepant results were found, especially between culture and NAATs, which were more frequent with rectal specimens, but the numbers of specimens from nongenital sites was too small to accurately assess the performance of the assays at these sites.

A CDC-sponsored multicenter study also evaluated the use of SDA and TMA using urine and genital swabs (vagina and urethra) in contrast to culture for diagnosis of *C. trachomatis* in children from birth to 13 years of age.[19] Cultures for *C. trachomatis* were performed at the laboratories of each center, according to their own protocols. Culture protocols at all sites included the isolation of *C. trachomatis* in cycloheximide-pretreated McCoy cells, in shell vials or 24-well or 96-well tissue culture plates. The fixed monolayers were stained to detect chlamydial inclusions with fluorescein-conjugated *Chlamydia* genus–specific or *C. trachomatis* species–specific monoclonal antibodies. All samples were processed and tested according to manufacturers' protocols, except for the TMA tests, which were performed on previously frozen urine or swabs collected in BD ProbeTec sample collection medium. Test results that were positive by SDA for *C. trachomatis* were confirmed using in-house PCR targeting the *ompA* gene performed at the CDC. Of 485 female participants, 15 (3.1%) had a positive result for *C. trachomatis* by any test (1.4% by culture; 2.3% by vaginal NAAT; 2.7% by urine NAAT). All participants who had a positive vaginal culture for *C. trachomatis* also had positive urine NAAT. Two girls had positive *C. trachomatis* cultures from rectal swab specimens, but negative vaginal swab specimens by both culture and NAATs and negative urine NAATs. No discrepant results were found in any of the participants tested by SDA and TMA for *C. trachomatis*. All *C. trachomatis*–positive results were confirmed by DNA sequence genotyping. The sensitivity of vaginal culture for *C. trachomatis* was 39% in all girls studied. In contrast, the sensitivities of urine and vaginal swab NAATs were 100% and 85% in all female children, respectively, for detection of *C. trachomatis*. The 2015 CDC Sexually Transmitted Diseases Treatment Guidelines recommend that NAATs can be used for detection of *C. trachomatis* in girls being evaluated for suspected sexual abuse, with important limitations[28,159]:

1. Because the prevalence of *C. trachomatis* in this population is low, additional testing is probably necessary.
2. Extrapolation cannot be made from these results to other NAATs or used in specimens other than vagina and urine in girls.
3. Specimens should be retained for further testing.

Some available commercial NAATs, such as TMA (Aptima Combo 2 Assay), offer an alternative target confirmation method that can be used on the same testing platform; however, no data exist on the use of this confirmatory test in this setting. Additional options include sending blinded specimens to an independent or reference laboratory for confirmation testing, confirming an NAAT-positive result by culture test (requires a separate, invasive specimen), or using a second, alternative technology commercial NAAT. Specimens collected from children for forensic applications should be retained in the laboratory for purposes of additional testing, in accordance with local policies and procedures and recent recommendations by the CDC.[28] Several new NAATs have been approved by the FDA for use in adolescents and adults but are not approved for use in children. Limited data suggest that they should perform as well as TMA and SDA in vaginal and urine specimens from children.[31]

Treatment

Chlamydial infections in older children may be treated with oral erythromycin 50 mg/kg per day orally four times daily, with a maximum of 2 g/day for 7 to 14 days.[28] Children older than 8 years may be treated with tetracycline 25 to 50 mg/kg per day orally four times daily for 7 days. Azithromycin 1 g orally as a single dose also may be used in children who weigh at least 45 kg, are 8 years or older, or both.[28] However, there are no data on the optimum dose or efficacy of the recommended regimens of azithromycin in children. Follow-up is extremely important to ensure that the infection has been effectively treated. One must also be careful to exclude possible reinfection.

The first-line treatment regimen recommended by the CDC for uncomplicated *C. trachomatis* genital infection in men and nonpregnant women is azithromycin 1 g orally as a single dose or doxycycline 100 mg orally twice daily for 7 days. Alternative regimens are erythromycin base 500 mg orally four times daily for 7 days, erythromycin ethylsuccinate 800 mg orally four times daily for 7 days, and levofloxacin 500 mg orally once daily for 7 days. The high erythromycin dosages may not be well tolerated. Doxycycline and ofloxacin or levofloxacin are contraindicated in pregnant women; quinolones are contraindicated in persons younger than 18 years. However, use of levofloxacin offers no advantages over doxycycline. For pregnant women, the recommended treatment regimen is also single-dose azithromycin. Alternative regimens are erythromycin base 500 mg orally twice daily for 7 days, amoxicillin 500 mg orally three times daily for 7 days, erythromycin base 250 mg orally four times daily for 14 days, and erythromycin ethylsuccinate 800 mg orally four times daily for 7 days or 400 mg orally four times daily for 14 days. Amoxicillin at this dosage is as effective as azithromycin or any of the erythromycin regimens and is much better tolerated.

INFECTION CAUSED BY *CHLAMYDIA PSITTACI*

Human infection with *C. psittaci* was described first probably by Juergensen in 1874 or Ritter in 1876. Ritter described seven cases of an unusual pneumonia that appeared to be caused by parrots and finches that were caged in the study of his brother's home in Switzerland. After these reports, several outbreaks of a similar disease in Europe established the association with exposure to birds. The term *psittacosis* was coined by Morange in 1892 from the Greek word for parrots, *psittakos.*

Organism

C. psittaci is a diverse species that affects psittacine and nonpsittacine birds.[2] The known host range includes 470 avian species.[27,30,87,140] Birds that have been reported to have *C. psittaci* infection contain six major domestic species: chickens, turkeys, Pekin ducks, Muscovy ducks, geese, and pigeons. Infections in these species have been associated with significant outbreaks in humans.[26,30,164] In the past, chlamydial infection in psittacine birds was termed *psittacosis,* whereas disease in wild and domestic fowl was called *ornithosis.* However, because *C. psittaci* strains isolated from psittacine or nonpsittacine species have been shown to produce identical disease in birds of either grouping, this distinction is artificial. The more universally applicable term *chlamydiosis* can be usefully employed to describe chlamydial infections of all animal species. New molecular assays using different gene targets have identified two new avian *Chlamydia* species, *C. avium* and *C. gallinacea.*[67,166] Both may have zoonotic potential in humans. *C. gallinacea* has been identified in chicken flocks in several European countries as well as Australia and China. Detection of infection with these species in humans may require development of new diagnostic tests because available EIA assays for *C. psittaci* will not detect antibodies to *C. avium* and *C. gallinacea.*[166]

Epidemiology

Chlamydial infections in birds represent a biologic hazard to human health and economic loss to the poultry industry.[27,30,164] *C. psittaci* has been recovered from symptomatic and apparently healthy birds. Infection principally involves the gastrointestinal tract, and the chlamydiae are shed in feces or through infectious respiratory tract discharges.[174] Clinically inapparent, latent infections may be the predominant state. Overt clinical disease may be activated by stress factors, including overcrowding, poor nutrition, other bacterial and viral infections, and transportation.

Apparently healthy birds shedding chlamydiae can infect other birds or humans through contact. Infectious chlamydiae in respiratory secretions or feces may remain viable for several months. Transmission of disease is mainly through aerosols of fecal or feather dust, but oral infection is an alternative route. Transmission through eggs has been shown in chickens, ducks, seagulls, and psittacine birds.[174] However, most infected eggs do not hatch. In the nest, parent birds may infect their young, which may carry the infectious agent for many years. Young birds are more susceptible to infection than are older birds, and some species seem to be more susceptible than others. Often, disease carriers may be identified by the transmission of disease to other susceptible birds or by the sudden death of young nestlings with apparently healthy parents.[152]

From 2003 through 2010, 94 human cases of psittacosis were reported to the CDC, a dramatic decrease from 935 cases reported from 1998 to 2003.[30] Eighty-five percent of cases of psittacosis in the United States were associated with exposure to birds; 70% of these reported cases were the result of exposure to caged pet birds.[164] Individuals at highest risk for acquiring psittacosis included bird owners or fanciers and pet shop employees. Since 1984, several major outbreaks of psittacosis have occurred in the United States in turkey-processing plants, in which approximately 300 persons were infected. Workers exposed to turkey viscera were at the highest risk for acquiring infection.[27,87] In 1995, the CDC investigated an outbreak of avian chlamydiosis in a shipment of more than 700 pet birds from a Florida bird distributor to the Atlanta area.[133] Affected birds included parrots, parakeets, finches, lovebirds, cockatiels, conures, and canaries. Clinical psittacosis or serologic evidence of *C. psittaci* infection was found in 30.7% of households with birds from the infected flock. An average of 21 days (range, 1–47 days) elapsed between purchase of the bird and the onset of symptoms. Most of the infected individuals had mild or asymptomatic illnesses. Among persons in exposed households, illness occurred more frequently if the recently purchased bird had become sick or had died. Kissing or nuzzling, handling, and feeding the bird all were significantly associated with the development of clinical psittacosis, but in contrast to earlier studies, cleaning the bird's cage was not. The risk for acquiring clinical psittacosis varied significantly by type of bird to which the individual was exposed. The attack rate was highest for individuals exposed to parrots.

Inhalation of infectious aerosols derived from the feces, fecal dust, or secretions of *C. psittaci*–infected animals is thought to be the primary route of infection. The source birds can be infected asymptomatically or can show signs of infection, such as anorexia, ruffled feathers, depression, and watery green droppings. Psittacosis frequently is a systemic infection in birds, and the turkey strains can induce severe pericarditis.[174]

Psittacosis is an uncommon occurrence in children. In a series of 135 cases from Australia observed during a 15-year period, the youngest patient was 17 years of age.[182] Children may be less likely to be exposed to birds. Bird keeping is more commonly a hobby of adults, and the parents are the ones who usually clean the cage of the family's pet bird. An outbreak of psittacosis involving two adolescents was reported from a small village in Scotland. The source of the infection appeared to be the local pet shop, which had taken delivery of four lovebirds, two of which died shortly after arrival.[134]

Clinical Manifestations

Infection with *C. psittaci* in humans may range from clinically inapparent to severe infection involving multiple organ systems, as well as pneumonia.[10,54,133,182] Symptomatic *C. psittaci* infection in humans may present as two forms: a severe atypical pneumonia or pneumonitis and a systemic toxic or septic form without respiratory involvement. In both cases, fever, chills, muscle aches and pains, and severe headache are typical. Other manifestations may be diarrhea, nausea, and vomiting. The mean incubation period is 15 days after exposure (range, 5–21 days). The onset usually is abrupt, with complaints of fever, cough, and headache. The fever is high and frequently associated with rigors and sweats. The headache can be so severe that meningitis can be considered a possibility; 33% of patients in the Australian series underwent lumbar puncture.[182] The cough usually is nonproductive, and rales may be heard on auscultation. Chest radiographs generally are abnormal, with variable infiltrates. Pleural effusions also may be present. In contrast, most of the individuals in the Atlanta outbreak had very mild disease characterized by fever, headache, and cough.[133]

Laboratory Findings

The white blood cell count usually is not elevated, but mild leukocytosis may be present. Almost 50% of patients in the Australian series had abnormal liver function test results, including elevated levels of aspartate aminotransferase, alkaline phosphatase, and bilirubin.[182]

Diagnosis

The CDC and the Council of State and Territorial Epidemiologists have established national case definitions for epidemiologic surveillance of psittacosis. The updated case definitions were published in 2010.[164] A patient is considered to have a confirmed case of psittacosis if clinical illness is compatible with psittacosis and the case is laboratory confirmed by one of two methods: isolation of *C. psittaci* from respiratory specimens (e.g., sputum, pleural fluid, or tissue) or blood, or a fourfold or greater increase in antibody (immunoglobulin G [IgG]) against *C. psittaci* by complement fixation or microimmunofluorescence (MIF) between paired acute- and convalescent-phase serum specimens obtained at least 2 to 4 weeks apart. A patient is considered to have a probable case of psittacosis if the clinical illness is compatible with psittacosis and one of the two following laboratory results is present: supportive serology (e.g., *C. psittaci* antibody titer [IgM] of 32 or greater in at least one serum specimen obtained after onset of symptoms) or detection of *C. psittaci* DNA in a respiratory specimen (e.g., sputum, pleural fluid, or tissue) through amplification of a specific target by PCR assay.

Most diagnoses are established by clinical presentation and positive antibodies against *C. psittaci* in paired sera using MIF methods. The MIF is more sensitive and specific than the previously used complement fixation tests; however, some cross-reactivity occurs with other chlamydiae (i.e., *C. pneumoniae, C. trachomatis,* and *C. felis),* so a titer result less than 1:128 should be interpreted with caution.[175] Acute-phase serum specimens should be obtained as soon as possible after the onset of symptoms, and convalescent-phase serum specimens should be obtained at least 2 weeks after the first specimen. Because antimicrobial treatment can delay or diminish the antibody response, a third serum sample

4 to 6 weeks after the acute sample might help confirm the diagnosis. To increase the reliability of serologic results, acute and convalescent sera should be analyzed simultaneously at the same laboratory.

C. psittaci also can be isolated from the patient's sputum, pleural fluid, or clotted blood during acute illness and before treatment with antimicrobial agents. Although *C. psittaci* will grow in the same culture systems used for the isolation of *C. trachomatis* and *C. pneumoniae,* very few laboratories culture for *C. psittaci,* mainly because of the potential biohazard.

Real-time PCR (rt-PCR) assays have been developed for use in the detection of *C. psittaci* in respiratory specimens.[10,125] These assays can distinguish *C. psittaci* from other chlamydial species and identify different *C. psittaci* genotypes. Although the assays appear to be highly sensitive and specific in avian samples, they have not yet been validated for use in human samples. Because proper sample collection techniques and handling are critical to obtain accurate test results, clinical laboratories performing these tests should be contacted directly for specifics on specimen submission.

Information about laboratory testing is available from state public health departments. Few commercial laboratories provide MIF testing, and manufacturing problems in 2009 resulted in limited availability of the MIF testing kits. Certain laboratories accept human specimens to confirm *C. psittaci* infection through culture, MIF, or PCR (Table 194.2).

Treatment

The recommended treatment of psittacosis in adults and children older than 8 years of age is tetracycline 500 mg orally four times daily for 7 to 10 days.[168] Erythromycin 50 mg/kg per day up to 2 g/day, for 7 to 10 days also can be used. The experience in the Australian series[182] and anecdotal reports suggest that tetracycline may be more effective than erythromycin. The initial infection does not appear to be followed by long-term immunity. Reinfection and clinical disease can develop within 2 months of treatment; two well-documented cases of reinfection are reported in the literature. A pet shop employee had two episodes of psittacosis 11 months apart. Each episode met the CDC's confirmed case definition.[26]

INFECTION CAUSED BY *CHLAMYDIA PNEUMONIAE*

Organism

The first isolates of *C. pneumoniae* were obtained serendipitously during trachoma studies in the 1960s.[64] After the recovery of a similar isolate from the respiratory tract of a college student,[66,169] the designation TWAR was applied, which refers to the first two isolates, TW-183 and AR-39. On the basis of inclusion morphology and staining characteristics in cell culture, *C. pneumoniae* initially was considered a *C. psittaci* strain. Subsequent analysis, however, has demonstrated that this organism is distinct from both *C. psittaci* and *C. trachomatis.*[24,65] Sequencing has revealed that *C. pneumoniae* differs significantly from *C. trachomatis* in several areas. *C. pneumoniae* encodes 21 polymorphic membrane proteins versus 9 in *C. trachomatis.* Polymorphic membrane proteins may be surface exposed in *C. pneumoniae.*[96,151] Ultrastructural studies have demonstrated an elementary body morphology distinct from that of *C. trachomatis* and *C. psittaci* (Fig. 194.2).[34] However, some isolates of *C. pneumoniae,* including IOL-207, have been found to have round elementary bodies.[25,141,144] Thus it may not be a consistent species characteristic. At this point, a strain-typing system for *C. pneumoniae* has not been developed. A plasmid has been detected in a single isolate obtained from a horse but not from any human isolate of *C. pneumoniae.*

Epidemiology

C. pneumoniae appears to be a common human respiratory pathogen. The organism also has been isolated from nonhuman mammalian species, including a horse, koalas, bandicoots, and reptiles and amphibians, although the role these infections may play in human disease is unknown.[22,48,94,96,110,129,146] The animal isolates are diverse and have DNA sequences that differ slightly from human *C. pneumoniae* isolates.[127] It

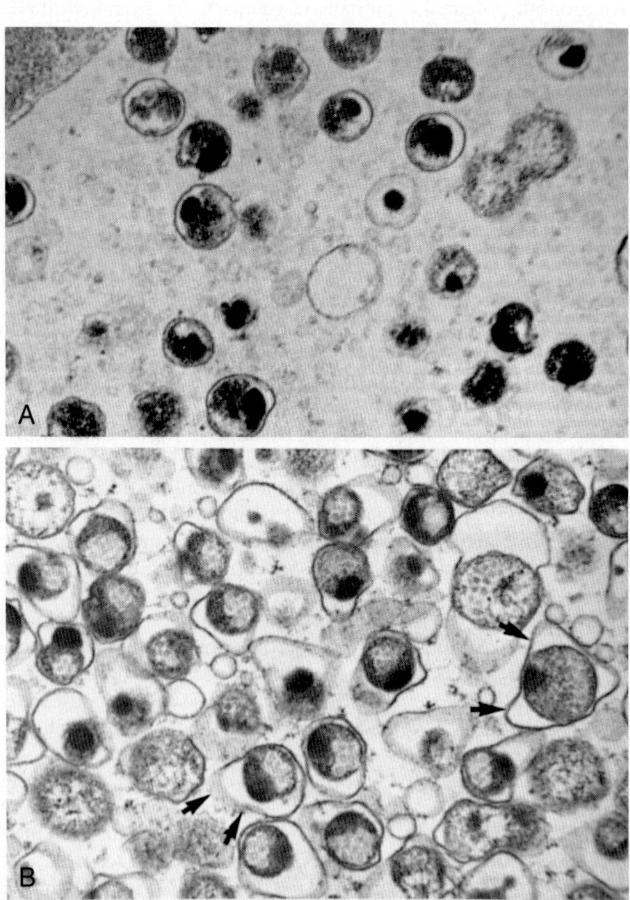

FIG. 194.2 Electron micrographs of (A) *Chlamydia trachomatis* and (B) *Chlamydia pneumoniae* inclusions demonstrating the morphology of the elementary body. The elementary bodies of *C. pneumoniae* have a pear shape because of a loose periplasmic membrane *(arrows),* unlike the typically round elementary bodies of *C. trachomatis* and *C. psittaci.*

TABLE 194.2 Laboratories That Test Human Specimens for *Chlamydia psittaci*[164]

Laboratory	Tests Performed	Contact Information
Focus Diagnostics Inc. (Quest subsidiary), Cypress, CA	Culture, MIF (IgM, IgA, IgG)	800-445-4032 http://www.focusdx.com
Laboratory Corporation of America, Burlington, NC	Culture, MIF (IgM, IgG)	800-222-7566 http://www.labcorp.com
Quest Diagnostics, Valencia, CA	MIF (IgM, IgG, IgA)	800-421-7110 http://www.specialtylabs.com
ViroMed Laboratories Minnetonka, MN	Culture, MIF (IgG, IgM)	800-582-0077 http://www.viromed.com
Response and Surveillance Laboratory, Respiratory Diseases Branch, CDC Atlanta, GA[a]	MIF (requires paired sera), PCR, culture, genotyping (multiple specimen types)	404-639-4921

[a]Centers for Disease Control and Prevention (CDC) is a reference laboratory; samples must be submitted through State Health Departments.
MIF, Microimmunofluorescence; *PCR,* polymerase chain reaction.

TABLE 194.3 **Selected Studies of *Chlamydia pneumoniae* Lower Respiratory Tract Infection in Children**

				NO. TESTED/NO. POSITIVE RESULTS (%)			
Study	**Year**	**Country**	**Age**	**No.**	**Culture**	**PCR**	**Serology**
Saikku et al.[156]	1988	Philippines	<5 y	220	ND	ND	14 (6.4)
Forgie et al.[51]	1991	Gambia	1-9 y	74	ND	ND	9 (12.1)
Jantos et al.[98]	1995	Germany	2 d–15 y	290	1 (0.3)	2/290 (0.7)	2/101 (2)
Block et al.[21]	1995	United States	3-12 y	260	34 (13)	ND	48 (18.5)
Harris et al.[84,85]	1998	United States	6 mo–16 y	456	31 (7.3)	ND	37 (8.8)
Principi et al.[146]	2001	Italy	2–14 y	613	ND	48 (7.8)	52 (11.4)
Baer et al.[7]	2003	Switzerland	1–18 y	50	1 (2)	1 (2)	2 (4)
Likitnukul et al.[117]	2003	Thailand	1 mo–18 y	333	ND	ND	149 (44.7)
Tsolia et al.[172]	2004	Greece	5–14 y	75	ND	0	2 (3)
Michelow et al.[126]	2004	United States	6 wk–18 y	154	ND	ND	14 (9)
Liu et al.[119]	2005	China	≤5 y	85	ND	4 (2.2)	ND

ND, Not done; *PCR,* polymerase chain reaction.

has been hypothesized that human *C. pneumoniae* may be zoonotic in origin.[127,129,135,137] Human isolates have been found to be relatively uniform.[19] Currently no strain typing system has been developed for *C. pneumoniae.* The mode of transmission remains unclear but probably involves infected respiratory tract secretions. Acquisition of infection by droplet aerosol was described during a laboratory accident.[89] *C. pneumoniae* can remain viable on Formica countertops for 30 hours and can survive small-particle aerosolization.[50,164] Spread of *C. pneumoniae* within families and enclosed populations such as military recruits and prisoners has been described. Outbreaks among these populations appear to becoming more frequent.[49,102,105,178] In contrast, the proportion of community-acquired pneumonia associated with *C. pneumoniae* infection in adults has ranged from 0% to 19%, varying with the geographic location, the age group examined, and the diagnostic methods used.* Three studies published after 2010, from diverse geographic areas (Europe, Africa, and Thailand), that used rt-PCR found prevalence of *C. pneumoniae* infection ranging from 0% to 3.8%.[43,99,104,160] This was compared with 11.4% in a Chinese study published in 2012 that only used MIF serology; 30% of the patients only had a single serum sample.[167]

Studies of the role of *C. pneumoniae* in lower respiratory tract infections in pediatric populations have found evidence of infection in 0.3% to more than 44% (Table 194.3). Most of these studies relied entirely on serology for diagnosis. Early studies that relied on serology suggested that infection in children younger than 5 years was rare[112,177]; however, in a study of Filipino children younger than 5 years with lower respiratory tract infection, nearly 10% had either acute or chronic antibody to *C. pneumoniae.*[152] In Brooklyn, the proportion of lower respiratory tract infections associated with *C. pneumoniae,* as determined by culture, increased from 9% in children younger than 5 years to 19% in children and adolescents 5 to 16 years of age.[35]

Studies that have used culture or PCR have found a poor correlation with serology, especially in children.[21,46,57,58,83,111,113] Although 7% to 13% of children 6 months to 16 years of age enrolled in two multicenter pneumonia treatment studies were culture positive and 7% to 18% met the serologic criteria for acute infection with the MIF test, they were not the same patients.[21,83] Only 1% to 3% of the culture-positive children met the serologic criteria, and approximately 70% were seronegative.

Prolonged culture positivity lasting several weeks to several years after acute infection has been reported.[35,46,75] Asymptomatic nasopharyngeal carriage also occurs in 2% to 5% of adults and children.[20,46,62,90,91,109] The role that asymptomatic carriage plays in the epidemiology of *C. pneumoniae* is not known, but possibly these persons could serve as a reservoir for spread of infection.

*References 7, 21, 51, 77, 111, 114, 115, 117, 124, 127, 144, 152, 155, 169, 170, 172, 177, 179.

Clinical Manifestations

Most *C. pneumoniae* respiratory infections are mild or asymptomatic. Longitudinal serologic data obtained during an epidemic among military recruits in Finland suggest that only approximately 10% of infections result in clinically apparent pneumonia.[102,105] Initial reports emphasized mild atypical pneumonia clinically resembling that associated with *Mycoplasma pneumoniae.*[63,64,153,156] In several subsequent studies, however, pneumonia associated with *C. pneumoniae* was clinically indistinguishable from other pneumonias.[21,83,85] Coinfection with other pathogens, especially *M. pneumoniae, Streptococcus pneumoniae,* and viruses, is frequent.[21,83,85,165,169] In one multicenter pneumonia treatment study, 20% of the children with positive *C. pneumoniae* cultures were coinfected with *M. pneumoniae;* they could not be distinguished from children who were infected with either organism alone.[21] In these cases, *C. pneumoniae* may not be the primary cause of the pneumonia but might disrupt the normal clearance mechanisms and enable other pathogens to invade. This may have been the case in an outbreak of pneumonia and fatal pneumococcal meningitis among US Army trainees.[40] Six of 12 trainees with pneumonia were infected with *C. pneumoniae,* which suggested a simultaneous outbreak of both infections. *C. pneumoniae* has been associated with severe illness and even death, although the role of preexisting chronic conditions as contributing factors in many of these patients is difficult to assess. In some cases, however, *C. pneumoniae* clearly appears to be implicated as a serious pathogen, even in the absence of underlying disease. *C. pneumoniae* was isolated from the respiratory tract and the pleural fluid of a previously healthy adolescent boy with severe pneumonia complicated by respiratory tract failure and pleural effusions (Fig. 194.3).[5]

C. pneumoniae appeared to be responsible for 14% to 19% of episodes of acute chest syndrome in children with sickle cell disease.[41,111,126,128] *C. pneumoniae* infection in these patients appeared to be associated with more severe hypoxia than was infection with *M. pneumoniae.*

C. pneumoniae may act as an inflammatory trigger for asthma. Several cases of culture-documented *C. pneumoniae* infection in patients with significant bronchospasm have been reported.[70,75] Asthmatic bronchitis was diagnosed in one patient who was receiving systemic and inhaled steroids.[75] This patient did not improve until her chlamydial infection was treated. Hahn and associates[70] reported an association between serologic evidence of acute *C. pneumoniae* infection and wheezing in adults seen for lower respiratory tract illness. However, they were able to isolate the organism from only one of 365 patients. As part of a study in children, *C. pneumoniae* was isolated from 13 of 118 children (11%) 5 to 15 years of age who were evaluated initially for either new or acute exacerbations of asthma.[46] Treatment of the infection appeared to result in both clinical improvement and improvement in pulmonary function test scores. Only five of the children with confirmed infection had detectable IgG antibody to *C. pneumoniae.* One child who did not comply with his antibiotic therapy was culture positive on five occasions during a 3-month period. Anti–*C. pneumoniae* antibody as determined

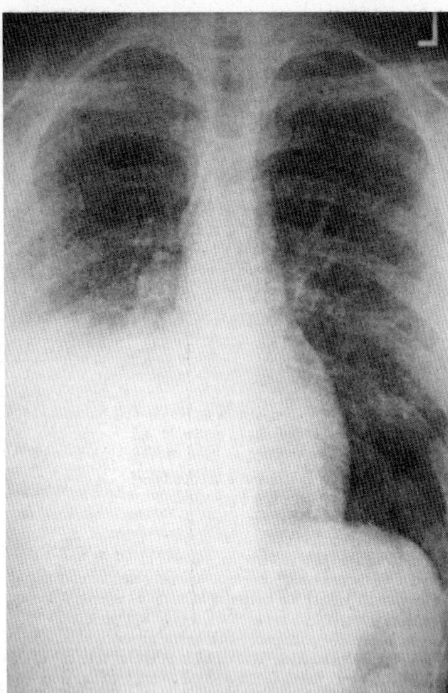

FIG. 194.3 Chest radiograph of a 19-year-old man with *Chlamydia pneumoniae* pneumonia demonstrating pleural effusion in the right lung. *C. pneumoniae* was isolated from the pleural fluid. (From Augenbraun MH, Roblin PM, Mandel LJ, et al. *Chlamydia pneumoniae* pneumonia with pleural effusion: diagnosis by culture. *Am J Med.* 1991;91:437-438.)

by MIF was never detected. Specific anti–*C. pneumoniae* IgE was, however, detected in 85.7% of the culture-positive asthmatic patients in contrast to 9% of the children with *C. pneumoniae* pneumonia who were not wheezing.[47] This finding suggests that the bronchial reactivity seen with *C. pneumoniae* infection may be IgE mediated. The potential prolonged, persistent *C. pneumoniae* infection may produce chronic inflammation and trigger bronchospasm in susceptible persons. *C. pneumoniae* has been demonstrated to induce in vitro ciliostasis in ciliated bronchial epithelial cells.[157,161] Animal studies also suggest that steroids can reactivate *C. pneumoniae* lung infection in mice.[119] In addition, immune-mediated phenomena, including erythema nodosum and iritis, have been described as complicating *C. pneumoniae* infection.[163,165,175,177]

The role of *C. pneumoniae* in upper respiratory tract infections is not as well defined. *C. pneumoniae* has been isolated from the middle ear fluid of children and adults with otitis media.[20,137-139] Block and colleagues[20] recovered *C. pneumoniae* from the middle ear fluid of eight children, 3 months to 14 years of age, with acute otitis media. *C. pneumoniae* was the sole pathogen isolated in two patients. Copathogens in the remaining six patients included β-lactamase–positive *Haemophilus influenzae* and *Moraxella catarrhalis,* along with penicillin-resistant and penicillin-sensitive *S. pneumoniae.* Five of the children who tested positive for *C. pneumoniae* responded favorably despite not being treated with antibiotics active against the organism, either a course of an oral β-lactam or single-dose intramuscular ceftriaxone. Symptoms suggestive of sinus involvement are not uncommon in patients with upper respiratory tract infection associated with *C. pneumoniae,* but only one case of isolation of the organism, from a 47-year-old man with sinusitis, has been reported.[85,86] Cultrara and colleagues[39] examined nasopharyngeal swabs, ethmoid and maxillary sinus biopsy samples, and adenoids from 20 children, 3 to 16 years of age, with chronic sinusitis. *C. pneumoniae* was not isolated from any sinus tissue but was isolated from the nasopharyngeal swab and adenoid tissue of a 6-year-old. The results of this study suggest that *C. pneumoniae* does not play a significant role in chronic sinusitis in children.

Diagnosis

A specific laboratory diagnosis of *C. pneumoniae* infection can be made by isolation of the organism from nasopharyngeal or throat swabs, sputum, or pleural fluid, if present. The nasopharynx appears to be the optimal site for isolation of the organism.[21] *C. pneumoniae* grows readily in cell lines derived from respiratory tract tissue, specifically HEp-2 and HL cells.[147,149] Culture with an initial inoculation and one passage can take 4 to 7 days.

Nasopharyngeal cultures can be obtained with Dacron-tipped, wire-shafted swabs. Each lot of swabs should be treated in a mock infection system to ensure that no inhibitory effects occur on either the viability of cells or recovery of chlamydiae. Specimens for culture should be placed in appropriate transport media, usually a sucrose phosphate buffer with antibiotics and fetal calf serum, and stored immediately at 4°C (39.2°F) for no longer than 24 hours. Viability decreases if specimens are held at room temperature. If the specimen cannot be processed within 24 hours, it should be frozen at −70°C (−94°F) until culture can be performed. After 72 hours of incubation, culture confirmation can be performed by staining with either a *C. pneumoniae* species–specific or a *Chlamydia* genus–specific (anti-LPS) fluorescein-conjugated monoclonal antibody.[129,130,131,147,149] Unfortunately, no commercially produced *C. pneumoniae*–specific culture-confirmation reagents are available. If a genus-specific antibody is used, *C. pneumoniae* should be confirmed by differential staining with a specific *C. trachomatis* antibody; if that result is negative, the isolate is either *C. pneumoniae* or *C. psittaci.* If the patient has not had avian exposure, psittacosis would be highly unlikely.

The most common method still used by investigators for the diagnosis of *C. pneumoniae* infection is serologic testing. Assays available for detection of *C. pneumoniae*–specific antibodies include MIF tests, enzyme-linked immunosorbent assays (ELISAs), and EIAs, each of which exists in a variety of in-house and commercial versions.[171] MIF is considered by the CDC to be the only currently acceptable serologic test, and therefore it is considered to be the reference standard for serodiagnosis, despite significant limitations.[42] The recommendations proposed by the CDC[42] in 2001 defined the criteria for serologic diagnosis of acute *C. pneumoniae* infection as a single IgM titer of 1 : 16 or greater or a fourfold increase in the IgG titer, as determined by MIF testing. The use of single IgG titers was discouraged. However, not only is the literature replete with studies that deviate widely from the proposed guidelines[112] but also several limitations exist that are inherent for serodiagnosis of *C. pneumoniae* infection, even when these guidelines are observed. The MIF assay has been repeatedly and conclusively demonstrated to be insensitive and have poor correlation with the detection of the organism by culture or PCR assay, particularly for children.[58,112] Seventy percent of children 6 months to 16 years of age in two multicenter pneumonia treatment studies and 7 of 12 (58.3%) children 5 to 16 years of age with acute wheezing who had culture-documented infection had seronegative results by MIF test.[21,46,83,84] Only 1% to 3% of culture-positive children in the former study and 25% in the latter met the serologic criteria for acute infection. Most of the children remained seronegative, even after 3 months of follow-up.[46]

Background rates of seropositivity also can be high in some populations. Hyman and associates,[91,92] as part of a study of asymptomatic *C. pneumoniae* infection in subjectively healthy adults in Brooklyn, found 81% to have IgG or IgM titers of 16 or higher. Seventeen percent had evidence of "acute infection" (i.e., IgG titer ≥512, IgM titer ≥16, or both). However, none of these persons was culture or PCR positive. Similar results were reported by Kern and associates[103] in healthy firefighters and policemen in Rhode Island. Some IgG antibody may result from a heterotypic response to other chlamydial species because cross-reactions with MOMP occur among the three species, as do cross-reactions caused by the genus LPS antigen. Moss and colleagues[135] reported that antibodies to *C. pneumoniae* and *C. psittaci* were found in as many as half of all chlamydial IgG–positive persons attending an STI clinic. This point is reinforced by the observation that studies from the early 1980s suggesting *C. trachomatis* as a cause of community-acquired pneumonia and pharyngitis in adults and children were probably detecting antibody to *C. pneumoniae* rather than *C. trachomatis*[59,105,106,108,142] or, in one outbreak in a boys school, *C. psittaci.*[140] Other organisms that have been reported as possibly causing cross-reactions on MIF are *Bartonella*[121,123] and *Bordetella pertussis.*[93,95] The latter could be significant because older children and adolescents with pertussis frequently have a chronic cough or severe bronchitis, which is a clinical feature often ascribed to *C. pneumoniae*. Other studies have found significant homology between human and *C. pneumoniae* heat shock protein 60 (HSP-60) and *Escherichia coli* GroEL.[136,138]

Moreover, the MIF test is not standardized, and reading of the slides has a large subjective component and requires an experienced microscopist. Littman and associates[118] evaluated the interlaboratory reliability of the MIF test for measurement of *C. pneumoniae*–specific IgA and IgG titers for 392 serum samples, using reagents and antigens obtained from a common source. The investigators reported the exact agreement of IgA and IgG titers to be 55% and 38%, respectively, and the agreement within a twofold dilution to be 75% and 66%, respectively. EIAs may overcome some of the limitations of the MIF test by being objective and less technically complex. However, the CDC did not endorse any EIA, pending demonstration of adequate sensitivity and specificity in contrast to the MIF test. None of the currently available EIAs has FDA approval. Herrmann and colleagues[88] compared seven commercial EIAs or ELISAs (one of which was genus-specific) with four MIF assays for detection of specific IgG antibodies, using serum samples from 80 healthy subjects; they reported sensitivities and specificities ranging from 88% to 100% and from 42% to 100%, respectively. Similar results have been reported by others with the same assays in different populations, including children.[111,120,139,170,171,173]

Multiple in-house NAAT methodologies (such as PCR) have been published, but the literature has been confounded by lack of standardization and validation. In 2000, a CDC workshop suggested a few assays that were considered to be validated enough to be used for research.[42] The advantages of these NAAT or PCR assays are their sensitivity, decreased possibility of contamination, and ability to quantify DNA. More than a decade later, however, many of these tests turned out to be highly prone to false-positive results.[4] Numerous in-house PCR-based tests still are performed, but these assays range from those that are well validated to those that are not validated at all. Although NAATs offer the promise of exquisite sensitivity, theoretically allowing detection of a single organism in a clinical sample, both false-negative and false-positive results can and do occur because of a large number of technical issues that were summarized recently.[4] Currently, rt-PCR technology for the detection of *C. pneumoniae* should be used.[15] rt-PCR offers significant advantages over conventional PCR in its rapidity, the ease with which it can be automated, the potential decreased risk for carryover contamination, and the potential provision of a quantitative result.

Until recently, there have been no commercially available NAAT assays. BioFire Technologies (formerly Idaho Technologies) developed a FilmArray assay for the detection of 17 viruses, which is FDA cleared.[143] The FilmArray system now includes assays on the same platform for some of the atypical agents of pneumonia, including *C. pneumoniae*, *M. pneumoniae*, and *B. pertussis*. This assay received FDA clearance in July 2012. The FilmArray system combines nucleic acid extraction, nested PCR, detection, and data analysis in a single-use pouch. However, data on the performance of this assay for detection of *C. pneumoniae* in clinical settings are limited. Most of the published studies that evaluated the performance of the BioFire FilmArray respiratory panel were limited to respiratory viruses or had very few patients with *C. pneumoniae* infection.[3,33,38,143] Several other similar assays are being developed by other companies.[33]

Treatment

Chlamydia spp. are susceptible to tetracyclines, macrolides, and quinolones.[72,107] *C. pneumoniae*, like *C. psittaci*, is resistant to sulfonamides.[72,107] To date, few published data have described the response of *C. pneumoniae* to antimicrobial therapy. Most of the treatment studies of pneumonia caused by *C. pneumoniae* published thus far have relied entirely on diagnosis by serology; consequently, microbiologic efficacy could not be assessed. Anecdotal reports have suggested that prolonged courses, up to 3 weeks, of either tetracyclines or erythromycin may be needed to eradicate *C. pneumoniae* from the nasopharynx of adults with influenza-like illness and pharyngitis.[75] The results of two pediatric multicenter pneumonia treatment studies found that 10-day courses of erythromycin and clarithromycin and 5 days of azithromycin suspension were equally efficacious; they eradicated the organism in 79% to 86% of children.[21,83,85,148] Quinolones, including levofloxacin and moxifloxacin, also have been demonstrated to have 70% to 80% efficacy in eradicating *C. pneumoniae* from adults with community-acquired pneumonia.[81,82,73] Most patients improved clinically despite persistence of the organism. Persistence does not appear to be secondary to the development of antibiotic resistance because the maximum inhibitory concentrations of the isolates obtained after treatment did not change.[72,73,82,84,107,148,150]

On the basis of these limited data, the following regimens for respiratory tract infection caused by *C. pneumoniae* can be suggested: in adults, doxycycline 100 mg twice daily for 14 to 21 days; tetracycline 250 mg four times daily for 14 to 21 days; azithromycin 1.5 g for 5 days; levofloxacin 500 mg/day orally or intravenously for 7 to 14 days; and moxifloxacin 400 mg/day orally for 10 days. For children, suggested regimens include erythromycin suspension 50 mg/kg per day for 10 to 14 days; clarithromycin suspension 15 mg/kg per day for 10 days; and azithromycin suspension 10 mg/kg on day 1 followed by 5 mg/kg per day once daily on days 2 to 5. Some patients may require retreatment.

NEW REFERENCES SINCE THE SEVENTH EDITION

1. Adachi K, Nielsen-Saines K, Klausner JD. *Chlamydia trachomatis* infection in pregnancy: The global challenge in preventing adverse pregnancy and infant outcomes in Sub-Saharan Africa and Asia. *Biomed Res Int.* 2016;2016:9315757.
3. Andersson ME, Olofsson S, Lindh M. Comparison of the FilmArray assay and in-house real-time PCR for detection of respiratory infection. *Scand J Infect Dis.* 2014;46:897-901.
15. Benitez AJ, Thurman KA, Diaz MH, et al. Comparison of real-time PCR and a microimmunofluorescence serological assay for detection of *Chlamydophila pneumoniae* infection in an outbreak investigation. *J Clin Microbiol.* 2012;50:151-153.
28. Centers for Disease Control and Prevention. Sexually transmitted diseases treatment guidelines. *MMWR Recomm Rep.* 2015;64(RR-3):1-140.
31. Centers for Disease Control and Prevention. Recommendations for the laboratory-based detection of *Chlamydia trachomatis* and *Neisseria gonorrhoeae*—2014. *MMWR.* 2014;63(RR #2):1-24.
33. Chen JH, Lam HY, Yip CC, et al. Clinical evaluation of the new high-throughput Luminex NxTAG respiratory pathogen panel assay for multiplex respiratory pathogen detection. *J Clin Microbiol.* 2016;54(7):1820-1825.
38. Couturier MR, Barney T, Alger G, et al. Evaluation of the FilmArray respiratory panel for clinical use in a large children's hospital. *J Clin Lab Anal.* 2013;27:148-154.
40. Dawood FS, Ambrose JF, Russell BP, et al. Outbreak of pneumonia in the setting of fatal pneumococcal meningitis among US Army trainees: potential role of *Chlamydia pneumoniae. BMC Infect Dis.* 2011;11:157.
43. Dumke R, Schnee C, Pletz MW, et al. *Mycoplasma pneumoniae* and *Chlamydia* spp. infection in community acquired pneumonia, Germany 2011-2012. *Emerg Infect Dis.* 2015;21:426-432.
44. Eberly MD, Eide MB, Thompson JL, Nylund CM. Azithromycin in early infancy and pyloric stenosis. *Pediatrics.* 2015;135:483.
49. Fajardo KA, Zorich SC, Voss JD, Thervil JW. Pneumonia outbreak caused by *Chlamydophila pneumoniae* among US Air Force Academy Cadets, Colorado, USA. *Emerg Infect Dis.* 2016;21:1049-1051.
80. Hammerschlag MR, Kohlhoff SA, Darville T. *Chlamydia pneumoniae* and *Chlamydia trachomatis*. In: Fratamico PM, Smith JL, Brogden KA, eds. *Sequelae and Long-Term Consequences of Infectious Diseases.* Washington, DC: American Society for Microbiology; 2009:27-52.
90. Huang W, Gaydos CA, Barnes MR, et al. Comparative effectiveness of a rapid point of care test for detection of *Chlamydia trachomatis* among women in a clinical setting. *Sex Transm Dis.* 2013;89:108-114.
97. Jacquier N, Viollier PH, Grueb G. The role of peptidoglycan in chlamydial cell division: towards resolving the chlamydial anomaly. *FEMS Microbiol Rev.* 2015;39(2):262-275.
99. Johansson N, Kalin M, Tiveljung-Lindell A, et al. Etiology of community-acquired pneumonia: increased microbiological yield with new diagnostic methods. *Clin Infect Dis.* 2010;50:202-209.
104. Kim C, Nyoka R, Ahmed JA, et al. Epidemiology of respiratory infections caused by atypical bacteria in two Kenyan refugee camps. *J Immigr Minor Health.* 2012;14:140-145.
107. Kohlhoff SA, Hammerschlag MR. Treatment of chlamydial infections: 2014 update. *Expert Opin Pharmacother.* 2014;16:2015-2212.
132. Moore DL, MacDonald NE. Canadian Paediatric Society, Infectious Diseases and Immunization Committee. Preventing ophthalmia neonatorum. *Paediatr Child Health.* 2015;20(2):93-96.
143. Pierce V, Elkan M, Leet M, et al. Comparison of the Idaho Technology FilmArray system to real-time PCR for detection of respiratory pathogens in children. *J Clin Microbiol.* 2012;50:364-371.

154. Sachse K, Baviol PM, Kaltenboeck B, et al. Emendation of the family *Chlamydiaceae*: proposal of a single genus, *Chlamydia*, to include all currently recognized species. *Syst Appl Microbiol.* 2015;38(2):99-103.
159. Seña AC, Hsu KK, Kellogg N, et al. Sexual assault and sexually transmitted infections in adults, adolescents and children. *Clin Infect Dis.* 2015;61(suppl 8):S856-S864.
166. Szymanska-Czerwinska M, Neimczuk K. Avian chlamydiosis zoonotic disease. *Vector-Borne Zoo Dis.* 2016;16(1):1-3.
167. Tao L, Hu B, He L, et al. Etiology and antimicrobial resistance of community-acquired pneumonia in adult patients in China. *Chin Med J.* 2012;125:2967-2972.

The full reference list for this chapter is available at ExpertConsult.com.

Rickettsial and Ehrlichial Diseases

195

Paul M. Lantos • Ross McKinney Jr

The Rickettsiaceae are a family of organisms that share a fascinating history and common biology. The critical steps in the epidemiology were first characterized by Howard T. Ricketts in the early 20th century. He was doing fieldwork in the Bitterroot Valley in Montana and described how Rocky Mountain spotted fever (RMSF) was transmitted by the Rocky Mountain wood tick. Interestingly, before he did his work demonstrating tick-dependent transmission using guinea pigs, the fact that human transmission was through a tick vector had already been proved. In the *Transactions of the Chicago Pathological Society*, Dr. Ricketts reported[150]:

> *At the time this work was done I had no knowledge of previous experiments which demonstrated the ability of the "wood tick" to transfer spotted fever. Recently I have had authoritative information that Dr. L. P. McCalla and Dr. H. A. Brereton, of Boise City, Idaho, transmitted the disease from man to man in two experiments. The tick was obtained "from the chest of a man very ill with spotted fever," and "applied to the arm of a man who had been in the hospital for two months and a half, and had lost both feet from gangrene due to freezing." On the eighth day the patient became ill and passed through a mild course of spotted fever, leaving a characteristic eruption. The experiment was repeated by placing the tick on a woman's leg, and she likewise was infected with spotted fever. Although these results received no publicity other than that given in reports to local societies, I take pleasure in according to Dr. McCalla and to his colleague, Dr. Brereton, the credit of having first shown that the tick may act as a carrier of spotted fever. Their experiments preceded by more than a year those of Dr. King and of myself, and they were performed with the full consent of the patients concerned.*

The study was more fully described by Dr. McCalla in 1908.[113]

Sadly, funding for Dr. Ricketts' RMSF research dried up, and he moved to Mexico to investigate an outbreak of tabardillo, a Mexican typhus fever, which he suspected was similar in biology to RMSF. He identified lice as the vector for the disease, but in his attempt to isolate the causative organism, he contracted typhus and died. Shortly before his death, he learned that the state of Montana was ready to resume funding of his research on RMSF. (This is, of course, a cautionary tale to all academics with insecure funding.)

Rickettsiae are small coccobacilli in the class Alphaproteobacteria,[65] visible by light microscopy, that cause their disease intracellularly. The challenging nature of their physical identification was borne out by the fact that Howard Ricketts thought the cause of RMSF was a viral infection. The organism eventually named *Rickettsia rickettsii* was first described by Simeon Burt Wohlbach in 1916, although it took several years for his identification of a 0.2- to 0.5-μm gram-negative organism to be confirmed.[72,197] Rickettsiae cause disease by multiplying in the vascular endothelium, producing a generalized vasculitis involving mostly small blood vessels and symptoms that can involve nearly the entire body.

The human rickettsiae are in the family Rickettsiaceae, which is divided into two genera, *Rickettsia* and *Orientia*.[29] The rickettsiae are the more important pathogens and consist of the spotted fever group and the typhus group.[169] *Orientia* includes only one pathogen, *Orientia tsutsugamushi*, the cause of scrub typhus. The Anaplasmataceae family is closely related and is divided into two genera, *Anaplasma* and *Ehrlichia*.[147]

All of the infections discussed in this chapter are transmitted by arthropod vectors. The spotted fever group of rickettsiae is predominantly transmitted by ticks, although rickettsialpox is spread by mites. Scrub typhus is spread by human body lice as well as by ticks, and murine typhus is spread by fleas (Table 195.1).

Rickettsiae are important causes of human disease and have, in fact, played a profound role in human history.[206] This chapter reviews the pediatric manifestations of diseases caused by the spotted fever and typhus groups of *Rickettsia*, *Ehrlichia*, and Anaplasmataceae.

SPOTTED FEVERS

The spotted fever group of the genus *Rickettsia* is composed of pathogens that are arthropod borne, mostly by ticks. The exception is rickettsialpox, caused by *Rickettsia akari*, which is a mite-borne infection. Disease produced by *R. rickettsii*, of which RMSF is the prototype, occurs throughout the Americas. There are a variety of other spotted fever illnesses seen around the world, most of which are less clinically severe. These diseases are distinguished by their geography and by variations in the causative organism, but they share their sensitivity to tetracyclines and their obligately intracellular life cycle.

Rocky Mountain Spotted Fever

Historical aspects. RMSF has an unusually fascinating history. It was originally recognized in the Bitterroot Valley of western Montana, nestled against the Idaho border. According to Howard Ricketts, the first description of "the so-called spotted fever of Idaho" was made by Edward E. Maxey of Boise City, Idaho, in 1899.[151] The description of the illness, like many clinical characterizations of disease in the prelaboratory era, was surprisingly consistent with our view today, "an acute, endemic, non-contagious, but probably infectious, febrile disease, characterized clinically by a continuous moderately high fever, severe arthritic and muscular pains, and a profuse petechial or purpuric eruption in the skin, appearing first on the ankles, wrists, and forehead, but rapidly spreading to all parts of the body."[151] The disease was soon recognized throughout the Rocky Mountain states. Whereas there were speculations that ticks were the vectors of RMSF, it was Ricketts who unequivocally proved the association through carefully performed experiments with a guinea pig model of disease. As noted earlier, he died before he was able to identify the causative organism of RMSF with certainty, a step performed by Simeon Burt Wohlbach in 1916. Wohlbach noted that the organism occurred in large numbers in the smooth muscle cells of arteries and veins. There were disputes between Wohlbach and researchers at the Rockefeller Institute in New York as to whether this new small organism was in fact the real pathogen. The dispute was sadly resolved when a laboratory technician working with RMSF at the Rockefeller Institute developed a fever, perhaps after a needle scratch, and died. The technician's blood was transported to Wohlbach's laboratory, where he inoculated guinea pigs and they became symptomatic with characteristic RMSF (in a guinea pig, fever, rash, and vasculitis). Wohlbach chose to name the organism after Howard Ricketts, whom he believed had, in fact, first seen the organism.

Another challenge was to grow the organism, then known as *Dermacentroxenus rickettsii*. It was originally thought that the organism could be grown only in cell cultures,[198] which led to confused debates about whether the organism was an intracellular bacterium or a virus. The answers came as Herald R. Cox discovered that rickettsiae could be grown in larger numbers in the yolk sacs of fertilized chicken eggs.[33]

Many mysteries remain about certain elements in the natural history of RMSF. For example, the preantibiotic era mortality rate of RMSF in

TABLE 195.1 **Classification, Primary Vector, and Reservoir Occurrence of Rickettsiae Known to Cause Disease in Humans**

Antigenic Group	Disease	Species	Vector	Animal Reservoirs	Geographic Distribution
Anaplasma	Human granulocytic anaplasmosis	*Anaplasma phagocytophilum*	Tick	Deer, elk, small mammals, and rodents	Worldwide
Ehrlichia	Human monocytic ehrlichiosis	*Ehrlichia chaffeensis*	Tick	Deer, wild and domestic dogs, domestic ruminants, and rodents	Worldwide
	Ehrlichiosis	*E. muris*	Tick	Deer and rodents	Western United States, Russia, Japan
	Ehrlichiosis	*E. ewingii*	Tick	Deer, wild and domestic dogs, and rodents	North America
Neorickettsia	Sennetsu fever	*Neorickettsia sennetsu*	Trematode	Fish	Japan, Malaysia, possibly other parts of Asia
Scrub typhus	Scrub typhus	*Orientia tsutsugamushi*	Larval mite (chigger)	Rodents	Asia-Pacific region from maritime Russia and China to Indonesia and North Australia to Afghanistan
Spotted fever	Rickettsiosis	*Rickettsia aeschlimannii*	Tick	Unknown	South Africa, Morocco, Mediterranean littoral
	African tick bite fever	*R. africae*	Tick	Ruminants	Sub-Saharan Africa, West Indies
	Rickettsialpox	*R. akari*	Mite	House mice, wild rodents	Countries of the former Soviet Union, South Africa, Korea, Turkey, Balkan countries, North and South America
	Queensland tick typhus	*R. australis*	Tick	Rodents	Australia, Tasmania
	Mediterranean spotted fever or boutonneuse fever	*R. conorii*[a]	Tick	Dogs, rodents	Southern Europe, southern and western Asia, Africa, India
	Cat flea rickettsiosis	*R. felis*	Flea	Domestic cats, rodents, opossums	Europe, North and South America, Africa, Asia
	Far Eastern spotted fever	*R. heilongjiangensis*	Tick	Rodents	Far East of Russia, northern China, eastern Asia
	Aneruptive fever	*R. helvetica*	Tick	Rodents	Central and northern Europe, Asia
	Flinders Island spotted fever, Thai tick typhus	*R. honei*	Tick	Unknown	Australia, Thailand
	Japanese spotted fever	*R. japonica*	Tick	Rodents	Japan
	Australian spotted fever	*R. marmionii*	Tick	Rodents, reptiles	Australia
	Mediterranean spotted fever–like disease	*R. massiliae*	Tick	Unknown	France, Greece, Spain, Portugal, Switzerland, Sicily, central Africa, and Mali
	Maculatum infection	*R. parkeri*	Tick	Rodents	North and South America
	Rocky Mountain spotted fever, febre maculosa, São Paulo exanthematic typhus, Minas Gerais exanthematic typhus, Brazilian spotted fever	*R. rickettsii*	Tick	Rodents	North, Central, and South America
	North Asian tick typhus, Siberian tick typhus	*R. sibirica*	Tick	Rodents	Russia, China, Mongolia
	Lymphangitis-associated rickettsiosis	*R. sibirica mongolotimonae*	Tick	Rodents	Southern France, Portugal, China, sub-Saharan Africa
	Tick-borne lymphadenopathy (TIBOLA), *Dermacentor*-borne necrosis and lymphadenopathy (DEBONEL)	*R. slovaca*	Tick	Lagomorphs, rodents	Southern and eastern Europe, Asia
Typhus fever	Epidemic typhus, sylvatic typhus	*R. prowazekii*	Human body louse, flying squirrel ectoparasites, *Amblyomma* ticks	Humans, flying squirrels	Central Africa; Asia; Central, North, and South America
	Murine typhus	*R. typhi*	Flea	Rodents	Tropical and subtropical areas worldwide

[a]Includes four different subspecies that can be distinguished serologically and by polymerase chain reaction assay and respectively are the etiologic agents of boutonneuse fever and Mediterranean tick fever in southern Europe and Africa (*R. conorii* subsp. *conorii*), Indian tick typhus in south Asia (*R. conorii* subsp. *indica*), Israeli tick typhus in southern Europe and Middle East (*R. conorii* subsp. *israelensis*), and Astrakhan spotted fever in the North Caspian region of Russia (*R. conorii* subsp. *caspiae*).

From Eremeeva ME, Dasch GA. Rickettsial (spotted & typhus fevers) & related infections (anaplasmosis & ehrlichiosis). In: *CDC Yellow Book Online.* http://wwwnc.cdc.gov/travel/yellowbook/2012/chapter-3-infectious-diseases-related-to-travel/rickettsial-spotted-and-typhus-fevers-and-related-infections-anaplasmosis-and-ehrlichiosis.htm.

Idaho was 5% to 7%, whereas in the Bitterroot Valley of Montana, it was 70%.[85] The molecular basis for this difference in virulence remains unclear even today.[29] The epidemiology of RMSF has evolved during the 20th century from being a disease predominantly recognized in the northern Rocky Mountains to a disease most commonly found in a band of contiguous states from Oklahoma to the Carolinas (Fig. 195.1). North Carolina, Tennessee, Arkansas, Missouri, and Oklahoma account for 60% of the reported RMSF cases in the United States.[163] The incidence of RMSF has been generally rising, whereas the case-fatality rate has been falling (Fig. 195.2). In 2008, there were roughly 2500 cases of RMSF in the United States, the largest number on record.[163] In 2008–12, passive surveillance reported 8.9 cases of RMSF per million persons in the United States.

For surveillance purposes the CDC has replaced RMSF with the label "spotted fever group rickettsia" because of the similarity between the clinical syndromes produced by *R. rickettsii*, *Rickettsia parkeri*, and

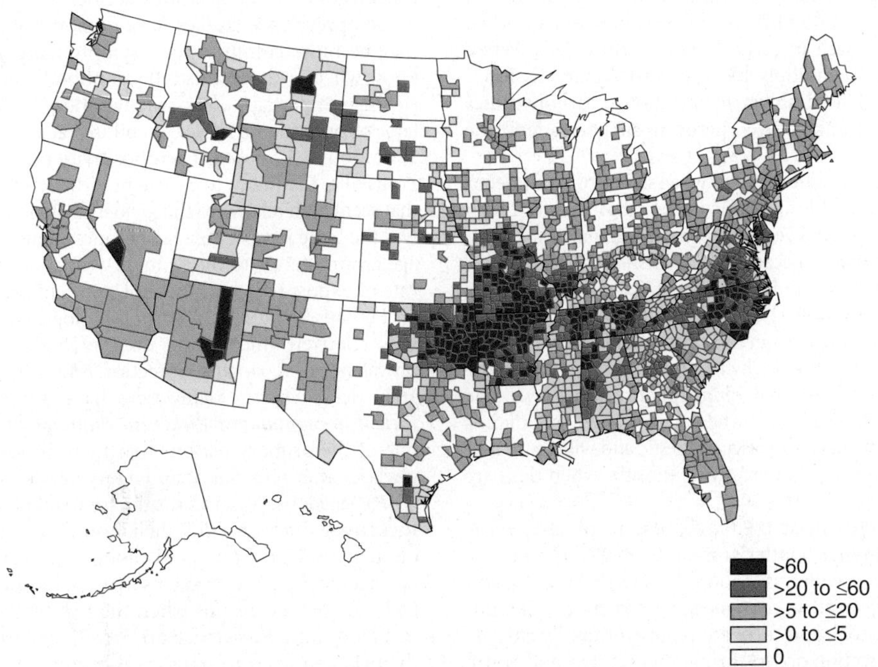

FIG. 195.1 Reported incidence rate of spotted fever rickettsiosis, by county—United States, 2000–13. As reported through national surveillance, per 1 million persons per year. Cases are reported by county of residence, which is not always where the infection was acquired. Includes Rocky Mountain spotted fever (RMSF) and other spotted fever group rickettsioses. In 2010, the name of the reporting category changed from RMSF to spotted fever rickettsiosis. (From Biggs HM, Behravesh CB, Bradley KK, et al. Diagnosis and management of tickborne rickettsial diseases: Rocky Mountain spotted fever and other spotted fever group rickettsioses, ehrlichioses, and anaplasmosis—United States. *MMWR Recomm Rep.* 2016;65[2]:1-44.)

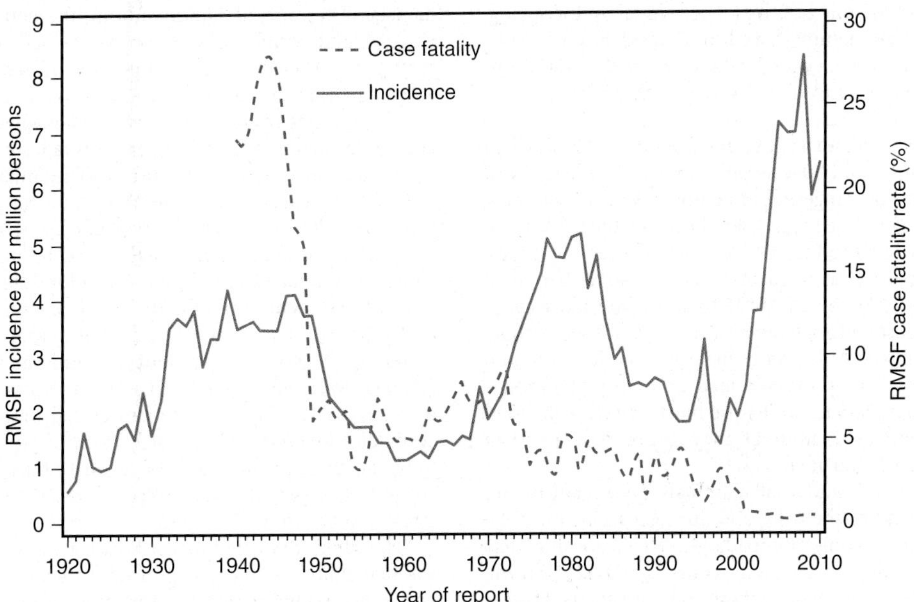

FIG. 195.2 Rocky Mountain spotted fever incidence and case fatality, 1920–2010. (From Centers for Disease Control and Prevention. Statistics and epidemiology: annual cases of RMSF in the United States. http://www.cdc.gov/rmsf/stats/.)

Rickettsia species 364D.[12] For the purposes of this chapter, we will use the traditional label of Rocky Mountain spotted fever, but it should be recognized there is some overlap with the other spotted fever group organisms.

Etiology, morphology, growth, and metabolism. *R. rickettsii*, the etiologic agent of RMSF, is a small, nonmotile, pleomorphic, weakly gram-negative coccobacillus measuring 0.3 to 0.5 μm in diameter and 0.3 to 4 μm in length. The cell wall and cytoplasmic membrane are fairly typical for gram-negative bacteria. Rickettsiae must penetrate into living cells to grow and multiply (i.e., they are obligately intracellular). They are grown most readily in the yolk sacs of embryonated eggs; but under special conditions, they also grow well in certain tissue culture cells. When inside a cell, rickettsial cells multiply by transverse binary fission.[75] The organisms lack the intrinsic ability to metabolize carbohydrates and amino acid substrates and derive energy from host adenosine triphosphate (ATP).[29]

Rickettsiae take on a characteristic red color when stained with Gimenez stain. *R. rickettsii* possess a soluble antigenic moiety that is shared with antigenic variants in the spotted fever group and rickettsialpox.

Epidemiology and transmission. Because *R. rickettsii* is transmitted to people through adult tick vectors, understanding of tick ecology explains much of the epidemiology of RMSF. The vectors for RMSF are *Dermacentor variabilis* (the American dog tick) in the eastern and central United States, *Dermacentor andersoni* (the Rocky Mountain wood tick) in the Rocky Mountain states and West, and *Rhipicephalus sanguineus* (the brown dog tick) in eastern Arizona.[163] These ticks prefer woodlands where small rodents share habitats with large domestic and wild animals.[23] RMSF is most common in spring and summer months when ticks are most active.

Regionally, RMSF is concentrated. Fifty-six percent of cases come from five states (North Carolina, South Carolina, Tennessee, Oklahoma, and Arkansas). However, it is widely distributed in North America, and cases have been reported from all 48 contiguous United States.[43] It tends to occur in hyperendemic foci, and there are reports of family clusters of disease.[51] *R. rickettsii* infection occurs throughout Central and South America via several different tick species; there are a variety of regional names for the infection, such as Tobia fever (Colombia) and São Paolo fever (Brazil).

The life cycle of *Dermacentor andersoni* ticks requires roughly 2 years. In the spring and early summer, adult ticks seek out hosts for a blood meal. Ticks that attach feed for 7 to 9 days, then mate. The engorged females drop off their hosts, laying 5000 to 7000 eggs each. After 35 days, the eggs hatch and the larvae seek out small mammals to which to attach. After 2 to 6 days of feeding, the larvae drop off, mature into nymphs, and become inactive for the winter. In the spring, the nymphs attach to small mammals, feed for 7 days, drop off, hide, and mature into adults. They generally hide for the duration of the summer, fall, and winter and in the spring seek out their adult blood meal.[23]

D. variabilis is similar to the Rocky Mountain wood tick but adapted to the climate of the central and eastern United States. The larvae and nymphs have a narrower host range and show a preference for meadow and white-footed mice. Dogs are the primary hosts for the adult ticks, but the adult ticks are willing to bite a wide range of large mammals, including humans, who are thus incidental victims. Larvae are most active in the early spring (March and April), then become active again in the late summer (August and September) if they did not successfully feed in the spring. Nymphs are also active in spring and late summer, with the spring nymphs having overwintered and the late summer nymphs a product of spring larvae. Adults also most actively seek blood meals from April to September, although they can become active in any month if the weather is warm enough.[23]

Rickettsiae multiply in ticks and small mammals. The organisms are found in the salivary gland of the ticks, and during a blood meal the organisms are activated and become more pathogenic. They are ultimately injected into the host by the tick during the course of the blood meal, although ticks can also transmit if they are squeezed during the process of tick removal.[29] Rickettsiae can be passed from one generation of tick to the next transovarially and can persist from hatching into the adult tick. This is particularly impressive because adult ticks can wait up to 4 years for a blood meal. However, infected ticks seem to have a biologic disadvantage, and relatively few *R. rickettsii*–infected larvae ultimately mature into adults.[49] The organisms are found in the salivary glands and the gastrointestinal tract of the ticks. Interestingly, RMSF is also a sexually transmitted disease; it can be spread from infected male ticks to uninfected females through infected spermatozoa.[76,132]

Although it is uncommon, RMSF can be spread through aerosolization in the laboratory, so care should be taken (a biosafety level 3 facility is required). In addition, there have been uncommon transmissions by transfusion[191] and needlestick accidents.[156]

Seroprevalence studies have demonstrated that subclinical disease may be more common than symptomatic, although it is difficult to know whether the results reflect antibodies to rickettsiae other than *R. rickettsii* or perhaps cross-reactive antigens from other organisms.[195] A large seroprevalence survey of children at sites in the southeastern United States found *R. rickettsii* seropositivity rates that varied from 3.5% in Louisville, Kentucky, to 21.9% in Little Rock, Arkansas. These are rates that seem high relative to the incidence of clinical RMSF. Also noteworthy was the large jump in overall seroprevalence from the 1- to 6-year-old age group (4.2%) to the 7- to 12-year-olds (13.9%), suggesting a high rate of exposure in early school-aged children.[112]

Perhaps because *R. rickettsii* is biologically disadvantageous for ticks, it is relatively uncommon even in highly endemic areas. The tick prevalence of *R. rickettsii* infection is less than one RMSF infection per 1000 ticks, whereas many ticks have nonpathogenic rickettsiae like *Rickettsia montana* or *Rickettsia rhipicephali*.[180] This low prevalence is one of the primary reasons that there is no role for doxycycline prophylaxis after removal of an engorged tick.

Pathogenesis. Vasculitis is the fundamental disease process in RMSF. Rickettsiae infect the endothelial cells lining blood vessels, particularly of small and medium-sized blood vessels, and the resultant cellular damage creates vascular lesions that can involve almost the entire vascular bed. The process begins when the tick bites an individual and begins its blood meal. Rickettsiae are introduced from the salivary glands of the tick, and the infectious cycle begins.

At a cellular level, rickettsiae are internalized by endocytosis into vacuoles. They are initially enclosed in a vacuolar membrane but are able to degrade the membrane and escape into the cytosol. Rickettsiae are obligate intracellular pathogens, and they require access to the cytoplasm to grow. They lack the ability to metabolize carbohydrates and amino acids and thus obtain their energy from host ATP molecules.[29] When in the cytoplasm, the organisms replicate by binary fission. They recruit host cell actin molecules, and they use the actin to spread from cell to cell, transported through cell membranes without producing damage. They spread rapidly among the endothelial cells lining the vascular and lymphatic systems. As the cells become injured by the rickettsiae, they lose their attachment to adjacent cells, and the smooth vascular surface becomes increasingly rough and leaky.

The immune response to *R. rickettsia* involves perivascular lymphocytic infiltrates. As the endothelial cells fail, small leaks in the capillary bed produce increased vascular permeability, microhemorrhages, localized edema, and local inflammation. With time, the problem becomes more generalized, involving a wide variety of organs, including the skin, brain, lungs, kidneys, and liver. Eventually the combination of leakage, edema, and inflammation can produce organ failure. On pathologic examination in affected patients, inflammation can be seen in the affected tissues.

Clearance of *R. rickettsii* is predominantly by cellular immunity, including cytotoxic T lymphocytes and interferon-γ. The immune response lyses infected cells, an action that may be the primary means by which rickettsial infection causes cell injury.[180] A broad range of antibodies are produced against *R. rickettsii*, and these antibodies appear to be the host's primary defense against reinfection. Although it is not absolutely certain, it is generally believed that people are not infected by *R. rickettsii* more than once.

The laboratory hallmarks of RMSF are also a product of this diffuse vascular injury, with often profound thrombocytopenia and mild to moderate hyponatremia. The thrombocytopenia is a result of platelet consumption along damaged vascular surfaces; the hyponatremia is probably a combination of shifting of electrolytes from the intracellular to the extracellular space, loss of sodium through excretion, exchange of sodium for potassium at the cellular level, and the syndrome of inappropriate antidiuretic hormone secretion.[89]

The extent of disease is dependent on several factors in addition to the timing of treatment initiation. For example, there is the regional variation noted earlier (Montana vs. Idaho). The inoculum size is almost certainly important and may relate to the duration of tick attachment. Most of the time, *R. rickettsii* in tick salivary glands are in a dormant, noncontagious state. During the blood meal, the rickettsiae become active and virulent, a process that may take as long as 4 to 6 hours. As a result, that duration is thought to be the necessary length of attachment for transmission to occur. Host factors that make RMSF potentially more severe include glucose-6-phosphate dehydrogenase (G6PD) deficiency (a sex-linked condition found in 12% of African American males), age (adults are at higher risk for severe disease), and gender (males more than females).[180]

Clinical manifestations. The classic manifestations of RMSF are fever, headache, myalgias, severe malaise, and rash. The illness is seldom subtle, and most children infected with *R. rickettsii* appear quite ill. Temperatures in the range of 40°C (104°F) are typical. In the early stages, rash may not be present or may be only pale, erythematous macules. In dark-skinned patients, the early rash may not be apparent. As the illness progresses, the fever persists, the degree of malaise becomes complete prostration, and the rash evolves from macules to petechiae. Eventually, the child can become hypotensive and obtunded and may die if not appropriately treated.

RMSF is transmitted by tick bite, but surprisingly only half of patients can recall being bitten by a tick.[21] This probably reflects the facts that ticks are stealthy and generally obtain their blood meal efficiently, without pain. They may attach in areas that are not easily seen. The consequence for physicians is that the historical review should focus not only on tick bites but also on behaviors that put someone at risk for tick exposure. These behaviors include walking in woods or high grass in the spring or summer or during a sustained warm spell. In terms of RMSF, the degree of regional incidence of *R. rickettsii* infection should also be considered; the southeastern and south-central United States have the highest incidence.

The incubation period for RMSF after the tick bite is 48 hours to 14 days, with a median of 4 days.[21,29] The first symptoms are usually fever, headache, myalgias, and malaise. These are obviously nonspecific findings, making the diagnosis of RMSF difficult. Fever is virtually a *sine qua non*, occurring in 98% of pediatric RMSF cases.[21] Profound malaise is also present from early in the illness, marking RMSF as more than the typical nonspecific virus infection. Sixty percent of children develop a headache, which is often severe. Lumbar punctures typically have a mild leukocytosis, with a median of 25 cells/mm^3.[21]

Rash is not reliably present in the early stages of disease, unfortunately. The rash typically appears in the second to fourth day of illness, which is generally after patients have first sought medical care.[28] Eventually 90% or more of children have rash. The early rash begins as faint macules, often on the arms and lower legs. At this stage, the lesions still blanch on pressure. Petechiae evolve during several days. Classically the rash evolves from the periphery toward the trunk and involves the palms and soles. However, neither the centripetal nature nor palm and sole involvement is a definitive or reliable finding. Generalized petechiae are seen around the fifth or sixth day of illness, at which point patients are severely ill. They are likely to have organ system dysfunction, and recovery will be slow even with treatment.[28]

Other common symptoms are myalgia (45% in the Buckingham series),[21] abdominal pain that can mimic appendicitis (36%), diarrhea (34%), conjunctival injection (33%), altered mental status (33%), lymphadenopathy (29%), and peripheral edema (25%). Less common findings include hepatomegaly, photophobia, seizures, meningismus, splenomegaly, periorbital edema, and coma. Of these symptoms, the conjunctival injection and peripheral edema are most likely to point in the direction of RMSF, although both usually occur in patients who already have extensive rash.

The laboratory findings are also only moderately helpful. As noted in the section on diagnosis, the only true acute diagnostic test is biopsy of petechial or macular lesions and demonstration of the organism by immunohistochemical staining or polymerase chain reaction (PCR) testing. Antibody tests have almost no utility acutely because the immunofluorescent antibody (IFA) assay titers will not rise into a diagnostic range until 10 days or more into the illness, days after treatment should have been started. The two most useful laboratory findings are thrombocytopenia and hyponatremia. Sixty percent of children have a platelet count below 150,000 cells/mm^3 at their initial presentation, and the median platelet count is 128,000 cells/mm^3. In regard to serum sodium, 52% have sodium concentrations below 135 mEq/L, with a median concentration of 133 mEq/L. Other laboratory values that can be abnormal include hepatic enzymes (alanine aminotransferase, aspartate aminotransferase), serum bilirubin, hemoglobin, cerebrospinal fluid cell count, glucose, and protein.

Some patients with RMSF have focal cardiac disease, in particular myocarditis, and rare patients have evidence of pneumonia.

Even with treatment, RMSF can leave patients with residual neurologic damage, as described later in the prognosis section. Conditions associated with more severe RMSF, in addition to delayed treatment, include G6PD deficiency and early treatment with sulfa drugs.

Diagnosis. Because the early manifestations of *R. rickettsii* infection are nonspecific, the challenge is to diagnose RMSF effectively and to avoid overtreating a multitude of children. In the right season (summer) in an endemic region, this can be a significant problem. If an error is made, it should be in overtreatment of patients in whom infection is suspected, given the relative risks of undertreatment of RMSF versus the potential for unnecessary exposure to doxycycline.

For confirmation of a diagnosis of *R. rickettsii* infection, the most widely used test is the indirect IFA assay. The sensitivity of this assay is inadequate to be useful in the first 10 to 12 days of illness. There is essentially no value in a negative test result; it does not rule out RMSF and should not be used for that purpose. The value of IFA assay comes to confirm whether an illness was RMSF ex post facto. The test is 94% sensitive by 14 to 21 days.[88] The diagnosis requires a fourfold rise in titer between acute and convalescent sera. A "probable" diagnosis is generally made on the basis of a single convalescent IFA titer of 1:64 or greater.

To make a diagnosis of RMSF more acutely, if a patient has a rash, a skin biopsy can be performed to sample petechial lesions. The lesion can be sent for either immunohistochemical staining or PCR testing, depending on availability. Immunohistochemical staining of biopsy material has been found to be 100% specific and 70% sensitive.[181] It is most useful either before or very early in treatment. PCR is less established as a diagnostic method but can be performed on either tissue or blood.

The other important but nonspecific diagnostic clues pointing toward RMSF are thrombocytopenia, hyponatremia, and the rash. One case series found the average platelet count at presentation to be 128,000 cells/mm^3; 41% had fewer than 100,000 platelets at initial presentation.[21] In terms of sodium, the median sodium concentration at presentation was 133 mEq/L, and 52% of children had a serum sodium concentration below 135 mEq/L. The rash, when present, is an important clue, but the absence of rash does not exclude RMSF. As noted before, the rash begins as faint macules, which become petechial as the disease progresses. They may be found on the palms and soles, but rashes in those locations are seen in only two-thirds of children.[21]

Differential diagnosis. Perhaps the greatest challenge to RMSF is making a clinical diagnosis in time for effective treatment. The characteristics that define early RMSF are fairly nonspecific: fever, headache, some photophobia, and severe malaise. The first critical clue is whether the patient has been in an endemic area, although RMSF has occurred in all of the lower 48 states, and whether the season is right (spring, summer, or a recent warm spell). A rash usually appears somewhere between the third and fifth day and can be a helpful clue, but roughly 10% of patients with confirmed RMSF never have a rash. Because of the lack of specificity to the symptoms, clinicians must begin with a high level of suspicion. Enteroviral infections (echovirus, coxsackievirus) appear similar to RMSF, have the same summer seasonality, and can produce a similar rash. In endemic regions, the practical reality is that quite a few enteroviral infections are "cured" with doxycycline.

A more problematic overlap is with *Neisseria meningitidis*. The early symptoms of meningococcemia are again similar to RMSF, with fever, headache, and malaise. Laboratory findings may also be similar, with thrombocytopenia and a leukocyte count that reflects a left shift. Because neither RMSF nor meningococcemia can be quickly confirmed, and because both require a rapid initiation of treatment, it is reasonable and appropriate to begin both doxycycline and penicillin (or some other appropriate β-lactam or cephalosporin) until the situation can be sorted out (primarily by blood culture).

The full differential diagnosis for RMSF includes enteroviral infections, adenoviral infections, meningococcemia, influenza, gram-negative bacterial sepsis, toxic shock syndrome, measles, rubella, secondary syphilis, leptospirosis, typhoid fever, disseminated gonococcal infection, immune thrombocytopenic purpura, thrombotic thrombocytopenic purpura, immune complex vasculitis (e.g., systemic lupus erythematosus), infectious mononucleosis, hypersensitivity reaction to drugs, murine typhus, rickettsialpox, recrudescent typhus, and sylvatic *Rickettsia prowazekii* infection that is enzootic in flying squirrels.[180]

During the summer in endemic regions, it is fairly common practice to see patients early in the course of a febrile illness. In the first 2 days of fever, practitioners often obtain screening laboratory tests (a complete blood count and chemistry) and, if the patient does not have severe malaise, opt to watch. If the fever persists into the third day, if the screening laboratory test results appear suggestive, or if the patient appears to be more ill than is usually the case with a viral illness, treatment with doxycycline is initiated. The worst outcomes with RMSF occur when a physician dogmatically holds to a preliminary diagnosis in the face of persisting illness, often because of the absence of a rash or laboratory test result pointing toward RMSF.

Treatment. RMSF is an easily treatable disease with a good prognosis if treatment is begun suitably early. However, therapeutic failures occur every summer because the diagnosis is not considered. The symptoms can mimic other diseases (e.g., enterovirus infection, meningococcemia, infectious mononucleosis, appendicitis, pharyngitis), prompting inappropriate treatment decisions. If doxycycline is initiated within the first 5 days of fever, the prognosis is excellent. The problem is deciding which patients to treat, which to observe. Even in areas where RMSF is endemic, 60% to 75% of patients with RMSF are given an alternative diagnosis at their first clinical visit. The probabilities of morbidity and mortality escalate rapidly with each day of treatment delay.

The other important challenge to treating RMSF is the need to begin treatment before the standard diagnostic test results become definitively positive. At the onset of fever, antibody titers against *R. rickettsii* will almost always be negative. In most cases, the IFA test result becomes positive between 7 and 10 days, and by 14 to 21 days, IFA titers are 94% sensitive. However, during the first week, when treatment needs to be initiated, antibody titers will be negative. Even defining who is at risk can be difficult. Because ticks are very good at their profession (blood sucking), in only 50% of cases do patients report a time-appropriate tick exposure.[21]

Doxycycline is the primary antibiotic used to treat RMSF. Historically, chloramphenicol was demonstrated to be equally effective, and it remains the only documented alternative treatment, but its side-effect profile, particularly in causing aplastic anemia, has made oral chloramphenicol unavailable in the United States. Doxycycline is dosed at 2.2 mg/kg per dose every 12 hours (maximum, 100 mg every 12 hours) for the duration of fever and an additional 3 days (at least 5 days, and typically 7 to 10 days). After the patient is improving, relapse is highly unlikely, and there is no chronic form of *R. rickettsii* infection. Doxycycline may be given intravenously or orally, depending on the degree of illness. Whereas tetracyclines have been associated with dental staining, doxycycline does not pose a significant risk (particularly in comparison to untreated RMSF).

Severe RMSF can require hospitalization and, at times, advanced life support: intravenous fluids, pressors, and assisted ventilation. In its severe form, RMSF includes a profound vasculitis that can mimic disseminated intravascular coagulopathy, with thrombocytopenia, generalized petechiae, hemorrhages, and shock. In many ways, it clinically resembles meningococcemia.

Whereas some children with RMSF are empirically treated with antibiotics other than doxycycline during the early phases of management, given the already noted similarity to meningococcemia, most of those antibiotics will have no effect on the course of RMSF. The one exception is sulfa drugs, including trimethoprim-sulfamethoxazole, which can make RMSF more severe. The mechanism for this observation is still unclear.[28]

Prognosis. The mortality rate in the modern era for untreated RMSF is 20%; for treated patients, it is roughly 5%.[28] Interestingly, in the preantibiotic era, the mortality rate for RMSF was highly variable. For example, RMSF in the Bitterroot Valley of Montana had a mortality rate of 75%, whereas in the Snake River Valley in southern Idaho it was 3%.[3] The reasons for differential rates like these have never been explained.[29] Most of the current mortality is in patients with delayed initiation of doxycycline. For patients treated with doxycycline in the first 5 days of symptoms, the prognosis is excellent.

In children who have had severe RMSF, there is a significant rate of residual problems. In one series, 13 of 89 surviving children were discharged from the hospital with neurologic deficits, including speech and swallowing dysfunction, global encephalopathy, ataxia or gait disturbances, and cortical blindness.[21] Many of the children with long-term follow-up continued to have neurologic problems. Two of the 89 children had loss of digits due to autoamputation.

Prevention. The most effective measures for control of RMSF are personal steps to avoid ticks. Wearing pants tucked into boots or socks is not a fashion statement, but it can be useful in tick avoidance. Permethrin-based insect repellants can be effective, although they should be applied to clothes rather than directly on skin (a caution for which users will be grateful after smelling permethrin-based repellants). Insect repellants containing 20% to 50% DEET applied to skin may have some effect, although they are probably more effective in deterring mosquitoes than ticks. Adults should perform regular tick inspections on themselves and on children for whom they are responsible because ticks require 4 to 6 hours of attachment to transmit *R. rickettsii*. Ticks are fond of high grasses, brushy areas, and mixed forests, so care should be taken to stay in the center of well-trodden trails. Pets can be protected with medications or flea and tick collars.[134]

Patients should be taught the art of removing ticks from skin. There are many old wives' tales about how to remove ticks: touching their backs with an extinguished match, applying clear nail polish to suffocate them, applying petroleum jelly. Given the effectiveness of these strategies, the surprise is that there are any old wives left to tell tales. To remove a tick, use tweezers, grasp the tick's head as close to the skin as possible, and twist out. The area should be scrubbed with soap or alcohol because any residual tick spit or fecal material has the potential to be infectious and to contaminate the bite wound. Incinerating a tick after removal is, however, perfectly appropriate, as is the more usual approach of flushing it into the sewer system.

Whereas vaccines against RMSF were in use for many years, they were probably marginally effective, if at all, and are no longer available.

Mediterranean Spotted Fever

Overview. Mediterranean spotted fever (MSF) is a tick-borne infection caused by *Rickettsia conorii*. The disease was first described by Conor and Bruch in 1910,[32] and the name "Mediterranean spotted fever" was adopted in 1932. In the Mediterranean region, this infection is also known as boutonneuse fever and Marseilles fever. Whereas the infection has been recognized for a century, until recently it was regarded as a benign disease. In 1982 the first case report of fatal MSF was published.[142] Its potential lethality has been demonstrated in numerous other studies, including one in which 32.3% of hospitalized patients died.[38] It is now regarded as comparable to RMSF in its potential for mortality.

Epidemiology. *R. conorii* infection occurs across a wide geographic swath that includes not only the Mediterranean region but also parts of central and southern Africa, the Middle East, and central and south Asia. Locale-specific names given to this infection include Astrakhan spotted fever, Kenya tick bite fever, African tick typhus, India tick typhus, and Israeli spotted fever. The geographic diversity of MSF is matched by its genetic diversity; there are numerous regional subspecies of *R. conorii* capable of causing human disease.[205] The only known vector is the brown dog tick, *Rhipicephalus sanguineus*. This tick is also the only known reservoir for *R. conorii*.

MSF occurs in all age groups of both sexes. The epidemiologic pattern is determined by the activity of the tick; consequently, a consistent seasonal peak occurs from June to October. The incidence of the disease appears to rise and fall periodically. The most recent decades have seen an increase in cases in a number of countries, including Portugal, Italy, France, Spain, Bulgaria, and Algeria.[154]

Clinical manifestations. The infecting bite is unnoticed in most cases. Conjunctival inoculation occurs occasionally. The incubation period ranges from 6 to 10 days. The primary lesion, tache noire (black spot), described and named by Pieri in the 1920s, develops at the site of the tick bite, is not painful, and is rarely pruritic.[183] It occurs most often on the head in children and on the legs in adults. The lesion develops central necrosis, then an eschar, and regional lymph nodes enlarge. The initial lesion heals slowly and resolves after 10 to 20 days without scarring, although residual pigmentation can persist indefinitely.

Tache noire is highly characteristic, but the lesion is identified in only 30% to 90% of patients. The occasional patient has multiple lesions. Formation of the lesion requires a substance secreted by the tick and another of rickettsial origin; it is not reproduced by a separate bite of an uninfected tick or by experimental inoculation of *R. conorii*. An inflammatory infiltrate, predominantly mononuclear, accumulates at the tache noire site, suggesting the importance of T cell–mediated immunity in local host defense.

The onset of disease usually is abrupt, with malaise and fever that reaches temperatures of 39°C to 40°C (102.2°F–104°F) within the first 2 or 3 days. The fever continues for 6 to 12 days, but antibiotics can shorten the febrile period. Severe and unremitting headache is a typical feature of the disease in adults.[5] On the other hand, headache occurs in less than one third of pediatric patients.[31] Arthralgia and myalgia, especially of the leg muscles, are prominent features in adults; in children, they are rarely of sufficient severity to restrict mobility.

By the third to fifth day of fever nearly all patients develop a maculopapular exanthem. Lesions first appear on the extremities, spreading within a day or so to the trunk, neck, face, buttocks, palms, and soles. The initial lesions are macular, pink, and irregularly defined but within hours become maculopapular. The rash can be intensely pruritic. Lesions generally measure 1 to 4 mm in diameter. The rash persists for 10 to 20 days after the illness has otherwise resolved. Atypical cutaneous manifestations include petechiae, purpura, or papulovesicular lesions.[31,57]

The cutaneous manifestations of MSF are caused by infection of the vascular structures of the dermis. Rickettsemia during the incubation period probably seeds the endothelial cells of the capillaries, arterioles, and venules. The vasculitis produced is much like that seen in RMSF. It gradually disappears during convalescence, and as the maculopapules fade, a brown discoloration of the skin may be noticed.

Cardiovascular and respiratory changes are transient and nonspecific. Bradycardia is the most consistent finding, but other dysrhythmias can occur. More seriously ill patients have developed pericarditis, heart failure, and myocarditis. The most important vascular complication is phlebitis of the lower extremities. Deep vein thrombosis is a recognized complication, particularly among pregnant patients. Other important complications include pneumonitis, pleuritis, pleuropericarditis, and the adult respiratory distress syndrome.

In addition to the headache that is characteristic of rickettsial illnesses, varying degrees of impaired consciousness can occur. Rarely, stupor, delirium, convulsions, and transient hypoacusis may be noted. Rickettsial encephalitis may be followed by long-term neurologic sequelae.

Renal function is not altered in most cases, although nephritis with acute renal failure has occurred occasionally. The liver is palpable in one-third of patients, and the spleen may be enlarged in 20% of children. Tests of hepatic function reveal an increase in serum transaminase levels in one-fourth to one-half of pediatric cases. Alkaline phosphatase levels are elevated in one-third of patients. Liver pathology reveals foci of hepatocellular necrosis and a predominantly mononuclear reaction to the necrosis at sites of infection by *R. conorii*. The lesions differ from true granulomas in that they are not aggregates of epithelioid macrophages.[184]

A variety of other systemic symptoms can occur. Photophobia and bilateral conjunctivitis have been reported. Severe unilateral conjunctivitis suggests that transmission of the disease occurs by the conjunctival route. Uveitis, choroiditis, retinal artery occlusion, and neuroretinitis are uncommon ocular disturbances.[2,41]

Hematologic abnormalities include isolated cases of autoimmune anemia and mixed cryoglobulinemia associated with MSF. Some studies report a high incidence of hypoproteinemia. Immune complex–mediated vasculitis associated with MSF has been described.[36]

On occasion, MSF can have a malignant, rapidly fatal course, even in previously healthy children. The illness is consistent with a widespread vasculitis characterized by irreversible shock, encephalopathy, disseminated intravascular coagulopathy, and renal failure.[203]

Diagnosis. Rickettsial organisms can be detected by immunofluorescence if biopsy is performed early in the course of disease or by restriction fragment length polymorphism analysis of a PCR product from the tache noire.[116,196] *R. conorii* cannot be isolated from blood cultures by routine laboratory procedures. The clinical findings, geographic location, and epidemiologic considerations help establish the diagnosis.

The diagnosis can be established by one of multiple serologic tests that include complement fixation, latex agglutination, microagglutination, Western blot, and indirect IFA assays.[57,79,173] An IFA assay for *R. conorii* is commercially available. Identification of specific immunoglobulin M (IgM) by immunofluorescence can identify acute infection, although some patients with proven MSF treated early with antibiotics have normal antirickettsial IgM levels.

Differential diagnosis. Before the rash appears, differentiation of MSF from other acute infections is difficult. Even after appearance of the rash, the disease can be confused with measles, meningococcemia, and secondary syphilis. Other rickettsial diseases should be considered, especially in the absence of a tache noire. Cross-reactions among rickettsiae occur with indirect immunofluorescence.

Treatment and prevention. MSF generally has a benign course, and fatalities rarely occur. Doxycycline is the drug of choice. Alternative regimens that have been effective in children include azithromycin 10 mg/kg daily for 3 days, clarithromycin 15 mg/kg twice daily for 7 days, and chloramphenicol 50 mg/kg 4 times daily for 7 days.[26,31,207] The optimal duration of therapy has not been definitively established, however, and regimens ranging from single doses to treatment for up to 15 days have been reported.[70]

The major effective methods of control involve avoidance of tick bites. Natural immunity occurs after infection, and antibodies persist for as long as 4 years after acute illness. Effective vaccines are not available.[109]

Rickettsialpox

Historical aspects. First described in New York City in 1946 by Sussman as "Kew Gardens spotted fever," rickettsialpox is a benign spotted fever group rickettsial disease caused by *R. akari*.[82,84,167] Reporting of rickettsialpox declined in the latter decades of the 20th century; fewer than 50 cases were reported by the New York City Department of Health between 1980 and 1999. At least 34 cases were confirmed in 2001 and 2002, possibly as the result of increased awareness and detection of the disease after the bioterrorism anthrax attacks of 2001.[125]

Organism. The etiologic agent, *R. akari*, is an obligate intracellular gram-negative coccobacillus that is morphologically identical to *R. rickettsii*. The principal vector is the house mouse mite, *Liponyssoides sanguineus*. Rodents, particularly the house mouse, *Mus musculus*, serve as a reservoir for *R. akari*.

Epidemiology and transmission. Most rickettsialpox in the United States has been reported from New York City, but cases also have occurred in many other cities in the United States and worldwide in Russia, Korea, and South Africa. Whereas house mice are the natural hosts of the mite transmitting rickettsialpox in the United States, rats have been shown to host the mite in Russia, and wild rodents are suspected of carrying the disease in South Africa. The reservoir for rickettsialpox may extend to additional, as yet unidentified, wild or domestic animals.

The disease has a natural cycle between the mite vector and the house mouse.[83] The mite passes the disease agent transovarially, and as such serves as both reservoir and vector. Depletion of rodent hosts from reduced food or pest control measures causes mites to feed on humans as an alternative host. The disease affects persons of all ages. Males and females are equally susceptible.[20,69]

Pathology. Biopsy specimens from eschars are characterized by variable degrees of epidermal and dermal necrosis. Ulcerated lesions typically have neutrophils and thrombosed vessels in the ulcer base. The primary pattern of inflammation is a deep perivascular mononuclear cell infiltrate. Immunohistochemical staining reveals spotted fever group rickettsiae predominantly within the macrophages or mononuclear cells of the perivascular infiltrates associated with eschars or papules.[97]

Clinical manifestations. The incubation period of rickettsialpox is 9 to 14 days after the usually painless mite bite occurs.[20,90] The primary lesion is a papule that develops at the site of the mite bite. This lesion progresses through a papulonodular stage to a tense 0.5- to 2-cm vesicle that ruptures to form an eschar with surrounding induration, which is the hallmark of the disease.[155] Two eschars may be seen. Regional lymph nodes related to the primary eschar are almost invariably enlarged.

Constitutional symptoms develop approximately a week after the mite bite. Fever and malaise are commonly present. The fever is irregular, with temperature fluctuating between 37.8°C and 39.5°C (100°F and 103°F), and rarely lasts longer than 6 or 7 days. It usually is accompanied by the frontal headache characteristic of rickettsial diseases. Rhinorrhea, cough, sore throat, nausea, vomiting, and abdominal pain are occasional findings.[68]

The rash is the most remarkable aspect of the disease. It usually develops within several days of the onset of fever as scattered nonpruritic macules, which rapidly become firm maculopapules. Within a day or two, vesicles develop on the summits of the papules. The lesions usually appear on the face, trunk, and extremities, with sparing of the palms and soles.[19] The number of lesions ranges from 5 or 6 to more than 100.

Diagnosis. The diagnosis can be made by immunohistochemical staining of skin biopsy specimens, by PCR analysis of amplified gene products from eschars or culture of *R. akari* from eschars, and by serologic assays. These tests, used singly or in combination to establish the diagnosis, are available through the Centers for Disease Control and Prevention (CDC). A fourfold increase in serum antibodies to *R. akari* between acute and convalescent sera or a single titer of more than a 1:64 dilution is considered diagnostic. Cross-reaction is seen between antibodies to *R. akari* and *R. rickettsii*, but titers are greater with *R. akari* than with *R. rickettsii* antigen.[125]

Differential diagnosis. Anthrax is a differential consideration. Rickettsialpox lacks the striking brawny, nonpitting edema surrounding the eschar that is characteristic of anthrax. Anthrax is not associated with the characteristic papulovesicular rash of rickettsialpox. The haphazard distribution of the characteristic papulovesicles is similar in appearance to chickenpox rash in an adult. Infectious mononucleosis, gonococcemia, and infection with echovirus or coxsackieviruses also should be considered.[104] Patients often give a history of having worked in basements, around incinerators, or in similar areas that might be infested by house mice and their mites.

Treatment. Rickettsialpox is a self-limited nonfatal disease that resolves within 7 to 10 days in untreated patients. Treatment shortens the duration of symptoms, usually to 24 to 48 hours.[20] Doxycycline is the drug of choice. A treatment course of 3 to 5 days is sufficient.

Other Spotted Fever Group Rickettsioses

A number of antigenically distinct *Rickettsia* spp. cause disease in humans. Among these, *R. parkeri* is perhaps the most important emerging rickettsial disease in the United States. This organism produces a mild spotted fever illness that may be difficult to clinically distinguish from mild RMSF.[124] In contrast with RMSF, an eschar is an important feature of *R. parkeri* infection. The vector for *R. parkeri* is the Gulf Coast tick, *Amblyomma maculatum*, which is most heavily concentrated in Gulf Coast and southeastern states. Whereas most cases occur in the Deep South, both infected *A. maculatum* ticks and at least one human case of *R. parkeri* infection have been reported from Virginia.[58,193,202] Serologic assays in clinical use cannot distinguish *R. parkeri* from *R. rickettsii*. Whereas *R. parkeri* infection may be self-limited, it would be prudent to treat all suspected *R. parkeri* cases as if they are RMSF.

Another notable member of the spotted fever group is *Rickettsia africae*, the cause of African tick bite fever (ATBF). Evidence suggests that this is one of the most common acute febrile illnesses experienced by travelers to Africa.[87] This disease has primarily been associated with travel to southern Africa and in particular travel in the game parks in this part of the continent.[59,141] Its known range is broader, however, and includes much of sub-Saharan Africa. It is also endemic on some eastern Caribbean islands. Cattle ticks from the genus *Amblyomma* are responsible for transmission of the organism. The clinical hallmarks of ATBF are fever, headache, neck muscle myalgias, and an inoculation eschar with regional lymphadenopathy. Up to 50% of patients have multiple eschars that ascend along the lymphatic drainage.[103] Rash is unusual in ATBF. This is a benign infection and is probably self-limited in most cases. Doxycycline has been associated with rapid resolution.

Many other *Rickettsia* species are known to infect humans. *Rickettsia japonica* is the etiologic agent of Japanese spotted fever, *Rickettsia sibirica* of Siberian tick typhus, and *Rickettsia australis* of Queensland tick typhus. Dogs are the principal mammalian reservoir; ticks also act as reservoirs by virtue of transovarial transmission. Other newly recognized tick-borne diseases, such as *Rickettsia slovaca* infection, for which the wild boar is the main host, have been described in Europe.[16] *Rickettsia felis* is transmitted by fleas, and its natural reservoirs are the opossum and the cat.[18] The diseases caused by these and other rickettsial species have similar clinical, pathologic, and epidemiologic patterns. As with other rickettsioses, doxycycline is the preferred therapy.

TYPHUS

The rather imprecise term *typhus* is most commonly used to refer to three rickettsial diseases: epidemic typhus, murine or endemic typhus, and scrub typhus. Whereas the respective agents of epidemic and murine typhus, *Rickettsia prowazekii* and *Rickettsia typhi*, are phylogenetically related, scrub typhus is caused by *Orientia tsutsugamushi*, which is not even a member of the genus *Rickettsia*. To make matters more confusing, various spotted fevers are referred to as tick typhus (e.g., Queensland tick typhus, Siberian tick typhus).

Rickettsia prowazekii Infection (Epidemic Typhus)

Overview. Epidemic typhus is a louse-borne infection caused by *R. prowazekii*. Explosive epidemics of typhus are seen under conditions of overcrowding and extreme squalor. Typhus has been the suspected cause of some human epidemics dating back to the Dark Ages, but the first known epidemic occurred during the Spanish siege of Moorish Granada in 1489. Most sizeable typhus epidemics have struck during times of war. Outbreaks of typhus occurred throughout the world during the 19th century, famously ravaging Napoleon's army as it retreated from Moscow. Typhus afflicted thousands of soldiers during World War I, particularly on the eastern front. A devastating outbreak struck Russia during its civil war between 1917 and 1925, afflicting an estimated 25 million people and killing 3 million. During World War II, typhus killed tens of thousands as a result of the deplorable conditions in the Nazi ghettos, concentration camps, and prisoner-of-war camps. Typhus also struck combatants in the North African and Eastern European theaters.

The use of dichlorodiphenyltrichloroethane (DDT) in the 1950s resulted in a dramatic worldwide decline in typhus. Since then, it has reemerged predominantly in highland regions of sub-Saharan Africa and to a lesser extent Central and South America. Rwanda, Burundi, and Ethiopia have been particularly affected, certainly as a result of the coexistence of poverty and war.[128] In 1997 approximately 100,000 persons in Burundi were affected and as many as 15% died.[14,144,146] A smaller outbreak occurred in Russia in 1997.[171] Although autochthonous cases in the United States are rare, there have been at least 30 cases since 1976. These are most likely due to exposure to the flying squirrel (*Glaucomys volans*), which is a sylvatic reservoir for *R. prowazekii*.[44,114,148]

Epidemiology and transmission. Humans are the primary reservoir for *R. prowazekii*. During interepidemic periods some people who previously survived typhus can be a reservoir of *R. prowazekii*. This is particularly true in persons with Brill-Zinsser disease, a form of relapsed typhus that can occur many years after the original infection.[64] The best established natural reservoir for *R. prowazekii* is the flying squirrel, *Glaucomys volans*, which is associated with sylvatic cases. These cases are recognized on rare occasion in the United States.[136] Lice that infest flying squirrels will not bite humans, suggesting that human infection results from direct exposure to aerosolized louse feces.

The vector for epidemic typhus is the human body louse, *Pediculus humanus corporis*. The body louse inhabits clothing, from which it will take blood meals from its host. Frequent blood meals are required because the louse is sensitive to dehydration. It is also sensitive to deviations from normal human body temperature, such as fever. Cold conditions, in which humans have more clothing and blankets, will increase louse habitat. Lice will not survive for long away from a suitable host, so impoverished persons who do not have changes of clothing will be most heavily parasitized. Lice will proliferate under these conditions, and a single person may be infested by thousands of lice. Lice will readily pass between people under crowded and unhygienic conditions. A heavily infested person who develops typhus can infect thousands of lice, which will promptly seek a new host once fever develops. Because each infected person can secondarily infect many others, there can be explosive epidemic potential under conditions of both high human density and heavy louse infestation.

R. prowazekii incubates in the louse for 5 to 10 days after it bites an infected person. Great numbers of rickettsiae are then shed in louse feces.[145] Because the louse defecates as it feeds, infectious feces can be rubbed into a louse bite wound. The bodies of crushed lice are also infectious. Dried louse feces can be aerosolized and cause infection through the eye or the respiratory tract.

Pathogenesis. The organism initially spreads through lymphatics and the blood to infect small vessel endothelial cells in a wide variety of target organs.[9] Intracellular proliferation of the organism results in mechanical cell lysis, producing widespread vasculitis and capillary leak.

Clinical manifestations. Illness begins after a 10- to 14-day incubation period. An initial period of malaise is followed by high fever, headache, and rash.[4] Body temperature generally rises rapidly to 40°C (104°F) or higher. In untreated patients, it remains at this level with minor fluctuations until death or recovery occurs. Headache is common and may be severe or intractable. Cough is also a frequent complaint. The rash usually appears on the trunk by the fourth to seventh day; it spreads peripherally to the extremities and typically spares the face, palms, and soles. Initially, the rash consists of macules that fade on pressure; they soon become fixed as maculopapules and later become petechial or hemorrhagic. Rash is less frequently recognized in individuals with dark skin. Central nervous system manifestations are described in up to 80% of patients, including delirium, coma, seizures, and hearing loss.[61] Other complications include parotitis, otitis media, pericarditis, myocarditis, pericardial effusion, pleural effusion, and pneumonia.[40,199,200] Severe cases of typhus can be manifested with shock or with tissue ischemia, including gangrene. Mortality was as high as 60% in the preantibiotic era and is higher in malnourished populations and elderly people. With appropriate antibiotics, the mortality is approximately 4%. Recrudescent infection (Brill-Zinsser disease) can occur years after the primary infection if it is not eradicated. Because of partial immunity, Brill-Zinsser disease is milder than primary typhus.

Diagnosis. Typhus is diagnosed with evidence of seroconversion. A fourfold rise in IgG antibody titer is considered diagnostic. This requires paired acute and convalescent sera. Several testing methods are available, but the preferred method is indirect IFA assay.[99,122] IFA assay will not discriminate epidemic from murine typhus (*R. typhi* infection); discrimination between the two infections requires Western blotting with cross-adsorption.[100] Shell vial culture can detect *R. prowazekii* from blood specimens.[13] The Weil-Felix agglutination test is no longer recommended because of lack of specificity (due to cross-reactivity) and poor sensitivity in Brill-Zinsser disease.

Differential diagnosis. Typhus may be difficult to distinguish from other acute febrile illnesses, especially early in the course of disease. Depending on the local epidemiology, these can include typhoid fever, dengue, malaria, influenza, leptospirosis, and other rickettsial illnesses. The rash of louse-borne typhus begins centrally on the trunk and spreads peripherally to the extremities, whereas the reverse is true for RMSF. Moreover, a rash on the palms and soles, a common event in RMSF, rarely is observed in typhus.

Treatment. Doxycycline is the treatment of choice for epidemic typhus.[98] Therapy is given until the patient is afebrile for at least 3 days and clinical improvement is evident; the usual duration is 7 to 10 days. Lack of defervescence after 3 days suggests an alternative diagnosis. Single-dose therapy with doxycycline 200 mg has been effective in epidemic settings.[129] Chloramphenicol is an alternative agent for those with a serious contraindication to doxycycline. As with other rickettsial infections, the risk for tooth staining is negligible for young children receiving this degree of doxycycline exposure; moreover, the potential lethality of typhus justifies the use of doxycycline in children in whom the diagnosis is plausible. Whereas fluoroquinolones have in vitro activity, there has been a treatment failure with ciprofloxacin resulting in death.[204]

Prevention. DDT was effective at limiting the burden of typhus in the 1950s. Its use has been long banned by many countries. Along with DDT, malathion and permethrin are also effective at eradicating lice from infested clothing and bedding. Lice will die within days if they do not have access to a host, so removal of infested clothing for 1 week may suffice.[145] Relief workers assisting persons at risk for typhus can pretreat their clothing with permethrin. Doxycycline prophylaxis appears to be effective in select populations at risk for scrub typhus; whether this is true for epidemic typhus remains unknown.

Rickettsia typhi Infection (Murine Typhus)

Overview. Murine typhus, also known as flea-borne or endemic typhus, is a flea-borne zoonosis primarily of rats, opossums, and cats. The disease occurs worldwide, especially in warm climates where rats or opossums are abundant. During the early 20th century, there were thousands of annual cases of murine typhus in the United States, particularly along the Gulf Coast and the southern Atlantic seaboard. In recent years, 60 to 80 cases have been reported annually, most of which are from southern California, the southeastern Gulf Coast including Texas, and Hawaii.[1,54] The actual incidence in the United States is unknown. Approximately 0.6% of children in south-central states have an *R. typhi* titer of greater than 1:64.[110] The seroprevalence in southeastern Texas may be as high as 15%. These figures suggest that murine typhus is considerably underrecognized in certain regions.[54,137,194]

Epidemiology and transmission. *R. typhi* infection is a vector-borne zoonosis that persists in a flea-mammal cycle in nature. The classically described cycle involves the Oriental rat flea, *Xenopsylla cheopis*, and peridomestic rats. Rat infestations, especially near granaries and ports, pose a risk for human contact. A more recently described transmission cycle involves the cat flea, *Ctenocephalides felis*, and opossums or domesticated cats as their primary mammalian host. This cycle seems primarily responsible for ongoing transmission of both *R. typhi* and *R. felis* in suburban regions of southern California and south Texas.[1,17,160] Uninfected fleas acquire the organism from infected mammals and can transmit it to new hosts, including humans; in turn, an infected mammal can serve as a reservoir for many fleas. Rickettsiae multiply and reside in both the digestive and reproductive tracts of the flea, which is unaffected by the organism. The flea goes on to produce highly infectious feces for the rest of its life. It can also pass the organism transovarially to its offspring. Humans are not the preferred hosts for fleas, but the cat flea in particular will readily bite humans. If the flea bites a person, infection typically occurs when flea feces are rubbed into the bite wound; it can also be inoculated by direct contact or by aerosol to mucous membranes.

Clinical manifestations. Murine typhus is clinically similar to epidemic typhus (*R. prowazekii* infection), but it is milder, of shorter duration, and less likely to be severe or fatal. Symptoms develop after a 5- to 10-day incubation period, although an antecedent flea bite is not always reported. All affected patients develop fever, and most have headache or rash.[192] The classic triad of fever, headache, and rash occurs in half of patients. This may be because rash typically appears between days 3 and 10 of illness and may not be present when patients first seek medical attention. Other common symptoms include malaise, myalgias, and vomiting. Rashes are typically macular or maculopapular; only in rare cases have they been described as petechial. Laboratory abnormalities are inconsistently reported, but the most common include elevated hepatic transaminases and mild hyponatremia.[54,160] Children who receive appropriate antibiotics undergo defervescence in 1 to 3 days. Even without appropriate treatment, murine typhus is generally self-limited, with recovery in 1 to 2 weeks and a very low rate of complications.[54,160]

Diagnosis. A fourfold change in titer between acute and convalescent sera by indirect IFA assay, latex agglutination, complement fixation, or enzyme immunoassay is diagnostic. Differentiation among antibodies produced in response to epidemic typhus is difficult but may be accomplished by use of an IgM-specific enzyme immunoassay, if needed. Immunohistochemical staining or PCR analysis of amplified gene product of tissues and culture, available through the CDC, also can be used for confirmation.

Differential diagnosis. Murine typhus is an undifferentiated acute febrile illness and resembles numerous other infections. In the United States, these include but are not limited to enteroviral disease, other viral exanthems, other rickettsial diseases, and group A streptococcal infection. A history of recent travel to tropical or developing countries could expand the differential diagnosis to include other febrile illnesses, such as malaria, dengue, typhoid fever, and leptospirosis.

Treatment. Doxycycline is the treatment of choice for murine typhus. Chloramphenicol is an alternative in patients with an important contraindication to tetracyclines. Whereas fluoroquinolones have been used successfully to treat *R. typhi* infection, at least one treatment failure has been documented. [101,165] Treatment should be continued for at least 3 days after defervescence and evidence of clinical improvement; this is typically 3 to 7 days.

Prevention. Rat control measures can lower the likelihood of human disease in areas where *R. typhi* is transmitted.

Scrub Typhus

Overview. Scrub typhus is a mite-borne rickettsial disease that exclusively occurs in the Asia-Pacific region. This infection may have been recognized as early as the 3rd century AD and was the subject of non-Western medical writing in Japan during the 19th century.[118] In the South Pacific theater of World War II, scrub typhus was second only to malaria as a cause of fever, affecting more than 16,000 Allied soldiers.[118,131] It remained an important pathogen among febrile American soldiers in the Vietnam conflict.[10,77]

Organism. The causative organism, *Orientia tsutsugamushi*, was formerly a member of the genus *Rickettsia*. In 1995 it was reclassified to the novel genus *Orientia* on the basis of distinctive phenotypic and genetic features.[165] *O. tsutsugamushi* is distinguished by remarkable antigenic heterogeneity. Strain differences also appear to contribute to striking differences in its severity.

Epidemiology and transmission. Scrub typhus is widely distributed throughout central, eastern, and southern Asia. It is transmitted as far north as Kamchatka in eastern Russia and as far west as Pakistan and Afghanistan. Its southern range includes the islands of Indonesia and Oceania as well as northern Australia.[91] The disease is distributed according to the habitat of its vectors, which in turn are distributed in widely diverse habitats. Scrub typhus has been described from sea level to alpine meadows above 3000 meters in elevation, in both arid and humid environments, in a variety of agricultural regions, and more recently in cities.[157,166,177,178] Humans are most likely to encounter chiggers in undergrowth in rural areas. Travelers engaged in outdoor activities, such as camping and trekking, are at risk for acquiring scrub typhus; some of these individuals do not become clinically ill until after return to their home country.[80,157]

Trombiculid mites from the genus *Leptotrombidium* are the vectors for scrub typhus. Only the six-legged larvae, known colloquially as chiggers, will feed on humans. The eight-legged nymphs and adults feed on plant matter and do not parasitize mammals. Wild rodents, particularly rats, are the preferred host for chiggers and are important in the ecology of scrub typhus. The rodents, however, are not thought to be a natural reservoir for *O. tsutsugamushi*, and in fact each mite feeds on a mammalian host only once in its life. Rather, the microorganism persists transstadially (across life cycle stages) within the mite and is passed transovarially to subsequent generations.[60,168,182] Thus the mite itself is the natural reservoir for this pathogen.

Pathogenesis. *O. tsutsugamushi* primarily infects endothelial cells and mononuclear leukocytes. Human autopsy specimens have shown endothelial cells infected with microorganisms in numerous organs, including brain, heart, kidney, and lung.[117] They have also been found in macrophages and in cardiac muscle cells. Dissemination from the inoculation site to target organs may occur through infected peripheral blood mononuclear cells.[186] Infection of monocytes induces a robust inflammatory cascade that may be responsible for tissue injury and both systemic and organ-specific disease manifestations.[96,170] There are marked differences in disease severity and mortality, and these are likely due to strain variations. The phenotypic factors responsible for this variability are poorly understood.

Clinical manifestations. In one-half to two-thirds of cases, the initial mite bite lesion develops into a necrotic eschar. In adults eschars are most commonly found on the trunk[94]; in children they are seen commonly in moist intertriginous areas such as the genitalia and perineum.[159] The incubation period is approximately 1 to 2 weeks, and characteristic features of the disease develop at approximately the same time that the eschar is noted. A scar often persists at the site of the eschar.[190]

Fever is nearly universal. Common clinical findings include hepatomegaly, respiratory distress, and lymphadenopathy. Among 30 children presenting with febrile illness of at least 5 days' duration in Thailand, common physical signs included lymphadenopathy (93%), hepatomegaly (73%), eschar (68%), conjunctival hyperemia (33%), maculopapular rash (30%), interstitial pneumonia (30%), and splenomegaly (23%).[159] In a separate series of 60 Sri Lankan children, the most common findings in patients with confirmed scrub typhus were hepatomegaly (95%), generalized lymphadenopathy (60%), respiratory distress (45%), and splenomegaly (35%).[37] Hepatomegaly was observed in 80% and cough in 73% of Indian children with scrub typhus.[126] Patients can present with either transudative or exudative pleural effusions.[92] Nervous system disease can manifest as aseptic meningitis, meningoencephalitis, or cranial or peripheral neuropathies. Severe complications include myocarditis, disseminated intravascular coagulation, and the acute respiratory distress syndrome.[119,126] The severity and lethality of scrub typhus can vary widely.

Diagnosis. The mainstay of scrub typhus diagnosis is serologic testing. The gold standard is the indirect IFA assay; however, there is little consensus in IFA methodology and positivity cutoff limits. Blacksell and colleagues reviewed the evidence base for various methodologies and the criteria for positive IFA assay results and concluded that the diagnosis should be based on a fourfold or greater increase in the IFA titer in paired serum specimens and on a single sample only when there is an adequate local evidence base.[15] The limited number of source strains used for IFA assay antigen may be inadequate given the enormous antigenic diversity and geographic heterogeneity of *O. tsutsugamushi*.[91]

Other tests, such as enzyme-linked immunosorbent assay, dot immunoassay, indirect immunoperoxidase, and Weil-Felix OX-K assay, are also used.[86,120] The last is the most commonly used diagnostic modality in developing countries; however, this assay lacks both sensitivity and specificity. OX-K agglutinins develop in only a little more than 50% of scrub typhus patients. Moreover, OX-K agglutinins also are produced in relapsing fever.

Identification of the rickettsial strain in infected patients by use of strain-specific monoclonal antibodies in an inhibition enzyme-linked immunosorbent assay or PCR with strain-specific primers offers potential to establish the diagnosis in the acute stage of the illness.[62,63] An eschar PCR assay, evaluated prospectively, demonstrated high sensitivity and specificity compared with IFA assay.[93] Cell culture and xenodiagnosis-based assays are expensive and laborious and are not available clinically.

Differential diagnosis. Scrub typhus can be suspected when a patient gives a history of recent exposure in a geographic area where scrub typhus occurs. If, in addition, a local eschar, evanescent rash, and general and regional lymphadenopathy along with fever, headache, and conjunctival suffusion are present, the physician should be alerted to suspect scrub typhus; however, it cannot be differentiated with certainty from other febrile illnesses that occur in the region. These include but are not limited to dengue, chikungunya, leptospirosis, malaria, typhoid fever, and other rickettsioses such as murine typhus.

Treatment. Doxycycline is the treatment of choice. Children have responded well to treatment for 4 to 7 days.[159] Doxycycline is rickettsiostatic, and patients with scrub typhus who are treated in the first week of illness can require sporadic short courses of antibiotic therapy for prevention of relapse.[179] Chloramphenicol, azithromycin, and rifampin are alternatives.[95,127,133] Strains with reduced susceptibility to antibiotics have been observed in northern Thailand.[187] In one study from this region, rifampin was found to produce a significantly faster clinical response than did doxycycline.[188]

Prognosis. The prognosis varies widely because of significant differences in the severity of disease caused by different strains in different populations and in various geographic areas. Mortality rates in the preantibiotic era ranged from 1% to 60%. With the use of antimicrobials, fatalities rarely occur. When treatment is begun early in the course of scrub typhus, relapses as well as definite second attacks of the disease can occur. The heterogeneity of scrub typhus strains probably accounts for reinfections.

Prevention. Vector control involves impregnating clothing and smearing exposed skin surfaces with dimethyl or dibutyl phthalate. Short-term vector control of camping grounds can be accomplished by cutting, burning, or bulldozing vegetation, along with heavy spraying with insecticides such as lindane. Chemoprophylaxis is feasible for persons with high-risk exposure for short periods. Doxycycline given once a week may provide effective chemoprophylaxis against naturally transmitted scrub typhus if the prophylaxis is started before exposure to infection and continued for 6 weeks after exposure.[179] A recent report, however, showed that prophylactic failures can occur and are not associated with antimicrobial resistance.[74] No satisfactory vaccine has been produced.

EHRLICHIOSIS AND ANAPLASMOSIS

Overview. Ehrlichiosis and anaplasmosis are tick-borne infections caused by rickettsial organisms from the genera *Ehrlichia* and *Anaplasma*. Strictly speaking, they are best thought of as anaplasmoses because both genera are members of the family Anaplasmataceae of the order Rickettsiales. Six members of this family are known to infect humans: *Ehrlichia chaffeensis*, *Ehrlichia ewingii*, *Ehrlichia canis*, *Ehrlichia muris*–like, *Anaplasma phagocytophilum*, and *Neorickettsia sennetsu*. The last two were formerly members of the genus *Ehrlichia*; *A. phagocytophilum* was reclassified to its own genus in 2001.[46]

Unlike many rickettsial infections, which have been recognized for decades if not centuries, ehrlichiosis and anaplasmosis are emerging diseases that have been only recently identified. From 1953 until the late 1980s, the only known human infection from this group was Sennetsu fever, a mild febrile illness in East Asia caused by *Neorickettsia* (formerly *Ehrlichia*) *sennetsu*. The disease that ultimately became known as human monocytic ehrlichiosis (HME) was first described in humans in 1986, and it was suspected that this was due to *E. canis*, a known veterinary pathogen.[50,107] It was not until 1991 that its primary cause, *E. chaffeensis*, was identified.[4] Human ehrlichiosis can also be caused by *E. ewingii*, *E. canis*, and an *E. muris*–like organism.[22,135] In the early 1990s, the syndrome now known as human granulocytic anaplasmosis (HGA) was identified in the upper Midwest; its cause, *A. phagocytophilum*, was recognized in 1994.[30]

Organisms. *Ehrlichia* and *Anaplasma* are small gram-negative obligately intracellular bacteria. *E. chaffeensis* propagates in macrophages; *A. phagocytophilum* and *E. ewingii* multiply in neutrophils.

Epidemiology and transmission. The incidence for both HME and HGA has increased substantially during the last decade, although this may be partly a function of increased recognition. These infections have also been reportable only since the late 1990s, which suggests that some of the increased incidence is a function of more complete reporting and case ascertainment practices. There is also annual variation in the incidence of both diseases, which lacks a satisfactory explanation. Nonetheless, hundreds of persons are affected annually. In 2009 there were 944 cases of HME and 1161 cases of HGA.[28] In 2010 there were 740 cases of HME and 1761 cases of HGA. The prevalence of *E. chaffeensis* titers of 1 : 160 or higher was 3% among children residing in the southeast and south-central regions of the United States, suggesting that exposure is far more common than is the incidence of recognized disease.[111]

The geographic distributions of both HME and HGA are tied to the distribution of their respective tick vectors. The lone star tick, *Amblyomma americanum*, is the principal vector of HME and *E. ewingii* ehrlichiosis. This aggressive tick is by far the most common "pest" tick in the southern and southeastern United States.[24,52,66,115] In low numbers, its range extends as far north as New England, but it is particularly abundant in Missouri, North Carolina, and states farther south. All active stages of the tick will readily bite humans. Individuals can become multiply parasitized by larval ticks (known colloquially as seed ticks). The adult female tick is easily recognized by a conspicuous light-colored spot, but this marking is not present on males or on immature ticks. HME is transmitted in the eastern half of the United States, from the Great Plains to the Atlantic Coast. Oklahoma, Arkansas, and Missouri together account for 35% of all cases.[105] Southeastern and mid-Atlantic states account for most of the remainder, but HME acquisition is well documented in Delaware and New Jersey and occasionally occurs even in coastal New England. There is also serologic evidence of HME transmission in Central and South America. The white-tailed deer is the most likely natural reservoir for *E. chaffeensis*.[105]

HGA, by contrast, is transmitted in North America, Europe, and Asia. In the United States, it primarily occurs in northeastern states, from New Jersey through northern New England, as well as in Minnesota and Wisconsin in the upper Midwest.[105] The black-legged or deer tick, *Ixodes scapularis*, is the vector for HGA. *A. phagocytophilum* is maintained in nature in a tick-mammal cycle that primarily involves small rodents.[27,172] Whereas adult *I. scapularis* ticks will occasionally feed on humans, it is primarily the nymph whose feeding habits make it a vector for human infections. The nymph is most active in late spring and early summer. Because this immature stage of the tick is quite small, a tick bite often will go unrecognized. HGA shares a vector with Lyme disease, and there is evidence that the endemic range for Lyme disease is expanding; this may portend further expansion of the anaplasmosis-endemic zone as well. HGA is rarely acquired in California, where the Western black-legged tick (*Ixodes pacificus*) is the responsible vector. In Europe, it is transmitted by *Ixodes ricinus*; in Asia, its vector is *Ixodes persulcatus*.

Both anaplasmosis and ehrlichiosis are predominantly transmitted from May through October, in conjunction with the peak activity of their tick vectors. In contrast to other tick-borne diseases such as Lyme disease and RMSF, in which children have among the highest incidence rates, it is older adults who suffer the highest incidence of HGA and HME.

Pathogenesis and pathology. The pathogenesis of ehrlichiosis is incompletely elucidated. Although it is capable of establishing infection in numerous organs and tissues, the primary target cell for HGA is the granulocyte; for HME, it is the macrophage. Granulomas of the bone marrow occur frequently in HME, suggesting that involvement of the reticuloendothelial system may be important in pathogenesis.[47]

Organisms enter the cytoplasm of host cells and proliferate in phagosomes into elementary bodies. These individual organisms multiply by binary fission into immature inclusions called initial bodies. Mature groups of elementary bodies form morulae, which are released by rupture of the cell to reinitiate the infecting process.[107]

Clinical manifestations. Most patients become clinically ill within 2 weeks of exposure. HME and HGA are acute febrile illnesses in which fever and malaise are universal symptoms.[45,48,56,130] Headache, myalgia, arthralgias, and nausea are also common. Confusion occurs in about 20% of patients with HME, primarily among older adults; this symptom is less common in HGA. Rash is more common in ehrlichiosis than in anaplasmosis and primarily occurs in children. Rashes can be macular, maculopapular, or petechial and seldom develop in adult infections. Rashes are reported in about 30% of cases of HME, compared with 10% or less in HGA.

Meningitis as a manifestation of HME has been reported in children. Symptoms can range from irritability and meningismus to obtundation with response only to painful stimuli.[11,42,67] Initial examination of cerebrospinal fluid reveals pleocytosis ranging from approximately 50 to 1400 white blood cells, usually with a predominance of mononuclear cells; a range of 5 to 40 red blood cells; mildly elevated protein concentration; and a normal to slightly low glucose value. Complete recovery is the rule. Central nervous system involvement is much less common in HGA.

The most common laboratory findings in both infections are hematologic abnormalities and elevated hepatic transaminases.[45] Thrombocytopenia is seen in three-fourths of patients, leukopenia in two-thirds, and anemia in one-half. In HME, the leukocyte abnormalities are primarily lymphopenia and monocytopenia. In HGA, neutropenia is more common, especially with illness of longer duration. Elevations of hepatic transaminases are seen up to 80% of the time in both HGA and HME.

A variety of complications may be seen in both infections. These include protracted fever, renal dysfunction occasionally of sufficient severity to require dialysis, acute respiratory distress syndrome, myocarditis, neuropathies and plexopathies, opportunistic infections, and a toxic shock–like syndrome.[45,55,153] Whereas persistent infection is much better documented in reservoir hosts, there has been a case report of fatal, treatment-refractory persistent infection in an older adult, although relapse after doxycycline therapy is thought to be otherwise unheard of.[123] There is one case report of fatal seronegative HME in a patient with advanced HIV infection.[123] Up to one-half of patients with HME or HGA require hospitalization. The mortality rate is 3% for ehrlichiosis and 0.5% for anaplasmosis.

Diagnosis. In contrast to RMSF and other infections with agents in the genus *Rickettsia*, anaplasmosis and ehrlichiosis are primarily infections of circulating leukocytes. This potentially allows the diagnosis to be made at the point of care or during the patient's clinical illness. Peripheral blood smear examination will reveal morulae in neutrophils in 25% to 75% of patients with HGA; intramonocytic morulae are seen in 10% or less of patients with HME.[6,7,162] Whereas the sensitivity of this examination is low, a positive blood smear is pathognomonic and will allow a real-time diagnosis. PCR amplification of a peripheral blood specimen is a more sensitive alternative for both anaplasmosis and ehrlichiosis; it is also the only modality available for the specific diagnosis of *E. ewingii* infection. Reported sensitivities range from 60% to 85% for HME and 67% to 90% for HGA.[6,7,81,121] These assays are available from some clinical laboratories. The sensitivity of both blood smear examination and PCR is abrogated by antecedent doxycycline treatment.

Serology by indirect IFA assay remains the most sensitive and widely used means to diagnose ehrlichiosis and anaplasmosis. Paired acute and convalescent sera must be obtained, and a fourfold rise in antibody titer is considered diagnostic. The reported sensitivity is 88% to 90% for HME and 82% to 100% for HGA.[35,121,185] Antibodies to *Ehrlichia* and *Anaplasma* may be cross-reactive, so simultaneous serologic testing for both infections is preferred. The use of paired acute and convalescent sera must be emphasized for two reasons: (1) a single acute serum specimen will yield a positive result in only 3% of cases; and (2) a positive titer at a single time point may be due to prior infection, asymptomatic seropositivity, or cross-reactivity to other infectious agents.[8,121,185]

Differential diagnosis. A variety of febrile illnesses can be indistinguishable from ehrlichiosis and anaplasmosis, especially early in infection. The most common symptoms of fever, headache, and malaise are generic. A careful history, exposure assessment, and physical examination can help limit the differential diagnosis. Differential considerations include but are not limited to viral infections (e.g., enteroviruses, adenoviruses) and bacterial infections (including septic and toxic shock syndromes and focal bacterial infections such as pneumonia that have not yet manifested focally). A number of tropical infectious diseases can have similar clinical presentations and laboratory findings; these include dengue virus infection, typhoid fever, malaria, and leptospirosis.

HME and HGA must be distinguished from other tick-borne diseases, in particular RMSF. Compared with RMSF, these infections are less likely to be accompanied by rash and more often are associated with leukopenia or pancytopenia. The similarity of ehrlichiosis and RMSF is emphasized by two retrospective serosurveys in which approximately 10% of specimens from patients lacking the serologic criteria for a diagnosis of RMSF fulfilled diagnostic criteria for ehrlichiosis.[73,152] Other tick-borne illnesses, such as babesiosis, Colorado tick fever, relapsing fever, and tularemia, should be included in the differential diagnosis. In fact, the only major tick-borne infection in North America that is unlikely to be confused for HGA or HME is Lyme disease because high fever and systemic toxicity would be unusual for this infection.

Treatment. The drug of choice for treatment of human ehrlichiosis and anaplasmosis is doxycycline. The recommended dosage is 2.2 mg/kg twice daily (maximum adult dose, 100 mg twice daily). Treatment should continue for at least 3 days after defervescence for a total course of 5 to 14 days.[174,201] Because both infections may be severe or fatal, doxycycline treatment should be initiated when the diagnosis is suspected, without regard for the age of the child. Severe cases can require a longer course of treatment. Rifampin is an alternative that can be used in pregnancy and in early childhood, particularly when the index of suspicion for anaplasmosis or ehrlichiosis is low. There is contradictory in vitro evidence about fluoroquinolones, and these are not recommended for the treatment of either infection. Prophylactic treatment after tick bites is discouraged for the prevention of HGA, HME, or other tick-borne rickettsial illnesses.

Coinfection. HGA shares the same tick vector and geographic distribution as *Borrelia burgdorferi* and *Babesia microti*, the agents of Lyme disease and human babesiosis. Simultaneous coinfection with two or even three of these pathogens occasionally occurs and is well described. Because Lyme disease is by far the most common of these three, one should consider coinfection in patients who have Lyme disease that is accompanied by atypically high fever, systemic toxicity, uncharacteristic laboratory abnormalities, or poor response to therapy. Doxycycline therapy for anaplasmosis will be active against *B. burgdorferi*, but the duration of therapy may be shorter than that recommended for early Lyme disease (typically 10–14 days). Treatment of babesiosis requires either clindamycin with quinine or atovaquone plus azithromycin.

Q FEVER

Historical aspects. Q fever (the "Q" is for "query") was first described by Edward Derrick as part of an investigation of an apparently infectious febrile illness in 1937.[39] The cause of Q fever was discovered in the late 1930s independently by Burnet and Freeman in Australia and by Cox in the United States. The organism was named *Coxiella burnetii* in honor of two of the discoverers. Infection with *C. burnetii* is worldwide in distribution and is often asymptomatic. When it causes symptoms, the disease is Q fever; it is typically an influenza-like acute illness characterized by fever, headache, fatigue, and myalgias.[176] It can also cause a difficult to diagnose chronic infection, particularly in patients with preexisting valvular heart disease.

Organism. *C. burnetii* is a small gram-negative coccobacillus that looks like most rickettsiae. However, it has recently been reclassified in the Gammaproteobacteria on the basis of 16s rDNA studies (order: Legionellales) and is now understood to be relatively closely related to *Legionella pneumophila*.[102,164] *C. burnetii* is an intracellular pathogen that multiplies within phagosomes in the cells it infects, in contrast to the rickettsiae, which can live independently in the cytoplasm or nucleus of infected cells. It is believed that *C. burnetii* is the only intracellular pathogen that is able to neutralize the acidic, degradative environment of eukaryotic polyphagolysosomes.[78] Its life cycle is distinctive in that it produces endospores that are similar to those seen in some gram-positive organisms.[158] These small cell variants protect the organism in the external environment, where it can survive for long periods.[176]

C. burnetii is also distinctive because it exhibits antigenic phase variation. Phase I variants are associated with mammalian infection and are highly contagious; phase II variants, of reduced virulence, follow propagation and are associated with a chromosomal deletion that results in a partial loss of lipopolysaccharide that makes the organism noninfectious.[143]

Epidemiology and transmission. Q fever is distinct from human rickettsial infections in that it is primarily a disease of animals that is transmitted to humans by contact with infected animals rather than by an arthropod bite. It infects a broad range of animals including mammals, birds, and arthropods (mostly ticks). The most common sources of human infection are cattle, goats, and sheep, but pets (including dogs, cats, rabbits, and pigeons) can be vectors.[176] *C. burnetii* organisms are found in very high concentration in the placentas of infected parturient animals and are shed into the environment after labor or abortion.[102] Transmission of infection to humans is through aerosols. Unfortunately, the organisms can be wafted by the wind and infect people with no known exposure.[175] Epidemics have occurred in a variety of situations like abattoirs, tanneries, and shearing camps in rural areas. Cases have been reported of schoolchildren who went to farms on field trips.[108] Laboratory outbreaks are also a concern,[71] and the organism should be cultivated only in a biosafety level 3 laboratory.[102]

Outbreaks of Q fever can occur and cause massive public health ramifications. There was, for example, an epidemic of more than 2200 cases in the Netherlands in 2009 that resulted in the prophylactic slaughter of 50,000 dairy goats in an attempt to end the outbreak.[106]

Pregnant women can transmit the infection to their infants, although the risk for abortion with Q fever is considerable. Those infants not aborted are likely to be delivered prematurely or to have low birth weight.[140]

The prevalence of human Q fever is unknown. The diagnosis is difficult to make, and systematic epidemiologic evaluations are few and overreliant on antibody testing in subjects with variable suspicion of disease. The number of reported cases (an average of 50 to 60 cases per year to the CDC) almost certainly substantially underestimates the actual incidence.[139] The disease has been diagnosed in children younger than 3 years and should be considered during an evaluation for fever of unknown origin.[149] However, Q fever is quite uncommon in the United States, with an average of 40 cases per year reported in the United States, and very few cases in children younger than 15 years.[34] In that 2015 survey, an exposure to raw milk was noted as a risk factor for Q fever disease.

Pathology. Mortality from Q fever is rare, so autopsy specimens are relatively uncommon. Pathologic series obtained during outbreaks described liver and bone marrow disease, in which distinctive fibrin-ring and lipid granulomas were seen. Granulomas have also been seen in the lungs at autopsy. The cellular response was thought to be primarily histiocytic.[161] Biologic control of *C. burnetii* requires a T-cell response, and patients with impaired cellular immunity (cancer patients, HIV-infected people) are at high risk for chronic infection.[102]

Clinical manifestations. Q fever is manifested in both acute and chronic forms. The most common outcome of *C. burnetii* infection is an asymptomatic seroconversion. Symptomatic Q fever is particularly uncommon in children; infected adults are more likely to be symptomatic than children.[176] Using standard diagnostic criteria, in 2002, Maltezou and Raoult could identify 46 published pediatric cases (many patients previously described did not meet current standards for diagnosis). The most common manifestations in children were fever and pneumonia. Other common manifestations were febrile seizures, meningeal irritation, malaise, lymphadenitis, and anorexia. The fever was typically sustained for 5 to 10 days.[108] Q fever myocarditis has been diagnosed in three pediatric patients.

In adults, acute Q fever is manifested as an influenza-like syndrome with the abrupt onset of high fever, fatigue, headaches, and myalgias. Atypical pneumonias can occur, but the chest radiograph is usually normal and the primary manifestation is a nonproductive cough. Hepatitis is common, although it appears to be regionally distributed (some areas have more pneumonia, some more hepatitis). Maculopapular and purpuric rashes are seen in 10%, and myocarditis (although rare) can be potentially fatal.[176]

Chronic Q fever most often occurs in patients with some form of immune compromise. In particular, patients with T-cell defects, pregnant women, and patients with abnormal heart valves are at risk for chronic Q fever. It occurs in 1% to 5% of *C. burnetii*–infected patients, symptomatic and not, and may develop months or years after the primary infection.[176] Q fever endocarditis is manifested with low-grade fever, nonspecific cardiac findings, and a positive antibody test response for *C. burnetii*. It occurs primarily in patients with preexisting valvular disease. A 2002 review article found five cases of pediatric Q fever endocarditis, all of which had vegetations on the child's heart valves. The diagnosis is made serologically. *C. burnetii* was demonstrated on the valves from two of the cases. Q fever osteomyelitis has also been rarely seen in normal children.

Q fever can be severe during pregnancy; 33 confirmed cases were investigated, and in only 5 cases was there a normal pregnancy and healthy term delivery.[108] A subsequent study identified 53 pregnant women with Q fever. Eighty-one percent of patients who were not treated with long-term trimethoprim-sulfamethoxazole therapy had complications: 5 had spontaneous abortions, 10 experienced intrauterine fetal deaths, 10 had fetal intrauterine growth restriction, and 10 were delivered prematurely. Patients treated with long-term trimethoprim-sulfamethoxazole therapy were protected from chronic maternal Q fever, placental infections, and obstetric complications.[25]

Diagnosis. *C. burnetii* can be diagnosed by several techniques, but for practical reasons the primary diagnostic modality is serology. The most commonly used test is an IFA assay. The test is actually directed at detection of antibodies against phase II antigens, the nonpathogenic form of the organism. Antibodies peak 4 to 8 weeks after the onset of disease. Detection of anti–phase I antigens is used in the diagnosis of chronic Q fever (e.g., endocarditis, osteomyelitis) because in chronic Q fever, the level of anti–phase I antibodies will exceed anti–phase II antibodies.[102] Culture of *Coxiella* is possible, but because of the high degree of transmissibility, culture should be undertaken only by reference laboratories with biosafety level 3 facilities. If culture is used, either blood or operative specimens of vegetations are acceptable, although the latter will be more sensitive.[189] PCR is also available from reference laboratories; tests on samples from vegetations will be more sensitive than those from blood. A variety of staining techniques can also be used to demonstrate *C. burnetii* in infected tissues.[102]

Differential diagnosis. Because Q fever is not common, routinely searching for it seems impractical, but it is almost certainly underdiagnosed. The acute form of Q fever is essentially self-resolving, and antibody titers do not peak for several weeks after the onset of disease, so diagnostic testing is generally unnecessary. In the correct situation, where there are outbreaks (as occurred in the Netherlands), or for individuals with animal exposure or living in rural areas (particularly with heavy sheep, goat, and cattle farming), *C. burnetii* infection should certainly be considered in the differential. Where the diagnosis becomes critical is in patients with classic fever of unknown origin, for which chronic Q fever should be strongly considered. For patients with known valvular disease or immune compromise, including pregnancy, the possibility of Q fever should be evaluated through the use of serologic screening.

Treatment. Because acute Q fever is generally self-resolving, particularly in children, treatment is usually not necessary. The classic therapy for adults is doxycycline, and alternatives include trimethoprim-sulfamethoxazole, fluoroquinolones, and clarithromycin.[108] The important exception in regard to treatment is the situation of valvular heart disease because 39% of cases of acute Q fever will result in endocarditis in patients with preexisting valvular disease.[53] In those cases, the acute treatment should include both doxycycline and hydroxychloroquine.

In contrast to acute disease, chronic Q fever requires prolonged treatment. Eighteen to 36 months of both doxycycline and hydroxychloroquine is recommended.[108] Valve replacement may unfortunately be necessary for cure in cases of endocarditis. Pregnant women should be treated throughout pregnancy with trimethoprim-sulfamethoxazole to prevent transmission and abortion or premature delivery.[140]

Prevention. A vaccine for Q fever was developed in Australia for use in people with occupational risks, but it is not available in the United States. Most of the preventive strategies involve minimizing contact with infected animals and postdelivery materials through the rapid and hygienic disposal of placentas and aborted fetuses.[138]

NEW REFERENCES SINCE THE SEVENTH EDITION

12. Biggs HM, et al. Diagnosis and management of tickborne rickettsial diseases: Rocky Mountain spotted fever and other spotted fever group rickettsioses, ehrlichioses, and anaplasmosis. *MMWR Recomm Rep*. 2016;65:1-44.
34. Dahlgren FS, McQuiston JH, Massung RF, et al. Q fever in the United States: summary of case reports from two national surveillance systems, 2000-2012. *Am J Trop Med Hyg*. 2015;92(2):247-255.
43. Drexler NA, Dahlgren FS, Heitman KN, et al. National Surveillance of Spotted Fever Group Rickettsioses in the United States, 2008-2012. *Am J Trop Med Hyg*. 2016;94(1):26-34.
74. Harris PN, Oltvolgyi C, Islam A, et al. An outbreak of scrub typhus in military personnel despite protocols for antibiotic prophylaxis: doxycycline resistance excluded by a quantitative PCR-based susceptibility assay. *Microbes Infect*. 2016;18(6):406-411.

The full reference list for this chapter is available at ExpertConsult.com.

196 Mycoplasma and Ureaplasma Infections

Natalie M. Quanquin • James D. Cherry

Mycoplasmas and ureaplasmas, the smallest free-living microorganisms, are ubiquitous in nature. More than 100 species have been recovered from many animals, including human beings.[965,1167,1215,1219] Of this group, 17 have been identified as human pathogens or as part of the normal human flora, with *Mycoplasma pneumoniae* causing respiratory disease as well as a protean array of other clinical manifestations and the genital mycoplasmas (*Mycoplasma hominis, Mycoplasma genitalium, Ureaplasma urealyticum,* and *Ureaplasma parvum*) having clinical significance in neonates and as sexually transmitted infections (STIs).

These organisms lack a cell wall, giving them the class name Mollicutes, which means "soft skin."[518] The genera name *Mycoplasma* is derived from Greek and Latin. *Myco* refers to the mycelial, or filamentous, characteristic and *plasma* indicates the plasticity and pleomorphism of the organism.[1136] *Urea* in *Ureaplasma* indicates the presence of urease,[379] and although this group is in its own genus, because of its shared history, it is commonly included as a "mycoplasma" in the literature.

HISTORY

In 1898, Nocard and Roux[880] recovered the first *Mycoplasma* organism from cattle with contagious pleuropneumonia. Shortly after the original discovery, many other mycoplasmas were recovered from several different animals.[466] These other mycoplasmas, which frequently were not associated with disease, originally were called *pleuropneumonia-like organisms*; this designation was abbreviated to PPLO. The term PPLO enjoyed general use until the early 1960s.

The first isolation of a mycoplasma from a human was reported in 1937 by Dienes and Edsall.[273] This organism, now recognized as *M. hominis,* was recovered from an abscessed Bartholin gland. In 1944, Eaton and colleagues[299] reported the recovery of an organism, originally called the Eaton agent, from persons ill with primary atypical pneumonia. For many years, the Eaton agent was considered to be a virus even though it was inhibited by streptomycin and chlortetracycline.[297,298] In 1961, Marmion and Goodburn[755] noted that the Eaton agent was morphologically similar to PPLOs. In 1962, the organism now known as *M. pneumoniae* was cultivated on a cell-free agar medium and was shown in human volunteer studies to be the etiologic agent of primary atypical pneumonia.[172,174,466]

In 1954, Shepard[1045] reported the recovery of PPLOs with a distinctive small-colony characteristic from men with and without nongonococcal urethritis. These T strains (T for tiny), as they were called, now are classified as *Ureaplasma.* Early literature referred to both ureaplasmas as *U. urealyticum*; however, sequencing techniques have shown sufficient differences that they are now recognized as a separate species—*U. parvum* (formerly biovar 1) and *U. urealyticum* (formerly biovar 2).[129,177,179] One center that rescreened respiratory and genital samples sent to them over the previous 10 years found that the majority of mollicutes isolated were *Ureaplasma* spp. and that the majority of those sequenced (67%) were actually *U. parvum.*[1040]

The observation in the 1970s that some men with nongonococcal urethritis and negative cultures still responded to tetracycline led to the closer examination of urethral smears and the discovery of small motile spiral forms that resembled the insect and plant pathogens of the genus *Spiroplasma.* In 1981, this new microbe was classified as *M. genitalium,* and with a 580-kb genome, it has been considered the smallest known organism capable of independent growth and reproduction.[1141,1142,1167,1170,1171] It served as a guide for the minimal requirements needed to create a synthetic genome, achieved by John Craig Venter and his team in 2010.[401]

CLASSIFICATION

Mycoplasma, Ureaplasma, and *Acholeplasma* are genera of the family *Mycoplasmataceae,* in the order *Mycoplasmatales,* which belongs to the class Mollicutes.[378,965,1215,1219] Both *Mycoplasma* and *Ureaplasma* require cholesterol for growth, have a genome with a molecular weight of approximately 4.5×10^8, and have nicotinamide adenine dinucleotide (NADH) oxidase localized in the cytoplasm. The limited size of their genomes prevents them from encoding many of the enzymes necessary for amino acid synthesis and energy production, making them slow-growing, fastidious organisms that are difficult to isolate in culture. They generate adenosine triphosphate (ATP) through carbohydrate fermentation (glycolysis), lactate oxidation to pyruvate, and/or arginine hydrolysis, depending on the species.[583] Members of the genus *Ureaplasma* are also able to hydrolyze urea.[1047,1048,1140]

The normal human mollicute flora includes 14 *Mycoplasma,* 2 *Ureaplasma,* and 1 *Acholeplasma* spp.[161,309,379,693,1154,1167] These organisms are listed by site of most common isolation and frequency of occurrence in Table 196.1. Most species do not invade submucosal tissues and do not cause disease in immunocompetent hosts unless this protective barrier is breached through surgery or trauma. *Mycoplasma salivarium* and *Mycoplasma orale* are commonly part of the normal respiratory flora and have not been associated with illness in nonimmunocompromised persons. *M. hominis, U. urealyticum,* and *U. parvum* also are recovered commonly from human genital tracts, and although they are considered normal flora, they can trigger inflammatory processes in pregnant women which have been linked to preterm labor. *M. genitalium* is also found in the genital tracts of sexually active individuals and is a cause of nongonococcal urethritis. Inflammatory processes resulting from the presence of *M. genitalium* and *Mycoplasma fermentans,* another colonizer of the genital tract, are possible; however, a link with adverse pregnancy outcomes has not been definitively established.[655,1137,1215,1217] Persistent infections in blood, bones, joints, and kidneys with *Mycoplasma penetrans, Mycoplasma pirum, M. fermentans, M. hominis,* and *U. urealyticum* have occurred in patients with immunodeficiencies (Tully JG. Personal communication. December 1, 1991).[67,817] *Mycoplasma buccale, Mycoplasma amphoriforme, Mycoplasma primatum, Acholeplasma laidlawii,* and *Mycoplasma lipophilum* are rarely isolated and are not thought to cause disease in nonimmunocompromised humans. *Mycoplasma faucium* has been rarely identified in brain abscesses caused by polymicrobial infections likely originating from the oropharynx, but its contribution to the infection is unclear.[303] *M. pneumoniae* is a common cause of respiratory and other human illness.

MYCOPLASMA PNEUMONIAE

Properties

Morphology

Because mycoplasmas lack a cell wall, they all tend to be pleomorphic. Kammer and colleagues[568] studied the morphologic characteristics of *M. pneumoniae* organisms grown in broth medium by scanning electron microscopy and grouped their observations by days of incubation. From 0.3 to 2 days, the predominant morphologic feature consisted of 0.51 ± 0.011 μm symmetric round forms in tightly packed clusters. During the

TABLE 196.1 Mollicute Flora of Humans Listed by Site of Most Common Isolation and Prevalence

Organism	Prevalence
Respiratory Tract	
Mycoplasma salivarium	Very common
Mycoplasma orale	Very common
Mycoplasma buccale	Rare
Mycoplasma faucium	Rare
Mycoplasma lipophilum	Rare
Mycoplasma pneumoniae	Common
Mycoplasma amphoriforme	Rare
Acholeplasma laidlawii	Rare
Genitourinary Tract	
Mycoplasma hominis	Very common
Mycoplasma genitalium	Rare
Mycoplasma fermentans	Rare
Mycoplasma primatum	Rare
Mycoplasma spermatophilum	Rare
Mycoplasma penetrans	Rare
Ureaplasma urealyticum	Very common
Ureaplasma parvum	Very common
Blood	
Mycoplasma pirum	Rare

Data from references 154, 693, 751, 1085, 1154, 1167, 1170, 1215, 1219.

interval from day 2 to day 6, branched and straight filaments and bulbs were the predominant forms. The bulbous elements had a diameter of 0.25 ± 0.006 µm, and the filamentous forms were 0.19 ± 0.005 µm in diameter. The filaments were intertwined, and occasional round forms were observed. From day 6 to day 10, the organisms had a rounded shape but were asymmetric. Their diameter was 0.72 ± 0.027 µm, and they occurred in groups of three or four cells. Biberfeld and Biberfeld[83] noted that *M. pneumoniae* filamentous forms varied in length from 1 to 5 µm.

The ultrastructure of *M. pneumoniae,* as well as that of all members of the family *Mycoplasmataceae,* is relatively simple and consists of a cell membrane and cytoplasm.[379,1166] In 7-day *M. pneumoniae* cultures, Domermuth and associates[277] noted the following characteristics: elementary bodies 105 to 120 nm in diameter, mature cells with a maximal diameter of 690 to 750 nm and an average diameter of 440 to 590 nm, asymmetry of the limiting membrane, electron-dense lines outside the limiting membrane, and dense bodies as cytoplasmic inclusions.

Wilson and Collier[1255] studied the ultrastructure of *M. pneumoniae* in hamster tracheal organ culture and noted filamentous organisms with three-layered membranes. The cells were polymorphic but each had a specialized terminal structure at the site of attachment to the organ culture. This terminal structure had a dense central core containing a denser central filament. Between the organism and the organ culture cell, fusion was not detected, but a loose network of fibrils was noted between the two surfaces. The bodies of the mycoplasmas contained densely stained fibrillar material and cytoplasmic granules, both of which contained nucleic acid.

Motility and Multiplication

Bredt[116] studied *M. pneumoniae* motility and multiplication on a glass surface in liquid medium by phase-contrast microscopy. The organisms were observed to multiply by binary fission; first, short filamentous structures were formed, which then separated into two cells. A growth cycle between two separations lasted approximately 3 hours. After division, the new cells moved by means of a gliding motion. The gliding speed has been noted to be approximately 0.2 to 0.5 µm/s, but maximal speeds of 1.5 to 2.0 µm/s have been observed.[957]

Composition

Mycoplasmas are composed of approximately 40% to 60% protein, 10% to 20% lipid, and a variable amount of carbohydrate. The *M. pneumoniae* genome is circular, double-stranded DNA with a contour length of 4.8×10^8 D and a size of 816 kb.[825] The guanosine plus cytosine content of the DNA is 38.6% to 40.8%.[108,863,965,1139]

Growth Characteristics and Physical Properties

M. pneumoniae grows in mycoplasma broth medium and on agar enriched with yeast extract and animal serum.[169,466,965,1136,1166] *M. pneumoniae* ferments carbohydrates and requires sterol for growth. It grows under both anaerobic and aerobic conditions, but growth is more consistent when it is incubated in nitrogen and 5% carbon dioxide. When compared with other mycoplasmas isolated from humans, *M. pneumoniae* grows relatively slowly, with visible formation of colonies rarely occurring in less than 1 week and possibly taking 3 weeks or more. Repeated agar passage results in more rapid growth, and laboratory strains thus treated produce colonies in 3 days.

M. pneumoniae colonies on agar generally appear different from the classic mycoplasma "fried egg" look noted with other types recovered from humans. The *M. pneumoniae* colony is spherical and dense, with a rough "mulberry" surface.

M. pneumoniae has the following enzyme systems: $NADH_2$ oxidase, nicotinamide adenine dinucleotide phosphate ($NADPH_2$) oxidase, lactate dehydrogenase, probably succinic dehydrogenase, and diaphorases.[466] In liquid medium, the following can be noted: acid color change in medium with added glucose and phenol red as a result of glucose metabolism, reduction of methylene blue in medium as a result of dehydrogenase activity, and reduction of 2-3-5 tetrazolium chloride to red formazan by dehydrogenase activity.[1136]

On agar, *M. pneumoniae* hemolyzes erythrocytes in an agar overlay by liberation of peroxide. Erythrocytes and other cells adsorb to *M. pneumoniae* colonies, and organisms in suspension cause hemagglutination. *M. pneumoniae* has also been found to create biofilms on abiotic surfaces,[622] which may help it survive in the environment.

Mycoplasmas, including *M. pneumoniae,* are heat sensitive. They have a half-life of less than 2 min at 50°C (122°F) and lose viability within 1 week at room temperature.[1166] They can be stored for several years at −20°C (−4°F), but −70°C (−94°F) is optimal for long-term storage.

Mycoplasmas are resistant to osmotic environmental changes but are sensitive to detergents. They are inhibited by gold salts and antibiotics not directed against cell wall synthesis.

Antigenic Composition

The following immunologic reactions have been noted in association with *M. pneumoniae*–host serum interactions: specific complement fixation; precipitation in gel; growth inhibition; indirect hemagglutination; metabolic inhibition; antigen–antibody union identified by immunofluorescence, enzyme-linked immunosorbent assay (ELISA), and radioimmunoassay; adherence inhibition assay; and nonspecific complement fixation (i.e., positive serologic test result for syphilis) and agglutination (i.e., cold and *Streptococcus* MG agglutinins).[135,506,533,693,949,1136] *M. pneumoniae* organisms have both membrane and cytoplasmic antigens.[338,589] Two membrane antigens can be identified by immunodiffusion,[938] with the major membrane antigen being found in the lipid fraction of the organism.[338,589] The antigens are glycolipids and are of major importance in complement fixation, metabolic inhibition, and mycoplasmacidal reactions.[146] The cytoplasmic (soluble) antigen, which also contains lipid, can be identified by complement fixation when the antigen is prepared by phenol extraction. Many surface lipoproteins are also differentially expressed on contact with epithelial cells[450] and are thought to play a role in both activating and evading the innate immune system.[124,519]

Humans have an immunoglobulin (Ig) G immune response to eight principal protein antigens.[15,108,177,251,252,377,631,641,1203,291] These eight polypeptides have the following molecular masses: 170, 130, 116, 90, 68, 45, 35, and 30 kDa. The 170-kDa antigen is the P1 protein. This protein is localized at the surface of the terminal organelle (terminal structure), is the major adhesin responsible for attachment, and is the cause of the gliding motility of the organism. Antibodies to P1 protein inhibit hemadsorption and adherence to respiratory epithelium.[502,504,505,532,564,632,1107] Other important adhesins include the 30-kDa protein (P30) and 116-kDa protein (P116). In addition, multiple accessory proteins are involved in the adherence of *M. pneumoniae* to host cells,[965] including P65, HMW1, HMW2, HMW3, and A, B, and C.[58,461]

The 68-kDa community-acquired respiratory distress syndrome (CARDS) toxin is a recently identified protein unique to *M. pneumoniae* but that shares some homology with pertussis toxin.[570,787] It possesses adenosine diphosphate (ADP) ribosyltransferase activity, is highly immunogenic, and has been associated with airway cellular damage.[72,106,571,787] Diagnostic assays based on this protein have recently been developed.[833]

M. pneumoniae strains can be divided into two groups based on the sequence variation in the P1 gene.[281,282,292] Within this classification system (types 1 and 2), multiple variant subtypes also exist, which can be distinguished by restriction fragment length polymorphism (RFLP)[1091] or polymerase chain reaction (PCR)–based denaturing gradient gel electrophoresis.[1266] Type 2 strains have been found to produce higher levels of CARDS toxin[709] and stronger biofilms[1064]; however, studies have not yet shown an association between strain type and worse clinical pathology.[873] Further molecular typing of strains by the number and location of tandem repeats in the gene is also possible and mostly used for epidemiologic tracking, although there is some disagreement regarding the classification system.[1115] Three prevalent "multilocus variable-number tandem-repeat analysis" types in recent years are 4-5-7-2, 3-5-6-2, and 3-6-6-2,[270] and one study in Hong Kong found that increasing macrolide resistance rates in *M. pneumoniae* were predominantly a result of mutations in 4-5-7-2, from 25% in 2011 to 59.1% in 2012, to 89.7% in 2013, and to 100% in 2014.[480,953]

Membrane determinants of *M. pneumoniae* cross-react with the erythrocyte glycoprotein containing the I antigen and the related sugar chain (F1)[474,537]; with pneumococcal serotypes 23 and 32[17]; with the glycolipids of spinach, parsnips, and carrots; with selected strains of *Staphylococcus aureus* and group A streptococci; and perhaps with the filamentous hemagglutinin of *Bordetella pertussis*.[432,527,590,1194]

Animal Susceptibility

M. pneumoniae grows and causes pneumonia in hamsters and cotton rats and causes inapparent infection of the bronchial epithelium of chicken embryos.[949]

Epidemiology

Epidemic Pattern

In large urban areas, *M. pneumoniae* is endemic; infection and disease occur throughout the year. Foy and associates[359,364] noted cultural or serologic evidence of *M. pneumoniae* infection in a Seattle, Washington prepaid medical care group during all seasons throughout an 11-year period. Similar endemicity has been reported in other studies.[816,821,879] Wan and colleagues[1222] tested air filters at a hospital in Taiwan and detected seasonal peaks of *M. pneumoniae* in the pediatric emergency department (July) and outpatient areas (August–January). In addition to the background endemic pattern, *M. pneumoniae* enjoys a cyclic epidemic pattern that is specific for a particular urban community. Epidemics have occurred at 3- to 7-year intervals,[321,364,560,696,879] most recently in Europe and Jerusalem from 2010 to 2012.[165,305,679,874,1176] Epidemics, which develop slowly, usually start in the fall and persist in the community for 12 to 30 months. While previous epidemics were thought to represent shifts in circulating P1 strain types,[591,904] there are conflicting reports regarding whether this most recent epidemic also saw a change in the pattern. Analysis of respiratory samples from *M. pneumoniae*-infected patients in Germany from 2003 to 2012 showed that 55% of strains were type 2, with no type shifts preceding or during the epidemic.[529] However, two towns in western Russia experienced *M. pneumoniae* outbreaks in 2013 solely with the type 2c strain, whereas samples from that region taken in 2006 to 2007 and 2010 showed that 41% were type 1, 52% were type 2a, and only 7% were type 2c.[302] Similarly, samples taken from patients in China showed that 20% were type 2 between 2008 to 2012, which increased to over 40% in 2013 and 2014.[1295] A retrospective analysis of 199 cases in the United States showed a similar pattern, with type 1 strains being predominant from 2006 to 2011, after which type 2 and variant strains each increased between 2011 and 2013.[270]

As part of an influenza surveillance program, Layani-Milon and associates[660] studied acute respiratory infections in outpatients for six winters in the Rhône-Alpes region of France by PCR plus a hybridization-based detection system. Each year from 1992 to 1997, at least one peak of *M. pneumoniae* infection was noted in the late fall. Overall, they studied 3897 children and adults with acute respiratory illnesses, and 7.3% were found to be infected with *M. pneumoniae*. The yearly rate of *M. pneumoniae* cases fell from 10.1% in 1992 to 1993 to 2.0% in 1995 to 1996; in the subsequent year (1996–97), it rose to 4.2%.

Incidence of Infection and Disease

In the past, most pediatricians and other physicians considered *M. pneumoniae* illness to be uncommon in the general population. The initial epidemiologic studies were concerned mainly with the occurrence of pneumonia in closed populations, such as the military and boarding schools.[173,816,997,1104,1106,1185] During the past 52 years, however, many large studies in civilian populations, coupled with more sensitive diagnostic techniques, have indicated that both infection and disease with *M. pneumoniae* occur commonly.*

Hornsleth[495] examined 367 serum samples collected from children hospitalized in Copenhagen from September 1963 to May 1965 for complement-fixing antibodies. He noted that 42% of infants 6 to 11 months of age had demonstrable antibody; from 1 to 9 years of age, more than two-thirds of the children had antibody. Suhs and Feldman[1113] found a similar high prevalence of hemagglutination-inhibiting antibody in the sera of residents of Point Barrow, Alaska, but only 5% of the serum samples from a children's home in Syracuse had measurable antibody. A study of 319 pediatric patients with chronic respiratory disease found that 32.6% had bronchoalveolar lavage fluid positive for mycoplasmas, of which only 31% represented *M. pneumonia*.[924] Brunner and associates[128] detected serum antibody by the sensitive radioimmunoprecipitation test in 28% of 7- to 12-month-old infants, 55% of 13- to 24-month-old children, 67% of 25- to 60-month-old children, and 97% of persons older than 17 years. The high antibody prevalence noted in this study and the findings in Copenhagen and Alaska suggest an infection incidence rate of approximately 20% to 30% per year in a susceptible population of young children. The prevalent antibody noted at an early age in these studies possibly is not caused specifically by *M. pneumoniae* infection but instead could be the result of exposure to the many cross-reacting antigens in nature.[17,399,590] However, studies by Fernald and colleagues,[340] in which infants and children in a daycare center were monitored systematically, indicated a yearly infection rate of approximately 12%.

Monto and colleagues,[821] in a large study involving 3243 persons, investigated the incidence of infection in six yearly cohort groups of children and adults. Infection was determined by significant rises in titer of complement-fixing antibody on three serum specimens collected during a 1-year period from each subject. The overall yearly infection rate was found to be 5.3%. The highest rate (8.8%) occurred in the 5- to 9-year-old group. Infants younger than 1 year had a rate of 2.8%.

Brunner and associates[128] noted that geometric mean antibody titers tended to increase with increasing age, which suggested that the older children were being reinfected. Fernald and colleagues[340] reported that 5 of 22 children infected with *M. pneumoniae* in their investigation experienced reinfections during the 5-year observation period. In the study by Monto and associates,[821] 24.4% of the 172 infections detected in subjects of all ages were reinfections. During a 12-year serologic surveillance period, Foy and coworkers[364] noted great variation in the incidence of *M. pneumoniae* infection; in the period from October 1965 to May 1966, only 0.2% of 398 children had fourfold rises in complement-fixation antibody titer, whereas during the May 1973 to May 1974 period, 35% of 246 subjects 10 to 20 years of age had serologic evidence of infection.

The incidence of disease caused by *M. pneumoniae* depends on the endemic or epidemic prevalence of the organism in the community and is age related. The incidence of *M. pneumoniae* by age for two epidemics and the surrounding endemic periods in Seattle was studied by Foy and associates.[364] The highest epidemic attack rate was 14 per

*References 51, 52, 87, 128, 154, 233, 269, 278, 287, 309, 318, 340, 363, 360, 361, 362, 364, 367, 369, 412, 416, 429, 495, 540, 549, 560, 696, 707, 715, 801, 821, 822, 870, 879, 910, 1044, 1113, 1165.

1000 children 5 to 9 years of age, and the highest endemic attack rate (4 per 1000) occurred in the same age group. Children 10 to 14 years of age had the second highest attack rate during both epidemic and endemic periods. The attack rate in children younger than 5 years was about twice that observed in young adults.

The ratio of symptomatic to asymptomatic infection has varied across studies. In family studies, both Balassanian and Robbins[57] and Foy and associates[363] noted that only 15% of infections were asymptomatic, whereas Saliba and associates[997] noted that 55% of the residents of a boys' home had asymptomatic infection. Chanock and colleagues[173] observed that only 1 in 30 infections in Marine recruits manifested as clinically apparent pneumonia. Recent studies on the human microbiome show that the presence of *M. pneumoniae* in the airway is more common than previously thought, although it is unclear how much represents acute versus chronic infection, reinfection, or asymptomatic carriage.[45] A study in the Netherlands found *M. pneumoniae* DNA in 21% of 405 asymptomatic children and 16.2% of children with upper respiratory symptoms, the latter persisting for up to 4 months after sampling.[1089]

Incubation Period

The reported incubation period has varied from a mean of approximately 1 week in volunteer studies and point-source epidemics to 3 weeks in community outbreaks.* In a volunteer study, Rifkind and colleagues[970] administered tissue culture–grown *M. pneumoniae* in a concentration of 320 to 1280 EID_{50} (mean egg-infective dose) into the nose and posterior pharyngeal area of 27 men with no demonstrable antibody. In this study, pneumonia occurred 9 to 12 days after inoculation, following 1 to 3 days of upper respiratory tract illness. In six volunteers, only upper respiratory tract illness was noted, and the incubation period varied from 4 to 9 days. In a similar study in which volunteers received 10^6 to 10^7 broth-grown organisms, the incubation period was 8 to 10 days.[1073]

In an interesting common-source outbreak caused by an intense 8-hour exposure at a party, the peak incubation period was 13 days and most of the cases occurred between days 11 and 14.[324] In another probable point-source outbreak, which may have resulted from a room aerosol, the incubation period varied from 4 to 9 days.[1005] In studies of case-to-case intervals in families, Foy and associates[363] reported a median incubation time of 23 days, with most of the cases occurring between days 16 and 25. In similar studies, Copps and colleagues[233] noted an average interval of 21 days, and Biberfeld and Sterner[87] found a modal value of 20 days. A point-source outbreak in a family unit was described in which all seven family members became ill 10 to 16 days after the onset of symptoms in the index case.[596]

The longer incubation period in the family situation than in the volunteer studies and the point-source outbreaks may be the result of larger inocula in the last instances. In contrast to other respiratory illnesses, such as measles and influenza, the spread of disease caused by *M. pneumoniae* in both closed populations (such as military training units and boarding schools) and open communities is usually slow. For example, the introduction of influenza or measles into a family most often results in infection of all susceptible persons from the primary case. In contrast, the spread of *M. pneumoniae* through a family of six people probably would require three or four passages. Foy and associates[363] noted secondary attack rates in families of 64% for children and 17% for adults. Biberfeld and Sterner[87] reported secondary infection rates of 41% and 84%, respectively, for adults and children in families. In contrast to family groups, the spread of *M. pneumoniae* in schools and other situations of brief exposure is low.[360,368] In one Seattle elementary school, the infection rate was 18%. Foy and Alexander[359] believe that neighborhood spread among playmates is more important than school exposure in community transmission of *M. pneumoniae*.

Transmission in families occurs during the acute phase of illness; transmission by persons with asymptomatic infection has not been documented.[360]

Geography

The endemic and epidemic presence of *M. pneumoniae* has been demonstrated in the urban areas of developed countries with temperate climates throughout the world.* Serologic investigations in more remote areas, including both arctic and tropical zones, also indicate the presence of *M. pneumoniae* infection. Suhs and Feldman[1113] found measurable antibody in the serum of 68% of 169 persons in Point Barrow, and Golubjatnikov and associates,[416] in a study of children in a remote Mexican highland community, detected seropositivity in 16% of 637 children. Serologic evidence of infection also has been noted in Cairo, Singapore, Hong Kong, the West Indies, and southern Africa.[170,560] Incidence studies have not been performed in rural areas, but patterns of infection probably would be characterized by epidemic periods of a year or so and then complete absence of *M. pneumoniae* circulation for several years.

Gender Difference

Although the results of studies have varied, the difference in the incidence of *M. pneumoniae* disease by sex is small. During the 11 years of study in Seattle, Foy and associates[364] noted that the rate of *M. pneumoniae* pneumonia was higher in women than in men in the 30- to 39-year age group (1.8 vs. 1.2 per 1000). In infants, boys were afflicted more often than girls; otherwise, the rates for children by gender were virtually identical. Jensen and associates[549] found that pneumonia, otitis media, and nasopharyngitis in various combinations occurred more commonly in boys than in girls. Monto and colleagues[821] noted that boys younger than 5 years of age had more infections, but that the reverse was true for children 5 to 14 years of age. In a review of Japan's National Surveillance Data, Eshima and colleagues[317] found a slightly greater female preponderance in symptomatic infection at all ages except those over 70 years old. In other studies involving all age groups, males have shown a slightly greater frequency of illness than females.[754,879] In the Seattle family studies, symptoms were more severe in boys than in girls.

Pathogenesis and Pathology

Sequence of Events in Infection

M. pneumoniae infection is acquired via the respiratory route from the respiratory secretions of an ill person infected with this agent. Spread can be accomplished by small-particle aerosols or large droplets of secretions coming in contact with the epithelial surface of the nasopharynx and perhaps the surfaces of the lower respiratory tract (i.e., trachea, bronchi, and bronchioles) as well. In volunteer studies, Couch[238] observed that the 50% human infectious dose by small-particle aerosol was 1 colony-forming unit (nasal instillation required a dose that was 100 times greater).

Because epidemiologic data indicate the need for close and perhaps prolonged personal contact for transmission of infection, transmission by small-particle aerosol probably occurs rarely under natural conditions. After acquisition of the infectious agent, multiplication occurs extracellularly on mucous membrane surfaces. The incubation period, which varies from 4 days to more than 3 weeks, probably depends strongly on the size of the original inoculum. The extent of the respiratory infection increases during the incubation period, and shedding of organisms in respiratory secretions can be observed 2 to 8 days before clinical illness.[238] Initial symptoms of infection include headache, malaise, fever, sore throat, and cough; evidence of lower respiratory tract disease is present within the succeeding 3 days.[269,970] The method of extension of infection within the respiratory tract is unknown. The extent of disease possibly depends totally on the initial distribution of the infectious agent at the time of acquisition rather than on spread of infection from a primary upper respiratory site.

After the onset of clinical symptoms, the concentration of *M. pneumoniae* in respiratory secretions peaks, remains high for approximately 1 week, and then persists for 4 to 6 weeks or longer.[238,269] The associated symptoms and signs in disease caused by *M. pneumoniae* (i.e., meningitis, arthritis, hemolytic anemia, rash, and pericarditis) suggest the possibility of frequent dissemination of the organism from the respiratory tract. Some reviews on the subject tend to discount the possibility of generalized *M. pneumoniae* infection and attribute the associated systemic clinical findings to immunologic events related to respiratory infection.[238,269,796] However, little published evidence indicates

*References 87, 233, 324, 363, 360, 366, 970, 1005, 1074, 1167.

*References 89, 269, 333, 360, 364, 540, 696, 732, 754, 849, 879, 1097.

that the organism has been sought carefully in the blood and other sites of dissemination. In many instances, *M. pneumoniae* has been recovered from or identified by PCR in the blood, pericardial fluid, middle ear fluid, vesicular skin lesions, pleural fluid, kidneys, brain, and cerebrospinal fluid (CSF).* In addition, the observation of low CSF glucose in *M. pneumoniae* meningoencephalitis suggests direct involvement by the organism.[612]

Pathology

Pathologic findings in *M. pneumoniae* disease in children have not been reported, and only minimal data from adults are available. However, a reasonable understanding of the pathologic process of *M. pneumoniae* disease can be constructed from studies in the hamster, various tracheal organ cultures, and human biopsy and postmortem material.† The primary damage in *M. pneumoniae* infection is to the epithelial lining of the mucosal surfaces of the respiratory tract. This damage has been observed on the surface of bronchi, bronchioles, and alveoli; clinical symptoms in children suggest that similar pathologic changes occur in the trachea and upper respiratory tract as well. Specifically conspicuous is destruction of the ciliated epithelium of the bronchi and bronchioles. Because of mucosal desquamation and ulceration, the lumina contain considerable debris; added to this debris is an inflammatory exudate consisting of fibrin, mononuclear cells, and neutrophils. The alveolar spaces contain similar exudate and edema fluid.

The walls of the bronchi and bronchioles are thickened by edema and contain an infiltrate of macrophages, lymphocytes, and plasma cells. The alveolar walls are also thickened and contain lymphocytes, mononuclear cells, and erythrocytes. Dilation of the septal capillaries occurs. Edema and cellular infiltration extend into the interstitial spaces. Gross examination of the lungs reveals areas of hemorrhage and congestion. The pleura may contain patches of fibrinous exudate, and pleural fluid may be present. The pneumonic areas may be discrete or widespread.

A biopsy specimen of a vesiculopustular skin lesion revealed an epidermis with mild acanthosis and marked edema that primarily was intracellular.[1146] The papillary and upper reticular dermis contained neutrophils and round cells, and hemorrhagic foci were present within the upper corium and epidermis. The blister fluid contained plasma protein and neutrophils. Findings in other organs include mesenteric lymphadenitis, focal hepatic necrosis, follicular splenitis, acute myocarditis, and hemorrhagic encephalitis.

Immunologic Events

Specific antibody. A specific serum antibody response usually occurs after infection with *M. pneumoniae*, which can be measured by many different serologic techniques: immunofluorescence, complement fixation, indirect hemagglutination, precipitation, growth inhibition, mycoplasmacidal antibody test, ELISA, radioimmunoassay, adherence inhibition assay, and radioimmunoprecipitation test.‡

Complement-fixing antibodies occur early in *M. pneumoniae* disease, reach a peak titer in approximately 1 month, and then decline slowly over a variable period. Fluorescent-staining antibodies and antibody determined by ELISA have temporal patterns similar to those of complement-fixing antibodies. Growth-inhibiting antibodies appear later (i.e., 2–3 weeks after the onset of illness), peak later, and persist longer than do complement-fixing antibodies. The initial serum immune response includes specific IgM, IgG, and IgA antibodies. After clinical illness and convalescence, specific antibody is located mainly in the IgG serum fraction. Occasionally, significant levels of IgM antibody persist for several months or years after infection.[82,129,312,557] Antibody titer responses in infected children are generally of a lesser magnitude than those in adults.[287] Asymptomatic infections in children may not be associated with a measurable serum antibody response. *M. pneumoniae*–specific IgE antibodies have been detected in the sera of patients with asthma, atopic dermatitis, or both conditions.[1157]

After infection, specific antibody is also present in nasal secretions and sputum.[81,126] In volunteer studies, Brunner and colleagues[126] noted that 42% and 73% of subjects had IgA nasal and sputum responses, respectively. Biberfeld and Sterner[88] found specific antibody in 44 of 55 sputum specimens from patients with *M. pneumoniae* infection of the lower respiratory tract. They noted IgA antibody in all specimens tested, IgG antibody in 24 of 31 specimens, and IgM antibody in 13 of 27 specimens.

Specific cell-mediated immunity. Fernald and coworkers[336,337] demonstrated that lymphocytes from adults previously infected with *M. pneumoniae* undergo blast transformation when cultured in vitro in the presence of *M. pneumoniae* organisms. In age-related studies, researchers noted that only one of nine children younger than 4 years of age with documented previous infection had evidence of specific cell-mediated immunity as measured by lymphocyte stimulation.[340] In contrast, 7 of 12 children older than 4 years and 87% of an adult group demonstrated specific lymphocyte stimulation. This study suggests that specific cell-mediated immunity increases as a function of age and depends on repeated infection. Koh and colleagues[614] noted high levels of interleukin (IL)-4 and a high IL-4/interferon (IFN)-γ ratio in the bronchoalveolar lavage fluid of children with *M. pneumoniae* pneumonia, thus suggesting a predominant T_H2-like cytokine response. Wang and coworkers[1226] found elevated IL-4 and decreased IL-2 levels in children infected with *M. pneumoniae*, and found that those with a particular IL-2 polymorphism had an increased risk of asthma and of a higher load of the pathogen. Martin and colleagues[757] found that leukocytes from volunteers with *M. pneumoniae* infection demonstrated chemotaxis in the presence of the organism, whereas leukocytes collected before infection did not. Patients infected with *M. pneumoniae* also respond with IFN-γ in their blood and nasopharyngeal secretions early in infection and with IFN-γ during convalescence.[850,851]

Nonspecific responses. Antibodies to several diverse antigens develop during human infection with *M. pneumoniae*. The best known of these antibodies are cold agglutinins, which are useful in the diagnosis of *M. pneumoniae* pneumonia.[236,330,467,540,1076] Cold agglutinins are directed against the I antigen of erythrocytes.[537,697,1076] Most pneumonias in which serum cold agglutinins are noted are caused by *M. pneumoniae*. Cold agglutinins are detected in the serum of approximately 75% of patients with *M. pneumoniae* pneumonia; they are less common in *M. pneumoniae* infection without pneumonia.[169]

Patients with *M. pneumoniae* also frequently develop antibodies to the MG strain of nonhemolytic streptococci[695] and occasionally to *M. genitalium*,[699] *M. hominis*,[1009] *M. salivarium*, *Mycoplasma hyorhinis*, *Mycoplasma orale*, *Mycoplasma pulmonis*, and *Mycoplasma mycoides* variety mycoides, the etiologic agent of contagious pleuropneumonia of cattle.[678] Cross-reacting antibodies to filamentous hemagglutinin and pertactin of *B. pertussis* also occur.[1194] Other heterologous antibodies found in the serum of patients with *M. pneumoniae* infection include those to smooth muscle, the mitotic spindle apparatus, brain, lung, liver, and Wasserman (WR) cardiolipin antigen.[81,89,698] In addition to these findings, Biberfeld and Norberg[85] detected immune complexes by the platelet aggregation technique in the sera of 16 of 39 patients with acute respiratory illness caused by *M. pneumoniae*. Mizutani[811] demonstrated the presence of circulating immune complexes in most patients with pneumonia caused by *M. pneumoniae*. The same investigator also detected rheumatoid factor in the sera of patients with *M. pneumoniae* disease.[812]

Possible Mechanisms of Disease Production

Numerous studies have been performed in an attempt to understand the pathogenesis of respiratory disease caused by mycoplasmas.[128,192,193,191,219,217,218,225,227–230] Of particular interest in human *M. pneumoniae* infection is the apparent high prevalence of infection in infants, children, adolescents, and young adults, but the frequently mild nature of disease in infants and young children in comparison with older patients. Some studies suggest that the more severe disease in older patients is associated with reinfection and is mediated somewhat by immunologic responses.[1008,1114]

Organ culture and animal studies indicate that damage at the site of primary infection—the respiratory epithelium—is the result of close

*References 2, 26, 68, 75, 93, 262, 353, 514, 574, 617, 657, 719, 720, 727, 844, 845, 848, 859, 860, 965, 1080, 1082, 1121, 1158.

†References 280, 514, 561, 617, 657, 735, 802, 920, 1146, 1304.

‡References 127, 128, 135, 286, 339, 467, 506, 533, 693, 705, 949, 1022, 1144.

organism–cell attachment.[191,228,230,503,701,702,840,943] This attachment of organism to cell uses neuraminic acid receptors on the cell.[1081] In an organ culture system with *M. mycoides* variety capri, ciliary damage was decreased when the cellular receptor sites were treated with receptor-destroying enzyme.[191] Lipman and associates[701,702] noted that one attenuated *M. pneumoniae* strain had lost its ability to cytadsorb. The close association of organism and cell allows the transport of specific damaging material to the cell. Although the precise nature of this substance is not known, the data available suggest that it might be hydrogen peroxide. It is liberated by *M. pneumoniae* in vitro; in organ culture studies, hydrogen peroxide has been shown to be the damaging factor in another *Mycoplasma* infection.[191,702,704] In cell culture, *M. pneumoniae* inhibits host–cell catalase activity.[20] This inhibition of catalase activity enhances the toxicity of the hydrogen peroxide generated by the microorganism. *M. pneumoniae* also enters host cells and persists intracellularly for at least 7 days.[65]

Once released in the cell, the CARDS toxin is able to mediate mono-ADP ribosylation and vacuolization, processes that lead to airway inflammation and damage to ciliated respiratory epithelial cells.[106,570,635,787] Another possible important component of *M. pneumoniae* pathogenicity is the induction of proinflammatory and other cytokines during infection.[444,455,643,1036,1054,1224,1273]

In addition to direct damage from inflammatory cytokines and bacterial cytotoxins, other mechanisms have been proposed in the development of extrapulmonary findings in *M. pneumoniae* infection.[856,1206] Autoantibodies are often detected in these cases, most likely as a result of cross-reactivity between host cell proteins and mycoplasma membrane antigens. Autoimmune mechanisms have been linked to findings as varied as arthritis, coagulopathies, and encephalitis in *M. pneumoniae* infection. Another mechanism of pathology commonly seen is vascular occlusion caused by either direct inflammation of the vessels or various coagulopathies associated with *M. pneumoniae* infection. This led to associated findings, such as stroke, pulmonary emboli, and coronary artery disease.[198,210,352,387,602,665,681] Although not directly proven, the ability of mycoplasma to bind to erythrocytes and disseminate through the bloodstream may contribute to the high frequency of extrapulmonary findings seen with these infections.[864]

Fernald and associates[340] noted that specific cell-mediated immunity to *M. pneumoniae* as measured by lymphocyte transformation becomes more prevalent with increasing age, as does specific antibody. Their studies suggest that more than one exposure to antigen may be necessary to elicit both humoral and cellular responses. Fernald and Glezen,[341] in an inactivated *M. pneumoniae* vaccine trial in children, noted that lymphocyte sensitivity developed in many recipients but not a humoral antibody response. In a trial of an inactivated vaccine in adults, Smith and associates[1073] found that on challenge infection, an exaggerated illness occurred in vaccinees who failed to form humoral antibodies after immunization. These findings have led to the consideration that persistent specific cell-mediated responsiveness might contribute to the pulmonary process in *M. pneumoniae* infection. However, the incubation period of illness in adults and children is similar, which argues against the sensitization theory.[213]

Foy and associates[365] noted that complement-fixing antibodies remained elevated for 2 to 9 years after infection with pneumonia but fell quickly after the second year in persons with mild illness. Protection against reinfection was better in those who previously had pneumonia than in those with mild symptoms.

Clinical Manifestations

Pneumonia

Pneumonia is the most important clinical manifestation of *M. pneumoniae* infection, and this agent is responsible for 10% to 20% of all cases of pneumonia.* The highest incidence of pneumonia caused by *M. pneumoniae* in Seattle occurred in children 5 to 14 years of age.[364] In a study in Chiba Prefecture, Japan, researchers noted that the peak age of lower respiratory tract illness caused by *M. pneumoniae* was 4 years.[846] In a prospective study of community-acquired pneumonia in Finland, 11% of the children with *M. pneumoniae* infection were younger than 5 years of age, 32% were between 5 and 9 years of age, and 57% were 10 to 14 years of age.[471] Although researchers frequently state that *M. pneumoniae* pneumonia rarely occurs in children younger than 5 years of age, in actuality, the incidence in this group was found to be about twice that noted in young adults in Seattle.[364] Pneumonia caused by *M. pneumoniae* occurs less commonly in children younger than 2 years of age and rarely in infants younger than 6 months of age. The apparent frequency of *M. pneumoniae* pneumonia is influenced by the relative occurrence of pneumonia caused by other pathogens. During the child's first 5 years of life, *M. pneumoniae* is only one of many agents (e.g., respiratory syncytial virus, adenoviruses, parainfluenza viruses, influenza viruses, *Streptococcus pneumoniae,* and *Haemophilus influenzae*) that cause pneumonia. During later childhood and adolescence, pneumonia as a consequence of infection with these other agents is a rare event; therefore *M. pneumoniae* is the leading cause of pneumonia in these persons.

Because isolation rates of *M. pneumoniae* during both endemic and epidemic periods do not vary greatly by season, as do those of common respiratory viruses, the proportion of patients with *M. pneumoniae* pneumonia increases during the summer months.

Symptoms and signs. Since 1961, a large number of studies have reported the frequency of signs and symptoms in *M. pneumoniae* infection.* Unfortunately, many studies have included only special populations, such as the military; with few exceptions, community investigations have failed to indicate differences by age. In only a small number of investigations have data regarding children been itemized separately.[122,265,371,1108,1225,1286] Table 196.2 presents the relative frequency of symptoms and signs as compiled from eight studies in which both children and adults were included. The hallmark of pneumonia caused by *M. pneumoniae* is fever and cough. The onset of illness usually cannot be demarcated clearly, but malaise, fever, and headache are early complaints. Cough has an onset 3 to 5 days after the beginning of illness and is initially nonproductive. Foy and colleagues[368] and Biberfeld and coworkers[86] noted that 77% and 100%, respectively, of the patients that they studied had maximal temperatures greater than 38.9°C (102°F). Copps and associates[233] found that 58% of the group that they evaluated had temperatures higher than 39.4°C (103°F) and 4% had temperatures higher than 40.6°C (105°F).

The reporting of headache in association with *M. pneumoniae* pneumonia has varied considerably. Nakao and associates[849] noted this report in only 8% of subjects, whereas Biberfeld and associates[86] and Foy and colleagues[368] reported it in two-thirds of those studied. Chills and the production of sputum are present in about 50% of ill patients. Again, great differences among investigations are noted, and they probably are related to the relative ages of the patients.

Coryza is unusual in *M. pneumoniae* pneumonia; therefore, its occurrence should suggest another etiologic agent for illness in a specific patient. In a study involving children exclusively, Stevens and colleagues[1108] noted that coryza occurred more commonly in young children; as might be expected, they found productive cough more frequently in their older patients. Hoarseness, earache, sore throat, gastrointestinal complaints, and chest pain occur in approximately 25% of patients.

On physical examination, approximately 75% of patients have auscultatory evidence of pneumonia and about half have pharyngitis. Remarkable lymphadenopathy, particularly with cervical involvement, is noted in approximately 25% of patients. Twenty-one percent of the patients studied by Foy and associates[368] had otitis media. In other studies, this manifestation was noted in about 5% to 10% of cases. Conjunctivitis was observed in almost half the patients reported by Fransen and associates.[374] In contrast, except for Jansson and colleagues,[541] who noted conjunctivitis in 3% of their study group, this finding was

*References 221, 265, 269, 368, 369, 375, 471, 499, 707, 896, 782, 801, 870, 910, 1165, 1285, 1286

*References 2, 8, 11, 22, 32, 34, 39, 42, 49, 52, 68, 74, 75, 84, 89, 93, 125, 145, 206, 220, 224, 261, 280, 288, 323, 331, 342, 351, 375, 415, 481, 482, 499, 526, 574, 585, 598, 606, 612, 618, 620, 621, 625, 636, 654, 675, 681, 700, 725, 758, 803, 828, 834, 857, 869, 877, 879, 884, 889, 906, 917, 942, 984, 996, 1020, 1049, 1069, 1082, 1098, 1102, 1108, 1132, 1135, 265, 1149, 1158, 1164, 1174, 1235, 1245, 1286, 1201

TABLE 196.2 Frequency of Clinical Findings in Children and Adults With *Mycoplasma* Pneumoniae Pneumonia

Finding	Frequency
Symptoms	
Fever	++++
Cough	++++
Malaise	+++
Headache	++
Sputum	++
Chills	++
Hoarseness	+
Earache	+
Coryza	+
Sore throat	+
Diarrhea	+
Nausea and/or vomiting	+
Chest pain	+
Signs	
Rales	+++
Pharyngitis	++
Lymphadenopathy	+
Conjunctivitis	±
Rash	±
Otitis media	±

Compiled from eight studies in which both children and adults were included (references 84, 86, 233, 367, 374, 541, 744, 849).
+ + + +, close to 100%; + + +, 75%; + +, 50%; +, 25%; ±, 0–10%.

not mentioned in the other reports. Similarly, rash was reported in 6%, 11%, and 17%, respectively, in studies in Minnesota, Wisconsin, and Seattle,[233,369,744] but it was not mentioned in the other studies.

The most common finding on chest auscultation is dry rales, but musical rales with expiration are noted occasionally. Rales usually persist for 2 weeks, and hearing them a month or more after the onset of disease is not unusual. Occasionally, patients have no auscultatory evidence of pulmonary disease throughout their illness in spite of the presence of abnormalities on chest radiographs. During illness, cough becomes increasingly prominent; initially, it is nonproductive but later it may produce a frothy white sputum in older children and adolescents. The sputum also may appear purulent and contain blood. Cough persists for 3 to 4 weeks and longer after nonrespiratory symptoms such as fever and headache have subsided.

In a study of 44 children with lower respiratory tract illness caused by *M. pneumoniae*, Stevens and associates[1108] noted the following frequencies of symptoms and signs: cough (97%), malaise (82%), vomiting (40%), abdominal pain (35%), headache (32%), rash (20%), fever higher than 38°C (>100.4°F; 78%); rales (78%), pharyngitis (32%), rhonchi (30%), bronchial breathing (27%), and otitis media (27%). Foy and coworkers[371] found that chills and productive cough were more common in adults than children and that temperatures tended to be higher in children.

In a large study involving 108 children with *M. pneumoniae* infection, wheezing occurred with the acute illness in 40%.[992] When the children in this study were evaluated 3 years after their acute illness, they were found to have three indicators of lung function that had mean values significantly lower than those in control children.

Few reports specifically describe pneumonia caused by *M. pneumoniae* in young children.[52,185,222,265,363,437,846,1067,1108,1286] However, a review of the case descriptions available indicates that illness, when it occurs, can be severe and relatively prolonged in contrast to common viral and bacterial infections. Singer and DeVoe[1067] reported a 3-year-old severely ill child who had a temperature of 39.4° C (102.9° F), a pulse of 150 beats/min, and a respiratory rate of 40 breaths/min. Diffuse pulmonary involvement of the right upper lobe and lingular segments of the left lower lobe was observed by radiography, although rales and altered breath sounds could not be heard. The patient's condition worsened over a 6-day period. At that point, specific therapy with erythromycin was instituted, and slow recovery followed. The child had a normal white blood cell count, transiently elevated serum aspartate aminotransferase and alanine aminotransferase values, and microscopic hematuria. Grix and Giammona[437] observed two 5-year-old children with extensive pneumonia, pleural effusions, and febrile periods of 10 and 16 days. Stevens and associates[1108] reported a 5-year-old boy with pulmonary consolidation and aseptic meningitis, and Clyde and Denny[222] described an asymptomatic 3-year-old boy with a "feathery infiltrate" in the right upper lung field. In a family study, Foy and colleagues[363] investigated four children younger than 6 years. In a 4-year-old child, the pneumonia persisted for more than 1 month, and in this child's brother, the illness lasted approximately 2 weeks. We have seen a 4.5 year-old girl with scattered infiltrates throughout both lung fields and febrile illness of 14 days' duration.[186]

Severe and extensive pulmonary disease occurs occasionally in *M. pneumoniae* infection.* Massive lobar pneumonia is noted on occasion, and pleural effusions are fairly common findings.† A number of cases of necrotizing pneumonitis with massive pleural effusions have been described.[62,201,1232] All of these children had protracted periods of fever and respiratory distress. Acute respiratory distress syndrome has been observed, and illness has suggested pulmonary embolism with infarction.[62,178,350,958,1063,1181] *M. pneumoniae* is a recognized cause of postinfectious bronchiolitis obliterans in children.[688,689,1227] Chronic intestinal pulmonary fibrosis and fulminant fatal diffuse interstitial fibrosis has been noted in two adults with *M. pneumoniae* pneumonia, and localized bronchiectasis developed in a 20-year-old man at the site of previous acute lung infection.[199,421,564,1122] Children who had a delay in onset or inadequate duration of macrolide treatment were found by Marc and associates[747] to have reduced lung diffusion capacity after contracting *M. pneumoniae* pneumonia. Barreira and associates[62] describe a previously healthy 8-year-old boy who developed necrotizing pneumonitis, septic shock, and meningoencephalitis from *M. pneumoniae.* A 5-year-old girl had severe necrotizing pneumonitis and a 4-year-old boy developed a necrotizing pulmonary cavity.[889,928] An adult had bronchiolitis obliterans–organizing pneumonia.[708] *M. pneumoniae* pneumonia is generally more severe in patients with preexisting cardiorespiratory problems, immunodeficiencies, and sickle-cell disease.[76,211,373,393,546,794,933,1057,1084]

Six patients—three children, one adolescent, and two adults—were found to have lung abscesses in association with *M. pneumoniae* infection.[199,680,686,903,1061] The illness in the adolescents and adults was characterized by productive cough and chest pain for 2 to 4 weeks. In one patient, clinical recovery and clearance of the pulmonary lesion were dramatic with tetracycline therapy; two other patients received suboptimal therapy but eventually recovered. One of the child cases was a 6-year-old girl who had a 7-day history of cough and a 4-day history of fever.[199] In addition to the abscess, she had pleural effusion, thrombocytopenia, and disseminated intravascular coagulation. Another child was a 10-year-old boy with fever and cough for 15 days refractory to treatment with amoxicillin and ceftriaxone, but with rapid improvement on clarithromycin.[680] The third child was a 10-year-old boy with West syndrome who developed high fevers, cough, and cytokine storms that did not resolve on antibiotics or steroids, requiring cyclosporine A. Fluid from the abscess was positive by PCR for *M. pneumoniae,* as was serology.[903] A 6-year-old boy with 15 days of chest pain, 2 days of fever, and positive serology to *M. pneumoniae* was also found to have a lung abscess, but given that his symptoms improved after several days of empiric vancomycin, ceftazidime, and clindamycin, it was presumed that his disease was caused by secondary infection with another organism.[987] One 18-year-old man with extensive consolidation of the right

*References 62, 187, 190, 199, 201, 211, 232, 347, 350, 360, 437, 442, 517, 579, 686, 708, 737, 794, 830, 848, 881, 889, 920, 958, 971, 1057, 1061, 1063, 1067, 1084, 1096, 1190, 1232.

†References 51, 164, 190, 196, 201, 223, 264, 347, 350, 437, 714, 719, 831, 845, 848, 881, 926, 1067, 1096, 1190, 1232.

lower lung field had residual pleural scarring 8 months after the acute illness.[831]

Newborns who contracted congenital pneumonia, probably via vertical transmission of *M. pneumoniae*, have been described.[1092,1179]

Clyde[221] reported factors that correlated with *M. pneumoniae* pneumonia in a study of 1139 subjects with community-acquired pneumonia. Positive factors were sore throat, headache, fever of 38.9°C (102°F) or higher, exanthem, family size of four or more, and ear infection. In the same study, pneumonia did not correlate with coryza, leukocytosis (15×10^9/L or more and 10×10^9/L or more), preexisting disease, recurrent pneumonia, hospitalization for treatment, or cigarette smoking.

Although recovery from *M. pneumoniae* pneumonia is usually complete, two studies suggest that persistent abnormalities in lung function can occur after illness.[819,992]

Radiography. Because the classic clinical entity primary atypical pneumonia has numerous causes but often is used as a synonym for *M. pneumoniae* pneumonia, much confusion has ensued about the spectrum of the radiographic appearance of the specific mycoplasmal infection. The radiographic pattern of primary atypical pneumonia is varied, but bilateral, diffuse, reticular infiltrates are common components.[718,1024,1071] Subsequent study has indicated that the diffuse interstitial pattern is an uncommon finding in *M. pneumoniae* infection and more often is the result of infection with other agents, such as viruses, fungi, and *Chlamydophila*.[121,398,861,951,1172]

Brolin and Wernstedt[121] carefully evaluated the radiographic findings in 56 patients with significant *M. pneumoniae* pneumonia; 21 of the patients were younger than 20 years. They noted the following distribution of different patterns: typical lobar pneumonia (8 patients); predominantly alveolar but not total consolidation (13); interstitial (either reticular or noduloreticular, 20); a combination of lobar pneumonia and other alveolar involvement without total consolidation (2); a combination of lobar involvement and interstitial (10); and a combination of alveolar involvement without total consolidation and interstitial (3). Alveolar patterns were more common in females; interstitial involvement was found more frequently in males. Twenty-two percent of patients had enlargement of the hilar or paratracheal lymph nodes and 14% had pleural effusion.

The persistence of radiographic changes is variable. Brolin and Wernstedt[121] noted that 13% of their patients who underwent follow-up studies had abnormal findings more than 4 weeks after the initial study. They observed that persistence tended to be longer in patients with alveolar disease than in those with interstitial patterns. The degree of clinical symptoms and pulmonary physical findings frequently correlates poorly with the apparent degree of involvement noted on radiographs. In many patients with significant symptoms, only minimal interstitial changes are observed. In other instances, patients with lobar pneumonia often have few clinical findings indicating pulmonary disease.

Lee and colleagues[666] reported the chest computed tomography (CT) features in 11 children and 5 adults with *M. pneumoniae* pneumonia. The children had the following findings: lobar or segmental consolidation (100%); pleural effusion (82%); lymphadenopathy (82%); and volume decrease of the involved lobe (73%). None of the children had diffuse nodules of ground-glass attenuation, septal thickening, or bronchial wall thickening. In contrast to the children, the adults had diffuse nodules of ground-glass attenuation (80%); septal thickening (40%); lymphadenopathy (40%); bronchial wall thickening (40%); and volume decrease of the involved lobe (20%). None of the adults had lobar or segmental consolidation and pleural effusion. In a retrospective analysis of 64 adult cases of *M. pneumoniae* pneumonia in Japan, the most common CT findings were bronchial wall thickening (81%), followed by centrilobular nodules (78%), ground-glass attenuation (78%), and consolidation (61%).[810]

Kim and associates[600] performed high-resolution CT on 38 children who had been hospitalized with *M. pneumoniae* pneumonia 1 to 2.2 years previously. Abnormalities in two or more lobes, which corresponded to the initial chest radiographic infiltrates, were found in 37% of the children. Young age (<8 years) at the time of hospitalization and high *M. pneumoniae* antibody titer were found to be risk factors for the subsequent abnormalities.

Nonspecific laboratory data. The total leukocyte count in patients with pneumonia caused by *M. pneumoniae* is most often normal, but variation is considerable.[84,233,321,368,371,375,540,816,1108,1172] In a group of more than 250 children younger than 15 years, Foy and associates[371] noted that 30% and 6% had total leukocyte counts greater than 10,000 and 15,000 cells/mm^3, respectively. In a group of 45 children, Stevens and colleagues[1108] observed leukocytosis in 33% of patients and leukopenia in one patient. Sixty-seven percent of the children had neutrophilia, and one patient had neutropenia. An increased percentage of band form neutrophils in *M. pneumoniae* pneumonia is an unusual finding.

The erythrocyte sedimentation rate is elevated in all cases,[84,233,540] and this elevation is usually marked. Biberfeld and colleagues[84] noted that 16 of 37 patients had erythrocyte sedimentation rates of 50 mm/h. Serologic tests for syphilis are found to be falsely positive on occasion, and serum cold agglutinins and antibodies to *Streptococcus* MG antigen are common findings.[82,169,173,269] Results of the direct Coombs test are frequently positive, and elevated levels of serum IgM are noted.[82,330] Urinalysis results are generally normal.

Respiratory Disease Other Than Pneumonia

Common cold and unspecified upper respiratory illness. By strict definition (i.e., significant nasal symptoms, no pharyngitis, and minimal fever), *M. pneumoniae* rarely causes the common cold. However, mild upper respiratory tract illness is noted frequently as the only manifestation of *M. pneumoniae* infection in children, adolescents, and young adults.* The frequency of unspecified upper respiratory tract illness as a manifestation of *M. pneumoniae* infection, in contrast to other manifestations resulting from infection with this agent, varies considerably among studies. Feizi[331] studied patients from a country practice in England and noted that 50% of the patients had upper respiratory tract symptoms. Illness in these persons often was prolonged, however, and lasted as long as 7 to 10 weeks. In a review in Scotland, only 3% of 596 *M. pneumoniae* infections were classified as upper respiratory tract illness. In studies of common respiratory tract illnesses in children in which viruses and other agents were sought, *M. pneumoniae* was noted in 2% to 5% of patients with upper respiratory tract illness.[170,269,715]

Pharyngitis and nasopharyngitis. As noted in Table 196.2, pharyngitis is observed in approximately half of all patients with *M. pneumoniae* pneumonia. However, pharyngitis as the major manifestation of *M. pneumoniae* infection occurs less commonly. Parrott[922] found that 12% of children admitted to the hospital with severe "bronchitis-pharyngitis" had *M. pneumoniae* infection. Jensen and associates[549] noted the frequent occurrence of pharyngitis and otitis media in children infected with *M. pneumoniae*. In a study of 715 children and adolescents with pharyngitis, Glezen and colleagues[411] reported that 36.8% had group A streptococcal infection and 3.1% were infected with *M. pneumoniae*. When the *M. pneumoniae* infections were grouped by age, the peak (11.4%) occurred in the 12- to 14-year-old group and none were observed in children younger than 6 years. Five patients with *M. pneumoniae* infection had concomitant group A streptococcal infection, but the illnesses in these cases could not be distinguished clinically from those caused by either agent alone. Cervical lymphadenopathy occurred in approximately 50% of those infected, and the pharyngeal lesion was exudative in 43%. In a study of 127 children with acute pharyngitis, 25 (20%) were found to have serologic evidence of *M. pneumoniae* infection.[318] Seven (28%) of these children had pharyngeal exudates and 10 (40%) had cervical lymphadenopathy. In a study involving 131 adult patients with pharyngitis, 10.6% were found to have serologic evidence of *M. pneumoniae* infection.[619]

Otitis media and bullous hemorrhagic myringitis. Although the incidence has varied across studies, otitis media is noted in approximately 5% of children and adolescents with *M. pneumoniae* pneumonia. The role of *M. pneumoniae* as an etiologic agent in common acute otitis media in children is unclear. Halsted and associates[451] noted that 12% of children with otitis media had serologic evidence of *M. pneumoniae* infection, but they were unable to recover the agent from middle ear fluid. In a study in which children were selected because of *M. pneumoniae* infection

*References 170, 235, 269, 287, 329, 331, 333, 340, 363, 368, 491, 660, 715, 816, 849, 869, 997

in a family member, 47 of 49 children with otitis media had *M. pneumoniae* infection.[549] Räty and Kleemola[962] used PCR to detect *M. pneumoniae* in 16 of 380 (4%) middle ear fluid samples from 138 children with acute otitis media.

In a volunteer study, myringitis developed in 13 of 52 subjects.[970] Findings were usually bilateral and associated with throbbing pain. The appearance of the tympanic membrane varied from mild injection to severe inflammation with edema. Hemorrhagic areas on the drum were noted in five subjects, and serous-appearing blebs containing blood were observed in two. Bullous myringitis also has been noted only occasionally with natural *M. pneumoniae* infection.[122,222,363,368,744,1080] In one study of 148 children and adults with *M. pneumoniae* pneumonia, 27 (18%) were found to have bullous myringitis.[744] Using PCR, Kotikoski and associates[626] studied middle ear fluid from 30 children and blister fluid from 12 children with acute meningitis and found no evidence of *M. pneumoniae* DNA.

Sinusitis. Although clinically recognized sinusitis has been reported rarely in patients with *M. pneumoniae* infection, Griffin and Klein[435] found radiographic evidence of sinusitis in approximately two-thirds of a group of Navy recruits with *M. pneumoniae* pneumonia. In general, the patients with sinusitis had more prolonged illness than did recruits without sinusitis. Savolainen and colleagues[1013] noted that 11 of 310 patients with acute maxillary sinusitis had fourfold or greater rises in complement-fixing antibody to *M. pneumoniae.* A 37-year-old man with chronic sinusitis that evolved into a Pott's puffy tumor was found to have a positive *M. pneumoniae* serology and was treated with doxycycline and surgical excision.[215] In chronic suppurative maxillary sinusitis, cultures for *M. pneumoniae* have been performed but no organisms were isolated.[80,1088]

Acute bronchitis. Acute bronchitis characterized by fever, cough, and rhonchi with or without associated pharyngitis is a frequent manifestation of *M. pneumoniae* infection.* Of 40 patients with *M. pneumoniae* infection, Feizi[331] reported that 6 had bronchitis, 3 had upper respiratory tract illness plus bronchitis, and 1 had sinusitis plus bronchitis. In contrast to these findings, Hornsleth[495] noted that only one of 25 patients with *M. pneumoniae* infection had acute bronchitis. In the differential diagnosis of acute bronchitis, *M. pneumoniae* infection accounts for 10% to 20% of cases.[171,175,269,322,938]

Croup. *M. pneumoniae* infection has been associated only occasionally with croup. Parrott[922] found no instances of *M. pneumoniae* infection in a large number of children with croup, and Chanock and Parrott[175] did not list this agent as an etiologic consideration in croup. In contrast, extensive studies in both Seattle and Chapel Hill, North Carolina, have revealed that approximately 2% of croup cases are associated with *M. pneumoniae* infection.[269,361,412,714] Because no descriptions of clinical illness are available, a reasonable assumption is that croup caused by *M. pneumoniae* infection is generally mild and without distinguishing characteristics.

Bronchiolitis and infectious asthma. The presence of *M. pneumoniae* in the lower airways can trigger a proinflammatory cytokine response similar to that seen in asthmatic and allergic patients.[460,599,787,792,1239,1277] *M. pneumoniae* pneumonia itself can cause bronchiolitis and wheezing[52,992]; however, it is also commonly found in asthmatics and is a cause of their symptomatic exacerbations.[79,509,834,910,1044] Approximately 5% of cases of bronchiolitis are caused by infection with *M. pneumoniae,* but the percentage varies across studies.[170,171,175,269,287,361,412,714,922] In two large studies, no instances of *M. pneumoniae*–associated bronchiolitis were reported.[491,495] Horn and associates[491] noted that *M. pneumoniae* was isolated from 6.6% of children with wheezy bronchitis, and Berkovich and associates[79] found *M. pneumoniae* infection in 7 of 33 episodes of wheezing in asthmatic children. Biscardi and coworkers[91] studied children 2 to 15 years of age hospitalized for severe asthma. Of 119 children with previously diagnosed asthma, 24 (20%) had *M. pneumoniae* infections during the exacerbation that caused their hospital admission. In 51 children with first asthma episodes, *M. pneumoniae* infection was demonstrated in 26 (50%). Children with a first attack of asthma associated with *M. pneumonia* infection were significantly more likely to have asthma recurrences than children whose primary episodes were not related to *M. pneumoniae* infection. Lehtinen and colleagues[674] studied 220 children with wheezing associated with viral infection and found that 5% were coinfected with *M. pneumoniae.* Freymuth and colleagues[379] identified *M. pneumoniae* in nasal aspirate samples by PCR in 3 of 132 children (2%) with acute exacerbations of asthma. Using a sensitive assay for the CARDS toxin, Wood and associates[1259] detected *M. pneumoniae* in 54% of their pediatric patients with acute asthma exacerbation, 65% with refractory asthma, and 56% of healthy controls. Compared to asthmatics with a negative CARDS screen, the former two groups were found to have poorer asthma control and quality of life scores. CARDS-positive asthmatics also had lower levels of IgM and IgG to *M. pneumoniae* than healthy controls. By contrast, a study looking at stable asthmatic pediatric patients without recent exacerbations found that they had higher IgM titers to *M. pneumoniae* than healthy controls.[1077]

Although a significant number of asthma exacerbations can be linked to *M. pneumoniae* infection, there is still conflicting evidence on the benefit of prophylactic or empirical antibiotic therapy in asthmatics.[623] Macrolides are sometimes advocated not only as an antibiotic but also for their antiinflammatory properties.[417] However, Shin and associates found that children with *M. pneumoniae* pneumonia and a history of atopic sensitization or asthma were also more likely to have infections refractory to macrolide treatment, requiring steroids.[1055]

Other. Exacerbations of chronic obstructive pulmonary disease have been associated with *M. pneumoniae* infection.[194,649,786,1075,1246] By culture, Cherry and associates[194] did not obtain any *M. pneumoniae* isolates from the bronchial specimens of adults with chronic bronchitis. However, more recently, Kraft and colleagues,[629] using PCR, detected *M. pneumoniae* in the bronchoalveolar lavage or bronchial biopsy specimens of nine of 18 adults with chronic asthma. Smith and associates[1075] were unable to show that patients with chronic obstructive pulmonary disease had increased susceptibility to infection in contrast to normal subjects. Illness suggestive of pertussis has been described in three children.[651,1108] Teig and associates[1145] studied nasal brush specimens and induced sputum from 38 children with stable chronic lung disease and 42 healthy controls for the presence of *M. pneumoniae* DNA by PCR. Specimens from four (10.5%) of the children with chronic lung disease had *M. pneumoniae* DNA, whereas none of the specimens from control patients were positive. In two provocative studies, Esposito and coworkers[319,320] found that *M. pneumoniae* infections may play a role in recurrent respiratory infections in children. In their studies, they found that children with tonsillopharyngitis or other respiratory infections caused by *M. pneumonia* who were treated with azithromycin 10 mg/kg per day for 3 days weekly for 3 weeks were significantly less likely to have recurrent respiratory tract infections than children with similar *M. pneumoniae* infections who did not receive azithromycin treatment.

Exanthem and Enanthem

Exanthem as a manifestation of *M. pneumoniae* infection is a common occurrence, but its incidence has varied considerably among different studies.* In large studies involving children in which *M. pneumoniae* infection was evaluated in a specific geographic area, the incidence of exanthem has varied from 3% to 33%.† Foy and associates[368] noted rash in 17% of 319 patients with *M. pneumoniae* pneumonia during a 5-year surveillance period. In a study involving only children, Stevens and colleagues[1108] noted exanthem in 9% of their patients. Copps and coworkers,[233] in a community outbreak in La Crosse, Wisconsin, found that 11% of their patients with pneumonia also had rash.

The cutaneous manifestations in *M. pneumoniae* infection are protean. Most common is an erythematous maculopapular rash that is most prominent on the trunk and back; the lesions may be discrete (rubelliform) or confluent (morbilliform). Although not the most common cutaneous manifestations of *M. pneumoniae* infection, erythema multiforme and Stevens-Johnson syndrome are the most often reported and the most

*References 170, 171, 175, 322, 331, 491, 495, 849, 869, 922, 997

*References 13, 146, 188, 190, 211, 232, 233, 321, 333, 355, 363, 365, 366, 368, 418, 429, 442, 491, 540, 578, 651, 656, 662, 723, 727, 732, 744, 848, 849, 869, 902, 964, 988, 1006, 1016, 1098, 1108, 1111, 1146, 1172.

†References 233, 333, 363, 368, 491, 540, 651, 732, 744, 849, 869, 1108, 1098.

TABLE 196.3 Selected Clinical Findings in 29 Patients With *Mycoplasma pneumoniae* Infection and Exanthem

Clinical Findings	No. Patients
Predominant Components of Exanthem	
Erythematous macular	4
Erythematous maculopapular	14
Vesicular	14
Bullous	6
Petechial	1
Urticarial	2
Discrete lesions	11
Confluent lesions	7
Pruritic	6
Predominant Distribution of Exanthem	
Hands	9
Arms	20
Feet	8
Legs	19
Trunk	19
Face	11
Buttocks	9
Genitals	8
Duration of Exanthem (Days)	
<7	2
7–14	11
>14	10
Time of Onset of Exanthem	
Before fever	2
With fever	4
During fever	17
After fever	1
Antibiotics Administered Before Exanthem	
Yes	17
No	10
Enanthem	
Generalized ulcerative stomatitis	14
Tonsillitis or pharyngitis	7
Conjunctivitis	
Severe	8
Mild	3
Pneumonia	
Yes	25
No	4

From Cherry JD. Anemia and mucocutaneous lesions due to *Mycoplasma pneumoniae* infections. *Clin Infect Dis* 1993;17(suppl 1):47–51.

serious.* Other unusual cutaneous manifestations include erythema nodosum, pityriasis rosea, varicella-like urticaria, subcorneal pustular dermatosis, acute hemorrhagic edema of infancy, papular purpuric gloves-and-socks syndrome, and Cockade purpura.† In Table 196.3, the clinical findings in 29 well-documented cases of *M. pneumoniae* infection with exanthem are presented. Of the total group, all but eight were male, 24 of 29 were younger than 20 years, and 12 of 20 were younger than 11 years. The duration of exanthem was longer than 7 days in all but two patients; all patients were febrile, and in 17 cases, the rash occurred during fever.

Enanthems are also common with *M. pneumoniae* and have been given their own name—*Mycoplasma pneumoniae*–associated mucositis.[1012,1162] Oral lesions appear most frequently, followed by ocular and urogenital involvement. Because concurrent cutaneous manifestations are often milder or completely absent, some also to refer to this syndrome as an "atypical Stevens-Johnson" or "Fuchs syndrome."[777,795,959,1017,1269] Extensive reviews of published cases of *M. pneumoniae*-related mucocutaneous disease have, in fact, caused some groups to protest against using descriptive terms like Stevens-Johnson syndrome and erythema multiforme.[144,947,1204] Canavan and associates propose instead the name "*Mycoplasma pneumoniae*-induced rash and mucositis."[144] They point out that in cases in which *M. pneumoniae* infection is strongly implicated, the patients tend to be younger (2–20 years old), mucositis is prominent with sparse cutaneous findings, and the course is milder and mortality rare (3%) in contrast to those other syndromes. They suggest that making this distinction may help in early management decisions. However, this should not eliminate *M. pneumoniae* from the diagnostic differential in cases of severe mucocutaneous disease. McDermott and associates reported a 19-year-old with mucositis and a diffuse muculopapular, bullous rash that extended to over 30% of his skin, also meeting histologic criteria for toxic epidermal necrolysis.[773] A community hospital in Colorado retrospectively analyzed their pediatric records for Stevens-Johnson syndrome cases, and while they found that those with *M. pneumoniae* infection were more likely to have radiographic pneumonia and fewer sites of skin involvement, the majority had severe disease and required prolonged hospitalization and surgical intervention.[902]

In Table 196.4, the specific mucocutaneous findings in 20 of 29 patients are itemized. Of these, 14 patients had generalized ulcerative stomatitis and 7 had tonsillitis or pharyngitis. Severe conjunctivitis was observed in 8 patients, and this manifestation was seen only in those with vesicular or bullous cutaneous lesions. All 8 patients with severe conjunctivitis also had generalized ulcerative stomatitis. Surprisingly, vesicular or bullous exanthems with oral and eye lesions rarely occurred in females.[51,764,1108] In an analysis of 42 cases of erythema multiforme seen during a 20-year period, Villiger and associates[1193] noted a presumptive or definite diagnosis of *M. pneumoniae* infection in 14 children. Nine of the children were boys (64%) and eight of the illnesses had mucous membrane involvement. Campagna and coworkers describe a 12-year-old boy with acute bronchitis, Stevens-Johnson syndrome, and positive *M. pneumoniae* serology and PCR, whose Stevens-Johnson syndrome findings recurred 8 months later.[143] Mucocutaneous findings also are present in vasculitic disorders such as Kawasaki disease and Behçet syndrome, both of which have also been associated with mycoplasma infection.[300,663,1198,1306]

The occurrence of rash as the major manifestation of *M. pneumoniae* infection is probably rare. As noted in Table 196.3, 25 of 29 patients had pneumonia. In a study of 112 patients who had suspected infectious exanthems without pneumonia, Cherry and associates[189] could find none with *M. pneumoniae* infection. However, Foy and colleagues[363] noted a 2-year-old child with only rash, and Stutman[1111] reported a 15-year-old boy with Stevens-Johnson syndrome but not pneumonia, from whom the organism was recovered from a vesicular lesion. Ruhrmann and Holthusen[988] observed frequent cases of mild erythema multiforme without pneumonia.

Many patients with *M. pneumoniae* infection and exanthem have a history of drug administration before development of the rash; this observation suggests the possibility that the rash is drug induced rather than a result of the infectious process.[1128] As noted in Table 196.3, 17 patients had received antibiotics before the rash appeared, yet the exanthem was present before the administration of antibiotic therapy in 10. In addition, *M. pneumoniae* has been recovered from the blister fluid of two patients with erythema multiforme.[727] Although these data incriminate the infection as a cause of exanthem, the large number of cases in association with the administration of antibiotic raises the possibility that the antibiotic intensifies the dermosensitive potential of the infectious agent in a manner similar to that noted between Epstein-Barr virus (EBV) and ampicillin in infectious mononucleosis.

Cardiac Manifestations

Cardiac involvement during *M. pneumoniae* infection generally is considered to be unusual.* However, studies of Pönkä[940] and Sands and

*References 51, 146, 190, 232, 331, 333, 365, 566, 578, 640, 723, 727, 746, 764, 869, 902, 964, 966, 976, 1006, 1018, 1027, 1060, 1108, 1111, 1172, 1193.

†References 105, 190, 274, 290, 418, 429, 430, 572, 656, 717, 848, 930, 960, 988, 1030, 1053, 1125, 1146, 1262.

*References 188, 232, 260, 332, 330, 346, 419, 499, 595, 735, 918, 975, 1033, 356, 464, 1014, 1065, 1108, 1133.

TABLE 196.4 Mucocutaneous Findings in 20 Patients With *M. Pneumoniae* Infections and Exanthem

Case	Reference	Age (y)	Sex	Distinguishing Characteristic of Exanthem	Generalized Ulcerative Stomatitis	Conjunctivitis
1	190	16	M	Fiery-red confluent maculopapular	0	0
2	190	17	F	Blotchy erythematous	0	0
3	185	4.5	F	Morbilliform	0	0
4	353	9	M	Erythematous maculopapular	+	0
5	353	8	M	Papulovesicular; "target" appearance	+	0
6	365	14	M	Symmetric macular and bullous	+	+
7	578	19	M	Erythematous maculopapular, vesicles; "iris" lesions	+	0
8	651	10	F	Macular and petechial	0	0
9	656	16	M	Varicella-like	+	+
10	1172	8	M	Macular	+	0
11	1172	6	M	Diagnosed as measles	0	0
12	723	16	M	Scattered vesicular; generalized	+	+
13	723	6	M	Vesicular; generalized	+	0
14	848	7	M	Urticarial	0	0
15	848	9	M	Maculopapular	0	0
16	1006	10	M	Vesiculobullous and maculopapular	+	+
17	1146	27	M	Vesiculopustular to papular; "pityriasis-like"	0	0
18	359	10	M	Vesiculobullous; generalized	+	0
19	662	5	M	Maculopapular	0	0
20	732	11	F	Papular; most marked on hands and feet	0	0

F, Female; *M*, male.
Modified from Cherry JD, Hurwitz ES, Welliver RC. *Mycoplasma pneumoniae* infections and exanthems. *J Pediatr* 1975;87:369–373.

associates[1007] and survey data of Noah[879] and Assaad and Borecka[42] indicate that *M. pneumoniae* myocarditis and pericarditis are important causes of both morbidity and mortality. In a study of fatal viral and mycoplasmal infections, Assaad and Borecka[42] noted six cardiovascular deaths related to *M. pneumoniae* infection during a 9-year period. Noah[879] found that 1% of 700 patients with *M. pneumoniae* infection had cardiac manifestations as the main clinical feature. Pönkä[940] published findings of a 7-year study involving 560 patients with serologic evidence of *M. pneumoniae* infection. In this group, 69 patients with cardiac manifestations were detected; of these 69 patients, 25 had carditis for which no causal agent other than *M. pneumoniae* could be incriminated. Pönkä[940] also reviewed the world literature and found a total of 33 other cases of carditis.

Of 25 carefully studied patients, 17 had respiratory symptoms before the diagnosis of carditis and 10 had radiologically confirmed pneumonia. All but four patients had fever. Of the 25 patients, two were younger than 10 years and two were in the 10- to 19-year-old age group. Of the 33 cases in the literature, seven were 20 years old or younger. Of this survey group, 25 of 33 had respiratory illness and in 19 it was recorded as pneumonia.

Of the 25 patients in Finland reviewed by Pönkä, six had pericarditis and the remainder had perimyocarditis. Antibiotic therapy in 11 patients did not appear to shorten the duration of illness or diminish the number of cardiac sequelae. At a 16-month follow-up, 11 patients had persistent cardiac damage. Another interesting aspect of this study was the finding of rises in *M. pneumoniae* complement-fixing antibody titer in five adults with myocardial infarcts.

Chergui and associates[184] described a 45-year-old man with bilateral interstitial infiltrates and second-degree heart block. He was treated with erythromycin; his heart block, fever, and respiratory distress cleared on hospital day 5. Hartleif and coworkers[459] describe at 16-year-old boy with severe acute onset chest pain with ST segment elevations and reduced myocardial contractility, with rising IgM and IgG titers to *M. pneumoniae*. His myocardial function normalized within days of starting doxycycline, although EKG abnormalities persisted for months.

Mycoplasma may also affect the heart through vasculitis, valvular disease, atherosclerosis, and coronary artery disease, although there are conflicting data on the subject.[58,223,377,615] Chung and colleagues[210] analyzed data from Taiwan's nationwide patient database and found that adults with newly diagnosed *M. pneumoniae* were 37% more likely to develop acute coronary syndrome within the following year compared to the general population.

Hematologic Manifestations

Severe hemolytic anemia has been reported on several occasions in patients with *M. pneumoniae* infection.* Most cases of *M. pneumoniae* hemolytic anemia have been associated with marked pulmonary involvement. Stevens-Johnson syndrome is a common associated finding, and myocarditis has been noted on two occasions.[232,332,331,595,1108] In general, severity of illness correlates with high titers of cold agglutinins. One unusual case of a 2-year-old boy with severe *M. pneumoniae* IgM-mediated hemolytic anemia without pulmonary symptoms was described.[627]

The hemolysis may be severe and acute, often with a 50% reduction in hemoglobin concentration. In contrast to uncomplicated pulmonary disease, the leukocyte count in patients with hemolytic anemia frequently is elevated markedly with a predominance of neutrophils. Results of the direct Coombs test are usually positive. Clinical experience suggests that administration of steroids in conjunction with proper antibiotic therapy may be beneficial in this illness. Boccardi and associates[104] observed a 7-year-old boy with hemolytic anemia and transitory paroxysmal cold hemoglobinuria.

Feizi[330] has demonstrated that clinically inapparent compensated hemolysis frequently is associated with *M. pneumoniae* pulmonary infection. Fiala and associates[346] noted that bone marrow suppression also contributed to the anemia in a patient whom they studied, and pancytopenia has also rarely been described.[446] Ruhrmann and Holthusen[988] reported a hemorrhagic variant of erythema multiforme (Cockade purpura) similar to Henoch-Schönlein disease in *M. pneumoniae* infection; they also noted severe thrombocytopenia not associated with hemolytic anemia. A woman in her third trimester of pregnancy with upper respiratory symptoms developed severe thrombocytopenia and was found to have acute *M. pneumoniae* infection.[876] Gill and Marrie[404]

*References 180, 184, 195, 326, 332, 385, 429, 440, 588, 594, 595, 627, 644, 651, 685, 716, 844, 878, 915, 1121, 1262.

reported a 27-year-old man who had hemophagocytosis with an *M. pneumoniae* infection. Several pediatric cases of hemophagocytic lymphohistiocytosis in association with *M. pneumoniae* infections have been reported.[520,615,1276] Also noted was a 4-year-old girl with neutropenia, thrombocytopenia, and acute hepatitis.[179] Severe *M. pneumoniae* infection with pneumonia, thrombocytopenia, and disseminated intravascular coagulation has been described.[199,207] Hypercoagulability resulting from *M. pneumoniae* infection with evidence of autoimmune antibodies has manifested as venous thrombosis, pulmonary embolisms, and priapism in several cases.[40,48,56,123,427,531,567,1303] Aviner and colleagues[48] also describe eight cases of *M. pneumoniae* infection with associated thrombocytopenia not related to disseminated intravascular coagulation. Khoury and colleagues[597] discuss the case of a 79-year-old woman with anemia and methemoglobinemia believed to be caused by *M. pneumoniae* infection.

Abdominal Manifestations

Nonspecific gastrointestinal findings. Approximately 25% of patients with *M. pneumoniae* pneumonia have nausea, vomiting, diarrhea, or some combination thereof (see Table 196.2). Aside from these complaints, gastrointestinal problems in association with *M. pneumoniae* infection are rare events. Stevens and associates[1108] found that 15% of a group of 44 children with infection had notable abdominal pain. Referred abdominal pain with pneumonia also has been observed.[331]

Liver involvement. Liver involvement in *M. pneumoniae* infection is a surprisingly rare event. Levine and Lerner[684] reported that mild increases in transaminases occur and that acute and chronic active hepatitis has been noted with respiratory symptoms and proven *M. pneumoniae* infection, but they provided no further information. Shin and colleagues[1056] did a retrospective analysis of 117 South Korean patients with positive *M. pneumoniae* serology and no other risk factor for hepatitis and found that 25 (21%) had greater than twofold the normal level of transaminases, with up to 40% having greater than fivefold alanine transaminase levels. MacLean[732] reported a 13-year-old girl who initially had a sore throat and 9 days later had clinical and laboratory evidence of hepatitis. Murray and associates[837] presented a case report of an adult with typical *M. pneumoniae* pneumonia in whom liver function and enzyme studies indicated hepatitis. Helms and colleagues[472] noted that six of 17 patients with *M. pneumoniae* pneumonia had elevated aspartate aminotransferase values. Enzyme changes have been observed in other case evaluations,[686,744,1067] some with coagulopathy,[167] and hepatic necrosis has occurred.[735,835]

Simonian and Janner[1065] reported a 12-year-old boy who had pleural effusion, hepatitis, and hemolytic anemia. Narita and associates[860] noted two children with lymphadenopathy and liver dysfunction. These two patients are of interest because both had mycoplasmemia and neither had pneumonia. Elevated liver enzymes without respiratory symptoms also have been found in young adults with elevated *M. pneumoniae* serologies.[663,956,980,1056] A prospective study of 80 pediatric patients with positive *M. pneumoniae* serology and hepatitis showed that these patients tended to have favorable outcomes and that further unnecessary evaluation of the hepatitis should be avoided.[603]

Splenic infarct. Two children (a 13-year-old girl and a 10-year-old boy) with pneumonia resulting from *M. pneumoniae* infection had splenic infarcts and transient antiphospholipid antibodies.[1257] A 24-year-old man with an elevated *M. pneumoniae* IgM titer developed hepatosplenomegaly and splenic infact.[919] A 19-year-old woman developed splenic infarct during a coinfection with *M. pneumoniae*, cytomegalovirus and EBV.[690]

Pancreatitis. In 1974, Märdh and Ursing[752] reported six patients with respiratory tract illnesses, serologic evidence of *M. pneumoniae* infection, and pancreatitis. In four patients, pancreatic symptoms began 1 to 2 weeks after the onset of respiratory tract illness; in the other two patients, the pancreatitis was subclinical. Diabetes developed in two patients, one of whom died. At postmortem examination, pneumonitis and pancreatitis were confirmed. Nakagawa and colleagues[847] report on an 8-year-old girl who developed necrotizing pancreatitis 10 days into her treatment for *M. pneumoniae* pneumonia. In a study of pancreatitis, Leinikki and Pantzar[676] noted that sera from 18 of 56 patients had rises in complement-fixing antibody titer to *M. pneumoniae*. Because none of the patients in this study had respiratory tract illness suggestive of *M. pneumoniae* infection, the investigators suggested that perhaps the antibody responses were not specific for *M. pneumoniae* infection but were caused by a cross-reacting infection or were the result of autoantigens from pancreatic damage. Leinikki and associates[677] have conducted further studies; their thought is that the antibody response is nonspecific, but their data neither confirm nor refute this assumption. In another study, Freeman and McMahon[377] also noted serologic evidence of *M. pneumoniae* infection in 33% of patients with pancreatitis. Oderda and Kraut[888] reported a 22-month-old girl with pancreatitis and a rise in complement-fixing antibody titer to *M. pneumoniae.* This child had no respiratory symptoms. Yang and associates[1274] report the case of a 6-year-old girl with fever, drowsiness, respiratory and gastrointestinal symptoms, with rising *M. pneumoniae* titers, who was found to have acute necrotizing pancreatitis with a large pseudocsyt.

Renal disease. Mycoplasma infection can lead to renal disease, thought to be due to immune complex deposition. Glomerulonephritis was reported in a few patients with pneumonia[9,941] or preceding upper respiratory infection symptoms.[35,181,669] Acute IgA nephropathy following *M. pneumoniae* infection has also been described.[1117] Hemolytic uremic syndrome was reported in a 1-year-old boy with *M. pneumoniae* respiratory infection, although the mechanism was unclear.[413]

Arthritis

Mycoplasmas are a common cause of arthritis in animals other than human beings.[226,539] Likewise, *M. pneumoniae* infection is associated occasionally with joint manifestations.* In a review of 1259 patients with *M. pneumoniae* infection, Pönkä[939] noted transient arthritis in 0.9%. Two patients were found to have Reiter syndrome. Hernandez and colleagues[477] reported seven instances of arthritis in 38 persons with *M. pneumoniae* respiratory disease. In one patient, the illness lasted 18 months and was associated with the development of rheumatoid factor.

Twenty-one instances of illness suggestive of rheumatic fever have been described.[77,214,556,650,823,844,855,1031,1243] In all 21 patients, large joints were involved; 18 patients had joint swelling or effusion, whereas three had only pain. Most patients had a history of preceding respiratory illness with sore throat, and 10 of 21 had radiographic evidence of pneumonia. The sedimentation rate was elevated in all patients in whom the test was performed. One child had an erythema marginatum–like rash, as well as polyarthritis and fever.[823] Poggio and colleagues[937] reported a child with reactive arthritis 3 weeks after the onset of diarrhea and a respiratory tract infection. Leukocytoclastic vasculitis and polyarthritis associated with *M. pneumoniae* infection has been described in a young adult.[934]

Muscular Disease

Berger and Wadowksy[78] reported a 15-year-old girl with right lower lobe pneumonia, hepatitis, and rhabdomyolysis associated with *M. pneumoniae* infection. Minami and associates[804] reported a 4-year-old boy with pneumonia and a rhabdomyolysis associated with a marked titer rise to *M. pneumoniae* using a passive agglutination assay. Oishi and associates[893] described a case of multidrug-resistant *M. pneumoniae* causing rhabdomyolysis in a 7-year-old girl. Rhabdomyolysis in a 25-year-old woman[804] and a 7-year-old boy[231] with *M. pneumoniae* respiratory infections have also been reported. Polymyositis has been noted in association with *M. pneumoniae* infection on six occasions.[932]

Ocular and Neurologic Disease

Conjunctivitis is a frequent mucocutaneous manifestation of mycoplasma infection; however, the eye may also be affected through cranial neuropathies, optic papillitis, or anterior uveitis.[706] A 15-year-old patient suffered bilateral optic disk edema and iritis during an acute *M. pneumoniae* infection.[999] An 8-year-old boy had bilateral optic neuritis resulting in blurred vision that resolved after 2 months of treatment.[197] A 15-year-old boy had headaches, diplopia, and blurred vision, with a CT angiogram demonstrating vasculitis of the middle cerebral arteries in an area with ischemic demyelination on magnetic resonance imaging.[138]

*References 44, 53, 77, 258, 393, 399, 477, 554, 556, 651, 650, 751, 840, 855, 939, 990, 1243.

Miller Fisher syndrome was described in a 38-year-old man and a 75-year-old woman during the course of an *M. pneumoniae* pneumonia, the former experiencing acute diplopia and the latter with ptosis and opthalmoplegia.[667,1068]

Several large community and military studies of *M. pneumoniae* pneumonia and other respiratory tract illnesses are notable in that neurologic disease is not described.[173,233,321,368,540,816,830] However, other studies, particularly those performed more recently, indicate a surprising spectrum of neurologic illness associated with *M. pneumoniae* infection.* The failure to find neurologic disease in the initial large studies mentioned was probably due not to its absence but to the orientation of the investigators; neurologic disease was not studied under the respiratory investigation protocols. In addition, when neurologic manifestations of *M. pneumoniae* infection occur, it is often in the absence of any respiratory symptoms.[26,138,858] In three large studies of *M. pneumoniae* illness involving 1856 cases, 2.6 to 4.8% had neurologic illness.[869,879,942] Assaad and Borecka[42] noted five fatal *M. pneumoniae* infections in which central nervous system findings were the major clinical manifestations.

In 1973, Lerer and Kalavsky[683] reported 5 cases of neurologic disease associated with *M. pneumoniae* infection and analyzed 45 cases from the literature. They noted the following frequencies of specific clinical involvement: generalized encephalitis (30%), spinal nerve roots (30%), meningitis (20%), cranial nerves (20%), focal encephalitis (16%), cerebellum (14%), psychosis (8%), and spinal cord (2%). Combined involvement was noted in 36% of cases; in 79%, a history of antecedent respiratory illness was elicited. Of the patients, 53% were 20 years old or younger, and 15% were younger than 10 years. Eighty percent of the children and adolescents were males. The onset of neurologic disease occurred 3 to 23 days after the onset of respiratory illness, with a mean value of 10 days. Five deaths were noted and 22% of the survivors had residual neurologic deficits.

In a review of 61 patients with *M. pneumoniae*–associated neurologic disease during a 24-year period in Helsinki, Finland, Koskiniemi[625] noted that 45 of the patients were children and that all these children had encephalitis. Of the total group, 5 patients (8%) died and 14 (23%) had severe sequelae.

In a study of acute childhood encephalitis in Toronto, Canada, nine of 50 children (18%) with adequate microbiologic study had evidence of *M. pneumoniae* infection.[618] Interestingly, four of the nine children also had evidence of concomitant viral infection. In a further study of encephalitis at the same center during a 5-year period, researchers noted that 50 of 159 children (31%) with encephalitis had evidence of *M. pneumoniae* infection[93]; in this analysis, 30 of the 50 cases (60%) had microbiologic evidence of other concomitant infections. Respiratory prodromal symptoms preceded the encephalitis in approximately 67% of the patients in whom the diagnosis was based on culture, PCR, or both. Two children had acute demyelinating encephalomyelitis. Long-term neurologic sequelae occurred in 48% to 64% of cases. From 1998 to 2006, 1988 patients with encephalitis of unclear etiology were referred to the California Encephalitis Project.[206] *M. pneumoniae* was the most common agent implicated; 111 patients had evidence of *M. pneumoniae* infection and 84 (76%) of these patients were children. In later years, the California Encephalitis Project began to detect an increasing number of cases of anti-*N*-methyl-D-aspartate receptor encephalitis among children,[381] an autoimmune process that in some cases has been linked to *M. pneumoniae* infection.[24,380,1186,1188]

In other studies, aseptic meningitis is reported more frequently; other less common findings include poliomyelitis-like syndrome, bilateral sensorineural deafness, Reye syndrome, cerebral infarction, opsoclonus-myoclonus syndrome, brainstem syndrome, transverse myelitis, psychosis, cerebellar syndrome, radiculopathy, brachial plexus neuropathy, demyelinating polyneuropathy with syndrome of inappropriate secretion of antidiuretic hormone (SIADH), acute disseminated encephalomyelitis, bilateral striatal necrosis, Kluver-Bucy syndrome, Tourette syndrome, obsessive-compulsive disorder, hydrocephalus and intracranial hypertension, Bell palsy, and Guillain-Barré syndrome. Specific examples include SIADH in a 6-year-old boy,[704] acute self-limiting parkinsonism in a 9-year-old boy and 12-year-old boy,[1134] a 4-year-old boy with acute disseminated encephalomyelitis,[259] Bickerstaff brainstem encephalitis in a 9-year-old boy,[797] hypertensive encephalopathy and Guillain-Barré syndrome in a 7-year-old girl,[23] and new-onset seizures in three pediatric cases that resolved with immunotherapy.[37] Arthur and Margolis[39] noted the appearance of mycoplasma-like structures in granulomatous angiitis of the central nervous system at postmortem examination of a 35-year-old man.

*References 2, 22, 32, 34, 47, 49, 59, 66, 74, 94, 198, 224, 280, 288, 313, 415, 454, 465, 481, 526, 573, 598, 606, 612, 621, 637, 654, 681, 700, 758, 798, 828, 834, 877, 883, 887, 917, 921, 945, 984, 996, 1020, 1025, 1029, 1049, 1066, 1098, 1108, 1132, 1149, 1161, 1164, 1174, 1201, 1235, 1245, 1256, 1279, 1280, 1289.

Mixed Infections

In many studies of *M. pneumoniae* infection, cultural or serologic evidence of concomitant or sequential infection with other infectious agents has been noted.* In a large study of patients hospitalized with acute respiratory illness, Fransen and associates[374] found that 64% of patients with rises in complement-fixing antibody titer to *M. pneumoniae* also had antibody titer rises to viral, chlamydial, or bacterial agents. In this group, the most common concomitant infections were with parainfluenza viruses. The occurrence of mixed infection did not appear to have a pronounced effect on clinical manifestations; the only significant difference between patients with mixed infection and those with single *M. pneumoniae* infection was the more common finding of a high erythrocyte sedimentation rate in the former group. In several other large studies of disease caused by *M. pneumoniae,* concomitant infections were common, but no evidence of synergistic or antagonistic roles of one agent for another was noted.[333,411,816,1097,1098] By contrast, Johansson and associates[552] did observe more severe disease in patients with mixed viral and bacterial infections, including *M. pneumoniae,* than those with bacteria alone. A different study of 59 children with *M. pneumoniae* pneumonia found 19 cases of coinfection with viruses and nine cases of coinfection with *S. pneumoniae.* While those with *S. pneumoniae* mixed infection were more likely to be younger and have higher durations of fever and hospitalization, those with combined viral and *M. pneumoniae* infection showed no significant clinical differences from those infected by only mycoplasma.[200] Hon and colleagues described a 4-year-old girl who succumbed to a severe pneumonia, septic shock, and hemolytic uremic syndrome while infected with *S. pneumoniae, M. pneumoniae*, and human metapneumovirus.[486]

Renner and associates[968] found a lower than expected frequency of seropositivity to *M. pneumoniae* in 91 serum pairs with seroconversion to influenza A virus.

The high rate of possible mixed infections in the large encephalitis study in Toronto is of particular interest.[93] In addition to common respiratory viruses and enteroviruses, they noted herpes group viruses, *Bartonella henselae,* and *Mycobacterium tuberculosis.* Similar to *M. pneumoniae, M. tuberculosis* is also able to induce cold-agglutinins and hemolytic anemia, and other cases of dual infection with both organisms have been described.[1263] In studies of *Bordetella pertussis* infection, evidence of mixed infection with *M. pneumoniae* or perhaps serologic cross-reactivity has been found repeatedly.[182,527,582,1194,1305] Vervloet and colleagues[1190] found that of 44 cases of *M. pneumoniae* pneumonia, 9 had concomitant *S. pneumoniae* infection.

The observation by Grady and Gilfillan[423] that 81% of patients with Legionnaires' disease also had serologic evidence of *M. pneumoniae* infection is interesting. In the same study, 29% of all patients seropositive for *M. pneumoniae* were also seropositive for the Legionnaires' disease antigen. Comparable studies performed by the Centers for Disease Control and Prevention failed to find a similar rate of high co-positivity in sera obtained in other Legionnaires' disease epidemics. Another study found no serologic relationship between *M. pneumoniae* and *Legionella pneumophila.*[967] Severe bacterial disease after *M. pneumoniae* infection has been reported occasionally. Stadel and colleagues[1093] noted *Hemophilus influenzae* pneumonia and bacteremia after a mild *M. pneumoniae* illness. Biberfeld and colleagues[86] reported staphylococcal septicemia in two cases of *M. pneumoniae* pneumonia, and Rykner and associates[990]

*References 13, 51, 93, 308, 333, 334, 375, 486, 581, 611, 411, 423, 433, 448, 527, 528, 618, 682, 697, 745, 756, 816, 857, 968, 1093, 1097, 1098, 1190, 1191, 1194, 1242, 1223, 1305

recovered pneumococci from the pleural exudate of a patient with *M. pneumoniae* pneumonia. Klein and coworkers reported a 16-year-old girl with *M. pneumoniae* pharyngitis followed by Lemierre syndrome with *Fusobacterium nucleatum* and later complicated by acute EBV infectious mononucleosis.[611]

Kleemola and Kayhty[608] found fourfold or greater increases in *M. pneumoniae* complement-fixing antibody titer in 40.7% of 54 patients with bacterial meningitis. However, they thought that this antibody response was not caused by specific *M. pneumoniae* infection but by cross-reactive glycolipids resulting from the bacterial infection.[608,609]

Lind and associates[700] reported that four of 19 patients with neurologic disease and *M. pneumoniae* infection had serologic evidence of concomitant viral infection. Wang and colleagues[1223] discovered that three of 22 children with *M. pneumoniae*–positive PCR assay also had a positive PCR for respiratory viruses.

Other Disease Associations

Foy and colleagues[363] noted that both ear involvement and pneumonia as manifestations of *M. pneumoniae* infection occurred more commonly in children with previous tonsillectomy. Putman and associates[950] found that in all but three of 31 patients with sarcoidosis, the serum complement-fixing antibody titer to *M. pneumoniae* was 1:32 or higher, whereas in a similar-sized control group without sarcoidosis, only two persons had titers of 1:32 and none had higher titers. Other interesting observations include multiple birth defects in a newborn exposed to *M. pneumoniae* in utero,[115] a tubo-ovarian abscess in a young woman from whom *M. pneumoniae* was isolated in pure culture,[1153] Lipschütz ulcers from three females with positive *M. pneumoniae* serology,[1192] and fever of unknown origin in a 32-year-old man.[638]

Recurrent Disease

The results of several investigations suggest that recurrent *M. pneumoniae* infection is a frequent finding.[126,342,1104] Repeat infections can be associated with severe disease, such as pneumonia. In the Seattle studies, second attacks of pneumonia have been documented and similar findings have been observed in England.[359,370,372,491] Recurrent *M. pneumoniae* infections also occurred throughout the lifetime of a child who was immunocompromised from both poorly controlled human immunodeficiency virus (HIV) and B-cell lymphoma therapy and who died at 8 years of age.[1240]

Disease in the Neonate

M. pneumoniae is a common cause of respiratory infection beyond the neonatal period; however, rare cases of intrauterine infection leading to pneumonia in infancy have been found.[1092,1179]

Diagnosis

Differential Diagnosis

Because the clinical manifestations of *M. pneumoniae* infection are protean and because infections occur commonly in children and adolescents, this agent should be considered in the differential diagnosis of most infectious illnesses. Most important is its consideration in patients with pulmonary disease, in whom illnesses caused by viruses (particularly adenoviruses, parainfluenza viruses, and influenza viruses); *Chlamydophila psittaci*, *Chlamydophila pneumoniae*, *Coxiella burnetii*, bacteria (particularly *Streptococcus pneumoniae*, *B. pertussis*, *H. influenzae*, and *M. tuberculosis*); and fungi (particularly *Histoplasma capsulatum* and *Coccidioides immitis*) are the main differential possibilities. Because the clinical manifestations, including the radiographic appearance of the lungs, are frequently similar in the various differential possibilities, the following other factors are important: the status of the host (i.e., normal or immunologically compromised), the environment (i.e., human, animal, or inanimate source), the age of the patient, the incubation period, and the season.

In otherwise healthy children, *M. pneumoniae* is a common cause of pneumonia in those older than 3 years and is the leading cause of pneumonia in older children and adolescents. The lack of coryza is sometimes useful in differentiating *M. pneumoniae* pneumonia from that caused by common viral agents, and elevation of the white blood cell count along with an increase in band form neutrophils is evidence against a mycoplasmal etiologic agent, except in patients with concomitant hemolytic anemia. The occurrence of exanthem and, in particular, Stevens-Johnson syndrome, should lead the physician to suspect *M. pneumoniae*; similarly, the occurrence of hemolytic anemia, joint manifestations, or neurologic signs and symptoms with pneumonia should lead the physician to strongly suspect *M. pneumoniae* as the etiologic agent. Because the pulmonary manifestations of *M. pneumoniae* infection are not always clinically apparent, a physician investigating an unusual acute or subacute case (i.e., aseptic meningitis or other neurologic illness; exanthem; enanthem; hepatitis; pancreatitis; pericarditis, myocarditis, or both; and arthritis) would be wise to consider the possibility of *M. pneumoniae* as the etiologic agent and to obtain appropriate chest radiographs, as well as definitive cultures and serologic studies.

Specific Diagnosis

Serum cold agglutinins. Despite the considerable confusion in the literature and by physicians in general regarding the diagnostic value of the serum cold agglutination test for *M. pneumoniae* infection, our opinion is that when it is used appropriately, the test is a simple and useful procedure. One cause for confusion was a report in 1966 in which only one of 28 children with positive cold agglutination titers actually had serologic evidence of *M. pneumoniae* infection by complement fixation.[1116] However, this report can be criticized because the study population consisted of 444 children younger than 4 years of age and only 170 of this group had pneumonia. Because cold agglutinins are noted occasionally in the sera of patients of all ages with a variety of illnesses, for useful results, their study should have been restricted to patients likely to have *M. pneumoniae* lower respiratory tract disease.[190,348,399,696] In various studies of pneumonia, serum cold agglutinins at a titer of 1:32 or higher were found in 50% to 90% of patients with *M. pneumoniae* infection.[89,169,173,375,399,540,830,1108,1185] In general, the cold agglutinin response correlates directly with the severity of pulmonary involvement; patients with extensive lobar involvement nearly always have positive titers[8] (1:32), whereas those with only minimal findings on radiographic study frequently have equivocal or negative titers. Positive cold agglutination titers have been observed in 18% of adenoviral pneumonias in a study involving a military population.[399] In general, the higher the cold agglutinin titer, the more likely that a particular illness is caused by *M. pneumoniae.*

A rapid screening test for cold agglutinins is available and useful.[393,434] This test is performed by adding 4 drops of blood to a tube containing sodium citrate or another anticoagulant. The tube is placed in ice water (0°C to 4°C [32°F to 39.2°F]) in a freezer for approximately 30 seconds and then examined immediately for coarse agglutination by tilting the tube on its side. When the tube is warmed, the agglutination should resolve, and it can be reproduced again by repeating the ice-water cooling procedure. A modified version of this rapid test was used in 126 children in an emergency department who had asthma exacerbations.[168] The test had a sensitivity of 78.3% and a specificity of 41.3% in contrast to an IgM ELISA.

Specific antibody determinations. Several specific antibody tests (i.e., growth inhibition, immunofluorescence, indirect hemagglutination, precipitation, mycoplasmacidal antibody, complement fixation, ELISA, adherence inhibition assay, radioimmunoassay, and radioimmunoprecipitation) can be used to measure serum antibodies to *M. pneumoniae.* In the past, only the complement-fixation test was available routinely. A fourfold rise in complement-fixation antibody titer indicates acute *M. pneumoniae* infection. Because complement-fixation antibody in *M. pneumoniae* infection is of relatively short duration, the observation of a fourfold fall in titer also can be useful on occasion in assigning etiologic significance in a particular illness. High single titers (≥1:256) usually indicate recent infection, but rarely can be used to relate the cause of an illness specifically to *M. pneumoniae.* Because *M. pneumoniae* infection is associated with a relatively long incubation period, the development of antibodies is occurring at the time of acute disease. As a consequence, fourfold changes in titer can occur in a short interval (5 days), and collection of paired sera 5 to 7 days apart usually reveals a significant rise in complement-fixation antibody titer.

Most diagnostic laboratories have replaced the complement-fixation test with commercial immunofluorescence or ELISA for demonstration of antibodies to M. pneumoniae antigens.* These tests, in addition to demonstrating rises in antibody values in paired sera, can identify specific IgM and IgA antibodies in single serum samples. In general, when used by experienced laboratory personnel, both immunofluorescence and ELISA have sensitivities and specificities similar to those of the complement-fixation test for determining significant increases in antibody values in paired serum specimens. In addition, demonstration of specific IgM or IgA antibody in a single serum sample suggests a recent infection. Today, the most common method used for diagnosing *M. pneumoniae* infection in clinical practice in the United States is the single serum IgM assay (although PCR assay is becoming more frequent in the hospital setting). It should be pointed out that most available serologic tests have low specificity and can be falsely positive in other acute infections so that overdiagnosis is common[73,136,166,247,295,647,875,1129]; therefore, new panels of antigens are being developed.[294] Furthermore, the specific IgM and IgA responses after infection may last for several months; therefore, demonstration of these antibodies in a single serum sample may be misleading with regard to the diagnosis of specific illness. Hence, in most instances, paired sera (i.e., 5 to 14 days apart) should be examined to confirm a clinical diagnosis. Also useful is the determination of cold agglutinin titers at the time of IgM ELISA. If an ELISA IgM test is positive and a cold agglutinin test is negative, the physician should be skeptical of the former value.

Culture. With proper media, experienced personnel have little difficulty isolating *M. pneumoniae* from throat swabs of infected patients.[18,1169] However, because *M. pneumoniae* is relatively slow growing, in most instances requiring more than 1 week of incubation, culture is of less use for diagnosis of routine cases than is serologic study. Cultures should be performed in all unusual situations; specifically, joint fluid, CSF, pericardial fluid, and biopsy material should be cultured. The modified SP-4 medium, which is more sensitive than conventional mycoplasma culture media, coupled with the agar plate immunofluorescence identification procedure, may assist the cultural diagnosis of *M. pneumoniae.*[979,1169] However, low yield and sensitivity have caused some to recommend abandoning this diagnostic method.[1041]

Detection by nucleic acid amplification and mass spectrometry Tests. A large number of studies have indicated the usefulness of PCR for demonstration of specific *M. pneumoniae* DNA in sputum, throat, nasopharyngeal, blood, CSF, urine, and tissue specimens.† Multiple primers have been used to identify gene sequences of the P1 cytoadhesin, ATPase operon, 16S rRNA, 16S-23 S rRNA spacer, tuf, parE, dnaK, pdhA, ptsI, repMp1 noncoding element, and the CARDS toxin.[1023,1205] In cases of treatment failure or in communities with high rates of macrolide resistance, specific primers can be made to target several well-characterized mutations.[551,691,886,1175] This is especially important in Asia, where the rate of resistance is high; however, rural areas may not have the resources to perform PCR. There have been multiple studies in China evaluating loop-mediated isothermal amplification as a simpler and less expensive screening test than standard PCR.[14,420,523,565,1294]

Using culture with serologic criteria as the comparative standard, several studies have shown excellent sensitivity and specificity using PCR. However, given the high carriage rate of *M. pneumoniae*,[1089] correlation of positive results with a clinical picture consistent with infection is critical. In addition, both serology and PCR will occasionally give nonoverlapping false-negative results; therefore a combination of these two diagnostic methods would be optimal.[575,952,1156]

In a hospital setting where patients may be in more urgent need of a diagnosis despite the broad differential of possible organisms, multiplex PCR has come into favor due to its ability to rapidly screen for multiple respiratory pathogens[44,886,1043] although this also raises its cost. Matrix-assisted laser desorption/ionization time-of-flight spectrometry can similarly screen for multiple panels of pathogens at once, with enough sensitivity and specificity to identify strain subtypes and the carriage of antibiotic resistance markers.[1268]

*References 5, 73, 150, 247, 294, 295, 301, 328, 349, 496, 616, 664, 829, 875, 961, 1062, 1072, 1129, 1151, 1150, 1177, 1234.

†References 2, 93, 100, 140, 263, 283, 293, 406, 487, 515, 550, 575, 736, 776, 800, 809, 826, 843, 858, 935, 963, 969, 1026, 1037, 1082, 1130, 1254, 1272, 1293.

Treatment

Antimicrobial Therapy

M. pneumoniae is sensitive in vitro to erythromycin, tetracyclines, chloramphenicol, clarithromycin, azithromycin, several aminoglycosides, and quinolones.[71,269,521,522,542,749,871,1070] It is resistant to all penicillins and for practical purposes to the cephalosporins. In spite of this demonstrated in vitro sensitivity of the organism and several studies that have shown clinical therapeutic effectiveness,* a common misconception of many physicians is that antibiotic therapy is of little value in the treatment of illness caused by *M. pneumoniae.* This idea had its origin before the present era, when many patients with viral pneumonia were given a diagnosis of primary atypical pneumonia and treated unsuccessfully with antibiotics.

In 1961, Kingston and associates[604] demonstrated the therapeutic effectiveness of demethylchlortetracycline for pneumonia caused by *M. pneumoniae.* Since then, several other antibiotics have been studied carefully and also have been found to be effective against *M. pneumoniae* pneumonia.[169,269,368,399,540,988,1035,1070,1074] The drugs of choice for pneumonia caused by *M. pneumoniae* are either erythromycins or tetracyclines. Because of the adverse effects of tetracyclines on teeth, a macrolide is the drug of choice in children. Fluoroquinolones are also effective, and have found an increased use in cases of macrolide resistance; however, they also carry a small risk for tendonitis. In *M. pneumoniae* pneumonia, the dose of erythromycin for children is 40 to 50 mg/kg every 24 hours administered every 6 hours for a minimum of 10 days. For adolescents and adults, the dosage of erythromycin or tetracycline is 2 g every 24 hours administered every 6 hours. In general, the effectiveness of antibiotic therapy correlates directly with the severity of pneumonia and the elapsed time of illness before the initiation of therapy.

Azithromycin and clarithromycin both are approved for the treatment of community-acquired pneumonia in children.[102,457] Their advantage is less frequent dosing, shorter duration of therapy, and less gastrointestinal disturbance in older patients. The azithromycin dosing schedule is 10 mg/kg per day (maximal dose, 1 g/d) on day 1, followed by 5 mg/kg per day (maximal dose, 500 mg/d) for 4 days. The clarithromycin dose is 15 mg/kg per day administered every 12 hours for 10 days (maximal dose, 1 g/d). Macrolide-resistant strains of *M. pneumoniae* were first noted from clinical isolates in Japan in 2000, and are associated with mutations in the 23S rRNA gene.[760,827] These strains have since spread worldwide, with a rate of 8.2% resistance found in the United States between 2007 and 2010[149,1270] and 10% to 13% between 2006 and 2014.[270,1163,1297] Predominantly in Asia, where the rate of resistance can be as high as 95%,[1296] studies have shown that macrolide resistance is associated with longer durations of fever, hospital stay, and treatment.[1233,1261,1281,1299] However, the clinical relevance is still debated as the overall outcome is usually the same.[148,808,1163] Even in cases in which resistant strains are present, mild or moderate respiratory infections frequently resolve on macrolide therapy.[946] This is thought to be due to the immunomodulatory properties of this class of drugs, since much of the disease pathology is caused by inflammatory damage.[1008] However, therapy for chronic or lower respiratory infections with *M. pneumoniae* should be prompty changed to effective antibiotics if analysis proves that the strain is resistant. Successful treatment of these strains has been shown using minocycline, doxycycline, or levofloxacin.[580,726,894] Ciprofloxacin has also be used[722,994] although it may display an elevated minimal inhibitory concentration.

In all other clinical manifestations of *M. pneumoniae* infection except pneumonia (e.g., nonpulmonary respiratory infection, neurologic disease, and Stevens-Johnson syndrome), antibiotic therapy has not been evaluated adequately. In general, otitis media, pharyngitis, croup, and bronchiolitis appear to be mild, self-limited illnesses that require no therapy. In more serious illness, such as Stevens-Johnson syndrome and neurologic disease, individual case studies have indicated little evidence of therapeutic benefit with either erythromycin or tetracycline therapy. However, our opinion is that, when diagnosed, most *M. pneumoniae* infections should be treated because there is little to lose and in vitro data suggest the possibility of efficacy.

*References 102, 169, 269, 363, 368, 391, 399, 540, 604, 988, 1028, 1035, 1070, 1074, 1090.

Corticosteroid Therapy

Steroids have been used in the management of severe pulmonary disease, Stevens-Johnson syndrome, encephalitis, and hemolytic anemia. Although definitive data are lacking, several case studies suggest associated clinical benefit, and one randomized clinical trial of severe pneumonia patients showed significantly faster resolution of symptoms in those who were treated with steroids within 24 hours of admission compared to after 72 hours.[508] Steroids seem to be particularly useful in treating severe hemolytic anemia.

Several groups[668,1131,1287] reported on the use of prednisolone or methylprednisolone in the treatment of children with *M. pneumoniae* pneumonia in whom the clinical course worsened while receiving appropriate macrolide therapy. Corticosteroid treatment in these children was related to clinical and radiologic improvement. Cimolai[212] noted dramatic improvement in a 7-year-old girl treated with methylprednisolone, and in 1964 Copps[232] noted dramatic improvement in an adolescent with persistent fever, severe pneumonia, and hemolytic anemia when treated with a corticosteroid and erythromycin. Lu and accociates[722] successfully treated six cases of macrolide-resistant *M. pneumoniae* infection with ciprofloxacin and corticosteroids.

Intravenous Immunoglobulin

Intravenous immunoglobulin (IVIG) therapy has been used successfully in certain cases of severe refractory *M. pneumoniae* infection, especially when there is suspicion of an autoimmune process.[46,120,1042,1285] It is also used in cases of mycoplasma-induced Kawasaki disease. A review of 10 pediatric Stevens-Johnson syndrome cases found that IVIG given in combination with steroids produced a better outcome than IVIG alone.[12]

A 6-year-old girl with brainstem and striatal encephalitis complicating *M. pneumoniae* pneumonia experienced neurologic improvement within 48 hours of administration of IVIG.[996]

Plasmapheresis

Plasmapheresis has been used rarely to treat severe manifestations of *M. pneumoniae* disease, including transverse myelitis with psychosis,[237] autoimmune encephalitis,[1188] glomerulonephritis,[9] and severe autoimmune hemolytic anemia.[454]

General Management

Children and adolescents with *M. pneumoniae* pneumonia should be discouraged from engaging in excessive physical activity during the acute illness and for a 2-week period during convalescence because clearance, as observed by radiography, is slow and lags behind apparent clinical well-being. Older children and adolescents should be advised of their contagiousness to others; this risk period exists as long as cough persists, even with successful antibiotic therapy.

Prevention

Because of the marked and prolonged morbidity associated with *M. pneumoniae* infection, which has been particularly troublesome in the military, much effort was directed toward the development of vaccines. In 1965, Jensen and associates[548] reported encouraging initial trials with an inactivated vaccine. In that study, significant rises in *M. pneumoniae* growth-inhibiting antibody titer developed in 25 of 30 volunteers. Later challenge studies with the same vaccine indicated that nine of 10 volunteers with serum antibody were protected, but illness more severe than that in the unvaccinated control group occurred in vaccinees who did not have an antibody response after initial immunization.[1073] This altered reactivity on challenge suggested a sensitization process perhaps similar to that observed with other inactivated antigen vaccines and indicated the need for caution in further trials.[242,342] Additionally, because of the large incidence of autoantibody formation in *M. pneumoniae* infection, autoimmune sequelae could potentially be a significant adverse effect with these vaccines.[553] Other trials of inactivated vaccines in both adults and children have had varying degrees of success.[553,694,793,815,1244]

A trial with a live attenuated vaccine (i.e., a temperature-sensitive mutant) gave encouraging results.[431] However, because further study of natural *M. pneumoniae* disease indicated that reinfection occurs commonly and because sensitization may play a role in pathogenesis, proceeding slowly in conducting further vaccine trials in children seems prudent.[340]

DNA vaccines encoding a fusion of the *M. pneumoniae* P1 protein with an *Escherichia coli* toxin were recently found to confer protection in mice.[1301,1302] A recombinant protein vaccine that included conserved regions of the P1 and P30 cytoadhesins was also shown to induce protective mucosal and systemic antibodies in guinea pigs.[463]

The degree of contagion of *M. pneumoniae* is relatively low, so isolation methods should be effective in preventing spread of disease. Jensen and colleagues[549] noted that prophylactic administration of oxytetracycline to family contacts prevented disease but not infection. Azithromycin prophylaxis has been used successfully in two hospital outbreaks of *M. pneumoniae* pneumonia.[513,607] These studies indicate that in certain circumstances (in particular, high-risk subjects such as patients with sickle-cell disease and high-risk populations), prophylactic administration of antibiotics may be justified.

UREAPLASMA

Properties

Ureaplasmas (formerly T-strain mycoplasmas) are distinguished from all other members of the order *Mycoplasmatales* by their production of urease and their ability to hydrolyze urea.[909,1047,1048,1140] The morphologic characteristics of *Ureaplasma* spp. in young liquid medium culture are similar to those of other mycoplasmas. Round-ovoid elements approximately 330 nm in diameter with a range of 100 to 850 nm are found; rod-shaped and filamentous structures also occur, and the latter have a length of 2 μm and a width of 50 to 300 nm.[97,1048,1250] In clinical material, short bacillary forms with monopointed ends are common findings. Organisms are surrounded by a single trilaminar membrane approximately 10 nm thick with pilus-like structures radiating from the surface. Multiplication occurs by a simple budding process and perhaps by binary fission.

On unbuffered standard mycoplasma agar with a pH of 6.0, *Ureaplasma* spp. colonies are small (20–30 μm) and circular, with irregular borders, and grow downward into the agar.[1048] On buffered agar, *Ureaplasma* spp. colonies are bigger and often have the "fried egg" appearance of typical large colony-forming mycoplasmas.[737]

Isolation of *Ureaplasma* spp. from clinical material is assisted by the demonstration of urease activity.[345,1046,1143] In liquid medium containing urea and phenol red, growth of *Ureaplasma* spp. results in the production of ammonia, with a resultant increase in pH and a change in color. Subculture from broth to agar medium that contains urea and manganese sulfate yields dark-brown ureaplasmal colonies.

Epidemiology

The main reservoirs of human strains of *Ureaplasma* spp. are the genital tracts of adult men and women.[36,366,767-769,771,1143,1167,1215,1170] *Ureaplasma* spp. are sexually transmitted organisms that colonize the urogenital tract of women at rates of 30% to 80%.[114,306,770,1143] One study found that pregnancy was associated with a higher rate of *U. urealyticum* carriage in the cervix in contrast to rates in nonpregnant women (26% vs. 15.3%).[50] High rates of colonization have been associated with younger age, lower socioeconomic status, sexual activity with multiple partners, black ethnicity, and use of oral contraceptives, although not with HIV status.[422]

In general, cervicovaginal colonization with *Ureaplasma* spp. and *M. hominis* during pregnancy is not predictive of adverse outcomes, such as premature delivery, low-birth-weight infants, and spontaneous abortion.[160,202,316,422,1215] However, preterm labor has been associated with the altered microbial environment found in bacterial vaginosis, although there have been conflicting reports on whether genital mycoplasmas may play a role as well.[279,670] High-density genital ureaplasmal colonization has been associated with chorioamnionitis and preterm delivery.[5,562,905] It is capable of invading the upper genital tract in a subpopulation of women, as evidenced by their isolation from the endometrium,[652] placenta,[311,468,638] and amniotic fluid.[151,156,159,357,428,497,1155,1282,1283] These organisms also have immunogenic surface lipoproteins that may trigger inflammatory reactions that lead to preterm premature rupture of membranes and/or preterm labor.[456,562,655,885,929]

Ureaplasma spp. have been strongly associated with histologic chorioamnionitis, postpartum fever, and endometritis.[30,31,152,159,160,468,488,1086]

Infants become colonized during passage through the birth canal of an infected woman.[371,610,671,1120,1215] With ruptured membranes, the infant can be infected in utero.[610] *Ureaplasma* spp. have been recovered from the following sites in newborn infants: throat, nose, genitourinary tract of girls, urine of boys, external auditory canal, umbilicus, and perineum. Not all infants of infected women become colonized, and neonatal colonization tends to not persist. In one study in which *Ureaplasma* spp. were recovered from 38% of girls and 6% of boys at birth, follow-up during a 2-year period revealed a decreasing prevalence of colonization; at 2 years, none of the children had positive cultures.[367] However, in one large study of pediatric patients with chronic respiratory disease, 8.8% carried *U. parvum* and 2.8% carried *U. urealyticum* in their respiratory tract.[924]

During prepubertal childhood, *Ureaplasma* spp. are recovered only rarely from urine or genital specimens.[364,671] After puberty, colonization is a common occurrence and is primarily the result of sexual contact.[765,767,769] Colonization in adults is related directly to sexual activity. In population studies, *Ureaplasma* spp. are rarely isolated from persons with no sexual experience, but they occur in approximately 50% of men and 75% of women for whom sexual intercourse with three or more partners is reported.

Clinical Manifestations

Because ureaplasma can be recovered with considerable frequency from the throat, eyes, and genitourinary tract of babies and from the genitourinary tract of postpubertal males and females who are well, establishing cause-and-effect relationships in disease frequently has been difficult. Studies suggest the following disease associations with ureaplasma in human genitourinary and reproductive disease: good to strong association with nongonococcal urethritis, prostatitis, and urethral syndrome; moderate association with epididymitis, involuntary infertility, repeated spontaneous abortion and stillbirth, chorioamnionitis, and low birthweight; weak association with urinary calculi, pyelonephritis, Reiter disease, and pelvic inflammatory disease; and no association with Bartholin gland abscess, vaginitis, cervicitis, postabortal fever, and postpartum fever.*

Adverse Pregnancy Outcomes and Infertility

There has been much debate regarding genital mycoplasmas and whether they play a role in spontaneous abortion and premature labor, although supporting evidence is growing.[315,838,1195,1215] A study at a Cincinnati hospital that included 443 moderate-to-late preterm (32–36 weeks' gestation) births found that 9.9% of those placentas were positive for infection by culture or PCR.[1118] Not only were *Ureaplasma* spp. the most commonly isolated organisms (>68% of all isolates), but their presence was significantly associated with choriomnionitis by histology and the presence of inflammatory markers, such as G-CSF. The Alabama Preterm Birth Study in 2008[414] examined umbilical cord blood cultures for genital mycoplasmas in very preterm newborn neonates (i.e., 23–32 weeks' gestation). They found *U. urealyticum*, *M. hominis*, or both in 23% of the samples and more commonly in infants of nonwhite mothers (27.9% vs. 16.8%, $P = .016$), mothers younger than 20 years of age, those having a spontaneous rather than an indicated preterm delivery (34.7% vs. 3.2%, $P = .0001$), and those delivering at an earlier gestational age. Infants with positive cultures were more likely to have had intrauterine infection and inflammation, as shown by positive placental cultures, elevated cord blood IL-6 levels, and placental histology. Positive growth for these genital mycobacteria in cord blood also was associated with systemic inflammatory response syndrome (41.3% vs. 25.7%, $P = .007$). No significant difference between groups was found for intraventricular hemorrhage or death. Romero and Garite[979] commented on particularly significant findings from this study, including that genital mycoplasmas caused bacteremia in 1in 4 of very preterm newborns, most commonly *U. urealyticum*, although a large number (i.e., 22% of those with positive umbilical blood cultures) had simultaneous colonization with *M. hominis*. They raise the question of whether these organisms should be screened for in routine prenatal and perinatal care, and whether standard neonatal sepsis antibiotic regimens should be adjusted to cover them. Kwak and colleagues[645] found that preterm infants born to mothers with vaginal cultures positive for both *U. urealyticum* and *M. hominis* were significantly more premature, had lower birth weights, and were more likely to have histologic chorioamnionitis and require NICU admission, compared to those born to mothers infected with ureaplasma alone. By contrast, a retrospective study of 153 births with preterm (24 to 36 weeks' gestation) premature rupture of membranes found *Ureasplasma* spp. and/or *M. hominis* involvement in only 15 cases, none of which showed a significant association between bacterial load and signs of a high fetal inflammatory response.[563] Waites and associates[1217] wrote a comprehensive review of the literature trying to support a link between genital mycoplasmas and adverse outcomes. Comparisons of recent findings in prophylactic antibiotic use to forestall these outcomes, however, were inconclusive, possibly as a result of the varied methods used.

Genital mycoplasmas can invade the upper genital tract and cause inflammation; this has been proposed as a potential cause of infertility.[445,516] In addition, some *Mycoplasma* spp. can bind and affect sperm; infertility in men has been associated with these infections.[272,395,998] These topics will not be discussed further because they are outside the scope of this text's pediatric focus.

Nongonococcal Urethritis

Nongonococcal urethritis (NGU) occurs more commonly than gonococcal urethritis in men in most developed countries.[458,530,763] Approximately 40% of cases of NGU are caused by *Chlamydia trachomatis*, and 20% to 30% are the result of ureaplasma infection.[109,110,239,483,768,1015] Clinical differentiation of disease caused by *C. trachomatis* and ureaplasma has not been studied, but NGU and gonococcal urethritis have been evaluated comparatively.[453,530,671,1200]

The incubation period in NGU is relatively long, with most cases occurring 10 to 20 days after exposure, whereas with gonorrhea the period is shorter, usually less than 1 week.[453] The onset of symptoms in NGU is generally more gradual than that associated with gonorrhea. Virtually all men with gonorrhea have a urethral discharge, and most have both discharge and dysuria. In contrast, Jacobs and Kraus[530] found that only 38% of men with NGU had both dysuria and discharge. In the same study, 15% of patients with NGU had only dysuria, whereas only 2% of those with gonococcal urethritis had a similar problem. On examination, Handsfield[453] found the discharge in NGU to be purulent in 36% of his cases, nonpurulent in 9%, and of an intermediate character in the remaining 55%. In contrast, 73% of patients with gonorrhea had a purulent discharge, 27% had an intermediate discharge, and none had a nonpurulent discharge. Because of the more gradual onset and the usually less severe symptoms, patients with NGU are less prompt in seeking medical care than those with gonorrhea. Jacobs and Kraus[530] found that 76% of patients with discharge and gonococcal infection came to the clinic within 4 days of onset, whereas only 43% of patients with similar NGU visited the clinic within 4 days of disease onset. Without treatment, nongonococcal urethritis symptoms subside gradually in some patients during a 1- to 3-month period.[907]

After penicillin, ampicillin, or spectinomycin treatment of men with urethral gonorrhea, urethritis recurs (postgonococcal urethritis) in many patients.[485] Studies of postgonococcal urethritis indicate an etiologic role for *C. trachomatis*; genital mycoplasmas are probably responsible for some cases,[908] especially as persistent urethritis after doxycycline treatment also has been reported.[1252]

A 7.5-year-old sexually inactive boy with recurrent urethritis associated with *U. urealyticum* infection has been described.[1039]

Other Infections

Ureaplasma has also been associated with postoperative mediastinitis in adults.[390,396,451] It was recovered from the synovial fluid of a 21-year-old woman on immunosuppression for juvenile idiopathic arthritis who developed a genitourinary infection, soft tissue abscesses, and septic arthritis of the knee and hip.[397]

Disease in the Neonate

Transmission. Vertical transmission of *Ureaplasma* spp. and *M. hominis* from a colonized mother to her newborn occurs in utero or during

*References 130, 156, 161, 311, 639, 648, 774, 1100, 1110, 1143, 1159, 1171.

delivery.[7,16,424,1001,1215] The relative frequency of occurrence at each time point is not fully known. Acquisition of mycoplasmas by newborns can occur at the time of delivery through contact with a colonized birth canal, but they also have been found on the mucosal surfaces of newborns delivered by cesarean section performed before the onset of labor and rupture of amniotic membranes.[1003,1120] In utero transmission occurs either transplacentally by the hematogenous route or via an ascending intrauterine infection from a colonized maternal genital tract. Mycoplasmas have been isolated from maternal blood at the time of delivery and from umbilical cord blood, amniotic fluid, endometrium, chorioamnion, placenta, and aborted fetal tissue. Specific IgM antibody responses have been detected in neonatal serum. Postpartum or nosocomial transmission probably occurs, but definitive proof is lacking. The idea was suggested by the finding of ureaplasmal colonization in infants at 3 to 4 weeks of age who were not previously shown to be colonized with *Ureaplasma* spp. while in a neonatal intensive care unit (NICU).[1003]

The rate of vertical transmission of *Ureaplasma* spp. ranges from 0.9% to 55% in full-term infants and 8.5% to 58% in preterm infants, depending on the number and type of mucosal surfaces sampled.[16,208,890,1001–1003,1120] *M. hominis* has been isolated from the nasopharyngeal aspirates and gastric secretions of 30% to 42%[208,209] and 8%,[424] respectively, of infants born to colonized mothers. The rate of vertical transmission of *Ureaplasma* spp. is not affected by the method of delivery or the duration of time after rupture of membranes. Vertical transmission is increased significantly in the presence of chorioamnionitis and intraamniotic infection.[276,1058] Colonization of newborn infants increases with decreasing gestational age and birthweight[10] and is highest in infants weighing less than 1000 g at birth.[1003] Female newborns are more likely than males to be colonized with ureaplasma because the vagina is a common site of colonization.[366,1002]

Colonization with ureaplasma persists through early infancy; 68%, 33%, and 37%% of full-term newborns colonized in the throat, eye, and vagina, respectively, are still colonized at 3 months of age.[940,1120] However, most of them lose colonization by the time they reach 2 years of age.[315,366] Among preterm infants, 65% remain colonized at the time of discharge from the NICU or at 28 days of life.[1003] Overall, the prevalence of ureaplasmal colonization varies from 2% to 86% among infants admitted to NICUs, and as many as 14% to 41% of infants have endotracheal aspirate cultures positive for *Ureaplasma* spp.[257,296,469,525,900,1001]

Clinical Manifestations

The role of *Ureaplasma* spp. in neonatal disease continues to be investigated and defined. *M. hominis* and *Ureaplasma* spp. have been recovered from the lungs, brain, heart, and viscera of aborted fetuses and stillborn infants, with histologic findings of bronchopneumonia present in the lungs.[734,1123] *Ureaplasma* spp. were isolated from blood in as many as 34% of infants younger than 34 weeks' gestational age.[899] *Ureaplasma* spp. were isolated from blood in as many as 34% of infants younger than 34 weeks' gestational age. Twenty-six percent of preterm infants had positive endotracheal aspirate cultures for *Ureaplasma* spp. in one study.[158] Genital mycoplasmas also have been isolated from the blood, urine, CSF, and lung tissue of infants with clinical signs of infection. These organisms frequently colonize the mucosal surfaces of newborns,[610,1002] and ascribing disease often is difficult. However, isolation from normally sterile body fluids in symptomatic infants has led to the recognition that these organisms are neonatal pathogens.

Chorioamnionitis

In a study of 249 puerperal women and their babies, Shurin and colleagues[1058] noted on histologic examination of the placentas that *Ureaplasma* spp. were recovered from 37.5% of babies whose placentas showed chorioamnionitis and from only 19% of those with normal placentas. In this study, no adverse effects could be attributed to either the placental lesions or colonization of the babies. Another group found that *U. urealyticum* and *M. hominis* in the umbilical cord was associated with funisitis, but the presence of these organisms in the placenta, tracheal aspirate, or gastric fluid of preterm infants did not show a significant difference in the presence of chorioamnionitis in the mother or chronic lung disease in the baby.[304] Caspi and associates[151] reported a 32-year-old woman with amnionitis in whom ureaplasma was recovered from blood. After delivery, the same organism was recovered from the blood of one of the twin infants.

Pneumonia

Fatal neonatal pneumonia in a term infant was documented by isolation of ureaplasma from lung tissue at autopsy, with demonstrated elevated serum IgG and IgM titers to the organism.[954] Afebrile pneumonitis was reported in infants younger than 3 months of age.[1094] Pneumonia and persistent pulmonary hypertension were documented in three infants from whom *Ureaplasma* spp. were isolated from blood, endotracheal aspirates, pleural fluid, or lung tissue (or any combination of these sites) at autopsy.[1211] Cultrera and colleagues[248] reported finding an association between colonization of the lower respiratory tract by *Ureaplasma* spp., particularly by *U. parvum* in preterm newborns, and respiratory distress syndrome. The potential role of ureaplasma in neonatal pneumonia[131,386,408,913] has been strengthened by demonstration of histologic evidence of pneumonia in the lungs of newborn mice and premature baboons; ureaplasmal isolates were obtained from the pleural fluid, lung biopsy specimens, and lung tissue of these experimental pneumonia models.[157,986,1220] Crouse and associates[243] demonstrated that pneumonia is produced in newborn mice, but significantly less often in mice older than 14 days, and is potentiated by oxygen therapy. *Ureaplasma* spp. have been shown to induce ciliostasis and mucosal lesions in human fetal tracheal organ cultures.[157] In addition, ureaplasma can induce the production of alveolar macrophage proinflammatory cytokines in vitro,[687] and both *Ureaplasma* spp. and *M. hominis* stimulate the production of tumor necrosis factor-α and inducible nitric oxide synthase from murine macrophages.[244] Viscardi and colleagues[1197] developed the first juvenile mouse model of ureaplasma pneumonia. Their data suggest that *Ureaplasma* alone may cause limited inflammation and minimal tissue injury in the early phase of infection but may promote a mild chronic inflammatory response in the later phase of infection (days 14–28), similar to the process that occurs in human newborns.

Chronic Lung Disease

Isolation of *Ureaplasma* spp. from endotracheal secretions, the nasopharynx, the throat, or gastric aspirates (or any combination of these sites) has been associated with chronic lung disease of prematurity. Development of chronic lung disease was described in low-birthweight infants whose respiratory tracts were colonized with *Ureaplasma* spp. in the first week of life.*

The results from a meta-analysis performed by Wang and colleagues[1229] involving 17 publications supported a significant association between ureaplasmal colonization and the subsequent development of chronic lung disease. Crouse and associates[245] noted that infants who weighed 1250 g or less at birth, had respiratory tract disease, and were colonized with *Ureaplasma* spp. in their tracheal secretions were more likely to have radiographic evidence of more severe pulmonary disease than were infants who were not colonized. Similar findings were made by Honma and coworkers,[488] who noted that infants younger than 32 weeks' gestational age with elevated white blood cell counts and *U. urealyticum* colonization were more likely to develop infection-related chronic lung disease. These findings were not supported by studies by Cordero and colleagues,[234] who did not detect any specific radiographic abnormalities in 183 infants with a birthweight of 1250 g or less and who had endotracheal colonization with *Ureaplasma* spp., gram-negative cocci, or gram-negative bacilli. However, Ollikainen and associates[896] found that preterm infants colonized with *Ureaplasma* spp. had higher leukocyte counts on the first 2 days of life and that they required high-frequency oscillatory ventilation more often than those not colonized. In addition, the isolation by Walsh and colleagues[1221] of *Ureaplasma* spp. from the lungs of infants with chronic lung disease implies an invasive bacterial process as part of the pathogenesis of lung injury. In a retrospective study of 60 ventilated babies born at less than 30 weeks' gestation, 25 of whom were ureaplasma culture–positive, Theilen and associates[1152] found that the ventilated babies with ureaplasma in their tracheal

*References 3, 15, 17, 34, 57, 68, 109, 128, 140, 150, 156, 161, 180, 220, 222, 223, 235, 254, 301, 309, 488, 630, 927.

secretions had a clinical and radiologic course different from that of the infants who were culture negative. Specifically, they had less acute lung disease but an earlier onset of chronic lung disease.

In contrast to these studies, Heggie and colleagues,[469] Da Silva and associates,[257] and Couroucli and colleagues[241] found no association between ureaplasma and the development of bronchopulmonary dysplasia (BPD). Bowman and colleagues[111] used erythromycin to treat extremely-low-birthweight infants colonized with ureaplasma and found no association between the initial colonization and the development of chronic lung disease. They also called attention to the fact that in the study by Heggie and coworkers,[469] a substantial proportion of the colonized infants were treated with erythromycin, which might explain the lack of an association between colonization and subsequent chronic lung disease. In 1997, van Waarde and associates[1187] noted that preterm infants who were at the highest risk for the development of chronic lung disease (i.e., those with the lowest gestational age and birthweight) also were the ones most likely to be colonized with *Ureaplasma* spp. Castro-Alcaraz and coworkers[162] found that a persistently positive colonization pattern, which accounted for 45% of the ureaplasma-positive infants, was associated with a significantly increased risk for the development of chronic lung disease.

One theory suggests that ureaplasma is not the primary cause of BPD but might be the cause of undetected pneumonia.[155] This pneumonia results in an increased requirement for supplemental oxygen, and BPD is the result of oxygen toxicity caused by the supplemental oxygen therapy. Viscardi and associates,[1196] using the preterm baboon model, suggested that a prolonged proinflammatory response initiated by intrauterine ureaplasma infection contributed to the early development of fibrosis and altered developmental signaling in the immature lung.

The possibility that ureaplasmal colonization of the respiratory tract induces an inflammatory response without direct pulmonary invasion and infection cannot be excluded.[438,729] It has been supported by the finding of elevated levels of tumor necrosis factor-α, IL-6, IL-8, and monocyte chemoattractant protein–1 in the tracheal secretions of colonized infants,[54,157,439,743,1101] as well as by elevated white blood cell counts and eosinophilia in infants whose respiratory tract is colonized by *Ureaplasma* spp.[892,896,916] The contribution of *U. urealyticum* and *U. parvum* was evaluated by Heggie and colleagues.[469] Both species colonized preterm infants with a birthweight of less than 1500 g; however, no association was seen between endotracheal colonization with either species and the development of chronic lung disease. In a study performed by Katz and colleagues,[577] *U. parvum* was detected more often than *U. urealyticum*, but the researchers found no significant difference or trend in the prevalence of either species between infants with or without BPD. Similarly, the Alabama Preterm Birth Study showed no association between ureaplasma infection and respiratory distress syndrome (RDS).[414] However, Cultrera and associates[248] did find a strong association in preterm infants of RDS development and colonization, especially with *U. parvum*.

In a meta-analysis, Schelonka and colleagues[1019] reviewed 36 articles in which cohorts of neonates were screened for the presence of ureaplasma by culture with or without PCR and monitored prospectively for the development of BPD. They concluded that colonization with ureaplasma was associated with higher reported rates of BPD. However, the greatest reported effect was seen in the small studies, and, therefore, reporting bias may be partially responsible for the higher rates of BPD in colonized infants. The Alabama study could also find no significant association with BPD when adjusted for maternal race, infant gestational age, and gender.[414]

Central Nervous System Infections

Both *Ureaplasma* spp. and *M. hominis* have been isolated from the CSF of both full-term and preterm infants.* The repeated isolation of these organisms from the CSF of predominantly preterm infants with suspected meningitis and their association with a CSF pleocytosis consisting of polymorphonuclear or mononuclear cells, hypoglycorrhachia, and elevated protein content support their role in causing neonatal meningitis. Waites and colleagues[1216] noted hemiplegia, hydrocephalus, and developmental delay in survivors. Glaser and associates[410] report the case of a 26-week-gestation infant born to a mother who underwent cerclage. The baby had progressive hydrocephalus and meningitis for over 200 days before diagnostic tests for mycoplasma were performed, which were positive for *U. parvum* by CSF culture and PCR.

Isolation of *Ureaplasma* spp. from the CSF of preterm infants also has been associated with severe intraventricular hemorrhage.[4,898,1216] However, Likitnukul and associates[692] cultured the CSF and blood of 203 infants with suspected sepsis and failed to isolate *Ureaplasma* spp. Primarily in full-term infants, isolation of *Ureaplasma* spp. and *M. hominis* often has been associated with minimal if any CSF abnormalities, and these infants have done well without receiving specific antimicrobial therapy.[470,862,1019,1180,1213] In such instances, the presence of these organisms remains of unclear clinical significance, and their role in producing disease is questionable.

Other Infections

Nonimmune hydrops fetalis was reported in a newborn at 32 weeks' gestation in whom *U. urealyticum* was isolated from bronchial secretions and lung and brain tissue at autopsy.[897] Osteomyelitis of the femur was associated with isolation of ureaplasma from the blood of a preterm infant.[407] Ureaplasma was recovered from a scalp abscess at the site of an internal fetal electrode monitor.[452]

Differential Diagnosis

In clinical practice, the most important differential consideration is between gonococcal infection and nongonococcal urethritis. Although the symptoms of the two illnesses are frequently different, sufficient overlap exists to render arriving at a specific diagnosis without laboratory aid hazardous. Microscopic examination of a urethral specimen is essential. In most instances, the observation of gram-negative cell-associated diplococci on Gram stain is sufficient for a diagnosis of *Neisseria gonorrhoeae* infection. When smears reveal polymorphonuclear neutrophils without organisms suggestive of gonococci, a specific bacterial culture should be performed. Because infection with multiple agents occurs commonly and postgonococcal urethritis is a frequent problem, thorough investigation of initial illnesses in adolescents with cultures for bacteria, chlamydia, and ureaplasma is advised.

Because of the frequent colonization of newborn infants with mycoplasmas, an etiologic role for these agents cannot be supported by detection of organisms on mucosal surfaces only. However, isolation from normally sterile sites would support further workup and possibly treatment.

MYCOPLASMA HOMINIS

Properties

Three basic morphologic forms of *M. hominis* have been observed by phase-contrast microscopy: coccoidal cells 30 to 80 nm in diameter, diploforms and filamentous forms with a thickness of 30 to 40 nm, and forms with variable lengths reaching 40 μm or more.[103,117,119,277] Bredt[118] studied newly isolated strains and noted that coccoid forms and ring- or disk-shaped cells were predominant; with some strains, filamentous forms of variable length also were noted. Multiplication occurs by binary fission, by fragmentation of filaments and rings, and by budding.[103,973]

Anderson and Barile[29] studied the ultrastructure of *M. hominis* and noted considerable variability in internal components. In some cells, ribosome-like granules in the cytoplasm and a more central area of net-like strands were present, suggestive of a nucleus. Other cells had only irregular densities within the cytoplasm. In some instances, dense cytoplasmic bodies were observed; in other cells, vacuoles were seen.

On mycoplasma agar, *M. hominis* colonies are approximately 200 to 300 μm in diameter and have the typical mycoplasmal "fried egg" appearance.[1143] *M. hominis* grows on ordinary blood agar and produces pinpoint nonhemolytic colonies. It metabolizes arginine to ammonia, so that arginine-supplemented liquid medium with a pH indicator (phenol red) can be used for primary isolation. *M. hominis* can be identified specifically and differentiated from other human mycoplasmas that metabolize arginine by growth inhibition by specific antibody.

*References 25, 135, 392, 403, 462, 479, 605, 750, 775, 862, 1038, 1059, 1095, 1180, 1213, 1216.

Multiple membrane proteins that mediate the adhesion of *M. hominis* to cells of the urogenital tract and to trichomonas have been identified.[475,489] Attachment is to sulfated glycolipids of the host cells.[901]

Epidemiology

M. hominis colonizes the urogenital tracts of sexually active adults,[371,765,767,769–771,1143,1215] with the rate of carriage in women estimated to be 20% to 50%.[114,770,1143] One study that found an association between pregnancy and ureaplasma colonization noted only minimal rates of *M. hominis* carriage and no significant difference in rate in pregnancy.[50] The rest of its epidemiology follows the same characteristics as those listed for the *Ureaplasma* spp. Similarly, the simple presence of *M. hominis* in the lower genital tract during pregnancy is not predictive of adverse outcomes[147,160,316,1215] and has a controversial role in causing spontaneous abortion and preterm delivery.[315,841,1215] One study suggests that genetic differences between strains may account for the variable outcomes seen.[19] Like the *Ureaplasma* spp., it can invade the upper genital tract. *M. hominis* has been shown to be a cause of pelvic inflammatory disease, postpartum septicemia, and endometritis,[157,586,772,866,936] and it has been associated with surgical wound infection after cesarean delivery.[624,731,972] It can be recovered from the oral cavity of 1% to 5% of normal adults.[1085] In one large study, it was found in the respiratory tract of 4.7% of pediatric patients with chronic respiratory tract disease.[924]

M. hominis has been identified inside *Trichomonas vaginalis*, where it is believed to play a symbiotic role.[271,824] *T. vaginalis* strains harboring *M. hominis* were found to have increased virulence behavior.[1182] Conflicting reports exist of metronidazole resistance being conferred by *M. hominis*.[137,253,1267] An unrelated, novel mycoplasma species isolated almost exclusively from women with *T. vaginalis* infection has also been described.[344]

Clinical Manifestations

Studies suggest the following disease associations with *M. hominis* in human genitourinary and reproductive diseases: good to strong association with pyelonephritis, pelvic inflammatory disease, postabortal fever, and postpartum fever; moderate association with prostatitis, vaginitis, and cervicitis; weak association with Bartholin's gland abscess and involuntary infertility[395,601]; and no association with nongonococcal urethritis, epididymitis, urinary calculi, Reiter disease, urethral syndrome, repeated spontaneous abortion and stillbirth, or chorioamnionitis.* With the exception of pelvic inflammatory disease and complications of pregnancy, which occur in adolescents, the other disease associations reported do not involve pediatric patients.

M. hominis has been recovered on two occasions from the CSF of a 2.5-year-old girl with a ventriculoperitoneal shunt.[1212] Because she had no complications from the infection and only minimal CSF inflammation, no treatment was initiated. Three months later, the organism could not be isolated from CSF and the child was doing well.

In volunteer studies in adults, researchers found that *M. hominis* could produce exudative pharyngitis.[173] Moffet and associates[814] isolated *M. hominis* from the throat of 1 of 174 infants and children with pharyngitis but made no similar isolation from a control group of children without pharyngitis. Neu and Ellner[867] recovered *M. hominis* from the throat of 1 child in a group of 56 with exudative pharyngitis. Other *M. hominis* infections include septicemia in a 10-month-old burned infant,[255] chronic multifocal osteomyelitis in an 8-year-old child,[511] arthritis and vulvitis in a 4-year-old girl and 13-year old girl,[43] septicemia after heart surgery in a 5-year-old girl,[254] severe pneumonia and pericarditis in a healthy 15-year-old girl,[923] and exudative vaginitis in a 10-year-old girl.[1207] In one study, 10 patients with sickle-cell disease were found to have acute chest syndrome in association with *M. hominis* recovery from sputum or bronchoscopy specimens.[868] A 4-year-old girl was found to have *M. hominis* endocarditis after biventricular repair of her congenital heart defect.[238] Surgical wound infections, including to the brain and spine, have been due to *M. hominis*.[634,972,1251]

In adult patients, the following clinical manifestations have been caused by *M. hominis*: rheumatoid arthritis[44]; mediastinitis[390,673,761,842]; endocarditis[335,382,500,512,535,981]; isolated pericarditis in a lung transplant recipient[679]; hyperammonemia believed to be directly generated by *M. hominis*, resulting in fatal encephalopathy and sepsis in a lung transplant recipient[1264]; pneumonia in a previously healthy man[995]; ICU-acquired infection in seven critically ill men[388]; soft tissue, cavity, spine, and meningeal infections at surgical sites[142,354,498,624,672,805,1271]; parapharyngeal abscess after EBV infection[587]; brain abscess[21,473,501,641,642,914,1298]; and bacteremia in a patient with multiple injuries.[441]

*References 101, 130, 156, 310, 311, 400, 442, 646, 911, 912, 983, 1052, 1100, 1143, 1170, 1171.

Disease in the Neonate

Infants become colonized during passage through the birth canal, but such colonization tends to not persist. In a recent study of 208 women at delivery, *M. hominis* was recovered from cervicovaginal specimens in 11% and the gastric secretions of 1% of newborns.[424] In prepubertal children, *M. hominis* only rarely is recovered from urine or genital specimens.

M. hominis also has been associated with neonatal pneumonia,[1178] septicemia,[157] and meningitis in premature infants.[468,1241] The Analyses of the Extremely Low Gestational Age Newborns study showed that infants born at less than 28 weeks' gestation with *M. hominis* recovered from the placenta were at an increased risk (odds ratio [OR], 2.5; 95% confidence interval [95% CI], 1.2–5.3) of later developing, emotional and behavioral dysregulation[376] or attention deficit/hyperactivity problems (adjusted relative risk [RR], 2.3; 95% CI, 1.1–4.8).[289] A review by Hata and colleagues[462] associated poor outcomes with delayed or infective initial therapy of *M. hominis* meningitis and presented a case in a premature infant that was successfully treated with moxifloxacin, promoting fourth-generation fluoroquinolones as an alternative treatment. A case was found of an infant sustaining birth-related eye injury who subsequently developed multiple subdural empyemas caused by *M. hominis*.[203] Other systemic presentations include brain and scalp abscesses, ventriculitis, submandibular adenitis, abscesses of subcutaneous tissue, pericarditis, and conjunctivitis.[1,409,558,802,944,993]

Differential Diagnosis

Illness caused by *M. hominis* infection rarely occurs in children. This organism should be considered an etiologic possibility in wound infections and a variety of illnesses in which routine cultures are negative. The possibility of *M. hominis* as an etiologic agent also should be considered in adolescent girls with urethritis or pelvic inflammatory disease.

MYCOPLASMA GENITALIUM

Properties

A thorough review by Taylor-Robinson and Jensen[1142] summarizes the recent characterization of *M. genitalium*. It is a pleomorphic organism most often found with a tapered end, giving it a flask or bottle shape. It has a length of 0.6 to 0.7 µm and a diameter of 0.3 to 0.4 µm at the broadest part and 0.06 to 0.07 µm at the tip. As in other mycoplasmas, the terminal rod-like structure is believed to play a role in motility, cytoadherence, and binary fission.

Colonies have the typical "fried egg" morphology on solid media. Growth is suppressed on *Mycoplasma* media containing thallous acetate, which is normally used to prevent bacterial contamination. In media containing phenol red and glucose, *M. genitalium* metabolism can be detected by a color change from red to yellow. *M. genitalium* does not metabolize arginine or urea.

M. pneumoniae is closely related to *M. genitalium* and is believed to contain all of the latter's open reading frames within its genome.[478] Because of similarities in their antigens, cross-reactivity between the two can occur in serologic testing. The genome of *M. genitalium* (580 kb) is much smaller, however, which necessitates efficiency. Rather than encode gene regulators, it is believed to rely on DNA supercoiling,[284] antisense RNA,[710] and environmental signals, such as osmotic stress[1292] and temperature,[839] to modify transcription. It is also able to produce unlimited variants of its genes through homologous recombination within its own genome and through gene exchange between different clones.[134,524,730]

Epidemiology

Over recent years, *M. genitalium* has become recognized as an STI that causes NGU in men and is strongly implicated in several inflammatory reproductive tract syndromes in women. A comprehensive review of the literature by McGowin and associates[780] found a worldwide incidence of 7.3% and 2.0%, in high- and low-risk female populations, respectively. Rates of infection are not associated with ethnicity, gender, isolation site, or previous pregnancies in women[659,982] but have occasionally been shown to be associated with younger age, thought to be related to sexual promiscuity and risky behavior.[555,813] *M. genitalium* infection was shown to be significantly reduced in circumcised versus uncircumcised men (8.2% and 13.4%, respectively).[788] Studies in the adult general population abroad have shown an asymptomatic carrier rate of 0.3% in Korea,[601] 0.6% in the United Kingdom,[982] and 1% in Japan,[1127] whereas in a study by the University of Illinois, investigators reported that of the 52 male patients with *M. genitalium* in their patient population in Kenya (9.9% prevalence), all but one were asymptomatic.[788]

In addition, multiple studies have shown elevated coinfection rates of *M. genitalium* with HIV.[394,555,762,854] It is unclear whether this relationship is pathologically significant or merely represents the elevated risk for multiple infections in people with high-risk sexual activity.[738,1142] Reports are conflicting about whether infection with *M. genitalium* is associated with increased vaginal HIV shedding.[394,742,780,853] A prospective study of women found that those positive for *M. genitalium* infection at that visit were 2-fold more likely to test positive for HIV at the next visit.[762] It has been proposed that inflammation caused by a high *M. genitalium* load may weaken defensive barriers and attract CD4 T cells to the area, facilitating HIV transmission.[256,267,779,781] In a study of Kenyan women, those with a high but not low burden of *M. genitalium* were more commonly found to have HIV shedding.[742]

The organism also has been recovered from the respiratory tract of patients with pneumonia who were participating in an *M. pneumoniae* vaccine trial.[64] Patel and colleagues[924] found that 9.1% of broncheoalveolar lavage fluid samples taken from a large pediatric population with chronic respiratory disease were PCR positive for *M. genitalium*.

Clinical Manifestations

As cases are often asymptomatic, the role of *M. genitalium* as a sexually transmitted pathogen was initially unclear and required careful characterization, including studies of disease in experimentally infected chimpanzees.[1141,1167,1171] With the use of PCR, Jensen and associates[547] presented evidence suggesting a causative role in some cases of NGU. *M. genitalium* is now generally accepted as an emerging STI[740] and a cause of mucopurulent cervicitis in women[267,739] and NGU in men.[790] Recent studies estimate that it is the most common etiology of NGU after *C. trachomatis*, responsible for 10% to 30% of the cases.[818] In addition, *M. genitalium* infection has been strongly associated with endometritis, pelvic inflammatory disease, preterm birth and spontaneous abortion, and infertility in both men and women.[95,395,447,703,741,778]

M. genitalium has been recovered from pediatric patients with pneumonia and chronic respiratory disease.[64,924] Respiratory colonization has been shown to occur during neonatal passage though the birth canal for other mycoplasmas. Hematogenous spread of *M. genitalium* is also possible and has been postulated as the mechanism for cases of arthritis with this organism.[1142,1168] A 29-year-old man with a lesion on the glans penis was PCR positive for *M. genitalium* and negative for *N. gonorrhea*, and developed symptomatic urethritis with discharge, inguinal lymphadenopathy, perianal intertrigo, aphthous lesions on the oral mucosa, and oligoarthritis in both ankles and the right elbow.[205]

Differential Diagnosis

M. genitalium presents most commonly as an STI causing pathology in the lower genital tracts of both men and women and a possible role in upper tract inflammation. It should be considered in the workup of adolescents with urethritis or pelvic inflammatory disease.

MYCOPLASMA FERMENTANS

M. fermentans originally was isolated from the genital tract of men and women over 50 years ago, but it has not been well established as a cause of genitourinary disease.[989,1138,1167] Horie and colleagues did describe three cases of nonsexually acquired genital ulcers (Lipschütz ulcers) in young women with positive serology for *M. fermentans*, indicating recent infection.[490] Although it has been identified by PCR in the peripheral blood mononuclear cells and lymph nodes of HIV-infected patients[465,576,631,1010] and was initially suspected as a cofactor in the development of AIDS,[1215] it was also detected in the blood of homosexual men without HIV infection.[576,631,733] In addition, it has been isolated from the respiratory tract, bone marrow, synovial fluid, and urine of healthy and immunocompromised patients.[65,99,713,751,820,836,1215,1238,1253] Its membrane surface carries highly immunogenic proteins and phosphoglycolipids[985] which could trigger inflammatory arthritic diseases, including rheumatoid arthritis.[402,554,1083] A lipid-associated membrane protein from *M. fermentans* named macrophage-activating lipopeptide-2 (MALP-2) was found to be an extremely potent natural macrophage stimulator, comparable to LPS.[383,832]

MYCOPLASMA PENETRANS

M. penetrans is a relatively newly recognized species originally isolated from the urogenital tract of patients with AIDS.[711,712] In a seroprevalence study, Wang and associates[1230] found that 35.4% of HIV-infected patients had antibody to *M. penetrans* versus only 0.4% of HIV-seronegative subjects. They subsequently noted a high prevalence of antibody to *M. penetrans* in the sera of homosexual men but not in the sera of other HIV transmission groups.[1231] In a more recent study, Grau and colleagues[426] found that 18.2% of HIV-infected patients had antibody to *M. penetrans*, whereas only 1.3% of HIV-seronegative persons had antibody. *M. penetrans* antibody seroprevalence increased with progression of HIV-associated disease, and it was associated predominantly with homosexual practices in the HIV-infected patients. No pediatric data relating to *M. penetrans* seroprevalence are available.

DIAGNOSIS OF GENITAL MYCOPLASMAS

M. hominis, *U. urealyticum*, and *U. parvum* are ubiquitous in the genital tracts of normal persons and frequent colonizers of mucosal surfaces in infants; therefore, assigning causation of disease based on isolation is difficult. *M. genitalium* is now widely recognized as an STI, and culture or PCR for mycoplasmas is warranted in cases of urethritis when smears reveal polymorphonuclear neutrophils without organisms suggestive of gonococci. Isolation of these species from a normally sterile site or suppurative focus warrants further investigation, especially in newborns and others with weakened immune systems. The clinical significance of isolation of genital mycoplasmas from urine obtained by suprapubic bladder aspiration in infants remains to be determined.[692] In such instances, analysis of urinary sediment has been normal.

Because of their fastidious growth, these species cannot be identified by routine bacteriologic culture methods; therefore, specific culture for mycoplasma must be requested. Genital mycoplasmas may be isolated on special broth and solid media that are available commercially. Shepard 10B broth and A8 agar have been used successfully for cultivation.[157] A recent study comparing different culture specimens found that urethral swabs were more accurate (specificity, 99.9%; positive predictive value [PPV], 99.6%) than vaginal swabs (specificity 95.1%; PPV, 67%) or urine cultures (specificity, 96%; PPV, 75%) for detecting *M. hominis* in women with lower urinary tract symptoms, with similar numbers for *U. urealyticum*.[510]

Cassell and colleagues[153,157] recommended that mucosal specimens be obtained with a Dacron or calcium alginate swab and be placed in a specific mycoplasmal transport medium, such as Shepard 10B broth. Specimens should be refrigerated at 4°C (39.2°F) until they are transported to the laboratory and should be protected from drying. Alternatively, specimens in appropriate transport media can be frozen at −70°C (−94°F) because mycoplasmas are stable for long periods under these conditions. Specimens should be diluted serially in 10B broth to at least 10^{-3} (preferably to 10^{-5}) to overcome any potential inhibitory substances or metabolites, and an aliquot of the original sample and dilution should be plated directly onto A8 agar. Body fluids (e.g., blood, CSF, and pleural fluid) should be inoculated into 10B broth in an approximate 1:10 ratio (usually 0.1 mL fluid/0.9 mL 10B broth). Blood should be collected free of anticoagulants. Broth cultures and agar plates are incubated under 95% nitrogen and 5% carbon dioxide. Cultures generally become positive within 2 to 5 days. The presence of mycoplasmal growth in 10B medium is indicated by a change in color from yellow to pink, which is caused by an alkaline shift in the media as a result of either the urease activity of ureaplasmas or arginine hydrolysis by other *Mycoplasma* spp. Growth of mycoplasmas in broth culture, as indicated by a change in color, should be confirmed by inoculation of a broth specimen onto A8 agar. Characteristic colonies can be identified readily on A8 agar after 24 to 72 hours of incubation.

Serologic tests have been used to measure antibody to genital mycoplasmas. Such tests include the metabolic inhibition assay, enzyme-linked immunosorbent assay, mycoplasmacidal test, indirect hemagglutination, indirect immunofluorescence, and IgG and IgM immunoblotting.[157,275,384,955] Because of the presence of maternal antibodies, as well as their own poorly functional immune system, use of these tests for establishing the diagnosis of mycoplasmal infection in infants remains problematic and is not well established. In these cases, diagnosis should rely on culture results and/or NAAT tests (PCR or transcription-mediated amplification).

PCR assays have become commercially available over recent years for detecting genital mycoplasmas.[98,974,1105,1284] Comparison studies show that PCR is a more rapid and sensitive method of detection for genital mycoplasmas than culture. On endotracheal secretions, Blanchard and associates[98] reported finding a sensitivity of 100% and a specificity of 99% for *Ureaplasma* spp.

PCR assays involving the urease gene, 16S RNA genes, and multiple-banded antigen genes have been used to detect *Ureaplasma* spp.* PCR detection of 16S rRNA and ribosomal DNA targets of *M. hominis*[6,425,724] and the 23S rRNA[543] and 16S rRNA[807] from *M. genitalium* are available in certain large medical centers and commercial laboratories, although they are not yet approved by the Food and Drug Administration (FDA) in the United States. Assays also exist that can screen for multiple *Mycoplasma*-related species simultaneously, using fluorescence polarization,[60] PCR-RFLPs,[807] multiplex PCR[783-785,1000] and oligonucleotide microarrays.[536] Ultimately, these methods may aid in identifying colonized or infected infants more readily (results available in 1 day) and reliably, given the fastidious nature of these organisms and the scarcity of microbiology laboratories that routinely perform mycoplasmal culture.

OTHER *MYCOPLASMA* SPECIES AND *MYCOPLASMA* RELATIONSHIPS

Mycoplasma salivarium

M. salivarium is part of the normal human oral flora. It contains a very potent macrophage- and fibroblast-stimulating lipoprotein that can induce inflammatory reactions in gingival cells[895,1112] and has been thought to occasionally play a role in oral and periodontal infections[1237]; however, it has rarely been associated with disease in other sites of the body. Examples include arthritic joints, such as the knee of a 39-year-old-woman with hypogammaglobulinemia,[1079] the knees of rheumatoid arthritis patients,[554] the synovial fluid of patients (including a 15-year-old girl and 16-year-old girl) with temporomandibular joint disorders,[1238] a submasseteric abscess in an 84-year-old woman,[436] and an empyema in a 39-year-old man with laryngeal cancer.[61] The organism was also found in the polymicrobial biofilm of an occluded biliary stent in a 71-year-old man with liver cirrhosis.[476]

Mycoplasma pirum

M. pirum originally was recovered from eukaryotic cell cultures, and its origin was traced to a human tumor cell line.[15,268,661] It has been recovered more recently from primary lymphocyte cells in patients with AIDS.[99]

Zoonotic *Mycoplasma*

Mycoplasma spp. have been identified that infect a wide variety of birds, reptiles, fish, and mammals. Human infection with these species is rare but can occur when there is close contact, such as in veterinary medicine, animal training, hunting, fishing, and agriculture. There have been reports of fishermen with open hand wounds or bites catching *Mycoplasma phocacerebrale* from seals. Commonly referred to as "seal finger," this disease involves cellulitis of the affected area with eventual joint involvement if not treated.[55,538,1249] One case of seal finger with a novel mycoplasma species caused disseminated infection and septic arthritis of the hip.[1247] Hemotropic mycoplasmas (also known as "hemoplasmas") cause hemolytic anemia in many domestic and farm animals, and cases have been described of humans being infected through arthropod vectors associated with pigs, sheep, cattle, dogs, and cats.[107,285,507,1119,1236,1290] In one case, a novel hemoplasma with no identified origin was found in a 60-year-old woman.[1103] Coinfections with *Bartonella* spp. are not uncommon. Outbreaks of hemoplasmas in China have been described, including a high prevalence of congenital infection with severe disease.[507,1275]

*References 6, 7, 27, 98, 183, 202, 250, 724, 729, 865, 974, 1021, 1147, 1284.

Acquired Immunodeficiency Syndrome–Associated Mycoplasmal Infections

The frequent identification of *M. fermentans*, *M. pirum*, and *M. penetrans* infections in HIV-infected patients led to the consideration that they may function as cofactors in the progression of HIV infection and immunodeficiency.[99,496,628,820] Although these mycoplasmas have the capacity to invade cells and to be potent immunomodulators, their pathogenic role, if any, in association with HIV has not yet been determined. Studies on *U. urealyticum*, *M. hominis*, *M. salivarium*, and *M. orale* infection rates in HIV-positive and HIV-negative subjects showed no significant differences.[176,653]

Mycoplasma and *Ureaplasma* Infections in Immunocompromised Patients

Patients with hypogammaglobulinemia are susceptible to severe persistent infection with *Ureaplasma* spp., *M. hominis*, *M. amphoriforme*, *M. pneumoniae*, *M. salivarium*, and *M. orale*.[41,358,374,405,817,948,978,1079] Clinical manifestations include osteomyelitis, arthritis, cellulitis, and chronic respiratory tract illness. Patients need to be treated for prolonged periods with high-dose intravenous immunoglobulin and antibiotics to which the specific agents are susceptible. Severe and persistent infections also have occurred in liver, kidney, and bone marrow transplant recipients, as well as other immunocompromised patients.[216,534,569,728,806,933,1087,1199]

Yechouron and associates[1278] reported a 64-year-old man with Hodgkin lymphoma who died of septicemia caused by *Mycoplasma arginini*, an animal pathogen. A similar case was described by Watanabe and colleagues.[1236] Three children with cancer had pneumonia in which bronchoalveolar lavage fluid specimens yielded *U. urealyticum*.[132] Two of the patients died; the survivor's improvement coincided with erythromycin treatment. A pregnant woman with controlled congenital HIV infection and hypogammaglobulinemia secondary to lymphoma treatment developed severe pneumonia with effusions, in which pleural and lymph node samples were PCR positive for *M. hominis*.[343] *M. hominis* infection has also been reported as a cause of septic arthritis in patients with hypogammaglobulinemia,[1011,1265] septic arthritis in a 15-year-old girl 2 months after renal transplantation,[799] osteomyelitis in a patient with Good syndrome,[882] and abdominal infection in a 9-year-old boy after liver transplantation.[721]

Mycoplasma and Cancer

Mycoplasma invasion into human cells and subsequent chronic inflammatory processes have been proposed as potential mechanisms of tumorigenesis, alone or in conjunction with other oncogenic infections. Studies have attempted to link mycoplasma infections with prostate cancer, lung cancer, oral cancer, and lymphomas.[141,314,925,977,1288,1291] Charles Rosser's laboratory has been able to induce malignant transformation of human prostate cells in vitro using mycoplasma.[852] Studies have also found an increased rate of *M. hominis* infection in patients with prostate cancer.[63] Studies in women with high-grade cervical dysplasia found that a majority were also infected with *Ureaplasma* spp. with or without *M. hominis*.[306] Genital mycoplasmas have been considered an important cofactor for human papillomavirus infection.[90,307,306] Also of concern is that some commensal mycoplasma species preferentially colonize neoplastic tissues and have been found to contain enzymes capable of inactivating certain chemotherapeutic agents.[1183,1184]

Mycoplasma as a Cell Culture Contaminant

When *Mycoplasma* spp. were still first being recognized as human pathogens, they were also being studied as a prevalent and serious contaminant in the research and biopharmaceutical industries.[38] Because they are slow growing, pleomorphic, and resistant to β-lactams and other antibiotics frequently used to eliminate bacteria from cell culture media, contamination is often difficult to identify. Possible sources of mycoplasma include animal- and plant-derived raw materials in culture media and the skin from workers with poor aseptic technique. Fortunately, with better antibiotic options and rapid detection by PCR, these issues are resolving.[753,1034]

TREATMENT OF GENITAL MYCOPLASMAS

Having no cell wall, mycoplasmas are naturally resistant to β-lactam antibiotics (i.e., penicillins, cephalosporins, monobactams, and carbapenems), polymyxins, sulfonamides, and vancomycin.[113,1209,1210,1214] Although they may have moderate sensitivity to the aminoglycosides, the MICs of these agents for genital mycoplasmas usually are too high for therapeutic use. Tetracyclines and macrolides have been the drugs of choice, although because of concern for tetracycline toxicities and the comparative ease of taking a short course of azithromycin, the latter has come more into favor. Azithromycin is also seen as having the added benefit of treating both gonococcal and chlamydial genital infections when the etiology is not yet identified or could be polymicrobial. However, antibiotic resistance is growing, and some *Mycoplasma* spp. now require alternative regimens.[240] Quinolones such as moxifloxacin and levofloxacin also have good activity against genital mycoplasmas and ureaplasmas,[70,633,1126] but resistant variants have already appeared. When possible, antibiotic susceptibility testing should be performed on all clinically significant isolates. If the site of the mutation is known, high-resolution melt analysis[1160,1173] or genetic amplification and sequencing[544,1258] can be used to rapidly identify antibiotic resistance at the time of the initial diagnosis and eliminate the risk for treatment failure. These mutations can also be carried on plasmids or transposable genetic elements, sometimes conferring resistance to multiple groups of antibiotics.[543,544,633,748,931,1050,1051,1124] Mutations in the 23S rRNA gene of genital mycoplasmas, just as in *M. pneumonie*, are conferring widespread macrolide resistance. The discovery that genital mycoplasmas may also create biofilms, protecting them from antibiotic activity, further complicates therapy.[389]

Ureaplasma spp. have retained susceptibility to macrolides, doxycycline, tetracycline, and chloramphenicol. Resistance to ciprofloxacin is developing; however, oxifloxacin and moxifloxacin are still effective and better than levofloxacin.[633] Historically, tetracycline has been used for empiric coverage in cases of NGU.[453,484] However, due to adverse effects, erythromycin was considered a preferable alternative in children, and would also cover *Chlamydia* and *Ureaplasma*. Although still commonly used, erythromycin is less favored as a result of growing resistance[633] and adverse effects. Cardiac toxicity, consisting of acute cardiorespiratory deterioration possibly secondary to cardiac arrhythmias, has been reported in neonates treated with intravenous erythromycin lactobionate for presumed ureaplasmal pneumonia.[327] Ototoxicity has been seen in adults but not in neonates.[246] Oral erythromycin has also been associated with hypertrophic pyloric stenosis in infants younger than 6 weeks.[163] Doxycycline has since become a preferred choice for ureaplasmal infections, while also being effective against coinfection with *M. hominis* or gonorrhea.* First-line therapy for NGU is doxycycline 100 mg twice daily for 7 days. In cases of treatment failure due to resistant strains, 5-day therapy with azithromycin is advised.[494] Azithromycin and clarithromycin are active in vitro against *Ureaplasma* spp.,[584,991,1078,1208] but their use in neonates has not been evaluated thoroughly. When given orally to infants with very low birthweight colonized with *Ureaplasma* spp., serum levels of clarithromycin at a dose of 7.5 mg/kg every 12 hours were subtherapeutic.[1004] For this reason, a dose of 15 mg/kg every 12 hours is recommended. Although the exact duration of therapy is not known, a 10- to 14-day course seems reasonable when clinical improvement and microbiologic eradication are observed during that period.

M. hominis has developed marked resistance to common macrolides, which are no longer recommended for treatment.[991,1208] By contrast, 16-membered ring macrolides, such as josamycin and related lincosamides, have shown effectiveness against *M. hominis*. However, they have not been extensively studied and are not approved by the FDA in the United States.[584,633,931,1300] Other therapies include chloramphenicol, clindamycin, rifampicin, quinolones (i.e., ofloxacin and moxifloxacin), and tetracyclines (doxycycline especially).[70,613,1209] *M. hominis* is usually sensitive to tetracyclines; these antibiotics should be used if the benefits outweigh the risk for toxicity.[113,139,1109,1136,1248] During the past decade, resistance of *M. hominis* to tetracycline itself has increased; however, doxycycline remains effective.[249,633,766]

M. genitalium remains sensitive to macrolides and newer-generation quinolones, such as moxifloxacin.[449,1099,1126,1148] A single 1-g dose of azithromycin has been a favored choice because it also treats both gonococcal and chlamydial genital infections when the etiology is not yet identified or could be polymicrobial. However, resistance of *M. genitalium* to azithromycin is becoming more common, with rates as high as 30% to 50% in some populations.[443,872,1260] The United States and United Kingdom 2015 treatment guidelines[494,1260] recommend 5-day dosing (500-mg dose followed by four 250-mg doses) over single-dose treatment, especially as some resistance mutations have been observed to develop de novo during therapy.[28,112,204,325,443,544,658,1051] Others suggest extended regimens that include at least one dose that is 1 or 1.5 g to also ensure coverage of chlamydia, although this could reduce patient compliance.[492] Extended dosing with azithromycin has been found to be significantly more effective than even multidose doxycycline.[28,96,789] Doxycycline efficacy is only 30% to 40%, and although the mechanism for its failure has not been identified, its use has not been found to promote resistance.[493,1032,1260] Moxifloxacin (400 mg daily for 7–14 days) is highly effective in cases of azithromycin resistance, but moxifloxacin resistance is also beginning to appear.[791,1050] Although not FDA approved, sitafloxacin[266] and pristinamycin[92] have been used to treat quinolone-resistant strains abroad, and solithromycin has been shown to be highly effective in vitro.[545]

Mycoplasmas are not susceptible to the antimicrobial agents routinely used to treat neonatal infections. The decision to cover for possible mycoplasmal infection should be based on the clinical picture and culture results. In general, isolation of mycoplasmas from a normally sterile site in an ill neonate is an indication for consideration of treatment. The possibility of mycoplasma infection also should be suspected when a child appears septic and is not responding to standard antibacterial or antiviral therapy, and appropriate samples for mycoplasma culture or PCR assay should be obtained. However, no large randomized clinical trials have determined the efficacy of treatment in neonates. Experience on which to base treatment decisions, the choice of drug, and the duration of therapy is very limited.[1228]

Isolation of mycoplasmas from endotracheal secretions is not diagnostic of pneumonia, and most of these infants do not require any antimycoplasmal therapy. However, if pneumonia is suspected and the infant's clinical condition is deteriorating, a trial of therapy may be indicated despite the unknown efficacy of treatment. Azithromycin has been used for its antiinflammatory properties to protect infants from BPD. However, the safety and efficacy of azithromycin in infants with very low birthweight has not yet been studied.

PREVENTION OF GENITAL MYCOPLASMAS

Tetracyclines and fluoroquinolones are contraindicated in pregnancy; therefore, erythromycin is often used to treat mothers with genital mycoplasma infection. However, one report found that erythromycin administered between 26 and 35 weeks' gestation to pregnant women colonized with *Ureaplasma* spp. was not effective in reducing adverse outcomes, such as preterm delivery, low birthweight, or premature rupture of membranes.[316] In the ORACLE I study,[592] in which the use of broad-spectrum antibiotics was evaluated in mothers with premature rupture of membranes, use of erythromycin was associated with prolongation of pregnancy, reduction in neonatal treatment with surfactant,

*References 69, 613, 633, 759, 995, 1010, 1069, 1189, 1209, 1218, 1300.

decrease in oxygen dependence at 28 days of age and older, fewer major cerebral abnormalities on ultrasonography before discharge, and fewer positive blood cultures. The ORACLE II study, which consisted of 6295 women with spontaneous preterm labor, intact membranes, and no evidence of clinical infection, showed that none of the trial antibiotics were associated with a lower rate of the composite primary outcome events than occurred in placebo recipients.[593] Smorgick and associates[1078] reported on a woman with preterm labor at 27 weeks' gestation and amniotic colonization with *U. urealyticum*, treated with 3 days of ciprofloxacin that was changed to 7 additional days of erythromycin after developing an allergic pruritic reaction. This regimen failed to eradicate the organism, and she was switched to 10 days of intravenous clindamycin and oral levofloxacin. Although there was no further testing of amniotic fluid for infection, the patient was able to delay delivery for 6 weeks and the infant was healthy despite placental pathology revealing chorioamnionitis with acute funisitis. Vouga and coworkers[1202] performed a retrospective analysis of 5377 women who were treated with clindamycin for *M. hominis* or *Ureaplasma* spp. infections in late pregnancy and found that they had reduced rates of premature labor and had newborns with fewer respiratory complications compared to uninfected, untreated patients. Because erythromycin therapy does not eliminate *Ureaplasma* spp. from the lower genital tract, it most likely also does not prevent neonatal ureaplasmal colonization.[891] Smorgick and associates[1078] support that in cases of *Mycoplasma* spp., intraamniotic colonization remote from term, expectant management is possible and that fluoroquinolones, clindamycin, or both may be more effective than erythromycin.

The effect of erythromycin on prevention of neonatal disease has not been evaluated fully.[33] Administration of erythromycin to preterm infants whose mothers had *Ureaplasma* spp. in their lower genital tract reduced respiratory tract colonization but did not decrease the duration of supplemental oxygen therapy[559] or chronic lung disease.[111,729] Treating infants with very low birthweight who have respiratory tract colonization with *Ureaplasma* spp. to prevent chronic lung disease cannot be recommended at present.[133]

With adolescent patients who test positive for genital mycoplasma infections, it is prudent to seek out and treat the sex partners whenever possible.

NEW REFERENCES SINCE THE SEVENTH EDITION

12. Ahluwalia J, Wan J, Lee DH, et al. Mycoplasma-associated Stevens-Johnson syndrome in children: retrospective review of patients managed with or without intravenous immunoglobulin, systemic corticosteroids, or a combination of therapies. *Pediatr Dermatol.* 2014;31(6):664-669.
14. Aizawa Y, Oishi T, Tsukano S, et al. Clinical utility of loop-mediated isothermal amplification for rapid diagnosis of *Mycoplasma pneumoniae* in children. *J Med Microbiol.* 2014;63(Pt 2):248-251.
19. Allen-Daniels MJ, Serrano MG, Pflugner LP, et al. Identification of a gene in *Mycoplasma hominis* associated with preterm birth and microbial burden in intraamniotic infection. *Am J Obstet Gynecol.* 2015;212(6):779.e1-779.e13.
23. Al-Mendalawi MD. Hypertensive encephalopathy as the initial manifestation of Guillain-Barre syndrome in a 7-year-old girl. *Neurosciences.* 2013;18(3):287.
24. Almuslamani A, Mahmood F. First Bahraini adolescent with anti-NMDAR-Ab encephalitis. *Qatar Med J.* 2015;2015(1):2.
26. Al-Zaidy SA, MacGregor D, Mahant S, et al. Neurological complications of PCR-proven M. pneumoniae infections in children: prodromal illness duration may reflect pathogenetic mechanism. *Clin Infect Dis.* 2015;61(7):1092-1098.
28. Anagrius C, Lore B, Jensen JS. Treatment of *Mycoplasma genitalium*. Observations from a Swedish STD clinic. *PLoS ONE.* 2013;8(4):e61481.
35. Arca M, Bellot A, Dupont C, et al. Two uncommon extrapulmonary forms of *Mycoplasma pneumoniae* infection. *Arch Pediatr.* 2013;20(4):378-381.
37. Arkilo D, Pierce B, Ritter F, et al. Diverse seizure presentation of acute *Mycoplasma pneumoniae* encephalitis resolving with immunotherapy. *J Child Neurol.* 2014;29(4):564-566.
43. Astrauskiene D, Griskevicius A, Luksiene R, et al. *Chlamydia trachomatis, Ureaplasma urealyticum,* and *Mycoplasma hominis* in sexually intact girls with arthritides. *Scand J Rheumatol.* 2012;41(4):275-279.
44. Ataee RA, Golmohammadi R, Alishiri GH, et al. Simultaneous detection of *Mycoplasma pneumoniae, Mycoplasma hominis* and *Mycoplasma arthritidis* in synovial fluid of patients with rheumatoid arthritis by multiplex PCR. *Arch Iran Med.* 2015;18(6):345-350.
45. Atkinson TP. Is asthma an infectious disease? New evidence. *Curr Allergy Asthma Rep.* 2013;13(6):702-709.
72. Becker A, Kannan TR, Taylor AB, et al. Structure of CARDS toxin, a unique ADP-ribosylating and vacuolating cytotoxin from *Mycoplasma pneumoniae*. *Proc Natl Acad Sci USA.* 2015;112(16):5165-5170.
92. Bissessor M, Tabrizi SN, Twin J, et al. Macrolide resistance and azithromycin failure in a *Mycoplasma genitalium*-infected cohort and response of azithromycin failures to alternative antibiotic regimens. *Clin Infect Dis.* 2015;60(8):1228-1236.
105. Bohelay G, Duong TA, Ortonne N, et al. Subcorneal pustular dermatosis triggered by *Mycoplasma pneumoniae* infection: a rare clinical association. *J Eur Acad Dermatol Venereol.* 2015;29(5):1022-1025.
106. Bose S, Segovia JA, Somarajan SR, et al. ADP-ribosylation of NLRP3 by *Mycoplasma pneumoniae* CARDS toxin regulates inflammasome activity. *MBio.* 2014;5(6).
134. Burgos R, Wood GE, Young L, et al. RecA mediates MgpB and MgpC phase and antigenic variation in *Mycoplasma genitalium*, but plays a minor role in DNA repair. *Mol Microbiol.* 2012;85(4):669-683.
136. Busson L, Van den Wijngaert S, Dahma H, et al. Evaluation of 10 serological assays for diagnosing *Mycoplasma pneumoniae* infection. *Diagn Microbiol Infect Dis.* 2013;76(2):133-137.
138. Butler AM, Vijayan V, Meehan C, et al. A persistently febrile adolescent with headache and vision changes. *Pediatr Ann.* 2014;43(10):402-405.
141. Caini S, Gandini S, Dudas M, et al. Sexually transmitted infections and prostate cancer risk: a systematic review and meta-analysis. *Cancer Epidemiol.* 2014;38(4):329-338.
143. Campagna C, Tassinari D, Neri I, et al. *Mycoplasma pneumoniae*-induced recurrent Stevens-Johnson syndrome in children: a case report. *Pediatr Dermatol.* 2013;30(5):624-626.
144. Canavan TN, Mathes EF, Frieden I, et al. *Mycoplasma pneumoniae*-induced rash and mucositis as a syndrome distinct from Stevens-Johnson syndrome and erythema multiforme: a systematic review. *J Am Acad Dermatol.* 2015;72(2):239-245.
147. Capoccia R, Greub G, Baud D. *Ureaplasma urealyticum, Mycoplasma hominis* and adverse pregnancy outcomes. *Curr Opin Infect Dis.* 2013;26(3):231-240.
148. Cardinale F, Chironna M, Chinellato I, et al. Clinical relevance of *Mycoplasma pneumoniae* macrolide resistance in children. *J Clin Microbiol.* 2013;51(2):723-724.
164. Cha SI, Shin KM, Jeon KN, et al. Clinical relevance and characteristics of pleural effusion in patients with *Mycoplasma pneumoniae* pneumonia. *Scand J Infect Dis.* 2012;44(10):793-797.
166. Chang HY, Chang LY, Shao PL, et al. Comparison of real-time polymerase chain reaction and serological tests for the confirmation of *Mycoplasma pneumoniae* infection in children with clinical diagnosis of atypical pneumonia. *J Microbiol Immunol Infect.* 2014;47(2):137-144.
181. Chen X, Xu W, Du J, et al. Acute postinfectious glomerulonephritis with a large number of crescents caused by *Mycoplasma pneumoniae*. *Indian J Pathol Microbiol.* 2015;58(3):374-376.
182. Cheon MK, Na H, Han SB, et al. Pertussis accompanying recent mycoplasma infection in a 10-year-old girl. *Infect Chemother.* 2015;47(3):197-201.
198. Chiang WY, Huang HM. Bilateral monosymptomatic optic neuritis following *Mycoplasma pneumoniae* infection: a case report and literature review. *Indian J Ophthalmol.* 2014;62(6):724-727.
200. Chiu CY, Chen CJ, Wong KS, et al. Impact of bacterial and viral coinfection on mycoplasmal pneumonia in childhood community-acquired pneumonia. *J Microbiol Immunol Infect.* 2015;48(1):51-56.
205. Chrisment D, Machelart I, Wirth G, et al. Reactive arthritis associated with *Mycoplasma genitalium* urethritis. *Diagn Microbiol Infect Dis.* 2013;77(3):278-279.
210. Chung WS, Hsu WH, Lin CL, et al. *Mycoplasma pneumonia* increases the risk of acute coronary syndrome: a nationwide population-based cohort study. *QJM.* 2015;108(9):697-703.
215. Ciobanu AM, Rosca T, Vladescu CT, et al. Frontal epidural empyema (Pott's puffy tumor) associated with *Mycoplasma* and depression. *Rom J Morphol Embryol.* 2014;55(3 suppl):1203-1207.
231. Consilvio NP, Rapino D, Scaparrotta A, et al. *Mycoplasma pneumoniae* infection with rhabdomyolysis in a child. *Infez Med.* 2014;22(1):48-50.
240. Couldwell DL, Lewis DA. *Mycoplasma genitalium* infection: current treatment options, therapeutic failure, and resistance-associated mutations. *Infect Drug Resist.* 2015;8:147-161.
253. da Luz Becker D, dos Santos O, Frasson AP, et al. High rates of double-stranded RNA viruses and *Mycoplasma hominis* in *Trichomonas vaginalis* clinical isolates in South Brazil. *Infect Genet Evol.* 2015;34:181-187.
256. Das K, De la Garza G, Siwak EB, et al. *Mycoplasma genitalium* promotes epithelial crossing and peripheral blood mononuclear cell infection by HIV-1. *Int J Infect Dis.* 2014;23:31-38.
259. Dawson E, Singh D, Armstrong C, et al. Asymptomatic mycoplasma infection causing acute demyelinating encephalomyelitis: case report and review of literature. *Clin Pediatr (Phila).* 2016;55(2):185-188.
266. Deguchi T, Kikuchi M, Yasuda M, et al. Sitafloxacin: antimicrobial activity against ciprofloxacin-selected laboratory mutants of *Mycoplasma genitalium* and inhibitory activity against its DNA gyrase and topoisomerase IV. *J Infect Chemother.* 2015;21(1):74-75.

267. Dehon PM, McGowin CL. *Mycoplasma genitalium* infection is associated with microscopic signs of cervical inflammation in liquid cytology specimens. *J Clin Microbiol.* 2014;52(7):2398-2405.
270. Di Lernia V. Mycoplasma pneumoniae: an aetiological agent of acute haemorrhagic oedema of infancy. *Australas J Dermatol.* 2014;55(4):e69-e70.
270. Diaz MH, Benitez AJ, Winchell JM. Investigations of *Mycoplasma pneumoniae* infections in the United States: trends in molecular typing and macrolide resistance from 2006 to 2013. *J Clin Microbiol.* 2015;53(1):124-130.
289. Downey LC, O'Shea TM, Allred EN, et al. Antenatal and early postnatal antecedents of parent-reported attention problems at 2 years of age. *J Pediatr.* 2015;166(1):20-25.
291. Duffy MF, Walker ID, Browning GF. The immunoreactive 116 kDa surface protein of *Mycoplasma pneumoniae* is encoded in an operon. *Microbiology.* 1997;143(Pt 10):3391-3402.
293. Dumke R, Jacobs E. Evaluation of five real-time PCR assays for detection of *Mycoplasma pneumoniae. J Clin Microbiol.* 2014;52(11):4078-4081.
302. Edelstein I, Rachina S, Touati A, et al. *Mycoplasma pneumoniae* monoclonal P1 Type 2c outbreak, Russia, 2013. *Emerg Infect Dis.* 2016;22(2):348-350.
303. Edouard S, Courtois GD, Gautret P, et al. High prevalence of Mycoplasma faucium DNA in the human oropharynx. *J Clin Microbiol.* 2016;54(1):194-196.
306. Ekiel A, Pietrzak B, Wiechula B, et al. Urogenital mycoplasmas and human papilloma virus in hemodialysed women. *ScientificWorldJournal.* 2013;2013:659204.
314. Erturhan SM, Bayrak O, Pehlivan S, et al. Can mycoplasma contribute to formation of prostate cancer? *Int Urol Nephrol.* 2013;45(1):33-38.
325. Falk L, Enger M, Jensen JS. Time to eradication of *Mycoplasma genitalium* after antibiotic treatment in men and women. *J Antimicrob Chemother.* 2015;70(11):3134-3140.
343. Fernandez S, Nicolas D, Pericas JM, et al. A case of *Mycoplasma hominis* disseminated infection in a human immunodeficiency virus-1-infected pregnant woman with hypogammaglobulinemia. *J Microbiol Immunol Infect.* 2017;50(1):118-119.
344. Fettweis JM, Serrano MG, Huang B, et al. An emerging mycoplasma associated with trichomoniasis, vaginal infection and disease. *PLoS ONE.* 2014;9(10):e110943.
352. Flateau C, Asfalou I, Deman AL, et al. Aortic thrombus and multiple embolisms during a *Mycoplasma pneumoniae* infection. *Infection.* 2013;41(4):867-873.
354. Flouzat-Lachaniette CH, Guidon J, Allain J, et al. An uncommon case of *Mycoplasma hominis* infection after total disc replacement. *Eur Spine J.* 2013;22(suppl 3):S394-S398.
376. Frazier JA, Wood ME, Ware J, et al. Antecedents of the child behavior checklist-dysregulation profile in children born extremely preterm. *J Am Acad Child Adolesc Psychiatry.* 2015;54(10):816-823.
382. Gagneux-Brunon A, Grattard F, Morel J, et al. *Mycoplasma hominis*, a rare but true cause of infective endocarditis. *J Clin Microbiol.* 2015;53(9):3068-3071.
383. Galanos C, Gumenscheimer M, Muhlradt P, et al. MALP-2, a *Mycoplasma* lipopeptide with classical endotoxic properties: end of an era of LPS monopoly? *J Endotoxin Res.* 2000;6(6):471-476.
389. Garcia AV, Fingeret AL, Thirumoorthi AS, et al. Severe Mycoplasma pneumoniae infection requiring extracorporeal membrane oxygenation with concomitant ischemic stroke in a child. *Pediatr Pulmonol.* 2013;48(1):98-101.
390. Garcia C, Ugalde E, Monteagudo I, et al. Isolation of *Mycoplasma hominis* in critically ill patients with pulmonary infections: clinical and microbiological analysis in an intensive care unit. *Intensive Care Med.* 2007;33(1):143-147.
391. Gardiner SJ, Gavranich JB, Chang AB. Antibiotics for community-acquired lower respiratory tract infections secondary to *Mycoplasma pneumoniae* in children. *Cochrane Database Syst Rev.* 2015;(1):CD004875.
397. George MD, Cardenas AM, Birnbaum BK, et al. Ureaplasma septic arthritis in an immunosuppressed patient with juvenile idiopathic arthritis. *J Clin Rheumatol.* 2015;21(4):221-224.
405. Gillespie SH, Ling CL, Oravcova K, et al. Genomic investigations unmask *Mycoplasma amphoriforme*, a new respiratory pathogen. *Clin Infect Dis.* 2015;60(3):381-388.
410. Glaser K, Wohlleben M, Speer CP. An 8-month history of meningitis in an extremely low birth weight infant? - Long-lasting infection with *Ureaplasma parvum. Z Geburtshilfe Neonatol.* 2015;219(1):52-56.
413. Godron A, Pereyre S, Monet C, et al. Hemolytic uremic syndrome complicating *Mycoplasma pneumoniae* infection. *Pediatr Nephrol.* 2013;28(10):2057-2060.
419. Goodman A. Pericardial mass and cardiac tamponade associated with *Mycoplasma pneumoniae. Clin Med (Lond).* 2015;15(1):106-107.
420. Gotoh K, Nishimura N, Ohshima Y, et al. Detection of *Mycoplasma pneumoniae* by loop-mediated isothermal amplification (LAMP) assay and serology in pediatric community-acquired pneumonia. *J Infect Chemother.* 2012;18(5):662-667.
430. Greco F, Catania R, Pira AL, et al. Erythema nodosum and *Mycoplasma pneumoniae* infections in childhood: further observations in two patients and a literature review. *J Clin Med Res.* 2015;7(4):274-277.
440. Gu L, Chen X, Li H, et al. A case of lethal hemolytic anemia associated with severe pneumonia caused by *Mycoplasma pneumoniae. Chin Med J.* 2014;127(21):3839.
443. Gundevia Z, Foster R, Jamil MS, et al. Positivity at test of cure following first-line treatment for genital *Mycoplasma genitalium*: follow-up of a clinical cohort. *Sex Transm Infect.* 2015;91(1):11-13.
444. Guo L, Liu F, Lu MP, et al. Increased T cell activation in BALF from children with *Mycoplasma pneumoniae* pneumonia. *Pediatr Pulmonol.* 2015;50(8):814-819.
454. Hanzawa F, Fuchigami T, Ishii W, et al. A 3-year-old boy with Guillain-Barre syndrome and encephalitis associated with *Mycoplasma pneumoniae* infection. *J Infect Chemother.* 2014;20(2):134-138.
455. Hao Y, Kuang Z, Jing J, et al. *Mycoplasma pneumoniae* modulates STAT3-STAT6/EGFR-FOXA2 signaling to induce overexpression of airway mucins. *Infect Immun.* 2014;82(12):5246-5255.
459. Hartleif S, Wiegand G, Kumpf M, et al. Severe chest pain caused by *Mycoplasma* myocarditis in an adolescent patient. *Klin Padiatr.* 2013;225(7):423-425.
463. Hausner M, Schamberger A, Naumann W, et al. Development of protective anti-*Mycoplasma pneumoniae* antibodies after immunization of guinea pigs with the combination of a P1-P30 chimeric recombinant protein and chitosan. *Microb Pathog.* 2013;64:23-32.
473. Henao-Martinez AF, Young H, Nardi-Korver JJ, et al. *Mycoplasma hominis* brain abscess presenting after a head trauma: a case report. *J Med Case Rep.* 2012;6:253.
480. Ho PL, Law PY, Chan BW, et al. Emergence of macrolide-resistant *Mycoplasma pneumoniae* in Hong Kong is linked to increasing macrolide resistance in multilocus variable-number tandem-repeat analysis type 4-5-7-2. *J Clin Microbiol.* 2015;53(11):3560-3564.
486. Hon KL, Ip M, Chu WC, et al. Megapneumonia coinfection: pneumococcus, Mycoplasma pneumoniae, and metapneumovirus. *Case Rep Med.* 2012;2012:310104.
489. Hopfe M, Deenen R, Degrandi D, et al. Host cell responses to persistent mycoplasmas–different stages in infection of HeLa cells with Mycoplasma hominis. *PLoS ONE.* 2013;8(1):e54219.
490. Horie C, Kano Y, Mitomo T, et al. Possible Involvement of *Mycoplasma fermentans* in the development of nonsexually acquired genital ulceration (Lipschutz Ulcers) in 3 young female patients. *JAMA Dermatol.* 2015;151(12):1388-1389.
493. Horner P, Blee K, Adams E. Time to manage *Mycoplasma genitalium* as an STI: but not with azithromycin 1 g! *Curr Opin Infect Dis.* 2014;27(1):68-74.
494. Horner P, Blee K, O'Mahony C, et al. 2015 UK National Guideline on the management of non-gonococcal urethritis. *Int J STD AIDS.* 2016;27(2):85-96.
492. Horner PJ. Editorial Commentary: *Mycoplasma genitalium* and declining treatment efficacy of azithromycin 1 g: what can we do? *Clin Infect Dis.* 2015;61(9):1400-1402.
498. Hos NJ, Bauer C, Liebig T, et al. Autoinfection as a cause of postpartum subdural empyema due to *Mycoplasma hominis. Infection.* 2015;43(2):241-244.
508. Huang L, Gao X, Chen M. Early treatment with corticosteroids in patients with Mycoplasma pneumoniae pneumonia: a randomized clinical trial. *J Trop Pediatr.* 2014;60(5):338-342.
512. Hussain ST, Gordon SM, Tan CD, et al. Mycoplasma hominis prosthetic valve endocarditis: the value of molecular sequencing in cardiac surgery. *J Thorac Cardiovasc Surg.* 2013;146(1):e7-e9.
523. Ishiguro N, Koseki N, Kaiho M, et al. Sensitivity and specificity of a loop-mediated isothermal amplification assay for the detection of *Mycoplasma* pneumonia from nasopharyngeal swab samples compared with those of real-time PCR. *Clin Lab.* 2015;61(5-6):603-606.
529. Jacobs E, Ehrhardt I, Dumke R. New insights in the outbreak pattern of *Mycoplasma pneumoniae. Int J Med Microbiol.* 2015;305(7):705-708.
531. Jacobs M, Lo MD, Lendvay TS. Painless pediatric priapism and cough. *Pediatr Emerg Care.* 2015;31(1):36-38.
545. Jensen JS, Fernandes P, Unemo M. In vitro activity of the new fluoroketolide solithromycin (CEM-101) against macrolide-resistant and -susceptible *Mycoplasma genitalium* strains. *Antimicrob Agents Chemother.* 2014;58(6):3151-3156.
551. Ji M, Lee NS, Oh JM, et al. Single-nucleotide polymorphism PCR for the detection of *Mycoplasma pneumoniae* and determination of macrolide resistance in respiratory samples. *J Microbiol Methods.* 2014;102:32-36.
563. Kacerovsky M, Pliskova L, Menon R, et al. Microbial load of umbilical cord blood *Ureaplasma* species and *Mycoplasma hominis* in preterm prelabor rupture of membranes. *J Matern Fetal Neonatal Med.* 2014;27(16):1627-1632.
565. Kakuya F, Kinebuchi T, Fujiyasu H, et al. Genetic point-of-care diagnosis of *Mycoplasma pneumoniae* infection using LAMP assay. *Pediatr Int.* 2014;56(4):547-552.
567. Kalicki B, Sadecka M, Wawrzyniak A, et al. Absence of inferior vena cava in 14-year old boy associated with deep venous thrombosis and positive Mycoplasma pneumoniae serum antibodies–a case report. *BMC Pediatr.* 2015;15:40.
571. Kannan TR, Krishnan M, Ramasamy K, et al. Functional mapping of community-acquired respiratory distress syndrome (CARDS) toxin of *Mycoplasma pneumoniae* defines regions with ADP-ribosyltransferase, vacuolating and receptor-binding activities. *Mol Microbiol.* 2014;93(3):568-581.
573. Karampatsas K, Patel H, Basheer SN, et al. Chronic meningitis with intracranial hypertension and bilateral neuroretinitis following *Mycoplasma pneumoniae* infection. *BMJ Case Rep.* 2014;2014.
581. Kazama I, Nakajima T. Dual infection of *Mycoplasma pneumoniae* and Chlaimydophila *pneumoniae* in patients with atopic predispositions successfully treated by moxifloxacin. *Infez Med.* 2014;22(1):41-47.
582. Kazama I, Tamada T, Nakajima T. Resolution of migratory pulmonary infiltrates by moxifloxacin in a patient with dual infection of *Mycoplasma pneumoniae* and *Bordetella pertussis. Infez Med.* 2012;20(4):288-292.

591. Kenri T, Okazaki N, Yamazaki T, et al. Genotyping analysis of *Mycoplasma pneumoniae* clinical strains in Japan between 1995 and 2005: type shift phenomenon of *M. pneumoniae* clinical strains. *J Med Microbiol.* 2008;57(Pt 4):469-475.
597. Khoury T, Abu Rmeileh A, Kornspan JD, et al. *Mycoplasma pneumoniae* pneumonia associated with methemoglobinemia and anemia: an overlooked association? *Open Forum Infect Dis.* 2015;2(1):ofv022.
602. Kim GH, Seo WH, Je BK, et al. *Mycoplasma pneumoniae* associated stroke in a 3-year-old girl. *Korean J Pediatr.* 2013;56(9):411-415.
601. Kim JH, Cho TS, Moon JH, et al. Serial changes in serum eosinophil-associated mediators between atopic and non-atopic children after *Mycoplasma pneumoniae* pneumonia. *Allergy Asthma Immunol Res.* 2014;6(5):428-433.
603. Kim KW, Sung JJ, Tchah H, et al. Hepatitis associated with *Mycoplasma pneumoniae* infection in Korean children: a prospective study. *Korean J Pediatr.* 2015;58(6):211-217.
615. Koike Y, Aoki N. Hemophagocytic syndrome associated with *Mycoplasma pneumoniae* pneumonia. *Case Rep Pediatr.* 2013;2013:586705.
635. Krishnan M, Kannan TR, Baseman JB. *Mycoplasma pneumoniae* CARDS toxin is internalized via clathrin-mediated endocytosis. *PLoS ONE.* 2013;8(5):e62706.
637. Kumar S, Kapoor S, Saigal SR. Hemorrhagic encephalitis caused by *Mycoplasma pneumoniae* in an 11-year-old boy: A rare case report. *Indian J Med Microbiol.* 2015;33(3):463-464.
643. Kurata S, Osaki T, Yonezawa H, et al. Role of IL-17A and IL-10 in the antigen induced inflammation model by *Mycoplasma pneumoniae*. *BMC Microbiol.* 2014;14:156.
644. Kurugol Z, Onen SS, Koturoglu G. Severe hemolytic anemia associated with mild pneumonia caused by *Mycoplasma* pneumonia. *Case Rep Med.* 2012;2012:649850.
645. Kwak DW, Hwang HS, Kwon JY, et al. Co-infection with vaginal *Ureaplasma urealyticum* and *Mycoplasma hominis* increases adverse pregnancy outcomes in patients with preterm labor or preterm premature rupture of membranes. *J Matern Fetal Neonatal Med.* 2014;27(4):333-337.
647. Lai CH, Chang LL, Lin JN, et al. High seroprevalence of *Mycoplasma pneumoniae* IgM in acute Q fever by enzyme-linked immunosorbent assay (ELISA). *PLoS ONE.* 2013;8(10):e77640.
658. Lau A, Bradshaw CS, Lewis D, et al. The efficacy of azithromycin for the treatment of genital mycoplasma genitalium: a systematic review and meta-analysis. *Clin Infect Dis.* 2015;61(9):1389-1399.
661. Le Guern R, Loiez C, Loobuyck V, et al. A new case of *Mycoplasma hominis* mediastinitis and sternal osteitis after cardiac surgery. *Int J Infect Dis.* 2015;31:53-55.
664. Lee EH, Winter HL, van Dijl JM, et al. Diagnosis and antimicrobial therapy of *Mycoplasma hominis* meningitis in adults. *Int J Med Microbiol.* 2012;302(7-8):289-292.
665. Lee H, Moon KC, Kim S. Cutaneous vasculitis and renal involvement in *Mycoplasma pneumoniae* infection. *Korean J Intern Med.* 2015;30(3):402-405.
668. Lee M, Joo IS, Lee SJ, et al. Multiple cerebral arterial occlusions related to *Mycoplasma pneumoniae* infection. *Neurol Sci.* 2013;34(4):565-568.
672. Lee SY, Lee YH, Chun BY, et al. An adult case of Fisher syndrome subsequent to *Mycoplasma pneumoniae* infection. *J Korean Med Sci.* 2013;28(1):152-155.
691. Li SL, Sun HM, Zhao HQ, et al. A single tube modified allele-specific-PCR for rapid detection of erythromycin-resistant *Mycoplasma pneumoniae* in Beijing. *Chin Med J.* 2012;125(15):2671-2676.
688. Li Y, Cheng H, Wang H, et al. Composite factors, including mycoplasmal pneumonia, hypersensitivity syndrome, and medicine, leading to bronchiolitis obliterans in a school-age child. *Clin Pediatr (Phila).* 2014;53(14):1409-1412.
689. Li Y, Pattan V, Syed B, et al. Splenic infarction caused by a rare coinfection of Epstein-Barr virus, cytomegalovirus, and *Mycoplasma pneumoniae*. *Pediatr Emerg Care.* 2014;30(9):636-637.
691. Li YN, Liu L, Qiao HM, et al. Post-infectious bronchiolitis obliterans in children: a review of 42 cases. *BMC Pediatr.* 2014;14:238.
703. Lis R, Rowhani-Rahbar A, Manhart LE. *Mycoplasma genitalium* infection and female reproductive tract disease: a meta-analysis. *Clin Infect Dis.* 2015;61(3):418-426.
706. Liu EM, Janigian RH. *Mycoplasma pneumoniae*: the other masquerader. *JAMA Ophthalmol.* 2013;131(2):251-253.
709. Lluch-Senar M, Cozzuto L, Cano J, et al. Comparative "-omics" in *Mycoplasma pneumoniae* clinical isolates reveals key virulence factors. *PLoS ONE.* 2015;10(9):e0137354.
713. Lo SC, Wear DJ, Green SL, et al. Adult respiratory distress syndrome with or without systemic disease associated with infections due to *Mycoplasma fermentans*. *Clin Infect Dis.* 1993;17(suppl 1):S259-S263.
717. Lombart F, Dhaille F, Lok C, et al. Subcorneal pustular dermatosis associated with *Mycoplasma pneumoniae* infection. *J Am Acad Dermatol.* 2014;71(3):e85-e86.
726. Lung DC, Yip EK, Lam DS, et al. Rapid defervescence after doxycycline treatment of macrolide-resistant *Mycoplasma pneumoniae*-associated community-acquired pneumonia in children. *Pediatr Infect Dis J.* 2013;32(12):1396-1399.
741. Manhart LE, Kay N. Mycoplasma genitalium: Is it a sexually transmitted pathogen? *Curr Infect Dis Rep.* 2010;12(4):306-313.
748. Mardassi BB, Aissani N, Moalla I, et al. Evidence for the predominance of a single tet(M) gene sequence type in tetracycline-resistant *Ureaplasma parvum* and *Mycoplasma hominis* isolates from Tunisian patients. *J Med Microbiol.* 2012;61(Pt 9):1254-1261.
773. McDermott AJ, Taylor BM, Bernstein KM. Toxic epidermal necrolysis from suspected *Mycoplasma pneumoniae* infection. *Mil Med.* 2013;178(9):e1048-e1050.
779. McGowin CL, Annan RS, Quayle AJ, et al. Persistent *Mycoplasma genitalium* infection of human endocervical epithelial cells elicits chronic inflammatory cytokine secretion. *Infect Immun.* 2012;80(11):3842-3849.
781. McGowin CL, Radtke AL, Abraham K, et al. *Mycoplasma genitalium* infection activates cellular host defense and inflammation pathways in a 3-dimensional human endocervical epithelial cell model. *J Infect Dis.* 2013;207(12):1857-1868.
791. Meng DY, Sun CJ, Yu JB, et al. Molecular mechanism of fluoroquinolones resistance in *Mycoplasma hominis* clinical isolates. *Braz J Microbiol.* 2014;45(1):239-242.
796. Meyer Sauteur PM, Jacobs BC, Spuesens EB, et al. Antibody responses to *Mycoplasma pneumoniae*: role in pathogenesis and diagnosis of encephalitis? *PLoS Pathog.* 2014;10(6):e1003983.
797. Meyer Sauteur PM, Relly C, Hackenberg A, et al. *Mycoplasma pneumoniae* intrathecal antibody responses in Bickerstaff brain stem encephalitis. *Neuropediatrics.* 2014;45(1):61-63.
798. Meyer Sauteur PM, Roodbol J, Hackenberg A, et al. Severe childhood Guillain-Barre syndrome associated with *Mycoplasma pneumoniae* infection: a case series. *J Peripher Nerv Syst.* 2015;20(2):72-78.
808. Miyashita N, Akaike H, Teranishi H, et al. Macrolide-resistant *Mycoplasma pneumoniae* pneumonia in adolescents and adults: clinical findings, drug susceptibility, and therapeutic efficacy. *Antimicrob Agents Chemother.* 2013;57(10):5181-5185.
818. Moi H, Blee K, Horner PJ. Management of non-gonococcal urethritis. *BMC Infect Dis.* 2015;15:294.
832. Muhlradt PF, Kiess M, Meyer H, et al. Isolation, structure elucidation, and synthesis of a macrophage stimulatory lipopeptide from *Mycoplasma fermentans* acting at picomolar concentration. *J Exp Med.* 1997;185(11):1951-1958.
838. Murtha AP, Edwards JM. The role of *Mycoplasma* and *Ureaplasma* in adverse pregnancy outcomes. *Obstet Gynecol Clin North Am.* 2014;41(4):615-627.
841. Musilova I, Pliskova L, Kutova R, et al. *Ureaplasma* species and *Mycoplasma hominis* in cervical fluid of pregnancies complicated by preterm prelabor rupture of membranes. *J Matern Fetal Neonatal Med.* 2016;29(1):1-7.
853. Napierala Mavedzenge S, Muller EE, Lewis DA, et al. *Mycoplasma genitalium* is associated with increased genital HIV type 1 RNA in Zimbabwean women. *J Infect Dis.* 2015;211(9):1388-1398.
872. Nijhuis RH, Severs TT, Van der Vegt DS, et al. High levels of macrolide resistance-associated mutations in *Mycoplasma genitalium* warrant antibiotic susceptibility-guided treatment. *J Antimicrob Chemother.* 2015;70(9):2515-2518.
873. Nilsson AC, Bjorkman P, Welinder-Olsson C, et al. Clinical severity of *Mycoplasma pneumoniae* (MP) infection is associated with bacterial load in oropharyngeal secretions but not with MP genotype. *BMC Infect Dis.* 2010;10:39.
882. Noska A, Nasr R, Williams DN. Closed trauma, *Mycoplasma hominis* osteomyelitis, and the elusive diagnosis of Good's syndrome. *BMJ Case Rep.* 2012;2012.
886. Nummi M, Mannonen L, Puolakkainen M. Development of a multiplex real-time PCR assay for detection of *Mycoplasma pneumoniae, Chlamydia pneumoniae* and mutations associated with macrolide resistance in *Mycoplasma pneumoniae* from respiratory clinical specimens. *Springerplus.* 2015;4:684.
894. Okada T, Morozumi M, Tajima T, et al. Rapid effectiveness of minocycline or doxycycline against macrolide-resistant *Mycoplasma pneumoniae* infection in a 2011 outbreak among Japanese children. *Clin Infect Dis.* 2012;55(12):1642-1649.
895. Okusawa T, Fujita M, Nakamura J, et al. Relationship between structures and biological activities of mycoplasmal diacylated lipopeptides and their recognition by toll-like receptors 2 and 6. *Infect Immun.* 2004;72(3):1657-1665.
902. Olson D, Watkins LK, Demirjian A, et al. Outbreak of *Mycoplasma pneumoniae*-associated Stevens-Johnson syndrome. *Pediatrics.* 2015;136(2):e386-e394.
903. Omae T, Matsubayashi T. Lung abscess caused by *Mycoplasma pneumoniae*. *Pediatr Int.* 2015;57(4):773-775.
904. Omori R, Nakata Y, Tessmer HL, et al. The determinant of periodicity in *Mycoplasma pneumoniae* incidence: an insight from mathematical modelling. *Sci Rep.* 2015;5:14473.
914. Pailhories H, Rabier V, Eveillard M, et al. A case report of *Mycoplasma hominis* brain abscess identified by MALDI-TOF mass spectrometry. *Int J Infect Dis.* 2014;29:166-168.
918. Park IH, Choi du Y, Oh YK, et al. A case of acute myopericarditis associated with *Mycoplasma pneumoniae* infection in a child. *Korean Circ J.* 2012;42(10):709-713.
925. Patil S, Rao RS, Raj AT. Role of *Mycoplasma* in the initiation and progression of oral cancer. *J Int Oral Health.* 2015;7(7):i-ii.
926. Patra PK, Thirunavukkarasu AB. Unusual complication of *Mycoplasma* pneumonia in a five-year-old child. *Australas Med J.* 2013;6(2):73-74.
928. Pellan M, Bastian C, Gaudelus J, et al. Pulmonary necrotizing cavity caused by Mycoplasma pneumoniae infection. *Arch Pediatr.* 2013;20(10):1158-1159.
946. Principi N, Esposito S. Macrolide-resistant *Mycoplasma pneumoniae*: its role in respiratory infection. *J Antimicrob Chemother.* 2013;68(3):506-511.
947. Prindaville B, Newell BD, Nopper AJ, et al. *Mycoplasma pneumonia*-associated mucocutaneous disease in children: dilemmas in classification. *Pediatr Dermatol.* 2014;31(6):670-675.

952. Qu J, Gu L, Wu J, et al. Accuracy of IgM antibody testing, FQ-PCR and culture in laboratory diagnosis of acute infection by *Mycoplasma pneumoniae* in adults and adolescents with community-acquired pneumonia. *BMC Infect Dis.* 2013;13:172.
953. Qu J, Yu X, Liu Y, et al. Specific multilocus variable-number tandem-repeat analysis genotypes of *Mycoplasma pneumoniae* are associated with diseases severity and macrolide susceptibility. *PLoS ONE.* 2013;8(12):e82174.
960. Rao M, Agrawal A, Parikh M, et al. Mycoplasmal upper respiratory infection presenting as leukocytoclastic vasculitis. *Infect Dis Rep.* 2015;7(1):5605.
976. Rock N, Belli D, Bajwa N. Erythema bullous multiforme: a complication of *Mycoplasma pneumoniae* infection. *J Pediatr.* 2014;164(2):421.
981. Romeu Prieto JM, Lizcano Lizcano AM, Lopez de Toro Martin Consuegra I, et al. Culture-negative endocarditis: *Mycoplasma hominis* infection. *Rev Esp Cardiol (Engl Ed).* 2015;68(11):1037-1038.
985. Rottem S. Unique choline-containing phosphoglycolipids in Mycoplasma fermentans. *Chem Phys Lipids.* 2015;191:61-67.
987. Ruffini E, De Petris L, Candelotti P, et al. Lung abscess in a child secondary to *Mycoplasma pneumoniae* infection. *Pediatr Med Chir.* 2014;36(2):87-89.
994. Saegeman V, Proesmans M, Dumke R. Management of macrolide-resistant *Mycoplasma pneumoniae* infection. *Pediatr Infect Dis J.* 2012;31(11):1210-1211.
1008. Saraya T, Kurai D, Nakagaki K, et al. Novel aspects on the pathogenesis of *Mycoplasma pneumoniae* pneumonia and therapeutic implications. *Front Microbiol.* 2014;5:410.
1023. Schmitt BH, Sloan LM, Patel R. Real-time PCR detection of *Mycoplasma pneumoniae* in respiratory specimens. *Diagn Microbiol Infect Dis.* 2013;77(3):202-205.
1025. Schmucker RD, Ehret A, Marshall GS. Cerebellitis and acute obstructive hydrocephalus associated with *Mycoplasma pneumoniae* infection. *Pediatr Infect Dis J.* 2014;33(5):529-532.
1029. Schuhfried G, Schuhfried G, Stanek G. Gilles de la Tourette syndrome caused by *Mycoplasma pneumoniae* successfully treated with macrolides. *Klin Padiatr.* 2014;226(5):295-296.
1032. Sena AC, Lensing S, Rompalo A, et al. *Chlamydia trachomatis, Mycoplasma genitalium,* and *Trichomonas vaginalis* infections in men with nongonococcal urethritis: predictors and persistence after therapy. *J Infect Dis.* 2012;206(3):357-365.
1036. Shao L, Cong Z, Li X, et al. Changes in levels of IL-9, IL-17, IFN-gamma, dendritic cell numbers and TLR expression in peripheral blood in asthmatic children with *Mycoplasma pneumoniae* infection. *Int J Clin Exp Pathol.* 2015;8(5):5263-5272.
1043. Shen H, Zhu B, Wang S, et al. Association of targeted multiplex PCR with resequencing microarray for the detection of multiple respiratory pathogens. *Front Microbiol.* 2015;6:532.
1053. Shimizu M, Hamaguchi Y, Matsushita T, et al. Sequentially appearing erythema nodosum, erythema multiforme and Henoch-Schonlein purpura in a patient with *Mycoplasma pneumoniae* infection: a case report. *J Med Case Rep.* 2012;6:398.
1054. Shimizu T, Kimura Y, Kida Y, et al. Cytadherence of *Mycoplasma pneumoniae* induces inflammatory responses through autophagy and toll-like receptor 4. *Infect Immun.* 2014;82(7):3076-3086.
1055. Shin JE, Cheon BR, Shim JW, et al. Increased risk of refractory *Mycoplasma pneumoniae* pneumonia in children with atopic sensitization and asthma. *Korean J Pediatr.* 2014;57(6):271-277.
1056. Shin SR, Park SH, Kim JH, et al. Clinical characteristics of patients with *Mycoplasma pneumoniae*-related acute hepatitis. *Digestion.* 2012;86(4):302-308.
1064. Simmons WL, Daubenspeck JM, Osborne JD, et al. Type 1 and type 2 strains of Mycoplasma pneumoniae form different biofilms. *Microbiology.* 2013;159(Pt 4):737-747.
1068. Sini V, Tegueu CK, Nguefack S, et al. [Miller Fisher syndrome with anti GQ1b negative in *Mycoplasma pneumoniae* pneumonia]. *Pan Afr Med J.* 2013;15:122.
1072. Smith-Norowitz TA, Silverberg JI, Kusonruksa M, et al. Asthmatic children have increased specific anti-*Mycoplasma pneumoniae* IgM but not IgG or IgE-values independent of history of respiratory tract infection. *Pediatr Infect Dis J.* 2013;32(6):599-603.
1089. Spuesens EB, Fraaij PL, Visser EG, et al. Carriage of *Mycoplasma pneumoniae* in the upper respiratory tract of symptomatic and asymptomatic children: an observational study. *PLoS Med.* 2013;10(5):e1001444.
1090. Spuesens EB, Meyer Sauteur PM, Vink C, et al. *Mycoplasma pneumoniae* infections–does treatment help? *J Infect.* 2014;69(suppl 1):S42-S46.
1091. Spuesens EB, Oduber M, Hoogenboezem T, et al. Sequence variations in RepMP2/3 and RepMP4 elements reveal intragenomic homologous DNA recombination events in *Mycoplasma pneumoniae. Microbiology.* 2009;155(Pt 7):2182-2196.
1112. Sugiyama M, Saeki A, Hasebe A, et al. Activation of inflammasomes in dendritic cells and macrophages by *Mycoplasma salivarium. Mol Oral Microbiol.* 2016;31(3):259-269.
1114. Sun H, Chen Z, Yan Y, et al. Epidemiology and clinical profiles of *Mycoplasma pneumoniae* infection in hospitalized infants younger than one year. *Respir Med.* 2015;109(6):751-757.
1115. Sun H, Xue G, Yan C, et al. Multiple-locus variable-number tandem-repeat analysis of *Mycoplasma pneumoniae* clinical specimens and proposal for amendment of MLVA nomenclature. *PLoS ONE.* 2013;8(5):e64607.
1118. Sweeney EL, Kallapur SG, Gisslen T, et al. Placental infection with ureaplasma species is associated with histologic chorioamnionitis and adverse outcomes in moderately preterm and late-preterm infants. *J Infect Dis.* 2016;213(8):1340-1347.
1124. Tagg KA, Jeoffreys NJ, Couldwell DL, et al. Fluoroquinolone and macrolide resistance-associated mutations in *Mycoplasma genitalium. J Clin Microbiol.* 2013;51(7):2245-2249.
1125. Taguchi K, Oka M, Bito T, et al. Acute generalized exanthematous pustulosis induced by *Mycoplasma pneumoniae* infection. *J Dermatol.* 2016;43(1):113-114.
1128. Takeo N, Hatano Y, Yamamoto K, et al. Case of *Mycoplasma pneumoniae* infection with maculopapular-type eruptions due to acetaminophen. *J Dermatol.* 2013;40(4):304-306.
1134. Tay CG, Fong CY, Ong LC. Transient parkinsonism following mycoplasma pneumoniae infection with normal brain magnetic resonance imaging (MRI). *J Child Neurol.* 2014;29(12):NP193-NP195.
1156. Thurman KA, Walter ND, Schwartz SB, et al. Comparison of laboratory diagnostic procedures for detection of *Mycoplasma pneumoniae* in community outbreaks. *Clin Infect Dis.* 2009;48(9):1244-1249.
1160. Touati A, Peuchant O, Jensen JS, et al. Direct detection of macrolide resistance in Mycoplasma genitalium isolates from clinical specimens from France by use of real-time PCR and melting curve analysis. *J Clin Microbiol.* 2014;52(5):1549-1555.
1161. Tran H, Allworth A, Bennett C. A case of Mycoplasma pneumoniae-associated encephalomyelitis in a 16-year-old female presenting to an adult teaching hospital. *Clin Med Insights Case Rep.* 2013;6:209-211.
1162. Trapp LW, Schrantz SJ, Joseph-Griffin MA, et al. A 13-year-old boy with pharyngitis, oral ulcers, and dehydration. *Mycoplasma pneumoniae*-associated mucositis. *Pediatr Ann.* 2013;42(4):148-150.
1163. Tsai V, Pritzker BB, Diaz MH, et al. Cluster of macrolide-resistant *Mycoplasma pneumoniae* infections in Illinois in 2012. *J Clin Microbiol.* 2013;51(11):3889-3892.
1175. Uh Y, Hong JH, Oh KJ, et al. Macrolide resistance of *Mycoplasma pneumoniae* and its detection rate by real-time PCR in primary and tertiary care hospitals. *Ann Lab Med.* 2013;33(6):410-414.
1183. Van Putten WK, Hachimi-Idrissi S, Jansen A, et al. Uncommon cause of psychotic behavior in a 9-year-old girl: a case report. *Case Rep Med.* 2012;2012:358520.
1186. Vande Voorde J, Balzarini J, Liekens S. Mycoplasmas and cancer: focus on nucleoside metabolism. *EXCLI J.* 2014;13:300-322.
1187. Vande Voorde J, Vervaeke P, Liekens S, et al. *Mycoplasma hyorhinis*-encoded cytidine deaminase efficiently inactivates cytosine-based anticancer drugs. *FEBS Open Bio.* 2015;5:634-639.
1188. Venancio P, Brito MJ, Pereira G, et al. Anti-N-methyl-D-aspartate receptor encephalitis with positive serum antithyroid antibodies, IgM antibodies against *Mycoplasma pneumoniae* and human herpesvirus 7 PCR in the CSF. *Pediatr Infect Dis J.* 2014;33(8):882-883.
1192. Vieira-Baptista P, Lima-Silva J, Beires J, et al. Lipschutz ulcers: should we rethink this? An analysis of 33 cases. *Eur J Obstet Gynecol Reprod Biol.* 2016;198:149-152.
1195. Viscardi RM. Ureaplasma species: role in neonatal morbidities and outcomes. *Arch Dis Child Fetal Neonatal Ed.* 2014;99(1):F87-F92.
1202. Vouga M, Greub G, Prod'hom G, et al. Treatment of genital mycoplasma in colonized pregnant women in late pregnancy is associated with a lower rate of premature labour and neonatal complications. *Clin Microbiol Infect.* 2014;20(10):1074-1079.
1204. Vujic I, Shroff A, Grzelka M, et al. *Mycoplasma pneumoniae*-associated mucositis–case report and systematic review of literature. *J Eur Acad Dermatol Venereol.* 2015;29(3):595-598.
1207. Waites KB, Brown MB, Stagno S, et al. Association of genital mycoplasmas with exudative vaginitis in a 10 year old: a case of misdiagnosis. *Pediatrics.* 1983;71(2):250-252.
1226. Wang K, Gill P, Perera R, et al. Clinical symptoms and signs for the diagnosis of *Mycoplasma pneumoniae* in children and adolescents with community-acquired pneumonia. *Cochrane Database Syst Rev.* 2012;(10):CD009175.
1224. Wang L, Chen Q, Shi C, et al. Changes of serum TNF-alpha, IL-5 and IgE levels in the patients of mycoplasma pneumonia infection with or without bronchial asthma. *Int J Clin Exp Med.* 2015;8(3):3901-3906.
1228. Wang M, Wang Y, Yan Y, et al. Clinical and laboratory profiles of refractory *Mycoplasma pneumoniae* pneumonia in children. *Int J Infect Dis.* 2014;29:18-23.
1226. Wang RS, Jin HX, Shang SQ, et al. Associations of IL-2 and IL-4 expression and polymorphisms with the risks of *Mycoplasma pneumoniae* infection and asthma in children. *Arch Bronconeumol.* 2015;51(11):571-578.
1227. Wang X, Liu C, Wang M, et al. Clinical features of post-infectious bronchiolitis obliterans in children undergoing long-term azithromycin treatment. *Exp Ther Med.* 2015;9(6):2379-2383.
1236. Watanabe H, Uruma T, Nakamura H, et al. The role of *Mycoplasma pneumoniae* infection in the initial onset and exacerbations of asthma. *Allergy Asthma Proc.* 2014;35(3):204-210.
1247. Westley BP, Horazdovsky RD, Michaels DL, et al. Identification of a novel *Mycoplasma* species in a patient with septic arthritis of the hip and seal finger. *Clin Infect Dis.* 2016;62(4):491-493.

1251. Whitson WJ, Ball PA, Lollis SS, et al. Postoperative *Mycoplasma hominis* infections after neurosurgical intervention. *J Neurosurg Pediatr*. 2014;14(2):212-218.
1256. Winikor JM, Kennedy JC, Leonard MS, et al. A 14-year-old boy with *Mycoplasma pneumoniae*-associated mucositis and intracranial hypertension. *Clin Pediatr (Phila)*. 2016;55(1):83-85.
1258. Wold C, Sorthe J, Hartgill U, et al. Identification of macrolide-resistant *Mycoplasma genitalium* using real-time PCR. *J Eur Acad Dermatol Venereol*. 2015;29(8):1616-1620.
1259. Wood PR, Hill VL, Burks ML, et al. *Mycoplasma pneumoniae* in children with acute and refractory asthma. *Ann Allergy Asthma Immunol*. 2013;110(5):328-334. e321.
1260. Workowski KA, Bolan GA, Centers for Disease Control and Prevention. Sexually transmitted diseases treatment guidelines, 2015. *MMWR Recomm Rep*. 2015;64(RR-03):1-137.
1261. Wu PS, Chang LY, Lin HC, et al. Epidemiology and clinical manifestations of children with macrolide-resistant *Mycoplasma pneumoniae* pneumonia in Taiwan. *Pediatr Pulmonol*. 2013;48(9):904-911.
1264. Wylam ME, Kennedy CC, Hernandez NM, et al. Fatal hyperammonaemia caused by *Mycoplasma hominis*. *Lancet*. 2013;382(9908):1956.
1265. Wynes J, Harris WT, Hadfield RA, et al. Subtalar joint septic arthritis in a patient with hypogammaglobulinemia. *J Foot Ankle Surg*. 2013;52(2):242-248.
1266. Xiao D, Zhao F, Zhang H, et al. Novel strategy for typing *Mycoplasma pneumoniae* isolates by use of matrix-assisted laser desorption ionization-time of flight mass spectrometry coupled with ClinProTools. *J Clin Microbiol*. 2014;52(8):3038-3043.
1266. Xiao J, Liu Y, Wang M, et al. Detection of *Mycoplasma pneumoniae* P1 subtype variations by denaturing gradient gel electrophoresis. *Diagn Microbiol Infect Dis*. 2014;78(1):24-28.
1269. Yachoui R, Kolasinski SL, Feinstein DE. *Mycoplasma pneumoniae* with atypical Stevens-Johnson syndrome: a diagnostic challenge. *Case Rep Infect Dis*. 2013;2013:457161.
1274. Yang A, Kang B, Choi SY, et al. Acute necrotizing pancreatitis associated with *Mycoplasma pneumoniae* infection in a child. *Pediatr Gastroenterol Hepatol Nutr*. 2015;18(3):209-215.
1276. Yasutomi M, Okazaki S, Hata I, et al. Cytokine profiles in *Mycoplasma pneumoniae* infection-associated hemophagocytic lymphohistiocytosis. *J Microbiol Immunol Infect*. 2016;49(5):813-816.
1277. Ye Q, Xu XJ, Shao WX, et al. *Mycoplasma pneumoniae* infection in children is a risk factor for developing allergic diseases. *ScientificWorldJournal*. 2014;2014:986527.
1279. Yimenicioglu S, Yakut A, Ekici A, et al. *Mycoplasma pneumoniae* infection with neurologic complications. *Iran J Pediatr*. 2014;24(5):647-651.
1281. Yoo SJ, Kim HB, Choi SH, et al. Differences in the frequency of 23S rRNA gene mutations in *Mycoplasma pneumoniae* between children and adults with community-acquired pneumonia: clinical impact of mutations conferring macrolide resistance. *Antimicrob Agents Chemother*. 2012;56(12):6393-6396.
1287. Youn YS, Lee SC, Rhim JW, et al. Early additional immune-modulators for *Mycoplasma pneumoniae* pneumonia in children: an observation study. *Infect Chemother*. 2014;46(4):239-247.
1288. Yow MA, Tabrizi SN, Severi G, et al. Detection of infectious organisms in archival prostate cancer tissues. *BMC Cancer*. 2014;14:579.
1289. Yuan ZF, Chen B, Mao SS, et al. Reversible bilateral striatal lesions following *Mycoplasma pneumoniae* infection associated with elevated levels of interleukins 6 and 8. *Brain Dev*. 2016;38(1):149-153.
1291. Zarei O, Rezania S, Mousavi A. *Mycoplasma genitalium* and cancer: a brief review. *Asian Pac J Cancer Prev*. 2013;14(6):3425-3428.
1295. Zhao F, Liu L, Tao X, et al. Culture-independent detection and genotyping of *Mycoplasma pneumoniae* in clinical specimens from Beijing, China. *PLoS ONE*. 2015;10(10):e0141702.
1295. Zhao F, Liu Z, Gu Y, et al. Detection of *Mycoplasma pneumoniae* by colorimetric loop-mediated isothermal amplification. *Acta Microbiol Immunol Hung*. 2013;60(1):1-9.
1296. Zhao F, Lv M, Tao X, et al. Antibiotic sensitivity of 40 *Mycoplasma pneumoniae* isolates and molecular analysis of macrolide-resistant isolates from Beijing, China. *Antimicrob Agents Chemother*. 2012;56(2):1108-1109.
1297. Zheng X, Lee S, Selvarangan R, et al. Macrolide-resistant *Mycoplasma pneumoniae*, United States. *Emerg Infect Dis*. 2015;21(8):1470-1472.
1299. Zhou Y, Zhang Y, Sheng Y, et al. More complications occur in macrolide-resistant than in macrolide-sensitive *Mycoplasma pneumoniae* pneumonia. *Antimicrob Agents Chemother*. 2014;58(2):1034-1038.
1303. Zhuo Z, Li F, Chen X, et al. *Mycoplasma* pneumonia combined with pulmonary infarction in a child. *Int J Clin Exp Med*. 2015;8(1):1482-1486.

The full reference list for this chapter is available at ExpertConsult.com.

197 Classification of Fungi

David Bruckner

Fungal infections are an important and growing cause of morbidity and mortality. This is largely because of an expanding population of immunosuppressed individuals who serve as susceptible hosts, including persons with human immunodeficiency virus (HIV) infections, recipients of solid organ or hematopoietic stem cell transplants, and patients with hematologic malignancies, burns, and indwelling medical devices. Less than 50 of the more than 100,000 currently identified species of fungi are known primary pathogens in humans, but many fungal organisms previously thought of as contaminants in clinical specimens are now recognized as etiologic agents of disease under the right circumstances. The challenging task of the clinical microbiologist is to learn to recognize and correctly identify clinically relevant fungi to guide proper patient treatment.

Medically important fungi belong to the kingdom called Fungi.[1–7] These organisms are classified by their basic growth pattern as yeasts or molds. Yeasts are unicellular fungi that reproduce by budding (e.g., *Candida* spp.) or by fission (e.g., *Schizosaccharomyces pombe*). The buds produced by infectious yeasts, called blastoconidia, can form chains called pseudohyphae. Molds are multicellular fungi that grow by means of filamentous cell projections called hyphae. The nuclei in different cells may or may not be separated by characteristic crosswalls or septa.

Some medically important fungi change from a multicellular hyphal form in the natural environment or in vitro to a budding single-celled yeast form or spherule with endospores in tissue. These pathogens are known as dimorphic fungi and include *Blastomyces dermatitidis*, *Coccidioides immitis*, *Coccidioides posadasii*, *Histoplasma capsulatum*, *Paracoccidioides brasiliensis*, and *Talaromyces marneffei* (formerly *Penicillium marneffei*).

Fungi may reproduce sexually or asexually. The sexual form of growth is called the teleomorph, and the asexual form is called the anamorph. Some fungi have more than one name because the anamorph and teleomorph forms were described and named at different times without the connection between them being recognized. As a result, the teleomorph and the anamorph forms of the same fungus have different names. *Emericella nidulans*, for example, is the teleomorph for the anamorph, *Aspergillus nidulans*. Some teleomorphic fungi can produce more than one asexual form of propagation. *Pseudallescheria boydii* is the teleomorph of two anamorphs, *Scedosporium apiospermum* and *Graphium eumorphum*. These three names refer to the same organism. Although the sexual means of reproduction forms the basis of the taxonomy of fungi, the anamorph is usually obtained in culture, and the anamorph name typically is used in reports from a clinical microbiology laboratory.

Until recently, fungi were allowed to carry multiple scientific names based on the sexual (teleomorph) and asexual (anamorph) stages of their life cycle. In many cases, it was difficult to establish the relationship of these forms. With the use of molecular genetics, dual naming is no longer necessary. Beginning in 2013, the dual naming was no longer permitted, and only one name is now used for a fungus. The main criteria for classification are genetic rather than phenotypic.[1,3–7]

The Kingdom Fungi is divided into eight phyla. The medically important fungi are contained within the phylum Ascomycota, phylum Basidiomycota, and what was previously named phylum Zygomycota, for which sexual spores and their mode of production form the main basis for classification. Accepted fungal scientific names are published by the International Code of Nomenclature for Algae, Fungi, and Plants (ICN). Accepted scientific name databases can be seen at MycoBank (http://www.mycobank.org) and Species Fungorum (http://www.speciesfungorum.org). The phylum names and the type of sexual spore formed by its members are as follows:

1. Ascomycota (ascospores)
2. Basidiomycota (basidiospores)
3. Glomeromycota (zygospores)

Organisms previously assigned to the phylum Zygomycota have been divided among subphylum Mucormycotina and subphylum Entomophthoromycotina within the phylum Glomeromycota. Current fungal taxonomy and classification into phyla and subphyla is based on the mode of sexual reproduction and concordant multilocus DNA sequences. Asexual fungi with no known teleomorph phase, previously characterized as a separate formal group known as the Fungi Imperfecti, have been designated in the familiar phyla based on molecular phylogenetics. The taxonomic scheme depicted is based on various sources. The higher-level classification of kingdom Fungi was revised by Hibbett and colleagues in 2007.[4]

The basic taxonomic units are the species, and they are grouped into a hierarchical system that includes genera, families, orders, classes, and phyla. The categories may be subdivided (e.g., subphylum, subclass, suborder) to indicate degrees of relationship. Populations within a given species that have some characteristics in common may be set apart as tribes, varieties, or some other subset designation. Delineation of the zoopathogen *Ajellomyces capsulatus*, the teleomorph of *Histoplasma capsulatum*, is as follows:

Kingdom: Fungi
- Phylum: Ascomycota (includes 80% of the medically important fungi)
  - Class: Ascomycetes
    - Order: Onygenales
      - Family: Onygenaceae
        - Genus: Ajellomyces
          - Species: Ajellomyces capsulatus (anamorph: Histoplasma capsulatum)
            - Variety (applies to the anamorph):
              - *H. capsulatum* var. *capsulatum*
              - *H. capsulatum* var. *duboisii*
              - *H. capsulatum* var. *farciminosum*

This chapter includes taxa known to contain medically important fungi. Classes, orders, and families not known to contain pathogens are omitted. More detailed information can be obtained by consulting the references.

Kingdom: Fungi
- Phylum: Ascomycota (The teleomorph consists of ascospores borne in an ascus. The anamorph may be unicellular yeasts or multicellular molds. This group accounts for 50% of all described fungi and 80% of the medically important fungi. Molecular phylogeny studies have been used to define this group, even when a known teleomorph for a given anamorph has not been described.)
  - Subphylum: Saccharomycotina
    - Class: Saccharomycetes
      - Order: Saccharomycetales (Ascomata are absent, asci are formed singly or in chains, and yeast cells divide by budding or fission.)
        - Family: Saccharomycetaceae
          - Genus: *Candida*
            - *Debaryomyces* (teleomorph)
            - *Kluyveromyces* (teleomorph)

Pichia (teleomorph)
Clavispora (teleomorph)
Issatchenkia (teleomorph)
Saccharomyces (teleomorph)
Subphylum: Pezizomycotina (>90% of Ascomycota are mold species)
Class: Eurotiomycetes
Order: Onygenales (ascomata are cleistothecia)
Family: Arthrodermataceae (agents of tinea [ringworm])
Genus: *Arthroderma* (teleomorph)
Microsporum (anamorph)
Trichophyton (anamorph)
Epidermophyton (anamorph)
Chrysosporium (teleomorph)
Family: Onygenaceae (agents of endemic pulmonary mycoses)
Genus: *Coccidioides* (anamorph)
Family: Ajellomycetaceae
Genus: *Ajellomyces* (teleomorph)
Histoplasma (anamorph)
Blastomyces (anamorph)
Emmonsia (anamorph)
Paracoccidioides (anamorph)
Order: Chaetothyriales
Family: Herpotrichiellaceae (agents of phaeohyphomycoses and chromoblastomycoses)
Genus: *Capronia* (teleomorph)
Cladophialophora (anamorph)
Exophiala (anamorph)
Fonsecaea (anamorph)
Phialophora (anamorph)
Rhinocladiella (anamorph)
Order: Eurotiales (ascomata are cleistothecia)
Family: Trichocomaceae (contains the largest number of human pathogens)
Genus: *Aspergillus* (anamorph)
Penicillium (anamorph)
Talaromyces (teleomorph)
Emericella (teleomorph)
Eurotium (teleomorph)
Neosartorya (teleomorph).
Paecilomyces (anamorph)
Order: Ophiostomatales (ascomata are perithecia with long necks)
Family: Ophiostomaceae
Genus: *Ophiostoma* (teleomorph)
Sporothrix (anamorph)
Class: Sordariomycetes
Order: Hypocreales (ascomata are mostly perithecia)
Family: Hypocreaceae (contains agents of mycoses)
Genus: *Gibberella* (teleomorph)
Nectria (teleomorph)
Acremonium (anamorph)
Fusarium (anamorph)
Trichoderma (anamorph)
Order: Microascales (ascomata are cleistothecia or perithecia)
Family: Microascaceae
Genus: *Pseudallescheria* (teleomorph)
Scedosporium (anamorph)
Microascus (teleomorph)
Scopulariopsis (anamorph)
Order: Sordariales (ascomata are cleistothecia or perithecia; rarely pathogens; contains many of the teleomorphs of the anamorph genus *Fusarium)*
Class: Dothideomycetes
Order: Dothideales (ascomata are cleistothecia)
Family: Dothioraceae
Genus: *Aureobasidium* (anamorph)
Family: Teratosphaeriaceae
Genus: *Hortaea*
Family: Davidiellaceae
Genus: *Cladosporium* (anamorph)
Family: Piedraiaceae
Genus: *Piedraia* (teleomorph)
Order: Pleosporales
Family: Pleosporaceae
Genus: *Cochliobolus* (teleomorph)
Exserohilum (anamorph)
Setosphaeria (teleomorph)
Curvularia (anamorph)
Alternaria (anamorph)
Ulocladium (anamorph)
Lewia (teleomorph)
Class: Pneumocystidomycetes (found as trophozoites, cysts, and intracystic bodies; originally considered members of the kingdom Protozoa)
Order: Pneumocystidales
Family: Pneumocystidaceae
Genus: *Pneumocystis*
Phylum: Basidiomycota (Teleomorphs are basidium-bearing basidiospores; anamorphs are yeasts or molds. Arthroconidia are propagules of some molds.)
Class: Tremellomycetes
Order: Filobasidiales
Family: Filobasidiaceae
Genus: *Filobasidiella* (teleomorph)
Filobasidium (teleomorph)
Cryptococcus (anamorph)
Trichosporon (anamorph)
Magnusiomyces (teleomorph)
Class: Malasseziamycetes
Order: Malasseziales
Family: Malasseziaceae
Genus: *Malassezia* (anamorph)
Class: Agaricomycetes
Order: Agaricales
Family: Schizophyllaceae
Genus: *Schizophyllum*
Phylum: Glomeromycota (Teleomorphs consist of zygospores; anamorphs consist of sporangiospores within a sporangium.)
Subphylum: Mucormycotina
Order: Mucorales
Family: Cunninghamellaceae
Genus: *Cunninghamella*
Family: Lichtheimiaceae
Genus: *Lichtheimia*
Rhizomucor
Family: Mucoraceae
Genus: *Actinomucor*
Cokeromyces
Mucor
Family: Rhizopodaceae
Genus: *Rhizopus*
Family: Saksenaeaceae
Genus: *Apophysomyces*
Saksenaea
Family: Syncephalastraceae
Genus: *Syncephalastrum*
Subphylum: Entomophthoromycotina (formerly phylum Zygomycota)
Order: Entomophthorales (agents of entomophthoromycoses)
Family: Ancylistaceae
Genus: *Conidiobolus*
Order: Basidiobolales
Family: Basidiobolaceae
Genus: *Basidiobolus*
Phylum: Microsporidia (unicellular organisms that are obligate spore formers and intracellular parasites invading host cells)
Subphylum: Apansporoblastina
Family: Enterocytozoonidae
Genus: Entercytozoon

Family: Nosematidae
Genus: *Nosema*
Vittaforme
Family: Encephalitozoonidae
Genus: *Encephalitozoon*
Subphylum: Pansporoblastina
Family: Pleistophoridae
Genus: *Pleistophora*
Trachipleistophora

NEW REFERENCES SINCE THE SEVENTH EDITION

1. Bittinger K, Charlson ES, Loy E, et al. Improved characterization of medically relevant fungi in the human respiratory tract using next-generation sequencing. *Genome Biol.* 2014;15:487-500.
2. Corradi N, Keeling PJ. Microsporidia: a journey through radical taxonomical revisions. *Fungal Biol Rev.* 2009;23:1-8.
3. de Hoog GS, Chaturvedi V, Denning DW, et al. Name changes in medically important fungi and their implications in clinical practice. *J Clin Micribiol.* 2015;53:1056-1061.
4. Hibbett DS, Binder M, Bischoff JF, et al. A higher-level phylogenetic classification of the Fungi. *Mycol Res.* 2007;111:509-547.
5. Jorgensen JH, Pfaller MA, eds. *Manual of Clinical Microbiology.* 11th ed. Washington, DC: ASM Press; 2015.
6. Rossman AY. Lessons learned from moving to one scientific name for fungi. *IMA Fungus.* 2014;5:81-89.
7. Stielow JB, Levesque CA, Seifert KA, et al. One fungus, which genes? Development and assessment of universal primers for potential secondary fungal DNA barcodes. *Persoonia.* 2015;35:242-263.

198 Aspergillosis

William J. Steinbach

Aspergillus is a versatile organism that can cause a broad spectrum of disease, including invasive disease in profoundly immunocompromised patients, saprophytic disease in immunocompetent people, and allergic disease in atopic individuals. Invasive aspergillosis (IA) is the leading cause of death due to major invasive mycoses. The high incidence of IA likely reflects the increasing number of severely immunosuppressed patients, more intensive immunosuppressive therapies for graft-versus-host disease (GVHD) and rheumatologic diseases, increased use of mismatched or unrelated donor transplants, newer preparative regimens used to avoid rejection or relapse, and increases in early posttransplantation survival due to better control of bacterial and cytomegalovirus (CMV) infections.[143,241]

ORGANISM

Established by the Italian botanist Pier Antonio Micheli in 1729, the genus *Aspergillus* was created to accommodate an asexual fungus that produces spores (i.e., conidia) in chains or columns radiating from central structures. As a priest, Micheli recognized the resemblance of the spore-forming structures to that of the aspergillum, the liturgical instrument used to sprinkle holy water during the Catholic Mass and therefore applied the name *Aspergillus* to the fungus. More than 100 years later, *Aspergillus fumigatus*, the most important pathogenic species of the genus, was named by Fresenius because it looked like a puff of smoke.

The role of aspergilli in human disease was first recognized by Virchow in 1856.[237] Virchow noticed the similarity between the aspergilli described from cases of animal infections and those he had observed in human disease. IA was recognized by Rankin in 1953, when he reported disseminated aspergillosis in a patient with aplastic anemia.[187] For the subsequent 60 years, the number of cases of IA increased substantially due to a rise in the number of immunocompromised patients.

The genus *Aspergillus* is characterized by the formation of flask-shaped or cylindrical phialides in a single or double series on the surface of a vesicle at the apex of a conidiophore.[188] Conidia are deciduous and globose, oblong to elliptical, and various colors.

In 1926, Thom and Church assembled all available information on *Aspergillus* in a monograph.[221] In 1965, Raper and Fennell expanded this work by adding many new species and provided descriptions of the species classified into 18 informal groups.[188] In 1985, Gams and colleagues revised the groups and assigned them to 18 sections as a formal taxonomic status.[78] Currently, there are approximately 250 species assigned to 17 sections in the family Aspergillaceae,[100] and this number will continue to grow as new species are described.

Most human disease is primarily caused by *A. fumigatus*, *Aspergillus flavus*, *Aspergillus niger*, *Aspergillus terreus*, and *Aspergillus nidulans*. The classification of the genus *Aspergillus* has been revised from the original taxonomy to incorporate phenotype, morphology, and newer molecular approaches; consequently, the taxonomy remains dynamic.[195] *A. fumigatus* causes approximately 70% to 80% of cases of IA,[209] but it is difficult to differentiate from the other closely related species based solely on morphology. *A. fumigatus* is responsible for most pulmonary disease, and most isolated sinus disease is caused by *A. niger* and *A. flavus*.[182] Specific determination of the species of *Aspergillus* is clinically important for therapeutic reasons (e.g., antifungal resistance). For example, a review of *Aspergillus* cultures found that *A. terreus* was seen in only 3% of isolates in cases of IA, but it was found exclusively in cases of invasive disease (i.e., no cases of colonization).[182]

Aspergillus is a ubiquitous organism, but its ecologic niche is the soil, where it functions as a saprophytic fungus growing on organic debris and recycling carbon and nitrogen.[254] A classic sexual stage has been identified for *A. fumigates*,[170] but the clinical relevance is unclear. Asexual reproduction is abundant and characterized by the production of green-pigmented, echinulate, asexual conidia (i.e., spores). *Aspergillus* aerosolize conidia, which immunocompetent people asymptomatically breathe every day; most people inhale several hundred *A. fumigatus* conidia each day.[84] Infection in immunocompromised patients is usually acquired through inhalation of airborne conidia.

Two lines of host defense exist against *Aspergillus*—macrophages and neutrophils—and it appears that both are required for resistance to invasive disease. First-line defense is offered by alveolar macrophages, and in vitro murine studies have suggested that resident pulmonary macrophages are responsible for eliminating inhaled *Aspergillus* conidia from the lung.[198,199] If conidia escape this defense mechanism, they develop into invasive *Aspergillus* hyphae and become susceptible to neutrophil killing by the release of toxic reactive oxygen species. The host can develop disease because of neutropenia, high-challenge doses of conidia that overcome macrophages, or corticosteroid suppression of macrophage conidiacidal activity.[63]

A. fumigatus is particularly successful at causing invasive disease in immunocompromised patients due to characteristics such as thermotolerance, small and abundant pigmented conidia, fast growth rate, production of toxic secondary metabolites, and numerous enzymes involved in breaking down complex polysaccharides. The ability to grow at 37°C is crucial for the development of human disease. Although some *Aspergillus* species can grow at this high temperature, it has been reported that *A. fumigatus* can survive at temperatures up to 75°C, and this thermotolerance is likely a major factor in its ability to cause human disease.[23]

Conidia are 2.5 to 3 μm in diameter, and this small size allows them to remain buoyant in the air for prolonged periods and to be inhaled deep into the lung alveoli. When inhaled by an immunocompetent person, conidia rarely have deleterious effects because they are cleared by phagocytic cells of the innate immune system. However, severe allergic disease can occur with repeated exposure to large doses of conidia or in atopic individuals.

Pigments found on the conidial surface are thought to play important roles in mediating the effects of damaging reactive oxygen species produced by phagocytic cells.[185] Mutants of *A. fumigatus* that lack these conidial pigments are more susceptible to killing by alveolar macrophages than their pigmented counterparts.[125] Whole-genome sequencing of several *Aspergillus* species has revealed that the fungi contain large numbers of enzymes involved in degrading complex polysaccharides.[77] The enzymes allow *Aspergillus* species to be enormously successful as saprophytes and contribute to their ability to cause invasive disease.

Species of *Aspergillus* are known for their production of secondary metabolites, including aflatoxin, which is produced by some strains of *A. flavus.* Although aflatoxin is extremely carcinogenic, its role in the development of human mycoses has not been thoroughly examined. Various putative *Aspergillus* virulence factors have been exhaustively reviewed,[128] and earlier gene-disruption studies examined proteases, toxins, hemolysins, melanin pigmentation, and other gene products with little success. The virulence of *A. fumigatus* likely depends on a combination of many attributes.

CLINICAL PRESENTATIONS

Aspergillus species are uncommon among pathogens because they are responsible for a gamut of infections, including primary allergic reactions, saprophytic involvement, and invasive disease.[145] The type of *Aspergillus* infection typically depends on the immunologic background of the infected host. Immunodeficient patients develop invasive disease, and immunoreactive patients develop allergic disease. The most frequently encountered presentations involve the lungs, such as allergic bronchopulmonary aspergillosis (ABPA) and acute or chronic invasive pulmonary aspergillosis (IPA). Other common infections include invasive acute or chronic sinusitis, cutaneous aspergillosis, aspergilloma, and cerebral aspergillosis.[49,145] The clinical manifestations of these infections in immunocompromised patients can be subtle and nonspecific, and they commonly occur late in the course of disease. A high index of suspicion must be maintained to ensure treatment in the early stages of disease. Unfortunately, the patients most vulnerable to *Aspergillus* infections are the least likely to display significant symptoms, adding to the difficulty of diagnosis.[49]

Invasive Pulmonary Aspergillosis

Aspergillus species are ubiquitous in the environment, and a major portal of entry is the respiratory tract. In some immunocompetent patients, inhalation can result in nonpathogenic saprophytic colonization, but in the immunocompromised patient, conidial acquisition likely results in establishment of invasive disease.[224] IPA is the most frequently documented form of IA, and it contributes considerably to morbidity and mortality among high-risk patients.[53] In a systematic review of the literature regarding the case-fatality rate of aspergillosis, 70% of infections were found to be invasive pulmonary disease.[130]

As with other forms of *Aspergillus* infections, the burden of IPA is sustained by immunocompromised patients, including those who have undergone hematopoietic stem cell transplantation (HSCT), solid organ transplant (SOT) recipients, cancer patients, patients with various congenital immune deficiencies such as chronic granulomatous disease (CGD), and patients treated for autoimmune diseases with immune modifiers.[192]

The clinical manifestation of IPA is heterogeneous; it can include fever unresponsive to broad-spectrum antibiotics, dry cough, shortness of breath, pleuritic chest pain, hemoptysis, and pulmonary infiltrates on radiography.[7] Although neutropenic patients more commonly have fever at presentation, for about 20% of patients (i.e., those receiving high-dose corticosteroid therapy), fever and cough are not evident for the first several days of infection.[98,145] Disease often manifests as bilateral, diffuse pulmonary infection, and dyspnea is a common presentation for these patients. Progression of infection is characterized by invasion of small vessels that causes hemoptysis, a leading symptom of IPA in some neutropenic patients. Two patterns of hemorrhage may be identified: hemorrhagic infarction due to vascular invasion and formation of mycotic aneurysms during recovery from neutropenia, which can rupture and cause fatal hemoptysis.[159]

Although cancer patients undergoing treatment account for most of those at risk for *Aspergillus* infections, IPA is the leading cause of death for another, largely pediatric patient population with underlying chronic granulomatous disease (CGD). Patients with CGD have an estimated 33% lifetime risk of IA, and IPA can be the first manifestation of CGD. Whereas disease in most patient groups is caused by *A. fumigatus*, most cases of *A. nidulans* infection have affected patients with CGD.[40] In one review, *A. nidulans* occurred in six patients with CGD but did not occur in any other patient group.[202] Although *A. fumigatus* was more common than *A. nidulans* in CGD patients, infection with *A. nidulans* was significantly more likely to be refractory to antifungal therapy and result in dissemination and death.

In addition to the epidemiologic variations of specific *Aspergillus* species, the clinical presentations of patients with CGD can be different from those of neutropenic patients. Unlike the acute, rapidly progressive illness described for other immunocompromised patients, the clinical course of patients with CGD is characterized by an insidious onset of fatigue, fever, increased sedimentation rate, and pneumonia.[202] The diagnosis for a patient with CGD often does not contain typical clinical symptoms (including no symptoms) and may consist of only an elevated erythrocyte sedimentation rate in the setting of no fever. In early-stage disease, there is an acute neutrophilic response in which the neutrophils surround hyphae. However, in patients with CGD, the hyphae remain intact due to impaired neutrophil-mediated killing. In this setting, IPA in a patient with CGD is a chronic, progressive infection that can spread locally to involve pleura, vertebrae, and the chest wall.

Aspergillus osteomyelitis involving a rib, vertebra, or femur is a common presentation for patients with CGD, but it is not commonly seen in other patient populations.[65] Thoracic wall extension of pulmonary IA has been reported.[253] In a study of 24 cases of osteomyelitis caused by *Aspergillus* species in 22 CGD patients, 14 isolates (58%) were caused by *A. nidulans,* and 10 were caused by *A. fumigatus.*[66]

In contrast to patients with neutropenia, hyphal angioinvasion is not a feature of disease in patients with CGD. The halo sign (i.e., angioinvasion with surrounding tissue ischemia), cavitated lesions, and pulmonary infarcts are not typical in patients with IA and CGD.

Invasive Aspergillus Sinusitis

Fungal sinusitis can manifest as allergic, saprophytic, or invasive disease. Invasive *Aspergillus* sinusitis is likely underdiagnosed because of its variable clinical presentation and difficulty in establishing the diagnosis,[49,98,145] possibly due to a decreased inflammatory response in affected patients. Patients can have nasal congestion, discharge, headache, facial pain or swelling, and abnormal nasal cavity findings such as pallor of the nasal septum or turbinate mucosa. Patients also can have epistaxis, orbital swelling, and high fever.[161]

A definitive diagnosis can best be established by endoscopic evaluation and selective biopsy. Common findings on endoscopy include pallor of the mucosa, discoloration or granulation of the mucosa due to ischemia from angioinvasion, and as the disease progresses, a blackened necrotic focus can be found (Figs. 198.1 and 198.2). Extension into bony structures can occur at the site of necrosis, spreading disease into adjacent structures such as the orbit and the brain, which carries a high mortality rate.

Although imaging is not diagnostic, it can aid in establishing the diagnosis because it can be used as a roadmap for endoscopy by identifying the involved sinuses (Fig. 198.3). In a review of 25 patients with rhinosinusitis, 44% showed evidence of invasion beyond the sinus cavities

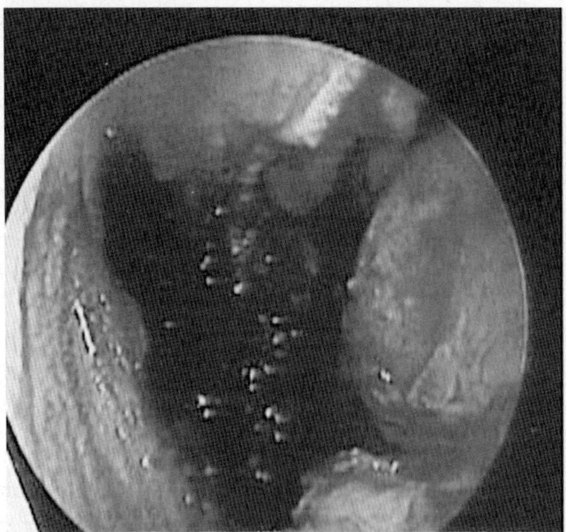
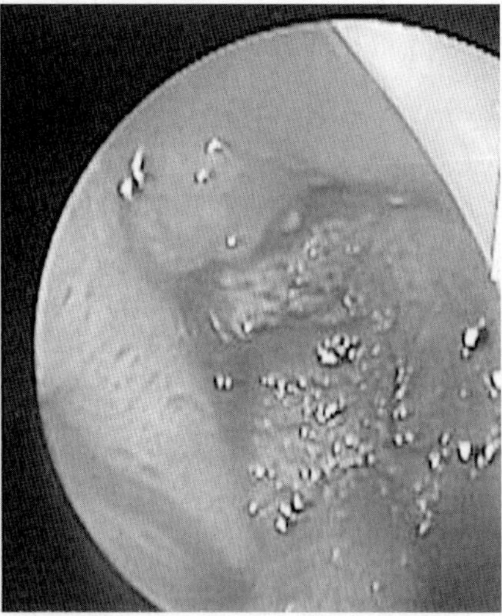

FIG. 198.1 A 12-year-old with acute myelogenous leukemia and unrelated cord blood transplant developed *A. fumigatus* sinusitis. Endoscopy shows classic pale mucosa.

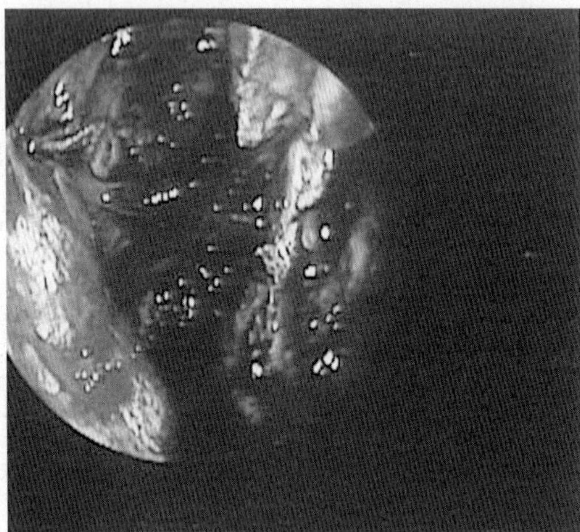
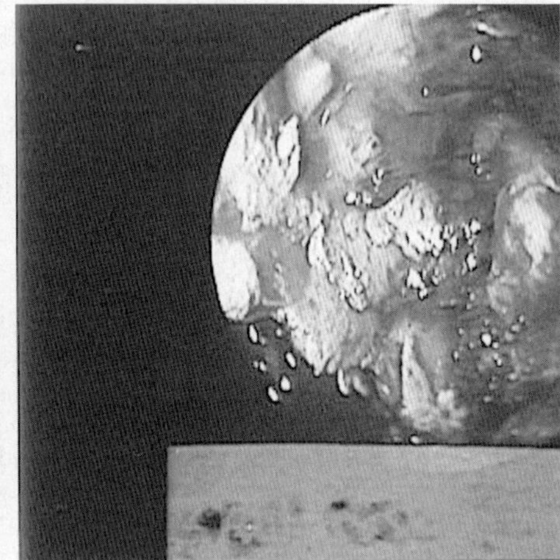

FIG. 198.2 In the same patient as in Fig. 198.1, endoscopy shows necrotic mucosa at the basilar skull area.

on computed tomography (CT).[82] In the same study, however, 12% of patients had negative CT scans, emphasizing the need for physicians to have a high index of clinical suspicion in making the diagnosis to ensure the best outcome.

Cerebral Aspergillosis

Aspergillus infections most commonly involve the lungs, but disease can disseminate through the bloodstream and involve distant organs. The central nervous system (CNS) is a common site of dissemination.[87] Cerebral aspergillosis may result from direct extension through the sinuses. Studies have estimated that CNS aspergillosis may be found in 40% to 50% of patients with IA and acute leukemia or allogeneic HSCT.[105,197] As with other *Aspergillus* infections, *A. fumigatus* is the most frequently encountered species in cerebral aspergillosis, although *A. flavus*, *A. niger*, and *A. nidulans* also have been implicated.[106]

The clinical presentation often does not include classic symptoms for an intracranial process such as headache, nausea, or vomiting. Patients instead have mental status alterations, convulsions, hemiplegia or hemiparesis, ophthalmoplegia, and loss of consciousness. Severely immunocompromised patients may not display these symptoms, and disease progresses more rapidly.

Aspergillus hyphae are angioinvasive and thrombose arteries to create hemorrhagic infarcts. CNS aspergillosis can manifest as solitary or multiple abscesses or, less commonly, as mycotic aneurysms and carotid artery invasion. Cerebral aspergillosis can also appear as meningitis or granuloma.[106] Cerebral aspergillosis is seen as multiple areas of low density and no enhancement even with contrast on CT, and lesions are usually located within the basal ganglia and gray-white matter junction. On magnetic resonance imaging (MRI), these abnormalities appear as foci of an intermediate T2-weighted signal surrounded by a rim of higher signal intensity.[171,223]

Because aspergillosis of the CNS carries a case-fatality rate of almost 90% [130] prompt diagnosis and treatment are key to survival. Unfortunately, a definitive diagnosis requires biopsy, and these patients typically are too coagulopathic to undergo the procedure.

Cutaneous Aspergillosis

Neonates, burn victims, HSCT recipients, SOT recipients, and other immunocompromised patients most frequently develop cutaneous aspergillosis. Cutaneous *Aspergillus* infection has a reported incidence between 4% and 11%.[48,248]

Cutaneous aspergillosis can be primary, as is more often seen in children as a result of skin injury or traumatic inoculation, or secondary, occurring as hematogenous spread or extension from infected underlying structures.[228] Primary cutaneous aspergillosis has been associated with intravenous access devices, adhesive dressings, and sites of burns or surgery. Although cutaneous aspergillosis is rare, premature infants are at particular risk because their skin is immature and vulnerable. HSCT recipients usually develop disease as a result of secondary hematogenous seeding from a primary source, usually the lungs.

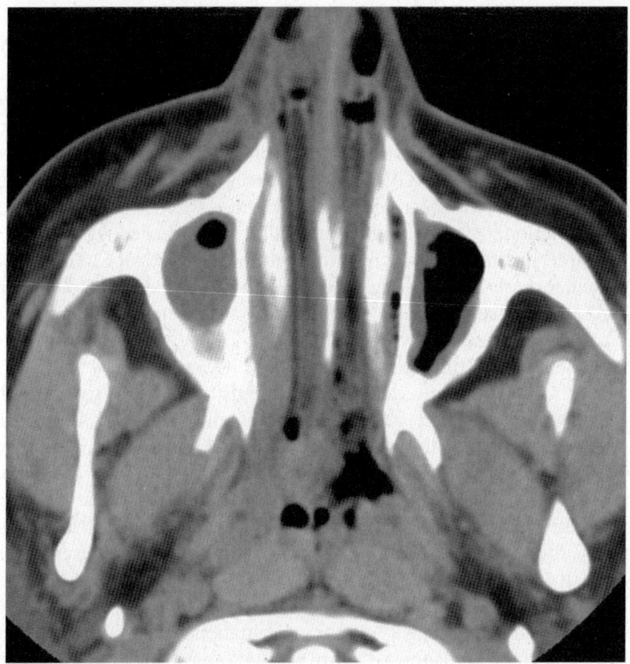

FIG. 198.3 In the same patient as in Figs. 198.1 and 198.2, computed tomography shows complete opacification of the right maxillary sinus.

Lesions often begin as erythematous, indurated papules that progress to ulcerative, painful, and necrotic lesions.[213] Treatment involves debridement and excision of necrotic tissue, which provides diagnostic material, and the use of systemic intravenous antifungals and topical preparations. Because cutaneous aspergillosis often heralds underlying, undiagnosed systemic disease, relying on topical antifungal coverage alone is likely inadequate.

Chronic Aspergillosis

Chronic aspergillosis is an important and distinct entity from IA. It typically affects immunocompetent or less immunocompromised patients, although some degree of immune suppression usually exists, and exposure to corticosteroids is common. Patients often have underlying pulmonary disease, such as cavitary tuberculosis, sarcoidosis, emphysema, or fibrotic lung disease.

The 2016 clinical guidelines for chronic pulmonary aspergillosis include consensus approaches to diagnosis and management.[51] Five categories are used to describe chronic pulmonary aspergillosis, and each has significantly overlapping clinical features: aspergilloma, chronic cavitary pulmonary aspergillosis (CCPA), chronic fibrosing pulmonary aspergillosis (CFPA), *Aspergillus* nodule, and subacute IA, which was previously called chronic necrotizing or semi-IA.

Diagnosis of chronic pulmonary aspergillosis requires a specific appearance in thoracic imaging (preferably CT), direct evidence of *Aspergillus* infection or an immunologic response to *Aspergillus*, exclusion of alternative diagnoses, and disease lasting for at least 3 months. If a fungal ball is observed, diagnosis requires only a positive assay for *Aspergillus* immunoglobulin G (IgG) or precipitins or the finding of *Aspergillus* in a bronchoscopic specimen. Due to the ubiquitous nature of *Aspergillus*, a positive sputum culture alone is not diagnostic.

Aspergillomas consist of a mass of tangled hyphae, cellular debris, fibrin, and few inflammatory cells. They develop as a complication of existing cavitary lesions and are typically found in the upper lobes, where there is poor drainage.[145,224] The cavitary lesions can be caused by tuberculosis infection, sarcoidosis, bullous emphysema, and other diseases associated with cavitary lung lesions. *A. fumigatus* typically causes pulmonary aspergilloma. Although some patients remain asymptomatic, many have recurrent hemoptysis. The earliest radiographic sign is pleural thickening of a preexisting lung cavity. As the fungal ball develops, CT or plain radiography shows a solid, round, radiolucent intracavitary mass that is separated from the thickened wall by a crescenteric volume of air (i.e., air crescent sign).[86]

Aspergilloma is a late manifestation, formed by the collapse of the fungal growth inside the cavity. Aspergillomas are designated as simple or complex based on radiologic criteria. The simple aspergilloma is a single cavity containing a fungal ball. Simple aspergillomas lack constitutional symptoms, paracystic lung opacities, cyst expansion, and progressive pleural thickening.[113] Serologic or microbiologic evidence implicates *Aspergillus* in immunocompetent patients with minor or no symptoms and no radiologic progression during at least 3 months of observation.

CCPA, previously called complex aspergilloma, is the most common form of chronic pulmonary aspergillosis. Multiple pulmonary cavities form and expand, and they may or may not contain solid or liquid material or a fungal ball. A positive *Aspergillus* IgG antibody test or microbiologic evidence implicates *Aspergillus* spp. as the cause. To meet the diagnostic criteria, significant pulmonary or systemic symptoms and overt radiographic progression (i.e., new cavities, increasing pericavitary infiltrates, or increasing pleural thickening) should be observed over at least 3 months. Left untreated, the cavities enlarge and coalesce.

A fungal ball seen on chest imaging supports the diagnosis of chronic pulmonary aspergillosis in the form of a single aspergilloma or CCPA. Confirmation is provided by *Aspergillus* IgG testing,[20,174] and the two forms are differentiated on the basis of symptoms and radiologic appearance. However, most CCPA patients do not have a fungal ball but instead have multiple empty cavities or cavities with an irregular internal wall with associated pleural thickening and pericavitary infiltrates. Most patients have negative results for sputum cultures. *Aspergillus* polymerase chain reaction (PCR) is more sensitive,[55] and bronchoalveolar lavage galactomannan (GM) testing is preferred over serum GM evaluation for diagnosis.[51] Biopsy of the wall of a cavity in cases of CCPA yields chronic inflammatory cells and fibrosis, sometimes with granulomas. Hyphae consistent with *Aspergillus* spp. are usually seen adjacent to the cavity wall, but they are not invasive. Percutaneous aspiration of a cavity with a positive *Aspergillus* culture is an alternative means of establishing the diagnosis. More than 50% of patients have an increased total and *Aspergillus*-specific IgE titer, and eosinophilia may be detected.[27]

CFPA, which is characterized by progression of the cavities to extensive pulmonary fibrosis is an end-stage complication of CCPA. It is severe fibrotic destruction of at least two lobes of the lung that complicates CCPA and causes major loss of lung function. Fibrosis usually manifests as a consolidation on imaging, but large cavities with surrounding fibrosis may be seen. Thoracic imaging usually shows one or more *Aspergillus* nodules (<3 cm in diameter) that do not cavitate. Tissue invasion is lacking, but necrosis may be seen.

Subacute IA was previously called chronic necrotizing pulmonary aspergillosis (CNPA), subacute IPA, or semi-IPA. It is an indolent pulmonary infection of patients with mild or moderate immune dysfunction, such as after prolonged corticosteroid use or after resolution of neutropenia.[145] Subacute IA is more progressive than CCPA

Clinical signs of subacute IA include cough, fever, fatigue, and weight loss. At presentation, patients often have pulmonary and general symptoms. Hemoptysis, shortness of breath, and productive cough are typical, but fever and chest pain are uncommon.[27] Patients are often mistakenly thought to have tuberculosis.

Allergic Bronchopulmonary Aspergillosis

ABPA occurs in asthmatic and cystic fibrosis (CF) patients. It is a pulmonary disease caused by type I and III hypersensitivity reactions to *A. fumigatus* allergens. Exposure and inhalation of *Aspergillus* conidia results in saprophytic (noninvasive) colonization of the bronchial airways, which triggers an IgE-mediated allergic inflammatory response. Over time, bronchial obstruction takes place, and patients develop productive cough, wheezing, and chest pain. Fever and malaise are other presenting symptoms.[214]

Diagnosis is based on eight primary criteria: history of bronchial obstruction (e.g., asthma), peripheral blood eosinophilia, elevated total serum IgE levels, serum IgE antibodies specific to *A. fumigatus*, immediate (type I) skin test reactivity to *Aspergillus* antigen, serum precipitin (specific IgG) antibodies to *A. fumigatus*, pulmonary infiltrates, and central bronchiectasis, often with peripheral tapering of the bronchi. The 2016 international consensus–proposed revised diagnostic criteria for ABPA included a predisposing condition (i.e., bronchial asthma or CF) and two obligatory criteria: a type I *Aspergillus* skin test positive result or elevated IgE levels against *A. fumigatus* and an elevated total IgE level. Two of three other required criteria include precipitating or IgG antibodies against *A. fumigatus* in serum, radiographic pulmonary opacities consistent with ABPA, and a total eosinophil count greater than 500 cells/μL in a steroid-naive patient.[51]

Radiologically, ABPA is characterized by bronchial wall thickening, pulmonary infiltrates, and central bronchiectasis, a result of the type III hypersensitivity reaction.[145,224] The diagnosis of ABPA in CF patients is difficult because many of the diagnostic criteria overlap with common manifestations of CF. In asthmatic patients, ABPA manifests as poorly controlled asthma, pneumonia that represents mucoid impaction, persistent eosinophilia, and bronchiectasis or with chronic pulmonary aspergillosis and lung fibrosis. In CF patients, ABPA manifests as exacerbations that are difficult to control.

EPIDEMIOLOGY

Aspergillus is ubiquitous in the environment. *Aspergillus* species are estimated to be responsible for more than 200,000 cases of IA annually, and global burdens suggest that more than 1.2 million patients have chronic pulmonary aspergillosis and 4.8 million patients suffer from ABPA.[50,56]

Those at risk for IA include patients with prolonged neutropenia, HSCT recipients, SOT recipients, patients receiving corticosteroids or other immune modifiers, and patients with CGD. In patients with hematologic malignancies, myelodysplastic syndrome, and other diseases associated with marrow failure (e.g., aplastic anemia), the intensity and duration of neutropenia predict the risk of IA.[81,251] Patients with refractory or relapsed acute leukemia treated with reinduction regimens are at particularly high risk for IA. In SOT recipients, the intensity of immunosuppression to prevent or treat allograft rejection, colonization, and coinfection with CMV influence the risk of IA. Lung transplant recipients have one of the highest risks of IA,[163,175] and one half of these cases of IA occur 1 year or more after transplantation.[64] Pretransplantation *Aspergillus* airway colonization is common among CF patients, and it increases the risk of IA after lung transplantation.[132]

IA also has been recognized in critically ill patients without traditional risk factors. One retrospective analysis[151] identified 127 patients of 1850 (6.9%) admitted to the intensive care unit (ICU) with evidence of *Aspergillus* infection; however, only 5 of these patients had proven IA without predisposing host factors. Nonclassic factors include chronic obstructive pulmonary disease (COPD) and cirrhosis,[24,150] and IA can follow other major infections, including influenza.[127,250]

IA was the most common invasive mold infection in a review of approximately 5500 patients who underwent HSCT; among the more than 7% of HSCT recipients who had mold infections, *Aspergillus* infections were the most common, followed by *Fusarium*, Zygomycetes, and *Scedosporium* infections.[143] The incidence of *Aspergillus* infection among HSCT recipients is 3% to 7%,[153,255] but the true incidence likely depends on many factors. In one study of HSCT recipients with IA, the risk of developing the disease was 12.8 times higher among recipients of allogeneic than autologous HSCT.[167] A retrospective review of 409 patients showed that 13.1% had IA, which represented 17.2% of all isolated pathogens for allogeneic transplant recipients and 3.8% for autologous transplant recipients.[120]

Allogeneic HSCT recipients have three periods of risk for IA: neutropenia after the conditioning regimen, exogenous immunosuppression for treatment of acute GVHD, and exogenous immunosuppression for treatment of chronic GVHD (i.e., day 100+ after transplantation). The level of allogeneic donor and recipient human leukocyte antigen (HLA) disparity is the major determinant for GVHD severity and intensity of immunosuppression needed to control GVHD, which is the major predisposing factor for IA. T-cell–depleted or CD34-selected stem cell products can increase the risk of IA.[142,227]

The well-characterized bimodal distribution of aspergillosis among HSCT recipients correlates with pre-engraftment neutropenia (median, 16 days after transplantation) and the peak of GVHD (median, 96 days after transplantation).[239] This distribution likely reflects the two major mechanisms of protection against IA: alveolar macrophages and granulocytes. Most patients (86%) with autologous transplants were diagnosed with IA while neutropenic, whereas patients with allogeneic transplants were at greatest risk after engraftment or during impairment of cell-mediated immunity due to CMV or GVHD.[239] In large reviews of patients undergoing allogeneic HSCT, the mean time to IA diagnosis was 88 to 115 days after transplantation,[147,167,191,197] and the mortality rate exceeded 80%.

A large, prospective French study analyzed 424 cases of IA and found an incidence of 0.9% among autologous and 8.1% among allogeneic HSCT patients, respectively,[131] highlighting a consistent finding that IA occurs much more readily in allogeneic HSCT recipients. Among SOT recipients with IA, the highest incidence of IA was for heart transplant recipients (4.8%), followed by lung recipients (4.1%), and significantly dropping for liver (0.8%) and kidney recipients (0.3%). These findings have been consistent in most larger studies. However, most patients with IA had a hematologic malignancy. The largest group had acute leukemia (35%), and the second largest group had chronic lymphoproliferative disorders (22%). For those with acute leukemia, IA occurred in 68% during the induction phase of chemotherapy, when the cytotoxic agents used typically are most intense, and in 27% during the consolidation phase.

The time to developing IA after transplantation was similar in different settings, with 68% diagnosed more than 100 days after HSCT and 18 of 27 SOT recipients with IA diagnosed at least 100 days after transplantation. Multivariate analysis showed factors independently associated with increased risk of death included older age, diagnosis based on positive culture with two positive GM assays, and pleural effusion or CNS involvement. The mortality rate for patients with acute leukemia was 38%, and allogeneic HSCT recipients had a staggering 56% overall mortality rate.

The Transplant-Associated Infection Surveillance Network (TRANSNET) study sponsored by the Centers for Disease Control and Prevention evaluated HSCT and SOT recipients from 23 US medical centers (2001–05) and included assessment of a total of 642 cases of IA.[15] The 12-month cumulative incidence of IA for all HSCT recipients was 1.6%, compared with 0.63% for SOT recipients. The 12-week all-cause mortality rate was 57.5% for HSCT recipients and 34.4% for SOT recipients. Multivariable analysis demonstrated that neutropenia, renal insufficiency, hepatic insufficiency, early onset (<30 days) IA, proven IA, and methylprednisolone use (often for GVHD) were independently associated with mortality. Analysis for SOT recipients revealed that hepatic insufficiency, malnutrition, and CNS disease were independently associated with an increased risk of death. Among HSCT and SOT recipients, receipt of voriconazole as part of the initial antifungal therapy was more common among survivors.

A TRANSNET study focused on only the 875 HSCT recipients found IA was the most common (43%) of all invasive fungal infections, followed by invasive candidiasis (28%).[118] The median time of developing IA after HSCT was 99 days. Of the 80 cases of IA in autologous HSCT, 50% occurred within 1 month after receipt of transplant, whereas among allogeneic HSCT recipients, only 22% of cases occurred within 1 month after transplantation. Autologous HSCT recipients had an all-cause mortality rate of 13% at 12 months, and allogeneic recipients had a rate of 36% at 12 months after transplantation. The 12-month cumulative incidence for IA for all HSCT recipients was 1.6%, compared with 1.1% for invasive candidiasis, and the overall 1-year survival rate for HSCT recipients with IA was only 25.4%.

Another large database, the Prospective Antifungal Therapy (PATH) Alliance, also found IA was most common among HSCT recipients, and approximately 70% of the HSCT recipients with IA had undergone allogeneic transplantation. The median time for development of IA after HSCT was similar (82 days), with a diagnosis at a median of 51 days after autologous transplantation and 83 days after allogeneic transplantation.[164] Another study of HSCT recipients found the prognostic factors at diagnosis that strongly correlated with death due to IA were dissemination of IA, pleural effusion, low monocyte count, corticosteroids within the previous 2 months and receipt of a dose of 2 mg/kg or more at the time of diagnosis, and uncontrolled GVHD.[43]

The TRANSNET database also analyzed all invasive fungal infections among SOT recipients and found that IA (19%) in this population was the second most common invasive fungal infection (unlike HSCT recipients) and invasive candidiasis (53%) was more common in SOT recipients.[175] The median time to onset of IA was 184 days after SOT transplantation, with a 1-year incidence of developing IA of 0.65% and a 12-month survival rate of 59%. The PATH Alliance analysis of SOT found that the likelihood of developing IA (25%) was second to that of invasive candidiasis but that IA was more common among lung transplant recipients (60%).[163] IA developed a median of 400 days after transplantation (including a median of 100 days after liver transplantation, 504 days after lung transplantation, and 384 days after heart transplantation). Most cases of IA among liver transplant recipients occurred less than 6 months after transplantation, whereas 62% of lung transplant recipients with IA developed the disease longer than 1 year after transplantation.

These findings contrasted with some of the results of a retrospective review of 158 cases of IA in Spanish SOT recipients, which found that 57% had early-onset IA (within 3 months after transplantation), but the mean time to development of IA was still 234 days.[79] The overall incidence of IA among their SOT recipients was 1.4%, with a similar distribution among specific organ transplant recipients, including an incidence of 3% for lung, 2.4% for heart, 2% for liver, and 0.2% for kidney transplantation. The overall mortality rate was 77%, with no significant differences found between SOT groups. Risk factors for developing early-onset IA included a complicated postoperative period, repeated bacterial infections or CMV disease, and renal failure.

One study found that 59% of patients with IA had neutropenia as risk factor, most of whom had hematologic or solid malignancies. Among the 41% of nonneutropenic patients, most had steroid-treated COPD, asthma, or rheumatologic disorders. Compared with neutropenic patients, the nonneutropenic patients were significantly less likely to have symptoms of IA and more likely to have frequent episodes of intercurrent pneumonia with another microorganism. The mortality rate was significantly higher among nonneutropenic (89%) compared with neutropenic patients (60%) with IA,[47] but the sensitivity of GM antigenemia was similar (approximately 65%) for neutropenic and nonneutropenic patients.

The risk of IA is expected to increase from 1% per day after the first 3 weeks of neutropenia to between 4% and 5% per day after 5 weeks,[201] with a 70% incidence after neutropenia exceeds 34 days.[81] Prolonged or marked macrophage dysfunctions that occur as a result of underlying disease and its treatment can also predispose patients to IA. Risk of infection is higher with advanced underlying disease, transplantation during relapse of malignancy or chemotherapeutic rescue therapy, GVHD, or concurrent infection such as CMV.[201] In a survey of 24 medical centers and 148 IA patients, 30% also had a bacterial infection, 20% had a viral infection, and 19% had another fungal infection.[182]

Corticosteroids are a major risk factor for the development of IA. They can suppress the ability of monocytes and macrophages to kill conidia through inhibition of nonoxidative processes and impairment of lysosomal activity. Corticosteroids also inhibit polymorphonuclear neutrophils in chemotaxis, oxidative bursts, and activity against hyphae.[68] Corticosteroids suppress macrophages, and cytotoxic chemotherapy decreases neutrophil number and function. Corticosteroids also greatly accelerate the growth of *A. fumigatus*, in one study decreasing the doubling time to 48 minutes.[165]

In several studies of HSCT patient risk factors, only moderate to severe GVHD and steroid prophylaxis for GVHD[21,147,191,257] or total-body irradiation[257] were significant variables in the multivariate analyses. In one study, the parameters found to influence survival in the period from HSCT to diagnosis of fungal infection were related to the cumulative dose of prednisolone. In the multivariate analysis, there was a relative risk (RR) of 8.78 of death from IA for patients with acute, active GVHD (i.e., grade 2 or higher) or extensive, chronic GVHD combined with a cumulative total prednisolone dose of more than 7 mg/kg in the 1 week before diagnosis.[191]

There is little specific information on the fundamental epidemiology of pediatric IA, and most epidemiologic investigations do not offer pediatric analyses.[46,76,120,257] One study found that the highest incidence of IA was seen among children who had undergone allogeneic HSCT (4.5%) and those with acute myelogenous leukemia (AML) (4%). The incidence of IA among patients with AML was significantly greater than the incidence among patients with acute lymphoblastic leukemia (ALL) (RR, 5.6; 95% confidence interval [CI], 4.6–7.0).[258]

The largest detailed analysis was a retrospective multicenter study of 139 children with IA. *A. fumigatus* was the species most frequently recovered (52.8%), and most children had a malignancy with or without HSCT. Significant risk factors that affected survival were immunosuppressive therapies and allogeneic HSCT.[32] Analysis of a large US pediatric inpatient database found an annual incidence of 0.4% of IA among immunocompromised children, and most had an underlying malignancy.[258] The incidence of IA was 4.5% among children who underwent allogeneic HSCT, 4% among patients with AML, and 0.3% for those who underwent autologous HSCT. Lung transplant recipients had the greatest incidence (5%) of IA among pediatric SOT recipients. Children with CGD had an incidence of 6.5%, and those with Wiskott-Aldrich syndrome ($n = 267$) had a staggering incidence of 30%. For pediatric patients with specific underlying diseases with or without IA revealed, the RR of death was increased for CNS tumors (RR, 21.6), ALL (RR, 14.9), and lymphoma (RR, 13.5), showcasing the overall good survival rates of those with common pediatric malignancies and the devastating effect of adding IA to reasonably curable underlying pediatric malignancies.

The largest international, prospective cohort study on invasive mold infections in children (2007–11)[249] included a total of 131 children and 98 (75%) with IA. Children with IA and those with other types of invasive mold infections had similar underlying risk factors, except that children with infections caused by non-*Aspergillus* species were more likely to have received mold-active antifungal agents preceding diagnosis. Among 43 patients who underwent HSCT, 27 (63%) underwent myeloablative conditioning. Of the 36 HSCT recipients who had complete information regarding timing of an invasive mold infection diagnosis from transplantation, five(14%) were diagnosed before or on the day of HSCT, and 31 (86%) were diagnosed at a median of 168 days after HSCT (interquartile range [IQR], 25–247). The distribution of the intervals from HSCT to invasive mold infection diagnosis was approximately bimodal, with 11 invasive mold infections diagnosed within the first 30 days and 2 diagnosed between 30 and 90 days.

DIAGNOSIS

The diagnosis of IA is often complicated. Due to myriad clinical manifestations, IA is categorized as proven, probable, or possible disease based on meeting certain clinical, microbiologic, and radiologic criteria designed and later revised by the European Organization for the Research and Treatment of Cancer and the Mycoses Study Group (EORTC/MSG).[12,59] These criteria have served as a standard in clinical trials to segregate patients with similar disease characteristics, but the criteria are not perfect, and the designers have cautioned against their implementation in routine clinical practice. Nonetheless, these distinctions have served the community well by establishing a common framework for discussion about disease in high-risk patients. Proven and probable IA diagnoses can be considered as one entity because numerous clinical trials have shown their general equivalency in patient outcomes.

Cultures

A proven diagnosis of IA requires isolation from an otherwise sterile culture and histologic demonstration (Fig. 198.4).[59] No histopathologic finding can definitively diagnose the pathogen, and confirmation by culture or nonculture techniques is necessary to differentiate *Aspergillus* from other filamentous fungi such as *Fusarium* spp. and *Scedosporium* spp. Unfortunately, this gold standard of tissue biopsy is often considered too invasive and is complicated by bleeding or secondary infection in high-risk patients.

An important distinction for a positive *Aspergillus* culture must be made between disease and colonization. A 1-year retrospective study found that only 12% of patients with *Aspergillus*-positive cultures met the criteria for IA. A positive culture was associated with IA in 50% to 65% of high-risk patients, 8% to 28% of intermediate-risk patients, and almost no low-risk patients.[182]

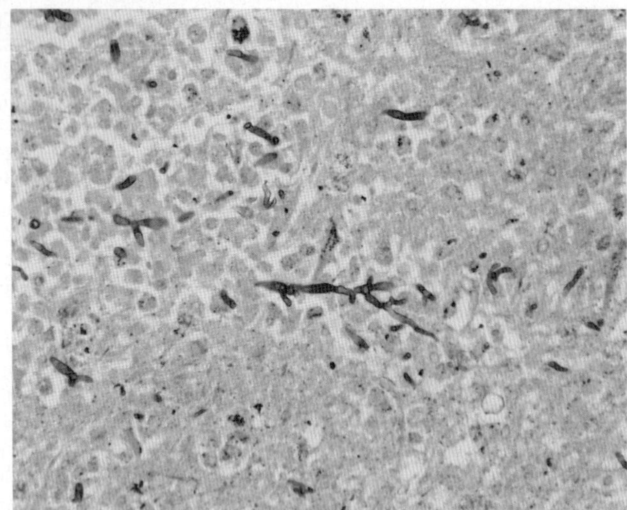

FIG. 198.4 Histopathologic findings of a lung biopsy show septate hyphae of invasive aspergillosis on Gomori methenamine silver stain. (Courtesy Thomas J Cummings, MD, Duke University Medical Center Pathology Department, Durham, NC.)

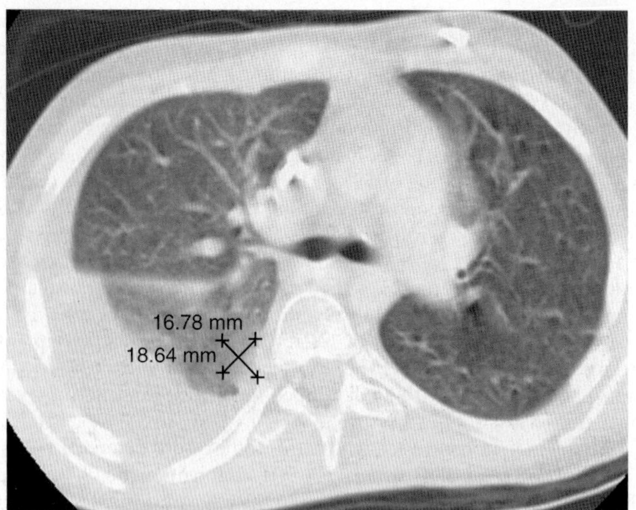

FIG. 198.5 In a 15-year-old adolescent with Schwachman-Diamond syndrome and acute myelogenous leukemia, computed tomography shows right lower lobe pulmonary nodules and a pleural effusion.

In one study, the predictive value of respiratory tract cultures from patients with IPA was 40% to 100%.[225] Even in patients with established disease the sputum specimens are commonly negative,[98,194] which is likely because IPA is predominantly infiltrative and does not have aerial growth in the bronchial tree.[98] Colonization with *Aspergillus* species has been a marker for reduced short-term survival because 12% of colonized patients died within 3 months of diagnosis. IPA was diagnosed in 12% of patients with a positive culture, but this figure is likely an underestimate because diagnosis was often made by radiographic imaging and culture specimens were not always obtained.[182]

During a 10-year period in one study, *Aspergillus* species were recovered during 30 episodes from 27 heart transplant recipients (incidence of 10.5%). The overall positive predictive value was 60% to 70%, but it increased to 88% to 100% when the organism was recovered from a respiratory specimen other than sputum and decreased to 50% to 67% when it was recovered from sputum. The sensitivities of fungal and conventional media for the recovery of *Aspergillus* species were 95% to 100% and 33% to 38%, respectively.[160]

Prior nasal colonization before transplantation has been a predictor of subsequent IPA in some studies,[3] but it has not been duplicated in others.[108] Prior IA does not eliminate the chance of a successful HSCT. In one study, there were recurrences in nine patients with IA before transplantation, and all patients showed no signs of delayed engraftment compared with transplant recipients without a history of IA.[203]

IA is rarely diagnosed by blood culture.[83] In a study of 1477 separate positive cultures, there were more than a dozen positive blood cultures, but most were associated with pseudofungemia or terminal events observed at autopsy.[182] The *Aspergillus* hyphal mass that develops in the lumen during angioinvasion typically remains in place until the force of blood flow causes hyphal breakage, which allows the mass to circulate. The likelihood of a blood culture capturing these irregularly and infrequently discharged units is small.

The difficulty in detecting *A. fumigatus* in blood culture contrasts with other angioinvasive filamentous fungi (e.g., *Fusarium* spp., *Paecilomyces lilacinus, Scedosporium prolificans, Acremonium* spp.), which have the ability to discharge a steady series of unicellular spores into the bloodstream and are more likely to be captured in a blood sample. This ability to sporulate in tissue and blood is called *adventitious sporulation*.[200] Because *A. terreus* also displays adventitious sporulation, histopathology and KOH examination of these spores can allow rapid, presumptive identification of *A. terreus*. A blood culture positive for *A. terreus* or another mold that demonstrates adventitious sporulation should not be ignored, and a blood culture positive for other *Aspergillus* species should be further evaluated.

Radiology

IPA characteristically manifests on radiographs as multiple, ill-defined, 1- to 3-cm peripheral nodules that gradually coalesce into larger masses or areas of subsegmental and segmental consolidation. Lobar or diffuse pulmonary consolidation is a common finding.[41] Chest radiographs can be abnormal, but in one series, they were normal for approximately 30% of patients in the week preceding death.[190]

There are two classic radiologic signs of IPA. The halo sign is observed in neutropenic patients with a hemorrhagic nodule due to angioinvasion. An early CT finding of the halo sign is a rim of ground-glass opacity surrounding the nodule. In one study, the halo sign was seen in all patients with biopsy-proven IPA, but it is so nonspecific that it was also seen in patients with mucormycosis, organizing pneumonia, or pulmonary hemorrhage.[256]

Early lesions change into a cavitary lesion or lesion with an air crescent sign 2 to 3 weeks later, when neutropenia recovers.[41,121] In one study, this was seen in 48% of patients 3 to 10 days after recovery of neutropenia.[197] Cavitation of the nodules or masses occurs in about 40% of patients and is characterized by an intracavitary mass composed of sloughed lung and a surrounding rim of air. A retrospective review of the CT finding for 47 autopsy-proven cases of IPA showed that nodular lesions and cavitation occurred significantly more often compared with controls.[91]

Just as the clinical presentation is nonspecific and heterogeneous, so are the findings in radiologic studies (Figs. 198.5 and 198.6). In most patients, disease is seen as round infiltrates, peripheral wedge-shaped lesions, and the typical halo sign early in the course of IPA during the neutropenic period, but in patients with CGD, hyphal angioinvasion is not a feature of disease, and the halo sign, cavitated lesions, and pulmonary infarcts therefore are not observed (Fig. 198.7). Instead, there are areas of tissue destruction due to acute and granulomatous inflammatory processes.[156]

Long-term CT follow-up of 40 immunocompromised patients with IPA showed that formation of cavitation most strongly predicted the time until radiologic remission and beneficial outcome. The natural history of early IPA lesions was evaluated, and it was found that 90% of patients had an increase in lesion size and number, followed by a plateau in size and a decrease in number. Lesion cavitation developed in 55% of patients, and complete radiologic remission within a median of 80 days was observed in 42.5% of patients. The number of days until remission without cavitation (50 days) was less than for those with cavitation (95 days), and no cavitation strongly predicted radiologic remission.[30]

In another study, the appearance of the air crescent sign had no relation to duration of neutropenia, and the sign had a tendency to

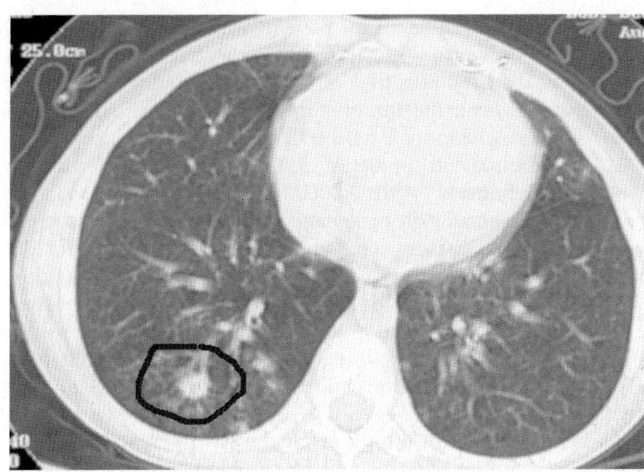

FIG. 198.6 In an 11-year-old child with cystic fibrosis after bilateral lung transplantation, computed tomography shows bibasilar nodular opacities. Encircled is a 1-cm opacity associated with some peripheral speculation.

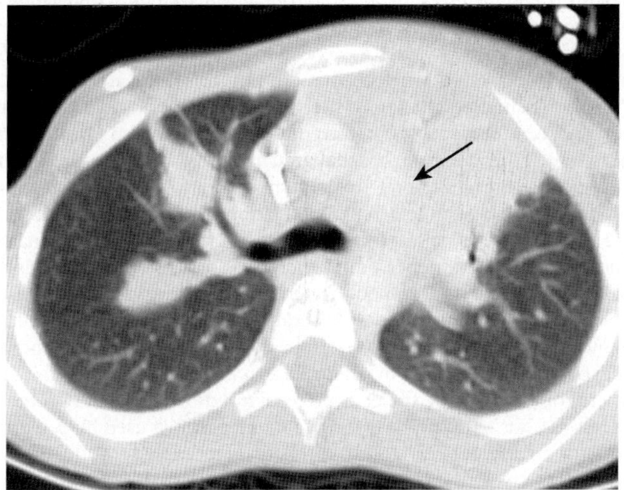

FIG. 198.7 In a 9-year-old child with chronic granulomatous disease, computed tomography shows a soft tissue mass *(arrow)* in the anterior mediastinum with heterogenous enhancement. The mass caused a convex deformity of the left anterior chest wall.

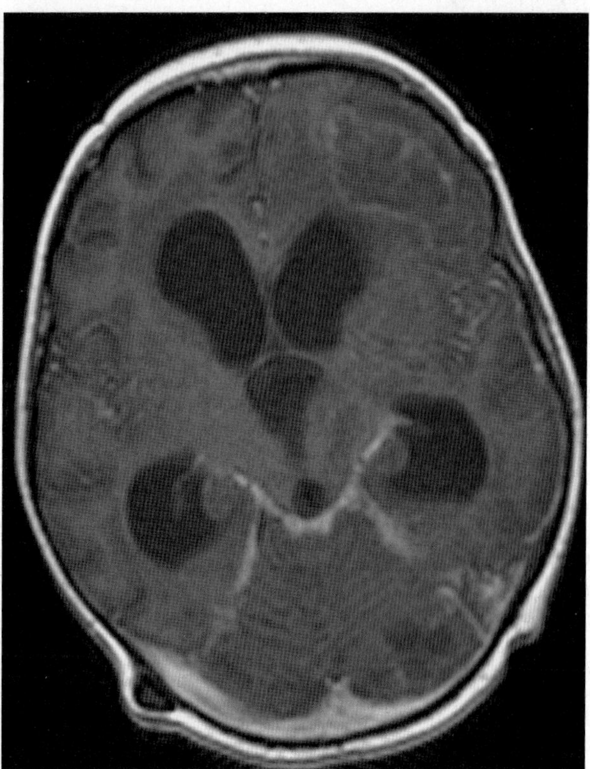

FIG. 198.8 A 3-year-old child with medulloblastoma who underwent chemotherapy and radiation therapy had new-onset acute mental status changes. T1-weighted axial magnetic resonance imaging showed multiple lesions in the subcortical area.

appear in large lesions such as consolidations or masses rather than small lesions such as nodules.[115] Repeat CT within 2 weeks of the start of treatment is not recommended unless the patient experiences clinical deterioration.[179] An exception is the finding of a nodule close to a large vessel because of the risk for massive hemoptysis if the lesion continues to increase in size. Routine use of contrast with CT is not recommended.

Adult and pediatric patients can have radiologic differences in IA. In adult series of IPA, approximately 50% of cases showed cavitation, and 40% had air crescent formation.[80] In one 10-year review of pediatric patients (mean age, 5 years), there was central cavitation of small nodules in only 25% and no evidence of air crescent formation in any area of consolidation.[223] In another pediatric report, a 22% rate (six of 27 patients) of cavitation was determined by chest radiography,[8] and in another, a 43% rate (six of 14 patients) of cavitation was demonstrated by CT.[220] In the latter two pediatric series, the mean ages were higher than the first report of lower rates of cavitation and no air crescent formation, suggesting that there is a spectrum of radiologic disease that is directly related to age, with cavitation and air crescent formation more likely to occur in older children and adults than in younger children.

A review of 27 pediatric patients showed that radiographic changes developed after HSCT but before the diagnosis of pulmonary fungal infection; it included unilateral infiltrates (52%) slightly more often than bilateral infiltrates. At the onset, the infiltrates were interstitial (41%), alveolar (41%), and mixed (18%). Hilar or mediastinal plural effusion or thickening and lymphadenopathy were rare. By the time of diagnosis of pulmonary fungal infection, the infiltrates were largely bilateral (66%) and alveolar or nodular (74%), and 22% of patients had cavitary lesions.[8] The largest series of contemporary pediatric IA cases found the most common clinical site of IA was the lungs (59%), and the most frequent diagnostic radiologic finding was nodules (34.6%).[32] Radiologic evaluation found the air crescent sign in only 2.2% of the children, the halo sign in 11%, and cavitation in 24.5%.[32]

Thoracic MRI findings are not as specific as chest CT findings. The typical MRI finding is the target sign, a nodular lesion with lower signal intensity in the center compared with a higher, contrast-enhancing signal intensity in the rim on T1-weighted images. This sign suggests late-stage disease.[25] MRI is the modality of choice for diagnosing cerebral aspergillosis because its sensitivity is better than that of CT (Fig. 198.8). Images often demonstrate multiple lesions located in the basal ganglia that show an intermediate signal intensity, lack of contrast enhancement, and absence of a mass effect.[154] CT of the head often reveals one or more hypodense, well-demarcated lesions. Findings of hemorrhage and mass effect are unusual, but for patients with adequate peripheral white blood cell counts, a ring enhancement and surrounding edema are more common.[49] T2-weighted MRI shows very decreased signal intensity compared with images of bacterial sinusitis, which show increased signal intensity.[49]

Serology

The *Aspergillus* IgG antibody test is the most sensitive microbiologic test for chronic pulmonary aspergillosis or ABPA in immunocompetent individuals, but unfortunately, serology plays little role in diagnosing the immunocompromised patient because *Aspergillus* growth does not correlate with an increase in anti-*Aspergillus* antibody titers.[128] For example, serologic examination of 18 patients with IA showed anti-*Aspergillus* antibody detection was negative in all cases, likely due to profound immunosuppression.[197]

Despite the historical lack of success with antibody testing, there is a movement to consider using antibody testing for patients before immunosuppression in an attempt to discern who is most likely to later develop IA. In a study to evaluate antibody responses using an enzyme-linked immunosorbent assay (ELISA) format for different types of aspergillosis, results showed that three recombinant antigens had diagnostic potential.[196] The candidate recombinant antigens are 18-kd ribonuclease (RNU), 360-kd catalase, and 88-kd dipeptidylpeptidase V (DPPV). For aspergilloma patients, all three of the antigens were equally useful for diagnosis, but only catalase was useful for immunocompetent and immunocompromised patients.

Galactomannan Antigen

GM is a major cell wall component of *Aspergillus*, and the highest concentrations of GM are released in the terminal phases of the disease.[128] An ELISA technique was developed using a rat anti-GM monoclonal antibody (EB-A2) that recognizes the 1→5-β-D-galactofuranoside side chains of the GM molecule.[138] A sandwich ELISA technique was introduced in 1995,[215] and by using the same antibody as a capture and detector antibody in the sandwich ELISA (Platelia *Aspergillus*, Bio-Rad, Marnes-La-Coquette, France), the threshold for detection can be lowered to 1 ng/mL. This technique is employed in the commercially available GM assay for the diagnosis of IA.

In a meta-analysis conducted to characterize the clinical utility of the serum GM assay, 27 studies were identified, and overall, the GM assay had a sensitivity of 71% and a specificity of 89% for proven cases of IA as defined by the specific clinical criteria.[184] There was considerable heterogeneity among the studies, and in subgroup analysis, performance of the test varied by patient population and by which reference diagnostic standard was used. The assay was most useful for patients with hematologic malignancy or those who had undergone hematopoietic transplantation, but for solid organ transplant recipients, the sensitivity and specificity were 22% and 84%, respectively.

The latest guidelines[179] recommend serum and bronchoalveolar lavage (BAL) specimens for detection of GM, which is an accurate marker for the diagnosis of IA in adult and pediatric patients when used in certain patient subpopulations (e.g., hematologic malignancy, HSCT). GM testing is not recommended for routine blood screening of patients receiving mold-active antifungal therapy or prophylaxis, but it can be applied to bronchoscopy specimens from those patients. For patients receiving mold-active antifungal prophylaxis, the use of serum GM levels as a screening tool has a very poor predictive value, with most positive test results being false positives in this setting.[67] GM testing is not recommended for screening of solid organ transplant recipients or patients with CGD due to the low predictive value and high false-negative rates, respectively.

When used, serial testing twice weekly during periods of greatest risk is recommended.[52] In one study, an increase in GM values during the first week of observation predicted treatment failure in allogeneic HSCT patients.[28] In a large, prospective study of hematology and HSCT patients with confirmed or probable IA, elevated GM values were detected in 65% of patients an average of 8.4 days before positive CT scans or cultures, and increased GM levels were detected in 40% of patients before the onset of clinical symptoms by a mean of 6.9 days. The test was performed easily, and results were available in 4 hours; two successive samples with elevated GM values were required for positivity.[216]

The GM assay has decreased sensitivity in the setting of treatment with anti-*Aspergillus* (mold-active) antifungals, but the specificity for detection does not change.[140] Reduced sensitivity results from the decreased fungal burden in patients receiving mold-active antifungals. Unfortunately, those are exactly the high-risk patients for whom the GM assay would be used. A subsequent study found that the GM test was best performed for patients not receiving antifungals, for whom the sensitivity was 89%, compared with 52% for patients who received empiric mold-active antifungals.[144]

Neutropenia also affects a GM-based diagnosis. GM values for patients with an absolute neutrophil count (ANC) less than 100 cells/μL and not receiving antifungal therapy were statistically higher than those for patients with an ANC greater than 100 cells/μL. However, GM values were not statistically different for patients with an ANC less than 100 cells/μL and receiving antifungal therapy compared with those with an ANC greater than 100 cells/μL.[42] This effect may result from a fungal burden that is higher at the time of initial IA in patients with neutropenia, or IA lesions may be more extensive in the setting of neutropenia.

The specific patient population tested is essential for optimizing GM testing usefulness.[179] Although GM has been extensively validated in patients with hematologic malignancy and those who have undergone HSCT, for unclear reasons, GM appears to be less useful for SOT recipients. When used for liver transplant recipients, there was a high false-positive rate, especially for patients with autoimmune liver disease or undergoing dialysis,[123] and in lung transplant recipients, sensitivity was greatly decreased, perhaps due to the pathophysiologic differences in *Aspergillus* tracheobronchitis and anastomotic disease seen in these patients.[102] The serum GM level was not sensitive (38%) for patients with aspergilloma, but it improved for those with hemoptysis.[176] It is also not sensitive (23%) for patients with chronic pulmonary aspergillosis [204] or COPD.[10] GM testing of patients with CF who were colonized with *Aspergillus* species was consistently negative.[247]

The GM assay result has been repeatedly negative for patients with CGD and IA,[155,235] potentially due to a lack of angioinvasion or immune complex formation with high levels of *Aspergillus* antibodies. One report described a nonneutropenic, 4-year old child with CGD and IA diagnosed by lung biopsy who had persistent false-negative serum GM testing.[234] Similarly, serum GM values have been higher for patients with angio-invasive IA than those with IA that did not invade the airway.[97]

False-positive results for GM testing can hamper its clinical utility and are seen for patients concurrently receiving some β-lactam antibacterials. Piperacillin-tazobactam was once the major cause of this false-positive reaction due to contamination with GM during the production process, but current formulations used in the United States are a rare cause of false-positive results.[231] One study that evaluated false-positive GM kinetics found a gradual increase in GM levels in patients receiving β-lactam antibacterials and an average of 5.5 days to a negative antigen test result.[13] Several years ago, there were concerns about increased false-positive results for children, and one theory suggested it was caused by *Bifidobacterium bifidum* spp. in the gut microflora that mimic the epitope recognized by the EB-A2 probe in the ELISA kit[152] and by GM-positive infant formula used by pediatric patients.[1] False-positive results probably are caused by the ELISA antibodies cross-reacting with specific antigens, many of which have not been defined, and this phenomenon is not associated with the patient's age.

Diagnosis of pediatric IA with GM, although originally reported to be less useful due to a higher false-positive rate,[95,218] has been validated as effective for children.[17,36,39,61,74,92,109,207] A study of 64 pediatric allogeneic HSCT recipients found that after excluding patients receiving piperacillin-tazobactam (previously known to cross-react because of GM contamination), the false-positive rate was only 1.6%, producing a specificity of 98.4% for this high-risk population. In that study, the GM test result was falsely positive for the first sample obtained after initiation of piperacillin-tazobactam, but cessation of piperacillin-tazobactam produced a negative test result in the subsequent samples obtained over 3 to 4 days.[207] Another report of 56 pediatric oncology patients found a sensitivity of 66% with a specificity of 87%, and in six of seven cases of IA, the GM test result was positive before clinical or radiographic evidence of disease.[92] A retrospective study found a similarly low false-positive rate (1.5%), and found that GM testing performed better in periods after aggressive chemotherapy than in those after allogeneic HSCT.[36]

Bronchoalveolar Lavage

Guidelines state that bronchoscopy with BAL is recommended for patients with a suspicion of IPA.[179] Because the yield of BAL is low for peripheral nodular lesions, percutaneous or endobronchial lung biopsy should be considered. BAL should include routine culture, cytologic analysis, and non–culture-based methods (e.g., GM levels).

BAL is often useful in diagnosing IA, but a negative BAL culture does not conclusively rule out disease. A thorough review of the diagnostic yield of BAL specimens for histologically proven IA patients found sensitivities of approximately 40% (range, 0–67%),[189] but in one study, BAL had a sensitivity of only 50%, even for patients with focal IA.[149] The sensitivity of respiratory tract culture specimens has been 15% to 69%,[182] and in one study, it increased to 50% to 70% for high-risk IA groups.

The sensitivity of BAL samples may be increased by the use of GM testing, amplifying the yield of bronchoscopy and possibly avoiding the need for further invasive procedures. Although the GM cutoff value in serum samples is 0.5, the cutoff is best set at 1.0 for BAL GM testing. A retrospective analysis of 99 high-risk hematology patients, including 58 with IA, who underwent BAL for the diagnosis of new pulmonary infiltrates found that a BAL GM value of 1.0 or more yielded an increased sensitivity (91.3%) compared with BAL culture (50%) or BAL microscopy (53.3%). The combined sensitivity of all three BAL methods was 98.2%.[134] Further analyses in that study found that the mean BAL GM value was not different for neutropenic and nonneutropenic patients.

A meta-analysis of BAL GM studies found sensitivities between 59% and 100% and specificities between 76% and 100%. Antifungal therapy did not significantly affect sensitivity, as it does with serum GM assays.[88] A retrospective study of patients with hematologic malignancies and HSCT recipients also found that BAL GM testing was more sensitive than serum GM assays for diagnosing IA and determined that BAL GM results were not affected by mold-active antifungals, suggesting that these findings might reflect the different levels of antifungals found in sera and alveolar fluid. This study supported the use of BAL GM testing to diagnose IA because the positive predictive value was optimized, whereas serum GM testing might be best applied as a screening test with the use of a lower cutoff value to maximize the negative predictive value.[166] A retrospective study of pediatric BAL GM testing found an optimal BAL GM cutoff of 0.98 to yield the best sensitivity (78%) and specificity (92%). Using a BAL GM value of 1.0 or higher and a concurrent serum GM value of 0.5 or higher yielded the best sensitivity (89%) and specificity (90%).[60]

(1→3)-β-D-Glucan

(1→3)-β-D-Glucan is an integral cell wall component, and in contrast to GM, it is not normally released from the fungal cell.[128] Factor G, a coagulation factor of the horseshoe crab, is a highly sensitive natural detector of (1→3)-β-D-glucan.[168] The G test detects the fungal call wall component (1→3)-β-D-glucan with a modified limulus endotoxin assay, but it does not identify the genus of the fungi detected.[168] Unlike the GM assay, this assay is nonspecific and detects several fungi, including *Aspergillus spp., Candida spp., Fusarium spp., Trichosporon spp., Saccharomyces cerevisiae, Acremonium, Coccidioides immitis, Histoplasma capsulatum, Sporothrix schenckii*, and *Pneumocystis jiroveci*. The (1→3)-β-D-glucan assay does not detect *Cryptococcus* and the yeast form of *Blastomyces dermatitidis,* which produce low levels of (1→3)-β-D-glucan, or *Absidia, Mucor*, and *Rhizopus,* which produce no (1→3)-β-D-glucan.

False-positive results can occur in a variety of contexts, such as through glucan-contaminated blood collection tubes, gauze, depth-type membrane filters for blood processing, and various drugs such as antibiotics, including some cephalosporins, carbapenems, and ampicillin-sulbactam, and possibly chemotherapeutics such as PEG asparaginase.[148] The Fungitell assay (Associates of Cape Cod) for detection of (1→3)-β-D-glucan is cleared by the US Food and Drug Administration (FDA) for the diagnosis of invasive mycoses, including aspergillosis, and it has been evaluated in high-risk patients with hematologic malignancies and allogeneic HSCT recipients.[169,172] A 1-year prospective study of patients with hematologic malignancies and controls found the sensitivities were 79% for real-time PCR, 58% for the GM assay, and 67% for the G test; specificities were 92%, 97%, and 84%, respectively.[111]

In one study comparing (1→3)-β-D-glucan and GM assays, the sensitivity, specificity, and positive and negative predictive values were identical. False-positive reactions occurred at a rate of 10.3% in both tests, but the patients with false-positive results were different in each test. Both tests anticipated the clinical diagnosis and CT abnormalities, but the (1→3)-β-D–glucan assay result tended to become positive earlier than for GM testing. A combination of the two tests improved the specificity to 100% and positive predictive value to 100% for each test without affecting the sensitivity and negative predictive values.[180] Another study compared GM, PCR, and (1→3)-β-D-glucan assays for patients with hematologic disorders, and the receiver operating characteristic (ROC) analysis showed that the area under the ROC curve was greatest for the GM assay using two consecutive positive results. This suggests that the GM assay was the most sensitive in predicting the diagnosis of IA for high-risk patients with hematologic disorders.[114] A meta-analysis of cohort studies of the (1→3)-β-D-glucan assay for IA revealed that using a single test resulted in a pooled sensitivity of 57% with a specificity of 97%.[124]

Comparative studies have shown that the Fungitell assay can be slightly more sensitive than GM testing for IA, but it is limited by its poor specificity,[217] whereas others have found that the Fungitell assay is not as helpful for diagnosing IA.[17] However, another study in a large cancer center that compared GM and (1→3)-β-D-glucan assays prospectively over a 3-year period for 82 patients (each for 12 weeks) found that the (1→3)-β-D-glucan assay was more sensitive than the GM assays for detection of IA and other mold infections in patients with hematologic malignancies.[90] One meta-analysis of β-glucan assays revealed limitations,[124] whereas another found similar deficiencies but improvement in diagnostic capabilities with the combination of both biomarkers.[180] The 2016 guidelines recommend serum assays for (1→3)-β-D-glucan for diagnosing IA in high-risk patients (e.g., hematologic malignancies, allogeneic HSCT), but they are not specific for *Aspergillus.*[179] Other organizations have recommended the GM over Fungitell assay for specifically diagnosing IA.[139]

Polymerase Chain Reaction

The exact clinical utility of blood-based PCR in diagnosing IA is unclear. The 2016 guidelines state that direct comparison studies have shown *Aspergillus* PCR to be substantially more sensitive than culture of blood and respiratory fluids.[179] In a meta-analysis of clinical trials evaluating the accuracy of serum or whole-blood PCR assays for IA, sensitivity and specificity were 84% and 76%, respectively.[11] These values are promising, but PCR of blood or serum alone is unable to confirm or exclude suspected IA in high-risk patients. The sensitivity of *Aspergillus* PCR for BAL fluid was higher than for blood samples, but in many instances, its specificity was lower.[14,93]

In a systematic review of nine cohort studies using reference IA definitions that strictly adhered to the 2002 or 2008 EORTC/MSG criteria, the summary sensitivity and specificity values for the diagnosis of proven or probable IPA by PCR of BAL fluid were 77.2% and 93.5%, respectively.[14] One difficulty is that the lungs are often colonized by *Aspergillus* (particularly in many high-risk populations, such as lung transplant recipients) and that PCR cannot differentiate colonization from disease or distinguish different *Aspergillus* spp. The high negative predictive value of BAL PCR (usually ≥95%) suggests a role in ruling out IPA. The data suggest that the diagnostic performance of blood or BAL PCR is comparable to that of serum and BAL GM index and that sensitivity for both tests is affected by antifungal use. Using both PCR and GM detection in serum improved sensitivity with no sacrifice of specificity.[14]

Despite promising results, *Aspergillus* PCR cannot be recommended for routine use in clinical practice because few assays have been standardized and validated, and the role of PCR testing in patient management is not established. Initiatives such as the European *Aspergillus* PCR Initiative (EAPCRI) have made significant progress in developing a consensus standard protocol for blood-based *Aspergillus* PCR.[252] This diagnostic method is not commercially available, and reports can be difficult to interpret due to the lack of experimental standardization between centers. Due to the ubiquitous nature of the mold, the value of this test will likely be its high negative predictive value.

TREATMENT

Overall success in treating IA depends on more than the choice of a specific antifungal. Detailed knowledge of host factors, underlying disease, concomitant infections, and degree and duration of immunosuppression are key to the overall management of IA in immunocompromised patients. Immune reconstitution is paramount for successful IA therapy, and continued exposure to certain immunosuppressive medications, such as corticosteroids, worsens IA. Antifungal prophylaxis used before the diagnosis of IA can affect the ultimate choice of empiric or targeted therapy. The diagnostic workup should be aggressive to confirm disease, but it should never delay antifungal therapy if IA is a concern.

The cornerstone of antifungal therapy for IA is prompt and aggressive institution of antifungal therapy based on diagnostic results and on clinical suspicion of infection if the diagnosis is not immediately made. Antifungal resistance is slowly increasing among *Aspergillus* isolates, and it continues to have specific geographic trends that influence antifungal choice, although for the moment, it seems to spare much of the United States. There also are questions about whether to use antifungal monotherapy or combination antifungal therapy and which classes of agents should be used.

Although immune reconstitution is paramount, the role and real benefit of adjunctive immunotherapy remains unclear. Treatment for most forms of IA follows the 2016 recommendations made for the more common IPA.[179] Most of the treatment section focuses on IPA, with additional comments provided on the more common chronic and allergic forms of IA.

Treatment for Invasive Aspergillosis

Primary Antifungal Therapy

The 2016 Infectious Diseases Society of America treatment guidelines[179] recommend primary (initial) treatment with voriconazole. These recommendations mirror guidelines from many other international groups, which recommend voriconazole for the primary treatment of IA[4,26,135,158,179,240] in all clinical sites. Alternative therapies include liposomal amphotericin B, isavuconazole, and other lipid formulations of amphotericin B. Combination primary antifungal therapy with voriconazole plus an echinocandin may be considered, but it is not necessarily recommended in selected patients with documented IA. Primary therapy with an echinocandin is not recommended, but an echinocandin can be used in the settings in which azole or polyene antifungals are contraindicated. Treatment of children with IA uses the same recommended agents as for adult patients, but the dosing is often very different, and for some antifungals, the exact dosing in children is unknown.

Treatment of IA should be continued for a minimum of 6 to 12 weeks, depending on the degree and duration of immunosuppression, site of disease, and evidence of disease improvement. Patients treated successfully who require subsequent immunosuppression should receive secondary prophylaxis to prevent recurrence. Many experts think treatment should continue until complete clinical and radiographic resolution of disease, often with an accompanying significant decrease in biomarkers (e.g., GM). If a patient remains substantially chronically immunosuppressed due to ongoing cytotoxic chemotherapy or lack of engraftment after HSCT, it is advisable to continue the antifungal therapy for IA until there is no evidence of disease, often 3 months or longer.

Surgical therapy may be useful for patients with lesions contiguous with the great vessels of the pericardium to avoid fatal hemoptysis. However, surgery to debulk disseminated lesions usually is not advised.

Since its approval for use in 1958, amphotericin B deoxycholate was the first-line therapy for IA and the gold standard against which other therapies were measured. However, with overall survival rates of about 35% among patients treated with amphotericin B for several decades and limited tolerance as a result of acute and chronic toxicities, there was a clear need to develop a better antifungal. Itraconazole became available in 1990 for the treatment of IA, but it was not without flaws, particularly decreased fungicidal activity compared with amphotericin B, unpredictable bioavailability of the capsular formulation in high-risk patients, and significant drug interactions.[211]

The next step taken in the search for a better antifungal was development of three lipid formulations of amphotericin B, whose advantages included an increased daily dose of the parent drug, high tissue concentrations with better delivery to reticuloendothelial organs, decreased infusion-related side effects, and decreased renal toxicity.[62] These three lipid formulations—amphotericin B lipid complex, amphotericin B colloidal dispersion, and liposomal amphotericin B—provided greater safety for patients who could not tolerate conventional amphotericin B.[211]

Voriconazole is a second-generation triazole and a synthetic derivative of fluconazole that was approved for use in the United States in May 2002 for treatment of IA. The global clinical trial that led to its approval prospectively showed that voriconazole had a superior response rate in the primary treatment of IA compared with amphotericin B deoxycholate (52.8% vs. 31.6%). Survival rates increased from 57.9% for amphotericin B to 70.8% for voriconazole.[94] A secondary analysis of the study's results, which employed the most recent consensus definitions of invasive fungal disease that were unavailable at the time of the original trial,[59] revealed slightly more favorable results for voriconazole compared with amphotericin B.[96] Although the original 2002 study was criticized for employing conventional amphotericin B as the comparator to voriconazole (due to approval indications at the time of study design), later analysis clearly showed that primary therapy with voriconazole was superior to primary therapy with amphotericin B, regardless of subsequent switching for intolerance of refractory disease to any other licensed antifungal therapies (e.g. liposomal amphotericin B, itraconazole, other agents).[178]

Later epidemiologic studies have confirmed the benefit of voriconazole compared with the decades of data on amphotericin B. Although controlled clinical trials have the benefit of rigorous evaluation, they often suffer certain biases because of enrollment of a generally healthier patient population. A Belgian multicenter observational study followed 113 adult patients with IA and found an overall successful response rate, typically viewed in antifungal clinical trials as the sum of the complete response rate and partial response rate, of 50.4% with voriconazole.[103] A French epidemiologic study found similar results by analyzing 393 adult patients with IA and concluded that any treatment regimen containing voriconazole, alone or in an antifungal combination, was superior in terms of survival to any antifungal regimen without voriconazole.[131]

The improved voriconazole response rate has translated well to the pediatric population, as shown by a review of 42 children treated for IA with voriconazole.[244] An analysis of the compassionate open-label use of voriconazole in children for refractory IA demonstrated a 43% complete or partial response rate. Voriconazole was also shown in these studies to be better tolerated and to have less toxicity than amphotericin B in adults and children.

The fundamental pharmacokinetics of voriconazole are different in children (i.e., linear) than in adults (i.e., nonlinear).[243] For instance, although the recommended starting dose of voriconazole for adult patients is 6 mg/kg twice daily for the first day and the maintenance dose is 4 mg/kg twice daily, the preferred pediatric dosage is substantially higher. Population pharmacokinetic analyses of voriconazole in children, adolescents, and adults, which are based on the area under the concentration-time curve, reveal that children should be given an intravenous 9 mg/kg loading dose to be comparable to the 6 mg/kg dose given to adults.[75] The maintenance intravenous dose for children of 8 mg/kg was comparable to the dose of 4 mg/kg for adults, and the oral pediatric dose of 9 mg/kg was found to be similar to that for adults receiving 200 mg of oral voriconazole twice daily.

Most adolescents can be dosed as adults, but for younger adolescents (12–14 years), the analysis found that body weight was more important than age in predicting voriconazole pharmacokinetics. During this age transition period, adolescents 12 to 14 years of age should be dosed as children if their weight is less than 50 kg and dosed as adults if their weight is 50 kg or higher.[75] The oral bioavailability of voriconazole, although thought to be greater than 95% in adults, is approximately 50% to 65% in children.[112,242] This is important for patients receiving oral voriconazole long after transplantation and during the second bimodal peak of disease at approximately day 100 after transplantation. Higher voriconazole doses may be needed in some cases. A population pharmacokinetic analysis of adult patients found that higher voriconazole doses were required to achieve adequate therapeutic serum trough levels.[177]

The triazole antifungals require therapeutic drug monitoring. Effective management of IA requires obtaining a voriconazole trough level, which has high interpatient variability that limits its extrapolation to a larger population but much lower intrapatient variability, allowing successive trough levels to be used to monitor dose adjustments for individual patients.[206] The exact voriconazole trough level for clinical efficacy against IA is uncertain because in several clinical studies, some patients have had undetectable voriconazole levels but had clinical responses. However, a serum trough level that is greater than the usual minimal inhibitory concentration (MIC) of the infecting *Aspergillus* species is preferable. Although individual studies have debated the exact cutoff, it is clear that the serum level should be a true trough level and not a random drug level.

Most experts advocate for a serum trough voriconazole level of 2.0 μg/mL or higher and stress the importance tailoring therapy for each patient. Inherent in the individualized treatment approach is the understanding that various populations metabolize voriconazole differently. Three major genotypes due to allelic polymorphisms in the human cytochrome P450 isoenzymes (largely CYP2C19) are responsible for voriconazole metabolism.[110]

The choice of primary antifungal therapy must address concerns about azole-resistant, often panazole-resistant, isolates in specific geographic regions of the world. An international (largely European) surveillance study of approximately 4000 isolates from 19 countries found the azole resistance rate for *A. fumigatus* was 3.2%, and azole resistance was documented in 5.1% of IA cases.[229] This is especially worrisome because approximately 70% of patients with azole-resistant IA have never received an azole antifungal. Of the many genotypes uncovered in azole-resistant species, TR_{34}/L98H and TR_{46}/Y121F/T289A are responsible for 80% of azole-resistant IA.[232] These genotypes denote mutations in the *cyp51A* gene, which encodes the target enzyme of the azoles, and a tandem repeat of 34 or 46 base pairs in the *cyp51A* promoter region.

Epidemiologic cutoff values have been established for determining likely clinical resistance for itraconazole (1 μg/mL), voriconazole (1 μg/mL), posaconazole (0.25 μg/mL), and preliminarily for isavuconazole (1 μg/mL).[69] An international expert opinion panel recommended azole susceptibilities for all *Aspergillus* isolates, and if an isolate is determined to be azole resistant, they advise switching to liposomal amphotericin B, using voriconazole plus echinocandin, or considering a non–azole-based regimen (e.g., echinocandin).[232] For empiric therapy, if the rate of environmental resistance is 10% or higher, voriconazole plus echinocandin or liposomal amphotericin B should be used initially.

Alternative Antifungal Therapy

An alternative for primary treatment of IA is liposomal amphotericin B. Although no randomized trial has been performed to evaluate effectiveness of this drug compared with voriconazole for primary therapy, a series of randomized trials suggest therapeutic effectiveness. Amphotericin B has always been considered a concentration-dependent antifungal, and one clinical trial compared liposomal amphotericin B at 3 mg/kg per day ($n = 107$ patients) and 10 mg/kg per day ($n = 94$ patients).[44] The favorable overall response for the lower dose (50%) and the higher dose (46%) were similar, with no demonstrable additional benefit for higher amphotericin B dosing and found higher rates of nephrotoxicity. Although these response rates are similar to the favorable response seen earlier with voriconazole,[94] most of the amphotericin B responses were partial responses and not complete treatment responses, suggesting that the triazole was overall more effective in disease eradication.

The results suggest that liposomal amphotericin B should be considered as alternative primary therapy for some patients, especially when hepatic toxicities or drug interactions warrant nonazole alternatives and when voriconazole-resistant molds (e.g., mucormycosis) remain a concern. Because conventional amphotericin B was shown to be inferior to voriconazole, few experts recommend conventional amphotericin B for IA management.

A pivotal randomized trial compared voriconazole with isavuconazole and demonstrated noninferiority in the treatment of IPA.[137] This multicenter, randomized, double-blind study of patients 18 years of age or older showed noninferiority (19% for isavuconazole vs. 20% for voriconazole) in terms of the primary end point of all-cause mortality at 6 weeks in the intent-to-treat population of patients with possible, probable, and proven aspergillosis. There were also fewer drug-related adverse effects for people who received isavuconazole (42% vs. 60%). Based on these data, isavuconazole was approved by the FDA for first-line therapy of IA and is recommended as an alternative primary therapy for IA.

Salvage Antifungal Therapy

Salvage therapy is defined as treatment after primary therapy, often because of ineffectiveness or patient intolerance. Guidelines recommend an individualized approach that considers the rapidity, severity, and extent of infection; patient comorbidities; and the need to exclude the emergence of a new pathogen.[179] There should be an aggressive and prompt attempt to establish a specific, correct diagnosis, which includes bronchoscopy with or without CT-guided biopsy. For example, mucormycosis and aspergillosis appear radiographically similar, but treatment of mucormycosis with voriconazole is unsuccessful. Assuming that the diagnosis of IA is correct, the first step in treating refractory disease is to establish that the correct dose of voriconazole is being used. Documentation of serum azole levels should also be verified if therapeutic drug monitoring is available because this has historically been a common cause of antifungal failure.

The general strategies for salvage therapy typically include changing the class of antifungal, tapering or reversal of underlying immunosuppression when feasible, susceptibility testing of any *Aspergillus* isolates recovered from the patient, and surgical resection of necrotic lesions in selected cases. In the context of salvage therapy, an additional antifungal agent may be added to current therapy, or combination antifungal drugs from different classes other than those in the initial regimen may be used. For patients currently receiving an antifungal and exhibiting an adverse event attributable to the agent, it makes sense to change to an alternative class of antifungal or the use of an alternative agent with a nonoverlapping side effect profile. For salvage therapy, agents include lipid formulations of amphotericin B, micafungin, caspofungin, posaconazole, and itraconazole.

Choosing appropriate antifungal therapy is especially important in the setting of prior azole exposure (i.e., antifungal prophylaxis before diagnosis) because of concerns about development of antifungal resistance. Itraconazole resistance was first described in 1997,[58] and resistance to echinocandins largely results from researchers genetically modifying the *fks1* gene (i.e., target of echinocandins) in *A. fumigates.*[193] However, azole resistance is increasing among clinical strains,[31] including multiazole- or panazole-resistant (e.g., voriconazole, posaconazole, itraconazole) strains. Azole resistance in *A. fumigatus* has emerged over the past decade, with a prevalence as high as 5% to 13% in the Netherlands and Great Britain.[101,230] The most common multiazole-resistance mechanism consists of mutations in the *cyp51A* gene, which is involved in ergosterol biosynthesis.[233]

Some *Aspergillus* species are more likely to be resistant to certain antifungals. *A. terreus* is a recalcitrant *Aspergillus* species due to its in vitro resistance to amphotericin B,[219] which has been confirmed in animal models.[245] A review of in vitro analyses, multiple animal models, and previously reported clinical cases showed almost uniform failure with amphotericin B against *A. terreus.*[210] A multicenter, retrospective analysis of more than 80 cases demonstrated that the mortality rate was decreased for patients who received voriconazole instead of amphotericin B therapy.[208] Other studies have shown that patients with *A. terreus* disease are more likely to be neutropenic,[89] more likely to have disseminated disease, and have a decreased response to all classes of antifungals compared with patients infected with *A. fumigatus.*[126]

Newer species, such as *Aspergillus lentulus,*[18] *Aspergillus udagawae* (formerly *Neosartorya udagawae*),[236] and *Aspergillus pseudofischeri,*[107] have been described, and many have reduced antifungal susceptibility.[6] Two studies that analyzed the MIC distribution of more than 5000 isolates showed that some species are significantly more susceptible to amphotericin B, itraconazole, or voriconazole.[70,71] In the case of *A. pseudofischeri* and *A. udagawae*, susceptibility to amphotericin B and itraconazole is somewhat controversial, but the general consensus is that these species are less susceptible to voriconazole than *A. fumigates.*[19,186] *Aspergillus calidoustus* is resistant to all azoles.[5,16] *A. lentulus* is overall less susceptible than *A. fumigatus* to amphotericin B, itraconazole, and voriconazole based on its high MICs.[19]

There are no randomized studies examining posaconazole for primary therapy of IA, but numerous in vitro and in vivo data suggest that this triazole can be as effective as voriconazole as a potential first-line agent against IA. A multicenter study of salvage therapy evaluated 107 patients with IA treated with posaconazole compared with 86 historical controls and found response rates of 42% and 26%, respectively, and found improved survival rates at 30 days of 74% and 49%, respectively.[246] This study was significant because all patients had salvage therapy (usually after failing amphotericin B products or itraconazole), demonstrating that the newer triazoles are the best treatment option for IA.

Additional studies support the argument for using triazoles. Voriconazole or posaconazole therapy was associated with fewer deaths compared with amphotericin B products or caspofungin in an Italian study of 140 patients with IA and AML.[173] Voriconazole therapy produced more survivors than caspofungin, amphotericin B formulations, or itraconazole among 642 patients with IA who were HSCT and SOT recipients in the United States.[15]

Three echinocandins are approved in the United States: caspofungin, micafungin, and anidulafungin. Several in vitro antifungal susceptibility studies have shown the general equivalency of all three echinocandins against *Aspergillus* species.[183] The echinocandin activity against *Aspergillus* is fungistatic compared with triazole fungicidal activity. Because it blunts the hyphal tip but does not kill the organism,[29] activity is reported as the in vitro minimal effective concentration (MEC), not the MIC.[122]

Caspofungin was first studied an open-label, noncomparative study of salvage therapy for immunocompromised patients with proven or probable aspergillosis.[136] Caspofungin produced a complete or partial response in 45% (37 of 83) of patients, which is significant because the patients were refractory to or intolerant of previous antifungal therapy. These findings were validated by two subsequent clinical trials in which caspofungin resulted in complete resolution or stabilization of disease in 74% patients ($n = 31$) in one, and in the other trial, caspofungin had an overall response rate of 56% ($n = 32$).[35,226] Few studies have evaluated caspofungin as primary therapy for IA. One phase II dose-escalation clinical trial evaluated 46 patients with caspofungin as primary therapy and found a favorable response rate of 54.3% but found no dose-dependent effect on efficacy for caspofungin.[45] A later observational study of caspofungin as primary or salvage therapy and as monotherapy or in a combination approach found an overall 56.4% favorable response rate, validating caspofungin as a viable therapeutic option.[133]

The largest study with micafungin was a noncomparative, open-label, multicenter study of adult and pediatric patients that examined the safety and efficacy of micafungin in the treatment patients with IA who had failed to respond to prior therapy or could not tolerate other therapies. Of the 225 patients who met diagnostic criteria, 35.6% (80 of 225) had a favorable response, and of those treated with only micafungin, a 50% (six of 12) of the primary therapy group and 40.9% (nine of 22) of the salvage therapy group had a favorable response.[54] Anidulafungin is approved in the United States for the treatment of candidemia and esophageal candidiasis. Although in vitro studies show activity against *Aspergillus* species isolates, there are no clinical studies of anidulafungin used against IA as primary or salvage monotherapy.

Combination Antifungal Therapy

Although no controlled clinical trial fully supports its efficacy for treating IA and use is not recommended by guidelines, clinicians who are desperately seeking new strategies to improve outcomes sometimes turn to combination antifungal therapy. With the surge in the development of newer antifungals for IA, more permutations of combination antifungal therapies are available. Drawing from treatments for other diseases such as human immunodeficiency virus (HIV) infection, tuberculosis, and cryptococcal meningitis (CM),[22] combination therapy for IA seems a plausible approach to optimize therapy. Unfortunately, the range of data from in vitro experiments, animal model studies, and small clinical series extend from synergy to antagonism and parallel the wide range of unproven treatment practices used by clinicians who are searching for the best care for their patients.

The largest analysis of combination therapy for IA reviewed 6281 cases of IA management from 1966 through 2001, focusing on 249 clinical uses of combination therapy reported in 128 articles.[212] Unfortunately, three combination regimens that are not commonly used now nor currently recommended (i.e., amphotericin B plus flucytosine, amphotericin B plus itraconazole, and amphotericin B plus rifampin) comprised most of the reported clinical experience at that time. Although these data helped to lay the foundation for combination therapy in the past, the drug combinations used historically are not those necessarily applied by clinicians in current practice.

Combination antifungal therapy has several likely advantages: a widened spectrum and potency of drug activity, more rapid antifungal effect, drug synergy, lowered dosing of toxic drugs, and a reduced risk of antifungal resistance.[129] Although each antifungal agent has limitations, combination regimens may prove more effective, as demonstrated by the highly active antiretroviral therapy (HAART) used for treating HIV patients. Without large-scale clinical trials, clinicians often derive treatment strategy information from experimental in vitro or in vivo data. Unfortunately, due to the extensive heterogeneity of experimentation and interpretation, firm conclusions cannot be drawn about the clinical relevance of the combination antifungal experiments. In vitro combination drug testing is useful for screening antagonistic interactions before investigating further in animal model or clinical studies.

Animal model testing is preferred over in vitro analysis because of greater predictive value for human pharmacokinetic and pharmacodynamic effects, including tissue penetration and achievable drug levels at the foci of infection, and for determining toxicities. In vivo testing also can be used to compare various disease location models and analyze different host immune states. Histologic examination is used to determine fungal sterilization. Although in vitro testing can suggest an effective antifungal, the dose needed to achieve the desired effect may be unachievable safely in vivo, or the drug may not penetrate infected tissue adequately.

For combination antifungal therapy to be viable, the combination treatment needs to be superior to any of the individual therapies. Voriconazole has made this task more complicated because the agent is quite effective at killing *Aspergillus*, sterilizing infected tissue in numerous animal models, and clinically curing patients who were once thought to be hopeless. Regardless of the continuous stream of data, the in vitro and in vivo interactions must continue to be questioned due to so many confounding patient variables. Clinical experience remains the most accurate tool, but clinical relevance may be related to patient factors (e.g., recovery of neutropenia, cessation of glucocorticoid therapy) and not intrinsically related to the susceptibility of the fungus to voriconazole.

Combination in vitro testing has many potential pitfalls, and the final fractional inhibitory concentration index (FICI), the mathematical foundation behind the commonly used checkerboard test, can be clinically deceiving. For example, the interaction between fluconazole and terbinafine in one study was reported to be synergistic against *A. fumigatus* strains (FICI, 0.38).[157] However, individually fluconazole is known to have zero anti-*Aspergillus* activity, and terbinafine has poor tissue penetrance,[99] and the combination would appear to be a poor clinical choice for IA. The individual MIC of fluconazole was 512 μg/mL, and that terbinafine was 8 μg/mL, but both improved in combination to 64 μg/mL and 2 μg/mL, respectively, mathematically achieving the definition of antifungal synergy. However, it could be argued that this result indicates that two already poor choices for treatment were made less poor in combination. It is unlikely clinicians would advocate combination fluconazole plus terbinafine for their IA patients despite a final result of synergy based on in vitro testing.

In vitro drug combination studies have inherent experimental variations, and there is no standardization in animal model experimentation. If a single antifungal offers as much as 50% protection or many infected control animals survive, it can be difficult to show improvement with combination therapy over single agents.[85] Many variables influence the outcome of animal model experiments (similar to patient cases), including the degree of neutropenia, route of infection determining which target organs are infected, timing of drug delivery, tissue processing, and fungal burden measurement.

In the clinical setting, the antifungal combination of voriconazole plus caspofungin has the most anecdotal experience, likely because of approval and availability and the presumed synergistic interaction due to the simultaneous inhibition of (1→3)-β-D-glucan synthesis in the fungal cell wall and ergosterol synthesis in the fungal cell membrane.[116,181] One clinical study analyzed voriconazole plus caspofungin in a retrospective review of 47 patients with proven or probable IA from 1997 to 2001 who experienced failure of primary therapy with amphotericin B formulations.[141] Salvage therapy was begun with voriconazole (n = 31) or with voriconazole plus caspofungin (n = 16) after 7 or more days of failed amphotericin B therapy. The overall survival rate 3 months after the day of diagnosis of IA was slightly higher among those who received combination therapy (P = .048). In the bivariate analysis (controlling for antifungal therapy and receipt of HSCT), the combination showed an improved 3-month overall survival rate (HR, 0.27; 95% CI, 0.09–0.78; P = .008). An accompanying editorial to the article pointed out that the preclinical data for combination therapy seemed promising but inconsistent.[238] The authors responded,[37] and in analyzing the patients at 1 year, found there was no difference in overall survival (P = .26).

The prevailing expert opinion is that if a combination antifungal therapy approach is beneficial for treating IA, the combination should include a cell membrane–active triazole and a cell wall–active echinocandin. It is unclear whether any combination therapy can produce the great advance seen with the use of voriconazole instead of conventional amphotericin B due to the increasing fragility of immunosuppressed patients with IA. Although the latest treatment guidelines state that primary combination antifungal therapy is not routinely recommended based on a lack of definitive clinical data, one retrospective study used voriconazole plus caspofungin primary combination therapy for lung transplant recipients because of the known delay in time to achieve an adequate voriconazole serum level, thereby using the second agent only during the initial early weeks of therapy.[222]

In a large, double-blind, placebo-controlled, randomized trial of combination antifungal therapy, voriconazole monotherapy was compared with combination therapy using voriconazole plus anidulafungin for primary therapy of IA.[146] A total of 454 patients with hematologic malignancies who were 16 years of age or older were randomized in a 1 : 1 ratio in the study and given voriconazole alone or combination therapy for a minimum of 2 weeks, followed by voriconazole monotherapy to complete 6 weeks of treatment. The primary efficacy end point was the 6-week, all-cause mortality rate for the patients with confirmed proven or probable IA. The mortality rates at 6 weeks were 19.3% for combination therapy recipients and 27.5% for monotherapy recipients (P = .087; 95% CI, −19 to 1.5). Although the results for combination therapy demonstrated a substantial benefit, the difference did not achieve the prespecified threshold for statistical superiority. In post hoc analyses of the subgroup of patients who were diagnosed as having probable aspergillosis based on radiographic abnormalities and positive GM assays, the difference in mortality rates was most notable (15.7% for combination therapy vs. 27.3% for monotherapy; P = 0.037; 95% CI, −22.7 to −0.4). However, global clinical responses at 6 weeks were lower for the combination group (33% vs. 43%), which was attributed to more patients in the combination group being unevaluable for this secondary end point due to missing data.

The combination antifungal drug study, likely never to be repeated due to the substantial costs involved, suggested potential benefits for combination therapy with voriconazole and an echinocandin. For this reason, the latest guidelines[179] suggest consideration of but not a definitive indication for an echinocandin with voriconazole for primary therapy in the setting of severe disease, especially for patients with a hematologic malignancy and those with profound and persistent neutropenia.

Adjunctive Therapies

Reducing doses of or eliminating immunosuppressive agents, when feasible, is strongly recommended. However, IA is not an absolute contraindication to additional chemotherapy or transplantation, and the risks and benefits of the antineoplastic treatment of underlying disease must be weighed against the risk of progressive IA if treatment if delayed. According to the 2016 guidelines,[179] colony-stimulating factors (CSFs) may be considered for neutropenic patients, but there is insufficient evidence regarding the value of granulocyte CSF versus granulocyte-macrophage CSF in this setting. Granulocyte transfusions can be considered for neutropenic patients with IA that is refractory or unlikely to respond to standard therapy for an anticipated duration of more than 1 week. Recombinant interferon-γ, although recommended as prophylaxis in CGD patients, is of unclear benefit as adjunctive therapy for IA.

Surgery for aspergillosis should be considered for localized disease that is easily accessible to debridement (e.g., invasive fungal sinusitis, localized cutaneous disease). The benefit for IA in other settings, such as in the treatment of endocarditis, osteomyelitis, or focal CNS disease, appears rational. Other indications are less clear and require consideration of the patient's immune status, comorbidities, confirmation of a single focus, and the risks of surgery.

Treatment for Chronic or Allergic Aspergillosis

According to the latest guidelines,[179] the objectives of therapy of CCPA are to improve symptoms, reduce hemoptysis, reduce progressive lung fibrosis (particularly to prevent CFPA), and prolong survival. Oral itraconazole or voriconazole is a first-line therapy, depending on tolerance and affordability.[2,9,33,34,104] Because resistance to itraconazole during treatment has been reported more frequently than with voriconazole, for patients with a large fungal load, voriconazole may be preferable, although clinical evidence to support this approach is lacking. Posaconazole is currently third-line therapy because of the general lack of data and cost over long periods.[73]

Treatment should be continued for a minimum of 6 months, and if well tolerated with a good response, it may be continued for years.[119] However, toxicity may develop with long-term triazole therapy.

Monitoring of therapy is critical and should be undertaken by physicians experienced with antifungal therapy. Standard monitoring includes assessing radiographic changes (every 3 to 12 months), inflammatory markers, and *Aspergillus* IgG titers and performing annual pulmonary function tests. Susceptibility testing of isolates obtained from patients on therapy should be tested for azole resistance. Acutely ill patients who fail therapy, are intolerant of treatment, or develop azole resistance may require an initial course of intravenous antifungal therapy. Amphotericin B deoxycholate, liposomal amphotericin B, and micafungin have been extensively used for CCPA, with modest response rates.[57,117,162]

Occasionally surgical resection is necessary for CCPA, typically for intractable hemoptysis, destroyed lung (CFPA) with poor quality of life, or azole resistance. The surgical outcomes are acceptable, but the risk of death and complications such as pleural space infection are higher for CCPA than for a single aspergilloma. Relapse rates up to 25% are documented,[72] which makes decision making difficult, especially in the knowledge that subtle immune deficits will persist after surgery.

Because ABPA is a hypersensitivity disease, therapy centers on corticosteroids to manage the allergic component of *Aspergillus*, coupled with adjunctive oral antifungal therapy to diminish the fungal burden. Itraconazole is the best antifungal agent for this disease, and clinical trials have shown a clear benefit for itraconazole treatment of patients with ABPA, including those with CF and ABPA.[205] Patients who fail itraconazole treatment or are intolerant of itraconazole may respond to voriconazole, posaconazole or inhaled amphotericin B.[38] Relapse after improvement during antifungal therapy is common; long-term suppressive therapy may be necessary. Because disease activity correlates with serum IgE levels, monitoring of IgE levels is used as one marker to define duration of therapy.

NEW REFERENCES SINCE THE SEVENTH EDITION

2. Agarwal R, Vishwanath G, Aggarwal AN, et al. Itraconazole in chronic cavitary pulmonary aspergillosis: a randomised controlled trial and systematic review of literature. *Mycoses*. 2013;56:559-570.
4. Al-Abdely HM, Alothman AF, Salman JA, et al. Clinical practice guidelines for the treatment of invasive *Aspergillus* infections in adults in the Middle East region: expert panel recommendations. *J Infect Public Health*. 2014;7:20-31.
5. Alastruey-Izquierdo A, Mellado E, Pelaez T, et al. Population-based survey of filamentous fungi and antifungal resistance in Spain (FILPOP Study). *Antimicrob Agents Chemother*. 2013;57:3380-3387.
9. Al-shair K, Atherton GT, Kennedy D, et al. Validity and reliability of the St. George's Respiratory Questionnaire in assessing health status in patients with chronic pulmonary aspergillosis. *Chest*. 2013;144:623-631.

10. Aquino VR, Nagel F, Andreolla HF, et al. The performance of real-time PCR, galactomannan, and fungal culture in the diagnosis of invasive aspergillosis in ventilated patients with chronic obstructive pulmonary disease (COPD). *Mycopathologia.* 2012;174:163-169.
11. Arvanitis M, Ziakas PD, Zacharioudakis IM, et al. PCR in diagnosis of invasive aspergillosis: a meta-analysis of diagnostic performance. *J Clin Microbiol.* 2014;52:3731-3742.
14. Avni T, Levy I, Sprecher H, et al. Diagnostic accuracy of PCR alone compared to galactomannan in bronchoalveolar lavage fluid for diagnosis of invasive pulmonary aspergillosis: a systematic review. *J Clin Microbiol.* 2012;50:3652-3658.
16. Baddley JW, Marr KA, Andes DR, et al. Patterns of susceptibility of *Aspergillus* isolates recovered from patients enrolled in the Transplant-Associated Infection Surveillance Network. *J Clin Microbiol.* 2009;47:3271-3275.
17. Badiee P, Alborzi A, Karimi M, et al. Diagnostic potential of nested PCR, galactomannan EIA, and beta-D-glucan for invasive aspergillosis in pediatric patients. *J Infect Dev Ctries.* 2012;6:352-357.
19. Balajee SA, Nickle D, Varga J, et al. Molecular studies reveal frequent misidentification of *Aspergillus fumigatus* by morphotyping. *Eukaryot Cell.* 2006;5:1705-1712.
20. Baxter CG, Denning DW, Jones AM, et al. Performance of two *Aspergillus* IgG EIA assays compared with the precipitin test in chronic and allergic aspergillosis. *Clin Microbiol Infect.* 2013;19:E197-E204.
24. Blot SI, Taccone FS, Van den Abeele AM, et al. A clinical algorithm to diagnose invasive pulmonary aspergillosis in critically ill patients. *Am J Respir Crit Care Med.* 2012;186:56-64.
26. Blyth CC, Gilroy NM, Guy SD, et al. Consensus guidelines for the treatment of invasive mould infections in haematological malignancy and haemopoietic stem cell transplantation, 2014. *Intern Med J.* 2014;44:1333-1349.
27. Boogaerts M, Winston DJ, Bow EJ, et al. Intravenous and oral itraconazole versus intravenous amphotericin B deoxycholate as empirical antifungal therapy for persistent fever in neutropenic patients with cancer who are receiving broad-spectrum antibacterial therapy. A randomized, controlled trial. *Ann Intern Med.* 2001;135:412-422.
33. Cadranel J, Philippe B, Hennequin C, et al. Voriconazole for chronic pulmonary aspergillosis: a prospective multicenter trial. *Eur J Clin Microbiol Infect Dis.* 2012;31:3231-3239.
34. Camuset J, Nunes H, Dombret MC, et al. Treatment of chronic pulmonary aspergillosis by voriconazole in nonimmunocompromised patients. *Chest.* 2007;131:1435-1441.
38. Chishimba L, Langridge P, Powell G, et al. Efficacy and safety of nebulised amphotericin B (NAB) in severe asthma with fungal sensitisation (SAFS) and allergic bronchopulmonary aspergillosis (ABPA). *J Asthma.* 2014;52:1-7.
39. Choi SH, Kang ES, Eo H, et al. *Aspergillus* galactomannan antigen assay and invasive aspergillosis in pediatric cancer patients and hematopoietic stem cell transplant recipients. *Pediatr Blood Cancer.* 2013;60:316-322.
42. Cordonnier C, Botterel F, Ben Amor R, et al. Correlation between galactomannan antigen levels in serum and neutrophil counts in haematological patients with invasive aspergillosis. *Clin Microbiol Infect.* 2009;15:81-86.
50. Denning DW, Bromley MJ. Infectious disease. How to bolster the antifungal pipeline. *Science.* 2015;347:1414-1416.
51. Denning DW, Cadranel J, Beigelman-Aubry C, et al. Chronic pulmonary aspergillosis: rationale and clinical guidelines for diagnosis and management. *Eur Respir J.* 2016;47:45-68.
55. Denning DW, Park S, Lass-Florl C, et al. High-frequency triazole resistance found In nonculturable *Aspergillus fumigatus* from lungs of patients with chronic fungal disease. *Clin Infect Dis.* 2011;52:1123-1129.
61. Dinand V, Anjan M, Oberoi JK, et al. Threshold of galactomannan antigenemia positivity for early diagnosis of invasive aspergillosis in neutropenic children. *J Microbiol Immunol Infect.* 2016;49:66-73.
64. Doligalski CT, Benedict K, Cleveland AA, et al. Epidemiology of invasive mold infections in lung transplant recipients. *Am J Transplant.* 2014;14:1328-1333.
67. Duarte RF, Sanchez-Ortega I, Cuesta I, et al. Serum galactomannan-based early detection of invasive aspergillosis in hematology patients receiving effective anti-mold prophylaxis. *Clin Infect Dis.* 2014;59:1696-1702.
69. Espinel-Ingroff A, Chowdhary A, Gonzalez GM, et al. Multicenter study of isavuconazole MIC distributions and epidemiological cutoff values for *Aspergillus* spp. for the CLSI M38-A2 broth microdilution method. *Antimicrob Agents Chemother.* 2013;57:3823-3828.
70. Espinel-Ingroff A, Cuenca-Estrella M, Fothergill A, et al. Wild-type MIC distributions and epidemiological cutoff values for amphotericin B and *Aspergillus* spp. for the CLSI broth microdilution method (M38-A2 document). *Antimicrob Agents Chemother.* 2011;55:5150-5154.
71. Espinel-Ingroff A, Diekema DJ, Fothergill A, et al. Wild-type MIC distributions and epidemiological cutoff values for the triazoles and six *Aspergillus* spp. for the CLSI broth microdilution method (M38-A2 document). *J Clin Microbiol.* 2010;48:3251-3257.
72. Farid S, Mohamed S, Devbhandari M, et al. Results of surgery for chronic pulmonary aspergillosis, optimal antifungal therapy and proposed high risk factors for recurrence—a National Centre's experience. *J Cardiothorac Surg.* 2013;8:180.
73. Felton TW, Baxter C, Moore CB, et al. Efficacy and safety of posaconazole for chronic pulmonary aspergillosis. *Clin Infect Dis.* 2010;51:1383-1391.
74. Fisher BT, Zaoutis TE, Park JR, et al. Galactomannan antigen testing for diagnosis of invasive aspergillosis in pediatric hematology patients. *J Pediatric Infect Dis Soc.* 2012;1:103-111.
78. Gams W, Christensen M, Onions AH, et al. Infrageneric taxa of *Aspergillus.* In: Samson RA, Pitt J, eds. *Advances in Penicillium and Aspergillus systematics.* New York: Plenum Press; 1985:55-62.
90. Hachem RY, Kontoyiannis DP, Chemaly RF, et al. Utility of galactomannan enzyme immunoassay and (1,3) beta-D-glucan in diagnosis of invasive fungal infections: low sensitivity for *Aspergillus fumigatus* infection in hematologic malignancy patients. *J Clin Microbiol.* 2009;47:129-133.
93. Heng SC, Morrissey O, Chen SC, et al. Utility of bronchoalveolar lavage fluid galactomannan alone or in combination with PCR for the diagnosis of invasive aspergillosis in adult hematology patients: a systematic review and meta-analysis. *Crit Rev Microbiol.* 2015;41:124-134.
96. Herbrecht R, Patterson TF, Slavin MA, et al. Application of the 2008 definitions for invasive fungal diseases to the trial comparing voriconazole versus amphotericin B for therapy of invasive aspergillosis: a collaborative study of the Mycoses Study Group (MSG 05) and the European Organization for Research and Treatment of Cancer Infectious Diseases Group. *Clin Infect Dis.* 2015;60:713-720.
97. Hidalgo A, Parody R, Martino R, et al. Correlation between high-resolution computed tomography and galactomannan antigenemia in adult hematologic patients at risk for invasive aspergillosis. *Eur J Radiol.* 2009;71:55-60.
104. Jain LR, Denning DW. The efficacy and tolerability of voriconazole in the treatment of chronic cavitary pulmonary aspergillosis. *J Infect.* 2006;52:e133-e137.
109. Jha AK, Bansal D, Chakrabarti A, et al. Serum galactomannan assay for the diagnosis of invasive aspergillosis in children with haematological malignancies. *Mycoses.* 2013;56:442-448.
117. Kohno S, Izumikawa K, Ogawa K, et al. Intravenous micafungin versus voriconazole for chronic pulmonary aspergillosis: a multicenter trial in Japan. *J Infect.* 2010;61:410-418.
119. Koyama K, Ohshima N, Suzuki J, et al. Recurrence of chronic pulmonary aspergillosis after discontinuation of maintenance treatment by antifungal triazoles. *J Infect Chemother.* 2014;20:375-379.
127. Lat A, Bhadelia N, Miko B, et al. Invasive aspergillosis after pandemic (H1N1) 2009. *Emerg Infect Dis.* 2010;16:971-973.
132. Luong ML, Chaparro C, Stephenson A, et al. Pretransplant *Aspergillus* colonization of cystic fibrosis patients and the incidence of post-lung transplant invasive aspergillosis. *Transplantation.* 2014;97:351-357.
133. Maertens J, Egerer G, Shin WS, et al. Caspofungin use in daily clinical practice for treatment of invasive aspergillosis: results of a prospective observational registry. *BMC Infect Dis.* 2010;10:182-189.
134. Maertens J, Maertens V, Theunissen K, et al. Bronchoalveolar lavage fluid galactomannan for the diagnosis of invasive pulmonary aspergillosis in patients with hematologic diseases. *Clin Infect Dis.* 2009;49:1688-1693.
135. Maertens J, Marchetti O, Herbrecht R, et al. European guidelines for antifungal management in leukemia and hematopoietic stem cell transplant recipients: summary of the ECIL 3–2009 update. *Bone Marrow Transplant.* 2011;46:709-718.
162. Nam HS, Jeon K, Um SW, et al. Clinical characteristics and treatment outcomes of chronic necrotizing pulmonary aspergillosis: a review of 43 cases. *Int J Infect Dis.* 2010;14:e479-e482.
179. Patterson TF, Thompson GR 3rd, Denning DW, et al. Practice guidelines for the diagnosis and management of aspergillosis: 2016 update by the Infectious Diseases Society of America. *Clin Infect Dis.* 2016;63:e1-e60.
229. van der Linden JW, Arendrup MC, Warris A, et al. Prospective multicenter international surveillance of azole resistance in Aspergillus fumigatus. *Emerg Infect Dis.* 2015;21:1041-1044.
231. Vergidis P, Razonable RR, Wheat LJ, et al. Reduction in false-positive *Aspergillus* serum galactomannan enzyme immunoassay results associated with use of piperacillin-tazobactam in the United States. *J Clin Microbiol.* 2014;52:2199-2201.
232. Verweij PE, Ananda-Rajah M, Andes D, et al. International expert opinion on the management of infection caused by azole-resistant *Aspergillus fumigatus. Drug Resist Updat.* 2015;21–22:30-40.
249. Wattier RL, Dvorak CC, Hoffman JA, et al. A prospective, international cohort study of invasive mold infections in children. *J Pediatric Infect Dis Soc.* 2015;4:313-322.
250. Wauters J, Baar I, Meersseman P, et al. Invasive pulmonary aspergillosis is a frequent complication of critically ill H1N1 patients: a retrospective study. *Intensive Care Med.* 2012;38:1761-1768.

The full reference list for this chapter is available at ExpertConsult.com.

Blastomycosis

199

Gregory M. Gauthier • Bruce S. Klein

Blastomyces dermatitidis and *Blastomyces gilchristii,* the etiologic agents of blastomycosis, belong to a group of ascomycete fungi that exhibit thermal dimorphism. Other pathogens in this group include *Histoplasma capsulatum, Coccidioides immitis, Coccidioides posadasii, Paracoccidioides brasiliensis, Paracoccidioides lutzii, Sporothrix schenckii,* and *Talaromyces marneffei* (formerly *Penicillium marneffei*). In the soil (at 22°C–25°C), these fungi grow as filamentous mold that produce infectious conidia (i.e., asexual spores). After disruption of soil by activities such as construction, conidia and mold fragments that are aerosolized and inhaled into the lungs of the host (37°C) convert into pathogenic yeast.

In the yeast form, *Blastomyces* can evade immune defenses by impairing the host's cytokine and immune cell responses. In 21% to 53% of patients, infection disseminates to other organs, such as the skin or bone. Diagnosis requires a high degree of clinical suspicion coupled with the use of culture and nonculture diagnostic tests. Treatment recommendations, which were updated in 2008 by the Infectious Diseases Society of America, include the use of polyene or azole antifungal agents. Echinocandins are not effective. Selection of antiinfective therapy is influenced by disease severity, site of infection, immunosuppression, and pregnancy.

HISTORICAL PERSPECTIVE

Blastomycosis was first described as "protozoan dermatitis" by Thomas Casper Gilchrist at the 1894 American Dermatological Association meeting in Washington, DC.[59] Two years later, Gilchrist published a detailed histologic analysis of the cutaneous findings in a manuscript titled "A case of Blastomycetic Dermatitis in Man."[60] In 1896 and 1898, Gilchrist and W.R. Stokes described a second case of blastomycetic dermatitis and named the pathologic agent *Blastomyces dermatitidis.*[61,62]

Almost a decade later in 1907, Walter W. Hamburger analyzed four clinical isolates and described the growth of *B. dermatitidis* as mold at room temperature and as budding yeast at 37°C.[72] During this time, heightened awareness of the disease resulted in the publication of several case reports and case series describing the clinical characteristics of blastomycosis, including invasive disease.[110,147] Most clinical cases were from the Chicago area, and the disease became known as Chicago disease or Gilchrist disease. In early publications, two distinct forms of the disease were recognized: cutaneous and systemic.[110,147]

In the early 1950s, Jan Schwarz and Gerald L. Baum performed a detailed clinicopathologic analysis of patients with blastomycosis and established that the primary portal of entry was pulmonary and that most cutaneous lesions were the result of dissemination from the lungs.[138] In the mid-1980s, *B. dermatitidis* caused an outbreak among children and was successfully isolated from the soil.[86] In 2013, phylogenetic analysis of 78 *Blastomyces* strains from the soil, humans, and dogs identified a new species, *Blastomyces gilchristii.*[25]

In 2015, the sequenced genomes of *B. dermatitidis* (i.e., strains ER-3, ATCC26199, and ATCC18188) and *B. gilchristii* (i.e., strain SLH14081) were published.[23,112] *B. dermatitidis* genes that are upregulated during infection were revealed through in vivo transcriptional profiling in a mouse model of pulmonary blastomycosis.[98,112]

MYCOLOGY

B. dermatitidis and *B. gilchristii,* the etiologic agents of blastomycosis, are haploid ascomycetes that exhibit thermal dimorphism by growing as yeast at 37°C and as mold at 22°C to 25°C (Fig. 199.1). *Blastomyces* yeast forms (8–20 μm) are characterized by a broad-based bud (4–5 μm) and a doubly refractile cell wall.[163] This appearance is unique among the dimorphic fungi; however, giant yeast forms (28–40 μm) have been reported, and they can be confused with *Coccidioides.*[164]

At environmental temperatures, *Blastomyces* grows as septate hyphae (1–2 μm in diameter) capable of producing asexual spores called *conidia.*[161,163] Conidia are small (4–5 μm) and are oval or piriform. Individual conidia are attached to hyphae by a short conidiophore and have the appearance of a lollipop.[161,163] Macroscopically, yeast colonies appear off-white and can have a smooth or rough appearance. Mold colonies initially appear off-white or tan.[163] The morphologic characteristics for *Blastomyces* mold are not pathognomonic, and definitive identification requires molecular confirmation or conversion to yeast at 37°C. The conversion between mold and yeast is reversible and can be induced in the laboratory by shifting the temperature between 22°C to 25°C and 37°C.

B. dermatitidis is considered the asexual or anamorph form. The sexual or teleomorph form is known as *Ajellomyces dermatitidis.*[104,105] In the sexual stage, *A. dermatitidis* exhibits heterothallic mating, which means that opposite mating types (+ and −) exchange genetic material to produce progeny. During mating, *A. dermatitidis* produces cleistothecia with coiled spirals that can give rise to spores known as *asci.* Individual asci are capable of forming hyphae with conidia (at 25°C) or converting to virulent yeast when inoculated into mice (at 37°C).[104,105] Sexual and asexual spores and both mating types (+ and −) are capable of causing infection.[103,106]

The genomes of clinical and environmental isolates of *B. dermatitidis* and *B. gilchristii* have been sequenced, annotated, and made available to the scientific community.[23,112] The size of the *Blastomyces* genome ranges from 66.6 to 75.4 Mb and contains 9180 to 10,187 genes.[23,112]

ECOLOGY AND EPIDEMIOLOGY

Blastomyces is endemic to North America and is geographically restricted to the Midwest, South Central, and Southeastern United States and several Canadian provinces (i.e., Saskatchewan, Manitoba, Ontario, and Quebec) (Fig. 199.2A). In endemic regions, *Blastomyces* spp. are not uniformly distributed but grow in an ecologic niche characterized by forested, sandy soils with an acidic pH that are located near water and contain decaying vegetation or organic matter.[86] Similar to *H. capsulatum,* a related dimorphic fungus, *Blastomyces* can grow in bird and animal excreta. Knowledge about the niche and conditions that promote growth of the mold form has been gleaned mostly from analysis of outbreaks of blastomycosis (Table 199.1). Occupational and recreational activities associated with infection involve disruption of soil and include construction of homes or roads, boating and canoeing, tubing on a river, fishing, exploration of beaver dams and underground forts, and use of a community compost pile (see Table 199.1).

Outside North America, blastomycosis is a rare cause of deep fungal infection, but autochthonous cases of culture-proven infections have been reported from India and 18 countries in Africa (see Fig. 199.2).[7,102,139] *Blastomyces* is not considered endemic to Central America, South America, Europe, Asia, or Australia. In the developing world, the ecologic niche inhabited by *Blastomyces* spp. has not been identified. *Blastomyces* has never been isolated from soil outside North America, nor have there been human or veterinarian outbreaks to help define the geographic distribution of this pathogen in Africa or India. Compared with North American strains, African *Blastomyces* isolates display unique features, including a decreased ability to convert to yeast after a shift in temperature from 25°C to 37°C, unique media requirements for maintenance of yeast growth in vitro, and a less antigenically complex cell surface.[80]

Information about the epidemiology of blastomycosis in North America is based on retrospective studies and passive surveillance. In the endemic zone, six states (i.e., Wisconsin, Minnesota, Michigan, Missouri, Arkansas, and Louisiana) and two provinces (i.e., Ontario and Manitoba) mandate reporting of new cases of blastomycosis. In North America, the annual incidence of blastomycosis ranges from 0.2 to 1.94 cases per 100,000 people (Table 199.2). Several geographic areas are considered to be hyperendemic: Kenora, Ontario (117.2 cases per 100,000 people); Vilas County, Wisconsin (40.4 per 100,000); Eagle River, Wisconsin (101.3 per 100,000); Washington Parish, Louisiana (6.8 per 100,000); and central and south central Mississippi (more than 5 per 100,000) (see Table 199.2).

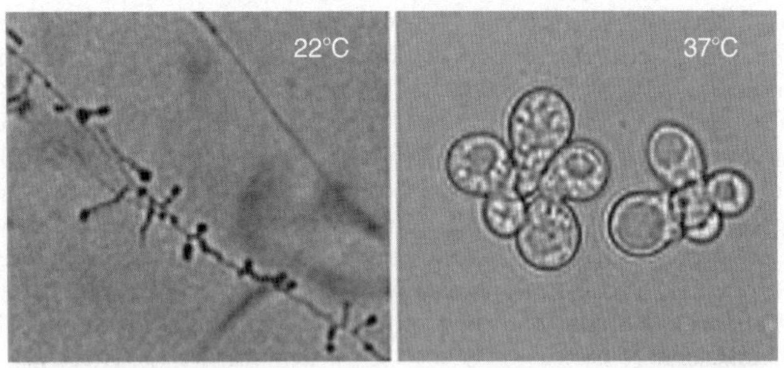

FIG. 199.1 Mold growing at 22°C and yeast growing at 37°C are forms of *B. dermatitidis*.

The true incidence of blastomycosis is likely much greater than the reported numbers. Reliable skin and serologic tests are not available, and about 50% of infected people develop subclinical or asymptomatic illness.[86] Epidemiologic analysis is limited to patients with clinically apparent infection that is recognized, diagnosed, and reported to public health agencies when required by law. Most epidemiologic studies show a slight male predominance for patients diagnosed with blastomycosis (see Table 199.2), which is also observed for coccidioidomycosis and histoplasmosis.

Although most patients with clinical disease have normal immune function, several medical conditions can be associated with the development of severe clinical disease, including immunosuppression due to solid organ transplantation, acquired immunodeficiency syndrome (AIDS),[118] and treatment with medications that block the activity of tumor necrosis factor-α (TNF-α).[134,141] A case report described severe pulmonary blastomycosis in a pediatric patient with GATA2 deficiency.[143] Most clinically recognized cases of blastomycosis are sporadic, but 17 well-defined outbreaks have been reported in North America (see Table 199.1). Hmong ethnicity increased susceptibility to infection according to an outbreak-related investigation in Wisconsin (see Table 199.1).[130]

In the developing world, blastomycosis is found mainly in Africa and India.[7,139] In Africa, almost 100 cases have been described from countries north and south of the equator [7,28,51] (see Fig. 199.2B). Only a few cases have been identified from western Africa and none from

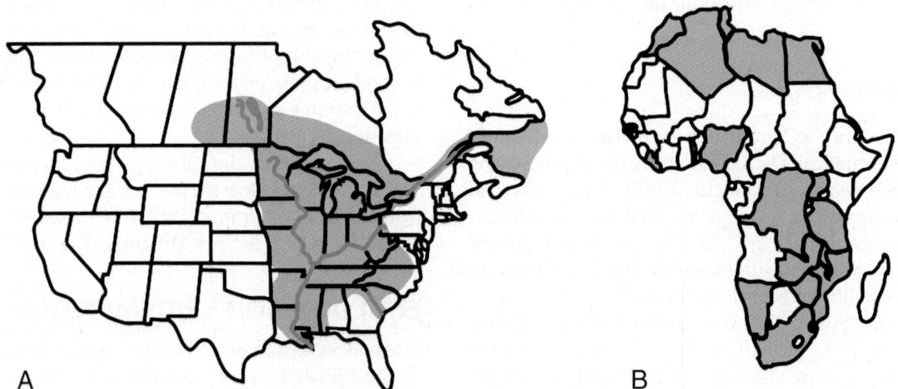

FIG. 199.2 Endemic regions *(brown)* of blastomycosis in (A) North America and (B) Africa.

TABLE 199.1 Outbreaks of Human Blastomycosis in North America

State	Years	No. of Cases	Source of Outbreak	Reference
North Carolina	1953–54	11	Not identified	142
Minnesota	1972	12	Cabin construction	153
North Carolina	1975	5	Peanut farm harvest	30
Illinois	1974–75	5	Apartment complex construction	79
Wisconsin	1979	8	Canoeing on Namekegon River	34
Wisconsin	1984	48	Abandoned beaver lodge	86
Virginia	1984	4	Raccoon hunting	5
Wisconsin	1985	14	Underground timber fort; fishing	84
Wisconsin	1988	32	Hotel construction near Eagle River	13
Tennessee	1989	3	Construction at a rayon factory	54
Wisconsin	1989–90	8	Not identified	124
Colorado	1998	2	Prairie dog relocation	39
Wisconsin	1998–2000	9	Likely related to construction or excavation	14
North Carolina	2001–02	8	Likely related to construction projects	94
Wisconsin	2006	21	Community yard waste site	121
Wisconsin	2009–10	55	Not identified	130
Wisconsin	2015	90	Tubing on the Little Wolf River	162

TABLE 199.2 **Incidence of Human Blastomycosis in the United States and Canada**

State or Province	Years Studied	Annual Incidence/ 100,000 People	Ratio (M:F)	Immune Suppression	Blastomycosis-Attributable Mortality Rate	Reference
Wisconsin	1973–82	0.48	1.8:1	NR	NR	82
	1986–95	1.4	1.5:1	NR	4.3%	31
	1984–90	40.4 for Vilas County; 101.3 for Eagle River area	1.6:1	6.7%	2.7%	12
Illinois	1981–89	1.94[a]	2.2:1	NR	NR	95
Indiana	2003–08	0.65[b]	1.8:1	23.7%	1.9%	27
Kentucky	1960–65	0.44	NR	NR	NR	55
Tennessee	1980–95	0.77[c]	2.3:1	12.5%	16.7%	155
	1996–2005	1.23[c]	2.5:1	19.7%	14.8%	75
Missouri	1992–99	0.2	2.1:1	14.8%	22%	26
Arkansas	1960–65	0.43	NR	NR	NR	107
Mississippi	1963–67	0.61	NR	NR	NR	55
	1979–88	1.3	1.7:1	17.2%	9.6%	33
Louisiana	1976–85	0.23 (6.8[d])	1.1:1	NR	16.6%[d]	92
Ontario	1997–99	117.2 for Kenora	1.1:1	6.5%	3.3%	45
	1994–2003	0.30	1.9:1	NR	NR	111
Manitoba	1988–99	0.62	1.9:1	1.4%	6.3%	37

[a]Data collected from Rockford, Illinois.
[b]Data collected from Indianapolis, Indiana.
[c]Data collected from northeastern Tennessee; incidence in Washington County is 3.01–3.5 cases/100,000 people.
[d]Data collected from Washington Parish, Louisiana.
NR, Not reported.

the island of Madagascar. This contrasts with *H. capsulatum* var. *duboisii*, which is endemic to western and central Africa and to Madagascar. In India, fewer than a dozen cases have been reported. Limitations in public health infrastructure and diagnostic capabilities likely contribute to underestimation of the true incidence of disease.

The clinical presentation of blastomycosis often mimics that of other pulmonary and cutaneous infections. Physicians in North America and the developing world confront a similar challenge in entertaining blastomycosis in the differential diagnosis, which is important because special stains and culture media are needed for the identification and growth of *Blastomyces*.

B. dermatitidis and *B. gilchristii* cause disease in children with normal and impaired immune defenses. Blastomycosis is uncommon in children, with an estimated 2% to 13% of cases occurring in the pediatric population.[37,38,46,55,90,107,111] Few studies have focused solely on the pediatric population.[3,22,47,52,123,137,144,] In these studies, the average age was 9.1 to 12.9 years, with a range of 18 days to 18 years of age, and gender distribution slightly favored male predominance.[3,22,52,47,89,123,137,144] Perinatal blastomycosis is rare, with only a few reported cases.[37,100,159,167] In two well-described cases, the mothers developed disseminated blastomycosis (during the first and third trimesters, respectively), and the neonates were admitted to the hospital for medical care at 18 and 21 days of life.[100,159,167] Both neonates died of respiratory failure from severe pulmonary blastomycosis.[100,159] Similar to the neonate population, blastomycosis in infants 1 to 12 months of age is exceedingly uncommon.[37,47,107,120,111,]

Although most cases of blastomycosis are sporadic, outbreaks are common and often result in clinical disease in children. Of the 17 reported outbreaks (see Table 199.1), 14 involved pediatric patients. The literature on pediatric blastomycosis suggests that risk of infection correlates with environmental exposure and is not influenced significantly by age or gender.[154]

PATHOGENESIS

The ability to convert from mold to yeast is an essential event in the pathogenesis of *Blastomyces* infection and other dimorphic fungi. In the soil (at 22°C to 25°C), *B. dermatitidis* and *B. gilchristii* are thought to grow as a mold that produces infectious conidia. After disruption of soil, aerosolized conidia and mold fragments inhaled into the lungs of a human host (at 37°C) convert into pathogenic yeast.[56] Temperature is the primary environmental stimulus that promotes this morphologic switch. The phase transition is a complex event that involves global changes in transcription, metabolism, cell signaling, cell wall composition, and plasma membrane lipid content.[56]

Over the past 2 decades, the molecular tools available to genetically manipulate the dimorphic fungi have expanded and enabled the discovery of genes that affect the phase transition, including genes for dimorphism regulating kinase 1 *(DRK1)* and siderophore biosynthesis repressor in *Blastomyces (SREB)*. *DRK1* encodes a histidine kinase that regulates the conversion of mold to yeast, production of conidia, cell wall carbohydrate composition, and expression of the essential virulence factor *Blastomyces* adhesion 1 (BAD1), formerly called Wisconsin 1 (WI1).[113] Genetic deletion of *DRK1* in *B. dermatitidis* and *H. capsulatum* resulted in hyphal growth at 37°C (and 22°C), reduced transcription of BAD1, failure to produce conidia at 22°C, and decreased cell wall glucan.[113] Moreover, *B. dermatitidis* and *H. capsulatum* with reduced *DRK1* transcripts were avirulent in a murine model of infection. These studies offered genetic proof that the conversion from mold to yeast is required for virulence of the dimorphic fungi.

SREB encodes a GATA transcription factor that promotes the conversion from yeast to mold after a drop in temperature to 22°C and regulates genes involved in iron homeostasis and lipid metabolism.[58,97] The defect in the conversion to hyphae in *SREB*-null mutants correlates with reduction in the biosynthesis of triacylglycerol and ergosterol and with impaired homeostasis of lipid droplets, which are specialized lipid storage organelles.[97] In addition to *SREB*, *N*-acetylglucosamine (GlcNAc) accelerates the morphologic switch of *Blastomyces* (and *Histoplasma*) to hyphae, which is mediated by NGT1 and NGT2 transmembrane transporters.[63]

B. dermatitidis and *B. gilchristii* are considered primary fungal pathogens because they cause disease in persons with intact or impaired immune defenses. Features that promote fungal growth in human tissue include the ability to survive at core human body temperature (37°C), convert to budding yeast, express yeast-phase–specific virulence factors, and evade killing by host immune cells.[19,20,21,49,50,113,145,146] The conversion of conidia to yeast is accelerated after phagocytosis of *Blastomyces* spores by alveolar macrophages.[146] Yeast survive and replicate within macrophages during the early stages of infection.[146] This intracellular lifestyle is similar to that of *H. capsulatum, Coccidioides spp., and Paracoccidioides* spp.

In the yeast phase, *Blastomyces* upregulates the expression of *BAD1*, which encodes a 120-kd protein that is secreted extracellularly and binds to chitin on the fungal cell wall.[20,49,50] Deletion of *BAD1* renders *Blastomyces* nonpathogenic in a murine model of pulmonary infection, demonstrating this yeast-phase–specific virulence factor is essential for virulence.[21] BAD1 has multiple functions. Cell wall and soluble BAD1 bind macrophage receptors (i.e., CR3 and CD14) to induce downregulation of TNF-α in a transforming growth factor-β (TGF-β)–dependent and –independent manner, respectively.[20,49,50] TNF-α is a critical cytokine for host defense against *Blastomyces*; antibody-mediated neutralization of TNF-α results in progressive pulmonary infection in animal models.[50] BAD1 impairs activation $CD4^+$ T cells, which results in decreased production of interleukin-17 (IL-17) and interferon-γ (INF-γ).[19] BAD1 also facilitates adhesion of yeast to lung tissue and T cells through interaction with heparan sulfate,[16,19] binds exogenous calcium,[18] and impedes binding of complement (C3) to the yeast cell surface.[169]

Blastomyces yeast also secrete dipeptidylpeptidase IVA (DPPIVA), which impairs recruitment and differentiation of inflammatory monocytes by cleaving host chemokines.[145] The loss of recruited inflammatory monocytes (and differentiated cells) to the lung enhances the virulence of *Blastomyces* yeast.[145] DPPIVA also cleaves granulocyte-macrophage colony-stimulating factor (GM-CSF), which promotes intracellular survival in macrophages and blunts neutrophil antifungal activity.[145]

Changes in cell wall carbohydrate composition associated with the phase transition may contribute to virulence and immune evasion. During the conversion from mold to yeast, the amount of α-(1,3)-glucan increases and that of β-(1,3)-glucan decreases. *Blastomyces* mutants deficient in α-(1,3)-glucan have impaired virulence in a murine model of infection.[73] Similarly, reduction or complete loss of α-(1,3)-glucan synthase activity in *H. capsulatum* renders this dimorphic fungal pathogen avirulent.[127] The concentration of cell wall β-(1,3)-glucan drops from 40% to 50% in mycelia to less than 5% in yeast.[77] Exposed β-(1,3)-glucan binds mannose-binding lectins (i.e., MBL-A and MBL-C).[87] Collectively, these events may block the recognition of *Blastomyces* β-(1,3)-glucan by the Dectin-1 receptors on innate immune cells (i.e., macrophages). Moreover, the reduction of β-glucan in the yeast cell wall precludes the use of the (1→3)- β-D-glucan test for diagnosis and of echinocandins for treatment of blastomycosis.[32,65]

To combat infection, the innate and adaptive immune responses are required, whereas humoral immunity is dispensable. After inhalation of aerosolized conidia, alveolar macrophages phagocytize and kill a large percentage of conidia and regulate transformation to the pathogenic yeast phase.[43,148,149] Neutrophils also can ingest and kill conidia.[43] Conidia that survive the initial assault by macrophages and neutrophils germinate into yeast. *Blastomyces* yeast cells are more difficult to kill because they fail to induce a robust oxidative response, are relatively resistant to reactive oxygen species, and suppress nitric oxide production in macrophages.[129]

The adaptive immune response, which is coordinated by T lymphocytes, is important for controlling infection in a manner that requires helper T-cell type 17 (Th17) responses (i.e., IL-17) and helper T-cell type 1 (Th1) cytokine responses (i.e., interferon-γ and TNF-α) to activate macrophages to enhance fungicidal activity and promote clearance.[17,165] After infection, patients develop specific cellular immunity to that persists for at least 2 years.[81]

CLINICAL MANIFESTATIONS

The heterogeneous clinical manifestations of blastomycosis range from asymptomatic infection to acute pneumonia to disseminated disease. The lung is the primary portal of entry for aerosolized conidia and mycelial fragments after disruption of soil. After evasion of pulmonary host defenses, *B. dermatitidis* can remain localized in the lung or disseminate to other organs. Less common routes of transmission in children include direct cutaneous inoculation and inhalation of infected vaginal secretions at birth.[100,159,167,168] Definitive evidence for transplacental transmission to the fetus is lacking but is theoretically possible; *Blastomyces* yeast have been isolated from placental tissue.[93] Transmission of *Blastomyces* through solid organ transplantation (i.e., infected allograft) has not been reported, but this route of transmission has been described for *H. capsulatum* and *Coccidioides* species.[96]

Based on studies during an epidemic,[85,86] onset of symptomatic (acute pulmonary) disease occurs 3 weeks to 3.5 months after exposure to *B. dermatitidis* or *B. gilchristii.*

Pulmonary Disease

Acute pneumonia is the most common clinical manifestation of blastomycosis, and symptomatic disease develops in approximately 50% of infected children.[86] Clinical manifestations resemble community-acquired pneumonia and include fevers, chills, headache, cough (which is often productive), dyspnea, chest pain, and malaise.[47,123,154,166] Severity of disease ranges from mild illness that can be managed in the outpatient setting to acute respiratory distress syndrome (ARDS) requiring intubation and mechanical ventilation.[3,38,57,84,86,123] Chronic pneumonia can develop and is often associated with extrapulmonary dissemination and a delay in diagnosis.[47,137,144]

The lung is the most common organ affected by *Blastomyces* and is involved in 79% to 86% of patients with symptomatic blastomycosis.[3,38,47,52,143,166] Consolidation, which can be unilobar, multilobar, or diffuse, is the most frequent radiographic pattern described for children with pulmonary blastomycosis (Fig. 199.3).[2,47,84,86,123,137] Consolidation from blastomycosis is indistinguishable from bacterial pneumonia. Nodular and interstitial infiltrates are the second and third most common findings on chest radiography, respectively.[2,46,47] Hilar lymphadenopathy, pleural effusion, and lung abscess are infrequently encountered (Fig. 199.4).[2,47,84,123] Cavitary disease and mass lesions are rare in children and can mimic tuberculosis or neoplasm.

After treatment of pulmonary blastomycosis, radiographic abnormalities can persist for several years, and functional pulmonary deficits (i.e., restrictive or obstructive disease) can be slow to normalize in patients with severe disease.[1,2,123] Fortunately, most patients experience a full recovery without long-term pulmonary sequelae.[1]

Disseminated Disease

After infection is established in the lung, *Blastomyces* can disseminate to almost any organ in the body. Based on retrospective studies, disseminated disease in children occurred in 21% to 53% of sporadic cases,[3,22,47,52,137] which is similar to the rate for adults with blastomycosis

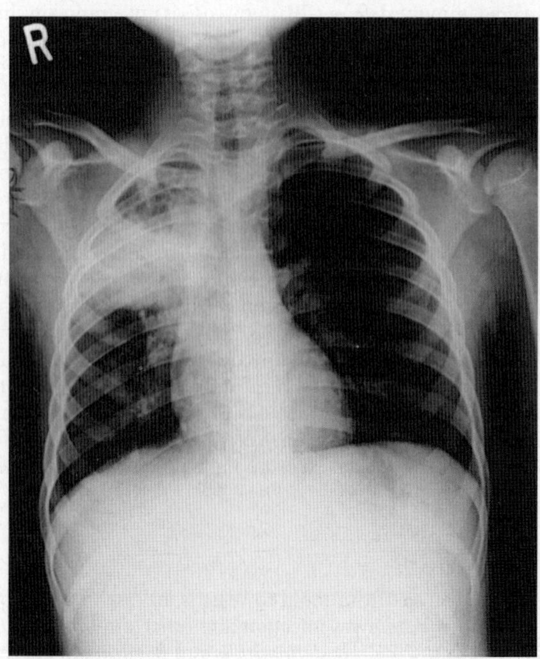

FIG. 199.3 Chest radiograph of a right upper lobe infiltrate due to blastomycosis.

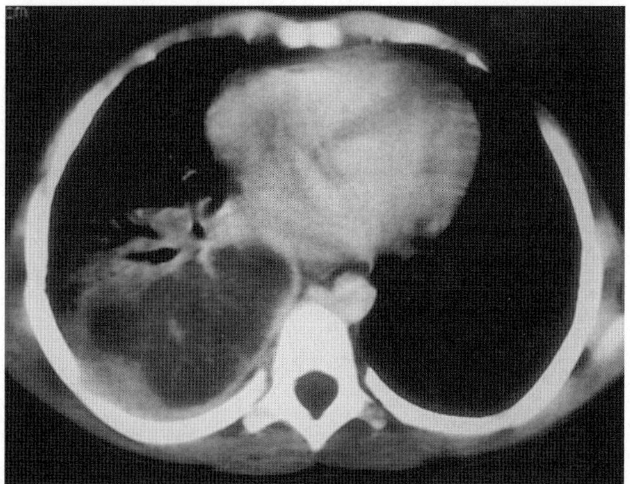

FIG. 199.4 Computed tomography of the chest reveals consolidation and abscess formation in the right lower lobe of the lung.

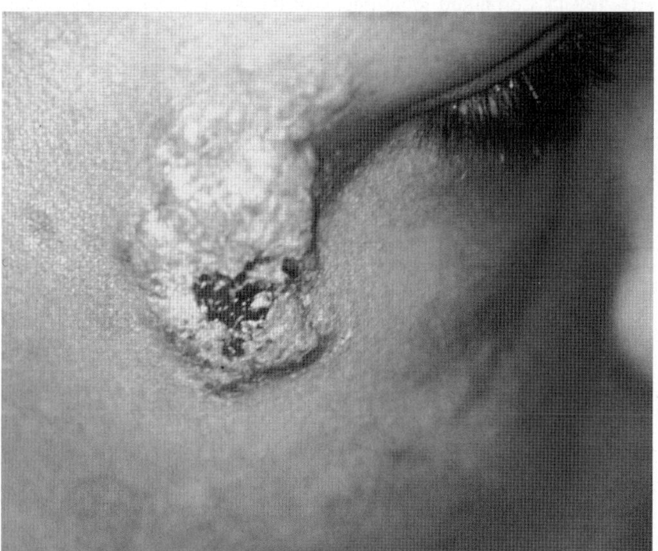

FIG. 199.5 Verrucous lesion of blastomycosis on the face of a child.

(25–40%).[32] In contrast, dissemination with acute pulmonary blastomycosis associated with point-source outbreaks occurred in a minority of patients.[154] The time from symptom onset to diagnosis is often delayed in patients who are diagnosed with disseminated disease.[47,137] Collectively, these data suggest that the duration of infection rather than age influences the risk for dissemination.[154]

Disseminated blastomycosis most commonly affects the skin and bone.[47,143,166] Cutaneous disease often begins as papulopustular lesions and progresses to ulcerative, verrucous, or crusted lesions (Figs. 199.5 and 199.6).[166] Erythema nodosum, which is common in patients with histoplasmosis and coccidioidomycosis, is rare in cases of blastomycosis.[166] Skin involvement can be associated with underlying osteomyelitis and manifests as pustules, abscesses, and ulcers (Figs. 199.7 and 199.8).[114] Invasion of *Blastomyces* into the bone results in lytic destruction that is often associated with a periosteal reaction and a sclerotic margin.[114] Although any bone can be infected, the most common sites include the long bones (e.g., tibia, humerus), skull, ribs, and vertebral bodies (Figs. 199.9 and 199.10).[47,114,131,166]

Clinical manifestations of osteomyelitis include bone pain and soft tissue swelling associated with a draining sinus, ulcer, or abscess.[114] Vertebral osteomyelitis can be complicated by extension into the soft tissues, resulting in paravertebral and psoas abscesses or invasion of the adjacent intervertebral disks and vertebral bodies.[131] These features

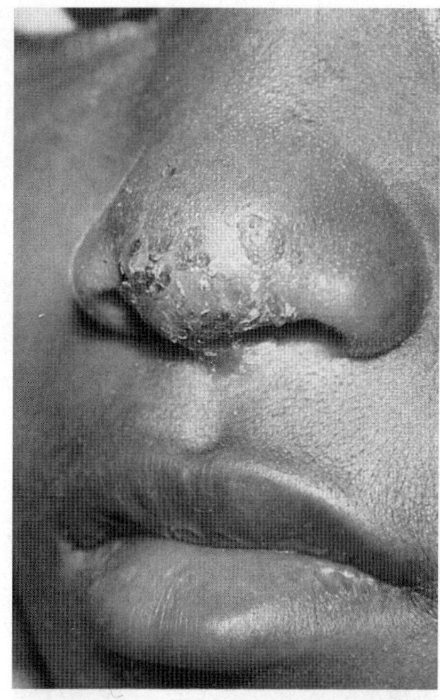

FIG. 199.6 Crusted skin lesion on the nose caused by *Blastomyces*.

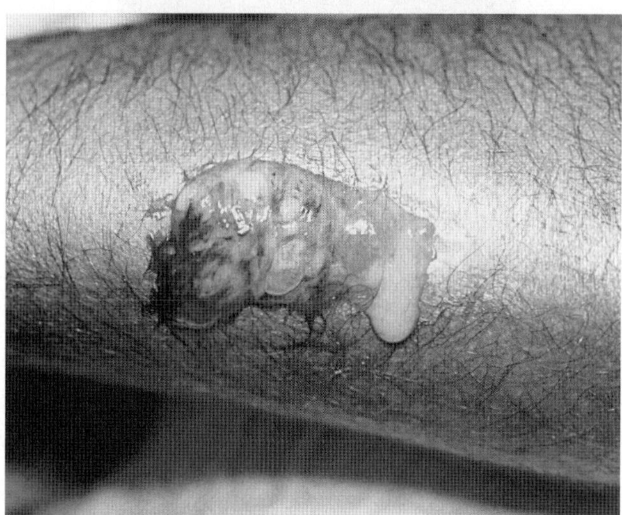

FIG. 199.7 Purulent wound drainage overlying a region of osteomyelitis due to blastomycosis.

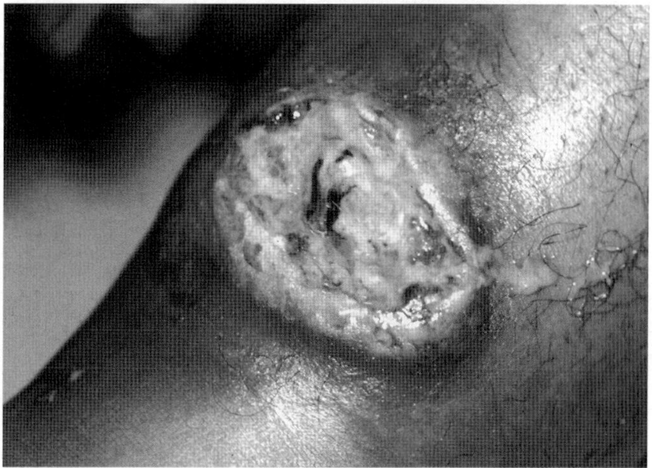

FIG. 199.8 Ulcerative lesion overlying a region of osteomyelitis due to blastomycosis.

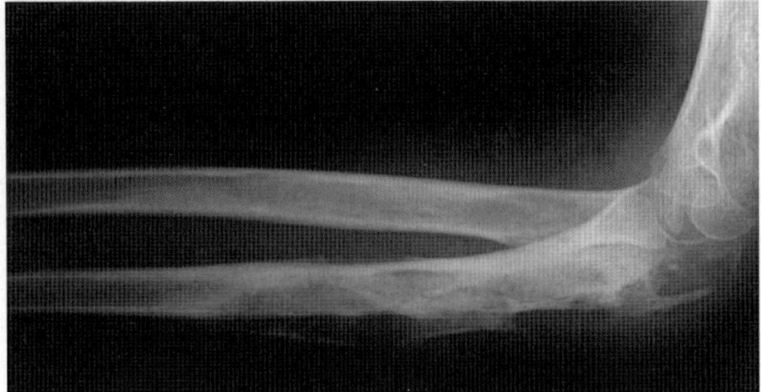

FIG. 199.9 Bone destruction of the ulna due to blastomycosis.

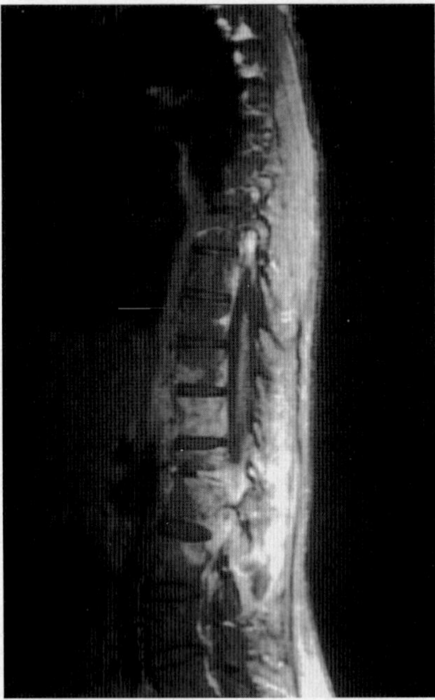

FIG. 199.10 Magnetic resonance imaging of the spine demonstrates signal abnormalities at T11 through L3, a severe compression deformity of the L1 vertebral body, and multiple oval lytic lesions caused by blastomycosis.

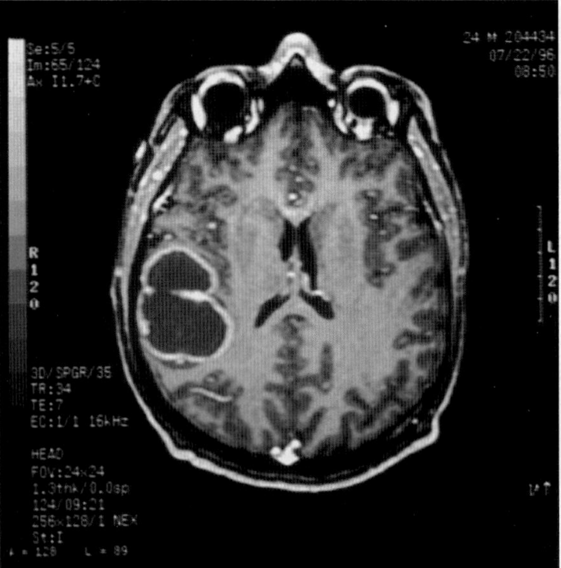

FIG. 199.11 Computed tomography of the brain demonstrates a multiloculated abscess in the right temporal lobe as a result of infection with *B. dermatitidis*.

can mimic *Mycobacterium tuberculosis* (i.e., Pott disease).[114] Progressive destruction of vertebral bone can result in compression fractures.[131] Similarly, osteomyelitis of the long bones can be complicated by pathologic fracture or extend into the joint space to cause septic arthritis.[89,114]

Blastomycosis rarely disseminates to the central nervous system (CNS) or other organs such as the liver, spleen, heart, or middle ear.[38,52,74,76,166] Otitis media from blastomycosis is an uncommon complication related to contiguous extension from an extra-auditory focus into the middle ear.[48,76] CNS blastomycosis is estimated to occur in less than 5% to 10% of nonimmunocompromised patients and results from hematogenous spread or direct invasion from untreated infection of the scalp or skull.[38,47,90] CNS blastomycosis manifests as meningitis, epidural abscess, or brain abscess involving the cerebrum or cerebellum (Fig. 199.11).[10,47,90] Some patients have concomitant meningitis and brain abscess.[10] Complications include hydrocephalus, mass effect from edema, cerebral herniation, infarction, seizures, panhypopituitarism, residual weakness, and impaired ability to function at school.[10,47] In patients with meningitis, cerebrospinal fluid (CSF) demonstrates a lymphocytic or neutrophilic pleocytosis associated with elevated protein levels and hypoglycorrhachia.[10] Forty-five percent of CSF cultures grow *B. dermatitidis.*[10]

Disease in Immunocompromised Patients

Information regarding the clinical course and treatment outcomes for blastomycosis in children with impaired immunity is limited to a few case reports.[141,157,168] Clinical studies have investigate blastomycosis in adults who have undergone solid organ transplantation, developed AIDS, or been diagnosed with malignancy.[57,70,118,119,152] Blastomycosis is estimated to occur in less than 0.2% of solid organ allograft recipients and manifests 0.4 to 250 months after transplantation, occurring in an almost equal distribution before and after the first year of transplantation.[57,70] Infection most commonly causes pneumonia, which is often complicated by respiratory failure or ARDS.[57,70] The frequency of extrapulmonary infection (33–50%) is similar to that in the general population (25–40%).[32,57,70] The mortality rate is 33% to 38%, but it increases to 67% for patients with ARDS.[57,70,119]

Blastomycosis in patients with AIDS is uncommon, and a single case series of 15 patients was published before the use of highly active antiretroviral therapy (HAART) that systemically investigated *Blastomyces* infection in this patient population.[118] The lung was infected in 87% of patients, and extrapulmonary disease occurred in 53%.[118] Invasion of *Blastomyces* into the CNS was common and occurred in 40% of patients. This clinical profile sharply contrasts to that of patients immunosuppressed by transplantation or malignancy, among whom the incidence of CNS blastomycosis is similar to that in the general population (<5–10%).[57,70,90,119] Approximately two thirds of AIDS patients with blastomycosis had prior opportunistic infections. The $CD4^+$ T-lymphocyte count at the time of diagnosis of blastomycosis was often less than 200 cells/mm^3.[118] The mortality rate attributable to blastomycosis was 53%.[118]

Blastomyces can infect patients with hematologic or solid organ malignancies, including those with lung carcinoma, squamous cell cancers of the head and neck, breast cancer, gastrointestinal neoplasms, chronic lymphocytic leukemia, acute myelogenous leukemia, Hodgkin disease, and multiple myeloma.[119,152] Similar to allograft recipients and those with AIDS, pneumonia was the most common clinical manifestation and was complicated by ARDS in some patients.[119] Extrapulmonary disease occurred in approximately 50%.[119] The high mortality rate was attributable to the underlying malignancy or blastomycosis.[119]

Blastomycosis is a rare complication for patients receiving TNF-α inhibitors.[29,101,134,141] In 2008, the US Food and Drug Administration issued an alert stating that patients taking TNF-α blockers such as etanercept, adalimumab, infliximab, and certolizumab are at risk for endemic mycoses, including histoplasmosis, coccidioidomycosis, and blastomycosis.[29] In this alert, seven cases of blastomycosis were reported. An analysis of health claims information from 2007 to 2009 with 30,772 unique patients who received TNF-α blockers identified 253 infections in 158 people, with only 4% due to blastomycosis.[134] However, no clinical data were provided about the patients with blastomycosis. The clinical information about blastomycosis in patients on TNF-α inhibitors is limited to a few case reports.[101,141]

Blastomycosis During Pregnancy and in Neonates

Blastomycosis is a rare complication of pregnancy, and clinical information is limited to sporadic case reports.[13,37,91] Women can be infected in any trimester, but the disease is most frequently diagnosed in the second or third trimester.[13,37,91] Disseminated disease is common (62%) and often involves the lungs, bone, and skin.[91] Isolated pulmonary infection occurs in 38% of patients.[91] Reliable information regarding the frequency of placental involvement is lacking because examination by histology or culture has been performed in only one third of clinical cases. However, dissemination to the placenta is possible.[91,93] Histologic analysis identified *B. dermatitidis* yeast in the placenta of a 23-year-old woman with pulmonary blastomycosis complicated by ARDS during the third trimester.[93] Her infant was delivered by cesarean section and did not develop blastomycosis.[93]

Although clinical data are limited, blastomycosis during pregnancy does not appear to increase the risk for congenital malformations. However, based on isolation of *Blastomyces* yeast from the placenta of one mother and two well-described clinical cases of neonatal blastomycosis, there is potential for transmission of blastomycosis during the peripartum period.[93,100,159] Both infants were admitted to the hospital for respiratory failure at 18 and 21 days of life. Infection was limited to the lungs, and both infants died of progressive pulmonary blastomycosis.[100,159] The underlying pathogenesis of neonatal blastomycosis is not well defined and may involve transplacental transmission or aspiration of infected vaginal secretions.

DIAGNOSIS

The diagnosis of blastomycosis requires a high index of suspicion because clinical and radiographic manifestations can mimic other diseases, including bacterial pneumonia, mycobacterial infections, and neoplasm. A detailed history focusing on potential exposures for the acquisition of *Blastomyces* can facilitate diagnosis in a timely fashion. The delay between symptom onset and diagnosis often exceeds 2 months.[47,137,144] Risks factors for endemic fungal infections include outdoor activities (i.e., canoeing, hiking, beaver dam exploration), home remodeling, construction (e.g., residential, commercial, road), playing in outdoor forts, hunting, fishing, use of a woodpile for a wood burning stove, and employment in a microbiology laboratory (see Table 199.1).[52,69,88]

The diagnosis of blastomycosis in a household pet, frequently a dog, suggests a common source of exposure.[5,13,15,24,52,64,108] Canine blastomycosis can serve as a harbinger of human blastomycosis.[136] In a retrospective analysis of 111 children with blastomycosis, 8.1% of patients had a dog with blastomycosis.[52] Airborne transmission of *Blastomyces* between animals and humans does not occur; however, primary cutaneous blastomycosis has been reported from bite injuries.[66,69] Microbiology laboratory workers are at risk for cutaneous infection from injuries caused by sharp implements such as needlesticks.[69,88]

Diagnostic evaluation for blastomycosis should be considered for patients with pneumonia or cutaneous lesions that fail to respond to antibiotic therapy. Pneumonia identified on chest radiography and cutaneous lesions on physical examination strongly suggest blastomycosis.

Definitive diagnosis of blastomycosis requires identification of *Blastomyces* in culture from sputum, skin, bone, or other clinical specimens. Commonly used culture media include Sabouraud dextrose agar and potato dextrose agar.[132] For culture of tissue specimens, supplementation of medium with brain-heart infusion agar is recommended.[132] Incubator temperatures used in most clinical laboratories (25°C–30°C) promote the growth of *Blastomyces* as mold. Because several other fungal species have a similar appearance, additional confirmatory tests are required, which can include use of chemiluminescent DNA probes that target specific rRNA sequences, polymerase chain reaction (PCR) assay, and conversion to yeast at 37°C.[132]

A presumptive diagnosis of blastomycosis can be made when yeast forms (8–20 μm) with broad-based budding and a doubly refractile cell wall are visualized by light microscopy from respiratory secretions, purulent material, or histopathologic sections. Visualization of *Blastomyces* requires special stains such as 10% potassium hydroxide, calcofluor white, Gomori methenamine silver (GMS), periodic acid–Schiff (PAS), or Papanicolaou (Fig. 199.12).[90] *Blastomyces* yeast can be difficult to visualize using Gram staining or hematoxylin and eosin stains. Neutrophilic infiltration with noncaseating granulomas (i.e., pyogranulomas) in tissue specimens can suggest the diagnosis of blastomycosis and should prompt detailed microscopic examination for *Blastomyces* yeast.

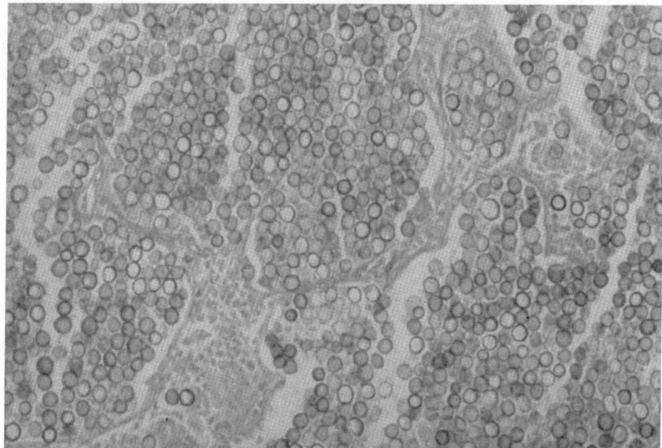

FIG. 199.12 Overwhelming infection with *B. dermatitidis* is demonstrated in lung tissue with a silver stain.

For patients with pulmonary disease, specimens can be obtained from sputum, tracheal aspirate, bronchoscopy with bronchoalveolar lavage (BAL), or open-lung biopsy. Sputum cultures can be diagnostic for *Blastomyces* in up to 75% of patients[99]; however, sputum specimens tend to be more useful in older patients because collection of high-quality sputum can be difficult to obtain in young children.[137] If sputum cannot be obtained or is nondiagnostic, a tracheal aspirate or bronchoscopy with BAL can be performed. Although the diagnostic yield for BAL has been reported as 92%, results in the pediatric population may be suboptimal because of technical limitations.[99,137] If specimens obtained from sputum and BAL fail to demonstrate *Blastomyces* and clinical suspicion remains high, open-lung biopsy is required. In some case series[137] but not others,[47] lung biopsy was needed for diagnosis of most children.

Nonculture diagnostic techniques are often used in conjunction with fungal smear and culture to facilitate the diagnosis of blastomycosis. An antigen test against a galactomannan component of the *Blastomyces* cell wall has become an important adjunctive test. Specimens for antigen testing can be collected from the urine, serum, BAL fluid, and CSF, but robust clinical data exist only for urine and serum specimens.[9,36,44] Sensitivity for the urine antigen test ranges from 76.3% to 92.9% and is influenced by the burden of infection.[9,36,53] For patients with localized pulmonary disease, sensitivity decreases to 50%, whereas for those with diffuse pulmonary disease, sensitivity increases to 87.5%.[9] Antigen levels tend to be higher in those with ARDS than those without.[36] Serum *Blastomyces* antigen sensitivity is 57% to 81.8%.[9,36] Because there is substantial cross-reactivity with *H. capsulatum* (96%), *P. brasiliensis* (100%), and *P. marneffei* (70%), the specificity of the antigen test is 76.9% to 79%.[9,44] Cross-reactions sometimes cause diagnostic difficulties because *Histoplasma* and *Blastomyces* exist in similar endemic regions in North America. However, this does not usually affect clinical management because treatment recommendations for blastomycosis and histoplasmosis are similar.[32,160] Diagnostic confusion related to cross-reactions with *P. brasiliensis* or *P. marneffei* are uncommon, unless the patient has resided in or visited Central or South America or Southeast Asia, respectively. Urine antigen detection has been successfully used in the pediatric population for diagnosis and monitoring the response to antifungal therapy.[53,109]

Classic serologic studies such as complement fixation (CF), immunodiffusion (ID), and enzyme immunoassays (EIA) have been largely supplanted by the *Blastomyces* antigen test. Although the specificity for CF and ID assays range from 97% to 100%, the sensitivity is 9% and 28%, respectively.[85] EIA has a sensitivity of 77% with a specificity of 92%.[85] All three serologic tests detect antibodies against the A antigen found in the *B. dermatitidis* cell wall. A radioimmunoassay for the BAD1 surface protein has a sensitivity of 85% and specificity of 98%, but the test is not commercially available.[83] A EIA that uses microplates coated with BAD1 protein has a sensitivity of 87% and specificity of 94% to 99% for patients with active blastomycosis.[128] Combined BAD1 EIA and antigen testing increased diagnostic sensitivity to 97%.[128] The BAD1 antibody EIA test is expected to become commercially available.

Molecular diagnostic assays using real-time PCR to amplify *BAD1* and *DRK1* genes have been developed, but they are not commercially available.[6,140]

TREATMENT

Treatment of blastomycosis is influenced by the severity of the infection, presence or absence of CNS dissemination, integrity of the immune system, and pregnancy (Table 199.3).[32] Antifungal therapy is recommended for all patients diagnosed with blastomycosis, including those with resolution of clinical symptoms before receiving therapy.[32] Although spontaneous resolution of symptomatic blastomycosis has been reported,[135] the frequency of this phenomenon remains unknown. Moreover, dissemination to organs such as the skin and CNS can occur after the spontaneous resolution of pulmonary disease. Because 31% to 53% of children with blastomycosis develop disseminated disease,[3,22,47,52,137] the decision to withhold therapy for pulmonary blastomycosis can be dangerous and lead to extrapulmonary spread of infection. The goal of therapy for patients with spontaneous resolution of acute pulmonary blastomycosis is to prevent extrapulmonary blastomycosis.[32]

For children with mild to moderate pulmonary blastomycosis, itraconazole in a dosage of 10 mg/kg per day (maximum, 400 mg/day) for 6 to 12 months of therapy is recommended (see Table 199.3).[32] For children with severe pulmonary blastomycosis (including ARDS), treatment consists of induction with amphotericin B for 1 to 2 weeks and consolidation with itraconazole (10 mg/kg per day; maximum, 400 mg/day) for 12 months (see Table 199.3).[32] Recommended amphotericin B formulations include amphotericin B deoxycholate (0.7–1 mg/kg per day) or liposomal amphotericin B (3–5 mg/kg per day).[32] Children tolerate the deoxycholate formulation better than adults.[32]

Treatment recommendations for children with impaired immunity from human immunodeficiency virus (HIV) infection or AIDS, transplantation, or malignancy involves induction therapy with amphotericin B followed by consolidation with itraconazole (see Table 199.3).[32] For some immunosuppressed patients, lifelong suppression may need to be considered if immune suppression cannot be reversed.[32] Specific recommendations regarding criteria for suppressive therapy are lacking, and the decision is left to the health care provider. Most adult transplant recipients adequately treated for blastomycosis do not experience relapse, and lifelong suppressive therapy is used only in selected patients.[57,70] Whether these clinical observations of adult transplant recipients are directly applicable to immunosuppressed pediatric patients is unknown.

Children with mild to moderate disseminated blastomycosis are treated with itraconazole in a dosage of 10 mg/kg per day (maximum, 400 mg/day) for 6 to 12 months (see Table 199.3).[32] Patients with severe disseminated disease are treated in a similar manner as those with severe pulmonary disease. This includes induction therapy with amphotericin B for 1 to 2 weeks followed by 12 months of itraconazole.[32]

Treatment of CNS blastomycosis requires a prolonged course of liposomal amphotericin B at 5 mg/kg per day for 4 to 6 weeks followed by high-dose azole antifungal therapy for at least 12 months.[32] Liposomal amphotericin B is the preferred formulation because of its superior CNS penetration compared with amphotericin B lipid complex (ABLC) or amphotericin B deoxycholate.[32,71] Recommended azoles include fluconazole (800 mg/day), itraconazole (200 mg two to three times daily), or voriconazole (200–400 mg twice daily).[32] The most effective azole for CNS disease remains to be determined.

Fluconazole has excellent CSF penetration (52–82% of serum levels), but minimal inhibitory concentrations are higher than those with itraconazole or voriconazole.[68,78] Itraconazole has been successfully used to treat some cases of CNS blastomycosis despite its poor penetration into the CSF at less than 10% of serum.[32,78] In contrast, voriconazole levels in the CSF are 38% to 68% of serum, and minimal inhibitory concentrations are similar to those of itraconazole.[68,78] There are several case reports of successful use of voriconazole to treat adults with CNS fungal infections, including blastomycosis.[8,150] Surgical

TABLE 199.3 Treatment of Blastomycosis in Children and Pregnant Women

Condition	Drug of Choice	Dosage	Duration
Pulmonary Blastomycosis			
Mild to moderate	Itraconazole	10 mg/kg/day[a]	6–12 mo
Severe or life-threatening	Amphotericin B deoxycholate	0.7–1 mg/kg/day	1–2 wk
	Lipid amphotericin B	3–5 mg/kg/day	1–2 wk
	Itraconazole[b]	10 mg/kg/day[a]	12 mo
Extrapulmonary (Non-CNS) Blastomycosis			
Mild to moderate	Itraconazole	10 mg/kg/day[a]	6–12 mo
Severe or life-threatening	Amphotericin B deoxycholate	0.7–1 mg/kg/day	1–2 wk
	Liposomal amphotericin B	3–5 mg/kg/day	1–2 wk
	Itraconazole[b]	10 mg/kg/day[a]	12 mo
Immunocompromised patient	Amphotericin B deoxycholate	0.7–1 mg/kg/day	1–2 wk
	Liposomal amphotericin B	3–5 mg/kg/day	1–2 wk
	Itraconazole[b]	10 mg/kg/day[a]	12 mo
CNS blastomycosis	Liposomal amphotericin B	5 mg/kg/day	4–6 wk
	Itraconazole[c]	400–600 mg/day	12 mo
	Fluconazole[c]	800 mg/day	12 mo
	Voriconazole[c]	400–800 mg/day	12 mo
Pregnant patient	Liposomal amphotericin B	3–5 mg/kg/day	
Neonate	Amphotericin B deoxycholate	1 mg/kg/day	

[a]Maximal dose of 400 mg/day.
[b]Itraconazole should be started after at least 1 to 2 weeks of therapy with amphotericin.
[c]Itraconazole, fluconazole, or voriconazole should be started after at least 4 to 6 weeks of therapy with amphotericin.
CNS, Central nervous system.

debridement should be considered for patients with intracranial masses, epidural abscesses, cranial osteomyelitis, and spinal osteomyelitis with instability.[158]

Pediatric patients of childbearing age with blastomycosis should undergo pregnancy testing before initiation of antifungal therapy. High-dose and prolonged treatment with triazoles increases the risk for fetal deformities and spontaneous abortion.[11,41,122,126,156] Administration of fluconazole to pregnant patients diagnosed with *C. immitis,* a dimorphic fungus related to *Blastomyces,* resulted in skeletal and craniofacial defects resembling Antley-Bixler syndrome (i.e., trapezoidocephaly–multiple synostosis syndrome).[126] Voriconazole and posaconazole can cause skeletal abnormalities in animal models.[122,156] Several human studies have demonstrated that itraconazole increases the risk of spontaneous abortion.[11,41] To minimize harm to the developing fetus, liposomal amphotericin B (3–5 mg/kg per day) is recommended.[32,35]

After delivery, the placenta should be examined histopathologically for *Blastomyces.* The neonate should be carefully assessed for infection and clinically monitored for the clinical signs and symptoms of blastomycosis. Amphotericin B deoxycholate (1 mg/kg per day) is the recommended antifungal agent for treatment of neonatal blastomycosis.[32]

Effective clinical management of patients with blastomycosis requires efforts to minimize toxicity, avoid drug-drug interactions, optimize bioavailability, and monitor drug levels. Amphotericin B deoxycholate and its lipid formulations are fungicidal against *Blastomyces* and achieve high rates of clinical cure.[33] However, these agents require intravenous administration, are nephrotoxic, and promote urinary wasting of potassium, magnesium, and bicarbonate. Hydration with normal saline before and after therapy with amphotericin and use of lipid-associated formulations can minimize the risk for nephrotoxicity.[133] Replacement of potassium and magnesium losses is needed in most patients. Bicarbonate replacement is rarely required. Frequent monitoring of electrolytes and creatinine is needed for patients receiving amphotericin.[32]

In contrast to amphotericin B, azole antifungal agents are fungistatic against *Blastomyces,* and clinical efficacy varies among the available agents. In a prospective, nonrandomized, open-label trial, itraconazole (200–400 mg/day) resulted in a 90% cure rate.[42] Itraconazole is available in capsule and liquid formulations. Absorption of the capsule formulation is enhanced with gastric acidity and coadministration with food.[32,40] The liquid formulation (100 mg/10 mL) has 30% better bioavailability than the capsule formulation and should be administered without food.[32,40]

Fluconazole is less efficacious than itraconazole and is not recommended by the 2008 guidelines published by the Infectious Diseases Society of America for pulmonary or non-CNS disseminated blastomycosis.[32] If fluconazole is used for treatment, 400 to 800 mg/day dosing is required to optimize clinical response. The success rate for 400 to 800 mg/day dosing was 87%, whereas it was 65% for 200 to 400 mg/day.[116,117] Approximately 50% of patients who received high-dose fluconazole experienced adverse events, including alopecia, xerosis, and elevated results of liver function tests.[117] Similar to fluconazole, ketoconazole is no longer recommended for the management of blastomycosis.[32]

The newest triazoles—voriconazole, posaconazole, and isavuconazole—have in vitro activity against *Blastomyces.*[68,67] Although clinical experience with voriconazole, posaconazole, and isavuconazole is limited, several case reports suggest that they can be an effective treatment option.[8,115,125,150,151] To optimize bioavailability, voriconazole needs to administered in the fasting state, whereas posaconazole liquid suspension requires coadministration with fatty foods and avoidance of proton pump inhibitors or histamine-2 (H_2) receptor blockers[122,156] Posaconazole delayed-release tablets and isavuconazole capsules can be administered without regard to food or stomach acidity. Voriconazole, posaconazole, and isavuconazole can also be administered parentally.

Therapeutic drug monitoring for itraconazole is recommended after steady-state levels are achieved, which is at the end of the second week of therapy. Given the long half-life of itraconazole (i.e., 24 hours), serum levels can be obtained independent of the time the drug was administered.[32] Goal therapeutic levels are more than 1 µg/mL (i.e., itraconazole and hydroxy-itraconazole levels are added together).[32] Serum concentrations greater than 10 µg/mL are not needed and can increase the risk of side effects. Therapeutic drug monitoring can also be performed for voriconazole; goal serum levels are between 1.0 and 5.5 µg/mL.[4]

In addition to therapeutic monitoring, liver function tests should be assessed at baseline, at 2 and 4 weeks into therapy, and then every 3 months for all azoles.[32] Careful review of all medications is needed to avoid drug-drug interactions with azoles. This is especially important for patients who are immunosuppressed by organ transplantation or receiving pharmacologic therapy for seizures.

Debridement for osteomyelitis or abscesses is not considered curative, and antifungal agents should always be administered after surgical intervention. Moreover, the duration of antifungal therapy should not be shortened.

Patients diagnosed with blastomycosis do not require isolation because person-to-person transmission through aerosols or respiratory droplets has not been reported. Standard barrier precautions (i.e., gloves) are needed in caring for patients with open wounds.

NEW REFERENCES SINCE THE SEVENTH EDITION

3. Anderson EJ, Ahn PB, Yogv R, et al. Blastomycosis in children: a study of 14 cases. *J Pediatric Infect Dis Soc.* 2013;2:386-390.
6. Babady NE, Buckwalter SP, Hall L, et al. Detection of Blastomyces dermatitidis and Histoplasma capsulatum from culture isolates and clinical specimens by use of real-time PCR. *J Clin Microbiol.* 2011;49:3204-3208.
16. Beaussart A, Brandhorst T, Dufrêne YF, Klein BS. Blastomyces virulence adhesion-1 protein binding to glycosaminoglycans is enhanced by protein disulfide isomerase. *MBio.* 2015;6:e1403-e1415.
19. Brandhorst TT, Roy R, Wüthrich M, et al. Structure and function of a fungal adhesion that binds heparin and mimics thrombospondin-1 by blocking T cell activation and effector function. *PLoS Pathog.* 2013;9:e1003464.
22. Brick KE, Drolet BA, Lyon VB, Galbraith SS. Cutaneous and disseminated blastomycosis: a pediatric case series. *Pedaitr Dermatol.* 2013;30:23-28.
25. Brown EM, McTaggart LR, Zhang SX, et al. Phylogenetic analysis reveals a cryptic species Blastomyces gilchristii, sp. nov. within the human pathogenic fungus Blastomyces dermatitidis. *PLoS ONE.* 2013;8:e59237.
29. Castillo CG, Kauffman CA, Miceli MH. Blastomycosis. *Infect Dis Clin North Am.* 2016;30:247-264.
38. Dalcin D, Ahmed SZ. Blastomycosis in northwestern Ontario, 2004-2014. *Can J Infect Dis Med Microbiol.* 2015;26:259-262.
52. Frost HM, Anderson J, Ivacic L, Meece J. Blastomycosis in children: an analysis of clinical, epidemiologic, and genetic features. *J Pediatric Infect Dis Soc.* 2017;6:49-56.
63. Gilmore SA, Naseem S, Konopka JB, Sil A. N-acetylglucosamine (GlcNAc) triggers a rapid temperature-responsive morphogenetic program in thermally dimorphic fungi. *PLoS Genet.* 2013;9:e1003799.
67. González GM. In vitro activities of isavuconazole against opportunistic filamentous and dimorphic fungi. *Med Mycol.* 2009;47:71-76.
97. Marty AJ, Broman AT, Zarnowski R, et al. Fungal morphology, iron homeostasis, and lipid metabolism regulated by a GATA transcription factor in Blastomyces dermatitidis. *PLoS Pathog.* 2015;11:e1004959.
101. McCann DA, Smith HL. Infliximab-associated Blastomyces dermatitidis in treatment of ulcerative colitis. *Colorectal Dis.* 2013;15:e102-e103.
112. Muñoz JF, Gauthier GM, Desjardins CA, et al. The dynamic genome and transcriptome of the human fungal pathogen Blastomyces and close relative Emmonsia. *PLoS Pathog.* 2015;11:e1005493.
120. Pelly L, Juaid AA, Fanella S. Severe blastomycosis in infants. *Pediatr Infect Dis J.* 2014;33:1189-1191.
128. Richer SM, Smedema ML, Durkin MM, et al. Development of a highly sensitive and specific blastomycosis antibody enzyme immunoassay using Blastomyces dermatitidis surface protein BAD-1. *Clin Vaccine Immunol.* 2014;21:143-146.
130. Roy M, Benedict K, Deak E, et al. A large community outbreak of blastomycosis in Wisconsin with geographic and ethnic clustering. *Clin Infect Dis.* 2013;57:655-662.
134. Salt E, Wiggins AT, Rayens MK, et al. Risk factors for targeted fungal and mycobacterial infections in patients taking tumor necrosis factor inhibitors. *Athritis Rheumatol.* 2016;68:597-603.
140. Sidamonidze K, Peck MK, Perez M, et al. Real-time PCR assay for identification of Blastomyces dermatitidis in culture and in tissue. *J Clin Microbiol.* 2012;50:1783-1786.
141. Smith RJ, Boos MD, Burnham JM, et al. Atypical cutaneous blastomycosis in a child with juvenile idiopathic arthritis on infliximab. *Pediatrics.* 2015;136:e1386-e1389.
145. Sterkel AK, Lorenzini JL, Fites JS, et al. Fungal mimicry of a mammalian aminopeptidase disables innate immunity and promotes pathogenicity. *Cell Host Microbe.* 2016;19:361-374.
151. Thomposn GR 3rd, Rendon A, Dos Santos R, et al. Isavuconazole treatment of cryptococcis and dimorphic mycoses. *Clin Infect Dis.* 2016;63:356-362.
162. Wisconsin Department of Health Services. Blastomycosis. https://www.dhs.wisconsin.gov/disease/blastomycosis.htm.

The full reference list for this chapter is available at ExpertConsult.com.

200 Candidiasis

Brian T. Fisher • P. Brian Smith • Theoklis E. Zaoutis

In the last 2 decades of the previous century, *Candida* species emerged as major human pathogens.[26,86,331,340] The increase in invasive candidiasis (IC) was likely the result of an expanding population of patients with immune systems compromised by prematurity, immunomodulatory therapies, and chemotherapeutic agents. Increased use of broad-spectrum antimicrobial therapy, administration of parenteral nutrition, and placement of invasive devices probably further contributed to a growing population of persons who are highly susceptible to IC. Although data suggesting a decline in IC at pediatric institutions in the United States are encouraging,[254] *Candida* remains the most common cause of invasive fungal disease and the second most common cause of central line–associated bloodstream infections (BSIs) in US health care settings. Furthermore, IC results in substantial attributable mortality rates among neonates and children with significant increases in health care resource use.[279,337] This chapter discusses the epidemiology, pathogenesis, clinical manifestations, diagnosis, and management of IC in the pediatric population. Because of notable differences in the pathogenesis, presentation, and management of IC in neonates, neonatal candidiasis is discussed separately.

ORGANISM

Candida spp. comprise a heterogeneous group of eukaryotic, diploid organisms that grow predominantly with yeast morphology (i.e., unicellular). Most members are able to produce pseudohyphae; however, only *C. albicans* and *C. dubliniensis* are able to produce true hyphae, thus making them the only polymorphic *Candida* species. *Candida* spp. are commensal organisms, commonly found in the gastrointestinal and genitourinary tracts of healthy humans. More than 150 species have been described; of these, more than 20 different species are associated with infection in humans.[48,130,277] *C. albicans* is the most frequent species isolated from humans; other more commonly isolated pathogenic species include *C. parapsilosis, C. tropicalis, C. glabrata* (previously known as *Torulopsis glabrata*), and *C. krusei.* Less commonly, IC may be caused by *C. guilliermondii, C. lusitaniae, C. dubliniensis, C. pelliculosa, C. kefyr, C. rugosa, C. famata, C. norvegensis, C. orthopsilosis, C. metapsilosis, C. nivariensis,* and *C. inconspicua.*

Candida spp. grow on routine agar and do not require special fungal media for isolation. The appearance of *Candida* colonies may vary from cream to yellow in color, with a texture that may vary from smooth to wrinkled, glistening or dry, depending on the species. Under optimal growth conditions, yeast grow in log phase as unicellular budding yeast forms (blastospores) that are spherical to ovoid and measure 2.5 to 6 μm in diameter.[122,277] Pseudohyphae are polarized growths that form when budding daughter cells remains attached to the parent cell wall, thereby forming elongated, often branching forms with constricted septal junctions between cells. In contrast, true hyphae are formed from yeast cells or as branches from existing hyphae and are characterized by defined septa that divide the hyphae into separate fungal units. True hyphae can be a feature of some *Candida* species such as *C. albicans* and *C. dubliniensis*. Growth of *Candida* hyphae can be precipitated in the presence of serum at 37°C and at pH 7.[184,277,293] Germ tube formation is a precursor to hyphae, and the presence of germ tube formation has been used to inform a presumptive identification of *C. albicans,* although false-positive and false-negative results may occur.[136,275]

Identification of the most common *Candida* species is possible on the basis of carbohydrate assimilation and fermentation testing, in addition to morphology. The use of commercially available kits such as API 20C AUX (bioMérieux-Vitek), the Auxacolor2 (Sanofi Diagnostics Pasteur), and the Uni-Yeast Tek kit (Remel Laboratories) use changes in turbidity or the production of color through enzymatic reactions to create specific biochemical profiles that permit the rapid identification of the more common *Candida* spp.[87] Chromogenic agar (e.g., CHROMagar Candida, Becton Dickinson), which incorporate substrates linked to chemical dyes in a solid medium, allows for presumptive identification of clinically important *Candida* spp. including *C. albicans* (green smooth colonies), *C. tropicalis* (metallic blue colonies with a pink halo), *C. krusei* (pale rose flat colonies), and *C. glabrata* (white or purple smooth glistening colonies), although misidentification of less common *Candida* spp. as *C. glabrata* has been reported.[87,136,238] Chromogenic agar permits identification in as early as 24 to 48 hours and is particularly valuable in detecting coinfection with different *Candida* spp., which may be ordinarily missed during conventional subculture on solid medium.[87,277]

EPIDEMIOLOGY

Candida is the most important cause of fungal infection in health care settings. It broadly affects a growing population of immunocompromised patients, in addition to patients with critical illness, prematurity, or complex chronic conditions. The incidence of IC in the United States has risen since the 1970s, with rates of nosocomial BSI with *Candida* quadrupling between 1980 and 1989.[24] An increase in adult candidemia-related hospitalizations was sustained in the United States between 2000 and 2005.[340] More recent publications have suggested a decline in IC among both pediatric and neonatal populations throughout the first decade of this century.[61,65,99] The cause of this decline is not known but is likely multifactorial and hypothesized to be related to improved adoption of infection control initiatives and use of targeted antifungal prophylaxis in high-risk groups. Nonetheless, data from the National Healthcare Safety Network still show *Candida* spp. as the second most common cause of central line–associated BSIs in the United States.[276]

IC is of particular concern in the pediatric population given its potential to cause significant morbidity and mortality. Crude mortality rates in children with candidemia range from 10% to 26%, with an attributable mortality rate of candidemia in children estimated to be 10%.[43,189,223,291,336,337] Evidence of dissemination has been estimated to occur in 8.3% to 17% of children with candidemia,[43,84,96,306,335] with organ involvement most commonly occurring in the lungs (45.2–58%), liver (23%), kidney (16%), brain (12%), heart (8–22.3%), spleen (8%), and eyes (3.2–8%).[84,335,339] In addition to severe clinical outcomes, candidemia in children results in a prolonged length of inpatient stay and considerable increase in monetary expenditures.[337]

C. albicans is the predominant *Candida* species colonizing the gastrointestinal genital mucosa and the mucous membranes of 30% to 60% of humans.[184] Not surprisingly, *C. albicans* is the most common cause of invasive fungal disease in children; however, on the basis of international data, non–*C. albicans* species now account for more than half of IC episodes in children.[291] Furthermore, the epidemiology of non-*albicans* species differs among children as compared with adults. Specifically, *C. parapsilosis* is the second most common species isolated from children with IC. International prospective pediatric cohort studies have identified *C. parapsilosis* in 22% to 34% of IC episodes,[223,291] thus corroborating the epidemiologic findings from single-center pediatric studies.[81,189,288,339] Experimental animal models have demonstrated that *C. parapsilosis* is associated with reduced virulence compared with that of *C. albicans* and *C. tropicalis,*[327] and clinical studies have also shown higher rates of treatment success in children and reduced mortality rates in adults with *C. parapsilosis* invasive disease compared with other *Candida* spp.[223,291]

Understanding the distribution of *C. glabrata* and *C. krusei* is necessary given their reduced susceptibility to triazole antifungal agents. *C. glabrata* exhibits variable susceptibility to fluconazole, with well-described cross-resistance with the extended spectrum triazoles,[232] whereas *C. krusei* is intrinsically resistant to fluconazole, with most isolates susceptible to voriconazole.[233,234] The epidemiology of *C. glabrata* differs between adults and children. In adults, *C. glabrata* accounts for more than one-fourth of the IC events,[43,137,223] but less than 9% of pediatric cases.[221] *C. krusei* is similarly infrequent in all age groups.

C. tropicalis is an infrequent cause of IC in children and predominantly occurs in oncologic populations.[175] Data from animal models indicate that *C. tropicalis* is similar in virulence to *C. albicans*, although *C. tropicalis* has been associated with an increased propensity for dissemination in neutropenic hosts than has *C. albicans*.[172,175]

Several cohort studies have been performed to elucidate specific risk factors for the development of IC in children. In a single-center case-control study examining risk factors for candidemia in a children's hospital, cases were more likely to occur in children with central venous catheters, use of topical antifungal agents before candidemia, and longer exposure to hyperalimentation compared with controls; however, only unadjusted analysis was performed, limiting interpretation of the results.[189] A single-center population-based case-control study examined risk factors for candidemia in pediatric patients admitted to a pediatric intensive care unit.[339] On multivariable analysis, receipt of vancomycin or an antimicrobial agent with anaerobic activity for 4 days or longer was both independently associated with a significant increased risk of candidemia (adjusted odds ratio [OR], 6.19; 95% confidence interval [CI], 2.40–15.99; and adjusted OR, 3.51; 95% CI, 1.47–8.38, respectively). Other significant risk factors included malignant disease (OR, 4.02; 95% CI, 1.23–13.11) and the presence of a central venous catheter (adjusted OR, 30.45; 95% CI, 7.76–119.49). Receipt of hyperalimentation was found to be significantly associated with candidemia on unadjusted analysis, but the association became nonsignificant after inclusion into the multivariable model.

Leveraging these individual risk factors, a clinical prediction rule was derived inclusive of the following factors: vancomycin, anaerobic-spectrum antibiotics, malignant disease, presence of a central venous catheter, and hyperalimentation. Children with three or more risk factors had between 10% and 46% predicted probability of developing candidemia.[339] Similar risk factors of the presence of central venous catheters, arterial lines, hyperalimentation, prolonged antibiotic exposure, and antibiotic exposure were identified in another study performed in a population of pediatric intensive care patients.[97] Unfortunately, an attempt to validate the aforementioned clinical prediction rule failed in a multicenter cohort. This failure highlights the challenges of leveraging factors that vary across institutions for a one-size-fits-all clinical prediction rule.[100]

Risk factors for disseminated candidiasis in children have been examined by several investigators.[84,95,335] In a case-control study of children with candidemia, persistently positive blood cultures for *Candida*, more than 3 days with a central venous catheter in place, and immunosuppression (neutropenia, use of immunosuppressant medications, or history of bone marrow transplant) were found to be independent risk factors for the development of disseminated candidiasis.[335] Another case-control study of children with candidemia identified receipt of vasopressors, prolonged candidemia (≥3 days) after central venous catheter removal, and neutropenia to be independently associated with disseminated candidiasis.[84] Similarly, in an unadjusted analysis of children hospitalized with candidemia, prolonged candidemia and the presence of an immunocompromising condition were found to be associated with dissemination.[95] Risk factors for mortality among pediatric patients have also been examined, with location in a pediatric intensive care unit at the time of infection, the presence of an arterial catheter, tracheal intubation, and neutropenia significantly associated with death.[223,336] With the exception of neutropenia, these risk factors are likely markers for severe illness.

Finally, investigators have studied risk factors for infection, specifically with *C. glabrata* and *C. krusei*, given the increased azole resistance among these pathogens. Age older than 2 years, recent surgical procedure, and prior fluconazole exposure were each identified as independent risk factors for infection from these species in children.[239]

PATHOGENESIS

Pathogen Factors

The virulence of a pathogen is an important determinant of the ability of a microorganism to inflict host cell damage and cause disease. Virulence factors have been best studied in *C. albicans* likely because this species is the most common cause of IC and is thought to be the most pathogenic.[277] Consequently *C. albicans* serves as the prototype for this discussion of virulence factors, with exceptions noted for other non-*albicans Candida* species where relevant. The pathogenicity of *C. albicans* is mediated by several virulence factors, including adhesion, biofilm formation, secretion of hydrolytic enzymes, and morphology switching, thus permitting it to become the most successful opportunistic fungal pathogen in humans.

The obligatory first step in the establishment of colonization and subsequent host invasion is the adherence of *C. albicans* to host surfaces and medical devices. Adherence is essential for initiating and maintaining a commensal relationship with the host,[255] and it is mediated by adhesion biomolecules present at the fungal surface that permit binding to host cells and host-cell ligands. Agglutinin-like sequence proteins (Als) are the most widely expressed adhesins in *C. albicans* and encode a group of glycosyl-phosphatidyl-inositol (GPI)–anchored proteins localized on the outer cell wall layer.[305] Among all Als proteins, Als1p, Als3p, and Als5p appear to play major roles in adherence to host cells.[305] Hyphal wall protein 1 (Hwp1p) is found exclusively at the germ tube surface and is another important adhesin, mediating tight binding to buccal epithelial cells.[287] Cell wall carbohydrates such as glycosylated mannoproteins and sialic acids may also contribute to adherence.[305] Among non–*C. albicans* species, *C. tropicalis* has been shown to produce Als proteins, whereas *C. glabrata* has been found to produce a group of adhesins encoded by the *EPA* (epithelial adhesin) gene family. Cell wall adhesin-like proteins have also been discovered in *C. parapsilosis*, although further work on the virulence associated with these proteins is limited.[277]

Biofilm formation is an important mechanism of virulence for several *Candida* species, including *C. albicans*, *C. parapsilosis*, *C. tropicalis*, and *C. glabrata*.[277] The capacity to establish a biofilm plays a significant role in infections involving medical devices such as central venous catheters, urinary catheters, cardiovascular devices, and prosthetic implants.[23,169] *Candida* biofilms are complex communities of yeast, pseudohyphae, and hyphae encased in a self-produced extracellular matrix. The formation, structure, and composition of the biofilm depend on the nature of the contact surface, environmental factors, and *Candida* species, the last of which can dictate ability to switch morphology from yeast to hyphae.[209,277] Several studies have demonstrated that biofilm growth can dramatically enhance resistance to antifungal agents. Minimum inhibitory concentrations (MIC) of amphotericin B, flucytosine, fluconazole, itraconazole, and ketoconazole against *C. albicans* growing in biofilms have all been shown to be significantly higher (up to 2000 times higher) than the MIC in planktonic *C. albicans*.[129,176,244,299] Investigators have suggested that biofilm-associated *Candida* acquire resistance because of a low growth rate and decreased drug penetration through the matrix; however, certain studies have not supported these conclusions.[4,18] Instead, antifungal resistance is thought to be conferred by contact-dependent upregulation of genes encoding efflux pumps during the course of biofilm formation, although multiple mechanisms may contribute to antifungal resistance of the *Candida* biofilm.[208,245]

Production of extracellular hydrolytic enzymes is an essential aspect of the pathogenicity of *Candida* species, facilitating tissue invasion by disruption of the host mucosal membranes and by degrading important immunologic and structural proteins, including IgG heavy chains, α_2-macroglobulin, β-lactoglobulin, C3 protein, lactoperoxidase, collagen, and fibronectin.[236,277] The three most important hydrolytic enzymes produced by *Candida* are the secreted aspartyl proteinases (Saps), phospholipase B enzymes, and lipases.[211,277] The Sap proteins are encoded by a family of 10 *SAP* genes and are considered key determinants of *Candida* virulence, with level of Sap activity in vitro appearing to correlate with the virulence of *C. albicans*, *C. tropicalis*, and *C. parapsilosis*.[211] Data are limited on the capacity of *C. glabrata* to produce proteinases.

Morphologic conversion between yeast and hyphal forms is believed to play an important role in the dissemination and tissue invasion of

C. albicans. Initial experiments using animal models suggested that the hyphal form represented the pathogenic state of the organism because mutant strains lacking hyphae exhibited impaired ability to invade tissue compared with wild-type *C. albicans.*[57,187] Subsequent data demonstrating constitutively filamentous mutant strains as avirulent led to the hypothesis that it was not the morphologic form per se, but rather the ability to undergo morphology switching, that contributed to the pathogenicity of *C. albicans.*[44] More recently, a mouse model of hematogenously disseminated candidiasis using a mutant *C. albicans* strain that permitted external modulation of morphology switching demonstrated that both yeast and hyphae were important stages in the development of IC.[266] Saville and coinvestigators[266] were able to demonstrate in a mouse model of disseminated candidiasis that mice injected with this strain under conditions permitting hyphal development succumbed to infection, whereas all mice injected under conditions inhibiting the formation of hyphae survived, thus indicating that filamentous formation was a critical factor in pathogenicity. However, fungal burdens were almost identical in animals injected with strains under hyphae-permitting and hyphae-repressing conditions, a finding suggesting that yeast forms were important for initial extravasation and dissemination in the host. Interestingly, histopathologic examination of kidneys recovered from mice exposed to hyphae-repressing conditions revealed no significant damage despite organ invasion, with all the invading fungal cells present only in yeast form.[266]

Host Factors

As previously noted, *Candida* spp. can cause infection in almost any anatomic location in either localized or disseminated presentations. The immune responses to these different compartments are distinct, as evidenced by the differing clinical presentations depending on a patient's risk factors and underlying immune compromise. Both innate and adaptive arms of the immune system play key roles in the immune response to *Candida* and are influenced by the site of infection. A detailed discussion of the host immune response to *Candida* is beyond the scope of this chapter, but several excellent reviews are available for more in-depth coverage.[70,119,312]

The initial host response to infection with *Candida* involves recognition of pathogen-associated molecular patterns (PAMPs) present on the fungal cell wall.[312] Pattern recognition receptors (PRR) on the surface of innate immune cells perform this function, and several classes of PRR have been identified in the induction of innate host responses to *Candida*, including the Toll-like receptors (TLRs), the C-type lectin receptors (CLRs), and the NOD-like receptors (NLRs).[119] Recognition of yeast and hyphae morphologic features is differential, with each form recognized by different host receptors.[80,311] TLR2, TLR4, and TLR9 have all been implicated as having key roles in recognition of *Candida* and induction of proinflammatory cytokines.[312] CLRs comprise a large family of receptors with a shared ability to recognize microbial polysaccharides, and they are thought to be the most important PRR family in the recognition of fungi.[119] Within this family, dectin 1, dectin 2, macrophage mannose receptor 1, dendritic cell–specific intercellular adhesion molecule 3 (ICAM3)–grabbing nonintegrin (DC-SIGN), and soluble mannose-binding lectin serve to recognize *C. albicans* and are involved in phagocytosis, production of inflammatory cytokines, neutrophil recruitment and activation, and complement activation.[119,312] Finally, NLRs located within the cytoplasm function to activate inflammosomes (protein platforms that induce the activation of interleukin [IL]-1β and IL-18 through caspase 1) and may have an important role in in T-helper 1 (T_H1)–type and T_H17-type responses against *C. albicans*, important for containing disseminated and mucosal infection, respectively.[313,319]

Beyond the role of PRRs in the innate immune response to *Candida*, neutrophils, macrophages, and monocytes are all critically important antifungal effector cells, as evidenced by the high risk of disseminated disease in neutropenic patients.[54,84,144,335] Phagocytes already residing in infected organs are involved in the killing of invading *Candida*, whereas neutrophils and monocytes are recruited to the site of infection. The large size of hyphae may preclude engulfment of *Candida* by these phagocytes; however, studies have demonstrated the important role of neutrophil extracellular traps (NETs) in the killing of both hyphal and yeast forms.[309,310]

The adaptive immune system plays a critical role in protecting against oropharyngeal candidiasis. Until recently, protective adaptive responses were thought to be mediated by $CD4^+$ T_H1 effector cells. However, with the discovery in 2005 of a subset of $CD4^+$ T_H17 cells,[127,178,227] investigators found that T_H17-type responses play a crucial role in controlling *C. albicans* at the mucosa.[70,119] This finding is supported by the observation that patients with chronic mucocutaneous candidiasis (CMC), either as isolated autosomal dominant CMC (AD-CMC) or as part of a primary immunodeficiency secondary to hyperimmunoglobulin E syndrome (HIES) or autoimmune polyendocrinopathy with candidiasis and ectodermal dystrophy (APECED), share a common defect related to an inadequate T_H17 response. The major genetic defect causing HIES is a mutation in the gene encoding STAT3 transcription factor, resulting in impaired T_H17 differentiation.[70] Most patients with AD-CMC have a defect in the STAT1 gene, which is involved in the IL-23/IL-23-R pathway crucial for induction of T_H17 responses. The mechanism of susceptibility to *Candida* infection in patients with APECED has been linked to neutralizing autoantibodies against T_H17-type cytokines in affected patients.[165,241]

With respect to hematogenously disseminated candidiasis, the portal of entry of *Candida* into the host bloodstream has been the source of much debate, with both the gastrointestinal tract and the skin proposed as the source of acquisition. In a remarkable experiment performed in 1969, an investigator ingested 10^{12} *C. albicans* cells and underwent serial blood and urine sampling. After experiencing a transient febrile reaction with chills, *C. albicans* was isolated from the blood and urine within 3 hours of ingestion, thus forming the only experimental human evidence to support the gut as a source of candidemia.[174] Animal models of candidal gut colonization and subsequent development of disseminated candidiasis after immunosuppression also support an intestinal source for candidemia.[210,264,308] In a systematic review of the literature investigating skin or intestinal colonization as the source of candidemia, the investigators identified more compelling data in support of intestinal colonization as the primary source.[215] This conclusion is consistent with findings of anaerobic spectrum antibiotics as significant risk factors for candidemia[339] because antibiotics with anaerobic activity have been shown to permit a higher and more sustained increase in intestinal colonization with yeasts.[263] However, other portals of entry besides the intestines are important for the development of IC, as evidenced by the increased incidence of candidemia in patients with burn injury[230] and in patients requiring intravascular devices.[169]

The Damage Response Framework (DRF) has been proposed as a novel construct to classify the interaction of a microbe and the host because it relates to the clinical presentation of infection in the host.[50] The DRF has six classifications that depend on whether the microbe is causing an infection in a host at a time when the immune system is weakened or robust. The details of this construct are beyond the scope of this chapter; however, the DRF has been used to explain the variety of clinical infections that result from *Candida* species such as oropharyngeal candidiasis, vulvovaginal candidiasis, candidemia and disseminated candidiasis, and intra-abdominal candidiasis.[143] More details on each of these clinical manifestations are provided in the following sections.

CLINICAL MANIFESTATIONS

Infections with *Candida* spp. have myriad presentations and depend largely on the immune status of the host as well as the existence of predisposing risk factors. The clinical manifestations of candidiasis in the neonatal population are unique and are discussed separately. Given the differences in pathogenesis of candidal diseases, the following discussion is subdivided into superficial (mucocutaneous) and invasive disease manifestations.

Superficial Candidiasis

Oropharyngeal Candidiasis

Oropharyngeal candidiasis is one of the most common manifestations of *Candida* infection. Pediatric populations in which oropharyngeal candidiasis can be seen most frequently include young infants, patients with primary or acquired immunodeficiency, and patients receiving chemotherapy for malignant diseases. Additionally, occurrence in healthy children with other risk factors (e.g., inhaled corticosteroid exposure,[109] broad-spectrum antibiotic exposure[286]) is not uncommon.

The most common manifestation of oropharyngeal candidiasis in children is pseudomembranous candidiasis, or thrush. Pseudomembranous candidiasis is characterized by the presence of white to creamy plaques on the buccal mucosa, tongue, and gums, although less frequently the soft palate, uvula, and tonsils may also be involved. These lesions may be associated with pain and dysphagia, although frequently they are asymptomatic.[314] These adherent plaques may be removed by gentle scraping, which discloses an erythematous base. Histologic examination of these membranes reveals epithelial cells together with yeast and filamentous forms of *Candida.*[330] Aside from pseudomembranous candidiasis, other forms include erythematous atrophic candidiasis and angular cheilitis. Erythematous atrophic candidiasis most frequently manifests as painful erythematous lesions on the dorsum of the tongue and palate, although the buccal mucosa may also be involved. This form is commonly associated with prior broad-spectrum antibiotic exposure and may spontaneously resolve once antibiotics are discontinued and normal bacterial flora is restored.[330] Angular cheilitis may appear alone or in conjunction with pseudomembranous or erythematous atrophic candidiasis, and it is characterized by painful erythema and fissuring at the angles of the mouth. *C. albicans* is the most common species isolated, although *C. tropicalis, C. parapsilosis,* and *C. glabrata* may also be seen.[34,111,142,201,218]

Esophageal Candidiasis

Esophageal candidiasis is most commonly seen in severely immunocompromised children and is an acquired immunodeficiency syndrome–defining illness in children infected with human immunodeficiency virus (HIV). Similar to oropharyngeal candidiasis, other risk factors include immunosuppression related to malignant disease, transplantation, or primary immunodeficiency, in addition to corticosteroid exposure (inhaled or systemic) and broad-spectrum antibiotics.[13,17,123,145,167,270] Although esophageal candidiasis is frequently accompanied by oropharyngeal candidiasis, the absence of oral involvement does not exclude *Candida* esophagitis. In a case-series of HIV-infected children receiving highly active antiretroviral therapy, 28% of *Candida* esophagitis episodes were not associated with concomitant oropharyngeal candidiasis.[60] Common presenting symptoms include odynophagia, retrosternal or epigastric pain, and dysphagia, although in severely immunocompromised children fever may occasionally occur.[59,60,314] Findings on endoscopic examination include the presence of white plaques, erythema, and edema of the esophageal mucosa, ulceration, and, in severe cases, strictures. *Candida* spp. may be cultured from endoscopic brushings, although positive isolation does not distinguish infection from commensal *Candida* colonization. Reliable diagnosis may be made by histologic evidence of tissue invasion in biopsy material.[314] In addition to esophageal endoscopy, barium contrast studies of the esophagus may reveal findings of shaggy mucosal irregularities and nodular filling defects suggestive of esophageal candidiasis, although other radiographic patterns can be seen.[116,180,181]

Vulvovaginal Candidiasis

Vulvovaginal candidiasis is extremely rare before menarche, but it increases in frequency during late adolescence and adulthood. Between 50% and 70% of women may be diagnosed with this condition during their lifetime.[104,285] Risk factors for the development of vulvovaginal candidiasis include diabetes mellitus, pregnancy, oral contraceptives, glucocorticoid exposure, and broad-spectrum antibiotics.[2,118,283] Unlike in other mucosal sites of *Candida* infection, HIV seropositivity is not a clear risk factor for vulvovaginal candidiasis, although rates of *Candida* vaginal colonization have been shown to be significantly higher in HIV-seropositive versus HIV-seronegative at-risk women.[2,269] Common symptoms include vaginal pruritus, erythema, dysuria, and an odorless, thick, white, curdlike discharge.[7] The diagnosis can be clinically supported by identification of yeast and pseudohyphae or hyphae seen with potassium hydroxide or saline on microscopy, although the sensitivity of microscopy varies between 38% and 83%.[7] Isolation of *Candida* from culture of vaginal secretions does not differentiate infection from colonization.

Cutaneous Candidiasis

Cutaneous candidiasis occurs in moist, occluded cutaneous sites that promote maceration of the skin and superficial invasion by *Candida.* Diaper dermatitis is a common manifestation that typically occurs in infants, with peak prevalence during the second to fourth months of life.[135] The lesions of *Candida* diaper dermatitis generally erupt in the perianal area, spreading to involve the perineum and inguinal folds, with confluent erosions, satellite pustules on an erythematous base, and marginal scaling. Evidence of *Candida* colonization in the stool is present in up to 90% of children,[247] a finding suggesting that the gastrointestinal tract is the most important source for *Candida* diaper dermatitis. Oropharyngeal candidiasis is accompanied by diaper dermatitis in 34% to 52% of patients, thus indicating that diaper dermatitis may be the result of successive oral and gastrointestinal colonization.[135] Cutaneous candidiasis may also manifest as intertrigo occurring in the inframammary, axillary, inguinal, perineal, intergluteal, and interdigital regions. Lesions may appear as pustules on an erythematous base with central confluence, satellite lesions, and associated pruritus and tenderness.[332] Folliculitis and balanitis are less common presentations of cutaneous infection.

Chronic Mucocutaneous Candidiasis

CMC is a clinical syndrome characterized by persistent or recurrent *Candida* infections of the oropharynx, skin, nails, and, uncommonly, esophagus and larynx.[164,168] In some patients, chronic localized *Candida* granulomas may occur, manifesting as thick, adherent, hyperkeratotic "warty" lesions on the scalp and face.[164,332] Rather than a single entity, CMC is a manifestation of several heterogeneous disorders unified largely by a common downstream defect in a mucosal *Candida*-induced T_H17-type response,[119] although some exceptions exist. CMC can manifest as an isolated disease (autosomal dominant CMC) or as part of a primary immunodeficiency disorder such as HIES, APECED, severe combined immunodeficiency, dedicator of cytokinesis 8 (DOCK8) deficiency, and deficiencies of IL-12, IL-17, and IL-23.[317] CMC typically appears in infancy or early childhood and may be associated with recalcitrant or relapsing candidal disease despite antifungal therapy. Despite extensive cutaneous and mucosal involvement, reports in the literature of IC are rare for children with CMC.

Invasive Candidiasis

Candidemia

The clinical manifestations of candidemia may vary from nonspecific signs of fever and malaise to septic shock and multiple organ dysfunction syndrome.[170] Additional manifestations may be apparent as a result of dissemination through the bloodstream to distal sites including the central nervous system (CNS) and musculoskeletal system, the lungs, the eyes, and the abdominal viscera, with the risk of dissemination increasing with the number of days of blood culture positivity and immunosuppression.[1,335]

Acute Disseminated Candidiasis

Endovascular candidiasis. Endovascular candidiasis manifests most commonly as infective endocarditis, although septic thrombophlebitis and mycotic aneurysm are less frequently seen.[204,265] *Candida* may be the most common cause of health care–associated infective endocarditis in children; a single-center study reported isolation of *Candida* spp. from 27% of children with nosocomial infective endocarditis.[196] Previous reports suggested an increasing rate of *Candida* endocarditis,[298,253] although no published data commenting on recent trends are available. Clinical manifestations are similar to those of non-*Candida* endocarditis and may include fever, onset of a new or changing murmur on auscultation, hepatosplenomegaly, and congestive heart failure, in addition to the embolic and immunologic phenomena seen with infective endocarditis. Transthoracic or transesophageal echocardiography may reveal the presence of an intracardiac thrombus or valvular vegetations.

Risk factors cited for *Candida* endocarditis include prematurity, congenital or acquired heart defects or endovascular prostheses, the presence of a central venous catheter, immunosuppression, broad-spectrum antibiotic exposure, and hyperalimentation.[204,298] In a literature review of pediatric *Candida* endocarditis, the frequency of involvement of right-sided intracardiac structures (e.g., right atrium, tricuspid valve) was three times that of left-sided structure for patients with a reported site of intracardiac lesion.[204] This finding likely reflects the contributory role of central venous catheters as both a source of endothelial trauma and a portal of entry of *Candida* in the development of this complication.

Cardiac candidiasis. *Candida* spp. may be a rare cause of pericarditis and myocarditis in children.[323] At least six cases of pediatric *Candida* pericarditis and five cases of *Candida* myocarditis have been reported in the English literature.[73,268,323] *Candida* pericarditis and myocarditis may occur in the setting of recent cardiothoracic surgical procedures, contiguous focus of pleural or mediastinal infection, contiguous intracardiac spread of infection (e.g., *Candida* endocarditis), or acute hematogenous dissemination.[268,323] Clinical symptoms of *Candida* pericarditis may be subtle but include fever, chest pain, and dyspnea, with evidence of pericardial rub and cardiac tamponade on examination, enlarged cardiac silhouette on chest radiography, and ST-T-wave changes on electrocardiography. Blood culture results may not be positive, thus complicating early recognition.[73,323] Echocardiography reveals the presence of pericardial effusion. Candidal invasion and necrosis of the myocardium may be extensive and produce associated signs of congestive heart failure, with electrocardiographic changes suggestive of myocarditis.[323] Mortality rates in the literature have been high, with only 1 of 11 patients with reported pediatric *Candida* pericarditis and myocarditis having survived. The high mortality rate may have reflected the lack of recognition of *Candida* as the origin because the diagnosis was made postmortem in the majority of these cases.[73,268,323]

Pulmonary candidiasis. Two different patterns of invasive pulmonary candidiasis have been described: primary *Candida* bronchopneumonia and secondary pulmonary disease in the setting of disseminated candidiasis.[126,151,228] Primary *Candida* bronchopneumonia is limited largely to immunocompromised patients and infants and is thought to occur by aspiration of *Candida* into the upper respiratory tract. In autopsy studies of adults with invasive pulmonary disease with no other sites of dissemination or antemortem candidemia, a distinct pattern of intra-alveolar hemorrhage, alveolar exudates, necrosis, and microabscesses with evidence of *Candida* may be present, with several cases also showing evidence of esophageal candidiasis.[126] A similar pattern was seen in autopsies of three infants with evidence of airspace IC concurrent with colonization of the upper respiratory tract and oropharynx.[151] Although *Candida* species are often cultured from respiratory specimens taken from critically ill patients, this finding typically represents colonization rather than true infection.[333] Only a small subset of patients with a positive respiratory specimen for a *Candida* species will have *Candida* bronchopneumonia.[267] Histologic demonstration of invasion of *Candida* within lung tissue is the only widely accepted criterion for the definitive diagnosis of primary *Candida* bronchopneumonia.[28] However, lung biopsy is not always possible to establish the diagnosis definitively, thereby making it difficult to know which patients should receive antifungal therapy. In general, antimycotic therapy for *Candida* bronchopneumonia should be reserved for patients with underlying immunocompromise, respiratory failure, and evidence of pneumonia without growth of another pathogen.

More commonly, invasive pulmonary candidiasis occurs as a secondary consequence of hematogenous dissemination in a patient with candidemia or from showering of septic thrombi from an infected central venous catheter, septic thrombophlebitis, or *Candida* endocarditis. In disseminated candidiasis, secondary pulmonary involvement is typically capillary invasive, with bilateral lung involvement. On microscopic examination pseudohyphae are seen to invade the pulmonary capillaries, arterioles, and small arteries and thus enter the lung parenchyma. Microabscesses may be present in the lungs as well as in other end-organ sites of dissemination. In embolic pulmonary candidiasis the lungs are seeded with infected emboli from an endovascular source, with resulting hemorrhagic infarcts in the periphery of the lungs and septic thrombi in the small and medium-sized pulmonary arteries. Extrapulmonary thrombi may also be seen in other sites.[151]

Secondary pulmonary candidiasis may be suspected in the setting of candidemia or other sites of disseminated disease. The radiographic appearance of secondary pulmonary involvement typically consists of multiple 3- to 30-mm nodules scattered throughout the lung parenchyma with consolidation found in advanced disease. Histologically these lesions have areas of central necrosis with pseudohyphae and budding yeast. Cavitation is not typically seen.[46,151,228]

Candidiasis of the peritoneum, gastrointestinal tract, and gallbladder. The most common cause of *Candida* peritonitis is peritoneal dialysis (PD)–associated peritonitis; other causes include perforation of an intra-abdominal viscus or surgery-related peritonitis resulting from an anastomotic leak. Fungal peritonitis has been reported to occur in 3% of all peritonitis episodes in children undergoing PD, with *Candida* spp. comprising most causes of fungal peritonitis.[206,243,325] Similar to other *Candida* health care device–associated infections, colonization or biofilm formation of the PD catheter is the presumed nidus of infection, and thus catheter removal is often an important component of source control. Early removal of the PD catheter has been associated with improved outcomes in adults.[53] Common presenting signs and symptoms include fever and abdominal pain; sepsis with hemodynamic instability may also be seen, although extraperitoneal dissemination is rare. An elevated leukocyte count of greater than100/mm^3 in the dialysate may be seen, whereas Gram stain may reveal budding yeast forms. Culture of the dialysate allows identification of the organism. Recent administration of systemic antibiotics has been consistently noted to be a risk factor for the development of PD-associated fungal peritonitis.[243,325] Outcomes are generally good, with a low mortality rate in children of 0% to 6% compared with the 13% to 53% mortality seen in adults. In addition, 50% to 70% of children are able to continue PD after treatment for fungal peritonitis.[243,325]

IC of the lower gastrointestinal tract is an uncommon but previously described entity in severely immunocompromised patients, although the literature has been limited to the adult population.[63,202,296,240] Clinical manifestations include invasive candidal enterocolitis with or without pneumatosis and infarction. Patients may present with fever, acute abdominal pain, distention, emesis, and bloody diarrhea. Grossly, hemorrhagic ulcerations and nodules may be seen, occasionally with transmural infarction. White plaques may be seen and mistaken for pseudomembranous colitis. On histopathologic examination, periodic acid–Schiff and Gomori methenamine silver stains may reveal budding yeast and filamentous forms invading the mucosa and submucosa.

In addition to peritonitis and intestinal IC, *Candida* has also been described to cause acalculous candidal cholecystitis, as well as biliary obstruction resulting from *Candida* mycetoma.[49,202]

Candidiasis of the urinary tract. In the majority of asymptomatic persons without a urinary catheter, the presence of yeast in the urine indicates contamination or colonization. The clinical significance of candiduria in the setting of an indwelling urinary catheter is less clear because *Candida* in the urine may signify either a catheter-associated urinary tract infection (UTI) or simply colonization and biofilm formation of the catheter in the absence of true infection. A repeat urine specimen from a newly placed catheter can help to distinguish candiduria from colonization of the catheter. Urinalysis should also be performed because the presence of pyuria, hematuria, or leukocyte esterase may be useful in distinguishing infection from colonization. However, longstanding catheters can elicit an abnormal urinalysis. Clinical manifestations of *Candida* UTI may be indistinguishable from those of bacterial UTIs, with dysuria, frequency, urgency, and, in the setting of pyelonephritis, fever and flank pain. In patients with indwelling catheters, symptoms may be less recognizable, either because of a lack of dysuria or as a result of sedation status that impedes the patient's ability to communicate symptoms in the intensive care unit, although suprapubic discomfort may be reported.[152]

In patients who are symptomatic, imaging with renal ultrasonography is the preferred modality for identifying renal parenchymal abnormalities resulting from ascending infection and for detecting urinary tract obstruction if present. Renal mycetomas may appear as hyperechoic, nonshadowing foci, whereas renal abscesses may appear as hypoechoic masses.[45,246] Other imaging modalities used to identify pyelonephritis, renal abscesses, and renal mycetomas include computed tomography (CT), magnetic resonance imaging (MRI), and renal cortical scintigraphy.

In patients with candidemia, isolation of *Candida* in the urine may signify infection from hematogenous seeding of yeast to the renal parenchyma, with subsequent development of renal abscesses, renal mycetomas (fungus balls), collecting system obstruction, and renal failure. In the setting of hematogenous seeding of the renal parenchyma, a urine culture may yield relatively low colony counts of *Candida*.[152] Patients with this clinical presentation should have further imaging such as renal ultrasonography to assess the renal parenchyma.

Osteoarticular candidiasis. *Candida* osteomyelitis is not common but is a well-described form of IC with *Candida* seeding the bone by hematogenous dissemination, direct inoculation, or contiguous infection.[110] Risk factors cited include the presence of a central venous catheter, a history of preceding candidemia, prior surgical intervention, broad-spectrum antibiotics, and immunosuppression.[110,278] The most common sites of involvement in children are (in descending order) the femur and humerus, with rib, vertebra, and sternum involvement much more infrequent. This is in contrast to adults, in whom the vertebra is the most common site of infection. Involvement of more than one site is common; 83% of cases in one study had two or more bones infected.[110] The clinical presentation of *Candida* osteomyelitis is indolent, with presenting symptoms lasting several weeks to months. Fever is less common, but most patients have tenderness with erythema or edema. Draining sinus tracts are common and are more likely to occur with nonvertebral osteomyelitis (32%). Laboratory markers such as erythrocyte sedimentation rate and C-reactive protein level are commonly elevated. Imaging with radionuclide scanning may reveal multiple sites of involvement; MRI may reveal bone destruction, soft tissue extension, and abscess formation, with decreased signal intensity on T1-weighted imaging and increased signal intensity on T2-weighted imaging.[110] However, inflammatory markers and imaging findings are nonspecific, and thus, in the absence of candidemia, a biopsy of the involved site with culture and histopathology stains may be necessary to secure the diagnosis.

Up to 85% of cases of pediatric fungal arthritis occur in infants younger than 6 months of age.[294] Arthritis concomitant with bone involvement has been reported to occur in 11% to 80% of cases, with the most common synovial joints infected being the knee (11%) and hip (5%).[89,110,294] Infection often originates from the bloodstream, with seeding of the synovium or metaphyseal vessels resulting in septic arthritis and osteomyelitis, respectively. *Candida* septic arthritis has been reported to manifest several months to a year after the initial episode of candidemia.[128,294] Although two-thirds of patients may have acute symptoms of fever and painful swelling of the joint, *Candida* arthritis may also manifest indolently. Arthrocentesis of the affected joint should be performed for diagnostic and therapeutic reasons. The synovial fluid typically reveals a with a neutrophilic predominant leukocyte count that can range from 7500 to 151,000/mm^3; *Candida* may be isolated from cultures of the synovial fluid. Histopathologic examination of the synovium may reveal a nonspecific mononuclear inflammatory infiltrate with thickening of the synovium. In contrast to other fungal arthritides, granuloma formation is uncommon with *Candida* arthritis.[89,294]

Central nervous system candidiasis. *Candida* infection of the CNS can involve any part of the brain or spinal cord and manifests as acute or chronic meningitis, ventriculitis, microabscesses, or macroabscesses. Fortunately, CNS involvement is not common. In a large international case series of culture-proven IC, only 1% of pediatric patients and 4% of neonates had a positive cerebrospinal fluid (CSF) culture result for a *Candida* species.[220] CNS involvement is typically the result of hematogenous spread; up to 66% of patients with *Candida* infection of the CNS have a recent or concurrent positive blood culture result at the time of diagnosis.[124,200,335] Involvement of the CNS through direct inoculation at the time of surgery or through infection of intracranial device (e.g., ventriculoperitoneal shunt, external ventricular drain) may also occur. Neonates, patients with hematologic malignant disease, hematopoietic transplant recipients, and neurosurgical patients are at increased risk for CNS disease; thus heightened clinical suspicion is needed in these patient populations.[113,124,200]

The clinical manifestations of CNS candidiasis vary depending on the patient population and the type of involvement. Importantly, profound immunosuppression with neutropenia and consequent limited ability to mount an inflammatory response may lead to subtle symptoms in oncologic patients and transplant recipients with candidal meningitis and brain abscesses. A single-center case series of 12 children with leukemia and candidal meningitis highlighted the subtle nature of this serious infection in immunocompromised patients. Among the 12 patients, 42% had fever as their only sign of systemic infection, and only 50% exhibited an altered level of consciousness.[200] Similarly, in a case series of 19 pediatric and adult bone marrow transplant recipients with *Candida* brain abscesses, only 42% had altered mental status, 26% had cranial nerve abnormalities, and 16% had seizures. Headache, papilledema, nausea, and vomiting were uncommon, and nearly one-third had no signs or symptoms, with diagnosis being made postmortem.[124] In both studies, the findings of CSF analysis were often unremarkable, with at least one-half of subjects in each series lacking pleocytosis and with mildly elevated protein levels and hypoglycorrhachia found in only a minority of patients. In those with CSF pleocytosis, a neutrophilic predominance is typically seen,[10,69,124,188] although a mononuclear predominance may be present in neutropenic patients.[200] MRI appears to be more sensitive than CT in the detection of brain abscesses; however, 60% of patients with *Candida* brain abscesses may have normal scans, likely related to the difficulty in detecting microabscesses on imaging. *Candida* frequently produces multiple brain lesions, with one-half of affected patients having three or more lesions, on the basis of autopsy evaluation.[124] Dissemination of *Candida* to other organs is frequently seen in addition to intracranial infection, and thus detection of lesions in other organs should prompt evaluation of the CNS as well. Outcomes of CNS *Candidiasis* are poor, with an associated 30% to 100% mortality rate.[113,124,141,200]

In patients with intracranial devices, isolation of *Candida* from the CSF may represent colonization of the device or true intracranial infection. In a case series of 21 neurosurgical patients from whom *Candida* was isolated from CSF, nine patients with a single CSF culture did not receive antifungal therapy, and four patients underwent removal of the intracranial drain as the only intervention.[113] These patients also had normal CSF parameters and were clinically asymptomatic. In contrast, 10 patients had multiple positive CSF cultures and were treated for *Candida* meningitis; most were symptomatic, with lethargy, fever, meningismus, focal neurologic signs, and neutrophilic pleocytosis. Isolation of *Candida* as a contaminant may occur even in the absence of an intracranial device. In a single-center case series of 23 infants and children from a single institution with fungi isolated from the CSF, six patients, the majority of whom did not have an intracranial device and five of whom had a negative CSF culture result on repeat sampling, were considered to have *Candida* as a contaminant and did not receive antifungal therapy, with a good outcome.[10] Both studies highlight the importance of considering underlying medical conditions as well as the presence of other clinical signs and symptoms in the interpretation of *Candida* isolated from the CSF.

Ocular candidiasis. *Candida* may involve the eye during the course of candidemia and subsequent disseminated disease. Review of cohorts of children with candidemia who had eye examinations found that 3% to 8% of children had ocular dissemination.[96,335] Endophthalmitis is thought to result from hematogenous seeding of the choroid and retina through the small vessels, with subsequent chorioretinitis manifesting as white chorioretinal lesions, or "fluff balls," on the posterior fundus.[20] Vitritis is marked by extension of inflammation into the vitreous. Hypopyon, scleritis, retinal detachment, and optic nerve involvement may also occur. In patients who are able to report symptoms, "floaters" and blurred vision are the most common.[274]

Chronic Disseminated Candidiasis

Chronic disseminated candidiasis (CDC), sometimes referred to as hepatosplenic candidiasis when limited to the liver and spleen, is a distinct form of IC seen primarily in patients with leukemia and treatment-induced neutropenia. Involvement predominantly occurs in the liver, spleen, and occasionally other organs. *Candida* colonization of the gastrointestinal tract with subsequent dissemination through the portal venous circulation during periods of neutropenia is thought to be the predominant cause of this disease entity, especially when the process is limited to the liver and spleen. Prolonged neutropenia is the most cited risk factor for CDC; other reported risk factors include younger age and exposure to quinolone prophylaxis.[198,262] Common symptoms of CDC include persistent fever and right upper quadrant pain. The most common laboratory finding is a significantly elevated and persistent serum alkaline phosphatase level (median duration, 130 days); serum bilirubin and transaminase levels may exhibit brief elevation.[295] CT has been shown to be more sensitive than ultrasound for the detection of hepatosplenic lesions, although MRI may be superior to both imaging modalities. Blood cultures are not often diagnostic, yielding positive results in less than 20% of patients with CDC. A biopsy for identification of *Candida* elements on histopathologic study or culture can confirm the diagnosis; however, the clinical, radiographic, and laboratory findings may be enough to direct therapy and avoid the need for an invasive diagnostic procedure.[198,272] Clinical symptoms (i.e., fever), laboratory abnormalities (i.e., elevated alkaline phosphatase), and radiographic findings of CDC may manifest during neutropenia but often persist well after neutrophil recovery. The persistence of fever and lesions on radiographs has been hypothesized to represent a form of immune reconstitution syndrome against *Candida* species.[295] Lesions are typically not apparent until neutrophil recovery, and they manifest on imaging as "wheel in wheel" target lesions, with biopsy showing histopathologic features of a central necrotic focus of yeast and filamentous forms with a surrounding rim of inflammatory cells.[295]

DIAGNOSIS

Culture

Isolation of *Candida* spp. from cultures of blood or other sterile sites is considered the gold standard of laboratory-based microbiologic confirmation of IC. However, the sensitivity of blood cultures is not ideal and varies depending on the clinical presentation of IC. The sensitivity of blood cultures for IC has been found to range from 60% to 83% in some studies and is even lower when considering when the specific clinical entity of CDC is considered.[35,64,219] On the basis of studies evaluating the yield of blood culture systems inoculated with *Candida*, the sensitivity of commercially available blood culture media to detect candidemia varies by the type of culture media (aerobic, anaerobic, mycologic), inoculum size, and blood culture system. One study demonstrated that even when aerobic blood culture bottles were deliberately spiked with 10^3 *Candida* yeast cells, the yield was only 90%.[138] Depending on the blood culture system used, mycologic blood culture bottles may provide a slight advantage in the recovery of *Candida* because of the added benefit of a lysing agent to release viable phagocytosed fungal cells, the addition of nutrients essential to fungal growth, and antibiotics to suppress competitive bacterial growth in case of coinfection.[139] Time to positivity depends on inoculum size as well as specific *Candida* species.[114] Using current automated blood culture systems, most *Candida* species have growth detected within approximately 24 to 36 hours, even at densities of 1 colony-forming unit(CFU)/mL, although *C. glabrata* has been shown to exhibit significantly longer time to positivity.[114,139]

Although *Candida* spp. can grow on routine sheep's blood agar, use of selective fungal media such as Sabouraud dextrose agar or chromogenic *Candida* agar may enhance isolation of organisms from other types of body fluid and tissue specimens. However, despite the presence of visible yeast and pseudohyphae in the specimen, tissue culture results may still be negative. The yield of culture may also vary depending on the type of IC. For instance, tissue cultures in patients with hepatosplenic candidiasis have a particularly low yield. One study of 45 oncologic patients with hepatosplenic candidiasis who underwent biopsy reported that biopsy culture results were negative in 56.5%.[295] Prior antifungal exposure, nonviable organisms in the specimen, and sampling error may contribute to negative culture results.

Histology

Histopathologic examination of tissue specimens may be an important alternative means to diagnose IC in suspected cases when culture results are negative, and they may be important in differentiating tissue invasion from surface colonization. Yeast, hyphae, and pseudohyphae may be visible on hematoxylin and eosin stain. Special fungal stains such as Gomori methenamine stain and periodic acid–Schiff should be used to enhance identification of *Candida* structures.

Antigen

In light of the poor sensitivity of blood cultures, the use of fungal biomarkers to establish a diagnosis of IC has been explored. One such biomarker is the (1→3) β-D glucan (BDG), which is a major cell wall component of most fungi (except *Mucorales* and *Cryptococcus* spp.), including *Candida*. Commercially available BDG assays harness the ability of BDG to activate a coagulation cascade in amebocyte lysate from the horseshoe crab in what is called the Limulus test, by allowing measurement of this reaction through colorimetric or turbidimetric methods.[146] BDG is released into the blood and tissues during invasive fungal infection, and thus the availability of commercial assays represents an opportunity for indirect diagnosis of IC. Unfortunately, the sensitivity of the BDG assay for detecting any proven or probable invasive fungal infection has been low, ranging from 49% to 76.8% in multiple adult meta-analyses.[79,146,177] Although these studies did not focus specifically on IC, the reported sensitivities do not appear substantially better than that of blood culture.

Furthermore, data on the use of BDG assays in children have been limited but call into question the applicability of adult data to pediatric populations. Mean serum BDG levels in healthy children have been found to be higher than that in adults (68 pg/mL vs. 48 pg/mL, respectively), thereby questioning whether the threshold of 80 pg/mL identified in the package insert for a positive test result is applicable to children.[280] In addition, a prospective study evaluating *Candida* colonization and BDG serum values in children with leukemia demonstrated that 30% of colonized children exceeded the assay manufacturer positive cutoff values. None of the children developed evidence of invasive fungal infection, and the investigators postulated that absorption of BDG through the gut, or other sources of false-positive results, may have contributed to this result.[205] Large prospective cohort studies are needed to assess the clinical utility of this test for diagnosing IC in the pediatric population.

A second biomarker, the mannan antigen and antimannan antibody assay, has been proposed as a tool for indirect diagnosis of IC. Mannan is an immunogenic polysaccharide that is a major component of the cell wall in *Candida* spp., and it can be found in serum during infection. Different assays have been developed to detect mannan antigen and antimannan antibodies, with enzyme-linked immunosorbent assays being the most frequently used in Europe.[203] However, none of these assays have yet been approved by the US Food and Drug Administration for use in the United States. A meta-analysis of 14 studies evaluating the test characteristics of the mannan and antimannan antibody assays for proven and probable IC (on the basis of European Organization for Research and Treatment of Cancer/Invasive Fungal Infections Cooperative Group and National Institute of Allergy and Infectious Diseases Mycoses Study Group criteria) demonstrated a pooled sensitivity of 58% and specificity of 93% for mannan antigen. The antimannan antibody assay had a pooled sensitivity of 59% and specificity of 83%, whereas the pooled sensitivity of using combined mannan antigen and antimannan antibody assays was 83%, with a specificity of 86%.[203] Significant heterogeneity of the studies in the meta-analysis was detected, however, and data have been extremely limited in the pediatric population. The increased sensitivity with the combination of mannan antigen and antimannan antibody assays make this an intriguing diagnostic tool, although the potential for false-positive results and the lack of pediatric specific data limit the ability to recommend these tests for routine clinical use in diagnosing IC.[231,273] As with the BDG assay, prospective pediatric-specific studies are needed.

Molecular-Based Testing

Polymerase chain reaction (PCR)–based assays have also been evaluated in the diagnosis of IC. The ribosomal RNA gene cluster contains the 18 Svedburg (S), internal transcribed spacer (ITS) 1 and 2, 5.8S, and 28S regions and is a popular amplification target.[173] The presence of multiple copies of this ribosomal RNA cluster in fungal cells increases the sensitivity of PCR. Given that blood samples may contain only a small number of fungal cells (1 cell/mL),[235] the ability of PCR-based assays to detect down to 0.22 cells/mL represents a potential advantage compared with conventional culture.[173] In addition, DNA derived from both dead and living *Candida* cells can be amplified. Numerous DNA amplification methods have been developed including nested PCR, multiplex PCR, and real-time (RT) PCR platforms. Most studies have reported sensitivities near or equal to 100%, with a specificity greater than 90%.[173] In a prospective study comparing *Candida* RT-PCR, BDG assay, and blood cultures in the diagnosis of IC in 73 hospitalized adults, RT-PCR outperformed BDG for the detection of deep-seated candidiasis (89% vs. 53%; $P = .004$).[212] Two studies examined the use of PCR to detect IC exclusively in the pediatric population. One study was conducted in neonatal and pediatric intensive care units, and the other was conducted in an oncologic population of patients presenting with fever and neutropenia. Both studies demonstrated high sensitivity.[77,297] PCR-based assays for the detection of *Candida* are promising test modalities, but larger pediatric prospective studies and standardization of PCR techniques are needed before these techniques are incorporated into clinical practice.

Other Novel Diagnostic Approaches

The advancement of novel technologies provides the potential for more rapid and accurate identification of Candida to the species level. Matrix-assisted laser desorption ionization–time of flight (MALDI-TOF) mass spectrometry uses a laser to irradiate a specimen resulting in charged ions of varying size that are then directed through a mass spectrometer. Particles are identified based on their time of flight, which depends on their mass-to-charge ratio. Comparison of MALDI-TOF mass spectrometry with biochemical identification by commercial assays revealed high agreement for species identification.[289] The T2Candida assay (T2 Biosystems) combines the patient sample with species-specific magnetic nanoparticles. Clustering of the species with the magnetic nanoparticles can then be measured by T2-weighted MRI. An initial small study of pediatric patients with candidemia suggested that the assay is capable of accurately identifying *Candida* to the species level[48] directly from the blood specimen before culture. Both the MALDI-TOF and T2Candida technologies offer distinct benefit compared with conventional blood culture and subsequent biochemical testing because they can significantly reduce the time to organism identification.[125,289] Whether these novel diagnostic tools will have improved overall sensitivity compared with blood culture is still not known.

ANTIFUNGAL PROPHYLAXIS AND TREATMENT

Prophylaxis

Consideration for antifungal prophylaxis has been given primarily to patients with the greatest risk for invasive fungal infection. Data from clinical trials on the efficacy of antifungal prophylaxis in the oncologic, liver transplant, intensive care unit, and surgical populations derive largely from studies in adults; antifungal prophylaxis in the neonatal population is a notable exception and is discussed later, in the neonatal candidiasis section.

Children undergoing chemotherapy for hematologic malignant diseases are at significantly high risk of developing invasive fungal infections, of which *Candida* spp. is most commonly identified. High-risk categories in this group can be refined further, with acute myeloid leukemia, relapsed acute lymphoblastic leukemia, allogeneic or autologous hematopoietic stem cell transplantation, and graft-versus-host disease associated with rates of invasive fungal infection ranging from 9% to 29%.[85] Severe aplastic anemia, although not an oncologic process, is also associated with a significant risk of invasive fungal infection because of bone marrow failure and prolonged neutropenia.[303] Given the notable frequency of invasive fungal infection and the high mortality rates associated with IC in these patients,[304] extrapolation from comparative data in adults with regard to the benefits of antifungal prophylaxis is reasonable. In a meta-analysis of 64 randomized controlled trials of antifungal prophylaxis in patients with cancer after chemotherapy or hematopoietic stem cell transplantation, antifungal prophylaxis led to a significant decrease in rates of all-cause mortality, fungal-related death, documented IC, and occurrence of any invasive fungal infection, compared with placebo, no treatment, or nonsystemically absorbed antifungal agents. The greatest benefit was seen in allogeneic and autologous hematopoietic stem cell transplant recipients.[251] Although there is a dearth of randomized controlled trial data in children, more recent pediatric observational data in children with acute myeloid leukemia have suggested a mortality benefit of antifungal prophylaxis compared with no prophylaxis.[98]

A detailed discussion of the comparative effectiveness of different antifungal prophylactic regimens is beyond the scope of this chapter. However, with regard to the type of antifungal prophylaxis, fluconazole is currently the most commonly recommended agent in high-risk children, given its proven survival benefit in adults, its low adverse effects, and its comparatively fewer common drug interactions compared with alternatives.[85,271,301] In patients for whom broader antifungal coverage may be indicated, the extended-spectrum triazoles and the echinocandins are alternative options.[85,302,304] Prophylaxis for high-risk patients is often administered for the duration of neutropenia in patients with prolonged neutropenia after a course of chemotherapy, for conditioning for hematopoietic stem cell transplantation, and in patients with severe graft-versus-host disease.[226]

Earlier studies in pediatric liver transplant recipients suggested a high rate of IC.[51,115] More contemporary publications report a relatively low rate of IC in the post–liver transplant period and argue against the routine use of antifungal prophylaxis in this population.[76] On the basis of reports in adults, the Infectious Diseases Society of America currently recommends fluconazole or a lipid or liposomal formulation amphotericin B (LFAmB) as postoperative prophylaxis for 7 to 14 days for liver transplant recipients with at least two of the following risk factors: repeat transplantation, creatinine level greater than 2.0 mg/dL, choledochojejunostomy, intraoperative use of more than 40 units of blood products, prolonged intraoperative time (>1 hour), and fungal colonization detected at least 2 days before and 3 days after transplantation.[226] Prolonged operative time and the need for intensive care before transplantation have also been identified as risk factors for IC in children, and thus antifungal prophylaxis in these higher-risk patients may be warranted, similar to the adult recommendations.[76]

Data on the benefit of antifungal prophylaxis for other pediatric organ transplant populations are limited. The adult expert consensus guidelines recommend fluconazole prophylaxis for small bowel transplant recipients for at least 2 weeks after transplantation.[226] Pediatric small bowel transplant recipients appear to be at high risk of invasive fungal infection,[103] and thus extrapolation of the adult recommendation to children may be warranted.

The benefit of antifungal prophylaxis in pediatric intensive care unit patients remains unclear because more data are needed to identify prospectively those patients at highest risk for IC, as well as to define the benefit of targeted antifungal prophylaxis in this population. On the basis of data from adults, current guidelines suggest that antifungal prophylaxis may be warranted in intensive care units with very high rates of IC and in patients who are at highest risk (>10%) of IC.[226]

Treatment

The approach to treatment of superficial and IC should take into consideration the source of infection (e.g., endovascular, medical device associated), the site of involvement, *Candida* species and susceptibility profile, prior antifungal exposure, and the clinical status of the host, as well as drug-specific factors such as pharmacokinetic and pharmacodynamic properties and the potential for drug-drug interactions. This section focuses on the management of superficial and IC in the non-neonatal pediatric population and relies heavily on updated clinical practice guidelines issued by the Infectious Diseases Society of America.[226] Detailed discussions of individual properties of antifungal agents are discussed in Chapter 240 and are not reviewed here.

The choice of antifungal therapy for *Candida* infections is influenced largely by the species causing the infection because certain *Candida* species exhibit characteristic antifungal susceptibility profiles. In general, the echinocandins are preferred for infection with *C. glabrata*, although transition to fluconazole or voriconazole is possible if susceptibility of the isolate is confirmed. Because the MIC values for echinocandins have been found to be higher for some *C. parapsilosis* isolates as a result of the presence of an intrinsic *FKS1* mutation encoding glucan synthase,[37] recommendations had been made to avoid echinocandins as first-line therapy for this pathogen.[226] However, the clinical significance of higher echinocandin MIC values in this species remains unclear. More recent adult epidemiologic data did not find a difference in outcomes between echinocandin and azole therapy among patients with *C. parapsilosis* infections,[58,94] and thus the most recent IC guidelines no longer specifically recommend avoiding echinocandins for this pathogen.[226]

Although the general guidance provided in the previous paragraph can be helpful for empiric antifungal therapy choices, it is ideal to base decisions on sensitivity testing. Fortunately, the Clinical Laboratory and Science Institute (CLSI) provides clinical breakpoints for sensitive and resistant threshold testing for several *Candida* species. These breakpoints were updated in 2012 and are species specific[66] (Box 200.1). Routine performance of resistance testing for *Candida* spp. isolated from sterile site cultures should be considered as the standard of care to guide definitive therapeutic choices.

Dosing recommendations for antifungal agents in children continues to be a moving target as more pediatric specific pharmacokinetic data become available. Specific treatment choices with recommendations for dosing are provided in the following subsections for each clinical indication as a guide for the reader. However, when choosing a dose for a specific clinical case, the clinician should confer with a pharmacist or infectious disease specialist with expertise in antifungal dosing.

Superficial Candidiasis

Oropharyngeal candidiasis. Most patients with oropharyngeal candidiasis respond to topical antifungal therapy, although in patients with moderate to severe disease, systemic antifungal therapy may be required. In children with mild cases of oropharyngeal candidiasis, 4 to 6 mL of nystatin suspension (100,000 U/mL) may be administered four times daily as a swish-and-swallow medication. Effort should be made to prolong contact time with the oral mucosa as long as possible before swallowing because nystatin does not adhere well to the oral mucosa.[135] Clotrimazole, 10 mg troches administered five times daily, or one to two nystatin pastilles (200,000 U each) administered four times daily, can be used as alternatives. For infants, 100,000 to 200,000 units can be painted onto the affected areas four times daily. When applicable, cleaning of bottle nipples and pacifiers after each use should be attempted to reduce reintroduction of *Candida* through colonized surfaces. Treatment should be administered for 7 to 14 days.

For moderate to severe disease, systemic antifungal therapy is warranted. Oral fluconazole, 6 to 12 mg/kg (maximum, 100–200 mg/dose), may be administered for 7 to 14 days.[222] For fluconazole-refractory disease, itraconazole solution, 2.5 mg/kg twice daily, has been shown to be effective and safe in phase II clinical trials in children with cancer, liver transplantation, or HIV infection for the treatment of oropharyngeal candidiasis. Use of itraconazole in children is off-label because it has not been approved for use in children younger than 18 years of age.[121] In children 2 to 11 years of age, or 12 to 14 years old and weighing less than 50 kg, voriconazole, 9 mg/kg (maximum, 350 mg) orally every 12 hours, may be administered, whereas children 12 to 14 years old and weighing 50 kg more, or children older than 14 years of age, should receive 200 mg orally every 12 hours as maintenance.[121,106] In the event of treatment failure, amphotericin B deoxycholate (AmB-d), given as an oral 1-mL suspension four times daily, may be tried. Intravenous therapies such as echinocandins and amphotericin B products should be considered as last resorts in children with persistent disease. In an otherwise healthy child, long-term suppressive therapy is often unnecessary. However, in children presenting with persistent or recurrent episodes, an underlying primary, acquired, or iatrogenic immune defect should be investigated. Long-term suppressive therapy can be considered in children with an immunodeficiency predisposing to persistent or recurrent oropharyngeal candidiasis. In such settings fluconazole three times weekly is considered the regimen of choice.[226]

Esophageal candidiasis. The treatment of esophageal candidiasis requires systemic antifungal therapy. Oral fluconazole, at 6 to 12 mg/kg daily (or 200–400 mg daily) for 14 to 21 days, is recommended.[222] For fluconazole-refractory disease, itraconazole, voriconazole, and caspofungin are suitable alternatives (see earlier for pediatric dosing). As in oropharyngeal candidiasis, long-term suppressive therapy with fluconazole three times weekly may be administered.[226]

BOX 200.1 Neonatal Cutaneous Candidiasis Definition

Definition: Extensive *Candida* rash covering ≥2 affected areas from A and/or B

Affected Areas

A. Skin
- Chest
- Abdomen
- Back
- Extremity
- Groin or perineal area
- Neck
- Face or scalp

B. Umbilical cord and placenta
- White plaques on umbilical cord
- Placenta with yeast invasion

Timing

CCC: Presenting in the first 48 h of life; usually present at birth
CC: Presenting after 2–7 days of life

Skin Rash

Macular-papular
Scaly, erythematous
Dry flaking
Desquamating
Burn-like erythematous

Presentation

Extensive
- Covering ≥2 affected areas (see below)
- Covering 1 affected area (see below); umbilical plaques or placental pathologic features (silver or H&E) would count as 1 affected area

Evaluation

CCC: Skin rash sites, placental and/or cord culture, and pathologic examination with silver stain for yeast blood culture and CSF (unless rash over lumbar area; if so, treat empirically for meningitis)
CC: Skin rash sites, blood, urine, CSF (unless rash over lumbar area; if so, treat empirically for meningitis)

Diagnosis

One or more of the following:
- Surface culture isolating *Candida* species
- Placental or cord identification (culture or silver stain) of yeast or *Candida* species for CCC
- Positive blood, urine, CSF cultures for *Candida* species

Treatment

Preterm infants (<37 weeks' gestation): 14-day course of IV antifungal therapy
Full-term infants: IV antifungal therapy pending culture results

CC, Cutaneous candidiasis; *CCC*, congenital cutaneous candidiasis; *CSF*, cerebrospinal fluid; *H&E*, hematoxylin and eosin; *IV*, intravenous.

Vulvovaginal candidiasis. The approach to the treatment of vulvovaginal candidiasis varies depending on the presence of complicated vulvovaginal disease (severe disease, four or more episodes of symptomatic vulvovaginal candidiasis in 1 year, non–*C. albicans* infection, or abnormal host).[82] For uncomplicated cases topical therapies are effective, and no data have revealed the superiority of any topical regimen.[248,282] In a meta-analysis of 19 randomized, controlled trials oral and topical antifungal regimens had similar effectiveness.[217] Topical therapies are often administered for 3 days. Uncomplicated vulvovaginal candidiasis can also be effectively treated with a single oral dose of fluconazole. In patients found to have vulvovaginal candidiasis from a fluconazole-resistant isolate, topical nystatin has been shown to be effective.[91] Complicated vulvovaginal candidiasis often requires extended therapy either with 1 week of a topical agent or three doses of oral fluconazole each separated by 3 days.[2] The management of recurrent vulvovaginal candidiasis was studied in a randomized controlled trial. All patients were started on three doses of fluconazole every 3 days and then randomized to once a week fluconazole for 6 months versus placebo. Patients in the former group had 90% response rate versus 36% in the placebo arm.[284] These data support a prolonged maintenance therapy phase for patients with recurrent disease.

Cutaneous candidiasis. Because moist, macerated skin promotes the development of cutaneous candidiasis, it is important to keep affected areas dry as much as possible; antifungal therapy alone usually does not produce a cure. For candidal diaper dermatitis, frequent diaper changes should be performed. Topical antifungal therapy with nystatin or azoles may be applied twice daily and continued until symptoms resolve.

Invasive Candidiasis

Candidemia. All pediatric patients with candidemia require systemic antifungal therapy. The adult guidelines support an echinocandin as the preferred therapy for candidemia on the basis of improved efficacy in adult trials likely related to the fungicidal activity against *Candida.*[226] Data comparing the effectiveness of antifungal therapies in children are limited. Retrospective data suggest similar outcomes among children treated with fungicidal and fungistatic agents.[316] However, until more definitive pediatric data are available, clinicians should defer to the adult guidelines. Certainly, for neutropenic patients, patients who are critically ill, or those with recent azole exposure, an echinocandin should be considered first-line therapy. LFAmB (3–5 mg/kg daily) may be given as an alternative option in these clinical situations. In children in clinically stable condition who do not meet any of the aforementioned criteria, fluconazole therapy may be given as a first-line agent at 12 mg/kg intravenously (IV) daily. Step-down therapy to fluconazole is recommended for patients with susceptible isolates, whereas voriconazole may be offered as step-down oral therapy for candidemia resulting from *C. krusei* or susceptible *C. glabrata.*[226] In children 2 to 11 years, or 12 to 14 years and weighing less than 50 kg, voriconazole may be given as a 9 mg/kg loading dose IV every 12 hours on day 1, followed by 8 mg/kg IV every 12 hours as maintenance. Oral dosing may be given as 9 mg/kg (maximum, 350 mg) every 12 hours. In children 12 to 14 years and weighing 50 kg or more, or children more than 14 years old, dosing should be as in adults and may be given as a 6 mg/kg loading dose IV every 12 hours on day 1, followed by 4 mg/kg IV every 12 hours as maintenance, whereas oral dosing may be given as 200 mg every 12 hours as maintenance.[121,106]

A dilated funduscopic examination should be performed in all patients with candidemia after initiation of antifungal therapy, and routine blood cultures should be performed to document clearance of *Candida* from the bloodstream. The eye examination should be reserved until after documented clearance of candidemia. In patients without evidence of disseminated disease, antifungal therapy should continue for 14 days from symptom resolution and documented bloodstream clearance of *Candida.* In patients with candidemia in the setting of neutropenia, therapy is often continued until neutrophil count recovery.

Current guidelines recommend that central venous catheters in patients with candidemia should be removed when possible because data from most observational studies in children and adults have shown fewer rates of complications, reduced mortality rates, and more rapid rates of response to antifungal therapy.[8,75,101,229,249] This recommendation comes with acknowledgment of potential residual confounding in these observational studies, specifically the possibility that patients whose central venous catheters were retained had significantly more severe illness compared with patients whose catheters were removed, thus precluding catheter removal.[216] Nonetheless, the consistent and cumulative observational data support line removal as early as possible.

Candidemia in the neutropenic patient is further complicated by the issue that the source of infection may be the gastrointestinal tract, and thus the significance of catheter removal when candidemia is documented is less clear. In a single-center study of 404 patients with cancer and central venous catheters in place at the time of candidemia, the investigators attempted to differentiate candidemia associated with the central venous catheter from candidemia associated with a non-catheter source and to define the benefit of timing of catheter removal on resolution of candidemia-associated symptoms and blood culture sterilization. In patients with evidence of catheter-associated candidemia, catheter removal up to 72 hours from first positive blood culture result was found to be significantly associated with improved response rates compared with removal after more than 72 hours, whereas patients with candidemia resulting from an alternate or undefined source did not have a statistically significant improvement in response rates with early catheter removal.[242] Other data have shown mixed results in support of early removal of catheters in candidemic patients with cancer.[186,315] Although the data are not definitive, central catheter removal should still be strongly considered when feasible in children with neutropenia.

Endovascular candidiasis. Data informing evidence-based practice for management of *Candida* endocarditis are limited, but endocarditis and IC guidelines support a multipronged approach including antifungal therapy and surgical intervention.[22,226] Fungicidal regimens are preferred for *Candida* endocarditis, and most experience in the literature involves the use of AmB-d with or without flucytosine. LFAmB is associated with less toxicity and permits higher dosages; thus LFAmB (3–5 mg/kg IV daily), with or without flucytosine (100–150 mg/kg per day in four divided doses enterally), is recommended for the treatment of native valve and prosthetic valve *Candida* endocarditis in the non-neonatal population. Echinocandins are considered a second-line option. In a small observational study, outcomes of patients receiving amphotericin B–based therapy versus echinocandin-based therapy were similar.[11] Data from case reports, case series, and a meta-analysis[90,290] suggest that surgery is an important adjunct to antifungal therapy, and these data serve as the basis for recommendation that patients with *Candida* endocarditis undergo surgical resection of the infectious process. The duration of antifungal therapy is recommended to be at least 6 weeks from surgical intervention for native valve endocarditis. In patients unable to have surgical resection or in those with initial prosthetic valve endocarditis, a transition to long-term suppressive therapy with an azole agent after completion of initial therapy is recommended.[16,226]

Cardiac candidiasis. Pericarditis and myocarditis caused by *Candida* spp. are both rare clinical entities, and thus data are limited to guide management. A report documented the successful use of amphotericin B for *Candida* pericarditis,[268] and the known lower toxicity profile seen with LFAmB suggests that pericarditis can be treated with LFAmB. An echinocandin or azole (assuming a susceptible isolate) is a logical alternative. Treatment should be continued for several months, in combination with either a pericardial window or pericardiectomy, because this appears to be the best approach for achieving cure.[268] Step-down therapy to fluconazole can be considered in patients in clinically stable condition who have shown an initial response to an amphotericin product or echinocandin.

Peritoneal candidiasis. As noted earlier, peritoneal candidiasis can manifest in various clinical forms, but in children it is most often related to presence of a peritoneal catheter. Most experts agree that peritoneal catheters should be removed in patients with peritoneal candidiasis; the basis of this recommendation is the high rates of treatment failure seen in case series of patients with retained catheters, as well as the known challenges involved in treating biofilm present on the device.[52,166,207] Recommendations call for prompt (<24 hours) removal of the peritoneal catheter on diagnosis of fungal peritonitis.[183] This recommendation is supported by observational data showing reduced mortality rates in adults with early catheter removal compared with delayed removal.[53] Peritoneal candidiasis requires systemic administration of an antifungal agent. No comparative data exist on the ideal antifungal agent, and data on the ability of available antifungal agents to reach the peritoneum are limited. Some reports suggest that fluconazole may be more able to penetrate the peritoneum than amphotericin B products.[199,42] Fluconazole may also be given intraperitoneally as a 75 mg/L concentration added daily to the dialysate after a systemic loading dose.[206] Intraperitoneal

AmB-d has been associated with severe peritoneal irritation, as well as fibrosis and membrane loss, and it should be avoided.[9] The role of echinocandins in fungal peritonitis is not yet well defined, and some data suggest that the fungicidal activity of the echinocandins may be reduced by PD fluid.[300]

Candidiasis of the urinary tract. No treatment is recommended for patients with asymptomatic candiduria. In patients with an indwelling catheter, removal of the device may be adequate to resolve the candiduria without antifungal therapy. Fluconazole is highly water soluble, is primarily excreted into the urine as active drug, and expected urinary concentrations are more than 10-fold those in serum, thereby exceeding the MIC even for susceptible dose-dependent *Candida* species.[102] Thus fluconazole is considered the drug of choice for both cystitis and pyelonephritis. LFAmB should not be used to treat *Candida* UTIs because of the low drug levels achieved in the renal parenchyma and urine. Although voriconazole was shown in an animal model of renal parenchymal candidiasis to be superior to AmB-d or fluconazole, urine voriconazole levels are low, with less than 5% of the active drug excreted, which limits the drug's utility in the treatment of UTIs. Similarly, the echinocandins have been shown in experimental models to clear renal parenchymal infections in the setting of disseminated candidiasis, but very little active drug is excreted in the urine, and clinical experience with treatment of UTIs is limited. For fluconazole-resistance organisms, AmB-d or oral flucytosine is an alternative. Continuous bladder irrigation with AmB-d has also been used to treat *Candida* cystitis, although relapse rates after local bladder irrigation are high.[102]

Mycetomas (fungus balls) in the urinary collecting system may not respond to medical management alone, and thus surgical intervention may be necessary for source control. Surgical procedures include options such as endoscopic removal or instillation of AmB-d into the mycetoma through a nephrostomy tube. Pediatric data to guide decisions on when to invoke a surgical intervention for mycetoma or what intervention is ideal are limited.

Osteoarticular candidiasis. The management of osteoarticular *Candida* infections is challenging because no pediatric-specific comparative data are available to guide antifungal therapy choices. Furthermore, regardless of the therapeutic option, the rate of disease relapse is high.[110,278] Therapeutic options include fluconazole, an echinocandin, or LFAmB. Adult guidelines favor fluconazole as primary therapy and offer an alternative regimen that includes either an echinocandin or LFAmB for a 2-week induction period with step-down therapy to fluconazole. Regardless of the therapeutic choice, a total duration of 6 to 12 months is recommended.[226] Fluconazole 12 mg/kg daily, or intravenous LFAmB, at 3 to 5 mg/kg daily for at least 2 weeks, followed by step-down therapy to fluconazole, at 6 mg/kg daily for 6 to 12 months, is currently recommended. Echinocandins may be a suitable alternative to upfront parenteral LFAmB administration. Adjunctive surgical debridement may be beneficial in select cases.

For septic arthritis, a minimum of 6 weeks of fluconazole or LFAmB or an echinocandin for at least 2 weeks followed by fluconazole is recommended. Adequate surgical drainage is a crucial aspect of the management of non-neonatal *Candida* arthritis, and it should be performed in all cases.[226]

Central nervous system candidiasis. Most experience in the literature regarding the treatment of *Candida* CNS infections has been with AmB-d, with or without flucytosine.[10,113] Liposomal formulation Amphotericin B has been preferred because of its lower toxicity profile and known tissue penetration in the brain. The combination of liposomal formulation Amphotericin B and flucytosine has demonstrated synergism in vitro, and flucytosine achieves excellent CSF concentrations, thus making combination therapy attractive. Limited experience with the echinocandins has revealed both treatment successes and failures, in addition to breakthrough CNS infections after therapy for candidemia. The echinocandins have poor CSF penetration, with low levels compared with serum.[78] As a result, this antifungal class is not recommended for CNS candidiasis. Current recommendations for treatment of *Candida* CNS infection are to administer intravenous LFAmB 3 to 5 mg/kg daily with or without flucytosine (100–150 mg/kg per day in four divided doses enterally) for the initial several weeks of treatment, followed by step-down therapy to fluconazole (12 mg/kg daily) once a treatment response to LFAmB has been established. The ultimate duration of therapy is not known, but antifungal therapy should continue until all clinical and radiographic evidence of disease has resolved. Removal of infected intracranial devices is strongly recommended.[226]

Ocular candidiasis. No prospective studies exist for the treatment of *Candida* endophthalmitis, but current guidance is contingent on presence or absence of vitritis. All cases of *Candida* endophthalmitis require systemic antifungal therapy. Options for systemic therapy include fluconazole, voriconazole, or LFAmB with or without flucytosine.[226] No comparative data exist to establish the superiority of any of these options for ocular disease. However, given that fluconazole and voriconazole achieve reasonable posterior segment eye concentrations, some investigators favor these agents as first-line options over AFAmB.[250] Patients with vitritis or macular involvement of the retina are recommended to have intravitreal therapy with either voriconazole or AmB-d. In severe cases of vitritis, vitrectomy may help reduce the burden of infection. The optimal duration of antifungal therapy is not determined, but therapy should be continued until clinical evidence of infection has resolved. At minimum therapy should be for at least 4 to 6 weeks.[226]

Chronic disseminated candidiasis. Treatment recommendations for CDC are made on the basis of case reports and series; however, most clinical experience has been with AmB-d, LFAmB, and fluconazole. In clinically stable patients, fluconazole is recommended. Echinocandins or an amphotericin B product can be used to treat acutely ill patients or patients nonresponsive to fluconazole, either as a 1- to 2-week induction period before fluconazole step-down therapy or as single therapy. The duration of therapy for CDC is variable, depending on the clinical situation and the patient's response to treatment, but typically it is prolonged, with a median duration of more than 3 to 5 months.[198] Most experts recommend that antifungal therapy continue until all lesions resolve or calcify.[226] Continuation of chemotherapy has been shown to be safe in these patients, and stem cell transplantation may be performed if indicated in patients whose disease is controlled.[40,324] The prolonged fever and persistence of lesions in patients with this chronic entity have been hypothesized to be secondary to a type of immune reconstitution inflammatory syndrome. As such in patients with persistent fevers, adjuvant low-dose corticosteroid therapy in addition to antifungal therapy has been proposed. This therapeutic approach has been shown to result in symptom resolution.[56,179] This intervention can be considered in select cases of persistent symptoms, but more data are needed for routine recommendation of corticosteroids.

NEONATAL CANDIDIASIS

Epidemiology

IC in neonatal intensive care units (NICUs) remains a serious health problem because it is associated with substantial morbidity and mortality. Strategies for prevention and management of IC are paramount for improving outcomes for neonates.[30,31,153,292,338] The incidence of candidiasis had increased in the NICU as advances in medical therapy allowed for increased survival of extremely low-birth-weight (ELBW) and low-gestational-age premature infants between the 1980s and 1990s and then remained stable until 2001, when a decreased incidence was observed.[5,62,107,171] More recent evident has shown that the incidence of candidiasis is decreasing, from 3.6 to 1.4 per 1000 NICU admissions between 1997 and 2010.[5] The decrease in candidiasis may be related to the increased use of fluconazole prophylaxis at high-incidence centers, decreased use of broad-spectrum antibiotics, and improved infection control practices.

C. albicans and *C. parapsilosis* infections account for 80% to 90% of neonatal IC in centers not using antifungal prophylaxis.[31] Centers using fluconazole prophylaxis are more likely to observe infections caused by non-*albicans Candida* species. Less common *Candida* species include *C. glabrata* and *C. tropicalis,* and a few infections are caused by *C. lusitaniae, C. guilliermondii,* or *C. dubliniensis.*

IC in the infant include congenital cutaneous candidiasis (CCC) and late-onset cutaneous candidiasis, candidemia, UTIs, meningitis, peritonitis, and infection of other sterile sites (bone and joint infections).

Prematurity is the predominant factor predisposing hospitalized infants to IC. The immune system of the premature infant has defects in chemotaxis, cytokine and antibody production, and phagocytosis.[55,182]

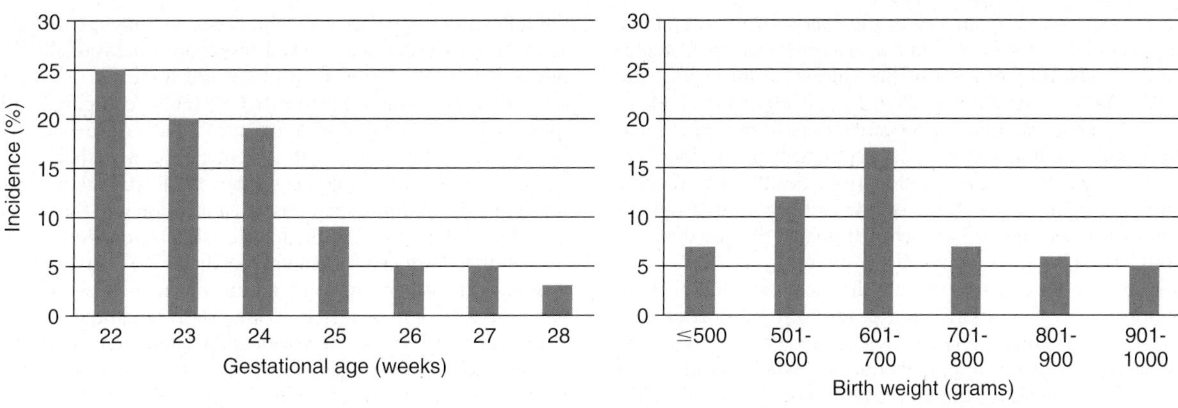

FIG. 200.1 Invasive candidiasis by gestational age and birth weight in infants weighing less than 1000 g. Invasive candidiasis: candidemia, urinary tract infection, meningitis, or peritonitis in infants weighing <1000 g at birth who were not receiving antifungal prophylaxis. Gestational age has a linear relationship with invasive candidiasis that aids in defining the highest-risk patients. (Data from 137 infections in 1515 infants weighing less than 1000 g from 19 centers of the National Institute of Child Health and Human Development Neonatal Research Network.)

In addition, invasive medical devices such as central venous catheters and endotracheal tubes compromise already underdeveloped skin and place the premature infant at an especially high risk for IC.

There is significant variation in the incidence of IC by NICU. This variation by NICU has been attributed to differences in patients' demographics, use of antifungal prophylaxis, surgical population, resuscitation of extremely preterm infants, feeding protocols, and antibiotic prescribing practices. The incidence has been reported to range between 3% and more than 23% among NICUs in infants weighing less than 1000 g.[31,107,71] Among 128 US NICUs using National Nosocomial Infections Surveillance (NNIS) system data from 1995 to 2004 (n = 130,523 infants),[107] the median incidence of candidemia was 7% for infants weighing less than 1000 g, and 25% of NICUs had rates of 13.5% or higher. The incidence of candidemia for infants with birth weights of 1001 to 1500 g was 1.3%, for weights of 1501 to 2500 g it was 0.4%, and for those weighing more than 2501 g it was 0.3%. The highest incidence of IC occurs in the most extremely preterm infants and is greater than 20% for infants at less than 25 weeks of gestation (Fig. 200.1).[31]

Infants with complex congenital anomalies or those requiring surgical procedures are also at high risk of IC. Feja and colleagues[93] found that candidemia was increased in patients with gastrointestinal disease (OR, 4.57; 95% CI, 1.62–12.92). Gastrointestinal disease was defined in their study as tracheoesophageal fistula, gastroschisis, omphalocele, Hirschprung disease, intestinal atresias, or episodes of necrotizing enterocolitis (NEC). Candidemia accounts for 9% of BSIs in patients with congenital heart disease cared for in NICUs in the first 4 months of life.[12] *Candida* BSI occurred in 6.3 per 1000 admissions and had an overall mortality rate of 21%. *Candida* species are the second most common causes of infection in infants on extracorporeal membrane oxygenation and are responsible for 10% of infections.[39]

Risk Factors

Given that neonatal candidiasis can be fatal among premature infants, an understanding of the risk factors that lead to infection within this high-risk group is critical. Conditions that facilitate fungal colonization and proliferation and increase the risk for invasive infection include gastrointestinal dysmotility or ileus, antibiotics, acid inhibition, steroids, and the patient's immune system immaturity. Several risk factors have been identified, with gestational age having the strongest effect. This correlates with the degree of the underdeveloped immune system, skin, and gastrointestinal tract in these infants.

The immature lymphocyte and antibody system predisposes premature infants to skin and mucosal fungal colonization, whereas deficient innate host defense mechanisms predispose them to dissemination and overwhelming infection. With compromise of the barrier defense system, IC may result from deficient neutrophil number and function. Neutrophils provide the major role in antifungal defense, ingesting and killing *Candida* in a process requiring production of oxygen metabolites, antibodies, and cytokines and activation of the C3 complement component, all of which are decreased in premature infants compared with term infants and adults. Also deficient are neutrophil granules and cytokines that play a critical role in the lysis of *Candida* hyphae and pseudohyphae, which are too large to be engulfed by phagocytosis. Macrophages have impaired adherence, phagocytosis, and oxidative killing in preterm infants, thus affecting their ability to contain fungal colonization and infection. In addition to cell-mediated defenses, cytokines contribute to innate immunity against fungal infection through enhancement of cell-mediated fungicidal activity. Pulmonary host defense is primarily through alveolar macrophages, cilia and mucus, and surfactant, all of which are deficient in preterm infants.

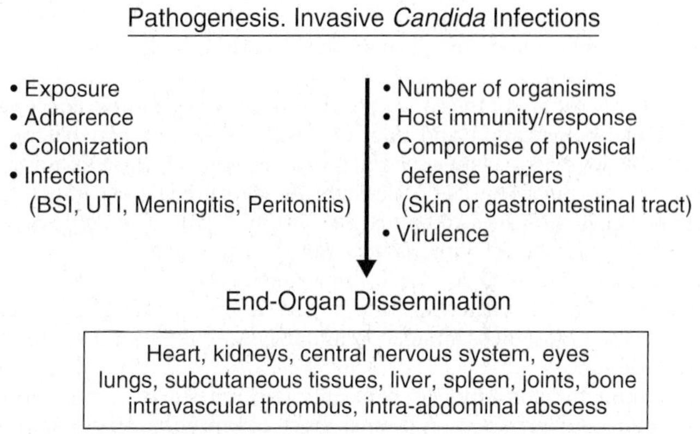

Pathogenesis. Invasive *Candida* Infections

- Exposure
- Adherence
- Colonization
- Infection
  (BSI, UTI, Meningitis, Peritonitis)

- Number of organisims
- Host immunity/response
- Compromise of physical defense barriers (Skin or gastrointestinal tract)
- Virulence

End-Organ Dissemination

Heart, kidneys, central nervous system, eyes lungs, subcutaneous tissues, liver, spleen, joints, bone intravascular thrombus, intra-abdominal abscess

FIG. 200.2 Pathogenesis of invasive candidiasis. *BSI,* Bloodstream infection; *UTI,* urinary tract infection.

Risk factors for *Candida* colonization and sepsis are similar.[260,261] Colonization of the skin, mucosal membranes, and vascular catheters commonly precedes infection. Biofilm formation on catheters inhibits the host's defense mechanisms and the penetration of antifungal agents.

Infants may be colonized through maternal transmission or acquire colonization during their admission in the NICU. Colonization in ELBW (<1000 g at birth) infants has been reported to be as high as 46% in the first 28 days of life.[166] Fungal colonization of the skin, respiratory tract, or gastrointestinal tract occurs in 10% of full-term infants compared with 27% to 62% of very low-birth-weight (VLBW; <1500 g at birth) infants in the first weeks of life.[155] Fungal colonization and subsequent infection depend on exposure, size of inoculum, host susceptibility, and properties of the pathogen (Fig. 200.2).

In a multicenter trial examining fungal colonization in six NICUs, *Candida* species were isolated on the hands of 29% (859 of 2989) of health care workers.[261] Although *C. albicans* was the more common fungal isolate in all NICU patients (14% vs. 7%), *C. parapsilosis* was the most common species isolated from the hands of NICU staff. *C. parapsilosis* was isolated from 19% (similar to a single-center incidence of 20%) and *C. albicans* from 5% of the cultures from health care personnel ($P < .001$). *C. lusitaniae* (2%), *C. guilliermondii* (1%), *C. tropicalis* (<1%), and *C. glabrata* (<1%) were also recovered from hand cultures. Increased handling required by sicker preterm infants increases the risk of acquiring fungal colonization from health care workers' hands, contaminated infusates, catheters, or catheter-related devices because there are an average of 32 touches of infants directly during a 12-hour shift.[67,261]

The skin and gastrointestinal tract are the most common sites for *Candida* colonization.[21,157] Colonization is inversely proportional to gestational age, and fungal colonization occurs on the skin and gastrointestinal tract before the respiratory tract. *Candida* species produce proteases that may be lytic for the thin keratin layer produced by the immature stratum corneum and phospholipases against lipid membranes that both may facilitate epithelial invasion.[88,155] Increased transepidermal water loss from preterm skin creates a moist environment that facilitates fungal colonization and growth. Because of the increased permeability of the preterm skin, substrates such as glucose may diffuse to the epithelial surface and facilitate *Candida* growth. *Candida* may alter its surface structure in the presence of high glucose, thus increasing its adherence and proliferative properties. Skin maturation occurs by 2 weeks of life in the extreme preterm infant, after which new fungal skin colonization occurs less frequently.

The microflora of the gastrointestinal tract plays an important role in fungal colonization and infection. Buccal candidal adherence is increased in preterm compared with term infants and facilitates colonization.[72] A normal bacterial flora inhibits *Candida* growth by competing for both adhesion sites and nutrients.[133,162] In a study of athymic mice given an oral challenge with *Candida*, fungal colonization was attenuated in mice with a normal gut flora compared with those with a germ-free microflora.[133] This finding highlights the fact that the intestinal microflora may be as important as an intact immune system in preventing fungal colonization.

Although colonization of skin and gastrointestinal tract is more common and precedes respiratory tract colonization, endotracheal colonization has a higher risk for infection.[159] Rowen and associates[256] demonstrated that with endotracheal fungal colonization, candidemia was 15.4 times more likely to occur compared with infants without any fungal colonization. Controlling for fungal colonization at other sites, endotracheal colonization alone increased the risk for fungal sepsis (risk ratio, 5.9; 95% CI, 1.34–26).

Use of broad-spectrum antibiotics enhance *Candida* colonization by destroying competing bacterial flora.[155] In a cohort of more than 6000 infants, cephalosporin or carbapenem use in the previous 7 days was associated with candidiasis.[27] Histamine-2 (H_2)–blocking and proton pump inhibiting agents have been shown to increase *Candida* overgrowth in the gastrointestinal tract of adults,[117] and their use is associated with candidiasis in infants.[262]

The extremely preterm infant has the unique combination of being immunocompromised (including an immature skin and gastrointestinal tract), requiring prolonged intensive care (parenteral nutrition, mechanical ventilation, central venous access), being exposed to medications that promote fungal growth (H_2-blocking agents, proton pump inhibiting agents, postnatal corticosteroids, and broad-spectrum antibiotics), and having an increased rate of gastrointestinal dysmotility and disease (NEC and focal bowel perforation).[31,93,260] Infants with complicated gastrointestinal diseases such as gastroschisis or NEC have combined risk factors of prolonged ileus, central venous access, parenteral nutrition, surgery, and exposure to prolonged or broad-spectrum antibiotics.[93]

Clinical Manifestations

Congenital Cutaneous Candidiasis

CCC is an uncommon clinical condition in which the infant at birth has a diffusely erythematous papular rash (Fig. 200.3; see also Box 200.1).[74] CCC is caused by an ascending infection into the uterus before birth. The papular rash becomes pustular, followed by the development of vesicles and bullae. The rash may also develop as bright red, burn-like dermatitis. The skin involvement covers one or more of the following areas: face or scalp, chest, abdomen, perineal area, one or more extremities, and back. These lesions occasionally lead to desquamation. ELBW infants with CCC are at greater risk of developing dissemination to blood, urine, or CSF (66%) compared with 33% in those 1000- to 2500-g or term infants (11%). For this reason, all these infants should be treated with systemic antifungal therapy.

In a study examining the pathogenesis and pathology of these infections, skin biopsies demonstrated invasion into the epidermis with an inflammatory process ranging from dermal invasion and granuloma formation to focal necrosis and hemorrhage.[257] These data from biopsies give insight into the invasive nature of cutaneous involvement and demonstrate that these infections are invasive and need prompt systemic antifungal therapy. Routine aerobic skin culture will isolate the *Candida* species and cause the cutaneous manifestations (skin biopsies are not needed.) By culturing for both fungal and bacterial organisms, the source of infection can be determined promptly and treatment started in a timely fashion. Differential diagnosis includes staphylococci, other bacteria, and other fungal skin infections. Pathologic examination with fungal staining of the umbilical cord and placenta can also aid in diagnosis.

Neonatal Candidemia

BSI with fungal species manifests with clinical signs and symptoms similar to those of bacterial sepsis. The following signs and symptoms occur, in order of their prevalence with candidemia[92]: thrombocytopenia of less than 100,000/μL (84%), immature-to-total neutrophil ratio of 0.2 or greater (77%), increase in apnea or bradycardia (63%), oxygen requirement (56%), assisted ventilation (52%), lethargy or hypotonia (39%), gastrointestinal symptoms (e.g., gastric aspirates, distention, bloody stools) (30%), hypotension (15%), hyperglycemia (13%), elevated white blood cell count greater than 20,000/μL (12%), metabolic acidosis (11%), and absolute neutrophil count lower than 1500/μL (3%). Most importantly, candidemia can be associated with disseminated disease. Evaluation of cardiac, renal, and ophthalmologic systems and the CNS is warranted.

Neonatal Urinary Tract Infection

Among infants with IC, up to 40% may have kidney involvement.[31] *Candida* infections of the renal system include cases of isolated candiduria, fungal debris within the renal collecting system, and renal parenchymal involvement.[147] If the urine culture result is positive for *Candida*, renal ultrasonography should be performed to assess for disease in the collecting system. Candiduria develops in approximately 2.4% of VLBW infants and in up to 6% of ELBW infants.[31,157] Studies have demonstrated similar mortality rates in infants with *Candida* UTIs alone (26%) compared with *Candida* BSIs (28%) in ELBWs.[31]

Neonatal Meningoencephalitis

Among infants, meningitis is found in approximately 15% of cases of candidemia, much higher than the incidence of meningitis observed in adults with candidemia.[28] This fact has important implications for diagnostic evaluation and therapeutic approaches because clinicians cannot assume that the CNS is not involved in otherwise seemingly straightforward candidemia. Candidiasis of the CNS is accurately described as meningoencephalitis because infection often results in granulomas, parenchymal abscesses, and vasculitis. Importantly, fungal abscesses of the CNS have been reported to be microscopic and not readily detectable by ultrasonography. Furthermore, CSF parameters in the presence of CNS infection may be normal.[108,155] In a study of 46 ELBW patients with fungal sepsis and/or meningoencephalitis, only six of 13 patients with fungal CNS abscesses (detected by ultrasound, CT scan, or autopsy) had abnormal results on lumbar puncture.[108] Studies have found an association between invasive fungal infection and periventricular leukomalacia in preterm infants, possibly related to release of cytokines that may damage the periventricular white matter.[108]

Neonatal Endocarditis and Infected Vascular Thrombi

Candida endocarditis has been reported in 5.5% to 15.2% of cases of fungal sepsis, with equal prevalence for *C. albicans* and *C. parapsilosis*.

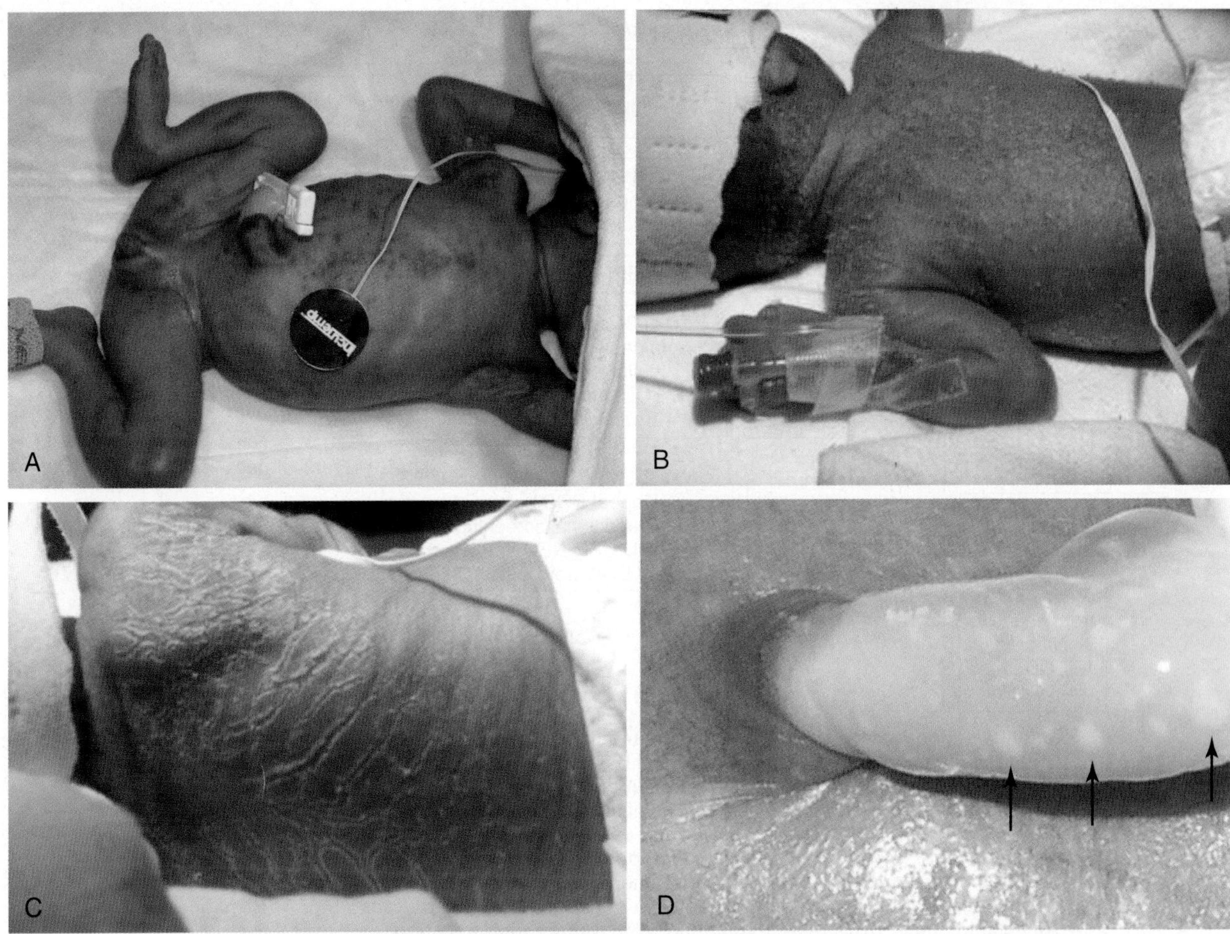

FIG. 200.3 Various presentations of congenital cutaneous candidiasis. (A) Macular papular rash. (B) Dry, flaky rash. (C) Dry, cracking scaly rash. (D) White plaques of the umbilical cord.

Candida endocarditis may be associated with higher mortality rates than candidemia alone.[55,213] Central vascular catheters place infants at increased risk for endocarditis and infected vascular thrombi. As discussed previously they can cause local trauma to valvular, endocardial, or endothelial tissue creating a nidus for thrombus and infection.

Neonatal Endophthalmitis and Retinopathy of Prematurity

The incidence of retinal endophthalmitis with candidemia has decreased over the years, likely because of more rapid diagnosis, treatment, and surveillance of systemic candidemia. In a retrospective study from 1989 to 1999, 6% (four of 67) of preterm infants with fungal sepsis who had indirect ophthalmoscopy examination had endophthalmitis.[213]

Even in absence of visible retinal abscesses or chorioretinitis, some epidemiologic evidence suggests that *Candida* sepsis may predispose preterm infants to severe retinopathy of prematurity (ROP). In a study of ELBW infants, threshold ROP developed in 33% (19 of 58) of infants with a history of candidemia compared with 10% (39 of 391) without candidemia, but this was not statistically significant when controlling for gestational age.[148] Conversely, Noyola and colleagues,[214] in a case-control study of VLBW infants and infants at less than 28 weeks of gestation, found that 52% (24 of 46) of infants with candidemia developed threshold ROP compared with 24% (11 of 46) of controls without candidemia ($P = .008$). Although the data on an association between fungal sepsis and ROP are conflicting, early and frequent screening for retinal disease is recommended in preterm infants with candidemia.

Neonatal Candida *End-Organ Dissemination*

At the time IC is clinically apparent, the organisms have often disseminated from the blood, urine, or CSF to adhere and proliferate in body fluids, tissues, and organs. *Candida* species can cause endocarditis, endophthalmitis, dermatitis, peritonitis, osteomyelitis, and septic arthritis, and abscesses may form in the CNS, kidneys, liver, spleen, skin, bowel, and peritoneum (Fig. 200.4). A review of 21 manuscripts found the following median prevalence rates for end organ involvement in the setting of IC in infants: endophthalmitis, 3% (interquartile range, 0–17%); endocarditis, 5% (0–13); and hepatosplenic abscesses, 1% (0–3%).[28] Dissemination may be higher in the lower-birth-weight infant.

Noyola and colleagues[213] and Chapman and associates[55] found that infants with candidemia for more than 5 and 7 days, respectively, were more likely to demonstrate ophthalmologic, renal, or cardiac abnormalities than infants with a shorter duration of candidemia. When amphotericin B was administered and central vascular catheters were removed within 2 days of the first positive blood culture, outcomes such as end-organ dissemination and mortality were not increased.[213] With improved blood culture methods, the majority of blood cultures that are a positive for a *Candida* species will be positive within 2 days of collection.

Diagnosis

Cultures of blood, urine, CSF, and peritoneal fluid or other sterile body fluids remain the best method for diagnosing IC (see Fig. 200.4). Focus on obtaining sufficient blood culture volumes (≥1 mL) and performance of urine and CSF cultures at the time of evaluation for sepsis remain critical to making a prompt diagnosis. In the setting of candidemia, dissemination can occur, and screening for end-organ dissemination is warranted. Most commonly, with BSI, an initial screen including a lumbar puncture, echocardiogram, abdominal ultrasound scan, cranial ultrasound scan, and ophthalmologic examination is needed.

Treatment and Prevention

Amphotericin B Preparations

AmB-d should be started at 1 mg/kg, and LFAmB should be started at 5 mg/kg.[19,47,227] Linder and colleagues[185] demonstrated that dosing of

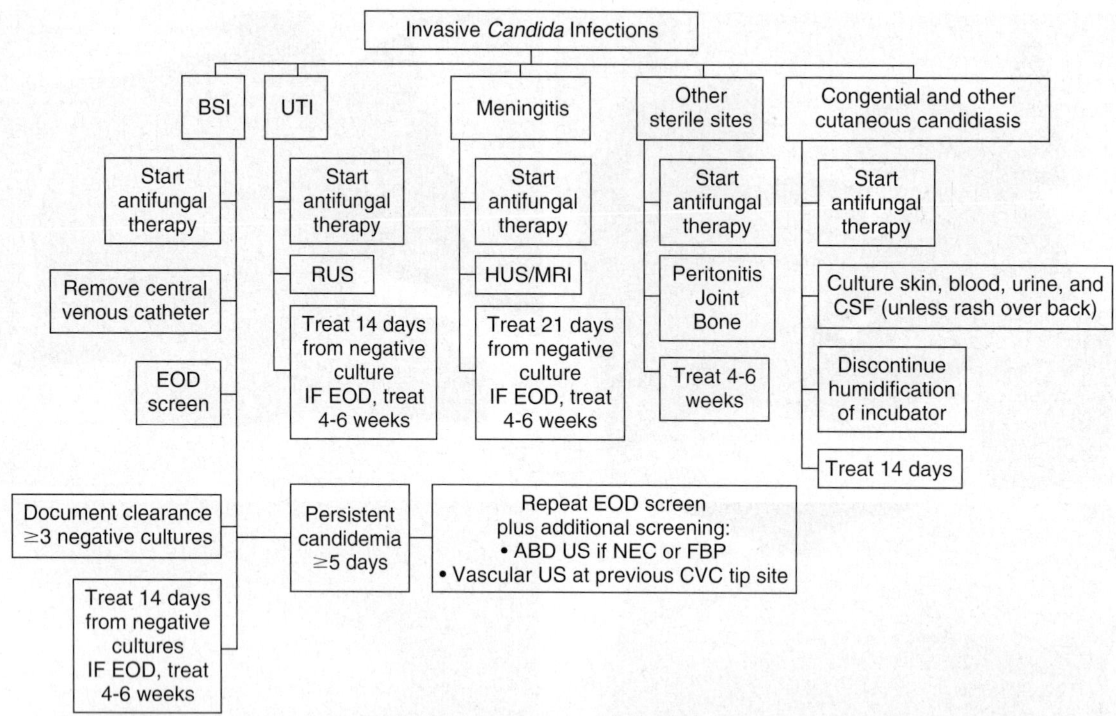

FIG. 200.4 Algorithm for evaluation and treatment of invasive candidiasis in neonates. Initial therapy pending susceptibilities: amphotericin B deoxycholate (*ABD;* 1 mg/kg/day). Alternatives: amphotericin B lipid preparations (5 mg/kg/day) or fluconazole (12 g/kg/dose). With meningitis or persistent candidemia lasting >7 days, combination therapy with a second antifungal (fluconazole) can be considered. With bowel disease such as necrotizing enterocolitis *(NEC)* or focal bowel perforation *(FBP):* complete abdominal ultrasound *(US)* for abscess should be performed. *BSI,* Bloodstream infection; *CCC,* congenital cutaneous candidiasis; *CSF,* cerebrospinal fluid; *CVC,* central venous catheter; *EOD,* end-organ dissemination; *HUS,* head ultrasound; *MRI,* magnetic resonance imaging; *RUS,* renal ultrasound; *UTI,* urinary tract infection.

1 mg/kg of AmB-d ($n = 34$) did not affect renal function. Creatinine levels (mg/dL) remained unchanged from the start of treatment (0.8 ± 0.4), at 24 hours after beginning treatment (0.8 ± 0.4), and again at the end of therapy (0.6 ± 0.2). This is an important difference compared with older children and adults, in whom infusion-related reactions and nephrotoxicity are frequent concerns with AmB-d. Lower "test" dosages of AmB-d are not needed in infants. Moreover, lower dosages in neonates only delay the time to achieve optimal therapy and may contribute to morbidity and mortality by delaying clearance of *Candida* species. LFAmB has less reliable penetration into the kidney,[334] and this property has led most experts to recommend these formulations only in the setting of negative urine culture results and without evidence of renal parenchymal involvement.

Azoles

Fluconazole is commonly used to treat candidiasis in infants.[329] The two most common species of *Candida* found in infants, *C. albicans* and *C. parapsilosis*, are almost always sensitive to fluconazole. However, 50% of *C. glabrata* and 100% of *C. krusei* isolates are resistant to fluconazole.[258] Infants require 12 mg/kg per day to achieve exposures similar to older children and adults,[320] and a loading dose of 25 mg/kg has been shown to achieve steady-state concentrations sooner than the traditional dosing scheme.[237,321] Voriconazole has a wider spectrum of activity against *Candida* than fluconazole and is active in vitro against some isolates of *C. glabrata* and *C. krusei* that are resistant to fluconazole. However, the pharmacokinetics of voriconazole has not been described in infants.[29,83,150]

Echinocandins

The echinocandins have efficacy against all *Candida* species, although the potential exists for resistance of *C. parapsilosis* isolates with acquired gene mutations. Of the echinocandins, the pharmacokinetics of micafungin is the most extensively described in infants.[134] In a rabbit model of *Candida* meningoencephalitis, adequate systemic exposure of micafungin (area under the curve during 24 hours [AUC_{0-24}]: >170 μg/mL per hour) was associated with 90% decreased fungal burden in brain tissue.[134] In a pharmacokinetic study, up to 15 mg/kg of micafungin was well tolerated in premature infants.[281] The recommended dose of micafungin in infants is 10 mg/kg per day to achieve adequate systemic exposure for the CNS.[134,32] In a study of infants less than 3 month of age who were administered caspofungin at 25 mg/m^2 per day, caspofungin peak concentrations were lower and trough concentrations were higher compared with older children receiving 50 mg/m^2 per day.[259] Anidulafungin has been studied in eight infants, but additional study is needed to determine appropriate dosing in infants.[68] Guidelines do not recommend echinocandins as initial therapy for neonatal candidiasis[226] because of concerns about penetration in the CSF, although multiple animal models have demonstrated brain parenchyma penetration.

Central Venous Catheter Removal With Bloodstream Infections

Several studies have demonstrated that prompt removal of a central venous catheter is associated with lower mortality rates, a shorter duration of infection, and reduced end-organ dissemination.[30,55,149,213] National Institute of Child Health and Human Development Neonatal Research Network data showed that the mortality rate was reduced from 37% to 21% ($P < .024$) when catheters were removed promptly (<24 hours) compared with delayed removal.[30] The combined outcome of neurodevelopmental impairment and death was associated with delayed removal or replacement of catheters.

Empiric Antifungal Therapy

The value of empiric therapy and its ability to improve outcomes in neonatal candidiasis continue to be investigated. Some studies have suggested that empiric antifungal therapy may lower mortality rates and improve outcomes in VLBW infants ultimately confirmed to have *Candida* sepsis, but these issues have not been investigated in controlled trials.[27,120,190] Clinicians have proven inaccurate in administering empiric therapy to infants who subsequently diagnosed with candidiasis. In a cohort of more than 1500 ELBW infants, only 29% of infants with candidiasis received empiric antifungal therapy.[31]

Prevention

As with other infectious diseases, prevention is key to achieving the best clinical outcomes. Morbidity and mortality rates are high, and for ELBW infants, 73% do not survive or survive with neurodevelopmental impairment.[31] To date, antifungal prophylaxis is the only intervention that has been subjected to evidence-based randomized controlled trials for the prevention of IC. Prophylactic antifungal therapy has been shown to reduce both colonization and IC in the high-risk preterm infants. At birth, most infants are not colonized or have low colony counts of yeast, thus making them ideal candidates for antifungal prophylaxis. In the absence of antifungal prophylaxis, up to 60% of ELBW infants become colonized in the first 2 to 3 weeks after birth.[157] Prophylaxis prevents IC by decreasing *Candida* colonization of the skin, gastrointestinal tract, and respiratory tract, and central venous catheter, as well as colonization at multiple (two or more) sites.[193,14,157,192,193]

Fluconazole prophylaxis. Currently there are more than 20 studies examining fluconazole prophylaxis for the prevention of IC in more than 5000 neonates consistently demonstrating efficacy with an overall reduction in IC of 70% to 80%.* The overall incidence of IC in the placebo or control (untreated) groups was 9.1% compared with 1.3% in the fluconazole prophylaxis groups ($P < .0001$).[156] Efficacy is highest in the smallest infants (<1000 g) and youngest infants (≤27 weeks) when prophylaxis is started shortly after birth and given to all high-risk patients. All these studies have demonstrated the safety of fluconazole prophylaxis and lack of emergence of resistance.[154,157,158,160,194]

The first study of fluconazole prophylaxis against fungal colonization and infection in premature infants was a prospective, randomized, double-blind clinical trial involving 100 ELBW infants requiring central venous access or endotracheal intubation.[157] Infants were randomly assigned during the first 5 days of life to receive either 3 mg/kg fluconazole IV or placebo for up to 6 weeks. Results demonstrated that fluconazole prophylaxis significantly decreased invasive fungal infection. None of the infants in the treatment group developed infection compared with 20% of infants in the placebo group ($P = .008$). The efficacy of a twice-weekly dosing regimen was studied as a simplified schedule in a randomized controlled trial compared with the more frequent dosing schedule. The randomized controlled trial demonstrated that 3 mg/kg administered twice weekly was as effective in preventing ICs as the more frequent dosing schedule used in the previous study.[158] Manzoni and colleagues[193] in Italy performed a multicenter, randomized, placebo-controlled trial investigating two different fluconazole doses (3 and 6 mg/kg) compared with a placebo group. In 322 VLBW infants, fungal colonization was significantly decreased from 29.2% in the placebo-treated patients to 7.7% and 9.8% in the 3 and 6 mg/kg groups, respectively. IC was decreased from 13.2% in the placebo-treated patients to 7.7% and 9.8% in the 3 and 6 mg/kg groups, respectively ($P = .005$ for the 6-mg group and $P = .02$ for the 3-mg group vs. the placebo group). Fluconazole prophylaxis had similar efficacy for both the 3 and 6 mg/kg groups. In a trial of 6 mg/kg twice weekly in infants weighing less than 750 g at birth, the incidence of IC was significantly decreased in the treatment arm, but when considering the combined outcome of death or IC, no significant difference was noted in the study arms. Additionally, rates of long-term neurologic impairment did not differ between the treatment and placebo groups.[33]

Safety of fluconazole prophylaxis. No significant adverse effects have been reported in randomized trials in infants treated with fluconazole prophylaxis compared with control patients. Preventing IC has not led to an increased incidence in other infections. The incidence of bacterial infections and NEC are similar in all studies between treatment and control groups. Fluconazole-related cholestasis has been examined closely in several studies. No cholestasis was seen between groups in the randomized controlled trials, and retrospective studies have shown by multivariate analysis that cholestasis is related to other factors such as NEC and bacterial infections and not fluconazole prophylaxis.[132,157,193,197]

Neurodevelopmental status and quality of life of survivors from the first randomized controlled trial were evaluated at 8 to 10 years of life.[161] No differences were found in the Vineland Adaptive Behavior Scales-II scores for the fluconazole-treated group compared with the placebo group. No differences were noted between groups regarding emotional difficulties or behavior problems. In a second trial of 361 infants weighing less than 750 g at birth, there was no significant difference in the incidence of neurodevelopmental impairment between patients in the fluconazole and placebo study arms (31% vs. 27%; $P = .60$). This finding remained in models that controlled for antenatal steroids, cesarean section, and level of maternal education ($P = .87$). The proportion of infants in each cohort who developed cerebral palsy, blindness, or deafness in each group was also not statistically different.

Nystatin prophylaxis. Nystatin, an enteral or orally administered nonabsorbable antifungal agent, was the first antifungal studied for prophylaxis in premature infants and has been the subject of several randomized or quasirandomized clinical trials and observational studies. These studies have added to our understanding of antifungal prophylaxis by demonstrating the benefits of prophylaxis even in NICUs with low rates of infection, thus confirming the greater effectiveness of prophylaxis when it is started early (by 72 hours after birth) versus later, after colonization is detected.

Two large retrospective studies of nystatin prophylaxis demonstrate the use of antifungal prophylaxis even in NICUs with low *Candida* bloodstream rates. In the largest multicenter observational study to date ($n = 14{,}778$) that compared preterm infants who received nystatin prophylaxis with those who did not receive any antifungal prophylaxis (1993–2006; Australia and New Zealand), oral nystatin prophylaxis was associated with a decrease in BSI or meningitis in infants weighing less than 1500 g (1.23%–0.54%; $P < .0001$) and in infants weighing less than 1000 g (2.7%–1.2%; $P < .0001$).[140] In a second study performed in a UK cohort of premature infants born at less than 33 weeks, nystatin prophylaxis was proven effective at reducing IC, and notably the all-cause mortality rate was significantly lower in the nystatin prophylaxis group (11.8%) compared with patients not receiving prophylaxis (17.8%) ($P < .0001$).[112]

Many questions regarding fluconazole and nystatin prophylaxis remain unanswered, but two studies have compared the two strategies. One randomized controlled trial of infants weighing less than 1500 g at birth compared oral fluconazole with oral nystatin prophylaxis started in the first 7 days and continued until full enteral feedings were achieved.[318] IC occurred in 2 of 38 (5.3%) fluconazole-treated infants compared with 6 of 42 (14.3%) nystatin-treated infants. No deaths occurred in the fluconazole-treated group compared with an all-cause mortality rate of 7.5% in the nystatin-treated group ($P = .03$). Of the six deaths, three were caused by NEC, one was caused by focal bowel perforation, and two were sepsis related. Only one of the six deaths was attributed to IC. One-third of the eligible patients for this study ($n = 44$) were excluded for hemodynamic instability or gastrointestinal concerns. The oral suspension of nystatin has a very high osmolarity of 3002 mOsm/L, and concern exists about the use of hyperosmolar medications and NEC.

Aydemir and associates,[14] conducted a three-arm randomized controlled trial of antifungal prophylaxis in infants weighing less than 1500 g. Patients were randomized to fluconazole ($n = 93$), nystatin (n = 94), or placebo ($n = 91$). This study demonstrated that fungal colonization was less common in the fluconazole (10.8%) and nystatin (11.7%) prophylaxis groups compared with the placebo arm (42.9%). The rate of IC was significantly lower in both the fluconazole (3.2%) and nystatin (4.3%) groups compared with the placebo-treated (16.5%) patients. Although a previous study had raised concerns regarding nystatin use and NEC and all-cause mortality,[318] this study demonstrated no differences among groups in the incidence of NEC (fluconazole, 8.6%; nystatin, 9.6%; placebo, 9.9%) or mortality rates (fluconazole, 8.6%; nystatin, 8.5%; placebo, 12.1%).

Although oral fluconazole for prophylaxis was used in one of the foregoing studies, almost all other fluconazole prophylaxis studies have

*References 3, 14, 15, 25, 36, 38, 131, 132, 157, 163, 191, 193, 197, 252, 307, 318, 328.

used intravenous administration in the first weeks. Even though enteral fluconazole is 90% absorbed, absorption characteristics in preterm infants are variable and not well studied. Additionally, as discussed earlier, enteral administration of fluconazole prophylaxis may not be an option if patients have an ileus, NEC, intestinal perforation, or hemodynamic instability. It is during these clinical situations that fungal colonization, proliferation, and dissemination are most likely to occur. For these reasons and to prevent colonization of central venous catheters, the intravenous route is recommended for fluconazole prophylaxis in preterm infants when peripheral or central intravenous catheters are present. In some studies, fluconazole was changed to enteral administration once patients achieved full enteral feedings and intravenous access was discontinued.

Assessing the evidence collectively, fluconazole is recommended as the preferred prophylaxis agent over nystatin, given the greater effectiveness of fluconazole in preventing IC (80–90% compared with 50–60%), safety in infants weighing less than 1000 g, twice-weekly administration, and ability to administer to all high-risk infants weighing less than 1000 g, even in the presence of gastrointestinal disease or hemodynamic instability.

Infection control measures to prevent neonatal invasive candidiasis

Prenatal detection and eradication of maternal vaginal candidiasis. In pregnancies complicated by preterm labor or prolonged rupture of membranes, screening and treatment of vaginal candidiasis may be beneficial in preventing candidal colonization and subsequent infection in the newborn (Box 200.2).[41,105,322]

Medication and feeding stewardship. Practices reducing medications that increase the risk for IC should be avoided if possible and instituted with stewardship, guidelines, tracking or auditing, and accountability.[156] Medications that increase risk for IC, as discussed previously, include: broad-spectrum antibiotics (third- or fourth-generation cephalosporins or carbapenems), gastric acid inhibitors (H_2 blockers and proton pump inhibitors), and postnatal dexamethasone.[156] Data from a multicenter randomized trial of postnatal hydrocortisone in infants weighing less than 1000 g did not associate hydrocortisone exposure with an increased rate of candidemia; both the hydrocortisone-treated group and the placebo group had an incidence of *Candida* BSIs of 10%.[326] Implementation of early feeding protocols (starting early and trophic and slow feed advances) and promoting breast milk feedings may aid in decreasing the risk for IC as well.

Central line–associated bloodstream infection bundles. Standardized protocols for insertion and management of central venous catheters, attention to sterile practices, hub and dressing care, and closed medication delivery systems may reduce central line–associated BSIs, including *Candida*-related BSIs.[6,62] Aly and colleagues[6] reported a significant reduction in all central line–associated BSIs and elimination of *Candida* infection by using a "bundled approach" that included antifungal prophylaxis in addition to line placement and maintenance interventions.

Lactoferrin. In a randomized controlled trial of bovine lactoferrin (bLF) in infants weighing less than 1500 g, the incidence of late-onset sepsis was significantly lower in the bLF and bLF plus probiotics groups than in the placebo-treated patients.[195] Subanalysis found that invasive fungal infections were also significantly less common with bLF alone compared with placebo. One limitation of the study was that it contained only between 9 and 18 infants weighing up to 750 g in each group. Confirmation of the findings in extremely preterm infants is needed.

BOX 200.2 Strategies to Reduce Neonatal Invasive Candidiasis Morbidity and Mortality

1. Use antifungal prophylaxis (IV fluconazole) while IV access is in use (central or peripheral) for infants with birth weight <1000 g and/or ≤27 weeks' gestational age
   a. There is A-I evidence for antifungal prophylaxis with nystatin but limited data in infants <750 g and <26 weeks' gestation. Because fluconazole prophylaxis has greater efficacy compared with nystatin, efficacy in the most immature patients, and can be given to infants not feeding, current evidence currently favors fluconazole prophylaxis in preterm infants weighing <1000 g.
2. Start treatment of documented infections with appropriate antifungal dosing and prompt catheter removal for candidal BSI.
   a. Consider starting empiric antifungal therapy if invasive candidiasis is suspected.
   b. Promptly treat congenital cutaneous candidiasis.
3. Decrease broad-spectrum antibiotic use. Restrict third- and fourth-generation cephalosporins and carbapenems to treatment of proven gram-negative infections.
4. Decrease H_2 blocker and proton pump inhibitor use. Use only for proven gastritis, and restrict use to 3 days or until symptoms resolved.
5. Decrease postnatal dexamethasone use. Use only for severe lung disease.
6. Institute central line associated bloodstream infection reduction bundles
7. Monitor rates of invasive candidiasis including candidemia, UTI, meningitis and peritonitis infections and feedback to staff.

Level of evidence. US Public Health Service Grading System for ranking recommendations in clinical guidelines: Strength of recommendation and levels of evidence. A: good evidence; B: moderate evidence; C: poor evidence. I: at least one randomized clinical trial; II: at least one well-designed but nonrandomized trial; III: expert opinions on the basis of experience or limited clinical reports.

BSI, Bloodstream infection; *IV*, intravenous; *UTI*, urinary tract infection.

Outcomes

Neurodevelopmental Impairment

IC may lead to significant neurodevelopmental impairment even in absence of documented fungal meningitis. Neurodevelopmental impairment in most studies is the presence of one or more of the following: low mental and motor development using Bayley Scales of Infant Development II, cerebral palsy, deafness, and blindness. Using these criteria, the incidence of neurodevelopmental impairment is 57% in patients with IC versus 29% in noninfected ELBW infants[292,30] (Fig. 200.5). The incidence of neurodevelopmental impairment was similar for the subset of patients with *Candida* meningitis (53%). These data are similar to those from a study from an earlier time period.[108] Neurodevelopment was intact in 41% of *Candida*-infected patients and in 65% of controls ($P = .02$). The frequency of periventricular leukomalacia was increased in the patients with IC, but this difference did not reach statistical significance (26% vs. 12%; $P = .06$). In this study neurodevelopmental outcome was related to timing of initiation of antifungal therapy. Commencement of antifungal therapy was 5.1 ± 3.0 days after blood culture was drawn in those infants who had severe disabilities or who died compared with 2.1 ± 1.3 days in those infants who were normal or mildly impaired ($P < .0001$).

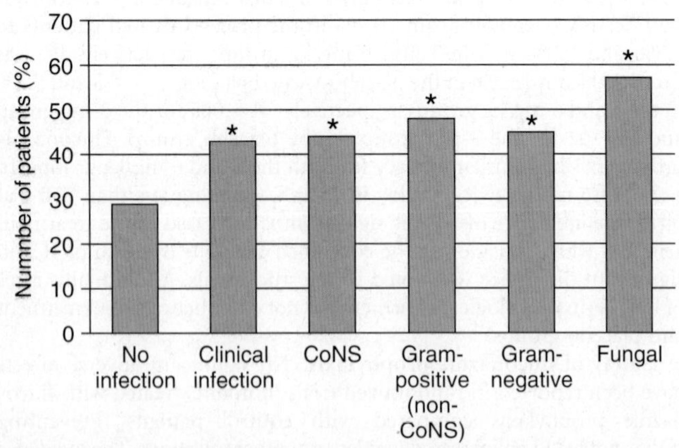

FIG. 200.5 Neurodevelopmental impairment and candidemia in infants weighing <1000 g. Neurodevelopmental impairment: one or more of the following: Bayley Scales of Infant Development II physical or mental developmental index <70, cerebral palsy, or visual or hearing impairment. Clinical infection: late-onset infection with negative culture results with antibiotic treatment for ≥5 days. *CoNS*, Coagulase-negative staphylococci; *$P \leq .001$ compared with the no-infection group.

Survival

Mortality rates are high among ELBW infants with IC. A multicenter study of patients weighing less than 1000 g found that the overall mortality rate was 34% for infants with IC compared with 14% without IC.[31] All-cause mortality rates were 28% for infants with candidemia, 26% for those with *Candida* UTI, and 50% for those with other sterile site infections (meningitis and peritonitis). If two or more culture sites tested positive (blood plus urine or urine plus CSF), the mortality rate rose to 57%.

There is a marked difference in overall and attributable mortality for IC between infants weighing less than 1000 g and those infants who are larger and more mature. In infants weighing less than 1000 g with IC, one analysis reported an all-cause mortality rate of 26% compared with 13% in infants without candidiasis. For infants weighing more than 1000 g with IC versus those without, the mortality rate was 2% compared with 0.4%.[338]

Candida-*Related Mortality*

Assessing attribution of death to *Candida* is difficult and varies by publication. Some researchers have linked attribution to death within a specified number of days from the onset of infection (3, 7, 14, or 30 days) or review each death and assign attribution by using predetermined definitions. Furthermore, published attributable mortality rates of IC vary depending on the study type. In observational cohorts of infants weighing less than 1000 g mortality rates have been documented to be between 13% and 15%,[31,338] whereas in the placebo or control arms of randomized trials of prophylaxis agents, the mortality rates range from 23% to 66%.[154]

NEW REFERENCES SINCE THE SEVENTH EDITION

2. Achkar JM, Fries BC. *Candida* infections of the genitourinary tract. *Clin Microbiol Rev*. 2010;23(2):253-273.
11. Arnold CJ, Johnson M, Bayer AS, et al. *Candida* infective endocarditis: an observational cohort study with a focus on therapy. *Antimicrob Agents Chemother*. 2015;59(4):2365-2373.
16. Baddour LM, Wilson WR, Bayer AS, et al. Infective endocarditis in adults: diagnosis, antimicrobial therapy, and management of complications: a scientific statement for healthcare professionals from the American Heart Association. *Circulation*. 2015;132(15):1435-1486.
22. Baltimore RS, Gewitz M, Baddour LM, et al. Infective endocarditis in childhood: 2015 update: a scientific statement from the American Heart Association. *Circulation*. 2015;132(15):1487-1515.
34. Berberi A, Noujeim Z, Aoun G. Epidemiology of oropharyngeal candidiasis in human immunodeficiency virus/acquired immune deficiency syndrome patients and CD4+ counts. *J Int Oral Health*. 2015;7(3):20-23.
50. Casadevall A, Pirofski LA. The damage-response framework of microbial pathogenesis. *Nat Rev Microbiol*. 2003;1:17-24.
53. Chang TI, Kim HW, Park JT, et al. Early catheter removal improves patient survival in peritoneal dialysis patients with fungal peritonitis: results of ninety-four episodes of fungal peritonitis at a single center. *Perit Dial Int*. 2011;31(1):60-66.
56. Chaussade H, Bastides F, Lissandre S, et al. Usefulness of corticosteroid therapy during chronic disseminated candidiasis: case reports and literature review. *J Antimicrob Chemother*. 2012;67:1493-1495.
58. Chiotos K, Vendetti N, Zaoutis TE, et al. Comparative effectiveness of echinocandins versus fluconazole therapy for the treatment of adult candidaemia due to *Candida parapsilosis:* a retrospective observational cohort study of the Mycoses Study Group (MSG-12). *J Antimicrob Chemother*. 2016;71:3536-3539.
61. Chitnis AS, Magill SS, Edwards JR, et al. Trends in *Candida* central line-associated bloodstream infections among NICUs, 1999–2009. *Pediatrics*. 2012;130:e46-e52.
65. Cleveland AA, Farley MM, Harrison LH, et al. Changes in incidence and antifungal drug resistance in candidemia: results from population- based laboratory surveillance in Atlanta and Baltimore, 2008–2011. *Clin Infect Dis*. 2012;55:1352-1361.
66. Clinical and Laboratory Standards Institute. CLSI 2012. Reference method for broth dilution antifungal susceptibility testing of yeasts; 4th informational supplement; 2012. CLSI document M27-S4. Wayne, PA: Clinical and Laboratory Standards Institute.
64. Clancy CJ, Nguyen MH. Finding the "missing 50%" of invasive candidiasis: how nonculture diagnostics will improve understanding of disease spectrum and transform patient care. *Clin Infect Dis*. 2013;56:1284-1292.
76. De Luca K, Green M, Symmonds J, et al. Invasive candidiasis in liver transplant patients: incidence and risk factors in a pediatric cohort. *Pediatr Transplant*. 2016;20:235-240.
82. Dovnik A, Golle A, Novak D, et al. Treatment of vulvovaginal candidiasis: a review of the literature. *Acta Dermatovenerol Alp Pannonica Adriat*. 2015;24:5-7.
91. Fan S, Liu X, Wu C, Xu L, Li J. Vaginal nystatin versus oral fluconazole for the treatment for recurrent vulvovaginal candidiasis. *Mycopathologia*. 2015;179:95-101.
94. Fernandez-Ruiz M, Aguado JM, Almirante B, et al. Initial use of echinocandins does not negatively influence outcome in *Candida parapsilosis* bloodstream infection: a propensity score analysis. *Clin Infect Dis*. 2014;58:1413-1421.
96. Fierro JL, Prasad PA, Fisher BT, et al. Ocular manifestations of candidemia in children. *Pediatr Infect Dis J*. 2013;32(1):84-86.
98. Fisher BT, Kavcic M, Li Y, et al. Antifungal prophylaxis associated with decreased induction mortality rates and resources utilized in children with new-onset acute myeloid leukemia. *Clin Infect Dis*. 2014;58:502-508.
99. Fisher BT, Ross RK, Localio AR, et al. Decreasing rates of invasive candidiasis in pediatric hospitals across the United States. *Clin Infect Dis*. 2014;58(1):74-77.
100. Fisher BT, Ross RK, Roilides E, et al. Failure to validate a multivariable clinical prediction model to identify pediatric intensive care unit patients at high risk for candidemia. *J Pediatric Infect Dis Soc*. 2016;5:458-461.
101. Fisher BT, Vendetti N, Bryan M, et al. Central venous catheter retention and mortality in children with candidemia: a retrospective cohort analysis. *J Pediatric Infect Dis Soc*. 2016;5:403-408.
118. Goncalves B, Ferreira C, Alves CT, et al. Vulvovaginal candidiasis: epidemiology, microbiology and risk factors. *Crit Rev Microbiol*. 2016;42:905-927.
125. Hamula CL, Hughes K, Fisher BT, et al. T2Candida provides rapid and accurate species identification in pediatric cases of candidemia. *Am J Clin Pathol*. 2016;145:858-861.
143. Jabra-Rizk MA, Kong EF, Tsui C, et al. *Candida albicans* pathogenesis: fitting within the host-microbe damage response framework. *Infect Immun*. 2016;84(10):2724-2739.
220. Steinbach WJ, Roilides E, Berman D, et al. Results from a prospective, international, epidemiologic study of invasive candidiasis in children and neonates. *Pediatr Infect Dis J*. 2012;31(12):1252-1257.
221. Palazzi DL, Arrieta A, Castagnola E, et al. Candida speciation, antifungal treatment and adverse events in pediatric invasive candidiasis: results from 441 infections in a prospective, multi-national study. *Pediatr Infect Dis J*. 2014;33(12):1294-1296.
222. Panel on Opportunistic Infections in HIV-Exposed and HIV-Infected Children. Guidelines for the Prevention and Treatment of Opportunistic Infections in HIV-Exposed and HIV-Infected Children. Department of Health and Human Services. Available at http://aidsinfo.nih.gov/contentfiles/lvguidelines/oi_guidelines_pediatrics.pdf.
226. Pappas PG, Kauffman CA, Andes D, et al. Clinical practice guideline for the management of candidiasis: 2016 update by the Infectious Diseases Society of America. *Clin Infect Dis*. 2016;62(4):e1-e50.
239. Prasad PA, Fisher BT, Coffin SE, et al. Pediatric risk factors for candidemia secondary to *Candida glabrata* and *Candida krusei* species. *J Pediatr Infect Dis Soc*. 2013;2(3):263-266.
250. Riddell J 4th, Comer GM, Kauffman CA. Treatment of endogenous fungal endophthalmitis: focus on new antifungal agents. *Clin Infect Dis*. 2011;52(5):648-653.
254. Fisher BT, Ross RK, Localio AR, et al. Decreasing rates of invasive candidiasis in pediatric hospitals across the United States. *Clin Infect Dis*. 2014;58(1):74-77.
267. Schnabel RM, Linssen CF, Guion N, et al. *Candida* pneumonia in intensive care unit? *Open Forum Infect Dis*. 2014;1(1):ofu026.
271. Science M, Robinson PD, MacDonald T, et al. Guideline for primary antifungal prophylaxis for pediatric patients with cancer or hematopoietic stem cell transplant recipients. *Pediatr Blood Cancer*. 2014;61:393-400.
276. Sievert DM, Ricks P, Edwards JR, et al. Antimicrobial-resistant pathogens associated with healthcare-associated infections: summary of data reported to the National Healthcare Safety Network at the Centers for Disease Control and Prevention, 2009–2010. *Infect Control Hosp Epidemiol*. 2013;34:1-14.
278. Slenker AK, Keith SW, Horn DL. Two hundred and eleven cases of *Candida* osteomyelitis: 17 case reports and a review of the literature. *Diagn Microbiol Infect Dis*. 2012;73(1):89-93.
284. Sobel JD, Wiesenfeld HC, Martens M, et al. Maintenance fluconazole therapy for recurrent vulvovaginal candidiasis. *N Engl J Med*. 2004;351:876-883.
289. Stefanuik E, Baraniak A, Fortuna M, Hryniewicz W. Usefulness of CHROMagar Candida medium, biochemical methods—API ID32C and VITEK 2 Compact and two MALDI-TOF MS systems for *Candida* spp. identification. *Pol J Microbiol*. 2016;65:111-114.
300. Tobudic S, et al. Comparative in vitro fungicidal activity of echinocandins against *Candida albicans* in peritoneal dialysis fluids. *Mycoses*. 2013;56(6):623-630.
316. Vendetti N, Bryan M, Zaoutis TE, et al. Comparative effectiveness of fungicidal vs. fungistatic therapies for the treatment of paediatric candidaemia. *Mycoses*. 2016;59:173-178.
333. Wood GC, Mueller EW, Croce MA, et al. *Candida* sp. isolated from bronchoalveolar lavage: clinical significance in critically ill trauma patients. *Intensive Care Med*. 2006;32:599-603.

The full reference list for this chapter is available at ExpertConsult.com.

201 Coccidioidomycosis

Kareem W. Shehab • Ziad M. Shehab

Coccidioidomycosis is an infection caused by a dimorphic fungus of the genus *Coccidioides*. The primary pulmonary infection produced by this organism usually is self-limited, but disseminated and fatal disease can occur. In the United States, coccidioidomycosis is an endemic disease of the southwestern states and results in 150,000 infections per year.[72] In other parts of the United States, it is seen in individuals who have traveled to or lived in the endemic areas of the Southwest or Mexico.[28,35,54] The disease is endemic in other areas of the Western Hemisphere, most notably in northern Mexico and in certain countries in South and Central America.[133]

Pulmonary disease is underrecognized even in areas of high endemicity.[107,171] With population growth in the endemic areas of the Southwest and increased population mobility, clinicians in nonendemic areas are likely to encounter this disease, particularly in its more severe or disseminated forms. Reactivation, especially in the immunocompromised host, can result in disease long after primary infection, emphasizing the need for a thorough travel history.

Coccidioidal granuloma, a form of disseminated coccidioidomycosis, was described first by Posadas in 1892 in Argentina.[88] The disease initially was thought to be a form of skin tumor. Rixford and Gilchrist associated it with what they thought was a protozoon resembling coccidia and named it *Coccidioides*. In 1900, Ophüls and Moffitt were the first to attribute coccidioidal granuloma to the fungus *Coccidioides immitis*. Although earlier investigators had observed fungal growth on cultures from pathologic specimens, they were dismissed as contaminants. Between 1900 and 1936, numerous reports of coccidioidal granuloma appeared in the medical literature, but the association between coccidioidal granuloma and acute pulmonary infection remained unrecognized. In 1936, Gifford[79] and Dickson were the first to designate *C. immitis* as the causative agent of what had previously been known in California as San Joaquin fever or valley fever.[74,88]

In the period that followed, the epidemiology of the disease[153,156] and ecology of the organism[61,117] were studied carefully by many investigators, led by the efforts of Charles Smith.[88] Many different therapies were attempted for disseminated disease during this era, but none proved satisfactory.[61] In 1957, with the use of amphotericin B, effective antifungal therapy became available, and the prognosis associated with disseminated disease improved.

As with many pathogenic fungi, the life cycle of *C. immitis* demonstrates two distinct phases: saprophytic, or vegetative, and parasitic. In nature and on most laboratory media, the organism grows as mycelia with branching, septate hyphae. After 5 to 7 days, the aerial mycelia show development of rectangular spores (i.e., arthrospores or arthroconidia) separated by empty, nonviable cells (Fig. 201.1). At this stage, the hyphae become fragile, and the arthroconidia easily become airborne. Their size (2–8 μm in diameter) allows them to reach the alveolar spaces of the lung when they are inhaled.

On gaining access to mammalian host tissues, the arthroconidia begin the parasitic phase of their life cycle. They enlarge and develop into spherules during the course of approximately 48 hours while undergoing internal segmentation to form endospores that are 2 to 5 μm in diameter. The spherules (Fig. 201.2) are round, double-walled structures measuring 20 to 100 μm in diameter. Endospores are released into the surrounding tissues by rupture of the spherule wall, where they mature into more spherules, repeating the tissue phase of the life cycle.[147]

Coccidioides spp. grow on laboratory media relatively easily, producing nonpigmented colonies that become visible in 3 to 4 days. They represent the mycelial phase of the fungus and appear as flat, smooth, and gray colonies from which spicules may project in some, whereas others have a velvety, membranous appearance. Colonies appear as tufts in the second week and then develop cobweb-like aerial hyphae. Pigmentation can be seen after 2 weeks and is observed best as a brownish undersurface. Variability in colony morphology can be significant.

Of the two species of *Coccidioides*, *C. immitis* is prevalent in California, and *C. posadasii* accounts for isolates from Arizona, Texas, Mexico, and parts of Central and South America.[67] No clinical differences have been recognized between the two species. Identification is accomplished using reliable techniques showing in vitro conversion to the spherule stage, demonstration of specific exoantigens, or identification of the organism by genetic probes, any of which obviate the need for animal inoculation.[147]

EPIDEMIOLOGY

Coccidioidomycosis is endemic in the Western Hemisphere between 40 degrees of latitude north and south. In the United States, these areas lie in the southwestern states, especially in Arizona, California, western Texas, and southern New Mexico. The organism also has been found in soil in areas not classically thought of as endemic, such as south central Washington state,[120] where a cluster of cases has been identified.[121] Other cases have occurred in nonendemic areas, such as Missouri.[170]

The areas in which coccidioidomycosis is prevalent generally correspond to the lower Sonoran life zone.[133] This life zone is characterized by an arid to semiarid climate, with hot summers and relatively short winters with limited rainfall and few freezes. Most fungal growth occurs during the rainy season in alkaline soil and at low altitude. The fungus is found in the soil to a depth of 20 cm, especially in the walls of rodent burrows. Environmental conditions in endemic regions apparently inhibit the growth of competitive organisms.[61,67] A variety of animals, including rodents, cattle, sheep, and dogs, are susceptible to naturally acquired infections.

Arthroconidia become airborne during wind storms or during disruption of soil by construction work, farming, and earthquakes.[34,68] Prolonged droughts followed by heavy rains also have resulted in an increased number of cases, as occurred in California in 1992 and 1993.[33] Archeologic excavations and digging by children in soil containing the organism have resulted in local outbreaks.[36,187] Transmission also has occurred by contaminated fomites, such as dusty clothing and farm products.[1,144]

The ease with which arthroconidia become airborne makes the organism dangerous to laboratory personnel. Epidemics have resulted from inadvertent opening of a single culture plate.[101] Guidelines for management of accidental laboratory exposures have been published.[162]

Primary coccidioidal infection occurs most frequently in summer and fall, after the rainy seasons. Arthroconidia are more likely to become dispersed during dry weather after promotion of greater hyphal growth by a wet environment.[61,153,154] Variations in seasonal incidence are partially explained by the occurrence of dust storms[133,135,154] and earthquake activity.[34]

Susceptibility to primary coccidioidal infection is unaffected by age, sex, or racial background.[66] Estimates of infection rates in endemic areas, which are based on the risk of infection in children, had declined as urbanization developed with dust abatement and paved roads. For example, infection rates measured by coccidioidin skin test reactivity declined from approximately 10% in 1937 through 1939 to 2% in 1959 and to less than 1% thereafter among kindergarten and first-grade students who had lived all of their 5 to 7 years in Kern County, California.[112] Similarly, the annual risk has been estimated to be between 2% and 4% among college students in Tucson, Arizona.[106] Incidence rates are higher for older male children, in rural areas, during wind

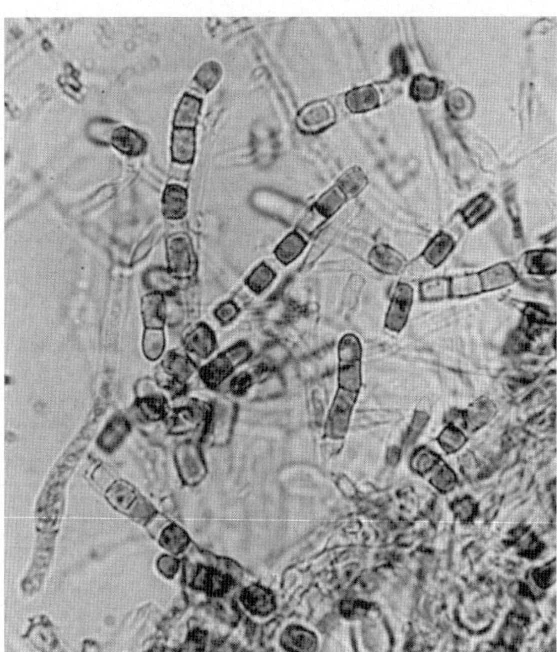

FIG. 201.1 In the mycelial form of *Coccidioides immitis,* arthroconidia are separated by vacuolated cells. (From Davis BD, Delbecco R, Eisen HW, et al., eds. *Microbiology, Including Immunology and Molecular Genetics*. 3rd ed. Hagerstown, MD: Harper & Row; 1980.)

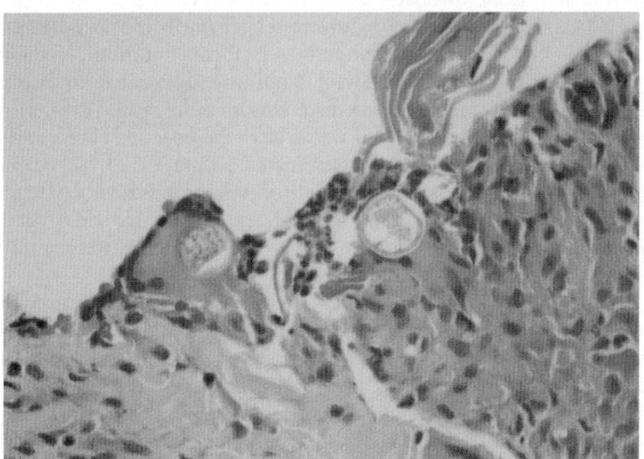

FIG. 201.2 Coccidioidal granuloma shows a multinucleated giant cell containing a spherule filled with endospores. The adjacent field consists of granulomatous inflammation.

storms, and for those with occupational exposure.[121,142,153] Significant increases in the number of reported cases have been observed in Arizona and California, from 5.3 per 100,000 in 1998 to 42.6 per 100,000 in 2011.[69,87]

In contrast to susceptibility to primary infection, the frequency of dissemination and severe disease varies considerably and is higher among infants,[42,43,97,153] Filipinos, Hispanics, and blacks. Immunosuppressed hosts also are at increased risk for disseminated infection. Persons receiving anti–tumor necrosis factor-α (TNF-α) therapy are at increased risk for severe pulmonary coccidioidomycosis.[13,127] In the era of potent antiretroviral therapy, the severity of the disease has decreased among human immunodeficiency virus (HIV)–infected individuals and is inversely associated with control of the infection.[123]

The tissue phase of the organism is the spherule, which is not infectious. Although mycelial growth can be found in cavities when they are carefully searched, no evidence exists of person-to-person spread of *C. immitis,*[84,186] except in special situations in which the fungus is allowed to revert to its airborne form, such as growth from wound drainage on a plaster cast.[60] Patients with coccidioidomycosis do not require isolation, even when draining wounds exist. In these circumstances, dressings should be changed frequently to prevent growth of the fungus and the formation of arthroconidia.

Once limited to the lower Sonoran life zone, the disease is seen throughout the country because of the ease and frequency of travel, increased populations in endemic areas, and reactivation of infection in immunocompromised hosts, including transplant recipients, patients with acquired immunodeficiency syndrome (AIDS), and recipients of TNF-α inhibitors. For these patients, delays in establishing the diagnosis can be fatal, and rapid recognition of the diagnosis and prompt institution of appropriate therapy mandate a timely and accurate diagnosis.

PATHOGENESIS AND PATHOLOGY

Acquisition of *Coccidioides* spp. infection usually occurs through the respiratory tract. It is surmised that most human infections result from exposure to only a single spore.[72] Growth of the organism stimulates an intense inflammatory response, and in most patients, the infection remains localized to the lung and hilar nodes. This bronchopneumonic process can occur in any lobe of the lung. In a few patients, clinically significant extrapulmonary dissemination occurs by way of lymphatics or the bloodstream. Rarely, direct cutaneous inoculation may occur by puncture of the skin with a contaminated object, which results in localized disease with occasional sporotrichoid spread.[39,130]

The initial inflammatory response of acute pulmonary coccidioidomycosis consists primarily of a neutrophilic reaction, possibly related to a chemotactic effect of endospores or complement activation from other *Coccidioides* antigens. Tissue necrosis, spherules, and a few mononuclear cells are present at this stage of the disease, but epithelial giant cells are infrequently seen. Although this response may slow the progress of the infection temporarily, it ultimately cannot arrest the disease process[72] because neutrophils do not kill coccidioidal forms.

Killing has been demonstrated with natural killer cells and mononuclear leukocytes. Numerous studies have demonstrated the importance of T-cell–mediated responses, particularly the Th1 response, in controlling the infection, as evidenced by delayed cutaneous hypersensitivity, peripheral lymphocyte transformation, and production of interleukin-12, interferon-γ, and TNF-α.[72] Dermal hypersensitivity correlates well with other measures of peripheral blood lymphocyte responsiveness, such as lymphocyte transformation and cytokine production.[3] In patients with progressive disease, cell-mediated immune defenses become defective, possibly because of defective antigen presentation, antigen overload, suppressor cells, immune complexes, or fungal immunomodulatory substances, resulting in an undesirable and ineffective Th2 response.[48] Cytokines, including interferon-γ and tumor necrosis factor-α, are important in protection and control of infection by enhancing Th1 and Th17 immune responses.[176] The role of the Th17 response in acute infection remains controversial, but it may have a beneficial effect in preventing primary infection in murine models.[92,180]

Disseminated coccidioidomycosis resembles progressive tuberculosis of childhood, which usually occurs within weeks or months after the initial infection develops. However, endogenous reactivation also can occur, particularly among individuals with immunosuppressive conditions.[3,21,73] Extrapulmonary spread can occur anywhere in the body, but lesions are found most frequently in bone, soft tissue, lymph nodes, liver, spleen, and meninges. Bone lesions resemble chronic osteomyelitis (Fig. 201.3). Infection of the brain parenchyma is a rare event, but meningitis occurs commonly and frequently localizes to the basilar area.[23,93]

The pathologic findings of fatal coccidioidomycosis have been reviewed extensively.[94] The tissue reaction in disseminated disease predominantly is granulomatous but can be accompanied by elements of acute inflammation. Typically, the granulomatous lesions contain abundant giant cells and histiocytes. Caseous necrosis is a common occurrence, and spherules usually can be identified lying freely and within macrophages or multinucleate giant cells (see Fig. 201.2). Fibrous tissue can surround areas of inflammation, but calcification is an infrequent occurrence.

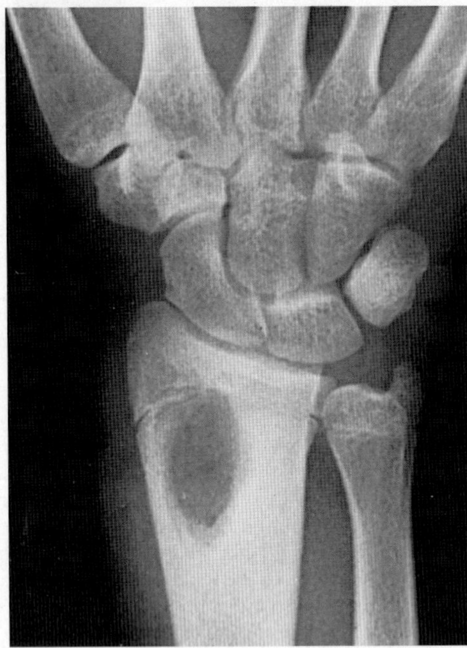

FIG. 201.3 An osteolytic lesion involving the distal radius in a 14-year-old boy with osteomyelitis and disseminated coccidioidomycosis.

Most cases of disseminated coccidioidal infection in the first months of life have been associated with heavy exposure to dust; these infants apparently acquire their infection by the respiratory route.[44,97] Most infants described have had severe disease,[42,43,97,167] but primary infection sometimes is unrecognized.[43] Although women who develop coccidioidomycosis late in pregnancy may be at increased risk for development of disseminated disease,[178] with a few exceptions,[40,115] their infants are born free of infection.[44,45,152,172] In several patients with apparent perinatal transmission, the mothers had coccidioidal endometritis, and infected amniotic fluid was the most likely source of their infants' infections.[14,115,149,160]

Dissemination of coccidioidomycosis occurs more frequently in immunosuppressed patients who have resided in an endemic area.[73,119] No specific immunologic abnormalities have been detected in other groups, such as Filipinos, who also are at high risk for disseminated disease. Gain-of-function mutations in the *STAT1* gene, resulting in aberrant regulation of the interferon-γ and interleukin-12 axis, have been identified in patients with disseminated disease.[146] After dissemination occurs, the patient's cell-mediated immunity is frequently impaired,[3,32,47,48,158] especially if infection is extensive.[10,156]

Dissemination can occur in patients who have a selective lack of response to coccidioidal antigens, as evidenced by negative skin test results to coccidioidin or spherulin, without evidence of generalized anergy. In vitro measurements of lymphocyte transformation to phytohemagglutinin or to specific cell wall antigens of *C. immitis* are also depressed.[10,47] In contrast, patients with disseminated disease with positive skin test results usually have normal in vitro lymphocyte responses that are similar to those found in healthy persons who have recovered from primary infection.[48,131,190] Patients who have recovered from severe disseminated disease may show return of specific and nonspecific cell-mediated immunity.[10,32,66,158] Infected children demonstrate immunologic findings similar to those described in adults, but they have not been studied as extensively.

CLINICAL MANIFESTATIONS

Primary Pulmonary Infection

The clinical features of acute coccidioidomycosis in children are thought to be similar to the manifestations observed in adults.[155] Studies of Air Force personnel indicate that infection is subclinical or indistinguishable from a mild upper respiratory tract infection in 60% of infected persons.[156,158] Twenty-five percent experience an influenza-like illness lasting 1 to 2 days, whereas the remainder have more severe lower respiratory illnesses, including lobar pneumonia, pleural effusions, and occasionally, pericarditis.[66,72,136] With intensive exposure, such as occurs during military field exercises, the attack rate may be high, and a large proportion of infections may be symptomatic.[50]

The disease may mimic bacterial pneumonia and sepsis.[6,116] When serologic studies are used routinely in the evaluation of adults with community-acquired pneumonia in endemic areas, 17% to 28% of cases are the result of coccidioidal infection.[107,171] However, only 2% to 13% of adults with community-acquired pneumonia are tested for coccidioidomycosis, even in highly endemic areas.[38] Although most symptomatic pulmonary infections are subacute and self-limited, some patients experience more complicated pulmonary infections or have extrapulmonary disease.[69] Outside of endemic areas, these patients are likely to undergo extensive workups, and delays in establishing the diagnosis can occur if coccidioidomycosis is not considered.[27,28,54] Severe disease is more likely to develop in individuals with diabetes, a recent history of cigarette use, or immunocompromising conditions.[143]

The usual incubation period is 10 to 16 days, but it may range from less than a week to almost a month.[66] In young adults, fatigue (77%), cough (64%), chest pain (53%), and dyspnea (17%) are the most common symptoms. Fever occurs in 46%, with arthralgias, myalgias, and headaches each reported for 22%.[166] Chest pain sometimes is severe and is usually pleuritic.[166] It may be followed by vague chest pain that persists for several months.[72] Primary pulmonary coccidioidomycosis resembles other lower respiratory illnesses, including those caused by viruses, bacteria, mycoplasma, *Mycobacterium tuberculosis*, and other fungi (e.g., *Histoplasma*). In infants, stridor rarely may be the result of primary infection of subglottic tissue.[78,85]

Transient rashes probably occur more frequently in children than in adults and are observed in slightly more than one half of symptomatic children.[56,90,140] The rash can manifests as erythema nodosum, erythema multiforme, toxic erythema, Sweet syndrome, or reactive interstitial granulomatous dermatitis. Erythema nodosum is the most characteristic lesion. It usually appears 1 to 3 weeks after the onset of illness and is associated with a lower risk of disseminated disease.[9,56,66,90,153] Erythema multiforme–like lesions are common in children, as is toxic erythema, a macular, papular, urticarial, or morbilliform rash that manifests within 48 hours of onset of symptoms. It may last for several weeks and is followed sometimes by palmar desquamation.[56]

Acute arthritis or arthralgia can accompany primary coccidioidal infection. These findings usually are transient, do not signify dissemination, and are thought to represent a hypersensitivity reaction.[58]

The radiographic appearance of primary coccidioidomycosis is nonspecific.[11,41,83,140] Bronchopneumonic infiltrates are the most frequent finding and often are associated with hilar lymphadenopathy. Segmental or lobar consolidation and nodular or patchy pulmonary infiltrates also can occur. Small pleural effusions or pleuropericardial reactions occur in 15% of hospitalized patients (Fig. 201.4) and are usually sterile.[126] These radiographic findings resolve in 90% to 95% of symptomatic cases, albeit slowly in some, and usually do not necessitate specific therapy. Mediastinitis with necrotizing mediastinal adenitis was diagnosed in 21% of children admitted for coccidioidomycosis to a central California hospital, a rate much higher than is reported for adults.[125]

In neonates, the constellation of radiographic findings of focal consolidation with diffuse nodular densities, nonspecific symptoms, and minimal clinical evidence of respiratory tract infection has been described but is not specific for coccidioidomycosis.[14,41] Chorioretinitis as a manifestation of systemic disease has also been reported.[80]

In some patients, cavitation, nodule formation, bronchiectasis, or calcification can develop at the site of the pulmonic infiltrate.[16] The cavities usually are asymptomatic and rarely require surgical therapy. Nodules and thin-walled cavities develop in 5% of patients with coccidioidal pneumonia. The well-circumscribed lesions are typically single and less than 6 cm in diameter. Many resolve spontaneously, but patients nonetheless require prolonged care and convalescence. Rarely, the cavities lead to pneumothorax (Fig. 201.5), empyema, or bronchopleural fistulas, which are more likely to occur in immunosuppressed patients or in diabetics.[98] In adults, nodules may be confused with carcinoma of the

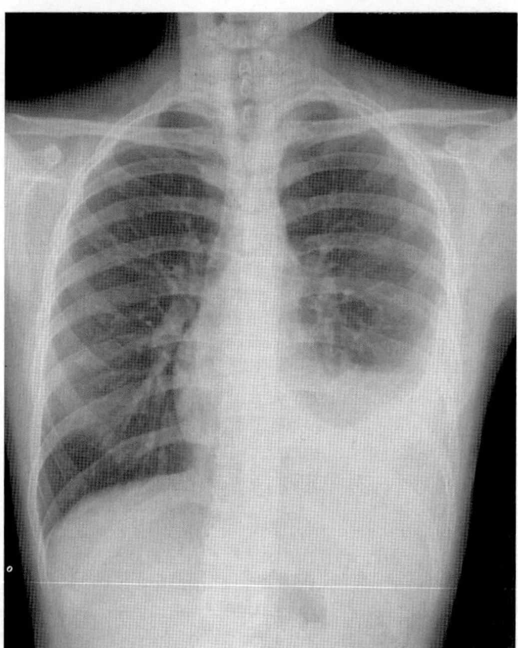

FIG. 201.4 Chest radiograph of a patient with acute pulmonary coccidioidomycosis showing pulmonary infiltrates, extensive pleural fluid, and enlargement of the left hilum. Drainage was not attempted, and the chest radiograph normalized after 3 months of treatment with fluconazole alone.

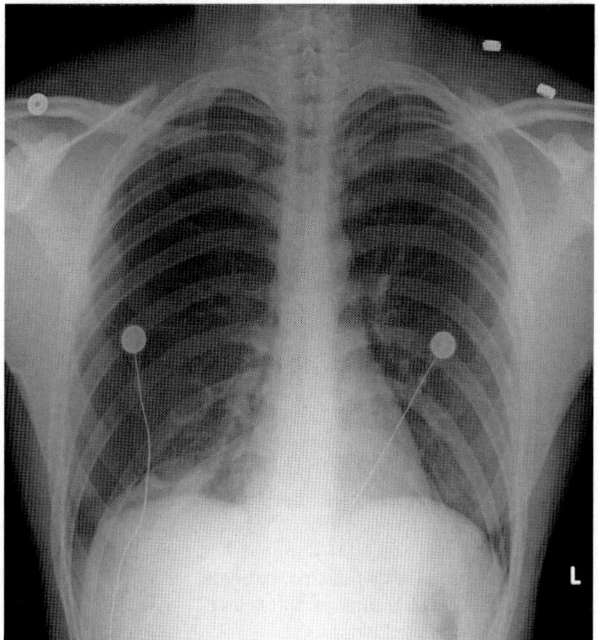

FIG. 201.5 A right lower lobe thin-walled cavity resulting in pneumothorax in an otherwise healthy 17-year-old boy.

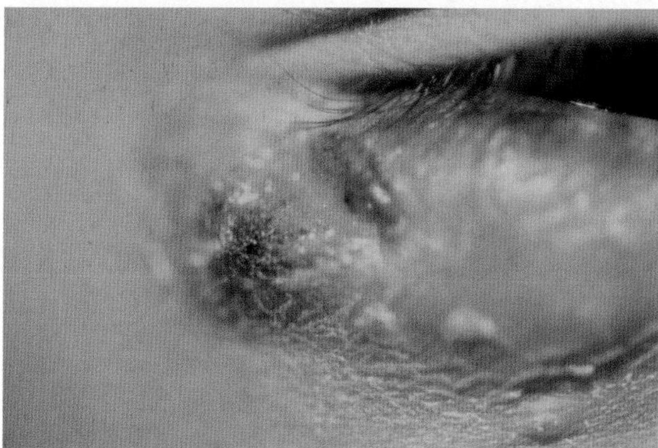

FIG. 201.6 A chronic, right lower eyelid lesion resulting from traumatic inoculation at the site several weeks earlier. Tissue cultures grew *Coccidioides* spp.

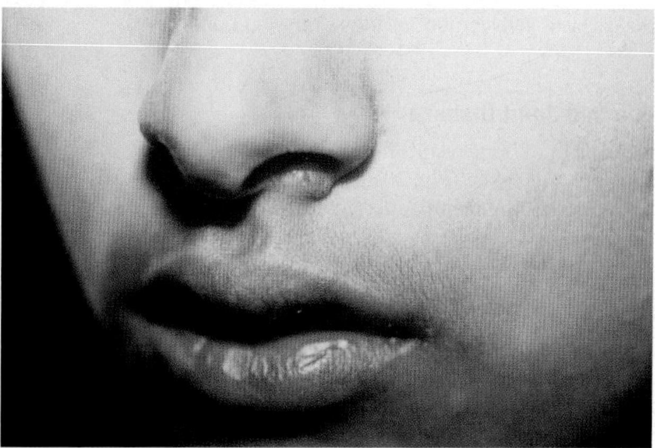

FIG. 201.7 Verrucous cutaneous lesion at the nasolabial fold from coccidioidal hematogenous dissemination.

lung, requiring excision or diagnostic fine-needle aspiration.[57] A miliary pattern, indicating hematogenous or lymphatic spread, sometimes can be appreciated in immunocompromised hosts and rarely in immunocompetent hosts.[8] Occasionally, endotracheal or endobronchial lesions can be demonstrated by endoscopy.[137]

The manifestations of primary coccidioidal disease vary. Because no constellation of symptoms and signs is specific enough to establish a diagnosis, specific laboratory tests are a requirement.

Primary Inoculation-Related Infection

Rarely, primary cutaneous coccidioidomycosis develops after direct inoculation of the skin (Fig. 201.6). Lesions develop 1 to 3 weeks after an injury and are often associated with localized lymphadenitis. Nodular lymphangitis mimicking sporotrichosis, cutaneous nocardiosis, and *Mycobacterium marinum* infection can occur.

In adults, constitutional symptoms usually are mild, and the process spontaneously resolves within 2 to 3 months. However, progressive and prolonged infection commonly occurs in children, and antifungal therapy may be necessary.[130,185] Transmission by cat bite has been reported.[71]

Disseminated Coccidioidomycosis

Except in very young children, dissemination appears to occur less frequently in pediatric patients than in adults (0.5%), although this view has been questioned.[102,151] Spread of infection usually becomes apparent within a few weeks to a few months after the initial infection occurs. It is heralded by persistent fever, toxicity, and insidious development of lesions outside the chest.

A few patients develop disseminated disease after having an asymptomatic primary infection.[52,64,102] Disseminated disease rarely can manifest with peritonitis, pericarditis, empyema, laryngeal lesions, endocarditis, or soft tissue abscesses.[25,51,91]

Skin Disease

The most common cutaneous manifestation of disseminated coccidioidomycosis is a verrucous granuloma that is characteristically located at the nasolabial fold (Fig. 201.7).[66,90] These lesions may heal or may continue to progress. They can also take the form of papules, nodules, subcutaneous abscesses, pustules, or sinus tracts. They can be single or multiple and can ulcerate. Rarely, they appear similar to mycosis fungoides. Cutaneous lesions result from bloodborne dissemination and contain the organism. These lesions mimic those caused by other fungi, tuberculosis, actinomycetes, and syphilis.[56]

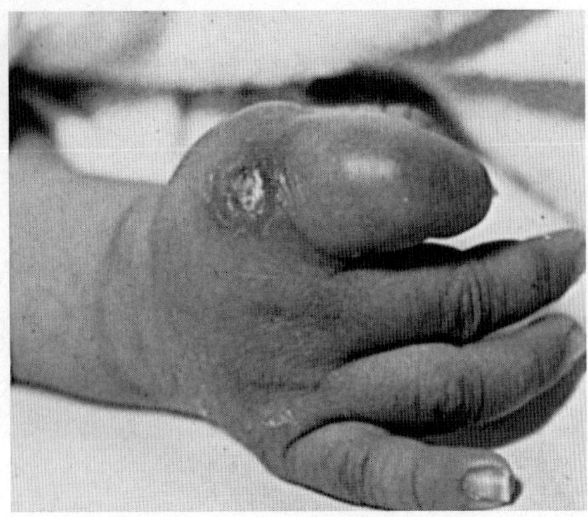

FIG. 201.8 Swelling and chronic draining sinus is seen over the proximal phalanx of the index finger. The infant has disseminated coccidioidomycosis with involvement of the underlying bone.

Bone and Joint Disease

Involvement of bone results in chronic osteomyelitis,[17,53,89,99] which can drain into soft tissue (Fig. 201.8) and fistulize to the overlying skin.[52] The bones most frequently infected are the vertebrae, tibias, metatarsals, skull, and metacarpals. The lesions are identified in a single bone in 60% of cases; two bones in 20%, three in another 10%, and four or more bones in the remainder. On radiographic examination, the lesions typically are lytic (see Fig. 201.3).

Involvement of the axial skeleton is common. Vertebral osteomyelitis is characterized by involvement of all parts of the vertebra with relative sparing of the disk, in contrast to tuberculosis. Spread of infection locally leading to meningitis is a serious concern with vertebral osteomyelitis. Skull involvement typically leads to erosion of the outer table. Arthritis has a waxing and waning course and usually involves the knee or ankle. It can result from direct inoculation of the joint, as in the case of a cactus spine. Periarticular disease, such as tenosynovitis, can also occur through inoculation or hematogenous dissemination.[30]

Meningitis

Coccidioidal meningitis may be the sole site of extrapulmonary disease, particularly in whites, but it also occurs as part of widespread dissemination.[23,100,150] It may manifest acutely with the primary infection or appear up to 6 months later.

The most common symptom is headache. Altered mental status, sluggishness, ataxia, and vomiting are other common symptoms. Children often lack signs of meningeal irritation and sometimes have focal neurologic deficits at presentation.

The pathologic process is that of granulomatous and suppurative basilar meningitis, with frequent parenchymal involvement with granulomas and abscesses of the spinal cord and brain.[63,128] Vasculitic complications with infarction and stroke-like findings may be abrupt in onset.[63,184] Hydrocephalus is common in children and is treated by placement of a ventriculoperitoneal shunt.[150]

Before amphotericin B became available, coccidioidal meningitis was uniformly fatal, and the average length of survival in children was 5.5 months. Death with coccidioidal meningitis has become an uncommon event. However, adults with neuroimaging abnormalities, especially hydrocephalus with or without cerebral infarction, have a high mortality rate.[7]

Examination of the cerebrospinal fluid (CSF) usually reveals moderate pleocytosis, usually between 100 and 500 white blood cells/mm^3 (with a range of a few to more than 10,000 white blood cells/mm^3) with mononuclear cell predominance, hypoglycorrhachia, and an elevated protein level.[105,150] Polymorphonuclear cell predominance may occur early in the course of the illness. These findings are typical for CSF sampled from the lumbosacral space. However, considerable variation occurs in the cell count, chemistry, and antibody content of fluid obtained from the ventricles, cisterna magna, or lumbosacral space.[81,86,150] The lumbosacral space exhibits the most severe changes, including a lower glucose concentration, higher protein level, higher cell count, and higher CSF coccidioidal complement fixation titer.

Eosinophilic pleocytosis in the CSF suggests coccidioidal meningitis and should prompt an appropriate diagnostic workup; it is of no prognostic value.[139] The CSF culture often is negative for the fungus, whereas CSF antibody is detectable in up to 95% of patients.[105] The diagnosis is confirmed by a positive CSF culture or serology and is supported by a positive serum serologic result or culture of *Coccidioides* spp. from a pulmonary or nonpulmonary site.

Coccidioidomycosis in Pregnancy

Like tuberculosis, coccidioidomycosis can involve the pelvic organs. Early studies had indicated an alarming risk of dissemination in and death of women who acquired coccidioidomycosis, especially during the third trimester of pregnancy. In a population-based study, Wack and colleagues[178] showed that coccidioidomycosis occurs infrequently during pregnancy but remains associated with serious complications when the disease develops in the third trimester or soon after delivery. This is thought to be the result of immunosuppression and increased hormonal levels that favor the growth of spherules.[161] Pregnant women with erythema nodosum are much less likely to experience disseminated disease than are those without.[9]

Wide variations are reported in the rates of dissemination and fatality for pregnant women, although all studies agree that the rate of dissemination for pregnant women is higher than that for the general population.[29,49] Maternal infection is more severe when it is acquired late in pregnancy and most severe in the immediate postpartum period.[12]

Coccidioidomycosis in the Immunocompromised Host

Control of coccidioidal infection depends primarily on cell-mediated immunity. Conditions that result in immune suppression, particularly T-lymphocyte dysfunction, such as those in patients who have undergone hematopoietic stem cell transplantation (HSCT) or solid organ transplantation, predispose the individual to more fulminant forms of coccidioidomycosis.[21,141] Infections may be primary or the result of reactivation. Solid organ transplant recipients are at the highest risk in the first year after undergoing transplantation, especially during primary infection. Dissemination also can occur late as a result of reactivation of a prior infection. The risk is increased by a prior history of coccidioidomycosis or a positive serologic reaction just before transplantation.[21] By use of targeted prophylaxis with fluconazole, however, the overall rate of coccidioidomycosis after liver transplantation (2.4%), renal transplantation (3%), and HSCT (1.5%) can be significantly reduced.[26,177]

An increased risk of acquiring severe symptomatic disease was described for patients receiving TNF-α antagonists.[13] In HIV-infected patients, the severity of pulmonary disease is related inversely to virologic control, with greatly increased risk of severe pulmonary and extrapulmonary disease when the CD4 count is less than 250 cells/µL. The morbidity rate for HIV-1–infected patients receiving antiretroviral therapy and with CD4 counts of 250 cells/µL or higher is similar to that in non–HIV-infected persons.[2,123]

In endemic areas, the risk of coccidioidomycosis among solid organ transplant recipients is 4% to 9%.[21,173,177] Most cases occur in the first year after solid organ transplantation. One-third of the patients have disseminated disease, with a mortality rate of 13% among those with posttransplantation coccidioidomycosis.[177] Genetic factors, such as deficiencies in interferon-γ receptor 1 or in interleukin-12 receptor β_1, have been recognized in some patients with refractory disseminated coccidioidomycosis.[174,175]

DIAGNOSIS

In endemic areas where an awareness of the disease exists, the diagnosis of coccidioidomycosis usually is established readily by obtaining appropriate laboratory studies. However, even in these areas, coccidioidal pneumonia may be more prevalent than previously thought and can be underdiagnosed.[107,171] Cases have occurred even after brief exposure in an endemic area. In nonendemic areas, the diagnosis is often not considered unless a travel history is obtained.

The hematologic findings for primary coccidioidal infection consist of elevation of the erythrocyte sedimentation rate, leukocytosis, and sometimes, eosinophilia. Eosinophilia may be observed, but it occurs in a minority of patients.[66,118] Hypercalcemia is occasionally diagnosed and is the result of aberrant production of parathyroid hormone–related peptide within coccidioidal granulomas.[65] Patients with coccidioidal infection may demonstrate cross-reactivity to the (1→3)-β-D-glucan assay, but the performance characteristics of this test in coccidioidomycosis cases are unknown.[188] Specific diagnosis is most often established serologically, but cultures, sputum examination, antigen testing, and histologic examination of tissue are often useful, particularly for immunocompromised patients, whose blunted antibody responses may yield false-negative serologic results.[125]

Culture and Identification of the Fungus

The organism is detected readily by direct examination and culture from purulent material. The yield from other sources, such as pleural fluid, blood, and gastric aspirate, is somewhat lower. Approximately one third of CSF samples are culture positive, and direct examination of the CSF usually yields negative results.[105,147] Detection of the fungus from the blood is an uncommon occurrence and is associated with severe forms of disseminated disease.[4] Tissue biopsies of pleura, cavities, synovium, or meninges often yield the organism by culture or by histologic demonstration of coccidioidal spherules or hyphae.[159]

In severe pulmonary or disseminated disease, microscopic examination of bronchoalveolar lavage specimens, exudates, or biopsy specimens is diagnostic if typical spherules containing endospores are seen. Hematoxylin and eosin–stained sections can be used to demonstrate spherules, but they are used mainly to show the inflammatory process. The periodic acid–Schiff stain is useful for demonstration of spherule contents (Fig. 201.9), whereas methenamine silver stains highlight the wall of the spherule. Potassium hydroxide stains are useful but lack sensitivity and specificity; calcofluor white fluorescent stains are more sensitive but require experienced technologists.[147] Cytologic examination of sputum is more sensitive than potassium hydroxide stains.[181]

Cytologic examination of bronchial wash or bronchoalveolar fluid is diagnostic for approximately one third of people with or without HIV infection and is less sensitive than culture.[57] The Gram stain is not useful because it is not picked up by the spherules.

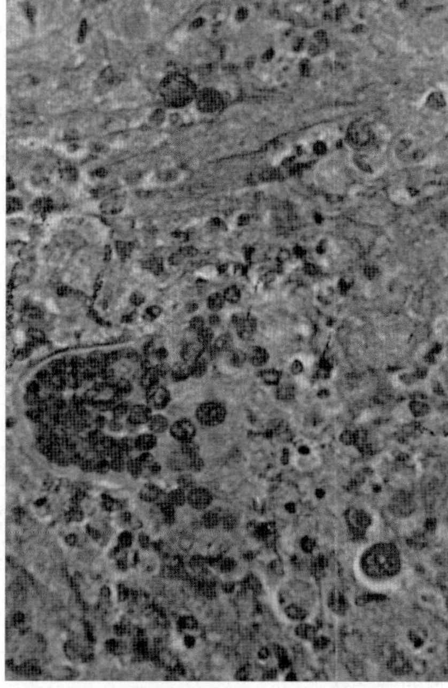

FIG. 201.9 A recently ruptured spherule is in the process of releasing endospores.

With the rare exception of individuals with primary cutaneous infection, the finding of spherules in tissues outside the thoracic cavity is evidence that the patient has disseminated disease. Biopsy may be useful to establish a diagnosis, particularly for patients with negative or low complement fixation antibody titers. Cultures of *Coccidioides* spp. from body fluids, sputum, or exudates can be performed on most laboratory media. If coccidioidomycosis is suspected, the use of mycologic media containing cycloheximide can be helpful.[101,164] The organism grows on routine bacterial, fungal, and *Legionella* media. Aerosolization of the organism is hazardous when handling cultures, and the use of biosafety level 3 practices is required. *Coccidioides* spp. are no longer designated as *select agents* by the Centers for Disease Control and Prevention (i.e., they do not pose a severe threat to public, animal, or plant health).

After a nonpigmented mold is grown, definitive identification of the organism is done typically by the use of genus-specific genetic probes.[132] The probes do not differentiate between *C. immitis* and *C. posadasii*, and it is not clinically relevant to differentiate the two species. Real-time polymerase chain reaction assays are being developed for rapid detection of *Coccidioides* spp. in a variety of clinical specimens but are not commercially available.[15,129]

Skin Test

Intradermal skin tests using lysates of the mycelial phase (i.e., coccidioidin) or the spherule phase (i.e., spherulin) have been used to elicit delayed-type hypersensitivity. Spherulin, unavailable since the late-1990s, was reintroduced in 2014.[1,179] Skin test conversion typically occurs by the first week after onset of symptoms in 83% of healthy subjects and in 99% by the third week.

Skin test reactions may be negative for immunocompromised individuals and those with disseminated disease, and false positives have been reported due to hypersensitivity to the preservative thimerosal, which has been replaced with phenol in the newer formulation. Skin tests have primarily been used as epidemiologic tools or to monitor for the development of a cellular immune response by delayed-type hypersensitivity in anergic patients with disseminated infection.

Serologic Studies

The initial antibody response to coccidioidal infection is predominantly in the immunoglobulin M (IgM) fraction and is responsible for the positive precipitin test result that accompanies primary infection. Samples from 50% of patients yield positive results in the first week, and 90% do so within 2 to 3 weeks. Thereafter, antibody reversion occurs, and by 5 months, only 10% of patients with uncomplicated infection remain positive for IgM.[157] In contrast to immunoglobulin G (IgG) titers measured by complement fixation, the magnitude of the IgM titer does not correlate with an increased risk of dissemination.[156] IgM may persist in some patients with disseminated infection or may reappear with reactivation of infection. IgM occasionally has been detected in the cord blood of newborns whose mothers had detectable antibody, but these infants had no evidence of infection on follow-up.[134]

IgM responses can be measured by tube precipitins, latex agglutination, enzyme immunoassay (EIA), or immunodiffusion methods.[134] Precipitating IgM antibody detected by the tube precipitin assay or by immunodiffusion usually indicates acute infection.[157] Latex agglutination is sensitive, rapid, and easy to perform but frequently yields false-positive reactions.[134] Positive results should therefore be confirmed by a second method. Latex agglutination produces false-positive results for CSF samples and diluted sera and should not be used for these specimens.[134]

The EIA is a rapid method for the detection of IgM. It does not suffer from the subjectivity required to interpret the other assays, is less labor intensive, and may be positive earlier in the course of illness than other methods.[70,104,122,183] Its reported sensitivity is 74%, but its initial reported specificity of 96% has been the subject of controversy, particularly in the absence of IgG positivity. Kuberski and colleagues found that 82% of patients with a positive IgM response and a negative IgG response had no evidence of coccidioidomycosis.[109] However, Blair and Currier detected few false-positive results among 706 EIAs, including 28 isolated IgM seropositives.[20] In a follow-up study of 1117 patients, of whom 102 patients (9%) had isolated IgM EIA positivity, IgM specificity ranged from 90% for the 60 patients with compatible symptoms to 45% for the 29 asymptomatic patients undergoing screening.[22] In Puerto Rico, which is not endemic for *Coccidioides* spp., isolated IgM positivity by EIA was observed in 1.5% to 3.4% of 534 samples (depending on the assay manufacturer), all of which were antibody negative for *Histoplasma*. Rates from 1218 samples from asymptomatic blood donors in Arizona were between 1.1% and 2.4%, suggesting that a proportion are falsely positive.[114]

Antibodies measured by complement fixation are slower to develop and primarily are in the IgG fraction.[134] They usually are not detected in serum samples obtained during the first week of illness, may appear as late as 3 months after onset of symptoms,[96,157] and typically last 6 to 8 months.[134] Early therapy with fluconazole may interfere with the development of IgG antibodies.[165] The antibodies are seen more commonly in symptomatic infections and are detected in 50% to 90% of patients by 3 months after the onset of symptoms. At least 90% of people show a positive IgM or IgG response after symptomatic primary infections.[134,147] The main methods of detection of IgG antibodies are complement fixation, quantitative immunodiffusion, and enzyme immunoassay.[122,134,182,189] These assays correlate well, and immunodiffusion is particularly useful for detection of antibody in patients whose sera are anticomplementary.[134]

The magnitude of the IgG titer correlates closely with the severity of infection and the likelihood of dissemination.[157] Although the antibody titer cannot be used as the sole indicator of dissemination, titers of 1:32 or greater in most laboratories strongly suggest extrapulmonary spread of infection[95,157]; 61% of these patients have a titer of at least 1:16, whereas 95% to 100% of those without dissemination have a titer lower than 1:16. The titer of complement fixation antibody parallels disease activity and is useful in following the progress of patients with disseminated disease. A few patients, especially those with extensive pulmonary involvement and pleural effusion, develop high titers without other clinical evidence of dissemination.[134] Conversely, some patients with dissemination, particularly those with single lesions in skin, bone, or meninges, have lower titers. These antibodies are measured by complement fixation or immunodiffusion.

The IgG enzyme immunoassay has a sensitivity of 92% and specificity of 97%. The assay is qualitative. Unlike complement fixation titers, reported optical density or EIA index values have no prognostic or therapeutic significance. The complement fixation antibody is detectable in the CSF of 70% of patients at the time of diagnosis of coccidioidal meningitis and eventually becomes detectable in almost all. The antibody measured is not a reflection of serum levels but rather indicates specific immunoglobulin biosynthesis by cells residing within or contiguous with the central nervous system (CNS). Some patients with vertebral osteomyelitis or epidural abscesses produce low complement fixation titers in the CSF without other evidence of meningeal involvement.[134] Some patients with immunodeficiency disease, in particular HIV infection, can have extensive disease with low or undetectable antibody levels.[2,134] Bone marrow transplant recipients may have no serologic or skin test response before or shortly after bone marrow transplantation, and aggressive attempts may be required to culture the fungus for diagnosis.[141]

Antigen Detection

Antigen detection assays have been developed for identification of *Coccidioides* galactomannan in urine, blood, respiratory secretions, and CSF.[3] On the basis of preliminary data, they have detection rates of 50% to 71% for antigenuria and up to 73% for antigenemia when the specimen is treated with heat in the presence of EDTA to dissociate immune complexes.[59] Antigen cross-reactivity was observed in patients with histoplasmosis.[110] A retrospective review of CSF coccidioidal antigen testing for 36 patients with coccidioidal meningitis revealed a sensitivity of 93% and specificity of 100%.[3,103] Sensitivity of CSF antibody detection by immunodiffusion or complement fixation alone was 67% to 70%.

TREATMENT

Primary Infection

In more than 90% of children, primary coccidioidomycosis is a self-limited illness, and antifungal therapy is not needed. In some children with severe primary disease, therapy with antifungals may be justified to abbreviate the period of morbidity or to lessen the chance of dissemination in those with an elevated complement fixation titer.

Whether patients with primary uncomplicated pulmonary infections should receive therapy remains controversial. When treatment is prescribed, the agent of choice is fluconazole, which is usually administered for 3 to 6 months. Evidence of severe infection or of concurrent risk factors such as immunosuppression should lead to the initiation of therapy. In adults, severe infections usually are heralded by weight loss of more than 10%, intense night sweats for a duration of longer than 3 weeks, infiltrates involving more than one half of one lung or portions of both lungs, prominent or persistent hilar adenopathy, complement fixation titers greater than 1:16, failure to develop normal skin test hypersensitivity to coccidioidal antigens, inability to work, or symptoms that persist for longer than 2 months.[75] Convalescence usually is prolonged with or without antifungal therapy.[19]

Diagnosis of primary coccidioidomycosis during the third trimester of pregnancy or immediately after delivery should prompt consideration of treatment. Amphotericin B is recommended for pregnant women in the first trimester because of the teratogenic potential of fluconazole, which is classified as a class D agent.[12] Thereafter, an azole antifungal or amphotericin B can be used. Fluconazole can be used in breastfeeding women, but other azoles should be avoided.[12]

Because of the high risk for dissemination, persons of African or Filipino ancestry should be considered for antifungal therapy. Immunocompromised patients, such as those with AIDS, recipients of solid organ transplants, patients receiving high-dose steroids, or those receiving TNF-α inhibitors, also warrant treatment.

When reticulonodular or miliary disease is seen, a more aggressive approach is warranted. Therapy usually is initiated with amphotericin B or high-dose fluconazole. Amphotericin B seems to yield a faster response and can be replaced by an azole after a few weeks.[75] The total course of therapy should last for at least 1 year and should be followed by oral azole therapy for secondary prophylaxis.[75]

Asymptomatic pulmonary cavities usually do not require therapy. Consideration should be given to excision of some cavities that persist for longer than 2 years, are progressively enlarging, or are adjacent to the pleural cavity. For patients with cavities that result in local discomfort, superinfection, or hemoptysis, therapy with oral azoles may alleviate the symptoms. Resection of localized cavities is an alternative to recurrent courses of antifungal therapy.[75] Pyopneumothorax results from rupture of a cavity into the pleural space. Its treatment is surgical resection and decortication with or without a course of antifungal therapy. Chronic fibrocavitary disease usually is treated with oral azoles for at least a year. For patients with inadequate responses, increasing the dose of azole, switching to a different azole, and administering amphotericin B are options. Surgical resection may be helpful in cases of localized disease or when significant hemoptysis has occurred.[75]

Asymptomatic pulmonary nodules resulting from coccidioidomycosis represent healed infection. They usually do not warrant therapy, except in immunocompromised patients.[75].

Disseminated Disease

Nonmeningeal Dissemination

Patients with disseminated disease who have clinically apparent lesions outside the thoracic cavity typically require antifungal therapy, usually with an azole (i.e., fluconazole or itraconazole). In fulminant infections, amphotericin B is the agent of choice because it is thought to produce more rapid improvement.[75]

The classic therapy consists of amphotericin B deoxycholate administered initially at a dose of 1 to 1.5 mg/kg per day and then tapered to 1 to 1.5 mg/kg per day three times per week. The usual duration of therapy is 3 months to 1 year. Local instillation or irrigation of abscesses and cavities with amphotericin B or other antifungal agents may be beneficial, but it has not been studied systematically.[17,99] Total duration of therapy is determined by the patient's response. Lipid-complexed amphotericin B preparations offer the possibility of administering higher doses with less toxicity and have largely replaced intravenous amphotericin B deoxycholate.

The azoles have been tested extensively in this form of the disease. The main agents used are fluconazole and itraconazole. In a randomized, double-blind study of progressive nonmeningeal coccidioidomycosis, a trend toward better efficacy with itraconazole, especially in the subgroup of patients with skeletal infections, was demonstrated.[77] For children, this approach must be weighed against the need for more frequent drug administration, dietary limitations related to the erratic absorption of itraconazole, and its higher cost. Itraconazole has important drug interactions, most notably with tacrolimus, cyclosporine, and phenytoin.[82] Reports suggest that voriconazole and posaconazole offer effective treatment for patients refractory to fluconazole therapy.[5,108,163] A single case report demonstrated beneficial results with the concurrent use of interferon-γ.[111]

The azoles are used for several months after resolution of symptoms or for at least 1 year of therapy. Fluconazole should not be used in the first trimester of pregnancy because cases of multiple craniofacial and skeletal malformations somewhat reminiscent of the Antley-Bixler syndrome have been described.[12] The role of echinocandins is currently unclear.

Treatment is recommended for all HIV-infected individuals with active coccidioidomycosis and CD4 counts of less than 250 cells/μL. After the infection is controlled, discontinuation of the therapy is reasonable if the CD4 count has risen to more than 250 cells/μL, except in cases of meningitis, for which therapy should be lifelong.

Meningeal Disease

Fluconazole is considered the drug of choice for coccidioidal meningitis.[75] Studies using 400 mg of fluconazole or itraconazole in the treatment of meningitis without concurrent use of amphotericin B have shown good results, with response rates of approximately 80%.[76,168,169] Some experts prefer starting at a dose of 800 to 1200 mg of fluconazole or 600 mg of itraconazole.[100] On the basis of limited data, the pediatric dose of fluconazole is approximately 12 mg/kg per day.[145] Patients usually respond clinically within 1 to 2 months, although for some patients, abnormalities of the CSF may persist for a prolonged period. When therapy has been stopped, increases in CSF cell count or complement fixation antibody titer may be the only indications of reactivation of meningeal disease and signify a need to intensify therapy.[58]

Before the availability of fluconazole, therapy with amphotericin B deoxycholate for coccidioidal meningitis was associated with a marked improvement in survival rates.[62,74] However, this requires prolonged intrathecal therapy through lumbar, ventricular, or cisternal administration. It is associated with significant side effects that include headache, nausea, vomiting, chills and fever, arachnoiditis, and occasionally, paralysis, seizures, and coma. The symptoms of arachnoiditis may be indistinguishable from those of microbiologic relapses.[86,100] For these reasons, routine use of amphotericin B deoxycholate has largely been supplanted by fluconazole therapy. Some investigators use intra-CSF administration of amphotericin in conjunction with an azole to achieve a faster response.

Significant attention should be paid to CSF flow dynamics because most children with coccidioidal meningitis develop obstructive hydrocephalus, which requires ventriculoperitoneal shunting and rarely a second shunt to drain a trapped fourth ventricle.[86,150] A systemically administered drug such as fluconazole obviates the problems of impaired CSF flow when intrathecal or intraventricular therapy is used. Monitoring CSF pressure is important in assessing the timing of CSF shunting; persistent pressures above 200 mm H_2O herald the need for shunting.[100]

Studies have indicated that the relapse rate after discontinuation of azole therapy is high. Of 14 persons treated for coccidioidal meningitis with azoles (i.e.., ketoconazole, itraconazole, or fluconazole) for periods ranging from 8 to 101 months, 11 (78%) had a relapse of disseminated coccidioidomycosis within 0.5 to 30 months after therapy was stopped. There were no clinical or laboratory predictors of patients at risk for relapse. The data indicate that moderately prolonged azole therapy for coccidioidal meningitis suppresses but does not eradicate the infection, suggesting the need for prolonged or lifelong therapy.[55]

The role of systemic corticosteroids in the management of coccidioidal CNS infection, particularly in the setting of vasculitis, is an area of controversy. Some experienced practitioners advocate the use of a short course of high-dose dexamethasone with a rapid taper, analogous to the regimen employed in tuberculous meningitis.[112] Whether this approach is beneficial or detrimental has not been studied systematically.

Surgical Management

Surgery seldom is required in patients with primary disease, but therapeutic thoracentesis may be indicated rarely when pneumonitis is complicated by large pleural effusions.[11] Surgery also is necessary when pericardial involvement is complicated by tamponade. Patients with persistent coccidioidal cavities (>2 years) may require lobectomy, especially if the lesions are symptomatic.[75] Coccidioidal lymphadenitis occasionally requires excision.

Bone and joint disease requires a combined surgical and medical approach. Coccidioidal arthritis typically responds poorly to systemic therapy, and synovectomy may aid in the control of symptoms.[17,18] Osteomyelitis optimally is dealt with by curettage and drainage of the involved bone, with the addition of amphotericin B therapy, itraconazole, or fluconazole.[17,31,53,77] Itraconazole appears to be more effective than fluconazole in skeletal infections but not for other forms of the disease.[77] The role of neurosurgical intervention to relieve elevated intracranial pressure in CNS disease was discussed previously.

Refractory or Progressive Disease

A variety of alternative regimens have been successfully used as salvage therapy in refractory or progressive disease, but data remain limited to case reports and small case series, with various definitions of what constitutes treatment failure. Regimens have included monotherapy with liposomal amphotericin B, voriconazole, or posaconazole. Combinations with purported efficacy include voriconazole with caspofungin (i.e., nine patients, two of whom had CNS disease, and one who did not survive)[124] and liposomal amphotericin B with an azole, sometimes with the addition of caspofungin.[113] The role of combination therapies in CNS infections has not been defined.[46,108,138,148,163]

PROGNOSIS

Primary pulmonary coccidioidal infection usually is self-limited, with complete recovery occurring as early as 1 to 3 weeks after starting treatment, but it often results in prolonged convalescence. Fatigue, sometimes severe, is commonly seen in individuals with symptomatic coccidioidomycosis.[24] A prospective cohort of healthy adults with mild to moderate primary disease reported an average time to complete resolution of symptoms of 4 months regardless of whether antifungals were prescribed.[19] In a few cases, localized complications of the primary infection, such as pleural effusion or pericarditis, prolong the clinical course.

Dissemination is a rare event among whites and is less likely to occur in patients with erythema nodosum. Until the late 1950s, no effective therapy was available for the more severe forms of coccidioidomycosis, and the mortality rate for patients with disseminated disease was approximately 50%.[66] The mortality rate for patients with multiple sites of dissemination and those with coccidioidal meningitis approached 100%. Current therapy with amphotericin B or azoles may cure some of these patients, and it prolongs useful life for many others.

Certain forms of disseminated infection, such as synovitis, are resistant to systemic therapy and may persist for many years without other signs of dissemination. For patients with HIV infection, therapy for disseminated coccidioidomycosis usually is not curative, and lifelong suppressive therapy with intermittent doses of amphotericin B or oral azoles may be required to prevent relapses in those with CD4 counts less than 250 cells/μL. Those with counts higher than 250 cells/μL have a clinical course that is similar to that of immunocompetent individuals.[123]

The prognosis for pregnant women has markedly improved with antifungal therapy.[12] The azoles are a major advance in the therapy for coccidioidal meningitis, although they are fungistatic and require lifelong administration, sometimes failing to maintain remission of disease. Solid organ transplant recipients remain at risk for disseminated disease and increased mortality rates due to primary or reactivation disease when coccidioidomycosis develops after transplantation.

PREVENTION

Prevention of primary coccidioidal infection with antifungal agents or physical barriers such as masking is not practical. In endemic areas, control of dust, avoidance of wind storms, and avoidance of soil digging can decrease the risk of infection. Vaccine efforts are continuing but have not yielded a viable candidate vaccine.

Within endemic areas, routine serologic screening and primary prophylaxis are not indicated for HIV-infected children[37] and those receiving TNF-α inhibitors.[75] Azoles have been used for primary and secondary prophylaxis in endemic areas for patients with solid organ transplants. Because of inhibition of the cytochrome P450 system, levels of cyclosporine and tacrolimus should be monitored.[21] The duration of primary prophylaxis usually is 6 to 12 months or more after transplantation, but the optimal dose and duration are unknown. For secondary prophylaxis in immunocompromised individuals, azoles are continued for the duration of immunosuppression due to a high risk of reactivation disease.[75]

NEW REFERENCES SINCE THE SEVENTH EDITION

19. Blair JE, Chang YH, Cheng MR, et al. Characteristics of patients with mild to moderate primary pulmonary coccidioidomycosis. *Emerg Infect Dis*. 2014;20:983-990.
22. Blair JE, Mendoza N, Force S, et al. Clinical specificity of the enzyme immunoassay test for coccidioidomycosis varies according to the reason for its performance. *Clin Vaccine Immunol*. 2013;20:95-98.
24. Bowers JM, Mourani JP, Ampel NM. Fatigue in coccidioidomycosis. Quantification and correlation with clinical, immunological, and nutritional factors. *Med Mycol*. 2006;44:585-590.
30. Campbell M, Kusne S, Renfree KJ, et al. Coccidiodal tenosynovitis of the hand and wrist: report of 9 cases and review of the literature. *Clin Infect Dis*. 2015;61:1514-1520.
65. Fierer J, Burton DW, Hachighi P, et al. Hypercalcemia in disseminated coccidioidomycosis: expression of parathyroid hormone-related peptide is characteristic of granulomatous inflammation. *Clin Infect Dis*. 2012;55:e61-e66.
69. Frieden RT, Jaffe HW, Stephens JW, et al. Increase in reported coccidioidomycosis—United States, 1998–2011. *MMWR Morb Mortal Wkly Rep*. 2013;62:217-221.
75. Galgiani JN, Ampel NM, Blair JE, et al. 2016 Infectious Diseases Society of America (IDSA) clinical practice guideline for the treatment of coccidioidomycosis. *Clin Infect Dis*. 2016;63:e112-e146.
88. Hirschmann JV. The early history of coccidioidomycosis: 1892–1945. *Clin Infect Dis*. 2007;44:1202-1207.
89. Ho AK, Shrader MW, Falk MN, et al. Diagnosis and initial management of musculoskeletal coccidioidomycosis in children. *J Pediatr Orthop*. 2014;34:571-574.
91. Horng LM, Yaghoubian S, Ram A, et al. Endocarditis due to *Coccidioides* spp: the seventh case. *Open Forum Infect Dis*. 2015;2:ofv086.
92. Hung CY, Jimenez-Alzate Mdel P, Gonzalez A, et al. Interleukin-1 receptor but not toll-like receptor 2 is essential for MyD88-dependent Th17 immunity to *Coccidioides* infection. *Infect Immun*. 2014;82:2106-2114.
103. Kassis C, Zaidi S, Kuberski T, et al. Role of *Coccidioides* antigen testing in the cerebrospinal fluid for the diagnosis of coccidioidal meningitis. *Clin Infect Dis*. 2015;61:1521-1526.
110. Kuberski T, Myers R, Wheat LJ, et al. Diagnosis of coccidioidomycosis by antigen detection using cross-reaction with a *Histoplasma* antigen. *Clin Infect Dis*. 2007;44:e50-e54.
113. Levy ER, McCarty JM, Shane AL, et al. Treatment of pediatric refractory coccidioidomycosis with combination voriconazole and caspofungin: a retrospective case series. *Clin Infect Dis*. 2013;56:1573-1578.
114. Lindsley MD, Ahn Y, McCotter O, et al. Evaluation of the specificity of 2 enzyme immunoassays for coccidioidomycosis by using sera from a region of endemicity and a region of nonendemicity. *Clin Vaccine Immunol*. 2015;22:1090-1095.
118. Lundergan LL, Kerrick SS, Galgiani JN. Coccidioidomycosis at a university outpatient clinic: a clinical description. In: Einstein HE, Catanzaro A, eds. *Coccidioidomycosis. Proceedings of the Fourth International Conference*. Washington, DC: National Foundation for Infectious Diseases; 1985:47-54.
120. Mardsen-Haug N, Hill H, Litvintseva AP, et al. *Coccidioides immitis* identified in soil outside its known range—Washington, 2013. *MMWR Morb Mortal Wkly Rep*. 2014;63:450.
121. Marsden-Haug N, Goldoft M, Ralston C, et al. Coccidioidomycosis acquired in Washington State. *Clin Infect Dis*. 2013;56:847-850.
124. McCarty JM, Demetral LC, Dabrowski L, et al. Pediatric coccidioidomycosis in central California: a retrospective case series. *Clin Infect Dis*. 2013;56:159-185.
125. Mendoza N, Blair JE. The utility of diagnostic testing for active coccidioidomycosis in solid organ transplant recipients. *Am J Transplant*. 2013;13:1034-1039.
127. Mertz LE, Blair JE. Coccidioidomycosis in rheumatology patients: incidence and possible risk factors. *Ann N Y Acad Sci*. 2007;1111:343-357.
129. Mitchell M, Dizon D, Libke R, et al. Development of a real-time PCR assay for identification of *Coccidioides immitis* by use of the BD Max system. *J Clin Microbiol*. 2015;53:926-929.
146. Sampaio EP, Hsu AP, Pechacek J, et al. Signal transducer and activator transcription 1 (STAT1) gain-of-function mutations and disseminated coccidioidomycosis and histoplasmosis. *J Allergy Clin Immunol*. 2013;131:1624-1634.
159. Sobonya RE, Yanes J, Klotz SA. Cavitary pulmonary coccidioidomycosis: pathologic and clinical correlates of disease. *Hum Pathol*. 2014;45:153-159.
170. Turabelidze G, Aggu-Sher RK, Jahanpour E, et al. Coccidioidomycosis in a state where it is not known to be endemic—Missouri, 2004–2013. *MMWR Morb Mortal Wkly Rep*. 2015;64:636-639.
176. Viriyakosol S, Jimenez Mdel P, Gurney MA, et al. Dectin-1 is required for resistance to coccidioidomycosis in mice. *MBio*. 2013;4:e00597-12.
179. Wack EE, Ampel NM, Sunenshine RH, et al. The return of delayed-type hypersensitivity skin testing for coccidioidomycosis. *Clin Infect Dis*. 2015;61:787-791.
180. Wang H, LeBert V, Hung CY, et al. C-type lectin receptors differentially induce Th17 cells and vaccine immunity to the endemic mycosis of North America. *J Immunol*. 2014;192:1107-1119.
183. Wieden MA, Lundergan LL, Blum J, et al. Detection of coccidioidal antibodies by 33-kDa spherule antigen, *Coccidioides* EIA, and standard serologic tests in sera from patients evaluated for coccidioidomycosis. *J Infect Dis*. 1996;173:1273-1277.
188. Zangeneh TT, Malo J, Luraschi-Mmonjagatta C, et al. Positive (1-3)-β-D-Glucan and cross reactivity of fungal assays in coccidioidomycosis. *Med Mycol*. 2015;53:171-173.

The full reference list for this chapter is available at ExpertConsult.com.

202 Paracoccidioidomycosis

Gil Benard • Maria José Soares Mendes-Giannini

Paracoccidioidomycosis, formerly known as South American blastomycosis, caused by *Paracoccidioides brasiliensis* and *Paracoccidioides lutzii*, is usually a progressive chronic disease that preferentially affects the lungs, skin, mucous membranes, adrenals, and reticuloendothelial system. Benign, self-limited infections also have been occasionally documented. Two types of clinical presentations are described: the acute-subacute (juvenile) and the chronic (adult) forms of the disease.[101] The prevalence of the disease is limited to the American continent, from Mexico to Argentina. The differences between the clinical forms may be related to multiple factors, among them, deforestation at agricultural frontiers, as occurs in some Brazil regions. Occupational exposure of children and young adults to different species of *Paracoccidioides* during agricultural work may be larger at these places.[92]

Children generally present with the acute form, which affects predominantly the reticuloendothelial system organs. Children account for about 5% to 10% of cases, and both sexes are infected*; the systemic form of paracoccidioidomycosis occurs in about 70% of episodes.[24,29,136,154,184] The disease is acquired by soil aerosolization and inhaling of infectious particles of *Paracoccidioides* spp.[40,100] The mycosis is limited geographically to various Latin American countries†, but some cases of paracoccidioidomycosis have been reported and diagnosed in countries outside Latin America.[40,43,57,118,127,133] This disease may be considered a traveler's disease in this condition[200] and now is included among the neglected diseases.[119]

The disease was described originally by Lutz in Brazil in 1908 and initially observed in children in 1911.[128]

ORGANISM

The *Paracoccidioides* genus consists of dimorphic fungi, the etiologic agents of paracoccidioidomycosis. Currently, phylogenetic studies divide the *Paracoccidioides* genus in two species, named *Paracoccidioides brasiliensis* (S1, PS2, PS3, and PS4 phylogenetic species) and *P. lutzii* (Pb01-like).[149,247,171,252]

The recognition of *Paracoccidioides* spp. as an anamorph in the phylum Ascomycota, order Onygenales, family Ajellomycetaceae has been accomplished by means of molecular tools.[28,261] *Paracoccidioides* spp. are phylogenetically closer to *Lacazia loboi* than to *Blastomyces dermatitidis, Emmonsia parva,* and *Histoplasma capsulatum.*[261]

The fungus has four or five DNA chromosomes showing molecular sizes ranging from 2 to 10 Mb.[50,93,164] The genomes range in size from 29.1 to 32.9 Mb and encode 7610 to 9132 genes,[1,82] which is in agreement with the estimated gene number for ascomycete fungi genomes. Genomic analysis of *P. brasiliensis* and *P. lutzii* pointed to important differences. Although the genome sizes of the two cryptic species (S1/Pb18 and PS2/Pb03) of *P. brasiliensis* are comparable (30 Mb and 29.1 Mb, respectively), the *P. lutzii* genome is almost 3 Mb larger (32.9 Mb). The total number of initial predicted genes varies between 7875 in *P. brasiliensis* and 9132 in *P. lutzii*. Transposons may be one of the reasons for the widening of *P. lutzii* genome because they constitute 16% of it, twice as much as that of *P. brasiliensis* S1/Pb18 and PS2/Pb03 genomes (8–9%).[82]

Differences between *P. lutzii* and *P. brasiliensis* (S1, PS2, and PS3 species) were also observed in their proteomic yeast profiles by means of two-dimensional electrophoresis and mass spectrometry. The expression levels of the enzymes related to glycolysis suggested the use of a more anaerobic metabolism for energy production from glucose in the *P. lutzii* (Pb01 isolate).[195]

Paracoccidioides spp. genome information is available at: http://www.broad.mit.edu/annotation/genome/paracoccidioides_brasiliensis.

Paracoccidioides spp., a thermally dimorphic fungus, appears as round to oval yeast cells of variable size (6–40 μm) in tissues and culture at 37°C, and in the environment or in vitro at temperatures lower than 24°C it changes its morphology to the mold form when cultured under starvation conditions in minimal media. Conidia and mycelial fragments are considered the infectious particles. When inhaled, they reach the alveoli, where, at the host tissue's temperature (37°C), they change from their saprophytic form to the parasitic multiple budding yeast form capable of producing disease.[128,198,199] Another important fact is that *P. brasiliensis* is able to form biofilm in vitro, which opens up new possibilities in understanding the infection process of these fungi[53,77] because biofilm formation is a condition that provides for the pathogen's protection against drugs and the host's immune system.[227]

Different groups have addressed the overall scenario of gene expression in *Paracoccidioides* spp. yeast versus mycelium, or undergoing phase transition in vitro, making use of different molecular methods.[14,94,108,117,126,138,179,185] Many genes were also described related to conidia,[116] in the parasitic phase in vitro[37,70,236] as well as in vivo models of infection.[10,9,70,88,111,134,151,159,160,178,194,237] Recently, this approach focused on identification of regulated transcripts analysis of *Paracoccidioides* spp. yeast cells treated with different drugs.[69]

In the mycelial phase, growth is slow, requiring approximately 3 to 4 weeks; the colony is white to tan and compact, with short aerial mycelia. On microscopic examination, hyphae are fine (0.8–2.5 μm in diameter), septate, interlaced, and hyaline. Chlamydoconidia (20–50 μm in diameter) that are round to subspherical, terminal, and intercalary, as well as arthroconidia, may be observed.[128,206,234] Some isolates can produce aleurioconidia, uninucleate pear-shaped pedunculated or terminal structures, after long periods of incubation and under nutritional deprivation (media with reduced carbohydrate content).[40,128,210] The small size of these conidia (<5 μm) renders them compatible with alveolar deposition; furthermore, such conidia have been shown to be infectious when they are inhaled.[152]

The mycelial phase is not distinctive, and subcultures at 37°C are required for complete identification. At this temperature, *P. brasiliensis* produces soft, wrinkled, cream-colored colonies that develop in approximately 6 to 10 days. On microscopic examination, the most characteristic feature is the presence of multiple budding yeast cells; the parental cell produces various peripheral buds and acquires the appearance of a pilot's wheel. *P. brasiliensis* may possess alternative control mechanisms during cell growth to manage multiple budding and its multinucleate nature.[1] Single buds and short chains also are produced, but they are not diagnostic. Cells are variable in size (2–40 μm) and have a thick cell wall and internal vacuoles.[40,199] Differences in daughter cells were observed in relation to the two species,[240,247,248,252] as well as in sporulation (concerning conidia amount and morphology) among the different cryptic species: S1 isolates produce a higher conidia amount compared with other *P. brasiliensis* and *P. lutzii*. The growth is identical to the one observed in tissue and pathologic materials.[40,102,128,199,206] The organism does not readily take most bacterial or hematologic stains. *P. brasiliensis* is aerobic, but to form biofilm in vitro it needs hypoxic conditions.[227] The fungus in mycelial phase grows well in the regular mycologic media to which antibiotics and cycloheximide have been added to reduce growth of bacteria and saprophytic fungi. Isolation should be attempted by the use of modified Sabouraud agar, yeast extract (15%) agar plus antibiotics and cycloheximide, yeast extract–phosphate agar, brain-heart infusion agar plus blood and antibiotics, or tryptic soy agar plus fungus water extract and horse serum, incubated at room temperature.[40,128]

TRANSMISSION

Paracoccidioidomycosis is not a contagious disease.[40,102,128,206,267] A single case of placental involvement that did not result in fetal infection has been reported.[32] Epidemic outbreaks have not been reported, and only a few cases in family members have been documented,[128,130,267] which could be attributed to the long periods of mycosis latency between the moment of infection and the appearance of overt clinical manifestations.[205] Consequently, the patient's memory of the activity contributing to the infection or of the accompanying individuals usually has been forgotten, which prompted Borelli[36] to coin the name "reservarea" for those places in the endemic areas where the fungus has its habitat and humans acquire the infection.[209] This concept differs from that of an endemic area, which implicates the place where the disease is diagnosed.

P. brasiliensis infection in animals as proved by culture or histologic examination has been shown consistently in armadillos, mammals that probably acquire the infection when they disturb the terrestrial habitat of the fungus,[7,45,204,215,238,249] and more recently in a dog.[74,212] The spatial distribution of the pathogens has been done by molecular detection from soil[4,86,239,267] and by their isolation from wild animals such as armadillos.[4,63,238] This approach is important for monitoring their environmental and geographical distribution.[4]

Unfortunately, the microniche of *P. brasiliensis* has not been identified properly; soil has been incriminated, but the number of isolates from this source is small.[204,251,267] The inhibitory effect of pesticides on *P. brasiliensis* may suggest that they can interfere with attempts to isolate *P. brasiliensis* from soil.[181] Recently, the role played by deforestation in increasing both exposure and incidence rates has been documented in Brazil in Amerindians and in children.[59,98,148,215]

Some studies are developed related to presence of the fungus in environmental aerosol samples[2] and related to climate change.[13,12] Species-specific inner primers derived from rDNA regions (internal transcribed spacer [ITS], 5.8S gene) have been described, and the nested

*References 11, 22, 25, 55, 86, 96, 98, 112, 115, 130, 173.

†References 7, 16, 33, 36, 40, 41, 43, 61, 128, 144, 184, 204, 234.

polymerase chain reaction (PCR) sensitivity was higher for the detection of *P. brasiliensis* in soil than in culture and animal inoculation. The fungus was detected in soil artificially seeded (positive soil control) and from environmental samples collected in an armadillo burrow.[251] This approach probably would improve the fungal microniche studies. *P. brasiliensis* S1 and PS2 species (São Paulo state, Brazil) and PS3 (Colombia) have been highly recovered from the armadillos *Dasypus novemcinctus* and *Cabassous centralis* in endemic areas, whereas no *P. lutzii* has been isolated from these animals yet.[4]

The ecologic factors that prevail in the reservarea also have been characterized, with the following being significantly associated with the disease: altitude 1000 to 1499 m above sea level, annual rainfall 2000 to 2999 mm, and presence of humid forests and of coffee and tobacco crops.[47] Environmental correlates (soil texture and precipitation) indicate that moisture availability plays an important role in paracoccidioidomycosis distribution.[239] The fertile regions of endemic areas have the highest incidence rates of paracoccidioidomycosis.[47,144,256]

Paracoccidioidomycosis was thought, and still is by some, to be acquired by trauma. However, clinical and experimental data indicate that infection is acquired most commonly by inhalation.[40,112,130,211]

EPIDEMIOLOGY

Paracoccidioidomycosis is a fungal diseases with high medical and social impact in areas of high endemicity because of the considerable number of cases, chronicity of the disease, treatment, and frequent sequelae that cause inability to work and poor quality of life. The epidemiology of this disease has some difficulties because of the noncompulsory notification, the difficulty in recognizing the recently acquired infection, and the absence of epidemic outbreaks.

INCIDENCE

The incidence of paracoccidioidomycosis was estimated at 0.71 to 9.40 per 100,000 inhabitants per year, depending on the region.[16,40,55,144] Some South America countries have a lower incidence of paracoccidioidomycosis, with the exception of Brazil and Colombia.[61] The incidence of the mycosis may temporarily reach higher rates in areas with major socioenvironmental changes.

Age

Patients with paracoccidioidomycosis vary in age from 2 to more than 80 years.[11,16,33,52,55,128,130,267] The prevalence is higher (>70%) in patients who are 30 years or older. The number of childhood cases was shown to vary from 2.1% to 12.7% in the first decade of life, depending on the region.[16,33,55,98,130,184] These series, some compilations,[25,177,191,189] several individual reports, and a thesis[11] have revealed that the disease occurs more frequently in individuals 12 to 15 years of age than in younger children (Table 202.1). More than 250 reports of paracoccidioidomycosis in children aged 3 to 14 years, including those analyzed by Londero and colleagues[130] have been found in a literature search. Bellissimo-Rodrigues and colleagues[16] described 1219 patients, among whom 196 (16%) were younger than 21 years, and 42 (3.4%) were 3 to 10 years of age. Other studies reported incidence rates of 15.4% to 20% in the Midwest or Southeast regions of Brazil.[33,184]

The intradermal application of *P. brasiliensis* antigens is used to measure delayed hypersensitivity and most frequently is used to detect asymptomatic infection with the fungus. In certain places, the infection rates measured by a positive skin test reaction also were high. In 1976, Pedrosa[188] found that 34% of the children tested positive for paracoccidioidin, a figure indicative of early exposure to the fungus. The prevalence of infection with *P. brasiliensis* was evaluated in a cross-sectional study of 298 asymptomatic schoolchildren in the Brazilian Amazon region. The skin test reactivity of children was 4.6% to two different *P. brasiliensis* antigen preparations, paracoccidioidin and a purified 43-kDa glycoprotein (gp43).[123]

TABLE 202.1 Age and Gender Distribution in 354 Children With Paracoccidioidomycosis

	AGE		
Gender[a]	***3–9 y***	***10–14 y***	**Total by Gender (%)**
Male	95	125	220
Female	63	71	134
Total by age	158 (41.8%)	196 (58.2%)	354 (100%)

[a]Male-to-female ratio = 1.6:1.
Data from references 33, 58, 60, 98, 162, 176, 188, 189, 216, 218.

The relative paucity of children with this mycosis in comparison with the figures reported in adults[40,128,267] may be explained, in part, by the effective control exerted by most hosts on the progression of the primary infection, by the long incubation period characteristic of the mycosis, and by the establishment of latent foci that may become apparent clinically many years after initial exposure.[20,40,101,106,205,267]

Benard and associates[22] consider that the association with different age groups is related to the epidemiology of paracoccidioidomycosis because in the endemic areas, as previously shown, children become exposed to the fungus at an early age. In healthy children, appropriate defenses usually curtail development of the mycosis, but in infants of low socioeconomic conditions, the transition from infection to overt disease may be accelerated and aggravated by the mycosis itself, by malnutrition, or by other associated conditions.[17,24,25,33,106,216] In addition, unknown susceptibility factors, the intensity of exposure to the infectious source, the virulence of certain isolates, and other factors may well contribute to the development of the disease in children.[20,60,97,98,114,130,267] The reduction in acute-subacute cases observed in the recent descriptions may be related to the lower exposure of children and adolescents to the fungus as a result of the intense public policy aimed at reducing child labor in agriculture.[92]

Gender

Adult men are afflicted with much greater frequency than are women, but the male-to-female ratio varies according to geographic region.[33,40,98,155,174] In children, however, the disease affects boys and girls in approximately equal proportions.[33,47,55,130,176,215,267] (see Table 202.1). These findings suggest that sex hormones, hormone-dependent immunologic factors, or both play a role in determining the outcome of the host-parasite interaction.[6,5,40] Researchers have shown in vitro that estrogens inhibit *Paracoccidioides* mycelium to yeast transition, thereby hindering the progression of the infection.[6,228] Analysis of the mortality profile from paracoccidioidomycosis according to gender and age showed similar death totals for both genders in the groups younger than 20 years. The majority of deaths among male patients (97.14%) occurred in individuals older than 15 years, with only 2.37% among individuals younger than 15 years. Among female patients, most deaths from paracoccidioidomycosis (89.21%) also occurred in those older than 15 years, but 9.75% did occur in those younger than 15 years; that rate is nearly 5 times the percentage observed in males. These findings corroborate the literature, according to which the infection and disease occur equally between the genders during childhood, with a slight predominance of males with the disease, compared with an absolute predominance of males among adults with the chronic form of the mycosis.[65]

Occupation and Race

Almost half of the reported cases in adults occur in individuals whose occupations require extensive exposure to the soil. Adult residents of areas in which paracoccidioidomycosis is endemic generally develop disease less severe than that seen in immigrants or in people who migrate to highly endemic settings. These people often develop disseminated infection, much like the juvenile cases do. The proportion of acute-subacute cases observed in the Bellissimo-Rodrigues study[16] (26.4%) might be explained by the higher proportion of children, women, and African descendants. The influence of genetic traits on the mycosis has not been elucidated,[84] but in patients with the unifocal chronic form of the disease, a mild clinical presentation in which lesions are restricted or localized, the HLA allele most commonly seen was DRB1*11, suggesting that the participation of HLA antigens may influence the outcome of the host-parasite interaction in paracoccidioidomycosis.[222]

Geographic Distribution

Paracoccidioidomycosis is restricted to Latin America, from Mexico to Argentina; some countries within this area (Chile and some of the Caribbean Islands), however, are free of the disease. In endemic countries, the disease distribution is uneven, and most cases occur in individuals living in regions corresponding to the humid tropical and subtropical forests. The endemic area is centered in Brazil (80% of the reported cases), followed by Venezuela, Colombia, Ecuador, and Argentina.[33,128,130,141,267] New endemic areas have been reported in the Amazon region, where the mycosis was considered to be rare. In Brazil, this fungal infection is considered to be a very important cause of mortality among infectious diseases, with a rate of 1.45 cases per 1 million inhabitants.[31,65,141,148] Paracoccidioidomycosis represented the most important cause of deaths among systemic mycoses[65,196] (approximately 51.2%).

Although paracoccidioidomycosis has been reported in patients not living in endemic areas, prior residence in Latin America has been documented in every cases.[43,45,118,124,133,239] In some of these patients, the interval between residence in the endemic area and clinical manifestations of the disease has been 10 to 40 years.[43,128] Within endemic areas, 2% (among children) to 82%, react to the intradermal administration of paracoccidioidin, suggesting previous contact or subclinical infection with *P. brasiliensis*.[40,45,59,61,123] Even though the mycosis is powerfully related to the rural environment, cases of paracoccidioidomycosis acquired in suburban areas have also been described.

P. brasiliensis is a complex species,[149,150] and phylogenetic studies have revealed that this species actually contains at least five cryptic phylogenetic species.[247,248] *P. brasiliensis* S1 is associated with most paracoccidioidomycosis cases and is widely distributed in South America by means of armadillos, soil, and penguin feces. Recently, S1 lineage was separated into two clades (S1a and S1b); S1b presented high recombination, and all of the S1b strains are clinical isolates and include virulent strains, although not differentiate clinical forms.[171] PS2 comprises a paraphyletic and recombining population that has been identified so far only in Brazil and Venezuela; PS3 comprises a monophyletic and clonal population that has been recovered in humans and armadillos in endemic regions of Colombia; and PS4 was recently identified and is composed of a monophyletic population of clinical isolates from Venezuela.[4,149,150,214,247,248,224,250] *P. lutzii* comprises a single monophyletic and recombining population found to date in central, southwest, and northern Brazil and Ecuador. Despite the apparently restricted ecologic niche, the habitat of the etiologic agent has not been determined precisely.[4,100,171,204]

PATHOGENESIS AND PATHOLOGY

The initial stages of the host-parasite interaction are unknown because of our inability to detect the precise moment when infection does occur.[17] However, through the study of many cases, including autopsies, what has become apparent is that pulmonary lesions are primary, with the infection taking place by inhalation of fungal propagules.[22,106,208] In experimental animals, the inhalatory route has been shown to give rise to disseminated disease.[152] In most cases, the initial pulmonary infection does not cause undue symptoms.[101,130] When the conidia reach the terminal bronchi or the alveolar spaces, yeast transformation ensues.[152] In some cases, the fungus promptly disseminates by the lymphohematogenous route, producing distant subclinical and quiescent foci. Apparently, the local defenses are capable of controlling fungal spread, but some viable yeast cells may remain dormant in such foci, most commonly in the pulmonary and mediastinal lymph nodes, and eventually in other organs.[41,23] Rarely, the initial pulmonary infection outweighs the host's immune defenses, causing an acute-subacute disease, the juvenile type, with predominant involvement of the reticuloendothelial system.[64,101] The disease in children falls into this category. Often, the quiescent foci remain so throughout life, as demonstrated by the high number of subclinical infections compared with the low disease incidence of this mycosis in the endemic regions.[99,267] Nevertheless, the most common clinical presentation of the disease is the chronic form, or adult-type disease, believed to result from fungal reactivation in these foci.[101] This reactivation frequently occurs when the patient has left the endemic area, as demonstrated by the cases reported outside Latin America, in countries where paracoccidioidomycosis is considered an imported pathology.[57] Of note, these cases may manifest decades after leaving the endemic area, leading to difficult and delayed diagnosis.[118]

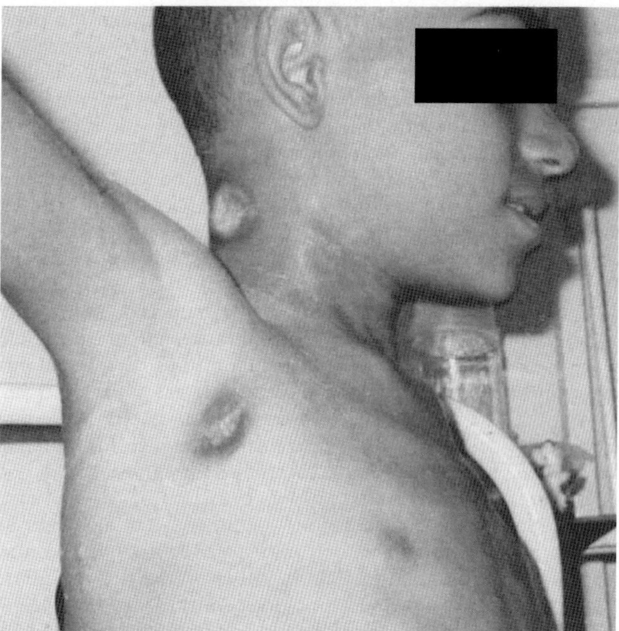

FIG. 202.1 An 11-year-old boy with a 5-month history of fever and cervical and axillary lymph node enlargement, with fistulization.

Thus, in the acute-subacute form, the initial lung infection may pass unnoticed but is followed by prompt dissemination to other organs and tissues.[22] In the chronic form, lung pathology frequently occurs. Pathology is restricted to the lungs in some of these patients, but in most, other organs also are afflicted. This may be caused by lymphohematogenous dissemination from reactivated pulmonary foci or directly from foci at virtually any organ.[23,41] Actually, paracoccidioidomycosis, in the acute-subacute or chronic forms, is more frequently a disseminated disease, even though clinical manifestations may appear to be restricted to a sole organ.[101,269] However, determination of the degree of dissemination certainly is influenced by the availability of diagnostic procedures. After appropriate therapy, residual lesions, mostly fibrotic, become established in a nonnegligible number of patients and represent the actual main challenge in this diasease.[64,102,154]

As already mentioned, the disease in children is acute-subacute and progressive (the juvenile form).[25,55,130] The time that elapses between infection and the onset of symptoms is not known precisely but has been estimated to be short in most cases, such as a few months according to the rare case reports with putative known date of infection.[41,101] The juvenile form is usually a severe, systemic disorder that involves preferentially the reticuloendothelial system (Fig. 202.1) to such an extent that it is the hallmark of the process.[11,25,130]

In adults, pulmonary lesions as seen on chest plain films may be defined as micronodular or miliary, nodular, infiltrative or interstitial, cavitary, fibrotic, and mixed types.[154,262] Emphysematous areas, pleural thickening, and enlarged hilar and mediastinal lymph nodes also can be observed. These alterations can be better visualized by computed tomography.[103,241] Lung involvement probably is secondary to a chronic lymphangitic process provoked by the fungus itself and the host's response represented by formation of granulomas and fibrosis, the latter of which predominates at the perihilar region. This aspect correlates with the butterfly-like (perihilar) micronodular and interstitial infiltration observed on plain films.[260] Obstruction and reversal of lymphatic flow would lead to the spread of the inflammatory process throughout the lungs.[260]

In children and adolescents, the pulmonary component tends to pass unnoticed, and neither clinical examination nor radiologic studies reflect the real damage.[106] Actually, only a minor proportion of the cases reported have included lung symptoms.[130,210] However, lack of notification may be more apparent than reality because the weight of the extrapulmonary lesions tends to minimize the less intense respiratory manifestations. Frequently, the mycosis is misdiagnosed, especially for tuberculosis and certain lymphomatous disorders.[130] Nonetheless, a careful search of pulmonary samples, including induced sputum, may reveal the characteristic multiple-budding *P. brasiliensis* yeast cells.[130,211] Moreover, gallium and computed tomography have allowed detection of incipient or discrete interstitial pulmonary lesions not revealed by plain radiographs.[103,269]

Lesions in the oropharyngeal and laryngeal mucosa occur frequently in the chronic form. They may be infiltrative, ulcerated, nodular, or vegetative and usually have a granulomatous aspect and may mimic squamous cell carcinoma.[29,154,161,226] The base of the ulcerated lesions usually is covered by small abscesses (the mulberry-like lesions) that probably represent fungal dissemination through the lymphatic system because they usually are accompanied by regional lymph node involvement.[54]

In children, such mucosal lesions are rather exceptional, but skin involvement occurs more commonly and tends to be multiple, in contrast with the adult chronic form.[154] In the latter, lesions are represented mostly by contiguous involvement of the periorificial mucosal lesions or draining lymph nodes. In children or young adults, and eventually in adults with the chronic severe disseminated disease, they represent hematogenous spread of the fungus. In this case, the lesions may appear as ulcerated or ulcerovegetative lesions, papules, or crust-covered ulcers and warts, usually at the same stage of development. Skin involvement may rarely present as sarcoid-like lesions.[60,173] Reports of septic shock caused by septicemia by *P. brasiliensis* show that the fungus can be bloodborne.[115]

The reticuloendothelial system is the target organ in both children and young adults.[11] Almost every child with paracoccidioidomycosis exhibits involvement of the superficial or deep lymph node chains. Lymph nodes vary in size, number, consistency, and location; with time, they may liquefy, forming abscesses or fistulas (Fig. 202.2). The spleen and liver frequently are involved in these same groups. Abdominal lymph node involvement also is a common occurrence in children.[11,130] Hypertrophied lymph nodes, usually generalized but particularly periaortic, around the hepatic hilum and retroperitoneally, can be detected by ultrasonography (see Fig. 202.2), computed tomography, or magnetic resonance imaging.[145] Coalescent masses may become palpable and may result in pathology caused by extrinsic compression of adjacent structures, such as jaundice by compression of the biliary duct,[33] pancreatitis,[33] or an intestinal obstruction.[146]

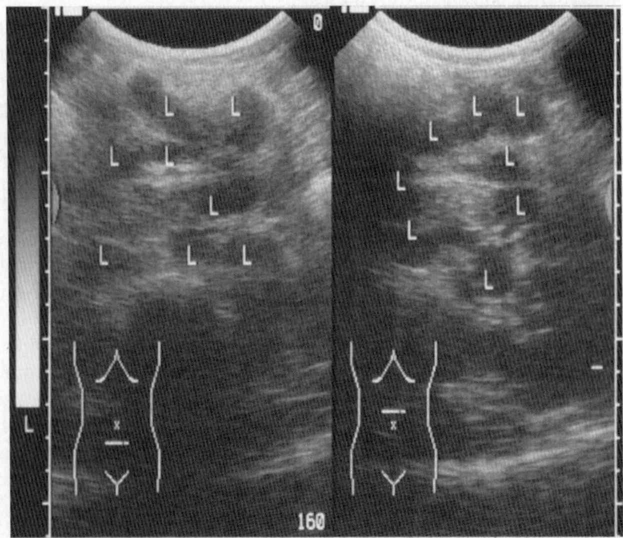

FIG. 202.2 Extensive mesenteric lymph node enlargement *(L)* in a 10-year-old boy as shown by ultrasonography imaging.

Splenic lesions are nodular or miliary. Gross hepatic lesions may not be apparent, but histopathologic examination regularly reveals fungal invasion of this organ.[11,25,34,130] In a series of fatal cases of paracoccidioidomycosis, 56.7% revealed the presence of yeast cells in the liver, associated with a granulomatous tissue response. Thirty percent of the patients had only widening of the portal tracts by fibrosis (31.6%), whereas 11.6% had an essentially normal liver.[246] Younger patients and those with severe hypoalbuminemia are more likely to present with liver involvement by *P. brasiliensis*.[39]

The intestinal mucosa may be affected, but similar to the lungs, its involvement is secondary to blockade of the regional lymphatic flow, with retrograde progression of *Paracoccidioides* spp. to the mucosa, a process resulting in mycotic enteritis.[33,97,146] In this case, the submucosal inflammatory process is granulomatous; fungal cells are visualized; and the intestinal changes may vary from dilated loops, edema, congestion, and nodule formation to multiple mucosal ulcers.[97,146]

Studies also have shown bone marrow infiltration mainly, but not exclusively, in the acute-subacute form of the disease: in a small case series report, 25.7% of the patients examined during active disease and 36.4% of those who died of paracoccidioidomycosis revealed this type of involvement.[202] Bone marrow necrosis has also been reported in the juvenile form.[203] The histology pattern was variable, but appropriate staining always displayed fungal cells. Bone marrow invasion frequently is associated with marked eosinophilia.[202,232] In addition, bone (Fig. 202.3) and joint lesions are frequent occurrences in the acute-subacute form of the disease[3,25,130,259] and appear closely related to bone marrow infiltration.[202]

The adrenals often are involved in patients with the chronic form of the mycosis, with a small proportion of the patients evolving to adrenal hypofunction or insufficiency (Addison disease). The glands contain multiple granulomatous foci, and diffuse necrosis may be seen in the most severe cases. Hyperplasia of the adrenal glands also occurs commonly.[154] Adrenal insufficiency has been documented in patients even after prolonged posttherapy follow up.[254]

Histologically, formation of granulomas is the rule, except in patients with severe disseminated disease such as those with the acute-subacute form.[102] The granulomatous inflammation is associated with a mixed pyogenic component, especially in the case of ulcerated skin lesions or ruptured lymph nodes.[183] Caseation and central necrosis may be present. In compact granulomas, abundant epithelial cells, Langerhans or foreign-body giant cells, plasmacytes, and lymphocytes are seen; often, phagocytosis of the yeast cells can be observed. $CD4^+$ lymphocytes dominate over $CD8^+$ lymphocytes and appear as peripheral mantles around aggregates of macrophages and histiocytes.[168] In the juvenile disseminated disease, the inflammatory reaction is diffuse, with abundance of both mononuclear and yeast cells but sparse formation of compact granulomas.[55,210] Loose granulomas appear unable to circumscribe fungal antigens, and at their periphery, *Paracoccidioides* spp. antigens may permeate throughout the intercellular space.[225] Skin and mucous membrane lesions usually exhibit pseudoepitheliomatous hyperplasia and intraepithelial microabscesses.[186,225] The role of neutrophils in the inflammatory response against *Paracoccidioides* spp. has recently been investigated, and it was shown that neutrophil extracellular traps are present in tegumentary lesions of patients.[79]

An interesting aspect drawn from the previously described histologic studies is the frequent description of areas of extremely active disease characterized by pyogenic reaction and loose granulomas, rich in budding fungal cells, intermingled with areas with compact granulomas, rare fungal cells, and variable degrees of fibrosis. This mixed aspect can be observed in lymph nodes, skin, or pulmonary lesions, suggesting that the disease evolves through localized new bouts of fungal multiplication and tissue invasion, whereas the adjacent older lesions are on their way to fibrotic resolution. Computed tomography of the lung confirmed this aspect by depicting areas with alveolar condensation along with fibrotic and emphysematous zones and the simultaneous presence of features of more recent and chronic lesions.[103,241]

Tissue reactions are nonspecific; thus diagnosis depends on finding *P. brasiliensis*. If the parasite is abundant, it may be identified by hematoxylin and eosin stains. Special fungal stains (e.g., Grocott silver methenamine), however, always should be employed, especially when

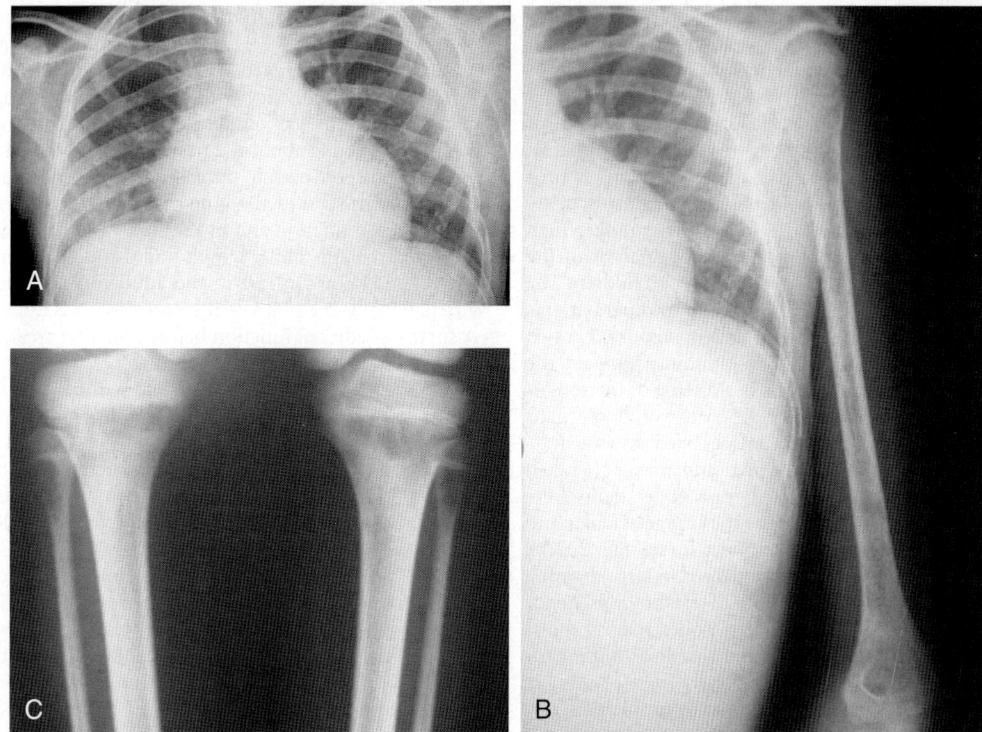

FIG. 202.3 Severe disseminated subacute paracoccidioidomycosis in a 9-year-old boy. (A) The chest radiograph shows mediastinal lymph node enlargement and mild bilateral infiltrates in the middle and lower fields. Osteolytic lesions of long bones: (B) humerus and (C) tibia and fibula bilaterally.

granulomas are examined. The typical multiple budding yeast cells must be found to establish a diagnosis. The presence of fungal cells of different sizes (2–40 μm) suggests the presence of *P. brasiliensis*. In some cases, short chains and cells with single buds also are observed, and in these patients, differentiation of *P. brasiliensis* from *Cryptococcus neoformans*, *Blastomyces dermatitidis*, and even *H. capsulatum* and *Pneumocystis jirovecii* must be made.[40,235] When the disease is chronic, most of the fungal cells are found inside the macrophages, but free yeast cells predominate in disseminated cases. Internalized yeast cells exhibit altered morphology.[205]

Like other chronic granulomatous diseases, paracoccidioidomycosis is also phenotypically a spectral disease, with the acute-subacute form of the disease characterized by poor cellular immune responses; high fungal burden; high anti-*Paracoccidioides* antibody titers, including those of the immunoglobulin E (IgE) subclass; and eosinophilia—all of which are typical of a predominance of helper T-cell subtype 2 (Th2) over Th1 immune responses.[17] Conversely, some patients with the chronic form have a localized disease, low fungal burden, compact granulomas, and low antibody titers, suggesting that they are still able to mount Th1 responses. The latter patients would eventually have a specific "protective" genetic background.[222] In between would stay the chronic multifocal patients with deficient Th1 responses without marked shift to Th2 responses.[17] However, the simplistic view of a Th1/Th2 paradigm of immune response has been complicated further by the description of new subtypes of helper T cells such as Th17 cells, Th9 cells, and Th22 cells. The clinical phenotypes presented by these patients have recently been associated with these subsets, and in the acute-subacute form a mixed Th2/Th9 response was detected predominantly, whereas in the chronic form there was a balance between Th1, Th17, and Th22 responses depending on the extent of the disease.[73]

CLINICAL MANIFESTATIONS

Paracoccidioidomycosis is a polymorphic disorder that at a particular time may involve more than one organ system (Table 202.2). Thus, making a topographic classification is unrealistic, and the classification of the mycosis currently accepted takes into consideration not only the organs involved but also the host's immune condition and the disease's natural history.[101] The infection is categorized as a subclinical form, and the overt process is subdivided into acute-subacute or chronic disease. The acute-subacute pattern predominates in children and young adults, although the disease is also called the *juvenile form*, whereas the chronic disease affects adults and aged people and is thus called the *adult form*. According to the severity of the process, juvenile patients are assigned to two subgroups: severe and moderate. The adult form may be localized to pulmonary lesions, be unifocal disease, or be disseminated from its primary foci, the multifocal process. Disseminated

TABLE 202.2 Clinical Findings on Admission Diagnosis in Children With Paracoccidioidomycosis

Clinical Findings	No. of Children (%)[a]
Lymph node enlargement	
Superficial	81.6
Thoracic	25
Abdominal	36.6
Abdominal masses	19.9
Hepatomegaly or splenomegaly	60.7
Ascites	19.1
Jaundice	10.5
Diarrhea, vomiting, abdominal pain, or distention	19.1
Joint or bone lesions	37.8
Skin lesions	29.1
Respiratory symptoms	9.1
Pulmonary consolidations or infiltrates	10.2
Pleural effusion	5.1
Oral and upper respiratory tract mucosa lesions	9.2

[a]Total number of children investigated for each clinical finding varied from 98 to 199.
Data from references 3, 16, 60, 89, 98, 133, 162, 176, 189, 208.

disease is characterized by involvement of the skin, mucosa, reticuloendothelial system, adrenal glands, and, less frequently, the gastrointestinal or the genitourinary tract, bones, and central nervous system.[11,106,154,162,210] The chronic form can be mild, moderate, or severe.[101]

Patients with acute or subacute disease develop signs and symptoms of a wasting process. Fever, malaise, listlessness, weight loss, and emaciation are recorded frequently. The severity of these symptoms is proportional to the degree of the organ involvement. Londero and associates reviewed the literature and found 269 cases in children younger than 14 years of age[130]; however, sufficient clinical data for analysis of the prominent organ involvement were provided for only 77 children. The clinical characteristics exhibited by these children and by other patients reported subsequently, including the series of patients reported at two other centers, are shown in Table 202.2. These findings support the notion that juvenile paracoccidioidomycosis is a disease of the reticuloendothelial system resulting in damage of the corresponding organs caused by severe macrophage dysfunction, as suggested previously.[102] Superficial lymph node enlargement was the predominant sign (81.6%) in these cases. Cervical and submandibular lymph node chains were involved most commonly, followed by those of the supraclavicular and axillary regions; however, any chain can be affected (see Fig. 202.1). Lymph nodes may vary in size from slightly enlarged to large, painful, coalescent masses; they may be mobile and of elastic consistency or fixed to the adjacent tissues; hypertrophied nodes may progress to fistulization and discharge purulent material rich in *P. brasiliensis* yeast cells.

The next most important finding was hepatomegaly or splenomegaly (60.7%), which usually was asymptomatic. In a recent report of 102 cases of paracoccidioidomycosis in children younger than age 16, liver involvement was detected in 40%, of whom 68% presented with hepatomegaly and 29% with jaundice.[219] Liver enzymes, especially alkaline phosphatase and γ-glutamyltransferase, were frequently but not markedly increased.[177] Portal hypertension also was a rare occurrence. Importantly, those with liver involvement were younger and had more severe anemia, hypoalbuminemia, and malnutrition, and eventually higher risk for death.[39] Findings and complaints relating to the abdomen and digestive tract, such as presence of abdominal masses, lymph node enlargement, diarrhea, vomiting, abdominal distention or pain, and ascites, also have also been recorded in a sizable proportion of patients (see Table 202.2 and Fig. 202.2). Signs and symptoms of an acute abdomen, caused by masses formed by hypertrophied lymph nodes or perforation, also have been reported; this problem may lead to intestinal occlusion, blockage of lymphatic drainage, and, later, ascites.[11,25,130,176,189]

In a series comprising predominantly patients with the juvenile form of the disease, abdominal radiographic studies (double-contrast barium) revealed ileal and jejunal alterations in 42% to 51%.[97,146,147] The main findings were distortion and coarsening of the mucosal pattern and loop dilation. However, part of these alterations was probably nonspecific because jejunal biopsies performed in a small number of patients revealed neither granulomatous response nor *P. brasiliensis* yeast cells.[147] On the other hand, histopathologic examination of autopsies (likely the more severe cases) showed a specific granulomatous enteritis in 80%.[97] Additionally, in a magnetic resonance imaging study of patients, mostly with the juvenile form, 48% had abdominal lymph node enlargement, even if no abdominal signs and symptoms had been recorded.[145] This lymph node involvement can cause mesenteric lymphatic stasis and enteric mucosal edema that may progress to fungal enteritis accompanied by abnormal intestinal function such as reduced absorption of fat.[147,176,189] Computed tomography and magnetic resonance imaging have proved helpful in determining the extent and nature of abdominal involvement.[147] Abdominal complications continue to be occasionally reported in more recent series.[136,176,189]

Bone damage and articular problems also are important components (37.8%) of disseminated disease, especially in younger children. In these patients, the long bones were frequently affected, with the lytic lesions located at the diaphyseal or metaphyseal-epiphyseal regions,[3,165] probably because of their higher vascularization, emphasizing the hematogenous dissemination that typically occurs in this form of the disease (see Fig. 202.3). Ribs, skull, phalanges, and vertebral lytic lesions also have been documented (see Fig. 202.3). Differently from the painful, motion-restriction joint lesions, the bone lesions can be silent or olygosymptomatic.[3,25,89,165] Pathologic fractures occasionally may occur.[163]

Skin lesions were noted in 29.1% of the juvenile cases, with a tendency toward higher frequency with increasing patient age. Distribution of cutaneous lesions was variable, but face and trunk were involved more frequently.[154] Lung abnormalities were recorded in a smaller proportion of cases. However, even in the absence of clinical and radiologic involvement, colonization of the lung by *P. brasiliensis* can be demonstrated by direct examination and by culture.[211] When chest radiographs were abnormal, enlarged hilar lymph nodes and miliary infiltrates predominated.[106,130,211] In contrast to the adult form of the disease, in which adrenal involvement is a serious concern, it is uncommon in children. A survey of adrenal function before and after treatment in 23 children has shown normal adrenal function.[190]

Anemia, an increased erythrocyte sedimentation rate, severe hypoalbuminemia, and hypergammaglobulinemia with high IgG serum concentrations are found regularly.[11,25,102,177] Nonetheless, anti-*Paracoccidioides* antibodies may prove undetectable in some patients with localized disease and low fungal burden or because of the production of low avidity antibodies.[175] Eosinophilia, as well as elevated IgE antibody titers, has been detected in most patients.[177,232,270]

The association between human immunodeficiency virus (HIV) infection and paracoccidioidomycosis has been investigated.[20,166] However, the youngest patient reported was a 15-year-old boy who had enlargement of superficial and mediastinal lymph nodes, skin nodules, and pulmonary infiltrates.[58] The mycosis was also diagnosed occasionally in other patients whose immune function was depressed by certain conditions or medications.[139,220] The incidence of this mycosis has not increased in HIV-infected patients as would have been expected.[20] No report of paracoccidioidomycosis and HIV coinfection in children has so far been published. In the chronic, progressive, adult form of paracoccidioidomycosis, signs and symptoms differ substantially from those found in children. Descriptions of the disease in adults are beyond the scope of this text but are referenced.[154,226]

DIAGNOSIS

Specific diagnosis depends solely on laboratory confirmation.[68] The gold standard for paracoccidioidomycosis diagnosis is the direct observation of characteristic multiple-budding cells in biologic fluids and tissue sections or the isolation of the fungus from clinical specimens, but it may take up to 6 weeks to produce some results. In this sense, as an adjunct to clinical and histologic findings, the immunodiagnosis based on the detection of antibodies or fungal antigens is frequently used and is of a special value.[68]

However, because of the discovery of different species, the serology of paracoccidioidomycosis is now a challenge for diagnosis because there is no universal antigen. This feature may have led to a substantial number of false-negative results.[15,105] Since the mid-2000s, several molecular methods, such as PCR, have been developed for the detection of DNA from both species in clinical samples, providing high sensitivity and specificity rates.[94] The large cell, with multiple exosporulation, resembling a pilot's wheel, is pathognomonic of the disease (Fig. 202.4). The direct microscopic observation of the characteristic *Paracoccidioides* spp. should be done in a drop of physiologic saline or potassium hydroxide test.[40,128] Usually, the sources of clinical specimens are sputum, secretion, and scraps or debris from ulcerated skin and mucosal lesions, draining material from suppurating lymph nodes or abscesses, bronchoalveolar fluid, biopsy tissue, and exfoliative cytology.[51,78,244] Bronchoalveolar, articular, cerebrospinal, or other fluids must be centrifuged before examination. Draining material from suppurating lymph nodes usually is rich in fungal cells with multiple buds. Sputum is one of the most important specimens used for diagnosis, and various procedures are used to improve the detection of the organism in this specimen. When the first examination of the sputum is negative, it can be homogenized with an equal volume of *N*-acetyl-L-cysteine and then centrifuged again. Sodium or potassium hydroxide can be used, but only in direct examination because this treatment reduces the fungus isolation. The sensitivity of the direct examination (wet mount, smears, and histopathologic examination) varies from 80% to 100% or less and depends

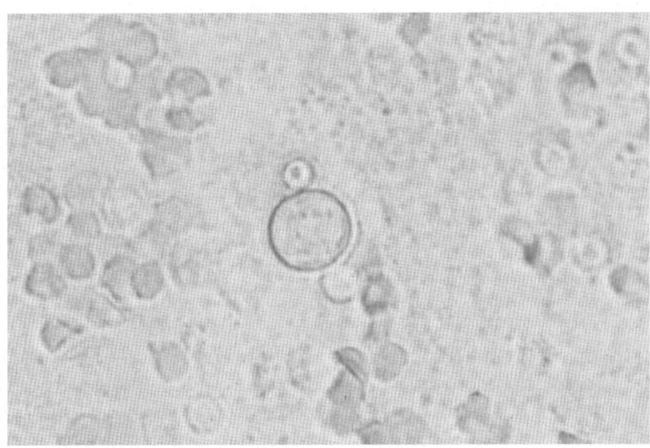

FIG. 202.4 Direct examination of a potassium hydroxide mount of a patient's sputum specimen showing a budding *Paracoccidioides brasiliensis* yeast form–like cell.

on the laboratory.[40,128,167] Biopsy samples should be taken only when routine direct examinations have failed, and the specimen should be placed in two separate flasks: one with sterile saline and the other with formalin buffered for mycologic and histopathologic examinations, respectively. Because the morphologic appearance of the parasitic forms of *P. brasiliensis* is pathognomonic, the diagnosis of the mycosis can be established by biopsy specimen and confirmed by either culture or serology. If the parasite is abundant, it may be identified by hematoxylin and eosin stain and confirmed by a special fungal stain such as periodic acid–Schiff or Gomori methods.[128,225] Pereira and colleagues[189] established the diagnosis of 63 children with paracoccidioidomycosis by the identification of *P. brasiliensis* in lymph node biopsy (84%), bone biopsy (9%), or skin biopsy (7%) specimens.

When the disease is chronic, most of the fungal cells are found inside the macrophages, but free yeast cells predominate in disseminated cases. Pauciparasitic forms of the *Paracoccidioides* spp. granuloma that show a sarcoid pattern with rare yeast forms may appear. In these cases, the diagnosis may rely on epidemiologic data plus serologic and molecular diagnostic tools such as PCR on paraffin-embedded tissue.[67,72,109,157,158] Visualization of the multiple budding yeast cells, in which the buds are connected to the parent cells by a narrow bridge with a well-defined refringent double wall, is mandatory because the *Paracoccidioides* spp. yeast cells may range from a few microns to 30 to 40 μm. Sometimes, in the lesions, the parasite is present as diminutive yeast cells, measuring about 3 to 5 μm.[128,205] For this reason, the multiple budding structures always should be found for specific diagnosis. *Paracoccidioides* spp blastoconidia may be confused with *Blastomyces dermatitidis,* capsule-deficient *Cryptococcus neoformans,* endospores and small *Coccidioides immitis* empty spherules, large *H. capsulatum* yeast cells,[40,128] or even *Pneumocystis carinii.*[235] In these cases, the molecular tests such as PCR and immunocytochemistry with specific polyclonal or monoclonal anti–*P. brasiliensis* antibody could be used.[49,71,104,107,109]

Disseminated and pulmonary paracoccidioidomycosis both can be confused with tuberculosis, histoplasmosis, leukemia, malignant neoplasms, or Hodgkin disease. When the skin or mucous membranes are affected, paracoccidioidomycosis must be differentiated from histoplasmosis, leishmaniasis, leprosy, syphilis, lupus erythematosus, and a variety of malignant neoplasms. In children, tuberculosis, acute abdominal syndrome, intestinal obstruction, osteomyelitis, and rheumatic fever also are important considerations in the differential diagnosis of this disorder. Paracoccidioidomycosis should be considered as a differential diagnosis in cases of hypereosinophilia associated to massive splenomegaly in endemic areas to this mycosis.[75,143]

Culture samples should be obtained to support the diagnosis and to establish the viability of the fungus. However, they are not always positive because the presence of other more rapidly growing microorganisms in the samples renders isolation difficult. At room temperature, *Paracoccidioides* spp. are a slow-growing fungus that can be overgrown readily by bacteria, yeasts (especially *Candida*), and contaminant molds. Isolation should be attempted by the concomitant use of modified Sabouraud agar and yeast extract agar plus antibiotics and cycloheximide. In noncontaminated samples, the use of brain-heart infusion agar plus blood and antibiotics (without cycloheximide), a hemoglobin-containing agar incubated at 37°C, or both, also is advisable. Cultures should be observed for 4 to 6 weeks, depending on temperature of incubation, with a definitive classification being accomplished only in the yeast phase. The isolation rate of the fungus in culture varies from 80% to 100% but may be less in other nonspecialized centers.[40,128] Because the mycelial form is not characteristic, subcultures in brain-heart infusion plus blood, Fava Netto's agar, or peptone–yeast extract–glucose agar, for up to 14 days at 35° to 37°C, allow yeast conversion to occur and definitive diagnosis to be established.[125,128,206]

The correct identification of the species of *Paracoccidioides* that cause infection is important for the correct diagnosis and understanding of the clinical aspects of paracoccidioidomycosis. Several molecular markers—microsatellite, hsp70 indel, and prp8 intein—as well as multilocus, coding, and noncoding genealogies of mitochondrial and nuclear genes have been described to distinguish between species of *Paracoccidioides.*[120,129,149,150,170,250,252] By using microsatellite marker system, *P. brasiliensis* S1 and PS2 can be differentiated,[150] but PS3 genotypes are not recognized, probably owing to the low diversity within this group.[149,150,252] A PCR-based assay targeting an indel region in the HSP70 locus can reportedly selectively amplify *P. lutzii* isolates,[247] and Theodoro and colleagues[252] successfully employed qPCR and SNaPshot reactions to detect single-nucleotide polymorphism among the cryptic groups in *P. brasiliensis* and *P. lutzii.* Recently, genotyping of *Paracoccidioides* has been applied using transposable elements (Trem A–H), and there is the possibility of differentiation between the two species, as well as using PCR restriction-fragment length polymorphism of the α-tubulin (*TUB1*) gene.[217]

The species-specific *gp43* gene of *P. brasiliensis* was detected by loop-mediated isothermal amplification in DNA from *P. brasiliensis* strains in 3 hours, suggesting that this method may be applied to rapid identification of this fungus.[91,245] Recently, the identity of the *P. brasiliensis* typical and atypical strains could be confirmed by its dimorphism, by the expression of gp43, and by PCR using specific primers for gp43 as well as ribosomal internal transcribed spacer regions.[35,197] However, an important note is that one sequence (483 base pairs) of the *L. loboi* gp43-like gene had 85% identity at the nucleotide level and 75% identity with the deduced amino acid sequences of the *P. brasiliensis* gp43 protein.[266]

Several *Paracoccidioides* spp. DNA sequences of potential diagnostic value have been reported,* but few have been applied to clinical samples, needing further study before they are introduced in diagnosis[28,43,104,109] *Paracoccidioides* spp. DNA sequences of potential diagnostic are a species-specific sequences of gp43 gene.[28,104,109,245] A PCR assay based on sequence of the gene coding for the gp43 antigen presented the highest sensitivity and specificity.[28,104,109] Although both species of *Paracoccidioides* express gp43 glycoprotein, there are some genetic differences in *P. lutzii* that hinder recognition by the primers used.[104] On the contrary, the Buitrago primers[43] apparently amplified both species.[149]

Patients with paracoccidioidomycosis not only have a polyclonal B-cell activation but also produce large amounts of anti–*P. brasiliensis* antibodies, which are long-lasting and generally correlate with the severity of the disease.[8,23,30,132,169,270] Assessment of the serologic response has long been used in paracoccidioidomycosis. It has been used as a diagnostic tool mainly because, in a significant proportion of the patients, it is difficult to obtain clinical specimens for visualization or cultivation of the fungus when only deep-sited lesions are present. On some occasions, a serologic result is the first indication of the mycotic nature of the patient's illness. In recent years, a great interest has been generated in the development of techniques to improve paracoccidioidomycosis diagnosis. These developments have come in the fields of either antibody or antigen detection. Thus serologic tests are of value for the diagnosis and may be useful in monitoring the evolution of the disease and its response to treatment. Antibodies are encountered in patients with clinical symptoms, and generally the titers of antibodies can be related

*References 28, 44, 71, 83, 104, 109, 127, 129, 213, 224, 245.

to the severity of the disease. Patients with paracoccidioidomycosis have a polyclonal activation of the humoral system with high serum concentrations of specific IgA, IgG, and IgE isotypes.[8,27,30,132,157,270] However, antibodies usually are impaired or absent in some patients with severe juvenile forms and in immunocompromised individuals.[80,264] On occasion, titer fluctuations may result in values below the level of detection by current methods, which may result in false-negative results. Experience over the years has resulted in various highly sensitive and widely employed serologic tests; the frequency of positive test results in patients with paracoccidioidomycosis varies from 70% to 95% and may even reach 100% in particular cases, depending on the type of test used and the stage of the disease. Of note is that discrepancies between serologic tests performed in different laboratories represent a problem because of the variation in reagents used, laboratory procedures adopted, and varying criteria used for evaluation of the results obtained.[72,265] Some of the most critical reasons for discrepancies are variations in the type of antigenic preparations, different strains, and, indeed, the mycelial or yeast cell phase chosen. Culture filtrates, cytoplasmic extracts, and antigens derived from the cell wall have been used as reagents in serologic tests for paracoccidioidomycosis, although culture filtrates are used in most laboratories.[15,48,72,81,122,158]

Various fractions that have been cloned, sequenced, and applied to the diagnosis include HSP60,[66] gp43,[197,257] gp70,[76] and 27-kDa fractions[62,182], P2,[46] peptide derived from gp70 as well as the combinations of the previously described 27-kDa recombinant antigen and the 87-kDa heat shock protein,[87] as well as rPb27 and rPb40 antigens, which showed a sensitivity of 96% with a specificity of 100% in relation to control normal human sera and to sera from patients with other systemic mycoses and 93.5% to sera from patients with diverse infections.[95]

Serologic methods that detect antigens or antibodies are extensively used and are useful for the diagnosis of paracoccidioidomycosis through the detection of gp43,[197,257] the main antigen used for the immunodiagnosis of this disease caused by *P. brasiliensis*.[49,157] However, the use of gp43 has become restricted because this marker is not identified in infections caused by *P. lutzii*.[15] Gegembauer and colleagues[105] proposed that all sera from patients suspected of paracoccidioidomycosis should be tested against the traditional exoantigen of *P. brasiliensis* (AgPbB339) and the purified gp43 molecule. Reactive sera are considered paracoccidioidomycosis due to *P. brasiliensis*, and the nonreactive sera are then tested against cell-free antigen of *P. lutzii*.[105] It should also be pointed out that it is not desirable to use a single antigen preparation to diagnose paracoccidioidomycosis, a disease that is caused by highly diverse pathogens.[131,149]

Many serologic tests have been developed and extensively studied. Agar gel immunodiffusion, complement fixation, and counterimmunoelectrophoresis tests have been employed extensively.[158] Also available are indirect immunofluorescence, indirect hemagglutination, enzyme-linked immunosorbent assay (ELISA), and dot-blot immunobinding and immunoblotting.[158,242] Some of the newer tests have employed purified antigens, such as gp43, which are well characterized and more specific. Immunodiffusion and counterimmunoelectrophoresis, which employ crude antigens derived from the yeast phase, can detect 90% or more of active cases.[72] Most authorities recommend the use of two different tests because none of these tests guarantees more than 90% sensitivity when it is employed alone. Immunodiffusion, for instance, is very simple and specific. Three precipitin bands, two of which are specific for *P. brasiliensis*, have been identified.[27,40]

A joint effort of several diagnostic centers assessing the value of this test with use of a reference crude antigen (Ag7) demonstrated it to be 84.3% sensitive and 98.9% specific.[72] Patients with very localized, benign disease may present negative results in these tests, but with more sensitive techniques (e.g., immunoblotting or gp43-ELISA), a diagnosis usually is reached. In our laboratory, three tests (immunodiffusion, counterimmunoelectrophoresis, immunoblotting) are used in a routine serologic diagnosis. The sensitivities of these tests were 85.3%, 92.9%, and 100%, respectively, evaluated against 120 paracoccidioidomycosis sera (data not published). Other studies have also described Western blot analysis as more a sensitive test.[90,193] Limitations of these tests include cross-reactivity to other mycotic disorders, especially histoplasmosis and *L. loboi* antigens, mainly in more sensitive tests,[197] and difficulties in standardization of the various tests and reagents.[48] The gp43 cross-reactivities were predominantly attributed to periodate-sensitive carbohydrate epitopes containing galactosyl.[197]

The severe juvenile form of paracoccidioidomycosis affects children, adolescents, and young adults. Patients with the severe form generally present with counterimmunoelectrophoresis titers of $\frac{1}{64}$ or greater and lack of intradermal reaction to paracoccidioidin. Patients with mild forms present with counterimmunoelectrophoresis titers of less than one-sixteenth and a positive intradermic paracoccidioidin reaction.[230]

The value of serologic tests in the follow-up of patients undergoing treatment also has been addressed by several centers.[155] The value of these tests in monitoring patients also is problematic, partly because of the diversity and complexity of the humoral response in patients with paracoccidioidomycosis. Serial serologic evaluations, usually done 3 months apart, together with the clinical, mycologic, and radiologic surveys, can guide the treatment schedule, and two negative results in two of the serologic tests routinely employed is an additional criterion that helps in the difficult decision of therapy discontinuation.[158,234]

The immunodiffusion, complement fixation, counterimmunoelectrophoresis, and ELISA tests were shown to be able to document the decline in antibody levels that parallels the clinical improvement; serum antibodies are cleared 1 to 2 years after cessation of therapy, depending on the clinical form.[42,81,158] Conversely, in these circumstances, rising antibody levels indicate a relapse. Nonetheless, a considerable number of patients maintain, sometimes lifelong, the so-called healing titers (i.e., the persistence of low serologic titers in the tests). This is seen more frequently in patients with the acute form or the chronic multifocal form of the disease.[81] The debate on the clinical relevance of this phenomenon—whether it represents the persistence of residual active lesions, thus predicting possible future relapses—is inconclusive. During treatment of paracoccidioidomycosis, an important consideration is to be able to establish cure or remission criteria. A significant fall in reactivity of anti-gp43 antibodies has been shown to correlate with clinical improvement. During relapses, the levels of specific antibodies rose, and some patients considered cured exhibited a residual reactivity. Some patients have a negative immunodiffusion and counterimmunoelectrophoresis test result but a residual reactivity with gp43 and gp70 by immunoblotting.[40,81,87,157]

On the other hand, gp43 and gp70 can be detected in the biologic fluids. Furthermore, several studies have shown that the detection of antigens in blood and urine instead of antibodies is a potent means of establishing a diagnosis, monitoring treatment, and maintaining cure control.[110,140,142,156,223,263] They allow a more precise diagnosis to be established for patients with disseminated childhood and adult multifocal disease, in which antibodies are undetectable because of their coupling to excess antigen or their incapacity to raise antibodies. Antigenemia follow-up studies permit a more precise determination of improvement because antigen load decreases with treatment response. The detection of circulating antigen may represent a more practical approach to the early and rapid diagnosis of the disease.[67] It also will be very helpful in establishing the diagnosis of immunocompromised patients, especially those with acquired immunodeficiency syndrome (AIDS), in which searching for an antibody response is not a completely reliable diagnostic tool.

The skin test with paracoccidioidin is not considered a diagnostic test because 30% to 50% of the patients are nonreactive when they are tested initially.[55,99,144] Conversely, a positive skin test result indicates previous contact with the fungus but not necessarily active disease. When histoplasmin skin test material is used, cross-reactions may be verified.[99] When the result of the skin test with paracoccidioidin is negative and the patient is treated, the skin test result may become positive, in which case the patient's prognosis is considered good.[40,128,174,206,230]

TREATMENT

Different classes of effective antifungal compounds are currently available that reduce the mortality of paracoccidioidomycosis. In addition to the prolonged use of antifungal drugs, an adequate humoral and cellular immune response is required to fully control the mycosis.[229] Cellular immunity, however, may be impaired in a large number of patients because of malnutrition or the disease process itself[11,25,169]; providing supportive therapy, therefore, is important. Rest, adequate nutrition, correction of anemia, and treatment of other concomitant infections are also recommended.[155] In children, the precise total duration of therapy is variable according to the severity of the disease and as such should also be dictated by the clinical and serologic responses of the patient to treatment. The importance of continuous treatment must be emphasized because relapses occur if the drug is not taken regularly.

Paracoccidioidomycosis is the only fungal disease that can be treated successfully with sulfa drugs. Sulfadiazine was largely employed in the past for patients with mild or moderately severe disease, or for patients who had been treated initially with amphotericin B,[155] but currently it is rarely used because of its inconvenient posology and side effects. However, in some centers sulfadiazine is still available and is provided orally at daily doses of 60 to 100 mg/kg divided in four to six equal parts to children; in adults, a maximum daily dose of 6 g can be used. Water intake and urine alkalinization (usually by bicarbonated water intake) should be encouraged during therapy to prevent crystalluria and tubular deposits of sulfadiazine.[155,231] Duration of the treatment is dictated by the patient's response after clinical and serologic improvements have been attained; in general, in the chronic form, at least 6 months are required. Treatment with sulfadiazine was in general followed by administration of slow-acting sulfa drug (sulfamethoxypyridazine or sulfadimethoxine) as maintenance treatment, at a maximum daily dosage of 1 g. Resistance to sulfonamides has already been documented.[207] Sulfadiazine has been replaced, especially in Brazil, which accounts for 80% of all cases in South America, by trimethoprim-sulfamethoxazole (80 mg of trimethoprim and 400 mg of sulfamethoxazole per tablet). This combination drug is also used in association with amphotericin B. Tolerability is good; myelotoxicity (leukopenia) is the main side effect and can be monitored and controlled by folinic acid administration without modification of the therapeutic regimen. The Brazilian consensus on paracoccidioidomycosis recommends 8 to 10 mg/kg of trimethoprim daily[234]; however, in adults it is given generally at a dose of two tablets administered orally at 12-hour intervals with satisfactory results. This combination has the advantage of permitting alternative parenteral administration whenever necessary; in this case it can be administered from 12- to up 6-hour intervals. Duration of the acute treatment with this drug varies in each case, but it usually lasts for 6 months. Maintenance treatment in these cases can be achieved by using one half the dose of the acute treatment or by using a slow-acting sulfa. Development of resistance to trimethoprim-sulfamethoxazole is occasionally clinically suspected but has rarely been documented in vitro. There is a single report of resistance of an isolate from an adult patient with the subacute form.[114]

Amphotericin B is effective but should be reserved for severely disseminated cases.[25,155] It also can be used by patients who relapse during the course of or after treatment with orally administered drug because gastrointestinal involvement may impair drug absorption in these cases. The effectiveness of therapy with azoles has curtailed the need for more aggressive regimens. More than one course of therapy may be required in some patients.

There is a report of the successful amphotericin B–sulfonamide combination treatment in adults.[137] Data regarding effectiveness of the new amphotericin B lipid formulations in paracoccidioidomycosis are still limited. A series of 28 patients with severe disease treated with amphotericin B lipid complex showed good results in all cases; however, only one child was included in this study.[85,187]

Ketoconazole is now rarely considered in the therapy of paracoccidioidomycosis because of its side effects and numerous drug interactions compared with other triazole derivatives for oral administration (itraconazole, fluconazole).[203,229] Today, more experience has been gained with itraconazole.[38,56,155,172] This triazole is more potent and less toxic than ketoconazole and is equally or even more effective than the parent compound. It is administered in 100-mg capsules that should be given with or shortly after a meal. One to two capsules, depending on the severity of the fungal process, taken daily for 6 months have been shown to be effective in reducing all active lesions. Most (98%) of the patients, including children and young adults, respond.[155,172] Posttherapy observations in predominantly adult series indicate variable proportions (ranging from 2.1% to 21%) of relapses depending on the severity of the disease, duration of therapy, and time of follow-up.[135,255] Side effects have been few and include transient elevation of hepatic enzymes.[155,172,255] The Brazilian consensus on paracoccidioidomycosis suggests itraconazole as a second option after trimethoprim-sulfamethoxazole, based on the more limited experience in children with this compound compared with the latter (or with amphotericin B),[234] but recent reports are encouraging, and itraconazole, at least for adult paracoccidioidomycosis, has become the first treatment choice in many reference centers. A randomized trial with sulfadiazine, ketoconazole, and itraconazole for the treatment of adult patients with disease of moderate severity failed to show higher efficacy of a particular regimen over the others.[231] However, two recently published studies with a larger number of patients and more extended follow-up suggested the superiority of itraconazole over trimethoprim-sulfamethoxazole; the most consistent difference between the two treatments was the shorter time to achieve cure with itraconazole.[38,56] Unfortunately again, both studies addressed mostly adult patients, and predominantly those with the chronic form of the disease. Itraconazole in children is recommended at a dose of 5 to 10 mg/kg daily, with a maximum dosage of 200 mg twice daily. A liquid formulation of itraconazole in cyclodextrin was initially suggested as a promising alternative for children treatment, but it has not been marketed in countries where the disease is endemic, and thus far no clinical experience could be gathered to support its recommendation.

Fluconazole is not as effective in this disorder; higher doses, up to 600 mg/day, and longer treatment periods should be considered. Recrudescence and relapse of disease apparently occur more frequently than when itraconazole is used.[25,155] Fluconazole may be useful in severely ill patients who must be treated intravenously.[155] No experience in children is available. The literature has only one report of the successful use of terbinafine in an adult patient.[180] Voriconazole is an extended-spectrum triazole antifungal agent that is available in both oral and intravenous formulations. In vitro susceptibility data show that *P. brasiliensis* is highly sensitive to voriconazole. A pilot open-label study showed that it is well tolerated and as effective as itraconazole for the treatment of chronic paracoccidioidomycosis.[201] However, this drug is not approved for pediatric use.

Isavuconazole, a new triazole agent, can be administered orally or intravenously and has been tested in few patients with paracoccidioidomycosis with promising results, in agreement with its good in vitro anti-*Paracoccidioides* activity. Further studies with larger number of patients with the juvenile form of the disease are required to determine its place in the treatment of children with the mycosis.[253]

Many questions remain to be answered regarding optimal treatment of paracoccidioidomycosis. The role of adjunct therapy with immunomodulators, such as peptides derived from the immunodominant glycoprotein form *P. brasiliensis* that act by augmenting the Th1-mediated immune responses, has been investigated mainly in experimental models of the disease and showed promising results.[221] Two studies demonstrated some reactivity of patients' T cells to these peptides.[121] Further studies are required to demonstrate their utility in promoting protective cell-mediated immune responses in the human host. α-Glucan obtained from *Saccharomyces cerevisiae* with immunoenhancing properties has been preliminary investigated, but further studies are needed.[153] In the opposite direction, some investigators have administrated short courses of corticosteroids as adjunct therapy to severe cases, based on the rationale that the failure to improve with antifungal therapy observed in these cases was due to uncontrolled or excessive inflammatory response.[18,113] Some fatalities were attributed to the exacerbated inflammatory response.[19,26] The clinical and laboratory criteria that allow reduction in the antifungal dose or that could be used to end treatment with the assurance that the patient is cured are not established. Progressive decrease in the titers of the serologic tests currently available is one of the laboratory parameters used most frequently. Newer methods (e.g., antigenemia detection and molecular biology approaches) still need further standardization and clinical studies and have not yet become widely available.[110,140,142] Meanwhile, most specialists agree that treatment decisions need to be tailored according to the patient.

PROGNOSIS

Paracoccidioidomycosis has no prophylaxis. Vaccine strategies are being developed but are still restricted to experimental models of the disease.[243,258] The mycosis can be fatal if left untreated, but currently this has seldom been observed.[19,26,115,192,219] On the other hand, sequelae remain a problem. Residual lesions have been observed in a few patients with no known history of active mycotic infection.[101,106,154]

Prognosis depends on the status of the patient at the time of diagnosis. Children and young adults in whom fungemia has taken place and who have multiple organ involvement may respond less well to therapy. The fatality rate in young patients at one time was reported to be 31%,[55] but it now is much lower as a result of earlier diagnoses and better treatments. Nevertheless, it remains a life-threatening disease with 6% fatalities in the most recent series.[39] This was attributed to delayed diagnosis or searching for medical assistance, irregular treatment, or treatment not monitored. Abdominal complications, especially liver involvement, ascites, and malnutrition, were associated with the lethal prognosis.[11,39,176,189] In the adult group, mortality rates are much lower. After specific treatment is instituted, lesions regress promptly; skin lesions may heal completely in 2 to 4 weeks.[155] Complete remission is expected for most patients with the acute-subacute and chronic form of the disease. Prognosis has improved as a result of earlier diagnosis, new antifungal drugs that facilitate compliance, and better knowledge of the disease. The latter has provided better clinical and laboratory follow-up and the notion that the disease needs prolonged surveillance, as shown by the decrease in positive mycologic tests during and after therapy.[155,255] Some investigators consider the term *cure* inappropriate because of the inability to confirm complete eradication of the organism; the term *apparent cure* should instead be used.[155]

Paracoccidioidomycosis persists as a disease with relatively low mortality but high morbidity. Complications vary and, like prognosis, their occurrence depends on the extent of fungal invasion. In the juvenile form, early complications that may lead to surgical intervention are intestinal obstruction and jaundice, both of which result from enlarged mesenteric lymph nodes. Disabsorptive syndromes may be associated, aggravating the nutritional status of the patients.[21,233] Patients also may present with ascites or chylothorax. Lymph nodes may suppurate, and fistulas can develop. A late complication that has been described is abdominal malakoplakia.[218] In the adult form, acute complications of mucosal involvement are dysphagia and dysphonia,[268] edema of the glottis, respiratory insufficiency, and Addison disease,[154] among others.[259] Sequelae are not as common in children as in adults. In general, fibrosis is the cause of serious problems in patients who respond to therapy, particularly when extensive pulmonary infiltrates are present. Despite the newer, very effective therapies, these sequelae preclude, in a proportion of the cases, the complete restoration of the patients' previous health status.[164,154,155,172,255] In the former group, scarring and fibrosis of the affected nodes and residual pulmonary fibrosis have been noted.[130] Malabsorption syndrome probably is the most serious sequela in the juvenile form because of the enteric loss of proteins and inflammatory cells that results in immunodeficiency and opportunistic infections.[21,233]

Acknowledgments

We thank Professor Angela Restrepo for her invaluable contribution to this version of the chapter and Drs. Ana Marisa Fusco Almeida, Maria Gorete Nogueira, and Ricardo Pereira for their comments and sharing unpublished material. We also thank Irani Coito for the bibliography revision.

NEW REFERENCES SINCE THE SEVENTH EDITION

1. Almeida AJ, Matute DR, Carmona JA, et al. Genome size and ploidy of *Paracoccidioides brasiliensis* reveals a haploid DNA content: flow cytometry and GP43 sequence analysis. *Fungal Genet Biol.* 2007;44(1):25-31.
3. Alves FL, Ribeiro MA, Hahn RC, et al. Transposable elements and two other molecular markers as typing tools for the genus *Paracoccidioides*. *Med Mycol.* 2015;53(2):165-170.
4. Arantes TD, Theodoro RC, Teixeira Mde M, Bosco Sde M, Bagagli E. Environmental mapping of *Paracoccidioides* spp. in Brazil reveals new clues into genetic diversity, biogeography and wild host association. *PLoS Negl Trop Dis.* 2016;10(4):e0004606.
18. Benard G. An overview of the immunopathology of human paracoccidioidomycosis. *Mycopathologia.* 2008;165:209-221.
38. Borges SR, Silva GM, Chambela Mda C, et al. Itraconazole vs. trimethoprim-sulfamethoxazole: a comparative cohort study of 200 patients with paracoccidioidomycosis. *Med Mycol.* 2014;52:303-310.
39. Braga Gde M, Hessel G, Pereira RM. Hepatic involvement in pediatric patients with paracoccidioidomycosis: a clinical and laboratory study. *Mycopathologia.* 2013;176:279-286.
42. Buccheri R, Khoury Z, Barata LC, Benard G. Incubation period and early natural history events of the acute form of paracoccidioidomycosis: lessons from patients with a single *Paracoccidioides* spp. exposure. *Mycopathologia.* 2016;181:435-439.
51. Cavalcante Rde S, Sylvestre TF, Levorato AD, de Carvalho LR, Mendes RP. Comparison between itraconazole and cotrimoxazole in the treatment of paracoccidiodomycosis. *PLoS Negl Trop Dis.* 2014;8:e2793.
64. Costa AN, Benard G, Albuquerque AL, et al. The lung in paracoccidioidomycosis: new insights into old problems. *Clinics (Sao Paulo).* 2013;68:441-448.
68. da Silva Jde F, de Oliveira HC, Marcos CM, et al. Advances and challenges in paracoccidioidomycosis serology caused by *Paracoccidioides* species complex: an update. *Diagn Microbiol Infect Dis.* 2016;84(1):87-94.
69. da Silva Neto BR, Carvalho PFZ, Bailão AM, et al. Transcriptional profile of *Paracoccidioides* spp. in response to itraconazole. *BMC Genomics.* 2014;15:254.
73. de Castro LF, Ferreira MC, da Silva RM, et al. Characterization of the immune response in human paracoccidioidomycosis. *J Infect.* 2013;67:470-485.
75. Della Coletta AM, Bachiega TF, de Quaglia e Silva JC, et al. Neutrophil extracellular traps identification in tegumentary lesions of patients with paracoccidioidomycosis and different patterns of NETs generation in vitro. *PLoS Negl Trop Dis.* 2015;9(9):e0004037.
76. de Macedo PM, Almeida-Paes R, de Medeiros Muniz M, et al. *Paracoccidioides brasiliensis* PS2: first autochthonous paracoccidioidomycosis case report in Rio de Janeiro, Brazil, and literature review. *Mycopathologia.* 2016;181(9-10):701-708.
78. de Oliveira HC, Assato PA, Marcos CM, et al. Paracoccidioides-host interaction: an overview on recent advances in the paracoccidioidomycosis. *Front Microbiol.* 2016;6:1319.
83. Dias L, de Carvalho LF, Romano CC. Application of PCR in serum samples for diagnosis of paracoccidioidomycosis in the southern Bahia-Brazil. *PLoS Negl Trop Dis.* 2012;6(11):e1909.
92. Fabris LR, Andrade UV, Ferreira dos Santos A, et al. Decreasing prevalence of the acute/subacute clinical form of paracoccidioidomycosis in Mato Grosso do Sul State, Brazil. *Rev Inst Med Trop Sao Paulo.* 2014;56:121-125.
100. Franco M, Bagagli E, Scapolio S, Lacaz CS. A critical analysis of isolation of *Paracoccidioides brasiliensis* from soil. *Med Mycol.* 2000;38(3):185-191.
104. Gaviria M, Rivera V, Muñoz-Cadavid C, Cano LE, Naranjo TW. Validation and clinical application of a nested PCR for paracoccidioidomycosis diagnosis in clinical samples from Colombian patients. *Braz J Infect Dis.* 2015;19(4):376-383.
105. Gegembauer G, Araujo LM, Pereira EF, et al. Serology of paracoccidioidomycosis due to *Paracoccidioides lutzii*. *PLoS Negl Trop Dis.* 2014;8(7):e2986.
115. Hahn RC, Rodrigues AM, Fontes CJ, et al. Fatal fungemia due to *Paracoccidioides lutzii*. *Am J Trop Med Hyg.* 2014;91:394-398.
119. Hotez PJ, Bottazzi ME, Franco-Paredes C, Ault SK, Periago MR. The neglected tropical diseases of Latin America and the Caribbean: a review of disease burden and distribution and a road map for control and elimination. *PLoS Negl Trop Dis.* 2008;2(9):e300.
131. Machado GC, Moris DV, Arantes TD, et al. Cryptic species of *Paracoccidioides brasiliensis*: impact on paracoccidioidomycosis immunodiagnosis. *Mem Inst Oswaldo Cruz.* 2013;108(5):637-643.
139. Marques SA. Paracoccidioidomycosis. *Clin Dermatol.* 2012;30(6):610-615.
143. Marques de Macedo P, de Oliveira LC, Freitas DF, et al. Acute paracoccidioidomycosis due to *Paracoccidioides brasiliensis* S1 mimicking hypereosinophilic syndrome with massive splenomegaly: diagnostic challenge. *PLoS Negl Trop Dis.* 2016;10(4):e0004487.
145. Martinez R. Epidemiology of paracoccidioidomycosis. *Rev Inst Med Trop Sao Paulo.* 2015;57 Suppl 19:11-20.
171. Muñoz JF, Farrer RA, Desjardins CA, et al. Genome diversity, recombination, and virulence across the major lineages of paracoccidioides. *mSphere.* 2016;1(5):pii:e00213-16.
175. Neves AR, Mamoni RL, Rossi CL, de Camargo ZP, Blotta MH. Negative immunodiffusion test results obtained with sera of paracoccidioidomycosis patients may be related to low-avidity immunoglobulin G2 antibodies directed against carbohydrate epitopes. *Clin Diagn Lab Immunol.* 2003;10:802-807.
187. Peçanha PM, de Souza S, Falqueto A, et al. Amphotericin B lipid complex in the treatment of severe paracoccidioidomycosis: a case series. *Int J Antimicrob Agents.* 2016;48:428-430.
196. Pigosso LL, Parente AF, Coelho AS, et al. Comparative proteomics in the genus *Paracoccidioides*. *Fungal Genet Biol.* 2013;60:87-100.
210. Restrepo A, Arango MD. In vitro susceptibility testing of *Paracoccidioides brasiliensis* to sulfonamides. *Antimicrob Agents Chemother.* 1980;18:190-194.

217. Roberto TN, Rodrigues AM, Hahn RC, de Camargo ZP. Identifying *Paracoccidioides* phylogenetic species by PCR-RFLP of the alpha-tubulin gene. *Med Mycol.* 2016;54(3):240-247.
219. Ruas LP, Pereira RM, Braga FG, et al. Severe paracoccidioidomycosis in a 14-year-old boy. *Mycopathologia.* 2016;181(11-12):915-920.
220. Ruiz e Resende LS, Yasuda AG, Mendes RP, et al. Paracoccidioidomycosis in patients with lymphoma and review of published literature. *Mycopathologia.* 2015;179:285-291.
227. Sardi Jde C, Pitangui Nde S, Voltan AR, et al. In vitro *Paracoccidioides brasiliensis* biofilm and gene expression of adhesins and hydrolytic enzymes. *Virulence.* 2015;6(6):642-651.
228. Siqueira IM, Fraga CL, Amaral AC, et al. Distinct patterns of yeast cell morphology and host responses induced by representative strains of *Paracoccidioides brasiliensis* (Pb18) and *Paracoccidioides lutzii* (Pb01). *Med Mycol.* 2016;54(2):177-188.
233. Shikanai-Yasuda MA. Paracoccidioidomycosis treatment. *Rev Inst Med Trop Sao Paulo.* 2015;57(suppl 19):31-37.
243. Taborda CP, Urán ME, Nosanchuk JD, Travassos LR. Paracoccidioidomycosis: challenges in the development of a vaccine against an endemic mycosis in the Americas. *Rev Inst Med Trop Sao Paulo.* 2015;57(suppl 19):21-24.
248. Teixeira MM, Theodoro RC, Nino-Vega G, Bagagli E, Felipe MSS. Paracoccidioides species complex: ecology, phylogeny, sexual reproduction, and virulence. *PLoS Pathog.* 2014;10:e1004397.
253. Thompson GR, Rendon A, Ribeiro Dos Santos R, et al. Isavuconazole treatment of cryptococcosis and dimorphic mycoses. *Clin Infect Dis.* 2016;63:356-362.
255. Tobón AM, Agudelo CA, Restrepo CA, et al. Adrenal function status in patients with paracoccidioidomycosis after prolonged post-therapy follow-up. *Am J Trop Med Hyg.* 2010;83:111-114.
265. Vidal MS, Del Negro GM, Vicentini AP, et al. Serological diagnosis of paracoccidioidomycosis: high rate of inter-laboratorial variability among medical mycology reference centers. *PLoS Negl Trop Dis.* 2014;8(9):e3174.

The full reference list for this chapter is available at ExpertConsult.com.

Cryptococcosis 203

David L. Goldman • John R. Perfect

Cryptococcus neoformans is an encapsulated yeast that causes meningoencephalitis and pneumonia in both immunocompetent and immunocompromised children. Since its identification as a pathogen in 1894,[122] great strides have been made in our understanding of the biology and the pathogenesis of cryptococcosis. The incidence of cryptococcosis greatly increased in association with both the acquired immunodeficiency syndrome (AIDS) epidemic and improvements in health care, which have resulted in an increased number of individuals at risk for cryptococcosis. We have also come to recognize *C. neoformans* comprises at least two separate species, *C. neoformans* and *Cryptococcus gattii,* that evolved from each other more than 40 million years ago.[46] Disease caused by these two species is similar in many ways, but there are important differences. Despite the availability of antifungal therapy, the mortality associated with cryptococcosis remains high, and new therapies and prevention strategies are needed.

ORGANISM

C. neoformans is an encapsulated basidiomycete that is evolutionarily distinct from yeasts like *Candida albicans* and more closely related to corn and grain plant fungal pathogens.[77] *C. neoformans* is a round yeast (5 to 10 μm diameter) that produces white (frequently mucoid) colonies on standard mycologic media. *C. neoformans* can also form giant cells (also known as titan cells) that can be as large as 80 to 100 μm diameter, which have been described primarily in the context of animal models of infection.[56] The capsule varies greatly in size among strains and its size is regulated by the local milieu. *C. neoformans* is capable of sexual reproduction in the laboratory, and mating types (alpha and A) have been identified. In the environment and during infection, the organism is typically haploid and replicates asexually.

C. neoformans was originally classified into five serotypes (A, B, C, D, and AD) based on its reaction with anticapsular serum. Serotypes B and C, formally known as *C. neoformans* var. *gattii,* are now collectively named *C. gattii.* This species is now further classified into four genotypes (VGI, VGII, VGIII, and VGIV), with VGII genotype being further classified into types, VGIIa, VGIIb, and VGIIc. Serotype A (also known as *C. neoformans* var. *grubii*) is responsible for the vast majority of *C. neoformans* disease and is now classified into three main genotypes (VNI, VNII, and VNB). Serotype D (*C. neoformans* var. *neoformans*) is primarily found in Europe, and occasionally hybrids such as serotype A/D and other diploid strains are found in nature.

C. neoformans and *C. gattii* can be distinguished by a variety of biochemical, serologic, and molecular typing techniques, although these are not routinely available in clinical microbiology laboratories. For instance, *C. gattii* (but not *C. neoformans*) produces blue coloration on L-canavanine, glycine, and bromothymol blue (CGB) medium. Recently, matrix-assisted laser desorption/ionization time-of-flight mass spectrometry (MALDI-TOF MS) has been demonstrated to be useful in making the distinction between these two cryptococcal species.[51] Other species of *Cryptococcus* (e.g., *Cryptococcus laurentii, Cryptococcus albidus*) are less virulent and rarely have been reported to cause disease.[12,57]

Virulence

Several important virulence traits common to *C. neoformans* and *C. gattii* include encapsulation, melanization, the ability to grow at 37°C, and both urease and phospholipase production. These characteristics are not uniformly present in other cryptococcal species. The emergence of some of these traits has been hypothesized to have been selected for because of survival advantages they confer in their natural environment, where these yeasts are exposed to invertebrate predatory scavengers such as nematodes and amebae.

Capsule

The impressive capsules of *C. neoformans* and *C. gattii* are composed of long unbranched polymers of xylose and glucuronic acid. The capsule plays a central role in cryptococcal virulence, and acapsular and hypocapsular mutants exhibit greatly reduced virulence.[23] Although capsules can be produced by other cryptococcal species, studies suggest that there are important differences in the biophysical properties between the capsule of virulent and nonvirulent species.[8] Capsule size is actively regulated in response to local conditions such as PCO_2, serum, and iron. In nature, the small capsule likely protects the yeast from desiccation and ingestion by soil amebae. However, entering the mammalian host environment signals the enlargement of the capsule around the yeast and gives the organism its distinctive appearance in India ink staining (Fig. 203.1). The substantial polysaccharide material forming the capsule is extensively shed into host tissue, cerebrospinal fluid (CSF), and blood during infection; and the detection of this shed polysaccharide forms

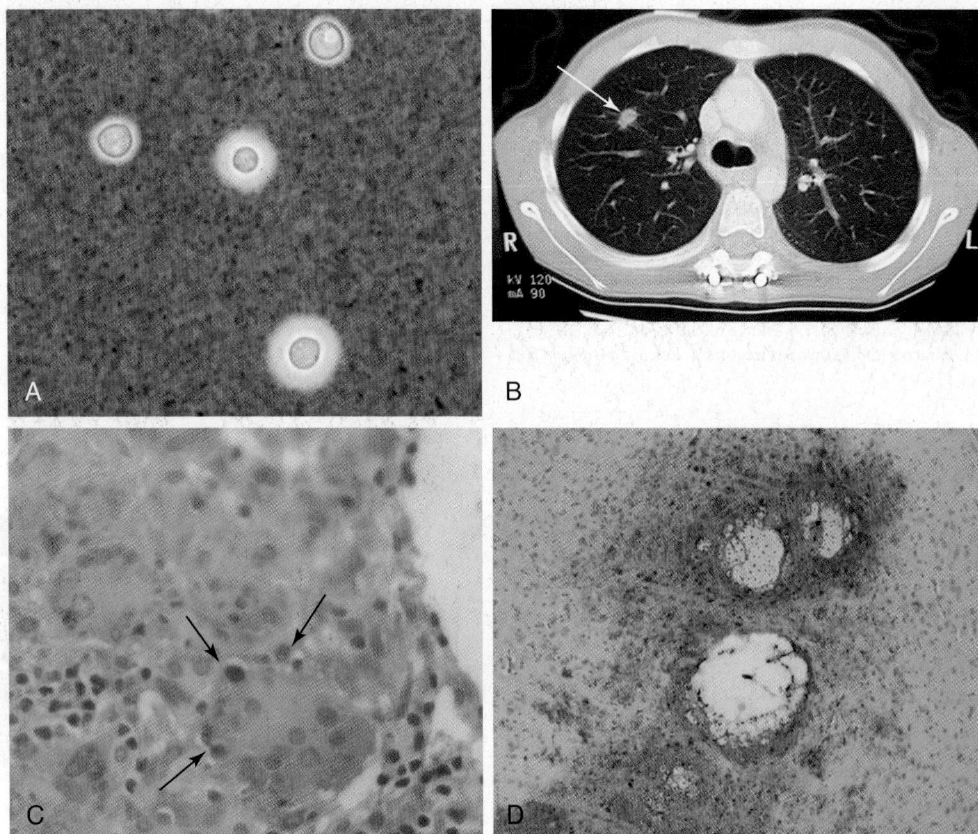

FIG. 203.1 (A) India ink staining of cerebrospinal fluid demonstrates *Cryptococcus neoformans* and capsule, which excludes the stain and results in a halo around the organism. (B) Computed tomography scan of a child with rhabdomyosarcoma reveals nodule *(white arrow)* secondary to *C. neoformans*. (C) Mucicarmine staining of a lung from a rat with experimentally induced pulmonary cryptococcosis shows granulomas containing *C. neoformans (black arrows)*. (D) Immunostaining for cryptococcal polysaccharide reveals extensive shedding of polysaccharide within the brain parenchyma and around cryptococcomas of a rat with experimentally induced cryptococcal meningoencephalitis.

the basis of the cryptococcal antigen (CRAG) testing. Similar to prototypical pediatric pathogens (e.g., *Streptococcus pneumoniae, Haemophilus influenzae, Neisseria meningitidis*), the cryptococcal capsule inhibits antibody- and complement-mediated phagocytosis and thereby interferes with the development of an effective immune response.[94] However, the capsule also exhibits a variety of other antiinflammatory properties, including inhibition of leukocyte migration,[44] enhanced interleukin-10 secretion,[173] inhibition of T-cell proliferation,[183] and induction of macrophage apoptosis.[178] In addition, the cryptococcal capsule also has been hypothesized to contribute to deadly cerebral edema[71] and to promote replication of the human immunodeficiency virus (HIV).[141] Given the central role of the capsule in cryptococcal pathogenesis, administration of capsular-specific antibody has been studied as potential adjunctive therapy in animal models to remove antigen and improve host elimination of the yeasts.[124,151] However, this therapeutic approach has so far found limited success in humans.[99]

Melanin

Melanin is a pigment that is synthesized from catechol precursors (e.g., dopamine, epinephrine) by the laccase enzymes of *C. neoformans* and *C. gattii*. The laccase enzyme is similar to enzymes produced by wood-rotting fungi and is capable of digesting lignin, an important constituent of trees, and may thereby promote growth of the yeast in decaying trees. Melanin is produced during cryptococcal infection and is localized to the cell wall.[147] Melanin content can vary significantly among individual *C. neoformans* strains.[181] However, yeast mutants lacking the ability to produce melanin are less virulent in animal models than their melanin-producing parental strains. Although melanin structure remains poorly understood, its chemistry endows it with the ability to stabilize free radicals and provides a stable framework even under extremely harsh environmental conditions. These characteristics likely play an important role in the capacity of melanin to protect against damage caused by nitrogen- and oxygen-derived host oxidants in addition to exogenous factors such as ultraviolet light and antifungal agents. Melanin also appears to promote disease through its immunomodulatory properties[76] and its ability to bind to host antimicrobial peptides.[127] One explanation for cryptococcal neurotropism relates to the hypothesis that high concentrations of catechol precursors within the brain promote cryptococcal melanization, which in turn protects the organism from the host immune response within the brain.[144]

Extracellular Enzymes

C. neoformans and *C. gattii* also produce a variety of extracellular enzymes that have been linked to virulence, including proteinase, phospholipase, and urease. Urease catalyzes the hydrolysis of urea to ammonia and carbamate. The importance of urease in virulence and during infection appears to depend on the infection site and may be more important for pulmonary infection than brain infection.[37] Urease production by *C. neoformans* has been associated with the accumulation of immature dendritic cells and the production of a disease-enhancing helper T-cell subtype 2 (Th2) inflammation.[130] It may also promote entry into the brain, across the blood-brain barrier.[156] *C. neoformans* strains vary in their phospholipase production, and high phospholipase production has been associated with increase fungal burden in animal models.[176] Conversely, lack of phospholipase production has been linked to reduced virulence of a cryptococcal strain[36] Phospholipases have also been implicated in promoting entry into the brain[35] by facilitating passage through brain endothelial cells.[115] Phospholipases may also promote intracellular growth by releasing arachidonic acid from host cells.[182] Other virulence factors that have been identified include mating type,[97] prostaglandin production,[50] calcineurin signaling,[161,129] and several stress response pathways involving protein kinase A and trehalose.[142]

Phenotypic Variation

Recent studies highlight several processes by which strains of *Cryptococcus* undergo significant phenotypic variation during infection, which in turn promotes disease pathogenesis. This includes the formation of giant or titan cells that can be 20 times the size of a typical cell (reviewed in reference 184). These Titan cells typically exhibit increased ploidy and are more resistant to phagocytosis.[38] Other processes by which *Cryptococcus* undergoes significant phenotypic changes include phenotypic switching,[58] replicative aging,[16] and quorum sensing.[4] These phenotypic changes are bolstered by vibrant genome plasticity during stresses in the host.[73,81] Furthermore, we can now begin to see how this yeast responds to the human environment by capturing its transcriptome at the site of infection.[30]

ECOLOGY AND EPIDEMIOLOGY

Cryptococcus neoformans

There are important differences in the ecology of *C. neoformans* and *C. gattii* (Table 203.1). *C. neoformans* (but not *C. gattii*) is well known for its association with bird droppings, including those from pigeons, canaries, and parrots. *C. neoformans* is capable of growth in the acidic environment of bird droppings. Nonetheless, birds are unlikely to be the primary environmental source for *C. neoformans* because their high internal temperatures inhibit *C. neoformans* growth and possibly possess innate avian host factors against this yeast. In addition, the *C. neoformans* density is much higher in aged pigeon droppings compared with fresh droppings, suggesting the possibility for secondary contamination as the mechanism for this ecologic niche.[109] Other primary environmental sources for *C. neoformans* include rotting trees and fruits.[31,111]

There are also important differences in the epidemiology of disease caused by these different species of *Cryptococcus*. *C. neoformans* is generally considered an opportunistic pathogen that causes central nervous system (CNS) and respiratory disease in patients with depressed cellular immunity. However, cryptococcosis secondary to *C. neoformans* also occurs in individuals without any identified risk factors. A dramatic increase in the prevalence of cryptococcosis occurred in association with the AIDS epidemic. In patients with HIV infection, cryptococcal meningoencephalitis (CME) is an AIDS-defining diagnosis, typically occurring in both adults and children with profound immunodeficiency, as evidenced by a finding of $CD4^+$ T cells less than 100/μL. In countries where highly active antiretroviral therapy (HAART) has been successfully introduced, the prevalence of cryptococcosis has greatly decreased. Unfortunately, cryptococcosis has emerged as a significant cause of disease in AIDS patients in countries with limited resources. Worldwide, most cases of cryptococcosis occur in sub-Saharan Africa and Southeast Asia, affecting an estimated 1 million individuals annually[135] and up to 30% of AIDS patients.[14] Although this number has shrunk with the widespread introduction of antiretroviral therapy worldwide, the prevalence remains high. In South Africa, *C. neoformans* is the leading cause of meningitis in adults, with an incidence more than twice that of tuberculous meningitis.[83] In developed countries, an increase in the incidence of *C. neoformans* disease among non–HIV-infected individuals has been recognized. This appears to be primarily associated with improvements in medical care and an increase in the number of individuals receiving immunosuppressive therapy, especially organ transplant recipients and other immunosuppressants such as steroids and anti–tumor necrosis factor therapies. Among solid-organ transplant recipients, cryptococcosis is the third most common invasive fungal infection. Among non–HIV-infected patients with cryptococcosis in the United States, 20% to 60% are transplant recipients.[177] Interestingly, *C. neoformans* var. *grubii* has been increasingly reported as a cause of disease in individuals from China (including children) without any recognized immune deficit.[75]

Overall, cryptococcosis secondary to *C. neoformans* is less common in children than adults but remains an important cause of pneumonia and meningoencephalitis, especially in certain parts of the world. Owing to the rarity of pediatric cryptococcosis, the precise prevalence is difficult to define and may vary by region. Studies of US children with AIDS in the 1990s estimated an incidence of cryptococcosis to be about 1%.[60] A more recent US series identified 63 cases of pediatric cryptococcosis from a consortium of 42 children's hospitals over a 5-year period, with an admission rate of 6.2 per million hospitalizations.[86] Most children (63.5%) in this cohort had underlying immunosuppression, whereas 21% were immunocompetent and 16% had AIDS. The 8-year point prevalence of cryptococcosis among Thai children with AIDS was 2.97%.[107] A study from South Africa reported 361 cases of pediatric cryptococcosis over a 3-year period, representing 2% of all cases of cryptococcosis over this time.[118] The reported median age at time of diagnosis of pediatric cryptococcosis varies from 7 to 12 years. In most series, pediatric cryptococcosis rarely occurs in children younger than age 1 year, although in the South African cohort an increased incidence was noted within the first year of life. In addition to AIDS, cryptococcosis has been identified in children with a variety of primary and secondary immunodeficiency states, including organ transplantation, lymphoma, leukemia, lupus, glucocorticoid therapy, sarcoma, hyperimmunoglobulin M syndrome, Bruton agammaglobulinemia, and severe combined immunodeficiency.[5,80,102,162,180] Neonatal cryptococcosis is rare but has been described (see later discussion).

Although the incidence of symptomatic cryptococcosis is disproportionately low in children, serologic studies suggest that children from certain regions of the country may be infected with *C. neoformans* at a very young age.[59] The basis for this discrepancy between serologic findings and clinical disease is unknown. It is likely that most pediatric infections are asymptomatic or misdiagnosed as viral disease. Potential reasons for the low incidence of symptomatic pediatric cryptococcosis

TABLE 203.1 Summary of Characteristics of *Cryptococcus gattii* and *Cryptococcus neoformans*

	Cryptococcus gattii	*Cryptococcus neoformans*
Microbiology	Serotypes B and C Molecular type VGI associated with Australia and VGIIa with outbreak in Pacific Northwest Bluish discoloration on CGB media Distinction can also be made by MALDI-MS	Serotypes A and D Molecular type VNI most common cause of *C. neoformans* diseases
Ecology	Eucalyptus and other trees	Bird droppings and trees
Epidemiology	Immunocompetent > immunocompromised Endemic in certain tropical/subtropical regions Outbreak in Pacific Northwest	Immunocompromised (especially AIDS and T-cell defects) > immunocompetent High incidence in sub-Saharan Africa and Southeast Asia Decreased incidence in regions where HAART is available
Clinical manifestations	Primary pulmonary infection and CNS cryptococcomas with associated complications	Meningoencephalitis and disseminated disease a common presentation, especially among AIDS patients

AIDS, Acquired immunodeficiency syndrome; *CGB,* L-canavanine, glycine, and bromothymol blue; *CNS,* central nervous system; *HAART,* highly active antiretroviral therapy; *MALDI-MS,* matrix-assisted laser desorption/ionization time of flight.

include the time needed to reactivate infection, the importance of repeated exposures, and differences in infecting strains.[120] Nonetheless, it remains a perplexing issue as to why many children appear to be infected but rarely develop disease.

Cryptococcus gattii

In contrast to *C. neoformans, C. gattii* was initially recognized as a disease of tropical regions and endemic in Australasia, where it is associated with eucalyptus trees (both river red and forest red gum trees). However, *C. gattii* has been increasingly recognized to cause disease outside Australasia and tropical regions. Over the past 15 years, *C. gattii* has been linked to an outbreak of disease in the Pacific Northwest. This outbreak was initially recognized on Vancouver Island with subsequent extension into the United States (including the states of Washington and Oregon). Cryptococcosis secondary to *C. gattii* may occasionally occur in travelers returning from the Pacific Northwest. Disease typically presents within weeks to months after travel but may occur as long as 1 year after travel.[66] In the Pacific Northwest, *C. gattii* has been isolated from non–eucalyptus tree species (Douglas fir, alder, and Garry oak), soil, air, fresh water, and sea water. There are also *C. gattii* cases being reported outside the geographic boundaries typically associated with *C. gattii* disease,[116] including areas east of the Mississippi in the United States.[96] This change in the environmental location of *C. gattii* may be the result of genetic changes in the yeast or climactic changes that allow the organism to successfully compete in new geographic regions

Cryptococcus gattii causes disease in both immunocompetent and immunocompromised individuals, although disease appears to be more common among immunocompetent individuals compared with *C. neoformans.* In the Pacific Northwest outbreak, corticosteroid use and older age (>50 years) have been associated with increased severity.[67] In an Australian study of *C. gattii* disease, 72% of patients were found to have no recognizable immune deficit.[29] Some investigators, however, have hypothesized that apparently "normal" individuals infected with *C. gattii* may have subclinical immune deficits,[114] including autoantibodies to granulocyte-macrophage colony-stimulating factor.[148] Because standard microbiologic techniques fail to distinguish between the two species, the precise prevalence of *C. gattii* disease is not yet known.

The incidence of cryptococcosis secondary to *C. gattii* in children is not well characterized. Of 218 cases of cryptococcosis secondary to *C. gattii* in British Columbia between 1999 and 2007, four cases (1.8%) occurred in children younger than 18 years.[53] In contrast, among 43 cases of *C. gattii* meningoencephalitis in a series from Brazil, 19% occurred in children younger than 12 years.[152]

PATHOGENESIS

C. neoformans and *C. gattii* infections are believed to be acquired through inhalation of infectious propagules within the environment. The precise infecting form remains to be understood and may involve either desiccated yeast cells or small basidiospores (1 to 2 μm), thus allowing alveolar deposition. Once within the lung, infection may cause disease through progression of pneumonia and dissemination to the CNS. Alternatively, infection may be contained in a dormant site within the lungs and reactivate in the setting of subsequent immunosuppression, such as HIV infection or corticosteroid use. Evidence for reactivation disease includes molecular typing[55] and pathologic[69] and serologic studies.[150] Furthermore, recent reports of very early cryptococcosis after organ transplantation highlight the tendency of *C. neoformans* to cause latent infections within transplanted organs.[164] Differences in the propensity for *C. neoformans* and *C. gattii* to cause primary progressive disease may exist. For example, molecular typing studies and cases of cryptococcosis among returning travelers to the Pacific Northwest highlight the potential for *C. gattii* to cause primary progressive disease.[19,22] These findings are consistent with findings from animal experimentation.[95] Within the lung, both innate and adaptive immune responses are essential to the effective control of yeasts that can survive in both the intracellular and extracellular environment of the host. *C. neoformans* can be recognized by the cells of the innate immune system through a variety of receptors, including toll-like, β-glucan, and mannose receptors. Both classically and alternatively activated macrophages play a central role in the host immune response.[154] Dendritic cells, natural killer cells, neutrophils, and activated macrophages can kill the yeast. *C. neoformans* is a facultative intracellular pathogen and is well adapted to survive and replicate within the acidic environment of the phagolysosome.[104] Unlike other intracellular pathogens, *C. neoformans* does not employ typical strategies to escape or modify the phagolysosomal compartment. However, intracellular yeast survival within the harsh environment of the phagolysosome is supported by virulence traits, including capsule production, melanization, secretion of extracellular enzymes, and prostaglandin production. Interestingly, *C. neoformans* can escape the macrophage through induction of cell lysis or phagosomal extrusion.[6] The latter process allows the transfer of yeasts between macrophages without inducing macrophage death and its associated inflammation. This novel mechanism likely promotes the intracellular persistence of *C. neoformans.*

Adaptive immunity and T-cell–mediated activation of macrophages are central to the successful host immune response. The critical importance of T-cell immunity in the protective host response to cryptococcosis is highlighted by the increased susceptibility of individuals with defective T-cell immunity to cryptococcosis, such as with HIV-infected individuals. Animal experimentation conclusively highlights the protective nature of Th1 immunity and the nonprotective (disease-enhancing) nature of Th2 immunity.[72,90] In this regard, *C. neoformans* and *C. gattii* virulence have been linked to their ability to actively modulate the inflammatory response and to elicit nonprotective Th2 inflammation.[2,39] It should also be noted that increasing evidence suggests that B cells and humoral immunity also play a part in the effective immune composite response against cryptococcal infection.[146]

PULMONARY CRYPTOCOCCOSIS

The lungs are the most commonly recognized body site of cryptococcal disease after the CNS. Pulmonary cryptococcosis can present as the primary manifestation of cryptococcosis (e.g., without extrapulmonary disease) or in association with disseminated disease or meningoencephalitis. Symptomatic pulmonary cryptococcosis typically occurs in individuals with underlying immunodeficiency or chronic lung disease. Nonetheless, pulmonary cryptococcosis in individuals without recognized risk factors is well described and appears to be more common for infection secondary to *C. gattii.* In one study of HIV-negative patients with cryptococcosis, 15% of patients with pulmonary cryptococcosis had no underlying disease.[134] Among AIDS patients with cryptococcal meningoencephalitis, pulmonary cryptococcosis has been reported to be present in a wide range (10–55%) of patients.[18] This variation may occur as a result of the nonspecific features of pulmonary disease along with differences in diagnostic evaluation within cohorts.

Case reports and series describing adults with primary pulmonary cryptococcosis first appeared in the 1960s. Initial descriptions of this disorder highlighted the chronic, nonspecific nature of pulmonary cryptococcosis and a tendency for it to occur in older white men.[20] Although primary pulmonary cryptococcosis occurs in apparently normal hosts, several underlying conditions (in addition to HIV) have been identified as risk factors. These include corticosteroid use, chronic lung disease, Cushing syndrome, diabetes mellitus, malignancy, tuberculosis, rheumatologic disease, and chronic obstructive pulmonary disease.[3,134] Among patients with cancer, a lymphoid malignancy is present in most patients with pulmonary cryptococcosis, as is corticosteroid use and lymphopenia.[93] In the mid-2000s reports highlighted the risk for anti–tumor necrosis factor therapies and pulmonary cryptococcosis, similar to that for tuberculosis and other endemic mycosis.[65] In a multicenter study of organ transplant recipients, 39% of patients with cryptococcosis had primary pulmonary disease.[132] Primary pulmonary cryptococcosis has also been reported to be disproportionately more common in the British Columbia *C. gattii* outbreak, where it is the most common form of presentation.[54] Nonetheless, the specific presentation of *C. gattii* disease may still be primarily dependent on host immune status.[29]

Pulmonary Cryptococcosis in Children

Pulmonary disease as the primary manifestation of cryptococcosis in children is uncommon but has been described and affects both immunocompetent and immunocompromised children.[60,131] Infected children usually have chronic respiratory tract symptoms (i.e., cough, fever, chest pain, and weight loss) and are initially treated for bacterial pneumonia before the diagnosis is suspected. In one review of pulmonary cryptococcosis in children, a predilection for lower lobe lung disease was apparent, with most children being asymptomatic, immunocompromised, and male.[167] Children may be asymptomatic and the diagnosis recognized as a result of imaging performed for other reasons. Several characteristic cases of pediatric pulmonary cryptococcosis in the context of soft tissue malignancy were diagnosed as a result of imaging to evaluate for metastasis.[5,167] These children all had lung nodules that were initially thought to represent metastatic disease, and they were often lymphopenic.

Clinical Manifestations

The typical symptoms of pulmonary cryptococcosis in all age groups include cough, chest pain, dyspnea, fever, and weight loss.[20,91] However, several studies indicate that a significant proportion of infected patients do not have respiratory symptoms. In a study of pulmonary cryptococcosis among solid-organ transplant recipients, 38% of the cases were asymptomatic.[157] Asymptomatic disease appears to be more common among immunocompetent individuals but, as previously noted, does occur in immunosuppressed patients and may be initially confused with cancer. In patients with recognizable pulmonary disease, symptoms are typically mild and often chronic. In immunocompetent individuals, primary pulmonary cryptococcosis is often self-limited. In contrast, pulmonary cryptococcosis among immunocompromised individuals is more likely to occur in the context of disseminated disease or progress to involve the CNS. Constitutional signs, especially fever, weight loss, and anorexia, have been described, particularly in association with the underlying immunosuppression. Rarely, pulmonary cryptococcosis can rapidly progress to acute respiratory distress syndrome in the severely immunocompromised patient. Coinfection with other pathogens, including *Mycobacterium tuberculosis* and *Aspergillus* spp., occasionally has been described.[49,172]

Radiology

The three most common radiologic appearances of pulmonary cryptococcosis are nodular (see Fig. 203.1), infiltrative, and interstitial, although pleural effusions and cavitary disease have also been described.[32,92] Nodules may be solitary or multiple and are nonspecific. Among AIDS patients, interstitial disease and large lobar infiltrates are the most common radiologic findings. Diffuse interstitial findings may be an indication of disseminated disease. Nodular densities or mass lesions are more likely to be asymptomatic or incidentally detected pulmonary cryptococcosis than pleural effusions and infiltrates.[157] Cavitation of cryptococcal nodules, progressive infiltrates, or acute respiratory distress syndrome may occur, especially immunocompromised individuals, and these features have been described in the context of immune reconstitution inflammatory syndrome (IRIS, see later discussion) in AIDS patients[84] and transplant recipients.

Diagnosis

Sputum culture has an extremely limited sensitivity in the diagnosis of pulmonary cryptococcosis. In one study, only 19 of 101 cases of pulmonary cryptococcosis in adults were confirmed by sputum culture.[20] Bronchoscopy with lavage fluid testing for fungal culture and cryptococcal polysaccharide antigen may aid in the diagnosis of cryptococcosis, although the sensitivity of this approach can be variable. Definitive diagnosis may require obtaining tissue directly through either transthoracic, transbronchial, or open-lung biopsy. Serum cryptococcal antigen is typically nondetectable in isolated pulmonary cryptococcosis, and the presence of serum antigenemia supports at least consideration of disseminated disease.

CRYPTOCOCCAL MENINGOENCEPHALITIS

CME typically involves the subarachnoid space or leptomeninges and is usually associated with brain parenchymal involvement even if cryptococcomas are not observed radiographically. Infection may extend through the Virchow-Robin space into the brain substance, most commonly affecting the midbrain and basal ganglia. Immunohistochemistry studies of brains from patients reveal extensive shedding of cryptococcal polysaccharide into the brain parenchyma (see Fig. 203.1).[100] Subarachnoid and parenchymal inflammation ranging from minimal to extensive granulomas may be present, depending on the host immune status and the fungal burden.[101] Increased intracranial pressure (ICP) often complicates CME and contributes significantly to the morbidity and mortality of this disease (see later). Cryptococcomas and CNS complications, including hydrocephalus and cranial nerve palsies, appear to be more common with *C. gattii* disease[123,160] but can occur with *C. neoformans*. Differences between CME in HIV-infected and non–HIV-infected individuals have also been described. These include a more acute presentation and the presence of a second site of infection in HIV-infected individuals,[105] with less associated inflammation.

The mechanisms by which *C. neoformans* and *C. gattii* enter the CNS are still incompletely understood. In general, organisms cross the blood-brain barrier by one of three mechanisms: transcellularly, paracellularly, or through infected phagocytes (Trojan horse). Evidence for both transcellular[24] and Trojan horse mechanisms exist for *Cryptococcus*. In this regard, *C. neoformans* adheres to and infects endothelial cells in vitro.[79] This process may be active and involve the secretion of enzymes (e.g., urease, phospholipase metalloprotease), which in turn induces cytoskeleton rearrangements, or signaling that results in movement across the blood-brain barrier.[115,179,85] Evidence supporting the Trojan horse model comes from experiments in which CNS infection was successfully produced by infection of mice with *C. neoformans*–infected monocytes.[27]

Clinical Manifestations

CME is a subacute to chronic process that generally presents symptomatically over weeks to even months. Occasionally, shorter and longer time intervals are described. Affected patients typically have a persistent headache with or without a variety of other nonspecific symptoms, including fever, lethargy, nausea, and vomiting. Meningismus and photophobia, which are typical of bacterial meningitis, are often absent in adults. Symptoms of encephalitis may also be present and even predominate, including personality changes, memory loss, and altered mental status. Patients with cryptococcomas can have signs of increased ICP and localizing neurologic symptoms and signs, consistent with an intracranial mass.

Pediatric Cryptococcal Meningoencephalitis

Because of the small number of cases, it is difficult to know if there are specific clinical differences in pediatric compared with adult meningoencephalitis in the presentation. The most common symptoms reported in the largest pediatric series to date are headaches and fever. Other commonly reported symptoms include nausea and vomiting. In one study of affected African children with AIDS, seizures were significantly more common in children compared with adults (38% vs. 11%); however, this high incidence of seizures has not been reported in other pediatric series.[64] Additional reported symptoms include altered mental status, focal neurologic deficits, photophobia, abdominal pain, and respiratory symptoms. In some studies, meningismus is present in the majority of children. In a recent study of Colombian children with cryptococcosis, the most common symptoms were headache (78.1%), fever (68.8%), nausea and vomiting (65.6%), confusion (50%), and meningeal signs (37.5%).[110] Like adults, it is common to see a relative lack of CSF inflammation in children with cryptococcal meningoencephalitis, and CSF profiles may be at almost normal. Increased ICP in pediatric CME is well described, but the precise incidence is not well documented. In one study, more than 80% of children with CME had increased ICP with or without symptoms.[107]

Diagnosis

Cerebrospinal Fluid Profile

The CSF profile of both adults and children with CME is characterized by a lack in both cellularity and alterations in biochemical profile, especially in HIV-infected individuals. In pediatric studies, mean CSF white blood cell counts vary from 4 to 16 cells/mm^3.[1,74,153] In another study, approximately 50% of infected children had normal CSF findings (with a normal white blood cell count of <7 cells/mm^3).[107] Likewise, CSF protein and glucose concentrations are often normal, although elevated protein concentrations may be present, especially with obstruction. In one study, decreased glucose or increased protein concentrations were present in 19% of infected children.[107] Given the normal appearance of CSF, a high suspicion and cryptococcal specific studies (see later discussion) are necessary for diagnosis.

Imaging

In cryptococcal meningoencephalitis, imaging often underrepresents the extent of disease, although magnetic resonance imaging results are more likely to be abnormal.[26] The presence of imaging abnormalities may be a marker of more extensive disease and high risk for death.[45] Meningeal enhancement is not uniformly present, which likely reflects the paucity of inflammation in this disease. In a study of solid-organ transplant recipients with cryptococcal meningoencephalitis, meningeal enhancement (the most common finding) was present in only 15% of patients.[158] A similar frequency of enhancement has been reported in patients with AIDS. Other imaging features that may occasionally be noted include parenchymal masses (see later discussion), dilation of the Virchow-Robin spaces, hydrocephalous, and cerebral edema.[41,145] Lesions of the Virchow-Robin spaces (called "soap bubble" lesions) are nonenhancing on magnetic resonance imaging and occur at the level of the thalamus, basal ganglia, periventricular white matter, and cerebellum. These lesions correlate with invasion through the perivascular Virchow-Robin spaces seen on autopsy and are characteristic of meningoencephalitis.[9]

India Ink Staining

India ink staining is based on the exclusion of the dye by the *C. neoformans* or *C. gattii* capsule, which creates a halo around the cell against a dark background. The sensitivity of India ink staining of CSF has been reported to vary from 50% to more than 80%. The sensitivity of this assay depends on the number of organisms in the CSF, which may in part be dependent on the immune state of the host.[34] False-positive results may be reported from leukocytes and tissue cells that can be removed by treatment with potassium hydroxide.

Culture and Histopathology

In adults with CME and HIV infection, CSF and blood cultures are positive in 75% to 90% and 70% of patients, respectively. Similar numbers have been reported in pediatric series.[1] For patients who undergo biopsy (e.g., brain biopsy for cryptococcoma), *C. neoformans* or *C. gattii* is best visualized with special stains, including silver stain and stains that label the capsule (e.g., mucicarmine and Alcian blue). As with other fungi, the cell wall of this organism can be visualized with fluorescence using calcofluor, whereas melanin can be detected with a Fontana-Masson stain. Detection of the organism by immunohistochemistry using capsule-specific antibody and polymerase chain reaction has also been described (see Fig. 203.1).[167,174] Although not part of routine clinical practice, quantitative CSF yeast counts and their serial measurements have been used on a research basis to predict prognosis and treatment success.[15]

Antigen Detection

The polysaccharide capsule is shed during infection and can be measured in serum, CSF, and bronchoalveolar lavage fluid using two different antibody-based technologies (latex agglutination and enzyme-linked immunosorbent assay). Currently, latex agglutination is the most commonly used assay in clinical laboratories. This is a semiquantitative assay, which is reported as a titer. The sensitivity and specificity of antigen detection (using CSF or serum) for patients with CME are both more than 95%. Antigen may also be detected in the serum in more than 90% of patients with disseminated disease.[11] As noted earlier, high CSF antigen titers have been associated with increased mortality, presumably reflecting a high fungal burden. In fact, CSF fungal burden can reach more than 1 million yeasts per milliliter of CSF in advanced cases. In patients with extremely high antigen titers, a false-negative agglutination test may result from a prozone phenomenon. This can be addressed by dilution of samples. Care should therefore be taken in interpreting negative result in patients in whom there is a high clinical suspicion. Rare false-positive results have been reported in patients with infections secondary to other fungal pathogens such as *Trichosporon* spp.[117,169] and other microbes.[25] Although antigen detection assays are useful in diagnosis, they have limited utility in following response to therapy. A lateral flow assay (LFA), which shows good agreement with standard antigen testing, has been developed for the diagnosis of cryptococcosis, especially in resource-limited countries.[108] This assay offers the advantages of rapidity, ease of use, and decreased cost. Like other antigen detection techniques, the LFA has limited utility in following the effectiveness of therapy. Interestingly, limited data suggest that initial LFA testing results may correlate with fungal burden and prognosis.[87] In resource-limited areas or areas with known high prevalence of cryptococcosis, the point-of-care, simple, cheap LFA may be integrated into a preemptive strategy for HIV-infected patients to identify and treat early disease.[175]

Complications

Mortality

Untreated CME is uniformly fatal. Despite the development of a variety of antifungal therapies, the mortality associated with cryptococcosis, particularly CNS and disseminated disease, remains high. Worldwide there are more than an estimated one-half million deaths annually, with the majority of these deaths occurring in sub-Saharan Africa and Southeast Asia.[135] Overall, cryptococcal meningitis is the fourth leading infectious cause of death in sub-Saharan Africa, surpassing even tuberculosis.[135] In solid-organ transplant recipients, the mortality associated with CME can approach 40%.[78] This is comparable to the 10% to 30% mortality for HIV-associated cryptococcal disease in developed countries. In pediatric series, mortality rates have been reported to range between 23% and 38%.[1,64,153] Mortality is affected by several variables, including the underlying immune status, the presence of brain involvement, and the availability of appropriate antifungal therapies. Predictors of mortality reflect host factors and yeast burden and thus include a high CSF cryptococcal antigen titer, increased ICP, altered mental status, positive India ink staining, and low CSF white blood cell counts at baseline (<10 cells/mm^3).[7,43,149]

Increased Intracranial Pressure

Increased ICP is an important and common complication of cryptococcal meningoencephalitis, occurring in as many as 60% of adult AIDS patients with this fungal infection. Increased ICP appears to be more common in patients with *C. gattii* disease, who also tend to have more cryptococcomas. The precise incidence of increased ICP in children with CME is not known but is likely to be similar to that in adults.[107] The entity is well described in children and includes cases of fulminant ICP.[125] The basis of increased ICP in CME remains unknown, but possible mechanisms include (1) inflammation, (2) osmotic effects of shed polysaccharide or mannitol, and (3) obstruction of normal CSF drainage pathways (e.g., arachnoid villi) by cryptococcal polysaccharide or obstructing yeasts. In support of this latter hypothesis, increased ICP has been associated in some studies with higher CSF fungal burden and CSF cryptococcal antigen levels but not with inflammation.[62] Furthermore, a difference in the tendencies of individual strains to elicit increased ICP has been demonstrated in animal models.[53]

Increased ICP is a recognized risk factor for early mortality in cryptococcal meningoencephalitis[62,171] and may correlate with increased CSF fungal burden, increased CSF cryptococcal antigen levels, and failure to sterilize CSF at 14 days. Patients with increased ICP may have symptoms (e.g., hearing loss, altered mental status, cranial nerve palsy), but increased ICP may not be clinically apparent. Furthermore, computed tomography usually does not reveal ventricular dilation, although occasional cases of obstructive hydrocephalous on presentation have been described. Appropriate treatment of CME therefore includes the documentation of CSF opening pressures at the initiation of therapy. Symptomatic increased opening pressure (≥250 mm^3 of H_2O) should be managed by serial lumbar punctures with daily withdrawal of CSF or a lumbar drain. Although there have been no controlled studies to determine the best approach to lowering ICP, the most recent Infectious Diseases Society of America (IDSA) guidelines suggest removal of enough CSF to decrease pressure by 50% if it is extremely high or to a normal pressure of less than 200 mm^3 H_2O.[139] Temporary percutaneous lumbar drains or ventriculostomy for persons who require repeated daily lumbar punctures should be considered. Permanent ventriculoperitoneal shunts may be indicated in patients who fail less-invasive methods. Acetazolamide and mannitol are not indicated in the treatment of increased ICP and may be detrimental.

Corticosteroids are also generally not indicated in the treatment of increased ICP associated with CME, although this paradigm is based primarily on data from HIV-infected cohorts.[63] A recent prospective double-blinded study for the use of dexamethasone during induction therapy for CME was conducted in Asia and Africa to better define the effects of adjunctive steroids on CME-associated mortality in HIV-infected individuals. In this study the tapering doses of dexamethasone had no benefit on mortality but did appear to have increased adverse events and reduced killing of cryptococci in the subarachnoid space.[13] Corticosteroid therapy should not be routinely used during induction therapy for CME. A potential role for corticosteroids in the treatment of severe, recalcitrant elevated ICP in association with *C. gattii* disease has been hypothesized, but more studies are needed before this practice is routinely accepted.[52] Importantly, successful treatment of increased ICP in association with IRIS with corticosteroids has been described in case reports and small series, and its use remains an important management strategy when IRIS is diagnosed during CME.[103]

Cryptococcoma

Intraparenchymal brain lesions (cryptococcomas) are a recognized complication of CME and have been associated with increased mortality.[26,158] Lesions may be singular or multiple, occur in 11% to 35% of patients,[145] and can be associated with focal neurologic symptoms and hydrocephalus. Cryptococcomas appear to be more common in non-AIDS patients and those with *C. gattii* disease. In a recent study of *C. gattii* meningoencephalitis in Australia, 37% of patients developed radiographic cryptococcomas.[29] The treatment of cryptococcomas has not been studied in a prospective manner, and current recommendations are based on small series and expert opinion. These recommendations highlight the importance of extended duration for therapy induction and prolonged maintenance antifungal therapies. In patients with large lesions (≥3 cm), consideration should be given to surgical debulkment.[139] Repeat imaging is helpful in monitoring the response of brain lesions to therapy, but lesions may persist radiographically for a long time and can develop surrounding edema in the context of effective antifungal therapy. This dynamic change can interfere with the assessment of size and evaluation of response to therapy. Intraparenchymal brain lesions also occur in the context of IRIS (see next discussion).

IMMUNE RECONSTITUTION INFLAMMATORY SYNDROME

IRIS is thought to occur as a result of improved immune function in the context of residual microbial antigens, which, in turn, produces symptoms secondary to enhanced inflammation. The current paradigm is that IRIS represents a dysregulated immune response with exaggerated Th1 response relative to Th2 inflammation. Support for this hypothesis comes from studies elucidating the CSF cytokine pattern in individuals with IRIS.[168] IRIS in association with cryptococcosis was initially described in AIDS patients treated with HAART, although it has subsequently been described in solid-organ transplant recipients,[165] pregnant patients,[48] and apparently normal hosts.[47] Cryptococcal IRIS may unmask a previously unrecognized infection (unmasking IRIS) or occur after treatment of cryptococcosis, resulting in a paradoxical worsening of symptoms (paradoxical IRIS). IRIS has not been particularly well documented in children. In a recent study of South Africa children, IRIS was felt to contribute to increased ICP and lymphadenopathy, leading to substantial morbidity and mortality in affected children.[68]

The lack of precise clinical criteria for a diagnosis of cryptococcal IRIS has hindered the study and management of this phenomenon. Several essential elements for this diagnosis have been proposed, including: (1) appearance or worsening of clinical or radiologic manifestations consistent with an inflammatory process; (2) symptoms occurring during receipt of appropriate antifungal therapy that cannot be explained by a newly acquired infection; and (3) negative results of cultures or stable or reduced biomarkers for the initial fungal pathogen during the diagnostic workup for the inflammatory process.[159] Physicians considering a diagnosis of IRIS should exclude progression of infection (owing to inadequate antifungal therapy, antifungal resistance, or worsening immune function) and alternative diagnoses (e.g., other infection, malignancy). Cryptococcal IRIS may present in the form of lymphadenitis, pneumonia, meningitis, or space-occupying lesions in the CNS. Histopathology of affected lymph nodes typically reveals granulomatous inflammation with necrosis and few or absent fungal forms. Cultures typically reveal no growth. Patients with CNS IRIS may develop headache, fever, neck stiffness, and increased ICP, and the associated morbidity and mortality may be significant.[88] In patients with AIDS, cryptococcal IRIS has been reported to occur days to years after initiation of HAART, but typically it occurs weeks to months after HAART is begun. There is usually an associated decline in HIV viral load (at least 1 $\log_{10}$), although changes in $CD4^+$ T cell counts are more variable. Risk factors for cryptococcal IRIS among HIV patients include lower baseline $CD4^+$ T cells, higher HIV viral load, and higher fungal burden at the initiation of therapy. With transplant recipients, IRIS may occur with rapid lowering of an immunosuppression regimen.

There is controversy on the role of early institution of HAART and the development of IRIS. Delayed initiation of HAART may be associated with progression of HIV disease as with other opportunistic infections. However, increasing evidence identifies early initiation of HAART in the context of cryptococcal meningitis as an important risk factor for IRIS.[112,113,155,166] In a recent randomized controlled trial of HIV-positive adults from South Africa and Uganda with CME, patients who received earlier HAART (1–2 weeks after CME diagnosis) had a 15% higher mortality rate at 26 weeks compared with patients for whom HAART was deferred for 5 weeks after diagnosis (45% vs. 30%).[17] Based on these observations, HAART is generally started after CME diagnosis and treatment initiation from 4 to 10 weeks.

Specific treatment of cryptococcal IRIS has not been well studied. Minor IRIS manifestations may resolve spontaneously without specific therapy. Recent IDSA guidelines suggest that prednisone 0.5 to 1 mg/kg in conjunction with antifungal therapy may be helpful for the treatment of CNS cryptococcal IRIS or the use of tapering doses of dexamethasone.[13]

OTHER FORMS OF CRYPTOCOCCOSIS

Besides the CNS and pulmonary tract, *C. neoformans* disease may affect a wide range of organ systems. Primary cutaneous disease may occasionally occur as a result of direct inoculation.[126] More commonly, cutaneous disease represents secondary dissemination, especially in immunocompromised hosts.[138,163] The clinical presentation varies and may include acneiform lesions, purpura, vesicles, nodules, abscesses, ulcers, granulomas, pustules, draining sinuses, and cellulitis. In patients with AIDS, cutaneous cryptococcosis may appear similar to molluscum contagiosum. A high clinical suspicion, along with tissue sampling, is therefore needed to make a diagnosis. The presence of skin disease should prompt an evaluation for disseminated disease. The prostate has been hypothesized to serve as a sanctuary for *C. neoformans* during antifungal therapy and thereby promote recurrent infection. *C. neoformans* has been isolated from prostatic secretions of AIDS patients with disseminated infection, during and after treatment.[98] The clinical significance of these observations, however, remains unclear, and routine surveillance of prostatic secretions is not indicated.

Congenital Cryptococcosis

Congenital cryptococcosis is rare. More than a dozen cases of cryptococcosis in early infancy (e.g., within the first 3 months of life) have been reported, with a mortality greater than 50%.[137] Disease is typically multisystemic, usually with involvement of the central nervous and respiratory systems. Early (e.g., within hours to days of life)[21] and late presentations[89] of cryptococcosis (weeks to months) have been described in neonates. Based on the timing of disease, it has been hypothesized that infection can be transmitted both transplacentally and perinatally, possibly through the aspiration of infected material. The rarity of congenital cryptococcosis among women with active cryptococcosis during pregnancy indicates that the placenta is extremely effective in limiting maternal-fetal transmission. This notion is further supported by several descriptions of cryptococcal placentitis without neonatal disease.[40]

TREATMENT

The treatment of cryptococcosis depends on both the type of disease and the underlying immune status of the host. Although there are clinical differences in cryptococcosis secondary to *C. neoformans* and *C. gattii*, there are no differences in treatment recommendations at the present time. There are no clinical trials addressing the treatment of cryptococcosis in children. Therefore, current pediatric recommendations are based on extrapolations from adult studies using known pharmacokinetic profile of antifungal drugs in children. Routine testing for antifungal susceptibility is not indicated because resistance to amphotericin B and fluconazole is rare. Furthermore, minimal inhibitory concentration (MIC) cutoffs for fluconazole susceptibility have not been established and do not always correlate with clinical outcome. In one study of 487 isolates, only 3 (0.6%) demonstrated a high fluconazole MIC (i.e., ≥16 μg/mL), and all isolates were inhibited by very low concentrations of amphotericin B and exhibited very low MICs to voriconazole and posaconazole.[61] The IDSA guidelines suggest testing for antifungal susceptibilities only in the context of relapsing disease.[139]

Pulmonary Disease

In patients with pulmonary disease, it is essential to determine whether there is associated extrapulmonary involvement. To this end, testing serum for cryptococcal antigen and CSF analysis should be considered in all patients with CNS symptoms and in those with underlying immunosuppression even without symptoms. Isolated pulmonary disease in an immunocompetent patient, which is not severe and asymptomatic, can be treated with fluconazole and without lumbar puncture. The dosage of fluconazole for pulmonary disease in children is 6 to 12 mg/kg per day for 6 to 12 months based on resolution of symptoms (not to exceed the adult dosage of 400 mg daily). Itraconazole is an alternative therapy for individuals who cannot tolerate fluconazole, and the successful use of extended-spectrum azoles (e.g., voriconazole, posaconazole, and isavuconazole) has been described.[140,143,170] Patients with evidence of extrapulmonary disease or severe pulmonary involvement should be treated with the same approach used to treat meningoencephalitis. Azoles are contraindicated in early pregnancy.

Central Nervous System Disease

The currently recommended treatment strategy for CME involves a staged approach using amphotericin B with flucytosine in combination for induction followed by consolidation treatment with fluconazole. The IDSA Guidelines for the Management of Cryptococcal Disease recommend amphotericin B at 0.7 to 1 mg/kg per day plus flucytosine 100 mg/kg per day for the treatment of cryptococcal meningitis.[139] In children, who tolerate amphotericin B better than adults, the higher dosage (e.g., 1 mg/kg per day) is preferred. In adults, there has been a significant shift toward lipid formulations of amphotericin B such as AmBisome 3 to 6 mg/kg per day because of amphotericin B deoxycholate nephrotoxicity. It is unclear in children whether the lipid formulation will carry this therapeutic advantage. The combination of amphotericin B and flucytosine has been demonstrated to be synergistic in vitro and result in improved outcomes in both animal models and clinical studies.[42] Both amphotericin B and flucytosine have significant toxicities, and patients must be closely monitored for these treatment complications. The duration of induction therapy is typically at least 2 weeks but should be individualized. A longer duration of induction should be considered under the following conditions: lack of clinical improvement, positive CSF cultures at 2 weeks, the inability to administer flucytosine, HIV negative, and non–transplant recipient. Most meningoencephalitis studies have been done in patients with AIDS and in transplant recipients, and the duration of induction therapy for other individuals with CME has not been well studied. Repeated CSF examination at 14 days should be considered to document CSF sterilization. Patients with persistently positive CSF cultures should continue induction therapy, and CSF analysis should be repeated every 2 weeks until CSF is sterile. If flucytosine cannot be administered, amphotericin B administered alone is an acceptable alternative or with high-dose fluconazole.[121] In patients whose renal function is impaired, lipid formulations of amphotericin B (liposomal amphotericin B 3 to 6 mg/kg per day, or amphotericin B lipid complex 5 mg/kg) may be substituted. Lipid formulations of amphotericin B are also recommended as first-line agents for solid-organ transplant recipients with cryptococcosis. In resource-limited regions where amphotericin B is not readily available, high-dose fluconazole (1200 mg/day) with flucytosine has been studied as an alternative in adults.[128] After successful induction therapy, children should be treated with fluconazole 12 mg/kg per day (adult dosage, 400 mg) for 8 weeks.

Secondary Prophylaxis

After successful therapy for pneumonia and meningoencephalitis, children with AIDS should be maintained on suppressive fluconazole therapy (6 mg/kg per day, not to exceed the adult dosage of 200 mg daily) to prevent recurrence of disease. In adults, the current recommendations are to continue fluconazole until patients demonstrate a response to HAART, as manifested by a CD4 cell count greater than 100/μL and a sustained undetectable or very low HIV RNA level for 3 months (with a minimum of 12 months of antifungal therapy).[139] Although this approach is generally applied to children, there are few clinical data to support this practice, and it should be undertaken with caution and with close observation for recurrence. A 6- to 12-month period of suppressive fluconazole therapy should also be considered in organ transplant recipients.[139]

Adjuvant Interferon-γ

Consistent with its action as a Th1 cytokine, interferon-γ (IFN-γ) plays a central role in the effective host response to cryptococcosis in animal models.[10,28] Furthermore, exogenously administered IFN-γ enhances resistance and potentiates the effects of amphotericin B in these models.[33,70] A phase II study demonstrated that adjuvant IFN-γ is well tolerated in patients with cryptococcal meningoencephalitis.[133] In another study it was suggested that the addition of IFN-γ to initial induction with amphotericin B or flucytosine results in quicker CSF sterilization, a marker that has previously been associated with clinical success.[82] This study, however, was not powered to detect differences in mortality. Current IDSA guidelines recommend that adjuvant IFN-γ should be considered in refractory cases.[139]

Primary Prophylaxis

In resource-limited regions where HAART is not widely available, there has been increased interest in fluconazole prophylaxis to prevent cryptococcosis. The rationale for this approach lies in the high incidence and mortality of cryptococcosis in these regions. Two different strategies have been applied with promising results. With the first preemptive approach, at-risk HIV-infected individuals are regularly screened for serum cryptococcal antigenemia and treated with fluconazole if they are antigenemic but without overt cryptococcosis.[119] Cryptococcal antigenemia is a marker for the subsequent development of symptomatic cryptococcosis and for death from cryptococcosis and other causes.[106] In essence, this approach represents treatment of incipient disease and is similar to the preemptive strategy used in cytomegalovirus disease in solid-organ transplant recipients. This approach may become more attractive with the recent development of the LFA for antigen detection. With the second approach, all at-risk individuals (i.e., those with CD4 T cells <200/μL) are prophylactically treated with fluconazole. In a Ugandan prospective, double-blind randomized controlled trial, fluconazole prophylaxis for all patients with CD4 T cells less than 200 μL was effective in preventing cryptococcosis and cryptococcosis-associated death,[136] but this strategy can be costly, increase adverse drug events, and potentially encourage drug-resistance development.

NEW REFERENCES SINCE THE SEVENTH EDITION

4. Albuquerque P, Nicola AM, Nieves E, et al. Quorum sensing-mediated, cell density-dependent regulation of growth and virulence in *Cryptococcus neoformans*. *MBio*. 2014;5(1):e00986-00913.
13. Beardsley J, Wolbers M, Kibengo FM, et al. Adjunctive dexamethasone in HIV-associated cryptococcal meningitis. *N Engl J Med*. 2016;374(6):542-554.
16. Bouklas T, Pechuan X, Goldman DL, et al. Old *Cryptococcus neoformans* cells contribute to virulence in chronic cryptococcosis. *MBio*. 2013;4(4).
17. Boulware DR, Meya DB, Muzoora C, et al. Timing of antiretroviral therapy after diagnosis of cryptococcal meningitis. *N Engl J Med*. 2014;370(26):2487-2498.
30. Chen Y, Toffaletti DL, Tenor JL, et al. The *Cryptococcus neoformans* transcriptome at the site of human meningitis. *MBio*. 2014;5(1):e01087-01013.
35. Cox GM, McDade HC, Chen SC, et al. Extracellular phospholipase activity is a virulence factor for *Cryptococcus neoformans*. *Mol Microbiol*. 2001;39(1):166-175.
38. Crabtree JN, Okagaki LH, Wiesner DL, et al. Titan cell production enhances the virulence of *Cryptococcus neoformans*. *Infect Immun*. 2012;80(11):3776-3785.
42. Day JN, Chau TT, Lalloo DG. Combination antifungal therapy for cryptococcal meningitis. *N Engl J Med*. 2013;368(26):2522-2523.
51. Firacative C, Trilles L, Meyer W. MALDI-TOF MS enables the rapid identification of the major molecular types within the *Cryptococcus neoformans/C. gattii* species complex. *PLoS ONE*. 2012;7(5):e37566.
52. Franco-Paredes C, Womack T, Bohlmeyer T, et al. Management of *Cryptococcus gattii* meningoencephalitis. *Lancet Infect Dis*. 2015;15(3):348-355.
62. Graybill JR, Sobel J, Saag M, et al. Diagnosis and management of increased intracranial pressure in patients with AIDS and cryptococcal meningitis. The NIAID Mycoses Study Group and AIDS Cooperative Treatment Groups. *Clin Infect Dis*. 2000;30(1):47-54.
68. Hassan H, Cotton MF, Rabie H. Complicated and protracted cryptococcal disease in HIV-infected children. *Pediatr Infect Dis J*. 2015;34(1):62-65.
73. Hu G, Wang J, Choi J, et al. Variation in chromosome copy number influences the virulence of *Cryptococcus neoformans* and occurs in isolates from AIDS patients. *BMC Genomics*. 2011;12:526.
74. Huang KY, Huang YC, Hung IJ, et al. Cryptococcosis in nonhuman immunodeficiency virus-infected children. *Pediatr Neurol*. 2010;42(4):267-270.
81. Janbon G, Ormerod KL, Paulet D, et al. Analysis of the genome and transcriptome of *Cryptococcus neoformans* var. grubii reveals complex RNA expression and microevolution leading to virulence attenuation. *PLoS Genet*. 2014;10(4):e1004261.
85. Jong A, Wu CH, Chen HM, et al. Identification and characterization of CPS1 as a hyaluronic acid synthase contributing to the pathogenesis of *Cryptococcus neoformans* infection. *Eukaryot Cell*. 2007;6(8):1486-1496.
87. Kabanda T, Siedner MJ, Klausner JD, et al. Point-of-care diagnosis and prognostication of cryptococcal meningitis with the cryptococcal antigen lateral flow assay on cerebrospinal fluid. *Clin Infect Dis*. 2014;58(1):113-116.
96. Kunadharaju R, Choe U, Harris JR, et al. *Cryptococcus gattii*, Florida, USA, 2011. *Emerg Infect Dis*. 2013;19(3):519-521.
110. Lizarazo J, Escandon P, Agudelo CI, et al. Cryptococcosis in Colombian children and literature review. *Mem Inst Oswaldo Cruz*. 2014;109(6):797-804.
121. Milefchik E, Leal MA, Haubrich R, et al. Fluconazole alone or combined with flucytosine for the treatment of AIDS-associated cryptococcal meningitis. *Med Mycol*. 2008;46(4):393-395.
140. Perfect JR, Marr KA, Walsh TJ, et al. Voriconazole treatment for less-common, emerging, or refractory fungal infections. *Clin Infect Dis*. 2003;36(9):1122-1131.
142. Petzold EW, Himmelreich U, Mylonakis E, et al. Characterization and regulation of the trehalose synthesis pathway and its importance in the pathogenicity of *Cryptococcus neoformans*. *Infect Immun*. 2006;74(10):5877-5887.
143. Pitisuttithum P, Negroni R, Graybill JR, et al. Activity of posaconazole in the treatment of central nervous system fungal infections. *J Antimicrob Chemother*. 2005;56(4):745-755.
146. Rohatgi S, Pirofski LA. Host immunity to *Cryptococcus neoformans*. *Future Microbiol*. 2015;10(4):565-581.
148. Rosen LB, Freeman AF, Yang LM, et al. Anti-GM-CSF autoantibodies in patients with cryptococcal meningitis. *J Immunol*. 2013;190(8):3959-3966.
156. Shi M, Li SS, Zheng C, et al. Real-time imaging of trapping and urease-dependent transmigration of *Cryptococcus neoformans* in mouse brain. *J Clin Invest*. 2010;120(5):1683-1693.
161. Steinbach WJ, Reedy JL, Cramer RA Jr, et al. Harnessing calcineurin as a novel anti-infective agent against invasive fungal infections. *Nat Rev Microbiol*. 2007;5(6):418-430.
170. Thompson GR 3rd, Rendon A, Dos Santos RR, et al. Isavuconazole treatment of cryptococcosis and dimorphic mycoses. *Clin Infect Dis*. 2016;63(3):356-362.
175. Vidal JE, Boulware DR. Lateral Flow Assay for cryptococcal antigen: an important advance to improve the continuum of HIV care and reduce cryptococcal meningitis-related mortality. *Rev Inst Med Trop Sao Paulo*. 2015;57(suppl 19):38-45.
179. Vu K, Tham R, Uhrig JP, et al. Invasion of the central nervous system by *Cryptococcus neoformans* requires a secreted fungal metalloprotease. *MBio*. 2014;5(3):e1101-e1114.
184. Zaragoza O, Nielsen K. Titan cells in *Cryptococcus neoformans:* cells with a giant impact. *Curr Opin Microbiol*. 2013;16(4):409-413.

The full reference list for this chapter is available at ExpertConsult.com.

Histoplasmosis 204

Martin B. Kleiman • Elaine G. Cox • John C. Christenson

Histoplasmosis is the most common pulmonary and systemic mycosis in humans, and it affects millions of people.[211,428] Although most infections occur in areas where the etiologic agent, *Histoplasma capsulatum,* is highly endemic, histoplasmosis is being recognized in areas not previously known to be endemic. Substantial proportions of infections with *H. capsulatum* occur in the United States, where approximately 500,000 persons are infected annually.[421] Of these, an estimated 55,000 to 200,000 infected persons become symptomatic.[70] During 2001 to 2012, histoplasmosis-associated hospitalizations in the United States were estimated to be 50,778.[31] Histoplasmosis was the primary diagnosis in approximately 20% of cases, with infection rates lowest in persons younger than 18 years old. The significance of *H. capsulatum* as a cause of opportunistic infection has escalated in proportion to the increasing numbers of persons who are immunosuppressed.[266] Although an increase in hospitalizations has been observed in transplant recipients and in those receiving biologic agents, the proportion of hospitalizations in patients with human immunodeficiency virus (HIV) infection or acquired immunodeficiency syndrome (AIDS) decreased from 2001 to 2012 (from 21.5% to 17.3%).[31]

H. capsulatum was described first in 1906 by Darling[88,89] during examination of autopsy specimens of a man who died of a chronic, wasting illness. He observed organisms within histiocytes and thought them to be encapsulated plasmodia. In 1932, Dodd and Tompkins described intracellular *H. capsulatum* in the peripheral blood smear of a febrile child, and DeMonbreum isolated the organism and correctly classified it as a fungus.

In 1944, Christie and Peterson[69] developed histoplasmin and, after cutaneous inoculation, showed a localized reaction in a child with histoplasmosis. In 1945, Parsons and Zarafonetis characterized the disease as rare and usually fatal after studying 71 patients with disseminated histoplasmosis. Broader use of histoplasmin skin testing by Christie and Peterson,[69] however, showed histoplasmosis to be a common and usually mild disease. They also determined that histoplasmosis was the cause of pulmonary calcifications in patients who were presumed to have had tuberculosis but whose tuberculin skin test results were negative. Demonstration of the organism in soil and air samples in the late 1940s and early 1950s confirmed the natural habitat and transmission of the pathogen.[5,120,478]

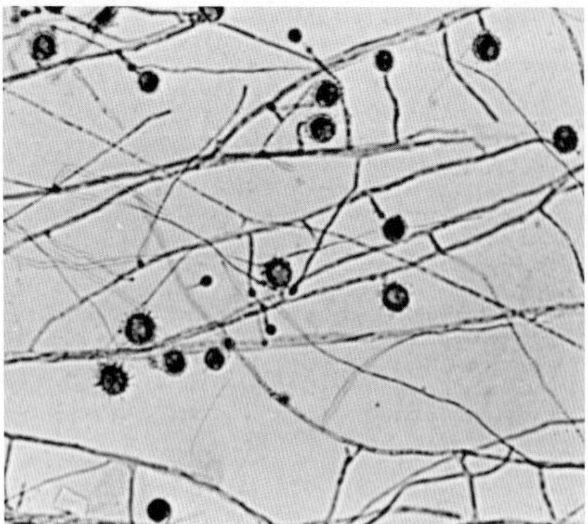

FIG. 204.1 Culture of *Histoplasma capsulatum* from sputum illustrating tuberculate macroaleuriospores and microaleuriospores (lactophenol cotton blue, ×52).

ORGANISM

Histoplasma capsulatum var. *capsulatum* is a thermally dimorphic, saprophytic fungus. At temperatures of 25°C to 30°C, the mold grows as a fluffy colony with an aerial mycelium that varies from white to buff brown. Mycelia, small oval microconidia (2–4 μm) that are attached laterally to hyphae, and tuberculate and nontuberculate macroconidia (8–6 μm) are seen microscopically (Fig. 204.1). Growth is slow, with 1 to 2 weeks required for laboratory strains and 8 to 12 weeks for growth from clinical specimens. When cultured at 37°C on enriched media containing cysteine, the mold transforms to the yeast form in 7 to 10 days. The small, heaped, yellow-white, pasty colonies appear microscopically as ovoid, budding yeasts (1–3 μm × 3–5 μm) with rare pseudohyphae.[294]

In its natural habitat, the soil, *H. capsulatum* exists as spore-bearing mycelia. Optimal survival is supported in moist (95–100% humidity), nitrogen-rich soil at temperatures of 37°C or greater and can be found 1 mile below the soil surface.[409,421] The droppings of chickens, blackbirds, and starlings contain nutrients that promote growth, and, at least in the case of chickens, may contain substances that discourage the growth of competitive organisms. Birds excrete the fungus in droppings yet remain uninfected, probably because of their high body temperature. Bats become infected and excrete the fungus in their guano, which contains substances that encourage fungal growth.[121,242,392] The migratory behavior of bats has been shown to be associated with genetic variation and both the geographic distribution and the ecotype dispersion of *H. capsulatum*.[393] *H. capsulatum* can remain viable in droppings or other contaminated sites for many years.[460]

Examinations of restriction fragment length polymorphisms of DNA have delineated three broad classes of this fungus that exhibit geographic and possibly clinical differences.[113,213,414] Class 1 strains are isolated almost exclusively from immunocompromised patients. Class 2 strains are found most frequently in North America, and class 3 strains are found in Central and South America. Individual strains within each class have been examined further with additional nucleic acid–based and genome-wide approaches to reveal considerable genetic diversity.[193,273,393] Such strain differences are useful for molecular epidemiologic investigations.[272,391,394,477] Additional investigations using molecular methodology have suggested that genetic differences in the pathogen may underlie clinical differences.[208,275] Studies have suggested that patients with AIDS may be infected with less virulent, temperature-sensitive variants of *H. capsulatum*.[379]

Histoplasma duboisii, the cause of African histoplasmosis, is a variant of *H. capsulatum*. *H. capsulatum* var. *duboisii* is indistinguishable from *H. capsulatum* var. *capsulatum* in its mycelial stage; in its tissue phase it appears as thick-walled, oval yeast forms that are 10 to 15 μm in diameter. Infections caused by *H. capsulatum* var. *duboisii* have been described across central and western Africa, and cases occur along with histoplasmosis caused by *H. capsulatum*.[160,244]

EPIDEMIOLOGY

Histoplasmosis is almost always acquired when sites contaminated with *H. capsulatum* are disturbed and spores are aerosolized and inhaled. The early understanding of its global epidemiology and clinical signs was skewed by analyses of localized outbreaks after exposure to large inocula. A more accurate picture emerged when skin test epidemiology, environmental cultures, vectors, and analyses of patients' exposures were considered.[59]

Histoplasmosis has been reported worldwide in tropical, subtropical, and, most frequently, temperate areas.[265] Most illnesses are sporadic and unassociated with exposure to a specific site or specific activity. They are presumed to result when environmental conditions are conducive to fungal growth and when dry, windy conditions or other events or activities facilitate the aerosolization of spores.

Although early reports emphasized that the infection usually was associated with occupational exposure in primarily rural environments, infection is recognized commonly in urban areas, where it may affect many people.[194,246,454] Asymptomatic infections are common in children and are usually clinically unrecognized.[45,164,185] In a highly endemic area, skin test reactivity was 34% in children younger than 2 years of age, 55% between 2 and 4 years of age, and 77% in 10-year-old children.[479] Rates accelerated in summer.

Regions with high rates of infection are considered endemic. The incidence of infection varies widely in these regions. Localized and very heavily contaminated sites, termed *microfoci,* may be found in which localized, sometimes severe, outbreaks occur. Because the droppings of birds and bats accelerate growth of the mycelial form in the environment, implicated sites have included blackbird and pigeon roosting areas, chicken houses, bat-infested caves,[22,187,248] attics, chimneys, old structures, and decaying woodpiles and trees. Activities that disturb these areas have been implicated in localized outbreaks.[185,319] Infections in children have been associated with exploring caves, playing in barns or hollow trees, cleaning abandoned buildings, cutting firewood or decayed tree stumps, renovation of older homes, digging in contaminated sites, excavation or demolition of buildings, cleaning seldom-used fireplaces, and exposure to fungal aerosols that gain access to air duct intakes.[63,246] An outbreak in Mexico was associated with contact with contaminated compost in potted plants.[394]

The geographic distribution of *H. capsulatum* skin test reactivity among 275,558 US Navy recruits was studied between 1958 and 1965.[114,115,253] The highest incidence was found in residents of the Ohio-Mississippi-Missouri, St. Lawrence, and Rio Grande River Valleys. In four states (Arkansas, Kentucky, Missouri, and Tennessee), the percentage of positive adult reactors ranged from 57% to 68%. In the adjacent states (Illinois, Indiana, Ohio, and Oklahoma), reactivity ranged from 50% to 73% among adults in farm areas. Of the other seven states in the endemic area, lifetime prevalence rates exceeding 50% were shown in one or more counties. Epidemiologic studies have not been repeated, and population shifts and changes in land use may alter these patterns. In Latin America,[60] areas of high prevalence include Venezuela,[256] Colombia,[19,274] Ecuador,[299] Brazil,[28] Paraguay, Uruguay, and Argentina.[79]

Analyses of point-source and sustained outbreaks offer some means of assessing the epidemiology and clinical spectrum of infections. An outbreak in Indianapolis, Indiana, affected an estimated 100,000 persons within a 400-square-mile area and lasted nearly 1 year.[453] Illnesses were identified in 435 persons (including 49 children <15 years), and disseminated disease developed in 46. Persons 15 to 34 years of age were more likely to become infected than were other age groups. An equal sex distribution of infections occurred before puberty; male patients predominated in a 3 : 1 ratio in older persons. Localized outbreaks related to high-risk sites and activities are well documented.[54,350,408] In one analysis, 105 reported outbreaks comprising 2850 cases were documented in the United States during 1938 to 2013.[32] In 70 outbreaks with complete data, 51% of cases occurred among children younger than 18 years of age, with a majority of cases associated with two large school-related outbreaks. Indiana had the most reported cases (790).

Infections acquired during travel and/or migration to endemic regions are being reported more frequently.* Infections acquired in areas not recognized as endemic, such as occurred in college students whose only known common exposure was vacationing at a hotel in Mexico,[270] require consideration of the diagnosis in patients with compatible clinical findings.[14,52,57,349] Isolated cases may not be associated readily with high-risk activities. Rarely, infections occur in nonendemic areas and may result from reactivation of quiescent infection in patients who become immunosuppressed.[15,48,189,403]

Vertical transmission, in an area not endemic for histoplasmosis, of both disseminated histoplasmosis and HIV infection was reported in the 5-week-old infant of a mother with both HIV infection and disseminated histoplasmosis.[11] In another case, mother-infant transmission with resulting dissemination was documented following exposure to tumor necrosis factor-α (TNF-α) blocker therapy.[62] Although a case of sexual transmission that resulted from exposure to mucosal lesions of a patient with disseminated histoplasmosis has been described,[370] human-to-human transmission is exceedingly rare. Transmission has been confirmed, with the use of molecular typing methodology, in the recipients of two cadaveric organs from a donor who had resided in an endemic area.[234] Although various wild and domestic animals may become infected, transmission of histoplasmosis to humans does not occur.[46] Infection of an infant after exposure to a pillow that contained contaminated feathers has been reported.[58] Infections caused by inoculation of contaminated material from either the environment or laboratory accidents are also rare.[50]

PATHOPHYSIOLOGY

H. capsulatum has unique interactions with human macrophages, dendritic cells, and neutrophils, the outcomes of which contribute to its success as a pathogen.[284,286,365] Key are its abilities to infect and gain access to macrophages; alter the intracellular environment, thereby allowing the organism to survive, replicate, and disseminate; remain viable during clinically unapparent infection; and become reactivated when host immune factors permit.[55,95,117,153,469] Inhalation of fungal spores induces a brisk innate immune response that is followed by an acquired immune response after about 2 weeks. During these events, the fungus induces an orderly modulation of the host inflammatory and cytokine and chemokine responses.[220] Production of cytokines begins within 24 hours of primary infection and continues for approximately 3 weeks, bridging both the innate and acquired immune responses. Successful clearance of the infection depends primarily on the functional integrity of cellular immunity.[21,206,293,329,481] The clinical manifestations and outcome are determined by this complex interplay of events.

The length of the incubation period of histoplasmosis varies inversely with the size of the inoculum, the integrity of the host immune response, the presence of immunity from previous infection, and strain-related differences in fungal virulence.[116,150,218] Although the range of incubation periods is reported to be 1 to 3 weeks in nonimmune hosts, it has been based largely on data from point-source outbreaks in which the time of the event leading to exposure is readily determined. In these settings, the size of the infecting inocula is probably larger, however, than those resulting in sporadic infections.[59] Because most infections occur sporadically and either are asymptomatic or result in nonspecific and self-limited flu-like illnesses that are not diagnosed, the upper range may be longer. In patients who retain specific cellular (protective) immunity from previous infection, reexposure results in milder symptoms and shorter incubation periods, usually 4 to 7 days.[59] A very few otherwise normal infants as well as persons of any age with primary or acquired cellular immune dysfunction are more likely to experience symptomatic illness after exposure.[150] In the most common situation, pneumonitis develops after inhalation of *H. capsulatum* microconidia or mycelial fragments.[29] Because of their smaller size, microconidia enter terminal alveoli and, within 2 to 3 days, germinate and convert to yeast forms. Dimorphism appears to be a major determinant of virulence; chemical blockage of the transition has been shown to impair virulence.[179,290] Progress in understanding the molecular cell biology and genetics of the mold-to-yeast transition has been reviewed.[186]

In the first week, a neutrophil response occurs at the site of the infection; it is followed in approximately 2 weeks by the accumulation of helper T lymphocytes and macrophages.[321] The yeast forms attach to integrins of the CD11/CD18 group of cell surface receptors and enter neutrophils[361,365] and macrophages.[51,389] This process enables the organism to evade the host oxidative burst response associated with host-directed opsonophagocytosis.[468] Human neutrophils possess fungistatic activity that resides within azurophilic granules.[47,285] Although neutrophils appear to play a role in the primary immune response, depletion of neutrophils in a systemic model of secondary infection did not alter the course.[483] Phagocyte-produced reactive oxygen species participate in the immune response, whereas superoxide dismutase facilitates pathogenesis by detoxifying host-derived reactive oxygen, thereby enabling survival of *Histoplasma*.[476]

The yeast forms seem to have a competitive advantage within the membrane-bound vacuoles of macrophages,[283,282] and the asylum seems to protect it from pulmonary collectin-mediated killing.[257] Both fungal growth and virulence are exquisitely sensitive to the availability of iron.[178] Zinc deprivation is also thought to be a host defense mechanism used by macrophages in a mouse model.[466] Lysis of infected cells releases additional yeasts and results in infection of increased numbers of macrophages. During this period of fungal sequestration and replication, lymphohematogenous dissemination distributes yeast from the lungs to the reticuloendothelial system and to other organs.

Although infection usually results in a brisk antibody response, humoral immunity does not contribute substantially to primary or secondary immunity.[251,290,351] Human dendritic cells that reside in the lung serve to link the innate and adaptive immune responses. Because they are more efficient antigen-presenting cells than alveolar macrophages, dendritic cells use the fibronectin receptor, phagocytose and rapidly degrade the organism, present *H. capsulatum* antigen for lymphocyte proliferation, and facilitate the induction of cell-mediated immunity.[143,283,388] Dendritic cells also have been shown to cross-present exogenous antigen through uptake of apoptotic macrophage-associated fungal antigens.[237] Destruction of yeast within human dendritic cells is an important role within the innate immune response.[283] Conidia transformation into yeast-like forms does not take place within dendritic cells.[286]

After they participate in the innate immune response, several endogenous cytokines,[220] induced by the development of cellular immunity,[283] activate macrophages, which then function as primary cellular effectors that control the infection.[95,282,365] Cytokines that play key roles in the resolution of primary or secondary infection (protective immunity) include TNF-α, interferon-γ (IFN-γ),[10,76,224,413] interleukin (IL)-4,[94] IL-12,[56,484,485] IL-1,[99] and granulocyte-macrophage colony-stimulating factor.[10,98,376]

In addition to macrophages, specific T-cell subpopulations also are capable of killing *H. capsulatum*. $CD4^+$ cells have been shown to be essential for fungal clearance in mouse models.[93,147,236] This comports with observations showing that the risk for severe histoplasmosis in adults with HIV infection increases when the $CD4^+$ count is lower than 200/μL.[436] $CD8^+$ cells also mediate immunity, but their contribution is not as significant as that of $CD4^+$ cells.[236,237,482] Natural killer cells participate to a limited degree in the immune response in immunocompetent animals and play a more substantial role in animals depleted of T cells.[283,308]

In immunocompetent hosts, cellular immunity is suppressed early in the course of histoplasmosis, especially in disseminated histoplasmosis of infancy.[21,72,293,312] Cellular immune function returns to normal after 4 to 6 weeks of treatment. T-cell immunity develops 10 to 21 days after exposure, and splenic suppressor T-cell numbers decrease, whereas helper T-cell numbers increase.[21] In one report, lymphoproliferative responses approached normal in patients with $CD4^+$ counts greater than 500 cells/μ; lymphoproliferative responses and IFN-γ production were depressed in patients with $CD4^+$ counts of 200 to 500 cells/μL.[407] In addition to having defective cellular immunity resulting from decreased numbers of $CD4^+$ cells, the macrophages of patients with HIV infection have impaired ability to control *H. capsulatum*. This results from a profound defect in

*References 15, 16, 17, 49, 123, 137, 188, 203 to 205, 270, 289, 304, 364, 420.

the ability of these macrophages to recognize and bind to yeast and from permissiveness for intracellular fungal growth.[65] The HIV envelope glycoprotein gp120 seems to play a role in inhibiting phagocytosis of *H. capsulatum* by macrophages, but it is not responsible for the capacity for accelerated growth of yeast within macrophages.[66]

PATHOLOGY

With the exception of patients who have severe, progressive, disseminated infection, particularly patients with preexisting primary or acquired cellular immune dysfunction, histopathologic findings in histoplasmosis are characterized by granulomatous inflammation, usually in association with caseating and noncaseating granulomas. The mature granuloma serves both to localize inflammation and to inhibit fungal growth. Another potential and clinically important outcome of this microenvironment is late reactivation of the infection in the event of acquired immune dysfunction.[175,410]

Granulomas appear after the development of an effective acquired immune response; the cellular elements consist primarily of mononuclear phagocytes and lymphocytes, largely T cells. Langerhans giant cells often are present; and typical yeast forms occasionally, but not consistently, are visible within macrophages. Inflammation ultimately progresses to fibrosis and often is accompanied by calcification.[150] The rate of calcification is age dependent, and it may occur within months in children and over several years in adults.[150,383] Exuberant granulomatous inflammation or fibrosis, or both, can result in obstruction or dysfunction of adjacent mediastinal or, less commonly, abdominal structures. In areas endemic for histoplasmosis, old granulomas in the lung, bone marrow, or other sites may be seen as incidental findings, the significance of which depends on clinical assessment. Yeasts are hardly ever observed in histologic sections of extensive fibrosis in late histoplasmosis.

In patients with acute progressive manifestations of histoplasmosis, especially patients with preexisting cellular immune dysfunction, or in otherwise normal infants, the inflammatory response is impaired, and granuloma formation is poor.[124,268] In these instances, extensive parasitization of macrophages by yeasts occurs, and organisms may be seen readily in various reticuloendothelial structures, especially the bone marrow, and sometimes within leukocytes in the peripheral blood.[293] Many other organ systems are often involved. The histopathologic findings in central nervous system (CNS) infection consist of granulomatous basilar meningeal and vascular inflammation, perineural inflammatory changes in cranial nerves, and the presence of many organisms at the periphery of mass lesions.[429] In disseminated infections, the adrenal glands frequently are affected.[24,387] A spectrum of pathologic abnormalities of the gastrointestinal tract may also occur.[23,78,223,305,334]

CLINICAL MANIFESTATIONS

Approximately 95% of infections caused by *H. capsulatum* occur in healthy persons and either are asymptomatic or cause brief, self-limited illnesses with no sequelae. The only residual findings are the incidental radiographic demonstration of typical granulomas in the lung parenchyma and calcifications in the hilar mediastinal lymph nodes or spleen (Fig. 204.2). In immunocompetent hosts, the size of the inoculum probably is the principal determinant of whether infection is accompanied by clinical symptoms. After exposure to small inocula, only 1% of persons develop symptoms, whereas after heavy exposure, 50% to 100% will become ill.[421] Additionally, the symptoms that develop are more severe in persons exposed to large inocula. Severity may be reduced in persons with preexisting immunity derived from previous infection. Protection is incomplete, however, and severe disease can occur after reexposure to a large inoculum.

A crucial determinant of susceptibility and disease severity also is host dependent. Persons with primary or acquired disorders of cellular immunity and otherwise normal infants younger than 1 year of age have a disproportionately high risk for developing symptoms after exposure. These groups are at far greater risk for progression of early dissemination. The precise factor or factors that predispose to a higher risk for progressive dissemination in infections acquired during infancy have not been determined.[231,293,328]

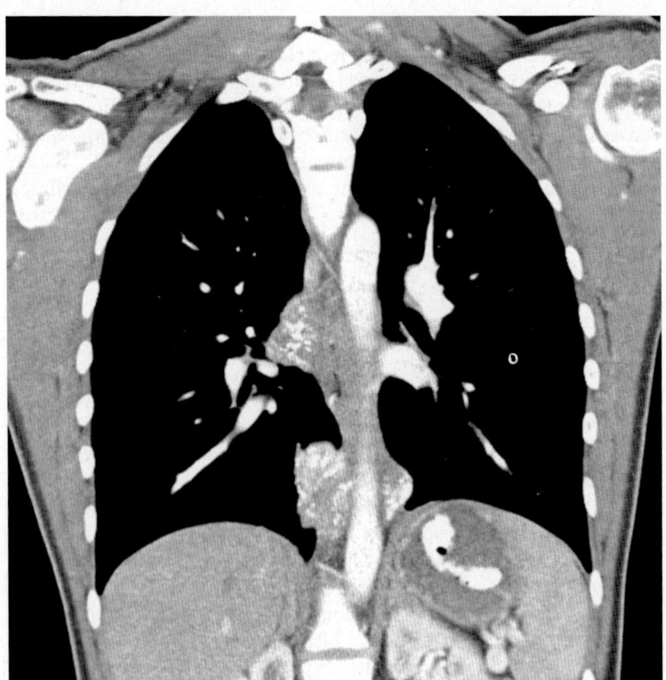

FIG. 204.2 Computed tomography scan of an asymptomatic previously healthy adolescent girl undergoing evaluation for idiopathic scoliosis is found to have multiple areas of lymph node calcifications secondary to histoplasmosis.

As with other endemic mycoses, histoplasmosis begins as acute inflammatory pneumonitis, undergoes self-limited or progressive dissemination, and requires an effective host immune response for its control. Clinical manifestations (Box 204.1) vary because they result from any or all of the following: the nonspecific systemic effects caused by the infection, symptoms resulting from either the primary inflammatory focus or perturbation of function of anatomic structures adjacent to primary sites of inflammation, hypersensitivity phenomena resulting from the acquired immune response, symptoms caused by hematogenously infected sites, life-threatening multisystem symptoms resulting from progressive parasitization of the reticuloendothelial and other organ systems, symptoms caused by chronically progressive forms of pneumonitis or dissemination, or exacerbation of quiescent disease. Recognition, confirmation of the diagnosis, and selection of prudent therapeutic options require understanding of these diverse clinical manifestations. Aside from patients with known preexisting conditions or those receiving therapy that impairs immune function, all patients with serious disseminated disease, persistent antigenuria after completion of therapy, relapse, or recurrent infections should undergo comprehensive assessment of immune function.

Pulmonary Histoplasmosis

The most common symptoms of acute primary histoplasmosis encompass a spectrum of respiratory and systemic complaints of varying severity.[262,432] Eighty percent of infections that are accompanied by symptoms are mild, undifferentiated, flulike illnesses with cough, myalgia, headache, and variable low-grade fever. Symptoms usually are self-limited and resolve in 3 to 5 days.[421] In patients with more significant fungal exposure, fever is present, and symptoms can include headache, myalgia, chills, persistent cough, and nonpleuritic chest pain.[150] Acute illness may persist for as long as 2 weeks and be associated with nausea, asthenia, weight loss, or fatigue. These manifestations are also self-limited, although fatigue and weight loss improve slowly after the fever resolves. In primary infections that last more than 2 weeks, fever persists and is often accompanied by greater weight loss, chills, night sweats, fatigue, or chest pain. The chest pain that occurs in histoplasmosis typically is nonpleuritic. It may be substernal, posterior, or lateralized, it usually is brief in duration, and it recurs frequently. This pattern of chest pain may last from a

BOX 204.1 Clinical Manifestations of Histoplasmosis

- Asymptomatic infection
- Pneumonia
- Progressive disseminated infection (HIV, immunocompromise, infancy)
- Mediastinal lymphadenopathy
- Cavitary pneumonia[a]
- Asthma-like illness
- Pleural effusion or granulomatous pleuritis[a]
- Obstruction or dysfunction of contiguous mediastinal structures (bronchi, esophagus) by granulomatous inflammation of lymph nodes (mediastinal granuloma)
- Isolated cervical or supraclavicular lymphadenopathy[a]
- Superior vena cava syndrome[a]
- Mediastinal fibrosis[a]
- Vocal cord granuloma
- Vocal cord paralysis
- Hemoptysis
- Broncholithiasis with lithoptysis[a]
- Chylothorax[a]
- Diaphragmatic weakness or paralysis
- Esophageal diverticulum or fistula
- Pericarditis
- Erythema nodosum
- Meningitis or focal cerebritis[a]
- Arthritis or arthralgias
- Parotitis
- Nephrocalcinosis
- Interstitial nephritis[a]
- Hypercalcemia
- Gastrointestinal tract ulceration or hemorrhage
- Gastrointestinal tract pseudomalignancy
- Crohn disease–like illness
- Biliary obstruction[a]
- Ocular histoplasmosis, choroiditis[a]
- Endocarditis[a]
- Adrenal mass[a]

[a]Rare in children.
HIV, Human immunodeficiency virus.

week to several months.[150] Wheezing may be an early symptom.[53,419] Hepatosplenomegaly occasionally is present, although its occurrence should raise suspicion of the early onset of progressive dissemination. In these prolonged illnesses, resolution without treatment may occur, but with the safe and effective oral antifungal agents available, most experts recommend treatment.

After development of the respiratory complaints that accompany primary infection, rheumatologic syndromes may be seen within several months of infection. They usually consist of erythema multiforme,[267] erythema nodosum (Fig. 204.3),[150,241,267,303,366] acute migratory polyarthritis, or any combination of these conditions.[74,344] Although histoplasmosis-induced erythema nodosum is seen during childhood and adolescence, arthritis is uncommon. The rheumatologic symptoms are immune mediated and usually self-limited or respond to mild antiinflammatory therapy.

Finally, in acute primary infections that occur after exposure to a large inoculum of spores, the resulting diffuse pneumonitis may be associated with severe symptoms, particularly dyspnea or adult respiratory distress syndrome early in the infection. In these instances, the ordinarily self-limited early dissemination has a high risk of becoming progressive, and treatment is required.

Various symptoms may result from complications arising from intrathoracic or, less commonly, intraabdominal lymphadenitis caused by *H. capsulatum*. One of the most problematic, often termed mediastinal lymphadenitis, is an acute primary infection accompanied by fever, weight loss, and a mediastinal mass visible on chest radiograph. The presence of mediastinal lymphadenopathy in the absence of any recognized clinical symptoms often requires a definitive diagnosis to exclude a neoplasm, especially lymphoma.[134,279] Pediatric series that have examined the definitive diagnosis of such manifestations have found rates of histoplasmosis to range from 1% to 57%, a discrepancy best explained by considering whether the study population lived in an endemic region.[40,134,418,470] In a highly endemic region, middle mediastinal masses were more likely to be features of histoplasmosis if the *Histoplasma* complement-fixation (CF) titers were 1:32 or greater, thereby obviating need for biopsy to determine likelihood of lymphoma.[134]

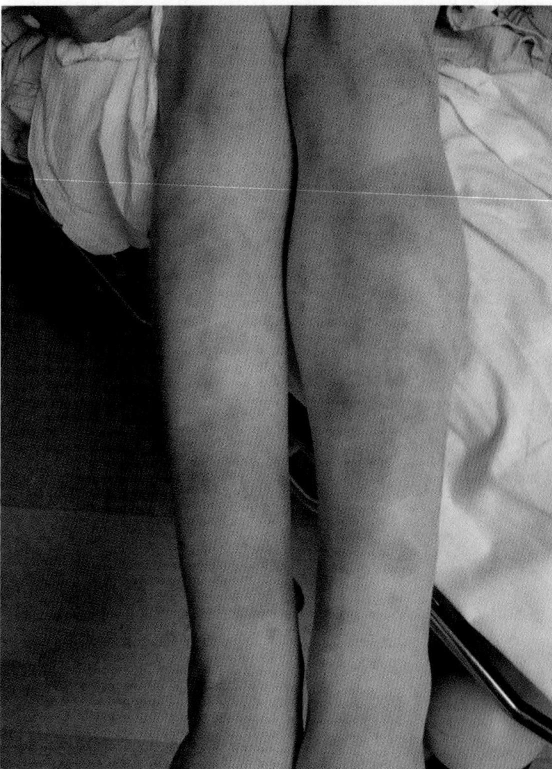

FIG. 204.3 Erythema nodosum in an adolescent boy with pulmonary histoplasmosis.

Complications of acute primary histoplasmosis may be seen when granulomatous lymphadenitis results in inflammation, compression, or obstruction of contiguous structures within the thorax; this manifestation occasionally is termed mediastinal granuloma.[339,404] Structures most commonly affected are, in decreasing order of frequency, the bronchi, trachea, pericardium, pulmonary vasculature and great vessels,[196] lymphatics, esophagus (Fig. 204.4),[112,381] nerves, and endovascular infections of prosthetic endografts or valves.[173,195] Symptoms include bronchial compression or obstruction, or both, which sometimes are associated with the following: distal pneumonitis; pericarditis; pulmonary infarction; esophageal diverticula,[381] fistula formation, or dysmotility, alone or in combination; tracheoesophageal fistula formation; phrenic or recurrent laryngeal nerve palsy; or, in endovascular infections, embolic phenomena. Presumably because of their more pliable airways, children are more susceptible than adults to tracheobronchial compression as a result of encroachment by enlarged lymph nodes.[136]

In highly endemic regions, histoplasmosis is the cause of 25% of acute pericarditis cases; approximately one-fourth of patients have symptoms of cardiac tamponade.[422] In almost all instances, pericardial effusion results from inflammation caused by infected lymph nodes adjacent to the pericardium and not by frank fungal pericarditis.[475] Rarely, contiguous adenitis or broncholiths erode through the pericardium and cause fungal contamination of the pericardial space.[150,475] The pericardial fluid is exudative, bloody, and almost always sterile.[453] Most patients with *Histoplasma* pericarditis quickly improve with

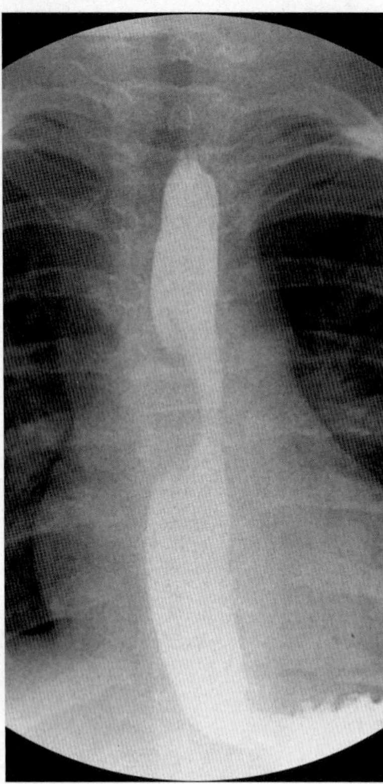

FIG. 204.4 Esophagogram of a young child with difficulty in swallowing and weight loss. Compression of the esophagus secondary to a large mediastinal granuloma is evident.

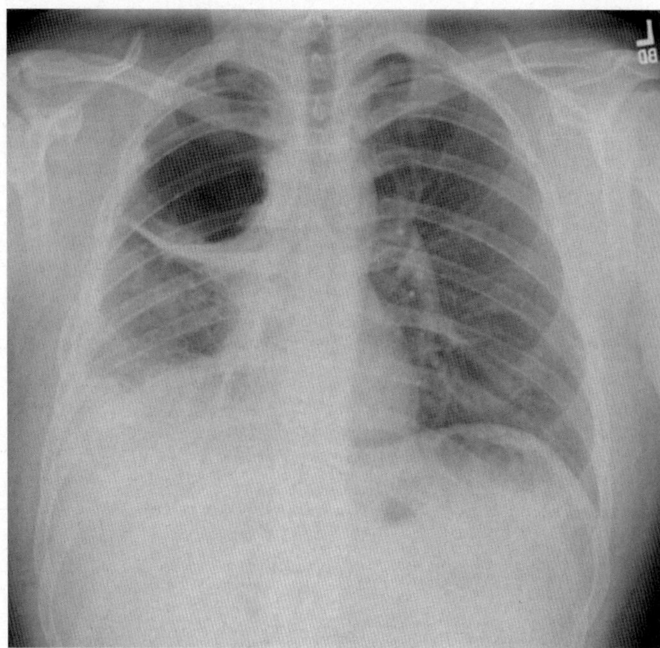

FIG. 204.5 Cavitary lung disease caused by histoplasmosis in a 16-year-old previously healthy boy presenting with cough and hemoptysis. Sputum was positive for *Histoplasma capsulatum*.

administration of nonsteroidal antiinflammatory drugs, and neither acute drainage nor pericardiectomy is needed.

Pleural effusions occur very rarely in children with histoplasmosis, and, similar to pericarditis, seem to result from pleural inflammatory reactions to adjacent granulomas; results of cultures of pleural fluid are negative.[327] Chylothorax caused by extrinsic compression of the thoracic duct by histoplasmosis-induced lymphadenitis was reported to occur in a 3-year-old child.[404] Broncholithiasis may result from calcifications that erode through bronchi but rarely occurs in children.[35] Lower cervical or supraclavicular adenitis is an infrequent manifestation of histoplasmosis and usually is seen in association with mediastinal involvement.[258] Lymphadenitis occasionally affects intraabdominal lymph nodes and has been reported to cause biliary tract obstruction in children.[7,309,334]

Subacute or chronic manifestations of intrathoracic histoplasmosis may occur in children, although they most commonly affect older adults. Of these entities, diffuse mediastinal fibrosis may affect adolescents, albeit infrequently. In these rare instances, granulomatous inflammation progresses to dense fibrosis and may cause stenosis, obstruction, or malfunction of contiguous critical mediastinal structures. Although symptoms are similar to those caused by active granulomatous inflammation that impairs the function of these structures, the fibrosis is progressive and irreversible and responds to neither antifungal therapy nor antiinflammatory agents.[245] Common complications include the superior vena cava syndrome or stenosis or obstruction of the trachea, bronchi, pulmonary artery, or esophagus. Late constrictive pericarditis has been reported in adults with *Histoplasma* pericarditis,[150,471] but it is a rare finding in children.

Additional late complications of intrathoracic histoplasmosis are seen primarily in adults and include pulmonary histoplasmomas (lung nodules), which are granulomas in the peripheral lung fields that become encased in dense fibrous tissue, often with concentric layers of calcification. These may enlarge over several years and cause symptoms of a mass lesion or may manifest as an isolated pulmonary mass.[152] Endobronchial lesions may result in stricture, obstruction, or hemoptysis and mimic bronchogenic neoplasms.[341,345]

Cavitary (also termed chronic) pulmonary histoplasmosis is rarely observed in children.[33,106] In an analysis of risk factors for cavitary disease in an outbreak estimated to have involved 150,000 persons, only 2 in 170 patients with cavitary disease were younger than 19 years of age (Fig. 204.5).[456] Cavitary disease was seen primarily in adults with chronic obstructive pulmonary disease. Symptoms include low-grade fever, productive cough, weakness, weight loss, and fatigue. Early pulmonary findings consist of apical interstitial pneumonitis that eventually progresses to fibrosis, cavitation, and gradual spread to uninvolved areas of the lung.[447] If chronic histoplasmosis is untreated, the disease is fatal.[211] Disseminated infection has been reported to develop in approximately 80% of patients with this disorder.[347]

Primary Cutaneous Histoplasmosis

Numerous reports describe immunocompetent patients who present with mucosal, corneal,[399] or cutaneous ulcerated lesions that show characteristic pathologic changes and morphologic and cultural documentation of *H. capsulatum* and resolve without treatment.[83,138,295,342,370,412,474] These lesions have been considered to be primary, localized infections.[397] Aside from several cases that reasonably may be attributed to documented instances of direct inoculation,[221,370] many of these reports fail to provide sufficient evidence to exclude low-grade, chronic dissemination with histoplasmosis.[8,122]

Progressive Disseminated Histoplasmosis

Progressive disseminated histoplasmosis (PDH) occurs most frequently in immunodeficient patients and patients at the extremes of age.[151,231,293,447] The clinical entity is defined as an illness that is accompanied by active replication of *H. capsulatum* in multiple organ systems. Symptoms are prolonged and usually last for more than 3 weeks. Laboratory evidence of dissemination may include the following: anemia, thrombocytopenia, or leukopenia, or a combination of these; persistent antigenuria or antigenemia, or both; demonstration of granulomas in extrapulmonary tissue; histopathologic demonstration of compatible yeast; or growth of the fungus in culture. The intense exposure to a large fungal inoculum results in severe primary infection that overwhelms the host's ability to mount an effective cellular immune response, thus allowing the usually self-limited primary dissemination to progress.

Distinct clinical presentations of PDH in adults permit subclassification into acute, subacute, and chronic forms. In contrast, PDH in children occurs almost exclusively as an acute, progressive, life-threatening infection.[231,293,328] Most of these infections develop in immunocompetent infants younger than 1 year of age or in children with acquired or primary cellular immunodeficiency. Rarely, PDH occurs in an immunocompetent child, usually in association with exposure to a large fungal inoculum.[90] Transplacental infection has been reported to occur in infants of women with PDH complicating HIV infection.[459]

PDH may result from exogenous exposure of a susceptible or immune host or from reactivation of endogenous quiescent foci of infection. Although reactivation of infection may occur in an immunosuppressed host,[190,403,410] epidemiologic data in immunosuppressed persons who reside in areas highly endemic for histoplasmosis favor a new episode of exogenous exposure as the most common mechanism. Supporting evidence consists of observations showing that rates of PDH in immunocompromised patients increase only during periods in which infection rates increase in the general population and do not increase in interepidemic periods.[314,357,360,407] Using the results of histoplasmin skin testing obtained at the time of diagnosis of malignancy in a large cohort of children, Hughes[184] found that skin test reactivity was absent in all children in whom PDH subsequently developed and that in none of those known to be skin test positive at the time of diagnosis of neoplastic diseases did PDH develop later.

Progressive Disseminated Histoplasmosis of Infancy

PDH of infancy usually affects children younger than 1 year of age.[231,293] It usually is a subacute illness in which symptoms often are reported to have been present for 1 to 12 weeks before the patient undergoes an initial evaluation; as the disease progresses, patients eventually become profoundly ill and usually die unless treated. Early symptoms include variable fever, failure to thrive, and hepatosplenomegaly in almost all instances.[380] Pallor, cough, tachypnea, oropharyngeal ulcerations, lymphadenopathy, gastrointestinal bleeding, or hemorrhagic skin lesions may develop. Abnormalities that are seen frequently in laboratory studies, and inexorably worsen, include anemia, thrombocytopenia, leukopenia,[151,231,328] disseminated intravascular coagulopathy, and marked depression of immunoregulatory cells.[72,293] These abnormalities reflect the overwhelming fungal parasitization of the reticuloendothelial system and often mimic the presenting signs of a lymphoreticular malignant disease.[2] The chest radiograph may show signs of focal pneumonitis, mediastinal adenopathy, or miliary disease, but more than 50% of chest radiographs are normal at the time of diagnosis. Anatomic sites commonly affected include the spleen, liver, bone marrow, lymph nodes, gastrointestinal tract, and adrenal glands. Abnormalities in the cerebrospinal fluid (CSF) were found in 62% of a series of infections in Costa Rican infants.[293]

PDH of infancy was uniformly fatal before effective antifungal agents became available,[231] but survival rates are now excellent. In a series of Costa Rican children that included some infants with malnutrition, 90% of patients treated with amphotericin B survived. In our experience, survival has been 100% in an Indiana series of PDH of infancy.

Progressive Disseminated Histoplasmosis in Immunocompromised Hosts

Immunocompromised persons, including those with either a preexisting medical condition or therapy that has depressed cellular immunity, are at risk for progressive dissemination if they acquire histoplasmosis. Common predisposing conditions include AIDS,[64] primary immunodeficiency disorders,[180,353,481] iatrogenic immunosuppressive therapy for reticuloendothelial malignant diseases,[184] organ transplantation,[158,259,288] rheumatologic disorders,[166] and chronic renal failure.[191] Severe PDH infections have been recognized in patients treated with TNF-α antagonists for inflammatory disorders.[166,467] This effect seems to be associated most closely with the use of infliximab, a TNF-α inhibitor.[108,118,133,229,233,411]

The most common initial symptom is persistent fever, usually without localizing symptoms and unassociated with toxicity. As the illness evolves, fever persists, and liver and spleen enlargement may occur. Laboratory abnormalities include progressively worsening anemia, leukopenia, and thrombocytopenia; disseminated intravascular coagulopathy may ensue. The chest radiograph may be normal. *Histoplasma* antibody assay results

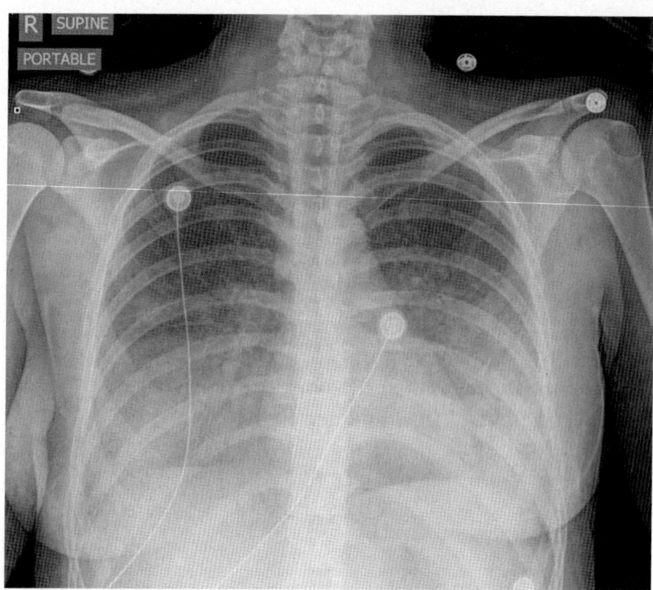

FIG. 204.6 Diffuse lung disease secondary to disseminated histoplasmosis in an adolescent girl with immunoglobulin A nephropathy treated with immunosuppressive therapy.

usually are negative, and the diagnosis is confirmed reliably by using the *Histoplasma* antigen assay of urine or serum.[2,184]

Another common symptom complex consists of respiratory complaints and tachypnea. In these instances, persistent fever is followed in several days by dyspnea. Chest radiographs, although occasionally normal at the onset of symptoms, show diffuse interstitial infiltrates that progressively worsen (Fig. 204.6).[2] Hypoxemia usually accompanies the symptoms and is progressive. This clinical complex is not specific for histoplasmosis and may be indistinguishable from those caused by *Pneumocystis jiroveci,* cytomegalovirus, various viral respiratory pathogens, other opportunistic fungi, and bacterial septicemia.

A subacute form of PDH is seen primarily in adults,[447] although in one report of 19 cases it was found in seven infants and one child.[151] The principal clinical features that distinguish the subacute from the acute form of PDH are a history of more prolonged symptoms at initial evaluation, a higher frequency of focal lesions, less pronounced fever, and fewer hematologic abnormalities in the subacute illness. Early complaints are nonspecific and may be present for 1 to 6 months; malaise and weight loss occur frequently. Hepatosplenomegaly is seen almost uniformly, and intestinal ulceration,[206] sometimes with perforation, occurs commonly.

Gastrointestinal histoplasmosis has protean manifestations, including perforation,[201] that may occur in association with mediastinal histoplasmosis[202] or in the setting of PDH.[201] An autopsy study of 93 adults with AIDS in an endemic region identified gastrointestinal histoplasmosis in 12% of cases.[161] The terminal ileum often is involved, and findings may mimic those of Crohn disease.[61,382] Colonic lesions may result in bleeding or obstruction,[177,367] and they may mimic neoplasms.[228] Isolated colonic lesions without evidence of dissemination are rare.[216] Oropharyngeal ulcerations often occur and are large and deep and can mimic neoplasms.[18,122,151] Seventy-five percent of patients have adrenal involvement, which sometimes is unilateral.[387] Adrenal insufficiency occurs less frequently but is reported in 15% to 50% of adults.[10,151,156,225,330,331,377] CNS infections are seen occasionally and may manifest as chronic meningitis, focal mass lesions, or focal areas of cerebritis. Reports suggest that patients with *STAT3*-mutated hyper–immunoglobulin E (Job) syndrome may be at high risk of disseminated infection involving the CNS and gastrointestinal systems.[292,382] Endovascular infections occur and may affect normal or native valves. The aortic or mitral valves or prosthetic valves most commonly are affected.[9,36,67,119,139,173] Valvular disease seen is typical of fungal endocarditis, with large vegetations and a high frequency of embolic phenomena.[101] Valve replacement was common.[338]

Vaginal and penile ulcerations, soft tissue nodules, recurrent panniculitis, tenosynovitis, carpal tunnel syndrome, osteomyelitis and arthritis, enteropathies, immune hemolytic anemia, and epididymitis all have reported.[200,212,215,301,322,344,370,384,419] Although the pace of subacute PDH is slower than that of acute PDH, the subacute form is nonetheless fatal in 2 to 24 months if untreated.[151]

Chronic disseminated histoplasmosis is seen almost exclusively in adults, usually in association with cavitary pulmonary lesions.[151] Oropharyngeal ulcers are accompanied by chronic, mild, intermittent constitutional symptoms. A chronic relapsing disseminated form of the disease was described in two younger patients, 9 and 20 years old, with chronic mucocutaneous candidiasis[124,268,310] and in a child with IFN-γ receptor-1 deficiency.[481]

Progressive Disseminated Histoplasmosis in Human Immunodeficiency Virus–Infected Patients

Before the development of effective antiretroviral therapy, disseminated infection developed in more than 90% of HIV-infected adults who acquired histoplasmosis.[436] In 1988, less than 0.5% of adult patients with AIDS had disseminated disease.[154] In endemic areas, it has been reported in approximately 5% of patients,[170,263] as well as in 21% to 53% of patients during epidemic periods.[39,424,436,455]

In a multivariate analysis of risk factors for the development of histoplasmosis in HIV-infected adults residing in endemic areas, receipt of antiretroviral therapy and triazole drugs was associated independently with decreased risk.[170,263] One study found the risk to be increased with positive baseline serologic findings, $CD4^+$ cell counts lower than 150/μL, and exposure to chicken coops.[263] Risk factors for death in two large cohorts of adults were also determined.[84,101,430] Mortality rates were greater in HIV-infected patients with PDH who were treated with antifungal therapy compared with HIV-negative patients with PDH; in HIV-positive patients receiving highly active antiretroviral (HAART) therapy in association with antifungal therapy, clinical outcomes were similar to those of patients with PDH unassociated with HIV infection.[400] Comparable studies have not been done in children. In Arkansas, a highly endemic area, histoplasmosis was the AIDS-defining illness in 8% of 40 children who acquired HIV infection in the perinatal period.[363] Histoplasmosis in this population is occasionally is seen in nonendemic regions, perhaps because of reactivation of quiescent foci of infection.[17,123,352,356] An adult series found that patients with AIDS complicated by disseminated histoplasmosis had a substantially higher mortality rate (32% vs. 14%) than did HIV-infected patients with other opportunistic infections.[86]

In HIV-infected adults with disseminated histoplasmosis, early symptoms often are nonspecific; prolonged unexplained fever and weight loss are seen almost uniformly, and respiratory complaints occur in approximately one-half of patients.[165,198,356,436] Features are not distinctive, and in areas in which *Talaromyces marneffei* (formerly known as *Penicillium marneffei*) also is endemic, clinical, laboratory, and radiographic findings often overlap.[227,269] In adults, initial chest radiographs are normal in approximately 40%, diffuse interstitial or reticulonodular infiltrates are seen in approximately 50%, and localized lesions are noted in approximately 5%. Diffuse abnormalities may appear during treatment of patients whose chest radiographs initially were normal.[356]

Gastrointestinal symptoms, including perforation and those caused by partial obstruction, are reported commonly and usually are nonspecific; abdominal pain, weight loss, and diarrhea occur in 50% to 70% of patients.[23,169,171,202,223,367,385] Coinfections do occur.[3,317] Enlargement of the liver and spleen occurs in approximately 25% of patients. Ten percent of patients are initially gravely ill with signs of a septic shock–like syndrome.[436] Mucocutaneous lesions occur in approximately 10% of adult patients and include nonspecific maculopapular rash, papules, nodules, pustules, ulcerative lesions, acneiform lesions, mucosal ulcers, and vegetative plaques.[18,129,130,167] Lesions may mimic those of secondary syphilis,[307] and histopathologic examination of skin biopsy specimens often is diagnostic. The frequency of skin lesions in a cohort of Brazilian adult patients with disseminated infection was 66%.[207]

CNS involvement, including meningitis, encephalitis, and focal brain lesions, occurs in approximately 18% of patients with PDH complicating HIV infection.[12,13,39,197,250,356,429] Symptoms include headache, encephalopathy, or complaints arising from focal neurologic abnormalities.

Published reports of histoplasmosis complicating HIV infection in children are few; in four HIV-infected children in Indiana, fever was present in all, and cutaneous lesions were absent; hepatosplenomegaly was found in one child, and an abdominal mass caused by an infected abdominal lymph node was seen in one child.

With the widespread use of HAART for treating advanced HIV infections, an immune reconstitution inflammatory syndrome has been described.[1,85,278,368] The immunopathogenesis is presumed to result from interaction between HAART-induced improvement of host immune function and residual microbial antigens.[239,340] *H. capsulatum* is among other granuloma-inducing pathogens reported to induce immune reconstitution inflammatory syndrome.[1,43,306,368]

Central Nervous System Infection

CNS manifestations occur in 5% to 10% of adults with PDH, but they also may occur as chronic meningitis without other signs of apparent dissemination.[34,217,429,452] Clinical manifestations are varied and include chronic meningitis and arachnoiditis, hydrocephalus, focal parenchymal lesions, cerebellar ataxia, cranial nerve neuropathy, vasculitis, stroke, and diffuse encephalitis. Isolated meningitis in immunocompetent adults has been associated with presenting signs that include headache, signs of meningeal irritation, and mental status changes.[359] Meningitis is seen in association with disseminated infections in children, especially if acquired during infancy.[293] Isolated meningitis is extremely unusual in an immunocompetent child. Isolated or multiple focal lesions affecting the brain[25,172] or spinal cord,[181] stroke syndromes,[75,287] and encephalitis constitute the balance of manifestations. Meningitis has been reported to occur years after apparent total resolution of PDH.[43,399] This may result from failure of antifungal agents to penetrate the CNS compartment sufficiently to eradicate the infection.[25,400,429] Symptoms of meningitis often are present within 6 months of diagnosis but have been reported to be present for 7 years.[140] Commonly associated symptoms include headache, altered level of consciousness, confusion, and cranial nerve deficits in 28% to 56% of cases.[429]

Diagnosis is problematic in patients with histoplasmal meningitis and no associated manifestations of localized or disseminated infection.[348] It is suspected ante mortem in only 40% of cases. A case was reported with the onset of symptoms 4 years before the diagnosis was confirmed.[34] Symptoms and findings often mimic those caused by other granulomatous infections, sarcoidosis,[429] cerebral vasculitis,[429] neoplasms,[197] or conditions leading to hydrocephalus. CSF findings are nonspecific and include mild pleocytosis, elevated protein, and depressed glucose concentration.[332] The diagnosis is confirmed by isolating *H. capsulatum* from CSF, detecting *Histoplasma* antigen or antibody in CSF, or identifying the organism in non-CNS sites. Although the specificities of culture and antigen methodologies are high, the sensitivity is variable. CSF antigen sensitivity is 38% in non–HIV-infected patients and 67% in HIV-infected patients. CSF antibody is present in 80% to 89% of cases; cross reactions with *Cryptococcus* occur in 28% of cases.[452]

Presumed Ocular Histoplasmosis Syndrome

The entity termed presumed ocular histoplasmosis syndrome consists of a triad of findings: (1) discrete atrophic choroidal scars in the macula or midperiphery ("histo spots"), (2) peripapillary atrophy, and (3) choroidal neovascularization[373] that can lead to loss of central vision.[71] In contrast to the acute endophthalmitis[149] or choroiditis[302] that occurs as a manifestation of disseminated infection, the abnormalities seen with presumed ocular histoplasmosis syndrome occur in the absence of inflammatory changes in the vitreous or anterior chambers. Smoking, level of educational attainment, and older age have been reported as risk factors for acquisition of presumed ocular histoplasmosis among a cohort of affected adults.[68]

Commonly diagnosed in endemic areas, the cause-and-effect relationship of the findings in presumed ocular histoplasmosis syndrome and histoplasmosis has been determined largely on the basis of a weak epidemiologic association with histoplasmin skin test reactivity.[42] The clinical syndrome also occurs in persons residing in nonendemic regions, however.[300,386,417] Little histopathologic evidence supports histoplasmosis as its cause.[214,298,324] A single report detected *H. capsulatum* DNA in cells of an enucleated eye from an affected patient; however, a nonstandardized polymerase chain reaction (PCR)–based methodology was used. Another isolated report of the ocular syndrome used a nested PCR assay to detect *H. capsulatum* in serum.[176] Presumed ocular histoplasmosis does not seem to occur in children younger than 10 years of age.[405] A good recovery of vision has been reported to follow surgical removal of the choroidal neovascularization that accompanies this entity. Scleritis, a rare manifestation of histoplasmosis, has been reported in immunocompetent adults.[87]

Illness Caused by Infection with *Histoplasma capsulatum* var. *duboisii*

In patients infected with *H. capsulatum* var. *duboisii,* focal lesions are seen more commonly in bones (usually the femur, ribs, or skull) and skin (cutaneous or subcutaneous).[4] The lungs, gastrointestinal tract, liver, spleen, and lymph nodes rarely are involved. A progressive disseminated form of infection with *H. capsulatum* var. *duboisii* occurs and is associated with pyogranulomatous inflammation involving multiple organs.[77,135,247,464] In addition, cases of isolated pulmonary histoplasmosis have been reported in immunocompetent persons years after departing an endemic region.[333,336]

Radiographic Findings

The radiographic findings seen most commonly in children with histoplasmosis are not pathognomonic and may mimic the findings seen in tuberculosis or other granulomatous processes and, in some instances, neoplastic conditions, especially lymphoma.[134,216,279,316] After small or moderate degrees of fungal exposure, the plain chest radiograph is normal in approximately 75% of skin test converters.[151,458] Computed tomography (CT) is more sensitive and likely to reveal parenchymal infiltrates that are not visualized in plain radiographs. The most common pulmonary parenchymal changes are "soft" single or multiple, poorly defined areas of airspace consolidation,[163] often found in the basilar portions of the lungs. CT may also reveal a "reversed halo" sign.[254] Findings either may fully resolve or consolidate into granulomas that persist, with or without calcification, in residents of, or travelers to, endemic areas.[296]

The appearance of enlarged hilar or mediastinal lymph nodes, either in association with pulmonary infiltrates or as isolated findings, also is a common radiographic finding in acute pulmonary histoplasmosis.[390] Isolated hilar or mediastinal adenopathy occurs in 20% of cases, 80% of which are asymptomatic.[81] With CT, low signal intensity within nodes sometimes is present; however, frank suppuration is unusual. Infected nodes may enlarge and compress or obstruct adjacent structures (Figs. 204.7A–B; see also Fig. 204.4). Nodes usually have reached their maximal size at the time of diagnosis and become smaller or return to normal in several months; calcification may occur, but not consistently. In infants and young children, clusters of small infiltrates occasionally coalesce into a larger bronchopneumonic lesion.[150] Although small pleural effusions are present in 10% of adults with acute histoplasmosis,[453] they occur infrequently in children.[2,325] Isolated calcifications may be seen in the spleen or liver months to years after infection. These calcifications result from the self-limited fungal dissemination that occurs during primary infection and often are appreciated as incidental findings in persons who have lived in or visited endemic regions.

Three distinct chest radiographic patterns have been described in persons who have had intense exposure to the fungus.[150] Persons from nonendemic areas initially may have scattered infiltrates that later evolve into "buckshot" calcifications. The second and most common pattern is the presence of smaller, nodular lesions. Finally, a diffuse miliary or interstitial pattern (Fig. 204.8) may occur, often in a patient with protective immunity. In PDH, the chest radiograph in adults may show abnormalities in only 25% to 50% of patients.[80] Diffuse abnormalities commonly appear during treatment of patients whose chest radiographs initially were normal.[356] Diffuse interstitial or reticulonodular infiltrates are present in approximately 50%, and localized lesions are present in the remainder. In immunocompromised children, diffuse interstitial infiltrates are the most common radiographic findings; they worsen rapidly and in concert with progressive hypoxemia, especially in patients with HIV infection or patients receiving immunosuppressive therapy.[80] The presence of interstitial infiltrates at admission was reported in 60% of children with PDH of infancy in a Costa Rican series.[293] Abdominal ultrasound evaluation or CT, or both, may show evidence of adrenal enlargement in chronic disseminated disease in adults.[24,465]

Fibrosing mediastinitis caused by histoplasmosis is seen radiographically as pronounced thickening of the mediastinum that often compresses

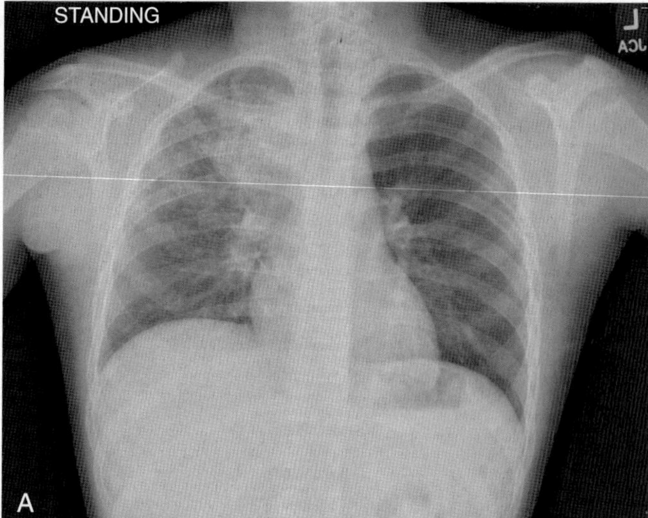

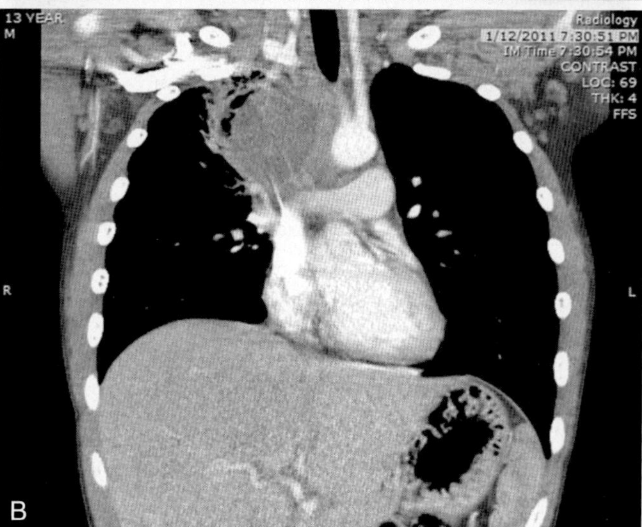

FIG. 204.7 Adolescent boy presenting with chest pain, difficulty in swallowing, fever, and weight loss. Upper mediastinal granuloma noted on (A) chest radiograph and (B) computed tomography scan of the chest.

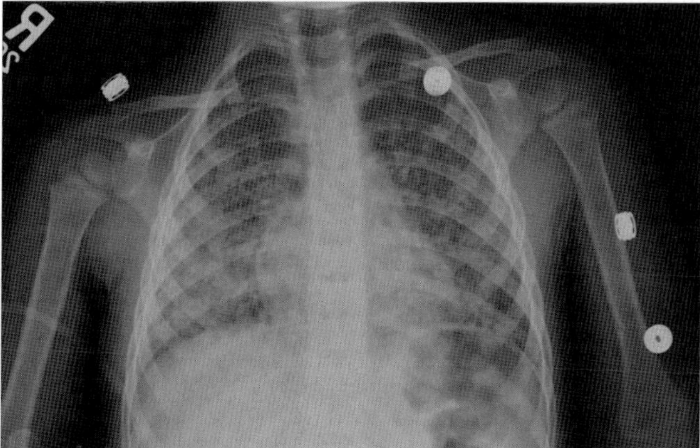

FIG. 204.8 Extensive pulmonary disease with a miliary pattern in an adolescent girl who cleaned a dusty barn contaminated with bird droppings and bat guano.

TABLE 204.1 Laboratory Test Results in Children With Histoplasmosis According to Clinical Manifestations

Clinical Manifestation	Antigen[a]	Complement Fixation: antibody	Immunodiffusion: Antibody	Culture	Comments
Acute histoplasmosis with severe pulmonary disease (high inoculum)	++[b]	++++	+++	+[c]	Antigen assay results are likely to be positive early in the disease
Acute histoplasmosis with mild pulmonary disease	++	++++	+++	–	Antigen assay results are likely to be positive early in the disease
Acute histoplasmosis with fever >1 month	+++	++++	+++	–	
Mediastinal granulomas with or without associated symptoms and signs of compression	–	++	++	–	Middle mediastinal mass plus CF ≥1 : 32: biopsy not needed Histoplasmosis is the most likely cause
Disseminated disease, infants	++++	++++	++++	+++[c]	
Disseminated disease, immunocompromised patient	++++	+++	++	+++[c]	Serologic assay results may be negative early in the infection
CNS histoplasmosis	+	+++[d]	++	–	
Pericarditis, erythema nodosum (other rheumatologic manifestations)	–	++	++	–	
Asymptomatic, history of histoplasmosis and/or presence of mediastinal calcified nodules, calcified hepatic or splenic nodules	–	+	+	–	

[a]Negative antigen: progressive disseminated infection is unlikely.
[b]Serum or urine, bronchoalveolar lavage fluid, or bronchial washings.
[c]Bone marrow and blood specimens.
[d]Antibody detection in cerebrospinal fluid.
–, Negative; +, rarely positive; ++, occasionally positive; +++, frequently positive; ++++, always positive. *CF,* Complement fixation; *CNS,* central nervous system.

or obstructs the superior vena cava, major bronchi, esophagus, or other critical structures. It can be found in a localized pattern that frequently contains calcification. This condition must be differentiated from idiopathic fibrosis or fibrosis not induced by infection, which may cause similar symptoms.[369] CT and magnetic resonance imaging help differentiate active inflammation from fibrosis and aid in monitoring progression.[343,346] Diffuse mediastinal fibrosis caused by histoplasmosis is rare in children.

DIAGNOSIS

Several laboratory tests play key roles in establishing the diagnosis of histoplasmosis. Although each has value, optimal use necessitates an understanding of their differing sensitivities and specificities in various clinical settings.[427] General guidelines for their interpretation are provided in Table 204.1.

Organisms Shown on Histology

In clinical and epidemiologic settings compatible with histoplasmosis, observation of 2- to 4-μm typical yeast forms[162] in histopathologic specimens demonstrating granulomatous inflammation[271] is strong supportive evidence of histoplasmosis. Rarely, typical yeast may be observed but result from past infection.[427] Care must be taken to differentiate *H. capsulatum* from the intracellular pathogens *Leishmania donovani* and *Toxoplasma gondii,* small variants of *Blastomyces dermatitidis,* endospores and young spherules of *Coccidioides immitis, P. marneffei,* and the yeast forms of *Cryptococcus neoformans.* Both Giemsa-stained and hematoxylin and eosin–stained specimens show intracellular yeasts in sputum, blood smears, bone marrow aspirates (Fig. 204.9), and biopsy specimens. The Gomori methenamine silver stain is the most sensitive reagent.[294] Test sensitivity is better in disseminated forms of histoplasmosis, in which yeasts are readily observed in bone marrow, in affected tissue, and often in blood smears (Table 204.2).[197] Tests are less sensitive in self-limited primary infections,[463] including acute pulmonary infection following heavy exposure, in which cytology and histopathology sensitivities are 25%.[427]

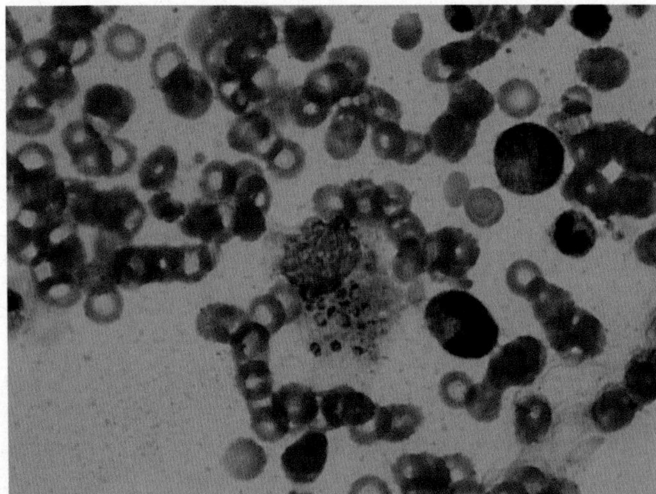

FIG. 204.9 Bone marrow aspirate from an immunocompromised girl presenting with a hemophagocytic-like syndrome with disseminated histoplasmosis illustrating intracellular yeast forms of *Histoplasma capsulatum.*

Histopathologic demonstration of typical yeast forms ranged from 18% to 62% in three large Indianapolis outbreaks.[427] The technique usually is unrewarding in patients with calcified or fibrotic lesions.[255,463]

Culture

Normally, sterile specimens and minced or homogenized tissue can be inoculated onto suitable media, such as brain-heart infusion agar, inhibitory mold agar, Sabouraud glucose (dextrose) agar, and enriched broth such as brain-heart infusion broth. The optimal method for recovery of *H. capsulatum* from blood is the lysis-centrifugation technique,[297] which lyses white blood cells, inhibits complement, and prevents coagulation. After processing is completed, the resulting

TABLE 204.2 Sensitivity of Diagnostic Studies in Different Histoplasmosis Syndromes

Test	Acute Pulmonary	Subacute Pulmonary	Progressive Disseminated
Antigen (%)	75–81	19–34	91–92
Antibody (%)	40–80	78–89	63–81
Histopathology (%)	47	9–38	12–43
Culture (%)	34	9–15	75–85

Modified from Wheat LJ. Improvements in diagnosis of histoplasmosis. *Expert Opin Biol Ther.* 2006;6:1207–1221.

concentrate is transferred to culture media. Specimens from nonsterile sites should be cultured on media that inhibit bacteria and saprophytic fungi; non–cycloheximide-containing media also should be used to permit the growth of other opportunistic pathogens. Cultures are incubated aerobically at 25°C to 30°C and held for at least 12 weeks before being considered negative. Most isolates grow in 3 to 4 weeks.[182] Use of the lysis-centrifugation system for blood culture has shortened the time required for identification of a positive culture result from approximately 16 days to 9 days.[38,311] Laboratory-based rapid identification and differentiation of fungal pathogens using PCR methodology have been developed.[128,323,326]

Recovery of *H. capsulatum* from a clinical specimen obtained from a symptomatic patient with a compatible illness confirms the diagnosis of active histoplasmosis. The only exception is the infrequent event in which an incidental granuloma is found to be culture positive, but active histoplasmosis is not a likely cause of the clinical symptoms. The sensitivity of culture varies in direct proportion to the severity of the infection and the fungal burden (see Table 204.2).[462] In primary acute, self-limited histoplasmosis, 40% of patients have positive culture results when samples are obtained from sputum (23%), bronchoalveolar lavage (BAL) fluid (39%), lung, and extrapulmonary sites (37%).[427] In contrast, culture results are positive in 75% to 85% of adults with PDH. In the latter patients, sites from which *H. capsulatum* commonly is recovered include the lower respiratory tract, blood, bone marrow, CSF, liver, spleen, skin lesions, and synovium of affected joints.[222,293] The highest yield in PDH is from bone marrow, which is positive in 75% of instances.[357,422] Urine is positive in 40% to 70%, and sputum is positive in 60%.[377] In adults with PDH, rates of positive lysis-centrifugation culture results in peripheral blood are 90% to 100% in acute dissemination and 50% in subacute dissemination; positive culture results are very rarely seen in chronic dissemination.

In forms of pulmonary histoplasmosis other than low-inoculum infection, sputum may be a reliable site for recovery of the organism in culture but not the best choice among diagnostic methods. High-inoculum infection after exposure to heavily contaminated sites usually results in moderate to severe infection in which patients seek medical attention within 2 weeks of exposure.[63] In these instances, the fungal burden is high, and specimens of respiratory secretions or lung tissue may show the organism, thus allowing the diagnosis to be made promptly. Culture results also may be positive, but the 2- to 4-week delay in achieving growth renders culture less desirable than other diagnostic methods, especially antigen detection. In adults with chronic cavitary pulmonary infection, sputum culture is positive in 50% to 85% of instances.[151,425] The sensitivity of sputum culture may be increased with multiple sampling. Bronchoscopy with BAL may be helpful in patients with pulmonary disease. In a study of bronchoscopy in 71 adults, BAL results were positive in only 4% of patients with a single pulmonary nodule, but it increased to 55% in the remainder of the patient group. The highest yield of 88% occurred in the presence of infiltrates or cavitary disease.[325] Bronchoscopy did not appear to be helpful in evaluating patients with adenopathy, chronic pleural effusion, or bronchopleural fistulas. In adults with mediastinal granuloma and fibrosis, culture results were positive in only 3.8% to 10%.[103,245] In children, culture plus staining of BAL fluid has been rewarding in diagnosing high–fungal burden infection in patients with HIV, but it is less sensitive than lung biopsy in other immunocompromised patients, especially those receiving chemotherapy for reticuloendothelial malignant disease. In patients with HIV infection, culture remains a value diagnostic tool with a positivity value of 75% compared with 35% in non–HIV-infected persons.[20]

Culture results usually are negative in rheumatologic manifestations of histoplasmosis, such as arthritis, erythema nodosum, erythema multiforme, and pericarditis. The reason is presumed to be that these reactive manifestations usually occur months after low-burden infection in patients whose acquired cellular immune response has controlled fungal replication. Isolated CNS infection is uncommon in children, but meningitis was reported in 25 of 40 cases of PDH of infancy; yeasts were observed in the CSF, and *H. capsulatum* was recovered in culture from 4 patients.[293] The number of organisms in CSF is small, so the yield is improved substantially by culturing large volumes (10–20 mL in adults) on at least two occasions.[452] In isolated CNS infections, culture is usually unrewarding.

Antibody and Antigen Detection

The serologic methods that are used most commonly for the diagnosis of histoplasmosis are immunodiffusion (ID) and CF. These tests are useful because, despite documentation of skin test reactivity in 50% to 70% of young, healthy adults residing in an endemic area, seropositivity in this population has been found to be 0.5% by ID and 2% by CF using the mycelial antigen and 4% with the yeast antigen. Therefore, if these test results are elevated, they serve to substantially increase the probability of acute or recent histoplasmosis when performed in a patient with a compatible illness.

Both serologic methods have equal sensitivity (75–85%); however, ID is slightly more specific (>95% vs. 85–90%).[422,423] In immunocompetent patients, either or both tests are positive in 95% of patients with acute primary pulmonary infection. CF titers often become positive 2 to 4 weeks earlier, usually within 4 to 6 weeks after exposure.[422] In patients with CF antibody, 25% have a negative ID result; only 1% of patients reactive by ID are CF negative.[91] When the ID test is reactive, however, it remains so for a longer period of time. In addition to the 4- to 6-week lag in developing elevated titers, an important limitation of both serologic assays is their reduced sensitivity in immunosuppressed patients. Only 50% of immunosuppressed children and adults with disseminated histoplasmosis are seropositive.[91] Of immunocompetent infants and young children with severe PDH during infancy and early childhood, 93% had elevated antibody titers.[293]

Cross reactivity with other fungal antigens affects CF and ID assays.[442] CF cross reactivity occurs most commonly with *B. dermatitidis* (40%) and *C. immitis* (16%). Cross reactions also occur, albeit rarely, with candidiasis, tuberculosis, aspergillosis, and cryptococcosis.[249,443,238] Cross reactivity also is seen occasionally in patients with chronic cavitary tuberculosis, although simultaneous infection with tuberculosis and fungal pathogens can occur.[132,443] Variability in the specificity of commercial reagents has been reported to cause false-negative results.[232]

Complement Fixation

CF uses sensitized sheep red blood cells, killed whole *H. capsulatum* yeast cells, and histoplasmin, a soluble mycelium-form filtrate antigen. In a common-source outbreak of acute primary pulmonary histoplasmosis, the titer becomes positive in 6% of individuals at 3 weeks, 73% at 4 weeks, and 77% at 6 weeks.[91,443] Upon resolution of infection, titers decrease to 1:8 to 1:16 within 4 to 6 months and, in most instances, become undetectable (<1:8) by 9 months. Reported sensitivities for a single titer vary from 70% to 95% and depend on the threshold for considering a result positive. Single titers of 1:32 or greater performed by an experienced laboratory are strong supportive evidence of acute or recent infection, especially when the accompanying clinical symptoms are compatible. One report showed that 12 of 28 patients with non-*Histoplasma* febrile pneumonia had false-positive CF titers of 1:32 or greater, so other laboratory and clinical data need to be considered.[396]

The demonstration of a fourfold increase between acute and convalescent sera provides the best serologic evidence of recent infection. The individual yeast (CF-Y) and mycelial (CF-M) phases can be measured.

The CF-Y phase is more sensitive than the CF-M phase when performed in recent or active infection. In a series of 11 children with acute pulmonary histoplasmosis, CF-Y was 1:32 or greater in nine children, but the CF-M titer was 1:32 or greater in only three children. In highly endemic areas, background low-titer CF serologic reactions may be present in 5% to 15% of adults but they have been reported to occur in as many as 30%.[141,150,444]

The serologic response seems to correlate with the severity of disease in immunocompetent individuals with acute infection.[226,447] During an extensive outbreak of histoplasmosis, seropositivity was 90% to 100% in severe acute histoplasmosis, 86% in moderate histoplasmosis, 75% in mild histoplasmosis, and 18% in asymptomatic histoplasmosis. Twenty-five percent of patients with acute histoplasmosis have CF titers that could be considered borderline positive, between 1:8 and 1:16.[91] Although they may result from previous infection, these titers should not be disregarded if clinical symptoms are compatible with acute infection. In adults with chronic pulmonary histoplasmosis, the CF titer is greater than 1:32 in almost all patients.[134,210,279] In children who present with middle mediastinal masses caused by histoplasmosis, 67% have CF titers of 1:32 or greater.[134] A newer enzyme immunoassay that measures *Histoplasma* IgM and IgG antibodies appear to have demonstrable higher sensitivity that CF and ID.[337]

The serologic diagnosis of patients with isolated meningitis caused by *H. capsulatum* often is problematic because no single test exhibits high sensitivity.[452] CF and ID can be positive in CSF, but half of patients with other chronic fungal meningeal infections may show false-positive results.[320,442] CF-M antibody seems to be the most sensitive and specific test for the diagnosis of meningitis caused by histoplasmosis. In one study, no false-positive CSF CF-M titers occurred in patients with cryptococcal meningitis but CF-Y was false positive in five of 18 patients.[442] Individuals with fibrosing mediastinitis or mediastinal granuloma generally have negative or very low levels of CF antibody.[447]

Immunodiffusion

The micro-ID method detects precipitins (reported as bands) against the H and M glycoprotein antigens of *H. capsulatum.*[444] The M band is present in 25% of infections by the fourth week of infection and in 50% to 86% by the sixth week.[30,91,315] It can persist for 18 to 36 months after recovery, but eventually it becomes nonreactive. In endemic areas, in which serologic surveys show that 24% of healthy adult blood donors have CF-Y titers of 1:8 or 1:16, ID serologic test results are positive in less than 1%.[141] Because it is more specific, ID can be of value to confirm the diagnosis of histoplasmosis in patients with *Histoplasma* CF titers in the borderline 1:8 to 1:16 range.[416]

The H band is present infrequently in patients with histoplasmosis; when seen, it is transient, and its presence suggests active infection.[150] In patients with active pulmonary histoplasmosis, one-half to three-fourths have an M band alone. The H band only is present in 10% to 20% of acute infections,[444] and only 10% of patients have both M and H bands present. The presence of both is highly suggestive of active histoplasmosis. The H band is detected less consistently in children with histoplasmosis.[419] In adults with disseminated disease, both bands are present in 25% of patients. The M band has been detected in 52% and 57% of patients with chronic pulmonary and disseminated disease.[155] The ID test is not approved for use in CSF specimens and has not been evaluated as a test for the diagnosis of meningitis.[427]

Antigen Detection

The development in 1986 and further refinements of the *Histoplasma* antigen assay have filled an important gap in laboratory diagnosis.[448] When performed on serum, urine, or other selected body fluids, antigen detection provides rapid, accurate, noninvasive diagnostic information for the most serious manifestations of disease. It is especially useful for the evaluation of infections in immunocompromised hosts, in whom serologic methods often produce negative results. Although evaluated almost exclusively in adults, antigen detection occupies the same diagnostic niche for managing infection during infancy and childhood.

Antigen detection is most sensitive in infections accompanied by high fungal burdens.[462] These include progressive disseminated infections in intensely exposed or immunocompromised hosts and primary pulmonary infection, in which antigen detection reflects the early hematogenous dissemination that occurs before being aborted by an effective cellular immune response. In addition to its usefulness in diagnosis, antigen assay provides a quantitative parameter with which to assess the pace and adequacy of response to therapy and, thereafter, a sensitive monitor that promptly detects relapse in patients who are at high risk for recurrence.[433,437–439]

The sensitivity of urine antigen detection (see Table 204.2) in patients with acute primary pulmonary infection is 75% to 81%, with the highest rates seen in patients tested within a few weeks of exposure, in those with large inoculum exposure, and in patients with extensive pulmonary involvement.[425,463] Sensitivity is less in subacute pulmonary and chronic cavitary infection in adults. The sensitivity of antigen detection is very high in manifestations of progressive disseminating manifestations of histoplasmosis. In adults with disseminated infections, antigen is detected in 91% to 92% of immunosuppressed and nonimmunosuppressed patients and in 95% to 100% of patients with AIDS.[448,449,463] In 22 children with PDH, urinary antigen test results were positive in 100%.[125]

Although *Histoplasma* antigen can be detected in serum, the sensitivity is substantially less than that of urine. In immunosuppressed adults with disseminated histoplasmosis, antigen was detected in 50% of serum samples and in 92% of urine specimens. Similarly, in patients with disseminated histoplasmosis complicating AIDS, antigenuria was seen in 95% versus 85% in serum.[448,463] Antigen often is found in BAL fluid of patients after high-inoculum exposure to histoplasmal spores and in immunocompromised patients with hematogenous dissemination and lung involvement.[436,440]

In adults with isolated meningitis, antigen detection in CSF may be the sole basis for confirming the diagnosis.[448,449,452] The range of antigen positivity in all cases of meningitis is 40% to 66%; the highest rates are found in severe infections with heavy fungal burdens, especially infections that occur in immunosuppressed patients.[452] In patients with clinical findings suggestive of meningitis but with no antigen present in CSF, antigen detected in extrameningeal sites sometimes can confirm the diagnosis.

Antigen concentration decreases during effective therapy.[168] Failure of the antigen concentration to decline or documentation of progressive increase may indicate treatment failure. Persistent but decreasing concentrations of antigenuria may be present after completion of an appropriate and effective course of antifungal therapy. Patients who have completed appropriate courses of therapy for serious infections and have had resolution of their clinical symptoms yet demonstrated persistent but decreasing concentrations of antigenuria have done well after the completion of the planned course of antifungal therapy. Infants with PDH who have been treated adequately, who have had a good clinical response, and whose urine antigen levels have substantially decreased during therapy often have persistence of low levels of urine antigen after completion of amphotericin B therapy.[328] Residual excretion of urine antigen after adequate treatment continues to decrease and eventually ceases; monitoring is recommended to confirm resolution of antigenuria.[125,328]

Conversely, the persistence of moderate antigenuria has been associated with a risk for recrudescence. This risk has been shown best, but not exclusively, in patients with AIDS and histoplasmosis, in whom significant antigenuria often persists after cessation of therapy.[437,438] Monitoring urine antigen in such patients has shown that increasing concentrations foretell recurrence of active infection.[437] The sensitivity of the antigen assay is high, however, and the pattern of antigen clearance has not been established firmly in other clinical settings.

Antigen concentrations in urine measured with a quantitative assay often exceed the upper end of the calibration curve, especially in disseminated infections. If urine concentration is too high and unable to quantitate, monitoring is more informative if antigen concentrations of serum are initially followed because concomitant serum concentrations are lower than those of concomitant urine samples and are more likely to be within the range in which differences in concentration could be measured accurately. Thereafter, when antigenemia is resolved, urine concentrations can be followed with the quantitative assay. Testing should be performed routinely at 3- to 4-month intervals during treatment, at the end of therapy, if symptoms recur, and periodically for another year to monitor for relapse.

Cross reactions in the *Histoplasma* antigen assay occur in paracoccidioidomycosis, African histoplasmosis caused by *H. capsulatum* var.

duboisii, blastomycosis, sporotrichosis, and infections caused by *P. marneffei*.[457] Because these infections have distinguishing epidemiologic and clinical features and because supportive diagnostic tests may aid further in differentiating them from histoplasmosis, such cross reactions usually create little difficulty in interpreting positive test results.

Skin Testing

A skin test for histoplasmosis that uses a standardized histoplasmin antigen prepared from a mycelial phase culture filtrate had been a valuable epidemiologic and investigational tool but provided limited diagnostic usefulness for distinguishing past from active infection; it no longer is commercially available.[131,150]

Molecular Methods

Epidemiologic studies have used restriction fragment length polymorphisms of DNA. Nucleic acid–based and genome-wide approaches have been used to explore the genetic diversity of the pathogen.[213,273,414] Molecular methods also have been used to examine strains recovered from patients with failed therapy and to identify relatedness in isolates recovered after organ transplantation.[235,450]

Molecular methods that reliably detect *H. capsulatum* in clinical samples are starting to show promise when compared with standard diagnostic tests.[67,276] PCR methodology has been evaluated for identifying *H. capsulatum*[26] in tissue and body fluids, but false-negative results were encountered in one-third of specimens.[37] PCR methodology used with clinical specimens (urine, serum, BAL, CSF) containing urine antigen showed specificities of 80% to 100% but sensitivities of only 0% to 22%.[426] More recent reports show promise for PCR methodology in laboratory identification of *H. capsulatum* in clinical samples.[26,128,354,371]

TREATMENT

Most patients with symptomatic histoplasmosis recover without receiving antifungal therapy.[150] Treatment is required for patients with severe symptoms, prolonged illness, congenital or acquired immune dysfunction, or signs or symptoms suggestive of progressive dissemination. Evidence-based, consensus practice guidelines for treatment of histoplasmosis have been published and include recommendations for treatment of children.[441]

No controlled therapeutic trials have been conducted in children. Chronic pulmonary infection and subacute and chronic dissemination syndromes rarely occur in children. Recommendations for treating the clinical manifestations of histoplasmosis seen most frequently in children are summarized in Table 204.3. These recommendations have been derived from anecdotal published reports, clinical experience, and extrapolation from experience in adults.

Medical Management for Manifestations Requiring Antifungal Therapy

Because most patients with light or moderate exposure to fungal spores recover without treatment, the first decision is to determine whether to observe the patient carefully or to begin administering an antifungal agent. The key criteria in making this decision are clinical assessment of the character, severity, and duration of symptoms and assessment of the adequacy of the patient's cellular immunity. When treatment with antifungal agents has been elected, a regimen is selected that is appropriate for the initial findings. Manifestations of histoplasmosis in children that most often require antifungal treatment are severe or protracted symptoms resulting from acute primary pulmonary infection, mediastinal adenitis that is causing compression of adjacent structures, disseminated infection of infancy, and infection in an immunocompromised host. Treatment recommendations are summarized in Table 204.3.

The antifungal agents that play primary roles in medical management include amphotericin B deoxycholate, liposomal amphotericin B, amphotericin B lipid complex, and itraconazole. Amphotericin B preparations are fungicidal for *H. capsulatum*, whereas itraconazole is fungistatic. Combined use of the two agents does not result in synergy. On the basis of its faster clearance of fungemia in patients with AIDS,[199,431] amphotericin B is more effective for severe infection than

TABLE 204.3 Summary of Treatment Recommendations for Children With Histoplasmosis

Manifestation	Moderately Severe or Severe Illness	Mild to Moderate Illness
Acute pulmonary manifestations	AMB[a] for 1–2 wk followed by ITR[b] for 12 wk Steroids appears to be beneficial in patients with high-inoculum disease	Symptoms <4 wk: none Persistent symptoms >4 wk: ITR for 6–12 wk[b] Alternative agents: FLU, POS[b]
Disseminated disease (non-HIV)	AMB[b] for 1–2 wk followed by ITR for at least 6 mo[c]	ITR for 6–18 mo or the same as for severe illness[b] Alternative agents: FLU, POS[c]
Disseminated disease (HIV)	LAB for 1–2 wk followed by ITR for life	
CNS histoplasmosis	LAB for 4–6 wk, followed by ITR for 12 mo[b]	
Granulomatous mediastinitis	AMB[a], then ITR for 6 mo	ITR for 6–12 mo Alternative agents: fluconazole and posaconazole[c]
Fibrosing mediastinitis	ITR for 3 mo[d]	Same as for severe illness
Pericarditis	Pericardial drainage for severe tamponade + an NSAID, for 2–12 wk[e]	NSAID 2–12 wk
Rheumatologic manifestations	NSAID for 2–12 wk	Same as for severe illness
Compression of contiguous structures by granulomatous lymphadenopathy	No treatment needed if symptoms <4 wk Symptoms >4 wk: ITR for 6–12 wk,g[f,g]	

[a]LAB or deoxycholate AMB. Many clinicians prefer LAB because it has a lower frequency of infusion-related adverse reactions and nephrotoxicity. Dosages: LAB: 3–5 mg/kg body weight, IV once daily; deoxycholate AMB: 0.7–1.0 mg/kg body weight, IV once daily.
[b]ITR drug level monitoring is needed. ITR suspension has higher bioavailability than the capsule form and is the preferred agent for follow-up ITR treatment. Dosages: FLU: 5–6 mg/kg body weight IV or PO per dose twice daily (max, 600 mg/day); ITRA: initial loading dose of 2.5–5 mg/kg body weight (max, 200 mg) per dose PO three times daily for first 3 days of therapy followed by 2.5–5 mg/kg body weight (max, 200 mg) per dose twice daily; POS: oral suspension, 400 mg twice daily (children ≥8 y).
[c]Serum concentrations of posaconazole should be monitored and achieve a level of ≥1 μg/mL at steady state.
[d]Therapy should continue until the *Histoplasma* antigen concentration in serum is undetectable and the *Histoplasma* urine antigen concentration is <2 μg/mL and stable. (Low urine concentrations can be present for extended periods following successful therapy.)
[e]Probably ineffective if fibrotic. When granulomatous mediastinitis could be present, it may be considered.
[f]Indomethacin is the preferred NSAID. Prompt administration may obviate need for drainage in non–life-threatening manifestations of pericarditis.
[g]Steroids may be beneficial in reducing the effect of compression. If steroids are used, ITR should be used.
AMB, Amphotericin B; *CNS*, central nervous system; *FLU*, fluconazole; *HIV*, human immunodeficiency virus; *ITR*, itraconazole; *IV*, intravenously; *LAB*, liposomal amphotericin B; *max*, maximum; *NSAID*, nonsteroidal antiinflammatory agent; *PO*, orally; *POS*, posaconazole.
Modified from Wheat LJ, Freifeld A, Kleiman MB, et al. Practice guidelines for management of patients with histoplasmosis. *Clin Infect Dis*. 2007;45:807–825.

is itraconazole.[445] Amphotericin B is used most commonly as "induction" therapy, especially in severe infections; after substantial clinical improvement has occurred, the drug is stopped, and itraconazole is begun to complete treatment. Monotherapy with itraconazole is effective for treating patients who have mild or only moderately severe symptoms. In addition to regimens that are used to treat acute infections, suppressive (secondary prophylaxis) regimens have been developed for treating patients with AIDS because of the high rate of relapse if antifungal treatment is stopped and if immune function has not been improved by HAART.[441] Primary prophylactic regimens also have been developed for use by patients with AIDS who live in highly endemic areas.[261]

A detailed discussion of the antifungal agents used to treat histoplasmosis is presented in Chapter 240. Amphotericin B deoxycholate usually is well tolerated and effective in children. Liposomal amphotericin B is the best evaluated of the lipid preparations. A comparative trial of amphotericin B deoxycholate and liposomal amphotericin B in adults with disseminated histoplasmosis and AIDS showed faster improvement and lower mortality rates with the liposomal preparation.[199]

For moderately severe or severe infections amphotericin B is administered for 1 to 2 weeks. This regimen is always followed by a course of itraconazole (see Table 204.3).[441] Because relapse has been observed in immunosuppressed patients, close follow-up with monitoring of urine antigen concentrations is required.

Itraconazole generally is well tolerated by children and, in adults, is more effective and less likely to induce resistance than the other azoles. Although formal trials using itraconazole have not been conducted in children, clinical experience has confirmed its effectiveness as the oral azole of choice. The erratic bioavailability of the capsule form can be improved when it is taken with liquids with low pH and caloric content (concomitant food and a cola drink are recommended).[192] Serum levels should be monitored, particularly if symptoms persist.[144] The liquid solution of itraconazole is better absorbed, particularly when it is taken on an empty stomach, but it may have adverse gastrointestinal effects that affect compliance. The 90% minimal inhibitory concentration (MIC_{90}) of itraconazole for *H. capsulatum* is less than 0.01 μg/mL; the optimal therapeutic level has not been determined, but serum concentrations greater than 2 μg/mL are effective, readily achieved, and well tolerated.[174] With the drug's long half-life, serum concentrations vary little after steady state is achieved (approximately 2 weeks). When used as monotherapy or as step-down treatment after amphotericin B induction, a loading dose of itraconazole consisting of 150% of the total daily dose is recommended for the initial 3 days of therapy. As with the other azoles, important drug-drug interactions need to be considered in patients receiving agents known to affect excretion of the azole or whose excretion is affected by the antifungal agent.

Fluconazole was less effective than itraconazole in treating adults with chronic pulmonary histoplasmosis[261] or disseminated histoplasmosis.[450] It also has been associated with relapse in disseminated infection,[451] is less effective than itraconazole for secondary prophylaxis in adults with disseminated infection,[264] and clears fungemia more slowly in adults with disseminated infection than does itraconazole.[433]

With the availability of newer azoles with high efficacy and improved safety profile, ketoconazole is no longer a recommended agent for the treatment of histoplasmosis.

Both voriconazole and posaconazole have in vitro activity against *H. capsulatum*. Posaconazole has shown greater activity,[82,435] and it seems to be more active in experimental models and several case reports. Six patients with severe forms of histoplasmosis (five with disseminated disease) received salvage treatment with posaconazole, all with favorable outcomes.[335] Resistance that seems to have been induced by fluconazole when the drug was used in patients with AIDS also was accompanied by an increase in MIC values to voriconazole, a finding suggesting that resistance may emerge during treatment with voriconazole.[435,434] However, a review of isolates from 208 cases found no development of drug resistance during a 4-year period.[44] Voriconazole and posaconazole have been effective in isolated reports describing differing manifestations of infection.[6,102,127,148,181,280,335,402] These agents and fluconazole remain second-line alternatives to itraconazole.[73,318] If these agents are elected for use, therapeutic drug monitoring is recommended.

Primary Pulmonary Infection

Primary pulmonary histoplasmosis that occurs after exposure to a large inoculum of spores may result in life-threatening illness.[110,151,150,166] Infection of this severity should be treated promptly; induction with amphotericin B is indicated and it is continued until substantial clinical improvement occurs. Anecdotal evidence indicates that concomitant use of corticosteroids may be beneficial in treating patients with severe inhalation and adult respiratory distress syndrome.[209,395,473] After improvement resulting from amphotericin B induction, itraconazole should be started and continued for at least 3 months. In patients who may not appear as ill, but with laboratory or clinical evidence suggestive of progressive primary dissemination, empiric therapy should be initiated.

Patients without respiratory distress but whose systemic complaints, such as fever, fatigue, and weight loss, persist for 2 to 4 weeks or longer also are candidates for antifungal therapy. In these instances, firm criteria to guide the timing of this decision are not established, and treatment must be individualized. Nonetheless, as observed when amphotericin B was the only effective treatment, and its toxicity and inconvenience resulted in deferring its use for longer than currently practiced, a significant proportion of these symptoms could be expected to undergo spontaneous resolution. The convenience of oral administration of antifungal agents renders the decision less problematic because these protracted but mild to moderately severe symptoms may be treated with itraconazole. Itraconazole should be used for at least 6 weeks in these instances (see Table 204.3).

Mediastinal Adenitis

One of the most common initial presentations of acute illness is the onset of symptoms caused by the mediastinal adenitis that commonly accompanies pulmonary infection with *H. capsulatum*. In this setting, affected lymph nodes enlarge, may coalesce, and often compress or obstruct adjacent structures. The illness is generally is self-limited, but symptoms may persist for several weeks. Although only anecdotal evidence supports the benefit of treatment, itraconazole may be helpful for patients with active inflammation. An elevated erythrocyte sedimentation rate and CF titer could be considered markers compatible with active inflammation. As also shown in a study involving dogs with mediastinal granuloma,[362] adjunctive treatment with corticosteroids sometimes is beneficial,[157,395,441] and, if effective, results in prompt improvement. If a corticosteroidal agent is used, it should be given in association with an effective antifungal agent because of the risk for dissemination resulting from corticosteroid-induced suppression of cellular immunity. Itraconazole should be continued for 6 to 12 weeks. Although fibrosing mediastinitis is a late complication of histoplasmosis, no evidence has shown that focal mediastinal adenitis is its precursor and that antifungal therapy prevents its occurrence.

Mediastinal granuloma describes a group of mostly caseous lymph nodes that coalesce into a single lesion usually located in the paratracheal region (Fig. 204.7). It is very infrequently seen in children. Lesions often are asymptomatic and discovered as incidental findings in imaging studies. Spontaneous drainage of caseous material may occur and result in fistulous tracts to the esophagus,[381] bronchi, or skin. In this setting, treatment with itraconazole is appropriate, although its efficacy in this situation is unproven. Operative intervention or stenting of the affected portion of the superior vena cava sometimes is indicated in the event that compression of vital structures occurs and fails to respond to antifungal therapy.[196]

Disseminated Infection

Progressive disseminated infections in children require treatment with antifungal agents. Treatment recommendations are summarized in Table 204.3.

Immunocompetent Patients and Immunosuppressed Patients Without Human Immunodeficiency Virus Infection

If not treated with antifungal agents, patients with acute PDH have a mortality rate approaching 100%.[105,151,231,240] Treatment with amphotericin B results in survival of more than 90% of infants with PDH.[184,231,293] In contrast to adults, in whom monotherapy with itraconazole for patients with nonsevere dissemination has been successful,[104,445] only one report has described the outcome of itraconazole monotherapy in children with disseminated histoplasmosis.[401] Seven children ranging from 2 to 14 years old were treated. A 2-year-old child died "shortly after" treatment was stopped at 1 month. "Marked improvement" was noted in patients treated for 3 months (four patients) and 6 months (one patient), and complete resolution was reported in one patient after 12 months of therapy. Monotherapy with itraconazole is not recommended for disseminated histoplasmosis.[441] Largely on the basis of its demonstrated effectiveness in clinical trials in adults, however, and its ease of administration and tolerability in children, itraconazole is recommended for step-down therapy after induction and clinical improvement with amphotericin B. Serum levels of itraconazole should be monitored along with serum or urine antigen concentrations during therapy and in follow-up to confirm that the fungal burden is decreasing. If amphotericin B is elected as monotherapy, a course of 4 to 6 weeks is recommended. In a retrospective study of 98 patients receiving TNF-α therapy, infliximab and corticosteroid use was associated with higher urine antigen levels and severe disease.[411] TNF-α was discontinued in almost all patients, and approximately 50% received amphotericin B for the first 2 weeks of treatment. Itraconazole was administered for 12 months. TNF-α therapy was resumed in one-third of patients with a low rate of disease recurrence (3%). Investigators concluded that resumption of TNF-α therapy appears to be safe in most patients, especially if they have received 12 months of itraconazole.[411]

Disseminated Infection in Patients With Acquired Immunodeficiency Syndrome

The severity of the initial signs of illness heavily influences the outcome and the treatment regimens selected for patients with disseminated histoplasmosis complicating HIV infection (see Table 204.3). Regimens are determined on the basis of trials conducted in adults. Amphotericin B was effective in 74% to 88% of all cases,[424,436] whereas patients treated for infections that were sufficiently severe to require hospitalization had a 50% mortality rate.[424] In adult patients with moderate to severe disseminated histoplasmosis, liposomal amphotericin B provided a survival benefit compared with that of amphotericin B deoxycholate.[199] Adults with only mild or moderate symptoms were treated successfully with itraconazole monotherapy in 85% of instances.[445]

Recommendations for children are similar to the recommendations for adults; amphotericin B deoxycholate usually is well tolerated in children and is recommended as monotherapy at a dose of 1 mg/kg per day given for 4 to 6 weeks. Alternatively, it may be used for 2 weeks as induction therapy and, after a satisfactory clinical response, discontinued and followed by itraconazole, 5 to 10 mg/kg per day for 12 months. Liposomal amphotericin B, a more costly preparation, may be substituted for the deoxycholate preparation with either regimen in the event of renal complications. Serum, followed by urine, antigen monitoring is recommended during therapy and for 1 year after its completion to confirm clearance and thereafter to assess for relapse. After the completion of therapy, the significance of low levels of antigenuria in the absence of antigenemia and clinical symptoms is unclear and is not an indication to prolong therapy. Prolonged follow-up is recommended in these instances.

Because of a high rate of relapse of histoplasmosis after cessation of antifungal therapy in patients with AIDS complicated by persistently impaired immune function, long-term maintenance therapy (secondary prophylaxis) is recommended.[198,436,453] In adults with mild to moderately severe disseminated infection, amphotericin B is effective in 81% to 97% of cases,[260,436] and itraconazole is effective in 90%.[174,446] Itraconazole is the azole of choice for mildly or moderately ill patients, in whom it may be used as both induction therapy and secondary prophylaxis. Fluconazole is not recommended for secondary prophylaxis but may be considered if patients received amphotericin B as induction therapy or if itraconazole is poorly tolerated or its cost precludes its use.

A prospective observational study of adults with AIDS and disseminated histoplasmosis found it safe to discontinue secondary prophylaxis after 12 months of primary antifungal therapy and the demonstration of sustained immunologic improvement resulting from HAART therapy.[145] Specific criteria for withholding secondary prophylaxis include negative blood culture results, low *Histoplasma* urine antigen concentration of less than 4 ng/mL, and $CD4^+$ T-cell counts greater than 150 cells/μL in patients continuing to receive HAART.[162] Primary prophylaxis with itraconazole is effective for patients with AIDS who live in hyperendemic areas (areas in which the incidence of histoplasmosis is more than 5 cases per 100 patients per year).[264]

Prophylaxis of Immunosuppressed Patients

Clusters of infection occasionally are reported in high-risk populations, sometimes in geographic regions with low background rates.[126] On the basis of results of a large clinical trial, however, the need for prophylaxis for patients residing in a hyperendemic area and who are undergoing immunosuppression for management of neoplasms, inflammatory syndromes, or transplantation of allogeneic bone marrow or solid organs[28,372] seems to be low.[407] Included were patients with CF titers to *H. capsulatum* of 1:8 or 1:16, positive M bands by ID, or radiographic evidence suggestive of past infection (calcified splenic or lung nodules). In contrast, patients receiving TNF-α antagonists seem to be at greater risk for developing disseminated histoplasmosis,[375,415,467] perhaps attributable to reactivation of latent infection. Although long-term use may appear to be costly, a study from French Guiana showed that primary prophylaxis in a selected patient population could be cost effective.[277]

Central Nervous System Infection

With the exception of CNS infections that accompany PDH of infancy, isolated histoplasmosis of the CNS in children rarely is seen. Death is almost certain if meningitis is untreated. Treatment is effective in only 20% to 40% of patients with meningitis, and 50% of responders experience relapse after cessation of treatment.[217]

Amphotericin B preparations enter the CSF poorly; however, liposomal amphotericin B concentrations are higher in brain parenchyma.[111,159,230] It is recommended that patients with CNS infections receive liposomal amphotericin B, 5 mg/kg per day for 4 to 6 weeks, followed by itraconazole for 1 year.

Meningitis was present in 25 of 40 children in a series of PDH.[293] All children received amphotericin B deoxycholate followed by ketoconazole for 3 months. The overall mortality rate in the series was 10%; however, two deaths were in children who failed to complete therapy, and two died within 4 days of presentation, findings suggesting that this regimen cured meningitis in most cases. In the rare setting of a child with meningitis as an isolated infection, recommendations reasonably could include the use of liposomal amphotericin B (in place of amphotericin B deoxycholate) followed by itraconazole for 12 months.

Despite isolated case reports that have documented success with ketoconazole, itraconazole, fluconazole, the combination of itraconazole and fluconazole, and voriconazole,[402,441] the efficacy of azole monotherapy for the treatment of CNS infections remains inadequately studied. Posaconazole has been used successfully as salvage therapy in a patient after therapeutic failure with prior regimens.[318,335] The evidence is insufficient to recommend azole monotherapy for CNS infection.

Medical Management of Manifestations That Do Not Require Antifungal Therapy

Several manifestations of histoplasmosis, both common and uncommon, do not require antifungal treatment. Apart from mild primary pulmonary infection, one of the most common is pericarditis. Because it rarely is associated with frank fungal infection of the pericardium, pericarditis usually resolves spontaneously or with nonsteroidal antiinflammatory drugs. Indomethacin usually is effective in rapidly reducing inflammation and can reverse signs of impending cardiac tamponade.[475] Corticosteroids have been reported to be effective, but, if used, they should be accompanied by antifungal therapy. Rheumatologic symptoms of arthritis, with or without erythema multiforme or erythema nodosum, also respond to nonsteroidal antiinflammatory drugs.[366] Fibrosing mediastinitis is a late complication of histoplasmosis, but it occurs occasionally in children. When granulomatous lesions evolve to become diffusely and densely fibrotic, both antifungal and antiinflammatory therapies are ineffective. The clinical and laboratory criteria that are used to assess whether active inflammation is present are inexact, however, and a trial of antifungal therapy often is warranted if clinical features or laboratory evidence of active inflammation, or both, are present. Treatment with antifungal agents almost always is unsuccessful, but improvement has been reported, albeit rarely.[406] Presumed ocular histoplasmosis is seen almost exclusively in adults and does not improve with antifungal therapy; its management has been reviewed extensively.[71]

Surgical Treatment

Operative intervention rarely is needed to manage patients with histoplasmosis. In a review of 94 patients, 10 to 40 years old, the most common reason for evaluation was obstruction of thoracic structures by mediastinal masses.[136] Seventy-five patients underwent surgical intervention or endoscopy to relieve obstruction of the pulmonary artery, superior vena cava, bronchus, or esophagus. Recurrent pneumonia, tracheoesophageal fistula, hemoptysis, carinal injury, and broncholithiasis were other indications for surgical procedures.[136,142,480] Because attempts to excise caseous nodes completely sometimes can damage contiguous structures, the preferable approach is to incise and evacuate debris from such lesions and leave the adherent portion of the capsule intact.[136,313,461]

Surgery has little place in the management of fibrosing mediastinitis caused by histoplasmosis. The dense fibrous consolidation of mediastinal structures coupled with the hypervascularity of mediastinal tissues renders the risk for development of hemorrhagic and other life-threatening operative complications high. Excisional biopsy carries a prohibitive risk.[92] Bronchoscopy coupled with coagulation of hyperemic vessels within bronchi in patients presenting with hemoptysis has been useful.[252] When calcification has occurred in fibrosing mediastinitis, surgical repair is not feasible, and the fibrosis continues postoperatively. Some success has been achieved with relief of vascular obstruction by percutaneous placement of intravascular stents,[109,196,398] but complications occur. Prophylactic excision of enlarged mediastinal nodes has not been shown to prevent fibrosis, and patients with large mediastinal lymph nodes who are otherwise asymptomatic rarely progress to develop mediastinal fibrosis.[447]

PROGNOSIS

Histoplasmosis is either unrecognized or self-limited in the majority of persons who acquire this most common of the endemic mycoses. Histoplasmosis causes serious illness in infants, immunocompromised patients, and older persons, particularly those with emphysematous pulmonary disease.[41] The cure rate for children who receive therapy for serious acute manifestations is high. Little prospective information is available about the long-term outcome in acute pulmonary histoplasmosis. A study that examined pulmonary function in six children and their parents after intense exposure found restrictive (three patients) and obstructive (two patients) patterns and a reduction in carbon monoxide diffusing capacity in five of six tested.[219] At 2 years, a diffusing capacity abnormality remained in three children, and hypoxemia persisted in the most severely affected patient.[250] No data that can help predict the occurrence of long-term complications, such as mediastinal fibrosis, are available. Because, by definition, mediastinal fibrosis impairs the function of both the airways and pulmonary vasculature,[374] its prognosis is influenced heavily by whether it affects one or both lungs.[92] The prognosis is poor in the latter instance.

PREVENTION

Complete prevention of histoplasmosis is currently impossible, but reasonable precautions can substantially decrease the exposure to persons with risk factors that predispose them to serious complications should they acquire the infection. Persons with impaired cellular immunity who reside in, or plan travel to, endemic regions should be counseled about the potentially serious consequences of infection. This should include education about areas that are endemic for histoplasmosis, sites likely to be heavily contaminated with *H. capsulatum*, and the circumstances, activities, and events that may aerosolize spores and result in inhalation and infection. Primary prophylactic regimens using itraconazole may be considered for HIV-infected patients with exposure to soil mixed with bird or bat droppings.[170] If such activities are unavoidable, the use of National Institute for Occupational Safety and Health–certified high-efficiency mask filtration devices should be encouraged; however, effective devices appropriate for use by young children may be unavailable. Sterilization of sites by formaldehyde spray have been attempted, but the toxicity of this agent renders its use undesirable and, in some settings, ineffective. When potentially contaminated sites, such as old or unused structures in which birds or bats have roosted, are disturbed, aerosols that may contain spores can be substantially reduced by thoroughly dampening the areas with water before they are manipulated.[27] Although educating and counseling high-risk patients affords some protection against acquiring infection from microfoci, some of which can result in intense exposure, this approach is not helpful in protecting against "sporadic" exposure to contaminated aerosols. For the general population residing in endemic areas, education also is beneficial, particularly for protecting persons whose occupational and recreational activities may increase their risk for exposure to sites likely to be contaminated with *H. capsulatum*.

Although long an active area of research, vaccines directed against any of the endemic mycoses have not yet been developed. Among the challenges in this effort are the need both to target the general population in an extensive geographic region and to develop a vaccine product that provides lifelong protection, perhaps necessitating repeat immunization.[378] Investigations in animal models[183,291,355] are ongoing in an attempt to identify vaccine targets[96,100,243,472] and to delineate the regulatory elements needed for developing immunity against *H. capsulatum*.[97,358] Investigations in such models have shown that monoclonal antibodies can alter the pathogenesis of histoplasmosis by targeting host costimulatory molecules or fungal cell surface proteins.[290] Another area of inquiry is that of identifying vaccine targets integral to dimorphism, a requisite for the pathogenicity of all the endemic fungi.[281] Additional efforts have explored the feasibility of developing vaccines against invasive fungal pathogens in the setting of severe immunodeficiency, including persons with $CD4^+$ T-cell deficiency.[472] An animal model has shown that immunization with apoptotic phagocytes that contain heat-killed *H. capsulatum* antigen activated functional $CD8^+$ T cells as well as $CD4^+$ T cells and protected against infection.[183] Biodegradable microspheres that contain leukotriene B_4 and cell-free antigens of *H. capsulatum* have been shown to activate murine bone marrow–derived macrophages.[107] A recombinant protein vaccine has been produced from cloned sequences of DNA coding for the cell wall glycoprotein HSP60 and found to be protective in a mouse model against a lethal intravenous inoculum of *H. capsulatum*.[146] This vaccine protected mice in a model of pulmonary infection.

NEW REFERENCES SINCE THE SEVENTH EDITION

3. Agudelo CA, Restrepo CA, Molina DA, et al. Tuberculosis and histoplasmosis co-infection in AIDS patients. *Am J Trop Med Hyg*. 2012;87:1094-1098.
5. Ajello L, Zeidberg LD. Isolation of *Histoplasma capsulatum* and *Allescheria boydii* from soil. *Science*. 1951;113:662-663.
20. Arango-Bustamante K, Restrepo A, Cano LE, et al. Diagnostic value of culture and serological tests in the diagnosis of histoplasmosis in HIV and non-HIV Colombian patients. *Am J Trop Med Hyg*. 2013;89:937-942.
32. Benedict K, Mody RK. Epidemiology of histoplasmosis outbreaks, United States, 1938-2013. *Emerg Infect Dis*. 2016;22:370-378.
31. Benedict K, Derado G, Mody RK. Histoplasmosis-associated hospitalizations in the United States, 2001-2012. *Open Forum Infect Dis*. 2016;3:ofv219.
62. Carlucci JG, Halasa N, Creech CB, et al. Vertical Transmission of histoplasmosis associated with anti-tumor necrosis factor therapy. *J Pediatric Infect Dis Soc*. 2016;5:e9-e12.
87. Dalvin LA, Thom SB, Garcia JJ, Fadel HJ, Baratz KH. Scleritis due to histoplasmosis. *Cornea*. 2016;35:402-404.
88. Darling ST. A protozoon general infection producing pseudotubercles in the lungs and focal necroses in the liver, spleen and lymph nodes. *J Am Med Assoc*. 1906;46:1283-1285.
89. Darling ST. The morphology of the parasite (*Histoplasma capsulatum*) and the lesions of histoplasmosis, a fatal disease of tropical America. *J Exp Med*. 1909;11:515-531.
102. Dhawan J, Verma P, Sharma A, et al. Disseminated cutaneous histoplasmosis in an immunocompetent child, relapsed with itraconazole, successfully treated with voriconazole. *Pediatr Dermatol*. 2010;27:549-551.
120. Emmons CW. Isolation of *Histoplasma capsulatum* from soil. *Public Health Rep*. 1949;64:892-896.

127. Freifeld AG, Wheat LJ, Kaul DR. Histoplasmosis in solid organ transplant recipients: early diagnosis and treatment. *Curr Opin Organ Transplant*. 2009;14:601-605.
130. Friedman A, Solomon G, Segal-Maurer S, Pereira F. Sudden onset of verrucous plaques to the face and trunk: a case of reactivation cutaneous histoplasmosis in the setting of HIV. *Dermatol Online J*. 2008;14:12.
148. Goncalves D, Ferraz C, Vaz L. Posaconazole as rescue therapy in African histoplasmosis. *Braz J Infect Dis*. 2013;17:102-105.
159. Groll AH, Giri N, Petraitis V, et al. Comparative efficacy and distribution of lipid formulations of amphotericin B in experimental *Candida albicans* infection of the central nervous system. *J Infect Dis*. 2000;182:274-282.
172. Hariri OR, Minasian T, Quadri SA, et al. Histoplasmosis with deep CNS involvement: case presentation with discussion and literature review. *J Neurol Surg Rep*. 2015;76:e167-e172.
196. Johansen M, Hoyer M, Kleiman M. Transcatheter treatment of SVC syndrome from histoplasmosis-related mediastinal fibrosis in a 9-year old male. *Catheter Cardiovasc Interv*. 2013;82:E708-E711.
247. Lucas AO. Cutaneous manifestations of African histoplasmosis. *Br J Dermatol*. 1970;82:435-447.
253. Manos NE, Ferebee SH, Kerschbaum WF. Geographic variation in the prevalence of histoplasmin sensitivity. *Dis Chest*. 1956;29:649-668.
277. Nacher M, Adenis A, Basurko C, et al. Primary prophylaxis of disseminated histoplasmosis in HIV patients in French Guiana: arguments for cost effectiveness. *Am J Trop Med Hyg*. 2013;89:1195-1198.
279. Naeem F, Metzger ML, Arnold SR, Adderson EE. Distinguishing benign mediastinal masses from malignancy in a histoplasmosis-endemic region. *J Pediatr*. 2015;167:409-415.
287. Nguyen FN, Kar JK, Zakaria A, Schiess MC. Isolated central nervous system histoplasmosis presenting with ischemic pontine stroke and meningitis in an immune-competent patient. *JAMA Neurol*. 2013;70:638-641.
288. Nieto-Rios JF, Serna-Higuita LM, Guzman-Luna CE, et al. Histoplasmosis in renal transplant patients in an endemic area at a reference hospital in Medellin, Colombia. *Transplant Proc*. 2014;46:3004-3009.
292. Odio CD, Milligan KL, McGowan K, et al. Endemic mycoses in patients with *STAT3*-mutated hyper-IgE (Job) syndrome. *J Allergy Clin Immunol*. 2015;136:1411-1413, e1-2.
299. Ollague Sierra JE, Ollague Torres JM. New clinical and histological patterns of acute disseminated histoplasmosis in human immunodeficiency virus-positive patients with acquired immunodeficiency syndrome. *Am J Dermatopathol*. 2013;35:205-212.
330. Rana C, Krishnani N, Kumari N. Bilateral adrenal histoplasmosis in immunocompetent patients. *Diagn Cytopathol*. 2011;39:294-296.
333. Regnier-Rosencher E, Dupont B, Jacobelli S, et al. Late occurrence of *Histoplasma duboisii* cutaneous and pulmonary infection 18 years after exposure. *J Mycol Med*. 2014;24:229-233.
336. Richaud C, Chandesris MO, Lanternier F, et al. Imported African histoplasmosis in an immunocompetent patient 40 years after staying in a disease-endemic area. *Am J Trop Med Hyg*. 2014;91:1011-1014.
337. Richer SM, Smedema ML, Durkin MM, et al. Improved diagnosis of acute pulmonary histoplasmosis by combining antigen and antibody detection. *Clin Infect Dis*. 2016;62:896-902.
338. Riddell JT, Kauffman CA, Smith JA, et al. *Histoplasma capsulatum* endocarditis: multicenter case series with review of current diagnostic techniques and treatment. *Medicine (Baltimore)*. 2014;93:186-193.
348. Saccente M, McDonnell RW, Baddour LM, Mathis MJ, Bradsher RW. Cerebral histoplasmosis in the azole era: report of four cases and review. *South Med J*. 2003;96:410-416.
353. Sampaio EP, Hsu AP, Pechacek J, et al. Signal transducer and activator of transcription 1 (*STAT1*) gain-of-function mutations and disseminated coccidioidomycosis and histoplasmosis. *J Allergy Clin Immunol*. 2013;131:1624-1634.
354. Sampaio Ide L, Freire AK, Ogusko MM, Salem JI, De Souza JV. Selection and optimization of PCR-based methods for the detection of *Histoplasma capsulatum* var. *capsulatum*. *Rev Iberoam Micol*. 2012;29:34-39.
355. Sa-Nunes A, Medeiros AI, Nicolete R, et al. Efficacy of cell-free antigens in evaluating cell immunity and inducing protection in a murine model of histoplasmosis. *Microbes Infect*. 2005;7:584-592.
364. Segel MJ, Rozenman J, Lindsley MD, et al. Histoplasmosis in Israeli travelers. *Am J Trop Med Hyg*. 2015;92:1168-1172.
411. Vergidis P, Avery RK, Wheat LJ, et al. Histoplasmosis complicating tumor necrosis factor-alpha blocker therapy: a retrospective analysis of 98 cases. *Clin Infect Dis*. 2015;61:409-417.
428. Wheat J, Wheat H, Connolly P, et al. Cross-reactivity in *Histoplasma capsulatum* variety capsulatum antigen assays of urine samples from patients with endemic mycoses. *Clin Infect Dis*. 1997;24:1169-1171.
432. Wheat LJ, Azar MM, Bahr NC, et al. Histoplasmosis. *Infect Dis Clin North Am*. 2016;30:207-227.
451. Wheat LJ, Wass J, Norton J, Kohler RB, French ML. Cavitary histoplasmosis occurring during two large urban outbreaks: analysis of clinical, epidemiologic, roentgenographic, and laboratory features. *Medicine (Baltimore)*. 1984;63:201-209.
478. Zeidberg LD, Ajello L, Dillon A, Runyon LC. Isolation of *Histoplasma capsulatum* from soil. *Am J Public Health Nations Health*. 1952;42:930-935.

The full reference list for this chapter is available at ExpertConsult.com.

Sporotrichosis 205

Bernhard L. Wiedermann

Sporotrichosis is an infection caused by the fungus *Sporothrix schenckii* species complex that is manifested most commonly as an ulcerating nodule at a site of local trauma, with spread occurring along regional lymphatic channels. Infection of other tissues or widespread dissemination is rare. It is an uncommon problem in children, but young adults seem to be infected more frequently, presumably owing to more frequent exposure to soil, plants, and decaying vegetable matter that harbor the organism. The disease was described first by a medical student, Schenck, in 1898, and most of what is known about the clinical syndrome has been learned from studies of large outbreaks, particularly one occurring in gold miners near Johannesburg, South Africa, in the early 1940s.[103,118]

ORGANISM

S. schenckii is a dimorphic fungus found principally in decaying vegetable matter or plant debris, although it does not seem to be a plant pathogen. In addition to *S. schenckii* sensu lato, *S. globosa* and *S. braziliensis* are important pathogens in some geographic areas, with *S. mexicana*, *S. lucrei*, and *S. albicans* having less clinical importance.[2,19,21,31] Molecular phylogenetic studies have demonstrated multiple clades that tended to group according to geographic origin.[21,79] The organism grows well on most culture media and is resistant to cycloheximide. Preferred culture media are Sabouraud glucose agar and blood agar, incubated at 25°C to 27°C. Most isolates grow readily from clinical material within 3 to 5 days, although occasional instances of slow growth have been reported, and cultures should be held at least 4 weeks before being considered negative. Incubation on blood agar at higher temperatures (37°C) allows growth of the yeast phase, which is necessary for specific identification of the organism in culture.[96]

EPIDEMIOLOGY

Most cases of sporotrichosis are reported from Central and South America, especially from Mexico and Brazil, and cases in the United States appear to cluster in the Midwest, particularly along the Mississippi and Missouri river areas.[50,90] Disease in humans usually results from inoculation of minor wounds by debris containing *S. schenckii,* and gardeners and nursery workers, forestry workers, miners, and other individuals exposed to contaminated plant materials are at higher risk for acquiring the disease.[20,25] Disseminated disease has been the initial presentation of some human immunodeficiency virus (HIV)-infected individuals, but the relative paucity of such reports probably reflects the low virulence of the organism.[4,82] Laboratory personnel working with the organism have become infected after incurring needlestick injuries.[116] The large South African epidemic in the gold mines of Transvaal probably resulted from the miners' brushing against rotting timbers in the mines, and a cluster of cases that occurred after a brick-throwing incident in Florida was traced to *S. schenckii* in the packing straw of the bricks.[99,118] Contaminated hay was the source of one outbreak linked to a Halloween haunted house.[32] Pulmonary disease may result from inhalation of spores.[90] Uncommonly, transmission of disease from animals, particularly domestic cats with cutaneous disease, or from family members occurs.[34,41,45,94] One adult acquired the disease after being bitten by a squirrel,[100] and a young girl developed cutaneous disease after a rodent bite.[57] In South America, armadillo hunters are at risk for development of sporotrichosis, but it is acquired from the decaying plant debris in armadillo nests rather than from the animals themselves.[78] Cats have been implicated in ongoing outbreaks in Brazil.[2,10,43,104,105] Molecular typing of isolates can be useful in investigations of outbreaks.[24,83,84]

PATHOGENESIS AND PATHOLOGY

As indicated, the most common mode of acquisition of sporotrichosis is by inoculation of the organism into skin structures, although disease also may develop from inhalation of spores of the organism. The incubation period varies considerably, commonly ranging from 7 to 30 days after cutaneous inoculation but possibly as long as 6 months.[96] The disease usually remains localized; of the 2825 cases of sporotrichosis in the Transvaal mine epidemic, none had systemic spread.[118]

S. schenckii, similar to other yeasts, seems to bind specifically to the glycosphingolipid lactosylceramide, which is present on the cell surface of animal cells.[61] This mechanism may be one by which the organism establishes a foothold in the host. Cell-mediated immune responses probably are important for containment of infection. One study documented intact responses in patients with cutaneous forms of the disease, whereas patients with systemic sporotrichosis had impaired cell-mediated immunity.[89] This study is supported by the observation that systemic disease tends to occur in individuals with underlying diseases or conditions that alter cell-mediated immunity. Deficiencies in toll-like receptor 4 have been suggested as contributing to severity of sporotrichosis.[9,101] Specific virulence factors also may contribute to likelihood of disseminated disease.[5,9,115,128]

Histopathologic examination of primary cutaneous lesions usually reveals changes in the epithelium, with hyperkeratosis, parakeratosis, and pseudoepitheliomatous hyperplasia. Intraepidermal microabscesses may be seen as well. In more established lesions, the pathologic process involves the dermis and below, with inflammatory infiltrate extending perivascularly.[75] The classic lesion on microscopic examination is a granuloma with an asteroid body at the center, although this picture is not pathognomonic for sporotrichosis. The asteroid body is an antigen-antibody complex deposited on the surface of the organism and may consist of several forms.[74,129] Visualization of fungi in tissue sections often is difficult, even with special staining techniques, because of the paucity of organisms in tissue. They may be seen on Gram stain as gram-positive but irregularly staining bodies, sometimes as cigar-shaped, 3- to 5-μm yeast forms. Periodic acid–Schiff and silver stains probably are better suited for detection of fungi in tissue sections.[75,96] Immunohistochemical staining techniques may prove superior to standard methods.[81,87]

CLINICAL MANIFESTATIONS

Sporotrichosis can occur in cutaneous and extracutaneous forms; the cutaneous varieties account for approximately 80% of all cases.[96] These categories can be broken down further into the organ system involved (Table 205.1).

TABLE 205.1 Clinical Forms of Sporotrichosis

Cutaneous	Extracutaneous
Lymphocutaneous	Osteoarticular
Fixed cutaneous	Pulmonary
	Muscular
	Ocular
	Genitourinary
	Central nervous system

Data from references 1, 53, 55, 70, 90, 97.

TABLE 205.2 Summary of 42 Cases of Pediatric Sporotrichosis

Duration of symptoms before diagnosis	3–10 weeks
Lymphatic involvement	28/47[a]
Culture positive	39/44[a]
Relapse after therapy	1/21[a]

[a]Numerator is number of patients positive; denominator is number of patients tested.
Data from references 17, 22, 27, 48, 76, 85.

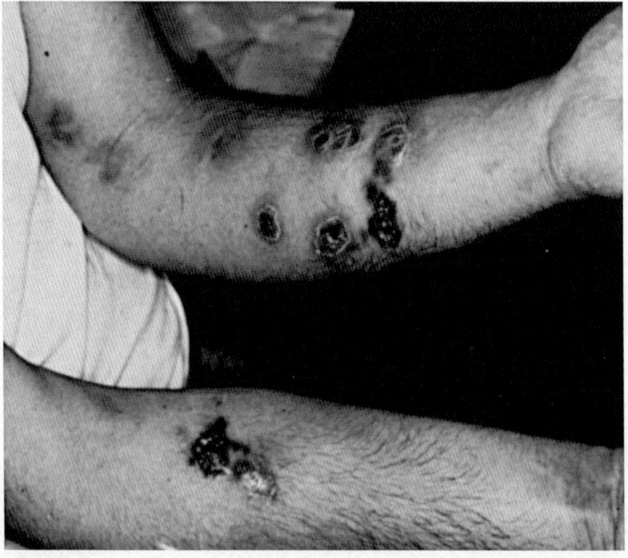

FIG. 205.1 Cutaneous lymphatic sporotrichosis of both arms. Note the characteristic involvement of lymphatics that drain the sites of the primary lesions. (Courtesy G. Medoff and G. S. Kobayashi.)

Cutaneous Sporotrichosis

Cutaneous disease with *S. schenckii* can be either lymphocutaneous or fixed cutaneous, the latter of which occurs less frequently. In lymphocutaneous cases, the initial lesion appears as a firm, slightly tender subcutaneous nodule. It progresses along local lymphatic channels, with multiple nodules appearing. The lesions typically enlarge and may ulcerate and suppurate (Fig. 205.1). Untreated, they may heal slowly during months or persist; recurrences are frequent. Differential diagnosis includes cutaneous nocardiosis, atypical mycobacterial disease, leishmaniasis, rosacea, syphilis, pyoderma gangrenosum, disseminated *Acanthamoeba* disease, and cutaneous manifestations of other fungal diseases.[29,68,93,113,126]

The fixed cutaneous form of the disease is just as the name implies, with no evidence of lymphatic spread. The primary lesions are identical to the lesions seen in the lymphocutaneous form. Although some researchers have suggested that sporotrichosis in children, compared with that in adults, is more likely to appear in the fixed cutaneous form, this theory has not been borne out in prior studies. Table 205.2 shows results from six reports of series of cases of sporotrichosis in children. The 60% rate for the lymphocutaneous form may not differ much from the 90% figure quoted for adults when one takes into account that many pediatric studies are reports of small numbers of cases and may have resulted from selection bias. A large series of patients from Peru documented a disproportionate number of children with facial lesions (86 of 143 children vs. 23 of 95 adults) but did not classify fixed versus lymphocutaneous forms by age.[88] Fixed cutaneous disease in children has been confused with impetigo.[17] A study from Peru also documented a predilection of children to develop lymphocutaneous lesions on the face and neck.[77] Risk factors for disease in children in this study included playing in fields, ownership of a cat, and residence in a house with dirt floors. Unusual dermatologic manifestations reported include molluscum-like lesions in a patient with alcoholic liver disease and Sweet syndrome in middle-aged women.[44,102]

Extracutaneous Sporotrichosis

Sporotrichosis occurring in extracutaneous sites either may be localized (related to an unusual area of trauma) or may represent disseminated disease. In the absence of trauma, the presence of extracutaneous sporotrichosis should raise suspicion of disseminated disease and consideration of immunodeficiency states. Overall, infection of bones and joints is the most common form of extracutaneous disease.[124] Sporotrichal arthritis usually is an indolent and slowly progressive disease that may occur with or without cutaneous or lymphatic disease, suggesting a hematogenous route of infection for most cases. Diagnosis generally requires synovial biopsy with culture to show the organism.[106,124] Two studies showed diagnostic delays averaging 17 and 25 months from the onset of symptoms.[11,26] Sporotrichal osteomyelitis usually occurs with concomitant arthritis, but isolated bone involvement has been recorded. Lytic lesions and periosteal changes are noted most frequently.[52,124]

Pulmonary sporotrichosis seldom occurs with cases of disseminated disease and probably develops after inhalation of spores, as with primary pulmonary histoplasmosis.[90] The presence of cavitary lesions in the upper lobes often leads to a diagnosis of tuberculosis, and fungal culture of sputum, bronchoscopic specimens, lung tissue, or gastric aspirate usually is needed to establish the diagnosis.[35,90,122] In addition to cavitary disease, noncavitary radiographic patterns also are reported.[6] Pleural involvement is uncommon (three of 47 cases in one review), and complications, such as massive hemoptysis, rarely occur.[37,56,90]

Sporotrichosis has been found to involve virtually every organ system in the body as part of disseminated disease.[124] Most commonly, underlying immunodeficiency states, such as diabetes, prolonged steroid therapy, alcoholism, immunosuppressive therapy, and acquired immunodeficiency syndrome (AIDS), are present.* In one Brazilian cohort of HIV-infected patients with sporotrichosis, 7 of 21 developed disseminated disease and 2 had meningitis.[42] Ocular and endocardial infection has been reported as well.[112] Disseminated disease, including meningitis, also has been reported as part of immune reconstitution syndrome in AIDS patients.[46,54] Fungemia in the absence of disseminated disease has been documented in one otherwise healthy adult with a lysis-centrifugation blood culture system, and laryngeal and cutaneous sporotrichosis has been reported in a healthy child.[67,69] Dissemination in patients with neoplasia seldom occurs. One child with chronic granulomatous disease and sporotrichal lymphadenitis has been reported.[121]

DIAGNOSIS

A high index of suspicion is necessary to establish the diagnosis of sporotrichosis. In the largest outbreak in the United States, which occurred in 1988 among horticulturists and forestry workers, only 15% of cases were diagnosed at the time of initial presentation to a physician.[23] Culture is the gold standard for diagnosis of sporotrichosis. Although organisms occasionally are seen on pathologic specimens, the yield is low enough to render biopsy unnecessary. If the diagnosis is suspected, scrapings of cutaneous lesions for culture should be sufficient to establish the diagnosis.[96]

A skin test antigen has been available for many years, but as with the histoplasmin skin test for histoplasmosis, it is useful mainly as an epidemiologic tool. Polymerase chain reaction may prove useful for diagnosis in the future.[63] Serodiagnosis has been explored in a few studies. Immunoprecipitation or commercially available slide latex agglutination can be useful when material for culture is difficult to obtain or cultures are negative, such as with sporotrichal meningitis.[30,107] In the ongoing Rio de Janeiro outbreak, an enzyme-linked immunosorbent assay detecting immunoglobulin G antibody to the SsCBF cell wall antigen has shown promising results.[12] Antibody titers in cerebrospinal fluid tend to decrease with successful therapy, and such tests might prove useful for monitoring of response to therapy.[13,107] Western blot testing has been used to detect sporotrichal antibody.[108] Using a crude antigen preparation, Scott and Muchmore[108] determined that detection of antibody to three antigens, 32 kDa, 40 kDa, and 70 kDa, seems to be sensitive and specific for diagnosis of active sporotrichosis. Patients with extracutaneous disease seemed to form antibody to a greater number of *S. schenckii* organisms than did patients with cutaneous disease. Further studies of the immune response in sporotrichosis should enable development of better serodiagnostic tests than those that now are routinely available.

TREATMENT AND PROGNOSIS

Sporotrichosis may resolve spontaneously, but treatment is indicated in most circumstances.[8,91] The Infectious Diseases Society of America has published practice guidelines for management of patients with sporotrichosis in 2007, reviewed and deemed current in 2013.[66]

Heat applied to the site of cutaneous disease has been reported anecdotally to cause resolution of lesions in patients in whom medical therapy was contraindicated.[47,97,119] One prospective study showed good results with use of benzene pocket warmers for heat therapy of facial lesions in children.[59] Surgical removal of infected skin and soft tissue has been used, but skin grafting may be required.[16] This form of treatment usually is unnecessary with the availability of medical management except possibly for some cases of pulmonary infection (particularly if it is confined to one lobe) and other extracutaneous disease.[26,52,90] Hyperthermia remains an option for treatment of sporotrichosis in pregnancy, in situations in which other agents may be contraindicated.[64]

A saturated solution of potassium iodide (SSKI), a proteolytic agent for which the mechanism of action against sporotrichosis is unclear,[65,72] can be used for uncomplicated sporotrichosis. The in vitro growth of *S. schenckii* is not inhibited appreciably by iodide, but free iodine has a marked inhibitory effect on growth.[123] The small amount of free iodine in a saturated solution of potassium iodide may be sufficient to cause resolution of disease. The pediatric dosage of a saturated solution of potassium iodide is empiric; it usually is given three times daily in juice or milk, starting at a low dose (e.g., 1 to 2 drops per year of age, up to 5 drops) and increasing the dose during the course of several days to a maximum of 30 to 40 drops per dose.[22,76,85] For younger children, lower dosages may be acceptable.[76,92] Treatment is continued until a few weeks after all lesions have resolved. Adverse reactions, such as salivary gland swelling, excessive lacrimation or salivation, nausea, vomiting, and abdominal pain, may resolve with temporary cessation of therapy followed by reinstitution at a lower dosage. SSKI currently is only an alternative treatment for lymphocutaneous and cutaneous forms of the disease.[64]

In vitro susceptibility testing is not used widely, and results may not always agree with clinical response.[98,120] The Clinical and Laboratory Standards Institute has proposed a microdilution test, whereas the European Committee for Antimicrobial Susceptibility Testing uses a similar assay with a different inoculum and test medium.[9] Breakpoints have not been established.

Itraconazole, an oral azole derivative, is the drug of choice for treatment of cutaneous, lymphocutaneous, and osteoarticular forms of sporotrichosis.[15,60,61,64,110] Restrepo and colleagues[95] showed clinical cures in all 17 patients with cutaneous forms of sporotrichosis treated with itraconazole (100 mg/day), with no major side effects. Borelli[14] reported a treatment failure, however, in a patient treated with 100 mg/day, who subsequently responded when the dose was increased to 200 mg/day. Systemic disease also has been treated with itraconazole with favorable clinical responses, although all information is from cases in adults.[7,71,86,110,125] Unfortunately, itraconazole resistance in *Sporothrix* has been reported.[49,114]

*References 1, 38, 51, 58, 62, 70, 111, 117, 124, 127.

Intravenous amphotericin B remains the drug of choice for treatment of patients with disseminated or severe sporotrichosis.[64,73,124] Duration of therapy in children has not been studied, but recommendations are to begin with liposomal amphotericin B at 3 to 5 mg/kg per day, with stepdown to itraconazole after clinical improvement to complete 12 months of total treatment.[66] On occasion, intraarticular amphotericin B is used to treat sporotrichal arthritis if response to other therapy is poor.[33] Amphotericin B therapy in patients with pulmonary sporotrichosis is less effective than with other forms of sporotrichosis, which has prompted many clinicians to use a combined medical-surgical approach.[66,90] Itraconazole is an alternative therapy and may be useful for long-term suppression.[66] Amphotericin B seems to be effective in treating sporotrichal meningitis when it is given early in the course of the disease, but adjunctive therapy with flucytosine or rifampin might be helpful.[106] Itraconazole and fluconazole also may have roles in treating meningitis.[60,66] Immunosuppressed individuals may require lifelong suppressive therapy with itraconazole to prevent recurrence, depending on the degree of immunosuppression and severity of disease.[66]

S. schenckii does not seem to be particularly susceptible to ketoconazole in vitro, and clinical experience with ketoconazole treatment of sporotrichosis has been mixed.[18,28,109] Possibly, relatively large doses of ketoconazole are needed to produce a good clinical response. Terbinafine, an allylamine, has looked promising in clinical studies.[39,40,60] Posaconazole has looked promising in a murine model of sporotrichosis, including in combination with amphotericin B.[36,80] Melanin production by *Sporothrix* strains appears to lessen the effects of antifungal agents such as terbinafine.[3]

Prognosis for cutaneous forms of disease is excellent, but the extracutaneous forms are associated with significant morbidity and mortality, in part related to the underlying conditions predisposing these patients to disseminated disease. Many cases of osteoarticular disease result in permanent disability.[26]

PREVENTION

The key to prevention of sporotrichosis is the elimination of exposure to the organism, particularly with regard to skin surfaces and mucous membranes. Usually, elimination of exposure can be accomplished by the use of protective clothing during high-risk activities, such as working with sphagnum moss or other decaying, moist plant material.[20,23] Nursery workers should be educated about the hazards and early signs of sporotrichosis, and physicians and veterinarians should be aware of the uncommon circumstances of spread of the infection from family members and domestic cats. The epidemic in the Transvaal gold mines was stopped when timbers in the mine shafts were sprayed with a fungicide.[118] Although reporting of individual cases of sporotrichosis is not required in the United States, reporting of clusters of cases can aid epidemiologic investigations and stop the spread of the disease.

NEW REFERENCES SINCE THE SEVENTH EDITION

2. Almeida-Paes R, de Olivera MME, Freitas DFS, et al. Sporotrichosis in Rio de Janeiro, Brazil: Sporothrix brasiliensis is associated with atypical clinical presentations. *PLoS Negl Trop Dis.* 2014;8:e3094.
3. Almeida-Paes R, Figueiredo-Carvalho MHG, Brito-Santos F, et al. Melanins protect Sporothrix brasiliensis and Sporothrix schenckii from the antifungal effects of terbinafine. *PLoS ONE.* 2016;11:e0152796.
6. Aung AK, Teh BM, McGrath C, et al. Pulmonary sporotrichosis: case series and systematic analysis of literature on clinic-radiological patterns and management outcomes. *Med Mycol.* 2013;51:534-544.
12. Bernardes-Engemann AR, de Lima Barros M, Zeitune T, et al. Validation of a serodiagnostic test for sporotrichosis: a follow-up study of patients related to the Rio de Janeiro zoonotic outbreak. *Med Mycol.* 2015;53:28-33.
19. Camacho E, Leon-Navarro I, Rodriguez-Brito S, et al. Molecular epidemiology of human sporotrichosis in Venezuela reveals high frequency of Sporothrix globosa. *BMC Infect Dis.* 2015;15:94.
21. Chakrabarti A, Bonifaz A, Gutierrez-Galhardo MC, et al. Global epidemiology of sporotrichosis. *Med Mycol.* 2015;53:3-14.
49. Gompertz OF, Rodrigues AM, Fernandes GF, et al. Case report: atypical clinical presentation of sporotrichosis caused by Sporothrix globosa resistant to itraconazole. *Am J Trop Med Hyg.* 2016;94:1218-1222.
80. Mario DN, Guarro J, Santurio JM, et al. In vitro and in vivo efficacy of amphotericin B combined with posaconazole against experimental disseminated sporotrichosis. *Antimicrob Agents Chemother.* 2015;59:5018-5021.
82. Moreira JAS, Freitas DFS, Lamas CC. The impact of sporotrichosis in HIV-infected patients: a systematic review. *Infection.* 2015;43:267-276.
114. Stopiglia CDO, Magagnin CM, Castrillon MR, et al. Antifungal susceptibilities and identification of species of the Sporothrix schenckii complex isolated in Brazil. *Med Mycol.* 2014;52:56-64.
121. Trotter JR, Sriaroon P, Berman D, et al. Sporothrix schenckii lymphadenitis in a male with X-linked chronic granulomatous disease. *J Clin Immunol.* 2014;34:49-52.

The full reference list for this chapter is available at ExpertConsult.com.

206 Mucormycosis and Entomophthoramycosis

Rachel L. Wattier • William J. Steinbach

Mucormycosis and entomophthoramycosis are invasive fungal infections once grouped together as "zygomycosis" based on a previous common classification within the phylum Zygomycota. However, they differ greatly in epidemiology and disease syndromes. Mucormycosis is the second most common invasive mold infection in immunocompromised hosts and tends to be rapidly progressive with extremely high mortality. Entomophthoramycosis occurs most commonly as indolent subcutaneous infection affecting immunocompetent hosts in tropical and subtropical regions.

Molecular phylogenetic analyses have since determined that the organisms previously grouped into the phylum Zygomycota did not share common evolutionary relationships, and thus the phylum has been abandoned. Currently those taxa conventionally classified in Zygomycota are now distributed among the new phylum Glomeromycota and four subphyla.[81] Causative agents of mucormycosis, within the order Mucorales, are grouped in the subphylum Mycoromycotina, and causative agents of entomophthoramycosis, within the order Entomophthorales, are grouped in the subphylum Entomophthoromycotina (Fig. 206.1).

It is now preferred to use the names "mucormycosis" to refer to disease caused by members of the order Mucorales (not by organisms from the genus *Mucor* as the name might suggest) and "entomophthoramycosis" for disease caused by members of the order Entomophthorales. As molecular phylogenetics continues to progress, these taxonomic definitions and clinical names may be subject to further change. This chapter focuses on mucormycosis, with a brief description of entomophthoramycosis.

MUCORMYCOSIS

Paltauf is credited with the first description of mucormycosis in humans in 1895 in his paper entitled "Mycosis Mucorina," describing a case of disseminated mycosis in a cancer patient.[119] The first English-language

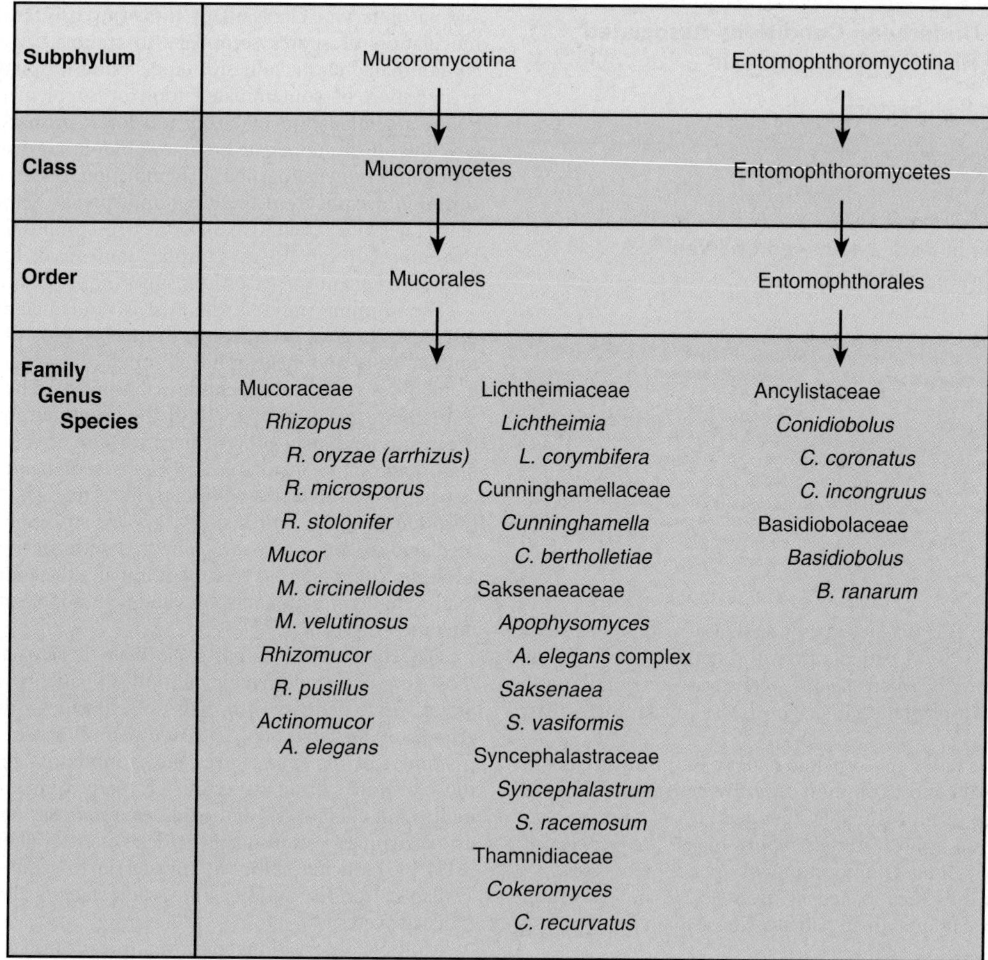

Subphylum
Mucoromycotina
Entomophthoromycotina
Class
Mucoromycetes
Entomophthoromycetes
Order
Mucorales
Entomophthorales
Family
Genus
Species
Mucoraceae
Rhizopus
R. oryzae (arrhizus)
R. microsporus
R. stolonifer
Mucor
M. circinelloides
M. velutinosus
Rhizomucor
R. pusillus
Actinomucor
A. elegans
Lichtheimiaceae
Lichtheimia
L. corymbifera
Cunninghamellaceae
Cunninghamella
C. bertholletiae
Saksenaeaceae
Apophysomyces
A. elegans complex
Saksenaea
S. vasiformis
Syncephalastraceae
Syncephalastrum
S. racemosum
Thamnidiaceae
Cokeromyces
C. recurvatus
Ancylistaceae
Conidiobolus
C. coronatus
C. incongruus
Basidiobolaceae
Basidiobolus
B. ranarum

FIG. 206.1 Taxonomy of human pathogens causing mucormycosis and entomophthoramycosis. Not all disease-causing species are represented. The orders Mucorales and Entomophthorales were previously grouped together in the class Zygomycetes, within the phylum Zygomycota; they are now classified in separate subphyla.

description of the disease appeared in 1940 when Wade and Matthews described a case of cutaneous mucormycosis of the face.[162]

ORGANISMS

The most common causative genera of Mucorales in humans are *Rhizopus, Mucor,* and *Lichtheimia* (formerly *Absidia*), which account for 70% to 80% of reported cases, with *Cunninghamella, Apophysomyces, Saksenaea, Rhizomucor, Cokeromyces, Actinomucor,* and *Syncephalastrum* species individually accounting for fewer than 1% to 5% of reported cases.[49] These organisms grow readily on common laboratory media but are inhibited by cycloheximide. Mucorales on solid media demonstrates rapid growth of woolly colonies, often with spores seen as tiny dark dots to the naked eye. Hyphae characteristically are large (10–30 μm in diameter), aseptate, and often twisted or ribbonlike. The lack of septation and the tendency of hyphae to branch at right angles usually serve to distinguish them from *Aspergillus* species, which are septate, smaller, and branch at acute angles.[5] Genera usually are differentiated from one another by examination of mycelia. Speciating the members of Mucorales is often difficult using conventional methods but can be improved by molecular methods.[37]

EPIDEMIOLOGY

Causative agents of mucormycosis are ubiquitous in nature and found in all parts of the world in soil and decaying organic material such as vegetation, bread, seeds, fruits, and manure. They are also occasionally isolated from the hospital environment, and acquisition of mucormycosis among immunocompromised hosts may be facilitated by hospital construction activities.[77,137,171] Recent hospital-acquired cases have been linked to contaminated linens and to a dietary supplement.[22,39,155] Mucormycosis has also been reported in association with environmental exposure during natural disasters.[115,170]

Mucormycosis is rare, with population-based incidence estimates of 1.7 cases per million population in the United States in 1992–93, and 0.09 cases per 100,000 population in France in 2001–10.[11,130] However, the incidence of mucormycosis in France increased by 7.3% per year, and mucormycosis-associated mortality increased by 9.3% per year between 2001 and 2010.[11]

Compared with other invasive mold infections, mucormycosis can affect hosts with a wider range of predisposing factors. In addition to the traditional immunocompromised risk groups (individuals with hematologic malignancy, transplant recipients), mucormycosis can affect individuals with diabetes mellitus and other metabolic disorders, breakdown of skin or soft tissue integrity such as in burn patients or surgical patients, and prematurity (Box 206.1).[87] Cases are occasionally reported in immunocompetent hosts with no known risk factors.[6,9,18,70]

The multicenter Transplant-Associated Infection Surveillance Network (TRANSNET) found that mucormycosis was rare, but second to invasive aspergillosis as a cause of invasive mold infection. Among 1208 invasive fungal infections (IFIs) identified among 1063 solid-organ transplantation (SOT) patients, mucormycosis accounted for only 2% of cases, compared with invasive aspergillosis (19%) and other non-*Aspergillus* molds (8%).[121] The median time from transplantation to diagnosis of mucormycosis

BOX 206.1 Underlying Conditions Associated With Increased Risk for Mucormycosis

Pediatric-Specific Risk Factors[177]

Prematurity
Methylmalonic aciduria
Malnutrition

Risk Factors Seen in Both Adults and Children[134,177]

Neutropenia or neutrophil dysfunction
Diabetes mellitus
Malignancy
Organ transplantation
Corticosteroid therapy
HIV infection
Deferoxamine therapy
Intravenous drug use
Trauma or surgery
Burns

was 312 days. Of 983 IFIs diagnosed among 875 hematopoietic stem cell transplantation (HSCT) patients from the same network, 8% of cases were mucormycosis, whereas 43% were invasive aspergillosis.[75] Median time from transplantation to diagnosis was 135 days, later than invasive aspergillosis.

In most large case series and systemic reviews of mucormycosis in adults and children, the most common causative genera are *Rhizopus* and *Mucor*, identified in approximately 50% and 20% of cases, respectively.[72,134,177] European cohort studies report higher frequencies of *Lichtheimia* (formerly *Absidia*), accounting for up to 29% of cases.[87,145] Less common organisms such as *Apophomyces elegans* and *Saksenaea vasiformis* occur more frequently in patients whose main predisposing factor is trauma.[70,92]

The most frequently reported predisposing conditions for mucormycosis vary based on setting and time period. In a systematic review of 929 reported cases from 1855 through 2003, diabetes mellitus was the most common predisposing factor, seen in 36% of cases.[134] Contemporary case series show greater disease burden among patients with hematologic malignancy, who account for approximately 45% to 60% of cases.[72,87,126,145] Overlapping risk factors are commonly observed; for example, patients with hematologic malignancy who have undergone HSCT are receiving immunosuppression and may also have hyperglycemia or iron overload.[72] In children, prematurity is an important risk factor, seen in 17% of cases in a large systematic review.[177]

Some centers have reported a rising incidence of mucormycosis among HSCT recipients and patients with hematologic malignancy.[74,101] Breakthrough infections with mucormycosis have been increasingly reported among patients receiving voriconazole as antifungal prophylaxis and as empirical, preemptive, and targeted antifungal therapy for invasive aspergillosis.[62,74,102,143] One hypothesis is that voriconazole, because of its lack of activity against the Mucorales, has exerted selective pressure favoring the emergence of mucormycosis. However, a longitudinal study evaluating the incidence of mucormycosis within well-defined populations of HSCT and SOT patients at multiple transplantation centers showed a stable incidence of mucormycosis within those populations before and after availability of voriconazole, although the absolute number of cases increased in direct proportion to the growing number of transplant recipients.[1] Increases in the reported number of cases of mucormycosis may in fact be related to increases in the number of immunocompromised individuals at risk and transplantation of higher risk individuals, with voriconazole as a surrogate marker for other risks associated with the development of mucormycosis.

PATHOGENESIS AND PATHOLOGY

Mucormycosis usually is acquired after inhalation of spores from environmental sources, and the organisms may colonize the sinuses and nasopharynx. Occasionally, mucormycosis results from cutaneous inoculation of spores secondary to trauma, as has occurred with contaminated elastic adhesive tape[31,47] and hospital linens,[22,39] as well as ingestion of contaminated food or supplement products.[89,114,155] Following inhalation of airborne spores, primary infection usually develops in the upper or lower respiratory tract and may spread by contiguous or hematogenous dissemination. Disseminated disease most commonly arises from the lungs and spreads hematogenously to the central nervous system (CNS), kidneys, gastrointestinal tract, and heart. Dissemination can also occur from cutaneous or subcutaneous sites of infection. Person-to-person transmission has not been documented.

The immune status of the host is fundamental to production of disease. In normal hosts, agents of mucormycosis are killed by mononuclear cells and neutrophils through the generation of oxidative metabolites and cationic peptide defensins.[34,165] The neutrophil appears to be the primary component of the immune response against these organisms and may prevent germination of inhaled spores.[33] Both neutropenia and qualitative deficiencies of neutrophil function are associated with an increased risk for mucormycosis.[134,177] *Rhizopus oryzae* (also known as *R. arrhizus*) displays less susceptibility to neutrophil-mediated oxidative damage, compared with *Aspergillus fumigatus*.[20] In addition, corticosteroid treatment impairs the ability of macrophages to prevent germination of spores and is an important clinical risk factor for mucormycosis.[134,164,177]

Diabetes mellitus, in particular diabetic ketoacidosis, is one of the most common underlying conditions in patients with mucormycosis. Serum from patients with diabetic ketoacidosis does not inhibit the growth of *Rhizopus* spp., but serum from those same patients after treatment of the ketoacidosis shows inhibitory properties similar to those of normal human serum.[46] Hyperglycemia and acidosis impair neutrophil chemotaxis and oxidative responses needed to damage *R. oryzae* hyphae.[23] Additionally, acidosis alters availability of serum iron, likely by reducing ability of transferrin to sequester iron in serum; available iron is another important factor altering virulence of mucormycetes.[7]

Multiple observations support a role for iron availability in pathogenesis of mucormycosis. Paradoxically, patients treated with the iron chelator deferoxamine have a markedly increased risk for mucormycosis, as demonstrated by the tendency for deferoxamine therapy to result in progression of both natural and experimental mucormycosis.[14,15,28,30,140,157] This phenomenon has been particularly observed in patients undergoing hemodialysis.[14,13,174] Studies in experimental models suggest that deferoxamine serves as a siderophore for *Rhizopus* spp., making previously unavailable iron available for use, with resultant increased fungal growth and increased mortality in a guinea pig model.[12,30,157] Enhanced iron uptake in the presence of deferoxamine appears to be a unique virulence factor among the Mucorales because the effect of deferoxamine is less pronounced for *A. fumigatus* and is minimal for *Candida albicans*.[12] Enhanced iron uptake and virulence of mucormycosis is unique to deferoxamine and has not been observed with other iron chelators.

The hallmark of histologic examination of mucormycosis is vascular invasion with resultant thrombosis and tissue necrosis and accompanying acute and chronic inflammation. Most of the clinical findings of progressive disease can be related to these effects on blood vessels. Septic emboli may affect all parts of the body. Perineural invasion also occurs commonly.[45] In the rhinocerebral form, the disease may progress along nerve roots during intracranial spread. Although relatively sparse, hyphal forms may be seen in tissue on routine hematoxylin and eosin staining more commonly than with silver or other special fungal stains[132] (Fig. 206.2).

CLINICAL MANIFESTATIONS

The clinical forms of mucormycosis are best considered by type of organ system involvement (Box 206.2). The primary site of infection at the time of initial diagnosis varies as a function of the host population (Table 206.1). The most common forms of mucormycosis are rhinocerebral, pulmonary, and cutaneous.[134] Historically, rhinocerebral infection was reported to be the most common form (39% of cases), but in contemporary series, a greater proportion of cases have been

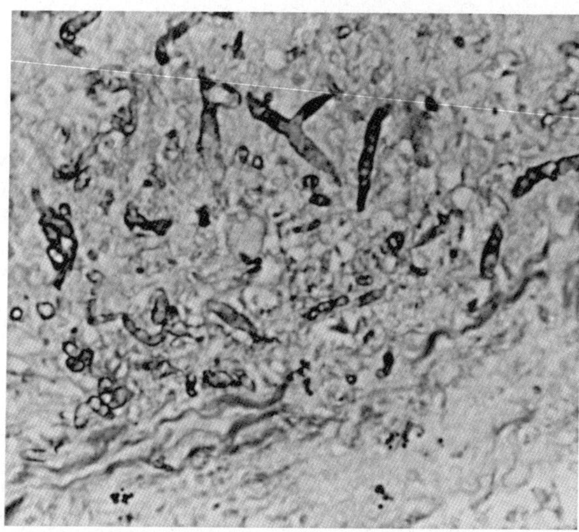

FIG. 206.2 Mucormycosis caused by *Rhizopus* species. Observe the varied morphologic features of the aseptate hyphae and large size. (Hematoxylin and eosin, original magnification ×64.)

BOX 206.2 Clinical Forms of Mucormycosis

Rhinocerebral	Gastrointestinal
Cutaneous/skin and soft tissue	Disseminated
Pulmonary	Miscellaneous

TABLE 206.1 Patterns of Mucormycosis by Host Population

Predisposing Condition	Predominant Sites of Infection (In Order of Frequency)
Diabetes mellitus	Rhinocerebral, pulmonary, sinoorbital, cutaneous
Malignancy with neutropenia	Pulmonary, sinus, cutaneous, sinoorbital
Hematopoietic stem cell transplantation	Pulmonary, disseminated, rhinocerebral
Solid-organ transplantation	Sinus, cutaneous, pulmonary, rhinocerebral, disseminated
Intravenous drug use	Cerebral, endocarditis, cutaneous, disseminated
Malnutrition	Gastrointestinal, disseminated
Deferoxamine therapy	Disseminated, pulmonary, rhinocerebral, cerebral, cutaneous, gastrointestinal
No underlying condition	Cutaneous, pulmonary, sinoorbital, rhinocerebral, gastrointestinal

From Kontoyiannis DP, Lewis RE. Invasive zygomycosis: update on pathogenesis, clinical manifestations, and management. *Infect Dis Clin North Am.* 2006;20(3):581-607.

pulmonary (28–46%), corresponding to the increase in disease burden among individuals with hematologic malignancy.[72,87,134,145] Other forms of invasive mucormycosis include gastrointestinal, disseminated, and other rare presentations.

Rhinocerebral Mucormycosis

The acute rhinocerebral form of mucormycosis, including sinus and sinoorbital infection, occurs most often in the setting of diabetes mellitus or hematologic malignancy.[134,145] Compared with invasive aspergillosis, mucormycosis is more likely to involve the orbit, versus only the sinuses.[152] Rhinocerebral mucormycosis spreads from the nares, palate, or sinuses to the paranasal sinuses, and then to the retroorbital region and brain by contiguous or hematogenous spread. Symptoms include facial pain, edema, and headache, with facial anesthesia in advanced infection.[122] Physical examination reveals brownish, blood-tinged nasal discharge, proptosis, or cranial neuropathies. Involved tissues become red, then violaceous, and finally black as vessels are thrombosed and tissues undergo necrosis.[122] Involvement of the orbital region can be manifested as proptosis or orbital edema, and ocular or optic nerve involvement can be suggested by pain, blurring, diplopia, or loss of vision.[122,147] Manifestations of invasive cerebral involvement include seizures,[116] encephalopathy, or stroke.[105]

Pulmonary Mucormycosis

Pulmonary mucormycosis may develop as a result of inhalation or by hematogenous or lymphatic spread. Pulmonary mucormycosis is the most common manifestation among patients with hematologic malignancy and HSCT patients.[72,87,134,145,176] Patients with pulmonary mucormycosis often present with fever, cough, chest pain, and rapidly progressive dyspnea, although findings can initially be subtle, with isolated fever.[150] Angioinvasion results in necrosis of lung tissue, which may lead to cavitation and hemoptysis. Massive pulmonary hemorrhage may result from vascular erosion.[53,169] Chest radiographs and computed tomography (CT) scans may reveal a focal consolidation, isolated masses, nodules, cavitation, or wedge-shaped areas of infarction.[66,76,106,150] Because of the lack of inflammatory cells that are capable of infiltrating the lung in neutropenic patients, however, radiography may not be dramatically abnormal.

Distinguishing pulmonary mucormycosis from invasive pulmonary aspergillosis is a clinical challenge, but certain epidemiologic, clinical, and radiographic features favor mucormycosis. Among patients with cancer, pulmonary mucormycosis is associated with previous exposure to voriconazole or other *Aspergillus*-active agents.[21] Among HSCT patients, acute graft-versus-host disease and history of invasive aspergillosis are associated with subsequent mucormycosis.[131] Clinical presentation with concomitant sinusitis and pulmonary disease is more often associated with mucormycosis.[21] Radiographic features suggestive of pulmonary mucormycosis include the presence of multiple nodules (≥10) and, to a lesser degree, pleural effusions on CT scans.[21] The reversed halo sign on CT, a central ground-glass opacity surrounded by a halo of dense consolidation, is seen more frequently with pulmonary mucormycosis than with other invasive mold infections (19% vs. <1% in one study, and 54% vs. 6% in another).[66,163] In contrast, pulmonary aspergillosis is associated with more airway invasive findings, such as clusters of centrilobular nodules, peribronchial consolidation, and bronchial wall thickening.[66]

Some atypical and more indolent presentations of pulmonary mucormycosis include chronic infection with constitutional symptoms in relatively immunocompetent hosts.[106] Rarely, fungus balls have been noted within a preexisting lung cavity.[83] Hypersensitivity pneumonitis caused by *Rhizopus* spp. has been described in farm workers as well as Scandinavian sawmill workers (so-called wood-trimmer's disease).[40]

Skin and Soft Tissue (Cutaneous) Mucormycosis

Cutaneous (also referred to as skin and soft tissue) mucormycosis represents approximately 20% of reported cases in adults and a slightly higher proportion of pediatric cases.[134,177] Primary cutaneous infection usually occurs at the site of trauma, burns, adhesive dressings, or invasive procedures in immunocompromised hosts.[25,47,71,154,172,173] Skin and soft tissue infection is the primary manifestation of mucormycosis that is reported among immunocompetent hosts, and typically is due to contamination of wounds with organic material.[18,70,92,115] Among neonates, the skin is a common point of entry, with involvement of adhesive tape, monitor leads, or central venous access sites predominating. Premature infants represent most of the neonatal cases.[96,133] Secondary cutaneous disease may be seen with hematogenous dissemination.[71] Primary disease may be very invasive locally and by direct extension affect adjacent bone and tissue. With vessel invasion, frankly disseminated disease may arise.

Primary cutaneous disease typically begins with a lesion that appears erythematous and indurated and progresses with ulceration and necrosis to form a black eschar (Fig. 206.3). In contrast, cutaneous disease arising

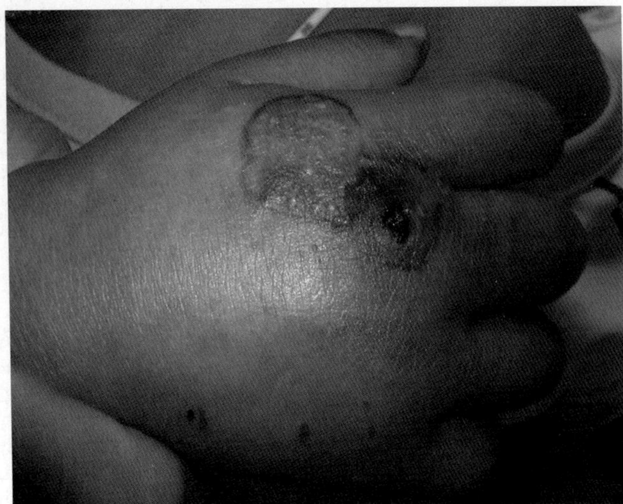

FIG. 206.3 Cutaneous mucormycosis in a child with neutropenia.

secondarily from disseminated disease usually manifests as nodular subcutaneous lesions, which may ulcerate. Skin and soft tissue infections associated with trauma can vary in presentation depending on the type and extent of original injury, with manifestations from superficial to deep, sometimes presenting as necrotizing fasciitis.[92,115]

Gastrointestinal Mucormycosis

Gastrointestinal mucormycosis is a rare manifestation that probably results from ingestion of fungal spores, either from the environment or from colonized upper airways. Occasionally, hematogenous or direct extension routes result in intestinal tract involvement. Immunosuppression, malnutrition, prematurity, uremia, and underlying gastrointestinal disease, such as typhoid fever or amebiasis, are predisposing factors.[35,110,114] Gastrointestinal mucormycosis is the most common clinical manifestation among neonates, representing two-thirds of neonatal cases.[177] Most gastrointestinal disease in neonates is seen in premature neonates, sometimes occurring in association with progressive necrotizing skin lesions and sometimes manifesting with necrotizing enterocolitis.[175,177]

All sites along the intestinal tract can be involved. Historically, the stomach and colon were the most common sites, but a recent review of cases in immunocompromised hosts suggests that localization varies based on host susceptibility.[35,114] Intestinal disease was more common among HSCT patients and patients with hematologic malignancy, and reported cases increased over time; gastric localization was more common among SOT patients.[35] Fever and nonspecific abdominal pain with hematemesis, hematochezia, or melena may occur. Dissemination to other sites may occur by hematogenous routes. Perforation after bowel wall necrosis is common. Among the forms of mucormycosis, gastrointestinal infection is associated with the longest diagnostic delays, and diagnosis is frequently made only at autopsy.[35]

Disseminated Mucormycosis

Disseminated mucormycosis, with infection occurring at two or more noncontiguous sites, is reported in 15% to 20% of cases.[72,87,134,145] Disseminated infection is most likely to occur in severely immunocompromised hosts, such as those with active hematologic malignancy or allogeneic HSCT patients.[134] Patients who develop mucormycosis in the setting of deferoxamine therapy may also present with widely disseminated infection, often without an apparent primary site.[13,14,174] Clinical manifestations vary depending on the sites involved and the extent of tissue invasion. Disseminated infection often stems from pulmonary infection as the primary site, with the central nervous system as a frequent secondary site. A subacute form of disseminated disease with a protracted but fatal course has been reported.[117] Disseminated mucormycosis is associated with extremely high mortality and is often not apparent premortem.[64,158]

Miscellaneous Forms of Mucormycosis

A variety of case reports of mucormycosis involving isolated areas of the body are found in the literature and include reports of endocarditis,[109,138,178] brain abscess,[134] peritonitis,[17,112,124] osteomyelitis,[41] mediastinitis,[104] tracheitis,[141] corneal infection,[151] otitis externa,[151] superior vena cava syndrome,[16] and renal disease.[99] Common to these disease manifestations is some type of local trauma or surgery that results in a ready access site for invasion of fungal organisms. Outcome varies highly and depends on the underlying condition of the host as well as the extent of disease.

DIAGNOSIS

The diagnosis of mucormycosis is established by identification of a causative organism by culture, direct microscopy, or histopathology in a patient with compatible clinical findings.[26,32,144] A high index of suspicion is needed to make the diagnosis, with appropriate radiographic imaging and sampling of tissue from affected clinical sites. Securing diagnostic samples from internal sites such as the lung can be challenging because of risks for invasive procedures in unstable and thrombocytopenic patients. Sites such as skin and sinuses are more amenable to sampling, leading to more definitive diagnoses in cutaneous and rhinocerebral infections. Even with adequate tissue samples, the diagnosis of mucormycosis can be difficult to establish owing to limitations of culture and histology. Because of these diagnostic challenges and the rapidly progressive nature of the disease, empiric therapy should be started as soon as mucormycosis is suspected.

Cultures may be negative in a large portion of cases, even when Mucorales hyphae are visualized in tissue, because the aseptate hyphae are prone to shearing during tissue processing. Many specimens, including blood, sputum, gastric fluid, or nasal swabs, are either difficult to culture or of minimal diagnostic value, and invasive mucormycosis is ideally diagnosed with tissue biopsy and culture.[43] Cultures from bronchoalveolar lavage fluid may grow Mucorales but are of lower yield than cultures from tissue. The presence of Mucorales in cultures does not always represent active infection. The spores from asexual reproduction are easily airborne and may be laboratory contaminants; some patients may be colonized. One study showed that 65% of patients with positive cultures for Mucorales did not meet criteria for proven or probable IFI.[86] Patients with hematologic malignancy were more likely to meet criteria for disease, whereas patients with chronic respiratory diseases were less likely to meet criteria and had a benign clinical course.[86]

It can be difficult to definitively identify Mucorales by histopathology because the appearance of hyphae may not be characteristic in damaged or necrotic tissue, or there may be insufficient hyphae present to characterize the morphology. It is not possible to identify Mucorales to the species level based on histopathology alone. Several methods show potential to improve identification of Mucorales within tissues, including immunohistochemistry,[67] polymerase chain reaction (PCR)–based methods,[3,37,38] and matrix-assisted laser desorption/ionization time-of-flight mass spectrometry (MALDI-TOF MS).[36] Many of these methods are technically specialized, and only Mucorales PCR and pan-fungal PCR (based on ribosomal RNA sequence) are available for clinical use.

There is no established noninvasive method to diagnose mucormycosis. β-D-Glucan and galactomannan are not released by Mucorales, and no other serum biomarkers have been identified for mucormycosis. There may be a future role for novel methods to improve diagnostic yield from less invasive sampling techniques. A study of PCR and high-resolution melt analysis conducted on bronchoalveolar lavage samples showed improved detection of probable pulmonary mucormycosis compared with culture and histopathology, but included only a small number of patients with mucormycosis.[93] One study showed that circulating Mucorales DNA was detectable in serum by PCR from 9 of 10 patients with proven or probable mucormycosis, with the first positive sample preceding diagnosis by 3 to 68 days.[108] None of the 10 healthy controls evaluated had detectable circulating Mucorales DNA. In a subsequent study, 36 of 44 (81%) patients with proven or probable mucormycosis had detectable circulating Mucorales DNA, with the first positive at a median of 9 days (range, 0–25 days) before diagnosis.[107]

Another investigational diagnostic method is the detection of Mucorales-specific T cells in peripheral blood. In a study of 204 patients screened during chemotherapy for hematologic malignancy, 21 (10.3%) had detectable Mucorales-specific T cells.[125] Six of these patients had clinical evidence of IFI and were distinguishable from patients without IFI based on high production of interleukin-10 and interleukin-4.[125] Although these noninvasive methods appear promising, they will require further evaluation to determine their performance characteristics in diverse clinical populations. There is currently a study in progress to establish a registry and biobank of mucormycosis cases and controls to facilitate development of novel diagnostic methods.[168]

TREATMENT

General Principles

Of overall great importance is the combination of early and aggressive surgical excision of necrotic lesions, reversal of predisposing conditions (immune dysfunction, neutropenia, hyperglycemia, acidosis), and early antifungal therapy. Because tissue infarction is a prominent feature, removal of devitalized tissue is critical because antifungals alone, especially in the setting of continued immunosuppression, will not elicit cure.[91,123] All necrotic-appearing tissue should be removed, and often patients require repeated surgical procedures for removal of devitalized tissue. Among 22 patients with rhinocerebral mucormycosis from a French registry, all of the patients who had complete local control of disease survived to 90 days, whereas 90-day survival was only 25% in the patients without complete local control.[161] Duration of therapy for mucormycosis is highly individualized; guidelines recommend continuation of therapy until resolution of clinical and radiographic manifestations and restoration of immune function.[26,144] Patients who remain immunocompromised may require long-term secondary prophylaxis to prevent recurrence.

Amphotericin B Formulations

Lipid formulations of amphotericin B, either liposomal amphotericin (L-AmB) or amphotericin B lipid complex, given at high doses (at least 5 mg/kg per day, up to 10 mg/kg per day) are recommended as first-line therapy for mucormycosis.[26,144] Conventional amphotericin B deoxycholate has been used historically but is highly nephrotoxic. Although different doses of lipid amphotericin B formulations have not been directly compared with one another in humans, higher doses of L-AmB were associated with better disease response in a murine model.[94] A single-arm clinical trial (AmBizygo) of high-dose (10 mg/kg) L-AmB (combined with surgery in 71% of cases) in 40 patients with mucormycosis showed favorable clinical responses in 36% of patients at week 4 and 45% at week 12.[88] However, doubling of creatinine occurred in 40% of patients.[88] Delayed amphotericin B–based therapy (treatment ≥6 days after diagnosis) was associated with a two-fold increase in mortality (83% vs. 49%) in one study, emphasizing the importance of early appropriate therapy.[19]

Triazoles

Most triazoles, including fluconazole and voriconazole, have no activity against Mucorales. This point is critically important because voriconazole is an excellent antifungal against invasive aspergillosis, but has no clinical activity in mucormycosis. Whether or not exposure to voriconazole actually enhances virulence of mucormycosis is debated. Prior exposure to voriconazole is associated with occurrence of breakthrough mucormycosis,[62,74,102,143] and some studies have shown higher mortality in patients with mucormycosis who previously received voriconazole.[72] Data from animal models show enhancement of *Rhizopus* and *Mucor* virulence following exposure to voriconazole.[10,84] However, a multicenter longitudinal cohort study of HSCT and SOT patients showed stable disease severity and mortality of mucormycosis over time, before and after availability of voriconazole.[1]

Posaconazole has activity against Mucorales and has shown efficacy in salvage therapy for patients intolerant of or unresponsive to amphotericin B formulations.[156,159] Reported clinical response rates range from 66% to 79% in salvage therapy.[50,156,159] These rates cannot be accurately compared with the success rate for primary therapy with L-AmB because patients who survive long enough to qualify for salvage therapy studies likely have more slowly progressive disease and may have benefited already from surgery or reversal of underlying conditions. Additionally, reporting bias likely inflates the success rates in case reports and series.

Posaconazole has not been systematically evaluated as primary monotherapy and should be used with caution, particularly in early phases of therapy.[26,144] Posaconazole has slower in vitro killing[80] and is active against a narrower range of clinical isolates[4] compared with amphotericin B. In vitro susceptibility to posaconazole among clinical isolates of *R. oryzae* and *Mucor circinelloides*, two of the most common causative agents of mucormycosis, is poor, with only 64% of *R. oryzae* isolates and none of six *M. circinelloides* isolates showing susceptibility.[4] Studies in murine models show zero or limited activity of posaconazole against experimental infection caused by *R. oryzae* and *M. circinelloides*.[29,61,135,139] Bioavailability of the posaconazole oral suspension is unreliable, particularly in patients with mucositis or diarrhea.[78,79,90,153] New oral tablet and intravenous formulations are now available but have not yet been evaluated in children. Posaconazole is currently recommended for salvage or stepdown therapy and secondary prophylaxis of mucormycosis, but not for primary antifungal therapy.[26,144]

Isavuconazole is a triazole with a broad spectrum of activity, including Mucorales. It shows favorable pharmacokinetics compared with other triazoles, with good oral bioavailability and linear elimination kinetics.[136] It is given orally or intravenously as a prodrug, isavuconazonium sulfate, which is converted to the active drug in vivo. In a murine model, it showed similar efficacy to amphotericin B in protecting against experimental mucormycosis.[98] In a single-arm open-label clinical trial (VITAL), adults with mucormycosis (21 receiving primary treatment, 11 refractory to other agents, 5 intolerant to other agents) treated with isavuconazole showed 11% partial response and 43% stable disease at day 42.[103] For assessment of the secondary endpoint, all-cause mortality, patients receiving isavuconazole as primary therapy were matched to contemporaneous controls from a registry (FungiScope) who received primary therapy with amphotericin B formulations. All-cause mortality at day 42 was similar in cases treated with isavuconazole (33%) compared with controls treated with amphotericin B–based therapy (39%).[103] Isavuconazole is now licensed for primary therapy of mucormycosis based on this study, but its ultimate place in therapy will depend on further clinical assessments. Pharmacokinetics and safety of isavuconazole have not yet been defined in children.

Combination Therapy

Poor outcomes of mucormycosis treated with monotherapy have prompted investigation of combination antifungal therapy; the data on this approach are conflicting. Although echinocandins lack significant activity against Mucorales, there is biologic plausibility for synergy in combination with amphotericin B–based therapy. *R. oryzae* expresses the gene encoding for the 1,3-β-D-glucan synthase complex, and its enzyme activity is inhibited by caspofungin.[57] Furthermore, caspofungin uncovers β-D-glucan in the cell wall of *R. oryzae*, enhancing activity of human neutrophils against the organism.[85] Murine models have shown benefit of combination amphotericin B and echinocandin therapy in experimental mucormycosis.[60,148] A clinical study of polyene-echinocandin combination therapy for mucormycosis found a benefit in patients who were predominantly nonneutropenic with diabetic ketoacidosis as the main predisposing factor.[129] However, this study was retrospective and small, with only 6 patients receiving combination therapy, compared with 31 who received amphotericin B–based monotherapy.

The effect of amphotericin B and posaconazole combination therapy in murine models is unclear, with one study suggesting benefit and another showing similar responses to L-AmB with or without posaconazole.[61,135] A report from two large prospective registries described responses to therapy in 32 patients with mucormycosis who were treated with combination L-AmB and posaconazole, mostly as salvage therapy.[118] At a median 3-month follow-up time, clinical improvement was seen in 18 patients (56%); the study was not controlled.

Subsequent observational studies incorporating strategies to control for bias and confounding have called the benefit of combination therapy into question. A longitudinal study showed that 90-day survival among HSCT and SOT patients with mucormycosis was not significantly different between two time periods, 1995–2003, during which amphotericin

B–echinocandin therapy was used in 5% of cases, and 2004–11, during which it was used in 31% of cases.[1] Another study used propensity scores to adjust for likelihood of receiving initial combination therapy (defined as two or more of L-AmB, posaconazole, or caspofungin) among patients with hematologic malignancies and mucormycosis.[82] There was no apparent impact of combination therapy on mortality, with or without propensity score adjustment. At this time, guidelines for treatment of mucormycosis suggest that combination therapy may be used for salvage of refractory cases, but there is insufficient evidence to support its use as primary therapy.[26,144]

Adjunctive Therapies

Iron chelation with agents other than deferoxamine has been evaluated as adjunctive therapy for mucormycosis and shows benefit in animal models.[59,58] A clinical trial of 20 patients randomized to adjunctive deferasirox versus placebo for treatment of mucormycosis (DEFEAT Mucor) showed higher mortality at 90 days in the deferasirox arm.[149] However, the trial was small and baseline characteristics were unbalanced, with higher frequency of active malignancy, neutropenia, and corticosteroid therapy in the deferasirox arm. At this time, clinical guidelines for mucormycosis do not recommend the use of deferasirox, particularly in patients with hematologic malignancies, but further studies are needed to determine whether there is a role for adjunctive deferasirox in other at-risk populations.[26,144]

Hyperbaric oxygen therapy has been used as an adjunct to surgical and antifungal therapy for some patients with mucormycosis in an attempt to limit the extent of gangrene and tissue necrosis.[27,44,68,127] The increased oxygen pressure achieved with hyperbaric therapy seems to improve the ability of neutrophils to kill organisms and inhibit fungal growth in vitro.[8] Although this regimen is apparently promising, the number of patients evaluated with this form of treatment is much too small to permit any firm conclusions on benefit.

The role of other adjunctive therapies for mucormycosis has not been well studied. Granulocyte transfusions, or cytokines that enhance phagocytic activity, such as interferon-γ and granulocyte-macrophage colony-stimulating factor, have been used occasionally to treat patients with mucormycosis.[2,48,146] Case reports have indicated favorable outcomes in patients treated with these adjunctive therapies,[2,146] but further studies are warranted to determine their role in therapy.

PROGNOSIS AND PREVENTION

The disease site and host factors are key determinants of prognosis for mucormycosis. The reported mortality rate is highest for disseminated disease (100%), followed by gastrointestinal (85%), cerebral (79%), pulmonary (76%), and rhinocerebral (46%) disease.[134] Localized cutaneous disease is associated with a low mortality rate of 10%. Significant risk factors for mortality include disseminated disease, renal failure, active malignancy, monocytopenia at diagnosis, and lymphopenia at diagnosis.[19,70,95,134] Patients who undergo surgery and those who receive early amphotericin B–based therapy are significantly more likely to survive.[19,56,72,134] Neutrophil recovery is also a favorable prognostic factor.[19] Among children, age younger than 1 year is associated with higher mortality.[177] Mucormycosis is sufficiently uncommon that primary prophylaxis is not routinely recommended.[26,144]

ENTOMOPHTHORAMYCOSIS

The name of the order Entomophthorales comes from the Greek and means "insect destroyer," highlighting the fact that many species in this order are insect pathogens. Few species are associated with human disease, which typically is seen in immunocompetent patients residing in tropical and subtropical areas of the world. Infections caused by Entomophthorales are usually chronic, subcutaneous, and localized without blood vessel invasion.[142]

ORGANISMS

The Entomophthorales organisms that cause human infection are confined to two genera, *Conidiobolus* and *Basidiobolus*. *C. coronatus* and *C. incongruus* are the major disease-causing species of *Conidiobolus*. *Basidiobolus ranarum* is the only human pathogen of the *Basidiobolus* genera; previously reported disease-causing species *B. haptosporus* and *B. meristosporus* are now known to be identical to *B. ranarum*.[142] Growth of Entomophthorales occurs readily on solid media, as flat, gray, or pale-yellow waxy colonies with velvety white mycelia on the surface. The hyphae may or may not have septae.

EPIDEMIOLOGY

Entomophthoramycosis occurs sporadically, with most cases reported in Africa and Asia, although cases have also been reported in Europe, North America, and South America.[142] Since the mid-1990s multiple cases of gastrointestinal basidiobolomycosis have been reported from Arizona; reasons for emergence there are unclear.[160] In a case-control study including seven adult patients in Arizona, infected patients tended to be more likely to use ranitidine and to have resided in Arizona for a longer time compared with controls.[100]

Members of Entomophthorales commonly are found in feces of reptiles, amphibians, and other animals as well as in decaying vegetable matter.[142] The mode of acquisition is not determined but is hypothesized to be through minor trauma, inhalation, or ingestion of environmental spores.[142]

PATHOGENESIS AND PATHOLOGY

The organisms causing entomophthoramycosis are of extremely low virulence, as manifested by the rare occurrence of these infections despite the ubiquitous nature of the fungi. Given their low virulence, some have proposed that infection with Entomophthorales is acquired during a state of transient immunosuppression, such as during a viral illness, or from repeated exposure.[142]

Conidiobolus spp. are characteristically associated with rhinofacial infections, and *B. ranarum* is more often associated with subcutaneous infections of the back, buttocks, and lower extremities.[142] However, both genera have been reported to cause both forms of subcutaneous disease.[52,54] Additionally, invasive and fulminant infection resembling mucormycosis has been reported to occur in immunocompromised hosts.[166,167]

Histopathologic examination of affected tissues shows areas of acute and chronic inflammation in association with broad hyphal elements that may or may not display septations. The hyphae are more visible with hematoxylin and eosin staining than with more specific fungal stains.[142] The tendency for vascular invasion typical of mucormycosis does not occur with entomophthoramycosis, and tissue necrosis is uncommon. A characteristic pathologic feature of the subcutaneous forms of entomophthoramycosis is the Splendore-Hoeppli phenomenon, consisting of organisms with inflammatory infiltrate surrounded by eosinophilic material in a stellate pattern.[142] The eosinophilic material is thought to consist of antigen-antibody precipitate on the organisms. The Splendore-Hoeppli phenomenon is not pathognomonic of entomophthoramycosis, however, and has been seen in other chronic fungal infections, as well as chronic bacterial and parasitic infections.[142]

CLINICAL MANIFESTATIONS

Chronic Rhinofacial Entomophthoramycosis

Chronic rhinofacial entomophthoramycosis, also called *entomophthoramycosis conidiobolae* because most infections are caused by *Conidiobolus coronatus*, is an indolent subcutaneous infection involving the nasal and paranasal structures.[55,111,113] Typically, painless bilateral intranasal swelling and obstruction eventually progress to invasion of the sinuses and nodular soft tissue swelling of the face, unaccompanied by fever or pain. Firm subcutaneous nodules can become deeply attached and feel anchored to underlying tissues.[142] Symptoms commonly persist for weeks or months. Deep tissue progression is unlikely to occur, but spread to the orbits, central nervous system, and mediastinal structures has been reported.[142]

Chronic Subcutaneous Entomophthoramycosis

Chronic subcutaneous entomophthoramycosis, also known as *entomophthoramycosis basidiobolae*, is similar to chronic rhinofacial disease with the exception that the lesions usually are on the trunk or extremities. The usual etiologic agent is *B. ranarum*. Painless subcutaneous nodules may progress to invade deeper soft tissues, and massive soft tissue swelling may develop. In contrast to subcutaneous lesions caused by *Conidiobolus* spp., subcutaneous nodules caused by *B. ranarum* are typically not anchored to underlying tissues and are freely mobile.[128,142] They are often misdiagnosed initially as soft tissue sarcomas.[128] With rare exceptions, most cases of subcutaneous entomophthoramycosis are slowly progressive, but they can cause lymphatic obstruction and elephantiasis and are occasionally deeply invasive.[65,142]

Gastrointestinal Basidiobolomycosis

Gastrointestinal basidiobolomycosis is an extremely rare condition resulting from *B. ranarum* infection of the gastrointestinal tract. Clinical features include fever, abdominal pain, leukocytosis, and eosinophilia; sometimes an abdominal mass is palpable.[42,120,160] Initial misdiagnosis as inflammatory bowel disease or colon cancer is common.[42]

DIAGNOSIS

Diagnosis of entomophthoramycosis relies on clinical suspicion and supportive findings from tissue biopsy. Histopathology shows typical findings including the Splendore-Hoeppli phenomenon. As with mucormycosis, cultures may have lower yield because hyphae are easily damaged during tissue processing.[42,142] Molecular methods may be used to identify organisms in tissues when cultures are negative.[142] Serodiagnosis by immunodiffusion is possible, but tests are not widely available for clinical use.[63,69]

TREATMENT

Evaluating therapy for this group of diseases is difficult because of their rarity and occasional reports of spontaneous resolution. Many agents have been tried, alone or in combination, with variable success, including potassium iodide, triazole antifungals, amphotericin B, and trimethoprim-sulfamethoxazole.[24,128,142] Most isolates of *Conidiobolus* and *Basidiobolus* spp. have relatively high minimum inhibitory concentrations (MICs) to amphotericin B.[51] *Conidiobolus* displays relatively high MICs to fluconazole, posaconazole, and itraconazole, whereas *Basidiobolus* tends to have lower MICs to these agents. A systematic review of therapies for *Conidiobolus* infections was unable to identify a clear benefit of any specific antifungal agent.[24]

Surgery is thought to be important for resolution of gastrointestinal basidiobolomycosis.[5] Surgery may be beneficial in early stages of rhinofacial entomophthoramycosis, but in advanced stages lesions may not be resectable.[24,142] Although surgery is frequently reported for subcutaneous entomophthoramycosis, some have reported frequent recurrence of disease after surgery.[128] Successful adjunctive therapy with hyperbaric oxygen has been reported.[44,97]

PROGNOSIS AND PREVENTION

Mortality caused by entomophthoramycosis is unlikely to occur, but morbidity and disfigurement are common. Adverse outcomes are associated with underlying immunocompromising conditions, atypical clinical presentation (e.g., orbital involvement with rhinofacial disease, visceral or perineal involvement with subcutaneous entomophthoramycosis), and absence of the Splendore-Hoeppli phenomenon on pathology, perhaps reflecting a poor immune response.[24,128,142] Among infections caused by *Conidiobolus* spp., mortality is higher in the setting of facial elephantiasis, female gender, and infections caused by non-*coronatus* species.[24] Specific means for preventing disease are unavailable because so little is known about factors predisposing individuals to these chronic infections.

NEW REFERENCES SINCE THE SEVENTH EDITION

1. Abidi MZ, Sohail MR, Cummins N, et al. Stability in the cumulative incidence, severity and mortality of 101 cases of invasive mucormycosis in high-risk patients from 1995 to 2011: a comparison of eras immediately before and after the availability of voriconazole and echinocandin-amphotericin combination therapies. *Mycoses*. 2014;57:687-698.
5. Al-Shanafey S, Alrobean F, Hussain IB. Surgical management of gastrointestinal basidiobolomycosis in pediatric patients. *J Pediatr Surg*. 2012;47:949-951.
3. Alanio A, Garcia-hermoso D, Mercier-Delarue S, et al. Molecular identification of Mucorales in human tissues: contribution of PCR electrospray ionization mass spectrometry. *Clin Microbiol Infect*. 2015;21:594.e591-594.e595.
4. Almyroudis NG, Sutton DA, Fothergill AW, et al. In vitro susceptibilities of 217 clinical isolates of zygomycetes to conventional and new antifungal agents. *Antimicrob Agents Chemother*. 2007;51(7):2587-2590.
6. Antony SJ, Parikh MS, Ramirez R, et al. Gastrointestinal mucormycosis resulting in a catastrophic outcome in an immunocompetent patient. *Infect Dis Rep*. 2015;7:60-65.
9. Beatty N, Al Mohajer M. Primary cutaneous mucormycosis developing after incision and drainage of a subcutaneous abscess in an immunocompetent host. *BMJ Case Rep*. 2016;2016.
10. Bellanger AP, Albert ND, Lewis RE, et al. Effect of preexposure to triazoles on susceptibility and virulence of *Rhizopus oryzae*. *Antimicrob Agents Chemother*. 2015;59:7830-7832.
11. Bitar D, Lortholary O, Strat YL, et al. Population-based analysis of invasive fungal infections. *Emerg Infect Dis*. 2014;20:1149-1155.
18. Burrell S, Ostlie D, Saubolle M, et al. *Apophysomyces elegans* infection associated with cactus spine injury in an immunocompetent pediatric patient. *Pediatr Infect Dis J*. 1998;17:663-664.
22. Cheng VCC, Chen JHK, Wong SCY, et al. Hospital outbreak of pulmonary and cutaneous zygomycosis due to contaminated linen items from substandard laundry. *Clin Infect Dis*. 2016;62:1-8.
24. Choon S-E, Kang J, Neafie RC, et al. Conidiobolomycosis in a young Malaysian woman showing chronic localized fibrosing leukocytoclastic vasculitis: a case report and meta-analysis focusing on clinicopathologic and therapeutic correlations with outcome. *Am J Dermatopathol*. 2012;34:511-522.
26. Cornely OA, Arikan-Akdagli S, Dannaoui E, et al. ESCMID and ECMM joint clinical guidelines for the diagnosis and management of mucormycosis 2013. *Clin Microbiol Infect*. 2014;20:5-26.
32. De Pauw B, Walsh TJ, Donnelly JP, et al. Revised definitions of invasive fungal disese from the European Organization for Research and Treatment of Cancer/Invasive Fungal Infections Cooperative Group and the National Institute of Allergy and Infectious Diseases Mycoses Study Group (EORTC/MSG) Consensus Group. *Clin Infect Dis*. 2008;46(12):1813-1821.
35. Dioverti MV, Cawcutt KA, Abidi M, et al. Gastrointestinal mucormycosis in immunocompromised hosts. *Mycoses*. 2015;58:714-718.
36. Dolatabadi S, Kolecka A, Versteeg M, et al. Differentiation of clinically relevant Mucorales *Rhizopus microsporus* and *R. arrhizus* by matrix-assisted laser desorption ionization time-of-flight mass spectrometry (MALDI-TOF MS). *J Med Microbiol*. 2015;64:694-701.
37. Dolatabadi S, Najafzadeh MJ, de Hoog GS. Rapid screening for human-pathogenic Mucorales using rolling circle amplification. *Mycoses*. 2014;57:67-72.
38. Drogari-Apiranthitou M, Panayiotides I, Galani I, et al. Diagnostic value of a semi-nested PCR for the diagnosis of mucormycosis and aspergillosis from paraffin-embedded tissue: A single center experience. *Pathol Res Pract*. 2016;212:393-397.
39. Duffy J, Harris J, Gade L, et al. Mucormycosis outbreak associated with hospital linens. *Pediatr Infect Dis J*. 2014;33:472-476.
42. El-Shabrawi MH, Kamal NM, Kaerger K, et al. Diagnosis of gastrointestinal basidiobolomycosis: A mini-review. *Mycoses*. 2014;57:138-143.
49. Gomes MZR, Lewis RE, Kontoyiannis DP. Mucormycosis caused by unusual mucormycetes, non-*Rhizopus*, -*Mucor*, and -*Lichtheimia* species. *Clin Microbiol Rev*. 2011;24:411-445.
50. Greenberg RN, Mullane K, van Burik JA, et al. Posaconazole as salvage therapy for zygomycosis. *Antimicrob Agents Chemother*. 2006;50(1):126-133.
51. Guarro J, Aguilar C, Pujol I. In-vitro antifungal susceptibilities of *Basidiobolus* and *Conidiobolus* spp. strains. *J Antimicrob Chemother*. 1999;44:557-560.
52. Hamid ME, Joseph MR, Al-Qahtani AS. Chronic rhinofacial basidiobolomycosis caused by *Basidiobolus ranarum*: Report of a case from Aseer Region, Kingdom of Saudi Arabia. *J Mycol Med*. 2015;25(4):306-309.
54. Hernandez MJ, Landaeta W, Salazar BN, et al. Subcutaneous zygomycosis due to *Conidiobolus incongruus*. *Int J Infect Dis*. 2007;11(5):468-470.
56. Hong H-L, Lee Y-M, Kim T, et al. Risk factors for mortality in patients with invasive mucormycosis. *Infect Chemother*. 2013;45:292-298.
66. Jung J, Kim MY, Lee HJ, et al. Comparison of computed tomographic findings in pulmonary mucormycosis and invasive pulmonary aspergillosis. *Clin Microbiol Infect*. 2015;21:684.e611-684.e618.
67. Jung J, Park YS, Sung H, et al. Using immunohistochemistry to assess the accuracy of histomorphologic diagnosis of aspergillosis and mucormycosis. *Clin Infect Dis*. 2015;61:1664-1670.
70. Kennedy KJ, Daveson K, Slavin MA, et al. Mucormycosis in Australia: contemporary epidemiology and outcomes. *Clin Microbiol Infect*. 2016;22(9):775-781.

72. Kontoyiannis DP, Azie N, Franks B, et al. Prospective antifungal therapy (PATH) alliance: Focus on mucormycosis. *Mycoses*. 2014;57:240-246.
75. Kontoyiannis DP, Marr KA, Park BJ, et al. Prospective surveillance for invasive fungal infections in hematopoietic stem cell transplant recipients, 2001-2006: overview of the Transplant-Associated Infection Surveillance Network (TRANSNET) Database. *Clin Infect Dis*. 2010;50:1091-1100.
82. Kyvernitakis A, Torres HA, Jiang Y, et al. Initial use of combination treatment does not impact survival of 106 patients with haematologic malignancies and mucormycosis: a propensity score analysis. *Clin Microbiol Infect*. 2016;22(9):811.e1-811.e8.
86. Langford S, Trubiano JA, Saxon S, et al. Mucormycete infection or colonisation: experience of an Australian tertiary referral centre. *Mycoses*. 2016;59:291-295.
88. Lanternier F, Poiree S, Elie C, et al. Prospective pilot study of high-dose (10 mg/kg/day) liposomal amphotericin B (L-AMB) for the initial treatment of mucormycosis. *J Antimicrob Chemother*. 2015;70:3116-3123.
92. Lelievre L, Garcia-Hermoso D, Abdoul H, et al. Posttraumatic mucormycosis: A nationwide study in France and review of the literature. *Medicine (Baltimore)*. 2014;93:395-404.
93. Lengerova M, Racil Z, Hrncirova K, et al. Rapid detection and identification of mucormycetes in bronchoalveolar lavage samples from immunocompromised patients with pulmonary infiltrates by use of high-resolution melt analysis. *J Clin Microbiol*. 2014;52:2824-2828.
94. Lewis RE, Albert ND, Ligo D, et al. Comparative pharmacodynamics of amphotericin B lipid complex and liposomal amphotericin B in a murine model of pulmonary mucormycosis. *Antimicrob Agents Chemother*. 2010;54:1298-1304.
95. Lewis RE, Georgiadou SP, Sampsonas F, et al. Risk factors for early mortality in haematological malignancy patients with pulmonary mucormycosis. *Mycoses*. 2014;57:49-55.
98. Luo G, Gebremariam T, Lee H, et al. Isavuconazole therapy protects immunosuppressed mice from mucormycosis. *Antimicrob Agents Chemother*. 2014;58:2450-2453.
103. Marty FM, Ostrosky-Zeichner L, Cornely OA, et al. Isavuconazole treatment for mucormycosis: a single-arm open-label trial and case-control analysis. *Lancet Infect Dis*. 2016;16(7):828-837.
107. Millon L, Herbrecht R, Grenouillet F, et al. Early diagnosis and monitoring of mucormycosis by detection of circulating DNA in serum: retrospective analysis of 44 cases collected through the French Surveillance Network of Invasive Fungal Infections (RESSIF). *Clin Microbiol Infect*. 2016;22(9):810.e1-810.e8.
108. Millon L, Larosa F, Lepiller Q, et al. Quantitative polymerase chain reaction detection of circulating DNA in serum for early diagnosis of mucormycosis in immunocompromised patients. *Clin Infect Dis*. 2013;56:e95-e101.
115. Neblett Fanfair R, Benedict K, Bos J, et al. Necrotizing cutaneous mucormycosis after a tornado in Joplin, Missouri, in 2011. *N Engl J Med*. 2012;367:2214-2225.
118. Pagano L, Cornely OA, Busca A, et al. Combined antifungal approach for the treatment of invasive mucormycosis in patients with hematologic diseases: A report from the SEIFEM and FUNGISCOPE registries. *Haematologica*. 2013;98:e127-e130.
120. Pandit V, Rhee P, Aziz H, et al. Perforated appendicitis with gastrointestinal basidiobolomycosis: a rare finding. *Surg Infect (Larchmt)*. 2014;15:339-342.
122. Payne SJ, Mitzner R, Kunchala S, et al. Acute invasive fungal rhinosinusitis: a 15-year experience with 41 patients. *Otolaryngol Head Neck Surg*. 2016;154:759-764.
128. Raveenthiran V, Mangayarkarasi V, Kousalya M, et al. Subcutaneous entomophthoromycosis mimicking soft-tissue sarcoma in children. *J Pediatr Surg*. 2015;50:1150-1155.
131. Riches ML, Trifilio S, Chen M, et al. Risk factors and impact of non-*Aspergillus* mold infections following allogeneic HCT: a CIBMTR infection and immune reconstitution analysis. *Bone Marrow Transplant*. 2016;51:277-282.
136. Roilides E. Isavuconazole: an azole active against mucormycosis. *Lancet Infect Dis*. 2016;16(7):761-762.
142. Shaikh N, Hussain KA, Petraitiene R, et al. Entomophthoramycosis: a neglected tropical mycosis. *Clin Microbiol Infect*. 2016;16(7):761-762.
144. Skiada A, Lanternier F, Groll AH, et al. Diagnosis and treatment of mucormycosis in patients with hematological malignancies: Guidelines from the 3rd European Conference on Infections in Leukemia (ECIL 3). *Haematologica*. 2013;98:492-504.
152. Trief D, Gray ST, Jakobiec FA, et al. Invasive fungal disease of the sinus and orbit: a comparison between mucormycosis and Aspergillus. *Br J Ophthalmol*. 2015;100(2):185-188.
155. Vallabhaneni S, Walker T, Lockhart S, et al. Fatal gastrointestinal mucormycosis in a premature infant associated with a contaminated dietary supplement—Connecticut, 2014. *Morb Mortal Wkly Rep*. 2015;64:155-156.
159. Vehreschild JJ, Birtel A, Vehreschild MJGT, et al. Mucormycosis treated with posaconazole: review of 96 case reports. *Crit Rev Microbiol*. 2012;39:310-324.
160. Vikram HR, Smilack JD, Leighton JA, et al. Emergence of gastrointestinal basidiobolomycosis in the United States, with a review of worldwide cases. *Clin Infect Dis*. 2012;54:1685-1691.
161. Vironneau P, Kania R, Morizot G, et al. Local control of rhino-orbito-cerebral mucormycosis dramatically impacts survival. *Clin Microbiol Infect*. 2014;20:O336-O339.
163. Wahba H, Truong MT, Lei X, et al. Reversed halo sign in invasive pulmonary fungal infections. *Clin Infect Dis*. 2008;46:1733-1737.
168. Walsh TJ, Skiada A, Cornely OA, et al. Development of new strategies for early diagnosis of mucormycosis: from bench to bedside. *Mycoses*. 2014;57:2-7.
170. Webb BJ, Blair JE, Kusne S, et al. Concurrent pulmonary *Aspergillus fumigatus* and *Mucor* infection in a cardiac transplant recipient: a case report. *Transplant Proc*. 2013;45(2):792-797.
176. Xhaard A, Lanternier F, Porcher R, et al. Mucormycosis after allogeneic haematopoietic stem cell transplantation: a French multicentre cohort study (2003-2008). *Clin Microbiol Infect*. 2012;18:e396-e400.
177. Zaoutis TE, Roilides E, Chiou CC, et al. Zygomycosis in children: a systematic review and analysis of reported cases. *Pediatr Infect Dis J*. 2007;26(8):723-727.

The full reference list for this chapter is available at ExpertConsult.com.

207 Fusariosis and Scedosporiosis

Damian J. Krysan • Melanie Wellington • William J. Steinbach

Fusarium and *Scedosporium* are species of molds that cause hyalohyphomycosis. Hyalohyphomycoses, although not as common as invasive aspergillosis or mucormycosis, are invasive fungal infections caused by nondematiaceous molds that lack cell wall melanin and thus are nonpigmented, in contrast to phaeohyphomycoses, which are fungal infections caused by pigmented molds. In profoundly immunocompromised patients, fusariosis and scedosporiosis are increasing in prevalence and are associated with high mortality. Recent guidelines on the diagnosis and management of invasive mold infections in immunocompromised hosts have included sections on *Fusarium* and *Scedosporium*,[5,47,73] and the first clinical practice guideline focused on management of *Fusarium* and *Scedosporium* disease was published in 2014.[73]

INFECTIONS CAUSED BY *FUSARIUM* SPECIES

Microbiology and Pathogenesis of Infection

Molds of the *Fusarium* genus are saprophytic environmental fungi that are well recognized as plant pathogens and, increasingly, as the cause of human infections.[18,51,54] *Fusarium* species are among the organisms that cause hyalohyphomycosis by virtue of their characteristic tissue form consisting of hyaline-like branching or nonbranching hyphal elements.[18] The most common clinical *Fusarium* isolates include *Fusarium solani* (50%), *Fusarium oxysporum* (20%), *Fusarium moniliforme* (10%), and *Fusarium verticillioidis* (10%).[18,51,54] In immunocompetent patients, *Fusarium* is the most common cause of fungal keratitis; *F. oxysporum* is the predominant organism.[18,51,54,78] Keratitis can progress to endophthalmitis, but this is more common in immunocompromised patients.[54] In addition, *Fusarium* is an important cause of onychomycosis.[52] Invasive fusarial disease can develop in immunocompetent patients who have had tissue breakdown due to trauma or burns[53] and in patients who have indwelling catheters, such as for vascular access, hemodialysis, or peritoneal dialysis.[21] Among immunocompromised patients, *Fusarium* is an emerging cause of infection[55]; *Fusarium* species are now the third most common cause of mold infections in hematopoietic stem cell and solid organ transplant recipients after *Aspergillus* and Mucorales.[30,46,58]

A limited set of case series describing invasive mold infections in children provides insights into the epidemiology of pediatric fusariosis. First, a prospective international study of invasive mold infections in children by the International Pediatric Fungal Network (IPFN) between 2007 and 2011 identified 4 children with invasive fusariosis among 131 total cases of invasive mold infection.[77] Second, Schwartz and colleagues reported a 15-year experience of invasive fusariosis at a single center that included five cases over that period.[66] Finally, an outbreak of fusariosis occurred in a children's cancer hospital in Brazil.[36] Over a 16-month period, a total of 10 confirmed cases of invasive fusariosis were identified; in the 5-year period before the outbreak period, no cases had been observed. The source of the outbreak was thought to be the water system, and instillation of 0.2-μm filters seemed to lead to resolution, although the last case occurred nearly 1 year after the instillation.

The portal of entry for most cases of disseminated *Fusarium* infections is the respiratory tract, but access to the patient may also be gained through vascular catheters.[1,7,20,51,55] *Fusarium* species have a propensity for vascular invasion, resulting in thrombosis and tissue necrosis, as well as for dissemination to extrapulmonary tissues.[53] One of the characteristics of *Fusarium* infections compared with other molds such as *Aspergillus* is that there is a high rate of fungemia. Many isolates of *Fusarium* species are capable of producing a yeast-like synanamorph when the microconidia enlarge; then, instead of germinating to form hyphae, these give rise directly to unicellular propagules, called adventitious sporulation (Fig. 207.1). This leads to a rapid dissemination and could explain the higher rate of positive blood cultures compared with other molds, such as *Aspergillus* species.[7] Another explanation for the high rate of positive blood cultures is the potential ability of *Fusarium* organisms to sporulate by forming phialides and phialoconidia within the human body.[65]

Risk Factors and Clinical Syndromes

One of the most common fusarial infections of immunocompetent patients is keratitis.[18,54,78] Indeed, fungal keratitis is one of the most important causes of monocular vision loss worldwide. *Fusarium* species are the dominant causative agent of fungal keratitis in tropical regions, whereas yeast are more common in temperate regions. In addition, an outbreak of fusarial keratitis occurred in 2006 in contact lens wearers[13,29] in association with a specific contact lens solution (ReNu with MoistureLoc) and resolved after the product was voluntarily removed from the market. Onychomycosis is a second common manifestation of fusarial infection in immunocompetent hosts and typically results from environmental contamination of the great toenail, presenting as proximal subungual onychomycosis.[74]

In immunocompromised patients, invasive fusariosis shares many characteristics with invasive aspergillosis, including the risk factors of neutropenia and corticosteroid exposure, which results in a similar bimodal distribution (before and after engraftment) in hematopoietic stem cell transplant recipients.[7,54,55] Among allogeneic hematopoietic stem cell transplant recipients with fusariosis, other risk factors identified in multivariate models include severe graft-versus-host disease and an underlying diagnosis of multiple myeloma.[43,54,55]

The incidence of fusariosis appears to be affected by both geography and season. A multicenter retrospective study found that fusariosis occurred more frequently in the summer and autumn months than in the winter and spring months. The infections were more likely to occur during the rainy season, which was thought to be due to the dispersal of the soil-borne fungi by the rain and wind.[51] As discussed earlier, increasing numbers of reports have suggested that this organism may also be acquired through hospital water supplies.[1]

Invasive fusariosis in hematopoietic stem cell transplant recipients most frequently is manifested as invasive pulmonary disease, with dissemination to the extrapulmonary organs in as many as 70% of cases.[43] Widespread skin lesions occur in approximately 70% of cases (Fig. 207.2), in sharp contrast to invasive *Aspergillus,* which has skin manifestations in less than 5% of cases.[53] Cutaneous lesions may take several forms, including painful, discrete, erythematous nodules; raised keratotic masses; and violaceous papules and nodules that break down to form black necrotic centers.[53] Although these skin lesions are typically larger, more erythematous, and more painful than those caused by *Aspergillus* species, the appearance is not specific for fusariosis. Other filamentous fungi, such as *Acremonium* and *Alternaria* species, can cause

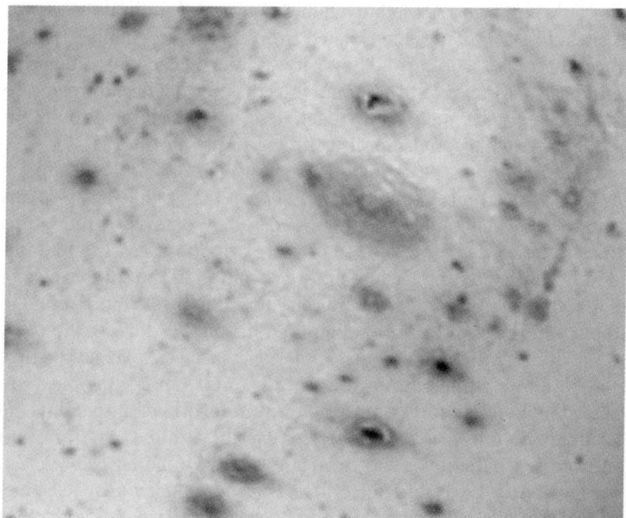

FIG. 207.1 Characteristic cutaneous lesions of disseminated fusariosis. (Courtesy Dr. John Perfect, Duke University.)

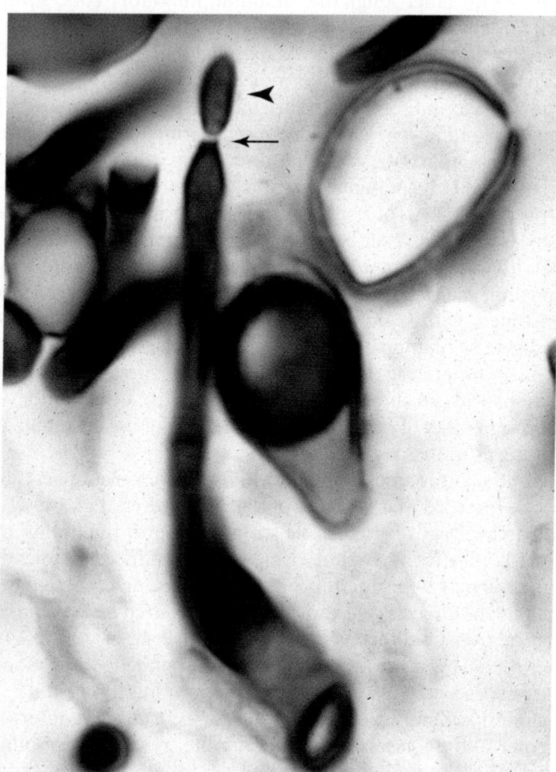

FIG. 207.2 Silver stain of a knee biopsy specimen from a patient with disseminated fusariosis showing adventitious sporulation. The *arrow* points to the phialide, and the *arrowhead* points to the released conidium. (Courtesy Wiley Schell, Duke University.)

similar skin lesions, in which the characteristic yeast-like structures are noted on histopathologic examination. However, culture of skin lesions was the most important basis for the diagnosis of fusariosis in a series of immunocompromised patients[53]; therefore, in this population of patients, biopsy specimens of all skin lesions should be taken and evaluated by both fungal culture and histology.

Localized cutaneous infections can also occur in immunocompromised patients; the most common manifestations are onychomycoses and cellulitis. Because localized infections may progress to involve cellulitis and may lead to disseminated infection, *Fusarium* isolated in nail cultures should not be dismissed as a contaminant in an immunocompromised patient.[3,7,51]

Diagnosis and Therapy

The clinical presentation of fusariosis has no features that reliably distinguish it from other invasive fungal infections. In addition, no specific diagnostic methods exist for fusariosis except for histopathology and the microbiologic examination of blood, sputum, and biopsy tissues. Major clues to *Fusarium* infections include blood cultures positive for mold and the presence of the characteristic skin lesions. In contrast to aspergillosis, *Fusarium* species are isolated from the bloodstream in approximately 50% of patients.[53] Non–culture-based methods have been developed for the diagnosis of invasive fungal disease by the detection of galactomannan and (1→3)-β-D-glucan in the serum.[34,56] Like most other fungi, *Fusarium* species are generally positive in the (1→3)-β-D-glucan assay.[56] Some *Fusarium* species have been reported to contain galactomannan in vitro, and a limited case series found that nine of 11 patients with fusariosis had positive galactomannan assays.[45,72]

In general, *Fusarium* species are relatively resistant to most clinically used antifungal agents on the basis of in vitro studies. Among currently available agents, voriconazole and amphotericin B are the most active.[54] Keratitis is typically treated with topical natamycin. Although initial studies of topical voriconazole indicated that it may be an alternative, a large clinical trial found that it is inferior to natamycin for the treatment of fungal keratitis largely owing to its reduced efficacy against *Fusarium*.[80] Echinocandins have very little in vitro activity against *Fusarium*.[76] Compared with other fungi, the minimum inhibitory concentrations (MICs) for amphotericin B–based agents are high (0.5–8 μg/mL); accordingly, animal studies indicate minimal therapeutic responses to lower doses of amphotericin B formulations.[23,39]

Reports have indicated that voriconazole and posaconazole have good in vitro and in vivo activity against experimental *Fusarium* infections.[23,39] Currently, both voriconazole and posaconazole are licensed by the Food and Drug Administration for salvage treatment of fusariosis.[48] A retrospective analysis of 73 cases of fusariosis treated with voriconazole suggested that voriconazole has efficacy that is comparable to the historical response rate reported for patients treated with amphotericin B.[38] Combination drug studies have also been reported, with in vitro synergy demonstrated with a combination of amphotericin B and either 5-flucytosine or rifampin.[68] Similarly, the combination of amphotericin B and caspofungin has been shown to yield synergistic or additive interactions with no antagonism observed in vitro.[37] In addition, there have been a number of case reports of the successful use of combinations of antifungals in the treatment of patients.[37]

High-dose intravenous amphotericin B lipid formulation has historically been regarded as a first-line option.[48] However, the case series of patients treated with voriconazole strongly support the notion that it is at least as effective as amphotericin B, and given its better tolerability, voriconazole may be a superior choice.[38] The first dedicated guidelines for hyalohyphomycosis give voriconazole a preferred treatment recommendation over lipid formulation amphotericin B.[73]

Neutropenia is a prime risk factor for disseminated infection, and without the recovery of neutrophils, *Fusarium* infection is fatal.[50,55] A large clinical review, which included 43 cases of invasive fusariosis at one center and 54 cases from the literature, reported a response to therapy of 30% and 48%, respectively. Cure was observed only in those patients showing resolution of myelosuppression.[7] This is further emphasized by the fact that the only pediatric patient who survived as reported in the Schwartz case series was a girl whose neutropenia resolved.[66] Attention to immune reconstitution is critical; granulocyte transfusions and the administration of colony-stimulating growth factors should be considered in all patients who are persistently neutropenic. Another review of fusariosis that was diagnosed among hematopoietic stem cell transplant recipients in nine centers in the United States and Brazil found that the survival rate after diagnosis was only 13%, with a median duration of 13 days.[55] The mortality rates from the pediatric series and the outbreak were 80% and 50%, respectively.[66,77]

In summary, invasive fusariosis can be extremely difficult to diagnose and treat. In the immunocompromised patient, the clinical presentation often mimics invasive aspergillosis, but it has some unique features. Because standard doses of amphotericin B do not appear to be consistently effective, voriconazole has emerged as an attractive option for the treatment of fusariosis. Similar to invasive aspergillosis, the attention to the recovery of neutrophils is paramount, and control of the underlying disease is essential to a favorable outcome. Surgery may decrease the fungal burden and may provide time for the recovery of immune function.[40] Because of the ability of *Fusarium* organisms to attach to and to degrade plastics, removal of infected catheters and prosthetic devices is, as always, strongly recommended.

INFECTIONS CAUSED BY *SCEDOSPORIUM* SPECIES

Microbiology and Pathogenesis

Scedosporium is a taxonomically complex genus, of which the three most medically significant species are *Scedosporium prolificans*, *Scedosporium auranticum*, and *Scedosporium apiospermum*.[16,31] Until recently, the anamorph (asexual stage) and teleomorph (sexual stage) forms of these fungi bore different names. For example, *S. apiospermum* is the anamorph, or asexual stage, of *Pseudallescheria boydii*. This dual naming system arose because the majority of fungi were initially identified based on their microscopic morphology, which is a function of the stage of the organism. With the advent of genetic analyses of the medically important fungi, the dual naming system became unnecessary. A series of nomenclature symposia were held to develop guidelines for a "one fungus, one name" system.[63] Currently, fungal nomenclature remains in transition, but the *Scedosporium* genus name is preferred for most of the organisms in this family. The taxonomy of *S. prolificans* remains a debate; this organism is also referred to by the synonymous names *Lomentospora prolificans* and *Lomentospora auranticum*. Some authors have begun to refer to all or some of this group of pathogens as the *Scedosporium/Lomentospora* complex, a designation that may serve to decrease nomenclature confusion.[14,81] However, care must be taken when grouping these organisms because the *Scedosporium* species differ significantly in their antifungal susceptibility.[32]

Scedosporium species are ubiquitous fungi recovered worldwide from polluted water, soil, and poultry and cattle manure.[16,24,28,31,42,64,71,79] This genus has morphologic characteristics of both hyaline and dematiaceous molds.[16] *S. prolificans* is a relatively new species of mold that was first described in 1984 after being isolated from a deep, subcutaneous lesion in the right foot of a 6-year-old boy[16]; it was initially named *Scedosporium inflatum*.[11,28,64] More recently, human infections involving a third species, *Scedosporium aurantiacum*, have been described in a large population-based survey of *Scedosporium* infections in Australia.[24]

S. apiospermum appears to be more prevalent in temperate climates compared with tropical regions.[16] *S. prolificans* has mainly been isolated in the Iberian peninsula, Australia, and in some areas of the United States. In the United States, for example, *S. prolificans*–associated bone and joint infections appear to be more common in the southern states and in California.[26] *S. prolificans* was also found to be the most abundant pathogen in the soils of potted plants in hospitals.[69]

Like other pathogenic molds, *Scedosporium* species cause disease in both immunocompetent and immunocompromised people, with localized infections most common in immunocompetent patients and disseminated infections almost exclusively limited to immunocompromised patients.[16] The first case of disseminated *S. prolificans* was reported in 1991, and since that time, *Scedosporium* species have emerged as the fourth most common cause of invasive mold infections in transplant recipients after *Aspergillus*, Mucorales, and *Fusarium*.[42,58] The mortality rates associated with disseminated *Scedosporium* infections in immunocompromised patients are extremely high, ranging between 58% and 100% in reported case series.[4,25,33,41,57-59]

The respiratory tract appears to be the portal of entry for disseminated infection in most cases, although the organism can also invade through ulcerative lesions in the gastrointestinal tract, through surgical wounds, or by inoculation from trauma.[16] In localized infection, the most common mechanism seems to be direct inoculation of wounds by organisms in the environment.[16,64] Germination into hyphae can result in hematogenous dissemination to other organs, particularly the kidneys, lungs, and brain. In the tissue, *Scedosporium* species form slender, septate hyphae with parallel cell walls that cannot reliably be distinguished from other molds, such as *Aspergillus* or *Fusarium* species, unless conidia are present.[16,39,42]

Risk Factors and Clinical Syndromes

In immunocompetent patients, *S. boydii* is an important cause of mycetoma, a clinical syndrome characterized by infection of soft and connective tissue, joints, and bone by soil-borne fungi.[44] *S. boydii* has been estimated to cause approximately 10% of mycetoma worldwide.[16] Case series in the United States and Brazil found that *S. boydii* is the most common cause of fungal mycetoma in these regions.[22,62] Mycetoma displays a characteristic triad of symptoms: tumefaction or edematous tissue; draining sinus track formation; and presence of "grains" (balls of fungal hyphae) in pus.[16] Although localized nonmycetomatous infections involving a wide range of anatomic sites in immunocompetent patients have been reported (Fig. 207.3), they are uncommon.[16]

An important clinical manifestation of *S. boydii* disease in immunocompetent patients is its association with sinopulmonary and central nervous system infection of victims of near-drowning incidents in polluted waters.[9,16] The syndrome affects previously healthy individuals and generally is manifested within days to weeks of the incident, although presentation has been delayed up to nearly 5 months.[16] Dissemination from the lungs to a range of anatomic sites has been reported, but the syndrome is most commonly characterized by the formation of brain abscesses.[9,19] Although *S. boydii* is the most common mold associated with near-drowning–related infections, *Aspergillus* can also cause a similar syndrome[33]; in contrast, *S. prolificans* has not been associated with near-drowning.[16,35] Unfortunately, near-drowning–associated *S. boydii* infections carry a very poor prognosis, with mortality rates higher than 70%.[16]

Consistent with the respiratory tract being the most common portal of entry, *Scedosporium* species also appear to be transient colonizers of the sinopulmonary tract. A model for the host-pathogen interaction in pulmonary scedosporiosis was proposed by Cortez and associates, in which transient colonization occurs that in the setting of a normal respiratory tract is clinically insignificant.[16] If the pulmonary tract has been altered by the presence of a fixed cavity, damage due to tuberculosis, or cystic fibrosis, persistent colonization can result.[6] The first report of this occurrence was in 1955 and involved a patient with a previous pyogenic abscess that was subsequently colonized by *S. Boydii*.[17] *S. apiospermum* appears to be a relatively common component of respiratory cultures isolated from patients with cystic fibrosis.[15,81] Although a case report has described the possible cerebral dissemination of *S. apiospermum* in a patient with cystic fibrosis, the clinical significance of this colonization is not entirely clear.[61,62] As with *Aspergillus*, persistent colonization of dysfunctional airways with *Scedosporium* species could trigger a syndrome similar to allergic bronchopulmonary aspergillosis; in fact, one multivariate analysis found that patients with cystic fibrosis who are colonized with *S. apiospermum* may have a higher risk for allergic bronchopulmonary disease (odds ratio, 13) than those colonized with *Aspergillus fumigatus* (odds ratio, 1.6).[60] However, the presence of molds such as *Scedosporium* species may be more relevant as more cystic fibrosis patients undergo lung transplantation, as illustrated by a case report describing the death of such a patient from disseminated *S. apiospermum* infection after double-lung transplantation.[70] This report emphasizes the notion that colonization of the airway can lead to dissemination when the immune status of the patient is altered.

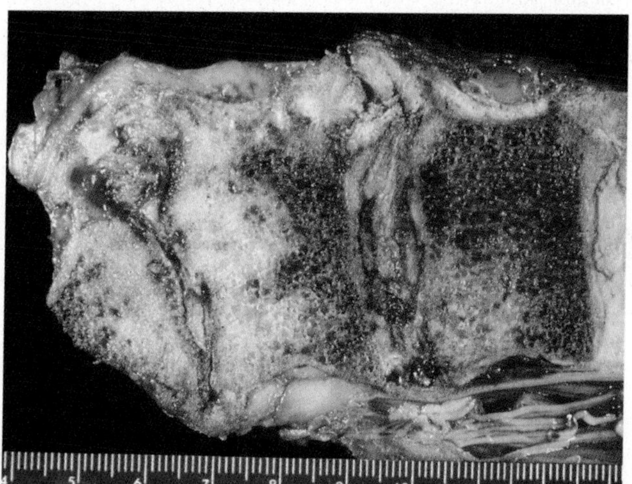

FIG. 207.3 Pathology specimen from a patient with lumbar vertebral *Scedosporium apiospermum* infection. (Courtesy Wiley Schell, Duke University.)

The role of *Scedosporium* species in mold infections of immunocompromised patients has become more apparent as an increasing number of case series and large multicenter surveillance data have become available.[4,16,24-26,31,33,57,58,67,79] *Scedosporium* is among the four most commonly isolated molds associated with invasive disease in immunocompromised patients. The rate of disseminated disease in one study was 69% for hematopoietic stem cell transplant recipients and 53% for solid-organ transplant recipients.[25] Risk factors and clinical manifestations parallel those caused by other filamentous molds, such as *Aspergillus* and *Fusarium* species.[4,16,24-26,33,57,58,67,79] Prognosis is similarly poor; for example, a large multicenter case series of infections involving transplant recipients found that the overall mortality rate was 58%.[25]

In general, although *Scedosporium* infection is often clinically and radiographically indistinguishable from other filamentous fungi infections in neutropenic patients, several unique, salient features are present that reflect a large amount of fungal replication in vivo. These include a high incidence of positive blood cultures, characteristic although not pathognomonic erythematous cutaneous lesions, frequent hematogenous spread to the central nervous system, and a high incidence of visual complaints because of endophthalmitis.[4,16,24-26,33,41,57-59,67,79]

Diagnosis and Therapy

Histologic findings are insufficient to distinguish *Scedosporium* from other filamentous fungi, such as the *Aspergillus* species. However, scedosporiosis is frequently characterized by a high frequency of positive blood cultures. In fact, from 1990 to 1999, *S. prolificans* was the most common filamentous fungus isolated from blood culture at one hospital in Spain.[26] In another report, 12 of 16 patients with *Scedosporium* infections had growth in blood culture, four of 16 had growth in respiratory tract specimens, and three of 16 had growth in skin biopsy specimens.[4] No specific studies evaluating β-glucan or galactomannan assays in the setting of proven *Scedosporium* infections have been reported, so the utility of these methods in detecting this species of mold is unclear.

Scedosporium species have low in vitro susceptibility to currently available antifungal drugs, a fact that certainly contributes to the dismal outcomes associated with these infections. The excellent review by Cortez and associates presented a large set of susceptibility data from a variety of isolates.[16] In general, *S. apiospermum* appears more susceptible than *S. prolificans*; the median MIC among *S. prolificans* isolates is above 8 μg/mL for most antifungals; of these, voriconazole is the most active agent. The agent most active against *S. apiospermum* is also voriconazole (median MIC_{50} of 0.25 μg/mL), whereas amphotericin B has poor activity with an MIC_{50} of 4 μg/mL.[16] As with other molds, a number of studies have examined the activity of combinations of antifungal drugs, but none yielded particularly encouraging results.[38] The in vitro activity of the newly approved antifungal drug isavuconazole, as well as several azoles currently under development (albaconazole[10] and ravuconazole) against *Scedosporium* species, has been reported.[11,49] Of these agents, albaconazole is the most active, with geometric mean MICs toward *S. prolificans* and *S. apiospermum* of 0.35 μg/mL and 1.0 μg/mL, respectively.[11] Encouragingly, albaconazole has been shown to have efficacy superior to that of amphotericin B in a rabbit model of disseminated *S. prolificans* infection.[10]

A case series describing the treatment of scedosporiosis with voriconazole collated from the global voriconazole clinical trials database suggested that voriconazole has promising activity against both *S. apiospermum* and *S. prolificans.*[75] In this uncontrolled observational series, an overall response to therapy rate was 57%, and the overall mortality rate was 40%. Although it is difficult to make conclusions from this study, these rates are much better than those reported in previous case series.[4,16,24-26,33,41,57-59,79] This case series also demonstrated that the difference in in vitro susceptibility of *S. apiospermum* and *S. prolificans* to voriconazole is clinically relevant; patients with *S. apiospermum* had higher survival rates than those with *S. prolificans*.

Because of the resistance of this fungus to antifungal drugs, immune function and surgical intervention play critical roles. The prognosis is particularly grim for patients with persistent neutropenia. For example, a case series of 16 patients with *S. prolificans* infections revealed that all patients who failed to recover neutrophils died.[4] Anecdotal reports of success have been noted with the adjunctive use of granulocyte colony-stimulating factor and interferon-γ.[8,27] These immunomodulation-based approaches are similar to those applied to other mold infections, but to date, none has progressed to the state at which it can be routinely recommended.[2] Surgical resection, combined with systemic antifungal therapy, should be pursued when feasible and was reported to be successful for a near-drowning victim.[12]

In summary, *Scedosporium* infections are difficult to treat and frequently occur in the immunocompromised host. The standard of care for localized infections in an immunocompetent host is surgical excision whenever possible, particularly because these organisms are highly resistant to antifungal therapy. In the immunocompromised host, in whom disseminated disease renders this approach useless, *Scedosporium* infections are generally rapidly fatal unless immune reconstitution occurs. Voriconazole appears to be the most active antifungal drug in this setting and should be considered the agent of choice. The current treatment guidelines on *Scedosporium* infections stress that there are not sufficient data to recommend specific therapies.[5,47,73] Nevertheless, given the dismal prognosis of the disease, treatment guidelines moderately consider combination therapy with voriconazole and terbinafine, based on in vitro data and case reports of patients who had good outcomes while on this regimen. It remains to be seen whether or not such combination therapy has a significant clinical impact on *Scedosporium* disease.

NEW REFERENCES IN THE SEVENTH EDITION

5. Blyth CC, Gilroy NM, Guy SD, et al. Consensus guidelines for the treatment of invasive mould infections in haematological malignancy and haemopoietic stem cell transplantation, 2014. *Intern Med J*. 2014;44(12b):1333-1349.
14. Chen M, Zeng J, De Hoog GS, et al. The "species complex" issue in clinically relevant fungi: a case study in *Scedosporium apiospermum*. *Fungal biology*. 2016;120(2):137-146.
15. Cimon B, Carrere J, Vinatier JF, et al. Clinical significance of *Scedosporium apiospermum* in patients with cystic fibrosis. *Eur J Clin Microbiol Infect Dis*. 2000;19(1):53-56.
28. Jeanmart L, Vollont GH, Hennebert A, et al. [Atypical bronchopulmonary aspergillosis]. *J Belge Radiol*. 1974;57(3):193-200.
30. Klingspor L, Saaedi B, Ljungman P, et al. Epidemiology and outcomes of patients with invasive mould infections: a retrospective observational study from a single centre (2005–2009). *Mycoses*. 2015;58(8):470-477.
32. Lackner M, de Hoog GS, Verweij PE, et al. Species-specific antifungal susceptibility patterns of *Scedosporium* and *Pseudallescheria* species. *Antimicrob Agents Chemother*. 2012;56(5):2635-2642.
33. Lamaris GA, Chamilos G, Lewis RE, et al. *Scedosporium* infection in a tertiary care cancer center: a review of 25 cases from 1989-2006. *Clin Infect Dis*. 2006;43(12):1580-1584.
36. Litvinov N, da Silva MT, van der Heijden IM, et al. An outbreak of invasive fusariosis in a children's cancer hospital. *Clin Microbiol Infect*. 2015;21(3):268.e1-268.e7.
46. Montagna MT, Lovero G, Coretti C, et al. SIMIFF study: Italian fungal registry of mold infections in hematological and non-hematological patients. *Infection*. 2014;42(1):141-151.
47. Mousset S, Buchheidt D, Heinz W, et al. Treatment of invasive fungal infections in cancer patients-updated recommendations of the Infectious Diseases Working Party (AGIHO) of the German Society of Hematology and Oncology (DGHO). *Ann Hematol*. 2014;93(1):13-32.
49. Munoz P, Guinea J, Bouza E. Treatment options in emerging mold infections. *Curr Infect Dis Rep*. 2008;10(6):473-479.
60. Paugam A, Baixench MT, Demazes-Dufeu N, et al. Characteristics and consequences of airway colonization by filamentous fungi in 201 adult patients with cystic fibrosis in France. *Med Mycol*. 2010;48(suppl 1):S32-S36.
63. Redhead SA, Demoulin V, Hawksworth DL, et al. Fungal Nomenclature at IMC10: Report of the Nomenclature Sessions. *IMA Fungus*. 2014;5(2):449-462.
64. Restrepo A, McGinnis MR, Malloch D, et al. Fungal endocarditis caused by *Arnium leporinum* following cardiac surgery. *Sabouraudia*. 1984;22(3):225-234.
66. Schwartz KL, Sheffield H, Richardson SE, et al. Invasive Fusariosis: A Single Pediatric Center 15-Year Experience. *J Pediatric Infect Dis Soc*. 2015;4(2):163-170.
67. Slavin M, van Hal S, Sorrell TC, et al. Invasive infections due to filamentous fungi other than *Aspergillus:* epidemiology and determinants of mortality. *Clin Microbiol Infect*. 2015;21(5):490.e1-490.e10.
68. Spader TB, Venturini TP, Cavalheiro AS, et al. In vitro interactions between amphotericin B and other antifungal agents and rifampin against *Fusarium* spp. *Mycoses*. 2011;54(2):131-136.
70. Symoens F, Knoop C, Schrooyen M, et al. Disseminated *Scedosporium apiospermum* infection in a cystic fibrosis patient after double-lung transplantation. *J Heart Lung Transplant*. 2006;25(5):603-607.
72. Tortorano AM, Esposto MC, Prigitano A, et al. Cross-reactivity of *Fusarium* spp. in the *Aspergillus* galactomannan enzyme-linked immunosorbent assay. *J Clin Microbiol*. 2012;50(3):1051-1053.
73. Tortorano AM, Richardson M, Roilides E, et al. ESCMID and ECMM joint guidelines on diagnosis and management of hyalohyphomycosis: *Fusarium* spp., *Scedosporium* spp. and others. *Clin Microbiol Infect*. 2014;20(suppl 3):27-46.
77. Wattier RL, Dvorak CC, Hoffman JA, et al. A Prospective, International Cohort Study of Invasive Mold Infections in Children. *J Pediatric Infect Dis Soc*. 2015;4(4):313-322.
80. Yadav MK, Babu BK, Saxena AK, et al. Real-time PCR assay based on topoisomerase-II gene for detection of *Fusarium udum*. *Mycopathologia*. 2011;171(5):373-381.
81. Ziesing S, Suerbaum S, Sedlacek L. Fungal epidemiology and diversity in cystic fibrosis patients over a 5-year period in a national reference center. *Med Mycol*. 2016;54(8):781-786.

The full reference list for this chapter is available at ExpertConsult.com.

208 Miscellaneous Mycoses

William J. Steinbach

The landscape of medical mycology is changing. Less common fungi that were once innocent or only contaminants are now emerging to lead to lethal disseminated disease in immunocompromised patients. While we are only beginning to learn about the full implications of some of these fungi, there is also the realization that nearly all of the current therapeutic evaluations in these emerging pathogens are in vitro analyses with limited case report clinical experience. Every miscellaneous mycosis and fungal opportunist cannot be listed, and the field of taxonomy is dynamic with genera always shifting. The field is filled with continued reports of previously nonpathogenic fungi now infecting severely immunocompromised patients. This chapter will highlight the most relevant miscellaneous fungi causing disease. Often these diseases can be classified as infection through trauma or inoculation, such as keratitis, mycetoma, or soft tissue infection, or as more invasive disease such as sinusitis, pneumonia, cerebral abscess, or disseminated infection.

YEASTS

Malassezia Species

There are 14 *Malassezia* species that have been isolated from normal and diseased human and animal skin, and *Malassezia furfur* is the most common species. Most microbiologists identify *Malassezia* as the "spaghetti and meatball" yeast that causes the prototypical recurrent skin disease tinea versicolor (also known as pityriasis versicolor), characterized by hypopigmented or hyperpigmented plaques covered in scales and generally distributed over the back, chest, and neck. Evidence also suggests that seborrheic dermatitis, a frequently relapsing skin disorder characterized by greasy, scaly, reddish patches, results from a nonspecific immune response to *Malassezia* yeasts; dandruff is linked to this yeast, and research continues on the role of this yeast in atopic eczema and psoriasis. *Malassezia* is also responsible for folliculitis in patients with underlying immunosuppression (including diabetes mellitus, transplantation, and malignancy) and intravascular catheter-related sepsis in immunocompromised patients, particularly neonates, receiving parenteral fat emulsions for nutrition.

Most invasive disease is caused by either *M. furfur* or *M. pachydermatis*. *M. furfur* is a lipophilic yeast that lacks the ability to synthesize long-chain fatty acids and requires an exogenous supply of lipids for growth, growing in culture only if C12 through C24 fatty acids are added to the medium. Most of the lipids in parenteral intralipid formulations are C16 and C18 fatty acids, chiefly linoleic acid, and oleic acid.[51] This absolute requirement for long-chain fatty acids leads to specific procedures required for isolation and identification. Although *M. furfur* is obligatory lipophilic, the other major species, *M. pachydermatis*, does not require lipids for growth and is the only of the 14 *Malassezia* species that is not dependent on lipid for growth.[5] *M. pachydermatis* is a zoophilic yeast associated with otitis externa and seborrheic dermatitis in dogs and is only occasionally isolated from human skin, but it has been implicated in invasive neonatal infection.[77] One outbreak of *M. pachydermatis* was associated with the colonized dogs of health care workers.[9]

The first invasive disease reported with *Malassezia* species was in a patient with chronic renal failure treated with peritoneal dialysis who had repeated episodes of "sterile" peritonitis, with high levels of cholesterol and triglyceride found in the peritoneal fluid after meals, thought to have originated from the small intestinal lymphatics. The yeast did not grow in culture until the agar was overlaid with olive oil.[84] Neonatal systemic *Malassezia* disease was first reported in 1981 in a 740-gram premature infant on long-term intralipid therapy through an indwelling central venous catheter.[60]

Lipophilic *Malassezia* species infections (such as *M. furfur*) can be divided in two major groups: the first comprising children and adults with various forms of immunosuppression, and the second involving infants on parenteral nutrition. Most published case reports and mini-epidemics have involved infants, children, and adults with profound immunosuppression, serious concurrent health problems, and the infusion of total parenteral nutrition with lipid supplementation through central vascular catheters.[25] There have been numerous outbreaks in neonates involving *M. furfur*, and fewer outbreaks involving *M. pachydermatis*. A review of 55 neonates infected with *Malassezia* species found that prematurity was the most common underlying condition, followed by short-gut syndrome, but that all infected infants were receiving intralipid supplementation.[42]

A study of the prevalence of *M. furfur* skin colonization of infants hospitalized in the intensive care unit found that of the 361 infants studied over 1 year, 133 (36.8%) had at least one positive culture for *M. furfur*. Colonized infants, compared with noncolonized infants, had younger mean gestational age, lower mean birth weight, a longer stay in the hospital, and more mean days' use of an incubator, lamb's wool, paper tape, and Op-Site tape, suggesting that hospitalization in an intensive care unit often leads to *M. furfur* colonization.[58] Another study reported isolation of *M. furfur* in 41% of critically ill newborns in the neonatal intensive care unit (NICU), whereas only 10% of hospitalized newborns in nonintensive care settings were colonized.[7] Another study reported colonization in 28% of infants in an NICU in the first week of life, but this increased to 84% in older infants.[6]

The use of intravenous fat emulsions appears to alter the microenvironment of the catheter and allows colonization and subsequent infection. Dissemination of the organism appears to be limited to the lungs, which at autopsy show lipid deposits in the arterial walls. Because of the serious underlying diseases of patients with *M. furfur* catheter sepsis, it is difficult to determine the exact role of the organism in the overall status of the patients.[41] In an effort to determine whether intralipid contamination was the source of these outbreaks, an experimental study found that six blood culture isolates of *M. furfur* from infected patients grew well in both 10% and 20% parenteral fat emulsions at 35°C for 6 days. Room-temperature growth was much slower, but there was no loss of viability. The authors concluded that intralipid solution provided more optimal supplementation than vegetable oils.[57]

Clinical signs and symptoms of *Malassezia* fungemia and sepsis are nonspecific, including fever, respiratory distress, lethargy, hepatomegaly, splenomegaly, and others.[77] A review of 16 infants infected with *M. furfur* revealed that most presented with classical signs of sepsis, including apnea and bradycardia, and nine had radiographic evidence of interstitial pneumonitis to accompany worsening pulmonary status. Abnormal laboratory tests included leukocytosis, elevated neutrophil band counts, and thrombocytopenia. Blood cultures were most commonly positive from the central catheter, with few peripheral (noncatheter) blood cultures positive and few organisms found on those positive cultures.[41]

Clinicians must maintain a high index of suspicion of *M. furfur* catheter sepsis in the appropriate clinical setting (generally central venous catheter and intralipids in a premature infant or immunocompromised patient), and laboratory investigators must be prepared to provide appropriate diagnostic methods.[41] Culture of biologic fluids and biopsy specimens in selective medium, as well as an increased incubation time (10–15 days), would increase the rate of isolation of lipophilic *Malassezia* species. The blood of infants receiving lipid emulsions probably contains sufficient lipid to support initial growth of the organism, but would not be sufficient for routine identification. On subculturing, a few drops of olive oil placed on the agar surface will help in isolation.[41] Therefore the frequency of infection may actually be much higher than previously reported because routine blood cultures will not detect the fungus easily. Unfortunately, *Malassezia* polymerase chain reaction (PCR) testing appears not yet ready for general use.[77]

The diagnosis should not be overlooked when evaluating symptomatic, low-birth-weight, premature infants receiving total parenteral nutrition with lipid supplementation because simple removal of the catheter after the identification of the causative agent can lead to clinical improvement. In fungemia, prompt removal of the catheter, along with temporary discontinuation of the parental intralipid nutrition, is the key to therapy for *M. furfur* catheter sepsis. Most treatments in the literature focus on topical or systemic agents for the minor skin infection and not on disseminated disease.

In vitro antifungal susceptibility testing against *Malassezia* has not been standardized, and significant variation has been reported. One report of 95 *Malassezia* spp. isolates (including 74 *M. furfur* strains) revealed excellent antifungal activity with itraconazole, voriconazole, and ketoconazole, and limited activity with fluconazole.[47] There is a poor response to amphotericin B,[46] supported by the in vitro high minimum inhibitory concentration (MIC) values of this agent,[41] which is in contrast to European guidelines that suggest amphotericin B.[5] All reported studies show that the echinocandins and flucytosine have no appreciable activity against *Malassezia*, and therefore these drug classes are not recommended.[5] Catheter removal or discontinuance of the fat emulsion therapy is required, and antifungal therapy without either of these two steps has not been shown to be efficacious.

Trichosporon Species

Fungemia caused by *Trichosporon* species is increasing in patients with hematologic malignancies and neutropenia, and has been reported as the second most common yeast infection in cancer patients after *Candida* species.[36] One study showed that 10% of all fungemias at one institution were caused by *Trichosporon* spp.[36] *Trichosporon* spp. are able to colonize and proliferate in different parts of human body, including the gastrointestinal system, respiratory tract, skin, and vagina. More than 10% of people have been shown to be colonized by *Trichosporon* species on their normal perigenital skin (scrotal, perianal, and inguinal sites of the body).[12] The opportunistic *Trichosporon* spp. are therefore part of the cutaneous fungal microbiota in humans, and this cutaneous position may be one of the routes through which deep-seated trichosporonosis is acquired. *Trichosporon* spp. may cause deep-seated, mucosa-associated, or superficial infections, with invasive trichosporonosis documented in patients with hematologic malignancies and other immunosuppressive states, whereas superficial infections and allergic pneumonia are found predominantly in immunocompetent hosts.[12]

The taxonomy of *Trichosporon* has been revised several times and now includes 50 species. Most frequently reported species are *T. asahii* (formerly *T. beigelii* and *T. cutaneum*), *T. pullulans*, and *T. capitatum* (formerly *Blastoschizomyces capitatus*).[48] Culture identification of *Trichosporon* spp. may be difficult because it is often morphologically confused with *Candida* spp., which is worrisome because *Trichosporon* has decreased susceptibility to amphotericin B and is intrinsically resistant to echinocandins.

The clinical presentation of superficial *Trichosporon* infection in humans is often benign superficial lesions of hair, called white piedra, characterized by the presence of irregular nodules on the affected hair. These nodules are loosely attached to the hair shaft, have a soft texture, and may be white or light brown. White piedra is a disease affecting children and adults from areas with tropical and temperate climates, and most cases have been reported in children and young adults, particularly females who frequently use headbands.[12]

The first case of invasive trichosporonosis was described in 1970.[86] Clinically, the genus often causes catheter-related fungemia, but there are reports of endocarditis,[10] peritonitis,[39] meningitis,[2] and pneumonitis.[70] Infections with invasive *Trichosporon* spp. are usually associated with central venous catheters, bladder catheters, and peritoneal catheter–related devices. The ability to form biofilms on implanted devices aids in the development of invasive trichosporonosis because it can promote escape from antifungals and host immune responses. Similar to biofilms of *Candida* spp., *T. asahii* cells are able to rapidly adhere to polystyrene after a 30-minute incubation.[15]

Trichosporon was the third most commonly isolated (10.7%) non-*Candida* yeast from one global antifungal surveillance program and was the second most common cause of yeast fungemia (after *Candida*) in patients with hematologic malignancy.[46] A multicenter retrospective Italian study was conducted to characterize cases of proven or probable invasive trichosporonosis diagnosed over the past 20 years in patients with hematologic diseases. Of 17 cases classified as *Trichosporon* spp. infections, acute myeloid leukemia accounted for 65.4% of the cases, leading to an incidence of 0.4% of *Trichosporon* spp. in acute leukemia patients, including 76.9% of cases with a positive blood culture. Pulmonary involvement was documented in 26.9% of cases, and death was reported for 64.7% of *Trichosporon* spp. infections. A literature review on 287 published trichosporonosis cases with any underlying disease revealed that *Trichosporon* spp. infections are seen with similar frequencies on all continents. Most published *Trichosporon* spp. infections occurred in patients with hematologic diseases (62.8%), with more than half suffering from acute leukemia (68% of all patients with *Trichosporon* spp.). Crude mortality rates were 77% for *Trichosporon* spp.[28]

A worldwide review of 185 cases from 1975 to 2014[37] found that most patients had a history of hematologic malignancy (especially acute leukemia), as well as neutropenia and a central venous catheter. The most commonly isolated species was *T. asahii* (75%). Antifungal therapy for this invasive yeast has gravitated since the 1970s from amphotericin B to a triazole, most commonly voriconazole, and overall positive outcomes have increased.

The only published guideline on treating trichosporonosis recommends voriconazole as the preferred agent.[5] One study of 39 *Trichosporon* clinical isolates showed high MICs for amphotericin B, with fluconazole and itraconazole relatively lower. Posaconazole and voriconazole appeared to be more active than amphotericin B or fluconazole and similar to itraconazole. There were also potential fungicidal effects with the triazoles.[53] An in vitro study with eight *Trichosporon* spp. isolates showed that voriconazole was most effective, being slightly more active than itraconazole, amphotericin B, and fluconazole.[80] Another study showed that voriconazole had excellent activity, superior to amphotericin B, itraconazole, and fluconazole.[20] In vitro activity against several *Trichosporon* species showed that voriconazole was far superior to amphotericin B, fluconazole, and itraconazole. Notably, *T. pullulans* was generally more resistant to antifungals, including total resistance to amphotericin B and fluconazole.[45]

Trichosporon species have limited susceptibility to amphotericin B, and earlier clinical studies and animal models showed that azoles were effective therapy[3] and that azoles plus polyenes were potentially additive.[4] In one study, five of 12 reported cases occurred while the patient was receiving itraconazole prophylaxis, and 11 of the 12 patients died despite amphotericin B therapy.[36] The mortality rate of hematogenous trichosporonosis was higher than candidiasis in that study, confirmed by a review of the published literature since the 1990s showing that *Trichosporon* spp. mortality rates were 64% to 80%[36] and central venous catheters were the most frequent risk factor for fungemia. Girmenia and colleagues reported the clinical outcomes for 55 patients with hematologic diseases and disseminated trichosporonosis who were treated with amphotericin B. A clinical response to amphotericin B was documented in only 13 of 55 patients (24%) evaluated.[28]

A head-to-head comparison of various triazole antifungals against *T. asahii* found that no agents achieved fungicidal killing by time-kill studies, and the most active agents, in order, were voriconazole, itraconazole, posaconazole, isavuconazole, and fluconazole.[31] However, no worrisome reports have been made of pan-azole resistance in *Trichosporon*[52] or of biofilm formation at levels similar to *Candida* species, and therefore there is no evidence of development of resistance to many antifungal agents.[33]

Echinocandins alone have little to no activity against *Trichosporon* spp. and are not recommended for trichosporonosis treatment. In vitro studies against the formerly named species *T. beigelii* showed that the echinocandins caspofungin and anidulafungin had no activity.[19] This inactivity was validated in further studies with micafungin[75] and anidulafungin.[81] Invasive *T. beigelii* infection developed in a bone marrow transplant recipient who was receiving caspofungin prophylaxis against *Aspergillus* infection.[29] Indeed, breakthrough trichosporonosis in immunocompromised patients after administration of amphotericin B and echinocandins, and more rarely after the use of triazoles, has been extensively reported.[12]

Rhodotorula mucilaginosa

Rhodotorula mucilaginosa (formerly *Rhodotorula rubra*) is considered to be ubiquitous because of its worldwide distribution in terrestrial, freshwater, and marine habitats and its ability to colonize a large variety of substrates. *Rhodotorula* is naturally found in soil, water, and plants and is a constituent of the normal human respiratory, gastrointestinal, and genitourinary flora.[67] Previously this organism was only considered a harmless colonizer when isolated from healthy individuals, but it is now reported in immunocompromised patients causing fungemia, endocarditis, meningitis, and peritonitis.[35] This is also the fungus that is chiefly responsible for the pink ring left in toilet bowls. The genus *Rhodotorula* contains 46 species, of which *R. mucilaginosa*, *R. glutinis*, and *R. minuta* cause human disease.[87]

In review of all 43 reported cases from 1960 to 2000, the most common risk factor was central venous catheter insertion. It appears that the yeast is already an inhabitant of the skin and mucosa and is introduced into the bloodstream following a disruption of normal anatomic barriers. In contrast to *Trichosporon*, mortality with *Rhodotorula* is uncommon. In a review, 10 of 36 survivors of infection were not treated with antifungals and appeared to respond to removal of the infected catheter.[67] This yeast has a strong affinity for plastic,[1] and almost all published cases involve a catheter inserted over a long period of time. One single series reported 23 cases of fungemia; only two of the patients were neutropenic, and outcome was favorable in all using various treatment strategies of line removal alone, removal with amphotericin B, or antifungal therapy alone.[35]

A review of 29 cases of *Rhodotorula* fungemia in Spain found that the most common underlying hematologic disorder was acute leukemia (65.5%). *Rhodotorula mucilaginosa* was the species found more frequently (79.3%), and the most common predisposing factors were the presence of central venous catheter (100%) and neutropenia (62.1%). Most patients (81.5%) were treated with amphotericin B, and the overall mortality rate was higher (13.8%) than that described in nonhematologic patients (5.8% in solid-organ neoplasms and 9% in patients with AIDS or other chronic diseases). Patients with acute leukemia had a higher mortality rate (15.7%) than patients with non-Hodgkin lymphoma (0%).[27]

A review of 25 Brazilian cases of *Rhodotorula* spp. isolated from blood cultures found that most patients (88%) had a central venous catheter and 40% were bone marrow transplant recipients; 80% of cases were classified as a bloodstream infection. Amphotericin B was the most common antifungal used, and the catheter was removed in 89.5% of the patients, whereas death occurred in four patients (17.4%). All strains were identified as *R. mucilaginosa,* and amphotericin B demonstrated good in vitro activity, whereas fluconazole had no activity.[13] Because of *Rhodotorula* species resistance to fluconazole and echinocandin antifungal agents, patients receiving fluconazole and caspofungin might be susceptible to the development of breakthrough *Rhodotorula* fungemia.[40]

In vitro testing of 35 clinical samples of *Rhodotorula* spp. showed low MICs against all agents tested, including amphotericin B, ketoconazole, flucytosine, and itraconazole. The azoles were generally less effective than amphotericin B, and fluconazole showed an MIC of more than 32 µg/mL against all isolates.[26] In vitro amphotericin B is slightly superior to voriconazole and itraconazole, with general fluconazole resistance.[20]

Guideline-recommended therapy for *Rhodotorula* infection is amphotericin B, and *Rhodotorula* species are considered generally resistant to azoles and echinocandins but susceptible to amphotericin B and flucytosine. Removal of the central venous catheter is strongly recommended.[5]

Talaromyces (Penicillium) marneffei

Talaromyces marneffei, renamed from *Penicillium marneffei* in 2015, is the only dimorphic and human pathogenic *Talaromyces* species and is endemic in tropical Asia, especially Thailand, China, and Vietnam. It has emerged as the third most common AIDS-defining illness in parts of Southeast Asia.[32] Incidence of this disease has increased markedly after the first reported natural infection in 1973 of an American minister with Hodgkin disease who resided in Southeast Asia.[16] From approximately 30 cases from 1973 to 1990, this infection has risen to more than 160 reported cases by 1995.[18] However, epidemiology is changing again somewhat with the increased control of HIV, so now there are a greater proportion of non–HIV-infected patient cases following newer immunosuppressive modalities such as T-lymphocyte–depleting agents, anti-CD20 monoclonal antibodies, and tyrosine kinase inhibitors.[8]

Some of the most common clinical features include fever, malaise, cough and dyspnea.[8] In approximately 85% of cases, disseminated disease can begin as numerous papules with central necrosis and located on the face and neck (Fig. 208.1).[83] Lesions can also appear on the upper extremities, trunk, and lower extremities. The disease can present with nonproductive cough, generalized lymphadenopathy, fever, anemia, and weight loss.[18] Approximately half of the cases involve fungemia.[18]

T. marneffei can mimic and often can be misdiagnosed as other infections such as tuberculosis, *Pneumocystis carinii* pneumonia, cryptococcosis, and histoplasmosis. Most patients with HIV have a low $CD4^+$ count. *T. marneffei* has temperature-dependent dimorphic growth, whereby below 37°C it grows as mycelia (mold) with the formation of septate hyphae and bearing conidia, but at 37°C it grows in a yeast-like form. *T. marneffei* is the only dimorphic *Talaromyces* species, and the conidia in the environment likely enter through the respiratory tract and convert to the yeast form, in which pulmonary alveolar macrophages appear to be the primary pulmonary host defense.

An in vitro study of 30 isolates revealed susceptibility to itraconazole and ketoconazole and intermediate activity to amphotericin B and fluconazole.[32] Two comparative in vitro studies showed terbinafine and itraconazole with similar activity,[44] and itraconazole and voriconazole possessed identical activity.[59] In another study, posaconazole showed better in vitro activity than itraconazole and amphotericin B against four isolates.[79] Micafungin showed the best in vitro activity compared with fluconazole, itraconazole, miconazole, and amphotericin B.[78]

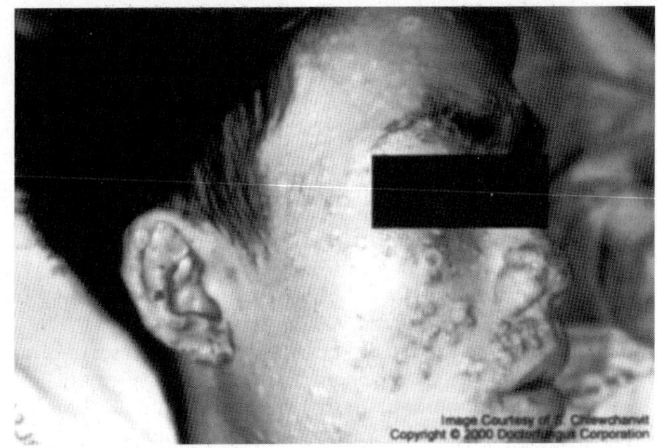

FIG. 208.1 Skin lesions from *Talaromyces marneffei.* (Courtesy S. Chiewchanvit, provided by http://www.doctorfungus.org.)

Amphotericin B has been used as successful initial management of disseminated penicilliosis in immunocompromised patients; however, it requires prolonged intravenous therapy, and relapse is common. Amphotericin B followed by itraconazole is also effective (97.3%),[71] but itraconazole takes an average of 57 days to clear fungemia.[72] A review of 74 clinical isolates showed that itraconazole generally possessed the best in vitro activity over amphotericin B, fluconazole, and ketoconazole, and thus it is generally recommended for treatment.[32]

For treatment of severe cases, initial induction treatment with amphotericin B is necessary for 2 weeks, followed by an oral azole, such as itraconazole, for the next 10 weeks.[82] Although itraconazole is presently the azole of choice, voriconazole can also be effective for chronic suppressive therapy.

MOLDS

Phaeohyphomycosis: *Cladophialophora bantiana* and *Bipolaris* Species and Others

Phaeohyphomycosis is a heterogeneous group of fungal species commonly found in the soil, distributed worldwide, and characterized by dematiaceous (darkly pigmented brown or black) hyphal forms in tissue. This staining can help distinguish between *Aspergillus* infections, and hyphae often appear more fragmented than those seen with *Aspergillus* infections.[88] The characteristic color of the hyphae is related to the presence of melanin in the fungal cell wall, which likely plays a role in fungal pathogenesis.[50] "Phaeo" comes from the Greek meaning "dark" and has been commonly used, particularly when describing infections due to these fungi as phaeohyphomycosis. It has been suggested that the term dematiaceous is not appropriate given its etymologic derivation from the Greek "deme," meaning bundle, although it has become fairly entrenched in medical mycologic literature. The term melanized has recently been used more frequently, given its specific meaning.[61] Infections can manifest as a range of clinical entities, including localized cutaneous infection and subcutaneous nodules, mycetomas (localized infections involving the cutaneous and subcutaneous tissue, fascia, and bone, often of the lower extremities, and characterized by mycotic granules), chromoblastomycosis (sclerotic bodies in tissues usually seen in tropical regions), keratitis, pulmonary infections, localized deep infections, cerebral abscesses, disseminated infection, allergic fungal sinusitis, and allergic bronchopulmonary mycosis.

Phaeohyphomycosis has been attributed to more than 150 species of fungi, spanning several orders in the kingdom Fungi. Among the most prevalent causes of human infection are *Alternaria alternata, Acrophialophora fusispora, Aureobasidium pullulans, Bipolaris* spp.,

Curvularia spp. (some were previously *Bipolaris*), *Chaetomium* spp., *C. bantiana, Exserohilum* spp., *Fonsecaea* spp., *Hortaea werneckii, Neoscytalidium dimidiatum, Verruconis gallopava* (previously *Ochroconis gallopava*), *Phaeoacremonium* spp., *Phoma* spp., *Pyrenochaeta* spp., *Rhinocladiella* spp. *Veronaea botryosa, Wangiella dermatitidis* (previously *Exophiala dermatitidis*), and *Phialophora* spp.[11,50]

Diagnosis of phaeohyphomycosis relies on pathologic examination of cultures and biopsies, often with expert gross and microscopic examination required. There are no simple serologic or antigen tests to detect these fungi in blood or tissue, and PCR is in its infancy for this group of organisms. Almost all allergic disease and eosinophilia is caused by either *Bipolaris* or *Curvularia* spp.[88]

Cladophialophora bantiana is the etiology for most cases of central nervous system (CNS) phaeohyphomycosis, including patients that may have no apparent immunosuppression.[17] Other common etiologies of phaeohyphomycotic brain abscess are *Ramichloridium mackenziei, O. gallopava*, and *W. dermatitidis*.[62] CNS disease commonly presents with a headache and a focal neurologic deficit, frequently a hemiparesis, or seizures. *Bipolaris* spp. are the most common cause of phaeohyphomycotic sinusitis, but they may also cause pneumonia, fungemia, and disseminated infections.[85]

The CDC-sponsored Transplant-Associated Infection Surveillance Network (TRANSNET) collected data on 56 patients with phaeohyphomycosis from 15 centers.[43] Median time to diagnosis after transplantation varied by underlying type of transplantation (hematopoietic stem cell transplantation, median of 100 days; solid organ transplantation, median of 685 days). The most frequent sites of infection were the lungs, skin, and sinuses, and the most frequently isolated pathogen was *Alternaria* species (32%), followed by *Exophiala* (11%). Overall, cutaneous disease was more common in solid-organ transplant recipients, whereas pulmonary disease was more common in hematopoietic stem cell transplant recipients. In this series, bloodstream and CNS infections were only seen in hematopoietic stem cell transplant recipients.

European guidelines highlight the sparse data on preferred therapy, including in vitro data, limited animal model studies, and expert opinion.[11] There are no clearly defined standard therapies, but the guideline panel generally recommended voriconazole, posaconazole, or itraconazole because those agents demonstrate the most consistent in vitro antifungal activity against this group of fungi. Specifically, voriconazole is likely the best for CNS infections because of its excellent penetration. For invasive infections, surgery is crucial to the overall treatment.

In vitro studies with *C. bantiana* show similarly low MICs for voriconazole, itraconazole, and amphotericin B.[22] One study showed that posaconazole had activity slightly worse than itraconazole but much better than either anidulafungin or caspofungin.[19] Another study showed that itraconazole MICs were better than those of voriconazole against seven isolates,[59] whereas in another set of experiments, voriconazole had superior in vitro activity to itraconazole and amphotericin B.[34]

The in vitro activity of drugs against *Bipolaris* species can give mixed results. Amphotericin B possessed better activity compared with voriconazole and itraconazole against *Bipolaris hawaiiensis* and *Bipolaris spicifera*.[22] However, in another study voriconazole showed the best in vitro activity compared with amphotericin B, fluconazole, and itraconazole.[45] In contrast, a study with six *Bipolaris* species isolates showed itraconazole with the best activity, followed closely by voriconazole and amphotericin B,[20] and another study with 43 isolates showed itraconazole had great in vitro activity.[44] In the evaluation of the echinocandins, itraconazole retained the best activity, with both voriconazole and posaconazole displaying good activity, and all were far better than caspofungin or anidulafungin.[19] Comparing all available triazoles, posaconazole had the most activity, followed by itraconazole, and lastly by voriconazole.[56]

Including only culture-positive cases of CNS phaeohyphomycosis, the survival rate for this infection is only 35%.[17] CNS lesions may be best managed surgically, and a series of 30 cases revealed that patients with single, encapsulated lesions did much better than those with multifocal disease. However, no patient who did not undergo surgery survived. Whether patients underwent neurosurgery alone or with antifungal therapy, the most important factor for cure was resectability of the lesion; antifungal therapy itself was not associated with improved survival.

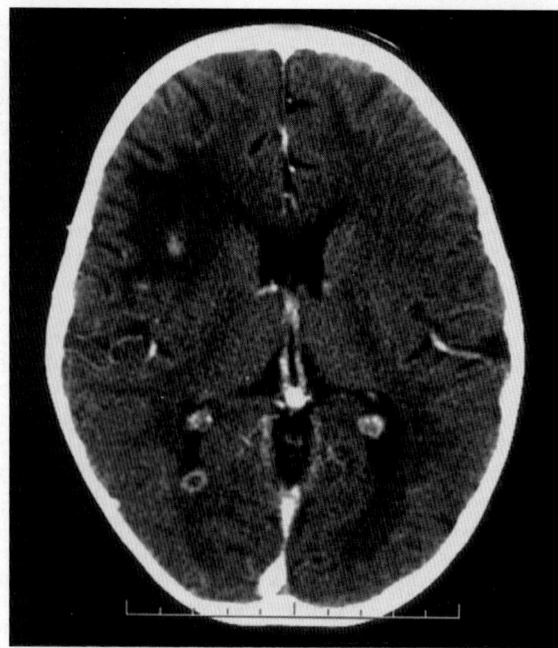

FIG. 208.2 Brain computed tomography image showing six enhancing lesions at initial diagnosis.

CNS phaeohyphomycosis continues to have a high mortality rate without surgical resection, and this may be the case for all localized cases of phaeohyphomycosis. The extended-spectrum triazoles such as voriconazole and posaconazole show good in vitro activity against *C. bantiana, Bipolaris* spp., and several other dematiaceous fungi, with some positive correlating clinical experience. Although the triazoles are probably more effective, the echinocandins do have some limited activity, and these agents will likely be tried in refractory cases as combination therapy. A review of 101 cases of culture-proven CNS phaeohyphomycosis found that the most frequently isolated species was *C. bantiana*, followed by *R. mackenziei*, which is seen exclusively in patients from the Middle East (Fig. 208.2). More than one-half of the cases occurred in patients with no known underlying immunodeficiency. Mortality rates were high, and therapy, although not standardized, was most successful with the combination of amphotericin B, flucytosine, and itraconazole. Complete excision of brain lesions may provide better results than simple aspiration, underscoring that a very aggressive medical and surgical approach is needed.[62]

Hyalohyphomycosis

In contrast to phaeohyphomycosis, hyalohyphomycosis refers to infections caused by hyaline (colorless, nonpigmented, nonmelanized) septate fungal hyphae. The major hyalohyphomycotic pathogens are *Fusarium* spp. and *Scedosporium* spp. (both covered in great detail in Chapter 207), *Paecilomyces* spp., *Trichoderma* spp., *Acremonium* spp., *Scopulariopsis* spp., and *Purpureocillium* spp.[76] These species are often misidentified as *Aspergillus* spp., but they can be differentiated by their conidia and phialide morphologies.[50] Similar to the phaeohyphomycoses, diagnosis requires culture or detailed expert microscopic examination.

Fungemia can be seen when *Fusarium* spp., *Paecilomyces* spp., and *Acremonium* spp. invade tissue, and they produce hyphae as well as adventitious structures similar to microconidia that hematogenously disseminate and are found in blood culture.[38] *Aspergillus* does not do this, except *A. terreus*, which can elaborate lateral conidia in vitro and in vivo.[55]

Paecilomyces Species

Paecilomyces species are common soil saprophytes and can be recovered from the air because they are resistant to common methods of sterilization.[50] The two most common species associated with clinical infection are *P. variotii* and *P. lilacinus*, but the latter is now reclassified as *Purpureocillium lilacinum*. They are often confused with the *Penicillium* species and are clinically difficult to identify because their presentation can mimic better-known fungi such as dematiaceous fungi and certain other hyalohyphomycoses.[66] They can cause keratitis, endophthalmitis, and subcutaneous infections in the healthy host. In immunocompromised patients they can manifest as cutaneous disease, catheter-related fungemia, sinusitis, and disseminated disease. Many immunocompromised patients obtain infection by integument breaks with intravascular catheters or chemotherapy.[55] In fact, contaminated skin lotion has caused a nosocomial outbreak of infection in a bone marrow transplantation unit.[73] Of the approximately 160 cases of invasive *Paecilomyces* spp. infection reported,[54] approximately 50% are in the form of keratitis or endophthalmitis.

Amphotericin B is very potent against *P. variotii* but has poor in vitro activity against the most common species, *P. lilacinum*. Voriconazole MICs are much lower than itraconazole against *P. lilacinum*, including superior fungicidal activity[22] which was confirmed in another study, but the reverse was true for *P. variotii* with itraconazole activity better than voriconazole.[59] In a study with posaconazole, it was found to have similar activity to itraconazole and better activity than amphotericin B against *P. variotii*. Posaconazole displayed significantly better activity against *P. lilacinum* compared with itraconazole, whereas amphotericin B showed no activity against that species.[79] Comparing all triazoles, posaconazole had the most activity, followed by itraconazole, ravuconazole, and finally voriconazole.[56] Caspofungin was inactive in vitro against *P. lilacinum* but showed excellent activity against *P. varioti*.[14] On the other hand, micafungin showed good in vitro activity against *P. lilacinum* and *P. variotii* and better activity than fluconazole, itraconazole, miconazole, and amphotericin B.[78]

In an immunosuppressed murine model of disseminated infection with *P. lilacinum*, voriconazole significantly prolonged survival with respect to the group treated with amphotericin B, reducing the fungal load in the spleen, kidneys, and liver of infected mice. Survival of mice treated with amphotericin B did not differ from that of the control group, and amphotericin B was not able to reduce the tissue burden in any organ with respect to the control group.[65] In another murine model of paecilomycosis, posaconazole was superior to amphotericin B or liposomal amphotericin B and was the only treatment able to significantly reduce fungal loads in the spleens, kidneys, and livers of the mice infected by each of the two strains.[64]

The cornerstone of therapy has been surgical resection and removal of any foreign object. In vitro data suggest that the triazoles might be effective treatment for *Paecilomyces* infection; however, large datasets of clinical experience are lacking to support the recommendation, and it remains even less clear whether the echinocandins have any place in the management of these infections.

Trichoderma longibrachiatum

Trichoderma species are an ubiquitous component of soil and play an important role decomposing plant material, with several species of the genus *Trichoderma* identified as etiologic agents of infection in immunocompromised hosts, including *T. longibrachiatum, T. citrinoviride, T. harzianum, T. koningii, T. pseudokoningii*, and *T. viride*.[63,68] *T. longibrachiatum* causes virtually all human infections and has been reported to cause pulmonary, cerebral, soft tissue, and disseminated disease in immunocompromised patients. It has been suggested that *T. longibrachiatum* can be acquired through the gastrointestinal tract, and prolonged therapy with fluconazole and antibacterial agents may selectively favor this filamentous fungi.[63] Another likely source may be aerosols or contaminated water.[50] The first case of *Trichoderma* infection in an immunocompromised patient was reported in 1976, and a review lists only 10 cases reported in immunocompromised hosts.[63]

Itraconazole displays the best in vitro activity among older antifungals.[24,49,69,74] Other studies showed itraconazole with no activity, and amphotericin B had better activity than voriconazole.[21] However, amphotericin B resistance is uniform in reported clinical cases. Extended-spectrum triazoles should be considered over the polyenes for treatment, but recovery from immunosuppression appears crucial to success. In one series, voriconazole had superior in vitro antifungal activity over posaconazole and itraconazole, amphotericin B showed nearly zero antifungal activity, and the echinocandins also showed excellent antifungal activity.[68] Stool surveillance cultures for early identification of this fungus remain unproved for clinical management but may play a role with future studies.

Acremonium Species

Acremonium species are ubiquitous in the environment and common in soil, plant debris, and rotting mushrooms; *A. kiliense* (now reclassified as *Sarocladium kiliense*) is the most important among the 10 species reported as infectious etiologies in vertebrates. *Acremonium* spp. grow slowly, so culture plates need to be incubated for at least 2 weeks for detection. The immunocompetent host can form a mycetoma or develop an ocular infection after sustaining a penetrating injury.[30] *Acremonium spp.* can lead to a wide range of infections from keratitis to disseminated disease, with the lung and gastrointestinal tract as apparent portals of entry.[85]

The first case of *Acremonium* spp. infection other than mycetoma or ocular infection was described in 1932, but most have arisen since 1985.[30] The largest review of 36 localized or disseminated cases showed that most disseminated cases occurred in immunocompromised patients and only approximately one-half could be cured, with complete resolution of disease dependent on neutrophil recovery.[30] Recognition of disseminated *Acremonium* infection is difficult because specific signs and symptoms do not exist. Patients may present with a cutaneous nodule, papular skin rash, or fungemia.

The rarity of *Acremonium* infections makes it difficult to adequately assess the best treatment regimen. Amphotericin B was previously recommended as initial therapy,[23] and despite the in vitro resistance to azole treatment, the combination of surgery and azoles has often been successful.[30] Voriconazole appears to have the greatest in vitro activity against *Acremonium*, and European guidelines recommend voriconazole as initial antifungal therapy.[76] Similar to other fungal pathogens, the status of the host defense system is crucial. *Acremonium* infections are still rare but deadly, and the limited amount of clinical experience makes firm recommendations difficult. The echinocandins appear to have limited activity, whereas the newer triazoles may be beneficial adjunctive therapy in concert with boosting the host immune response.

In one study, itraconazole had no activity and voriconazole had a marginally effective MIC for *A. kiliense*.[59] Another study showed voriconazole with the best in vitro activity compared with amphotericin B, fluconazole, and itraconazole for *A. alabamensis* and *A. strictum*.[45] Anidulafungin has no activity against *Acremonium* species, but posaconazole and caspofungin both possess some fungistatic activity against *A. strictum*.[19] A more recent study showed that voriconazole and ravuconazole had similar activity and had superior activity to posaconazole, whereas the strains tested were resistant to amphotericin B and itraconazole.[56]

NEW REFERENCES SINCE THE SEVENTH EDITION

5. Arendrup MC, Boekhout T, Akova M, et al. ESCMID and ECMM joint clinical guidelines for the diagnosis and management of rare invasive yeast infections. *Clin Microbiol Infect*. 2014;20(suppl 3):76-98.
6. Aschner JL, Punsalang A Jr, Maniscalco WM, et al. Percutaneous central venous catheter colonization with *Malassezia furfur*: incidence and clinical significance. *Pediatrics*. 1987;80(4):535-539.
7. Bell LM, Alpert G, Slight PH, et al. *Malassezia furfur* skin colonization in infancy. *Infect Control Hosp Epidemiol*. 1988;9(4):151-153.
8. Chan JF, Lau SK, Yuen KY, et al. *Talaromyces (Penicillium) marneffei* infection in non-HIV-infected patients. *Emerg Microbes Infect*. 2016;5:e19.
11. Chowdhary A, Meis JF, Guarro J, et al. ESCMID and ECMM joint clinical guidelines for the diagnosis and management of systemic phaeohyphomycosis: diseases caused by black fungi. *Clin Microbiol Infect*. 2014;20(suppl 3):47-75.
31. Hazirolan G, Canton E, Sahin S, et al. Head-to-head comparison of inhibitory and fungicidal activities of fluconazole, itraconazole, voriconazole, posaconazole, and isavuconazole against clinical isolates of *Trichosporon asahii*. *Antimicrob Agents Chemother*. 2013;57(10):4841-4847.
33. Iturrieta-Gonzalez IA, Padovan AC, Bizerra FC, et al. Multiple species of *Trichosporon* produce biofilms highly resistant to triazoles and amphotericin B. *PLoS ONE*. 2014;9(10):e109553.

37. Liao Y, Lu X, Yang S, et al. Epidemiology and Outcome of *Trichosporon* fungemia: a review of 185 reported cases from 1975 to 2014. *Open Forum Infect Dis.* 2015;2(4):ofv141.
43. McCarty TP, Baddley JW, Walsh TJ, et al. Phaeohyphomycosis in transplant recipients: Results from the Transplant Associated Infection Surveillance Network (TRANSNET). *Med Mycol.* 2015;53(5):440-446.
46. Miceli MH, Diaz JA, Lee SA. Emerging opportunistic yeast infections. *Lancet Infect Dis.* 2011;11(2):142-151.
87. Wirth F, Goldani LZ. Epidemiology of *Rhodotorula*: an emerging pathogen. *Interdiscip Perspect Infect Dis.* 2012;2012:465717.
88. Wong EH, Revankar SG. Dematiaceous Molds. *Infect Dis Clin North Am.* 2016;30(1):165-178.

The full reference list for this chapter is available at ExpertConsult.com.

Classification and Nomenclature of Human Parasites

209

Lynne S. Garcia

Although common names frequently are used to describe parasitic organisms, these names may represent different parasites in different parts of the world. To eliminate these problems, a binomial system of nomenclature in which the scientific name consists of the genus and species is used.[1,4,5,13,17,18,22] These names generally are of Greek or Latin origin. In certain publications, the scientific name often is followed by the name of the person who originally named the parasite. The date of naming also may be provided. If the name of the individual person is in parentheses, it means that the person used a generic name no longer considered to be correct.

On the basis of life histories, morphologic characteristics, and molecular techniques, systems of classification have been developed to indicate the relationships among the various parasite species. Closely related species are placed in the same genus, related genera in the same family, related families in the same order, related orders in the same class, and related classes in the same phylum, one of the major categories in the animal kingdom. As one moves up the classification schema, each category becomes broader; however, each category still has characteristics in common.

Parasites of humans are classified in several major divisions. They include the Protozoa (amebae, flagellates, ciliates, sporozoans, and coccidia), the Fungi (microsporidia), the Platyhelminthes or flatworms (cestodes, trematodes), the Acanthocephala or thorny-headed worms, the Nematoda or roundworms, and the Arthropoda (insects, spiders, mites, ticks, and so on). Although these categories appear to be well defined, often considerable confusion occurs in attempting to classify parasitic organisms. One of the primary reasons is the lack of known specimens. Some organisms recovered from humans are very rare; difficulty thus arises in determining morphologic and physiologic variations among such groups. Type specimens must be deposited for study before a legitimate species name can be given. Even when certain parasites are numerous, they may represent strains or races of the same species with slightly different characteristics.

Generally, reproductive mechanisms are valid in determining definitions of species, but so many exceptions exist within parasite groups that taking into consideration properties such as sexual reproduction, parthenogenesis, and asexual reproduction is difficult. Other difficulties in recognition of species are the ability and the tendency of the organisms to alter their morphologic forms according to age, host, or nutrition, changes that often result in several names given to the same organism. An additional problem involves alternation of parasitic and free-living phases in the life cycle. These organisms may be very different and difficult to recognize as belonging to the same species. Despite these difficulties, newer, more sophisticated molecular methods of grouping organisms often have confirmed taxonomic conclusions reached hundreds of years earlier by experienced taxonomists.

As investigations continue in parasitic genetics, immunology, biochemistry, and molecular studies, the species designation will be defined more clearly. Originally, these species designations were determined primarily by morphologic differences, resulting in a phenotypic approach. With the use of highly sophisticated molecular techniques, the approach will continue to be more genotypic. Benefits of these studies also include the development of highly specific and sensitive diagnostic tests and the ability to diagnose parasitic infections on the basis of molecular parameters, rather than merely phenotypic characteristics.

Although gaps in our knowledge concerning classification of all human parasites remain, the binomial system has allowed the classification of 1.5 million species of organisms in the animal kingdom such that all published information can be retrieved, regardless of the language spoken. The difficulty for the clinician arises when one considers the rapid increase in information concerning microbiology during the past few years and changing considerations such as the role of immunosuppression in the host-parasite interaction and the modified definitions of "normal flora" and "nonpathogenic" in this patient population.

The classification of parasites is presented in tabular form. Although certain designations of species may be somewhat controversial, this classification scheme is designed to provide some order and meaning to a widely divergent group of organisms. No attempt has been made to include every possible organism, and only those organisms considered clinically relevant in the context of human parasitology are included. The main groups that are presented include protozoa and fungi (Box 209.1), nematodes (roundworms; Box 209.2), cestodes (tapeworms; Box 209.3), and trematodes (flukes; Box 209.4). Some relevant information on Acanthocephala (Box 209.5) and arthropods (Tables 209.1 and 209.2) is also presented. The hope is that this information will provide some insight into the parasite groupings, thus leading to a better understanding of parasitic infections and the appropriate diagnostic and clinical approach.

BOX 209.1 Protozoa

Amebae—Intestinal

These organisms are characterized by having pseudopods (motility) and trophozoite and cyst stages in the life cycle and include some exceptions in which a cyst form has not been identified. Amebae usually are acquired by humans through fecal-oral transmission or mouth-to-mouth contact *(Entamoeba gingivalis)*.

Current Name

Entamoeba histolytica[a]
Entamoeba dispar[a]
Entamoeba hartmanni[b]
Entamoeba coli
Entamoeba polecki
Entamoeba moshkovskii
Entamoeba bangladeshi
Entamoeba gingivalis
Endolimax nana
Iodamoeba bütschlii
Blastocystis spp.[c]

Flagellates—Intestinal

These organisms move by means of flagella and are acquired by fecal-oral transmission. With exception of the genera *Trichomonas* and *Pentatrichomonas*, they have trophozoite and cyst stages in the life cycle. *Trichomonas* and *Pentatrichomonas* spp. do not have a cyst stage.

Current Name

Giardia lamblia[d]
Chilomastix mesnili
Dientamoeba fragilis[e]
Pentatrichomonas hominis
Trichomonas tenax
Enteromonas hominis
Retortamonas intestinalis

Ciliates—Intestinal

These organisms, which move by means of cilia, are acquired by humans through fecal-oral transmission. They have both trophozoite and cyst forms in the life cycle.

Current Name

Balantidium coli

Apicomplexa, Sporozoa (Intestinal)

These organisms are acquired by humans by ingestion of various meats or through fecal-oral transmission through contaminated food or water.

Current Name

Apicomplexa

Cryptosporidium hominis[f]
Cryptosporidium parvum[f]
Cryptosporidium spp.
Cyclospora cayetanensis[23,24]
Cystoisospora (Isospora) belli
Sarcocystis hominis
Sarcocystis suihominis
Sarcocystis bovihominis
Sarcocystis heydorni[g]

Fungi (Microsporidia[g])—Intestinal

Enterocytozoon bieneusi
Encephalitozoon (Septata) intestinalis[h]

Amebae, Flagellates—Other Body Sites

The amebae are pathogenic, free-living organisms that may be associated with warm, freshwater areas. They have been found in the central nervous system, the eye, and other sites. *Trichomonas vaginalis* usually is acquired by sexual transmission. This particular flagellate is found in the genitourinary system.

Current Name

Amebae

Naegleria fowleri
Acanthamoeba spp.
Hartmannella spp.
Balamuthia mandrillaris
Sappinia diploidea

Flagellates

Trichomonas vaginalis

Apicomplexa, Sporozoa (Coccidia)—Other Body Sites

The coccidia are particularly important in the compromised patient. They also may infect many persons who have no apparent symptoms.[11,12] On the basis of molecular studies, the microsporidia are linked more closely to the fungi and have been reclassified with those organisms. However, during this transition phase, their classification will remain with the parasites.

Current Name

Coccidia

Toxoplasma gondii

Fungi (*Pneumocystis*,[i] Microsporidia)—Other Body Sites

Microsporidia

Anncaliia (Brachiola) connori
Anncaliia (Brachiola) algerae
Anncaliia (Brachiola) vesicularum
Encephalitozoon cuniculi
Encephalitozoon hellem
Encephalitozoon intestinalis[j]
Enterocytozoon bieneusi[k]
Microsporidium africanum
Microsporidium ceylonensis[l]
Nosema ocularum
Pleistophora ronneafiei
Trachipleistophora hominis
Trachipleistophora anthropophthera
Tubulinosema acridophagus
Vittaforma corneae[m]

Sporozoa, Flagellates—Blood and Tissues

All these organisms are arthropod borne. The diagnosis may be somewhat more difficult to make than that of infection with the intestinal protozoa, particularly if automated blood differential systems are used. The *Leishmania* genus has undergone extensive revisions in classification. However, from a clinical perspective, recovery and identification of the organisms still are related to body site. Recovery

BOX 209.1 Protozoa—cont'd

of the organisms is limited to the site of the lesion in infections other than those caused by the *Leishmania donovani* complex (visceral leishmaniasis).

Current Name

Apicomplexa, Sporozoa (Malaria, Babesiosis)

Malaria

- *Plasmodium vivax*
- *Plasmodium ovale*
- *Plasmodium malariae*
- *Plasmodium falciparum*
- *Plasmodium knowlesi*[n]

Babesiosis[o]

- *Babesia microti*
- *Babesia divergens*
- *Babesia duncani*
- *Babesia* spp.

Flagellates (Leishmaniasis, Trypanosomiasis)

Leishmaniasis

- *Leishmania tropica* complex (cutaneous leishmaniasis)
- *Leishmania infantum* complex (cutaneous leishmaniasis)
- *Leishmania major* complex (cutaneous leishmaniasis)
- *Leishmania mexicana* complex (cutaneous leishmaniasis)
- *Leishmania braziliensis* complex (mucocutaneous leishmaniasis)
- *Leishmania donovani* complex (visceral leishmaniasis)

Trypanosomiasis

- *Trypanosoma brucei gambiense* (West African trypanosomiasis)
- *Trypanosoma brucei rhodesiense* (East African trypanosomiasis)
- *Trypanosoma cruzi* (American trypanosomiasis)
- *Trypanosoma rangeli*

[a]*E. histolytica* is being used to designate the true pathogen, whereas *Entamoeba dispar* is being used to designate a nonpathogen. Unless trophozoites containing ingested red blood cells (*E. histolytica*) are seen during microscopic examination, or a specific immunoassay for the pathogen (*E. histolytica*) is used, the two organisms cannot be differentiated on the basis of morphology seen in permanent stained smears of fecal specimens and will be reported as *E. histolytica/E. dispar*. Some laboratories are now using the term *E. histolytica/E. dispar* group; other organisms share a typical morphology (*E. moshkovskii, E. bangladeshi*). Fecal immunoassays for antigen detection are available commercially for differentiating *E. histolytica* from *E. dispar* and for detecting the *E. histolytica/E. dispar* group.[12] Because the differences in pathogenicity are genetic and not just phenotypic, the decision to treat is one that must be determined by the physician. The finding of organisms of the *E. histolytica/E. dispar* group in patients' specimens must continue to be reported to state and county departments of public health (follow your particular state reporting regulations).

[b]*E. hartmanni* is nonpathogenic and is totally different from *E. histolytica*. "Small race *E. histolytica*" is incorrect and should not be used at any time to designate *E. hartmanni*.

[c]Currently, this organism is classified as an anaerobic, single-celled stramenopile (brown algae; Kingdom Chromista, class Blastocystea).[27] *Blastocystis* is comprised of a number of subtypes, approximately half of which are pathogenic and half are nonpathogenic. However, from organism morphology seen microscopically, these subtypes cannot be differentiated. Therefore the diagnosis of this organism should be considered potentially pathogenic for the patien.

[d]Although some investigators have changed the species designation for the genus *Giardia* to *G. duodenalis* or *G. intestinalis*, no consensus exists. Therefore, for this listing, we retain the name *G. lamblia*. However, molecular and epidemiologic evidence suggests that at least two assemblages of *Giardia* infect humans, one of which is *G. duodenalis* and the other, possibly a new species, *G. enterica*.[21]

[e]The cyst stage has been confirmed in *D. fragilis*.[25] On the basis of electron microscopy studies, *D. fragilis* has been reclassified as an ameboflagellate rather than an ameba and is closely related to *Histomonas* and *Trichomonas* spp. However, it is normally referred to as a flagellate.

[f]*C. parvum* infects cattle, sheep, goats, and humans as primary hosts, but *C. hominis* infects only humans and primates.

[g]The microsporidia are now thought to be more closely related to fungi than to protozoa; however, clinical parasitologists have been reluctant to part with this group, whereas mycologists have been equally reluctant to accept it. Consequently, the microsporidia are retained within this list for parasites, although they are classified within the Fungi.[3,16,28,29]

[h]Formerly called *Septata intestinalis*.[15,20]

[i]*Pneumocystis carinii* has been reclassified with the fungi and renamed *Pneumocystis jirovecii*.[10,18,26] Consequently, it will be removed from future parasite listings. An unusual group of spore-forming fungi, and the earliest-diverging clade of sequenced fungi,[3] microsporidia lack mitochondria or mitochondrial remnants and are obligate intracellular eukaryotic unicellular parasites. Microsporidia can rapidly extrude their polar tubes, which penetrate the host plasma membrane. The sporoplasm is transferred into the host cells, where the spores develop and complete their life cycles. At this point parasitologists are reluctant to relinquish these organisms, whereas mycologists are reluctant to accept them; consequently they are included in this parasite classification list.

[j]Formerly called *Septata intestinalis*.

[k]*E. bieneusi* has been recovered from sites other than the intestinal tract.

[l]This designation is now written as a true genus, but it remains a "catch-all" for those organisms that have not been (or may never be) identified as belonging to the true genus or species levels.

[m]Formerly called *Nosema corneum*.

[n]*P. knowlesi*, a malaria parasite of macaque monkeys in Southeast Asia that is now established as a naturally transmitted parasite of humans in Malaysia and other parts of Southeast Asia, has been responsible for a number of deaths.[6,19] Thus, five species of malaria pathogens now that infect humans.

[o]Molecular studies confirm that humans can also harbor several *Babesia* parasites that have not yet been identified.[14]

BOX 209.2 Nematodes

Intestinal

These organisms normally are acquired by ingestion of eggs or penetration of the skin by larval forms from the soil.

Current Name

- *Ascaris lumbricoides*
- *Enterobius vermicularis* (pinworm)
- *Ancylostoma duodenale* (Old World hookworm)
- *Necator americanus* (New World hookworm)
- *Strongyloides stercoralis*
- *Strongyloides fuelleborni*
- *Trichostrongylus* spp.
- *Trichuris trichiura* (whipworm)
- *Capillaria philippinensis*
- *Oesophagostomum spp.* (*O. bifurcum* most common in humans—West Africa)
- *Ternidens diminutus* (as high as 80% in Zimbabwe)

Tissue

For the most part, these organisms rarely are seen within the United States; however, the first three are more important.

Continued

BOX 209.2 Nematodes—cont'd

Current Name

Trichinella spiralis
Trichinella spp.
Toxocara canis or *T. cati* (visceral or ocular larva migrans)
Ancylostoma braziliense or *A. caninum* (cutaneous larva migrans)
Ancylostoma ceylanicum[2]
Baylisascaris procyonis (severe systemic visceral larva migrans, neural larva migrans)
Dracunçulus medinensis
Angiostrongylus cantonensis
Angiostrongylus costaricensis
Gnathostoma spinigerum
Gnathostoma spp.
Anisakiasis (larvae from salt-water fish)
- *Anisakis* spp.
- *Phocanema* spp.
- *Contracaecum* spp.
- *Pseudoterranova* spp.
- *Hysterothylacium* spp.
- *Porrocaecum* spp.

Capillaria hepatica
Dioctophyma renale
Thelazia spp.

Filarial Worms—Blood, Other Body Fluids, Skin

These organisms also are arthropod borne. The adult worms tend to live in the lymphatic tissues. The diagnosis is made on the basis of the recovery and identification of the larval worms (microfilariae) in the blood, other body fluids, or skin. Elephantiasis may be associated with some of the organisms listed.

Current Name

Wuchereria bancrofti
Brugia malayi
Brugia timori
Loa loa
Onchocerca volvulus
Mansonella ozzardi
Mansonella streptocerca
Mansonella perstans
Dirofilaria immitis ("coin" lesion in the lung) (dog heartworm)
Dirofilaria spp. (may be found in subcutaneous nodules)

BOX 209.3 Cestodes

Intestinal

The adult form of these organisms is acquired by humans through ingestion of the larval forms contained in poorly cooked or raw meats or freshwater fish. In the case of *Dipylidium caninum*, infection is acquired by the accidental ingestion of dog fleas. Both *Hymenolepis nana* and *H. diminuta* are transmitted by ingestion of certain arthropods (fleas, beetles). Also, *H. nana* can be transmitted through egg ingestion (life cycle in the human can bypass the intermediate beetle host). Humans can serve as both the intermediate and definitive hosts in *H. nana* and *Taenia solium* infections.

Current Name

Diphyllobothrium latum (broad, fish tapeworm)
Dipylidium caninum (dog tapeworm)
Hymenolepis (Rodentolepis) nana (dwarf tapeworm)
Hymenolepis diminuta (rat tapeworm)
Taenia solium (pork tapeworm)
Taenia saginata (beef tapeworm)
Taenia asiatica (Taiwanese variant of *T. saginata*)

Larval Forms—Tissue

The ingestion of certain tapeworm eggs or accidental contact with certain larval forms can lead to the diseases shown in parentheses.

Current Name

Taenia solium (cysticercosis)
Echinococcus granulosus (hydatid disease)
Echinococcus canadensis[7]
Echinococcus multilocularis (alveolar hydatid disease)
Echinococcus oligarthrus (polycystic hydatid disease)
Multiceps multiceps (coenurosis)
Diphyllobothrium spp. (sparganosis)
Spirometra mansonoides (sparganosis)

BOX 209.4 Trematodes

Intestinal

These organisms are uncommon within the United States, except for four species of *Alaria*, which are endemic within North America.

Current Name

Fasciolopsis buski (giant intestinal fluke)
Echinostoma ilocanum
Eurytrema pancreaticum
Heterophyes heterophyes
Metagonimus yokogawai
Alaria spp.

Liver, Lung

These organisms are not seen commonly within the United States; however, some Southeast Asian refugees do harbor some of these parasites.

Current Name

Clonorchis (Opisthorchis) sinensis (Chinese liver fluke)
Opisthorchis viverrini
Fasciola hepatica (sheep liver fluke)
Paragonimus westermani (lung fluke)
Paragonimus kellicotti (lung fluke endemic in the United States)
Paragonimus spp.
Metorchis conjunctus (North American liver fluke)

Blood

The schistosomes are acquired by penetration of the skin by the cercarial forms that are released from freshwater snails. Although they are not endemic within the United States, occasionally patients are seen who may have these infections.

Current Name

Schistosoma mansoni
Schistosoma haematobium
Schistosoma japonicum
Schistosoma intercalatum
Schistosoma mekongi

TABLE 209.1 Human Vector-Borne Infections

Infection (Disease)	Causative Agent	Vector (Common Name)
Protozoal		
Malaria	*Plasmodium* spp.	Mosquitoes
Leishmaniasis	*Leishmania* spp.	Sandflies
Chagas disease	*Trypanosoma cruzi*	Triatomid bugs
East African trypanosomiasis	*Trypanosoma brucei rhodesiense*	Tsetse flies
West African trypanosomiasis	*Trypanosoma brucei gambiense*	Tsetse flies
Babesiosis	*Babesia* spp.	Ticks
Helminthic		
Filariasis	*Wuchereria bancrofti*	Mosquitoes
Filariasis	*Brugia malayi*	Mosquitoes
Filariasis	*Dirofilaria* spp.	Mosquitoes
Filariasis	*Mansonella perstans*	Biting midges
Filariasis	*Mansonella streptocerca*	Biting midges
Filariasis	*Mansonella ozzardi*	Biting midges
Onchocerciasis	*Onchocerca volvulus*	Black flies
Loiasis	*Loa loa*	Deer flies
Dog tapeworm infection	*Dipylidium caninum*	Dog lice and fleas, human fleas
Rat tapeworm infection	*Hymenolepis diminuta*	Rat fleas, beetles, grain beetles
Dwarf tapeworm	*Hymenolepis nana*	Grain beetles (rare)

TABLE 209.2 Medically Important Arthropods

Local or Systemic Problems	Vector (Common Name)
Skin reaction to bites	Sucking lice
	Bedbugs
	Kissing bugs
	Biting midges
	Sandflies
	Black flies
	Mosquitoes
	Deer flies
	Tsetse flies
	Soft ticks
	Hard ticks
Painful bite	Horseflies
	Fire ants
	Centipedes
Intense itching	Human itch mites
	Chiggers
Painful sting, potential anaphylaxis	Honeybees
	Bumblebees
	Wasps, hornets, yellow jackets
	Fire ants
	Scorpions
Dermatitis, ulcerations	Fleas
Nodular ulceration with subsequent secondary infection	Chigoe flea
Blistering of skin after contact with adult beetles	Blister beetles
Bite, usually painless, delayed systemic reaction	Black widow spiders
Initial blister followed by extensive necrosis and slow healing	Brown recluse spiders
	South American brown spider

BOX 209.5 Acanthocephala

The Acanthocephala or thorny-headed worms are normally parasites of fish. Although two species are found in humans, these infections tend to be somewhat rare.

Moniliformis moniliformis
Macracanthorhynchus hirudinaceus
Macracanthorhynchus ingens[8]

NEW REFERENCES SINCE THE SEVENTH EDITION

2. Brunet J, Lemoine JP, Lefebvre N, et al. Bloody diarrhea associated with hookworm infection in traveler returning to France from Myanmar. *Emerg Infect Dis.* 2015;10:1878-1879.
3. Capella-Gutierrez S, Marcet-Houben M, Gabaldon T. Phylogenomics supports microsporidia as the earliest diverging clade of sequenced fungi. *BMC Biol.* 2012;10:47.
5. Cox FEG. Taxonomy and classification of human parasitic protozoa and helminths. In: Jorgensen JH, Pfaller MA, Carroll KC, et al, eds. *Manual of Clinical Microbiology.* 11th ed. Section VIII *Parasitology*. Washington, DC: ASM Press; 2015:2285-2292.
7. Cucher MA, Macchiaroli N, Baldi G, et al. Cystic echinococcosis in South America: systematic review of species and genotypes of *Echinococcus granulosus* sensu lato in humans and natural domestic hosts. *Trop Med Int Health.* 2016;21:166-175.
8. Dingley D, Beaver PC. *Macracanthorhynchus ingens* from a child in Texas. *Am J Trop Med Hyg.* 1985;34:918-920.
9. Dubey JP, van Wilpe E, Calero-Bernal R, et al. *Sarcocystis heydorni*, m. sp. (Apicomplexa: Sarcocystidae) with cattle (*Bos taurus*) and human (*Homo sapiens*) cycle. *Parasitol Res.* 2015;114:4143-4147.
12. Garcia LS. *Diagnostic Medical Parasitology.* 6th ed. Washington, DC: ASM Press; 2016.
19. Millar SB, Cox-Singh J. Human infections with *Plasmodium knowlesi:* zoonotic malaria. *Clin Microbiol Infect.* 2015;217:640-648.
25. Stark D, Garcia LS, Barratt JL, et al. Description of *Dientamoeba fragilis* cyst and precystic forms from human samples. *J Clin Microbiol.* 2014;52:2680-2683.

The full reference list for this chapter is available at ExpertConsult.com.

210 Amebiasis

Shinjiro Hamano • William A. Petri Jr

Diarrheal diseases continue to be major causes of morbidity and mortality in children in developing countries. In Bangladesh, 10% of children in the first year of life have amebic diarrhea, and one in 30 children dies of diarrhea or dysentery by age 5 years.[85] Amebiasis is an infection caused by the protozoan parasite *Entamoeba histolytica*. Infection occurs by ingestion of the parasite's cyst from fecally contaminated food, water, or hands. Approximately 55,500 deaths, 50 million illnesses, and 2.24 million disability-adjusted life years occur annually from amebiasis, thereby rendering it the third leading cause of death by parasitic disease in humans.[79,85] Although amebiasis is present worldwide, it occurs most commonly in developing areas, especially Asia, sub-Saharan Africa, and Central and South America. In the United States and other developed countries, cases of amebiasis are most likely to occur in immigrants from and travelers to endemic regions, but amebiasis can affect populations of the developed world, as shown by the epidemic in Tbilisi in the Republic of Georgia that was caused by contaminated municipal water.[13] Currently, there is no vaccine to prevent the childhood morbidity and mortality resulting from infection with *E. histolytica*.

ETIOLOGY

E. histolytica is the cause of amebiasis and was named for the pathologic evidence of "lysis" of tissues. Additional *Entamoeba* spp. that infect humans and that are identical in appearance microscopically to *E. histolytica* include the following: *E. dispar*, which is nonpathogenic; *E. moshkovskii*, which may cause diarrhea[104]; and the more recently identified enteric parasite *E. bangladeshi*.[100] The first demonstration of the organism in human tissues was made by Lambl in 1859 in the postmortem examination of the colon of a child who died as a result of excessive diarrhea.[16,81] No connection of the organism with the disease was made until 1875, when Losch,[63] in St. Petersburg, Russia found the organism at autopsy in the colon of a woodcutter. Losch induced diarrhea and ulcerations in a dog given feces from the patient. He did not think, however, that a connection existed between the organism and the disease. The first patient described in the United States was a physician treated by Osler[81] for an amebic liver abscess in 1890. Councilman and Lafleur[28] described the organism and the disease in 1891.[21,46] Further investigation of the disease was delayed until a better understanding of the life cycle of *E. histolytica* could be obtained. In more recent years, the application of modern molecular biology techniques to the study of *E. histolytica* and *E. dispar* has resulted in an explosion of information about the mechanisms of virulence, pathogenicity, and immune responses to these organisms.[96,98]

E. histolytica is the pathogenic species, with the capacity to invade tissue and cause symptomatic disease, whereas *E. dispar* (and *E. histolytica*) is associated with the asymptomatic carrier state.[6,32,96] More recently, a study revealed that all genotypes of *E. histolytica* are not equally capable of causing disease.[6] Morphologically distinct members of the genus *Entamoeba*, such as *Entamoeba coli* and *Entamoeba hartmanni*, also are nonpathogenic. *Entamoeba moshkovskii*, *Dientamoeba fragilis*, and *Entamoeba polecki* have been associated with diarrhea, and *Entamoeba gingivalis* has been associated with periodontal disease.

Members of the genus *Entamoeba*, which are protozoan organisms belonging to the subphylum Sarcodina and close to *Dictyostelium discoideum* on one of the lowest branches of the eukaryotic tree, have trophozoite and cyst forms.[40] The cysts of *E. histolytica, E. dispar, E. moshkovskii*, and *E. bangladeshi* are almost spherical, surrounded by a cell wall composed of chitin. The cysts may have one to four nuclei, although quadrinucleate cysts are most typical. This feature allows differentiation from *E. coli*, which usually has six to eight nuclei in the cysts and may have 32 nuclei.[82] Cysts of *E. histolytica* are 5 to 20 μm in diameter (average, 12 μm) and have a greenish tint in the unstained condition.[64] Young cysts contain chromatoid bodies, which are composed of ribosome particles in crystalline arrays.[12] The cysts of *E. hartmanni* appear identical to those of *E. histolytica* except for being smaller (4–10 μm). *E. histolytica* cysts can survive for days in the dried state at 30°C or for months at 0°C to 4°C. They can be killed by temperatures greater than 50°C retained for 5 minutes.[46] They are completely resistant to the concentrations of chlorine used in water supplies but may be killed with hyperchlorination or with iodine solutions.[64,82] They are filtered from water supplies that pass through a sand filtration phase. They resist acids well.

When these quadrinucleate cysts are ingested, they resist the acid pH of the stomach and ultimately excyst in the alkaline environment of the bowel. The process of excystation results in the release of four trophozoites that divide by binary fission to produce eight trophozoites. The usual trophozoites have a diameter of 25 μm (range, 10–60 μm).[28,96] They have a single nucleus that is 3 to 5 μm in diameter and contains fine peripheral chromatin with a slightly eccentric karyosome. They have a granular endoplasm that typically contains vacuoles in which bacteria and debris can be seen. Some glycogen is present and can be stained with periodic acid–Schiff stain.

Although amebae were thought to lack organelles, such as mitochondria, endoplasmic reticulum, and Golgi apparatus, evidence to the contrary is coming to light. The existence of nuclear-encoded mitochondrial genes and a remnant mitochondrial organelle was reported more recently.[65,74,111] The presence of ingested erythrocytes is a characteristic feature of *E. histolytica* but not *E. dispar*.[96] Movement is accomplished by extension of clear pseudopodia. Replication is by binary fission. These protozoa live in the colon of humans and other mammals. Trophozoites die quickly outside the body and are quite sensitive to acid. Therefore they generally are not considered to be infective.[33] When cooled (as when feces are expelled and gradually cooled from body temperature) or stimulated by as yet undefined luminal conditions, the trophozoites form cysts that can remain viable for weeks to months on excretion.[96]

Trophozoites of *E. coli* are 15 to 50 μm in diameter; they have much more sluggish motility than the trophozoites of *E. histolytica;* and they have blunt pseudopodia, rather than the sharp, finger-like pseudopodia of *E. histolytica*. Trophozoites of *E. hartmanni* are 4 to 14 μm in diameter and have much less glycogen than the trophozoites of *E. histolytica*.[28]

EPIDEMIOLOGY

Amebiasis is distributed throughout the world. The number of people infected with either *E. histolytica* or *E. dispar* per year is estimated to be 500 million. Although most people remain asymptomatic, thus perpetuating the natural cycle of the organism through fecal excretion of infective cysts, approximately 50 million people experience the severe morbidity associated with invasive disease, with an estimated 55,500 deaths annually and 2.24 million disability-adjusted life years.[85,108] In the United States, 50% of cases of amebiasis are observed in Hispanics, Asians, and Pacific Islanders. Travelers from developing countries, malnourished persons,[76] men, and residents of institutions for the

BOX 210.1 Risk Factors for Amebiasis in the United States

Hispanic/Asian/Pacific Islanders: 50% of US cases reported to the Centers for Disease Control and Prevention
Travelers to endemic regions of the world: 0.3% incidence in one study
Institutions for intellectually disabled
Men who have sex with men
Men: 90% amebic liver abscesses found in men; rare in children

intellectually disabled are considered to be at higher risk for amebiasis (Box 210.1). In parts of Asia and Australia, *E. histolytica* is also common in men who have sex with men and can be sexually transmitted.[48] A study in Japan detected antibodies to *E. histolytica* in 21% of 1303 patients with human immunodeficiency virus infection; 88% of *E. histolytica* infections were in men who has sex with men.[67]

During the 1990s, enough evidence had accumulated to support the formal separation of two morphologically identical species of ameba, the nonpathogenic *E. dispar* from the potentially pathogenic *E. histolytica*.[1,14,31,32,39,108] Morbidity and mortality data in absolute numbers that existed before this time pertaining to cases of invasive disease were not greatly affected by this reclassification because all invasive disease was known to be caused by *E. histolytica*.[108] Because most prevalence and incidence data previously collected pertained to asymptomatic persons, however, and it was clear that most asymptomatic persons with cysts detected in their stool were infected with nonpathogenic *E. dispar*, the true prevalence and incidence of *E. histolytica* became a matter of speculation.[108]

Estimates of *E. histolytica* infections have been made primarily on the basis of examinations of stool for cysts and parasites, but these tests are insensitive and cannot differentiate *E. histolytica* from morphologically identical species, such as *E. dispar* organisms that are nonpathogenic and *E. moshkovskii* and *E. bangladeshi*.[5,23] Specific and sensitive means to detect *E. histolytica* in stool are now available and include antigen detection and polymerase chain reaction (PCR) analysis.[1,45,60]

A prospective study of preschool children in a slum of Dhaka, Bangladesh showed *E. histolytica*–associated diarrhea in 9% and *E. histolytica*–associated dysentery in 3% of the children annually.[43] Not all people are equally susceptible to amebiasis; a leptin receptor polymorphism and certain human leukocyte antigen (HLA)-DR and HLA-DQ alleles are associated with resistance to infection and disease.[24,25,80] The annual incidence of amebic liver abscess was reported to be 21 cases per 100,000 inhabitants in Hue City, Vietnam.[14] Carefully conducted serologic studies in Mexico, where amebiasis is endemic, showed antibody to *E. histolytica* in 8.4% of the population.[18] In the urban slum of Fortaleza, Brazil, 25% of all residents tested carried antibody to *E. histolytica;* the prevalence of antiamebic antibodies in children 6 to 14 years old was 40%.[15]

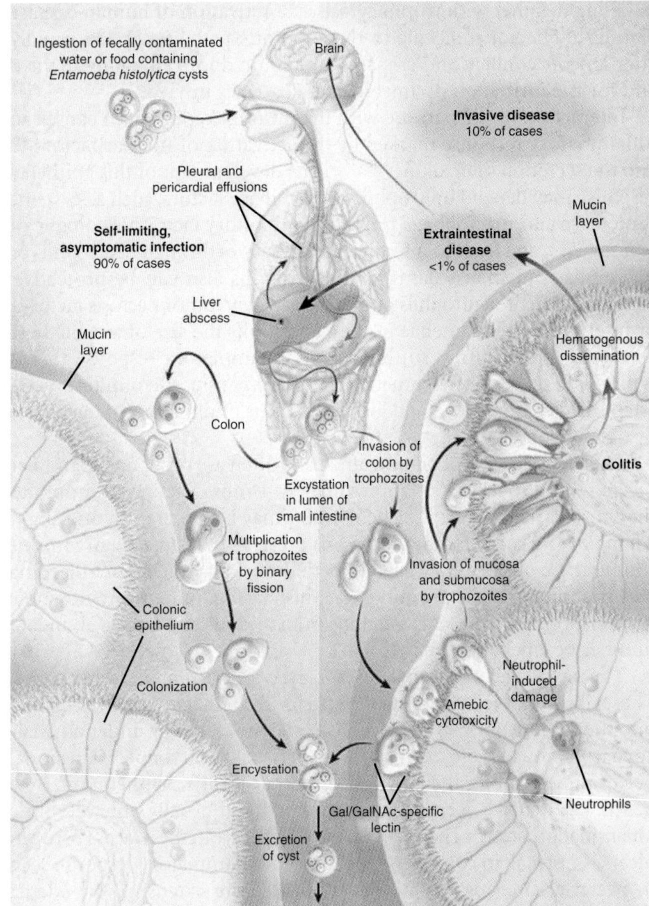

FIG. 210.1 Life cycle of *Entamoeba histolytica*. Infection normally is initiated by the ingestion of fecally contaminated water or food containing *E. histolytica* cysts. The infective cyst form of the parasite survives passage through the stomach and small intestine. Excystation occurs in the bowel lumen, where motile and potentially invasive trophozoites are formed. In most infections, the trophozoites aggregate in the intestinal mucin layer and form new cysts, resulting in a self-limited and asymptomatic infection. In some cases, adherence to and lysis of the colonic epithelium, mediated by the galactose and *N*-acetyl-D-galactosamine (Gal/GalNAc)–specific lectin, initiates invasion of the colon by trophozoites. Neutrophils responding to the invasion contribute to cellular damage at the site of invasion. When the intestinal epithelium is invaded, extraintestinal spread to the peritoneum, liver, and other sites may follow. Factors controlling invasion, as opposed to encystation, most likely include parasite "quorum sensing" signaled by the Gal/GalNAc-specific lectin, interactions of amebae with the bacterial flora of the intestine, and innate and acquired immune responses of the host. (From Haque R, Huston CD, Hughes E, et al. Amebiasis. *N Engl J Med.* 2003;348:1565–73.)

PATHOGENESIS AND PATHOLOGY

The cysts are transported through the digestive tract to the intestine, where they release their mobile, disease-producing form, the trophozoite. *E. histolytica* trophozoites can live in the large intestine and form new cysts without causing disease. They also can invade the lining of the colon, where they kill host cells and cause diarrhea, amebic colitis, acute dysentery, or chronic diarrhea.[91] The trophozoites also can be carried through the blood to other organs, most commonly the liver and occasionally the brain, where they form potentially life-threatening abscesses (Fig. 210.1). Important virulence factors include the trophozoite cell-surface galactose and *N*-acetyl-D-galactosamine (Gal/GalNAc)–specific lectin that mediates adherence to colonic mucins and host cells,[84,97] cysteine proteinases that likely promote invasion by degrading extracellular matrix and serum components, pore-forming proteins involved in killing of bacteria and host cells, and trophocytosis.[61,91,101]

The interface of the Gal/GalNAc lectin with the host mucins lining the intestine is the defining moment of the infection.[20] If the parasite lectin attaches to the host mucin glycoproteins that line the intestinal lumen, a noninvasive gut infection ensues. The life cycle continues as the trophozoites reproduce by clonal expansion in the mucin layer. Subsequently, the Gal/GalNAc lectin, along with mucin glycoproteins or other gut bacteria, initiates the developmental pathway leading to encystment.[27,108]

Colitis is caused when the trophozoite penetrates the intestinal mucous layer, which otherwise acts as a barrier to invasion by inhibiting amebic adherence to the underlying epithelium and by slowing trophozoite motility.[20] Invasion is mediated by the killing of epithelial cells, neutrophils, and lymphocytes by trophozoites, an action that occurs only after the parasite lectin engages host GalNAc on O-linked cell surface oligosaccharides.[85,91] The interaction of the lectin with glycoconjugates is stereospecific and multivalent.[117] The identity of the high-affinity intestinal epithelial cell receptor is unknown. Secretion of amebapore, a 5-kDa pore-forming protein, by the ameba may contribute to killing together with trophocytosis.[59,91] Activation of human caspase 3, a distal effector molecule in the apoptotic pathway, occurs rapidly after amebic contact, and caspases are required for cell killing in vitro and for the formation of amebic liver abscesses in vivo.[49,116]

Interaction of the parasite with the intestinal epithelium causes an inflammatory response marked by the activation of nuclear factor-κB and the secretion of cytokines.[26,77,102] The development of this epithelial response may depend on trophozoite virulence factors, such as cysteine proteinase and macrophage migration inhibitory factor homologue of *E. histolytica*, and leads to intestinal abnormalities through neutrophil- or macrophage-mediated damage.[77] Neutrophils also can be protective, and activation of neutrophils or macrophages by tumor necrosis factor-α or interferon-γ kills amebae in vitro and limits the size of amebic liver abscesses.[7,22] In contrast to the intense inflammatory response that is typical of early invasive amebiasis, inflammation surrounding well-established colonic ulcers and liver abscesses is minimal, given the degree of tissue damage.[16]

The initial lesions of clinical amebiasis often are small interglandular ulcers with a diameter of approximately 1 mm. They extend only to the muscularis mucosa.[16,69] The margins may be hyperemic, and slight edema of the surrounding mucosa is present. *E. histolytica* organisms seen in these ulcers stain well with periodic acid–Schiff stain.[86] Bleeding and friability are not prominent at this stage, although proctoscopic examination may find mucus coming from these ulcers, with an abundant number of amebae present.

The next stage of intestinal disease is the production of deeper ulcers. These "buttonhole" ulcers may be 1 cm in diameter and may extend into the submucosa.[16,86] The ulcer often extends laterally under normal-appearing mucosa, to form a characteristic flask shape. Occasional perforation through the serosa leads to peritonitis or pneumoperitoneum.[107] Extensive necrosis may be present, but usually only very little inflammation occurs. The edema is more intense, but the mucosa between ulcers is normal, in contrast to the marked inflammatory response seen in bacterial enteritis. When ulceration is more extensive, the edema surrounding the ulcers becomes confluent, and the mucosa appears gelatinous. In young children, this condition can progress to fulminant necrotizing colitis associated with transmural necrosis. The pathologic events associated with this phenomenon are not understood. Rarely, an inflammatory response is present, resulting in granulation of the tissue with a fibrous outer wall.[82] It is given the name ameboma. Occasionally, an ameboma fills a significant portion of the lumen and causes stricture or obstruction. Other complications of intestinal amebiasis result from direct extension of the ulcers. This extension may result in cutaneous involvement of the perianal area or lesions of the penis, vulva, vagina, or cervix.[2,82] Cutaneous and ophthalmologic amebiasis also is caused by fecal contamination of the face.[72]

Amebae disseminate to the liver in 50% of patients with fulminant amebiasis.[2,3] Dissemination to other organs directly from the intestine probably does not occur, but dissemination from the liver to lung, heart, brain, spleen, scapula, larynx, stomach, and aorta has been described.[16] Amebic abscess of the liver occurs more often in men than in women by a ratio of 16:1 but occurs equally often in prepubertal children of both sexes.[3,16] Abscesses occur more commonly in adults but occur in children as young as 4 months of age.[78] These abscesses vary from microscopic lesions to massive necrosis of 90% of the liver. Fever, right upper quadrant pain, and the presence of serum antibodies to amebae point to amebic liver abscess.[95] Examination of the fluid from such an abscess frequently reveals a reddish, "anchovy paste" fluid that rarely may appear white or green. The fluid is acidic, with a pH ranging from 5.2 to 6.7.[93] Amebae are found in the walls of the abscess and only rarely in the fluid of the abscess. Many patients with amebic liver abscess also have anaerobic bacteria in the abscess fluid.[94] The walls are composed of a thin connective tissue capsule. The right lobe of the liver is involved with amebic liver abscess about six times as often as the left lobe. Abscesses in the right lobe can perforate and cause disease below the diaphragm or in the thoracic cavity. Abscesses in the left lobe can lead to pericardial effusions, which are less common than pleural effusions.[34,51]

Pleural effusions can remain loculated or lead to cutaneous fistulas or to bronchopleural fistulas. Drainage from these fistulas is acidic, in contrast to the neutral secretions in the normal lung. Seeding of the cardiac valves and of the brain has been described.[16] Cerebral abscesses have the same microscopic findings as do liver abscesses, with a thin capsule of connective tissue surrounding a fluid with little or no associated inflammatory response.

IMMUNITY

Protection from amebiasis, including acquired immunity to infection and invasion by *E. histolytica*, is associated with a mucosal immunoglobulin A antibody response against the carbohydrate recognition domain of the parasite Gal/GalNAc lectin.[35,38,40,57] Cell-mediated immunity in protection from invasive amebiasis, but not infection per se, also has been shown. Substantial evidence from an in vivo animal model and more recently from human studies indicates an important role for interferon-γ and interleukin-17 in protection from amebic colitis, by acting in part by activating of macrophages to kill the parasite.[17,35,44,47] Invasive amebiasis rarely occurs in persons with human immunodeficiency virus infection or acquired immunodeficiency syndrome, even in areas where amebiasis is common; this finding suggests that an important role also exists for natural immunity or innate immune responses, or both, in protection from infection.[7,37,39]

CLINICAL MANIFESTATIONS

Intestinal Amebiasis

Asymptomatic Intraluminal Amebiasis

The most common type of amebic infestation is an asymptomatic cyst-passing carrier state. All *E. dispar* infections and 90% of *E. histolytica* infections are asymptomatic, manifesting as only *Entamoeba* cysts in the feces.[31,32,88]

Entamoeba histolytica–Associated Diarrhea

Diarrhea is the most common manifestation of amebic disease, present in 9% of children in the Mirpur cohort each year, compared with only 3% of children having amebic colitis each year.[43] *E. histolytica*–associated diarrhea is defined as three or more unformed stools in a 24-hour period accompanied by a new episode of *E. histolytica* infection. This definition was validated previously in the cohort by the following: (1) showing that diarrhea was approximately five times more common in the setting of a new infection (age-adjusted odds ratio for the association of new *E. histolytica* infection with diarrhea of 4.7; 95% confidence interval, 2.9 to 7.6); and (2) showing by a complete bacteriologic, virologic, and parasitic workup that only 32% of patients with *E. histolytica*–associated diarrhea were coinfected with another pathogen compared with identification of an enteropathogen in 59% of all cases of diarrhea.[40]

Acute Amebic Colitis

Amebic dysentery is defined by a diarrheal stool sample containing occult or gross blood that is positive for *E. histolytica* antigen. Seventy percent of patients have a gradual onset of symptoms over 3 or 4 weeks after infestation, with increasingly severe diarrhea as the primary complaint, accompanied by general abdominal tenderness. Occasionally, the onset may be acute or may be delayed for several months after infestation. This onset differs from bacterial causes of dysentery, in which patients usually have symptoms of only 1 to 2 days' duration. The diarrhea is usually associated with pain in children. Pain may be of such severity that an acute abdomen is suspected.[52,86] The stools contain blood and mucus in virtually all cases.[2,86,87] Fever is present in only a few patients with amebic colitis. Abdominal distention and dehydration occur in less than 10% of patients. In young children, intussusception, perforation, peritonitis, or necrotizing colitis may develop rapidly.[10,52,107] Amebic colitis has been shown to be associated with cognitive disability as a long-term sequela.[110]

Ameboma

Unusual manifestations of amebic colitis include toxic megacolon (0.5% of cases, usually requires surgical intervention), ameboma (granulation tissue in colonic lumen mimicking colonic cancer in appearance), and a chronic nondysenteric form of infection that can manifest as years of waxing and waning diarrhea, abdominal pain, and weight loss (easily misdiagnosed as inflammatory bowel disease).

Extraintestinal Amebiasis

Amebic Liver Abscess

The typical patient with an amebic liver abscess in the United States is an immigrant, usually Hispanic, Asian, or a Pacific Islander; is male; is 20 to 40 years old; and has fever, right upper quadrant pain, leukocytosis, abnormal serum aminotransferase and alkaline phosphatase levels, and a defect on hepatic imaging study. Roughly 90% of patients with liver abscesses are men. The abscess usually is single and is in the right lobe of the liver 80% of the time.[53] Most frequently, patients have liver abscess without concurrent colitis. Amebae are infrequently seen in the stool at the time of diagnosis of liver abscess.[3] Liver abscess can manifest acutely as fever and right upper abdominal tenderness and pain or subacutely as prominent weight loss and, less frequently, fever and abdominal pain. The peripheral white blood cell count is elevated, as is the alkaline phosphatase level, in many patients.

Early evaluation of the hepatobiliary system by ultrasonography or computed tomography (CT) is essential to show the abscess in the liver. The differential diagnosis of the lesion in the liver includes pyogenic abscess, hepatoma, and echinococcal cyst. Aspiration of the abscess occasionally is required to diagnose amebiasis (although amebae are visualized in the pus in only a few cases; if the abscess is pyogenic, the responsible bacteria are seen or cultured). Antibodies to *E. histolytica* are present in the serum of 70% to 90% of patients on acute presentation with amebic liver abscess and are useful diagnostically, especially in combination with antigen detection or PCR tests.[42] Unusual extraintestinal manifestations of amebiasis include direct extension of the liver abscess to pleura or pericardium and brain abscess. In a patient who has right upper quadrant pain, ultrasonography, CT, or magnetic resonance imaging (MRI) should be performed to examine the liver and gallbladder.

If a space-filling defect in the liver is observed, the differential diagnosis includes the following: (1) amebiasis (most common in men with a history of travel or residence in a developing country); (2) pyogenic or bacterial abscess (suspected in women, patients with cholecystitis, older persons, patients with diabetes, and patients with jaundice); (3) echinococcal abscess (an incidental finding because echinococcal abscess should not cause pain or fever); and (4) cancer. Most patients with amebic liver abscess have detectable circulating antigen in serum and serum antiamebic antibodies.[1]

In children, abdominal pain is infrequently reported with amebic liver abscess.[36,73] More commonly, high fever, abdominal distention, irritability, and tachypnea are noted. Some children are admitted to the hospital with a fever of unknown origin. Hepatomegaly occurs frequently, but elicitation of hepatic tenderness is not well documented. In one report, four of five children younger than 5 years of age died of amebic liver abscesses because the diagnosis was not suspected.[58] Death usually results from rupture of the liver abscess into the peritoneum, thorax, or pericardium, but it may follow extensive hepatic damage and liver failure.[3,92]

Metastatic Amebiasis

Extra-abdominal amebiasis presumably follows direct extension from liver abscesses, rather than direct dissemination from the intestine.[3,16] Thoracic amebiasis is the most common type of extra-abdominal amebiasis and occurs in less than 10% of patients with amebic liver abscess.[16,51] Symptoms depend on the type of involvement. Empyema, bronchohepatic fistulas, or extension of a pleuropulmonary abscess into the pericardium may occur.

Pericardial amebiasis is the next most common form of extraintestinal involvement and may result from rupture of a liver abscess in the left lobe of the liver into the pericardium or through the extension of the right-sided pleural amebiasis.[16,29,30,34] It is estimated to occur in 3% of patients with hepatic abscesses.[30] It manifests as acute pericarditis with cardiac tamponade and, occasionally, as pneumopericardium.[29] Amebic liver abscess in the left lobe also may rupture directly into the left side of the chest.[68]

Cerebral amebic abscesses are seen only in persons with amebic liver abscess and were found in 8% of patients with liver abscess discovered at autopsy in one study.[62] In other studies, lower rates of 0.66% to 4.7% of patients with amebic liver abscess and brain abscesses were reported.[50,106] Patients with cerebral amebiasis frequently are so ill from the intestinal, liver, and possibly lung involvement that neurologic signs are not always assessed easily. In 18 patients with proven cerebral amebiasis, the initial neurologic examination was normal in 13, and only one patient later developed seizures.

Other foci of infection are rare findings, but amebic rectovesical fistula formation and involvement of pharynx, heart, aorta, and scapula have been reported. Cutaneous extension after the adherence of perforated, inflamed bowel to the skin is an extremely painful and rare complication.[16,82] This situation also may arise after invasion of the skin occurs from trophozoites emerging out from the rectum.[72]

DIAGNOSIS

The prevalence of diarrhea caused by *E. histolytica* in the first year of life in impoverished children in the developing world may be as high as 10%.[75] A heightened suspicion of amebiasis should be present if the patient has been in a developing country as a resident or traveler. The diagnosis of amebiasis should be considered in any child with risk factors who has the following: diarrhea, bloody stools, or stools with mucus; a hepatic abscess; or right upper quadrant pain, abdominal distention, or tachypnea.[58,73] In a patient with diarrhea, if blood is present in the stool (grossly bloody or occult blood positive), infectious (Shiga toxin–producing *Escherichia coli, Salmonella, Shigella, Campylobacter,* and *E. histolytica*) and noninfectious (inflammatory bowel disease, diverticulosis, arteriovenous malformations, cancer) causes should be considered.

Microscopic Examination of Stool

Before the development of newer antigen detection tests and PCR analysis, amebiasis was diagnosed by examining a stool sample under a microscope to determine whether *E. histolytica* cysts were present. This method often requires more than one specimen, however, because the number of cysts in the stool varies greatly. In addition, stool microscopy has limited sensitivity and specificity. The body's immune system produces macrophage cells that can look like the amebae. Four different amebae (*E. histolytica,* which causes amebiasis; *E. dispar,* which does not cause disease; and *E. moshkovskii* and *E. bangladeshi,* which may cause diarrhea) look identical under a microscope.[23,100,104]

Polymerase Chain Reaction, Real-Time Polymerase Chain Reaction, and Antigen Detection Tests

Single and multiplex real-time PCR assays have replaced microscopy as the gold standard for the detection of this parasite. Simultaneously, several microplate enzyme-linked immunosorbent assays (ELISAs) and rapid immunochromatographic assays have been developed to detect amebic antigen in stool[114]; these tests vary in their sensitivities and specificities and often cannot reliably distinguish between *E. histolytica* and *E. dispar*. The *E. histolytica* II ELISA (TechLab) is the only Food and Drug Administration–approved commercially available microplate ELISA known to detect specifically *E. histolytica* Gal/GalNAc-specific lectin and exclude infection by other *Entamoeba* species.[42] This ELISA exhibits a greater sensitivity than that of the combination of microscopy and culture but a lower sensitivity (79%) and specificity (96%) than that of real-time PCR.[99] The *E. histolytica* antigen test can be performed rapidly and cheaply, and it can detect infection before symptoms appear. Early presymptomatic treatment can prevent the development of invasive amebiasis and minimize the spread of infection. Moreover, follow-up tests can be performed to confirm eradication of intestinal infection.

Serologic Tests

Serologic tests for antiamebic antibodies also are a very useful tool in diagnosis, with a sensitivity of 70% to 80% early in the disease and approaching 100% on convalescence.[105,109] The combined use of serologic tests and stool antigen detection or PCR analysis offers the best diagnostic approach.

Noninvasive Diagnosis of Extraintestinal Amebiasis

Amebiasis outside the intestine has been even more difficult to diagnose. Clinical manifestations of extraintestinal disease vary widely, and less than 10% of patients with amebic liver abscesses have identifiable *E. histolytica* in their stools. The TechLab *E. histolytica* II test was reported to detect Gal/GalNAc lectin in the sera of 22 of 23 (96%) patients with amebic liver abscess tested before treatment with the anti-amebic drug metronidazole and 0 of 70 (0%) controls. After 1 week of treatment with metronidazole, more than 80% of patients became serum lectin antigen negative. Detection of *E. histolytica* Gal/GalNAc lectin in the sera using the TechLab *E. histolytica* II kit is sensitive to diagnose hepatic and intestinal amebiasis before the institution of metronidazole treatment.[42] One report noted that a real-time PCR assay detected *E. histolytica* DNA in 49%, 77%, and 69% of blood, urine, and saliva specimens, respectively, from patients with amebic liver abscesses.[41]

Noninvasive diagnostic procedures such as ultrasound, CT, and MRI can detect extracolonic amebiasis in the liver, paracecal masses, brain, and other sites, but they cannot distinguish between abscesses caused by amebae and those caused by bacteria, thus hampering proper treatment of the condition. Most patients with amebic liver abscess have a single abscess in the right lobe of the liver, although multiple lesions also can occur.[4] Chest radiographs show the elevation of the right diaphragm in 56% of patients with hepatic abscess.[3] The diagnosis of cerebral amebiasis requires careful neurologic evaluation and radiographic evaluation with either CT or MRI.[16,50,62] In one case, *E. histolytica* DNA was detected by PCR in the central nervous system to make the diagnosis.[106] Because of the risk for perforation, barium studies are relatively contraindicated in patients with amebic colitis.

Biopsy Studies

The colonic and rectal mucosa in amebic colitis usually reveals ulcerations with a diameter of 1 to 10 mm. Amebic trophozoites often are at the periphery of these necrotic areas, which can be sampled through a biopsy specimen taken during sigmoidoscopy or colonoscopy.[46,53] Because of the potential for perforation, colonoscopy should be undertaken with caution.

In patients with amebic liver abscesses, amebic trophozoites are found near the capsule of the abscess. Until more recently, the most accurate diagnostic test involved examination by microscopy of a sample collected from the abscess tissue by needle aspiration, a procedure that is relatively insensitive and risky and that identifies amebic trophozoites only 20% of the time. PCR, in contrast, is a sensitive and specific means to identify *E. histolytica* in liver abscess material.[41]

Differential Diagnosis

Invasive amebic colitis may resemble ulcerative colitis, Crohn disease of the colon (inflammatory bowel disease), bacillary dysentery, or tuberculous colitis.[11,19,46,102] Stool *E. histolytica* antigen or PCR analysis, colonoscopic examination with biopsies, and serologic examination should be able to differentiate amebic colitis from these diseases. Histologic examination of involved colonic mucosa should differentiate amebic colitis, with its lack of inflammation and rare granulation tissue, from the inflammatory responses seen in ulcerative colitis, bacillary dysentery, and Crohn disease of the colon. Tuberculous colitis and Crohn disease are more likely to show granuloma formation than amebiasis. Ileocecal or small bowel involvement as seen on barium studies would suggest Crohn disease or tuberculosis of the gastrointestinal tract, rather than amebiasis. Tuberculous colitis is usually associated with pulmonary tuberculosis and with a strong reaction to tuberculin skin testing. In some cases, differentiating between invasive amebic colitis and inflammatory bowel disease may be impossible. If a patient with this differential diagnosis is administered corticosteroids and his or her condition deteriorates, the corticosteroids should be stopped, and repeat investigation for amebiasis should be performed.[19,73,82]

Amebic liver abscess must be differentiated from pyogenic abscesses and neoplastic lesions. Detection of *E. histolytica* Gal/GalNAc lectin in the sera using the TechLab *E. histolytica* II kit was helpful in one study to diagnose hepatic and intestinal amebiasis before the institution of metronidazole treatment.[42] Total leukocyte counts and cultures of blood may help to differentiate pyogenic and amebic abscesses. Many children with pyogenic liver abscesses have negative blood culture results, however. Often, amebic and pyogenic liver abscesses show similar features on CT and MRI. Occasionally, nuclear imaging with gallium is helpful because, in contrast to a pyogenic abscess, very few neutrophils are contained within an amebic liver abscess.[96,98] Gallium scanning of an amebic liver abscess may reveal a cold spot, possibly with a bright rim. For someone with risk factors for amebiasis, several investigators recommend instituting treatment for amebic abscess for 3 or 4 days while serologic, antigen detection, or PCR results are awaited.[41,73] Patients with amebic liver abscess should respond to treatment in this length of time by becoming afebrile. No change in size of the liver or size of the abscess should be noted at this time because resolution of the abscess usually takes 2 months to several years.[4,89,90,103,115]

COMPLICATIONS

Complications of amebiasis may be prevented by early establishment of diagnosis and initiation of treatment with appropriate agents.[50,73] When complications occur, the prognosis generally is worse.

Invasive intestinal amebiasis has been associated most commonly with perforation and peritonitis,[8,10,52,73,107,113] which apparently are end results of "necrotizing" or "toxic" amebic colitis. In children, perforation may be heralded by the appearance of an acute abdomen or pneumoperitoneum, with rapid progression to death, presumably from sepsis.[8,73,113] Surgical resection and therapy for endotoxic shock improve the prognosis.[113] This complication is not rare and accounts for more than 30% of deaths from amebiasis in children.[11,54] Massive intestinal hemorrhage causes approximately 3% of deaths from amebiasis. Multiple colonic strictures also can occur and cause obstructive symptoms. Fistulas to other organs or to the skin may develop.

Liver abscesses are unusual manifestations of amebiasis in children, but their resultant complications account for approximately 40% of all deaths from amebiasis.[54] Liver abscess also was found in 13% of patients with amebiasis at postmortem examinations. Liver abscess with rupture into the abdomen was present in 8% of patients who died of amebiasis, and rupture of a liver abscess into the right pleural space was found in 12%.[54] Many patients with amebic liver abscess also have anaerobic bacteria in the abscess fluid.[94] In cases free of bacterial contamination, the fluid has few inflammatory cells and an acidic pH. Amebic pericarditis or pneumopericardium occurs rarely and is found in only 1% of patients whose deaths were caused by amebiasis.[29,30,34,54] The fluid is similar to that found in the pleural space. A cerebral abscess was found in 4% of patients with amebiasis who died.[54] It has been reported in fewer than 10 children, only one of whom survived.[9,16,50,62] Other complications include infections of the retroperitoneal space, stomach, spleen, esophagus, and duodenum.[62]

TREATMENT

Intestinal Amebiasis

Asymptomatic Intraluminal Amebiasis

Therapy for asymptomatic colonization differs from therapy for invasive infection. Asymptomatic infections may be treated with intraluminal agents, such as paromomycin or diloxanide furoate. Each agent has a high rate of success for the eradication of cyst passage.[70,71] Paromomycin is a nonabsorbable aminoglycoside that is active against the cyst and trophozoite stages. High cure rates have been reported with a 7-day oral dose of paromomycin at 25 to 35 mg/kg per day in three divided doses (Table 210.1). Diloxanide furoate (Furamide), which is not approved by the Food and Drug Administration, is a poorly absorbed agent that is quite active against only intraluminal amebiasis.[66] Cure rates have been greater than 90% with a 10-day oral course of diloxanide furoate at 20 mg/kg per day in three divided doses (maximum, 1500 mg/day).[70,71,83]

Acute Amebic Colitis

Nitroimidazoles, particularly metronidazole, are the mainstays of therapy for invasive amebiasis.[40] The oral dosage of metronidazole is 35 to 50 mg/kg per day (maximum, 2250 mg/day) in three divided doses for

TABLE 210.1 Pediatric Dosage of Drugs for Amebiasis

Type of Disease	Drug	Dosage
Asymptomatic colonization	Paromomycin	25–35 mg/kg/day in 3 doses × 7 days
Mild to moderate intestinal disease	Metronidazole	35–50 mg/kg/day in 3 doses × 7–10 days
	Tinidazole	50 mg/kg/day (maximum, 2000 mg) × 3 days
Severe intestinal and extraintestinal disease	Metronidazole	35–50 mg/kg/day in 3 doses × 7–10 days
	Tinidazole	50 mg/kg/day (maximum, 2000 mg) × 3 days

7 to 10 days for severe intestinal or extraintestinal amebiasis. Metronidazole is concentrated in the ameba, probably by reduction of its nitro group by ferredoxin or flavodoxin-like electron transport proteins, which maintain a gradient for the entry of the unchanged drug. Metabolic intermediates of metronidazole damage DNA and possibly other macromolecules, and they deprive the organism of reducing equivalents by acting as an electron sink. Nitroimidazoles with longer half-lives (tinidazole, secnidazole, and ornidazole) are better tolerated and allow shorter periods of treatment.[42] For children 3 years of age or older, the oral dosage of tinidazole is 50 mg/kg per day (to a maximum of 2000 mg/day) for 5 days for severe intestinal or extraintestinal amebiasis (see Table 210.1).

Approximately 90% of patients who present with mild to moderate amebic dysentery have a response to nitroimidazole therapy. In the rare case of fulminant amebic colitis, adding broad-spectrum antibiotics to treat intestinal bacteria that may spill into the peritoneum is prudent; surgical intervention occasionally is required for acute abdomen, gastrointestinal bleeding, or toxic megacolon.[40] Agents such as metronidazole that are active against invasive and extraintestinal amebiasis are well absorbed and do not stay in the lumen long enough to have an effect on intestinal amebiasis. Parasites persist in the intestine in 40% to 60% of patients who receive nitroimidazole. Nitroimidazole treatment should be followed with paromomycin or the second-line agent diloxanide furoate to cure luminal infection.[42] Metronidazole and paromomycin should not be given at the same time because diarrhea, which is a common side effect of paromomycin, may render assessing the patient's response to therapy difficult.[54–56]

Extraintestinal Amebiasis

Amebic Liver Abscess and Metastatic Amebiasis

Extraintestinal and severe intestinal amebiasis must be treated with tissue-active agents. Metronidazole, 35 to 50 mg/kg per day in three divided doses for 7 to 10 days, is preferred because it is effective and relatively free of serious side effects (see Table 210.1).[2,3,66,96,98] It is effective for extraintestinal amebiasis in any location, although amebic brain abscesses usually are not treated successfully with any medications. Most patients with amebic liver abscess respond to metronidazole within 72 hours. For amebic colitis, follow-up therapy with a luminal agent is very important because of the high rates of asymptomatic intestinal colonization in patients with amebic liver abscess.

Therapeutic aspiration of an amebic liver abscess occasionally is required as an adjunct to antiparasitic therapy. Drainage of the abscess should be considered in patients who have no clinical response to drug therapy within 5 to 7 days or patients with a high risk of experiencing a rupture of the abscess, as defined by a cavity with a diameter of more than 5 cm or by the presence of lesions in the left lobe.[112] Because many patients with amebic liver abscess also have anaerobic bacteria in the abscess fluid,[94] the addition of antibiotics, drainage, or both to the treatment regimen in the absence of a prompt response to nitroimidazole therapy is reasonable. Image-guided percutaneous treatment (needle aspiration or catheter drainage) has replaced surgical intervention as the procedure of choice for reducing the size of an abscess.[112]

PROGNOSIS

The invasive disease develops in 50 million people each year, and 50,000 to 100,000 deaths result.[88,95,96] The case-fatality ratio is between 1:500 and 1:1000 diagnosed cases. Among patients with illness severe enough to require hospitalization, the case-fatality ratio is higher. One small study in children reported a 9% mortality rate and a 27% morbidity rate.[73]

Bowel necrosis or perforation is the cause of death from purely intestinal amebiasis, and early surgical intervention can reduce the mortality rate of these complications from 100% to 28%.[113] Amebic liver abscess has a case-fatality rate of 10% to 15% in combined figures of adults and children.[58,78,92] The mortality rate, when pleural involvement is noted, is 14%.[51,58] Amebic pericarditis has a case-fatality rate of 40%.[34] Cerebral amebiasis is fatal if untreated.[106]

FUTURE CONSIDERATIONS

Amebiasis could be prevented by eradicating fecal contamination of food and water. Providing sanitation and safe food and water for all children in developing countries is an important and achievable goal but will require massive societal changes and monetary investments. An effective amebiasis vaccine is a desirable and feasible goal to help the approximately 1 billion people living in unsanitary conditions. The high incidence of amebiasis in community-based developing country studies of infants, who bear the brunt of morbidity and mortality from diarrhea, suggests that an effective vaccine would improve children's health.

The finding that humans naturally acquire partial immunity against intestinal infection indicates that barriers to stimulating an effective acquired immune response should not be insurmountable. Aiding vaccine design is the demonstration that several recombinant antigens, including the Gal/GalNAc-specific lectin, provide protection in animal models of amebiasis and that human immunity is linked to intestinal immunoglobulin A against the lectin.[35,38,40] The high degree of sequence conservation of the Gal/GalNAc-specific lectin suggests that a vaccine could be broadly protective. Finally, the absence of epidemiologically significant animal reservoirs suggests that herd immunity could interrupt fecal-oral transmission in humans. The challenges will be to design vaccines capable of eliciting durable mucosal immunity, to understand the correlates of acquired immunity, and, most important, to enlist the continued support of industrialized nations to combat diarrheal diseases of children in developing countries.

NEW REFERENCES SINCE THE SEVENTH EDITION

17. Burgess S, Buonomo E, Carrie C, et al. Bone marrow dendritic cells from mice with an altered microbiota provide IL-17A-dependent protection from *E. histolytica* colitis. *MBio*. 2014;5:e01817.
48. Hung CC, Chang SY, Ji DD. *Entamoeba histolytica* infection in men who have sex with men. *Lancet Infect Dis*. 2012;12:729-736.
67. Marie C, Petri WA Jr. Regulaton of virulence of *Entamoeba histolytica*. *Annu Rev Microbiol*. 2014;68:493-520.
74. Mi-Ichi F, Miyamoto T, Takao S, et al. *Entamoeba* mitosomes play an important role in encystation by association with cholesteryl sulfate synthesis. *Proc Natl Acad Sci USA*. 2015;112:E2884-E2890.
77. Moonah SN, Abhyankar MM, Haque R, et al. The macrophage migration inhibitory factor homolog of *Entamoeba histolytica* binds to and immunomodulates host macrophages. *Infect Immun*. 2014;82:3523-3530.
79. Murray CJL, Vos T, Lozano R, et al. Disability-adjusted life years (DALYs) for 291 diseases and injuries in 21 regions, 1990–2010: a systematic analysis for the Global Burden of Disease Study 2010. *Lancet*. 2012;380:2197-2223.
80. Naylor C, Burgess S, Madan R, et al. Leptin receptor mutation results in defective neutrophil recruitment to the colon during *Entamoeba histolytica* infection. *MBio*. 2014;5:e02046-14.
91. Ralston KS, Solga MD, Mackey-Lawrence NM, et al. Trogocytosis-like ingestion by *Entamoeba histolytica* contributes to human cell killing and tissue invasion. *Nature*. 2014;508:526-530.
99. Roy S, Kabir M, Mondal D, et al. Real-time-PCR assay for diagnosis of *Entamoeba histolytica* infection. *J Clin Microbiol*. 2005;43:2168-2172.
114. Verkerke HP, Hanbury B, Siddique A, et al. Multisite clinical evaluation of a rapid test for *Entamoeba histolytica* in stool. *J Clin Microbiol*. 2015;53:493-497.

The full reference list for this chapter is available at ExpertConsult.com.

211 *Blastocystis hominis* and *Blastocystis* spp. Infection

Peter J. Hotez

Blastocystis hominis and related *Blastocystis* species are among the most common gastrointestinal protists of humans, with a worldwide prevalence that may be greater than 50%.[36,39] The infection is believed to be more common in low- and middle-income countries. Other *Blastocystis* spp. have been described from numerous other vertebrates and insects.[38] Although new information about the molecular and cell biology of this organism has been acquired in recent years, considerable controversy about its true taxonomy and life cycle remains.[5,36,39,42,43] The pathogenicity of *B. hominis* and its ability to cause gastrointestinal illness in humans are equally controversial. Some evidence links *B. hominis* infection to irritable bowel syndrome (IBS),[28] but emerging evidence also indicates a role of this protist in the normal human microbiome.[3,12,13,15,19,33] Investigators have also suggested that *B. hominis* infection may cause human gastrointestinal disease indirectly through the process of dysbiosis, including alteration of normal microbiota.[28]

ETIOLOGY AND PATHOGENESIS

Since its discovery in the early part of the 20th century by Alexeieff[1] and then Brumpt,[7] *B. hominis* has been assigned to many different phyla in animal and plant kingdoms. Early on, it was identified by various workers as vegetable material, a yeast, a fungus, or a protozoan. Although the organism was identified as a polymorphic protozoan parasite in 1967, its subphylum status bounced between the Sporozoa and the Sarcodina.[5] Nucleic acid sequencing data now suggest that *B. hominis* does not belong to either category,[18,16] but instead it probably constitutes its own group (class Blastocystea) more closely related to the stramenopiles, a heterogeneous group of unicellular and multicellular protists that includes slime nets, water molds, and brown algae.[39] Additional molecular taxonomic data suggest that the intraspecific variation among stocks of *B. hominis* is sufficiently different to warrant multiple separate species assignments for the organism.[6,39] Currently at least 19 subtypes are recognized within the *Blastocystis* genus, including 9 subtypes found in humans (ST1-9),[41] with ST1 and ST3 the most common subtypes isolated from humans.[35] The differences among the subtypes ultimately may have a bearing on the current controversies surrounding the pathogenicity of the organism and its different modes of transmission (i.e., zoonotic and human to human).[39] ST3 is believed to be of human origin, whereas the others may be zoonotically transmitted to humans from a variety of animal sources.[38] The genome of the ST7 subtype has been completed and shown to have an incomplete oxidative phosphorylation chain and a partial Krebs cycle despite the presence of mitochondria-like organelles.[9] These mitochondria-like organelles have been shown to increase in number after metronidazole treatments.[30]

Ultrastructural data gathered from light and electron microscopy on organisms obtained from in vitro culture and from fresh fecal material indicate the existence of at least six different parasite forms. These include cyst forms; ameboid forms; and the so-called granular, avacuolar, vacuolar, and multivacuolar forms.[5,35] The *B. hominis* vacuolar cell is the most distinctive and appears as a thin peripheral band of cytoplasm surrounding a large, membrane-enclosed central vacuole.[5] The central vacuole may have a storage function. Although *B. hominis* is thought to have predominantly anaerobic metabolism, structures that look like mitochondria have been identified on transmission electron microscopy. As noted earlier, *Blastocystis* mitochondria may function in only lipid biosynthesis and not oxidative phosphorylation.[5,42] Several highly speculative life cycles of *B. hominis* have been proposed.[5,16] The infective stage probably is a dormant cyst form that undergoes excystation in response to host gastric acid and intestinal enzymes. Excystation may result in the release of avacuolar forms that can undergo facultative transformation to either an ameboid form or a multivacuolar form. The multivacuolar form either may encyst to an infective stage or may coalesce to the vacuolar form.[5] These stages are thought to predominate in the large intestine, although organisms also have been recovered from duodenal aspirates. Which, if any, of these life cycle stages invades tissue or causes disease is unknown. Acquisition of knowledge in this area has been hampered by the lack of a suitable animal model, although infection of gnotobiotic guinea pigs with this organism was reported to result in mild intestinal hyperemia and superficial invasion of *B. hominis* into the mucosa of the cecum. Nonspecific inflammation (infiltration of lymphocytes and plasmocytes) and edema of the colonic mucosa have been seen during sigmoidoscopy with biopsy in some patients.[5] So far, except in a subset of patients with IBS who reportedly show elevated immunoglobulin G2 antibody,[14] no serologic antibody response to the organism has been shown.[8] Evidence for the role of *B. hominis* in the pathogenesis of IBS has been reviewed.[28] Among the proposed mechanisms are proteases either secreted by *B. hominis* or on the surface of the microorganism that are proinflammatory, glycosyltransferases that perturb intestinal tight junctions, and indirect mechanisms in which *B. hominis* causes dysbiosis of the gut microbiome.[28] The possibility remains that *B. hominis* is entirely commensal in humans or represents a normal component of the human microbiome.

EPIDEMIOLOGY AND CLINICAL MANIFESTATIONS

B. hominis has a worldwide distribution in tropical and temperate regions, with infection rates of 54% among some populations.[2,4,5,10,11,26,25,33,40] Developing countries, including Brazil, Egypt, and Indonesia, appear to have a higher prevalence than developed countries.[4,38,38] High rates of infection also have been reported in persons with a recent history of travel,[32] with exposure to pets or farm animals,[10] and living in institutionalized settings.[5] In many of these people, however, *B. hominis* probably is a commensal parasite. Although *B. hominis* is found commonly in preschool-age and school-age children,[26,25,27] children overall do not seem to be at increased risk for acquisition of infection.[5] Contaminated water may represent the most common source of *B. hominis* transmission.[38]

Most studies investigating the association between *B. hominis* infection and disease primarily have as their basis clinical laboratory isolates of the organism in patients exhibiting gastrointestinal symptoms. Common clinical complaints include abdominal discomfort, bloating, cramping, diarrhea, and vomiting.[2] Seroconversion to *B. hominis* antigens has been linked to IBS.[14,24] The presence of *Blastocystis* nucleic acids from ST3 to ST5 have been linked to increase interleukin levels in patients with IBS.[29] Weight loss associated with protein-losing enteropathy also has been described. Infective arthritis also has been reported.[19] Because *B. hominis* commonly is found in symptomatic and asymptomatic persons, some investigators proposed that only very heavy infections result in disease.[20,34] Many of these studies were not controlled, however. Overall, the most common symptoms ascribed to *B. hominis* infection are abdominal pain and diarrhea.[38]

Shlim and colleagues[34] conducted a large, prospective controlled study in a population of expatriates and tourists in Katmandu, Nepal who were at high risk for development of traveler's diarrhea. These investigators concluded that *B. hominis* in high concentrations was not associated with diarrhea and that the presence of higher concentrations of the organism in stool was not associated with more severe symptoms.[34] In a subsequent editorial, several design features were cited that may "weaken the authors' conclusions."[18] At least four other prospective trials have been conducted; one supported *B. hominis* as a cause of diarrhea, one argued against it, and two others were inconclusive.[32] The confusion may be resolved partly by the increasing recognition of separate human subtypes of *Blastocystis*,[6,16] which may lead to improved molecular diagnostic techniques to distinguish pathogenic from nonpathogenic species. This situation is somewhat analogous to the morphologically identical species of *Entamoeba* (*Entamoeba histolytica* and *Entamoeba dispar*, only the former of which causes colitis). Some investigators believe that by distinguishing among the different subtypes, at least one or more may be identified as pathogenic, especially among immunocompromised patients, including patients who have undergone spenectomy.[17,38]

DIAGNOSIS

Examination by light microscopy of wet preparations of fresh or concentrated stool usually identifies *B. hominis*. Staining of preparations with iodine or trichrome also is beneficial. Many laboratories attempt to identify the characteristic vacuolar forms, which may be underrepresented in clinical material.[5] Under these circumstances, the services of an experienced technologist are required to identify the less distinctive fecal cyst form.[39] Organisms also can be recovered from biopsy material obtained during sigmoidoscopy and colonoscopy.

TREATMENT

Given the controversy surrounding the pathogenicity of *B. hominis*, a prudent approach is to refrain from treating asymptomatic immunocompetent persons.[21] In patients who have gastrointestinal illness, including IBS, and in whom other pathogens have been excluded, administering a course of antiprotozoal chemotherapy may be reasonable. The results of several drug studies, including three that were placebo controlled, indicate that therapeutic improvements with parasite clearance in symptomatic patients were noted with the use of metronidazole (15–30 mg/kg per day for 7 to 10 days), nitazoxanide (200 mg twice daily for children 4–11 years old and 100 mg twice daily for children 1–3 years old for 3 days), and trimethoprim-sulfamethoxazole (6 mg/kg trimethoprim and 30 mg/kg sulfamethoxazole daily in two equal doses for 7 days in children; 320 mg trimethoprim and 1600 mg sulfamethoxazole daily in two equal doses for 7 days in adults).[22,38] However, because these drugs are broad spectrum, it is possible that clinical improvement may have been a consequence of treating an unidentified enteric pathogen.[38] To date, the scientific community has been unable to fulfill the Koch postulates for members of the genus *Blastocystis*.[38] Some investigators have reported symptomatic improvement in patients receiving either metronidazole or tinidazole.[5,11]

Using an in vitro assay that used metabolic labeling, researchers found that the drugs emetine, satranidazole, furazolidone, and quinacrine were superior in activity to either metronidazole or tinidazole.[5] These authors cautioned, however, that the in vitro assay does not take into account the pharmacokinetic properties of the drugs. More recent in vitro testing of ST1, ST3, ST4, and ST8 found that *B. hominis* exhibits minimal sensitivity to metronidazole, paromomycin, and triple therapy consisting of furazolidone, nitazoxanide, and secnidazole; however, sensitivity to trimethoprim-sulfamethoxazole and ivermectin was observed.[31] A clinical pilot study from Australia reported on the efficacy of triple antibiotic therapy in 10 adult patients with *Blastocystis*-positive IBS.[23] The three-drug (or drug combination) regimen comprised diloxanide furoate, trimethoprim-sulfamethoxazole, and secnidazole for 14 days, and it was shown to clear *Blastocystis* infection in 60% of patients, but with inconclusive effects on IBS in this small pilot study, such that larger studies may be required.[23] Ultimately, additional studies that examine drug sensitivities of different *Blastocystis* subtypes may help clarify this situation, but for now the status of treating human *Blastocystis* infection remains controversial.[35]

NEW REFERENCES SINCE THE SIXTH EDITION

3. Andersen LO, Stensvold CR. *Blastocystis* in health and disease: are we moving from a clinical to a public health perspective? *J Clin Microbiol*. 2016;54:524-528.
9. Denoeud F, Roussel M, Noel B, et al. Genome sequence of the stramenopile *Blastocystis*, a human anaerobic parasite. *Genome Biol*. 2011;12:R29.
17. Karasartova D, Gureser AS, Zorlu M, et al. Blastocystosis in post-traumatic splenectomized patients. *Parasitol Int*. 2016;65:802-805.
23. Nagel R, Bielefeldt-Ohmann H, Traub R. Clinical pilot study: efficacy of triple antibiotic therapy in *Blastocystis* positive irritable bowel syndrome patients. *Gut Pathog*. 2014;6:34.
24. Nagel R, Traub RJ, Kwan MM, et al. *Blastocystis* specific serum immunoglobulin in patients with irritable bowel syndrome (IBS) versus healthy controls. *Parasit Vectors*. 2015;8:453.
28. Poirier P, Wawrzyniak I, Vivares CP, et al. New insights into *Blastocystis* spp.: a potential link with irritable bowel syndrome. *PLoS Pathog*. 2012;8:e1002545.
29. Ragavan ND, Kumar S, Chye TT, et al. *Blastocystis* sp. in irritable bowel syndrome (IBS): detection in stool aspirates during colonoscopy. *PLoS ONE*. 2015;10:e0121173.
30. Raman K, Kumar S, Chye TT. Increase number of mitochondrion-like organelle in symptomatic *Blastocystis* subtype 3 due to metronidazole treatment. *Parasitol Res*. 2016;115:391-396.
31. Roberts T, Bush S, Ellis J, et al. In vitro antimicrobial susceptibility patterns of *Blastocystis*. *Antimicrob Agents Chemother*. 2015;59:4417-4423.
35. Stensvold CR, Smith HV, Nagel R, et al. Eradication of *Blastocystis* carriage with antimicrobials: reality or delusion? *J Clin Gastroenterol*. 2010;44:85-90.
37. Sungkar S, Pohan AP, Ramadani A, et al. Heavy burden of intestinal parasite infections in Kalena Rongo village, a rural area in South West Sumba, eastern part of Indonesia: a cross sectional study. *BMC Public Health*. 2015;15:1296.
38. Tan KSW. New insights on classification, identification, and clinical relevance of *Blastocystis* spp. *Clin Microbiol Rev*. 2008;21:639-665.
41. Yason JA, Tan KS. Seeing the whole elephant: imaging flow cytometry reveals extensive morphological diversity within *Blastocystis* isolates. *PLoS ONE*. 2015;10:e0143974.

The full reference list for this chapter is available at ExpertConsult.com.

Entamoeba coli Infection 212

Peter J. Hotez

Until recently, *Entamoeba coli* was considered to be entirely nonpathogenic and was of interest to the clinician only because of its morphologic similarities to *Entamoeba histolytica* that could result in misdiagnosis. In 1991, several case reports from northern Europe appeared, however, that implicated *E. coli* as a possible cause of infectious diarrhea.[2,5,10] Two cases of diarrhea associated with *E. coli* have been described in children.[2]

ETIOLOGY AND PATHOGENESIS

E. coli, similar to other members of the genus *Entamoeba*, has trophozoite and cyst forms. The trophozoite is similar in size to that of *E. histolytica* (15–50 μm) but has a more sluggish motility with short pseudopodia.[4] The cytoplasm is described as granular, coarse, or frothy and contains numerous bacteria, yeasts, and other food materials.[4,8] Occasionally, red blood cells are seen in the cytoplasm, but their occurrence is not nearly as common as in pathogenic strains of *E. histolytica.* During passage through the colon, the trophozoite rounds up and synthesizes a chitin-containing cyst wall. *E. coli* cysts measure 10 to 35 µm and usually contain 8 to 16 nuclei, although occasionally 32 nuclei are seen.

Transmission of *E. coli* infection occurs through the fecal-oral route in the same manner as *E. histolytica* infection. On cyst ingestion, the total number of excysting trophozoites usually is lower than eight.[4] The *E. coli* trophozoites colonize the lumen of the large intestine. Very little is known about the events by which *E. coli* trophozoites occasionally cause human gastrointestinal illness. Even with a pathogenic *E. coli* strain, the invasive potential of this organism is presumed not to be nearly as great as that of *E. histolytica* because diarrheal disease in patients infected with *E. coli* is not associated with dysentery or accompanied by leukocytosis or elevated serum immunoglobulin A level.[10]

EPIDEMIOLOGY AND CLINICAL MANIFESTATIONS

E. coli is worldwide in distribution, although it occurs more commonly in warmer climates, especially in tropical urban slums, and in some populations of homosexual men.[4,6] In 1991, Wahlgren[10] described eight patients from Sweden with mild or persistent diarrhea who harbored *E. coli.* Before receiving specific antiamebic chemotherapy, all eight patients had their stools examined repeatedly by the following means: (1) light microscopy, to exclude other protozoa and helminths; (2) electron microscopy, to exclude the presence of some pathogenic viruses; and (3) aerobic and anaerobic culture, to exclude pathogenic bacteria. These patients typically had a long history of loose but not watery stools (without blood or mucus), flatulence, and colicky pain. One patient was a parasitology laboratory technician who had symptoms for more than 15 years. Every patient responded to specific antiamebic chemotherapy.[10] Two children with similar symptoms who also responded to antiamebic chemotherapy subsequently were described in Ireland.[2] In a more recent study, children in Mexico infected with *E. coli* were shown to exhibit higher percentages of body fat,[11] such that *E. coli* amebiasis may contribute to childhood obesity.

DIAGNOSIS AND TREATMENT

E. coli sometimes is difficult to distinguish from *E. histolytica,* particularly because the nuclear structures of their trophozoite stages are similar.[3] Some differences exist, however, including the karyosome, which is eccentric in *E. coli* but central in *E. histolytica,* and the cytoplasm, which is coarse and seldom contains red blood cells in *E. coli,* in contrast to *E. histolytica.*[3] The differences between the cyst stages of *E. coli* and *E. histolytica* (and *Entamoeba dispar*) are more apparent. The *E. coli* cyst typically has two to four times more nuclei than cysts in *E. histolytica.* The *E. coli* cyst has been reported to become more refractive during fixation so that it often is visualized better in a wet preparation.[4] With use of the polymerase chain reaction assay it is possible to distinguish *E. coli* from other pathogenic amebas.[7] A newer Luminex assay has also been developed to distinguish among different ameba species found in human stool.[9]

Generally, *E. coli* still is regarded by most investigators as a commensal organism. In patients with persistent diarrhea whose diagnostic fecal evaluation reveals only the presence of *E. coli,* administering a course of specific antiamebic therapy is reasonable.[1] All the Swedish patients were reported to respond to a 10-day course of diloxanide furoate in a dose of 500 mg three times daily.[7] Children also may respond to an equivalent pediatric dose of 20 mg/kg per day in three divided doses for 10 days. As of 1994, diloxanide furoate was available in the United States from the Centers for Disease Control and Prevention Drug Service. Alternatively, two children from Ireland (where diloxanide furoate was unavailable) were treated successfully for *Entamoeba coli*–associated diarrhea with metronidazole.[2]

NEW REFERENCES SINCE THE SEVENTH EDITION

6. Korkes F, Kumagai FU, Belfort RN, et al. Relationship between intestinal parasitic infection in children and soil contamination in an urban slum. *J Trop Pediatr.* 2009;55:42-45.
7. Proctor EM. Laboratory diagnosis of amebiasis. *Clin Lab Med.* 1991;11:829-859.
9. Santos HL, Bandyopadhyay K, Bandea R, et al. LUMINEX(R): a new technology for the simultaneous identification of five *Entamoeba* spp. commonly found in human stools. *Parasit Vectors.* 2013;6:69.
11. Zavala GA, Garcia OP, Campos-Ponce M, et al. Children with moderate-high infection with *Entamoeba coli* have higher percentage of body and abdominal fat than non-infected children. *Pediatr Obes.* 2016;11:443-449.

The full reference list for this chapter is available at ExpertConsult.com.

213 Giardiasis

Tina Q. Tan

Giardiasis is caused by an infection with the flagellated, binucleated protozoan parasite *Giardia lamblia* (also known as *Giardia duodenalis* or *Giardia intestinalis*). Worldwide, it is one of the most prevalent and important infectious causes of diarrheal illness in humans.[98] Anton van Leeuwenhoek first described the parasite when examining his own stool under a microscope in 1681. Vilem Lambl described the trophozoite in 1859, and Grassi described the cyst in 1879.[82] This flagellated parasite, which belongs to the genus *Giardia,* family Hexamitidae, and supergroup Excavata,[118] is one of the most ancient eukaryotes and lacks many organelles, including Golgi apparatus, peroxisomes, and mitochondria.[43] In 2003, however, mitochondrial genes were discovered in the organism; and the organism has been shown to possess specialized membrane structures, known as mitosomes, that perform the respiratory chain activities of the inner mitochondrial membrane. This finding lends support to the theory that *Giardia* organisms have become highly evolved and have lost many ancestral characteristics.[1,4,75,76,99,126,127] For centuries, *Giardia* organisms were thought to be nonpathogenic, but data since the 1980s have shown that *G. lamblia* can be a pathogen that causes both sporadic and epidemic disease.[34,54]

ORGANISM AND ETIOLOGY

This organism has two morphologic forms: the infectious cyst, which is relatively resistant to chemicals and environmental stresses; and the motile trophozoite, which is responsible for the disease. The trophozoite is pear shaped, with a dorsal convexity and a spiral organelle on its ventral surface. The spiral organelle or sucking disk is the way in which the organism attaches to the epithelial microvillus of the upper small intestine.[93] The trophozoite usually measures 10 to 21 μm in length and 5 to 15 μm in width. It has a complex cytoskeleton that maintains the shape of the parasite and anchors the four pairs of flagella, which emerge ventrally, anterolaterally, posterolaterally, and caudally from the cell body. It also has two diploid oval symmetric nuclei surrounded by nuclear envelopes. These nuclei are each approximately 1 μm in diameter and are located in the anterior half of the cell, at the right and left sides of the longitudinal axis. They live in the small intestine and divide by binary fission. The cyst form is most commonly seen in stool samples and is oval, measuring 8 to 12 μm in length and 5 to 10 μm in width. It contains two to four nuclei and remnants of organelles. Cysts can remain viable for long periods of time (≥3 months) in cold water and are resistant to killing by iodine and chlorine, but they can be destroyed by heating to 50°C and by desiccation. This form of the parasite is responsible for transmission among susceptible hosts.[2,16,17] Six species of *Giardia* have been identified on the basis of the morphologic characteristics of the trophozoite: *G. duodenalis, G. agilis, G. muris, G. ardeae, G. psittaci,* and *G. microti. G. lamblia,* also called *G. duodenalis,* is the primary pathogenic species in humans and other mammals. All the other species primarily infect animal species and cause no significant disease in humans. The species that infects humans is morphologically indistinguishable from that of other mammals.[2,54] Isoenzyme and genetic analyses indicate that isolates from infected individuals exhibit high levels of genetic diversity and comprise a large number of genotypes, which can be placed in four groups.[18] The different isolates within groups demonstrate some specificity for infection in various mammals versus humans, but no consistent genetic differences exist between isolates that cause symptomatic versus asymptomatic disease. The genotypes are grouped into two major genetic assemblages (assemblage A and assemblage B) and several minor assemblages (assemblages C, D, E, F, and G) that have very strong host specificities and narrow host ranges. It is believed that humans are infected only with assemblages A and B.[34] Studies have demonstrated that in symptomatic infection the correlation between isolate assemblage type and severity of infection is strong; however, the infectivity and pathogenicity of *Giardia* genotypes seem to vary depending on the age, clinical and nutritional status, and immune responses of the host.[2,59,88,102]

EPIDEMIOLOGY

Giardia infections are ubiquitous, and outbreaks occur in developed and developing countries throughout the world. Cross-transmission and infection occur between domestic and wild animals and humans and between humans.[30,113] Transmission involves the fecal-oral, waterborne, and foodborne transmission of cysts; thus the level of sanitation and a high intradomiciliary or peridomiciliary concentration of domestic animals are directly related to the prevalence of infection.[36,61,66,77,111,117] *Giardia* is one of the most common parasites in the United States; it affects persons of all ages and is found in 4.2% to 7% of specimens submitted to the laboratory for examination.[65] The populations that are affected most frequently include children from birth to 5 years of age, adults 31 to 40 years of age, and backpackers, campers, hunters, and travelers to areas where the disease is endemic.[60,85] Data from the National Giardiasis Surveillance System of the Centers for Disease Control and Prevention estimate that 2.5 million cases occur each year in the United States.[141] Cases per 100,000 population range from 1.4 to 30, with seven states reporting more than 15 cases per 100,000 population. In 2005, Vermont had the highest incidence, with 30 cases per 100,000 population. Cases are more prevalent in boys and men, and rates are highest in children 1 to 4 years of age (children in day care and their close contacts), followed closely by children 5 to 9 years of age and adults 31 to 39 years of age. Most cases are reported in the early summer through early fall.[141]

Giardia is a frequent cause of diarrhea in day care centers around the world, with infection rates of 1% to 55%.[3,9,68,89,92,97] Most children are symptomatic, and long-term passage of cysts in some preschool-aged children in day care centers may last for as long as 5 to 6 months after the initial diagnosis. Transmission from these infants and children to adult family members is not an uncommon occurrence; up to 25% of the children have *Giardia*-positive stools. The prevalence rates are highest in centers with many non–toilet-trained children and staff members who change diapers and prepare food without adequate hand washing. Prevalence rates decline after children are toilet trained.[9] Sexual transmission may occur with both heterosexual and homosexual contact, but male homosexual behavior is an established risk factor for acquiring *G. lamblia* infection, and cyst passage rates may be as high as 20%.[57,67,73] Other persons at risk include campers, backpackers, hunters, and other travelers to national parks, wilderness areas, and disease-endemic areas because of vertical transmission from animals and ingestion of untreated drinking water.[137] Patients who were infected during travel had longer exposures in countries where the prevalence was high.[63] *Giardia* has been found to be the most common cause of diarrhea in travelers presenting to travel clinics.[107,110] In addition, many outbreaks have been reported in municipal water supplies that have not been treated with flocculation or filtration. From 1985 to 1994, *Giardia* was responsible for 44% of the outbreaks of waterborne diarrheal illness in which a cause could be determined. Sixty-four percent of these outbreaks were associated with unfiltered water. According to a sample survey of 66 reservoir sites in Canada and the United States, 81% contained *Giardia* cysts at a concentration of 3 cysts/L before treatment and 1.7 cysts/L after treatment.[69,70] Treatment of water with iodine preparations kills most cysts, but the cysts are relatively resistant to chlorination. Swimming pools may be another source of infection when pools are used by diapered infants and developmentally delayed persons.[100] A less common mode of transmission is through ingestion of contaminated food, in which as few as 10 cysts may be required to establish infection.[84,104] Transmission has also been documented through ingestion of green leafy vegetables and culinary bivalves harboring *G. lamblia* shed from coastal and marine life.[42,114]

PATHOGENESIS

Humans are infected by the oral ingestion of as few as 10 to 25 cysts.[104] If symptoms develop, the onset usually begins after a 6- to 15-day incubation period that often precedes detection of parasites in stool. Excystation occurs in the stomach and small intestine, and the trophozoites are found in large numbers in the upper part of the small intestine, where they closely apply their sucking disks to the mucosa (Fig. 213.1). They may penetrate into the secretory tubules of the mucosa and at times are found in the gallbladder and in the biliary drainage. Scanning electron micrographs of the intestinal mucosa (Fig. 213.2) demonstrate the mechanical damage caused by the presence of the organisms on the mucosal surface. The histologic changes seen in the tissues do not always correlate with the presence or absence of symptoms. Biopsy specimens of the small intestine in children and adults show normal histologic features despite the presence of diarrhea and other symptoms.[28] Conversely, flattening of the brush border, damage to mucosal epithelial cells, and slight flattening of the

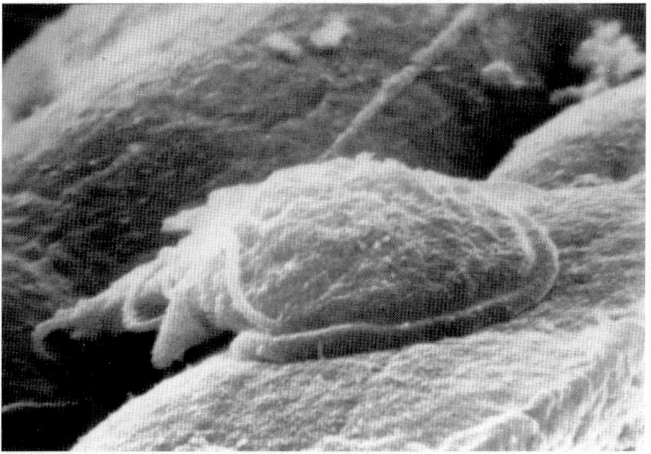

FIG. 213.1 Trophozoite of *Giardia lamblia* adhering to the intestinal surface.

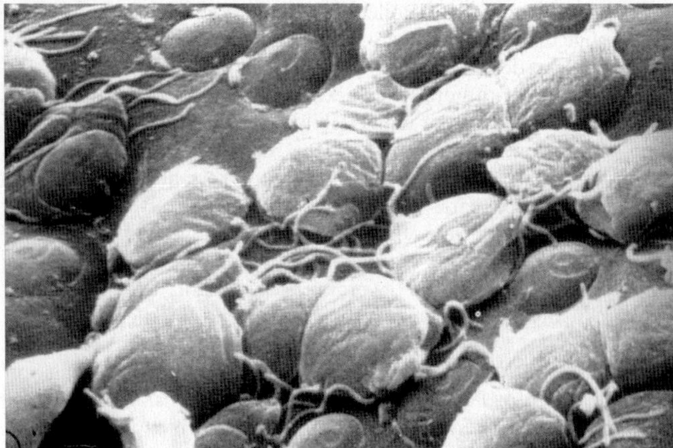

FIG. 213.2 Scanning electron micrograph of trophozoites of *Giardia lamblia* from an intestinal biopsy. Note the indentations left on the mucosal surface by the parasite's sucking disk.

villi with increased mitotic index, increased goblet cells, alteration of bile content or duodenal flora, and infiltration with inflammatory cells also may be present.[29,90,105,140] Studies have demonstrated that *Giardia* disrupts the tight junctional zona occludens, increases permeability, and induces apoptosis in small intestinal epithelial cells. Disruption of the intestinal epithelial cell brush border and inhibition of brush-border enzymes and trypsin may explain the lactose intolerance that commonly develops.[12,20] In vivo and in vitro studies have established that *Giardia* causes malabsorption of glucose, sodium, and water and hypersecretion of chloride and reduces disaccharidase activity, secondary to shortening of the microvilli in a $CD8^+$ lymphocyte–dependent manner, thus resulting in loss of epithelial absorptive surface area.[6,7,11,22,23,115,116] Disruption of digestion by bile and proteases may produce malabsorption, diarrhea, and resultant malnutrition.

Giardia-infected persons may have a spectrum of manifestations ranging from asymptomatic carriage to acute or chronic diarrheal disease, the causes of which are not well understood. Hypotheses include the following: (1) the parasite as a physical barrier to absorption; (2) disruption of the brush border with loss of enzymatic activity; (3) elaboration of toxins by the parasite; (4) changes in fat absorption in the small intestine; (5) activation of cytokines with mucosal inflammation after damage to enterocytes; (6) luminal competition for nutrients; (7) induction of epithelial cell damage, arrested proliferation, and tight-junctional abnormalities; (8) disaccharidase deficiency; (9) nutrient-dependent growth impairment and decreased villus-to-crypt ratios; and (10) translocation of microbiota across the mucosa.[19,94,121,122,125] However, it appears that the primary cause of diarrhea in giardiasis is malabsorption.

Host immunity, both the humoral and cellular components, is important in the variable manifestations of giardiasis and in clearance and protection against reinfection with *Giardia.* Persistence of infection in nude mice suggests a role for T-cell activity.[31,106,124] Humans produce serum immunoglobulin (Ig) G, IgM, IgA, IgE, mast cells, T cells, dendritic cells, and nitric oxide in response to infection.* Studies have shown that IgM and IgG antibody with complement is lethal to *Giardia* trophozoites. In the intestinal lumen, the secretory IgA response appears to play a role in the modulation of infection, as does the migration of infiltrating lymphocytes in the intestinal mucosa.[27,78,112] The absence of secretory IgA is associated with the inability to clear *Giardia* infection and is associated with the development of chronic giardiasis in humans.[18,101] Eighty-four percent of human volunteers experienced self-cure in 18.4 days, whereas the remainder became chronically infected.[104] Human milk has been shown to kill the trophozoites of *G. lamblia* by generating toxic lipolytic products.[43,44,103]

Infection may be severe and difficult to eradicate in immunodeficient persons with antibody deficiencies (e.g., common variable immunodeficiency, X-linked agammaglobulinemia) or in patients with reduced gastric acidity. Giardiasis long has been associated with hypogammaglobulinemia, nodular lymphoid hyperplasia of the small intestine, and chronic diarrhea.[55] Patients with hypogammaglobulinemia, absence of plasma cells in the intestinal lamina propria, cystic fibrosis, protein-calorie malnutrition, and human immunodeficiency virus infection (or acquired immunodeficiency syndrome) and patients who are receiving immunosuppressive therapy are more likely to develop chronic giardiasis than are patients with X-linked hypogammaglobulinemia, selective IgA deficiency, and Wiskott-Aldrich or Nezelof syndrome.[62,91,119]

*References 38, 41, 44, 47, 88, 95, 104, 109, 117, 120, 135.

TABLE 213.1 Symptoms of Giardiasis

Symptom	Frequency (%)
Flatulence	56–74
Anorexia	40–64
Abdominal cramps	55–80
Foul-smelling stool	57–72
Abdominal distention	31
Bloating	55–69
Nausea	58–68
Malaise	84
Diarrhea	89
Belching	30
Weight loss	48–64
Fever	17–28

TABLE 213.2 Stool Characteristics of Giardiasis

Characteristic	Frequency (%)
Mushy	52
Formed	33
Watery	12
Mucous	3
Blood	0

CLINICAL MANIFESTATIONS

Infection with *Giardia* can result in asymptomatic infection (5–15%), an acute self-limited diarrheal illness (25–50%), or chronic diarrhea and malabsorption, depending on host susceptibility and pathogen genotype virulence.[6,52,60] The incubation period for giardiasis is 7 to 14 days. Symptoms may vary from mild abdominal discomfort and diarrhea to severe cramping, bloating, and severe, explosive, watery, greasy, foul-smelling diarrhea (Table 213.1).[57] Patients and caretakers describe a constellation of signs and symptoms, including abdominal bloating, flatulence, and frequent foul-smelling diarrhea. Young infants may exhibit anorexia, weight loss, or a malabsorption syndrome that resembles sprue. Symptoms usually last for more than 7 to 10 days and in the majority of cases clear spontaneously. Stooling patterns vary from normal to mushy, foul-smelling diarrhea (Table 213.2). Gross blood, pus, and mucus are usually not present in the stool, and signs of inflammatory diarrhea, such as tenesmus and bloody diarrhea, do not occur. *Giardia* infection also may lead to disorders at extraintestinal sites. Extraintestinal symptoms may involve the eyes (iridocyclitis, choroiditis, retinal hemorrhages, and "salt and pepper" degeneration involving the retinal pigmented epithelium),[21,96] joints (reactive arthritis most commonly involving the joints of the lower limbs, particularly the knee and ankle),[15,58] muscles (hypokalemic myopathy), skin, and circulation and may cause micronutrient deficiencies, iron deficiency anemia, protein-energy malnutrition, and growth and cognitive retardation.[23,51] One study estimated that one-third of patients infected with *Giardia* will express long-term extraintestinal symptoms, a finding suggesting that this involvement is not as uncommon as previously believed.[14]

TABLE 213.3 **Drugs for the Treatment of Giardiasis**

Drug	Dose	Efficacy (%)	Side Effects
Metronidazole	15 mg/kg/day orally divided 3 times a day for 5–10 days (maximum, 750 mg/day)	80–100	Metallic taste, headache, nausea, vomiting, rash, peripheral neuropathy, neutropenia, disulfiram-like effects
Tinidazole	50 mg/kg, single dose (maximum, 2 g)	80–96	Metallic taste, nausea, vomiting, headache, rash, peripheral neuropathy, neutropenia, disulfiram-like effects
Ornidazole[a]	40–50 mg/kg, single dose (maximum, 2 g)	96–100	Metallic taste, nausea, vomiting, headache, rash, peripheral neuropathy, neutropenia, disulfiram-like effects
Secnidazole	2 g, single dose	90	Nausea, anorexia, abdominal pain
Albendazole[b]	15 mg/kg per day for 5–7 days (maximum, 400 mg/day)	94–100	Anorexia, constipation, neutropenia, elevated liver function test results
Furazolidone	6 mg/kg per day orally divided 4 times a day for 10 days	81–96	Allergic reactions, headache, nausea, vomiting, diarrhea, brown discoloration of urine, hemolysis, disulfiram-like effects
Paromomycin	30 mg/kg per day divided 3 times a day for 5–10 days (maximum, 1.5 g/day)	55–88	Nausea, vomiting, ototoxicity, nephrotoxicity
Quinacrine[a]	6 mg/kg per day divided 3 times a day for 7 days	92–95	Nausea, vomiting, dizziness, headache, yellow or orange skin and mucous membrane discoloration, hemolysis, toxic psychosis
Nitazoxanide	1–3 years: 200 mg/day divided 2 times a day for 3 days 4–11 years: 400 mg/day divided 2 times a day for 3 days ≥12 years: 1000 mg/day divided 2 times a day for 3 days	85–90	Nausea, abdominal pain, diarrhea, anorexia, flatulence, headache, yellow eyes, discolored urine, increased creatinine and serum glutamic-pyruvic transaminase levels

[a]No longer produced in the United States. Can be obtained from Panorama Pharmacy, Panorama City, CA.
[b]Not approved by the US Food and Drug Administration for this indication in the United States.

A few patients develop persistent, chronic infection that is associated with severe malaise, headache, weight loss, and diffuse abdominal and epigastric discomfort that is exacerbated by eating. Episodes of diarrhea typically alternate with periods of normal bowel movements and may persist over a period of months. Lactose intolerance may develop in 20% to 40% of patients and persist for weeks after the infection has been eradicated.[119,138] Children with symptomatic giardiasis may develop steatorrhea and malabsorption of vitamin A, vitamin B_{12}, protein, D-xylose, and iron.[46,51,123] Anecdotal reports have attributed a variety of other symptoms, including rash, urticaria, arthralgia, reactive arthritis, constipation, biliary tract disease, and gastric infection to giardiasis, but no firm evidence supports *G. lamblia* as the cause of these symptoms.

Cyst passers may be asymptomatic and may serve as a reservoir of infection for others. This fact is particularly important for food handler and day care center outbreaks. Severe, prolonged illness that requires hospitalization occurs in 2 per 100,000 cases, a rate similar to that seen in shigellosis.[72] Hospital admission for young children and pregnant women usually is required because of volume depletion and failure to thrive.[123]

Parasitic infection, including giardiasis, should be considered in the evaluation of the child who fails to thrive and in immunocompromised infants and children who have diarrhea or gastrointestinal complaints. It also should be considered in the differential diagnosis of any child who is in day care or who has traveled outside the United States and has gastrointestinal symptoms.[53,89]

DIAGNOSIS

Obtaining a thorough travel and potential exposure history is important in making the diagnosis of giardiasis. Recent travel to wilderness areas or a national park and travel to developing areas or other endemic areas of the world where fecal-oral hygiene is a problem are important parts of the history in any patient with persistent diarrhea. Demonstration of trophozoites or cysts in the stool on ova and parasite examination is the traditional standard of diagnosis.[83] Examination of preserved fecal specimens reveals cysts or trophozoites in most infections. Organisms are excreted in a highly variable pattern; therefore, multiple samples taken on different days are required for detection.[26] A single stool sample misses 20% to 40% of the infections, whereas three stool samples miss less than 10% of infections.[56]

Commercially available tests to detect antigen by an enzyme-linked immunosorbent assay (ELISA) have been shown to be rapid and highly sensitive and specific, but they are qualitative and are unable to distinguish among genotypes or detect low levels of infection.[64,136] The ELISA may be particularly useful in screening during mass outbreaks and assessing cure. Monoclonal antibodies usually are used to detect antigen either by an ELISA or an immunofluorescence assay. Some of these assays have a sensitivity of 91% to 95% and specificities of more than 98%.[33,79,136] Antigen may be best detected when the stool is preserved in formalin.[33] These tests do not replace microscopic examination of the stool, which is considered to be the standard, because of the possibility of infection with multiple organisms in travelers.

Molecular techniques such as polymerase chain reaction (PCR) are alternative methods that may be used for the specific detection of *Giardia* in the stool. These techniques, in combination with restriction fragment length polymorphism or nested PCR, may be used to genotype the organisms. The sensitivity of detection by PCR is greater than that of microscopy, and PCR is much better for detection of low number of parasites in stool samples.[8] An advance in PCR-based technology for the detection of *G. lamblia* in stool is the use of real-time PCR. This method, using dual-labeled fluorescent probes targeting the β-giardin gene, is sensitive, is rapid, and may be used to detect *G. lamblia* in stool and to differentiate the major genotypes of the organism. Real-time PCR can be adapted to high-throughput detection for the screening of large numbers of samples, especially in outbreak situations.[13,49]

Even with the available diagnostic tests, infections may be missed in some patients; and in cases with a high index of suspicion, the organism may be recovered by duodenal biopsy or duodenal aspiration. Invasive techniques may be important diagnostic adjuncts in immunosuppressed patients and in patients with sprue, for whom histologic examination of the bowel also may be important in planning therapy.

TREATMENT

All patients with either cysts or trophozoites in the stool should be treated. Multiple classes of drugs are available for the treatment of giardiasis, each with different clinical properties and efficacies, as shown in Table 213.3.[5,39,139] The nitroimidazole class of agents includes metronidazole, tinidazole, ornidazole, and secnidazole and is the mainstay of therapy for the treatment of giardiasis. These drugs are administered orally in their inactive probiotic form.[39] Of the nitroimidazoles, metronidazole has been the most extensively studied and widely used worldwide. The mechanism of killing of *Giardia* by the nitroimidazoles involves use of the anaerobic metabolic pathways of the organism. The drug diffuses into the trophozoite, where it is activated and inhibits trophozoite respiration and causes cellular damage by the production of toxic radicals and loss of DNA helical structure, with resulting trophozoite death.[45,132] Of the nitroimidazoles, tinidazole and metronidazole have demonstrated the greatest in vitro activity.[25,48] Metronidazole is considered the drug of choice for treatment, with tinidazole as an alternative.[37,39] Although albendazole has been shown to be curative either in single doses or a 5-day course, it is not approved for use in giardiasis in the United States.[50,143] Quinacrine, which is inexpensive and has excellent efficacy, also is no longer available in the United States.[39] It may cause hemolysis in children with glucose-6-phosphate dehydrogenase deficiency. Furazolidone is an effective alternative and is available in a liquid form. However, it is administered four times a day for 7 to 10 days and is associated with side effects that include rash, nausea, and vomiting. Tinidazole has been shown to eliminate the parasite after single-dose therapy.[37] Another member of the 5-nitromidazoles, secnidazole has been shown to be well tolerated at 30-mg/kg per day (maximum, 2 g) and is an option for therapy.[45] Paromomycin, an aminoglycoside that is not well absorbed, is the only drug that can be used in a pregnant patient. It is not as effective as other medications in eradicating the parasite but may induce clinical improvement. A 3-day course of nitazoxanide has been shown to treat successfully 85% of children with diarrhea caused by *Giardia.*[35,108] Although outbreaks in day care centers are common, treating all children in the day care center is not efficacious because recurrence rates are high and a chance of a drug reaction always exists. Treatment is reserved for symptomatic children.

Treatment failures and the development of drug resistance have been reported with all the common agents used to treat *Giardia,* including albendazole, furazolidone, metronidazole, and quinacrine.[5,71] The prevalence of clinical metronidazole-resistant cases is reported to be up to 20%,[10,32,128,131,133] with recurrence rates up to 90%.[142] Metronidazole-resistant *Giardia* strains have also manifested cross-resistance to tinidazole.[128,131,133] Furazolidone-resistant *Giardia* species can be induced both in vitro and in vivo, and this may induce the organism to become resistant more easily to quinacrine.[80,129,134] *Giardia* resistant to albendazole has been reported to develop rapidly in vitro. Albendazole resistance also develops more easily in *Giardia* strains that are furazolidone resistant, giving rise to multidrug-resistant phenotypes.[74,130]

Patients with clinically resistant strains have been treated with longer repeat courses or higher doses of the initial agent.[40,87] However, the most effective means of eradicating these infections seems to be the use of an anti-*Giardia* agent from a different class to avoid potential cross-resistance.[9,24,41,81,86] For *Giardia* strains that are phenotypically considered to be multidrug resistant, the administration of anti-*Giardia* drugs in combination is a method that may be used for successful treatment of the infection.

NEW REFERENCES SINCE THE SEVENTH EDITION

6. Ankarklev J, Jerlstrom-Hultqvist J, Ringqvist E, et al. Behind the smile: cell biology and disease mechanisms of *Giardia* species. *Nat Rev Microbiol.* 2010;8:413-422.
7. Bartelt LA, Sartor RB. Advances in understanding *Giardia*: determinants and mechanisms of chronic sequelae. *F1000Prime Rep.* 2015;7:62.
14. Cantey PT, Roy S, Lee B, et al. Study of nonoutbreak giardiasis: novel findings and implications for research. *Am J Med.* 2011;124:1175.e1-1175.e8.
15. Carlson DW, Finger DR. Beaver fever arthritis. *J Clin Rheumatol.* 2004;10:86-88.
16. Carranza PG, Lujan HD. New insights regarding the biology of *Giardia lamblia. Microbes Infect.* 2010;12:70-80.
19. Chen TL, Chen S, Wu HW, et al. Persistent gut barrier damage and commensal bacterial influx following eradication of *Giardia* infection in mice. *Gut Pathog.* 2013;5:26.
21. Corsi A, Nucci C, Knafelz D, et al. Ocular changes associated with *Giardia lamblia* infection in children. *Br J Ophthalmol.* 1998;82:59-62.
22. Cotton JA, Amat CB, Buret AG. Disruptions of host immunity and inflammation by *Giardia* duodenalis: potential consequences for co-infections in the gastro-intestinal tract. *Pathogens.* 2015;4:764-792.
23. Cotton JA, Beatty JK, Buret AG. Host-parasite interactions and pathophysiology of *Giardia* infections. *Int J Parasitol.* 2011;41:925-933.
27. Dann SM, Manthey CF, Le C, et al. IL-17A promotes protective IgA responses and expression of other potential effectors against the lumen-dwelling enteric parasite *Giardia. Exp Parasitol.* 2015;156:68-78.
34. Feng Y, Xiao L. Zoonotic potential and molecular epidemiology of *Giardia* species and giardiasis. *Clin Microbiol Rev.* 2011;24:110-140.
42. Giangaspero A, Papini R, Marangi M, et al. *Cryptosporidium parvum* genotype IIa and *Giardia duodenalis* assemblage A in *Mytilus galloprovincialis* on sale at local food markets. *Int J Food Microbiol.* 2014;171:62-67.
51. Halliez MCM, Buret AG. Extra-intestinal and long term consequences of *Giardia* duodenalis infection. *World J Gastroenterol.* 2013;19:8974-8985.
58. Hill Gaston JS, Lillicrap MS. Arthritis associated with enteric infection. *Best Pract Res Clin Rheumatol.* 2003;17:219-239.
71. Leitsch D. Drug resistance in the microaerophilic parasite *Giardia* lamblia. *Curr Trop Med Rep.* 2015;2:128-135.
78. Lopez-Romero G, Quintero J, Astiazaran-Garcia H, et al. Host defences against *Giardia lamblia. Parasite Immunol.* 2015;37:394-406.
81. Meltzer E, Lachish T, Schwartz E. Treatment of giardiasis after nonresponse to nitroimidazole. *Emerg Infect Dis.* 2014;20:1742-1744.
86. Munoz Gutierrez J, Aldasoro E, Requena A, et al. Refractory giardiasis in Spanish travelers. *Travel Med Infect Dis.* 2013;11:126-129.
94. Panaro MA, Cianciulli A, Mitolo V, et al. Caspase-dependent apoptosis of the HCT-8 epithelial cell line induced by the parasite *Giardia intestinalis. FEMS Immunol Med Microbiol.* 2007;51:302-309.
96. Pettoello Mantovani M, Giardino I, Magli A, et al. Intestinal giardiasis associated with ophthalmologic changes. *J Pediatr Gastroenterol Nutr.* 1990;11: 196-200.
98. Pires SM, Fischer-Walker CL, Lanata CF, et al. Aetiology-specific estimates of the global and regional incidence and mortality of diarrhoeal diseases commonly transmitted through food. *PLoS ONE.* 2015;10:e0142927.
99. Plutzer J, Ongerth J, Karanis P. *Giardia* taxonomy, phylogeny and epidemiology: facts and open questions. *Int J Hyg Environ Health.* 2010;213:321-333.
101. Prucca CG, Lujan HD. Antigenic variation in *Giardia lamblia. Cell Microbiol.* 2009;11:1706-1715.
107. Ross AG, Olds GR, Cripps AW, et al. Enteropathogens and chronic illness in returning travelers. *N Engl J Med.* 2013;368:1817-1825.
110. Ryan ET, Wilson ME, Kain KC. Illness after international travel. *N Engl J Med.* 2002;347:505-516.
114. Schets FM, van den Berg HH, de Roda Husman AM. Determination of the recovery efficiency of *Cryptosporidium* oocysts and *Giardia* cysts from seeded bivalve mollusks. *J Food Prot.* 2013;76:93-98.
121. Solaymani-Mohammadi S, Singer SM. Host immunity and pathogen strain contribute to intestinal disaccharidase impairment following gut infection. *J Immunol.* 2011;187:3769-3775.
122. Solaymani-Mohammadi S, Singer SM. *Giardia duodenalis*: the double-edged sword of immune responses in giardiasis. *Exp Parasitol.* 2010;126:292-297.
125. Teoh DA, Kamieniecki D, Pang G, et al. *Giardia lamblia* rearranges F-actin and alpha-actinin in human colonic and duodenal monolayers and reduces transepithelial electrical resistance. *J Parasitol.* 2000;86:800-806.
126. Touz MC, Rivero MR, Miras SL, Bonifacino JS. Lysosomal protein trafficking in *Giardia lamblia*: common and distinct features. *Front Biosci (Elite Ed).* 2012;4:1898-1901.

The full reference list for this chapter is available at ExpertConsult.com.

Dientamoeba fragilis Infections

214

Damien Stark

Dientamoeba fragilis is a protozoan parasite of the human bowel, commonly reported throughout the world in association with gastrointestinal (GI) symptoms.[63] Although discovered in 1908, it was not described in the scientific literature until 1918, by Jepps and Dobell,[34] and at that time it was considered to be a rare intestinal commensal. Despite its discovery more than 100 years ago, we know less about this organism than about any other of the commonly encountered enteric protozoan of humans. The details of its life cycle, mode of transmission, and potential as a human pathogen are all poorly defined or lacking completely. Controversy therefore still surrounds the pathogenicity of *Dientamoeba*, with conflicting reports on the pathogenic potential of this organism.[24]

ORGANISM

Dientamoeba was classified initially in the genus *Entamoeba*. The similarity of *D. fragilis* to flagellates, however, specifically to *Histomonas meleagridis*, the cause of "blackhead" enterohepatitis in fowl, was noted on careful examination under the light microscope.[19] Later studies using various techniques, including microscopic, immunologic, antigenic, electron microscopic, and molecular studies, resulted in the reclassification of *D. fragilis* as a nonflagellated trichomonad.[6,17,21,20] Genetic studies confirmed recent evolution with trichomonads,[7,27] with two genotypes detected in DNA encoding ribosomal RNA.[35] Genotype 1 seems to predominate in epidemiologic studies.[52,66] Investigators have proposed that *D. fragilis* could be a heterogeneous species, with variants having similar morphology but different virulence.[74]

Although *D. fragilis* was initially thought to occur only as a trophozoite lacking a cyst stage, more recent studies identified distinct morphologic forms, a putative precystic form and a cyst form in both rodent models and human clinical samples.[44,70] The frequency in which cysts are found in human clinical samples would lead us to believe that they may not be an aberrant form in this host.[70]

D. fragilis infects the mucosal crypts of the large intestine in close proximity to mucosal epithelium from the cecum to the rectum. The organism ranges in size from 3 to 18 μm in diameter, but usually it is 7 to 12 μm (Fig. 214.1A–C). Although the organisms are found most commonly in the binucleate form, approximately 20% are in the uninucleate form, and a few are multinucleate.[24] Each nucleus contains a large, fragmented (four to eight granules) karyosome surrounded by a clear zone with no peripheral chromatin and a fine nuclear membrane.[63]

Humans seem to be the natural hosts of *D. fragilis*, with only a limited number of reports of nonhuman hosts, including apes, monkeys, and pigs.[13,32,71] Munasinghe and colleagues[44] described the successful establishment of a rodent model of *Dientamoeba* infection, and wild rats have subsequently been described as natural hosts of *D. fragilis*.[50]

EPIDEMIOLOGY AND TRANSMISSION

Despite the discovery of *D. fragilis* more than a century ago, both its life cycle and its mode of transmission are unknown; however, two mechanisms of transmission have been postulated.[11] One hypothesis is that *D. fragilis* is transmitted in the eggs of *Enterobius vermicularis* (pinworm) in a manner similar to the transmission of *H. meleagridis* in the eggs of the avian nematode *Heterakis gallinae*.[11] In support of this theory, many investigators have noted a high frequency of concomitant infection with *D. fragilis* and *E. vermicularis*.[4,28] Ockert[47,48] provided the most convincing support for this theory when, by ingesting eggs of *E. vermicularis*, which he had washed with water and exposed to pepsin and hydrochloric acid, he became infected with *E. vermicularis* and *D. fragilis* The role of *E. vermicularis* as a vector of *D. fragilis* transmission is supported by two more recent studies that detected *D. fragilis* DNA in DNA extracted from surface sterilized *E. vermicularis* ova.[49,56] Other investigators, noting a high rate of concomitant infection of *D. fragilis* with organisms causing intestinal infections and negative test results for *E. vermicularis*, have suggested fecal-oral transmission.[39–41,64,66,79] A study using laboratory rodents demonstrated fecal-oral transmission between mice and from mice to rats, thereby indicating that vectors play no role in the transmission of this organism.[44]

D. fragilis was thought to be uncommon until improved diagnostic techniques were used for detection, including prompt fixation for preserving the organism[25,29,59] and molecular methods.[52,65,78] However, when appropriate diagnostic methods are used, *D. fragilis* is found to be more prevalent than *Giardia*.[12] The trophozoites of *D. fragilis* have been noted to be quite sensitive to an aerobic environment.[10] They die and disintegrate within 1 hour in an isotonic salt solution at room temperature; when smeared on slides, they round up and become granular within 15 minutes during microscopic examination at room temperature and low humidity.[10]

D. fragilis has been reported worldwide with a prevalence in selected populations of 0.9% to 71%,[63] with the higher rates reported in crowded living conditions, such as institutions and communal groups,[2,40,41] in extended families in close contact,[72] and in persons traveling outside the United States.[57,69] A serologic survey in Canada that used indirect immunofluorescence techniques detected antibodies to *D. fragilis* in 87% to 100% of healthy children 1 to 19 years old, a finding suggesting that infection is common during childhood.[9] Although the antibodies detected in this survey did not absorb when incubated with *Klebsiella pneumoniae* or *Bacteroides vulgatus*, known to contaminate the antigen source of *D. fragilis*, additional studies are needed to confirm the specificity of the assay and to define the seroprevalence in other populations.

CLINICAL MANIFESTATIONS

An overwhelming body of evidence dates back several decades and indicates that treatments that eliminate *D. fragilis* result in significant clinical improvement of patients experiencing GI symptoms.* This finding suggests that *D. fragilis* plays some role in the development of GI disease. Clinical presentation of infection ranges from asymptomatic carriage to various GI symptoms including altered bowel motions, abdominal pain, and diarrhea, often in association with eosinophilia, which is reported in up to 50% of patients.[14,51,53,68]

However, some reports from Northern Europe support a very different trend. In a study from the Netherlands,[18] *D. fragilis* was detected more frequently in the stools of healthy control subjects (14.6%) than in the stools of subjects with GI complaints (10.3%). A large, case-control comparison study comprising 1515 symptomatic patients and 1195 healthy control subjects detected *D. fragilis* in 390 symptomatic patients at a prevalence of 25.7% and in 446 in the control group at a prevalence of 37.3%.[3] This study found that *D. fragilis* was more common in healthy, nonsymptomatic groups than in symptomatic patients. Another study, by de Jong and associates,[16] found higher rates of *D. fragilis* in healthy control subjects when compared with pediatric patients presenting with chronic abdominal pain. These investigators found no differences in symptoms when comparing children with and without *D. fragilis*

*References 1, 5, 10, 14, 30, 31, 36, 37, 42, 52–55, 60, 61, 73, 80–82, 84, 85.

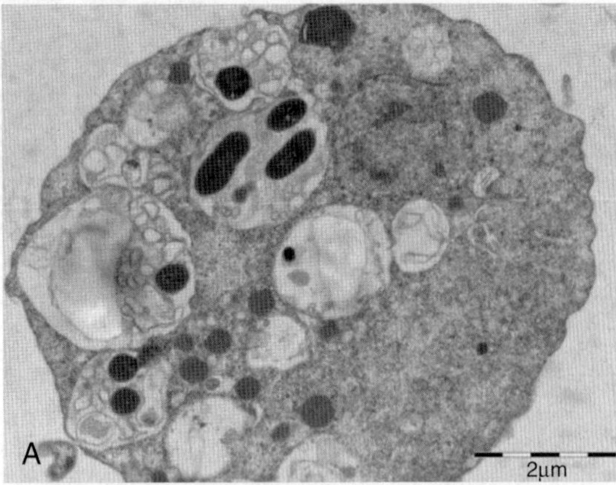

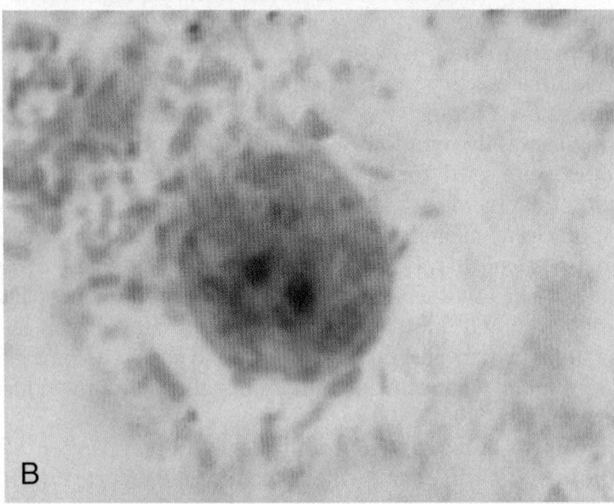

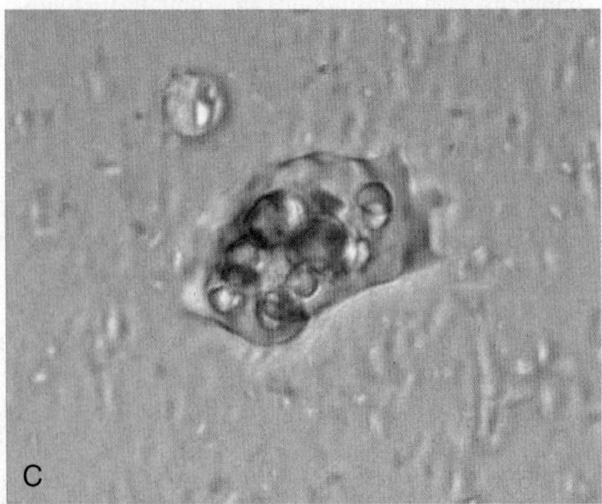

FIG. 214.1 (A) *Dientamoeba fragilis* trophozoites on electron micrography. (B) Light microscopy of trophozoite on modified iron-hematoxylin stain. (C) Phase contrast microscopy of trophozoite in culture (with ingested rice starch).

infection, a finding suggesting no association between chronic abdominal pain and *D. fragilis* infection.

DIAGNOSIS

Infection with *D. fragilis* should be considered in patients with abdominal pain, diarrhea, or both, persisting beyond 1 week when all other causes are ruled out. The diagnosis of dientamoebiasis may be problematic if inadequate laboratory methods are used. Investigation for *D. fragilis* infection should include the collection of at least three stool specimens that are immediately placed in a stool preservative such as polyvinyl alcohol stool preservative to retain the morphologic characteristics of the delicate trophozoite.[33,59,76] The diagnosis also can be made by permanent stained smear of a fresh or purged fecal specimen.[29] Detection

TABLE 214.1 Treatment Options for Dientamoebiasis

Drug of Choice	Alternative Drugs
Iodoquinol	**Paromomycin**
Adults: 650 mg PO 3 times daily × 20 days	Adults: 500 mg PO 3 times daily × 7 days
Pediatric: 30–40 mg/kg/day (maximum, 2 g) PO in 3 doses × 20 days	Pediatric: 25–35 mg/kg/day PO in 3 doses × 7 days
	Tetracycline
	Adults: 500 mg PO 4 times daily × 10 days
	Pediatric: 40 mg/kg/day (maximum, 2 g) PO in 4 doses × 10 days
	Metronidazole
	Adults: 500–750 mg PO 3 times daily × 10 days
	Pediatric: 35–50 mg/kg/day PO in 3 doses × 10 days

PO, Orally.

of the organism seems not to be compromised by use of an "environmentally friendly" mercury-free stool preservative and stain (EcoFix and EcoStain).[26]

Examination of three fecal specimens properly collected and stained leads to the identification of this intestinal protozoan in 70% to 93% of infected persons.[33] Stool specimens should be collected on alternate days because excretion of *D. fragilis* seems to manifest a cyclic pattern.[63] Stool samples should be collected before radiologic studies with barium are done because barium interferes with detection of the protozoa. Other medications interfering with parasite identification include antibiotics, mineral oil, antimalarial agents, antiprotozoal agents, nonabsorbable diarrheal preparations, and bismuth. These substances may interfere with the detection of parasites for 3 weeks.[23]

After arrival in the laboratory, stool specimens are processed with the use of a formalin-ether sedimentation concentration technique and are stained with either iron hematoxylin or trichrome and examined by qualified and experienced personnel for the proper identification of *D. fragilis.*[24] Diagnostic characteristics of *D. fragilis* on a permanently stained smear include a high percentage of binucleate trophozoites and nuclei without peripheral chromatin, but with four to eight chromatin granules in a central mass.[63]

Other methods used for the detection of *D. fragilis* include indirect immunofluorescence,[8] xenic culture,[43,58,83] and conventional and real-time polymerase chain reaction methods that show excellent sensitivity and specificity, in contrast to microscopy.[15,62,65,67,78] One serologic test has been developed; however, it is not commercially available, and the high seroprevalence of *D. fragilis* precludes its use as a diagnostic tool.[9]

TREATMENT

Several agents have been used in the treatment of *D. fragilis* infection. However, most treatment data are based only on a small number of case reports. No large-scale double-blind, randomized placebo-controlled trials testing the efficacy of antimicrobial agents against *D. fragilis* have been undertaken.[45] At present, one of four drugs is recommended for the treatment of *D. fragilis* infection (Table 214.1): iodoquinol, tetracycline, paromomycin, or metronidazole.[38,53,77,75] However, because of the paucity of clinical studies, tetracycline and paromomycin are considered investigational by the US Food and Drug Administration. Among newer agents, the 5-nitroimidazole derivatives secnidazole and ornidazole seem effective in limited studies, and they have the advantage of longer half-lives, single doses, and fewer side effects.[38] Laboratory studies have found that ronidazole, tinidazole, and nitazoxanide are active in vitro.[22,46]

Iodoquinol, 650 mg three times daily for 20 days, is recommended for adults, and a regimen of 30 to 40 mg/kg per day in three divided doses is recommended for children. The tablets should be taken with meals. Side effects include abdominal discomfort, diarrhea, anal irritation and pruritus, headache, and dysesthesias of the hands and feet. Paromomycin, 500 mg three times daily for adults and 25 to 35 mg/kg per day in three divided doses in children for 7 days may be more effective than iodoquinol.[45] Adverse reactions to paromomycin include nausea, abdominal cramps, and diarrhea. It is absorbed poorly after oral administration and is no longer available in syrup form in the United States.

Recrudescence or relapse has been reported after one or more 7-day courses of paromomycin in some children.[75] Alternative therapy consists of tetracycline hydrochloride or metronidazole. Tetracycline is recommended at a dosage of 500 mg four times daily for adults and 40 mg/kg per day in four divided doses for children for 10 days. Tetracycline may cause GI and central nervous system symptoms. It should not be given to children younger than 9 years of age because it may cause discoloration of the teeth. Metronidazole treatment is recommended at a dosage of 500 to 750 mg three times daily for 10 days for adults and 20 to 40 mg/kg per day divided into three doses for children.[45] Treatment with metronidazole may cause GI and central nervous system symptoms. Because of the adverse reactions associated with these drugs, the clinician should evaluate the need for therapy carefully in each case and discuss treatment options with the child's family.

NEW REFERENCES SINCE THE SEVENTH EDITION

3. Bruijnesteijn van Coppenraet LE, Dullaert-de Boer M, Ruijs GJ, et al. Case-control comparison of bacterial and protozoan microorganisms associated with gastroenteritis: application of molecular detection. *Clin Microbiol Infect.* 2015;21(6):592.e9-592.e19.
7. Cepicka I, Hampl V, Kulda J. Critical taxonomic revision of Parabasalids with description of one new genus and three new species. *Protist.* 2010;161(3):400-433.
11. Clark CG, Roser D, Stensvold CR. Transmission of *Dientamoeba fragilis:* pinworm or cysts? *Trends Parasitol.* 2014;30(3):136-140.
13. Crotti D, Sensi M, Crotti S, et al. *Dientamoeba fragilis* in swine population: a preliminary investigation. *Vet Parasitol.* 2007;145(3-4):349-351.
15. De Canale E, Biasolo MA, Tessari A, et al. Real Time PCR for *Dientamoeba fragilis:* a comparison between molecular and microscopical approach. *Microbiol Med.* 2009;24(3):133-138.
16. de Jong MJ, Korterink JJ, Benninga MA, et al. *Dientamoeba fragilis* and chronic abdominal pain in children: a case-control study. *Arch Dis Child.* 2014;99(12):1109-1113.
18. de Wit MA, Koopmans MP, Kortbeek LM, et al. Etiology of gastroenteritis in sentinel general practices in the Netherlands. *Clin Infect Dis.* 2001;33(3):280-288.
23. Garcia LS. Clinical diagnostic parasitology. *Am J Med Technol.* 1981;47(1):53-69.
24. Garcia LS. *Dientamoeba fragilis,* one of the neglected intestinal protozoa. *J Clin Microbiol.* 2016;54(9):2243-2250.
30. Hakansson EG. *Dientamoeba fragilis,* a cause of illness: report of a case. *Am J Trop Med Hyg.* 1936;1936(16):175-178.
31. Hakansson EG. *Dientamoeba fragilis*: some further observations. *Am J Trop Med.* 1937;17:349-362.
32. Helenbrook WD, Wade SE, Shields WM, et al. Gastrointestinal parasites of Ecuadorian mantled howler monkeys (*Alouatta palliata aequatorialis)* based on fecal analysis. *J Parasitol.* 2015;101(3):341-350.
42. Mollari M, Anzulovic JV. Cultivation and pathogenicity of *Dientamoeba fragilis,* with a case report. *J Trop Med Hyg.* 1938;41:246-247.
44. Munasinghe VS, Vella NG, Ellis JT, et al. Cyst formation and faecal-oral transmission of *Dientamoeba fragilis:* the missing link in the life cycle of an emerging pathogen. *Int J Parasitol.* 2013;43(11):879-883.
46. Nagata N, Marriott D, Harkness J, Ellis JT, Stark D. Current treatment options for *Dientamoeba fragilis* infections. *Int J Parasitol Drugs Drug Resist.* 2012;2:204-215.
48. Ockert G. [Epidemiology of *Dientamoeba fragilis* Jepps and Dobell, 1918. 3. Further studies on *Enterobius* transmission through eggs]. *J Hyg Epidemiol Microbiol Immunol.* 1975;19(1):17-21, [in German].
49. Ogren J, Dienus O, Lofgren S, et al. *Dientamoeba fragilis* DNA detection in *Enterobius vermicularis* eggs. *Pathog Dis.* 2013;69(2):157-158.
50. Ogunniyi T, Balogun H, Shasanya B. Ectoparasites and endoparasites of peridomestic house-rats in ile-ife, Nigeria and implication on human health. *Iran J Parasitol.* 2014;9(1):134-140.
51. Oxner RB, Paltridge GP, Chapman BA, et al. *Dientamoeba fragilis:* a bowel pathogen? *N Z Med J.* 1987;100(817):64-65.
54. Preiss U, Ockert G, Bromme S, et al. *Dientamoeba fragilis* infection, a cause of gastrointestinal symptoms in childhood. *Klin Padiatr.* 1990;202(2):120-123.
55. Robertson A. Specimens from a human case of infection with *Dientamoeba fragilis,* Jepps and Dobell, 1917. *Proc R Soc Med.* 1923;16(Sect Trop Dis Parasitol):48.
56. Roser D, Nejsum P, Carlsgart AJ, et al. DNA of *Dientamoeba fragilis* detected within surface-sterilized eggs of *Enterobius vermicularis. Exp Parasitol.* 2013;133(1):57-61.
57. Sapero JJ, Johnson CM. *Entamoeba histolytica* and other intestinal parasites: incidence in variously exposed groups of the Navy. *U S Navy Med Bull.* 1939;37:297-301.
60. Shein R, Gelb A. Colitis due to *Dientamoeba fragilis. Am J Gastroenterol.* 1983;78(10):634-636.
63. Stark D, Barratt J, Chan D, et al. *Dientamoeba fragilis,* the neglected trichomonad of the human bowel. *Clin Microbiol Rev.* 2016;29(3):553-580.
64. Stark D, Barratt J, Roberts T, et al. A review of the clinical presentation of dientamoebiasis. *Am J Trop Med Hyg.* 2010;82(4):614-619.
69. Stark D, Garcia LS, Barratt JL, et al. Description of *Dientamoeba fragilis* cyst and precystic forms from human samples. *J Clin Microbiol.* 2014;52(7):2680-2683.
68. Stark DJ, Beebe N, Marriott D, et al. Dientamoebiasis: clinical importance and recent advances. *Trends Parasitol.* 2006;22(2):92-96.
73. Steinitz H, Talis B, Stein B. *Entamoeba histolytica* and *Dientamoeba fragilis* and the syndrome of chronic recurrent intestinal amoebiasis in Israel. *Digestion.* 1970;3(3):146-153.
75. van Hellemond JJ, Molhoek N, Koelewijn R, et al. Is paromomycin the drug of choice for eradication of *Dientamoeba fragilis* in adults? *Int J Parasitol Drugs Drug Resist.* 2012;2:162-165.
80. Wenrich DH, Stabler RM, Arnett JH. *Entamoeba histolytica* and other intestinal protozoa in 1060 college freshmen. *Am J Trop Med.* 1935;15:331-345.
81. Wenrich DH. Studies on *Dientamoeba fragilis* (Protozoa). IV. Further observations, with an outline of present days knowledge of this species. *J Parasitol.* 1944;30:322-338.
84. Yang J, Scholten T. *Dientamoeba fragilis:* a review with notes on its epidemiology, pathogenicity, mode of transmission, and diagnosis. *Am J Trop Med Hyg.* 1977;26(1):16-22.

The full reference list for this chapter is available at ExpertConsult.com.

215 *Trichomonas* Infections

Joan S. Purcell • Mariam R. Chacko

Trichomonas spp. are found in animals and humans. The most widely studied member of this species is *Trichomonas vaginalis* because it is the trichomonad most relevant to human disease. Donne first described *T. vaginalis* in 1836 as motile microorganisms in the purulent frothy leukorrhea of women with vaginal discharge and genital irritation.[20] Epidemiologic information concerning *Trichomonas* infection is most detailed in the adult population; nonetheless, studies that document the epidemiology of *T. vaginalis* in children and adolescents are available.

MICROBIOLOGY

Trichomonads are acellular flagellated protozoans. The Trichomonadidae family is characterized as mononucleate with an axial organelle that has an undulating membrane. The *Trichomonas* genus includes protozoans that have organelles with three to four anterior flagella and an undulating membrane comprising the posterior flagellum. Five *Trichomonas* spp. infect humans, and three *Trichomonas* spp. infect animals. In humans, the five species of *Trichomonas* are *T. tenax, T. ardin delteili, T. faecalis, T. hominis,* and *T. vaginalis.*[69] *T. vaginalis* is the most clinically relevant human trichomonad; the other four species are nonpathogenic. *T. vaginalis* consists of four anterior flagella and a posterior flagellum incorporated into the undulating membrane. *T. vaginalis* can survive but cannot multiply at room temperature. In contrast, *T. hominis* has five anterior flagella and a trailing posterior flagellum, and it can survive and multiply at room temperature. Only *T. hominis* can survive in media without serum and in feces for 24 hours.[69]

EPIDEMIOLOGY

Prevalence

Trichomonas infection is not a notifiable sexually transmitted infection (STI) in the United States. This infection is found in all age groups, from neonates to adults, and is the most common nonviral STI, affecting up to 3.7 billion persons.[53] The absence of screening programs and variations in diagnostic tests influence prevalence data, but the emergence of point-of-care and nucleic acid amplification tests (NAATs) has enhanced epidemiologic information in this field of study. For details on newborns, infants, and premenarcheal children, see Chapter 42.

The prevalence of *T. vaginalis* varies greatly, from 5% to 74% in women with the highest rates reported from STI clinics and other high-risk populations.[13,49,71] In adolescent girls, the prevalence rate ranges from 3.6% to 18% depending on the population studied.[19,24,38,66] The 2003 to 2004 National Health and Nutrition Examination Survey, which randomly samples the noninstitutionalized civilian population in the United States, found a 3.6% weighted prevalence rate for *T. vaginalis* in sexually active girls and women 14 to 19 years of age by polymerase chain reaction testing.[19] In an inner-city primary care clinic the prevalence of *T. vaginalis* was 14.4% by wet mount and culture in 13- to 19-year-old female patients.[38] In an urban pediatric emergency department a prevalence rate of *T. vaginalis* by OSOM Trichomonas Rapid enzyme test (Sanofi Genzyme) was 9.9% in 14- to 19-year-old female patients; 25% of the positive test results occurred among 14- and 15-year-olds.[24] In another emergency department–based study, using NAAT and rapid antigen testing, the prevalence of *Trichomonas* was 18.4%.[66]

In contrast to girls and women, the prevalence in boys and men is not well studied. Data in adolescent boys are limited. In men attending STI clinics, the prevalence of *T. vaginalis* was 22% to 29% in sexual contacts of women with trichomoniasis, and it was 6% in male patients who had sex with male partners.[29,40] *T. vaginalis* was found in 58% of 85 young black men 16 to 22 years of age who were sexually active, of whom 69% previously had an STI.[54] An Internet-based study of self-collected penile swabs was conducted among 1699 men; 42% were African American, 9% were younger than 20 years, and 32% were 20 to 24 years of age. The overall prevalence rate of *T. vaginalis* in swabs returned after requesting kits was 3.7%; it was 2% in 15 to 19 year olds and 6% in 20- to 24-year-olds.[23]

Risk Factors

A large epidemiologic neighborhood study isolated *T. vaginalis* in young adults living in neighborhoods with a higher concentration of low-income African Americans. Factors such as immigrant concentration and residential instability were not associated with *T. vaginalis.*[18] Trichomoniasis apparently does not have a seasonal pattern of infection.[45]

Urogenital trichomoniasis occurs more commonly in women than in men and in inner-city patients 20 to 30 years of age.[45] The rate of *T. vaginalis* infection is increased in the following: African American women; women with other STIs, including gonococcal cervicitis; a vaginal pH shift greater than 4.5; pregnancy; menarche; and after menopausc.[48,69]

Infection with *T. vaginalis* increases in direct relation to the number of sexual partners, and the number of sexual partners, in turn, increases the risk for coinfection with other sexually transmitted organisms, including, but not limited to, *Chlamydia trachomatis, Neisseria gonorrhea, Mycoplasma hominis,* and human immunodeficiency virus (HIV). Oral contraceptives diminish the rate of infection with *T. vaginalis,* in contrast to an intrauterine device or tubal ligation.[45] The use of nonoxynol-9 spermicidal cream was not related significantly to a decrease in *Trichomonas* infection.[6] In another study of 226 women attending an STI clinic, no association was found with patients' age, frequency of coitus, date of most recent coitus, day of menstrual cycle, antibiotic use, contraceptive methods, or symptoms of discharge or pruritus.[48] The risk for *T. vaginalis* is decreased in the wives of circumcised men.[26]

Other risk factors for women may involve a change in the normal vaginal flora, such as overgrowth of *Gardnerella vaginalis, Bacteroides,* or *Peptostreptococcus.* These bacteria may serve as sources of nutrients for trichomonads and allow them to thrive. In men, sexual contact with a woman infected with *T. vaginalis,* nongonococcal urethritis, or nongonococcal nonchlamydial urethritis was associated with an increased risk for acquiring infection with *T. vaginalis.*[41]

In men, age older than 30 years, black race, younger age of sexual debut, and the presence of urethral symptoms are all significant predictors of *Trichomonas* infection.[23]

TRANSMISSION

The likelihood of perinatal transmission is high in infants younger than 1 year. In a child or an infant younger than 1 year, *T. vaginalis* may have resulted from transmission within a family without sexual abuse, although the probability of sexual abuse must be considered. Perinatal transmission and transmission of infection through fomites should not be assumed without an investigation for sexual abuse. For details see Chapter 42.

T. vaginalis usually is transmitted sexually in adolescents and adults. In an STI clinic, 60% of husbands of women ($n = 30$) who had chronic, repeated *T. vaginalis* infections had positive culture results for *T. vaginalis,* in contrast to 8% in a control group of 50 men attending the same clinic. *T. vaginalis* has been isolated in two men reporting receptive anal intercourse,[14] as well as in a lesbian couple who denied using penetrative sex toys or having male partners, a finding suggesting that transmission may occur through mutual masturbation.[29]

PATHOLOGY AND PATHOGENESIS

As noted previously, five species of *Trichomonas* have been identified in humans; the most clinically important is *T. vaginalis. T. vaginalis* is not part of the normal flora, but is found in the human vagina, urethra, and prostate. Inoculation experiments with *T. vaginalis* in the mouth and intestines failed to establish infection in these sites.[69] *T. tenax* is found in the mouth, and *T. hominis, T. ardin delteili,* and *T. faecalis* are found in the bowel. *T. tenax* is detected in approximately 5% of patients with *T. vaginalis. T. tenax, T. ardin delteili,* and *T. faecalis* are part of the normal flora and are nonpathogenic. *T. hominis* can infect humans and is associated with gastrointestinal dysentery. The incidence of *T. hominis* in humans is 0.4% to 3.5%. *T. hominis* is found only rarely in the stools of patients who concomitantly have *T. vaginalis.*[69]

Virulence factors associated with *T. vaginalis* infection have been defined and include adherence, contact-independent factors, hemolysis, and host macromolecule acquisition. Epithelial cell adherence depends on an intact cytoskeleton and *Trichomonas* protein ligands and proteases, which are necessary to activate adherence molecules.[15,22] Cell contact–independent factors include pH variability and cell-detaching factor, which in vitro inhibit reorganization of cells infected with *T. vaginalis. T. vaginalis* produces lactic and acetic acid as by-products of glucose metabolism.[15] These acids lower the pH, which is cytotoxic to epithelial cells. Another metabolic by-product of *T. vaginalis* is cell-detaching factor, which has a cytopathic effect on epithelial cells and increases subepithelial vascularity, thus producing the clinical sign of "strawberry cervix."[15] The activity of cell-detaching factor is optimal at pH 5.0 or greater. Hemolysis is seen only in the presence of live trichomonads. Cysteine proteases seem to be important for hemolysis because introduction of their inhibitors in vitro eliminates hemolysis by *T. vaginalis.*[11,15]

The addition of metronidazole reduces levels of hemolysis by 50%.[15] The hemolytic activity of *T. vaginalis* is temperature dependent, with maximal hemolysis at 37°C (98.6°F). Hemolysis is inhibited by separation of trichomonads from erythrocytes by a 3-mm filter, a finding suggesting a contact-dependent mechanism.[15] As a parasite, *T. vaginalis* also depends on host macromolecules for nutrition, including plasma proteins and lactoferrin.

The host responds to *T. vaginalis* infection at the cellular level with polymorphonuclear cells and lymphocyte activity. *T. vaginalis* secretes proteases that are chemotactic to polymorphonuclear leukocytes, with resultant phagocytosis and killing of the trichomonad by oxidative mechanisms.[15] *T. vaginalis* secretions are mitogenic to lymphocytes; they enhance phagocytosis by polymorphonuclear cells and may suppress the host immune response if numerous suppressor lymphocytes are activated.

Estrogen levels in female patients directly correlate with infection at peak estradiol levels, and symptoms may be influenced by vaginal concentration of estrogen.[22] In an early study of premenarcheal vaginitis in children 3 months to 9 years of age, *T. vaginalis* infection accounted for only 2.8% to 4.4% of cases of vaginitis in unestrogenized vaginas, in contrast to 50% of infections in fully estrogenized vaginas of patients nearing puberty.[25] In asymptomatic male subjects infected with *T. vaginalis,* the prostate gland serves as a reservoir. Men may remain asymptomatic because of the concentration of zinc salts in prostatic fluid, which is cytocidal for trichomonads.[40] In symptomatic male patients, *T. vaginalis* may be isolated in specimens from urine, urethral discharge, and semen.[33,40]

In the host, trichomonads may serve as a vector for bacteria and viruses, as shown by the high coinfection rate with *T. vaginalis* and human papillomavirus. Although bacteria contaminate trichomonads externally, trichomonads are thought to ingest virus-infected cells and destroy them, with the active virus left intact.[27] *T. vaginalis* has been implicated in pelvic inflammatory disease (PID) through ascension from the vagina to the fallopian tubes. In vitro studies have shown *Escherichia coli* strains, a part of the normal vaginal flora, intimately attached to trichomonads by glycoprotein strands.[34] Trichomonads contaminated with bacteria serve as vectors for the bacteria to produce pelvic infection on reaching the uterus, fallopian tubes, or peritoneum.[34] Similarly, a more recent study involving Dutch women attending an STI treatment clinic found that 71% of the women infected with *T. vaginalis* were coinfected with *M. hominis*. Because of the small sample size, however, whether infection with *T. vaginalis* predisposes female patients to infection with *M. hominis* or whether this coinfection reflects the sexual behavior of the individual person remains unclear.[7]

In contrast, vaginal colonization with *Lactobacillus* spp. was thought to inhibit trichomonal invasion by lowering vaginal pH. In a study of 336 African women 15 to 49 years of age, 199 of whom were pregnant, 31% had positive culture results for *T. vaginalis,* and only 40% of the patients tested positive for *Lactobacillus.* Although the rate of *Lactobacillus* colonization in these African women was low, the high rate of *T. vaginalis* infection was not related to the absence of *Lactobacillus.* Trichomonads may not alter the vaginal flora substantially.[47] In women infected with *T. vaginalis* in the lower genital tract, however, the aggressive inflammatory response with resultant punctate hemorrhages allows transmission and infection with HIV-1.[60]

A spectrum of severity of disease exists in patients infected with *T. vaginalis.* Some patients are asymptomatic, whereas others experience severe symptomatic inflammation and discomfort. The virulence of *T. vaginalis* isolates varies; whether this variance is caused by the host response or inherent properties of the parasite is unknown. The Golgi apparatus in *T. vaginalis* is a prominent structure and seems to be a key station in the production of adhesins.[8] Evidence indicates, however, that the dramatic heterogeneity that exists on the surface of the parasite leads to antigenic diversity among different isolates of *T. vaginalis.* In one study, prominent immunogens absent on the surface of *T. vaginalis* isolates led to an enhanced ability of the parasite to cause cytoadherence-dependent killing of HeLa cells in monolayer culture. In addition, only the adherent parasites possessed adhesins, which directly affected cytoadherence and cytotoxicity of the parasites.[2] The cysteine proteases of *T. vaginalis* may be responsible for the cytoadherence, nutrient acquisition, and cytotoxicity of *T. vaginalis.* These proteinases are shed during the life cycle and growth of *T. vaginalis.* One hundred percent of serum samples from women infected with *T. vaginalis,* but none from normal uninfected women, possessed immunoglobulin (Ig) G to numerous trichomonad cysteine proteinases. This serum antiproteinase antibody disappeared after the women received effective therapy for the infection.[3]

Some studies provide insight into the relationship between *T. vaginalis* and HIV infection. Potentially biologic synergy is present between *T. vaginalis* and HIV infection, with a 1.5- to 1.7-fold increased risk for HIV acquisition when *T. vaginalis* is present. *T. vaginalis* probably alters the cervicovaginal epithelium by several interacting mechanisms mediated by toll-like receptors, cytokines, chemokines, and innate immune factors, thereby increasing the risk for HIV infection.[67] Women with HIV infection with *T. vaginalis* are found to have a higher prevalence of HIV RNA in vaginal secretions than women without *T. vaginalis* infection. A decrease in mean HIV RNA genital shedding among HIV-infected women also has been noted after *T. vaginalis* treatment and over a 1- to 3-month period.[5] HIV-infected women with *T. vaginalis* alone or with gonorrhea and *Chlamydia* infection also have a 1.9 times higher risk for PID.[5]

IMMUNOLOGY

The interaction between *T. vaginalis* and host immunoglobulins is unclear. In women infected with *T. vaginalis,* specific local antibodies—IgG and IgA—are seen in vaginal secretions. IgA may serve to increase opsonization of the parasite by IgG and result in enhanced phagocytosis. IgG specific for *Trichomonas* cysteine proteases and surface proteins is seen, but it does not help rid the host of infection.[3] *T. vaginalis* synthesizes high-molecular-weight proteins with variable surface expression.[4] Of samples obtained from women infected with *T. vaginalis,* 70% of vaginal washes and 80% of vaginal mucus samples had IgG to a specific *T. vaginalis* surface protein immunogen with a molecular mass of 230,000 Da (P230). In contrast, no antibody to P230 was detected in uninfected women or in detergent extract depleted of P230, a finding suggesting a highly specific antibody.[4] Clinically, this finding may account for the lack of resistance to repeated *Trichomonas* infections and variable host antibody titers in infected persons.

CLINICAL MANIFESTATIONS

Trichomonas has been isolated from the tracheal aspirates in preterm neonates with respiratory failure and from nasal secretions in a full-term newborn with suppurative nasal discharge and respiratory distress.[52,64,65] The vagina of an infant may serve as a reservoir of infection that goes unnoticed until the infant is evaluated for fever 5 to 6 weeks after birth. Motile trichomonads and pyuria are seen on examination of the urine. Symptoms resolve after treatment with metronidazole.[55] Vaginitis, with a purulent foul-smelling discharge and itching, is the most common manifestation of infection with *T. vaginalis* in premenarcheal girls; in some patients, trichomonads may be found in the urine initially, with the development of frank signs of vaginitis 7 to 28 days later.[27,44]

In adolescent girls *T. vaginalis* causes an infection of the vagina, the urethra, the Bartholin and Skene glands, and the cervix. However, 50% of adolescent girls infected with *T. vaginalis* are asymptomatic.[63] *T. vaginalis* infection is associated significantly with purulent discharge, vulvar itching, a "strawberry cervix" (punctuate hemorrhagic spots), and vaginal and vulvar erythema. The sensitivity of the other signs and symptoms of *Trichomonas* vaginitis, including vaginal burning, dysuria, urinary frequency, dyspareunia, frothy discharge, and cervical friability, is low.[70] Although frothy leukorrhea is associated most frequently with *Trichomonas* infection, 29% of the patients with frothy discharge in one study did not have *Trichomonas* infection.[70] Colpitis macularis or strawberry cervix is pathognomonic of *T. vaginalis* infection, but it is noted in only 2% to 3 of patients. Thus this finding cannot be depended on to establish a clinical diagnosis of *T. vaginalis* vaginitis in most patients.[70] Using an NAAT, *T. vaginalis* has been isolated from the anorectal canal in 8.8% of women and 0.9% of men who reported anorectal intercourse. The significance of this finding is not completely understood, but it is possible that in women perianal contamination from the vagina occurred.[14] Trichomonads may ascend the fallopian tubes and, if contaminated with bacteria, can produce PID.[11,34] In HIV-infected girls and women, the risk for developing PID increases significantly with *T. vaginalis* vaginitis.[51]

In male patients *T. vaginalis* causes an infection of the urethra, urine, semen, Skene glands, epididymis, and prostate and may manifest as symptomatic urethritis with dysuria secondary to urethral inflammation and discharge, balanitis, and rarely prostatitis. However, 90% of adolescent boys and men infected with *T. vaginalis* are asymptomatic.[63] On examination, the discharge often is not visualized. When a discharge is present, it is clear to cloudy, but not grossly purulent. On microscopy, numerous inflammatory cells are seen.[39,43]

T. vaginalis also may be a cause of chronic nonbacterial prostatitis and may manifest as chronic prostatitis resistant to standard therapy.[32,43,68] Large numbers of trichomonads have been isolated by culture of prostatic secretions of husbands of women with recurrent *T. vaginalis* infection,[68] with the highest yield (83%) from prostatic secretions, followed by urethral and urine specimens.[68] *T. vaginalis* has been reported to be an etiologic agent of epididymitis in men, with purulent urethral discharge, scrotal swelling, and enlargement of the epididymis.[17] Although a rare finding, *T. vaginalis* has been reported to infect the median raphe of the penis.[61]

CLINICAL DIAGNOSIS

In girls and women, report of vaginal discharge, the presence of a frothy purulent discharge, vulvar or vaginal erythema, and a strawberry cervix should be suggestive of *Trichomonas* infection. Boys and men tend to be asymptomatic or, if symptomatic, have a purulent urethral discharge and urethral inflammation. If the physician relies on clinical examination alone, 80% of infections may be missed.[20,62]

Screening and Diagnosis

No recommendations have been provided by the Centers for Disease Control and Prevention (CDC) regarding routine screening of asymptomatic female and male patients because of the lack of studies that adequately tested screening for these populations. However, the agency states that decisions about routine screening may be informed by the local epidemiology of *T. vaginalis* infection. Screening can be considered in high-prevalence settings such as STI clinics and correctional facilities and in persons with multiple sex partners, exchange of sex for payment, illicit drug use, or a history of STI. However, data are lacking on whether screening and treatment using these criteria can reduce any adverse health events or community burden of infection.[71]

Routine screening for *T. vaginalis* infection in asymptomatic HIV-positive female patients is recommended by the CDC.[71] Routine screening for *T. vaginalis* infections among adolescent girls in foster care should be considered as a best practice measure in pediatric settings.[1,28]

Because of the high prevalence of *Trichomonas* infections in girls and women, testing should be performed in symptomatic female patients seeking care for vaginal discharge. In a study that assessed testing practices for *T. vaginalis,* only 45% of symptomatic women at STI clinics were tested.[49] Local testing policies may be influencing the variations in clinical practice, including the availability of microscopy in clinical settings.

Laboratory Tests

Several tests are currently available, including culture, point-of-care tests, and NAATs.

Point-of-Care Tests

Vaginal microscopy of vaginal secretions continues to be a popular and efficient point-of-care test, especially in urban clinics. However, wet mount examinations are tests that are regulated by the Clinical Laboratory Improvement Amendments (CLIA), may have become a barrier to performing these tests in office-based laboratories.

Wet mount preparations are obtained by swabbing the lateral and anterior vaginal fornices to obtain discharge material with vaginal epithelial cells; the secretions are placed in a tube with normal saline and are mounted on a slide as soon as possible to detect motile trichomonads with flagella. These preparations are easy to perform, and the method is cost effective, but in women its sensitivity is only approximately 51% to 65%.[71] The sensitivity of wet mount preparations has also been shown to decrease from 57% to 22% after douching.[20] In addition, the validity of the result depends on the technical skill of the examiner and the rapidity with which the specimen is examined; cooling greatly affects the motility of trichomonads.[42] The sensitivity has been found to decrease by up to 20% within 1 hour after collection.[71]

Other Food and Drug Administration–cleared point-of-care diagnostic tests for *T. vaginalis* in adolescent and adult women include an immunochromatographic capillary flow dipstick technology (the OSOM Trichomonas Rapid Test, Genzyme) and a direct nucleic acid probe hybridization test for *T. vaginalis*, *Gardnerella vaginalis*, and *Candida* spp. (Affirm VP III Microbial Identification System, Becton Dickinson, Franklin Lakes, NJ).[10] Results of these tests can be obtained in 10 and 45 minutes, respectively. Although the sensitivity of both tests on vaginal secretions is greater than 83% and the specificity is greater than 97%, false-positive test results may occur in low-prevalence populations.[7,71] These point-of-care tests have not been validated or approved for use in genital specimens from prepubertal girls or male urethral specimens.[28,71]

A positive attitude toward home testing by adolescent female patients 14 to 22 years of age predicted high self-test acceptability, and tampon use was associated with increased self-test comfort.[30] Results of patient-collected swabs were in 100% agreement with swabs and tests conducted by a physician.[31] This finding is helpful for purposes of clinical research and home-based clinical services.

Culture

Culture using Diamond medium (Remel) was the gold standard for detecting *T. vaginalis* infections in vaginal secretion before the NAATs became available.[71] The sensitivity of the culture method is 75% to 96%, and the specificity is 100%.[71] However, the cost of and time taken to process this test in the laboratory, the storage requirements, and the transport requirements of using culture media may be prohibitive for routine office use.

In contrast to wet mount examination, the InPouch (Biomed Diagnostics) method also was found to be significantly more sensitive and specific in one study conducted in young adolescent girls (median age, 13.6 years). This finding underscores the need for accurate testing when using culture-based testing and using InPouch or Diamond medium in cases of sexual abuse.[21] In men, the combination of prostatic massage before collection of the specimen and culture of urethral samples and urinary sediment has a sensitivity of 94% to 98%.[41,54]

Nucleic Acid Amplification Tests

NAATs are the gold standard today because they detect T. vaginalis infection three to five times more than the wet mount examination.[71] The Aptima *T. vaginalis* test (analyte-specific reagent assay; Hologic) is commercially available, and it is frequently combined with tests for bacterial vaginosis, yeast infection, gonorrhea, and *Chlamydia* infection. The sensitivity and specificity of this test in detecting *T. vaginalis* in vaginal specimens, endocervical swabs, and urine specimens are 95% to 100%.[71] The BD Probe Tec TV Q[x] Amplified DNA Assay (Becton Dickinson) is also cleared by the Food and Drug Administration for detection of *T. vaginalis* from endocervical, vaginal, or urine specimens from women.[71] However, no data are available in children.[28]

Papanicolaou Smear

T. vaginalis may be an incidental finding on a Papanicolaou test, but neither conventional nor liquid-based Pap tests are considered diagnostic tests for trichomoniasis, because false-negative and false-positive results can occur.[71]

Other Diagnostic Tests

Acridine orange stain is rarely used in the United States; however, this technique continues to be useful in clinical settings around the world with very basic laboratory resources. Acridine orange stains may permit a rapid, accurate diagnosis of *T. vaginalis* infection and seem to be at least as sensitive as wet mount examination.[9,56] The dye stains DNA (yellow-green) and RNA (bright red). *T. vaginalis* stains brick red with an oval, yellow-green nucleus. The flagella do not stain. Unfixed smears are kept at room temperature for 24 hours; fixed slides may be kept for 5 days.

TREATMENT

Metronidazole or tinidazole is the treatment of choice for *T. vaginalis* infection, and these drugs are available in the United States. Worldwide, other drugs used for trichomoniasis include nifuratel, nimorazole, secnidazole, and carnidazole. Despite the availability of these other drugs, metronidazole remains the standard therapy for trichomoniasis. Metronidazole enters the trichomonad by passive diffusion, and its nitro group is reduced to a cytotoxic intermediate that reacts with DNA and causes cell death. Metronidazole is 93% to 95% bioavailable; after oral administration, peak serum levels are attained in 1 to 3 hours, and a steady state is attained in 2 to 3 days. Metronidazole is metabolized by the liver, with only 20% protein bound; the drug is distributed well in the body.[46]

Side effects reported with the use of metronidazole include nausea, vomiting, anorexia, a metallic taste, headache, dizziness, diarrhea, and darkening of the urine. Urticaria, reversible peripheral neuropathy, seizures, and ataxia have been reported with intravenous use. The side effects tend to be dose related and self-limited.[46] In a study of 1199 women with *T. vaginalis* infection who were treated with metronidazole, only 4% to 5% experienced symptoms of nausea, coated tongue, dryness of the mouth, anorexia, or diarrhea. All symptoms disappeared within a few days of completion of treatment, and in only one case was treatment discontinued because of side effects. In addition, relative and absolute leukopenia was not observed in these subjects. Metronidazole enhances or reactivates the growth of *Candida albicans* in the vagina. Metronidazole may potentiate the actions of anticonvulsant agents and warfarin. Because a significant disulfiram-like effect is produced when the drug is combined with moderate intake of alcohol, alcohol should be avoided during and for 48 hours after completion of a course of therapy with metronidazole.[46]

In the United States, two treatment regimens are recommended for treatment of *T. vaginalis*. The first is metronidazole, 2 g orally in a single dose in adolescents. This regimen is 90% to 95% effective.[71] The second regimen is tinidazole, 2 g orally in a single dose. This regimen is 86% to 100% effective. An alternative regimen is metronidazole, 500 mg twice daily for 7 days. Some strains of *T. vaginalis* have reduced susceptibility to metronidazole, with low-level metronidazole-resistant strains reported in 2% to 5% of infected cases. Metronidazole vaginal gel is less efficacious than oral metronidazole and is therefore not recommended.[71] Although rare, higher-level resistance also has been reported.[50,57,59] Treatment options for metronidazole-resistant cases are limited. If the infection fails to respond to metronidazole, it should be re-treated with tinidazole or metronidazole at 500 mg twice daily for 7 days.[71] If treatment failure continues, the patient can be re-treated with 2 g of metronidazole or tinidazole once daily for 5 days.[71]

Treatment of *T. vaginalis* in an HIV-positive adolescent is the same as the standard treatment.[71] However, a randomized clinical trial has demonstrated that the 7-day regimen of metronidazole, 500 mg twice daily for 7 days, is better than the single-dose regimen in HIV-positive patients.[36] Metronidazole is a pregnancy category B drug. To date, studies have not been able consistently to show an association between metronidazole use during pregnancy and teratogenic effects in infants. In addition, although some data suggest an increased risk for having a premature or low-birth-weight infant after undergoing metronidazole treatment, limitations of the studies prevent definitive conclusions regarding risks involved in treatment.[37,71] Treatment during pregnancy may relieve symptoms and prevent pregnancy and perinatal complications. The CDC recommends counseling all pregnant patients on the potential risks and benefits of treatment. Treatment of all symptomatic women is recommended. In asymptomatic women, deferring treatment after 37 weeks of gestation is an option.[71]

Tinidazole is a pregnancy category C drug, and its safety in pregnancy has not been evaluated. It is not offered during pregnancy.[71] A breastfed infant consumes approximately 1% of a single 2-g oral dose of metronidazole; infants of mothers who are breastfeeding and who are treated with a single dose of metronidazole for trichomoniasis should be removed from the breast for at least 24 hours after treatment of the mothers.[46,71] In the case of treatment with tinidazole, breastfeeding can be resumed 3 days after the last dose.

In children weighing less than 45 kg with *T. vaginalis* vulvovaginitis, metronidazole, 45 mg/kg per day orally in three divided doses (maximum 2 g/day) for 7 days, is recommended. Metronidazole syrup, 200 mg/5 mL, is available.[35]

The CDC has not recommended partner treatment for *Trichomonas* infection because of inadequate data to support this approach.[12,71] Nonetheless, it is not unusual for practitioners to prescribe expedited partner therapy for *T. vaginalis*. As more data emerge to demonstrate a decrease in repeat infection with partner treatment, a national policy on expedited partner therapy for *T. vaginalis* may be reconsidered.[58]

PROGNOSIS

If untreated, *T. vaginalis* can lead to chronic inflammation of the Bartholin and Skene glands in adolescent girls and to prostatitis and urethritis with urethral stricture formation in adolescent boys.[16] *T. vaginalis* has been associated with adverse pregnancy outcomes, primarily premature rupture of membranes, preterm labor, and low-birth-weight infants.[37] Complete resolution of symptoms in addition to eradication of *T. vaginalis* usually is noted when treatment is provided promptly in all situations. *Trichomonas* infection is also associated with a two- to threefold risk for HIV infection. HIV-positive female patients with *Trichomonas* infections are at increased risk for pelvic inflammatory disease.[71]

NEW REFERENCES SINCE THE SEVENTH EDITION

23. Gaydos DA, Barnes MR, Quinn N, et al. *Trichomonas vaginalis* infection in men who submit self-collected penile swabs after Internet recruitment. *Sex Transm Infect.* 2013;89:504-508.
35. Kimberlin DW, Brady M, Jackson MA, Long SS. American Academy of Pediatrics. Red Book On Line 2015: Report of the Committee on Infectious Diseases. http://www.redbook.solutions.aap.org.
49. Meites E, Llata E, Braxton J, et al. *Trichomonas vaginalis* in selected U.S. sexually transmitted disease clinics: testing, screening, and prevalence. *Sex Transm Dis.* 2013;40:865-869.
53. Satterwhite CL, Torrone E, Meites E, et al. Sexually transmitted infections among U.S. women and men: prevalence and incidence estimates. *Sex Transm Dis.* 2008;40:187-193.
66. Territo HM, Wrotniak BH, Bouton S, et al. A new strategy for *Trichomonas* testing adolescents in the emergency department. *J Pediatr Adolesc Gynecol.* 2016;29:378-381.
71. Workowski KA, Bolan GA; Centers for Disease Control and Prevention. Sexually transmitted diseases treatment guidelines, 2015. *MMWR Recomm Rep.* 2015;64(RR-03):1-137.

The full reference list for this chapter is available at ExpertConsult.com.

216 *Balantidium coli* Infection

Peter J. Hotez

Balantidium coli is the largest protozoan parasite and the only ciliate to infect humans.[10,15,23] The organism has a worldwide distribution, but usually it is found in less developed nations of the tropics. Because pigs are the principal animal reservoir, most human infections have been reported in tropical regions where swine have close contact with humans, such as Southeast Asia and the islands of East Asia and the South Pacific (including Thailand, the Philippines, Papua New Guinea, and West Iran) and Central and South America (including the Altiplano of Bolivia).[3,16,17] High prevalence rates of this infection can be found among pig farmers in this region. Balantidiasis occurs in areas where other swine-associated parasitic zoonoses (e.g., taeniasis, trichinellosis, ascariasis) also are prevalent, although infection with *B. coli* occurs rarely. In Iran, where pig raising no longer is permitted, wild boars serve as an animal reservoir.[18] The organism first was described in 1857 by Malmsten, who observed the ciliates from two patients in Sweden.[5]

ETIOLOGY AND PATHOGENESIS

The organism has trophozoite and cyst stages. The trophozoite is a large, pear-shaped organism covered with cilia. Estimates of size range from 50 to 100 μm in length and 40 to 70 μm in width.[10] This enormous protozoan organism typically can be seen by light microscopy using only low-power magnification.[10] Subcellular organelles, such as a cytostome and many large vacuoles containing bacteria and debris, are visualized under higher magnification. Similar to many other ciliates, *B. coli* trophozoites have a macronucleus and a micronucleus. The trophozoites colonize the large intestine, where ultimately they round up and secrete a cyst wall as they pass down the lumen. The cysts measure 50 to 70 μm and also contain a macronucleus and a micronucleus. The cyst stages can survive in the outside environment and are infectious to a wide range of animals, including humans (see later discussion).

Frequently, *B. coli* does not invade human tissues and does not cause clinical disease. Under conditions that are not well understood, however, *B. coli* also has the potential for highly aggressive invasion and destruction of tissue. Whether the invasive potential of *B. coli* results from parasite virulence, compromised host defenses, or some combination of these two factors is unclear. The observation that invasive disease occurs more commonly in debilitated patients and in patients with polyparasitism suggests that host defenses have an important role in limiting tissue destruction by *B. coli*.[1,15]

When parasite invasion occurs, it begins in the colonic mucosa, where ulcerations and secondary microabscesses can result. Extensive tissue damage in the cecum and appendix results in clinical presentations of typhlitis and appendicitis.[7,8,15] Histopathologic examination of these tissues reveals flask-shaped ulcerations and necrosis with an extensive inflammatory infiltrate composed predominantly of polymorphonuclear leukocytes.[7,15] *B. coli* probably creates mucosal ulcerations through the release of histolytic enzymes similar to those described from *Entamoeba histolytica*.[19] Ulcerations can lead to hemorrhage or even colonic perforation. A second type of histopathology has been reported in which patients harboring *B. coli* develop inflammatory polyposis of the rectum and sigmoid colon.[14]

When tissue invasion is extensive, the organism can metastasize to extraintestinal sites and cause hepatic and pulmonary involvement. Polymorphonuclear inflammatory cell infiltration results in abscesses at these sites.[5,8,14] Most patients with metastatic balantidiasis have recognizable defects in host defenses.[14]

EPIDEMIOLOGY

As noted earlier, human balantidiasis has a worldwide distribution, but epidemic foci have been reported in the swine-producing areas of Papua New Guinea, West Irian, Micronesia, the Seychelles Islands, the Philippines, and Central and South America.[5,16,21] Incidence rates can be high among swine farmers and slaughterhouse workers. The potential for development of human *B. coli* infections is thought to be high in areas of poor hygiene where extensive contact occurs between humans and pigs. The major risk factors include close contact between pigs and humans, inadequate sanitation, and subtropical or tropical climates that favor survival of the infective cyst stages.[17] A notorious outbreak of human balantidiasis occurred after a devastating typhoon on the Pacific island of Truk caused widespread contamination of ground and surface water supplies with pig feces.[21] Many other animals, including nonhuman primates, guinea pigs, horses, cattle, and rats, also potentially can serve as reservoir hosts. *B. coli* also colonizes many great apes, including baboons, orangutans, chimpanzees, and gorillas, and clinical balantidiasis has been reported in these primates when they are maintained in captivity.[15] Human epidemics also have been described in institutional settings, especially where crowding mixes with low levels of personal hygiene.[21] In these instances, human-to-human spread has been postulated. Although *B. coli* is not known as an opportunistic pathogen in patients infected with human immunodeficiency virus, at least one case of *B. coli* in this setting has been described.[5]

CLINICAL MANIFESTATIONS

Asymptomatic Infection

Most infections are asymptomatic or cause occasional loose stools. This situation probably accounts for 85% of patients harboring *B. coli*.[15] Asymptomatic infection may occur more commonly in children than in adults.[22]

Diarrhea

The next most frequent presentation of *B. coli* infections is in patients who have intermittent diarrhea, abdominal pain, and weight loss.[22] Sometimes, discrete ulcerations can be observed during sigmoidoscopy.[15] Chronic diarrhea has been described in a patient with acquired immunodeficiency syndrome.[4] A subset of patients with balantidiasis subsequently develops invasive disease.

Invasive Colonic Balantidiasis

The hallmark of *Balantidium* colitis is dysentery with bloody and mucous stools, colonic tenderness, leukocytosis, and fever. Sigmoidoscopy and colonoscopy of these patients reveal ulcerations and formation of mucosal granulomas.[1,15,21] Involvement of the large intestine can be diffuse, although in some cases, right-sided colonic lesions predominate. Right-sided colonic lesions can progress to typhlitis or appendicitis.[7,8,15] Transmural involvement of the colon frequently results in intestinal obstruction, hemorrhage, and balantidial peritonitis. Colonic perforation is an ominous complication that is associated with extremely high mortality rates.[15]

Metastatic and Extraintestinal Balantidiasis

Highly invasive balantidiasis leading to metastatic disease of the mesenteric lymph nodes, liver, and lung is a rare complication that can occur in malnourished, debilitated, and immunocompromised patients. Pulmonary infection with *B. coli* has been described.[17] A case of extraintestinal disease associated with pulmonary hemorrhage and iron deficiency was described, possibly as a result of inhalation of pig manure.[13] *B. coli* has been rarely reported as a urinary tract pathogen linked to hematuria[2,12] and as a cause of vertebral osteomyelitis.[6]

DIAGNOSIS

Stools from patients harboring *B. coli* have been described as having a pigpen odor.[22] The examination of wet preparations of fresh or concentrated stools usually reveals cyst and trophozoite forms of *B. coli.* Cilia motility and rapid rotary motion of the trophozoites occasionally can be appreciated under low-power magnification. Because the organism takes up heavy concentrations of dye, stained preparations typically do not reveal internal structures or even cilia.[10] These large organisms can be confused with helminth ova, especially on stained preparations.[10] As an adjunct to direct fecal examinations, sigmoidoscopy can show ulcerations from which abundant trophozoites may be obtained for diagnosis.[22] Bronchoalveolar wash fluid containing *B. coli* has been reported; investigators have suggested that diagnosing such lung infections can be problematic because of the potential to confuse ciliated *B. coli* with ciliated pulmonary epithelial cells.[17]

TREATMENT

For the treatment of intestinal balantidiasis, numerous chemotherapeutic regimens have been tried, usually with some improvement. In many cases, the parasite is not eradicated, however.[15] For children older than 8 years of age, tetracycline, 40 mg/kg per day in four doses for 10 days (maximum, 2 g/day), is the treatment of choice.[20] Tetracycline is considered to be investigational for this condition by the US Food and Drug Administration. Also considered investigational for balantidiasis are the drugs iodoquinol, 30 to 40 mg/kg per day (maximum, 2 g) in three doses for 20 days, and metronidazole, 35 to 50 mg/kg per day in three doses for 5 days (maximum dosage, 2 g).[9,11] Nitazoxanide also may be effective.[17] Alternative chemotherapeutic agents that have been tried with variable success include paromomycin and chloroquine.[15] Surgical intervention often is required for gastrointestinal invasive complications of *B. coli,* such as typhlitis, appendicitis, and peritonitis.

NEW REFERENCES SINCE THE SEVENTH EDITION

2. Bandyopadhyay A, Majumder K, Goswami BK. *Balantidium coli* in urine sediment: report of a rare case presenting with hematuria. *J Parasit Dis.* 2013;37(2):283-285.
3. Boonjaraspinyo S, Boonmars T, Kaewsamut B, et al. A cross-sectional study on intestinal parasitic infections in rural communities, northeast Thailand. *Korean J Parasitol.* 2013;51(6):727-734.
6. Dhawan S, Jain D, Mehta VS. *Balantidium coli:* an unrecognized cause of vertebral osteomyelitis and myelopathy. *J Neurosurg Spine.* 2013;18(3):310-313.
9. *Drugs for Parasitic Infections From the Medical Letter.* 2nd ed. New Rochelle, NY: The Medical Letter; 2010.
13. Koopowitz A, Smith P, van Rensburg N, Rudman A. *Balantidium coli*-induced pulmonary haemorrhage with iron deficiency. *S Afr Med J.* 2010;100:534-538.
17. Schuster FL, Ramirez-Avila L. Current world status of *Balantidium coli. Clin Microbiol Rev.* 2008;21:626-638.
12. Karuna T, Khadanga S. A rare case of urinary balantidiasis in an elderly renal failure patient. *Trop Parasitol.* 2014;4(1):47-49.
20. The Medical Letter. Drugs for parasitic infections, 3rd edition. *Treat Guidel Med Lett.* 2013;11(suppl).

The full reference list for this chapter is available at ExpertConsult.com.

Cryptosporidiosis 217

Poonum S. Korpe • A. Clinton White Jr

Cryptosporidium is an important cause of acute diarrhea in normal hosts worldwide, of persistent diarrhea in children in developing countries, and of chronic diarrhea in immunocompromised hosts, including patients with acquired immunodeficiency syndrome (AIDS).[42,83,124,195,218] These protozoan parasites were identified first in the stomach of mice in 1907,[209] and for decades they were considered to be veterinary pathogens. The first human cases of cryptosporidiosis were reported in 1976.[140,160] In the early 1980s, large numbers of cases were noted with the emerging epidemic of AIDS.[51] Thereafter, *Cryptosporidium* was identified in animal handlers and children,[51,223] and it was associated with large waterborne outbreaks of diarrhea.[53,130] Studies have shown that *Cryptosporidium* is a common cause of diarrheal disease in immunocompetent and immunocompromised hosts. More recent studies using more sensitive techniques suggest that it is an under-recognized cause of moderate to severe diarrhea in Africa and Asia. *Cryptosporidium* is thought to be second to rotavirus as a cause of diarrhea morbidity worldwide.[113,195]

MICROBIOLOGY

Cryptosporidium spp. are ubiquitous, small (4–6 μm), obligate intracellular protozoan parasites that infect the epithelium of the gastrointestinal tract of vertebrates. *Cryptosporidium* was previously classified within the subclass Coccidia, along with *Cystoisospora*, *Cyclospora*, and *Toxoplasma*, but this may soon change.[218] Species names were given according to the animal that they infected.[61] Initial cross-transmission studies revealed that little host specificity exists. Subsequent genetic studies have identified at least 26 accepted species of *Cryptosporidium* and more than 45 *Cryptosporidium* genotypes.[33,122] At least 15 species have been documented to cause human infection.[19,33] Most human infections are caused by separate species, *C. hominis* and *C. parvum*. *C. hominis* is found mainly in humans (but can infect gnotobiotic pigs), and *C. parvum* is found in a wide range of animals (particularly cattle and sheep) and in humans. The relative frequency of *C. hominis* and *C. parvum* in humans differs in geographic regions, probably as the result of differences in transmission routes. In European countries, *C. parvum* was initially found more commonly in human cases than *C. hominis,* although several more recent *C. hominis* outbreaks have been reported throughout Western Europe.[75,120,184,221] In the rest of the world, *C. hominis* has been the predominant species in humans.[23,25,225] *C. meleagridis* has been identified in most case series. Humans are less frequently infected with *C. cuniculus, C. canis, C. felis, C. muris, C. ubiquitum,* and *C. viatorum.*[24,37,58,59,70–72] Rare infections have been noted with six other species and four other genotypes.[33]

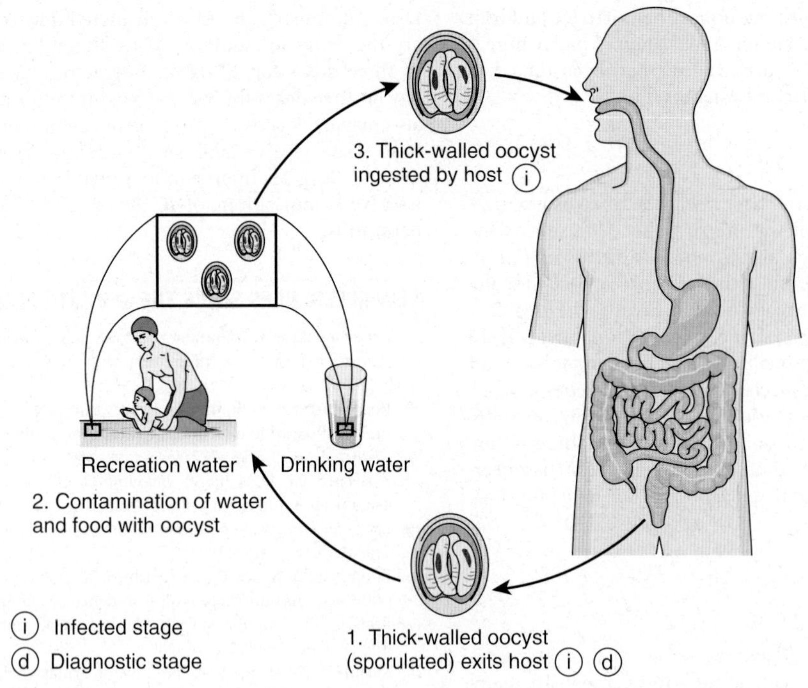

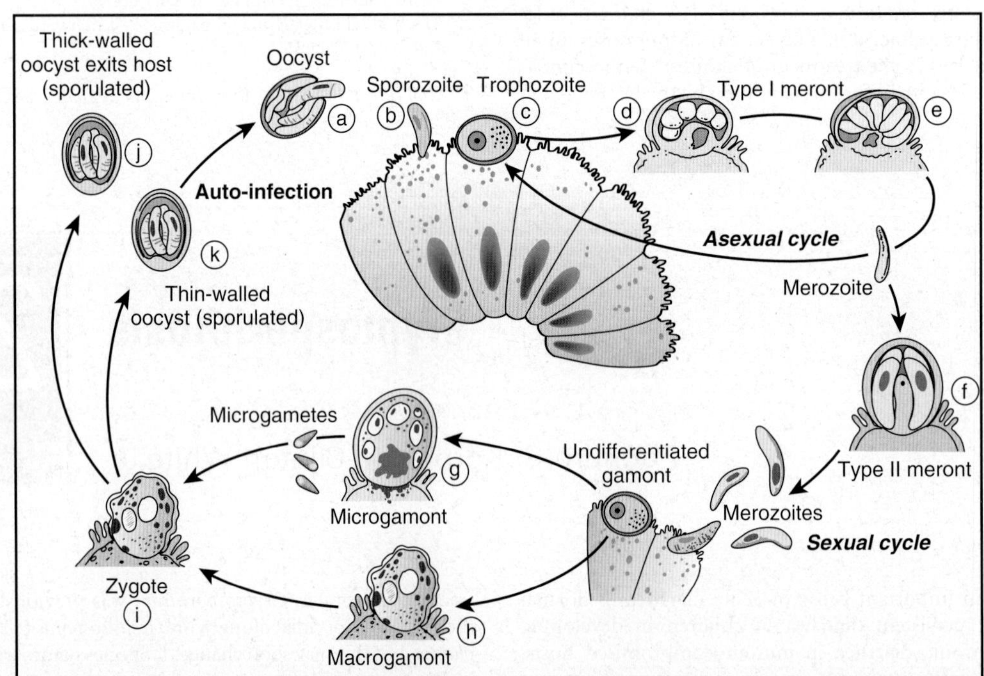

FIG. 217.1 Life cycle of oocyst. After ingestion, the oocysts *(a)* release the sporozoites *(b)*, which attach to and are engulfed by the epithelial cell. Inside the parasitophorous vacuole, the organisms enlarge to form trophozoites *(c)* and divide to form meronts *(d, e, f)*. After reinvasion, they may differentiate into the sexual forms (microgamont *[g]* and macrogamont *[h]*), which fuse to form the zygote *(i)*. The zygote releases the thin-walled oocysts *(k)*, which cause autoinfection, or thick-walled oocysts *(j)*, which are the infectious form.

LIFE CYCLE

Cryptosporidium spp. can complete their entire life cycles, including asexual (merogony) and sexual (sporogony) reproductive cycles, within a single host (homoxenous). The life cycle is characterized by six major developmental stages: (1) excystation, or release of infective sporozoites; (2) merogony, or asexual replication in the host; (3) gametogony, or the formation of microgametocytes and macrogametocytes; (4) fertilization, or the union of microgametocytes and macrogametocytes; (5) oocyst formation; and (6) sporogony, or the formation of infectious sporozoites within the oocyst wall (Fig. 217.1).[19,61,163]

The life cycle begins with ingestion of the infectious oocyst. The oocysts are activated in the stomach (temperature and acid) and upper intestines (bicarbonate, bile, and pancreatic enzymes). This process allows the organisms to excyst, releasing four infective sporozoites.[163] The motile sporozoites glide over the surface of the epithelium and bind to receptors on the surface of the intestinal epithelium, thus inducing actin polymerization and protrusion of the intestinal epithelial cell membrane.[163] The membrane surrounds the sporozoite and fuses to form the parasitophorous vacuole, which remains in the microvillus layer on the surface of the epithelium. Inside the parasitophorous vacuole the parasites undergo asexual reproduction (merogony). They enlarge into trophozoite forms and divide to form type I meronts, which mature and rupture to release the motile merozoites. The merozoites bind to receptors on the epithelial cells and are engulfed by the cells. They then either repeat the process of merogony or undergo sexual differentiation (sporogony).

In the case of sexual differentiation, the merozoites differentiate into the microgametocytes and macrogametocytes. The microgametocyte releases the microgametes, which penetrate the cells infected with macrogametocytes. The macrogametocytes and microgametes fuse to form the zygote form, which then undergoes meiosis to form the oocyst, containing four sporozoites. Two morphologic forms of the oocyst have been described: thin-walled oocysts, which excyst within the same host in a process of self-infection; and thick-walled oocysts, which are shed into the environment.

EPIDEMIOLOGY

Cryptosporidium is distributed worldwide. Infection generally is more common in warm, humid months. Prevalence rates generally are higher in resource-poor countries than in industrialized countries.[124] Older surveys not involving patients with human immunodeficiency virus (HIV) infection documented oocysts in 1% to 3% of specimens from industrialized countries of Europe and North America and in approximately 10% to 15% of specimens from developing countries.[124] Most studies on the prevalence of infection have relied on detection of oocysts in fecal samples using acid-fast stains, which are insensitive. However, with the development of improved diagnostic techniques, such as antigen detection, immunofluorescence, and polymerase chain reaction (PCR), the true burden of cryptosporidiosis is being uncovered.[5,24,42,154,171,190,208] Cryptosporidiosis has been identified as a leading cause of severe diarrhea among young children in low-income countries.[113] A multicenter case-control study of causes of moderate to severe diarrhea estimated 2.9 million cases of cryptosporidiosis in children less than 2 years of age in sub-Saharan Africa and 4.7 million cases in South Asia, with approximately 200,000 *Cryptosporidium*-attributable deaths in these regions.[199]

Studies from Peru, Brazil, India, Bangladesh, Guinea-Bissau, and Zimbabwe have documented frequent infections in children during their first 2 years of life.[4,5,41,104,111,145,151,158,177,213] In a Peruvian birth cohort study of diarrheal disease, the incidence rate of cryptosporidiosis as determined by a serologic assay was higher than the rate determined by stool microscopy (0.77 vs. 0.41 infection/child-year of surveillance).[177] Similarly high seroprevalence rates were noted along the United States–Mexico border.[118] Young children in day care centers are at high risk for acquiring infection. Outbreaks of cryptosporidiosis in day care centers have been reported from numerous countries.[10,46,78,142,214]

Cryptosporidium is also a common cause of persistent diarrhea in immunocompetent and immunocompromised children in developing countries.[72,152,158,161,198,207,208] A study in West African children investigated episode-specific determinants for the progression of an acute episode of diarrhea to chronic diarrhea; current infection with *C. parvum* was the most significant risk factor.[198] Among 243 children with persistent diarrhea in Uganda, 76 (31%) had *Cryptosporidium* infection.[207] Of the 243 children, 91 had HIV infection, of whom 67 (74%) had *Cryptosporidium*. Children with CD4$^+$ cell counts less than 25% were more likely to have *Cryptosporidium* infection.[207]

In wealthy countries, cryptosporidiosis is an important but underdiagnosed problem. The number of cases reported in the United States tripled in the early 2000s, in part because of increased use of diagnostic tests. Currently, approximately 8000 cases are reported per year in the United States (incidence of ~2.6 in 100,000).[168,226,227] However, the actual number of cases is estimated to be 100-fold higher because of underdiagnosis and underreporting.[42,192] In England and Wales, more than 4000 cases are reported per year (incidence of eight in 100,000 per year).[38] In both countries, more cases are detected when laboratories use routine testing for *Cryptosporidium* in all stools from children and when more sensitive immunologic techniques are used (instead of stool microscopy).[34,42,135,174]

Cryptosporidium is a common cause of diarrhea in patients infected with HIV. Cryptosporidiosis occurs in an estimated 10% to 15% of patients with AIDS in developed countries and in 30% to 50% of patients with AIDS in developing countries.[124] Among patients with HIV infection, the infection rate is proportional to the CD4$^+$ cell count. In a longitudinal study of patients with HIV infection, the infection rate varied from 23% of patients with CD4$^+$ cell counts greater than 1000/μL to 46% with cell counts less than 100/μL.[175] The widespread use of highly active antiretroviral therapy has resulted in the restoration of immune function and a reduction in the incidence of cryptosporidiosis and other opportunistic infections.[117]

Cryptosporidiosis also has been noted in other immunodeficient hosts, including patients with primary immunodeficiencies, organ transplantation, cancer, and diabetes.[97] A particularly high prevalence of cryptosporidiosis occurs in patients with X-linked hyper–immunoglobulin (Ig) M syndrome. In two case series of hyper-IgM syndrome, the prevalence of cryptosporidiosis was 24%.[88,121] Cryptosporidiosis is also increasingly recognized after solid organ or stem cell transplantation.[18,114,119]

TRANSMISSION

Humans can acquire *Cryptosporidium* infections through several transmission routes, such as direct contact with infected people (person-to-person transmission) or animals (zoonotic transmission) and ingestion of contaminated water (waterborne transmission) and food (foodborne transmission). The relative importance of these transmission routes varies by species and from country to country.[19,38,226] For example, foodborne disease has been noted more frequently in Scandinavia than in other regions.[76] Transmission dynamics are modulated by the low infectious dose, the fact that oocysts are immediately infectious when shed, the resistance of oocysts to chlorination, the stability of oocysts in the environment (especially in water), and the different dynamics of anthroponotic and zoonotic species.

The infectious dose of *Cryptosporidium* is low. In human challenge studies (including *C. hominis*, *C. parvum*, *C. ubiquitum*, and *C. meleagridis*), all organisms demonstrated a low infectious dose, but considerable variability was noted among isolates, ranging from approximately 1000 oocysts (UCP strain) to 10 oocysts (Texas isolate, *C. hominis*).[39,57,164,165] Because the infectious dose is low, *Cryptosporidium* is transmitted easily from person to person. This route of transmission was recognized initially in outbreaks associated with contact with day care centers[46,223] and with nosocomial transmission.[63,109,157,191] Secondary transmission within households also is common.[131] During the acute diarrheal illness, large quantities of oocytes are excreted in stool and are highly infectious. Asymptomatic shedding of oocytes may continue for 5 weeks after an acute episode of diarrhea.[201] Contact with an ill person is a major risk factor for cryptosporidiosis.[19,226] Sexual transmission has been postulated to occur in association with anogenital sex.[89]

Cryptosporidium parasites are well adapted to waterborne transmission.[12,33,94] *Cryptosporidium* oocysts are resistant to environmental conditions; oocysts can remain infectious for at least 6 months if they are kept moist, but viability decreases rapidly with desiccation.[12,61,163] Oocysts are killed by heat, pasteurization, hydrogen peroxide, ozone, and ultraviolet radiation.[61,106,163] Oocysts are highly resistant to chlorination, however.[110] Surveys have shown that most surface sources of drinking water are contaminated with oocysts before treatment, and even low-grade contamination has been documented in samples of treated water.

Waterborne outbreaks of cryptosporidiosis have been linked to contaminated drinking water, such as water from artesian wells, surface water, and filtered public drinking water,[54,62] and to contaminated recreational water, such as swimming pools, water parks, lakes, rivers, beaches, and fountains.[33,94] The largest documented waterborne outbreak of diarrhea occurred in Milwaukee, Wisconsin in 1993, affecting an estimated 400,000 people.[130] Many of the waterborne outbreaks, including the outbreak in Milwaukee, have been caused by *C. hominis*. However, both *C. hominis* and *C. parvum* have been implicated in spread by drinking water.[38,33,115] With improvements in filtration, drinking water is less often implicated in cases in the United States and Europe, but *Cryptosporidium* remains the main cause of illness associated with recreational water (e.g., swimming pools, rivers, lakes, fountains).[33,94]

The epidemiology varies considerably by parasite species. Studies in the United Kingdom demonstrated that *C. hominis* is associated with the population of young children, international travel, and recreational water.[38] Incidence peaks in the fall. By contrast, *C. parvum* infection peaks in the spring and is associated with animal contact, surface water, and private water supplies. Numerous outbreaks have been attributed to animal contact.[19,38,115] Other species are more frequent in older patients, immunosuppressed hosts (e.g., patients with AIDS), and persons with animal contact.[25,58,59,70,178]

Foodborne infections occur less commonly.[226] Outbreaks have been associated with contaminated apple cider, unpasteurized milk, chicken salad, and raw produce. Oocysts are found commonly on vegetables in developing countries.[167] *Cryptosporidium* is associated with international travel and causes approximately 6% of traveler's diarrhea.[156]

PATHOLOGY AND PATHOGENESIS

In immunocompetent hosts, the organisms are localized primarily to the distal small intestines and proximal colon. In immunodeficient hosts, the parasites have been identified throughout the gut, in the biliary tract, and in the respiratory tract.[45,80,103] Studies using PCR suggest that respiratory involvement may be underappreciated in children with cryptosporidiosis.[153] Children with persistent cryptosporidiosis may have villous atrophy and a mild increase in lamina propria lymphocytes.[173] Heavier infection is associated with the following: villous atrophy; crypt hyperplasia; marked infiltration with lymphocytes, plasma cells, and neutrophils[45,74,79,80,129]; and extraintestinal involvement.

Cryptosporidium causes watery diarrhea, malabsorption, and weight loss. These symptoms are thought to result from sodium malabsorption, electrogenic chloride secretion, and increased intestinal permeability.[124] In vitro studies demonstrated that *Cryptosporidium* infection directly induces defects in intestinal epithelial cell barrier function in vitro.[2,81,182] Cryptosporidiosis also is characterized by defects in intestinal permeability.[79,125,194,228] Increased permeability may result in decreased absorption of fluids and electrolytes and solute fluxes into the gut. Studies in children with cryptosporidiosis have shown a correlation between the severity of disease and altered intestinal permeability.[228] Increased permeability is associated with circulating endotoxin and childhood malnutrition.[151]

Infection of intestinal epithelial cells leads to activation of nuclear factor-κB.[141,181,188] Toll-like receptors and MyD88 are key mediators of this pathway.[43,185] The main effect of this activation is to inhibit apoptosis of the infected cells. This signaling pathway leads to modulation of microRNAs and secretion of defensins.[43,163] Increased expression of proinflammatory cytokines and markers of inflammation also occurs, including tumor necrosis factor-α and increased expression of proinflammatory CXCL8, CXCL10, and lactoferrin.[107,124,163,170] The chemokines and cytokines recruit inflammatory and immune cells into the intestines. Infection also leads to increased expression of cyclooxygenase-2, production of prostaglandins by the epithelial cells, and production of neuropeptides by the inflammatory cells.[90,116,181] Prostaglandins are thought to mediate decreased sodium absorption and to stimulate chloride secretion. However, prostaglandin inhibitors have not proved to be effective in therapy of human cryptosporidiosis. The neuropeptide substance P correlates with severity of diarrhea in patients with cryptosporidiosis and AIDS and causes many of the defects associated with cryptosporidiosis in a monkey model.[90,181] Octreotide, a substance P antagonist, partially suppresses diarrhea in patients with chronic cryptosporidiosis.[68]

Cryptosporidiosis leads to villous atrophy and crypt hyperplasia.[47,79,129,173] Increased epithelial cell apoptosis has been shown in cells from tissue cultures and in biopsy specimens from infected intestines.[129] Loss of villous surface area is associated with malabsorption.[45,79,194]

IMMUNOLOGY

Both innate immunity and acquired immunity are important in the defense and clearance of *Cryptosporidium*.[170] Innate responses play a key role in clearance of initial infections.[136] Some host factors have been implicated in innate responses, including mannose-binding lectins, complement, defensins, natural killer cells, and nonspecific inflammatory responses.[27,29,43,52,172]

CD4$^+$ T cells play a key role in the control of cryptosporidiosis, mainly associated with acquired immunity. Among patients with HIV infection, cryptosporidiosis is self-limited in patients with CD4$^+$ cell counts greater than 180/μL, chronic in patients with cell counts lower than 100/μL, and fulminant in some patients with cell counts lower than 50/μL.[17,64,86,133] Resolution of cryptosporidiosis in patients with AIDS in response to highly active antiretroviral therapy is associated with an influx of CD4$^+$ cells into the intestines.[193] Similarly, Kirkpatrick and colleagues[108] noted an association between major histocompatibility class (MHC) II types (which present antigen to CD4 cells) and susceptibility to cryptosporidiosis.

Interferon-γ (IFN-γ) is an important mediator of the immune clearance of *Cryptosporidium* in murine models.[12,14,15,19,139,206,211] Similarly, lymphocytes from persons who have recovered from cryptosporidiosis produced IFN-γ after antigen stimulation in vitro.[2,77] Although seropositive volunteers challenged with *C. parvum* expressed IFN-γ in the intestinal mucosa, biopsy samples from seronegative volunteers in human challenge studies, lymphocytes obtained during active cryptosporidiosis, and stool from children with active cryptosporidiosis lacked IFN-γ expression, even though all had self-limited disease.[2,5,16,77,107,176,220] Thus the role of IFN-γ in human infections is predominantly in acquired immunity and memory responses. CD8 cells may be important in human infection because they produce IFN-γ in response to parasite antigen, MHC I polymorphisms are associated with risk of infections, and in vitro studies suggest that CD8 T cells clear infection in vitro.[6,10,12,13,108,169,170,176]

Some IFN-γ–seronegative, normal volunteers were experimentally infected, and in patients with AIDS who were recovering from cryptosporidiosis, interleukin-15 was expressed in the intestines in association with IFN-γ–independent control of infection.[166,180] This effect likely is mediated by activation of natural killer cells.[52,136]

The role of antibody in the immune response to cryptosporidiosis is controversial.[170] High levels of serum and fecal antibodies to *C. parvum* have been found in patients with AIDS with chronic cryptosporidiosis and in volunteers challenged with *C. parvum*.[11,14,48] The presence and timing of antibody correlated with shedding of oocysts, however, rather than with clearance or resistance to infection, and cryptosporidiosis has not been associated with immunoglobulin defects.[97] However, more recent studies suggest that maternal antibodies in breast milk may be protective.[112]

Hyper-IgM syndrome, because of defects in CD40 ligand, is associated with increased frequency and severity of *Cryptosporidium* infection.[3,7,88,122] This susceptibility is thought to result from profound defects of antigen-presenting cells, production of interleukin-12 and tumor necrosis factor-α, and defective stimulation of IFN-γ production.[4,98] Other primary immunodeficiencies associated with cryptosporidiosis include CD4 cell deficiency, deficient MHC II, and combined immunodeficiencies.[97,137,224]

CLINICAL MANIFESTATIONS

The clinical spectrum of disease caused by *Cryptosporidium* is broad and depends on the immunologic status of the host, prior exposure, and parasite species (Table 217.1). Symptoms of cryptosporidiosis develop after a prepatent period, during which the parasites invade the intestinal epithelium and proliferate. The prepatent period, determined from point-source exposures and human challenge studies, is approximately 1 week (range, 1–30 days).[36,130] However, this period varies considerably with parasite strain and intensity of exposure. Regardless of the immunologic status of the patient, diarrhea is the most common clinical manifestation of cryptosporidiosis. Children present with an acute diarrheal syndrome characterized by watery diarrhea, cramps, and

TABLE 217.1 **Clinical Manifestation of Cryptosporidiosis**

Host	Clinical Manifestations	Comments
Normal host	Acute watery diarrhea	Relapses common Persistent diarrhea common
Children in developing countries	Acute watery diarrhea Persistent diarrhea	Diarrhea more severe in children with malnutrition Persistent diarrhea affecting nutritional status, growth, and intellectual function
Immunocompromised host	Acute watery diarrhea Relapsing diarrhea Persistent or chronic diarrhea Cholera-like illness Extraintestinal involvement	Transient, self-limited, similar to disease in normal host Very common Usually found in patients with low CD4 count or malnutrition Voluminous watery diarrhea, only with very low CD4 count Respiratory tract, biliary tract, and pancreas

TABLE 217.2 **Diagnosis of *Cryptosporidium* Infection**

Test Type	Method	Comments
Microscopic examination of stools	Modified acid-fast stain of stools Fluorescent stains (auramine O, auramine-rhodamine) Immunofluorescent assays	Inexpensive and widely available diagnostic test Faster than other acid-fast stains and may improve sensitivity More sensitive than acid-fast staining but also more expensive
Antigen-detection assays	Enzyme immunoassay and immunochromatographic tests: direct and indirect immunofluorescence assay	Good sensitivity (66–100%) and excellent specificity (93–100%), but occasional lots associated with false-positive test results
Molecular methods	Polymerase chain reaction	Increased sensitivity in contrast to microscopic or antigen-detection studies

abdominal pain.[35,124,218] Other, less common clinical findings include fever, flatulence, nausea, vomiting, shortness of breath, and cough. The stools are occasionally described as foul-smelling, bulky, or containing mucus, but they rarely contain blood and fecal leukocytes. Respiratory symptoms are not uncommon, and lung involvement has been noted frequently.[153] In immunocompetent patients, the onset of diarrhea is often abrupt, and the illness usually is self-limited. Recurrent symptoms develop in 40% of patients after initial resolution. Relapses may occur after a diarrhea-free period of several days to weeks.[130,131,158] Forty-five percent of patients have diarrhea lasting more than 14 days.[159,198]

Cryptosporidium is one of the most common causes of prolonged and persistent diarrhea in developing countries and is responsible for about one-third of cases.[104,123,152,158,161,198] Children with persistent diarrhea, especially if caused by *Cryptosporidium*, are at high risk for additional gastrointestinal infections after the initial illness, weight loss, and premature death.[3,7,123,149,150] A long-term follow-up study of children with an onset of cryptosporidiosis before 1 year of age suggests an association with poorer physical fitness and poorer cognitive development that persists for years.[84]

Cryptosporidiosis is more severe in children with malnutrition, and malnourished children tend to have a protracted course and shed oocysts longer.[148,150,151,189] They often require hospitalization, and the disease may have a fatal outcome.[8,49,191] Prospective cohort studies of children followed from birth have shown significant differences in nutritional status before acquisition of *Cryptosporidium* infection.[3,40,148] In addition, the onset of cryptosporidiosis is associated with growth faltering. Older children eventually recovered and experienced catch-up growth, but children infected before 1 year of age often never recovered.[3,40,148] Asymptomatic infection can lead to malnutrition even without diarrhea.[15,41,111] A cohort study of Bangladeshi infants found that even a single asymptomatic infection in the first 24 months of life was associated with increased risk of stunting at age 2 years.[111]

The clinical manifestations also vary somewhat by parasite species. In general, *C. hominis* causes more severe disease than other species. Cama and colleagues[24] noted more nausea, vomiting, and malaise with *C. hominis* than with zoonotic species. Hunter and colleagues[96,97] noted that *C. hominis* was more strongly associated with extraintestinal sequelae (e.g., joint pain, eye pain, fatigue).[36,96]

The clinical manifestations of cryptosporidiosis in patients with HIV vary. Four distinct gastrointestinal syndromes have been described in HIV-infected patients: (1) transient, self-limited diarrhea, similar to diarrhea in normal hosts, usually in patients with $CD4^+$ cell counts greater than 150/µL; (2) voluminous watery diarrhea or cholera-like illness that requires rehydration, seen in a few cases, usually in patients with $CD4^+$ cell counts lower than 50/µL; (3) relapsing diarrhea; and (4) a chronic diarrheal illness resulting in wasting, usually in patients with $CD4^+$ cell counts lower than 150/µL.[17,86,129,133,207] The severity and duration of illness in both patients with AIDS and other patients with immunodeficiencies generally depend on the degree of immunodeficiency.

In immunocompromised patients, extraintestinal involvement may occur in the respiratory tract, biliary tract, and pancreas.[44,86,128,143,212] Respiratory tract involvement often is asymptomatic, but it may cause cough, shortness of breath, wheezing, croup, and hoarseness. *Cryptosporidium* has been reported as a cause of laryngobronchitis in children.[85] Biliary tract involvement in cryptosporidiosis has been limited to patients with profound immunodeficiency.[86,212] Patients may have acalculous cholecystitis or cholangitis and, less frequently, sclerosing cholangitis or hepatitis.[86,203,212] Pancreatitis is an uncommon finding, but it has been reported in adults and children infected with HIV.[87,128,146] Concomitant infection with cytomegalovirus can occur and frequently is associated with irregularities of the intrahepatic duct.[13,93,101]

DIAGNOSIS

Many laboratories do not test for *Cryptosporidium* unless the tests are specifically requested (Table 217.2). *Cryptosporidium* infection usually is diagnosed by microscopic examination of stools. Fresh, preserved, and frozen stools can be used for testing, but preservatives may interfere with some assays.[30,35,197] Numerous concentration methods have been attempted to improve the yield, but formalin-ethyl acetate concentration is the most widely used.[30,197] The oocysts are small, 4 to 6 µm, and similar in size and shape to yeast forms, and stains that are used routinely to detect other intestinal parasites (i.e., iodine, trichrome, and iron hematoxylin) do not detect *Cryptosporidium*. The method most commonly used by clinical laboratories to detect *Cryptosporidium* oocysts in stools has been the modified acid-fast stain.[34,174] Oocysts stain pink or red, whereas yeast cells and fecal debris stain green or blue (Fig. 217.2).[32,37] The sensitivity of stool examination with acid-fast staining is poor, requiring an oocyst concentration of greater than 500,000/mL in formed stools,[216] with fewer cases detected than with other methods.[35] Fluorescent stains (e.g.,

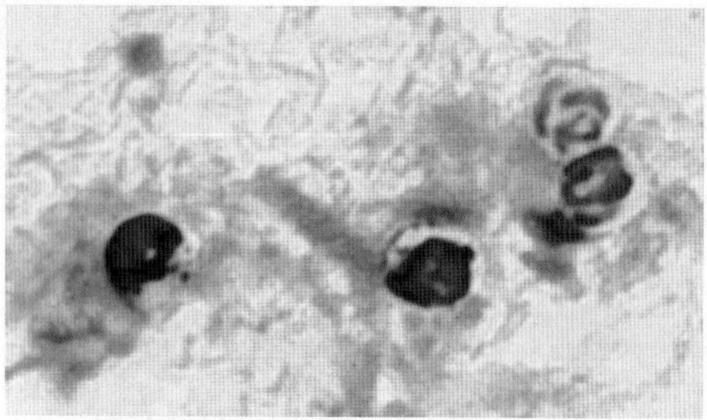

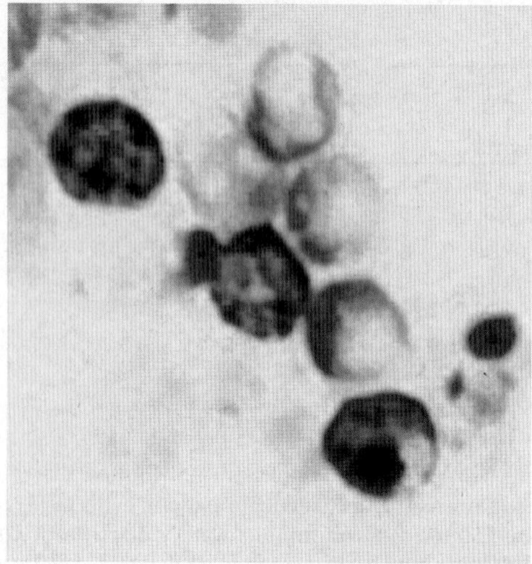

FIG. 217.2 Staining of oocysts.

auramine O, auramine-rhodamine) can be read more quickly than other acid-fast stains and may have improved sensitivity, but positive results require confirmation by a second method.[35,105,197] Immunofluorescent assays are more sensitive than other microscopic methods.[35,66,105]

Antigen-detection assays are being used increasingly for diagnosis. Commercial kits for *Cryptosporidium* are available in enzyme-linked immunosorbent assay (ELISA) and immunochromatographic formats. The ELISA kits for *Cryptosporidium* have good sensitivity (66–100%) and excellent specificity (93–100%).[35,67,66,197] The sensitivity has been poor in some studies, however, and pseudo-outbreaks from false-positive results have been reported.[31,56] Commercial ELISA kits also may test for *Giardia* and *Entamoeba* antigens. Immunochromatographic tests are rapid tests for *Cryptosporidium* and *Giardia* antigen.[67,99] The sensitivity is less than with other assays, and results are available in minutes.[67,99] The specificity was initially reported to be excellent, but a more recent study from Minnesota suggested a poor positive predictive value.[67,99,179] Antigen assays as a group have the advantage of not requiring skill in microscopic identification of organisms.

Molecular methods such as PCR for *C. parvum* DNA also have been used to detect organisms. These methods have increased sensitivity, in contrast to microscopic or antigen-detection studies of stool.[5,137,156,197,204] In one study of children with primary immunodeficiencies, PCR was able to detect significantly more cases of biliary cryptosporidiosis than were detected by stool studies.[137] In general, the number of cases detected increases significantly with molecular methods. Multiplex assays, including for a wide range of enteric pathogens, are in development.[126] A multiplex assay for enteric pathogens using polymerase amplification and detection with probes attached to beads has been approved in the United States.[202]

Biopsy of the intestine typically is unnecessary for the diagnosis of intestinal infection, although the unique apical location within the intestinal epithelium is distinctive. The parasite can be visualized by light microscopy after staining with hematoxylin and eosin or by electron microscopy.[50]

MANAGEMENT

Replacement of fluids and electrolytes is a crucial first step in management, as with all cases of diarrhea. Oral rehydration is preferred, but severely ill patients may require parenteral fluids. Glutamine supplementation may improve fluid absorption.[26] Dietary management is crucial in cryptosporidiosis, especially if it is associated with persistent diarrhea. Supportive care should include initially a lactose-free diet because lactase activity is decreased on the apical border of epithelial cells.[173]

Cryptosporidiosis is associated with increased intestinal transit, which could interfere with absorption of fluids, electrolytes, and drugs.[20,194] Antimotility and antisecretory agents (i.e., tincture of opium, loperamide, octreotide, and acetorphan) have roles in therapy, but their use generally is limited to refractory cases in adults with AIDS.[68,196] These agents may control the diarrhea, but they do not eradicate the parasite.

In immunocompromised hosts, management of intestinal cryptosporidiosis is problematic. For patients with AIDS with chronic cryptosporidiosis, effective antiretroviral therapy can result in dramatic improvement in diarrhea.[28,65,82,132,144,166] The HIV protease inhibitors have anticryptosporidial activity in vitro and reduced infection by 90% in an animal model,[95,141] and most of the studies reporting responses have used protease inhibitors. In contrast, cryptosporidiosis is associated with malabsorption of nucleosides.[22] Similarly, reversal of immunosuppression may be a key component of management of severe cryptosporidiosis in transplant recipients.[114,119] Patients with X-linked immunodeficiency with hyper-IgM syndrome may respond to a CD40 agonist antibody.[60]

The role of antiparasitic therapy in cryptosporidiosis is controversial. Because cryptosporidiosis usually is self-limited in immunocompetent hosts and can be variable in compromised hosts, controlled trials are crucial. No agent has proved reliably curative in patients with advanced AIDS. A meta-analysis of seven randomized controlled clinical trials found no clear evidence for efficacy of antiparasitic agents in the management of cryptosporidiosis in compromised hosts.[1]

Nitazoxanide is a nitrothiazolyl-salicylamide derivative with a broad spectrum of antiprotozoal and anthelmintic activity.[162] Nitazoxanide is active against *Cryptosporidium* in vitro and in animal models.[69,205] A placebo-controlled study of nitazoxanide in patients with cryptosporidiosis showed significant clinical improvement in apparently immunocompetent children and adults with persistent diarrhea.[186] By day 7, diarrhea had resolved in 39 of 49 (80%) patients treated with nitazoxanide, in contrast to 20 of 49 (41%) patients treated with placebo. Nitazoxanide also reduced the duration of shedding of oocysts. In parallel randomized studies in severely malnourished HIV-infected and HIV-negative children in Zambia with chronic cryptosporidiosis, a 3-day course of therapy not only led to clinical and parasitologic improvement, but also improved survival in HIV-negative children.[8] All children were treated with nitazoxanide suspension (100 mg twice daily for 3 days) or matching placebo. Among non–HIV-infected patients, resolution by day 7 was noted in 14 of 25 (56%) patients treated with nitazoxanide, in contrast to 5 of 22 (23%) in the placebo group. Similar findings were reported in immunocompetent patients 12 years of age and older. A good clinical response was seen in 27 of 28 (96%) patients receiving nitazoxanide, in contrast to 11 of 27 (41%) patients receiving placebo.[187] Among the HIV-infected children, most with severe malnutrition, no significant response occurred.[8] A second study using higher doses and prolonged therapy in children with HIV and cryptosporidiosis also did not demonstrate efficacy.[9]

Nitazoxanide suspension was approved in the United States in 2002 for treatment of cryptosporidiosis and giardiasis in children. For most indications, it is administered every 12 hours for 3 days. The recommended dose is 100 mg (5 mL) for children 12 to 47 months of age, 200 mg for children 4 to 11 years old, and 500 mg for patients age 12 years and older (~15 mg/kg per day).[217] Safety data for use of nitazoxanide in children younger than 12 months are lacking; thus its use in infants is not recommended at this time. Nitazoxanide generally is well tolerated; adverse events occur at a frequency similar to that for placebo and include abdominal pain, diarrhea, vomiting, and headache.[217] Although unproved, nitazoxanide and other antiparasitic drugs should be considered as adjuncts to antiretroviral agents or reversal of immunosuppression in children with severe cryptosporidiosis.[147] Combinations of nitazoxanide with other agents (e.g., paromomycin and azithromycin) have been used in some severely compromised patients.

Paromomycin is an orally administered nonabsorbable aminoglycoside. Initial in vitro studies noted poor activity against *C. parvum*. When patients with AIDS and cryptosporidiosis were treated with available antiparasitic drugs, however, some improved when treated with paromomycin.[73] Three randomized, controlled trials examined the effects of paromomycin in patients with AIDS and cryptosporidiosis.[91,102,219] Paromomycin was associated with a significant reduction in shedding of oocysts and decreased stool frequency, but not cure.[219] In another study, no significant difference was found between groups.[91]

Macrolide antibiotics, including spiramycin, azithromycin, roxithromycin, and clarithromycin, have some activity against *Cryptosporidium*.[16] In one study, children treated with spiramycin had shorter duration of symptoms and shedding of oocysts,[188] but a second trial showed no effect.[222] Case series noted improvement in cryptosporidiosis in patients with HIV infection and cancer who were treated with azithromycin,[55,92,100,155] but subsequent trials in patients with AIDS did not show changes in frequency of stools or shedding of oocysts.[16] A study in Egyptian school children suggested that resolution of symptoms was faster with azithromycin.[6] Roxithromycin treatment was associated with improvement in AIDS-associated cryptosporidiosis in two uncontrolled studies.[200,210]

PREVENTION

In hospitals and day care centers, hand washing is the most important measure to prevent the spread of any enteric pathogen. Alcohol rubs may not be adequate. Enteric precautions (i.e., washing hands, wearing gloves, and wearing gowns if soiling is likely) are important measures to prevent nosocomial spread.

Swimming pools are important sources of infection. Contamination of treated recreational water, such as a fecal accident in a swimming pool, should prompt aggressive measures, including closing the pool temporarily.[32,33] Recreational waters, such as lakes, may pose a danger for compromised hosts, who should avoid contact with untreated water.[147]

Control of waterborne transmission of cryptosporidiosis is a major public health concern. This issue is complicated by the ability of *Cryptosporidium* to escape the filtration system used in most public water facilities and its resistance to chlorination. The Centers for Disease Control and Prevention (CDC) recommends that during outbreak situations, compromised patients boil tap water for 1 minute or filter tap water using a filtration system to remove particles 1 μm or larger, or use bottled water prepared by distillation or reverse osmotic filtration.[30] In situations not associated with an outbreak, no special measures are recommended. However, routinely using the outbreak measures outlined earlier for severe immunosuppressed patients may be prudent.[147] The CDC website contains an excellent patient fact sheet about *Cryptosporidium* and its prevention (http://www.cdc.gov/parasites/crypto). Currently, no vaccine is available to protect against *Cryptosporidium*. Vaccines for cryptosporidiosis are in developmental stages, but, as of this writing, no vaccines have progressed to human trials.[21,127,134,138,183,215]

NEW REFERENCES SINCE THE SEVENTH EDITION

11. Bartelt LA, Sevilleja JE, Barrett LJ, et al. High anti-*Cryptosporidium parvum* IgG seroprevalence in HIV-infected adults in Limpopo, South Africa. *Am J Trop Med Hyg*. 2013;89:531-534.
42. Checkley W, White AC Jr, Jaganath D, et al. A review of the global burden, novel diagnostics, therapeutics, and vaccine targets for *Cryptosporidium*. *Lancet Infect Dis*. 2015;15:85-94.
47. Costa LB, JohnBull EA, Reeves JT, et al. *Cryptosporidium*-malnutrition interactions: mucosal disruption, cytokines, and TLR signaling in a weaned murine model. *J Parasitol*. 2011;97:1113-1120.
75. Gertler M, Durr M, Renner P, et al. Outbreak of *Cryptosporidium hominis* following river flooding in the city of Halle (Saale), Germany, August 2013. *BMC Infect Dis*. 2015;22:88.
96. Hunter PR, Hughes S, Woodhouse S, et al. Health sequelae of human cryptosporidiosis in immunocompetent patients. *Clin Infect Dis*. 2004;39:504-510.
111. Korpe PS, Haque R, Gilchrist C, et al. Natural history of cryptosporidiosis in a longitudinal study of slum-dwelling Bangladeshi children: association with severe malnutrition. *PLoS Negl Trop Dis*. 2016;10:e0004564.
162. Ochoa TJ, White AC Jr. Nitazoxanide for treatment of intestinal parasites in children. *Pediatr Infect Dis J*. 2005;24:641-642.
168. Painter JE, Hlavsa MC, Collier SA, et al. Cryptosporidiosis surveillance: United States, 2011–2012. *MMWR Surveill Summ*. 2015;64:1-28.
184. Roeslfsema JH, Sprong H, Caccio SM, et al. Molecular characterization of human *Cryptosporidium* spp. isolates after an unusual increase in late summer 2012. *Parasit Vectors*. 2016;9:138.
199. Sow SO, Muhsen K, Nasin D, et al. The burden of *Cryptosporidium* diarrheal disease among children < 24 months of age in moderate/high mortality regions of sub-Saharan Africa and South Asia, utilizing data from the Global Enteric Multicenter Study (GEMS). *PLoS Negl Trop Dis*. 2016;10:e0004729.
221. Widerström M, Schönning C, Lilja M, et al. Large outbreak of *Cryptosporidium hominis* infection transmitted through the public water supply, Sweden. *Emerg Infect Dis*. 2014;20:581-589.

The full reference list for this chapter is available at ExpertConsult.com.

Cyclosporiasis, Cystoisosporiasis, and Microsporidiosis 218

Martin Montes • Seher Anjum • A. Clinton White Jr

CYCLOSPORA CAYETANENSIS

Cyclospora cayetanensis is an intestinal coccidian protozoan parasite, related to *Toxoplasma, Cryptosporidium, Sarcocystis,* and *Cystoisospora*. This parasite infects the gastrointestinal tract of returning travelers and immunocompromised patients, causing acute diarrheal disease.[3,67,68,136,194] In 1979, *C. cayetanensis* was first identified by Ashford[11] in the stool of a woman and two children from Papua New Guinea. *C. cayetanensis* was identified in four patients with diarrhea after travel to Mexico and Haiti.[165] The organisms were identified in stools from travelers and expatriates in Nepal. Subsequent studies noted an association with diarrhea in patients with acquired immunodeficiency syndrome (AIDS) patients.[3,136,162,193,194]

Microbiology and Life Cycle

The oocysts of *C. cayetanensis* found in stool are round, measuring 8 to 10 μm.[128] In reports from the late 1980s and early 1990s, the taxonomy was in doubt and the organisms were referred to as *Cyanobacterium*-like body, a blue-green algae, a coccidian-like body, *Cryptosporidium*-like, or big *Cryptosporidium*.[12,18,74,128,131,132,134,143,161,166] Ortega and colleagues[128,132] demonstrated sporulation and excystation of the organisms, characterizing them as a coccidian species and suggesting the name *C. cayetanensis*.[193] Molecular studies have confirmed that the organisms are coccidian parasites closely related to the *Eimeria*.[141] Humans are the only known host of *C. cayetanensis*.

Infected patients pass unsporulated oocysts into the environment. A period of 1 to 2 weeks in a warm, moist environment is required for maturation into an infectious, sporulated oocyst.[164,169] In vivo, excystation of mature sporulated oocysts most likely occurs in the small bowel. In vitro, a combination of bile salts, sodium taurocholate, and mechanical pressure is required for excystation.[169] After excystation, the sporozoites invade the intestinal epithelial cells, where they undergo first asexual and later sexual reproduction. Sexual and asexual stages of *Cyclospora* are found in jejunal biopsy specimens from infected individuals, showing that this coccidian parasite can complete its entire life cycle in a single host.[130]

Epidemiology and Transmission

Cyclospora is found worldwide. Most reports of cyclosporiasis in wealthy countries involve residents of or travelers returning from resource-limited countries.[72,122,128,132,143,161] The organism has been acquired in numerous geographic areas, including North, Central, and South America; the Caribbean islands; Europe; Turkey; northern, central, and southern Africa; southwest, southern, and eastern Asia; and Papua New Guinea and Australia.[7,6,22,55,79,110,121,158,164,169,195,196] In one study of diarrheic stool from subjects returning from tropical areas, *C. cayetanensis* was identified in 5% of samples, rendering it the second most common pathogen after *Giardia*.[180] Seasonal variation has been described.[72,86,128,197] In Nepal, most cases occur during the rainy season, between May and October.[72] In Peru, the peak is during the fall, between April and June.[128] The prevalence in endemic regions varies with the age and immunologic status of the host. Prevalence rates in children from Peru and Nepal are reported to range from 2% to 18%.[72,128] In a Venezuelan review, Chacin-Bonilla and associates[31] report a prevalence that ranges from 0% to 41.6%. A report from Mexico identified *Cyclospora* in 0.7% of children under age 15.[127] In Kathmandu, the overall prevalence in children ages 3 to 14 years was 4%, with higher prevalence among 3- to 5-year-olds (10%).[20] In one series from Haiti, *Cyclospora* was reported in 11% of adults infected with human immunodeficiency virus (HIV), but was not detected in non–HIV-infected adults or infants younger than 6 months.[136]

Hall and associates[67] published an active surveillance of *C. cayetanensis* cases in the United States. They noted 370 cases and significant association to travels and outbreaks.[67]

Direct person-to-person transmission is unlikely to occur because a period outside the host is required for maturation into a sporulated oocyst.[169] Contamination of the environment with oocysts plays a major role in the transmission of *Cyclospora*. Foodborne and waterborne transmission of *Cyclospora* have been described.[65,78,115,169] Waterborne outbreaks have been reported in Chicago and Nepal.[75,134,193] In one area of Egypt, the average prevalence of *Cyclospora* spores in stool samples was 5.6% in patients with diarrhea, in contrast to 2.3% in asymptomatic subjects, with higher prevalence in places with higher water contamination.[55] High levels of aquatic contamination also were documented in Hanoi (Vietnam), reaching 63.6% in certain areas, again emphasizing the important role of contaminated water in the spread of the pathogen.[114]

Foodborne outbreaks have been reported frequently.[65,69,70,68,78,115] Eleven foodborne outbreaks occurred in North America between 1990 and 2000, affecting 3600 people.[109] For example, widespread outbreaks of cyclosporiasis occurred in the United States and Canada in 1996 and 1997 associated with the consumption of raspberries imported from Guatemala.[69,70,68] Researchers postulated that the raspberries were contaminated with insecticide or fungicides that were mixed with contaminated water or that the irrigation water was contaminated with *Cyclospora* oocysts.[133,164] During 1997, clusters of cases were identified in which fresh basil and mesclun lettuce were implicated.[145] Recent multistate outbreaks of cyclosporiasis occurred in the United States. associated with imported fresh cilantro and romaine lettuce.[1,25] *Cyclospora* oocysts contaminating vegetables are not removed easily by routine washing.[130]

Clinical Manifestations

Cyclospora affects both immunocompetent and immunocompromised patients.[79,110,121,128,136,143,161,180,193] The incubation period typically is 2 to 11 days.[134] In an immunocompetent host, diarrhea may last up to 7 weeks.[193] Relapsing diarrhea alternating with constipation is the rule.[164] Resolution of symptoms usually correlates with disappearance of the organism from stool.[72,137] Asymptomatic oocyst shedding also occur.[18,143] In one prevalence study in a Venezuelan community, *C. cayetanensis* oocysts were identified in 6.1% of subjects, of whom 84.6% were asymptomatic.[32]

In immunocompromised hosts especially onset of watery diarrhea may be abrupt or gradual. Malaise, myalgia, and anorexia are common.[35,193] Low-grade fever is reported in approximately 25% of patients.[72,134,161,193] Vomiting may occur but is less common than diarrhea. Other associated symptoms include abdominal cramping, heartburn, and indigestion.[164] Weight loss and malabsorption occur with prolonged illness.[72,73,165,194]

The median duration of disease in various US outbreaks has been 10 to 20 days (range, 1 to 60 days).[68] In HIV-infected patients, *Cyclospora* causes symptoms that are indistinguishable from symptoms of *Cryptosporidium* and *Cystoisospora* infection.[193] Biliary disease was reported in two patients with AIDS who were infected with *Cyclospora*. These patients had clinical and radiographic confirmation of biliary disease and did not have evidence of infection with other pathogens. Both patients had acalculous cholecystitis that was responsive to therapy with trimethoprim-sulfamethoxazole (TMP-SMX).[165] *Cyclospora* also has been identified in respiratory secretions of immunocompromised patients.[77]

Diagnosis

Cyclospora can be visualized by light microscopy on wet mounts or after formol-ether concentration of the stool. In fresh stool, the oocysts are unsporulated. They appear as refractile spherical bodies measuring 8 to 10 μm and have a central greenish morula that contains six to nine refractile globules.[132] Safranin staining enhances the outline of the membrane, but does not stain internal structures. Galvan-Diaz and colleagues[63] compared safranin and Ziehl-Neelsen stains using as gold standard the direct visualization of the parasite. They found a sensitivity of 95% and specificity of 98% with safranin staining and a sensitivity of 90% and specificity of 100% for Ziehl-Neelsen staining.[63]

The sensitivity of wet mounts is 75%.[136] Oocysts exhibit bright blue autofluorescence when exposed to ultraviolet light. Auramine-rhodamine staining enhances the visualization of internal structures. Staining is variable with modified Ziehl-Neelsen stain (Fig. 218.1).[128] *Cyclospora* is not visualized by Gram, Giemsa, Grocott-Gomori methenamine–silver nitrate, Lugol iodine, periodic acid–Schiff, or hematoxylin and eosin staining.[138,193]

A direct comparison of formalin-ether sedimentation, direct smear examination, and sucrose centrifugal flotation yielded the highest recovery of *Cyclospora* oocysts in stool with the last method.[91] Nucleic acid tests such as polymerase chain reaction (PCR)[76,95,97,178,180] and flow cytometry[54] have been studied as more sensitive detection methods. More recently, multiplex nuclei acid tests, such as FilmArray, have been approved for commercial use with 100% sensitivity and specificity compared to PCR.[26]

Treatment

When treatment is indicated because of the severity or persistence of symptoms, TMP-SMX is the drug of choice.[73,105,106,179] No clear alternatives are available in patients who are intolerant of TMP-SMX. Ciprofloxacin was inferior to TMP-SMX in patients with AIDS.[179] Nitazoxanide has been used in a limited number of patients.[198] Prophylaxis with TMP-SMX 3 days per week seems to prevent recurrent episodes in HIV-infected patients.[136]

CYSTOISOSPORIASIS

Cystoisospora belli (previously known as *Isospora belli*) is an intestinal coccidian parasite (Fig. 218.2). Human infection was first recorded in

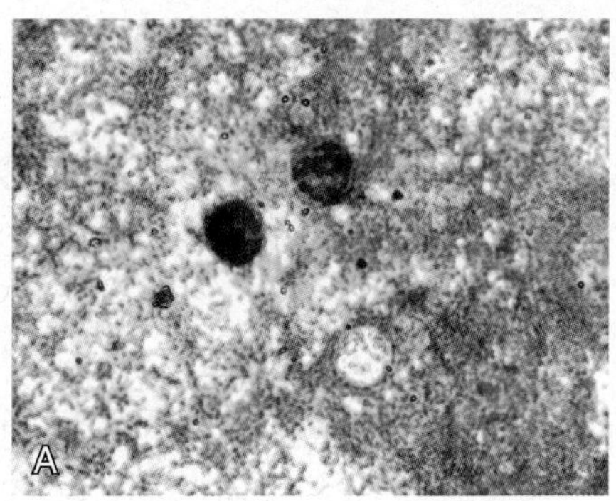
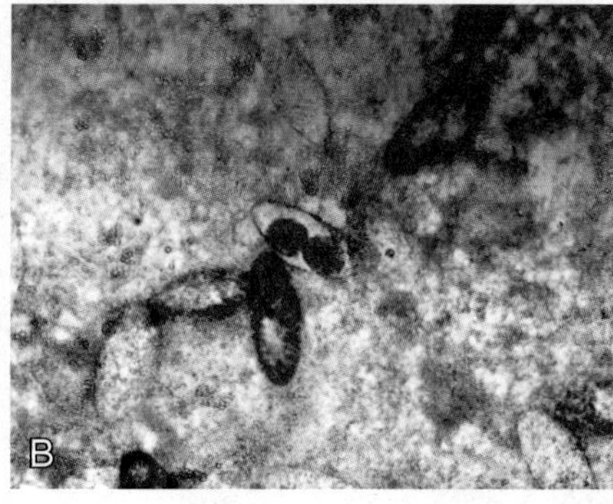

FIG. 218.1 Oocysts of (A) *Cyclospora cayetanensis* and (B) Cystoisopora *belli* stained with a modified acid-fast stain. Note the variable staining. Note two *Cystoisorpora* sporocysts are visible within the shell of one of the oocysts.

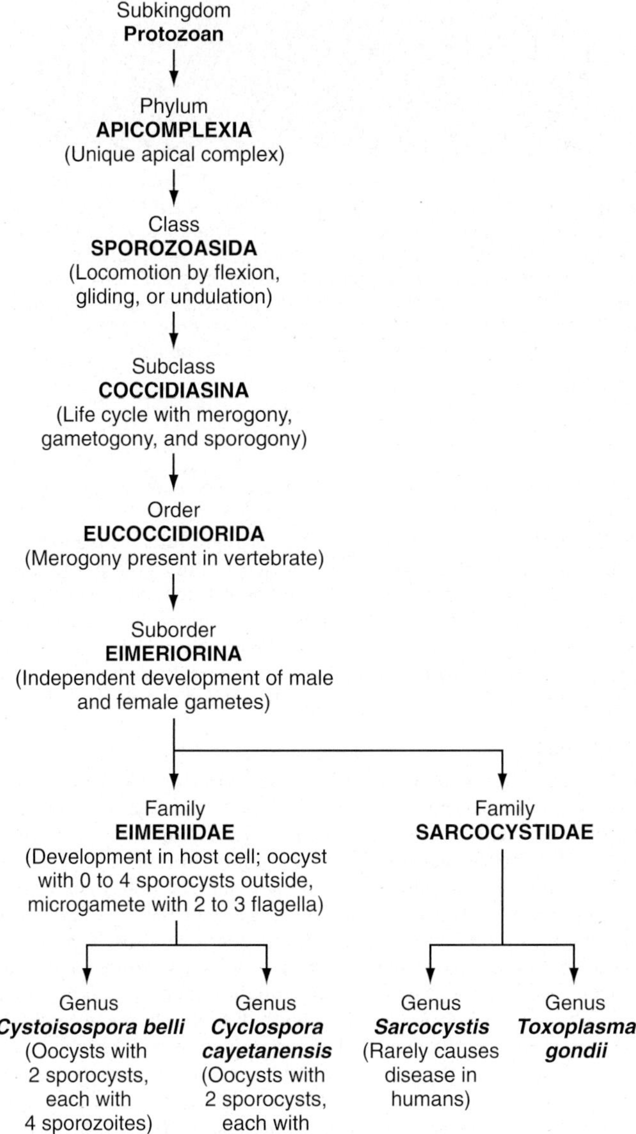

FIG. 218.2 Taxonomic classification of *Cryptosporidium, Isospora, Cyclospora,* and *Sarcocystis.*

US military personnel during World War I. The first US cases were described in children with chronic diarrhea and malnutrition.[24] *C. belli* causes acute and chronic diarrhea in immunocompetent children but can cause prolonged, life-threatening diarrhea and volume depletion in patients with compromised cellular immunity, particularly among patients infected with HIV.[71,151]

Microbiology and Life Cycle

C. belli is a coccidian parasite.[101] The taxonomy was recently revised, separating the genus *Isospora*, with organisms that infect birds reclassified as *Atoxoplasma* and those infecting mammals as *Cystoisospora*.[16] Some species of *Cystoisospora* infect other mammals, but only *C. belli* infects humans.[101] Mature oocysts of *C. belli* are oval, measure 10 to 20 mm × 20 to 33 μm, with a translucent thin wall that contains two round sporoblasts, each with four crescent-shaped sporozoites.[36] Humans acquire the infection by ingesting food or water contaminated with the mature sporulated oocyst. Excystation occurs in the proximal part of the small intestine, leading to the release of sporozoites that invade enterocytes of the distal duodenum and proximal jejunum and develop into trophozoites. The trophozoites reproduce asexually to form merozoites. The merozoites undergo asexual replication (schizogony or merogony) or sexual replication (gametogony) that results in the production of an immature unsporulated oocyst. This latter form is excreted in stool and requires 12 to 48 hours to mature into the infectious form, a sporulated oocyst.[101]

Epidemiology and Transmission

C. belli is distributed worldwide, but most cases are reported from tropical and subtropical regions. Travel to or immigration from resource-poor areas is the main risk factor for infection among cases in Europe and North America, including in patients with HIV and AIDS.[5,66,94,159,167] The incidence of *C. belli* among HIV-infected patients with chronic diarrhea in the developing world varies markedly, with very high rates of 13% to 26% of patients with diarrhea in Venezuela, Haiti, and India.[2,30,46,182] Infection is also common in Egypt, sub-Saharan Africa, Brazil, and other parts of Asia, but recorded rates have been lower.[163,186,192] On the other hand, *C. belli* is less common among HIV-infected patients taking cotrimoxazole prophylaxis.[29,66]

Transmission is by the fecal-oral route. However, direct person-to-person transmission is considered very uncommon, because the immature oocysts shed by humans require at least 1 to 2 days in the environment to become infectious.[46,101] The incubation period is thought to be 3 to 14 days.[101] The infectious dose is largely unknown. The oocysts of *C. belli* are resistant to commonly used disinfectants and may remain viable for months.

Pathophysiology

The pathologic findings are nonspecific. Typical histopathologic findings include shortening of the villi; hypertrophy of the crypts; and infiltration

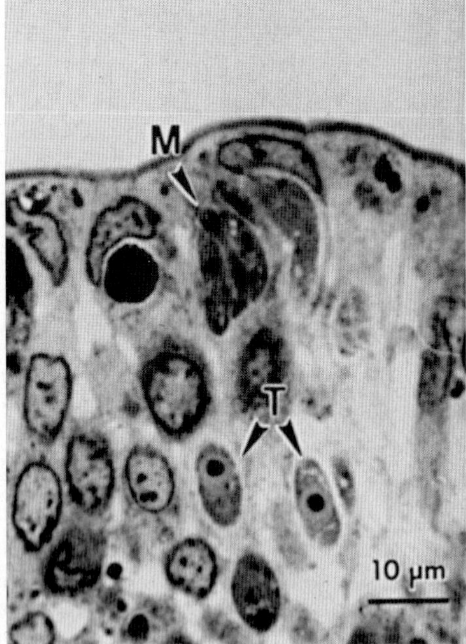

FIG. 218.3 *Isospora* infecting the jejunum of a patient with severe diarrhea. Trophozoites *(T)* divide within enterocytes by schizogony to form merozoites *(M)*. (From Garcia LS, Owen RL, Current WL. Isosporiasis. In: Balows A, Hausler WJ Jr, Ohashi M, Turano A, eds. *The Laboratory Diagnosis of Infectious Diseases: Principles and Practice.* Vol 1. New York: Springer-Verlag, 1988:899-903.)

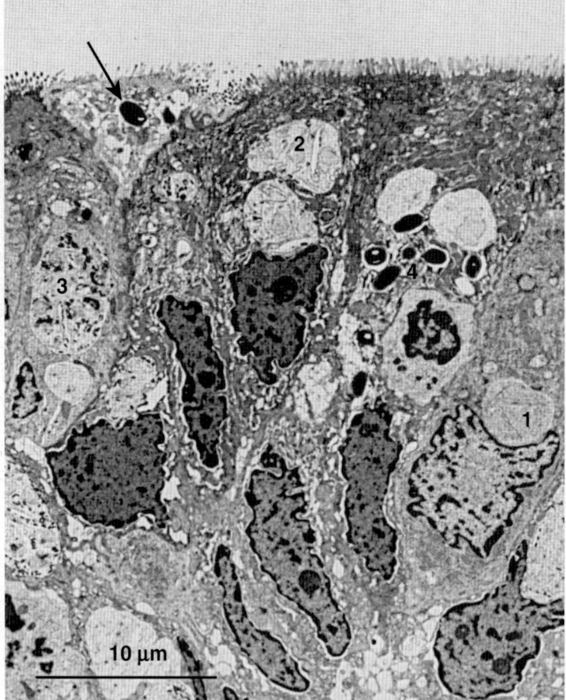

FIG. 218.4 Jejunal biopsy from a patient with AIDS and severe diarrhea. Various developmental stages of the intestinal microsporidian *Enterocytozoon* infect almost every enterocyte. Stages include proliferative plasmodia *(1)*, early sporogonial plasmodia *(2)*, late sporogonial plasmodia *(3)*, and mature spores *(4)*. A spore *(arrow)* can be seen within a necrotic enterocyte, which appears ready to slough into the lumen. (From Cali A, Owen RL. Intracellular development of *Enterocytozoon:* a unique microsporidian found in the intestine of AIDS patients. *J Protozool.* 1990;37:145.)

of the lamina propria with plasma cells, lymphocytes, polymorphonuclear leukocytes, and eosinophils.[58,120] All stages of the life cycle have been identified within the villous epithelium (Fig. 218.3). *C. belli* also can cause biliary tract infection.[183] The pathophysiology of cystoisosporiasis has not been defined, but the organisms are strongly associated with diarrhea and malabsorption syndromes.[10,17,177]

Clinical Manifestations

The main clinical manifestation of cystoisosporiasis is nonbloody, watery diarrhea. However, the spectrum of disease ranges from asymptomatic infection to life-threatening diarrhea. Immunocompetent patients usually have a self-limited illness, although diarrhea may not resolve for several weeks.[88,116,177] Some children have chronic malabsorption.[17] Headache, malaise, vomiting, fever, and dehydration may be noted. The disease is more severe in infants and children than in adults. In contrast to other protozoan parasites, *C. belli* is strongly associated with peripheral eosinophilia, which can be marked.[30,85]

The clinical course of cystoisosporiasis in immunosuppressed children depends on their cellular immunity. HIV-infected patients with CD4 cell counts below 200 cells/mm^3 are particularly at risk for becoming infected and for presenting symptoms, usually for prolonged periods with intermittent bouts of reactivation.[10,14,94] Patients who have a reconstituted immune system as a result of effective antiretroviral therapy are seldom symptomatic.[15] Seasonality has been observed in some but not all studies from developing countries.[30,44] Other conditions associated with depressed cellular immunity, including lymphomas and organ transplantation, predispose to a more severe illness.[149,150] The onset of illness is insidious and is associated with nonspecific symptoms, such as low-grade fever, headache, malaise, myalgia, and anorexia. Nausea, vomiting, and diffuse abdominal pain may be present as well. The diarrhea is typically watery. Severe dehydration, hypokalemia, metabolic acidosis resulting from bicarbonate losses, and azotemia may occur.[151,190] Marked weight loss, reaching 30% of body weight, has been reported in a patient with a 9-month clinical course.[151] Elevated stool osmolality and steatorrhea are also common findings.

Extraintestinal manifestations of *C. belli* are rare; gallbladder and biliary tract infections have been reported in both HIV-infected and immunocompetent patients.[21,60,183] Cholangitis, defined as elevation of alkaline phosphatase and dilation of the common bile duct detected by ultrasound, was found in 4 of 28 chronically infected patients in France.[94] The organism has been identified in tracheobronchial, mediastinal, and mesenteric lymph nodes; the spleen; and the liver.[113]

Diagnosis

C. belli infection is usually diagnosed by observing oocysts in a stool wet-mount preparation or using modified acid-fast or auramine-rhodamine stain (http://dpd.cdc.gov/dpdx/Html/Cystoisosporiasis.htm).[99,129] Concentration techniques such as zinc sulfate, hypertonic sodium chloride, formalin-ether sedimentation, and Sheather sucrose solution are recommended to increase the sensitivity. Multiple stool samples may be required to make the proper diagnosis. The oocysts are oval, contain one or two sporoblasts, and are 10 times larger than *Cryptosporidium* oocysts. Like *Cyclospora,* the oocysts of *C. belli* exhibit autofluorescence with an ultraviolet epifluorescent illuminator (450- to 490-nm excitation filter). Histologic examination of the small bowel shows nonspecific findings, but asexual and sexual stages of the parasite can be observed within the enterocytes[24] (Fig. 218.4). *C. belli* can be found infecting the small and large intestine in patients with HIV and AIDS. Peripheral blood eosinophilia and Charcot-Leyden crystals in stool specimens are present in most cases.[37] PCR can increase detection of *C. belli,* and multiplex PCR methods allow for detection of other coccidian parasites at the same time.[120,173,174] However, these methods are expensive and not widely available.

Treatment

Treatment includes careful attention to fluid replacement, nutritional support, antimicrobial therapy, and, in patients with HIV, antiretroviral therapy. Immunosuppressed patients tend to experience higher degrees of dehydration than immunocompetent patients. In addition, the presence of *C. belli* and other coccidian parasites among HIV and AIDS patients has been associated with higher mortality rates.[53] Patients with severe dehydration require intravenous fluids and electrolyte support, with particular consideration to correction of hypokalemia, metabolic acidosis, and children coinfected with *C. belli* and other coccidian parasites, hypoalbuminemia, and malabsorption of vitamins and fats are commonly described. Hence, careful nutritional support is highly advised in these patients. Patients with mild-to-moderate dehydration who can tolerate the oral route should be offered oral rehydration solutions.

TMP-SMX (TMP 10 mg/kg per day and SMX 50 mg/kg per day in two divided doses, or TMP 160-mg and SMX 800-mg tablet for adolescents twice daily) is the drug of choice.[99] For immunocompetent hosts, one dose two times per day for 7 to 10 days is curative in most cases.[46,179] Patients with HIV or AIDS may require higher doses. The current recommendations for these patients are to start with TMP 5 mg/kg and SMX 25 mg/kg two times per day and observe the response, which usually occurs within 2 to 3 days; if no response is observed, the recommendation is to increase the dose to one tablet four times per day for 7 to 10 days. Children who do not respond may have malabsorption of the drug, and, in these patients, parenteral therapy may be considered. Patients with HIV or AIDS present more frequent drug reactions to the sulfa component (SMX) than normal hosts.[84] Clinical data are very limited on treatment alternatives to TMP-SMX. Ciprofloxacin may have some activity, but it is inferior to TMP-SMX.[179] Pyrimethamine with or without a long-acting sulfonamide is an alternative agent and has worked in some cases refractory to TMP-SMX.[80,187] Nitazoxanide has in vitro activity, but clinical data are limited to case reports with both successes and failures.[21,126] Recurrences are very common among patients with HIV or AIDS; therefore, secondary prophylaxis is indicated. Current recommendation includes either TMP 5 mg/kg and SMX 25 mg/kg three times per week or pyrimethamine (25 mg) plus sulfadoxine (500 mg) once a week. Prophylaxis should be continued until the CD4 cell count is out of the AIDS range. However, failure to eradicate *C. belli* even in patients with immune reconstitution has been reported.[23]

MICROSPORIDIOSIS

Microsporidiosis comprises a diverse group of infectious diseases caused by the single-cell eukaryotic pathogens from the phylum Microsporidia, formerly termed Microspora.[52,188,191] Microsporidia were first identified in 1857 as pathogens of silkworms. The first human infection was described only in 1959, when the organisms were found in the spinal fluid of a Japanese child with seizures. Widespread human infection was initially recognized during the 1980s in AIDS patients. For over a century, the organisms were misclassified as protozoan parasites. However, molecular studies have clarified that the organisms are a unique phylum, closely related to the fungi. Microsporidia have been associated with a wide range of human infections, but most cases present with keratoconjunctivitis or diarrheal disease.

Microbiology and Life Cycle

The phylum Microsporidia includes over 170 genera with more than 1200 species.[188] Eight genera and 14 species have been identified in human infections (Table 218.1). Recent classification schemes reflecting emerging genomic sequences include them with fungi in the Opisthokonta supergroup. All are obligate intracellular pathogens. Their hosts include every animal phylum and some protozoa. Their genomes are highly compact, ranging from 2.3 to 19.5 Mb, with some of the smallest eukaryotic genomes, with few introns, high gene density, and shorter protein sequences than noted for corresponding genes in *Saccharomyces cerevisiae*.[40,89,140,144] Although the organisms were initially thought to be primitive eukaryotic organisms, recent studies have demonstrated that they are a highly evolved and divergent group of fungal organisms that are highly adapted and specialized for intracellular parasitism. Review of microsporidian genomics indicates that as they adapted to live intracellularly, they have lost genes and now use host proteins for their energy metabolism.[27,38,56,168] This phenomenon has been associated with increased ability to multiply rapidly within their host.

Microsporidia form characteristic unicellular spores (ranging in size from 1.0 × 3.0 μm to 1.5 × 4.0 μm) with a proteinaceous exospore, an endospore made of chitin and protein, and a plasma membrane. All spores contain a nucleus, a polaroplast, and a coiled microtubular extrusion apparatus, termed the polar filament, which is anchored to one end of the spore. The host is infected by ingestion or inhalation of spores. Within the host, the spores undergo extrusion of the polar tube and injection of the sporoplasma into the host cell cytoplasm. Within the host cells, the pathogen undergoes cell division by either binary or multiple fission (merogony). This leads to formation of spores (sporogony), during which meront cell membranes thicken and divide to form spores. The spores are usually released by lysis of the host cell.

Epidemiology

Microsporidiosis has been identified on all continents except Antarctica.[188] Microsporidia infection appears to be common, with mainly asymptomatic or mild self-limited illnesses in normal hosts.[51,52,108,123,152-154,188] Prevalence is variable and can be as high as 80% in some populations

TABLE 218.1 Microsporidia Implicated in Human Disease

Genus	Species	Main Clinical Manifestation
Enterocytozoon	*E. bieneusi*	Chronic diarrhea
Encephalitozoon	*E. intestinalis* (syn *Septata*)	Chronic diarrhea
	E. hellem	Keratoconjunctivitis, disseminated infection
	E. curriculi	Disseminated infection, seizure
Trachipleistophora	*T. anthropophthera*	Disseminated infection
	T. hominis	Myositis
Pleistophora	*Pleistophora* spp.	Myositis
Anncaliia (syn. *Brachiola*)	*A. vesicularum*	Myositis
	A. connori	Disseminated infection
	A. algerae	Keratoconjunctivitis
Nosema	*N. ocularum*	Keratoconjunctivitis
Vittaforma	*V. corneae*	Keratoconjunctivitis
Microsporidium	*M. africanus*	Corneal ulcer
	M. ceylonensis	Corneal ulcer

and not detected in others. Clinical disease was initially recognized in compromised hosts, especially patients with AIDS. Microsporidia, especially *Enterocytozoon bieneusi,* are commonly detected in stools from HIV-infected children with persistent diarrhea who are not on effective antiretroviral therapy (up to 77% of cases, but typically about 15%).[176] Microsporidiosis is increasingly recognized in children on immunosuppression for organ transplantation, particularly renal transplant recipients.[4,62,90,93,96] Among transplant patients, *Enterocytozoon bieneusi* is the most commonly isolated species in stool,[64,90] but *Encephalitozoon* can cause systemic infection.[90,147] Recent studies have suggested underdiagnosis in normal hosts, including travelers and children, especially those living in resource-limited countries.[8,48,102,104,135,155,189] Even a minor increase in economic status can protect against disease.[125] However, a foodborne outbreak was associated with diarrhea in normal hosts in Sweden.[45,52]

Most human infections appear to be acquired by ingestion or inoculation in the eye.[51,52] Sources of ingested organisms include other people, food, and water. Person-to-person transmission was documented in an orphanage.[98] Pathogenic microsporidial spores are commonly found in surface and drinking water.[34,61] A foodborne outbreak has been described.[35] *Encephalitozoon* species are common in mammals and birds.[49,48,111,171] *Enterocytozoon bieneusi* has also been reported from pigs and a number of other mammalian and avian hosts.[49,48,111,156,171]

Clinical Manifestations

Microsporidiosis has been associated with a wide range of clinical manifestations. Most cases present with either diarrhea or keratoconjunctivitis. Less common manifestations include disseminated infection (including neurologic disease) and myositis. Infection of a wide range of other organs has been rarely described, including kidney, liver, central nervous system, and sinuses.

Intestinal and Biliary Tract Microsporidiosis

Human microsporidiosis was first recognized as a cause of chronic diarrhea in patients with AIDS. Most cases of intestinal microsporidiosis are caused by *E. bieneusi* and, less frequently, Encephalitozoon *intestinalis.* Other species have rarely been identified as causes of diarrhea. Cases typically present with severe immunodeficiency (AIDS patients with $CD4^+$ cell count <50/mm^3 or transplant patients on immunosuppression).[13,39,56,64,90,92,93,146,176,184,188] AIDS patients typically have chronic diarrhea, often with 3 to 10 loose or watery bowel movements per day. Stools are not typically bloody or mucoid. Affected children also may have anorexia, wasting or failure to thrive, and abdominal pain. Fever is unusual. Intestinal biopsies typically reveal villus atrophy and crypt hyperplasia, and malabsorption of carbohydrates (e.g., D-xylose), zinc, and fats frequently occurs.[13,100] By contrast, only a limited degree of inflammation is noted.[155] Infection may be fatal without aggressive treatment, but may also be self-limited or asymptomatic, especially in children with higher CD4 cell counts or those on combination antiretroviral therapy.[19,135] Children with malignancies or who have undergone organ transplantation also may have chronic diarrhea.[2,4,9,102] In immunocompetent children, most cases are either asymptomatic or self-limited.[124,152] However, intestinal microsporidiosis has been associated with stunting in some series.[60,119,142]

Disease may spread to the biliary tract. Biliary tract disease with acalculous cholecystitis and sclerosing cholangitis have been associated with very low CD4 counts.[60,142] Children have abdominal pain, fever, and right upper quadrant tenderness. Imaging studies may reveal dilation of the intrahepatic and common bile ducts or irregularities of the bile duct and gallbladder wall. AIDS cholangiopathy is similar to cholangiopathy associated with cytomegalovirus and cryptosporidial infection.[164]

Ocular Infection

Ocular involvement is also a common manifestation of microsporidiosis. The main manifestations are keratoconjunctivitis and stromal keratitis. Keratoconjunctivitis was initially recognized in patients with AIDS and subsequently in other compromised hosts. However, recent studies from Asia have demonstrated that it is a common and usually self-limited illness.[42,82,103,148,157,160,175] Most patients have a history of local trauma or exposure to contaminated water or dirt. Many cases were previously treated with topical steroids. Immunocompetent individuals usually experience a gradual onset in the week before presentation. Most complain of tearing and redness. Other frequent symptoms include the sensation of a foreign body in the eye, ocular pain, and decreased visual acuity, Most cases are unilateral. On examination, all patients have nonpurulent conjunctivitis. Most have a coarse punctate keratitis often accompanied by a superficial scar. Most cases have a full recovery without loss of visual acuity. The clinical presentation of keratoconjunctivitis in AIDS patients and other compromised hosts is more often chronic and bilateral. However, the clinical presentation is still typically with a superficial keratoconjunctivitis.[160,172,188] Most cases in AIDS patients are thought to be caused by *Encephalitozoon* spp. However, *Anncaliia, Nosema, Vittaforma,* and *Trachipleistophora* also have been identified in immunocompetent patients with keratoconjunctivitis.

Stromal keratitis often with corneal ulceration is a more severe but less frequent form of ocular microsporidiosis.[160] Stromal keratitis has been described only in hosts thought to be immunocompetent. Cases have been attributed to *Microsporidium* spp., *Vittaforma corneae,* and *Trachipleistophora hominis.* Patients have redness, tears, eye pain, and decreased visual acuity. Cases are often confused with herpetic keratitis. Cure usually requires surgery.

Other Clinical Presentations

Disseminated infection has been described commonly with *Encephalitozoon* spp. Many people are seropositive for *Encephalitozoon* spp., and infection has been associated with seizures, hepatitis, brain abscesses, endocarditis, sinusitis, and respiratory infection.[188] Spores are frequently found in urine, reflecting common involvement of the urinary tract, even in patients with diarrhea. *Pleistophora* spp., *T. hominis, Brachiola* spp., *Tubulinosema,* and *Anncaliia* spp. have been associated with myositis.[28,41,57,139,170,185] Patients present with myalgia, weakness, and elevated muscle enzymes. Cases have been reported in HIV patients with $CD4^+$ less than 100/mm^3 and patients receiving immunosuppressive therapy for rheumatoid arthritis or solid organ transplants. Anti–tumor necrosis factor agents and corticosteroids have specifically been shown to increase risk.[185]

Diagnosis

The mainstay of diagnosis is the demonstration of spores or intracellular organisms in specimens from appropriate tissues.[56] Stool microscopy remains the most commonly used technique for diagnosis in patients with diarrhea. The spores are similar in size to bacteria and do not readily stain with routine parasitologic stains, so demonstration of the organisms in stool requires special stains. Chromotrope 2R (modified trichrome), Uvitex 2B, calcofluor white, and the quick hot Gram-chromotrope stains have been used to visualize spores in the stool.[50,112,188] The fluorescent stains (Uvitex 2B and calcofluor white) are more sensitive but less specific than the chromotrope stains. Fluorescent antibody kits are commercially available for identification of *Encephalitozoon* and *E. bieneusi* in water and stool. Urine specimens are frequently positive in cases with *Enterocytozoon* infection.

Organisms are sometimes identified in tissues.[147] Spores can be identified in conjunctival scrapings by Giemsa, Gram-chromotrope, or calcofluor white staining.[42,83] Tissue Gram stains or chromotrope 2R can be used to stain the organisms in biopsy or autopsy tissues. Occasionally, organisms are identified in intestinal biopsies when missed on stool studies. Electron microscopy can provide more precise anatomic detail but is rarely required.

Molecular assays such as PCR are increasingly being used to diagnose microsporidiosis.[59,81,148,181] The assays are more sensitive than microscopic methods. Primers are available to identify organisms to the species level.

Treatment

Microsporidiosial diarrhea is usually self-limited in immunocompetent hosts. Thus, when possible, reconstitution of the immune response plays a critical role in management. Children with AIDS should be treated with effective combination antiretroviral therapy, which often will lead to resolution of illness.[87,107]

Albendazole 400 mg twice daily is effective therapy for some microsporidial species, including a small randomized trial in intestinal infection with *E. intestinalis*.[117] It has been used in intestinal and systemic infections.[188] However, albendazole does not work for *E. bieneusi*, the most common cause of intestinal microsporidiosis.[188]

Fumagillin is active in vitro against most microsporidial species. A small randomized trial demonstrated efficacy of fumagillin 20 mg three times daily in diarrhea caused by *E. bieneusi,* mainly in AIDS patients.[118] There have been recent case reports of successful fumagillin use in the pediatric age group in transplant recipients suffering from E. *bieneusi* diarrhea.[33,47] Thrombocytopenia frequently occurs during therapy. Fumagillin is licensed in France, but with limited availability. It is not licensed in the United States, but can be obtained for compassionate use.

Keratoconjunctivitis may be self-limited or respond to minor debridement, although debridement alone has not shown any benefits in resolution of corneal lesions or improvement in vision.[43] Topical fumagillin is available for ocular use in cases of severe keratoconjunctivitis.[42] Topical quinolone antibiotics also may be effective. Systemic albendazole may improve some cases and is recommended with *Encephalitozoon* infections, which may be associated with systemic infection. Most patients with stromal keratitis require keratoplasty and may require corneal transplantation.[172]

There have been studies showing progression of myositis to bulbar involvement and dysphagia if not treated aggressively. In places lacking resources to accurately identify Microsporidia species, triple therapy with albendazole, pyrimethamine, and sulfadiazine has been used successfully.[139]

NEW REFERENCES SINCE THE SEVENTH EDITION

1. Abanyie F, Harvey RR, Harris JR, et al. 2013 multistate outbreaks of *Cyclospora cayetanensis* infections associated with fresh produce: focus on the Texas investigations. *Epidemiol Infect.* 2015;143(16):3451-3458.
12. Ashford RW, Warhurst DC, Reid GD. Human infection with cyanobacterium-like bodies. *Lancet.* 1993;341(8851):1034.
20. Bhandari D, Tandukar S, Parajuli H, et al. *Cyclospora* infection among school children in Kathmandu, Nepal: prevalence and associated risk factors. *Trop Med Health.* 2015;43(4):211-216.
25. Buss BF, Joshi MV, Dement JL, et al. Multistate product traceforward investigation to link imported romaine lettuce to a US cyclosporiasis outbreak—Nebraska, Texas, and Florida, June-August 2013. *Epidemiol Infect.* 2016;144(13):2709-2718.
26. Buss SN, Leber A, Chapin K, et al. Multicenter evaluation of the BioFire FilmArray gastrointestinal panel for etiologic diagnosis of infectious gastroenteritis. *J Clin Microbiol.* 2015;53(3):915-925.
27. Calderon EJ, Cushion MT, Xiao L, et al. The 13th International Workshops on Opportunistic Protists (IWOP13). *J Eukaryot Microbiol.* 2015;62(5):701-709.
28. Cali A, Takvorian PM. Ultrastructure and development of *Pleistophora ronneafiei* n. sp., a microsporidium (Protista) in the skeletal muscle of an immune-compromised individual. *J Eukaryot Microbiol.* 2003;50(2):77-85.
37. Centers for Disease Control. *Cystoisosporiasis.* Available at: https://www.cdc.gov/parasites/cystoisosporiasis.
38. Corradi N. *Microsporidia*: Eukaryotic intracellular parasites shaped by gene loss and horizontal gene transfers. *Annu Rev Microbiol.* 2015;69:167-183.
41. Curry A, Beeching NJ, Gilbert JD, et al. *Trachipleistophora hominis* infection in the myocardium and skeletal muscle of a patient with AIDS. *J Infect.* 2005;51(3):e139-e144.
47. Desoubeaux G, Maakaroun-Vermesse Z, Lier C, et al. Successful treatment with fumagillin of the first pediatric case of digestive microsporidiosis in a liver-kidney transplant. *Transpl Infect Dis.* 2013;15(6):E250-E259.
50. Didier ES, Orenstein JM, Aldras A, et al. Comparison of three staining methods for detecting microsporidia in fluids. *J Clin Microbiol.* 1995;33(12):3138-3145.
56. Field AS, Milner DA. Intestinal microsporidiosis. *Clin Lab Med.* 2015;35(2):445-459.
57. Field AS, Paik JY, Stark D, et al. Myositis due to the microsporidian *Anncaliia* (*Brachiola*) *algerae* in a lung transplant recipient. *Transpl Infect Dis.* 2012;14(2):169-176.
86. Kaminsky RG, Lagos J, Raudales Santos G, et al. Marked seasonality of *Cyclospora cayetanensis* infections: ten-year observation of hospital cases, Honduras. *BMC Infect Dis.* 2016;16:66.
90. Kicia M, Wesolowska M, Kopacz Z, et al. Prevalence and molecular characteristics of urinary and intestinal microsporidia infections in renal transplant recipients. *Clin Microbiol Infect.* 2016;22(5):462.e465-462.e469.
93. Ladapo TA, Nourse P, Pillay K, et al. Microsporidiosis in pediatric renal transplant patients in Cape Town, South Africa: two case reports. *Pediatr Transplant.* 2014;18(7):E220-E226.
99. Legua P, Seas C. *Cystoisospora* and *Cyclospora. Curr Opin Infect Dis.* 2013;26(5):479-483.
122. Nichols GL, Freedman J, Pollock KG, et al. *Cyclospora* infection linked to travel to Mexico, June to September 2015. *Euro Surveill.* 2015;20(43).
127. Orozco-Mosqueda GE, Martínez-Loya OA, Ortega YR. *Cyclospora cayetanensis* in a pediatric hospital in Morelia, México. *Am J Trop Med Hyg.* 2014;91(3):537-540.
134. Outbreak of diarrheal illness associated with *Cyanobacteria* (blue-green algae)-like bodies-Chicago and Nepal, 1989 and 1990. *MMWR Morb Mortal Wkly Rep.* 1991;40(19):325-327.
139. Patel AK, Patel KK, Chickabasaviah YT, et al. *Microsporidial* polymyositis in human immunodeficiency virus-infected patients, a rare life-threatening opportunistic infection: clinical suspicion, diagnosis, and management in resource-limited settings. *Muscle Nerve.* 2015;51(5):775-780.
147. Ramanan P, Pritt BS. Extraintestinal microsporidiosis. *J Clin Microbiol.* 2014;52(11):3839-3844.
168. Stentiford GD, Becnel JJ, Weiss LM, et al. *Microsporidia*—emergent pathogens in the global food chain. *Trends Parasitol.* 2016;32(4):336-348.
170. Suankratay C, Thiansukhon E, Nilaratanakul V, et al. Disseminated infection caused by novel species of *Microsporidium*, Thailand. *Emerg Infect Dis.* 2012;18(2):302-304.

The full reference list for this chapter is available at ExpertConsult.com.

Babesiosis 219

Peter J. Krause

The first reference to babesiosis may have been in the Bible, where a widespread murrain or plague in cattle and other domestic animals is described in Exodus 9:3: "Behold, the hand of the Lord is upon thy cattle which is in the field, upon the horses, upon the asses, upon the camels, upon the oxen, and upon the sheep: there shall be a very grievous murrain." The word *murrain* has been used to describe red-water fever, a form of babesiosis found in cattle in parts of Ireland.[31] Babesiosis long has been recognized as an important disease in livestock and has a significant economic impact in many parts of the world; the health burden of babesiosis on humans has been recognized only more recently.[31,43,157]

Babesiosis is a disease caused by intraerythrocytic protozoa that are transmitted by ticks from animal reservoirs. Babesiosis has many clinical features similar to those of malaria. The parasite first was described in cattle in 1888 by Babes.[5] In 1893, it became the first microorganism shown to be transmitted by arthropods when Smith and Kilbourne[139] identified a tick as the vector for a species of babesiosis (*Babesia bigemina*) in Texas cattle. The first human case was described in 1957.[136] During the past 60 years, the epidemiology of the disease has changed from a few isolated cases to the establishment of endemic areas in the northeastern and northern Midwestern United States and in northeastern China, with reports of cases from a wide geographic range in North America, Europe, Asia, Africa, Australia, and South America.[65,157] Evidence indicates that the disease is more common in children and adults than is currently reported.[78,81,157]

EPIDEMIOLOGY

Worldwide, more than 100 species in the genus *Babesia* infect a wide variety of wild and domestic animals. *B. bigemina, B. bovis, B. divergens,* and *B. major* are found in cattle; *B. equi* is found in horses; *B. canis* is found in dogs; *B. felis* is found in cats; and *B. microti* is found in rodents.[90] Each species previously was thought to be host specific, but the host range of some species now is recognized to be quite broad.[56,89,90,143,150] Some confusion has occurred in taxonomy because the identification of different *Babesia* spp. has been based largely on morphology and the vertebrate host.[54] Most *Babesia* spp. are small (1 to 5 µm in length) and pear-shaped, round, or oval.[54,89] Several *Babesia* spp. have been found to cause disease in humans, including *B. microti, B. divergens, B. duncani, B. venatorum,* and KO1, as well as several other *Babesia* that are genetically related (e.g., *B. divergens*–like, *B. duncani*–type, *B. microti*–like).[28,48,59,84,113,134,157] The complete genome of *B. microti* has been sequenced. It has the smallest nuclear genome of all parasites in the phylum Apicomplexa, including *Plasmodium, Toxoplasma,* and *Cryptosporidium*, and has the minimal metabolic requirement for intraerythrocytic protozoan parasitism.[29] These and other data suggest that *B. microti* should be renamed, but additional phenotypic and genotypic characterization of this organism and of *B. microti*–like strains or isolates is needed.

Human babesiosis is a zoonotic disease transmitted by a tick vector from an infected animal reservoir (Fig. 219.1). Humans are an uncommon and terminal host for *Babesia* spp., which depend on other species for survival. The primary reservoir for *B. microti* in eastern North America is the white-footed mouse (*Peromyscus leucopus*), but the parasite also has been found in shrews, chipmunks, voles, and rats.[55,143,151] Two thirds of *P. leucopus* have been found to be parasitemic in endemic areas.[144] *Babesia* spp. are transmitted by hard-bodied (ixodid) ticks. The primary vector in the northeastern United States is *Ixodes scapularis* (also known as *Ixodes dammini*). This same tick transmits five other pathogens: *Borrelia burgdorferi* (the etiologic agent of Lyme disease), *Anaplasma phagocytophilum* (the agent of human granulocytic anaplasmosis), *Borrelia miyamotoi*, Powassan virus, and *Ehrlichia muris*–like agent.[35,66,70,75,140,142–145,149,158] *I. scapularis* ticks, *P. leucopus* mice, and humans may be infected simultaneously with two or more of these agents.[95,109,158,7,9,81,84,92,101,152]

Each of the three active stages in the life cycle of *I. scapularis* (i.e., (larva, nymph, and adult) takes a blood meal from a vertebrate host to

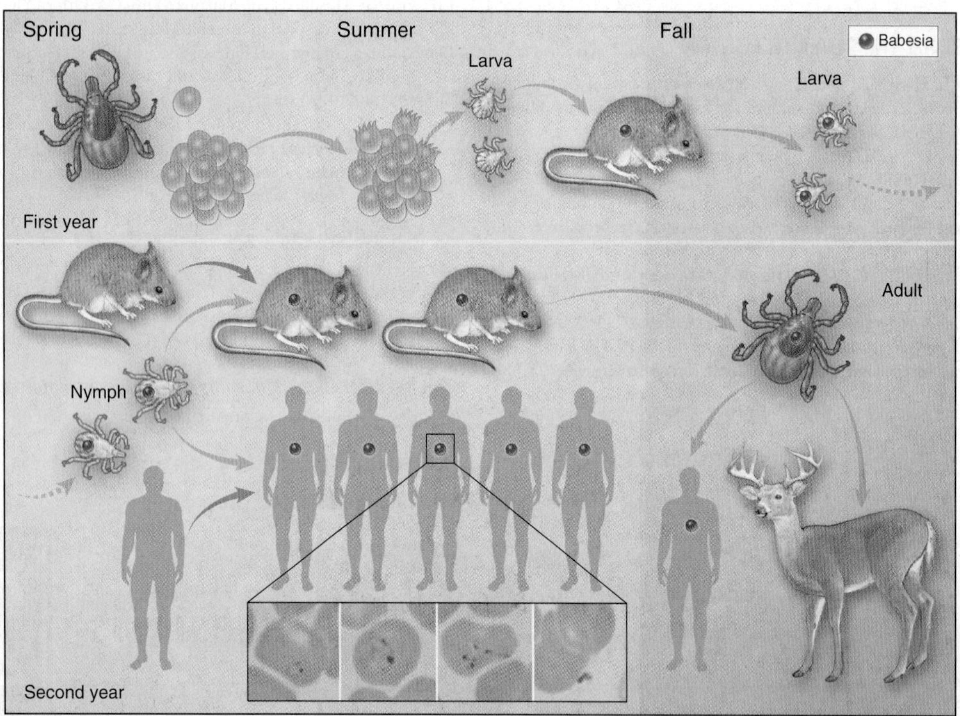

FIG. 219.1 Transmission of *Babesia microti* by the *Ixodes scapularis* tick. Adult female ticks lay eggs in the spring *(first year, top left panel)*. Larvae hatch in the early summer and become infected with *B. microti (red circle)* as they take a blood meal from infected white-footed mice *(Peromyscus leucopus)* in late summer. White-footed mice are the primary reservoir host, but other small rodents can carry *B. microti*. Larvae molt to nymphs the next spring *(second year, bottom left panel)*. When infected nymphs feed on mice or humans in late spring or early summer, the hosts may become infected. Humans are accidental hosts, and most cases occur from late spring through summer *(row of infected people)*. In the fall, nymphs molt to adults that feed on white-tailed deer *(Odocoileus virginianus)* but rarely on humans. White-tailed deer do not become infected with *B. microti* but amplify the tick population by providing a blood meal for adult ticks. The next spring, adult female ticks lay eggs that are free of *B. microti* (i.e., no transovarial transmission), and the cycle is repeated. *B. microti* are obligate parasites of erythrocytes. Infection can be detected on Giemsa-stained, thin blood smears *(inset)*. From left to right, the blood smears show a ring form with a nonstaining vacuole surrounded by cytoplasm *(blue)* and a small nucleus *(purple)*, an amoeboid form, a tetrad (i.e., Maltese cross sign), and an extracellular form. (Modified from Vannier E, Krause PJ. Human babesiosis. *N Engl J Med.* 2012;366:2397–2407.)

mature to the next stage.[144] Ingested babesial organisms infect intestinal tissue of the tick and subsequently travel to the salivary glands, from which they may be introduced into a new vertebrate host.[110] *Babesia* spp. are transmitted to the subsequent tick stage (transstadial passage). In some species of *Babesia,* such as *B. bovis,* the organisms may invade the ovaries and pass transovarially to the larvae. The tick transmission cycle begins in late summer, when newly hatched larvae ingest the parasite with a blood meal from an infected rodent and maintain the parasite to the nymphal stage (see Fig. 219.1). Nymphs transmit the *Babesia* spp. to rodents in late spring and summer of the following year.[144,141] Larvae, nymphs, and adults can feed on humans, but the nymph is the primary vector.[110] All active tick stages also feed on the white-tailed deer (*Odocoileus virginianus*), which is an important host for the tick but is not a reservoir for *B. microti.*[111,144] An increase in the deer population during the past few decades is thought to be a major factor in the spread of *I. scapularis* and the resulting increase in human cases.[144,141] Domestic animals such as the dog may carry the adult *I. scapularis,* but they do not seem to be important hosts for the tick and are not infected with *B. microti.*[128,142]

Since the 1980s, human babesiosis has been described with increasing frequency at mainland sites, and studies suggest that the endemic range continues to expand.[34,37,68,82,157] At certain sites, in years of high transmission, babesiosis may constitute a significant public health burden.[78] *B. microti* has been identified in rodent populations in several regions of the United States,[2,3,44,122,143] and human cases have been reported along the East Coast from Maryland to Maine and in Minnesota and Wisconsin (Fig. 219.2).[20,32,35,37,68,82,99,122,132,146] Moderate to severe illness caused by *B. duncani* and *B. duncani*–type organisms have been reported on the Pacific Coast from northern California to Washington State.[28,72,107,113] Cases of human babesiosis caused by *B. divergens*–like organisms have been reported in Arkansas, Kentucky, Missouri, and Washington.[6,57,59,171] The tick vectors and reservoir hosts for *B. duncani* and *B. divergens*–like organisms have not been definitively identified.[62,157] In Europe, *B. divergens* and *B. venatorum* infections are transmitted primarily by the cattle tick *Ixodes ricinus.*[14,42,41,48,63] *B. venatorum* has been found to be endemic in northeastern China, and the likely vector is *Ixodes persulcatus.*[65] Human babesiosis cases also have been reported in Africa, Australia, and South America.[16,118,133,134,157,160] An absence of clinical cases of babesiosis in the tropics may be due to cross-immunity from other endemic protozoal diseases.[69] Most human cases of babesiosis occur in the summer and in areas where the vector tick, rodents, and deer exist in close proximity to humans.[143,141,146]

Babesiosis also may be acquired through blood transfusion; more than 200 cases have been identified.[4,13,47,50,51,58,87,88,93,106,137,154,170] *B. microti* is the most common transfusion-transmitted pathogen reported in the United States.[58,87,170,172] Whole blood, frozen erythrocytes, and platelets have been implicated. The incubation period in these cases is usually 6 to 9 weeks but may be as long as 6 months. Transfusion-transmitted babesiosis has been reported throughout the year and in nonendemic areas. About a fifth of the cases have been fatal.[58,154,170] Although most cases of babesiosis in neonates have been acquired through blood transfusion, a few cases of transplacental transmission of babesiosis have been described.[36,39,67,157] The outcome in these cases has been good after treatment with appropriate antibiotic therapy.

PATHOGENESIS AND PATHOLOGY

Understanding of the pathogenesis and pathology of babesiosis in humans is incomplete and is based largely on information gathered from human case studies and studies of babesiosis in other animals. Rudzinska and colleagues studied the life cycle of *B. microti* in erythrocytes using electron microscopy.[70,120,121] After adhesion and entry into the erythrocyte occurs, the organism multiplies by asexual budding into two to four daughter cells, or merozoites. In contrast to *Plasmodium*

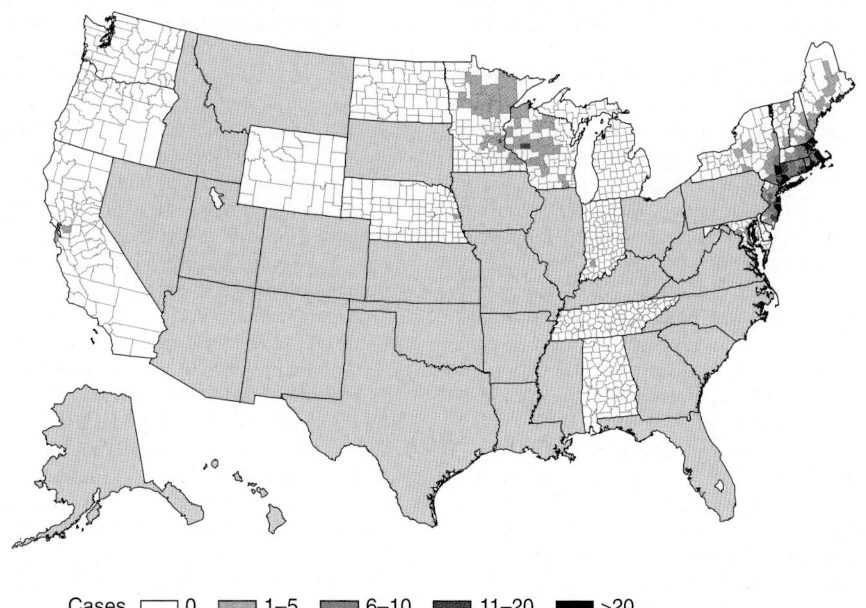

FIG. 219.2 Geographic distribution of human cases of babesiosis in the United States. Babesiosis became a nationally notifiable condition in January 2011. As of 2014, babesiosis was reportable in 22 states and the District of Columbia. The incidence of babesiosis (number of cases per 100,000 people) is shown by county of residence in 2014. Human babesiosis caused by *B. microti* has long been reported from the Northeast, particularly Massachusetts to New Jersey, and it recently became endemic in northern New England (i.e., Maine and New Hampshire) and in the northern mid-Atlantic states (i.e., Pennsylvania to Maryland). *B. microti* also causes disease in the upper Midwest, particularly in Wisconsin and Minnesota. *B. duncani* has been the etiologic agent along the northwest Pacific Coast. Cases of *B. divergens*–like infection have been reported from the states of Arkansas, Kentucky, Missouri, and Washington. (Modified from Centers for Disease Control and Prevention. Surveillance for babesiosis—United States. Available at http://www.cdc.gov/parasites/babesiosis/data-statistics.html; and Vannier E, Diuk-Wasser M, Ben Mamoun C, Krause PJ. Babesiosis. *Infect Dis Clin North Am.* 2015;29:357–70.)

spp. merozoites, which are released from the erythrocytes all at once (synchrony), *Babesia* spp. merozoites are released at varying intervals. New erythrocytes are infected, and the cycle is repeated.

The pathogenesis of babesial infection is closely linked to the host response to infection and modification of the erythrocyte membrane.[74] Investigation of *Babesia rodhani* suggests that activation of the alternative complement pathway allows entry of the parasite into red blood cells through the C3b receptor.[63] It is unknown whether the initial merozoite release leads to destruction of the host erythrocyte, but alteration of the erythrocyte membrane and eventual lysis occur.[120,147] Erythrocyte lysis is associated with many of the clinical manifestations and complications of the disease, including fever, hemolytic anemia, jaundice, hemoglobinemia, hemoglobinuria, and renal insufficiency. The absence of synchrony decreases the possibility of massive hemolysis and may explain why patients heavily parasitized with *Babesia* spp. may be less ill than patients with *Plasmodium* spp.[147]

Babesia spp. are intraerythrocytic protozoa, and extracellular forms are seen only in heavily parasitized cases.[1,147] *Babesia* organisms do not invade fixed tissue, and evidence in animals suggests that disease results from the excessive production of proinflammatory cytokines (e.g., tumor necrosis factor), as is thought to occur with malaria.[26,27,74] The release of proinflammatory cytokines in patients with babesiosis may be initiated by contact with an important surface protein, glycosylphosphatidylinositol (GPI).[24,29] These cytokines subsequently stimulate release of downstream mediators, such as nitric oxide, which kill parasites, but also may cause direct cellular damage if produced in excess.[23,26]

In addition to proinflammatory cytokine release, obstruction of blood vessels may be caused by adherence of parasitized erythrocytes to vascular endothelium. The accompanying ischemia and necrosis may result in cerebral abnormalities, hepatomegaly and hepatic dysfunction, and splenomegaly.[31,117,124] Although such cytoadherence appears to occur in cattle infected with *B. bovis*, it has yet to be demonstrated in human babesial infection.[25,74] A report of fatal human babesiosis with cerebral involvement was not associated with erythrocyte adherence and vascular occlusion.[25] Clinical manifestations such as hypotension, vascular congestion, and anoxia also may result from the activation of fibronectin, kallikreins, and complement.[33,168,167]

Innate and adaptive immune mechanisms limit the severity of babesial infections. The spleen plays a critical role in protection against *Babesia* spp. by removing parasites from infected erythrocytes through a process known as pitting, by ingesting parasites (by means of resident reticuloendothelial cells and macrophages), and by producing antibabesial antibody.[9,18,30,33,119,157,167] It long has been known that splenectomized animals have more severe babesiosis than animals with intact spleens. Animals that have recovered from babesiosis with negative blood smears have developed parasitemia again after undergoing splenectomy.[91,129] Many fatal cases of babesiosis in humans have occurred in splenectomized individuals, although asplenia does not always result in death or even severe illness.[17,119] Other host defense mechanisms that may help limit babesial infection include macrophages and macrophage products, such as tumor necrosis factor,[26,33,157,167] B lymphocytes,[98] T lymphocytes,[18,98,126,164] polymorphonuclear leukocytes,[135] antibody,[18] and complement.[9,167]

Age is an important factor in host defense against babesial disease in animals and humans. Most clinically apparent cases are reported in adults, but serologic surveys indicate that children are equally susceptible to infection and presumably are exposed to ticks to the same extent.[81,128,122] Almost all of the pediatric cases reported have been in neonates.[39,96,163] Data from a murine model of babesiosis suggested that resistance to *B. microti* infection conferred by the adaptive immune system is genetically determined and associated with age.[155] Immunity is incomplete because parasitemia may exist for months to years in animals and up to 27 months in humans after recovery from the initial illness.[80] Reinfection may occur, although it is uncommon.

CLINICAL MANIFESTATIONS

Clinical manifestations of babesiosis range from subclinical illness to fulminating disease resulting in death. Overt signs and symptoms begin after an incubation period of 1 to 6 weeks from the beginning of tick feeding or 6 weeks to 6 months after transfusion.[58,128] The unengorged *I. scapularis* nymph is about 2 mm in length, and the patient often has no recollection of having a tick bite. In most cases, the patient has a gradual onset of malaise, anorexia, and fatigue followed by intermittent fever as high as 40°C (104°F) and one or more of the following: chills, sweats, myalgia, arthralgia, nausea, and vomiting.[1,41,77,84,96,127,122,146] Less commonly noted are emotional lability and depression, hyperesthesia, headache, sore throat, abdominal pain, conjunctival injection, photophobia, weight loss, and nonproductive cough.[73,124,146,147] In contrast to other tickborne illnesses such as Lyme disease, Rocky Mountain spotted fever, and tularemia, rash seldom is noted.[32] Ecchymoses and petechiae have been described.[71,147]

The findings on physical examination usually are minimal, often consisting only of fever.[1,59,84,127,146] Mild splenomegaly, hepatomegaly, or both are noted occasionally.[124,163] Slight pharyngeal erythema, jaundice, and retinopathy with splinter hemorrhages and retinal infarcts also have been reported.[73,96,104] Several abnormal laboratory findings in patients with babesiosis reflect the invasion and subsequent lysis of erythrocytes by the parasite.[73,96,124,122] Mild to moderately severe hemolytic anemia occurs, with an elevated reticulocyte count. Elevated liver enzyme levels may be detected in serum.[122] The leukocyte count is normal, increased, or decreased. Neutropenia may occur.[173] Thrombocytopenia is common.[124] The erythrocyte sedimentation rate is elevated. Proteinuria and elevated levels of blood urea nitrogen and creatinine also may be noted.[71,73,93,124] The illness usually lasts a week to several months, with prolonged recovery taking up to 18 months.[1,8,80,124,127,146] Parasitemia may continue even after the patient feels well. Persistent parasitemia and relapse of illness, as noted with malaria, has been described 27 months after the initial episode.[80] Highly immunocompromised patients may experience a prolonged relapsing course of illness despite standard antibiotic therapy.[76]

Some patients, especially patients who are immunocompromised and those with *B. divergens* or *B. duncani* infection, have a more severe form of the disease consisting of fulminant illness lasting approximately 1 week and ending in death or a prolonged convalescence.[42,52,62,71,72,92,147] Severe *B. microti* illness requiring hospital admission is common in patients with splenectomy; malignancy; HIV infection; chronic heart, lung, or liver disease; organ transplantation; or acquisition of babesiosis through blood transfusion, as well as in newborn infants and the elderly.[156,157] Signs and symptoms include high fever, hemolytic anemia, hemoglobinemia and hemoglobinuria, jaundice, ecchymoses, petechiae, congestive heart failure, pulmonary edema, renal failure, adult respiratory distress syndrome, and coma.[45,46,52,71,76,146,147,161] Patients coinfected with babesiosis and Lyme disease experience more severe acute illness than patients with Lyme disease alone but not patients with babesiosis alone.[49,84,92,152] Coinfected patients usually experience moderate to severe acute illness, often followed by persistent fatigue. Between 10% and 66% of patients with antibody to *B. burgdorferi* also have antibody to *B. microti*.[7,81,84]

Inapparent infection occurs in approximately one quarter of adults and one half of children with babesiosis.[78] Serosurveys provide evidence of asymptomatic infection because of the disparity between seroprevalence rates and the number of indigenous reported cases of babesiosis. In a survey on Nantucket Island in Massachusetts, 2% of 577 random blood samples and 7.5% of 133 blood samples from patients with a history of tick bite or fever had *B. microti* indirect immunofluorescent antibody (IFA) titers of 1:64 or greater.[127] A survey of adults living on Shelter Island, New York, showed that 6 (4.4%) of 136 study subjects and seven (6.9%) of 102 subjects had *B. microti* IFA titers of 1:64 or greater.[38] In a survey of Massachusetts blood donors, 29 (37%) of 779 donors from Cape Cod had *B. microti* IFA titers of 1:16, compared with seven (4.7%) of 148 donors from metropolitan Boston.[112] In a serosurvey in Connecticut, 72 (9.5%) of 735 residents who were seropositive for *B. burgdorferi* had positive *B. microti* IFA titers of 1:64, compared with eight (2.7%) of 299 residents who were seronegative for *B. burgdorferi*.[82] Serosurveys in Mexico, Nigeria, and Taiwan also showed high *B. microti* seroprevalence rates compared with the number of indigenous reported cases of babesiosis.[60,86,105]

DIAGNOSIS

Specific diagnosis of babesiosis is made by microscopic identification of the organism by Giemsa or Wright staining of thick or thin blood smears and by detection of babesial antibodies by one of several serologic tests. *Babesia* spp. are round, oval, or pear shaped and have a blue cytoplasm with a red chromatin. The ring form is most common and is similar to the rings of *Plasmodium falciparum*.[54] *Babesia* spp. can be distinguished from *Plasmodium* spp. by (1) the absence of hemozoin pigment, which is present in older trophozoites of *Plasmodium* spp.; (2) the absence of identifiable gametocytes; (3) the absence of synchronous stages within the erythrocytes; and (4) the presence of the infrequently noted tetrad or Maltese cross form, in which four compact masses, each containing nuclear material, are joined by strands of cytoplasm[54] (see Fig. 219.1, inset).

Only a few erythrocytes are infected in the early stage of the illness, when most people seek medical attention, so multiple thick and thin blood smears should be examined.[54] Rapid automated differential blood analyzers may fail to distinguish erythrocytic inclusions.[15] In thick smears, the *Babesia* organism appears as a tiny red-to-purple nucleus with a thin tail of light blue cytoplasm. Maximum erythrocyte infection is approximately 10% in normal hosts but up to 85% in asplenic individuals.[146] Usually less than 1% of erythrocytes are parasitized early in the course of the illness, so the laboratory investigation of possible babesiosis should include more than an examination of blood smears.

If the presence of *Babesia* spp. is suspected but not detected by blood smears, babesial DNA can be amplified and detected using the polymerase chain reaction (PCR).[83,108,148,159,175] Blood from the patient also can be injected by the intravenous or intraperitoneal route into small laboratory animals such as hamsters or gerbils. If *B. microti* is present in the patient, it usually appears in the blood of the inoculated animal within 2 to 4 weeks.[10] This diagnostic technique is less sensitive and more time-consuming and costly than the PCR.[83]

Several serologic tests have been developed to detect babesial antibodies, including IFA, ELISA, and Western blot.[27,79,85,124,131,176] During the acute phase of the illness, titers usually exceed 1:1024, but they decline to 1:64 or less within 8 to 12 months. A babesial IFA titer of 1:1024 or greater usually signifies active or recent infection.[21,125] Although cross-reactions occur to different *Babesia* spp. and *Plasmodium* spp. with the IFA test, these titers almost always are low (≤1:16).[21,22] The problem of cross-reactivity with *Plasmodium* spp. is minimized in areas that have no indigenous malaria. Enzyme-linked immunosorbent assays for detection of *B. divergens* and *B. major* have been found to be superior to complement fixation and IFA procedures.[11,116,150,153]

PREVENTION AND TREATMENT

The combination of atovaquone plus azithromycin for 7 to 10 days is the recommended therapy for patients with babesiosis. Clindamycin plus quinine is an alternative choice.[77,174] In patients with severe babesiosis, IV azithromycin plus oral atovaquone should be given; IV clindamycin plus oral quinine is an alternative option.[174] In such patients, exchange transfusion should be considered. The dosage recommendations are as follows[19,39,45,114,165]:

- Atovaquone—children, 20 mg/kg every 12 hours (maximum of 750 mg per dose); adults, 750 mg orally every 12 hours
- Azithromycin—children, 10 mg/kg given intravenously once a day (maximum 500 mg/dose) or 10 mg/kg once on day 1 (maximum of 500 mg per dose) and 5 mg/kg once per day (maximum of 250 mg per dose) orally thereafter; adults, 500 mg given intravenously once a day or 500 to 1000 mg on day 1 and 250 mg orally once per day thereafter; immunocompromised adults, 600 to 1000 mg/day
- Clindamycin—children, 7 to 10 mg/kg given intravenously or orally every 6 to 8 hours (maximum of 600 mg per dose); adults, 300 to 600 mg every 6 hours intravenously or 600 mg every 8 hours orally
- Quinine—children, 8 mg/kg given orally every 8 hours (maximum of 650 mg per dose); adults, 650 mg every 6 to 8 hours orally

The clindamycin and quinine combination first was used for an 8-week-old infant girl who contracted babesiosis from a blood transfusion.[163] Initially she was thought to have malaria. Clindamycin and quinine were given after failure with chloroquine. Her favorable outcome suggested the prospective use of this combination in adults. Since then, numerous children and adults have been treated with clindamycin and quinine, with prompt clearing of parasitemia and resolution of clinical signs and symptoms.[20,19,84,96,146]

The successful use of atovaquone and azithromycin for the treatment of malaria and for babesiosis in hamsters prompted a clinical trial to determine whether the combination would be effective in human babesiosis.[61,77,162] In the first prospective trial of antibabesial therapy in humans, atovaquone and azithromycin were compared with clindamycin and quinine in adults.[77] Adverse effects were reported in 15% of subjects who received atovaquone and azithromycin compared with 72% of subjects who received clindamycin and quinine. In approximately one third of subjects taking clindamycin and quinine, the apparent drug reactions were severe enough that the drugs were discontinued or the dosages decreased; this occurred in only 2% of subjects taking atovaquone and azithromycin. Both drug combinations were equally effective in clearing symptoms and parasitemia. Although rare cases of resistance to atovaquone and azithromycin have been reported, this combination is effective in children and adults and is the antimicrobial combination of choice.[39,114,165,166,174]

Other antimicrobial agents that have been used to treat babesiosis generally are ineffective or found to be useful in only a few cases.[76] Although chloroquine may give some symptomatic relief of fever and myalgia through its antiinflammatory action, it often fails to clear parasitemia in guinea pigs and humans and is not recommended.[19,100] Other antimalarial drugs, such as quinacrine, primaquine, pyrimethamine, sulfadiazine, combined pyrimethamine and sulfadiazine, and tetracycline, have no effect on parasitemia in animals. Pentamidine isothionate has been found to decrease fever and parasitemia, but the organisms are not eradicated, and the drug has proved to be ineffective in animals and humans.[40] Diminazene aceturate was effective in clearing parasitemia and clinical symptoms in one patient, but he developed Guillain-Barré syndrome during recovery, possibly as a result of receiving the drug.[130] Pentamidine and trimethoprim-sulfamethoxazole were used successfully to treat a case of *B. divergens* infection in France.[115]

Additional therapeutic measures may be necessary for people with severe babesiosis, especially those who are immunocompromised. Partial or complete red blood cell exchange transfusion is an important adjunctive therapy that can decrease the degree of parasitemia rapidly and remove toxic byproducts of babesial infections.[17,64,147,157] Exchange transfusion is indicated for patients with severe babesiosis, which is characterized by high-grade parasitemia (≥10%), significant hemolysis, or renal, hepatic, or pulmonary compromise.[165] No data are available to determine whether partial or complete exchange transfusion is preferable. For highly immunocompromised patients who experience therapeutic failure with an initial course of standard antibiotic therapy, resolution of infection may require at least 6 weeks of antimicrobial therapy, including 2 weeks after the parasites are no longer detected on blood smears.[76]

Babesiosis can be prevented by avoiding areas where ticks, deer, and mice are known to thrive from May through September. It is especially important for asplenic individuals and other immunocompromised patients who are at increased risk of severe babesiosis and who live or travel in endemic areas to avoid tall grass and brush where ticks may abound. Use of clothing that covers the lower part of the body and that is sprayed or impregnated with diethyltoluamide, dimethyl phthalate, or permethrin (Permanone) is recommended for individuals who travel into the foliage of endemic areas.[31,138] A search for ticks on people and pets should be carried out and the ticks removed as soon as possible.[31] Tick removal is accomplished best with tweezers by grasping the mouth parts and gently pulling.[32,103] Landscape-management approaches such as keeping grass mowed, clearing leaf litter, and spraying property where there is high tick density may help reduce the risk of infection.[53,94] Reduction of deer on islands has been shown to decrease the number of *I. scapularis* ticks and the incidence of Lyme disease.[95,138,141,177–179] It is recommended that prospective blood donors who reside in endemic areas and who present with a history of fever within the preceding 1 to 2 months be excluded from giving blood to prevent transfusion-related cases.[123] Blood donors who have a history of babesiosis are permanently deferred from donating.[97,170] Effective *B. bovis* and *B. bigemina* vaccines have been developed for use in cattle, but no *B. microti* vaccine has been developed.[102,169]

Babesiosis is a worldwide tickborne zoonosis that is endemic in the northeastern and northern midwestern United States and in northeastern China. The incidence is increasing and is greater than currently recognized. Babesiosis manifests as a viral-like illness with generalized nonspecific symptoms, and diagnosis may be delayed. The diagnosis is confirmed by visualizing the organism on blood smears, or detection of *B. microti* DNA with PCR, or indirectly by detection of *B. microti* antibody. The disease can be severe or fatal, primarily in immunocompromised hosts, but complete recovery with antibabesial chemotherapy is the rule.

NEW REFERENCES SINCE THE SEVENTH EDITION

34. Diuk-Wasser M, Liu L, Steeves T, et al. Monitoring human babesiosis emergence through vector surveillance New England USA. *Emerg Infect Dis.* 2014;20:225-231.
35. Diuk-Wasser M, Vannier E, Krause PJ. Coinfection by *Ixodes* tick-borne pathogens: ecological, epidemiological, and clinical consequences. *Trends Parasitol.* 2016;32:30-42.
65. Jiang JF, Zheng YC, Jiang RR, et al. Epidemiological, clinical, and laboratory characteristics of 48 cases of "*Babesia venatorum*" infection in China: a descriptive study. *Lancet Infect Dis.* 2015;15:196-203.
156. Vannier E, Diuk-Wasser M, Ben Mamoun C, Krause PJ. Babesiosis. *Infect Dis Clin North Am.* 2015;29:357-370.
170. Wang G, Wormser GP, Zhuge J, et al. Utilization of a real-time PCR assay for diagnosis of *Babesia microti* infection in clinical practice. *Ticks Tick Borne Dis.* 2015;6:376-382.

The full reference list for this chapter is available at ExpertConsult.com.

220 Malaria

Rosemary M. Olivero • Elizabeth D. Barnett

Malaria is a disease of global importance. In 2015 there were an estimated 214 million new cases of malaria resulting in 438,000 deaths.[122] Worldwide, despite declines in malaria cases and deaths, the majority of deaths from malaria continue to occur in children.[122] Regular transmission of malaria occurs in parts of Africa, Asia, the Middle East, Central and South America, Hispaniola, and Oceania. The infection has been imported by travel to nearly every part of the world. Because of the ubiquity of the infection and the increasing volume of international travel, recognizing the signs and symptoms of malaria and knowing about methods of prevention and treatment are important for health care professionals wherever they practice.[46,55]

Malaria usually is transmitted from one person to another through bites of infected female *Anopheles* mosquitoes. Disease typically results from infection with one or more of the four species of *Plasmodium* (*Plasmodium falciparum*, *P. vivax*, *P. ovale*, or *P. malariae*) that commonly infect humans. A fifth species, *P. knowlesi*, which is a malaria parasite of monkeys, has also been identified as causing human malaria by zoonotic transmission.[29] These protozoa have complex life cycles involving arthropod and vertebrate hosts. If untreated, *P. falciparum* can progress to coma, renal failure, pulmonary edema, and death. Asymptomatic carriage may last decades in the case of infection with *P. malariae*. Relapses are common after infection with *P. vivax* and *P. ovale*. Resistance of the parasites to antimalarial agents and incomplete success in developing and maintaining programs to eradicate the mosquito vectors have contributed to making malaria a persistent worldwide challenge.

HISTORY

Malaria has been known since antiquity and probably affected prehistoric humans. Fossilized mosquitoes have been found in geologic strata 30 million years old. Descriptions of the signs and symptoms of malaria have been found in early Hindu and Chinese writing, and Hippocrates described seasonal and geographic aspects of the disease.[164] Numerous references to malaria occur in literature, ranging from Shakespeare's *The Tempest* to Laura Ingalls Wilder's *Little House on the Prairie*. The name is derived from the Italian *mal aria* ("bad air") based on recognition of the connection between malaria and swamps. One of the first methods of malaria control, draining swamps, was based on this association.

The first malaria treatment known to Europeans was bark of the cinchona tree, which was identified in the early 17th century almost 200 years before the active ingredient (quinine) was isolated. Not until the late 1800s was the vector-borne nature of malaria understood and described; for their roles in this discovery, Laveran, a French military surgeon working in Algeria, and Ross, a British military physician working in India, were awarded Nobel prizes. Further work by many investigators rounded out the current understanding of the life cycle of the malaria parasites and the complex interrelationship with vector mosquitoes.

During the 20th century, parallel efforts directed toward vector control and discovery and development of drugs to treat malaria were undertaken. The development of larvicides and insecticides permitted control of the mosquito vector. The spectacular success of house spraying with dichlorodiphenyltrichloroethane (DDT) was instrumental in eradicating malaria from most of North America and Europe and in decreasing its prevalence significantly in the Mediterranean area, the Middle East, the Far East, and parts of southern Africa.[145] The development of antimalarial drugs, stimulated largely by the need to protect soldiers during World Wars I and II during shortages of the standard antimalarial agent quinine, allowed for successful treatment of malaria cases.

The World Health Organization (WHO) launched a global campaign for eradication of malaria in 1957. Early successes, attributable to the efficacy of DDT and development of new antimalarial agents, subsequently were hindered by resistance of mosquito vectors to DDT and resistance of the parasites to antimalarial drugs. In 1969, the WHO philosophy on malaria was altered to emphasize the development of health services and research. The goals of malaria control since then have been refined and broadened to include implementation of selective and sustainable preventive measures, early diagnosis and prompt treatment, early detection or prevention of epidemics, and strengthening of local infrastructures to allow better understanding of the determinants of local transmission and malaria control.[145,164]

During 2000 through 2010, reductions of more than 50% in malaria cases have occurred in almost half (43 of 99) of the countries with ongoing transmission; eight additional countries showed downward trends. These successes are likely due to renewed global commitment to financing of malaria programs, allowing increased access to insecticide-treated mosquito nets (from <2% in 2000 to 55% in 2015 in sub-Saharan Africa), and indoor residual spraying, as well as increased availability of rapid diagnostic tests and artemisinin-based combination therapies.[122] Reductions in malaria control have proven most challenging in countries with the most intense transmission, such as the Democratic Republic of Congo and Nigeria.[122] Ongoing challenges to global malaria elimination include maintaining local control measures; resistance to antimalarial drugs, especially to artemisinin derivatives; changes in climate; and population movement as a result of urbanization, mass displacement of populations, and international travel.[17,86,92,97,122,146]

Mortality from malaria, particularly in adults, increased around the turn of the 21st century, with increases in malaria deaths from 995,000 in 1980 to a peak of 1,817,000 in 2004. Corresponding to the increases in malaria cases attributed to financing of global malaria programs, mortality rates decreased to 1,238,000 in 2010. The majority of malaria deaths continue to be reported from Africa.[107,122]

Despite reductions in many areas of the world, in the United States in 2011 there were 1925 reported cases of malaria; this represents the highest number of cases since 1980. The number of reported cases declined to 1687 in 2012 then increased to 1727 in 2013.[32,33] These figures emphasize the impact of international travel on malaria prevalence in travelers from the United States, and the need for increased prevention measures in this population.

ORGANISM

The life cycle of malaria parasites is complex and requires a suitable population of *Anopheles* mosquitoes and infected humans for completion (Fig. 220.1). To begin the cycle, the female anopheline mosquito injects sporozoites along with saliva in preparation for taking a blood meal

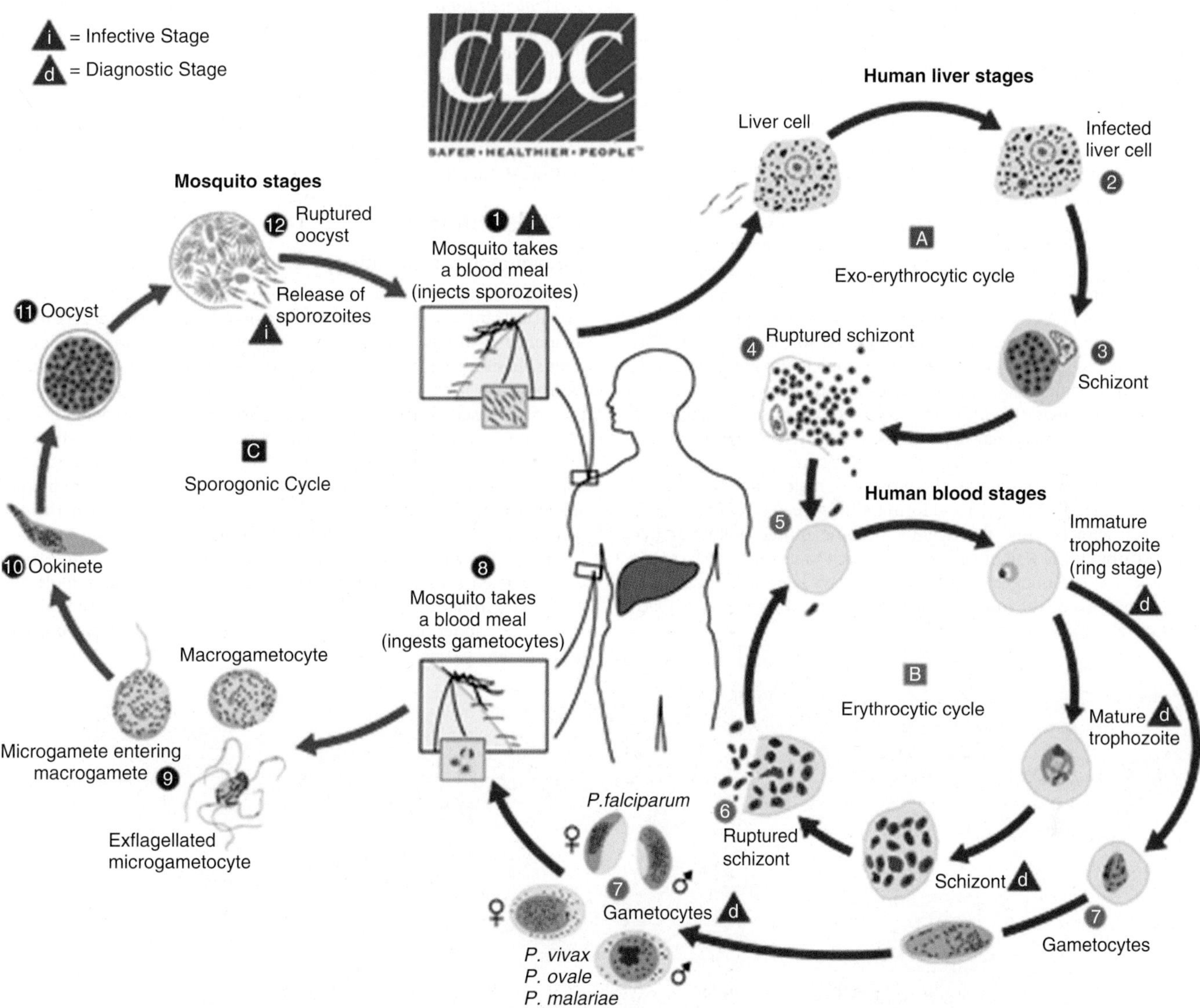

FIG. 220.1 Life cycle of the human malaria parasites. The malaria parasite life cycle involves two hosts. During a blood meal, a malaria-infected female *Anopheles* mosquito inoculates sporozoites into the human host *(1)*. Sporozoites infect liver cells *(2)* and mature into schizonts *(3)*, which rupture and release merozoites *(4)*. (Of note, in *P. vivax* and *P. ovale* a dormant stage [hypnozoites] can persist in the liver and cause relapses by invading the bloodstream weeks, or even years, later.) After this initial replication in the liver (exo-erythrocytic schizogony *[A]*), the parasites undergo asexual multiplication in the erythrocytes (erythrocytic schizogony *[B]*). Merozoites infect red blood cells *(5)*. The ring stage trophozoites mature into schizonts, which rupture, releasing merozoites *(6)*. Some parasites differentiate into sexual erythrocytic stages (gametocytes) *(7)*. Blood stage parasites are responsible for the clinical manifestations of the disease. The gametocytes, male (microgametocytes) and female (macrogametocytes), are ingested by an *Anopheles* mosquito during a blood meal *(8)*. The parasites' multiplication in the mosquito is known as the sporogonic cycle *(C)*. While in the mosquito's stomach, the microgametes penetrate the macrogametes, generating zygotes *(9)*. The zygotes in turn become motile and elongated (ookinetes) *(10)* and invade the midgut wall of the mosquito, where they develop into oocysts *(11)*. The oocysts grow, rupture, and release sporozoites *(12)*, which make their way to the mosquito's salivary glands. Inoculation of the sporozoites *(1)* into a new human host perpetuates the malaria life cycle. (From Centers for Disease Control and Prevention. About Malaria: Biology; http://www.cdc.gov/malaria/about/biology/)

from a vertebrate host. Sporozoites, the infective stage of *Plasmodium,* remain in the circulation for less than 1 hour and then migrate to the liver, where they invade hepatocytes and multiply asexually. Proliferation within hepatocytes takes approximately 1 week for *P. falciparum* and *P. vivax* and approximately 2 weeks for *P. malariae.* At the end of this period, mature tissue schizonts rupture and release thousands of merozoites, which then invade red blood cells (RBCs). *P. vivax* and *P. ovale* have a second type of exoerythrocytic form, the hypnozoite, which can remain dormant for weeks to years. Dormant hypnozoites may develop weeks, months, or years later into merozoites, which then can enter RBCs and cause relapse of malaria. The factors that influence which exoerythrocytic form develops are not understood. Complete details of the erythrocytic phases of *P. knowlesi* in humans are not yet known.[82]

Merozoites released from tissue schizonts invade RBCs, where the erythrocytic phase of the life cycle occurs. Two pathways exist in the erythrocytic, or blood, phase: asexual and sexual. In the asexual phase, development of the parasite begins with the youngest stage, the trophozoite or ring form. The parasite undergoes nuclear division to form schizonts and then merozoites in the asexual multiplication process, called erythrocytic schizogony/merogony. Lysis of RBCs releases the merozoites, which invade other RBCs, perpetuating the asexual erythrocytic cycle. The cycle continues until interrupted by treatment or by the host's immune response.

In the sexual phase, subpopulations of merozoites in the erythrocytic phase differentiate into gametocytes, or sexual forms, which then are available for ingestion by mosquitoes to complete the life cycle within the mosquito. Female macrogametocytes and male microgametocytes appear in the circulation within 3 to 15 days of the onset of symptoms. Gametocytes of *P. vivax* may appear in 4 days, whereas gametocytes of *P. falciparum* may require 10 days for development.

In the stomach (midgut) of the mosquito, male gametocyte nuclei divide into four to eight nuclei and form motile gametocytes that fertilize the female gametocytes. The zygotes become motile ookinetes that migrate through the wall of the midgut, attach to its outer surface, and form oocysts. The oocysts rupture 9 to 14 days later and release sporozoites that invade the mosquito salivary glands, where they are ready for inoculation into the next vertebrate host.

EPIDEMIOLOGY

Transmission of malaria occurs in large parts of Africa, the Indian subcontinent, Southeast Asia, the Middle East, Oceania, and Central and South America (Fig. 220.2). Although indigenous transmission of malaria has been eradicated almost completely from the United States, Canada, Europe, most of the Caribbean, parts of South America, Israel, Turkmenistan, Morocco, the United Arab Emirates, Armenia, Lebanon, Reunion, Singapore, Hong Kong, Japan, Korea, Taiwan, Brunei, and Australia, many cases of imported malaria occur in these countries each year.[122]

P. falciparum is the major malaria species in sub-Saharan Africa and the island of Hispaniola, with *P. malariae* assuming a more minor role. *P. vivax* occurs alongside *P. falciparum* in the Indian subcontinent, Central and South America, Mexico, Southeast Asia, and Oceania. *P. ovale* occurs mainly in Africa. *P. vivax* occurs rarely in sub-Saharan Africa because most Africans lack the Duffy blood group antigen necessary for parasite invasion.[76] *P. knowlesi* has been isolated only in Southeast Asia.[122]

TRANSMISSION

Epidemiologic Terminology

Patterns of transmission of malaria include stable endemic malaria (natural transmission occurring over many years, with a predictable incidence of illness and prevalence of infection) and unstable malaria (transmission rates vary from year to year in areas of low immunity, with a greater likelihood of epidemics occurring). The degree of endemic malaria is based on the parasite rate in children 2 to 9 years old. Types of endemic malaria include hypoendemic (parasite rate of 0–10%), mesoendemic (parasite rate of 11–50%), hyperendemic (parasite rate consistently >50%, with a high proportion of adults having enlarged spleens), and holoendemic (parasite rate consistently >75%, with a low proportion of adults having enlarged spleens).[164]

Autochthonous malaria is acquired locally and may be indigenous or introduced. Introduced malaria may occur when migrant populations with asymptomatic infection provide blood meals for feeding anopheline mosquitoes under conditions that allow for the life cycle to be completed

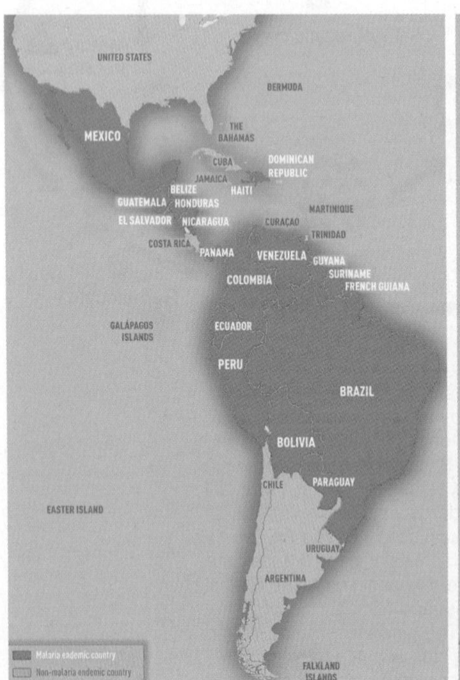

A

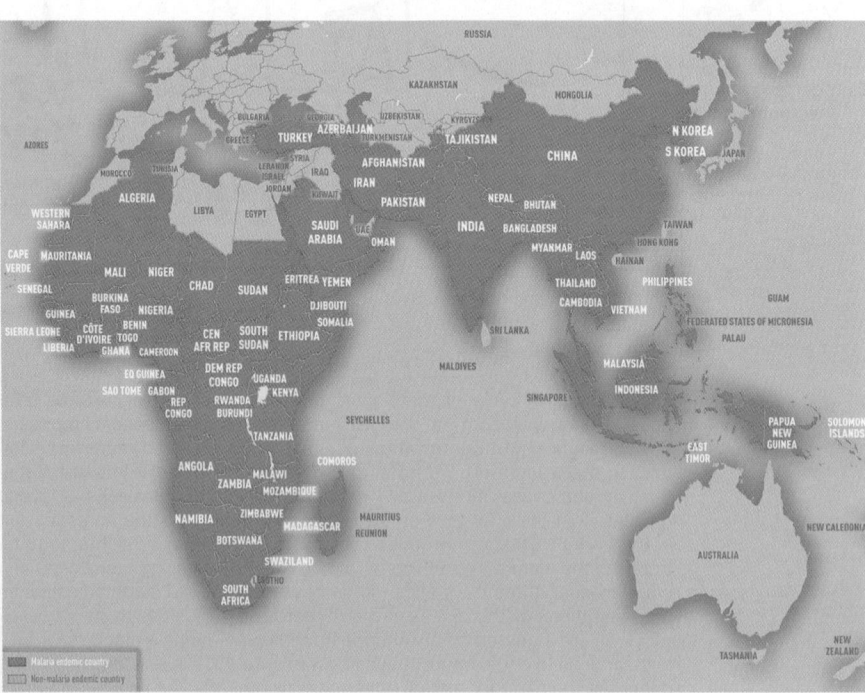

B

FIG. 220.2 Malaria-endemic countries in the (A) Western and (B) Eastern Hemispheres, 2016. (From Centers for Disease Control and Prevention. *Health Information for International Travel 2016,* http://wwwnc.cdc.gov/travel/yellowbook/2016/infectious-diseases-related-to-travel/malaria.)

in the mosquito, enabling the mosquito to infect others. Imported malaria cases may occur in nonendemic areas but result from infection in an endemic area. Induced malaria is acquired by exposure to infected blood, such as from blood transfusion, needlestick injury, laboratory accident, or, historically, medical treatments. Cryptic malaria cases are cases for which no explanation can be found and no epidemiologic link to other cases can be identified.

Mosquito-borne Transmission

The most typical means of transmission of malaria is through the bite of an infected female anopheline mosquito. Although more than 450 species of *Anopheles* mosquitos exist, only approximately 60 have been shown to be effective vectors of malaria.[25] A population of infected humans is necessary to sustain transmission because of the short life span of mosquitoes (5–20 days) and the long incubation period required in the mosquito (8 to ≥10 days).

Bloodborne Transmission

Transmission of malaria via blood transfusion is well documented.[106,123] Transmission also may occur through organ donation or needlestick injury.[32,57] Relapses of malaria cannot occur with bloodborne transmission, even if the infecting species is *P. vivax* or *P. ovale,* because the infection is produced by the transmission of infected RBCs rather than by forms that invade the liver.

Congenital Malaria

Infants can acquire malaria from their mothers during pregnancy. Transplacental transmission of parasites has been proposed as the most likely route of transmission, although breakdown of placental barriers allowing transmission of maternal blood cells to the infant during labor or delivery also has been suggested as a mechanism of transmission.[64,94,102] *P. vivax* most often is associated with this phenomenon, but it may occur with all species. Congenital malaria is less likely to occur in infants of semi-immune mothers because of transplacental passage of maternal antibody during the third trimester. As with transfusion-associated malaria, relapses do not occur. An important sequela of infection that occurs in pregnancy is fetal growth restriction and increased risk of morbidity and mortality.[169]

Cryptic Malaria

The category of cryptic malaria includes cases for which no source of infection can be identified. Typical cases include confirmed malaria in US residents who have never traveled to or resided in malarial areas, who have not received blood transfusions, and who are not linked epidemiologically with other cases.[32,81,136] Airport malaria, one kind of cryptic malaria, occurs in proximity to international airports and is thought to occur when mosquitoes arriving with airplanes from endemic areas infect individuals working in or living near airports.[75]

HOST-PARASITE INTERACTION

The intensity of transmission of malaria depends on factors that affect the density of vectors and the extent of vector-human contact. Transmission of malaria may be continuous or seasonal, or it may depend on local site-specific factors, such as the presence of irrigation projects or intermittent flooding. Mosquito vectors differ in their efficiency in transmitting malaria; the principal vector in sub-Saharan Africa, *Anopheles gambiense,* is known for being a highly effective vector. Variations in climate may affect the viability of mosquitoes.

The incidence and severity of malaria are affected by the intensity of exposure, the presence of immunity, and genetic factors. Distinction must be made between malaria infection (presence of parasitemia) and malaria illness. A major puzzle in malaria is why individuals with similar degrees of parasitemia may exhibit radically different clinical manifestations.

Individuals who reside in endemic areas and are exposed continually to infected mosquitoes acquire some degree of immunity to malaria illness. Adults in these areas continue to become infected, but they have lower levels of parasitemia. Infants born to mothers with acquired immunity may be protected transiently by transplacental passage of maternal antibody. The highest incidence of infection with malaria occurs in infants and young children who are no longer protected by maternal antibody but who are too young to develop sufficient acquired immunity. The lack of acquired immunity in infants and young children accounts partly for their increased risk for acquiring disease and having severe manifestations such as cerebral malaria. Acquired immunity diminishes during pregnancy, and pregnant women are at high risk for development of severe complications of malaria. Individuals in the population who remain asymptomatic but harbor gametocytes in their blood are reservoirs of infection when bitten by mosquitoes. With the exception of *P. knowlesi,* which infects monkeys, there are no significant animal reservoirs of malaria.

Clinical manifestations of malaria may be severe in nonimmune patients. Malaria is the most common life-threatening infection acquired by travelers to malaria-endemic regions. Individuals with acquired immunity who then leave endemic areas for long periods may lose their immunity and be at risk for severe disease if reexposed.

Genetic factors determine the risk for acquiring malaria and having severe infection. Individuals who have a Duffy-negative blood type lack the most important specific receptors for invasion of the merozoites of *P. vivax,* and these individuals have markedly reduced susceptibility to infection with this species.[76,103] This resistance is the basis for the low incidence of vivax malaria in Africa. Specific human leukocyte antigens present in individuals from West Africa may protect against the development of severe complications of malaria, including cerebral malaria and severe anemia. The best-known example of the relationship between malaria and genetics is the association between sickle hemoglobinopathies and protection against severe falciparum malaria. This balanced polymorphism is thought to have helped ensure survival of the gene for hemoglobin S in the population because of the selective advantage provided on a population basis to those who are heterozygous for sickle-cell disease. Individuals with sickle hemoglobinopathies still may be infected and manifest signs and symptoms of malaria, although the risk for acquiring severe malaria or dying of malaria may be 60-fold to 70-fold less in children with hemoglobin AS than in children with hemoglobin AA.[168]

PATHOPHYSIOLOGY

Pathophysiologic changes in malaria are caused by destruction of RBCs, production of cytokines, stimulation of intravascular synthesis of nitric oxide, and sequestration of infected erythrocytes.

Lysis of RBCs leads to anemia, which may be acute and severe, and its attendant hemodynamic consequences. Anemia may develop as a result of hemolysis, impaired erythropoiesis, or bone marrow depression secondary to folic acid deficiency.[127] Intravascular hemolysis may be so severe that it results in pronounced hemoglobinuria (blackwater fever), which may be a precipitating event in the development of renal failure. This complication has been noted in association with treatment using quinine. Hematopoiesis is suppressed during acute infection, and such suppression may not be reversed as readily in iron-deficient individuals, contributing to the development of chronic anemia.

Cytokines such as tumor necrosis factor (TNF) and interleukin-1 have important roles in the pathogenesis and severity of malaria infection.[14,77,79] Severe disease has been associated with higher concentrations of TNF, and TNF polymorphisms may play a role in the development of specific complications.[99,100] Higher TNF concentrations have been observed in those with cerebral malaria and those who have required longer hospitalizations for malaria.[77] Parasite factors responsible for release of cytokines have not been identified. A possible mechanism for the role of TNF in malaria pathogenesis is the binding of TNF to its receptors, causing signaling to amplify cytokines of inflammatory cascades.[138] Another possible role of TNF in malaria is to stimulate production of nitric oxide, a short-lived neurotransmitter. Nitric oxide may have a role in cerebral malaria pathogenesis, and its transient nature may provide a partial explanation for the complete recovery noted in some patients with severe cerebral malaria. TNF and nitric oxide have both harmful and beneficial roles in the pathogenesis of malaria; both have been shown to be correlated with clearance of parasites and eventual recovery and with severity of illness.

Sequestration of infected RBCs has long been thought to contribute to the clinical manifestations of malaria, particularly that caused by *P. falciparum*. Late-stage parasites induce host cells to develop knobs on the surface of erythrocytes that facilitate adherence of these cells to vascular endothelium. The effects of these sequestered RBCs on the perfusion, nutrition, and oxygenation of surrounding tissues may be responsible for the complications of *P. falciparum* infection, including cerebral malaria, renal failure, and watery diarrhea.[109,132] Consumption of glucose by metabolically active late-stage parasites contributes to hypoglycemia and lactic acidosis. Despite these changes, the majority of histopathologic appearances of tissue is remarkably benign, consistent with the reversible nature of the changes and supportive of the role of cytokines and secondary messengers in the pathogenesis of complications of cerebral malaria.[164,168] Recent postmortem microscopy of brain sections from adults who died of malaria confirmed that sequestration of cerebral microvasculature was significantly higher in patients with cerebral malaria and was also correlated with deeper levels of premortem coma and shorter time to death.[133]

CLINICAL MANIFESTATIONS AND LABORATORY FINDINGS

The clinical manifestations of malaria depend on the species causing the infection, the immune status of the individual, the mode of transmission of infection, whether the individual was taking prophylaxis, and host immune factors (Table 220.1). Acute malaria generally is understood to refer to the signs and symptoms associated with disease caused by infection with malaria parasites.

Recurrent infections are of three types: relapse, recrudescence, and reinfection. Relapses occur as a result of delayed maturation of the dormant liver stages (hypnozoites) of *P. vivax* or *P. ovale*. Recrudescence occurs when parasitemia caused by the same parasite responsible for the initial infection recurs after clearance or a significant reduction in the initial parasitemia, and occurs most commonly with *P. falciparum* because of drug resistance. Reinfection with different parasites and infection with more than one type of *Plasmodium* occur especially in areas with a high intensity of transmission. Persistent infection is noted with *P. malariae*; hypnozoites have not been identified with *P. malariae*, so the organism is thought to persist as a low-level parasitemia that can exist for years without causing symptoms.

A classic description of malaria includes features of the malaria paroxysm resulting from lysis of parasitized RBCs and release of merozoites into the circulation at the completion of asexual reproduction. The paroxysm is characterized by fever and chills accompanied by constitutional symptoms of headache, body ache, fatigue, dizziness, and malaise. Gastrointestinal symptoms include nausea and vomiting, abdominal pain, and diarrhea. Cough and dyspnea may accompany an attack. Although periodicity of the paroxysms in primary attacks is thought to be pathognomonic for malaria species, this periodicity may take several days to become established, may not occur at all in asynchronous infections, or may be modified by previous immunity or treatment.

In children, fever and headache may be the sole symptoms or gastrointestinal symptoms may predominate. Physical signs of malaria include pallor, jaundice, and hepatosplenomegaly. Rash and lymphadenopathy typically are not associated with malaria, although malaria may precipitate recrudescence of latent herpes infections.

Anemia is the most common laboratory abnormality in malaria. Thrombocytopenia is common and may be the first manifestation in patients with uncomplicated malaria.[168] Leukopenia also may occur, and leukocytosis is less common and should provoke investigation for other conditions. Liver function test abnormalities may be present and can be mistaken for infectious hepatitis, especially in patients with jaundice and tender hepatosplenomegaly. Hypoglycemia occurs frequently with falciparum malaria and may develop before or as a consequence of treatment with quinine. When present in children before treatment, hypoglycemia is associated with a poor prognosis.[165] Hyponatremia may occur as part of the syndrome of inappropriate secretion of antidiuretic hormone. Serum creatinine and blood urea nitrogen values may be elevated transiently or may increase significantly with acute renal failure.

Malaria stimulates a polyclonal increase in immunoglobulins associated with rapid production of malaria-specific antibodies and reduced complement levels. False-positive tests for syphilis, rheumatoid factor, heterophil agglutinins, and cold agglutinins may occur.[164]

Severe and Complicated Malaria

Nonimmune individuals are most susceptible to severe complications of falciparum malaria, which include cerebral malaria, pulmonary failure or acute respiratory distress syndrome, renal failure, and severe anemia.[90] Hypoglycemia and metabolic acidosis may occur. Falciparum malaria in nonimmune patients should be considered a medical emergency, and treatment of *P. falciparum* should be initiated in all ill patients with malaria until the species can be confirmed. The highest mortality is seen in those who have a combination of severe respiratory distress, impaired consciousness, and severe anemia. The Centers for Disease Control and Prevention (CDC) and WHO criteria for the diagnosis of severe malaria are outlined in Table 220.2.

Severe Anemia

Children younger than 1 year old, especially in sub-Saharan Africa, are those most likely to experience severe malarial anemia. This complication is thought to occur most often in areas with year-round transmission. Clinical consequences of anemia are determined by rate of development and severity of the anemia, with high risk for complications as hemoglobin decreases to less than 5 g/dL.[112] Hemolysis has been reported as a consequence of treatment with artemisinin derivatives, most commonly IV artesunate, approximately 2 weeks after initiation of treatment[142]; it

TABLE 220.1 Characteristics of the *Plasmodium* Species Responsible for Human Malaria

	SPECIES				
Characteristic	***P. falciparum***	***P. vivax***	***P. ovale***	***P. malariae***	***P. knowlesi***
Incubation period in days (range)	12 (8–25)	14 (8–27)	17 (15 to ≥18)	28 (15 to ≥40)	11 (9 to >12)
Periodicity of febrile attacks (hours)	None	48	48	72	24
Earliest appearance of gametocytes (days)	10	3	?	?	?
Relapse	No	Yes	Yes	No	No
Duration of untreated infection (years)	1–2	1.5–4	1.5–4	3–50	?
RBC preference	Younger cells (but can invade cells of all ages)	Reticulocytes	Reticulocytes	Older cells	?
Characteristic morphology	Ring forms Multiply infected cells Banana-shaped gametocytes	Schüffner dots Enlarged RBCs	Schüffner dots Enlarged RBCs	Normal-sized cells Band or rectangular forms of trophozoites	Ring forms Occasional multiply infected cells Band forms

RBC, Red blood cell.

TABLE 220.2 **Manifestations of Severe Malaria**

Centers for Disease Control and Prevention Definition[a]	World Health Organization Definition[162]
Cerebral malaria	Prostration, impaired consciousness, coma (cerebral malaria) or multiple convulsions
Severe anemia	Severe anemia
Acute renal failure	Renal impairment
Hemoglobinuria	Hemoglobinuria
Hypoglycemia	Hypoglycemia (<40 mg/dL)
Metabolic acidosis	Acidosis or hyperlactatemia
Hypotension caused by cardiovascular collapse	Circulatory collapse or shock
Acute respiratory distress syndrome	Respiratory distress or pulmonary edema
Coagulopathy	Abnormal bleeding
Hyperparasitemia (>5% infected RBCs)	Hyperparasitemia (>2% infected RBCs in low-transmission areas or >5% in high-transmission areas)
	Jaundice
	Failure to feed

RBCs, Red blood cells.
[a]From www.cdc.gov/malaria/about/disease/html#severe.

is unclear whether this hemolysis is a complication of artemisinin treatment rather than the severity of malaria in these cases.

Hypoglycemia

Hypoglycemia (blood glucose <40 mg/dL) may be present on initial evaluation in 20% of children with severe malaria and is associated with a poor prognosis. The etiology of pretreatment hypoglycemia is thought to be a combination of parasite consumption of glucose and inadequate gluconeogenesis in the liver. Hypoglycemia also can occur as a result of treatment, most typically with quinine. Intravenous or oral administration of quinine may lead to hypoglycemia by stimulating insulin secretion. Pregnant women seem to be especially susceptible to this complication.

Acid-Base Changes

Metabolic acidosis is a marker of malaria illness severity and clinically may manifest as hyperpnea. Acidosis often is associated with hypoglycemia. Fluid resuscitation and treatment with antimalarial drugs often result in rapid resolution of acidosis, although persistence of acidosis may occur in patients who eventually die of malaria.

Renal Complications

Acute renal failure is a potentially life-threatening consequence of acute malaria that occurs more commonly in adults than in children. It typically is oliguric and often is reversible if the patient can be supported by dialysis through the oliguric phase. Acute renal failure is a rare development in residents of endemic areas and long has been thought to occur more frequently in patients treated with quinine or quinidine (blackwater fever). The histologic changes resemble those of acute tubular necrosis.

Nephrotic syndrome and chronic renal failure occur more frequently in areas where malaria is endemic and usually are associated with infection with *P. malariae.* Symptoms occur in individuals younger than 15 years old in approximately half of cases, with gradual progression to renal failure over 3 to 5 years. Most patients have asymptomatic proteinuria and the gradual development of hypertension and deterioration in renal function. Adults more commonly have hematuria and azotemia; adults and children may have hematuria. The disease does not respond to antimalarial agents. Treatment with corticosteroids, cyclophosphamide, and azathioprine has had variable results, with remission occurring only in patients with mild changes on renal biopsy.[164]

Respiratory Complications

Pulmonary edema typically develops late in the course of severe malaria when other complications are already present, and it may occur when parasitemia has resolved and the patient appears to be improving clinically. Pulmonary edema occurs more commonly in adults than in children, and the pathogenesis is consistent with capillary leak syndrome. Supplemental oxygen or mechanical ventilation with positive end-expiratory pressure may be necessary to manage respiratory complications. A well-characterized pulmonary inflammatory response driven by alveolar macrophages can lead to respiratory distress in severe malaria.[118] Respiratory distress is the most dangerous presentation of severe malaria, especially in combination with severe anemia and cerebral malaria.[52]

Cerebral Malaria

Cerebral malaria is the most common complication of falciparum malaria in children and occurs most often in children 3 to 6 years old.[66,128] It presents as alteration of consciousness and diffuse encephalopathy with prolonged multiple seizures in a patient with no other explanation. Patients may be comatose without response to stimuli and may assume an opisthotonic posture. Generalized convulsions may occur, and focal findings are uncommon. Serial electroencephalographic monitoring of 65 Kenyan children uncovered a large range of clinical and electrographic seizures with diffuse background slow-wave activity, which are nonspecific features; electrical seizure activity consistently arose from the posterior temporoparietal region.[30] Intracranial pressure often is increased in children with cerebral malaria, and the presence of increased intracranial pressure was recently found to be associated with increased mortality.[152] Factors associated with neurologic sequelae include prolonged coma, severe anemia, and multiple seizures. Mortality rates range from 15% to 30% of affected children; most survivors recover completely, though approximately 10% may have neurologic sequelae. The most common neurologic sequelae in children noted in a study in the Gambia were hemiplegia, cortical blindness, aphasia, and ataxia.[19]

Many factors, including hypoglycemia, anemia, microvascular obstruction, acidosis, and elaboration of inflammatory mediators, contribute to the syndrome of cerebral malaria. Histopathologic features are minor, with occasional hemorrhages and perivascular infiltrates.

Malarial retinopathy is a more recently described phenomenon in children with falciparum cerebral malaria. The retinal changes seen in malarial retinopathy include retinal whitening, vessel discoloration, retinal hemorrhages, and papilledema, and the severity of retinal findings has been found to have prognostic value in predicting risk of death and length of coma in survivors of severe malaria.[12]

Hyperreactive Malarial Syndrome (Tropical Splenomegaly Syndrome, Hyperreactive Malarial Splenomegaly)

Hyperreactive malarial syndrome is characterized by massive splenomegaly, high concentrations of total serum IgM and malarial antibodies of multiple immunoglobulin classes, and clinical and immunologic response to antimalarial agents.[84,183] Hyperreactive malarial syndrome is correlated with malaria endemicity, with an incidence ranging from 0.5% to 80% of the adult population. The pathogenesis is unknown but seems to involve chronic exposure to malaria, resulting in chronic stimulation of the immune system and genetic factors. Findings on physical examination include a huge spleen (>10 cm below the costal margin) and an enlarged liver. Laboratory findings include anemia and an increased reticulocyte count, elevated IgM (>2 standard deviations above the mean), and high antibody levels of antimalarial antibodies.[157] Some patients have thrombocytopenia or neutropenia. Patients may have an increased risk for acquiring bacterial infections, and some researchers have suggested that hyperreactive malarial syndrome is a premalignant condition.[10] Lifelong treatment with antimalarial agents is the treatment of choice for patients who reside in endemic areas.[84] Treatment of patients who have left endemic areas has not been standardized; several case reports show success with a single short (≤7 days) treatment course of antimalarial agents followed by close monitoring of the size of the spleen.[84,157]

Malaria in Special Populations

Malaria in Children

The signs and symptoms of malaria in children range from asymptomatic infection to life-threatening illness. Severe anemia is most likely to develop in children younger than 2 years old, whereas cerebral malaria is most likely to occur in older children (mean age, 3.5 years). The greatest burden of disease is borne by infants and young children, although the impact of disease on adolescents has not been studied extensively. Malaria in pregnant adolescents may be of particular concern.[80]

In endemic areas, lack of diagnostic facilities, limited resources, and encroaching drug resistance complicate the ability to make a rapid, accurate diagnosis and provide expedient treatment to children with malaria. Malaria often is difficult to distinguish from other common illnesses such as pneumonia. Clinical algorithms that can distinguish children with malaria from children with pneumonia or other illnesses have been developed and studied but do not eliminate completely the overlap with conditions having similar clinical manifestations.[139,140,148] Risk factors for a fatal outcome in children with malaria were studied in Kenya; the presence of coma or respiratory distress, or both, at initial evaluation identified children at high risk for dying.[52,96]

Imported malaria occurs in children in many nonendemic countries. The diagnosis often is delayed because of lack of consideration of malaria as a cause of illness and unfamiliarity with the disease. In children with acquired immunity, the signs and symptoms of disease may be subtle and nonspecific, but fever or a history of fever is universal.[40,89] Other symptoms include anorexia, vomiting, diarrhea, headache, lethargy, and abdominal pain. Laboratory findings include anemia, thrombocytopenia, and leukopenia. The diagnosis of malaria should be considered in every child with fever or a history of recent fever who has visited an area where malaria occurs.

Congenital Malaria

P. falciparum, P. malariae, P. vivax, and *P. ovale* can be transmitted congenitally, but the disease most often is associated with *P. vivax*. Congenital malaria has not been reported with *P. knowlesi*. That congenital malaria is not seen more frequently is due partly to the effective barrier function of the placenta. Congenital malaria develops in infants of approximately 0.1% of immune mothers and 10% of nonimmune mothers in endemic areas, although placental infection occurs in one third of pregnant women.[70] In endemic areas, distinguishing malaria acquired congenitally from malaria acquired by transmission from mosquitoes is difficult. In non–malaria-endemic countries, congenital malaria is very rare; only five cases have been reported in the United States since 2000.[27]

The onset of symptoms is insidious and usually occurs at 2 to 8 weeks of age. The typical malaria paroxysm is absent, with the infant instead having poor feeding, fever, vomiting, diarrhea, irritability, and hepatosplenomegaly on physical examination.[64] The most common laboratory finding is anemia, but thrombocytopenia and hyperbilirubinemia also occur. Therapy for the infecting species of malaria is curative, and the infant does not need treatment of the exoerythrocytic stages of the parasite (although the mother does).

Malaria in Pregnancy

The effects of malaria on the mother depend on the degree of immunity that she has attained and her parity.[102] Relapses and recrudescence of malaria are common during pregnancy, as acquired immunity diminishes with the pregnant state. Malaria can exacerbate the anemia occurring during pregnancy, and hypoglycemia and renal insufficiency may complicate falciparum malaria during pregnancy.[51]

Placental infection during pregnancy is associated with delivering low-birth-weight infants, particularly in primigravidas. Fetal growth restriction begins early in gestation and can occur even in asymptomatic parasitemia.[144] An in vitro study showed that placental falciparum malaria results in inhibition of transplacental amino acid transport and that this is a plausible mechanism of fetal growth restriction.[15] Vivax malaria has been linked to maternal anemia and low birth weight in multigravidas and primigravidas.[113] Severe falciparum malaria is harmful to the fetus because of fetal tachycardia and distress secondary to maternal fever; disruption of maternal-fetal blood flow and exchange of metabolic substrates by malaria parasites trapped in the placenta; and the potential for reduction in fetal glucose supply, which may be exacerbated by treatment with quinine, a drug that is able to stimulate the release of insulin.[88] Heavy infection of the placenta interferes with transfer of tetanus antibodies from the mother to the fetus, but the effect on other antibodies is unknown.[18] Prompt treatment of pregnant women with malaria is critical to survival of the mother and the fetus, as fetal growth restriction and low birth weight are associated with high infant mortality and morbidity rates.[15,169]

DIAGNOSIS

The most important first step in establishing the diagnosis of malaria is to consider the diagnosis in all individuals with febrile illness, especially febrile individuals with a history of travel to endemic areas. Having a high index of suspicion for the diagnosis of malaria cannot be overemphasized. Failure to diagnose and treat malaria promptly contributed to fatal outcomes in US civilians who died of malaria between 1963 and 2001.[111] In one series of fatal falciparum malaria cases in the United States, 40% of patients were not recognized as having malaria during their initial contact with a physician.[50] Manifestations of the disease are most classic in nonimmune individuals or in individuals in areas where malaria transmission is seasonal. Signs and symptoms of disease may be nonspecific in semi-immune individuals, those who have received malaria prophylaxis, or individuals who have been partially treated.

In nonendemic areas, a history of travel to an endemic area should suggest the diagnosis in all individuals with a febrile illness, regardless of the accompanying signs and symptoms.[179] Common diagnoses mistakenly assigned to patients ultimately determined to have malaria include gastroenteritis and viral syndrome. The course of disease may be modified by exposure to antimalarial drugs, such as agents that may have been used for prophylaxis, and the incubation period may be prolonged after the administration of antimalarial chemoprophylaxis. Because malaria may be transmitted by blood transfusion or an organ transplant, may be congenitally acquired, and, rarely, occurs cryptically, the diagnosis also should be considered in patients with compatible signs and symptoms of malaria, anemia, or thrombocytopenia and no other explanation for their illness.

Microscopy is the technique traditionally used for establishing the diagnosis of malaria. Rapid diagnostic tests to detect parasite antigens are important tools in centers lacking around-the-clock expertise in malaria diagnostic microscopy. Other alternatives to microscopic diagnostic techniques for malaria include tests using fluorescent microscopy, DNA probes, polymerase chain reaction (PCR), antibody detection, and flow cytometry. Only a few of these methods meet the requirements of low cost, high reliability and reproducibility, and rapid turnaround time. Some of them are suitable for use in field conditions, however, and have been used in endemic areas and for self-diagnosis.

Diagnosis of cerebral malaria is largely clinical. Patients with cerebral malaria typically do not have marked cerebrospinal fluid (CSF) pleocytosis, differentiating this entity from bacterial meningitis. In comparing CSF parameters in children with cerebral malaria to those with viral encephalitis, those with cerebral malaria have a lower CSF glucose level and higher protein and lactate dehydrogenase (LDH) levels, CSF-to-blood LDH ratio, and CSF-to-serum adenosine deaminase ratio.[68] The clinical finding of malarial retinopathy shows promise in aiding in the diagnosis of severe falciparum malaria complicated by coma,[12] but use of this finding is limited to settings where indirect ophthalmoscopy is available.

Microscopy

Microscopy is the gold standard for establishing the diagnosis of malaria. Identification of typical parasite forms by an experienced microscopist is the mainstay of diagnosis worldwide (Figs. 220.3 through 220.7). There are many advantages of using light microscopy: it can be performed at low cost, it can be done rapidly, it typically allows identification of the infecting species and estimation of parasite load, and it can be

Text continued on p. 2167

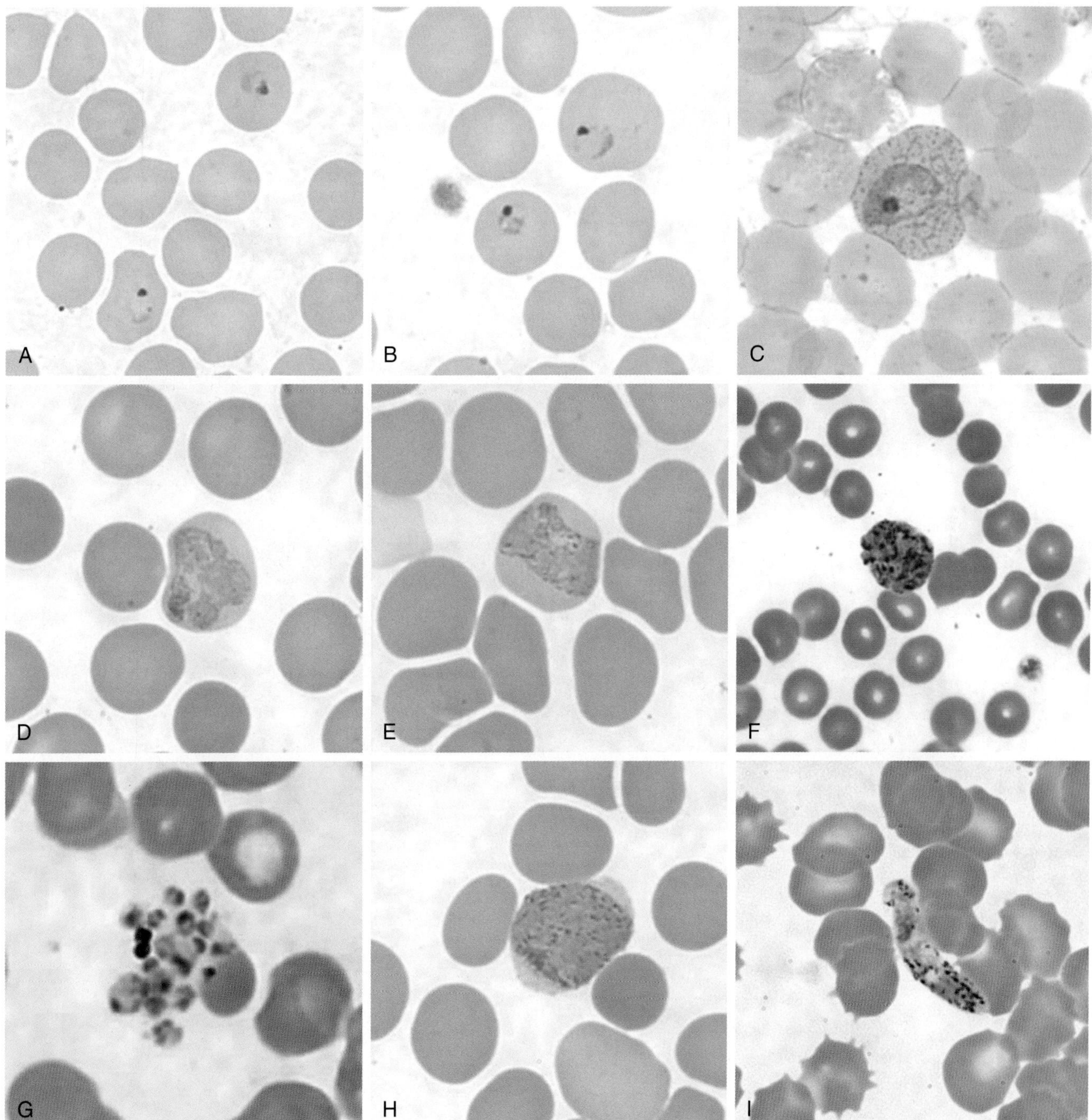

FIG. 220.3 *Plasmodium vivax.* (A–B) Ring trophozoites. (C–E) Trophozoites. (F–G) Schizonts. (H) Macrogametocyte. (I) Ookinete. (From Centers for Disease Control and Prevention, DPDx: Laboratory Identification of Parasitic Diseases of Public Health Concern: Malaria. www.cdc.gov/dpdx/malaria/gallery.html.)

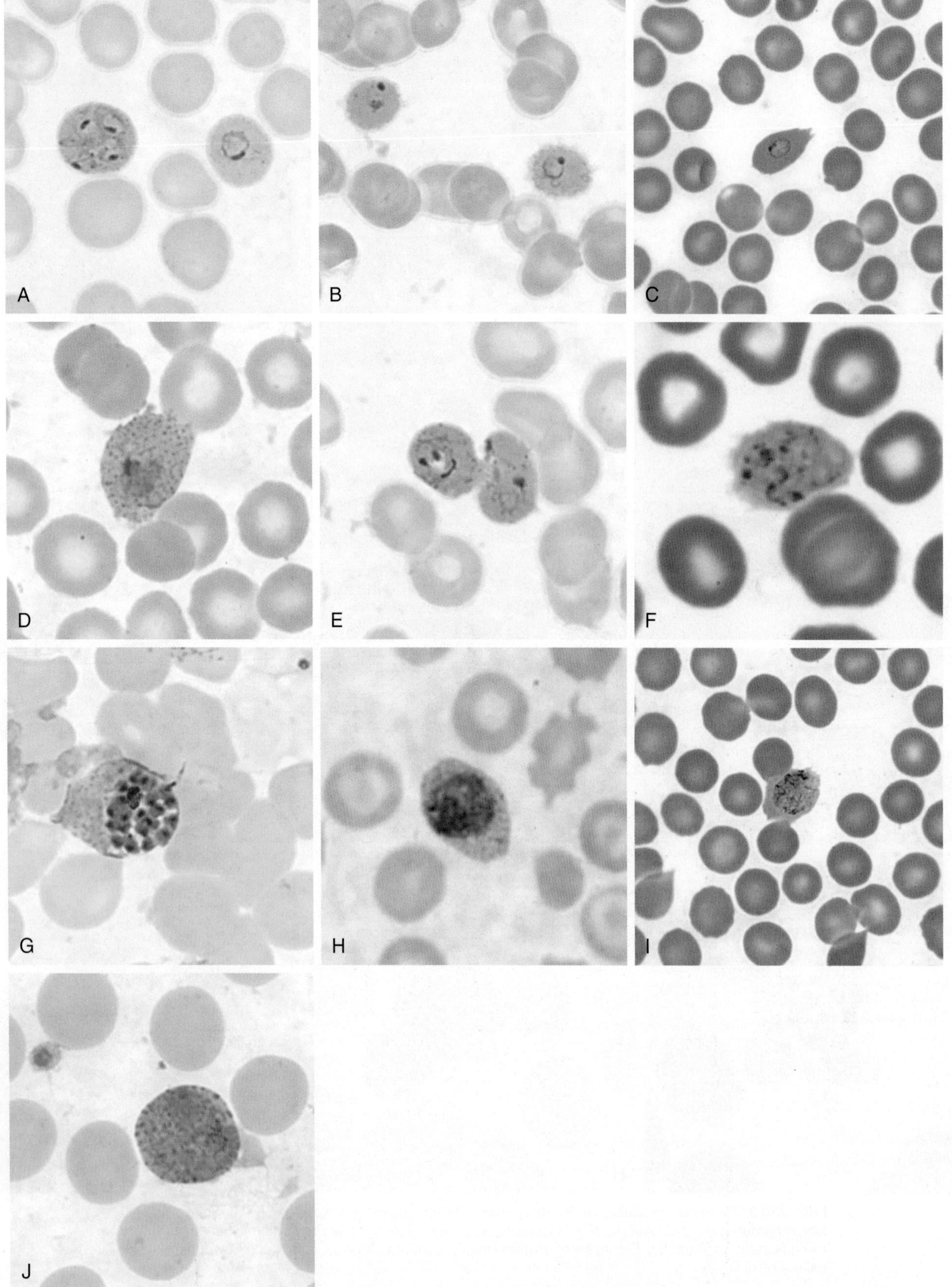

FIG. 220.4 *Plasmodium ovale.* (A–B) Ring trophozoites. (C–E) Trophozoites. (F–G) Schizonts. (H–I) Macrogametocytes. (J) Microgametocyte. (From Centers for Disease Control and Prevention, DPDx: Laboratory Identification of Parasitic Diseases of Public Health Concern: Malaria. www.cdc.gov/dpdx/malaria/gallery.html.)

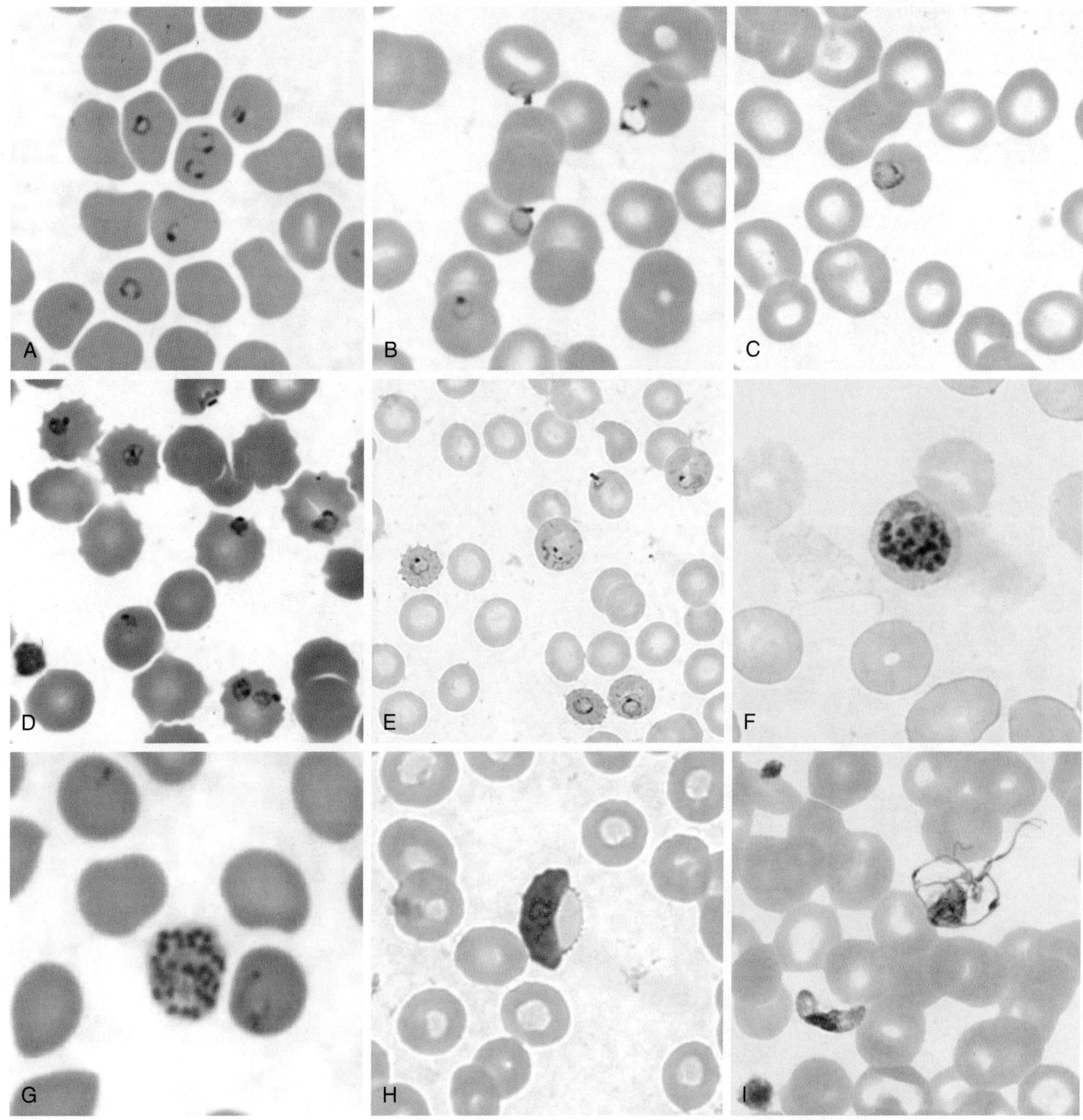

FIG. 220.5 *Plasmodium falciparum.* (A–C) Ring trophozoites. (D–E) Trophozoites. (F–G) Schizonts. (H–I) Gametocytes. (From Centers for Disease Control and Prevention, DPDx: Laboratory Identification of Parasitic Diseases of Public Health Concern: Malaria. www.cdc.gov/dpdx/malaria/gallery.html.)

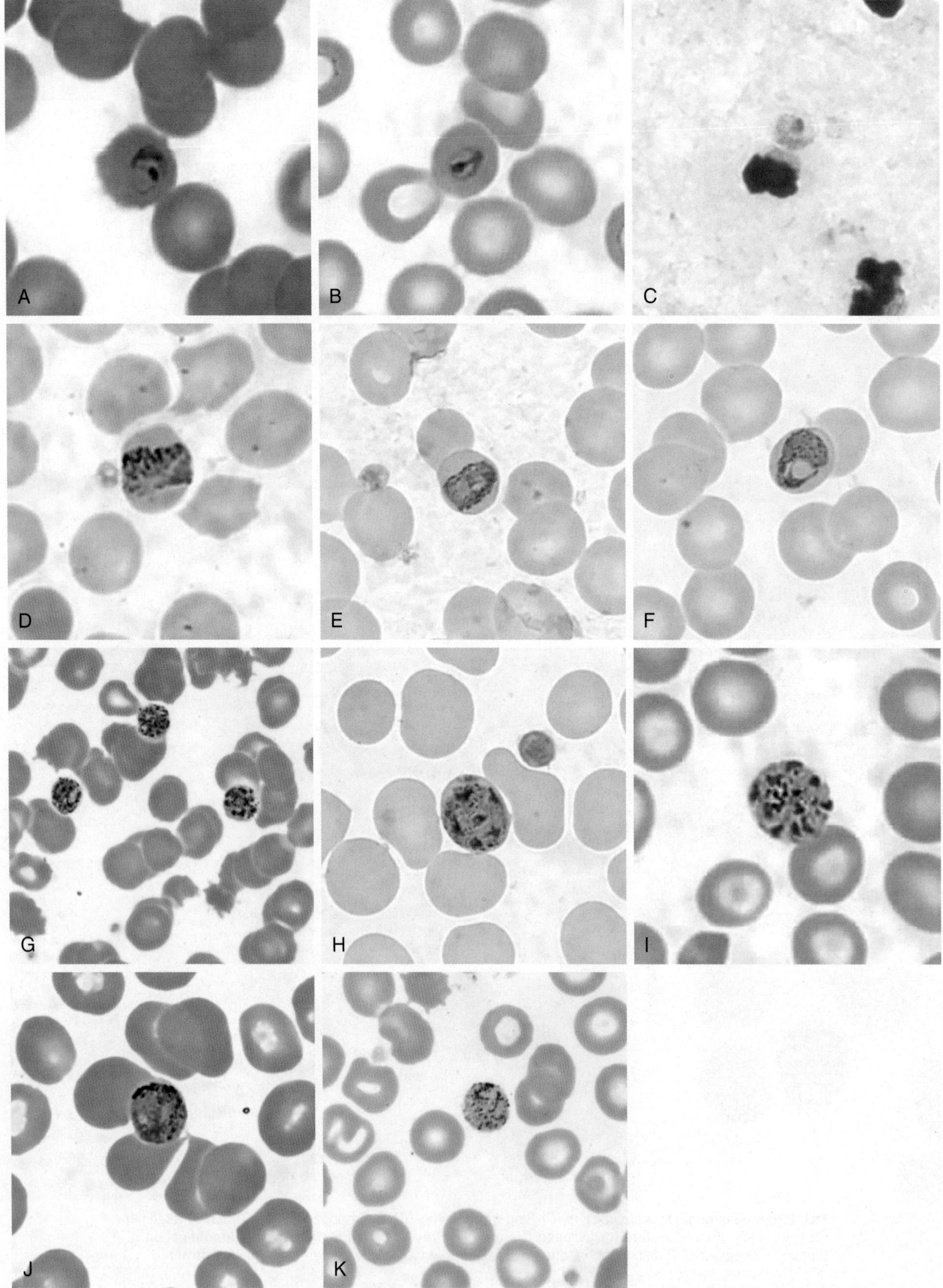

FIG. 220.6 *Plasmodium malariae.* (A–B) Ring trophozoites. (C–F) Trophozoites. (G–I) Schizonts. (J–K) Macrogametocytes. (From Centers for Disease Control and Prevention, DPDx: Laboratory Identification of Parasitic Diseases of Public Health Concern: Malaria. www.cdc.gov/dpdx/malaria/gallery.html.)

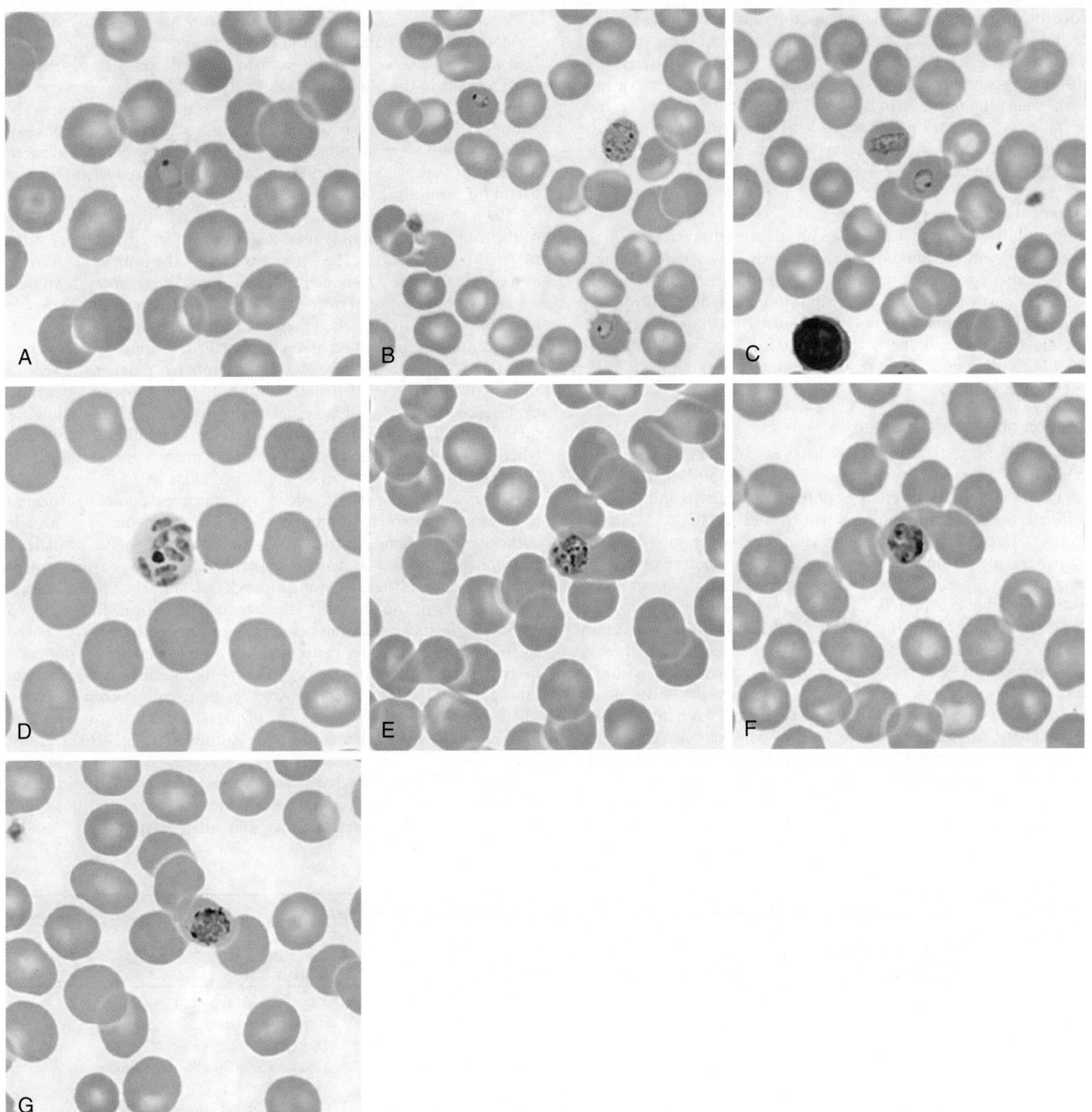

FIG. 220.7 *Plasmodium knowlesi.* (A–B) Ring trophozoites. (C) Trophozoites. (D–F) Schizonts. (G) Gametocyte. (From Centers for Disease Control and Prevention, DPDx: Laboratory Identification of Parasitic Diseases of Public Health Concern: Malaria. www.cdc.gov/dpdx/malaria/gallery.html.)

performed with a small sample of blood. The major disadvantage of microscopy is the need for an experienced microscopist. In settings where malaria is not endemic, the need for specialists to review microscope slides may lead to a delay in establishing the diagnosis.

Thin smears are the most useful in diagnosing malaria. They are easy to prepare, with only a single drop of blood required. The drop of blood is placed at one end of the slide, and the edge of a second slide is placed at the edge of the blood smear and drawn across the slide.[119] RBC morphology is preserved by methanol fixation, so invasion of large RBCs by the parasites can be identified and speciation of the organism is possible (see Table 220.1). Oil-immersion magnification (×1000) should be used for viewing the slide because many young asexual intraerythrocytic parasites are only 2 to 3 μm in diameter and may be missed when using high-dry (×440) magnification. The microscopist begins by looking at the thin edge of the blood film farthest from where the drop of blood was placed. Giemsa stain is preferred to Wright stain when available because it preserves details such as Schüffner dots in *P. vivax* and *P. ovale* infections. When individual RBCs can be seen at low magnification (×100), switching to oil immersion allows examination for parasites within the cells. The major disadvantage of thin films is low sensitivity. With low parasite loads (<100 to 300/μL), the amount of blood on the smear may be too small to allow detection of the parasites.

Thick smears have greater sensitivity than thin smears as a result of the larger quantity of blood used. Because the RBCs are lysed during preparation of the slide, the types of cells containing parasites cannot be identified. To make a thick smear, a drop of blood is placed on the slide and spread in a circle. The slide is stained without using methanol fixation so that RBCs lyse.

Estimating parasite density is useful for assessing degree of parasitemia and for evaluating response to therapy. The density of parasites can be determined on thick or thin smears.[168] When thin smears are used, the proportion of RBCs infected is counted while the smear is viewed under an oil-immersion lens.

Fluorescent Microscopy

The quantitative buffy-coat test relies on identification of parasitized RBCs stained with acridine orange in the RBC layer of centrifuged blood.[161] Experienced personnel can perform the test rapidly, but the reagents are costly when compared with those needed for microscopy, and the species of parasite cannot be identified. If a fluorescent microscope is available, identification of parasitized RBCs can be accomplished by staining a thick smear with acridine orange and examining it under fluorescent light.

Detection of Parasite Antigen

Rapid diagnostic tests (RDTs) for diagnosis of malaria have been developed. These tests are immunochromatographic assays using monoclonal antibodies directed against target malaria antigens and require only 5 to 15 μL of blood, with results obtained in 5 to 20 minutes.[180] Depending on the combinations of target antigens used, certain RDTs detect only *P. falciparum* antigens, whereas others can distinguish *P. falciparum* from *P. vivax, P. ovale*, and *P. malariae*. Assays detecting histidine-rich protein 2 (HRP-2) are specific for *P. falciparum*, whereas assays based on parasite LDH or HRP-2 and aldolase can identify four species of *Plasmodium*.[37,91,105]

Compared with PCR, HRP-2 assays performed well, with sensitivity of 88% to 95% and specificity of 95% to 97%; when the HRP-2 assays were compared with microscopy, sensitivity ranged from 80% to 95% and specificity ranged from 85% to 100%.[119] The tests also performed well when used in nonimmune travelers; a meta-analysis of 21 studies identified sensitivity of 88% to 98% and specificity of 95% to 100% for detection of *P. falciparum*.[98] The HRP-2/aldolase-based assays can detect four species of malaria, but they have a lower sensitivity for diagnosis of vivax malaria, although this assay has a higher sensitivity for detection of malaria than the HRP-2 assays.[26,67,105] A limitation of HRP-2-based assays is that they remain positive after therapy because HRP persists in the blood after acute infection. LDH-based assays are able to distinguish between *P. falciparum* and other malaria species, although the test is unreliable in detecting *P. vivax* in the presence of *P. falciparum*.[137] An advantage of LDH-based assays is the ability to distinguish between viable and nonviable parasites, rendering the test useful for monitoring response to therapy.[23,28,67,105,125]

The target antigens, malaria species detected, sensitivity, and specificity of the four most commonly used RDTs in the United States are summarized in Table 220.3. The Binax Now test is the only RDT licensed in the United States.[44] Although RDTs including Binax Now offer timely results without the use of microscopy, false-negative results are possible and can be problematic when there is low parasitemia. For this reason, many centers in the United States will perform diagnostic microscopy as a follow-up to a negative RDT; this approach reduces the risk of missing the diagnosis of malaria and should be performed when an experienced microscopist is available. Because RDTs do not allow for quantification of parasitemia, diagnostic microscopy should be pursued where available when a diagnosis of severe malaria is entertained, so that response to therapy can be monitored closely.

Dipstick tests may have a role in cost-effective diagnosis of malaria in situations in which laboratory services are inadequate, in mobile clinics or sites lacking electricity,[180] in locations where levels of malaria transmission are low and drug resistance is high, when the cost of treatment exceeds the cost of the dipstick test, and when blood smears are negative and determining the diagnosis is critical. In developed countries, dipstick assays can benefit laboratories with less experienced microscopists by helping them establish a rapid diagnosis, confirm a diagnosis made by microscopy, or determine the infecting species. Current limitations of the tests are decreased sensitivity compared with expert microscopy, especially at low levels of parasite density, cost, and lack of approval by the US Food and Drug Administration (FDA) of most of the tests.

Dipstick malaria tests have been proposed for use by travelers for self-diagnosis of malaria and have been tested for this purpose. The accuracy of both test performance and interpretation of results by

TABLE 220.3 Malaria Rapid Diagnostic Tests Available in the United States[a]

RDT Name	Malaria Antigen Target	Malaria Species Detected	Sensitivity	Comment
Binax Now	HRP-2 and aldolase	*P. falciparum, P. vivax, P. malariae*, and *P. ovale*	94% for *P. falciparum* 84% for non-*P. falciparum* 87% for pure *P. vivax* infections 62% for pure *P. ovale* and *P. malariae* infections	Sensitivity increased to 96% for pure *P. falciparum* infection Overall specificity of 99%[44] FDA approved for use in the United States
Parasight F	HRP-2	*P. falciparum*	96.5–100 in Kenya when >60 parasites/μL, lower with less parasitemia[11] 40% in travelers when <50 parasites/μL, >93% when >100 parasites/ μL[65]	Antigen persists for 6–7 days 6 in 11.9–20% of subjects whose blood smears had cleared[11,65] Not FDA approved for use in the United States
ICT Malaria Pf/Pv	HRP-2 and aldolase	*P. falciparum* and *P. vivax*	97% for *P. falciparum* 44% for *P. vivax*	Specificity of 90% for *P. falciparum* Specificity of 100% for *P. vivax*[131] Not FDA approved for use in the United States
OptiMAL-IT	LDH	*P. falciparum, P. vivax, P. malariae*, and *P. ovale*	85-95%; decreased with lower parasite density[63]	Specificity of 100% *P. falciparum*, 75–85% for *P. vivax* Not FDA approved for use in the United States
Clearview	LDH	*P. falciparum, P. vivax, P. malariae*, and *P. ovale*	93% specificity of 100%, with sensitivities of 99%, 90.0%, 86%, and 60%, respectively, for *P. falciparum, P. vivax, P. malariae*, and *P. ovale*[63]	Specificity of 100% for *P. falciparum*, 99% for *P. vivax*, 90% for *P. malariae*, and 60% for *P. ovale*[63] Not FDA approved for use in the United States

[a]Direct microscopy should be performed where available with a negative RDT given higher false-negative rates with low parasitemia, and when severe malaria is suspected.
HRP-2, Histidine-rich protein-2; *RDT*, rapid diagnostic test.

travelers has not been demonstrated as high enough to recommend this strategy routinely for travelers. Most experts suggest using the test to guide initial treatment while the traveler is heading to a source of health care for more definitive diagnosis and treatment.[69,117]

DNA Probe

Specific DNA probes for identification of *P. falciparum* have been developed and tested in field conditions in Thailand.[8] The technique compared favorably with microscopy and could be used to test large numbers of samples at a time, but it had the disadvantage of needing a radiolabeled probe. Nonisotope probes have been used in other field trials in Madagascar, where an enzyme-linked probe was compared with microscopy for diagnosis of falciparum malaria. Results were comparable to examination of thick smears by microscopy for *P. falciparum* infection, but the assay could not identify infection with *P. vivax, P. ovale,* or *P. malariae* alone.[101]

Polymerase Chain Reaction

PCR-based techniques used for establishing the diagnosis of malaria are highly sensitive and now are able to detect mixed infections. Compared with thick and thin smears, sensitivity and specificity are nearly 100%. PCR techniques can be useful for determining the species of an infection when microscopy is equivocal. Early detection of resistance to antimalarial drugs is another benefit of PCR-based techniques, which have been used to detect a mutation of *P. falciparum* associated with resistance to chloroquine.[43,72] Currently, PCR is the only definite and validated means of diagnosing *P. knowlesi,* because this species may be confused with *P. malariae* on microscopy.[82]

Major disadvantages of the PCR assay include the need for expensive equipment, reagents, and significant technical expertise and the length of time required to perform the testing. At this time, the PCR assay may be better suited for use in large-scale epidemiologic surveys, rather than for establishing the diagnosis of acute malaria in the clinical setting.

Flow Cytometry

Automated blood cell analyzers based on flow cytometry have been shown to display cells containing malaria pigment as a population of cells distinct from other blood components. To date, this discovery has been serendipitous in patients not suspected to have malaria and the diagnosis must be confirmed by conventional methods.[55,73] A future application of this technology could be to modify automated blood cell analyzers to flag specimens that need to be examined further by thin or thick smears (or both).[73]

Antibody Detection

Malaria antibodies develop rapidly after infection and remain present for years; they are of limited value in diagnosing malaria in individual patients. Occasionally, antibody tests might prove useful in the diagnosis of nonimmune individuals with cryptic febrile illnesses or on a population basis to assess the degree of community-wide immunity. Measurement of antibody may have a role in the diagnosis of hyperreactive malarial syndrome.[183]

TREATMENT

Treatment of malaria depends on identification of the species of *Plasmodium* causing infection, knowledge of the presence of resistance to chloroquine and other drugs in the area in which malaria was contracted, and therapeutic goals (treatment of acute illness versus eradication of the exoerythrocytic phase of malaria). Drugs and classes of drugs currently in use for treating malaria include 4-aminoquinolines and related compounds (chloroquine, mefloquine [Lariam], amodiaquine); primaquine; sulfadoxine-pyrimethamine (Fansidar); halofantrine; atovaquone-proguanil (Malarone); artemisinin (qinghaosu) and other artemisinins (artemether, artesunate) and artemisinin drugs in combination with other agents; cinchona alkaloids (quinine, quinidine); and the antimicrobial agents doxycycline, tetracycline, and clindamycin. Investigational compounds and combination drugs are in various stages of development. Drugs that may be used for the treatment of malaria in the United States are listed in Table 220.4. Drugs used for the prevention of malaria are discussed in a subsequent section.

The choice of agent to treat symptomatic malaria depends on the presence of resistance to chloroquine and other antimalarial drugs, the availability of drugs in the local area, and the age of the patient. Local and national guidelines for the treatment of malaria differ, and practitioners treating patients with malaria should consult local resources and experts. Country-specific information on the local areas with malaria, the estimated risk for malaria, whether there is chloroquine-resistant malaria, and which malaria species are present is available in the United States from the CDC (www.cdc.gov/malaria/travelers/country_table/a.html) and outside the United States from local and national health organizations and the WHO (www.who.int/malaria/diagnosisandtreatment.html).

In malaria-endemic areas, strategies such as intermittent treatment of infants and pregnant women are being employed in combination with use of insecticides and treated bed nets to prevent and treat malaria.[150] A full discussion of these programs is beyond the scope of this chapter.

Antimalarial Agents Available for Use in the United States

Chloroquine

Chloroquine is the drug of choice for chloroquine-susceptible malaria caused by *P. falciparum* and *P. vivax* and for all infections with *P. ovale* and *P. malariae.* Chloroquine is a 4-aminoquinoline with rapid schizonticidal activity. It is not effective against exoerythrocytic forms of the parasite, and patients treated with chloroquine after acquiring *P. vivax* or *P. ovale* infection need to have additional treatment to eliminate these forms. Chloroquine is most active against late ring stages and mature trophozoites. Response to treatment is rapid, with disappearance of parasitemia within 48 to 72 hours after initiation of treatment when the parasite is susceptible.

Chloroquine is available as an oral preparation and, outside the United States, as intramuscular and intravenous formulations. Oral absorption is excellent, and the drug is safe and effective when given by nasogastric or orogastric tube in comatose children.[177] Intramuscular and intravenous administration may be associated with an increased risk for cardiac arrhythmias, hypotension, and circulatory failure, and its use is discouraged by experts. There is a current prolonged shortage of chloroquine in the United States, and alternate medications for the treatment of malaria should be pursued without delay until this shortage is resolved.

Adverse reactions to chloroquine rarely occur at the doses used for prevention or treatment of malaria. Side effects include gastrointestinal symptoms such as nausea, vomiting, and diarrhea; dizziness; headache; and fatigue. Pruritus may be a troubling adverse event, especially in black patients. Chloroquine has no known teratogenic effects, and it may be used in pregnant and lactating women. The drug is not contraindicated in glucose-6-phosphate dehydrogenase (G6PD)-deficient individuals. Psychotic symptoms occur rarely with chloroquine.[48] Oral doses are absorbed rapidly. The lethal dose of chloroquine is 1 g in children and 4 g in adults. Cumulative doses exceeding 100 g are associated with an increased risk for development of retinopathy. Dose reduction is required for patients with severe renal impairment, and chloroquine should be used with caution in patients with hepatic impairment, alcoholism, or concurrent use of hepatotoxic drugs.

Artemether-Lumefantrine

Artemisinin (qinghaosu) is a sesquiterpene lactone that, along with its derivatives (artemether, artesunate, arteether, and others), has antimalarial activity thought to be due to the ability to cause free radical damage in parasite membrane systems.[59] These compounds are unique in their ability to cure malaria more rapidly than other agents, with rare adverse events. Significant hemolysis has been reported 13 to 15 days after treatment with artemisinin derivatives; this has occurred most frequently after treatment of patients with high parasite loads with parenteral artesunates.[142] There is no consensus on the mechanisms through which artemisinin derivatives kill malaria parasites. Lumefantrine, a dichlorobenzylidine derivative, also has an unclear mechanism of action. The

TABLE 220.4 Guidelines for Treatment of Malaria in the United States[a]

Clinical Diagnosis and *Plasmodium* spp.	Region Infection Acquired	Recommended Drug and Adult Dose[b]	Recommended Drug and Pediatric Dose[b] *Pediatric dose should NEVER exceed adult dose*
Uncomplicated malaria: *P. falciparum* or species not identified If "species not identified" is subsequently diagnosed as *P. vivax* or *P. ovale*: see *P. vivax* and *P. ovale* (below) for treatment with primaquine.	**Chloroquine-resistant or unknown resistance**[c] (All malarious regions except those specified as chloroquine-sensitive listed below.)	**A. Atovaquone-proguanil (Malarone)**[d] Adult tab = 250 mg atovaquone/100 mg proguanil: 4 adult tabs PO daily × 3 days	**A. Atovaquone-proguanil (Malarone)**[d] Adult tab = 250 mg atovaquone/100 mg proguanil Pediatric tab = 62.5 mg atovaquone/25 mg proguanil 5–8 kg: 2 pediatric tabs PO daily × 3 days 9–10 kg: 3 pediatric tabs PO daily × 3 days 11–20 kg: 1 adult tab PO daily × 3 days 21–30 kg: 2 adult tabs PO daily × 3 days 31–40 kg: 3 adult tabs PO daily × 3 days >40 kg: 4 adult tabs PO daily × 3 days
		B. Artemether-lumefantrine (Coartem)[d] 1 tablet = 20 mg artemether and 120 mg lumefantrine A 3-day treatment schedule with a total of 6 oral doses is recommended for both adult and pediatric patients based on weight. The patient should receive the initial dose, followed by the second dose 8 h later, then 1 dose PO twice daily for the following 2 days. 5–15 kg: 1 tablet/dose 15–25 kg: 2 tablets/dose 25–35 kg: 3 tablets/dose ≥35 kg: 4 tablets/dose	
		C. Quinine sulfate plus one of the following: doxycycline tetracycline, or clindamycin **Quinine sulfate:** 542 mg base (= 650 mg salt)[e] PO 3 times a day × 3 or 7 days[f] **Doxycycline:** 100 mg PO twice daily × 7 days **Tetracycline:** 250 mg PO 4 times a day × 7 days **Clindamycin:** 20 mg base/kg/day PO divided 3 times a day × 7 days	**C. Quinine sulfate**[e] **plus one of the following: doxycycline,**[g] **tetracycline,**[g] **or clindamycin** **Quinine sulfate:** 8.3 mg base/kg (= 10 mg salt/kg) PO × 3 or 7 days[f] **Doxycycline:** 2.2 mg/kg PO q12h × 7 days **Tetracycline:** 25 mg/kg/day PO divided 4 times a day × 7 days **Clindamycin:** 20 mg base/kg/day PO divided 3 times a day × 7 days
		D. Mefloquine (Lariam and generics)[h] 684 mg base (= 750 mg salt) PO as initial dose, followed by 456 mg base (= 500 mg salt) PO given 6–12 h after initial dose Total dose = 1250 mg salt	**D. Mefloquine (Lariam and generics)**[h] 13.7 mg base/kg (= 15 mg salt/kg) PO as initial dose, followed by 9.1 mg base/kg (= 10 mg salt/kg) PO given 6–12 h after initial dose. Total dose = 25 mg salt/kg

Uncomplicated malaria: *P. falciparum* or species not identified	**Chloroquine-sensitive (Central America west of Panama Canal; Haiti; the Dominican Republic; and most of the Middle East)**	**Chloroquine phosphate (Aralen and generics)**[i] 600 mg base (= 1000 mg salt) PO immediately, followed by 300 mg base (= 500 mg salt) PO at 6, 24, and 48 h Total dose: 1500 mg base (= 2500 mg salt) *or* **Hydroxychloroquine (Plaquenil and generics)** 620 mg base (= 800 mg salt) PO immediately, followed by 310 mg base (= 400 mg salt) PO at 6, 24, and 48 h Total dose: 1550 mg base (= 2000 mg salt)	**Chloroquine phosphate (Aralen and generics)**[i] 10 mg base/kg PO immediately, followed by 5 mg base/kg PO at 6, 24, and 48 h Total dose: 25 mg base/kg *or* **Hydroxychloroquine (Plaquenil and generics)** 10 mg base/kg PO immediately, followed by 5 mg base/kg PO at 6, 24, and 48 h Total dose: 25 mg base/kg
Uncomplicated malaria: *P. malariae* or *P. knowlesi*	**All regions**	**Chloroquine phosphate**[i]**:** treatment as above *or* **Hydroxychloroquine:** treatment as above	**Chloroquine phosphate**[i]**:** treatment as above *or* **Hydroxychloroquine:** treatment as above
Uncomplicated malaria: *P. vivax* or *P. ovale*	**All regions** For suspected chloroquine-resistant *P. vivax*, see below.	**Chloroquine phosphate**[i] **plus primaquine phosphate**[j] **Chloroquine phosphate:** treatment as above **Primaquine phosphate:** 30 mg base PO daily × 14 days *or* **Hydroxychloroquine plus primaquine phosphate**[j] **Hydroxychloroquine:** treatment as above **Primaquine phosphate:** 30 mg base PO daily × 14 days	**Chloroquine phosphate**[i] **plus primaquine phosphate**[j] **Chloroquine phosphate:** treatment as above **Primaquine:** 0.5 mg base/kg PO daily × 14 days *or* **Hydroxychloroquine plus primaquine phosphate**[j] **Hydroxychloroquine:** treatment as above **Primaquine phosphate:** 0.5 mg base/kg PO daily × 14 days
Uncomplicated malaria: *P. vivax*	**Chloroquine-resistant**[k] (Papua New Guinea and Indonesia)	**A. Quinine sulfate plus either doxycycline or tetracycline plus primaquine phosphate**[j] **Quinine sulfate:** treatment as above **Doxycycline or tetracycline:** treatment as above **Primaquine phosphate:** treatment as above **B. Atovaquone-proguanil plus primaquine phosphate**[j] Atovaquone-proguanil: treatment as above Primaquine phosphate: treatment as above **C. Mefloquine plus primaquine phosphate**[j] Mefloquine: treatment as above Primaquine phosphate: treatment as above	**A. Quinine sulfate plus either doxycycline**[g] **or tetracycline**[g] **plus primaquine phosphate**[j] **Quinine sulfate:** treatment as above **Doxycycline or tetracycline:** treatment as above **Primaquine phosphate:** treatment as above **B. Atovaquone-proguanil plus primaquine phosphate**[j] Atovaquone-proguanil: treatment as above Primaquine phosphate: treatment as above **C. Mefloquine plus primaquine phosphate**[j] Mefloquine: treatment as above Primaquine phosphate: treatment as above

Continued

TABLE 220.4 **Guidelines for Treatment of Malaria in the United States[a]—cont'd**

Clinical Diagnosis and *Plasmodium* spp.	Region Infection Acquired	Recommended Drug and Adult Dose[b]	Recommended Drug and Pediatric Dose[b] *Pediatric dose should NEVER exceed adult dose*
Uncomplicated malaria: alternatives for pregnant women[l,m,n]	**Chloroquine-sensitive** (see uncomplicated malaria sections above for chloroquine-sensitive species by region)	**Chloroquine phosphate:** treatment as above *or* **Hydroxychloroquine:** treatment as above	Not applicable
	Chloroquine-resistant (see sections above for regions with chloroquine-resistant *P. falciparum* and *P. vivax*)	**Quinine sulfate plus clindamycin** **Quinine sulfate:** treatment as above **Clindamycin:** treatment as above *or* **Mefloquine:** treatment as above	Not applicable
Severe malaria[o,p,q]	**All regions**	**Quinidine gluconate[o] plus one of the following: doxycycline,[e] tetracycline,[e] or clindamycin** **Quinidine gluconate:** 6.25 mg base/kg (= 10 mg salt/kg) loading dose IV over 1–2 h, then 0.0125 mg base/kg/min (= 0.02 mg salt/kg/min) continuous infusion for at least 24 h. An *alternative regimen* is 15 mg base/kg (= 24 mg salt/kg) loading dose IV infused over 4 h, followed by 7.5 mg base/kg (= 12 mg salt/kg) infused over 4 h q8h, starting 8 h after the loading dose (see package insert). Once parasite density <1% and patient can take oral medication, complete treatment with oral quinine, dose as above. Quinidine/quinine course = 7 days in Southeast Asia; = 3 days in Africa or South America. **Doxycycline:** treatment as above. If patient not able to take oral medication, give 100 mg IV q12h and then switch to oral doxycycline (as above) as soon as patient can take oral medication. For IV use, avoid rapid administration. Treatment course = 7 days. **Tetracycline:** treatment as above **Clindamycin:** treatment as above. If patient not able to take oral medication, give 10 mg base/kg loading dose IV followed by 5 mg base/kg IV q8h. Switch to oral clindamycin (oral dose as above) as soon as patient can take oral medication. For IV use, avoid rapid administration. Treatment course = 7 days. ***Investigational new drug (contact CDC for information):*** **artesunate followed by one of the following: atovaquone-proguanil (Malarone), doxycycline (clindamycin in pregnant women), or mefloquine**	**Quinidine gluconate[o] plus one of the following: doxycycline,[e] tetracycline,[e] or clindamycin** **Quinidine gluconate:** same mg/kg dosing and recommendations as for adults. **Doxycycline:** treatment as above. If patient not able to take oral medication, may give IV. For children <45 kg, give 2.2 mg/kg IV q12h and then switch to oral doxycycline (dose as above) as soon as patient can take oral medication. For children >45 kg, use same dosing as for adults. For IV use, avoid rapid administration. Treatment course = 7 days. **Tetracycline:** treatment as above **Clindamycin:** treatment as above. If patient not able to take oral medication, give 10 mg base/kg loading dose IV followed by 5 mg base/kg IV q8h. Switch to oral clindamycin (oral dose as above) as soon as patient can take oral medication. For IV use, avoid rapid administration. Treatment course = 7 days. ***Investigational new drug (contact CDC for information):*** **artesunate followed by one of the following: atovaquone-proguanil (Malarone), clindamycin, or mefloquine**

[a]Based on drugs currently available for use in the United States. If outside the United States, contact national authorities about current recommendations.
CDC, Centers for Disease Control and Prevention; *G6PD,* glucose-6-phosphate dehydrogenase; *IV,* intravenous; *PO,* by mouth.
[b]If a person develops malaria despite taking chemoprophylaxis, that particular medicine should not be used as part of their treatment regimen. Use one of the other options instead.
[c]Three options (A, B, C, or D) are available for treatment of uncomplicated malaria caused by chloroquine-resistant *P. falciparum.* Options A, B, and C are equally recommended. Because of a higher rate of severe neuropsychiatric reactions seen at treatment doses, we do not recommend option D (mefloquine) unless the other options cannot be used. For option C, because there are more data on the efficacy of quinine in combination with doxycycline or tetracycline, these treatment combinations are generally preferred to quinine in combination with clindamycin.
[d]Take with food or whole milk. If patient vomits within 30 minutes of taking a dose, they should repeat the dose.
[e]US manufactured quinine sulfate capsule is in a 324 mg dosage; therefore 2 capsules should be sufficient for adult dosing. Pediatric dosing may be difficult due to unavailability of noncapsule forms of quinidine.
[f]For infections acquired in Southeast Asia, quinine treatment should continue for 7 days. For infections acquired elsewhere, quinine treatment should continue for 3 days.
[g]Doxycycline and tetracycline are not indicated for use in children age <8 years. For children age <8 years with chloroquine-resistant *P. falciparum,* atovaquone-proguanil and artemether-lumefantrine are recommended treatment options; mefloquine can be considered if no other options are available. For children age <8 years with chloroquine-resistant *P. vivax,* mefloquine is the recommended treatment; if it is not available or is not being tolerated and if the treatment benefits outweigh the risks, atovaquone-proguanil or artemether-lumefantrine should be used.
[h]Treatment with mefloquine is not recommended in persons who have acquired infections from Southeast Asia due to drug resistance.
[i]When treating chloroquine-sensitive infections, chloroquine and hydroxychloroquine are recommended options. However, regimens used to treat chloroquine-resistant infections may also be used if available, more convenient, or preferred.
[j]Primaquine is used to eradicate any hypnozoite forms that may remain dormant in the liver and thus prevents relapses in *P. vivax* and *P. ovale* infections. Because primaquine can cause hemolytic anemia in G6PD-deficient persons, G6PD screening must occur prior to starting treatment with primaquine. For persons with borderline G6PD deficiency or as an alternate to the above regimen, primaquine may be given 45 mg orally one time per week for 8 weeks; consultation with an expert in infectious disease and/or tropical medicine is advised if this alternative regimen is considered in G6PD-deficient persons. Primaquine must not be used during pregnancy.
[k]Three options (A, B, or C) are available for treatment of uncomplicated malaria caused by chloroquine-resistant *P. vivax.* High treatment failure rates due to chloroquine-resistant *P. vivax* have been well documented in Papua New Guinea and Indonesia. Rare case reports of chloroquine-resistant *P. vivax* malaria have also been documented in Myanmar (Burma), India, and Central and South America. Persons acquiring *P. vivax* infections outside Papua New Guinea or Indonesia should be started on chloroquine. If the patient does not respond, the treatment should be changed to a chloroquine-resistant *P. vivax* regimen and CDC should be notified. For treatment of chloroquine-resistant *P. vivax* infections, options A, B, and C are equally recommended.
[l]For pregnant women diagnosed with uncomplicated malaria caused by chloroquine-resistant *P. falciparum* or chloroquine-resistant *P. vivax,* treatment with doxycycline or tetracycline is generally not indicated. However, doxycycline or tetracycline may be used in combination with quinine (as recommended for nonpregnant adults) if other treatment options are not available or are not being tolerated, and if the benefit is judged to outweigh the risks.
[m]Atovaquone-proguanil and artemether-lumefantrine are generally not recommended for use in pregnant women, particularly in the first trimester due to lack of sufficiency safety data. For pregnant women diagnosed with uncomplicated malaria caused by chloroquine-resistant *P. falciparum,* atovaquone-proguanil or artemether-lumefantrine may be used if other treatment options are not available or are not being tolerated and if the potential benefit is judged to outweigh the potential risks.
[n]For *P. vivax* and *P. ovale* infections, primaquine phosphate for radical treatment of hypnozoites should not be given during pregnancy. Pregnant patients with *P. vivax* and *P. ovale* infections should be maintained on chloroquine prophylaxis for the duration of their pregnancy. The chemoprophylactic dose of chloroquine phosphate is 300 mg base (= 500 mg salt) orally once per week. After delivery, pregnant patients who do not have G6PD deficiency should be treated with primaquine.
[o]Persons with a positive blood smear *or* history of recent possible exposure and no other recognized pathology who have one or more of the following clinical criteria (impaired consciousness/coma, severe normocytic anemia, renal failure, pulmonary edema, acute respiratory distress syndrome, circulatory shock, disseminated intravascular coagulation, spontaneous bleeding, acidosis, hemoglobinuria, jaundice, repeated generalized convulsions, and/or parasitemia of >5%) are considered to have manifestations of more severe disease. Severe malaria is most often caused by *P. falciparum.*
[p]Patients diagnosed with severe malaria should be treated aggressively with parenteral antimalarial therapy. Treatment with IV quinidine should be initiated as soon as possible after the diagnosis has been made. Patients with severe malaria should be given an intravenous loading dose of quinidine unless they have received more than 40 mg/kg of quinine in the preceding 48 hours or if they have received mefloquine within the preceding 12 hours. Consultation with a cardiologist and a physician with experience in treating malaria is advised when treating malaria patients with quinidine. During administration of quinidine, blood pressure monitoring (for hypotension) and cardiac monitoring (for widening of the QRS complex and/or lengthening of the QTc interval) should be done continuously and blood glucose (for hypoglycemia) should be monitored periodically.
[q]Pregnant women diagnosed with severe malaria should be treated aggressively with parenteral antimalarial therapy.Modified from Centers for Disease Control and Prevention. Guidelines for Malaria Treatment in the United States. www.cdc.gov/malaria/resources/pdf/treatmenttable.pdf.

fixed dose combination of artemether (20 mg) and lumefantrine (120 mg) (Coartem) is available in the United States, is FDA approved, and is considered a first-line agent for treatment of uncomplicated falciparum malaria in countries where it is available. Artemether-lumefantrine is well tolerated and effective against multidrug-resistant falciparum malaria.[141] A six-dose regimen compared favorably with other agents in African children and adults with uncomplicated falciparum malaria.[108,130] Its side effect profile along with rapid parasite clearance and high cure rate for uncomplicated falciparum malaria in African infants and children make this regimen favorable.[42] Bioavailability of lumefantrine is enhanced when it is taken with food.[41]

Artemether-lumefantrine is not approved for use in treatment of infection with *P. vivax, P. ovale,* or *P. malariae* because there are few data on its efficacy for infection with these species. There may be a role for the use of artemether-lumefantrine in treating chloroquine-resistant vivax malaria, because this drug combination produces rapid clearance of the blood stage. The short half-life of lumefantrine may, however, allow for a shorter time to relapse by dormant hypnozoites.[9,182]

Atovaquone-Proguanil

A fixed-dose combination (available in adult and pediatric formulations) of atovaquone and proguanil hydrochloride is available for treatment of malaria caused by *P. falciparum* for individuals who were not taking this agent for prophylaxis. The combination is significantly more effective than either drug alone and is effective for treatment of malaria strains resistant to other antimalarial drugs. It has fewer reported adverse events than quinine-based regimens. The combination also is likely to be active against the blood stages of *P. vivax, P. ovale,* and *P. malariae,* but the regimen does not have activity against the hypnozoites of *P. vivax.* Atovaquone-proguanil is significantly more effective than mefloquine, chloroquine, amodiaquine, or pyrimethamine-sulfadoxine in locations where parasites are resistant to these drugs.[87]

Mefloquine

The development of mefloquine was a major advance in the treatment of chloroquine-resistant malaria, although resistance has developed rapidly in some parts of the world where it is used widely. Mefloquine is a 4-quinolone-carbinolamine whose exact mechanism of action is unknown. Its main target is early trophozoites. Similar to chloroquine, it is not active against exoerythrocytic phases. Mefloquine has been associated with neurologic and psychiatric side effects when used for treatment or prophylaxis,[164] and in 2013 the US FDA updated their warnings regarding these potentially serious side effects. Vomiting occurs commonly when mefloquine is given to children younger than 5 years old and may decrease its efficacy.[159] Mefloquine should not be administered concurrently with quinine, quinidine, or halofantrine due to increased risk of developing arrhythmias. Pregnancy is not a contraindication to treatment in any trimester, although with the development of other well-tolerated medications, mefloquine is no longer the first choice for treatment of malaria in pregnancy.

Quinine and Quinidine

Quinine has been used for the treatment of malaria for centuries.[164] It is active against the mature asexual erythrocytic forms of all four species of human malaria and against the gametes of all species except *P. falciparum,* where it has activity only against immature gametes. It is not effective against exoerythrocytic forms. It may be given orally, intravenously, or intramuscularly. Quinine crosses the placenta easily and may be used in the treatment of pregnant women, although close monitoring for hypoglycemia is warranted.[88]

Adverse reactions to quinine include tinnitus, headache, nausea, visual and hearing disturbances, and tremors, a constellation of symptoms called cinchonism. Symptoms may appear during the first 1 to 3 days of therapy and stop when treatment is terminated. Hypoglycemia may occur, particularly when the drug is used to treat pregnant women. Severe adverse events are rare but may occur idiosyncratically. Blackwater fever (hemoglobinuria) seems to occur after treatment with quinine, but the causal mechanism is unknown.

Recrudescence rates may be high when quinine is used alone because of the presence of quinine-resistant strains of *P. falciparum,* and a second drug is needed to treat the remaining parasites. Drugs that may be used with quinine include doxycycline, tetracycline, and clindamycin.

Quinidine is a related drug that may be given intravenously; in countries where intravenous quinine is unavailable, it is a treatment option for severe malaria. The mechanisms of action and adverse events are similar, although cardiac arrhythmias occur more commonly with quinidine and cardiac monitoring is advised.[176]

Primaquine

Primaquine, an 8-aminoquinoline derivative that is effective against exoerythrocytic hypnozoites, is used primarily to prevent relapses of infections with *P. vivax* and *P. ovale,* although it may not be completely effective against some strains of *P. vivax.* Despite adequate treatment with primaquine, relapses of infections with *P. vivax* and *P. ovale* do occur[16]; in some instances this may be due to inadequate dosing. It is not an effective blood schizonticide but is an active gametocidal and sporontocidal drug for the four main species of *Plasmodium* that cause human malaria. Primaquine can cause intravascular hemolysis in individuals with G6PD deficiency, and patients should be confirmed to have normal G6PD activity before using primaquine. Other adverse events include gastrointestinal symptoms such as nausea, epigastric pain, anorexia, and abdominal cramps. Rare side effects include methemoglobinemia, hemoglobinuria, and bone marrow suppression. Safety in pregnancy has not been established, and the drug should not be used by pregnant women. After delivery, women with *P. vivax* or *P. ovale* infections and without G6PD deficiency may be treated with primaquine.

Tetracycline and Doxycycline

Tetracycline, doxycycline, and the related drug minocycline have very slow activity against malarial schizonts.[164] Doxycycline and minocycline may be given once daily. They are active against chloroquine-resistant and pyrimethamine-sulfadoxine-resistant *P. falciparum.* Resistance to tetracycline has not been shown. Because of their slow activity, these agents should be given in combination with a rapidly acting drug such as quinine. These drugs should not be used in children younger than 8 years old or by pregnant or nursing women.

Antimalarial Agents Not Currently Available or Recommended for Treatment of Malaria in the United States

Other Artemisinin Derivatives

Aside from artemether-lumefantrine, the only artemisinin derivative available in the United States is parenteral artesunate, which is available on an emergency basis only from the CDC. Further study of late hemolysis especially after use of parenteral artesunate in high levels of parasitemia is needed.[142] Other artemisinin derivatives are available in other parts of the world. When used alone, recrudescence rates are high, and the drug class has limited potential for prophylaxis. Oral preparations, suppositories, and oil-based preparations for intramuscular injection are available, although standardization of preparations is lacking.[141] Combinations including artemisinins are the preferred antimalarial agents worldwide[121] and have shown major utility in areas of multidrug-resistant *P. falciparum.*[1,59] In clinical trials in the Gambia, artemether was as effective as quinine and chloroquine for treatment of cerebral malaria in children.[172,178] When used in sequence with mefloquine, the combination was effective and tolerated well by patients with acute, uncomplicated falciparum malaria in Thailand, an area with multidrug resistance.[76] Later studies showed that the use of this combination may have helped halt the progressions of mefloquine resistance in the region.[116] Artemisinin-based combination treatments of falciparum malaria have been shown to be better tolerated and more effective than quinine and non-artemisinin combination therapies.[20] The use of artemisinin-based combination therapies has contributed to significant reductions in malaria burden in many parts of the world. There is, however, reduced susceptibility of *P. falciparum* to artemisinin derivatives in the Cambodia-Thailand border region, likely owing to use of the artemisinins as single-drug therapy as opposed to combination therapy, leading to a WHO-led program to contain artemisinin resistance in this region.[39] Emerging resistance to artemisinin derivatives in Southeast Asia has been documented; longer courses of artemisinin-based combination therapy may be required in these areas to achieve cure.[7]

Pyrimethamine-Sulfadoxine

The combination pyrimethamine-sulfadoxine, a sulfonamide plus a dihydrofolate reductase inhibitor, exhibits synergy in its action against malaria parasites; the combination is active even against strains resistant to the individual drug components. Although pyrimethamine-sulfadoxine has been used for presumptive treatment of malaria in travelers who are taking other drugs for prophylaxis in areas where chloroquine resistance occurs, widespread resistance to the drug combination and its slow action limits its use in nonimmune individuals with falciparum malaria. The CDC no longer recommends pyrimethamine-sulfadoxine for treatment of malaria. Although safety has not been established in pregnancy, the drug has been used widely and effectively for intermittent presumptive treatment of pregnant women in endemic areas to decrease the risk for severe anemia and placental malaria.[36,156,158]

Amodiaquine

Amodiaquine, similar to chloroquine, is a 4-aminoquinolone. It has similar efficacy but may have increased activity compared with chloroquine for the treatment of strains of *P. falciparum* resistant to chloroquine.[120] It is available in an oral preparation and is more palatable than chloroquine. Significant adverse events, including agranulocytosis, hepatotoxicity, and death, when used as a prophylactic agent have limited its use as a first-line agent. It is not licensed or marketed in the United States, though its use is increasing outside the United States.

Halofantrine

Halofantrine is a 9-phenanthrene-methanol that has been used to treat malaria caused by chloroquine-resistant *P. falciparum*. Its major side effect is dose-related prolongation of the QT interval, and it has been associated with cardiac arrhythmias and sudden death, especially in individuals taking mefloquine prophylaxis.[115,163] Its major use was in uncomplicated malaria in areas of multidrug resistance, but cardiac toxicity at the doses required to be effective and mounting resistance limit its widespread use.[166] It is contraindicated in pregnant and lactating women because of embryotoxic effects. Travelers who are taking mefloquine for prophylaxis should be cautioned against accepting treatment with halofantrine if they are diagnosed with malaria during their travels. Halofantrine is unavailable in the United States.

Supportive Therapy

Malaria is a potentially fatal illness even in patients who may have developed partial immunity. Children and those without prior immunity with falciparum malaria should have immediate treatment and generally should be admitted to the hospital, especially in nonendemic countries such as the United States. Patients with severe malaria should be managed in intensive care units, and experts in treatment of malaria and its complications should be consulted. Blood smears should be examined at least every 12 to 24 hours (and every 4 to 6 hours for severe malaria) until parasitemia is less than 1%. Patients with uncomplicated malaria can be treated with oral medication, although patients should be switched promptly to parenteral medication if oral medication is not tolerated. CDC (www.cdc.gov/malaria/pdf/treatmenttable.pdf) and WHO (www.who.int/malaria/diagnosisandtreatment.html) guidelines for treatment of malaria, including management of severe malaria, are available.

Goals of supportive therapy are to maintain oxygenation and treat acidosis and hypoglycemia. Treatment with dextrose infusion, oxygen, and blood transfusion may be necessary. Mechanical ventilation with positive-pressure ventilation may be needed to manage acidosis and acute respiratory distress syndrome. In some cases, hemodialysis may be needed. A high index of suspicion should be maintained for other concomitant or nosocomial infections, such as meningitis or septicemia.

Investigational Drugs and Adjunctive Therapy

Targets for new antimalarial drugs include malaria proteases and protein kinases, which play a crucial role in malaria pathogenesis.[38,147] These drugs are largely in the development phase.

A novel primaquine analogue, tafenoquine, is currently under investigation for use in prophylaxis and treatment of *P. falciparum* and *P. vivax* malaria in African countries. The advantages of this drug are its long half-life, activity against liver-stage malaria parasites, and favorable therapeutic and safety profile.[83,110,154] As with primaquine, G6PD activity must be measured prior to its use.

Adjunctive therapies that have been shown to be beneficial include antipyretic and anticonvulsant drugs. Exchange transfusion remains a controversial option[168,176] largely owing to the lack of sufficient randomized controlled trials. Exchange transfusion may decrease parasite clearance times compared with quinine alone,[171] but there is a lack of clear survival benefit with exchange transfusion.[143] Adjunctive therapies that would modify or prevent the deleterious effects of inflammatory mediators, oxidative stress, iron overload, acidosis, and hypercoagulability in severe and cerebral malaria have been proposed, but limited clinical studies have not shown significant benefit.[71] A randomized study of inhaled nitric oxide in severe malaria is ongoing.[56] Some therapies, such as high-dose corticosteroids for cerebral malaria or heparin, have been shown to be harmful.[176,181] The search for effective adjunctive therapy for severe and complicated malaria continues.

PREVENTION

Prevention of malaria can be accomplished by reducing the mosquito population, using personal protection methods to prevent mosquito bites, and using chemoprophylaxis. Reduction of mosquito vectors is most successful when locally controlled programs are developed and maintained.[78] Strategies that combine personal protective measures with community-based control measures, such as distribution of insecticide-treated mosquito nets and indoor residual spraying, are most likely to be successful.[122] Most programs in endemic areas require a combination of preventive strategies and effective treatment modalities. Many nonendemic countries have developed recommendations for prevention of malaria in travelers.

Personal Protective Measures

A significant reduction in the incidence of malaria in children in communities where bed nets, especially when impregnated with insecticide, are used consistently has been reported from many countries.[34,49,160] In northern Ghana, community-wide use of bed nets was associated with a reduction in all-cause child mortality in young children.[14] Use of bed nets, especially those impregnated with insecticide, is recommended for travelers to malarial areas. Other personal protective measures include using mosquito repellents and insecticide-impregnated clothing or gear; wearing clothing that covers areas likely to be bitten; and residing in air-conditioned or well-screened areas during times when mosquitoes are biting. Diethyltoluamide (DEET)-containing repellents are recommended most commonly for prevention of mosquito bites and are highly effective.[45] Other agents, such as picaridin, oil of lemon eucalyptus, and IR3535, are available. Picaridin is available in a 20% formulation, which may be used as an alternative to DEET.[129] Other agents have not been studied extensively against *Anopheles* mosquitoes.

Chemoprophylaxis

Country-specific information regarding recommendations for the use of antimalarial drugs may differ, and readers are urged to seek recommendations from national or local authorities. In the United States, these recommendations are available widely in publications from the CDC[134] or national health information sources. Many excellent sources of health information for travelers include discussions of malaria prevention.[21,22,24,95,149,155,162] The Infectious Diseases Society of America has published detailed pre-travel guidelines that include recommendations for malaria prevention.[60] A list of drugs available for malaria prevention is presented in Table 220.5. Prevention of malaria for travelers is best discussed in the context of providing complete pre-travel services, advice, and information.

Antimalarial Agents Available in the United States for Prevention of Malaria

Chloroquine and Hydroxychloroquine

A major determinant of appropriate chemoprophylaxis is whether a patient is to travel to an area of chloroquine resistance. In areas of the

TABLE 220.5 **Drug Regimens Used for Prevention of Malaria**

Drug	Adult Dosage	Pediatric Dosage	Comments
Chloroquine-Sensitive Areas			
Chloroquine phosphate (drug of choice)	500 mg salt (300 mg base) orally once/wk	8.3 mg/kg salt (5 mg/kg base) once/wk, up to adult dose of 300 mg base	Begin 1–2 wk before exposure, continue during exposure, and continue for 4 wk after exposure May be used in pregnant women
Hydroxychloroquine sulfate	400 mg salt (310 mg base) orally once/wk	6.5 mg/kg salt (5 mg/kg base) orally once/wk	Begin 1–2 wk before exposure, continue during exposure, and continue for 4 wk after exposure An alternative to chloroquine for use only in areas with chloroquine-sensitive malaria
Chloroquine-Resistant Areas			
Atovaquone-proguanil	250 mg/100 mg (1 tablet) daily	5–8 kg: ½ pediatric tablet daily 9–10 kg: ¾ pediatric tablet daily 11-20 kg: 1 pediatric tablet daily 21-30 kg: 2 pediatric tablets daily 31-40 kg: 3 pediatric tablets daily >40 kg: 1 adult tablet daily	Begin 1–2 days before exposure, continue during exposure, and continue for 7 days after exposure Pediatric tablets contain 62.5 mg atovaquone and 25 mg proguanil hydrochloride See text for contraindications
Mefloquine	250 mg salt (228 mg base) orally once/wk	≤9 kg: 5 mg/kg salt (4.6 mg/kg base) orally once/wk 10-19 kg: ¼ tablet orally once/wk 20-30 kg: ½ tablet orally once/wk 31–45 kg: ¾ tablet orally once/wk >45 kg: 1 tablet orally once/wk	Begin 1–2 wk before exposure, continue during exposure, and continue for 4 wk after exposure See text for contraindications
Or			
Doxycycline	100 mg daily	2.2 mg/kg/day up to 100 mg/day	Begin 1–2 days before exposure, continue during exposure, and for 4 wk after exposure; not to be used in children >8 yr or pregnant women
Or			
Alternative			
Primaquine	52.6 mg salt (30 mg base) orally daily	0.8 mg/kg salt (0.5 mg/kg base) up to adult dose orally daily	Begin 1–2 days before exposure, continue during exposure, and continue for 7 days after exposure Contraindicated in people with G6PD deficiency, in pregnancy, and during lactation Prophylaxis to areas principally with *P. vivax*

world that have no resistance to chloroquine, the drug of choice for prevention of malaria is chloroquine or hydroxychloroquine. This drug class is tolerated well and may be given to children and adults of all ages, including infants. Dosing of chloroquine and hydroxychloroquine in children is based on the child's weight and can be found in Table 220.4. In the United States, chloroquine is available only in tablets that have a very bitter taste. Pharmacies can also prepare appropriate doses in capsules, and the contents of the capsule can be mixed with a small amount of liquid or semisolid food for administration. Although liquid preparations are widely available overseas and are stable for long periods,[104] many US pharmacies are reluctant to prepare them. If patients are considering purchasing liquid preparations overseas, the family should be given information with the child's medication dose calculated as the base and the salt because concentrations of liquid preparations may vary. Families also should be cautioned about the greater incidence of ineffective or counterfeit medications available in some areas. In 2015, the US FDA issued a drug shortage alert for chloroquine, and this has yet to be resolved, limiting its current use. Hydroxychloroquine was recently on shortage, but the shortage has since been resolved.

Adverse events caused by chloroquine are uncommon when the medication is used at doses needed for malaria prophylaxis. Minor side effects include gastrointestinal upset, headache, dizziness, blurred vision, and pruritus. Adverse events rarely require discontinuation of medication. Chloroquine may be taken during pregnancy and is not contraindicated in children with G6PD deficiency.

The choice of antimalarial agents in locations where drug-resistant parasites have been identified is more challenging. Chloroquine-containing regimens are not recommended for travel to areas with known chloroquine-resistant *P. falciparum*, and deaths from malaria have occurred when these regimens have been used.[93] The choice of regimen depends on the type of drug resistance, length of stay, age of the traveler, and individual medical history. Drugs currently available in the United States include mefloquine, doxycycline, atovaquone-proguanil, and primaquine.

Atovaquone-Proguanil

Atovaquone-proguanil is the most common choices for malaria chemoprophylaxis because of the favorable side effect profile and the need to take the medication once daily for only 1 to 2 days before and 7 days after leaving the area of risk for malaria. Once-weekly dosing of atovaquone-proguanil for prophylaxis may be possible, but larger field trials are needed before this can be recommended.[35] The drug is effective against most *P. falciparum*, including resistant strains. It is available in adult and pediatric dosing formulations and is administered daily. Adverse events most commonly reported with atovaquone-proguanil are abdominal pain, nausea, vomiting, and headache. Some of these adverse events can be mitigated by taking the drug with food; absorption is also better when taken with a fatty meal. It is not recommended at this time for prophylaxis of infants weighing less than 5 kg, for mothers nursing such infants, or for pregnant women.

Mefloquine

Mefloquine generally is well tolerated in children and can be given to infants. Dosing is based on weight, and no liquid preparation is available. Doses for older children can be supplied by breaking tablets; when small fractions of tablets are needed, pharmacists can provide individual doses in capsules. The medication has a pasty consistency but does not taste as bitter as chloroquine. Infants tend to swallow doses better when given liquids or semisolid foods after the medication. Adverse events with mefloquine are self-limited in most cases and include gastrointestinal disturbance, insomnia, and dizziness.[85] Withdrawal rates in adults, presumably caused by the incidence of these adverse events, may impair the efficacy of mefloquine.[31] Rarely, serious adverse events, such as psychosis or seizures, have occurred after prophylactic doses of mefloquine, prompting an updated warning from the US FDA in 2013. This black box warning requires that providers review an information sheet and read the details of the warning prior to prescribing mefloquine and has decreased the use of mefloquine for malaria prophylaxis. Mefloquine should not be used in individuals who have seizures or neuropsychiatric disorders or in individuals who have had previous adverse events with mefloquine. Mefloquine also is contraindicated in patients with cardiac conduction abnormalities, although it may be used in individuals concurrently taking β-blockers for indications other than arrhythmias.

Mefloquine must be taken weekly, beginning 1 to 2 weeks before travel (with some experts recommending initiation up to 4 weeks before travel) and continued for 4 weeks after leaving the malarial area. Families may be counseled to choose a day of the week to take the medicine and to take their first dose or doses on that day of the week 1 to 2 weeks before departure. Mefloquine may be used by pregnant women in any trimester of pregnancy.[114,173]

Doxycycline

Doxycycline is an effective antimalarial drug in parts of the world where chloroquine resistance is present. It also has been shown to be effective in areas where mefloquine-resistant *P. falciparum* exists, such as portions of Cambodia, Myanmar (Burma), Vietnam, and Thailand. Limitations in the use of this drug include that it is contraindicated in children younger than 8 years, need for daily dosing, and photosensitivity. In women, daily use of doxycycline may be associated with an increased risk for *Candida* vulvovaginitis. Gastrointestinal side effects, including nausea and vomiting, can be limited by taking the medication with meals and by avoiding bedtime dosing. Doxycycline must not be used by pregnant or lactating women. Prophylaxis with doxycycline needs to begin 1 to 2 days before travel and should be continued daily for 4 weeks after leaving the malarial area.

Primaquine

Primaquine is used most often to eradicate exoerythrocytic stages of *P. vivax* and *P. ovale.* The CDC recommends primaquine for chemoprophylaxis primarily in regions with predominantly vivax malaria. Individuals must be tested and shown not to be deficient in G6PD before they take this drug. Efficacy of primaquine compared favorably with that of mefloquine, doxycycline, and chloroquine plus proguanil in children in the holoendemic area of western Kenya.[47,151,175] It cannot be used in pregnant women.

Antimalarial Agents Not Available or Recommended in the United States for Prevention of Malaria

Tafenoquine

Tafenoquine is an investigational long-acting primaquine analogue that kills parasites in the liver and in blood. It is thought to be more effective and less toxic than primaquine, but it cannot be used by individuals with G6PD deficiency or by pregnant women. No dosing regimen has been established, and it is not licensed for use,[54,153,174] but it may be available in the future.[62,74,153]

Proguanil

Proguanil has been used in combination with chloroquine to prevent chloroquine-resistant *P. falciparum,* but it is less effective than mefloquine and is not recommended or available as a single agent in the United States.

Pyrimethamine-Sulfadoxine

Pyrimethamine-sulfadoxine has been used for prevention of malaria in areas of chloroquine-resistant *P. falciparum.* An unacceptably high incidence of Stevens-Johnson reactions (fatalities in one in 11,000 to 25,000 users) resulted in withdrawal of the indication for using this drug for malaria prophylaxis.

Standby Emergency Self-Treatment

Standby emergency treatment (SBET) is the self-administration of antimalarial drugs when malaria is expected and prompt medical attention is unavailable within 24 hours of the onset of symptoms. The goal of SBET is to prevent death or severe malaria. This strategy is intended for emergency use only and is considered when the risks of toxicity from chemoprophylactic drugs outweigh the benefit of avoided infection. SBET should not be recommended for travelers to high-risk *P. falciparum*-endemic areas, where chemoprophylaxis is the preferred strategy. SBET is an option for clearly defined situations, and its use must be weighed carefully with the traveler's ability to use SBET as directed.[124,135]

Intermittent Preventive Treatment

Intermittent preventive treatment in infants (IPTi) and children (IPTc) is a strategy entertained in sub-Saharan Africa to reduce malaria disease burden especially in children who are at higher risk of fatal disease. The impact of IPTi and IPTc on the development of immunity, transmission of malaria parasites and the development of antimalarial resistance are yet to be defined in the field[3] but are areas of current study.

Vaccine

Vaccination against malaria has been a subject of active research for several decades, but a licensed vaccine is not yet available. Development of a vaccine is challenging because of the complexity of the parasite life cycle, heterogeneity of the host immune response, lack of animal models, and absence of surrogate markers of protection. Testing of vaccines is difficult because vaccine efficacy depends on conditions of transmission and the degree of immunity present in the population being studied.[167] Targets for development of a vaccine include the sporozoite (prevention of infection), the merozoite (prevention of disease manifestations by preventing invasion of RBCs), and the gametocyte (prevention of transmission by interfering with development of the parasite within the mosquito). Hundreds of candidate vaccine antigens have been identified by the *P. falciparum* genome project; choosing the most promising ones is challenging.[53]

The first malaria vaccines were directed against circumsporozoite antigen, an antigen present over most of the surface of the sporozoite. Development of these vaccines was based on the concept that sporozoites should be susceptible to antibody-mediated destruction in the extracellular space. Results of early studies with these vaccines were disappointing, with inadequate protection provided against sporozoite challenge, inconsistent relationships between antibody response and clinical efficacy, and numerous local side effects.[58,61] More recently, the candidate vaccines RTS,S/AS02A and RTS,S/ASOIE have shown promise in trials in Mozambique[5] and Kenya.[13] The candidate vaccine RTS,S/AS01, currently being studied in a phase III trial in seven African countries, has shown vaccine efficacy of 50.4% against malaria, with efficacy against severe malaria of 45.1%.[2] Recent phase II data in African children have shown that anti-circumsporozoite protein IgG avidity is similar after second and third doses of RTS,S/ASO1 vaccines, and further study relating the IgG avidity to vaccine efficacy is needed.[4] Merozoite surface proteins are another group of antigens that have been studied in connection with the development of a blood-stage, or asexual, malaria vaccine.[126] The SPf66 vaccine, derived from three merozoite proteins linked to a 4-amino acid from a *P. falciparum* circumsporozoite protein, has been tested in clinical trials in Colombia, Tanzania, and the Gambia.[6,34,170] Although initial studies in countries in South America with low malaria endemicity showed promise, investigations in African countries with high endemicity have been disappointing, with protective efficacy ranging from 31% (95% confidence interval [CI], 0–52%) in Tanzania to 8% (95% CI, 18–29%) for first or only clinical episodes and 3% (95% CI, −24% to 24%) in overall incidence of clinical episodes in the Gambia.

Vaccines that block transmission from humans to mosquitoes would reduce the reservoir of infected mosquitoes and reduce transmission on a population level. The poor immunogenicity and diversity of gametocyte antigens have proved challenging to this approach to the development of a vaccine, and no vaccines of this type have been used yet in clinical trials. Future vaccines are likely to use a combination approach that incorporates target antigens from all three stages of the parasite. To have a significant impact on decreasing worldwide burden of malaria, vaccines ultimately may need to be combined with other prevention strategies, including protection against mosquito bites with insecticides and treated bed nets and intermittent preventive treatment with antimalarial drugs.[53]

NEW REFERENCES SINCE THE SEVENTH EDITION

3. Aguas R, Lourenço JM, Gomes MG, White LJ. The impact of IPTi and IPTc interventions on malaria clinical burden—in silico perspectives. *PLoS ONE.* 2009;4(8):e6627.
4. Ajua A, Lell B, Agnandji ST, et al. The effect of immunization schedule with the malaria vaccine candidate RTS,S/AS01E on protective efficacy and anti-circumsporozoite protein antibody avidity in African infants. *Malar J.* 2015;14:72.
7. Ashley EA, Dhorda M, Fairhurst RM, et al. Spread of artemisinin resistance in *Plasmodium falciparum* malaria. *N Engl J Med.* 2014;371:411-423.
12. Beare NA, Taylor TE, Harding SP, et al. Malarial retinopathy: a newly established diagnostic sign in severe malaria. *Am J Trop Med Hyg.* 2006;75(5):790-797.
15. Boeuf P, Aitken EH, Chandrasiri U, et al. *Plasmodium falciparum* malaria elicits inflammatory responses that dysregulate placental amino acid transport. *PLoS Pathog.* 2013;9(2):e1003153.
20. Burger RJ, van Eijk AM, Bussink M, et al. Artemisinin-based combination therapy versus quinine or other combinations for treatment of uncomplicated *Plasmodium falciparum* malaria in the second and third trimester of pregnancy: a systematic review and meta-Analysis. *Open Forum Infect Dis.* 2015;3(1):1-12.
32. Cullen KA, Arguin PM. Malaria surveillance—United States, 2012. *Morb Mortal Wkly Rep Surveill Summ.* 2014;63(SS12):1-22.
33. Cullen KA, Mace KE, Arguin PM. Malaria surveillance—United States, 2013. *Morb Mortal Wkly Rep Surveill Summ.* 2016;65(SS2):1-22.
77. Kinra P, Dutta V. Serum TNA alpha levels: a prognostic marker for assessment of severity of malaria. *Trop Biomed.* 2013;30(4):645-653.
82. Lee KS, Cox-Singh J, Singh B. Morphological features and differential counts of *Plasmodium knowlesi* parasites in naturally acquired human infections. *Malar J.* 2009;8:73.
83. Lell B, Faucher JF, Missinou MA, et al. Malaria chemoprophylaxis with tafenoquine: a randomized study. *Lancet.* 2000;355(9220):2041-2045.
84. Leoni S, Buonfrate D, Angheben A, et al. The hyper-reactive malarial splenomegaly: a systemic review of the literature. *Malar J.* 2015;14:185.
110. Nasveld P, Kitchener S. Treatment of acute vivax malaria with tafenoquine. *Trans R Soc Trop Med Hyg.* 2005;99(1):2-5.
121. World Health Organization. *Guidelines for the Treatment of Malaria, WHO 3rd Ed.pdf.* Geneva: Author; 2015.
122. World Health Organization. *World Malaria Report 2015.* Geneva: Author; 2015.
131. Playford EG, Walker J. Evaluation of the ICT malaria Pf/Pv and the OptiMAL rapid diagnostic tests for malaria in febrile returned travelers. *J Clin Microbiol.* 2002;40(11):4166-4171.
142. Rehman K, Lotsch F, Kremsner PG, et al. Haemolysis associated with the treatment of malaria with artemisinin derivatives: a systematic review of current evidence. *Int J Infect Dis.* 2014;29:268-273.
144. Rijken MJ, Papageorghiou AT, Thiptharakun S, et al. Ultrasound evidence of early fetal growth restriction after maternal malaria infection. *PLoS ONE.* 2012;7(2):e31411.
152. Seydel KB, Kampondeni SD, Valim C, et al. Brain swelling and death in children with cerebral malaria. *N Engl J Med.* 2015;372:1126-1137.
154. Shanks GD, Oloo AJ, Aleman GM, et al. A new primaquine analogue, tafenoquine (WR 238605), for prophylaxis against *Plasmodium falciparum* malaria. *Clin Infect Dis.* 2001;33(12):1968-1974.
169. Umbers AJ, Aitken EH, Rogerson SJ. Malaria in pregnancy: small babies, big problem. *Trends Parasitol.* 2011;27(4):168-175.

The full reference list for this chapter is available at ExpertConsult.com.

221 Leishmaniasis

Lynne S. Garcia

Leishmaniasis is a parasitic disease affecting more than12 million people in over 95 countries, with 350 million more at risk and 2 to 2.5 million new cases reported each year.[22,36,53] The infection consists of a group of diseases that may affect the skin, mucous membranes, and/or viscera, with a wide range of clinical presentations caused by obligate intracellular hemoflagellates of the genus *Leishmania.* Infection is transmitted by several genera and species of phlebotomine sandflies. Four major clinical syndromes usually are recognized: cutaneous (CL), mucocutaneous (MCL), visceral (VL), and American tegumentary (cutaneous) (ATL) leishmaniasis. Macrophages of the skin, mucous membranes, and/or spleen, liver, and bone marrow (reticuloendothelial system) are parasitized. New species continue to be identified, particularly in the New World. However, the taxonomy of leishmaniasis is controversial, and species differentiation is currently based on molecular techniques rather than morphology and clinical presentation.[12]

Studies on the components of sandfly saliva suggest that substances may partially influence the tropism of the parasite and therefore the resulting disease. The amount of a vasodilatory peptide, maxadilan, in sandfly saliva appears to correlate with the type of human infection.[60] Sandflies in Brazil that transmit *Leishmania chagasi* VL have relatively large amounts of maxadilan, in their saliva, which causes marked vasodilation and may encourage visceralization of the parasites. The same complex of sandflies in Costa Rica, which have relatively small amounts of the vasodilatory peptide in their saliva, transmit organisms that produce a nonulcerating and nonvisceralizing *L. chagasi* infection that is limited to the dermis.

The clinical manifestations of leishmaniasis appear to depend on a complex set of factors, including tropism and virulence of the parasite strain, as well as the susceptibility of the host, which may be determined genetically.[10] Cell-mediated immune mechanisms appear to be the major factors in modulating these diseases (Table 221.1). However, specific pathway factors responsible for the generation of virulent amastigotes in human infections are still poorly understood.[10,50] Disease syndromes range from self-healing cutaneous lesions to debilitating mucocutaneous infections, subclinical viscerotropic dissemination, and fatal visceral involvement.

In CL, *Leishmania tropica* (with some notable exceptions), *Leishmania major, Leishmania aethiopica,* and *Leishmania mexicana* tend to be restricted to reticuloendothelial cells of the skin, and infections generally are self-limited, with spontaneous healing. Similarly, in MCL *Leishmania braziliensis* can invade the reticuloendothelial cells of the skin and the mucous membranes of the nose, mouth, and pharynx, resulting in serious disfigurement, if not death. Some strains of *L. tropica* may cause viscerotropic disease. In cases of VL (kala-azar), *Leishmania donovani, Leishmania chagasi,* and *Leishmania infantum* invade cells of the reticuloendothelium of viscera, usually causing splenomegaly and occasionally hepatomegaly and pancytopenia; untreated, the disease is progressive and generally fatal.[46]

In ATL, *Leishmania (Viannia) braziliensis* and *L. (Leishmania) mexicana* have an annual incidence of 1 to 1.5 million cases. Some patients, when self-cure of the cutaneous lesions does not occur, will develop the disseminated form of the disease.[71–73]

Individuals with acquired immunodeficiency syndrome (AIDS) may have atypical manifestations. Dermotropic strains of *L. infantum* are known to cause visceral infection in immunocompromised patients with AIDS.[57] VL is quite prevalent among AIDS patients in certain

TABLE 221.1 Clinical Syndromes Caused by Leishmania Species and Their Geographic Distribution[a]

Clinical Syndromes	Leishmania Species[b]	Location
Visceral Leishmaniasis		
Kala-azar: Generalized involvement of the reticuloendothelial system (i.e., spleen, bone marrow, liver)	*L. (L.) donovani*	Indian subcontinent, northern and eastern China, Pakistan, Nepal
	L. (L.) infantum	Middle East, Mediterranean littoral, Balkans, Central and southwestern Asia, northern and northwestern China, northern and sub-Saharan Africa
	Canine visceral leishmaniasis	Foxhounds in 18 states (United States)
	L. (L.) donovani (archibaldi)	Sudan, Kenya, Ethiopia
	L. (L.) spp.[a]	Kenya, Ethiopia, Somalia
	L. (L.) chagasi	Latin America
	L. (L.) amazonensis	Brazil (Bahia State)
	L. (L.) tropica	Israel, India, and viscerotropic disease in Saudi Arabia (US troops)
Post–kala-azar dermal leishmaniasis	*L. (L.) donovani*	Indian subcontinent, East Africa
Old World Cutaneous Leishmaniasis		
Single or limited number of skin lesions	*L. (L.) major*	Middle East, northwestern China, northwestern India, Pakistan, Africa
	L. (L.) tropica	Mediterranean littoral, Middle East, western Asiatic area, Indian subcontinent
	L. (L.) aethiopica	Ethiopian highlands, Kenya, Yemen
	L. (L.) infantum	Mediterranean basin
	L. (L.) donovani (archibaldi)	Sudan and East Africa
	L. (L.) spp.	Kenya, Ethiopia, Somalia
Diffuse cutaneous leishmaniasis	*L. (L.) aethiopica*	Ethiopian highlands, Kenya, Yemen
New World Cutaneous Leishmaniasis (Includes American Tegumentary Leishmaniasis[c])		
Single or limited number of skin lesions	*L. (L.) mexicana* (chiclero ulcer)	Central America, Mexico, Texas, Oklahoma, Arizona
	L. (L.) amazonensis	Amazon basin and neighboring areas, Bahia and other states in Brazil
	L. (V.) braziliensis	Multiple areas of Central and South America
	L. (V.) guyanensis (forest yaws)	Guyana, Suriname, northern Amazon basin
	L. (V.) peruviana (uta)	Peru (western Andes) and Argentinean highlands
	L. (V.) panamensis	Panama, Costa Rica, Colombia
	L. (V.) pifanoi	Venezuela
	L. (V.) venezuelensis	Venezuela
	L. (V.) colombiensis	Colombia and Panama
	L. (L.) chagasi	Central and South America
Diffuse cutaneous leishmaniasis	*L. (L.) amazonensis*	Amazon basin and neighboring areas, Bahia and other states in Brazil
	L. (V.) pifanoi	Venezuela
	L. (L.) mexicana	Mexico and Central America
	L. (L.) spp.	Dominican Republic
Mucosal leishmaniasis	*L. (V.) braziliensis* (espundia)	Multiple areas in Latin America

[a]This table contains the most common species; not every organism is listed above.
[b]>*(L.)* subgenus *Leishmania; (V.)* subgenus *Viannia.*
[c]These two organisms are the primary cause of American tegumentary leishmaniasis from the southern United States to the southern part of Argentina.
Data from Laison R, Shaw JJ. Evolution, classification and geographic distribution. In: Peters W, Killick-Kendrick R, eds. *The Leishmaniases in Biology and Medicine.* London: Academic Press; 1987:1–120; modified from Pearson RD, Sousa AQ. Clinical spectrum of leishmaniasis. *Clin Infect Dis* 1996;22:1–13; from Pearson RD, Jeronimo SMB, de Queiroz A. Leishmaniasis. In: Guerrant RL, Walker DH, Weller PF, eds. *Tropical Infectious Diseases: Principles, Pathogens and Practice.* Philadelphia: Churchill Livingstone; 1999; and Alva J, Vélez ID, Ber C, et al. Leishmaniasis worldwide and global estimates of its incidence. *PLoS One.* 2012;7:e35671.

geographic areas (southern Spain), with a high proportion of cases being subclinical. Like other opportunistic infections, subclinical VL can be found at any stage of HIV-1 infection, but symptomatic cases appear mainly when severe immunosuppression is present.[52] HIV-*Leishmania* coinfection is being seen more and more frequently in the Mediterranean basin, especially in Spain, France, and Italy.

ORGANISM

In vertebrate hosts, *Leishmania* spp. are obligate intracellular parasites that exist only in the amastigote stage. The species that infect humans are usually morphologically indistinguishable from one another at both the light microscopic and ultrastructural levels. The organisms are round to oval bodies approximately 2 to 4 μm in diameter with a single nucleus, a specialized mitochondrial structure that has extranuclear DNA termed a *kinetoplast*, and no free flagellum. Amastigotes are engulfed by macrophages and reside within the parasitophorous vacuole of the macrophage host. They multiply by binary fission and eventually destroy the host cell. Subsequently, they are phagocytized, and the process occurs repeatedly.[27]

When the vector, a female sandfly, feeds on an infected person, it may ingest an infected cell from blood or tissue. Amastigotes are liberated in the fly's midgut, and within a few hours, transformation to the promastigote stage occurs. Promastigotes are elongated flagellates 15 to 25 μm long by 1.5 to 3.5 μm wide, each with an anterior, free flagellum that measures approximately 15 to 28 μm in length and may vary morphologically from a short and stumpy to an elongated form. Binary fission then begins, and large numbers of promastigotes are produced and gradually move forward to the pharynx, buccal cavity, and mouth parts. Depending on temperature and the species of sandfly, at 8 to 20 days, the mouth parts of the fly may be blocked partially or completely by huge numbers of promastigotes. These organisms may be dislodged into the bite wound when the female sandfly (*Phlebotomus, Lutzomyia*) next takes a blood meal. Promastigotes have surface molecules that bind to several macrophage receptors. The phagocytized promastigote forms transform into amastigotes within the parasitophorous vacuole, and multiplication takes place.

Amastigotes can be seen in Giemsa- or Wright-stained tissues or smears by light microscopy with the nucleus and kinetoplast staining bright red and the cytoplasm pale blue. Other blood stains are also acceptable. In Novy-MacNeal-Nicolle (NNN) culture medium at 24°C, the organisms grow readily and assume the promastigote or insect form.

In the past, specific and subspecific taxonomy designations have been determined by the clinical syndrome caused by an isolate in a particular geographic area. Also, various molecular techniques have been used to characterize the strains and species of clinical isolates: endonuclease restriction studies of kinetoplast DNA (K-DNA), buoyant density of K-DNA and mitochondrial DNA (M-DNA) on cesium chloride, leishmanial isozyme patterns, monoclonal antibody specificity, exoantigen secretory factor 4 serotyping, polymerase chain reaction (PCR) real-time PCR, nucleic acid sequence-based amplification (NASBA), and loop-mediated isothermal amplification (LAMP).[5,21]

EPIDEMIOLOGY

Leishmaniasis is mainly a zoonosis, although in certain areas of the world there is primarily human-vector-human transmission. The World Health Organization (WHO) estimates that 1.5 million cases of CL and 500,000 cases of VL occur every year, with 62,500 yearly deaths.[2,30] From 2005 to 2013, the number of Disability Adjusted Life Years (DALYs) for leishmaniasis increased to 4.283 million.[29] With recent outbreaks in many areas of the world, including Brazil, India, Italy, Spain, Sudan, and Kenya, leishmaniasis has become more widely recognized as an important emerging infectious disease in many developed as well as underdeveloped countries.[58,61] As of 2013, there were 3.914 million prevalent cases of CL and 113,700 prevalent cases of VL.[28] Although the parasite usually is transmitted via the bite of the sandfly vector, it may be transmitted also as a result of a laboratory accident, direct person-to-person transmission, and blood transfusion.[27,45] In addition, evidence indicates that it may be transmitted either in utero or during the peripartum period.

The phlebotomine sandfly, the vector for leishmaniasis, was first identified in 1691 by Bonanni.[23] The name of the genus, however, *Phlebotomus*, was coined in 1840 by Rondani and Berte. In 1907, the first description of an American phlebotomine sandfly was made by Coquillet. In 1909 Gaspar Vianna in Brazil identified the parasites responsible for cutaneous leishmaniasis, later identified as *Leishmania braziliensis* in 1911.[19] Concurrently Lutz and Neiva identified the first three species of sandflies in Brazil. *Lutzomyia* sandflies were later named after Adolfo Lutz. To date 229 species have been identified. It was not until 1921, however, that the Sergent brothers implicated the phlebotomine sandflies in the transmission of cutaneous leishmaniasis in Algeria. The evidence was substantiated by the work of Aragao in 1922 and Pessoa and Pestana in Brazil, in 1940. Later in 1950, it was discovered that the different forms of leishmaniasis infesting the American continent were caused by distinct species of the parasite. The research on leishmaniasis and sandflies has shed light on the transmission of other zoonotic illnesses, including trypanosomatids (*Crithidia*, *Endotrypanum*, *Trypanosoma*), and several viruses including Rhabdoviridae, Bunyaviridae, and Reoviridae, all isolated from phlebotomine sandflies. Sixty-nine different serotypes of arboviruses isolated from sandflies have been identified in the Amazon region.[23]

OLD WORLD CUTANEOUS LEISHMANIASIS

Definition and Epidemiology

Old World CL is caused by *L. major* (rural), *L. tropica* (urban), and *L. aethiopica*. It is found throughout the Middle East, along the Mediterranean basin and islands, and in East and West Africa, India, and southwestern Asia.[27] There has been a large increase in *L. tropica* cases in Afghanistan and Syria due to the military conflicts in occupied territories.[40] In humans, infection by *L. tropica* usually produces skin ulcers in which intracellular (amastigote) parasites can be found within macrophages in and around the lesions. These organisms are rarely found in spleen, liver, or bone marrow; however, several recent reports have described *L. tropica* isolates from patients with VL. In many areas, dogs or rodents are found to be naturally infected and are thought to be the natural reservoirs of infection. Various *Phlebotomus* spp. transmit the infection, although person-to-person transmission is possible and is the basis of the long-time practice in middle and central Asia of immunizing inoculation, that is, "leishmanization" to prevent possible disfigurement by a natural infection (Fig. 221.1).

Old World leishmaniasis, or Oriental sore (Delhi boil, Aleppo button) can be classified into "wet" and "dry" types. The wet or rural form is caused by *L. major* and is found chiefly in various rodents on the edge of deserts.[15,44] The dry or urban type is caused by *L. tropica* and is transmitted by phlebotomine species that frequently feed on humans and dogs. The dry or urban form of Oriental sore has a long incubation period, long duration of active infection, and large numbers of parasites in the dermis. The moist or rural type has a short incubation period, with rapid healing and few parasites in the skin. *L. aethiopica* is restricted to the mountain valleys of the Rift Valley of Ethiopia and Kenya, where rock and tree hyraxes are infected regularly. Humans become infected when they intrude in these areas. This form of CL is usually self-limited, although in a small number of individuals (1 per 100,000), nonhealing diffuse cutaneous (DCL) disease has been reported.[66]

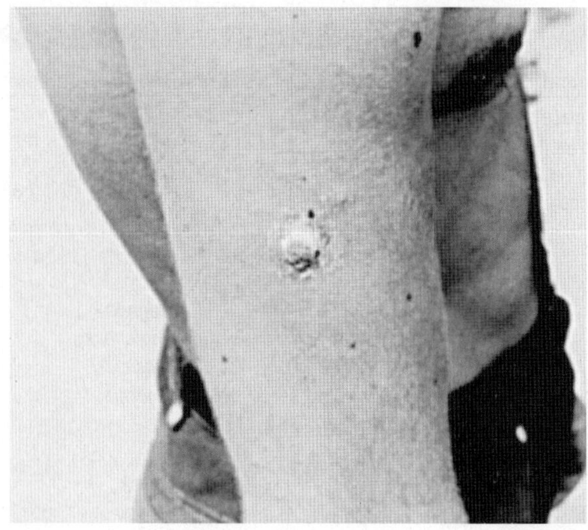

FIG. 221.1 *Leishmania tropica*. Immunization by an induced lesion. (From a nonprofit cooperative endeavor by numerous colleagues under the editorship of Dr. Herman Zaiman, New York.)

Pathology

At the bite site, promastigotes are engulfed by histiocytes, in which they multiply. The histiocytes are destroyed, and amastigotes are released into tissues, where the process is repeated. Lymphocytic and plasma cell infiltration along with histiocytic hyperplasia occurs, and in some lesions, epithelioid and giant cells may be seen. Hypertrophy of the stratum corneum and hyperplasia of dermal papillae occur early, usually followed by necrosis of the area caused by capillary obstruction and endothelial proliferation. The epithelium overlying the center of the lesion becomes necrotic and is sloughed, with the formation of a characteristic ulcer. Secondary neutrophil infiltration also occurs. At this point, a depressed ulcer with a raised purpuric indurated border and a base of friable granulation tissue is present. Amastigotes are located within the cells, although during the period of necrosis, organisms may be seen outside cells but division does not occur.

With *L. tropica*, development of the cutaneous lesion may take weeks to months, with large numbers of parasites present in nests of macrophages. In *L. major* infection, the onset is rapid, with an outpouring of lymphocytes and plasma cells; parasites are sometimes difficult to find. In some cases, satellite lesions form close to the primary lesion so that local spread is seen. The pathologic reaction may be florid, with marked pseudoepitheliomatous hyperplasia that can be mistaken for carcinoma. Secondary bacterial infection may complicate the lesion and delay healing. Once the ulcer heals, however, usually by fibrosis, the patient has long-lasting immunity (Fig. 221.2).

Several manifestations of CL have been described and seem to be associated with the ability of the patient to respond to the infection by cell-mediated immune mechanisms. Whether these mechanisms are directly responsible for protection in humans is still not certain. However, in a small number of patients, the inability to mount a suitable cell-mediated immune reaction is associated with specific anergy to leishmanin and an indolent nonhealing lesion.[35] This condition is known as DCL, or diffuse cutaneous leishmaniasis. Characteristically, lesions in DCL are

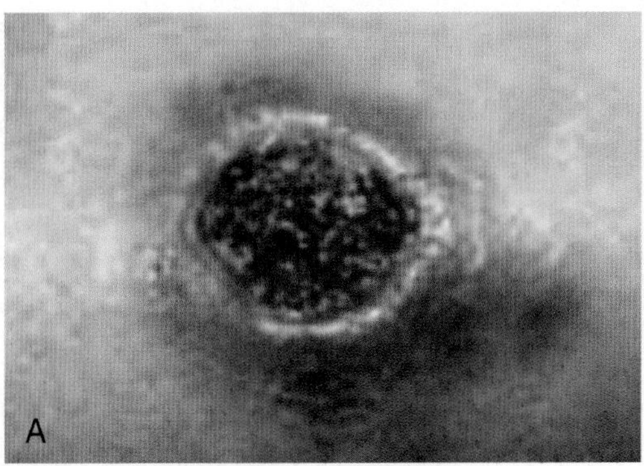

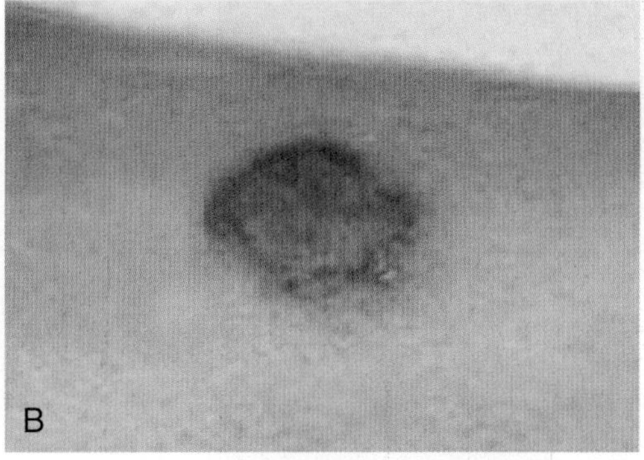

FIG. 221.2 (A) Typical cutaneous leishmaniasis ulcer. (B) Healed cutaneous leishmaniasis ulcer.

filled with large, parasite-containing histiocytes, and lymphocytes are absent. Recent studies of DCL from the Dominican Republic suggest that immune suppression plays an important role in this form of the disease.

At the other extreme is a small group of patients whose cell-mediated immune response to infection with leishmanial organisms is exaggerated and whose lesions heal by scarring. At the edge of the scar, however, new lesions appear, so the disease seems to extend from the margins. Eventually, tissue damage may be rather extensive. On histologic examination, many lymphocytes, plasma cells, epithelioid cells, and large multinucleated giant cells are seen. Organisms are difficult to locate but sometimes can be cultured from these lesions. This form of CL is called leishmaniasis recidivans. Patients exhibit marked delayed hypersensitivity to leishmanin. Cutaneous leishmaniasis may represent a spectrum of diseases analogous to leprosy.[63] DCL is at one end of the spectrum and represents anergy, and leishmaniasis recidivans is at the other end and represents marked delayed hypersensitivity; an ordinary Oriental sore represents the center of the spectrum.

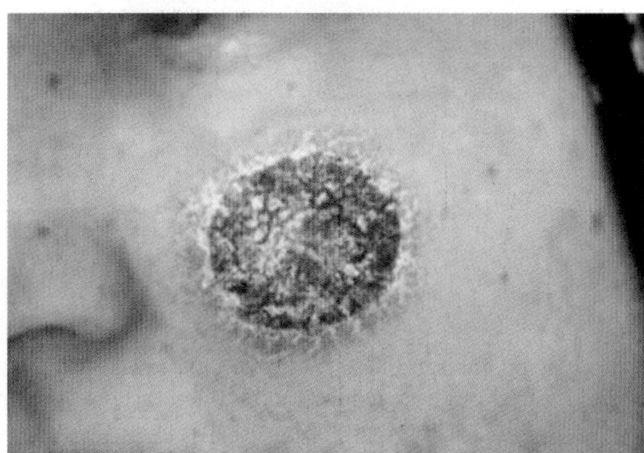

FIG. 221.3 Healing cutaneous leishmaniasis in a patient from Venezuela.

Clinical Manifestations

The disease usually begins with the appearance of a pruritic, red, vesicular papule that appears weeks to months after the bite of a sandfly. The papule gradually enlarges, often measuring 1 to 2 cm in diameter. When the surface of the papule dries, it encrusts and drops off to reveal a shallow ulcer. The ulcer may or may not enlarge progressively and characteristically has raised, sharp, indurated, deep purpuric margins. Healing usually occurs in 3 to 18 months, with an obvious hypopigmented or hyperpigmented depressed scar frequently remaining (Fig. 221.3). However, single or multiple papules often heal directly without extensive ulceration. If the lesions do not become infected secondarily, usually no complications occur.

Diagnosis

Definitive diagnosis depends on demonstrating the amastigotes in tissue specimens or the promastigotes in culture. Microscopic examination of Giemsa-, Wright-, or other rapid blood-stained smears of tissue obtained from nonnecrotic areas of the ulcer or from the base should be performed. Aspiration and culture of tissue fluid taken from the ulcer margin can be positive; however, biopsy material taken from the edge of the ulcer is preferred and should be examined histologically, as should small fragments macerated in saline and inoculated into NNN medium or Schneider's insect medium supplemented with antibiotics. It is very important to make sure the lesion is cleaned thoroughly to remove all secondary infectious organisms (contaminating bacteria and/or fungi) prior to taking the punch biopsy specimen for culture. The specimen of choice would be a collection of several punch biopsy specimens taken from the most active lesion areas. Clinically, the lesions are often characteristic, so the diagnosis should be suspected in a patient who has visited an endemic area.

Although the leishmanin test is usually positive in patients with ulcerated lesions, the material is not readily available in the United States. However, a positive leishmanin skin test may help distinguish a variety of skin lesions such as syphilis, tropical phagedenic ulcer, yaws, tuberculosis, and various fungal diseases. The indirect fluorescent antibody test or direct agglutination test may be positive in this infection, although often at low titer and, therefore, of little value.

Treatment

Uncomplicated *L. tropica* lesions generally respond well to chemotherapy or to conservative management. Because Old World CL usually remains a local lesion, if the ulcer is not disfiguring and appears to be healing, allowing the lesion to heal spontaneously is appropriate. In most cases, systemic therapy with stibogluconate sodium is effective.[37]

Ambisome (liposomal amphotericin B) has been used for treatment of visceral leishmaniasis, and more recently for treatment of cutaneous leishmaniasis.[32] However, a healthy 38-year-old man treated with liposomal amphotericin B for cutaneous leishmaniasis acquired during military duties in Iraq reported memory difficulties and confusion after completion of his therapy. Extensive evaluation revealed no other source, and his cognitive issues were attributed to liposomal amphotericin B toxicity (mentioned in the package insert). The patient's symptoms resolved over a few weeks, which is consistent with published data about the drug's tissue penetration and metabolism. This is a potential side effect of liposomal amphotericin B that can be observed in otherwise healthy patients.[32]

Various imidazoles (e.g., ketoconazole, itraconazole) have been used and appear to have limited antileishmanial activity. An ointment containing paromomycin (aminosidine) and methylbenzethonium chloride (Leshcutan) has been reported to show some promise in treating cutaneous lesions, especially in Israel.[12,63]

A 31-year-old man who had suffered since age 3 years from diffuse cutaneous leishmaniasis (DCL), a disease with profound physical and psychosocial repercussions and no effective treatment at present, was treated with miltefosine.[70] The patient was treated for 120 days, 100 mg/day for 1 week, then 150 mg/day subsequently. Lesions were free of parasites at 43 days, and no signs of infiltration were present at day 76. No adverse side effects were observed. The dramatic clinical effect of miltefosine in this patient appears to fully justify further evaluation of this experimental therapy in DCL.

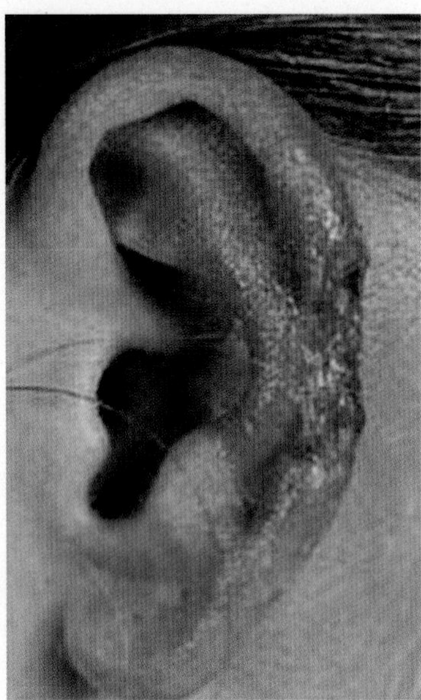

FIG. 221.4 Chiclero ulcer *Leishmania (mexicana) mexicana.* A typical chronic lesion of the external ear is evident. Such lesions never metastasize.

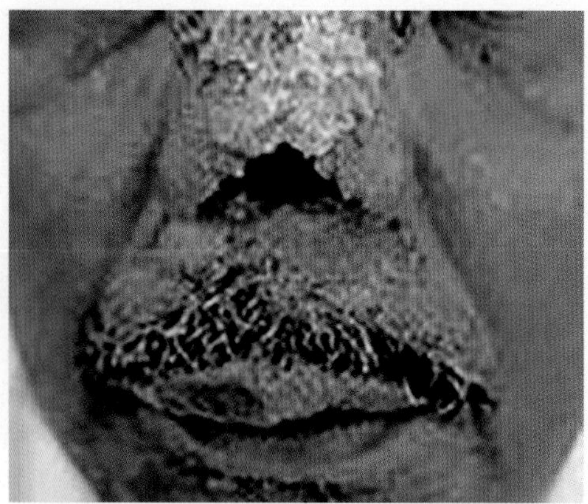

FIG. 221.5 Mucocutaneous leishmaniasis: *Leishmania (braziliensis) braziliensis.* The entire nasal septum has been eroded. Few organisms could be found by smear or biopsy; however, promastigote forms were cultured from the lesion.

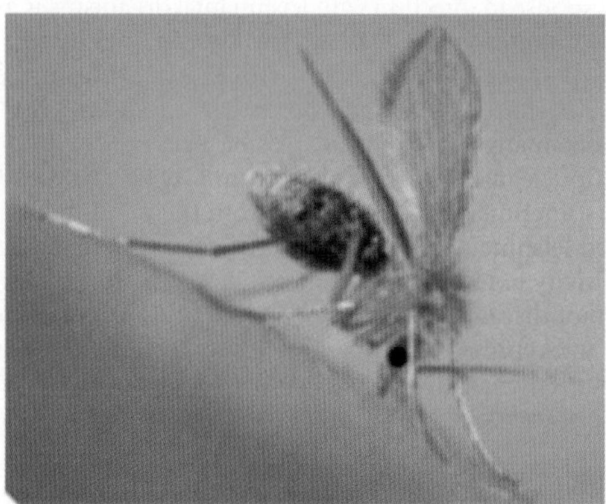

FIG. 221.6 Sandfly.

Prevention

Residual spraying for sandflies, eradication of reservoir hosts, and vaccination procedures have reduced and limited this disease in many areas of the Middle East and central Asia. Because of the indolent nature of the healing with vaccination and the possibility of visceralization, this practice has been discontinued in Israel. The customary method for controlling leishmaniasis and sandfly bites in Israel involves the spraying of large quantities of residual insecticides on walls of houses and neighboring surfaces. However, the high summer temperatures, strong radiation, and dust limit the efficacy of the method.[20]

AMERICAN CUTANEOUS LEISHMANIASIS

The epidemiology and etiology of American CL are quite complex. In South and Central America, many varieties of leishmaniasis exist, including the mucocutaneous form, or espundia. In contrast to Old World CL, American cutaneous disease is tied closely to the forests of South and Central America, and each variety has its own distinct epidemiologic, pathologic, and clinical picture.[33,35] Whether designating each of the clinical types of American CL by a separate species of *Leishmania* is justified remains unclear. With regard to the American cutaneous forms, two main groups of organisms are distinguished: the *L. mexicana* and *L. braziliensis* complexes (Figs. 221.4 and 221.5). The former are often characterized by rapid growth in culture medium and in hamsters, and the latter are organisms that grow slowly in culture and hamsters. These cases occur from the southern United States to the southern part of Argentina.

Leishmania Mexicana Complex

L. (mexicana) mexicana is transmitted by species of sandflies of the genus *Lutzomyia* (Fig. 221.6). Many rodent reservoir hosts exist. This species is found in Mexico, Guatemala, and Belize. It causes mild infection, often a single cutaneous lesion that is self-limited, or persistent chronic ear lesions, as well as chiclero ulcer.[4] One case of disseminated disease has been reported. This species is probably responsible for the occasional cases of CL and ATL found in the southern portion of the United States. The range of endemic infection has now been expanded within the United States to include areas that are farther north than the southern Texas site previously identified.[25,69] Apparently, wood rats serve as the primary wild reservoir hosts in these two states.

Cutaneous leishmaniasis is endemic within south-central Texas and appears to be spreading northward into the Dallas–Fort Worth metropolitan area, affecting humans, cats, and dogs. Multiple vectors and rodent reservoir hosts exist within Texas; vector-borne sandfly-based transmission is probably the primary means of disease spread in this area. Because of poor surveillance and infrequent diagnosis in the United States, leishmaniasis may have been present within at-risk canine and feline populations before the more recently recognized "outbreaks" in foxhounds or people. Evidence suggests that this disease may continue to emerge as a result of changes in the environment and closer contact between pets and sylvatic ecosystems.[55,69]

L. (mexicana) amazonensis is found along the Amazon basin and in Trinidad. It rarely infects humans but is transmitted by various species of *Lutzomyia* in rodents. In humans, it causes a mild and self-limited skin lesion. Reportedly, disseminated disease occasionally develops.[34]

Leishmania Braziliensis Complex (Mucocutaneous Leishmaniasis)

L. (braziliensis) braziliensis or *L. (Viannia) braziliensis* is transmitted by various species of *Lutzomyia* in Brazil and the forest areas east of the Andes. It was originally described by Gaspar Vianna in Brazil as the cause of Bauru ulcer.[19] This organism is the "prototype" of American CL/ATL or MCL, or espundia. It may cause destructive ulcerative lesions of the naso-oropharynx as a result of early or late metastases from a more superficial site.

L. (braziliensis) guyanensis is transmitted by species of *Lutzomyia* in Guyana, Suriname, Brazil, and Venezuela. It causes single or multiple spreading cutaneous ulcers over many parts of the body and is believed to metastasize along the lymphatics but does not visceralize. The organism sometimes spreads to the naso-oropharynx and causes mucosal disease. It sometimes is referred to as pian bois, or forest yaws.

L. (braziliensis) panamensis is transmitted by species of *Lutzomyia* in Panama and possibly farther north and south. It may cause single to several superficial ulcers and may metastasize along the lymphatics to the naso-oropharynx. A cluster of five cases was reported of CL with *L. (Viannia) panamensis* among men attempting emigration from East Africa, who acquired the infection while traveling from Central America to the United States. Species identification of the infecting species revealed important information related to a well-defined human smuggling route with potential public health consequences from this emerging infectious disease risk.[13] High rates of *L. (braziliensis) panamensis* have been found among Cuban immigrants trafficked through the Darien jungle, Panama.[6]

L. (braziliensis) peruviana is seen in Peru on the western slopes of the Andes to an altitude of 3000 m. It causes a single or a few self-healing ulcers. No oronasopharyngeal spread occurs. Often, it is referred to as uta. Dogs are regarded as the reservoir hosts.

In MCL as represented by espundia, researchers estimate that nasal involvement may occur in as many as 80% of infections, up to 30% of which eventually mutilate the mucous membranes of the mouth, nose, palate, larynx, and trachea. These cases are often fatal because of the intervening sepsis. Lesions of the mucous membranes often occur years to decades after a cutaneous ulcer has healed. Once mucous membrane involvement occurs, the infection may be difficult to cure using chemotherapy.

Diagnosis

The discussion of Old World CL includes the various methods for diagnosis. In mucocutaneous disease, the fluorescent antibody test using amastigote antigen is most useful in that it is positive in 75% to 85% of cases, with declining titers after therapeutic cure.[35] A direct agglutination test using promastigotes also is used frequently, as is enzyme-linked immunosorbent assay (ELISA).[35] A DNA-DNA hybridization or dot-blot test that is highly sensitive and species-specific in tissue or biopsy specimens has been used.[47] Isozyme analysis of isolated organisms currently is being used to help identify the species causing the infection.

Treatment

As in Old World CL, treatment of most lesions is effective using pentavalent antimonials. Because prompt and adequate therapy for primary cutaneous lesions may reduce the risk of subsequent metastatic disease in potentially mucocutaneous infections, pentavalent antimony should be used. If lesions should prove unresponsive to antimony therapy, amphotericin B should be tried. Liposomal amphotericin treatment has been useful in selected studies.[17] Relapses with this form of leishmaniasis are common and must be retreated. Pentavalent antimonials are moderately effective in treating mild mucosal disease but are often unsatisfactory with severe mucosal involvement. Diffuse cutaneous leishmaniasis, a disseminated form of the disease, should be treated with stibogluconate sodium[37]; when relapses occur, amphotericin B should be used next because this disease is usually refractory to further antimony therapy.[17,35] Pentamidine also has been used with limited success when lesions have proved resistant to antimony compounds. Pentavalent antimony-resistant cutaneous disease, such as leishmania recidivans, has been treated with limited success with ketoconazole, 400 to 600 mg daily for 4 weeks. Miltefosine, an oral antileishmanial agent effective against VL, has shown promise for the treatment of ATL *(L. panamensis/ amazonensis).*[16]

Prevention

This disease is extremely difficult to prevent because it is a forest disease. It can be avoided only by sleeping in tents under fine-mesh netting, wearing long-sleeved clothing, and using insect repellents. The presence of *Leishmania* parasites in the unaffected skin and peripheral-blood monocytes of a high proportion of patients even after treatment and the acquisition of infection by sandflies supports the plausibility of anthroponotic transmission of American cutaneous leishmaniasis.[68] As travel to Latin America has become increasingly common, cutaneous leishmaniasis is increasingly seen among returning travelers—for instance, the number of observed cases has doubled in the Netherlands and tripled in the United Kingdom in the past decade.[62] A high proportion of cases are acquired in rural or jungle areas of the Amazon basin. In children acquiring cutaneous *Leishmania (Viannia) braziliensis* infections, the major risk factor for acquisition of disease was the presence of an adult in the household with cutaneous leishmaniasis within the previous year.[3] Humans may serve as both reservoir and source of infection for young children. Vaccine development against American cutaneous leishmaniasis is underway.[38,56]

VISCERAL LEISHMANIASIS

VL is caused by various organisms in the *L. donovani* spp. complex in Asia and Africa, as well as by *L. infantum* in southern Europe and North Africa and the related *L. chagasi* in Brazil and elsewhere in the new world. Strains of *L. tropica* from the Middle East and *L. amazonensis* from Latin America have also been found to cause this syndrome.[43]

VL, or kala-azar, is found in a broad belt that extends from the Strait of Gibraltar across the Mediterranean through Asia to the east coast of China, at latitude between 30 and 48 degrees north. It is transmitted by various species of sandfly, although congenital and blood-borne infections can also occur.[45] VL has been reported from 47 countries, but the Sudan and India account for more than half of cases. In the Western Hemisphere, it is found in Brazil, northern Argentina, Paraguay, Venezuela, Colombia, Guatemala, and Mexico. Kala-azar appears to exist in at least three epidemiologic forms.

The Mediterranean type of VL, with a canine reservoir, infects young children (1 to 4 years of age); dogs, foxes, or feral animals are the reservoirs *(L. infantum).* This type extends from the Mediterranean littoral through central Asia into China; it is also present in parts of South America *(L. chagasi),* where foxes and dogs are reservoir hosts. In Brazil, young males are infected most often. Infected dogs are the primary reservoir for zoonotic visceral leishmaniasis in endemic regions and are the most significant risk factor predisposing humans to infection.[55] Dogs have a wide range of clinical presentation due to infection with *L. infantum*, ranging from asymptomatic to fatal visceral disease.

An Indian type *(L. donovani)* of VL with a human reservoir predominates in Indian children between 5 and 15 years of age; humans are the only known reservoir. Though sought, evidence of natural infection in dogs has not been found. No evidence of rodent reservoirs exists.

The African type of VL has rodents for the reservoir hosts. The Nile rat in the Sudan and probably the gerbil in Kenya are the reservoirs. In Kenya, researchers have noted that kala-azar often is related to old or eroded termite mounds where young males often congregate (see Fig. 221.5).

Pathology

The main pathologic lesions are the result of reticuloendothelial cell hyperplasia, especially in the spleen and liver (Fig. 221.7). Later, the bone marrow and lymph nodes are filled with infected macrophages, and a concomitant leukopenia and anemia develop (i.e., pancytopenia). Also, the kidneys may be filled with infected macrophages, and invasion of the submucosa and mucosa of the duodenum and jejunum results in hypertrophic congested and edematous villi. Small ulcerations and hemorrhages may occur. The spleen gradually enlarges, sometimes assuming enormous proportions, and eventually extends into the pelvis. Splenic infarcts are a frequent development. The capsule is thickened, and more deeply, the sinuses are dilated. Erythrophagocytosis by histiocytes is seen commonly, and the anemia so typical of kala-azar may in part be the result of such sequestration of red cells. Kupffer cells of the liver, filled with amastigotes, are swollen and hyperplastic, and centrilobular necrosis or fatty infiltration of the hepatic parenchyma often is observed. In late-stage or chronic disease, increased hepatic fibrosis may give a nodular cirrhotic appearance. Lymphadenopathy, especially of the mesenteric glands, is an early finding, and large numbers of parasite-filled macrophages are present. The bone marrow often is filled with parasitized histiocytes that replace the normal marrow elements; such replacement results in myelophthisic anemia.

The immunologic response to kala-azar infection is imperfectly understood. At the bite site, a small, pea-sized, dermal lesion may form (i.e., a leishmanioma); the parasites, initially localized in dermal macrophages, disseminate within the macrophages to the spleen, liver, bone marrow, and lymph nodes.

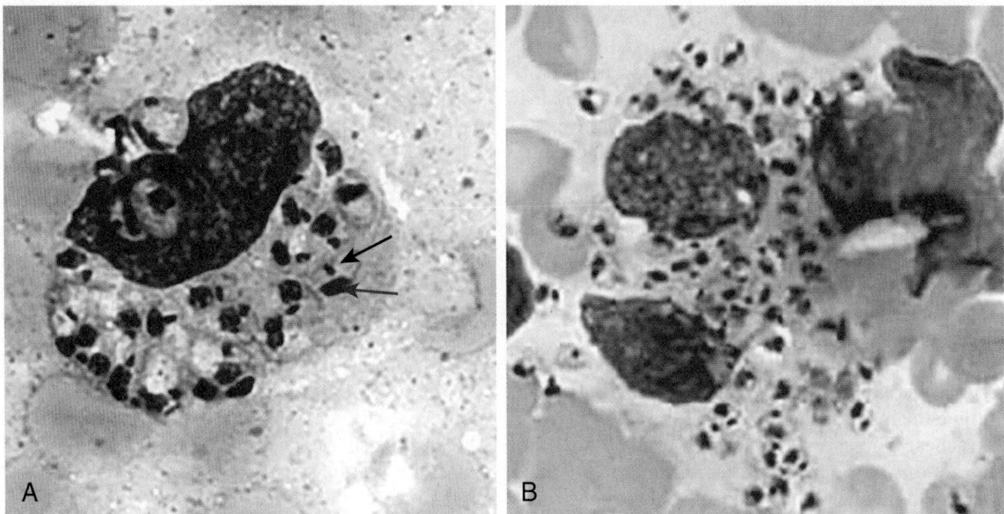

FIG. 221.7 (A) *Leishmania tropica* in a macrophage. The *red arrow* indicates the nucleus in the amastigote; the *black arrow* indicates the kinetoplast (small bar). (B) *Leishmania donovani* in a liver touch preparation.

The infection outcome depends on the host's ability to raise a suitable cell-mediated immune response and the virulence of the invading organism. Experimentally, resistance in mice appears to be determined by a single autosomal gene. Researchers have shown in experimental infections that the disease is controlled by the T_H1 subset of $CD4^+$ and $CD8^+$ T cells; these cells are related to the production of cytokines such as interferon-γ (IFN-γ), interleukin-2, and tumor necrosis factor-α. Infection with *L. donovani* amastigotes induces a Th1 cytokine milieu in both dendritic cells and T cells.[31] Cytokines activate macrophages to kill intracellular amastigotes by oxidative and nonoxidative mechanisms. Studies in mice indicate that nitric oxide is an important factor in killing amastigotes. If the infection is not eliminated or controlled by the host's cellular immune response, it then becomes clinically evident. Lymphocytogenesis and histiocytogenesis occur in affected organs, with resultant hepatosplenomegaly and lymphadenopathy. Polyclonal B-cell activation ensues and causes hyperglobulinemia. This outpouring of humoral antibodies, chiefly IgG and largely nonspecific, is not protective and may represent more than half the total serum proteins of the patient. The specific antibodies produced during active disease have diagnostic significance. Fluorescent antibody, ELISA, indirect hemagglutination, and complement-fixation tests are reasonably reliable diagnostic procedures.

Resistance to kala-azar is essentially absent once the infection has become evident clinically. However, after chemotherapeutic cure, acquired immunity emerges; delayed hypersensitivity, as demonstrated by the Montenegro (leishmanin) skin test (see later), also becomes apparent. Moreover, the hypergammaglobulinemia abates concomitant with chemical cure and the appearance of delayed hypersensitivity. Usually, immunity to VL is complete and long lasting after chemotherapeutic cure. However, relapse, as seen in post–kala-azar dermal leishmaniasis (PKDL), is characterized by delayed hypersensitivity, dermal localization of parasites, and moderate hypergammaglobulinemia. Although macrophage activation results in enhanced phagocytosis of parasites, macrophages remain unable to eliminate parasites. The appearance of dermal delayed hypersensitivity at the time that acquired immunity appears suggests that cell-mediated immunity plays an important role in protection. Further work on this aspect of VL is needed. The genetics of resistance in humans remains unclear.

Clinical Manifestations

The incubation period varies widely from 6 weeks to 6 months but has been reported to be as short as 10 to 14 days and as long as 10 years. A primary skin nodule is rarely seen, although in African leishmaniasis, it is a more regular feature. Infantile VL may begin either suddenly with high fever and vomiting or insidiously with irregular daily fever, anorexia, weight loss, lassitude, and pallor. When fever is present, double daily spikes are a characteristic sign, with temperatures reaching 40° to 40.6°C. The spleen gradually enlarges so that by the end of the first month, it can be palpated. If the symptoms continue unabated, the spleen may extend to the umbilicus or even into the pelvis. Diarrhea or frank dysentery is not unusual, and blood sometimes is observed. A general bleeding diathesis often becomes evident shortly before death. After several months, if the disease is untreated, patients usually die. Acute fulminant disease is seen more often in infants and young children.

In other cases, the clinical course is more protracted and generally ends fatally after a year or two. In older age groups, the disease tends to assume a more chronic course, with marked emaciation, brittle hair, massive splenomegaly, lymphadenopathy, and a dusky slate-gray complexion. Hyperglobulinemia, leukopenia, and anemia typically are found. As a result of general debility, death often results from concurrent infections such as pneumonia, amebic or bacillary dysentery, malaria, or cancrum oris in more than 90% of cases. Infantile VL has been associated with alterations in lipoprotein metabolism.[7] A handful of cases of presumed congenital VL have been reported.[26] These infants were born of infected mothers, and in some, evidence of parasitism of the placenta was found.[26] However, whether these cases represent congenital infection or peripartum infection is unclear because sophisticated serologic techniques were not available.

Infantile visceral leishmaniasis in the Mediterranean basin may begin with a high fever and vomiting or with irregular daily fevers, anorexia, and splenomegaly. In a small group of patients, an unusual echographic pattern of multiple nodules associated with splenomegaly was reported.[48] The authors strongly suggested that splenic nodules may represent a signature finding in infants.

In another pediatric study reviewing characteristics of visceral leishmaniasis-associated hemophagocytic lymphohistiocytosis (HLH), disease onset occurred before age 2 years and the symptoms could not be distinguished from other HLH causes. With therapy, 11 of 12 patients had a long-term remission. Several cases were treated with prolonged L-AmB therapy.[11]

In a study of hormonal disturbances in visceral leishmaniasis, primary adrenal insufficiency was observed in 45.8% of patients; low aldosterone/renin plasma ratio in 69.4%; low daily urinary aldosterone excretion in 61.1%; and low transtubular potassium gradient in 68.0%. All patients had normal plasma antidiuretic hormone (ADH) concentrations, hyponatremia, and high urinary osmolality. Plasma parathyroid hormone was low in 63%; hypomagnesemia was present in 46.4%, and increased urinary magnesium excretion in 100%. Primary thyroid insufficiency was observed in 24.6%, and secondary thyroid insufficiency in 14.1%. Normal follicle-stimulating hormone plasma levels were present in 81.4%; high luteinizing hormone and low testosterone plasma levels were found in 58.2% of men. There were also hypothalamus-pituitary-adrenal axis abnormalities, inappropriate aldosterone and ADH secretions, and presence of hypoparathyroidism, magnesium depletion, and thyroid and testicular insufficiencies.[67] Patient ages ranged from 15 to 58 years.

Cutaneous manifestations of kala-azar are encountered frequently. In India, the dark gray appearance of the skin is known as kala-azar (black sickness). In some cases of inadequately treated VL, PKDL may ensue. In Indian VL, this complication is encountered in 15% to 20% of cases and appears several years after therapy. Individuals with kala-azar and individuals with PKDL are considered to be reservoirs of transmission of *L. donovani* in India.[64] In African disease, PKDL occurs much less commonly, often during therapy in approximately 2% to 3% of cases, and it heals spontaneously in a few months. The lesions are characterized by the appearance of hypopigmented, erythematous, or nodular lesions on the skin of the face, chest, neck, and buttocks. At times, the nodular lesions of the face may resemble lepromatous leprosy. The lesions are thought to represent a modified form of *L. (L.) donovani* infection in which the parasites no longer invade the viscera and are localized to the skin. These lesions seem to be related to the host's immune response. This change to dermal tropism is said to coincide with recovery from visceral disease and to disappear with relapse. Infection with *L. (L.) chagasi* causes VL in young children. Atypical CL has been reported in older children with this infection.[8]

Pancytopenia is not unusual. Characteristically, anemia is always evident, with hemoglobin levels below 8 g/dL. Survival of red cells is shortened as a result of several possible factors, including Coombs-positive hemolytic anemia and hypersplenism. Leukopenia of 2000 to 3000 cells/mm^3 typically is found with neutropenia, relative lymphocytosis, an almost total absence of eosinophils, and thrombocytopenia. Serum albumin is usually less than 3 g/dL, and globulin levels (mostly IgG) are often greater than 5 g/dL (5 to 10 g/dL).

Kala-azar has been reported as an important opportunistic infection in patients infected with human immunodeficiency virus type 1 (HIV-1) and not known to have contracted *Leishmania* infection previously. These patients appear to have a more severe and fulminant form of kala-azar. In this regard, inapparent *Leishmania* infection may become evident after immunosuppression, such as chemotherapy for malignant disease. The diagnosis may be particularly difficult to make, inasmuch as the findings are often atypical and consist of low-grade fever, fatigue, cough, and gastrointestinal complaints. Certainly in AIDS patients, VL is a recurrent disease that is highly prevalent and whose clinical course is modified by HIV. VL is very prevalent among HIV-1-infected patients in southern Spain, with a high proportion of cases being subclinical.[1] Symptomatic cases appear mainly when severe immunosuppression is present. There is also an association between VL, the male sex, and intravenous drug use. Similarly, atypical visceral disease caused by *L. tropica* was seen in individuals who participated in Operation Desert Storm in the Persian Gulf.[42]

Diagnosis

VL is diagnosed by finding the organism in stained smears of spleen aspirate,[27] peripheral blood, or bone marrow (Fig. 221.7). In Indian kala-azar, the parasites may be found regularly in peripheral blood monocytes (i.e., buffy coat), but in the African and Mediterranean forms, they may be difficult to find by this technique. Blood and marrow cultures grown on NNN medium or in Schneider insect medium with 15% to 20% fetal calf serum are most useful (Fig. 221.8). Some investigators regard splenic rather than bone marrow aspiration as the most sensitive procedure, although it can be especially hazardous in individuals with a bleeding diathesis. Contraindications include a soft or diffluent, acutely enlarging spleen. Patients with low platelet counts or a prolonged prothrombin time (or both) should not undergo the needle biopsy procedure. In children younger than 5 years, splenic aspiration should be performed only by a physician fully experienced in the procedure.

Spleen and bone marrow aspirates should be placed in culture medium and smeared on slides, and saline-diluted aspirates should be inoculated into the peritoneal cavity of hamsters (see Fig. 221.6).

In a study conducted in pediatric patients in the Mediterranean region, antibody detection techniques, the antigen detection in urine (KAtex kit), and *Leishmania* nested PCR (LnPCR) analysis of the blood were useful for diagnosis of the first clinical episode.[18] After treatment, clinical improvement was associated with negative NNN cultures and microscopy of bone marrow aspirate, KAtex test, and LnPCR blood analysis results. New noninvasive techniques tested showed high diagnostic sensitivity. However, LnPCR analysis of the bone marrow was the most sensitive and was able to detect the persistence of parasites and predict potential relapses.[18]

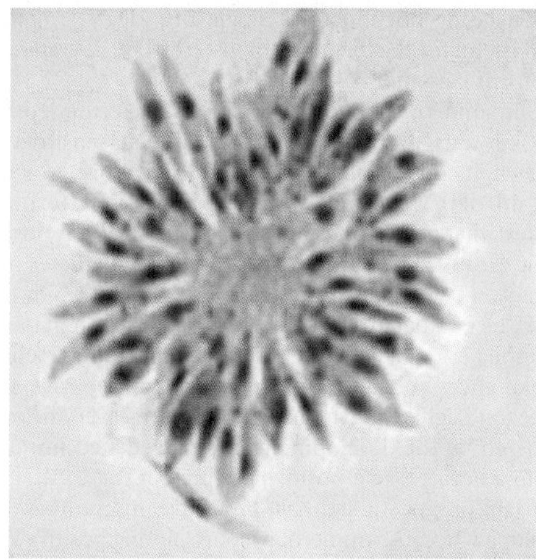

FIG. 221.8 *Leishmania* sp. promastigotes from culture system.

Diagnostic approaches for visceral leishmaniasis have been improved in the past decade with the development of serological and molecular tests. However, in many parts of the world, a definitive diagnosis still relies on the older parasitological methods. Recombinant antigens have led to improved performance of serodiagnostic methods. Serology-based tests, rk39 antigen dipstick, and direct agglutination test are highly sensitive methods; however, they fail to distinguish present from past infections. Molecular approaches have become increasingly relevant because of their remarkable sensitivity, specificity, and flexibility in sample selection. Quantitative PCR is a highly sensitive and specific tool used in referral labs for detection and assessment of parasite load in VL patients and in monitoring treatment response. This method has the potential to distinguish asymptomatic patients in endemic areas. Techniques such as loop-mediated isothermal amplification offer a reliable molecular diagnostic method for field application.[59,65]

Nonspecific tests detecting the markedly elevated serum globulins, such as the formol gel test, are helpful in acute disease and are performed readily in the field. Antileishmanial antibodies are usually present and can be used to aid in the diagnosis. The fluorescent antibody test is highly specific, as are the indirect hemagglutination and gel diffusion tests. The complement-fixation test, however, is positive in only 65% to 70% of cases. Sera from patients with VL are known to give false-positive results when antibodies to *T. cruzi* are present; consequently, in the Western Hemisphere, absorbing out these antibodies may be necessary. It is important to recognize that fluorescent antibody titers usually fall after complete cure, so a negative titer often is regarded as a sign of successful therapy. DNA-DNA hybridization tests are being evaluated and promise exquisite specificity and sensitivity for the diagnosis of leishmaniasis.[47] Serologic tests may be positive as a result of past or subclinical inapparent infection. An ELISA that detects antibodies to a cloned recombinant antigen, K39, of *L. chagasi* has been shown to be specific in active VL and could detect antibodies in AIDS patients. A recent study has demonstrated that this test could be applied to field situations.

In HIV-1-infected patients with active VL, the sensitivity of a peripheral blood smear is about 50%, because of a high parasitemia in these patients. However, in patients with HIV-1 and subclinical VL, the sensitivity of a routine blood smear is less than 10%.[1] Unfortunately, in these patients serology and *Leishmania* skin tests have low sensitivities and are not very helpful. Cultures have proven to be effective in VL patients who are coinfected with HIV-1. The usual diagnostic tests may also be negative in patients with *L. tropica* infection or in otherwise profoundly immunocompromised patients. However, two genomic fragments encoding portions of a single 210-kDa *L. tropica* protein have proved useful for the diagnosis of viscerotropic *L. tropica* infection in Desert Storm patients.[24]

The leishmanin or Montenegro skin test, like the lepromin and tuberculin skin tests, is a measure of delayed hypersensitivity to leishmanial antigen. It consists of 10^6 phenol-killed, culture-grown promastigotes in 1 mL of 0.5% phenol in saline. The test is performed like the tuberculin test, that is, 0.1 mL is injected intradermally. A positive result is a palpable area of induration at least 5 mm in diameter in 48 to 72 hours. Because the leishmanin test can be positive in CL or VL, the results must be evaluated carefully. In VL, the test remains negative throughout the period of active disease. Once chemotherapeutic control starts to take effect and immunocompetent lymphocytes are able to respond, the test begins to turn positive.[14] Thus, recovery from kala-azar is characterized by the development of cell-mediated immunity. The change from a negative to a positive leishmanin test in VL is regarded as an important prognostic sign that protective immunity is developing or has developed. Because numerous reports noting positive leishmanin tests in individuals who have had no history of VL have appeared, researchers have postulated that many individuals in an endemic area may become immune by previous inapparent infection.

Prognosis

Untreated VL is fatal in 75% to 85% of infantile and 90% of adult cases. Properly treated at an early stage, it can be cured in 85% to 95% of cases. The prognosis for patients in whom pancytopenia or bleeding diatheses develop or in whom a delayed hypersensitivity skin reaction fails to develop usually is poor.

Patients can be initially misdiagnosed as having an autoimmune disease because visceral leishmaniasis may mimic diseases such as systemic lupus erythematosus, autoimmune hepatitis, dermatomyositis, or other disorders. In pediatric patients, the risk of life-threatening complications is very high; thus, leishmaniasis must be considered in order to avoid an incorrect diagnosis and inappropriate immunosuppressive therapy.[51]

Treatment

VL generally responds to treatment with pentavalent antimonials such as stibogluconate sodium (Pentostam, Triostam), which is the usual drug of choice in the United States and is available through the Drug Service of the Centers for Disease Control and Prevention.[37] Meglumine antimoniate (Glucantime) is available in French-speaking countries and Latin America.[16] The pediatric and adult dose is 20 mg/kg daily administered intramuscularly or intravenously for 28 days. Treatment can be repeated. In areas where leishmanial parasites may have acquired relative resistance to pentavalent antimonials, such as India, Nepal, and East Africa, extending therapy for more than 4 weeks may be necessary.[41] Side effects occur commonly and include nausea, vomiting, headache, anorexia, and abdominal pain. Elevated levels of serum amylase and lipase, indicative of pancreatitis, are encountered occasionally and can be severe. Electrocardiographic changes are seen, including decreased T-wave amplitude and T-wave inversion, prolongation of the QTc, and nonspecific ST-T wave changes. They resolve shortly after therapy is concluded. (Treatment should be discontinued if the QTc interval exceeds 0.5 second.) Deaths, presumably caused by arrhythmias, have been reported in patients who were receiving more than 20 mg per day. Primary antimony resistance, as well as relapses after receiving pentavalent antimony therapy, occurs with all types of VL but is most often encountered with the Indian form. The mechanism of antimonial resistance is unclear. In HIV-infected patients, almost 25% fail to respond to antimony therapy, and almost 40% of responders subsequently relapse.[49,54]

Liposomal amphotericin B (AmBisome) has been approved by the US Food and Drug Administration for the treatment of VL. This compound is taken up by cells of the reticuloendothelial system, where amastigotes reside, and is less nephrotoxic, thereby allowing for higher daily doses with shorter courses of therapy. The approved, recommended regimen for immunocompetent VL patients is 3 mg/kg per day on days 1 through 5 and days 14 and 21. In immunosuppressed and HIV patients, treatment of VL with AmBisome has resulted in an almost 100% response rate. However, most of these patients relapse.[49,54] The recommended treatment is 4 mg/kg per day on days 1 through 5, 10, 17, 24, 31, and 38. Without maintenance therapy, almost all these patients relapse. Because resistance to pentavalent antimonials has developed, amphotericin B is used and is highly efficacious. Several recent studies have used liposomal amphotericin B successfully for the treatment of VL presumably caused by *L. infantum* in immunocompetent children.[35]

Parenteral pentamidine isethionate (Pentam 300) is administered intramuscularly (4 mg/kg is given three times weekly for up to 15 doses, depending on side effects such as hypotension, vomiting, and blood dyscrasias). Pentamidine occasionally may exacerbate diabetes mellitus or precipitate latent diabetes. Shock and liver and renal damage have been reported.

In several clinical trials, miltefosine, an oral alkyl phospholipid agent initially developed as an oral antineoplastic drug, has been used as an effective agent for the treatment of antimony-resistant Indian VL.[9,39] The treatment dose was 2.5 mg/kg per day for 4 weeks.

Patients may require hospitalization for therapy; supportive and corrective measures should be instituted in the event that other infections are present. An occasional patient may be encountered who may require splenectomy to relieve the profound hypersplenism and the resulting anemia. Response to therapy often can be assessed by return of the patient's temperature to normal, a brisk reticulocytosis, a gradual reduction in spleen size, and the reappearance of eosinophils on the peripheral blood smear.

Allopurinol has been used with pentavalent antimonials to treat cases of VL that did not respond to pentavalent antimonials alone. Several reports suggest that recombinant IFN-γ is helpful, along with pentavalent antimonial drugs, in successfully treating this disease. Because assessing whether a cure has been achieved is difficult, patients must be monitored at 6-month intervals for as long as 2 years. Fluorescent antibody titers should be absent by the end of 1 year and complement-fixation titers by 6 to 8 months. If PKDL occurs, treatment should be reinstituted.

Prevention

Control of VL has many aspects. Sandflies *(Phlebotomus* and *Lutzomyia)* can be eliminated readily by residual spraying. Because sandflies ordinarily do not fly very high, sleeping quarters should be above ground level. Permethrin-impregnated bed nets can be highly effective in preventing sandfly bites. Animal reservoirs, such as infected dogs and rodents, should be destroyed. Early therapy will prevent family and neighborhood transmission. A vaccine against different forms of leishmaniasis should be feasible, considering the wealth of information on genetics and biology of the parasite, the clinical and experimental immunology of leishmaniasis, and the availability of vaccines that can protect experimental animals against challenge with different *Leishmania* species. At the present time, however, there is no vaccine for human use against any form of leishmaniasis.[38] One major obstacle is the lack of a conceived market for human leishmaniasis vaccines. Ninety per cent of visceral leishmaniasis occurs in five countries (Bangladesh, Brazil, India, Nepal, and Sudan). Nonetheless, local studies for vaccine development are ongoing in India and Brazil.

NEW REFERENCES SINCE THE SEVENTH EDITION

6. Barry MA, Koshelev MV, Sun GS, et al. Cutaneous leishmaniasis in Cuban immigrants to Texas who traveled through the Darien Jungle, Panama. *Am J Trop Med Hyg*. 2014;91:345-347.
28. GBD 2013 Collaborators. Global, regional and national incidence, prevalence and years lived with disability for 301 acute and chronic diseases and injuries in 188 countries, 1990-2013: a systematic analysis for the Global Burden of Disease Study 2013. *Lancet*. 2015;386:743-800.
29. GBD 2013 DALYs and HALE Collaborators, Murray CJ, et al. Global, regional, and national disability-adjusted life years (DALYs) for 306 diseases and injuries and healthy life expectancy (HALE) for 188 countries, 1990-2013: quantifying the epidemiological transition. *Lancet*. 2015;386:2145-2149.
30. GBD 2013 Mortality and Causes of Death Collaborators. Global, regional and national age-sex specific all-cause and cause-specific mortality for 240 causes of death, 1990-2013: a systematic analysis for the Global Burden of Disease Study 2013. *Lancet*. 2015;385:117-171.
40. Karimkhani C, Wanga V, Coffeng LE, et al. Global burden of cutaneous leishmaniasis: a cross-sectional analysis from the Global Burden of Disease Study 2013. *Lancet Infect Dis*. 2016;16(5):584-591.

The full reference list for this chapter is available at ExpertConsult.com.

Trypanosomiasis 222

Louis V. Kirchhoff

Trypanosomes are protozoan parasites that are widely distributed in nature.[121] They are found in a broad range of cold- and warm-blooded vertebrates, as well as in a large number of invertebrate species that frequently act as vectors.[87] It is fair to say that if an animal has blood or a blood-like substance, it is likely that it acts as a host for trypanosomes. The striking diversity of animals infected with trypanosomes suggests that these parasites may confer a survival advantage to their hosts. Trypanosomes were first seen by Valentin, who in 1841 saw them through a microscope in the blood of a trout. Shortly thereafter Gluge and Gruby saw trypanosomes in toad blood and, upon observing their undulating membranes, named the genus *Trypanosoma* (Greek: *trypanon* means auger or screw, and *soma* means body). Lewis, while studying rats, was the first to see trypanosomes in mammalian blood, and trypanosomes were first seen in human blood in 1901 by an English boat captain named Forde who was traveling on the Gambia River with a febrile passenger. The following year that organism was named *Trypanosoma gambiense* by Dutton. Around that time sleeping sickness became a defined illness in Africa (today more broadly called human African trypanosomiasis [HAT]), and by 1905 its cause had been found, its vectors had been identified, and the first therapeutic drug (atoxyl) had been found. This remarkable progress resulted from the efforts of a number of investigators, and in recognition of Bruce's prominent role in the process the infecting species was named *Trypanosoma brucei*.[100]

Within a few years the Brazilian physician, Carlos Chagas, discovered the cycling of trypanosomes between wild mammals and insect vectors and also observed the organism in the blood of an ill 2-year–old child.[34,41] Chagas named the organism *Schizotrypanum cruzi* (later renamed *Trypanosoma cruzi* by others) after his mentor Oswaldo Cruz, and the disease ultimately became known as Chagas disease (now also referred to as American trypanosomiasis). Chagas presented detailed descriptions of the organism, its presence in insect and mammalian hosts, and the acute illness it can cause in humans in a monumental publication in German in 1909.[41]

Only three species of trypanosomes infect humans. The first is *Trypanosoma rangeli,* which is endemic in areas of Central and South America, does not appear to cause persistent infection, and is not known to be pathogenic. *T. cruzi* has a much larger endemic range, including Mexico as well as all the countries of Central and South America, establishes lifelong infection, and is a major cause of morbidity and death in humans. Two subspecies of *T. brucei*, *T. b. gambiense* and *T. b. rhodesiense*, which are endemic in West and East Africa, respectively, also cause persistent infection and often result in serious illness and death in infected persons. In areas endemic for Chagas disease or HAT, children are at risk for becoming infected. Despite the similarity of the organisms that cause Chagas disease and HAT, they are quite different when viewed from biologic, epidemiologic, and clinical perspectives and thus are considered separately in this chapter.

AMERICAN TRYPANOSOMIASIS (CHAGAS DISEASE)

Biology, Life Cycle, and Mechanisms of Transmission of *Trypanosoma cruzi*

American trypanosomiasis, Chagas disease, and *T. cruzi* infection are synonyms and simply indicate infection with *T. cruzi*. *T. cruzi* is a single-celled protozoan hemoflagellate parasite (order Kinetoplastida, family Trypanosomatidae) (Fig. 222.1). The molecular tools developed in recent decades have been applied in extensive studies of *T. cruzi* genetics and biochemistry. Notably, the complete sequence of the *T. cruzi* genome was published in 2005, as were those of the closely related species *T. brucei* and *Leishmania major*.[18,64,65,94] Molecular work on *T. cruzi* has focused on a broad range of basic and applied issues, including extensive molecular epidemiologic studies. In the latter, genetic analyses of *T. cruzi* isolates from geographically diverse vectors and mammalian hosts, including humans, have shown that there are six lineages, designated TcI to TcVI.[134] Unfortunately, no crisp associations between the lineages and pathogenicity or drug susceptibility have been found. In general, the extensive genetic and more recently proteomics data generated to date, including the framework of the lineages, have not yet led to new tools to reduce transmission, advances in the management of clinical disease, the development of new drugs, or the development of a vaccine.

In contrast, in the area of diagnosis the results of molecular work on *T. cruzi* has led to advances that directly affect persons at risk for or having *T. cruzi* infection. Application of DNA sequence data, generated for the most part in the late 1980s and 1990s, has led to the development of polymerase chain reaction (PCR) assays for detecting *T. cruzi*.[140,157,178,193] By far the most important application of these assays is for testing infants born to *T. cruzi*–infected mothers for congenital Chagas disease. In addition, to a limited extent these assays are used for diagnosing other acute *T. cruzi* infections, including reactivation in immunosuppressed persons, and for detecting treatment failure in chronically infected patients. In a second instance, *T. cruzi* molecular data have been productively exploited in the development of serodiagnostic assays for chronic *T. cruzi* infection. Several assays based on recombinant *T. cruzi* proteins are available commercially in the endemic countries and in other areas to which at-risk persons have emigrated (particularly the United States and Europe), and to date tens of millions of persons have been tested accurately with these assays.[43,47,156]

T. cruzi has a complex life cycle and can infect a variety of mammalian species, both omnivores and carnivores, as well as many species of insect vectors [family Reduviidae (assassin bugs), subfamily Triatominae (kissing bugs or triatomines)] (Fig. 222.2). The vectors are sometimes called reduviid bugs but more correctly should be referred to as triatomines.[120,191] Notably, the parasites go through distinct developmental stages in both insect and mammalian hosts. Vectors become infected when they take blood meals from mammalian hosts that contain nondividing trypomastigote forms of the parasite (Fig. 222.3). Once in the midgut of the vectors, the trypomastigotes transform into epimastigotes, which then multiply and ultimately move into the hindgut, where they become nondividing infective metacyclic trypomastigotes that are discharged with the feces at the time of a subsequent blood meal. Transmission then takes place to another mammalian host when breaks in the skin, conjunctivae, or mucous membranes (e.g., the nares or oral mucosa) are contaminated with bug feces containing infective forms. The latter can enter a wide variety of cell types, and after doing so transform to amastigotes, which are dividing intracellular forms (Fig. 222.4). The host cells soon fill with dozens of dividing amastigotes and then, likely in response to biochemical stress or specific signals, transform to bloodstream trypomastigotes. These parasites are released as the infected cell ruptures, and they presumably invade adjacent cells or find their way into the lymph and bloodstream and thus spread throughout their host. The vector-borne cycle is completed when circulating parasites end up in a blood meal of a vector.

Other routes of transmission of *T. cruzi* merit mention. Congenital transmission of *T. cruzi* has long been recognized as an important problem. Studies have shown that the overall risk of congenital transmission of the parasite from chronically infected mothers to their infants is about 5%, with a range in various studies of 2% to 10%.[90] Transfusion

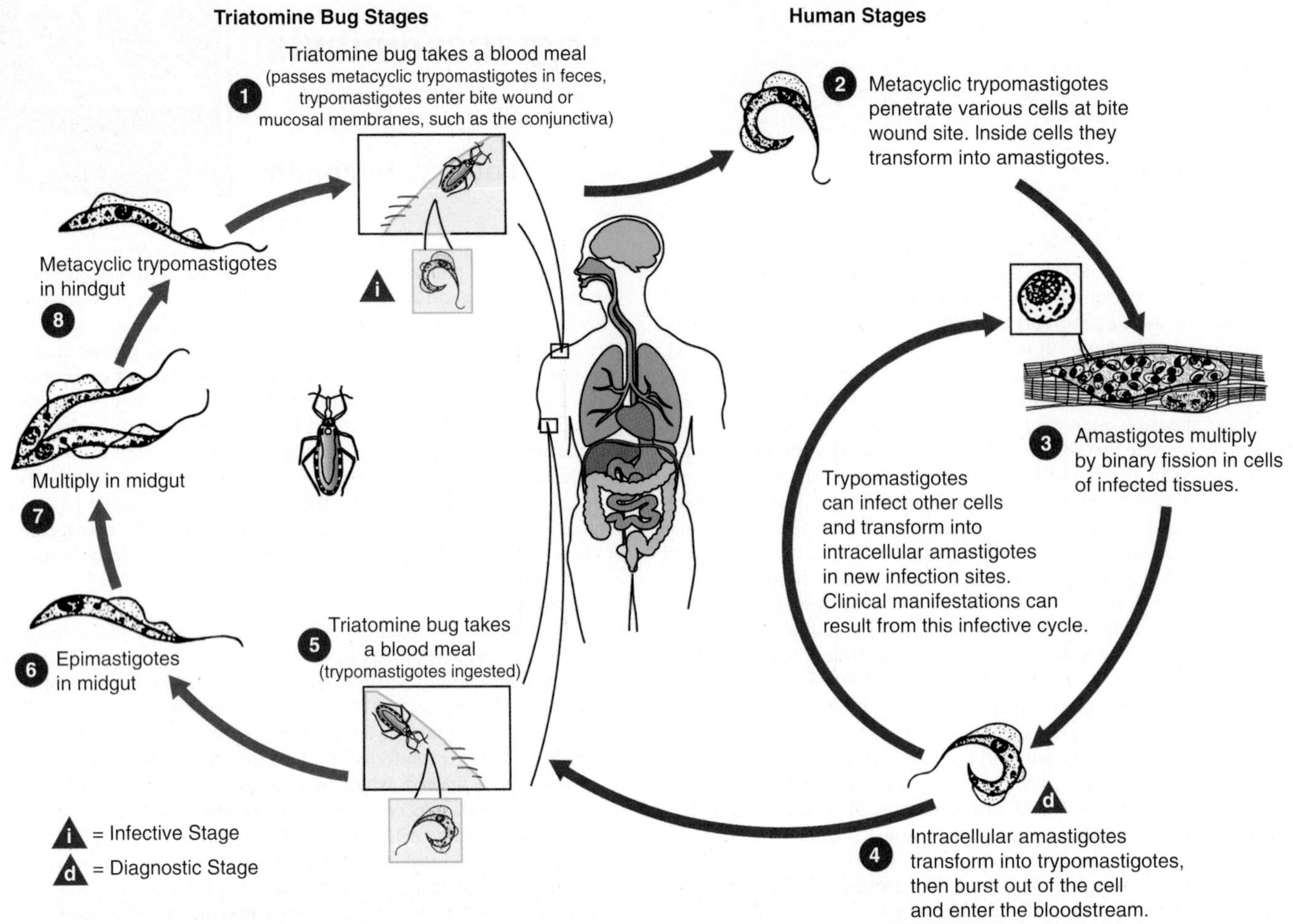

Triatomine Bug Stages

Human Stages

1 Triatomine bug takes a blood meal (passes metacyclic trypomastigotes in feces, trypomastigotes enter bite wound or mucosal membranes, such as the conjunctiva)

2 Metacyclic trypomastigotes penetrate various cells at bite wound site. Inside cells they transform into amastigotes.

3 Amastigotes multiply by binary fission in cells of infected tissues.

Trypomastigotes can infect other cells and transform into intracellular amastigotes in new infection sites. Clinical manifestations can result from this infective cycle.

4 Intracellular amastigotes transform into trypomastigotes, then burst out of the cell and enter the bloodstream.

5 Triatomine bug takes a blood meal (trypomastigotes ingested)

6 Epimastigotes in midgut

7 Multiply in midgut

8 Metacyclic trypomastigotes in hindgut

i = Infective Stage

d = Diagnostic Stage

FIG. 222.1 Life cycle of *Trypanosoma cruzi* in its insect vectors and mammalian hosts. (Courtesy Centers for Disease Control and Prevention, Atlanta, GA.)

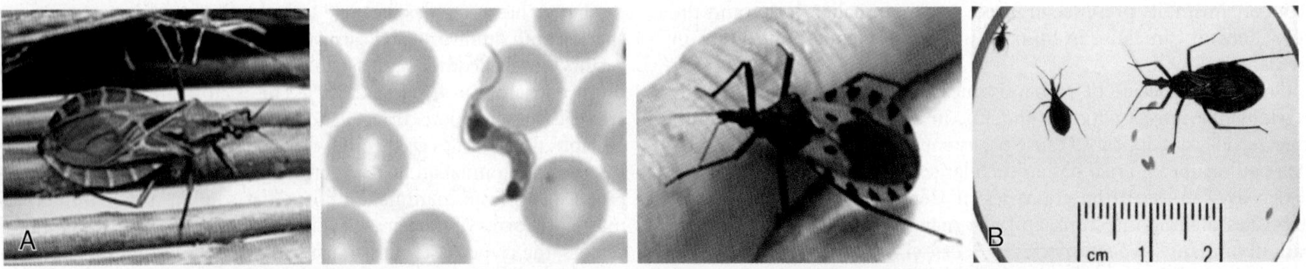

FIG. 222.2 Triatomine vectors of *Trypanosoma cruzi*. (A) *Triatoma infestans*. (B) *Rhodnius prolixus*. (A, Courtesy Centers for Disease Control and Prevention, Atlanta, GA. B, From Kirchhoff LV. *Trypanosoma* species (American trypanosomiasis, Chagas' disease): biology of trypanosomes. In: Bennett JE, Dolin R, Blaser MJ, eds. *Mandell, Douglas, and Bennett's Principles and Practice of Infectious Diseases*, 8th ed. Philadelphia: Elsevier; 2015.)

of blood from *T. cruzi*–infected donors can result in transmission of the parasite,[15,109,180] as can transplantation of organs obtained from infected donors.[48,38,189] Several outbreaks have been reported of acute Chagas disease caused by ingestion of food and drink contaminated with infected vector excreta or by the insects themselves, and finally dozens of laboratory accidents involving transmission have been described.

Epidemiology

T. cruzi is enzootic from southern Chile and Argentina to the southern tier of states in the United States. In spotty distributions within this range large numbers of at least a dozen species of triatomine insects capable of harboring *T. cruzi* are found,[77,111] as are large populations of potential mammalian hosts.[52,146] *T. cruzi* has been isolated from more than a hundred mammalian species, and armadillos, opossums, wood rats, raccoons, and canines are among those most commonly parasitized. Infected vectors live in the burrows and nesting places of the mammals, and contact with *T. cruzi*–infected feces in such places may be an important mechanism of transmission. Ingestion of infected insects also may be a common means of transmission, and the eating of infected mammals by carnivores may be important as well. Congenital transmission also occurs in these mammalian hosts,[9] but there is no direct evidence that sheds light on the relative importance of these routes of transmission in the sylvatic cycle. It is fair to say that most *T. cruzi* parasites are in infected wild mammals and insect vectors. Humans and domestic animals are only incidental hosts and have little to do

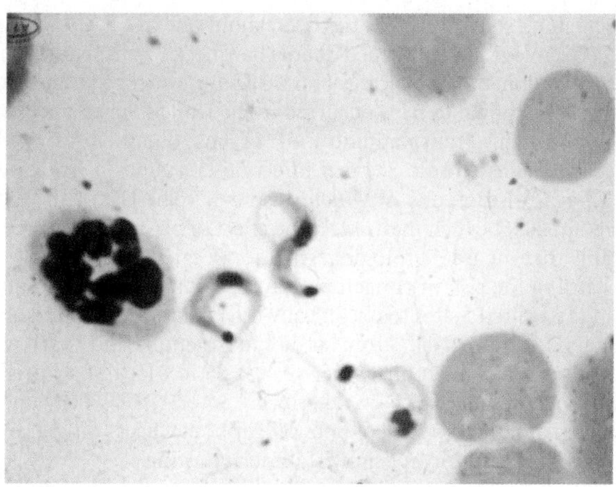

FIG. 222.3 ***Trypanosoma cruzi*** **trypomastigotes in rat blood smear (Giemsa, ×625).** (Courtesy Dr. Herbert B. Tanowitz, New York, NY.)

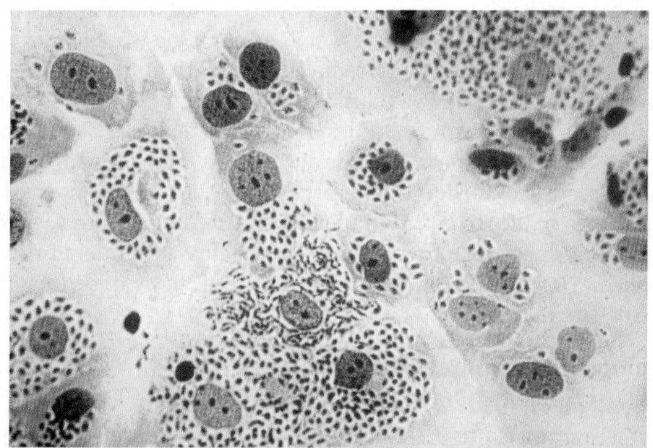

FIG. 222.4 ***Trypanosoma cruzi*** **amastigotes and trypomastigotes in mouse macrophages in liquid culture.** (Courtesy Dr. James A. Dvorak, Bethesda, MD.)

with the long-term persistence of the enormous reservoir of *T. cruzi* in the wild. Given the existence of the wildlife reservoir, the elimination of *T. cruzi* is not a realistic goal. Rather, resolution of the problem of human Chagas disease will result primarily from reducing contact with vectors, eliminating transmission by transfusion and organ transplantation, and treating infants with congenital transmission, and major progress along these lines has been made in recent decades.

The endemic range of Chagas disease includes all the countries of Central and South America as well as Mexico, a total of 21 nations. It is often stated that all of Latin America is endemic, but strictly speaking this is incorrect because there is no Chagas disease in Haiti, Cuba, the Dominican Republic, or Puerto Rico, which certainly are part of Latin America, whereas Belize, Surinam, and Guyana are not part of Latin America but are endemic. There is no Chagas disease in any of the Caribbean islands.

Historically, in the endemic range humans have become involved in the sylvatic cycle of *T. cruzi* transmission when they move into enzootic areas and infected vectors take up residence in the primitive wood, mud, and stone houses that are typical in rural areas. Native Americans who live in enzootic areas typically are affected as well.[73,125] The massive migrations that have been going on for decades from rural areas with vector-borne transmission to cities, where little if any such transmission occurs, has served to urbanize the disease in a major way. Similarly, Chagas disease has become globalized as many millions of persons from endemic countries have emigrated to nonendemic nations, and increased recognition of the consequent risk of chagasic cardiac and gastrointestinal (GI) disease, as well as congenital transmission, has occurred in these areas as well.[40,92,129,165,168,187]

The World Health Organization (WHO) estimated that 6 to 8 million persons are infected with *T. cruzi* in the endemic countries, and that annually about 12,000 deaths can be attributed to Chagas disease.[42] In addition, estimates have put the number of new *T. cruzi* infections per year at 28,000, of which approximately 15,000 result from congenital transmission.[33] Studies have shown that the overall risk of congenital transmission of the parasite from chronically infected mothers to their infants is about 5%, with a range in various studies of 2% to 10%.[90]

Epidemiologic data have long indicated that most new vector-borne *T. cruzi* infections occur in children. However, children are not known to be intrinsically more susceptible than adults to acquiring *T. cruzi* infection. They become infected early simply because their exposure to infected vectors often begins as soon as they are born. Risk is thought to be simply a function of the likelihood of infective parasites coming in contact with vulnerable host cells, independent of age.

The aggregate economic impact of Chagas disease in the endemic countries has been estimated to be in the range of US$8 billion per year.[117,179] When viewed from a global perspective, the death toll attributable to Chagas disease, which is roughly equal to the death toll attributable to intestinal helminths, ranks third among neglected tropical diseases, after malaria and leishmaniasis.[139]

In contrast to this gloomy situation resulting from the prevalence of chronic Chagas disease in the endemic countries, the outlook regarding secular patterns of transmission of the parasite is markedly much brighter. Starting decades ago, vector control programs were quite successful in some areas (e.g., São Paulo State in Brazil). In 1991, moreover, the six countries of the Southern Cone of South America (Uruguay, Paraguay, Argentina, Bolivia, Chile, and Brazil), in cooperation with the WHO and the Pan American Health Organization, began an ambitious program aimed at interrupting the vector-borne transmission of *T. cruzi* called the Southern Cone Initiative (SCI).[135] Spraying of residual insecticides, improvement of housing, and education of at-risk populations are the core elements of the SCI. During the 25 years that the SCI has been in place, a striking level of success has been achieved. Ongoing population-based serologic surveillance in many areas has revealed major reductions in *T. cruzi* prevalence in younger age groups, as well as a gradual decrease in seropositivity rates among blood donors, clear evidence of the success of the program.[124,130,171] Uruguay was certified free of vector-borne transmission in 1997, Chile followed 2 years later, and certification followed in Brazil in 2006. Major successes also have been achieved in Paraguay, Bolivia, and Argentina in the context of the SCI. In addition, programs similar to the SCI have been implemented in the Andean countries and in Central America, and major progress is being made in these regions as well.[35,80] The broad successes of all these vector control programs in reducing transmission of *T. cruzi*, the expectation of their continued impact in the coming years, and the largely effective implementation of donor screening for Chagas disease mandated by statute in all 21 endemic countries constitute grounds for reasonable optimism regarding the ultimate elimination of *T. cruzi* transmission in the next decade or so as foreseen by the WHO.

The epidemiology of Chagas disease in Mexico is of special interest because historically it has been less well studied there than in the other endemic countries, and proportionally fewer public health resources have been dedicated to the problem. Moreover, the situation of Chagas disease in Mexico should be of particular interest because roughly 17 million Mexican immigrants currently live in the United States.[190] In the mid-1990s a national survey carried out in Mexico among blood donors showed an overall prevalence rate of *T. cruzi* infection of 1.5%. In 2006 Kirchhoff and coworkers[109] reported a confirmed prevalence of *T. cruzi* infection of 0.8% among donors in five blood banks in the states of Jalisco and Nayarit. Moreover, in that study four of nine recipients of *T. cruzi*–tainted blood products were found to be infected with the parasite, thus demonstrating clearly that transfusion transmission was taking place. These data, along with the results of other serologic surveys of donors, were carefully considered in the writing of the new national regulations for blood products that became law in 2012,[143] under which the screening of donated blood for Chagas disease is mandated nationally.[174]

As far back as 1966, outbreaks in the endemic countries of *T. cruzi* transmission to groups of people through ingestion of food or drink presumably contaminated with infectious parasites from vectors have been reported.[59,167,202,208] There is no doubt that reports of such outbreaks have appeared more frequently in recent years. It is not clear, however, whether this increase results from an actual increase in *T. cruzi* transmission by this route or from a growing awareness of its possibility and an enhanced ability to investigate such outbreaks by public health authorities in the endemic countries. In either event, in terms of preventing such outbreaks it is important to recognize that they result not from a narrow *T. cruzi* problem but rather from the much broader problem related to a lack of adequate food safety standards that also results in the transmission of a variety of other pathogens.

Several dozen cases of *T. cruzi* transmission in laboratory settings were reported in the past, despite the negative publication bias relating to such incidents.[84] The fact that only one such report[106] has appeared during the last 15 years, however, suggests that accidental transmission may have been largely eliminated as increasingly stringent biosafety practices have been implemented in laboratories in which infective forms of *T. cruzi* are produced.

Despite the presence of the sylvatic cycle of *T. cruzi* in large areas of the southern and western United States, as noted earlier, only seven cases of vector-borne transmission to humans here have been described.[61] In addition, in the 5 years following implementation of blood donor screening in the United States in 2007, during which time more than 40 million donors were screened, only 17 seropositive donors were identified who appeared to have chronic *T. cruzi* infection acquired from vectors in the United States.[32] These data suggest that autochthonous transmission in the United States may be a bit more common than it had appeared to be. It is important to keep in mind, however, that these 17 donors with presumably autochthonously acquired chronic *T. cruzi* infection came to light through what is essentially a cross-sectional prevalence study that looked back over their entire lives. Thus their identification presents a limited perspective of the general incidence of vector-borne transmission and certainly says nothing regarding the secular trend of such transmission. In a review focused solely on Chagas disease and *T. cruzi* in Texas,[75] the results of earlier heterogeneous prevalence studies published over several decades were tabulated. Recognizing the obvious methodologic heterogeneity of the studies cited therein and the inherent risks of drawing inferences from such aggregated information, the data do suggest that in Texas at least autochthonous transmission of *T. cruzi* may be more common than previously thought. As in the case of the 17 infected blood donors, no inferences can be drawn from these data regarding a secular trend of such transmission, and overall it is still clear that vector-borne transmission is a rare event in Texas and other enzootic areas in the United States.[136,137] Importantly, the last reported autochthonous case of acute *T. cruzi* infection acquired in the United States from vectors occurred in the early 2000s.[61]

Since the 1980s, roughly 15 laboratory-acquired and imported cases of acute *T. cruzi* infection have been reported to the Centers for Disease Control and Prevention (CDC), but only one imported case occurred in a tourist returning to the United States from a Chagas-endemic country.[36] Three instances of tourists returning to Europe from endemic regions with acute *T. cruzi* infection have been reported, however, as has a similar case in Canada.[39] It is clear from this paucity of imported cases of acute Chagas disease, especially when viewed against the backdrop of the many millions of tourists who visit the Chagas-endemic countries each year, that the risk of acquiring acute *T. cruzi* infection while visiting these areas is extremely low.

The number of people with chronic *T. cruzi* infections who live in the United States has grown considerably in recent decades. More than 23 million persons born in Chagas-endemic countries reside in the United States. Moreover, it merits mention that most of the 6 million non-Mexican immigrants from endemic countries who currently live here were born in regions where the prevalence of chronic Chagas disease is higher than it is in Mexico. The CDC estimated that 300,000 persons with chronic *T. cruzi* infection currently live in the United States, essentially all of whom were already infected when they emigrated from their home countries.[16] Before donor screening began in 2007 a total of seven cases of transfusion transmission of *T. cruzi* had been reported in the United States and Canada,[210] and two additional instances were found in trace-back investigations done after screening was implemented.[105] The confirmed rate of *T. cruzi* infection in blood donors since screening started in 2007 has been about one in 13,300, and more than 2000 serologically confirmed donors have been permanently deferred from further donation.[53] No cases of transfusion-associated transmission of *T. cruzi* are known to have occurred in the United States since donor screening began. Transplantation of organs obtained from three immigrants with chronic *T. cruzi* infections resulted in five cases of acute Chagas disease, one of which was fatal.[37] The last of these cases occurred in 2006, which may reflect the effect of organ donor screening programs that include serologic testing for *T. cruzi*.

Regarding the risk of congenital transmission of *T. cruzi* to infants born in the United States to chronically infected mothers, a reasonable estimate based on risk data from studies in Argentina and Brazil would put the number of such births per year at 63 to 315, but surprisingly only one such instance has been described.[40] Several issues likely underlie this enigma, but the low level of knowledge about Chagas disease among caregivers may result in substantial underreporting.[201]

Hardly any information has been published that sheds light on the question of whether the rate of congenital transmission can be reduced by prophylactically treating women of childbearing age with either nifurtimox or benznidazole before they become pregnant. In the one investigation relevant to this question,[67] only a small number of women in the study group received treatment as adults. One would expect that parasitemias would have been reduced by the treatment, as was the case in the Benznidazole Evaluation for Interrupting Trypanosomiasis (BENEFIT) trial and other studies, and some of the treated women may have been cured parasitologically, but no data relevant to these questions were provided in the report. None of the infants born to any of the women in the study had congenital Chagas disease, thus suggesting that this prophylactic approach may be effective in reducing the rate of congenital transmission. A larger study needs to be done to address this issue adequately.

Pathology and Clinical Manifestations

Acute and Indeterminate Phases of Chagas Disease

The first sign of acute *T. cruzi* infection, which is seen much more commonly in children than in adults, can be a chagoma, which is an indurated and erythematous lesion at the site where the parasite entered host cells 10 to 14 days earlier.[13] If the organisms entered through the conjunctivae, the patient may develop painless unilateral periorbital edema, which is called Romaña sign (Fig. 222.5). In either case, local histologic changes include infiltration of lymphocytes, interstitial edema, intracellular parasitism of myocytes and a variety of other cells, and reactive swelling of adjacent lymph nodes. Fever and malaise, in addition

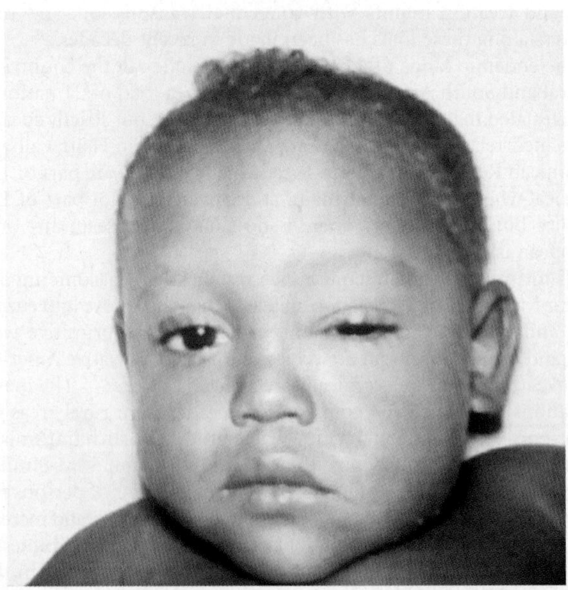

FIG. 222.5 Romaña sign in an Argentinean child with acute Chagas disease. (Courtesy Dr. Humberto Lugones, Santiago del Estero, Argentina.)

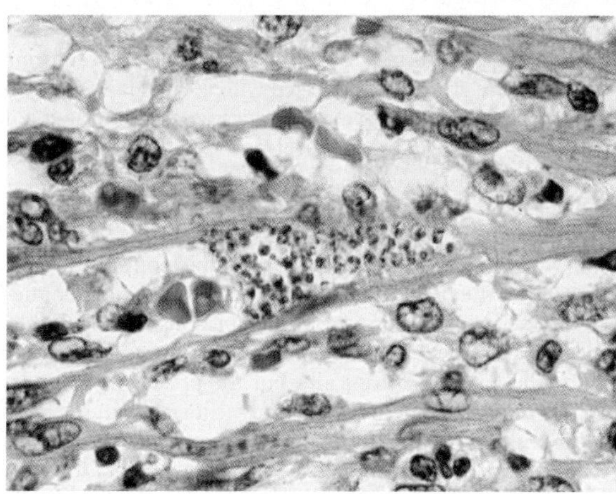

FIG. 222.6 **Intracellular *Trypanosoma cruzi* amastigotes in the cardiac muscle of a child with acute Chagas disease who died of acute myocarditis in Texas (H&E, ×900).** (From Kirchhoff LV. *Trypanosoma* species (American trypanosomiasis, Chagas' disease): biology of trypanosomes. In: Bennett JE, Dolin R, Blaser MJ, eds. *Mandell, Douglas, and Bennett's Principles and Practice of Infectious Diseases,* 8th ed. Philadelphia: Elsevier; 2015.)

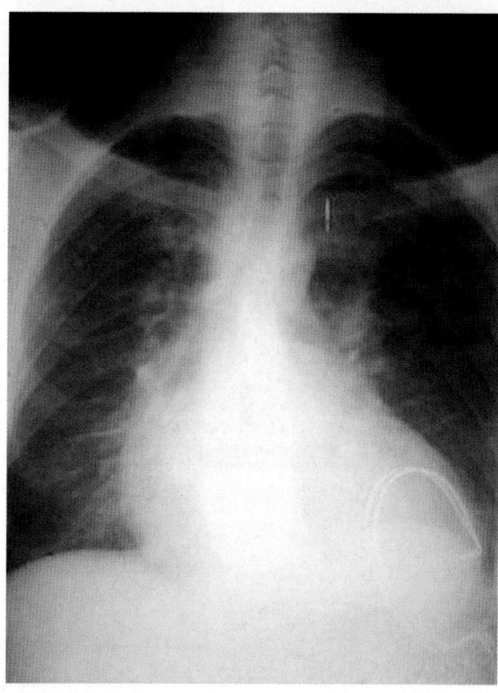

FIG. 222.7 **Chest radiograph of a Bolivian patient with chronic *Trypanosoma cruzi* infection, congestive heart failure, and rhythm disturbances. Pacemaker wires are present in the area of the left ventricle.** (From Kirchhoff LV. *Trypanosoma* species (American trypanosomiasis, Chagas' disease): biology of trypanosomes. In: Bennett JE, Dolin R, Blaser MJ, eds. *Mandell, Douglas, and Bennett's Principles and Practice of Infectious Diseases,* 8th ed. Philadelphia: Elsevier; 2015.)

to edema of the face and lower extremities, widespread lymphadenopathy, and hepatosplenomegaly, may develop as the parasites spread through the lymphatics and bloodstream from the site of initial multiplication. Occasionally patients with acute Chagas disease develop diffuse morbilliform rashes called *schizotrypanides*. Muscle cells can become heavily parasitized, and clinically manifest myocarditis develops in a small proportion of patients, occasionally precipitating fatal congestive heart failure[144,149] (Fig. 222.6). On histologic examination of cardiac tissue from patients with acute myocarditis, patchy areas of parasitized cells are present, in addition to intense infiltration of mononuclear cells and necrosis. The pathognomic *pseudocysts* also often seen in cardiac tissue are actually aggregates of *T. cruzi* amastigotes inside cardiomyocytes. Nonspecific electrocardiographic abnormalities may be present in tracings from patients with acute chagasic myocarditis, but the life-threatening dysrhythmias that can develop in patients with chronic cardiac Chagas disease usually do not occur.

Patients with acute Chagas disease can also have central nervous system (CNS) involvement, which was first described by Carlos Chagas.[41] It is not known how often the parasites actually invade extravascular spaces of the CNS in acutely infected patients, but in general, neurologic findings are uncommon in patients with acute Chagas disease. In a particularly noteworthy study related to this issue, parasites were found in the cerebrospinal fluid of eight of 11 patients examined, but none had neurologic symptoms.[88] Nonetheless, meningoencephalitis does occur rarely in patients with acute Chagas disease, mostly in infants, and generally it is associated with a poor outcome.[203] At a cellular level, focal presence of parasites accompanied by mononuclear cell infiltration has been described in all anatomic areas of the brain. Macrophages and glial cells can be heavily parasitized, but parasites are rarely seen in neurons. The clinical findings in patients with acute chagasic meningoencephalitis are indistinguishable from those found in acute CNS infections caused by other agents. Seizures can occur in variable patterns, and spasticity and hyperreflexia often develop.

In almost all patients with acute Chagas disease the signs and symptoms resolve spontaneously in 4 to 8 weeks, after which they enter the indeterminate phase of *T. cruzi* infection. This phase is characterized by a lack of symptoms, lifelong subpatent parasitemias, and detectable specific antibodies to *T. cruzi* antigens.

Congenital *T. cruzi* infection can be associated with premature rupture of membranes and preterm delivery, but there is no proven association with stillbirths and miscarriages. Most infants with congenital Chagas disease, which is a form of acute Chagas disease, are asymptomatic in the days after birth, and in the following months they evolve uneventfully into the indeterminate phase of *T. cruzi* infection. Infected neonates often display nonspecific signs and symptoms reminiscent of the TORCH syndrome.[142] Meningoencephalitis, heart disease, and megaesophagus have occasionally been reported in congenitally infected infants.[13,23,40,72,197]

Chronic Chagas Heart Disease

Fortunately, only 10% to 30% of persons with long-standing *T. cruzi* infections ever develop clinically manifest chronic Chagas disease. When associated signs and symptoms do develop, they typically first appear many years or even decades after initial infection. Nonetheless, rhythm disturbances and other cardiac abnormalities have been documented in chronically infected children.[50,55] Cardiac problems are the most common clinical expressions of long-term *T. cruzi* infection, and since the 1990s, convincing experimental evidence has accumulated showing that the persistence of parasites in heart muscle stimulates chronic inflammation that leads to organ dysfunction and, in many cases, death.[10,99,211] The inflammatory process can lead to a variety of cardiac rhythm disturbances, including atrial bradyarrhythmias and atrial fibrillation; premature ventricular contractions; bundle branch blocks, often of the right bundle; and complete atrioventricular block. These dysrhythmias can cause dizziness and syncope, and sudden death is common.[86,160,195] Fibrosis, cardiomyopathy, and biventricular dilatation can develop as well, leading to congestive heart failure, thrombus formation, and strokes; strokes sometimes represent the first expression of the underlying disease, and they occasionally occur even in young persons (Fig. 222.7).

Chronic Gastrointestinal Chagas Disease (Megadisease)

The GI tract is the second most frequently affected organ system in patients with clinically manifest chronic Chagas disease, and it is estimated that 10% of persons with chronic Chagas disease eventually develop GI tract symptoms. The most common clinical manifestations of megadisease are caused by megaesophagus (Fig. 222.8), but problems related to megacolon (Fig. 222.9) are also common. Patients with megaesophagus have symptoms similar to those of idiopathic achalasia such as cough, odynophagia, dysphagia, regurgitation, and chest pain.[58,164]

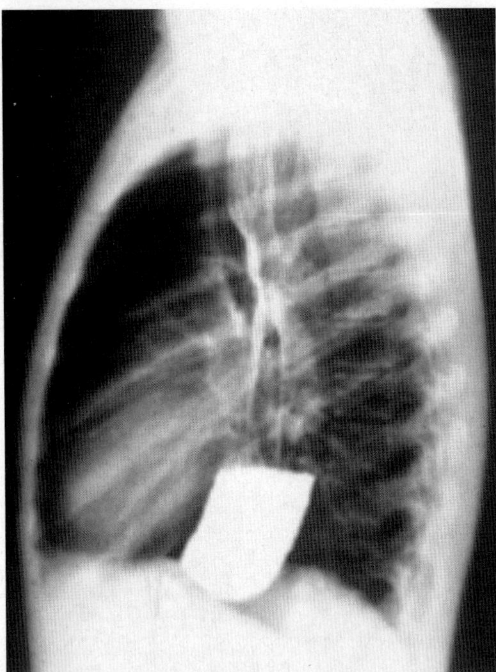

FIG. 222.8 Barium swallow radiographic study of a Brazilian patient with chronic *Trypanosoma cruzi* infection and megaesophagus. The markedly increased diameter of the esophagus as well as its failure to empty are typical findings in chagasic patients with megaesophagus. (Courtesy Dr. Franklin A. Neva, Bethesda, MD.)

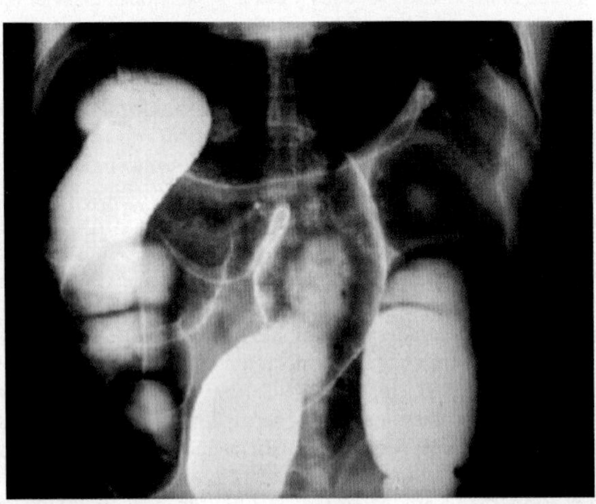

FIG. 222.9 Air-contrast barium enema of a constipated Bolivian patient with megacolon and chronic Chagas disease. Markedly increased diameters of the ascending, transverse, and sigmoid segments of the colon are readily apparent. (From Kirchhoff LV. *Trypanosoma* species (American trypanosomiasis, Chagas' disease): biology of trypanosomes. In: Bennett JE, Dolin R, Blaser MJ, eds. *Mandell, Douglas, and Bennett's Principles and Practice of Infectious Diseases.* 8th ed. Philadelphia: Elsevier; 2015.)

Hypersalivation often accompanies all these symptoms, and substantial parotid gland hypertrophy has been observed in some untreated patients with megaesophagus. Aspiration can become a problem, and recurrent episodes of aspiration pneumonia are common in patients with untreated severe chagasic esophageal dysfunction. Malnutrition can combine with pneumonia to cause death in patients with megaesophagus, although this is not common today because of the availability of effective symptomatic treatment. The typical symptoms of patients with megacolon are chronic constipation and abdominal pain. Patients with severe megacolon can go for weeks without a bowel movement, and acute obstruction, sometimes associated with volvulus, can result in perforation, septicemia, and death, but this scenario also is uncommon because of the widespread availability of surgical treatment.[93,115] Children and adolescents who are chronically infected with *T. cruzi* have been known to develop cardiac dysfunction and/or megadisease, but the incidence is very low.

Trypanosoma cruzi *Infection, Immunosuppression, and Transplantation*

In patients with chronic Chagas disease immunosuppression can result in reactivation of the indolent *T. cruzi* infection in a manner and with a severity not seen in immunocompetent persons.[12,19,96,153] In general, reactivation occurs in a small proportion of immunosuppressed persons who harbor the parasite chronically, but the precise incidence is not known. Immunosuppression is the only clinical context in which encephalitis and brain abscesses occur in persons with chronic *T. cruzi* infection. Reactivation after kidney and liver transplantation has been described, and in rare cases, abscesses in the CNS were involved.[49,76,119,166,169] Reactivation of *T. cruzi* infections and associated CNS encephalitis or brain abscesses also have been reported in patients who become immunosuppressed in association with other illnesses. One patient was described in whom a tumor-like CNS lesion caused by *T. cruzi* was found at the same time chronic lymphocytic leukemia was diagnosed.[172] Much more common, however, is the occurrence of *T. cruzi* reactivation in persons co-infected with *T. cruzi* and human immunodeficiency virus (HIV); dozens of such patients have been described, for the most part before HIV protease inhibitors became available.[28,51,56,83,175] A large percentage of these patients had CNS mass lesions caused by *T. cruzi*, lesions that, as noted, simply do not occur in immunocompetent persons chronically infected with the parasite. Myocarditis also has been observed commonly in dually infected persons in whom *T. cruzi* has reactivated.[176] It is noteworthy that reactivation of chronic *T. cruzi* infection overall occurs only in a small minority of patients who also harbor HIV.

A panel of experts reviewed the limited available data relating to the transplantation of organs obtained from *T. cruzi*–infected donors.[48] These experts and others[132] concluded that with informed consent, transplantation of kidneys and livers from infected donors is reasonable, but they emphasized that careful postoperative and long-term monitoring for *T. cruzi* infection in the recipients should be carried out, perhaps with guidance from staff at the CDC. Hearts from *T. cruzi*–infected donors should not be transplanted.[114] Seropositive transplant recipients should be monitored similarly for acute or reactivation infection. Unfortunately, no information is available on which to base guidance for prophylactic trypanocidal treatment of patients in either of these situations.

Diagnosis

There are no specific epidemiologic or clinical markers for Chagas disease, and thus the diagnosis must be made by laboratory studies. In acute Chagas disease, the diagnosis is parasitologic, and the highly motile parasites often can be seen on microscopic examination of wet smears of anticoagulated blood or buffy coat. Parasites also can sometimes be seen microscopically in the pellets of spun cerebrospinal fluid (CSF),[88] but a brain biopsy is unlikely to be diagnostic if a careful search in blood and other fluids is negative. Moreover, determining whether a parasitologically positive patient has CNS involvement is not critically important because its presence does not alter the recommended treatment regimen, as is the case in HAT. PCR assays are sensitive and specific in acute Chagas disease, but they are not used widely because of their limited availability and technical complexity.[110,178] Hemoculture and xenodiagnosis should not be attempted because they are prohibitively cumbersome, require several weeks to complete, and have sensitivities of only 50% to 70% even in the best of hands. Assays for *T. cruzi*–specific immunoglobulin M (IgM) lack accuracy and should not be used for diagnosing acute Chagas disease.

The approach to diagnosing congenital Chagas disease in infants merits special attention. As indicated schematically in (Fig. 222.10), all pregnant women with geographic or maternal risk should be tested serologically for *T. cruzi*. Among at-risk women in the nonendemic countries, the prevalence of chronic *T. cruzi* infection may vary considerably, depending on the countries from which the women have emigrated.

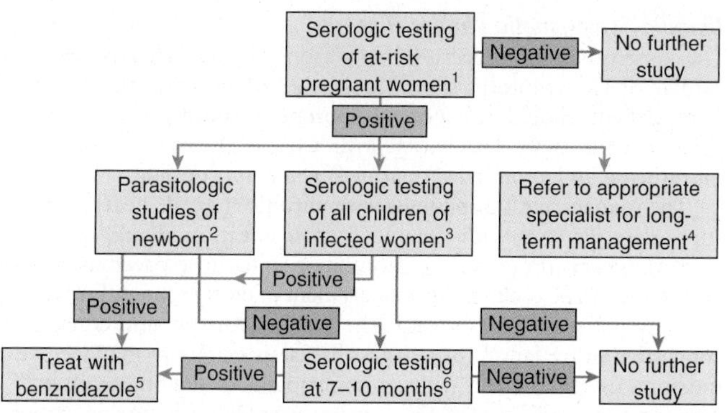

FIG. 222.10 Diagnosis and management of congenital Chagas disease. [1]Mexico as well as all the nations of Central and South America are endemic for Chagas disease. Chagas disease is not endemic in any of the Caribbean Islands. Women born in Chagas disease–endemic countries, or who have resided therein for substantial periods of time, are at geographic risk for having Chagas disease. In addition, women who are not themselves at geographic risk, but whose mothers have such risk and are not known to be seronegative, are in turn considered to be at risk for Chagas disease. [2]The two approaches useful in this regard are microscopic examination of anticoagulated blood and polymerase chain reaction (PCR). Serologic testing of newborns is not useful because assays for specific immunoglobulin (IgG) will be positive, reflecting the mothers' chronic infection, and because IgM assays lack acceptable levels of sensitivity and specificity. [3]All children born to at-risk women should be tested serologically because several studies indicate that the rate of congenital Chagas disease in babies born to infected mothers is 2% to 10%. [4]The latter should include periodic monitoring for signs and symptoms of chronic cardiac and gastrointestinal Chagas disease followed by appropriate interventions when indicated. The usefulness or specific drug treatment in adults with chronic *Trypanosoma cruzi* infections has not been clearly demonstrated and is a matter of ongoing debate. [5]The parasitologic cure rate in babies with congenital Chagas disease approaches 100% when a full course of treatment is given during the first year of life. [6]The sensitivities of microscopic examination of anticoagulated blood and PCR are less than 100%. Thus an occasional baby who tests negative in these approaches right after birth may actually be infected with *T. cruzi.* Serologic testing for specific IgG should be delayed until maternal IgG has disappeared.

For example, in a study done among Hispanic immigrant women in Barcelona, Spain, where there is a substantial population of Bolivians, the seroprevalence rate was 3.5%,[148] whereas the rate among Hispanic immigrant women in Houston, Texas, who were mainly from Mexico and Central America, was only 0.25%.[63]

No drugs or other measures are available for reducing the rate of congenital transmission. Thus having made the diagnosis of chronic *T. cruzi* infection in a pregnant woman, efforts then need to be focused on looking for evidence of congenital infection in the infant right after birth. Guidance on this process can be obtained at parasites@cdc.gov and by speaking with CDC staff at 404-718-4745. The general approach is to examine wet mounts and buffy coat of cord or whole blood obtained from the infant right after birth, and if parasites are not seen, to test the samples by PCR assay. The results of one study indicate that PCR assay on cord blood is more sensitive than microscopic examination.[17] If results of these parasitologic approaches are negative, blood obtained from the infant 7 to 10 months after birth should be tested serologically. If all these assay results are negative, no further testing for congenital Chagas disease is warranted. If any of the assays gives a positive result that is confirmed on repeat testing, the infant is deemed to have congenital Chagas disease and should be treated with benznidazole as outlined later. Such treatment will result in parasitologic cure in nearly 100% of the infants treated, thus presumably eliminating the risk of their developing chronic symptomatic Chagas disease years later. It will also break the chain of congenital transmission in that the treated female infants will not pass the infection on to their infants years later, unless of course they become reinfected in the interim through vector-borne transmission. An additional issue of importance is that other children of a pregnant woman found to be infected with *T. cruzi* should be tested serologically and, if positive, treated with benznidazole as indicated later.

With rare exceptions chronic Chagas disease is diagnosed by detecting IgG antibodies that bind specifically to *T. cruzi* antigens. It appears that detectable levels of such antibodies are universally present in persons chronically infected with *T. cruzi*. There is no credible evidence from properly structured studies that supports the concept of "seronegative Chagas disease." At present, at least a couple dozen serologic assays for chronic Chagas disease are available commercially,[43,62,78,147,173] and they are used widely for screening donated blood and clinical diagnosis in the endemic countries, as well as in other areas to which persons with geographic risk have emigrated. As with all assays, the sensitivities and specificities are less than 100%, and false-positive results can occur with specimens from patients with leishmaniasis, syphilis, malaria, and other infectious and autoimmune diseases. Although historically serodiagnostic tests for Chagas disease have been plagued with false-positive and false-negative results, the validated tests commercially available today in general are at a par with tests for other infectious diseases. The WHO recommends that samples be tested in two assays based on different methodologies before diagnostic decisions are made.[207] In Brazil the use of a single assay for both screening and diagnostic testing has been recommended officially. In the United States serologic testing is usually done in a single screening assay, followed by supplemental or confirmatory testing. Unvalidated in-house serodiagnostic tests for *T. cruzi* infection should not be used in any clinical or research context.

In the United States two assays are approved by the US Food and Drug Administration (FDA) for clinical testing (Chagatest Recombinante, Laboratorios Wiener, Rosario, Argentina; Chagas Kit, Hemagen Diagnostics, Inc., Columbia, MD). The Abbott Architect Chagas assay (Abbott Laboratories, Inc., Abbott Park, IL),[1,156] which is an accurate chemiluminescence assay based on a mixture of four chimeric recombinant *T. cruzi* proteins, is not approved in the United States. It is approved and used widely for both donor and clinical testing in a majority of the Chagas-endemic countries. The Abbott Prism Chagas assay,[43] a high-throughput automated chemiluminescence assay based on the four recombinant proteins employed in the Architect Chagas, and the Ortho *T. cruzi* ELISA Test System (Ortho-Clinical Diagnostics, Raritan, NJ), an enzyme-linked immunosorbent assay (ELISA) based on a lysate of parasites grown in culture,[78] are the only assays approved by FDA for donor testing and are currently used to screen the US blood supply. A radioimmune precipitation assay (Chagas RIPA),[108,147] which is approved under the Clinical Laboratories Improvement Act (CLIA) for testing clinical and research samples, is available in my laboratory. This assay is also approved by FDA for confirmatory testing of donor samples that are positive in the Abbott Prism Chagas assay or the Ortho *T. cruzi* ELISA Test System. Finally, the Abbott ESA Chagas (Enzyme Strip Assay), also based on the group of recombinant antigens used in the Architect Chagas assay, is FDA approved for confirmatory testing of screen-positive donor samples.[47] Unfortunately, PCR assays do not have consistently high levels of sensitivity that would allow their use for confirmatory testing of screen-positive donor samples.[178]

Treatment

Nifurtimox (Lampit, Bayer 2502) and benznidazole (Rochagan, Roche 7-1051) are the only two drugs available for treating patients with *T. cruzi* infection. There are no data from properly structured trials that justify the use of other drugs, either alone or in combination with each other or with nifurtimox or benznidazole, for treating any form of *T. cruzi* infection.[162] Both nifurtimox and benznidazole are unsatisfactory from several perspectives.[11] Nifurtimox has been used to treat *T. cruzi* infection for more than 4 decades. It reduces the severity and duration of acute Chagas disease and decreases mortality. Substantial proportions of patients treated with nifurtimox experience bothersome side effects.[95] GI complaints include nausea, vomiting, abdominal pain, anorexia, and weight loss. Neurologic complaints related to nifurtimox can include restlessness, twitching, paresthesias, and insomnia. Fortunately, these symptoms usually disappear when the dosage is reduced or treatment is stopped.

The recommended daily dosage for nifurtimox is 15 to 20 mg/kg for children up to 10 years of age, 12.5 to 15 mg/kg for adolescents, and 8 to 10 mg/kg for adults. The drug should be given orally in four divided doses, and treatment should be continued for 90 to 120 days.

Benznidazole is viewed as the drug of choice by most specialists in the endemic countries.[126] Side effects include rash, granulocytopenia, and peripheral neuropathy.[3,154] Overall it is fair to say that benznidazole is better tolerated by patients than nifurtimox, likely because of its lower incidence of bothersome GI side effects.

The recommended daily dosage for benznidazole is 5 to 10 mg/kg for children and 5 mg/kg for adults, in two or three divided doses, for 60 days. Thus the dosages of both nifurtimox and benznidazole vary as a function of the patient's age and weight, but generally not as a function of infection history, the levels of parasitemia, the presence of CNS disease, or other clinical manifestations. In the United States both nifurtimox and benznidazole are available only from the CDC Drug Service (404-639-3670), and specific guidance for the use of these drugs can be obtained from staff there as well.

The question of which groups of *T. cruzi*–infected persons should be given specific therapy has been the focus of intense discussion for decades. This is a thorny issue because benznidazole generally is effective in infants and children in all stages of *T. cruzi* infection, but it has limited efficacy in adults with long-standing chronic infection.[68] In general the efficacies of benznidazole and nifurtimox are similar. The consensus of experts in the endemic countries is that all persons with acute *T. cruzi* infection, including infants with congenital Chagas disease and patients with reactivated chronic infections caused by natural or iatrogenic immunosuppression, should be treated with either nifurtimox or benznidazole. An estimated 70% of immunocompetent acute patients will be cured parasitologically. Importantly, moreover, considerable data from benznidazole trials in congenitally infected infants in Argentina and Brazil indicate that the cure rate approaches 100% if treatment is given in the first year of life.[2,145,177] Moreover, in most immunosuppressed patients the often life-threatening reactivations will be suppressed, although the likelihood of parasitologic cure is quite low and the risk of later reactivations will persist if immunosuppression continues.

In terms of how to treat persons who harbor *T. cruzi* chronically, the current evidence-based consensus is that chronically infected children and adolescents up to 18 years of age should receive specific treatment. Clinical trial data indicate clearly that a large proportion of patients in this group will be cured parasitologically.[14,177,188]

In contrast, in adults with long-standing *T. cruzi* infection, including persons in the indeterminate phase as well as those with manifest chagasic symptoms, most of whom presumably were infected while quite young, the probability of parasitologic cure with either drug is less than 10%.[27,116,204] Determining which treated patients are cured is challenging, moreover, because treatment suppresses parasitemias, as reflected in reduced rates of positivity in post-treatment PCR assays, and levels of anti–*T. cruzi* antibodies can remain positive for years.[4,157] Until more recently, moreover, data from properly structured randomized clinical trials that assessed the effect of specific treatment in chronically infected adults have been lacking. A segment of this void was filled by the results of the BENEFIT trial.[128,138] In this blinded, placebo-controlled trial of benznidazole versus placebo that was performed in Colombia, Argentina, and Brazil, 2854 *T. cruzi*–infected patients with mild cardiac disease were followed for a mean of 5.4 years. Unfortunately, although as expected parasite detection by PCR assay was reduced, benznidazole did not significantly reduce cardiac clinical deterioration or death. In view of these results, specific treatment of adults with long-standing *T. cruzi* infection and demonstrable cardiac disease cannot be recommended. Moreover, as noted, no adults in the indeterminate phase of chronic *T. cruzi* infection were included in the BENEFIT trial, and thus randomized clinical trial data that shed light on the potential usefulness of treatment of persons in this group are still lacking.[127] A panel of experts convened by the CDC in 2006,[14] as well as the Ministries of Health in Brazil[152] and Argentina,[79] recommended that treatment should be offered to adults with indeterminate phase disease and that, after discussion of the risks and possible benefits, a decision should be made by the treating physician and each patient.

Chronic Symptomatic Chagas Disease

The consensus among experts is that persons who have already developed cardiac or GI symptoms should not be given antiparasitic treatment. These patients should be referred to appropriate subspecialists, preferably persons with some familiarity with Chagas disease, for long-term monitoring and supportive treatment when appropriate.

The management of patients with chronic chagasic heart disease is supportive. Persons with chronic *T. cruzi* infection should have electrocardiograms done every 6 months or so because pacemakers have been shown to be useful in the management of dysrhythmias that develop in many patients in this group. The cardiomyopathy and consequent congestive heart failure of Chagas disease is generally managed with measures used in patients with cardiomyopathies from other causes.[160,161] The usefulness of implantable cardioverter-defibrillators in patients with advanced chagasic heart disease is controversial and is the focus of a large, ongoing trial in Brazil.[8,158]

Cardiac transplantation is an option in patients with end-stage Chagas heart disease, and hundreds of patients have had this procedure in Brazil, Argentina, and the United States.[6,60,69,107] As might be expected, *T. cruzi* has been found in endomyocardial biopsies of transplant recipients, thus raising the possibility of early destruction of the new hearts by invasion of parasites. Nonetheless, long-term survival is greater in patients with Chagas disease who have undergone heart transplantation than in patients who have had heart transplants for diseases caused by other processes. It also merits mention that chagasic patients who have undergone cardiac transplantation may develop skin lesions containing high numbers of intracellular parasites. Conversely, encephalitis or cerebral abscess resulting from *T. cruzi* reactivation is rare after heart transplantation,[19] even though this occurs commonly in HIV-infected patients with chronic *T. cruzi* infection in whom reactivation occurs.

Chagasic megaesophagus generally should be treated in the same way as idiopathic achalasia.[82,159,164] Balloon dilation of the lower esophageal sphincter is the first approach to relieving symptoms, and patients in whom this approach fails generally are treated with laparoscopic surgical myotomy with a partial fundoplication. In patients with advanced megaesophagus esophagectomy with gastroplasty is often performed.[155]

Chronically infected patients in the early stages of colonic dysfunction are generally managed with a high-fiber diet and occasional laxatives and enemas. Fecal impaction requiring manual disimpaction can occur, as can toxic megacolon and volvulus, both of which require surgery. Several surgical procedures have been used to treat advanced megacolon resulting from Chagas disease, and all involve removal of part of the rectum and resection of the sigmoid colon.[74]

Prevention and Control

No vaccine or prophylactic drug is available for preventing transmission of *T. cruzi*.

The following measures are key elements in continuing the enormous progress that has been made to date in controlling Chagas disease:

- Control vector-borne transmission of *T. cruzi* by development of public health infrastructure capable of identifying areas where transmission occurs and implementing programs focused on the three core elements of the SCI: (1) housing improvement, (2) spraying of residual insecticides, and (3) education of populations at risk for acquiring *T. cruzi* infection.
- Serologically screen blood donors for chronic *T. cruzi* infection, and permanently defer seropositive donors.
- Serologically screen organ donors and transplant recipients for chronic *T. cruzi* infection.
- Serologically screen all pregnant women who have geographic or maternal risk for *T. cruzi* infection. Test all infants born to seropositive mothers parasitologically and, if need be, serologically, and treat infants with congenital Chagas disease with benznidazole.
- Educate tourists planning to travel to Chagas-endemic countries regarding the risk of *T. cruzi* transmission. Urge them to avoid sleeping in dilapidated dwellings and outdoors, but if they must, to take measures for reducing contact with vectors, such as screens and insect repellents.[113,122] Special precautions beyond the usual measures

for reducing the insect exposure of campers, hunters, and others engaging in outdoor activities in the United States are not warranted.

- Serologically screen all children and adolescents through age 18 years who have geographic or maternal risk for *T. cruzi* infection.[205] Treat seropositive persons so identified, and in the majority who will be cured parasitologically, the risk of their developing clinically manifest Chagas disease later in life and the risk of congenital transmission to their children presumably will be eliminated.
- Serologically screen all adults who have geographic or maternal risk for *T. cruzi* infection. Refer all seropositive persons to appropriate subspecialists, who ideally will have some knowledge of Chagas disease, for appropriate long-term monitoring and symptomatic treatment when necessary.
- Given the rarity of transmission of *T. cruzi* by ingestion of contaminated food or drink, reducing its risk in endemic areas cannot be productively approached with a sole focus on the parasite and its vectors. Rather, a reduction in its incidence can be achieved only through broad improvement in food safety standards and education.
- *T. cruzi* is classified as a risk group 2 agent in the United States. and a risk group 3 agent in some European countries. To avoid accidental transmission, laboratory staff who work with *T. cruzi* in culture or in infected vectors and mammals should strictly apply containment levels consist with the risk group classification in their areas.[20,91]

AFRICAN TRYPANOSOMIASIS (SLEEPING SICKNESS)

Biology, Life Cycle, and Mechanisms of Transmission of African Trypanosomes

HAT, also known as sleeping sickness, results from infection with flagellated protozoan parasites that are transmitted to humans by tsetse flies. The infecting trypanosomes first cause a febrile illness that in untreated patients is followed months or years later by progressive neurologic impairment and death. *T. brucei gambiense* and *T. b. rhodesiense*, two subspecies of the *T. brucei* complex, cause the West African *(gambiense)* and East African *(rhodesiense)* forms of sleeping sickness, respectively. These subspecies are morphologically identical, but nonetheless cause illnesses that are clinically and epidemiologically distinct (Table 222.1). These trypanosomes are transmitted by blood-sucking tsetse flies that belong to the genus *Glossina*.[206] They become infected when they suck blood from infected mammalian hosts that have parasites circulating in their bloodstream (Fig. 222.11). In the midgut of the vectors the parasites go through many cycles of multiplication and ultimately migrate to the salivary glands. Transmission occurs when parasites are inoculated into a mammalian host during a subsequent blood meal. The trypanosomes so injected then multiply in the blood and other extracellular spaces (Fig. 222.12). In contrast to *T. cruzi*, African trypanosomes do not have an intracellular phase in their mammalian hosts. They evade immune destruction indefinitely in a given mammalian host through a process called antigenic variation, which involves sequential gene switching that results in periodic changing of the antigenic structure of the parasites' predominant glycoprotein surface coat.[45,89]

TABLE 222.1 Comparison of West African and East African Trypanosomiases

	West African *(Gambiense)*	East African *(Rhodesiense)*
Organism	*Trypanosoma brucei gambiense*	*Trypanosoma brucei rhodesiense*
Vectors	Tsetse flies (*palpalis* group)	Tsetse flies (*morsitans* group)
Primary reservoir	Humans	Antelope and cattle
Human illness	Chronic (late CNS disease)	Acute (early CNS disease)
Duration of illness	Months to years	<9 months
Lymphadenopathy	Prominent	Minimal
Parasitemia	Low	High
Epidemiology	Rural populations	Tourists in game parks; workers in wild areas; rural populations

CNS, Central nervous system.
From Kirchhoff LV. Agents of African trypanosomiasis (sleeping sickness). In: Bennett JE, Dolin R, Blaser MJ, eds. *Mandell, Douglas, and Bennett's Principles and Practice of Infectious Diseases.* 8th ed. Philadelphia: Elsevier; 2015.

Essentially all transmission of African trypanosomes to both wild and domestic animals, and to humans, occurs in the cyclic fashion outlined earlier. It has not been shown that these trypanosomes can be transmitted by vectors other than tsetse flies, and similarly, mechanical transmission is not thought to be important. Transmission by blood transfusion is possible but appears to be extremely rare. The rate of congenital transmission is unknown, but such transmission also is thought to occur rarely.[57,123,131,198] A few incidents of laboratory transmission of the parasites have been reported, but none since the 1990s.[84,163]

Epidemiology

The endemic range of sleeping sickness is limited to sub-Saharan Africa.[70] It was much more of a problem in the past than at present, with major epidemics involving hundreds of thousands of persons described in the late 19th and the early 20th century.[85,100,104,185] The problem was nearly eliminated by the mid-1960s, but after the end of the colonial era, as control programs fell by the wayside, there was a gradual resurgence in the number of new cases in several countries that peaked in the 1990s, primarily in Angola, Sudan, Uganda, the Democratic Republic of the Congo, and the Central African Republic. In response, control activities organized by national health authorities, nongovernmental organizations, and the WHO were intensified, and by 2009 fewer than 10,000 cases were reported annually to the WHO. By 2014 that number had come down to 3796, which was the lowest level since surveillance throughout the endemic range had started 75 years earlier. All told, 85% of these cases occurred in the Democratic Republic of the Congo. It is recognized that underreporting is a persistent reality, however, and it is estimated that the actual total number of cases in 2014 was around 20,000. Notwithstanding the latter figure, there is no doubt that barring major political and economic upheavals, sleeping sickness is headed for the history books. Consistent with this view, based on successes of the control programs, in 2009 a panel of experts summoned by the WHO developed a vision for the eradication of sleeping sickness, and in 2012 the WHO Neglected Tropical Diseases Roadmap targeted the elimination of sleeping sickness as a public health problem by 2020.[71,103,118,181,183,192,200]

Human infection with *T. b. gambiense* occurs in widely distributed endemic foci in tropical rain forests of West and Central Africa. *Gambiense* trypanosomiasis is primarily a problem in rural populations, and tourists rarely become infected. Importantly 98% of reported cases of sleeping sickness are caused by *T. b. gambiense* infection, and humans are the only important reservoirs of this subspecies. These two facts are important elements that will facilitate the eventual elimination of sleeping sickness. In contrast, trypanotolerant antelope species in woodland areas and savannas of East and Central Africa are the principal reservoirs of *T. b. rhodesiense*. Importantly, cattle can also be infected with this and other trypanosome species, and they generally succumb to the infection.[5,209] Because the risk for acquiring *T. b. rhodesiense* mostly results from contact with tsetse flies that primarily feed on wild animals, humans acquire *T. b. rhodesiense* infection only incidentally, usually while working in or visiting areas where the cycle of transmission involving vectors and natural reservoirs is present. About one or two imported cases of sleeping sickness are reported to the CDC each year, and almost all of them are in persons who acquired the infection in East African game parks.[98,186] Patients with imported sleeping sickness occasionally are diagnosed in Europe and other nonendemic areas as well.[54,133,184,194]

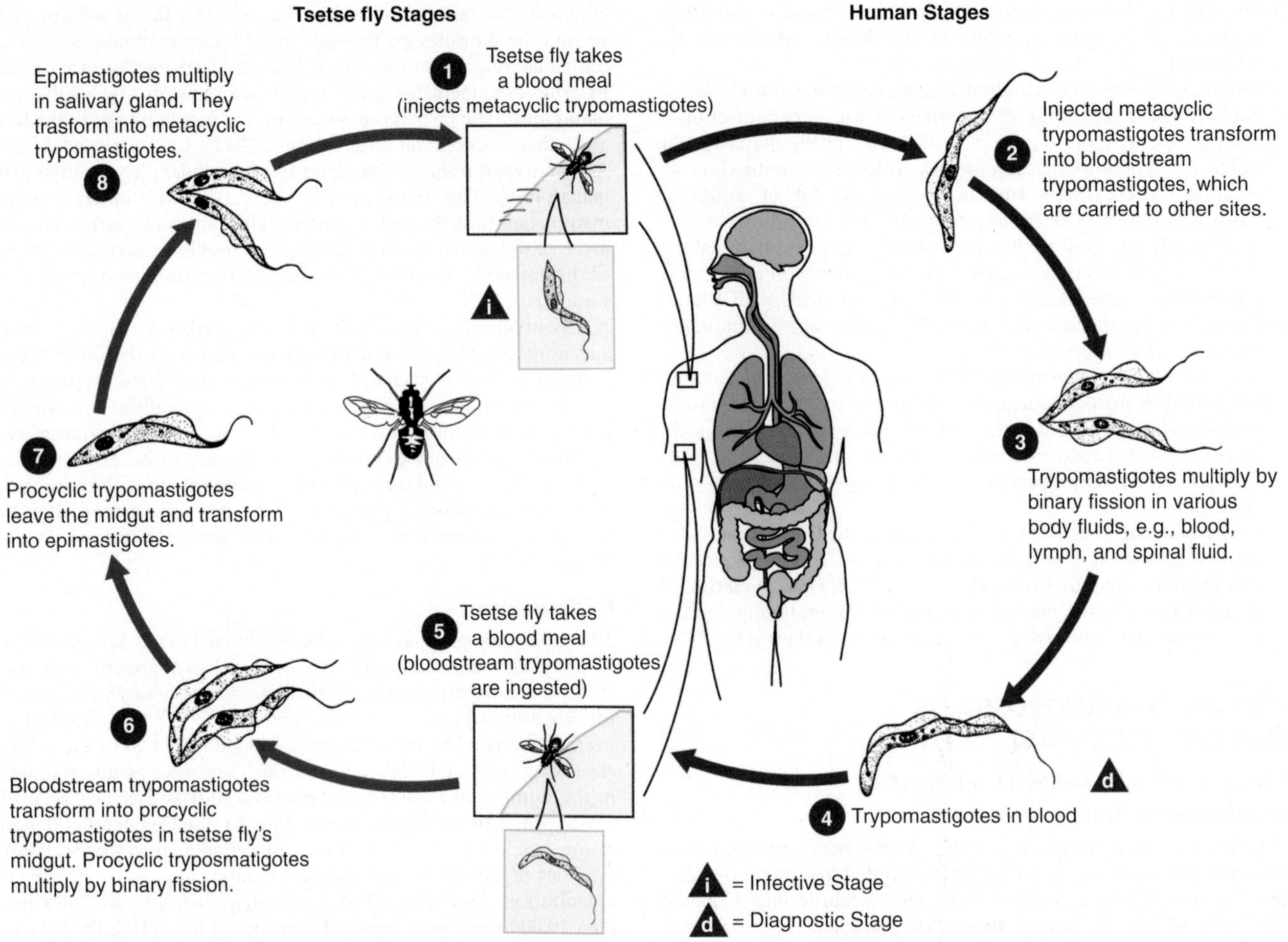

Tsetse fly Stages

Human Stages

1 Tsetse fly takes a blood meal (injects metacyclic trypomastigotes)

2 Injected metacyclic trypomastigotes transform into bloodstream trypomastigotes, which are carried to other sites.

3 Trypomastigotes multiply by binary fission in various body fluids, e.g., blood, lymph, and spinal fluid.

4 Trypomastigotes in blood

5 Tsetse fly takes a blood meal (bloodstream trypomastigotes are ingested)

6 Bloodstream trypomastigotes transform into procyclic trypomastigotes in tsetse fly's midgut. Procyclic tryposmatigotes multiply by binary fission.

7 Procyclic trypomastigotes leave the midgut and transform into epimastigotes.

8 Epimastigotes multiply in salivary gland. They trasform into metacyclic trypomastigotes.

i = Infective Stage

d = Diagnostic Stage

FIG. 222.11 Life cycle of *Trypanosoma brucei* in its insect vectors and mammalian hosts. (From Centers for Disease Control and Prevention, Atlanta, GA.)

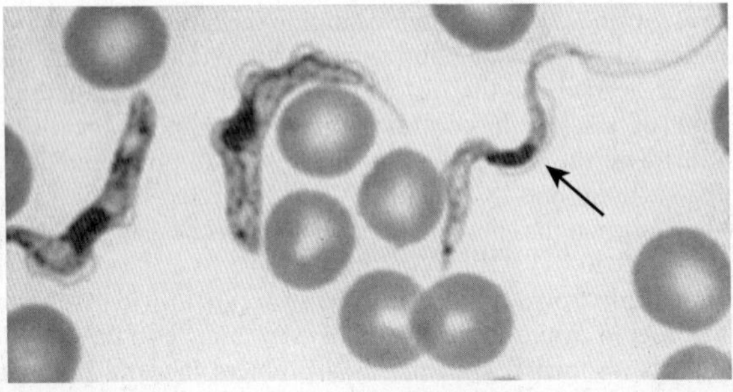

FIG. 222.12 *Trypanosoma brucei rhodesiense* parasites in rat blood. The slender parasite *(arrow)* is thought to be the form that multiplies in mammalian hosts, whereas the stumpy forms are nondividing and are capable of infecting insect vectors (Giemsa, ×1200). (From Kirchhoff LV. *Trypanosoma* species (American trypanosomiasis, Chagas' disease): biology of trypanosomes. In: Bennett JE, Dolin R, Blaser MJ, eds. *Mandell, Douglas, and Bennett's Principles and Practice of Infectious Diseases.* 8th ed. Philadelphia: Elsevier; 2015.)

Pathology and Clinical Manifestations

A painful inflammatory lesion (trypanosomal chancre) may appear a week or so after inoculation of the parasites through the bite of an infected tsetse fly. Systemic sleeping sickness without invasion of the CNS is referred to as stage 1 disease. In this stage, the parasites multiply as they disseminate through the lymphatics and bloodstream, and a systemic febrile illness develops. Typically, bouts of high temperatures lasting days are separated by periods without fever. There can be splenomegaly and widespread lymphadenopathy that can be prominent in stage 1 *T. b. gambiense* disease. The lymph nodes are often movable, discrete, and nontender. Cervical nodes are often readily apparent, and lymph node enlargement in the posterior cervical triangle, or Winterbottom sign, is a classic finding in *T. b. gambiense* disease. Maculopapular rashes and pruritus are common. Variable findings include headache, malaise, arthralgias, edema, weight loss, and tachycardia. These findings can develop in children as well as in adults.

Hematologic findings in stage 1 disease often include leukocytosis, anemia, and thrombocytopenia. In addition, high levels of immunoglobulins, consisting mainly of polyclonal IgM, as well as heterophile antibodies, anti-DNA antibodies, and rheumatoid factor, often are present. Inflammatory cytokines appear to have important roles in the pathogenesis of HAT.[101] Antigen-antibody complexes may play a role in vascular damage and increased permeability that facilitate dissemination of the parasites. Endarteritis, with perivascular infiltration of both lymphocytes and parasites, may develop in lymph nodes and the spleen. Myocarditis often develops in patients with stage 1 disease and is much more common in *T. b. rhodesiense* infections than in *T. b. gambiense* infections.

Stage 2 sleeping sickness is defined as invasion of the CNS by trypanosomes that is accompanied by the insidious appearance of a wide variety of signs and symptoms. With time a picture of progressive daytime somnolence and indifference can develop (hence the name "sleeping sickness"), sometimes alternating with insomnia and restlessness at night.[45,102] Speech may become halting and indistinct, and a listless gaze accompanies a loss of spontaneity. Extrapyramidal signs may include fasciculations, choreiform movements, and tremors. Ataxia is common, and the patients may appear to have Parkinson disease, with tremors, hypertonia, and a shuffling gait. In untreated patients, progressive neurologic impairment ends in coma and death.

The presence of parasites in perivascular areas in the CNS is accompanied by intense infiltration of mononuclear cells. Abnormalities in CSF can include increased intracranial pressure, increased total protein concentration, and pleocytosis. In addition, trypanosomes are frequently found in CSF in patients with stage 2 disease.

The most notable difference between the East African and West African forms of sleeping sickness is that the latter generally follows a more acute course. Typically, tourists with *rhodesiense* disease develop systemic signs of infection before returning home or shortly thereafter. As the illness progresses persistent tachycardia unrelated to fever is common in *T. b. rhodesiense* trypanosomiasis, and death may result from congestive heart failure and arrhythmias before stage 2 disease develops. In general, the historical record indicates that untreated *T. b. rhodesiense* trypanosomiasis can lead to death in a matter of weeks to months, sometimes without a clear distinction between the hemolymphatic and CNS stages. In contrast, *T. b. gambiense* infection persists subclinically for many months or even years before life-threatening neurologic manifestations develop. A comparison of the epidemiologic and clinical features of East and West African trypanosomiases is presented in Table 222.1.

Infants and Children

HAT may manifest in any age group. Abortion or perinatal death of infected babies may occur but not be reported as HAT. As noted, congenital transmission does occur but appears to be quite rare. Nonetheless, recommendations regarding the screening of pregnant women and the infants born to infected mothers in endemic areas have been published. In community screening programs women found to have HAT who are of childbearing age should undergo pregnancy testing. The newborns of mothers with HAT should be evaluated by parasitologic methods including examination of cord or other blood as early as possible. The card agglutination test for trypanosomes (CATT) should not be used in infants. If the result of initial testing in at-risk infants is negative, the test should be repeated in 6 months. In addition, because cases often occur in family clusters, all children in a family unit in which an infected adult has been identified should be evaluated for HAT even if they are asymptomatic. Overall, the incidence in young children appears to be lower than in adults.

Children with HAT may be asymptomatic or may present with nonspecific signs and symptoms that in general are similar to those observed initially in adults.[31,66,112] Lymphadenopathy is less frequently reported in children younger than 7 years compared with adults.[25] In infected small children headache, sleeping disorders, or motor weakness may be difficult to evaluate, and such findings may be accompanied by neuropsychiatric manifestations. There appears to be a higher incidence of stage 2 disease in children younger than 2 years of age. The reason may be that nonspecific clinical manifestations are difficult to differentiate from other common co-endemic febrile illnesses of childhood in endemic areas, such as malaria. This delay in diagnosis and treatment can result in CNS damage.

Diagnosis

In contrast to Chagas disease, a definitive diagnosis of sleeping sickness always requires detection of parasites.[26] In a patient at risk for sleeping sickness, the search can begin with microscopic examination of Giemsa-stained smears or wet preparations of fluid expressed from a chancre or aspirated from a lymph node. If no parasites are seen by these approaches, similar study of serial blood samples should be the next step. If no trypanosomes are seen initially in blood samples, microscopic examination of centrifuged microhematocrit tubes containing acridine orange or a buffy coat wet preparation may be useful. In general, the likelihood of finding parasites in blood is higher in patients with *T. b. rhodesiense* disease than in persons infected with *T. b. gambiense* and is greater in stage 1 disease than in stage 2. Parasites can sometimes be seen in bone marrow aspirates. In addition, this material can be inoculated into liquid culture medium, and lymph node aspirates, CSF, blood, and buffy coat can be processed similarly.

CSF must be examined in all patients suspected of having sleeping sickness. In a patient in whom parasites have been found in other sites, any abnormality in CSF parameters must be viewed as pathognomic for stage 2 disease and prompt the use of a treatment regimen appropriate for that stage. Parasites also may be seen in the pellet of spun CSF. In at-risk patients with abnormal CSF parameters in whom trypanosomes have not been found, HIV-associated CNS infections such as cryptococcosis and tuberculous meningitis should be included in the differential diagnosis.

Several serologic tests, such as CATT, for *T. b. gambiense*, are commercially available.[44,97,199] Their ease of use makes them valuable for epidemiologic surveys, but their variable sensitivity and specificity restrict their use to surveys, and decisions regarding the treatment of individual patients must be based on parasitologic diagnoses. New serologic assays are being developed.[21,170] Sensitive and specific PCR assays for detecting African trypanosomes in humans have been developed and when available can be productively used to examine all the samples mentioned earlier,[150] and other molecular assays are in the pipeline.[29,81,141] Unfortunately, however, in most endemic areas the lack of necessary technical and human resources stands in the way of the widespread use of these methods.

Treatment

The drugs used for treatment of HAT are pentamidine, suramin, eflornithine, melarsoprol, and nifurtimox (see Table 222.2). In the United States, these drugs can only be obtained from the CDC Drug Service (404-639-3670). Therapy for HAT must be individualized on the basis of the infecting subspecies, the stage of the infection, adverse reactions, and rarely drug resistance. Guidance for the use of these drugs for treating HAT is presented Table 222.2.

Pentamidine is the drug of choice for treating stage 1 *gambiense* HAT. The dose for adults as well as children is 4 mg/kg per day, given intramuscularly or intravenously for 7 to 10 days. Common, immediate adverse reactions include nausea, vomiting, hypotension, and tachycardia. These reactions are usually transient and do not warrant cessation of treatment. Other adverse reactions include nephrotoxicity, abnormal liver function tests, neutropenia, hypoglycemia, rashes, and sterile abscesses. Suramin is an alternative for stage 1 *T. b. gambiense* infection.

Suramin is highly effective against stage 1 *rhodesiense* HAT. It can cause serious adverse effects, however, and must be given under the close supervision of a physician. A 100- to 200-mg intravenous dose should be given initially to test for hypersensitivity. The dosage for adults is 20 mg/kg on days 1, 5, 12, 18, and 26. Suramin is given by slow intravenous infusion of a freshly prepared 10% aqueous solution. Roughly one patient in 20,000 has an immediate, severe, and potentially fatal reaction to the drug that can involve nausea, vomiting, shock, and seizures. Less severe reactions include photophobia, fever, arthralgias, pruritus, and skin eruptions. Nephrotoxicity is the most common important side effect of suramin, and transient proteinuria frequently appears during treatment. Urinalysis should be performed before each dose, and therapy should be discontinued if proteinuria increases or if

TABLE 222.2 Drugs Recommended for Treatment of the African Trypanosomiases

	CLINICAL STAGE	
Causative Agent	**1**	**2**
Trypanosoma brucei gambiense	Pentamidine	Eflornithine
	Alternative: suramin	Alternatives: eflornithine/nifurtimox; melarsoprol
Trypanosoma brucei rhodesiense	Suramin	Melarsoprol

From Kirchhoff LV. Agents of African trypanosomiasis (sleeping sickness). In: Bennett JE, Dolin R, Blaser MJ, eds. *Mandell, Douglas, and Bennett's Principles and Practice of Infectious Diseases.* 8th ed. Philadelphia: Elsevier; 2015.

red blood cells and casts appear in the sediment. Suramin should not be given to patients with any degree of renal insufficiency.

Eflornithine is highly effective for treating both stages of *gambiense* HAT. In the trials on which the FDA based its approval, eflornithine cured more than 90% of 600 patients with stage 2 *T. b. gambiense* disease. The recommended dosage schedule is 400 mg/kg per day, given intravenously in four divided doses, for 2 weeks. Adverse reactions include diarrhea, anemia, thrombocytopenia, seizures, and hearing loss. The high dosage and length of therapy required are serious disadvantages that make the widespread use of eflornithine a challenge. A randomized trial comparing the standard eflornithine regimen (400 mg/kg per day infused over 6 hours for 14 days) with nifurtimox-eflornithine combination therapy (oral nifurtimox, 15 mg/kg per day in three divided doses, plus intravenous eflornithine, 200 mg/kg per day in two divided doses, both for 7 days) in adults with stage 2 *gambiense* HAT showed greater efficacy and reduced side effects with combination therapy, thereby making this approach suitable for first-line use.

The arsenical melarsoprol is the drug of choice for the treatment of *T. b. rhodesiense* HAT with CNS involvement (stage 2 disease) and is an alternative agent for stage 2 *gambiense* disease.[7] The "short course" of melarsoprol that is currently recommended has been shown to be noninferior to the decades-old course of therapy for *T. b. rhodesiense*, which was administered over several weeks and was much more toxic.[22,46] The recommended short-course regimen involves melarsoprol in 10 daily doses of 2.2 mg/kg intravenously, each dose given with prednisolone (1 mg/kg).

Melarsoprol is very toxic and should be administered with close medical supervision. As noted, patients being treated with melarsoprol should also receive prednisolone to reduce the likelihood of drug-induced encephalopathy.[24,151] Without prednisolone prophylaxis, the incidence of reactive encephalopathy in treated patients was as high as 18% in some studies. Signs of reactive encephalopathy include high fever, tremor, headache, seizures, impaired speech, and even coma and death. Treatment with melarsoprol should be stopped at the first sign of encephalopathy but can be resumed cautiously at lower doses a few days after signs have resolved. Extravasation of the drug results in serious local reactions. Abdominal pain, vomiting, nephrotoxicity, and myocardial damage can occur as well.

Prevention

Trypanosomiasis in Africa has long presented complex enzootic and public health challenges. As noted earlier, enormous progress has been made in endemic areas through programs that focus on vector control, combined with early diagnosis and treatment of infected persons. In more recent years, increasingly integrated programs run by the WHO, along with its governmental and nongovernmental partners, have served as a framework for advancing the control of tsetse fly populations and for reducing transmission to humans, and the number of reported cases has reached historic lows. Major elements underlying the optimism regarding the ultimate elimination of HAT are the facts that humans are the only important reservoirs for *T. b. gambiense* and that 98% of HAT cases currently reported are caused by *T. b. gambiense.* Importantly, moreover, although many challenges lie ahead, no major scientific discoveries are necessary for the elimination of HAT. In this context, there is no doubt that, barring major political and economic upheavals in the endemic countries, HAT is headed for the history books. The process of its elimination likely will be facilitated by the application of new technologies, such as the electronic geospatial database, HAT-Atlas,[182] and progress additionally may be enhanced by the development of novel rapid individual diagnostic tests,[30] as well as simple oral treatment regimens.[196] Based on successes of the control programs, in 2009 a panel of experts convened by the WHO developed a vision for the elimination of sleeping sickness, and in 2012 the WHO Neglected Tropical Diseases Roadmap targeted the elimination of sleeping sickness as a public health problem by 2020.[71,103,118,181,183,192,200]

Tourists can reduce their risk of becoming infected with African trypanosomes by avoiding areas known to be endemic or enzootic and by using insect repellent along with protective clothing. Neither chemoprophylaxis nor a vaccine is available to prevent transmission of the parasites.

SELECTED REFERENCES

4. Alvarez MG, Bertocchi GL, Cooley G, et al. Treatment success in *Trypanosoma cruzi* infection is predicted by early changes in serially monitored parasite-specific T and B cell responses. *PLoS Negl Trop Dis.* 2016;10(4):e0004657.
7. Balasegaram M, Young H, Chappuis F, et al. Effectiveness of melarsoprol and eflornithine as first-line regimens for *gambiense* sleeping sickness in nine Medecins Sans Frontieres programmes. *Trans R Soc Trop Med Hyg.* 2009;103(3):280-290.
13. Bern C, Martin DL, Gilman RH. Acute and congenital Chagas disease. *Adv Parasitol.* 2011;75:19-47.
14. Bern C, Montgomery SP, Herwaldt BL, et al. Evaluation and treatment of Chagas disease in the United States: a systematic review. *JAMA.* 2007;298(18):2171-2181.
22. Bisser S, N'Siesi FX, Lejon V, et al. Equivalence trial of melarsoprol and nifurtimox monotherapy and combination therapy for the treatment of second-stage *Trypanosoma brucei gambiense* sleeping sickness. *J Infect Dis.* 2007;195(3):322-329.
25. Blum J, Schmid C, Burri C. Clinical aspects of 2541 patients with second stage human African trypanosomiasis. *Acta Trop.* 2006;97(1):55-64.
31. Buyst H. Sleeping sickness in children. *Ann Soc Belge Med Trop.* 1977;57:201-212.
32. Cantey PT, Stramer SL, Kamel H, et al. The U.S. *Trypanosoma cruzi* Infection Study: evidence for autochthonous *Trypanosoma cruzi* transmission among United States blood donors (abstract S70-030F). *Transfusion.* 2010;50(suppl):32A.
43. Chang CD, Cheng KY, Jiang L, et al. Evaluation of a prototype *Trypanosoma cruzi* antibody assay with recombinant antigens on a fully automated chemiluminescence analyzer for blood donor screening. *Transfusion.* 2006;46(10):1737-1744.
47. Cheng KY, Chang CD, Salbilla VA, et al. Immunoblot assay using recombinant antigens as a supplemental test to confirm antibodies to *Trypanosoma cruzi. Clin Vaccine Immunol.* 2007;14(4):355-361.
66. Eperon G, Schmid C, Loutan L, et al. Clinical presentation and treatment outcome of sleeping sickness in Sudanese pre-school children. *Acta Trop.* 2007;101(1):31-39.
67. Fabbro DL, Danesi E, Olivera V, et al. Trypanocide treatment of women infected with *Trypanosoma cruzi* and its effect on preventing congenital Chagas. *PLoS Negl Trop Dis.* 2014;8(11):e3312.
81. Hayashida K, Kajino K, Hachaambwa L, et al. Direct blood dry LAMP: a rapid, stable, and easy diagnostic tool for human African trypanosomiasis. *PLoS Negl Trop Dis.* 2015;9(3):e0003578.
86. Hidron A, Vogenthaler N, Santos-Preciado JI, et al. Cardiac involvement with parasitic infections. *Clin Microbiol Rev.* 2010;23(2):324-349.
102. Kato CD, Nanteza A, Mugasa C, et al. Clinical profiles, disease outcome and co-morbidities among *T. b. rhodesiense* sleeping sickness patients in Uganda. *PLoS ONE.* 2015;10(2):e0118370.
103. Keating J, Yukich JO, Sutherland CS, et al. Human African trypanosomiasis prevention, treatment and control costs: a systematic review. *Acta Trop.* 2015;150:4-13.
109. Kirchhoff LV, Paredes P, Lomeli-Guerrero A, et al. Transfusion-associated Chagas' disease (American trypanosomiasis) in Mexico: implications for transfusion medicine in the United States. *Transfusion.* 2006;46(2):298-304.
115. Lara Romero C, Ferreiro Arguelles B, Romero Perez E. Acute colonic complications in a patient with Chagas disease. *Rev Esp Enferm Dig.* 2016;108.
118. Lehane M, Alfaroukh I, Bucheton B, et al. Tsetse control and the elimination of Gambian sleeping sickness. *PLoS Negl Trop Dis.* 2016;10(4):e0004437.
125. Lucero RH, Bruses BL, Cura CI, et al. Chagas' disease in Aboriginal and Creole communities from the Gran Chaco region of Argentina: seroprevalence and molecular parasitological characterization. *Infect Genet Evol.* 2016;41:84-92.
127. Maguire JH. Treatment of Chagas' disease—time is running out. *N Engl J Med.* 2015;373(14):1369-1370.
138. Morillo CA, Marin-Neto JA, Avezum A, et al. Randomized trial of benznidazole for chronic Chagas' cardiomyopathy. *N Engl J Med.* 2015;373(14):1295-1306.
141. Mumba Ngoyi D, Ali Ekangu R, Mumvemba Kodi MF, et al. Performance of parasitological and molecular techniques for the diagnosis and surveillance of *gambiense* sleeping sickness. *PLoS Negl Trop Dis.* 2014;8(6):e2954.
147. Otani MM, Vinelli E, Kirchhoff LV, et al. WHO comparative evaluation of serologic assays for Chagas disease. *Transfusion.* 2009;49:1076-1082.
153. Pinazo MJ, Espinosa G, Cortes-Lletget C, et al. Immunosuppression and Chagas disease: a management challenge. *PLoS Negl Trop Dis.* 2013;7(1):e1965.
156. Praast G, Herzogenrath J, Bernhardt S, et al. Evaluation of the Abbott ARCHITECT Chagas prototype assay. *Diagn Microbiol Infect Dis.* 2011;69(1):74-81.
159. Rassi A Jr, Rassi A, Marcondes de Rezende J. American trypanosomiasis (Chagas disease). *Infect Dis Clin North Am.* 2012;26(2):275-291.
158. Rassi A Jr, Rassi A. Another disappointing result with implantable cardioverter-defibrillator therapy in patients with Chagas disease. *Europace.* 2013;15(9):1383.
178. Schijman AG, Bisio M, Orellana L, et al. International study to evaluate PCR methods for detection of *Trypanosoma cruzi* DNA in blood samples from Chagas disease patients. *PLoS Negl Trop Dis.* 2011;5(1):e931.

181. Simarro PP, Cecchi G, Franco JR, et al. Monitoring the progress towards the elimination of *gambiense* human African trypanosomiasis. *PLoS Negl Trop Dis.* 2015;9(6):e0003785.
184. Simarro PP, Franco JR, Cecchi G, et al. Human African trypanosomiasis in non-endemic countries (2000-2010). *J Travel Med.* 2012;19(1):44-53.
204. Villar JC, Perez JG, Cortes OL, et al. Trypanocidal drugs for chronic asymptomatic *Trypanosoma cruzi* infection. *Cochrane Database Syst Rev.* 2014;(5):CD003463.
205. Wagner N, Jackson Y, Chappuis F, et al. Screening and management of children at risk for Chagas disease in nonendemic areas. *Pediatr Infect Dis J.* 2016;35(3):335-337.

The full reference list for this chapter is available at ExpertConsult.com.

Naegleria, Acanthamoeba, and *Balamuthia* Infections 223

Tina Q. Tan

Interest in free-living amebae has increased since demonstration of their pathogenicity and, more recently, their role as reservoirs and vectors for potentially pathogenic bacteria, such as *Legionella pneumophila, Vibrio* spp., *Listeria* spp., and *Mycobacterium avium.* Small free-living amebae of the genera *Naegleria, Acanthamoeba,* and *Balamuthia* cause severe central nervous system (CNS) infections in humans and animals that are characterized by few distinguishing symptoms and an almost uniformly poor prognosis. Although these severe infections are uncommon, for optimal treatment it is important to recognize and diagnose them early.[153,158]

Although small free-living amebae share structural and pathogenic similarities, the infections they cause have distinctive epidemiology, clinical presentation and course, neuroimaging, immunology, and pathology. Primary amebic meningoencephalitis caused by *Naegleria fowleri* is an acute fulminant illness that affects healthy children and young adults and usually results in death within 1 week of presentation. Almost invariably, the patient has a recent history of swimming in bodies of warm fresh water, although there are recent reports of acquiring the infection through nasal irrigation using a neti pot sinus rinse. In contrast, granulomatous amebic encephalitis caused by *Acanthamoeba* spp. or *Balamuthia mandrillaris* (formerly leptomyxid amebae) is an insidious, subacute, and protracted illness that affects primarily, but not exclusively, immunocompromised or debilitated patients and leads to death in weeks to months. Typically, the patient has no history of recent exposure to fresh water. One other species of ameba belonging to the genus *Sappinia* has also been identified as a cause of severe encephalitis.[154]

Despite these differences, the prognosis of CNS infection caused by *N. fowleri, Acanthamoeba* spp., and *B. mandrillaris* is similarly dismal, with few reports of survival. In the handful of cases that survived from the hundreds reported, recognition, early diagnosis, and timely administration of appropriate antimicrobial treatment were crucial to achieving a successful outcome. *Acanthamoeba* spp. also are associated with disseminated cutaneous, pulmonary, or sinus infection in immunocompromised hosts and with chronic painful and potentially sight-threatening keratitis in association with use of contact lenses or corneal trauma in otherwise healthy patients.

The pathogenic potential of small free-living amebae was recognized first during polio vaccine trials in the 1950s, when they were found to cause cytotoxicity in contaminated cell cultures.[29,64] Subsequently, the fulminant fatal encephalitis that followed intracerebral injection or intranasal instillation of tissue culture fluid in experimental mice and monkeys showed pathogenicity and a potential route for human infection.[22,28,29] The first cases of human infection caused by small free-living amebae were recognized in four children from southern Australia by Fowler and Carter[46] in 1965 and soon afterward by Butt[14] in Florida.

More recently, Visvesvara and colleagues[157,159] isolated and named *B. mandrillaris,* a new agent of amebic meningoencephalitis, from the brain of a mandrill baboon. The first reported human case of *B. mandrillaris* encephalitis was in a patient with acquired immunodeficiency syndrome (AIDS).[3] Reports of infection in immunocompetent hosts have followed.[7,36,48,70,117] Subsequently, infections caused by free-living amebae have been reported worldwide.[4,72,86,87,97,120] Finally, the first case report of nonfatal CNS disease, in an otherwise healthy adult, caused by *Sappinia diploidea,* a free-living ameba normally found in soil contaminated with elk and buffalo dung, adds to the list of pathogenic small free-living amebae and suggests that others may be identified in the future.[51,110,161]

EPIDEMIOLOGY

Pathogenic and opportunistic free-living amebae are found worldwide and are cosmopolitan in their distribution, living primarily in soil, but also in seawater, drinking water, swimming pools, sewage, eyewash solutions, contact lenses, dialysis units, dental treatment units, in dust, inside vertebrates, on plants, and in the air.[38,102,116,135] They are spread readily by wind and water currents. In humans, infection with free-living amebae causes primary amebic meningoencephalitis, granulomatous amebic meningoencephalitis, disseminated granulomatous disease (cutaneous, pulmonary, kidney, or sinus), and keratitis.[86,87,130]

Although they are rare, cases of infection caused by *N. fowleri* have been reported throughout the world.[45] As of 2015, well over 200 cases of primary amebic encephalitis have been documented worldwide, with approximately half occurring in the United States.[25,130] In the United States between 1962 and 2008, 135 fatal cases of primary amebic meningoencephalitis were reported to the Centers for Disease Control and Prevention (CDC).[101,169] Most of them occurred in the summer and in young children. Increased water temperatures, whether from thermal pollution or sunlight, provide the ideal environment for proliferation of *N. fowleri.*[148,162] Cases typically are associated with a history of swimming, diving, or playing in bodies of warm fresh water, brackish habitats with a soil and water interface, artificial lakes, hot springs, and thermally polluted rivers and streams.[25,32,45,90,101,148] Researchers have postulated that thermal pollution, particularly from overflow of power plants, or inadequate chlorination of water kills off normal thermosensitive and chlorine-sensitive fauna, shifting the balance in favor of thermotolerant, less chlorine-sensitive, pathogenic *N. fowleri.*[130] In North America, cases of primary amebic meningoencephalitis tend to be clustered in the warmer southern states and Mexico.[130] In one study, almost 50% of freshwater lakes in Florida contained *N. fowleri* when the temperature was 30°C or higher.[162] *N. fowleri* may be found in colder areas, however. In temperate regions, distribution of *N. fowleri* is limited by seasons, being greatest during summer and early fall.[148] *N. fowleri, Acanthamoeba* spp., and *B. mandrillaris* were present year-round in lakes in the Tulsa region of Oklahoma.[67] Although it is most prevalent in areas where water temperatures are higher, *N. fowleri* has the ability to overwinter, in cyst form, in sediment at the bottom of lakes.[162] Cases of fatal *N. fowleri* infection acquired in Minnesota have been reported.[73]

Small outbreaks of primary amebic meningoencephalitis have been described. Over a 3-year period, from 1962 to 1965, 16 swimmers died after being exposed to warm contaminated and inadequately chlorinated water in an indoor pool in Czechoslovakia.[18,130] Similarly, eight cases of fulminant meningoencephalitis associated with exposure to the water of an artificial lake in Richmond, Virginia, were recognized retrospectively as being caused by *N. fowleri.*[16] Finally, five cases of primary amebic meningoencephalitis caused by *N. fowleri* occurred in 1990 in people swimming in a drainage canal in Mexicali, Mexico.[80]

Disease also has been documented in patients with no history of exposure to fresh water. Atypical exposures have included bathing in domestic bath water, playing in a warm muddy puddle, and being baptized by full-body immersion.[4,9,89] *N. fowleri* also has been shown in domestic tap water.[39,89] Although cases of infection have not followed ingestion of drinking water contaminated by amebae, fatal infection was associated with washing in tap water heated to high temperatures in pipes by the summer sun in South Australia and with exposure to contaminated domestic water in Arizona.[2,39,89] Recently, the CDC reported the first case of fatal primary amebic meningoencephalitis, occurring in a 4-year-old child, associated with culturable *N. fowleri* in tap water from a treated public drinking water system. The only water exposure that this child had was the water in a lawn water slide on which they had played.[26]

Infections occur far more frequently in previously healthy children and young adults than in other age groups, presumably because youngsters are most likely to remain in water for prolonged periods and to disturb sediment containing amebae by diving and swimming underwater.[25,101] In one series of primary amebic meningoencephalitis cases, boys outnumbered girls 12 to 1, presumably because boys are more likely than girls to engage in aquatic horseplay.[156] The incubation period in natural human infection is 2 to 15 days after exposure.[9,25,101] Death usually ensues within 1 week of presentation (generally within 72 hours).

Acanthamoeba spp. are among the most prevalent protozoa found in the environment, being found in soils from tropical to arctic regions. They are important components of the food chain and promote plant growth by predation on soil bacteria. *Acanthamoeba* spp. are prevalent in natural and artificial habitats that include fresh, brackish, sea, potable, or stagnant water; in sewage; in improperly treated swimming pools; and in taps, sinks, hot tubs, air-conditioning units, aquaria, flowerpots, showers, dialysis units, dental units, ventilators, and ventilation units in homes and hospitals.[19,43,87,127,130] Although warm waters might enhance their numbers, pathogenic amebae may be isolated year-round from water samples in the United States.[162] Their distribution and viability are governed primarily by availability of a bacterial food source; soil texture; water temperature, pH, and salinity and by ultraviolet light and desiccation.[116,130] Growth of *Acanthamoeba* spp. is inhibited by temperatures of 35°C to 39°C. Although *Acanthamoeba* spp. seemingly are ubiquitous in water, *Acanthamoeba* infections generally are not associated with a history of recent swimming or water activities.[130] Acquisition occurs by inhalation or direct contact with contaminated soil or water.

In contrast to *N. fowleri, Acanthamoeba* spp. are opportunistic pathogens. Granulomatous amebic encephalitis and disseminated disease caused by *Acanthamoeba* spp. generally are seen in immunocompromised hosts or in patients with underlying disease or debilitation, such as that due to malignancy, cancer chemotherapy, corticosteroid treatment, organ transplantation, human immunodeficiency virus, diabetes, or malnutrition.[86,87] *Acanthamoeba* spp. cause keratitis in otherwise healthy individuals by directly attacking the corneal surface, usually in association with poor contact lens care or corneal trauma. Although cases of CNS or disseminated *Acanthamoeba* infection are extremely rare, in 2015, the estimated prevalence of amebic keratitis worldwide was one to nine per 100,000.[85,130] However, in recent years, the number of *Acanthamoeba* keratitis cases has been increasing in developing countries, correlating with the increased number of contact lens wearers.

Comparatively less is known about *B. mandrillaris.* It is closely related to *Acanthamoeba* and causes a similar spectrum of infections that includes granulomatous amebic encephalitis and cutaneous and sinus disease.[130] Although initial cases of *B. mandrillaris* infection were confined to immunocompromised and debilitated hosts, its ability to cause disease in apparently healthy children is well documented.[7,36,49,70,117] By 2012, more than 200 cases of human infection had been reported.[12,84,130] *Balamuthia* inhabits soil and water; it has been isolated in soil from a flowerpot associated with a case of amebic encephalitis in a child from northern California.[123]

As with *Acanthamoeba* spp., granulomatous encephalitis caused by *B. mandrillaris* seems to occur after inhalation of airborne cysts or soil contamination of breaks in the skin. The patient generally has no history of recent exposure to fresh water. To date, 50% of cases of *Balamuthia* infection reported in the United States have occurred in patients of Hispanic ethnicity.[7,125] The majority of cases worldwide have also been reported in children and young men of Hispanic ethnicity. Although this statistic most likely is a result of environmental exposure, a genetic predisposition may exist. Among California cases of balamuthiasis, most cluster in the southern part of the state. Researchers have postulated that the area's dry, warm soil is conducive for the amebae and that large-scale agriculture in these areas increases the likelihood of workers being exposed to soil or wind-blown particles. Cases of *B. mandrillaris* infection linked directly to incidental exposure to soil or to blowing soil while traveling in an open car or by motorcycle are reported.[36,70,123,127] Although *Balamuthia* encephalitis is a zoonosis, animals do not represent a source of infection for humans.

Despite their seeming ubiquity in the environment and ample opportunity for contact with humans compared with other parasitic protozoa, such as *Entamoeba,* malaria and trypanosome infections caused by free-living amebae are extremely rare. Given the enormous number of exposures to water containing *Naegleria,* why so few individuals become infected remains unknown. Only seven cases of primary amebic meningoencephalitis were reported in Florida during a 14-year period, despite estimates of billions of potential exposures in contaminated freshwater lakes during that time period.[162] Epidemiologic investigations of cases typically find that many other individuals swam in the same water at the same time but did not become ill. Factors other than the presence of amebae, such as host susceptibility, anatomy, inoculum size, and activity at the time of exposure, have been implicated.[162] Nonetheless, in recent years, an increase in the number of diagnoses of primary amebic meningoencephalitis cases has been noted.[82,168] The increase probably reflects a combination of greater recognition of the pathogenic potential of free-living amebae, improved diagnostic techniques, and a growth in the numbers of immunocompromised hosts.

Acanthamoeba organisms can infect the cornea directly, after trauma, or, most commonly, in association with the combination of extended-wear soft contact lens use and subsequent exposure to contaminated water.[132,143] Major risk factors for development of amebic keratitis include poor compliance with care of daily-wear soft contact lenses, particularly use of homemade saline solutions using nonsterile tap water that may be contaminated with amebae; use of chlorine release lens disinfection systems; and inadequate cleansing of lens cases, which encourages growth of a bacterial biofilm that acts as a nidus and a food source for amebae.[113,142] Wearing contact lenses while swimming or in hot tubs, which potentially may be contaminated with amebae, is similarly risky.[118]

Since the first cases of amebic keratitis were described in the early 1970s, the incidence has increased dramatically. Between 1973 and 1984, slightly more than 200 cases of amebic keratitis were reported to the CDC. By 2002, in the United States, more than 3000 cases had been reported and 1 in 250,000 people were estimated to be affected.[68,79,105,130] The increased incidence most likely is due to increased use of contact lenses, particularly of the soft, extended-wear variety. Although many of these lenses were marketed as products requiring "low care," many patients interpreted this designation as meaning "no care."[113]

ORGANISMS

In contrast to the related true parasite protozoa *Entamoeba* spp., *Naegleria, Acanthamoeba,* and *Balamuthia* spp. are amphizoic protozoa, capable of existing as free-living amebae and as parasitic pathogens.[130] *Naegleria* spp. are ameboflagellates found primarily in moist soil and warm fresh water.[90] Although more than 27 separate *Naegleria* spp. have been identified, to date only *N. fowleri* is associated with human infections.[32,130] *Naegleria* spp. can exist in three forms: an active feeding trophozoite, a rarely seen dormant cyst (Fig. 223.1), and a flagellate form (Fig. 223.2).[90]

Of these forms, only the trophozoite is found in tissue or cerebrospinal fluid (CSF). The trophozoite of *N. fowleri* is smaller than that of *Acanthamoeba* spp., measuring 8 to 15 μm in diameter, with a conspicuous nucleus containing a large, dense central karyosome without peripheral chromatin lining the membrane.[94] *Naegleria* trophozoites move slowly by extension of broad, rounded anterior pseudopodia (lobopodia). This feature may be noted on a warm saline preparation or in CSF specimens. *Naegleria* cysts are spherical, measure 7 to 12 μm in diameter, and have a single-layered outer membrane.

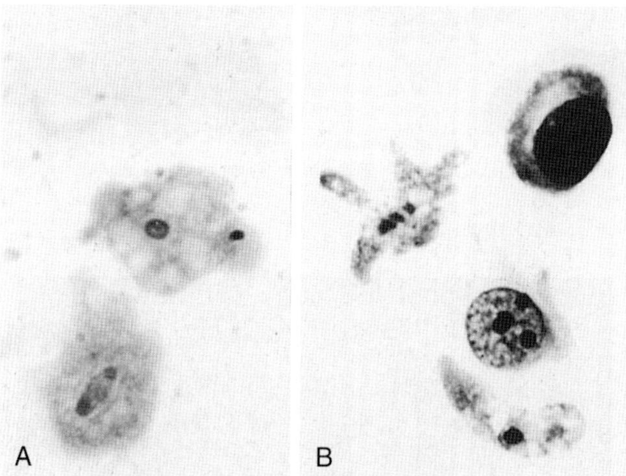

FIG. 223.1 Trophozoites of *Naegleria.*

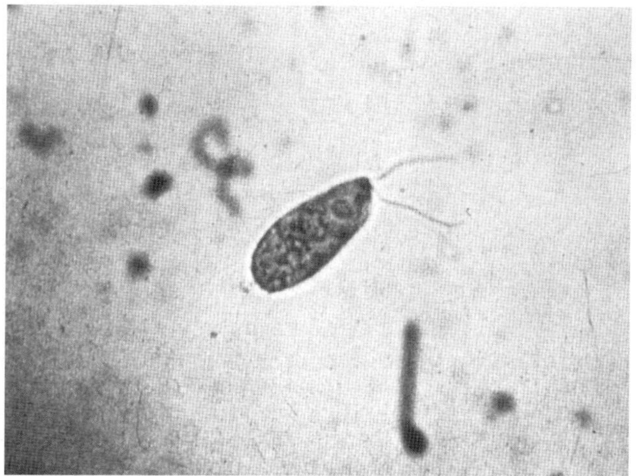

FIG. 223.2 Flagellate form of *Naegleria fowleri.*

Approximately 20 *Acanthamoeba* spp. are identified by morphologic criteria.[130] Because morphologic distinctions do not always correlate with results of molecular typing, however, classification is complex and is currently under review.[87] Molecular classification is ongoing. The life cycle of *Acanthamoeba* spp. consists of two stages: an actively feeding and dividing trophozoite and a dormant cyst stage (Fig. 223.3).[107] The trophozoite is 15 to 40 μm. The nucleus is vesicular; has a large, dense central "targetoid" nucleolus; and is surrounded by vacuolated cytoplasm. Locomotion typically is sluggish, by extrusion of multiple fine spiny pseudopodia (acanthopodia).[94] *Acanthamoeba* trophozoites feed on bacteria, yeasts, and algae. *Acanthamoeba* cysts are smaller, 15 to 20 μm, with a distinct, wrinkled, thick double wall. Encystation occurs in response to adverse environmental conditions, such as desiccation, scarcity of food, and changes in pH or temperature. *Acanthamoeba* cysts are particularly hardy; they are intrinsically resistant to chlorination and sterilization of potable water, to biocides used for disinfecting bronchoscopes and contact lenses, and to antibiotics; they may remain viable for decades after freezing.[34,76,99] *Acanthamoeba* is the only pathogenic free-living species isolated from marine water. *Naegleria* spp. do not tolerate sea water.

Few *Acanthamoeba* spp. have been associated with human infections. Among the potentially pathogenic species, *Acanthamoeba culbertsoni, Acanthamoeba castellanii, Acanthamoeba astronyxis,* and *Acanthamoeba polyphaga* are prominent.[97] On the basis of 18S rRNA gene sequences, *Acanthamoeba* spp. are divided into 15 genotypes (T1 through T15). At present, no clear consensus has been reached regarding which genotypes are pathogenic. Genotypes T1, T4, T7, T10, and T12 are found among cases of granulomatous encephalitis, whereas isolates associated with keratitis fall into genotypes T3, T4, and T11.[11,44,87,145] Genotype T4 makes up 94% and 80% of keratitis and nonkeratitis *Acanthamoeba* isolates, respectively,[11] presumably reflecting the preponderance of this genotype in the environment. Rare genotypes, such as T1, T10, and T12, are found only in CNS disease and are not found in the environment.

B. mandrillaris is the only pathogenic *Balamuthia* spp. identified to date.[130,136] It exists as either an active trophozoite or a dormant cyst (Fig. 223.4). The cysts are highly resistant to physical and chemical conditions. Trophozoites are similar in appearance to *Acanthamoeba* spp. but larger (50 to 60 μm in diameter), and the spherical cyst stage (10 to 30 μm in diameter) has a triple-layered wall on electron microscopy consisting of an outer thin and irregular ectocyst, an inner thick endocyst, and a middle amorphous fibrillary mesocyst. *Balamuthia* trophozoites typically have a single vesicular nucleus, often with multiple large, dense nucleoli. Movement occurs by extension of broad pseudopodia. *Balamuthia* has been isolated more recently from environmental soil samples.[41] Because of its slow growth, it may have been obscured in environmental cultures by overgrowth of more rapidly growing bacteria, fungi, or other amebae. In contrast to *Naegleria* and *Acanthamoeba* spp., *Balamuthia* feeds on smaller amebae and protozoa and does not prey on bacteria.

Sappinia diploidea is a species of free-living ameba that is found worldwide and has been isolated from soil, fresh water, forest litter, and

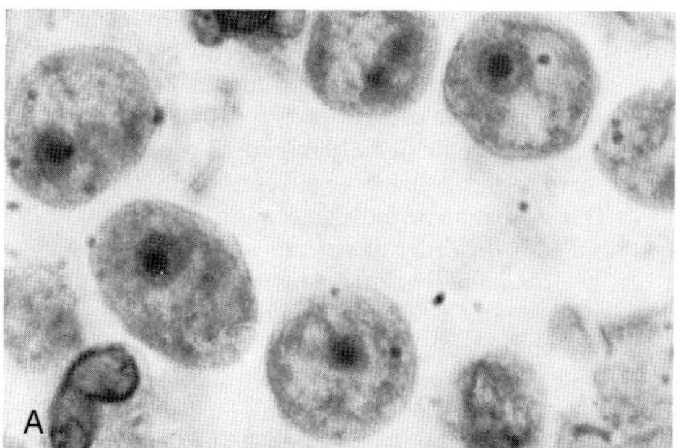

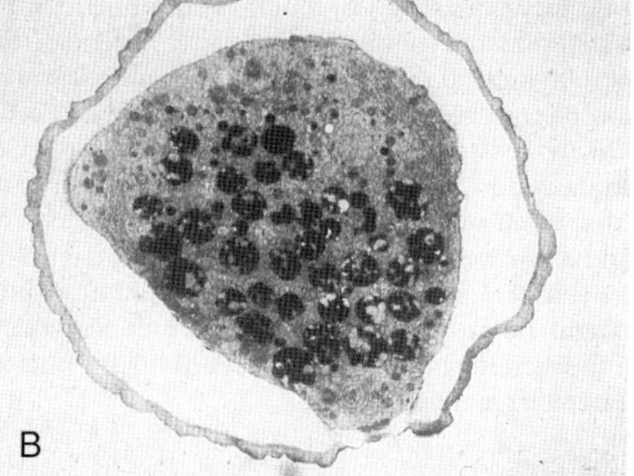

FIG. 223.3 (A) Trophozoite of *Acanthamoeba.* (B) Cyst of *Acanthamoeba* (scanning electron micrograph). (A, From Jager BV, Stamm WP. Brain abscesses caused by free-living amoeba probably of the genus *Hartmannella* living in a patient with Hodgkin disease. *Lancet* 1972;2:1343-5.)

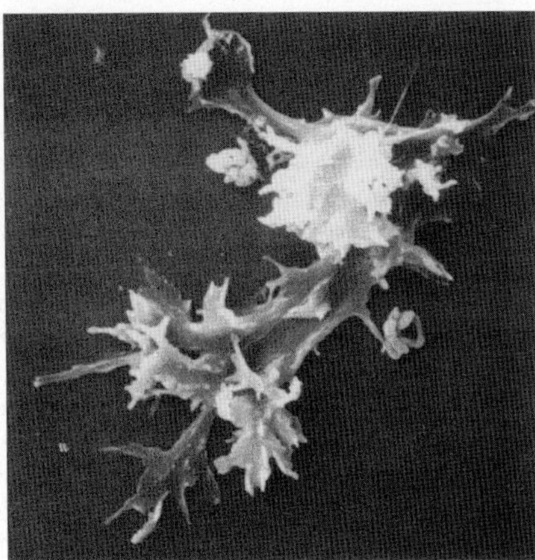
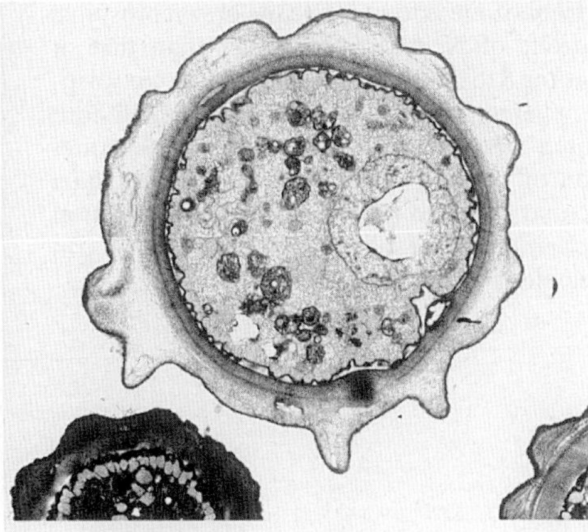

FIG. 223.4 Trophozoite and cyst of *Balamuthia mandrillaris*. (Courtesy Dr. G.S. Visvesvara, Centers for Disease Control and Prevention.)

mammalian feces. The life cycle of this organism involves animal feces. Both the trophozoite and cyst stages are binucleate. The trophozoites are 40 to 80 μm in diameter and can be distinguished by the presence of a large cytoplasmic contractile vacuole and food vacuoles, mitochondria with characteristic tubular crystal patterns, a juxtanuclear Golgi-like network, and a double nucleus.[51] The cyst is round and measures 15 to 30 μm.[161]

CLINICAL MANIFESTATIONS

Naegleria Fowleri

Primary amebic meningoencephalitis caused by *N. fowleri* is an acute, rapidly progressive illness occurring principally in healthy children and young adults that almost uniformly is fatal. Patients have an abrupt onset of severe bifrontal or bitemporal headache, high fever, nausea and vomiting, malaise, rhinitis, nuchal rigidity and other meningeal signs, neurologic abnormalities, irritability, and other changes in mental status 1 to 15 days after exposure (typically 5 to 8 days), most frequently after swimming or bathing in warm contaminated fresh water.[45,86,101,134] A history of disturbances of taste and smell has been noted in many cases, although for the most part the early clinical features of primary amebic meningoencephalitis are not distinctive.[59] Progression from fever to signs of meningitis and encephalitis is unrelenting and rapid. Seizures are common. Coma is present at or develops soon after hospital admission. In the absence of early diagnosis and appropriate treatment, the illness characteristically progresses rapidly to death within 1 week of onset of symptoms (median, 72 hours).[9] The cause of death is usually from increased intracranial pressure with brain herniation, leading to cardiopulmonary arrest and pulmonary edema.

Other than the clue of a recent history of exposure to warm fresh water, there is little to distinguish primary amebic meningoencephalitis from fulminant bacterial meningitis. A high peripheral polymorphonuclear leukocytosis may be present. CSF findings are similarly nonspecific, with increased pressure, elevated protein level (ranging from 100 mg/100 mL to 1000 mg/100 mL), a normal to low glucose value, and modest polymorphonuclear pleocytosis (ranging from 300 cells/mm^3 to as high as 26,000 cells/mm^3), but no bacteria, mycobacteria, or fungi are identified on culture. Patients with a suggestive history and CSF indices suggestive of purulent meningitis, but without bacteria on Gram stain, should have a wet mount examined for the presence of motile trophozoites (Fig. 223.5). Smear of the CSF should be stained with Giemsa or Wright stains to identify the trophozoite, if present. The ameba can be clearly differentiated from host cells by the nucleus with its centrally placed large nucleolus.

Acanthamoeba *Species*

Acanthamoeba spp. and *B. mandrillaris* cause granulomatous amebic encephalitis. The course typically is prolonged, with progression from focal neurologic signs to diffuse meningoencephalitis over weeks to months after exposure.[87,130] Patients most susceptible to contracting this disease include very young, old, debilitated, immunosuppressed (HIV/AIDS, organ transplantation), and chronically ill patients (diabetics). The clinical picture resembles that of a bacterial brain abscess or brain tumor, with insidious onset of headache, intermittent low-grade fever, nausea, vomiting, lethargy, stiff neck, and symptoms of increased intracranial pressure. Altered mental status is particularly prominent. As the infection progresses, depending on the area of the brain affected, focal neurologic signs, hemiparesis, drowsiness, aphasia, ataxia, cranial nerve palsies, behavioral and personality changes, and seizures develop. The incubation period after exposure to onset of CNS disease is unknown but is of the order of several weeks to months.

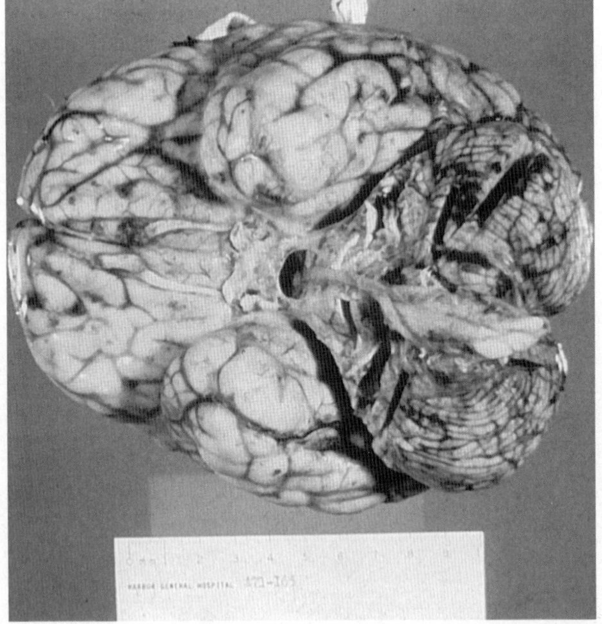

FIG. 223.5 Brain from a fatal case of *Naegleria* meningoencephalitis. Note the areas of necrosis on the basilar surface.

Acanthamoeba skin lesions often have been present for months before the onset of CNS disease. Routine CSF findings frequently are abnormal but nonspecific, with elevated protein level, low glucose value, and, typically, a mononuclear pleocytosis. *Acanthamoeba* spp. also may cause cutaneous, pulmonary, bone, and nasopharyngeal or sinus disease.[52,83,96] Cutaneous *Acanthamoeba* infection is characterized by pustules, papules, skin ulcerations, and hard erythematous nodules, which develop into nonhealing indurated draining ulcers or subcutaneous abscesses.[47,87] The most affected sites where lesions occur are the face, trunk, and extremities. Disseminated disease without CNS involvement has a slightly better prognosis. In patients with AIDS, mortality rates of 70% and 100% are reported for *Acanthamoeba* skin disease alone and in association with CNS disease, respectively.[69]

Acanthamoeba *Keratitis*

In contrast to its role as an opportunistic pathogen in CNS and skin disease, most cases of *Acanthamoeba* keratitis occur in otherwise healthy individuals who wear contact lenses or who have a history of corneal trauma. Contact lenses of any type, including daily wear and disposable soft and extended-wear lenses, have been implicated in infection. All soft contact lenses contain 50% to 75% water. These lenses can absorb pathogens from contaminated cleaning solutions, carrying cases, and hands. When the lens comes into contact with the contaminated fluid, the amebae quickly adhere to the lens surface. *Acanthamoeba* must be in the trophozoite stage to bind to human corneal epithelial cells. If corneal trauma is present, the organisms invade the corneal tissue and produce parasite-mediated cytolysis of the cornea.[66] The infection causes destruction of the corneal epithelium and stroma, infiltration of inflammatory cells, and formation of descemetocoele and perforation. The nidus for infection most likely is trauma to the cornea but also may be related to preexisting herpesviral or bacterial conjunctivitis (Fig. 223.6). Amebic keratitis characteristically is painful, progressive, and sight threatening and fails to respond to conventional antibacterial or antiviral treatment.[5,87] Typically, only one eye is involved; however, bilateral keratitis has been reported. Early symptoms include severe eye pain, lacrimation, foreign body sensation, conjunctival hyperemia, and photophobia. *Acanthamoeba* keratitis frequently is misdiagnosed, initially, as herpetic, bacterial, or fungal infection. The course usually is more indolent, however. Periods of temporary remission delay establishing the diagnosis further. Recurrent corneal epithelial breakdown with dendritic infiltrates progresses to nonsuppurative keratitis, which waxes and wanes over several months and ends in a characteristic ring-shaped stromal abscess with secondary uveitis leading to loss of the cornea.[5,150] Infection that follows severe trauma deteriorates more rapidly than that which follows contact lens wear. In addition, complications of infection include iritis, cataracts, corneal epithelial ulceration, hypopyon, glaucoma, scleritis, loss of visual acuity, blindness, and penetrating keratitis.[5]

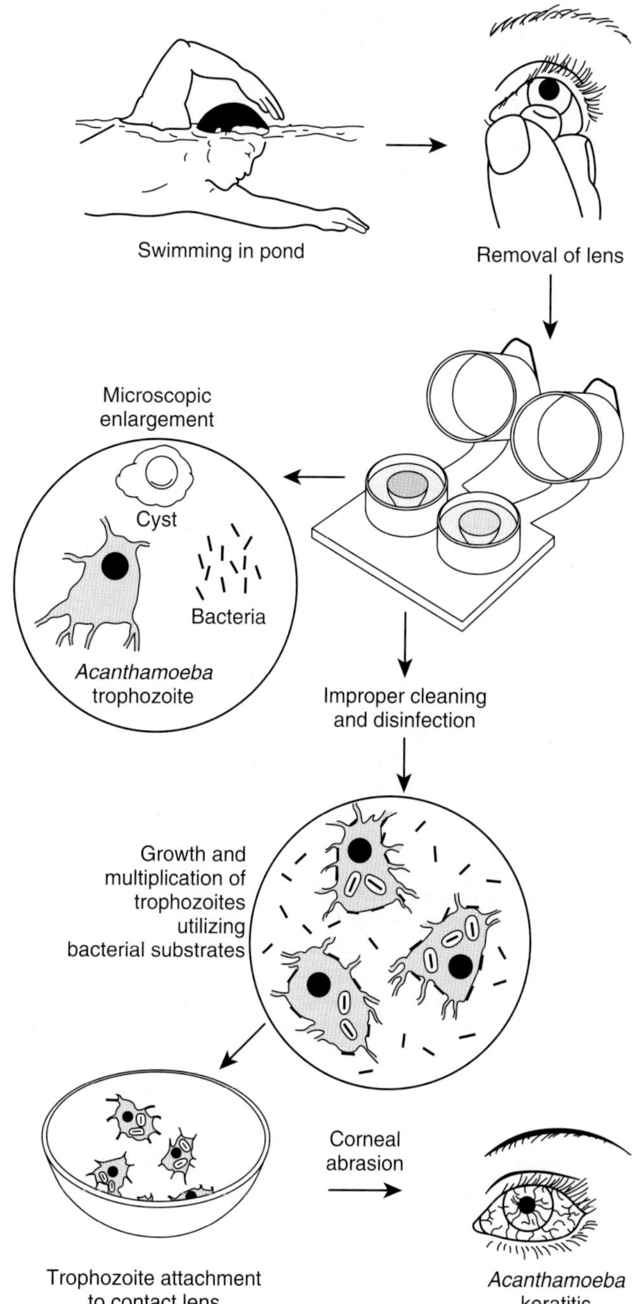

FIG. 223.6 Proposed mechanism for *Acanthamoeba* keratitis. Bacterial contaminants in the water on the lens support the growth of amebae, which leads to an increased number of invading organisms. The organisms adhere to the contact lens and enter tissue through the damaged cornea, with the subsequent development of keratitis.

Balamuthia Mandrillaris

B. mandrillaris causes granulomatous encephalitis and cutaneous, sinus, and nasopharyngeal disease.[130] The portal of entry is skin lesions contaminated by soil, or cysts transported by air currents to the respiratory tract.[119] The incubation period of CNS disease is unknown but is thought to be weeks to months (not <10 days).[97] In animal models, extensive CNS necrosis develops 1 to 3 weeks after inoculation.[93] This ameba is known to be extremely encephalotropic and cytopathic, causing extensive damage to the brain tissues. The infection is chronic, and the time between the appearance of skin lesions and neurological symptoms ranges from 1 month to 2 years. Onset of symptoms of granulomatous encephalitis is insidious, with low-grade fever, severe frontal headache, photophobia, nausea and vomiting, meningismus, personality change, and prominent focal neurologic signs that have included cranial nerve palsies, hemiparesis, dysarthria/aphasia, focal seizures, and ataxia.[7,57] A history of recent otitis was noted by many authors.[7,57] A slow relentless deterioration to coma and death ensues over several weeks to months (as long as 2 years afterward). Death usually results from cardiorespiratory failure secondary to severe cerebral edema. In many reports, manifestation of cutaneous lesions (facial, nasal, and limb) has preceded development of CNS disease.[36,63,109,114,163] Although normal CSF parameters have been described in *B. mandrillaris* CNS infection, the typical findings are moderately increased protein levels (may be >1 g/dL), normal or mildly decreased glucose values, and a pleocytosis (about 500 cells/mm^3), which commonly but not invariably has a mononuclear predominance.[7,49,57,93,130]

NEUROIMAGING

Neuroimaging findings in infections caused by free-living amebae are nonspecific and alone do not provide clues to an earlier diagnosis. In addition, in the early stages of infection, results of computed tomography (CT) and magnetic resonance imaging (MRI) may be normal. In primary amebic meningoencephalitis, cranial CT and MRI show obliteration of basal cisterns and signs of diffuse brain edema, hydrocephalus, focal and basilar meningeal enhancement, and infarction.[78,121,137] In granulomatous encephalitis, neuroimaging reveals variable but nondiagnostic abnormalities that include, alone or in combination, discrete corticomedullary lesions; large, solitary, masslike lesions (which may be confused with brain abscess or tumor); large arterial occlusions; and spinal cord infarctions.[78,121,137] Similarly, in *Balamuthia* infection, neuroimaging is helpful but nondiagnostic; CT scans show a focal enhancing mass or ring-enhancing cystic lesions or both, vascular occlusion, and diffuse edema that frequently progresses to communicating hydrocephalus.[7,36,57]

MRI shows ring-enhancing lesions or low-density abnormalities mimicking one or multiple space-occupying masses.

PATHOGENESIS

Naegleria trophozoites or cysts enter the body through the nasal cavity by aspiration of water or inhalation of soil. The trophozoites penetrate the olfactory mucosa and, after active phagocytosis by sustentacular neuroepithelial cells of the olfactory nerve, migrate along the nerve, pass through the cribriform plate, and gain entry to the CNS at the level of the olfactory bulbs.[6,65,97] From the olfactory bulb, which is bathed in CSF and lies in the highly vascularized subarachnoid space, *N. fowleri* disseminate throughout the CSF and CNS. *Naegleria* induce an intense inflammatory response associated with lytic necrosis hemorrhage surrounded by purulent exudates. Numerous superficial hemorrhagic areas also occur in the cortex, around the base of the brain, hypothalamus, midbrain, pons, medulla oblongata, and the upper portion of the spinal cord.[6,30] Only *Naegleria* trophozoites are found in the CNS lesions. In contrast, most *Acanthamoeba* spp. infections seem to follow hematogenous dissemination from a primary lower respiratory or cutaneous focus.[97] Researchers have postulated that *Acanthamoeba* spp. are inhaled or inoculated through skin in the cyst phase. *Acanthamoeba* most likely enters the CNS through the blood-brain barrier, particularly through the endothelial lining of cerebral capillaries.[6,74,95] Less commonly, *Acanthamoeba* is capable of causing CNS infection directly via the olfactory neuroepithelium. The pathogenic mechanisms of infections caused by *B. mandrillaris* are unclear, but it is believed that the organisms migrate either through tissue or via hematogenous spread to the location or locations where disease becomes manifest.[6] For CNS disease, studies using a mouse model indicate that the organism is inhaled through the nasal passages, adheres to the nasal epithelium, and then travels along the olfactory nerve in to the central nervous system as is seen with both *Naegleria* and *Acantamoeba*.[77]

Virulence factors described for free-living amebae include the ability to adhere to brain microvascular epithelium, production of extracellular metalloprotease and elastases, release of a pleiotropic cytokine, IL-6, and phagocytosis by food cups or amebostomes.[1,43,58,75,87,90] Among *Naegleria* spp., pathogenicity is closely related to thermotolerance.[32] *N. fowleri*, the only species pathogenic for humans, is unusually thermophilic and can tolerate temperatures of 45°C.[130] In addition, *N. fowleri* has less demanding growth requirements than nonpathogenic *Naegleria* spp. Trophozoites of pathogenic *Acanthamoeba* spp. also are thermophilic, being able to tolerate temperatures of 37°C, relative to their nonpathogenic counterparts.[130,128] Thermotolerance seems to be less important for *Acanthamoeba* strains that cause keratitis, presumably because corneal temperatures are lower (32°C–35°C).[130]

PATHOLOGY

Pathologic changes of infection with small free-living amebae are most marked in the CNS. The pathology of primary and granulomatous amebic encephalitis differs fundamentally.[97] Macroscopically, *N. fowleri* produces diffuse meningoencephalitis, most severely affecting the cortical gray matter. It is characterized by marked cerebral edema and purulent leptomeninges, particularly adjacent to the olfactory bulbs, at the base of the frontal and temporal lobes, and at the hypothalamus.[94] Frequently, the olfactory bulbs are necrotic and hemorrhagic. Microscopically, an acute mononuclear and polymorphonuclear (PMN) fibrinopurulent leptomeningeal inflammatory infiltrate is seen throughout the cerebrum, brain stem, and cerebellum and the upper spinal cord. Trophozoites tend to concentrate in the perivascular spaces and adventitia of arteries, and they may contain ingested erythrocytes and brain tissue. Large numbers of amebic trophozoites, without the presence of PMNs, are seen within edematous and necrotic neural tissue. Trophic amebae are also seen deep in Virchow-Robin spaces, usually around blood vessels with no inflammatory response. Characteristically, only trophozoites are seen in the CSF or brain tissue.[97] Presumably, *N. fowleri* cysts are not found in clinical specimens because progression of *Naegleria* infection is so rapid and fatal that the patient dies before transformation from trophozoite into the cyst can occur.[86]

CNS infections caused by *Acanthamoeba* spp. and *B. mandrillaris* are characterized macroscopically by diffuse cerebral edema and hemorrhage, with areas of softening and abscess formation. The meninges are spared except for areas overlying involved cerebrum. Additional areas of hemorrhagic necrosis are concentrated in the posterior fossa, brain stem, cerebellum, midbrain, cerebral cortex, and basal ganglia.[7,36,37,86] Narrowing of the sulci and flattening of the gyri are noted in areas of active infection. Microscopic changes consist of multinucleated giant cells, with trophozoites and cysts seen within the lesions.[94] The olfactory bulbs and spinal cord are relatively spared.

Microscopically, necrotizing hemorrhagic encephalitis and subacute or chronic necrotizing granulomatous infiltrates and multinucleate giant cells are scattered throughout the CNS, particularly in the cerebral hemispheres, basal ganglia, midbrain, and brain stem. Typically, trophozoites and cysts of *Acanthamoeba* spp. or *B. mandrillaris* are present within necrotic cerebral tissue, particularly in perivascular spaces. Invasion of blood vessels causes severe necrotizing arteritis and hemorrhagic necrosis. The angiotropic distribution of *Acanthamoeba* or *Balamuthia* infection supports a hematogenous mechanism of spread. In severely immunocompromised patients, the inflammatory reaction may be negligible and lacks a granulomatous component.[10,93] In the absence of a vigorous granulomatous response, hemorrhagic necrosis that resembles primary amebic meningoencephalitis may occur.[164]

Skin lesions of acanthamebiasis and balamuthiasis are characterized by nodules, ulcers, and abscesses and by the presence of amebic trophozoites, cysts, and granulomas in tissue.[97,96,163] Amebic keratitis is characterized by moderate chronic inflammation of corneal stroma, a mixed polymorphonuclear and lymphocytic infiltrate, and the presence of amebic trophozoites and cysts within the corneal ulcerations.[156]

DIAGNOSIS

Previously, most cases of amebic meningoencephalitis were diagnosed with certainty only at autopsy or by brain biopsy.[10] Routine laboratory tests did not distinguish amebic meningoencephalitis from other causes of meningoencephalitis. The first and most important diagnostic step is to recognize the possibility that small free-living amebae may cause infection in the appropriate clinical setting. Among the few reported therapeutic successes, all are notable for early diagnosis and timely institution of appropriate antimicrobial therapy.[36,71,104,108]

Primary amebic meningoencephalitis should be included in the differential diagnosis of any child or young adult with meningoencephalitis. A history of recent exposure to fresh water should be sought, and a wet mount should be performed on centrifuged CSF. *Naegleria* is isolated most readily from CSF but also may be isolated from brain tissue, particularly olfactory lobes. In contrast, *Acanthamoeba* trophozoites characteristically are absent from CSF, and *B. mandrillaris* has yet to be seen in CSF. *Acanthamoeba* spp. are more likely to be isolated from brain tissue or skin biopsy or from corneal scrapings in cases of keratitis.[128] Diagnostic techniques include direct microscopy of wet-mount and stained CSF specimens, histologic stains of tissue, fluorescent and immunofluorescent antibody stains of CSF and tissue, direct immunohistochemical stains of tissue, serology, molecular diagnostics, and culture.[155]

Direct Microscopic Identification

If amebic infection of the CNS is suspected, a wet-mount preparation of fresh CSF should be examined for the presence of motile amebae.[86,97,94,155] This method remains the most rapid means of diagnosis. Ideally, the CSF specimen should be kept at room temperature and examined soon after it has been collected. *Naegleria* is particularly fragile. Although the specimen may be kept at 4°C for short periods, it never should be frozen.[155] If present, amebae tend to attach to the test tube wall or surface of the container, so gentle shaking and low centrifugation at 150*g* for 5 minutes is recommended to dislodge and concentrate the amebae.[94,155] The supernatant should be placed gently on a slide. The wet mount is examined best by light microscopy under low power (×10 and ×40 objectives), phase-contrast microscopy, or darkfield illumination and may be warmed to promote amebic motility. *Naegleria* trophozoites move in a characteristic "sluglike" fashion by extrusion of a few broad pseudopodia (lobopodia) anteriorly.[130] Leftover specimens can be frozen at −20°C for later antigen or antibody testing. Although *N. fowleri* may be shown by histologic stains of fixed CSF smears, Gram stain is not useful because it does not stain amebae and the heat fixation causes lysis.

Naegleria, Acanthamoeba spp., and *Balamuthia* may be shown in fixed sections of brain tissue biopsy or autopsy specimens by hematoxylin and eosin, Masson trichrome, periodic acid–Schiff, Wright-Giemsa stain, and Gomori-methenamine silver stains (Fig. 223.7).[86,87,97,94] Reliably differentiating *Acanthamoeba* and *Balamuthia* by histology alone is difficult. In addition, *Acanthamoeba* trophozoites have been variously mistaken for macrophages or "atypical mononuclear" or epithelial cells on routine histology.[94,164]

Immunofluorescent stains using monoclonal and polyclonal anti-*Acanthamoeba* and anti–*B. mandrillaris* antibodies (available at the CDC), immunoperoxidase staining, and electron microscopy of tissue sections have been used to confirm the diagnosis (Fig. 223.8).[36,69,91,155,154] Amebic keratitis may be diagnosed by direct detection of trophozoites or cysts in smears of deep corneal scraping or biopsy using Wright-Giemsa, trichrome, periodic acid–Schiff, calcofluor white, or indirect fluorescent antibody stains.[86,94,165]

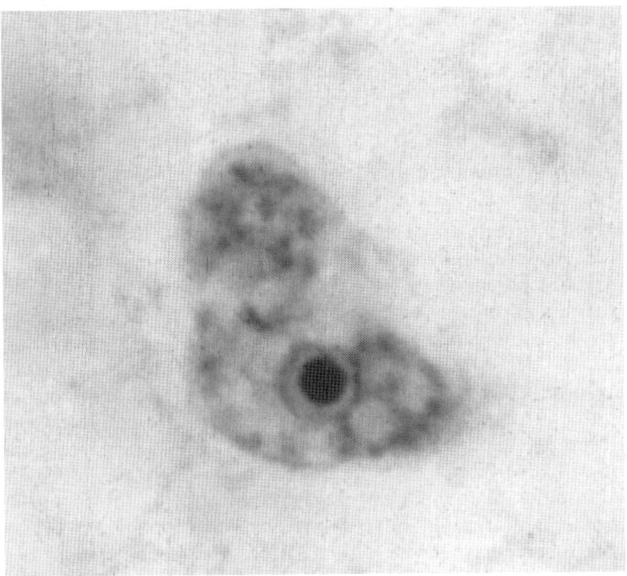

FIG. 223.7 Trichrome stain of a trophozoite of *Naegleria fowleri.*

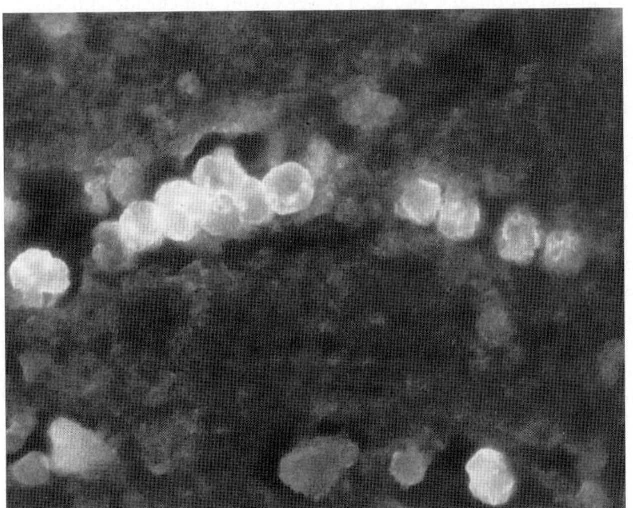

FIG. 223.8 Indirect fluorescent antibody examination of *Naegleria fowleri.* (Courtesy Dr. G.S. Visvesvara, Centers for Disease Control and Prevention.)

Culture

Culture has a limited role in diagnosis but is useful for confirmation, speciation, and antimicrobial susceptibility testing. *N. fowleri* and *Acanthamoeba* spp. can be cultivated using bacteria as a food source (xenic cultures) or without bacteria, in an enriched cell-free nutrient (axenic) medium that contains antimicrobial agents to inhibit growth of contaminating bacteria.[27,128,133,155] *N. fowleri* and *Acanthamoeba* spp. are readily cultured from CSF, brain, and lung tissue on various non-nutrient agars or with low concentrations of nutrients, in the presence of a lawn of living or killed bacteria (e.g., most commonly nonmucoid strains of *Escherichia coli* or *Enterobacter* spp.).[94,128,155] Amebae feed on the lawn of bacteria and grow to cover the plate after 1 to 2 days' incubation at 37°C. Culture plates are incubated at 37°C and examined under low power daily for 10 days.[94,155]

Amebae can be visualized directly through the back of the inverted agar plate with a conventional microscope under low power.[128] The characteristic slow, sluglike movement of *Naegleria* trophozoites that is readily seen in a wet mount of CSF is difficult to distinguish on an agar plate.[128] The ability of *Naegleria* to transform into the flagellated stage after suspension in distilled water is useful diagnostically.[128,155] Trophozoites of *Acanthamoeba* spp. move slowly by extrusion of multiple, finger-like pseudopodia (acanthopodia).

Culture and isolation of *Balamuthia* is more challenging. Generally, *B. mandrillaris* is more fastidious, does not use bacteria as a food source, grows slowly, and requires a heavily enriched basic medium. *N. fowleri, Acanthamoeba* spp., and *B. mandrillaris* all grow vigorously, however, and produce detectable cytopathic effects in mammalian cell cultures (monkey kidney, HeLa, and lung fibroblast tissue), which can be examined for cytopathic effect.[94,157] Typically, *Balamuthia* grows slowly and may require several weeks to proliferate.[157] Use of a positive control culture is advised to ensure correct methodology and to aid recognition.[128] In culture, the organism is sensitive to changes in osmolarity and does not readily tolerate either hypoosmotic or hyperosmotic conditions. *Sappinia diploidea* can be cultivated on non-nutrient agar plates coated with bacteria.

Although no outbreaks of infection in laboratory workers caused by free-living amebae have been reported, care must be taken when handling specimens to avoid getting culture materials on skin and in cuts or abrasions. Specimens should be handled in a biologic safety cabinet by technologists wearing masks and gloves.[94,155]

Serology

Although specific *N. fowleri* antibody has been shown in survivors of primary encephalitis, serologic tests are of no use diagnostically.[134] Onset of primary amebic meningoencephalitis is rapid, and almost all patients die before significant antibody production can occur. In contrast, because the clinical courses of *Acanthamoeba* spp. and *B. mandrillaris* infections usually are chronic, robust antibody responses have time to develop. Detection of serum or CSF antibody against *Acanthamoeba* spp. or *Balamuthia* by indirect immunofluorescence staining has helped establish the diagnosis in many cases.[36,70,130,149] By this method, amebae fixed on a slide bind antibody present in the patient's serum or CSF, which then is detected by fluorescein-conjugated anti-human antibody.

Serologic testing has been most useful as an epidemiologic tool. Although the incidence of infection with free-living amebae seems low, results of seroepidemiology studies suggest that human exposure to amebae occurs frequently. Sera from healthy adults and children contain antibody against *N. fowleri, Acanthamoeba* spp., and *B. mandrillaris.*[31,61,88,124,127] Detection of antibodies to *N. fowleri* and *Acanthamoeba* spp. in asymptomatic adult and pediatric populations from North Carolina, Virginia, and Pennsylvania in the United States and from Czechoslovakia and New Zealand presumably reflects unavoidable environmental contact with these ubiquitous organisms.[20,88] All specimens from a group of 93 asymptomatic patients from New Zealand contained anti-*Naegleria* and anti-*Acanthamoeba* IgG and IgM antibodies.[31] Antibodies were neutralizing against *Acanthamoeba* spp. but not against *N. fowleri.* In virtually all cases of infection caused by *Acanthamoeba* spp., disease occurs in the setting of immunocompromise or in an immunologically privileged site, such as the cornea. Whether neutralizing antibodies play a role in the very low incidence of infections in healthy individuals, despite seemingly frequent environmental exposure, is unknown.

Immunofluorescent antibody staining of serum for antibodies against *Acanthamoeba* spp. and *B. mandrillaris* has proved to be a rapid non-invasive diagnostic test in many clinical cases.[39,70,165] Potentially, this test may be useful clinically for establishing an earlier definitive diagnosis and initiation of therapy. Because the presence of *Balamuthia* antibodies may represent asymptomatic environmental exposure, confirmation of results of immunofluorescent antibody testing by histology, indirect immunofluorescent staining of tissue, or polymerase chain reaction (PCR) of CSF is advised. More recently, immunofluorescent antibody staining of serum from patients with encephalitis, predominantly from California, revealed seven previously unrecognized or misdiagnosed cases of *Balamuthia* and one case of *Acanthamoeba* encephalitis.[127] Most serum specimens showed some evidence of antibody (<1:64), which was attributed to cross-reactivity or subclinical exposure to contaminated soil. A cutoff value of greater than 1:64 for *Balamuthia* serology was considered positive pending results of confirmatory tests (e.g., histology, immunohistochemistry, or PCR).[127] Low levels of antibody may reflect preceding subacute disease or contact with environmental amebae.[127]

Molecular Diagnostics

Although microscopic assessment of a wet-mount preparation or histology may be useful in experienced hands, definitive identification in most centers awaits results of specimens sent out for immunofluorescence tests. Advances in molecular diagnostics offer the real possibility, however, of sensitive, specific, and rapid diagnosis being made by any laboratory with the capability to perform PCR. PCR of DNA extracted from frozen brain tissue has been used to confirm *N. fowleri* infection diagnosed by histopathology and immunofluorescent staining.[25] Similarly, nested and real-time PCR provide rapid, sensitive, and specific screening of environmental and recreational water sources for the presence of *N. fowleri.*[89,115] PCR, using mitochondrial 16S rRNA gene DNA as the target, has been used to detect *B. mandrillaris* in clinical samples of CSF and formalin-fixed brain and lung tissue of patients with encephalitis.[144,167] These assays have the ability to detect a single ameba per reaction mixture.[167]

The development of a multiplex real-time PCR assay for simultaneous detection of *N. fowleri, Acanthamoeba* spp., and *B. mandrillaris* in clinical specimens of CSF and brain tissue offers the possibility of highly sensitive and specific rapid confirmatory diagnosis of CNS infection by free-living amebae and the chance of initiating earlier, more effective treatment.[112] The assay is sensitive down to detection of a single ameba in a specimen and is species specific for *N. fowleri* and *B. mandrillaris* and genus specific for *Acanthamoeba.*[33,112] A recently developed real-time multiplex PCR assay identifies *N. fowleri* DNA in the CSF and brain tissue samples obtained from primary amebic encephalitis patients antemortem. This tests identifies all three genotypes known to be present in the United States. The time taken to identify *N. fowleri* from the time the specimen arrives in the laboratory is about 5 hours and can be cut down to 2 hours if the specimen is CSF.[112]

Finally, the development and use of metagenomic deep sequencing for the diagnosis of *Balamuthia mandrillaris* encephalitis and other unusual or novel organisms that may cause encephalitis is a powerful diagnostic tool that has the potential for rapid and precise identification of pathogens. This will allow for the initiation of treatment earlier in the course of the patient's illness, improving patient outcome.[166]

TREATMENT

Mortality among patients with primary and granulomatous amebic encephalitis is greater than 95%.[9,131] Indeed, there are only a handful of known survivors of primary amebic meningoencephalitis.[23,24,59] The high fatality rate undoubtedly is due partly to late diagnosis or misdiagnosis and late initiation of potentially effective treatment. Inclusion of amebic infection in the differential diagnosis, in the appropriate clinical setting, and timely administration of effective antiamebic treatment are emphasized in successful cases.[13,108] In the future, availability of real-time PCR may facilitate accurately establishing an early diagnosis. Although no randomized trials of optimal treatment for infection caused by free-living amebae have been performed, potentially effective treatment is available if the condition is recognized early.

If infection is suspected, treatment should not be withheld pending the results of confirmatory testing. Treatment regimens are based on results of in vitro susceptibility, in vivo animal experiments, and empirical treatment of individual cases. If amebic infection is suspected, accurate determination of the species is important to ensure optimal treatment. No one drug is effective against all free-living amebae (e.g., amphotericin is the drug of choice for *N. fowleri* infection but is neither amebistatic nor amebicidal for *Acanthamoeba* spp. and varies in its efficacy against *Balamuthia*).[40,129] Previously, authors have suggested initiating treatment with a combination of agents such as amphotericin B and flucytosine; pentamidine with sulfadiazine, clarithromycin, an azole compound, and flucytosine; flucytosine with an azole compound, azithromycin, pentamidine, and sulfadiazine; and pentamidine, an azole compound, sulfadiazine, amphotericin B, azithromycin, and rifampicin, which have activity against *Naegleria* and *Acanthamoeba* or *Balamuthia,* until amebae can be identified definitively.[36,98,153,164] Among newer antibiotics, miltefosine and voriconazole are potentially attractive as treatments for infection caused by free-living amebae. Both drugs penetrate brain tissue and have a low toxicity profile. Although differences in susceptibility exist among strains, voriconazole has activity in vitro against *Acanthamoeba* spp. and *N. fowleri,* whereas miltefosine has in vitro activity against *Acanthamoeba* spp. and *Balamuthia.*[126] Miltefosine is currently available via expanded access IND directly from the Centers for Disease Control and Prevention (CDC) in the United States for the treatment of infections with free-living amebae.[17]

Amebic Meningoencephalitis

N. fowleri is exquisitely susceptible in vitro to amphotericin B, which remains the treatment of choice for primary amebic meningoencephalitis.[131] All successfully treated cases have included amphotericin B in the treatment regimen. *Naegleria* also is susceptible in vitro to azithromycin and miconazole, with synergism in vitro and in the animal model with the combination of amphotericin and miconazole or tetracycline.[40,53,134,140,151] Treatment regimens in cases with successful outcomes have included intravenous amphotericin, high-dose intravenous and intrathecal amphotericin and miconazole, oral rifampin, intravenous sulfisoxazole, and intravenous and intrathecal amphotericin in combination with oral rifampin.[4,13,134] In at least one reported case, intravenous and intrathecal amphotericin B was combined with intravenous and intrathecal miconazole and with oral rifampin.[59] Rifampin has yielded conflicting results in in vitro testing.[54] Liposomal amphotericin B seems less effective in vitro and in the animal model than conventional amphotericin (10-fold higher minimum inhibitory concentration) and is not recommended.[54] Promising results in mice have been reported with chlorpromazine and to a lesser extent miltefosine and voriconazole.[154] In contrast to *Acanthamoeba* spp. and *B. mandrillaris, N. fowleri* remains a trophozoite and does not encyst in tissues, so after it is destroyed by antimicrobial therapy, infection with *N. fowleri* should not recur.

Optimal treatment for CNS disease caused by *Acanthamoeba* spp. has not been established, and the prognosis remains grim, with few reports of survivors.[131] Most cases are diagnosed at autopsy or a few days before death, leaving little time to evaluate treatment. Treatment successes have been attributed to initiation of treatment before spread of infection into the CNS. Combination treatment is favored because no single drug is active against trophozoites and cysts, and many drugs are amebistatic rather than amebicidal.[87] Among the few reports of successful treatment, orally administered trimethoprim-sulfamethoxazole, ketoconazole, and rifampin were associated with a favorable outcome in two apparently immunocompetent children with CNS disease.[138] Fluconazole, rifampin, metronidazole, and sulfadiazine were used successfully in a 64-year-old immunocompetent host with early disease.[108] Still other regimens have included pentamidine isethionate, 5-fluorocytosine, and itraconazole.[154]

Similarly, Slater and colleagues[139] reported successful treatment of disseminated cutaneous acanthamebiasis in a renal transplant recipient using 4 weeks of intravenous pentamidine, topical chlorhexidine, and

2% ketoconazole followed by maintenance oral itraconazole. A combination of pentamidine, 5-fluorocytosine, itraconazole, and topical chlorhexidine gluconate/ketoconazole cream was used to treat disseminated acanthamebiasis successfully in a lung transplant recipient.[106] Pentamidine is considered the most suitable treatment before CNS invasion has occurred because of its low penetration into the CNS. Because of its low penetration across the blood-brain barrier and nephrotoxicity, 5-fluorocytosine was preferred to pentamidine for CNS infection and in renal transplant recipients.[40,87] The anti-*Leishmania* drug miltefosine has been found to be useful both for systemic infections and for amebic keratitis.[154]

Optimal treatment for *B. mandrillaris* infection also remains to be determined. Reports of successful treatment for granulomatous encephalitis caused by *Balamuthia* based on empirical regimens are few. If it is recognized early in its course, however, a more favorable outcome apparently is possible. According to Visvesvara, in the 100 cases reported only seven patients have survived, including four patients treated with a combination of flucytosine, pentamidine isethionate, fluconazole, sulfadiazine, and a macrolide such as azithromycin switched to clarithromycin (better CSF penetration), whereas some patients also received a phenothiazine (thioridazine or trifluoperazine).[36,154] Pentamidine treatment frequently was discontinued or interrupted because of side effects. Treatment failures have been reported in patients treated with similar regimens, however, possibly because of late initiation of treatment.[49] Pentamidine and azithromycin were more effective in vitro than fluconazole, flucytosine, or sulfasalazine.[131] Some researchers have postulated, however, that some of these drugs may be synergistic in vivo.[131] Because of concern about reactivation from dormant cysts in the brain, both patients remained on long-term fluconazole and on sulfadiazine or clarithromycin prophylaxis. The drug miltefosine has also been used. One patient underwent excision of a brain abscess while undergoing treatment.

Use of corticosteroids to treat cerebral edema and inflammation seems to exacerbate *Acanthamoeba* infection. A precipitous decline in the clinical condition of one patient has been reported after administration of corticosteroid therapy.[49] At present, the risk of corticosteroid treatment probably outweighs any potential benefit and is best avoided.[49,87,117]

Amebic Keratitis

If untreated, amebic keratitis invariably progresses to visual loss and enucleation. Although amebic keratitis is more amenable to antimicrobial treatment than systemic infection, treating it is still difficult. The presence of *Acanthamoeba* cysts in deeper corneal layers renders exposure to adequate drug levels problematic. In addition, *Acanthamoeba* cysts are resistant to most antibacterial agents at concentrations that are achievable but nontoxic to the cornea. As with systemic infection, establishing the diagnosis early is required for treatment to be most effective.

In the early stages of infection, prolonged frequent application of drug is recommended. Combination treatment is preferred during prolonged treatment because of concerns for development of resistance. Nonetheless, cures have been reported with a variety of topical agents; the cationic antiseptic chlorhexidine gluconate and 0.02% polyhexamethylene biguanide (PHMB), a swimming pool disinfectant, alone or in combination with propamidine are among the drugs of choice for amebic keratitis.[42,81,131,132] Both drugs are effective against trophozoites and are well tolerated in the eye.[81] Alternatively, two diamidines, propamidine isethionate and hexamidine, can be used, or chlorhexidine can be used along with diamidine.[154] Visvesvara reports that they should be used hourly as drops day and night for 48 hours initially, followed by hourly drops by day only for another 72 hours and, then, because of epithelial toxicity, tapered to 2 hours by day 5 for 3 to 4 weeks. Neomycin and oral azoles (e.g., miconazole or itraconazole) also have proved useful. Newer agents, such as myristamidopropyl dimethylamine and miltefosine, are effective *Acanthamoeba* cysticidal agents, possess excellent antifungal and antibacterial activity and show promise in treating recalcitrant keratitis.[62,122,131]

Many cases of keratitis, particularly when chronic or where medical treatment alone fails, require keratoplasty and corneal grafting. In these cases, prolonged medical treatment aims to cure or control disease to allow for successful transplantation. Timing of surgery is controversial. Antiamebic drugs usually are continued for months after surgery to prevent late excystation of residual dormant cysts.[5] Use of topical or systemic corticosteroid to treat severe pain or inflammation is controversial. Severe complications have been described in clinical cases, and dexamethasone induces encystment and increases cytopathogenicity of emerging trophozoites in animal models.[100,145]

ROLE OF *ACANTHAMOEBA* SPECIES AS RESERVOIRS OF INTRACELLULAR PATHOGENS

Although most bacteria are prey for free-living amebae, some bacteria have evolved to survive uptake by amebae. Many *Acanthamoeba* spp. act as environmental reservoirs of recognized intracellular pathogens for humans, including *Coxiella burnetii, Legionella pneumophila, Mycobacterium* spp., *Pseudomonas aeruginosa,* and *Cryptococcus neoformans,* and for potential emerging pathogens, such as *Rickettsia*-like organisms and *Parachlamydia* spp.[56,55,60,92,147] Some ameba-resistant microorganisms coexist with amebae as endobacterial symbionts, whereas others exploit the amebae as hosts for survival, for multiplication, or as vectors of disease.[8] Free-living amebae act as a "Trojan horse" in the transmission of bacterial passengers, such as for *L. pneumophila* or *M. avium,* or as an "evolutionary crib" for the selection of virulence traits and for adaptation of microorganisms to life within human macrophages, such as for *C. neoformans*.[8,56]

For *L. pneumophila,* prior multiplication within free-living amebae, principally *Acanthamoeba* spp., seems to be a prerequisite for acquisition of infection in humans.[146] In addition, many bacteria, such as *M. avium,* survive protected from chlorination, biocides, antibiotics, and desiccation within ameba cysts.[91,144] Similarly, growth of *M. avium* in amebae results in enhanced survival in macrophages. Researchers also have postulated that free-living amebae may have adapted some microorganisms for successful intracellular survival within macrophages.[50,141] Free-living amebae also apparently promote virulence traits and antimicrobial resistance in *L. pneumophila, M. avium,* and *C. neoformans*.[21,22,103] Researchers have postulated that capsule formation evolved in *C. neoformans* in response to selective pressure to resist environmental amebae. Production and maintenance of a capsule allows *Cryptococcus* to survive in human macrophages.[141] Some microorganisms resistant to amebae seem to behave as endosymbionts and to influence development and maintenance of virulence traits that enhance pathogenicity of free-living amebae.[48,56] Clinical and environmental *Naegleria* spp. do not support bacterial endosymbionts.

PREVENTION

Infections caused by free-living amebae are reported to be characterized by an absence of distinguishing symptoms, delayed diagnosis or misdiagnosis, and an almost uniformly poor prognosis without early appropriate treatment. Prevention of infection is of paramount importance. Strategies to prevent *Naegleria* infection exist; *N. fowleri* is susceptible to 1 μg/mL or less of chlorine, and adequate chlorination of water in swimming pools or hot tubs is a simple and sensible preventive measure. If water temperatures are higher, use of increased concentrations of chlorine (>2 to 3 mg/L) is recommended.[97] In certain parts of the world, environmental levels of *N. fowleri* are monitored to ensure that it is safe to swim and that the probability of acquiring an infection is low.[15] A prudent measure is to educate the public on the potential dangers associated with exposure to warm bodies of fresh or thermally polluted water, especially when temperatures are high and water levels are low, and to avoid immersion, diving, jumping, or horseplay that might force water up the nasal passages or disturb sediment.[168] If a neti pot is used for nasal irrigation, only bottled or filtered water should be used.

Prevention of infection caused by *Acanthamoeba* spp. or *B. mandrillaris* is problematic and involves regular inspections of hot-water tanks, plumbing, and eye-wash stations. *Acanthamoeba* keratitis associated with use of contact lenses is preventable, however. Contact lens wearers should be aware of the importance of proper care of the lenses. Lenses should be cleansed in sterile benzalkonium-preserved saline or disinfected by heat. Use of homemade cleansing solutions and wearing lenses while swimming are contraindicated.

Although the incidence of infections caused by free-living amebae is small at present, the number of these infections is likely to grow with increasing numbers of transplant patients and patients with AIDS. Similarly, some researchers have predicted that climate change associated with global warming may further increase the numbers of free-living amebae in the environment.[25]

NEW REFERENCES SINCE THE SEVENTH EDITION

6. Baig AM. Pathogenesis of amoebic encephalitis: are the amoebae being credited to an "inside job" done by the host immune response? *Acta Trop*. 2015;148:72-76.
12. Bravo FG, Seas C. *Balamuthia mandrillaris* amoebic encephalitis: an emerging parasitic infection. *Curr Infect Dis Rep*. 2012;14:391-396.
17. Centers for Disease Control and Prevention. Investigational drug available directly from CDC for the treatment of infections with free-living amebae. *MMWR Morb Mortal Wkly Rep*. 2013;62(33):666.
23. Kato H, Mitake S, Yuasa H, et al. Successful treatment of granulomatous amoebic encephalitis with combination antimicrobial therapy. *Intern Med*. 2013;52:1977-1981.
24. Moriarty P, Burke C, McCrossin D, et al. *Balamuthia mandrillaris* encephalitis: survival of a child with severe meningoencephalitis and review of the literature. *J Pediatric Infect Dis Soc*. 2013;3(1):e4-e9.
26. Cope JR, Ratard RC, Hill VR, et al. The first association of a primary amebic meningoencephalitis death with culturable *Naegleria fowleri* in tap water from a U.S. treated public drinking water system. *Clin Infect Dis*. 2015;60(8):e36-e42.
30. Shuster FL, Visvesvara GS. Free-living amoebae as opportunistic and non-opportunistic pathogens of humans and animals. *Int J Parasitol*. 2004;34:1001-1007.
33. De Jonckheere JF. Molecular definition and the ubiquity of species in the genus *Naegleria*. *Protist*. 2004;155:89-103.
36. Deetz TR, Sawyer MH, Billman G, et al. Successful treatment of *Balamuthia* amoebic encephalitis: presentation of two cases. *Clin Infect Dis*. 2003;37:1304-1312.
38. Dendena F, Sellami H, Jarraya F, et al. Free-living amoebae: detection, morphological and molecular identification of *Acanthamoeba* genus in the hydraulic system of an hemodialysis unit in Tunisia. *Parasite*. 2008;15:137-142.
71. Kato H, Mitake S, Yuasa H, et al. Successful treatment of granulomatous amoebic encephalitis with combination antimicrobial therapy. *Intern Med*. 2013;52:1977-1981.
73. Kemble SK, Lynfield R, DeVries AS, et al. Fatal *Naegleria fowleri* infection acquired in Minnesota: possible expanded range of a deadly thermophilic organism. *Clin Infect Dis*. 2012;54:805-809.
74. Khan NA. *Acanthamoeba* and the blood-brain barrier: the breakthrough. *J Med Microbiol*. 2008;57:1051-1057.
77. Kiderlen AF, Tata PS, Ozel M, et al. Cytopathogenicity of *Balamuthia mandrillaris*, an opportunistic causative agent of granulomatous amebic encephalitis. *J Eukaryot Microbiol*. 2006;53:456-463.
84. Lorenzo-Morales J, Cabello-Vilchez MC, Martin-Navarro CM, et al. Is *Balamuthia mandrillaris* a public health concern worldwide? *Trends Parasitol*. 2013;1-6.
85. Lorenzo-Morales J, Khan NA, Walochnik J. An update on *Acanthamoeba* keratitis: diagnosis, pathogenesis and treatment. *Parasite*. 2015;22(10):1-20.
95. Martinez AJ. Infection of the central nervous system due to *Acanthamoeba*. *Rev Infect Dis*. 1991;13:S399-S402.
98. Martinez DY, Seas C, Bravo F, et al. Successful treatment of *Balamuthia* mandrillaris amoebic infection with extensive neurological and cutaneous involvement. *Clin Infect Dis*. 2010;51:e7-e11.
102. Mergeryan H. The prevalence of *Acanthamoeba* in the human environment. *Rev Infect Dis*. 1991;13(suppl 5):S390-S391.
104. Moriarty P, Burke C, McCrossin D, et al. *Balamuthia mandrillaris* encephalitis: survival of a child with severe meningoencephalitis and review of the literature. *J Pediatric Infect Dis Soc*. 2014;3(1):e4-e9.
110. Qvarnstrom Y, da Silva AJ, Schuster FL, et al. Molecular confirmation of *Sappinia pedata* as a causative agent of amoebic encephalitis. *J Infect Dis*. 2009;199:1139-1142.
112. Qvarnstrom Y, Visvesvara GS, Sriram R, et al. A multiplex real-time PCR assay for simultaneous detection of *Acanthamoeba* spp., *Balamuthia mandrillaris* and *Naegleria fowleri*. *J Clin Microbiol*. 2006;44:3589-3595.
119. Schafer KR, Shah N, Almira-Suarez MI, et al. Disseminated *Balamuthia mandrillaris* infection. *J Clin Microbiol*. 2015;53(9):3072-3076.
135. Shoff ME, Rogerson K, Dessler K, et al. Prevalence of *Acanthamoeba* and other naked amoebae in south Florida domestic water. *J Water Health*. 2008;6:99-104.
136. Siddiqui R, Khan NA. *Balamuthia mandrillaris*: morphology, biology, and virulence. *Trop Parasitol*. 2015;5(1):15-22.
153. Trabesi H, Dendana F, Sellami A, et al. Pathogenic free-living amoebae: epidemiology and clinical review. *Pathol Biol (Paris)*. 2012;60:399-405.
158. Visvesvara GS, Moura H, Schuster FL. Pathogenic and opportunistic free-living amoebae: *Acanthamoeba* spp., *Balamuthia mandrillaris*, *Naegleria fowleri*, and *Sappinia diploidea*. *FEMS Immunol Med Microbiol*. 2007;50:1-26.
161. Walochnik J, Wylezich C, Michel R. The genus Sappinia: history, phylogeny, and medical relevance. *Exp Parasitol*. 2010;126:4-13.
166. Wilson MR, Shanbhag NM, Reid MJ, et al. Diagnosing *Balamuthia mandrillaris* encephalitis with metagenomics deep sequencing. *Ann Neurol*. 2015;78:722-730.
169. Yoder JS, Eddy BA, Visvesvara GS, et al. The epidemiology of primary amoebic meningoencephalitis in the USA, 1962-2008. *Epidemiol Infect*. 2010;138:968-975.

The full reference list for this chapter is available at ExpertConsult.com.

224 Toxoplasmosis

Kenneth M. Boyer • Santhosh M. Nadipuram

Toxoplasma gondii is an obligate intracellular protozoan parasite (phylum Apicomplexa, class Sporozoasida, order Eucoccidiida).[195,204,254] It is the only species in the genus. Infection may be clinically inapparent or latent, or it may result in actual disease, called toxoplasmosis. Latent *Toxoplasma* infection is common, involving approximately a third of the world's population. Overt toxoplasmosis is relatively uncommon and ranges in severity from subtle, self-limited disease to devastating and life-threatening illness.

Toxoplasma gondii was observed first in 1908 by Nicolle and Manceaux[70,186] in mononuclear cells in the spleen and liver of a North African rodent, the gundi (*Ctenodactylus gundi*). The organism soon was identified as a cause of disease in other animals, and in 1923 Janku[115] first recognized a case in a human. He described a parasite found in the retina of an infant; it was recognized later by Levaditi[139] as *Toxoplasma*. In 1937, Wolf and Cowen[261] reported a case of congenital granulomatous encephalitis that they considered to be caused by an "encephalitozoon." Albert Sabin,[216,217] who previously had encountered *T. gondii* in virologic work in guinea pigs, made the correct diagnosis of congenital toxoplasmosis in this case, and it was confirmed by serial passage of the parasite in laboratory animals.[262]

The discovery of *Toxoplasma* as a cause of disease acquired later in life has been credited to Pinkerton and Weinman,[197] who in 1940 described a generalized fatal illness caused by this organism in a young man. In retrospect, a case of acquired toxoplasmosis had been reported in 1908 by Darling.[56] In 1948, Sabin and Feldman[215] described a serologic test, the dye test, that allowed numerous investigators to study the epidemiologic and clinical aspects of toxoplasmosis and to define the spectrum of disease in humans. In 1969, some 60 years after the parasite was discovered, Frenkel, Dubey, and Miller[73,83–85] established that *Toxoplasma* is a coccidian protozoan and that its definitive hosts are the domestic cat and related members of the felid family.

ORGANISM AND TRANSMISSION

T. gondii exists in three forms or stages: the proliferative stage, or tachyzoite; the latent stage, a tissue cyst that contains bradyzoites; and a sexual form, the oocyst, within which sporozoites develop. The oocyst is formed during the intestinal epithelial stage of infection, exclusively in members of the cat family, the definitive host. The tachyzoite and tissue cyst are found in the extraintestinal tissues of cats and also in many other mammalian and avian hosts. Each stage of the organism has antigens in common with the other stages as well as unique antigens. Many of these antigens have been cloned, sequenced, and localized to microanatomic structures.[168,254] Humans may become infected from any of the three forms, as detailed later.

The tachyzoite form (Fig. 224.1A–C) is crescent shaped or oval, is approximately 3 by 7 μm, and is seen during the acute stage of infection. It stains well with Wright or Giemsa stain. Ultrastructural features

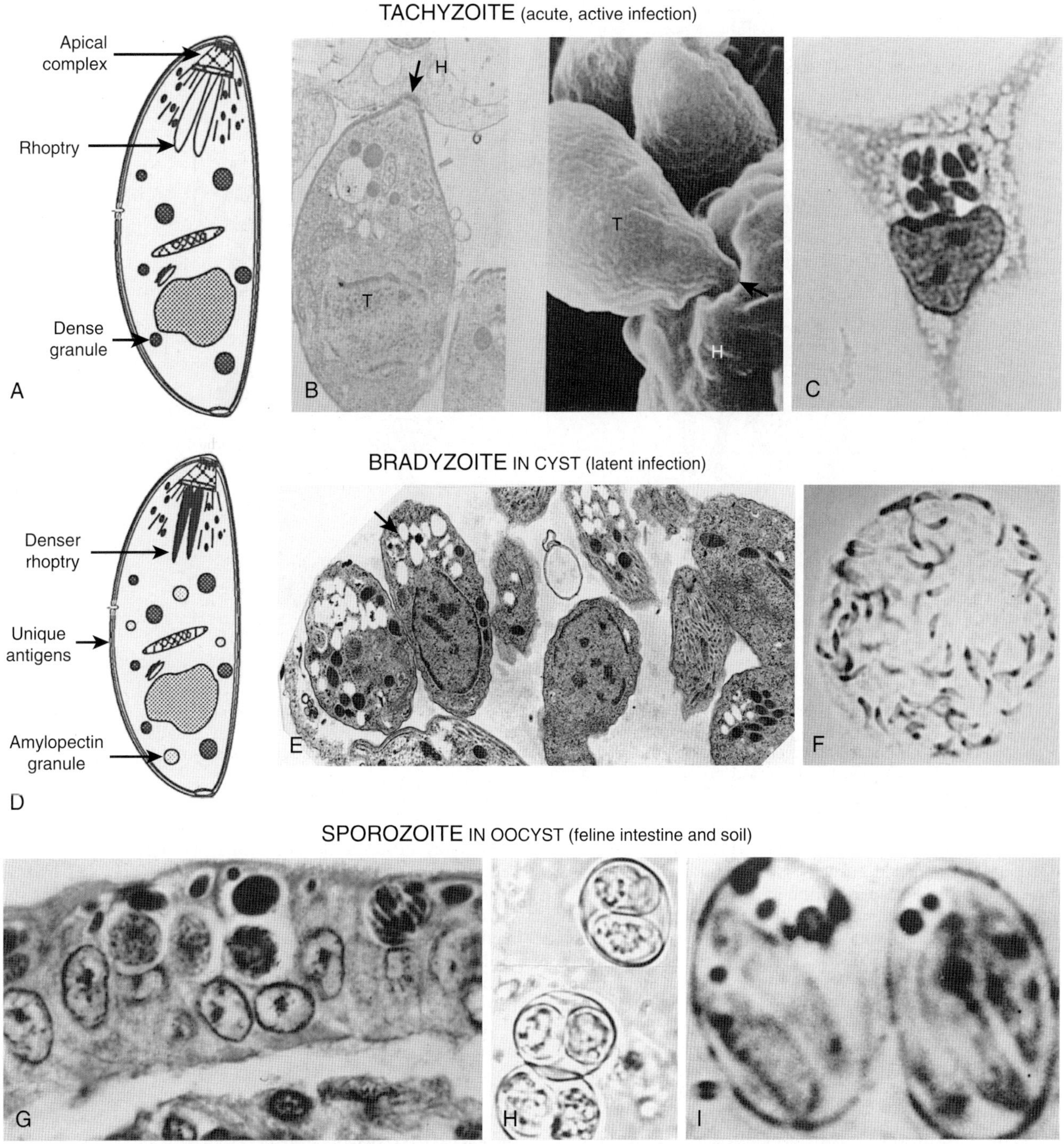

TACHYZOITE (acute, active infection)

Apical complex
Rhoptry
Dense granule
A
H
T
B
C

BRADYZOITE IN CYST (latent infection)

Denser rhoptry
Unique antigens
Amylopectin granule
D
E
F

SPOROZOITE IN OOCYST (feline intestine and soil)

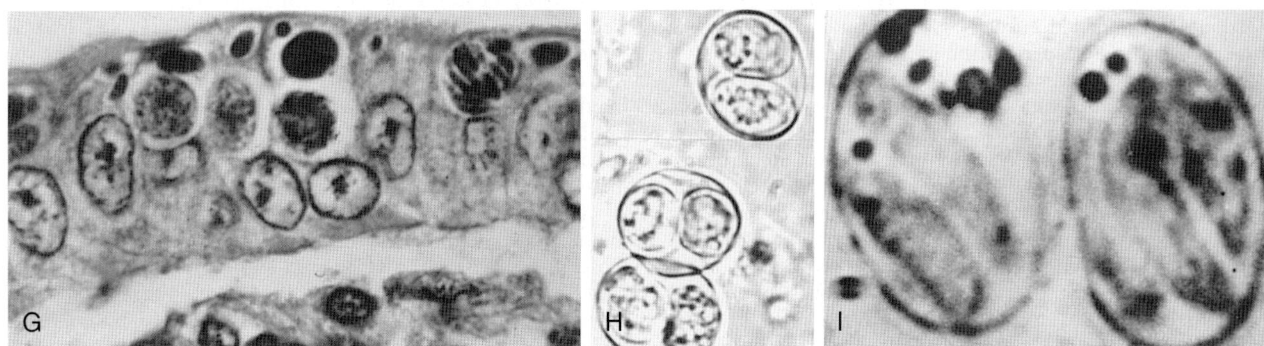

FIG. 224.1 Stages of *Toxoplasma gondii.* (A) Schematic diagram of a tachyzoite. (B) Transmission and scanning electron micrographs of a tachyzoite *(T)* invading a host cell *(H)*. *Arrow* indicates invagination of the host cell at the point of invasion. (C) Light micrograph of tachyzoites replicating within a parasitiferous vacuole in the host cell cytoplasm. (D) Schematic diagram of a bradyzoite. (E) Transmission electron micrograph of a cyst containing bradyzoites (*arrow* indicates amylopectin granules). (F) Light micrograph of a cyst containing bradyzoites. (G) Development of oocysts in cat intestine. (H) Oocysts in the lumen of cat intestine. (I) Sporulating oocysts that contain sporozoites. *A,* Apical complex; *H,* host cell; *T,* tachyzoite. (From Boyer KM, McLeod RL. *Toxoplasma gondii* [toxoplasmosis]. In: Long SS, Pickering LK, Prober CG, editors. *Principles and Practice of Pediatric Infectious Diseases.* New York: Churchill Livingstone; 1997:1423.)

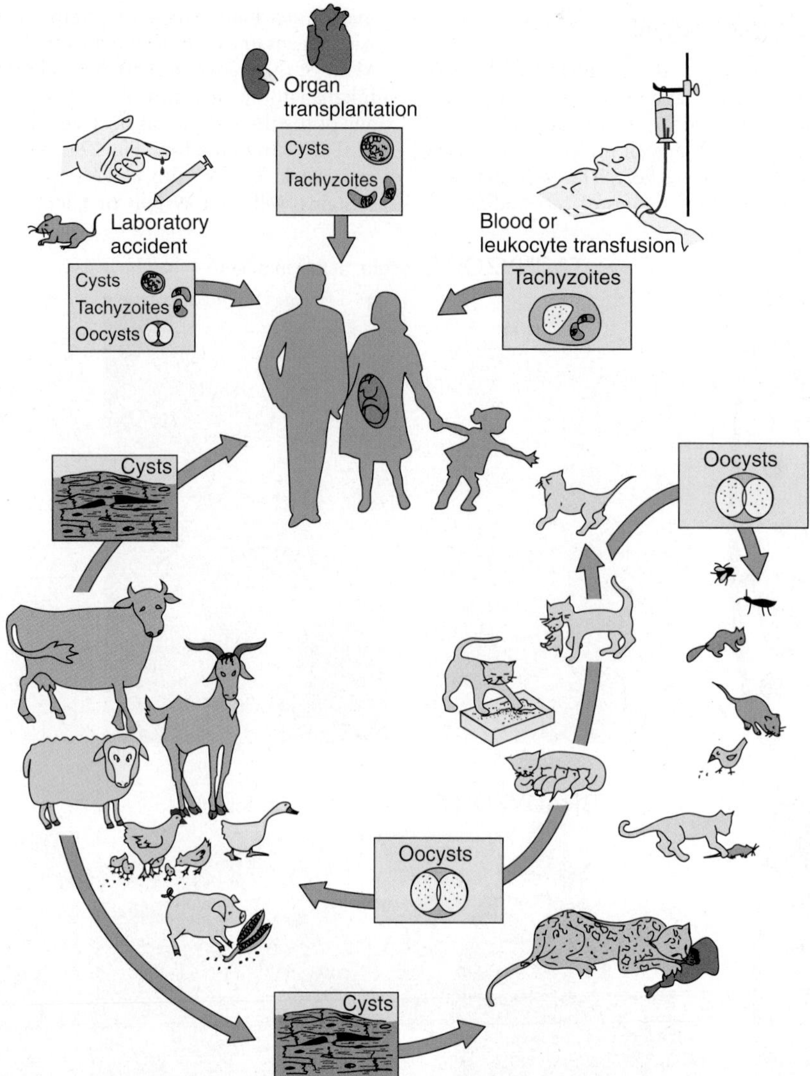

FIG. 224.2 Life cycle of *Toxoplasma gondii.* Cats are definitive hosts, with humans and other mammals being intermediate hosts. (From Remington JS, McLeod R. Toxoplasmosis. In: Braude AI, editor. *International Textbook of Medicine: Medical Microbiology and Infectious Disease.* vol. II. Philadelphia: Saunders; 1981:1818.)

include the apical complex of microtubules and rings, secretory organelles called rhoptries, micronemes and dense granules, and a chloroplast-like structure, called the apicoplast, with its own unique DNA.[36,74,254] Tachyzoites can invade all mammalian cells except perhaps nonnucleated red blood cells. They cannot withstand freezing and thawing, desiccation, or brief exposure to gastric or duodenal digestive juices. After penetration occurs, the tachyzoite multiplies by endodyogeny within a nonfusogenic vacuole, ultimately causing disruption of the cell and cell death. Hematogenous spread of tachyzoites to the placenta with secondary spread to the fetus results in congenital toxoplasmosis in humans and fetal infection and abortion in other susceptible animals.

The bradyzoite (see Fig. 224.1D–F) is able to persist in encysted form in all tissues and cause a chronic (latent) infection for the entire lifespan of the infected host. Cysts are demonstrable in tissues the first week of infection and range in size from approximately 10 to 100 μm. They have an argyrophilic wall but stand out most clearly from surrounding tissue when stained with periodic acid–Schiff stain. Usually, no inflammatory reaction occurs around cysts. Because this form can persist for many years in the tissues of clinically normal children and adults, its demonstration in histologic sections does not signify recent infection. Peptic or tryptic digestive fluids immediately disrupt the cyst wall, but the liberated bradyzoites (which have apical nuclei but otherwise resemble the tachyzoite form under light microscopy) can survive in these fluids for several hours, which allows time for invasion of local cells. Cysts can be destroyed by heating to 66°C (150°F), by freezing (below −20°C [−4°F]) and thawing, and by desiccation. They can survive for some months at refrigeration temperatures (4°C [39°F]) if they are in tissue. Infection in humans may be acquired by eating raw or inadequately cooked meat that contains cysts (Fig. 224.2). In carnivorous animals, infection may be acquired by eating raw meat or prey species that contain encysted organisms.

The oocyst form (see Fig. 224.1G–I) is found only in feces of members of the cat family (from household cats to mountain lions), the definitive hosts for *Toxoplasma,* and is the result of sexual reproduction (gametogony and schizogony), which occurs in the intestinal epithelium.[85,109] Oocysts are ovoid and approximately 10 to 12 μm. Infected cats may shed 10 million oocysts each day, which may be excreted for 3 weeks after primary (acute) infection but rarely thereafter. Excreted oocysts become infectious only after they undergo sporulation (eight sporozoites form in each oocyst); sporulation occurs 1 to 21 days (most commonly 2–8 days) after excretion, depending on temperature and the availability of oxygen. The oocyst is far more resilient than the other life cycle forms and can survive for months in water and for 1 year or more in moist soil. Ingestion of sporulated oocysts transmits the infection. Oocysts play a major role in transmission by the fecal-oral route in animal reservoirs and by inadvertent ingestion in humans.

The genome of *T. gondii* consists of 8 × 10^7 base pairs distributed among 12 chromosomes. Much of the genome has been sequenced, a genetic linkage map has been constructed, and three major clonal genotypes (I, II, and III) have been identified.[55,107,130,144,226,254] Some of the factors that regulate stage conversion from tachyzoite to bradyzoite have been defined.[168,254] Understanding of the regulation of life cycle stages and the unique pathways of intermediary metabolism in *T. gondii* and related apicomplexans (e.g. *Plasmodium*) may provide new approaches to therapy.

EPIDEMIOLOGY

Acquired Infection

Cats are central in the parasite's life cycle, and humans and other mammals are intermediate hosts. If infected tissue (e.g., a mouse) is consumed by a susceptible cat, the sexual cycle is induced in the cat intestine; oocysts are excreted and are infectious for mammals and birds, in which the life cycle (tachyzoites and encysted bradyzoites) is perpetuated. Cats shed oocysts for only brief durations (days to weeks) but in extremely large numbers (1 × 10^7/day). A cat is more likely to become infected if it is an outdoor (feral) cat or a predator or is fed fresh, uncooked table scraps. Humans come in contact with cat excrement either directly (e.g., emptying the litter pan, eating uncooked vegetables) or by more insidious means (e.g., cleaning a horse stall, weeding the garden, playing in a sandbox). Accidental ingestion may occur under circumstances that are unsuspected. In a recent report, only 49% of women with acute primary toxoplasmosis during pregnancy who gave birth to infected children could identify significant risk factors for sporozoite acquisition, although 78% had humoral antibodies against sporozoites.[22]

Meat for human consumption that contains tissue cysts may also serve as a source of infection if it is eaten raw or undercooked. Examples of inadvertent exposures include an Amish farm wife preparing sausage, a couple consuming steak tartare in an expensive restaurant, and a rancher butchering a deer.[22] Mode of infection probably varies internationally according to climate, cultural, dietary, and soil exposure practices. In Chile, for example, 43% of women with recent infection had antibody to sporozoite-specific protein (oocysts), suggesting ingestion of undercooked infected meat as the more common mode of acquisition.[181]

Infection with *Toxoplasma* occurs commonly in humans. It is estimated that 2 billion of the world's population are infected.[195] In the United States, the prevalence of seropositivity (synonymous with latent infection) has been determined from studies of military recruits, from surveys in major cities, and most comprehensively from the National Health and Nutrition Examination Surveys (NHANES). In the early 1960s, the overall prevalence in military recruits was 14%, with the lowest rates in the Mountain (3%) and Pacific (8%) states and the highest rates in the Northeast (20%) and East South Central (19%) states.[228] A more recent study from the late 1980s showed a similar geographic distribution, but prevalence rates were approximately a third lower throughout the country.[228]

The NHANES are periodic cluster sample surveys representing the entire population of the United States. The 1988 to 1994 NHANES showed an overall seroprevalence in individuals of childbearing age (12–49 years old) of 14.1% compared with rates of 9.0% for the same age cohort in the 1999 to 2004 NHANES[121] and 6.7% in the 2009 to 2010 study.[120] Higher prevalences of *Toxoplasma* infection in the United States are associated with foreign birth, low educational level, living in crowded conditions, and having a soil-related occupation.[122]

Dietary exposure is probably a declining mode of acquisition in the United States.[122] Previous estimates were that approximately 8% of commercial beef, 20% of commercial pork, and 25% of commercial lamb contained encysted *Toxoplasma* bradyzoites.[179] More recent data suggest much lower levels of viable tissue cysts in commercial meat, although "free range" and "organic" meats have higher prevalences.[72,101,118] An indirect mechanism of exposure to cysts derived from livestock, especially goats and sheep, is consumption of unpasteurized dairy products such as raw milk and cheese.[218] A "niche" meat source with high prevalence of *Toxoplasma* infection is game. Studies in Ohio yielded prevalences of 73% to 76% in white-tailed deer.[71] We are aware of two "miniepidemics" of acute toxoplasmosis (including congenital infections) related to consumption of deer and elk "tartare."

During these decades of declining prevalence of *Toxoplasma* infection, the rate of cat ownership has actually increased in the United States.[121,122] The net overall decline in prevalence may be explained partly by improved agricultural safety, but also by the common practice of freezing commercial meat before releasing it for sale. Combined with the use of home freezers, these practices may be having a significant beneficial effect.[101,118]

Additional modes of transmission, such as waterborne,[12,20,69] have been described. Their exact contribution to the overall prevalence of toxoplasmosis in the United States is unclear, however. During the decades of the NHANES studies, increasing proportions of US water supplies have added filtration to decrease *Giardia* and *Cryptosporidium* transmission. This filtration also is likely to eliminate *Toxoplasma* oocysts.[122]

Internationally, prevalence rates vary considerably. Rates in studies include the following: United Kingdom, 9%; China, 11%; Poland, 41%; France, 44%; Belgium, 49%; and Brazil, 60% to 77%.[192,195,240] The prevalence of infection is determined partly by climate; colder regions and regions that are hot and dry or at high altitude have lower rates of human infection than warmer and moister regions do. Prevalences are declining in Europe, notably in France,[188] because of educational efforts and improved meat safety. Tropical South American countries, particularly Brazil, continue to have high prevalences, with correspondingly high rates of congenital and ocular infection.[2,18,31,58,128,227,243]

Despite declining prevalence in the United States, it is estimated that more than 1 million new infections occur each year, with resultant ocular lesions in more than 21,500 persons, of which approximately 4800 are symptomatic.[119] An analysis of International Classification of Diseases, Ninth Revision (ICD-9) codes in private insurance records resulted in an estimate of 6856 cases per year.[149] The rate of hospitalization for human immunodeficiency virus (HIV)–associated toxoplasmosis has declined since the advent of effective antiretroviral therapy; however, hospitalization for non–HIV-associated toxoplasmosis has remained steady from 1993 to 2008.[123]

Common-source outbreaks of acute acquired *Toxoplasma* infection have been authenticated. Unique and clear-cut sources that have been documented to be highly likely include exposure to contaminated municipal water systems,[20,58] aerosolized cat excrement in a riding stable,[238] and consumption of unpasteurized goat milk.[218] In other circumstances, extensive investigations have failed to yield convincing answers.[151,223] Because of the possibility of common-source exposure, however, families of patients with acute acquired infection should be evaluated for subclinical infection.[43,147]

Accidental self-inoculation with a needle contaminated with *Toxoplasma* has resulted in acquired infections in laboratory workers. Infections also have been ascribed to blood transfusions, stem cell transplantation, and organ transplantation.[142,146,173]

Congenital Infection

Infection of the fetus occurs during maternal parasitemia, with subsequent infection of the placenta caused by tachyzoites.[84,165,195,204] Placental infection represents an important intermediary step between maternal and fetal infection. A delay of 16 weeks between placental infection and subsequent infection of the fetus has been noted and is termed the prenatal incubation period.[204] Congenital infection is thought to occur, with rare exception, only after primary maternal infection with *Toxoplasma*.[61,62,204] The only two well-documented exceptions to this rule occurred in immunodeficient pregnant women.[176,204] Maternal reinfection leading to congenital toxoplasmosis also has been reported very rarely.[88,204] In a large series that carefully studied more than 800 women who had given birth to congenitally infected children, not a single congenital infection occurred in subsequent pregnancies.[204] A general consensus is that only acute infection beginning during pregnancy can lead to congenital infection. Despite the existence of a few well-documented cases of biopsy-proven lymphadenopathic toxoplasmosis occurring 2 months before conception that resulted in congenitally infected infants, this pattern of occurrence also seems to be extremely rare.[88,246] Congenital toxoplasmosis has occurred in twins and triplets, with occasional discordance.[45,204]

The incidence of congenital toxoplasmosis in a population is determined by the risk of a woman's experiencing primary infection while she is pregnant. This incidence depends on three factors: (1) the age-specific incidence of primary infection during the childbearing years, (2) the age distribution of pregnant women in the population, and (3) the fetal transmission rate in primary infection. A theoretical analysis by Frenkel[83,204] that was based on these three factors, assuming a childbearing age group of 20 to 29 years and an overall fetal transmission rate of 40%, showed that maximal risk occurs when the age-specific incidence rate in a population is 3% to 5% per year, a rate that corresponds to a seropositivity prevalence of 50% to 80% in women of childbearing age. In such a population, the predicted incidence of congenital toxoplasmosis would be 4.4 to 4.6 per 1000 pregnancies. (A study from Brazil yielded prevalence and mother-to-infant transmission rates remarkably similar to these predictions.[243]) At higher age-specific incidences, rates of congenital toxoplasmosis would be lower because nearly all pregnant women already would be infected chronically. At lower incidences, rates also would be lower but because of less frequent acquisition of maternal infection.

Studies in the early 1970s revealed an incidence of congenital toxoplasmosis in the United States of approximately two per 1000 births.[1,13,204] More recently, the incidence of congenital infection in the United States has been documented to be 0.08 per 1000 births (one in 12,000 births) by immunoglobulin M (IgM) screening of blood specimens collected on filter paper from newborns in Massachusetts and New Hampshire.[100] This is a conservative estimate because the methodology detects approximately 75% of infections. (A corrected figure would be one in 9000.) In this experience from Massachusetts, a case-control study involving 14 years of newborn screening for congenital toxoplasmosis found that birth of the mother outside the United States, particularly in Cambodia and Laos, was the strongest predictor, whereas live birth rate of the mother (≥3) and both extremes of educational level were also predictors of congenital infection.[116] A global perspective is provided by a systematic review from the World Health Organization.[240] Incidences of congenital toxoplasmosis in Europe ranged from 0.5 to 1.6 per 1000 and 0.6 to 3.4 per 1000 in Central and South America. The estimated global incidence was 190,000 cases per year.

PATHOLOGY

After intracellular multiplication at the site of entry occurs, tachyzoites are disseminated in blood and may invade all organs and tissues. The severity of infection probably is a function of strain virulence, host susceptibility, tissue tropism, the strain's ability to transit endothelial barriers, and the immune privilege of the eyes and central nervous system (CNS).[97,98,150,195,204] Proliferation of tachyzoites results in death of the invaded cells and, eventually, small necrotic foci surrounded by intense cellular reaction. With recovery, cysts without an inflammatory response around them may persist in the brain, retinas, cochlea, bone marrow, lymph nodes, liver, spleen, and lungs, as well as in skeletal, heart, and smooth muscle.[82–84]

In active infection of the CNS, *Toxoplasma*-filled cells are scattered throughout the gray matter, where they produce diffuse meningoencephalitis with miliary microglial nodules and foci of perivascular inflammation.[42] Large lesions may mimic cerebral tumors. Areas of basal ganglial and periventricular inflammation may calcify in the fetus.[67,193] Obstruction of the aqueduct of Sylvius or the foramen of Monro may result in hydrocephalus in congenital infection.[110]

The enlarged lymph nodes in acute acquired toxoplasmosis show characteristic pathologic changes that may warrant making a presumptive diagnosis.[68,246] Such changes include reactive follicular hyperplasia, epithelioid histiocytes encroaching on and blurring the margins of germinal centers, and distention of subcapsular and trabecular sinuses by monocytoid cells. Tachyzoites and cysts rarely are seen.[68]

In the eye, active chorioretinitis begins in the retina with severe inflammation and necrosis and exudation into the vitreous. Single or multiple foci occur, and secondary involvement of the choroid is always present. Tachyzoites and cysts have been found in these lesions.[24,204,208,209]

In immunocompromised hosts, widespread necrotizing lesions may be seen in the heart, muscle, brain, and other organs. These lesions, particularly those involving the CNS, have been found frequently with reactivation of toxoplasmosis in patients with acquired immunodeficiency syndrome (AIDS).[145]

IMMUNOLOGY

Cell-mediated immune responses are the major immunologic mechanisms that prevent reactivation of *T. gondii* in a chronically infected normal host.[37,53] Numerous effector mechanisms contribute to protection in murine models and human infection: $CD8^+$ cytotoxic T lymphocytes, $CD4^+$ T lymphocytes, monocyte oxidative mechanisms, production of interferon-γ by natural killer cells, and activation of macrophages by interferon-γ and tumor necrosis factor-α.[91,102,125,127,224,233] Killing of the parasite within activated macrophages is associated with the release of interferon-γ and intracellular production of nitric oxide. Interleukin-2 and interleukin-12 enhance host resistance to *T. gondii;* interleukin-10 impairs the ability of macrophages to kill the parasite.[90]

In murine models, evidence exists for genetic determination of host resistance to infection.[26,25,150,161] Genetic and epigenetic factors at COL2A1, ABCA4, P2RX7, and ALOX12 influence susceptibility and clinical outcomes in human toxoplasmosis.[112–114,260] Presence of the DQ3 allele also seems to be associated with toxoplasmic encephalitis in patients with AIDS and hydrocephalus in infants with congenital toxoplasmosis.[25,26]

Successful immunization of mice[27] and sheep[28,29] with *T. gondii* components and live tachyzoites of an "incomplete" strain raises the possibility of developing a human vaccine.[117,162,252,254,266]

CLINICAL SYNDROMES

The disease in children may be considered in three categories: postnatally acquired, congenital, and ocular (which may be congenital or acquired).[203] Clinically apparent infection in older children may have been acquired recently or caused by reactivation of latent congenital or postnatally acquired infection. Congenital and acquired infections usually are subclinical, but untreated or briefly treated congenital infection ultimately leads to serious sequelae in most cases.[132]

Acute Acquired Toxoplasmosis

Acquired *Toxoplasma* infection is asymptomatic in most cases and frequently goes unrecognized because only 10% to 15% of infected individuals have clinical symptoms and signs. In certain outbreaks related to infection by oocysts, however, more than one-half of infected patients have been symptomatic.[238] The most common findings are lymphadenopathy and fatigue without fever.[154] The nodes are discrete and may or may not be tender. They do not suppurate. The groups of nodes most commonly involved are the cervical, suboccipital, supraclavicular, axillary, and inguinal. The adenopathy may be localized or involve multiple areas, including the retroperitoneal and mesenteric nodes. Uncommonly, the lymphadenopathy is accompanied by fever, malaise, fatigue, sore throat, and myalgia, a picture that closely simulates that of infectious mononucleosis but without serologic evidence of acute Epstein-Barr virus or cytomegalovirus (CMV) infection. The differential diagnosis of the lymphadenopathy often includes lymphoma, necessitating excisional biopsy. Chorioretinitis may develop during acute acquired infection, but, in the United States, it does not occur commonly and is seldom vision threatening.[151,180] For example, among mothers of congenitally infected infants in the National Collaborative Chicago-based Congenital Toxoplasmosis Study (NCCCTS), 10 of 130 mothers (7.7%) were found to have chorioretinal lesions (8 small, 2 medium-sized, all unilateral).[187] Ocular involvement is much more common and more severe in acquired disease in Brazil, a reflection of more virulent genotypes.[2,128,227] The liver may be involved, and liver function test results may reflect hepatocellular damage. In individuals with normal immunologic function and no severe underlying disease in the United States and Europe, the infection usually is self-limited and seldom requires treatment.

In contrast, more severe and frequently fulminant infections are seen in patients receiving immunosuppressive therapy, in patients who have disease of the bone marrow or reticuloendothelial system, in recipients of bone marrow or stem cell transplants, and in patients with AIDS.[59,89,111,141,142,145,152,214,245] Encephalitis and rarely pneumonitis and myocarditis are the most important localized forms that may be encountered in immunocompromised patients. In toxoplasmic encephalitis, the predominant neurologic symptoms are headache, disorientation, and drowsiness. These symptoms may simulate aseptic meningitis or a mass lesion. In view of the various clinical manifestations of CNS involvement, it is important to consider toxoplasmosis whenever evidence of acute CNS disease is present in the setting of immunocompromise.

Epidemiologic studies have suggested a correlation between *Toxoplasma* infection and a variety of neurologic and psychiatric illnesses in adults, including schizophrenia, suicide rates in women, and Alzheimer disease.[9,134,143,232] These intriguing findings require additional research before any conclusions can be reached.

Congenital Toxoplasmosis

Congenital infection usually is the result of an asymptomatic acute infection in the mother.[23,78] In a small proportion of cases, spontaneous abortion, prematurity, or stillbirth may result. Congenital toxoplasmosis has a wide spectrum of clinical manifestations but is subclinical (i.e., not recognized in the usual neonatal examination) in approximately 70% of infected newborns. When it is clinically apparent, it may mimic other diseases of the newborn.

Involvement of the eyes and CNS involvement are the hallmarks of congenital *Toxoplasma* infection. The presence of chorioretinitis, intracranial calcifications, and hydrocephalus is referred to as the "classic triad" of congenital toxoplasmosis. Fever, hydrocephalus or microcephaly, hepatosplenomegaly, jaundice, convulsions, chorioretinitis (usually bilateral), cerebral calcifications, and cerebrospinal fluid (CSF) abnormalities (markedly increased protein concentration and mononuclear pleocytosis) are considered the classic features of severe congenital toxoplasmosis.[67,172,204] These manifestations occurred commonly in an early series of patients from New York reported by Eichenwald[77] (Table 224.1). The case-fatality rate was 12%. In survivors in this series, sequelae included mental retardation in 86%; convulsions, spasticity, and palsies in almost 75%; and severely impaired vision in 60%.[77,210] Other occasional findings included rash (maculopapular, petechial, or both), myocarditis, pneumonitis and respiratory distress, hearing defects, an erythroblastosis-like picture, thrombocytopenia, lymphocytosis, monocytosis, and nephrotic syndrome. *Toxoplasma* has been detected in the inner ear and mastoid, with the associated inflammation resulting in deafness.[219] Ascending flaccid paralysis with myelitis also has been reported.[204] These signs now are known to be most typical of the severe form of the infection in the absence of treatment.

The risk for transmission to the fetus varies significantly with the trimester of gestation in which the mother becomes infected. The rates are approximately 15% in the first trimester, 30% in the second trimester, and 60% in the third trimester,[48,61,62] rates that have been confirmed in data from the Systematic Review on Congenital Toxoplasmosis (SYROCOT) study group in Europe.[239] In contrast, the severity of clinical disease in congenitally infected infants is related inversely to the gestational age at the time of primary maternal infection (Table 224.2). In the original studies from France,[62] disease that was clinically apparent at birth occurred in 8 of 11 (73%) infected live-born infants whose mothers had first trimester infection, in 19 of 68 (28%) with second trimester infection, and in only 8 of 76 (11%) with third trimester infection. Overall, 72% of live-born infected infants were asymptomatic. These findings were confirmed in subsequent studies from Paris[103] and the SYROCOT group.[239]

A later French prospective study of 210 congenitally infected infants born to mothers who were identified to have primary infection acquired during pregnancy (45% of whom were treated with spiramycin) revealed significant morbidity in 94 newborns.[48] Overall, 2 (0.9%) cases were fatal, 21 (10%) were severe, and 71 (34%) were mild; 116 (55%) cases were asymptomatic. These observations confirm that most congenital *Toxoplasma* infections are "subclinical" at birth. Obvious manifestations occur infrequently. Of the 116 infants in the same study with a normal routine newborn physical examination, however, 39 (34%) were found to have one or more abnormalities on closer scrutiny. Twenty-two of the 116 (19%) had abnormal CSF findings on lumbar puncture, 17 (15%) had chorioretinitis on indirect ophthalmoscopic examination, and 10 (9%) had intracranial calcifications on head radiographs or computed tomography (CT) scans. Guerina and colleagues[100] made remarkably similar observations in the congenitally infected newborns whom they identified in New England by heel-stick blood sampling.

Some infected children without overt disease as neonates may escape serious sequelae of the infection. However, a significant number (24% to 85%) will develop chorioretinitis, strabismus, blindness, hydrocephalus or microcephaly, cerebral calcifications, developmental delay, epilepsy, or deafness that will manifest months or years later. Three studies provide data that define the occurrence of these late sequelae.[131,132,135]

In a study from Paris,[135] 26,402 apparently healthy infants were tested routinely for serologic evidence of *Toxoplasma* infection at 10 months of age. Of these infants, 51 (1.9 of 1000 births) had positive serologic results for *Toxoplasma,* indicative of congenital infection. None had been treated for *Toxoplasma* infection in infancy. Of the 51, five were found to have chorioretinal scars by ophthalmologic examination, and chorioretinal lesions had developed in another four children by the time they reached 4 years of age, the longest period of follow-up. Some children eventually lost functional vision in one eye. Three had intracranial calcifications.

Similarly, in a study from Holland in which a cohort of 1821 pregnant women were screened serologically, 12 congenitally infected infants were detected, and 11 of them were monitored for 20 years.[131,132] Of the 11 children, five were treated as neonates for 1 month only, and six were not. Of the five treated infants, four had eye disease as neonates and one had parasites in CSF, which prompted therapy. Of the 11, nine (82%) had chorioretinal scars by the time they reached 20 years of age, and four of them, including two who were initially normal, had severe visual impairment or blindness in one eye. The onset of disease leading

TABLE 224.1 Vertical Transmission and Severity of Congenital Toxoplasmosis by the Timing of Maternal Infection During Pregnancy

	TRIMESTER OF MATERNAL INFECTION[a]			
	First	Second	Third	All[b]
Vertical transmission rate	17/126 (13)	73/246 (30)	76/128 (59)	166/500 (33)
Proportion of infected newborns with specific disease severity				
Subclinical (asymptomatic)	3/17 (18)	49/73 (67)	68/76 (89)	120/166 (72)
Mild disease	1/17 (6)	13/73 (18)	8/76 (11)	22/166 (13)
Severe disease	7/17 (41)	6/73 (8)	0/76 (0)	13/166 (8)
Stillborn or perinatal death	6/17 (35)	5/73 (7)	0/76 (0)	11/166 (7)

[a]Data are presented as n/N (%).
[b]A total of 42 of 542 pregnancies excluded because timing of infection was not ascertained.
Modified from Desmonts G, Couvreur J. Congenital toxoplasmosis: a prospective study of the offspring of 542 women who acquired toxoplasmosis during pregnancy: pathophysiology of congenital disease. In: Thalhammer O, Baumgarten K, Pollak A, eds. *Perinatal Medicine. Sixth European Congress, Vienna 1978.* Stuttgart, Germany: Georg Thieme; 1979.

TABLE 224.2 Signs and Symptoms Occurring Before Diagnosis or During the Course of Untreated Acute Congenital Toxoplasmosis[a]

	FREQUENCY OF OCCURRENCE[b] IN PATIENTS WITH	
Signs and Symptoms	**Neurologic Disease[c]**	**Generalized Disease[d]**
Infants	N = 108	N = 44
Chorioretinitis	102 (94)	29 (66)
Abnormal spinal fluid	59 (55)	37 (84)
Anemia	55 (51)	34 (77)
Jaundice	31 (29)	35 (80)
Splenomegaly	23 (21)	40 (90)
Convulsions	54 (50)	8 (18)
Fever	27 (25)	34 (77)
Intracranial calcification	54 (50)	2 (4)
Hepatomegaly	18 (17)	34 (77)
Lymphadenopathy	18 (17)	30 (68)
Vomiting	17 (16)	21 (48)
Hydrocephalus	30 (28)	0 (0)
Diarrhea	7 (6)	11 (25)
Pneumonitis	0 (0)	18 (41)
Microcephalus	14 (13)	0 (0)
Eosinophilia	6 (4)	8 (18)
Rash	1 (1)	11 (25)
Abnormal bleeding	3 (3)	8 (18)
Hypothermia	2 (2)	9 (20)
Cataracts	5 (5)	0 (0)
Glaucoma	2 (2)	0 (0)
Optic atrophy	2 (2)	0 (0)
Microphthalmos	2 (2)	0 (0)
Children ≥4 Years Old	N = 70	N = 31
Mental retardation	62 (89)	25 (81)
Convulsions	58 (83)	24 (77)
Spasticity and palsies	53 (76)	18 (58)
Severely impaired vision	48 (69)	13 (42)
Hydrocephalus or microcephalus	31 (44)	2 (6)
Deafness	12 (17)	3 (10)
Normal	6 (9)	5 (16)

[a]In 152 infants and 101 of these same patients after ≥4 years of follow-up.
[b]Data indicate numbers of patients, with percentages in parentheses.
[c]Patients with central nervous system diseases in the first year of life.
[d]Patients with nonneurologic diseases during the first 2 months of life.
Modified from Eichenwald HG. A study of congenital toxoplasmosis, with particular emphasis on clinical manifestations, sequelae, and therapy. In: Siim JC, ed. *Human Toxoplasmosis.* Copenhagen, Denmark: Munksgaard; 1960:44.

to blindness occurred as late as 18 years of age. No neurologic or cognitive sequelae were observed.

The results of this Dutch study are similar to those previously reported by Wilson and associates[259] from Alabama in a retrospective analysis of patients from the United States. During a mean follow-up period of 8.3 years, sequelae developed in 11 of 13 congenitally infected children (85%) who had no signs of disease on detailed examination in the newborn period. Sequelae included chorioretinal lesions in 11 children (85%), severe neurologic disability in one child (8%), and mental retardation in two children (15%). Sequelae first were noted at ages ranging from 1 month to 9 years. These 13 children were detected either as a result of routine screening of cord serum for IgM antibodies to *Toxoplasma,*[1] performed because acute *Toxoplasma* infection was diagnosed in the mother,[259] or as a result of nonspecific findings in the neonatal period (two were small for gestational age, and one had transient borderline thrombocytopenia).

That treatment may decrease the frequency or severity of sequelae is suggested by the Alabama and Paris studies, in which chorioretinitis developed only in untreated infants between 10 months and 4 years old. Taken together, these data indicate that most congenitally infected children who receive no or brief treatment, including children with inapparent infection as neonates, experience untoward sequelae during childhood. Current treatment regimens—prolonged for at least 1 year and often initiated before birth—are associated with substantially less frequent and less severe sequelae (see section on treatment).

Congenital toxoplasmosis may mimic or coexist with infection by other organisms. It must be differentiated from other perinatal infections caused by CMV, herpes simplex virus (HSV), rubella virus, *Treponema pallidum* (syphilis), HIV-1, lymphocytic choriomeningitis (LCM) virus, Zika virus, and certain bacteria (e.g., *Listeria*). HSV, CMV, LCM, and Zika virus infections, syphilis, and rubella may cause chorioretinitis; CMV, LCM, HSV, and Zika virus and HIV-1 infections may cause encephalopathies associated with cerebral calcifications. Degenerative encephalopathies and storage diseases in older children also may resemble congenital toxoplasmosis.

Infants or preschool children with coexisting HIV infection and toxoplasmosis have been described.[174,176] In at least six of these patients, HIV and *Toxoplasma* infections seem to have both been acquired in utero. Of these six patients, all but one had clinical evidence of CNS disease, and in most of these children, the CNS disease was associated with other findings common in congenital infection. These findings included hepatosplenomegaly, fever, and chorioretinitis and were evident at birth (one infant) or developed by the time the infant reached 4 months of age. Two of the other infants remained asymptomatic; one was treated for *Toxoplasma* infection, and the other was not treated. One additional infant who acquired HIV infection at 18 months of age from a blood transfusion died at 5 years of age of toxoplasmic encephalitis. The findings in this patient resembled those in adults with AIDS and toxoplasmic encephalitis.[145] The advent of highly active antiretroviral therapy (HAART) and the widespread use of trimethoprim-sulfamethoxazole for *Pneumocystis jiroveci* pneumonia prophylaxis (which has a prophylactic effect on *Toxoplasma*) have greatly decreased the frequency of clinical toxoplasmic encephalitis in children and adults with HIV infection.

Ocular Toxoplasmosis

In active congenital toxoplasmosis, the retinal lesions usually are bilateral.[172,189] In older children, chorioretinitis may involve only one eye and may be the sole manifestation of congenital toxoplasmosis. Toxoplasmic chorioretinitis in Europe and the United States, even in older children and adults, usually is considered to be the result of congenital infection.[180] A report of 38 children diagnosed with symptomatic chorioretinitis between 2002 and 2004 in the United Kingdom confirmed that 58% of cases were the result of congenital infection.[93] In some studies, *Toxoplasma* infection has accounted for 5% of severe visual impairments in children.[126] Active lesions in the fundus appear as white or yellowish foci with elevated, edematous margins surrounded by a zone of hyperemia (Fig. 224.3). Cells and fibrinous exudate in the vitreous may obscure the fundus. Older lesions appear as glial scars, and in areas in which the retina has been destroyed, the choroid and sclera are visible. Around the depigmented areas, deposition of pigment from the destroyed retina is present. The position of the lesion may be macular, juxtapapillary, or peripheral; 58% of congenital lesions involve the macula.[172]

Patients may experience loss of central vision (caused by a macular lesion), hazy vision (caused by accumulated exudate), or "floaters" (caused by reactivation of peripheral foci). Neonates or infants with toxoplasmic eye disease may have microphthalmos, small corneas, posterior cortical cataract, anisometropia, strabismus, and nystagmus.[172,249] Strabismus and nystagmus in a child of any age should raise the possibility of congenital toxoplasmosis. The appearance of lesions in the fundus is not specific for toxoplasmosis. Similar lesions may occur with other less common granulomatous diseases in the eye, such as toxocariasis, congenital LCM and Zika virus infection, cat-scratch disease, and tuberculosis. Chorioretinitis may be recurrent, most commonly with reactivation at the margins of preexisting lesions.

LABORATORY DIAGNOSIS

Acute infection can be diagnosed by isolation of *T. gondii* from blood or body fluids; demonstration of tachyzoites in histologic sections of tissue or cytologic preparations of body fluids; characteristic lymph node histologic findings; demonstration of *Toxoplasma* cysts in the placenta, fetus, or neonate; detection of the *Toxoplasma* genome by polymerase chain reaction (PCR) in body fluids; or characteristic serologic test results.[21,164,177–179,199,205,257] Each of these methods is discussed, but serologic tests are emphasized because they are the most common and readily available methods to establish the diagnosis (Table 224.3).[257]

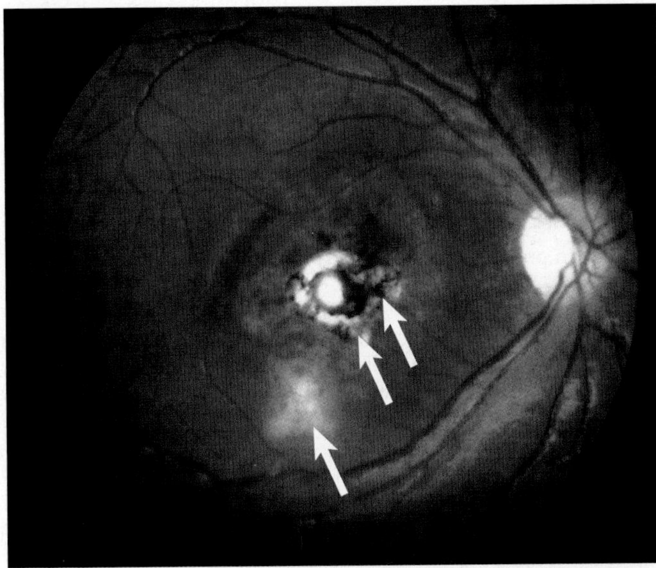

FIG. 224.3 Active and quiescent chorioretinitis caused by congenital toxoplasmosis in a 12-year-old patient. The active lesion *(single arrow)* is a satellite of an old chorioretinal scar *(double arrows)*. (From Mets M, Holfels E, Boyer KM, et al. Eye manifestations of congenital toxoplasmosis. *Am J Ophthalmol.* 1996;122:309–24.)

Serologic Methods

Measurements of IgG Antibody

The most useful tests for detection of IgG antibodies to *Toxoplasma* include the Sabin-Feldman dye test (the reference standard),[140,215] indirect immunofluorescent antibody (IFA) test, agglutination tests, and enzyme-linked immunosorbent assay (ELISA). Titers in ELISA are expressed in different terms for different commercial kits, thus precluding a discussion of IgG ELISA titers in relation to the diagnosis of acute infection.[65,251,257,267] In these tests, IgG antibodies appear within the first week of primary infection and reach peak titers (usually ≥1:500) within 1 to 2 months; detectable titers usually persist for life. Although the dye test is the most reliable method, it is available in only a few reference laboratories. Immunoblot compares well with the dye test and may detect antibody slightly earlier than other methods, but it is also not widely available.[124,138]

The IFA test and ELISA are the most widely available and, when properly performed, yield results similar to those obtained with the dye test; however, many laboratories use commercially available kits that are not consistently reliable. Because the performance of kits varies greatly, clinicians must be familiar with the variations if they are comparing results from different laboratories.[138] Some sera that contain antinuclear antibodies yield false-positive IFA test results.[3] The direct agglutination tests that currently are available use formalin-fixed tachyzoites or antigen-coated latex particles, are simple to perform, and are accurate.[228,257]

Initially after primary infection occurs, the avidity of IgG antibody for *T. gondii* antigen is low. Urea dissociates low-avidity antibodies, and a test has been developed that determines the percentage of antibodies that resist elution by 6 mol/L urea. This test is useful in the first 12

TABLE 224.3 Guidelines for Interpretation of Serologic Tests for Toxoplasmosis

IgG	IgM	IgG Avidity	Interpretation
Positive	Negative	—	Remote infection, immune. IgG avidity testing is best used when both IgG and IgM are positive and timing of infection is crucial, as in pregnancy (see below). For evaluation of infection in the newborn, false-negative IgM results occur in approximately 25% of cases. If infection is suspected in this setting, further testing (dye test, IgM EIA, IgA EIA, IgE EIA/ISAGA, PCRs, ideally with paired maternal serology tests—see text) is necessary in a reference laboratory (*Toxoplasma* Serology Laboratory, PAMF Research Institute, 795 El Camino Real, Ames Building Palo Alto, CA, 94301; 650-853-4828).
Positive	Positive or equivocal	High	Infection within the past 18 mo but likely >12 wk ago. If pregnant and beyond first trimester, consider sending specimen to reference laboratory for dye test, repeat IgG avidity and IgM EIA, IgA EIA, IgE EIA/ISAGA, and AC/HS testing (see above).
Positive	Positive or equivocal	Low	Infection within the past 12 wk. Consider sending specimen to a reference laboratory (see above) to time infection more accurately (dye test, repeat IgG avidity and IgM EIA, IgA EIA, IgE EIA/ISAGA, and AC/HS) in the setting of pregnancy.
Equivocal	Negative	—	Indeterminate. Test a new specimen or consider a different assay (IFA or ELISA).
Equivocal	Equivocal	—	Indeterminate. Test a new specimen or consider a different assay (IFA or ELISA).
Equivocal	Positive	—	Acute infection or false-positive IgM result. Test a second specimen; if IgG becomes positive or remains equivocal, consider sending specimen to a reference laboratory to time infection more accurately (dye test, IgG avidity, IgM EIA, IgA EIA, IgE EIA/ISAGA, AC/HS—see text) in the setting of pregnancy.
Negative	Negative	—	No evidence of *Toxoplasma* infection; not immune.
Negative	Equivocal	—	Either false-positive IgM result or possible recent infection. Obtain a new specimen and retest. If infection is recent, IgM and IgG should become positive, with low IgG avidity. If repeated testing is still IgG negative and IgM equivocal, patient is likely uninfected. Consider IgM ISAGA.
Negative	Positive	—	Acute infection or false-positive IgM result. Repeat testing on new specimen. If the result is the same, it is likely a false-positive IgM result. Consider IgM ISAGA.

AC/HS, Differential agglutination test; *EIA,* enzyme immunoassay; *ELISA,* enzyme-linked immunosorbent assay; *IFA,* immunofluorescence assay; *Ig,* immunoglobulin; *ISAGA,* immunosorbent agglutination assay; *PCR,* polymerase chain reaction.

weeks of gestation in that the presence of high-avidity antibodies excludes the acquisition of infection in the previous 3 months.[30,182,257,265]

Other tests vary in their reliability. Indirect hemagglutination is widely available, but the results frequently are negative in newborns with congenital infection.[257] This test should not be used for screening of pregnant women because detectable increases in titer are delayed compared with the increases detected by ELISA and by the dye, IFA, and agglutination tests. Meaningful interpretation of changes in titer on sequential sera requires that assays on each sample be performed in the same run by a reliable laboratory.[257]

Measurements of IgM Antibody

IgM antibodies are detected most commonly by the IgM IFA test, IgM immunosorbent agglutination assay (ISAGA), or IgM ELISA. IgM antibodies appear in the first week of primary infection and peak within 1 month.[185] Depending on the sensitivity of the method used, IgM antibodies may be demonstrable for 2 to 3 months or 1 year or longer. This prolonged presence of IgM leads to the most common diagnostic error in pregnant women—the assumption that a positive IgM result indicates fetal exposure, when the maternal infection may have occurred well before pregnancy began.[66] IgM ELISA and IgM ISAGA are much more sensitive than the IgM IFA test. Absence of IgM ELISA or IgM ISAGA antibodies in an immunologically normal older child (>1 year old) or adult essentially rules out a recently acquired infection.[257] A negative IgM IFA test result is not as sensitive in ruling out recently acquired infection. Of sera that were negative with the IgM IFA test and obtained from adults who had acquired toxoplasmosis recently, 93% were strongly positive in IgM ELISA.[184] IgM IFA testing detects specific IgM antibody in only 25% of infants with proven congenital infection, whereas IgM ELISA detects antibody in approximately 75% of such cases.[184]

The presence of rheumatoid factor or antinuclear antibodies may cause false-positive results in IgM IFA testing.[3] The "double-sandwich" IgM ELISA avoids the false-positive results caused by the presence of rheumatoid factor, which the infant can produce in utero, and the false-negative results caused by competition from the high levels of maternal IgG antibody that occur in the IgM IFA test.[183,257] In addition, the false-positive results in the IgM IFA test caused by antinuclear antibodies are not found in IgM ELISA.[3,183]

ISAGAs are used widely in Europe. Similar to IgM ELISA, they capture IgM on a solid surface, detect specific IgM, and involve the addition of whole formalin-fixed organisms or *Toxoplasma* antigen–coated latex particles.[64,202] These assays are available commercially and give results comparable to those of IgM ELISA, are simpler to perform, and do not require expensive equipment.

Measurements of IgA and IgE Antibodies

Demonstration of IgA and IgE antibodies in the fetus or newborn by ELISA and ISAGA seems to be at least comparable to the demonstration of IgM antibody in sensitivity for the diagnosis of congenital *Toxoplasma* infection.[57,198,230,263] The IgA test also seems to be more sensitive than the IgM test for detection of acquired infection. Specificity remains an issue, however, so neither IgA/IgE ELISA nor IgA/IgE ISAGA has superseded the IgM test for diagnosis of acquired infection. IgA and IgE antibodies persist longer than IgM antibodies and may be useful in cases of subacute illness or when IgM titers are low.

Differential Agglutination

Acetone-fixed and formalin-fixed *T. gondii* tachyzoites may yield differing agglutination titers, depending on the acuity of the infection. The test based on this phenomenon is called the AC/HS differential agglutination test.[52] In general, a disproportionately high agglutination titer with acetone-fixed organisms suggests acute infection; a disproportionately high titer with formalin-fixed organisms suggests chronic infection. Interpretative norms for this test have been established.[52] This test, when it is combined with the dye test, IgM ELISA, IgA ELISA, IgE ELISA/ISAGA, and avidity studies, yields a "toxoplasmic serologic profile" that permits the most accurate evaluation of infection acuity in pregnant women,[179,257,264] and often it can resolve any inconclusive or discrepant results obtained in a hospital or commercial laboratory.

Multiplexed Serologic Assays

A multiplex assay for anti-*Toxoplasma* IgG, IgM, and IgA antibodies uses microarray nanotechnology with plasmonic gold chips and near-infrared fluorescence enhancement.[140,200] It has yielded high levels of sensitivity and specificity on small whole blood or serum samples when compared with the dye test (IgG) or double-sandwich ELISAs (IgM and IgA.) This newer technology may enable an accurate and cost-effective means of screening of mothers during gestation with single or small numbers of samples.

Point of Care Testing

The development of technology that would permit screening of maternal sera for IgG and IgM antibodies in an office setting by nontechnical personnel at the "point of care" has generated interest. One such system yielded 97% sensitivity and 96% specificity when random and selected specimens from obstetric practices in France were used.[41] Because cost-benefit considerations must be taken into account in any systematic screening program, the application of this low-cost technology could make such programs more practical in the United States.

Nonserologic Methods

Nonserologic methods are now used less commonly to establish the diagnosis of *Toxoplasma* infection because they are not widely available, are labor intensive, and may require tissue specimens.

Isolation of the Organism

Isolation of *Toxoplasma* from blood or body fluids (e.g., CSF) establishes that the infection is acute. In the case of a neonate, isolation from the placenta or the infant's tissues is sufficient to diagnose congenital *Toxoplasma* infection. In 90% of placentas from which *T. gondii* is isolated, congenital infection has occurred.[204] Sensitivity of placental detection of *Toxoplasma* by isolation for the diagnosis of congenital infection appears to vary, with reports from 25% to 67%, and depends on the trimester of acquisition of infection.[80,206] Isolation of *Toxoplasma* from the tissues of older children or adults may reflect, however, only the presence of latent infection (cyst form). The organism may be isolated by inoculation of body fluids, leukocytes, or tissue specimens into the peritoneal cavities of mice or into tissue cultures. Specimens should be processed and inoculated immediately; however, tissue and blood may be stored at 4°C (39°F) overnight. Freezing and thawing or formalin treatment will kill the organism. Establishment of definitive diagnosis by isolation of *Toxoplasma* from tissues usually takes 4 to 6 weeks by mouse inoculation; tissue culture is less sensitive for recovery of *Toxoplasma*, but the results are available sooner.

Histology

Demonstration of tachyzoites, but not cysts, in tissue sections or smears of body fluids (e.g., CSF) establishes a diagnosis of acute infection. The organism may be difficult to see with routine stains. The peroxidase-antiperoxidase technique is exquisitely sensitive and has been used with a high degree of sensitivity and specificity to show the organism in biopsy specimens of the CNS in patients with AIDS.[42] In older children and adults, the histopathologic changes in toxoplasmic lymphadenitis are sufficiently distinctive to enable pathologists to make a presumptive diagnosis of acute acquired toxoplasmosis (see section on pathology).[68,246] Histologic demonstration of cysts establishes that a patient has *Toxoplasma* infection, but these findings are diagnostic of toxoplasmosis only in the placenta, fetus, or newborn.

Antigen-Specific Lymphocyte Transformation

Lymphocyte transformation in response to *Toxoplasma* antigens is a specific and sensitive indicator of previous *Toxoplasma* infection in adults and has been used successfully to diagnose congenital *Toxoplasma* infection in infants 2 months old or older.[158,167,256] Lymphocyte transformation often is absent in the newborn period, however, particularly in more severely affected infants, because of specific immune tolerance.[158,167]

Polymerase Chain Reaction

Amplification of the B1 gene of *T. gondii* DNA by PCR permits detection of the parasite in body fluids or tissues such as CSF, amniotic fluid, and lymph nodes.[38,99,104,191,212,213,219] Experience with the test in France, where PCR analysis of amniotic fluid was compared with the results of percutaneous umbilical blood sampling in 339 pregnant women, has shown that agreement of the two methods is almost 100% for the diagnosis of intrauterine infection.[103] In view of the considerably lower risk accompanying amniocentesis than with percutaneous umbilical blood sampling and the fact that amniocentesis potentially can be performed earlier in gestation, this diagnostic procedure has replaced umbilical sampling for prenatal diagnosis. An early prospective study in France showed, however, that only 48 (64%) of 75 amniotic fluid specimens from congenitally infected infants were positive by PCR analysis of a single sample obtained soon after maternal seroconversion. The test had a 100% positive predictive value, but a single negative assay did not rule out fetal infection.[213] However, a more recent report from the same institutions, using real-time PCR and the more repetitive REP-529 sequence as primer, for analysis of amniotic fluid of 261 acutely infected pregnant women yielded an overall sensitivity of 92% and a negative predictive value of 98%, with specificity and positive predictive values of 100%.[248]

A more recently developed nucleic acid amplification test, the loop-mediated isothermal amplification method (LAMP), uses the same general principle as conventional PCR but may offer a simpler and less expensive alternative if initial encouraging reports are confirmed prospectively.[136]

Interferon-γ Release Assay

Interferon-γ release assays on whole blood have been approved for the diagnosis of latent tuberculosis infection. Two reports from France suggest that this same technique, using *T. gondii* instead of *Mycobacterium tuberculosis* antigens to stimulate white blood cells and then measuring the release of interferon-γ, has a sensitivity of 94% and a specificity of 98% for diagnosis of congenital toxoplasmosis.[39,40]

Diagnosis in Specific Clinical Situations

Acute Acquired Toxoplasmosis

If IgM and IgG antibodies are not detectable, the diagnosis of acute *Toxoplasma* infection in an immunocompetent child virtually is excluded.[255,257] The diagnosis of recently acquired infection is confirmed if seroconversion from a negative to a positive titer is noted or if a serial fourfold increase in titer to high levels is observed when sera drawn at 3-week intervals are run in parallel. A single high titer in any test is not diagnostic. A dye test or IFA titer of 1:500 or greater in the presence of a high IgM antibody titer probably is diagnostic of recent acute infection. Because IgM can remain positive for 18 months after acute infection, a serum IgG avidity test can be performed to time the infection more accurately. Low IgG avidity suggests that infection has occurred within the past 12 weeks, whereas high avidity suggests more remote infection.[257,265] The absence of IgM antibodies in IgM ELISA or IgM ISAGA essentially excludes the diagnosis of acute infection. In contrast, the absence of IgM antibodies in the IgM IFA test does not mean that the infection is not acute; in one series, 25% of results in adults with acute infection were negative by the IgM IFA test.[184]

Toxoplasma Infection in Immunodeficient Children

Serologic tests should be done to identify individuals at risk for acquiring toxoplasmosis, such as recipients of organ, stem cell, and bone marrow transplants. In candidates for transplantation, knowing the status of both donor and recipient is relevant. The available serologic tests may be inadequate to detect acute active infection in some immunodeficient patients because their antibody response may be abnormal, which is especially the case in stem cell and bone marrow transplant recipients.[60,152] Experience in the Palo Alto, California, reference laboratory has revealed that acute infection may be present in patients with AIDS and in bone marrow transplant recipients without any demonstrable IgM antibody and in some immunocompromised patients who have little or no IgG antibody.[146] In patients with AIDS and active *Toxoplasma* infection, antibody titers in the modified direct agglutination test[65] may be elevated in the presence of low or undetectable titers in the dye or IFA test.[155] These and other immunodeficient patients can have progressive, lethal toxoplasmosis. In almost all cases, focal encephalitis, brain abscesses, or both are the predominant findings; hepatic involvement, pneumonitis, and myocarditis may also be present. A high index of suspicion is necessary in these patients, and immunoperoxidase staining of appropriate biopsy specimens often is required to establish the diagnosis.[42] Real-time PCR may be a valuable aid in these situations, although tissue immunoperoxidase staining remains the most reliable test.[38]

Toxoplasma Infection in Pregnant Women

Toxoplasma infection acquired during pregnancy is associated with clinical signs (e.g., lymphadenopathy) in only 10% to 15% of patients. The fetus is at risk, however, for contracting the infection regardless of whether the mother is symptomatic. The best way to detect acute infection in a pregnant woman is a routine screening program in which serologic tests are performed periodically throughout pregnancy, as has been mandated in France since 1992.[250] A suitable test for IgM antibody (IgM ELISA or IgM ISAGA) should be performed if a single random or clinically indicated serologic test result is positive at any titer. This is the common situation in countries such as the United States where screening is not mandated. If a suitable IgM antibody test is unavailable and the original serum contains IgG antibodies, the IgG antibody test should be repeated in 3 weeks, in parallel with the original serum, to determine whether the titer is stable or increasing.[205,257] More recent experience with IgG avidity testing on a single maternal specimen suggests that this additional tool may be helpful in attempting to define maternal infection as acute (within the previous 12 weeks) or remote.[30,54,182,199,205] The multiplex IgG, IgM, and IgA serologic screening test may be an accurate and economical newer approach to analyzing a single specimen during pregnancy.[140,200]

If the IgM ELISA or IgM ISAGA result is negative and the IgG antibody titer is stable and less than 1:500, no further evaluation is necessary. Because IgG titers usually stabilize at high levels (e.g., the dye test or IFA titer ≥1:500) at 6 to 8 weeks or longer after acquisition of the infection, if the dye test or IFA titer is less than 1:500 and stable (regardless of IgM antibody titer), infection was acquired at least 4 weeks and probably more than 8 weeks before the serum was obtained. In the United States, an asymptomatic woman commonly is evaluated for the first time more than 8 weeks after conception, however. If her dye test or IFA titer is 1:500 or greater, her IgM ELISA or IgM ISAGA result is negative, her IgG avidity is high, and no significant increase in titer in any test can be shown, her infection almost certainly was acquired before conception. In women with elevated IgM titers, low IgG avidity, or increasing IgG titers, infection possibly was acquired during pregnancy. In that case, a complete toxoplasmic serologic profile[179] in a reference serologic laboratory is recommended to settle the question.

Fetal Diagnosis

As noted earlier, severe congenital disease almost always is associated with primary maternal infection in the first or second trimester of pregnancy, but only 15% and 30%, respectively, of such maternal infections result in fetal infection.[48,61,62] These rates in exposed fetuses may be reduced by half by maternal treatment with spiramycin.[62] Identification of cases in which the fetus already is infected permits a parental decision to terminate the pregnancy or to treat the fetal infection more aggressively with pyrimethamine-sulfadiazine.

Studies by workers in Paris established an approach that allows definitive diagnosis and treatment of fetal infection in utero.[50,63,103] After maternal seroconversion, these researchers initially sought to establish the diagnosis of fetal infection at 20 to 29 weeks of gestation by isolation of *Toxoplasma* from amniotic fluid or from fetal blood obtained by percutaneous umbilical blood sampling and use of the sensitive mouse inoculation method. Prenatal diagnosis was attempted in 746 pregnancies in which seroconversion occurred near the time of conception or before the 26th week of gestation. In 39 of these pregnancies, fetal infection was diagnosed in utero. *Toxoplasma* was isolated from fetal blood alone in 12 cases, from amniotic fluid alone in seven cases, and from both in 15 cases, for a total of 34. *Toxoplasma*-specific IgM antibodies were detected in fetal blood in only nine cases with the highly sensitive ISAGA, and no result was positive before 24 weeks of gestation. By follow-up examination until 3 months post partum or by examination of aborted fetal tissue, a total of 42 cases were proved to have been infected. These researchers were able to detect 39 (93%) of 42 cases of fetal infection occurring before the 26th week of gestation; no false-positive diagnoses occurred.

These investigators subsequently extended their series and reported that a definitive diagnosis of infection was established in utero in 80 (90%) of 89 cases in which the fetus was infected.[104] However, the risks involved and technical expertise required in umbilical cord blood sampling have led to development of safer and less invasive, but equally sensitive, approaches to fetal diagnosis.

With the use of PCR to amplify the B1 gene of *Toxoplasma* in amniotic fluid obtained after 18 weeks of gestation, these same investigators were able to achieve sensitivity and specificity for the diagnosis of fetal infection that approached 100%.[103] In the most recent multicenter collaborative French study, in which a single specimen was prospectively studied in 261 pregnant women with acute toxoplasmosis, the specificity and positive predictive value remained 100%, with a sensitivity of 92% and a negative predictive value of 98%.[248]

These data demonstrated the value of specifically identifying exposed fetuses that truly are infected and are at risk for acquiring severe disease, thus enabling optimal maternal treatment. Negative results, conversely, allowed reassurance of parents and successful completion of pregnancies in which fetal infection had not occurred.

The current "state of the art" for management of maternal and fetal infection during pregnancy is described in the landmark study reported in 2013 from Lyon, France (the "Lyon Cohort").[195,250] This study included outcomes from 2576 women with gestational or periconceptional seroconversion who were studied between 1987 and 2008. Their protocols changed in 1992, when serologic screening was mandated in France, and again in 1995, when PCR analysis of amniotic fluid replaced umbilical cord venous sampling and mouse inoculation studies. All mothers with acute infection were treated with either spiramycin or alternating spiramycin and pyrimethamine-sulfadiazine/folinic acid until fetal involvement was evaluated. If fetal infection was documented, maternal pyrimethamine-sulfadiazine/folinic acid was given until delivery. If results of fetal studies were negative, spiramycin alone was given until delivery. After birth, all babies were treated with combinations of pyrimethamine and a sulfonamide for 12 months.

The risk of infection in exposed babies in the Lyon Cohort (before and after mandated screening in 1992) decreased from 59.4% to 46.6% (P = .038). The risk of clinical signs of infection (before and after diagnosis by PCR in 1995) decreased from 11.0% to 4.0% (P = .012). Of 207 infected children evaluated serially up to age 3 years, 46 (22.2%) had sequelae—five (2.4%) had hydrocephalus, 22 (10.6%) had intracranial calcifications, and 32 (15.4%) had chorioretinitis.[250] By way of comparison, of 210 children with congenital toxoplasmosis referred to the NCCCTS in Chicago, 65 (31%) had hydrocephalus; these outcomes are a dramatic improvement.[110,170] Because postnatal management in the two populations is very similar, the differences in outcome most likely are the result of the differences in obstetric and prenatal management in France.

Diagnosis of Congenital Toxoplasmosis After Birth

A thorough clinical and laboratory examination is necessary to evaluate fully the existence and extent of congenital toxoplasmosis in a newborn (Box 224.1). Demonstration of IgM, IgA, or IgE antibody in an infant's blood or CSF at any time is diagnostic of congenital infection if contamination by maternal blood can be reasonably excluded.[257] Specimens obtained after the infant reaches 10 days of age are more reliable in this regard. If the much less sensitive IgM IFA test is used, the presence of antinuclear antibody and rheumatoid factor also must be excluded. As mentioned earlier, the detection rate in congenitally infected infants is 25% for the IgM IFA test and 75% for IgM ELISA and IgM ISAGA. Data are insufficient for predicting how often IgA and IgE antibodies are detected. IgM antibodies may be demonstrable in the first few days of life or may appear at variable times after birth. Investigators from France reported on their use of likelihood ratios of the various tests used to confirm congenital infection in 767 children born after acute maternal toxoplasmosis during pregnancy. The probability of a child's being infected was essentially 100% if the amniotic fluid was PCR positive and the IgM test result was positive in the newborn baby.[201] If both test results were negative, there was still a 10% probability of infection in their cohort.

If toxoplasmosis is suspected clinically but *Toxoplasma* is not isolated and IgM, IgA, or IgE antibodies are not detected, follow-up serologic testing is the only means of establishing the diagnosis. Maternally transmitted IgG antibodies may persist for 6 to 12 months or longer, depending on the original titer. The higher the original titer, the longer maternal antibody may be detectable in the infant. Synthesis of IgG *Toxoplasma* antibody usually can be shown by the third month of life if the infant is not treated; it may be delayed until the sixth or ninth month if the infant is treated. At the time that the infant begins to synthesize IgG antibody, infection may be documented by computing the specific "antibody load"—the ratio of specific serum antibody titer to the level of serum IgG in the infant.[204] In the absence of infection, the antibody load decreases in the second or third month as the infant begins to produce IgG that does not contain specific *Toxoplasma* antibodies. In the presence of *Toxoplasma* infection, the infant produces specific antibodies, and the antibody load remains the same or increases. Most infected infants who are treated during the first year of life have a substantial increase in antibody after termination of therapy (serologic rebound).[153,247] This phenomenon permits the diagnosis to be confirmed retrospectively in some uncertain cases.

Ocular Toxoplasmosis

Toxoplasma has been estimated to cause 35% of cases of chorioretinitis in the United States and Central and Western Europe.[106,220,236] In these

BOX 224.1 Evaluation of a Neonate When Serology of the Mother or Illness of the Neonate Indicates That a Diagnosis of Congenital Toxoplasmosis Is Suspected or Probable

In addition to a careful general examination, the infant is examined by the following:

Clinical Evaluation and Nonspecific Tests

Pediatric ophthalmologist
Pediatric neurologist
Brain CT (data suggest excellent agreement between CT and ultrasonography,[121] which can be obtained more quickly and without the need for sedation)
Blood tests
Complete blood cell count with differential and platelet counts
Serum total IgM, IgG, IgA, and albumin
Serum alanine aminotransferase, total and direct bilirubin
CSF cell count, glucose, protein, and total IgG

***Toxoplasma Gondii*–Specific Tests**

Newborn serum analyzed for antibody detected by Sabin-Feldman dye test, IgM ISAGA, IgA EIA, IgE EIA/ISAGA (0.5 mL serum to *Toxoplasma* Serology Laboratory, PAMF Research Institute, 795 El Camino Real, Ames Building, Palo Alto, CA, 94301; 650-853-4828)
Newborn blood for inoculation into mice (1–2 mL clotted whole blood in red-topped tube to *Toxoplasma* Serology Laboratory)
Lumbar puncture: CSF dye test and IgM EIA (0.5 mL CSF to *Toxoplasma* Serology Laboratory); consider PCR (1 mL frozen CSF to *Toxoplasma* Serology Laboratory)
Sterile placental tissue (100 g in saline, from fetal side near insertion of cord, no formalin, to *Toxoplasma* Serology Laboratory for subinoculation)
Maternal serum analyzed for antibody detected by dye test, IgM EIA, IgA EIA, IgE EIA/ISAGA, and AC/HS

AC/HS, Differential agglutination test; *CSF,* cerebrospinal fluid; *CT,* computed tomography; *EIA,* enzyme immunoassay; *Ig,* immunoglobulin; *ISAGA,* immunosorbent agglutination assay; *PCR,* polymerase chain reaction.

Modified from McLeod R, Wisner J, Boyer K. Toxoplasmosis. In: Krugman S, Katz SL, Gershon AA, editors. *Infectious Diseases of Children.* St. Louis: Mosby; 1992:539.

regions, where clonal genotype II strains predominate, acquired toxoplasmosis usually is not accompanied by chorioretinitis.[180,187] Most cases are thought to result from congenital infection that does not become clinically apparent until after reactivation. This event occurs most commonly in adolescence. In Central and South America, clonal genotype III organisms predominate, as well as other more virulent clones. In these regions, acquired toxoplasmosis may be severe and often is accompanied by acute vision-threatening chorioretinitis.[2,18,31,227]

Although the presence of chorioretinitis should prompt a search for *Toxoplasma* infection, proof that *Toxoplasma* caused the eye disease may be lacking. The titer of antibody in serum often does not correlate with the presence of active lesions in the fundus. Low titers of IgG antibody are the usual finding in patients with reactivation *Toxoplasma* chorioretinitis. IgM antibodies generally are absent. *Toxoplasma* probably is excluded as a cause of chorioretinitis if the results of serologic tests are negative in undiluted serum. If the retinal lesions are characteristic and serologic test results are positive, the diagnosis is probable. If the retinal lesions are atypical and the serologic test results are positive, the diagnosis of *Toxoplasma* chorioretinitis is less certain because of the increasing prevalence of *Toxoplasma* antibodies with age in the normal population. Finding *Toxoplasma* antibodies in the child's mother supports the possibility of congenital infection, as does detection of intracranial calcification on CT scan of the patient. Demonstration of local antibody production or *Toxoplasma* DNA by PCR in aqueous humor obtained by paracentesis of the anterior chamber can be used to establish the diagnosis of *Toxoplasma* chorioretinitis in equivocal cases, but neither test is fully sensitive.[19,204,257] Thus, the risk of this procedure when vision is threatened must be weighed against the relatively low risk of a course of empiric treatment.

TREATMENT

The need for therapy and the duration of therapy are determined by the nature and severity of the clinical illness and by the immune status of the infected patient. Antibody titers are not useful indicators of therapeutic response, and an increasing antibody titer soon after discontinuation of therapy (serologic rebound) is not an indication of therapeutic failure. Specific therapy acts primarily against the tachyzoite form; the drugs currently available do not eradicate the encysted form containing bradyzoites. Close, longitudinal follow-up and supportive interventions are crucial contributors to therapeutic success.

Therapeutic Agents

The therapeutic agents used, their dosages, and indications for their use in the management of toxoplasmosis are included in Table 224.4 and discussed next.

Spiramycin

Spiramycin is a macrolide that has been used extensively in Europe (but also in the United States) to reduce transmission of infection from an acutely infected mother to the fetus in utero.[45] It is typically prescribed initially if there is documentation of seroconversion and is continued (1) until delivery if amniotic fluid studies are negative or (2) until initiation of pyrimethamine-sulfadiazine/folinic acid if fetal infection is documented.[195,250] It is concentrated in the placenta and is reported to reduce transmission by 50% to 60%. It reduces the ability to isolate the organism from the placentas of definitively infected newborns from 95% to 80%.[47] Spiramycin is less effective than pyrimethamine-sulfadiazine in the treatment of congenital infection and toxoplasmic

TABLE 224.4 Treatment of Toxoplasmosis

Disease	Medication	Dosage	Length of Therapy
Acute acquired—generally not treated unless severe or persistent symptoms, vital organ damage, or host is immunosuppressed[a]	Pyrimethamine *plus*	2 mg/kg/day for 2 days, then 1 mg/kg/day	4–6 wk or 2 wk after symptoms resolve for normal host; 4–6 wk beyond resolution for immunosuppressed hosts. In AIDS, treat until CD4+ count >200
	Sulfadiazine *plus*	75–100 mg/kg/day divided twice daily (maximum 4 g/day); consider the lower dose in children >20 kg (see text)	
	Folinic acid	5–20 mg 3 times weekly; use higher doses if marrow suppression	
Ocular, older child	Pyrimethamine *plus*	2 mg/kg/day for 2 days, then 1 mg/kg/day (maximum 50 mg/day)	4–6 wk or 2 wk after symptoms resolve
	Sulfadiazine *plus*	75–100 mg/kg/day divided twice daily (maximum 4 g/day); consider the lower dose in children >20 kg (see text)	Prednisone should be continued until resolution of sight-threatening active chorioretinitis
	Folinic acid *plus*	5–20 mg 3 times weekly	
	Prednisone	1 mg/kg/day divided twice daily	
Congenital	Pyrimethamine *plus*	2 mg/kg per day for 2 days, then 1 mg/kg/day for 6 mo, then 3 times weekly (M-W-F) for 6 mo	1 y
	Sulfadiazine *plus*	100 mg/kg per day divided twice daily	
	Folinic acid *plus*	5–10 mg 3 times weekly	
	Prednisone	1 mg/kg/day divided twice daily	Until resolution of elevated CSF protein level or sight-threatening active chorioretinitis
Pregnant women—acute infection first 21 wk of gestation	Spiramycin	3 g/day divided twice daily without food	Until fetal infection documented or excluded at 21 wk of gestation; if fetus infected, change to pyrimethamine plus sulfadiazine plus folinic acid until delivery
Pregnant women—fetal infection confirmed (amniotic fluid PCR positive)	Pyrimethamine *plus*	100 mg/day divided twice daily for 2 days, then 50 mg/day	Until delivery
	Sulfadiazine *plus*	3 g/day divided twice daily	
	Folinic acid	5–20 mg/day	

[a]For more detailed recommendations for patients with human immunodeficiency virus infection/AIDS, see http://aidsinfo.nih.gov/guidelines.
AIDS, Acquired immunodeficiency syndrome; *CSF,* cerebrospinal fluid; *PCR,* polymerase chain reaction.

encephalitis.[46,47,61,221,222] Toxoplasmic encephalitis has developed in patients receiving spiramycin and has been treated effectively with pyrimethamine-sulfadiazine. Toxicities include allergic manifestations, gastrointestinal intolerance, and paresthesias.

Spiramycin apparently does not treat manifestations of *T. gondii* infection in the fetus in utero.[47,61,104,221] It formerly was used in alternate-month regimens with pyrimethamine and sulfadiazine for postnatal treatment of congenital toxoplasmosis in France.[204] Spiramycin is not approved by the US Food and Drug Administration but may be obtained with compassionate clearance by calling 301-796-1400. The manufacturer (Aventis-Pasteur, 800-633-1610) provides the drug after the diagnosis has been documented and Food and Drug Administration forms have been completed.

Pyrimethamine

Pyrimethamine is a folate antagonist that has been shown to be effective against *T. gondii* in vitro,[169,166] in animal models,[86] and in human infections.[49,51,86,148,169,264] It is considered the drug of choice for *T gondii* infection. When this drug is used in conjunction with sulfadiazine, based on their inhibition of sequential steps in folate metabolism, synergy can be shown. The pharmacokinetics of pyrimethamine has been studied in infants and adults.[169,253] Pyrimethamine is metabolized in the liver. The pharmacokinetics is not altered by renal insufficiency but is affected by concomitantly administered drugs (e.g., phenobarbital). Pyrimethamine toxicities include reversible marrow suppression (most commonly) and allergy. Aplastic anemia, hepatotoxicity, and various allergic manifestations (including Stevens-Johnson syndrome) also have been listed as toxicities of this medication. Pyrimethamine always should be administered in conjunction with leucovorin (i.e., folinic acid) because human cells can use folinic acid for synthesis of nucleic acids, but *T. gondii* cannot.[169]

Leucovorin

Leucovorin (folinic acid) always is administered during treatment with pyrimethamine. Folinic acid has a protective effect for human cells that folic acid does not. (Confusion of the two in prescribed regimens can be harmful.) Increased doses of leucovorin are used in the event of marrow suppression. Because of the long half-life of pyrimethamine (60 hours in infants), continuation of leucovorin therapy for 1 week after discontinuation of a course of pyrimethamine is recommended.

Sulfadiazine

The three sulfonamides sulfadiazine, sulfamerazine, and sulfamethazine (known as triple sulfa when used in combination) are the three most active of the sulfonamides against *T. gondii* and are synergistic with pyrimethamine in their activity against *T. gondii*. Of the three drugs, however, only sulfadiazine is available in the United States. All other sulfonamides are less active in vitro.[166] The sulfonamides are excreted by the kidney, and the dosage must be adjusted for patients with renal insufficiency. Nephrolithiasis can occur in older children and adults, in whom urinary acidification is more effective, and fluid requirements are lower on a weight basis than in infancy. The risk for development of stones in these groups can be reduced by aggressive fluid supplementation (1–2 L above maintenance) and urine alkalinization.[34] In older children who weigh more than 20 kg, a dose of 75 mg/kg per day (rather than the conventional 100 mg/kg per day) should be considered because this dose more closely approximates the calculated adult dose based on body surface area. Other sulfonamide toxicities include allergy (including Stevens-Johnson and DRESS [drug reaction with eosinophilia and systemic symptoms] syndromes), marrow suppression, and hepatotoxicity.[163] Sulfonamide pharmacokinetics have been studied in infants.[204]

Clindamycin

Although the effect of clindamycin is delayed, it does have an effect in vitro against *T. gondii* with prolonged time in culture.[196] The drug also has been shown to be effective in murine models. Clindamycin has been found to be comparable in efficacy to sulfadiazine for the treatment of toxoplasmic encephalitis in adult patients with AIDS when it is used in a combined high-dose regimen with pyrimethamine.[51,148]

Other Antimicrobial Agents

Because the activity of sulfamethoxazole is less than that of sulfadiazine, trimethoprim-sulfamethoxazole has been considered less effective and is not used for treatment of congenital toxoplasmosis. Many investigators have used this combination successfully, however, to treat toxoplasmic encephalitis in adults with AIDS.[241] Prophylactic doses of trimethoprim-sulfamethoxazole, as used to prevent *P. jiroveci* pneumonia, also seem to prevent episodes of reactivated toxoplasmosis.[32,79] A randomized controlled trial showed that trimethoprim-sulfamethoxazole is as effective as pyrimethamine-sulfadiazine in the treatment of isolated ocular toxoplasmosis in young adults.[229] In vision-threatening disease, however, pyrimethamine-sulfadiazine is preferred.

Pyrimethamine combined with sulfadoxine, despite having lower in vitro activity than pyrimethamine-sulfadiazine, is widely used in Europe to treat both reactivated and congenital infection.[15,166,194,195,237,250] Sulfadoxine has an even longer half-life than pyrimethamine, thus enabling it to be used in weekly or 10-day dosing regimens. It has the added advantage of availability in suspension form, a convenience in prescribing for infants and children. Its long half-life is a disadvantage, however, in the event of sulfonamide hypersensitivity. Numerous other antimicrobial agents have been shown to be effective in vitro or in animal models against either tachyzoites or encysted bradyzoites,[4–8,105,106] but their role, if any, in the treatment of human disease remains to be defined. Atovaquone (5-hydroxynaphthoquinone) was effective against bradyzoites within cysts in vitro.[108] However, 13% of patients with AIDS had progression of toxoplasmic encephalitis while being treated with this antimicrobial agent,[242] so it does not appear to have the desired effect in vivo. Other antimicrobial agents with an effect on *T. gondii* tachyzoites in vitro or in vivo include cycloguanil[105]; artemisinin[105]; rifabutin[8]; and the macrolides clarithromycin, azithromycin, and roxithromycin.[4,6,7] Isolated reports of clinical use of some of these agents, most typically when standard agents are not available or not tolerated, have appeared in the literature with mixed results. In patients with vision-threatening recurrent chorioretinitis, long-term prophylaxis with azithromycin has been safe and effective in some cases (R. McLeod, personal communication).

The major unsolved therapeutic problem in toxoplasmosis is the lack of a safe agent that could eliminate encysted bradyzoites, a therapeutic approach which would be analogous to isoniazid treatment of latent tuberculosis infection. Investigational agents that target calcium-dependent protein kinase 1 and the cytochrome bc_1 complex in encysted bradyzoites have recently shown promise in model systems.[171,244]

Therapy in Specific Clinical Settings

Acquired Toxoplasmosis

Most immunologically normal patients with the lymphadenopathic form of toxoplasmosis do not require specific treatment. Indications for treatment in these cases are the presence of severe and persistent symptoms and damage to vital organs. Because of the high incidence of severe morbidity and mortality in immunocompromised patients, toxoplasmosis should be treated in this population. Most immunocompromised patients in whom the diagnosis is established ante mortem improve when specific therapy is administered. The major problem lies in establishing the diagnosis early enough to institute treatment.

The optimal duration of specific therapy for toxoplasmosis is unknown. Patients who seem to be immunologically normal but who have severe and persistent symptoms or damage to vital organs should receive specific therapy for 2 to 6 weeks, provided symptoms resolve. In immunocompromised patients, therapy should continue at least 4 to 6 weeks beyond complete resolution of all signs and symptoms of active disease. Careful follow-up of these patients is imperative because relapses may occur and require prompt reinstitution of therapy. In patients with AIDS in whom toxoplasmosis develops, suppressive therapy with pyrimethamine-sulfadiazine, pyrimethamine-clindamycin, or trimethoprim-sulfamethoxazole should be continued for life or until immune reconstitution has been sustained for at least 6 months.[225]

Treatment of Pregnant Women

Treatment of an acutely infected woman during pregnancy may prevent transmission of the infection to her fetus. The rationale for such treatment is derived from the observation that the incubation period between the onset of maternal infection and acquisition of infection in the fetus may be significant. Data from France,[61,62] where women with seroconversion were treated with spiramycin, and from Austria[10,11] and Germany,[133] where women were treated with pyrimethamine and sulfonamides, indicate that the incidence of congenital infection in the children of mothers treated during gestation is at least 50% less than that in the children of untreated mothers. None of these studies was controlled rigidly. A meta-analysis including 20 cohorts with 1721 infected mothers and 506 infected children suggested that a reduction in the incidence of transmission (odds ratio: 0.48; 95% confidence interval: 0.28–0.80) was achieved if therapy was started within 3 weeks of maternal seroconversion.[239] These results, combined with the numerous women studied by the groups from France, strongly suggest that intrauterine treatment does reduce the incidence of transmission of maternal infection to the fetus.[62,195,250] A more recent report of an observational cohort included in the analysis from the European Multicentre Study on Congenital Toxoplasmosis (EMSCOT) showed a significant reduction not only in transmission but also in serious neurologic sequelae for children with congenital toxoplasmosis who were treated prenatally, with the most significant impact for those women who seroconverted in the first 10 weeks of gestation.[44] The studies from Lyon, mentioned earlier, also revealed a marked reduction in clinically significant manifestations of congenital infection in babies treated prenatally and postnatally with combinations of pyrimethamine and sulfonamides (sulfadiazine and sulfadoxine.)[250] Long-term follow-up of congenitally infected young adults who were treated antenatally and postnatally in the Lyon cohort showed remarkably normal quality of life and visual function.[194] An additional report from a different center in France similarly found minimal disability (74% asymptomatic, 26% with chorioretinitis, and one child with serious neurologic involvement) in 107 children treated both prenatally and postnatally.[16]

Postnatal treatment of congenital infection. Data regarding the efficacy of postnatal treatment of infants with congenital *Toxoplasma* infection are becoming available.[94,160] However, as discussed previously, the improved outcomes reported from several centers in France generally include prenatal treatment as well as postnatal therapy. Nevertheless, uncontrolled studies in humans and controlled studies in experimental animals[204] have indicated beneficial effects of postnatal treatment on the development of sequelae in both symptomatic and asymptomatic infants with congenital *Toxoplasma* infection. The controlled NCCCTS has been in progress since 1981.[153,159] This study seeks to define optimal postnatal therapeutic regimens. Physicians treating patients in the United States with congenital *Toxoplasma* infection who are younger than 2.5 months of age may wish to contact this multidisciplinary group about potential enrollment of their patients in that study (773-834-4152).

Outcomes to date from the NCCCTS have been substantially better for most but not all infants treated from the neonatal period for 12 months with pyrimethamine-sulfadiazine and leucovorin than for historical controls receiving no or short-course therapy.[153,159] Signs of active infection resolve within weeks of initiation of treatment. In many children, the appearance of brain CT scans has improved remarkably. Cerebral calcifications have diminished in size or resolved in most such treated children.[193] In conjunction with this improvement in brain CT scans, cognitive function has been in the normal range (including the high normal range) for 69% of treated children.[211,234] Overall, 18 (27%) of 66 children in the NCCCTS have intelligence quotient (IQ) results lower than 70 compared with 86 (85%) of 101 untreated or briefly treated children in the reported literature (see Table 224.1).[77,159]

No significant diminution in cognitive function occurs over time, and most treated children function well in regular school classrooms. Although the number of children compared is limited, for a small subset of these children measures of cognitive function seem to be less than those for their siblings. No sensorineural hearing loss has been ascribable to congenital toxoplasmosis in treated children.[153,157,159] Despite the much improved neurologic outlook for most of these children, a subset of children with significant irreversible neurologic damage already present in the perinatal period has manifested profound developmental delay, motor impairment, and seizures. For the most part, these were children with hydrocephalus, high CSF protein concentration, minimal improvement in brain CT scans after shunting, and often substantial delays in shunt placement or needed revision for shunt failure or other intercurrent medical problems.[110,234] This experience emphasizes the importance of recognizing hydrocephalus and managing it aggressively.

Although treatment during the first year of life arrests all signs of active disease, results in normal cognitive and motor outcomes for most children, and may result in resolution of seizures without recurrence for some treated children, the drugs currently available do not eradicate all cysts containing bradyzoites. In most children, serologic titers of *T. gondii*–specific antibodies rebound in the 3 to 4 months after treatment is discontinued.[153,159,247]

To date, new retinal lesions have occurred in 17 of 58 children in the NCCCTS during 3 to 10 years' follow-up after the 1-year course of treatment.[159] These active lesions have responded to brief courses of treatment with pyrimethamine, sulfadiazine, and leucovorin without subsequent loss of visual acuity. Although follow-up durations are shorter, this result contrasts with the almost uniform eventual development of retinal lesions in studies of untreated or briefly treated children in the United States and Europe.[45,77,131,132,247] We recommend that infected children undergo retinal examination each month for 3 months after discontinuing treatment around their first birthday, then every 3 months until they are old enough to describe visual symptoms accurately, and then every 6 months. In addition, an ophthalmologic evaluation should be performed promptly for any acute visual signs or symptoms (e.g. "floaters," acuity changes) that may be related to recrudescence of congenital ocular toxoplasmosis.[172]

Sequential fetal and postnatal treatment. Several studies[44,76,87,96] have described outcomes in patients treated in utero with continuing treatment during the first year of life. As noted earlier, however, some pregnancies in France in which fetuses had obvious manifestations on ultrasound examination and most pregnancies with definite first trimester fetal infection were terminated. For example, in the study from Toulouse,[16,17] of 676 women with seroconversion, 10 (1.5%) chose termination based on these criteria. However, of the 107 infected babies in the same cohort who were tested, treated, and followed for an average of 9 years, 79 (74%) were asymptomatic and free of eye disease. Similarly, in the analysis of data from the Lyon cohort,[250] of 207 treated babies followed up to age 3 years, 80% were free of *Toxoplasma*-related symptoms.

These findings contrast starkly with the presence of retinal or neurologic involvement in 50% of asymptomatic newborns detected in the newborn period by serologic screening in Massachusetts[100] and in 75% of children whose pediatricians referred them to our NCCCTS for treatment in the postnatal period.[159,170] A prospective study (as part of the NCCCTS) is under way to compare outcomes in infants identified by obstetricians, as detected prenatally and treated in utero, with those identified by pediatricians after birth and then referred and treated postnatally.

Coexistent HIV Infection

Active toxoplasmosis with coexistent HIV infection in children is increasingly rare since the advent of HAART and effective prevention of vertical HIV transmission.[75,175,190] Most children described with toxoplasmosis and HIV infection in the past have had congenital toxoplasmosis and have been symptomatic. For such children, concomitant therapy with HAART and pyrimethamine-sulfadiazine/folinic acid is recommended in the doses described in Table 224.4.[225] HIV-infected adult and adolescent patients receiving secondary prophylaxis with trimethoprim-sulfamethoxazole (i.e., long-term maintenance therapy) after toxoplasmic encephalitis are at low risk for recurrence when they have successfully completed initial therapy, remain asymptomatic with regard to signs and symptoms of toxoplasmic encephalitis, and have sustained increases in $CD4^+$ T lymphocyte counts of more than 200 cells/μL after effective HAART.[225]

Although the numbers of patients with toxoplasmic encephalitis who have been evaluated remain limited and occasional recurrences have been reported, on the basis of these observations and inference from more extensive cumulative data indicating the safety of discontinuing secondary prophylaxis for other opportunistic infections during advanced HIV disease, discontinuation of long-term maintenance therapy among such patients is a reasonable consideration.[225] (Also see http://aidsinfo.nih.gov/guidelines/ for the latest Department of Health and Human Services recommendations regarding treatment and prophylaxis of toxoplasmosis in AIDS.) The highest risk for relapse seems to occur within the first 6 months of discontinuing secondary prophylaxis. Many specialists would obtain a magnetic resonance image of the brain as part of their evaluation to determine whether it is appropriate to discontinue therapy. Zidovudine is known to antagonize the toxoplasmacidal effect of pyrimethamine and its in vitro synergy with sulfonamide. Whether this effect occurs in vivo is unknown.[137]

Recurrent Ocular Toxoplasmosis

Because currently available therapies do not eradicate bradyzoites, recurrences of toxoplasmic chorioretinitis are a lifelong threat for children with congenital infection. Prompt initiation of specific treatment in reactivated ocular toxoplasmosis is mandatory to preserve vision. Inflammatory reactions in the vitreous are a frequent clinical finding in patients with reactivation, and in such cases coadministration of corticosteroids *in addition* to specific anti-*Toxoplasma* therapy is recommended strongly.[172] The use of corticosteroids also is recommended for cases of vision-threatening retinochoroiditis involving the macula, maculopapillary bundle, or optic nerve. The initial daily dosage of prednisone is 1 mg/kg orally to a maximum of 75 mg in 24 hours. The equivalent dosage of another corticosteroid may be given. The dosage of corticosteroid may be reduced gradually when the lesion appears to be well demarcated and pigmentation has begun. Some physicians have administered systemic or intraocular clindamycin to treat patients in whom the use of corticosteroids and pyrimethamine plus sulfadiazine has failed[235]; the efficacy of this approach has not been proved in humans. Choroidal neovascular membranes and subretinal hemorrhages resulting from reactivated toxoplasmic chorioretinitis have been treated successfully with intravitreal anti–vascular endothelial growth factor monoclonal antibody preparations.[14]

BOX 224.2 Prevention of Toxoplasma Infection

Prevention of Acquired Infection (Primary Prevention)

Cook meat to medium (66°C [150°F]), smoke it, or cure it in brine.

Wash fruits and vegetables before consumption.

Avoid touching mucous membranes of the mouth and eyes while handling uncooked meat or unwashed fruits or vegetables.

Wash hands and kitchen surfaces thoroughly after contact with raw meat or unwashed fruits or vegetables.

Prevent access of flies, cockroaches, and other coprophagous insects to fruits and vegetables.

Avoid contact with materials that potentially are contaminated with cat feces, such as cat litter boxes, or wear gloves when handling such materials and when gardening.

Disinfect cat litter boxes for 5 minutes with nearly boiling water.

Prevention of Congenital Infection (Secondary Prevention)

Identify women at risk by serologic testing.

Treatment of acute maternal infection with spiramycin during pregnancy results in an approximately 50% reduction in the incidence of infection in infants.

Maternal treatment with pyrimethamine, sulfadiazine, and leucovorin, when fetal infection is documented by amniotic fluid PCR, significantly improves clinical outcome.

Therapeutic abortion may prevent birth of a severely affected infant—consider for PCR-proven fetal infection in the first two trimesters with abnormalities documented by ultrasound or MRI.

MRI, Magnetic resonance imaging; *PCR*, polymerase chain reaction.

Modified from Remington JS, Wilson CB. Toxoplasmosis. In: Kass EH, Platt R, editors. *Current therapy in infectious disease: 1983-1984.* Philadelphia: BC Decker; 1983:149-153.

PREVENTION

The entire issue of congenital infection may be avoided by preventing primary *Toxoplasma* infection during pregnancy.[81,156,258,265] This approach has come to be known as primary prophylaxis. The responsibility of all physicians caring for pregnant women at risk is to inform them of specific hygienic measures (Box 224.2) for avoiding *Toxoplasma* infection. Similar measures are useful for prevention of acquired infection in other settings as well. The effectiveness of a 10-minute education program, offered as part of prenatal care, to reduce the risk of acquiring *Toxoplasma* infection by modifying the behavior of pregnant women with regard to cats, food, and personal hygiene has been shown.[33] Internet resources that describe methods to prevent toxoplasmosis in pregnant women are available from the March of Dimes (www.marchofdimes.org/pregnancy.toxoplasmosis.aspx) and from the Centers for Disease Control and Prevention (www.cdc.gov/parasites/toxoplasmosis/resources/ToxoWomen_2.2003.pdf).

When primary maternal infection has occurred, several problems are inherent in the secondary prevention of congenital toxoplasmosis by pregnancy termination or by treatment of the pregnant woman.[35] Because 80% to 90% of women with primary *Toxoplasma* infection are asymptomatic, most primary infections are overlooked, unless sequential serologic testing is performed routinely in pregnant women. The cost effectiveness of routine screening in the prevention of congenital toxoplasmosis is abundantly clear in some European countries where screening is mandated by law.[61,62] In countries with a significantly lower incidence, cost efficacy is more difficult to prove.[92,95,207] An analysis of the cost of a universal screening program for pregnant women in the United States modeled after the French approach suggests cost savings for the US population even with current levels of congenital infection of approximately one case per 10,000 live births.[100,129,207,231] In the absence of national guidelines, physicians may choose to screen patients on an individual basis.[258] If screening is undertaken, a reliable serologic test for IgG antibodies (see section on laboratory diagnosis) should be performed before conception occurs or as soon as possible thereafter and then repeated every 2 to 3 months until the time of delivery. Serologic test results that suggest the acquisition of primary infection during pregnancy (IgG seroconversion and/or IgM or IgA antibodies) should be confirmed by a reference laboratory. Decisions about treatment or therapeutic abortion should be based on a consideration of whether the fetus is infected or affected, as determined by amniocentesis and ultrasonography.

Acknowledgments

We acknowledge Drs. Jack Remington, Rima McLeod, and James McAuley as contributors to work in the previous edition from which this chapter was constructed.

NEW REFERENCES SINCE THE SEVENTH EDITION

2. Arantes TE, Silviera C, Holland GN, et al. Ocular involvement following postnatally acquired *Toxoplasma gondii* infection in southern Brazil: a 28 year experience. *Am J Ophthalmol.* 2015;159:1002-1012.
14. Benevento JD, Jager RD, Noble AG, et al. *Toxoplasma*-associated neovascular lesions treated successfully with ranizumab and antiparasitic therapy. *Arch Ophthalmol.* 2008;126:1152-1156.
18. Bossi P, Bricaire F. Severe acute disseminated toxoplasmosis. *Lancet.* 2009;364:579.
19. Bourdin C, Busse A, Kouamou E, et al. PCR-based detection of *Toxoplasma gondii* DNA in blood and ocular samples for diagnosis of ocular toxoplasmosis. *J Clin Microbiol.* 2014;52:3987-3991.
31. Carme B, Demar M, Ajzenberg D, et al. Severe acquired toxoplasmosis caused by wild cycle of *Toxoplasma gondii,* French Guiana. *Emerg Infect Dis.* 2009;15:656-658.
40. Chapey E, Wallon M, L'Olivier C, et al. Place of interferon-gamma assay for diagnosis of congenital toxoplasmosis. *Pediatr Infect Dis J.* 2015;34:1407-1409.
41. Chapey E, Wallon M, Peyron F. Evaluation of the LDBIO point of care test for the combined detection of toxoplasmic IgG and IgM. *Clin Chim Acta.* 2017;464:200-201.
43. Contopoulos-Ionnidis D, Wheeler K, Ramirez R, et al. Clustering of *Toxoplasma gondii* infections within families of congenitally-infected infants. *Clin Infect Dis.* 2015;61:1815-1824.
54. Dard C, Fricker-Hidalgo H, Brenier-Pinchart M-P, et al. Relevance of and new developments in serology for toxoplasmosis. *Trends Parasitol.* 2016;32:492-506.
58. DeMoura L, Bahia-Oliviera LMG, Wada MY, et al. Waterborne toxoplasmosis, Brazil: from field to gene. *Emerg Infect Dis.* 2006;12:326-329.

66. Dhakal R, Gujarel K, Pomares C, et al. Significance of a positive *Toxoplasma* immunoglobulin M test result in the United States. *J Clin Microbiol.* 2015;53:3601-3605.
73. Dubey JP. The history of *Toxoplasma gondii*—the first 100 years. *J Eukaryot Microbiol.* 2008;55:467-475.
69. Dubey JP, Dennis PM, Verma SK, et al. Epidemiology of toxoplasmosis in white-tailed deer *(Odocoileus virginianus)*: occurrence, congenital transmission, correlates of infection, isolation, and genetic characterization of *Toxoplasma gondii*. *Vet Parasitol.* 2014;202:270-275.
79. Felix JPF, Lira RPC, Zacchia RS, et al. Trimethoprim-sulfamethoxazole versus placebo to reduce the risk of recurrences of *Toxoplasma gondii* retinochoroiditis: randomized controlled clinical trial. *Am J Ophthalmol.* 2014;157:762-766.
101. Guo M, Dubey JP, Hill D, et al. Prevalence and risk factors for *Toxoplasma gondii* infection in meat animals and meat products destined for human consumption. *J Food Prot.* 2015;78:457-476.
107. Howe DK, Sibley LD. *Toxoplasma gondii* comprises three clonal lineages: correlation of parasite genotype with human disease. *J Infect Dis.* 1995;172:1561-1566.
110. Hutson SL, Wheeler KM, McLone D, et al. Patterns of hydrocephalus caused by congenital *Toxoplasma gondii* infection associated with parasite genetics. *Clin Infect Dis.* 2015;61:1831-1834.
112. Jamieson SE, Cordell H, Peterson E, et al. Host genetic and epigenetic factors in toxoplasmosis. *Mem Inst Oswaldo Cruz.* 2009;104:162-169.
113. Jamieson SE, deRoubaix LA, Cortina-Borja M, et al. Genetic and epigenetic factors at COL2A1 and ABLA4 influence clinical outcome in congenital toxoplasmosis. *PLoS ONE.* 2008;3:e2285.
114. Jamieson SE, Peixoto-Rangel AL, Hargrove AC, et al. Evidence for association between the purinogenic receptor P2RX7 and toxoplasmosis. *Genes Immun.* 2010;11:374-383.
120. Jones JL, Kruszon-Moran D, Rivera HN, et al. *Toxoplasma gondii* seroprevalence in the United States 2009-2010 and comparison with the past two decades. *Am J Trop Med Hyg.* 2014;90:1135-1139.
140. Li X, Pomares C, Gonfrier G, et al. Multiplexed anti-*Toxoplasma* IgG, IgM, and IgA assay on plasmonic gold chips: toward making screening possible with dye-test precision. *J Clin Microbiol.* 2016;54:1726-1733.
144. Lorenzi H, Khan A, Behnke MS, et al. Local admixture of amplified and diversified secreted pathogenesis determinants shapes mosaic *Toxoplasma gondii* genomes. *Nat Commun.* 2016;7:10147.
149. Lykins J, Wang K, Wheeler K, et al. Understanding toxoplasmosis in the United States through "large data" analyses. *Clin Infect Dis.* 2016;63:468-475.
147. McAuley JB, Boyer KM, Patel D, et al. Early and longitudinal evaluations of treated infants and children and untreated historical patients with congenital toxoplasmosis. *Clin Infect Dis.* 1994;18:38-72.
164. McLeod R, Lee D, Clouset F, Boyer K. Diagnosis of congenital toxoplasmosis. In: Stevenson D, Sunshine P, Cohen R, van Meurs K, eds. *Neonatology: Clinical Practice and Procedural Atlas.* New York, NY: McGraw-Hill; 2015:[Chapter 116].
165. McLeod R, Lee D, Clouset F, Boyer K. Toxoplasmosis in the fetus and newborn infant. In: Stevenson D, Sunshine P, Cohen R, van Meurs K, eds. *Neonatology: Clinical Practice and Procedural Atlas.* New York, NY: McGraw-Hill; 2015:[Chapter 57].
170. McLeod R, Wheeler KM, Boyer K. Reply to Wallon and Peyron (Letter.). *Clin Infect Dis.* 2016;62:812-814.
171. McPhillie M, Zhou Y, El Bissati K, et al. New paradigms for understanding and step changes in treating active and chronic, persistent apicomplexan infections. *Sci Rep.* 2016;6:29179.
173. Michaels MG, Wald ER, Fricker J, et al. Toxoplasmosis in recipients of heart transplants. *Clin Infect Dis.* 1992;14:847-851.
182. Murat J-B, Dard C, Fricker-Hidalgo H, et al. Comparison of the Vidas system and two recent fully automated assays for diagnosis and follow-up of toxoplasmosis in pregnant women and newborns. *Clin Vaccine Immunol.* 2013;20:1203-1212.
187. Noble AG, Latkany P, Kusmierczyk J, et al. Chorioretinal lesions in mothers of children with congenital toxoplasmosis in the National Collaborative Chicago-based Congenital Toxoplasmosis Study. *Sci Med (Porto Alegre).* 2010;20:20-26.
188. Nogareda F, Le Staat Y, Villena I, et al. Incidence and prevalence of *Toxoplasma gondii* infection among women in France. 1980-2020: model-based estimation. *Epidemiol Infect.* 2014;142:1662-1670.
191. Olariu TR, Remington JS, Montoya JG. Polymerase chain reaction in spinal fluid for the diagnosis of congenital toxoplasmosis. *Pediatr Infect Dis J.* 2014;35:561-570.
192. Pappas G, Ronssos N, Fologos ME. Toxoplasmosis snapshots: global status of *Toxoplasma gondii* seroprevalence and implications for pregnancy and congenital toxoplasmosis. *Int J Parasitol.* 2009;39:1385-1394.
195. Peyron F, Wallon M, Kieffer F, Garweg J. Toxoplasmosis. In: Wilson CB, Nizet V, Maldonado YA, Remington JS, Klein JO, eds. *Remington and Klein's Infectious Diseases of the Fetus and Newborn Infant.* 8th ed. Philadelphia, PA: Saunders Elsevier; 2016:949-1042.
199. Pomares C, Montoya JG. Laboratory diagnosis of congenital toxoplasmosis. *J Clin Microbiol.* 2016;54:2448-2454.
200. Pomares C, Zhang B, Arulkumar S, et al. Validation of IgG, IgM multiplex plasmonic gold platform in French clinical cohorts for the serodiagnosis and follow-up of *Toxoplasma gondii* infection. *Diagn Microbiol Infect Dis.* 2017;87:213-218.
216. Sabin AB, Olitsky PK. Toxoplasma and intracellular parasitism. *Science.* 1937;85:336-338.
219. Salviz M, Montoya JG, Nadol JB, et al. Otopathology in congenital toxoplasmosis. *Otol Neurotol.* 2013;34:1165-1169.
225. Siberry GK, Absug MJ, Nachman S, et al. Guidelines for the prevention and treatment of opportunistic infections in HIV-infected children: recommendations from the NIH, CDC, IDSA, PIDS, and AAP. *Pediatr Infect Dis J.* 2013;Suppl 2:C1-C13.
227. Silveira C, Mucciolo C, Holland GN, et al. Ocular involvement following an epidemic of *Toxoplasma gondii* infection in Santa Isabel do Ivai, Brazil. *Am J Ophthalmol.* 2015;159:1013-1021.
232. Sutterland AL, Fond G, Kuin A, et al. Beyond the association. *Toxoplasma gondii* in schizophrenia, bipolar disorder, and addiction: systematic review and metaanalysis. *Acta Psychiatr Scand.* 2015;132:161-179.
237. Teil J, Dupont D, Charpiat B, et al. Treatment of congenital toxoplasmosis: safety of sulfadoxine-pyrimethamine combination in children based on a method of causality assessment. *Pediatr Infect Dis J.* 2016;35:634-638.
230. Torgerson PR, Mastroiacovo P. The global burden of congenital toxoplasmosis: a systematic review. *Bull World Health Organ.* 2013;91:501-508.
241. Torre D, Casari S, Speranza F, et al. Randomized trial of trimethoprim-sulfamethoxazole versus pyrimethamine-sulfadiazine for therapy of toxoplasmic encephalitis in patients with AIDS. *Antimicrob Agents Chemother.* 1998;42:1346-1349.
242. Torres RA, Weinberg W, Stansell J, et al. Atovaquone for salvage treatment and suppression of toxoplasmic encephalitis in patients with AIDS. *Clin Infect Dis.* 1997;24:422-429.
243. Varella IS, Canti IC, Santos BR, et al. Prevalence of acute toxoplasmosis infection among 41,112 pregnant women and the mother-to-child transmission rate in a public hospital in South Brazil. *Mem Inst Oswaldo Cruz.* 2009;104:383-388.
244. Vidadala RSR, Rivas KL, Ojo KK, et al. Development of an orally available and central nervous system (CNS) penetrant *Toxoplasma gondii* calcium-dependent protein kinase 1 (*Tg*CDPK1) inhibitor with minimal human ether-a-go-go related gene (hERG) activity for the treatment of toxoplasmosis. *J Med Chem.* 2016;59:6531-6546.
250. Wallon M, Peyron F, Vinault S, et al. Congenital *Toxoplasma* infection: monthly prenatal screening decreases transmission rate and improves clinical outcome at age 3 years. *Clin Infect Dis.* 2013;56:1223-1231.
252. Wang Y, Wang G, Cai J, et al. Review on the identification and role of *Toxoplasma gondii* antigenic epitopes. *Parasitol Res.* 2016;115:459-468.
260. Witola WH, Lin SR, Monpetit A, et al. ALOX2 in human toxoplasmosis. *Infect Immun.* 2014;82:2670-2679.
262. Wolf A, Cowen D, Paige B. Human toxoplasmosis: occurrence in infants as an encephalomyelitis verification by transmission to animals. *Science.* 1939;89:226-227.
266. Zhang NZ, Chen J, Wang M, et al. Vaccines against *Toxoplasma gondii:* new developments and perspectives. *Expert Rev Vaccines.* 2013;12:1287-1299.

The full reference list for this chapter is available at ExpertConsult.com.

225 *Pneumocystis* Pneumonia

Francis Gigliotti • Terry W. Wright

Pneumocystis pneumonia (PCP) is a life-threatening pneumonia that occurs in immunocompromised infants, children, and adults. Even with modern medical management, mortality is significant. Although the organism has been identified in a variety of tissues, the pathologic process is generally limited to the lungs. Infection in the normal child is common, with most children infected by 2 years of age with a mild or asymptomatic respiratory tract infection. Chemoprophylaxis is highly effective in preventing PCP in at-risk patients.

ORGANISM

Pneumocystis was originally identified in 1909 by Chagas, who believed it was a form of *Trypanosoma cruzi.*[9] It is now known to be a unique and ubiquitous pathogen of mammals. The first description of *Pneumocystis* infecting a human was reported in 1942.[76] The taxonomic placement of *Pneumocystis* has been difficult and has varied over time. The organism has features of both protozoa and fungi. Protozoan features include morphology with three distinct forms, termed cyst, sporozoite, and trophozoite; sensitivity to antimicrobial agents with activity against protozoal organisms; and resistance to most antifungal drugs. Fungal features include the structure of the cyst wall, which contains chitin and β-1,3-glucan, and its genetic structure is more typical of that of fungi.[20,21]

Because *Pneumocystis* cannot be maintained in culture, definitive knowledge of its life cycle is limited. The thick-walled cyst is 5 to 8 μm in diameter and contains up to 8-μm sporozoites (or intracystic bodies), which on leaving the cyst become trophozoites (or tropic forms) varying in size from 1 to 4 μm (Fig. 225.1). There is some evidence for a sexual cycle in *Pneumocystis* based largely on the presence of homologs of genes involved in sexual cycles in fungi.

Pneumocystis strains or species have the remarkable biologic feature of only being able to infect a single mammalian species[27]; for example, organisms isolated from mice are incapable of infecting other mammals, even those as closely related as the rat. This restricted transmission is consistent with studies demonstrating unique phenotypes and genotypes of *Pneumocystis* isolated from each mammalian host studied to date.[25,29,58,69,84] The obvious implication of this biologic property is that the source of *Pneumocystis* causing PCP in humans must be other humans.

The host species specificity and restricted transmission have led to discussions regarding whether these features represent distinct species of *Pneumocystis.* Efforts have been made to adopt new nomenclature for *Pneumocystis,* primarily to distinguish between strains derived from humans and strains from lower mammals. In 1976, Frenkel suggested *Pneumocystis jiroveci* n. sp. for isolates from humans.[23] During the ensuing three decades this term was not used. In 1988, Hughes and Gigliotti[37] proposed a nomenclature merely designating the host from which the organism was obtained (e.g., *Pneumocystis carinii, humanus; P. carinii, rattus*). In 1994, Stringer and the *Pneumocystis* Workshop[71] used DNA sequence data to employ a "special forms" designation (e.g., *P. carinii* f. sp. *hominis*). A subsequent system put forth in 2002 by Stringer and colleagues[70] is currently used by some investigators and designates the human form as *P. jiroveci* Frenkel. *P. jiroveci* is being increasingly used to designate *Pneumocystis* that infects humans. However, because issues have been raised regarding this new nomenclature, some authors use only the genus name when describing this organism.[26,34,43,70]

TRANSMISSION AND EPIDEMIOLOGY

Transmission

Pneumocystis is spread by the airborne route.[35] *Pneumocystis* has been isolated from a wide variety of animal species from all over the world. Because *Pneumocystis* organisms isolated from different mammalian hosts are morphologically quite similar, it was initially thought that PCP in humans was a zoonotic infection stemming from contact with infected animals. As noted earlier, it is now clear that transmission between two different mammalian species is highly unlikely. Longitudinal serologic studies starting just after birth demonstrate that most children are infected with *Pneumocystis* by 2 years of age.[77] These serologic data are substantiated by the finding of *Pneumocystis* in the lungs of many infants who have died of sudden infant death syndrome.[54,78] Infection of a normal host early in life could result in the establishment of a latent infection, as happens in the case of tuberculosis. This was believed to be the case with *Pneumocystis* when infection in the immunocompromised host was postulated to be the result of reactivation of a latent *Pneumocystis* infection.[13] However, under controlled experimental conditions, normal mice were shown to control *Pneumocystis* after infection in a typical pattern of infection, immune response, and resolution of infection.[3] Furthermore, latent infection does not occur after immune-mediated resolution of infection.[10] When infected, but before resolution of infection, immunologically normal mice can transmit *Pneumocystis* to another mouse.[30] If the recipient mouse is normal, a subclinical infection occurs. This cycle, if repeated, would serve to maintain *Pneumocystis* in the population. If instead the recipient mouse is immunocompromised, then full PCP results.

By using information gained from animal models and observational studies, it is possible to propose a likely transmission cycle for *Pneumocystis.* Seronegative infants who are continuously introduced into the population present a large pool of susceptible humans who become transiently infected. Infection can be either asymptomatic or mildly symptomatic.[77] In either case, the infection is transmissible. Continued passage from normal host to normal host would serve as a reservoir of *Pneumocystis* that when transmitted to an immunocompromised individual results in life-threatening PCP. Consistent with this model, molecular studies suggest that a second case of PCP occurring more than 6 months after the first episode is most likely the result of reinfection with a new strain of *Pneumocystis.*[45] It is not known whether subclinical reinfection of adults can serve as another reservoir of *Pneumocystis,* but the finding of microscopically visible organisms rarely has been documented in adults.

Pneumocystis Pneumonia and AIDS

AIDS was brought to the attention of the medical community in the United States as a result of a small cluster of cases of PCP in previously healthy young men,[8] and PCP remains the most common AIDS-defining illness. It was reported in 39% of 2786 pediatric AIDS patients reported to the Centers for Disease Control and Prevention (CDC) through 1990 and in 75% of untreated adults with AIDS, and more than half of adults dying with AIDS have had at least one episode of PCP.[43,67] The key determinant in host defense against PCP is the $CD4^+$ T cell. Although the precise role of $CD4^+$ T cells in protection against PCP has not been defined, it is clear that any condition that interferes with $CD4^+$ T-cell number or function puts the patient at risk for developing PCP. Because the pathogenesis of AIDS involves the destruction of $CD4^+$ T cells, it is easy to identify at-risk patients simply by checking $CD4^+$ T-cell counts. Adults whose $CD4^+$ T-cell counts fall below 200/μL are at high risk for developing PCP. The determination of risk for PCP in children with AIDS is based on age because $CD4^+$ T-cell counts are very high at birth, fall rapidly during the first year of life, and then fall more slowly to reach adult levels around 6 years of age. Thus children with AIDS are at high risk for developing PCP if they are younger than 1 year with $CD4^+$ T-cell counts less than 1500/μL; 1 to 5 years of age

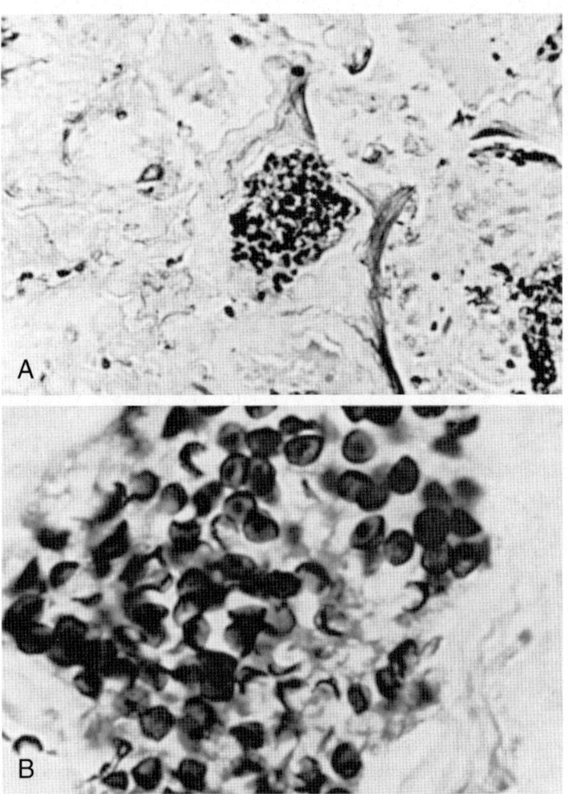

FIG. 225.1 Typical cyst forms shown by Gomori silver methenamine stain of lung tissue obtained by open lung biopsy from a 20-month-old child with severe combined immunodeficiency disease (A, ×100; B, ×100).

with counts less than 500/μL; and older than 5 years with counts less than 200/μL.

Pneumocystis Pneumonia Not Associated With AIDS

The other large group of patients at risk for PCP is those with congenital immunodeficiencies involving T- and B-cell function and those with medical conditions requiring immunosuppressive therapy, such as malignancies. For this latter group, it is important to remember that it is generally the therapy and not the underlying disease that puts the patient at risk for developing PCP. This was clearly demonstrated in children with acute lymphocytic leukemia when those receiving one, two, or three chemotherapeutic agents had an incidence of PCP between 2% and 5%, whereas in those receiving four drugs the incidence was 22%.[30] Likewise, the addition of radiation therapy to a three-drug chemotherapeutic regimen increased the incidence of PCP to as high as 35%.[37] Thus it is important to keep in mind that as therapies change, so, too, does the risk for developing PCP. For example, PCP was rarely seen in patients with Crohn disease receiving conventional immunosuppressive therapy. However, PCP is now a well-recognized complication of Crohn disease since the addition of anti–tumor necrosis factor (TNF) therapy to the treatment regimen.[44]

The incidence of PCP seems to be increasing, possibly owing to the increasing use of biologic response modifiers, such as anti-TNF agents, and newer, more potent immunosuppressive drugs. Reports from cancer centers show that the incidence or prevalence, or both, of PCP has increased in this population.[58,85] Similar increases are reported among patients receiving organ transplants, those with autoimmune diseases, and those who have had a bone marrow transplantation.[4,57,75]

In contrast to patients with AIDS, in which there is consensus on the guidelines for starting PCP prophylaxis, the risk for developing non–AIDS-associated PCP can be more difficult to predict. This is because the immunosuppressive regimen affects not only cell number but also cell function. Thus a patient on chemotherapy may have a $CD4^+$ T-cell count above the risk threshold seen in AIDS patients, but if function is suppressed then the risk for PCP increases. Because T-cell function is not routinely measured in clinical laboratories, physicians must rely on cumulative clinical experience when judging the need for PCP prophylaxis.

IMMUNOPATHOGENESIS

Pneumocystis is the classic opportunistic pathogen: it is incapable of producing overt pneumonia in the immunologically normal host, yet in the immunocompromised host PCP is universally fatal if untreated. Even with treatment the mortality is high, ranging from 5% to 25%, depending on the patient population.

The occurrence of PCP in patients with AIDS and pure T-cell deficiency disease provides indirect evidence of the potential importance of cellular immunity in protecting the host against this opportunist. Direct evidence for the necessity of $CD4^+$ T cells comes from mouse studies showing that depletion of this cell population renders the mouse susceptible to PCP. Less well appreciated is the evidence for the importance of humoral immunity in protection against *Pneumocystis.* For example, PCP occurs in patients with agammaglobulinemia or hyperimmunoglobulin M syndrome and mice with a variety of genetically engineered defects in antibody response pathways have been demonstrated to be susceptible to PCP.

The host response to *Pneumocystis* is likely the critical determinant of the severity of lung injury occurring as a result of PCP.[28] Three clinical observations support the importance of the inflammatory response in the outcome of PCP: (1) neutrophil number, but not organism counts, in lung secretions correlates with higher morbidity and mortality[50]; (2) the differential in mortality between AIDS-related and non–AIDS-related PCP[51]; and (3) the ability of PCP to trigger the immune reconstitution inflammatory syndrome (IRIS).[56]

In recent years, the application of molecular technology has provided a vast amount of information to aid in understanding the immunopathogenesis of PCP.[28] When *Pneumocystis* reaches the lungs of a normal host by the airborne route, the organism elicits what we have termed a balanced immune response and the subject remains asymptomatic or mildly symptomatic while the infection is cleared. Alternatively, if the host is severely immunocompromised owing to insufficient $CD4^+$ cells, a life-threatening pneumonitis develops, driven by $CD8^+$ T cells. Because $CD8^+$ T cells are a critical determinant of the lung injury, without controlling organism burden, we have termed this response *ineffective inflammation.* Finally, in the setting of return of $CD4^+$ T cells, such as after institution of treatment for human immunodeficiency virus (HIV) infection or during engraftment after bone marrow transplantation, one may see an exaggerated but effective response, as seen in IRIS, that clears the *Pneumocystis* but at the expense of significant lung injury.

Alveolar macrophages play a critical role in pulmonary host defense and contribute to both innate and adaptive immune responses. Alveolar macrophages have long been thought to serve as the effector cell for clearing *Pneumocystis* organisms from the lung, but these cells are not capable of controlling *Pneumocystis* infection in hosts with impaired $CD4^+$ T-cell function. A recent study utilizing an animal model of PCP has demonstrated that macrophage phagocytosis is the effector mechanism for the $CD4^+$ T-cell–mediated clearance of *Pneumocystis* organisms from the lung, indicating that the adaptive immune response must direct the macrophage-mediated clearance of this fungal pathogen.[81] In addition to host defense, macrophages also likely contribute to the immunopathogenesis of PCP. Macrophages are significant sources of proinflammatory cytokines, including TNF-α and interleukin-1 (IL-1), and *Pneumocystis* β-glucan is a potent stimulator of the alveolar macrophage cytokine response.[47] Therefore, in addition to their function in host defense, alveolar macrophages may also contribute to PCP-related lung injury through elaboration of inflammatory mediators.

The proinflammatory cytokines TNF-α and IL-1 are required for host defense against *Pneumocystis* infection[11,12] but also contribute to the immunopathology associated with PCP. These cytokines, acting through chemokine signals, promote neutrophil, lymphocyte, and monocyte recruitment to the lung, which may cause alveolar damage and diminished gas exchange, resulting in respiratory failure. Importantly, mice lacking TNF receptors are partially protected from PCP-related respiratory impairment and weight loss.[83] Other cytokines associated with helper T-cell type 1, 2, or 17 responses may also modulate host defense and PCP-related immunopathogenesis by regulating alveolar macrophage phenotype and activation state, but these issues need further clarification.

Surfactant phospholipids and apoproteins are critical to lung function and are adversely affected by *Pneumocystis* infection. Patients with PCP display dramatic alterations in surfactant function and composition,[65] which is likely an important determinant of disease severity. In vitro studies have determined that *Pneumocystis* organisms interact directly with pulmonary surfactant to reduce its surface tension–lowering properties.[80] Furthermore, studies in animal models have found that *Pneumocystis*-driven inflammation also contributes to surfactant dysfunction in the setting of PCP.[5,82] Anecdotal reports describe some benefit from the administration of exogenous surfactant to patients with PCP.[15]

PATHOLOGY

The pathologic findings of *Pneumocystis* infections are, with rare exceptions, limited to the lungs. Rarely, *Pneumocystis* organisms have been detected in the lymph nodes, spleen, liver, retina, bone marrow, gastrointestinal tract, pancreas, heart, adrenals, and peripheral blood.[73]

In the infantile "epidemic" form of disease, essentially all alveoli contain large numbers of organisms. Extensive interstitial plasma cell infiltrates distend the alveolar walls five to 20 times over their normal thickness, and almost no intraalveolar fibrinous exudate is noted.[33]

The progression of disease in childhood and adult forms of PCP can be divided into three pathologic stages.[33,61] An initial stage is characterized by the presence of cysts and trophozoites attached, possibly by fibronectin, to the alveolar walls.[60] No septal inflammatory or cellular response is evident, and no clinical disease is associated with this stage. A second stage, which may or may not be associated with clinical signs and symptoms, is characterized by desquamation of alveolar cells and an increase in the number of cysts within alveolar macrophages. TNF may be a major mediator involved in the killing of *Pneumocystis* by activated alveolar macrophages and may be induced by oxidative stress in the alveoli.[59] The final stage is typified by extensive reactive and desquamative alveolitis manifested by marked cytoplasmic vacuolization of macrophages, mononuclear and plasma cell infiltrates within alveolar septa, and clusters of organisms located predominantly within macrophages in the lumen of alveoli. The histopathology of this final stage definitely is associated with clinical manifestations of pneumonitis.[61]

CLINICAL MANIFESTATIONS

Hypoxia is the hallmark of PCP. The natural course of *Pneumocystis* infection varies greatly and depends primarily on the status of host defenses in individual patients. The onset may be insidious, with a clinical course of 3 weeks or more, or may be fulminant and rapidly progressive over a few days. For example, AIDS patients are probably more immunocompromised than oncology patients at the point in time when they develop PCP, as evidenced by typically higher organism burdens, yet AIDS patients are more likely to have a longer history of symptoms and a lower mortality rate than non-AIDS patients.[51,72]

Symptoms in immunosuppressed children or adults without AIDS may be more abrupt in onset and rapidly progressive, but, even with these patients, the course varies greatly.[6,31] The mortality rate approaches 100% in untreated cases. In cases in children and adults, in contrast to infantile cases, fever generally is present and of high grade. It often precedes the onset of nonproductive cough, tachypnea, and severe dyspnea. Fever, tachypnea, and the radiographic appearance of pulmonary infiltrates, in that sequence, 1 to 21 days before diagnosis was established, occurred in a group of children with malignancies. The time of onset of clinical disease in non-AIDS, high-risk patients is unpredictable, but disease often occurs after discontinuance or a reduction in the dose of corticosteroid therapy.[6] Patients with severe combined immunodeficiency disease who receive a bone marrow transplant subsequently may contract fulminant PCP when apparent immunologic reconstitution has occurred.[6]

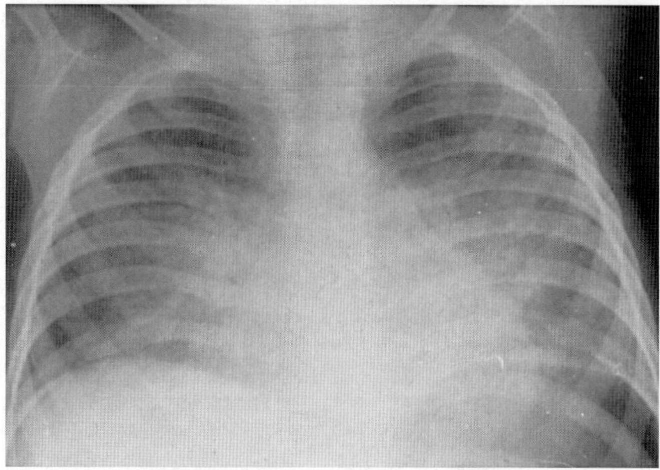

FIG. 225.2 Typical diffuse interstitial infiltrates seen in a 20-month-old child with severe combined immunodeficiency disease at the time of evaluation for clinical *Pneumocystis carinii* pneumonitis.

These observations support the hypothesis that the clinical features early in the course of PCP are dependent to a large extent on the patient's ability to mount an inflammatory response.

Infants and children with AIDS may have a more insidious onset of PCP and therefore may come to medical attention later than non-AIDS patients. In this scenario, the patient is usually acutely ill with fever, cough, dyspnea, tachypnea, and an alveolar-arterial oxygen gradient greater than 30 mm Hg at the time of diagnosis.[14]

In children and adults with and without AIDS, physical examination at the time of initial evaluation may reveal tachypnea; nasal flaring; and intercostal, subcostal, or suprasternal retractions. An ashen color or cyanosis may be present or may develop rapidly. Auscultation of the chest frequently is characterized by a conspicuous absence of adventitious sounds despite the presence of rapid (80–100 breaths/min), shallow respirations. Scattered rales, rhonchi, or wheezes most often are detected later in the clinical course as resolution occurs. Aside from variable elevation in temperature, few other physical abnormalities are noted except those referable to pulmonary disease or secondary to the patient's underlying disease or treatment.[6,31]

Various radiographic abnormalities have been observed in documented cases of isolated PCP.[19,22] These variations result partly from observations at different stages in the course of disease. Bilateral diffuse parenchymal infiltrates (Fig. 225.2) occur most commonly, but no pattern is sufficiently specific either to exclude or to confirm a diagnosis of PCP. Although initially a reticulogranular interstitial process, *Pneumocystis* pneumonitis progresses to a predominantly alveolar process with coalescence and air bronchogram formation. Late in the course of the disease, lung fields may opacify completely. Unusual radiographic findings, including an asymmetric distribution, consolidated lobar infiltrates, pneumothorax and pneumomediastinum, localized parenchymal nodular densities, and pleural effusion, have been documented.[19] During treatment, radiographs show gradual clearing after a variable latent period, during which they may appear worse. Residual interstitial fibrosis occurs in a small percentage of patients.

DIAGNOSIS

The clinical features associated with PCP are not sufficiently specific to differentiate it from other opportunistic pulmonary infections. Mixed infections with viral, bacterial, fungal, or parasitic agents have been documented along with *Pneumocystis*. Implicit in these observations is the importance and urgency of establishing a definitive diagnosis before the institution of specific therapy. An etiologic diagnosis can be ascertained only by the demonstration of *Pneumocystis* organisms in lung tissue or respiratory secretions.

Numerous techniques have been used to obtain suitable material for diagnostic purposes. Specimens obtained by noninvasive methods, especially from induced sputum or tracheal aspirate, have been used to reveal *Pneumocystis,* and the sensitivity of these methods is 50% to 60%. Bronchoalveolar lavage is quite reliable, with a sensitivity of 90% to 95%.[16] Other methods of obtaining a specimen, such as endobronchial brush biopsy, transbronchial lung biopsy, or percutaneous needle aspiration, have been used successfully to establish a diagnosis of PCP, but are not commonly used since the advent of bronchoalveolar lavage.

If PCP remains a possibility after using the just-noted diagnostic methods, one should proceed to an invasive technique such as open-lung biopsy. Open-lung biopsy provides the most dependable specimen from which identification of the organism and the extent of the infection can be ascertained.[1] The chief disadvantage is the need for general anesthesia.

For diagnostic purposes, the methenamine silver nitrate method of Gomori and the less widely used, but more rapid, toluidine blue O and calcofluor white stains are most useful for showing cyst forms in tissue sections, aspirates, or imprints. For more detailed morphologic study of intracystic sporozoites and trophozoites, polychrome stains, including Giemsa, Wright, Gram, and methylene blue stains, are more suitable. In tissue sections, the Gomori stain, in combination with hematoxylin and eosin staining, allows study of the organism and host tissue. A direct immunofluorescent monoclonal antibody technique has become commercially available.[62] Serologic methods are not useful for diagnostic purposes.

There are a large number of studies describing detection of *Pneumocystis* DNA by polymerase chain reaction. Although this has proved to be a valuable laboratory technique, it has had limited use in clinical situations. Reported sensitivities are excellent, but specificities can be less than 85% to 90%.[2,74] At this time, polymerase chain reaction remains a research tool and is not widely used in general clinical practice.

Hematologic studies are of no diagnostic value, primarily because of baseline abnormalities reflecting the underlying disease of affected patients. Eosinophilia has been reported in isolated cases but usually is not present. Depressed serum total protein and albumin values frequently are noted because of the poor nutritional status of representative patients. Lactate dehydrogenase activity is increased, but it is not a specific marker for PCP and is of little diagnostic benefit.[79]

PROGNOSIS

Before the availability of specific therapeutic agents, the overall prognosis of patients with PCP was poor. Despite supportive care, almost 100% of infected patients with underlying neoplastic or immunodeficiency disorders died, whereas approximately 50% of infants in the European epidemics died as a result of this pulmonary infection. With modern medical management, the prognosis for patients with PCP depends to some extent on the underlying risk factor for PCP. For example, the mortality for PCP in cancer patients (25–40%) is four to five times higher than for those with AIDS (5–10%).[51] Patients who require mechanical ventilation have mortality rates in excess of 60% to 70%. A similar high mortality is seen in infants with PCP whose disease progresses and who then require mechanical ventilation.[66]

TREATMENT

Trimethoprim-sulfamethoxazole is the drug of choice for both the treatment and prevention of PCP.[38,46] A minimum of 2 weeks of therapy is recommended for non-AIDS patients; 3 weeks may be optimal for patients with AIDS. The CDC, the National Institutes of Health, and the Infectious Diseases Society of America have provided consensus guidelines for the treatment and prevention of PCP in immunosuppressed patients (Table 225.1).[7] Atovaquone, a hydroxynaphthoquinone approved by the US Food and Drug Administration, is effective and has few side effects (rash, nausea, and diarrhea). It can be administered only by the oral route.[42] The sulfone dapsone has been evaluated in children[24] and may be used alone but is synergistic with trimethoprim[49] against *P. jiroveci.* Dapsone may cause rashes, neutropenia, thrombocytopenia, anemia, and methemoglobinemia. Clindamycin plus primaquine has also been used.[64]

Some studies in adults with AIDS and PCP suggest that the administration of corticosteroids early in the course of moderately severe pneumonitis reduces the occurrence of respiratory failure and improves

TABLE 225.1 Dosing Recommendations for the Prevention and Treatment of *Pneumocystis* Pneumonia

Indication	First Choice	Alternative	Comments/Special Issues
Primary prophylaxis	Trimethoprim 5 mg/kg with sulfamethoxazole 25 mg/kg (TMP-SMX) daily generally divided into two doses. The total daily dose should not exceed 1600 mg SMX and 320 mg TMP. Several dosing schemes have been used successfully: given 3 days per week on consecutive days or on alternate days; given 2 days per week on consecutive days or on alternate days; or given every day.	Dapsone (children ≥1 mo), 2 mg/kg (maximum, 100 mg) orally daily or 4 mg/kg (maximum, 200 mg) orally weekly. Atovaquone (children aged 1 to 3 mo and >24 mo, 30 mg/kg orally daily; children aged 4 to 24 mo, 45 mg/kg orally daily) Aerosolized pentamidine (children aged ≥5 y), 300 mg every month via Respirgard II nebulizer	*Primary prophylaxis indicated for:* All HIV-infected or HIV-indeterminate infants aged 4–6 wk to 12 mo regardless of CD4 count/percentage; HIV-infected children aged 1–5 y with CD4 count <500 cells/mm^3 or CD4 percentage <15%; HIV-infected children aged 6–12 y with CD4 count <200 cells/mm^3 or CD4 percentage <15%. *Criteria for discontinuing primary prophylaxis:* Do not discontinue in children aged <1 y. After ≥6 mo of HAART and Age 1–5 y, CD4 percentage or count is ≥15% or ≥500 cells/mm^3 for >3 consecutive months *or* Age ≥6 y, CD4 percentage or count is ≥15% or ≥200 cells/mm^3 for >3 consecutive mo *Criteria for restarting primary prophylaxis:* Age 1–5 y with CD4 percentage <15% or count <500 cells/mm^3 Age ≥6 y with CD4 percentage <15% or count <200 cells/mm^3
Secondary prophylaxis (prior *Pneumocystis* pneumonia [PCP])	Same as for primary prophylaxis	Same as for primary prophylaxis	Secondary prophylaxis indicated for children with prior episode of PCP. *Criteria for discontinuing secondary prophylaxis:* same as for primary prophylaxis. *Criteria for restarting secondary prophylaxis:* same as for primary prophylaxis.

Continued

TABLE 225.1 Dosing Recommendations for the Prevention and Treatment of *Pneumocystis* Pneumonia—cont'd

Indication	First Choice	Alternative	Comments/Special Issues
Treatment	TMP-SMX 15–20 mg/kg TMP *plus* 75–100 mg/kg SMX daily given orally in three to four divided doses given for 21 days (followed by prophylaxis dosing)	*If TMP-SMX intolerant or clinical treatment failure after 5–7 days of TMP-SMX therapy:* Pentamidine 4 mg/kg IV once daily is first-choice alternative regimen (pentamidine may be changed to atovaquone after 7–10 days IV therapy) Atovaquone 30–40 mg/kg (maximum, 1500 mg/day) orally in two divided doses with food for patients from birth to 3 mo and ≥24 mo. For infants from 3–24 mo, an increased dose of 45 mg/kg daily in two divided doses with food is needed.	After acute pneumonitis resolved in mild-moderate disease, IV TMP-SMX may be changed to oral dosing. Dapsone 2 mg/kg orally once daily (maximum, 100 mg/day) *plus* trimethoprim 15 mg/kg/day orally divided into three doses has been used in adults, but data in children are limited. Primaquine base 0.3 mg/kg orally once daily (maximum, 30 mg/day) *plus* clindamycin 10 mg/kg IV or by mouth (maximum 600 mg given IV and 300–450 mg given orally) every 6 h has been used in adults, but data in children are not available. *Indications for corticosteroids:* Pa_{O_2} <70 mm Hg at room air or alveolar-arterial oxygen gradient >35 mm Hg. Prednisone dose: 1 mg/kg orally twice daily for 5 days, then 0.5–1 mg/kg orally twice daily for 5 days, then 0.5 mg/kg orally once daily for days 11 to 21. Chronic suppressive therapy (secondary prophylaxis) with TMP/SMX is recommended in children and adults after initial therapy.

oxygenation.[55] Other studies show no benefit from corticosteroids.[18] Limited studies of this supportive therapy have been reported to increase survival in children.[68] When used, a reasonable approach seems to be to withdraw corticosteroid therapy as soon as pulmonary function has become stabilized.

PREVENTION

PCP can be prevented in more than 95% of patients at high risk for acquiring the disease.[41,32,39] Patients in high-risk groups, such as patients with cancer, acquired and congenital immunodeficiency disorders, and organ or bone marrow transplants or those receiving intensive immunosuppressive therapy, should be placed on a chemoprophylaxis regimen throughout the risk period (see Table 225.1).

Because of the high risk for acquiring PCP during the first year of life, often before HIV infection is recognized, PCP prophylaxis should be initiated at 4 to 6 weeks of age in all infants born of HIV-infected women, regardless of $CD4^+$ lymphocyte cell counts. The use of chemoprophylaxis in this age group has been highly effective in HIV-infected infants.[63] When infants are shown not to be infected with HIV, prophylaxis may be discontinued. HIV-infected infants and infants with undetermined status should be continued on prophylaxis during the first year of life. At 1 year of age and subsequently, the use of chemoprophylaxis is based on the $CD4^+$ lymphocyte count and other AIDS-defining features.

Trimethoprim-sulfamethoxazole given 3 days per week is the preferred drug for chemoprophylaxis. For patients unable to take trimethoprim-sulfamethoxazole, dapsone 2 mg/kg per day or 4 mg/kg per week is suggested.[24] Studies in adults show that daily doses of dapsone[53] or one dose of dapsone per week[40] is effective prophylaxis.[52] An alternative to dapsone is aerosolized pentamidine 300 mg monthly through Respirgard II inhaler.[48] The dosage for aerosolized pentamidine is the same as the dosage for adults.[48] Atovaquone has been shown to be effective and safe in children.[17] A controlled study compared prophylaxis with atovaquone and azithromycin with trimethoprim-sulfamethoxazole in 366 high-risk, HIV-infected children.[36] The regimens were similar in effectiveness in prevention of bacterial infections, and PCP occurred with equal frequency.

Studies in adults and children show that PCP prophylaxis can be discontinued safely in patients responding to highly active antiretroviral therapy with a sustained increase in $CD4^+$ T lymphocytes to levels above the risk threshold for PCP (see Table 225.1).

Patients are protected from pneumonitis only while receiving chemoprophylaxis and become susceptible again when use of the drugs is discontinued. No vaccine is available.

The full reference list for this chapter is available at ExpertConsult.com.

Parasitic Nematode Infections 226

Peter J. Hotez

INTESTINAL NEMATODES

The three major intestinal nematodes of children, *Ascaris lumbricoides, Trichuris trichiura,* and the hookworms (led by *Necator americanus*), together have a substantial impact on the health and well-being of children living in less-developed nations of the world.[5] This "unholy trinity" of soil-transmitted helminths (STHs), or "geohelminths," deprives hundreds of millions of young children of their full intellectual and growth potential. Some estimates suggest that 2 billion people are infected with STHs, 300 million of whom have severe morbidity. According to the World Health Organization (WHO) an estimated 800 million children are at risk for STHs in low- and middle-income countries.[33] Building on studies from the early part of the 20th century,[24,25] extensive data from many different geographic regions confirm that chronic intestinal nematode infections acquired during childhood suppress cognitive and intellectual development[7,22,25] and impair physical growth and fitness.[9,29,30,28] Through these mechanisms the STH infections can actually cause poverty in the world's developing countries.[13] Because many of these detrimental effects are reversible with the use of anthelmintic drugs to eliminate nematodes from the intestinal tract,[29,30] several investigators and international relief agencies have advocated the administration of benzimidazole anthelmintics (sometimes known as "deworming") as a cornerstone of public health programs directed at school-aged children.[5,6,23]

A 2001 World Health Assembly resolution urges its member states to "deworm" at least 75% and up to 100% of school-aged children at risk for acquiring STH infections through programs of mass drug administration (MDA). Additional studies also point to the benefits of deworming preschool-aged children.[2] For both populations single-dose benzimidazole drugs, either albendazole (400 mg) or mebendazole (500 mg), are most commonly used. Globally, efforts are under way to link deworming for STH infections with MDA for other neglected tropical diseases, including lymphatic filariasis, onchocerciasis, and trachoma,[13,16,10] as well as linking deworming to the control of human immunodeficiency virus (HIV) infection and acquired immunodeficiency syndrome (AIDS), malaria, and tuberculosis.[15]

In some highly endemic areas, reinfection with *A. lumbricoides, T. trichiura,* and hookworms occurs within 6 months of receiving anthelmintic treatment.[3] Therefore, MDA is not always a practical means of control, unless the drugs are used frequently. Newer information suggests that the efficacy of single-dose anthelmintic drugs used for MDA may not be as high as believed previously.[19] Thus, although single-dose benzimidazoles are generally highly effective against pediatric ascariasis, they are less effective against hookworm infection or trichuriasis.[1,26] Such observations may explain why a Cochrane analysis inconsistently demonstrated the health benefits of deworming,[31] as well as why over the last 2 decades there have been dramatic decreases in the global prevalence of ascariasis, but not hookworm infection and trichuriasis.[8] Concern about the potential for emerging anthelmintic drug resistance also exists. Some researchers have pointed to the use of genetically engineered anthelmintic vaccines, especially for hookworm, as one possible solution to the problem of worm reinfection and disease during childhood.[12,34]

Still another public health concern about the long-term effects of STH infections is evidence suggesting that they may promote the susceptibility to, or worsen the severity of, malaria and HIV infection or AIDS.[17] Interest has developed in examining the impact of large-scale deworming on these killer diseases.[15,20] Information also indicates the potential impact of parasitic infections, including the STH infection toxocariasis, in developed countries such as the United States and Europe.[14,10,21,27] In the United States, hardly any of the therapeutic regimens for STH infections are approved by the US Food and Drug Administration, in part because there have been few if any incentives for pharmaceutical companies to pursue indications for these orphan diseases. Also of concern is the high cost of some of these anthelmintic drugs, many of which are generic but monopolized by just a few companies.[4]

In addition to the long-term effects seen when children harbor numerous intestinal nematodes are the increasingly recognized unique neonatal and infantile syndromes that information indicates may result from vertical transmission of the infective stages of some intestinal nematodes, probably in colostrum and breast milk.[5,11] The best-documented example of vertical transmission in infants results in the "swollen belly syndrome" caused by *Strongyloides fuelleborni kellyi,* although other perinatal nematode infections probably also occur (see later). Another emerging pediatric neurologic syndrome (and cause of epilepsy) of great concern (but of unknown etiology) is so-called "nodding syndrome" that has become endemic among some school-aged children and adolescents living in onchocerciasis-endemic areas of South Sudan and Uganda.[32] Finally, children experience significant morbidity during zoonotic transmission of the infective stages of intestinal nematodes in companion animals such as dogs and cats. The resultant aberrant migration of these foreign nematode larvae has become a major pediatric public health problem in large urban areas of the United States and Europe.[14,18]

Ascaris lumbricoides

Ascariasis is one of the most prevalent infections in the world,[44,45] with an estimated 804 million people chronically infected with *A. lumbricoides.*[5,8] Currently, the greatest numbers of cases of ascariasis occur in East Asia, Southeast Asia, and the Indian subcontinent.[5,59] Surveys conducted in rural southern communities of the United States during the 1970s indicated that the prevalence of ascariasis was 20% to 67%.[37] Those rates most likely have declined significantly over the past decades, however.[10,27]

Ascaris infection, when relatively light, is usually not apparent until the patient passes an adult worm through the rectum or a worm emerges from the nasopharynx. In heavy infections, constitutional symptoms may occur during the early phase, and intestinal malabsorption and obstruction may occur in the later phase. The infection is acquired by ingestion of the infective eggs, which hatch in the upper part of the small intestine and free the larvae. The larvae penetrate the intestinal wall, reach venules or lymphatics, and pass through the portal circulation to the liver, the right ventricle, and the lungs.

In the lungs, the larvae break out of the capillaries and begin ascending through the respiratory radicles until they reach the glottis; passing over the epiglottis, they enter the esophagus and are carried down to the small intestine, where they mature and become adult worms. The adult female *Ascaris* produces huge numbers of eggs—possibly 200,000 a day. To ensure adequate quantities of egg-requiring cholesterol, the parasite sequesters oxygen through a specially modified hemoglobin.[47] The entire cycle, beginning with the infective eggs and resulting in ovipositing females, lasts approximately 2 months. Infection is maintained in the community by the deposition of human stool in soil, which permits embryonated eggs to develop into the infective stage. This process takes approximately 2 weeks. The high prevalence of infection results not only from deficient sanitary facilities for disposal of human excreta but also from the deliberate use of human feces as fertilizer.

Epidemiology

In many regions of the developing world, *Ascaris* eggs are almost ubiquitous in the environment. All ages are affected by the parasite; young children, who are exposed more often to the contaminated soil, are affected most frequently. These children usually harbor greater numbers of adult worms in their intestine than do adults living under similar conditions.[29,30,28,43] High worm burdens in children also occur with *Trichuris* infections (see later). Because the phenomenon of heavy *Ascaris* and *Trichuris* worm burdens in childhood is found throughout most of the developing world, pediatric predisposition to "worminess" is widely thought to have a possible genetic or immunologic basis.[9]

Ascaris eggs are extremely hardy and resistant to extremes of temperature and desiccation, features that may explain the common finding of high rates of ascariasis in impoverished urban environments (e.g., Guatemala City, Mexico City) and in rural environments. The eggs also are resistant to chemical disinfectants and are not destroyed readily by sewage treatment. In some areas, pigs may serve as a reservoir for zoonotic *Ascaris* infection.[36]

Pathophysiology

During the migratory phase of the infection, the larvae evoke an inflammatory response associated with eosinophilic infiltration. *Ascaris* antigens—so-called ABA-1 allergen—released during the molting of larvae evoke an immune response, and immunoglobulin E (IgE) antibodies directed against ABA-1 may be associated with parasite resistance.[55] However, through these mechanisms ascariasis is considered a major cause of asthma in impoverished areas of the world.[35,38,63] *Ascaris* larvae also release immunomodulatory glycosphingolipids that inhibit T-helper type 1 (Th1) responses.[5,43] Chronic ascariasis and trichuriasis may suppress host inflammation and even responses to vaccines by promoting a Th2-type cytokine profile.[60] There are also data to support a role for ascariasis in promoting susceptibility to malaria,[20] although not all studies confirm this finding, and some even suggest a possible protective effect.[57] During the intestinal stage of infection, symptoms derive primarily from the physical presence of the worms in the gut, from aberrant migration into other lumina, or from perforation into the peritoneum. As a protective mechanism for its own survival, *Ascaris* secretes peptides that block the action of pancreatic digestive enzymes (trypsin, chymotrypsin, elastase),[48,51] a feature that may play a role in parasite-associated nutrient malabsorption, including the malabsorption of vitamin A.[42] Ascariasis also results in lactose intolerance.[42] Whether these phenomena provide the basis of observed *Ascaris*-associated physical growth retardation during childhood is unknown.[7,29,30,28,43,56]

Clinical Manifestations

The degree of disease induced by the migratory phase of *Ascaris* is related directly to the number of larvae migrating simultaneously. In light infections, this phase is typically unrecognized. Heavy infection, such as that induced in himself by Koino,[53] who swallowed 2000 infected eggs, may cause severe pneumonitis. In some regions of the world, pediatric *Ascaris* pneumonitis is seasonal and can resemble a seasonal form of asthma associated with eosinophilia.[5,46]

In the lumen of the intestine, *Ascaris* adult worms may become matted together and form a bolus large enough to cause intestinal obstruction, sometimes leading to bowel infarction and intestinal perforation. This is a particular problem in very young children because of the small luminal diameter of their intestines.[52] The incidence of this complication has been estimated at 2 per 1000 infected children per year.[37] Children with *Ascaris* obstruction exhibit a toxic appearance, often with signs and symptoms of peritonitis.[5] When recognized early, the obstruction can be treated with medical management, but in many cases surgical intervention is mandatory. Ascariasis has also been linked to chronic intussusception.[58]

Hepatobiliary and pancreatic ascariasis (HPA) results from blockage of the bile duct and pancreatic duct. Patients with HPA are subject to cholecystitis, acute cholangitis, "biliary colic," acute pancreatitis, or hepatic abscess.[52] In contrast to intestinal obstruction, HPA tends to be more common in adults, especially women.[52] Certain irritants, such as halogenated hydrocarbons (e.g., carbon tetrachloride and tetrachloroethylene, used in the past to treat certain hookworm infections), elevation of body temperature, and general anesthesia, have been known to precipitate aberrant migration. *Ascaris* screening by fecal examination should be considered before performing elective surgery on a child who may have immigrated recently from an impoverished area of the tropics.

Whatever the mechanism of interference by *Ascaris* with growth or nutrition, treatment with anthelmintics leads to substantial catch-up growth in previously parasitized children.[7,29,30,28,54,56] Ascariasis in pregnant women results in intrauterine growth retardation.[62] Most individuals with light infections rarely are symptomatic (they become aware of the parasites by passage of adult worms in stool or through regurgitating and vomiting the adult worms), although researchers have conjectured that even these individuals may exhibit subtle deficits in cognitive and intellectual development.[7]

Several cases of neonatal ascariasis have been described in the literature.[39,41] The mode of acquisition of these infections is unknown, but canine and feline ascarid infections commonly are acquired by a transplacental route, suggesting the possibility that this route also may occur in humans.

Diagnosis and Differential Diagnosis

The differential diagnosis of pneumonia caused by *Ascaris* suggests a parasitic etiology because of the peripheral eosinophilia. Any nematode with a migratory phase through the lungs can mimic this infection, however. *Ascaris* must be considered as a cause of intestinal obstruction in any geographic locale where its prevalence is high.

The diagnosis of intestinal ascariasis is established by identifying the characteristic ascarid eggs through microscopic examination of stool. Efforts have been made more recently to detect *Ascaris* metabolites in the urine by gas-liquid chromatography[49,50] or parasite DNA.[40] HPA is suspected in heavily infected children who have signs of biliary obstruction. Ultrasonography and endoscopic retrograde cholangiopancreatography are useful adjunctive diagnostic procedures for these conditions.[52]

Treatment

For an ordinary *Ascaris* infection, either albendazole administered at a fixed dose of 400 mg once or mebendazole administered at a fixed dose of 100 mg twice daily for 3 days is effective. A single fixed dose of 500 mg of mebendazole also may be effective, but it may be unsuitable for the treatment of other STH coinfections. As an alternative, pyrantel pamoate or ivermectin is effective. In a systematic review it was shown that single-dose oral albendazole, mebendazole, and pyrantel pamoate result in ascariasis cure rates of 88%, 95%, and 88%, respectively.[19] The benzimidazoles and pyrantel pamoate are not approved for children younger than 2 years old, and printed statements caution against the use of these drugs in the younger age group. An examination of the use of benzimidazoles in children 12 to 24 months old concluded, however, that these agents are probably safe and should be used if the circumstances warrant it.[56] In such cases, the dose of albendazole in these young children should be reduced to 200 mg.[3] The risk for treatment in this younger age group currently is undergoing more rigorous investigation because of mounting evidence that the growth and cognitive delay caused by STHs may be corrected with albendazole or mebendazole.[29,30,28,56,61] These drugs have a potential for embryotoxicity, however, so judicious use in young children is warranted. The WHO is evaluating the use of benzimidazoles during pregnancy, particularly for use during the second and third trimesters.

In cases of intestinal obstruction, piperazine citrate may be effective because this drug paralyzes the myoneural junction of *Ascaris* and may result in relaxation of the matted bolus of worms. Piperazine citrate is frequently unavailable, however, and it is antagonistic to pyrantel pamoate, so these two drugs should not be administered together.

Management of intestinal obstruction or HPA often is surgical. For some patients, biliary decompression may be performed with endoscopic retrograde cholangiopancreatography.[52]

Prognosis

The prognosis is excellent in most cases of ascariasis. In patients with obstruction or perforation, the prognosis depends entirely on the speed of recognition and therapy.

Prevention

Ascaris infection could be eliminated entirely through proper disposal of human excreta. As an isolated means of health improvement in the absence of economic development, this approach seldom is successful. Elimination of *Ascaris* from a community or a substantial reduction in the incidence of this infection usually occurs after general efforts in poverty reduction and improvements in the standard of living have been achieved. Periodic administration of community-wide therapy with anthelmintics has been effective in reducing worm burden as a short-term strategy. However, reinfection can occur within 6 months after treatment in areas of high transmission.[3] Ultimately, of all the STH infections caused by the exquisite sensitivity of *A. lumbricoides* to benzimidazole anthelmintics and the concentration of *Ascaris* infections among children, ascariasis may offer the best chance of being eliminated through frequent and periodic MDA programs.

Trichuris trichiura

Trichuriasis has a prevalence of approximately 477 million cases worldwide,[8] with the largest number of cases in South and Southeast Asia, and sub-Saharan Africa.[2,59] Heavy infections, however, lead to colitis and sometimes dysentery. Light infections are often asymptomatic but may still result in deficits in cognition, however.[7,22,78]

The infection is acquired by the ingestion of embryonated eggs acquired from the soil on hands or through contaminated food. The eggs hatch in the upper part of the small intestine, and the liberated larvae penetrate the villi. In contrast to the larvae of *Ascaris, Trichuris* larvae do not undergo extraintestinal migration but remain in situ for approximately 1 week, at which time they begin a progressive descent into the cecum and the colon. They mature there, and the attenuated anterior end of the adult worm embeds itself in the colonic mucosa. Creation of syncytial tunnels (derived from the columnar epithelium of the colon) is facilitated by the release of a parasite-derived, pore-forming protein.[68] The parasites derive their nourishment from these colonic mucosal tunnels. The entire cycle from the ingestion of embryonated ova to the development of sexually mature adults takes approximately 2 months. Persistence of the infection in a community depends on continual contamination of the soil with human feces.

Epidemiology

These parasites are found most commonly throughout the developing countries of the tropics and subtropics. The distribution of this worm often parallels that of *Ascaris.* In addition, as in the case of *Ascaris,* children with trichuriasis usually harbor greater numbers of worms than adults living under similar conditions.[65,66] Consequently, children have greater morbidity from trichuriasis than adults do. The mechanistic basis of added worminess in children is unknown, although researchers have observed that for all of the soil-transmitted helminthiases, including trichuriasis, infections are aggregated, with a few children having particularly heavy infections. These heavily infected children seem to have a genetic or immunologic predisposition to *Trichuris* infection.[65,66] Children also are the major source of *Trichuris* eggs in the environment; when the eggs are deposited in the soil, they become infective in approximately 1 month and remain viable for several months. They are killed by exposure to temperatures greater than 40°C within 1 hour. Freezing temperatures less than −8°C also destroy these eggs. Similar to ascarid eggs, *Trichuris* eggs are resistant to chemical disinfectants.

Pathophysiology

At the site of attachment, the adult worm elicits characteristic changes in the colonic mucosa, as noted earlier. Inflammatory cells also are found at these sites, but they do not seem to account entirely for the clinical resemblance of trichuriasis to some forms of inflammatory bowel disease.[65,74] Similar to many other intestinal worms, *Trichuris* is expelled through the action of the host's immune system. This expulsion results from a combined effect of antibody and lymphoid cells.[80] Regulation of *Trichuris* populations in the gut has been ascribed to a carefully orchestrated balance of host-derived cytokines.[69] Although anemia has been attributed to trichuriasis,[72] the amount of blood loss caused by this parasite is much less than hookworm-associated blood loss and is insufficient to account for anemia.[73] One possibility is that *Trichuris*-induced anemia results from chronic inflammation, similar to the anemia of inflammatory bowel disease.[65,66]

Clinical Manifestations

Two major disease syndromes are caused by heavy *Trichuris* infection during childhood.[65,66] *Trichuris* dysentery syndrome (TDS) is associated with severe diarrhea with blood and mucus. It can also be associated with chronic iron-deficiency anemia,[70] although anemia should be considered first and foremost a hallmark of human hookworm infection. Children with TDS are anemic and frequently manifest growth retardation and failure to thrive.[67] Infants and toddlers with TDS are at risk for protracted tenesmus, which leads to rectal prolapse. *Trichuris* colitis is a more chronic manifestation of moderate to heavy infection that is characterized by a form of inflammatory bowel disease similar to what occurs in Crohn disease or ulcerative colitis. Children with this form of colitis also can have chronic malnutrition and short stature. Moderately and heavily infected (and possibly even lightly infected) children are at risk for having deficits in cognition and intellectual development.[78]

Diagnosis and Differential Diagnosis

The diagnosis is established by identification of the characteristic barrel-shaped eggs through microscopic examination of stool. Clinically, heavily infected children with TDS may resemble children with amebic or bacillary dysentery. Children with *Trichuris* colitis may have signs and symptoms that resemble other forms of inflammatory bowel disease. The erythrocyte sedimentation rate is not elevated in children with *Trichuris* colitis, however. Among other diagnostic modalities, *Trichuris* colitis has been detected by Doppler ultrasonography,[64] whereas the presence of adult worms can also be seen on colonoscopy.[77]

Treatment

In the past, when noxious or toxic drugs had to be used, only patients with heavy infection were treated. Currently, any patient with this infection can be treated by the administration of either albendazole, administered as a single fixed dose of 400 mg in MDA programs or on 3 successive days otherwise, or mebendazole, at 100 mg twice daily for 3 days.[75] A single dose of albendazole (400 mg) mebendazole (500 mg) also is used for MDA in some developing countries, although this practice is often not efficacious for trichuriasis. A systematic review revealed that cure rates after single-dose oral albendazole and mebendazole are only 28% and 36%, respectively.[19] Studies indicate that the efficacy can be improved by using a double dose of albendazole or mebendazole given 8 hours apart.[76] A combination of albendazole and mebendazole has also been effective,[76] as is adding ivermectin to either albendazole or mebendazole.[71] Because albendazole is frequently combined with ivermectin in MDA efforts to eliminate lymphatic filariasis in Africa, this practice could have important collateral benefits for trichuriasis. As alternatives, the drug oxantel pamoate is effective for the treatment of trichuriasis. In some countries, oxantel pamoate is formulated with pyrantel pamoate, and it has been reported that albendazole formulated with oxantel pamoate is highly effective in treating trichuriasis.[65] As noted earlier, the safety of the benzimidazoles in very young children has not been established, but this may not preclude its use in the practice of pediatrics.[51,79]

Prevention

As in the case of other nematodes, sanitary disposal of excreta—but more important, improvement in the standard of living—tends to reduce the incidence of infection. Frequent mass treatments with mebendazole reduce the worm burden in a community.

Hookworms

Hookworm infection is one of the most important infections of adults and children in the developing world, with an estimated prevalence of approximately 472 million cases.[5,8,12] Hookworms are the predominant STH in sub-Saharan Africa[99] where they frequently cause coinfections with schistosomiasis and falciparum malaria.[86,87,102] Hookworm infection is also widespread in Asia and Latin America.[59] Hookworms exert their pathogenic effect by causing intestinal blood loss, which leads to iron-deficiency anemia.[95] By considering the average daily blood loss induced by each worm, a moderate hookworm infection comprising 25 adult hookworms produces 1 mL of blood loss per day, often sufficient blood loss to rob a child of his or her daily iron requirement.[92] Because loss of blood represents loss of erythrocytes and plasma, heavy infections also contribute to protein malnutrition.[100]

Two major species of hookworms infect the human intestine: *Ancylostoma duodenale* and *Necator americanus,* although *N. americanus* is found more commonly worldwide (responsible for more than 80% of the global hookworm burden), especially in sub-Saharan Africa, Southeast Asia, and the Americas.[95] Two other zoonotic members of the genus *Ancylostoma,* the dog and cat hookworm *A. ceylanicum* and the dog hookworm *A. caninum,*[103] are much less frequent causes of intestinal pathology in humans.[94] *A. ceylanicum* causes hookworm infection in focal rural areas of the Asia-Pacific region,[97] whereas *A. caninum* is a rare cause of eosinophilic enteritis.[91]

The infection is acquired either by exposure of skin to moist soil infested with the larvae of these worms (*A. duodenale* and *N. americanus*) or by ingestion of the infective larvae (*A. duodenale* only). The most propitious circumstances for infection are shady areas and sandy or loamy soil. Infection is particularly likely to occur early in the morning, when the ground is moist with dew, or after a rainfall. After the larvae enter the host, they initiate a developmental program that continues until they enter the intestine.[9,95] This process is coupled with the release of parasite-derived proteases and other virulence factors.[109] Larvae that enter through the skin are carried by the venous circulation to the right ventricle and there follow the route described for *Ascaris,* whereas larvae that are ingested may develop entirely within the gastrointestinal tract.

On reaching the small intestine, the larvae mature to adult worms, which become attached with their mouth parts to the intestinal mucosa. Eosinophilia begins during this phase of the infection. The adult worms sustain themselves by releasing hydrolytic enzymes that degrade the intestinal mucosa and then feed on cellular and connective tissue debris.[95] During this process, capillaries and arterioles are eroded and lacerated, with subsequent extravasation of blood. The adult worms also ingest hemoglobin in blood through the action of parasite gut brush border proteases.[107] Anticoagulants that block the activity of host factor Xa and VIIa/tissue factor facilitate blood flow and are responsible for continued bleeding from the original site after the worm has moved to a new one.[90]

The entire cycle from penetration of the skin or ingestion of larvae to the development of mature worms usually takes 6 to 8 weeks. At that time, hookworm eggs appear in the feces. *A. duodenale* larvae also may undergo a period of developmental arrest within the human host that lasts weeks or months. Intestinal ancylostomiasis can occur up to 1 year (and possibly longer) after initial exposure to infective larvae has occurred.[105,104] Investigators have conjectured that the reservoir of arrested *A. duodenale* larvae enters the mammary glands and breast milk.[94] This sequence of events may account for cases of infantile ancylostomiasis noted in Africa, India, and China.[85,89,94] Humans are the major reservoir of these organisms, and this infection is maintained by continual contamination of soil by human feces.

Epidemiology

Although in ancient times these parasites had a worldwide distribution, they currently are most prevalent in areas of rural poverty in the tropics and subtropics. *N. americanus* is the predominant hookworm in the world, especially in the Western Hemisphere, most of Africa, China south of the Yangtze River, Southeast Asia and Indonesia, and certain islands of the Pacific. In Asia, *A. duodenale* predominates in many parts of the Indian subcontinent and focal areas of China north of the Yangtze River.[9] *A. duodenale* also is a major parasite in Egypt and other parts of the Mediterranean region, Africa, and a few focal areas in South America, including Paraguay and northern Argentina. A small Central American focus also exists in southern Honduras and El Salvador, and one exists among aboriginal populations in Australia. This differential distribution is not always absolute, and small numbers of either parasite can be present where the other predominates. Mixed infections with both species are common. *A. ceylanicum* occurs in focally endemic areas of southern Asia,[95] whereas the dog hookworm *A. caninum* has been described as a cause of human eosinophilic enteritis in Australia and possibly elsewhere.[100]

Larvae survive in soil for 6 weeks. They are destroyed by drying, freezing temperatures, and heat greater than 45°C. Hookworm infection occurs in areas with high agricultural intensity and is not found frequently in urban areas, where *Ascaris* and *Trichuris* may predominate. Because shade and moisture are essential for survival at the infective larval stage, a not surprising finding is high rates of hookworm infection in families that harvest tea in India and Bangladesh, mulberry leaves (for the silkworm industry) in eastern China, sweet potatoes and corn in western China, coffee and bananas in Central and South America, and rubber in Africa.

Similar to other STHs, hookworm infections usually are aggregated such that most individuals harbor light worm burdens, whereas a substantial minority harbors moderate or heavy infections.[95,105] Even after receiving specific anthelmintic chemotherapy, moderately and heavily infected individuals seem to be predisposed to the reacquisition of heavy infection.[105] A predisposition to hookworm infection may have a genetic or immunologic basis.

In contrast to the other STHs, high rates of hookworm infection occur in adults and children. In some regions, the age-associated prevalence and intensity increase linearly, with the heaviest infections occurring in older adult populations.[93] Hookworm coinfections with strongyloidiasis,[83] schistosomiasis,[12,108] and malaria[86,87] have been described and are believed to be common in low- and middle-income countries.

Pathophysiology

During the migratory phase of the infection, the larvae evoke an inflammatory response. Immune responses to the infection have been difficult to study in humans, but in an animal model a dog infected with *A. caninum* was rendered immune to challenge infection by receiving repeated dosing with the infective larvae. This observation provided a means of producing a live attenuated larval vaccine in the laboratory, but it is unsuitable for humans. An infective hookworm larval antigen known as ASP-2 has been identified as an immunodominant antigen linked to hookworm larval vaccines.[82,84]

Host eosinophilia occurs as larvae enter the gut and mature into adult hookworms. Adult hookworms feed on human blood and have the capacity to lyse red blood cells and degrade host hemoglobin.[101] The major source of injury to the host is loss of blood, with *A. duodenale* producing greater blood loss than *N. americanus.* Rarely, massive bleeding has been reported.[103] Iron-deficiency anemia results when iron loss exceeds the host's iron reserves. Because children and women of reproductive age generally have lower iron reserves than do other populations, they are at the highest risk for developing hookworm disease and anemia.[95] Systematic reviews have confirmed the association between anemia and hookworm infections in children and pregnant and nonpregnant adults.[88,106] Long-standing moderate and heavy infections result in the characteristic features of severe iron deficiency. Loss of protein contributes further to malnutrition. Together, the iron deficiency and protein malnutrition result in impaired growth and physical fitness.[24,29,30,28,95] In some cases, hypoproteinemia can be corrected by a high-protein diet without deworming the patient,[103] although the World Food Program and other international agencies now frequently incorporate deworming into their nutritional supplementation programs. In addition to the physical deficits noted earlier, hookworms may affect cognitive development because iron is important for the development of dopaminergic neurons and for the biosynthesis of some neurotransmitters.[95] An experimental human hookworm vaccine for *N. americanus* infections is under development; the vaccine targets key parasite enzymes involved in blood digestion and heme detoxification.[12]

Clinical Manifestations

Penetration by larvae causes "ground itch" or "dew itch," a type of pruritus that occurs after walking in the morning dew. These cutaneous manifestations can occur on almost any part of the body. This phase of early infection is followed within days to weeks by pneumonitis, which typically is less pronounced than *Ascaris* pneumonitis.

The acute intestinal phase in heavy infections is characterized by abdominal pain, diarrhea, nausea, and anorexia.[94] Eosinophilia occurs approximately at the onset of the intestinal phase. Subsequently, well-nourished individuals with light infections have mild gastrointestinal symptoms, but no evidence of anemia or malnutrition. At the other extreme, children with moderate hookworm infections can show signs and symptoms of iron-deficiency anemia, whereas heavily infected children can have hemoglobin values of 2 g/dL and edema or anasarca caused by hypoproteinemia. Infants with severe ancylostomiasis can exhibit failure to thrive, profound pallor, and melena.[85,89,94]

Deficits in physical and intellectual growth as a result of chronic hookworm infection in childhood have been reported since the early part of the 20th century.[7,9,24,25,95] Some recovery has been described after "deworming," although some deficits occurring in infancy may be irreversible.

Diagnosis and Differential Diagnosis

Hookworm pneumonitis resulting from the early migratory stages typically is nonspecific in its presentation and difficult to diagnose. Hookworm anemia is caused by blood loss; it must be distinguished from all other causes of intestinal loss of blood. In developing countries, where severe hookworm anemia is common, the probability of the occurrence of rarer causes of intestinal blood loss, such as Meckel diverticulum and polyps, is low. The opposite holds true for regions where hookworm infections are light or infrequent. In sub-Saharan Africa, the distribution of hookworm overlaps with other significant causes of so-called agricultural anemias, including malaria, schistosomiasis, malnutrition, and hemoglobin polymorphisms.[17]

The diagnosis is established by identifying the characteristic eggs by microscopic examination of stool. The eggs of *A. duodenale* and *N. americanus* cannot be distinguished from each other by morphologic criteria, but the worms can be differentiated by direct examination of the infective larvae or adults, or the polymerase chain reaction.[40] One must assume that it is one or the other species on the basis of the geographic origin of the patient. Although this decision is not of paramount importance, it does have some therapeutic implications, including the possibility that arrested larvae of *A. duodenale* would become reactivated and either repopulate the intestine at some point after treatment or enter breast milk during or after parturition. Hookworms have been detected visually by endoscopy.[98]

Treatment

For *N. americanus* infection, the drug of choice is either albendazole, administered at a fixed dose of 400 mg, or mebendazole, given as 100 mg twice daily for 3 days. In settings of MDA for low-income countries, mebendazole is sometimes given as a single 500-mg dose. Pyrantel pamoate, given as a dose of 11 mg/kg, not to exceed 1 g, for 3 days is a suitable alternative drug. One meta-analysis and systematic review found that the efficacy of single-dose oral albendazole for hookworm infection was 72%, whereas single-dose mebendazole results in a cure rate of only 15% and pyrantel pamoate in a cure rate of 31%.[19] In a systematic review single-dose mebendazole was shown not to improve hookworm anemia.[83] Therefore, albendazole should be considered the first-line treatment of hookworm infection. However, even single-dose albendazole frequently has failed to reduce hookworm burdens in some endemic settings.[1,26,81] In areas endemic for ancylostomiasis, the health care provider should be aware of the potential of arrested tissue larvae to repopulate the intestine or enter breast milk and infect infants during the perinatal period. Iron supplementation and transfusion are occasional important adjunctive therapies for severe hookworm disease.

Prevention

As in all cases of STH infections, the sanitary control of the disposal of excreta represents an important public health control measure. Accomplishing effective sanitation in resource-poor settings has not been feasible in most of the developing world. The popular recommendation to wear shoes is naïve because *N. americanus* larvae also enter through the upper extremities, torso, and legs and because *A. duodenale* also is orally infective. Studies to develop and test a first-generation recombinant hookworm vaccine are in progress.[12,96] The human hookworm vaccine is in clinical trials in Brazil and Gabon. Unlike first-generation larval vaccines, this new vaccine targets adult blood-feeding hookworms.

Enterobius vermicularis

Pinworm infection (enterobiasis), or oxyuriasis (the older term), is one of the most frequent of all human helminth infections and one that is common in North America and Europe.[120] Some investigators believe that the overall prevalence of enterobiasis is declining in the United States, however. Most infected individuals are children, and the infection is found in all socioeconomic classes. It is acquired by the ingestion of infective eggs picked up on the perianal skin, in the air, or on bedclothes and underwear. Swallowed eggs, transmitted to the mouth by fingers or through inhalation, hatch in the duodenum, and the liberated larvae undergo additional maturational steps in the small intestine before reaching the cecum. There, the sexually mature worms copulate and proceed to the rectum and eventually to the perianal skin, where the gravid females lay eggs. The eggs become infective within 2 to 4 hours after deposition.

The entire cycle from ingestion of the egg to the egg-laying phase of the gravid female is 4 to 6 weeks. Rarely, a retrograde infection occurs in which eggs hatch on the anal mucosa and the larvae migrate up the bowel and mature to adult worms. Sexual transmission from oral-anal contact has also been reported.[110] Although enterobiasis is a human infection, anthropoid apes can be infected experimentally.

Epidemiology

The infection is worldwide in distribution, and children are infected most frequently. Communal living, especially assembling in school gymnasia and living in crowded households, promotes transmission of the infection. Adults tend to be infected through their contact with children; parents and teachers are the most vulnerable. Orphanages and day care centers frequently are affected.[120]

Pathophysiology

No intestinal reactions occur during the migratory phase, and because no tissue migration takes place, no eosinophilia occurs to the degree seen with some other nematodes. Occasionally, hypersensitive individuals may have a slight increase in eosinophils. The deposited ova induce pruritus on the perianal skin. No evidence indicates that some individuals are more susceptible than others to this infection.

Enterobius occasionally has been found in vermiform appendixes removed at surgery.[112] A causal relationship with appendicitis has not been established, but some evidence points to the possibility that this worm induces granuloma formation and may cause obstruction of this vestigial structure.[111,113] When the adult gravid female migrates along the perineal skin into the vagina, it may cause vulvitis as a reaction to the eggs deposited in that region.[115] Some investigators speculate that migrating pinworms may introduce bacteria into the lower urinary tract and result in urinary tract infection.[119] *E. vermicularis* has also been reported from the fallopian tube and as a cause of infertility.[122] Other aberrant infections, such as those causing hepatic granuloma and renal disease, occur more infrequently.[114,118]

Clinical Manifestations

Pruritus is the most common symptom; its intensity varies from mild perianal itching to acute, intractable pain. Secondary cellulitis also may occur in severely pruritic cases.[117] Perianal abscess has also been described.[96] Vaginal discharge and vulval itching are symptoms in the rare cases in which a worm has migrated into the vagina. Insomnia, restlessness, irritability, loss of appetite, loss of weight, and grinding of teeth all have been reported anecdotally in individuals with pinworm infection, but no evidence has shown that any of these symptoms is related causally to *Enterobius* infection. Enuresis also has been blamed on the pinworm, but one epidemiologic study failed to determine causality.[121] An unusual form of eosinophilic ileocolitis resulting from massive infestation with many *E. vermicularis* larvae was described in a homosexual man.[116] Various clinical manifestations resulting from ectopic infections, including appendicitis and infertility, have been reported.[112,122]

Diagnosis

E. vermicularis eggs are identified readily by low-power microscopic examination of transparent adhesive tape previously applied to the perianal skin and then affixed to a microscope slide.

Treatment

Single-dose therapy with mebendazole (100 mg), albendazole (400 mg), or pyrantel pamoate (11 mg/kg, not to exceed 1 g) is effective. With the current availability of these three highly effective drugs, the intensive laundering of underwear and bed clothing, recommended in the older literature, no longer is necessary. Treating all members of the household is advisable, however, because they all must be presumed to be infected. Repeat treatment in 2 or 3 weeks to destroy any adult worms that have hatched from the eggs swallowed at the time of initial therapy may be necessary. None of these drugs destroys the eggs.

One of the most important aspects of management of this infection is reassurance that in some areas its ubiquity virtually precludes effective eradication. Reinfection can be anticipated in any family infected with pinworms because of the high prevalence of this worm in the community. It also is important to reassure families that the presence of pinworms does not suggest poor hygienic standards in the family.

Strongyloides stercoralis and *Strongyloides fuelleborni kellyi*

Strongyloides stercoralis and *Strongyloides fuelleborni kellyi* are among the most virulent helminthic pathogens of humans, although human strongyloidiasis is believed to be less prevalent than *Ascaris* or hookworm, with some estimates indicating 30 to 100 million cases worldwide, but there is an urgent need to refine global disease burden estimates.[149] High rates of infection are found in Southeast Asia (especially rural Cambodia),[144] as well as selected areas of Africa and Latin America. Foci of strongyloidiasis are also believed to occur still in parts of the southern United States, including Appalachia.[153] *S. stercoralis* has the unusual ability to cause autoinfection, which can lead to hyperinfection and disseminated infection in immunocompromised hosts.[106,110,113–117,119,125,126] *S. fuelleborni kellyi* causes an aggressive infantile protein-losing enteropathy that leads to ascites and high mortality rates.[123,124]

S. stercoralis infection is acquired by the exposure of skin to infective larvae in the soil, much as in the case of hookworm infection. Similar circumstances that promote the survival of hookworm larvae in soil (i.e., moisture, sandy or loamy soil, and shade) promote the survival of *Strongyloides*. Larvae penetrate skin, facilitated by a potent histolytic protease that they secrete.[126,148] From the moment of penetration of the skin to the arrival of the worms in the intestine, the cycle commonly is thought to be similar to that of hookworms, although experimental evidence suggests that *S. stercoralis* also may explore routes of migration that bypass the lungs.[155] Within the intestine, the small adult worms do not attach to the mucosa as hookworms do but instead lie embedded in its folds. The cycle from penetration of skin to development of mature worms in the intestine is approximately 28 days.

No parasitic adult male worms exist to fertilize the eggs. Instead, the mature eggs may develop by parthenogenesis. In addition, in contrast to the eggs of other parasitic nematodes, these eggs usually are not found in feces but instead embryonate within the intestine and develop into larvae, which are deposited in soil with human stool. These so-called rhabditiform larvae must molt before they become infective.

This cycle has two variations. One permits the development of nonparasitic male and female adults in soil, which can maintain infestation of the soil for a certain period; this free-living phase sometimes is called the heterogonic life cycle. The second variation has much greater clinical relevance. Under certain conditions that are not well defined, the rhabditiform larvae molt to new infective larvae while they are still in the intestine. These new infective larvae can penetrate the intestine and set up a new cycle, commonly called autoinfection or the autoinfective cycle.[139] In this fashion, this nematode, in contrast to most other intestinal nematodes of humans, actually can increase in number without reinfection from the outside world. This phenomenon also is responsible for persistence of this infection for decades in an untreated host.[141] Some investigators think that low levels of autoinfection occur in most patients with strongyloidiasis, but this concept requires further investigation.

When host defenses are impaired, especially through use of high-dose corticosteroids (discussed later), *S. stercoralis* can undergo multiple rounds of autoinfection, leading to the production of thousands to hundreds of thousands of adult parasites in the intestine. This phenomenon is known as hyperinfection.[128,134,140,151] One possible consequence of hyperinfection is disseminated infection, in which larval and adult worms are identified at extraintestinal sites.

S. fuelleborni kellyi larvae are passed to infants by ingestion in breast milk.[123,127] Transmammary infection by nematode larvae is an extremely common route of transmission in nonhuman nematode infections[23]; although not well studied, it probably also occurs commonly in humans.

Epidemiology

S. stercoralis infection has worldwide distribution, but it is most prevalent in tropical and subtropical regions.[149] The difficulty in diagnosing strongyloidiasis has hindered efforts to understand the global disease burden of this important illness more clearly. The highest prevalence is likely in Southeast Asia, but strongyloidiasis also is endemic in Brazil and Jamaica and presumably elsewhere in Latin America, as well as in sub-Saharan Africa.[135,149,152] In North America, strongyloidiasis is focally endemic in some parts of Appalachia,[130,153] and it is common in Southeast Asian immigrants.[142] In one study, 76.6% of Kampuchean immigrants and 55.6% of Laotian immigrants were seropositive for *S. stercoralis* infection.[142] Between 1991 and 2006 an estimated 347 deaths from strongyloidiasis occurred in the United States, mostly among older white men and those living in the southeastern states.[133] The seroprevalence in rural Appalachian Kentucky was estimated to be 1.9%.[153] Because of the possibility of autoinfection and, by extension, infection through contamination of skin by infested feces, strongyloidiasis is highly prevalent in mental hospitals, prisons, and homes for mentally disabled children. Dogs and anthropoid apes may serve as animal reservoir hosts for *S. stercoralis*. *S. fuelleborni kellyi* infection is endemic in Papua New Guinea and parts of sub-Saharan Africa.[123,124,145]

Pathophysiology

During the migratory phase of the infection, the larvae of *S. stercoralis* evoke an inflammatory response associated with eosinophilic infiltration. The adult phase in the intestine, even in moderate infection, may be associated with an inflammatory reaction sufficient to be symptomatic. Some evidence suggests that *Strongyloides* induces a malabsorption syndrome, which has been treated effectively by deworming.[130,150] It also has been noted, however, that the diarrhea associated with strongyloidiasis in young children occurs more frequently in those children with underlying malnutrition.[134] Young children with *S. stercoralis*–induced malabsorption experience stunted growth and failure to thrive.[130]

The deficits in host defense that promote hyperinfection and disseminated strongyloidiasis are not well understood. Although cell-mediated immune deficits, such as those occurring in immunosuppression, organ transplantation, severe malnutrition, and cytotoxic chemotherapy for neoplasms and collagen vascular disease, are associated with this phenomenon, certain established deficits in cell-mediated immunity, such as those in HIV infection, do not trigger hyperinfection.[139] Researchers have suggested that patients receiving large doses of corticosteroids are particularly susceptible to hyperinfection because the corticosteroids themselves function as direct signals or ligands for the parasite to undergo autoinfection.[139] Patients with human T-cell lymphotropic virus type I seem to be at high risk for acquiring opportunistic strongyloidiasis,[137,143] possibly because of a specific deficit in their effector IgE immune response.[152] The pathogenesis of the marked protein-losing enteropathy that leads to ascites in the swollen belly syndrome of *S. fuelleborni kellyi* infection has not been established.

Clinical Manifestations

During the migratory phase of larval strongyloidiasis, patients may be susceptible to the development of pneumonitis associated with eosinophilia. Larval migration through the skin can result in larva currens. Although most patients harboring *S. stercoralis* in their intestine are asymptomatic, patients with moderate or heavy infection classically have intense diarrhea productive of watery, mucous stool. Periods of alternating diarrhea and constipation may occur. Anorexia and cachexia, which lead to failure to thrive and other deficits in physical growth, are common features of pediatric strongyloidiasis.[130] Eosinophilia is also common, although among pediatric refugees this sign was not considered predictive of *S. stercoralis* infection.[136] Chronic strongyloidiasis has been linked to nephrotic syndrome.[132]

In disseminated strongyloidiasis caused by the hyperinfective cycle, larvae may invade all tissues, including the central nervous system (CNS). Because larvae penetrate the intestine, they may carry with them enteric flora and cause sepsis or meningoencephalitis.[128] Although diarrhea is the most commonly recognized consequence of *Strongyloides* infection, the hyperinfective cycle has the greatest portent for immunosuppressed patients. Infants with *S. fuelleborni kellyi* infection may manifest the swollen belly syndrome, with marked abdominal ascites and pleural effusions that can be fatal. In older children *S. fuelleborni* kellyi infection can be associated with malnutrition.[145]

Diagnosis and Differential Diagnosis

Strongyloides pneumonitis can resemble the clinical manifestations associated with the lung migration of other nematode parasites, such as *Ascaris* and hookworm. The differential diagnosis of diarrhea must include causes of chronic diarrheal disease. In some patients, eosinophilia is a presenting sign of strongyloidiasis, either in patients with diarrhea or even in asymptomatic immigrants from developing countries.

The diagnosis is established by identification of the characteristic larvae during microscopic examination of stool, which is not easy because rhabditiform larvae usually are not produced in abundance. Specific stool concentration techniques are available to increase the sensitivity of fecal examination, although they are not as effective as amplifying the heterogonic life cycle by the Baermann technique or by looking for characteristic larval tracks on nutrient agar plates.[156] The stool of all immunosuppressed individuals, including those given corticosteroids for any reason, who have ever been in a region where *Strongyloides* is found must be examined to rule out this infection. If routine stool examination results are negative, the stool should be processed as outlined earlier. In addition, examination of duodenal contents can be attempted by the string test (Enterotest). This examination divulges only the contents of the duodenum, however, and can miss the larvae in the lower part of the small intestine. An enzyme-linked immunosorbent assay (ELISA) for detection of *Strongyloides*-specific antibodies is available on a research basis, as is a polymerase chain reaction–based assay.[40,142,152] The accuracy of five serologic assays including the different ELISA assays has been compared.[129]

Children with the swollen belly syndrome from *S. fuelleborni kellyi* infection shed eggs rather than larvae in their feces. Large numbers of eggs are common findings in clinical cases.

Treatment

Previously, the drug of choice for *S. stercoralis* and *S. fuelleborni kellyi* infection was thiabendazole.[131] The drug has high toxicity, however, which frequently includes nausea, vomiting, and vertigo and sometimes requires interruption of therapy. Rarely, it induces leukopenia, rash, and Stevens-Johnson syndrome. Because the drug is detoxified in the liver, its dose may have to be reduced for patients with liver failure. Another benzimidazole used with increasing frequency is albendazole 400 mg twice daily for 7 days. Studies have shown that ivermectin is equivalent to thiabendazole in terms of its efficacy, but ivermectin has a much better safety profile.[125] Similarly, single and double doses of oral ivermectin are more effective than a 7-day course of high-dose albendazole for patients with *S. stercoralis* chronic infection.[157]

Ivermectin is considered the treatment of choice for strongyloidiasis. It is administered at a dose of 200 μg/kg per day for 2 days. Treatment with ivermectin gives a cure rate of 80%.[143,147] The safety of the drug in young children (<15 kg) and pregnant women remains to be established. Because the mortality rate of patients with disseminated strongyloidiasis remains high despite specific anthelmintic therapy, a common practice is to treat with a prolonged course or with a repeat course of therapy. In addition, several case reports have now described the use of veterinary parenteral formulations in patients too ill to take oral medications[147] or the use of ivermectin combined with albendazole.[150] Secondary bacterial complications, such as sepsis and meningitis, are common with disseminated strongyloidiasis, so judicious use of broad-spectrum antimicrobial agents frequently is indicated for this condition. As an additional supportive measure, patients who have hyperinfective strongyloidiasis and are receiving high-dose corticosteroid therapy will probably benefit from steroid taper. Patients with transplants and cyclosporine immunosuppression may benefit from some of the direct helminthotoxic properties of this compound.[154]

Prognosis

The prognosis is excellent in patients who do not have disseminated infection and are treated promptly. Unrecognized disseminated infection can be lethal.

Prevention

Proper disposal of human excreta substantially reduces the prevalence of strongyloidiasis in any community. In closed institutions, where control of direct spread is not likely to be achieved, identification in addition to treatment of infected individuals is the only feasible control.[138] There have been calls to incorporate strongyloidiasis control more effectively in MDA activities for ascariasis, trichuriasis, and hookworm infection.[146]

ABERRANT INFECTIONS WITH INTESTINAL NEMATODES

Toxocara canis and *Toxocara cati*

One of the most dramatic examples of an aberrant infection with an STH is visceral larva migrans and a related syndrome, ocular larva migrans, caused by infection with *Toxocara canis.* This species of roundworm causes intestinal infection in the dog, in which its cycle resembles that of *A. lumbricoides* in humans. Humans become infected by *Toxocara* through the ingestion of an embryonated egg, much as in human infection with *Ascaris.* Larvae hatch in the small intestine, penetrate the villi, and begin a migration that takes them through every organ and tissue of the body. Because they cannot mature, the larvae tend to migrate for months until they are overcome by the inflammatory reaction of the host and die. Although visceral larva migrans and ocular larva migrans are the most dramatic manifestations of toxocariasis, these are relatively rare conditions. In contrast, a covert form associated with eosinophilia together with either cognitive or pulmonary deficits may be widespread in the Western Hemisphere, including North America, as well as in Europe, Africa, and other regions. There are no published global disease burden estimates.

Although larvae of other toxocarids such as *Toxocara cati* and *Toxascaris leonina* have been suggested as possible causes of visceral larva migrans, they may be less important as zoonotic pathogens in humans. However, the more recently noted association between toxocariasis and toxoplasmosis seroprevalence has reopened the possibility that *T. cati* may also be an important environmental cause of *Toxocara* egg contamination in the environment.[146]

Because population-based serologic testing is limited to only a handful of research studies,[21,159,171,181,182] the prevalence of toxocariasis in North America and elsewhere may be underestimated. According to some investigators, *T. canis* infection may have replaced *E. vermicularis* as the most common helminth parasite in the United States.[18] A critical question regarding toxocariasis in North America and elsewhere is the potential contribution of the covert form of this disease to cognitive and learning deficits among socioeconomically disadvantaged children.[174]

Epidemiology

The prevalence of toxocariasis is difficult to assess because of the failure of establishing the diagnosis in many cases. The disease has been reported from many parts of the world, including temperate climates, and one can assume that it is found wherever humans and dogs coexist. High prevalence rates of the infection have been reported from Brazil, Africa, Eastern Europe, and the United States and Mexico[14,18,10,21,165]; toxocariasis may represent one of the most common helminth infections worldwide.[18]

Young children often come into contact with *Toxocara* eggs while playing in sandboxes and on playgrounds that were contaminated by stray dogs or cats or a family pet.[173,176] The level of contamination of public areas also is difficult to ascertain. In several studies, ova were present in 5% to 25% of soil samples obtained, and surveys of dogs in urban communities have shown the occurrence of frequent infections, particularly in puppies, which are infected almost universally with *T. canis* (canine infection occurs transplacentally).[168,169]

Subsequent dissemination of *Toxocara* eggs in the environment probably is aided by migrating earthworms and other soil invertebrates.[164] The seroprevalence of toxocariasis in the United States is high, and the parasite should be considered an emerging pathogen in some poor rural and urban areas. In some groups of socioeconomically disadvantaged black children, the seroprevalence is 30%,[172,180] with even higher rates occurring among US inner-city Hispanic children.[182] In the United States, the disease is linked to being poor and of African American or Hispanic ethnicity.[18,10,166,188] It has been estimated that up to 2.8 million African Americans have toxocariasis, so this disease represents a major but neglected health disparity.[10] Toxocariasis is endemic to Puerto Rico. Major risk factors for acquiring toxocariasis include having a litter of puppies in the home and the habit of geophagia.[177] The latter risk factor probably accounts for the observed association between toxocariasis and elevated lead levels.[177] In the poorest areas of the United States, including impoverished rural areas and in degraded urban environments, it is possible that *Toxocara* eggs are ubiquitous, and this accounts for the high seroprevalence of this infection among vulnerable populations. In Ireland, the prevalence of ophthalmologist-diagnosed ocular toxocariasis is 9.7 per 100,000, whereas in the United States it was determined that 68 patients were newly diagnosed with ocular toxocariasis between September 2009 and September 2010.[163,173]

The presence of a positive skin test result for toxocariasis is associated with poliomyelitis statistically.[189] No direct causal relationship exists; possibly, the circumstances leading to ingestion of *Toxocara* ova also are conducive to ingestion of poliomyelitis virus. *Toxocara* and *Toxoplasma* coinfections have also been noted; possibly these are from *T. cati* infection reflecting concurrent exposure from cats.[175] Several provocative studies have linked *Toxocara* exposure to neurologic and pulmonary disease. For example, seizures, cognitive deficits, pulmonary dysfunction, and asthma are correlated with seropositivity for *Toxocara* antibodies, but a causal relationship has not been established.[18,159,186,187,185] Some investigators have postulated that toxocariasis may be an important cause of asthma, idiopathic seizures, and cognitive delays in young children.[18,170,173] Given the link to poverty, important questions need to be addressed regarding *Toxocara* eggs as an environmental cause of asthma and developmental delays among socioeconomically disadvantaged children.[174]

Pathophysiology

The entire infection is restricted to the migratory phase and bears some clinical resemblance to the symptoms found during the early phases of *A. lumbricoides* infection. Symptoms are protean and depend on which organ or tissue is infected. For unknown reasons, visceral migration through the liver, lungs, and brain occurs more commonly in toddlers and children younger than 5 years old, whereas older children are more likely to exhibit only ocular involvement.[173,176] Epidemiologic evidence suggests that this infection produces two distinct syndromes, visceral and ocular, because involvement of one tends to occur in the absence of the other.[171] Visceral migration elicits eosinophilic granuloma formation in the target organs and leads to hepatitis, pneumonitis, or cerebritis. Larval migration in the retina results in ocular larva migrans, which includes granuloma formation in the retina.[160,167,183] The lesion can resemble retinoblastoma so that it often is confused with it. Endophthalmitis[167] or papillitis[164] also may develop. Invasion of other organs and tissues induces granuloma formation. The third and perhaps most common pathophysiologic process results in a covert form of the disease linked to larval migrations but without ocular or obvious visceral findings. These individuals exhibit positive *Toxocara* antibody titers often accompanied by eosinophilia. The covert form may be linked to pulmonary and neurologic deficits, including lung dysfunction and cognitive delays, respectively. The factors responsible for whether children develop visceral or ocular larval migrans versus the covert form of the disease are not known.

Clinical Manifestations

Most patients infected with *T. canis* are thought to be asymptomatic. Some of these individuals have isolated findings, including eosinophilia, or wheezing and asthma. The term *covert toxocariasis* is used by some investigators to describe these patients, who often are identified by their circulating anti–*T. canis* antibody titers. An association between asthma and covert toxocariasis has been well described in Europe, but as yet this association is unproven in North America.[182] Potentially, this association would represent an important avenue for investigation, given the high prevalence rates among African American and Hispanic children who live in poverty in the United States and are considered at high risk for asthma.[18]

Visceral larva migrans, the extreme form of toxocariasis, typically occurs in a toddler with the symptoms and signs of a multisystemic disease. It is associated with fever, hepatosplenomegaly, lung infiltrates accompanied by wheezing, a high degree of eosinophilia (approaching 80%), and elevated immunoglobulin levels, particularly of the IgM class.[170,173,176,177] Seizures and neuropsychiatric disturbances also are common. In one case report, the child's major neurologic manifestation was static encephalopathy.[170]

In contrast, ocular larva migrans is characterized by a unilateral vision deficit and, sometimes, strabismus. Ophthalmologic examination frequently reveals one or more posterior poles or peripheral pole granulomas.[167,176,183] More global eye inflammation also can occur (discussed earlier). Children with ocular involvement usually have few, if any, systemic manifestations. Often, no laboratory abnormalities are detected.

In covert toxocariasis, the individual is often asymptomatic, except some persons develop wheezing or other evidence of lung dysfunction. Alternatively, they may exhibit cognitive deficits or epilepsy. Both the pulmonary and neurologic sequelae of covert toxocariasis may or may not be accompanied by eosinophilia. The extent and clinical importance of covert toxocariasis still require further clinical investigations.

Diagnosis and Differential Diagnosis

Visceral larva migrans must be distinguished from the migratory phase of the other nematode infections. Because of hepatosplenomegaly and hypereosinophilia, eosinophilic leukemia occasionally has been suspected, but it can be ruled out readily by examining bone marrow.

T. canis larvae can be identified in tissues in liver biopsy specimens, but the diagnostic yield is low. One must resort to indirect means and be aware that a multisystemic disease with elevated IgM and hypereosinophilia fits the diagnostic criteria. An ELISA available at the Centers for Disease Control and Prevention is highly specific and diagnostic.[176,181,180] However, the exact interpretation of being seropositive to *T. canis* is considered controversial; some investigators are of the opinion that this finding reflects previous exposure, whereas others believe it indicates the presence of actively migrating larvae. Efforts to improve the existing ELISA by substituting antigens prepared from living larvae with recombinant protein-based reagents (to make testing kits more widely available) are in progress.[158,190]

Ocular larva migrans usually is diagnosed by an experienced ophthalmologist who recognizes the characteristic granulomas and larval tracks on retinal examination. Presumably because of minimal antigen presentation by a few migrating larvae in the eye, often no measurable immune response occurs in this condition. For this reason, ELISA frequently is unreliable for establishing the diagnosis of ocular larva migrans.[172,176,177,181,180]

The full clinical spectrum of the third form of toxocariasis, covert toxocariasis, is still under active investigation. There is no single case definition of covert toxocariasis, but it has been loosely defined as exposure to *Toxocara* eggs and larval migrations that are either asymptomatic or with physical findings confined to evidence of pulmonary or neurologic on further testing, together with a positive ELISA result. Covert toxocariasis generally requires a high index of suspicion on the part of the clinician; most cases go undiagnosed.

Treatment

Traditionally, treatment of visceral larva migrans was primarily symptomatic, especially because much of the morbidity is associated with immunopathologic responses against dying parasites. In the 1960s, thiabendazole and diethylcarbamazine were determined to be effective against migrating larvae.[179] Since then, newer agents of the benzimidazole class have been claimed to be equally effective but associated with fewer drug toxicities.[173] In a comparative study with thiabendazole, albendazole 10 mg/kg per day in two divided doses for 5 days was shown to be well tolerated and less toxic.[184] Another benzimidazole, mebendazole, also may be effective when given in doses high enough to achieve significant extraintestinal levels.[161] Albendazole 400 mg twice daily for 5 days is the treatment of choice.[178] As in almost all drug treatments for parasitic infections using albendazole this indication is not approved by the US Food and Drug Administration. Although anecdotal experience with albendazole and mebendazole overseas suggests that these drugs are safe in children,[162] the large doses required for the treatment of larva migrans may be associated with hepatic and other toxicities (including embryotoxicities), and they have not been approved for this purpose.

Treatment of ocular larva migrans often requires surgical management, particularly in cases associated with tractional retinal detachment.[167,183] Specific anthelmintic adjunctive chemotherapy seems to be beneficial in some cases.[168,173,183]

Prognosis

Except for patients in whom blindness develops as a consequence of retinal damage and a rare fatal case resulting from the intensity of the acute clinical reaction, most patients recover. The recovery phase may be slow, however, and may take 2 years.

Prevention

Theoretically, the disease can be prevented by elimination of dog and cat feces from the human environment, but in practice that is no less difficult to achieve than control of human excrement disposal. Animal control for stray dogs and cats, especially in degraded urban environments, is also needed.

OTHER ABERRANT INFECTIONS WITH INTESTINAL NEMATODES

Baylisascaris procyonis, a parasite of raccoons, also can cause visceral larva migrans, as well as an emerging eosinophilic meningitis.[198] *Baylisascaris* infection occurs when humans accidentally ingest parasite eggs that are shed in barn lofts and attics accessible to raccoons.[177,196,197,200,202] In at least one reported human case, the infection was fatal in an infant.[200] Similar to *Toxocara* infection, *Baylisascaris* larvae within aberrant hosts cannot complete their cycle and continue their aimless migration through the tissues of these hosts. Baylisascariasis is probably more severe because of the propensity of the larval stages of the parasite to invade the CNS, however, along with the continued growth of the larvae during migration resulting in greater mechanical damage.[196,197] The lesions caused by the larvae are eosinophilic granulomas, which tend to be concentrated in the CNS and result in eosinophilic meningitis. The disease is characterized by a severe eosinophilic pleocytosis in the cerebrospinal fluid and nonspecific diffuse white matter lesions seen on magnetic resonance imaging.[198] Neither the frequency nor the range of severity of this infection in humans is known. Most human cases have been diagnosed at autopsy. Because baylisascariasis is so uncommon, no studies are available to evaluate different anthelmintic chemotherapy regimens systematically. Some clinicians have recommended prolonged treatments with high doses of albendazole.[196,197] Given the potential severity of infection, some investigators propose administering postexposure prophylaxis after intimate contact with raccoon feces or soil contaminated with raccoon feces (albendazole 25 mg/kg per day orally for 20 days) as soon as possible after exposure and up to 3 days after possible infection.[178] Prolonged albendazole treatment requires monitoring of blood cell counts and liver function.

Other, less severe aberrant infections of importance to humans are those caused by the dog hookworm, primarily *Ancylostoma braziliense,* but possibly also *Uncinaria stenocephala.*[94,196,199,210] Infection with the larvae of *A. braziliense* and *U. stenocephala* cannot be completed, and larvae remain viable and migrate in the skin (usually between the epidermis and dermis); hence the terms *cutaneous larva migrans* and *creeping eruption* are used. In North America, cutaneous larva migrans is common along the Gulf Coast and along the Atlantic seaboard.[95] It also is common in the Caribbean. Failure of these zoonotic hookworms to complete entry through the human skin may reflect differences in the hydrolytic enzymes released.[199] Infection is acquired in the same fashion as that of the human hookworms. Children who expose their whole bodies to contaminated soil may be infected at any site. Adults are most likely to have infection in the lower extremities, but plumbers in the tropics, who often must crawl beneath houses, acquire infection on the elbows and knees.

The interval from exposure to appearance of the first symptoms is approximately 2 weeks; papules 2 mm in diameter then begin to appear on the skin. Behind them usually are serpiginous, erythematous, intracutaneous tunnels. The entire area itches intensely. If left untreated, cutaneous larva migrans tends to last 2 months. Albendazole, 400 mg daily for 3 days, or ivermectin, 200 µg/kg daily for 1 to 2 days, is effective treatment when administered orally. Topical therapy with a 15% aqueous suspension of thiabendazole was successful in one reported series. Forty-seven of 50 patients achieved permanent cure in 2 weeks, and 2 more patients were cured after a third week of treatment.[213] Placebo-treated patients were used as controls in this study. In contrast to skin penetration of zoonotic hookworms, oral ingestion of the dog hookworm *A. caninum* results in an eosinophilic enteritis syndrome (see the earlier discussion of hookworm infection).

Rarer aberrant infections include those caused by various species of *Trichostrongylus, Oesophagostomum, Angiostrongylus, Capillaria,* and *Anisakis. Trichostrongylus* is a common parasite of many mammals, and it has been found in the small intestine of humans, mainly in Asia, Africa, and Australia. Ingestion of larvae leads to the development of adult worms in the small intestine. Whether this development results in any disease remains a moot point because infections tend to be mild and usually are associated with other helminth infections.[197] *Oesophagostomum bifurcum* is a common nematode of subhuman primates in Africa and has been reported to be a common intestinal nematode that causes nodular disease of the intestines in humans living in West Africa.[204,207] Human esophagostomiasis has been treated successfully with pyrantel pamoate.[204]

Land snails and slugs serve as intermediate hosts for *Angiostrongylus* spp. *Angiostrongylus cantonensis* is a cause of eosinophilic meningitis (neuroangiostrongyliasis) throughout eastern Asia and Hawaii[193,203,208,209]; *A. cantonensis* has also emerged in the mainland United States, especially on the Gulf Coast after importation of infected rats and African land snails on container ships.[195] *Angiostrongylus costaricensis* is a cause of mesenteric arteritis and abdominal pain in Central and South America and in Latin American immigrants to the United States.[201] The rat serves as the natural host of these parasites, which live either in the lung *(A. cantonensis)* or in mesenteric arteries *(A. costaricensis).* The rat eats the infected mollusks and ingests the larvae, which migrate to their final destination. An incomplete infection develops in individuals who ingest either the mollusks or food contaminated by the mollusks. *A. cantonensis* infection usually is limited to the CNS and is manifested as eosinophilic meningitis.[193,203,208,209]

Signs and symptoms of neuroangiostrongyliasis include meningismus, severe headache, paresthesias, and, less commonly, cranial nerve palsies. No specific treatment is available (although anthelmintics are effective in some experimental animal models[193]), but the disease is self-limited and lasts no longer than 2 weeks. Symptomatic relief has been reported with the use of prednisone. Some investigators have reported success in treating neuroangiostrongyliasis with albendazole and prednisone, together with repeated spinal taps to decrease intracranial pressure.[198] However, the treatment of *A. canontensis* infection is considered controversial and "varies across endemic areas" because no anthelmintic has proven to be effective.[178] In contrast, *A. costaricensis* infection typically is manifested as abdominal or right iliac fossa pain, fever, and eosinophilia. In children with this condition, appendicitis or Meckel diverticulum may be diagnosed.[201] High doses of mebendazole have been tried as therapy for this condition, as well as albendazole.

Capillaria philippinensis is a common parasite of water fowl in the Philippines.[192] The mode of transmission of this parasite to humans is unknown, but human cases have been reported in which 40,000 adult worms were found embedded in the crypts of the small intestine. *C. philippinensis,* similar to *S. stercoralis,* can undergo autoinfection and hyperinfection in humans.[192] No associated inflammatory reaction occurs, but flattening of villi, loss of epithelial surface area, and severe malabsorption have been reported.[192,194,212] In a series of 1000 cases of *C. philippinensis* infection, a mortality rate of 10% was reported.[194] Thiabendazole may be effective in shortening the course of the infection,[212] although albendazole has become the treatment of choice more recently.[192] At least one recommended regimen of albendazole includes 400 mg daily for 10 days, whereas for mebendazole 200 mg twice a day for 20 days is administered.[178] Neither regimen is approved by the US Food and Drug Administration. Another member of the genus, *Capillaria hepatica,* a rare zoonosis of humans, has been known to disseminate to the lungs, liver, and other viscera.[206]

Anisakis spp. are nematode parasites of marine mammals, with fish being intermediate hosts. When the infective larvae of the parasite are ingested as a result of eating raw or poorly cooked fish, they may become embedded in the gastric mucosa and cause eosinophilic granuloma.[76,157,171,177,181,185] In adults, the infection may resemble carcinoma of the stomach clinically and radiographically. Human anisakiasis occurs frequently in Japan, where raw marine fish are eaten commonly, and in Holland, where lightly pickled herring is considered a delicacy.

FILARIAL PARASITES

Except for rare instances of zoonotic *Brugia* infection, the filarial worms parasitizing humans affect people within the geographic area almost entirely limited to the developing world, especially sub-Saharan Africa, India, and Southeast Asia. Although accurate data are lacking, approximately 115 million people are infected with lymphatic filariasis, more than 40 million of whom are symptomatic, and 17 million are infected with onchocerciasis.[8,217] The various human parasites in this category have certain characteristics in common. They all are spread by vectors, and the adults invade and occupy the lymphatics, skin, connective tissue, or blood. They produce live embryos called microfilariae that enter the bloodstream or skin, where they can survive for months or years without further development. The range of disease caused by these worms is wide; some produce no symptoms, whereas others can be responsible for severe clinical disorders.

The life cycles of the filarial worms are similar in that infections are acquired through an insect bite, during which transmission is effected by introduction of infective larvae onto the skin of the host from the mouth parts of the insect. The larvae enter the wound in the skin and make their way to the respective tissue, where they mature into adult worms. The adults mate and produce live microfilariae, which, in lymphatic filariasis, migrate to the blood through the walls of the lymphatics or through the thoracic duct. To complete the life cycle, the microfilariae are ingested by blood-sucking insects, in which they undergo metamorphosis through two larval stages until they reach the third, infective stage. The interval from the infective bite to the appearance of microfilariae in the blood of the host can be 6 to 12 months.

MDA with ivermectin alone (for onchocerciasis), or ivermectin together with albendazole (for lymphatic filariasis), or diethylcarbamazine with albendazole (also for lymphatic filariasis) can reduce the microfilarial load of human populations living in endemic regions.[218]

For onchocerciasis, reductions in microfilarial loads lead to reductions in chronic morbidity, with marked improvement in the serious skin manifestations of the infection and the prevention of blindness. MDA using ivermectin can result in the elimination of onchocerciasis Such programs of MDA for onchocerciasis are in progress in 19 sub-Saharan African countries, under the auspices of the WHO in collaboration with its African Programme for Onchocerciasis Control (APOC),[221] whereas in the Western Hemisphere onchocerciasis is close to being eliminated in 5 countries through the activities of the Onchocerciasis Elimination Program for the Americas (OEPA), leaving only foci of infection among indigenous populations living near the border of Brazil and Venezuela.[222]

For lymphatic filariasis, widespread implementation of MDA one day may reduce transmission to the point of elimination, and a target for the year 2020 has been set for elimination. Through the WHO and the Global Programme to Eliminate Lymphatic Filariasis, such programs are currently under way in many countries in Asia, sub-Saharan Africa, and in Haiti.[220] For example, in Egypt, five rounds of mass drug distribution already may have effectively eliminated transmission.[219] Because the major manifestations of both lymphatic filariasis and onchocerciasis occur mainly in adults rather than children, both topics are treated only briefly here. An important exception is the emergence of a "nodding syndrome" affecting children in some of the onchocerciasis-endemic areas of South Sudan and Uganda, and possibly elsewhere in East Africa.

Lymphatic Filariasis: *Wuchereria Bancrofti* and *Brugia* Species

Epidemiology

Wuchereria bancrofti is prevalent primarily between the Tropic of Cancer and the Tropic of Capricorn but also is encountered north of the Tropic of Cancer in Africa. An estimated 115 million infections exist in 80 countries worldwide, with approximately one-half of the infected individuals living in sub-Saharan Africa.[217,219,228] In each of its geographic locales, it has a specific anopheline, culicine, or aedine mosquito vector. In the Caribbean area, South America, Asia, East and West Africa, and Papua New Guinea, the microfilariae of this worm exhibit nocturnal periodicity; in the South Pacific, their periodicity is diurnal. *W. bancrofti* has no animal hosts.

Brugia malayi occurs in India, Malaysia, and other parts of Southeast Asia. Some strains of *B. malayi* are associated with animal reservoirs, as are certain other members of the genus *Brugia,* such as *Brugia timori.* In the United States, zoonotic *Brugia* infections caused by *Brugia beaveri* and *Brugia lepori* may infect humans but cannot develop patent infections.[216,226,227]

Pathophysiology

The pathology of lymphatic filariasis is caused principally by the adult-stage parasite, the host response, and an unusual type of bacterial coinfection of tissues (resulting from helminth endosymbiotic bacteria of the genus *Wolbachia*), which together produce compromised lymphatic function. In children the adult worms initially induce lymphatic dilation that over time results in lymphatic dysfunction, lymphedema, and further sequelae, although the exact mechanisms responsible for these processes are still under investigation. The consequent inflammation, in addition to that caused by host responses to dying parasites, damages the delicate lymphatic vessels further and compromises lymphatic function further. When such processes occur in the lymphatic vessels of the scrotum, hydrocele develops. As tissue pathology progresses, some patients develop severe morbidity from elephantiasis. Microfilaremia often is "asymptomatic" but frequently is associated with immune complex nephritis; more rarely, the microfilariae can be the target of immunologic hyperresponsiveness and result in a severe "tropical pulmonary eosinophilia" syndrome.[224]

Clinical Manifestations

Asymptomatic microfilaremia often develops in children living in endemic areas. By using highly sensitive diagnostic tests, including antigen detection and ultrasound ("dancing filarial sign"), one-third of children living in endemic areas can be seen to be infected before age 5 years. Damage to the lymphatics of these young children frequently is subclinical, however.[229] With repeated exposure, these children begin to have episodes of acute adenolymphangitis, sometimes associated with fever and lymphangitis. These "filarial fevers" may reflect either an inflammatory response to dying parasites (with "retrograde" lymphangitis) or *Wolbachia* endosymbiotic bacterial coinfection.[215] Progression to lymphedema of the upper and lower extremities, the most common sequela of chronic lymphatic filariasis, is an uncommon occurrence in children until after the age of puberty. Arthritis has also been noted as an occult manifestation of lymphatic filariasis in India.[223] Benign lymphedema has been described in a few patients in the United States with zoonotic *Brugia* infection.[216,227] Chronic, recurrent eosinophilic pneumonitis associated with wheezing, cough, chest pain, pulmonary infiltrations, and hypereosinophilia (tropical pulmonary eosinophilia) is an IgE-mediated hypersensitivity reaction to microfilariae trapped in the lungs and, if left untreated, leads to debilitating interstitial pneumonitis.[224]

Diagnosis and Differential Diagnosis

The differential diagnosis of lymphatic obstruction in children should rule out other, more likely conditions before focusing on filariasis. In older children and adults, familial lymphedema (Milroy disease) can mimic filariasis.

In endemic regions, lymphatic filariasis typically is diagnosed on the basis of appropriate clinical findings in a region with known endemicity for the disease. In young children living in endemic areas, however, early infection is largely subclinical.[229] A definitive diagnosis of lymphatic filariasis still relies on detecting adult parasites in the lymphatics through ultrasonography or by recovering microfilariae from the blood. In the past, in view of the circadian periodicity of the appearance of numerous microfilariae in blood, a specimen was collected at the appropriate time, in many regions of the world between 10 PM and 2 AM, for microscopic examination by a staining or concentration technique. Increasingly, an immunochromatographic card test that measures specific filarial antigen is being used, especially in amicrofilaremic individuals.[215]

Treatment

New agents or drug regimens are needed that would be more effective against the adult filarial worm (a "macrofilaricide") and at the same time elicit minimal immunopathologic damage. Currently, the major drugs used are especially effective against microfilariae. Diethylcarbamazine is the treatment of choice and typically is given in a 12-day course (6 mg/kg per day in three doses) for a total dose of 72 mg/kg. In the United States, for patients with microfilariae in the blood, it is common practice to administer first small doses of 1 to 2 mg/kg (maximum of 50 to 100 mg) before beginning this regimen. One regimen includes beginning 50 mg on day 1, followed by 50 mg three times per day on day 2, 100 mg three times per day on day 3, and 6 mg/kg per day in three doses on days 4 to 14. More recently, a single dose of 6 mg/kg has been recognized to produce a similar therapeutic result (presumably following the test doses as just outlined).[215] Diethylcarbamazine is available under an investigational new drug protocol from the Centers for Disease Control and Prevention (CDC Drug Service: 404-639-3670 [evenings, weekends, or holidays: 770-488-7100]).

Side effects of specific antifilarial therapy include allergic and febrile reactions that are caused by the inflammatory response to dying microfilariae, rather than by the drug itself, and that occur primarily in patients with high levels of circulating microfilariae. These systemic manifestations can be treated symptomatically with antihistamines or corticosteroids. Some of the allergic manifestations also may be avoided by administering diethylcarbamazine in a graded, stepwise manner. For patients with *Loa loa* coinfections, the presence of microfilariae presents a particular problem because high levels of microfilaremia can lead to encephalopathy after treatment with antiparasitic drugs. Diethylcarbamazine also is the treatment of choice for tropical pulmonary eosinophilia, a syndrome caused by circulating microfilariae. Ivermectin also may have a role in the medical treatment of lymphatic filariasis because it is very effective in clearing circulating microfilariae.[225] Albendazole, in high doses, is effective in killing adult worms and, in lower doses, inhibits microfilarial production, but it is not registered for use in lymphatic filariasis in the United States.[219]

The difficulty in management of filariasis by drugs is that late symptoms, such as elephantiasis, do not abate. The main usefulness of chemotherapy is in cases recognized early, before the anatomic abnormalities develop. Hydrocele can be treated surgically. Of critical importance to the management of lymphedema and elephantiasis are attention to hygiene, wearing shoes to prevent injury, and reduction of lymphostasis with exercise and elevation of the lower extremity.

The more recent discovery that *W. bancrofti* harbors bacterial endosymbionts has led to efforts to use tetracycline and related antimicrobial agents as part of the therapeutic regimen for lymphatic filariasis.[227] The therapeutic use of such regimens is under active investigation. The Centers for Disease Control and Prevention (see earlier) and the Clinical Center of the National Institutes of Health have extensive experience and expertise in the management and treatment of human filarial infections, including *W. bancrofti, L. loa,* and *Onchocerca volvulus* infections.

Prevention

Prevention in the past depended principally on vector control, which was successful in some settings and unsatisfactory in others, primarily because of the difficulty in developing effective insecticides that also would be nontoxic to the rest of the environment. Successful experience in China has shown that large-scale chemoprophylaxis approaches to prevention are possible in endemic countries. Currently, through the Global Programme to Eliminate Lymphatic Filariasis, the international community is directing a large-scale lymphatic filariasis control campaign on this principle. Typically, this control is being accomplished through a single-dose combination of albendazole 400 mg with either ivermectin 200 μg/kg or diethylcarbamazine 6 mg/kg. On this basis, lymphatic filariasis has been eliminated in more than 20 countries, and long-term targets for the global elimination of this infection have been proposed.[217–219] The finding of extensive subclinical infection among children living in endemic regions highlights the importance of targeting this group for MDA, as well as adults.[229]

Loa Loa

L. loa infection is limited to a focal area of western and central Africa and is spread by *Chrysops* flies. Periodicity in *L. loa* microfilariae is diurnal. The parasite elicits numerous allergic inflammatory responses that are most evident in expatriates.[230,231] Infection leads to high eosinophilia and recurrent angioedema, which when localized develop into painful, pruritic, subcutaneous swellings on the extremities and the face known as Calabar swellings. Rarely, some cases of lymphatic obstruction of the lower extremities and hydroceles have been reported.

The most dramatic manifestation of this infection is the occasional appearance of a migrating *L. loa* adult under the conjunctiva of the eye. It does not damage the eye and can be removed surgically. Because of the genuine risk of encephalopathy, treatment with diethylcarbamazine, as indicated earlier, effectively destroys the adults, but reactions may be more intense than in the treatment of *Wuchereria* and *Brugia* infections. Diethylcarbamazine should be administered in a gradual, stepwise manner as described earlier, particularly in patients with high levels of circulating microfilariae. The recommended dose is higher than that used for lymphatic filariasis (9 mg/kg per day in three doses for 12 days). Coadministration of corticosteroids often is required during treatment. Encephalopathy has been described in patients receiving diethylcarbamazine, especially when they are heavily infected.[230] Ivermectin elicits fewer inflammatory symptoms during treatment and may be less toxic in general, but encephalopathy still can occur in patients with heavy *Loa* infections.[232] Moreover, because of the risk for encephalopathy, patients with loasis should be treated in consultation with an expert in this infection. Approaches to treatment may include plasmapheresis or a single 50-mg dose of diethylcarbamazine as for lymphatic filariasis (see earlier), gradually building to the final dose of 9 mg/kg per day over 2 weeks. In the United States, the Clinical Center of the National Institutes of Health has the greatest experience with treating *Loa* infections.

Onchocerca volvulus (and "Nodding Syndrome")

Onchocerca volvulus infection is acquired through the bite of a *Simulium* fly, which tends to breed along rivers and streams (hence the name of the disease "river blindness").

Epidemiology

Disease is limited to sub-Saharan Africa, where approximately 99% of the world's 17 million cases occur (approximately one-half of the cases occur in Nigeria and Congo),[217] and focal pockets near the border between Venezuela and Brazil. In view of human dependence on water and the establishment of settlements along rivers, the frequency of infection tends to be high in areas where *Simulium* prevails. The development of hydroelectric power based on the construction of large dams can increase the breeding sites of *Simulium* and increase the incidence of *Onchocerca* infection. A neurologic syndrome associated with seizures and known as "nodding syndrome" has emerged in *O. volvulus*–endemic areas of South Sudan and Uganda. The etiology of nodding syndrome is under investigation.

Pathophysiology

Larvae deposited by a *Simulium* bite remain in the subcutaneous tissue and develop into adult worms there. Adult worms tend to become coiled, and worms of both sexes become enveloped by fibrous tissue and form nodules within which they reproduce. The larvae produced by fertilized females invade the skin, where they remain until they are picked up by a *Simulium* bite, or they die about 30 months later. In addition to the skin, microfilariae penetrate the eye and affect every layer from the conjunctiva to the optic nerve. In African onchocerciasis, chorioretinitis and optic atrophy occur commonly.

The probability of the development of eye disease is related to the location of the adult worms. When the nodules are situated around the head, eye lesions are common; when they are in the lower parts of the body, eye lesions occur less frequently. In Africa, the nodules tend to be distributed primarily in the lower parts of the body, but because of the high prevalence of the infection, onchocercal blindness is common. Hypotheses surrounding nodding syndrome are discussed in the next section.

Clinical Manifestations

The appearance of the skin nodules and the presence of live microfilariae within the eye (readily seen with a slit-lamp ophthalmoscopic examination) are the manifestations of early and intermediate disease. Later, eye involvement includes keratitis, iridocyclitis, chorioretinitis, and, eventually, blindness. Microfilariae in the skin cause an inflammatory reaction that includes acute papular onchodermatitis and chronic changes such as edema, lichenification, atrophy, and depigmentation.[228] Because long-standing infection with *O. volvulus* is required to see these ocular and skin changes, these changes are often found in adults rather than in children.

However, an unusual neurologic syndrome related to onchocerciasis in children, known as nodding syndrome, has been noted in in South Sudan, northern Uganda, and Tanzania.[32] Nodding syndrome is a seizure-type disorder associated with unresponsiveness and paroxysms of 5 to 20 head nods/min, sometimes progressing to generalized tonic-clonic seizures, but also linked to long-term mental and developmental disabilities.[32] It most commonly appears among school-aged children and adolescents.[32] There is an epidemiologic association between nodding syndrome and onchocerciasis, but so far no direct causal relationship has been determined. Some investigators have hypothesized that nodding syndrome is related to host immunologic responses to *O. volvulus*,[32] whereas others have suggested that blackflies may simultaneously transmit a virus that causes this condition.[234]

Diagnosis and Differential Diagnosis

Because skin invasion is associated with itching, the pruritus of onchocercal infection must be differentiated from that caused by contact dermatitis, prickly heat, insect bites, and scabies. Onchocerciasis is identified by examination of a skin snip. Examination of sectioned and stained tissue or a stained impression smear reveals microfilariae. Nodding syndrome should be distinguished from other forms of epilepsy on the basis of clinical criteria and analysis of cerebrospinal fluid and radiographic imaging. One of the challenges of nodding syndrome is that it mostly occurs in extremely resource-poor areas of East Africa that often do not have access to diagnostic modalities.

Treatment

Surgical removal of all visible nodules may radically extirpate the source of new microfilariae that invade the eye. The routine use of nodulectomy is still controversial, however. Chemotherapy with ivermectin (single oral dose of 150 µg/kg administered every 6 to 12 months) until asymptomatic is the treatment of choice. Ivermectin reduces the number of microfilariae in the skin within days, and subsequently the number of microfilariae in the eye, and prevents the onset of blindness.[233] Ivermectin also can be used in mass treatment to diminish transmission by the vector and control the incidence of this infection.[217,218,233,236] Diethylcarbamazine is contraindicated for patients with onchocerciasis because it can lead to severe allergic symptoms, a condition sometimes known as the Mazzotti reaction.

The optimal treatment for nodding syndrome is under investigation, but it is believed that patients benefit from anticonvulsants, together with nutritional and emotional support.[31]

Prevention

Today the mainstay of river blindness control is MDA with ivermectin, which has led to the elimination of onchocerciasis in Mali and Senegal and has led to the near elimination of the disease in the six remaining Latin American countries.[217] Through The Onchocerciasis Vaccine Initiative for Africa (TOVA), a first-generation vaccine to prevent river blindness is also under development.[235]

Mansonella Perstans and *Mansonella Ozzardi*

Neither *Mansonella perstans* nor *Mansonella ozzardi* is known to cause significant human pathology, but the microfilariae present in blood must be distinguished morphologically from the microfilariae of the other more pathogenic filariae. *M. ozzardi* is found throughout the Caribbean (especially Haiti) and Central America. It has been suggested as a cause of chronic arthritis in these regions. *M. perstans* also is found in Africa, where it has been identified as a cause of painless nodules in the conjunctiva and secondary eyelid swelling. For that reason, it sometimes is called the Kampala or Ugandan eye worm.[237] Albendazole or mebendazole is the treatment of choice for *M. perstans* infection.

Dirofilaria immitis

Dirofilaria immitis is a filarial worm commonly found in dogs, in which it occupies the right ventricle of the heart. The microfilariae produced circulate in blood and are transmitted to new animals through the bite of culicine mosquitoes. Fewer than 100 cases of human infection have been reported, none of them in children. Most human hosts infected with *Dirofilaria* were asymptomatic, but individuals who had symptoms complained of chest pain, wheezing, and cough. All infected individuals had coin lesions detected on pulmonary radiographs.[238,239] Human infection is transmitted through a mosquito bite. As with visceral larva migrans and the zoonotic *Brugia* infections, *D. immitis* cannot complete its life cycle in humans. No microfilariae of this worm have ever been shown in human peripheral blood.

All patients evaluated for pulmonary dirofilariasis have had mild peripheral eosinophilia, usually not exceeding 10%. Because the radiographic picture is not diagnostic, and in view of the potential seriousness of a coin lesion,[238] the lesion must be examined histologically. If a worm is found, the diagnosis of dirofilariasis can be made; if it is not found, the diagnosis is still tenable. In the presence of eosinophilia and pneumonitis, however, a whole range of other diagnostic possibilities must be considered, including eosinophilic pneumonia, polyarteritis nodosa, Wegener granulomatosis, and histiocytosis X. No treatment is necessary for this infection in humans.

Dracunculus medinensis

Infection with *Dracunculus medinensis* (guinea worm) is limited largely to sub-Saharan Africa. As of 2017, fewer than 100 cases remain worldwide, all in Sahelian Africa.[240]

Because filtering of drinking water can prevent this infection effectively, authorities from the WHO and the Carter Center are optimistic that this parasite will soon be eradicated through appropriate control measures.[217]

NEW REFERENCES SINCE THE SEVENTH EDITION

Intestinal Nematodes

1. Adegnika AA, Zinsou JF, Issifou S, et al. Randomized, controlled, assessor-blind clinical trial to assess the efficacy of single- versus repeated-dose albendazole to treat *Ascaris lumbricoides, Trichuris trichiura,* and hookworm infection. *Antimicrob Agents Chemother.* 2014;58(5):2535-2540.

4. Alpern JD, Stauffer WM, Kesselheim AS. High-cost generic drugs—implications for patients and policymakers. *N Engl J Med.* 2014;371(20):1859-1862.
8. Global Burden of Disease Study Collaborators. Global, regional, and national incidence, prevalence, and years lived with disability for 301 acute and chronic diseases and injuries in 188 countries, 1990-2013: a systematic analysis for the Global Burden of Disease Study 2013. *Lancet.* 2015;386(9995): 743-800.
21. Lee RM, Moore LB, Bottazzi ME, et al. Toxocariasis in North America: a systematic review. *PLoS Negl Trop Dis.* 2014;8(8):e3116.
26. Soukhathammavong PA, Sayasone S, Phongluxa K, et al. Low efficacy of single-dose albendazole and mebendazole against hookworm and effect on concomitant helminth infection in Lao PDR. *PLoS Negl Trop Dis.* 2012;6(1):e1417.
31. Taylor-Robinson DC, Maayan N, Soares-Weiser K, et al. Deworming drugs for soil-transmitted intestinal worms in children: effects on nutritional indicators, haemoglobin, and school performance. *Cochrane Database Syst Rev.* 2015;(7):CD000371.
32. Wamala JF, Malimbo M, Tepage F, et al. Nodding syndrome may be only the ears of the hippo. *PLoS Negl Trop Dis.* 2015;9(8):e0003880.
33. World Health Organization. Soil-transmitted helminthiases: number of children treated in 2013. *Wkly Epidemiol Rec.* 2015;90(10):89-94.
34. Zhan B, Beaumier CM, Briggs N, et al. Advancing a multivalent 'pan-anthelmintic' vaccine against soil-transmitted nematode infections. *Expert Rev Vaccines.* 2014;13(3):321-331.

Ascaris lumbricoides

35. Ahumada V, Garcia E, Dennis R, et al. IgE responses to *Ascaris* and mite tropomyosins are risk factors for asthma. *Clin Exp Allergy.* 2015;45(7):1189-1200.
38. Buendia E, Zakzuk J, Mercado D, et al. The IgE response to *Ascaris* molecular components is associated with clinical indicators of asthma severity. *World Allergy Organ J.* 2015;8(1):8.
40. Cimino RO, Jeun R, Juarez M, et al. Identification of human intestinal parasites affecting an asymptomatic peri-urban Argentinian population using multi-parallel quantitative real-time polymerase chain reaction. *Parasit Vectors.* 2015;8:380.
46. Gelpi AP, Mustafa A. Seasonal pneumonitis with eosinophilia: a study of larval ascariasis in Saudi Arabs. *Am J Trop Med Hyg.* 1967;16(5):646-657.
57. Nacher M, Gay F, Singhasivanon P, et al. *Ascaris lumbricoides* infection is associated with protection from cerebral malaria. *Parasite Immunol.* 2000;22(3):107-113.
59. Pullan RL, Smith JL, Jasrasaria R, et al. Global numbers of infection and disease burden of soil transmitted helminth infections in 2010. *Parasit Vectors.* 2014;7:37.
63. Weatherhead JE, Hotez PJ. Worm infections in children. *Pediatr Rev.* 2015;36(8):341-352, quiz 353-344.

Trichuris trichiura

79. Speich B, Ame SM, Ali SM, et al. Oxantel pamoate-albendazole for *Trichuris trichiura* infection. *N Engl J Med.* 2014;370(7):610-620.

Hookworms

81. Adegnika AA, Zinsou JF, Issifou S, et al. Randomized, controlled, assessor-blind clinical trial to assess the efficacy of single- versus repeated-dose albendazole to treat *Ascaris lumbricoides, Trichuris trichiura,* and hookworm infection. *Antimicrob Agents Chemother.* 2014;58(5):2535-2540.
82. Asojo OA, Goud G, Dhar K, et al. X-ray structure of Na-ASP-2, a pathogenesis-related-1 protein from the nematode parasite, *Necator americanus,* and a vaccine antigen for human hookworm infection. *J Mol Biol.* 2005;346(3):801-814.
84. Bethony J, Loukas A, Smout M, et al. Antibodies against a secreted protein from hookworm larvae reduce the intensity of hookworm infection in humans and vaccinated laboratory animals. *FASEB J.* 2005;19(12):1743-1745.
91. Croese J, Fairley S, Loukas A, et al. A distinctive aphthous ileitis linked to *Ancylostoma caninum. J Gastroenterol Hepatol.* 1996;11(6):524-531.
96. Hotez PJ, Diemert D, Bacon KM, et al. The human hookworm vaccine. *Vaccine.* 2013;31(suppl 2):B227-B232.
97. Inpankaew T, Schar F, Dalsgaard A, et al. High prevalence of *Ancylostoma ceylanicum* hookworm infections in humans, Cambodia, 2012. *Emerg Infect Dis.* 2014;20(6):976-982.
99. Karagiannis-Voules DA, Biedermann P, Ekpo UF, et al. Spatial and temporal distribution of soil-transmitted helminth infection in sub-Saharan Africa: a systematic review and geostatistical meta-analysis. *Lancet Infect Dis.* 2015;15(1):74-84.
102. Raso G, Vounatsou P, Singer BH, et al. An integrated approach for risk profiling and spatial prediction of *Schistosoma mansoni*-hookworm coinfection. *Proc Natl Acad Sci USA.* 2006;103(18):6934-6939.

Enterobius vermicularis

111. Ahmed MU, Bilal M, Anis K, et al. The frequency of *Enterobius vermicularis* infections in patients diagnosed with acute appendicitis in Pakistan. *Glob J Health Sci.* 2015;7(5):196-201.

Strongyloides stercoralis* and *Strongyloides fuelleborni

129. Buonfrate D, Sequi M, Mejia R, et al. Accuracy of five serologic tests for the follow up of *Strongyloides stercoralis* infection. *PLoS Negl Trop Dis.* 2015;9(2):e0003491.
144. Khieu V, Schar F, Forrer A, et al. High prevalence and spatial distribution of *Strongyloides stercoralis* in rural Cambodia. *PLoS Negl Trop Dis.* 2014;8(6):e2854.
146. Krolewiecki AJ, Lammie P, Jacobson J, et al. A public health response against *Strongyloides stercoralis:* time to look at soil-transmitted helminthiasis in full. *PLoS Negl Trop Dis.* 2013;7(5):e2165.
153. Russell ES, Gray EB, Marshall RE, et al. Prevalence of *Strongyloides stercoralis* antibodies among a rural Appalachian population—Kentucky, 2013. *Am J Trop Med Hyg.* 2014;91(5):1000-1001.

Aberrant Infections With Intestinal Nematodes

158. Anderson JP, Rascoe LN, Levert K, et al. Development of a Luminex bead based assay for diagnosis of toxocariasis using recombinant antigens Tc-CTL-1 and Tc-TES-26. *PLoS Negl Trop Dis.* 2015;9(10):e0004168.
174. Hotez PJ. Neglected infections of poverty in the United States and their effects on the brain. *JAMA Psychiatry.* 2014;71(10):1099-1100.
178. Medical Letter. Drugs for Parasitic Infections. 3rd Edition. *Treat Guidel Med Lett.* 2013;11(suppl). New Rochelle, NY: The Medical Letter.
185. Walsh MG. *Toxocara* infection and diminished lung function in a nationally representative sample from the United States population. *Int J Parasitol.* 2011;41(2):243-247.
186. Walsh MG, Haseeb MA. Reduced cognitive function in children with toxocariasis in a nationally representative sample of the United States. *Int J Parasitol.* 2012;42(13-14):1159-1163.
187. Walsh MG, Haseeb MA. Toxocariasis and lung function: relevance of a neglected infection in an urban landscape. *Acta Parasitol.* 2014;59(1):126-131.
190. Zhan B, Ajmera R, Geiger SM, et al. Identification of immunodominant antigens for the laboratory diagnosis of toxocariasis. *Trop Med Int Health.* 2015;20(12):1787-1796.

Filarial Parasites

220. Ramaiah KD, Ottesen EA. Progress and impact of 13 years of the global programme to eliminate lymphatic filariasis on reducing the burden of filarial disease. *PLoS Negl Trop Dis.* 2014;8(11):e3319.
221. World Health Organization. African Programme for Onchocerciasis Control: progress report, 2014–2015. *Wkly Epidemiol Rec.* 2015;90(49):661-674.
222. World Health Organization. Progress toward eliminating onchocerciasis in the WHO Region of the Americas: verification of elimination of transmission in Mexico. *Wkly Epidemiol Rec.* 2015;90(43):577-581.

Onchocerca volvulus

234. Colebunders R, Hendy A, Nanyunja M, et al. Nodding syndrome: a new hypothesis and new direction for research. *Int J Infect Dis.* 2014;27:74-77.
235. Hotez PJ, Bottazzi ME, Zhan B, et al. The Onchocerciasis Vaccine for Africa—TOVA—Initiative. *PLoS Negl Trop Dis.* 2015;9(1):e0003422.

The full reference list for this chapter is available at ExpertConsult.com.

227 Cestodes

Jose A. Serpa • Miguel M. Cabada • A. Clinton White Jr

OVERVIEW OF CESTODES AND THEIR IMPORTANCE FOR CHILDREN

Cestodes are multicellular helminth parasites.[284] Children may harbor the adult worms (tapeworms) or larval stages (e.g., cysticercosis or hydatid disease). The adult tapeworms are segmented worms that contain a scolex (attachment organ); a neck region, where the segments are formed; and segments termed *proglottids*.[324] The scolex contains either sucking grooves (*Diphyllobothrium* and *Spirometra*) or round suckers (other species). In some species (e.g., *Taenia solium*), the scolex is armed with rows of hooks, which also aid in attachment. The proglottids develop in the neck region and move distally as they are displaced by newer proglottids. Eventually, chains of proglottids form and compose the body of the adult worm. The external surface of the proglottid forms an absorptive surface that functions as the parasite gut. As the proglottids are displaced from the scolex, they gradually mature, with both male and female sexual organs developing in each proglottid. The terminal proglottids contain the uterus, which is full of ova. The ova of *Spirometra* and *Diphyllobothrium* are shed into water, where they infect a series of aquatic intermediate hosts. The ova of other species infect the immediate host after being ingested. Both larval and adult forms of *Hymenolepis nana* live in the human intestines, and the entire life cycle can take place in a single host. Humans are dead-end hosts for numerous zoonotic tapeworms, including *T. solium* (cysticercosis), *Echinococcus* spp. (hydatid disease), and *Spirometra* (sparganosis). The term cysticercosis (literally, "bladder tail") refers to infection of tissues with an intermediate form of the parasite containing a cystic parasite with one (or a small number of) invaginated scolex. Human cysticercosis usually is caused by *T. solium*. However, human cysticercosis is also rarely caused by *Taenia crassiceps* or *Taenia multiceps*. *Hydatid disease* refers to infection of tissues with the intermediate form of the parasites of the genus *Echinococcus*, which form cystic lesions filled with innumerable protoscolices, each of which can turn into a tapeworm or another hydatid lesion, depending on the tissues. Infections with cestodes have been common human infections since antiquity and have been found in mummies.[23,125] Currently, approximately 200 million people worldwide are infected by cestodes.

TAENIA SAGINATA (BEEF TAPEWORM) INFECTION

The different life cycle forms and designation of species of the beef tapeworm were identified in the 18th and 19th centuries.[312] Although other species names have been used in the past, *Taenia saginata* is accepted now as an inclusive term for all of the species of tapeworms acquired from beef. In recent years, however, *Taenia asiatica* has been identified as a distinct species similar to *T. saginata* but acquired from pork. Differentiation of these species morphologically, however, is difficult, and identification of species is aided by DNA analysis.[46,125]

Organism

The scolex of *T. saginata* measures 1 to 2 mm in diameter and has four muscular suckers but bears no hooks. The length of the parasite usually varies from 4 to 10 m but may reach 25 m. The size of the proglottids depends on their stage of development and their state of muscular relaxation. Gravid proglottids typically are 16 to 20 mm in length and 5 to 7 mm in width. The linear, central uterine stem has 12 to 30 main lateral branches on each side. The eggs measure 30 to 40 μm in diameter. The six-hooked embryo is surrounded by a brown, radially striated embryophore. When the bovine host ingests the ova, embryos hatch and burrow through the intestinal mucosa, where they gain access to the circulation. After lodging in capillaries, the embryo develops into a larval cysticercus. This cystic, ovoid structure measures 7 to 10 mm × 4 to 6 mm and contains an invaginated scolex.

Cattle are the principal intermediate hosts. Humans are the only definitive host. Ingestion of *T. saginata* eggs is of no particular danger to children because humans are not susceptible to development of the cysticercus stage.

Transmission

The life cycle of *T. saginata* requires transmission of the infection to the intermediate host and subsequently to humans, who in turn transmit the organism to other intermediate hosts. Contamination of pastures or feed lots with human feces or untreated sewage leads to bovine cysticercosis. When humans ingest raw or poorly cooked beef containing viable cysticerci, the scolex evaginates from the cysticercus and attaches to the intestinal wall. Proglottids develop from the neck region and gradually enlarge to form the adult tapeworm. Gravid proglottids, which are at the distal end of the worm, appear only 84 to 120 days after infection.[286] Infection may persist for years. In most geographic areas, parasitism is with a single worm, but in highly endemic areas, multiple infections may be found.[286]

Ova may be found within feces. However, eggs are shed more frequently when gravid proglottids actively migrate from the anus. As these muscular proglottids crawl about, eggs are expressed from the anterior margin. The ova of *T. solium* and *T. saginata* are not distinguishable on morphologic grounds.

Epidemiology

Worldwide, 45 to 60 million people are thought to be infected with *T. saginata*. Infection is most important in tropical and subtropical cattle-raising areas of Africa, the Middle East, Europe, Asia, and South America.[46,153] The prevalence of human taeniasis caused by *T. saginata* is poorly understood. In general, the prevalence of human infections is less than 1% of stool examinations in all but highly endemic areas, but because of the poor sensitivity of the assays, this figure may understate the prevalence. In recent studies, prevalence rates of more than 20% have been noted in East Africa, Bali, and Tibet.[50] Although the incidence of taeniasis in the United States is low, transmission does occur. However, less than 0.1% of fecal specimens examined in state health laboratories were positive for *Taenia* eggs.[139] With socioeconomic changes, improvements in the cattle industry, and decreasing instances of ingestion of undercooked beef, the prevalence of intestinal taeniasis likely will continue to drop in much of the world.

Pathology and Pathogenesis

Little is known of the pathology or pathogenesis of intestinal taeniasis. Speculation about local mucosal trauma, irritation, production of toxic substances, or induction of clinically significant hypersensitivity has scant documentation. Rare, ectopic localization of worms or proglottids may stimulate local inflammatory reactions. Some have speculated that adult worms compete with the infected host for nutrients causing malnutrition, but no good evidence exists to support this possibility.

Clinical Manifestations

A variety of symptoms have been attributed to *T. saginata,* but the parasite infection likely is often merely coincidental to the concurrently observed symptoms in the child.[46,324] The most common complaint is the discomfort caused by the migration of gravid proglottids from the anus. Some studies of *T. saginata* infection revealed abdominal pain, nausea, weakness, and loss of weight as the most common symptoms recorded.[46,311] Alterations in appetite and bowel habits were reported inconsistently. Intestinal obstruction and symptoms related to ectopic localization of proglottids are extremely rare. Although taeniasis usually is not associated with significant eosinophilia, some patients occasionally have significant eosinophilia between the sixth and ninth weeks after the initial infection occurs. One study reported that by the time the patients first began passing proglottids, the eosinophil counts had returned to normal or nearly normal.[107] Another series of observations showed a syndrome of marked eosinophilia and severe colicky abdominal pain that occurred approximately 1 month before the patients passed *Taenia* proglottids.[11] A single experimental infection produced symptoms of nausea, headache, and disturbed sleep at approximately the time that gravid proglottids appeared in the stool, 84 days after infection. A 10.5% increase in the number of eosinophils and a 13% increase in the number of lymphocytes were noted.[286]

Diagnosis

The scolex of *T. saginata* lacks hooks and is differentiated easily from the scolex of *T. solium,* which bears a circle of hooks. However, the scolex usually is not recovered, even after successful treatment. Studies suggest that use of polyethylene glycol salts as a purgative may improve recovery of proglottids.[137] Eggs may be seen on routine fecal wet mounts, but the likelihood of their being detected is enhanced by concentration methods. Even then, ova are shed only intermittently, and the yield of a single stool examination is low. Cellulose tape swabs applied to the anal and perianal skin, as used for the diagnosis of *Enterobius* infection, have been found to be even more efficient than fecal concentration.[292]

The eggs of *T. saginata, T. asiatica,* and *T. solium* cannot be differentiated morphologically. Thus examination of gravid proglottids is the usual method for determining species. The patient is instructed to collect proglottids in a vial of saline and to deliver the specimen to the laboratory as soon as possible. Fixatives such as alcohol and formalin tend to render the proglottids rigid and opaque. The proglottid should be compressed between two microscope slides. If the uterus contains enough ova, counting the main branches of the uterine stem is relatively easy. The uterus is more readily identified by injecting a small amount of India ink into the midportion. A count of 13 or fewer branches on one side of the stem is considered diagnostic for *T. solium.* If the count is 14 or more, the species is designated *T. saginata.* Because of morphologic variations, this method has been criticized, particularly when the decision is based on gravid proglottids with counts in the range of 12 to 15. Analysis of many specimens of *Taenia,* as identified by their scolex, showed that mature proglottids with fully developed sex organs could be differentiated by several characteristics. The most prominent features are a vaginal sphincter seen only in *T. saginata* and a third ovarian lobe that is present only in *T. solium.* To define these and other features, the proglottids require painstaking staining and clearing as well as examination by a skilled parasitologist.

Antigen detection tests are becoming increasingly useful for the identification of *T. saginata.* Tests for *T. solium* currently are more specific than tests for *T. saginata.*[3] Polymerase chain reaction (PCR) testing has been useful in diagnosis of *T. saginata* in field situations.[46] On occasion, the diagnosis of tapeworm is established when larger portions of a worm appear as a ribbon-like defect in the barium column during contrast studies of the gastrointestinal tract. In plain films of the abdomen, a tapeworm may be seen as a linear density in a gas-filled loop of bowel.

Treatment

Praziquantel, a pyrazinoisoquinoline derivative, is the primary medication used to treat *T. saginata.* It is given as a single oral dose of 5 to 10 mg/kg. An alternative to praziquantel for treatment of intestinal taeniasis is niclosamide (marketed as Yomesan in parts of Europe but not consistently available in the United States), which is given as a single oral dose of 50 mg/kg (up to 2 g for large children or for adults). Nitazoxanide, a thiazolide agent approved for use in children with other parasitic infections, has been effective in treating taeniasis that has been incompletely responsive to both praziquantel and niclosamide.[153]

Because infection with *T. saginata* is not contagious, no routine follow-up is needed after treatment. If, however, proglottids are noted through the anus or in the stool more than a week after treatment is completed, subsequent therapy may be considered, perhaps with an alternative agent.

Prognosis

Symptoms, when present, may be annoying but do not usually alter health significantly. Treatment is highly effective, and the prognosis is excellent.

Prevention

T. saginata infection can be prevented by avoiding the ingestion of raw or undercooked beef. In addition, visual meat inspection is effective in detecting all but light infections. Cooking beef to a temperature of 56°C (133°F) kills cysticerci. Education of workers in the cattle-raising industry, coupled with detection and prompt treatment of human infection, may reduce the incidence of transmission. Vaccines to prevent bovine *T. saginata* cysticercosis are feasible, but development has been slowed by limited commercial interest.[160]

TAENIA ASIATICA (ASIAN PORK TAPEWORM)

T. asiatica was identified in East and Southeast Asia, where humans become infected by eating small cysts contained in raw porcine liver. The ova and proglottids are morphologically similar to those of *T. saginata,* such that it was not recognized as a separate species until 1993.[46,133]

Organism

Although adult tapeworm proglottids of *T. asiatica* are morphologically similar to those of *T. saginata,* the scolex contains a rostellum (like *T. solium*) but no hooks (like *T. saginata*). Proglottids usually contain 16 to 21 uterine branches, similar to *T. saginata.* The larval cysticercus stage is also similar to that of *T. saginata,* but the cysticerci generally are smaller. The cysticerci also are located primarily in the liver, not generally in muscle. *T. asiatica* cysticerci are found mainly in pigs but have been identified in cattle, goats, monkeys, and wild boar.[133]

Transmission

Pigs (and also cattle, wild boar, and goats) become infected by ingesting *T. asiatica* eggs, which hatch, releasing the larvae, which in turn invade and develop into the cysticercal stage primarily in the liver. Animals, including humans, become infected when they ingest cysticerci (usually in raw porcine liver) and then develop the intestinal adult forms of infection. An experimental human infection demonstrated that a period of 76 days transpired between ingestion of the cysticercus and the appearance of gravid proglottids.[74]

Epidemiology

Asian taeniasis has been identified in Taiwan, Korea, China, Philippines, Vietnam, Thailand, Indonesia, and Malaysia.[46,74] It may be that other parts of the Asia-Pacific region also are endemic for *T. asiatica* but that previous surveys incorrectly identified the offending organism as *T. saginata.* The prevalence of infection varies among regions, probably related to religious and cultural choices about food; 0% to 21% of people in various parts of Indonesia are infected.[305]

Pathology and Pathogenesis

Observations in humans and studies in mice suggest that the pathogenesis of infection by *T. asiatica* is similar to that of *T. saginata.*[134] No human cysticercal form has been identified.

Clinical Manifestations, Diagnosis, Treatment, and Prognosis

The clinical manifestations, diagnosis, treatment, and prognosis of *T. asiatica* have not been described completely, but they appear to be similar or identical to those of *T. saginata*.

Prevention

Human *T. asiatica* infection can be prevented by avoiding ingestion of undercooked liver and other viscera (especially porcine).

TAENIA SOLIUM

Cysticercosis was first described in ancient Greece, where cysticerci were noted in infected pork.[57] The life cycle was clarified by the 19th century. The main clinical manifestation results from infection of the central nervous system (CNS) and is termed neurocysticercosis. Large case series describing most of the clinical manifestations were published in the early 20th century.[64] Neurocysticercosis, however, was diagnosed only rarely until the late 1970s. Subsequent advances in neuroimaging led to a dramatic increase in recognition.[228] Neurocysticercosis is now recognized as among the more common causes of neurologic disease worldwide.[24,45,83,188,193]

Organism

T. solium, referred to as the pork tapeworm, takes two distinct forms in the human host: taeniasis (tapeworm infection of the gut lumen) and cysticercosis (infection of tissues with the larval cysticercus form).[83] Neurocysticercosis refers to cysticercosis involving the CNS (including the subarachnoid space, spinal cord, and eyes). Humans develop the adult tapeworm after ingesting undercooked pork containing the cysticercus. The scolex evaginates in the intestines, attaches, and develops chains of proglottids. The tapeworms can be several meters long. Eggs and gravid proglottids are shed intermittently into stool. The off-white proglottids appear as flattened segments 1 mm thick and up to 2 cm in length and 1 cm in width. Pigs are infected after ingesting eggs or proglottids from human fecal material. Once ingested, the larval oncospheres emerge from the eggs, penetrate the wall of the gut, enter the bloodstream, and migrate to the tissues, where they develop into cysticerci during a period of a few weeks.

Transmission

Field studies of both taeniasis and cysticercosis are associated with tight clustering.[89,90,156,194,200,250] Taeniasis is acquired by ingestion of undercooked pork and is closely tied to pig-raising areas in endemic countries. Most carriers are from families that raise pigs and butcher them informally in the household. Cysticercosis is acquired from the human tapeworm carriers, who not only shed eggs into the environment but also harbor eggs on their hands and fingernails. These eggs can then autoinfect the tapeworm carrier or infect other people. Thus most transmission occurs among close contacts of tapeworm carriers. Human cysticercosis is not always acquired directly from pork, as illustrated by outbreaks noted among vegetarians in India and orthodox Jews in the United States.[252,264] In both cases, transmission has been associated with domestic servants who were tapeworm carriers, a factor also seen in urban areas lacking infected pigs.[127]

Epidemiology

The global prevalence of human cysticercosis is not clearly defined. Between 50 and 100 million people are thought to be infected with cysticercosis, but far fewer with intestinal taeniasis.[24,45,193]

In the 2015 Global Burden of Disease study,[63] cysticercosis was reported to affect 1,931,000 (95% uncertainty interval: 1,597,000–2,312,000) people worldwide, which resulted in 286,700 (95% uncertainty interval: 194,200–392,800) years lived with disability.

Epidemiologic studies to determine the burden of neurocysticercosis have demonstrated associations between lifetime and active epilepsy with serologic and imaging findings of neurocysticercosis.[59,180,182,193,195,220] For instance, in Latin America more than 30% of people with epilepsy have findings compatible with neurocysticercosis [22]

Nearly all areas where pigs are raised that have access to human fecal material are endemic for cysticercosis.[45] In endemic areas, pigs often are reared on small farms, where they are allowed to forage for food rather than being fed. Improved sanitation, meat inspection, and animal husbandry led to the eradication of cysticercosis from western Europe, which previously was highly endemic. However, similar approaches have not proved sustainable in poorer countries. Currently, porcine cysticercosis remains highly endemic in Latin America, sub-Saharan Africa, and South and Southeast Asia, as well as parts of Korea, China, Indonesia, and Papua New Guinea.[133,194]

In the United States, porcine cysticercosis is a very rare occurrence. In contrast, human neurocysticercosis is widespread among immigrants from endemic countries.[61,197,201,258,259,274,297] Limited transmission occurs in the United States, mainly linked to tapeworm carriers infected in endemic areas.[53,199,259,276] Although infrequently reported, locally acquired infection has also been documented in the United States.[275]

In the United States, health care expenditure associated with neurocysticercosis is mainly due to hospitalization costs, which totaled approximately $1 billion for the period 2003 to 2012.[49,197,198]

Pathology and Pathogenesis

Cysticerci can develop in a wide range of tissues. In most tissues the cysticerci cause few symptoms, and their survival appears to be limited. For example, many of those infected have cigar-shaped calcifications noted on radiographs of skeletal muscle, despite the absence of musculoskeletal symptoms. By contrast, infection of the CNS often lasts for years and can cause severe symptoms.

Cysticerci mature to their full size (typically 10–20 mm in diameter) within a few weeks after infection occurs, but as illustrated in studies of British subjects returning from India and Hispanic immigrants to the United States, symptoms do not develop for several years.[61,64] This delay may reflect the parasites' complex array of molecules used to modulate the host inflammatory response.[83] When the parasites lose the ability to evade immune attack, the cysticerci are attacked by a granulomatous response with a mixed cell population, including lymphocytes and mononuclear cells, with variable numbers of eosinophils and neutrophils.[102,119,225,226,230,260] This granulomatous host response to the parasite, when it is present in the brain parenchyma, is thought to be the cause of seizures, the characteristic clinical feature of parenchymal neurocysticercosis.[279] During the course of several months, the inflamed parasite is invaded by inflammatory cells, the cyst cavity collapses, and the parasite material is replaced by the host granulomatous response.[119] The lesion eventually either resolves or is replaced by a small calcified granuloma. The calcified lesions contain a mixture of fibrosis and residual parasitic debris. An intermittent inflammatory response to persistent parasitic antigen may manifest as perilesional edema in calcified lesions,[82] and it may be the cause of recurrent seizures in patients with cerebral calcifications.[186,189] Rarely, massive infection is accompanied by a diffuse cerebral edema.[223,290]

Extraparenchymal neurocysticercosis is associated with a poorer prognosis, largely because of production of hydrocephalus.[99] Parasites can cause obstructive hydrocephalus by lodging in the outflow tracks of the cerebral ventricles. Cysticerci in the basilar cisterns often are associated with chronic arachnoiditis. This basilar inflammation may lead to chronic meningitis (with headache and nuchal rigidity but usually without fever), vasculitis and strokes, or communicating hydrocephalus. Less frequently, cysticerci in fissures enlarge to 5 cm or larger (termed giant cysticerci). The parasites, along with accompanying cerebral edema, may cause a mass effect. In patients with multiple cysticerci, several forms of the disease can be present at the same time.

Clinical Manifestations

Taeniasis

Taeniasis typically causes few symptoms. Cases have been associated with vague abdominal complaints and occasionally pruritus. The most specific symptom is the passage of proglottids in the stool. The proglottids appear flattened (typically 0.3–0.5 cm wide × 1 to 2 cm long and 1 mm thick). Each segment has 13 or fewer uterine branches. Unlike *T. saginata*, the proglottids usually are single and seldom are noted to be motile.

Cysticercosis

The clinical manifestations of cysticercosis are variable,[99,326] depending on the location of the parasites, their number, and the host inflammatory response. Experts now group neurocysticercosis into a range of syndromes that differ in pathogenesis, clinical manifestations, prognosis, and management.[83,88,99,188]

Single enhancing lesions. The most common presentation in children with neurocysticercosis is with seizures and a single enhancing lesion on neuroimaging studies.[95,238,240,244,260,265,282,302] Most cases are manifested with seizures, which can be isolated or recurrent. The seizures typically are focal with secondary generalization, although they may be focal or generalized.[263,268,269,302] Some children experience only severe headaches,[216] which can resemble either tension headaches or migraines. Imaging studies of children reveal either a focal area of enhancement or a ring-enhancing lesion, often with surrounding edema. Lesions typically are found within the cortex.

Multiple cystic (viable) lesions. Similar to children with single enhancing lesions, patients with multiple parenchymal cysticerci also have seizures. The seizures more often are generalized or focal with secondary generalization but also may be focal.[30,101,268] Neuroimaging studies demonstrate edema, contrast enhancement, or both for one or more parasites, and symptoms are thought to result from the host inflammatory response. Noninflamed cysts cause few symptoms, even when they are numerous,[84] but they pose a risk for development of recurrent symptoms when they degenerate.

Other symptoms include headaches. Infection has been associated with learning disabilities,[42,157,231,240,304] but these findings may be the result of either poorly controlled seizures or hydrocephalus.[285] An association of cysticercosis with depression and occasionally psychotic episodes also may exist.[79]

Cysticercal encephalitis. Some children have diffuse cerebral edema from large numbers of inflamed cysticerci, termed cysticercal encephalitis. The clinical presentation includes signs or symptoms of raised intracranial pressure, seizures, and altered mental status.[223,290] Cysticercal encephalitis is thought to result from a brisk inflammatory response to a massive infection and is seen more frequently in children and women than in adult men. This pathogenesis is the direct result of the host inflammatory response, and the key to management is to address inflammation and cerebral edema. Antiparasitic drugs are contraindicated because they can worsen the cerebral edema.

Parenchymal calcifications. Resolution of neurocysticercosis can be associated with the formation of calcified granulomas within the brain parenchyma.[188] The calcifications appear as well-defined calcified nodules measuring 2 to 10 mm. The calcified lesions contain fibrotic reactions, parasite debris, and calcium deposits, with variable degrees of inflammation.[186] Patients frequently present with seizures.[187-190,266] The most common imaging finding from neurocysticercosis in population-based studies in endemic villages is with focal calcifications.[59,78,180,220] Few patients will have focal abnormalities on electroencephalographic studies.[34] Among patients with seizures, calcified lesions are a risk factor for having recurrent seizures.[27,105,190,220] Patients with seizures and calcifications should be treated with antiepileptic therapy indefinitely. About half of patients with calcified neurocysticercosis and seizures have associated enhancement and edema on magnetic resonance imaging (MRI) studies.[10,190] Rather than revealing viable parasites, the enhancement may result from breakdown of the calcified granulomas, with release of antigen resulting in restimulation of the host inflammation.[118,190]

Ventricular neurocysticercosis. Approximately 10% to 20% of adult patients with cysticercosis have cysticerci in the ventricles,[83,191,224,245,259] but the numbers often are lower in children.[244] Cysticerci are found in any of the ventricles, but symptoms are particularly associated with obstruction of the outflow of the third or fourth ventricle at the cerebral aqueduct or foramina of Luschka and Magendie. In contrast to parenchymal disease that largely results from the host inflammatory response, symptoms of ventricular disease result from mechanical obstruction typically caused by viable parasites.[142] Within the thin-walled viable cysticerci, the cyst fluid often is isodense with cerebrospinal fluid (CSF), rendering them difficult to detect. Computed tomography (CT) scanning may show only obstructive hydrocephalus or distortion of the shapes of the involved ventricle. Even on MRI, the findings may be subtle and can be missed by inexperienced observers unless the patients have concomitant parenchymal cysticerci.[122,317,319] Newer three-dimensional MRI sequences (e.g., FIESTA, 3D CISS) may improve visualization of cysts in the ventricles or subarachnoid space.[32,115]

Symptoms from ventricular neurocysticercosis usually result from raised intracranial pressure and include headache, nausea or vomiting, altered mental status, papilledema with visual changes, or dizziness. The onset is extremely variable from chronic intermittent headache to sudden loss of consciousness.[296]

Subarachnoid cysticercosis. Subarachnoid cysticercosis can also be quite variable. Small cysticerci in the gyri have a clinical presentation and prognosis similar to those of parenchymal cysts, although they are associated more often with CSF pleocytosis, may be slightly larger, and respond less well to antiparasitic drugs.[83,245] Cysticerci in the basilar cisterns can cause arachnoiditis, leading to CSF outflow obstruction, communicating hydrocephalus, vasculitis, and strokes.[83,277] In the era before antiparasitic drugs were available, this form carried a high case-fatality rate.[277] By contrast, more recent case series have been characterized by low mortality rates.[45,54,191,224,259]

Most patients with cysticerci in the basilar cisterns are infected with large numbers of parasites, and they frequently have coexisting ventricular or parenchymal as well as subarachnoid disease. Symptomatic cysticerci in the basilar cisterns typically are accompanied by chronic arachnoiditis. This arachnoiditis may present as meningitis with headache, stiff neck, and CSF pleocytosis, but it usually is not accompanied by fever. Patients often develop communicating hydrocephalus (headaches, nausea, vomiting, and dizziness). Basilar cysticercosis frequently involves the basilar vasculature either by direct invasion or by inducing vasculitis. Thus patients may present with cerebrovascular accidents, which may involve either small vessels with lacunar infarctions from vasculitis or large vessel strokes (associated with invasion of the vessel wall by the parasite).[13,56,86] Some patients present with intracerebral hemorrhages.[303]

Giant cysticerci. Cysticerci can develop in the fissures (especially the sylvian fissure) and may enlarge to more than 5 cm in diameter; these are called giant cysticerci.[211] In some cases, the cysticerci can lose the scolex and may grow as clusters of cyst walls (termed racemose cysticercosis). Giant cysticerci not only are associated with symptoms of parenchymal inflammation but also can cause mass effects such as midline shift. Frequently, giant cysticerci are accompanied by cysticerci in the parenchyma or basilar cisterns. Giant cysticerci are readily visualized by CT or MRI, but the accompanying basilar cysticerci may not be seen as easily.

Other forms of cysticercosis. Neurocysticercosis rarely is limited to the spine, but spinal disease is common with subarachnoid disease.[29] Most patients present with radicular pain and, less frequently, myelitis. In most cases, cysticerci are in the spinal fluid, but they also can be intramedullary cysticerci.[155] The intramedullary form typically presents with myelitis. Orbital involvement includes subconjunctival cysticerci and involvement of the extraocular muscles.[39,215,257] Intraocular disease may be subretinal, intravitreal, or within the anterior chamber. Skeletal muscle involvement typically is asymptomatic, but it may result in pseudohypertrophy or weakness with massive infection. Subcutaneous lesions typically present as one or more painless mobile cystic lesions. Subcutaneous disease is more commonly noted in Asia and Africa than in the Western Hemisphere.

Diagnosis

Taeniasis

Taeniasis has been diagnosed traditionally by examination of the stool for proglottids, ova, or both. The ova and proglottids are shed only intermittently, and collection of stool specimens from children can prove difficult. Furthermore, the sensitivity of stool microscopy for ova is only 26%,[5] and the ova of *T. solium* and *T. saginata* are indistinguishable, which limits the specificity of the assay. Identification of species requires collection of the proglottids, which can be facilitated by treating the patient with polyethylene glycol.[137] The proglottids of the two species can be distinguished by counting the number of uterine branches. *Taenia saginata* proglottids usually have 15 or more uterine branches, compared with less than 13 branches in those of *T. solium*.

More sensitive and specific techniques are available only as research tools. Antigen-detection assays have a specificity of 99.2% and a sensitivity of 70% to 92%,[4,5,233] but most cannot distinguish *Taenia* spp. Enzyme-linked immunotransfer blot to identify serum antibodies to *T. solium* tapeworm-stage antigens may be more sensitive than are stool-based tests and seem to be specific for the *T. solium* tapeworm stage.[120,158,308] However, the antibody may persist after treatment. PCR techniques can be used to improve sensitivity and specificity compared with stool microscopy and to differentiate *Taenia* species.[114,171]

Neurocysticercosis

Establishing the diagnosis of neurocysticercosis is more difficult than with many other parasitic infections. The major clinical presentations are nonspecific, and the location of the parasites within the CNS usually precludes their being observed directly. Serologic tests using crude antigens (including a number of commercially available enzyme-linked immunosorbent assays [ELISAs]) are plagued by poor sensitivity and specificity. However, computerized imaging methods (e.g., CT and MRI) have led to a dramatic increase in the ability to recognize cases and are now the mainstay of diagnosis (Figs. 227.1 to 227.3), although even these techniques cannot always distinguish neurocysticercosis from other neurologic processes.

An expert group proposed diagnostic criteria based on neuroimaging studies, serologic tests, clinical history, and exposure.[58,325] The presence of either a single absolute criterion or two major criteria along with two minor or epidemiologic criteria is considered diagnostic. One major criterion plus two other criteria or three minor criteria along with exposure define a probable diagnosis.

Direct visualization of the parasite on ophthalmoscopic examination or histology is considered diagnostic of neurocysticercosis.[58] However, biopsy or autopsy material demonstrating *T. solium* parasites rarely is available, and parasites seldom are visualized in the eye. The neuroimaging pattern of a cystic lesion with a mural nodule measuring 1 to 3 mm (consistent with a scolex) is thought to be pathognomonic for cysticercosis.[317,318] However, rare cases have been reported in which similar findings have been noted in other diseases, and even in neurocysticercosis, the scolex cannot be visualized in most cases.

The main major diagnostic criterion for neurocysticercosis is one or more lesions on neuroimaging studies highly suggestive of neurocysticercosis.[58,55] Viable cysticerci appear on CT or MRI scans as rounded fluid collections typically 1 to 2 cm in diameter. The cyst fluid is isodense with CSF (hypodense in contrast to brain tissue on CT or T1 imaging). The scolex sometimes is visible as a small nodule found attached to the cyst wall. The wall of the cysticercus initially is isodense with the parenchyma and not easily visualized. On T2-weighted and fluid-attenuated inversion recovery images, the fluid is seen as hyperintense. Inflamed cysticerci are characterized by perilesional edema and contrast enhancement.[279] Subsequently, the cyst fluid increases in density and becomes infiltrated by host inflammatory cells. The cyst cavity eventually collapses, forming a solid area of focal enhancement. At that point, the granulomatous inflammation either resolves or leads to the formation of a calcified nodule typically measuring 2 to 6 mm in diameter. CT is better than MRI to detect calcifications; however, MRI is superior to detect associated perilesional edema. In addition, MRI, especially 3D sequences, is the imaging procedure of choice for intraventricular cysts and cysts located in the basilar cisterns, posterior fossa, and brain convexity.[32,85]

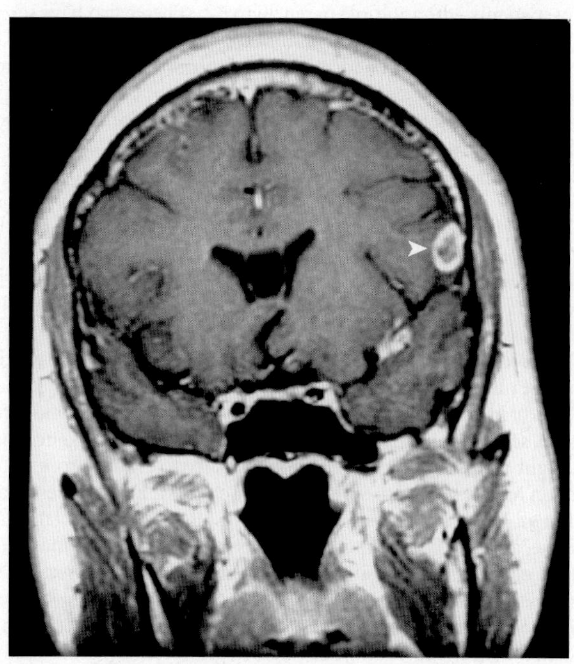

FIG. 227.2 Neurocysticercosis with subarachnoid involvement. (Courtesy C. Mark Mehringer, MD, Harbor-UCLA Medical Center.)

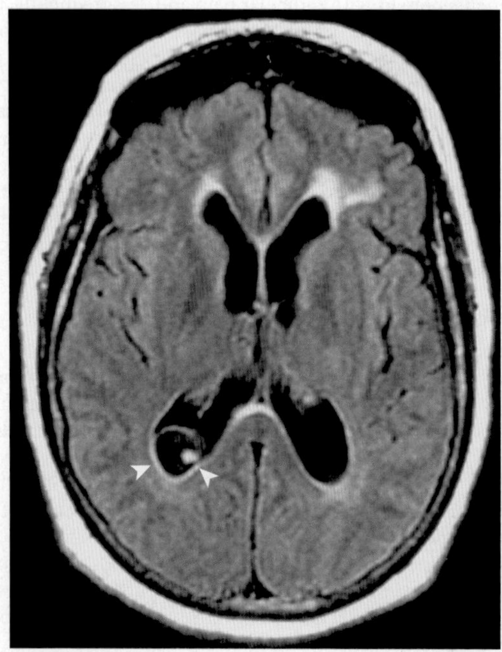

FIG. 227.1 Ventricular neurocysticercosis. (Courtesy C. Mark Mehringer, MD, Harbor-UCLA Medical Center.)

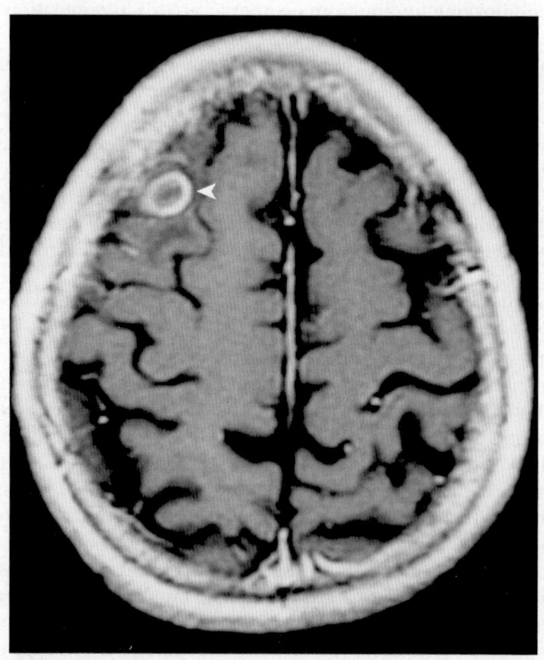

FIG. 227.3 Neurocysticercosis with parenchymal involvement. (Courtesy C. Mark Mehringer, MD, Harbor-UCLA Medical Center.)

Although enhancing lesions are typical of neurocysticercosis, similar lesions can be noted with tuberculomas, brain abscesses, and tumors. Rajshekhar and Chandy[218] noted that cysticercal lesions typically have a diameter smaller than 20 mm and rarely cause midline shift. A single, round, enhancing lesion less than 20 mm in diameter without midline shift on imaging studies in patients lacking signs or symptoms of systemic disease, focal neurologic deficits, or increased intracranial pressure was highly suggestive of neurocysticercosis in a prospective study of 401 patients in southern India.[218] However, the results are less specific in areas with a lower prevalence of cysticercosis. Spontaneous resolution or resolution achieved with antiparasitic drugs is another major criterion.

Serodiagnosis has proved problematic for cysticercosis. ELISAs employing unfractionated antigens, such as cyst fluid, have poor sensitivity and specificity.[212,221] The preferred serodiagnostic test is the enzyme-linked immunotransfer blot employing semipurified parasite glycoproteins.[298] A positive reaction to any one of seven glycoprotein bands is considered positive. ELISAs using recombinant versions of these antigens are being developed.[87,120,121,254] Studies have confirmed a specificity of nearly 100% in suspected cases, but the sensitivity is limited in subjects with either a single lesion or only calcified lesions.[108,212,253,310] For this assay, tests of serum are more sensitive than tests of CSF.[310] Assays to detect parasite antigens may prove to be important diagnostic studies in the near future.[75,94,97,100,205] Minor criteria include (1) lesions on neuroimaging studies consistent with neurocysticercosis but less suggestive (e.g., isolated basilar meningitis, hydrocephalus without demonstration of cystic lesions, or filling defects in the spinal subarachnoid space without discrete cysticerci), (2) symptoms suggestive of seizures or hydrocephalus, and (3) cysticercosis outside the nervous system (e.g., cigar-shaped muscle calcifications or subcutaneous nodules).[58] Epidemiologic criteria include residence or prolonged visits to endemic areas and contact with a tapeworm carrier. Since the guidelines were published several publications have reported detection of parasite antigens in CSF, serum, and urine.[52,184,232,306] Currently no commercial or well-standardized assays are available. Antigen is more frequently detected with viable cysticerci and with a larger parasite burden. They appear to be particularly useful for determining length of therapy in complicated subarachnoid cases. PCR assays have been reported on CSF, but these are also not well standardized.[175]

Numerous other tests may prove useful in excluding other illnesses but are not diagnostic of neurocysticercosis. These tests include blood counts, lumbar puncture for testing of CSF, and stool studies. Lumbar CSF frequently has elevated protein levels and may show hypoglycorrhachia. Cell counts are variable and may demonstrate a predominance of lymphocytes, neutrophils, or eosinophils.

Treatment

For patients with seizures caused by neurocysticercosis, initial management should focus on control of the seizures, which usually can be accomplished with a single antiepileptic drug.[326] Most published studies describe use of phenytoin or carbamazepine. Newer agents (e.g., valproate, lamotrigine, levetiracetam, topiramate, oxcarbazepine, or clobazam) may be more effective, but they are not affordable in endemic areas.[141] Breakthrough seizures usually occur with subtherapeutic antiepileptic drug levels, often from poor adherence to medication therapies.[81] Seizure therapy can be tapered off for many patients after they have a seizure-free period if radiographic resolution of the lesion is seen. However, a substantial risk exists for recurrence of seizures if residual inflamed or calcified lesions are present.[30,101,190,219,302] Antiepileptic drugs should be continued indefinitely if calcifications develop.

Patients with obstructive hydrocephalus usually require surgery.[83,88,188,191,224] For patients with mild or intermittent symptoms (e.g., a cysticercus in the lateral ventricles not associated with midline shift), elective endoscopic removal of the cysticercus is the treatment of choice.[217,224] Cases with altered mental status or impending herniation should undergo emergency CSF diversion by a ventriculostomy or placement of a ventriculoperitoneal shunt. A high rate of shunt failure exists if shunting is not followed by administration of antiparasitic therapy or corticosteroids.[83,142,224,277] Patients with communicating hydrocephalus often require placement of a ventriculoperitoneal shunt.[142] In some patients, cysticerci and associated edema may lead to mass effects. If the symptoms are life-threatening or if the cysticercus is easily approachable (e.g., in the sylvian fissure), surgical decompression of the cysticercus is the preferred approach.

A consensus is emerging among experts about the proper role of antiparasitic drugs and corticosteroids in the management of neurocysticercosis.[83] Experts agree that neurocysticercosis represents a spectrum of diseases that differ in optimal management.

Single Enhancing Lesions

The most common presentation of children with neurocysticercosis is seizures and a single enhancing lesion. Seizures generally can be controlled with antiepileptic medications.[141,219,302] Controlled trials of antiparasitic drugs in patients with single enhancing lesions have demonstrated a favorable prognosis with symptomatic therapy. However, the length of time until radiologic resolution is achieved and the duration of time for risk for experiencing seizures appear to be somewhat shorter with antiparasitic drug treatment.[204,265,267,293,321] By contrast, these treatments do not appear to affect the formation of calcified lesions or development of chronic epilepsy. The role of steroids is better defined; several studies showed clear benefit in reducing seizure activity and faster resolution of the lesion on CT when steroids were used in conjunction with antiepileptic medications.[104,106,150,168,209] Overall, the best evidence points to a small benefit achieved from use of antiparasitic drugs (e.g., albendazole 15 mg/kg per day for 7–14 days)[321] accompanied by corticosteroids (e.g., prednisone 1 mg/kg per day during antiparasitic therapy). A single study that used combinations of praziquantel 75 mg/kg per day and albendazole 15 mg/kg per day suggested enhanced cysticidal activity in children with single enhancing lesions compared with albendazole alone.[140]

Multiple Parenchymal Lesions

Patients with seizure activity with multiple cysticerci usually will have one or more lesions in the process of degeneration (e.g., edema or contrast enhancement on imaging studies). However, other cysticerci may be in the viable stage, posing a prolonged risk for having seizures. A placebo-controlled trial from Peru showed a modest reduction in the number of generalized seizures in patients treated with albendazole and corticosteroid,[101] but no decrease occurred in the development of chronic calcifications. A second study from Ecuador demonstrated similar results.[31,237] Overall, the current expert consensus is that patients with multiple parenchymal cysticerci usually should be treated with a course of an antiparasitic agent (albendazole 15 mg/kg per day in two daily doses for 7 to 10 days) and a simultaneous course of corticosteroids.[191] More recent data from randomized clinical trials demonstrated that the combination of praziquantel and albendazole was more effective than albendazole alone. Combination therapy led to higher cystic resolution at 6 months in patients with multiple cysts (e.g., those with more than two parenchymal cysts).[91,98] Even so, symptomatic therapy (e.g., antiepileptic drugs) remains a key to management. A study evaluating the effect of antiparasitic therapy in addition to corticosteroids showed that a 4-week course of dexamethasone compared with a 10-day course resulted in fewer seizures early after starting therapy. However, the beneficial effect was not significant after 3 weeks of follow-up.[92]

Cysticercal Encephalitis (Numerous Cysticerci With Cerebral Edema)

In this context of diffuse cerebral edema (cysticercal encephalitis), antiparasitic drugs are contraindicated because of their potential to exacerbate host inflammatory responses.[88,222,289] Most cases will resolve spontaneously with antiinflammatory medications.

Calcified Parenchymal Cysticerci

Parenchymal brain calcifications can be seen in more than 10% of residents in some neurocysticercosis endemic areas.[188,220] These parenchymal calcifications are a significant risk factor for having continued seizure activity.[103,219,302] If a patient with a history of seizures has a calcified lesion, that patient should be treated with antiepileptic therapy indefinitely. Recurrent seizures may be due to concomitant mesotemporal sclerosis.[301] Antiparasitic medications and antiinflammatory drugs are not indicated. Surgical removal of the calcified focus has been used in some cases of intractable seizures.[307] By contrast, most cases can be managed with a single antiepileptic medication. About half of cases demonstrate perilesional edema or enhancement on MRI. Some have tried antiinflammatory therapy, but steroid withdrawal can actually precipitate symptoms.[174]

Ventricular Neurocysticercosis

Patients with obstructive hydrocephalus usually require surgery.[326] As mentioned earlier, for mild or intermittent symptoms (e.g., a cysticercus in the lateral ventricles not associated with midline shift), elective endoscopic removal of the cysticercus is the treatment of choice.[88,128,214,217,224,281] Cases with altered mental status or impending herniation should undergo emergency CSF diversion by a ventriculostomy or placement of a ventriculoperitoneal shunt. A high rate of shunt failure exists if shunting is not followed by administration of antiparasitic therapy. Cysticerci in the lateral and third ventricles usually can be removed through a rigid endoscope. A flexible endoscope is required to approach the fourth ventricle or basilar cisterns.[129,296,322] Many surgeons, however, prefer a suboccipital craniotomy for removal of cysticerci in the fourth ventricle. Endoscopic foraminotomy and third ventriculostomy often can be used to treat residual hydrocephalus. Antiparasitic medications should not be given before the procedure is performed because they can cause the cysticerci to be friable or to adhere to the ventricular wall. The cysticerci frequently rupture during removal, but this rupture has not been associated with any adverse effects. Endoscopic third ventriculostomy has been used as an alternative to shunting procedures.[128,151,213]

A ventriculoperitoneal shunt may be used to treat hydrocephalus. The rate of shunt failure is high in patients treated only with ventriculoperitoneal shunting. However, shunt failure appears to occur less frequently when patients receive adjunct therapy with corticosteroids and antiparasitic drugs. Although some patients have been treated with only chemotherapy and steroids, a substantial risk exists for development of acute hydrocephalus from cysticerci or accompanying inflammation causing obstruction of the foramina.

Subarachnoid Neurocysticercosis

Basilar subarachnoid cysticercosis is perhaps the most severe form of infection and carries risks for communicating hydrocephalus, vasculitis, and strokes.[83,188] Data on how best to treat this form are limited, but most experts agree that patients should be treated with antiparasitic drugs, corticosteroids, and, in most cases, CSF diversion procedures.[211,326] Most experts recommend treatment with albendazole, typically 15 mg/kg per day in divided doses for at least 28 days, but cure rarely is achieved with a single course of albendazole. Repeated courses, prolonged therapy, higher doses, switching to praziquantel, and combination of the two drugs have been tried in some cases.[112,169] Improved responses have been noted with endoscopic debulking of some of the parasites,[116,191] but this approach has not yet been studied systematically.

Inflammation seems to drive much of the pathogenesis, and the residual symptoms may reflect a chronic inflammatory response to cysticercal antigens rather than viable cysticerci. Prednisone up to 60 mg/day or dexamethasone up to 24 mg/day should be used along with the antiparasitic drugs. After 2 to 4 weeks, the dose often can be tapered. In cases that require more prolonged steroid therapy, methotrexate has been used as a steroid-sparing agent.[177]

Giant Subarachnoid Neurocysticercosis

Some cysticerci, particularly in the sylvian fissure or basilar cisterns, may enlarge to more than 5 cm in diameter, causing mass effect either directly or by surrounding edema. If mass effect cannot be reversed quickly by corticosteroids, surgical decompression may be required. In the absence of symptomatic mass effect, however, giant cysticerci can be treated similarly to other subarachnoid cysticerci.[191,211]

Other Forms of Neurocysticercosis

Cysticercosis of the eye, spine, or subcutaneous tissue generally is treated by surgical removal.[83] Anecdotes of medical therapy also exist.

Prognosis

The prognosis of neurocysticercosis is extremely variable, depending on the type of infection. Patients with single enhancing lesions generally do well and often are seizure free and discontinue therapy within 1 to 2 years. Patients with calcified lesions may require chronic antiepileptic therapy. Patients with numerous subarachnoid cysticerci often require repeated courses of therapy and even repeated surgeries. However, with optimal management of hydrocephalus, cases are rarely fatal.

Prevention

Cysticercosis was eliminated from western Europe by improved sanitation, animal husbandry, and meat inspection.[93,113] For example, porcine cysticercosis can be prevented by not allowing pigs access to human feces.[300] However, confined pigs must be fed, which is not affordable for peasant farmers. Human infection with adult tapeworms also can be prevented by adequate cooking or freezing of infected pork, but meat inspection has not been successful in areas where pigs are slaughtered informally.[287] Mass chemotherapy of endemic populations for carriage of the human tapeworm or porcine cysticercosis has resulted in significant short-term decreases in prevalence,[4,113,249] but prevalence rates rapidly return unless mass treatment is continued. A recent study demonstrated sustained elimination of cysticercosis from northern Peru by the combined use of mass chemotherapy to eliminate human tapeworm carriage, mass chemotherapy of pigs to eliminate porcine cysticercosis, and vaccination of pigs.[96]

COENUROSIS (*TAENIA MULTICEPS*, OTHERS) AND CYSTICERCOSIS CAUSED BY *TAENIA CRASSICEPS*

Several species of *Taenia* have a larval stage called a *coenurus* that consists of a cystic membranous structure measuring up to 6 cm in diameter from which multiple scolices bud internally or externally.[119,131] On the basis of this morphologic appearance, the parasite was given the species name *multiceps*. Currently the preferred genus name is *Taenia* because of the morphology of the adult worms and the inability to justify a genus designation based solely on the form of larvae. The following species generally are accepted for purposes of discussion. The adult tapeworm of *T. multiceps* is found in dogs, and the larval stages occur in herbivores. The larvae often develop in the CNS in sheep. In sheep-raising areas of Europe and Asia, the infection is still endemic in animals. *Taenia serialis* adult worms are found in dogs and other canids, but common intermediate hosts are rabbits, hares, and rodents. The coenurus develops in subcutaneous and intramuscular tissue. *T. serialis* has been reported from the United States, Canada, France, and Africa. *Taenia brauni* is the name given to the tapeworms of dogs, jackals, foxes, and genets found in tropical Africa. The larvae develop in gerbils and other rodents. Humans are a rare accidental host for the larval stages of these worms. Fewer than 100 human infections have been recorded. Most infections are from Africa, with many occurring in children. Giving a species designation based solely on the morphologic features of organisms recovered from human tissue is nearly impossible. The infection is presumed to be acquired by the ingestion of eggs excreted by the definitive hosts, usually dogs. Because of the subcutaneous and subconjunctival locations of cysts in infections in tropical Africa, some researchers have suggested that direct contact of the eggs on skin or the conjunctiva is a mode of transmission. A review of the six human infections in North America has been published.[119,131]

The clinical manifestations of coenurosis are related to the location of the parasite. Involvement of the CNS produces a spectrum of illness that resembles that of cysticercosis (discussed earlier), including meningeal reactions. Larvae have been seen in the subconjunctival and subretinal tissue, the extraocular muscles, the anterior chamber, and the vitreous. Subcutaneous and intramuscular lesions occur most commonly in the abdomen and chest wall. A definitive diagnosis is made by demonstrating the characteristic morphologic features of the larva recovered at surgery. The multiple scolices that bud from the delicate cyst membrane have double rows of hooklets of a typical shape, size, and number. In instances in which no scolices are found, differentiation of a coenurus from a cysticercus of *T. solium* is impossible. The diagnosis of intramuscular coenurosis has been made by examination of fine-needle aspirates.[119,131] Radiographic studies such as CT are useful in cerebral coenurosis but do not differentiate the parasite from other cystic lesions. The metabolic changes of magnetic resonance spectroscopy in an adult with cerebral coenurosis have been reported.[7] Treatment is surgical. Mortality rates in cerebral disease are high. Organisms in other locations, with the exception of subretinal lesions, are removed easily. A combination of praziquantel and a corticosteroid administered to a patient with a subretinal coenurus caused death of the parasite, which resulted in a severe inflammatory reaction, retinal detachment, and permanent loss of vision.[130] Severe reactions were reported in the two additional cases described in this review. Praziquantel should be used with great caution, if at all, in cases of human coenurosis. Nonetheless, postoperative praziquantel and albendazole have been used without apparent complication.[14,73] Although the exact mode of infection in humans has not been identified, avoidance of close contact with dogs and dog excreta, which are the most likely sources of infection, is prudent.

T. crassiceps cysticerci usually are found in field mice, with the tapeworm found in foxes, other canids, and felines. There have been a few reported human cases with ocular disease or mass lesions in compromised hosts (e.g., patients with acquired immunodeficiency syndrome).[35,40,81,110,124,167] Experimental *T. crassiceps* infection induces a helper T-cell subtype 2 (Th2) response that can also modulate immune responses to subsequent pathogenic challenges.[227] Fluid from *T. crassiceps* vesicles has been used to develop ELISA tests, but these tests are not specific for *T. crassiceps* infection and are rather used for seroprevalence studies of neurocysticercosis resulting from *T. solium* infection.[132,210] The diagnosis and management of *T. crassiceps* infection require surgery, but anthelmintic treatment might play a helpful role.[110]

DIPHYLLOBOTHRIUM SPECIES (FISH TAPEWORM)

Diphyllobothriasis can occur in children who ingest raw, pickled, or undercooked fresh-water fish.[324] The prevalence of infection increases with age in endemic areas. Nonspecific gastrointestinal complaints may occur in infected individuals, and megaloblastic anemia has been described particularly among elderly people in northern Europe and Chile.[46,138,203,256,312]

Several species of *Diphyllobothrium* have been reported in humans. *Diphyllobothrium latum*, the most common, was described first in 1592 from specimens found in Switzerland; it is now estimated to infect approximately 9 million individuals worldwide, with most cases occurring in Europe.[68] *Diphyllobothrium pacificum* is a similar fish tapeworm found infecting humans in Japan and South America, and *Diphyllobothrium nihonkaiense* has been described in humans from the North Pacific Basin including Japan, China, and Korea.[38,46] The *Diphyllobothrium* spp. typically have dogs, cats, foxes, bears, fish-eating birds, and marine mammals as definitive hosts, but children living in endemic areas may be infected when they eat raw or undercooked fish.

Organism

The scolex of *D. latum* possesses neither discrete suckers nor hooks but has two deep grooves called *bothria*. The worm may be as long as 15 m. The gravid proglottids have a characteristic rosette-shaped central uterus. Eggs measure 55 to 61 μm by 37 to 56 μm and have light-brown, operculated shells. The eggs are shed in an unembryonated state from a uterine pore into the fecal stream. The embryos develop within the eggs in fresh water. The ciliated embryos hatch and are ingested by copepods to develop further. After the fish have ingested the infected copepod, the larval stages develop into the plerocercoid stage in the muscles of fish. As the smaller fish are eaten by larger species, the larvae parasitize the muscles of the new host. Eventually, the larvae are found in fish that are sources of food for humans, such as species of pike, perch, turbot, lake trout, and whitefish. The plerocercoid larvae or spargana are white, ribbon-like worms approximately 5 cm in length.

Transmission

Children can be infected by ingesting the infectious plerocercoid forms in raw or undercooked fish muscle. Cooking and freezing kill the larvae, but smoking and pickling fish does not. The cycle of infection is perpetuated by the discharge of untreated human sewage into fresh-water lakes and streams. Diphyllobothriasis is a problem in the aquaculture industry, with some countries reporting high rates of plerocercoid forms in feral fish in lakes where salmon is farmed.[28,239] Outbreaks of diphyllobothriasis associated with the consumption of raw imported farmed salmon have been described.[247,248]

Some fish-eating mammals also may serve as definitive hosts for *D. latum* and maintain the cycle of infection in the absence of humans. Other *Diphyllobothrium* species (e.g., *D. pacificum*) have a life cycle involving the marine environment and use marine fish and mammals like seals and sea lions as intermediate and definitive hosts, respectively. Because *Diphyllobothrium* spp. requires intermediate hosts, direct transmission cannot occur, and no techniques of isolation or special precautions are required for infected patients.

Epidemiology

The prevalence of infection increases with age in endemic areas. However, infections have been reported in children younger than 1 year of age.[46] The disease has a worldwide distribution, but a higher prevalence is described in areas where fresh-water fish is eaten raw, lightly salted, pickled, smoked, or partially cooked. Infection occurs frequently in the Baltic countries and Russia; Scandinavia; Switzerland and the adjacent lake regions of Italy, France, and Germany; the Danube River delta; the lake areas of the northern United States and river deltas of Alaska; and Canada, South America, and China.[117] Pediatric infection by *D. latum* has also been identified in school-aged children in India, Taiwan, Korea, Argentina, and Hawaii. Salmonid fish (i.e., salmon, trout, whitefish) transmit *D. nihonkaiense* to humans in Japan, China, and Korea.[38,320] Infection of humans with *D. pacificum* has been reported from Peru and Chile after the ingestion of salt water fish such as bonito and lorna drum.[138,256]

Pathology and Pathogenesis

Little is known about the direct effects of the parasite on the host. Megaloblastic anemia has been described in infected individuals in Northern Europe and Chile, but not in other regions.[206] The following factors may be significant in the pathogenesis of "tapeworm anemia": (1) the strains of *D. latum* found in Finland, where anemia occurs, absorb seven times more vitamin B_{12} than do strains from North America, where anemia has not been reported; (2) interference with absorption of vitamin B_{12} occurs in nonanemic carriers as well as in those with anemia, and deficient stores of vitamin B_{12} plus malabsorption of vitamin B_{12} may contribute to the anemic state; (3) dietary intake of vitamin B_{12} may be low in anemic patients, and oral vitamin B_{12} has been shown to cause reticulocytosis in the presence of the worm; (4) worms found in anemic patients take up more of an oral dose of vitamin B_{12} than do worms in asymptomatic carriers, and worms are attached more proximally in the small intestine in anemic patients; and (5) secretion of intrinsic factor is reduced in anemic patients. Thus host and parasite factors likely play a role in the development of megaloblastic anemia in diphyllobothriasis.

Clinical Manifestations

Most infections are asymptomatic, but patients may notice proglottids or tapeworm segments in the stool. In Finland, comparison of symptoms between nonanemic infected patients and uninfected controls revealed an increase in fatigue, weakness, craving for salt, lack of well-being, dizziness, and numbness of the extremities in the infected group.[241] Significant gastrointestinal symptoms occur infrequently. However, an experimental infection with seven larvae produced nausea, severe periumbilical pain, and marked weight loss. Episodes of intestinal obstruction associated with the vomiting of masses of tapeworms have been reported. Eosinophilia is an uncommon finding. Patients with *D. pacificum* reported abdominal pain, vomiting, diarrhea, and flatulence.[164] Megaloblastic anemia caused by *D. latum* infection is extremely rare outside Finland and neighboring endemic areas. In addition, no other *Diphyllobothrium* species have been associated with anemia. Usually, it is seen in patients older than 50 years of age (and may occur in as many as 2% of adult tapeworm carriers), but it has been reported in children as young as 9 years.

Diagnosis

Identification of the characteristic eggs (oval, operculated, approximately 60 μm across) or proglottids provides the diagnosis. The parasite produces nearly 1 million eggs per day, and ova usually are detected easily by fecal examination.

Treatment and Prevention

Treatment with praziquantel (5 to 10 mg/kg as a single oral dose) is highly effective. An alternative medical treatment is niclosamide (50 mg/kg as a single oral dose). Tapeworm-related anemia is reversible by treatment of the infection, but the affected child should receive supplementation with vitamin B_{12} initially.

A significant reduction in the transmission of *D. latum* has been accomplished in many areas through the introduction of sewage treatment and targeted drug treatment of human infections. Raw and undercooked fresh or chilled fish should not be consumed in areas where a possibility of larval infection exists. Also, caution should be used when consuming raw fresh or chilled imported farmed fish from endemic countries.[247] Larvae do not survive in fish that either is cooked for 5 minutes or more at temperatures of at least 55°C or frozen at temperatures of at least −10°C for 8 to 72 hours.[68]

DIPYLIDIUM CANINUM (DOG TAPEWORM)

Dipylidium caninum, the common tapeworm of dogs and cats, also infects infants and young children.[46,312] Transmission occurs through the accidental ingestion of infected dog, cat, or human fleas (*Ctenocephalides* spp.) and less often body lice (*Trichodectes* spp.). Although it usually is asymptomatic, infection may be associated with decreased appetite, abdominal discomfort, or, perhaps, diarrhea.

Organism

D. caninum adult worms have a scolex with four cup-shaped suckers and a rostellum that bears one to seven rows of small hooks. The worm ranges from 10 to 50 cm in length. The gravid proglottids resemble cucumber seeds in size and shape. The proglottids have two pairs of sex organs, and a genital pore opens on each lateral margin. The eggs measure 35 to 65 μm in diameter and appear in packets of 5 to 30 enclosed in a membrane. The motile gravid proglottids are excreted in feces or migrate actively from the anus. The eggs are liberated as the proglottid disintegrates in the environment. The flea larvae ingest the eggs of *D. caninum*. Development of the tapeworm's larval stages leading to a cysticercoid takes place as the flea metamorphoses into an adult. When the flea is ingested by the definitive host, the adult tapeworm develops in the small intestine.

Transmission and Epidemiology

Humans acquire the infection by the accidental ingestion of infected fleas. Because of the motility of the proglottids, eggs may be disseminated widely in the environment. Fleas are so ubiquitous that transmission to the intermediate host is accomplished readily.

Infection of dogs and cats is a common occurrence worldwide. *D. caninum* also has been found in a variety of wild canines and felids. Reports of dipylidiasis in humans in the United States, however, are uncommon and include almost exclusively infants.[33,179]

Clinical Manifestations, Diagnosis, Prognosis, and Treatment

Although the incubation period in humans is unknown, infection has been seen in infants aged 5 weeks. Frequently, the only evidence of infection is the finding of proglottids in stool or in an infant's diapers. Varying degrees of abdominal pain, diarrhea, irritability, and even pruritus have been recorded in symptomatic children.

The characteristic proglottids must be differentiated from other parasites. A frequent error is to assume, from the parents' description, that the small, motile proglottids that migrate from the anus are pinworms or fly larvae.[246] Examination of stool specimens may be spuriously negative because proglottids tend to migrate from the fecal mass and disintegrate on the walls of the specimen container. Treatment with praziquantel 5 to 10 mg/kg as a single oral dose is effective. An alternative treatment is niclosamide 50 mg/kg as a single oral dose.

Infected dogs and cats also should be treated. Flea control requires the use of appropriate insecticides on pets. In addition, particular attention must be given to carpets and areas where pets sleep because these are the sites of development of the larval fleas.

HYMENOLEPIS NANA (DWARF TAPEWORM)

Infection with *Hymenolepis nana*, the dwarf tapeworm, occurs worldwide and probably is maintained by direct fecal-oral transmission from person to person.[46,312,323] Insects may serve as intermediate hosts. Infection may be asymptomatic, but gastrointestinal, neurologic, and allergic symptoms have been reported.

Organism

Adult worms of *H. nana* measure 1 to 5 cm in length and are less than 1 mm in width. The tiny scolex has four cup-shaped suckers and a rostellum with a circle of 20 to 30 small hooks. Gravid proglottids disintegrate within the intestine, and eggs are found in the feces. The oval eggs measure 30 to 50 μm in diameter and contain a six-hooked embryo within two envelopes. The space between the two envelopes contains filaments that extend from two small polar protrusions on the inner envelope. Larval stages develop in insect intermediate hosts after they have ingested the eggs. However, if the definitive host ingests eggs, larval stages invade the intestinal villi and develop a cysticercoid larva in 4 to 5 days. Then larvae break into the lumen and develop into adult worms. Ova appear in feces 2 to 4 weeks after infection occurs. Autoinfection with *H. nana* causes long-term infections and occurs when eggs hatch in the intestinal lumen and larvae go through the rest of the lifecycle without ever being shed in to the environment. A morphologically identical organism found in rodents may be a separate species. The rodent strains are alternatively called *Hymenolepis fraterna* or *H. nana* var. *fraterna*.[46,166] The rodent strain occasionally infects humans.

Transmission

Human infection is acquired most commonly by the ingestion of eggs from the feces of infected persons or by autoinfection. Humans serve as both intermediate and definitive hosts in this direct cycle. Poor hygienic habits, overcrowding, lack of running water, and poor management of human excreta enhance transmission through the fecal-oral route. The rodent strains of *H. nana* are infectious for humans, and food contaminated by rodent feces is a possible source of infection. Eggs may be produced for periods longer than 1 year, but the possibility of recurrent autoinfection obscures the determination of the duration of the initial infection.

Epidemiology

H. nana is a common parasite of rats and mice worldwide, and 50 to 75 million people are thought to be infected.[46,312] The distribution of infection in humans is worldwide, with an increased prevalence in some urban areas. Stool surveys from endemic areas commonly show prevalence rates of 5% to 25%, which may approach 50% in children aged 4 to 10 years.[50] Children in slums and refugee camps are at high risk for infection.[1,176] In the United States, 1.5% of stool samples of subjects with gastrointestinal symptoms harbored *H. nana* eggs in the Rocky Mountain region.[41] Older reports showed a prevalence of up to 15% in institutionalized individuals in New York.[316]

Pathology and Pathogenesis

Little is known of the pathogenesis and pathology of *H. nana* infection in humans. The larval stage of *H. nana* is a cystlike structure called a *cysticercoid* that is approximately 250 μm in diameter. Local reactions consisting of mucosal inflammation or atrophy may occur at the site of attachment of the adult worms in the small intestine. Rare cases of disseminated infection in children and adults with depressed cellular immunity have been reported.[163,183]

Clinical Manifestations

A wide variety of symptoms have been ascribed to *H. nana* infection, but few well-controlled clinical studies have been presented. However, a significant number of cross-sectional studies suggest an increased prevalence of diarrhea in children with hymenolepiasis.[1,176,235,280,323] Heavy burdens of worms have been associated with abdominal pain, malnutrition, retardation of growth, and lethargy, whereas children with low burdens did not have significant symptoms.[36,37,270] In addition, a few studies have associated *H. nana* infection and anemia in children.[176,309]

Diagnosis

Detection of the characteristic eggs in fecal material by examination of direct saline wet mounts or by concentration techniques usually is not difficult. However, a single examination is not always adequate to rule out infection.

Treatment and Prognosis

Praziquantel 25 mg/kg as a single oral dose is effective in treating *H. nana* infection. However, under some conditions a second dose at least 10 days apart may be recommended to prevent relapses because praziquantel is less effective against the cysticercoid stage *H. nana.*[51] Nitazoxanide 100 mg by mouth twice daily for 3 days for children 1 to 3 years of age, 200 mg by mouth twice daily for 3 days for children 4 to 11 years of age, and 500 mg by mouth twice daily for 3 days for older children is a reasonable alternative therapy; efficacy is approximately 75% to 82%.[36,202] Family members should be examined and treated if they are infected. Infection with *H. nana* rarely is severe and responds well to appropriate treatment.

Prevention

Transmission of *H. nana* infection could be prevented by treating infected subjects, improving personal hygiene, promoting the consumption of safe water, and disposal of human waste. Infected food handlers always should be treated and monitored to ensure that treatment has been successful. Stored food should be protected from rodents and insects.

HYMENOLEPIS DIMINUTA (RAT TAPEWORM)

Hymenolepis diminuta is a rat tapeworm that only rarely presents as a human infection. Adult worms are 20 to 90 cm long, and the eggs are round.[46,312] Children become infected after ingesting larva-infected insects. Infection often is asymptomatic, but abdominal discomfort and pruritus have been reported. Treatment is with praziquantel 25 mg/kg in a single oral dose or niclosamide.

SPARGANOSIS (INTERMEDIATE-STAGE *SPIROMETRA* SPECIES INFECTION)

Sparganosis is a zoonotic infection seen most frequently in eastern Asia.[119,161,312] Recent cases have been recognized from Africa.[70] It occurs when humans are infected with a metacestode larval stage of *Spirometra* spp. and is often caused by *Spirometra erinaceieuropaei* in Asia and *Spirometra mansonoides* in the Americas.[8]

Organism

Evidence indicates that the amorphous, thin, ribbon-like *Spargana* organisms recovered from human infections belong to the genus *Spirometra.*[119,312] The adult tapeworms are found in dogs, cats, and a variety of wild carnivores. Eggs passed in the feces of these definitive hosts hatch in fresh water. The embryo that emerges from the egg is ingested by a copepod, where it undergoes larval development as a procercoid. When a second intermediate host ingests the infected copepod, the larva develops into a sparganum (plerocercoid). The range of second intermediate hosts includes amphibians, reptiles, birds, and mammals. When the second intermediate host is eaten by the definitive host, the sparganum attaches to the intestinal mucosa and develops into the adult tapeworm. A rare form of sparganosis that buds, branches, and multiplies asexually to massive numbers in humans is called *Sparganum proliferum.*[185]

Transmission

Sparganosis can be acquired by ingestion of copepods infected with procercoids or fish, reptiles, or frogs containing plerocercoids. In parts of Asia, application of poultices of amphibian or reptile flesh to wounds or sores is a common practice, and children can be infected when the *Spargana* organisms migrate from the poultice into human tissues. Human sparganosis in the United States often is associated with drinking well water or untreated surface water that could contain the minute copepods containing the procercoid form. Transmission by ingestion of the raw or inadequately cooked flesh of second intermediate hosts has been demonstrated experimentally in humans. Animal sources such as snakes, frogs, chickens, and pigs have been incriminated in human infection. Asymptomatic cats, especially those living outdoors, are infected in some areas.[123,135,242]

Epidemiology

Human infection is not uncommon in Thailand.[161] It is also reported from China, Korea, Japan, India, Indonesia, the Philippines, Australia, Africa, Italy, South America, and the former Soviet Union.[119,159,312,313] With changes in lifestyle and environmental control, the rate of sparganum seropositivity among patients suspected of having parasitic disease in South Korea dropped from 2.6% in 1993 to 1.6% in 2006.[154] However, the infection still seems to be a bit less uncommon in North Korea.[262] In the United States, almost all reports have come from the southern or southeastern states and from Puerto Rico or were reported in persons who had been in these areas, but one infected child was reported from southern California.[44]

Pathology, Pathogenesis, and Clinical Manifestations

Ocular sparganosis, usually acquired by contact, may involve conjunctival, retroorbital, or palpebral tissues and cause conjunctivitis, periorbital and palpebral edema, exophthalmos, chemosis, and corneal ulceration.[119,312,313] Subcutaneous sparganosis is the most common form of the infection, with the trunk frequently being involved. The lesion usually is nodular. Tenderness and inflammation may be absent, intermittent, or constant. Some lesions are migratory. Eosinophils may or may not be present. Some infections have had an associated peripheral eosinophilia, but it is not a constant finding. Spargana have been identified in a wide range of other tissues. Sparganosis of the CNS may be associated with a variety of neurologic manifestations.[119,149,273,312,313] Brain imaging of patients with cerebral sparganosis shows edema and degeneration of cerebral white matter commonly with a "tunnel sign" of hypodensity and ring enhancement.[273] Sequential MRI has revealed migration of larva between various regions of the brain in some children.[16,111] The disease caused by *S. proliferum* consists of progressive replacement of host tissues by the multiplying organisms.

Diagnosis

The diagnosis may be suspected in persons with typical subcutaneous lesions and a suggestive epidemiologic background. Usually, however, the diagnosis is made during surgical removal of a painful or cosmetically disturbing lump without anticipation of the parasitic etiology. *Spargana* organisms vary considerably in width and length. They usually are several centimeters in length, whitish, and opaque, and they may have the grooved indentations on the anterior end that are precursors of the bothria, or suckers of the scolex, of the adult worm. Small portions of *Spargana* are difficult to distinguish grossly or microscopically from cysticerci and other less common larval cestodes. Neuroimaging may yield characteristic findings in cerebral sparganosis.[149,273] Performing an ELISA or serum and CSF antibody appears to be useful in endemic areas, but this test is not generally available.[312]

Treatment and Prevention

Surgical removal is the only known form of therapy. Stereotactic aspiration and microsurgery have been effective, but care to remove all larval material is essential.[62] Praziquantel has been used in some cases, but no convincing evidence of clinical activity exists. Filtration of water prevents the ingestion of copepods from wells or ponds. Proper cooking of meat eliminates second intermediate hosts as sources of infection. Educational effort should be made to warn of the dangers of applying raw flesh poultices in areas where it is a cultural practice.

ECHINOCOCCUS GRANULOSUS AND RELATED SPECIES (CYSTIC HYDATID DISEASE)

Humans may be infected with the larval stages of parasites of the genus *Echinococcus*.[18,19,47,48,71,72,136,251,325] The infection is acquired by the ingestion of ova from the feces of carnivorous definitive hosts. The disease in humans and other intermediate hosts is called hydatid disease and is characterized further according to the morphologic features of each species larval stage: cystic echinococcosis caused by *Echinococcus granulosus* sensu stricto and related organisms, alveolar echinococcosis caused by *Echinococcus multilocularis,* and polycystic echinococcosis caused by *Echinococcus vogeli* or *Echinococcus oligarthrus*. The prevalence of hydatid disease in markedly higher in adults than in children, and most pediatric cases present with cystic echinococcosis, which is the focus of this section of the chapter.[18,47,48,71,72,136,251]

Organisms

Cystic echinococcosis is caused by *E. granulosus* sensu lato. Genetic studies have demonstrated 10 separate genotypes grouped into different clusters that infect different intermediate and definitive hosts.[71,136,251,288,325] Significantly different strains are found in sheep, Tasmanian sheep, cattle, pigs, horses, camels, and cervids (e.g., deer, reindeer, moose, elk). Thus the genotypic clusters include *E. granulosus* sensu stricto (genotypes 1–3), *E. equinus* (genotype 4), *E. ortleppi* (genotype 5), and *E. canadensis* (genotypes 6–10).[6] Most human infections are caused by *E. granulosus* sensu stricto genotype 1 (the sheep strain). *E. orleppi* and *E. canadensis* have been reported to infect humans, with *E. canadensis* genotype 6 being the second most common genotype to infect humans. *E. equinus* is regarded as not infective to humans, and no cases have been reported.[6] The life cycles of the species of *Echinococcus* are similar, but the geographic distributions, types of hosts, and clinical and morphologic features of the parasites differ significantly. Adult tapeworms of *E. granulosus* sensu stricto are found in dogs. *E. canadensis* tapeworms infect primarily wolves, but dogs also may be infected. The adult tapeworm is only 3 to 8 mm long and has two to five segments. Dogs often are hosts to thousands of adult worms. When sheep or humans ingest eggs from the feces of infected dogs, the embryos hatch in the intestine and burrow through the intestinal wall to gain access to the portal circulation. The embryos that survive are able to develop in many tissues, but they do so most commonly in the liver or lungs, where they become the cystic larval structures called *hydatid cysts*. A hydatid cyst is composed of an outer laminated, acellular membrane that is lined by a thin, cellular germinal membrane. Spherical structures called *brood capsules* grow from the germinal membrane. Protoscolices develop within the brood capsules. Each protoscolex has suckers and hooks and the potential to become the scolex of an adult worm if it is eaten by a dog. Compression and reaction from growth of the cyst produce a "pericyst" of compact, collagen-rich host tissue around its exterior. In older cysts, so-called daughter cysts may develop within the primary cyst cavity.

Transmission

Humans acquire cystic hydatid disease by ingestion of ova shed by the definite host, typically dogs.[48,71,173,181,243,251] Close contact with dogs can result in infection because tapeworm eggs can be found on the dog's perianal hair, muzzle, and paws. Contaminated food, drink, or fomites (e.g., flies and other insects) may disseminate the eggs from dogs' feces. However, most cases occur in pastoral families and are associated with close contact with infected dogs.

Epidemiology

E. granulosus sensu stricto is found worldwide in most areas where sheep are raised.[18,48,71,136,173,181,251] Studies of the global burden of disease and economic impact of cystic hydatid disease suggest that the impact is significantly underestimated in contrast to other illnesses.[20] The disease is endemic in the sheep-raising areas of South America, the Middle East, the Mediterranean basin, China, and the former Soviet Union.[21,48,71,136,173,181,243,251] One of the highest morbidity rates is seen in rural Africans in Kenya and Uganda, where people live in close association with their dogs. The custom of feeding sheep viscera to sheepdogs maintains foci of infection. Up to 79% of stray dogs were tapeworm carriers in one study in Peru, and 100% of sheepdogs were infected in study from Libya.[25,162] In the United States, Basques in central California, Mormon ranchers in Utah, and Native Americans in Arizona and New Mexico have been infected. In Alaska and Canada, human infection usually is limited to Eskimos and Native Americans who have working dogs that are fed moose and reindeer viscera.[291] The strain found in this region often is manifested as giant pulmonary cysts.

Pathology and Pathogenesis

In cystic hydatid disease, the pathologic process is related to compression or displacement of the host's tissue.[71,207,251] Cyst growth is variable and depends on (1) the organism involved being slower in the liver than in the lung; (2) the *Echinococcus* species, with *E. canadensis* usually being slow growing; and (3) the age of the subject, with cyst growth being faster in younger individuals.[236] Rates of up to 4 to 5 cm per year have been reported, but growth may be more rapid in the lung. The cyst may exceed 35 cm in diameter in the abdominal cavity. When rupture or leakage of a cyst occurs, an allergic reaction caused by the antigenic cyst contents may develop. Cysts may calcify after many years, which usually signifies death of the parasite. Hydatid cysts may form foci for secondary bacterial infection causing liver and lung abscesses.

Clinical Manifestations

Most children with *E. granulosus* infection have a single unilocular cyst, but multiple cysts are seen in 15% to 30% of patients, usually in a single organ system.[71,207,251,325] The most common site of the cysts is in the liver. In clinical series, approximately one in five children with a pulmonary cyst also has a concurrent liver cyst, but the proportion outside the liver is lower in population-based screening.[60] Approximately 10% of cysts are found in sites other than the liver or lung, including the spleen, kidney, peritoneum, genitourinary tract, bone, muscles, heart, eye, and brain. *E. canadensis* in Canada and Alaska characteristically produces slowly growing pulmonary cysts.[71,207,251] CNS hydatid disease occurs much more commonly in children than in adults.[43,66,67,146,178,196] Bone cysts, which may be seen in preschool children, occur most frequently in vertebral and long bones.[207,251] Unlike cysts in other sites, bone cysts characteristically are multilocular and contain little fluid. Eye, bone, and brain cysts typically are small when they are discovered, whereas cysts in other sites may exceed 35 cm in diameter before being detected. Complications usually occur only if cysts become large, and compress or erode into adjacent structures. Cyst leakage or rupture is one of the most common complications and may result in seeding of body cavities with fertile protoscolices, local inflammatory reactions (e.g., pneumonitis), infection of the cyst cavity, and type 1 allergic reactions, including hypotension, urticaria, and eosinophilia. Rupture may occur spontaneously or secondary to trauma or surgery, but it generally is considered to be an uncommon complication of hydatid disease in children.

The wide spectrum of symptoms in cystic hydatid disease depends on the number, size, and location of the cysts.[71,207,251] Slowly growing cysts in liver or lung often are asymptomatic for years. Symptomatic intrahepatic cysts cause constant or intermittent right upper quadrant or epigastric pain, enlargement of the liver, or nausea and vomiting. Unruptured cysts rarely cause fever. Rupture of a cyst may be precipitated by a traumatic event and may cause a range of symptoms, including fever, abdominal pain, hypotension, and allergic manifestations, including eosinophilia, urticaria, and anaphylaxis. Rupture into the biliary tract may cause cholangitis with fever and right upper quadrant pain. Some children with hydatid disease also have retarded growth patterns.[172]

Intact pulmonary cysts typically do not cause symptoms.[71,207,251,261,295] Rupture or leakage, however, may cause cough, chest pain, dyspnea, hemoptysis, and a salty taste. Fever may be present, but it is often a marker for secondary bacterial infection. As many as one-third of pulmonary cysts rupture into the pleural space or into a bronchus. In the latter case, the patient may describe coughing up portions of the membranes, which may resemble grape skins, or noting a characteristic salty taste. Bone cysts are seen in patients with bone pain or pathologic fracture. Vertebral hydatid disease causes signs and symptoms of spinal cord and radicular compression; severe pain on palpation of the affected portion of the spine is characteristic. Of intracranial cysts, 50% to 75% are seen in children.[43,109,146,299] Increased intracranial pressure with headache, vomiting, and focal neurologic symptoms are common findings. Seizures also may occur.

Diagnosis

The diagnosis of cystic echinococcosis usually is suspected on the basis of clinical or radiologic findings plus a history of residence in an endemic area.[18-20] Physical examination rarely is definitive. Only half of patients with hepatic cysts have abnormal liver enzyme results. Eosinophilia typically is low grade or absent. The initial diagnosis of cystic hydatid disease often is based on imaging findings. An unruptured pulmonary hydatid cyst has a sharply demarcated, round or oval smooth border. In the lung, it has a homogeneous cannonball appearance and sometimes is surrounded by a layer of atelectatic lung.[71,207,251] After the cyst has ruptured into a bronchus, a crescent-shaped air layer may be seen that is virtually diagnostic. In addition to the arc of air between the parasite and the host cyst wall, air in the cyst lumen also may be present. The membrane of a collapsed cyst floating on the surface of the fluid in a ruptured pulmonary cyst has a characteristic "water lily" appearance.

Cysts in the liver usually are visualized easily and measured with ultrasonography, CT, or MRI. Ultrasound techniques are useful for defining most cysts within the abdomen and can differentiate fluid-filled cysts from solid tumors. Because ultrasonography is portable and relatively inexpensive, it has been the main technique used in epidemiologic studies and clinical cases in developing countries. A World Health Organization staging system has been developed to define management (Fig. 227.4).[9,234] Stage CL cysts are unilocular collections without a discrete wall and with uniform anechoic contents. This appearance is not specific for *Echinococcus*. Stage CE1 cysts have a dense wall and may have internal echoes. This so-called hydatid sand is caused by protoscolices within the cyst. CE2 cysts have internal septa or daughter cysts, forming honeycomb patterns that are highly characteristic of hydatid cysts. CE3 cysts may demonstrate detachment of the cyst wall or early collapse (CE3a) or a mixed image with defined cystic and solid lesions (CE3b). CE4 cysts demonstrate inhomogeneous material instead of a cyst cavity sometimes showing collapsed membranes. CE5 cysts demonstrate a thick rim of calcification. Radiographically apparent cyst wall calcification occurs only in liver or spleen cysts and generally takes more than 5 to 10 years to develop. Bone cysts typically produce radiolucencies without periosteal reaction. MRI offers little advantage over CT for the imaging of cysts except in the CNS and for demonstration of biliary fistulas.[126]

Fine-needle aspiration of cysts for establishment of the diagnosis can cause spillage of hydatid fluid, which may induce anaphylactic shock and possibly secondary cyst development. The percutaneous route has been used for both diagnosis and treatment, with few untoward events. A review of 765 PAIR (*p*ercutaneous *a*spiration, *i*ntroduction of scolicide, and *r*easpiration) procedures showed that anaphylaxis and spillage occurred in 0.5% in each case. However, 14% of the subjects had other complications that included fever, abscesses, and biliary fistulas.[77] The fluid obtained should be examined for evidence of protoscolices, hooks, or antigen.

Serologic tests can be useful in confirmation of the diagnosis.[71,207,251] Antibody tests using crude antigen of either *E. granulosus* or *E. multilocularis* tested by ELISA, indirect hemagglutination, and fluorescent antibody assays are positive in 50% to 90% of cases. False-negative results are more common in patients with pulmonary, brain, and splenic cysts. Commercial rapid tests for the detection of *Echinococcus* antibodies are available, but their sensitivity and specificity are low, especially in subjects with inactive liver cysts.[283] Because the tests available may cross-react with cysticercosis or other parasitic infections, positive results should be confirmed by a more specific test, either an immunoblot assay or a gel diffusion assay.

Treatment and Prognosis

The treatment of cystic echinococcosis is in evolution.[19,20,325] Surgery was the traditional treatment of choice for nearly all cases of cystic echinococcosis, but a range of different approaches have been accepted gradually, including surgery, antiparasitic chemotherapy, percutaneous drainage (e.g., PAIR), and "watch and wait."[20,208,229] Currently expert opinion suggests that treatment should vary on the basis of the location of the cyst or cysts, the nature and size of the cysts, the condition of the patient, and the available expertise, with surgery required by only a minority of cases. A conservative management (watch-and-wait approach) with regular follow-up of the patients is acceptable under some circumstance. For example, in a prospective study, only 10% of children with hepatic cysts detected in a population-based ultrasound survey required surgery during the subsequent 5 years.[60,152] In a cohort of subjects diagnosed with 47 inactive liver cysts (CE4 and CE5) managed with a watch-and-wait approach and followed for a median of 52 months,

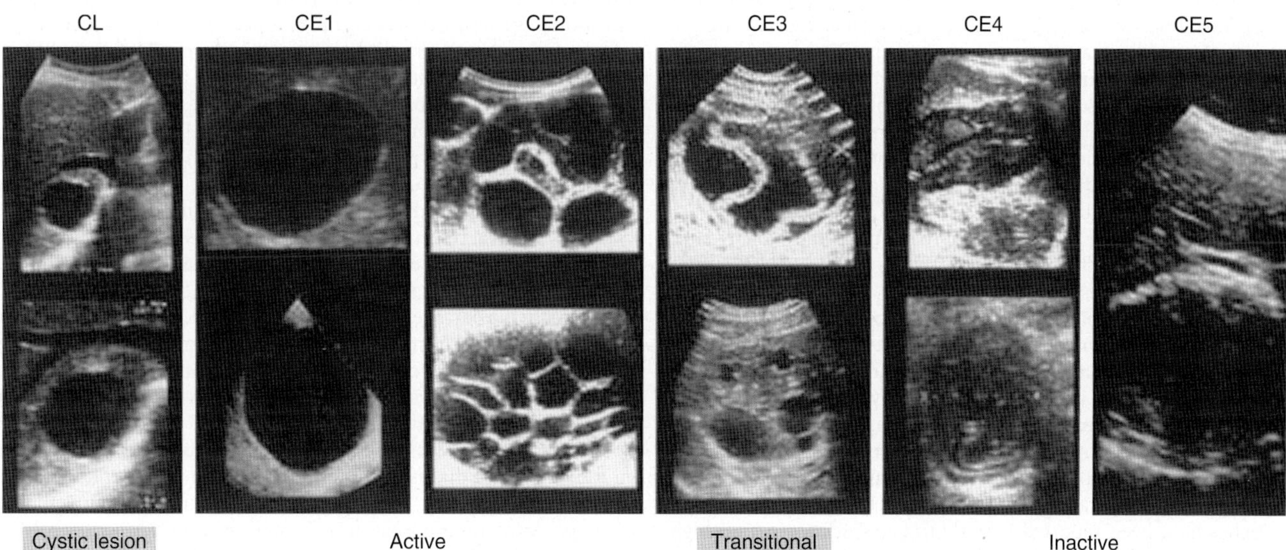

FIG. 227.4 Staging of echinococcosis. (Courtesy World Health Organization Informal Working Group on Echinococcosis: international classification of ultrasound images of cystic echinococcosis.)

only 1 case reactivated during the observation period.[208] The watch-and-wait approach was compared with albendazole treatment for 27 liver CE3b cysts. Although subjects treated with albendazole reached an inactive cyst stage faster than untreated subjects, the time to relapse of the cystic lesions was not different between the groups.[229]

The benzimidazoles albendazole and mebendazole have been used for chemotherapy.[71,76,80,145,152,251,278,294] Approximately one-third of hepatic cysts will resolve in response to benzimidazoles, and 30% to 50% will improve. Many of the residual cystic lesions considered treatment failures were shown subsequently to be inactive. The response to chemotherapy is better with smaller lesions. It is now thought to be the treatment of choice for small (<5 cm) CE1 and perhaps CE3a lesions.[20,71,251] Chemotherapy also has proved to be successful for treatment of small pulmonary cysts.[65] However, a high failure rate exists with chemotherapy alone for larger lesions in either the liver or the lung.[20] Albendazole is thought to be more effective than mebendazole. Albendazole typically is dosed at 10 to 15 mg/kg per day in two daily doses continued for 3 to 6 months. Side effects may include neutropenia, elevated liver enzymes, and alopecia. Prospective studies of surgically removed specimens show that protoscolices can remain viable for as long as 3 months, which is the minimum duration of chemotherapy.[15,76] Treatment failures have been successfully managed by further chemotherapy, PAIR, or surgery. In some cases, PAIR may demonstrate that protoscolices no longer are viable, even with persistent lesions. Because chemotherapy can be associated with relapses or treatment failure, children should receive follow-up imaging studies every 6 to 12 months for years after receiving chemotherapy. Chemotherapy also is an important adjunct to surgical therapy.

The PAIR technique offers a less invasive option than the traditional surgical approaches.[20,21,77,148,192,251,272,314,315] Results have been similar to those with surgery, but with fewer perioperative complications. PAIR is thought to be the treatment of choice for uncomplicated CE1 lesions larger than 5 cm and CE3a lesions. CE2 lesions can be treated with a modification of PAIR that employs a larger bore catheter and drainage combined with albendazole.[21,255] The treatment of CE3b lesions is usually surgical unless there is a reason precluding an invasive approach, in which case the watch-and-wait approach may be used. Although the data comparing different treatments are limited, PAIR was associated with similar efficacy and less morbidity than surgery in one randomized trial. PAIR should be performed after initiation of albendazole chemotherapy for at least 4 hours but preferably for several days. In a controlled trial, PAIR plus chemotherapy was superior to either chemotherapy or PAIR alone.[147,192] Aspiration generally should go through solid tissue (e.g., liver) rather than directly into the cyst (to limit spillage). The cyst fluid should be examined for protoscolices or hooks (to confirm the diagnosis). Before scolicidal agents are injected, the cyst fluid should be checked for bilirubin by dipstick, which suggests the presence of a biliary fistula. Injection of contrast medium to further characterize the biliary tract communication is necessary in positive cases because scolicidal agents can cause sclerosing cholangitis if they are injected into the biliary tract. Alcohol and hypertonic saline have been used as scolicidal agents in this procedure. Contrast material also is mildly scolicidal. Contraindications to PAIR include communication with the biliary tract, inaccessibility, superficial cysts, and cysts that are free in the abdomen, heart, brain, or spine.

Surgery has been the traditional approach to therapy for hydatid disease and remains the treatment of choice for complicated infections, lung lesions, and CE3b lesions.[20,71,207,251] The goal of surgery is to remove the entire cyst without spilling its contents. Rupture of the cyst contents at the time of surgery carries a risk for causing disseminated echinococcosis and a small risk for anaphylaxis occurring at the time of operation. Surgical approaches have included pericystectomy (removal of the entire cyst and a rim of surrounding tissues), resection of the involved organ, simple drainage, omentoplasty, and capitonnage. In general, the more radical procedures have been associated with fewer relapses, but at the cost of more perioperative complications. However, laparoscopic approaches have been reported recently to be associated with a high success rate and less morbidity.[26,69,165,315] Chemotherapy with albendazole with or without praziquantel is performed routinely.[12,76,251] With administration of chemotherapy, pressure within the cyst may be reduced, and removal of cyst membranes and contents will be facilitated. In addition, treatment decreases the likelihood of development of secondary cysts. With albendazole alone, cysts remain viable for as long as 3 months.[15] The preoperative administration of praziquantel combined with a benzimidazole has been suggested because of the scolicidal properties of praziquantel.[12] The practice of injecting the cyst with scolicidal drugs before removing it is associated with complications and is not thought to be necessary in the setting of preoperative and postoperative chemotherapy.[251]

Pulmonary cysts have been treated successfully surgically, medically, and with PAIR.[2,20,65,143,170,271] No controlled trials of these different strategies have been performed. However, retrospective series suggest that smaller cysts often respond to antiparasitic chemotherapy.[65] Larger cysts may be treated with surgery. *E. canadensis* from Alaska and Canada do not produce anaphylaxis on rupture, and pulmonary cysts spontaneously resolve after evacuating into bronchi. If the cyst wall remains in place after the patient has undergone chemotherapy or PAIR, residual parasite material can serve as a nidus for bacterial superinfections.[206] Thus many experts recommend against PAIR for pulmonary disease.[20]

The prognosis of hydatid disease varies widely from self-limited asymptomatic infection to fatal infection associated with rupture of the cyst. All of the modes of therapy are associated with relapse during the first few years of treatment. Thus careful follow-up is essential. With appropriate therapy, however, few cases are fatal.

Prevention

Control programs for cystic hydatid disease have met with variable success.[46,47,251] *E. granulosus* was eliminated from Iceland by banning home slaughter of sheep. Banning of home slaughter, education, arecoline purging of dogs, and treatment of infected dogs with praziquantel led to eradication in New Zealand and Tasmania. However, these eradication programs required significant resources and have been less successful elsewhere. A recombinant vaccine has proved to be highly effective in field studies but awaits implementation.[47] Other tools in developmental stages include coproantigen tests to detect infected dogs and improved therapy for ovine infection.

OTHER *ECHINOCOCCUS* SPECIES

Echinococcus multilocularis is the cause of alveolar hydatid disease.[71,136,144,207,251] Humans are an incidental host in a life cycle that typically involves foxes as definitive hosts (but also wolves and occasionally domestic dogs) and rodents as intermediate hosts. The larval parasite does not form a large cystic structure but grows by progressive external budding. The laminated membrane and host pericyst are thin. The larval mass slowly enlarges and replaces liver tissue much as a malignant neoplasm does. *E. multilocularis* is endemic in arctic and alpine areas, including western China, central Europe, and scattered foci in North America. In recent years, disease is emerging in much of central Europe. The larvae may invade contiguous structures and rarely metastasize. Human infection almost invariably involves the liver, but it may spread to adjacent tissues or metastasize to the brain. Because the larval mass grows slowly, with a typical latent period of 5 to 15 years before clinical presentation, clinical disease is a rare finding in children. Diagnosis involves imaging studies with serologic confirmation. Management requires surgical resection along with prolonged chemotherapy. Comprehensive reviews of epidemiology, clinical manifestations, diagnosis, and management are available.[17,71,136,144,207,251]

E. vogeli is a parasite of bush dogs and feral dogs in South America.[251] The intermediate hosts are rodents (i.e., pacas, agoutis, spiny rats). When humans are infected, the germinal membrane grows externally to form additional cysts, and septa develop within the original cyst. This manifestation is the "polycystic" variety of hydatid disease. A rare polycystic hydatid disease in humans has been attributed to *E. oligarthrus*, a fourth species that is found as adult tapeworms in wild felids such as pumas and jaguars. The intermediate hosts are the same as those for *E. vogeli*. Most infections occur in Central and South America. Polycystic hydatid disease is limited to South and Central America, where fewer than 100 human infections have been reported. Initial management should include administration of albendazole.

NEW REFERENCES SINCE THE SEVENTH EDITION

25. Buishi IE, Njoroge EM, Bouamra O, Craig PS. Canine echinococcosis in northwest Libya: assessment of coproantigen ELISA, and a survey of infection with analysis of risk-factors. *Vet Parasitol.* 2005;130:223-232.
29. Callacondo D, Garcia HH, Gonzales I, et al. High frequency of spinal involvement in patients with basal subarachnoid neurocysticercosis. *Neurology.* 2012;78:1394-1400.
31. Carpio A, Kelvin EA, Bagiella E, et al. Effects of albendazole treatment on neurocysticercosis: a randomised controlled trial. *J Neurol Neurosurg Psychiatry.* 2008;79:1050-1055.
32. Carrillo Mezo R, Lara Garcia J, Arroyo M, Fleury A. Relevance of 3D magnetic resonance imaging sequences in diagnosing basal subarachnoid neurocysticercosis. *Acta Trop.* 2015;152:60-65.
39. Chowdhary A, Bansal R, Singh K, Singh V. Ocular cysticercosis: a profile. *Trop Doct.* 2003;33:185-188.
49. Croker C, Reporter R, Mascola L. Use of statewide hospital discharge data to evaluate the economic burden of neurocysticercosis in Los Angeles County (1991–2008). *Am J Trop Med Hyg.* 2010;83:106-110.
51. de Castro Mde L, de Rezende GL. [Therapeutic efficacy of praziquantel and morphological changes in *Hymenolepis nana* eggs after its administration in 2 dosage schedules]. *Rev Inst Med Trop Sao Paulo.* 1985;27:40-45.
54. Del Brutto OH, Garcia HH. *Taenia solium* cysticercosis: The lessons of history. *J Neurol Sci.* 2015;359:392-395.
70. Eberhard ML, Thiele EA, Yembo GE, et al. Thirty-seven human cases of sparganosis from Ethiopia and South Sudan caused by *Spirometra* spp. *Am J Trop Med Hyg.* 2015;93:350-355.
82. Fujita M, Mahanty S, Zoghbi SS, et al. PET reveals inflammation around calcified *Taenia solium* granulomas with perilesional edema. *PLoS ONE.* 2013;8:e74052.
91. Garcia HH, Gonzales I, Lescano AG, et al. Efficacy of combined antiparasitic therapy with praziquantel and albendazole for neurocysticercosis: a double-blind, randomised controlled trial. *Lancet Infect Dis.* 2014;14:687-695.
92. Garcia HH, Gonzales I, Lescano AG, et al. Enhanced steroid dosing reduces seizures during antiparasitic treatment for cysticercosis and early after. *Epilepsia.* 2014;55:1452-1459.
98. Garcia HH, Lescano AG, Gonzales I, et al. Cysticidal efficacy of combined treatment with praziquantel and albendazole for parenchymal brain cysticercosis. *Clin Infect Dis.* 2016;62:1375-1379.
99. Garcia HH, Nash TE, Del Brutto OH. Clinical symptoms, diagnosis, and treatment of neurocysticercosis. *Lancet Neurol.* 2014;13:1202-1215.
102. Garcia HH, Rodriguez S, Friedland JS, Cysticercosis Working Group in P. Immunology of *Taenia solium* taeniasis and human cysticercosis. *Parasite Immunol.* 2014;36:388-396.
111. Gong C, Liao W, Chineah A, Wang X, Hou BL. Cerebral sparganosis in children: epidemiological, clinical and MR imaging characteristics. *BMC Pediatr.* 2012;12:155.
114. Gonzalez LM, Montero E, Puente S, et al. PCR tools for the differential diagnosis of *Taenia saginata* and *Taenia solium* taeniasis/cysticercosis from different geographical locations. *Diagn Microbiol Infect Dis.* 2002;42:243-249.
115. Govindappa SS, Narayanan JP, Krishnamoorthy VM, et al. Improved detection of intraventricular cysticercal cysts with the use of three-dimensional constructive interference in steady state MR sequences. *AJNR Am J Neuroradiol.* 2000;21:679-684.
117. Guo AJ, Liu K, Gong W, et al. Molecular identification of *Diphyllobothrium latum* and a brief review of diphyllobothriosis in China. *Acta Parasitol.* 2012;57: 293-296.
121. Hancock K, Pattabhi S, Whitfield FW, et al. Characterization and cloning of T24, a *Taenia solium* antigen diagnostic for cysticercosis. *Mol Biochem Parasitol.* 2006;147:109-117.
161. Liu Q, Li MW, Wang ZD, Zhao GH, Zhu XQ. Human sparganosis, a neglected food borne zoonosis. *Lancet Infect Dis.* 2015;15:1226-1235.
162. Lopera L, Moro PL, Chavez A, et al. Field evaluation of a coproantigen enzyme-linked immunosorbent assay for diagnosis of canine echinococcosis in a rural Andean village in Peru. *Vet Parasitol.* 2003;117:37-42.
174. Mejia R, Nash TE. Corticosteroid withdrawal precipitates perilesional edema around calcified *Taenia solium* cysts. *Am J Trop Med Hyg.* 2013;89:919-923.
176. Mirdha BR, Samantray JC. *Hymenolepis nana:* a common cause of paediatric diarrhoea in urban slum dwellers in India. *J Trop Pediatr.* 2002;48:331-334.
182. Moyano LM, Saito M, Montano SM, et al. Neurocysticercosis as a cause of epilepsy and seizures in two community-based studies in a cysticercosis-endemic region in Peru. *PLoS Negl Trop Dis.* 2014;8:e2692.
183. Muehlenbachs A, Bhatnagar J, Agudelo CA, et al. Malignant transformation of *Hymenolepis nana* in a human host. *N Engl J Med.* 2015;373:1845-1852.
190. Nash TE, Pretell J, Garcia HH. Calcified cysticerci provoke perilesional edema and seizures. *Clin Infect Dis.* 2001;33:1649-1653.
195. Nicoletti A, Bartoloni A, Reggio A, et al. Epilepsy, cysticercosis, and toxocariasis: a population-based case-control study in rural Bolivia. *Neurology.* 2002;58:1256-1261.
198. O'Neal S, Noh J, Wilkins P, et al. *Taenia solium* Tapeworm infection, Oregon, 2006–2009. *Emerg Infect Dis.* 2011;17:1030-1036.
199. O'Neal SE, Flecker RH. Hospitalization frequency and charges for neurocysticercosis, United States, 2003-2012. *Emerg Infect Dis.* 2015;21:969-976.
203. Osorio G, Daiber A, Donckaster R, et al. [Severe megaloblastic anemia due to *Diphyllobotrium latum.* First case identified in Chile]. *Rev Med Chil.* 1974;102:700-703.
204. Otte WM, Singla M, Sander JW, Singh G. Drug therapy for solitary cysticercus granuloma: a systematic review and meta-analysis. *Neurology.* 2013;80:152-162.
206. Pathogenesis of the tapeworm anaemia. *Br Med J.* 1976;2:1028.
208. Piccoli L, Tamarozzi F, Cattaneo F, et al. Long-term sonographic and serological follow-up of inactive echinococcal cysts of the liver: hints for a "watch-and-wait" approach. *PLoS Negl Trop Dis.* 2014;8:e3057.
229. Rinaldi F, De Silvestri A, Tamarozzi F, et al. Medical treatment versus "watch and wait" in the clinical management of CE3b echinococcal cysts of the liver. *BMC Infect Dis.* 2014;14:492.
235. Romero-Cabello R, Godinez-Hana L, Gutierrez-Quiroz M. [Clinical aspects of hymenolepiasis in pediatrics]. *Bol Med Hosp Infant Mex.* 1991;48:101-105.
236. Romig T, Zeyhle E, Macpherson CN, Rees PH, Were JB. Cyst growth and spontaneous cure in hydatid disease. *Lancet.* 1986;1:861.
237. Romo ML, Wyka K, Carpio A, et al. The effect of albendazole treatment on seizure outcomes in patients with symptomatic neurocysticercosis. *Trans R Soc Trop Med Hyg.* 2015;109:738-746.
239. Rozas M, Bohle H, Sandoval A, et al. First molecular identification of *Diphyllobothrium dendriticum* plerocercoids from feral rainbow trout *(Oncorhynchus mykiss)* in Chile. *J Parasitol.* 2012;98:1220-1226.
246. Samkari A, Kiska DL, Riddell SW, et al. *Dipylidium caninum* mimicking recurrent enterobius vermicularis (pinworm) infection. *Clin Pediatr (Phila).* 2008;47:397-399.
247. Sampaio JL, de Andrade VP, Lucas Mda C, et al. Diphyllobothriasis, Brazil. *Emerg Infect Dis.* 2005;11:1598-1600.
248. Santos FL, de Faro LB. The first confirmed case of *Diphyllobothrium latum* in Brazil. *Mem Inst Oswaldo Cruz.* 2005;100:585-586.
249. Sarti E, Schantz PM, Avila G, et al. Mass treatment against human taeniasis for the control of cysticercosis: a population-based intervention study. *Trans R Soc Trop Med Hyg.* 2000;94:85-89.
250. Sarti-Gutierrez EJ, Schantz PM, Lara-Aguilera R, Gomez Dandoy H, Flisser A. *Taenia solium* taeniasis and cysticercosis in a Mexican village. *Trop Med Parasit.* 1988;39:194-198.
254. Scheel CM, Khan A, Hancock K, et al. Serodiagnosis of neurocysticercosis using synthetic 8-kD proteins: comparison of assay formats. *Am J Trop Med Hyg.* 2005;73:771-776.
263. Singh G, Prabhakar S, Ito A, Cho SY, Qiu D-C. *Taenia solium* taeniasis and cysticercosis in Asia. In: Singh G, Prabhakar S, eds. *Taenia solium cysticercosis: from basic to clinical science.* Oxford: CABI Publishing; 2002.
269. Singhi P, Singhi S. Neurocysticercosis in children. *Indian J Pediatr.* 2009;76:537-545.
274. Sorvillo F, Wilkins P, Shafir S, Eberhard M. Public health implications of cysticercosis acquired in the United States. *Emerg Infect Dis.* 2011;17:1-6.
280. Suarez Hernandez M, Bonet Couce E, Diaz Gonzalez M, Ocampo Ruiz I, Vidal Garcia I. [Epidemiological study on *Hymenolepis nana* infection in Ciego de Avila Province, Cuba]. *Bol Chil Parasitol.* 1998;53:31-34.
282. Talukdar B, Saxena A, Popli VK, Choudhury V. Neurocysticercosis in children: clinical characteristics and outcome. *Ann Trop Paediatr.* 2002;22:333-339.
283. Tamarozzi F, Covini I, Mariconti M, et al. Comparison of the diagnostic accuracy of three rapid tests for the serodiagnosis of hepatic cystic echinococcosis in humans. *PLoS Negl Trop Dis.* 2016;10:e0004444.
308. Wilkins PP, Allan JC, Verastegui M, et al. Development of a serologic assay to detect *Taenia solium* taeniasis. *Am J Trop Med Hyg.* 1999;60:199-204.
309. Willcocks B, McAuliffe GN, Baird RW. Dwarf tapeworm *(Hymenolepis nana):* characteristics in the Northern Territory 2002-2013. *J Paediatr Child Health.* 2015;51:982-987.
316. Yoeli M, Most H, Hammond J. Scheinesson GP. Parasitic infections in a closed community. Results of a 10-year survey in Willowbrook State School. *Trans R Soc Trop Med Hyg.* 1972;66:764-776.
319. Zee C-S, Segall HD, Destain S, Ahmadi J, Apuzzo MLJ. MRI of intraventricular cysticercosis: surgical implication. *J Comput Assist Tomogr.* 1993;17:932-939.
320. Zhang W, Che F, Tian S, Shu J, Zhang X. Molecular identification of *Diphyllobothrium nihonkaiense* from 3 human cases in Heilongjiang Province with a brief literature review in China. *Korean J Parasitol.* 2015;53:683-688.
321. Zhao BC, Jiang HY, Ma WY, et al. Albendazole and corticosteroids for the treatment of solitary cysticercus granuloma: a network meta-analysis. *PLoS Negl Trop Dis.* 2016;10:e0004418.

The full reference list for this chapter is available at ExpertConsult.com.

228 Foodborne Trematodes

Miguel M. Cabada • Philip R. Fischer • A. Clinton White Jr

An estimated 56 million people are infected with foodborne trematodes, referred to as flukes. Almost 8 million have heavy infections.[42] Approximately 10% of the world's population is at risk for acquiring a trematode infection.

Flukes are flatworms (members of the phylum Platyhelminthes and of the subphylum Trematoda) (Figs. 228.1 to 228.3).[58,75,103] The adult forms of foodborne trematodes are flat and leaf shaped, with an oral and a ventral sucker for feeding and attachment, respectively, and a bifurcated, blind-ended gastrointestinal tract. Foodborne trematodes are hermaphroditic, producing operculated eggs that typically are passed in host feces. Eggs possess an operculum at one end, the opening through which a ciliated larva or miracidium will hatch. Specific species of freshwater snails are intermediate hosts for trematodes and are infected by either direct penetration by the ciliated larva or by ingestion of the unhatched egg. Complex larval development and multiplication occur within the snail host, with large numbers of larvae called cercariae ultimately produced. In most trematode life cycles, the cercariae emerge from the snails and swim about until they are ingested by or attach to the second intermediate host, which may be fish, crustaceans, mollusks, or aquatic vegetation. After attachment occurs, the larvae develop into metacercariae within protective cyst walls. Humans are typically infected by ingestion of the metacercariae. In Southeast Asia and the western Pacific region, foodborne trematodiasis has become an emerging public health problem, associated with the growth of aquaculture.[41,57] Many of the medically important flukes have a wide range of definitive hosts. Diagnosis of fluke infections typically is accomplished by examination of fecal specimens (or sputum in the case of *Paragonimus* spp.) for characteristic ova. Immunodiagnostic tests are available to aid in establishing the diagnosis of some flukes and are becoming the preferred method of diagnosis for certain species. Common liver, intestinal, and lung flukes are reviewed in this chapter.

LIVER FLUKES

Clonorchiasis and Opisthorchiasis

Three similar trematodes of the genus *Opisthorchis* infect the bile ducts of humans.[41,43,58,75] Although the name *Opisthorchis sinensis* is proper parasitologically, this organism is commonly referred to as *Clonorchis sinensis,* and the name of the infection, clonorchiasis, is well entrenched in the clinical literature. *Opisthorchis viverrini* and *Opisthorchis felineus* have similar life cycles and produce similar lesions and illnesses in humans.

Organisms

The adult flukes measure 4 to 25 mm in length and 2 to 5 mm in breadth and have an anterior oral sucker. The life cycle involves primarily humans, but dogs and cats also act as definitive hosts. Freshwater snails and fish participate as first and second intermediate hosts. In the definitive hosts, parasites are found mainly in the intrahepatic biliary ducts and occasionally in the extrahepatic and pancreatic ducts. *Opisthorchis* spp. and *Clonorchis* spp. produce small operculated eggs (30 × 16 μm), which are nearly identical morphologically. The ova are shed into bile and excreted in feces. The snail host ingests the embryonated eggs, and after a complex cycle of asexual reproduction, free-swimming cercariae emerge 6 to 8 weeks later. The cercariae encyst under the scales or in the muscle of freshwater fish as metacercariae. Humans and other definitive hosts are infected by ingestion of raw, inadequately cooked, or pickled fish infected with metacercariae. The larvae excyst in the intestine and migrate to the intrahepatic bile ducts through the ampulla of Vater. Juvenile flukes travel along the biliary tree against bile flow and attach to the bile duct epithelium with their suckers. Adult worms begin producing eggs approximately 4 weeks after ingestion and can survive for as long as 30 years.

Transmission and Epidemiology

Transmission is through the ingestion of raw or inadequately cooked freshwater fish infected with metacercariae. Cats, dogs, civet cats, and other fish-eating mammals serve as definitive hosts in nature. The expansion of aquaculture in China and other Asian countries and poor sanitation practices allow the contact of human feces with snails in ponds where fish are raised. This situation increases the risk for parasite transmission and hinders control efforts.[38,46]

An estimated 600 million people are at risk for *O. sinensis* infection, 67 million for *O. viverrini,* and 12 million for *O. felineus.*[42] *O. sinensis* is endemic in China, Japan, Korea, Taiwan, and Vietnam. Some of the highest infection rates are reported in endemic areas of China (16%) and Vietnam (26%).[49] *O. viverrini* is endemic to Thailand, Lao People's Democratic Republic, Vietnam, and Cambodia. In northern Thailand, infection rates may reach 60%, and it is estimated that 7 million residents are infected in that area.[98] *O. felineus* is endemic in central Siberia and in eastern and southeastern Europe. Sporadic infections with *O. felineus* have been reported from several Asian countries. Also, the infection is an emerging problem in Mediterranean countries, especially in Italy, where outbreaks of the disease have been reported among local populations and travelers.[88,106] Eating habits and snail presence are the major determinants for the geographic distribution of the infection. The three species of *Opisthorchis* follow similar patterns of infection in most areas. The lowest prevalence and intensity of infection is found in the youngest age groups and in women; whereas intensity of egg excretion often increases with age and male gender.[95] The prevalence peaks in older persons, as shown in studies in China and Korea.[27,123]

Pathology and Pathogenesis

The epithelium of infected bile ducts reacts with desquamation, adenomatous hyperplasia, and metaplasia of goblet cells, accompanied by an increase in mucus production. The pathogenesis of the hepatobiliary damage may be due to the induction of an immunologic response in the host by mechanical action and secreted products from the flukes. Fibrosis and ductal dilation and obstruction are the consequence of the inflammatory reaction elicited by the parasites. Bile stasis in turn may lead to bacterial cholangitis and further inflammation in the bile ducts. The severity of the changes relates to the intensity of infection, host susceptibility, and number of reinfections. Chronic infection may lead to extensive periportal and periductal fibrosis, a process in which interleukin-6–mediated responses seemed to play a key role.[101,103,104]

The infection is a significant risk factor for cholangiocarcinoma in endemic areas.[102,103] Experiments in hamsters have shown that repeated infection with *O. viverrini* induces overproduction of nitric oxide, which may play a significant role in the development of cholangiocarcinoma through oxidative and nitrosyl DNA damage.[87] In addition, a granulin-like growth factor in excretory and secretory products from *O. viverrini* induces proliferation of fibroblasts.[71,107] The excretory and secretory products induce the production of retinoblastoma and cyclin D1 proteins in the hamster model, both of which have been implicated in the mechanism of *Opisthorchis*-induced cholangiocarcinoma.[14] *O. viverrini*

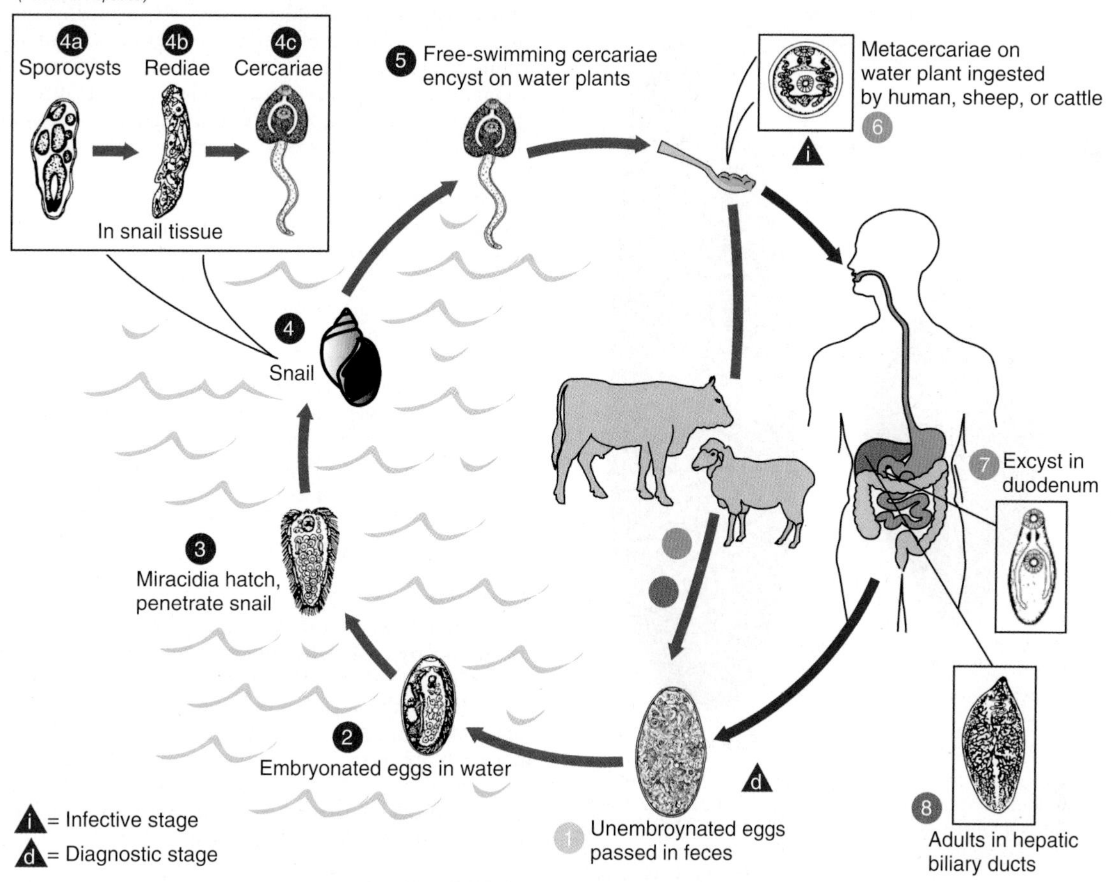

FIG. 228.1 Life cycle of foodborne trematodes including intestinal flukes (*Echinostoma, Fasciolopsis, Heterophyes*), a liver fluke (*Opisthorchis sinensis*), and a lung fluke (*Paragonimus*). (From Keiser J, Utzinger J. Food-borne trematodiasis. *Clin Micro Rev.* 2009;22:466-483.)

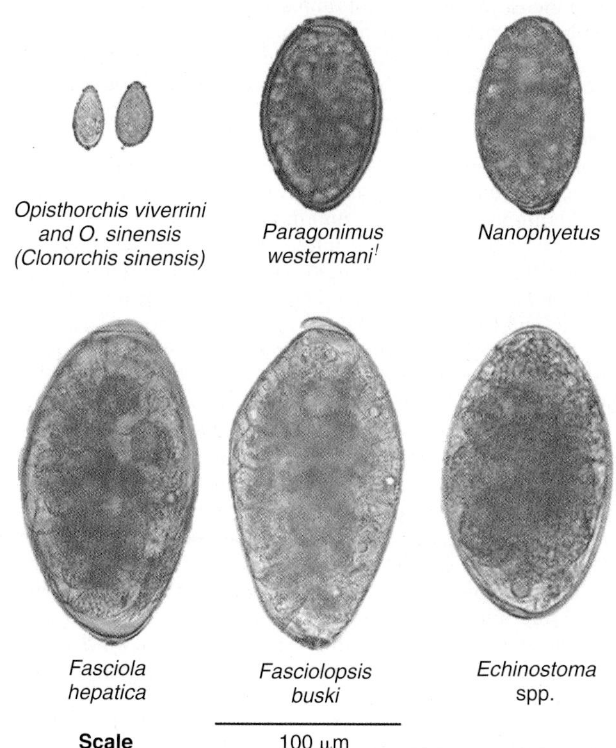

FIG. 228.2 Foodborne trematode ova found in human stool. (Modified from http://www.dpd.cdc.gov/dpdx/HTML/MorphologyTables.htm.)

infections involve the gallbladder and may lead to complications such as gallbladder sludge, cholecystitis, and formation of gallstones.[76,77] The parasites may be found in the pancreatic ducts, where reactions of the epithelium are similar to those in the bile duct. Pancreatitis occurs infrequently in these liver fluke infections and is usually mild.

Clinical Manifestations

In endemic areas, infections may begin early in life and often are asymptomatic.[77,103] The occurrence of symptoms correlates with the intensity of infection. Patients with higher fluke burdens are more likely than those with lower burdens to have right upper quadrant pain, abdominal discomfort, and jaundice. They are also more likely to have abnormalities on ultrasound examination, such as intrahepatic bile duct dilation and periductal liver fibrosis.[95] Other findings may include weakness, malaise, and liver enlargement. A community-based study showed significant improvement of symptoms, laboratory test results, and ultrasound abnormalities after treatment of infected subjects.[89]

An acute febrile syndrome starting 2 to 3 weeks after exposure has been reported with *O. sinensis* and *O. felineus* infections.[43,103] In *O. felineus* outbreaks, up to 80% of those infected may develop acute symptoms of infections and a cholestatic pattern in liver enzymes elevation.[109] The symptoms include fever, malaise, anorexia, diarrhea, and tender hepatomegaly. Eosinophilia, which is not as common in the chronic phase, is typically found during the acute illness.

Complications are more likely to occur in heavy infections. Relapsing cholangitis, cholecystitis, bilirubin gallstones, and pancreatitis all have been associated with infection.[76,95] Clonorchiasis has been cited as a cause of pancreatitis in individuals from endemic areas.[61] *O. viverrini* and *O. sinensis* are considered carcinogenic to humans and have been included in the World Health Organization list as group I carcinogens.[49]

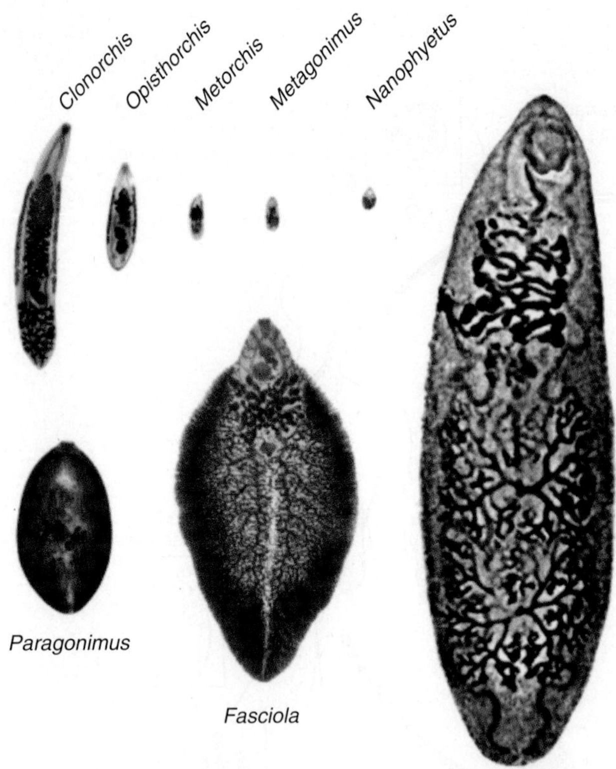

FIG. 228.3 Adult worms of foodborne trematodes. This is a threefold magnification of selected adult flukes illustrating their relative sizes. Actual lengths: *Nanophyetus salmincola,* 0.8–2.5 mm; *Opisthorchis viverrini,* 5–10 mm; *Paragonimus westermani,* 7–16 mm; *Fasciola,* 20–30 mm; and *Fasciolopsis,* 20–75 mm. (From Mahanty S, MacLean JD, Cross JH. *Liver, Pathogens, and Practice.* 3rd ed. Philadelphia: Saunders; 2011:854-867.)

O. viverrini and *O. sinensis* are associated with cholangiocarcinoma in adults, and the former is presumed to be responsible for more than 60% of liver tumors in northeastern Thailand.[40]

Diagnosis

Symptoms of acute infection may develop 3 to 4 weeks before eggs appear in the stool. Immunologic tests are useful to establish the diagnosis during this phase. Antibody-based tests are in use in some endemic areas but suffer from high rates of cross-reactions with antibodies to other parasites.[53,64,103] The sensitivity and specificity vary depending on the antigens used. Enzyme-linked immunosorbent assay (ELISA) using excretory and secretory products performs better than crude antigen ELISA, but cost precludes widespread use.[30,52] Demonstration of *O. viverrini* antigen in stool using a monoclonal antibody–based ELISA appeared to be specific and highly sensitive.[53,97,103] A novel urine antigen test for the diagnosis of opisthorchiasis has proved to be more sensitive than stool egg concentration tests, but further evaluation of the test specificity is needed.[117]

In chronic infections, eggs are evident on fecal microscopy examination. The Kato Katz test is widely used but lacks sensitivity, especially in patients with very low parasite burdens. Concentration techniques such as the formalin-ether test are more sensitive than the Kato Katz test.[8,41,43] Microscopy is useful in the clinical setting and in epidemiologic studies because it provides information regarding intensity of infection. Nonetheless, microscopic differentiation of *O. viverrini* and *O. sinensis* eggs is not easy. In addition, differentiation of these eggs from eggs of small heterophyid flukes is also difficult. Polymerase chain reaction (PCR)-based tests have shown promising results for the diagnosis of *O. viverrini* and *O. sinensis.*[62,93] The loop-mediated isothermal amplification test, based on DNA polymerase with strand displacement at a constant temperature, may be even more sensitive.[5,17,49,67]

Imaging studies may aid in the diagnosis of these flukes. Ultrasound findings include intrahepatic bile duct dilation, increased periductal echogenicity, and gallbladder sludge.[28,76] Cholangiography often shows multiple cystic dilations of the ducts, elliptic or filamentous filling defects within the peripheral intrahepatic ducts, and intrahepatic duct haziness.[29] A combination of large cystic dilations and small cystic ectasias or mulberry-like dilations is considered diagnostic. The adult worms also may be visible on endoscopic retrograde cholangiopancreatography.

Treatment and Prognosis

All three *Opisthorchis* infections respond well to treatment with praziquantel.[41,43,73,103] The recommended individual dose is 25 mg/kg given three times a day for 2 days. A single dose of 40 mg/kg also can be used, especially in control programs. At the recommended doses, praziquantel cures more than 80% of infected people.[73] Side effects of headache and dizziness are common occurrences. Treatment may decrease the risk for development of cholangiocarcinoma in those infected because regression of the bile duct lesions has been documented after praziquantel administration. Preliminary studies suggest that there may be efficacy for tribendimidine.[100] Two recent parallel dose-ranging phase II trials with tribendimidine for the treatment of *O. viverrini* showed that doses of 100 mg or higher were highly efficacious and safe among children (cure rate 98%) and adults (cure rate 77%) with light infections.[94]

Prevention

The main barriers to prevention are deep-seated eating habits of raw or improperly cooked fish in endemic areas.[118] Thus preventing contamination of fish ponds with human stool and decreasing the snail population in these settings helps decrease the prevalence of fish-borne fluke infections. An approach in which infected humans and other mammals are treated, sanitation is improved to avoid contamination of fishponds with raw human sewage, and health-promotion activities are carried out to decrease raw fish consumption is likely to have an impact on the incidence of infection.[98]

Fascioliasis

Fascioliasis is a parasitic disease caused by the flukes *Fasciola hepatica* and *Fasciola gigantica.* With 91 million people at risk for acquiring infection, human fascioliasis is an important public health problem with an increasing incidence of human cases in 51 countries.[16,41,42,75,81] Fascioliasis is primarily a zoonosis of ungulates (e.g., cattle and sheep). Although humans are considered an incidental host, the epidemiology of the disease is driven by human infection in hyperendemic areas.

Organisms

Fascioliasis is caused by two foodborne trematodes from the genus *Fasciola, F. hepatica* and *F. gigantica. F. hepatica* adult worms measure up to 30 mm in length and 13 mm in width. *F. gigantica* measures up to 75 mm.[75,103] During chronic infection adult parasites reside in the bile ducts, where eggs are produced. They reach the intestine through the bile and are excreted in feces. Eggs measure 130 µm in length and 90 µm in width and are indistinguishable from those of *Fasciolopsis buski*, an intestinal fluke. After maturing in water for several days, the ciliated miracidium hatches and penetrates the freshwater snail host, where it undergoes a complex cycle of asexual multiplication. Cercariae leave the snail and encyst on freshwater vegetation, including watercress and alfalfa. These encysted metacercariae initiate infection when the mammalian host ingests the raw aquatic vegetation or water contaminated with metacercariae. The metacercariae excyst in the intestine, and the larvae penetrate the intestinal wall and migrate from the peritoneal cavity to the liver. The developing worms penetrate the liver capsule and slowly burrow through the parenchyma to the bile ducts, where they mature into the adult worms. Adult *Fasciola* attach to the bile ducts epithelium causing inflammation and ulceration, which facilitates feeding on the host blood.[105] The life span of the adult fluke in humans ranges from 9 to 13 years.

Transmission and Epidemiology

Epidemiologic studies suggest that human *Fasciola* infection is transmitted through ingestion of infected raw aquatic plants, such as watercress and alfalfa, and by drinking untreated water with metacercariae.[58,78,81] Herbivorous mammals, such as sheep, cattle, goats, and camelids, act as definitive hosts in nature. Fascioliasis has a worldwide distribution, with human infection reported from at least 51 countries in South America, the Caribbean, Africa, and Asia.[81] The number of human cases is estimated between 2.6 million and 17 million, with more than half of the burden of infection reported from the Andean region and the Caribbean.[42] More recent data suggest that those studies may have significantly underestimated the burden of disease. For example, reports from Bolivia and Peru showed a prevalence as high as 70% in some hyperendemic areas.[16] The highest fascioliasis prevalence in the Andean region is observed in children, whereas in the rest of the world the infection prevalence is more evenly distributed among different age groups. Fascioliasis is emerging as a serious public health problem in Vietnam, with thousands of cases diagnosed in recent years.[81,103,108] Similarly, outbreaks have occurred in Iran, with more than 17,000 clinical cases.[47,91,92]

Pathology and Pathogenesis

Fascioliasis has an acute phase caused by juvenile flukes that migrate through the liver parenchyma and a chronic phase caused by the adult flukes that start egg production in the biliary tract. The pathogenesis of acute fascioliasis is related to direct liver damage caused by the migrating flukes and to the inflammatory reaction triggered by the fluke antigens. Linear necrotic lesions containing eosinophils form as flukes progress through the liver parenchyma. Flukes that die before reaching the bile ducts may produce necrotic cavities that eventually evolve into fibrous scar tissue. During the chronic stage, adult worms in the bile ducts cause inflammation and adenomatous changes in biliary epithelium, leading to duct thickening and dilation. Ductal and periductal fibrosis occurs. The gallbladder and extrahepatic ducts may be invaded and undergo similar inflammatory and fibrotic reactions. Adult worms may migrate back into the liver parenchyma through eroded biliary epithelium and cause formation of abscesses. Liver cirrhosis has been described in severe forms of fascioliasis. The inflammation associated with infection is probably associated with the anemia and weight loss that occurs with fascioliasis.

Clinical Manifestations

It is estimated that 15% of fascioliasis cases have high-intensity infections. As with other helminthes, those with a heavy burden of parasites are more likely to be symptomatic.[42] Even those considered asymptomatic may suffer from anemia.[72] Thus approximately 85% of *Fasciola* infections may remain subclinical and undiagnosed. Symptoms appear approximately 4 to 6 weeks after infection. The duration of this latent period depends on host response and the intensity of infection. The acute phase is characterized by right upper quadrant or generalized abdominal pain, tender hepatomegaly, fever, and anemia, typically associated with marked eosinophilia.[6,12,43,56] Sweating, dizziness, wheezing, and urticaria may occur. This stage lasts 1 to 3 months. The chronic form of the disease is associated with symptoms of biliary system obstruction. These symptoms frequently are identical to those of gallbladder disease, cholangitis, and pancreatitis caused by nonparasitic conditions. Elevation in alkaline phosphatase levels is a common manifestation.[6,12] Heavy and repeated infections eventually may cause liver damage sufficient to produce cirrhosis. Eosinophilia is not uncommon in chronic infections but is usually low grade. Juvenile flukes that fail to migrate into the liver may wander about and cause ectopic fascioliasis. The most common ectopic localization of immature *F. hepatica* flukes is in the subcutaneous tissues of the thorax, back, and extremities but also has been observed in lungs, heart, brain, and intestinal wall.[103] Blancas-Torres and colleagues reviewed a large series of fascioliasis patients (37 acute and 240 chronic) admitted to a hospital in Peru. A significant finding among these patients was the prevalence of weight loss (40%) and anemia (30%).[12] Severe acute disease may follow massive exposure and present with fever, eosinophilia, subcapsular hematoma, and tracks on imaging studies.[79]

Diagnosis

The acute manifestations of human fascioliasis may precede the appearance of eggs in the stool by 7 to 12 weeks. The triad of fever, abdominal pain, and eosinophilia, combined with compatible exposures, helps to suggest the diagnosis. Multiple immunodiagnostic tests are available to detect *Fasciola* during the acute phase of infection. Differences in sensitivity vary according to the antigens and antibodies used. The Fas2 ELISA test has a sensitivity of 92% and a specificity of 83%.[35] A commercially available sandwich ELISA using excretory-secretory antigens had a sensitivity and specificity of more than 95% when tested using serum of chronically infected individuals.[112] Serologic tests are also useful in the diagnosis of ectopic fascioliasis.

During chronic infection, *Fasciola* eggs may be detected in the stool. The Kato Katz and the rapid sedimentation tests are commonly used for microscopy diagnosis of fascioliasis, with the former being a quantitative test and the latter being significantly more sensitive.[8,54] Because of the inconsistent egg production and intrinsic low sensitivity of microscopy testing, multiple stool specimens are often required. False-positive stool examination results may occur if the patient recently ingested raw infected liver containing *Fasciola* eggs. Serum and stool antigen tests are available for diagnosis in veterinary medicine, and studies in humans suggest that these tests are highly sensitive and specific, but no commercial versions for human use are available[16,31,111] PCR-based tests are at least as sensitive as coproantigen tests and may detect the infection as early.[90] In addition, they have the potential to differentiate *Fasciola* species. PCR targeting the ITS-2 region of the ribosomal DNA gene has shown the highest sensitivity and specificity. A loop-mediated isothermal amplification test has been used to successfully detect *Fasciola* DNA with 10^4 times more sensitivity than conventional PCR in laboratory specimens.[3] The loop-mediated isothermal amplification test could also differentiate *F. hepatica* from *F. gigantica*.[3] However, no PCR-based test is available commercially for the diagnosis of fascioliasis in humans, and implementation of these in the traditional laboratory formats is unlikely in endemic areas.

Adult flukes may be seen on ultrasonography and appear as curvilinear lucent areas in the contrast medium in cholangiography. Endoscopic retrograde cholangiopancreatography may directly visualize the adult flukes, which are leaf shaped and bile stained. Eggs also may be identified in bile aspirates by microscopy. Radiologic imaging of the liver may demonstrate slowly evolving lesions, including track lines, small abscesses, and subcapsular hematomas.[21,34,56,65,80]

Treatment and Prognosis

Unlike other trematode infections, fascioliasis is resistant to praziquantel. The drug of choice is triclabendazole at a dose of 10 mg/kg with a meal once or twice in 24 hours. The formulation manufactured for human use as Egaten is not approved by the US Food and Drug Administration and is only available through the Centers for Disease Control and Prevention under an investigational protocol in the United States. Triclabendazole (Fasinex) has been used for many years by veterinarians for treatment of livestock in endemic areas. Anecdotally, it has been used safely in humans. Triclabendazole has been used successfully in a variety of open clinical trials in adults and children for both acute and chronic fascioliasis.[79,113] The drug is effective against both migrating flukes and established infections by adult parasites. However, resistance is a well-established problem in the livestock industry, with widespread resistance reported from several countries like Ireland, Australia, Spain, Argentine, and Peru.[60] Although not well studied and likely underreported, triclabendazole resistance is starting to emerge in human cases. Winkelhagen and colleagues[115] reported a possible case of triclabendazole resistance in an elderly sheep farmer who failed several courses of treatment. Several cases of treatment failures to multiple ascending doses of triclabendazole have been reported in humans from Peru.[15] Artemisinins have been used for the treatment of fascioliasis in two trials, with disappointing results.[59] Nonetheless, the combination of triclabendazole and artemisinins or ketoconazole showed promising results to overcome resistance in animal studies.[81] Nitazoxanide may be used as an alternative to treat chronic fascioliasis, but reports about its effectiveness are inconclusive, and subjects with Triclabendazole-resistant infection did not respond to 7 days of treatment.[15,36]

Prevention

Education and communication on safe growing of water plants for human consumption to avoid contamination with fecal material should be promoted.[81,103] Consumption of wild water plants in the field should be discouraged. Water purification systems should be implemented in highly endemic areas. The World Health Organization advocates the use of mass treatment with triclabendazole of children in endemic areas, but data are limited on safety and efficacy of this approach, especially in a setting of possible emerging resistance.[113,118]

LUNG FLUKE

Paragonimiasis

The parasites of the genus *Paragonimus* are zoonotic parasites with felines, canines, and other carnivores as definitive hosts, snails as intermediate hosts, and crabs or crayfish as second intermediate hosts.[10,41,58,75,103] More than 40 species of *Paragonimus* have been identified, at least 9 of which have been recovered from humans. The species causing human disease vary by region.

Organisms

The adult forms of *Paragonimus* form flattened leaf-like structures that measure about 7 to 16 mm long and 3.5 to 6 mm wide with anterior and ventral suckers.[10,75] The adult worms typically are located in the lungs of the definitive host. The ova are large (80–120 µm × 48–65 µm), yellow-brown in color, and contain a single operculum. Ova are shed into the bronchi and are either expectorated or swallowed and excreted in feces. After an incubation period of at least 2 weeks in fresh water, the free-living miracidia emerge and penetrate the snail intermediate host. After several weeks, the cercariae emerge and invade or are ingested by freshwater crabs and crayfish, forming cystic metacercaria in the tissues. Humans and other mammalian hosts are infected by ingestion of undercooked crab or crayfish. Larvae released from the metacercaria penetrate the wall of the intestines and migrate through the diaphragm to reach the lungs. In some instances, the worms may lodge in ectopic sites within the abdomen, liver, subcutaneous tissue, or central nervous system (CNS). The worms usually are found singly or in pairs within a capsule or cyst of reactive host tissue. Approximately 2 to 3 months are required from the time of ingestion until the worms are fully mature. Diploid forms reproduce sexually and triploid forms by parthenogenesis. In most infections, the worms die within 10 years; however, production of eggs for 20 years after the individual has left the endemic area has been reported.

In the past, most cases of paragonimiasis were attributed to infection with *P. westermani*, but molecular studies have revealed that more than nine different species of *Paragonimus* infect humans.[10,11,50,75] Molecular characterization has shown that typical pleuropulmonary infections in China, Japan, and Korea were largely due to *P. westermani*.[10] However, *P. skrjabini* and the related *P. skrjabini myazakii* cause atypical clinical disease in those areas.[103,10,11] Although *P. westermani* is endemic in India and Southeast Asia, nearly all clinical isolates are *P. heterotremus*.[32,33,96,122] Endemic areas with *P. africanus* and *P. uterobilateralis* can be found in Central Africa (Cameroon and Nigeria)[4,85] and with *P. mexicanus* also the Pacific rim from Peru to Central America, with the major focus in Ecuador.[10,51] Endemic cases have also been increasingly recognized in Missouri and are due to *P. kellicotti*.[37]

Transmission and Epidemiology

The endemic areas for paragonimiasis are largely limited to areas where the ecology allows for infection of all of the hosts, including infection of freshwater snails, spread to freshwater crabs and crayfish, and ingestion of the crabs and crayfish by the definitive hosts.[10,75] Human infection is acquired by eating freshwater crabs, crayfish, or shrimp that are raw, inadequately cooked, salted, or pickled. Recent cases acquired in the United States have been traced to ingestion of raw crayfish (*P. kellicotti*) or imported crabs (*P. westermani*).[13,66] A number of autochthonous cases have been described associated with freshwater canoe trips in which raw crayfish were ingested on a dare.[66] Infection has also been associated with ingestion of undercooked wild boar meat, with the boar serving as a paratenic host. There are also reports of infection from ingestion of water contaminated with metacercaria from crabs.

The global prevalence of human infection is estimated at more than 20 million persons infected, with 293 million at risk.[10,41,42] Overall, prevalence has been decreasing in much of east Asia such that disease is uncommon in Japan, Korea, Taiwan, Philippines, and eastern China, which once were highly endemic.[10,42,69] However, recent studies demonstrate ongoing transmission in Kyushu Island Japan.[84] A study in the Zamboanga del Norte, Philippines noted a prevalence of 6.7% of subjects.[7] Nevertheless, a recent national survey in China revealed a seroprevalence of paragonimiasis in 1.7%, with disease found in 21 different provinces.[69] Disease appears to be increasing in some areas after construction of the Three Gorges Dam.[125] Paragonimiasis remains endemic in much of Southeast Asia (including Vietnam, Thailand, and the Lao People's Democratic Republic). For example, seroprevalence ranged from 0% to 12.7% in parts of Vietnam,[33] and disease is described in all countries of southeast Asia as well as eastern India,[32,96] where more than half of children were seropositive in one focus. *Paragonimus* is endemic in central and western Africa, but most human cases are reported from Cameroon and Nigeria, with up to 14.8% of the population seropositive in some regions of southwestern Cameroon.[4,85] *P. mexicanus* is endemic in Latin America, with the primary focus in Ecuador and northern Peru, but case series have been reported from Colombia and Venezuela, in Central America, and as far north as Mexico.[10,19,20,51]

Pathology and Pathogenesis

Larvae are released after ingestion of ova. The larvae penetrate the duodenum and enter the abdominal cavity aided by excretory proteases.[10] Larvae may penetrate the diaphragm to the pleura soon thereafter, or the larvae may linger in the abdominal cavity or liver. After penetration of the pleura, the larvae burrow into the lung parenchyma and lodge near larger bronchioles or bronchi surrounded by an exudate of neutrophils and eosinophils. In time, this inflammatory response around the parasite organizes into a fibrotic wall that may measure up to several millimeters thick. The cysts usually are 1 to 2 cm in diameter and often are filled with a brownish material that likely contains hematin. Ova are released through communications with bronchioles or bronchi into sputum. Complications of paragonimiasis include bronchiectasis, fibrosis, interstitial pneumonia, and secondary bacterial infections.

Parasites can also be found in ectopic locations such as the CNS or subcutaneously. Ectopic parasites are more common for species that are less well adapted to the human host, especially *P. skrjabini*. Up to 31% of cases may involve the CNS in some areas.[23,121] All areas of the brain and meninges are susceptible to invasion. The adult worms and the eggs cause areas of central necrosis and granuloma formation with dense collagenous walls surrounded by lymphocytes, plasma cells, eosinophils, and Charcot-Leyden crystals. The lesions vary in size and may be several centimeters in diameter and may appear cystic. Eventually, the wall may calcify. Spinal cord lesions are similar. The organisms can also cause a migratory subcutaneous nodule. Other sites at which worms may cause cysts or abscesses are the intestinal wall, mesentery, peritoneal cavity, liver, diaphragm, and myocardium.

Clinical Manifestations

Classical (pleuropulmonary) paragonimiasis. The classical presentation of paragonimiasis is with pleural or pulmonary disease.[41,43,75] Pulmonary disease is more common with species better adapted to the human host (e.g., *P. westermani*, *P. heterotremus*, or *P. africanus*)[32,33,69,85] than species less adapted to the human host (e.g., *P. skrjabini*).[10] Migration of the worms from the intestinal tract to the lungs does not usually cause symptoms but has rarely been associated with fever, abdominal pain, diarrhea, and eosinophilia. However, if the parasites migrate across the liver, patients frequently present with abdominal pain and eosinophilia.[68] As the parasites enter the pleura, patients may present with fever, chest pain, dyspnea, cough, malaise, and night sweats. The pulmonary clinical manifestations are mainly a chronic cough. Cough may be dry or associated with sputum production, which may be described as mucoid, rust colored, or blood streaked. Hemoptysis usually is intermittent and occasionally may be severe. Eosinophilia is a common finding in the early stages of infection but may return to normal over a period of months or years. Complications may include pneumothorax, pleural effusion, empyema, and pneumonia. The presence of hemoptysis and cavitary lung lesions can be confused with tuberculosis, but tuberculosis typically has more systemic symptoms (e.g., fevers, night sweats, and weight loss). However, systemic symptoms have been noted in most recent cases from North America.[66]

Nonclassical presentations. Paragonimiasis may also infect other sites, including the subcutaneous tissues, brain, liver, abdomen, pericardium, and abdominal cavities. Extrathoracic disease is more common with parasites less adapted to the human host, especially *P. skrjabini*, but has been described from all endemic areas.[125]

Up to 31% of cases may involve the CNS.[26] Cerebral involvement is more common in children than adults.[121] Most cases present with headache, nausea, and vomiting. Others may present with focal findings (e.g., aphasia, motor involvement, or sensory abnormalities). Patients also may have seizures, which are usually described as generalized. They may or may not have coexisting pleuropulmonary disease. Spinal cord lesions often are extradural and mimic mass lesions caused by tumors or infection.

Cutaneous paragonimiasis presents with subcutaneous nodules, which may be fixed or slowly migrate. Cutaneous nodules can account for up to 42% of cases in areas endemic for *P. skrjabini* but are also noted in other areas. Worms recovered from these lesions are immature.

Diagnosis

Most patients have pleuropulmonary symptoms, and initial evaluation includes a chest radiograph. Radiographs initially may be normal but more typically demonstrate pleural effusions, nodules, or infiltrates.[32,48,55,63,85] Other radiographic findings include cavitations and fibrosis. Nodules and cysts can be found in any part of the lungs, but tend to localize in the periphery of the middle and lower lung fields. A common radiographic diagnostic feature is a "ring shadow." This finding represents the circular or oval thin-walled cyst with a crescent-shaped opacity along one side. Chest computed tomography (CT) findings vary by region (and thus likely by parasite species). Studies from Korea noted infiltrates and nodules in most cases.[63] Studies from Laos and India were more likely to show multiple cavitary lesions.[32,55] North American series noted more pleural effusions, pericardial involvement, and lymph nodes.[48]

Cerebral paragonimiasis may be seen as either an avascular mass or a hemorrhage on CT or magnetic resonance imaging.[1,23,26,120] Findings may include low-density, irregular shadows in most cases or, less frequently, hemorrhages. Either can be associated with edema and contrast enhancement. The ring enhancement may involve clusters of rings. In long-standing cerebral infections, the cystlike structures may calcify and be seen as a cluster of "soap bubbles." The individual oval or spherical bubbles may measure 2 to 40 mm in diameter, and a cluster of these structures may extend 10 cm.

Nearly all cases of paragonimiasis will present with eosinophilia. There can be some variability such that some authorities recommend repeating blood counts if eosinophilia is not present on the initial examination. Radiologic studies play a key role in diagnosis.

Pulmonary paragonimiasis is diagnosed definitively by finding the characteristic eggs in sputum or stool from a patient with symptoms suggesting the infection. Ova are more readily visualized with concentration or Ziehl-Neelsen staining.[99] Eggs are not present until 2 to 3 months after infection develops. Concentration techniques may help identify eggs in patients with light infections. Eggs have also been identified by percutaneous aspiration of lung nodules.[124] Several immunodiagnostic tests, including ELISA and immunoblotting, have been developed, which may assist with confirming the presence of infections. Immunodiagnosis is especially useful in infections in which eggs are not demonstrated easily, such as in cerebral paragonimiasis. The immunoblot assay performed with a crude antigen extract of *P. westermani* has a sensitivity of 96% and specificity of 99% and is the serodiagnostic test of choice.[86] Tests that amplify parasite DNA, including loop-mediated amplification, may improve sensitivity but are not widely available.[25]

Treatment and Prognosis

Praziquantel 75 mg/kg divided into three doses is given daily for 2 or 3 days.[41,43] Triclabendazole has been studied as an alternative treatment for humans infected with *Paragonimus* spp.[18] One study demonstrated 84% to 90% efficacy with single-day regimens of one or two doses of triclabendazole for the treatment of pulmonary paragonimiasis.[18,41]

The prognosis is good in most pulmonary infections, even if they go untreated, although symptoms may persist for many years. Treatment effectively resolves the pulmonary lesions and symptoms. The prognosis for CNS involvement depends on the location and extent of the lesions but is usually grave.

Prevention

The key in prevention is education of the population in endemic areas concerning the source of infection. Crabs and crayfish, prepared in a manner that transmits paragonimiasis, are delicacies in many parts of the world. However, education about preparation of these foods has led to dramatic reductions in the number of cases in Japan, Korea, the Philippines, and eastern China. Mass chemotherapy is being used to try to help prevent infections. Because paragonimiasis is a zoonosis, however, it is less amenable to control by mass treatment of human populations or improved sanitation.[118]

INTESTINAL FLUKES

Approximately 40 to 50 million people are thought to be infected by one or more of the 70 species and 14 families of intestinal flukes.[22,58,75] They are diverse morphologically, ranging in size from the *F. buski* (7.5 cm in length) to the tiny heterophyids (1–2.5 mm in length). Most cases cause few symptoms. However, heavy infections have been associated with a number of gastrointestinal symptoms. The most widely recognized organisms include *F. buski, Heterophyes* spp., *Metagonimus yokogawai*, and *Echinostoma* spp.

Fasciolopsiasis

Life Cycle

Fasciolopsiasis is a foodborne intestinal zoonosis caused by *F. buski*, the giant intestinal fluke.[22,44,45,75,103] The adult fluke measures up to 7.5 cm in length and attaches to the duodenum and jejunum walls. The life span of adult *Fasciolopsis* is approximately 6 months. Egg production starts about 3 months after infection, and these are 130 to 150 μm in length by 80 to 85 μm in breadth. A single parasite may excrete 25,000 eggs daily. The eggs are released in the feces, and after several weeks in fresh water, ciliated larvae hatch from the eggs and penetrate snails, where they reproduce asexually undergoing several larval stages. Cercariae emerge from the snail approximately 1 to 2 months later and encyst as metacercariae on a wide variety of aquatic vegetation and debris as well as on the water surface. Mammalian hosts are infected after ingestion of the metacercariae. Pigs are common reservoir hosts. Water chestnuts, caltrop, and water bamboo are common sources of human infection. Ingestion of larvae also can occur through drinking untreated water or handling water-derived plants (e.g., peeling contaminated water chestnuts with the teeth).

Epidemiology

Fasciolopsiasis occurs most often in Asia and the Indian subcontinent, with high prevalence rates recorded in parts of south Asia and Thailand.[2,22,44,45,103,116] Pigs are the definitive host, and the prevalence of fasciolopsiasis is higher in areas where pigs are raised and aquatic plants are consumed. Fasciolopsiasis is most prevalent in school-aged children, in whom high worm burdens are not uncommon findings.

Pathology

The parasites infect the duodenum and jejunum, but in heavy infections they can be observed in the stomach, ileum, and colon. Inflammation, ulceration, and small abscesses sometimes develop in the intestinal mucosa where the parasite is attached. Increased mucus secretion and mild bleeding can result. Light infections typically are asymptomatic. Massive infections can lead to intestinal obstruction and perforation.

Complications such as malabsorption and protein-losing enteropathy are common occurrences in heavy infections and can lead to generalized edema and ascites.

Clinical Manifestations

The severity of symptoms is correlated with the burden of parasites. Epigastric discomfort has been reported as early as 30 days after exposure. Diarrhea and abdominal pain may be intermittent and may occur separately. Patients may note passing fleshy masses in stool.[2] In heavy infections, nausea and vomiting may develop. Facial edema, anasarca, ileus, and intestinal perforation are encountered in severe infections. Eosinophilia with counts greater than 30% is not an uncommon occurrence. Leukocytosis and mild anemia may be noted.

In endemic areas, fasciolopsiasis contributes to malnutrition in children, especially when associated with other helminth infections. Fasciolopsiasis adds an additional burden to the host and in concert with other chronic helminth infections may be responsible for significant morbidity.

Diagnosis

The eggs of *Fasciolopsis* are demonstrated easily by routine fecal examination, but they are virtually indistinguishable from those of the liver fluke *F. hepatica* and the echinostomes. Epidemiologic information, such as travel history and exposure to sources of infection, may be helpful in determining the diagnosis. Because the life span of adult *Fasciolopsis* is short, anyone who has been out of an endemic area for longer than 9 months is not likely to have fasciolopsiasis. Incidentally, fasciolopsiasis can be diagnosed by upper endoscopy.

Treatment and Prognosis

Praziquantel 75 mg/kg divided into three doses given in 1 day is effective and safe. Infections treated early and most light infections, even when they are untreated, have an excellent prognosis. Heavy infections in children, especially when they are complicated by intestinal obstruction, edema, or concomitant secondary infections, portend a much poorer prognosis.

Prevention

Avoiding raw water plants and untreated water may be a practical approach to prevent fasciolopsiasis. Cooking aquatic vegetation or immersing the plants or nuts briefly in boiling water usually is sufficient to prevent infection. Also, discouraging the use of human feces as fertilizer and promoting the institution of modern pig farming both can aid in the control of fasciolopsiasis. Successful efforts in health education or mass chemotherapy have reduced the transmission of this parasite in some endemic areas[103,114]; however, in areas where fasciolopsiasis was presumed controlled, such as Uttar Pradesh, reemerging infection has been reported.[9]

Heterophyiasis

More than 11 different species of the family Heterophyidae have been reported to cause human infection.[22] *Heterophyes* spp., *Haplorchis* spp., and *M. yokogawai* are common human parasites, whereas other organisms are uncommon.

Organism

Heterophyes spp., *Haplorchis* spp., and *M. yokogawai* adult worms attach to the mucosa of the small intestine. The parasites are minute, measuring 1 to 2.5 mm in length and less than 1 mm in width. They often burrow deeply into the mucosa. The eggs measure 26 to 30 μm in length and 15 to 17 μm in width. The eggs are nearly identical. Eggs excreted in the stool are fully embryonated. The snail intermediate host becomes infected by ingesting the trematode egg. After multiplication in the snail, cercariae emerge and encyst as metacercariae under the scales or skin or in the muscle of a variety of freshwater fish. After being ingested by the definitive host, the metacercariae are freed from their cysts and develop into adults in as little as 5 days.

Transmission and Epidemiology

Humans acquire the infection by eating freshwater fish that is raw or inadequately cooked. Transmission may have a seasonal pattern, with the highest fish infection rates found during the summer.[24,70,110] Heterophyiasis occurs worldwide. Areas of endemic infection are Southeast Asia, the Middle East, the Nile Delta, China, Japan, Taiwan, the Philippines, and parts of the former Soviet Union. Many reservoir hosts, such as dogs, cats, and fish-eating birds, may play an important role in maintenance of infection in some endemic areas.

Pathology

The small heterophyid flukes cause variable degrees of inflammation in the intestinal wall.[22] Superficial inflammation and erosions are found at the sites of mucosal attachment. Eggs deposited beneath the mucosa cause eosinophilic granulomatous lesions. Eggs may invade the circulatory system through the intestinal capillaries or lymphatics. Eggs may reach distant sites such as the heart, brain, and spinal cord, causing significant morbidity and even mortality. The embolized eggs induce a granulomatous response, with the eventual production of fibrosis in the infected areas. The complications of embolic heterophyiasis appear to be particularly frequent in the Philippines, where heart disease often is attributed to heterophyiasis.

Clinical Manifestations

Light infections without the deposition of ectopic eggs usually are asymptomatic, although eosinophilia may be noted. In heavier infections, epigastric pain, diarrhea, malabsorption, and weight loss may occur. Seizures may result from eggs carried to the brain. Congestive heart failure or arrhythmias may occur after cardiac involvement.

Diagnosis

Routine fecal microscopy may demonstrate eggs. Nonetheless, differentiating morphologically heterophyid eggs from those of the liver flukes may be difficult. Eggs recovered from patients who have been exposed more than 2 years before presentation are very likely to be from *Opisthorchis* or *Clonorchis* because the life span of heterophyids is usually less than a year.

Treatment and Prognosis

Praziquantel 75 mg/kg per day in three divided doses for 1 day is the recommended treatment. With the exception of the complication of egg emboli to distant organs, the prognosis is excellent.

Metorchiasis

M. conjunctus, endemic in North American; *M. bilis,* in Russia; and *M. orientalis,* in China and Korea, are members of the Opisthorchiidae family. They have a life cycle similar to that of the other opisthorchids. A wide variety of fish-eating mammals may serve as definitive hosts. This infection is a significant cause of morbidity and mortality in sled dogs in Canada. It is an occasional incidental finding on fecal examination in native communities in northern Canada. An outbreak of 19 cases of *Metorchis* infection was related to fish prepared raw as sashimi.[74] The epidemiology of metorchiasis outside North America seems to be far from an incidental illness. In areas where the epidemiology of *O. felineus* and *M. bilis* overlap, the difficulties differentiating *M. bilis* from *O. felineus* eggs have led to overdiagnosis of opisthorchiasis and the impression that it is much more common than metorchiasis.[83] National surveys in China have identified some foci of human *M. orientalis* infection in the Fujian province. The severity and duration of the symptoms probably correlate with parasite burden. The symptoms during acute infection are fatigue, upper abdominal tenderness, fever, epigastric abdominal pain, headache, weight loss, anorexia, nausea, diarrhea, vomiting, muscle pain, backache, cough, and rash.[74] The degree of eosinophilia and elevation in liver enzymes are proportional to the intensity of infection. Eggs are noted in stool 10 days after infection develops. Praziquantel is effective during acute metorchiasis and in the chronic phase.

NEW REFERENCES SINCE THE SEVENTH EDITION

2. Achra A, Prakash P, Shankar R. Fasciolopsiasis: Endemic focus of a neglected parasitic disease in Bihar. *Indian J Med Microbiol.* 2015;33:364-368.
7. Belizario V Jr, Totanes FI, Asuncion CA, et al. Integrated surveillance of pulmonary tuberculosis and paragonimiasis in Zamboanga del Norte, the Philippines. *Pathog Glob Health.* 2014;108:95-102.

15. Cabada MM, Lopez M, Cruz M, et al. Treatment failure after multiple courses of triclabendazole among patients with fascioliasis in Cusco, Peru: A case series. *PLoS Negl Trop Dis*. 2016;10:e0004361.
18. Calvopina M, Guderian RH, Paredes W, Chico M, Cooper PJ. Treatment of human pulmonary paragonimiasis with triclabendazole: clinical tolerance and drug efficacy. *Trans R Soc Trop Med Hyg*. 1998;92:566-569.
20. Calvopina M, Romero D, Castaneda B, Hashiguchi Y, Sugiyama H. Current status of *Paragonimus* and paragonimiasis in Ecuador. *Mem Inst Oswaldo Cruz*. 2014;109:849-855.
23. Chai JY. Paragonimiasis. *Handb Clin Neurol*. 2013;114:283-296.
24. Chai JY, Jung BK, Kim DG, et al. Heterophyid trematodes recovered from people residing along the Boseong River, South Korea. *Acta Trop*. 2015;148:142-146.
54. Lopez M, Morales ML, Konana M, et al. Kato-Katz and Lumbreras rapid sedimentation test to evaluate helminth prevalence in the setting of a school-based deworming program. *Pathog Glob Health*. 2016;110(3):130-134.
60. Kelley JM, Elliott TP, Beddoe T, et al. Current threat of triclabendazole resistance in *Fasciola hepatica*. *Trends Parasitol*. 2016;32:458-469.
71. Smout MJ, Sotillo J, Laha T, et al. Carcinogenic parasite secretes growth factor that accelerates wound healing and potentially promotes neoplasia. *PLoS Pathog*. 2015;11(10):e1005209.
77. Mairiang E, Mairiang P. Clinical manifestation of opisthorchiasis and treatment. *Acta Trop*. 2003;88:221-227.
88. Pozio E, Armignacco O, Ferri F, Gomez Morales MA. Opisthorchis felineus, an emerging infection in Italy and its implication for the European Union. *Acta Trop*. 2013;126:54-62.
90. Robles-Perez D, Martinez-Perez JM, Rojo-Vazquez FA, Martinez-Valladares M. The diagnosis of fasciolosis in feces of sheep by means of a PCR and its application in the detection of anthelmintic resistance in sheep flocks naturally infected. *Vet Parasitol*. 2013;197:277-282.
94. Sayasone S, Odermatt P, Vonghachack Y, et al. Efficacy and safety of tribendimidine against *Opisthorchis viverrini:* two randomised, parallel-group, single-blind, dose-ranging, phase 2 trials. *Lancet Infect Dis*. 2016.
101. Sripa B. Pathobiology of opisthorchiasis: an update. *Acta Trop*. 2003;88:209-220.
105. Sukhdeo MV, Sangster NC, Mettrick DF. Permanent feeding sites of adult *Fasciola hepatica* in rabbits? *Int J Parasitol*. 1988;18:509-512.
106. Wunderink HF, Rozemeijer W, Wever PC, et al. Foodborne trematodiasis and opisthorchis felineus acquired in Italy. *Emerg Infect Dis*. 2014;20(1):154-155.
109. Traverso A, Repetto E, Magnani S, et al. A large outbreak of *Opisthorchis felineus* in Italy suggests that opisthorchiasis develops as a febrile eosinophilic syndrome with cholestasis rather than a hepatitis-like syndrome. *Eur J Clin Microbiol Infect Dis*. 2012;31:1089-1093.
117. Worasith C, Kamamia C, Yakovleva A, et al. Advances in the diagnosis of human opisthorchiasis: development of *Opisthorchis viverrini* antigen detection in urine. *PLoS Negl Trop Dis*. 2015;9:e0004157.
120. Xia Y, Chen J, Ju Y, You C. Characteristic CT and MR imaging findings of cerebral paragonimiasis. *J Neuroradiol*. 2016;43:200-206.
121. Xia Y, Ju Y, Chen J, You C. Cerebral paragonimiasis: a retrospective analysis of 27 cases. *J Neurosurg Pediatr*. 2015;15:101-106.

The full reference list for this chapter is available at ExpertConsult.com.

Schistosomiasis 229

Philip R. Fischer • A. Clinton White Jr

Approximately 260 million individuals are infected with parasites of the genus *Schistosoma*,[38,88,157,167,210] and another 700 million people are at risk for infection.[175,210,209] Many are unaware of their infection, although approximately 20 million people have severe disease with potentially fatal portal hypertension, urinary tract involvement, renal failure, and bladder cancer. Initial infection usually occurs during childhood. The prevalence typically peaks in the teen years, and, although most of the morbidity occurs in adults, symptomatic disease develops in millions of children.

There is historical evidence of schistosomiasis occurring as early as the second millennium BCE.[186,188] For example, *Schistosoma* eggs have been found in mummies from the 20th dynasty in ancient Egypt and in ancient China. In 1851, Theodor Bilharz identified the parasitic etiology of endemic hematuria. At the same time, the association between *Schistosoma* and Katayama fever was recognized in Japan. The complete life cycle was identified during the first decades of the 20th century. Before the development of effective curative medication in the 1970s, schistosomiasis was considered the "most dreadful of the remaining plagues of Egypt."[88,89] Nonetheless, it had been reported in 1919 that "it is now quite within the bounds of possibility that the disease may be largely controlled"[156]; even in this new millennium, success with disease control and eradication is still quite limited. Of 259 million people requiring treatment for schistosomiasis in 2014 (of whom 48% were school-aged children), only 62 million individuals actually received treatment.[167]

EPIDEMIOLOGY

Schistosomiasis is caused by helminth parasites of the class Trematoda, which includes the flukes. Schistosomes differ from other human flukes in that they live within the vascular system and have separate male and female sexes. Humans are the definitive host for six species within the *Schistosoma* genus.[186,188] *Schistosoma haematobium* is the cause of urinary schistosomiasis. *Schistosoma japonicum* and *Schistosoma mansoni* are common causes of disease resulting from infection of the intestinal vasculature. *Schistosoma mekongi* (in Asia), *Schistosoma guineensis* (in West Africa), and *Schistosoma intercalatum* (in Central Africa) also cause infection along the intestinal tract but are found only in small geographic areas.[40] Other mammalian *Schistosoma* species occasionally infect humans.

Each species of *Schistosoma* uses fresh-water snails as obligate intermediate hosts,[186,188] and the geographic distribution of *Schistosoma* is limited by the habitat of these snails (Fig. 229.1). Oncomelania snails transmitting *S. japonicum* live in the moist soil along slow-flowing streams and irrigation canals, limited primarily to parts of China, the Philippines, and Indonesia. The *Bulinus* snails associated with *S. haematobium* and the *Biomphalaria* snails associated with *S. mansoni* live in shaded, slow-flowing, shallow water. *S. haematobium* is seen primarily in tropical Africa, along the Nile River, and in the Middle East. In addition, however, *S. haematobium* has recently been identified in Corsica, France.[18] *S. mansoni* is found across tropical Africa, along the Atlantic coast of South America, and on some Caribbean islands. *Tricula,* the snail host for *S. mekongi,* is limited to the Mekong River in Laos and Cambodia. *S. intercalatum* and its snail host *Bulinus* spp. are found only in Cameroon and the Democratic Republic of Congo. Most human infections occur when children come into contact with fresh-water streams, rivers, or lakes inhabited by infected snails (Fig. 229.2).[188] Thus transmission typically occurs during routine activities such as obtaining water for household use, bathing, fishing, and irrigation. Humans are infected by the fork-tailed schistosomal cercariae. Cercariae penetrate the skin with the aid of secretory serine proteases.[114,166] During

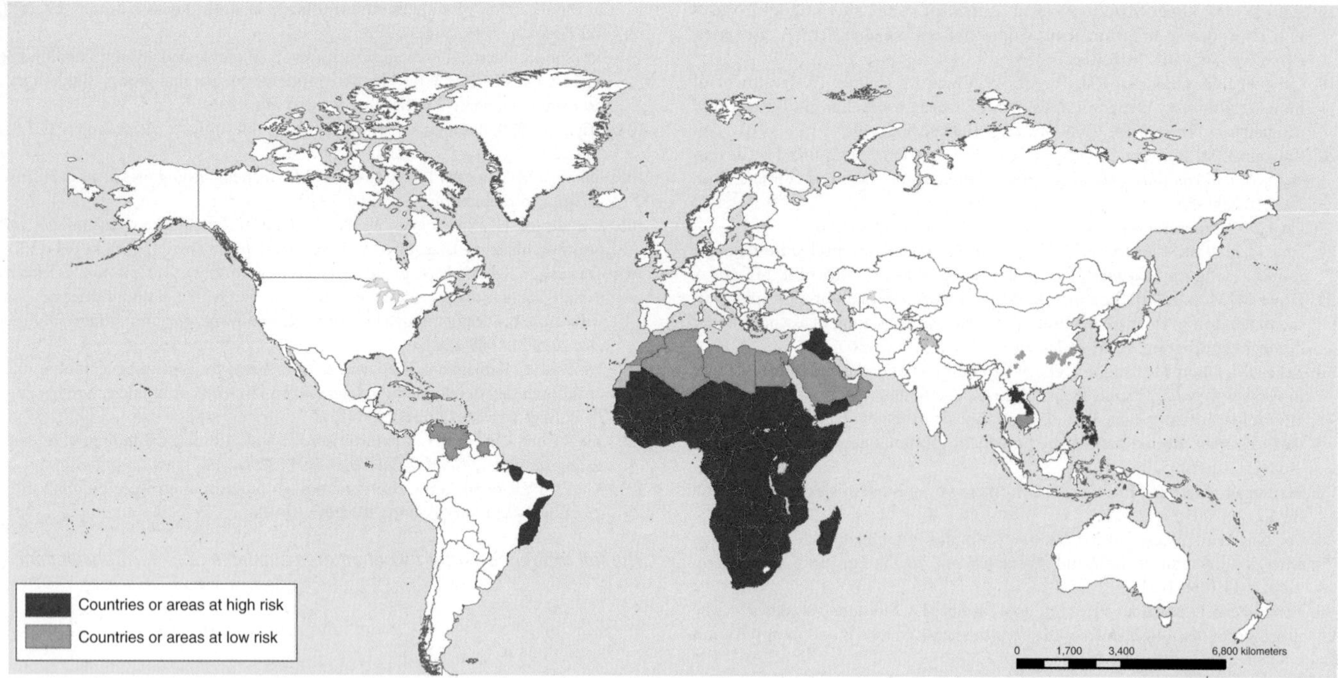

The boundaries and names shown and the designations used on this map do not imply the expression of any opinion whatsoever on the part of the World Health Organization concerning the legal status of any country, territory, city or area or of its authorities, or concerning the delimitation of its frontiers or boundaries. Dotted and dashed lines on maps represent approximate border lines for which there may not yet be full agreement.

Data Source: World Health Organization International Travel and Health

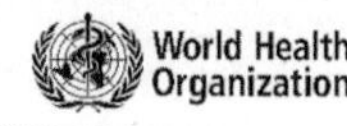

FIG. 229.1 Countries or areas at risk for schistosomiasis (2014). (From World Health Organization. http://gamapserver.who.int/mapLibrary/Files/Maps/Global_ShistoPrevalence_ITHRiskMap.png?ua=1.)

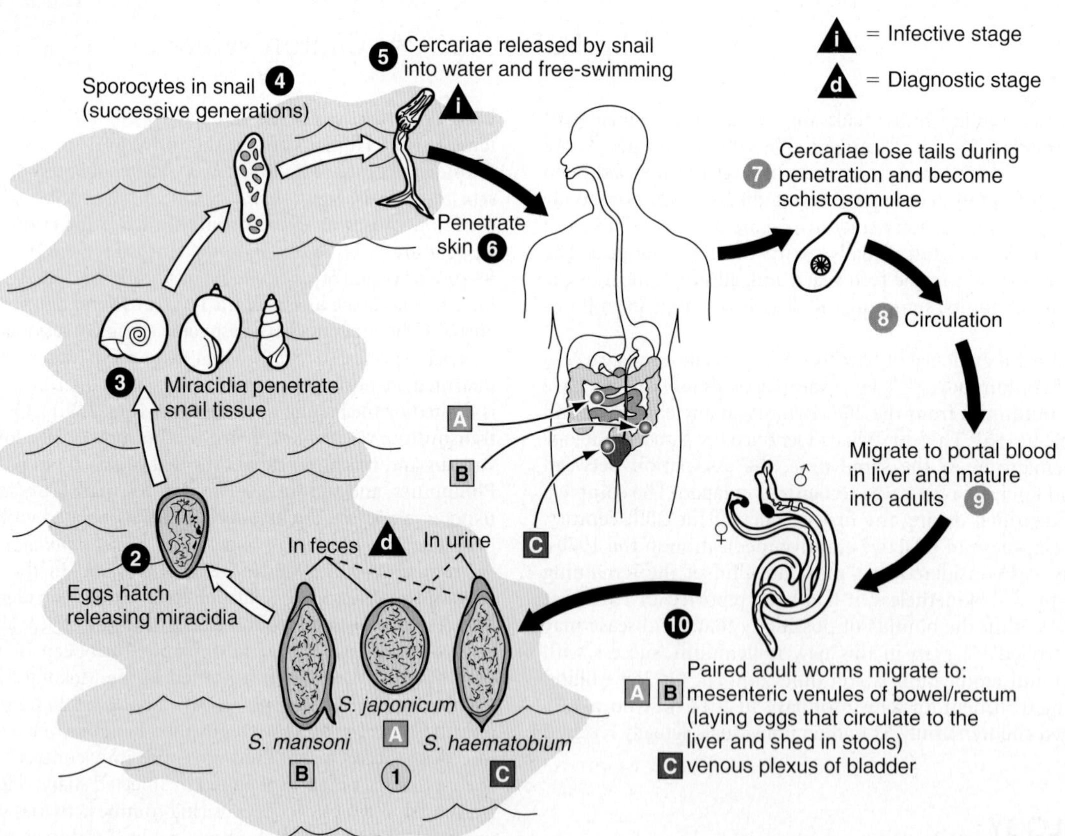

FIG. 229.2 Life cycle of the human schistosome species. (From Centers for Disease Control and Prevention: Schistosomiasis. http://www.dpd.cdc.gov/dpdx/HTML/Schistosomiasis.htm.)

penetration, the parasites lose their tails and modify their tegument to form the schistosomula stage. Schistosomulas enter the bloodstream and then migrate to the lungs. They move from the pulmonary arterial circulation to the venous circulation without exiting the vessels. The parasites then travel through the systemic circulation until they reach splanchnic vessels and gain access to the portal system.

During the course of a few weeks, the schistosomulas develop into mature male and female adults that mate continuously.[187,188] Adult worms are 1 to 3 cm in length and usually live for 3 to 7 years. *S. haematobium* localizes to the venules of the urinary bladder, *S. japonicum* goes to the superior mesenteric vessels, and *S. mansoni* goes to the inferior mesenteric vessels. The gravid females migrate upstream to lay eggs near the bladder or intestines. Each adult female can produce hundreds (in the case of African species) to thousands (for Asian species) of eggs per day.[75] Most of the eggs become embedded in the walls of the peripheral vessel where they were laid. However, some of them flow with the blood and can stimulate reactions and cause disease at other sites. A localized granulomatous response allows the eggs to pass through the wall of the bladder (for *S. haematobium*) or the intestine (for other species) to be released in urine or stool. Released eggs mature in a week's time and then hatch to release miracidia. The miracidia penetrate the snail to continue their life cycle and eventually develop into hundreds of cercariae.

Infection is seen in children as young as 6 months; exposure to cercariae often is greatest in boys between the ages of 5 and 10 years.[88,96,186] In lakeside Ugandan villages, however, nearly half of the children are infected during the first 3 years of life,[140] and in a western Kenya town, infection was noted in 14% of 1-year-olds, 63% of 5-year-olds, and 90% of 10-year-olds.[201] The peak intensity of infection, as measured by excretion of eggs, occurs in children 8 to 12 years old in heavily infected areas and takes place during the teenage years in more lightly infected areas. The intensity and the incidence of excretion of eggs decline after the adolescent years, and hormonal changes during puberty are associated with increased resistance to infection.[101]

PATHOGENESIS AND IMMUNITY

Within hours of penetration of the skin, local erythema and inflammation may result from the activity of parasite proteases.[113,165,192] In individuals previously sensitized, a delayed immune reaction may cause papular or vesicular lesions.[97,186] Infiltration of the epidermis and dermis with a mixture of mononuclear cells and eosinophils causes papules. This reaction (termed swimmer's itch) is more pronounced for avian schistosomes, which are unable to penetrate into the human circulation and die in situ. During the initial migration of schistosomes through the lungs, patients may develop fever, pneumonitis, pulmonary infiltrates, and eosinophilia. However, these reactions resolve spontaneously.

Acute schistosomiasis typically begins 2 to 12 weeks after exposure, at the time the female parasites begin to produce eggs.[53,159] This condition was initially recognized with *S. japonicum* but is now described with all species.[97,106,118,186] Patients characteristically have marked eosinophilia, along with immunoglobulin E (IgE) and IgG antibodies to the parasites, consistent with an active helper T-cell subtype 2 (Th2) response.[97,186] However, studies suggest that proinflammatory cytokines play an important role.[50,133] The antibodies react with egg antigens, which cross-react with antigens from the cercaria or schistosomula stages.[10,82,83] During early production of eggs, the quantity of antigen exceeds that of antibody, and soluble immune complexes are formed. Immune activation and immune complex deposition lead to the clinical manifestations, including fever, myalgia, urticarial rash, and bloody diarrhea. Pulmonary nodules and infiltrates may be noted during acute infection.[43,168] In addition, acute infection can be complicated by ectopic egg production. Patients with acute *S. mansoni* or *S. haematobium* infection occasionally can have neurologic involvement.[32,60,149] Interestingly, acute disease occurs rarely in endemic populations, perhaps because of modulation of the immune response from exposure to parasite antigens in utero.

Chronic Schistosomiasis

Despite the fact that the adult worms live within the bloodstream, they cause little host response. The parasite surface incorporates blood group glycoproteins and major histocompatibility antigens and downregulates expression of its own surface proteins, which may help the adults evade immune system attack.[72,146,177]

Chronic infection is characterized by localized granulomas surrounding the parasite eggs.[97,157,186] Excretory products of the eggs (termed soluble egg antigens) are the major antigens. The egg antigens are cytotoxic to host cells, such that infection of mice lacking T cells results in increased localized necrosis surrounding the eggs; the granulomas help protect the host from the ravages of the eggs. Interleukin-17 (IL-17) mediates the formation of granulomas in the liver.[218] The granulomas also facilitate transit of the eggs into stool and urine, as illustrated by the fact that immunodeficient hosts tend to have lower rates of shedding of eggs despite having high concentrations of eggs in tissues.[52,92,135] High levels of vasoactive endothelial growth factor and angiogenesis are associated with initial granuloma formation.[173]

The granulomas also contribute to the pathologic process. They are composed of a mixture of eosinophils, lymphocytes, macrophages, and granulocytes.[20] Late-stage granulomas also contain fibroblasts, collagen, and giant cells. Initially, antigen-presenting cells stimulate $CD4^+$ T cells to produce IL-2, tumor necrosis factor-α (TNF-α), and interferon-γ (IFN-γ).[134] Early expression of TNF-α plays a key role in the initial formation of granulomas.[5] A subsequent shift occurs toward production of Th2 cytokines (e.g., IL-4, IL-5, IL-10, and IL-13) along with antibody.[147] This event is accompanied by eosinophil recruitment. IL-4 and IL-13 also play a primary role in the development of hepatic granulomas, and IL-13 expression is linked closely to the development of fibrosis in murine models.[36,37,41] Subsequent immunomodulation, largely mediated by IL-10 and transforming growth factor-β (TGF-β), results in downsizing of the granuloma and suppression of the inflammation.[9,57,63,84,121,133,174,204] However, depletion of IL-4 results in tissue damage.[41] When granulomas are limited to the intestines, the cytokine response is dominated by antiinflammatory cytokines (e.g., IL-10 and TGF-β), and patients have few symptoms.[45] By contrast, patients with granulomas in the liver are more likely to be symptomatic. They express more inflammatory cytokines, including IL-13 and TNF-α. TGF-β also is associated with fibrosis in primate models,[57] whereas Th1 cytokines (e.g., IFN-γ and IL-12) suppress fibrosis.[22,211,219] Macrophages activated by IL-4 and IL-13 (alternative rather than classical IFN-γ–based activation) seem to protect mice against schistosomiasis-induced inflammation and fibrosis with the acute infection while later promoting fibrosis with chronic infection.[13] Eosinophils modulate peripheral blood mononuclear responses to adult worm antigens.[196]

IL-13 in particular stimulates the formation of fibrosis in the portal tracts,[36] probably through the induction of expression of fibrosis-associated genes.[117] Portal fibrosis, in turn, leads to the development of portal hypertension (i.e., hepatosplenomegaly, ascites, and esophageal varices).[97] Death from hepatic schistosomiasis typically results from gastrointestinal bleeding. Overt bleeding is an uncommon occurrence in children, but it can occur in adolescents and young adults. In patients with isolated schistosomiasis, hepatocellular function is surprisingly normal.[20] Patients are thought to tolerate even gastrointestinal bleeding better than do those with cirrhosis. By contrast, progressive hepatocellular damage and rapid progression to liver failure develop in patients coinfected with hepatitis viruses, particularly hepatitis C.[7,42,91] The immunomodulation that develops in response to schistosomiasis is thought to suppress immune control of the hepatitis virus. Whether schistosomiasis-associated immune changes alter susceptibility to or expression of human immunodeficiency virus is unknown.[200]

Reinfection after treatment is more common in children younger than 10 years and with higher IgG4 levels.[128] In some settings, boys are more likely to be reinfected than girls,[125] but this is not uniformly true.[128] Higher IgE levels are associated with less reinfection.[128]

Interestingly, patients with schistosomiasis are less susceptible to allergies.[28,139,199] Evidence indicates that asthmatic patients with schistosomiasis produce lower levels of IL-5 and greater levels of IL-10 than do asthmatic patients without schistosomiasis, and it is this suppression of Th2 responses that might modulate the expression of asthma and atopic disease in patients with schistosomiasis.[8] Alternatively, it is possible that a common genetic predisposition alters the risk for subsequent development of both atopic disease and schistosomiasis.[12,120] A population-based study in Zimbabwe identified a negative correlation between atopy and the intensity of schistosomal infection in a village with a high frequency of schistosomiasis but not in a village with lower infection frequency,[162] indicating the interrelatedness of schistosomal antigenic stimulation and the development of allergic disease.

Several means exist by which schistosomiasis might be related to anemia, and the exact pathologic mechanisms are not fully understood.[66] At least sometimes, however, the anemia is due to inflammation rather than iron deficiency.[104,126] Generalized undernutrition is associated with schistosomiasis; proinflammatory cytokines (IL-1β) and generalized inflammation (as manifested by elevated levels of C-reactive protein) are contributing factors.[47] Even without acute inflammation, schistosomal infection and periportal fibrosis are associated with reduced vitamin A status and high oxidative stress (increased serum hydroperoxides).[17] Schistosomiasis-affected children have lower levels of regulatory T cells with altered cytokine responses; this seems to provide some protection against concurrent malaria infection.[119] Similarly, parasite-induced changes in the Th1/Th2 balance are hypothesized to explain how young children with underlying schistosomiasis are less likely to develop malaria.[120]

Approximately 40,000,000 women of childbearing age are infected with schistosomes. Although mechanisms are not clear, some evidence indicates that schistosomiasis during pregnancy is associated with decreased birth weight and a higher risk for preterm delivery.[67]

Urinary Schistosomiasis

Genital and urinary schistosomiasis also is the result of granuloma formation. Severity of disease correlates with increased production of TNF-α and decreased production of IL-10.[99] Direct inflammatory responses to eggs along the ureters or from obstruction to ureteral drainage caused by space-occupying granulomas in the bladder wall block ureteral emptying.[95,178] All tissue layers may be involved, but pathologic changes are usually most extensive in the submucosal layer.[94] Abnormal ureteral flow, dilatation, and hydronephrosis develop.[178] In some communities where *S. haematobium* is common, ureteral deformities demonstrable on intravenous pyelography are noted in half of affected children and hydronephrosis develops in more than 10%.[98] Eventually, scarring and calcifications form and may be associated with chronic hydronephrosis, even with resolved or light chronic infection.[99,178] The hydronephrosis and urinary stasis predispose patients to chronic bacteriuria and urinary tract infections.

In *S. mansoni* infection, immune complexes may mediate glomerulonephritis, as evidenced by the finding of schistosome-derived immune complex deposits in glomeruli.[15,180] Nephrotic syndrome has been reported in association with chronic schistosomiasis.[123,124] Amyloid deposits have been found in the kidneys of children with chronic schistosomiasis, and this condition probably is caused by immune responses that are altered by the chronic parasitic infection.[14,202]

Squamous cell carcinoma of the bladder is a common occurrence in areas of heavy infection with *S. haematobium*, but otherwise it is a rare form of bladder cancer.[99,178,186] The prolonged irritation of bladder epithelium by schistosome eggs and the resulting immune response are thought to trigger hyperplasia and subsequent malignant disease.[105] In an animal model, direct exposure to schistosomal antigens stimulates increased proliferation and decreased apoptosis of endothelial cells along with downregulation of tumor suppressor p27 and upregulation of antiapoptotic molecule Bcl-2.[24] This condition could be aggravated by urinary stasis in the bladder with secondary increases in pH that favor malignant transformation of epithelial cells. Carcinogenic tryptophan metabolites also have been postulated to link the nutritional activities of parasites near the bladder with subsequent carcinogenesis. Schistosoma-related bladder cancers have biomarker prevalence different from that of nonschistosomal bladder cancers, and this might influence eventual treatment choices.[2]

CLINICAL MANIFESTATIONS

The main clinical manifestations of schistosomiasis vary with the stage of the parasite's life cycle and also differ among species. Many patients remain asymptomatic. Patients with asymptomatic schistosomiasis may be identified during community screening programs in an endemic area, through immigrant or returned traveler evaluations in a nonendemic area, or when diagnostic tests such as urine or stool microscopy are performed to evaluate other, seemingly unrelated symptoms. The minority of infected children, those with heavy infections, are most likely to develop early symptoms and also are at greatest risk for subsequent major health complications.

Cercarial Penetration

Within a few minutes of coming into contact with cercariae, some children develop pruritus. This response to initial contact with the parasite occurs more commonly in nonimmune visitors to endemic areas than it does in indigenous residents of endemic areas, but it seems to be more pronounced after repeated exposure to cercariae than on the first exposure. It may occur after contact with any of the human *Schistosoma* spp. but more commonly results after contact with the cercariae of avian schistosomes. An erythematous and sometimes papular rash may develop.[97,186] The rash usually subsides during a period of 2 to 10 days without scarring, regardless of whether specific treatment is given.

Acute Schistosomiasis (Katayama Fever)

Acute schistosomiasis, referred to as Katayama fever, typically begins 2 to 12 weeks after exposure, when the adult worms begin to produce eggs.[52,87,159] Clinical manifestations of acute schistosomiasis usually include high fever, chills, myalgia, headache, and a general ill appearance.[50,53] An urticarial rash, which may include giant urticaria, and diffuse lymphadenopathy may be seen.[154,221] Cough, rales, and pulmonary infiltrates may be noted, even in the absence of fever.[43,168] Gastrointestinal symptoms of anorexia, abdominal pain, and loose stools sometimes are observed. Bloody diarrhea may be seen acutely with heavy infections by *S. japonicum* and *S. mansoni*. Tender hepatomegaly and mild splenic enlargement develop in approximately 30% of children with Katayama fever. Some reports suggest that myelopathies are a common accompaniment of acute schistosomiasis.[60,149] Genital symptoms (primarily hematospermia) also are frequent initial symptoms.[44,153] Marked eosinophilia often is seen with acute schistosomiasis.

Urinary Schistosomiasis

Hematuria is the classical finding of *S. haematobium* infection.[26,51,95,186,207] In some highly endemic areas, for boys nearing puberty not to display this evidence of "male menstruation" is considered abnormal. Typically, hematuria results from the release of blood from irritated, inflamed areas around granulomas in the bladder wall as the bladder contracts during micturition.[178] Thus the blood is most obvious at the end of the urine stream ("terminal hematuria"). The hematuria usually is not associated with pain or discomfort, but dysuria can be present.[1,26] With chronic infection in children who either were not treated initially or were reinfected, obstructive uropathy can develop. In community surveys in endemic areas, as many as 40% of children were found to have significant renal or ureteral abnormalities (or both).[1,79,203] Hematuria and dysuria occur more commonly in children than in adults, presumably because they have heavier parasite loads. However, hydronephrosis, which develops more slowly, is seen more often in adults.[95,98,131,178]

Bacterial urinary tract infection may coexist with urinary schistosomiasis, probably secondary to obstruction of urinary outflow.[178] Chronic infection can lead to renal failure. Obstructive uropathy, with or without incident or recurrent urinary tract infections, can lead to loss of renal function. Children with schistosomal infection also can have glomerulonephritis and nephrotic syndrome. Bladder cancer, when it occurs, typically develops in the setting of untreated, heavy chronic urinary schistosomiasis.

Genital Schistosomiasis

Studies have emphasized the genital tract as an important site of schistosomiasis in both men and women.[29,107,149,150] In women, egg granulomas may be found in the cervix, uterus, or fallopian tubes.[58,107,108,150] Cervical irritation and ulceration, vaginal bleeding, or ectopic pregnancy may develop. Genital schistosomiasis can be confused with cancer.[190] Adolescent boys may have involvement of the prostate and seminal vesicles.[107,153] Eggs were noted in semen from 43% of men in an area endemic for *S. haematobium*.[107] The main clinical finding is hematospermia,[107] which may occur with acute infection or during chronic disease. Approximately 48% of 10- to 12-year-old girls with heavy urinary *Schistosoma* infection report genital symptoms.[80] Girls with genital schistosomiasis can experience bloody vaginal discharge, genital itch, burning genital sensations, malodorous discharge, and nodular or ulcerated lesions.[80] On pelvic and colposcopic examination, older adolescent girls and young adult woman with urinary schistosomiasis can have rubbery lesions (containing viable ova) and grainy or sandy patch lesions (containing calcified ova) on mucosal surfaces.[151] In females, genital schistosomiasis increases transmission of human immunodeficiency virus infection threefold to fourfold.[139,176]

Intestinal Disease

Most children with intestinal schistosomiasis do not have intestinal symptoms.[186,184] Thus even finding eggs in stool does not mean that symptoms are related to the schistosomiasis.[77] Nonetheless, both the small and large intestines may be involved with schistosomal disease. Irritation of the bowel wall from inflammatory reactions induced by eggs may lead to diarrhea that sometimes contains blood or mucus.[34,35,184-186] Crampy abdominal pain and generalized malaise may occur. Endoscopy can reveal granular inflammation with hyperemic areas, ulceration, and hemorrhage. Polyps, which may develop around granulomas, may be identified by contrast radiography or endoscopy. Protein-losing enteropathy and blood loss can result in malnutrition and iron deficiency, especially in cases with significant small bowel disease. The role of schistosomiasis in malnutrition was illustrated by studies of mass chemotherapy, which resulted in improved nutrition and a lower prevalence of anemia.[11,141,191]

Hepatosplenic Disease (Hepatomegaly, Splenomegaly, and Portal Hypertension)

The life-threatening complications caused by *S. japonicum* and *S. mansoni* are the result of eggs that remain in the venous vasculature and migrate back to the liver.[20] Egg burden seems to be the greatest predictor of hepatic involvement with schistosomiasis, but some link with human leukocyte antigen type has been suggested.[127,129,170,205]

Children with compensated disease initially have few symptoms. These symptoms may include anorexia, malaise, and abdominal fullness.[20,35,103,144,153,207] Children have hepatomegaly even without significant portal hypertension. The hepatomegaly generally is firm and either minimally tender or nontender. Splenic enlargement usually is noted as well. Liver function is affected only late in the course of hepatic schistosomiasis, so jaundice and liver enzyme elevations are unusual findings.

As fibrosis develops around eggs in the liver, portal hypertension ensues. Liver function usually remains intact, but esophageal varices can cause death during the late adolescent and early adult years.[20,35,143] Ascites gradually develops during a period of years, and the spleen may become very large. Bleeding esophageal varices are a common cause of demise in individuals who had heavy schistosomal infections in childhood. Such patients may come to medical attention for melena or hematemesis. Initial episodes are well tolerated. However, with progressive liver decompensation, variceal bleeding can be fatal.

Children with severe hepatosplenic schistosomiasis do not grow as well as other children. Debate has ensued about whether this deficiency is due to a direct effect of the parasitic infection or poor nutritional intake caused by poor general health. Some data suggest that a decrease in insulin-like growth factor-1 activity is linked to hepatic schistosomiasis.[145] Extensive formation of hepatic granulomas may hinder the liver's structure and function in such a way that growth-promoting factors are not produced normally.

Pneumonitis and Cor Pulmonale

Sometimes, children initially have low-grade fever and cough as schistosome larvae migrate through their lungs. This condition can occur with an initial heavy infection (when eggs will not be detectable) or a heavy reinfection (when eggs will be detectable in urine or stool from the preceding underlying infection). This larval pneumonitis can be manifested on lung examination as basilar rales and wheezing.[43,168] Radiographs may show basilar mottling in the lung fields. Eosinophilia is a common occurrence with this type of pneumonitis. Resolution, even without treatment, usually occurs in 2 to 4 weeks. Similar symptoms also may be seen as a reactive pneumonitis when patients with heavy parasite burdens are treated.

In children with advanced hepatosplenic schistosomiasis and portal hypertension, eggs may bypass the liver and flow from the abdominal and pelvic veins into the small lung vessels. Localized granulomas form around eggs lodged in the lungs. Over time, children may be subject to fatigue, cough, and right-sided heart failure. Medical therapy stops the progress of disease and may decrease the ongoing inflammatory responses, but right-sided heart failure, after it is established, is not fully reversible.

Central Nervous System Involvement

Neurologic manifestations of schistosomiasis may be dramatic, even if not common.[30,60,61,138,149,158,169] Worms do not always follow the typical routes described for urinary and intestinal schistosomiasis. On occasion, worms migrate to cerebral blood vessels. Production of eggs in that location can cause seizures and headaches in children.[149,169] Sometimes, optic field defects and dysarthria are noted; these findings seem to result from localized space-occupying inflammatory reactions that develop around worms or eggs. Magnetic resonance imaging (MRI) evaluation reveals a mass or masses of multiple intensely enhancing nodules.[116] Spinal fluid pressure may be elevated, and both protein concentrations and lymphocyte counts in spinal fluid may be increased. This cerebral schistosomiasis occurs more commonly with *S. japonicum* infection[61] and is thought to develop in as many as 2% of infected children.

S. mansoni infection and, to a lesser extent, *S. haematobium* infection can produce eggs that embolize to the spinal cord. The eggs or associated granulomas can cause transverse myelitis. Paraplegia along with urinary and fecal incontinence often is the initial problem in children with spinal schistosomiasis.[60,169]

Chronic or Recurrent Salmonellosis

In endemic areas, some children have salmonellosis and schistosomiasis concurrently and experience chronic low-grade fever, fatigue, malaise, and poor growth.[71,102,103,155,164,215] Blood cultures frequently demonstrate *Salmonella* bacteremia, but stool may not contain these bacteria. Some children have chronic *Salmonella* bacteriuria. Sepsis and mortality are unusual findings despite these persistent bacterial infections. Relapse of the *Salmonella* infection occurs commonly unless the coexisting schistosomal infection is treated. The bacteria are thought to hide within the parasitic worms, where antibiotic penetration is poor, and thereby evade host defenses.

DIAGNOSIS

A clinical diagnosis of schistosomiasis should be entertained in the presence of typical clinical features. These features might be as obvious as painless hematuria in a child in a region endemic for *S. haematobium*, or portal hypertension may be noted late in the second decade of life in an otherwise healthy adolescent from an area known to be endemic for *S. mansoni* or *S. japonicum*.[153,166] The other clinical findings described also should prompt the clinician to consider a diagnosis of schistosomiasis when the child has resided in or traveled through a *Schistosoma*-endemic area.[189] In traveling children, the index of suspicion must be particularly high because patients may be asymptomatic or have atypical symptoms, they may not have clear history of exposure to contaminated water, and parasitologic examination findings often are negative.[19,153]

Outside endemic areas, reinfection is not expected. Thus a reasonable approach is to test all children, including asymptomatic children, who have returned or emigrated from an endemic area where they had potentially significant exposure to fresh water. Such testing would involve all travelers who swam in, waded in, or even touched suspicious water, and it could involve immigrants who have spent long periods in endemic areas. Certainly, any child outside an endemic area who has even a remote history of having had possible contact with cercariae and clinical findings suggestive of any form of schistosomiasis should be tested.

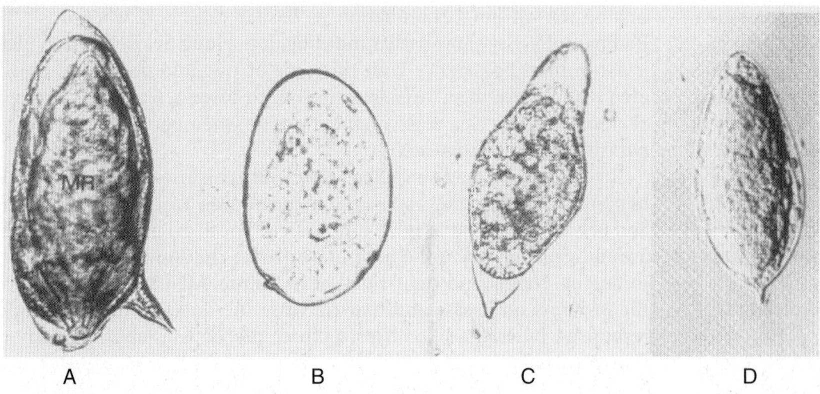

FIG. 229.3 Human schistosome eggs. (A) *Schistosoma mansoni.* (B) *Schistosoma japonicum.* (C) *Schistosoma intercalatum.* (D) *Schistosoma haematobium.* (From Mahmoud AAF, ed. *Schistosomiasis.* London: Imperial College Press; 2001.)

Testing is appropriate because even late therapy can favorably alter the course and outcome of schistosomiasis.

In some highly endemic areas, diagnostic testing is of limited feasibility, questionable reliability, or both, and curative medications are readily available. In such settings, establishing a proved diagnosis might be less necessary. For example, in a highly endemic setting, a urine paper strip test result positive for hematuria could provide sufficient suspicion of infection to warrant administration of specific antischistosomal therapy.[206] In populations with known high rates of infection, mass treatment (without expensive diagnostic testing) is reasonable.

In established heavy infections, eggs usually are readily apparent on microscopic examination of urine or stool. For lighter infections, concentrating techniques are useful. Urine can be centrifuged and filtered to increase the yield of eggs. The result of urine examination is most likely to be positive when urine is voided at midday and when it is collected at the end of the urine stream. In the event of high suspicion and negative urine findings, bladder wall biopsy can be performed. The procedure usually is not necessary, however, because urine microscopy, especially with filtered or concentrated samples, generally is positive. Examination of multiple samples increases the yield.

The eggs of *S. haematobium* and *S. mansoni* are approximately 90 mm in diameter, whereas the eggs of *S. japonicum* and *S. mekongi* are somewhat smaller. As demonstrated in Fig. 229.3, identification of species is aided by observation of the spine—small for *S. japonicum* and *S. mekongi,* at one end for *S. haematobium,* lateral for *S. mansoni,* and broad at each end for *S. intercalatum.* Eggs usually are detectable in voided urine. Plain radiographs might demonstrate some calcification in the bladder wall around chronic granulomas. Cystoscopy, if it is performed, reveals bladder wall hyperemia and, subsequently, nodular lesions and fibrosis that give rise to "sandy patches" on the bladder wall. Granulomas may protrude from the bladder wall into the lumen. Both edema and granulomas may be seen obstructing ureteral orifices.

In light infections, examination of stool or urine samples may not reveal ova because of intermittent or low-volume shedding. Thus negative stool or urine test results do not adequately rule out intestinal schistosomiasis.[20,153] When stools repeatedly are negative for ova, rectal biopsy may be performed. Samples may be obtained by random punch biopsy, but the yield is increased when samples are taken from inflamed sites under direct visualization. Eggs are detected in unstained smears made by pressing the tissue sample between a coverslip and a glass slide, but eggs also can be seen with standard histologic stains.

Nonviable eggs may be excreted for months or years after therapy has been successful. With good medical treatment, eggs usually are not viable when they are passed more than a week after the initiation of therapy. With ineffective treatment or reinfection, however, viable eggs may continue to be passed. On microscopic examination, living ova contain transparent miracidia within the egg, which often are motile. For further documentation of their viability, the eggs may be hatched by placing them in fresh water exposed to light for 20 minutes; observation with a hand lens then can reveal swimming miracidia.

Serologic tests may be needed in acute infection, which may occur before the eggs are excreted or with eggs in ectopic locations.[78,195] For travelers with limited exposure and the likelihood of having either an acute or a limited chronic infection, serologic examination is the main diagnostic tool. A common screening serologic test is the Falcon assay screening test–enzyme-linked immunosorbent assay (FAST-ELISA) using *S. mansoni* adult worm microsomal antigen.[194] This test also cross-reacts with *S. haematobium* but is less sensitive for *S. japonicum* or *S. mekongi* infection. Indirect hemagglutination tests are 70% to 80% sensitive for Katayama syndrome, and ELISA tests do not add to the diagnostic value when an indirect hemagglutination test has already been positive.[159] The species can be confirmed by use of an immunoblot assay (enzyme-linked immunotransfer blot).[195] An immunoblot assay also is available for *S. japonicum.* New tests hold promise in easily identifying antischistosomal antibodies in serum[216] and urine.[56] Antigen-detection assays may be helpful.[3,206] In a small study of European travelers with acute schistosomiasis from Rwanda, serum DNA detection performed better than parasitologic and serologic tests in confirming the diagnosis.[39]

Ultrasonography is the main imaging procedure used in schistosomiasis.[79] It can document involvement of the portal and urinary tracts and, in selected cases, be diagnostic of schistosomiasis. Ultrasonography can identify bladder polyps, ureteral dilation, hydronephrosis, and calcifications within the urinary tract. When resources are available, an ultrasound evaluation of the urinary tract should be performed in any child found to be infected with *S. haematobium.* Ultrasonography can be readily implemented in clinical settings in developing countries to follow lesions of urinary schistosomiasis.[21] For children with persistent urinary symptoms (i.e., dysuria, suprapubic pain, and hematuria) despite having received good medical treatment, cystoscopy should be considered, in part to screen for bladder cancer. Other radiographs and tests of renal function and excretion generally are not indicated unless the ultrasound evaluation reveals significant urologic disease.

Portal ultrasonography is the imaging study of choice for hepatic involvement. The presence of periportal fibrosis with thickening of the portal tracts and vein walls (so-called clay pipestem or Symmers fibrosis) correlates with parasite burden and hepatic disease. In experienced hands, schistosomiasis can be distinguished reproducibly from cirrhosis and other chronic liver diseases.

MRI is helpful in diagnosing neuroschistosomiasis.[61] A variety of cerebral changes may be identified; although not specific for *S. japonicum* neuroschistosomiasis, large masses containing enhancing nodules may be seen in the brain.[61,116] Focal cerebral white matter hyperintensities and hyperintense basal ganglia may be seen in children with hepatosplenic schistosomiasis even when they do not have overt neurologic symptoms.[122] Spinal schistosomiasis, usually caused by *S. mansoni* or *S. haematobium,* can cause spinal pseudotumors with heterogeneous enhancement as well as signal changes extending up and down the spinal cord from the thoracic level.[48,81]

TREATMENT

Optimal treatment of schistosomiasis varies with the stage of the disease. Cercarial dermatitis resolves spontaneously and requires no antiparasitic treatment. Oral antihistaminic agents, however, may be given for severe itching. Medical therapy for schistosomiasis caused by the human schistosomes is effective and well tolerated, without significant complications. No good medical reason exists to allow schistosomiasis to go untreated. The cost of therapy, however, is a limiting factor in resource-limited areas of the world. Several medications can be considered for curative treatment.

Praziquantel, a mixture of stereoisomers of pyrazinoisoquinoline ring structures, is a broad-spectrum oral anthelmintic agent that is effective against each of the human schistosome species.[33] The mechanism of action was thought to involve unmasking of parasite antigens with subsequent killing by the host immune response.[25] However, patients with acquired immunodeficiency syndrome respond well to praziquantel, raising questions about this hypothesis. Praziquantel is given in divided doses on a single day as full curative treatment. For infection with *S. haematobium, S. mansoni,* and *S. intercalatum,* the dose is 40 mg/kg in two divided doses given on the same day. For children infected by *S. japonicum* or *S. mekongi,* the recommended dose had been 60 mg/kg in three divided doses given on the same day,[4,6,160] but recent evidence and recommendations suggest that 40 mg/kg is appropriate for infection with all species of schistosomiasis in people of all ages.[33,142,222] Heavily infected children sometimes experience nausea, vomiting, and abdominal cramping with treatment. Rare side effects, including headache, pruritus, bloody stools, and fever, are transient and resolve within 1 to 2 days after the initiation of treatment. Because praziquantel primarily kills mature adult worms,[74] repeat testing with or without a second course 6 to 12 weeks later is recommended for the treatment of acute infection.[158] In endemic area settings of school-based and community-based mass treatment, adding a second dose of praziquantel 2 to 8 weeks after the initial dose improves reduction in egg counts.[100] Praziquantel is effective in more than 90% of treated children. Some studies suggested that resistance may be emerging.[33,110,111] However, those studies were performed in areas with frequent reinfection and with high parasite burden. Thus the poor response may have been because juvenile forms are not as susceptible to praziquantel. Ongoing work suggests that praziquantel is still effective in endemic areas.[33,132,172] Studies from nonendemic areas also continue to demonstrate excellent efficacy.[207] In addition to curing infection, treatment with praziquantel is associated with improved growth and reduction in anemia.[46] In endemic areas with high rates of infection, school-based and community-based (when many children in the area do not regularly attend school) treatment strategies (without confirmatory diagnostic testing) are effective; cost issues, however, raise concerns of program sustainability.[68,100] Praziquantel not only decreases infection rates but also reduces subsequent reinfection in some[171] but not all[137] areas.

An alternative treatment effective only against *S. mansoni* is oxamniquine, a tetrahydroquinoline compound.[182] The mechanism by which this agent acts is unknown. The effective dose has varied with the geographic origin of the schistosomal infection, but some resistance has been reported. Current recommendations are that children treated with oxamniquine be given 40 to 60 mg/kg divided into two doses administered on 1 day or four separate doses given during the course of 2 days. Mild side effects include nausea, headache, and fever. Seizures are a rare side effect, so administration of this medication should be avoided in children with seizure disorders. Cure rates of more than 90% are reported with oxamniquine.

Metrifonate is an organophosphate compound that causes paralysis of the parasite. It is 70% to 80% effective against *S. haematobium* when used at a dosage of 10 mg/kg orally once every 2 weeks for 6 weeks. It does decrease the child's own plasma and erythrocyte cholinesterase activity, but actual cholinergic symptoms seldom occur. This medication is less expensive than the other options, but it generally is not used when praziquantel is available.

Further exploration of new antischistosome agents and medication combinations continues.[54,93,214]

Medical therapy usually is effective for children with schistosomiasis,[161] even with advanced disease.[112,163,181,217] Clear improvement in the patient's disease burden occurs when treatment is given. Even established uropathy and portal hypertension often are reversible.[114,163,181] Surgical procedures usually are reserved for children with complications related to long-term infection, such as persistent portal hypertension. Propranolol prophylaxis and sclerotherapy or banding can reduce rebleeding from esophageal varices.[55] Some cases require surgical decompression of portal hypertension. Splenorenal shunts are associated with high rates of hepatic encephalopathy. Comparative studies suggest that in experienced hands, esophagogastric devascularization with splenectomy is the procedure of choice.[62,70]

Systemic steroids may be useful for severely ill children with Katayama fever or severe larval pneumonitis. Treatment of neuroschistosomiasis often involves a combination of corticosteroids and praziquantel, with surgery being reserved for those with medullary compression or hydrocephalus.[158] The role of steroids is significant[60,65] but controversial[31] and incompletely tested. Some experts suggest that glucocorticoids be started before the initiation of antiparasitic therapy, to prevent increased inflammatory responses triggered by dying worms.[158] Phenobarbital and phenytoin (but not levetiracetam) can alter metabolism of praziquantel; when used for neuroschistosomiasis-induced seizures, these medications might prompt upward adjustment of the praziquantel dose.[158] Corticosteroids have not been proved effective treatments in other forms of the disease.

PREVENTION

Schistosomiasis has been considered controllable or even eradicable for nearly 100 years.[156] However, control is still not quite within reach. Further multifaceted interventions are needed if we are to be rid of the scourge of schistosomiasis.[85,156] Nonetheless, successful programs in some countries such as Egypt and Brazil demonstrate that control and elimination of schistosomiasis are feasible.[167]

Travelers and expatriates in endemic areas can prevent disease by limiting exposure to infectious fresh water. In endemic areas, they should avoid swimming in fresh-water streams and lakes. In addition, the cercariae can be eliminated by chlorination or by allowing water to settle for 24 hours before bathing or washing.

The use of effective medical therapy coupled with improved urine and stool hygiene has the potential to eradicate schistosomiasis from endemic areas.[208] Elimination of the snails that serve as intermediate hosts also would be effective, but attempts at implementation of programs administering molluscicides have been unsuccessful to date. Historically, national control programs in China focusing on snail control, sanitation, and improved water supplies led to sustained reductions in infection rates, even apart from the influence of chemotherapy.[198,212] For specific populations, health education can lead to significant favorable changes in knowledge about the illness, water-exposure activities, and reinfection rates in school-aged children.[76] Recently, control efforts have focused on mass chemotherapy, with particular emphasis on school-based therapy.[11,77,141,144,208] Similar treatment of preschoolers, especially combined with nonpharmacologic control efforts, is also effective.[136,183] Treatment programs in which the entire school-aged population is treated, typically with praziquantel, have resulted in overall improvement in levels of nutrition and in a reduction in the prevalence of anemia. In areas where reinfection commonly occurs, however, the effects of mass treatment programs are of limited duration, and treatment must be repeated every 6 months to 1 year. Sadly, only about 10% of persons who could benefit from antischistosomiasis treatment are able to receive it each year.[85] Sustainability of national control programs and of favorable outcomes remains challenging in Africa.[59,69,86,90]

Several studies suggest that artemisinin derivatives can prevent development of infection and decrease the worm burden in those exposed to *S. mansoni* and *S. japonicum.*[109,115,157,197] With ongoing exposure to cercariae, prophylactic artemether or artesunate may be given as a 6 mg/kg dose every 1 to 2 weeks.[115] However, these medications are less effective for chemotherapy than is praziquantel,[23,49,158] probably because parasitologic activity is limited to the juvenile forms. Furthermore, the public health role of chemoprophylaxis in the prevention of infection has not been established.[158]

Immunization of experimental animals with irradiated cercariae can prevent experimental schistosomiasis.[179] Thus development of a vaccine to prevent human schistosomiasis is theoretically possible. Several potentially protective antigens have been identified on schistosomes, and they are being used as targets for vaccine development. Animal studies with the Sm-p80 vaccine show promise with some favorable effects on worm reduction, worm egg production reduction, and decreased acute schistosomiasis.[175] Murine studies with Sm-TSP-2 show some efficacy, and chimerization with a hookworm vaccine antigen (Na-APR-1) increases the antischistosomal effectiveness of the vaccine.[148] Human studies are in progress with Sh-28-GST for *S. haematobium*[152] and Sm-14 for *S. mansoni*.[27,193] However, the correlates of protective immunity in humans are not well defined.[27,213] Vaccines related to several *S. japonicum* antigens also are being studied in animals, but efficacy is limited.[130,159,220] No vaccine is yet ready for clinical use,[16,73] but progress continues.[64]

NEW REFERENCES SINCE THE SEVENTH EDITION

18. Berry A, Mone H, Iriart X, et al. *Schistosomiasis haematobium*, Corsica, France. *Emerg Infect Dis.* 2014;20:1595-1597.
33. Chai JY. Praziquantel treatment in trematode and cestode infections: an update. *Infect Chemother.* 2013;45:32-43.
40. Colley DG, Bustinduy AL, Secor WE, et al. Human schistosomiasis. *Lancet.* 2014;383:2253-2264.
41. Colley DG, Secor WE. Immunology of human schistosomiasis. *Parasite Immunol.* 2014;36:347-357.
54. Dong L, Duan W, Chen J, et al. An artemisinin derivative of praziquantel as an orally active antischistosomal agent. *PLoS ONE.* 2014;9:e112163.
64. Fonseca CT, Oliveira SC, Alves CC. Eliminating schistosomes through vaccination: what are the best immune weapons? *Front Immunol.* 2015;6:95.
80. Hegertun IEA, Gundersen KMS, Kleppa E, et al. *S. haematobium* as a common cause of genital morbidity in girls: a cross-sectional study of children in South Africa. *PLoS Negl Trop Dis.* 2013;7:e2104.
93. Keiser J, Silue KD, Adiossan LK, et al. Praziquantel, mefloquine-praziquantel, and mefloquine-artesunate-praziquantel against *Schistosoma haematobium*: a randomized, exploratory, open-label trial. *PLoS Negl Trop Dis.* 2014;8: e2975.
106. Leshem E, Meltzer E, Marva E, et al. Travel-related schistosomiasis acquired in Laos. *Emerg Infect Dis.* 2009;15:1823-1826.
118. Logan S, Armstrong M, Moore E, et al. Acute schistosomiasis in travelers: 14 years' experience at the Hospital for Tropical Diseases, London. *Am J Trop Med Hyg.* 2013;88:1032-1034.
125. Masaku J, Madigu N, Okoyo C, et al. Current status of *Schistosoma mansoni* and the factors associated with infection two years following mass drug administration programme among primary school children in Mwea irrigation scheme: a cross-sectional study. *BMC Public Health.* 2015;15:739.
126. Matangila JR, Doua JY, Linsuke S, et al. Malaria, schistosomiasis and soil transmitted helminth burden and their correlation with anemia in children attending primary schools in Kinshasa, Democratic Republic of Congo. *PLoS ONE.* 2014;9:e110789.
128. Mbanefo EC, Huy NT, Wadagni AA, et al. Host determinants of reinfection with schistosomes in humans: a systematic review and meta-analysis. *PLoS Negl Trop Dis.* 2014;8:e3164.
132. Mendonca AMB, Feitosa APS, Veras DL, et al. The susceptibility of recent isolates of *Schistosoma mansoni* to praziquantel. *Rev Inst Med Trop Sao Paulo.* 2016;58:7.
137. Nalugwa A, Nuwaha F, Tukahebwa EM, et al. Single versus double dose praziquantel comparison on efficacy and *Schistosoma mansoni* re-infection in preschool-age children in Uganda: a randomized controlled trial. *PLoS Negl Trop Dis.* 2015;9:e0003796.
139. Obeng BB, Amoah AS, Larbi IA, et al. Schistosome infection is negatively associated with mite atopy, but not wheeze and asthma in Ghanaian schoolchildren. *Clin Exp Allergy.* 2014;44:965-975.
151. Randrianasolo BS, Jourdan PM, Ravoniarimbina P, et al. Gynecological manifestations, histopathological findings, and *Schistosoma*-specific polymerase chain reaction results among women with *Schistosoma haematobium* infection: a cross-sectional study in Madagascar. *J Infect Dis.* 2015;212:275-284.
167. Schistosomiasis: number of people treated worldwide in 2014. *Weekly Epidemiol Record.* 2016;91:53-60.
171. Senghor B, Diaw OT, Doucoure S, et al. Efficacy of praziquantel against urinary schistosomiasis and reinfection in Senegalese school children where there is a single well-defined transmission period. *Parasit Vectors.* 2015;8:362.
176. Simon GG. Impacts of neglected tropical disease on incidence and progression of HIV/AIDS, tuberculosis, and malaria: scientific links. *Int J Infect Dis.* 2016;42:54-57.
196. Tweyongyere R, Namanya H, Naniima P, et al. Human eosinophils modulate peripheral blood mononuclear cell response to *Schistosoma mansoni* adult worm antigen in vitro. *Parasite Immunol.* 2016;38(8):516-522.
206. Weerakoon KGAD, Gobert GN, Cai P, et al. Advances in the diagnosis of human schistosomiasis. *Clin Microbiol Rev.* 2015;28:939-967.
214. Yepes E, Varela-M RE, Lopez-Aban J, et al. *In vitro* and *In vivo* antischistosomal activity of the alkylphospholipid analog edelfosine. *PLoS ONE.* 2014;9:e109431.
222. Zwang J, Olliaro PL. Clinical efficacy and tolerability of praziquantel for intestinal and urinary schistosomiasis: a meta-analysis of comparative and non-comparative clinical trials. *PLoS Negl Trop Dis.* 2014;8:e3286.

The full reference list for this chapter is available at ExpertConsult.com.

SUBSECTION V Arthropods

230 Arthropods

Jan E. Drutz

Arthropods comprise nearly three-fourths of the world's animal species. Although some arthropods are capable of producing damage to agriculture and homes and others serve as reservoirs, hosts, and vectors of human and animal pathogens, most have no significant impact in causing human disease.[76] However, among the more significant diseases transmitted to humans by arthropods are Chagas disease, malaria, dengue, and bubonic plague. In the United States, ticks transmit more vector-borne diseases caused by bacteria, rickettsia, viruses, and protozoa than do any other species.

TICKS

Ticks, mites, spiders, and scorpions all belong to a class of arthropods known as Arachnida. Two of three families of ticks belonging to this class contain species capable of transmitting pathogens to humans. Ixodidae, the hard tick family, and Argasidae, the soft tick family, serve as both vectors and reservoirs for many rickettsiae (Table 230.1). By use of a fluorescent technique, these rickettsiae can be identified in the tick hemolymph.

However, no rapid laboratory test is currently available to diagnose early-stage rickettsial disease. Possible confirmation of a clinical diagnosis can be obtained by polymerase chain reaction (PCR) testing or immunohistochemical staining of punch biopsy specimens. The expertise required is limited, available only at certain reference laboratories or the Centers for Disease Control and Prevention (CDC). A number of other tests have been used, but the time to diagnostic confirmation can be a disadvantage. Based on the physician's clinical judgment and expertise, treatment of the patient should not be delayed.

Hard ticks are so named because of their scutum, a dorsal sclerotized shield. Owing to the limited scutum coverage of the female, she is more capable of becoming engorged with blood than is the male, a factor significant in the reproductive process. During feedings, these ticks

TABLE 230.1 **Human Infectious Diseases for Which Ticks Are a Vector**

Disease	Agent
Relapsing fever	*Borrelia duttonii*
Q fever	*Coxiella burnetii*
Tularemia	*Francisella tularensis*
Queensland tick typhus	*Rickettsia australis*
Fièvre boutonneuse	*Rickettsia conorii*
Rocky Mountain spotted fever	*Rickettsia rickettsii*
Asian tick typhus	*Rickettsia sibirica*
Colorado tick fever	Arbovirus
Encephalitis	Arbovirus
Lyme disease	*Borrelia burgdorferi*
Human monocytic ehrlichiosis	*Ehrlichia chaffeensis*
Human granulocytic ehrlichiosis	*Ehrlichia* spp.
Babesiosis	*Babesia microti*

remain attached to the host for hours or days at a time.[21,66] Three genera of Ixodidae are known to transmit disease to humans in the United States: *Amblyomma, Dermacentor,* and *Ixodes*.[67]

Soft ticks have no scutum and tend to live for long periods, often surviving for years without eating. Both the nymph form and the adult tick have a tendency to eat often but for brief periods often lasting less than 30 minutes.[21,66] Of the family Argasidae, only ticks of the genus *Ornithodoros* are known to transmit pathogens to humans in the United States.[67] Specifically, they are the vectors of tick-borne relapsing fever.

Local reaction from tick bites appears to be mediated by complement. The reaction from these bites may persist and subsequently develop into a so-called tick bite granuloma. Systemic reactions such as fever, chills, nausea, vomiting, abdominal pain, and headache can be associated with tick bites.

As noted, tick-borne diseases can result from infection with pathogens that include bacteria, rickettsia, viruses, and protozoa.[68] The major tick-borne diseases occurring in the United States include tick paralysis (discussed here), tularemia (see Chapter 132), tick-borne relapsing fever (Chapter 195), Lyme disease (Chapter 140), Colorado tick fever (Chapter 185), Rocky Mountain spotted fever (Chapter 195), ehrlichiosis (Chapter 195), and babesiosis (Chapter 219).

Tick-borne rickettsial diseases are clinically similar yet epidemiologically and etiologically distinct illnesses. In the United States, they include Rocky Mountain spotted fever, human monocytotropic (or monocytic) ehrlichiosis, human granulocytotropic (or granulocytic) anaplasmosis (formerly known as human granulocytotropic ehrlichiosis), *Ehrlichia ewingii* infection, and other emerging tick-borne rickettsial diseases.[13] Mediterranean spotted fever, a tick-borne disease caused by *Rickettsia conorii* (Chapter 195), is found almost exclusively in the Mediterranean area.

Since 2007, five tick-borne diseases have been reported as occurring most often in the United States: Lyme disease, Rocky Mountain spotted fever, ehrlichiosis, anaplasmosis, and babesiosis. Lyme disease, babesiosis, and anaplasmosis are all transmitted by the *Ixodes scapularis* tick. Among contributing factors possibly accounting for the prevalence of these diseases are an increase in the number of ticks, geographic spread, climatic change, improved physician awareness and reporting, and improved local and state surveillance.[24]

Tick Paralysis

Tick paralysis is a neurologic syndrome characterized primarily by an ascending flaccid paralysis. The etiologic agent is a potent neurotoxin produced by an attached, engorged tick.[34] A well-known disease of animals, it was reported to occur in humans in North America first in 1912.[72] Most cases have been reported in the Pacific Northwest and Rocky Mountain states, during spring and summer.[68] It occurs more frequently in children than in adults, especially in girls between 2 and 5 years of age. Patients present with paresthesias and leg weakness, but have no fever. Within 1 to 2 days, weakness in the legs ascends to the trunk musculature, resulting in an inability of the patient to sit or walk without assistance.[34]

Numerous genera of ticks are known to be associated with tick paralysis. In North America, *Dermacentor andersoni* (wood tick) and *Dermacentor variabilis* (dog tick) are the primary species responsible.[48] In Australia, the ticks implicated most commonly are *Ixodes holocyclus* and *Ixodes cornuatus*. Both male and female adults, as well as immature ticks, have been implicated as vectors for this disease.

Pathogenesis

Tick paralysis is thought to be caused by a neurotoxin (holocyclotoxin) produced in the tick's salivary glands.[46] It usually is released by gravid female ticks at the site of attachment, generally the scalp. The neurotoxin is a protein with temperature-dependent activity.[19] The exact mechanism and location of the toxin's action are not known but may include decreased entry of calcium into motor nerve terminals or interference with presynaptic excitation–secretion coupling, which leads to a reduction of acetylcholine release at the motor end plate.

Investigations in children with tick paralysis have implicated peripheral nerve dysfunction, attributable to somewhat site-specific diminished nerve conduction velocities.[41,69] Compound muscle action potentials that are abnormally low or low-normal in amplitude when the patient has maximal neurologic deficits, generally are reversed rapidly once the tick is removed.[48] Swift and Ignacio[69] postulated that the major effect of the toxin is to prevent depolarization in the terminal portions of the motor neurons.

Clinical Manifestations

Onset of tick paralysis usually occurs 5 to 7 days after the female tick attaches to the skin. Until mating occurs with the male, engorgement of the female tick is relatively limited. Mating leads to rapid engorgement, fertilization of the eggs, and production of the neurotoxin. In turn, production of neurotoxin coincides with initial paralytic symptoms, and continual feeding accelerates production of toxin, accounting for rapid clinical deterioration. When the female becomes engorged, she disengages from the skin to deposit her eggs.[34]

Ascending paralysis, along with hyporeflexia or areflexia, progresses to arms, and then to the bulbar structures involved in speech, swallowing, and facial expression.[34] Sensory function usually is spared, and the sensorium remains clear.[68] Alternatively, the disease can present as acute ataxia without muscle weakness.[49] Nystagmus, strabismus, and seizures may occur.[41] After tick removal, symptoms tend to resolve within several hours or days. Left untreated, tick paralysis can be fatal, with reported mortality rates of 10% to 12%.[63]

Routine laboratory tests are not helpful in establishing the diagnosis. The white blood cell count, urine analysis, cerebrospinal fluid, and erythrocyte sedimentation rate are usually normal.

Diagnosis

The diagnosis of tick paralysis can be established when the patient has the typical clinical picture and then improves rapidly after tick removal. A fine-toothed comb can aid in the detection of ticks attached to the scalp. The differential diagnosis of tick paralysis includes Guillain-Barré syndrome, botulism, poliomyelitis, myelitis, spinal cord neoplasm, syringomyelia, and porphyria. Botulism is characterized by slow, descending paralysis involving cranial nerves first, along with a usual extraocular palsy and large, poorly reactive pupils.[34]

The neurologic impairment caused by the *I. holocyclus* tick in Australia is more severe than that caused by *Dermacentor* spp. in North America. With exposure to *I. holocyclus* neurotoxin, the weakness and bulbar symptoms often intensify during the first 24 to 48 hours after tick removal. Clinical recovery is much slower than with *Dermacentor*-related paralysis. *I. holocyclus* antitoxin must be administered before removal of the ticks, and a longer observation period is required.[34]

Treatment

The earlier the tick is removed in the course of the illness, the more promptly the signs and symptoms will resolve. Forceps, not fingers, should be used to remove the tick. The tick's head should be gently but firmly grasped, and slow, reverse traction should be applied to remove all body parts. Recovery generally is complete within 1 to 5 days. In one reported case, weakness did not resolve for several months.[26] Intensive supportive care is required if the patient has cranial nerve dysfunction. Ineffective ventilation and ensuing respiratory failure require assisted ventilation.

Myiasis

Myiasis is the invasion of a host's tissues by the larval stage (maggot) of nonbiting flies. Because of the immaturity of maggots, differentiating the various species is difficult. Myiasis can be classified according to the anatomic site of infestation (i.e., aural myiasis, ophthalmomyiasis, or cutaneous myiasis) or on the basis of the clinical syndrome (i.e., furuncular cutaneous myiasis, migratory cutaneous myiasis, or wound myiasis).[65] In the past, parasitic diseases were limited to their endemic areas. However, with the relative ease of worldwide travel, they are appearing with increasing frequency in the United States and other developed countries.[40]

Etiology

The true flies of the order *Diptera* undergo metamorphosis in four stages: egg, larva, pupa, and adult. To different degrees, some larvae of the suborder Cyclorrhapha have adapted to a parasitic relationship with humans. Some are classified as obligate, facultative, or accidental parasites in humans. In each case, the larval stage of the fly is able to invade the tissues of the host and progress in the stages of metamorphosis.

Epidemiology

The occurrence of human myiasis has been linked to humid and warm climates that favor the breeding of flies. Epizootics in livestock, marginal housing, poor disposal of refuse, and undernutrition also are important factors in the development of human myiasis.[52] In the United States, myiasis has been reported both from flies native to North America and from the larvae of flies acquired during foreign travel. More than 50 species of flies have been reported to cause human myiasis.

Pathogenesis

The pathogenesis of human myiasis differs with the degree of parasitic adaptation by each fly. *Dermatobia hominis* (the human botfly) uses a bloodsucking insect as a vector to deposit its eggs on a warm-blooded host. The larvae emerge from the eggs and then penetrate the host's skin, frequently using the puncture site of the carrier insect. The larvae develop within the dermal layer of skin, which leads to a boil-like swelling. During this period, the human host develops clinical symptoms. *D. hominis* and *Cochliomyia hominivorax,* the primary screwworm, are examples causing obligate myiasis.[52] *C. hominivorax* can be responsible for aural or nasal myiasis.

The genus *Sarcophaga* (flesh flies) is capable of causing facultative myiasis. The adult fly is attracted to wounds or ulcers containing purulent and necrotic material. The adult fly deposits eggs in the open wound, where the larvae hatch.

Maggots seldom are found in the human intestinal or urinary tract.[65] Accidental myiasis can occur when humans ingest eggs or larvae and the larvae remain in the intestinal tract. Genitourinary myiasis is thought to occur by the deposition of eggs around the external urethral orifice. The larvae then may migrate into and up the urethra. Such situations should be called *pseudomyias*[81] because the maggots are not living parasitically.

Clinical Manifestations

The lesions of cutaneous myiasis generally are located over the exposed area of the body. Early in the course of cutaneous myiasis, pruritus is the predominant symptom. As the larvae grow after the first week of infestation, a serous exudate may drain from the penetrating site. At this point, pain and pruritus are prominent symptoms and the lesion appears as a small furuncle (furuncular myiasis).[27] Tissue destruction by the larvae may continue, and secondary bacterial infection can occur. *Staphylococcus aureus,* group A streptococci, and gram-negative organisms have been isolated from infected cutaneous myiasis wounds.

Abdominal pain, diarrhea, and anal bleeding are the symptoms of intestinal myiasis, which is self-limited and may last 2 to 6 weeks. Larvae within the genitourinary tract may lead to proteinuria, dysuria, hematuria, and pyuria. Nasal myiasis can extend into bone, sinus cavities, and even the meninges.[4] Aural myiasis has been described in a child without underlying disease.[20] Ophthalmomyiasis is characterized by an acute catarrhal conjunctivitis.[27] Penetration into the brain has been associated with intracerebral hematomas.[47]

Diagnosis

A careful history of travel, occupation, and exposure is necessary to establish the diagnosis when the physician is confronted with unusual skin lesions that are pruritic and have not resolved with usual local care.[39,44] Myiasis is confirmed if larvae are demonstrated within the wound. A parasitologist or entomologist may be able to identify the species of larvae responsible.

Treatment

The removal of the larvae is necessary in any of the forms of myiasis. Endoscopic removal of nasal infestation is recommended. Surgical intervention may be required to expose the larvae in the wound. Forceps are used to pick out the larvae; the application of 5% chloroform in olive oil may facilitate removal. Occlusive coverings of the wound opening are helpful in extruding *Dermatobia* larvae because this tends to diminish the oxygen supply for the larvae. A thick layer of petrolatum jelly (Vaseline) effectively interrupts the airflow.[53] Local or systemic antibiotics may be required if secondary bacterial infection is present.

The prevention of human myiasis requires good wound care, adequate personal hygiene, screening to protect against flies, and the prevention of myiasis in domestic animals.

MITES

As mentioned earlier, mites belong to the same class of arthropods (Arachnida) as ticks, spiders, and scorpions. They, too, can be vectors for infectious agents. The house mite, *Liponyssoides sanguineus,* is the vector for rickettsialpox (Chapter 195) agent. Chiggers, which are larvae of mites (family Trombiculidae), transmit to humans the agent responsible for scrub typhus, *Rickettsia tsutsugamushi.*

Some mites transmit no specific disease but can cause an annoying pruritic rash. In 2004, the microscopic itch mite *(Pyemotes herfsi)* was identified as a likely cause of an intensely pruritic skin reaction in individuals living in several Midwestern states, as well as Texas and Oklahoma. Skin lesions were papular and erythematous and occurred primarily on the face, neck, and limbs.[12]

Scabies, an extremely pruritic skin infestation, has been known for more than 2500 years. The etiologic agent for this condition, *Sarcoptes scabiei* var. *hominis,* is an obligate human parasite that burrows into the epidermis, no deeper than the stratum granulosum.[17] Scabies appears to have an increased incidence in 15-year cycles[64] and is transmitted person to person through direct and usually prolonged contact.

Pathogenesis

Mites of all developmental stages tunnel into the stratum corneum and deposit feces (scybala) behind them. Characteristically, the gravid female lays eggs in the tunnels.[38] Clothing and bed linens are thought to be less important in the transmission of the *Sarcoptes* mite. Because scabies is transmitted by skin-to-skin contact, sexual transmission occurs commonly, as does nonsexual spread in family settings.[17] Epidemic outbreaks of scabies have been reported in hospitals and other institutions where people were living closely together and especially where poor sanitation predominated.[6]

Hypersensitivity of both immediate and delayed types has been implicated in the development of lesions other than burrows.[17] Papulovesicular scabies is characterized by perivascular lymphohistiocytic infiltrates with eosinophils. The papillary dermis is edematous. The histologic appearance of nodular scabies is one of a dense, superficial, and deep perivascular lymphohistiocytic infiltrate with many plasma cells and eosinophils. Various vascular changes also may be apparent.

Clinical Manifestations

Scabies is characterized by moderate to severe pruritus that starts several weeks to months after infestation, at which time the host has become hypersensitive to the mite or its products. Itching, most evident at night, is the primary symptom of infection. A papular or vesicular eruption with pustules and linear burrows occurs and classically involves the webs between the fingers, flexures of the arms, axillae, and genital regions of adults. In infants and children, scabetic lesions more typically occur on the palms, soles, head, and neck in the form of vesicles, pustules, or nodules. In this age group, scabies often is not suspected because of the atypical skin lesions that result from vigorous scratching and secondary infection.[42]

Acute glomerulonephritis may be associated with pyoderma in scabies. A careful history may reveal that other family members or child caretakers have pruritus and skin lesions consistent with scabies. Examination of the skin of family members for signs of scabies frequently is helpful. Crusted scabies, previously known as Norwegian scabies, occurs in immunocompromised patients, especially those on immunosuppressive medications or those with HIV or human T-lymphotropic virus type 1 infection.[35] In this condition, mite replication is uncontrolled by the host's immune system.[22,35] It is a psoriasiform dermatitis, frequently associated with a generalized or localized nonspecific hyperkeratosis.[28,35]

Diagnosis

Definitive diagnosis can be made by microscopic identification of the mites, eggs, or mite feces.[43] To obtain this material, skin scrapings should be taken from papules or the end of a burrow or from underneath the surface of fingernails. In some cases, a variety of biopsy techniques can be useful.[9] The diagnosis should be considered when the physician is faced with an unusual papular or bullous rash. The differential diagnosis of scabies in children includes impetigo, atopic eczema, seborrheic or contact dermatitis, psoriasis, histiocytosis, and chickenpox.[42,43]

Treatment

The management of scabies involves the application of a topical scabicide to all areas of skin, including the face and scalp, with subsequent removal in 8 to 24 hours, depending on the product applied. An effective scabicide used in the past was gamma-hexachlorocyclohexane (lindane). It is no longer recommended for use in children because of concerns regarding neurotoxicity.[22,50] Currently, effective topical scabicides licensed in the United States include 5% permethrin and 10% crotamiton. Although 5% malathion lotion is approved in the United States for treatment of head lice (see later discussion of head lice treatment), it has not received US Food and Drug Administration (FDA) approval to be used as a scabicide.[38]

The agent of choice for infants and young children is 5% permethrin topical cream, applied in the evening to the entire head, neck, and body of the infant and left on overnight.[42] It is indicated and safe for use in newborns and young children, as well as pregnant and lactating women.[38] A second application generally is recommended 1 to 2 weeks after the first dose.[22,38] All family members should be treated simultaneously.[58] Antibiotics may be necessary if secondary bacterial infection is present.

The CDC has recommended the off-label use of oral ivermectin 200 μg/kg per dose given with food for the treatment of scabies, although the FDA has yet to grant such approval.[22] Ivermectin is considered to be highly efficacious as an oral therapy for scabies in a single dose for otherwise healthy or HIV-infected adults.[54] Some have recommended two doses, with the second dose given 1 to 2 weeks after the first dose, especially for crusted scabies.[22] In an Australian study involving more than 2000 participants, enrollees were randomly assigned to treatment with either topical permethrin or an oral dose of ivermectin. From baseline to 12 months, scabies prevalence declined for all participants, with the greatest reduction in the ivermectin group.[60]

It works against several different parasites by interrupting gamma-aminobutyric acid–induced neurotransmission.[17] The CDC recommends not using ivermectin in pregnant or lactating women and states that safety has not been determined in children who weigh less than 15 kg.

A pharmaceutical preparation (moxidectin), currently being used to treat mange in animals, is under consideration for possible treatment of human scabies. Pending study results as to efficacy and safety in humans, this may become available as a single-dose treatment in the near future.[55]

From a global perspective, the International Alliance for the Control of Scabies was established in 2012. The organization is committed to the control of human scabies infestation and to promoting the health and well-being of all those living in affected communities. Priority areas have included advocacy, epidemiology, control strategies, and biological research.[32]

Articles of clothing and bed linens should be machine washed in hot water at 60°C (140°F). Insecticidal powder or aerosol should be reserved for materials that cannot be washed.[17] Pruritus often persists for some time after successful treatment with a scabicide and may be relieved by an oral antihistamine or mild to moderate topical steroids.[9,58] In hospitalized patients, contact isolation is recommended to lessen the potential for nosocomial transmission.

LICE

Pediculosis

Arthropods of the order Anoplura (sucking lice) are important as vectors of rickettsial or spirochetal illnesses. The body louse, *Pediculus humanus humanus,* is the vector for epidemic typhus *(Rickettsia prowazekii),* trench fever *(Bartonella quintana),* and louse-borne relapsing fever *(Borrelia recurrentis).* The body louse, head louse *(Pediculus humanus capitis),* and crab louse *(Phthirus pubis)* all are capable of achieving human infestation. Pediculosis has been a problem for humans for more than 10,000 years.[17]

Pathogenesis

Head lice are the most common type of louse, affecting more than 100 million people worldwide each year.[16] Tiny, they measure no more than 1 to 4 mm in length. They have six legs, each with powerful claws allowing firm attachment. Mouth parts consist of stylets (retracted when not in use) modified for piercing and sucking. When they are not feeding, lice are translucent, with gray-white bodies, but when engorged with blood, they become red. Each female is capable of laying as many as 300 eggs (nits) in a brief lifetime of 1 to 3 months. These eggs are less than 1 mm in diameter and hatch in 6 to 10 days, giving rise to nymphs. During a period of 10 days, the nymphs become adults. Schoolchildren of all socioeconomic groups are affected, with head-to-head contact being the most common means of transmission.

Clinical Manifestations

Children or adults with head lice usually have white or opalescent nits attached to individual strands of hair. The lice themselves firmly adhere to the base of the hair shaft, millimeters from the scalp. After a louse pierces the skin, a poisonous salivary secretion is exuded, resulting in pruritic dermatitis. Itching is the primary symptom in acute cases.

Body lice occur when socioeconomic conditions are poor. Infestation occurs when people fail or are unable to wash their clothes regularly, such as those living in refugee camps. Intense itching is a major problem, with noticeable excoriations and occasional secondary infections.

Pubic lice are transmitted primarily through sexual contact, although not exclusively so. In children, pubic lice generally occur from nonsexually transmitted contact with an infected parent. Again, itching is a major presenting symptom. Pubic lice may become attached to other hairy areas of the body, such as the axillae of adolescents, the eyelashes of children, and the scalp hair of any age group.[17]

As mentioned, body lice can function as vectors for the transmission of several diseases. One of these is trench fever, caused by *B. quintana.* Although some patients may have no symptoms, others may have fever, myalgias, headache, meningoencephalitis, transient maculopapular rashes, or chronic adenopathies. A second potentially transmitted disease is epidemic typhus, caused by *R. prowazekii.* Signs or symptoms of this infection may include fever, pruritic rash, headache, and confusion. Relapsing fever caused by *B. recurrentis* is the third disease known to be transmitted by the body louse.[17]

Diagnosis

Head, body, and pubic lice are visibly recognizable. The nits of head lice are attached firmly to hair shafts and are distinguished readily from dandruff flakes, lint, and other debris, which can be easily removed from the hair. Viable nits, located close to the scalp, are oval and gray-white to yellow-white. Empty nonviable nits, attached at some distance from the scalp, are almost completely clear. Although difficult to see with the naked eye, nits visibly fluoresce yellow-green under Wood lamp. PCR helps identify host DNA from lice through their blood meal, providing valuable information for rape, homicide, and child abuse cases.[51]

The body louse has been demonstrated as the true vector of trench fever by using PCR to detect within them the *B. quintana* DNA from infected patients.[8] Detection of rickettsial DNA in body lice has confirmed the presence of human typhus.

Treatment

Head lice. Numerous forms of treatment for the eradication of head lice have been used. Over the course of time, resistance developed to several of these forms of therapy. Gamma-hexachlorocyclohexane (lindane) shampoo was used almost exclusively until the early 1970s. Because of concern about potential neurotoxic effects for the patient, it no longer is recommended as a first-line medication for children.[50]

A systematic review (1995) concluded that sufficient evidence existed only for the use of a pyrethroid insecticide, 1% permethrin cream rinse.[16,73] This biodegradable and generally very safe product remains the recommended first-line therapy. It should be applied to wet hair and left in place for about 10 minutes before rinsing. Because of variable reports of head lice resistance to 1% permethrin, the current recommendation is two treatment applications 7 to 14 days apart, or even three treatments at 0, 7, and 15 days, based on the life cycle of head lice.[5] Some success has been reported with use of a 5% permethrin preparation and wearing a shower cap overnight.[61] To remove the firmly adherent nits, a fine-toothed stainless steel comb (LiceMeister) has been recommended.

Malathion lotion 0.5%, an organophosphate, has been an excellent alternative to the use of permethrin in areas where head lice resistance has occurred. When applied to the hair and left in place for 8 to 12 hours, it provides residual protection. The intent is to use it for those older than age 6 years. Live lice will be killed, but not all eggs. A second treatment 7 to 9 days later can be used if live lice remain. Caution should be taken because it is potentially flammable. Those treated should not be exposed to open flames or electric heat sources, including hair dryers and electric curlers.[1,5]

Cases of resistance to the malathion-containing formulation have been reported in Europe, but that product is different from the one licensed in the United States. The latter contains additional synergistic agents, including 78% isopropanol. Because it is hydrolyzed and detoxified by plasma carboxylesterases much more rapidly in mammals than in insects, it is considered safe. Although it is contraindicated for use in infants, the American Academy of Pediatrics considers it safe for use in children 2 years and older.[1,5]

Ivermectin has been used when other medications have failed. For those at least 6 months of age, ivermectin lotion 0.5% was approved by the FDA in 2012. A single application to dry hair is considered effective in most patients. Although not approved by the FDA for the treatment of head lice, ivermectin in a single oral dose of 200 μg/kg has been effective. If needed, a second dose of 400 μg/kg 9 to 10 days later can be given. Concern exists when the drug is used in patients weighing less than 15 kg or in those who are pregnant or breast-feeding.[10]

As a result of reports of difficult-to-treat head lice infestation, authors in one cluster-randomized, double-blind, double-dummy, controlled trial compared ivermectin 400 μg/kg to the application of 0.5% malathion lotion, each given on days 1 and 8. Ivermectin was reported to have superior efficacy. However, the malathion product was not the one licensed in the United States.[16]

In addition to malathion, two other topical pediculicides have received FDA approval for pediatric use. Labeled for use in children 6 months or older, benzyl alcohol should be applied to dry hair for at least 10 minutes. If live lice persist, a second application should be administered 7 days later. For children 4 years of age or older, spinosad should be applied in the same way as benzyl alcohol.

There have been other recommended approaches to the treatment of head lice, all with somewhat limited success. A short course of oral trimethoprim-sulfamethoxazole had been recommended in the past with the intent of destroying essential lice gut bacteria, responsible for the production of vitamin B, essential for continued life. A nonchemical approach to treatment has been the application of a topical lotion (Cetaphil Skin Cleanser) to the hair, with subsequent use of a blow dryer to "shrink-wrap" and ultimately suffocate lice.[57] Although this approach may result in significant success, the original study was not sufficiently rigorous to prove its effectiveness.

The use of a high-volume, hot-air blow dryer alone has been reported to have killed 94% to 98% of lice eggs and 76% to 80% of hatched lice.[37] When examined 1 week later, virtually all of the patients were completely cured. Although promising, this approach necessitates further testing by independent investigators. If proved efficacious, it could potentially eliminate the use of chemicals, to which some lice have become resistant.

Body lice. A general recommendation has been thorough washing of the body with soap and water followed by the application of a pyrethrin or pyrethroid or malathion for 8 to 24 hours. Again, caution should be taken in the use of these preparations in children. Decontamination of clothing and bed linens is essential by either washing them in hot soapy water at a temperature of 54°C (130°F) for 10 minutes or placing them in a hot clothes dryer for 20 minutes.

Pubic lice. Treatment should be similar to that used for managing head lice. Clothes and bed linens should be decontaminated. In the case of children, parents also should be treated; and in the case of adolescents, sexual partners require treatment.

BED BUGS

Numerous recent reports have documented the reemergence of bed bugs *(Cimex lectularius)* as a cause of pruritic, erythematous papules.[14,70] Although they are known to harbor pathogens (e.g., plague and hepatitis B), bed bugs are considered incapable of transmitting those diseases to humans[45,74] and therefore are not thought to pose a medical threat. Secondary skin infections, however, can develop as a result of persistent scratching, and allergic reactions are a possibility.

The upsurge in bed bug infestation has been attributed to various factors, including increased international travel and transport, exchange of secondhand furniture, insecticide resistance, and changes in insecticide use.[23] The primary result of contending with these annoying insects has been both social and psychological. Hotels, department stores, apartment buildings, and homeowners have encountered a significant economic loss in their efforts to eliminate these pests.

Pathogenesis and Clinical Manifestations

Bed bugs tend to be nocturnally active and are attracted to humans by warm body temperature and the exhalation of carbon dioxide. Most can be found within 5 feet of the bed. Survival depends on blood extracted from their respective hosts, which is achieved by piercing the skin with their beadlike proboscis containing a set of two hollow tubes. Online videos are available for viewing actual bed bug feeding.[25] Through one of these tubes, they inject saliva containing both anticoagulants and anesthetics; through the other one, blood is withdrawn.[70] Although they can live for up to 18 months without feeding, bedbugs typically seek blood every 5 to 10 days.

Feeding time generally takes place in the early morning hours, when the host is most calm and least likely to sense the presence of a crawling insect. Because bed bugs are opportunistic feeders, shift workers, who sleep during the daytime, also are vulnerable.

Total feeding time can range from as short as 5 minutes to as long as 30 minutes, after which the insect abandons the skin surface and seeks seclusion among bed sheets, blankets, mattresses, floorboard cracks, or other crevices.[70] The host generally does not experience itching or skin irritation until several minutes or hours after the insect has fed. In some cases, no skin reaction occurs at all.

Diagnosis

Suspicion for the possible presence of bed bugs occurs when the host awakens with itching and visible bites not present before going to sleep. Clues to the presence of bed bugs include discrete red-brown bloodstains on sheets and mattresses, as well as flecks of excrement at the portals of hiding places.[68] Confirmation requires finding and identifying these bugs. Current approaches to early detection include the use of various lures or traps and training dogs to pick up the scent of certain bed bug pheromones.[23]

Treatment

Treatment of bites is relatively conservative, directed toward symptomatic relief of itching, irritation, and secondary infection. Antipruritic medication, either topical or oral preparations, may be considered. First-generation antihistamines can help alleviate the itching but may be sedating. Topical corticosteroids can help reduce the erythema and itching. Oral antibiotics alone are sufficient to treat secondary bacterial skin infections.

Eradication

Insecticides containing pyrethroids are used widely as a control measure; however, pyrethroid-resistant bed bug populations have been found in some states. Nonchemical methods to effectively control bed bugs include heating infested rooms to 48°C (118°F) for 1 hour or cooling rooms to −16°C (3°F) for 1 hour; encasing mattresses and box springs with bed bug–excluding covers; and vacuuming, steaming, laundering, and disposing of infested items. Any effective control measure for bed bugs requires support from all residents in affected buildings and ongoing monitoring for infestation from other housing units. In addition, multiple inspections and treatments frequently are needed.

In a relatively recent report, a total of 111 illnesses, representing seven different states, were associated with bed bug–related insecticide use. The majority of the illnesses were of low severity (81%). One fatality was confirmed. The most common factors contributing to illness were excessive insecticide applications, failure to wash or change pesticide-treated bedding, and inadequate notification of pesticide application.[15] To rid the living environment of bed bugs, a professional exterminator should be consulted.

SPIDERS

Of the thousands of species in the United States, only a few pose a threat to humans. Species of the genus *Loxosceles* are the spiders predominantly responsible for necrotic arachnidism in the United States. The two most common species are the black widow spider *(Loxosceles mactans)* and the brown recluse spider *(Loxosceles reclusa)*. Both prefer dark, undisturbed habitats, such as outdoor lavatories, woodpiles, underside of stones, or dark corners of garages and attics. The black widow has a characteristic red hourglass shape on its ventral surface. The brown recluse has a violin-shaped marking over its dorsal surface. In the Pacific Northwest area of the United States, the hobo spider *(Tegenaria agrestis)* produces an envenomation similar to that of the brown recluse spider.[11]

Pathogenesis

Venom from the black widow contains a neurotoxin (α-lactrotoxin), not a tissue toxin. The main effect is at the presynaptic membrane of the neuromuscular junction. Venom from the brown recluse spider contains sphingomyelinase D, a phospholipase that induces dermal necrosis and also causes systemic effects through its interaction with red blood cells, platelets, and endothelium.[62] The necrosis caused by the venom depends on neutrophils, but the neutrophils are not activated by the venom itself. Rather, the venom is a potent stimulus for the inflammatory response of endothelial cells, which in turn activates the polymorphonuclear neutrophils to cause tissue destruction.[56]

Clinical Manifestations

The bite of the black widow spider generally is painless, but a target lesion may develop. Within 30 to 120 minutes, some patients complain of regional lymph node tenderness.[80] The primary symptom that follows the bite is muscle cramping, generally involving the abdomen, chest, or back, depending on the location of the bite. Autonomic symptoms, including profuse sweating, nausea, vomiting, and tachycardia, may occur.[62] Hypertension can be a significant problem. The degree of systemic symptoms depends on the amount of venom injected and the number of bites. Severe cases may progress to internal hemorrhage, paralysis, and, rarely, even death.

The brown recluse spider bite may produce a mild or sharp stinging sensation. After several hours, the pain intensifies and itching occurs.[2] Eventually, a blister with surrounding erythema forms at the site. In the course of time, the lesion becomes larger, and central necrosis develops. Systemic signs developing in the first 24 to 48 hours may include headache, fever, nausea, vomiting, and joint pain. Disseminated intravascular coagulation, multiorgan failure, and death have been reported in children.[36,78]

Like that of the brown recluse spider, the bite of the hobo spider may result in a central necrotic area. The most common systemic symptom is a severe headache. Protracted systemic effects, including aplastic anemia, intractable vomiting, and profuse secretory diarrhea, are rare occurrences but may be associated with death.[75]

Treatment

For the patient who has been bitten by a black widow spider, analgesia is the mainstay of care.[62] An antivenin is available, but only for the most severe cases of envenomation, unresponsive to other measures.[7]

For bites of brown recluse spiders, numerous treatments have been used, including hyperbaric oxygen therapy, early excision, antibiotics, dapsone, and corticosteroids. Careful supportive care, including monitoring of electrolytes and renal function, is required if symptoms are severe.[62] Systemic corticosteroid therapy may be of some benefit if the patient has considerable symptoms. Dapsone, an inhibitor of neutrophil function, appears to decrease the development of wound complications and subsequent need for surgical excision.[59]

SCORPIONS

Scorpions, like ticks, mites, and spiders, belong to the Arachnida class of arthropods.[30] The striped bark scorpion *(Centruroides vittatus)* is the most common type of scorpion found in the United States.[29] The most dangerous and perhaps the most lethal scorpion in this country is *Centruroides exilicauda* (former species name, *sculpturatus*), occasionally referred to as the bark scorpion.[31,62] It is indigenous to the desert Southwest, particularly Arizona. Depending on the species, scorpions tend to reside in cracks and crevices, in cupboards and closets, or under loose tree bark. They inject their venom when disturbed or threatened.

Pathogenesis and Clinical Manifestations

C. vittatus produces a neurotoxic venom stored in poison glands in the tip of the tail. The venom of these scorpions is deadly to insect prey and produces a painful sting for humans. For those allergic to the sting, an anaphylactic reaction may occur.[29] The venom from the *Vaejovis carolinianus* (plain eastern stripeless scorpion) is considered to be mild, similar to that of a honeybee sting. Anecdotal reports indicate that on occasion, a severe reaction may occur.[30] The *C. exilicauda* scorpion produces a neurotoxic venom that can lead to cardiac failure, respiratory paralysis, agitation, paresthesias, hypersalivation, hypertension, and gastrointestinal symptoms. Although tachycardia and hypertension are frequent reactions, opposite effects are a possibility when the venom activates the parasympathetic nervous system.[59] The absence of local tissue reaction is helpful in distinguishing *C. exilicauda* stings from those of other scorpions found in Arizona.[31] Children and elderly adults are most at risk as a result of envenomation from *C. exilicauda*.[29]

Treatment

Most scorpion stings necessitate only nonprescription analgesic medication. For the management of *C. exilicauda* envenomation, atropine can be used to control hypersalivation, although it could be contraindicated when the sting has been produced by scorpions foreign to the United States. In some of those cases, the use of atropine can exacerbate an adrenergic toxicity reaction created by the sting of the scorpion. Treatment of *C. exilicauda* envenomation with an antivenin (available in Arizona only; not approved by the FDA) has been reported to provide relief from the neurotoxic effects. It has the unfortunate potential of causing both immediate and delayed hypersensitivity reactions.[31,62]

FLEAS

Murine Typhus

Also known as endemic typhus fever, murine typhus is a worldwide flea-borne infection of humans. It is caused by *Rickettsial felis* and *Rickettsial typhi*. The disease most commonly occurs among people in contact with rats or areas where rats live, but also occurs among people who live near or have contact with other small mammals (e.g., opossums and cats). Cases reported in the United States are usually confined to suburban areas of Texas and Southern California, as well as several Hawaii islands. The cat flea *Ctenocephalides felis* is considered to be the primary vector.[18] The disease is often difficult to diagnose because of its nonspecific clinical presentation. Clinicians are led to believe that patients have other, more commonly seen vector-borne infections, such as dengue fever, ehrlichiosis, West Nile virus, and Rocky Mountain spotted fever, or non–vector-borne infections (e.g., bacterial or viral meningitis disease, Kawasaki disease, or secondary syphilis).[18]

Pathogenesis and Clinical Manifestations

Like other rickettsiae, *R. typhi* is a small (0.4–1.3 mm) gram-negative obligate intracellular bacterium depending on hematophagous arthropods (e.g., fleas and ticks) and mammals to maintain its life cycle. *R. typhi* multiplies in the epithelial cells of the flea midgut and subsequently are shed into the feces, which in turn are deposited on the host skin surface while the flea is feeding.[18] Humans and other mammals acquire the bacteria when the flea bites or feces are inoculated into the bite site.[3] *R. felis* has been identified as the cause of typhus-like illness in the United States (Texas), Mexico, France, and Brazil. Molecular studies have found that *R. felis* and *R. typhi* are indistinguishable serologically and require separate identification using PCR analysis.[18]

Following an incubation period of 1 to 2 weeks, the most common symptoms include 3 to 7 days of fever, headache, exanthema, and arthralgia. The exanthema can be variable from patient to patient. It can be macular or maculopapular and nonpruritic, beginning on the trunk, eventually spreading to the arms and legs, but sparing the palms and soles. It appears about 7 days after the onset of fever and remains unchanged for a period of 1 to 4 days.[18]

The mortality rate for murine typhus is low with use of appropriate antibiotics (1%) and about 4% without the use of antibiotics. In most cases, it will present as an acute, self-limited illness without complications. However, serious complications have been associated with acute infection, including endocarditis, splenic rupture, and aseptic meningitis.[18]

Diagnosis

Most rickettsial infections are diagnosed using serologic methods such as IFA, often considered to be the most ideal test. Unfortunately, serologic studies are rarely diagnostic when blood specimens are collected at the onset of symptoms. A convalescent-phase specimen, yielding a fourfold increase in titer between the acute- and convalescent-phase samples, is usually required to confirm the diagnosis.[18,79]

Other available serologic assays include the indirect immunoperoxidase assay, latex agglutination, line blot, and Western immunoblot. Isolation of rickettsiae from blood cultures is rarely successful and usually necessitates the expertise of a specialized research laboratory. Diagnosis has been made by PCR with the use of peripheral blood, buffy coat, and plasma specimens and occasionally with fresh-frozen or paraffin-imbedded tissue specimens or with arthropod vectors acquired during ecologic surveillance (i.e., cat fleas).[18,79]

Treatment

Antimicrobial testing is not routinely performed on rickettsiae. As with other rickettsial diseases, the preferred antibiotic is a tetracycline, particularly doxycycline for children 9 years and older. The course of treatment is usually a week or less, limiting the risk for dental staining.[13,77]

Tungiasis

Tungiasis, also known as sand flea disease, is a parasitic skin infestation. It is indigenous to parts of South America and sub-Saharan Africa. The population most vulnerable are children and elderly people, living in impoverished, resource-poor areas. *Tunga penetrans* and *Tunga trimamillata* belong to the genus *Tunga* of the order Siphonaptera. They are unique among other fleas in that the nonfertilized females of these species burrow into the skin, but only minimally advance further. Staying in situ, they subsequently die off in 4 to 6 weeks. During this time, their distal segment remains exposed to the open environment, allowing them to breathe, defecate, copulate, and expel eggs. The entry site becomes a portal for access by infectious microorganisms.[33]

The primary penetrance site is the sole of a bare foot. However, any body part is vulnerable, especially if the person is sleeping on the floor or ground. Marked erythema, pain, edema, and itching are present. Aerobic and anaerobic bacteria, adherent to the flea or introduced by scratching the skin site, are provided a pathway for producing a subsequent infection. Particularly in impoverished areas of the world lacking appropriate immunization access, tetanus is not an uncommon occurence.[33]

In addition to humans, a broad spectrum of domestic and sylvantic animals is also susceptible to infiltration by the sand flea. Treatment to eliminate the burrowed flea has met with limited success. Many individuals have attempted removal using nonsterile sharp instruments or sharpened pieces of wood. One field application involved a combination of 10% imidacloprid and 50% permethrin, providing temporary reduction in the parasite load. Another preventive had been the application of a plant-based repellent, Zanzarin. More recently, the topical application of a mixture of two low-viscosity dimethicones has met with some degree of success.[33,71]

Despite the large number of people affected by sand flea infestation, especially in resource-poor countries, and limited treatment options, tungiasis remains unlisted by the World Health Organization as a neglected tropical disease.

NEW REFERENCES SINCE THE SEVENTH EDITION

32. Engelman D, Kiang K, Chosidow O, et al. Toward the global control of human scabies: introducing the international alliance for the control of scabies. *PLoS Negl Trop Dis*. 2013;7:e2167, 1-4.
33. Feldmeier H, Heukelbach J, Ugbomoiko US, et al. Tungiasis: a neglected disease with many challenges for global public health. *PLoS Negl Trop Dis*. 2014;8:e3133.
55. Mounsey KE, Bernigaud C, Chosidow O, McCarthy JS. Prospects for moxidectin as a new oral treatment for human scabies. *PLoS Negl Trop Dis*. 2016;10(3):e0004389.
60. Romani L, Whitfield MJ, Koroivueta J, et al. Mass drug administration for scabies control in a population with endemic disease. *N Engl J Med*. 2015;373(24):2305-2313.
71. Thielecke M, Nordin P, Ngomi N, Feldmeier H. Treatment of tungiasis with dimeticone: a poof-of-principle study in rural Kenya. *PLoS Negl Trop Dis*. 2014;8:e3058.

The full reference list for this chapter is available at ExpertConsult.com.

Global Health

231

Holly E. McBride • Peter J. Hotez • Gail J. Harrison

The keys to success as a global health professional are compassion, competence, critical thinking, and creative adaptability.

Chunhuei Chi

This chapter provides an introduction to the definition, evolution, disciplinary perspectives, interventions, and contemporary challenges associated with global health. For information on specific health conditions and infectious diseases of global concern, such as human immunodeficiency virus (HIV) infection and acquired immunodeficiency syndrome (AIDS), malaria, tuberculosis, parasites, or specific circumstances, such as international adoptions, the reader is referred to the individual chapters for each of these entities.

DEFINITION OF GLOBAL HEALTH

The term global health is widely used and very popular among academic institutions, humanitarian and government agencies, nongovernment organizations (NGOs), and nonprofit organizations around the world.[30] Global health is increasingly mentioned as an area of public health and medical professional interest, as well as a philanthropic goal, but it is rarely defined by a definition agreed on by even the most influential health organizations.[2,4,27] Many organizations and institutions have used the term global health as a state of being or condition, as a goal, or as a field of study that relates to education, research, and practice. Uniformity of definition is desirable because it sets the foundation for collaborative efforts of global purpose, clear objectives for action, and reliable instruments for measuring achievements. Fragments of public health and international health definitions, which evolved from hygiene and tropical medicine, have been used to assemble a concept of global health that is becoming universally accepted.[5–7] Global health often overlaps in the fundamental purpose and initiatives of both public and international health and can be seen as evolving from both disciplines. An understanding of the history and evolution of definitions of health, public health, and international health is helpful in understanding the overall objective of global health.[27]

The World Health Organization (WHO), one of the leading authorities for health, has defined health as "a state of complete physical, mental and social well-being and not merely the absence of disease or infirmity."[8] This definition was the basis from which the WHO worked their evolving and emerging projects toward the goals to improve the overall health of the world. This definition is broad and all inclusive. It includes the larger picture of overall health for one person, or a whole community, and covers not only the administration of medical attention, but also prevention of disease through public health, policy, mental well-being, research, and many more factors influential in health.

The current public health concepts emerged in mid-19th-century Europe and the United States. During this time, medical advances in the cause, management, and prevention of infectious diseases and the growth of social reform movements helped establish the discipline of public health with four main concepts: (1) decision making based on data and evidence gathered through vital statistics, surveillance, outbreak investigations, and scientific method; (2) focus on populations or groups rather than individuals; (3) action rooted in social justice and equity; and (4) prevention of disease rather than treatment or cure of established disease. In 1988, the Institute of Medicine reconfirmed public health as a preventive discipline that uses a community approach and involves multiple partners working toward a common good of public health. The American Public Health Association (APHA) defines public health in contemporary terms as "the practice of preventing disease and promoting good health within groups of people, from small communities to entire countries," including the well-being of the population of a specific country or community within a country.[5] Public health practice emerged from the works of many pioneering scientists and physicians and the early discoveries about quarantine, sanitation, and housing; public knowledge on sexually transmitted infections and diseases; and vaccinations. Eventually, the practice of public health evolved from early efforts of individuals to organized efforts among societies and nations.

The field of international health was further developed from public health, hygiene, and tropical medicine disciplines as medical missionaries, scientists, and other humanitarians traveled and shared their discoveries and new ideas. The specific focus of international health and international medicine currently lies in the differences among countries, peoples, and regions. International health applies the well-established public health principles of industrialized countries to assist the health problems and challenges of low-income populations in developing countries, through foreign aid activities and missionary work (Table 231.1). It often includes "diseases of the developing world" and "health work abroad," with a focus on infectious and tropical diseases, water and sanitation, malnutrition, and maternal-child health.[5–7] Previously, international health and global health were considered interchangeable terms, whereas now most experts recognize them as distinct disciplines and practices.[27]

Global health transcends the individual nations and borders and emphasizes worldwide improvement of health, reduction of disparities, and protection against threats to health of the people of all nations (see Table 231.1). Global health focuses on the similarities throughout the world and the issues that cross nations.[27] It blurs the borders to create a sense of unity and understanding of how people, cultures, and the environment interact and affect each other. It emphasizes both the individual and the population and strives for equity among people of all nations. It also is highly interdisciplinary and multidisciplinary in its approach to problem solving and strives to provide creative and sustainable solutions for resource management in resource-poor regions (see Table 231.1).

Current global health issues involve not only the direct health impact, but also other disciplinary perspectives that indirectly influence health, such as climate change and natural disasters, economics, politics, conflict, war, migration, food crisis, energy crisis, and neglected diseases.[1] The political perspective of global health emphasizes the influences of war and economy on the health of the world. The educational and research perspectives of global health are evident when global health is taught as curriculum in both medical and sociologic disciplines and are an educational goal of many institutions of higher learning. The epidemiologic perspective of global health identifies and follows trends of major global health threats and partners with the medical perspective to describe the pathologic factors, clinical manifestations, diagnosis, treatment, and prevention of these diseases. From an economic perspective, global health emphasizes cost-effectiveness and cost-benefit approaches for population health and includes the measurement of health burden, including life expectancy; adult, maternal, infant, and child mortality; disability; and quality of life.[11,12,14] Many experts also view global health from the ethical and societal perspective and include educational disparities, reproductive health, violence against women and children, and child labor and hawking laws as global health concerns.

TABLE 231.1 Comparison of Global, International, and Public Health

Comparison Factors	Global Health	International Health	Public Health
Geographic reach	Focuses on issues that directly or indirectly affect health but that can transcend national boundaries	Focuses on health issues of countries other than one's own, especially those of low and middle income	Focuses on issues that affect the health of the population of a particular community or country
Level of cooperation	Development and implementation of solutions often require global cooperation	Development and implementation of solutions usually require binational cooperation	Development and implementation of solutions do not usually require global cooperation
Individual or populations	Embraces both prevention in population and clinical care of individuals	Embraces both prevention in populations and clinical care of individual	Mainly focused on prevention programs for populations
Access to health	Health equity among nations and for all people is a major objective	Seeks to help people of other nations	Health equity within a nation or community is a major objective
Range of disciplines	Highly interdisciplinary and multidisciplinary within and beyond health sciences	Embraces a few disciplines but has not emphasized the multidisciplinary	Encourages multidisciplinary approaches, particularly within health sciences and with social sciences

From Koplan JP, Bond TC, Merson MH, et al. Towards a common definition of global health. *Lancet.* 2009;373:1993–5.

HISTORY AND EVOLUTION OF GLOBAL HEALTH

The beginnings of the contemporary concepts surrounding global health evolved from European colonization and colonial enterprises. Colonialism affected the public health of the world at the time through the introduction and rapid spread of non-native diseases, such as measles, smallpox, and malaria to previous nonimmune indigenous people in Saint Domingue, Haiti, and the Americas. In addition, the extraction of wealth prevented the indigenous people from exiting the cycle of poverty and disease. Furthermore, colonization of Africa, India, and the Americas by the British and other Europeans created urban centers and crowding that bred infectious diseases such as cholera, tuberculosis, and smallpox and fueled the HIV/AIDS epidemic. In contemporary terms, international spread of disease, such as influenza pandemics, through international travel or potentially by bioterrorism, is a global health concern.

Medicine underwent a dramatic change in the late 19th century with the discovery of the germ theory of disease and the awareness of it in the public health consciousness.[5] Proponents of the germ theory included Louis Pasteur, the father of the germ theory and early vaccinology; Robert Koch, father of Koch's postulates to establish a list of criteria to determine the cause of a disease; and John Snow, the father of modern epidemiology, who discovered the transmissibility of cholera and its prevention. In 1902, a model international collaboration to fight yellow fever created the Pan American Health Organization. After World War I, the League of Nations Health Committee changed its focus on infectious diseases to include nutrition and maternal and infant health. In 1947, the WHO was created by the United Nations to serve as a single global entity charged with fostering collaboration among member nations to work toward the new definition of health as a state of well-being and not merely the absence of disease. During this time the social determinants of health began to coexist with the advent of health care delivery and treatment of infections and other diseases.

This history of global health also has included disease eradication efforts. Smallpox, the first global disease to be eradicated, was declared eradicated in 1980 through the successful efforts of the WHO Smallpox Eradication Campaign. The achievement of smallpox eradication resulted not only from the possession of an effective smallpox vaccine but also through global cooperation that used intensive surveillance, disease reporting, and aggressive focus on immunization in every local community. Malaria, a disease demonstrated first by Ronald Ross to be transmitted by mosquitoes, was targeted for eradication by the Malaria Eradication Campaign of the WHO, using basic strategies of personal protection, mosquito reduction, and treatment of malaria disease. Unfortunately, despite these effective means of prevention and treatment of malaria, malaria remains a global health problem because most rural or resource-poor communities have not adopted these preventive and curative health measures. This failure demonstrates the complexity of global health problems and highlights the interrelationships among health, infrastructure, culture, politics, and economics, and it emphasizes the importance of culturally sensitive programs. Other infectious diseases also now targeted for global eradication programs include poliomyelitis, trachoma, tuberculosis, rabies, and HIV/AIDS.[43]

In the 1970s, a movement emphasizing primary health care in rural communities became increasingly popular. An example of such a movement were the "barefoot doctors" in China during the Cultural Revolution, who emphasized rural care and community-based health programs. In 1971, the NGO Doctors Without Borders was founded by French physicians who understood the importance of sociopolitical determinants of health. In 1978, the International Conference on Primary Health Care took place in Alma-Ata, the capital of the Soviet Republic of Kazakhstan, in the Soviet Union. From this conference emerged the Declaration of Alma-Ata, which stated that health was a fundamental human right and an important worldwide social goal and supported "Health for All by the Year 2000." It also emphasized the importance of culturally sensitive, local, community-based programs as opposed to the top-down vertical programs that were previously used in the smallpox and malaria eradication campaigns.

From the broad concepts of primary health brought forth from the Declaration of Alma-Ata came selective and targeted goals for primary health care implementation. These programs included goals for measles and diphtheria-pertussis-tetanus vaccination, treatment of malaria, oral rehydration for diarrhea in children, encouragement of breastfeeding, and family planning. The goals, implementation, and success of targeted and focused strategies on specific disease prevention and treatment could also then be measured and assessed for political and philanthropic funding. Donations for global health were estimated to be more than $10 billion dollars in 2000, and governments, agencies, companies, and individuals who fund global health initiatives now increasingly demand performance data in return for their financial aid.

Modern global health challenges include the ongoing balancing act between preventive public health initiatives and medical treatment interventions. A diagonal approach that synergistically incorporates both types of interventions is likely to be most successful. In addition, as industrialized development and economic progress spread globally, the challenge will be to emphasize the importance of local cultural sensitivity and avoid resource exploitation that may occur at the expense of the health of the local people. Global health indicators to monitor changes in the health of various populations are being advocated for both developed and developing countries.[11,12,14] These indicators should be well defined and applied internationally in a uniform manner. They also should be valid, reliable, and readily interpretable measurements that can be feasibly gathered and affordably ascertained even in developing countries, and they should be useful to decision makers who can easily act on the indicators at the local, national, and international level. Health indicators in developed countries often reflect lifestyles and individual behavior, such as diet, exercise, and smoking, whereas health indicators in developing countries focus on morbidity, mortality, and severe disease precursors of both these indicators.[29,28] Global health indicators present a contemporary challenge, especially in resource-poor areas with little or no access to electrical power and where records of birth, growth, lifestyle, medical illness, or death are not systematically documented and kept.[29,28]

Global health communication, public health awareness, and humanitarian efforts are also now facilitated through Internet use, mobile cellular phones, mobile applications, and social media. Through the power of the periphery that social media and mobile cell phones provide, people are able to expand their community and access not only information but also health care and transportation. In addition, many global health care organizations use cellular phones in remote or resource-poor locations to collect research data for social health projects or instantaneously log information into surveillance systems for outbreak investigations.

SOCIAL DETERMINANTS OF HEALTH

The social determinants of health reflect where people are born, grow, live, work, and age and represent a powerful influence on the global health and the global disease burden of all nations.[49] Disease is often directly and indirectly influenced by other social, political, economic, and environmental factors, which in turn are responsible for ongoing health inequalities or acute and urgent health crises. These social determinants of health include broad and general political, socioeconomic, cultural, and environmental conditions; social and community networks; individual and family lifestyle factors; and individual characteristics such as age, gender, and genetic or constitutional factors (Box 231.1).[49]

MILLENNIUM DEVELOPMENT GOALS FOR GLOBAL HEALTH AND THE NEW SUSTAINABLE DEVELOPMENT GOALS

The Millennium Development Goals (MDGs) consist of 8 broad global health goals established and agreed on by all UN Member States and 23 supporting organizations of the world during a UN summit in 2000 (Box 231.2).[45,46] The United Nations Millennium Declaration was adopted as a 15-year commitment to address the challenges facing human health globally and promote global development by improving social and economic conditions in the poorest countries, the "bottom billion," by the year 2015.[48,50,51] Goal 5 (MDG 4) "to reduce child mortality" and goal 5 (MDG 5) "to improve maternal health" specifically address pediatrics, and the sixth goal (MDG 6), "to combat HIV-AIDS, malaria, and other diseases," specially addresses infectious diseases (Fig. 231.1).[26,38,43,45]

Progress on the MDGs has been assessed through an initiative known as the Global Burden of Disease Study (GBD) based at the Institute for Health Metrics and Evaluation (IHME) at the University of Washington but ultimately involving hundreds of investigators internationally.[34–36] MDG 4 and MDG 6 showed some of the greatest gains. For instance, for MDG 4 there was an international effort to increase access to the major childhood vaccines available at the turn of the 21st century, as well as to accelerate the development of pneumococcal and rotavirus vaccines. Many of these activities were led by Gavi, the Vaccine Alliance, a UN agency headquartered in Geneva, Switzerland. According to the GBD 2013, which examined progress from the years 1990 to 2013, there was a 50% to 80% decrease in the number of childhood deaths from measles, tetanus, whooping cough, *Haemophilus influenzae* type B pneumonia, and rotaviral enteritis, whereas deaths from pneumococcal pneumonia were reduced by more than one-third.[34]

Similarly, with regard to MDG 6, there were also substantial gains for HIV/AIDS, tuberculosis, and malaria through the establishment of an international (and also Geneva-based) Global Fund to Fight AIDS, Tuberculosis, and Malaria (GFATM), as well as large-scale US government

BOX 231.1 Social, Environmental, and Individual Determinants of Health

Socioeconomic, Political, and Cultural

Government
Politics
War
Refugees and displaced populations
Food security
Global connectivity through travel and the Internet
Epidemics and pandemics both facilitated by travel and aborted by information exchange

Environmental

Global warming
Influences ecology and vector life cycles for hemorrhagic fevers
Natural disasters
Earthquakes, tsunami, hurricanes, volcanoes, floods, drought
Pollution
Industrial, fuel, wood-burning smoke
Water and sanitation
Agriculture and food production

Social and Community

Personal economic status
Housing or homelessness
Access to electrical power
Education opportunities, language, literacy
Child labor and child hawking practices
Transportation
Gender and age discrimination
Violence
Overcrowding
Access to health care and immunizations

Family and Individual Lifestyle

Employment or unemployment
Economic status
Chronic stress
Healthy food choices
Exercise
Smoking
Alcohol use or addiction
Drugs and addiction
Reproductive health and birth control

Individual Constitutional Factors

Prematurity and birth characteristics
Age
Gender
Physical health conditions
Sickle cell hemoglobinopathy
Anemia
Malnutrition
Other chronic conditions
Mental health conditions

From World Health Organization. *Social determinants of health.* http://www.who.int/social_determinants/en/.

initiatives such as the President's Emergency Plan for AIDS Relief (PEPFAR) and the President's Malaria Initiative for HIV/AIDS. GFATM and PEPFAR placed unprecedented numbers of people in low-income countries on antiretroviral drugs, whereas people with malaria in Africa and elsewhere had unprecedented access to antimalarial drugs and insecticide-treated nets. GBD 2013 found that through such efforts we

BOX 231.2 Millennium Development Goals Adopted by World Leaders at the United Nations in 2000 to Be Achieved by 2015

1. Eradicate extreme poverty and hunger
   a. Halve the proportion of people living on less than US$1 per day
   b. Achieve decent employment
   c. Halve the proportion of people suffering from hunger
2. Achieve universal primary education
   a. Allow all children, regardless of gender, to complete a full course of primary schooling
3. Promote gender equality and empower women
   a. Eliminate gender disparity in primary and secondary education
4. Reduce child mortality
   a. Reduce the "under 5" mortality rate by two-thirds from the year 1990
5. Improve maternal health
   a. Reduce the maternal mortality rate by three-fourths from the year 1990
   b. Achieve universal access to reproductive health
6. Combat HIV/AIDS, malaria, and other diseases
   a. Begin to reverse the spread of HIV/AIDS by 2015
   b. Achieve universal access to treatment of HIV/AIDS by 2010
   c. Begin to reverse the incidence of malaria and other major diseases by 2015
   d. Reduce tuberculosis worldwide
7. Ensure environmental sustainability
   a. Integrate the principles of sustainable development into country policy programs and reverse the loss of environmental resources
   b. Reduce biodiversity loss and achieve a significant reduction in the rate of loss
   c. Halve the proportion of the population without sustainable access to safe drinking water and basic sanitation
   d. Achieve a significant improvement in the lives of at least 100 million slum dwellers
8. Develop a global partnership for development

HIV/AIDS, Human immunodeficiency virus/acquired immunodeficiency syndrome.
Data from references 45 and 46.

have reversed the alarming rise of deaths from HIV/AIDS in Africa and elsewhere while simultaneously reducing deaths from malaria by approximately one-third, in addition to reducing the case-fatality rate from tuberculosis.[35] There have also been important reductions in the "other diseases" component of MDG 6, sometimes referred to as the neglected tropical diseases (NTDs), which includes the major helminth infections and trachoma.[16] Most of these gains have resulted from widespread use of a "rapid impact" package of essential NTD medications administered in programs of integrated mass drug administration.[16] It is estimated that almost one-half billion people have received partial or complete packages with substantial reductions in NTDs such as lymphatic filariasis, onchocerciasis, and trachoma,[47] to the point where it is believe that elimination of these diseases may be possible in the coming decade. For other NTDs, such as dengue fever, hookworm, and schistosomiasis, additional interventions may be required.

According to IHME, the impact of these reductions in deaths and morbidities from infectious diseases has been associated with a commensurate rise in noncommunicable diseases, especially diabetes, cardiovascular diseases, and cancer.[36] These findings have led to the formation of a Lancet Commission to establish a "Global Health 2035" initiative calling for new legislation and other activities to reduce the risk for noncommunicable diseases including policies aimed at limiting access to tobacco, alcohol, and other risk factors.[25] Still another important global health trend that has been noted are the high rates of neglected diseases, including NTDs, and HIV/AIDS, tuberculosis, and malaria noted among poor people living in wealthy Group of 20 countries. The term "blue marble health" has been coined to describe a changing global paradigm in which many economies are rising but leaving behind the poor with these diseases.[18,19,22,23] This finding explains why more than 10 million Americans live in poverty with an NTD in the United States,[19] as well as the high rates of these diseases among the poor in areas such as Europe, Australia, and of course the large middle-income countries that comprise the Group of 20 such as Brazil, China, India, and Indonesia.

With the ending of the MDGs, a new set of 17 Sustainable Development Goals (SDGs) has been launched (Box 231.3). The SDGs include a goal for health that includes targets for universal coverage, but they also emphasize heavily the environment and calls to reduce carbon emissions to slow climate change and global warming. The new SDGs

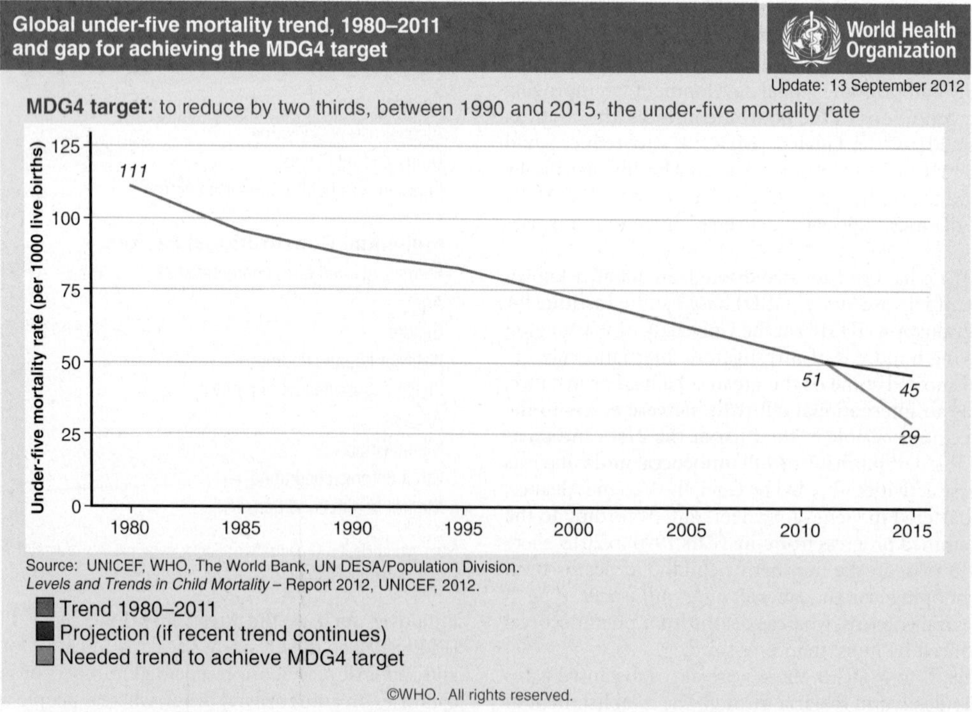

FIG. 231.1 Millennium Developmental Goal 4 to reduce child mortality. (From World Health Organization. Child health. Available at: http://www.who.int/gho/child_health/en/index.html.)

BOX 231.3 Sustainable Development Goals

1. **No poverty:** End poverty in all its forms everywhere
2. **Zero hunger:** End hunger, achieve food security and improved nutrition, and promote sustainable agriculture
3. **Good health and well-being:** Ensure healthy lives, and promote well-being for all at all ages
4. **Quality education:** Ensure inclusive and equitable quality education, and promote lifelong learning opportunities for all
5. **Gender equality**: Achieve gender equality, and empower all women and girls[37]
6. **Clean water and sanitation:** Ensure availability and sustainable management of water and sanitation for all
7. **Affordable and clean energy:** Ensure access to affordable, reliable, sustainable, and modern energy for all
8. **Decent work and economic growth:** Promote sustained, inclusive, and sustainable economic growth, full and productive employment, and decent work for all
9. **Industry, innovation, and infrastructure:** Build resilient infrastructure, promote inclusive and sustainable industrialization, and foster innovation
10. **Reduced inequalities**: Reduce income inequality within and among countries
11. **Sustainable cities and communities:** Make cities and human settlements inclusive, safe, resilient, and sustainable
12. **Responsible consumption and production:** Ensure sustainable consumption and production patterns
13. **Climate action:** Take urgent action to combat climate change and its impacts by regulating emissions and promoting developments in renewable energy
14. **Life below water:** Conserve and sustainably use the oceans, seas, and marine resources for sustainable development
15. **Life on land:** Protect, restore, and promote sustainable use of terrestrial ecosystems, sustainably manage forests, combat desertification, and halt and reverse land degradation and halt biodiversity loss
16. **Peace, justice and strong institutions:** Promote peaceful and inclusive societies for sustainable development, provide access to justice for all, and build effective, accountable, and inclusive institutions at all levels
17. **Partnerships for the goals:** Strengthen the means of implementation, and revitalize the global partnership for sustainable development

From United Nations. Sustainable development goals. http://www.un.org/sustainabledevelopment/sustainable-development-goals/.

reflect a need for physicians and other health care providers to become broadly trained and consider interdisciplinary approaches to solving global health problems.

FUTURE DIRECTION OF GLOBAL HEALTH

The rise of noncommunicable diseases by no means implies any reduction in the importance of infectious diseases in the coming years. Indeed, quite the opposite. For instance, the catastrophic epidemic of Ebola virus infection in Guinea, Liberia, and Sierra Leone in 2014 to 2015 dramatically highlighted our global vulnerability to emerging and neglected diseases. Among the forces that promoted the spread of Ebola virus infection in West Africa were poverty and the collapse of health systems in those countries because of long-standing civil conflict and war, together with deforestation, urbanization, human migrations, and climate change.[3] Today, these socioeconomic and environmental forces are not unique but are being replicated in several parts of the world, including the Middle East and North Africa, where we have seen the emergence or re-emergence of Middle Eastern respiratory syndrome coronavirus infection, leishmaniasis, and schistosomiasis, among other diseases.[20] A second and important alarming trend is the dramatic increase in vector-borne diseases, especially the arbovirus infections. There has been an explosion of dengue fever cases, especially in India, Indonesia, Brazil, and elsewhere,[32] as well as the emergence of chikungunya[31] and Zika virus in Latin America. Southern Europe has also seen new and unprecedented cases of dengue, chikungunya, and West Nile virus infection. Pandemic influenza and related viral infections also remain of enormous concern, as does the threat of widespread emergence of antimicrobial drug resistance of gram-negative bacteria and *Mycobacterium tuberculosis.*

In response the US Government has initiated a Global Health Security Agenda in partnership with the major UN agencies committed to health and ministries of health of dozens of countries globally, whereas globally the WHO and other organization are looking to lessons learned from the 2014 to 2015 Ebola epidemic to revise and update policies, including the International Health Regulations, for streamlined global epidemic response capabilities.[13,15,33] In parallel there is recognition that we need to identify mechanisms to accelerate the development of new countermeasures, including vaccines for many of the diseases highlighted earlier.[21] Thus the future directions of global health include collaborative progress by medical and public health teams, industry, world leaders, governments, NGOs, and private nonprofit philanthropic organizations in the context of the new SDGs (Figs. 231.2 through 231.11).[1]

In addition, future directions include advances in technology for diagnosis, treatment, and prevention of diseases of global importance; application of new technologies into global public health practice; education of new generations of global health scientists and global public health experts to develop and apply these new technologies to global health; and expansion of Internet and mobile applications to reach and educate people in developing world.[24]

An example of a rapidly emerging development in diagnostics in the field is "lab-on-a-chip" (LOC) technology, which may soon become an important part of efforts to improve global health, particularly through development of point-of-care testing devices. In poorly equipped clinics in resource-poor countries, treatable infectious diseases soon may be accurately diagnosed by clinicians using immunoassays and nucleic acid assays performed by microfluidic LOC technology, thereby allowing appropriate treatments to be administered. For example, accurate diagnosis of HIV infection and measuring the number of CD^+ T lymphocytes, with resultant antiretroviral treatment, may soon be possible with LOC brought to resource-poor areas where most of the untested, untreated HIV-infected individuals reside.[9,38] For the chips to be used in areas with limited resources, many challenges must be overcome. In developed nations, the most highly valued traits for diagnostic tools include speed, sensitivity, and specificity, but in countries where the health care infrastructure is less well developed, attributes such as ease of use and shelf life must also be considered. If LOCs are to be used in the resource-poor areas of the developing world, their reagents must have a long shelf life at tropical room temperatures, as well as have low cost, scalability, and recyclability.

Trainees in undergraduate and postgraduate courses in public health, medical schools, and medical residencies and fellowships, as well as students in schools of nursing and physician assistant training, have a growing interest in understanding the major factors that influence global health of individuals and populations worldwide.[39–42] Most medical schools and public health institutions are developing global health essential core competencies to provide their students with basic understanding of the complexity of global health issues, especially in low-resource settings, and the control of diseases of importance to global health.[10,39] In addition to studies in the classroom, many institutions now provide practical experience in international settings and global health career path training (Fig. 231.12).[42] A National School of Tropical Medicine was established in 2012 in Houston, Texas, thus providing a North American counterpart to the century-old Liverpool School of Tropical Medicine and the London School of Hygiene and Tropical Medicine.[17] The future of communication and information technology also includes global health. Social media provide unprecedented connectivity because even in the most resource-poor areas of the world, fragmented levels of power and Internet access are available (Fig. 231.13).[46] Social media are being used by philanthropic

Text continued on p. 2286

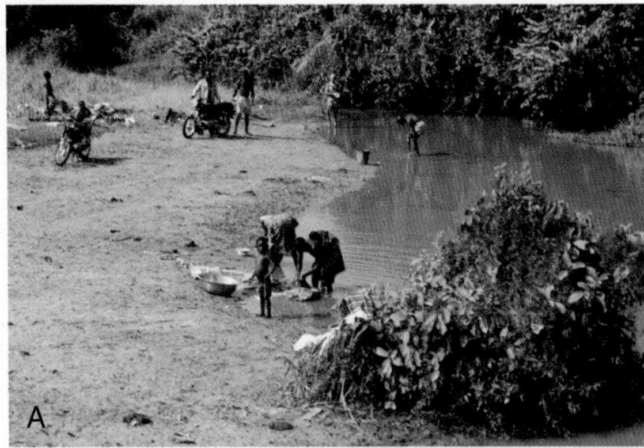

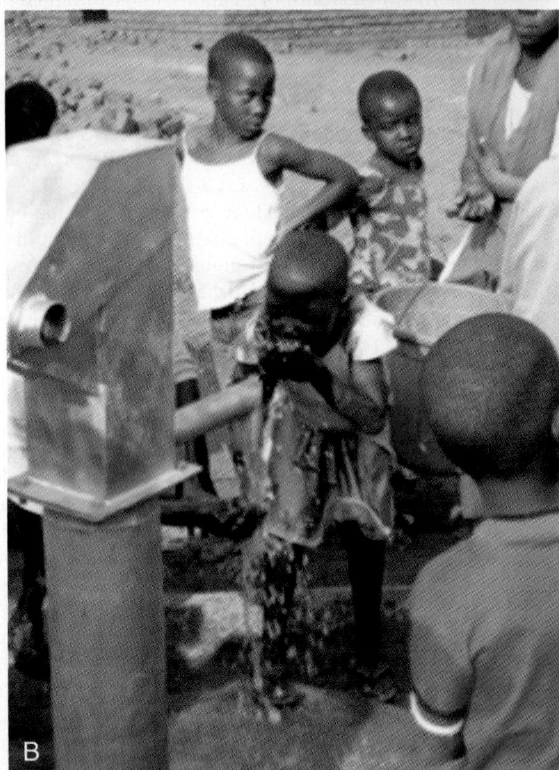

FIG. 231.2 (A) River scene near the rural town of Doma, Nasarawa State, Nigeria showing men, women, and children using river water for washing. The river also may be used to wash motorcycles and cars and even for drinking. Providing access for the world's people to safe and clean water for drinking and washing is one of the Millennium Developmental Goals for 2015. (B) Orphan girl at the Kang'oma orphanage and day care center near Mzuzu, Malawi takes a drink from a new water well and hand pump built by United Nations volunteers in August 2012. The well provides access to clean water for drinking and washing and helps prevent diarrheal diseases, dehydration, trachoma, and other diseases. Malawi is one of the poorest host countries in the "bottom billion." To halve the number of people without access to clean water and sanitation is one of the Millennium Development Goals to be achieved by 2015. (A, Courtesy Dr. Gail J. Harrison. B, Courtesy Byron McCord and Holly McBride.)

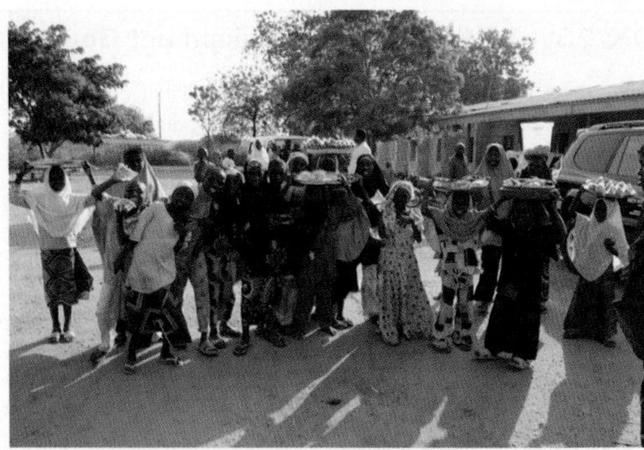

FIG. 231.3 Children gathered in front of the medical and surgical cottage hospital in Doma, Nasarawa State, Nigeria. Many children are shown with water, melons, and cashews in baskets balanced on their head, which they sell to local people through street trading or hawking. This practice is common in Nigeria; although it allows a means to make an income for their family's survival, it also often keeps the children from attending school and receiving an education, thereby perpetuating the cycle of poverty. To achieve universal primary education is one of the Millennium Development Goals for 2015. (Courtesy Dr. Gail J. Harrison.)

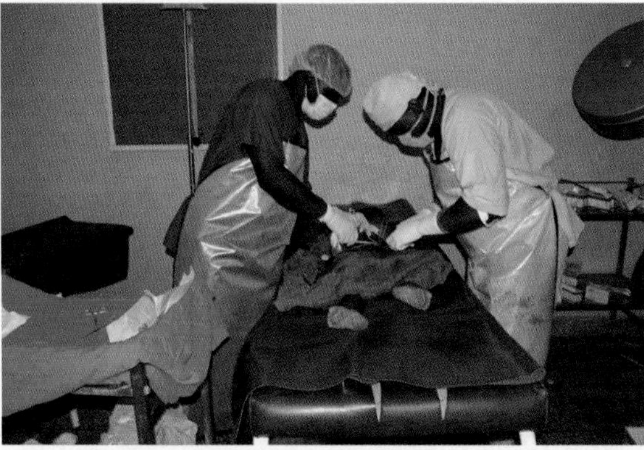

FIG. 231.4 Surgical procedures performed in remote areas of the world often must be done under stark and challenging conditions. This 3-year-old boy from Doma, Nasarawa State, Nigeria is having a right inguinal herniorrhaphy performed, under ketamine anesthesia, by local physicians in an operating room in Doma Hospital, Nasarawa State, Nigeria. The procedure was successfully completed, he awakened, and he received a postoperative intramuscular injection of an antibiotic to prevent infection. (Courtesy Dr. Gail J. Harrison.)

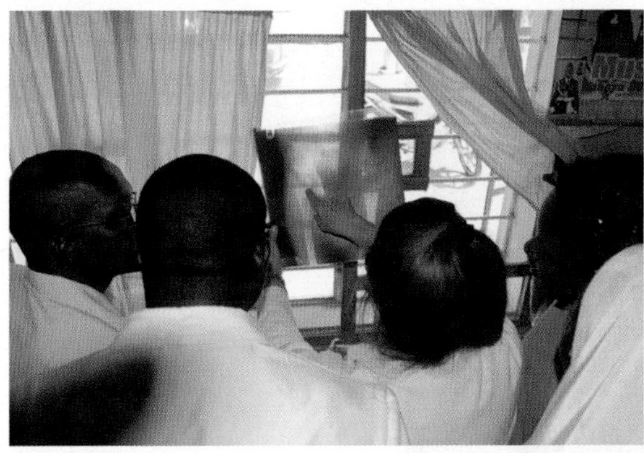

FIG. 231.5 The evaluation and treatment of patients for infectious diseases in remote rural areas are challenging efforts because microbiologic cultures, laboratory tests, diagnostic imaging, biopsies, and intravenous infusions are not available. In this photograph, the clinician, using natural light provided through a window, explains the findings of a plain radiograph showing destructive bone changes of the proximal right femur, consistent with chronic osteomyelitis. The patient, an 11-year-old boy, had a 2-year history of painful limp, chronic draining fistulous tracts, and tenderness over the proximal femur. Lack of money and access to transportation precluded accessing medical care with specialists in an urban hospital. The child was provided with crutches to help ease pain and facilitate mobility, as well as a 3-month supply of oral antibiotics. He also was given a "written referral" to a specialist in the medical center in Abuja, Nigeria, but unless he is able to travel to the larger urban center, his next follow-up will be in 1 to 2 years at the next medical mission. (Courtesy Dr. Gail J. Harrison.)

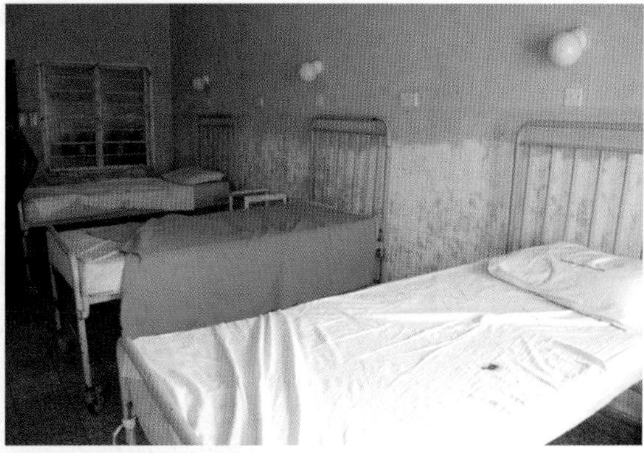

FIG. 231.6 Medical wards in hospitals in remote, resource-poor, rural areas of the "bottom billion" countries are often stark, are maintained as well as possible with available resources, and lack modern equipment to which health care providers in resource-rich countries are accustomed. (Courtesy Dr. Gail J. Harrison.)

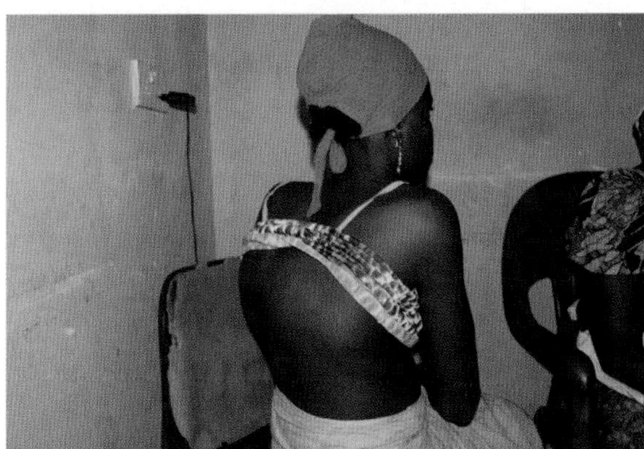

FIG. 231.7 This 13-year-old Nigerian girl had a several-year history of increasing kyphosis. A soft, nontender mass was palpated along her spine. The presumptive diagnosis was Potts disease, a presentation of extrapulmonary tuberculosis that most commonly affects the lower thoracic and upper lumbar vertebrae of the spine. The sixth goal "to combat HIV/AIDS, malaria, and other diseases" of the Millennium Development Goals specifically addresses the health and economic impact of infectious diseases on global health. It includes programs specifically targeted to combat tuberculosis.[43] (Courtesy Dr. Gail J. Harrison.)

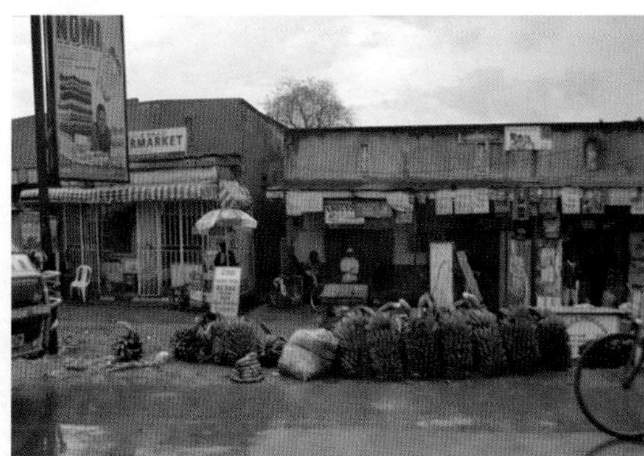

FIG. 231.8 Street scene with market and plantains, also called "cooking bananas," laid out for sale in Katende, in the Mpigi District, Uganda. Uganda is a developing country with more than 41 million people that is located on the Equator in East Africa. It is experiencing fast population growth, and most crops are still cultivated and produced by local farmers and sold in local markets. The common cultivated crops in Uganda include maize, cassava, yams, and sweet potato, which are all high-carbohydrate-content foods, and groundnuts and beans, which are high in protein and eaten to complement the starch crops. Meat or fish protein is a rare luxury. The high-carbohydrate diet consumed on a daily basis is contributing to a rising prevalence of type 2 diabetes mellitus in the adult population of Uganda. Millennium Development Goal 1 called to end or reduce extreme poverty and hunger. Sustainable Development Goal 2 or Zero Hunger calls to end hunger and achieve food security and improved nutrition and promote sustainable agriculture. (Courtesy Dr. Gail J. Harrison.)

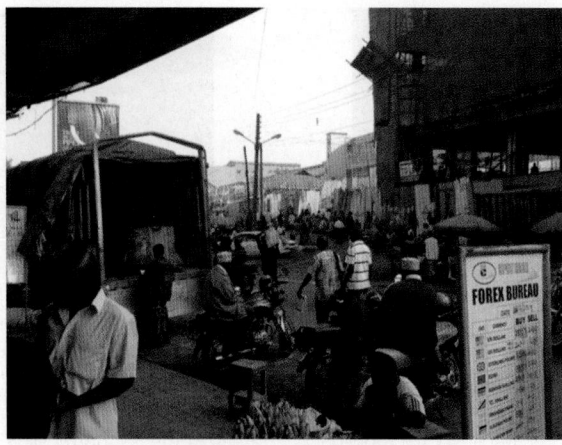

FIG. 231.9 Market street scene, outside of Kampala, in the Mpigi District, Uganda, with many people traveling on foot. Also notice the motorcycles, which are a common mode of transportation in Uganda, and the delivery truck. The motorcycles may be used for personal transportation for families that can afford to own their own, or as motorcycle taxis or "boda boda" for public transportation. Increasing population in Uganda has led to an increasing demand for public transportation. "Boda boda" provide an affordable means of public transportation and also vital job opportunities for entrepreneurial young men. They are also a frequent cause of road accidents, injuries, and death. In addition, the rapid urbanization and economic growth of cities in Uganda have given rise to air pollution, which is one of the biggest challenges faced in urban centers of developing countries. The main cause of air pollution is transportation exhaust fumes. The effects of this pollution on people is now becoming evident, with rising incidences of chronic lung diseases such as asthma, chronic obstructive pulmonary disease, and lung cancer. It has been estimated that 14% of children between 8 and 14 years of age who are living in Kampala have asthma. Millennium Development Goal 7 called to ensure environmental sustainability and to integrate the principles of sustainable development into country policy programs and reverse the loss of environmental resources. The new Sustainable Development Goal 13 is Climate Action. It calls to take urgent care to combat climate change and its impacts by regulating emissions and promoting development of renewable energy. (Courtesy Dr. Gail J. Harrison.)

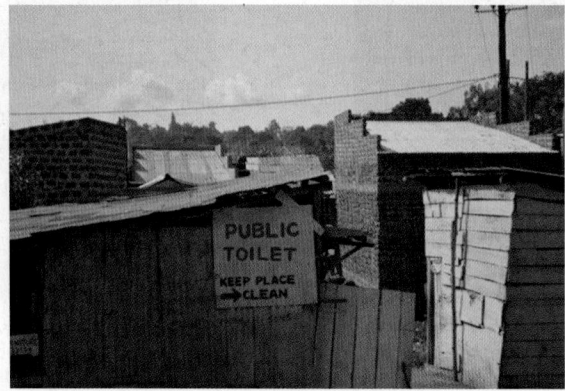

FIG. 231.10 A public toilet in the area of Kampala, in the Mpigi district of Uganda in East Africa. It is estimated less than 20% of the population in Uganda has access to toilets that are not shared and that are made with improved sanitation mechanisms that separate waste from human contact. Public sewer systems with water-borne flush toilets are still rare in Uganda and are present only in the wealthy residential and business districts. Open urination and defecation, or elimination into plastic or polythene bags ("flying toilets"), which are disposed of by throwing the bags into drainage channels, are sometimes the only options for the resource-poor areas. More fortunate areas may have public toilets, "outhouses," or pit latrines. These public toilets often overflow, and in the rainy season, sewage runs into the water-trapping gullies in the town, thus providing a source of disease such as typhoid and cholera. Women and girls often do not use public toilets, or do so in groups, because they often experience humiliation and have been victims of violent crimes such as assault and rape. Millennium Development Goal 7 called to ensure environmental sustainability and to halve the proportion of the population without sustained access to safe drinking water and basic sanitation. The new Sustainable Development Goal 6 calls for clean water and sanitation to ensure availability and sustainable management of water and sanitation for all. (Courtesy Dr. Gail J. Harrison.)

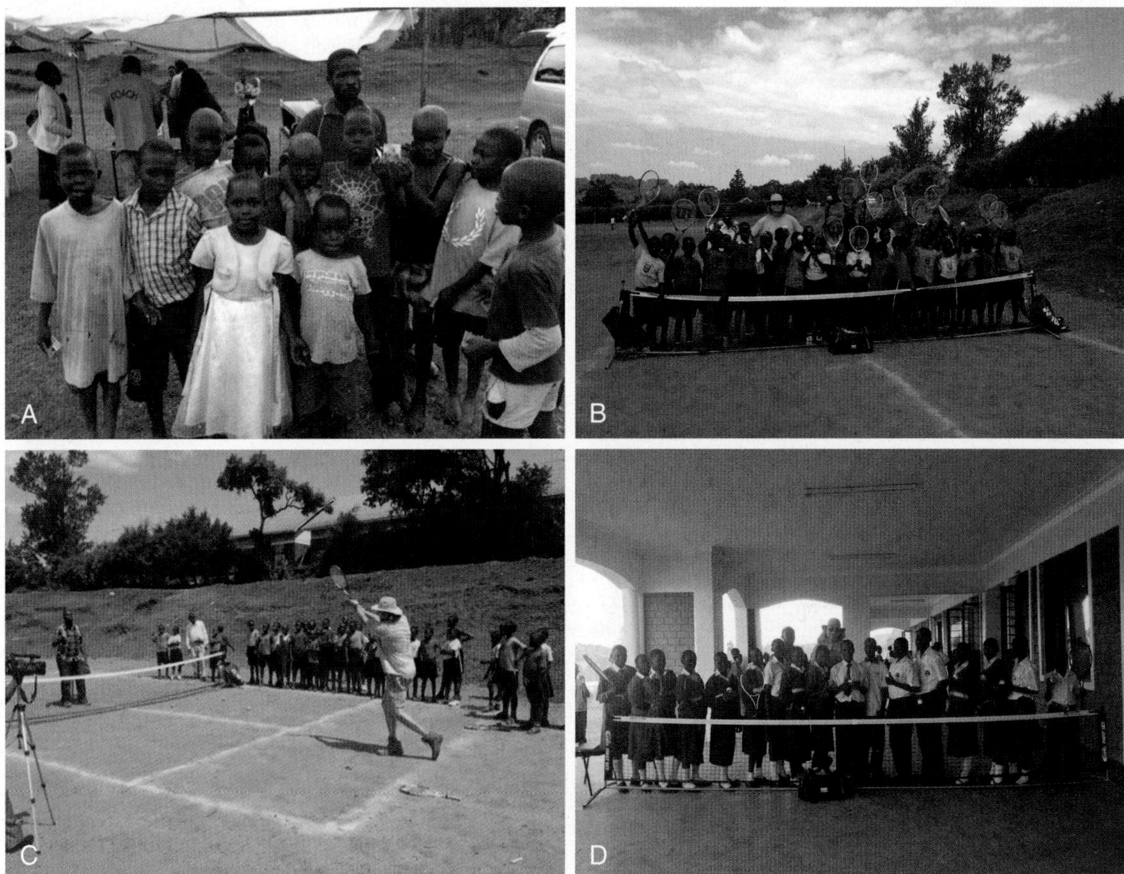

FIG. 231.11 Ugandan children. Millennium Development Goal 2 called for primary education allowing all children regardless of gender to complete a full course of primary education schooling and to promote gender equality and empower women and eliminate gender disparities in primary and secondary education. Sustainable Development Goal 4 calls for quality education to ensure inclusive and equitable quality education and promote lifelong learning opportunities for all. (A) These children came to the medical mission camp set up in a field near Katende, Uganda. All were fit and healthy appearing, except notice the boy on the left with a facial palsy of unknown cause. These children were "out of school." Education is a human right for all children, yet many children in resource-poor areas of the world do not receive an education. Even though Uganda is one of the first African countries to introduce universal primary education (both government and private schools), many children have never enrolled in school ("nonenrolled children") or drop out of primary school ("out of school" children). These children are often socially and economically disadvantaged, and their parents cannot afford the costs of scholastic materials such as pens, books, or a school lunch or uniform. Many children drop out of school to help support their family financially. Moreover, when girls start their menstrual period, they often drop out of school because they lack access to sanitary pads and other personal hygiene supplies. (B) and (C), These children are from St John's Bosco Katende Primary School located in Katende, about 15 miles from Kampala, Mpigi District, Uganda. It is a government-sponsored local primary school. The students participated in group tennis instruction as part of the "A Court Everywhere" (ACE) outreach program, sponsored by Neil Harrison Serves Tennis. A tennis court was fashioned from local resources: the clay dirt in the open field formed the court base, and tennis lines were made from ashes from the local open fire kitchens. Seven years of primary school (government or private) are provided in the education system in Uganda, from grades 1 to 7 (ages 7 to 13 years). On completion of their first 7 years, students must pass their "Leaving Exams" to continue to the next level of secondary education. (D) These children are from a local private secondary school near Kampala, Uganda. They participated in group tennis instruction as part of the ACE outreach program. Four years of secondary school (government of private) for middle-level education is provided in the education system in Uganda, from ages 14 to 17 years. Following the British model of education, Ugandan students who pass their O-Level examinations may proceed to Upper Secondary, advanced-level education. If students continue to be successful in school, and pass their A-Level examinations, they may attend Tertiary Education Universities at 1 of the 5 state universities, 11 religious-affiliated universities, or 1 private secular university in Uganda. For those students who do not perform well on their examinations, they may still attend technical colleges. (Courtesy Dr. Gail J. Harrison.)

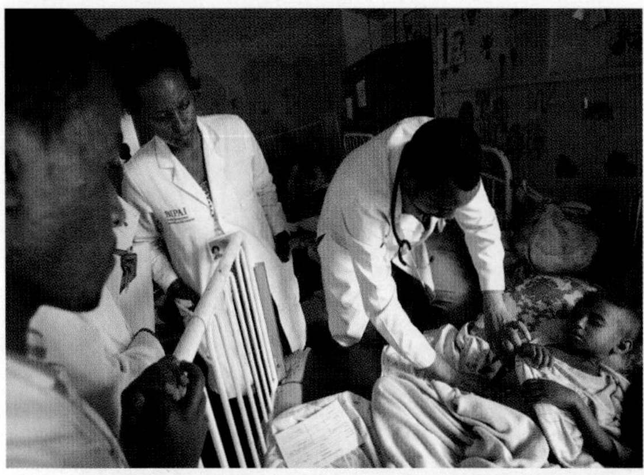

FIG. 231.12 Dr. Gelane Workneh *(left)* works with residents and medical students as she make rounds in the pediatric ward at University of Gondar Hospital (October 11, 2011) in Ethiopia. Dr. Workneh is one of three doctors the Texas Children's Hospital Global Health Corps physicians and the Baylor College of Medicine Pediatric AIDS Initiative provide to work with the Jewish Joint Distribution Committee and Gondar University College of Health Sciences in Gondar as part of a 3-year grant. These doctors work to expand pediatric medical capacity in Ethiopia by teaching medical students and interns from Gondar University and by training local health care professionals. Global health experiences have become an important part of medical education curriculum in many major medical centers. (Courtesy Smiley N. Pool and Baylor International Pediatric AIDS initiative, Houston, Texas.)

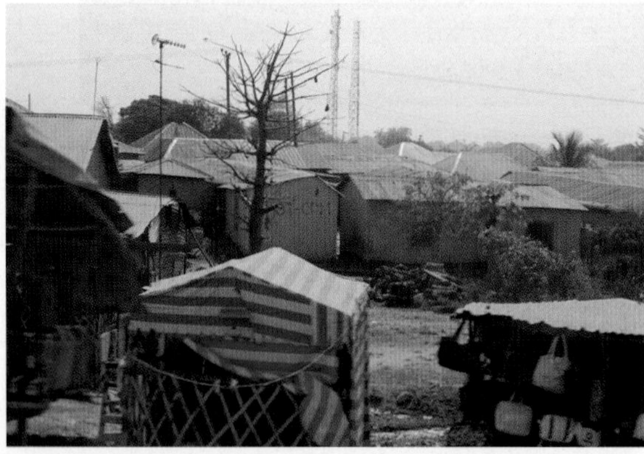

FIG. 231.13 Internet access through personal computers, local Internet cafes, and handheld mobile devices has reached even the most remote areas of the world and provides creative opportunities to improve global health and awareness in these remote communities. (Courtesy Dr. Gail J. Harrison.)

organizations, such as the Bill & Melinda Gates Foundation, to update their donors and partners on measureable markers of progress toward defined global health goals.[30] Mobile global health education applications, linking smart phones and pico projectors and other mobile technology, have the potential to be inexpensive, sustainable, ubiquitous, acceptable, and therefore effective in disseminating information on a global scale and linking resource-rich areas with remote, resource-poor areas of the world. In addition, mobile devices may be used for surveillance[44] of infectious diseases, as well as chronic conditions such as heart disease, hypertension, and diabetes. Mobile devices also may be used for global health surveys and health information systems management. Mobile technology is also ideal for providing rapid scientific, epidemiologic, and public health knowledge at the time of a disaster. Mobile technologies may soon revolutionize global health care because individuals who are patients in resource-poor remote areas also may own or borrow mobile phones, thereby allowing communication to access health care when needed and reducing mortality.[45] As an example of creative adaptability, in "light-poor" communities and villages without reliable electrical power at night, the light provided by individual cell phones allows health care providers to assist in medical procedures, including deliveries of babies at night.[46]

NEW REFERENCES SINCE THE SEVENTH EDITION

3. Bausch DG, Schwarz L. Outbreak of Ebola virus disease in Guinea: where ecology meets economy. *PLoS Negl Trop Dis.* 2014;8(7):e3056.
13. Gostin LO, DeBartolo MC, Friedman EA. The International Health Regulations 10 years on: the governing framework for global health security. *Lancet.* 2015;386(10009):2222-2226.
15. Heymann DL, Chen L, Takemi K, et al. Global health security: the wider lessons from the west African Ebola virus disease epidemic. *Lancet.* 2015;385(9980):1884-1901.
18. Hotez PJ. NTDs V. 2.0.: "Blue marble health"—neglected tropical disease control and elimination in a shifting health policy landscape. *PLoS Negl Trop Dis.* 2013;7(11):e0002570.
19. Hotez PJ. Neglected parasitic infections and poverty in the United States. *PLoS Negl Trop Dis.* 2014;8(9):e3012.
20. Hotez PJ. Vaccine science diplomacy: expanding capacity to prevent emerging and neglected tropical diseases arising from Islamic State (IS)–held territories. *PLoS Negl Trop Dis.* 2015;9(9):e0003852.
21. Hotez PJ, Bottazzi ME, Strych U. New vaccines for the world's poorest people. *Annu Rev Med.* 2016;67:405-417.
22. Hotez PJ. Blue marble health and "the big three diseases": HIV/AIDS, tuberculosis, and malaria. *Microbes Infect.* 2015;17(8):539-541.
23. Hotez PJ. Blue marble health redux: neglected tropical diseases and human development in the Group of 20 (G20) nations and Nigeria. *PLoS Negl Trop Dis.* 2015;9(7):e0003672.
25. Jamison DT, Summers LH, Alleyne G, et al. Global health 2035: a world converging within a generation. *Lancet.* 2013;382(9908):1898-1955.
31. Lwande OW, Obanda V, Bucht G, et al. Global emergence of Alphaviruses that cause arthritis in humans. *Infect Ecol Epidemiol.* 2015;5:29853.
32. Messina JP, Brady OJ, Scott TW, et al. Global spread of dengue virus types: mapping the 70 year history. *Trends Microbiol.* 2014;22(3):138-146.
33. Moon S, Sridhar D, Pate MA, et al. Will Ebola change the game? Ten essential reforms before the next pandemic. The report of the Harvard-LSHTM Independent Panel on the Global Response to Ebola. *Lancet.* 2015;386(10009):2204-2221.
34. Mortality Global Burden of Disease, Causes of Death Collaborators. Global, regional, and national age-sex specific all-cause and cause-specific mortality for 240 causes of death, 1990-2013: a systematic analysis for the Global Burden of Disease Study 2013. *Lancet.* 2015;385(9963):117-171.
35. Murray CJ, Ortblad KF, Guinovart C, et al. Global, regional, and national incidence and mortality for HIV, tuberculosis, and malaria during 1990-2013: a systematic analysis for the Global Burden of Disease Study 2013. *Lancet.* 2014;384(9947):1005-1070.
36. Murray CJ, Vos T, Lozano R, et al. Disability-adjusted life years (DALYs) for 291 diseases and injuries in 21 regions, 1990-2010: a systematic analysis for the Global Burden of Disease Study 2010. *Lancet.* 2012;380(9859):2197-2223.
47. USAID. USAID's NTD Program. Trachoma. https://www.neglecteddiseases.gov/usaid-target-diseases/trachoma.

The full reference list for this chapter is available at ExpertConsult.com.

International Travel Issues for Children

232

Nava Yeganeh • Michelle Weinberg •
Nicholas Weinberg • Susan A. Maloney

During the past half-century, the number of persons traveling internationally has increased tremendously. Between 1980 and 2011, the number of international arrivals worldwide more than tripled, growing from 277 million to 983 million. In 2015, US residents took more than 32 million trips overseas, 28 million trips to Mexico, and 12.5 million trips to Canada. Among the overseas US resident travelers, 12.5 million (17%) visited Europe, 10.4 million (10%) visited the Caribbean, 6.6 million (6.6%) visited Asia, 4.6 million (6.3%) visited Central and South America, 2 million (2.8%) visited the Middle East, 350,000 (0.5%) visited Africa, and 640,000 (0.9%) visited Oceania.[161,162,181] Although the exact number of children traveling is unknown, 2.2 million US travelers (8%) were adults and children traveling together and 3.1 million (11%) reported their occupation as students.[160] Worldwide, Mexico and Asia were the fastest growing destinations in terms of international tourist arrivals, with each growing more than 6% in 2015.

Study abroad by since the 1990s in the last 20 years; more than 289,000 US students studied abroad during the 2013 to 2014 school year. The United Kingdom, Italy, Spain, France, and China were the top host destinations; however, the numbers of students studying in Mexico, Chile, and Greece each increased by double digits.[102]

International travelers may be exposed to a variety of health risks, depending on the travel destination, trip itinerary, duration of stay, planned travel activities (i.e., business vs. adventure), individual risk factors, and preventive measures taken. For persons from industrialized countries visiting developing countries, travel may expose them to a variety of infectious pathogens and environmental hazards, some of which they may rarely encounter at home. Other infectious agents (e.g., chikungunya) may present a potential threat to public health by extending their presence into the United States.[135] Despite the well-documented health risks associated with international travel, surveys have shown that many travelers do not seek pretravel health advice or obtain appropriate travel-related preventive medications or vaccinations. As a result of global patterns of human migration, children are increasingly likely to accompany their parents on trips to lower income destinations, particularly to visit friends and family. Children have been repeatedly shown to be more vulnerable to preventable outcomes. Evaluation of data reported to the GeoSentinel Surveillance Network between 1997 and 2007 revealed that compared with adults, children disproportionately presented for medical care within 7 days of return, required hospitalization, lacked pretravel health advice, and had traveled for the purpose of visiting friends and family.[90] Surveys of US, European, and Australian travelers have shown that only 31% to 52.1% of the travelers sought travel advice before the trip. In an airport survey of 203 US passengers traveling to high-risk, malaria-endemic areas, only 46% were carrying antimalarial medications with them,[91,165,173] and few were vaccinated for their travel—only 11% for tetanus, 14% for hepatitis A, 13% for hepatitis B, and 5% for yellow fever.[91] Among 1704 respondents from the 2008 YouthStyles survey, an annual mail survey of demographics and health knowledge, attitudes, and practices of youth age 9 to 18 years, 131 (7.7%) traveled in the past 12 months; of these travelers, only 16.7% reported seeking pretravel medical care, mostly (84%) from a family doctor.[92] In a survey of 318 American students studying abroad, the primary source of travel health information was reported to be youth-oriented travel guidebooks (85%).[93]

TRAVELERS VISITING RELATIVES AND FAMILY

Travelers who are visiting friends and relatives are at high risk for acquiring a variety of illnesses, are more likely to travel for longer periods of time, and are less likely to seek pretravel medical advice.[10,11,15,37,116] A review of 3332 children seeking care through the Global TravEpiNet between 2009 and 2012 showed that children visiting relatives and family tend to be younger when they travel and are more likely to have a travel-related visit less than 14 days before departure.[88,116] In another study of children visiting families and relatives who required medical care after travel, only 33% to 50% had received pretravel advice.[90] Systemic febrile illnesses (including malaria), nondiarrheal intestinal parasitic infections, respiratory syndromes, tuberculosis, and sexually transmitted infections (STIs) were more commonly diagnosed among immigrants visiting friends and relatives than in other travelers, whereas acute diarrhea was less frequent. In contrast to other travelers, the immigrants who were visiting friends and relatives were more likely to travel to sub-Saharan Africa or Latin America and to take a trip lasting longer than 30 days.[116] In a review of travelers presenting at one GeoSentinel Surveillance Network clinic site, the proportion of travelers with malaria who had been visiting friends and relatives was eight times greater than among tourists (16.9% vs. 2.1%).[114]

Compared with adults, children are more likely to have illness after visiting relatives.[90] Given that children tend to be the least likely to seek care and the most likely to become ill, every effort must be made to encourage this particularly vulnerable group of travelers to receive appropriate care. Reasons for lack of care are likely multifactorial and include lack of access to care because of barriers at the health system level as well as lack of perception of risk.[11,15] Possible ways to encourage travelers to receive preventative services include asking parents during regular well-child care visits about any future planned travels; encouraging insurance companies to fully cover the cost of travel vaccines and travel-related medications, including malaria prophylaxis; and improving access to care for immigrant families.[114,116]

PEDIATRIC TRAVELERS AND HEALTH RISKS ABROAD

Recent studies have identified several major categories of morbidity among pediatric travelers: diarrheal illnesses, respiratory diseases, dermatologic conditions, and systemic febrile illnesses. In a multicenter study evaluating the morbidities of 1561 children returning from 218 global destinations presenting after travel, Hagmann and colleagues found that diarrheal syndromes were most common (28%), followed by dermatologic conditions (25%), systemic febrile illnesses (23%). and respiratory disorders (11%).[90] Dermatological conditions were twice as common after exposure to Latin America, and travel to the Middle East or North Africa was associated with greater risk for diarrheal disorder.[90] Herbinger and colleagues[95] reviewed data from 890 children younger than 20 years at an outpatient travel clinic at the University of Munich, Germany after travel to Africa (46%), Asia (35%), and Latin America (19%). The most frequent syndromes were acute diarrhea (25%, especially in children 0–4 years of age), dermatologic conditions (19%, especially in children 0–9 years of age), febrile and systemic diseases (20%), respiratory disorders (8%), chronic diarrhea (5%), and genitourinary disorders (3%). The 10 most frequently diagnosed infectious diseases were giardiasis (8%), schistosomiasis (4%), superinfected insect bites (4%), *Campylobacter* enteritis (4%), *Salmonella* enteritis (4%), cutaneous larva migrans (3%), amebiasis (3%), dengue fever (2%), mononucleosis (2%), and malaria (2%).[82] Hunziker and colleagues[98] reviewed data from 328 children 16 years and younger with travel-associated illness at the emergency department of the University of Zürich Children's Hospital. The main conditions were diarrheal illness

(39%), respiratory illness (28.7%), and systemic febrile illness (13.4%). No deaths were reported. Among 36 children with more serious diseases requiring hospitalization, 12 (3.7% overall) had potentially serious diseases: malaria ($n = 2$), *Salmonella typhi* ($n = 3$), *Salmonella paratyphi* ($n = 2$), meningococcal meningitis ($n = 1$), tuberculosis ($n = 2$), visceral leishmania ($n = 1$), and hepatitis A ($n = 1$). Eleven of the 12 children with serious diseases were visiting friends and family or immigrant children.[98] Van Rijn and colleagues[166] conducted a prospective observational cohort study of 152 children and their parents traveling to the tropics and subtropics; 85% of all children reported some kind of aliment during travel, with a mean aliment rate of 7 ailments per person-month of travel. The most frequently reported ailments were skin problems, including insect bites, sunburn, and diarrhea.[166]

Other authors have reported substantial health risks for pediatric travelers from noninfectious causes such as injuries. Most deaths are associated with swimming or automobile accidents.[97,118] One study of British children drowning abroad while traveling showed that an average of eight British children drown each year abroad, primarily in swimming pools without adequate lifeguards.[69]

Although some data from adult travelers can be extrapolated to use in the management of pediatric travelers, infants and children have special vulnerabilities and needs when preparing for travel abroad. These needs include (1) up-to-date and appropriate vaccinations (at times through accelerated or altered routine childhood vaccine schedules and also including special travel-related vaccines); (2) appropriate malaria and other chemoprophylaxis regimens tailored for use in pediatric travelers; (3) prevention counseling, particularly in the areas of food and water safety, insect barriers, and injury prevention; and (4) anticipatory guidance for the management of potential illness and successful location of medical resources overseas. This chapter provides recommendations for conducting a pediatric pretravel assessment to ensure that the child has received the appropriate vaccination and chemoprophylaxis regimens, pretravel prevention counseling, and means of accessing additional sources of travel information about health risks and the availability of medical resources at specific travel destinations.

GENERAL APPROACH TO PRETRAVEL ASSESSMENT FOR CHILDREN

Before embarking on international travel, children should have a pretravel health assessment performed by a health care provider. The number of physicians who specialize in travel medicine for children is relatively limited, and many pretravel assessments are performed by general pediatricians, pediatricians who specialize in infectious diseases, or travel medicine specialists without specific pediatric training. A study performed by members of the International Society of Travel Medicine (ISTM) Pediatric Interest Group found that even doctors who professed an interest in travel medicine often did not follow appropriate travel guidelines to prevent travel-associated morbidities in pediatric travelers.[89] Hence there need to be renewed attempts to train even those self-declared health professionals interested in travel medicine in order to prevent travel-related illnesses. Depending on the destination and the vaccinations recommended or required, the assessment should be conducted optimally 6 to 8 weeks before travel. Because families may not be aware of the need for multiple vaccinations and medications, health care providers should be proactive and routinely ask patients and their families if they are anticipating any international travel in the next several months, especially before holiday periods.

During the pretravel assessment, the provider should do the following:

1. Review the child's current and past medical history, including the status of routine childhood vaccinations.
2. Obtain specific details about the travel itinerary and planned activities. Review endemic diseases and recent outbreaks in travel destinations.
3. Administer indicated routine and travel-related vaccinations.
4. Prescribe antimalarial, other prophylactic, or self-treatment medication (based on risk assessment from the medical history, travel itinerary, and planned activities).
5. Counsel about prevention of travel-related illnesses, especially focusing on infectious diarrhea and mosquito-borne illnesses.
6. Provide guidance about seeking medical assistance for travel-related illness.

The pretravel assessment should include a detailed review of the trip itinerary. On the basis of risk assessment, preventive health counseling should include information about food and water safety, prevention of vector-borne illnesses, and other infectious and noninfectious illnesses, such as STIs and automobile accidents. General and specific prevention counseling recommendations are addressed later in the chapter. In addition, families should clarify with their health insurance company whether they are covered for health care provided abroad. If not, insurance can be purchased from several companies; such insurance may include coverage for health care providers in a specific country and airlift medical evacuation. If assistance for illness acquired abroad is needed, the US embassy or consulate can provide names and addresses of English-speaking health care providers at the travel destination. This information can be obtained before departure by accessing embassy Internet sites or by calling the embassy. In addition, names of physicians abroad can be obtained from some worldwide directories (see the discussion on international travel information resources). Parents should be told to carry all health-related documents with them for easy retrieval, including written prescriptions for medications, health insurance information, and medical contacts abroad. Counseling on ensuring the use of sterile needles and the safety of the local blood supply also should be included in pretravel prevention counseling topics; blood screening and infection control practices may not be as stringent in some countries as in the United States.

Special consideration must be given to children who have chronic diseases. Children with medical conditions should take a summary of their medical history and treatment record. If the child has cardiac disease, the family should consider taking a copy of the child's recent electrocardiogram and echocardiography report. Children with diabetes who are traveling through more than one time zone should consult their pediatrician or endocrinologist for guidance on the need for altering insulin dosing. Prescription medications should be carried in original bottles, and a sufficient supply for the length of the planned trip and a few extra doses should be packed. Required medications should be carried on the plane rather than packed in luggage because bags may be lost or exposed to unfavorable environmental conditions. Families should be counseled about the potential hazards of obtaining medications in pharmacies in developing countries, where many medications can be purchased over-the-counter without a prescription and where the names, content, and concentration of medications may be different from those of US products. Parents carrying medical equipment (such as nebulizers) should remember to take adaptors for foreign electric current and bring a letter from a physician that documents the need for the equipment.[36] Similar documentation is encouraged for anaphylaxis kits or other medications that require syringes.

VACCINATION FOR INTERNATIONAL TRAVEL

The provider should consider three categories of vaccinations: routine childhood vaccinations, required travel-related vaccinations, and recommended travel-related vaccinations. Some routine vaccinations should be administered at an earlier age or after an accelerated schedule in preparation for international travel. In addition, the provider should review and administer travel-related vaccinations that are required for entry by various countries to prevent the importation of disease and development of outbreaks, as well as vaccinations recommended for the prevention of illness in the individual traveler.[41] Currently, only two vaccines—yellow fever and meningococcal—are required for entry by selected countries; however, these requirements may change in the future. Vaccination recommendations change rapidly. Whereas this section provides guidance as of publication date, clinicians should obtain the most current recommendations available on the Centers for Disease Control and Prevention (CDC) website (see the discussion on international travel information resources).

Routine Childhood Vaccinations for Pediatric Travelers

For children who will be traveling internationally, having their routine immunizations brought up to date is essential because many vaccine-preventable diseases are more prevalent in countries outside the United

States. In particular, children who have nonmedical exemptions to routine vaccinations may be at high risk for acquiring vaccine-preventable diseases, such as measles and rubella, that no longer are endemic in the United States but still occur frequently in other countries, including many European destinations. The pretravel visit also may give the health care provider a unique opportunity to update the routine vaccination status of a patient who has fallen behind schedule. In certain cases, routine vaccinations may need to be accelerated to maximize protection, particularly against polio, diphtheria-tetanus-pertussis, varicella, hepatitis A, hepatitis B, and measles (e.g., measles vaccination is recommended for children 6–11 months of age).[7,113] Many vaccine series can be initiated as early as 6 weeks of age. The management plan for routine vaccinations will be determined by the travel destination and itinerary. For example, diphtheria and pertussis are prevalent in Eastern Europe and many developing countries, and measles is still endemic in the developing world and some European countries; therefore, if travel to these countries is planned, ensuring immunity is imperative, and accelerated schedules should be considered. In addition, parents should check their own immune status because traveling with children can increase their risk for exposure to measles and other vaccine-preventable diseases.[99,100]

Measles

Measles was declared eliminated in the United States in 2000. However, travelers to Europe, Asia, the Pacific, and Africa continue to be at risk. High two-dose mumps, measles, and rubella (MMR) vaccine coverage is essential for travelers to prevent measles importation and outbreaks in the United States. In 2014, the United States experienced a record number of measles cases, with 667 cases reported from 27 states. One large multistate outbreak involved Disneyland Parks and likely started from a traveler who became infected overseas because the measles virus type (B3) was identical to the virus type that caused an outbreak in the Philippines in 2014. In this widely publicized outbreak, at least 125 US citizens were diagnosed with measles between December 2014 and February 2015, with 110 cases in California alone. Thirty-nine (35%) of the Californians infected visited Disneyland parks during December 17 to 20, 34 (31%) were secondary cases, and 37 (34%) had an unknown exposure source. Most of the secondary cases were household contacts. Forty-nine affected individuals (45%) were unvaccinated, 5 (5%) had one dose of measles-containing vaccine, seven (6%) had two doses, 1 (1%) had three doses, and 47 (43%) had unknown or undocumented vaccination status.[51,182] Similarly, measles outbreaks in 2011 were associated with travelers returning from overseas, with most cases occurring in undervaccinated or unvaccinated individuals.[44] Numerous cases of serologically confirmed measles also have occurred among internationally adopted children and their new parents and siblings who had traveled to China to accompany them home. Data suggest that the exposure to measles occurred in China, probably at the orphanage, where an outbreak of measles was occurring.[33,34]

The MMR vaccine is administered routinely to children starting at 12 months of age. However, the MMR vaccine should be administered to children 6 to 11 months of age who are traveling internationally. These children should be revaccinated with two doses of MMR vaccine—the first at ages 12 through 15 months and at least 4 weeks after the previous dose and the second at ages 4 through 6 years. Children older than 12 months of age who are traveling internationally should receive the second dose, as long as 4 weeks have passed since the previous dose; even if administered before 4 years of age, this second dose counts toward the routine vaccination and does not need to be repeated at a later age. Providers should remind their patients who plan to travel internationally of the increased risk for measles and potential exposures during bus, train, or air travel and at large international events or gatherings.

Hepatitis A

Hepatitis A is endemic in most of the world, and travelers are at risk in any area where sanitation is poor. In 2006, hepatitis A vaccination became part of routine childhood recommendations in the United States for all children at 1 year of age (12–23 months), supplementing recommendations in 1999 for vaccination of children 2 to 18 years of age residing in states and communities with high incidence of disease and other high-risk groups. In addition, hepatitis A vaccine is now routinely recommended for all previously unvaccinated children aged 24 months or older for whom immunity is desired. Vaccination is recommended for pediatric travelers 1 year or older who will be visiting countries with intermediate to high endemicity, such as in Mexico, Central and South America, Asia, Africa, and eastern Europe.[3,36,45] Hepatitis A vaccine is administered as a two-dose series. The first dose of hepatitis A vaccine should be administered at least 14 days before travel. Limited data are available about the timing of the appearance of neutralizing antibody. Among a sample of vaccinated persons, 54% to 62% were positive for neutralizing antibody 14 days after the first dose, and 94% to 100% were positive at 1 month.[3] The second dose can be administered 6 months after the first dose. Intramuscular immunoglobulin is recommended for immunoprophylaxis against hepatitis A in children younger than 1 year. In addition, for children 1 year or older who will be departing sooner than 2 weeks after the pretravel visit (and therefore may not have sufficient time for immunity to develop after hepatitis A vaccination), both immunoglobulin and vaccine can be given concurrently at different sites to ensure more immediate protection. Shortages of immunoglobulin have occurred in the past, so obtaining it for hepatitis A prophylaxis may be difficult.[45] Hepatitis A outbreaks also have occurred among adoptees and their contacts, leading to American Academy of Pediatrics and the Advisory Committee on Immunization Practices recommendations for hepatitis A vaccination for all household members and close contacts, including babysitters, when children are adopted from countries with high or intermediate rates of hepatitis A infection. All nonimmune, unvaccinated people who will have close exposure to international adoptees during the 60 days after their arrival (regardless of whether they travel) should receive hepatitis A immunization, ideally 2 or more weeks before arrival of the adopted child.[2,9]

Polio

Worldwide polio eradication efforts have decreased the number of countries where travelers are at risk for acquiring polio. In 2015, 74 cases of wild poliovirus were reported, representing a decrease of 99% from 1988, when the Global Polio Eradication Initiative was launched. Wild poliovirus is considered endemic in two countries: Afghanistan and Pakistan. Of the three strains of wild poliovirus (1, 2, and 3), wild poliovirus type 2 was eradicated in 1999 and the last case of wild poliovirus 3 was reported in Nigeria in 2012.[183] To ensure protection, pediatric travelers visiting countries where polio is epidemic or still endemic should be fully immunized, and young adults 18 years or older should receive one booster dose of inactivated polio vaccine (IPV) if traveling to areas with risk for transmission. Clinicians should obtain up-to-date information about areas of transmission from the World Health Organization (WHO) or CDC (see discussion on international travel information resources).

Influenza

Respiratory tract infections caused by influenza are a major cause of illness among travelers.[115] Influenza can occur throughout the year in tropical countries. Peak influenza rates in temperate regions of the Southern Hemisphere occur from April through September. In North America, influenza vaccine may not be available during the summer months. All children 6 months and older should have routine influenza vaccination annually. Travelers to the Southern Hemisphere should be vaccinated by the spring, if possible. Influenza vaccinations should be considered for travelers who are at high risk for complications from influenza for travel to (1) the tropics any time of year, (2) the Southern Hemisphere from April through September, (3) any destination with large groups of tourists at any time of year, or (4) any destination where influenza outbreaks are occurring.[3] In 2009, pandemic H1N1 outbreak emerged in Mexico and spread quickly around the world through travel. Protection against H1N1 is included in seasonal influenza vaccine.[39,40]

Neisseria meningitis

Meningococcal disease occurs sporadically worldwide. Epidemic disease has been reported in India, Saudi Arabia, and sub-Saharan Africa; indeed, recurrent epidemics of meningococcal disease occur in sub-Saharan Africa, mainly from December to June (the dry season). Serogroup A is the most common cause of epidemics outside the United States, but serogroup C and other serogroups also have been associated with epidemics. Serogroup W-135 meningococcal infection has been reported in travelers returning from Saudi Arabia after visiting the Hajj.[161] Three meningococcal vaccines, a polysaccharide vaccine (MPSV4) and two conjugate vaccines (MCV4-D and MCV4-CRM), are available in the United States. Both conjugate vaccines are quadrivalent and effective against serogroups A, C, Y, and W-135. MCV4-D is licensed for use in children starting at 9 months of age, and MCV4-CRM can be used for children starting at 2 months of age. MCV4 (either MCV4-D or MCV4-CRM) is recommended for routine childhood vaccination in the United States for (1) all children at the 11- to 12-year-old visit, with a booster at 16 years of age; and (2) unvaccinated adolescents at 13 through 18 years of age, with a booster at 16 through 18 years. For infants aged 8 weeks to 6 months with functional/anatomic asplenia or complement deficiency, MCV-CRM can be given at 2, 4, 6, and 12 months. For infants and children 7 to 23 months old, MCV-CRM can be given in two doses administered at least 3 months apart, with the second dose given after 12 months. For children older than 2 months with functional/anatomic asplenia, complement deficiency, or HIV, either MCV-CRM or MCV4-D can be administered as a two-dose series given 2 months apart.[148] Meningococcal vaccination is recommended for pediatric travelers age 2 months or older who are visiting sub-Saharan Africa during the dry season or any country that is hyperendemic or where an epidemic caused by a vaccine serogroup is occurring using the above schedule. For children traveling to areas with risk for transmission, revaccination with MCV4 is recommended after 3 years for children who were previously vaccinated at 2 months to 6 years of age. Revaccination with MCV4 is recommended after 5 years for people who were previously vaccinated at 7 years or older and every 5 years thereafter for people who are at continued risk. Although it is less immunogenic than when it is administered to older children and adults, MPSV4 also can be used in children as young as 3 months to provide protection against serogroup A, such as travelers to areas with an epidemic or during seasonal transmission. These children should have two doses, 3 months apart.[66,122,148] Furthermore, two US Food and Drug Administration (FDA)-approved vaccinations against serotype B, Trumenba and Bexsero, can be used in a two-dose series in children older than 10 years who are traveling to an area with an outbreak. Of note, they are used effectively in much younger populations in Europe.[80,79]

Others Vaccine-Preventable Diseases

Hepatitis B, *Haemophilus influenzae* type b, rotavirus, *Streptococcus pneumoniae,* varicella, and human papillomavirus are endemic in many developing countries, and vaccination should be ensured.[70] For persons 18 years and older, a combination hepatitis A and hepatitis B vaccine (Twinrix) can be administered to travelers who need both vaccines. It is administered as a standard three-dose schedule at 0, 1, and 6 months after the first dose or can be accelerated at 0, 7, or 21 to 30 days, followed by a booster dose at 12 months.[38] Travel in large groups on conveyances such as cruise ships can facilitate the transmission of infectious and vaccine-preventable diseases.[124] The CDC has provided consultation on managing outbreaks of varicella and meningococcal disease in pediatric travelers on international cruise ships (CDC, unpublished data, 2013). For detailed information about accelerating routine childhood vaccinations and indications for use in pediatric travelers, see Table 232.1.

Common Travel-Related Vaccines for Children

An important consideration in determining travel vaccination needs is "required" versus "recommended" vaccinations. The most recent travel requirements and recommendations for vaccinations can be obtained from the CDC Travelers' Health Internet site (see the discussion on international travel information resources). Currently, there are only two vaccines that are required for entry into a country; yellow fever and meningococcal vaccines. Many countries in South America and Africa may require proof of vaccination against yellow fever for entry, especially if the traveler is arriving from a country where yellow fever is present. Yellow fever vaccine is available only from certified yellow fever vaccination centers; providers can contact their state public health department to locate certified centers in their areas. Saudi Arabia requires meningococcal vaccine for travelers visiting Mecca for the Hajj or for the Umrah.[29,35,43] The United States does not require arriving travelers to have any vaccinations for entry or return to the United States. However, immigrants, refugees, asylum seekers, and internationally adopted children migrating to the United States for permanent residence have different requirements. Some countries previously have required cholera vaccination, but currently no countries require vaccination as a condition of entry.[180]

Tables 232.1 and 232.2 provide general guidelines and indications for the use of routine and selected travel-related vaccines based on US recommendations.[7,43,46,96,101,102,104] WHO recommendations may differ.[180] Depending on the complexity of the travel itinerary and the patient's medical history, the vaccination plan may need to be developed in consultation with a travel medicine or infectious disease specialist. Travel-related vaccine recommendations should be tailored carefully to the trip itinerary and based on the travel destination, season when the travel will occur, duration of the trip, and activities to be undertaken.

Yellow Fever

Yellow fever occurs year-round in the predominantly rural areas of sub-Saharan Africa and South America; however, outbreaks have been increasing in incidence, particularly in Africa.[153] Infection occurs primarily through the bite of an infected mosquito, usually *Aedes* or *Haemagogus* spp. Transmission occurs in a human-to-vector-to-human cycle with monkeys, mosquitoes, and humans in three patterns: sylvatic (jungle), intermediate (savannah), and urban transmission. The resurgence of yellow fever in urban areas, in association with *Aedes aegypti* mosquitoes, has raised concern about increased risk in Brazil and urban areas of Latin America.[43,167,168] Although a rare disease, yellow fever continues to be reported in travelers, particularly unvaccinated travelers, and is usually fatal. From 1970 through 2010, nine cases of yellow fever were reported in unvaccinated travelers from the United States and Europe who traveled to West Africa (five cases) or South America (four cases); eight (88%) of these travelers died. One case of yellow fever in a vaccinated traveler, who survived infection, has been reported.[43,128] Preventive measures taken against yellow fever should include the use of personal protection against mosquitoes and vaccination. As discussed previously, some countries require yellow fever vaccination for travelers arriving from endemic regions; current requirements and recommendations for vaccination based on travel destination can be obtained from the CDC Travelers' Health website.

Yellow fever vaccine is largely considered to be a safe and effective vaccine. However, the vaccine has been found to be associated with an increased risk for development of yellow fever vaccine–associated neurologic disease (YEL-AND), which includes meningoencephalitis, Guillain-Barré syndrome, and other severe reactions in young infants.[7] The incidence is 0.8/100,000 doses. The vaccine should not be used in children younger than 6 months. It should be used with caution in children age 6 to 9 months after discussion with a travel medicine expert to weigh the risks and benefits.[43] Two cases of YEL-AND have been reported in children 6 to 8 months of age. Whenever possible, travel to yellow fever–endemic countries should be postponed for children younger than 9 months. Medical waivers can be given to children who are too young for vaccination and to those who have other contraindications to vaccination, such as immunodeficiency. Breastfeeding is a precaution for yellow fever vaccination. Three cases of transmission to infants have been associated with breastfeeding. None of the cases had permanent sequelae, but until more information is available, yellow fever vaccination should be avoided in breastfeeding women, if possible. Since 2001, yellow fever vaccine–associated viscerotropic disease (YEL-AVD), a life-threatening severe illness with major organ system failure similar to wild-type disease, has been reported in more than 50 confirmed and suspected cases worldwide. The syndrome usually consists of fever, jaundice, and multiple organ system failure. The case fatality ratio is 65%. The usual onset is 3 days (range, 1–8 days) after vaccination. The incidence of YEL-AVD cases in the United States is 0.4 per 100,000 doses of vaccine administered. The rate is higher in people 60 years

Text continued on p. 2297

TABLE 232.1 **Routine Childhood Vaccinations and Accelerated Schedules and Modifications for Pediatric Travelers**

Vaccine	Minimum Age	Routine Schedule[a]	Accelerated Schedule and Modifications[b]	Indications for Use and Other Information[c]
DTaP, DT	6 wk	5 doses at ages 2, 4, 6, 15–18 mo and 4-6 y	5 doses MI from dose 1 to dose 2: 4 wk MI from dose 2 to dose 3: 4 wk MI from dose 3 to dose 4: 6 mo Minimum age for dose 4: 12 mo MI from dose 4 to dose 5: 6 mo Minimum recommended age for dose 5: 4–6 y Dose 5 is not necessary if dose 4 was administered after the fourth birthday	Use for children ages 6 wk–7 y. Use DT for children age <7 y for primary series (instead of DTaP) when pertussis vaccination is contraindicated. The fourth dose may be administered as early as age 12 mo, provided at least 6 mo have elapsed since the third dose.
Tdap	10–11 y, depending on brand	One dose		Only 1 dose of Tdap is recommended. All subsequent doses of tetanus-diphtheria booster should be administered as Td. Tdap should be substituted for a single dose of Td in the catch-up series for children 7–10 y. If additional doses are needed, use Td. Tdap can be administered regardless of the interval since the last tetanus and diphtheria toxoid–containing vaccine.
Td	7 y	1 booster dose every 10 y Children ≥11 y should receive 1 dose of Tdap, followed by booster doses of Td every 10 y	MI for booster for travel: 5 y	Td should be used rather than Tdap if Tdap is not available and for: Anybody who has already received Tdap Additional doses for children 7–10 y in the catch-up series (one dose of Tdap should be administered) See information for Tdap regarding timing of Td vs. Tdap.
Haemophilus influenzae type b (Hib)	6 wk	4 doses at ages 2, 4, 6, and 12–15 mo *or* 3 doses at ages 2, 4, and 12–15 mo (PRP-OMP vaccines only) Unvaccinated child >15 mo: 1 dose	Accelerated schedule is available but varies by vaccine brand; see package insert for vaccine used MI between doses: 4–8 wk	MI between doses depends on age. Children receiving the first dose of vaccine at age ≥7 mo require fewer doses to complete the series. See *MMWR Morb Mortal Wkly Rep* 2005;54:Q1-4, for indications. Vaccinate all children <5 y and children >5 y with special indications (e.g., asplenia, immunodeficiency).
Hepatitis A	1 y	2 doses at ages 12 and 18 mo	MI from dose 1 to dose 2: 6 mo	Recommended for all children at 1 y (12–23 mo). Recommended for unvaccinated children ≥24 mo at high risk (see *MMWR Morb Mort Wkly Rep* 2006;55[RR-7]), and anyone ≥24 mo, previously unvaccinated, for whom immunity against hepatitis A virus infection is desired. Recommended for all persons ≥12 mo traveling to endemic areas, including Mexico, Central and South America, Asia (except Japan), Africa, and eastern Europe.[d] Immunogenicity: limited data are available for the timing of the appearance of neutralizing antibody. Among a sample of vaccinated persons, 54–62% were positive for neutralizing antibody 14 days after the first dose, and 94–100% were positive at 1 mo.[c]

Continued

TABLE 232.1 Routine Childhood Vaccinations and Accelerated Schedules and Modifications for Pediatric Travelers—cont'd

Vaccine	Minimum Age	Routine Schedule[a]	Accelerated Schedule and Modifications[b]	Indications for Use and Other Information[c]
Hepatitis B[e]	Birth	3 doses at 0–2, 1–4, 6–18 mo For children not previously vaccinated: 3 doses at 0-, 1-, and 4-mo intervals For unvaccinated adolescents 11–15 y: 2-dose vaccine series (only Recombivax HB, adult dose) at 0, 4–6 mo or 3 doses of other vaccine brands	3 doses (except 2 doses of Recombivax HB, adult dose for adolescents) MI from dose 1 to dose 2: 4 wk MI from dose 2 to dose 3: 8 wk MI from dose 1 to dose 3: 16 wk Minimum age for dose 3: 6 mo	Use for travelers to endemic areas, including Africa, Asia, Latin America, who plan to: Travel abroad for ≥3 mo Have intimate or sexual contact with local population Work in health care setting or may have contact with blood, blood products, or body fluids Count all doses; do not restart series even if time lapse between doses is greater than recommended interval. Accelerated schedule: 4 doses at 0, 7, 21–30 days and booster at 1 y
Human papillomavirus vaccine (HPV)	9 y For females and males 9–26 y Use HPV4 or HPV2 for females and HPV4 for males.	3 doses at 11–12 y at 0-, 2-, and 6-mo intervals	Recommended interval dose 1 to dose 2: 1–2 mo MI dose 1 to dose 2: 4 wk Recommended interval dose 1 to dose 3: 6 mo Recommended interval dose 2 to dose 3: 4 mo MI dose 2 to dose 3: 3 mo	
Influenza, trivalent or quadrivalent inactivated vaccine (TIV or QUID)	TIV and QID: 6 mo; however, check product because minimum age varies by vaccine manufacturer.	Recommended annually for children ≥6 mo. Children aged 6 mo–8 y who are receiving influenza vaccine for first time: 2 doses Children >8 y and persons who previously received influenza vaccine: 1 dose	TIV and QID: MI dose 1 to dose 2: 4 wk	Influenza can occur throughout the year in tropical countries. Peak influenza in temperate regions of the Southern Hemisphere occurs from April through September. In North America, influenza vaccine may not be available during the summer months. Travelers to the Southern Hemisphere should be vaccinated by the spring, if possible. Consider for travelers who are at high risk for complications from influenza for travel to tropics any time of year Southern Hemisphere from April through September Any destination with large groups of tourists at any time of year Any destination where influenza outbreaks are occurring
Measles, mumps, rubella (MMR)	6 mo	2 doses at ages 12–15 mo and 4–6 y	Children 6–11 mo: 1 dose, then revaccinate at 12–15 mo and 4–6 y of age Children >12 mo vaccinated with 1 prior dose: 1 additional dose at least 4 wk after dose 1 Unvaccinated children >12 mo: 2 doses separated by 4 wk MI between doses: 4 wk	Do not administer MMR for 3 mo after immunoglobulin for hepatitis A prophylaxis; see *MMWR Morb Mortal Wkly Rep* 2005;54:Q1-4, for deferral times for blood products and immunoglobulin administered for other indications. Defer immunoglobulin administration for 2 wk after MMR vaccination. Monovalent vaccines are available for measles, mumps, and rubella. Combination MMRV (measles-mumps-rubella-varicella vaccine) can be used for children 12 mo–12 y but is associated with higher risk for fever and febrile seizures 5–12 days after the first dose among children 12–23 mo.

Meningococcal (quadrivalent A, C, Y, W135) Conjugate vaccine (MCV4) Polysaccharide vaccine (MPSV4)	MCV4-D (Menactra): 9 mo MCV4-CRM (Menveo): 2 mo MPSV4: 3 mo for serogroup A protection, standard recommended minimum age: 2 y (see indications)	MCV4-D or MCV4-CRM: routine vaccination, 1 dose for children at age 11–12 y and booster at 16 y. Administer 1 dose at 13–18 y of age if not previously vaccinated MCV4-D: 2 doses for travelers to risk areas ideally at 9 and 12 mo or at least 8 wk apart for children 9–23 mo MCV4-D or MCV4-CRM: 2 doses for travelers to risk areas at least 8 wk apart for children 24 mo–10 y MCV4-CRM: Can be given at 2, 4, and 12 mo		Meningococcal vaccination is required for travelers to annual Hajj in Mecca, Saudi Arabia. Vaccination is recommended for travel to sub-Saharan Africa during dry season (December through June) or for travel to any countries where epidemic is occurring. Recommended for all children with certain medical conditions. See *MMWR Morb Mort Wkly Rep* 2011;60:72-6.
Pneumococcal conjugate: 13-valent (PCV13)	6 wk	4 doses at ages 2, 4, 6, and 12–15 mo 1 dose for all healthy children 24–59 mo who are not completely vaccinated for age 1 supplemental dose of PCV13 for certain children who received 1 dose of PCV7: (1) all children 14–59 mo and (2) children 60–71 mo with underlying medical conditions	MI between doses: 4–8 wk, depending on age Number of doses varies with age at first dose administered and current age.	MIs between doses depend on age. Children receiving the first dose of vaccine at ≥7 mo require fewer doses to complete the series. Pneumococcal polysaccharide vaccine (PPV23) is routinely recommended for high-risk persons aged ≥2 years. See *MMWR Morb Mortal Wkly Rep* 2010;59(RR 11).
Polio: inactivated poliovirus vaccine (IPV)	6 wk	4 doses at ages 2, 4, 6–18 mo and 4–6 y	Previously unvaccinated children: 3 doses MI between doses: 4 wk Preferred interval between dose 2 and dose 3: 2 mo Minimum age for dose 2: 10 wk Minimum age for dose 3: 14 wk Minimum age for dose 4: 18 wk Previously unvaccinated children <4 y at completion of dose 3: 4 doses Previously unvaccinated children ≥4 y at completion of dose 3: 3 doses MI between doses: 4 wk If ≥4 doses are administered before 4 y, an additional dose should be given at 4–6 y. The final dose in the series should be administered on or after the fourth birthday and at least 6 mo after the previous dose.	Primary series is recommended for all travelers; booster dose for persons ≥18 y is recommended for travelers to some areas of Africa, Asia, and the Middle East; not routinely recommended for travel to Latin America. Single booster of IPV for previously vaccinated adults confers lifetime immunity. Oral poliovirus vaccine (OPV) is no longer recommended or available in the United States. For use in other countries, the World Health Organization recommends birth as the minimum age of administration. The MI between doses is 4 wk. OPV can be used for children younger than 6 wk traveling to areas with polio transmission.

Continued

TABLE 232.1 **Routine Childhood Vaccinations and Accelerated Schedules and Modifications for Pediatric Travelers—cont'd**

Vaccine	Minimum Age	Routine Schedule[a]	Accelerated Schedule and Modifications[b]	Indications for Use and Other Information[c]
Rotavirus (RV): RV1 (Rotarix) and RV5 (Rota Teq)	6 wk	RV1: 2 doses at ages 2, 4 mo RV5: 3 doses at 2, 4, and 6 mo	MI between doses: 4 wk; there is no maximum interval between doses Minimum age for dose 2: 10 wk Minimum age for dose 3: 14 wk	Maximum age for first dose in series is 14 wk, 6 days; and 8 mo, 0 days for final dose in series. Can be administered before, concurrently, or after administration of immunoglobulin. See CDC website for information about risk for intussusception with rotavirus vaccine.
Varicella	12 months	2 doses at 12–15 mo and 4–6 y	MI between dose 1 and dose 2 for children <13 y: 12 wk MI between dose 1 and dose 2 for persons ≥13 y: 4 wk Minimum age for dose 2: 15 mo	Do not administer varicella vaccine for 3 mo after immunoglobulin for hepatitis A prophylaxis; see *MMWR Morb Mortal Wkly Rep* 2005;54:Q1-4, for deferral times for blood products and immunoglobulin administered for other indications. Defer immunoglobulin administration for 2 wk after varicella vaccination. Combination MMRV can be used for children 12 mo–12 y but is associated with higher risk for fever and febrile seizures 5–12 days after the first dose among children 12–23 mo.

[a]Number of doses and recommended ages. Minimum age is the US recommendation unless otherwise noted. Recommendations in the US schedule may be different from those of the World Health Organization and other countries.
[b]Number of doses and MI between doses. *Note:* Interval represents time to dose.
[c]Contraindications: Anaphylactic reaction to prior dose or to any vaccine component or moderate-to-severe acute illness is a contraindication for all vaccines.
[d]See MMWR Recomm Rep 2006;55(RR-7):1-23.
[e]Combination hepatitis A–hepatitis B (Twinrix) is available for use in persons ≥18 years. The vaccine, which is composed of inactivated viral components, is administered intramuscularly. The schedule involves 3 doses at 0, 1, and 6 months. It can be administered at an accelerated schedule of 4 doses at 0, 7, and 21–30 days and 1 year.
CDC, Centers for Disease Control and Prevention; *DTaP,* diphtheria and tetanus toxoids and acellular pertussis, vaccine; *DT,* diphtheria-tetanus (toxoid); *IPV,* inactivated poliomyelitis vaccine; *MI,* minimal interval; *MMR,* mumps, measles, rubella; *PRP-OMP,* PRP-outer membrane protein conjugate vaccine; *Tdap,* tetanus, diphtheria, and pertussis; *Td,* tetanus and diphtheria (toxoid).

TABLE 232.2 Common Travel-Related Vaccines and Immunoglobulin for Children

Vaccine[a]	Vaccine Type	Route	Minimum Age	Primary Series[b]	Booster or Revaccination[c]	Accelerated Schedule	Protection After	General Indications for Use[d]
BCG	Live, attenuated bacteria	ID, SC	Birth	1 dose	None	None	2 mo after dose (WHO)	Consider for children <1 y who will be long-term travelers residing in high-risk areas to protect against meningeal and miliary tuberculosis.
Immunoglobulin	Antibody from pooled human plasma	IM	Birth	1 dose	3–6 mo	None	Immediate	Use to prevent hepatitis A infection in children <1 y who are traveling to risk areas or for persons departing within 4 wk. Defer MMR and varicella vaccination for 3 mo after IG administered for hepatitis A prevention; defer the administration of IG for hepatitis A prevention for 2 wk after MMR or varicella vaccination. Defer rotavirus vaccine (RV) administration for 6 wk if possible. However, if 6-wk deferral would cause the first dose of RV to be scheduled for age ≥13 wk, a shorter deferral interval should be used to ensure that the first dose of RV is administered no later than age 13 wk.
Japanese encephalitis (IXIARO)	Inactivated virus	SC	2 mo	2 doses on days 0 and 28	Yearly for children age >17 y Booster: 1 dose	None	7 days after dose 2	Recommended for travelers who plan to spend a month or longer in endemic areas during the JEV transmission season. Consider for short-term travelers (<1 mo) to endemic areas during JEV transmission season if they plan to travel outside of urban areas and have an itinerary or activities that will increase their risk for JEV exposure; travelers to areas with an ongoing JEV outbreak; and travelers to endemic areas who are uncertain of specific destinations, activities, or duration of travel. Not recommended for short-term travelers whose visit will be restricted to urban areas or times outside of a well-defined JEV transmission season. See CDC website for further information. Clinicians should review updated data about risk areas because transmission varies by country and season. Destinations with transmission include to selected areas of Asia, Oceania (Australia and Papua New Guinea), Russia, especially long-term travelers to rural, agricultural endemic areas or epidemic regions during seasonal transmission (usually May to September). Mild adverse reactions (headache, myalgia, fatigue, influenza-like illness) reported in 13%–26% of vaccinees. There are no data on the use of IXIARO as a booster dose after a primary series with JE-VAX. Persons who received JE-VAX should receive the primary 2-dose series of IXIARO.
Rabies Human diploid cell vaccine (HDCV) Purified chick-embryo cell culture vaccine (PCEC)	Inactivated virus; cell culture derived	IM	United States: None	3 doses at 0, 7, and 21 or 28 days	No boosters or serologic testing recommended for routine international travelers. Boosters and/or serologic testing recommended for high-risk groups. See CDC website for additional information.	None	14 days after dose 3	Use for travelers to rabies-endemic countries. Vaccination is recommended for long-term travel in rural areas or in areas with limited access to health care. Travelers with extensive unprotected outdoor, evening, and nighttime exposure in rural areas, such as backpacking, should consider vaccination even for trips of short duration. Widespread worldwide rabies distribution. See Health Information for Travelers for list of countries that have not reported cases of rabies recently.

Continued

TABLE 232.2 Common Travel-Related Vaccines and Immunoglobulin for Children—cont'd

Vaccine[a]	Vaccine Type	Route	Minimum Age	Primary Series[b]	Booster or Revaccination[c]	Accelerated Schedule	Protection After	General Indications for Use[d]
								Postexposure vaccination is required even for persons who receive vaccination before exposure. After exposure in vaccinated person: 2 doses at 0, 3 days (no rabies immunoglobulin required). After exposure in unvaccinated person: Rabies immunoglobulin (RIG) (20 IU/kg) plus vaccination with 4 doses at 0, 3, 7, and 14 days. RIG can be administered up to and including day 7 of the postexposure prophylaxis series.
Typhoid (ViCPS)	Capsular polysaccharide	IM	2 y	1 dose	2 y	None	14 days after dose	Use recommended for travelers to Africa, Asia, and Latin America for long-term stays, travel outside usual tourist destinations, or travelers who desire maximal protection. Patients should be counseled about protective efficacy of vaccine (approximately 50–74% when studied in endemic areas) and importance of other preventive measures.
Typhoid oral (Ty21a)	Live, attenuated bacteria	Oral	6 y	4 doses at 0, 2, 4, 6 days	5 y	None	7–10 days after last dose	See indications for typhoid ViCPS. Patients should be counseled about protective efficacy of vaccine (approximately 60–85% when studied in endemic areas) and importance of other preventive measures. Must be swallowed (cannot be chewed) 1 h before meal, and vaccine must be refrigerated until administration. Do not administer within 72 h of any antibacterial agent, including doxycycline. Mefloquine, atovaquone-proguanil, and chloroquine can be administered concurrently. Contraindicated for immunocompromised patients.
Yellow fever	Live, attenuated virus	SC	6 mo	1 dose	10 y	None	10 days after dose	Use for travelers to selected areas of Africa and South America. Yellow fever has not been reported in Asia; however, some countries require proof of vaccination if the traveler is arriving from a yellow fever–endemic country. Yellow fever vaccination for children 6–9 mo should be discussed with an expert to weigh risk for adverse events against risk for yellow fever. Reports of rare serious adverse events of multiple organ system failure after vaccination. Contraindicated for patients who are immunocompromised or have allergy to eggs.

[a]Cholera vaccine is not available in the United States. Tick-borne encephalitis vaccine is not available in the United States. It is administered as a 4-dose series at 0, 28-day, 42-day, and 1-y intervals, with booster doses required every 3 to 5 y. The vaccine is available in Europe.

[b]Number of doses and recommended ages and intervals. *Note:* interval represents time from dose.

[c]Number of doses and recommended ages and intervals.

[d]Contraindications: Anaphylactic reaction to prior dose or to any vaccine component or moderate-to-severe acute illness is a contraindication for all vaccines.

BCG, bacille Calmette-Guérin; *CDC,* Centers for Disease Control and Prevention; *ID,* intradermal; *IG,* immunoglobulin; *IM,* intramuscular; *JEV,* Japanese encephalitis virus; *MMR,* measles, mumps, rubella; *SC,* subcutaneous; *WHO,* World Health Organization.

and older, with a rate of one per 100,000 doses in people 60 to 69 years of age and 2.3 per 100,000 doses in people 70 years and older. The risk is thought to be approximately one per 200,000 to 300,000 doses in persons younger than 60 years and one per 40,000 to 50,000 doses in persons 60 years and older. The risk is greater in persons with a history of thymus disorder associated with abnormal immune cell function such as thymoma, myasthenia gravis, or DiGeorge syndrome.[47] Further studies are being conducted.[63,126,167] In the interim, the CDC has recommended that, given the risk for serious illness and death from yellow fever,[118] evidence of increasing transmission of the disease,[147] and the known effectiveness of the vaccine, clinicians should continue to use yellow fever vaccine.[43] Health care providers should carefully review travel itineraries to ensure that only people traveling to areas endemic for yellow fever or areas where yellow fever activity is reported receive yellow fever vaccine.[25,27,43,180]

Japanese Encephalitis Virus

Japanese encephalitis is a viral infection transmitted by *Culex* mosquitoes that bite from dusk to dawn in an enzootic cycle between mosquitoes and vertebrate hosts, primarily pigs and wading birds. Japanese encephalitis virus (JEV) is primarily a disease of childhood, with most cases occurring among children younger than 15 years. Disease develops in less than 1% of infected persons.[81] JEV occurs year-round in tropical regions and primarily from May through October in temperate zones. The risk is greatest for travelers to rural Asia, where the mosquito breeds in rice fields and other agricultural areas. Clinicians should consult the CDC Travelers' Health website for the current list of areas with endemic and epidemic transmission. JEV is associated with high rates of case fatalities and severe neurologic sequelae, especially in young children and older adults. Among an estimated 35,000 to 50,000 annual cases worldwide, approximately 20% to 30% of patients die, and 30% to 50% of survivors have neurologic or psychiatric sequelae.[58] However, JEV is rare among travelers, estimated at less than 1 per 1 million travelers. During 1973 to 2008, 55 cases of travel-associated JEV among persons from nonendemic countries were reported in the literature. Five (9%) of the cases occurred in children 10 years or younger.[43] Expatriates and travelers who stay for prolonged periods in rural areas likely have a risk similar to that of the local population in affected areas (5 to 50 per 100,000/year).[43] All travelers to risk areas should use personal protective measures, such as repellent and long-sleeved clothing, to minimize mosquito bites. Vaccination is recommended for travelers who plan to spend a month or longer in endemic areas during the JEV transmission season. Vaccination should be considered for travelers who will spend 30 days or longer in endemic areas during transmission season if they plan to travel outside of an urban area and have an itinerary or activities that will increase their risk for exposure; travelers to an area with an ongoing outbreak; and travelers to endemic areas who are uncertain of specific destinations, activities, or duration of travel. Consider vaccination for short-term travelers (<1 month) to endemic areas during transmission season if they plan to travel outside of urban areas and have an itinerary or activities that will increase their risk for exposure. Vaccination is not generally recommended for short-term travelers (<30 days) whose visit will be restricted to urban areas or times outside of a well-defined transmission season.[43] IXIARO, an inactivated JEV vaccine, has been licensed for use in children 2 months and older in the United States since 2013.[49] IXIARO is administered as a two-dose series, with the second dose administered 28 days after the first dose. In children older than 17 years, if the primary series of IXIARO was administered 1 year or more previously, a booster dose should be given before potential reexposure or if there is a continued risk for JEV infection. The safety of a booster dose in children younger than 17 years has not been established. JE-Vax, an inactivated mouse brain–derived vaccine, was licensed in the United States in 1992 for use in travelers 1 year and older. In 2006, JE-Vax production was discontinued, and all remaining doses expired in May 2011. Other inactivated and live, attenuated JEV vaccines are manufactured and used in Asia but are not licensed for use in the United States.

Rabies

Rabies virus, which causes a progressive fatal encephalomyelitis, occurs worldwide, except in Antarctica. In certain areas of the world, including (but not limited to) parts of Africa, Asia, and Central and South America, canine rabies remains highly endemic. Rabies also occurs in other wild animals, including bats. The three-dose preexposure rabies vaccine should be considered for children visiting rabies-endemic countries for longer than 1 month, those undertaking extensive outdoor activities such as backpacking or camping in endemic countries, or children traveling to areas where access to health care is limited. Persons who completed the three-dose preexposure vaccine series or the full post-exposure prophylaxis and are considered preimmunized do not require routine boosters. Routine booster doses and/or serologic testing are recommended for certain high-risk persons working with rabies virus or for persons, such as cavers, with frequent exposure to mammals, such as bats. To reduce the risk for acquiring rabies, children and their families should be counseled to stay away from stray dogs and other animals, especially if traveling to Latin America, Asia, or Africa.[43] Exposure is considered a medical emergency. Wound management should include thorough cleansing with soap, water, and povidone-iodine, if available, and suturing delay of a few days, if possible. Postexposure prophylaxis should be administered as soon as possible; travelers who received preexposure vaccination should receive two booster doses on days 0 and 3 after exposure, whereas persons who did not receive preexposure vaccination should receive rabies immunoglobulin and a series of four injections of rabies vaccine over 14 days.[125,149]

Typhoid

Typhoid infection is an acute, life-threatening illness caused by *Salmonella enterica* serotype Typhi, which is usually acquired through contaminated food and water. Serotypes Paratyphi A, Paratyphi B, and Paratyphi C can also cause a protracted bacteremic illness referred to as paratyphoid fever. Enteric fever can be severe and even life-threatening, with a case-fatality rate of more than 10% if not recognized and treated appropriately.[156] The incubation period is 6 to 30 days, and illness onset is insidious with gradually increasing fatigue, fever, malaise, headache, and anorexia. A transient malar rash can occur.

Approximately 90% of US cases occur among persons returning from foreign travel, with more than 75% with travel to India, Bangladesh, or Pakistan.[55] Vaccination is recommended for pediatric travelers visiting developing countries, especially for prolonged periods, or traveling outside the usual tourist destinations. Travelers visiting friends and relatives are at increased risk. Two vaccines are available in the United States: (1) an attenuated, live oral vaccine that can be administered to children 6 years of age and older and (2) an injectable Vi capsular polysaccharide vaccine that can be administered to children starting at 2 years of age and that requires a booster every 2 years. The oral vaccine consists of four capsules, one taken every other day, and should be completed 1 week before travel. Boosters should be administered every 5 years. Because the oral typhoid vaccine is a live, attenuated vaccine, it should not be administered to individuals with immunodeficiency, acute febrile illness, or gastrointestinal disease.[12,103] Furthermore, the oral typhoid vaccine should not be administered within 72 hours of antibiotics. However, antimalarials, including atovaquone/proguanil, can be given concurrently with oral typhoid vaccine because this medication did not appear to diminish antibody titers after vaccination in a double-blind, placebo-controlled study involving 330 Gabonese school children.[77] There are no efficacy studies among travelers from nonendemic areas, but both vaccines have moderate efficacy in populations where typhoid disease is endemic, with efficacy rates ranging from 30% to 80% depending on the location and the age range studied.[12,157] Therefore parents should be cautioned that vaccination is not 100% effective, and precautions regarding safe food and water should be followed.[43]

Cholera

Cholera is a diarrhea illness caused by *Vibrio cholerae,* a gram-negative bacteria that can cause watery diarrhea leading to severe dehydration. Cholera primarily affects individuals in resource-limited settings with inadequate access to clean water and is mostly endemic in parts of Africa and Asia. However, massive epidemics do occur with the introduction of *V. cholera* into a naïve population. Most recently, there was a large outbreak in Haiti beginning in October 2010 with the introduction of *V. cholera* O1 variant El Tor strain, possibly through the United Nations stabilization forces after a large earthquake. Within 3 years, there were 692,098 cholera cases, of which 386,652 patients were hospitalized and 8470 died, giving a case-fatality rate of 1.2%.[64,140] Cholera is easily treatable with oral rehydration salts. In severely dehydrated patients, antibiotics diminish the duration of diarrhea and reduce the volume of rehydration fluids required. In June 2016, Vaxchora, a live, attenuated oral vaccine, was approved by the FDA for prevention of cholera caused by serogroup O1 in adults 18 to 64 years old traveling to affected areas, showing an efficacy of 90% 10 days after administration of one dose. Efficacy waned to 80% 3 months after vaccination.[163] Outside the United States, two different killed whole-cell oral vaccines exist with studied efficacy in children. Dukoral can be administered to adults and children aged 6 years or older in two doses. It can be given to children older than 2 years but younger than 6 years in three doses, and it provides protection 1 week after the last dose. Field trials in Bangladesh and Peru have shown that this vaccine is safe and effective, conferring protection with 85% efficacy for 4 to 6 months. Shanchol is given as two doses 2 weeks apart in children older than 1 year and provides 67% protection against clinically significant O1 cholera for 2 years.[86,179] As of 2013, an oral cholera stockpile was established for outbreak control and emergencies, and this has been used in a reactive campaign during cholera outbreaks as well as in preemptive vaccination campaigns in patients at high risk for cholera due to humanitarian crises.

PREVENTION OF MOSQUITO-BORNE ILLNESS

During a travel assessment, recommendations to prevent vector-borne diseases, including malaria, yellow fever virus, JEV, chikungunya virus, and dengue virus, should be determined by a comprehensive review of the travel itinerary and planned activities. The risk for acquiring an infectious disease differs and is probably greater for an adolescent who is participating in a rural home-stay program for 3 months than for a 5-year-old child traveling with parents to a beach resort. Furthermore, expatriates who live abroad and foreign-born persons, especially immigrants, refugees, and their children visiting friends and relatives in their home country, have health risks different from those of short-term travelers who are visiting tourist destinations.

Malaria

Malaria is a parasitic infection caused by one of four species of *Plasmodium: Plasmodium falciparum, Plasmodium vivax, Plasmodium ovale,* or *Plasmodium malariae.* It is transmitted by the bite of an infective female *Anopheles* mosquito. Malaria is endemic in more than 100 countries on five continents; transmission occurs primarily in the tropic and subtropical regions of sub-Saharan Africa, Asia, Latin America, the Caribbean, the Middle East, and Oceania. Globally, malaria is responsible for 250 million clinical infections and nearly 1 million deaths annually, with most caused by *P. falciparum,* principally in young children and pregnant women.[184,176]

An estimated 10,000 to 30,000 travelers from industrialized countries are thought to contract malaria each year, but these numbers probably are underestimated because they do not include travelers in whom malaria was diagnosed and treated abroad.[105,106,120,175] The number of malaria cases reported in 2010 in the United States was the largest since 1980. In 2010, 1691 cases of malaria, including nine fatal cases, were reported to the CDC. All fatal cases were *P. falciparum,* and seven were acquired in West Africa. Among the 898 cases in US civilians for whom information on chemoprophylaxis use and travel area was known, only 45 (5%) reported that they had followed and adhered to a chemoprophylactic drug regimen recommended by the CDC for the areas to which they had traveled. Among the 1573 cases among patients for whom age was known, 232 (15%) occurred in persons younger than 18 years. Among the 232 cases among persons younger than 18 years, 108 (47%) occurred among US civilian children, 101 (44%) occurred among children of persons categorized as having a foreign resident status at the time their malaria infection was acquired, and 23 (10%) occurred among children of unknown resident status. Of the 108 cases among US civilian children, four (4%) were younger than 24 months, 10 (9%) were 2 to 4 years, 54 (50%) were 5 to 12 years, and 40 (37%) were 13 to 17 years of age. Of these cases among US civilian children for whom country of exposure was known, 75 (75%) were attributable to travel to Africa. Among the 83 US civilian children for whom reason for travel was known, 69 (83%) were visiting friends and relatives, 10 (12%) were traveling for educational purposes, two (2%) were traveling for missionary work, and two were either tourists or specified as other. Of the 85 children for whom chemoprophylaxis information was known, 26 (31%) were reported as having taken prophylaxis, of whom 16 (62%) had taken an appropriate regimen; however, only five (31%) of these patients reported adherence.[32]

Reviews of deaths attributed to malaria in the United States indicate that failure to take or to adhere to recommended antimalarial chemoprophylaxis, promptly seek medical care for posttravel illness, and promptly diagnose and treat suspected malaria contributed to fatal outcomes.[28,123,137] Retrospective reviews of malaria in children also have found that a substantial proportion of cases occurred in recent immigrants and the children of former immigrants who had traveled to visit their family's country of origin.[18,96,146] These data highlight the importance of pretravel assessment and counseling, particularly for foreign-born persons, who may assume they are protected by natural immunity or do not perceive the risk for acquisition of malaria by their children who accompany them on returning to visit their home country. The CDC recommends that prevention messages directed toward Africa-bound travelers, particularly those whose destination is West Africa, should be emphasized in early spring, accompanied with a reminder in late fall through early winter. Malaria prevention messages directed toward Asia-bound travelers, specifically those bound for India, should be intensified in late spring.[123]

Dengue

A variety of pathogens increasingly are being recognized as emerging infectious diseases in travelers. In addition to malaria, other vector-borne infectious diseases are among the important diseases for consideration in travelers. Dengue is one of the most significant vector-borne viral infections worldwide. It is endemic in at least 100 countries in Asia, the Pacific, Africa, Latin America, and the Caribbean and occurs sporadically in the Middle East. Worldwide, an estimated 50 to 100 million cases of dengue fever occur annually, including 500,000 dengue hemorrhagic fever cases and 22,000 deaths, mostly among children.[53] Dengue fever has been reported among 2% to 14% of ill travelers.[16,85,138,171] Epidemics of dengue hemorrhagic fever, the more severe clinical form of dengue fever, occur every 3 to 5 years in Southeast Asia and are an emerging problem in Latin America.[139] Epidemics caused by all four serotypes (1–4) have become progressively more frequent and larger in the past 25 years. In addition, most tropical urban centers in endemic regions have multiple dengue virus serotypes cocirculating (hyperendemicity), which increases the risk for dengue transmission and the risk for dengue hemorrhagic fever.[42] Outbreaks of dengue fever also have occurred in Hawaii, Puerto Rico, the US Virgin Islands, Samoa, and Guam and along the United States–Mexico border.[53,57,58,143] In a recent short report by Krishnan and associates,[112] eight children were diagnosed with dengue between 2007 and 2010 at Bronx-Lebanon Hospital Center in New York City. The cases had a median age of 13.6 years (range, 0.3–17.6 years). All of the children were visiting friends and relatives in Puerto Rico (12%) or the Dominican Republic (88%). Of the eight children, three (38%) developed complications, including dengue shock syndrome in one infant.[112] Dengue is transmitted primarily by day-biting *Aedes aegypti* mosquitoes, which breed in flower vases, barrels, and discarded tires that collect water. Transmission occurs in rural and urban areas, but the risk is greatest in urban areas. Prevention should focus on protection against mosquito bites. Travelers to areas of risk should be counseled to apply repellent during the day, even while visiting cities. No vaccine is available, and previous infection with one of the four serotypes does not protect against infection with another serotype. The risk for contracting dengue hemorrhagic fever increases after subsequent infection with a different serotype.[159]

Chikungunya

Chikungunya virus is an alphavirus that exists in tropical Africa and is transmitted by the bite of an infected mosquito. Because chikungunya fever epidemics are sustained by human-mosquito-human transmission, the epidemic cycle is similar to the cycles of dengue and urban yellow fever. Infection is associated with fever, headache, severe joint pain, and, in approximately half of the cases, a generalized maculopapular rash similar to that of dengue virus infection. Complications are more common in children younger than 1 year. Large outbreaks of chikungunya have been reported recently on several islands in the Indian Ocean and in India, and the disease has now been locally transmitted in 45 countries. The first cases of locally transmitted disease in the United States occurred in Florida in 2014, and this disease has been widely reported in Puerto Rico.[109,154] Almost 1.8 million cases have been reported as of 2016.[50] No vaccines or specific preventive medications are available; therefore, prevention measures should focus on personal protection against mosquito bites and awareness of local epidemics.[36]

Zika Virus

Zika virus is an arthropod-borne flavivirus transmitted by the *Aedes* mosquito. It can also be transmitted sexually, through blood transfusions, or through vertical transmission from mother to child. Outbreaks have occurred in the past in Africa, Southeast Asia, and the Pacific Islands. Beginning in 2014, Zika virus was detected in Chile, and it continues to contribute to an epidemic that involves 41 countries and territories in the Americas and Caribbean.[13] More than 80% of infected individuals do not have symptoms. In the 20% who do have symptoms, they are often nonspecific and include low-grade fevers, pruritic rash, nonpurulent conjunctivitis, and arthralgia of the hands and feet. The two complications of Zika virus infection include Guillain-Barré syndrome and neurologic complications in infants born to infected mothers, including congenital microcephaly.[19] Although Zika virus has been detected in Puerto Rico and the Virgin Islands, all the cases in the continental United States have been imported.[52] There is no specific treatment recommended for infection, and prevention of disease largely depends on mosquito avoidance through personal protective measures. Pregnant women and their partners are discouraged from traveling to locations where there is local transmission of Zika virus, and men are encouraged to abstain from sex or to use condoms during a woman's pregnancy because the virus can persist in semen for weeks if not months.[14]

Personal Protection Methods

Prevention of mosquito-borne illnesses in pediatric travelers depends first on obtaining current and accurate information about the risk for acquiring these diseases in proposed travel destinations and determining whether planned activities, such as rural versus urban travel and the season of travel, place the traveler at increased risk for exposure. Information on the geographic- and country-specific risks for acquiring infections is available from multiple sources. Selected websites with information about the country-specific risk for acquiring diseases are listed in this chapter in the discussion on international travel information resources.

The first mainstay of prevention of mosquito-borne illnesses is appropriate and effective use of personal protection measures. All travelers to malaria-endemic areas should be counseled on recommended measures to avoid bites from *Anopheles* mosquitoes, which typically are evening and nighttime feeders, versus the *Aedes* mosquitos, which are daytime feeders. Such measures include wearing clothing that reduces the amount of exposed skin (e.g., long-sleeved shirts, long pants tucked into socks, hats, stroller nets) and, whenever possible, remaining in well-screened or enclosed air-conditioned areas. Travelers staying overnight in facilities without air conditioning or screens should use insecticide-treated mosquito nets over the beds. Stroller nets can be used for children in strollers. Bed nets that have been treated with insecticide such as permethrin are more effective in preventing malaria than are untreated bed nets and are safe for children.[136] Travelers can purchase permethrin to spray on the bed nets or purchase pretreated (or impregnated) bed nets. Permethrin also can be sprayed on clothing, but it should not be applied directly to skin. Permethrin remains effective through multiple washings. Clothing and bed nets should be retreated according to the product label. Permethrin should not be applied to the skin. Although permethrin provides longer duration protection, recommended repellents that can be applied to skin (DEET [*N,N*-diethyl-*m*-toluamide], picaridin, oil of lemon eucalyptus [OLE], or *para*-menthane-3,8-diol [PMD, the synthesized version of OLE]), and IR3535 can also be used on clothing and mosquito nets. During the evening, insecticide also can be sprayed inside rooms.

Another important focus of counseling for personal protection measures is appropriate use of insect repellent on exposed skin. The CDC recommends the use of repellent products with active ingredients registered with the US Environmental Protection Agency (EPA). Products containing the following active ingredients provide long-lasting protection (DEET, picaridin (KBR 3023), IR3535, and OLE or PMD, the synthesized version of OLE. Note that "pure" oil of lemon eucalyptus (essential oil) is not the same product as OLE insect repellent. Some controversy has occurred regarding the recommended concentration of DEET for pediatric use. In 1998, the EPA conducted an extensive review of DEET safety. The agency concluded that no evidence indicates that DEET is toxic to infants or children. Additional evaluations have not demonstrated a link between seizures and topical use.[43,54]

Most repellents can be used on children older than 2 months, with the following considerations: (1) products containing OLE specify that they should not be used on children younger than 3 years; (2) repellent products must state any age restriction (if none is stated, the EPA has not required a restriction on the use of the product); and (3) many repellents contain DEET as the active ingredient. DEET formulations of up to 50% can be used for children older than 2 months. The concentration of DEET affects the duration of protection. Higher concentrations provide longer protection; however, the duration of protection reaches a plateau at approximately 30% to 50%. Therefore most clinicians recommend products having up to 30% for children. The American Academy of Pediatrics recommends that 30% or lower DEET should be used on children older than 2 months and that repellents with DEET should not be used on infants younger than 2 months (https://www.epa.gov/insect-repellents).[3] In a laboratory study, a product with 23.8% DEET provided an average of 5 hours of protection (range, 3–6 hours) and a product with 6.65% DEET provided an average of 2 hours of protection (range, 1.5–2.8 hours). Duration of protection may be affected by the environmental temperature, sweating, and wind conditions.[25,54,83,87] Products that contain repellents and sunscreen generally are not recommended because of the need to reapply sunscreen more frequently than repellent.[6,8,134] Mosquito coils should be used with extreme caution in the presence of children to avoid burns and inadvertent ingestion.[60]

Clinicians are encouraged to stress to parents and children alike the importance of using personal protection measures. Despite the demonstrated efficacy of these measures, studies have found that only 17% of adult travelers with malaria reported using insect protection methods and only 11% took the recommended chemoprophylaxis.[105]

Antimalarial Medication

Other than personal protective measures, patients traveling to malaria-endemic regions should be encouraged to further protect themselves by using chemoprophylaxis. Selection of the appropriate drug for antimalarial chemoprophylaxis must be based on numerous factors: the most recent information available about malaria in the proposed travel destinations; the trip itinerary; the age, weight, and medical history of the traveler; the personal preference for the frequency of dosing and the duration of chemoprophylaxis on return from the trip; and the cost of medication. These decisions can be challenging for primary care providers and clinicians with limited experience in infectious disease and travel medicine, so when in doubt, clinicians should seek the advice of a travel medicine or infectious disease expert. In addition, the CDC provides resources with guidance on appropriate use of and recommended regimens for antimalarial chemoprophylaxis (listed in the section on international travel information resources).

Fig. 232.1 outlines an algorithm for determining appropriate antimalarial chemoprophylaxis regimens for pediatric travelers. Because data on the distribution of drug-resistant malaria are evolving constantly, clinicians always should obtain the most recent information about the risk for malaria and zones of drug resistance from the CDC website or other sources of information before prescribing malaria chemoprophylaxis.[38,43,153]

The first decision point in selecting appropriate antimalarial chemoprophylaxis is whether travel is occurring in a region of chloroquine-sensitive or chloroquine-resistant malaria. For travel to areas with

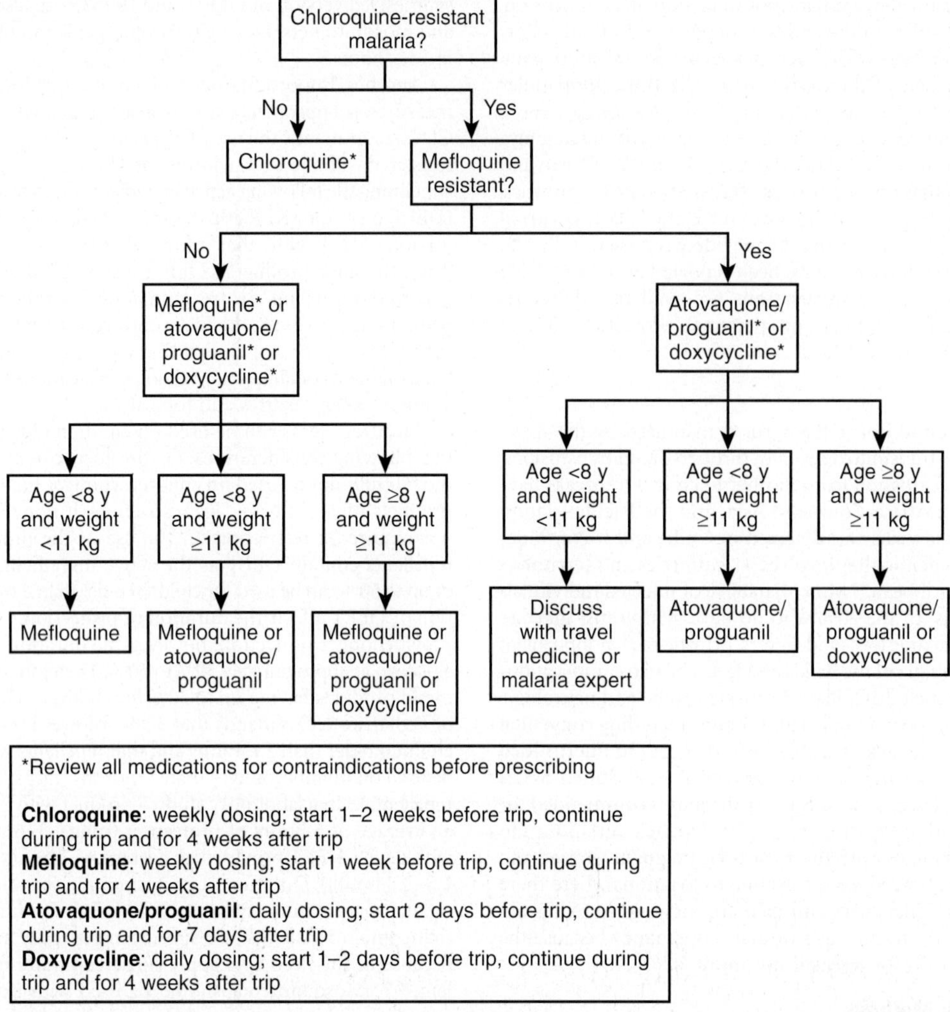

FIG. 232.1 Algorithm for determining appropriate antimalarial chemoprophylaxis regimens for pediatric travelers.

chloroquine-sensitive malaria, chloroquine is the drug of choice for antimalarial chemoprophylaxis. *P. ovale, P. malariae,* and most *P. vivax* are widely sensitive to chloroquine; however, chloroquine-resistant *P. vivax* is an emerging problem and has been reported from Guyana, Papua New Guinea, India, Burma (Myanmar), and areas of Indonesia.[42,105] In addition to chloroquine-resistant *P. vivax,* chloroquine-resistant *P. falciparum* has been reported from these areas, and consequently chloroquine would not be recommended as chemoprophylaxis for travelers to these regions. Chloroquine-sensitive *P. falciparum* exists in parts of the Caribbean, Central America, the Middle East, and China.[43,107]

If the traveler is visiting a region with chloroquine-resistant malaria, the next decision point is whether travel will include regions with chloroquine-resistant malaria only or both chloroquine- and mefloquine-resistant malaria. In some regions, *P. falciparum* may be resistant to both chloroquine and mefloquine; these areas currently are limited to the borders of Thailand with Myanmar (Burma) and Cambodia, the western provinces of Cambodia that border Thailand, and the eastern states of Myanmar (Burma) on the border between Burma and China, along the borders of Laos and Burma, the adjacent parts of the Thailand-Cambodia border, and southern Vietnam.[43,107] For travel to areas with chloroquine-resistant malaria, three current antimalarial chemoprophylaxis options are mefloquine (Lariam), atovaquone/proguanil (Malarone), and doxycycline. The CDC no longer recommends the use of chloroquine-proguanil for chemoprophylaxis in chloroquine-resistant areas. For travel to areas with chloroquine-resistant and mefloquine-resistant malaria, either atovaquone-proguanil or doxycycline can be used. Primaquine can be used as an option for primary prophylaxis in special circumstances. Clinicians should contact the CDC Malaria Hotline (770-488-7788 or 1-855-856-4713) for additional information. Primaquine also can be used for terminal prophylaxis to prevent relapses of *P. vivax* or *P. ovale.* In general, terminal prophylaxis is indicated only for persons who have had prolonged exposure to malaria-endemic areas (e.g., missionaries and expatriates).[43]

In evaluating options for antimalarial chemoprophylaxis, physicians should review each medication for contraindications and weight and age restrictions (Table 232.3). Pediatric doses of medications used for treatment should be calculated on the basis of body weight. Medications used for infants and young children are the same as those recommended for adults, except under the following circumstances: doxycycline should not be given to children younger than 8 years because of the risk for teeth staining, and atovaquone-proguanil should not be used for prophylaxis in children weighing less than 5 kg because of lack of data on safety and efficacy.

Chloroquine is relatively well tolerated in children. In the United States, chloroquine is available in tablet form; in Europe and other countries, it is also available as a syrup. Mefloquine can be used safely in children weighing less than 9 kg and may be useful for longer trips because it is administered once weekly.[121] However, it must be continued for 4 weeks after leaving the malarious area, and no liquid preparation is available. Doses for children are one-fourth, one-half, and three-fourths of a tablet, depending on weight. Mefloquine has been associated with rare but serious adverse reactions (e.g., psychoses and seizures) at prophylactic doses; these reactions are more frequent with higher doses used for treatment. Other side effects that have occurred

TABLE 232.3 Antimalarial Chemoprophylaxis Regimens for Pediatric Travelers

Medication	Regimen	Dose	Contraindications and Precautions	Side Effects	General Indications and Information for Use
Chloroquine (Aralen)	Weekly starting 1–2 wk before trip Continue weekly during trip and for 4 wk after trip	5 mg base/kg (8.3 mg salt/kg) up to 300 mg base (500 mg salt) Tablets: 300 mg base (500 mg salt)	Prior retinal or visual field changes Psoriasis (may be exacerbated by chloroquine)	Gastrointestinal symptoms, seizures, rash, headache, dizziness, pruritus (especially in dark-skinned persons), blurred vision, decreased hearing, tinnitus, retinal damage at high cumulative doses[a] High toxicity in overdoses, keep out of reach of children	Use only in areas of chloroquine-sensitive malaria. Limited usefulness because of widespread chloroquine resistance. Bitter taste.
Mefloquine (Lariam)	Weekly starting 1 wk before trip Continue weekly during trip and for 4 wk after trip	≤9 kg: 5 mg/kg/dose once weekly 9–19 kg: 62.5 mg (¼ of 250 mg tablet) once weekly 20–30 kg: 125 mg (½ of 250 mg tablet) once weekly 31–45 kg: 187.5 mg (¾ of 250 mg tablet) once weekly ≥45 kg: 250 mg once weekly Tablets: 228 mg base (250 mg salt)	Psychiatric conditions, cardiac conduction disorders, seizure disorders, persons with known hypersensitivity to mefloquine Should not take with quinine-like drugs	Gastrointestinal symptoms, dizziness, insomnia Occasional serious adverse effects: seizures, nightmares, depression, anxiety, psychosis, especially in persons with these preexisting medical conditions	Use in areas with chloroquine-resistant malaria. Advantageous for long-term travelers because of weekly dosing and less costly than atovaquone-proguanil. Bitter taste.
Atovaquone-proguanil (Malarone)	Daily starting 1–2 days before trip Continue daily during trip and for 7 days after trip	5–8 kg: ½ pediatric tablet once daily 8–10 kg: ¾ pediatric tablet once daily 10–20 kg: pediatric tablet once daily 20–30 kg: 2 pediatric tablets once daily 30–40 kg: 3 pediatric tablets once daily ≥40 kg: 1 adult tablet daily Pediatric tablets: 62.5 mg atovaquone and 25 mg proguanil hydrochloride Adult tablets: 250 mg atovaquone and 100 mg proguanil hydrochloride	Contraindicated in severe renal failure Not recommended or use with caution for children <11 kg, pregnant or lactating women Do not take with tetracycline, metoclopramide, rifampin, or rifabutin (all reduce concentrations of atovaquone)	Gastrointestinal symptoms, headache, loss of appetite, dizziness, pruritus	Use in areas with chloroquine-resistant or mefloquine-resistant malaria. Advantageous for short-term travelers because prophylaxis can be stopped 1 week after leaving malaria area. Available in pediatric tablets. Take with food or milk.
Doxycycline	Daily starting 1–2 days before trip Continue daily during trip and for 4 wk after trip	2 mg/kg up to 100 mg daily Tablets: 50 mg, 100 mg	Do not use for children <8 y, pregnant or lactating women Do not give within 3 h of antacids, iron or Pepto-Bismol Do not administer oral typhoid vaccine within 72 h of doxycycline	Gastrointestinal symptoms, photosensitivity, increased blood urea nitrogen level, hypersensitivity reactions, blood dyscrasias, vaginal candidiasis May decrease the effectiveness of oral contraceptives	Use in areas with chloroquine-resistant and mefloquine-resistant malaria (borders of Thailand with Myanmar (Burma) and Cambodia, the western provinces of Cambodia that border Thailand, and the eastern states of Myanmar (Burma), on the border between Burma and China, along the borders of Laos and Burma, the adjacent parts of the Thailand-Cambodia border, and in southern Vietnam. Take with food; taking with food or milk can decrease gastric irritation (absorption of doxycycline is not significantly decreased by simultaneous administration of milk or food).

[a]Despite the use of chloroquine as an antimalarial chemoprophylaxis agent for decades and the use of high-dose chloroquine for certain chronic diseases, the literature is inconclusive about the potential risk for retinopathy associated with long-term use of chloroquine for antimalarial prophylaxis. Retinopathy has rarely been reported in patients receiving weekly prophylaxis. Retinopathy appears to be related to dosage and accumulated dosage.

in chemoprophylaxis studies include depression, anxiety disorder, mood changes, panic attacks, and other neuropsychiatric symptoms. Mefloquine is contraindicated in travelers with active depression, a recent history of depression, generalized anxiety disorder, psychosis, schizophrenia, other major psychiatric disorders, or seizures. It carries a US Boxed Warning that it may cause neuropsychiatric adverse effects that can persist after mefloquine has been discontinued. During prophylactic use, if symptoms occur, an alternative medication should be used. It should be used with caution in people with a history of depression or psychiatric disorders. For children who weigh 5 kg or more and are at risk for acquiring chloroquine-resistant *P. falciparum* infection, atovaquone-proguanil can be advantageous for short trips because it is started 1 to 2 days before the trip commences and can be stopped 7 days after the trip. However, the patient or parent must remember to take or to administer the medication daily. It is available in pediatric tablet form. Doxycycline is contraindicated in children younger than 8 years because of concern about the propensity of tetracyclines to stain growing teeth or potentially affect developing bones. For older children, doxycycline must be administered daily and continued for 4 weeks after departing the malaria-endemic area.[43,107]

Chloroquine, mefloquine, and atovaquone-proguanil have a bitter taste. Before departure, pharmacists can be asked to pulverize tablets and prepare gelatin capsules with calculated pediatric doses. Mixing the powder in a small amount of food or drink can facilitate the administration of antimalarial drugs to infants and children. Additionally, any compounding pharmacy can alter the flavoring of malaria medication tablets so that they are more willingly ingested by children. Assistance with finding a compounding pharmacy is available on the International Academy of Compounding Pharmacists' website (http://www.iacprx.org). Because overdose of antimalarial drugs, particularly chloroquine, can be fatal, medication should be stored in childproof containers and kept out of the reach of infants and children.

The importance of determining appropriate antimalarial chemoprophylaxis regimens for travelers and counseling to improve compliance cannot be overemphasized. In retrospective reviews of pediatric malaria cases, between 75% and 100% of infected children had received inadequate or no chemoprophylaxis.[43,146,169] Finally, effective pretravel malaria prevention counseling includes anticipatory guidance for parents about recognition of and response to symptoms of malaria infection in young pediatric travelers. Parents should be counseled that although compliance with personal protection measures and chemoprophylaxis will decrease the risk, it cannot guarantee prevention of malaria infection. They should be instructed about the symptoms of malaria infection, such as fever, headache, vomiting, diarrhea, and myalgia, and be counseled to seek immediate medical attention if symptoms occur. Delay in recognition and treatment of malaria is associated directly with an increase in rates of morbidity and mortality; therefore prompt and appropriate initiation of effective therapy is paramount.[43,91,106,158,175] Parents also should be advised that some types of malaria can become symptomatic several weeks to months after exposure, and therefore prompt medical attention should be sought even if illness develops in a child months after international travel to malaria-endemic areas.

PREVENTION OF TRAVELER'S DIARRHEA IN CHILDREN

Epidemiology of Traveler's Diarrhea

One of the most difficult tasks faced by international travelers of any age is ensuring the safety of food and water. Traveler's diarrhea refers to diarrhea that develops during travel or within 14 days of travel, and is most often caused by the ingestion of contaminated food and water. It is typically defined as the occurrence of three or more unformed stools within a 24-hour period with at least one of the following signs or symptoms: temperature higher than 38°C (100.4°F), abdominal cramping, nausea, vomiting, fecal urgency, tenesmus, or blood or mucus in stools.[74,76,82,141] Traveler's diarrhea affects approximately 20% to 50% of adult travelers and 10% to 41% of children and is the health problem most frequently reported by travelers to developing countries.[73,74,82] It can occur any time during travel but typically occurs within the first week or two of the trip. The illness usually is self-limited, and for adults the average duration of illness has been reported to be 3 to 5 days.[76] Analysis from the GeoSentinel Surveillance Network shows that among 1840 children returning from 218 global destinations, diarrhea was the most common complaint with 28% of children listing it as their travel-related health issue, with bacteria causing 29% of the cases.[90] During 2004 to 2009, 24% of all travel-related enteric infections in the United States occurred in children. The main causative agents included *Campylobacter* (42%), nontyphoidal *Salmonella* (32%), and *Shigella* (13%). Of 328 children who sought care for travel-associated illness at the emergency department of the University of Zürich Children's Hospital, 129 (39%) had a diarrheal illness, including three with *Salmonella typhi* and two with *Salmonella paratyphi* infection. The proportion of children with diarrhea increased with age—33% in children age 0 to younger than 2 years, 39% in children 2 to 5 years and younger, and 45% in children 6 to 16 years of age. Among the ill pediatric travelers visiting family and relatives, 41% had diarrhea.[98] In a study of 890 children younger than 20 years presenting to the outpatient travel clinic of the University of Munich after travel to the tropics and subtropics and their associates, 25% had acute diarrhea, the most frequent syndrome among all ill travelers. The most frequently diagnosed infectious enteric pathogens were giardiasis (8%), *Campylobacter* enteritis (4%), *Salmonella* enteritis (4%), and amebiasis (3%).[95] A retrospective study of Swiss children who had visited the tropics or subtropics reported finding similar incidence rates of traveler's diarrhea in children—40%, 8.5%, 21.7%, and 36% in children aged 0 to 2, 3 to 6, 7 to 14, and 15 years and older, respectively. In this study, the authors also found that young children (0–2 years old) most frequently were affected with traveler's diarrhea and that the clinical course tended to be more severe and prolonged than in older children. Overall, children were found to have longer lasting illness than that noted in adults, with an average duration of 11 days for all children combined and 29 days for small children.[142]

Enteric pathogens typically are isolated from approximately 50% to 75% of stool specimens from adult travelers with diarrhea; in the remainder, usually no pathogen is isolated. Pathogen varies by location of travel, but in general, *Escherichia coli,* especially enterotoxigenic *E. coli,* is the most common overall cause of traveler's diarrhea, especially in Latin America and Africa, followed by *Campylobacter, Salmonella,* and *Shigella.* Other, less common causes of etiologic agents include pathogenic bacteria, such as *Aeromonas* and *Plesiomonas;* protozoa (e.g., *Giardia lamblia, Entamoeba histolytica, Cryptosporidium* spp., and *Cyclospora cayetanensis*); viruses, such as rotavirus and Norwalk-like viruses; and, rarely, helminths.[141] Numerous risk factors for traveler's diarrhea, including the consumption of certain high-risk foods (i.e., raw foods such as meats, seafood, and vegetables; unpasteurized dairy products; and ice and tap water) and travel to certain destinations, also have been identified.[155] Other authors previously categorized destinations by high, intermediate, and low levels of risk for acquiring traveler's diarrhea. Destinations generally considered to have the highest associated risk for contraction of traveler's diarrhea include most of Asia, Africa, Mexico, and Central and South America; destinations with intermediate risk include Eastern Europe, South Africa, and some of the Caribbean islands; and low-risk travel destinations include countries in North America, Northern and Western Europe, Australia, New Zealand, and Japan.[43] The location of food preparation also is a recognized risk factor for acquiring traveler's diarrhea, with a higher risk shown for travelers eating from street vendors and in local restaurants and a lower risk in luxury hotels and private homes. Although fewer data on traveler's diarrhea in children are available, children (especially toddlers) are probably more vulnerable to foodborne and waterborne pathogens for many reasons, including their propensity to touch multiple surfaces and to mouth objects. Of note, one study found that only 40% of parents said that they had practiced dietary prevention measures consistently and that only 5% reported using oral rehydration solutions (the mainstay of treatment of diarrhea in children).[142]

Preventive Counseling for Traveler's Diarrhea

Counseling parents of pediatric travelers about appropriate preventive behavior to avoid traveler's diarrhea and anticipatory guidance to ensure successful management of diarrhea is an important aspect of the pretravel assessment. Rotavirus vaccine and hepatitis A vaccine should be administered before travel if indicated, and cholera and typhoid vaccines should be considered if appropriate, as discussed earlier. However, adherence to hygiene measures and food and beverage precautions are the most important aspects of prevention.

Food and Beverage Precautions

The most important aspect of preventive counseling for parents of pediatric travelers is appropriate food and beverage precautions. In addition to preventing the diarrheal diseases already listed, compliance with food and water precautions also will decrease the risk for contracting other foodborne diseases, such as hepatitis A. Parents should be counseled that in areas where chlorinated tap water is not available or where hygiene and sanitation are poor, tap water (including ice cubes) should be considered contaminated and hence should be avoided. In addition, travelers also should be advised to avoid brushing their teeth with tap water. Breastfeeding, boiled or bottled water, and bottled carbonated beverages are recommended as typically safe beverages for children; powdered drink mixes made with boiled water (e.g., formula or tea) also generally can be considered safe. Parents should dry wet cans and bottles before opening and wipe drinking surfaces clean before serving.[104]

In areas where access to bottled water is poor, water may be boiled for 1 minute (or for 3 minutes at altitudes above 2000 m [6562 ft]). These procedures will kill bacterial, parasitic, and viral pathogens. Chemical disinfection with halogens (iodine or chlorine) is an alternative method for water treatment when the water cannot be boiled; however, some common waterborne parasites, such as *Cryptosporidium*, are poorly inactivated by iodine disinfection, even after extended contact time. Chlorine also can be used for chemical disinfection, but its germicidal activity varies with pH, temperature, and organic content of the water; therefore it can provide less consistent levels of disinfection in many types of water. Thus chemical disinfection with iodine or chlorine should be supplemented with filtration to remove these organisms. However, chlorine dioxide, which is more potent than equivalent doses of chlorine, is effective against all waterborne pathogens, is simple to use, and is available in liquid or tablet form.[40] Tablets for water disinfection are available at pharmacies, sporting goods stores, and camping outfitters. Ultraviolet (UV) light is effective against all waterborne pathogens. Some portable devices are available; however, clear water is required to ensure that the UV rays can reach the pathogens in the water. Portable filters are available and provide various degrees of protection against microbes. Reverse-osmosis filters afford protection against viruses, bacteria, and protozoa, but they are large and expensive, and the small pores can be plugged by cloudy or muddy water. Microstrainer filters with pore sizes in the 0.1- to 0.3-μm range can remove bacteria and protozoa from drinking water, but they do not remove viruses. To kill viruses, parents using microstrainer filters should be advised to chemically disinfect water with iodine after filtration. Data are inadequate at present to evaluate the efficacy of specific brands or models of filters, and therefore the CDC cannot recommend specific brands or models of filters most likely to remove bacteria, viruses, and parasites.[43]

Parents of pediatric travelers also should be counseled on the importance of advance planning for food and beverage items, especially for infants and young children. Breastfeeding infants are considered relatively safe from contracting traveler's diarrhea because they are not exposed to local food and water; therefore traveling mothers should be encouraged to continue breastfeeding for as long as practical. For infants receiving formula, formula concentrate and powdered forms are the most convenient for travel, but a clean water supply must be available or water must be boiled or chemically disinfected before preparation. For feeding toddlers and older children, the travel adage of "boil it, cook it, peel it, or forget it" applies. In general, unless beverages and food come from a can or can be completely cooked or peeled, they should be considered unsafe (including raw fruits and vegetables). Travelers should avoid unpasteurized dairy products, including cheese and ice cream. In addition, travelers should be advised not to consume raw seafood, shellfish, and meats. Freshly prepared steaming hot food, breads and cereals, hot pasta (including rice and noodles), and well-cooked meat or fish generally can be considered safe for consumption. Bringing crackers and peanut butter is a good suggestion for parents of hungry children when the availability of safe foods is uncertain. The incidence of traveler's diarrhea in children also can be reduced potentially by advising parents to encourage or supervise frequent hand washing, including the use of alcohol-based hand sanitizer, and to try to prevent children from placing objects in their mouths.

Some species of fish and shellfish can contain poisonous biotoxins, such as ciguatoxin and scombrotoxin, even when they are well cooked. Ciguatera poisoning is a potential risk in all subtropical and tropical regions of the West Indies and the Pacific and Indian oceans where the implicated fish are consumed; such fish include barracuda, red snapper, grouper, amberjack, and sea bass. Symptoms of ciguatera poisoning include gastroenteritis and neurologic manifestations such as dysesthesias and weakness. Scombroid poisoning occurs in tropical and temperate regions and is caused by high levels of histidine in the flesh of fish such as bluefin, yellowfin tuna, mackerel, bonito, mahi-mahi, herring, amberjack, and bluefish; if improperly refrigerated, histidine is converted to histamine, which can cause flushing, headache, nausea, vomiting, diarrhea, and urticaria.[43]

Managing Traveler's Diarrhea in Children

Adults traveling with children should be counseled about the signs and symptoms of dehydration and the proper use of WHO oral rehydration solution (ORS). Immediate medical attention is required for an infant or young child with diarrhea who has signs of moderate to severe dehydration, bloody diarrhea, temperature higher than 38.5°C (>101.5°F), or persistent vomiting. ORS should be provided to the infant by bottle or spoon while medical attention is being obtained.

The greatest risk to the infant with diarrhea and vomiting is dehydration. Fever or increased ambient temperature increases fluid losses and speeds dehydration. Parents should be advised that dehydration is best prevented and treated by use of ORS, in addition to the infant's usual food. Rice-based and other cereal-based ORSs, in which complex carbohydrates are substituted for glucose, also are available and may be more acceptable to young children. Adults traveling with children should be counseled that sports drinks, which are designed to replace water and electrolytes lost through sweat, do not contain the same proportions of electrolytes as those of the solution recommended by WHO for rehydration during diarrheal illness.

ORS packets are available at stores or pharmacies in almost all developing countries as well as most pharmacies in the United States. ORS is prepared by adding one packet to boiled or treated water. Travelers should be advised to check packet instructions carefully to ensure that the salts are added to the correct volume of water. ORS should be consumed or discarded within 12 hours if it is held at room temperature or 24 hours if it is kept refrigerated. A dehydrated child will drink ORS avidly; travelers should be advised to give it to the child as long as the dehydration persists. An infant or child who vomits the ORS usually will keep it down if it is offered by spoon, oral syringe, or straw in frequent small sips.[41,112,153]

Children weighing less than 10 kg who have mild to moderate dehydration should be administered 60 to 120 mL (2–4 oz) of ORS for each diarrheal stool or vomiting episode. Children who weigh 10 kg should receive 120 to 240 mL (4–8 oz) of ORS for each diarrheal stool or vomiting episode. Severe dehydration is a medical emergency that usually requires administration of fluids by intravenous or intraosseous routes.[43,72,111,151]

Travelers should be advised to give ORS to the child as long as the dehydration persists. As dehydration lessens, the salty-tasting ORS solution may be refused, and another liquid can be offered. Severely dehydrated children, however, often will be unable to drink adequately. Severe dehydration is a medical emergency that usually requires administration of fluids by intravenous or intraosseous routes.

Breast-fed infants should continue nursing on demand. Formula-fed infants should continue their usual formula during rehydration. They should receive a volume sufficient to satisfy energy and nutrient requirements. Lactose-free or lactose-reduced formulas usually are unnecessary. Dilution of formula may slow resolution of diarrhea and is not recommended. Older infants and children receiving semisolid or solid foods should continue to receive their usual diet during the illness. Recommended foods include starches, cereals, yogurt, fruits, and vegetables. Foods that are high in simple sugars, such as soft drinks, undiluted apple juice, gelatins, and presweetened cereals, can exacerbate diarrhea by osmotic effects and should be avoided. In addition, foods high in fat may not be tolerated because of their tendency to delay gastric emptying. The practice of withholding food for 24 hours or longer is inappropriate. Early feeding can decrease changes in intestinal permeability caused by infection, reduce illness duration, and improve nutritional outcome. Highly specific diets (e.g., the BRAT [bananas, rice, applesauce, and toast] diet) frequently have been recommended; however, similar to juice-centered and clear-fluid diets, such severely restrictive diets used for prolonged periods can result in malnutrition and should be avoided.[111]

Parents should be particularly careful to wash hands well after changing diapers of infants with diarrhea to avoid spreading infection to themselves and other family members.

Oral syringes available in most pharmacies for oral medications can be useful for the administration of ORS and can be included as part of the traveler's health kit for young children. Straws also can be useful for older children.

Bismuth subsalicylate (BSS), which is the active ingredient in Pepto-Bismol, can be used to prevent travelers' diarrhea in children 12 years of age and older. BSS can cause blackening of the tongue and stool and may cause nausea, constipation, and, rarely, tinnitus. BSS should be avoided by travelers with aspirin allergy, renal insufficiency, and gout and by those taking anticoagulants, probenecid, or methotrexate. In travelers taking aspirin or salicylates for other reasons, the use of BSS may result in salicylate toxicity. Because of the association between salicylates and Reye syndrome, BSS is not generally recommended to treat diarrhea in children younger than 12 years; however, some clinicians use it off-label, with caution in certain circumstances. Caution should be taken in administering BSS to children with viral infections, such as varicella or influenza, because of the risk for Reye syndrome. BSS is not recommended for children younger than 3 years. Studies have not established the safety of BSS use for periods longer than 3 weeks.[40] Insufficient data are available at this time to recommend the use of probiotics for the prevention of travelers' diarrhea in children.[43,75]

The use of antimotility agents (e.g., loperamide [Imodium] or dyphenoxylate and atropine [Lomotil]) in children younger than 2 years is not recommended and should be avoided because it can lead to serious adverse events, including toxic megacolon and central nervous system depression.[108] Because overdose of these types of drugs can be fatal, they should be used with extreme caution in children. Side effects of these drugs in adults include opiate-induced ileus, drowsiness, and nausea. Lomotil has been associated with fatal overdoses and other severe complications, including coma and respiratory depression. Antinausea medications, such as promethazine and prochlorperazine, are not recommended routinely. They are contraindicated for use in children younger than 2 years. Fatal respiratory depression in children has been reported with use of promethazine. Children with an acute illness, including gastroenteritis and dehydration, are more susceptible than are adults to neuromuscular reactions, especially dystonias, associated with prochlorperazine. The extrapyramidal side effects associated with these medications can be confused with symptoms of other undiagnosed primary diseases associated with vomiting, such as Reye syndrome. These medications should not be prescribed routinely for empirical treatment of children with possible traveler's diarrhea. Adults traveling with children should be fully counseled about the indications, dosage, frequency, and possible side effects if these medications are prescribed.[43,111]

Antibiotics

Prophylactic antibiotics are not recommended for most travelers. Many clinicians will prescribe antibiotics to be administered as empirical self-treatment. Trimethoprim-sulfamethoxazole was used previously for empirical treatment of traveler's diarrhea in children; however, widespread drug resistance has reduced its effectiveness, and it is no longer routinely recommended. Fluoroquinolones are used frequently for the empirical treatment of traveler's diarrhea in adults. In children, the American Academy of Pediatrics suggests some special circumstances for fluoroquinolone use, including the treatment of gastrointestinal infection caused by multidrug-resistant *Shigella* spp., *Salmonella* spp., *V. cholerae*, or *Campylobacter jejuni*.[67] For young adults 19 years and older, the fluoroquinolones are generally prescribed as 1- to 3-day regimens. Clinicians should be aware that fluoroquinolone resistance in gastrointestinal organisms has been reported from some countries, particularly in Southeast Asia.

Azithromycin has been found to be as effective as fluoroquinolones in treating traveler's diarrhea in adults.[1] In adults, some clinicians prescribe azithromycin as a single dose, which has been found to be highly effective. In children, most clinicians prescribe 10 mg/kg (maximum, 500 mg) for 3 days for empirical treatment of suspected *Shigella, Campylobacter,* and certain *E. coli* infections. Flavored oral suspension of azithromycin is available. The suspension does not require refrigeration; however, it should be used within 10 days of mixing. The non-reconstituted form of azithromycin has a longer expiration period. In certain circumstances, the non-reconstituted form can be provided with clear instructions for preparation and may be useful for children traveling for more than 10 days.

PREVENTION OF OTHER INFECTIOUS DISEASES IN PEDIATRIC TRAVELERS

Because the epidemiology of many diseases is evolving, prevention hinges on the clinician being knowledgeable about information on current outbreaks and risk in planned travel destinations, evaluating risk based on planned activities and the season of travel, and providing appropriate counseling and vaccination, if available. Information about specific infectious disease risks can be obtained from numerous sources listed in the section on international travel information resources. More detailed information about specific vaccinations is included in the section on vaccination for international travel.

Middle East coronavirus syndrome (MERS) was first reported in September 2012 and should be considered in individuals who have a syndrome of pneumonia and travel to the Arabian Peninsula or neighboring countries within the past 14 days. Common symptoms include fever (temperature >38°C [100.4°F]), cough, and shortness of breath, often leading to severe pneumonia and/or acute respiratory distress syndrome. Patients can also have acute kidney injury, gastrointestinal symptoms (anorexia, nausea, vomiting, abdominal pain), pericarditis, and disseminated intravascular coagulation.[48] There is one published description of MERS-CoV infection of children infected with MERS. In this series, the median age of patients was 13 years (range, 2–16 years). Nine children did not have symptoms, one patient died, and one patient who had symptoms recovered. Both patients with symptoms had underlying conditions.[130]

Avian influenza A (H5N1) has become a panzoonotic infection affecting regions of Asia, Africa, and the Middle East. Between 2003 and July 6, 2012, the WHO reported 607 human cases and 358 deaths caused by avian influenza from 15 countries, primarily from Indonesia, Vietnam, Egypt, China, Cambodia, and Thailand. Most of these cases were associated with direct contact with infected poultry.[59,124] Risk to travelers is low. However, clinicians should obtain up-to-date information about affected countries and counsel travelers going to those areas. Persons visiting areas with reports of outbreaks of H5N1 among poultry or of human H5N1 cases can reduce their risk for infection by (1) avoiding direct contact with poultry, including touching well-appearing, sick, or dead chickens; (2) avoiding poultry farms and bird markets; (3) avoiding handling surfaces contaminated with poultry feces or secretions; (4) practicing frequent and careful hand washing; and (5) consuming all foods from poultry, including eggs and poultry blood, only if they have been thoroughly cooked. Because influenza viruses are destroyed by heat, the cooking temperature for poultry meat should be 74°C (165°F).[59]

African trypanosomiasis (sleeping sickness), a parasitic infection transmitted by the bite of a tsetse fly, occasionally has been reported in travelers, including children. Infection can result in severe neurologic sequelae and is 100% fatal if untreated.[56] Infection is caused by two species of *Trypanosoma brucei: T. brucei rhodesiense,* which is found in eastern and southeastern Africa (primarily Tanzania, Uganda, Malawi, and Zambia), and *T. brucei gambiense,* which is found predominantly in central Africa and limited areas of West Africa. Most infections in US residents are caused by *T. brucei rhodesiense* and occur among travelers to East Africa game parks. In 2001, significant increases in cases were reported among US and European travelers to game parks in Tanzania and Kenya. Between 1967 and 2000, an imported case occurred on average every 1 to 2 years; however, in 2001, seven cases were reported in US travelers.[17,31,76,78,131-134] Travelers should use insect repellent and long-sleeved clothing in neutral colors of medium-weight material because tsetse flies are attracted to bright or dark clothes and can bite through lightweight clothing.[43]

Schistosomiasis, another parasitic infection caused by flukes that live part of their life cycle in fresh-water snail hosts, affects more than 200 million people worldwide. Schistosomiasis has been reported in travelers to endemic areas of Africa, Asia, South America, and the Caribbean who participated in high-risk activities such as swimming and wading in fresh water.[43,47,62,68] Most travel-associated infections occur among travelers to sub-Saharan Africa. Because most acute infections are asymptomatic, preventive counseling is critical. While in schistosomiasis-endemic areas, children should not swim in fresh, unchlorinated water such as lakes or ponds.[43]

More than 9 million new tuberculosis (TB) cases and 2 million TB-related deaths occur annually worldwide. A rate of tuberculin skin test seroconversion of 1.8% was reported among travelers to areas endemic for TB.[65] Of 357 travelers to the Hajj for pilgrimage, 10% had evidence of seroconversion when tested with use of QuantiFERON, a whole-blood assay for TB antigens.[172] Multidrug-resistant TB has been increasing in incidence worldwide. Cases of extensively drug-resistant TB have been reported from several countries, including Estonia, Latvia, Lesotho, Peru, the Philippines, South Africa, Swaziland, and the United States.[177,178] Travelers who may have prolonged exposure to TB should have two-step tuberculin skin test (TST) or a single interferon-γ release assay (IGRA), either the QuantiFERON TB test (Gold or Gold In-Tube versions) or T-SPOT TB test, before leaving the United States. If the predeparture test is negative, a single TST or IGRA should be repeated 8 to 10 weeks after returning from travel. IGRA is preferred for children who have received bacille Calmette-Guérin (BCG) vaccine.[43] According to reports, US children who had traveled to countries with a high prevalence of TB within the previous 12 months were 3.9 times more likely to have positive tuberculin skin test results than were children who lived in the same US areas but had not traveled.[119] BCG vaccine is a live vaccine prepared from attenuated strains of *Mycobacterium bovis;* BCG is used primarily in young infants to prevent disseminated and other forms of life-threatening disease caused by TB, such as tuberculous meningitis. BCG is recommended by the WHO for administration at birth. Vaccination of a young pediatric traveler (non–HIV infected and with a negative tuberculin skin test response) might be considered if long-term stay (e.g., children of missionaries or expatriates) is planned in a country with a high prevalence of TB, particularly multidrug-resistant or extensively drug-resistant TB, and prolonged contact with persons with active TB is thought to be a potential problem.[4,5,7] BCG vaccine can be obtained from the Canadian subdivisions of Sanofi Pasteur (http://www.sanofipasteur.ca).

Tick-borne encephalitis is transmitted primarily by the bite of *Ixodes* ticks. It also can be transmitted by the ingestion of unpasteurized dairy products from infected livestock. Transmission occurs during the summer months in western and central Europe, Scandinavia, and parts of the former Soviet Union. Russia has the highest incidence. Most cases occur from April through November, when ticks are most active.[43] Travelers to affected areas should use measures to avoid tick bites and avoid consuming unpasteurized dairy products. Persons who will be traveling for longer than 3 weeks in endemic rural areas or travelers who will be engaging in high-risk activities, such as camping, should be considered for vaccination. The vaccine is not available in the United States but can be obtained in Europe and Canada.[43]

Adventure travel can increase the risk for acquiring a variety of infectious diseases. Examples of recent outbreaks or cases of unusual pathogens affecting adventure travelers include fungal organisms (e.g., histoplasmosis and coccidioidomycosis), leptospirosis, and leishmaniasis. Histoplasmosis is a fungal infection acquired by the inhalation of spores, usually through exposure to bat, bird, or chicken droppings in barnyards and caves. The organism is endemic in the United States, Latin America, eastern Asia, parts of Europe, Africa, and Australia. Coccidioidomycosis, a fungal infection associated with the inhalation of organisms in soil from high-risk areas, is endemic in the southwestern part of the United States and Latin America. Both infections can cause a spectrum of illness from asymptomatic infection to acute pulmonary infection to severe, disseminated disease, especially in immunocompromised persons. Several outbreaks of histoplasmosis have been reported in groups of US visitors who entered a cave with bats in Costa Rica,[22] Ecuador,[164,176] Peru,[21] and Nicaragua.[170] More than 200 college students became infected with histoplasmosis during a spring break trip to Acapulco, Mexico.[31,141,180] Two outbreaks of coccidioidomycosis have been reported in youth missionary groups involved in construction work in Mexico.[20,24] Most of these fungal outbreaks have two common features: high-risk group activities and high attack rates, even in young, nonimmunocompromised individuals. Because no vaccine is available, prevention involves counseling travelers to avoid exposure or to use special masks for high-risk individuals who cannot avoid exposure.[32]

Leptospirosis is a zoonotic infection transmitted by exposure to water or soil contaminated with organisms excreted by domestic and wild animals. Outbreaks have been reported in white-water rafters in Costa Rica[23] and in athletes from 26 countries who participated in the Eco-Challenge multisport expedition race in Borneo, Malaysia, in 2000.[26,30] Because no vaccine against leptospirosis exists, persons engaging in high-risk activities with exposure to recreational water activities or exposure to contaminated surface waters and soil should be counseled to avoid exposure to water that may be contaminated or to wear protective clothing, especially footwear, and to cover cuts and abrasions with occlusive dressings. They should avoid contact with, submersion in, or swallowing potentially contaminated water. The CDC recommends that persons engaging in high-risk activities consider the use of doxycycline (4 mg/kg per dose, to a maximum of 200 mg/kg per dose every week), begun 1 to 2 days before exposure and continuing through the period of exposure for prophylaxis; doxycycline should not be used routinely for children younger than 8 years.[43] Travelers at increased risk for leptospirosis and in need of malaria chemoprophylaxis should consider using doxycycline for both indications.

Leishmaniasis, a parasitic infection transmitted by the bite of a sandfly, can lead to cutaneous or visceral infection. It has been reported in students who traveled to the rainforest in Costa Rica and other travelers.[94,96,129,174] The appropriate use of insect repellent and other personal protection measures against sandfly bites is the only prevention tool available.

Finally, studies of sexual practices among travelers have shown that 5% to 50% of short-term travelers engage in casual sex while abroad; 40% to 60% of long-term travelers have reported engaging in casual sex while abroad.[127,144,145] A study of British travelers reported that 18.6% had had new sexual partners, two-thirds of those who were sexually active did not use condoms on every occasion, and 5.7% contracted STIs.[155] Adolescents should be counseled about the risks for and prevention of STIs, hepatitis B, and HIV infection associated with sexual contact, sharing needles, or receiving acupuncture or tattoos. Patients should be asked about high-risk behaviors including sex without condoms, injection drug use, and sex while using drugs. Preexposure prophylaxis (PrEP) for HIV should be offered if deemed necessary. Before giving PrEP, patient should have HIV testing, a serum creatinine level and if female, a pregnancy test. At this point, the most widely studied medication used for PrEP two oral antiretroviral medications (tenofovir and emtricitabine) coformulated as a single pill (Truvada) taken once daily. Based on pharmacokinetic data, patients should initiate the drug 1 week before high-risk activity for a male patient and 3 weeks before high-risk activity for a female patient and continue PrEP for 1 month afterward.[152] Testing for STIs should be offered on return from the trip.

GENERAL TRAVEL HEALTH COUNSELING FOR CHILDREN

During the pretravel assessment, the clinician should provide the parents with general advice and preventive counseling to avoid health risks and injuries in children. Simple personal protection measures can prevent children from incurring many types of travel-associated injuries and conditions. One of the most common skin conditions reported by travelers is sunburn. To prevent sunburn and the subsequent risk for skin malignant neoplasms later in life, children should avoid sun exposure during peak hours and use sunscreen appropriate for the child's age. When sunscreen and insect repellent are used concomitantly, the sunscreen should be applied first. There is no evidence that air travel exacerbates the symptoms or complications associated with otitis media.[71] Travel to different time zones, "jet lag," and schedule disruptions can disturb sleep patterns in infants and children, as well as adults.[43]

Motor vehicle collisions, injuries, and drownings pose a great risk for morbidity and mortality among international travelers.[43,144] Vehicle-related incidents are the leading cause of death in children who travel. While traveling in automobiles and other vehicles, children shorter than 4 feet, 9 inches in height should be restrained in age-appropriate car seats or booster seats, as described earlier. In general, children are safest traveling in the rear seat; no one should ever travel in the bed of a pickup truck. Families should be counseled that in many developing countries, cars may lack front or rear seat belts. Parents traveling with infants or young children should be advised to bring their own child safety restraint seats for use during travel. Night driving can be more hazardous, especially outside urban areas in developing countries, and should be avoided.[43] Use of a helmet is imperative for bicycle travel. Fire injuries can be prevented by advising parents to inquire whether hotels have smoke detectors and sprinkler systems (they also may consider bringing their own smoke detector). Conditions at hotels and other lodging may not be as safe as those in the United States, and accommodations should be carefully inspected for exposed wiring, pest poisons, paint chips, or inadequate stairway or balcony railings.[43] Drowning is the second leading cause of death in young travelers. Children may not be familiar with hazards in the ocean or in rivers. Swimming pools may not have protective fencing to keep toddlers from falling into the pool. Close supervision of children around water is essential. Appropriate water-safety devices such as life vests may not be available abroad, and families should consider bringing these from home. Parents and children participating in boating activities should be counseled to be aware of weather conditions and forecasts, and parents should be advised that an adult should accompany children at all times when swimming. Personal floatation devices should be used when boating or water-skiing, regardless of the distance to be traveled or swimming ability.[150] Swimming in contaminated water can result in skin, eye, ear, and some intestinal infections; for prevention of infectious diseases, generally only pools that contain chlorinated water can be considered safe. Parents also should be advised that swimming in fresh-water lakes and streams in developing countries carries a risk for contracting schistosomiasis, leptospirosis, and primary amebic meningoencephalitis.[43] In saltwater bodies, biting and stinging fish, corals, and jellyfish also can be a risk. In general, children should wear covered footwear rather than sandals, including when wading on reefs and swimming.[43,150] Children should avoid walking barefoot, particularly in rural areas, to prevent cutaneous larva migrans, hookworm, and *Strongyloides* infections. Children are more likely than adults to have contact with soil or sand and therefore may be exposed to diseases caused by infectious stages of parasites present in soil, including ascariasis, hookworm infestation, cutaneous or visceral larva migrans, trichuriasis, and strongyloidiasis. Children and infants should wear protective footwear and play on a sheet or towel rather than directly on the ground. Clothing should not be dried on the ground. When traveling in countries with a tropical climate, clothing or diapers dried in the open air should be ironed before use to prevent infestation with fly larvae. Parents of pediatric travelers, especially to areas endemic for rabies, should be reminded to warn children that they should not attempt to pet, handle, or feed domestic or wild animals (including monkeys). Travelers also should avoid snakes because most bites are the direct result of handling, harassing, or trying to kill snakes.[43]

Travelers to high-altitude destinations should be counseled about the risk and prevention of altitude illness, including acute mountain sickness, high-altitude cerebral edema, and high-altitude pulmonary edema. Altitude sickness generally occurs at 2500 to 2700 m (8000–9000 ft), and acclimatization generally takes 3 to 5 days. Susceptibility and resistance are genetic traits, and no screening tests are available to predict risk. Children and adults are equally susceptible. Travelers to high-altitude destinations should be advised to ascend gradually, if possible, and those travelers going to destinations higher than 8000 to 9000 ft should be advised to acclimate at 8000 to 9000 ft for a few days before moving to higher altitudes. For higher altitudes, travelers should move sleeping altitude no higher than 500 m (1600 ft) per day and to plan on spending an extra day for acclimatization for every 1000 m (3300 ft), if possible. For abrupt ascent, pediatric travelers may require acetazolamide, prescribed as 2.5 mg/kg per dose every 12 hours, up to the standard adult dose of 125 mg twice per day. Travelers should begin acetazolamide 1 day before ascent and continue for the first 2 days at altitude. Dexamethasone is generally reserved for treatment of altitude illness.[43]

PEDIATRIC TRAVELER'S HEALTH KIT

Children traveling to developing countries may have unique exposures, particularly if they are traveling to remote locations or will have close contact with other children. Depending on the travel itinerary, children may need prescriptions for malaria chemoprophylaxis, antibiotic for self-treatment of travelers' diarrhea, and medication to prevent high-altitude sickness. Consideration should be given to inclusion of the following medications as part of the traveler's health kit: rectal preparations (suppositories) of selected medications, such as acetaminophen; topical treatments for lice and scabies for pediatric travelers to developing countries who may have extensive contact with local children; and a topical antibiotic, such as mupirocin, for bacterial skin infections.[43,117] Children with a history of anaphylaxis or serious allergic reactions should have a sufficient number of epinephrine pens and antihistamines in tablet or liquid form. Any medications purchased abroad should be obtained from a reliable pharmacy because of concern about counterfeit drugs, especially in developing countries. Adults accompanying these children and teenagers should consider obtaining basic first aid and safety training before departure. Although air travel is safe for healthy newborns, infants, and children, a few issues should be considered in preparation for travel. Children with chronic heart or lung problems may be at risk for hypoxia during flight, and a physician should be consulted before travel. Insurance coverage for illnesses and accidents while abroad should be verified before departure.[71] Consideration should be given to purchasing special travel insurance for airlifting or air ambulance to an area with adequate medical care.[43]

INTERNATIONAL TRAVEL INFORMATION RESOURCES

One of the most important functions a clinician can fulfill in preparing a pediatric patient and parents for international travel is to provide up-to-date and accurate travel health information and recommendations for preventing illness. Many varied sources of information are available, including software packages and databases designed specifically for use in travel medicine and pretravel care.[84,110] Increasingly, the Internet and computer-based travel resources are being used by practitioners and consumers alike because they provide current information to appropriately and effectively counsel and treat international travelers. Two reviews have provided comprehensive summaries of travel medicine resources.[84,110] Table 232.4 is a summary of selected travel health resources that can be useful for providing health care professionals and parents with essential information on health risks in specific travel destinations (including endemic or epidemic diseases) and current travel health recommendations (including immunizations and chemoprophylaxis). Travelers also should be aware of the need for health insurance and emergency evacuation coverage during travel and medical assistance in the event of a travel-related illness; a variety of companies offer these services, and travelers should investigate options before making any purchases. This summary is not meant to be comprehensive; because resources are constantly changing, clinicians are advised to review and to compare sites for availability and updated information and recommendations.

TABLE 232.4 **International Travelers' Health Information, Recommendations, and Outbreak Notices**

Resource	Contact Information	Information and Services Provided
Centers for Disease Control and Prevention (CDC) Travelers' Health Information Destination-Specific Information	http://wwwnc.cdc.gov/travel/	US travelers' health recommendations by destination region and country, including malaria chemoprophylaxis and vaccinations; links to other sites, travel health warnings, advisories, and outbreak notices
CDC Health Information for International Travel (Yellow Book)	http://wwwnc.cdc.gov/travel/page/yellowbook-home-2012	General travelers' health information, region- and destination-specific recommendations, including malaria chemoprophylaxis and vaccinations
CDC Malaria Branch	http://wwwnc.cdc.gov/travel/diseases/malaria 770-488-7788 or 1-855-856-4713 (9:00 AM to 5:00 PM EST, Monday through Friday) 770-488-7100 (after hours, on weekends and holidays)	Information about malaria prophylaxis and treatment, intended for use by health care professionals
CDC *Morbidity and Mortality Weekly Report, Recommendations and Reports, Surveillance Summaries*	http://www.cdc.gov/mmwr	Reports on US and international outbreak investigations, disease surveillance summaries, reports, and recommendations
CDC National Immunization Program	http://www.cdc.gov/vaccines/	Immunization information
US Immunization Schedules	http://www.cdc.gov/vaccines/schedules/index.html	Immunization schedules for children, adolescents, and adults
Immunization Action Coalition	http://www.immunize.org	Immunization information and educational material for practitioners and parents
National Network for Immunization Information (NNii)	https://www.immunizationinfo.net/	Information for public and health professionals about immunization Site includes immunization news, a vaccine information database, and a guide to evaluating vaccination information on the web
US State Department	http://www.travel.state.gov	General information about travel, including safety, visa requirements, links to individual embassies and consulates
World Health Organization (WHO) Health Topics	http://www.who.int/topics/en/	Information and maps of health topics and diseases
WHO Yellow Book, International Travel and Health	http://www.who.int/ith/en/	General travelers' health recommendations; country-specific malarial risks and recommendations
WHO, Outbreak News	http://www.who.int/csr/don/en/	Notifications of recent infectious disease outbreaks
WHO, Weekly Epidemiological Record	http://www.who.int/wer/en/	Global disease surveillance and WHO program updates
Health Canada, Travel Health	http://www.phac-aspc.gc.ca/tmp-pmv/index-eng.php	Canadian recommendations for travelers' health; outbreak information
EuroSurveillance	http://www.eurosurveillance.org	Surveillance and outbreak information for European nations; weekly and monthly surveillance reports and outbreak notices
ProMED (Program for Monitoring Emerging Diseases)	http://www.promedmail.org	Email postings; verified and unverified reports on emerging diseases and outbreaks
University of Texas at Austin	http://www.lib.utexas.edu/maps	World maps online
American Society of Tropical Medicine and Hygiene (ASTMH)	http://www.astmh.org 847-480-9592	Directory of travel medicine clinics and practitioners certified by ASTMH
International Society of Travel Medicine (ISTM)	http://www.istm.org	Directory of travel medicine clinics and practitioners with ISTM affiliation
NSF International	http://www.nsf.org/consumer	Information about water filters

NEW REFERENCES SINCE THE SEVENTH EDITION

2. Advisory Committee on Immunization Practices, Fiore AE, Wasley A, et al. Prevention of hepatitis A through active or passive immunization: recommendations of the Advisory Committee on Immunization Practices (ACIP). *MMWR Recomm Rep*. 2006;55(RR-7):1-23.
3. Advisory Committee on Immunization Practices, Smith NM, Bresee JS, et al. Prevention and Control of Influenza: recommendations of the Advisory Committee on Immunization Practices (ACIP). *MMWR Recomm Rep*. 2006;55(RR-10):1-42.
8. American Academy of Pediatrics. *Red Book: Report of the Committee on Infectious Diseases*. 29th ed. Elk Grove Village, Illinois: American Academy of Pediatrics; 2012.
12. Anwar E, Goldberg E, Fraser A, et al. Vaccines for preventing typhoid fever. *Cochrane Database Syst Rev*. 2014;(1):CD001261.
13. Armstrong P, Hennessey M, Adams M, et al. Travel-associated Zika virus disease cases among U.S. Residents—United States, January 2015–February 2016. *MMWR Morb Mortal Wkly Rep*. 2016;65(11):286-289.
14. Atkinson B, Hearn P, Afrough B, et al. Detection of Zika virus in semen. *Emerg Infect Dis*. 2016;22(5):940.
19. Brasil P, Pereira JP Jr, Raja Gabaglia C, et al. Zika virus infection in pregnant women in Rio de Janeiro: preliminary report. *N Engl J Med*. 2016;375(24):2321-2334.
23. Centers for Disease Control and Prevention. Chikungunya Virus. 2016; www.cdc.gov/chikungunya/geo/index.html.
34. Centers for Disease Control and Prevention. Measles–United States, 2011. *MMWR Morb Mortal Wkly Rep*. 2012;61:253-257.
35. Centers for Disease Control and Prevention. Measles (Rubeola) Outbreaks. 2016; www.cdc.gov/measles/cases-outbreaks.html.
38. Centers for Disease Control and Prevention. National Typhoid and Paratyphoid Surveillance. http://www.cdc.gov/nationalsurveillance/typhoid-surveillance.html.
39. Centers for Disease Control and Prevention. Notice to readers: FDA approval of an alternate dosing schedule for a combined hepatitis A and B vaccine (Twinrix®). *MMWR Morb Mortal Wkly Rep*. 2007;56(40):1057.
40. Centers for Disease Control and Prevention. Outbreak of acute febrile illness among participants in EcoChallenge Sabah 2000—Malaysia, 2000. *JAMA*. 2000;284(13):1646.
45. Centers for Disease Control and Prevention. Recommended immunization schedules for persons aged 0 through 18 Years—United States, 2012. *MMWR Morb Mortal Wkly Rep*. 2012;61(5):1-4.

52. Centers for Disease Control and Prevention. Update: novel influenza A (H1N1) virus infections—worldwide, May 6, 2009. *MMWR Morb Mortal Wkly Rep.* 2009;58(17):453-458.
55. Centers for Disease Control and Prevention. Update: severe respiratory illness associated with Middle East Respiratory Syndrome Coronavirus (MERS-CoV)—worldwide, 2012–2013. *MMWR Morb Mortal Wkly Rep.* 2013;62(23):480-483.
58. Centers for Disease Control and Prevention. Use of Japanese encephalitis vaccine in children: recommendations of the advisory committee on immunization practices, 2013. *MMWR Morb Mortal Wkly Rep.* 2013;62(45):898-900.
60. Environmental Protection Agency. *Repellents: Protection against mosquitos, ticks and other arthropods.* https://www.epa.gov/insect-repellents.
64. Chin CS, Sorenson J, Harris JB, et al. The origin of the Haitian cholera outbreak strain. *N Engl J Med.* 2011;364(1):33-42.
66. Cohn AC, MacNeil JR, Clark TA, et al. Prevention and control of meningococcal disease: recommendations of the Advisory Committee on Immunization Practices (ACIP). *MMWR Recomm Rep.* 2013;62(RR-2):1-28.
69. Cornall P, Howie S, Mughal A, et al. Drowning of British children abroad. *Child Care Health Dev.* 2005;31(5):611-613.
77. Faucher JF, Binder R, Missinou MA, et al. Efficacy of atovaquone/proguanil for malaria prophylaxis in children and its effect on the immunogenicity of live oral typhoid and cholera vaccines. *Clin Infect Dis.* 2002;35(10):1147-1154.
79. FDA News Release. FDA approves a second vaccine to prevent serogroup B meningococcal disease. 2015; www.fda.gov/NewsEvents/Newsroom/PressAnnouncements/ucm431370.htm.
80. FDA News Release. First vaccine approved by FDA to prevent serogroup B Meningococcal disease. 2014; http://www.idsociety.org/FDA_20141029.
81. Fischer M, Lindsey N, Staples JE, et al. Japanese encephalitis vaccines: recommendations of the Advisory Committee on Immunization Practices (ACIP). *MMWR Recomm Rep.* 2010;59(RR-1):1-27.
82. Fox TG, Manaloor JJ, Christenson JC. Travel-related infections in children. *Pediatr Clin North Am.* 2013;60(2):507-527.
86. Global Task Force on Cholera Control. *Oral Cholera Vaccine Use in Complex Emergencies: What's Next.* WHO Meeting: Cairo, Egypt; 2005.
88. Hagmann S, LaRocque RC, Rao SR, et al. Pre-travel health preparation of pediatric international travelers: analysis from the Global TravEpiNet Consortium. *J Pediatric Infect Dis Soc.* 2013;2(4):327-334.
90. Hagmann SH, Leshem E, Fischer PR, et al. Preparing children for international travel: need for training and pediatric-focused research. *J Travel Med.* 2014;21(6):377-383.
92. Han P, Balaban V, Marano C. Travel characteristics and risk-taking attitudes in youths traveling to nonindustrialized countries. *J Travel Med.* 2010;17(5):316-321.
102. Institute of International Education. Open Doors: International Students in the U.S. 2015 Fast Facts. www.iie.org/Research-and-Publications/Open-Doors/Data/Fast-Facts. Accessed 21 April 2016.
103. Jackson BR, Iqbal S, Mahon B, et al. Updated recommendations for the use of typhoid vaccine: Advisory Committee on Immunization Practices, United States, 2015. *MMWR Morb Mortal Wkly Rep.* 2015;64(11):305-308.
108. Kendall ME, Crim S, Fullerton K, et al. Travel-associated enteric infections diagnosed after return to the United States, Foodborne Diseases Active Surveillance Network (FoodNet), 2004-2009. *Clin Infect Dis.* 2012;54(suppl 5):S480-S487.
109. Kendrick K, Stanek D, Blackmore C, et al. Notes from the field: transmission of chikungunya virus in the continental United States—Florida, 2014. *MMWR Morb Mortal Wkly Rep.* 2014;63(48):1137.
110. Keystone JS, Kozarsky PE, Freedman DO. Internet and computer-based resources for travel medicine practitioners. *Clin Infect Dis.* 2001;32(5):757-765.
113. Kroger AT, Atkinson WL, Marcuse EK, et al. General recommendations on immunization: recommendations of the Advisory Committee on Immunization Practices (ACIP). *MMWR Recomm Rep.* 2006;55(RR-15):1-48.
122. MacNeil JR, Rubin L, McNamara L, et al. Use of MenACWY-CRM vaccine in children aged 2 through 23 months at increased risk for meningococcal disease: recommendations of the Advisory Committee on Immunization Practices, 2013. *MMWR Morb Mortal Wkly Rep.* 2014;63(24):527-530.
123. Mali S, Kachur SP, Arguin PM, et al. Malaria surveillance—United States, 2010. *Morb Mortal Wkly Rep Surveill Summ.* 2012;61(2):1-17.
125. Manning SE, Rupprecht CE, Fishbein D, et al. Human rabies prevention—United States, 2008: recommendations of the Advisory Committee on Immunization Practices. *MMWR Recomm Rep.* 2008;57(RR-3):1-28.
130. Memish ZA, Al-Tawfiq JA, Assiri A, et al. Middle East respiratory syndrome coronavirus disease in children. *Pediatr Infect Dis J.* 2014;33(9):904-906.
135. Nappe TM, Chuhran CM, Johnson SA. The Chikungunya virus: an emerging US pathogen. *World J Emerg Med.* 2016;7(1):65-67.
139. Pan American Health Organization. Epidemiological Update, Cholera. 2013; www.paho.org/hq/index.php?option=com_docman&task=doc_view&gid=23749&Itemid=.
140. Pan American Health Organization. Re-emergence of dengue in the Americas. *Epidemiol Bull.* 1997;18(2):1-6.
148. Robinson CL, Advisory Committee on Immunization Practices ACAIWG. Advisory Committee on Immunization Practices Recommended Immunization Schedules for Persons Aged 0 Through 18 Years—United States, 2016. *MMWR Morb Mortal Wkly Rep.* 2016;65(4):86-87.
149. Rupprecht CE, Briggs D, Brown CM, et al. Use of a reduced (4-dose) vaccine schedule for postexposure prophylaxis to prevent human rabies: recommendations of the advisory committee on immunization practices. *MMWR Recomm Rep.* 2010;59(RR-2):1-9.
152. Seifert SM, Glidden DV, Meditz AL, et al. Dose response for starting and stopping HIV preexposure prophylaxis for men who have sex with men. *Clin Infect Dis.* 2015;60(5):804-810.
154. Sharp TM, Roth NM, Torres J, et al. Chikungunya cases identified through passive surveillance and household investigations—Puerto Rico, May 5–August 12, 2014. *MMWR Morb Mortal Wkly Rep.* 2014;63(48):1121-1128.
156. Stuart BM, Pullen RL. Typhoid; clinical analysis of 360 cases. *Arch Intern Med.* 1946;78(6):629-661.
157. Sur D, Ochiai RL, Bhattacharya SK, et al. A cluster-randomized effectiveness trial of Vi typhoid vaccine in India. *N Engl J Med.* 2009;361(4):335-344.
162. US Department of Commerce, ITA, Office of Travel and Tourism Industries. United States Citizen Traffic to Overseas Regions, Canada and Mexico 2015. 2010; tinet.ita.doc.gov/view/m-2015-O-001/index.html.
163. US Food and Drug Administration, US Department of Health and Human Services. FDA approves vaccine to prevent cholera for travelers. 2016; www.fda.gov/NewsEvents/Newsroom/PressAnnouncements/ucm506305.htm?source=govdelivery&utm_medium=email&utm_source=govdelivery%20.
176. World Health Organization. *Roll Back Malaria. Fact sheet No. 94.* Geneva: World Health Organization; 2006.
179. World Health Organization. Cholera. 2015; www.who.int/mediacentre/factsheets/fs107/en/.
180. World Health Organization. International Travel and Health: Vaccination requirements and health advice. http://www.who.int/ith/en/.
182. Zipprich J, Winter K, Hacker J, et al. Measles outbreak—California, December 2014–February 2015. *MMWR Morb Mortal Wkly Rep.* 2015;64(6):153-154.
183. World Health Organization. Poliomyelitis. 2016; www.who.int/mediacentre/factsheets/fs114/en/.
184. World Health Organization. Malaria. http://www.who.int/malaria/en/.

The full reference list for this chapter is available at ExpertConsult.com.

233 Infectious Disease Considerations in International Adoptees and Refugees

Mary Allen Staat

Each year thousands of children immigrate to the United States to begin a new life (Fig. 233.1). The focus of this chapter will be on two groups of immigrants—refugees and internationally adopted children. Refugees are noncitizen immigrants who are unable or unwilling to return to their country of origin because of persecution or fear of persecution. Internationally adopted children are immigrants who are classified as orphans; however, most of these children are not truly orphaned, but have been abandoned by or separated from both parents.[111] These children generally will be given United States citizenship as they arrive or shortly after they arrive in the United States to join their new families.

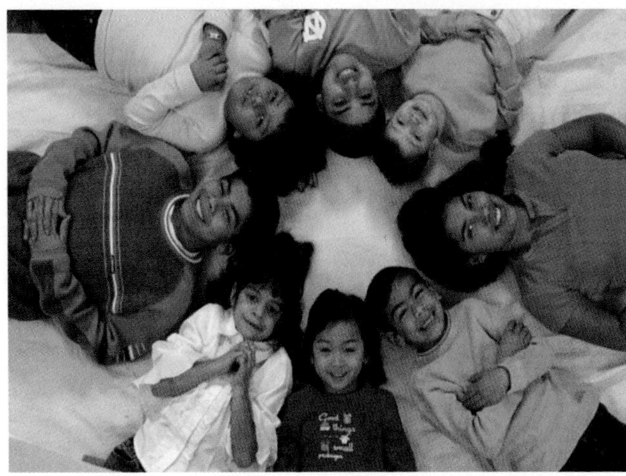

FIG. 233.1 A group of internationally adopted children.

In 2015, a total of 69,920 refugees arrived in the United States.[111] Of these, 80% came from just six countries: Burma (26%), Iraq (18%), Somalia (13%), Democratic Republic of the Congo (11%), Bhutan (8%), and Iran (4%). Although these are the most prevalent countries, refugees have come to the United States from countries all around the world, with the exception of northern Europe, Australia, New Zealand, and Canada. Of refugees immigrating to the United States in 2015, 43% were younger than 20 years and 48% were female. The ages of the children were fairly evenly distributed—younger than 5 years (26%), 5 to 9 years (27%), 10 to 14 years (24%), and 15 to 19 years (23%). Only 1% of refugee children were younger than 1 year.

In recent decades, international adoption has been a popular way to build families. Since 1999, more than 261,000 children have been internationally adopted to families in the United States.[120] The peak of international adoptions was in 2004, with 22,990 children immigrating to the United States; 83% of children came from just five countries: China (31%), Russia (26%), Guatemala (14%), South Korea (8%), and Kazakhstan (4%).[120] However, since 2004, a dramatic decline has occurred in the number of adoptions, and the countries where children are adopted from are far more diverse. In 2015, only 5648 children were adopted internationally, with 81% of children coming from 11 countries: China (42%), Ethiopia (6%), South Korea (6%), the Ukraine (5%), Uganda (4%), Bulgaria (3%), Latvia (3%), the Democratic Republic of the Congo (3%), Colombia (3%), Nigeria (3%) and the Philippines (3%).[120] Several countries that once allowed adoption, such as Romania, Vietnam, Cambodia, and Guatemala, are now closed to adoptions or have dramatically decreased the number of international adoptions from their countries. For example, in 2008, the largest numbers of adopted children were from Guatemala, with 4123 adoptions. In contrast, after the United States stopped processing Guatemalan adoptions, only 13 children were adopted from Guatemala in 2015.[120] In addition, there has been a change in the medical needs of internationally adopted children. In recent years, China has shifted to primarily referring children with special needs such as congenital heart disease, cleft lip and palate, limb deficiencies, anorectal malformations, spina bifida, and cerebral palsy, whereas in prior years, most children referred to families from China were healthy infants without known medical conditions.

Other demographic features have changed in international adoption as well. In 2015, 50% of internationally adopted children were female, 54% of children were younger than 5 years, and 1% were younger than 1 year at the time of adoption.[120] In contrast, in 2004, 65% of adopted children were girls, mainly because of the large number of girls available in China. Children were also much younger, with 86% of children younger than 5 years and 41% younger than 1 year.[120] With the arrival of older children, health care providers need to be aware that these children will have an increased risk for malnutrition, infectious disease exposures, unmet medical needs, and psychological traumas that often results in a more difficult transition to joining their families.

Children available for international adoption generally have resided all or most of their lives in orphanages before coming to the United States. The exception is South Korea and Guatemala, where nearly all children were placed in foster care until their adoption. In more recent years, some children from China have also been placed with foster families until adopted.

Because refugees and internationally adopted children come from resource-poor countries, physicians and other health care providers need to be aware of the global prevalence of infectious diseases that are seen less commonly in native-born North Americans. Both refugees and internationally adopted children are at increased risk for common infectious diseases such as tuberculosis (TB), intestinal parasites, dermatologic infections, and infestations. In addition, in countries where resources are few and infrastructure is limited for screening and prevention programs for hepatitis B, hepatitis C, human immunodeficiency virus (HIV), and syphilis, the prevalence is higher than in the United States.

Although many similarities exist in the infectious disease considerations for refugees and internationally adopted children, several important differences are seen.[6,10,12,35,37] Refugee and internationally adopted children differ in terms of the general medical screening they receive before their arrival to the United States.[10,137] Most refugees undergo organized screening evaluations before emigration visas are issued. Children have predeparture screening and a physical examination, and, depending on their country of departure, they may receive predeparture treatment for malaria, intestinal parasites, or tissue parasites. In contrast, only adoptees from certain countries with high rates of TB, such as China and Ethiopia, have been required to undergo this organized screening procedure for TB. Second, because medical screening for refugees is usually sponsored by responsible medical organizations, results of testing are typically accurate. In internationally adopted children, medical testing may be incomplete and is typically done shortly after birth or on entrance to the orphanage. However, families should expect to receive results for HIV, syphilis, and hepatitis B surface antigen testing with their referral information. For some countries, such as Ethiopia, HIV polymerase chain reaction (PCR) and hepatitis C test results also are provided. For Russian referrals, hepatitis C testing is often done as well. Although the reliability of testing done in the child's birth county has been a concern in the past, in recent years the testing has generally proved to be accurate when repeated in the United States. Third, preventive measures such as immunizations, vitamin supplementation, and dental care are provided for most refugee children while still in refugee camps; in adoptees, no standard approach is followed in the provision of these measures from country to country or even within a given country. Differences also exist in the types of infectious diseases and risks for acquiring these diseases in refugee children in contrast to internationally adopted children. Although both groups are susceptible to a variety of infectious agents, because the countries of origin and the living conditions differ, refugee children are more likely to have been exposed to infections such as typhoid fever, malaria, filariasis, flukes, and schistosomiasis, which are less commonly seen in internationally adopted children from countries outside of Africa.

Health care professionals will inevitably have the opportunity to provide care for these children as they immigrate to the United States and should therefore be knowledgeable of the infectious disease issues they may encounter and the need for screening for infectious diseases in these populations.

OVERALL EVALUATION

Because of the predominance of infectious diseases in resource-poor countries, recommendations for screening tests in refugees and internationally adopted children have been weighted toward infectious disease processes; thus this will be the focus of this chapter. It is important, however, that the initial assessment include all aspects of general health, including evaluation of growth and development and vision, hearing, and dental evaluations.[6,10,12,35,37] For internationally adopted children, several others tests are recommended, including testing for blood lead concentration, complete blood cell count with red blood cell indices, and differential of white blood cells to evaluate for eosinophilia,

TABLE 233.1 **Infectious Disease Screening for Refugee and Internationally Adopted Children**

Condition or Test	Refugee Children	Internationally Adopted Children
Hepatitis A Virus (Acute Infection)		
Hepatitis A IgM antibody	Not recommended	All
Hepatitis B Virus		
Hepatitis B surface antigen (HBsAg)	All	All[a]
Hepatitis B surface antibody (anti-HBs)	All	All[a]
Hepatitis B core antibody (anti-HBc)	All	All[a]
Hepatitis C Virus		
Hepatitis C antibody	Some	All[a]
Syphilis		
Nontreponemal test (RPR, VDRL, or ART)	≥15 years	All
Treponemal test (TPPA, MHA-TP, or FTA-ABS)	Not recommended	All
Human Immunodeficiency Virus		
Human immunodeficiency virus 1 and 2 antibody	≥13 years	All[a]
Recommended	<13 years	
Tuberculosis		
Tuberculin skin test (TST)	All	All[a]
or		
Interferon-γ release assay	≥5 years	≥5 years
Intestinal Parasites		
Microscopic evaluation of stool for ova and parasites	All (2 specimens)[b]	All (3 specimens)
Giardia intestinalis and *Cryptosporidium* antigen	All (1 specimen)[b]	All (1 specimen)
Bacterial Enteric Infection		
In children with diarrhea: bacterial stool culture	All	All
Chagas (Endemic Areas)		
Trypanosoma cruzi serologic testing	All	All
Complete Blood Count	All	All
Eosinophilia With Negative Stool Ova and Parasite for Helminths		
Strongyloides serologic testing	All	All
Schistosoma serologic testing (endemic countries)[c]		
Lymphatic Filariasis (Endemic Areas)		
Filaria serology	All	≥2 years
Chagas (Endemic Areas)		
Trypanosoma cruzi serologic testing	All	All
Malaria Screening (Endemic Areas)		
Malaria polymerase chain reaction	All without pretreatment	Not recommended
Hematuria (Schistosomiasis)		
Urinalysis	All	Not recommended

[a]Consider reassessing 6 months after arrival.
[b]All should be screened if there was no presumptive treatment before arrival to the United States; see guidelines for evaluation for intestinal parasites in refugees with presumptive treatment (http://cdc.gov/immigrantrefugeehealth/guidelines/domestic/intestinal-parasites-domestic.html).
[c]Some experts recommend serologic testing regardless of whether eosinophilia is present.
ART, Automated reagin test; *FTA-ABS*, fluorescent treponemal antibody absorption; *MHA-TP*, microhemagglutination–*Treponema pallidum*; *RPR*, rapid plasma reagin; *TPPA*, *Treponema pallidum* particle agglutination; *VDRL*, Venereal Disease Research Laboratory.

glucose-6-phosphate dehydrogenase screening, hemoglobin electrophoresis, measurement of thyroid-stimulating hormone concentration, and examination for congenital anomalies (including fetal alcohol syndrome). Similar to adoptees, a complete blood count and a lead level are recommended for refugees. Additional tests, such as a urinalysis to determine whether there is hematuria (for schistosomiasis) and screening for sexually transmitted infections, are recommended. Mental health screening is encouraged if services are available.

Although many immigrant children may appear healthy on arrival, children should be evaluated by a health care professional within 2 weeks after arrival to ensure that their initial health care needs are addressed, initial screening is done, and a plan for receiving preventive services such as immunizations is initiated. Table 233.1 outlines the infectious disease screening tests recommended for refugee and internationally adopted children, and details for each condition are outlined in the following discussion.

INFECTIOUS DISEASE SCREENING

Viral Hepatitis

Hepatitis A

Virtually all people residing in resource-poor countries have contracted hepatitis A by early adulthood and have hepatitis A immunoglobulin G (IgG) antibodies.[1,7,34] The prevalence of past hepatitis A infection varies by country and age. In a study examining the prevalence of acute and past hepatitis A infection in internationally adopted children, 1% of children had acute hepatitis A infection (positive hepatitis A IgM) on arrival to the United States and 29% had evidence of prior infection (positive total hepatitis A antibody).[1] In this study, the prevalence of prior infection increased with age; 13% of children younger than 2 years were immune, in contrast to 80% of children 12 to 17 years of age. The highest region-specific prevalence was in Africa (72%), and the lowest was in the Asia and Pacific Rim Region (17%).

Given the high prevalence of hepatitis A virus (HAV) in these countries, there is an ongoing risk for infection of children while in their country of origin. In internationally adopted children, children may be incubating HAV infection at the time of adoption and could transmit the virus to their adoptive families and others while in country or after arrival to the United States. Several cases have been reported of HAV transmitted from internationally adopted children to family members and close contacts.[1,48,123,138] Therefore adoptive parents and any accompanying family members should be immunized against hepatitis A or have documented immunity to HAV infection before international travel to receive their child.[1,7,17,31,47] It is also recommended that hepatitis A vaccine be administered before the arrival of the adoptee to all susceptible nontraveling people who plan to have close contact with an internationally adopted child from a country with high or intermediate hepatitis A endemicity.

In the United States, hepatitis A vaccine is recommended for all children 12 months of age and older.[7,31] Hepatitis A vaccine is not routinely administered to children or adults in resource-poor countries. Because the prevalence of past HAV infection is high in these countries, antibody testing can be done to determine HAV immunity. Hepatitis A antibody testing (total or IgG) should be considered in children older than 1 year for both refugees and internationally adopted children to determine the need for this vaccine.[9,10]

Infection with hepatitis A is often difficult to diagnose clinically in children; as many as 90% of children younger than 6 years and 50% to 60% of older children are anicteric.[7] Thus most young children will not have signs or symptoms of hepatitis A, yet those who are infected may shed the virus for months. To identify hepatitis A infection in children who do not have symptoms, hepatitis A IgM antibody testing should be done.[1,7,10] When acute infection is found in a child, secondary cases can be prevented by providing hepatitis A vaccine to unvaccinated family members and close contacts of the case.[7,31,47] Although most children do not have symptoms, viral hepatitis should be considered in children with symptoms such as vomiting and loss of appetite, when accompanied by fever and an enlarged, tender liver even in the absence of jaundice.

Hepatitis B

Routine screening for hepatitis B virus (HBV) infection is recommended for all refugees and internationally adopted children.[6,10,12,35,37] Most children who are hepatitis B carriers do not have symptoms. Therefore screening is important to identify these children so that appropriate management can be initiated and unvaccinated household contacts and caregivers can be vaccinated or be given hepatitis B immunoglobulin if they have had a significant exposure to blood of a hepatitis B carrier. The prevalence of hepatitis B infection is higher in resource-poor countries than in the United States. In Asia, Africa, and Central and South America, the prevalence of hepatitis B ranges from 2% to 7%, in contrast to only 0.5% in the United States.[34] Several studies have shown that rates of infection in refugee* and internationally adopted children† mirror the reported rates in their country of origin. Immigrant children have typically acquired HBV by vertical transmission, although bloodborne infection and horizontal transmission also have been implicated. In international adoptees, the highest reported rates were in Romanian adoptees from the early 1990s, with 53% having evidence of past or present infection and 20% with active infection.[60,71,73,100,104] Recent studies have consistently shown a lower range of prevalence (1–5%).[4,15,57,66,87,89,90,93,94,106,119,131] Several reasons explain the high prevalence of hepatitis B infection in Romanian adoptees. During that period, Romania had an overall high prevalence of hepatitis B, and therefore many children in orphanages were infected with hepatitis B. Needles were commonly reused for immunizations and other injections. Transmission was facilitated through contaminated needles and close contact with children infected with hepatitis B. Hepatitis B vaccine was not used during that period. In addition, hepatitis B screening was not routinely done in children available for adoption; thus many children arrived in the United States with unsuspected hepatitis B. In more recent years, hepatitis B vaccine in infants and screening for hepatitis B infection are routinely done and reported in the referral information. Thus the diagnosis of hepatitis B infection is nearly always known before adoption, and this condition is considered to be a special need.

Hepatitis B screening tests, including the hepatitis B surface antigen (HBsAg) and antibodies to surface (anti-HBs) and core (anti-HBc) antigens, are recommended in the medical evaluation of both internationally adopted children and refugees.[6,10,12,35,37] All three tests should be done to determine whether the child is immune as a result of immunization (anti-HBs positive only), has recovered from infection (anti-HBs and anti-HBc positive), or has acute or chronic hepatitis B (HBsAg and anti-HBc positive).[8] Patterns of hepatitis B serology can be found in Chapter 157. In a child found to be HBsAg positive, repeat testing should be done 6 months later. If the HBsAg persists for longer than 6 months, the child has chronic hepatitis B infection. If the child no longer has HBsAg and has developed anti-HBs, the child had acute infection and has recovered and is no longer able to transmit the virus to others. Children with acute or chronic hepatitis B (positive HBsAg) can transmit hepatitis B to others. A positive hepatitis B IgM differentiates acute hepatitis B from chronic hepatitis B. Children with acute or chronic hepatitis B should have additional testing done, including testing for HBeAg, HBeAb, and serum hepatic enzyme levels. HBsAg-positive children should be followed closely by a hepatologist for management.

Hepatitis D virus (HDV), which is seen only in patients with hepatitis B infection, occurs in North Africa, parts of South America, and the Mediterranean Basin.[8] Testing for HDV is not widely available but is recommended in patients from these regions who are found to have hepatitis B infection; however, a positive test does not change clinical management. For children who initially test negative for HBsAg, HBsAb, and HBcAb, some experts recommend repeat testing for hepatitis B approximately 6 months after arrival to ensure the child was not infected just before arrival to the United States.[10] Children with acute or chronic hepatitis B should have serologic testing for hepatitis A to determine the need for immunization with hepatitis A vaccine and for hepatitis C for overall management and treatment considerations.

Ideally, the family members of internationally adopted children should be vaccinated against hepatitis B before the child joins the family. If this has not been done, the household contacts of children with acute or chronic hepatitis B (HBsAg positive) must be vaccinated promptly. Hepatitis B is easily transmitted to unvaccinated household contacts. Up to 20% of household contacts will become HBsAg positive with 5 or more years of exposure within the home,[43,60] and transmission of hepatitis B from newly adopted children to their parents has been documented.[50,60,67,113]

Hepatitis C

Screening for hepatitis C is recommended for all internationally adopted children because most children with hepatitis C do not have symptoms, screening for risk factors is generally not possible, effective treatment and close follow-up of patients with hepatitis C are available, and there are high rates of hepatitis C in the countries of origin of adoptees.[6,10] In refugees, testing is recommended based on a history of specific risk factors, such as current or former injection drug use, receipt of blood products, or residence in settings with a documented high prevalence of hepatitis C.[6,10,37] Data on the prevalence of hepatitis C in both refugee[53,54,91,92,102] and internationally adopted children[57,70,104,106,110,131] are limited. In all families with internationally adopted children, the prevalence of hepatitis C was less than 1%.[106] In studies in refugees, the prevalence ranged from less than 2%[53,54,91,92,102] to 7% in Thai Hmong refugees.[91] Antibody testing with an enzyme immunoassay (EIA) should be done with the initial screening. If the antibody is positive, PCR should be done to confirm infection. Maternal antibody may be present until a child is 18 months of age. Children found to have hepatitis C infection should be immunized for hepatitis A and B and should be referred to a hepatologist for further management (see Chapter 177).

Human Immunodeficiency Virus 1 and 2 Infections

In the past, as part of the required overseas medical assessment, HIV testing was required for all immigrants and refugees 15 years of age

*References 12, 21, 22, 39, 45, 56, 62, 67, 85, 91, 92, 97, 99, 102, 127, 130.
†References 4, 10, 15, 57, 60, 64, 63, 65, 66, 71, 74, 75, 87, 89, 90, 93, 94, 106, 110, 119, 131.

and older. Children younger than 15 years of age were tested for HIV if history or examination raised concern about possible HIV infection (e.g., maternal history of HIV infection or history of rape or sexual assault). Since January 2010, HIV testing is no longer required for immigration medical assessment. The exception is that HIV testing still is recommended for people diagnosed with active TB. For refugees, HIV testing is recommended after arrival in the United States for persons age 13 to 64 years and encouraged for those younger than 13 years (http://www.cdc.gov/immigrantrefugeehealth/guidelines/domestic/screening-hiv-infection-domestic.html).[35]

The decision to screen children younger than 13 years depends on history and risk factors (e.g., receipt of blood products and maternal drug use), physical examination findings, and prevalence of HIV infection in the child's country of origin. If there is a suspicion of HIV infection, testing should be performed before administration of live vaccines.[37]

In contrast, most internationally adopted children have been tested for antibodies to HIV-1 by EIA in their birth country. In Ethiopia, an HIV-1 PCR test is generally also done. In children born to mothers with HIV and found to have antibodies to HIV in their country of origin, HIV-1 PCR testing is generally done. In more recent years, children known to be exposed to HIV have been given antiretroviral drugs when diagnosed in their birth country. For internationally adopted children, routine screening by EIA is recommended after they have arrived to the United States.[6,10]

Reports of HIV infection in internationally adopted children were uncommon until recent years. In the early 1990s, two cases of Romanian adoptees with HIV infection were reported.[73] Subsequently, Romania was found to have high rates of HIV in institutionalized children that were not felt to be maternally transmitted.[59] The high prevalence was found to be associated with transmission through contaminated needles and blood products. In a more recent case series, there have been no reports of HIV infection in adoptees.[106] In contrast to past years when children infected with HIV were not permitted to be adopted internationally, these children may now be adopted by families in the United States. Many children with HIV infection have now joined their new families through adoption, and they have generally been treated with antiretrovirals before arrival.[139]

For internationally adopted children, HIV testing with an enzyme-linked immunosorbent assay (ELISA) is recommended shortly after their arrival. Positive or indeterminate results should be resolved with use of HIV DNA PCR to detect HIV-1 virus (see Chapter 192B). If antibody testing by EIA is negative and clinical suspicion exists for HIV infection, HIV DNA PCR testing should be done. Some experts recommend PCR for any infant younger than 6 months on arrival. If PCR testing is done, two negative results from tests done 1 month or more apart with at least one done after 4 months of age are needed to exclude infection. Retesting children older than 6 months of age after arrival to the United States should be considered.[5] Clinicians should be prepared to provide care and resources for children arriving to the United States with HIV infection.

Preadoptive testing for HIV-2 infection is not performed routinely. HIV-2 infection is prevalent in some African nations and is now recognized on several other continents; perinatal transmission appears to be limited. Symptoms suggestive of HIV infection with negative ELISA results for HIV-1 should prompt testing for HIV-2.[5]

Bacterial Infections

Syphilis

Refugees and internationally adopted children 15 years and older are routinely screened for syphilis before coming to the United States.[6,9,37] Immigrants with positive results are required to complete treatment before arriving to the United States. On arrival to the United States, screening of all refugees 15 years and older is recommended regardless of the overseas results.[6,35] Children who are younger than 15 years should be screened if there is a history of sexual activity or sexual assault or a history of maternal syphilis.[6,37] In addition, all refugees emigrating from a country endemic for other treponemal infections such as yaws, bejel, or pinta should also be screened. Refugees of any age should be tested if there is clinical suspicion for syphilis.

Most internationally adopted children will have documentation of syphilis screening done in their birth country. For children with a history of syphilis or syphilis exposure, it is difficult to determine when the birth mother contracted syphilis and if she was treated and followed appropriately. In addition, in children with suspected syphilis exposure, details of the evaluation and prescribed treatment regimens are often incomplete or uninterpretable. Even though syphilis has rarely been reported in adoptees,[4,15,57,63–66,71,87,89,90,94,106,110,131] all internationally adopted children should be screened on arrival with both a nontreponemal test (rapid plasma reagin, Venereal Disease Research Laboratory, automated reagin test) and a treponemal test (microhemagglutination–*Treponema pallidum*, fluorescent treponemal antibody absorption, or *T. pallidum* particle agglutination) (see Chapter 144).[5] A positive treponemal test result warrants a complete and thorough evaluation to document the extent of the disease and to ensure adequate treatment regardless of a report of prior treatment. Because a positive treponemal test may be seen in pinta, bejel, yaws, and syphilis, it is important to consult with a specialist with expertise in these infections if the child is from a country where other treponemal infections are endemic.

Tuberculosis

TB is highly prevalent in the countries of origin for both refugees and internationally adopted children.[6,9,35,37] Therefore screening on arrival to the United States is recommended for both groups.[5,12,36,37] In the United States, 60% of all TB cases in the United States are among foreign-born people.[98] The rate of TB in foreign-born persons in the United States is 18.1 per 100,000; in US-born persons, the rate is 1.6 per 100,000. In addition, in the United States in 2009, the majority (89.4%) of multidrug-resistant TB cases were in foreign-born persons. In children, 22% of TB cases were in foreign-born patients. Case rates were significantly higher in foreign-born children (12.2 per 100,000) than in children born in the United States (1.1 per 100,000).[33,96]

Both refugees and internationally adopted children are at increased risk for TB infection. In immigrants and refugees, a high prevalence of latent tuberculosis infection (LTBI) was found in studies conducted in Minnesota (49%),[134] San Francisco (40%),[44] Buffalo (20%),[85] and Maine (35%).[56] A study in San Diego County found that 7% of immigrants screened had active pulmonary TB and 76% had LTBI.[80]

Overall, LTBI in internationally adopted children* appears to be lower (~20%) than that seen in refugees, which has been as high as 70% in certain populations.† This is likely due to the younger age and lower risk of living conditions of in this group of children. However, with the increased numbers of children coming from Ethiopia, a country with higher rates of tuberculosis, the rate of LTBI and tuberculosis in internationally adopted children is likely to increase. In two large studies in which all tuberculin skin tests (TSTs) were evaluated by a health care professional, 14% to 21% of international adoptees had LTBI.[82,129] The highest proportion with LTBI was seen in children from Russia and Eastern Europe (29%), and the lowest was in children adopted from China (10%).[129] Of note, very few children from Africa were included in these studies. Children with initially negative TSTs had their TSTs repeated at least 3 months later, and 13% to 20% of the TSTs were positive, suggesting that a high proportion of children initially had false-positive TSTs. The authors postulate that this could be due to anergy, testing too soon after infection, or boosting from TB infection or bacille Calmette-Guérin (BCG).

TB disease in international adoptees has rarely been reported.[42,57,75,76] In the first series of Korean adoptees, the overall prevalence was less than 1%, but two children had active TB and both had nonreactive TSTs.[75] One child had pneumonia caused by *Mycobacterium tuberculosis* and recovered. The other child had TB meningitis and died. These cases illustrate the importance of considering TB in the differential diagnosis even in children with negative TSTs. In the second case report,[42] a child with TB adopted from the Marshall Islands infected his female guardian and 20% of the contacts identified. On arrival in the United States, he had a TST done, but the test was never read. He had cavitary TB, but

*References 4, 52, 57, 63–66, 71, 75, 81, 82, 87, 89, 90, 94, 101, 106, 115, 129, 131, 132.

†References 12, 21, 39, 44, 56, 79, 80, 85, 97, 99, 102, 105, 125.

it was not diagnosed until his guardian developed TB. In a 2016 study examining the health status of internationally adopted children from Ethiopia, 6 of 315 children (2%) were found to have active tuberculosis.[131]

In the past, refugees older than 15 years and children younger than 15 years with concern about TB exposure or disease were screened with a chest radiograph before arriving in the United States. If the chest radiograph was abnormal, microscopic evaluation of sputum or gastric aspirate for acid-fast bacilli is performed. Refugees who were sputum positive were banned from entry until sputum smears were negative. In 2007, a major revision of the overseas TB screening requirements for immigrants and refugees bound for the United States was implemented that required TB screening for all people.[35] International adoptees from certain countries with high rates of TB (China and Ethiopia) now fall under the same requirements as other immigrants and refugees. For other adoptees, screening in the country of origin appears to be inconsistently done and generally is documented only in older children.

For both refugees and internationally adopted children, screening for TB should be done shortly after arrival to the United States.[6,9,12,35,37] Testing can be done at the initial assessment by placement of a TST (5 tuberculin units purified protein derivative) (Fig. 233.2). The test should be read 48 to 72 hours later by a health care professional. A reading of 10 mm or greater of induration is considered positive for both refugees and internationally adopted children arriving from a country endemic for TB. A reading of 5 mm or more is considered positive if there is a known contact with a person with active TB, an abnormal chest radiograph finding, signs or symptoms suggestive of TB, or evidence of immunosuppression. Children with a positive TST should have a thorough physical examination and chest radiograph performed to assess for *M. tuberculosis* disease. If the chest radiograph and physical examination are normal and the skin test is 10 mm or greater of induration, the diagnosis of LTBI is made and treatment with a 9-month course of isoniazid is begun. Similarly, a child with 5 to 9 mm of induration who has known exposure to someone with active TB or who is receiving immunosuppressive therapy or has an immunosuppressive condition, including HIV, with no evidence of disease, should receive isoniazid therapy as well. Retesting of TST-negative children 6 months or longer after arrival should be considered for all children given the high rate of false-negative TSTs shortly after arrival to the United States.[9,82,129]

Interferon-γ release assays (IGRAs), such as QuantiFERON Gold and T-SPOT.TB, are acceptable alternatives to the TST but are not currently recommended for children younger than 5 years, because of the lack of published data for younger children.[6,9] These assays use antigens that are secreted by *M. tuberculosis*–complex organisms but not by the Calmette-Guérin bacillus from the BCG vaccine. For TB disease, their sensitivity is comparable to that of the TST in children 5 years or older. For TB infection, the specificity of these tests is higher

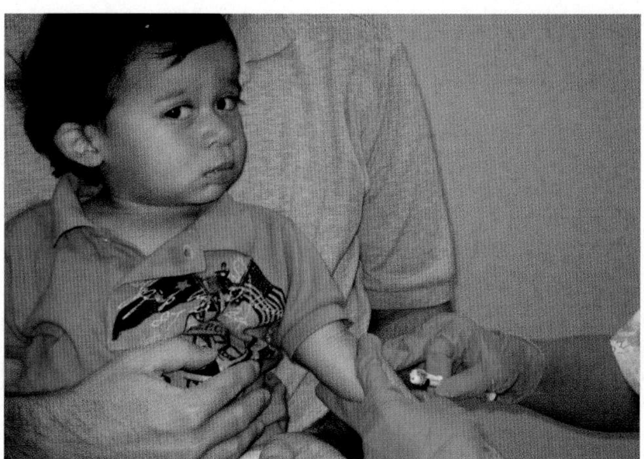

FIG. 233.2 Internationally adopted child from Guatemala having a tuberculin skin test placed.

than that of TSTs, but the sensitivity is not known. Logistical issues exist with the use of these tests because the test relies on stimulation of live blood mononuclear leukocytes with antigen, in vitro. In addition, these tests are more expensive than TSTs. For immunocompetent children 5 years and older, IGRAs can be used in place of a TST to confirm cases of TB or cases of LTBI. Similar to a positive TST, a child with a positive result from an IGRA should be considered infected with *M. tuberculosis* complex; however, a negative result from an IGRA cannot definitively rule out TB infection. IGRAs have the advantage of not requiring a follow-up visit for reading the TST or individual interpretation of the TST result. Studies done comparing TST with IGRAs in immigrant populations have found poor concordance with positive tests, with fewer positive results using the IGRA tests.[115,125]

Although most refugees and internationally adopted children with *M. tuberculosis* infection have LTBI, disease should be considered in children with pneumonia or nonspecific symptoms such as fever, malaise, growth delay, weight loss, cough, night sweats, and chills. In children, pulmonary TB is the most common site of infection, accounting for 77% of cases, followed by lymphatic TB in 16% of children.[96] Chest radiographs may reveal adenopathy, segmental or lobar infiltrates, or pleural effusion. Cavitary lesions and miliary disease are less commonly seen. Extrapulmonary manifestations of the central nervous system, middle ear and mastoids, lymph nodes, bone, joints, and skin also can be seen. Every effort should be made to recover the organism in children with suspected disease to determine the susceptibilities of the organism. Many children arrive from countries in which drug-resistant *M. tuberculosis* is common. Gastric aspirates, bronchoscopy, or both can be useful adjuncts in a child too young or too ill to expectorate sputum.

Initial management of active TB disease in refugees or internationally adopted children should include isoniazid, rifampin, pyrazinamide, and at least one other agent to ensure bactericidal coverage while culture results and susceptibility testing are pending (see Chapter 96).[11] The most recent resistant patterns from the child's country of origin should be considered along with any other epidemiologic information that can be obtained when making treatment decisions, especially if the cultures are negative.

Vaccination with BCG is common in most resource-poor countries. A history or evidence of BCG vaccine receipt is not a contraindication to the placement of a TST.[9,11] Studies have demonstrated that placement of a TST after BCG vaccination fails to elicit induration of 10 mm or greater.[78,108] Thus the history of BCG vaccine should not affect the interpretation of purified protein derivative.

BCG vaccination can be recognized by a 2- to 4-mm scarification, often seen on the left deltoid. Documentation of vaccination should be made in the child's vaccine record, and the scar, if present, should be documented on the physical examination record. Occasionally, complications from BCG vaccination can occur. These may include enlargement of regional lymph nodes or a nodule or ulcer that may or may not be draining at the vaccination site (Fig. 233.3). The lesion is granulomatous; culture of the lesion will yield *Mycobacterium bovis*. No consensus exists regarding the management of this condition. The outcome of these lesions varies. Some lesions resolve without treatment. Other lesions have been excised for diagnostic reasons, and others have been reported to require excision. Medical treatment with isoniazid, erythromycin, or clarithromycin has been used with success.[49,128]

Enteric Bacterial Infections

In contrast to intestinal parasites, bacterial enteric pathogens appear to be less common in immigrants and adoptees; however, most studies have not assessed systematically for bacterial causes. Children with bloody diarrhea or diarrhea associated with high fever should have stool examined for bacterial enteropathogens (e.g., *Salmonella, Shigella, Yersinia,* and *Campylobacter*) as part of the initial evaluation. Some experts also recommend obtaining stool cultures in newly arrived adoptees with diarrhea.[5] However, if a bacterial pathogen is identified, treatment may not be indicated or needed if symptoms have resolved.

Intestinal Parasites

Intestinal parasites are common in both refugee[14,18,21,77,79,92,102,105,107,122,127,137] and internationally adopted[4,57,71,75,87,89,90,94,106,110,116,131] children (Table 233.2).

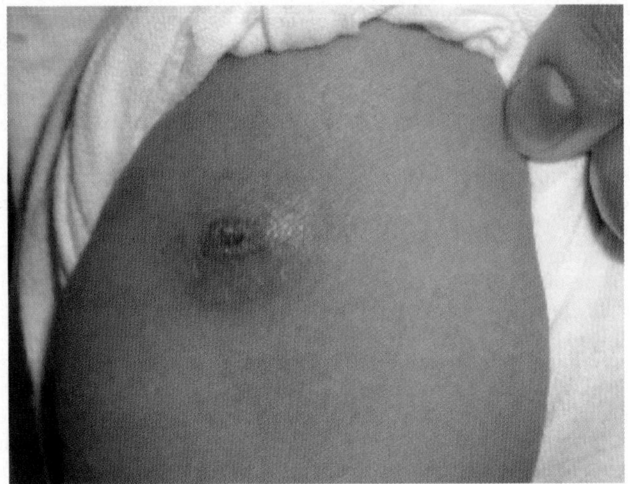

FIG. 233.3 Internationally adopted child from Vietnam with a bacille Calmette-Guérin granuloma on the shoulder.

TABLE 233.2 Pathogenic and Nonpathogenic Intestinal Parasites

Parasite Type	Pathogens	Nonpathogens
Protozoa	*Giardia intestinalis*	*Endolimax nana*
	Entamoeba histolytica	*Entamoeba coli*
	Dientamoeba fragilis[a]	*Entamoeba gingivalis*
	Balantidium coli	*Entamoeba hartmanni*
	Blastocystis hominis[a]	*Entamoeba polecki*
	Isospora belli	*Iodamoeba bütschlii*
	Cryptosporidium parvum	*Chilomastix mesnili*
	Cyclospora cayentensis	*Enteromonas hominis*
	Microsporidium spp.	*Retortamonas intestinalis*
		Trichomonas hominis
		Trichomonas tenax
Helminths		
Nematodes	*Ascaris lumbricoides* (roundworm)	
	Trichuris trichiura (whipworm)	
	Strongyloides stercoralis (threadworm)	
	Enterobius vermicularis (pinworm)	
	Necator americanus (hookworm)	
	Ancylostoma duodenale (hookworm)	
Cestodes	*Hymenolepsis* spp.	
	Taenia saginata (beef tapeworm)	
	Taenia solium (pork tapeworm)	
	Schistosoma spp.	

[a]Controversy exists regarding the pathogenicity of this organism.

Rates of infection vary by age and country of origin. Most children typically have not had testing before coming to the United States. However, presumptive treatment of refugees from certain regions before departure to the United States has been recommended since 1999, and screening strategies for these two groups are different.[6,35,37,83,122] Presumptive treatment has been found to be cost-effective in refugee populations.[69,83,122] Specifically, all refugees from the Middle East and South and Southeast Asia are recommended to receive a single dose of albendazole for round worms and ivermectin for *Strongyloides*. African refugees also should receive presumptive treatment for *Strongyloides*, and for those originating from areas endemic for schistosomiasis, presumptive treatment with praziquantel should be given. In African countries where Loa Loa is endemic, ivermectin should not be given for *Strongyloides* because treatment with this drug in the presence of Loa Loa has been associated with encephalopathy. Therefore in Loa Loa–endemic areas, 7 days of albendazole should be given. Additional details of the country-specific recommendations, timing, dosing, and duration of treatment can be found in the Centers for Disease Control and Prevention (CDC) guidelines for refugee and immigrant care.[35,37]

In internationally adopted children, the reported prevalence of intestinal parasites has varied from 9% to 51%, depending on the age of the child and country of origin.[4,57,71,75,87,89,90,94,106,110,116,131] Older children and children originating from countries other than Korea have been found to be at highest risk for intestinal parasites. *Giardia intestinalis* has been the most commonly identified pathogen in all studies, with as many as 19% of children infected. Helminthic infections have been less frequently identified (<3%), with *Hymenolepsis* spp., *Ascaris lumbricoides*, and *Trichuris trichiura* most often reported. In the largest study, the overall prevalence of intestinal parasites in internationally adopted children was 29%.[116] In this study, the prevalence of intestinal parasites was similar in children with and without gastrointestinal symptoms, and no significant difference was seen in malnourished children in contrast to children who were not malnourished.

Several studies report the prevalence of intestinal parasites in refugees, but few give pathogenic-specific data by age and country. In a large study of 26,956 refugees from Southeast Asia and Africa, the prevalence of intestinal parasites was examined.[122] The median age was 19 years, and 30% were children 2 to 14 years of age. For African refugees who were not pretreated, 7% had *Giardia* and 24% had at least one nematode, with *Trichuris* being most commonly identified. For Southeast Asian refugees, 12% had *Giardia* and 19% had at least one nematode, but hookworms were the most prevalent, at 11%. Children 2 to 14 years of age were significantly more likely than adults to have *Ascaris, Trichuris,* and *Giardia,* whereas hookworms were found more often in adults. In contrast, in another study, 17% of refugee children were found to have *Giardia* and 19% had helminthes, with hookworms most commonly seen.[14] This study found a high rate of hookworm in Bosnian refugees and found different rates of overall and pathogenic-specific recovery by region. Interestingly, this study found that refugees who reported gastrointestinal symptoms were significantly less often infected than those without symptoms ($P < .001$). In a study conducted from 2013 to 2015 evaluating unaccompanied minor Syrian refugees, 7% were found to have *Giardia* and 1.4% were diagnosed with schistosomiasis.[92]

Both refugees and adoptees should be screened for intestinal parasites on arrival to the United States.[6,9,12,19,35,37] The diagnosis for most intestinal parasites is done by examination of stool preserved in formalin and polyvinyl alcohol or sodium-acetate formalin for ova and parasite testing. Testing multiple stool specimens increases the sensitivity of microscopic examination for ova and parasites.[19,61,116] In one study in internationally adopted children, the sensitivity was 79% using one specimen and 92% for two specimens, and a third specimen identified parasites in an additional 8% of children.[116] Examination by an experienced technologist is critical in identifying intestinal parasites. One stool specimen should also be evaluated for *G. intestinalis* and *Cryptosporidium parvum* using antigen testing.[6,9] Repeat stool samples are essential to assess the effectiveness of treatment for the identified parasite or determine the presence of new (or newly found) pathogens. If the child remains persistently symptomatic, additional stool sample examinations are warranted, and testing for other parasites such as *Cyclospora* and *Strongyloides stercoralis* should be considered.

Eosinophilia and Tissue Parasites

In refugees or internationally adopted children who have negative stool ova and parasite examinations and in whom eosinophilia (absolute eosinophil count exceeding 450 cells/mm^3) is found on complete blood count, additional serologic testing should be done.[6,9,12,37,84,112] Children infected with these parasites often do not have symptoms.[95] In refugees, several studies have found eosinophilia to be very common, with a range of prevalence from 12% in asymptomatic refugees[112] to 9% to 28% in refugees with and without symptoms.[20,95,97,99] In one study conducted in international adoptees, 21% of children were found to have eosinophilia.[57] In both refugees and internationally adopted children, the most common cause of the eosinophilia was a helminth infection diagnosed by ova and parasite testing, or *Strongyloides,* schistosomiasis, or filariasis diagnosed by serology.

Serologic testing for *S. stercoralis* should be performed on all children with eosinophilia and no identified pathogen commonly associated with an increased eosinophil count, regardless of country of origin. Serologic testing for *Schistosoma* spp. should be performed in children with eosinophilia and no identified pathogen commonly associated with eosinophilia from sub-Saharan Africa, Southeast Asia, or areas of Latin America where schistosomiasis is endemic.

Testing for filariasis should be done for children older than 2 years with eosinophilia who come from areas where filariasis is endemic. Multiple parasites cause filariasis; therefore, if testing is positive, consultation with an infectious disease specialist with expertise in this disease should be done to ensure the correct treatment is given. Serologic testing for *Strongyloides, Schistosoma* spp., and filariasis is available through the CDC.

While eosinophilia should prompt clinicians for evaluation for helminths and tissue parasites, it is important to realize that these parasites may be present without eosinophilia.[95,114] Some experts will perform serologic tests for all refugees and international adoptees regardless of the presence of eosinophilia if children immigrated from an area endemic for these parasites.

Chagas Disease (American Trypanosomiasis)

Chagas disease is endemic throughout much of Mexico, Central America, and South America (Chapter 221) and is caused by *Trypanosoma cruzi.*[9] The risk for Chagas disease varies by region within countries with endemic infection. Although no studies have been done to assess the prevalence of Chagas disease in refugees or internationally adopted children, screening is warranted because treatment of infected children is highly effective in contrast to treatment in adults.[5,26,37,38] Children may become infected by vertical exposure or from vectors. Countries with endemic Chagas disease include Argentina, Belize, Bolivia, Brazil, Chile, Colombia, Costa Rica, Ecuador, El Salvador, French Guiana, Guatemala, Guyana, Honduras, Mexico, Nicaragua, Panama, Paraguay, Peru, Suriname, Uruguay, and Venezuela. Serologic testing should only be performed in children 12 months of age or older because of the potential presence of maternal antibody. Testing can be done through the CDC.

Malaria

For internationally adopted children, routine screening for malaria is not recommended.[4] In refugees who do not have a contraindication, predeparture presumptive antimalarial therapy with artesunate-combination therapy should be given to all sub-Saharan African refugees arriving from countries endemic for *Plasmodium falciparum.*[35,37] Refugees from these countries without presumptive treatment before departure should have postarrival testing done using malaria PCR. If PCR is not available, traditional blood films or a rapid antigen test may be used, recognizing that these tests are much less sensitive, especially in persons who do not have symptoms. Alternatively, presumptive treatment can be provided instead of testing. Refugees from malaria-endemic regions outside sub-Saharan Africa do not require postarrival testing or treatment. However, any refugee or internationally adopted child from a malaria-endemic region with signs or symptoms of malaria should be thoroughly evaluated.

Routine screening for malaria is not recommended for internationally adopted or refugee children.[6,9,37] Screening of symptom-free children from endemic areas may be indicated in children with splenomegaly. A study done in internationally adopted Ethiopian children from 2006 to 2011 found that 14% of children who had past or current hepatomegaly or splenomegaly and previously lived in a malaria-endemic area had asymptomatic parasitemia by microscopy or PCR.[2]

Multidrug-Resistant Organisms

Routine screening for carriage of multidrug-resistant organisms is not recommended in internationally adopted or refugee children. Several studies, however, have demonstrated high rates of carriage and in some cases transmission of drug-resistant bacteria, including extended spectrum β-lactamase (ESBL)-producing organisms.[13,15,16,51,55,57,58,124,126,133] A study of adoptees from Mali found that 24 of 25 children screened carried at least one ESBL-producing organism on arrival to France.[124] In another study of adoptees from Mali, ESBL was produced by 26 of 41 *Salmonella* species isolated from 30 families.[16] A study conducted in pediatric refugees hospitalized in Germany from 2015 to 2016 found that 34% of the 325 children had multidrug-resistant organisms.[126] Additional information is needed to determine whether recommendations for screening should occur. For now, health care providers should be aware that immigrant children might have high rates of multidrug-resistant organisms.

Other Testing

A complete blood count is recommended for refugees and internationally adopted children.[6,9,37] The hemoglobin and red blood cell indices may identify children with anemia, iron deficiency, hemoglobinopathies, or malaria. Low white blood cell counts and lymphopenia may indicate HIV infection or malnutrition. Eosinophilia is common among refugees and suggests parasitic infection. The prevalence of eosinophilia has not been reported in internationally adopted children. For refugees, a urinalysis is recommended to assess for hematuria and pyuria. Hematuria may indicate schistosomiasis, and pyuria may reflect a urinary tract infection or renal TB.

Elevated blood lead levels have been reported in internationally adopted children[23] and refugees,[29] and both groups should have a blood lead concentration as part of their initial evaluation.[6,9,37]

OTHER VACCINE-PREVENTABLE DISEASES

In addition to hepatitis A and hepatitis B, other vaccine-preventable diseases have been transmitted or brought into the United States by immigrants. One case of pertussis in an internationally adopted child from Russia has been reported,[25] along with several cases of measles imported by refugees[32] and internationally adopted children.[24,26-28,30] Clinicians should be aware of the signs and symptoms of measles and do proper testing if measles is suspected.

Dermatologic Infections and Infestations

Lice, scabies, fungal infections, and molluscum contagiosum are common in both refugees and internationally adopted children. The prevalence of these conditions has not been well documented. In three studies conducted with international adoptees, 35% to 70% had dermatologic conditions, including tinea, scabies, staphylococcal infections, and molluscum.[57,103,131] In refugee populations, the reported dermatologic conditions included these same conditions but were broader with leishmaniasis, tungiasis, and leprosy were also reported.[39,41,72,97,121] The physical examination should include careful evaluation for these entities so that appropriate treatment is given.

IMMUNIZATION GUIDELINES

Making immunization recommendations can be challenging for clinicians providing care for immigrant children. Most refugees arrive in the United States without immunization records, and most international adoptees have some documentation of receipt of immunizations. Refugee and internationally adopted children have typically had the opportunity to have received BCG, diphtheria-tetanus-pertussis–containing vaccines, poliovirus vaccine, hepatitis B, and measles vaccines in their countries of origin. In internationally adopted children, there has been an increase in documentation of *Haemophilus influenzae* type b vaccine, especially for children from South Korea, Guatemala, India, and China. For measles vaccine, most children will have received and have documentation of a monovalent measles vaccine. Mumps and rubella vaccines, in combination with measles vaccine as MMR, have been documented for adoptees from South Korea and Guatemala or as monovalent vaccines in older children from Eastern Europe and Russia. Pneumococcal conjugate and varicella vaccines are not routinely given but have been documented in records for children from South Korea and Guatemala. Although

TABLE 233.3 Serologic Testing for Verifying Immunization or Past Infection

Age	Test	Protective Level
Children ≥5 Months		
Diphtheria antibody (IgG)	ELISA	>0.10 IU/mL
Tetanus antibody (IgG)	ELISA	>0.10 IU/mL
Poliovirus antibody (serotypes 1–3)	Neutralizing antibody	Detectable antibody
Hepatitis B surface antibody (IgG)	ELISA	≥10 mIU/mL
Haemophilus influenza type b, (IgG) polyribosylribitol phosphate antibody	ELISA	≥1.0 IU/mL
Children ≥12 Months		
Rubeola (measles) antibody (IgG)	IFA or ELISA	[a]
Mumps antibody (IgG)	IFA or ELISA	[a]
Rubella antibody (IgG)	ELISA	[a]
Varicella antibody (IgG)	ELISA	[a]
Hepatitis A antibody (Total or IgG)	EIA	[a]

[a]Value for positive result varies by test and laboratory.

children may have documentation of some vaccine-preventable diseases, a clinical diagnosis of measles, mumps, rubella, varicella, or hepatitis A from the child's country of origin should not be accepted as evidence of immunity.

The Immigration and Nationality Act (INA) of 1996 requires immigrant visa applicants to provide proof of vaccination with at least the first dose of vaccines recommended by the Advisory Committee on Immunization Practice (ACIP) before entry into the United States.[3,6,9,37] These regulations apply to most immigrant children entering the United States; however, internationally adopted children who are 10 years or younger may obtain an exemption from these requirements. Adoptive parents are required to sign a waiver indicating their intention to comply with the ACIP immunization requirements within 30 days after the child's arrival in the United States. Refugees are not required to meet immunization requirements of the INA at the time of initial entry into the United States, but they must show proof of immunization when they apply for permanent residency—typically 1 year after arrival. Information about immunization requirements for immigrants is available on the CDC website (http://www.cdc.gov/ncezid/dgmq/).

People immunized in other countries, including refugees and internationally adopted children, should be immunized according to the US recommended schedule for healthy infants, children, and adolescents.[3,6,9,37] Only written documentation should be accepted as evidence of previous immunization. The written records may be considered valid if the vaccines, dates of administration, numbers of doses, intervals between doses, and age of the patient at the time of immunization are comparable to current US or World Health Organization (WHO) schedules (http://apps.who.int/immunization_monitoring/en/globalsummary/countryprofileselect.cfm). Overall, most vaccines used around the world are produced with adequate quality-control standards and are generally considered reliable. Immunization is one of the most important measures used to prevent diseases in resource-poor countries, and immunization of children is a priority worldwide. However, some vaccines with inadequate potency have been produced in other countries. In addition, immunization records may be difficult to interpret or have dates that appear inaccurate, causing concern that the records may not be valid and accurately reflect protection. Therefore, for children who do not have a record or who have an unknown or uncertain immunization status, serologic testing and reimmunization are both reasonable approaches. If serologic testing is not or cannot be done, any immunizations that are not documented or do not adhere to the US or WHO standards should be repeated.

For children whose immunizations are not up to date, but who have a valid, written immunization record for the vaccines documented, vaccines as recommended for their age should be administered. For children without documentation of immunizations or who have a record that does not adhere to US or WHO standards, a new vaccine schedule may be initiated or measurement of antibody concentrations to any or all of the following vaccine antigens can be done: diphtheria, tetanus, poliovirus (each serotype), measles, mumps, rubella, varicella, and hepatitis A (Table 233.3). Hepatitis B serology will be done to assess the child's hepatitis B status, which will also allow for determination of immunity. *H. influenzae* type b polyribosylribitol phosphate antibody also can be done; however, fewer data exist to support this testing to determine protection. Testing for measles, mumps, rubella, varicella, and hepatitis A should only be done in children older than 12 months because of the possible presence of maternal antibody. Because antibody testing for one vaccine may not be predictive for others, a combination of reimmunization and antibody testing also can be used. Serologic testing is not recommended for making vaccine decisions for pertussis, pneumococcus, or influenza. Because there are not reliable correlates of protection for pertussis, diphtheria and tetanus levels may be used to guide decision making. Age-appropriate immunization for conjugate pneumococcal and influenza vaccines is recommended.

Some caveats for interpreting antibody results should be reviewed. First, in general, antibody levels do not differentiate past disease from immunization. Measles, mumps, rubella, hepatitis A, varicella, and *H. influenzae* type b are prevalent in many of the countries of origin for refugees and internationally adopted children, so protective levels of antibody may be due to past immunization of infection. Poliovirus from oral poliovirus vaccine could be transmitted from another child, providing protection to children without documentation of poliovirus vaccine. For HBV, however, serology will distinguish between past disease and immunization. The presence of anti-HBc with anti-HBs reflects past, recovered disease, whereas anti-HBs alone is due to immunization. Second, if protective antibody is found, additional age-appropriate immunizations should still be given for some vaccines. For example, if a 9-month-old infant has protective antibody for diphtheria and tetanus, the 15- and 18-month and 4- to 6-year DTaP doses should still be given. In contrast, if a 3-year-old child has protective antibody to measles, mumps, and rubella, an additional MMR is not needed when the child is 4 to 6 years of age. Third, it is important to consider age, along with the antibody levels for diphtheria and tetanus. In a 3-year-old child with a protective level of 0.20 IU/mL for tetanus, a dose of DTaP should be given to boost the tetanus level and hopefully provide higher levels of protection for pertussis. Finally, if a child does not have protective antibody for measles, mumps, or varicella, two doses are needed. However, if measles and mumps antibody levels are protective and the rubella antibody is nonprotective, only one MMR dose is needed for rubella.

Several studies have been published examining antibody testing to verify the immunization status or immunity to vaccine-preventable diseases in internationally adopted children.* The results of these studies differ; some studies show inadequate protection, whereas others show good levels of protection. Differences in study design and laboratory methods likely account for the different results from the various studies. In the largest study to date, in internationally adopted children with three or more vaccine doses, overall protection was found to be high for diphtheria (85%), tetanus (95%), polio (93%), hepatitis B (77%),

*References 1, 40, 86, 87, 88–90, 94, 106, 109, 117–119, 132, 135, 136.

and *H. influenzae* type b (67%).[117] Of children 12 months and older with more than one dose of measles, mumps, or rubella vaccine, 95%, 72%, and 94%, respectively, were immune. In contrast to children without documentation for a given vaccine antigen (i.e., no doses), a lower proportion of children had protective levels of antibody: diphtheria (69%), tetanus (76%), polio (83%), hepatitis B (42%), *H. influenzae* type b (67%), measles (58%), mumps (31%), or rubella (30%). However, many of these children were still protected, suggesting that children either had a history of disease or had received vaccines and did not have documentation. In that same study, 33% of adoptees had protective levels of varicella antibody (with or without vaccine documentation), and 83% of children with a history of varicella had protective antibody. Few data exist on verifying immunization status by antibody testing in refugees, with most focusing on measles, mumps, rubella, and varicella, and protective antibody increased with age and varied by country.[46,68,105]

CONCLUSION

Providing care for refugees and internationally adopted children can be rewarding. Screening for infectious diseases and determining immunization needs is critical not only for the health and prevention of disease in these immigrants but also for the prevention of disease in their families and communities.

NEW REFERENCES SINCE THE SEVENTH EDITION

2. Adebo SM, Eckerle JK, Andrews ME, et al. Asymptomatic Malaria and Other Infections in Children Adopted from Ethiopia, United States, 2006–2011. *Emerg Infect Dis*. 2015;21(7):1227-1229.
3. Akinsanya-Beysolow I, Advisory Committee on Immunization Practices (ACIP); ACIP Childhood/Adolescent Immunization Work Group; Centers for Disease Control and Prevention (CDC). Advisory Committee on Immunization Practices recommended immunization schedules for persons aged 0 through 18 years—United States, 2014. *MMWR Morb Mortal Wkly Rep*. 2014;63(5):108-109.
5. American Academy of Pediatrics. AAP. Policy Statement: Providing care for immigrant, migrant, and border children. *Pediatrics*. 2013;131(6):e2028-e2034.
6. American Academy of Pediatrics. Hepatitis A. In: Kimberlin DW, Brady MT, Jackson MA, Long SS, eds. *Red Book: 2015 Report on the Committee on Infectious Diseases*. 30th ed. Elk Grove Village, IL: American Academy of Pediatrics; 2015:391-393.
7. American Academy of Pediatrics. Hepatitis B. In: Kimberlin DW, Brady MT, Jackson MA, Long SS, eds. *Red Book: 2015 Report on the Committee on Infectious Diseases*. 30th ed. Elk Grove Village, IL: American Academy of Pediatrics; 2015:400-423.
8. American Academy of Pediatrics. Immunization in Special Circumstances: refugees and immigrants. In: Kimberlin DW, Brady MT, Jackson MA, Long SS, eds. *Red Book: 2015 Report of the Committee on Infectious Diseases*. 30th ed. Elk Grove Village, IL: American Academy of Pediatrics; 2015:68-107.
9. American Academy of Pediatrics. Medical evaluation for infectious diseases for internationally adopted, refugee and immigrant children. In: Kimberlin DW, Brady MT, Jackson MA, Long SS, eds. *Red Book: 2015 Report of the Committee on Infectious Diseases*. 30th ed. Elk Grove Village, IL: American Academy of Pediatrics; 2015:192-201.
11. American Academy of Pediatrics. Tuberculosis. In: Kimberlin DW, Brady MT, Jackson MA, Long SS, eds. *Red Book 2015: Report of the Committee on Infectious Diseases*. 30th ed. Elk Grove Village, IL: American Academy of Pediatrics; 2015:805-831.
13. Bekal S, Lefebvre B, Bergevin M, et al. CTX-M-15 type ESBL-producing *Salmonella* Havana associated with international adoption in Canada. *Can J Microbiol*. 2013;59(1):57.
15. Blanchi S, Chabasse D, Pichard E, et al. Post-international adoption medical follow-up at the Angers University Hospital between 2009 and 2012. *Med Mal Infect*. 2014;44(2):69-75.
16. Boisrame-Gastrin S, Tande D, Munck MR, et al. *Salmonella* carriage in adopted children from Mali: 2001–08. *J Antimicrob Chemother*. 2011;66(10):2271-2276.
17. Brady MT, Bernstein HH, Byington CL, et al. Policy Statement. Recommendations for Administering Hepatitis A Vaccine to Contacts of International Adoptees. *Pediatrics*. 2011;128(4):803-804.
20. Caruana SR, Kelly HA, Ngeow JY, et al. Undiagnosed and potentially lethal parasite infections among immigrants and refugees in Australia. *J Travel Med*. 2006;13(4):233-239.
22. Centers for Disease Control and Prevention. CDC Health Information for International Travel 2016; 2016. http://www.cdc.gov/travel/content/yellowbook/home-2016.aspx.
24. Centers for Disease Control and Prevention. Elevated blood levels among internationally adopted children—United States. *MMWR Morb Mortal Wkly Rep*. 1998;49:97-100.
25. Centers for Disease Control and Prevention. General Refugee Health Guidelines; 2016. http://www.cdc.gov/immigrantrefugeehealth/guidelines/general-guidelines.html.
30. Centers for Disease Control and Prevention. Medical examination of immigrants and refugees; 2016. http://www.cdc.gov/immigrantrefugeehealth/exams/medical-examination.html.
31. Centers for Disease Control and Prevention. Multistate investigation of measles among adoptees from China—April 9, 2004. *MMWR Morb Mortal Wkly Rep*. 2004;53(14):309-310.
32. Centers for Disease Control and Prevention. Pertussis in an infant adopted from Russia—May 2002. *MMWR Morb Mortal Wkly Rep*. 2002;51(18):394-395.
33. Centers for Disease Control and Prevention. Refugee health guidelines: domestic intestinal parasite guidelines; 2016. http://www.cdc.gov/immigrantrefugeehealth/guidelines/domestic/intestinal-parasites-domestic.html.
36. Centers for Disease Control and Prevention. Update: measles among adoptees from China—April 14, 2004. *MMWR Morb Mortal Wkly Rep*. 2004;53(14):309.
39. Chai SJ, Davies-Cole J, Cookson ST. Infectious disease burden and vaccination needs among asylees versus refugees, District of Columbia. *Clin Infect Dis*. 2013;56(5):652-658.
40. Cilleruelo MJ, de Ory F, Ruiz-Contreras J, et al. Internationally adopted children: what vaccines should they receive? *Vaccine*. 2008;26(46):5784-5790.
41. Crogan J, Gunasekera H, Wood N, et al. Management of Old World cutaneous leishmaniasis in refugee children. *Pediatr Infect Dis J*. 2010;29(4):357-359.
43. Davis LG, Weber DJ, Lemon SM. Horizontal transmission of hepatitis B virus. *Lancet*. 1989;1(8643):889-893.
45. Dorman K, Bozinoff N, Redditt V, et al. Health status of North Korean refugees in Toronto: a community based participatory research study. *J Immigr Minor Health*. 2017;19(1):15-23.
46. Figueira M, Christiansen D, Barnett ED. Cost-effectiveness of serotesting compared with universal immunization for varicella in refugee children from six geographic regions. *J Travel Med*. 2003;10(4):203-207.
47. Fiore AE, Wasley A, Bell BP. Prevention of hepatitis A through active or passive immunization: recommendations of the Advisory Committee on Immunization Practices (ACIP). *MMWR Recomm Rep*. 2006;55(RR-7):1-23.
51. Georgakopoulou T, Mandilara G, Mellou K, et al. Resistant Shigella strains in refugees, August–October 2015, Greece. *Epidemiol Infect*. 2016;144(11):2415-2419.
52. George SA, Ko CA, Kirchner HL, et al. The role of chest radiographs and tuberculin skin tests in tuberculosis screening of internationally adopted children. *Pediatr Infect Dis J*. 2011;30(5):387-391.
53. Greenaway C, Ma AT, Kloda LA, et al. Correction: The Seroprevalence of Hepatitis C Antibodies in Immigrants and Refugees from Intermediate and High Endemic Countries: A Systematic Review and Meta-Analysis. *PLoS ONE*. 2015;10(12):e0144567.
54. Greenaway C, Thu Ma A, Kloda LA, et al. The Seroprevalence of Hepatitis C Antibodies in Immigrants and Refugees from Intermediate and High Endemic Countries: A Systematic Review and Meta-Analysis. *PLoS ONE*. 2015;10(11):e0141715.
55. Hagleitner MM, Mascini EM, van Berkel S, et al. Foreign adopted children are a source of methicillin-resistant *Staphylococcus aureus* transmission to countries with low prevalence. *Pediatr Infect Dis J*. 2012;31(6):655-658.
57. Henaff F, Hazart I, Picherot G, et al. Frequency and characteristics of infectious diseases in internationally adopted children: a retrospective study in Nantes from 2010 to 2012. *J Travel Med*. 2015;22(3):179-185.
58. Hendriksen RS, Mikoleit M, Kornschober C, et al. Emergence of multidrug-resistant *Salmonella* Concord infections in Europe and the United States in children adopted from Ethiopia, 2003-2007. *Pediatr Infect Dis J*. 2009;28(9):814-818.
62. Hirani K, Payne D, Mutch R, et al. Health of adolescent refugees resettling in high-income countries. *Arch Dis Child*. 2016;101(7):670-676.
65. Hostetter MK, Iverson S, Dole K, et al. Unsuspected infectious diseases and other medical diagnoses in the evaluation of internationally adopted children. *Pediatrics*. 1989;83(4):559-564.
63. Hostetter MK. Infectious diseases in internationally adopted children: findings in children from China, Russia, and Eastern Europe. *Adv Pediatr Infect Dis*. 1999;14:147-161.
64. Hostetter MK. Infectious diseases in internationally adopted children: the past five years. *Pediatr Infect Dis J*. 1998;17(6):517-518.
67. Hurie MB, Mast EE, Davis JP. Horizontal transmission of hepatitis B virus infection to United States-born children of Hmong refugees. *Pediatrics*. 1992;89(2):269-273.
68. Jablonka A, Happle C, Grote U, et al. Measles, mumps, rubella, and varicella seroprevalence in refugees in Germany in 2015. *Infection*. 2016;44(6):781-787.
69. Jazwa A, Coleman MS, Gazmararian J, et al. Cost-benefit comparison of two proposed overseas programs for reducing chronic hepatitis B infection among refugees: is screening essential? *Vaccine*. 2015;33(11):1393-1399.
70. Johansson PJ, Lofgren B, Nordenfelt E. Low frequency of hepatitis C antibodies among children from foreign countries adopted in Swedish families. *Scand J Infect Dis*. 1990;22(5):619-620.
72. Kopel E, Amitai Z, Sprecher H, et al. Tinea capitis outbreak in a paediatric refugee population, Tel Aviv, Israel. *Mycoses*. 2012;55(2):e36-e39.

73. Kurtz J. HIV infection and hepatitis B in adopted Romanian children. *BMJ.* 1991;302(6789):1399.
74. Lange WR, Kreider SD, Warnock-Eckhart E. Hepatitis B surveillance in Korean adoptees. *Md Med J.* 1987;36(2):163-166.
75. Lange WR, Warnock-Eckhart E. Selected infectious disease risks in international adoptees. *Pediatr Infect Dis J.* 1987;6(5):447-450.
83. Maskery B, Coleman MS, Weinberg M, et al. Economic analysis of the impact of overseas and domestic treatment and screening options for intestinal helminth infection among US-bound refugees from Asia. *PLoS Negl Trop Dis.* 2016;10(8):e0004910.
84. Meltzer E, Percik R, Shatzkes J, et al. Eosinophilia among returning travelers: a practical approach. *Am J Trop Med Hyg.* 2008;78(5):702-709.
91. Mixson-Hayden T, Lee D, Ganova-Raeva L, et al. Hepatitis B virus and hepatitis C virus infections in United States-bound refugees from Asia and Africa. *Am J Trop Med Hyg.* 2014;90(6):1014-1020.
92. Mockenhaupt FP, Barbre KA, Jensenius M, et al. Profile of illness in Syrian refugees: A GeoSentinel analysis, 2013 to 2015. *Euro Surveill.* 2016;21(10).
95. Naidu P, Yanow SK, Kowalewska-Grochowska KT. Eosinophilia: A poor predictor of *Strongyloides* infection in refugees. *Can J Infect Dis Med Microbiol.* 2013;24(2):93-96.
97. O'Brien DP, Leder K, Matchett E, et al. Illness in returned travelers and immigrants/refugees: the 6-year experience of two Australian infectious diseases units. *J Travel Med.* 2006;13(3):145-152.
98. Pang J, Teeter LD, Katz DJ, et al. Epidemiology of tuberculosis in young children in the United States. *Pediatrics.* 2014;133(3):e494-e504.
99. Parenti DM, Lucas D, Lee A, et al. Health status of Ethiopian refugees in the United States. *Am J Public Health.* 1987;77(12):1542-1543.
101. Priya Dhar C, Elena Gonzalez B, Dragga T, et al. Testing International Adoptees for Tuberculosis. *Pediatr Infect Dis J.* 2015;34(10):1138-1139.
102. Redditt VJ, Janakiram P, Graziano D, et al. Health status of newly arrived refugees in Toronto, Ont: Part 1: infectious diseases. *Can Fam Physician.* 2015;61(7):e303-e309.
103. Rigal E, Nourrisson C, Sciauvaud J, et al. Skin diseases in internationally adopted children. *Eur J Dermatol.* 2016;26(4):370-372.
105. Rungan S, Reeve AM, Reed PW, et al. Health needs of refugee children younger than 5 years arriving in New Zealand. *Pediatr Infect Dis J.* 2013;32(12):e432-e436.
108. Santiago EM, Lawson E, Gillenwater K, et al. A prospective study of bacillus Calmette-Guérin scar formation and tuberculin skin test reactivity in infants in Lima. *Peru Pediatrics.* 2003;112(4):e298.
110. Sciauvaud J, Rigal E, Pascal J, et al. Transmission of infectious diseases from internationally adopted children to their adoptive families. *Clin Microbiol Infect.* 2014;20(8):746-751.
111. US Department of Homeland Security. Security yearbook of immigration statistics: 2015; 2016. http://www.dhs.gov/immigration-statistics.
114. Soriano-Arandes A, Sulleiro E, Zarzuela F, et al. Discordances Between Serology and Culture for *Strongyloides* in an Ethiopian Adopted Child With Multiple Parasitic Infections: A Case Report. *Medicine (Baltimore).* 2016;95(10):e3040.
115. Spicer KB, Turner J, Wang SH, et al. Tuberculin skin testing and T-SPOT.TB in internationally adopted children. *Pediatr Infect Dis J.* 2015;34(6):599-603.
120. US Department of State. Immigrant visas issued to orphans coming into the US; 2016. http://adoption.state.gov/about_us/statistics.php.
121. Swaminathan A, Gosbell IB, Zwar NA, et al. Tungiasis in recently arrived African refugees. *Med J Aust.* 2005;183(1):51.
123. Sweet K, Sutherland W, Ehresmann K, et al. Hepatitis A infection in recent international adoptees and their contacts in Minnesota, 2007–2009. *Pediatrics.* 2011;128(2):e333-e338.
124. Tande D, Boisrame-Gastrin S, Munck MR, et al. Intrafamilial transmission of extended-spectrum-beta-lactamase-producing *Escherichia coli* and *Salmonella enterica* Babelsberg among the families of internationally adopted children. *J Antimicrob Chemother.* 2010;65(5):859-865.
125. Taylor EM, Painter J, Posey DL, et al. Latent Tuberculosis Infection Among Immigrant and Refugee Children Arriving in the United States: 2010. *J Immigr Minor Health.* 2016;18(5):966-970.
126. Tenenbaum T, Becker KP, Lange B, et al. Prevalence of Multidrug-Resistant Organisms in Hospitalized Pediatric Refugees in a University Children's Hospital in Germany 2015–2016. *Infect Control Hosp Epidemiol.* 2016;37(11):1310-1314.
127. Theuring S, Friedrich-Janicke B, Portner K, et al. Screening for infectious diseases among unaccompanied minor refugees in Berlin, 2014–2015. *Eur J Epidemiol.* 2016;31(7):707-710.
130. Ugwu C, Varkey P, Bagniewski S, et al. Sero-epidemiology of hepatitis B among new refugees to Minnesota. *J Immigr Minor Health.* 2008;10(5):469-474.
131. Van Kesteren L, Wojciechowski M. International adoption from Ethiopia: An overview of the health status at arrival in Belgium. *Acta Clin Belg.* 2017;72(5):300-305.
133. Vanhoof R, Gillis P, Stevart O, et al. Transmission of multiple resistant *Salmonella* Concord from internationally adopted children to their adoptive families and social environment: proposition of guidelines. *Eur J Clin Microbiol Infect Dis.* 2012;31(4):491-497.
134. Varkey P, Jerath AU, Bagniewski SM, et al. The epidemiology of tuberculosis among primary refugee arrivals in Minnesota between 1997 and 2001. *J Travel Med.* 2007;14(1):1-8.
139. Wolf ER, Beste S, Barr E, et al. Health Outcomes of International HIV-infected Adoptees in the US. *Pediatr Infect Dis J.* 2016;35(4):422-427.

The full reference list for this chapter is available at ExpertConsult.com.

PART

IV

Therapeutics

234 Antibiotic Resistance

Latania K. Logan • Jeffrey L. Blumer • Philip Toltzis

Soil bacteria developed mechanisms of resistance to antibiotics millions of years ago as a means of protecting themselves against other antibiotic-producing microorganisms or their own antimicrobial products. The current crisis of antibiotic resistance was prompted by the intense selective pressure posed by the worldwide use of antibiotics during the past 70 years. The problem of antimicrobial resistance in humans has been exacerbated by the widespread administration of antibiotics to farm animals.[290,445,510] Resistant zoonotic bacteria selected by this practice contaminate the food supply and thereby spread to human consumers.

To understand antibiotic resistance fully, a distinction must be made between the in vitro phenomenon of resistance and the less frequently observed clinical consequences of the in vitro phenomenon. Much of the discussion of bacterial resistance to antibiotics derives from the apparent changes in susceptibility of pathogenic bacteria to the concentrations of antibiotic achieved in blood after standard antibiotic dosing. These concentrations have been established as breakpoints based on integration of data derived from clinical and animal studies along with the measurement of plasma and serum drug concentrations associated with successful outcomes. Unfortunately, such breakpoints are not absolute. Rather, they depend on an intricate interrelationship between the pharmacokinetics and pharmacodynamics of the drug.[74] As such, if one component of this complex association is changed, the apparent breakpoint distinguishing susceptibility from resistance possibly and mostly likely will also change. Consequently, in presenting information concerning the mechanisms of antibiotic resistance and their clinical contexts, one must remember that the discussion derives in part from certain artificial pretexts. Changes in a drug-dosing paradigm (e.g., dose, infusion duration, formulation) can affect the clinical relevance of the in vitro observations dramatically.

RESISTANCE GENETICS

Bacteria develop resistance to antimicrobial agents through three principal cellular mechanisms (Box 234.1). Two or more mechanisms of resistance to a given agent can exist simultaneously in the same microorganism.

Antibiotic resistance is spreading at an alarming rate across international boundaries. In some instances, antibiotic resistance spreads when a resistance-conferring mutation occurs in the bacterial chromosome and the mutated organism then disseminates throughout the community and beyond. Perhaps even more importantly, antibiotic resistance is spread through the acquisition of exogenous DNA encoding the resistance determinant. These nucleic acid elements can mobilize; that is, move from one genetic location within the bacterium to another or from one organism to another (i.e., conjugation) (see Box 234.1). Mobilization frequently results in a reduction in the fitness of the host organism,[202,377] primarily through increased energy expenditure or from the insertion and disruption of other genes important to the bacterium's health. Consequently, mobilization typically is tightly controlled and is a relatively uncommon event,[472] occurring mostly when the environment surrounding the bacterium, particularly antibiotic exposure, clearly confers a survival benefit. Conversely, insertion and disruption of important bacterial genes may occasionally improve the organism's chance for survival. Disruption of DNA repair enzymes, for example, may render the bacterium hypermutable and thus better able to rapidly adapt to hostile surroundings through random mutation events.[472]

The genetic elements important in mobile antiobiotic resistance, from largest to smallest, are termed plasmids, transposons/integrative and conjugative elements, integrons, and insertion sequences.

Plasmids

The largest of the mobilization antibiotic-resistance elements and the first to be appreciated historically are called *plasmids*. Plasmids are extrachromosomal segments of double-stranded DNA and are unique among the antibiotic resistance elements in being able to replicate independent of the bacterial chromosome. The smallest plasmids are less than 1000 bp and contain only the machinery to replicate. Larger plasmids additionally contain the genes for conjugation plus numerous accessory genes. These latter genes are inserted into the plasmid and express resistance to antibiotics and other bacteriocides and virulence factors, but they are unrelated to the replication and conjugative functions of the plasmid. The largest plasmids contain more than 500 accessory genes and approach the size of the bacterial chromosome. A given bacterial isolate can harbor many different plasmids simultaneously. Groups of plasmids containing homologous replicative sequences, however, usually are unable to be maintained in the same bacterial cell. This property has enabled them to be categorized as incompatibility groups, which are designated by lettered or numbered names with the prefix *Inc*. With the definition of many plasmids at the sequence level, some authorities have proposed categorizing them by more precise characteristics such as homology of critical plasmid genes.[440]

Plasmids are transmitted from microorganism to microorganism vertically during bacterial division and horizontally through conjugation. Conjugation of plasmids occurs through binding of the plasmid-encoded relaxase to a sequence called the *origin of transfer (oriT)*. The relaxase carries a single strand of the plasmid to the plasmid-encoded type IV secretion system on the inner surface of the bacterial cell wall. The strand then is transferred to the recipient cell through an ATPase-dependent process, after which the complementary strand is synthesized and the element recircularizes as a double-stranded structure in the new host.[440]

Transposons and Integrative and Conjugative Elements

Transposons are mobile segments of nucleic acid that can transfer from one location to another, such as from different sites on the bacterial chromosome or from a chromosome to a plasmid.[422,426] Transposons do not replicate independently and therefore must be integrated into the chromosome or a plasmid to propagate. Like plasmids, transposons include accessory genes that express antibiotic resistance and other products beneficial to the survival of the host. Movement of transposons is catalyzed by a transposon-encoded integrase[417,427] located upstream from the accessory genes, which excises the segment from the surrounding nucleic acid. The transposon then forms a circularized intermediate before being integrated at an *attachment (att) site* in a different nucleic acid location through the action of the integrase.[417,427]

Some transposons also carry genes that enable them to conjugate. They are included under the broad rubric of mobile genes called *integrative and conjugative elements* (ICEs). In silico analysis of ever-enlarging databases of bacterial whole-genome sequences has revealed that ICEs are very widespread and enormously varied. Although most previously described conjugative transposons exhibited low specificity regarding their insertion site, many ICEs characteristically display a strong preference for insertion into specific conserved loci on the host chromosome, such as the tRNA or the peptide release factor gene.[202,377,472,516] ICEs vary in size between 100 and 500 kb.[202,377] Their accessory genes are preferentially inserted into hot spots within the ICE, which allows integration of new genetic material such as new antibiotic resistance genes with minimal disruption of ICE or host chromosomal function.[377]

BOX 234.1 Cellular Mechanisms of Antibiotic Resistance and Their Transfer

Mechanisms

- Genes that encode enzymes that modify or degrade antibiotics
- Genes that modify the molecular targets for antibiotics
- Genes that code for changes in cell wall channels or active pumping mechanisms

Transfer

- Plasmids: extrachromosomal genetic elements made of circular double-stranded DNA <10 to >400 kb pairs; autonomous and self-reproducing; may be conjugative or nonconjugative
- Transposon/integrative and conjugative elements: mobile genetic elements in the bacterial chromosome or plasmid that confer a recognizable phenotype characteristic; incapable of self-replication
- Integrons: DNA sequences on bacterial chromosome or plasmid often linked to a resistance gene, which facilitate recombination among nonhomologous DNA sequences
- Insertion sequences: small mobile elements that carry no antibiotic resistance genes themselves but may facilitate the activation or mobilization of nearby resistance determinants

ICEs usually do not excise and conjugate unless exposed to some stimulating factor, such as induction of the bacterial SOS stress response to chromosomal DNA damage or through quorum sensing interactions of surrounding bacteria. When conjugation does occur, the mechanism of intercellular transfer in many ICEs is similar to that identified in plasmids—a single strand is bound to an ICE-encoded relaxase attached to an *oriT* sequence, and the complex engages a type IV secretion system for transfer to the recipient cell.[202,516] Some ICEs employ other conjugative machinery, and in some instances, the mechanism of cell-to-cell transfer is unknown.[516]

The organization of ICEs is similar to antibiotic resistance *genetic islands* on the bacterial chromosome found in organisms such as *Acinetobacter* spp., *Salmonella* spp., and *Pseudomonas* spp. Genetic islands are composed of complexes of resistance genes congregated on a single portion of the bacterial chromosome.[377,472] Similar to ICEs, new resistance genes can be inserted into genomic islands with little disruption of chromosomal function.[472] Genomic islands are distinct from ICEs in that they do not include the genetic modules enabling them to conjugate independently. However, many genomic islands include cryptic ICE-like *oriT* sequences that can be recognized by the conjugative machinery of coresident ICEs, which then can promote horizontal transfer of the islands in *trans*. Indeed, genomic islands may be remnants of ICEs that have lost their conjugative functions.

Integrons

The accessory genes on plasmids and transposons are encoded by elements called *integrons*. Integrons are composed of segments of DNA that can capture and excise gene cassettes coding antibiotic-resistance genes. To disseminate, the integron first must insert into a plasmid or transposon.[121,370,392] Integrons contain an integrase that catalyzes the incorporation and excision of the cassette into the integron and a promoter that mediates the expression of the resistance determinant; both are situated 5′ to the cassette. The cassettes are small segments that usually encode a single antibiotic-resistance determinant. Hundreds of antibiotic-resistance cassettes have been characterized.[86,121,370,392] At the 3′ end of each cassette is a variable region called the *cassette attachment (attC) site*, which contains the sequences recognized by the integrase for incorporation of the gene cassette into the integron.[286,392]

Several classes of integrons have been defined based on the sequence of the integrase and their preference for certain transposons. Most antibiotic-resistance integrons belong to class 1.[86,286,392] A single integron may contain multiple antibiotic-resistance cassettes in tandem, all of which are controlled by the single integron promoter. However, transcription of tandem cassettes can terminate prematurely, such that the cassettes closest to the integron promoter are transcribed at the highest level.[370,392]

Insertion Sequences

The smallest elements involved in antibiotic resistance are called *insertion sequences* (ISs).[271] ISs are found in a broad variety of bacterial species. They are less than 2.5 kb and are composed exclusively of an integrase, the enzyme responsible for their insertion into other genetic material, plus terminal inverted repeats on either end. ISs usually are designated numerically (e.g., IS1, IS2).

ISs do not replicate or conjugate independently and do not contain accessory genes, but they can influence antibiotic resistance expression or mobilization in several indirect ways. For example, their insertion can disrupt a regulatory gene that normally suppresses the transcription of an antibiotic resistance determinant.[271,472] In other circumstances, the IS integrase reads through its right-sided terminal sequence and then continues through downstream genes, which sometimes encode antibiotic resistance, before encountering a surrogate termination sequence; excision of the IS mobilizes the accessory gene.[271,472] In addition, two ISs can insert on either side of an antibiotic-resistance gene, resulting in mobilization of the intervening sequence. These structures are called *composite transposons*, although they are structurally distinct from conventional unit transposons.[271,472]

Summary

The importance of mobile resistance genes in promoting the explosive spread of antibiotic resistance cannot be overstated. If each bacterial cell had to develop antibiotic resistance mechanisms independently, the process would be dauntingly inefficient because the likelihood of a particular strain undergoing even two advantageous mutations spontaneously is extremely remote. However, the clustering of antibiotic resistance genes on mobile elements has given bacteria a profound survival advantage in the age of antibiotics by enabling the instant acquisition of multiple, ready-made resistance determinants. In this way, bacteria can become resistant to a host of antibiotics almost immediately after exposure and can efficiently transmit the resistance phenotypes to bacteria coresiding in the same host and to bacteria colonizing or infecting multiple hosts in the same community.

RESISTANCE TO SPECIFIC ANTIBIOTICS

The language of antibiotic resistance includes an ever-increasing array of abbreviations denoting specific resistance determinants. A glossary of the abbreviations of those determinants is provided in Table 234.1.

β-Lactam Antibiotics

The β-lactam antibiotics are a diverse, highly effective family of drugs with broad activity against a wide variety of hospital- and community-acquired pathogens. The β-lactams are composed of four subgroups: penicillins, cephalosporins, monobactams, and carbapenems. Resistance to the β-lactams is mediated by one of two principal mechanisms: production of enzymes capable of hydrolyzing the β-lactam ring and alteration of the target bacterial molecules, the penicillin-binding proteins (PBPs).

β-Lactamase Production

Clinical relevance. The explosive development in antimicrobial therapeutics since the mid-20th century has been driven to a great extent by the impact of β-lactamases in the clinical setting. Shortly after penicillin became incorporated into the clinical armamentarium for the treatment of systemic infections, clinical failures were reported in patients treated for infections caused by *Staphylococcus aureus*. On further analysis, the failures were attributed to penicillinase, an enzyme elaborated and excreted by the bacteria that inactivated the antibiotic before it could produce its clinical effect. This finding led to the development of numerous new antistaphylococcal penicillins (i.e., isoxazolyl penicillins) that were not substrates for the enzyme.

At the same time, a newer class of β-lactam agents, the cephalosporins, was developed. A criterion for moving candidate drugs from this class to the clinic was resistance to inactivation by the penicillinase elaborated

TABLE 234.1 Glossary of Resistance Determinant Abbreviations

Resistance Determinant[a]	Resistance Phenotype
SHV, TEM	Early generation β-lactams
AmpC,* CMY	All β-lactams except cefepime and carbapenems
ESBL[b]	All β-lactams except carbapenems
KPC, OXA	All β-lactams
VIM, NDM, IMP	All β-lactams
mecA	Methicillin resistance in *S. aureus*
erm	Macrolides (MLS$_B$ phenotype)
mef	Macrolides (M phenotype)
dhps, dhfr[c]	Trimethoprim-sulfamethoxazole
AAC, ANP, APH	Aminoglycosides
rmt	Aminoglycosides
van	Glycopeptides
cfr	Linezolid
optrA	Linezolid
mprF	Daptomycin
gyrA, parC** mutations	Fluoroquinolones
micF	Fluoroquinolones
Qnr	Fluoroquinolones
acc(6′)-Ib-cr	Aminoglycosides and fluoroquinolones
OqxAB, QepA	Fluoroquinolones
PmrA/PmrB,* PhoP/PhoQ mutations*	Colistin
*mgrB**	Colistin
mcr-1	Colistin
CAT	Chloramphenicol

[a]Determinants in italics indicate genes; those not italicized indicate proteins. Determinants marked with an asterisk are encoded primarily on the bacterial chromosome; all others are encoded primarily on mobile elements.

[b]Includes late-generation SHV and TEM, CTX-M, and others.

[c]Transmissible mutations of *dhps* conferring sulfonamide resistance in Enterobacteriaceae are designated *sul1, sul2,* and *sul3.*

by staphylococci. Further development of penicillins, cephalosporins, monobactams, and carbapenems was influenced significantly by the recognition that the penicillinase elaborated by staphylococci was representative of a larger class of enzymes that also existed in gram-negative organisms.

As gram-negative organisms such as *Escherichia coli* emerged as important clinical pathogens, their emerging resistance to aminopenicillins on the basis of β-lactamase elaboration spawned the development of a group of enzyme inhibitors, including clavulanic acid,[391] sulbactam, and tazobactam,[8] each of which was structurally a β-lactam that could bind to and inactivate many β-lactamases. As it became necessary to expand the spectrum of the penicillins and cephalosporins to include some of the more itinerant gram-negative organisms (e.g., *Serratia* spp., *Enterobacter* spp., *Pseudomonas* spp.), β-lactamase stability emerged as a necessary attribute for clinical success. This expansion was accomplished through the addition of one of the β-lactamase inhibitors to members of the carboxy and acylureido class of penicillins or through structural engineering, such as that seen in the development of the second- and third-generation cephalosporins and carbapenems.

The inexorable challenges to antimicrobial susceptibility posed by the increasing number and specificity of β-lactamases has driven medicinal chemists to seek newer β-lactamase inhibitors that in combination with effective β-lactam antibiotics preserve their effectiveness in the face of bacterial adaptation.[46,345] The first group of these non–β-lactam β-lactamase inhibitors, the diazabicyclooctananes (DBOs), were synthesized to expand the range of activity of the β-lactamase inhibitors beyond the serine-based, Bush-Jacoby group 2/Ambler class A β-lactamases that were inhibited by clavulanic acid, sulbactam, and tazobactam. The first to reach clinical practice was the tight-binding reversible inhibitor avibactam.[107] This molecule also inhibited serine-based Amp C and carbapenem-hydrolyzing β-lactamases[70,112] (classifications of β-lactamases are described later), none of which were suppressed by the prior inhibitors. This finding was followed by the development of other DBO inhibitors, which are in clinical trials.[345] Simultaneously, a second group of non–β-lactam β-lactamase inhibitors was synthesized, leveraging the known effectiveness of boronic acids against a broad range of serine-based β-lactamases.[160]

Three sentinel clinical events were most responsible for establishing β-lactamase as a prominent clinical problem in pediatric practice. In 1974, the first case of bacterial meningitis caused by ampicillin-resistant *Haemophilus influenzae* type b was reported.[319] This report resulted in marked changes in clinical practice. First, all infants and children with suspected bacterial meningitis were treated empirically with ampicillin and chloramphenicol (i.e., a drug not susceptible to degradation by bacterial β-lactamase) instead of with ampicillin alone. In addition, several newer antibiotics, particularly the second- and third-generation cephalosporins, were evaluated for their efficacy in this clinical setting. From these studies, ceftriaxone or cefotaxime emerged as the drug of choice for the empiric treatment of suspected or proven bacterial meningitis in children. This selection was based on greater potency against *H. influenzae* type b and β-lactamase stability.

The second circumstance resulting in the affirmation of β-lactamase as an important clinical problem in pediatrics was the recognition of *Moraxella catarrhalis,* a β-lactamase–producing organism, as the third leading cause of acute otitis media in infants and children and the emergence of amoxicillin resistance among the nontypeable strains of *H. influenzae.* β-Lactamase production in *H. influenzae* was thought to be particularly associated with therapeutic failure, spawning the development of oral second- and third-generation cephalosporins and newer macrolides as therapeutic alternatives for treating childhood otitis media.

By the early 1980s, β-lactamase–producing bacteria garnered additional attention from pediatricians because of their role as nosocomial pathogens. These bacteria became prominent as children with severe but survivable conditions (e.g., hematologic malignancies, solid organ transplantation) required immunosuppressive therapy and prolonged hospitalization, both of which predisposed children to hospital-acquired infections. With each succeeding decade, the number and variety of β-lactamase–producing, hospital-acquired bacteria increased. By the early 21st century, virtually all nosocomial *S. aureus,* coagulase-negative staphylococci, and enteric and nonenteric gram-negative pathogens elaborated β-lactamase. These organisms commonly encode multiple, distinct β-lactamases and express them simultaneously. Consequently, many bacterial infections currently acquired in the hospital are resistant to all β-lactam agents except for the higher-generation β-lactam–β-lactamase inhibitor combinations, the advanced-generation cephalosporins, or the carbapenems.

Mechanisms of resistance. The β-lactamases constitute a broad array of enzymes that hydrolyze the β-lactam ring of selected antibiotics (Fig. 234.1). Most β-lactamases are structurally similar to the PBPs, and the consensus is that at least some of the β-lactamases were derived evolutionarily from them.[295] β-Lactamases can be identified in gram-positive and gram-negative bacteria. In gram-positive bacteria, the enzyme is secreted into the cell-free environment, whereas in gram-negative organisms, most of the enzyme is confined and concentrated in the periplasmic space between the cell wall and the outer membrane.

More than 2000 β-lactamases have been cataloged,[47,45,194] and doubtless many more exist in nature. The β-lactamases have been categorized according to substrate preference, isoelectric focus, whether they are encoded on the bacterial chromosome or an episome, their ability to be inhibited by clavulanate, and their molecular structure. The molecular classification proposed in the 1980s by Ambler[5] is still widely employed. Based on conserved and distinguishing amino acid motifs, this classification divides the β-lactamases into four classes: A through D. Ambler classes A, C, and D are categorized as serine β-lactamases; their three-dimensional structures are similar, and they all possess a serine-based catalytic site.[348] Ambler class B enzymes, which require a metal cofactor, do not.

The classification system of Bush, Jacoby, and Medeiros, proposed in 1995[48] and updated by Bush and Jacoby in 2010,[47] divides these enzymes into three groups (with subcategories) and principally uses

TABLE 234.2 **Properties of the Major Groups of β-Lactamases**

	Bush-Jacoby Group		
Properties	**1**	**2**	**3**
Ambler class	C	A, D	B
Substrate preference	All but carbapenems	Varies[a]	Varies (carbapenems)
Chromosomal/plasmid	C/P	P	C/P
Distribution	Gram negative	Gram negative or positive	Gram negative or positive
Clavulanate inhibition	No	Yes	No
Inducible[b]	Yes	No	No

[a]Can be divided into subgroups, including penicillinases, cephalosporinases, cloxacillinases, and carbapenemases. Enzymes frequently hydrolyze more than one group of β-lactam.
[b]Indicates that normally repressed β-lactamase production can be induced by β-lactam exposure.
Data from Bush K, Jacoby GA, Medeiros AA. A functional classification scheme for β-lactamases and its correlation with molecular structure. *Antimicrob Agents Chemother.* 1995;39:1211–33.

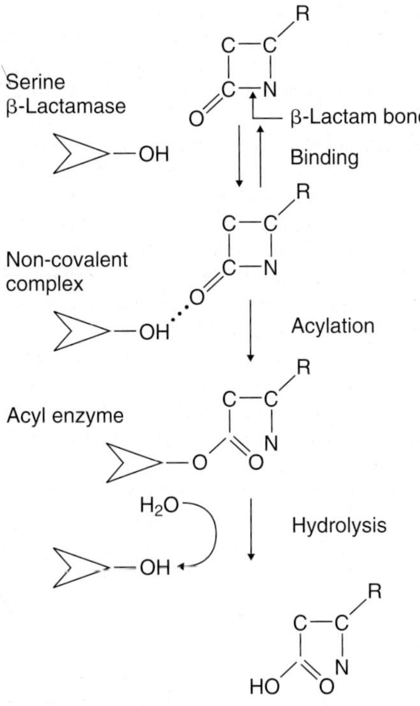

FIG. 234.1 Mode of action of β-lactamases of Ambler classes A, C, and D.

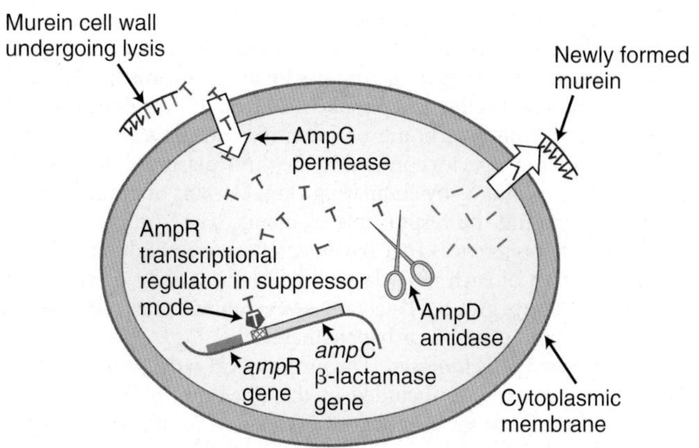

FIG. 234.2 Model for peptidoglycan recycling and β-lactamase induction in enterobacteria. The lytic transglycosylases in the periplasm cleave the bond between *N*-acetylglucosamine (GlcNac) and *N*-acetylmuramic acid (MurNac) and form the peptidoglycan degradation product, *N*-acetylglucosaminyl-1,6-anhydro-*N*-acetylmuramyl-L-alanyl-D-glutamyl-meso-diaminopimelic acid (T). The AmpG permease transports T into the cytoplasm. The AmpD amidase recognizes specifically substrate containing anhydromuramic acid and cleaves the bond between it and L-alanine, releasing the stem tripeptide, L-Ala-D Glu-m-A_2pm (I). Unprocessed T activates the AmpR transcriptional regulator, inducing β-lactamase production. Conversely, the tripeptide (I) recycles to form new peptidoglycan. By regulating the relative amounts of T and I, AmpD can control peptidoglycan composition. The regulatory function of the AmpC β-lactamase, if any, is unknown. (From Medeiros AA. Evolution and dissemination of beta-lactamases accelerated by generations of beta-lactam antibiotics. *Clin Infect Dis.* 1997;24[suppl 1]:S19-S45.)

substrate and inhibitor profiles to classify enzymes in a manner that correlates with their expressed phenotype in clinical isolates. The properties of these groups are described here and outlined in Table 234.2.

Bush-Jacoby group 1 (Ambler class C) AmpC β-lactamases. The group 1 enzymes (i.e., AmpC β-lactamases) hydrolyze virtually all β-lactam antibiotics, although to various degrees. The preferred substrates of AmpC β-lactamases are cephalosporins (including oxyiminocephalosporins), but the enzymes also hydrolyze benzylpenicillins, cephamycins, and monobactams. Hydrolysis rates are low against the fourth-generation cephalosporins (i.e., cefepime and cefpirome) and carbapenems due to low enzyme affinity, and these antibiotics remain therapeutic options.

The AmpC β-lactamases are resistant to inhibition by clavulanate. These enzymes typically are chromosomally encoded on a sequence labeled *amp*C present in a wide range of gram-negative bacteria; however, the AmpC β-lactamases are expressed in quantities sufficient to produce clinically important resistance only in selected species, including *Enterobacter cloacae, Serratia marcescens, Citrobacter freundii, Pseudomonas aeruginosa, Acinetobacter baumannii*, and *Morganella morganii.* In the absence of drug exposure, expression of the group 1 AmpC β-lactamases in these species is repressed by an upstream sequence labeled *amp*R (Fig. 234.2).[295,361] Exposure of the bacteria to a β-lactam leads to the production and intracellular incorporation of a bacterial cell wall metabolite that is processed by the enzyme AmpD.[190,257] In sufficient quantity, the AmpD substrate interacts with *amp*R, reversing the repression, and relevant quantities of the AmpC β-lactamase are thereby synthesized.

β-Lactam antibiotics induce AmpC β-lactamases by this mechanism to different degrees. Ampicillin, cefoxitin, and imipenem are potent inducers, whereas most of the third-generation cephalosporins are weak. However, spontaneous mutations leading to a dysfunctional AmpD enzyme that occur at high frequency in nature result in permanent de-repression of the *amp*C gene, which results in constitutive production of large quantities of the AmpC β-lactamase (see Fig. 234.2). De-repressed organisms are rendered highly resistant after this single mutational step. The third-generation cephalosporins are particularly prone to selecting AmpD mutants, and the clinical emergence of resistant de-repressed isolates during the course of treatment with a third-generation cephalosporin has been documented.[67,218,466]

In organisms lacking or poorly expressing chromosomal AmpC β-lactamase genes, such as *E. coli*, *K. pneumoniae*, and *Proteus mirabilis*, genes mediating AmpC β-lactamase resistance can be acquired by transmissible plasmids that often harbor other antibiotic-resistance determinants. The CMY-2 gene, which is genetically related to the AmpC β-lactamases of *C. freundii*, encodes the most common plasmid-based AmpC (pAmpC) β-lactamase recovered from isolates of human and animal origin. However, several other pAmpC genes are circulating worldwide in gram-negative bacteria, including those encoding FOX, ACT, MIR, DHA, ACC, CFE, and LAT enzymes, all of which have unique origins.[193,260]

Bush-Jacoby group 2 (Ambler class A and D) β-lactamases. The group 2 β-lactamases represent the largest and fastest-growing group of β-lactamases, largely due to the proliferation of newer enzymes with broad substrate specificities (see Table 234.2).[45,47] The group 2 β-lactamases are encoded primarily on mobile genetic elements such as plasmids and transposons.[162,229,349] These elements commonly contain resistance determinants to other antibiotic classes.

The plasmids are stable and frequently are maintained within the bacteria even in the absence of antibiotic pressure. Moreover, they can be transmitted by conjugation from organism to organism and across species, sometimes leading to a plasmid outbreak in a confined environment, such as a nursing home or intensive care unit (ICU), that is caused by different species containing the same plasmid. Alternatively, spread can be facilitated by circulating clonal strains of gram-negative bacteria containing the responsible elements. The group 2 enzymes have substrate preferences that have become increasingly broad with the introduction of each new class of β-lactam antibiotic and can be categorized as early group 2 β-lactamases, extended-spectrum group 2 β-lactamases, and group 2 carbapenemases.

Early group 2 β-lactamases. The prototypical early group 2 Ambler class A β-lactamases are included in the TEM and SHV families of enzymes, although large numbers of early enzymes not belonging to either of these families have been characterized. TEM-1, first identified in Europe in 1963, hydrolyzed ampicillin. During the ensuing decades, the TEM sequence mutated in a stepwise fashion (with each new iteration labeled sequentially: TEM-2, TEM-3, and so on), resulting in the ability of each new enzyme to degrade an ever-increasing number of β-lactam antibiotics.[105,192,295] Many of these mutations widen a critical cavity, formed by the three-dimensional configuration of the molecule, containing the serine-active site at its bottom that is key to hydrolysis of the β-lactam ring.[194]

Extended-spectrum β-lactamases. Of great importance among the group 2 Ambler class A enzymes are the extended-spectrum β-lactamases (ESBLs). ESBL-producing organisms are distributed worldwide, but their incidence varies geographically.[360] Initially, bacteria elaborating ESBLs infected primarily critically ill, hospitalized patients,[350] but these enzymes are being reported in increasing numbers in the community.[304,368]

ESBLs confer a common resistance phenotype, namely, reduced susceptibility to benzylpenicillins, cephalosporins (i.e., first through fourth generation, including oxyiminocephalosporins), and monobactams, but to varying degrees. Susceptibility to the cephamycins and carbapenems is preserved.[350] Common to other group 2 β-lactamases, hydrolytic activity typically is suppressed by the β-lactamase inhibitors.

The first ESBLs were molecular descendants of TEM-1 and SHV-1 and were found in *E. coli*, *K. pneumoniae*, and to a lesser extent, in *P. mirabilis*.[162] Other families of ESBLs have been described.[368] Concomitant with their molecular evolution, ESBLs have been identified in an ever-widening range of bacteria, including *Pseudomonas spp.*, *Acinetobacter spp.*, and multiple species of Enterobacteriaceae.[349]

Among the more important ESBLs are the heterogenous CTX-M family of enzymes, which are particularly active against cefotaxime and are responsible for the current pandemic of ESBL-producing *E. coli* infections.[55] The main contributor to this worldwide dissemination of ESBLs is the multidrug-resistant clone, multilocus sequence type (ST) 131 *E. coli* harboring the CTX-M-15 type ESBL.[14] ST131 *E. coli* are a lineage of extraintestinal pathogenic *E. coli* (ExPEC) and are responsible for a significant proportion of urinary tract and invasive infections worldwide. There are three major ST131 clades (i.e., A through C), which have different mobile genetic elements and recombinations of associated regions. The ST131 clade C strains make up the largest proportion circulating globally, and these strains possess several virulence determinants (i.e., ExPEC-associated genes), including the type 1 fimbriae FimH30 allele, and additional antibiotic resistance determinants, including those conferring resistance to fluoroquinolones.[14,359]

Although most ESBL-producing bacteria are overtly resistant, the third-generation cephalosporins have minimal inhibitory concentrations (MICs) against some ESBL-producing organisms that fall into the high end of the susceptible range. Consequently, the incidence of ESBL-producing bacteria is underestimated when conventional MIC breakpoints for resistance are used. Growing numbers of reports, however, indicate that infections caused by organisms expressing susceptible MICs are clinically unresponsive to the third-generation cephalosporins.[389] Many hospital microbiology laboratories therefore screen all *E. coli*, *Klebsiella*, and *P. mirabilis* clinical isolates for reduced susceptibility to ceftazidime and cefotaxime and alert the clinician accordingly.

The optimal therapy for infection caused by ESBL-producing gram-negative bacteria is not established. However, many authorities recommend a carbapenem for invasive ESBL-producing gram-negative bacterial infections.[194,349,389]

Group 2 carbapenemases. The latter half of the 2000s witnessed the alarming spread of a new set of group 2, Ambler class A β-lactamases composed of carbapenemases, including the enzyme labeled *Klebsiella pneumoniae* carbapenemase (KPC)[33,38,442] and advanced-generation group 2, Ambler class D OXA carbapenemases. This phenomenon has undermined the effectiveness of the class of antibiotics that had become the therapy of choice for previously encountered highly resistant organisms expressing AmpC β-lactamases and ESBLs.

KPC was first identified in an isolate of *K. pneumoniae* in the late 1990s from a patient in North Carolina.[33,442] Because of the presence of KPC on readily transmissible and promiscuous genetic elements, organisms expressing this enzyme spread rapidly up the American Atlantic Coast. By the mid-2000s, KPC-bearing *K. pneumoniae* had caused a city-wide epidemic among hospitalized patients in New York City[380]; soon thereafter, the organisms were discovered throughout the United States (i.e., reported in 48 states and Puerto Rico) and globally.[54,168,314,378] (http://www.cdc.gov/hai/organisms/cre/TrackingCRE.html#CREmapNDM).

Infections by KPC-expressing organisms have been identified primarily in critically ill adults in acute care hospitals[129,148,344] and residents of long-term care facilities,[64,354,515] without a significant representation in community-acquired disease. KPC-harboring organisms have been reported only sporadically in children,[261] but their presence in the pediatric age group may be underappreciated. A survey of resistant-organism colonization in a long-term care facility for neurologically impaired children and young adults in Ohio, for example, revealed an unrecognized high prevalence of KPC colonization among the residents.[489]

Virtually all reports document that infection by a KPC-bearing bacterium is associated with increased risk of death, with crude mortality rates frequently about 40% to 50%.[188,261,447,483] In vitro data and clinical experience with adults have indicated that treatment with at least two agents is better than monotherapy, including regimens containing a carbapenem when the MIC is in the lower range of resistance.[197,384,527]

The KPCs are extraordinarily broad-spectrum enzymes and are able to hydrolyze every class of β-lactam. Like other group 2 β-lactamases, the KPC enzymes have a serine-based active site for hydrolysis of the β-lactam ring. Their broad activity likely is the result of a more shallow position of the catalytic active site within the enzymatic cavity, rendering it more accessible to its antibiotic substrates.[380] Their activity is resistant to most β-lactamase inhibitors; the only commercially available exception is the DBO non–β-lactam β-lactamase inhibitor avibactam.[104] Unfortunately, organisms expressing KPC are almost always multidrug resistant. Tigecycline, colistin, one or more aminoglycosides, and the β-lactam/β-lactamase inhibitor combination of ceftazidime-avibactam are the antibiotics with the most consistent activity,[104,314] although some strains have emerged as resistant to colistin.[25,313]

The KPC family of enzymes is composed of multiple molecularly similar homologues that have been numbered sequentially as they have been discovered and characterized.[227,380] Most disease has been caused by *K. pneumoniae* expressing KPC-2 and KPC-3. Dominant lineages of KPC-producing *K. pneumoniae* have been identified through multilocus sequence typing (MLST). The sequence type ST258 has been an especially prominent clone in the United States.[148,227] ST258 has at least two distinct genetic clades, clade I and clade II. Although clade II is most often associated with KPC-3, clade I typically harbors KPC-2. Depending on KPC gene copy number or mutations in outer-membrane porin channels, the expressed level of carbapenem resistance can vary from susceptible to highly resistant.[62] In any given geographic location, however, organisms expressing KPC can be found in a variety of *K. pneumoniae* sequence types and less frequently in species and genera of Enterobacteriaceae other than *K. pneumoniae,* indicating that KPCs have spread by person-to-person transmission of dominant clones and by bacteria-to-bacteria transmission of enzyme-bearing plasmids.[227,243,283] The means of KPC acquisition in children may be of a more polyclonal epidemiology than adults in the same region.[264,265,454]

The Ambler class D OXA β-lactamases, originally named for their ability to hydrolyze oxacillin, are a diverse group of enzymes that are particularly prominent in *Acinetobacter* and *Pseudomonas* spp.[240] The first carbapenem-hydrolyzing OXA carbapenemase (OXA-23) was recovered from a clinical isolate in Scotland in 1985 before the introduction of carbapenems.[355] The OXA β-lactamases, particularly OXA-23, OXA-48, and OXA-181 variants, can inactivate carbapenems to varying degrees. Their activity is resistant to most β-lactamase inhibitors; the only commercially available exception is β-lactam combination therapy with avibactam.[104] The OXA-carbapenem hydrolyzing enzymes are increasingly identified globally in a broadening array of genera, including those belonging to the Enterobacteriaceae.[47,372] The OXA-48 enzymes, discovered in Turkey in 2001 in *K. pneumoniae*, hydrolyze penicillins at a high level and carbapenems at a low level, while sparing extended-spectrum cephalosporins; however, the coexpression of extended-spectrum β-lactamases results in broad-spectrum hydrolysis of all β-lactams.[57,371,372,374]

Bush-Jacoby group 3 (Ambler class B) metallo-β-lactamases. The group 3 β-lactamases are composed of the metallo-β-lactamases (MBLs) (see Table 234.2).[44,498] MLBs are genetically heterogeneous and structurally dissimilar to the serine β-lactamases. The MBLs are not suppressed by commercially available β-lactamase inhibitors, and the three subclasses (i.e., B1, B2, and B3) have different amino acid sequence homologies. Almost all clinically relevant, acquired MBLs belong to subclass B1. The active site requires the participation of zinc, and MBLs catalyze the hydrolysis of β-lactam drugs through a noncovalent mechanism; the zinc-dependent catalysis is inhibited by chelators such as ethylene diamine tetraacetic acid (EDTA). The active site itself is composed of a wide plastic groove that can accommodate many β-lactam substrates, including carbapenems. Some genes encoding MBLs are chromosomal (e.g., in *Stenotrophomonas*), but many are embedded in complex integrons that are inserted on transferable elements such as transposons and plasmids containing multiple antibiotic resistance genes.[498]

MBLs were originally identified in the middle to late 1980s in *P. aeruginosa*. The landscape dramatically changed in the 1990s and early 2000s with increasing reports of clinical infections and nosocomial outbreaks of gram-negative bacteria (including Enterobacteriaceae) harboring transferable genes encoding MBLs. The IMP (active on imipenem) and VIM (Verona integron encode D) types of MBLs were originally identified in Japan, Italy, and France and since have spread globally. VIM- and IMP-type MBLs continue to be prominent mechanisms of resistance in *A. baumannii* and *P. aeruginosa*.[29,355] Additional transmissible MBL-harboring gram-negative bacilli have remained generally restricted to certain regions (e.g., SPM).[138,380]

In 2008, attention to the MBL-producing Enterobacteriaceae epidemic increased with the discovery of a *K. pneumoniae* containing a new plasmid-borne MBL gene labeled New Delhi metallo-β-lactamase (NDM), identified in a Swedish patient who had previously received health care in India.[235] The introduction into Enterobacteriaceae is thought to have originated from *A. baumannii*. Organisms harboring NDM genes subsequently were identified throughout the Asian subcontinent and the United Kingdom, followed by global dissemination. Bacteria expressing NDM-type MBLs have been identified in patients in all age groups, including children, and in some instances have been the cause of community-associated infection.[235,262] Plasmids carrying NDM-type MBLs are diverse in size and incompatibility group, and as in the case of other acquired carbapenemases, there frequently is concomitant carriage of multiple antibiotic-resistance determinants, including other β-lactamases and carbapenemases, and genes encoding resistance to fluoroquinolones, aminoglycosides, polymyxins, and other antibiotic classes,[326] severely limiting therapeutic options.

For many of the β-lactamases described above, the degree of resistance exhibited by an organism expressing a specific enzyme frequently depends not only on its in vitro substrate specificity and kinetics but also on the amount of enzyme produced. Hyperproduction of β-lactamase usually is the result of some alteration of a controlling sequence or an increase in number of copies of the β-lactamase gene within the bacterium.[134,342,519] High-level resistance results, and the susceptibility of the organism diminishes, with increasing numbers of bacteria. Consequently, the organism may appear clinically unresponsive to a β-lactam antibiotic if hyperproduction occurs in the context of a high-inoculum disease. In some circumstances, hyperproduction operates in concert with other mechanisms to produce a resistant phenotype. For example, some isolates of *E. cloacae* and *P. aeruginosa* have been rendered carbapenem resistant through a combination of hyperproduction of an AmpC β-lactamase, which normally is ineffective in hydrolyzing the carbapenems, and the simultaneous loss of the outer-membrane porin through which carbapenems traverse to reach the PBP.[208,316,379]

Alteration of Penicillin-Binding Proteins

Clinical relevance. Two species of clinical importance to pediatricians express resistance to β-lactam drugs through the alteration of PBPs: penicillin-resistant *Streptococcus pneumoniae* and methicillin-resistant *Staphylococcus aureus* (MRSA). The precise clinical importance of penicillin resistance in *S. pneumoniae* remains unclear. Initially, their emergence was alarming because they frequently exhibited coincident resistance to other antibiotics, particularly trimethoprim-sulfamethoxazole (TMP-SMX) and the macrolides,[93,97,189,395,473] which were commonly used to treat respiratory tract bacterial pathogens. Because the basis for this type of β-lactam resistance is akin to altered enzyme affinity, investigators posited in the mid-1990s that overcoming the apparent decrease in efficacy could be possible by increasing the dose of β-lactam used.[212,288,289] On the basis of pharmacokinetic and pharmacodynamic calculations, it was predicted that a high-dose amoxicillin regimen (for outpatient therapy) or high-dose intravenous penicillin, ampicillin, or ceftriaxone (for inpatient therapy) would be curative in most nonmeningeal infections caused by *S. pneumoniae* with penicillin MICs of 2 to 4 μg/mL or less, well above traditional nonsusceptible breakpoints. This prediction subsequently was confirmed by several observational studies of children with acute otitis media and for adults and children with pneumonia and bacteremia due to nonsusceptible *S. pneumoniae*.[78,212,341,358,366,518,525]

In response to these observations, in 2008, the Clinical Laboratories Standards Institute, the organization responsible for defining susceptible and resistance MIC breakpoints in the United States, raised the penicillin MIC breakpoint designating resistance in nonmeningitis isolates from 2 μg/mL or higher to 8 μg/mL or higher,[66,506] validating and encouraging the use of β-lactams in infections by organisms expressing penicillin MICs beneath the new breakpoint.

In contrast, in patients with pneumococcal meningitis caused by organisms with decreased penicillin susceptibility, there is a delay in sterilization of cerebrospinal fluid in the setting of standard treatment due to the difficulty in delivering drug into the central nervous system.[144,253] The MIC breakpoint defining pneumococcal resistance in meningitis isolates therefore has remained unchanged (>0.12 μg/mL). Moreover, the current recommendations for empiric treatment of bacterial meningitis in infants and children consist of a combination of high-dose ceftriaxone or cefotaxime plus vancomycin[40] until the organism is identified and its antibiotic susceptibility is known.

The challenge of penicillin-resistant *S. pneumoniae* was also addressed by the introduction of the conjugated pneumococcal vaccines, first the 7-valent vaccine (PCV7), which became available in the United States in 2000, and then the 13-valent vaccine (PCV13) in 2010. The serotypes included in the 7-valent vaccine accounted for most of the pneumococci responsible for invasive infection in the United States at that time.[31] Coincidentally, the same serotypes were responsible for most of the penicillin resistance.

Surveys conducted by the Centers for Disease Control and Prevention (CDC) indicated that the incidence of invasive *S. pneumoniae* infection caused by penicillin-resistant strains decreased by more than 50% in the years immediately after the introduction of PCV7.[468] The decrease was most pronounced among children younger than 2 years of age, but the herd immunity created by universal PCV7 immunization resulted in a reduction of pneumococcal infection in all age groups. This benefit was mitigated in part by increases in disease caused by resistant serotypes not included in the vaccine, most notably serotype 19A.[17,180,236] In response to this phenomenon, PCV13 was developed, which included all seven serotypes represented in PCV7 plus six additional serotypes, including 19A, that accounted for most residual invasive and antibiotic-resistant pneumococcal infection encountered during the post-PCV7 era.[346,467]

Surveys conducted in the 5 years after the introduction of PCV13 indicate a further reduction in antibiotic resistance among isolates from invasive and noninvasive disease,[49,210,308,398,475] and most of the benefit resulted from reduction of infection caused by serotype 19A. Although residual resistance has been documented among non-PCV13 strains, no prominent resistant serotype has emerged.[79,90] However, *S. pneumoniae* has proved facile in evading population immunity through serotype replacement,[455] and assessment of the effectiveness of PCV13 in reducing invasive disease and penicillin resistance will need to be monitored throughout its use.

Like penicillin-resistant pneumococcus, the epidemiology of MRSA is fluid and constantly changing.[92,458] Most MRSA isolates have been derived from a finite number of pandemic clones that have emerged in separate waves and have settled in different worldwide geographic regions [92,334,458] A given strain may predominate regionally, only to be subsequently replaced by another. Historically, MRSA was isolated first from hospitalized adult patients in 1961, and through clonal expansion, it became a prominent pathogen among critically ill patients during the ensuing decades. Two additional international clones of hospital-associated MRSAs (HA-MRSAs) emerged in the 1980s. By the early 2000s, more than one half of *S. aureus* infections in patients in ICUs in the United States were caused by MRSA.[436]

Compared with those in adults, MRSA infections occurred relatively infrequently among hospitalized children. In the mid-1990s, however, MRSA infections were identified among otherwise healthy children with no prior contact with hospitals or hospitalized patients, first in Western Australia and soon thereafter in the United States.[163,184] These strains of community-associated MRSA (CA-MRSA) were molecularly distinct from all of the strains of MRSA previously identified in the hospital environment.

By the second decade of the new millennium, CA-MRSA had established a worldwide presence in children and adults.[323] These organisms cause primarily skin and soft tissue infection but occasionally cause bone and joint infection, severe necrotizing pneumonia, and other invasive, deep tissue disease. CA-MRSA infections are especially common in populations inhabiting close quarters and engaging in skin-abrading activities, including athletes participating in competitive sports, military personnel, and prison populations.[503] They increasingly are being identified in patients acquiring the infection in the hospital,[181,375,430] blurring the epidemiologic distinctions that had once characterized HA-MRSA and CA-MRSA lineages.

Several systems have been proposed to categorize the principal MRSA clonal groups to help track their spread. The system established by the CDC is based on *Sma*I macrorestriction patterns of bacterial DNA visualized after separation by pulsed-field gel electrophoresis (PFGE). The PFGE types defined have been labeled USA100 through USA1200.[186,292] Most American CA-MRSAs are included in the USA300 group, with a few derived from the USA400 and USA1100 groups.[226,323] American HA-MRSA strains are derived mostly from the USA100 pulsed-field type.[92,458]

MRSA strains also have been categorized by the MLST technique,[109] which distinguishes bacterial lineages based on polymorphisms found in seven housekeeping genes. Each PFGE type includes multiple MLSTs. MLSTs are catalogued online (http://www.mlst.net), facilitating the publication of new strains and the tracing of established ones across the globe.[92] The frequently encountered American HA-MRSA USA100 isolates belong primarily to MLST sequence type ST5, and the predominant USA300 belongs to ST8, but other MLST types are found within each of these groups of American isolates,[82] and altogether different MLST types of MRSAs dominate in other regions of the world.[85,323] Further strain discrimination is achieved through polymorphisms of the *S. aureus* protein A gene *(spa)*, which similarly are catalogued electronically (http://www.spaserver.ridom.de).

Mechanism of resistance. β-Lactam antibiotics must bind to PBPs to confer their activity, and alteration of the structure of PBPs results in diminished affinity for drug and in antibiotic resistance. The PBPs are a family of molecules on the bacterial cell surface. Although different species possess different numbers of PBPs, they historically have been designated numerically within each species by molecular weight and ordered largest to smallest.[133,153] The molecules also have been categorized by function and sequence,[421] with the high-molecular-mass PBPs (historically named PBP1 and PBP2) responsible for transglycosylation and transpeptidation, the final two steps of peptidoglycan synthesis, and the low-molecular-mass PBPs contributing to cell wall remodeling and cell division.[201,421,529] The β-lactams confer their activity by binding to the transpeptidase domain of the large-molecular-mass PBPs, interrupting peptidoglycan cross-linkage and reducing the tensile strength of the bacterial surface, which results in bacterial cell swelling and death.

Examination of PBP-mediated β-lactam resistance in *S. pneumoniae* and *S. aureus* exemplifies some of the features of this mechanism of resistance. Detailed investigations indicate that penicillin resistance in pneumococci is associated with alternations in PBP1A, 1B, 2A, 2X, and 2B; cephalosporin resistance has been correlated with structural abnormalities in PBP1A, 2A, and 2X.[15,69,142,312] Confirmation that the resistant phenotype is related directly to structural abnormalities in various pneumococcal PBPs has been achieved through transformation experiments.[15,69,142,312] In these studies, penicillin-susceptible strains are converted to penicillin-resistant strains by addition of amplified DNA encoding the putative resistant PBPs. Patterns of PBPs from resistant pneumococci vary considerably from geographic location to location, a finding indicating that PBP-related pneumococcal resistance probably arose independently in various parts of the world.[152]

PBPs from penicillin-resistant *S. pneumoniae* contain blocks of amino acid sequences that are remarkably divergent from those seen in susceptible pneumococci. These sequences are homologous to those encoding for PBPs from other streptococcal species (e.g., *Streptococcus oralis, Streptococcus mitis*), a finding suggesting that the resistant pneumococci contain mosaic PBPs that arose after transformation and recombination of homologous genes from closely related bacteria.[103,151,239] These sequences then developed point mutations that conferred resistance. A similar pattern of resistance blocks of amino acids has been identified in the PBPs of penicillin-resistant *Neisseria gonorrhoeae,* which appear to have originated from other *Neisseria* spp.[153] The degree of resistance conferred by a single mutated PBP is relatively small.[133,142] Acquisition of multiple abnormal PBPs results in incremental resistance and, ultimately, in an organism that can survive routine β-lactam therapy.

In distinction to β-lactam resistance in *S. pneumoniae,* the resistance in MRSA is conferred by the predominance of a single abnormal PBP. Whether associated with the hospital or the community, all isolates of MRSA contain the *mecA* gene, a 2130-bp chromosomal sequence encoding the PBP2A, which has low affinity for β-lactam antibiotics, unlike the other staphylococcal PBPs.[83,84] The *mecA* gene is carried on a mobile element designated the *staphylococcal cassette chromosome mec* (SCC*mec*) sequence. All MRSA strains contain an SSC*mec* complex, but their size and organization vary, allowing them to be grouped into eleven distinct SCC*mec* types, which are designated by roman numerals I through XI.[186,333,530] Most hospital-acquired (HA)-MRSA strains contain SCC*mec* types I to III, whereas CA-MRSA strains characteristically harbor type IV.[186]

In most HA-MRSA isolates, the SCC*mec* sequence contains resistance determinants in addition to *mecA*, including those conferring resistance to clindamycin, the aminoglycosides, and the fluoroquinolones.[89,530] These organisms possess a selective advantage in ICUs, where exposure to multiple classes of antibiotics commonly occurs. The CA-MRSA SCC*mec* type IV encodes a smaller SCC*mec* sequence usually lacking the multiple antibiotic-resistance genes found in their hospital-associated counterparts.[89,530] Although a growing number of American strains of CA-MRSA are emerging resistant to fluoroquinolones and a small but growing number are resistant to clindamycin, only a few CA-MRSA bacteria express resistance to other antibiotics.[291,470] However, USA300 CA-MRSAs express a number of virulence factors not common in other strains. Most notable among these is the Panton-Valentine leukocidin, possibly important for soft tissue breakdown and destruction, but a number of other virulence factors and altered genetic elements called *accessory genetic regulator (agr)* sequences controlling their expression have been identified.[470] The smaller SCC*mec* sequences allow CA-MRSA to replicate more rapidly than HA-MRSA[332] because they can be maintained by the bacterium at a lower metabolic cost. The relatively small size of the CA-MRSA SCC*mec* sequences further enables efficient transfer to co-colonizing susceptible *S. aureus.*[530]

SCC*mec* elements likely originated in coagulase-negative staphylococci. Type IV SCC*mec* sequences, for example, have been identified in isolates of *Staphylococcus epidermidis* from the 1970s.[513] Sequences have been found in *S. epidermidis* and *Staphylococcus hominis* strains that contain the regulatory genes and insertion sequences of the SCC*mec* elements found in MRSA but that lack the *mecA* gene itself.[3]

Macrolides, Lincosamides, and Streptogramins

Clinical Relevance

The macrolides are compounds that contain 14-member (e.g., erythromycin, clarithromycin), 15-member (e.g., azithromycin), or 16-member (e.g., spiramycin) lactone rings. Their activity is directed primarily against gram-positive organisms and some gram-negative respiratory tract pathogens. In many bacteria, resistance to macrolides occurs concomitantly with that of the structurally unrelated lincosamides (including clindamycin) and streptogramin B families of antibiotics, two classes with activity primarily against gram-positive bacteria. Because these three families of antibiotics interact competitively for ribosomal binding, they probably are associated with the same ribosomal site.

Resistance to the macrolides was identified in staphylococcal species soon after the introduction of erythromycin. More recently, macrolide resistance in streptococcal pathogens, particularly *S. pneumoniae* and *Streptococcus pyogenes,* emerged and assumed major clinical importance. Macrolide resistance among pneumococci is a result of international dissemination of resistant clones and horizontal transmission of resistance determinants.[131,416]

The late 20th century witnessed dramatic increases in the incidence of macrolide resistance in *S. pneumoniae* in many areas of the world.[167] In Southeast Asia, surveys indicated that almost 40% of pneumococcal isolates were resistant to all macrolide antibiotics, and samplings of organisms from Europe and the Western Hemisphere showed similar but less extreme trends.[167,224] Perhaps most troubling, resistance to macrolides among pneumococci occurred frequently in isolates coexpressing resistance to penicillin and other oral antibiotics.[97,185]

Similar to penicillin-resistant pneumococcus, the prevalence of macrolide-resistant *S. pneumoniae* was reduced during the first decade of the 21st century by the introduction and widespread administration of the conjugated pneumococcal vaccines, which include serotypes that most commonly express β-lactam and macrolide resistance.[474] Studies performed in Atlanta, Georgia, before release of the 7-valent vaccine, for example, documented that 31% of pneumococcal isolates causing invasive disease were resistant to erythromycin.[130] Follow-up studies performed after the introduction of that vaccine recorded a drop in incidence of macrolide-resistant invasive pneumococcal disease by more than two thirds.[450]

Similar to *S. pneumoniae,* macrolide resistance in *S. pyogenes* has been unevenly distributed geographically.[217] By the start of the 21st century, most surveys in the Western Hemisphere, including the United States, indicated a prevalence of resistance less than 10%.[143,340,399,508] Macrolide resistance in *S. pyogenes* is on average more prevalent in Europe, but the prevalence there also varies substantially from area to area, ranging in the mid-2000s from 3% in Norway[258] to 13% in Belgium[272] and to more than 20% in Spain and France.[24,356] Molecular analysis of macrolide-resistant group A streptococcal isolates from geographically diverse regions suggested that the resistance genes were acquired multiple times by many lineages, some of which then disseminated worldwide.[404]

The increase in macrolide resistance has occurred concomitant with increased worldwide consumption of these compounds for respiratory tract infections beginning in the 1980s,[22,68,185,429] a finding suggesting a biologic association between these two phenomena. A nationwide survey of macrolide susceptibility among pneumococcal isolates in the United States, for example, documented an increase in erythromycin resistance from 10.6% in 1995 to 20.4% in 1999, a time when the number of prescriptions for macrolides increased by 13% across the board and by 320% for pediatric patients.[185] Seppälä and colleagues[429] reported an increase in resistance among *S. pyogenes* isolates in Finland from 5% in 1988 to 13% in 1990 after national macrolide consumption doubled during the 1980s. In response, a national campaign to reduce macrolide prescribing practices in Finland was launched in the early 1990s, after which macrolide resistance fell by one half.[429] A similar campaign in Taiwan yielded similar results.[179]

Although the epidemiologic trends in macrolide resistance are alarming, the clinical consequences of the increases in macrolide resistance among streptococci are largely unknown. The newer macrolide compounds achieve tissue and intracellular concentrations that are much higher than the recommended MIC breakpoints.[110,328] Italian investigators, for example, reported a very high incidence of erythromycin resistance among group A streptococcal throat isolates, but neither clinical nor microbiologic failures were clearly associated with macrolide treatment.[488] The macrolides do not distribute in high concentrations to the blood compartment, however, and several reports document poor outcomes when this class of drugs is used for bacteremic pneumonia caused by macrolide-resistant pneumococcus.[223,268]

Despite these apparent shortcomings, the macrolides remain an attractive group of drugs because of their activity against atypical organisms and their safety profiles. As such, they have continued to attract the attention of the medicinal chemists. The second-generation drugs clarithromycin and azithromycin were introduced to overcome some of the resistance issues.[428] They were followed by the short-lived introduction of the ketolides, telithromycin and cethromycin, which have not been thoroughly evaluated for pediatric patients but do confer resistance protection through their binding to a second ribosomal site, which renders them effective against organisms resistant to first- and second-generation macrolides.[116,434]

Further structural engineering led to the synthesis and clinical evaluation of solithromycin, the first of the fluoroketolides.[117] Its introduction addressed a number of deficiencies of its predecessors, including a pharmacokinetic profile that provides antimicrobially significant concentrations of drug in plasma, tissues, and intracellularly and a pharmacodynamic profile that precludes many of the limiting side effects that hampered the earlier ketolides. It also has a third ribosomal binding site determined by the fluorine domain that ensures activity against organisms resistant to other macrolide antibiotics.

Mechanism of Resistance

Two principal resistance phenotypes to macrolides and related antibiotics have been detected. The first, the MLS_B phenotype, is characterized by resistance to all macrolides, regardless of the size of the ring, and to the lincosamides and the type B streptogramins. Most organisms expressing the MLS_B phenotype remain susceptible to the combination streptogramins.[154,424] The second phenotype, the M phenotype, is associated with resistance to the 14- and 15-member macrolides (including erythromycin, azithromycin, and clarithromycin) but not those with 16-member rings. The degree of resistance to the affected macrolides is lower on average than that seen with MLS_B resistance. In organisms with the M phenotype, susceptibility to clindamycin is preserved.[284,460]

Most MLS_B resistance results from methylation of the 23S ribosomal RNA (rRNA) in the 50S subunit of the bacterial ribosome within the peptidyltransferase circle in domain V.[88,196,469,509] The methylases are encoded on transposons, with sequences found on plasmids and in the bacterial chromosome.[137] Methylation of the 23S rRNA is encoded by a family of related genes called *erm* (i.e., *e*rythromycin *r*esistance methylases).[88,196,469,509] Historically, these methylases have been described and named in a haphazard fashion, although some investigators have proposed renaming many of the enzymes using a classification scheme based on genetic homology.[401]

Methylation is both inducible and constitutively expressed. Unlike many other inducible antibiotic-resistance factors, the mechanism of MLS_B resistance induction is at the level of translation rather than transcription.[507] In the uninduced state, the leader sequence of the mRNA encoding ErmC, one of the methylases found in *S. aureus,* forms two stem loop structures that stall the ribosome's movement along the message, thereby preventing synthesis of the methylase enzyme. The attachment of erythromycin to the ribosome leads to a conformational alternation of the leader sequence that uncovers the appropriate ribosomal binding sites and allows the stalled ribosomes to proceed to translation.[507]

Inducible macrolide resistance is detected in the clinical microbiology laboratory by the double-disk diffusion test (D test). In this assay, an erythromycin disk and a clindamycin disk are placed side by side on a lawn of the test organism. Induction of clindamycin resistance in the presence of erythromycin manifests by increased growth of bacteria on the erythromycin side of the clindamycin disk, producing a D-shaped zone of inhibition. Through the 1990s, greater numbers of *erm*-containing bacteria produced the rRNA methylase constitutively, a consequence of mutation of the leader sequence.[99,465]

In the mid-1990s, macrolide resistance mediated through a genetically transferable efflux pump was identified.[460] Most organisms expressing the M phenotype are resistant through this mechanism. Most macrolide-resistant pneumococci in North America express the macrolide efflux pump, and much of the expansion of macrolide resistance that occurred through the 1990s was the result of the appearance of organisms exhibiting this mechanism.[185,204,256,468] A family of related genes *(mef)* encodes the macrolide efflux pumps. The *mef* genes are included on transposons encoding associated functions, particularly an adenosine triphosphate (ATP)–binding protein.[130,131,137,284] As expected, ribosomes isolated from organisms resistant through *mef* genes bind to macrolide antibiotics as readily as do ribosomes from susceptible organisms. Radiolabeled erythromycin is excluded from the intracellular space in *mef*-positive bacteria, a phenomenon that is reversed by compounds that poison ATP-dependent pumps.[460]

Mechanisms of macrolide resistance besides rRNA methylation and efflux pumps have been identified but are uncommon. Some organisms modify the antibiotic by hydrolysis, acetylation, phosphorylation, or esterification.[401] Some evidence indicates that some erythromycin resistance is caused by altered ribosomal proteins and results in the production of ribosomes with diminished affinity for drug.[65]

Trimethoprim and Sulfamethoxazole

Clinical Relevance

The combination antibiotic TMP-SMX inhibits bacterial folate synthesis at two successive steps. This mechanism accounted for its broad activity against a wide variety of gram-positive and gram-negative bacteria when it was first introduced in 1968. Despite the dual activity of this combination, resistance to TMP-SMX has risen steadily during the decades of its use and is now common. Acquisition of resistance is potentiated by recent exposure to TMP-SMX.[115,449,517] When resistance occurs, the MIC expressed usually is very high,[183,182] and the affected organisms frequently are coresistant to multiple other classes of antibiotics.

TMP-SMX resistance is sufficiently widespread that it precludes the use of the drug as a first-line antibiotic in clinical circumstances in which it was formerly the agent of choice, such as respiratory tract infections and *Shigella*-associated dysentery. Its utility in urinary tract infection (UTI) also may be limited when the community prevalence of TMP-SMX resistance is sufficiently high. Ironically, its continued activity against CA-MRSA has rejuvenated the use of TMP-SMX among many practitioners as the incidence of infections caused by CA-MRSA organisms has mushroomed.

Respiratory tract infections: otitis media and pneumonia. The frequency of TMP-SMX resistance in organisms causing respiratory tract infections has increased significantly. Among *S. pneumoniae* organisms, resistance to TMP-SMX was identified during the 1990s in many geographic locations, with resistance detected in 12% to more than 50% of isolates.[97,167,178,189,277,347,456] A worldwide survey conducted in the late 1990s found the highest incidence of TMP-SMX pneumococcal resistance in the Asian Pacific region and in Latin America.[167] In surveys of US isolates, TMP-SMX resistance is the most common resistance phenotype found in *S. pneumoniae,*[511] although the incidence of resistance varies widely from region to region.[96]

TMP-SMX resistance is strongly associated with resistance to other classes of antibiotics commonly used in respiratory tract infections, particularly penicillin and the macrolides. Among other organisms implicated in respiratory tract infections, TMP-SMX resistance also has been documented with increasing frequency in *H. influenzae,* to which resistance ranges from 7% in Finland[277] to more than 50% in Taiwan.[178] The susceptibility of *M. catarrhalis* to TMP-SMX varies little from region to region. Although most *M. catarrhalis* organisms remain susceptible to TMP-SMX, the MICs cluster near achievable respiratory tract concentrations.[189]

The clinical consequences of TMP-SMX resistance in respiratory tract pathogens are not well defined. For example, direct evidence of the association between isolation of a TMP-SMX–resistant organism from the middle ear and failure of therapy by TMP-SMX in acute otitis media is lacking, but the association is assumed to exist. The issue of the clinical relevance of TMP-SMX resistance in respiratory tract infections is particularly pressing in developing countries, where World Health Organization (WHO) guidelines recommend TMP-SMX as a first-line agent for pneumonia. A comparison of amoxicillin and TMP-SMX for treating pneumonia in Pakistan demonstrated superiority of amoxicillin in producing clinical cure, but treatment failure was not associated with resistance in the infecting organism.[457] These data and others[220,390,406] support the continued use of TMP-SMX therapy of pneumonia in the developing world.

Shigellosis. Resistance of *Shigella* spp. to TMP-SMX rose dramatically during the 1980s in many parts of the world, including Bangladesh,[21] Thailand,[169] Somalia,[58] Israel,[10] and Canada.[156] In these surveys, the incidence of disease from TMP-SMX–resistant *Shigella* increased twofold to threefold, accounting for more than one half of the isolates. By 1998, more than 90% of *Shigella* organisms in Thailand[169] and *Shigella* cultured from patients with acquired immunodeficiency syndrome (AIDS) in Kenya[234] were resistant to TMP-SMX. Many of these *Shigella* organisms express extraordinarily high levels of resistance, with MICs to TMP exceeding 1000 μg/mL.

In the United States, TMP-SMX resistance among *Shigella* isolates initially was confined to closed populations.[144] A survey in Oregon, however, indicated that by the late 1990s the incidence of TMP-SMX resistance among *Shigella* isolates in that state approached 60%. Resistant isolates were found disproportionately frequently in migrant workers traveling from Mexico and other areas of Latin America,[396] a finding emphasizing the importance of geographic spread of resistance in modern society. Subsequent surveys performed by the CDC in the early 2000s revealed that TMP-SMX–resistant *Shigella* had spread nationwide, with the prevalence highest in the East and West.[438] The incidence of TMP-SMX resistance in *Shigella* mirrors the increased TMP-SMX resistance among other enteric species,[144] notably *Salmonella.*[1]

TMP-SMX resistance in *Shigella* is virtually always borne on conjugative plasmids, and these plasmids frequently contain resistance determinants to several other antibiotic classes.[58,144,234,254,438,485] Coresistance to four or more unrelated antibiotics, including β-lactams, chloramphenicol, tetracycline, and the aminoglycosides, is a common finding. Molecular analyses in a given geographic environment usually indicate fluid epidemiology, with multiple dominant chromosomal genotypes containing a variety of resistance plasmids.[37,254]

Urinary tract infections. Through the 1990s and 2000s, TMP-SMX resistance in urinary tract isolates of *E. coli,* the most prominent pathogen implicated in UTIs, rose to between 15% and 25% in the developed world and to as high as 60% in nonindustrialized countries.[147,149,216,275,532,533] Studies in the 1980s indicated that TMP-SMX–resistant *E. coli* can be transmitted to household contacts.[408] Although urinary concentrations of TMP and SMX are several-fold higher than concomitant concentrations in serum, resistance to TMP-SMX nonetheless is associated with treatment failure in UTIs. Bacterial and clinical response rates to TMP-SMX are 80% to 95% for cystitis and pyelonephritis caused by susceptible organisms, but the response falls to approximately 50% when the infecting agent is resistant to TMP-SMX.[287,463]

Considering all urinary tract pathogens together, the clinical and microbiologic response to TMP-SMX is almost equivalent to comparator agents, and most experts continue to recommend this drug as a first-line therapy for uncomplicated UTIs based on its low cost.[118,147,175] Analyses have indicated that the total expense of treatment of UTIs with TMP-SMX begins to exceed that incurred by therapy with more expensive antibiotics when the community TMP-SMX–resistance rates of urinary pathogens exceed approximately 20% as a result of the additional expense of clinical treatment failure.[242,463] Alternatives to TMP-SMX also should be considered when the patient possesses risk factors for acquisition of infection with a TMP-SMX–resistant strain, such as recent hospitalization, diabetes, or therapy with TMP-SMX within the previous 3 months.[146,175]

***Community-associated methicillin-resistant* Staphylococcus aureus.** Despite the explosive emergence of methicillin resistance in community-associated *S. aureus* infections in the latter half of the 1990s, these organisms have remained almost uniformly susceptible to TMP-SMX.[39,211,309] Most infections caused by CA-MRSA are skin and soft tissue infections that can be treated without hospitalization, and TMP-SMX offers an inexpensive, oral therapeutic option in this setting. The clinical effectiveness of TMP-SMX in CA-MRSA infection relative to other oral agents is uncertain; whether any antibiotic is superior to incision and drainage, particularly in mild cases, is not clear.[302,386,451] Accumulated reports, however, support the use of TMP-SMX as a therapeutic option for purulent cellulitis when CA-MRSA is suspected or confirmed.[300,451,462]

Mechanisms of Resistance

In susceptible bacteria, TMP-SMX inhibits sequential steps in the de novo synthesis of folate (Fig. 234.3). SMX inhibits the enzyme dihydropteroate synthetase (DHPS), which catalyzes the conversion of *para*-aminobenzoic acid to dihydrofolate. TMP inhibits the next enzyme in the pathway, dihydrofolate reductase (DHFR), which catalyzes the conversion of dihydrofolate to tetrahydrofolate. The resulting depletion of folate in the bacterium interrupts the synthesis of critical cellular substrates, including purine nucleotides.[405] Eukaryotic DHFR is resistant to the activity of the sulfonamides, and eukaryotic cells do not express DHPS activity at all, accounting for the selective activity of these drugs against bacteria.[182,183,405]

The principal mechanism of resistance to TMP-SMX is alteration of the target enzymes. Altered genes for DHFR with reduced susceptibility to TMP have been identified on the chromosomes of intrinsically resistant organisms from a variety of species[367] and on mobile elements. Many of the transferable resistance genes are encoded on transposons that can shuttle between plasmids and chromosomal DNA. Approximately 20 mobile *dhfr* resistance genes have been identified.[183] Resistance usually is conferred by a single-point mutation that results in a disruption of the three-dimensional conformation of DHFR, thereby interrupting a hydrogen bond normally available for binding the antibiotic but leaving the affinity for its natural substrate intact.[81,183,367] These structural changes can occur in concert with mutations of controlling sequences and lead to overproduction of the altered DHFR.[367] Similarly, sulfonamide resistance usually is the result of mutated *dhps* genes. Transmissible mutations of *dhps* conferring sulfonamide resistance in Enterobactgeriaceae have been designated *sul1*, *sul2*, and *sul3*.

In TMP-SMX–resistant *Neisseria meningitidis,* the abnormal chromosomal *dhps* sequence is different compared with that found in susceptible isolates over a large portion of the gene, a finding implying that resistance resulted from a recombination event after horizontal transfer from an unrelated *Neisseria* spp.[385] Similar recombination events may account for sulfonamide resistance in pneumococcus. In other species, the abnormal *dhps* gene is the result of a single amino acid mutation, and the resistance gene is encoded on a conjugative transposon,[339] which frequently is linked to a *dhfr* resistance gene.[183]

Some organisms, particularly *P. aeruginosa,* are intrinsically resistant to TMP-SMX on the basis of the expression of multidrug efflux pumps.[230] The same pumps are responsible for resistance to a wide variety of other antibiotics, including fluoroquinolones, chloramphenicol, and β-lactams. Homologous pumps occasionally have been identified in other gram-negative species. In some isolates, the mechanism of resistance

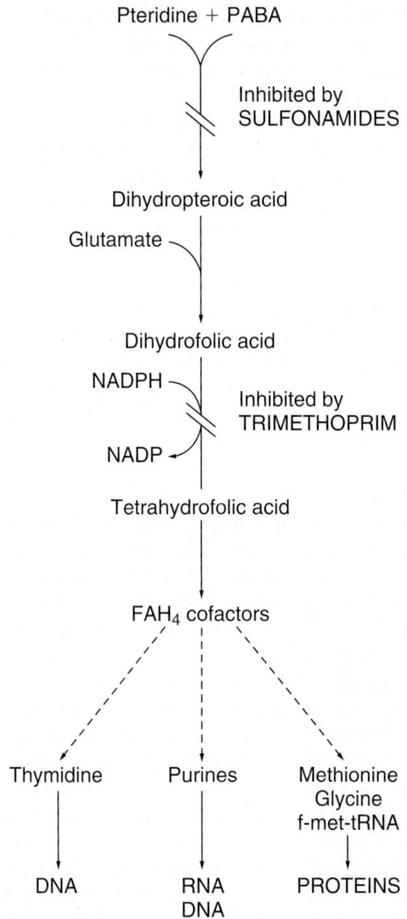

FIG. 234.3 Trimethoprim-sulfamethoxazole inhibition of de novo folate synthesis. *NADP,* Nicotinamide adenine dinucleotide phosphate; *NADPH,* reduced form of nicotinamide adenine dinucleotide phosphate; *PABA,* *para*-aminobenzoic acid.

to TMP-SMX is not attributable to any of those previously listed and remains undefined.[339]

Aminoglycosides

Clinical Relevance

The aminoglycosides are parenteral antibiotics that are employed primarily for serious infections in hospitalized patients. Resistance to aminoglycosides is encoded on transmissible elements that have disseminated throughout the world among gram-negative and gram-positive pathogens. Among gram-negative species, resistance to the aminoglycosides varies widely according to geographic location,[423,487] but it is especially prevalent among hospital-acquired bacteria that are multidrug resistant.[13,207,310]

Surveys of international hospital isolates conducted throughout Europe and North America in the late 1990s and the first decades of the 2000s indicated resistance rates of 1% to 15% for enteric bacilli and 10% to 50% for non–lactose fermenters.[28,120,164,207,299,321,412,423] In most cases, the incidence of resistance was lowest to amikacin. Few data exist for the endemic incidence of aminoglycoside resistance in gram-negative organisms specifically among hospitalized children. However, outbreaks caused by gram-negative rods resistant to aminoglycoside have been reported from numerous neonatal ICUs since the early 1980s.[71,293,419] Not surprisingly, fecal colonization with aminoglycoside-resistant bacilli is an uncommon finding among healthy persons.[248,335,381]

Although the aminoglycosides have no utility in the treatment of infections with gram-positive organisms when used alone, they improve bacterial killing in vitro when they are employed in combination with cell wall–active agents. For this reason, these drugs frequently are added to β-lactam agents or vancomycin in the treatment of difficult or persistent infections caused by *S. aureus,* coagulase-negative staphylococci, or enterococci. However, resistance to aminoglycosides has been documented in all these gram-positive microorganisms. Surveys in Europe indicated 20% to 30% resistance to aminoglycosides among hospital isolates of *S. aureus*.[423] The occurrence of aminoglycoside resistance is much higher among MRSA isolates than in bacteria that are methicillin susceptible.[87,120] Aminoglycoside resistance in hospital acquired coagulase-negative staphylococci also is a common finding.[95,228,423]

Since the 1970s, proliferation of enterococci that express MICs to the aminoglycosides exceeding 2000 μg/mL has occurred, rendering the organisms resistant to all synergistic effects when the aminoglycosides are used with a cell wall–active agent.[108,351] Such high-level aminoglycoside resistance has been recorded in approximately 30% of enterococcal samples from hospitals throughout the world.[269,528] Organisms expressing high-level aminoglycoside resistance frequently also test highly resistant to ampicillin.[351] High-level aminoglycoside resistance is a common finding in vancomycin-resistant enterococci, especially those identified in the United States.[269]

Mechanism of Resistance

The aminoglycosides are hydrophilic sugars composed of one to four rings, with amino groups substituting some of the hydroxyl groups at sites that vary from drug to drug. The amino groups render the drugs polycationic and allow them to bind with high affinity to selected sequences of nucleic acid.[394] The antibacterial activity of these drugs results from their binding to the A-site on the 16S ribosomal RNA responsible for the matching of tRNA and mRNA in the process of protein synthesis. Interaction with aminoglycosides results in a conformational change of the ribosome that results in diminished proofreading and missense translation.[19,233,388,394] The affinity of the aminoglycosides for ribosomal RNA is 10-fold higher in prokaryotes than in eukaryotes.[393]

The principal mechanism of resistance to the aminoglycosides is through the expression of aminoglycoside-modifying enzymes.[19,388] The modifications conferred by these enzymes result in altered electrostatic qualities of the antibiotic and consequent reduced ability to interact with rRNA. Many of these enzymes are encoded on transposons that reside in plasmids along with other resistance determinates.

Three groups of modifying enzymes have been identified: acetyltransferases (AAC), nucleotidyltransferases (ANT), and phosphotransferases (APH), each of which adds its respective moieties to selected side groups of the aminoglycoside sugar rings (Fig. 234.4).[19,233,388,432] Most members of each group of modifying enzymes share structural homologies, with minor amino acid variations resulting in specific substrate profiles.[432]

In the most commonly used nomenclature scheme, the enzymes are designated by the site they modify, by the resistance profile they confer, and by a lowercase letter identifying the specific enzyme within each group.[19,388] For example, AAC(6′)-IIa denotes an AAC that substitutes an acetyl group for the amino group at the 6′ site of the aminoglycoside, with a resulting resistance pattern II (including resistance to gentamicin, tobramycin, and sisomicin but not amikacin in this case); the letter *a* at the end denotes the specific enzyme within the group of AAC(6′)-II molecules. Several enzymes within the AAC(6′) group in particular have formed fusion proteins with other aminoglycoside-modifying enzymes through recombination events[388]; AAC(6′)-Ie-APH(2″)-Ia, for example, expresses AAC and APH activity. In the mid-2000s, a plasmid-borne AAC enzyme (i.e., AAC[6′]-Ib-cr) was characterized that could acetylate moieties on ciprofloxacin and norfloxacin as well as on aminoglycosides.[403] Although the degree of fluoroquinolone resistance conferred by this enzyme is small, coexpression of other quinolone resistance determinants results in clinically relevant reduction in susceptibility.[403]

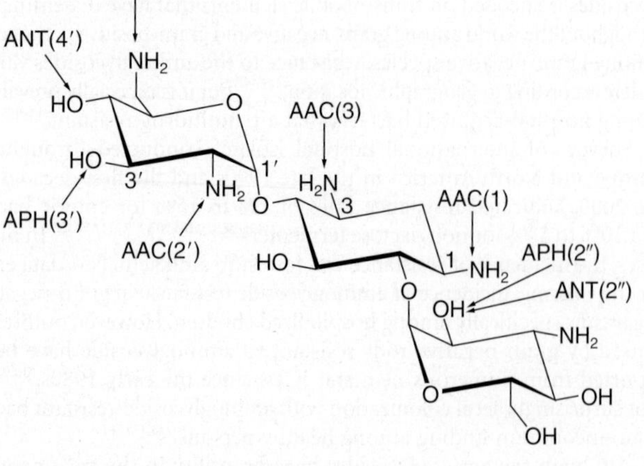

FIG. 234.4 Sites of modification on kanamycin B by various aminoglycoside-modifying enzymes. The *arrows* point to the sites of modification by the specific enzymes acetyltransferases (AAC), phosphotransferases (APH), and nucleotidyltransferases (ANT).

In the early 2000s, acquired 16S ribosomal RNA methyltransferases were discovered that interfered with the binding of aminoglycosides to the A-site, resulting in high-level resistance.[98] Two families of 16S rRNA methylases are defined. The N7-G1405 16S-RMTases have multiple subcategories and confer resistance to gentamicin, tobramycin, and amikacin but not to neomycin. The less frequently encountered N1-A1408 16-RMTase confers resistance to all aminoglycosides. These methylases have been identified in a wide variety of enteric and nonenteric gram-negative pathogens. They characteristically coreside on mobile elements encoding multiple other resistance determinants, including the ESBL, KPC, and especially NDM broad spectrum β-lactamases.[164] The 16S rRNA methylases have been found in isolates from around the globe, but they appear to be most frequently encountered in Southern and East Asia; their epidemiologic impact is not fully defined.[98,164,376]

Moderate-level resistance to the aminoglycosides has been achieved by some bacteria through decreased intracellular concentration of drug by reduced permeability of the cell membrane or efflux.[19,303] These mechanisms have been identified most frequently in *Pseudomonas* spp. Mutations of ribosomal proteins also have been associated with aminoglycoside resistance.[19,388] Modifications of the ribosomal A-site binding sequences have been identified only rarely as a mechanism of resistance to aminoglycosides.[19] The sequences involved in aminoglycoside binding likely are sufficiently critical to the survival of the organism that mutations within this site usually are fatal.[233]

Glycopeptides

Clinical Relevance

Vancomycin is one of two glycopeptides available for clinical use. The second, teicoplanin, is licensed in Europe but not the United States. Since the late 1980s, the prevalence of vancomycin resistance in organisms belonging to the genus *Enterococcus* (i.e., vancomycin-resistant enterococci [VREs]) has risen alarmingly. VREs frequently are highly resistant to many other antibiotics.

VREs appeared coincident with an increased use of vancomycin in the United States and the use of the glycopeptide avoparcin as a growth promoter in animal feed in Europe, a practice banned by the European Union in 1997.[315] The incidence of VREs colonization and disease is much more prevalent in the United States than in other areas of the world,[94,269] but these organisms occur globally.[177,512] Between 10% and 20% of US enterococcal isolates investigated in surveys in the late 1990s and early 2000s were resistant to vancomycin.[94,269] Disproportionate numbers of VREs in the United States are found in patients hospitalized in ICUs in large urban medical centers, especially people with prolonged hospitalizations and severe disease.[159,270,433] A high incidence of VREs is seen among oncology patients,[282] transplant recipients,[106,294] and those with chronic renal failure who are receiving dialysis.[11,471,492] Some surveys have documented VREs among adults in chronic care facilities, who exported the organism into the community after acquisition in an acute care setting.[478] In contrast, the prevalence of VREs is relatively low in US hospitals serving rural areas.[453]

Surveys of European centers also indicate a concentration of VREs in ICUs, although in smaller numbers compared with the United States.[413,425] The occurrence of VREs in Europe varies widely from country to country. In 2010, the proportion of blood isolates of *E. faecium* that were resistant to vancomycin ranged from 0% in Sweden and Finland to more than 20% in Portugal, Greece, and Ireland.[59] VREs also have been reported in Asia and Latin America but at rates approximately one half of those found in the United States.[59]

The genetic machinery conferring vancomycin resistance in enterococci is complex, and resistance does not develop de novo by spontaneous mutation under antibiotic pressure.[315] The initial event in the appearance of VREs in a given unit is the importation of the resistant organism into the environment. The association between antecedent treatment with vancomycin and acquisition of VREs has been documented by many[123,433] but not all investigators.[56,101] Some researchers have established a stronger connection between the appearance of VREs and the use of extended-spectrum cephalosporins[30,337] and antibiotics with potent antianaerobic activity,[100,270] but it is likely that exposure to any broad-spectrum antimicrobial increases the risk of VREs acquisition.[301]

Horizontal transmission of VREs is prominent in any closed environment and may outweigh antecedent antibiotic exposure as the principal determinant for acquisition.[30,159] Patient-to-patient spread in an ICU, presumably through the hands of caregivers, has been documented repeatedly, as has contamination of the immediate environment of the VRE-positive patient.[301,337,439] The most significant risk factor for acquisition of a VRE may be the number of neighboring patients colonized with the organism at the same time.[12,30]

In many American ICUs, multiple clones of VREs are present at any given time. Some are imported into the unit, and others spread after admission has occurred,[337] rendering control and containment difficult to achieve. Extreme barrier isolation precautions, including surveillance for VREs on admission to a unit, single-room isolation with dedicated medical instruments, and strict use of gowns and gloves, frequently are necessary to contain a VRE after it has established an endemic presence, and even these measures may not be entirely effective.[199,238,439]

With some exceptions,[141,482] VREs have been less of a threat to pediatric patients than to adults, despite the wide use of vancomycin among hospitalized pediatric patients and their geographic proximity in many hospitals to sick adults colonized with the organism. Several VRE outbreaks in the newborn nursery have been reported,[245,273] but they have resulted primarily from dissemination of a single clone within the unit and have been successfully eradicated with implementation of relatively simple barrier isolation and cohorting measures.

In the latter half of the 1990s, a second phenomenon involving reduced susceptibility to vancomycin was identified: vancomycin-intermediate *S. aureus* (VISA).[122,443] These organisms express MICs to vancomycin in the intermediate range of approximately 8 μg/mL. Virtually all of these isolates are coresistant to methicillin, but several have retained susceptibility to numerous other antimicrobial agents. VISA isolates have been identified primarily in patients who have been treated with prolonged courses of vancomycin for MRSA infection. Disproportionate numbers of these patients have been undergoing dialysis.[443] Cure of the VISA-infected patient has been difficult but achievable with high doses of vancomycin in combination with other antibiotics.[122,443]

In 2002, the first two cases of true vancomycin-resistant *S. aureus* (VRSA) in the United States were reported, one from Michigan and the other from Pennsylvania (MICs to vancomycin were >128 μg/mL and 32 μg/mL, respectively).[255] Both patients were suffering from chronic foot ulcers, from which the organisms were isolated. In both instances, the bacteria were susceptible to alternative agents, and the patients remained clinically stable. The potential for VRSA to emerge as a major public health hazard is substantial, but subsequent cases have been rare.[255,499] Almost all VRSA organisms have been derived from MRSA lineages associated with hospital-acquired strains, particularly USA100, but in contrast to other HA-MRSAs, surveys of close contacts of the index cases have failed to detect person-to-person transmission.[255,499]

Mechanisms of Resistance

By 2015, eight genotype clusters of vancomycin resistance in enterococci had been defined, labeled VanA through VanE and VanG, VanL, VanM, and VanN, each associated with phenotypic nuances.[73,301,315] The genotypes vary in the species of enterococci affected, the relative resistance conferred to vancomycin and teicoplanin, and whether they are inducible or constitutively expressed (Table 234.3). The VanC phenotype is distinct from the others in that it is an intrinsically expressed, species-specific product of *Enterococcus gallinarum, Enterococcus casseliflavus,* and *Enterococcus flavescens*.[318] The other vancomycin genotypes are acquired, although several are not readily transferable (see Table 234.3). Most human isolates are derived from the VanA group.

In susceptible bacteria, the glycopeptides are large molecules that interfere with cell wall peptidoglycan synthesis at a point proximal to that targeted by the β-lactam antibiotics. Specifically, the synthesis of peptidoglycan in vancomycin-susceptible bacteria includes the incorporation of a D-alanyl-D-alanine dipeptide onto the carboxyl end of the growing glycopeptide chain to form a pentapeptide precursor. The pentapeptide is translocated from the cytoplasm to the outer surface of the bacteria.[73] The D-Ala-D-Ala carboxyl-terminal end of the pentapeptide is critical for the continued synthesis of the peptidoglycan chain and ultimately for peptidoglycan cross-linking and the formation of a stable cell wall. Vancomycin, which never enters the cell, binds to the D-Ala-D-Ala moiety of the pentapeptide through several hydrogen bonds along the outer surface of the cell wall,[16] blocking synthesis of the remaining macromolecule.

The molecular basis for vancomycin resistance results from the complex, coordinated interactions of multiple genes that usually are on a single genetic element. These interactions have been defined best for the VanA phenotype, although genetic homologues are found in organisms expressing the other vancomycin-resistant phenotypes. The genetic machinery for VanA resides on the 10,851-bp transposon Tn*1546*.[9,496] The molecules central to conferring the resistant phenotype

TABLE 234.3 Types of Resistance to Glycopeptides in Enterococci

	ACQUIRED RESISTANCE								Intrinsic Resistance
	High Level		**Variable**	**Moderate**	**Low Level**				**Low Level**
Susceptibility	***VanA***	***VanM***	***VanB***	***VanD***	***VanE***	***VanG***	***VanL***	***VanN***	***VanC***
Vancomycin	R	R	r-R	R	r	r	r	r	r
Teicoplanin	R	R	S	r-R	S	S	S	S	S
Transferability	+	+	+	–	–	+	–	+	–
Main enterococcal species	A/B[a]	A	A/B	A/B	B	B	B	A	G/D
Expression	1	?	I	C	I/C	I	I	C	C/I
Genetic location	Plasmid (Chr)	Plasmid (Chr)	Chr (plasmid)	Chr (plasmid)	Chr	Chr	?	Chr	Chr
Precursors end	D-Ala-D-Lac	D-Ala-D-Lac	D-Ala-D-Lac	D-Ala-D-Ser	D-Ala-D-Ser	D-Ala-D-Ser	D-Ala-D-Ser	D-Ala-D-Ser	D-Ala-D-Ser

[a]Also other *Enterococcus* species.

A, E. faecium; B, E. faecalis; C, constitutive; *Chr,* chromosome; *D, E. casseliflavus; D-Ala-D-Lac,* D-alanyl-D-lactate; *D-ala-D-Ser,* D-alanyl-D-serine; *G, E. gallinarium; I,* inducible; *R,* high level of resistance (MIC > 16 mg/L); *r,* low level of resistance (MIC = 8–16 mg/L); *S,* susceptible; *Van,* vancomycin resistance in various enterococci; +, yes; –, no.

From Cattoir V, Leclercq R. Twenty-five years of shared life with vancomycin-resistant enterococci: is it time to divorce? *J Antimicrob Chemother.* 2013;68:731–42.

are encoded by the contiguous genes labeled *vanH, vanA,* and *vanX,* all of which are essential for expression of vancomycin resistance.

The *vanA* gene encodes a ligase that, unlike the native enterococcal ligase, produces an abnormal D-alanyl-D-lactate dimer over the normal D-alanyl-D-alanine.[41] This process results in the formation of the peptidoglycan precursor uridine diphosphate–MurNAc–L-Ala-D-Gl u-L-Lys-D-Ala-D-Lac, the carboxyl terminus of which has profoundly reduced affinity for vancomycin.[42,59] The homologous ligase in VanC-, VanE-, and VanG-expressing organisms synthesizes D-Ala-D-Ser (see Table 234.3) with similar consequences,[73,315] although the degree of resistance conferred by formation of D-Ala-D-Ser is less profound than that conferred by D-Ala-D-Lac. VanH catalyzes the reaction taking pyruvate to D-Lac and increases the availability of this substrate to VanA for production of the D-Ala-D-Lac dimer.[42] The *vanX* gene and a second gene labeled *vanY* encode a cleaving enzyme for the D-Ala-D-Ala dipeptide, reducing the natural cellular substrate for the D-Ala-D-Ala by adding enzyme and resulting in greater relative incorporation of D-Ala-D-Lac into the peptidoglycan precursor.[397]

Between 2002 and 2016, 14 adult American patients were described who had fully vancomycin-resistant MRSA infections, and small numbers of other VRSAs were detected in South Asia and Europe.[255] Among those VRSAs that were molecularly analyzed, the isolates harbored the TN*1546* transposon found in VREs,[255,499] and several patients were coincidentally colonized with VREs.[255,499] This finding indicates that true VRSA likely results from the conjugal transfer of the vancomycin-resistance transposon from VRE to MRSA, a phenomenon that can be replicated in vitro.[324]

VISA isolates do not contain the resistance genes found in VRE; these isolates acquire unusual extracellular material around the cell wall as detected by electron microscopy.[43,443] This layer represents accumulated peptidoglycan with reduced levels of cross-linking, exposing an excess of D-Ala-D-Ala moieties that bind to vancomycin before it can reach the cell wall.[497]

Other vancomycin-resistance phenomena in *S. aureus* have been described and include those in which subpopulations express MICs twofold to eightfold higher than those in the parent population (i.e., heteroresistance)[122,209] and those in which *S. aureus* can be inhibited but not readily killed by vancomycin (i.e., tolerance).[285] Some investigations indicated that isolates of *S. aureus* expressing vancomycin heteroresistance develop into VISA with continued exposure to the drug.[497]

Issues surrounding reduced susceptibility to vancomycin have been partially addressed by the introduction of the lipoglycopeptides (Table 234.4). These agents have a hydrophobic moiety added to the glycopeptide core, which anchors the agents into the cell wall close to the peptidoglycan molecular target, accounting for their increased potency compared with vancomycin.[531] In the case of oritavancin and telavancin, the interaction with the bacterial cell surface also alters cellular permeability and disrupts membrane potential, increasing their antibacterial effect. The lipoglycopeptides have very good activity against VISA and some of the infrequently encountered genotypes of VRE. Only oritavancin has activity against the *vanA* genotype[531]; hence, it exhibits in vitro activity against this most common VRE genotype and against VRSA (see Table 234.4)

Resistance to oxazolidinone daptomycin, and ceftaroline. Two antibiotics introduced in the early 2000s, linezolid and daptomycin, were developed to address the increasingly important problem of antibiotic-resistant gram-positive pathogens, especially VRE and MRSA. In both instances, the antibiotic represented a novel class of molecules, and it was hoped that resistance would be slow to develop. The fifth-generation cephalosporins, ceftaroline and ceftobiprole (the latter is not licensed in the United States), were introduced several years later to provide additional therapies, particularly for MRSA. Antibiotic resistance was identified for all of the newer classes of antibiotics after their introduction.

Oxazolidinones. Linezolid, the first of the oxazolidinone antibiotics, has activity against all important human gram-positive pathogens, including MRSA, VISA, coagulase-negative staphylococci, and VRE. Gram-negative organisms are intrinsically resistant to linezolid because they express efflux pumps that extrude the drug from the cytoplasm.[267] The molecular target of the oxazolidinones is domain V of the 23S rRNA of the 50S bacterial ribosomal subunit. Binding to this domain results in the inhibition of the initial steps of translation.[461] Although there is some overlap with the binding sites of other antibiotics whose activity is directed against the ribosome,[267] linezolid's binding site is unique to the oxazolidinones.

Resistance to linezolid in vivo has been an uncommon occurrence. Regional, national, and international surveys conducted during the 2010s, the second decade of the drug's licensure, identified remarkably few linezolid-resistant organisms among staphylococci, despite the widespread use of the agent. In most surveys, more than 98% of *S. aureus* (including MRSA) and coagulase-negative staphylococci were linezolid susceptible.[76,205,241,297] Resistance in enterococci occurs more frequently; in some regions, susceptibility of vancomycin-resistant enterococci has fallen below 90%.[437] The few endemic linezolid-resistant clinical isolates usually have been encountered after prolonged exposure to drug.[32,145] Intrahospital and regional epidemics of linezolid-resistant coagulase-negative staphylococci and vancomycin-resistant enterococci also have been reported; resistance resulted from clonal spread of resistant organisms.[213,327,329,330,539]

Four principal mechanisms of linezolid resistance have been defined. Most linezolid-resistant organisms possess a mutation in the gene encoding domain V of the 23S rRNA.[267,296,382] Most bacteria have multiple copies of this gene. The degree of resistance depends on the gene dose, and the MIC of linezolid usually remains in the susceptible range after a single mutation occurs but increases incrementally as each allele is affected.[296] In other linezolid-resistant organisms, the resistant phenotype is conferred through mutations of the ribosomal proteins L3 and L4.[267]

Through a third mechanism, ribosomal binding of linezolid is inhibited by methylation of the rRNA; this mechanism is mediated through the plasmid-borne enzyme Cfr methylase.[20,50,58,267,382] Methylation results in cross-resistance to clindamycin and the streptogramin A antibiotics.[267] In some instances, Cfr-bearing plasmids include several other antibiotic-resistance determinants.[140] Fourth, a transmissible ABC transporter gene *(optrA)* that can confer linezolid resistance was identified in enterococci in China in the mid-2010s.[51,502] This efflux gene also extrudes phenicol antibiotics, which have been used in animal husbandry for years. Organisms carrying the *optrA* gene were isolated before the introduction of linezolid in China, presumably arising in the phenicol-exposed food chain.[502]

Daptomycin. Daptomycin, a fermentation product of *Streptomyces roseoporus,* is a unique antimicrobial with activity against a full range of gram-positive bacteria. The compound is a cationic cyclic lipopeptide that interacts with the cell membrane in a manner similar to related cationic peptides that constitute part of the natural human host defense mechanisms against microbes. In the presence of calcium, this event disrupts the transmembrane electrical potential with a secondary interruption of ATP and macromolecular synthesis.[448] As with linezolid, laboratory surveys of large numbers of gram-positive clinical isolates

TABLE 234.4 Activity of the Lipoglycopeptide Antibiotics

Antibiotic	VISA	VRSA	VanA VRE	VanB VRE	VanC VRE
Dalbavancin	+	–	–	+	+/–
Oritavancin	+	+	+	+	+
Telavancin	+	–	–	+	+/–

Van, Vancomycin resistance in various enterococci genotypes (A, B, C); *VISA,* vancomycin-intermediate *S. aureus; VRE,* vancomycin-resistant enterococci; *VRSA,* vancomycin-resistant *S. aureus;* +, active; –, inactive.

from many areas of the world indicate that daptomycin resistance is rare.[76,410,437,481] Soon after daptomycin was introduced in the early 2000s, however, several cases were reported documenting the emergence of *S. aureus* and enterococci with reduced susceptibility to daptomycin during prolonged therapy.[7,221,276,280] In these cases, the infection emanated from a bony or endovascular focus into which penetration of the drug might have been limited.

Daptomycin resistance has been linked to mutations in multiple genes that regulate the composition and integrity of the bacterial cell membrane.[124,305] The mutations implicated in daptomycin resistance are different in *S. aureus* and enterococci, but in sum, they result in alterations in the phospholipid content of the bacterial cell surface, changing its charge and thereby decreasing the affinity of the drug to its target.[7,221,305,407,477] In *S. aureus*, ultrastructural analysis of daptomycin-resistant isolates reveals a thickened envelope, and several reports have correlated vancomycin-intermediate resistance in *S. aureus* and reduced susceptibility to daptomycin.[7,75,244] At the molecular level, an accumulation of gain-in-function mutations results in coincident reduction in susceptibility to both drugs. Chief among these are single-point mutations in the regulatory apparatus for the staphylococcal multiple protein resistance factor gene *(mprF)* [521], which results in an enhanced bacterial surface positive charge.[18,61]

Ceftaroline. The fifth-generation cephalosporin ceftaroline was introduced into clinical practice in the latter part of the 2000s. Unlike all prior cephalosporins, ceftaroline exhibits a high affinity for the penicillin-binding protein PBP2A responsible for conferring methicillin resistance in staphylococci,[420] rendering the drug active against MRSA. It also has activity against multidrug-resistant pneumococci and against staphylococci with intermediate resistance to vancomycin and reduced susceptibility to linezolid and daptomycin.[420]

Several surveys testing ceftaroline against a wide range of staphylococcal and pneumococcal clinical isolates in the first decade of the 2000s demonstrated almost uniform in vitro activity,[114,119] but continued surveillance into the next decade indicated a growing proportion of nonsusceptible isolates among MRSAs, ranging between 5% and 10%, from a wide variety of lineages and geographic regions.[113,215,409,411] Resistance rates approaching 50% were documented in Southeast Asia.[23]

The principal mechanism of resistance in MRSA strains is mutation of PBP2A.[298] Mutation in the ceftaroline binding pocket of the transpeptidase region of this penicillin-binding protein renders the organism highly resistant,[157,222,237,266] whereas mutations in other domains of PBP2A and alterations of other PBPs result in milder elevations of MIC.[4,237] Some analyses of archived MRSAs have documented ceftaroline resistance in isolates identified in the 1990s, well before the fifth-generation cephalosporins were introduced into clinical practice.[222]

Quinolones

Clinical Relevance

The quinolone family of antibiotics possesses activity against a broad variety of microorganisms. The safety profile for children of the more recently developed quinolones (i.e., fluoroquinolones) is similar to that recorded for adults.[132,198] This class of antibiotics has been effectively employed in selected children with serious infections caused by bacteria resistant to alternative agents. The following sections discuss clinical circumstances in which quinolone resistance is relevant to pediatric infections.

Bacterial enteritis. Antibiotic therapy, including treatment with quinolones, for bacterial enteritis usually is not indicated.[514] That said, with the exception of *Campylobacter,* most agents that cause bacterial enteritis have remained susceptible to the quinolones by in vitro testing, although epidemic strains of *Shigella* and *Salmonella* expressing quinolone resistance have been identified worldwide.[127,139,464] *Salmonella typhimurium* DT104, which spread rapidly throughout Europe and the United States in the late 1990s, is resistant to nalidixic acid, but most isolates (except for some identified in the United Kingdom) are susceptible to the newer fluoroquinolones.[139,161,306] Similarly, surveys of other non-*typhi Salmonella* conducted in the early 2000s indicated that few were ciprofloxacin resistant, although as many as one fifth of the strains had reduced susceptibility to the drug.[278,452]

In contrast to resistance among other enteritis-associated bacteria, high-level quinolone resistance among *Campylobacter* isolates from many parts of the world has become prominent.[169,362] *Campylobacter* can acquire quinolone resistance shortly after exposure to the antibiotic, and clinical relapse with quinolone-resistant organisms after therapy for *Campylobacter* enteritis is relatively common.[362]

The introduction of quinolones into poultry feed for animals bred for food has exacerbated the spread of *Campylobacter* resistance in humans.[320] In chickens obtained from several different supermarkets in Minnesota in the mid-1990s, almost 90% of samples were culture positive for *Campylobacter,* and approximately 20% of these samples were resistant to ciprofloxacin.[441] These circumstances prompted a US Food and Drug Administration (FDA) ruling withdrawing the use of quinolones in poultry in 2005. It is likely, however, that quinolone-resistant *Campylobacter* has found a stable ecologic niche in animals and humans and will continue to be encountered despite this intervention.[320]

Unlike most other bacteria, *Campylobacter* becomes highly resistant to the quinolones after a single mutation.[136,501] Most quinolone-resistant clinical isolates demonstrate MICs of 32 μg/mL or more, much higher than the conventional cutoff for defining quinolone resistance.

Urinary tract infections. Quinolone resistance in enteric gram-negative rods, particularly among uropathogens, was an uncommon occurrence in North America until the emergence of the multidrug-resistant extraintestinal pathogenic *E. coli* (ExPEC) clonal strains in the late 1990s and 2000s, predominately affecting health care–associated infections in adult patients. In a report on antimicrobial-resistant pathogens in device-related infections by the US National Healthcare Safety Network (NHSN), the percentage of pathogenic fluoroquinolone-resistant (FQR) *E. coli* associated with catheter-associated urinary tract infections (CAUTIs) was 24.8% in 2006 through 2007.[165] This percentage increased to 31.2% in the 2009-2010 NHSN report.[436]

Increases also have been reported in community-acquired UTIs, particularly in association with the pandemic ST131 *E. coli* strain, which encodes ESBLs and plasmid-mediated resistance to fluoroquinolones.[359] In a national study of third-generation cephalosporin-resistant (G3CR) and ESBL-producing pediatric Enterobacteriaceae isolates, most of which were recovered from the urinary tract, coresistance to quinolone antibiotics was demonstrated in 32.8% and 54.3% of isolates, respectively.[263] The U.S. data are consistent with trends in quinolone-resistant gram-negative urinary tract pathogens worldwide. In the 2009-10 global surveillance Study for Monitoring Antimicrobial Resistance Trends (SMART), of 1116 FQR gram-negative UTI pathogens, the regional rates of FQR were 23.5% in North America, 25.5% in the South Pacific, 29.4% in Europe, 33.2% in Asia, and 38.7% in Latin America.[31]

Cephalosporin antibiotics remain effective overall in pediatric uncomplicated UTIs, and the consensus is that routine use of quinolone will needlessly promote quinolone resistance to an even greater degree without clinical benefit.[118,146,175] The current recommendation from the American Academy of Pediatrics Committee of Infectious Diseases is to reserve quinolone use to cases of complicated UTI and pyelonephritis for which typical agents are not appropriate based on susceptibility data, allergy, or history of adverse events.[36]

Community-acquired respiratory tract infections. The applicability of quinolones to respiratory tract infections has been shadowed by the marginal activity of the first modern quinolones—ciprofloxacin, ofloxacin, and norfloxacin—against *S. pneumoniae.* MICs of these antibiotics against most clinical isolates of *S. pneumoniae* average 1 to 2 μg/mL, concentrations that are close to those achievable in bronchial secretions.[364] Several reports of clinical treatment failures were reported when ciprofloxacin was administered for pneumococcal disease in the respiratory tract.[231,246] Even when *S. pneumoniae* was not the intended target of therapy, the widespread use of the early quinolone agents in treating community-acquired infections during the 1990s resulted in the inadvertent exposure of respiratory tract colonizers, including *S. pneumoniae,* to these agents. This was associated with a gradual increase in the MICs of community-acquired *S. pneumoniae* isolates to ciprofloxacin.[63,203,415]

Most of the recently introduced fluoroquinolones are substantially more potent against *S. pneumoniae* than is ciprofloxacin, and they express MICs that are easily achieved in the respiratory tract. Susceptibility usually is maintained, even in isolates resistant to the older quinolone agents.[206,364] However, MICs against the newer quinolones roughly correlate with those expressed against ciprofloxacin. Consequently, clinically relevant resistance also has begun to emerge against these newer agents, particularly levofloxacin.[2,91,369,400] Susceptibility of other respiratory tract pathogens, including *H. influenzae, M. catarrhalis,* and the bacterial agents causing atypical pneumonias, remains very good to all the fluoroquinolones, although exceptions, particularly in *Haemophilus* spp., have been reported (http://cddep.org/sites/default/files/swa_2015_final.pdf).

Beyond issues of promoting resistance, in 2016, the FDA advised against the use of fluoroquinolones for uncomplicated infections such as routine respiratory tract disease, stating that the serious adverse effects of quinolones outweigh their benefits. (http://fda.gov/Drugs/DrugSafety/ucm500143.htm). For children, fluoroquinolone antibiotics are recommended only as alternative therapy for acute otitis media, sinusitis, and lower respiratory tract infections.[35,36,495]

Nosocomial infections. The quinolones traditionally have been mainstays of treatment for nosocomial infections in adult patients with severe illness. During the late 1990s and early 2000s, however, quinolone resistance in nosocomial gram-negative pathogens increased in many areas of the world among Enterobacteriaceae and non–lactose fermenters.[125,207,216,322] In several instances, quinolone resistance in gram-negative bacilli increased more rapidly than any other resistance phenotype.[125,207] Many of these hospital-acquired pathogens coexpress ESBLs and other resistance determinants.

Mechanisms of Resistance

The two principal molecular targets of the quinolone antibiotics are the topoisomerases DNA gyrase and topoisomerase IV. These enzymes mediate the three-dimensional topologic configuration of the bacterial duplex DNA ring during cell division and transcription and allow the repair and replication of nucleic acids and the separation of daughter chromosomes in the cramped intracellular environment.[158,170] Several reactions are mediated by these two bacterial DNA topoisomerases, including negative supercoiling and catenation.[171,459] In DNA gyrase and topoisomerase IV, the enzymes are heterotetramers with two subunits; gyrase is constructed as $GyrA_2B_2$ and topoisomerase IV as $ParC_2E_2$.[173,171,459] The GyrA subunit is homologous to ParC, as the GyrB subunit is homologous to the ParE subunit.[500] Quinolones bind reversibly to the GyrA and ParC subunit of the DNA gyrase and topoisomerase IV-DNA-ATP complexes near the active site tyrosine and prevent further progress of the enzyme along the nucleic acid.[171] Bacterial cell death is enhanced by the release of toxic DNA ends from the quinolone-topoisomerase complexes.[158,172]

Quinolone resistance is conferred through several molecular mechanisms (described later). Multiple mutations commonly occur in the same isolate, each one resulting in a higher MIC.

Mutations of topoisomerase. Most organisms resistant to the fluoroquinolones demonstrate one or more mutations in DNA gyrase or topoisomerase IV, or both. Resistance to quinolones among gram-negative bacteria usually is mediated through mutations in DNA gyrase, whereas resistance in gram-positive organisms is primarily the result of alterations of topoisomerase IV.[158,343] However, this pattern varies from organism to organism (e.g., the primary target in *S. pneumoniae* appears to be DNA gyrase) and from quinolone to quinolone.[158,172]

The mutations are clustered in the amino-terminal domains of GyrA or ParC, which reside near the active-site tyrosines of the enzymes. These domains are called the *quinolone-resistance determining region* (QRDR).[173,522,523] Hybrid DNA gyrase molecules composed of the A subunit from a resistant bacterial strain and the B subunit from a susceptible isolate exhibit quinolone resistance.[52] Within the QRDR, most mutations involve the substitution of a serine for a bulkier, nonpolar amino acid at a single, specific site. This mutation, first identified in *E. coli,*[490,522] has since been documented in a variety of organisms, and it reduces quinolone affinity for the target enzyme-DNA complex.[187,232,307,387] Other amino acid substitutions near this site also have been described, with multiple-site mutations resulting in increased quinolone resistance compared with a single mutation alone.[490]

Mutations of the GyrB and ParE subunits, which result in a quinolone-resistant phenotype, also have been identified in quinolone-resistant clinical isolates but remain less common than mutations in GyrA and ParC. Mutations affecting the GyrB subunit usually result in lower levels of resistance than those seen with GyrA.[523] As with GyrA mutations, those affecting GyrB preferentially localize to specific amino acids.[523]

Altered outer-membrane porin. Another mechanism of quinolone resistance involves decreased entry of antibiotic into the cell due to alterations in porin composition, a mutation that usually results in only moderate drug resistance and that affects individual quinolones differentially, depending on their hydrophilicity.[418] Attention has focused on alterations in outer-member protein F (OmpF).[174,534] This mutation, identified principally in *E. coli,* frequently is associated with resistance to other classes of antibiotics, including chloramphenicol, tetracycline, and some of the β-lactams. The diminished expression of OmpF in these resistant isolates does not appear to result from mutations in the corresponding structural gene or its regulatory sequences. Rather, the decreased expression of this outer-membrane protein is mediated through the enhanced expression of the gene *micF,* which transcribes an antisense RNA complementary to the 5′ end of the *ompF* message,[6] thereby destabilizing its binding to the ribosome. Occasional mutants involving additional strains of Enterobacteriaceae have demonstrated other alterations in outer-membrane porin composition.[52]

Efflux. Quinolone-resistant species can also mediate their resistance through increased drug efflux.[250,251] Bacterial and eukaryotic cells normally encode several efflux pumps that provide protection from a range of potential exogenous toxins.[352] The overexpression of an efflux pump resulting from the mutation of a controlling sequence accounts for reduced susceptibility to quinolones in many clinical isolates.[191,279] In gram-positive bacteria, the largest contributors of quinolone efflux transporters are members of the major facilitator superfamily (MFS); in gram-negative bacteria, most quinolone-related efflux pumps are derived from the resistance-nodulation-division (RND) superfamily.[253]

Individual efflux pumps select substrates based on their physical chemical properties (e.g., hydrophobicity, net charge), rather than their gross structural similarities. The various quinolone compounds, which vary in these properties, can be differentially susceptible to organisms expressing these pumps.[352]

The genes encoding the Nor MFS pumps in *S. aureus,* called *norA, norB, and norC,*[173,524] have been cloned, sequenced, and comprehensively analyzed. Transformation of susceptible bacteria with the putative gene results in a resistant phenotype, which can be abolished by the addition of inhibitors of energy-dependent cellular pumps.[524] NorA can transport only hydrophilic quinolones (e.g., norfloxacin, ciprofloxacin); intracellular accumulation of the hydrophobic drugs sparfloxacin and moxifloxacin, for example, are unaffected. NorB and NorC have broad substrate profiles and can transport hydrophilic and hydrophobic quinolones.[252,479,480,484,526]

Several other MFS efflux transporters affect quinolone resistance in *S. aureus.*[173] Additional transporter families such as the ATP-binding cassette (ABC) family and the multiple antibiotic and toxin extrusion (MATE) family can confer quinolone resistance.[173] A range of additional genes encoding efflux pumps capable of producing quinolone resistance has been identified in other species, such as *prmA* in *S. pneumoniae,*[363] *acrAB-TolC* complex in *E. coli,*[274] and the *mexAmexB-oprM* complex in *P. aeruginosa.*[281] This third complex gene encodes components that transport the drug through the cell wall and across the periplasmic space as well as an outer-membrane protein.[352] Most pumps can extrude a wide variety of exogenous substances, such as detergents, dyes, and other antibiotics, from the bacterial cytoplasm.[191] Therefore reduced susceptibility to quinolones may be selected by exposures unrelated to the quinolones themselves.

Plasmid-mediated quinolone resistance. The first decade of the 2000s witnessed the rapid emergence of transmissible plasmid-mediated quinolone resistance (PMQR). All previously defined mechanisms of quinolone resistance were chromosomal. Organisms exhibiting the transmissible mechanism have been identified in several countries worldwide.[402] The three main mechanisms of PMQR are production of proteins that protect DNA gyrase and topoisomerase IV from inhibition by quinolones; acetylation of quinolones by variants of aminoglycoside acetyl transferases; and efflux pumps.

Qnr proteins. The first PMQR products discovered, called *Qnr proteins,* are a group of molecules that bind to topoisomerase and protect it from the inhibitory effects of the quinolones.[325,402] Although all the Qnr molecules described belong to the pentapeptide-repeat family of proteins, a finding suggesting similar three-dimensional conformations, distinct families of Qnr proteins with largely nonhomologous amino acid sequences have been characterized.[325,402] These families have been named QnrA, QnrB, QnrC, QnrD, and QnrS, with subtypes identified within each.

Qnr homologues are encoded on the chromosomes of gram-positive and gram-negative bacteria, suggesting distinct and widely different origins of Qnr genes. The variety of plasmid and integron structures carrying Qnr proteins and the multiplicity of sequences of the proteins themselves support the notion that Qnr-mediated resistance arose through many independent molecular events before the introduction of quinolones in geographically distinct regions of the world.[195] The plasmids encoding the Qnr proteins have been found in multiple species belonging to the Enterobacteriaceae, but they are infrequently identified in nonenteric bacteria such as *Pseudomonas* and Acinetobacter.[402,476]

***AAC(6′)-Ib-cr* gene.** Qnr plasmids frequently carry other antibiotic-resistance genes, most notably those encoding ESBLs and the aminoglycoside-modifying gene *aac(6′)-Ib-cr,* which also can acetylate selected quinolones.[195,402] The *aac(6′)-Ib-cr* variant requires two unique amino acid substitutions (i.e., Asp179Tyr and Trp102Arg) for the acetylation of quinolones. Plasmids harboring the *aac(6′)-Ib-cr* gene are often located on an integron that is associated with other plasmid-mediated quinolone-resistance genes and additional antibiotic-resistance genes. The plasmids can be found, for example, in the multidrug-resistant epidemic *E. coli* ST131 strain. The *aac(6′)-Ib-cr* genes have been recovered from multiple members of the Enterobacteriaceae family and have been reported in *P. aeruginosa.*[173,195,359,402]

OqxAB and QepA efflux pumps. OqxABs are efflux pumps in the RND family. Genes for OqxAB are frequently found on the chromosomes of gram-negative organisms (e.g., *K. pneumoniae, Enterobacter* spp.). Plasmid-mediated variants were originally described in 2003 in association with a conjugative plasmid conferring resistance to a growth-enhancing food additive in pigs (i.e., olaquindox).[446] This was later discovered to be a multidrug efflux pump, conferring resistance to quinolones, trimethoprim, nitrofurantoin, and chloroamphenicol.[155,166] PMQR due to OqxAB variants is expressed at higher levels than the chromosomal counterpart. In countries where olaquindox is used in agriculture, such as China, stool colonization with OqxAB harboring *E. coli* in farm animals (40%) and farm workers (30%) is common.[155,166,537,538]

QepAs are efflux pumps in the MFS family that increase resistance to hydrophilic quinolones. The QepA variants, originally reported in 2007 in *E. coli,* have been found worldwide. They are most commonly located on plasmids in association with genes encoding the aminoglycoside ribosomal methylase *(rmtB)*. QepA expression varies, accounting for differences in the levels of quinolone resistance in QepA-harboring isolates.[150,195,357,520,538]

Polymyxins

Clinical Significance

The polymyxin antibiotics are represented by two agents: polymyxin B and polymyxin E; the latter is more commonly known as colistin. The drugs were introduced in the 1950s for parenteral therapy against a wide variety of gram-negative pathogens. Because of the high incidence of nephrotoxicity and, to a lesser extent, neurotoxicity, intravenous use of these drugs was relegated to a minor role when alternative agents became available.

By the early years of the new millennium, a growing number of hospital-associated organisms worldwide had become simultaneously resistant to multiple classes of parenteral antibiotics, including all available β-lactams, aminoglycosides, and fluoroquinolones, severely limiting therapeutic options during a period when new drug development against gram-negative bacteria was almost at a standstill. These circumstances led to a resurgence of intravenous colistin use.[111,249] The rejuvenation of parenteral colistin as an antibiotic of last resort was met with the sobering recognition that optimal dosing regimens in adults had never been established and the subsequent documentation that conventional dosing developed decades before could lead to subtherapeutic concentrations of the drug at the infected site.[317] Pharmacokinetics and pharmacodynamics in children were even less defined.[176]

With broader use of intravenous colistin, there has been a growing recognition of resistance to the drug.[383] When expressed in multidrug-resistant, carbapenemase-expressing organisms, this has sometimes resulted in an infection for which there are few or no therapeutic options.[486] The species most frequently associated with colistin resistance include *P. aeruginosa, A. baumannii,* and *K. pneumoniae;* all are virulent pathogens whose primary targets are fragile, critically ill people.

The frequency of colistin resistance is poorly defined because accurate susceptibility testing to colistin requires the time-consuming broth microdilution technique[77] and usually is reserved for the subset of clinical isolates expressing multiple-resistance phenotypes. A partial picture of the frequency of colistin resistance was presented in a survey of 19,719 international Enterobacteriaceae isolates published in 2015[34]: 1.6% were colistin resistant, but the incidence increased to 12% in carbapenem-resistant organisms, mostly in *K. pneumoniae*. The incidence of colistin resistance among all gram-negative species likely will increase significantly within a short period.

Until recently, colistin resistance was exclusively expressed chromosomally and was spread through clonal expansion and person-to-person transmission of selected strains. In the 2010s, outbreaks in hospitals and in long-term care facilities caused by one or a small number of genetically related organisms were described,[135,331] sometimes involving interinstitutional spread. In early 2016, a plasmid-borne transmissible form of colistin resistance was identified in *E. coli* in China.[259] This alarming finding generated multiple international surveys, which revealed that organisms bearing the resistance plasmid had already spread throughout the world.[353,373,426,493]

Agricultural use of polymyxins has been ongoing for decades. A high incidence of organisms expressing transmissible colistin resistance have been found in farm animals, particularly pigs and poultry, and in meats coming to market for human consumption, strongly suggesting a zoonotic origin of this resistance determinant.[373,426]

Mechanisms of Resistance

The polymyxins are amphipathic molecules that initially bind to the lipid A component of lipopolysaccharide. The antibiotic then mediates fusion with the cytoplasmic membrane underneath, resulting in cell surface disruption, osmotic imbalances, and death.[219] Chromosome-encoded resistance results from the synthesis of normally repressed products (e.g., 4-amino-4-deoxy-L-arabinose or phosphoethanolamine, depending on the species) that modify the lipopolysaccharide, reducing its affinity for the polymyxin.[26]

Synthesis of these molecules is regulated by a two-component system composed of a cell surface kinase and the resistance-determinant gene itself (i.e., PmrA/PmrB or PhoP/PhoQ). Phenotypic resistance may result from mutations of the kinase or the resistance gene.[219] Disruption of an additional negative regulator, the *mgrB* locus in *K. pneumoniae,*[53,338] also results in the resistant phenotype.

Transmissible resistance is mediated by the *mcr-1* gene that has been identified in *E. coli* on a particularly promiscuous conjugative plasmid.[259] The MCR-1 product is a phosphoethanolamine transferase enzyme that mediates the addition of that molecule to lipid A. Sequence analysis suggests that this enzyme initially was derived from a gene on the chromosome of a bacterium that naturally produces polymyxin, which then became incorporated onto a plasmid and transferred to *E. coli.*[259]

Chloramphenicol

Clinical Relevance

In industrialized nations, chloramphenicol has been supplanted by other agents with similar or improved antibacterial potency and less toxicity. However, the antibiotic remains a staple for pediatric bacteremia and meningitis in the developing world because of its broad antibacterial activity, low cost, favorable achievable serum concentrations after oral or intramuscular administration, and excellent penetration across the blood-brain barrier.

The incidence of resistance to chloramphenicol among the principal organisms causing bacteremia and meningitis in children—*H. influenzae, S. pneumoniae, N. meningitidis,* and *Salmonella*—varies greatly by geographic location. Between the late 1980s and the early 2000s, surveys of type b and non–type b *H. influenzae* were completed in several areas of the world. In vitro resistance to chloramphenicol was between 0% of isolates (i.e., Central African Republic and various locations in South America) and more than 50% (i.e., India and Kenya).[200,225,336,406,414,505] Studies in 2001 and 2003 of *H. influenzae* isolates in Canada and the United States, where infection by these organisms is almost always treated with an alternative agent, indicated chloramphenicol resistance in less than 0.5% of tested bacteria.[167,535]

International surveys completed in the middle to late 1990s that measured in vitro susceptibility of *S. pneumoniae* to chloramphenicol indicated resistance exceeding 10% to 20% in many areas of the world.[189,247,336,406] Chloramphenicol resistance was identified in approximately 10% of European isolates of *S. pneumoniae* and in 5% of isolates in the United States and Canada.[167] Resistance to chloramphenicol is seen more commonly and is of a higher grade in penicillin-resistant pneumococci than in isolates that are penicillin susceptible.[167] Even in penicillin-intermediate or penicillin-resistant strains that retain in vitro susceptibility to chloramphenicol, the clinical response to chloramphenicol in cases of meningitis is poor. Some investigators have suggested that the bacteria express high minimal bactericidal concentrations to chloramphenicol; as a result, concentrations of drug achieved in the cerebrospinal fluid with routine dosing are lower than those required for good outcomes in central nervous system infections.[126]

Chloramphenicol retains excellent activity against most strains of *N. meningitidis*. However, investigators described meningococcal strains from Vietnam, Paris, and Australia that possessed high-level resistance to the drug.[128,435] Chloramphenicol resistance in *Salmonella* spp., a fourth group of organisms that causes disseminated disease and meningitis in pediatric patients, varies geographically. Resistance with a prevalence exceeding 50% usually is detected in developing countries,[214] where chloramphenicol has been a readily available oral agent for typhoidal and nontyphoidal *Salmonella* infections for decades. In most *Salmonella* isolates, chloramphenicol resistance occurs coincident with resistance to many other antibiotics, particularly ampicillin, sulfonamides, tetracycline, and some of the older aminoglycosides. Chloramphenicol resistance has become increasingly common in industrialized nations.[72,444,504] In the United States, the strain *Salmonella typhimurium* DT104, which similarly coexpresses resistance to several classes of antibiotics, including chloramphenicol, has become a widespread health hazard.[1,491]

Mechanisms of Resistance

The antibacterial activity of chloramphenicol is conferred by its interference with the peptidyl transferase region of the 50S prokaryotic ribosome. The principal mechanism of resistance is expression of the modifying enzyme chloramphenicol acetyltransferase (CAT), which catalyzes the acetylation of the C3-hydroxy group of the drug and prevents its binding to the bacterial ribosome.[431]

CATs represent a family of enzymes. Many CATs share chemical properties and structural homologies, especially around the active site.[431] CATs frequently reside on plasmids or transposons that carry other antibiotic-resistance determinants.[494] In *Salmonella*, the chloramphenicol-resistance gene frequently is encoded on a class 1 integron incorporated in the *Salmonella* genomic island 1 (SGI1), which includes multiple antibiotic-resistance cassettes.[102,311] SGI1 is transmissible and has been identified in many different *Salmonella* serovars.

Alternative mechanisms of resistance to chloramphenicol have been identified in certain gram-negative species. In most of these organisms, resistance is linked to decreased intracellular accumulation of drug. In chloramphenicol-resistant *Pseudomonas,* this phenomenon has been associated with the overproduction of an approximately 50-kd outer-membrane protein,[251] which in the past led to the speculation that entry of drug into the bacterium was diminished by an abnormal porin. However, cell membrane proteins of this size have also been identified as components of a complex efflux apparatus that include the pump and proteins that channel the extruded substance across the periplasmic space and through the outer membrane.[352] More direct evidence of multidrug-resistant efflux pumps has been identified in chloramphenicol-resistant *E. coli,*[155] *Pseudomonas,*[251] *Stenotrophomonas,*[536] and *Salmonella.*[27,60,365] Usually, these pumps result in coresistance to multiple antimicrobial agents, including tetracycline, sulfonamide, aminoglycosides, quinolones, and selected detergents.

NEW REFERENCES SINCE THE SEVENTH EDITION

4. Alm RA, McLaughlin RE, Kos VN, et al. Analysis of *Staphylococcus aureus* clinical isolates with reduced susceptibility to ceftaroline: an epidemiological and structural perspective. *J Antimicrob Chemother.* 2014;69:2065-2075.
8. Aronoff SC, Jacobs MR, Johenning S, Yamabe S. Comparative activities of the beta-lactamase inhibitors YTR 830, sodium clavulanate, and sulbactam combined with amoxicillin or ampicillin. *Antimicrob Agents Chemother.* 1984;26:580-582.
10. Ashkenazi S, May-Zahav M, Sulkes J, et al. Increasing antimicrobial resistance of *Shigella* isolates in Israel during the period 1984 to 1992. *Antimicrob Agents Chemother.* 1995;39:819-823.
14. Banerjee R, Johnson JR. A new clone sweeps clean: the enigmatic emergence of *Escherichia coli* sequence type 131. *Antimicrob Agents Chemother.* 2014;58:4997-5004.
18. Bayer AS, Mishra NN, Cheung AL, et al. Dysregulation of mprF and dltABCD expression among daptomycin-non-susceptible MRSA clinical isolates. *J Antimicrob Chemother.* 2016;71:2100-2104.
19. Becker B, Cooper MA. Aminoglycoside antibiotics in the 21st century. *ACS Chem Biol.* 2013;8:105-115.
20. Bender J, Strommenger B, Steglich M, et al. Linezolid resistance in clinical isolates of *Staphylococcus epidermidis* from German hospitals and characterization of two cfr-carrying plasmids. *J Antimicrob Chemother.* 2015;70:1630-1638.
23. Biedenbach DJ, Alm RA, Lahiri SD, et al. In vitro activity of ceftaroline against *Staphylococcus aureus* Isolated in 2012 from Asia-Pacific countries as part of the AWARE Surveillance Program. *Antimicrob Agents Chemother.* 2016;60:343-347.
26. Boll M, Radziejewska-Lebrecht J, Warth C, et al. 4-Amino-4-deoxy-L-arabinose in LPS of enterobacterial R-mutants and its possible role for their polymyxin reactivity. *FEMS Immunol Med Microbiol.* 1994;8:329-341.
28. Bonelli RR, Moreira BM, Picao RC. Antimicrobial resistance among Enterobacteriaceae in South America: history, current dissemination status and associated socioeconomic factors. *Drug Resist Updat.* 2014;17:24-36.
29. Bonomo RA, Szabo D. Mechanisms of multidrug resistance in *Acinetobacter* species and *Pseudomonas aeruginosa. Clin Infect Dis.* 2006;43(suppl 2):S49-S56.
31. Bouchillon S, Hoban DJ, Badal R, Hawser S. Fluoroquinolone resistance among gram-negative urinary tract pathogens: global smart program results, 2009-2010. *Open Microbiol J.* 2012;6:74-78.
34. Bradford PA, Kazmierczak KM, Biedenbach DJ, et al. Correlation of beta-lactamase production and colistin resistance among Enterobacteriaceae isolates from a global surveillance program. *Antimicrob Agents Chemother.* 2016;60:1385-1392.
35. Bradley JS, Byington CL, Shah SS, et al. The management of community-acquired pneumonia in infants and children older than 3 months of age: clinical practice guidelines by the Pediatric Infectious Diseases Society and the Infectious Diseases Society of America. *Clin Infect Dis.* 2011;53:e25-e76.
36. Bradley JS, Jackson MA, Committee on Infectious Diseases, American Academy of Pediatrics. The use of systemic and topical fluoroquinolones. *Pediatrics.* 2011;128:e1034-e1045.
40. Buckingham SC, McCullers JA, Lujan-Zilbermann J, et al. Pneumococcal meningitis in children: relationship of antibiotic resistance to clinical characteristics and outcomes. *Pediatr Infect Dis J.* 2001;20:837-843.
45. Bush K. The ABCD''s of beta-lactamase nomenclature. *J Infect Chemother.* 2013;19:549-559.
46. Bush K, Bradford PA. β-lactams and β-lactamase inhibitors: an overview. *Cold Spring Harb Perspect Med.* 2016;6:pii: a025247.
49. Cabaj JL, Nettel-Aguirre A, MacDonald J, et al. Influence of childhood pneumococcal conjugate vaccines on invasive pneumococcal disease in adults with underlying comorbidities in Calgary, Alberta (2000-2013). *Clin Infect Dis.* 2016;62:1521-1526.
50. Cafini F, Nguyen le TT, Higashide M, et al. Horizontal gene transmission of the cfr gene to MRSA and Enterococcus: role of *Staphylococcus epidermidis* as a reservoir and alternative pathway for the spread of linezolid resistance. *J Antimicrob Chemother.* 2016;71:587-592.
51. Cai J, Wang Y, Schwarz S, et al. Enterococcal isolates carrying the novel oxazolidinone resistance gene optrA from hospitals in Zhejiang, Guangdong, and Henan, China, 2010-2014. *Clin Microbiol Infect.* 2015;21:1095 e1-1095 e4.
53. Cannatelli A, Giani T, D'Andrea MM, et al. MgrB inactivation is a common mechanism of colistin resistance in KPC-producing *Klebsiella pneumoniae* of clinical origin. *Antimicrob Agents Chemother.* 2014;58:5696-5703.
55. Canton R, Coque TM. The CTX-M beta-lactamase pandemic. *Curr Opin Microbiol.* 2006;9:466-475.
57. Carrer A, Poirel L, Yilmaz M, et al. Spread of OXA-48-encoding plasmid in Turkey and beyond. *Antimicrob Agents Chemother.* 2010;54:1369-1373.
59. Cattoir V, Leclercq R. Twenty-five years of shared life with vancomycin-resistant enterococci: is it time to divorce? *J Antimicrob Chemother.* 2013;68:731-742.
64. Chitnis AS, Caruthers PS, Rao AK, et al. Outbreak of carbapenem-resistant enterobacteriaceae at a long-term acute care hospital: sustained reductions in

transmission through active surveillance and targeted interventions. *Infect Control Hosp Epidemiol.* 2012;33:984-992.

66. Choi SH, Chung JW, Sung H, et al. Impact of penicillin nonsusceptibility on clinical outcomes of patients with nonmeningeal *Streptococcus pneumoniae* bacteremia in the era of the 2008 clinical and laboratory standards institute penicillin breakpoints. *Antimicrob Agents Chemother.* 2012;56:4650-4655.
70. Coleman K. Diazabicyclooctanes (DBOs): a potent new class of non-beta-lactam beta-lactamase inhibitors. *Curr Opin Microbiol.* 2011;14:550-555.
76. Cuny C, Layer F, Werner G, et al. State-wide surveillance of antibiotic resistance patterns and spa types of methicillin-resistant *Staphylococcus aureus* from blood cultures in North Rhine-Westphalia, 2011-2013. *Clin Microbiol Infect.* 2015;21:750-757.
77. Dafopoulou K, Zarkotou O, Dimitroulia E, et al. Comparative evaluation of colistin susceptibility testing methods among carbapenem-nonsusceptible *Klebsiella pneumoniae* and *Acinetobacter baumannii* clinical isolates. *Antimicrob Agents Chemother.* 2015;59:4625-4630.
78. Dagan R, Hoberman A, Johnson C, et al. Bacteriologic and clinical efficacy of high dose amoxicillin/clavulanate in children with acute otitis media. *Pediatr Infect Dis J.* 2001;20:829-837.
79. Dagan R, Juergens C, Trammel J, et al. Efficacy of 13-valent pneumococcal conjugate vaccine (PCV13) versus that of 7-valent PCV (PCV7) against nasopharyngeal colonization of antibiotic-nonsusceptible *Streptococcus pneumoniae. J Infect Dis.* 2015;211:1144-1153.
82. David MZ, Taylor A, Lynfield R, et al. Comparing pulsed-field gel electrophoresis with multilocus sequence typing, spa typing, staphylococcal cassette chromosome mec (SCCmec) typing, and PCR for panton-valentine leukocidin, arcA, and opp3 in methicillin-resistant *Staphylococcus aureus* isolates at a U.S. Medical Center. *J Clin Microbiol.* 2013;51:814-819.
85. DeLeo FR, Otto M, Kreiswirth BN, Chambers HF. Community-associated meticillin-resistant *Staphylococcus aureus. Lancet.* 2010;375:1557-1568.
86. Deng Y, Bao X, Ji L, et al. Resistance integrons: class 1, 2 and 3 integrons. *Ann Clin Microbiol Antimicrob.* 2015;14:45.
90. Desai AP, Sharma D, Crispell EK, et al. Decline in pneumococcal nasopharyngeal carriage of vaccine serotypes after the introduction of the 13-valent pneumococcal conjugate vaccine in children in Atlanta, Georgia. *Pediatr Infect Dis J.* 2015;34:1168-1174.
92. Deurenberg RH, Vink C, Kalenic S, et al. The molecular evolution of methicillin-resistant *Staphylococcus aureus. Clin Microbiol Infect.* 2007;13:222-235.
98. Doi Y, Wachino J, Arakawa Y. Aminoglycoside resistance: the emergence of acquired 16S ribosomal RNA methyltransferases. *Infect Dis Clin North Am.* 2016;30:523-537.
104. Drawz SM, Papp-Wallace KM, Bonomo RA. New beta-lactamase inhibitors: a therapeutic renaissance in an MDR world. *Antimicrob Agents Chemother.* 2014;58:1835-1846.
107. Ehmann DE, Jahic H, Ross PL, et al. Avibactam is a covalent, reversible, non-beta-lactam beta-lactamase inhibitor. *Proc Natl Acad Sci USA.* 2012;109:11663-11668.
109. Enright MC, Day NP, Davies CE, et al. Multilocus sequence typing for characterization of methicillin-resistant and methicillin-susceptible clones of *Staphylococcus aureus. J Clin Microbiol.* 2000;38:1008-1015.
111. Falagas ME, Kasiakou SK. Colistin: the revival of polymyxins for the management of multidrug-resistant gram-negative bacterial infections. *Clin Infect Dis.* 2005;40:1333-1341.
112. Falcone M, Paterson D. Spotlight on ceftazidime/avibactam: a new option for MDR gram-negative infections. *J Antimicrob Chemother.* 2016;71:2713-2722.
113. Fang H, Froding I, Gian B, et al. Methicillin-resistant *Staphylococcus aureus* in Stockholm, Sweden: molecular epidemiology and antimicrobial susceptibilities to ceftaroline, linezolid, mupirocin and vancomycin in 2014. *J Glob Antimicrob Resist.* 2016;5:31-35.
115. Feikin DR, Dowell SF, Nwanyanwu OC, et al. Increased carriage of trimethoprim/sulfamethoxazole-resistant *Streptococcus pneumoniae* in Malawian children after treatment for malaria with sulfadoxine/pyrimethamine. *J Infect Dis.* 2000;181:1501-1505.
116. Fernandes P. Use of core structures to generate new and useful macrolide antibiotics. In: Demain AC, Sanchez S, eds. *Antibiotics: Current Innovations and Future Trends.* Norfolk, UK: Carster Academic Press; 2015:375-393.
117. Fernandes P, Martens E, Bertrand D, Pereira D. The solithromycin journey—it is all in the ichemistry. *Bioorg Med Chem.* 2016;24:6420-6428.
135. Giani T, Arena F, Vaggelli G, et al. Large nosocomial outbreak of colistin-resistant, carbapenemase-producing *Klebsiella pneumoniae* traced to clonal expansion of an mgrB deletion mutant. *J Clin Microbiol.* 2015;53:3341-3344.
138. Glasner C, Albiger B, Buist G, et al. Carbapenemase-producing Enterobacteriaceae in Europe: a survey among national experts from 39 countries, February 2013. *Euro Surveill.* 2013;18:pii: 20525.
146. Gupta K, Hooton TM, Naber KG, et al. International clinical practice guidelines for the treatment of acute uncomplicated cystitis and pyelonephritis in women: a 2010 update by the Infectious Diseases Society of America and the European Society for Microbiology and Infectious Diseases. *Clin Infect Dis.* 2011;52:e103-e120.
150. Habeeb MA, Haque A, Iversen A, Giske CG. Occurrence of virulence genes, 16S rRNA methylases, and plasmid-mediated quinolone resistance genes in CTX-M-producing *Escherichia coli* from Pakistan. *Eur J Clin Microbiol Infect Dis.* 2014;33:399-409.
157. Harrison EM, Ba X, Blane B, et al. PBP2a substitutions linked to ceftaroline resistance in MRSA isolates from the UK. *J Antimicrob Chemother.* 2016;71:268-269.
160. Hecker SJ, Reddy KR, Totrov M, et al. Discovery of a cyclic boronic acid beta-lactamase inhibitor (RPX7009) with utility vs class A serine carbapenemases. *J Med Chem.* 2015;58:3682-3692.
161. Helms M, Ethelberg S, Molbak K, DT104 Study Group. International *Salmonella typhimurium* DT104 infections, 1992-2001. *Emerg Infect Dis.* 2005;11:859-867.
164. Hidalgo L, Hopkins KL, Gutierrez B, et al. Association of the novel aminoglycoside resistance determinant RmtF with NDM carbapenemase in Enterobacteriaceae isolated in India and the UK. *J Antimicrob Chemother.* 2013;68:1543-1550.
165. Hidron AI, Edwards JR, Patel J, et al. NHSN annual update: antimicrobial-resistant pathogens associated with healthcare-associated infections: annual summary of data reported to the National Healthcare Safety Network at the Centers for Disease Control and Prevention, 2006-2007. *Infect Control Hosp Epidemiol.* 2008;29:996-1011.
166. Ho PL, Ng KY, Lo WU, et al. Plasmid-mediated OqxAB is an important mechanism for nitrofurantoin resistance in *Escherichia coli. Antimicrob Agents Chemother.* 2016;60:537-543.
173. Hooper DC, Jacoby GA. Topoisomerase inhibitors: fluoroquinolone mechanisms of action and resistance. *Cold Spring Harb Perspect Med.* 2016;6:pii: a025320.
176. Hsu AJ, Tamma PD. Treatment of multidrug-resistant gram-negative infections in children. *Clin Infect Dis.* 2014;58:1439-1448.
180. Huang SS, Hinrichsen VL, Stevenson AE, et al. Continued impact of pneumococcal conjugate vaccine on carriage in young children. *Pediatrics.* 2009;124:e1-e11.
183. Huovinen P, Sundstrom L, Swedberg G, Skold O. Trimethoprim and sulfonamide resistance. *Antimicrob Agents Chemother.* 1995;39:279-289.
188. Jacob JT, Laxminarayan R, Beldavs Z, et al. Vital signs: carbapenem-resistant Enterobacteriaceae. *MMWR Morb Mortal Wkly Rep.* 2013;62:165-170.
191. Jacoby GA. Mechanisms of resistance to quinolones. *Clin Infect Dis.* 2005;41(suppl 2):S120-S126.
193. Jacoby GA. AmpC beta-lactamases. *Clin Microbiol Rev.* 2009;22:161-182.
195. Jacoby GA, Strahilevitz J, Hooper DC. Plasmid-mediated quinolone resistance. *Microbiol Spectr.* 2014;2:10.1128/microbiolspec.PLAS-0006-2013.
201. Johnson JW, Fisher JF, Mobashery S. Bacterial cell-wall recycling. *Ann N Y Acad Sci.* 2013;1277:54-75.
202. Johnson CM, Grossman AD. Integrative and conjugative elements (ICEs): what they do and how they work. *Annu Rev Genet.* 2015;49:577-601.
205. Jones RN, Flonta M, Gurler N, et al. Resistance surveillance program report for selected European nations (2011). *Diagn Microbiol Infect Dis.* 2014;78:429-436.
210. Kaplan SL, Center KJ, Barson WJ, et al. Multicenter surveillance of *Streptococcus pneumoniae* isolates from middle ear and mastoid cultures in the 13-valent pneumococcal conjugate vaccine era. *Clin Infect Dis.* 2015;60:1339-1345.
213. Karavasilis V, Zarkotou O, Panopoulou M, et al. Wide dissemination of linezolid-resistant *Staphylococcus epidermidis* in Greece is associated with a linezolid-dependent ST22 clone. *J Antimicrob Chemother.* 2015;70:1625-1629.
215. Karlowsky JA, Biedenbach DJ, Bouchillon SK, et al. In vitro activity of ceftaroline against bacterial pathogens isolated from patients with skin and soft tissue and respiratory tract infections in African and Middle Eastern countries: AWARE global surveillance program 2012-2014. *Diagn Microbiol Infect Dis.* 2016;86:194-199.
218. Kaye KS, Cosgrove S, Harris A, Eliopoulos GM, Carmeli Y. Risk factors for emergence of resistance to broad-spectrum cephalosporins among *Enterobacter* spp. *Antimicrob Agents Chemother.* 2001;45:2628-2630.
219. Kaye KS, Pogue JM, Tran TB, et al. Agents of last resort: polymyxin resistance. *Infect Dis Clin North Am.* 2016;30:391-414.
222. Kelley WL, Jousselin A, Barras C, et al. Missense mutations in PBP2A affecting ceftaroline susceptibility detected in epidemic hospital-acquired methicillin-resistant *Staphylococcus aureus* clonotypes ST228 and ST247 in Western Switzerland archived since 1998. *Antimicrob Agents Chemother.* 2015;59:1922-1930.
237. Lahiri SD, McLaughlin RE, Whiteaker JD, et al. Molecular characterization of MRSA isolates bracketing the current EUCAST ceftaroline-susceptible breakpoint for *Staphylococcus aureus*: the role of PBP2a in the activity of ceftaroline. *J Antimicrob Chemother.* 2015;70:2488-2498.
241. Larru B, Gong W, Vendetti N, et al. Bloodstream infections in hospitalized children: epidemiology and antimicrobial susceptibilities. *Pediatr Infect Dis J.* 2016;35:507-510.
244. Lee HY, Chen CL, Liu SY, et al. Impact of molecular epidemiology and reduced susceptibility to glycopeptides and daptomycin on outcomes of patients with methicillin-resistant *Staphylococcus aureus* bacteremia. *PLoS ONE.* 2015;10:e0136171.
249. Levin AS, Barone AA, Penco J, et al. Intravenous colistin as therapy for nosocomial infections caused by multidrug-resistant *Pseudomonas aeruginosa* and *Acinetobacter baumannii. Clin Infect Dis.* 1999;28:1008-1011.
252. Li XZ, Nikaido H. Efflux-mediated drug resistance in bacteria: an update. *Drugs.* 2009;69:1555-1623.
253. Li XZ, Plesiat P, Nikaido H. The challenge of efflux-mediated antibiotic resistance in gram-negative bacteria. *Clin Microbiol Rev.* 2015;28:337-418.

255. Limbago BM, Kallen AJ, Zhu W, et al. Report of the 13th vancomycin-resistant *Staphylococcus aureus* isolate from the United States. *J Clin Microbiol.* 2014;52:998-1002.
259. Liu YY, Wang Y, Walsh TR, et al. Emergence of plasmid-mediated colistin resistance mechanism MCR-1 in animals and human beings in China: a microbiological and molecular biological study. *Lancet Infect Dis.* 2016;16:161-168.
260. Livermore DM. Current epidemiology and growing resistance of gram-negative pathogens. *Korean J Intern Med.* 2012;27:128-142.
262. Logan LK, Bonomo RA. Metallo-beta-lactamase (MBL)-producing Enterobacteriaceae in United States children. *Open Forum Infect Dis.* 2016;3:ofw090.
263. Logan LK, Braykov NP, Weinstein RA, Laxminarayan R, Program CDCEP. Extended-spectrum beta-lactamase-producing and third-generation cephalosporin-resistant Enterobacteriaceae in children: Trends in the United States, 1999-2011. *J Pediatric Infect Dis Soc.* 2014;3:320-328.
264. Logan LK, Hujer AM, Marshall SH, et al. Analysis of beta-lactamase resistance determinants in Enterobacteriaceae from Chicago children: a multicenter survey. *Antimicrob Agents Chemother.* 2016;60:3462-3469.
265. Logan LK, Renschler JP, Gandra S, et al. Carbapenem-resistant Enterobacteriaceae in children, United States, 1999-2012. *Emerg Infect Dis.* 2015;21:2014-2021.
266. Long SW, Olsen RJ, Mehta SC, et al. PBP2a mutations causing high-level ceftaroline resistance in clinical methicillin-resistant *Staphylococcus aureus* isolates. *Antimicrob Agents Chemother.* 2014;58:6668-6674.
271. Mahillon J, Chandler M. Insertion sequences. *Microbiol Mol Biol Rev.* 1998;62:725-774.
297. Mendes RE, Hogan PA, Jones RN, et al. Surveillance for linezolid resistance via the Zyvox(R) annual appraisal of potency and spectrum (ZAAPS) programme (2014): evolving resistance mechanisms with stable susceptibility rates. *J Antimicrob Chemother.* 2016;71:1860-1865.
299. Mikulska M, Viscoli C, Orasch C, et al. Aetiology and resistance in bacteraemias among adult and paediatric haematology and cancer patients. *J Infect.* 2014;68:321-331.
300. Miller LG, Daum RS, Creech CB, et al. Clindamycin versus trimethoprim-sulfamethoxazole for uncomplicated skin infections. *N Engl J Med.* 2015;372:1093-1103.
301. Miller WR, Murray BE, Rice LB, Arias CA. Vancomycin-resistant enterococci: therapeutic challenges in the 21st century. *Infect Dis Clin North Am.* 2016;30:415-439.
308. Moore MR, Link-Gelles R, Schaffner W, et al. Effect of use of 13-valent pneumococcal conjugate vaccine in children on invasive pneumococcal disease in children and adults in the USA: analysis of multisite, population-based surveillance. *Lancet Infect Dis.* 2015;15:301-309.
314. Munoz-Price LS, Poirel L, Bonomo RA, et al. Clinical epidemiology of the global expansion of *Klebsiella pneumoniae* carbapenemases. *Lancet Infect Dis.* 2013;13:785-796.
317. Nation RL, Garonzik SM, Li J, et al. Updated US and European dose recommendations for intravenous colistin: how do they perform? *Clin Infect Dis.* 2016;62:552-558.
326. Nordmann P, Poirel L, Walsh TR, Livermore DM. The emerging NDM carbapenemases. *Trends Microbiol.* 2011;19:588-595.
329. O'Connor C, Powell J, Finnegan C, et al. Incidence, management and outcomes of the first cfr-mediated linezolid-resistant *Staphylococcus epidermidis* outbreak in a tertiary referral centre in the Republic of Ireland. *J Hosp Infect.* 2015;90:316-321.
330. O'Driscoll C, Murphy V, Doyle O, et al. First outbreak of linezolid-resistant vancomycin-resistant *Enterococcus faecium.* in an Irish hospital, February to September 2014. *J Hosp Infect.* 2015;91:367-370.
331. Oikonomou O, Sarrou S, Papagiannitsis CC, et al. Rapid dissemination of colistin and carbapenem resistant *Acinetobacter baumannii* in Central Greece: mechanisms of resistance, molecular identification and epidemiological data. *BMC Infect Dis.* 2015;15:559.
338. Oteo J, Perez-Vazquez M, Bautista V, et al. The spread of KPC-producing Enterobacteriaceae in Spain: WGS analysis of the emerging high-risk clones of *Klebsiella pneumoniae* ST11/KPC-2, ST101/KPC-2 and ST512/KPC-3. *J Antimicrob Chemother.* 2016;71:3392-3399.
345. Papp-Wallace KM, Bonomo RA. New beta-lactamase inhibitors in the clinic. *Infect Dis Clin North Am.* 2016;30:441-464.
348. Patel G, Bonomo RA. "Stormy waters ahead": global emergence of carbapenemases. *Front Microbiol.* 2013;4:48.
353. Payne M, Croxen MA, Lee TD, et al. Mcr-1-positive colistin-resistant *Escherichia coli* in travelers returning to Canada from China. *Emerg Infect Dis.* 2016;22:1673-1675.
355. Perez F, Hujer AM, Hujer KM, et al. Global challenge of multidrug-resistant *Acinetobacter baumannii. Antimicrob Agents Chemother.* 2007;51:3471-3484.
357. Perichon B, Courvalin P, Galimand M. Transferable resistance to aminoglycosides by methylation of G1405 in 16S rRNA and to hydrophilic fluoroquinolones by QepA-mediated efflux in *Escherichia coli. Antimicrob Agents Chemother.* 2007;51:2464-2469.
359. Petty NK, Ben Zakour NL, Stanton-Cook M, et al. Global dissemination of a multidrug resistant *Escherichia coli* clone. *Proc Natl Acad Sci USA.* 2014;111:5694-5699.
364. Piddock LJ. Mechanisms of fluoroquinolone resistance: an update 1994-1998. *Drugs.* 1999;58(suppl 2):11-18.
365. Piddock LJ. Quinolone resistance and *Campylobacter* spp. *J Antimicrob Chemother.* 1995;36:891-898.
366. Piglansky L, Leibovitz E, Raiz S, et al. Bacteriologic and clinical efficacy of high dose amoxicillin for therapy of acute otitis media in children. *Pediatr Infect Dis J.* 2003;22:405-413.
371. Poirel L, Bonnin RA, Nordmann P. Genetic features of the widespread plasmid coding for the carbapenemase OXA-48. *Antimicrob Agents Chemother.* 2012;56:559-562.
372. Poirel L, Naas T, Nordmann P. Diversity, epidemiology, and genetics of class D beta-lactamases. *Antimicrob Agents Chemother.* 2010;54:24-38.
373. Poirel L, Nordmann P. Emerging plasmid-encoded colistin resistance: the animal world as the culprit? *J Antimicrob Chemother.* 2016;71:2326-2327.
374. Poirel L, Potron A, Nordmann P. OXA-48-like carbapenemases: the phantom menace. *J Antimicrob Chemother.* 2012;67:1597-1606.
376. Potron A, Poirel L, Nordmann P. Emerging broad-spectrum resistance in *Pseudomonas aeruginosa* and *Acinetobacter baumannii*: mechanisms and epidemiology. *Int J Antimicrob Agents.* 2015;45:568-585.
377. Poulin-Laprade D, Carraro N, Burrus V. The extended regulatory networks of SXT/R391 integrative and conjugative elements and IncA/C conjugative plasmids. *Front Microbiol.* 2015;6:837.
382. Quiles-Melero I, Gomez-Gil R, Romero-Gomez MP, et al. Mechanisms of linezolid resistance among staphylococci in a tertiary hospital. *J Clin Microbiol.* 2013;51:998-1001.
383. Qureshi ZA, Hittle LE, O'Hara JA, et al. Colistin-resistant *Acinetobacter baumannii*: beyond carbapenem resistance. *Clin Infect Dis.* 2015;60:1295-1303.
386. Raff AB, Kroshinsky D. Cellulitis: a review. *JAMA.* 2016;316:325-337.
388. Ramirez MS, Tolmasky ME. Aminoglycoside modifying enzymes. *Drug Resist Updat.* 2010;13:151-171.
391. Reading C, Cole M. Clavulanic acid: a beta-lactamase-inhiting beta-lactam from *Streptomyces clavuligerus. Antimicrob Agents Chemother.* 1977;11:852-857.
398. Richter SS, Diekema DJ, Heilmann KP, et al. Changes in pneumococcal serotypes and antimicrobial resistance after introduction of the 13-valent conjugate vaccine in the United States. *Antimicrob Agents Chemother.* 2014;58:6484-6489.
403. Robicsek A, Strahilevitz J, Jacoby GA, et al. Fluoroquinolone-modifying enzyme: a new adaptation of a common aminoglycoside acetyltransferase. *Nat Med.* 2006;12:83-88.
409. Sader HS, Farrell DJ, Flamm RK, Jones RN. Activity of ceftaroline and comparator agents tested against *Staphylococcus aureus* from patients with bloodstream infections in US medical centres (2009-13). *J Antimicrob Chemother.* 2015;70:2053-2056.
411. Sader HS, Mendes RE, Farrell DJ, Flamm RK, Jones RN. Ceftaroline activity tested against bacterial isolates from pediatric patients: results from the assessing worldwide antimicrobial resistance and evaluation program for the United States (2011-2012). *Pediatr Infect Dis J.* 2014;33:837-842.
412. Sader HS, Rhomberg PR, Farrell DJ, Jones RN. Arbekacin activity against contemporary clinical bacteria isolated from patients hospitalized with pneumonia. *Antimicrob Agents Chemother.* 2015;59:3263-3270.
416. Sa-Leao R, Tomasz A, Sanches IS, et al. Carriage of internationally spread clones of *Streptococcus pneumoniae* with unusual drug resistance patterns in children attending day care centers in Lisbon, Portugal. *J Infect Dis.* 2000;182:1153-1160.
419. Saravolatz LD, Arking L, Pohlod D, Fisher EJ, Borer R. An outbreak of gentamicin-resistant *Klebsiella pneumoniae*: analysis of control measures. *Infect Control.* 1984;5:79-84.
421. Sauvage E, Kerff F, Terrak M, Ayala JA, Charlier P. The penicillin-binding proteins: structure and role in peptidoglycan biosynthesis. *FEMS Microbiol Rev.* 2008;32:234-258.
426. Schwarz S, Johnson AP. Transferable resistance to colistin: a new but old threat. *J Antimicrob Chemother.* 2016;71:2066-2070.
428. Seiple IB, Zhang Z, Jakubec P, et al. A platform for the discovery of new macrolide antibiotics. *Nature.* 2016;533:338-345.
434. Shi J, Montay G, Bhargava VO. Clinical pharmacokinetics of telithromycin, the first ketolide antibacterial. *Clin Pharmacokinet.* 2005;44:915-934.
436. Sievert DM, Ricks P, Edwards JR, et al. Antimicrobial-resistant pathogens associated with healthcare-associated infections: summary of data reported to the National Healthcare Safety Network at the Centers for Disease Control and Prevention, 2009-2010. *Infect Control Hosp Epidemiol.* 2013;34:1-14.
437. Simner PJ, Adam H, Baxter M, et al. Epidemiology of vancomycin-resistant enterococci in Canadian hospitals (CANWARD study, 2007 to 2013). *Antimicrob Agents Chemother.* 2015;59:4315-4317.
440. Smillie C, Garcillan-Barcia MP, Francia MV, et al. Mobility of plasmids. *Microbiol Mol Biol Rev.* 2010;74:434-452.
444. Soler P, Gonzalez-Sanz R, Bleda MJ, et al. Antimicrobial resistance in non-typhoidal *Salmonella* from human sources, Spain, 2001-2003. *J Antimicrob Chemother.* 2006;58:310-314.
446. Sorensen AH, Hansen LH, Johannesen E, Sorensen SJ. Conjugative plasmid conferring resistance to olaquindox. *Antimicrob Agents Chemother.* 2003;47:798-799.
451. Stevens DL, Bisno AL, Chambers HF, et al. Practice guidelines for the diagnosis and management of skin and soft tissue infections: 2014 update by the infectious diseases society of America. *Clin Infect Dis.* 2014;59:147-159.

454. Stillwell T, Green M, Barbadora K, et al. Outbreak of KPC-3 producing carbapenem-resistant *Klebsiella pneumoniae* in a US pediatric hospital. *J Pediatric Infect Dis Soc*. 2015;4:330-338.
455. Stockmann C, Ampofo K, Pavia AT, et al. Clinical and epidemiological evidence of the red queen hypothesis in pneumococcal serotype dynamics. *Clin Infect Dis*. 2016;63:619-626.
458. Stryjewski ME, Corey GR. Methicillin-resistant *Staphylococcus aureus*: an evolving pathogen. *Clin Infect Dis*. 2014;58(suppl 1):S10-S19.
466. Tamma PD, Girdwood SC, Gopaul R, et al. The use of cefepime for treating AmpC beta-lactamase-producing Enterobacteriaceae. *Clin Infect Dis*. 2013;57: 781-788.
471. Tokars JI, Frank M, Alter MJ, Arduino MJ. National surveillance of dialysis-associated diseases in the United States, 2000. *Semin Dial*. 2002;15:162-171.
472. Toleman MA, Walsh TR. Combinatorial events of insertion sequences and ICE in gram-negative bacteria. *FEMS Microbiol Rev*. 2011;35:912-935.
475. Tomczyk S, Lynfield R, Schaffner W, et al. Prevention of antibiotic-nonsusceptible invasive pneumococcal disease with the 13-valent pneumococcal conjugate vaccine. *Clin Infect Dis*. 2016;62:1119-1125.
476. Tran QT, Nawaz MS, Deck J, Nguyen KT, Cerniglia CE. Plasmid-mediated quinolone resistance in *Pseudomonas putida* isolates from imported shrimp. *Appl Environ Microbiol*. 2011;77:1885-1887.
479. Truong-Bolduc QC, Dunman PM, Eidem T, Hooper DC. Transcriptional profiling analysis of the global regulator NorG, a GntR-like protein of *Staphylococcus aureus*. *J Bacteriol*. 2011;193:6207-6214.
480. Truong-Bolduc QC, Hsing LC, Villet R, et al. Reduced aeration affects the expression of the NorB efflux pump of *Staphylococcus aureus* by posttranslational modification of MgrA. *J Bacteriol*. 2012;194:1823-1834.
484. Ubukata K, Itoh-Yamashita N, Konno M. Cloning and expression of the norA gene for fluoroquinolone resistance in *Staphylococcus aureus*. *Antimicrob Agents Chemother*. 1989;33:1535-1539.
486. van Duin D, Doi Y. Outbreak of colistin-resistant, carbapenemase-producing *Klebsiella pneumoniae*: are we at the end of the road? *J Clin Microbiol*. 2015;53:3116-3117.
488. Varaldo PE, Debbia EA, Nicoletti G, et al. Nationwide survey in Italy of treatment of *Streptococcus pyogenes* pharyngitis in children: influence of macrolide resistance on clinical and microbiological outcomes. Artemis-Italy Study Group. *Clin Infect Dis*. 1999;29:869-873.
493. von Wintersdorff CJ, Wolffs PF, van Niekerk JM, et al. Detection of the plasmid-mediated colistin-resistance gene mcr-1 in faecal metagenomes of Dutch travellers. *J Antimicrob Chemother*. 2016;71:3416-3419.
495. Wald ER, Applegate KE, Bordley C, et al. Clinical practice guideline for the diagnosis and management of acute bacterial sinusitis in children aged 1 to 18 years. *Pediatrics*. 2013;132:e262-e280.
499. Walters MS, Eggers P, Albrecht V, et al. Vancomycin-resistant *Staphylococcus aureus*—Delaware, 2015. *MMWR Morb Mortal Wkly Rep*. 2015;64:1056.
500. Wang JC. DNA topoisomerases. *Annu Rev Biochem*. 1996;65:635-692.
502. Wang Y, Lv Y, Cai J, et al. A novel gene, optrA, that confers transferable resistance to oxazolidinones and phenicols and its presence in *Enterococcus faecalis* and *Enterococcus faecium* of human and animal origin. *J Antimicrob Chemother*. 2015;70:2182-2190.
506. Weinstein MP, Klugman KP, Jones RN. Rationale for revised penicillin susceptibility breakpoints versus *Streptococcus pneumoniae*: coping with antimicrobial susceptibility in an era of resistance. *Clin Infect Dis*. 2009;48:1596-1600.
513. Wisplinghoff H, Rosato AE, Enright MC, et al. Related clones containing SCCmec type IV predominate among clinically significant *Staphylococcus epidermidis* isolates. *Antimicrob Agents Chemother*. 2003;47:3574-3579.
516. Wozniak RA, Waldor MK. Integrative and conjugative elements: mosaic mobile genetic elements enabling dynamic lateral gene flow. *Nat Rev Microbiol*. 2010;8:552-563.
520. Yamane K, Wachino J, Suzuki S, et al. New plasmid-mediated fluoroquinolone efflux pump, QepA, found in an *Escherichia coli* clinical isolate. *Antimicrob Agents Chemother*. 2007;51:3354-3360.
521. Yang SJ, Mishra NN, Rubio A, Bayer AS. Causal role of single nucleotide polymorphisms within the mprF gene of *Staphylococcus aureus* in daptomycin resistance. *Antimicrob Agents Chemother*. 2013;57:5658-5664.
524. Yoshida H, Bogaki M, Nakamura S, et al. Nucleotide sequence and characterization of the *Staphylococcus aureus* norA gene, which confers resistance to quinolones. *J Bacteriol*. 1990;172:6942-6949.
537. Zhao J, Chen Z, Chen S, et al. Prevalence and dissemination of oqxAB in *Escherichia coli* isolates from animals, farmworkers, and the environment. *Antimicrob Agents Chemother*. 2010;54:4219-4224.
538. Zhao L, Zhang J, Zheng B, et al. Molecular epidemiology and genetic diversity of fluoroquinolone-resistant *Escherichia coli* isolates from patients with community-onset infections in 30 Chinese county hospitals. *J Clin Microbiol*. 2015;53:766-770.
539. Zhou W, Niu D, Cao X, et al. Clonal dissemination of linezolid-resistant *Staphylococcus capitis* with G2603T mutation in domain V of the 23S rRNA and the cfr gene at a tertiary care hospital in China. *BMC Infect Dis*. 2015;15:97.

The full reference list for this chapter is available at ExpertConsult.com.

The Pharmacokinetic-Pharmacodynamic Interface: Determinants of Antiinfective Drug Action and Efficacy in Pediatrics

235

Jennifer L. Goldman • Susan M. Abdel-Rahman • Gregory L. Kearns

The *pharmacokinetic-pharmacodynamic interface* reflects an association between two determinants of drug effect—delivery of drug to the site of action and the intrinsic activity of a drug to alter cellular function after it reaches that site. The conjoint consideration of drug disposition (i.e., pharmacokinetics) and drug action (i.e., pharmacodynamics) is of critical importance in the selection and evaluation of any antiinfective drug regimen. In much of the contemporary clinical pharmacology and therapeutics literature, *kinetics* generally is associated with a description of the rate processes associated with drug absorption, distribution, metabolism, and excretion (ADME). Although accurate in its definition concerning the movement of drugs into and out of the body, kinetics as a determinant of drug effect must be viewed in a much broader context, specifically, the sojourn and fate of a drug molecule in both the extracellular and intracellular milieus. Although understanding this facet of drug behavior admittedly is difficult because of a relative inability in the clinical context to track the intracellular fate of a drug in humans, achieving a high degree of control over antiinfective therapy by the application of well-characterized and understood kinetic principles is quite possible.

The focus of this chapter is on the pharmacologic considerations necessary for the prudent use of antiinfective agents in pediatric patients, specifically, the pharmacokinetic and pharmacodynamic principles that, if embraced, can be the key to optimizing drug treatment and maximizing therapeutic efficacy and safety. The pediatric patient presents a particular challenge to the clinician. Although pediatric practitioners recognize that "children are not just miniature adults," more difficult to appreciate are the dramatic changes associated with normal human growth and development that can, and many times do, exert a profound influence on drug disposition, drug action, and, ultimately, therapeutic outcome of antiinfectives.[119] Failure to compensate for developmental differences in pharmacokinetics in the context of therapeutic drug use in pediatrics can increase the risk for occurrence of adverse drug effects associated with either overdose (i.e., drug toxicity) or underdose (i.e., lack of efficacy).[82,119]

In the following sections of this chapter are basic principles required to understand the pharmacokinetic-pharmacodynamic interface in pediatrics, namely, general principles in pharmacokinetics, the impact of development on drug disposition, the pharmacokinetic determinants of drug action, and methods to facilitate clinical integration of the pharmacokinetic and pharmacodynamic properties necessary to optimize antiinfective therapy.

PHARMACOKINETIC DETERMINANTS OF EXPOSURE

Implicit in the production of any pharmacologic effect is the association of a drug molecule with one or more receptors and the subsequent propagation of intracellular events that ultimately translate into drug action. In general terms, successful drug-receptor interactions are characterized by three principles: (1) *avidity,* the ability of a drug to combine with a receptor; (2) *affinity,* the physical combination of a drug with a receptor, and (3) *intrinsic activity,* the ability of the drug-receptor combination to generate one or more "impulses" or "signals" capable of activating biologic effector systems. The primary determinants of both avidity and affinity reside with the maintenance of structural specificity of both the drug and receptor to ensure that an association with one or more physicochemically distinct, active sites can occur. Simply stated, a drug molecule must fit into a receptor as a key fits into a lock before intrinsic activity becomes a possibility. The receptor or receptors thus will function in the role of cellular targets for drug molecules when an effective combination is required for drug effect and, ultimately, therapeutic efficacy.

The onset and offset of drug action are determined not only by receptor-modulated intrinsic activity but also by receptor occupancy. In almost all instances, these events are both concentration and time dependent. Hence the disposition of a drug in the body (e.g., ADME) becomes the "driver" for its pharmacodynamics. This action is particularly true for antiinfective drugs when the therapeutic target, the infecting organism, must be exposed to a sufficient concentration of pharmacologically active (i.e., free) drug for a period sufficient for drug binding to critical cellular elements (e.g., penicillin-binding proteins [PBPs], intracellular enzymes) to occur and for subsequent disruption of normal cellular function (e.g., inhibition of protein biosynthesis, inhibition of cell wall synthesis) to result in cellular demise. Thus the clinical determinants of drug efficacy (and safety), such as proper selection of both dose and dosing interval relative to the intrinsic sensitivity of the infecting pathogen or pathogens, and factors that determine delivery of the drug to the site or sites of infection embody the importance of pharmacokinetics in the selection and clinical use of antiinfective drugs.

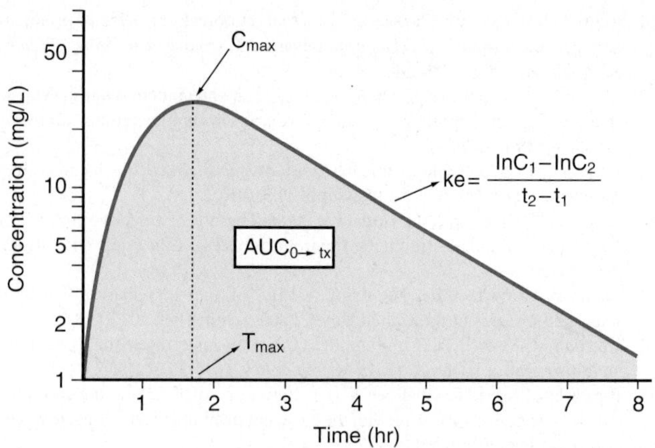

FIG. 235.1 Representative plasma concentration versus time curve. Illustrated are commonly referenced pharmacokinetic parameters. *AUC,* Area under the curve; C_{max}, maximal plasma concentration; *ke,* elimination rate constant; and T_{max}, time to achieve maximal plasma concentration.

BASIC TERMS

A complete discussion of pharmacokinetics is beyond the scope of this chapter because it would require a description of theory and a presentation of relatively sophisticated mathematical concepts. This information can be found in many excellent textbooks that provide both theoretical[81] and conceptual[119,194,242] presentations of pharmacokinetics and through Internet-based programmed instruction courses.[29] However, well within the scope of this chapter are a definition and glossary of pharmacokinetic terms sufficient to equip the reader with a conceptual, working knowledge of this pharmacotherapeutic tool. These definitions and concepts are presented as follows:

Absolute bioavailability (F) is the extent or fraction of drug absorbed after extravascular administration. It is determined by comparing the area under the plasma concentration versus time curve (AUC) after administration of an oral dose of a drug with the AUC after administration of an intravenous dose (e.g., $F = AUC_{PO} \times dose_{IV}/AUC_{IV} \times dose_{PO}$).

Relative bioavailability reflects the extent of drug absorbed from one dosage form given by an extravascular route of administration in comparison to a dose of a "reference" drug formulation administered by the same route. Generally, it reflects the relative extent of systemic availability (F) and is calculated by comparing the AUC of the test regimen relative to the reference formulation (e.g., $F = AUC_{test} \times dose_{reference}/AUC_{reference} \times dose_{test}$).

Absorption of drugs describes the process of drug uptake from a site of extravascular administration (e.g., oral, intramuscular, subcutaneous, intraperitoneal, intraosseous, intratracheal, intravaginal, intraurethral, sublingual, buccal, rectal, and dermal) into the systemic circulation. Drug absorption is conceptualized most accurately by considering both rate (e.g., absorption half-life, time to peak concentration) and extent (e.g., bioavailability), either of which can be influenced by biopharmaceutical (e.g., drug formulation), physicochemical (e.g., pH, solubility, hydrophilicity and lipophilicity, protein binding, complexation characteristics with food or drugs), and physiologic (e.g., barrier integrity, motility, volume and pH of body fluids at the absorptive site, protein-binding capacity, degradation/biotransformation potential) factors.

Area under the curve (AUC) is, conceptually, a measure of both the extent of drug absorbed and its persistence in the body. It is the integral of drug blood levels over time from zero to either a predetermined postdose time point (i.e., $AUC_{0\rightarrow n}$), the end of the dosing interval (i.e., $AUC_{0\rightarrow\tau}$), or extrapolated to infinity (i.e., $AUC_{0\rightarrow\infty}$) by using the apparent terminal elimination rate constant (similarly calculated from the observed plasma concentration versus time plot) (Fig. 235.1). AUC is therefore a pharmacokinetic parameter that is both time and concentration dependent.

Bioequivalence of a drug product is achieved if its extent and rate of absorption are not significantly different (i.e., within 80–125%) from those of a reference standard drug product when administered at the same molar dose. Bioequivalence is a pharmacokinetically determined parameter and does not entail a relative comparison of drug action or efficacy. Therefore, if a drug product (e.g., a generic drug) produces a rate and extent of absorption sufficiently similar to those of the reference formulation, the effect and toxicity profiles of the two drugs are assumed to be virtually identical.

Biopharmaceutics deals with the physical and chemical properties of the drug substance, the dosage form, and the body, as well as the biologic actions of a drug or drug product after administration. Biopharmaceutical considerations (e.g., rate and extent of the disintegration or dissolution of a dosage form, liberation of the active drug from a dosage form, solubility or binding of the drug at the site of absorption) can be rate limiting for drug absorption or bioavailability, or for both, and thus may limit the efficacy of drug therapy.

Clearance (Cl) of a drug is represented conceptually by the volume of blood from which a certain amount of unmetabolized drug is removed (i.e., cleared) per unit of time by any and all pathways capable of drug removal (e.g., renal, hepatic, biliary, pulmonary, breast milk, sweat). In pharmacokinetics, clearance generally is represented as total body (or plasma) clearance, renal clearance (Cl_{ren}), or nonrenal clearance (Cl_{nr}). Clearance is determined easily from knowledge of the drug dose, and AUC and can be calculated as follows:

$$Cl = Dose\,(mg/kg)/AUC\,(mg/L \times hour)$$

where AUC can represent either the $AUC_{0\rightarrow\tau}$ for single-dose administration, or the AUC from time zero to the end of the dosing interval at steady state (i.e., $AUCss_{0\rightarrow\tau}$). Calculation of renal clearance requires a complete, quantitative collection of urine (usually over the course of 24 hours) to determine the amount of drug excreted (Ae) unchanged. Nonrenal clearance generally is determined as the difference between total body clearance and renal clearance. For drug administration *by any extravascular route,* calculation of clearance yields an apparent value (e.g., Cl/F) in that it must be corrected for the extent of the drug dose absorbed (i.e., the bioavailability) from the site of administration.

A *compartment* in pharmacokinetics represents a *hypothetical space* into and out of which drug partitions as a function of time. Compartment *models* are used in pharmacokinetics to characterize the relationship between drug dose and concentration as a function of time. The most simple of all pharmacokinetic models is a *one-compartment open model* in which the only applicable rate processes represent drug ingress and egress from a single theoretical or central space. A *two-compartment model* has been used to characterize the disposition of many antiinfective agents in both pediatric and adult subjects. This particular model is composed of a central compartment and a peripheral compartment, both of which represent the various fluids and tissues where a drug may reside. Although a compartment often may not correspond to a true physiologic space that can be characterized by a specific volume of biologic fluid, compartment models can be used to conceptualize both drug distribution between physiologic spaces and elimination from the body. In the two-compartment model, for example, the central compartment often is used to represent a drug resident within the intravascular space and the highly exchangeable extracellular fluid of tissues and organs that are well perfused, whereas the peripheral compartment represents drug distribution to intracellular fluid and tissues and organs that are less well perfused and, in some instances, the association of the drug (e.g., binding) to specific tissues or tissue components. In all instances, compartmental models oversimplify the true processes of ADME. However, they have been demonstrated repeatedly to be useful as a reliable means to model, and therefore predict, the relationship between drug dose and concentration in both plasma and tissue.

Disposition refers collectively to the processes of ADME, all of which occur simultaneously after administration of a drug, as opposed to being discrete pharmacologic events.

Dose-response curve is a graphic representation of the pharmacologic effect as a function of either the drug dose or the concentration of the drug. A log dose-response curve is often sigmoidal, whereas a cartesian concentration-effect curve is hyperbolic (Fig. 235.2). Theoretically, a drug concentration of zero indicates no drug effect (i.e., E_0). As a drug travels to and interacts with a receptor, the effect (E) increases in a concentration-dependent manner (i.e., E $[(E_{max}\ C)/(E_{50} + C)]$) to a point at which a maximal effect (E_{max}) is attained and above which higher drug concentrations fail to enhance the effect. A pharmacologically important term that can be derived easily from a concentration-effect curve is the EC_{50}, or the drug concentration for which the observed effect is 50% of the E_{max}.

Elimination half-life of a drug is the time necessary to reduce the drug concentration (in blood serum or plasma) by 50% after absorption is complete and distribution between body compartments has attained equilibrium. Loss of drug from the body, as represented by the elimination half-life, reflects elimination of the administered parent drug molecule (i.e., not its metabolites) by metabolism, urinary excretion, or other pathways capable of resulting in elimination of drug. Accordingly, many individuals use elimination half-life as a surrogate indicator of drug clearance. Such a determination should be made cautiously because this particular pharmacokinetic parameter is dependent on both clearance and the apparent volume of distribution (VD), as illustrated by the following equation: $t_{1/2}$ elimination = $[(0.693 \times VD)/Cl]$, where $t_{1/2}$ is half-life. Practically speaking, the elimination half-life is an important pharmacokinetic parameter because it can be used to determine the period of time required for a drug dosing regimen to produce steady-state plasma concentrations (e.g., $5 \times t_{1/2}$ elimination) and the dosing interval required to produce a desired excursion (i.e., peak and trough) in plasma drug concentrations.

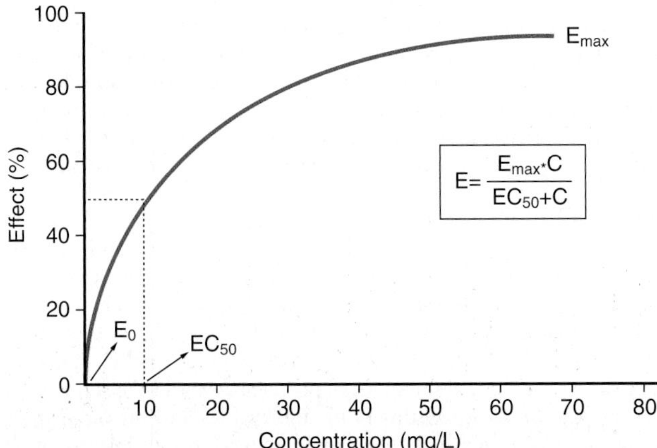

FIG. 235.2 Representative nonlinear concentration (C) versus effect profile. *E_{max},* Maximal effect; *EC_{50},* drug concentration for which the observed effect is 50% of the maximal effect.

Steady state reflects the level of drug accumulation in the blood and tissue after multiple doses when input (i.e., the amount of drug placed into the systemic circulation) and output (i.e., drug clearance) are at equilibrium. When drugs are given at fixed doses and dosing intervals, the steady-state concentrations fluctuate between a maximum (C_{max}) and minimum (C_{min}) within a given dose interval that are identical between doses, provided that the size of the dose, method of administration, dosing interval, or drug pharmacokinetics (or any combination of these parameters) does not change. For drugs that follow first-order pharmacokinetics, steady-state plasma concentrations for a given dosing regimen are attained over a period of time that corresponds to four to five times the elimination half-life. In general, the pharmacokinetics of a drug at steady state provides the most accurate correlate for examining drug effect.

First-pass effect describes a phenomenon whereby drugs may be metabolized or chemically degraded (or both) after extravascular administration before they reach the systemic circulation. Specific examples include biotransformation of selected drugs (e.g., cytochrome CYP3A4 substrates) in the enterocyte and nonenzymatic hydrolysis of an active drug (e.g., penicillin) in the lumen of the gastrointestinal tract (e.g., stomach, intestine, rectum). Drugs subject to a first-pass effect generally have a reduced rate or extent of relative bioavailability, or both, when compared with that achieved by parenteral administration.

Protein binding is the phenomenon that occurs when a drug (or metabolite) combines with plasma or extracellular or tissue proteins to form a drug-protein complex. In general, drug-protein binding usually is nonspecific and depends on the drug's affinity for the protein molecule (i.e., binding site), the number of protein-binding sites, and the drug and protein concentrations. With few exceptions, drugs that are bound to proteins are pharmacologically inactive and cannot be metabolized or excreted readily. The pharmacokinetic consequences of drug-protein binding can influence the drug dose versus the plasma concentration versus the effect relationship. For example, drugs with extensive tissue binding have apparent volumes of distribution that are far in excess of the total body water space and, in general, have relatively long elimination half-lives. Conditions in which intravascular proteins escape to extravascular sites (e.g., nephrotic syndrome, severe burns, ascites) can increase the apparent volume (and elimination half-life) of drugs that are extensively (i.e., >70%) bound to albumin.

Volume of distribution (apparent volume of distribution) (VD) represents a hypothetic volume of body fluid that would be required to dissolve the total amount of a drug at the same concentration as that found in the blood and is illustrated by the following equation:

$$VD = Dose/Cp^0$$

where Cp^0 represents the highest attainable plasma concentration after the administration of a single dose. As a proportionality constant, the VD is a determinant of plasma drug concentrations attained after administration of a given drug dose. For drugs that are not distributed extensively or that bind with great affinity to proteins and tissues, the apparent VD may correspond dimensionally to physiologic or anatomic body spaces (e.g., VD <0.1 L/kg approximates the intravascular space, 0.1–0.3 L/kg approximates the extracellular space, 0.6–0.7 L/kg approximates the total body water space), which, when altered by disease or

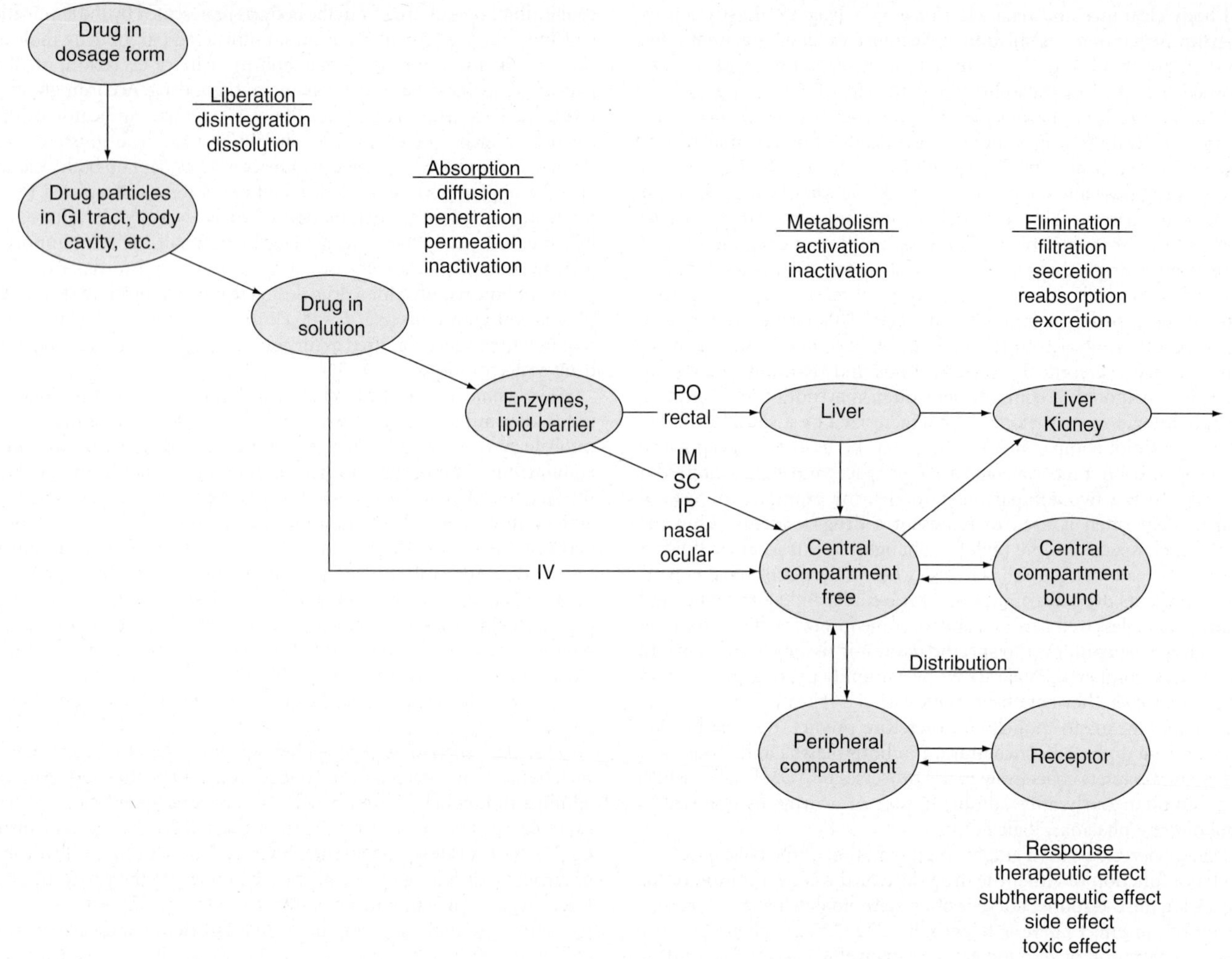

FIG. 235.3 Representation of the pharmacokinetic-pharmacodynamic interface. *GI,* Gastrointestinal; *IM,* intramuscular; *IP,* intraperitoneal; *PO,* oral; *SC,* subcutaneous.

development, or by both, will influence the apparent VD and thus the achievable concentration for a given drug.

A working knowledge of these pharmacokinetic definitions allows one to have an understanding of the relationships among drug dose, concentration, and effect. The use of knowledge related to the physicochemical and pharmacologic properties of a drug, the impact of isolated or concurrent variables on drug disposition, and predictors of pharmacodynamics or drug response enables the clinician to optimize the selection of agents and dosing regimens and thus individualize drug therapy. To accomplish this goal, it is imperative that the relationship between drug pharmacokinetics and pharmacodynamics not be compartmentalized, but rather, as illustrated in Fig. 235.3, be conceptualized as multifactorial, in which the determinants of drug concentration and effect are dynamic and change as a function of a disease state and drug therapy.

IMPACT OF ONTOGENY ON PHARMACOKINETICS

Development represents a continuum of biologic events that enable adaptation, somatic growth, neurobehavioral maturation, and, eventually, reproduction. The impact of development on the pharmacokinetics of a given drug is determined, to a great degree, by age-related changes in body composition and the acquisition of function in organs and organ systems that are important in determining drug metabolism and excretion. Although classifying pediatric patients on the basis of postnatal age (e.g., neonates, ≤1 month of age; infants, 1–24 months of age; children, 2–12 years of age; and adolescents, 12–18 years of age) often is convenient for providing drug therapy, recognizing that the changes in physiology are not linearly related to age and may not correspond to these age-defined breakpoints is important. In fact, the most dramatic changes in drug disposition occur during the first 18 months of life, when the acquisition of organ function is most dynamic. Additionally, the pharmacokinetics of a given drug may be altered in pediatric patients as a result of intrinsic (e.g., gender, genotype, ethnicity, inherited diseases) or extrinsic (e.g., acquired disease states, xenobiotic exposure, diet) factors that may occur during the first 2 decades of life.

Selection of an appropriate drug dose for a neonate, infant, child, or adolescent requires an understanding of the basic pharmacokinetic properties of a given compound and how the process of development affects each facet of drug disposition. Accordingly, conceptualizing pediatric pharmacokinetics by examining the impact of development on the physiologic variables that govern ADME is most useful.

Drug Absorption

The rate and extent of gastrointestinal absorption depend primarily on pH-dependent passive diffusion and motility of the stomach and small intestine, both of which control transit time. In full-term neonates, gastric pH ranges from 6 to 8 at birth and drops to 2 to 3 within the first few hours. After the first 24 hours of extrauterine life, gastric pH increases to 6 to 7 as a result of immaturity of the parietal cells. A relative state of achlorhydria remains until adult values and diurnal patterns of gastric pH are reached at approximately 20 to 30 months of age. Although basal gastric acid output can be quite similar in neonates, young infants, and adults, stimulated acid output can be threefold to fourfold higher than that seen in adults.[57,58]

TABLE 235.1 **Summary of Drug Absorption in Neonates, Infants, and Children**[a]

	Neonates	Infants	Children
Physiologic Alteration			
Gastric emptying time	Irregular	Increased	Slightly increased
Gastric pH	>5	2–4	Normal (2–3)
Intestinal motility	Reduced	Increased	Slightly increased
Intestinal surface area	Reduced	Near adult	Adult pattern
Microbial colonization	Reduced	Near adult	Adult pattern
Biliary function	Immature	Near adult	Adult pattern
Muscular blood flow	Reduced	Increased	Adult pattern
Skin permeability	Increased	Increased	Near adult pattern
Possible Pharmacokinetic Consequences			
Oral absorption	Erratic: reduced	Increased rate	Near adult pattern
Intramuscular absorption	Variable	Increased	Adult pattern
Percutaneous absorption	Increased	Increased	Near adult pattern
Rectal absorption	Very efficient	Efficient	Near adult pattern
Presystemic clearance	Less than adult	Greater than adult	Greater than adult (increased rate)

[a]The direction of alteration is given relative to the expected normal adult pattern.
Modified from Ritschel WA, Kearns GL. Pediatric pharmacokinetics. In: Ritschel WA, Kearns GL, eds. *Handbook of Basic Pharmacokinetics.* 6th ed. Washington, DC: American Pharmaceutical Association; 2004:227-240.

In neonates, gastrointestinal transit time is prolonged as a result of reduced motility and peristalsis. Gastric emptying is both irregular and erratic and only partially dependent on feeding. Gastric emptying rates approximate adult values by the time the infant reaches 6 to 8 months of age. During infancy, intestinal transit time generally is reduced relative to adult values because of increased intestinal motility.[119] In contrast to developmental changes in motility, histologic examination of the luminal absorptive surface suggests that the adult pattern of architecture (and hence absorptive surface area relative to body size) is present at birth.[86,238] In neonates and young infants, additional factors, including diminished splanchnic blood flow, immature biliary function, variable microbial colonization, and an apparent reduction in the activity of intestinal drug-metabolizing enzymes, may play a role in intestinal drug absorption.[44,187]

These developmental changes in gastrointestinal function and structure in the neonatal period and early infancy produce alterations in drug absorption that are quite predictable. In general, the oral bioavailability of acid-labile compounds (e.g., β-lactam antibiotics) is increased, whereas that of weak organic acids (e.g., phenobarbital, phenytoin) is decreased. For orally administered drugs with limited water solubility (e.g., phenytoin, carbamazepine), the rate of absorption (i.e., T_{max}) can be altered dramatically as a result of changes in gastrointestinal motility.[187] The pharmacokinetics of the antiviral agent pleconaril similarly provides an example of developmental differences in drug absorption. After administration of a 5 mg/kg dose, the AUC was much lower in neonates than either children or adults, thus demonstrating that the extent of pleconaril bioavailability in neonates was reduced. The reason for this difference may be attributed to the lipid-based pleconaril formulation and to developmental differences in the ability to absorb lipids as a consequence of biliary immaturity and reduced lipase secretion in neonates.[121]

In neonates and young infants, both rectal and percutaneous absorption is highly efficient for properly formulated drug products. The bioavailability of many drugs administered by the rectal route is increased as a result of not only efficient translocation across the rectal mucosa but also a reduced first-pass effect caused by the immaturity of a number of drug-metabolizing enzymes in the liver. Both the rate and extent of percutaneous drug absorption are increased because of the thinner and better hydrated stratum corneum in young infants. As a consequence, systemic toxicity can occur with the percutaneous application of some drugs (e.g., hexachlorophene) to seemingly small areas of skin during the first 8 to 12 months of life. In contrast to older infants and children, the rate of bioavailability for drugs administered by the intramuscular route may be altered (i.e., delayed T_{max}) more than the extent of absorption in a neonate. This developmental pharmacokinetic alteration is the consequence of relatively low muscular blood flow in the first few days of life, the relative inefficiency of muscular contractions (useful in dispersing an intramuscular drug dose), and an increased percentage of water per unit of muscle mass.[187]

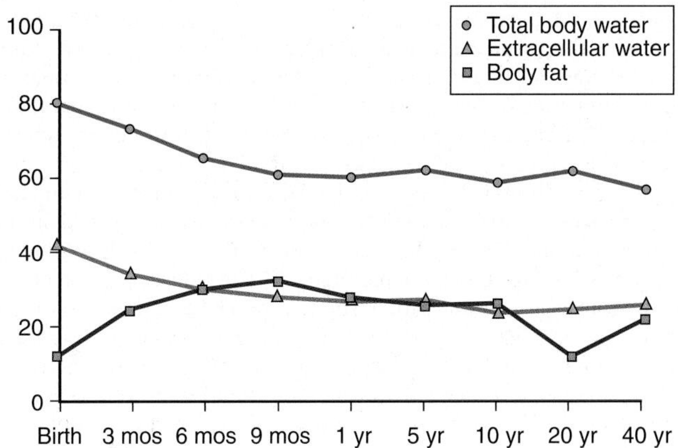

FIG. 235.4 Body composition reflected as a percentage (*y*-axis) of total body mass for total body water, extracellular water, and body fat as a function of age (*x*-axis). (From Ritschel WA, Kearns GL. Pediatric pharmacokinetics. In: Ritschel WA, Kearns GL, eds. *Handbook of Basic Pharmacokinetics.* 6th ed. Washington, DC: American Pharmaceutical Association; 2004:227-240.)

Developmental differences in drug absorption among neonates, infants, and older children are summarized in Table 235.1. The data contained therein reflect developmental differences that may be expected to occur in healthy pediatric patients. Certain conditions or disease states that could modify the function or structure, or both, of the absorptive surface area, gastrointestinal motility, or systemic blood flow can further affect either the rate or the extent of absorption for extravascularly administered drugs in pediatric patients.

Distribution

Development is associated with marked changes in body composition as reflected by examination of total body water, extracellular water, and stores of body fat (Fig. 235.4). The most dynamic changes occur in the first year of life, with the exception of total body fat, which has a distinctly different pattern in male and female children. Furthermore, the adipose

TABLE 235.2 Plasma Protein Binding and Drug Distribution[a]

	Neonates	Infants	Children
Physiologic Alteration			
Plasma albumin	Reduced	Near normal	Near adult pattern
Fetal albumin	Present	Absent	Absent
Total protein	Reduced	Decreased	Near adult pattern
Serum bilirubin	Increased	Normal	Normal adult pattern
Serum free fatty acids	Increased	Normal	Normal adult pattern
Blood pH	7.1–7.3	7.4 (normal)	7.4 (normal)
Possible Pharmacokinetic Consequences			
Free fraction	Increased	Increased	Slightly increased
Apparent volume of distribution			
Hydrophilic drugs	Increased	Increased	Slightly increased
Hydrophobic drugs	Reduced	Reduced	Slightly decreased
Tissue-to-plasma ratio	Increased	Increased	Slightly increased

[a]The direction of alteration is given relative to the expected normal adult pattern.Modified from Ritschel WA, Kearns GL. Pediatric pharmacokinetics. In: Ritschel WA, Kearns GL, eds. *Handbook of Basic Pharmacokinetics.* 6th ed. Washington, DC: American Pharmaceutical Association; 2004:227-240.

tissue of neonates may contain as much as 57% water and 35% lipids, whereas values in adults approach 26% and 72%, respectively.[187]

In addition to age-related alterations in body composition, several physiologic changes that occur during the neonatal period are capable of altering the plasma protein binding of drugs (Table 235.2). In neonates, the free fraction of drugs that are bound extensively to circulating plasma proteins is increased markedly, largely because of lower concentrations of drug-binding proteins, reduced binding affinity of these proteins, the presence of a relatively acidic plasma pH, and endogenous competing ligands (e.g., bilirubin, free fatty acids). This consideration is exemplified by ceftriaxone, a weak acid that is approximately 95% bound to albumin in adults but only 70% bound in neonates and thus is capable of producing significant displacement of bilirubin.[96,153] The reduced plasma protein binding, in combination with absolute and relative differences in the size of various body compartments (e.g., total body water, extracellular fluid, composition of body tissues), frequently influences (i.e., increases) the apparent VD for many drugs and also their localization (i.e., both uptake and residence) in tissue, which, in turn, can alter their plasma elimination half-life.

Renal Excretion

The renal excretion of many drugs is directly proportional to age-dependent patterns in the acquisition of renal function, primarily glomerular filtration and active tubular secretion. Accordingly, developmental differences in renal function may serve as a major determinant of drug clearance in neonates and young infants for compounds that are not metabolized extensively.[187]

In preterm infants, renal function is reduced dramatically because of the continued development of functioning nephron units (i.e., nephrogenesis). In contrast, the acquisition of renal function in a term neonate represents, to a great degree, the recruitment of fully developed nephron units. In both term neonates and preterm infants who have birth weights greater than 1500 g, glomerular filtration rates increase dramatically during the first 2 weeks of postnatal life (Fig. 235.5). This particular dynamic change in function is a direct consequence of postnatal adaptations in the distribution of renal blood flow (i.e., medullary distribution to the corticomedullary border) and results in a dramatic recruitment of functioning nephron units.[119] In addition, a glomerular-tubular imbalance exists in which the maturation of the glomerular function is more advanced than is the proximal tubular secretion. This imbalance may persist for up to 6 to 10 months of age, when both tubular function and glomerular function approach values approximately equal to those observed in healthy, young adults.[187]

The impact of development on each of the components of renal function can be characterized by a definable pattern during the first year of life (see Fig. 235.5).[172] Accordingly, the renal handling and, hence, excretion and elimination characteristics of virtually any drug

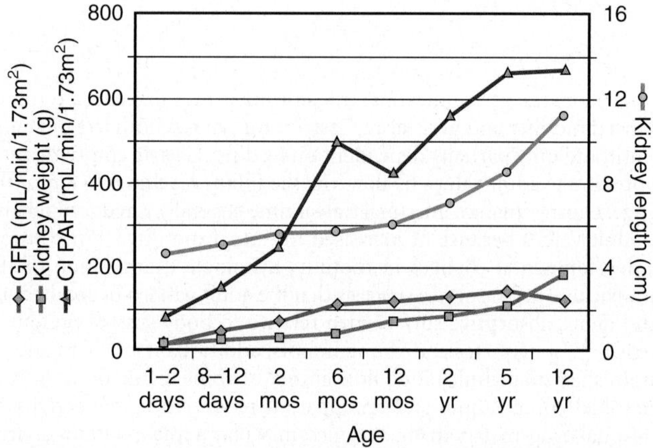

FIG. 235.5 Ontogeny of renal function. *Cl,* Clearance; *GFR,* glomerular filtration rate; *PAH, p*-aminohippuric acid. (Modified from Papadopoulou ZL, Tina LU, Sandler P, et al. Size and function of the kidneys. In: Johnson TR, Moore WM, Jeffries JE, eds. *Children Are Different: Developmental Physiology.* 2nd ed. Columbus, OH: Ross Laboratories; 1978:97-104.)

in neonates, infants, and children can be predicted largely by considering the ontogeny of renal function and the specific pharmacologic characteristics of a given drug with regard to its renal excretion (e.g., routes of renal excretion, the percentage of a given dose excreted unchanged in urine) in adults. For antimicrobial agents, the impact of the ontogeny of the renal function on pharmacokinetics is reflected largely by alterations in the plasma drug clearance. As summarized by van den Anker and Kearns,[228] the elimination half-life of antimicrobial agents from different classes that share predominantly renal pathways of excretion is increased substantially in neonates and young infants (Table 235.3). This increase is not the case for antimicrobial and other agents that are not excreted primarily by the kidneys (e.g., ceftriaxone).

Metabolism

Simply stated, drug metabolism (or biotransformation) involves the modification of a drug molecule by one or more enzymes such that the hydrophilicity of the product is increased relative to the parent drug, thus enhancing elimination and excretion. In most instances, drug metabolism creates products that are either less pharmacologically active than is the parent drug (e.g., desacetyl cefotaxime) or devoid of pharmacologic activity altogether (e.g., cefotaxime lactone metabolites).[118] In other instances, metabolism can result in drug bioactivation and produce metabolites with pharmacologic activity from an inactive parent drug (i.e., prodrug), such as inactive valganciclovir activated to

TABLE 235.3 **Impact of Ontogeny on the Elimination Half-Life of Drugs With Predominant Renal Routes of Excretion**[a]

Drug	Cl (mL/h/kg)	VD (mL/kg)	ELIMINATION $t_{1/2}$ (h) Neonate	Adult
Gentamicin	35–72	350–500	4.4–11.4	2.5
Tobramycin	41–74	590-840	8.2–11.3	2.0
Amikacin	50	570	8.4	2.5
Cefotaxime	50–100	310–790	3.4–6.4	1.2
Ceftriaxone	44–60	530–610	7.7–8.4	6.5
Ceftazidime	31–42	292–363	5.0–8.7	1.8
Vancomycin	36–78	480–680	8.0–17	6.0

[a]Data represent average or a range of average values reported from individual studies and summarized by van den Anker and Kearns[228] (for preterm infants) and Ritschel and Kearns[187] for adults.
Cl, Total plasma clearance; $t_{1/2}$, half-life; *VD*, apparent volume of distribution.

ganciclovir, or the generation of metabolites that can result in cellular toxicity in the host (e.g., sulfamethoxazole's nitroso and hydroxylamine reactive metabolites, acetaminophen's NAPQI reactive metabolite).

Virtually every tissue has some ability to carry out drug biotransformation reactions. Although the liver is quantitatively the most important organ capable of drug metabolism, the small intestine, lungs, skin, and kidneys also have substantial drug biotransformation activities. In infants, children, and adolescents, developmental variations in drug metabolism have been associated with age, sex, maturation, and genetic constitution. For compounds that are extensively metabolized, developmental differences in drug metabolism can serve as the primary determinant for age-appropriate dose selection.[137] Much of the existing information regarding the impact of ontogeny on drug metabolism has been derived as a byproduct of pharmacokinetic investigations designed, in part, to determine whether age-dependent differences in drug disposition were evident.[119] The following paragraphs highlight important general issues regarding drug metabolism and its relationship with development.

PHASE I PATHWAYS

Phase I biotransformation reactions include oxidation, reduction, and hydrolysis reactions that, in general, introduce or unmask a functional group (e.g., hydroxyl, amine, sulfhydryl) that renders a drug more polar. Quantitatively, the P-450 cytochromes are the most important of the phase I enzymes and represent a superfamily of heme-containing proteins that catalyze the metabolism of many lipophilic endogenous substances (e.g., steroids, fatty acids and fat-soluble vitamins, prostaglandins, leukotrienes, and thromboxanes) and exogenous compounds. In humans, the P-450 cytochromes can be divided functionally into two distinct classes: steroidogenic enzymes expressed in specialized tissues, such as the adrenal glands, gonads, and placenta; and enzymes involved in the metabolism of drugs, pesticides, and environmental contaminants. P-450 cytochromes that have been identified as important in human drug metabolism are found predominantly in the *CYP1, CYP2,* and *CYP3* gene families.[137]

As reviewed by Leeder and Kearns,[137] considerable interindividual variability exists in the hepatic expression of P-450 enzymes, and, for a given individual, the pathway and rate of a compound's metabolic clearance constitute that individual's unique phenotype with respect to the forms and amounts of P-450 isoforms expressed. Of the P-450 cytochromes involved in drug biotransformation, CYP2C19, CYP2C9, and CYP2D6 are examples of isoforms that are polymorphically expressed in humans. Polymorphic expression of CYP1A2 and CYP3A4 has been reported in the literature but not definitively established with regard to functional consequences. Within a P-450 subfamily, several isoforms can exist (e.g., CYP3A4, CYP3A5, and CYP3A7), each of which can demonstrate substrate specificity and a distinct developmental pattern with regard to enzyme activity. In addition, certain P-450 cytochromes (e.g., CYP3A4) can work cooperatively with transporters (e.g., MDR-1 or P-glycoprotein) located in distinct cells or tissues to alter the availability of specific drugs to the systemic circulation (e.g., first-pass metabolism of CYP3A4 substrates in the enterocyte). Moreover, for certain polymorphically expressed P-450 cytochromes (e.g., CYP2C19, CYP2D6), enzyme activity has been shown to vary as a consequence of racial or ethnic origin[183] and, within a given phenotypic distribution (e.g., extensive metabolizers for CYP2D6), as a function of single nucleotide polymorphisms that exist in either the gene or its regulatory regions.[181] Finally, throughout development, the activities of the P-450 cytochromes can vary widely (e.g., 5- to 25-fold) among individuals of the same phenotype,[137] an important factor with respect to the ability for induction or inhibition and, thus, the prediction of drug-drug or drug-xenobiotic interactions in vivo.

PHASE II PATHWAYS

In general, phase II reactions involve the coupling of a drug or drug metabolite with an endogenous substance to enhance its hydrophilicity further and to facilitate drug excretion in either urine or bile. These reactions require the participation of specific transferase enzymes (e.g., epoxide hydrolase, glucuronosyltransferases, glutathione *S*-transferases, sulfotransferases, *N*-acetyltransferases, methyltransferases, transacylases) and high-energy, activated endogenous substances. Although most conjugation reactions result in drug detoxification, examples of bioactivation by phase II enzymes do exist.[186] Similar to what has been found for certain of the P-450 cytochromes, different isoforms of phase II enzymes also occur in humans. This finding is exemplified by the review of de Wildt and colleagues,[45] who described substrate specificity for 10 different glucuronosyltransferase isoforms in humans and known polymorphisms in five different isoforms of this enzyme. The impact of age on the disposition of several glucuronosyltransferase substrates (e.g., morphine, acetaminophen, zidovudine, chloramphenicol) suggests that isoform-specific, age-related differences in activity occur to a degree sufficient to produce profound effects on drug clearance that translate directly into age-specific differences in a drug dose.[45]

Normal growth and development can have a profound effect on the activity of drug-metabolizing enzymes. Failure to recognize important developmental differences in drug biotransformation and to appropriately compensate for them by individualizing drug dosing can lead to serious consequences. This is exemplified by the "gray baby syndrome" previously associated with chloramphenicol, which is a life-threatening adverse drug reaction that was associated with supratherapeutic systemic drug exposure and, in some infants, produced cyanosis and cardiovascular collapse. The genesis of this particular toxicity resided with normal developmental reductions in the activity of the glucuronosyltransferase isoforms responsible for metabolizing chloramphenicol and the failure to appropriately adjust the dosing schedule to compensate for reductions in systemic clearance.[61,239]

Traditionally, the impact of ontogeny for all enzymes was viewed as being extremely limited in neonates, rapidly increasing in the first year of life to levels in toddlers and older children that may exceed adult capacity, and declining to adult levels by the conclusion of puberty. Experimental and clinical data previously reviewed demonstrated that this theory is not accurate.[119,137] As illustrated by the summary data contained in Table 235.4, the impact of ontogeny on the activity of both phase I and phase II drug-metabolizing enzymes is very much a substrate- and isoform-specific event; development is one dynamic factor in a multitude of conditions (e.g., nutritional status, gender, diurnal variation, menstrual cycle, disease states/organ dysfunction, pregnancy, concomitant drug therapy) capable of altering the activity of drug-metabolizing enzymes and, thus, the clearance of drugs (and their metabolites) from plasma. Although discussion of the impact of ontogeny on the disposition (pharmacokinetics) of specific drugs is beyond the scope of this chapter, the clinician can use much of the information concerning specific enzymes provided in Table 235.4 as a tool to facilitate inquiry or clinical decision making, or both. It can be done simply by using readily available, updated information describing which enzymes are responsible for drug metabolism and then searching the published or unpublished (e.g., information available from

TABLE 235.4 Developmental Patterns for the Ontogeny of Important Drug-Metabolizing Enzymes in Humans

Enzyme(s)	Known Developmental Pattern
Phase I Enzymes	
CYP2D6	Low to absent in fetal liver but present at 1 wk of age; poor activity (i.e., 20% of adult) by 1 mo; adult competence by 1 to 3 y of age
CYP2C9	Apparently absent in fetal liver; low activity in first 2 to 4 wk of life, with adult activity reached by approximately 6 mo; activity may exceed adult levels during childhood and declines to adult levels after conclusion of puberty
CYP1A2	Not present in appreciable levels in human fetal liver; adult levels reached by approximately 4 mo and exceeded in children at 1 to 2 y of age; adult activity reached after puberty
CYP3A7	Fetal form of CYP3A that is functionally active (and inducible) during gestation; virtually disappears by 1 to 4 wk of postnatal life when CYP3A4 activity predominates but remains present in approximately 5% of individuals
CYP3A4	Extremely low activity at birth, reaching 30% to 40% of adult activity by 1 mo and full adult activity by 6 mo; may exceed adult activity between 1 and 4 y of age and decrease to adult levels after puberty
Phase II Enzymes	
NAT2	Some fetal activity by 16 wk of gestation; poor activity between birth and 2 mo of age; adult phenotype distribution reached by 4 to 6 mo, with adult activity reached by 1 to 3 y
TPMT	Fetal levels approximately 30% of adult values; in newborns, activity approximately 50% higher than in adults, with phenotype distribution approximating that of adults; exception is Korean children, in whom adult activity is seen by 7 to 9 y of age
UGT	Ontogeny isoform specific; in general, adult activity reached by 6 to 24 mo of age
ST	Ontogeny isoform specific and appears faster than that for UGT; activity for some isoforms may exceed adult levels during infancy and early childhood

CYP, Cytochrome P-450; *NAT2, N*-acetyltransferase-2; *ST,* sulfotransferase; *TPMT,* thiopurine methyltransferase; *UGT,* glucuronosyltransferase.

Modified from Leeder JS, Kearns GL. Pharmacogenetics in pediatrics: Implications for practice. *Pediatr Clin North Am.* 1997;44:55–57.

pharmaceutical companies for drugs under development) literature for information describing the pharmacokinetics of the drug being considered.

Clinicians must recognize that age-dependent differences in the activity of enzymes that catalyze drug biotransformation are not limited solely to P-450 cytochromes or the host of transferase enzymes responsible for phase II drug metabolism, and, in many cases, these differences represent a critical determinant for successful antiinfective drug therapy. This factor is exemplified by considering the example of two antimicrobial agents that have unique places in pediatric therapy: cefotaxime and linezolid. In the case of cefotaxime, non–P-450 enzymes (probably an esterase) capable of generating the active desacetyl cefotaxime metabolite appear to be present and fully active by the third trimester of gestation.[123] Nonetheless, the elimination half-life of cefotaxime in neonates is approximately threefold greater (i.e., 3–4 hours) than that observed in older infants and children (i.e., 1–1.5 hours), a difference that permits extension of the dosing interval for the use of cefotaxime in neonates. The reasons for this developmental difference reside not with the enzymes responsible for generation of an active metabolite; instead, age-associated reductions in the activity of enzymes appear to be responsible for the generation of inactive metabolites of cefotaxime (e.g., cefotaxime lactone) and pathways involved in the renal clearance of desacetylcefotaxime.[122] Linezolid, an oxazolidinone antimicrobial approved in the United States for use in pediatric patients, undergoes extensive biotransformation in humans, not through a cytochrome P-450 enzyme, but rather by nonselective chemical oxidation.[125] As demonstrated by Kearns and associates,[120] the mean plasma clearance of linezolid in children was approximately threefold higher than that observed previously for adults, with the greatest increase noted in infants younger than 1 year. Given the mechanism of action for linezolid and properties that reflect time-dependent killing,[125] the clinical implications of the age-dependent pattern of increased plasma clearance for this drug in young infants and children suggest that for infections with selected pathogens that have relatively high (90%) minimal inhibitory concentration (MIC_{90}) values for the drug, shorter dosing intervals (e.g., every 8 hours) may be necessary to ensure sufficient exposure of the organism in blood and tissue through most of a dosing interval.[120]

PHARMACOKINETIC DETERMINANTS OF EFFECT

Collectively, the most important determinants of efficacy for antiinfective agents are the pharmacokinetic profile of the drug, the physicochemical and biochemical characteristics of the local environment (i.e., site of infection), and the susceptibility of the infecting organisms under local growth conditions. As previously reviewed by Barza,[17] the mechanisms and pharmacokinetics of drug transport to and accumulation at the site or sites of infection, as well as the subcellular localization of drugs, are critical to success and are poorly understood. In many circumstances, plasma drug concentrations may not be reflective of those in tissue. Pathophysiologic processes related to the host, the infection, and the physicochemical properties of the drug work in concert to regulate distribution into and retention of active drug at the site of infection. Because these considerations should be embraced by the clinician when a particular antiinfective drug is selected for treatment and its therapy is monitored for clinical evidence of success, some general examples are presented as follows.

In addition to age (as discussed earlier), many disease processes (e.g., trauma, malignancy, renal or hepatic disease) have an impact on both the quantity of circulating plasma proteins (e.g., albumin, α_1-acid glycoprotein) and their affinity to bind antiinfective agents. Given that only free drug is available to enter tissue, the degree of binding to protein components in the blood will affect tissue concentrations. Thus, despite the presence of total (i.e., free and bound) plasma drug concentrations well in excess of the MIC, these concentrations may not be predictive of concentrations of highly bound (i.e., >70%) drug at the site of infection. Properties of the capillary bed feeding the site of infection also dictate drug penetration. Highly vascularized tissue with a large ratio of capillary surface area to volume can be expected to accumulate higher drug concentrations than can tissue that is poorly vascularized, principally because of the rate and extent to which drug can be delivered to the site. As with protein binding, variability in capillary density may be a function of disease (e.g., severe atherosclerosis, diabetes), infection (e.g., abscess, cardiac vegetation), and age, and it should be expected to have an impact on drug delivery. Similarly, tissues with tight junctions and few fenestrations (e.g., eye, central nervous system [CNS]) afford lower tissue concentrations, given that drug entry is restricted to transport across the lipid bilayer of the endothelial cell (i.e., transcellular vs. paracellular transport). Here, adequate drug penetration is restricted to agents with a favorable lipid-water partition coefficient and ionization constant. As such, many infectious processes warrant direct instillation of antibiotic at the site of infection (e.g., intracisternal, intrathecal, intraarticular). Additionally, cellular transporters (e.g., P-glycoprotein at the blood-brain barrier, organic anion and cation transporters at the choroid plexus) capable of pumping drug from the cell can limit distribution and retention of drug at the tissue level. The pH at the site of infection (e.g., in tissue fluids, exudates, transudates) relative to the pH in plasma also can govern distribution of a drug. For example, in cases of bacterial meningitis, the pH that occurs in the CNS is lower relative to plasma. Weak acids (e.g., penicillin) are more highly ionized in plasma than in cerebrospinal fluid (CSF) and pass more readily from the CSF into plasma than in the reverse direction. Similarly, when the pH of the local environment drops in the presence of infection, as occurs in lung abscesses, aminoglycoside efficacy is reduced because of chemical inactivation of the drug by ionization and the formation of stable adducts with high DNA concentrations found in purulent secretions. Finally, the physicochemical association of an intact (i.e., unmetabolized) drug with a particular physiologic fluid as part of its normal excretion profile can serve to localize drug at the site of infection (e.g., accumulation of drugs excreted by the biliary route in patients with cholangitis and in the urine in patients with nephritis). It is important to recognize that such interactions modify the activity of antimicrobial agents. For example, in vitro data demonstrate that daptomycin interacts with pulmonary surfactant, which in turn decreases the activity of the antibiotic. Hence the drug is not currently indicated in the treatment of pulmonary infections.[207] When drug-tissue and drug–body fluid interactions occur, different approaches, including dose modification or combination therapy, may need to be considered to optimize therapy.

PHARMACODYNAMIC DETERMINANTS OF EFFECT

The desired effect of any drug is realized when sufficient concentrations are achieved and maintained at the active site for an adequate period. In many models of disease for which the treatment targets of modern chemotherapy remain fixed, the concentration-effect (i.e., pharmacodynamic) relationships can be described with relatively modest effort. In contrast, evaluating the concentration-effect relationship for antimicrobial agents can be anything but straightforward, given the dynamic nature of infection. The intended target of the antiinfective agent is in constant flux as the number of organisms changes, the quantity and affinity of target receptors evolve, and the contribution of the host response adapts accordingly during the course of infection. Moreover, antimicrobial agents demonstrate variable effects at different concentrations and under different physicochemical environments. In fact, evaluating whether an organism survives in the presence of antibiotic is only one criterion by which to predict or define drug effect. Rather, a variety of effects related to antimicrobial concentration—from the extremes of complete eradication to complete survival—can be observed in the invading organism. The previous sections of this chapter review the principles of pharmacokinetics, specifically, factors that link dose to concentration. The sections that follow include a discussion of the pharmacodynamics of antiinfective therapy and the multitude of factors that link concentration with effect.

Effects Described by Pharmacokinetic Parameters and Conventional Susceptibility End Points

Among the many decision-making tools that clinicians have at their disposal to guide in the selection of antimicrobial therapy are qualitative (e.g., breakpoints) and quantitative (e.g., MIC, minimal bactericidal concentration [MBC]) estimates of susceptibility. Although numerous studies and years of clinical evidence support the correlation between qualitative end points and clinical outcome, their predictive power is diminished in the presence of immunocompromise, severe underlying disease, mixed infections, and infection with organisms demonstrating heterogeneic resistance patterns.[34,40,64,146,155] Quantitative end points provide a better assessment of dose-effect relationships, with antibiotic concentration serving as a surrogate for the dose. However, these data alone do not reveal the complete picture relative to the anticipated bacterial response because laboratory-based quantitative tests contain a notable number of artificial aspects. Factors appreciated to influence the activity of antimicrobial agents in vivo (e.g., protein binding, fluctuating drug concentrations, serial drug exposure, inoculum size, immune defense status, physicochemical environment, compound stability) essentially are neglected when determining MIC values. As such, agents with comparable MIC values in vitro may, in fact, demonstrate markedly different effect profiles in a patient.[3,33,70,113,130]

In an attempt to move beyond reliance on quantitative tests as the sole marker for predicting antimicrobial activity in vivo, the integration of susceptibility information with population- and patient-specific pharmacokinetic data continues to be explored. Surrogate end points,

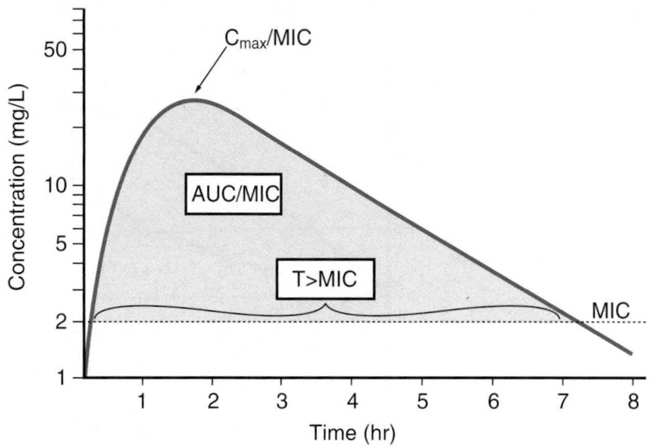

FIG. 235.6 Representative plasma concentration versus time curve illustrating commonly referenced pharmacodynamic parameters. *AUC,* Area under the curve; *C_{max},* maximal plasma concentration; *MIC,* minimal inhibitory concentration; *T,* time.

defined by a combination of pharmacokinetic parameters and quantitative susceptibility data, have been suggested to predict more reliably the efficacy of different antimicrobial agents. By far, pharmacodynamic determinants of antimicrobial effect most frequently link attainable drug concentrations or estimates of total body exposure, or both, with in vitro estimates of pathogen sensitivity. For antimicrobial agents for which the mechanism of action is determined to be time dependent (concentration independent), the percentage of time that plasma or tissue concentrations remain above the MIC has been closely linked to therapeutic response (Fig. 235.6). By comparison, the ratio of C_{max} to MIC has demonstrated a similar relationship for drugs with concentration-dependent killing (see Fig. 235.6). Furthermore, the ratio of AUC to MIC, which reflects the concentration profile over the course of time, has been used with both classes of agents (see Fig. 235.6).

Evidence to support the application of specific pharmacodynamic surrogates is reviewed in the following paragraphs. However, a large degree of interdependence exists among these pharmacokinetic parameters. With few exceptions, when the dose of a drug is increased, C_{max} and the total AUC increase, and with no change in clearance, so, too, does the percentage of time that plasma drug concentrations remain above the MIC. Accordingly, making distinctions among the various pharmacokinetic parameters in an attempt to determine the optimal pharmacodynamic end point can be misleading. Given that many studies evaluate a limited number of doses or dosing intervals, restrict the number of pharmacokinetic parameters that are calculated, or neglect to perform multivariate analysis on the data, clear distinctions between parameters cannot always be made, and an appropriate degree of caution should be exercised when evaluating such data.[233]

Time Above the Minimal Inhibitory Concentration

Among the first class of antimicrobial agents to be discussed in the context of their concentration-effect relationships were the β-lactams, specifically penicillin. Although limited supporting evidence existed at the time, investigators were concerned with maintaining adequate blood levels of the drug in the host for a fixed period of time. This concern was reflected in their attempts to inhibit clearance pathways and formulate sustained-release preparations designed specifically for the purpose of extending the time spent above some minimal concentration (T > MIC).[21,190] As it turns out, in vitro studies support the relative concentration independence of penicillin and demonstrate that a maximal rate of killing can be observed that is quickly saturated at reasonably low multiples of the MIC (Fig. 235.7A). As concentrations increase above this maximal level, no faster rates of kill can be demonstrated.[37] Rather, penicillin displays time-dependent killing in which the duration of time spent above some minimal concentration (typically ±1 to 2 dilutions of the MIC or MBC) appears to be the most important determinant of activity.[53] As newer antimicrobial agents with putative time-dependent

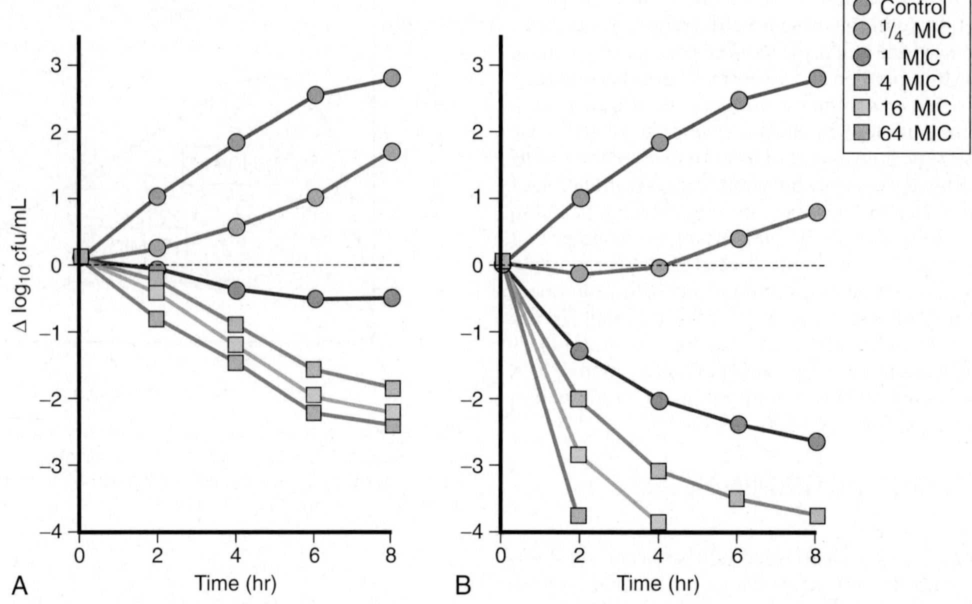

FIG. 235.7 Representative log-kill curves. These curves illustrate the response to (A) concentration-independent (time-dependent) and (B) concentration-dependent antimicrobial agents. *MIC,* minimal inhibitory concentration. (Modified from Craig WA, Ebert SC. Killing and regrowth of bacteria in vitro: A review. *Scand J Infect Dis.* 1991;74[Suppl]:63-70.)

activity became available for evaluation, those with longer plasma and tissue terminal elimination half-lives demonstrated enhanced bactericidal activity compared with similar drugs. Those that simply resulted in higher maximal peak concentrations, with no extension of the time above the MIC, produced minimal if any differences in effect.[12,87,197,240] This time-dependent activity has been observed in vitro with virtually all β-lactams (e.g., cephalosporins, carbapenems, monobactams) against both gram-positive and gram-negative organisms.[65,87,212,247] Similarly, other drug classes, namely, the macrolides, azalides, glycylcyclines, glycopeptides, ketolides, and oxazolidinones, appear to possess this same characteristic.[10,93,150,229,231]

When evaluating whether the time-dependent activity observed in vitro can be reproduced in vivo by evaluating intrinsic antibiotic activity in the host (through restriction of observations to animals in which the element of both humoral and cell-mediated immunity has been removed), the strongest relationship between antimicrobial concentration and effect for the aforementioned agents remains the time spent above the MIC.[193] Elegant studies evaluating extensive numbers of dosing regimens and drug-microbe combinations demonstrated that β-lactam and macrolide efficacy correlates best with the percentage of time spent above the MIC, irrespective of whether gram-positive or gram-negative pathogens are involved.[233] Given the same total daily dose, therapy administered at more frequent intervals is required for a successful outcome.[14,138] Even when the drug-microbe interaction is such that only bacteriostatic activity results, a regimen consisting of more frequent doses is able to maintain an environment of no net growth, whereas positive net growth is observed with larger doses administered less frequently.[79] From such data, the efficacy of time-dependent agents appears to be maximized by maintaining antibiotic concentrations above the MIC for as much of the dosing interval as possible.

When evaluating whether these agents obey the same relationship in the presence of a competent immune system, animal models similarly demonstrate a significant correlation between antimicrobial efficacy and the percentage of time spent above the MIC.[4,71] In contrast to immunocompromised animals, animals with a functional immune system do not require that virtually 100% of the dosing interval be spent above the MIC to achieve adequate antimicrobial activity. Although the bactericidal activity of penicillin ceases when concentrations fall below the MIC, the remaining organisms do not resume multiplication for many hours, well in excess of the time observed for the same organisms in vitro.[55,114] This difference may reflect the time required for the organism to recover from the initial antibiotic insult, coupled with the complementary activity of subinhibitory antibiotic concentrations and the immune system (these pharmacodynamic principles are explored later in further detail).[76] Irrespective of the mechanism by which the protracted antimicrobial effect occurs, the pharmacodynamic goals for time-dependent agents are not as stringent in vivo as they are in vitro. However, the persistent suppression of bacterial growth is not indefinite, and a maximal amount of time can be spent below the MIC before a reduction in efficacy becomes apparent. Thus a maximal dosing interval for these agents appears to exist in immunocompetent hosts, beyond which a decrease in efficacy can be expected.[54,202]

Clinical studies further confirm that for the agents discussed earlier, time above the MIC is a suitable pharmacodynamic end point in patients. In clinical studies of upper respiratory tract infection, the highest bacterial eradication rates for the β-lactams are observed when the time above the MIC exceeds 40% to 50% of the dosing interval.[41] For cefuroxime, cure rates drop from greater than 90% to approximately 75% when the time above the MIC falls to less than 40%.[74,83] Patients infected with a susceptible organism show 92% efficacy with a continuous-infusion regimen of cefamandole versus 63% efficacy with intermittent administration of the agent. Finally, in neutropenic patients, an overall efficacy rate of 65% was observed after continuous infusion of cefamandole as opposed to 21% efficacy in patients receiving intermittent administration.[28] For macrolide-susceptible pathogens, cure rates approaching 100% were observed when concentrations remained above the MIC for greater than 80% of the dosing interval.[41] As the MIC increases such that the percentage of time spent above the MIC falls, so, too, do cure rates. Macrolide concentrations rarely exceed the MIC for *Haemophilus influenzae,* and cure rates are comparable to those seen in placebo-treated individuals.[41] A few studies appear to contradict the aforementioned data, findings indicating that little difference in clinical response is observed when the same total daily dose of selected agents is administered as a continuous infusion or with increased frequency versus less frequent intermittent administration; however, a prolonged postantibiotic effect (PAE) or protracted half-life, such that both of the regimens evaluated spend nearly 100% of the dosing interval above the MIC, may explain these discrepancies.[32,133,234]

A natural extension of the considerations just discussed relates to the utility of continuous infusions for antimicrobial agents that exhibit time-dependent killing, a topic that has historically been controversial. Theoretically, continuous drug administration would ensure that serum concentrations and potentially those at the site of action would never fall below the MIC. This would be of particular value for antimicrobial agents with a short half-life, in patients in whom drug exposure is limited based on increased volumes of distribution or clearance rates, and in patients who have a significant degree of immunocompromise. Although the benefits appear obvious, the clinical findings are often equivocal, with data both supporting and refuting improvement in clinical outcomes related to continuous antimicrobial administration. Because of the relative dearth of new antimicrobial development and the ever-increasing cases of multidrug-resistant organisms encountered, application of extended or continuous infusions in clinical care continues with attempts of more rigorous evaluation of pharmacodynamic and clinical outcome results. These studies include designed randomized control trials, with further evaluation in different patient populations, including children.[50,59] Variability in antibiotic dosing, disease severity, causative bacterial pathogens, and susceptibility patterns all add to the complexity of accurately assessing prolonged infusions.[189] Moreover, challenges encountered with the administration of continuous infusions of antimicrobial agents include obtaining adequate serum concentrations, drug stability, practicality of administration, and potential adverse reactions associated with prolonged drug exposure. Consequently, clinical guidelines for the application of continuous infusions are lacking, and additional data are needed to better understand the potential advantages and disadvantages of continuous infusions, particularly in the setting of more highly resistant pathogens and in complex pediatric patient populations.

Concentration Above the Minimal Inhibitory Concentration

In contrast to the aforementioned agents, a smaller group of agents demonstrate concentration dependence, with the magnitude of antimicrobial effect increasing in direct proportion to increasing drug concentrations (Fig. 235.7B).[20,152] The aminoglycoside and fluoroquinolone antibiotics are the prototypic drugs of this pharmacodynamic class; however, concentration-dependent activity also has been observed with the lipopeptides, metronidazole, and the echinocandins.[7,43,149,180,211,230] Unlike the time-dependent agents, for which shortening the dosing interval results in increased efficacy, extending the dosing interval for concentration-dependent drugs affords an ability to increase the dose and results in a greater reduction in bacterial inoculum and, for some agents, a diminution in adaptive resistance.[42] Although highly variable, optimal ratios of peak plasma concentration to MIC that result in complete killing have been defined for many drug-microbe combinations. Similarly, ratios of C_{max} to MIC (C_{max}/MIC) can be defined, below which the organism is afforded the opportunity to regrow with increased selection of resistant subpopulations.[26,48,49]

Concentration-dependent killing for many of these agents has been demonstrated in both animal models and human clinical trials. In neutropenic mice with pseudomonal soft tissue infection, dosing schemes that deliver larger aminoglycoside doses less frequently result in greater killing than do schemes with the same total daily dose administered more frequently, even though all regimens achieved serum concentrations in excess of the MIC.[79] Additionally, once-daily dosing of aminoglycosides has been associated with less toxicity compared with multiple daily dosing.[18,209] In patients receiving quinolone therapy for the treatment of respiratory tract, urinary tract, and skin and soft tissue infections, several pharmacodynamic parameters proved to correlate with clinical response; however, the best correlation was observed with the C_{max}/MIC ratio.[178] In clinical trials in which patients received aminoglycoside therapy for gram-negative infections, the strongest association between pharmacokinetic indices and clinical response was observed with the C_{max}/MIC ratio. In fact, the relationship between the C_{max}/MIC ratio and clinical response appeared to be linear over the range of clinically relevant plasma concentrations. No significant difference occurred in the time to achieve C_{max} between responders and nonresponders; therefore the improved response rates in patients achieving higher peak plasma concentrations were not simply an artifact of drug accumulation as a result of longer duration of therapy.[159,160]

In addition to the absolute peak plasma concentration, the time that optimal peak levels are achieved appears to play a critical role in the response to concentration-dependent antimicrobial agents. A significant correlation with clinical improvement and reduction in mortality is observed if therapeutic peak plasma concentrations are reached early during the course of treatment.[161,164] The probable reason for this effect is that the response of the bacterial population to the same antibiotic concentration can change with subsequent doses. As alluded to earlier, subtherapeutic peak plasma concentrations serve to select out fewer susceptible variants within the population.[26,27,78] Based on these data, a key goal of therapy (i.e., in addition to proper drug selection) for concentration-dependent agents appears to be the attainment of high peak plasma concentrations early in therapy to afford rapid initial killing and minimize adaptive resistance.

Although prolonging the dosing interval affords the luxury of increasing the dose to optimize killing, the law of diminishing returns applies even for concentration-dependent agents, and it is possible to increase the dosing interval to excess and decrease efficacy. Despite the clear concentration dependence with escalating doses of fluoroquinolones, a simulated every-12-hour regimen was less effective than was a regimen using the same total daily dose administered every 8 hours.[19] Similarly, animal models of gram-negative lung and soft tissue infection suggest that delayed clearance of the infecting organism is observed in response to aminoglycoside and fluoroquinolone therapy when administered in protracted dosing regimens (e.g., dosing interval much greater than the half-life) as opposed to shorter dosing intervals.[138,163,191] Again, scattered studies appear to contradict these findings; however, they use agents with a longer half-life, and therefore the dosing interval may, in fact, not exceed the time spent above the MIC plus the residual PAE.[46] Thus, despite their concentration dependence, an element of time appears to be involved in the response to these agents. Unless peak concentrations are achieved in excess of those necessary to obtain maximal kill rates and the dosing interval does not markedly exceed time above the MIC plus the PAE, the efficacy of such agents is not only dose dependent but also dose interval dependent.

Total Body Exposure Above the Minimal Inhibitory Concentration

The AUC, a reflection of total body exposure, is a pharmacokinetic parameter that integrates both time and drug concentration. Estimates of AUC reflect the magnitude of the dose received and the drug half-life relative to the dosing interval. Accordingly, researchers have proposed that the ratio of AUC to MIC (AUC/MIC ratio) may serve as a better surrogate of pharmacodynamic activity for both time- and concentration-dependent agents. In several studies, the AUC/MIC ratio serves as the best correlate of the reduction in number of organisms for aminoglycosides, quinolones, streptogramins, rifamycins, isoniazid, evernimicin, echinocandins, and azole antifungal agents.[6-9,47,60,115,116,173] Because of the interdependence between AUC and the pharmacokinetic parameters previously noted, studies also can be identified that demonstrate a relationship between clinical or microbiologic outcome and the AUC/MIC ratio for agents with time-dependent activity (e.g., the β-lactams and glycopeptides). Often, however, these studies fail to evaluate multiple pharmacokinetic parameters.[158,201]

In an elegant study evaluating certain aminoglycoside dosing regimens against *Pseudomonas aeruginosa* and *Escherichia coli* infection, the log-normalized AUC provided the best correlation with efficacy. However, as was observed with concentration-dependent agents, when the dosing interval exceeded the time above the MIC plus the residual PAE, the best correlation with efficacy was the percentage of time spent above the MIC, thus reaffirming that the dosing interval can be too long with the aminoglycosides.[233] A meta-analysis of 19 studies evaluating eight quinolones and six different organisms in experimental endocarditis similarly demonstrated a correlation between the AUC/MIC and reduction in $\log_{10}$ colony-forming units (CFUs) per vegetation. However, given the relationship between the pharmacokinetic parameters, C_{max}/MIC and time greater than MIC also proved to correlate with a decrease in the size of the inoculum.[5] In human investigations, AUC/MIC appears to serve as the best predictor of clinical response, microbiologic response, and bacterial eradication for the fluoroquinolones. Nonetheless, C_{max}/MIC and time greater than MIC can be linked similarly to bacterial eradication for this class of agents.[68,69,175]

Clearly, the optimal AUC/MIC ratio will be different for different organisms despite sharing a similar quantitative susceptibility end point.

Similarly, optimal AUC/MIC ratios are highly variable and depend on the antimicrobial agent being evaluated. For example, effective eradication of organisms implicated in nosocomial pneumonia is observed with an AUC/MIC ratio of 540 for cefmenoxime, 34 for tobramycin, and 23 for ciprofloxacin.[200] Consequently, attempts have been made to standardize this pharmacodynamic end point, and investigators have proposed a value of 125 as the cutoff below which a reduction in efficacy and increase in resistance may be expected.[106,199] However, optimal AUC/MIC ratios may differ, depending not only on a given organism and agent but also on the desired outcome and the disease state. A ratio greater than 125 resulted in bacterial eradication roughly 7 days after the initiation of β-lactam and quinolone therapy; however, an AUC/MIC ratio of 250 resulted in eradication of the pathogen within 1 to 2 days after initiating quinolone therapy.[199] For patients with acute exacerbations of chronic bronchitis who are receiving fluoroquinolones, an AUC/MIC ratio less than 276 was associated with longer time to clinical success, whereas a ratio greater than 576 was associated with a reduction in coughs per day and a ratio greater than 212 with decreasing days to a reduction in the volume of sputum.[156] In an animal model of bacterial endocarditis, significantly lower numbers of organism were found in the vegetation after 3 to 6 days of therapy when the AUC/MIC ratio exceeded 100.[5] Moreover, a value of 100 appeared to be the cutoff below which an increased risk for resistance was observed in a retrospective review of 107 acutely ill patients with lower respiratory tract infection.[223] Furthermore, in vitro models evaluating fluoroquinolone activity against *Streptococcus pneumoniae* demonstrated effective eradication with an AUC/MIC ratio between 30 and 65, much lower than the value of 125 reported as optimal for other pathogens.[132,142]

Although this hybrid parameter bridges concentration and time (i.e., extent of systemic drug exposure from a given dose) and has been demonstrated to correlate with efficacy for numerous drug classes, optimal criteria appear to vary with the organism, agent, disease state, and desired outcome. In addition, established relationships no longer may hold for some agents when a protracted dosing interval is used in therapy. As such, a general classification and standard outcome are not straightforward, and agents need to be evaluated with respect to known mechanisms of activity and the specific clinical and microbiologic situations in which they are used.

Optimal Surrogates for Drugs in Combination

Combination antimicrobial therapy is initiated in numerous circumstances: to ensure broad-spectrum coverage early in therapy, to treat polymicrobial infections, and to combat organisms that require multiple agents for effective eradication. Often, combination therapy entails the use of agents from different classes or agents that have different mechanisms of action (or both). This particular situation raises the question of how one applies the aforementioned pharmacodynamic principles to selecting or evaluating the efficacy of drug therapy when confronted with the combined use of agents that do not share similar pharmacodynamic targets. Although optimization of combination therapy may be possible by choosing the interval for one agent,[80] efficacy appears to be explained best when a combination of both pharmacodynamic properties is considered.[79,162]

Reasonable models of a concentration-effect relationship have been proposed for numerous agents alone and in combination; however, optimal ratios remain to be defined for many drug-microbe combinations. Moreover, it is probably more complex than simply defining the optimal ratio for specific combinations. Even though one can define the best correlate, killing rates, in fact, may vary with the site of infection because penetration of a drug into or clearance from tissue varies from site to site. For example, logAUC proves to be the best predictor for clearance of organisms from the lung regardless of the dosing interval used. In contrast, given faster drug clearance from the thigh, the time above the MIC was a more important predictor of eradication when a longer dosing interval was used, whereas the logAUC was the best predictor of clearance of organisms with the use of shorter dosing intervals.[139] Similarly, in animal models of bacterial meningitis, greater kill rates were observed as time greater than MBC increased. However, when concentrations remained above the MBC for the entire dosing interval, which may not be unexpected in situations in which the antibiotic half-life is longer in CSF than in plasma, kill rates were directly proportional to both peak/MBC and AUC/MBC ratios.[151] These data suggest that we may need to expand the characterization of pharmacodynamic surrogates to look at the pharmacokinetic-pharmacodynamic interface at the site of infection rather than simply defining dosing strategies based on in vitro susceptibility data and the disposition characteristics of drugs in plasma. Without question, many data need to be collected and verified in the human host. The maximal dose and dosing regimen ideally are selected so that the resultant pharmacokinetic profile affords optimal pharmacodynamic activity without causing unnecessary adverse events, therapeutic failure, or both, as may be observed with inappropriate dosing. Development of a successful therapeutic strategy requires the following: incorporation of knowledge regarding the infecting pathogen; the physicochemical, pharmacologic, and pharmacokinetic properties of the antiinfective agent; and specific factors of the host or disease that are capable of altering either drug disposition or action. Such an approach enables the clinician to make clearer distinctions among agents with similar susceptibility profiles yet different mechanistic or pharmacokinetic profiles and to select an optimal drug regimen that will be most likely to result in successful therapy.

Effect of Suprainhibitory Antimicrobial Concentrations (Eagle Effect, Paradoxical Zone Phenomenon, Concentration Quenching)

In simplest terms, one typically thinks that antiinfective activity increases with increasing antimicrobial concentration. More sophisticated models describe increasing activity with increasing drug concentration to a maximal effect until activity reaches a plateau and remains relatively constant despite further increases in drug concentration (see Fig. 235.7). However, for many antibiotics, an increase in drug concentration can, in fact, result in a reduction in antimicrobial activity (Fig. 235.8).[101] This paradoxical effect was observed as early as 1945 and described 3 years later by Eagle and Musselman, who reported the existence of antibiotic concentrations above the maximally effective concentration at which the killing rate of bacteria is paradoxically reduced.[56,128] This phenomenon has been described with a host of organisms and although originally observed with penicillin has been confirmed with other β-lactams, glycopeptides, aminoglycosides, and fluoroquinolones.[148,166,176,218,243] Given the diversity of agents that demonstrate a paradoxical reduction in activity with increasing drug concentration, this phenomenon probably cannot be explained by a single mechanism; and although they are not definitively elucidated, numerous mechanisms have been proposed to explain these observations.

For certain β-lactam antimicrobials, induction of β-lactamase may be responsible for the paradoxical effects observed in selected organisms. In vitro experiments performed with *Proteus vulgaris* suggested that

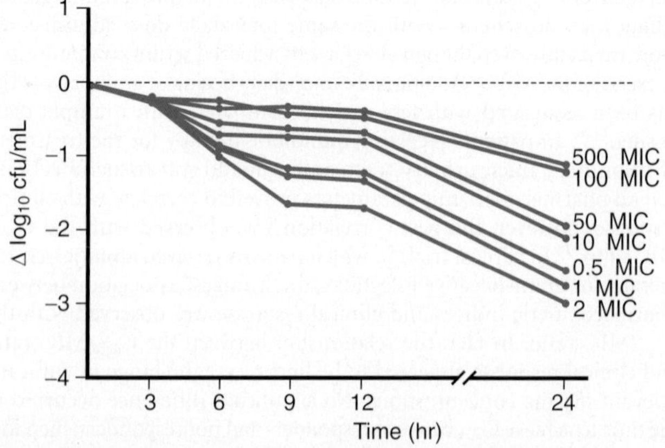

FIG. 235.8 Representative log-kill curve demonstrating the paradoxical effects that can be observed with suprainhibitory antimicrobial concentrations. *MIC*, Minimal inhibitory concentration. (Modified from Holm SE, Odenholdt-Tornqvist I, Cars O. Paradoxical effects of antibiotics. *Scand J Infect Dis Suppl.* 1991;74:113-117.)

the greatest paradoxical response seen with β-lactams was observed with agents that demonstrated the highest β-lactamase–inducing capacity and the poorest stability to degradation by this enzyme. When a mutant strain of this organism that was unable to induce β-lactamase production was evaluated, no paradoxical effect was noted.[110] In animal models of peritoneal infection, antibiotics with strong dose-dependent induction of β-lactamase similarly demonstrated a paradoxical effect against β-lactamase–positive strains of *P. vulgaris.* However, no paradoxical effect was observed against β-lactamase–negative strains. Agents that were only weak inducers of β-lactamase demonstrated no evidence of a paradoxical effect, regardless of whether the *P. vulgaris* strains produced β-lactamase.[108]

Because this paradoxical effect can be demonstrated with the β-lactams against organisms that do not produce β-lactamase, other mechanisms must also be responsible. One such mechanism may involve dysregulation of the bacterial autolytic system, which often confers tolerance to an organism but also may uncover an Eagle-type effect.[95] A paradoxical reduction in antimicrobial activity at high doses may be related to differences in regulation or expression of these autolytic enzymes. In *Enterococcus* strains that fully express only one of two recognized autolytic enzymes, diminished or deficient production of the second enzyme resulted in a paradoxical response to penicillin. Strains in which both enzymes were produced remained susceptible to the antibiotic irrespective of concentration, thus suggesting that a proportional dose-response relationship may require the synergistic activity of both enzymes.[66,67] Further investigation into the paradoxical effect observed in tolerant organisms suggests that organisms in the exponential growth phase demonstrate this response more consistently than do those in the stationary phase.[177,179] Animal models of *Staphylococcus aureus* endocarditis provide in vivo confirmation of the paradoxical response observed with tolerant organisms in vitro. Administration of continuous-infusion cloxacillin to animals infected with a nontolerant strain produced a dose-proportional reduction in bacterial density ($\log_{10}$CFUs/g) within the vegetation, whereas animals infected with a tolerant strain demonstrated a reduction and subsequent paradoxical increase in bacterial density with increasing dose. No statistical difference was observed in bacterial density within other organs or in overall survival, which raises questions regarding the in vivo significance of these observations.[235]

For antibiotics that demonstrate polyfunctional activity at supratherapeutic concentrations, a paradoxical response may occur as a result of secondary alterations in cellular functions that are requisite for antimicrobial activity. Despite a principal mechanism of action for the fluoroquinolones at the site of DNA gyrase, these agents appear to be bactericidal only in cells able to synthesize protein. As quinolone concentrations increase above those that are bactericidal, RNA synthesis and therefore protein synthesis are progressively inhibited, thus explaining the reduced rate of bactericidal activity observed at high quinolone concentrations.[188] Incompletely characterized genetic modifications also may confer a paradoxical response to antibiotics. β-Lactam resistance in methicillin-resistant *S. aureus* (MRSA) is mediated by de-repressing the production of a low-affinity PBP. However, because the modified PBP serves as an inefficient transpeptidase, it is regarded as an internal selective pressure in the bacterium, and a countermutation has arisen. Although it is not completely understood, the phenotypic expression of this countermutation is manifested as an Eagle-type resistance to methicillin.[129,196] Finally, an observed paradoxical response may not be a result of the drug-microbe combination alone but a result of the chemical environment as well. A paradoxical effect with penicillin, in which both cell count and the rate of killing were affected, was demonstrated in *Streptococcus agalactiae* when the pH was reduced under in vitro conditions.[109]

Most studies investigating the Eagle effect have been conducted in vitro, and the clinical implications of the paradoxical phenomenon have yet to be fully elucidated. However, anecdotal evidence appears to suggest that the clinical efficacy of antimicrobial agents can be compromised by high-dose antibiotic therapy. Case reports of β-lactam–susceptible streptococcal endocarditis and staphylococcal pneumonia describe patients who failed to respond to high-dose β-lactam therapy (plasma concentrations >100 times the MIC in one case), with subsequent improvement in each case when the dose was lowered.[77,88,221] For many agents, it is clearly advantageous to establish high peak drug concentrations early, the benefits of which include increasing log kill, preventing the selection of resistant mutants, overcoming refractoriness, and enhancing penetration of tissue. However, the relative safety of many drug classes (e.g., the β-lactams) often results in the use of doses that may be higher than necessary. When clear evidence is lacking for enhanced bactericidal activity at higher concentrations and the potential for diminished efficacy exists, escalation of antibiotic doses should be considered judiciously.

Effects of Subinhibitory Antimicrobial Concentration

Individuals may be exposed to subtherapeutic antimicrobial concentrations for many reasons, including underdosing, poor compliance, and, perhaps most commonly, the inability of the pharmacokinetic profile of the agent in question to afford adequate penetration to the site of infection. Exposure of bacteria to antibiotic concentrations below the MIC can have variable effects, depending on the organism and the antimicrobial agent. In fact, the effects observed with subinhibitory levels are not simply a milder extension of those observed at inhibitory concentrations but, instead, are qualitatively different from the effects observed at concentrations that equal or exceed the MIC.[144] Subinhibitory concentrations can have the following effects: enhance or impair opsonization and phagocytosis; affect the virulence of the bacteria by modifying the bacterial cell surface; alter adherence properties, antigen expression, or the excretion of enzymes and toxins (or any combination of these effects); and inhibit bacterial growth.[168,169,226] The result can be an increase or decrease in responsiveness to therapy, both of which are discussed later in this section. Before reviewing the current data, however, one should note that this discussion does not refer to subinhibitory concentrations occurring after initial suprainhibitory drug levels. These particular effects are distinguished as PAE and are addressed separately.

Even though antibiotic concentrations may fail to reach or exceed the MIC, these agents still can affect the growth of an invading organism adversely.[144,145,147] In fact, the term *minimal antibacterial concentration* (MAC), usually a fraction of the MIC, was coined to describe the lowest concentration of antibiotic required to produce either structural changes in the bacterium, a 1 $\log_{10}$ decrease in the number of organisms present, or a 10% delay in turbidimetric growth in vitro.[75,217] Rather than resulting in treatment failure, subinhibitory antimicrobial concentrations in concert with defenses in an immunocompetent host may be sufficient to clear the infection.[226] Many effects have been observed to occur as a result of exposure to subinhibitory antimicrobial concentrations, and they are mediated by a variable number of mechanisms.

Increased susceptibility to phagocytosis may be seen with subinhibitory antibiotic concentrations and can occur in many ways. Subinhibitory concentrations may induce morphologic changes in the bacterium such that its size and shape are altered markedly, and, as a result, the immune system is signaled to clear the bacterium.[13,217,236] However, subinhibitory concentrations of drugs that share a common intracellular target cannot be expected to have the same effects on bacterial morphology. Even though both penicillins and cephalosporins act through PBPs, subinhibitory concentrations of penicillins induce filaments in *Proteus mirabilis,* whereas cephalosporins induce the formation of globules.[145,147,221] A likely explanation lies in their different affinity for the various PBPs, whereby they can be expected to bind selectively at low concentrations and rather nonspecifically at therapeutic or supratherapeutic concentrations. The preferential binding of ceftibuten to PBP-3 of *E. coli* at subinhibitory concentrations results in filamentation because this PBP allows crosswall but not sidewall synthesis.[30] Similarly, subinhibitory concentrations of the same drug applied to different organisms can produce different morphologic changes. In *S. aureus,* subinhibitory concentrations of loracarbef induce no morphologic changes, whereas similar concentrations lead to elongated forms and short-chain forms in *E. coli* and elongated and filamentous forms in *H. influenzae.*[227]

Although size may be one factor stimulating enhanced clearance of the organism, increased uptake by the immune system can be demonstrated even for cells with little gross morphologic alteration. Subinhibitory antibiotic concentrations can impair the synthesis of antiphagocytic surface factors or liberate their release, thereby enhancing complement binding, opsonization, phagocytosis, and, ultimately, bacterial killing.[97,103,135] Production of the antiphagocytic A protein of *S. aureus* can be repressed by subinhibitory concentrations of selected protein synthesis inhibitors and fluoroquinolones.[154,210] Subinhibitory concentrations of β-lactam agents, but not vancomycin or protein synthesis inhibitors, increase the susceptibility of *S. agalactiae* to uptake by polymorphonuclear leukocytes (PMNs) because of the loss of antiphagocytic capsular material.[102] Carbapenems and cephalosporins at subinhibitory concentrations increase the serum sensitivity of K1-positive *E. coli* by reducing expression of the K1 capsular polysaccharide.[219]

Even drugs with no inherent bacteriostatic or bactericidal activity against a specific organism can induce sufficient changes in the cell surface to affect serum sensitivity. Preincubation of *P. aeruginosa* with subinhibitory concentrations of certain macrolides decreases cell surface hydrophobicity and enhances the sensitivity of the organism to human serum bactericidal activity.[222] Subinhibitory β-lactam concentrations are capable of sufficiently altering the peptidoglycan structure in MRSA to enhance susceptibility of the organism to the lysozyme present in sputum, even though the organism, because of altered PBP production, is no longer susceptible to the bactericidal activity of these agents.[107] Although most effects stimulating bacterial clearance by the host occur as a direct result of cellular changes in the organism, immune cells also can be altered by subinhibitory antibiotic concentrations. Erythromycin does not affect the generation of serum-derived leukoattractants, nor does it increase PMN cell numbers, yet it appears capable of stimulating the migration of PMNs. Researchers suggested that this effect probably results from the ability of erythromycin to sustain cellular migration by reducing the level of leukoattractant-induced autooxidation mediated by the myeloperoxidase–hydrogen peroxide–halide system.[63]

In addition to enhancing bacterial clearance, subinhibitory antibiotic concentrations also can impair bacterial virulence mechanisms. For many organisms, pili, fimbriae, and fimbriae-associated adhesins are responsible for the initial events surrounding adherence and colonization at the site of entry or infection.[198] Subinhibitory quinolone and clindamycin concentrations are capable of decreasing the adherence of nosocomial pathogens (e.g., *Staphylococcus epidermidis*) to the synthetic materials of implantable catheters.[35,206] Subinhibitory concentrations of penicillins, cephalosporins, azalides, and quinolones all have demonstrated the ability to decrease the formation of fimbriae or alter structures that mediate adherence. Specific examples include decreased adherence to oral and urinary tract epithelial cells for organisms such as *Porphyromonas gingivalis, E. coli, Salmonella typhimurium*, and *P. aeruginosa*.[30,143,210,220,236] Moreover, these effects do not appear to be growth phase specific for select drug-microbe combinations.[31]

Subtherapeutic antibiotic concentrations also can have an impact on virulence by downregulating bacterial toxin production. Subinhibitory concentrations of clindamycin can inhibit toxin production in *S. epidermidis* markedly without appreciably altering bacterial growth.[206] *Pseudomonas* exoenzymes that facilitate disease pathogenesis (e.g., exotoxin A, exoenzyme S, phospholipase C, total protease, elastase) are suppressed after exposure to subinhibitory concentrations of ciprofloxacin, tobramycin, and ceftazidime.[89] Finally, given the ability of subinhibitory fluoroquinolone concentrations to disrupt DNA structure sufficiently to interfere with effective mRNA production, continuous exposure of *S. aureus* to fluoroquinolones at subinhibitory concentrations decreases the production of nuclease and hemolytic α-toxin production.[210]

Although discerning which of these effects, alone or in combination, are responsible for the subinhibitory effects is difficult, one may see in vivo that the impact of the sum total of these effects can be observed at the level of the host. In a nonneutropenic rat model of *Klebsiella pneumoniae* pneumonia, a continuous infusion of ceftazidime resulting in steady-state concentrations of 0.06 mg/L protected all the animals from death, despite an MIC for the pathogen of 0.2 mg/L. The same could not be said, however, for immunocompromised animals, which required steady-state concentrations of 0.38 mg/L for adequate protection.[192,193] In a similar model of intraperitoneal *K. pneumoniae* infection, subinhibitory clindamycin concentrations resulted in an increase in bacterial clearance and a decrease in the $\log_{10}$CFUs in blood at 72 hours.[11] In humans, low-dose ampicillin (such that concentrations in urine were no greater than one-fourth to one-half times the MIC), combined with large water intake, was demonstrated to clear documented *E. coli* urinary tract infection in 16 of 20 patients within 2 days of initiating therapy, whereas none of the 18 control subjects receiving the fluid intervention alone demonstrated resolution of the infection.[185] Despite the resistance of *Pseudomonas* in patients with cystic fibrosis, the fluoroquinolones remain capable of eliciting a significant reduction in sputum colony counts and improvement in clinical signs and symptoms.[204,208]

Subinhibitory antimicrobial concentrations can be as potentially disadvantageous to the host as they can be beneficial. These concentrations can impair the ability of the host to respond to the bacterial inoculum, can augment bacterial defenses, and can serve to inactivate the antibiotic. For organisms that are susceptible to β-lactamase induction, strong inducers can upregulate β-lactamase synthesis at concentrations below the MIC. Although β-lactamase induction typically is a reversible phenomenon, many antibiotics demonstrate the ability to select out genetically de-repressed mutants at subinhibitory concentrations.[205,214] Irrespective of whether this induction is phenotypic or genotypic, many antibiotics to which the organism originally may have been susceptible no longer retain their efficacy in light of β-lactamase production. This type of adaptive resistance, observed in response to sublethal antibiotic concentrations, also can be nonenzymatic. A single, one-time exposure of *P. aeruginosa* to subinhibitory concentrations of chlorhexidine results in unstable resistance, and repeated exposure leads to stable expression of altered cell surface macromolecules or efflux systems responsible for resistance.[224] In a clinical strain of this same organism exposed to subinhibitory concentrations of fluoroquinolones and carbapenems for 5 days, a 16- to 32-fold increase in MIC was observed in concert with an alteration in overall protein expression.[36]

Sublethal antibiotic concentrations also can stimulate the production of toxins that may be detrimental to the host. Exposure of enterohemorrhagic *E. coli* to subinhibitory concentrations of fluoroquinolones, cephalosporins, tetracyclines, and inhibitors of folic acid synthesis induces enhanced expression of a *Shiga*-like toxin (SLT-1), which is proposed to mediate events surrounding the development of hemolytic uremic syndrome. Subinhibitory fluoroquinolone concentrations also can stimulate the production of verotoxins in this same organism.[237,244] Lincomycin and tetracycline at subinhibitory concentrations stimulate the production of heat-labile enterotoxin in enterotoxigenic *E. coli*, as well as *Vibrio cholerae* enterotoxin, even though these agents are principally protein synthesis inhibitors. Prior data suggest that the copy number of plasmids does not increase and proposed that the rate of enterotoxin liberation is enhanced as a result of antibiotic inhibition of the synthesis of proteins responsible for degrading the toxin.[141,245] The α-toxin of *S. aureus* is demonstrated to be hemolytic, dermonecrotic, and antichemotactic and appears to be upregulated in the presence of subinhibitory nafcillin concentrations, irrespective of whether the isolate is susceptible to the agent. Greater hemolytic activity and increased lethality of the broth filtrate in a murine intraperitoneal model are observed, and this activity is ablated when incubated with anti–α-toxin antibody.[126] Other β-lactams (with the exception of aztreonam), ofloxacin, and trimethoprim are similarly capable of inducing α-toxin expression at subinhibitory concentrations.[170]

The upregulation of protein expression by subinhibitory antibiotic concentrations not only is responsible for contributing to antibiotic and cellular destruction but also can enhance the binding of pathogens to host proteins and implantable devices. Subinhibitory concentrations of ciprofloxacin increase the transcription of fibronectin-binding proteins in *S. aureus* isolates and thereby result in greater adhesion to immobilized fibronectin and fibronectin-coated polymers, a particular concern with subcutaneously implanted devices that have polymer surfaces.[23,24] Subinhibitory concentrations of antibiotic also can alter the immunogenicity of the pathogen such that the host can no longer mount the same degree of immune response. *S. aureus* isolates coincubated with subinhibitory concentrations of oxacillin demonstrated a diminished capacity to stimulate proinflammatory cytokine production (e.g., tumor necrosis factor-α, interleukin-1β [IL-1β], and IL-6) in human monocytes. Given that activation of the complement system and cytokine release are stimulated by peptidoglycan molecules of a certain size or tertiary structure, subinhibitory β-lactam concentrations probably distort the peptidoglycan structure sufficiently that the immune system no longer effectively responds to these immunostimulatory components.[203] The impact of subtherapeutic antimicrobial exposure has widely been examined in the agriculture industry because of the common use of antimicrobials for prophylaxis and growth promotion in livestock. With continuous administration of low, subtherapeutic antimicrobial doses, multiple mechanisms of bacterial resistance have been detected among exposed livestock.[1,2]

Unless unusual circumstances prevail, the goal of therapy probably will not be to target plasma concentrations below the MIC. However, given the reality of encountering this situation in the clinical setting, practitioners certainly need to be aware of the potential implications for therapeutic response associated with subinhibitory concentrations of antimicrobial agents.

Effects That Persist After Antimicrobial Exposure (Postantibiotic Effect, Postantibiotic Leukocyte Enhancement, and Post–β-Lactamase Inhibitor Effect)

Early investigations into antibiotic activity described a delay in the recovery and regrowth of penicillin-exposed staphylococci and streptococci when the drug was removed by enzymatic inactivation or the organism was removed to drug-free media.[22,52,174] In addition, in vivo evaluations of penicillin activity suggested that the effects of penicillin in an immunocompetent animal lasted well beyond the time when blood levels remained above quantifiable concentrations. Despite a half-life of minutes, many hours can elapse after the administration of a dose of penicillin before bacterial growth resumes.[55,114,202] The term *postantibiotic effect* was coined to describe the suppression of bacterial growth that persists after brief exposure of the organism to an antimicrobial agent.[39] Unlike the subinhibitory effects discussed earlier in the chapter, the PAE occurs as a result of residual antimicrobial activity after initial exposure at inhibitory concentrations, as opposed to the subinhibitory concentrations themselves. The PAEs described to date typically are reversible; and although the mechanisms have not been elucidated fully, they probably are caused by either nonlethal damage or persistence of antibiotic at the site of action. In the same vein as the PAEs, the term *post–β-lactamase inhibitor effect* (PLIE) was coined to describe the residual effects of β-lactamase inhibitors after exposure to inhibitory concentrations.[225] Similarly, one encounters the term *postantibiotic leukocyte enhancement* (PALE), which is used to account for a PAE in vivo that lasts longer than that observed in vitro and is defined as exposure to subinhibitory concentrations of an antibiotic that render the organism more susceptible to the phagocytic and bactericidal action of neutrophils.

The PAE depends on many factors, the most discernible being the drug-microbe combination.[112] Since the initial descriptions with penicillin were reported, similar observations have been noted for a broad range of organisms, and essentially all antibiotic classes demonstrate a PAE against select organisms.[39] Virtually all agents evaluated demonstrate a PAE against susceptible gram-positive cocci. Inhibitors of protein and nucleic acid synthesis produce longer lasting PAEs in vitro than do cell wall–acting agents, with an average of 1 to 2 hours for β-lactams, 1 to 3 hours for fluoroquinolones, and 3 to 5 hours for protein synthesis inhibitors. For resistant gram-positive cocci, descriptions of a PAE are mixed. Against gram-negative bacilli, no appreciable PAE is observed for trimethoprim or the β-lactams in vitro, with the exception of the carbapenems, which demonstrate a PAE of 1 to 2 hours. The fluoroquinolones and protein synthesis inhibitors have PAEs of roughly 1 to 3 hours and 3 to 8 hours, respectively. Within this group of organisms, *P. aeruginosa* serves as an exception, and the fluoroquinolones and protein synthesis inhibitors display slightly shorter PAEs—1 to 2 hours and 2 to 3 hours on average for the respective drug classes. Similar observations have been described for the gram-negative anaerobes, with little or no PAE seen with the β-lactams but a measurable PAE observed for protein synthesis inhibitors.[39]

Given that most drug classes demonstrate a PAE, multiple mechanisms must exist by which this effect arises. For the β-lactams, researchers proposed that the PAE corresponds to the time required for the organism to synthesize new PBPs. The initial high β-lactam concentrations are thought to bind irreversibly to and thus inactivate the PBPs. As such, cell multiplication subsequently is prolonged until a critical number of PBPs are resynthesized and cell division can resume.[226] Within the large class of β-lactam agents, however, further distinctions can be made based on the specific PBP bound and the subsequent morphologic alteration that is induced. Against *E. coli*, the longest lasting PAEs are observed for agents that induce the formation of spheroplasts and the shortest for agents that induce the formation of filaments. On drug removal, filaments (which may contain a biomass corresponding to more than 20 bacteria) readily separate into individual bacteria, whereas spheroplasts require a longer period to resynthesize a normal cell wall and resume replication.[94] Analogous to the β-lactams, the time required for the resynthesis or recovery of ribosomal proteins is probably responsible for the PAEs observed after the administration of an aminoglycoside. Evaluation of the intracellular events taking place in *E. coli* during aminoglycoside-induced PAEs suggests that both DNA and RNA synthesis resume immediately after drug removal; however, synthesis of structural and functional protein does not resume for nearly 5 hours.[16,112] For the fluoroquinolones, the proposed mechanism behind the PAE is not as consistent with the antimicrobial activity of these agents. A progressive increase in ^{3}H-thymidine incorporation in *S. aureus* during the PAE suggests that DNA synthesis continues to occur, and, thus, the PAE may represent the time needed to repair the damage to DNA gyrase, the time required to reestablish the function of DNA gyrase after dissociation of the antibiotic from the enzyme, or the time required to synthesize new DNA gyrase.[84]

In addition to the specific drug-microbe combination, the magnitude and duration of drug exposure also have an impact on the PAE. Cell wall–acting agents (e.g., β-lactams and glycopeptides) demonstrate a concentration-dependent PAE. Increases in the concentration and duration of exposure (i.e., increasing AUC) prolong the PAE in both gram-positive and gram-negative organisms to a point of maximal effect, typically 2 to 6 hours, although the time may be shorter for some members of this class. In fact, the PAE appears to be related to the log-normalized AUC in a sigmoidal manner.[38,94,131] Similarly, an increasing concentration of protein synthesis inhibitors is associated with progressive prolongation in PAE to a point of maximal effect. However, it can be difficult to establish with the aminoglycosides and fluoroquinolones because complete killing at supratherapeutic concentrations can obscure accurate determination of the PAE.[39,112] Bacteriostatic agents generally demonstrate concentration-independent PAEs such that increasing the duration of antibiotic exposure, but not the concentration, results in an increase in PAE to some maximal effect.[39]

As expected, the magnitude of the PAE also depends on whether antimicrobial agents are administered alone or in combination. Indifferent, additive, and synergistic PAEs all have been described with the use of combination therapy.[72,90,112] However, for some drug-microbe combinations, the magnitude of the PAE may differ with the phenotypic expression of resistance. For *Enterococcus faecalis* isolates that demonstrate only low-level resistance to streptomycin or gentamicin, the effect of a penicillin-aminoglycoside combination on the PAE is markedly synergistic. In contrast, for isolates with high-level resistance to the aminoglycosides, no synergistic PAE is observed.[241] Additionally, physicochemical factors can affect in vitro determination of PAEs and, although the in vivo relevance is questionable, some are worthy of consideration. In *S. aureus*, the PAEs of penicillin and gentamicin are markedly protracted at the slightly acidic pH 6 compared with a physiologic pH of 7.4. Given that a relatively acidic pH can occur at the site of active infection, a disease-PAE interaction is possible. A similar pH-dependent effect on PAE is not observed with the fluoroquinolones or macrolides against *S. aureus*, nor is it noted for *E. coli* and *P. aeruginosa* with the β-lactams, fluoroquinolones, and macrolides.[73,91] An increase in PAE in vitro also is observed as temperature drops, a finding that raises the question whether the PAE is truly altered or the generation time is lengthened. Regardless, the temperatures evaluated were much lower than physiologic temperatures and probably have no clinical impact in the presence of infection. Finally, anaerobic conditions are observed to increase the PAE for ciprofloxacin/*E. coli* and gentamicin/*S. aureus* combinations, but not with other combinations.[73]

The attention paid to PAE of late highlights its significance, which lies in the flexibility that it affords to extend the dosing interval before reexposure to drug, essentially redosing, is necessary. Researchers suggested that agents with a small PAE require that a dosing interval be selected that will maintain concentrations above the MIC throughout most of the interval. Agents with a more protracted PAE can be given less often and thus at higher doses, thereby supporting the argument for once-daily dosing with drugs such as the aminoglycosides. However, many nuances can be identified between the in vitro conditions under which PAEs are determined and the in vivo conditions of infection such that the ultimate clinical (i.e., therapeutic) implications of these data have yet to be determined. In vitro, attempts are made to remove the drug completely (i.e., abruptly terminate drug exposure to the microbe) after initial exposure when determining the PAE. In contrast, drug concentrations fall in a more controlled, typically first-order fashion in vivo. The impact of this distinction on PAEs in patients remains unknown. Variable growth rates or metabolic states of the organism when growing in vivo similarly may have an impact on the PAE. In vitro, a prolonged PAE is observed when *Enterococcus faecium* is exposed to the combination of gentamicin and penicillin; yet, when the same drug concentrations and the same inoculum size are achieved in the vegetation of a murine aortic valve endocarditis model, no prolongation of PAE can be observed.[99] Similarly, a rat model of *P. aeruginosa* endocarditis failed to demonstrate a PAE in vivo for the combination of imipenem and gentamicin despite a PAE of nearly 5 hours determined in vitro; however, an observable PAE in vitro and in vivo was noted in the same model when ciprofloxacin was evaluated.[98,111]

Impact of Inoculum Size on the Concentration-Effect Relationship

The antimicrobial effect observed at any given drug concentration may vary with the number of organisms at the site of infection. Accordingly, the size of the inoculum can be a primary determinant of drug efficacy. Early investigations clearly demonstrated that the duration of the infection before treatment is a significant predictor of clinical response.[51] When therapy is delayed, presumably leading to a larger inoculum, the efficacy of that therapy often is affected adversely. In nonneutropenic rats, larger doses of antibiotic were needed to treat *K. pneumoniae*, whether administered by continuous or intermittent infusion, when the infection was allowed to progress 34 hours before therapy was initiated versus 5 hours.[192] Many potential mechanisms have been proposed to account for this event. Large inocula perhaps generate a higher local density of enzymes that effectively reduce active (i.e., functional) antibiotic concentrations at the site of infection. Large bacterial populations also are statistically more likely to contain resistant organisms that arise by spontaneous mutation and predominate within the population as a result of the selective pressure posed by the antibiotic. One such example has been observed in a murine model of group A streptococcal myositis, in which the activity of penicillin is compromised most severely in the presence of a large inoculum (10^8–10^9 CFUs/mL), with relatively little impact on the activity of clindamycin. Given that the isolate did not produce β-lactamase and that any residual PAE was irrelevant because both regimens maintained drug concentrations above the MIC for the duration of the dosing interval, this effect of the inoculum was attributed in part to the selection of a cell wall–deficient mutant.[215] Clindamycin, however, is not devoid of susceptibility to the inoculum effect for all organisms; an increase in the size of the inoculum or an increase in the time until therapy resulted in a lower reduction in $\log_{10}$CFUs in a murine *Bacillus fragilis* abscess model.[117] Another proposed mechanism for the effect of the inoculum lies in the finding that dense populations of organisms may grow at a slower rate or be metabolically inactive compared with their less dense counterparts. An effect arising by this mechanism probably will not affect antimicrobial agents that are bactericidal against both rapidly growing and stationary-phase organisms (e.g., fluoroquinolones). However, for agents that exert their bactericidal effects primarily on rapidly dividing organisms (e.g., β-lactams), activity may be compromised in the presence of an established infection in which the bacterial population is large and as many as 90% of the organisms may be slowly dividing and, thus, metabolically inactive. For clinical isolates of group G streptococci, time-kill studies demonstrated rapid complete bacterial killing when the organism was primarily in log-phase growth, regardless of whether 10^4 or 10^7 organisms were involved. In contrast, when the organism was principally in the stationary phase, rapid and complete killing was observed only for the smaller inoculum (10^4 organisms), with no appreciable killing at 10^8 organisms. Furthermore, in patients with a protracted clinical course of infection or recalcitrant infection, therapy failed despite high drug doses and the presence of a susceptible isolate.[134]

Attempting to link multiple pharmacodynamic effects in evaluating the outcome of antiinfective therapy poses an arduous task from both theoretical and practical perspectives, and, hence, a complete discussion is not undertaken in this chapter. Nonetheless, the combination of such effects has received some attention in the literature and merits mention. Specifically, large inocula appear to be capable of modulating the PAE and subinhibitory effects observed with numerous agents. Exposure of *E. coli* to subinhibitory sparfloxacin concentrations produced a pronounced inoculum-dependent subinhibitory effect. At a dose that was 0.3 times the MIC, growth of the organism was delayed by 0.3, 0.9, and 3.3 hours with inocula of 10^8, 10^6, and 10^4 CFUs, respectively, with similar observations noted for other drug-microbe combinations.[38,167]

Concentration-Dependent Combination Effects (Synergy and Antagonism)

As discussed earlier and elsewhere in this text, antimicrobial combinations are used for many purposes: to prevent or delay the emergence of resistance, to enable dosage reduction and thereby minimize dose-related toxicities, and to treat polymicrobial infections. Combination therapy can be designed with the goal of synergistic or additive activity in mind, or, alternatively, these effects can occur without conscious consideration or forethought. Moreover, the undesirable outcomes of indifference or antagonism similarly can result through the combination of agents. Although a complete review of antagonism and synergy is beyond the scope of this section, we would be remiss not to mention concentration-dependent combination effects. We provide this brief discussion specifically to point out that a simple classification of drug combinations as synergistic, antagonist, and so forth is not always feasible. As discussed elsewhere, disagreement in the classification certainly can arise when different methods are used for evaluation.[25,165]

However, even when restricted to evaluations using the same experimental methods, certain combinations can be classified differently, depending on antibiotic concentration. Synergy is observed with cefoperazone and low imipenem concentrations against MRSA; however, higher concentrations of imipenem antagonize the activity of cefoperazone. Although antagonism with imipenem often is explained away as being β-lactamase mediated, the concentration-dependent antagonism observed remains unexplained by this mechanism because antagonism was shown for strains that lacked β-lactamase production.[182] The combination of penicillin and clindamycin at subinhibitory concentrations demonstrates synergy against group A β-hemolytic streptococci. At concentrations ranging from two to four times the MIC, the combination demonstrates antagonism, and at clinically relevant concentrations (≈100 times the MIC), indifference is observed, with the combination exhibiting no advantage over either agent alone.[216] Against isolates of vancomycin-intermediate *S. aureus*, antagonism is observed when methicillin and vancomycin are combined at subinhibitory concentrations. However, when the methicillin concentration exceeds the MIC, synergy is observed with the same combination. Although the mechanism behind this differential activity remains unclear, researchers proposed that the antagonism observed at lower methicillin concentrations results from an increase in the density of non–cross-linked D-alanyl-D-alanine side chains, the target site for vancomycin and a substrate for the PBPs. This increase would decrease the efficacy of methicillin as a PBP inhibitor by substrate competition.[104] For certain strains of methicillin-sensitive *S. aureus*, a combination of rifampin and methicillin below the MIC is synergistic, but above the MBC it is antagonistic. Similarly, a rifampin-vancomycin combination is synergistic at concentrations close to the MBC but indifferent as concentrations rise.[248] Furthermore, for some drug-microbe combinations, it is not the classification per se that is affected by the concentration but rather the magnitude of the effect observed. Against *E. faecium,* fixed piperacillin and variable teicoplanin concentrations are synergistic. However, the degree of synergy depends on the teicoplanin concentration; comparable synergistic activity occurs at teicoplanin concentrations of 2, 4, or 8 mg/L; reduced synergistic activity occurs at teicoplanin concentrations of 16 and 32 mg/L; and the greatest degree of synergy is observed at a concentration of 64 mg/L.[184]

Thus the available data support the finding that, in many cases, the clinical assignment or "expectation" of synergy, additivity, or antagonism by specific combinations of antiinfective agents cannot be assumed simply by virtue of the drug class or drug-specific mechanisms of action, or both. With drug combinations for which the activity against an infecting pathogen is potentially concentration dependent, prediction of therapeutic outcome must entail some assessment, be it actual or theoretical (e.g., the use of pharmacokinetic modeling), of the time-dependent drug concentration profile at the site or sites of infection.

PHARMACOGENETIC-PHARMACOGENOMIC DETERMINANTS OF EFFECT

Although this chapter is designed to detail the pharmacokinetic and pharmacodynamic determinants of antiinfective drug response, we would be remiss not to introduce the emerging role of pharmacogenetics as a predictor of drug response and a driver of antiinfective drug therapy. Although the application of molecular biology to infectious diseases traditionally has been limited to diagnostics (e.g., polymerase chain reaction–based assays for the detection of viral pathogens and slow-growing microorganisms) and disease monitoring (e.g., viral loads), molecular tools increasingly are finding application with identifying the likelihood of drug response a priori and determining optimal treatment strategies for infectious pathogens. Genotyping strategies are used to identify mutations that confer drug resistance and guide the selection of antiretroviral therapy in management of human immunodeficiency virus infection.[140,232] Similarly, viral genotyping appears to be among the most robust predictors of response to combination therapy in the treatment of hepatitis C virus,[136,195] and it has prompted similar investigations for hepatitis B virus.[92,124] Commercially available molecular-based assays have been developed for the determination of methicillin resistance in *S. aureus,* multidrug resistance in *Mycobacterium tuberculosis,* and vancomycin resistance in *Enterococcus* in clinical isolates. These methods appear to perform well compared with conventional phenotype-based methods,[127,157,171] and the integration of these tools into clinical care has resulted in optimization of targeted antimicrobial therapy and improvement in patient care.[15,62]

Currently, genetic testing is rarely indicated before initiation of antiinfectives. However, there are cases for which gene testing has proved to directly enhance the safety of prescribing. An abacavir black box warning for *HLA-B*5701* allele screening before drug initiation is recommended. This haplotype is commonly associated with idiosyncratic adverse drug reactions, with approximately 50% of those patients exposed to abacavir with the allele experiencing an adverse reaction compared with less than 5% without the allele.[105] Caution is also recommended when prescribing drugs (e.g., dapsone, nitrofurantoin, sulfasalazine) that could be affected by polymorphisms associated with glucose-6-phosphate 1-dehydrogenase (G6PD) variants because the enzyme is involved in protecting erythrocytes from oxidative stress and hemolysis can occur in those with enzyme deficiency; thus genetic testing should be considered if G6PD deficiency is suspected.[246] Although the application of genotyping for specific enzymes related to the metabolism of antimicrobials is not routinely performed, in cases in which overall drug exposure is quite variable, genotyping has the potential to enhance dosing strategies. The antifungal agent voriconazole is case in point; CYP2C19 contributes to the metabolism of voriconazole, and poor CYP2C19 metabolizers have up to fourfold higher voriconazole levels compared with extensive metabolizers. Although CYP2C19 alone cannot explain variability in exposure, evaluation of CYP2C19 genotype can assist clinicians in the assessment of cases for which therapeutic concentrations of voriconazole cannot be achieved and guide dosing strategies.[100] The integration of genetic testing to optimize antimicrobial therapy will likely only continue to be used more commonly in the future as studies demonstrate clinical benefit.

CONCLUSION

With a recognized decline in the development of new antimicrobial therapies since the 1980s and the emergence of multidrug-resistant organisms (e.g., gram-negative organisms, *M. tuberculosis*), a continued need persists for the repurposing of older agents while awaiting the future development of newer therapies.[213] Unfortunately, there remains a relative paucity of pharmacokinetic-pharmacodynamic information for many of the currently available antimicrobial agents in children (e.g., antitubercular agents); and for older agents that continue to hold important places in pediatric therapeutics (e.g., metronidazole, clindamycin), complete profiles of their clinical pharmacology (i.e., absorption, biotransformation) in infants and children are lacking.[85] For both existing and emerging drug therapies, pharmacokinetics provides a powerful and valuable tool. The clinical scientist can use pharmacokinetics to characterize a given drug by providing a profile of its absorption, distribution, metabolism, and excretion in individuals with and without disease, during normal alterations of human physiology (e.g., pregnancy), as well as under conditions of normal altered organ function or body composition (e.g., growth and development, senescence). For the clinical practitioner, the tool of pharmacokinetics can provide a means to individualize drug therapy by characterizing the relationship between drug dose and resultant drug concentrations in plasma or other relevant biologic fluids (e.g., urine, CSF, synovial fluid, pleural fluid, peritoneal fluid). When linked with information regarding the pharmacodynamic behavior of the antibiotic, the susceptibility of the organism, and the status of the host, the application of pharmacokinetics affords the practitioner the ability to exercise some degree of adaptive control over drug therapy by selecting a drug and dosing regimen that have the greatest likelihood of producing both efficacy and safety.

Practicing Precision Medicine in Infectious Disease

For decades, practitioners who treat infectious diseases have had at their disposal specific, detailed information on most pathogens (e.g., in vitro sensitivity), antiinfective agents (e.g., killing characteristics, biopharmaceutical information, drug biotransformation, and pharmacokinetic data), and the host-infection interface (e.g., information regarding disease location, general physical condition of the patient, information pertaining to the intersection of development and disease). Consequently, the goal of "individualized therapy" has been the mantra of pediatric infectious disease. In the current genomic era, we can now quickly and relatively cheaply obtain genetic and genomic data about a patient and their pathogens that is not simply informative but also, in many cases, as illustrated previously, can be predictive. It is the synthesis of this information (much of which is presented in this chapter) and the application of tools such as pharmacokinetics that can reliably be used in an adaptive fashion to determine the proper antiinfective dose for a given patient and, most important, control the dose-exposure relationship that will enable the practice of true precision medicine in treating infectious diseases in infants, children, and adolescents.

NEW REFERENCES SINCE THE SEVENTH EDITION

1. Aarestrup FM. Association between the consumption of antimicrobial agents in animal husbandry and the occurrence of resistant bacteria among food animals. *Int J Antimicrob Agents.* 1999;12(4):279-285.
2. Alexander TW, Yanke LJ, Topp E, et al. Effect of subtherapeutic administration of antibiotics on the prevalence of antibiotic-resistant *Escherichia coli* bacteria in feedlot cattle. *Appl Environ Microbiol.* 2008;74(14):4405-4416.
15. Banerjee R, Teng CB, Cunningham SA, et al. Randomized Trial of Rapid Multiplex Polymerase Chain Reaction-Based Blood Culture Identification and Susceptibility Testing. *Clin Infect Dis.* 2015;61(7):1071-1080.
18. Barza M, Ioannidis JP, Cappelleri JC, et al. Single or multiple daily doses of aminoglycosides: a meta-analysis. *BMJ.* 1996;312(7027):338-345.
50. Dulhunty JM, Roberts JA, Davis JS, et al. Continuous infusion of beta-lactam antibiotics in severe sepsis: a multicenter double-blind, randomized controlled trial. *Clin Infect Dis.* 2013;56(2):236-244.
59. Falagas ME, Tansarli GS, Ikawa K, et al. Clinical outcomes with extended or continuous versus short-term intravenous infusion of carbapenems and piperacillin/tazobactam: a systematic review and meta-analysis. *Clin Infect Dis.* 2013;56(2):272-282.

62. Felsenstein S, Bender JM, Sposto R, et al. Impact of a Rapid Blood Culture Assay for Gram-Positive Identification and Detection of Resistance Markers in a Pediatric Hospital. *Arch Pathol Lab Med*. 2016;140(3):267-275.
105. Hughes AR, Spreen WR, Mosteller M, et al. Pharmacogenetics of hypersensitivity to abacavir: from PGx hypothesis to confirmation to clinical utility. *Pharmacogenomics J*. 2008;8(6):365-374.
209. Smyth AR, Bhatt J. Once-daily versus multiple-daily dosing with intravenous aminoglycosides for cystic fibrosis. *Cochrane Database Syst Rev*. 2014;(2):CD002009.
246. Youngster I, Arcavi L, Schechmaster R, et al. Medications and glucose-6-phosphate dehydrogenase deficiency: an evidence-based review. *Drug Saf*. 2010;33(9):713-726.

The full reference list for this chapter is available at ExpertConsult.com.

236 Antibacterial Therapeutic Agents

Ruston S. Taylor • Debra L. Palazzi

This review of antibacterial agents is divided into two sections: (1) the clinical pharmacology of currently available antibacterial drugs and (2) the various aspects of administration of antimicrobial agents to infants and children. The second section includes dosage schedules and routes, prophylactic use of antibacterial agents, considerations in writing orders and prescriptions, and other aspects of administration. Other antimicrobial agents used for the treatment of viruses, fungi, mycobacteria, and parasites are discussed in other chapters dealing with these pathogens. For the most part, only antimicrobial agents approved for use in infants and children by the US Food and Drug Administration (FDA) are discussed, although promising new agents that are likely to be approved for use in pediatrics are mentioned where relevant.

CLINICAL PHARMACOLOGY

The antibacterial agents of value in treating infectious diseases in infants and children may be classified into three major groups:

1. Agents that target cell wall or cell membrane, including the following:
   The β-lactams, including penicillins, cephalosporins, carbacephems, monobactams, and carbapenems
   The glycopeptides (e.g., vancomycin)
   The lipopeptides (e.g., daptomycin)
   The polymyxin: colistin
2. Agents that interfere with protein synthesis, including the following:
   Agents that bind the 30S subunit, including aminoglycosides, chloramphenicol, and tetracyclines
   Agents that bind the 50S subunit, including macrolides, clindamycin, and linezolid
   Other mechanisms: Rifamycins
3. Agents that target nucleic acids, including fluoroquinolones, sulfonamides, and metronidazole

The following properties that govern the use of each group of drugs in infants and children are considered: mechanism of action, mechanisms of resistance, in vitro activity, pharmacokinetics, indications for use, side effects, and toxicity.

AGENTS THAT TARGET THE CELL WALL

β-Lactams

Biochemical Structure

The β-lactams are a large group of compounds that have in common a four-membered β-lactam ring. The subclasses of β-lactams differ from one another with regard to their side chains and the presence of other ring structures: the penicillins contain a five-membered thiazolidine β-ring fused to the β-lactam ring,[193] the cephalosporins have a six-membered dihydrothiazine instead of the thiazolidine ring, and the carbacephems have a methylene group replacing the sulfur atom in the dihydrothiazine ring of the cephalosporin nucleus. The β-lactam ring is essential for antibacterial activity, whereas the side chains influence the pharmacologic properties of the β-lactam and the spectrum of antibacterial activity.

Mechanism of Action

Our understanding of the mechanism of action of the β-lactams has evolved over the past several decades. Researchers initially thought that binding of β-lactam to a bacterial cell membrane-associated enzyme (transpeptidase) blocked the terminal step in synthesis of the peptidoglycan layer of the bacterial cell wall. Cell death would ensue because the weakened cell wall could not withstand the osmotic and mechanical pressure resulting from a growing bacterium.[349] Additional evidence suggested that it is a more complex process involving activation of endogenous autolytic systems[249,351] and inhibition of bacterial enzymes called the penicillin binding proteins (PBPs), which include transpeptidase, carboxypeptidase, and endopeptidase. These enzymes are located beneath the cell wall and are responsible for cell wall synthesis by achieving cross-linkage between peptide chains of peptidoglycans. PBPs are vital for cell division, cell shape, and structural integrity. Because the specific PBPs within each bacterial species and the affinity of each β-lactam antibiotic for a particular PBP differ, some β-lactams have better activity than others against particular bacteria. The various β-lactam antibiotics can have different morphologic effects on the same bacterial species; this property is thought to be related to specific functions of the PBP to which the β-lactam binds.[330] Some bacteria have a deficiency in the system of autolytic enzymes that results in inhibition, but not killing, of the bacteria by a β-lactam that otherwise would be bactericidal. This phenomenon is termed tolerance and is demonstrated in vitro by a minimal inhibitory concentration (MIC) in the susceptible range and a ratio of minimal bactericidal concentration (MBC) to MIC of 32 or greater.[147]

β-Lactam antibiotics are bactericidal against most susceptible bacteria. The nature of the bactericidal activity has been described as time-dependent, as opposed to the concentration-dependent bactericidal activity of aminoglycosides.[211] Bactericidal activity is thought to be optimal when the concentration of β-lactam antibiotic at the site of infection is 4 to 10 times greater than that of the MIC (or MBC) of the infecting organism. The rapidity and extent of killing are not increased when concentrations exceed that ratio. A more important determinant of bactericidal activity for β-lactams is the length of time during the dosing interval for which the concentration of antibiotic exceeds the MIC (time >MIC) for the infecting organism. Optimal bacterial killing correlates with time greater than MIC that exceeds 40% to 50% of the dosing interval.[91]

Penicillins

Although first discovered by Fleming in the late 1920s, penicillin G was not available for general use in the United States for another 20 years. Since that time, numerous semisynthetic penicillins have been developed. The penicillins can be classified into four groups (natural penicillins,

BOX 236.1 Microorganisms for Which Penicillin G or V Is the Drug of Choice

Actinomyces israelii	*Spirillum minus*
Bacillus anthracis	*Staphylococcus aureus*[a,b]
Clostridium spp.	*Streptobacillus moniliformis*
Corynebacterium diphtheriae	*Streptococcus* groups A, B, C, D, G; viridans group[b]; anaerobic strains
Erysipelothrix rhusiopathiae	*Streptococcus pneumoniae*[b]
Leptospira spp.	*Treponema pallidum*
Neisseria gonorrhoeae[a]	
Neisseria meningitidis[a]	
Pasteurella multocida	

[a]Strains that do not produce lactamase.
[b]Only those without altered penicillin binding proteins.

penicillinase-resistant penicillins, aminopenicillins, and extended-spectrum penicillins) based on their antimicrobial activity, with some overlap. The spectrum of activity among the compounds within each group usually is similar; the differences are attributable to their pharmacologic properties.

Natural Penicillins: Penicillin G and Penicillin V

Despite the more than 70 years that penicillin G has been in use, some bacteria continue to be exquisitely susceptible. Resistant strains of *Streptococcus pyogenes* (group A streptococcus) and *Streptococcus agalactiae* (group B streptococcus) have not emerged. Penicillin G remains the drug of choice for the treatment of disease caused by a wide variety of microorganisms (Box 236.1).

Most bacteria have acquired resistance to penicillin G by producing β-lactamases; resistance caused by altered PBPs occurs less commonly. Most strains of *Staphylococcus aureus* and *Staphylococcus epidermidis* produce penicillinase. *Neisseria gonorrhoeae* gradually developed resistance to penicillin G beginning in the late 1960s by various mechanisms, including plasmid-mediated production of a TEM1-like β-lactamase, as well as chromosomal mutations in at least four genes (*penA, penB, ponA,* and *mtrR*) that encode increased expression of an efflux pump and alterations in PBPs and porins.[270] Mechanisms of β-lactam resistance in *Bacteroides* spp. and other gram-negative anaerobes include production of class A β-lactamases (penicillinase or cephalosporinase) and class B metallo-β-lactamases that hydrolyze carbapenems, as well as alteration of PBPs.[20] Historically, penicillin has been the antibiotic of choice for treatment of *Neisseria meningitidis* infections, but strains with reduced susceptibility to penicillin have been reported in Europe, South America, Asia, Australia, and less frequently in the United States, where approximately 15% of strains have alterations in PBP2 encoded by the *penA* gene that likely results from mosaic genes derived through transformation with DNA from commensal *Neisseria* spp. in the nasopharynx of colonized individuals. Although penicillin resistance resulting from production of β-lactamase has been reported, such strains are rare.[179]

Of particular concern is the global dissemination of strains of *Streptococcus pneumoniae* resistant to penicillin G as a result of altered PBPs. Surveillance data in the United States estimated the average rate of penicillin nonsusceptibility to be 33% (high-level resistance, 16%), with the highest incidence of 44% reported in the south-central region.[173] However, with the introduction of the 7-valent pneumococcal conjugate vaccine (PCV7) in 2000, invasive pneumococcal disease in young children caused by vaccine serotypes decreased by approximately 90%. Conversely, invasive disease caused by nonvaccine serotypes increased.[202] The incidence of disease caused by 19A serotype increased, and these isolates are associated with β-lactam antibiotic resistance (including penicillin and third-generation cephalosporins).[158,341] The Active Bacterial Core Surveillance (ABC) report from 2014 showed penicillin nonsusceptibility of 5.3% and cefotaxime nonsusceptibility of 3.3%.[70] From 1999 to 2003, approximately 6% of pneumococci were reported in the United States to exhibit a multidrug-resistance phenotype defined as resistance to penicillin, trimethoprim-sulfamethoxazole (TMP-SMX), erythromycin, clindamycin, and tetracycline.[173] Although penicillin-resistant pneumococcal meningitis has developed in patients who were receiving vancomycin for pneumococcal sepsis,[78] no treatment failures have been documented when the appropriate dosage of vancomycin was administered. In 2010, the 13-valent pneumococcal vaccine (PCV13), which includes serotype 19A, replaced PCV7 in the United States. The introduction of PCV13 has resulted in a decrease in antibiotic-nonsusceptible invasive pneumococcal disease across all age groups, with the most dramatic reductions in children less than 5 years of age. Several antibiotic nonsusceptible serotypes have emerged following the introduction of PCV13, but no single nonvaccine serotype is predominant as was witnessed following the introduction of PCV7.[352]

In 2008, the Clinical and Laboratory Standards Institute (CLSI; formerly the National Committee for Clinical Laboratory Standards) published new *S. pneumoniae* breakpoints for penicillin because of a reevaluation showing that clinical response to penicillin was being preserved in clinical studies of pneumococcal infection, despite reduced susceptibility in vitro. Under the former criteria, susceptible, intermediate, and resistant MIC breakpoints for penicillin were less than 0.06, 0.12, and greater than 2 μg/mL, respectively, for all pneumococcal isolates, regardless of clinical syndrome or route of penicillin administration. Those breakpoints remain unchanged for patients without meningitis who can be treated with oral penicillin. However, for patients without meningitis who are treated with intravenous penicillin, the new breakpoints are less than 2, 4, and greater than/equal to 8 μg/mL, respectively. Furthermore, isolates from patients with meningitis are now categorized as either susceptible or resistant, with intravenous penicillin breakpoints of less than 0.06 or greater than 0.12 μg/mL, respectively. Use of narrow-spectrum agents, such as penicillin, is encouraged to prevent the spread of antimicrobial-resistant *S. pneumoniae* and also the spread of methicillin-resistant *S. aureus* and *Clostridium difficile*, which can result from use of broader spectrum antimicrobials.

Several oral and parenteral forms of penicillin G are available. Selection of a preparation is based on the pattern of antimicrobial activity, including the peak and duration of activity in serum and tissues, and factors that reflect absorption, distribution, and excretion of the drug. These characteristics of penicillins are as follows:

1. Aqueous (water-soluble) penicillin G produces high peak concentrations of antibacterial activity in serum within 30 minutes after intramuscular administration but is excreted rapidly; thus, the concentration in serum is low within 2 to 4 hours. If aqueous penicillin G is given by the intravenous route, the peak is higher and occurs earlier, and the duration of antibacterial activity in serum is shorter (≈2 hours). Aqueous penicillin G given intravenously is used for severe disease such as meningitis, complicated pneumonia, and endocarditis caused by susceptible pathogens. In such cases, the drug should be administered at frequent intervals, usually every 4 hours, until the infection has been controlled.
2. Procaine penicillin G given intramuscularly produces lower concentrations of serum antibacterial activity (≈10% to 30% of the peak concentration achieved by the same dosage of the aqueous form), but activity persists in serum for as long as 12 hours. Intramuscular administration of procaine penicillin G should be reserved for patients with mild-to-moderate disease who cannot tolerate oral preparations. A 10-day course of this agent may be used as an alternative to intravenously administered aqueous penicillin G for infants with documented or suspected congenital syphilis.[370]
3. Benzathine penicillin G given intramuscularly is a repository preparation that provides low concentrations of serum activity (≈1% to 2% of the peak concentration achieved by the same dosage of the aqueous form). After administration of this drug, concentrations of penicillin are measurable in serum for 3 weeks or more and in urine for several months. Pain at the site of injection is the major deterrent to widespread use of this unique antibiotic. A combination of the benzathine and procaine salts (900,000 and 300,000 U, respectively) is a less painful treatment and is comparable in efficacy to benzathine alone (1,200,000 U) for the treatment of streptococcal pharyngitis.[28] Benzathine penicillin G is appropriate for only highly susceptible organisms present in tissues that are well vascularized so that the drug can diffuse readily to the site of infection. Thus, benzathine

penicillin G is suitable for treatment of children with group A streptococcal pharyngitis or impetigo and for prophylaxis of streptococcal infection in children who have had rheumatic carditis. Current recommendations by the Centers for Disease Control and Prevention (CDC)[370] for management of syphilis include the use of benzathine penicillin G for primary, secondary, and early latent syphilis (<1 year's duration). Benzathine penicillin G also is recommended for infants with suspected congenital syphilis who do not meet the criteria for therapy with a 10-day course of aqueous or procaine penicillin G and whose follow-up can be ensured for repeat serologic testing.

4. Oral preparations of buffered penicillin G (no longer available in the United States) and phenoxymethylpenicillin (penicillin V) are absorbed well from the gastrointestinal tract. The peak concentration of serum activity of penicillin V is approximately 40%, and that of buffered penicillin G is approximately 20% of the concentration achieved by the same dosage of aqueous penicillin G administered intramuscularly. Therefore, oral penicillins may be satisfactory for treating mild to moderately severe infections caused by susceptible organisms. Penicillin V and penicillin G have equivalent activity in vitro against gram-positive cocci, but penicillin V is less active than is penicillin G against *N. meningitidis, N. gonorrhoeae,* and susceptible strains of *Haemophilus influenzae.*[193] The benefit of treating streptococcal tonsillopharyngitis with a 10-day regimen of penicillin V for the prevention of acute rheumatic fever is based on indirect evidence derived from rates of pharyngeal eradication of *S. pyogenes* equivalent to those of injectable penicillin, the treatment with proven efficacy.[100,320]

All penicillins are excreted by both glomerular filtration and tubular secretion. The concomitant use of probenecid, a drug that blocks tubular secretion of organic acids, and a penicillin can produce higher peaks and more sustained concentrations of antimicrobial activity. Dosages and dosing intervals may need adjustment when penicillins are administered to persons with altered renal function.

Penicillinase-Resistant Penicillins

The semisynthetic penicillinase-resistant penicillins (cloxacillin, dicloxacillin, methicillin, nafcillin, and oxacillin) were developed in response to the emergence of penicillinase-producing staphylococci. The acyl side chain, by means of steric hindrance, prevents hydrolysis of the β-lactam ring by penicillinases. Most strains of *S. aureus* produce penicillinase, regardless of whether the infection is health care–associated or community acquired. In areas of low rates of resistance to β-lactams, penicillinase-resistant penicillins are the β-lactams of choice for the initial management of patients with suspected staphylococcal disease. However, alternative effective antimicrobials should be substituted or added if endemic rates of antibiotic resistance exceed 10% to 15% or if the severity of the disease warrants empirical treatment of methicillin-resistant *S. aureus* (MRSA).[136] With the exception of methicillin, these agents are active against streptococci and can be used for empirical treatment of infections commonly caused by both staphylococci and streptococci. Because these agents are less active than penicillin G against streptococci, penicillin G should be used instead of these agents if streptococci alone are isolated from culture. Penicillinase-resistant penicillins have no activity against gram-negative bacteria or enterococci.[232]

Methicillin was the first penicillinase-resistant penicillin to be introduced and was available in parenteral form only. Oxacillin and nafcillin are available in both parenteral and oral preparations. Cloxacillin and dicloxacillin are available in oral forms only and are absorbed more efficiently from the gastrointestinal tract than the other oral drugs. Differences among these five penicillins include routes of elimination, degree of binding to proteins, degradation by β-lactamases, and in vitro susceptibility.[262] However, all are effective in the treatment of susceptible strains of staphylococcal isolates, and clinical studies have shown them to be equivalent when used at appropriate dosage schedules. Suspension formulations are poorly tolerated because of their unpleasant taste. Disease caused by methicillin-resistant staphylococci was reported shortly after introduction of the drug in the 1960s. Resistance is caused by alterations in PBPs, rather than production of β-lactamase. The *mecA* gene encodes a PBP2a that has low affinity for β-lactams, thereby resulting in resistance to most β-lactam antibiotics currently available, including penicillinase-resistant penicillins, cephalosporins (first to fourth generation), and carbapenems. The mechanisms of resistance to other antibiotics are unrelated to PBPs and may be plasmid mediated or chromosomal.[228] Coagulase-negative staphylococci, including *S. epidermidis,* are residents of the normal microbial flora of the skin and are occasional contaminants of body fluid cultures. These organisms can be pathogens in certain settings, such as in neonates, or in infections of prosthetic devices, such as heart valves or cerebrospinal fluid (CSF) shunts. Most strains of coagulase-negative staphylococci produce a penicillinase that inactivates penicillin G, penicillin V, and ampicillin, and many strains have *mecA*-mediated altered PBP2a, leading to methicillin resistance. In addition, these methicillin-resistant, coagulase-negative staphylococci frequently are resistant to cephalosporins, erythromycin, and clindamycin. Vancomycin is the drug of choice for pathogenic coagulase-negative staphylococci and severe disease known or suspected to be caused by MRSA. Some experts advocate the addition of nafcillin or oxacillin for empirical therapy for suspected MRSA until susceptibility results are known in patients who are severely ill, although toxicity may be increased with combination therapy.[120,136]

Aminopenicillins

The aminopenicillins (ampicillin, amoxicillin, amoxicillin-clavulanate, and ampicillin-sulbactam) are semisynthetic β-lactam antibiotics formed by the addition of an amino group to benzylpenicillin. Amoxicillin differs from ampicillin by the presence of a hydroxyl group on the phenyl side chain. The aminopenicillins were the first penicillins that had activity against some gram-negative organisms, including *H. influenzae, Escherichia coli, Proteus mirabilis, Salmonella* spp., and *Shigella* spp., while retaining activity against penicillin-susceptible, gram-positive bacteria.[261]

In contrast to penicillin G, aminopenicillins are significantly more active against *Listeria monocytogenes*; slightly more active against enterococci; equally active against *Actinomyces, N. meningitidis,* and clostridial and corynebacterial species; and slightly less active against group A streptococci, group B streptococci, and pneumococci. Aminopenicillins are the drugs of choice for the treatment of infections caused by *L. monocytogenes* and enterococci. Other organisms susceptible in vitro to ampicillin and amoxicillin include non–penicillinase-producing strains of *H. influenzae, Moraxella catarrhalis, N. gonorrhoeae, S. aureus, E. coli, Salmonella,* and *Shigella.* A survey of health care–associated and community-acquired *H. influenzae* and *M. catarrhalis* strains isolated from the blood and respiratory tracts of children in North America documented ampicillin resistance rates of 34% and 99%, respectively.[178] The in vitro spectrum of activity for amoxicillin and ampicillin is identical, except that amoxicillin is two times less active against *Shigella* and two to four times more active against enterococci and *Salmonella* than ampicillin.[261]

As seen with penicillin G, the primary means of acquired resistance to aminopenicillins is the production of β-lactamase. However, organisms that are resistant to penicillin G or to methicillin because of altered PBPs—*S. pneumoniae* and *S. aureus,* respectively—also are resistant to aminopenicillins. β-Lactamase-negative, ampicillin-resistant strains of *H. influenzae* have been identified in the United States much less frequently than in Japan (0.2% vs. 2.6%, respectively).[165]

The broad-spectrum bactericidal activity of ampicillin and amoxicillin provides the basis for the use of these drugs as empirical therapy for lower respiratory tract infections and acute otitis media, for which amoxicillin remains the drug of choice.[11] Ampicillin or penicillin G is the recommended initial empirical therapy in community-acquired pneumonia in a fully immunized infant or school-aged child admitted to a hospital ward if the local epidemiology reveals no substantial high-level resistance for invasive *S. pneumoniae.*[51] Aminopenicillins are indicated for treatment of susceptible strains of *Shigella*-associated or *Salmonella*-associated enteric infections as well as susceptible acute and chronic infections of the urinary tract. By bacteriologic and clinical measures, amoxicillin is significantly less effective than ampicillin for the treatment of shigellosis.[259]

Both drugs are available for oral administration; ampicillin alone is available in a parenteral form. Amoxicillin provides higher and more prolonged serum concentrations than those achieved with equivalent dosages of ampicillin; thus, amoxicillin can be given in lower dosage, two or three times per day, rather than four times, as required for ampicillin. An additional advantage of amoxicillin is that absorption is not altered when the antibiotic is administered with food, whereas absorption of ampicillin is decreased significantly when it is given with food. Ampicillin is associated more frequently with diarrhea than is amoxicillin.

β-Lactam–β-Lactamase Inhibitor Combinations

β-Lactamase inhibitors are compounds that have weak antibacterial activity but can bind irreversibly to the catalytic site of many β-lactamases and render them inactive. The inhibitors currently in use are clavulanic acid, sulbactam, and tazobactam, the last of which is halogenated penicillanic acid derivative. All three inhibitors are identical in their mode of activity but differ to some degree in their potency and spectrum of enzyme inhibition. These agents primarily inhibit the plasmid-encoded β-lactamases and less frequently the chromosomally encoded β-lactamases. β-Lactamase inhibitors have been formulated in a fixed ratio with a β-lactam antibiotic. The spectrum of activity of each combination is determined primarily by the spectrum of activity of the β-lactam. However, many determinants of the inhibitor influence its activity, including its affinity for the β-lactamase and its ability to traverse the gram-negative cell wall to bind to periplasmic β-lactamases.[217] From a clinical perspective, all three β-lactamase inhibitors are considered therapeutically equivalent. The β-lactamase inhibitors are most effective against *S. aureus, H. influenzae, M. catarrhalis, Bacteroides* spp., *E. coli,* and other Enterobacteriaceae. The main indication for the use of these combination antimicrobial agents is for the treatment of health care–associated infections or infections caused by susceptible β-lactamase-producing pathogens.

Amoxicillin-clavulanic acid. Amoxicillin combined with potassium clavulanate was introduced in 1984 for oral administration. The pharmacokinetic properties of the two drugs are similar; both are absorbed rapidly and are not affected when taken with meals. Gastrointestinal side effects, including nausea, vomiting, and diarrhea, occur more commonly with amoxicillin-clavulanate than with amoxicillin alone.[192]

The combination drug is equivalent to amoxicillin alone in activity against amoxicillin-susceptible organisms. The addition of clavulanic acid extends the activity of amoxicillin to include β-lactamase-producing strains of *S. aureus* (but not methicillin-resistant strains), *H. influenzae, M. catarrhalis, N. gonorrhoeae, E. coli, Proteus, Klebsiella, Providencia, Haemophilus ducreyi,* and some anaerobic bacteria, including *B. fragilis.* Some β-lactamase-producing, gram-negative bacilli are resistant to amoxicillin-clavulanic acid because of either hyperproduction of β-lactamase or production of a β-lactamase that is not susceptible to clavulanate. Amoxicillin-clavulanate is not active against penicillin-resistant *S. pneumoniae* or vancomycin-resistant enterococci.

Amoxicillin is considered the preferred therapy for low-risk children with uncomplicated, mild to moderately severe disease of the respiratory tract, including initial empirical therapy for otitis media. In children who are at risk for penicillin-nonsusceptible pneumococcal acute otitis media, a 90-mg/kg daily regimen in two divided doses is recommended. Alternative therapy, including amoxicillin-clavulanic acid, should be considered if a β-lactamase-producing organism is known or suspected to be the cause of the disease based on risk factors, treatment experience, or microbiologic results. In 2001, high-dose amoxicillin-clavulanic acid suspension (Augmentin ES600; 600 mg of amoxicillin/5 mL and 42.9 mg of clavulanic acid/5 mL) was approved for use in children in the United States. The recommended dosage of this formulation is 90 mg/kg per day divided every 12 hours for the treatment of high-risk patients with acute otitis media.[11] The high ratio (14:1) of amoxicillin to clavulanate optimizes the amoxicillin dose without intensifying the risks for undesirable adverse effects associated with the β-lactamase inhibitor. The combination drug is useful in areas where the proportion of β-lactamase-producing strains of *H. influenzae* is large (40%) and *M. catarrhalis* organisms (most of which are β-lactamase producers) are identified more frequently as pathogens in otitis media, sinusitis, and other respiratory tract infections. Amoxicillin-clavulanate also has been used successfully for the oral treatment of urinary tract, skin, and soft tissue infections, as well as for the treatment of human and animal bite wounds.[64]

Ampicillin-sulbactam. Ampicillin combined with sulbactam as a parenteral β-lactam and β-lactamase inhibitor combination was approved in 1987. The spectrum of activity of ampicillin-sulbactam is similar to that of amoxicillin-clavulanate. It is most useful as monotherapy for potential polymicrobial intra-abdominal or gynecologic infections and is effective for treatment of soft tissue, urinary tract, and respiratory tract infections. Ampicillin-sulbactam has been shown to be safe and efficacious for the treatment of skin and skin structure infections caused by susceptible organisms in children aged 3 months to 12 years.[21] The combination of ampicillin-sulbactam and an aminoglycoside has efficacy equivalent to that of a combination of ampicillin, clindamycin, and an aminoglycoside for empirical treatment of intra-abdominal infections in children.[85] Ampicillin-sulbactam is potentially useful for multidrug-resistant health care–associated infections caused by *Acinetobacter baumannii-calcoaceticus* complex.[253] Carbapenems and third-generation cephalosporins are comparatively more active against members of the Enterobacteriaceae. Because ampicillin-sulbactam has no activity against certain strains of the Enterobacteriaceae that produce Bush group 1 β-lactamases and *P. aeruginosa,* it should not be used as empirical single-agent therapy for febrile neutropenic patients or severely ill patients with probable bacteremia.

Piperacillin-tazobactam. Piperacillin and piperacillin tazobactam, which are extended-spectrum penicillins, are semisynthetic derivatives of ampicillin that have better activity against gram-negative organisms because of a higher affinity for PBPs and greater penetration through the gram-negative outer membrane. Piperacillin combined with tazobactam was approved for use in adults in 1993 and was approved for pediatric use (2 months to 17 years of age) in the United States in 2007.[353] It extends the spectrum of activity of piperacillin to include β-lactamase-producing strains of oxacillin-susceptible *S. aureus,* many members of the Enterobacteriaceae, and virtually all gram-positive and gram-negative anaerobes; its spectrum of activity is superior to that of ceftazidime and other β-lactam and β-lactamase inhibitor combinations. It has equivalent activity against gram-positive bacteria in contrast to ampicillin-sulbactam. Tazobactam, however, does not increase the activity of piperacillin against bacteria with resistance that is mediated by altered cell wall permeability to piperacillin, including certain strains of *P. aeruginosa.* Penicillin-resistant pneumococci, methicillin-resistant staphylococci, *Corynebacterium jeikeium,* most *Enterococcus faecium* strains, and most gram-negative bacteria that produce Bush group 1 β-lactamases (*Citrobacter, Enterobacter, Morganella,* certain strains of *Pseudomonas,* and *Serratia* spp.) are resistant to piperacillin-tazobactam.[64] Although studies have shown piperacillin-tazobactam to be safe and effective for the treatment of lower respiratory tract, intra-abdominal, pelvic, skin and skin structure, bone, and diabetes-related foot infections in adults, as well as for empirical treatment of febrile episodes in neutropenic adults,[49] there is less experience in children. It is a potentially useful agent that has been administered for the treatment of serious or complicated polymicrobial infections in children, especially in febrile neutropenic children, as initial empirical treatment. Piperacillin-tazobactam has been proposed as an alternative treatment to carbapenems for single-agent therapy in community-acquired intra-abdominal infections.[329] Monte Carlo simulations have predicted achieving more time above the MIC_{50} with prolonged infusions of piperacillin-tazobactam (i.e., 4 hours) in contrast to conventional dosing, for MIC range MIC 4 to 16 mg/L. Similar results have been observed with other β-lactams, including meropenem, doripenem, cefepime, and ceftazidime. Clinical studies have not been conclusive.[229] Clinicians also should be aware that administration of piperacillin-tazobactam has been shown to cause false-positive *Aspergillus galactomannan* test results for up to 5 days after cessation of treatment[19] but that newer formulations of piperacillin-tazobactam used in the United States are rarely associated with false-positive results.[363]

Adverse Effects and Sensitization

The penicillins are unique among antimicrobial agents in having little dose-related toxicity (Table 236.1). Seizures may occur under circumstances that result in high concentrations of penicillin in nervous tissue:

TABLE 236.1 Adverse Reactions to Penicillins

Type of Reaction	Frequency (%)	Most Frequent[a]
Electrolyte Disturbance		
Hyperkalemia, acute	Rare	PCN G
Gastrointestinal		
Diarrhea	2–5	Ampicillin
Enterocolitis	<1	Ampicillin
Hematologic		
Hemolytic anemia	Rare	PCN G
Neutropenia	1–4	PCN G, Naf, Ox, Pip
Hepatic		
Elevated AST	1–4	Ox, Naf
Neurologic		
Seizures	Rare	PCN G
Bizarre sensations	Rare	Procaine penicillin
Renal		
Interstitial nephritis	1–2	Methicillin
Hemorrhagic cystitis	Rare	Methicillin
Allergic		
IgE-mediated	0.004–0.4	PCN G
Cytotoxic antibody	Rare	PCN G
Immune complexes	Rare	PCN G
Delayed hypersensitivity	4–8	Ampicillin

AST, Aspartate transaminase; *Naf*, nafcillin; *Ox*, oxacillin; *PCN G*, penicillin G; *Pip*, piperacillin.

[a]All reactions can occur with any penicillin.

Modified from Chambers HF, Neu HC. Penicillins. In: Mandell GL, Bennett JE, Dollin R, eds. *Mandell, Douglas and Bennett's Principles and Practice of Infectious Diseases.* 4th ed. New York: Churchill Livingstone; 1995.

rapid intravenous infusion of single large doses, substantial dosages for prolonged periods in patients with impaired renal function, or high concentrations given by the intrathecal route. Confusion, dizziness, seizures, and psychosis caused by toxic concentrations of procaine have been associated with the administration of procaine penicillin G.[324] Nephritis has been associated with the administration of some penicillins, most frequently after the use of methicillin. Bleeding because of drug-induced platelet aggregation has been noted after the administration of penicillin G.

Although toxicity may not be a significant concern with the penicillins, sensitization is an important factor.[214] Penicillins are haptens, that is, they are low-molecular-weight compounds too small to elicit an immune response alone, but when bound to a carrier molecule (e.g., host tissues or proteins), they are highly immunogenic in humans. The native penicillin molecule can bind to a protein, as can its major (benzylpenicilloyl) and minor (benzylpenicillin, benzylpenicilloate, benzylpenilloate) determinants. Four types of immune-mediated reactions can occur after the administration of a penicillin (or any drug or antigen): immediate hypersensitivity (immunoglobulin E [IgE]-mediated) reactions, cytotoxic antibody reactions, immune complex reactions (Arthus reaction), and delayed (cell-mediated) hypersensitivity reactions. Allergic reactions also can be classified as (1) immediate (onset ≤1 hour), accelerated (1–72 hours), or delayed (>72 hours). Researchers have estimated that an immediate serious reaction occurs in 2 per 10,000 courses, and fatal reactions occur in 1 per 100,000 treatment courses.[30,347]

1. Type 1 immediate hypersensitivity reactions usually occur within 30 minutes after administration and are life-threatening events. The interaction of preformed mast cell–bound IgE antibody to the antigenic determinants of penicillin results in the release of mast cell mediators.[44] Clinical signs include hypotension or shock, urticaria, laryngeal edema, and bronchospasm. Acute anaphylaxis is a rare event after the administration of penicillin, but significant numbers of fatalities occur each year because of the extensive use of these drugs. Children are thought to have fewer systemic reactions than do adults, presumably because of fewer previous exposures to penicillin antigens. Oral preparations are less likely to result in an immediate reaction than are parenteral forms, perhaps because antigens are altered in the gastrointestinal tract, absorption is slower, dosages are smaller, or a combination of these factors.
2. Type 2 cytotoxic antibody reactions can occur after passive absorption of the benzylpenicilloyl hapten by the membrane of circulating blood cells or by renal interstitial cells, especially when high dosages of penicillins are used for prolonged periods. IgM antibody, IgG antibody, or both antibodies to the benzylpenicilloyl antigen bind to the altered cell surface; complement can be activated, and damage to the cell ensues. Cytotoxic antibody reactions usually are manifested more than 72 hours after initiation of antibiotic therapy and include hemolytic anemia, leukopenia, thrombocytopenia, and drug-induced interstitial nephritis.
3. Type 3 immune complex (Arthus) reactions occur after the formation of immune complexes between soluble penicillin antigens and IgG and IgM antibodies. The complexes lodge in the skin, joints, kidneys, or other tissue sites. Complement activation occurs, and the clinical manifestations of serum sickness ensue—cutaneous symptoms (i.e., urticaria, maculopapular rash, and erythema multiforme), polyarthralgia, and fever. The onset typically is 7 to 21 days after initiation of penicillin therapy but can occur after use of the antibiotic has been discontinued. Although serum sickness has been associated with the administration of penicillins, it occurs more frequently after administration of cefaclor.
4. Type 4 delayed hypersensitivity reactions involve cellular rather than humoral immunity. On exposure to certain antibiotics, T lymphocytes become sensitized in a major histocompatibility restricted fashion and they mediate mild-to-severe reactions that include contact dermatitis, some maculopapular rashes, fixed drug eruption at sites of previous tinea infections, and toxic epidermal necrolysis. Diagnostic tools to detect an antibiotic that induces a type 4 reaction include the delayed reading (>6 hours) intradermal skin test, patch test, and in vitro lymphocyte transformation test. However, these tests have not been adequately standardized for routine use.[347]

Idiopathic reactions are those for which an immune-mediated mechanism has not been proved, but more recent data suggest that these reactions may represent a type 4 hypersensitivity reaction.[347] Included in this category are the morbilliform exanthems, erythema multiforme, photosensitivity reactions, exfoliative dermatitis, and pruritus. Approximately 4% of courses of penicillin and up to 9% of courses of ampicillin or amoxicillin therapy are associated with a maculopapular rash. In some of these patients, the rash is a manifestation of a primary viral infection such as infectious mononucleosis, for which the penicillin was prescribed inappropriately.

Identifying patients who will have a significant reaction if penicillin is administered remains difficult. Serologic assays (radioallergosorbent tests) for the detection of IgE antibodies to major and minor penicillin determinants are available but are time consuming, expensive, and less sensitive than skin testing. Because the immediate reaction is mediated largely by IgE reagin or skin-sensitizing antibody, patients who are likely to respond subsequently with a life-threatening reaction can be identified by the use of intradermal tests with appropriate antigens. However, selecting the most appropriate antigens to be used for skin testing has been problematic because many different antigens may play roles in the allergic reaction. Penicillin is degraded to various clinical products. At least 10 metabolic breakdown products of the penicillin nucleus have been identified. Other potential antigens include macromolecular impurities present in solutions of the drug, high-molecular-weight penicillin polymers found in poorly buffered penicillin solutions standing for prolonged periods, side chains of the various penicillins, and the bacterial enzymes (amidases) used to prepare semisynthetic penicillins. Thus, investigators have had difficulty choosing sensitive and specific antigens to use for skin testing. When these products are used in penicillin skin testing, the predictive value of testing for drug-specific IgE antibodies is high. However, skin testing evaluates IgE-mediated allergy only. For antibiotics other than penicillin it is not clear if the appropriate antigenic determinants are being used, for which a negative test should be interpreted with caution.[141]

The most informative studies of skin test antigens have been those of Levine,[209] who identified two antigens, benzylpenicilloyl poly-L-lysine (PrePen) and a "minor determinant mixture," a preparation of a dilute solution of aqueous crystalline penicillin G that includes metabolic breakdown products. Only the PrePen reagent is available commercially in the United States. The CDC currently recommends the use of benzylpenicilloyl poly-L-lysine and, if available, a freshly prepared mixture of dilute minor determinant precursors, including benzylpenicillin G, benzylpenicilloate, and penicilloyl propylamine, as well as a positive control (histamine) and a negative control (usually glycerinated saline) after a protocol prepared by Beall.[30] Of the minor determinants, only benzylpenicillin G (penicillin G) is available commercially in the United States. For patients with immediate systemic reactions to amoxicillin or ampicillin (i.e., aminopenicillins), aminopenicillins should be included in the skin testing panel.

An epicutaneous (prick) test is performed first. If the patient's history of penicillin allergy is that of a mild reaction, the skin test reagent can be used at full strength; however, if the previous history is suggestive of anaphylaxis, a 1 : 100 dilution of the reagent should be used for the first prick test, followed by a full-strength test if no reaction with the diluted reagent occurs. If the prick test result is negative, an intradermal test is performed using duplicate 0.02 to 0.05 mL volumes of antigen solutions, and the skin is observed for 20 minutes. A positive result is indicated by a wheal-and-flare reaction that is more than 3 mm larger than the negative control; this result suggests a significant chance that a reaction will occur on subsequent administration of a penicillin. A negative result suggests that a significant allergic reaction will not take place. Although much effort has gone into clinical tests of these antigens, the predictive value of positive and negative results in children remains uncertain. Because of the risk for severe life-threatening reactions when a skin test is performed, having a physician present and resuscitation equipment and medications readily available is prudent.

At present, the physician must rely on the patient's history of an adverse reaction after administration of a penicillin to identify who is likely to be allergic. If the reaction appears to be related to the administration of a penicillin, the drug should be avoided for minor infections. More recent experience suggests that fewer than 10% of adults with a history of penicillin allergy have positive skin tests. Of those individuals with negative skin tests, IgE-mediated reactions occur in 4% or fewer if these patients receive penicillin, a rate that is similar to that in individuals with no history of penicillin allergy.[347] Because no proved alternative therapies to penicillin are available for treating patients with neurosyphilis, congenital syphilis, or syphilis in pregnancy, the CDC recommends skin testing and desensitization of patients considered to have reacted positively to the skin test antigens.[370] If a life-threatening infection should occur and penicillin is clearly the drug of choice, the physician may choose to administer the drug under carefully controlled conditions after desensitization. All penicillins are cross reactive with regard to sensitization; allergy to any one implies sensitization to all, although cross sensitivity is considerably less than 100%.

Cephalosporins

The cephalosporins have a broad range of activity that includes gram-positive cocci, gram-negative enteric bacilli, and anaerobic bacteria. Most cephalosporins are relatively resistant to hydrolysis by β-lactamases produced by *S. aureus,* but many are susceptible to gram-negative β-lactamases. Unlike other antimicrobial agents, this group has a high therapeutic-toxic index. For simplicity, the cephalosporins have been categorized as first-, second-, third-, fourth-, and fifth-generation agents (Table 236.2), based on the pattern of in vitro activity. Newer generation cephalosporins have been evaluated recently. Ceftaroline is approved by the FDA for the treatment of acute skin and soft tissue infections and community-acquired bacterial pneumonia in adults and children older than 2 months of age.

Pharmacokinetics

The cephalosporins are available as parenteral and oral products. Most of the parenteral drugs can be administered by the intravenous or intramuscular routes. Most of the oral products are absorbed well from the gastrointestinal tract. Esterification of the base compounds of cefuroxime and cefpodoxime is required to enhance gastrointestinal absorption. The presence of food does not alter absorption and, for some antibiotics, even can enhance absorption. Cephalosporins penetrate most tissues and body fluids well, except CSF. The first- and second-generation cephalosporins do not achieve therapeutic CSF concentrations. CSF penetration of third-generation drugs varies but is generally adequate for most major meningeal pathogens, except cefotaxime/ceftriaxone-nonsusceptible pneumococci, for which vancomycin is added in the initial empirical regimen.[196] Cefepime, a fourth-generation cephalosporin, reaches adequate CSF concentrations for the treatment of most common invasive pathogens. There are no data regarding CSF penetration of ceftaroline, a fifth-generation cephalosporin. Because glomerular filtration and tubular secretion are the major modes of excretion, the urinary concentrations achieved are sufficient for the treatment of urinary tract infections. Ceftriaxone has dual excretion by the kidneys and the biliary tract and achieves high concentrations in urine and bile. The presence of moderate-to-severe renal insufficiency may require adjustment of the dosage or dosing interval for all cephalosporins, except those agents with biliary excretion. Hepatic insufficiency can affect the metabolism of cephalosporins that undergo biliary excretion; however, adjustments in ceftriaxone dosage or dosing interval are required only in the presence of both hepatic and renal insufficiency.

Therapeutic advantages of cephalosporins include concentration-independent bactericidal activity, broad-spectrum antibacterial activity, lack of significant dose-related toxicity, and relative stability against staphylococcal β-lactamases. Certain cautions must be kept in mind when prescribing cephalosporins: none is effective against enterococci, methicillin-resistant staphylococci (except ceftaroline), *L. monocytogenes,* chlamydial species, and *C. difficile,* and resistance may develop rapidly in closed communities, such as neonatal or pediatric intensive care units, because of inducible chromosomal β-lactamases produced by gram-negative bacteria. The new-generation cephalosporin ceftaroline has minimal activity against *Enterococcus faecalis* and no activity against *E. faecium.*[32,331]

TABLE 236.2 Classification Scheme and Route for Cephalosporins

First Generation	Third Generation
Cefadroxil (PO)	Cefdinir (PO)
Cefazolin (IM, IV)	Cefditoren pivoxil (PO)
Cephalexin (PO)	Cefixime (PO)
Second Generation	Cefotaxime (IM, IV)
Cefaclor (PO)	Cefpodoxime proxetil (PO)
Cefoxitin (IM, IV)	Ceftazidime (IM, IV)
Cefotetan (IM, IV)	Ceftazidime/avibactam (IV)
Cefuroxime (IM, IV)	Ceftriaxone (IM, IV)
Cefuroxime axetil (PO)	**Fourth Generation**
Cefprozil (PO)	Cefepime (IM, IV)
Ceftibuten (PO)	**Fifth Generation**
	Ceftaroline (IV)

IM, Intramuscularly; *IV,* intravenously; *PO,* orally.

First-Generation Cephalosporins

First-generation cephalosporins are effective against gram-positive cocci, including β-lactamase-producing *S. aureus,* and they have variable activity against gram-negative enteric bacilli. Three first-generation cephalosporins currently are available for infants and children: the parenteral drug cefazolin and the oral products cephalexin and cefadroxil. Cephalothin is not available in the United States. Cefazolin produces higher concentrations in blood than previously available parenteral first-generation drugs. Cefadroxil can be administered in twice-daily doses because of its longer serum half-life. None of these agents will attain appreciable concentrations in the central nervous system (CNS).

These drugs are of value as alternatives to penicillin for disease caused by *S. aureus, S. pyogenes,* and susceptible *S. pneumoniae,* and they are active against some strains of community-acquired gram-negative enteric bacilli such as *E. coli, P. mirabilis,* and *Klebsiella pneumoniae.* The oral preparations have comparable activity in vitro and in vivo. First-generation cephalosporins are valuable in children who have a history of nonanaphylactic allergy to penicillin. These drugs have been used to treat staphylococcal and streptococcal skin and skin structure infections, bone and joint infections, pharyngitis, and uncomplicated community-acquired urinary tract infections caused by susceptible bacteria. A meta-analysis revealed that many first-generation and other-generation cephalosporins (i.e., cephalexin, cefadroxil, cefuroxime, cefprozil, cefdinir, cefixime, cefpodoxime, and ceftibuten) have equivalent or superior bacteriologic and clinical cure rates in contrast to penicillin for treatment of group A streptococcal pharyngotonsillitis.[68] Experts disagree on the significance of the results of this meta-analysis. Cefadroxil is effective for the treatment of streptococcal pharyngitis in a once-daily dosage schedule. Cephalexin has been used for sequential parenteral-oral treatment of staphylococcal osteomyelitis and arthritis occurring after surgical intervention and an initial period of parenteral antibiotic therapy. Cefazolin and cefuroxime are the antibiotics of choice for perioperative prophylaxis in selected surgical procedures.[56] Because first-generation cephalosporins have minimal, if any, activity against *H. influenzae* and *M. catarrhalis* and inadequate activity against penicillin-resistant *S. pneumoniae,* they should not be used for empirical treatment of respiratory tract infections. First-generation cephalosporins should not be used for empirical therapy of suspected severe gram-negative health care–associated infections; a third- or fourth-generation cephalosporin in combination with an aminoglycoside, or other classes of antibiotics, should be selected for this purpose.

Second-Generation Cephalosporins

The second-generation cephalosporins that are approved for use in children consist of one parenteral drug (cefuroxime) and three oral preparations (cefaclor, cefuroxime axetil, and cefprozil). Also classified with the second-generation cephalosporins are the cephamycins, of which only one, cefoxitin, is approved for use in children. When compared with the first-generation cephalosporins, the second-generation agents have similar or somewhat less activity against gram-positive cocci but better activity against *H. influenzae, M. catarrhalis, N. meningitidis, N. gonorrhoeae,* and some members of the Enterobacteriaceae. The cephamycins are more active than first- or other second-generation cephalosporins against gram-negative enteric bacteria and *B. fragilis,* but they have poor activity against gram-positive cocci.

Cefaclor. Cefaclor is more active than cephalexin against *H. influenzae, M. catarrhalis, E. coli,* and *P. mirabilis* and has activity against staphylococci similar to that of cephalexin. Cefaclor is an unstable compound and is destroyed within 2 hours in human plasma. It is susceptible in vitro to hydrolysis by the β-lactamases produced by approximately 40% of *H. influenzae* and nearly all *M. catarrhalis* isolates; presumed rates of resistance of *H. influenzae* are considerably higher when pharmacokinetic and pharmacodynamic parameters are taken into account.[165] Although cefaclor is effective therapy for susceptible bacteria causing otitis media, sinusitis, and mild-to-moderate cases of pneumonia, it is not the preferred empirical agent for these indications because it is not effective against penicillin-nonsusceptible strains of *S. pneumoniae.* The rare but potential risk for serum sickness, as well as the poor stability of this drug to some β-lactamases, has limited its use. The safety and efficacy of cefaclor have not been established for infants younger than 1 month of age, although the drug has been used successfully to treat neonatal otitis media.

Cefoxitin. Cefoxitin has excellent activity against anaerobic organisms and is the most active cephalosporin against *B. fragilis.*[34] It has selective activity against gram-negative enteric bacilli, but *Enterobacter* or *Pseudomonas* spp. are inherently resistant. Cefoxitin is resistant to hydrolysis by the β-lactamases produced by gram-positive bacteria and some of the gram-negative β-lactamases. Because it is a potent inducer of Bush group 1 chromosomal β-lactamases, its indiscriminate use should be avoided. Cefoxitin has been shown to be effective for infections involving facultative gram-negative bacilli and anaerobes, such as intra-abdominal, pelvic, and gynecologic infections. When combined with doxycycline, cefoxitin is effective for the treatment of pelvic inflammatory disease.[370] The use of β-lactam and β-lactamase inhibitor combinations or metronidazole, rather than cefoxitin, should be considered for empirical treatment of patients with life-threatening anaerobic infections because as many as 25% of *B. fragilis* strains can be resistant to cefoxitin.[5] Higher doses of cefoxitin have been associated with an increased incidence of eosinophilia and elevated aspartate transaminase (AST) concentration. A diminished zone of inhibition in cefoxitin disk diffusion assays is useful in the clinical microbiology laboratory to detect inducible or constitutive (stably derepressed) AmpC Bush group 1 β-lactamase production among strains of *Citrobacter, Enterobacter, E. coli, Klebsiella, Morganella, Providencia, Pseudomonas,* and *Serratia.* Identification of this phenotype in vitro is important because these strains have high-level resistance to many classes of β-lactam antibiotics that may not be detected by standard susceptibility assays. Fourth-generation cephalosporins and carbapenems are potentially effective antimicrobial agents for these multidrug-resistant pathogens.[175]

Cefprozil. Cefprozil has a structure similar to that of the first-generation cephalosporin cefadroxil. It is more active than the oral first-generation agents against *S. pyogenes, S. pneumoniae, Neisseria* spp., *H. influenzae, M. catarrhalis, E. coli, P. mirabilis, Klebsiella,* and, to a lesser extent, staphylococci. This drug is hydrolyzed by the β-lactamases produced by approximately 40% of *H. influenzae* and nearly all *M. catarrhalis* isolates; rates of resistance of *H. influenzae* are likely considerably higher when pharmacokinetic and pharmacodynamic parameters are taken into account.[148] The rate of resistance among all *S. pneumoniae* isolates in the United States is approximately 30%.[148] Because of its relatively long serum half-life, cefprozil can be administered twice daily. Cefprozil is comparable to penicillin, cefaclor, and erythromycin in the treatment of pharyngitis,[235] and it is equivalent or superior to cefaclor and erythromycin in the treatment of mild-to-moderate skin and skin structure infections.[265] Cefprozil is approved for the treatment of acute otitis media, mild lower respiratory tract infections, acute sinusitis, and skin and skin structure infections. However, it is not the preferred antibiotic for these indications because it is unlikely to be effective in children with penicillin-nonsusceptible *S. pneumoniae, H. influenzae,* or *M. catarrhalis,* on the basis of unfavorable pharmacodynamic parameters.[354] Cefprozil is safe and effective as part of a parenteral-oral antibiotic regimen for the treatment of suppurative skeletal infections in children.[355] The safety and efficacy of cefprozil have not been established for infants younger than 6 months of age.

Cefuroxime. In contrast to first-generation cephalosporins, this parenteral second-generation cephalosporin is slightly less active against staphylococci but is more active against group A streptococci, pneumococci, and many members of the Enterobacteriaceae. Its stability to β-lactamases is greater than that of first-generation agents, and it is the only first- or second-generation antibiotic that achieves substantial CSF concentrations. However, cefuroxime is not recommended for treatment of suspected or proved bacterial meningitis because of suboptimal CSF pharmacologic characteristics, particularly in the context of infections caused by *H. influenzae* or nonsusceptible *S. pneumoniae,* for which third-generation cephalosporins (cefotaxime and ceftriaxone) are indicated.[318] Cefuroxime has been approved for the treatment of skin and skin structure infections, lower respiratory tract infections, bone and joint infections, uncomplicated gonorrhea, and uncomplicated urinary tract infections caused by susceptible bacteria. Cefuroxime is most useful for the treatment of infections sufficiently severe to warrant parenteral therapy, in which susceptible *S. aureus, S. pneumoniae, S. pyogenes,* encapsulated or nonencapsulated *H. influenzae,* and *M. catarrhalis* are probable pathogens. Cefuroxime offers the advantage of single-drug therapy for these diseases. The safety and efficacy of cefuroxime have not been established for infants younger than 3 months of age.

Cefuroxime axetil. Cefuroxime axetil is an oral form of cefuroxime with a similar spectrum of activity. It is an ester prodrug of cefuroxime that is metabolized to the active drug by intestinal esterases. Oral absorption is increased by the presence of food. When crushed, the tablet has a bitter taste that renders it unpalatable. The suspension has an unpleasant flavor that makes it difficult for some children to tolerate and therefore may limit adherence. The drug may be considered a suitable alternative to amoxicillin for the treatment of otitis media[11] and sinusitis when coverage must include β-lactamase-producing bacteria. Cefuroxime axetil has limited activity against penicillin-nonsusceptible pneumococci and *M. catarrhalis*, of which approximately 30% and 60%, respectively, of isolates are resistant.[165,173] This agent has been approved for the treatment of uncomplicated urinary tract infection, skin and soft tissue infection, acute bacterial maxillary sinusitis, and lower respiratory tract infection caused by susceptible bacteria. Cefuroxime axetil is an effective alternative to doxycycline and amoxicillin for the treatment of early Lyme disease.[371] The safety and efficacy of cefuroxime axetil have not been established for infants younger than 3 months of age.

Third-Generation Cephalosporins

Third-generation cephalosporins approved for use in children include the parenteral agents cefotaxime, ceftriaxone, and ceftazidime and the oral agents cefixime, cefpodoxime proxetil, ceftibuten, cefdinir, and cefditoren pivoxil. Third- and fourth-generation cephalosporins are the most potent cephalosporins against gram-negative enteric bacteria.[178] Most of these agents have excellent activity against *H. influenzae, M. catarrhalis, N. gonorrhoeae, N. meningitidis*, group A streptococci, and penicillin-susceptible pneumococci but relatively poor activity against staphylococci. Ceftazidime is the only third-generation cephalosporin, excluding the recently approved cephalosporin/β-lactamase combinations, with activity against *P. aeruginosa*. A serious global health concern has emerged because members of the Enterobacteriaceae have developed increased resistance to third-generation cephalosporins on the basis of plasmid-mediated production of extended-spectrum and AmpC β-lactamases.[277] The parenteral cephalosporins provide high concentrations of drug in serum and adequate concentrations in CSF.

In 2010, the CLSI released revised breakpoints for Enterobacteriaceae for third-generation cephalosporins and the first-generation cefazolin. The current MIC breakpoints in micrograms per milliliter are 1 and less for susceptible, 2 for intermediate, and 4 and greater for resistant organisms for cefazolin, cefotaxime, and ceftriaxone. For ceftazidime the MIC breakpoints are 4 and less, 8, and 16 or greater for susceptible, intermediate, and resistant organisms, respectively. Similarly, breakpoints for aztreonam (a monobactam) were revised. The revised breakpoints seek to eliminate the need to perform an extended-spectrum β-lactamase (ESBL) screen to direct patient care.[367]

Cefotaxime. Cefotaxime has excellent activity against group A streptococci, susceptible pneumococci, *H. influenzae, N. meningitidis*, and *N. gonorrhoeae*. Because cefotaxime can be hydrolyzed by AmpC Bush group 1-inducible chromosomal β-lactamases and by ESBLs, it is not active against strains of Enterobacteriaceae that produce these β-lactamases. Cefotaxime is metabolized in the liver to desacetyl cefotaxime, a less active metabolite that may act synergistically with cefotaxime. Although it is metabolized in the liver, cefotaxime is excreted by the kidneys. High serum, tissue, and CSF concentrations of cefotaxime can be achieved at the recommended dosages. The rapid development of resistance by colonizing gram-negative enteric bacilli when cefotaxime was used extensively for initial treatment of neonatal sepsis raised concern that extensive use of newer cephalosporins in the nursery or intensive care units could lead to more rapid emergence of drug-resistant bacteria than had been identified with the traditional regimens of a penicillin and an aminoglycoside. Because of its broad spectrum of activity against many of the common pathogens causing pediatric infections, cefotaxime is used widely for inpatient treatment of lower respiratory tract infections, urinary tract infections, sepsis, intra-abdominal infections, bone and joint infections, and meningitis or ventriculitis caused by susceptible organisms. Studies in neonates have raised concern that when cefotaxime is used routinely as part of an empirical regimen for neonatal sepsis, colonizing gram-negative enteric bacilli can rapidly develop resistance and certain neonates have adverse outcomes.[80,99] Therefore, it is prudent to reserve cefotaxime for appropriate clinical and microbiologic indications. In 2003, the CLSI published new breakpoints for defining the susceptibility of *S. pneumoniae* isolates to cefotaxime and ceftriaxone. The former breakpoints were based on attainable concentrations of these antibiotics in CSF and the level at which it was presumed that meningitis treatment failed because of elevated MICs. According to the former criteria, susceptible, intermediate, and resistant MIC breakpoints for cefotaxime and ceftriaxone were 0.5 µg/mL or less, 1 µg/mL, and 2 µg/mL or more, respectively, for pneumococci. Based on the newer criteria, the original breakpoints should be used for isolates from CSF in patients with suspected meningitis, but isolates causing nonmeningeal syndromes have breakpoints of 1 µg/mL or less, 2 µg/mL, and 4 µg/mL or more, respectively.[72]

Ceftriaxone. The antibacterial spectrum of ceftriaxone is similar to that of cefotaxime, with activity against β-hemolytic streptococci (including groups A, B, C, F, and G), susceptible pneumococci, *H. influenzae, M. catarrhalis, Neisseria* spp., and many members of the Enterobacteriaceae. Surveillance data from pediatric patients in the United States revealed that no significant resistance has been reported against ceftriaxone among oxacillin-susceptible strains of *S. aureus*.[178] Nonetheless, this drug should not be used as empirical monotherapy for severe infections presumed to be caused by staphylococci, because it has minimal activity against MRSA and its efficacy for treatment of susceptible strains has not been established in children. Ceftriaxone is not active against most strains of *Pseudomonas*. It differs from cefotaxime in pharmacokinetic properties. Ceftriaxone undergoes extensive protein binding and has a long serum half-life. Because of its broad spectrum of activity against many of the pathogens that commonly cause sepsis, meningitis, and respiratory tract infections in older infants and children, along with its unique pharmacokinetic features, ceftriaxone has been used excessively for outpatient management of febrile infants and young children being evaluated for possible systemic bacterial infection. Whereas single-dose therapy was approved for the treatment of acute otitis media in 1997, a 3-day regimen is recommended as alternative therapy for patients with refractory cases caused by penicillin-resistant *S. pneumoniae*.[11,207]

Ceftriaxone is effective for various sexually transmitted diseases (STDs), including chancroid, proctitis, epididymitis (in combination with doxycycline), and different forms of gonococcal disease (e.g., neonatal ophthalmia); uncomplicated urethral, endocervical, rectal, or pharyngeal gonorrhea (in combination with doxycycline for treatment of possible coexisting chlamydial infection); and disseminated gonococcal infection, meningitis, or endocarditis.[370] Short-course ceftriaxone therapy for typhoid fever in children is comparable in effectiveness to chloramphenicol therapy.[246] However, duration of ceftriaxone therapy longer than 5 days has been associated with fewer confirmed bacteriologic relapses.[339] Ceftriaxone (or cefotaxime) is recommended for treatment of acute Lyme disease with advanced heart block (14 to 21 days) or meningitis (14 to 28 days).[371] Administering an aminoglycoside in addition to a third-generation cephalosporin to severely ill patients with suspected infection caused by gram-negative bacteria often is prudent pending culture data because of the risk for encountering plasmid-mediated ESBL resistance or inducing the expression of chromosomally mediated AmpC Bush group 1 β-lactamases.

For infections requiring prolonged therapy (e.g., suppurative arthritis, osteomyelitis, and brain abscess) and caused by susceptible organisms, ceftriaxone therapy is cost-effective for use outside of the hospital. Once the acute signs of disease have diminished and the child remains in the hospital for only parenteral therapy, discharge and daily administration of ceftriaxone in the home or clinic can be considered.

Because of its extensive protein binding, ceftriaxone can displace bilirubin from albumin-binding sites, with the potential risk for inducing kernicterus, although to date this adverse clinical effect has not been reported. Cefotaxime is administered to neonates more often than ceftriaxone because considerably more information is available on its safety and pharmacokinetics. Ceftriaxone is excreted and concentrated in bile. Gallbladder "sludge," diagnosed by abdominal sonography (and not identifiable by other radiographic techniques), has been demonstrated in some patients who received ceftriaxone. The material appears to be a calcium-ceftriaxone complex and resolves on cessation of the drug. Most patients with ceftriaxone-associated sludge are asymptomatic, but occasionally patients have symptoms of gallbladder disease, and incidents of acute cholecystitis have been reported in a few children.

Ceftazidime. In contrast to cefotaxime and ceftriaxone, ceftazidime has poor antibacterial activity against *S. aureus*, is less active against penicillin-susceptible *S. pneumoniae*, and is slightly less active against group A streptococci, but it is more active against *P. aeruginosa*. It frequently is active in vitro against *P. aeruginosa* strains that are resistant to antipseudomonal penicillins. Resistance to ceftazidime can develop in gram-negative bacteria by the production of ESBLs or because of decreased bacterial cell permeability, as seen with *P. aeruginosa, Acinetobacter,* and some *Serratia* strains. Ceftazidime is indicated for use in the following circumstances: infections suspected to be caused by *Pseudomonas,* including acute exacerbations of chronic pulmonary infections in patients with cystic fibrosis, chronic suppurative otitis media, or malignant otitis externa; thermal injuries; puncture wound infections of the foot; and complicated health care–associated infections.

Cefixime. Cefixime has a vinyl group instead of a chlorine atom at position 3 of the cephem nucleus and an aminothiazole oxime group, rather than a phenyl glycine side chain. These biochemical changes result in potent gram-negative activity. Cefixime was introduced in 1989 as an oral third-generation cephalosporin with a broad spectrum of activity, including activity against group A streptococci, *H. influenzae, M. catarrhalis,* susceptible *S. pneumoniae,* and many members of the Enterobacteriaceae, including *Shigella, Salmonella, E. coli, Klebsiella,* and *P. mirabilis.*[27] Cefixime, like ceftibuten, is distinguished from other extended-spectrum oral cephalosporins by its lack of activity against *S. aureus.* It also is inactive against *Citrobacter freundii, Enterobacter, P. aeruginosa,* and *Serratia.* Although cefixime has in vitro activity against penicillin-susceptible pneumococci, lower bacteriologic cure rates occurred with cefixime than with amoxicillin when cefixime was used to treat children with pneumococcal acute otitis media.[157] Cefixime is resistant to degradation by certain β-lactamases. Administration of cefixime is facilitated by once-daily dosing,[112] pleasant taste, and stability of the suspension at room temperature. Cefixime is effective therapy for uncomplicated urinary tract infections caused by *E. coli* or *P. mirabilis,* for shigellosis, and for acute otitis media or sinusitis caused by *H. influenzae* or *M. catarrhalis.*[39] Because of increasing minimum inhibitory concentrations required to inhibit growth of *N. gonorrhoeae*, the Centers for Disease Control and Prevention no longer recommend the routine use of cefixime for the treatment of gonococcal infections[370] Clinical studies indicate that the rate of laboratory-confirmed eradication of *Shigella sonnei* in an epidemic setting is higher with a 5-day than with a 2-day cefixime regimen,[234] cefixime alone is equally effective as sequential therapy with intravenous and oral antibiotics in selected febrile infants with urinary tract infections,[37,153] and a 14-day cefixime regimen for treatment of multidrug-resistant *Salmonella typhi* septicemia in children has efficacy comparable to that of a 5-day course of ceftriaxone therapy.[131] Cefixime is not recommended for the treatment of infections frequently caused by staphylococci, such as skin or soft tissue infections, and it is not the most effective agent for the treatment of pneumococcal infections. The safety and efficacy of cefixime have not been established for infants younger than 6 months of age.

Cefpodoxime proxetil. The antibacterial activity of cefpodoxime proxetil is similar to that of cefixime, with the exception of improved activity against staphylococci. Cefpodoxime is active against group A streptococci; susceptible pneumococci; β-lactamase-producing strains of *N. gonorrhoeae, H. influenzae,* and *M. catarrhalis;* oxacillin-susceptible *S. aureus;* and many members of the Enterobacteriaceae. It is not active against *Enterobacter, Pseudomonas, Serratia,* or *Morganella.* Cefpodoxime proxetil, the ester prodrug of cefpodoxime, is cleaved by intestinal esterases to the active drug. Oral absorption is increased by the presence of food. Because of its longer serum half-life, cefpodoxime proxetil can be administered in twice-daily dosing intervals. Cefpodoxime is hydrolyzed by some ESBLs. The unfavorable palatability of cefpodoxime proxetil may adversely affect adherence.[332]

Treatment of group A streptococcal pharyngitis with a 5-day cefpodoxime proxetil regimen is equivalent to therapy with penicillin V and has been approved for this indication by the FDA.[93] A 5-day regimen is approved for the treatment of acute otitis media based on clinical outcomes that are comparable or superior to those with therapy with amoxicillin-clavulanate, cefaclor, or cefixime.[81] Cefpodoxime is not likely to be effective for the treatment of acute otitis media caused by penicillin-nonsusceptible pneumococci because of its unfavorable pharmacodynamic parameters.[359] It also has been approved for outpatient treatment of community-acquired respiratory tract infections, uncomplicated urinary tract infections, and mild skin and skin structure infections. The safety and efficacy of cefpodoxime proxetil have not been established for infants younger than 2 months of age.

Ceftibuten. Ceftibuten was approved by the FDA for pediatric use in 1995. The primary active component is formulated as a *cis*-isomer that is converted in serum to the less active *trans*-isomer. The chemical structure and spectrum of antimicrobial activity are similar to those of cefixime. Ceftibuten, like cefixime, is distinguished from other extended-spectrum oral cephalosporins by its lack of activity against *S. aureus.* Its antimicrobial activity against groups A, C, F, and G β-hemolytic streptococci is good, whereas its activity against groups B and D, as well as viridans streptococci, is poor. Ceftibuten exhibits MICs for penicillin-susceptible pneumococci in the susceptible range, whereas penicillin-nonsusceptible strains are ceftibuten-resistant. In contrast to other oral cephalosporins, ceftibuten is the most stable to hydrolysis by β-lactamases produced by Neisseriaceae, *Moraxella, Haemophilus,* and Enterobacteriaceae, including most strains of *E. coli* and *K. pneumoniae* that produce Ambler class A plasmid-mediated, ESBLs of the TEM, SHV, and OXA types. Ceftibuten is variably active against strains of *Citrobacter, Serratia,* and *Morganella,* but it is inactive against *Acinetobacter, Pseudomonas, Enterobacter, Bordetella,* and anaerobic species. It is also a weak inducer of AmpC Bush group 1 β-lactamases produced by *S. marcescens, E. cloacae,* and *Enterobacter aerogenes.*[142]

Ceftibuten has excellent bioavailability and a favorable pharmacokinetic profile that facilitates a once-daily dosing schedule.[25] Treatment regimens of 10 days have been approved for streptococcal tonsillopharyngitis and acute otitis media caused by *H. influenzae, M. catarrhalis,* or *S. pyogenes* because of superior clinical and microbiologic efficacy data for ceftibuten in comparison with penicillin V in children with streptococcal tonsillopharyngitis[280] and comparable clinical efficacy data for ceftibuten versus amoxicillin, amoxicillin-clavulanate, cefaclor, and cefprozil for the treatment of children with clinically defined acute otitis media with or without effusion. However, cumulative data from clinical trials indicate that microbiologic cure rates of pneumococcal otitis media are lower for ceftibuten than for comparable antimicrobial agents.[142] Because of the increasing prevalence of nonsusceptible *S. pneumoniae* isolates, ceftibuten has almost no place in the treatment of acute otitis media, especially in young or otherwise at-risk infants and children.

Ceftibuten also should be considered as alternative therapy for sinusitis caused by susceptible organisms. Although not approved for this indication, ceftibuten achieved clinical success equivalent to and bacterial eradication superior to those reported with trimethoprim-sulfamethoxazole in the treatment of complicated or recurrent urinary tract infections in children.[24] Adverse reactions to ceftibuten, which are limited mainly to the gastrointestinal tract, occur in approximately 10% of children, a rate similar to comparable oral β-lactam antibiotics. The safety and efficacy of ceftibuten have not been established for infants younger than 6 months of age.

Cefdinir. Cefdinir was approved in 1999 for the treatment of acute otitis media in children. It has a broad spectrum of in vitro antimicrobial activity, favorable pharmacokinetics, a convenient once-daily or twice-daily dosage schedule, superior palatability, a low rate of adverse events, and proved clinical efficacy against common childhood pathogens.[155,194] In contrast to cephalexin, cefaclor, cefuroxime, cefixime, and cefpodoxime, cefdinir has equivalent or superior MICs for groups A, B, C, F, and G streptococci, viridans streptococci, and oxacillin-susceptible staphylococci. Its in vitro activity against penicillin-susceptible and penicillin-nonsusceptible strains of *S. pneumoniae* is equivalent to that of cefuroxime and cefpodoxime but superior to that of other oral cephalosporins. Cefixime and cefpodoxime have superior activity against *H. influenzae* (including β-lactamase-producing strains), whereas cefdinir and cefuroxime have comparable activity against this pathogen. The activity of cefdinir against *M. catarrhalis* is similar to that of cefixime, cefpodoxime, and cefuroxime but superior to that of earlier-generation cephalosporins. Cefdinir is stable to hydrolysis by many common Enterobacteriaceae-produced β-lactamases. However, activity against these pathogens is variable. Cefdinir is inactive against strains of enterococci, methicillin-resistant staphylococci, *Legionella, Listeria, Acinetobacter, Citrobacter, Enterobacter, P. aeruginosa, Serratia, Stenotrophomonas,* and most anaerobes.[143]

Based on comparative clinical and microbiologic efficacy trials, administration of cefdinir should be considered for children with (1) acute bacterial otitis media caused by β-lactamase-positive or β-lactamase-negative strains of *H. influenzae* and *M. catarrhalis* or penicillin-susceptible strains of *S. pneumoniae* as either a 5- or 10-day regimen; cefdinir has efficacy equivalent to that of cefuroxime and cefpodoxime but superior palatability and therefore should be considered as an alternative to other second-line regimens; however, use of amoxicillin-clavulanate or three single daily doses of parenteral ceftriaxone is recommended if penicillin-nonsusceptible pneumococci are suspected or proved[11,15,194]; (2) group A streptococcal tonsillopharyngitis in 5- or 10-day dosage schedules; (3) acute maxillary sinusitis caused by susceptible organisms; and (4) uncomplicated skin and skin structure infections caused by oxacillin-susceptible *S. aureus* or group A streptococci.[176] Although cefdinir is not approved for treatment of urinary tract infections, microbiologic data support its potential utility for community-acquired uncomplicated urinary infections.[46] The safety and efficacy of cefdinir have not been established for infants younger than 6 months of age.

Cefditoren pivoxil. Cefditoren pivoxil was approved by the FDA in 2002 for oral treatment of acute exacerbations of chronic bronchitis, pharyngitis, tonsillitis, and uncomplicated skin and soft tissue infections in adults and adolescents 12 years of age and older. Cefditoren is similar to cefdinir and cefpodoxime in its antibacterial activity. It is stable to hydrolysis by many common Enterobacteriaceae-produced β-lactamases. Cefditoren has the greatest in vitro antimicrobial activity of all oral cephalosporins against *S. pneumoniae.* The inactive metabolite pivalate is eliminated by the kidneys in combination with carnitine as pivaloylcarnitine. Although cefditoren transiently decreases serum concentrations of carnitine, the clinical significance of this is not clear, but no adverse effects have been reported.[233]

Third-Generation Cephalosporin, β-Lactamase Combinations

Ceftazidime-avibactam. Ceftazidime-avibactam was approved by the FDA in 2015 for the treatment of complicated intra-abdominal infection and complicated urinary tract infection in adults who have limited or no alternative treatment options. Ceftazidime is a third-generation cephalosporin having activity against select gram-positive cocci and gram-negative bacilli, including *Pseudomonas aeruginosa.* Avibactam is a novel non–β-lactam, β-lactamase inhibitor exhibiting activity against Ambler class A (e.g., CTX-M, KPC, ESBL), C (e.g., FOX, AmpC), and select class D (e.g., OXA-48) β-lactamases. Ceftazidime-avibactam is available in a fixed 4:1 combination.[203,373,379]

Mechanisms of action. As with other β-lactam antibiotics, ceftazidime exerts its bactericidal activity by binding with PBPs of susceptible bacteria, which results in inhibition of cell wall synthesis. Ceftazidime is distinct among third-generation cephalosporins because of its activity against *Pseudomonas aeruginosa.* This activity is secondary to distinct side chains attached at positions 3 and 7 of the cephem nucleus. Ceftazidime specifically inhibits PBP3 of gram-negative bacteria, which results in a compromised peptidoglycan cell wall, ultimately leading to bacterial lysis and death. Avibactam exerts inhibition by covalently acylating the active site, a serine residue, of susceptible β-lactamases. After initial acylation, slow deacylation has been shown to occur, which fully restores the activity of the five-membered urea ring for additional activity. This differs from existing β-lactamase inhibitors, as previous inhibitors bind irreversibly to substrate and are subsequently decomposed.[203,373,379]

Mechanisms of resistance. Gram-negative bacteria demonstrate resistance to antimicrobial agents through numerous distinct resistance mechanisms, which can broadly be defined as either inherent or acquired. Organisms that possess or acquire β-lactamases classified as Ambler class B enzymes (e.g., NDM, VIM, IMP) and most OXA enzymes will exhibit resistance to avibactam. Resistance to avibactam, in combination with several different β-lactams, has also been shown to occur when (1) isolates of *P. aeruginosa* have decreased membrane permeability; (2) organisms have efflux pumps able to excrete antimicrobial agents after entry into the cell membrane; and (3) existing β-lactamases undergo point mutations resulting in resistant mutants with reduced inhibitor affinity. Avibactam has been reported not to induce expression of the chromosomal ampC in *Enterobacter cloacae.*[203,373,379]

In vitro activity. Avibactam has been shown to restore the activity of ceftazidime against Enterobacteriaceae producing the most common β-lactamases in US hospitals, which includes ESBLs and *Klebsiella pneumoniae* carbapenemases (KPCs).[69] Avibactam inhibits class A enzymes at least as well or better than clavulanate and tazobactam. The activity of avibactam against KPCs has been shown to be substantially greater than that of either clavulanate or tazobactam.[379] Avibactam also inhibits class C enzymes but does not inhibit β-lactamases such as NDM, VIM, or IMP due to their lack of a serine residue at the active site.[373,379] Sader and colleagues tested more than 10,000 clinically significant gram-negative bacilli, including Enterobacteriaceae, *Pseudomonas aeruginosa, and Acinetobacter* isolates, gathered from US hospitals and found that ceftazidime-avibactam had activity against ESBL producers (e.g., *Escherichia coli* and *Klebsiella pneumoniae*), *K. pneumoniae* not susceptible to meropenem, and *Enterobacter cloacae* not susceptible to ceftazidime alone. More than 95% of *P. aeruginosa* isolates were inhibited by ceftazidime-avibactam compared to an 80% susceptibility rate with meropenem, ceftazidime alone, and piperacillin-tazobactam. For ESBL-producing *K. pneumoniae,* greater than 99% were susceptible to ceftazidime-avibactam, whereas only 60% were susceptible to meropenem. *Acinetobacter* species, as with many other antibiotic agents, shows high resistance rates to ceftazidime-avibactam.[305]

Pharmacokinetics. Ceftazidime and avibactam each demonstrate nearly linear pharmacokinetics over a broad dosing range in adults; increases in dosage result in proportional increases in the peak plasma concentration. The pharmacokinetics associated with the concomitant administration of ceftazidime and avibactam do not result in altered pharmacokinetic profiles of either agent. Ceftazidime and avibactam each demonstrate low protein binding—21% for ceftazidime and 8% for avibactam—and are predominantly cleared by the kidney with a half-life of approximately 2.7 hours. The dosage should be reduced in adults with renal impairment. Although there are currently no labeled recommendations for patients receiving dialysis, both of these agents are efficiently cleared by hemodialysis; therefore, administration should occur after dialysis in patients with no alternative treatment options. Ceftazidime pharmacodynamic properties are optimized when the free drug concentration exceeds the MIC (%*f*T > MIC) of the target pathogen for approximately 40% to 50% of the dosing interval.[373] Pharmacodynamic parameters appear to be best optimized for avibactam when the free inhibitor concentration is above threshold concentration (%*f*T > C_T), where the threshold concentration for both inhibitor and β-lactam is that which inhibits organism growth. The adult dosing recommendations are ceftazidime 2 g, avibactam 0.5 g as a 2-hour prolonged infusion every 8 hours.[373,379]

Indications for use. During a phase II clinical trial for complicated intra-abdominal infection, ceftazidime-avibactam plus metronidazole demonstrated similar microbiologic and clinical response rates when compared to meropenem.[224] Similarly, ceftazidime-avibactam recipients in a phase II clinical trial of patients with complicated urinary tract infection found the efficacy and safety of ceftazidime-avibactam was similar to the comparator, imipenem-cilastatin.[361] A phase III study comparing the safety and efficacy of ceftazidime-avibactam to doripenem in adults hospitalized for complicated urinary tract infection, including pyelonephritis, found ceftazidime-avibactam to be non-inferior to doripenem.[365] Thus, the FDA approved ceftazidime-avibactam with available in vitro, in vivo, phase II trial data and preliminary phase III trial results for the treatment of complicated intra-abdominal infections, in combination with metronidazole, and complicated urinary tract infections, including pyelonephritis, in adults who have limited or no alternative treatment options.[74] Clinical trials are underway in pediatric patients.

Adverse effects. Data from phase I and II clinical trials indicate that ceftazidime-avibactam is generally well tolerated, with the rate of adverse and serious adverse events being similar between adult patients receiving ceftazidime-avibactam and those receiving comparator group agents.[373] In a phase II trial for complicated intra-abdominal infection, the overall rate of adverse events was similar between groups receiving either ceftazidime-avibactam plus metronidazole or meropenem. However, patients in the ceftazidime-avibactam group did experience higher rates of nausea, vomiting, and abdominal pain.[224] Additionally, a phase II trial for complicated urinary tract infection found that adverse drug event rates between patients randomized to either ceftazidime-avibactam or imipenem-cilastatin were similar between groups. Of those patients receiving ceftazidime-avibactam, the most commonly reported adverse events included headache, gastrointestinal symptoms, and injection-site reactions.[361] Data currently suggest that the safety profile of ceftazidime-avibactam appears similar to that of ceftazidime alone.

Ceftolozane-tazobactam. Ceftolozane-tazobactam was approved by the FDA in 2014 for the treatment of complicated intra-abdominal infection and complicated urinary tract infection in adults. Ceftolozane is a novel third-generation cephalosporin with activity against select gram-positive and many gram-negative organisms, including potent activity against multidrug-resistant *Pseudomonas aeruginosa.*[79,215,335] However, similar to other third-generation cephalosporins (e.g., ceftriaxone and ceftazidime), ceftolozane is vulnerable to attack by ESBLs and carbapenamases. Tazobactam, an established β-lactamase inhibitor, extends the spectrum of activity to include ESBLs and select anaerobes. Ceftolozane-tazobactam is available in a fixed 2:1 combination.[79,333]

Mechanisms of action. Ceftolozane exhibits bactericidal activity through inhibition of PBPs, impairment of peptidoglycan cross-linking, aberrant cell wall synthesis, and finally the initiation of cell lysis. Ceftolozane has a chemical structure most similar to that of ceftazidime; however, the heavier side chain at position 3 of ceftolozane offers increased stability against AmpC β-lactamase production of *P. aeruginosa.* Tazobactam, a β-lactamase inhibitor, extends the spectrum of ceftolozane to include ESBLs and some anaerobes. Tazobactam stimulates ring opening at the active site of susceptible β-lactamases, resulting in the formation of an irreversible covalent bond between the β-lactamase and tazobactam, thereby inactivating the β-lactamase.[79,306,333]

Mechanisms of resistance. Resistance mechanisms commonly used by *Pseudomonas aeruginosa* include use of efflux pumps, loss of cell wall porin proteins (OprD), and hyperproduction of efflux pumps and AmpC β-lactamases.[250,335] Takeda and colleagues found that ceftolozane, in comparison to ceftazidime, demonstrated enhanced stability in the presence of AmpC β-lactamases. Further, ceftolozane activity is not hindered by the presence of efflux pumps or by loss of OprD, which are known to be primary resistance mechanisms used by *P. aeruginosa* against fluoroquinolone and carbapenem agents.[333,335] In an effort to assess the propensity of ceftolozane to induce resistance in *P. aeruginosa* isolates, Takeda and colleagues performed serial passage experiments where ceftolozane demonstrated decreased rates of spontaneous mutation in *P. aeruginosa* isolates compared to that seen with ceftazidime, imipenem, and ciprofloxacin. Investigators suggest that resistance to ceftolozane is difficult to induce secondary to increased structural durability in the presence of AmpC β-lactamases. Ceftolozane activity is, however, hindered by organisms producing metallo-β-lactamases, carbapenemases, and ESBLs.[215,333,335,340] The addition of tazobactam to this novel third-generation cephalosporin broadens coverage to include organisms producing ESBLs, a common resistance mechanism employed by many Enterobacteriaceae.[333,335]

In vitro activity. Ceftolozane demonstrates a spectrum of activity similar to ceftazidime. It has select activity against gram-positive organisms, including streptococci, but less activity against staphylococci. It is active against gram-negative organisms, including drug-resistant isolates of *Pseudomonas aeruginosa* and Enterobacteriaceae.[335] The addition of tazobactam, an irreversible inhibitor of β-lactamases, does not significantly impact the activity of ceftolozane against gram-positive cocci, but does extend the spectrum of ceftolozane to include select anaerobic organisms (i.e., *B. fragilis*)[327] and gram-negative organisms producing ESBLs.[215,333,340,377] It is important to note that tazobactam does not add significantly to the activity of ceftolozane against *P. aeruginosa,* as ESBL production is not a resistance mechanism commonly used by this organism. Farrell and colleagues analyzed the activity of ceftolozane/tazobactam against 7071 Enterobacteriaceae, with the most common pathogens being *Escherichia coli* and *Klebsiella pneumoniae,* and 1971 *Pseudomonas aeruginosa* isolates obtained from US hospitals.[110] Of 2691 *E. coli* isolates, ceftolozane/tazobactam inhibited all non–ESBL-producing isolates at a MIC less than 2 μg/mL and overall inhibited 99% of isolates, including ESBL producers, at a MIC less than 4 μg/mL. Similarly, non–ESBL-producing *K. pneumoniae* isolates were 100% inhibited by ceftolozane/tazobactam at a MIC less than 2 μg/mL; however, decreased activity occurred in ESBL-phenotype *K. pneumoniae,* likely secondary to destruction of these agents by carbapenemase production. Although ceftolozane/tazobactam demonstrates overall good activity against Enterobacteriaceae, its anti-pseudomonal activity is most striking, as it is more potent than ceftazidime, cefepime, piperacillin/tazobactam, and meropenem. Importantly, ceftolozane/tazobactam retains potency even in the presence of multidrug and extensively drug-resistant *P. aeruginosa.*[111] Ceftolozane/tazobactam, as is the case with β-lactams, demonstrates poor activity against *Acinetobacter* spp. and *Stenotrophomonas maltophilia.*

Pharmacokinetics. In adults, ceftolozane and tazobactam each demonstrate nearly linear pharmacokinetics over broad dosing ranges; increases in dosage result in proportional increases in the peak plasma concentrations. The pharmacokinetics associated with concomitant administration of ceftolozane and tazobactam do not result in altered pharmacokinetic profiles of either agent. Ceftolozane and tazobactam demonstrate low protein binding at approximately 20% for ceftolozane and 30% for tazobactam. Ceftolozane is predominantly excreted unchanged in the urine with a half-life of 2.3 hours. Approximately 80% of tazobactam is excreted unchanged, the remaining 20% as an inactive metabolite into the urine.[79,333,377] Because both ceftolozane and tazobactam are cleared primarily through renal filtration, dosage reductions are necessary when creatinine clearance is 50 mL/min or less. In patients receiving hemodialysis, ceftolozane/tazobactam should be administered upon completion of dialysis.[333] For ceftolozane and ceftolozane/tazobactam, pharmacodynamic properties are optimized when the free drug concentration exceeds the MIC (%*f*T > MIC) of the target pathogen for approximately 40% to 50% of the dosing interval.[79] Adult ceftolozane/tazobactam dosing recommendations are ceftolozane 1 g–tazobactam 0.5 g administered via a 60-minute infusion every 8 hours.

Indications for use. In a phase III clinical trial for the treatment of complicated intra-abdominal infection in adults, ceftolozane/tazobactam plus metronidazole, even in the presence of multidrug-resistant pathogens, was found to be non-inferior to meropenem.[328] Adverse events, most commonly nausea and diarrhea, were found to occur at similar rates between treatment arms. Ceftolozane/tazobactam also was found to be superior to high-dose levofloxacin in a phase III clinical trial for the treatment of complicated urinary-tract infections in adults, where more than 80% of the microbiologic modified intention-to-treat cohort (those with one or two uropathogens) had pyelonephritis.[366] The frequency of adverse events, most commonly headache and gastrointestinal symptoms, was found to be similar between groups. With these data, ceftolozane/tazobactam received FDA approval for the treatment of complicated intra-abdominal infections in combination with metronidazole, and complicated urinary tract infections including pyelonephritis, in adult patients.[375] Ceftolozane/tazobactam studies are underway to evaluate plasma pharmacokinetics and lung penetration in critically ill adult patients as well as a pharmacokinetic and safety evaluation in pediatric patients with proved or suspected gram-negative infection or for perioperative prophylaxis (NCT02387372 and NCT 02266706). A phase III clinical trial is underway to evaluate the safety and efficacy of ceftolozane/tazobactam versus meropenem in the treatment of ventilated nosocomial pneumonia (NCT02070757), and a phase IV study is evaluating population pharmacokinetics and safety of this agent in adult patients with cystic fibrosis (NCT02421120).

Fourth-Generation Cephalosporins

Cefepime. Cefepime, the prototypic agent of this class of antibiotics, was approved by the FDA in 1996. It is distinguished from other cephalosporins by the rapid penetration of outer-membrane porins into the periplasmic space of gram-negative bacteria, facilitated by its net neutral charge; enhanced stability against hydrolysis by inducible or constitutively expressed chromosomally mediated AmpC Bush group 1 β-lactamases and Ambler class A plasmid-mediated SHV- and TEM-type ESBLs; and increased binding affinity to multiple PBPs. These factors contribute to cefepime's expanded spectrum of activity and improved efficacy against gram-negative pathogens in contrast to third-generation cephalosporins.

The in vitro activity of cefepime encompasses a broad range of gram-positive and gram-negative organisms, including oxacillin-susceptible staphylococci; approximately 75% of penicillin-resistant strains of *S. pneumoniae;* viridans streptococci; most strains of Enterobacteriaceae, including, most notably, ESBL-producing strains of *E. coli* and *K. pneumoniae;* and AmpC-mediated resistant *Enterobacter* spp. and *Citrobacter* spp., as well as approximately 90% of *P. aeruginosa* isolates. Furthermore, bacteria in which resistance to third-generation cephalosporins develops by means of single-step mutations usually remain susceptible to cefepime. Clinical and laboratory data also indicate that selection of cefepime resistance, specifically among *Enterobacter* spp. and *P. aeruginosa,* is uncommon. As with other cephalosporins, cefepime is inactive against enterococci, methicillin-resistant staphylococci, *S. maltophilia,* and many anaerobic organisms.[178,189]

Cefepime is indicated for the parenteral treatment of lower respiratory tract, urinary tract, skin and skin structure, and intra-abdominal (in combination with anaerobic antibacterial agents) infections, as well as for empirical monotherapy in pediatric patients with cancer who have fever and neutropenia, for whom cefepime has been shown to be as effective as meropenem, piperacillin-tazobactam, or ceftazidime with or without an aminoglycoside. In comparative clinical and microbiologic efficacy trials, cefepime as a single antibacterial agent was equivalent to third-generation cephalosporins for the most common childhood pathogens. In addition, cefepime is as safe and well tolerated, as are other cephalosporin antibiotics.[50,256,317]

Cefepime should be reserved for complicated community-acquired, health care–associated, or polymicrobial infections; penicillin-resistant and third-generation cephalosporin-resistant pathogens; and patients with cystic fibrosis and *P. aeruginosa* lung infections. Cefepime concentrations in CSF reach approximately 3 to 6 μg/mL (9% of the peak plasma concentration) in children with bacterial meningitis. Therefore, achievable CSF concentrations exceed the MICs of common CNS pathogens by at least 10-fold, except for penicillin- and cephalosporin-nonsusceptible *S. pneumoniae.*[43] Currently, data are insufficient to recommend cefepime as single-agent therapy for meningitis. The safety and efficacy of cefepime have not been established for neonates, but data extrapolated from pharmacokinetic studies among preterm and term infants support a dose of 30 mg/kg every 12 hours for infants younger than 14 days of age, regardless of gestational age. This dosage should provide antibiotic exposure equivalent to or greater than the approved dose of 50 mg/kg every 8 to 12 hours in older infants and children.[67]

Fifth-Generation Cephalosporins

Ceftaroline. Ceftaroline fosamil is a prodrug that is rapidly biotransformed when administered intravenously to the active agent, ceftaroline. Ceftaroline is a broad-spectrum, advanced-generation cephalosporin initially approved by the FDA in 2010 for the treatment of community-acquired pneumonia and skin and skin structure infections in adult patients. This agent distinguishes itself from other cephalosporins with its activity against multiple gram-positive organisms known to exhibit resistance to existing β-lactam agents including *Streptococcus pneumoniae* as well as methicillin-resistant *S. aureus,* including those isolates found to be vancomycin-intermediate and resistant. Ceftaroline also has select activity against gram-negative organisms, including those prevalent in the respiratory tract (e.g., *M. catarrhalis* and *H. influenzae*), but has restricted activity against *P. aeruginosa* and exhibits instability in the presence of those organisms producing either extended-spectrum or AmpC-type β-lactamases.[331]

Mechanisms of action. Similar to other β-lactam antibiotics, ceftaroline exerts its bactericidal activity by binding with PBPs of susceptible bacteria, which results in inhibition of cell wall synthesis. Ceftaroline has high affinity for PBPs 1, 2, and 3 for methicillin-susceptible strains of *S. aureus* (MSSA). However, this agent also contains a side chain with an alkoxyimino group in the C7 acyl moiety that provides in vitro activity for MRSA with high affinity for the PBP2a and another side chain with a 2-thiazolythio spacer group modification that optimizes the anti-MRSA activity. Because of its potent binding to PBP2x, ceftaroline also is active against *Streptococcus pneumoniae* resistant to penicillins and other cephalosporins.[331]

Mechanisms of resistance. During in vitro single-step selection investigation, where the goal was to detect the frequency of mutation occurrence, Mushtaq and colleagues failed to detect ceftaroline-resistant *S. aureus,* including isolates of MSSA, MRSA, vancomycin-intermediate *S. aureus* (VISA), or *S. pneumoniae,* regardless of penicillin susceptibility. Multistep selection investigation also was unable to detect isolates of mutant *S. aureus.*[255] However, ceftaroline resistance has been described by Alm and colleagues, who identified four isolates of MRSA with MIC values greater than 2 mg/L from medical centers located in Thailand and Spain. They characterized ceftaroline resistance in isolates as occurring secondary to (1) mutations in PBP2a that resulted in decreased ceftaroline binding affinity, and (2) alterations in the non–penicillin-binding domain (nPBD), the dimerized portion, of PBP2a. Mutation in the nPBD portion of PBP2a weakens the dimerization between PBP2a and PBP2, which leads to binding of PBP2 with other proteins and ultimately allows cell wall production to occur.[6] In addition to potent activity against multidrug-resistant gram-positive organisms, ceftaroline also demonstrates activity against many Enterobacteriaceae where the spectrum of activity of this agent resembles that of other extended-spectrum cephalosporins. Ceftaroline activity is, however, lost against those organisms producing extended-spectrum or AmpC-type β-lactamases.[255,381]

In vitro activity. In addition to this agent's anti-MRSA activity, ceftaroline also retains activity against isolates with reduced susceptibility to vancomycin (glycopeptide-intermediate *S. aureus* [GISA], heterogeneous GISA [hGISA], and glycopeptide-resistant *S. aureus* [GRSA]) or linezolid.[32,331] This antibiotic has in vitro activity against gram-positive organisms, including *S. aureus,* both MSSA and MRSA; coagulase-negative staphylococci; group A and group B β-hemolytic streptococci; and *S. pneumoniae,* including multidrug-resistant strains. It also has modest activity against *E. faecalis.* Ceftaroline has no activity against *E. faecium* (MIC_{90} >1632 μg/mL). It has activity against penicillin-nonsusceptible viridans group streptococci. Ceftaroline is active against non-ESBL enteric gram-negative organisms, including *E. coli* and *K. pneumoniae;* respiratory gram-negative organisms (including *M. catarrhalis* and *H. influenzae* and β-lactamase-positive strains); and *N. gonorrhoeae.* It has limited activity against nonfermenting gram-negative organisms, including *P. aeruginosa* and *A. baumannii* (with MIC >16 mg/L for both). Ceftaroline can induce expression of AmpC β-lactamases in a degree similar to that of ceftriaxone and cefotaxime based on in vitro induction assays.[331]

Pharmacokinetics. Ceftaroline fosamil is a prodrug that is converted into its active form by plasma phosphatases. Data from single- and multidose studies demonstrate nearly linear pharmacokinetics of ceftaroline over a broad dosing range; an increase in dosage results in proportional increases in peak plasma concentrations (C_{max}) and area under the concentration-time curve (AUC).[288,381] Protein binding of this agent is minimal and was found to range from 1% to 19% over different concentrations. Ceftaroline and its inactive metabolite, ceftaroline-M-1, are eliminated predominantly via renal excretion with half-lives of 2.6 hours and 4.5 hours, respectively. Dosage adjustment is required for moderate renal impairment and for patients receiving hemodialysis. Optimal pharmacodynamic parameters, similar to other cephalosporins, are achieved when the free drug concentration exceeds the MIC (%*f*T > MIC) for 50% of the time interval for staphylococci and 60% of the time interval for gram-negative bacilli.[288,381] Adult ceftaroline dosing recommendations are 600 mg administered via a 60-minute infusion every 12 hours.[118] In 2016, ceftaroline was FDA approved for the treatment of community-acquired pneumonia and bacterial skin and skin structure infections in children.

Indications for use. In phase III clinical trials for the treatment of skin and skin structure infections, ceftaroline proved to be non-inferior to a combination of vancomycin and aztreonam with similar clinical cure and bacterial eradication rates.[89,336] Two randomized, double-blind, multicenter, phase III trials showed similar cure rates when comparing ceftaroline and ceftriaxone (± clarithromycin) for the treatment of community-acquired pneumonia in adults.[115,222] A phase II/III clinical trial evaluated the safety and efficacy of ceftaroline versus intravenous comparators (either vancomycin or cefazolin with the option to add aztreonam) for the treatment of acute bacterial skin and skin structure infections in pediatric patients 2 months to 17 years of age and found ceftaroline to be well tolerated and as effective as the comparator regimens.[198] In a phase II/III clinical trial evaluating the safety, tolerability, and effectiveness of ceftaroline versus ceftriaxone in pediatric patients between the ages of 2 months and 18 years with community-acquired pneumonia, ceftaroline was found to be well tolerated, with similar rates of adverse events between groups, and as effective as ceftriaxone.[65] Ceftaroline is dosed at 8 mg/kg every 8 hours in children 2 months to less than 2 years of age; at 12 mg/kg every 8 hours in children weighing less than 33 kg and more than 2 years of age; and at 400 mg every 8 hours in those weighing more than 33 kg.[65,198] Higher doses were used in a phase IV clinical trial evaluating the safety and effectiveness of ceftaroline versus ceftriaxone with vancomycin in pediatric patients aged 2 months to 17 years with complicated community-acquired pneumonia, and ceftaroline again was found to be well tolerated, with similar rates of adverse events between groups, and as effective as treatment with ceftriaxone and vancomycin.[41]

Adverse effects. Ceftaroline has been well tolerated with no safety concerns reported in multiple studies in adults and children.[41,65,89,198,336] In adults, the most common adverse effects were diarrhea, nausea, headache, and insomnia. Ceftaroline may cause changes in urine color or smell. Ceftaroline did not cause QTc interval prolongation.[89,336] Although no case of hemolytic anemia was reported during pediatric investigations, the rate of direct Coombs test seroconversion among patients receiving ceftaroline in late-phase pediatric studies has ranged from 17% to 26%.[41,65,198] This seroconversion may come secondary to changes and/or nonspecific binding of IgG to the red blood cell membrane.[41,198] Case reports in children and adults have described patients who have experienced agranulocytosis while concurrently receiving ceftaroline. Until more is known about the association between ceftaroline and hematologic disturbances, providers should routinely (e.g., weekly) monitor peripheral white and red blood cell counts and differentials while treating patients with this agent.[322,360]

Adverse effects associated with cephalosporins in general. The cephalosporins, like the penicillins, are safe for children and have almost no dose-related toxicity. The most common reactions are local, including pain at the injection site or thrombophlebitis with parenteral administration and mild gastrointestinal complaints with oral dosing. Hypersensitivity reactions occur in approximately 1% to 3% of treatment courses and include morbilliform rash, urticaria, and pruritus. Drug fever has been associated with the administration of cephalosporins. Nonspecific antibiotic-associated diarrhea and, less commonly, *C. difficile* toxin–mediated colitis can occur after use of a cephalosporin.

Other adverse effects are rare, and some are unique to one or a few cephalosporins. Physicians should be alert for uncommon reactions, including reversible neutropenia, which can occur after prolonged use of high-dosage cephalosporins; Coombs-positive hemolytic anemia; and bleeding. Altered hemostasis because of hypoprothrombinemia can result when using any cephalosporin that contains a methylthiotetrazole side chain (cefotetan). These agents act as competitive inhibitors of vitamin K–dependent carboxylase, which converts clotting factors II, VII, IX, and X to their active forms. Gallbladder sludging, biliary pseudolithiasis, and symptomatic obstructive biliary disease rarely have been associated with the administration of ceftriaxone.[383]

The cephalosporins may produce allergic reactions similar to those caused by the penicillins. Cross sensitization exists among the cephalosporins, and allergy to one cephalosporin implies allergy to all. Various degrees of immunologic cross reaction of penicillins and cephalosporins have been demonstrated in vitro and in animal models.[276] Previously quoted studies suggest that the frequency of allergic reactions to cephalosporins ranges from 5.4% to 16.5% in adult patients with a history of penicillin allergy and 1.0% to 2.5% in those without such a history. The incidence of hypersensitivity to unrelated drugs is increased in some patients who are allergic to penicillin, a finding suggesting that excipients in antibiotic preparations may be responsible for these reactions.[314] Most patients who are thought to be allergic to penicillin receive cephalosporins without adverse reaction. Data indicate that the risk for an allergic reaction to a cephalosporin challenge among penicillin-allergic subjects with positive skin test responses is 4%. Therefore, the following options are available for individuals with positive skin test responses for penicillin hypersensitivity: administration of an alternative non-β-lactam antibiotic, administration of a cephalosporin by graded challenge, or desensitization to the cephalosporin. Individuals with a history of penicillin allergy who have negative penicillin skin test responses may receive cephalosporins because they are at no higher risk than the general population for experiencing allergic reactions.[213] In the absence of penicillin skin testing, a cephalosporin may be used with caution as an alternative to penicillin in children who have an ambiguous history of rash; however, cephalosporins should be avoided in patients with a known immediate or accelerated reaction to a penicillin. Currently, skin testing to evaluate for cephalosporin hypersensitivity is not possible because the potential cephalosporin haptens are unknown, and no standardized antigen exists.

Some products may cause unexpected reactions, such as bile sludge attributed to ceftriaxone and serum sickness–like disease described with cefaclor. A generalized pruritic rash, similar to erythema multiforme, developed in some children treated with cefaclor, along with fever, purpura, and arthritis with pain and swelling in the knees and ankles. The signs appeared 5 to 19 days after the start of therapy and generally disappeared within 4 to 5 days after discontinuing use of the drug. The children had no previous history of allergy to a penicillin or cephalosporin.[254] Levine[210] compared adverse reactions in children who received cefaclor (1017 patients and 2513 courses) or amoxicillin (1009 patients and 2358 courses). Serum sickness (defined as arthritis or arthralgia in addition to a rash or urticaria) or erythema multiforme occurred in 11 children (1.1%) who received cefaclor but in none of those who received amoxicillin. Studies suggest that serum sickness–like reactions to cefaclor are associated with lymphocyte sensitization.[186]

Monobactams

Aztreonam is the prototype monobactam, a name that refers to the unique monocyclic nucleus. This drug has aerobic, gram-negative antibacterial activity similar to that of ceftazidime, but it has no significant gram-positive activity. Unlike most β-lactam antibiotics, aztreonam has the advantage of not inducing β-lactamase activity, and its molecular structure confers a high degree of stability to hydrolysis by β-lactamases. The mechanisms of antibiotic resistance of some gram-negative bacteria include expression of efflux pumps, reduced expression of outer-membrane porin proteins, and production of AmpC-type β-lactamases or ESBLs. In a study conducted from 1998 to 2003, approximately 15% of Enterobacteriaceae in North America were resistant to aztreonam.[307] However, of 442 ESBL-producing Enterobacteriaceae collected between June 2013 and September 2014 from adult patients in US hospitals, only 7% were susceptible to aztreonam.[334] Although it is a β-lactam, aztreonam is weakly immunogenic and can be used in patients with minor forms of β-lactam allergy. Its use in pediatrics is indicated as a secondary agent for the intravenous treatment of lower respiratory tract, skin and soft tissue, urinary tract, and intra-abdominal infections caused by susceptible pathogens. Higher doses of aztreonam may be warranted for pediatric patients with cystic fibrosis. Aztreonam and aminoglycosides are synergistic in vitro against most strains of *P. aeruginosa,* many strains of Enterobacteriaceae, and other aerobic gram-negative bacilli. The safety and efficacy of aztreonam have not been established for infants younger than 9 months of age or for children with impaired renal function. However, aztreonam has been used with favorable outcomes in premature and term neonates, as well as in young infants. Updated breakpoints for enteric gram-negative organisms to aztreonam were released in 2010. The revised breakpoints include 4 μg/mL or less, 8 μg/mL, and 16 μg/mL or greater for susceptible, intermediate, and resistant organisms, respectively.[367] Aztreonam lysinate for inhalation is a novel monobactam formulation approved by the FDA in February 2010 for patients with cystic fibrosis who are colonized with *P. aeruginosa.* For children 7 years of age or older and adults, the dose recommended for inhaled aztreonam is 75 mg three times daily for 28 days.[281,374]

Carbapenems

Carbapenems differ from penicillin by virtue of the substitution of a sulfur atom by a carbon atom at position 1 of the β-lactam ring and possession of an unsaturated bond between carbon atoms at positions 2 and 3 in the structure. The carbapenem class of antimicrobial agents exhibits the broadest spectrum of activity of all β-lactam antibiotics;

these agents are active against most clinically significant gram-positive and gram-negative pathogens, including anaerobic organisms. Because they are acid-labile in the stomach, they must be administered parenterally.[90] Three carbapenems, imipenem-cilastatin, meropenem, and ertapenem, are approved for use in children.

Imipenem-Cilastatin

Imipenem-cilastatin was the first carbapenem evaluated for the treatment of severe bacterial infections in children. Extensive hydrolysis of imipenem by dehydropeptidase I occurs in the proximal renal tubule and results in the production of a potentially nephrotoxic inactive metabolite. Consequently, imipenem must be administered with cilastatin, an inhibitor of dehydropeptidase I. Despite favorable in vitro efficacy against a broad spectrum of bacterial pathogens, the clinical suitability of this antibiotic is limited because of the drug's epileptogenic potential, especially in children with bacterial meningitis. Imipenem causes seizures presumably by acting as a competitive inhibitor of ?-aminobutyric acid, an inhibitory neurotransmitter.[90] Of concern is that imipenem acts as a strong inducer of production of ESBL and may select for β-lactam resistance.[94] Imipenem-cilastatin is indicated for children with severe non-CNS infections caused by susceptible organisms. The dose must be reduced for children with impaired renal function. With the advent of meropenem, imipenem-cilastatin has been used less frequently in pediatrics.

Meropenem

Meropenem was approved for use in children in 1996. It is structurally related to imipenem. However, it is more stable against degradation by renal dehydropeptidase I and therefore does not require coadministration with cilastatin. On the basis of its superior safety and efficacy, meropenem generally is considered the preferred carbapenem for treatment of childhood infections.

Mechanisms of action. As with other β-lactam antibiotics, meropenem is bactericidal against susceptible bacteria because it inhibits bacterial cell wall synthesis. The *trans* configuration of the hydroxyethyl side chain and hydrogen atoms protect the parent β-lactam structure from inactivation by the most common β-lactamases: almost all Bush groups 1 and 2 (Ambler classes A, C, and D) β-lactamase-producing organisms, including those that produce ESBLs (*Citrobacter, Enterobacter, E. coli, Klebsiella* spp., and *P. mirabilis*) or AmpC β-lactamases (*Citrobacter, Enterobacter, Pseudomonas,* and *Serratia*). In addition, the pyrrolidine side chain enhances the compound's antipseudomonal activity.[94]

Mechanisms of resistance. Resistance may be intrinsic or acquired and is mediated by numerous mechanisms: (1) some strains of *P. aeruginosa* are deficient in the cell wall porin proteins (OprD) that usually facilitate intracellular penetration; (2) efflux pumps in some gram-negative bacteria are capable of excreting carbapenems; (3) *S. maltophilia* and some other gram-negative pathogens possess uncommon metallo-β-lactamases, the so-called carbapenemases (i.e., Bush groups 3a and 3b and Ambler class B), which form a diverse group of β-lactamases comprising the IMP and VIM families, and SPM1 and GIM1 enzymes; these carbapenemases have the ESBL and AmpC antibiotic substrate profile; (4) some gram-negative bacteria possess clavulanic acid–inhibited carbapenemases consisting of the *K. pneumoniae* carbapenemases (KPCs) (i.e., Bush group 2f and Ambler class A) or OXA enzymes (i.e., Bush group 2d and Ambler class D); and (5) MRSA strains and *E. faecium* have altered PBPs, which account for their inherent resistance. Furthermore, meropenem acts as a weak inducer of ESBLs.[54,94] At present, the risk that a single-step spontaneous mutation causes resistance among *Pseudomonas* spp. appears to be low.

In vitro activity. Meropenem has equivalent or slightly less in vitro potency than imipenem against gram-positive pathogens, but it is significantly more active against gram-negative organisms. The spectrum of activity of meropenem encompasses streptococci (excluding many strains of penicillin- and cefotaxime-nonsusceptible *S. pneumoniae*), oxacillin-susceptible staphylococci, ampicillin-susceptible enterococci, *L. monocytogenes, H. influenzae, N. meningitidis,* Enterobacteriaceae, most strains of *P. aeruginosa,* and anaerobes (including β-lactamase-positive strains of *B. fragilis*). Pathogens resistant to meropenem are *Stenotrophomonas,* MRSA, *E. faecium,* approximately 10% of *Pseudomonas* strains, and most strains of penicillin and cefotaxime-nonsusceptible *S. pneumoniae.*[54,55,61,358] In vitro tests indicate that meropenem acts synergistically with aminoglycoside antibiotics against some isolates of *P. aeruginosa.*[162]

Pharmacokinetics. Meropenem exhibits nearly linear pharmacokinetics; increases in dosage result in approximately proportional increases in the peak plasma concentration and AUC.[40] Only 2% of the drug is bound to plasma proteins, and the drug is distributed widely into tissues and fluids.[90] The elimination half-life declines with increasing age (premature neonates, 2.9 hours; term neonates, 2 hours; children, 1.1 hours; adults, 1 hour) and is longer than that for imipenem. Because meropenem is cleared primarily by glomerular filtration, the dosage should be reduced in children with renal dysfunction.[54] Furthermore, meropenem is cleared efficiently by hemodialysis; therefore, it should be administered after the patient undergoes this procedure. Pharmacodynamic studies indicate that a favorable bacteriologic outcome is best predicted by the duration of the dosing interval for which the meropenem plasma concentration exceeds the MIC_{90} of the target pathogen.[90] Accordingly, a dose of 20 mg/kg every 8 hours achieves optimal plasma concentrations (50 to 60 μg/mL) for systemic infections that do not involve the CNS,[42] whereas a dose of 40 mg/kg every 8 hours is recommended for patients with cystic fibrosis because of accelerated drug excretion.[154] Penetration of meropenem through inflamed meninges is approximately 8% of the mean plasma concentration. Consequently, a dose of 40 mg/kg every 8 hours is required to achieve mean peak CSF concentrations of 0.9 to 6.5 μg/mL and ensure effective treatment of bacterial meningitis.[90,268] An administration schedule of every 12 hours probably is appropriate for neonates because of their immature renal function.[40]

Indications for use. The FDA has approved meropenem as monotherapy for susceptible organisms causing intra-abdominal infections and bacterial meningitis in children older than 2 months of age. Meropenem should be reserved for treatment of cephalosporin-resistant nosocomial pathogens, severe polymicrobial infections with favorable susceptibility profiles, and infections that fail to respond to other antimicrobial agents. Meropenem monotherapy has clinical and microbiologic efficacy equivalent to that of third-generation cephalosporin-based regimens for septicemia and infections of the CNS, abdominal cavity, lower respiratory tract, urinary tract, and skin.[52,268] In addition, meropenem monotherapy has been shown to be equivalent to ceftazidime and amikacin and to piperacillin-tazobactam for empirical treatment of febrile children with neutropenia.[86,275] Clinical efficacy against cephalosporin-resistant pathogens also has been demonstrated in patients with cystic fibrosis.[154] In view of increasing resistance of pneumococci to β-lactam antibiotics, it is prudent to administer vancomycin with meropenem for empirical treatment of suspected bacterial meningitis until CSF microbiologic results are available. Given the significant emergence of multidrug-resistant gram-negative pathogens, empiric combination therapy with an aminoglycoside should be considered for suspected *P. aeruginosa* infections or infections caused by Enterobacteriaceae in critically ill or immunocompromised patients in view of emerging resistant strains and potential antibiotic synergy until microbiologic data become available. The effectiveness of meropenem for neonatal infections has been assessed in small, noncomparative studies that demonstrated a favorable clinical response in neonates.[83,162] Results from an open-label randomized controlled trial comparing the efficacy of meropenem with ampicillin plus gentamicin or cefotaxime plus gentamicin for the treatment of late-onset sepsis in neonates and young infants are awaited.[227]

Adverse effects. Data from well-designed clinical trials indicate that meropenem has clinical and laboratory adverse event profiles that are equivalent to those of comparable antibiotic regimens. In contrast to treatment with imipenem-cilastatin, no increased risk for seizures exists in children with or without meningitis who are treated with meropenem,[195] presumably because meropenem has less affinity than imipenem for the γ-aminobutyric acid receptor. Meropenem can be given intravenously as small-volume bolus injections (over a course of 3 to 5 minutes) without inducing nausea or vomiting. The most common adverse reactions include diarrhea (4%), rash (2%), and vomiting (1%).[54]

Ertapenem

Ertapenem is a newer, long-acting, parenteral carbapenem that initially was approved for use in adults in 2001. An indication for children was approved in 2005. However, clinical experience with this agent in children is limited. Ertapenem is distinctive because it is administered in a single daily dose in adolescents and adults and is stable against hydrolysis by many β-lactamases, except metallo-β-lactamases produced by certain bacterial nonfermenters, particularly *Pseudomonas* and *Acinetobacter*.[233] Apart from these organisms, its antimicrobial spectrum is similar to that of meropenem. Ertapenem has restricted activity against methicillin-resistant staphylococci, penicillin-nonsusceptible pneumococci, enterococci, *Pseudomonas* spp., and *Acinetobacter* spp.[187] The agent may be administered by intravenous or intramuscular routes. It exhibits nonlinear pharmacokinetics because of its concentration-dependent protein binding. The drug is excreted renally, and dosages need to be adjusted in patients with renal insufficiency.

Ertapenem is indicated for the treatment of patients 3 months of age and older with complicated intra-abdominal infections, complicated skin and soft tissue infections, community-acquired pneumonia, complicated urinary tract infections, and acute pelvic infections. Ertapenem is not recommended for the treatment of meningitis because drug concentrations in the CSF are subtherapeutic. The recommended dose in patients 3 months to 12 years of age is 15 mg/kg given parenterally twice daily, up to a maximum of 1 g/day. In older children and adults, the recommended dose is 1 g given once daily. The recommended duration is up to 14 days for intravenous administration. The most common adverse reactions, which include diarrhea, vomiting, and pain at the site of infusion, have rates comparable to those of other parenteral broad-spectrum β-lactam antimicrobials. Seizures have been reported in patients receiving ertapenem and may occur more commonly in individuals with underlying seizure disorders, brain lesions, or renal dysfunction.

Doripenem

Doripenem is a parenteral carbapenem approved in 2007 for use in adults with complicated intra-abdominal infections and complicated urinary tract infections and is currently under review for treatment of hospital-acquired pneumonia, including ventilator-associated pneumonia, and catheter-related bacteremia. Doripenem has activity against gram-positive organisms, including MSSA, penicillin-susceptible and non-susceptible *S. pneumoniae*, and *E. faecalis*. Activity against gram-negative bacteria is similar to that of meropenem and includes ESBL-producing strains. It also has good anaerobic coverage, including *B. fragilis*.[75,274]

Mechanisms of Resistance to β-Lactam Antibiotics

Bacteria can acquire resistance to an antibiotic by at least four mechanisms: (1) alteration in the antimicrobial target, (2) decreased uptake of the antibiotic by expression of efflux pumps or by reduction of cell membrane permeability that is determined by porin channels, (3) production of an enzyme that inactivates the antibiotic, and (4) production of an alternative metabolic pathway that bypasses the action of the drug.[342] With respect to β-lactam antibiotics, resistance involves alterations in PBPs, leading to decreased affinity for the β-lactam (this mechanism of resistance is observed in methicillin-resistant strains of *S. aureus* and penicillin-resistant strains of *S. pneumoniae*); decreased permeability of the bacterial cell wall, resulting in diminished amounts of β-lactam reaching the PBPs; or production of β-lactamases that hydrolyze the β-lactam ring. Hydrolysis of β-lactams is the mechanism that is most significant clinically. Gram-positive bacteria excrete their β-lactamases outside the cell wall, whereas the β-lactamases of gram-negative bacteria remain in the periplasmic space. The spectrum of β-lactamase activity involves (1) narrow-spectrum penicillinases that preferentially hydrolyze penicillins; (2) broad-spectrum β-lactamases that hydrolyze penicillins and cephalosporins equally well; (3) cephalosporinases that preferentially hydrolyze cephalosporins and are resistant to inhibition by clavulanic acid; (4) ESBLs that hydrolyze first-, second-, and third-generation cephalosporins but are susceptible to inhibition by clavulanic acid; and (5) carbapenemases that inactivate all β-lactams, including imipenem-cilastatin.[63]

Broad-spectrum β-lactamases were initially recognized in clinical isolates in the 1980s. Currently, the spread of ESBLs among enteric gram-negative organisms in both hospital and community settings has become an important public health problem. Rates of ESBL production have been high in Latin America, Asia and the Pacific region, Europe, and North America. For Latin America, the rates of ESBL production for *E. coli* and *K. pneumoniae* were 24.5 and greater than 40%, respectively, from 2004 to 2012.[188] β-Lactamases are classified on the basis of their (1) responses to β-lactamase inhibitors, (2) spectrum of antibiotic substrates (Bush-Jacoby-Medeiros classification, groups 1 to 4), or (3) primary molecular structure (i.e., Ambler classification: serine β-lactamases, which are class A, C, or D; and metallo-β-lactamases, which are class B). Bush group 2 corresponds to Ambler classes A and D, which are encoded frequently by genes carried on plasmids and easily spread among different species, whereas Bush groups 1 and 3 (Ambler classes C and B, respectively) are frequently encoded by chromosomal genes and therefore confined to certain species.[94,273] Chromosomally mediated, inducible Bush group 1 β-lactamases that are produced by certain species of *Citrobacter, Enterobacter, Morganella, Pseudomonas,* and *Serratia* are not inhibited by the β-lactamase inhibitors, and, consequently, they remain resistant to the accompanying β-lactam. However, *Bacteroides, Klebsiella, Legionella,* and *Moraxella* spp. produce chromosomally mediated β-lactamases that are effectively inactivated. Clavulanic acid and tazobactam are more potent inhibitors of β-lactamases. Furthermore, clavulanate induces Bush group 1 enzymes. Disks containing β-lactamase inhibitors can be used in the clinical microbiology laboratory to detect pathogens that produce Ambler class A ESBLs of the TEM and SHV types that may be overlooked otherwise.[64]

The ESBLs are classified in the Ambler class A and the functional (Bush group) 2be. ESBLs are present in various members of the Enterobacteriaceae family, particularly *E. coli* and *K. pneumoniae,* but they are also found in nonfermentative gram-negative bacteria, including *P. aeruginosa* and *A. baumannii.* Traditionally, β-lactamases derived mainly from the type A (Ambler) or 2be (Bush) groups, most commonly TEM (1 and 2) and SHV (1), derived by point mutations of the parent enzymes. These β-lactamases degrade penicillin, ampicillin, antipseudomonal penicillins, and narrow-spectrum cephalosporins (i.e., cefazolin and cefuroxime). They are inhibited by clavulanic acid, and this allows for laboratory detection of these enzymes. Another type of class A ESBL is the expanded-spectrum CTXM, which is becoming more prevalent, particularly in *E. coli* and *K. pneumoniae.* It preferably hydrolyzes cefotaxime in contrast to ceftazidime and degrades aztreonam and the same products hydrolyzed by TEM and SHV; for some enzymes cefepime may be a substrate. More than 100 enzymes on the CTXM group have been identified, and they can be divided into five groups on the basis of amino acid changes (i.e., CTXM1, CTXM2, CTXM8, CTXM9, and CTXM25). This enzyme has been disseminated on plasmids and is also inhibited by clavulanic acid. Carbapenemases of the type KPC (*Klebsiella pneumoniae* carbapenemases 1, 2, and 3) are also included on the Ambler class A β-lactamases, and they have the same substrates hydrolyzed by CTXM as well as cephamycins and carbapenems. They are inhibited by amoxicillin-clavulanate. Ambler class B (Bush group 3) requires divalent cations, particularly Zn^{2+}, at the active site. These enzymes can be chromosomally encoded or transferred by plasmids. This group includes the IMP and VIM families, as well as GIM1 and SPM1 β-lactamase. These β-lactamases are included in the group of carbapenemases and degrade the same products hydrolyzed KPC. They are not inhibited by clavulanic acid. Ambler class C (Bush group 1) β-lactamases are encoded by chromosomes. They are referred as AmpC and degrade substrates of the TEM and SHV, oxyiminocephalosporins (i.e., cefotaxime, cefpodoxime, ceftazidime, and ceftriaxone), monobactams, and cephamycins (i.e., cefotetan and cefoxitin). These enzymes are not inhibited by clavulanic acid. The OXA family β-lactamase (Ambler class D) has higher rates of hydrolysis for oxacillin in contrast to penicillin and also degrades substrates of CTXM. These enzymes are resistant to β-lactamase inhibitors. Plasmid-encoded OXA enzymes have been found in *P. aeruginosa*.[108,168,292]

Laboratory detection of ESBL includes phenotypic and genotypic tests. Phenotypic tests include screening tests by testing for resistance to cefpodoxime (hydrolyzed by all TEM, SHV, and CTXM ESBLs), cefotaxime, ceftazidime, ceftriaxone, and aztreonam. Then a confirmatory step is performed by demonstrating synergy between these agents and clavulanic acid (double-disk synergy test, combination disk method, or ESBL E tests). Genotypic tests consist of polymerase chain reaction amplification of specific genes.[108]

Treatment of ESBL-producing organisms represents a challenge. In vitro sensitivity may not correlate with effective treatment in vivo. Organisms producing TEM and SHV-type ESBL may appear susceptible to cefepime and piperacillin-tazobactam in vitro but may be nonsusceptible when the inoculum is increased to 10^5 to 10^7 organisms. In these circumstances it may be difficult to ensure good concentrations of the antibiotic at the site of the infection (above the MIC). A carbapenem remains the antibiotic of choice for treatment of ESBL-producing organisms. AmpC-producing strains are typically susceptible to carbapenems; however, diminished porin expression can make it a carbapenem-resistant strain. Bacteria expressing IMP, VIM, or OXA-type carbapenemases usually remain susceptible to aztreonam. Care should be taken in selecting the correct antibiotic because resistance to fluoroquinolones and aminoglycosides can occur.[168]

Glycopeptides

Vancomycin

Vancomycin, first isolated from *Amycolatopsis orientalis* (formerly called *Streptomyces,* then *Nocardia*) in soil samples from Borneo, is a high-molecular-weight, complex, soluble glycopeptide.[278] Because of a lack of adequate therapy for penicillinase-producing staphylococci, vancomycin was approved expeditiously by the FDA in 1956 before exhaustive pharmacologic and toxicologic studies had been performed. Original preparations contained fermentation by-products that caused significant toxicity. Once the penicillinase-resistant penicillins were developed, vancomycin use decreased until the emergence of methicillin-resistant staphylococci in the late 1970s.

Mechanisms of action. Vancomycin is slowly bactericidal against most susceptible gram-positive bacteria, except enterococci, for which it is bacteriostatic. It forms complexes with the D-alanyl-D-alanine portion of peptide precursor units and thus prevents polymerization of the phosphodisaccharide pentapeptide lipid complex and cross-linking of peptidoglycan during the second stage of cell wall synthesis. Because the site of action of vancomycin is distinct from that of β-lactam antibiotics, no cross resistance among the drugs and no competitive inhibition exist. Like penicillin, vancomycin exerts its antimicrobial effect on bacteria in the active growth phase. Additionally, vancomycin alters cytoplasmic membrane permeability and impairs RNA synthesis. Animal infection models suggest that the drug exhibits time-dependent bactericidal activity against susceptible organisms, as well as a moderately long in vitro postantibiotic effect. The most important pharmacokinetic and pharmacodynamic parameter that correlates with antimicrobial efficacy is the ratio of the 24-hour AUC to the MIC (24-hour AUC/MIC).[91] A lag phase before the onset of rapid killing has been demonstrated in serum killing studies.[3]

Mechanisms of resistance. Resistance can be categorized into three types: tolerance, acquired resistance, and inherent resistance. Some susceptible gram-positive bacteria, especially enterococci, are tolerant to the bactericidal activity of vancomycin; that is, vancomycin inhibits but does not kill the bacteria (MBC/MIC ratio >32). Staphylococci tolerant to vancomycin can have autolysin deficiencies. Although most resistance to vancomycin by gram-positive bacteria is acquired, three genera of gram-positive organisms are inherently resistant to vancomycin: *Erysipelothrix, Leuconostoc,* and *Pediococcus.* Nine gene clusters currently are known to be associated with vancomycin resistance in enterococci.[145] The *vanA, vanB, vanD,* and *vanM* gene clusters that cause vancomycin resistance by altering the terminal amino acids of peptidoglycan precursors from D-Ala-D-Ala to D-Ala-D-lactate (i.e., high-level resistance), while the *vanC, vanE, vanG, vanL,* and *vanN* gene clusters cause resistance through the formation of D-Ala-D-serine (i.e., low-level resistance).[145] The most clinically relevant vancomycin resistance determinants are *vanA* and *vanB*. The *VanA* gene encodes the VanA phenotype (vancomycin MIC >256 and teicoplanin resistance), which is on a plasmid that is easily transferable by conjugation to other enterococci. The VanB phenotype also is transferable and encodes vancomycin but not teicoplanin resistance. The presence of an inducer such as vancomycin or teicoplanin, another glycopeptide that has not been approved for use in the United States, activates the transcription of genes that encode ligases necessary for resistance to vancomycin. Some enzymes make cell wall precursors ending in D-alanyl-D-lactate located at the end of the pentapeptide side chain, to which vancomycin binds with very low affinity. Other enzymes inhibit or alter the synthesis of endogenous cell wall precursors ending in D-alanyl-D-alanine, to which vancomycin is unable to bind. The finding that vancomycin resistance genes can be transferred experimentally from vancomycin-resistant enterococci (VRE) to staphylococci highlights the potential risk for spread of resistance by means of naturally occurring plasmid or transposon-mediated conjugative systems.[252] Although vancomycin resistance can affect susceptibility to other investigational glycopeptides, no cross resistance exists between vancomycin and other unrelated antibiotics. Resistance to vancomycin rarely develops during appropriate therapy, perhaps because of its multiple mechanisms of action, but prolonged or indiscriminate use of the drug can contribute to selective pressure and result in the development of vancomycin-resistant enterococci colonizing the gut. Of great concern is the emergence of invasive strains of multidrug-resistant enterococci (≤14% of health care–associated enterococcal strains)[226] and staphylococci, for which only a few therapeutic options exist, including linezolid and other antimicrobials not approved for use in children such as quinupristin-dalfopristin, daptomycin, and tigecycline (a novel glycylcycline antibiotic). The first strains of *S. aureus* with intermediate resistance to vancomycin/glycopeptide (VISA/GISA) were detected in the United States in 1997. Soon thereafter, three cases of vancomycin-resistant *S. aureus* were isolated. The mechanism for this high-level vancomycin resistance involves the horizontal transfer of a transposon containing *VanA* and associated genes from vancomycin-resistant enterococci.[294] Glycopeptide-resistant isolates were found to have thicker extracellular matrices, a characteristic that may cause vancomycin to become trapped in the outer layers of the cell wall and may limit access to the cytoplasmic membrane where the functional targets are located. Pneumococci tolerant to vancomycin were described first in 1999.[267] These strains escape lysis and killing by vancomycin because of an alteration in the regulation of autolysin. Their prevalence is 4% to 10% of nasopharyngeal and invasive isolates, and they are associated with increased mortality when etiologic in meningitis.[301] In 2006, the CLSI modified the MIC breakpoints for *S. aureus* to vancomycin: from 4 μg/mL or less to 2 μg/mL or less for "susceptible," from 8 to 16 μg/mL to 4 to 8 μg/mL for "intermediate," and from 32 μg/mL or greater to 16 μg/mL or greater for "resistant." This change was made to increase the detection of heterogeneously resistant isolates and based on clinical data showing less response to vancomycin when the MIC is 4 μg/mL or greater.[343] The CDC recommends that the use of vancomycin be restricted appropriately to reduce the risk for inducing vancomycin resistance.[71]

In Vitro activity. The in vitro spectrum of activity for vancomycin is limited to gram-positive aerobic and anaerobic bacteria, with little, if any, activity against aerobic or anaerobic gram-negative bacilli, except *Chryseobacterium meningosepticum.* Group A streptococci, pneumococci, *Corynebacterium* spp., and *C. difficile* are highly susceptible to vancomycin, whereas *L. monocytogenes,* microaerophilic and anaerobic streptococci, enterococci, coagulase-positive and coagulase-negative staphylococci, *Bacillus anthracis* and other spp., *Lactobacillus, Actinomyces,* and other *Clostridium* spp. have higher MIC values that are still in the susceptible range. Pathogens resistant to vancomycin include *Erysipelothrix* and *Leuconostoc* and *Pediococcus* spp., which can cause serious infections in immunocompromised patients. The bactericidal activity of vancomycin combined with gentamicin has been shown to be synergistic in vitro against strains of enterococci (provided there is no high-level gentamicin resistance; MIC >2000 μg/mL), nonenterococcal group D streptococci, viridans streptococci, and most methicillin-susceptible *S. aureus* and MRSA. Addition of rifampin, gentamicin, or both results in improved cure rates for *S. epidermidis* prosthetic valve endocarditis.[226] Although vancomycin has activity against many gram-positive bacteria, it is not the most active agent for these organisms, but it is the drug of choice for multidrug-resistant bacteria such as methicillin-resistant staphylococci and highly penicillin-resistant and cephalosporin-resistant pneumococci.

Pharmacokinetics. Intravenous administration of vancomycin is preferred because intramuscular injection causes pain and tissue necrosis. Intravenous preparations must be diluted further in normal saline or dextrose solutions before beginning slow infusion. Vancomycin is approximately 55% bound to serum proteins and diffuses well into most body tissues, with adequate concentrations achieved in pericardial, pleural, ascitic, bone, and synovial fluids, but not in aqueous humor or bile. Vancomycin does not diffuse well into CSF in the absence of inflamed meninges, but CSF concentrations of 7% to 21% of concomitant serum levels can be achieved during therapy for meningitis when higher doses (15 mg/kg every 6 hours) are administered. The bone-to-serum ratio of vancomycin is 10%, but this figure increases up to 30% in infected bone. Vancomycin remains active at pH 6.5 to 8, and concentrations achieved in abscess fluid approximate serum levels.[226] Intrathecal or intraventricular administration has been used infrequently for CNS infections that are difficult to eradicate.[225] Vancomycin is not metabolized significantly and is excreted by glomerular filtration. The mean serum elimination half-life in adults with normal renal function is 6 hours. For children, it ranges from 5 to 10 hours in newborns and 4 hours in older infants to 2 to 3 hours in children. In anephric patients, the elimination half-life extends to 7 or more days. Hemodialysis removes small amounts of vancomycin, whereas peritoneal dialysis may reduce serum concentrations by approximately 40%. Nomograms and patient-individualized bayesian dosing regimens have been used for vancomycin dosing in renal failure in adults.[204,243]

Current recommendations for vancomycin monitoring in adult patients include checking trough concentrations rather than peak values as the most accurate method for vigilance over efficacy and toxicity. Trough values should be checked before the fourth dose of the antibiotic (steady state). Minimal concentration should be maintained above 10 μg/mL, and target concentrations of 15 to 20 μg/mL are preferred for complicated infections secondary to *S. aureus* in adults (bacteremia, endocarditis, osteomyelitis, meningitis, and hospital-acquired pneumonia).[216,303]

Indications for use. Because of the potential for development of resistance, vancomycin should be reserved for patients with moderate-to-severe infections caused by vancomycin-susceptible bacteria that are resistant to other antibiotics. Vancomycin can be used for the treatment of infections caused by β-lactam-susceptible and vancomycin-susceptible bacteria in patients with hypersensitivity reactions to β-lactam antimicrobial agents. Empirical therapy for patients with ventricular shunt–related and catheter-associated infections frequently includes vancomycin to provide activity against coagulase-negative staphylococci and MRSA. Vancomycin can be used in combination with gentamicin, rifampin, or both for bactericidal synergistic activity to treat documented prosthetic device–related *S. epidermidis* infections, methicillin-resistant staphylococcal endocarditis, or endocarditis caused by high-level penicillin-resistant, aminoglycoside-susceptible strains of enterococci. *S. epidermidis* infections of long-term intravenous catheters usually can be cured without removal of the device.[226] In addition, vancomycin is the drug of choice in patients with immediate-type hypersensitivity to penicillins and other β-lactam antibiotics for prophylaxis (e.g., in gastrointestinal or genitourinary procedures) or treatment of endocarditis caused by streptococci, enterococci, and staphylococci.[22,369] Empirical treatment of bacterial meningitis suspected or proved to be caused by *S. pneumoniae* in children 1 month of age or older should consist of vancomycin in addition to a third-generation cephalosporin until susceptibility data are available; if cephalosporin resistance is documented, rifampin should be added to the regimen. Vancomycin also is indicated for the treatment of infections with penicillin-resistant streptococci, *C. jeikeium,* and *Bacillus* spp. and penicillin-resistant enterococci, as well as for bacteremia, pneumonia, cellulitis, and osteomyelitis caused by methicillin-resistant staphylococci. Some experts advocate the addition of nafcillin, oxacillin, gentamicin, or rifampin for optimal coverage of oxacillin-susceptible *S. aureus* in severely ill patients who are receiving empirical treatment with vancomycin because certain strains of staphylococci are tolerant to vancomycin.[136] Proof of enhanced efficacy in children with combination therapy in this setting is lacking. Although nonabsorbable oral vancomycin is effective therapy for *C. difficile* colitis, oral metronidazole represents first-line therapy; vancomycin should be given only for metronidazole treatment failures, to limit the development of vancomycin-resistant enterococci. Vancomycin is among the agents of choice for the treatment of meningitis caused by *C. meningosepticum.*

Adverse effects. The purification of vancomycin allegedly decreased the frequency of adverse reactions noted several decades ago. The most common adverse effect is "red man" or "red neck" syndrome or glycopeptide-induced anaphylactoid reaction manifested as flushing of the face and upper part of the trunk, pruritus during vancomycin infusion, angioedema, and, rarely, hypotension. Vancomycin directly causes release of histamine from mast cells by non–immune-mediated mechanisms. Because it is a dose- and rate-dependent reaction, administering doses less than 500 mg, prolonging the infusion period to at least 1 hour, or both decreases the risk for occurrence. Pretreatment with histamine-1-receptor antagonists (i.e., diphenhydramine or hydroxyzine) prevents the development of this reaction, and symptoms usually resolve promptly after discontinuation of the infusion.

Controversy surrounds the issue of vancomycin-induced ototoxicity and nephrotoxicity.[60] Such toxicity has not been demonstrated in experimental animal models. Although numerous cases of toxicity in humans have been reported, the literature is difficult to interpret because of confounding variables, including recent or concurrent use of aminoglycosides or other ototoxic or nephrotoxic agents, lack of identification of antecedent otologic or renal disease, and inconsistencies in sampling methods when measuring serum vancomycin concentrations. Tinnitus and high-tone hearing loss have been associated with the administration of vancomycin, particularly when the peak serum levels exceed 50 μg/mL. If vancomycin is ototoxic, whether toxic peak or toxic trough serum concentrations are responsible is not clear. Several studies suggest an increased risk for nephrotoxicity when aminoglycosides are used concurrently with vancomycin, especially when they are administered in critically ill patients.[132,287] Other adverse effects seen occasionally with the use of vancomycin include reversible neutropenia, thrombocytopenia, drug fever, and macular rash.

The usefulness of serum vancomycin concentration determinations is controversial because a definitive relationship between vancomycin concentration and clinical outcome has not been proved, and several recent studies have suggested that higher vancomycin troughs did not improve outcomes but were associated with increased nephrotoxicity.[26,238] Until the significance of vancomycin serum concentration determinations has been clarified, monitoring has been suggested for the following clinical situations only: (1) patients with altered renal function, including premature infants; (2) patients receiving larger than normal dosages, especially those with meningitis in whom adequate CSF values are necessary; (3) anephric patients undergoing hemodialysis (to avoid subtherapeutic vancomycin concentrations during prolonged dosing intervals); and (4) patients receiving concomitant therapy with nephrotoxic agents.[303] Because serum vancomycin values commonly are subtherapeutic in the first days of treatment for severe sepsis, presumably because of larger volumes of distribution of vancomycin in these ill children, we recommend an initial dosage of 60 mg/kg per day in four divided doses.

Glycopeptides

Telavancin

Other semisynthetic glycopeptides approved for adults include telavancin and dalbavancin. They may have some advantage over vancomycin and daptomycin in that resistance of MRSA is less likely because of their dual mechanisms of action. Telavancin was approved by the FDA in 2009 for treatment of complicated skin and skin structure infections caused by susceptible gram-positive bacteria in adults. It is a lipoglycopeptide that contains a hydrophobic side chain linked to the vancosamine sugar and a hydrophilic group on the 4 position of amino acid

7. The hydrophobic chain provides improved binding activity for D-alanine-D-alanine-containing peptidoglycan intermediates. Its dual mechanism of action includes binding the peptidoglycan precursor at the D-alanine-D-alanine terminus with subsequent inhibition of transglycosylation (peptidoglycan polymerization) and then inhibition of transpeptidation. The second mode of action includes binding to the cell membrane and triggering rapid concentration-dependent dissipation of cell membrane potential with leakage of cytoplasmic adenosine triphosphate (ATP) and potassium loss. Telavancin is active against MSSA, MRSA, GISA, hGISA, coagulase-negative staphylococci, streptococci (including group A and group B β-hemolytic streptococci and *S. pneumoniae*), *Clostridium* spp., and *Actinomyces israelii*. It does not have activity against VRE (both VanA and VanB). It has high level of protein binding (~93%) and small volume of distribution. It is not inactivated by surfactant. Telavancin is mainly eliminated by renal excretion.[313]

Dalbavancin

Dalbavancin is a lipoglycopeptide antibiotic originating from modifications to a teicoplanin-like antibiotic, which is an analogue to vancomycin. Dalbavancin gained FDA approval in 2014 for use in adult patients with acute bacterial skin and skin structure infections. Similar to vancomycin, dalbavancin demonstrates activity against gram-positive pathogens including MRSA, streptococci, and enterococci. However, this agent has a half-life of greater than 1 week, which is an advantageous pharmacokinetic parameter allowing once-weekly dosing.[53,181,325]

Mechanisms of action. Similar to other lipoglycopeptide members of the glycopeptide antimicrobial family, the heptapeptide core of dalbavancin facilitates inhibition of key steps in bacterial cell wall synthesis, namely transglycosylation and transpeptidation.[181,325,376] Modifications to the heptapeptide core result in differences in the spectrum of coverage between lipoglycopeptides and the degree of activity of these agents against select gram-positive organisms. In the case of dalbavancin, increased activity against staphylococci originates from the addition of a basic amide group to the heptapeptide core. Along with modifications of the heptapeptide core, the addition of a lipophilic side chain results in the extended half-life of dalbavancin and also serves to anchor the molecule to the bacterial cell membrane. This anchoring of dalbavancin enhances antimicrobial activity due to increased binding affinity at the site of inhibition, the growing peptidoglycan chain.[376]

In vitro activity. Dalbavancin demonstrates 8- to 16-fold greater in vitro potency against susceptible streptococci and staphylococci when compared to the activity of vancomycin and daptomycin.[177,325] Further, the in vitro potency of dalbavancin against *Staphylococcus aureus* is unaffected by the presence of methicillin resistance amongst isolates [independent of the isolates sensitivity to beta-lactam agents]. Even in those *S. aureus* isolates found to be vancomycin-intermediate (VISA), dalbavancin continues to demonstrate MIC values four- to eightfold lower than those reported for vancomycin.[177] Dalbavancin is active against both vancomycin-susceptible *Enterococcus faecalis* and *faecium* with an MIC of 0.125 μg/mL. While dalbavacin demonstrates in vitro activity against organisms with the VanB resistance gene, it is inactive against those with the VanA resistance gene. Thus, VRE harboring the VanA resistance gene, the majority of VRE isolates in the United States, have much higher dalbavancin MIC values compared to those isolates demonstrating vancomycin-resistance secondary to the presence of the VanB resistance gene.[325] At present, the clinical utility of dalbavancin for treating infections caused by enterococci remains unknown, as only limited in vitro data exist.[181]

Pharmacokinetics. Dalbavancin demonstrates nearly linear pharmacokinetics over a broad dosing range; increases in dosage result in proportional increases in peak plasma concentrations. Similar to other glycopeptides, dalbavancin requires administration intravenously, as oral bioavailability is poor.[376] One unique pharmacokinetic parameter associated with dalbavancin, documented in both adolescent and adult patients, is an elimination half-life of greater than 1 week, allowing for once-weekly dosing.[53,325] The extended half-life of dalbavancin occurs as a result of substantial protein binding (approximately 95%) and intracellular retention.[325,376] Only 33% of dalbavancin is excreted in the urine unchanged; however, hepatic clearance does not appear to play an appreciable role in further drug metabolism.[208,230,325] It remains unknown how the drug is further metabolized. Adult patients with significant renal impairment (CrCl <30 mL/min) have been shown to require dose reductions due to increased AUCs on dalbavancin.[325] However, data from Marbury and colleagues suggest that patients on scheduled hemodialysis do not require dosage adjustment as they have levels of dalbavancin similar to those of patients with normal renal function.[230] Like other glycopeptide antimicrobials, dalbavancin exhibits bactericidal activity against pneumococci and staphylococci, where the pharmacokinetic parameter associated with efficacy is ratio of 24-h AUC to MIC.[13,325] In adult patients, dalbavancin is recommended as a two-dose regimen of 1000 mg in one dose to be followed a week later by a single dose of 500 mg, each administered via a 30-minute infusion.[106]

Indications for use. Dalbavancin has been studied mainly in adult patients with skin and soft tissue infections. Jauregui and colleagues completed one phase III study of dalbavancin, administered as a single intravenous 1000-mg dose on day 1 followed by a 500-mg dose on day 8, versus linezolid, administered as a 600-mg intravenous or oral dose twice daily for 14 days, in adult patients with suspected or confirmed complicated skin and skin structure infections.[170] Patients were randomized in a 2 : 1 ratio to receive either dalbavancin or linezolid. Within this study cohort, *Staphylococcus aureus* was identified as at least one of the organisms causing infection in 89% of patients, with 51% of isolates reported as MRSA. The two-dose regimen of dalbavancin was found to be both well tolerated and as effective as a 14-day course of either oral or intravenous linezolid. Boucher and colleagues also completed a phase III trial in adult patients with acute bacterial skin and skin structure infections who were randomized into one of two arms of the study: dalbavancin, 1 g initially followed by 500 mg on day 8, or vancomycin, 1 g every 12 hours for 3 or more days, with the option to switch to oral linezolid to complete a 10- to 14-day course of therapy. Dalbavancin administered weekly was shown to be equally efficacious both early in therapy and at the end of therapy in individual and pooled analyses when compared to intravenous vancomycin followed by linezolid.[48] In older pediatric patients between 12 and 17 years of age, a phase I study of dalbavancin 1000 mg, the standard adult dose, or 15 mg/kg in those patients weighing less than 60 kg, resulted in similar terminal half-lives and plasma exposures between pediatric weight cohorts.[53] When compared to previous adult studies, the plasma exposure to dalbavancin was found to be slightly lower in pediatric patients. A phase I pharmacokinetics and safety trial is underway to evaluate a single-dose of dalbavancin in pediatric patients 3 months to 11 years of age. In this study, patients greater than 5 years of age received a dalbavancin dose of 15 mg/kg up to a dose of 1000 mg and patients less than 5 years of age received a dose of 25 mg/kg (NCT0194658). Other pediatric dalbavancin studies not yet recruiting participants include (1) a phase I study in neonates and infants up to 3 months of age assessing the safety and tolerability of a single dalbavancin dose of 22.5 mg/kg (NCT02688790) and (2) a phase III study in pediatric patients receiving dalbavancin or comparator agents (i.e., cefazolin, nafcillin, oxacillin, or vancomycin) for the treatment of acute hematogenous osteomyelitis. The dalbavancin dose to be used in this study is 15 mg/kg/dose, not to exceed 1500 mg in patients greater than 12 years of age and 1000 mg in patients less than 12 years of age (NCT02344511).

Adverse effects. Data from multiple trials indicate that dalbavancin is safe and well tolerated, with the majority of adverse events across studies reported as mild. During an initial phase I study of dalbavancin in adult patients, the most commonly reported adverse events included pyrexia, headache, and nausea.[208] A phase I study in 10 pediatric patients also reported adverse events as mild, with the exception of one moderate event reported as headache.[53] Jauregui and colleagues found that gastrointestinal symptoms were the most common adverse events, whereas Boucher and colleagues found that adverse events occurred less frequently in those patients receiving dalbavancin versus the comparator group.[48,170] Although multiple studies involving dalbavancin report a favorable adverse event profile, additional clinical experience with this agent will allow identification of the true rate of adverse events.

Daptomycin

Daptomycin is a cyclic lipopeptide derived from the fermentation of *Streptomyces roseosporus.* It has been approved for treatment of adults with complicated skin and soft tissue infections, endocarditis, and sepsis. It is a parenteral lipopeptide that disrupts cell membrane potential, and, unlike vancomycin, it is rapidly bactericidal against MRSA strains. Daptomycin demonstrates activity secondary to calcium-dependent insertion into the bacterial cell membrane resulting in rapid depolarization. This membrane depolarization results in cell death, without cell lysis, in a concentration-dependent manner. Daptomycin is active against *S. aureus* (including MRSA, MSSA, and GRSA), streptococci, and *Enterococcus* spp. This antibiotic is not effective for the treatment of pneumonia because it is inactivated by surfactant. Daptomycin demonstrates time-independent and nearly linear pharmacokinetics over a broad dosing range; increases in dosage result in proportional increases in the peak plasma concentration and AUC. This agent demonstrates high reversible protein binding, at 92%, and is primarily renally excreted with a half-life of approximately 8 to 9 hours. Renal dose adjustment is recommended with significant renal impairment (CrCl <30 mL/min).[134] Daptomycin is administered once daily. A retrospective review of 16 pediatric cases with invasive gram-positive bacterial infections (MRSA, $n = 14$; MSSA, $n = 1$; and VRE, $n = 1$) showed clinical improvement after the addition of daptomycin to conventional therapy in patients with persistent bacteremia and severe clinical disease.[14] A pharmacokinetic analysis evaluated single-dose daptomycin for children 2 to 6 years of age. A dose of 8 to 10 mg/kg was shown to be well tolerated and reached appropriate systemic exposure, comparable to that in adults receiving doses of 4 to 6 mg/kg.[1] Single-dose pharmacokinetics were also evaluated in young infants, with a postnatal age range of 23 to 40 weeks, using a daptomycin dose of 6 mg/kg. Within this infant cohort, daptomycin was well tolerated with no reported adverse events, and clearance was found to be similar to that reported in children 2 to 6 years of age but faster than observed in adolescents/adults.[84] A retrospective, multicenter review of 46 pediatric patients treated with daptomycin for various gram-positive bacterial infections including sepsis (central venous catheter related, $n = 13$; non–central venous catheter related, $n = 7$), osteomyelitis ($n = 12$), complicated skin and soft tissue infections ($n = 11$), and endocarditis ($n = 3$) found that clinical cure occurred in 56.8%, clinical improvement in 29.6%, and failure in 13.6% of patients. Daptomycin was well tolerated with a median dose and duration of 7 mg/kg per day and 14 days, respectively.[127] Studies focusing on the inverse relationship between age and the required per-kilogram dose of daptomycin in children are ongoing. Side effects of daptomycin reported in adults include prolongation of prothrombin time and myopathy, with elevation of the serum creatinine kinase, which should be monitored weekly during treatment.

Colistin (Colistimethate Sodium: Polymyxin E)

Colistin is a cationic, cyclic polypeptide antibiotic that is structurally and pharmacologically related to polymyxin B. Colistin is less active in vitro and less toxic than is polymyxin B. Colistin was discovered in 1949 and is obtained from cultures of *Bacillus polymyxa* subsp. *colistinus.* The polymyxins have been used extensively for decades in topical ophthalmic and otic solutions. However, because of reports of common and serious nephrotoxicity and neurotoxicity, parenteral use of these drugs was abandoned in the early 1980s, except for treatment of multidrug-resistant, gram-negative bacterial infections in children and adults with cystic fibrosis. The emergence of gram-negative bacteria resistant to most classes of antibiotics and the lack of effective new antimicrobial agents led to the reconsideration of colistin as a valuable therapeutic option. Studies of patients who received intravenous polymyxins for the treatment of serious multidrug-resistant *P. aeruginosa* and *A. baumannii* infections, including pneumonia, bacteremia, and urinary tract infections, led to the conclusion that these antibiotics have acceptable effectiveness and considerably less toxicity than was reported previously.[185]

Mechanisms of Action

Colistimethate sodium is inactive until it is hydrolyzed to sulfomethylated derivatives and colistin, which acts as a cationic detergent with both lipophilic and lipophobic components. It damages the cytoplasmic membrane by displacing calcium and magnesium and binding to anionic lipopolysaccharide molecules, leading to permeability changes in the cell membrane, leakage of osmotically active intracellular metabolites and nucleosides, and cell death. Furthermore, colistin binds and neutralizes the lipid A portion of lipopolysaccharide in vitro; however, the clinical implications of this antiendotoxin activity are unknown.[109]

Mechanisms of Resistance

Gram-negative bacteria can develop resistance to colistin by means of inherited or acquired mechanisms. Inherited mutations occur infrequently and are not influenced by exposure to colistin. Acquired resistance rarely may be induced by prolonged exposure to the drug. Studies of polymyxin-resistant *P. aeruginosa* suggest that the development of resistance arises from modifications of the cell membrane, such as reductions in lipopolysaccharide, certain proteins or lipids, or magnesium or calcium. Currently, no evidence of efflux pump or enzyme-mediated resistance exists. Complete cross resistance occurs between colistin and polymyxin B, but not other antimicrobial agents.

In Vitro Activity

Colistin is highly active against many strains of aerobic gram-negative bacteria, including *Acinetobacter, Citrobacter, E. coli, Enterobacter, H. influenzae, Klebsiella, Morganella morganii, P. aeruginosa, Salmonella, Shigella,* and variable numbers of *Stenotrophomonas* strains. However, the antibiotic is inactive against most strains of *Brucella, Burkholderia cepacia, Edwardsiella, Proteus, Providencia, Serratia,* gram-negative cocci, gram-positive bacteria, and anaerobic bacteria. The CLSI defined bacterial resistance to colistin as an MIC of 4 μg/mL or greater. However, the sulfate form of colistin, which usually is used for in vitro testing, often is fourfold to eightfold more active than the sulfomethyl form, which is used in the parenteral formulation. Limited in vitro and clinical data suggest that synergism exists with colistin and other antimicrobial agents such as aminoglycosides, antipseudomonal β-lactams, fluoroquinolones, rifampin, and TMP-SMX.[109,185]

Pharmacokinetics

The pharmacologic evaluation of the polymyxins was performed decades ago. Consequently, pharmacokinetic and pharmacodynamic information is limited. Colistin is not absorbed from the gastrointestinal tract and must be given parenterally. The drug is distributed widely in the body, except for bones and synovial, pleural, and pericardial fluids. In a reported case of multidrug-resistant *A. baumannii* meningitis in an adolescent, parenterally administered colistin achieved a concentration in the CSF that was 25% of the serum concentration, and it cured the infection.[172] More than 50% of the agent binds to serum proteins. Colistimethate sodium and its metabolites are excreted mainly by the kidneys through glomerular filtration. Therefore, the dosage and frequency of administration should be decreased in children with renal impairment. Colistin is rapidly bactericidal against susceptible bacteria in a concentration-dependent manner, and it has a postantibiotic effect.[109,185] Considering these pharmacologic parameters, there may be a theoretical benefit in administering colistin less frequently with higher doses, but no clinical data validate this hypothesis.

Indications for Use

Colistin has been administered intravenously to infants and children of all ages for the treatment of acute or chronic infections caused by susceptible gram-negative organisms, particularly multidrug-resistant strains of *Pseudomonas* and *Acinetobacter* in patients with cystic fibrosis or complicated health care–associated infections. Colistin should be reserved for use when other more effective and less toxic antimicrobial agents are contraindicated or ineffective. The dosage of colistimethate sodium is expressed in terms of colistin. The usual parenteral dosage for adults and children with normal renal function is 2.5 to 5 mg/kg (75,000 to 150,000 IU/kg)/day divided into two to four doses, depending on the severity of infection (maximum, 300 mg/day). Intramuscular administration is not recommended because it causes severe pain at the injection site. Experience with the use of colistimethate sodium administered by nebulization for multidrug-resistant, gram-negative respiratory infections in patients with cystic fibrosis is extensive. Successful use of colistimethate sodium by the intraventricular route also has been reported. Colistin sulfate in combination with neomycin sulfate and hydrocortisone acetate is available in the United States for otic use. Colistin sulfate for oral administration no longer is available in the United States. Polymyxin B sulfate is available for topical use.[109]

Adverse Effects

Nephrotoxicity and neurotoxicity are the most serious adverse effects and occur most frequently when the drug is administered in higher than recommended doses, in patients with renal insufficiency, or in combination with other nephrotoxic agents. Progressive azotemia or acute tubular necrosis may occur, but renal dysfunction usually is reversible when the antibiotic is discontinued. Renal function should be monitored closely during therapy, and colistin should be discontinued immediately if urine output diminishes or concentrations of blood urea nitrogen or creatinine increase. Transient effects on the nervous system may occur, including dizziness, weakness, paresthesia, numbness, vertigo, ataxia, blurred vision, and slurred speech, but these symptoms are reversible and may be alleviated by reducing the dosage of colistin. Coma, psychosis, seizures, and noncompetitive neuromuscular blockade causing apnea also have been reported and warrant prompt discontinuation of the drug.

AGENTS THAT TARGET PROTEIN SYNTHESIS

Aminoglycosides

Aminoglycosides are natural and semisynthetic compounds that consist of at least two amino sugars bound by a glycosidic linkage to a hexose nucleus, the aminocyclitol ring. Streptomycin, isolated from *Streptomyces griseus,* was the first aminoglycoside and was available for use in 1944. Many aminoglycosides have been isolated or developed since that time. The suffix denotes the origin of the aminoglycoside—those ending with the suffix *mycin* were derived from *Streptomyces* spp., whereas those ending with *micin* were derived from *Micromonospora* spp. Currently, seven aminoglycosides are available for use in the United States (Table 236.3), and several more are available in other countries. Despite the development of less toxic antibiotics with broad-spectrum activity, aminoglycosides continue to fulfill an essential role in the treatment of severe infections caused by aerobic gram-negative bacilli and enterococci.

Mechanisms of Action

Against susceptible bacteria, aminoglycosides demonstrate rapid, concentration-dependent bactericidal activity.[105,357] They exert their effect by binding irreversibly to the 30S subunit of the bacterial ribosome, which results in inhibition of protein synthesis and induction of translational errors. Bacterial uptake of aminoglycosides can be facilitated by concomitant therapy with cell wall–active antibiotics such as β-lactams or vancomycin. Penetration of the outer membrane of gram-negative bacteria is mediated by a self-promoted uptake process involving aminoglycoside-induced disruption of magnesium bridges between adjacent lipopolysaccharide molecules. Passage through porin channels is unlikely because of the large size of aminoglycosides. Subsequent transport into cytoplasm and attachment to the 30S ribosomal subunit require two energy- and oxygen-dependent steps, energy-dependent phases I and II (EDPI and EDPII), that use an electrochemical proton gradient. EDPI is inhibited by hyperosmolarity, low pH, and anaerobic conditions. Unlike other protein synthesis inhibitors, which usually are bacteriostatic, aminoglycosides are bactericidal. Binding of aminoglycosides to the 30S subunit does not prevent formation of the initiation complex of peptide synthesis. However, it disrupts elongation of the peptide chain by impairing the proofreading process, an impairment that results in translational inaccuracy. Aberrant protein products may be inserted in the cell membrane and cause altered permeability. The primed amino sugar and 2-deoxystreptamine groups are essential for the ribosome-specific activity of aminoglycosides.[240]

TABLE 236.3 Classification Scheme for Aminoglycosides

Aminocyclitol Ring	Family	Member
Streptidine	Streptomycin	Streptomycin
2-Deoxystreptamine	Kanamycin	Kanamycin
		Amikacin
		Tobramycin
2-Deoxystreptamine	Gentamicin	Gentamicin
2-Deoxystreptamine	Neomycin	Neomycin
		Paromomycin

Mechanisms of Resistance

The prevalence of acquired aminoglycoside resistance is relatively low, and its development during therapy is an unusual event. Bacteria can acquire resistance to aminoglycosides because of alterations in the bacterial target, reduced bacterial cell permeability or uptake, or modification of the antibiotic by bacterial enzymes, the last being most significant clinically.[96] Mutations in the aminoglycoside-binding site of the 30S ribosome have been associated with high-level resistance to streptomycin but not to other aminoglycosides, possibly because, unlike in streptomycin, they bind to multiple sites on the ribosome. Facultative aerobic bacteria causing infection in sites with reduced oxygen tension, anaerobic bacteria, and such fermentative bacteria as streptococci are inherently resistant to aminoglycosides because they are unable to generate an electrochemical proton gradient sufficient for aminoglycoside transport into the cytoplasm. Other bacteria can acquire resistance because of reduced permeability or lack of transport, as demonstrated in staphylococci, in which resistance to aminoglycosides quickly develops when monotherapy is administered. *P. aeruginosa,* other nonfermenting gram-negative bacilli, and, less frequently, members of the Enterobacteriaceae can acquire a moderate level of resistance to all aminoglycosides as a result of various mechanisms that interfere with uptake, cytoplasmic transport, or regulation of the anaerobic respiratory pathway. Plasmid-mediated production of aminoglycoside-modifying enzymes is the most common mechanism of acquired resistance. Many enzymes have different substrate specificities, several of which can be elaborated simultaneously in the same bacterium. These acetyltransferases, nucleotidyltransferases, and phosphotransferases interact with amino or hydroxyl groups on the aminoglycoside and modify the aminoglycoside so that it binds poorly to the 30S ribosome, thereby usually resulting in high-level resistance.[240] Gentamicin and tobramycin are each susceptible to at least five modifying enzymes, whereas amikacin possesses an aminohydroxybutyryl group that prevents enzymatic modification at multiple sites. Consequently, more than 80% of gentamicin-resistant strains of Enterobacteriaceae and 25% to 85% of gentamicin-resistant *P. aeruginosa* strains are susceptible to amikacin.[199]

In Vitro Activity

The in vitro antibacterial spectrum of aminoglycosides includes a wide range of aerobic gram-negative bacilli, many oxacillin-susceptible staphylococci, many enterococci, and some mycobacteria.[242] Some gram-negative bacilli, including *B. cepacia* and *S. maltophilia,* are consistently resistant to all aminoglycosides. The spectra of activity of gentamicin and tobramycin are similar, and strains resistant to one usually are resistant to the other. The major advantage of tobramycin currently is its activity against some strains of *Acinetobacter* and indole-positive Proteae (*Morganella* spp., *Proteus* spp., *Providencia* spp.) that are resistant to gentamicin.[293] Because many aminoglycoside-modifying enzymes are active against gentamicin and tobramycin but inactive against amikacin, amikacin frequently is prescribed for empirical treatment of nosocomial gram-negative bacillary infections. Amikacin also has activity against the *Mycobacterium avium* complex (MAC), some rapidly growing mycobacteria, and *Nocardia asteroides.* Although gentamicin, tobramycin, and amikacin have similar spectra of activity, susceptibility testing is recommended because of geographic and interhospital variation in resistance patterns. Lack of activity against *P. aeruginosa, Klebsiella,* and *Serratia* has limited the use of kanamycin, which is no longer available in the United States. Streptomycin is inactive against many gram-negative enteric bacilli but does have activity against *Francisella tularensis, Yersinia pestis,* and *Mycobacterium tuberculosis.*

Pharmacokinetics

Aminoglycosides have in common many pharmacokinetic characteristics. They are highly polar, water-soluble compounds that are positively charged cations at neutral pH. Their antibacterial activity is pH dependent, with increased activity at higher pH. They are relatively resistant to degradation at various temperatures and pH values. After parenteral administration, aminoglycosides are distributed rapidly in extracellular body water, with slow accumulation in tissues. The volume of distribution is decreased (with respect to total body weight) in obese patients and is increased in patients with illnesses associated with edema, such as severe infections, burns, congestive heart failure, and ascites. With the exception of proximal renal tubular cells and possibly inner ear hair cells, penetration into other body compartments is impaired because of lipid insolubility, polycationic charge, and size of the aminoglycoside. Proximal renal tubular cells absorb aminoglycosides through carrier-mediated pinocytosis, and, as a result, renal cortical concentrations exceed those in plasma. Aminoglycosides do not penetrate the blood-brain barrier in the absence of meningeal inflammation, but with inflammation, approximately 20% to 25% of the serum concentration penetrates the CSF. These CSF concentrations are low in relation to the MIC of the meningeal pathogen for which it is given. Thus, because of this narrow therapeutic-toxic index, monotherapy for gram-negative bacillary meningitis with aminoglycosides is not recommended. Aminoglycosides are not metabolized and, after parenteral administration, are excreted unchanged in the kidney by glomerular filtration, with approximately 5% of excreted drug reabsorbed in the proximal tubular cells. Minimal amounts are excreted in saliva and feces. Urine concentrations exceed those in plasma by 25 to 100 times.

After intramuscular injection, aminoglycosides are absorbed completely, and peak serum concentrations are achieved within 90 minutes, except in some disease states that interfere with tissue perfusion, such as hypotension. When administered intravenously, the infusion should be given slowly over the course of 30 to 60 minutes to avoid the development of potential adverse effects. Peak serum concentrations are achieved within 30 to 60 minutes after infusion. Because of the polar nature of these drugs, absorption after oral administration is insignificant and inadequate to treat systemic infections, but aminoglycosides can accumulate in the presence of renal failure and result in concentrations sufficient to cause toxicity. Although aminoglycosides are nonirritating when they are instilled into pleural or peritoneal spaces, their absorption is rapid and can result in significant toxicity. In contrast, instillation into the lateral ventricles or irrigation of the bladder has not been associated with significant systemic absorption. In contrast to parenteral administration, aerosol administration of aminoglycoside results in higher concentrations in bronchial secretions and less toxicity.[289] Indiscriminate use of topical aminoglycosides in the form of ointments, creams, or ophthalmic solutions may lead to the rapid development of aminoglycoside resistance, especially in immunocompromised patients.

Antimicrobial dosing in newborns and young infants differs from that in older children and adults because of developmental changes in renal function and increased total body water composition. Neonates and young infants have a larger volume of distribution and a reduced glomerular filtration rate; these differences are more pronounced in premature neonates with very low birth weight.[282] Therefore, once- to twice-daily regimens have been the standard of care in newborn infants for years. Once-daily gentamicin dosing of 4 mg/kg in term neonates has been studied extensively and is used routinely in many nurseries; no differences in effectiveness or toxicity have been observed.[357] The aminoglycoside dosing schedule currently approved for use in older infants and children is a three-times-daily regimen. Because aminoglycosides demonstrate concentration-dependent bactericidal activity, higher peak serum concentrations result in more extensive and more rapid killing.[357] Aminoglycosides also demonstrate a postantibiotic effect against susceptible aerobic gram-negative bacilli in vitro and in vivo.[378] Furthermore, host leukocytes display enhanced phagocytosis of aminoglycoside-exposed bacteria in vitro, referred to as *postantibiotic leukocyte enhancement*.[117] The higher the peak serum concentration, the longer the duration of the postantibiotic effect. In the presence of normal renal function, the serum concentration is low or undetectable before the administration of the next dose (trough value), but antibacterial activity persists because of the postantibiotic effect. These characteristics favor single-daily dosing. Numerous studies in adults have shown that once-daily dosing of aminoglycosides (i.e., amikacin, gentamicin, or tobramycin) is either equivalent or superior to multiple-daily dosing with regard to clinical and bacteriologic effectiveness, nephrotoxicity, ototoxicity, mortality, and cost effectiveness.[357] The Hartford nomogram originally described by investigators from Hartford, Connecticut, commonly is used to guide extended-interval aminoglycoside dosing for adults. In adults, a single serum concentration of gentamicin or tobramycin is obtained 8 to 12 hours after the start of the infusion of the first dose and plotted on the nomogram to determine the appropriate dosing interval.[122] Similar nomograms for children have not been validated. Nonetheless, published guidelines support 7.5 mg/kg per dose of gentamicin for infants and children up to 10 years of age; for adolescents and adults, 6 to 7 mg/kg per dose is appropriate.[88,357] Extended-interval aminoglycoside dosing is contraindicated if the patient's volume status is altered (e.g., third spacing, thermal injury >20% total body surface area), if optimal dosing regimen is predefined (e.g., in cystic fibrosis and endocarditis), if renal function is impaired, or if immune status is compromised.

Indications for Use

The major use of aminoglycosides in children (usually in combination with other antibacterial agents) is for serious infections caused by gram-negative enteric bacilli, including neonatal sepsis, sepsis in a child with malignant disease or an immunologic defect, abdominal and systemic infections associated with spillage of fecal contents into the peritoneum, endocarditis caused by certain susceptible bacteria, and complicated urinary tract infections. Because gentamicin is the least expensive aminoglycoside and the one with which physicians have the most experience, it often is considered the first-line agent for empirical treatment of suspected aerobic gram-negative bacillary infections in institutions with minimal background resistance. Combinations of an aminoglycoside and a cell wall–active antibiotic have been used for synergistic bactericidal activity. Gentamicin or streptomycin, in combination with penicillin G, ampicillin, or vancomycin, is recommended for the treatment of endocarditis caused by susceptible enterococci, viridans streptococci, or *Streptococcus bovis.* Administration of gentamicin for 3 to 5 days, in combination with an antistaphylococcal agent, should be considered for the treatment of staphylococcal endocarditis.[22] An aminoglycoside combined with an acylureidopenicillin, ceftazidime, cefepime, or a carbapenem may be considered for serious infections suspected to be caused by *P. aeruginosa* or other gram-negative pathogens pending susceptibility data. Amikacin often is used for empirical treatment of nosocomial aerobic, gram-negative bacillary infections in patients in institutions having significant resistance to gentamicin and tobramycin. Streptomycin is indicated for use alone or in combination with other antibiotics for the treatment of tularemia and plague and in combination with other agents for the treatment of tuberculosis, brucellosis, and enterococcal endocarditis. For such purposes, gentamicin could be a more suitable agent for some of these conditions, such as brucellosis, tularemia, and plague. Paromomycin is too toxic for parenteral use, but when administered orally, it has been useful in the treatment of asymptomatic intestinal amebiasis, *Dientamoeba fragilis* infection, and *Giardia lamblia* infection during pregnancy. Tobramycin inhalation solution is approved by the FDA for twice-daily dosing in patients with cystic fibrosis.

Adverse Effects

Although aminoglycosides have intrinsic toxicity, allergic reactions are uncommon. All aminoglycosides can injure the proximal renal tubules, the cochlea, the vestibular apparatus, or a combination thereof and can cause neuromuscular blockade, but the risk varies with each agent. Because aminoglycosides do not induce a significant inflammatory response, pain at intramuscular injection sites and phlebitis at intravenous infusion sites are unusual. Hypersensitivity reactions and drug fever are rare events.

Many theories have been postulated regarding the mechanism of nephrotoxicity,[241] including inhibition of lysosomal phospholipases within the proximal renal tubules. Clinical findings include a mild, nonoliguric decrease in the glomerular filtration rate that typically is reversible. In contrast to traditional dosing, once-daily dosing causes similar or lower rates of nephrotoxicity.[88,357] In humans, nephrotoxicity has been associated with prolonged duration of therapy at high dosages, previous aminoglycoside therapy, administration of drugs to critically ill patients with intravascular volume depletion or hyponatremia and to those with impaired kidney function, and concomitant administration of other potentially nephrotoxic agents such as amphotericin B and loop diuretics.[98]

The mechanism by which aminoglycosides cause vestibular and cochlear ototoxicity has not been elucidated fully. Cochlear damage is manifested as tinnitus or high-frequency hearing loss, whereas vestibular toxicity is associated with vertigo, nystagmus, and ataxia.[18] Damage can be unilateral or bilateral. Occasionally, the ototoxicity is reversible, but permanent damage occurs commonly. Mild cochlear damage may not be recognized because the high-frequency hearing range is affected first. Conventional audiograms that do not test high-frequency ranges may not detect cochlear injury. Delayed onset of high-frequency hearing loss has been observed in humans. Factors that increase the risk for development of aminoglycoside ototoxicity in humans include impaired renal function and prolonged duration of treatment. Neuromuscular blockade can occur after rapid intravenous infusion, after extensive peritoneal irrigation, or during routine parenteral aminoglycoside administration in patients with underlying conditions that affect the neuromuscular junction, such as myasthenia gravis and botulism, or during concomitant administration of agents that act on the neuromuscular junction, such as succinylcholine. Hypomagnesemia in the neonate may predispose to hearing loss.

To avoid toxicity and ensure therapeutic values, concentrations of aminoglycosides in serum should be monitored in all patients who have impaired renal function or who receive other nephrotoxic medications or prolonged treatment; such monitoring is particularly relevant to preterm, low-birth-weight infants. Monitoring also should be considered in obese and undernourished children, children with severe burns, and those with chronic disease, for which the volume of distribution of the drug can be altered (e.g., cystic fibrosis).

Macrolides

Erythromycin, isolated from *Streptomyces erythreus* found in a soil sample in the Philippines, was the first macrolide and was available for use in 1952. Many natural and semisynthetic erythromycin derivatives have been developed since then, three of which are approved for use in pediatrics: erythromycin, clarithromycin, and azithromycin. Macrolide antibiotics consist of a large lactone ring attached by a glycosidic bond to one or more amino or neutral sugar moieties. Erythromycin and clarithromycin have 14-member lactone rings, whereas azithromycin, an azalide antibiotic that is grouped with the macrolides, has a tertiary amino group inserted in its 15-member ring. In addition to similarities in chemical structure, these macrolides have similar antibacterial spectra, mechanisms of action, and mechanisms of resistance, but they differ in their pharmacokinetic characteristics. Ketolides are a new class of macrolides with in vitro activity against macrolide-resistant gram-positive organisms, including *S. pneumoniae.* Telithromycin received FDA approval in 2004 for use in adults, but use is limited to mild-to-moderate community-acquired pneumonia after increasing reports of hepatotoxicity.[384]

Mechanisms of Action

Macrolide antibiotics reversibly bind to the 50S ribosomal subunit and inhibit protein synthesis. Initial studies suggested that the antibacterial activity of erythromycin usually was bacteriostatic, but against some actively growing, susceptible bacteria, large concentrations of erythromycin were bactericidal.[146] Clarithromycin and azithromycin usually are bacteriostatic, but they are bactericidal against *S. pyogenes, S. pneumoniae,* and *H. influenzae.*[385] Macrolides cause dissociation of peptidyl-tRNA from bacterial ribosomes, which results in accumulation of intracellular peptidyl-tRNA and depletion of the free tRNA pool, with toxic effects for bacteria.[344] The specific target appears to be the 23S ribosomal RNA. Macrolides block the entrance to the tunnel in the 50S ribosomal subunit through which many, if not all, nascent peptide chains exit the ribosome. By blocking the exit tunnel, macrolides induce premature dissociation of peptidyl-tRNAs from the ribosome just after initiation of protein synthesis. Erythromycin interferes with binding to the 50S ribosome by chloramphenicol and clindamycin, thus suggesting common or overlapping binding sites for these agents.

Mechanisms of Resistance

Many gram-negative bacteria are inherently resistant to macrolides because of the relative impermeability of their outer membrane. Other bacteria can acquire resistance by production of enzymes that modify and inactivate the macrolide, active efflux of the antibiotic, and alteration of their ribosomal targets.[206] Two mechanisms by which bacteria can alter their ribosomes and acquire macrolide resistance have been identified. High-level resistance because of an altered protein component in domain V of the 50S ribosomal subunit has occurred after a one-step chromosomal mutation. Such resistance has been demonstrated in *M. avium, Helicobacter pylori, Treponema pallidum,* and *Propionibacterium* spp. Plasmid-mediated macrolide, lincosamide, and streptogramin B (MLS_B) resistance occurs when a single adenine residue within a conserved region of domain V of the nascent 23S rRNA component of the 50S ribosomal subunit is methylated. Such methylation results in an altered common target that confers cross resistance to macrolides (i.e., erythromycin and clarithromycin), azalides (i.e., azithromycin), lincosamides (i.e., clindamycin), and streptogramin B (i.e., quinupristin-dalfopristin).[206] The production of methylases is encoded by a class of genes referred to as *erm* (erythromycin ribosome methylation), approximately 40 of which have been characterized in a wide range of microorganisms, including gram-positive species, spirochetes, and anaerobes. Twenty-one classes of *erm* genes with less than 80% sequence homology have been designated unique letters. Pathogenic bacteria are one of four major classes: bacteria in classes erm(A) and erm(C) typically are in methicillin-resistant or methicillin-susceptible strains of staphylococci, respectively; members of class erm(B) are mostly in streptococci and enterococci; and class erm(F) usually is associated with anaerobic pathogens.[299] These genes are exchanged easily among different strains by plasmids, transposons, or bacterial conjugation. Resistance mediated by erm can be constitutive or inducible. When bacteria with inducible MLS_B resistance are exposed to a macrolide inducer (i.e., erythromycin, clarithromycin, or azithromycin), inactive methylase mRNA undergoes rearrangements that permit ribosomes to translate the methylase coding sequence. The diversity of inducible macrolide-resistant genotypes results in complex phenotypes, particularly among streptococci and enterococci with *erm(B)* genes, whereas constitutive production of a methylase generally confers a predictable high-level cross resistance to all MLS_B antibiotics. Staphylococci that are resistant in vitro to 14- and 15-membered ring macrolides but susceptible to 16-membered ring macrolides, clindamycin, and streptogramins B should routinely undergo further testing with a double-disk diffusion test to screen for an erythromycin-induced, "D"-shaped zone of bacterial inhibition around a clindamycin disk. A positive D-test indicates that the *Staphylococcus* isolate has inducible MLS_B resistance and that use of clindamycin can result in clinical treatment failure, presumably related to selection of constitutive mutants in patients with severe infections and large bacterial inocula.[206] Similar inducible resistance phenotypes may be observed among various strains of streptococci for which the use of clindamycin should be discouraged.

Macrolide resistance associated with active efflux is caused by two classes of pumps: a plasmid-mediated, ATP-binding cassette (ABC) transporter encoded by the *msr(A)* gene and found in *Staphylococcus* spp., and a protein of the major facilitator superfamily found in streptococci and enterococci and encoded by the *mef(A)* gene. The MsrA pump confers a macrolide and streptogramin B (MS_B) pattern of resistance that can be distinguished from the MLS_B-inducible phenotype by the double-disk diffusion D-test. The Mef(A) pump affects only 14- and 15-membered ring macrolides (M phenotype).[206] Less commonly, bacteria produce enzymes that inactivate macrolides, including acetyltransferases, esterases, phosphotransferases, or glycosylases found in some strains of Enterobacteriaceae, but macrolides are not used to target these pathogens. Therefore, this mechanism of low-level resistance is not clinically important.[299] A causal association between erythromycin resistance and antibiotic use, probably mediated by selection pressure, was suggested by a nationwide epidemiologic study in Finland in which reduction of the use of erythromycin over the course of time was associated with a steady decline in erythromycin resistance among *S. pyogenes* isolates from throat swabs and pus specimens.[321] Conversely, increased consumption of macrolides in Spain since 1995 was related to an increase in macrolide resistance.[137] Pneumococcal resistance to macrolides has also increased to about 35% as reported in prospective multicenter monitoring studies. In the United States, 6% of the macrolide-resistant isolates exhibited low-level erythromycin resistance by expression of the *mef(A)* gene and about 20% expressed the *mef(A)* and the *erm(B)* gene, resulting in high-level resistance.[171,384]

In Vitro Activity

Erythromycin is effective in vitro against a diverse group of microorganisms, including *Bacteroides* spp., *Bordetella pertussis, Chlamydophila* spp., *Corynebacterium diphtheriae, H. pylori,* the bacterium of Legionnaires disease *(Legionella pneumophila),* mycoplasmas (*Mycoplasma pneumoniae* and *Ureaplasma urealyticum*), spirochetes *(T. pallidum),* and anaerobic and aerobic gram-positive cocci (*S. pneumoniae, S. pyogenes,* and penicillinase-producing and non–penicillinase-producing strains of oxacillin-susceptible *S. aureus*). Erythromycin is active against *Campylobacter jejuni, N. meningitidis, N. gonorrhoeae,* and, to a lesser extent, *H. influenzae.* Macrolide resistance among diverse pathogens is increasing worldwide, and the clinical consequences are topics of active research.[128,166,197]

The newer macrolides have spectra of activity similar to that of erythromycin. In contrast to erythromycin, clarithromycin has equivalent or greater activity against *M. catarrhalis, H. influenzae, M. pneumoniae, Chlamydia pneumoniae, Chlamydia trachomatis, L. pneumophila, U. urealyticum,* and *N. gonorrhoeae.* Clarithromycin is two to four times more active against most erythromycin-susceptible streptococci and staphylococci. However, pneumococci that are resistant to erythromycin (≤48% in certain regions[195]) also are resistant to clarithromycin and azithromycin; rates of macrolide resistance among pneumococci tend to correlate with rates of penicillin resistance.[385] Clarithromycin also has activity against organisms that are resistant to erythromycin, including *H. pylori, Toxoplasma gondii, Mycobacterium leprae,* MAC, and *Mycobacterium chelonae.*

In contrast to erythromycin, azithromycin has less activity against gram-positive bacteria, including *S. pneumoniae,* but has better activity against gram-negative bacteria, including *Vibrio cholerae* and some Enterobacteriaceae such as *Shigella* spp. The in vitro activity of azithromycin against *M. pneumoniae, C. pneumoniae,* and *L. pneumophila* is similar to that of erythromycin and clarithromycin. Azithromycin is more active than erythromycin against *C. trachomatis* and *U. urealyticum* and twofold to eightfold more active than erythromycin or clarithromycin against *M. catarrhalis, H. influenzae,*[23,237] *N. gonorrhoeae,* and *H. ducreyi.* Azithromycin has activity against *T. gondii* and, although less than that of clarithromycin, against MAC organisms. Azithromycin and clarithromycin are highly effective in vitro against *Borrelia burgdorferi, Bartonella henselae,* and *Bartonella quintana.*

Pharmacokinetics

The macrolides differ in pharmacokinetic properties. Clarithromycin[144] and azithromycin[135] are gastric acid stable and relatively well absorbed from the gastrointestinal tract, whereas erythromycin is acid labile and absorption varies with the oral preparation. Macrolides undergo metabolism by the hepatic microsomal cytochrome P450 (CYP450) system. Erythromycin and clarithromycin, but not azithromycin, are inhibitors of the CYP450 enzyme system (CYP3A and CYP1A subclasses) and can interact with other drugs that are metabolized by this system.[271] Most of the metabolites are inactive, with the exception of 14-(*R*)-hydroxyclarithromycin, an active metabolite that can act additively or synergistically with clarithromycin. The lipophilic macrolides are distributed well in tissues and fluids, except CSF. High intracellular concentrations are achieved, but, with the exception of azithromycin, the macrolides rapidly diffuse out of cells when extracellular concentrations are low. Clarithromycin and azithromycin are transported actively into leukocytes and macrophages. High concentrations of clarithromycin are present in the nasal mucosa, tonsils, and pulmonary epithelial lining fluid and alveolar cells.[87] Tissue concentrations of clarithromycin and azithromycin exceed those found in plasma by 2 to 20 times and 10 to 100 times, respectively. The favorable cellular penetration probably contributes to the efficacy of clarithromycin and azithromycin in the treatment of intracellular pathogens. Furthermore, sustained intracellular concentrations of azithromycin facilitate short-course therapy for pharyngitis and acute otitis media and single-dose therapy for chlamydial STDs.[135] Isolated cases of intravascular bacterial infections developing during macrolide therapy for focal infections have been reported and evoke concern that, despite elevated tissue concentrations, low serum concentrations may not treat systemic infections consistently.[197] Erythromycin and azithromycin are eliminated primarily by biliary excretion, whereas clarithromycin is excreted predominantly by the kidneys. A reduction in the dosage of clarithromycin may be required in patients with moderate-to-severe renal insufficiency. Because of their longer serum half-life, azithromycin and clarithromycin can be administered in a once- and twice-daily regimen, respectively, in contrast to the three- or four-times-daily dosing necessary for erythromycin.

Because erythromycin base is unstable at the low pH of the stomach, better-absorbed products were prepared by the addition of protective enteric coating or by alteration of the chemical structure through the formation of salts and esters. Salt and ester derivatives include ethylsuccinate or propionate (esters), stearate (a salt), and estolate (salt of an ester). Estolate provides the highest concentration of antimicrobial activity in serum, but controversy continues about which preparation provides the most biologically active drug at the site of infection. Because the base is the active component, all erythromycin preparations must be hydrolyzed to the base after absorption. Formulations of erythromycin base include tablets, delayed-release tablets, and capsules. Erythromycin estolate is marketed in capsule form, suspension, and tablets. Erythromycin ethylsuccinate is available in suspension, tablets, and chewable tablets. Erythromycin stearate is in tablet form only in the United States. Parenteral preparations of erythromycin include the lactobionate and gluceptate derivatives. Intramuscular administration of these forms is painful and should be avoided. Clarithromycin can be taken without regard to food, whereas azithromycin should be taken at least 1 hour before or 2 hours after a meal. Clarithromycin is available in suspension (125 and 250 mg/5 mL) and in tablet (250 and 500 mg) forms. Azithromycin is manufactured in 250-mg tablets and as a suspension (100 and 200 mg/5 mL). Azithromycin for intravenous injection has not been approved for use in children younger than the age of 16 years, although pharmacokinetic data are available.[167]

Indications for Use

Erythromycin is approved for the treatment of chlamydial conjunctivitis, pneumonia and urethritis, mycoplasmal and *Legionella* pneumonia, group A streptococcal sinusitis and pharyngitis, mild pneumococcal pneumonia, uncomplicated skin and soft tissue infections caused by susceptible organisms, diphtheria, pertussis, erythrasma, listeriosis, and nongonococcal urethritis and as second-line therapy for gonococcal urethritis. It also is approved for use as a preoperative bowel preparation, for penicillin-allergic persons as prophylaxis for bacterial endocarditis and rheumatic fever, and for the treatment of syphilis in nonpregnant individuals. In the context of increasing prevalence of erythromycin resistance among common pathogens, newer macrolides or other classes of antibacterial agents may be more effective for certain infections.

Clarithromycin is approved for treatment of bacterial exacerbations of bronchitis; streptococcal pharyngitis; mycoplasmal, chlamydial, and pneumococcal community-acquired pneumonia; acute maxillary sinusitis; and uncomplicated skin and soft tissue infections caused by susceptible bacteria. However, increasing rates of clarithromycin resistance among common pathogens of the respiratory tract and skin structures have been associated with treatment failure.[123,166] Clarithromycin and amoxicillin or metronidazole in combination with bismuth compounds, H_2-receptor antagonists, or proton pump inhibitors is recommended for the treatment of *H. pylori*–associated peptic ulcer disease. Clarithromycin also is approved for prophylaxis of disseminated MAC infections in children and adults with advanced human immunodeficiency virus (HIV) infection. Furthermore, clarithromycin, in combination with other antimycobacterials, is an effective therapeutic agent for disseminated MAC infections, but safety has not been established for this indication in children younger than 20 months of age. The safety and efficacy of clarithromycin have not been established for infants younger than 6 months of age.

In adults, azithromycin is approved for treatment of bacterial exacerbations of bronchitis; chlamydial and gonococcal cervicitis and urethritis; chancroid; streptococcal tonsillitis and pharyngitis; uncomplicated skin and soft tissue infections caused by susceptible bacteria; and acute otitis media and pneumonia caused by *H. influenzae, M. catarrhalis,* and *S. pneumoniae.* It also is approved in adults for prophylaxis of disseminated MAC infection in patients with advanced HIV infection. Pediatric indications include group A streptococcal pharyngitis; acute otitis media caused by *H. influenzae, M. catarrhalis,* and *S. pneumoniae;* and mild community-acquired pneumonia caused by *S. pneumoniae, H. influenzae, M. pneumoniae,* or *C. pneumoniae.*

Five-day regimens have been approved for the treatment of pharyngitis (single dose of 12 mg/kg per day followed by 6 mg/kg per day) and otitis media (single dose of 10 mg/kg followed by 5 mg/kg per day). A randomized clinical trial comparing azithromycin with high-dose (90/6.4 mg/kg per day) amoxicillin-clavulanate for the treatment of acute otitis media revealed that the lactam-containing regimen achieved superior bacteriologic and clinical outcomes for all bacterial pathogens, including penicillin-resistant *S. pneumoniae* and *H. influenzae.*[152] Consequently, consensus guidelines do not recommend azithromycin or clarithromycin for empirical treatment of acute otitis media unless the patient has a type 1 hypersensitivity reaction to penicillins.[11] Shorter courses of azithromycin for uncomplicated group A streptococcal pharyngitis (20 mg/kg per day for 3 days)[82] or acute otitis media (single dose of 30 mg/kg)[16] have been found to be as effective as standard therapy but have not been approved by the FDA. A clinical study suggested that a 5-day course of azithromycin for localized cervical lymphadenopathy caused by *B. henselae* (cat scratch disease) is beneficial.[29] The CDC recommends azithromycin for the treatment of chlamydial genital infections, nongonococcal urethritis, and chancroid (a single 20-mg/kg dose; maximum dose, 1 g)[370] and for prophylaxis of disseminated MAC infection in HIV-infected children.[73] The American Thoracic Society and Infectious Disease Society of America guidelines for treatment and prevention of nontuberculous mycobacteria recommend a combination regimen including a macrolide (either clarithromycin or azithromycin) with ethambutol and rifampin for patients with nodular, bronchiectatic, or fibrocavitary lung disease caused by MAC.[139] Data supporting the use of azithromycin for treatment of ophthalmia neonatorum caused by *C. trachomatis* are limited to one small study in which a single oral dose of 20 mg/kg per day for 3 days appeared effective.[370]

Although the safety and efficacy of azithromycin and clarithromycin have not been determined for infants younger than 6 months of age (or for pregnant or lactating women), these antimicrobials are recommended as first-line agents for treatment and postexposure prophylaxis of pertussis in individuals older than the age of 1 month, based on their in vitro effectiveness, safety and efficacy in older children, and more convenient dosing schedule. Duration of therapy or prophylaxis for pertussis is 14 days for erythromycin (40 to 50 mg/kg per day in four divided doses), 7 days for clarithromycin (15 mg/kg per day in two divided doses), and 5 days for azithromycin (10 mg/kg as single daily doses for infants <6 months of age; 10 mg/kg as a single dose on day 1, then 5 mg/kg per day on days 2 to 5 for infants and children ≥6 months of age). Azithromycin is the preferred macrolide for postexposure prophylaxis and treatment of pertussis in neonates because it has fewer adverse effects in contrast to erythromycin.[350] Infants younger than 6 weeks of age treated with either oral erythromycin or azithromycin should be closely monitored because there is an association between receipt of these oral agents and the development of infantile hypertrophic pyloric stenosis.[107] A multicenter study established that children with cystic fibrosis chronically infected with *P. aeruginosa* had significantly improved lung function and clinical endpoints associated with azithromycin treatment three times per week.[311] This effect may not persist. Studies in endemic regions showed that a single dose of azithromycin is as effective as standard therapy with erythromycin for treatment of cholera in children.[190] A 5-day course of azithromycin (20 mg/kg per day; maximum dose, 1 g) is an effective treatment for uncomplicated typhoid fever in children and adolescents.[124] One to six doses of azithromycin for trachoma have been shown to be equivalent to prolonged topical treatment with oxytetracycline polymyxin ointment.[97]

Adverse Effects

The macrolides usually are well tolerated and relatively safe. The most common adverse effect is gastrointestinal disturbance, which can occur with the administration of any macrolide but is associated most commonly with the use of erythromycin. It is a dose-related phenomenon. Because it acts as a motilin receptor agonist, gastrointestinal symptoms (i.e., nausea, vomiting, diarrhea, flatulence, and abdominal cramps) can occur with orally or parenterally administered erythromycin. Enteric coating of erythromycin does not decrease the incidence. Rapid intravenous infusions of erythromycin can result in thrombophlebitis. Cholestatic hepatitis is an unusual, but serious, macrolide toxicity. It occurs more commonly in adults and possibly in pregnant women and is associated most frequently with the estolate preparation.[57] The onset typically begins approximately 16 days after initiation of therapy and is manifested as fever, pruritus, jaundice, elevated liver function tests, and, occasionally, rash, leukocytosis, and eosinophilia. Signs and symptoms resolve after discontinuation of the macrolide but recur with subsequent therapy. Transient hearing loss has been described after the administration of large dosages of erythromycin lactobionate. Torsades de pointes is an uncommon reaction to intravenous infusions of erythromycin. A sevenfold increase in the rate of infantile hypertrophic pyloric stenosis was temporally associated with and probably causally related to the prophylactic use of erythromycin in neonates during a pertussis outbreak in a community hospital.[156] Azithromycin exposure in the first 2 weeks of life was associated with an eightfold increased risk of developing pyloric stenosis in a retrospective review using the US military health system database.[107] Postmarketing experience with the use of intravenous azithromycin reported two cases of infantile pyloric stenosis. Gastrointestinal disturbances occur less frequently with clarithromycin and azithromycin, principally because lower dosages are required for effective therapy.

A common and potentially serious toxicity is that of drug interactions.[271] Macrolides are metabolized by hepatic microsomal CYP450 enzymes. Drug interactions can occur during concomitant therapy with two or more drugs that undergo hepatic microsomal P450 metabolism. One proposal for this drug interaction suggests that the macrolide is N-demethylated to a nitrosoalkane that interacts with and inactivates the microsomal enzyme. Toxicity can occur because of interference with metabolism and consequent accumulation of the second drug. The ability to inactivate the enzyme varies with each macrolide; erythromycin is a more potent inhibitor than is clarithromycin. Azithromycin has not yet been associated with nitrosoalkane formation and resulting drug interactions, but caution should be exercised with concomitant administration of warfarin, digitoxin, and antacids. Drugs with which macrolides can interact include astemizole, benzodiazepines, buspirone, carbamazepine, cimetidine, cisapride, cyclosporine, digoxin, methylprednisolone, rifampin, tacrolimus, terfenadine, theophylline, triazolam, verapamil, warfarin, zidovudine, and certain protease inhibitors, among others.[271]

Chloramphenicol

Chloramphenicol, originally derived from *Streptomyces venezuelae* obtained from soil near Caracas, Venezuela, in 1947, now is prepared synthetically. It is a chemically unique agent that contains an aromatic nitro group, an N-dichloroacetyl substituent, and two chiral centers. The availability of less toxic and equally or more effective agents has limited the usefulness of chloramphenicol in the United States.

Mechanisms of Action

Chloramphenicol reversibly binds to the 50S subunit of 70S bacterial ribosomes and thereby inhibits protein synthesis. The mechanism of action involves suppression of peptidyltransferase activity, with a resultant inability to form peptide bonds and elongate the peptide chain.[319,372] Because the ribosomal binding sites of chloramphenicol overlap with those of macrolides, clindamycin, and linezolid, concomitant use of these antibiotics can result in antagonism and should be avoided. Chloramphenicol usually is bacteriostatic, but it can be bactericidal when high concentrations are achieved against highly susceptible organisms such as meningococci and *H. influenzae.*

Mechanisms of Resistance

The most common mechanism of acquired resistance is plasmid-mediated production of chloramphenicol acetyltransferases (CATs), which acetylate chloramphenicol and render it unable to bind to the ribosomal target. Numerous CAT genes encode classic (type A) or novel (type B) CATs and may be associated with multidrug resistance phenotypes. This resistance has been documented in many different genera of bacteria, including *H. influenzae,* members of the Enterobacteriaceae, *Neisseria,* streptococci, and *S. aureus.* Less commonly, multiple specific or multidrug transporter mechanisms (efflux pumps) and chromosomal or plasmid-mediated alterations in permeability have resulted in chloramphenicol resistance in a wide range of bacteria, including *B. cepacia, E. coli, H. influenzae, P. aeruginosa,* and *S. typhi* (in the absence of OmpF protein). More recently described alterations in bacterial 23S rRNA have been associated with chloramphenicol resistance by inducing frameshift mutations and readthrough of stop codons.[348] In addition, isolated cases of resistance in *Bacillus subtilis* because of altered ribosomes and in anaerobes because of inactivation of chloramphenicol by nitroreduction have been reported.[319]

In Vitro Activity

Chloramphenicol has broad-spectrum activity against aerobic and anaerobic gram-positive and gram-negative bacteria, chlamydiae, mycoplasmas, spirochetes, and rickettsiae.[295] It is bactericidal against susceptible strains of *H. influenzae, N. meningitidis,* and penicillin-susceptible *S. pneumoniae,* whereas it is bacteriostatic against most other susceptible microorganisms.[288] Frequently susceptible aerobic gram-positive cocci include groups A and B β-hemolytic streptococci, viridans streptococci, and penicillin-susceptible pneumococci. Because penicillin-resistant pneumococci may be tolerant to chloramphenicol in vitro, meaning that concentrations of drug necessary to kill these pneumococci are approximately 30-fold higher than necessary to inhibit the organism, verifying chloramphenicol susceptibility by MBC testing is prudent, especially when treating meningitis.[125] Usually, chloramphenicol is active against oxacillin-susceptible *S. aureus,* but susceptibility patterns vary with the use of chloramphenicol, and more suitable alternatives for therapy exist. Susceptible gram-positive bacilli include *Bacillus* spp., *L. monocytogenes, C. diphtheriae, Clostridium* spp., and *Eubacterium.* Most *N. meningitidis* and *N. gonorrhoeae* organisms are susceptible.[179] However, several high-level chloramphenicol-resistant strains of meningococcus belonging to serogroup B were isolated from the CSF of children in Vietnam.[126] The susceptibility of Enterobacteriaceae, including for *Salmonella* and *Shigella* spp., is variable. Other gram-negative bacilli frequently susceptible to chloramphenicol include *B. pertussis, B. cepacia, Brucella* spp., *C. jejuni, F. tularensis, H. influenzae, Pasteurella multocida, Pseudomonas pseudomallei, V. cholerae,* and *Y. pestis.* Virtually all obligate anaerobes are susceptible.

Pharmacokinetics

After oral administration, absorption of chloramphenicol is rapid and complete. Bioavailability is approximately 80% after oral administration, but it is only 70% after an intravenous dose because approximately 30% of the parenterally administered dose is excreted in urine before hydrolysis of the succinate ester to the active form. Intramuscular injection results in peak serum concentrations comparable to those achieved after intravenous infusion. Because of its lipid solubility, chloramphenicol diffuses rapidly and widely into tissues and fluids.[295] The highest concentrations are achieved in the liver and kidneys, with high concentrations present in urine, and therapeutic concentrations are achieved in aqueous and vitreous humor. CSF concentrations range from 21% to 50% and from 45% to 89% of serum values in the presence of uninflamed and inflamed meninges, respectively. Brain tissue concentrations exceed those in plasma. Chloramphenicol also is distributed into pleural, ascitic, and synovial fluids, as well as saliva and breast milk. Protein binding ranges from 32% in premature newborns to 50% to 60% in adults. Chloramphenicol palmitate and chloramphenicol sodium succinate are esterified prodrugs of chloramphenicol. Orally administered chloramphenicol palmitate is hydrolyzed to active drug by pancreatic esterases in the small intestine before absorption. After intravenous infusion, chloramphenicol sodium succinate is hydrolyzed rapidly to active drug in the kidneys, liver, and lungs. Ninety percent of active chloramphenicol is conjugated to the inactive glucuronide primarily by the liver. Immature metabolic function of the liver in the fetus and newborn results in inadequate conjugation of chloramphenicol, with subsequent accumulation of toxic concentrations of active drug. Peak serum concentrations in children after a dose of 25 mg/kg range from 19 to 28 µg/mL, whereas in adults receiving doses of 12.5 mg/kg, peak serum values of 11 to 18 µg/mL can be achieved. Although metabolized to inactive metabolites by the liver, chloramphenicol is excreted by the kidneys: 5% to 10% as active drug and 80% as inactive metabolites. The elimination half-life is significantly longer but variable, and serum concentrations are unpredictable in neonates.[295] Dosage adjustments should be considered in persons with severe hepatic insufficiency or combined hepatic and renal insufficiency and in patients receiving drugs that compete for hepatic CYP450 oxidases, such as phenytoin, phenobarbital, and rifampin. Chloramphenicol is not removed by peritoneal dialysis or hemodialysis, but charcoal hemoperfusion may lower serum concentrations.

Indications for Use

Because of its low therapeutic-toxic index, use of chloramphenicol should be reserved for serious infections for which less toxic agents are ineffective or contraindicated. In developed countries, chloramphenicol has been replaced by third-generation cephalosporins for the treatment of bacterial meningitis and by clindamycin or metronidazole for the treatment of anaerobic infections. Ceftriaxone is a safe and effective alternative to (1) chloramphenicol for the treatment of acute typhoid fever[246] and (2) long-acting oily chloramphenicol for epidemic meningococcal meningitis in sub-Saharan Africa.[258] Infections for which chloramphenicol may be indicated include pneumococcal, meningococcal, and *H. influenzae* meningitis in β-lactam-allergic individuals; brain abscesses caused by susceptible anaerobic bacteria resistant to other agents; acute typhoid fever; and rickettsial infections (i.e., typhus, Q fever, Rocky Mountain spotted fever). Doxycycline is preferred for treatment of rickettsial infections in children, even those younger than 9 years of age. Chloramphenicol is not indicated for the treatment of trivial infections, prophylaxis of infections, or treatment of typhoid carrier states.

Adverse Effects

Hematologic adverse events associated with the use of chloramphenicol include hemolytic anemia in patients with the Mediterranean type of glucose-6-phosphate dehydrogenase deficiency, reversible bone marrow suppression, and aplastic anemia. Reversible bone marrow suppression is a dose-related phenomenon. It usually occurs when serum concentrations exceed 25 µg/mL, as can be seen when administering large dosages, during prolonged therapy, or in patients with impaired liver function. Although mammalian cells contain 80S ribosomes, rather than the 70S ribosomes found in prokaryotes, mitochondria possess 70S ribosomes. A proposed mechanism of myelosuppression involves inhibition of mitochondrial protein synthesis in host bone marrow stem cells.[319] Dose-related bone marrow suppression is manifested by peripheral anemia with or without reticulocytopenia, leukopenia, and thrombocytopenia and bone marrow findings of increased cellularity, cytoplasmic vacuolization, and maturation arrest of erythroid and myeloid precursors. In contrast, aplastic anemia is a rare, often fatal idiosyncratic reaction that is unrelated to the dosage, duration, or route of therapy. The pathogenesis is understood less well but possibly is related to DNA damage from toxic metabolites of chloramphenicol produced by nitroreduction.[372] The incidence ranges from 1 per 25,000 to 1 per 40,000 courses. Onset can begin during therapy but typically occurs weeks to months or, rarely, years after therapy has been discontinued. Manifestations include peripheral pancytopenia and hypoplastic or aplastic marrow.

Gray syndrome, or gray baby syndrome, is a rare but serious and potentially fatal adverse event that usually occurs in newborn and young infants, but has been described in older children and adults with hepatic insufficiency. Most often, this syndrome occurs when serum chloramphenicol concentrations exceed 40 μg/mL and is thought to be a result of inhibition of mitochondrial electron transport in liver, skeletal muscle, and myocardium. The onset typically begins 2 to 9 days after initiating therapy. Manifestations include hypothermia, tachypnea, blue-gray skin color (cyanosis), abdominal distention, emesis, unresponsiveness, and refractory metabolic acidosis that can progress to vasomotor collapse and death within 2 days.

Uncommon side effects include hypersensitivity reactions such as drug fever, rash, urticaria, anaphylaxis, and a Herxheimer-like reaction during therapy for syphilis, typhoid fever, and brucellosis; gastrointestinal symptoms, including nausea, emesis, diarrhea, and an unpleasant taste; and neurologic symptoms such as peripheral neuritis, headache, mental confusion, and optic neuritis, the last of which may not be entirely reversible.

Chloramphenicol can inhibit the metabolism of other drugs metabolized by the hepatic microsomal CYP450 system and thus result in the accumulation of alfentanil, barbiturates, cyclophosphamide, phenytoin, antidiabetic sulfonylureas (more common with chlorpropamide and tolbutamide than with glyburide and glipizide), and warfarin during concomitant therapy.[7] Because some agents such as rifampin, phenobarbital, and phenytoin are potent inducers of hepatic microsomal enzymes, when they are given concomitantly with chloramphenicol, metabolism is enhanced, and serum concentrations of active chloramphenicol are reduced. Other drug interactions include a reduction in the effectiveness of estrogen-containing oral contraceptives when used concurrently with chloramphenicol and a delay in the response to vitamin B_{12}, folic acid, and iron. A mild disulfiram-like reaction can occur when alcohol is ingested during chloramphenicol therapy. Both cimetidine and chloramphenicol have rare associations with aplastic anemia; a few reports of concomitant use resulting in aplastic anemia have been documented, thus suggesting a potential for additive or synergistic risk. Concomitant acetaminophen therapy has been the subject of controversy; some studies suggest that coadministration can prolong the elimination half-life of chloramphenicol, but other reports suggest no effect or enhanced metabolism of chloramphenicol. Lincosamides and macrolides can have an antagonistic effect when they are administered concurrently with chloramphenicol because of competition for ribosomal binding sites. Chloramphenicol is physically incompatible in solution with many drugs, including tetracyclines and vancomycin.

Because of considerable variability in serum chloramphenicol concentrations, the narrow therapeutic-toxic index, and the potential for drug interactions, monitoring serum concentrations of chloramphenicol and peripheral blood counts during therapy is prudent, particularly for neonates.

Tetracyclines

Chlortetracycline (Aureomycin) was the first natural tetracycline discovered when isolated from *Streptomyces aureofaciens* in 1948.[116] Many tetracyclines have been developed since then. Those currently marketed include the natural agents tetracycline and demeclocycline and the semisynthetic agents doxycycline and minocycline. Their basic structure consists of a hydronaphthacene nucleus with four fused rings. They differ from each other biochemically by substituent variations at carbons 5, 6, or 7. Their mechanisms of action and mechanisms of resistance, as well as their spectra of activity, are similar, but the analogues differ in the degree of activity and pharmacokinetic properties. Tigecycline is a novel intravenously administered glycylcycline that is related structurally to minocycline. It is approved for use in adults with complicated skin and skin structure infections, community-acquired pneumonia, and complicated intra-abdominal infections. It is bacteriostatic, with improved activity against multidrug-resistant bacteria, and it has no cross resistance with other classes of antimicrobial agents. Tigecycline has activity against *S. aureus* (including MRSA), enterococci (including VRE), and multidrug-resistant gram-negative bacteria, including ESBL-producing enteric gram-negative organisms. It is also active against rapidly growing, nontuberculous mycobacteria. It is not recommended for serious infections caused by *P. aeruginosa*.[266]

Mechanisms of Action

Tetracyclines passively diffuse through outer-membrane porins and then traverse the cytoplasmic membrane by energy-dependent active transport. Tetracyclines are actively concentrated by most bacterial cells, but not by mammalian cells, a characteristic that explains the selective action of these drugs against bacteria. Tetracyclines are bacteriostatic agents that reversibly bind to the 30S subunit of 70S bacterial ribosomes and inhibit protein synthesis. Because attachment of aminoacyl-tRNA to the ribosome acceptor site is prevented, the bacteria are unable to add amino acids to the growing peptide chain.

Mechanisms of Resistance

In many bacteria, including members of the Enterobacteriaceae, *P. aeruginosa*, staphylococci, streptococci, and *Bacteroides*, resistance to tetracyclines has developed. Resistance in most bacteria results from the acquisition of new genes often associated with mobile elements such as plasmids or transposons, but it also can be chromosomally mediated. The genes encoding for acquired resistance are called tet (tetracycline)-resistance or otr (oxytetracycline)-resistance determinants. Resistance to one tetracycline usually implies resistance to all; however, many tetracycline-resistant bacteria are susceptible to doxycycline, minocycline, or both. At least 38 acquired tetracycline and oxytetracycline resistance genes have been identified that mediate (1) energy-dependent efflux of tetracycline (the most common type of resistance mechanism), (2) protection of the ribosomes from the action of tetracycline, or (3) enzymatic inactivation of tetracycline.[297] Tet genes that encode membrane efflux proteins are different in gram-positive and gram-negative bacteria. Efflux has been found in a wide range of bacteria, including *Acinetobacter, Aeromonas, Chlamydia,* the Enterobacteriaceae, *Haemophilus, Moraxella, Neisseria, Pseudomonas,* staphylococci, *Stenotrophomonas, V. cholerae,* and others. Less commonly, ribosomal protection by a soluble ribosomal protection protein encoded by different tet and otr genes has been found in a wide variety of aerobic and anaerobic gram-positive and gram-negative bacteria. The precise mechanism by which ribosomal protection protein mediates resistance to tetracyclines is being investigated. Researchers have hypothesized that these protection determinants produce allosteric disruption of the primary tetracycline binding site that causes the tetracycline molecules to be released from the ribosome. Enzymatic inactivation of tetracycline, encoded for by other tet genes, has been demonstrated in in vitro studies of *Bacteroides,* and *E. coli,* but the clinical significance has not been established.[297] Susceptibility of staphylococci to this class of agents typically is tested using tetracycline. However, this approach may overestimate the prevalence of resistance to doxycycline and minocycline. Although the prevalence of tetracycline resistance remains relatively low among CAMRSA isolates, resistance in some strains has been associated with tetK, a finding indicating that doxycycline and minocycline may be effective treatment options. However, because data are sparse on clinical outcomes associated with the use of minocycline or doxycycline to treat infections caused by tetracycline-resistant *S. aureus* strains, these agents are not recommended.[136] Tigecycline overcomes two major resistance mechanisms, including drug efflux and protection of ribosomes.

In Vitro Activity

Tetracyclines are broad-spectrum antibiotics with activity against aerobic and anaerobic gram-positive and gram-negative bacteria, chlamydiae, mycoplasmas, rickettsiae, and spirochetes. Activity against gram-negative bacteria has been limited by the emergence of tetracycline-resistant strains. Most *P. aeruginosa* and many *Shigella* and *Salmonella* organisms are resistant. Penicillin-susceptible strains of *N. gonorrhoeae* and *N. meningitidis* usually are susceptible to tetracyclines, but penicillin-resistant strains of *N. gonorrhoeae* are not. Gram-negative organisms with continued susceptibility to tetracyclines include *Aeromonas hydrophila, Brucella, Campylobacter,* some *Haemophilus* organisms, *Helicobacter, P. multocida, Plesiomonas shigelloides,* and *Vibrio.* Tetracyclines are active against some gram-positive bacilli, including *A. israelii, B. anthracis,* many clostridia, *Listeria,* and *Nocardia.* Tetracyclines have excellent activity against *C. pneumoniae, M. pneumoniae,* and rickettsiae. Other organisms for which tetracyclines have activity include *Mycobacterium marinum* and *Borrelia burgdorferi.* The more lipophilic agents doxycycline and minocycline generally are more active than the others. Minocycline has excellent activity against susceptible staphylococci, and both doxycycline and minocycline are more active than tetracycline against *S. aureus* and some streptococci, but they have no activity against enterococci and group B streptococci. Because of extensive plasmid-mediated resistance in pneumococci, therapy with tetracycline should be avoided. Doxycycline and minocycline are more active in vitro than the other agents against anaerobic bacteria, but alternative antimicrobials are preferred for anaerobic infections because more than 50% of *B. fragilis* isolates are resistant, and susceptibility among other anaerobes is highly variable.[296]

Pharmacokinetics

The four tetracycline compounds available for systemic use can be classified by duration of activity: tetracycline is a short-acting agent, demeclocycline is intermediate acting, and doxycycline and minocycline are long-acting agents. Oral administration is the preferred route because thrombophlebitis is associated with intravenous infusion and pain is associated with intramuscular injections. Oral absorption ranges from 58% for the short-acting agents to 100% for the long-acting ones. The presence of food decreases the absorption of demeclocycline and tetracycline. Because tetracyclines form insoluble complexes in the gut with aluminum, calcium, iron, magnesium, zinc, and other bivalent and trivalent cations, coadministration with milk and other dairy products, antacids, calcium or iron supplements, cathartics, and other agents can reduce absorption and should be avoided. Differences in lipid solubility affect penetration of tissues by the various tetracyclines. All agents readily penetrate many tissues and fluids, among which are pleural, ascitic, and synovial fluids, sinus secretions, sputum, bone, teeth, and breast milk. Tetracyclines can cross the placenta. The highest concentrations are achieved in bile and can exceed serum concentrations by 5 to 20 times. Therapeutic concentrations of doxycycline can be achieved in tonsillar and pulmonary tissues, the eye, and the prostate, and high concentrations are achieved in myometrial and endometrial tissue and the kidney.[312] Minocycline penetrates into sputum, saliva, and tears, as well as into cells of the vestibular apparatus.[174] Minocycline is biotransformed to inactive metabolites by the liver; the other tetracyclines are not metabolized, although whether doxycycline is metabolized is not clear. Demeclocycline and tetracycline are eliminated unchanged in urine. Approximately 10% of minocycline is excreted unchanged in urine, 20% to 35% is excreted unchanged in feces, and the remainder is excreted as inactive metabolites in urine and feces. Thirty percent to 40% of doxycycline is excreted in urine; the remainder is excreted by the biliary tract and by diffusion through the intestinal wall, where some of it is chelated and prevented from reabsorption and enterohepatic cycling. Dosing of short- and intermediate-acting tetracyclines must be adjusted for renal failure.

Systemic formulations available in the United States include tablets, capsules, delayed-release capsules, and suspensions for many of the tetracyclines, as well as parenteral preparations of doxycycline and minocycline. Ophthalmic and topical preparations also are available. Tigecycline is available only as a parenteral formulation.

Indications for Use

With few exceptions, tetracyclines no longer are the drugs of choice for many infections because of the availability of cephalosporins and semisynthetic penicillins with equivalent or greater activity and less frequent side effects. As a result of the potential for dental toxicity, tetracyclines are not recommended for use in children younger than 8 years of age, except for specific infections for which alternative therapy is potentially more toxic, such as chloramphenicol for Rocky Mountain spotted fever and ehrlichiosis.[2] Approved indications in the United States include treatment of actinomycosis, anthrax, brucellosis, inclusion conjunctivitis, psittacosis, Q fever, rickettsialpox, Rocky Mountain spotted fever, typhus, relapsing fever, syphilis, trachoma, yaws, and Vincent necrotizing gingivostomatitis caused by *Fusobacterium,* as well as infections caused by *Bacteroides* spp., *Bartonella bacilliformis, Campylobacter fetus, F. tularensis, M. pneumoniae, V. cholerae, Y. pestis,* and others. Because of its excellent tissue penetration and spectrum of activity, doxycycline is the preferred tetracycline for treatment of atypical pneumonia caused by *M. pneumoniae* and *C. pneumoniae,* intra-abdominal or pelvic infections, and several STDs, including granuloma inguinale, chlamydial infections, *U. urealyticum* infection, nongonococcal urethritis, pelvic inflammatory disease (plus cefotetan or cefoxitin, ampicillin-sulbactam or single-dose ceftriaxone with or without metronidazole), acute epididymitis (plus ceftriaxone), proctitis (plus ceftriaxone), and prostatitis.[370] Doxycycline is an alternative drug for (nonpregnant) penicillin-allergic patients with primary, secondary, or late latent syphilis. Although minocycline is effective in eradicating nasopharyngeal carriage of meningococcus, its potential for vestibular toxicity precludes its use for this purpose. For prevention of Lyme disease after a recognized tick bite, a single dose of doxycycline may be offered to adults (200 mg dose) and to children older than 8 years of age (4 mg/kg, up to a maximum dose of 200 mg), provided the following criteria are met: (1) the attached tick can be identified reliably as an adult or nymphal *Ixodes scapularis* tick that is estimated to have been attached for more than 36 hours on the basis of the degree of engorgement of the tick, (2) prophylaxis can be started within 72 hours of tick removal, and (3) the local rate of infection of these ticks with *B. burgdorferi* is more than 20%. Doxycycline (4 mg/kg per day in two divided doses, up to 100 mg per dose) is indicated in children older than 8 years of age and adults for treatment of erythema migrans, isolated cranial nerve palsy, uncomplicated cardiac disease, and uncomplicated arthritis.[371] Topical tetracyclines have been used extensively for the treatment of acne vulgaris and other dermatologic illnesses.[160]

Adverse Effects

Gastrointestinal disturbances are the most common side effects associated with tetracycline and include anorexia, nausea, emesis, flatulence, and diarrhea. These symptoms occur less frequently with minocycline. Esophageal ulceration has been associated with the oral administration of tetracyclines.[119] All tetracyclines except doxycycline can cause a negative nitrogen balance, with an elevation in blood urea nitrogen that usually is not significant except in the presence of underlying renal insufficiency. Demeclocycline can cause nephrogenic diabetes insipidus and, for this reason, has been used for treatment of the syndrome of inappropriate antidiuretic hormone secretion. Rarely, tetracyclines have been associated with hepatic injury, as manifested by elevated transaminases and diffuse vacuolar fatty metamorphosis on biopsy, with or without pancreatitis. The effect is dose related, and the risk is increased with pregnancy, malnutrition, and preexisting renal or hepatic disease and in patients receiving other hepatotoxic agents. The use of tetracyclines in children younger than 8 years of age is relatively contraindicated because tetracyclines chelate with calcium and can be deposited in developing bones and teeth and lead to a transient decrease in bone growth, permanent tooth discoloration, and enamel hypoplasia. The risk that these side effects will occur with one course at an appropriate dosage is low; the degree of tooth discoloration is associated with the total dosage administered.[140] Minocycline has been associated with reversible vestibular toxicity. All tetracyclines have been noted to cause pseudotumor cerebri, a benign elevation in intracranial pressure that is reversible after discontinuation of the drug. Some data suggest that an increased risk may exist with the concurrent use of tetracycline and isotretinoin. Tetracyclines have been associated with an exaggerated sunburn reaction after sun exposure. This risk occurs most frequently with demeclocycline and rarely with minocycline. Hypersensitivity reactions occur infrequently and include morbilliform rash, urticaria, exfoliative dermatitis, and, rarely, anaphylaxis. Hyperpigmentation of the mucosal membranes, skin, and nails has been reported with the use of tetracycline, particularly minocycline.

Drug-drug interactions are numerous. A decrease in absorption of tetracyclines can occur with the coadministration of oral antacids, bismuth subsalicylate, iron, kaolin or pectin, zinc sulfate, and other divalent or trivalent cations that chelate the antibiotic. A reduced effect of tetracyclines because of increased metabolism is associated with the concomitant use of doxycycline with barbiturates, carbamazepine, phenytoin, rifampin, and alcohol in heavy drinkers. Coadministration with tetracyclines can increase the effect of oral anticoagulants, digoxin, lithium, and theophylline and can decrease the effect of oral contraceptive agents and oral iron. Tetracyclines can inhibit the in vitro bactericidal activity of penicillins and aminoglycosides. Other drug-drug interactions include benign intracranial hypertension with the concomitant administration of vitamin A, severe nephrotoxicity with the coadministration of methoxyflurane and tetracycline, and localized hemosiderosis with amitriptyline and minocycline.

Lincosamides

Lincosamide antibiotics consist of an amino acid linked to an amino sugar. Lincomycin, elaborated by *Streptomyces lincolnensis* var. *lincolnensis*, originally isolated from a soil sample near Lincoln, Nebraska, was the first lincosamide available for use. Clindamycin, a semisynthetic derivative of lincomycin produced by the substitution of a chlorine atom for a hydroxyl group at position 7, was available for use in the early 1970s. Because clindamycin has increased antibacterial activity and better oral absorption than lincomycin, lincomycin rarely is used.

Mechanisms of Action

Lincosamides bind to the 50S subunit of susceptible bacterial ribosomes close to the peptidyl transferase center and thereby inhibit protein synthesis. Data indicate that clindamycin causes dissociation of peptidyl-tRNAs from the ribosome, depletion of free tRNA pools, and prevention of the egress of nascent peptides through a tunnel in the 50S subunit.[344] Because the ribosomal binding sites for lincosamides overlap with those of chloramphenicol and erythromycin, concurrent use of these agents can result in antagonism and should be avoided. Lincosamides usually are bacteriostatic but can be bactericidal against highly susceptible microorganisms in the presence of high lincosamide concentrations.

Mechanisms of Resistance

Some bacteria, including members of the Enterobacteriaceae and *Pseudomonas* and *Acinetobacter* spp., are inherently resistant to lincosamides, most likely because of relative impermeability of the outer membrane of the cell wall. Acquired resistance can develop as a result of altered ribosomal targets and, less commonly, lincosamide inactivation, whereas resistance as a result of reduced lincosamide uptake has not been described. Two mechanisms by which bacteria can alter their ribosomes and acquire lincosamide resistance have been identified. High-level resistance because of an altered protein component of the 50S ribosomal subunit after a one-step chromosomal mutation confers resistance to erythromycin and often to the lincosamides. Plasmid-mediated MLS_B resistance occurs when adenine residues on the 23S RNA component of the 50S ribosomal subunit are methylated, and an altered target is created that confers cross resistance to macrolides, lincosamides, and streptogramin B. The production of ribosomal methylases is encoded by the erm class of genes.[299] This resistance can be constitutive or inducible and can be seen in staphylococci, streptococci, and *Bacteroides* spp. Erythromycin is the most potent inducer of MLS_B resistance in staphylococci, whereas any macrolide, lincosamide, or streptogramin B can be an inducer in streptococci. Some strains of *B. fragilis* can have inducible MLS_B resistance that is not detected easily by disk agar diffusion susceptibility testing[337] but is recognizable because of frequently concurrent high-level erythromycin resistance. A macrolide-spectrogramin-B pattern of resistance that is plasmid mediated results in macrolide resistance as a result of active ATP-dependent efflux pumps encoded by the *mef(A)* and *msr(A)* genes. Isolates with these resistance genotypes are resistant to 14- and 15-membered ring macrolides and streptogramin B but not to clindamycin.[231] Rarely, staphylococci produce a plasmid-mediated, nonconjugative nucleotidyltransferase that inactivates lincosamides and results in high-level resistance to lincomycin and tolerance to clindamycin (MBC/MIC ratio >32).

In Vitro Activity

Both lincosamides are effective in vitro against gram-positive cocci, whereas clindamycin also is active against a wide range of anaerobic bacteria. Clindamycin is many times more active than lincomycin and is as active as or slightly more active than erythromycin against staphylococci, pneumococci, group A streptococci, and viridans streptococci. Unlike erythromycin, the lincosamides do not have clinically significant activity against *H. influenzae, M. pneumoniae,* or *Neisseria* spp. Clindamycin is active against many gram-positive cocci, including penicillinase-producing and non–penicillinase-producing staphylococci and groups A, B, C, and G β-hemolytic streptococci and pneumococci, but it is not active against enterococci or most health care–associated methicillin-resistant staphylococci. Rates of in vitro inducible erm-mediated MLS_B resistance among CAMRSA isolates vary widely, ranging from 4.5% in Houston[184] to 94% in Chicago.[121] Presence of this type of resistance can be detected in erythromycin-resistant strains of *S. aureus* with the use of the double-disk diffusion assay (D-test), in which clindamycin- and erythromycin-impregnated disks are placed 15 to 20 mm apart on Mueller-Hinton agar that has been inoculated with a standardized (0.5 McFarland) suspension of *S. aureus.* The finding of a D-shaped blunting of the circular zone of inhibition around the clindamycin disk on the side closest to the erythromycin disk indicates the presence of in vitro–inducible MLS_B resistance. These isolates have a high rate of mutation to constitutive clindamycin resistance, a trait that would confer a selective advantage during clindamycin therapy. The use of clindamycin for D-test-positive *S. aureus* infections has been reported to result in treatment failure in a few patients. Therefore, alternative effective antimicrobial agents should be sought, or, if empirical clindamycin therapy has been initiated, response to therapy should be carefully monitored.[136,231] Erythromycin and lincosamide resistance in pneumococci and group A streptococci has been increasing. Surveillance studies revealed rates of clindamycin resistance among multidrug-resistant pneumococci to be 12% and 19% in the United States and Europe, respectively.[173] Most facultative aerobic gram-negative bacilli, with the exception of *Campylobacter* spp. (including *C. jejuni* and *C. fetus*) and *H. pylori,* are inherently resistant to clindamycin. Anaerobes frequently susceptible to clindamycin include the anaerobic gram-negative bacilli *Bacteroides, Fusobacterium, Prevotella,* and *Porphyromonas* spp.; the non–spore-forming gram-positive bacilli *Propionibacterium, Eubacterium,* and *Actinomyces;* the anaerobic gram-positive cocci *Peptococcus, Peptostreptococcus,* and microaerophilic streptococci; and many *Clostridium* organisms, excluding *C. difficile, Clostridium sporogenes,* and *Clostridium tertium.* Clindamycin resistance does occur, especially in *Fusobacterium varium,* the non-fragilis *Bacteroides* group, an increasing proportion of *B. fragilis* isolates (about 30% or less in some series),[5] and as many as 20% of anaerobic gram-positive cocci. When combined with other agents, clindamycin is active against certain other pathogens such as *Babesia, Plasmodium, Pneumocystis jiroveci,* and *T. gondii.*

Pharmacokinetics

Oral absorption of lincosamides occurs rapidly. The presence of food delays but does not decrease the absorption of clindamycin, but it does reduce the absorption of lincomycin. Concomitant administration of kaolin or attapulgite-containing antidiarrheal agents can decrease absorption; therefore, these agents should not be administered within 2 hours before or 3 to 4 hours after oral lincosamides are given. Lincosamides are distributed rapidly and widely to most tissues and fluids, including saliva, sputum, respiratory tissue, pleural fluid, soft tissues, bones and joints, brain, prostate, semen, appendix, and peritoneal fluid.[257,272] Lincosamides are transported actively into macrophages and polymorphonuclear leukocytes, and high concentrations are achieved in bile, urine, and bone. Penetration into CSF is limited, unless inflammation is present. In experimental pneumococcal meningitis, concentrations of clindamycin in CSF were approximately 10% of the corresponding serum values. Lincosamides are highly protein bound, with values ranging from 70% to 75% for lincomycin and 92% to 94% for clindamycin. The inactive palmitate and phosphate esters are hydrolyzed in the liver to clindamycin, the active agent. Clindamycin undergoes hepatic biotransformation to active and inactive metabolites. Ten percent of absorbed lincomycin is excreted unchanged in urine, 3% is excreted unchanged in feces, and the remainder is excreted as inactive metabolites, primarily in the biliary system. Elimination is delayed in the presence of severe hepatic insufficiency alone or severe concurrent renal and hepatic impairment, and therefore adjustments in dosages may need to be made. Formulations of lincosamides available for use include lincomycin hydrochloride solution for parenteral use. Clindamycin phosphate, a water-soluble ester of clindamycin and phosphoric acid, is available for parenteral use. Oral formulations include clindamycin palmitate hydrochloride granules reconstituted to 75 mg base/5 mL and clindamycin hydrochloride capsules containing 75, 150, and 300 mg of the base compound. Clindamycin also is available as a topical solution, gel, lotion, foam, pad, and vaginal cream and suppository.

Indications for Use

Lincomycin can be used for the treatment of serious infections caused by susceptible strains of staphylococci, pneumococci, other streptococci, or anaerobic organisms, but it rarely is used in pediatric patients. Clindamycin is effective against and has been approved for treatment of susceptible strains of staphylococcal bone and joint infections[113]; anaerobic pelvic infections, including pelvic inflammatory disease, nongonococcal tubo-ovarian abscess, and postsurgical vaginal cuff infections; anaerobic intra-abdominal infections, including peritonitis and abscesses; pneumonitis, empyema, and lung abscesses caused by anaerobes and as a second-line agent for infections caused by susceptible strains of pneumococci and staphylococci; anaerobic septicemia; and skin and soft tissue infections caused by anaerobes, susceptible strains of staphylococci, and streptococci. Clinical prediction rules relating to resistance among community-acquired, community-onset health care–associated and traditional nosocomial staphylococcal isolates are becoming less reliable because certain strains with distinctive genetic determinants of virulence (e.g., *pvl* genes) and antibiotic resistance (e.g., SSCmec) are tending to predominate.[159,248] Prevalences of constitutive and inducible MLS_B resistance in community-associated *S. aureus* infections generally are increasing in the United States, although rates vary geographically and temporally as a function of predominant circulating clones.[76] Based on current experience, clindamycin should not be used for empirical therapy of suspected *S. aureus* infections if the local clindamycin resistance rate exceeds 10% to 15%. Conversely, clindamycin is effective in treating serious infections caused by clindamycin-susceptible (D-test-negative) CAMRSA infections, including bacteremia, osteomyelitis, suppurative arthritis, pleural empyema, and skin and soft tissue infections.[182,231] Clindamycin also is effective and has been approved as a topical agent for acne vulgaris. Unconfirmed retrospective data suggest that clindamycin in combination with a β-lactam antibiotic, with surgery if indicated, may be the most effective treatment of invasive *S. pyogenes* infections.[382] Other infections for which clindamycin may be effective but has not been approved for therapy include acute otitis media caused by penicillin-resistant pneumococci that has failed to respond to other antibacterial agents,[11] chronic suppurative otitis media or chronic sinusitis in which anaerobes may play a role, chronic pharyngeal carriers of group A streptococci,[338] odontogenic infections, toxoplasmosis of the CNS (in combination with pyrimethamine), uncomplicated *falciparum* malaria[200] or babesiosis (in combination with quinine), and mild-to-moderate *P. jiroveci* pneumonia in patients with acquired immunodeficiency syndrome (AIDS) (in combination with primaquine).[35] Because of poor penetration into CSF, this drug is not approved for the treatment of meningitis. Clindamycin is a third-line agent for endocarditis prophylaxis for upper respiratory tract, dental, or oral procedures in persons allergic to or intolerant of amoxicillin and erythromycin. Oral and intravenous formulations of clindamycin are approved for use in infants and children of all ages. The bitter taste of the oral suspension may limit compliance.

Adverse Effects

The most frequent side effects include generalized morbilliform-like rash and mild, self-limited diarrhea occurring in as many as 10% and in 2% to 20% of patients, respectively. Other gastrointestinal disturbances include anorexia, nausea, vomiting, flatulence, abdominal pain, and a metallic taste. Pseudomembranous colitis, a serious and sometimes fatal illness, is the adverse event posing the most concern. Most antibiotics have been associated with pseudomembranous colitis, but those most frequently implicated include ampicillin, lincosamides, and cephalosporins. The incidence of lincosamide-associated pseudomembranous colitis varies from 0.1% to 10%. Antibiotic-associated pseudomembranous colitis is caused by overgrowth of toxin-producing strains of *C. difficile;* at least two extracellular toxins are elaborated: toxin A, a potent enterotoxin; and toxin B, a cytotoxin.[58]

Other less common adverse events include hypersensitivity reactions such as urticarial rash, drug fever, and eosinophilia; transient neutropenia, agranulocytosis, or thrombocytopenia; and a mild, reversible elevation in hepatic transaminases. Caution must be exercised when administering lincosamides to newborns; fatal gasping syndromes have been described that possibly are related to the preservative benzyl alcohol.

Drug interactions include incompatibility with many agents in solution, including ampicillin, barbiturates, calcium gluconate, phenytoin, and magnesium sulfate, as well as interaction with hydrocarbon-containing inhalational anesthetics. Lincosamides are weak neuromuscular blockers,[326] but they can enhance neuromuscular blockade when they are administered concurrently with neuromuscular blockers. Chloramphenicol and macrolides can have an antagonistic effect when they are administered concurrently with lincosamides because of competition for ribosomal binding sites.

Linezolid

Linezolid is the first of a new class of oxazolidinone antibiotics that was approved for use in children by the FDA in 2002. Linezolid is a totally synthetic compound with favorable activity against multidrug-resistant, gram-positive bacteria.[102]

Mechanisms of Action

Linezolid inhibits an early stage of ribosomal protein synthesis by binding to a unique site, domain V on the bacterial 23S ribosomal RNA of the 50S subunit, and prevents formation of a functional 70S initiation complex. Inhibition of this process interferes with the bacterial translation process. Furthermore, linezolid causes ribosomes to shift reading frames and to read through stop codons, thereby affecting translational fidelity.[348]

Mechanisms of Resistance

Rarely, mutations conferring resistance have been reported in the peptidyl transferase region of the 23S rRNA genes. Cross resistance between linezolid and chloramphenicol is caused by a single nucleotide mutation in the peptidyl transferase center.[348] Cross resistance between linezolid and other classes of antibiotics that target the ribosome, such as aminoglycosides, macrolides, lincosamides, and streptogramins, rarely occurs because these agents target a distinct mechanism of protein elongation. Resistance to linezolid has been reported in enterococci, particularly *E. faecium, S. aureus,* and coagulase-negative staphylococci.[104] Predisposing factors include indwelling devices, undrained abscesses, and prolonged administration of linezolid, particularly if subtherapeutic antibiotic concentrations are achieved.[298]

In Vitro Activity

Time-kill studies demonstrated that linezolid is bacteriostatic against enterococci and staphylococci and bactericidal against most strains of streptococci. Linezolid is active against MRSA, coagulase-negative staphylococci, and vancomycin-resistant enterococci. Furthermore, linezolid has broad activity against *Nocardia* and rapidly growing mycobacteria, as well as slowly growing tuberculous and nontuberculous mycobacteria.[59]

Pharmacokinetics

Dosage adjustment is not necessary when switching from intravenous to oral formulations because the oral bioavailability is approximately 100%. Absorption is not significantly affected by food. The antibiotic is distributed to well-perfused tissues and has a relatively low protein binding (31%) that contributes to the high degree of penetration into bone, muscle, fat, alveolar cells, lung extracellular lining fluid, and CSF. Linezolid is metabolized primarily by oxidation and has no interaction with the CYP450 enzymes. The elimination half-life in children is less than 5 hours and is shorter than in adults. The disposition of linezolid varies as a function of age, with faster clearance and greater volume of distribution in children less than 11 years of age. The AUC values for children are lower than those for adults, whereas preterm neonates (gestational age <34 weeks) within the first week of life have larger AUC values than many full-term neonates and older children. The pharmacokinetics of linezolid in adolescents 12 years of age and older is not significantly different from that of adults. Dosage adjustment is not necessary for patients with renal insufficiency or mild-to-moderate hepatic insufficiency.[180]

Indications for Use

The safety and effectiveness of linezolid have been established for pediatric patients from birth through 17 years of age. Intravenous and oral linezolid is indicated for treatment of children with (1) uncomplicated and complicated skin and skin structure infections caused by oxacillin-susceptible or oxacillin-resistant *S. aureus,* or by group A or group B β-hemolytic streptococci; (2) community- and health care–associated pneumonia caused by penicillin-susceptible strains of *S. pneumoniae* or oxacillin-susceptible or oxacillin-resistant *S. aureus;* and (3) infections caused by vancomycin-resistant enterococci.[183] The recommended dosage for newborns (≥34 weeks' postconceptional age) and children up to the age of 11 years is 10 mg/kg intravenously or orally every 8 hours for 10 to 14 days for pneumonia and complicated skin and skin structure infections and for 14 to 28 days for pneumonia or bacteremia caused by vancomycin-resistant enterococci. The 10-mg/kg dose is administered every 12 hours for 5- to 11-year-old children with uncomplicated skin and soft tissue infections and for premature neonates (gestational age <34 weeks) within the first week of life. The dose for adolescents older than 11 years and adults is 600 mg every 12 hours, with a 1200-mg daily limit. Linezolid offers a safe therapeutic alternative to vancomycin for multidrug-resistant, gram-positive bacteria and has the additional advantage of being available in an oral liquid preparation (100 mg/5 mL), which facilitates sequential intravenous and oral therapy.[101,169,180,183] Safety and efficacy of therapy for longer than 28 days have not been evaluated in controlled clinical trials. Currently, no indication exists for treatment of mycobacterial infections, although linezolid has been used successfully for certain nontuberculous infections.

Adverse Effects

Data from multiple trials indicate that linezolid is safe and well tolerated, with adverse events similar to those of comparative drugs. The most common drug-related adverse events are diarrhea, nausea, vomiting, rash, and headache.[310] However, dose- and duration-dependent reversible myelosuppression, including mild-to-moderate anemia and thrombocytopenia and rarely neutropenia, have been reported in children treated with linezolid.[239,310] Therefore, weekly monitoring of complete blood counts is recommended in patients who receive linezolid for longer than 2 weeks, have preexisting myelosuppression, or receive other myelosuppressive antibiotics. Other rare adverse effects that warrant prompt evaluation include peripheral and optic neuropathy, lactic acidosis, and the serotonin syndrome in patients receiving concomitant selective serotonin reuptake inhibitors. The oral suspension formulation contains phenylalanine, which is contraindicated in children with phenylketonuria.

Tedizolid

Tedizolid became the second commercially available compound to be added to the oxazolidinone drug class with FDA approval in 2014 for use in patients more than 18 years of age. Similar to the spectrum of activity of linezolid, tedizolid has activity against MRSA and VRE; however, tedizolid also has potent activity against staphylococcal and enterococcal multidrug-resistant isolates demonstrating linezolid resistance.[304,380]

Mechanisms of Action

Similar to linezolid, tedizolid binding occurs at the 23S ribosomal RNA, called the V domain, of the 50S portion of the ribosome. This interaction prevents protein synthesis secondary to the inability to form a functional 70S initiation complex. The enhanced activity of tedizolid against linezolid-resistant strains occurs secondary to additional interactions between the side chain of tedizolid, also called the D-ring, and conserved areas of the ribosomal subunit.[304,380]

Mechanisms of Resistance

Oxazolidinone resistance occurs via mutations or modifications of the ribosomal binding site secondary to (1) genetic mutation of 23S rRNA, (2) genetic mutation of ribosomal proteins L3 or L4, or (3) the presence of the *cfr* (i.e., chloramphenicol-florfenical resistance) methyltransferase. The majority of linezolid-resistant isolates are a result of mutation to the 23S ribosomal subunit, where each additional mutation results in increased linezolid and tedizolid MICs for gram-positive organisms.[304,309] The G2576T mutation is an important exception as only a single mutated copy results in increased oxazolidinone MICs. Oxazolidinone resistance has also been shown to occur via mutation to either the L3 or L4 ribosomal proteins, which results in two- to fourfold increases in linezolid MICs. When additional mutations are present with an L3 or L4 mutation, even larger MIC changes occur; however, tedizolid MICs are consistently four times lower than MIC elevations seen with linezolid.[309] The *cfr* gene is horizontally transferrable because of its location on plasmids. The *cfr* gene confers resistance not only to linezolid but to additional antimicrobial agents including lincomycins, macrolides, aminoglycosides, fluoroquinolones, streptogramins, and amfenicols.[304] Linezolid resistance due to the *cfr* gene mutation is thought to occur secondary to steric hindrance associated with its large side chain, but tedizolid has a compact side chain and its activity has not been shown to be impacted by *cfr* gene mutation alone.[380] Overall, available surveillance data demonstrated 0.19% of 6884 gram-positive isolates with tedizolid MIC values greater than 1 μg/mL.[309]

In Vitro Activity

Tedizolid demonstrates 4- to 16-fold greater potency when compared with linezolid against key gram-positive organisms such as staphylococci, streptococci, and enterococci where in vitro activity is bacteriostatic. Tedizolid is active against linezolid-resistant MRSA and VRE. In addition to its gram-positive activity, tedizolid also demonstrates twofold greater activity, when compared with linezolid, against select gram-negative organisms including *H. influenzae* and *M. catarrhalis.*[218,283] In vitro tedizolid data demonstrate activity against *Nocardia brasiliensis* and *Mycobacterium tuberculosis*, even for *M. tuberculosis* isolates resistant to isoniazid and rifampin.[245]

Pharmacokinetics

Tedizolid phosphate is an inactive prodrug that undergoes rapid hydrolysis by serum phosphatases to the active compound, tedizolid.[191,218] As a monophosphate ester, tedizolid phosphate demonstrates increased bioavailability, increased water solubility, and compound stability across a wide pH range.[218] Tedizolid exhibits near linear pharmacokinetics with increasing dosages demonstrating corresponding increases in AUC. The AUC of tedizolid phosphate via oral and intravenous administration has been shown to be similar between adult, including the elderly, and adolescent patients.[191] Tedizolid demonstrates high protein binding at approximately 90% and has a volume of distribution of greater than 100L.[304,380] Metabolism of this agent predominantly occurs via conjugation and excretion by the liver as an inactive compound with the remainder, less than 20%, being excreted as unchanged drug in the urine.[380] The elimination half-life in adults is approximately 11 hours for both the oral and intravenous formulations.[304,380] Renal dosing adjustments are not required with this agent in patients exhibiting advanced renal failure, as the drug half-life and AUC of tedizolid were not significantly different between normal patient cohorts and patients in renal failure. Further, dosage adjustments are not required in patients receiving hemodialysis, as pharmacokinetics were not significantly impacted because this agent is not removed.[380] The tedizolid adult dosing recommendation is 200 mg administered daily via either the oral or intravenous route.

Indications for Use

Phase II evaluation of tedizolide evaluated three different oral dosages (200, 300, or 400 mg) administered daily for 5 to 7 days in adult patients with suspected or confirmed complicated skin and skin structure infection. A daily 200-mg oral dose was determined to be the lowest effective dose for the treatment of complicated skin and skin structure infection.[284] During a phase III clinical trial enrolling adult patients with acute bacterial skin and skin structure infections, a 6-day course of oral tedizolid phosphate proved to be non-inferior to a 10-day course of oral linezolid with early and sustained clinical response rates that were similar between groups.[285] Similarly, a phase III clinical trial enrolling patients older than 12 years with acute bacterial skin and skin structure infections found a 6-day course of intravenous tedizolid phosphate to be non-inferior to a 10-day course of linezolid.[247] With these data, tedizolid phosphate received FDA approval for the treatment of acute bacterial skin and skin structure infections in adults. A phase III study is underway to compare the safety of intravenous to oral tedizolid (200 mg) for 6 days versus a 10-day course of comparator antibiotic agents in adolescent patient (12 to <18 years of age) with complicated skin and soft tissue infection (NCT02276482). A phase III study is investigating intravenous tedizolid for the treatment of ventilated adult patients with presumed gram-positive hospital-acquired bacterial pneumonia or ventilator-associated bacterial pneumonia (NCT02019420).

Adverse Effects

Data from multiple trials indicate that tedizolid is safe and well tolerated, with the majority of adverse events across studies being reported as either mild or moderate. Prokocimer and colleagues reported the most commonly experienced adverse events included nausea, diarrhea, vomiting and headache. No patients were found to have significant alterations in hematologic parameters, including platelet and neutrophil counts, or changes in electrocardiograms.[284] In two phase III studies, fewer patients in the tedizolid groups had decreases in platelet count, neutrophil count or hemoglobin levels that were below the lower limit of normal as compared to patients in the linezolid groups.[247,285,323] However, additional experience with tedizolid is required to more appropriately assess differences in the risk of myelosuppression between tedizolid and linezolid, as studies to date have not been adequately powered to fully investigate this issue.

Rifamycins

The rifamycins are a group of complex macrocyclic antibiotics that were isolated from *Streptomyces mediterranei* in the early 1960s. Rifampin (rifampicin) and rifabutin are structurally related, semisynthetic broad-spectrum antibiotics derived from rifamycin B and S, respectively. These agents avidly bind to the subunit of the DNA-dependent RNA polymerase, prevent attachment of the enzyme to DNA, and thus block initiation of RNA transcription and protein synthesis. Rifabutin was approved in 1992 for prevention of disseminated MAC disease in adults with advanced HIV infection. Single-point mutations that determine resistance develop rapidly when rifamycins are used alone. Therefore, these antibiotics should be administered in combination with other antimicrobial agents when indicated. Rifaximin also is a semisynthetic derivative of rifamycin that was approved by the FDA in 2004 for the treatment of individuals 12 years of age or older who have nondysenteric and afebrile traveler's diarrhea caused by noninvasive strains of *E. coli*.[4]

In Vitro Activity

Rifampin usually is bactericidal, but it may be bacteriostatic, depending on the organism and drug concentration. Rifamycins have excellent in vitro activity against many gram-positive cocci, including many methicillin-resistant staphylococci and penicillin-nonsusceptible *S. pneumoniae* (enterococci are notable exceptions); some gram-negative organisms, including meningococci, gonococci, and *H. influenzae; Legionella; C. trachomatis; T. gondii; M. tuberculosis;* and *M. leprae.* Rifampin is active against *Mycobacterium kansasii,* but not against most other species of atypical mycobacteria. In contrast, rifabutin is active against most atypical mycobacteria, except *M. chelonae.* Rifabutin also is more active than rifampin against rifampin-susceptible strains of *Mycobacterium tuberculosis* and is active against approximately one third of rifampin-resistant strains.[219,244] Resistance to rifampin is mediated by point mutations in the *rpoB* gene that encodes the subunit of the DNA-dependent RNA polymerase, as well as alterations in membrane permeability. Surveillance data documented that 3% of meningococcal isolates in the United States are resistant to rifampin.[185] Rifaximin has activity against most enteric bacterial pathogens, including *C. difficile, C. jejuni, E. coli, H. pylori, Salmonella* spp., *Shigella* spp., *V. cholera,* and *Yersinia enterocolitica.*[4]

Pharmacokinetics

Rifampin and rifabutin are highly lipid soluble and highly protein bound molecules (72% to 89%). Consequently, they are well absorbed from the gastrointestinal tract and have excellent intracellular penetration. The drugs reach therapeutic concentrations in the CSF (≈10% to 20% of simultaneous serum concentrations), particularly in the presence of inflammation of the meninges. They are metabolized primarily by the liver through deacetylation, and 30% to 40% of the drug is excreted by the biliary system. In the presence of hepatic dysfunction, dosage adjustments are necessary, whereas no alteration in dosage is required for children with renal dysfunction. In adults, rifabutin has a significantly longer mean terminal half-life than rifampin (45 vs. 2 to 5 hours).[291] Rifampin, however, has a very long postantibiotic effect. Rifaximin is poorly absorbed, with a bioavailability of less than 0.4%. Therefore, dosage adjustment of rifaximin for hepatic or renal dysfunction is not necessary, and the agent is unlikely to interact with medications metabolized by the CYP450 system.

Indications for Use

The only situation in which rifampin should be considered for use as a single antibacterial agent is for prophylaxis of infection, because resistance to rifampin can develop rapidly when this agent is used alone for therapeutic purposes. Prophylaxis with rifampin monotherapy is indicated to eradicate nasopharyngeal colonization in close contacts of individuals with infections caused by *H. influenzae* type b[138,251] and *N. meningitidis,*[33] as well as index cases with these infections, unless they were treated with third-generation cephalosporins.

The use of rifampin, combined with two or three other bactericidal antituberculosis agents for the treatment of active tuberculosis, as well as its combined use with clofazimine and dapsone for the treatment of leprosy, is considered an essential component of effective regimens. The effect of adding rifampin to certain antibiotics for treatment of other infections often is unpredictable and may result in synergistic, additive, indifferent, or antagonistic activity. In some patients, rifampin can be considered part of a combination regimen for the treatment of (1) meningitis caused by penicillin- and cephalosporin-resistant *S. pneumoniae* in combination with a third-generation cephalosporin and vancomycin; (2) shunt- or catheter-associated staphylococcal infections, often with removal of the foreign material; (3) *S. aureus* implant-related orthopedic infections in combination with an effective agent; (4) non–life-threatening susceptible MRSA skin and skin structure infections in combination with TMP-SMX with the theoretical benefit of eradicating MRSA carriage, considering that rifampin achieves high concentrations on mucosal surfaces; (5) prosthetic valve endocarditis caused by staphylococci; (6) complicated or severe *B. henselae* infection (cat-scratch disease); (7) brucellosis in combination with TMP-SMX, a tetracycline, or an aminoglycoside[223]; (8) MAC-associated disseminated disease or lymphadenitis, if not completely resectable, in combination with ethambutol and azithromycin or clarithromycin; (9) *L. pneumophila* pneumonia in combination with a macrolide if response to macrolides alone is poor; and (10) multidrug-resistant *S. maltophilia* in combination with colistin (i.e., colistimethate sodium or polymyxin E) based on favorable in vitro data.[185,219] Furthermore, rifampin and minocycline-impregnated central venous catheters have been used successfully in adults to prevent catheter colonization and bloodstream infection with gram-positive and gram-negative pathogens, as well as with *Candida* spp. Data regarding the use of these catheters in children is limited.[269] Many physicians use rifampin combined with antistaphylococcal agents for treatment of disseminated MRSA infection without evidence from controlled studies of its effectiveness.

Rifabutin is effective for the treatment of most mycobacterial species, *H. pylori,* and *T. gondii* in adults. Limited data are available for the treatment of MAC infections in children with HIV infection. Clinical studies in adults with advanced HIV infection indicate that administration of daily clarithromycin or weekly azithromycin is superior to rifabutin alone for prophylaxis of MAC infection.[244] The use of rifabutin as an alternative to azithromycin or clarithromycin for prophylaxis of MAC infection in children is limited by drug interactions and lack of efficacy data.[73]

Rifampin is available in capsule (150 and 300 mg) and intravenous formulations. Rifabutin is available only in capsule (150 mg) form. A suspension can be compounded by the pharmacy, or the capsule contents can be mixed with thick, sweet food for infants and young children. Absorption of rifampin is optimal if administered 1 hour before or 2 hours after a meal, whereas a high-fat meal decreases the rate, but not the total amount, of absorption of rifabutin. The use of fixed-dose combinations of rifampin, isoniazid, and pyrazinamide is not recommended for children. Although the safety and efficacy of rifapentine, a rifamycin antibiotic similar in structure and activity to rifampin and rifabutin, have not been established for children younger than 12 years of age, a pharmacokinetic study indicated that dosages in children need to be greater than those for adults to achieve comparable systemic exposure.[36] Combination treatment with rifapentine and isoniazid given once weekly for 3 months for the treatment of latent tuberculosis infection was found to be as effective as daily therapy with isoniazid alone, safe and associated with a higher treatment completion rate in children 2 to 17 years of age.[364] The approved dosage of rifaximin for the treatment of traveler's diarrhea in adolescents and adults is 200 mg three times per day for 3 days. A dosage of 400 mg twice per day for 3 days apparently is equally effective and may be better tolerated by patients. Rifaximin should not be used to treat systemic infections or mucosally invasive enteric infections. Rifaximin is not indicated currently for the treatment of dysenteric diarrhea secondary to *Shigella, Salmonella,* or *Campylobacter* spp. infection or for the treatment of complicated diarrhea with fever, systemic toxicity, or bloody stools. The role of this agent for prophylaxis of traveler's diarrhea is being studied.[4,17]

Adverse Effects

Adverse events associated with rifampin include gastrointestinal disorders, rash, hepatotoxicity, hypersensitivity, and a flulike syndrome. Adverse reactions to rifabutin include gastrointestinal disorders, rash, leukopenia, neutropenia, and, rarely, uveitis, although safety data in children are limited. The parenteral form of rifampin is associated with thrombophlebitis. Routine determination of serum aminotransferase concentrations is not recommended for children receiving brief or prolonged courses of therapy, except for those with clinical evidence of hepatitis or severe or disseminated tuberculosis. In these situations, at least monthly measurements should be performed. In addition, patients should be warned that rifamycins discolor urine, tears, sweat, and feces and permanently stain soft contact lenses. Because rifamycins induce hepatic CYP450 enzyme activity, they may interact with other medications administered concurrently and cause decreased concentrations of some antiretroviral agents, particularly protease inhibitors, azole antifungal agents, barbiturates, oral contraceptives, clarithromycin, cyclosporine, digoxin, sulfonylureas, thyroxine, and warfarin (Coumadin). Conversely, rifamycin serum drug concentrations may increase if it is administered with other drugs that inhibit hepatic enzymes, and the dose of rifamycin antibiotic may need to be reduced by as much as 50%. Rifabutin induces hepatic enzymes to a lesser extent than does rifampin and therefore has less potential for drug interactions.[219,244] Rifaximin is well tolerated and has an excellent safety profile.

Antibiotics Interfering With Protein Synthesis Not Approved for Use in Children

Fidaxomicin is a macrocylic antibody isolated from the fermentation broth of *Dactylosporangium aurantiacum* that inhibits the bacterial sigma subunit involved in protein synthesis. It has a narrow spectrum of activity with bactericidal effect against gram-positive anaerobes, including *C. difficile,* and demonstrated activity for the NAP1/BI/027 strain. It received FDA approval in 2011 for treatment of *C. difficile*–associated diarrhea in adults. Fidaxomicin was shown to be non-inferior to vancomycin for the treatment of *C. difficile* infection and was effective in preventing recurrences. It has minimal systemic absorption and appears to be well tolerated.[92,114,368]

AGENTS THAT TARGET NUCLEIC ACID

Fluoroquinolones

Fluoroquinolone antibiotics are derivatives of nalidixic acid. In contrast to nalidixic acid, fluoroquinolones have (1) a broader spectrum of activity that includes aerobic gram-negative enteric organisms, particularly Enterobacteriaceae, *Haemophilus* spp., *Neisseria* spp., *M. catarrhalis,* nonenteric gram-negative bacilli such as *P. aeruginosa,* oxacillin-susceptible staphylococci, some streptococci, bacteria associated with atypical pneumonia, certain genital pathogens, and certain strains of mycobacteria; (2) better penetration into tissues; (3) good intracellular penetration; and (4) rapid bactericidal activity.

Mechanisms of Action

Fluoroquinolones are the only class of antibacterial agents in clinical use that directly inhibit DNA synthesis. They bind to bacterial DNA gyrase and topoisomerase IV. Inhibition of bacterial gyrase causes relaxation of the supercoiled DNA that leads to termination of chromosomal replication and interference with cell division and gene expression. Inhibition of the activity of topoisomerase IV leads to separation of two united DNA molecules and subsequent interference with cellular replication.

Mechanisms of Resistance

A growing concern is that widespread use of fluoroquinolones among adult populations has been associated with resistance rates, especially among Enterobacteriaceae, that exceed 50% in some regions. Mechanisms of resistance include chromosomal mutations in genes that encode fluoroquinolone target enzymes (i.e., DNA gyrase and topoisomerase IV), efflux pumps, or porin (i.e., outer-membrane diffusion) channels. Identified plasmid-mediated resistance determinants in strains of *K. pneumoniae, E. coli, Enterobacter,* and other enteric bacteria include (1) Qnr, a protein that protects DNA gyrase from quinolone action and is associated with multidrug resistance and (2) a variant of the aminoglycoside acetyltransferase found in gram-negative bacteria that is capable of inactivating ciprofloxacin.[212,300] Fluoroquinolone-resistant strains of *N. gonorrhoeae* are common findings in many parts of the world and are spreading in the United States, especially in California and Hawaii. The CDC no longer recommends fluoroquinolones for treatment of gonorrhea in the United States.[370] Other bacteria with increasing rates of resistance include *S. pneumoniae* and intestinal pathogens such as *Campylobacter jejuni, Shigella* spp., *Salmonella* spp., certain strains of *Klebsiella pneumoniae, E. coli,* and *P. aeruginosa,* among others.[9]

In Vitro Activity

Levofloxacin and moxifloxacin have greater potency than ciprofloxacin against gram-positive cocci, and moxifloxacin has enhanced activity against anaerobic bacteria, although in some series, approximately 50% of invasive *Bacteroides* spp. are resistant to moxifloxacin.[133] Ciprofloxacin remains the most potent marketed fluoroquinolone against gram-negative bacteria, particularly against some strains of *P. aeruginosa, Providencia* spp., *Proteus* spp., and *S. marcescens.* In vitro studies of newer and investigational fluoroquinolones against penicillin and cephalosporin-resistant pneumococci indicate excellent activity, whereas activity of ciprofloxacin, norfloxacin, and ofloxacin is limited. Fluoroquinolone use for MRSA and oxacillin-resistant, coagulase-negative staphylococci is limited because resistant mutants can be selected relatively easily, thus leading to treatment failure and relapse. Constitutive high-level resistance exists among MRSA isolates from patients with CAMRSA infections in some areas of the United States. Although MICs tend to be lower for newer (e.g., moxifloxacin and gatifloxacin) in contrast to older (e.g., ciprofloxacin and levofloxacin) fluoroquinolones, genes conferring fluoroquinolone resistance in *S. aureus* confer resistance to the entire class of agents.[136] Activity against enterococci is marginal or absent. Fluoroquinolones are effective against atypical pneumonia pathogens (i.e., *Chlamydophila pneumoniae, L. pneumophila,* and *M. pneumoniae*) and certain genital pathogens (i.e., *C. trachomatis, U. urealyticum,* and *Mycoplasma hominis*). Ciprofloxacin, levofloxacin, and moxifloxacin are active in vitro against certain strains of *M. tuberculosis, Mycobacterium fortuitum, M. kansasii,* and *M. chelonae* and are less active against MAC. No quinolone antibiotic has been shown to be active against *T. pallidum.*

Pharmacokinetics

The fluoroquinolones generally have excellent bioavailability that is not substantially affected by food, with values of 70% for ciprofloxacin, 85% for moxifloxacin, and greater than 95% for ofloxacin and levofloxacin. These drugs have large volumes of distribution, and they concentrate in the kidneys and in urine (except moxifloxacin, which undergoes hepatic metabolism and biliary excretion). This class of agents has favorable pharmacokinetic properties in children, and their efficacy correlates best with the 24-hour AUC/MIC ratio because of a combination of concentration-dependent killing and postantibiotic effect. These properties suggest that large doses given at relatively infrequent intervals would be most effective.[315] However, based on pharmacokinetic studies, doses for patients with cystic fibrosis should be higher and more frequent than for patients without cystic fibrosis, and the dosage should be decreased in proportion to increasing body weight. Fluoroquinolones can interact with a variety of other drugs, including caffeine, cyclosporine, dideoxyinosine, nonsteroidal antiinflammatory drugs, theophylline, and other agents that prolong the QT interval. Coadministration with antacids, ferrous sulfate, and multivitamins containing zinc can reduce oral bioavailability.

Indications for Use

Fluoroquinolones have been used extensively in adults for the treatment of skin and soft tissue, skeletal, and intra-abdominal infections, as well as infections of the urogenital, gastrointestinal, and respiratory tracts. Fluoroquinolones commonly used in adults include the second-generation agents ciprofloxacin and levofloxacin and the fourth-generation agent moxifloxacin. Other agents with limited indications include ofloxacin, norfloxacin (second generation), and gemifloxacin (third generation). Four agents have been withdrawn from the market in the United States: gatifloxacin, grepafloxacin (causes cardiac toxicity), sparfloxacin, and trovafloxacin (causes hepatotoxicity). Ciprofloxacin, levofloxacin, and moxifloxacin are FDA approved for the treatment of uncomplicated skin infections caused by susceptible organisms in adults. However, none of these fluoroquinolones are FDA approved for treatment of MRSA infections.

Use in pediatric patients has been limited because of the potential for inducing cartilage damage that leads to arthropathy, as demonstrated in juvenile animal studies. However, no convincing evidence exists that quinolone-induced arthropathy occurs in humans. Reversible arthralgia and tendinopathy have a temporal association with fluoroquinolone use. Fluoroquinolones are not approved for use in children and adolescents younger than 18 years, except in the following situations: (1) complicated urinary tract infections and pyelonephritis attributable to *E. coli* in children 1 year of age and older (approved by the FDA in 2004) and (2) exposure to aerosolized *B. anthracis* to prevent onset or progression of disease. However, these drugs have been used in certain clinical settings, such as cystic fibrosis, primarily because they are the only oral antibiotics with activity against *P. aeruginosa.* Furthermore, ciprofloxacin and levofloxacin are available in suspension formulations. In 2002 alone, approximately 500,000 prescriptions for fluoroquinolones were written in the United States for individuals younger than 18 years old.[9] These agents, particularly ciprofloxacin, have been used to treat exacerbations of chronic pseudomonal pulmonary infections in patients with cystic fibrosis; complicated urinary tract infections caused by multidrug-resistant bacteria; chronic suppurative otitis media associated with *P. aeruginosa;* osteochondritis attributable to *P. aeruginosa;* shigellosis, *C. jejuni,* and other bacterial causes of enteritis; multidrug-resistant typhoid fever; cholera; infections in neutropenic patients with cancer; in combination with other agents to treat multidrug-resistant mycobacterial disease; and multidrug-resistant gram-negative bacillary septicemia or meningitis (no controlled trials in children with meningitis have been reported using currently licensed agents).[9,66,308,316] Fluoroquinolones also effectively eradicate nasopharyngeal carriage of susceptible meningococci. One study showed that children with acute otitis media and otorrhea through tympanostomy tubes had better clinical outcomes with fewer adverse effects when they were treated with ciprofloxacin-dexamethasone otic suspension in contrast to high-dose amoxicillin-clavulanic acid suspension.[103] Although gatifloxacin is not approved for use in children and currently is not available in the United States, noncontrolled studies confirmed that it is safe and effective for treatment of recurrent acute otitis media and acute otitis media when therapy with standard antimicrobials has failed.[279]

The current recommendation is that parenteral and oral fluoroquinolones should be reserved for situations in which no effective, safe, and nonrestricted alternative antimicrobial agents are available to treat complicated or multidrug-resistant bacterial infections. Appropriate uses should be limited to the following clinical situations: exposure to aerosolized *B. anthracis;* urinary tract infections caused by *P. aeruginosa* or other multidrug-resistant, gram-negative bacteria; chronic suppurative otitis media or malignant otitis externa caused by *P. aeruginosa;* acute or chronic osteomyelitis or osteochondritis caused by *P. aeruginosa;* exacerbations of pulmonary disease in patients with cystic fibrosis who have *P. aeruginosa* colonization and for whom oral therapy is appropriate; susceptible mycobacterial infections as part of a combination regimen; gram-negative bacterial infections in immunocompromised hosts in whom oral therapy is appropriate or resistance to alternative agents is present; gastrointestinal infections caused by multidrug-resistant *Shigella* spp., *Salmonella* spp., *V. cholera,* or *C. jejuni;* and proved bacterial septicemia or meningitis caused by multidrug-resistant pathogens that are susceptible only to fluoroquinolones, that have failed to respond to approved agents, or that require use of a fluoroquinolone because of life-threatening hypersensitivity to alternative agents.[9]

Adverse Effects

Adverse events associated with fluoroquinolone therapy occur in 3% to 17% of adult and pediatric patients and cause discontinuation of treatment in 1% to 2%. The most common reactions are gastrointestinal, minor CNS disorders, and allergic rashes.[315] Other infrequent adverse reactions include photosensitivity; disorders of glucose homeostasis; prolongation of the QT interval, with rare cases of torsades de pointes, particularly among patients with long QT syndrome; leukopenia; and anaphylactoid reactions. Reversible tendonitis and tendon rupture occur uncommonly in adults.

Sulfonamides

Sulfonamides, discovered in the 1930s, are broad-spectrum antimicrobial agents derived from sulfanilamide (*p*-aminobenzene sulfonamide) and are structural analogues of *p*-aminobenzoic acid (PABA); they compete with PABA and result in interference with nucleotide synthesis. Sulfanilamide was manipulated to form other compounds with expanded antimicrobial activity and reduced toxicity. Sulfonamides are distributed widely in fluids and tissues. The preparations currently available have greater solubility than earlier compounds and are less likely to cause crystalluria. Sulfadiazine is available for single-agent use. Sulfonamide combinations, including trimethoprim-sulfamethoxazole (TMP-SMX) and erythromycin ethylsuccinate-sulfisoxazole acetyl (EES-SSX), are used frequently in pediatrics.

Trimethoprim-Sulfamethoxazole

TMP is a diaminopyrimidine antibiotic available for single-agent use. Combinations of TMP and sulfonamides were used in the late 1960s because of presumed synergistic antibacterial activity, although clinical evidence of synergy is equivocal. Because SMX has rates of absorption and elimination similar to those of TMP, it was the sulfonamide selected for combination. Iclaprim is a novel diaminopyrimidine with a broad spectrum of activity that includes TMP-resistant strains of *S. aureus* (including MRSA and vancomycin-resistant *S. aureus*), *S. pneumoniae* (including penicillin-nonsusceptible strains), *P. jiroveci, Neisseria, M. catarrhalis,* and *C. pneumoniae.*[149] Iclaprim inhibits bacterial dihydrofolate reductase; it has been evaluated in clinical trials, including a multicenter, double-blind, phase II, randomized study comparing safety and efficacy with vancomycin but has not been approved by the FDA.[201]

Mechanisms of action. SMX competitively inhibits dihydropteroate synthetase, the bacterial enzyme that assimilates PABA into dihydrofolic acid; such inhibition results in a reduction in dihydrofolic acid synthesis and therefore a reduction in the amount of tetrahydrofolic acid, a cofactor for nucleotide synthesis.[151] Only bacteria that must synthesize folic acid are potentially susceptible. SMX is bacteriostatic when used alone and can be inhibited by PABA and its derivatives (procaine and tetracaine). TMP reversibly binds and inhibits dihydrofolate reductase, an enzyme that reduces dihydrofolic acid to tetrahydrofolic acid; this activity results in diminished amounts of folic acid, an essential cofactor in nucleic acid production.[62] TMP is bacteriostatic when used alone, but in combination with SMX against susceptible bacteria, bactericidal activity can be achieved by blockade of sequential steps in folic acid metabolism. The effect of sulfonamide on bacteria is circumvented in mammals, which obtain folate from food sources. The reaction inhibited by TMP is similar in bacteria and mammals but differs quantitatively in the extent of binding of the drug to the enzyme; mammalian dihydrofolate reductase is 60,000 times less sensitive to TMP than is the enzyme in susceptible bacteria.

Mechanisms of resistance. Bacteria can be inherently resistant to either agent or can acquire resistance to TMP, SMX, or both agents. Resistance to SMX and other sulfonamides is associated with hyperproduction of PABA, as demonstrated in strains of *Neisseria* and staphylococci, or is caused by an altered dihydropteroate synthetase enzyme with lower affinity for sulfonamides, as found in *E. coli, N. meningitidis,* and *S. pneumoniae.*[346] Chromosomally mediated resistance to TMP on the basis of mutations in the *dhfr* gene has been observed in strains of *S. pneumoniae, H. influenzae, E. coli, Pediococcus, B. fragilis,* and *Nocardia* and *Clostridium* spp. Furthermore, *P. aeruginosa, K. pneumoniae,* and *S. marcescens* are inherently resistant to TMP because of cell wall impermeability. Acquired resistance to TMP can be plasmid-mediated or chromosomally mediated and occurs in members of the Enterobacteriaceae and in staphylococci and streptococci. Mechanisms of acquired TMP resistance include cell wall impermeability, thymine auxotrophy, resistant dihydrofolate reductase, and overproduction of dihydrofolate reductase, the most common being plasmid-mediated production of dihydrofolate reductases, which are encoded by at least 20 genes. Resistance to sulfonamides is encoded by the dhps family of genes that include the *folP* and *sulI* and *sulII* genes. The *sulI* gene usually is linked to other transferable resistance genes, often in the transposons that belong to the Tn21 family. Despite the reduced use of sulfonamides, the genetic determinants for sulfonamide resistance probably persist because of the efficient integron transfer mechanisms.[161] Bacterial resistance to both TMP and SMX can develop as a result of altered cell wall permeability or alternative metabolic pathways (e.g., thymine auxotrophy), whereby they obtain thymine or thymidine from the environment.[346]

In vitro activity. TMP-SMX has activity against a broad spectrum of gram-positive cocci and gram-negative enteric pathogens. TMP is more active than the sulfonamide, but the mixture is significantly more effective than either drug alone. Synergism is more likely to occur when the bacteria are susceptible to both drugs, but it can occur even when the bacteria are resistant to only one agent. Bacteria with potential susceptibility to the combination include *Aeromonas hydrophila, Brucella, B. cepacia, Campylobacter, E. coli, H. influenzae, M. catarrhalis, Kingella kingae,* some environmental mycobacteria, *N. gonorrhoeae, Nocardia, P. jiroveci, Proteus, Salmonella, S. marcescens, Shigella,* oxacillin-susceptible and methicillin-resistant *S. aureus, S. maltophilia* (usually with a β-lactam-lactamase inhibitor combination), penicillin-susceptible *S. pneumoniae,* and *Yersinia enterocolitica.* However, high levels of resistance to TMP-SMX among strains of penicillin-nonsusceptible *S. pneumoniae, M. catarrhalis, H. influenzae, Neisseria, E. coli, Klebsiella, Salmonella, Shigella, Campylobacter, P. aeruginosa, Acinetobacter, Actinomyces,* *mycobacteria, Bacteroides, Clostridium,* and *C. pneumonia* limit the usefulness of this antibacterial agent.[161]

Pharmacokinetics. Optimal synergistic activity occurs when a 1:20 ratio of TMP and SMX serum concentrations is attained, as can be achieved after the administration of a fixed 1:5 ratio of TMP to SMX. Both agents are absorbed rapidly and fairly well when administered alone and in combination. Both penetrate most body fluids and tissues, although TMP frequently penetrates extravascular tissues to a greater degree than SMX. Both agents cross the placenta, are excreted in breast milk, and diffuse into pleural, peritoneal, and synovial fluid and CSF. Protein binding varies from 40% to 60% for TMP and from 60% to 70% for SMX. Both drugs are metabolized in the liver to inactive metabolites. The primary route of elimination is by the kidneys, with small amounts excreted in bile and feces. Dosage adjustments are required for renal impairment.

Available preparations include an oral suspension containing 40 mg of TMP and 200 mg of SMX per 5 mL, tablets containing 80 mg of TMP and 400 mg of SMX, double-strength tablets consisting of 160 mg of TMP and 800 mg of SMX, and a parenteral solution.

Indications for use. TMP-SMX is approved for the treatment of acute exacerbations of chronic bronchitis in adults, enterocolitis caused by susceptible *Shigella* organisms, acute otitis media caused by susceptible strains of *H. influenzae* or pneumococcus, *P. jiroveci* pneumonia, traveler's diarrhea caused by *Shigella* and enterotoxigenic *E. coli,* and acute or chronic urinary tract infections. Although the combination is not approved for use and not usually prescribed as a first-line antibiotic, TMP-SMX has been effective therapy for typhoid fever, brucellosis, nocardiosis, sinusitis, biliary tract infections, and bone and joint infections caused by susceptible organisms. Because early studies did not evaluate the effect of prolonged or recurrent therapy on somatic growth or bone marrow function in children, TMP-SMX was not approved for prophylaxis or prolonged treatment of otitis media. It is not recommended for treatment of group A streptococcal tonsillopharyngitis because it does not eradicate the organism or reliably prevent the nonsuppurative sequelae. TMP-SMX is not recommended as first-line monotherapy for community-acquired pneumonia, acute otitis media, or skin infections caused by *S. pyogenes* because of frequent resistance among the etiologic pathogens and absence of efficacy data. TMP-SMX is not FDA approved for the treatment of any form of staphylococcal infection. However, the medical literature contains reports of the successful use of TMP-SMX alone or in combination with one or more agents such as rifampin in the treatment of *S. aureus* infections, including MRSA.[136,163] TMP-SMX is recommended as an alternative agent to macrolides for treatment of pertussis in individuals 2 months of age or older.[350] TMP-SMX also is an important prophylactic agent that is indicated to prevent bacterial, *P. jiroveci,* and other infections in the following clinical settings: immunosuppressed oncology or posttransplant patients, individuals with HIV who meet clinical and hematologic criteria or certain infants who are exposed in utero to HIV, patients with urinary tract infections who are at risk for recurrent disease, and patients with chronic granulomatous disease or other congenital immunodeficiency syndromes.

Adverse effects. Most of the side effects occurring during administration of TMP-SMX are caused by the sulfonamide. Gastrointestinal disturbances and hypersensitivity reactions are the adverse events most commonly observed. Anorexia, nausea, vomiting, diarrhea, drug eruption, and photosensitivity reactions can occur in 1% to 4% of patients. Hypersensitivity reactions that develop less frequently include erythema nodosum, erythema multiforme (including Stevens-Johnson syndrome), urticaria, anaphylaxis, and thyroid damage. Drug-induced hepatitis has been described but is an unusual event. CNS side effects include vertigo, ataxia, headache, and aseptic meningitis. TMP-SMX can affect renal function when it is administered to persons with underlying renal disease, but the side effect usually is reversible after discontinuation of therapy. Crystalluria occurred more commonly with earlier preparations because of low solubility. SMX has a greater tendency to cause crystalluria than other sulfonamides that are currently available, because of slower absorption and excretion. However, with adequate fluid intake, alkalinization of the urine usually is unnecessary. Interstitial nephritis and tubular necrosis seldom are associated with the use of TMP-SMX. Blood dyscrasias can be a limiting factor to the administration of TMP-SMX. Acute hemolytic anemia has been described after the use of TMP-SMX in patients with glucose-6-phosphate dehydrogenase deficiency. Although they are uncommon in patients with normal hematopoietic systems, aplastic anemia, agranulocytosis, leukopenia, and thrombocytopenia can occur. Prolonged use can result in megaloblastic anemia because of impaired folate use. Administration of sulfonamide can trigger an acute attack of porphyria. Sulfonamides can displace bilirubin from albumin binding sites. In neonates, especially premature infants, the activity of sulfonamides can be increased as a result of reduced conjugation by the immature liver. Because of the increased risk for development of kernicterus from sulfonamide displacement of bilirubin, the use of sulfonamides during the last month of pregnancy and in the first 2 months of life is discouraged.

Drug-drug interactions with TMP-SMX are numerous. Sulfonamides can displace other drugs from albumin binding sites and thereby result in increased effective activity of the second drug, as can be seen with the concurrent administration of methotrexate, phenytoin, sulfonylurea hypoglycemic agents, thiazide diuretics, and warfarin. Drugs that, when coadministered, can displace sulfonamides from binding sites and lead to increased effective sulfonamide activity include indomethacin, probenecid, and salicylates. Agents that reduce the effect of sulfonamides include methenamine, which results in insoluble urinary precipitates of the sulfonamide, and derivatives of PABA. Sulfonamides are physically incompatible with many drugs, among them aminoglycosides, chloramphenicol, insulin, lincomycin, methicillin, tetracycline, and vancomycin.

Erythromycin Ethylsuccinate–Sulfisoxazole Acetyl

The combination of EES and SSX in a fixed ratio expands the spectrum of antibacterial activity. The mechanism of action, mechanisms of resistance, pharmacokinetics, and adverse events for EES-SSX are the same as those for each individual drug. Because EES-SSX is effective in vitro against common pathogens causing otitis media in children, it was approved for the treatment of acute otitis media.[45] However, it is not effective against many strains of pneumococci and no longer is recommended for empirical therapy of acute otitis media.[11] Although it is not approved for use, it can be effective therapy for sinusitis caused by *H. influenzae,* susceptible pneumococci, and *M. catarrhalis.* Albeit uncommon, its principal use today in pediatrics is for the treatment of acute otitis media caused by susceptible pathogens in patients with β-lactam hypersensitivity.

Metronidazole

Metronidazole is a synthetic imidazole available since 1959. It was first introduced for the treatment of *Trichomonas vaginalis.* Metronidazole has antiprotozoal and anaerobic activity.

Mechanisms of action. Metronidazole enters the cells by passive diffusion, and the nitro side chain undergoes chemical reduction by the pyruvate-ferredoxin reductase complex into a toxic nitro radical that subsequently causes DNA destabilization and rupture with cell death. It has been postulated that metronidazole has antiinflammatory and immunomodulator effects by decreasing neutrophil generation of hydrogen peroxide and hydroxyl radicals.

Mechanisms of resistance. Bacteria become resistant to metronidazole by changes in the enzymes implicated in the activation of the antibiotic. Some bacteria contain *nim* genes that code for an inactivating enzyme that reduces the nitro group into an inactive amine. These genes may be present in plasmids and chromosomes.

Pharmacokinetics. Metronidazole has good oral absorption with a bioavailability of at least 90%. It is available in oral (i.e., tablets and capsules) and parenteral forms. It is also available for topical use (i.e., vaginal and rectal). It has good penetration and a low degree of protein binding (<20%), for which it has wide distribution, including good concentrations in CSF. Its half-life is approximately 8 hours. Metronidazole is eliminated mainly by renal clearance (60% to 80%), and 6% to 15% is eliminated unchanged in feces. It is cleared by hemodialysis but does not require dose adjustment with renal insufficiency. In cases of severe hepatic dysfunction, the dose should be adjusted secondary to reduced clearance.

Indications for use. Metronidazole is the treatment of choice for *T. vaginalis, Giardia duodenalis, Entamoeba histolytica,* bacterial vaginosis, and *C. difficile*–associated disease. Metronidazole has been widely used in pediatrics for the treatment of anaerobic infections, including intra-abdominal and head and neck infections (including brain abscess), despite its lack of FDA approval for these indications. For these infections a combination regimen should be used because metronidazole does not have aerobic activity. Metronidazole is used for the treatment of *H. pylori* ulcerative disease, in combination with other antibiotics and a proton pump inhibitor.[220] Safety and effectiveness of metronidazole in children have not been established, except for the treatment of amebiasis with oral metronidazole.

Adverse effects. Gastrointestinal disturbances are the most frequent adverse effects, including nausea and diarrhea. Less frequently, dizziness, headache, loss of appetite, emesis, and abdominal pain have been reported. Other rare effects include taste changes, constipation, dry mouth, glossitis or stomatitis, headache, dark urine, pruritus, rash, insomnia, arthralgias, fever, and reversible hematologic disturbances, including leukopenia and thrombocytopenia. The parenteral form may cause phlebitis at the site of injection. With high doses, neurologic effects may be seen, including ataxia, confusion, and irritability.[47] The neurologic side effects require discontinuation of the drug. In older patients, the concomitant consumption of metronidazole and alcohol can produce a disulfiram effect.

SELECTED ASPECTS OF THE ADMINISTRATION OF ANTIMICROBIAL AGENTS

Dosage Schedules for Infants and Children

Dosage schedules of antimicrobial agents commercially available in the United States for infants (beyond the newborn period) and children are listed in Table 236.4. The list is subdivided into dosage schedules for mild-to-moderate and for severe disease. Oral regimens are used for mild-to-moderate infections caused by susceptible organisms in areas that are well vascularized and in which adequate concentrations of drug are achieved at the site of infection. Parenteral administration should be considered for severe infections, especially those caused by less susceptible organisms that produce disease in areas in which diffusion of drug is limited.

Dosage Schedules for Newborn Infants

The clinical pharmacology of antimicrobial agents administered to newborn infants is unique and cannot be extrapolated from data derived from older children or adults. The physiologic and metabolic processes that affect the distribution, metabolism, and excretion of drugs undergo rapid changes during the child's first few weeks of life. The increased efficiency of kidney function after the infant's first 7 days requires an increase in dosage and a decrease in the interval between doses of penicillins and aminoglycosides for maintaining therapeutic concentrations of drug in blood and tissues. Thus, different dosage schedules are provided for the first week of life and for the subsequent weeks of the neonatal period (Tables 236.5 and 236.6). With survival of premature infants with very low birth weights, more data are needed on the use of antimicrobial agents in these infants with immature metabolic and physiologic mechanisms.[282] Dosages of antibiotics in these preterm infants, especially those weighing less than 1000 g, are unclear for many agents, and measurement of serum concentrations should be considered for drugs such as vancomycin and the aminoglycosides.

Should Dosages Be Determined by Weight or by Surface Area?

In most standard pediatric texts and in the package inserts prepared by manufacturers, dosages of antibiotics for children are based on body weight. Body surface area correlates more closely with extracellular fluid volume. Some investigators suggest that more predictable serum concentrations can be achieved by using calculations of dosages based on surface area than by using those based on weight.[150] This method may be more reliable for drugs that are distributed in extracellular fluid, such as aminoglycosides, especially when they are prescribed for obese or malnourished children. Currently, however, the convenience of calculating dosage on the basis of weight appears to be the more important consideration.

Use of Oral Preparations for Serious Infections

Oral preparations of antimicrobial agents vary in their degree of absorption within and between individuals, depending on the illness being treated and the formulation used. Because higher and more consistent serum concentrations of drug are achieved after parenteral administration, parenteral routes are preferable for serious infections. Sequential parenteral-oral antimicrobial therapy may be an option in patients with uncomplicated pneumonia, pyelonephritis, or intra-abdominal, skin and soft tissue, or suppurative skeletal infections.[236] Results of studies of orally administered antibiotics in children with skeletal infections indicate that this mode of administration can be used successfully for a portion of the therapeutic course.[260,345]

Specific guidelines for oral treatment of serious infections are recommended: (1) the patient should be able to swallow and retain the medication; (2) the dosage should be sufficiently large to provide adequate bactericidal concentrations of drug at the site of infection for at least 50% of the dosing interval for β-lactams; and (3) when possible, it is

TABLE 236.4 **Daily Dosage Schedules for Antimicrobial Agents in Pediatric Patients Beyond Newborn Period**

Agent, Generic (Trade Name)	Route	Mild-to-Moderate Infections[a]	Severe Infections[a]
Penicillin G, crystalline (numerous)	IV, IM	100,000-250,000 U ÷ into 4 doses	250,000–450,000 U ÷ into 6 doses
Penicillin G, procaine (numerous)	IM	50,000 U once daily (congenital syphilis); 300,000 (<60 lb) or 600,000–1,000,000 U (≥60 lb) ÷ into 1 or 2 doses for group A streptococcal infections	Inappropriate
Penicillin G, benzathine (Bicillin)	IM	300,000–600,000 U (<60 lb)[b] or 900,000 U (≥60 lb)[b] for group A streptococcal infections; 50,000 U/kg (up to 2,400,000 U)[b] for syphilis	Inappropriate
Penicillin V, phenoxymethyl penicillin (numerous)	PO	25-50 mg ÷ into 3 or 4 doses	Inappropriate
Penicillinase-resistant Penicillins			
Dicloxacillin	PO	25–50 mg ÷ into 4 doses	Inappropriate
Nafcillin (Nallpen)	IV, IM	50–100 mg ÷ into 4 doses	100–200 mg ÷ into 4 to 6 doses
Oxacillin (Bactocill)	IV, IM	100–150 mg ÷ into 4 doses	150–200 mg ÷ into 4 to 6 doses
Aminopenicillins			
Amoxicillin (numerous)	PO	25–90 mg ÷ into 2 or three doses	Inappropriate
Amoxicillin + clavulanate (Augmentin)	PO	45–90 mg ÷ into 2 or 3 doses	Inappropriate
Ampicillin (numerous)	IV, IM	100–200 mg ÷ into 4 doses	200–400 mg ÷ into 4 to 6 doses
	PO	50–100 mg ÷ into 4 doses	Inappropriate
Ampicillin + sulbactam (Unasyn)	IV	100–200 mg of ampicillin ÷ into 4 doses	200–400 mg of ampicillin ÷ into 4 to 6 doses
Extended-Spectrum Penicillins			
Piperacillin + tazobactam (Zosyn)	IV	Inappropriate	240–300 mg of piperacillin ÷ into 3 to 4 doses
Monobactams			
Aztreonam (Azactam)	IV, IM	90 mg ÷ into 3 doses	120 mg ÷ into 4 doses
Cephalosporins			
Cefadroxil (Duricef)	PO	30 mg ÷ into 2 doses	Inappropriate
Cefazolin (Ancef, Kefzol)	IV, IM	50 mg ÷ into 3 doses	50–100 mg ÷ into 3 or 4 doses
Cephalexin (Keflex, Keftab)	PO	25–100 mg ÷ into 4 doses	Inappropriate
Cefaclor (Ceclor)	PO	20–40 mg ÷ into 2 or three doses	Inappropriate
Cefoxitin (Mefoxin)	IV	Inappropriate	80–160 mg ÷ into 4 to 6 doses
Cefprozil (Cefzil)	PO	15–30 mg ÷ into 2 doses	Inappropriate
Ceftibuten (Cedax)	PO	9 mg once daily	Inappropriate
Cefuroxime (Kefurox, Zinacef)	IV, IM	Inappropriate	100–150 mg ÷ into 3 or 4 doses
Cefuroxime axetil (Ceftin)	PO	20–30 mg ÷ into 2 doses	Inappropriate
Cefdinir (Omnicef)	PO	14 mg ÷ into 1 or 2 doses	Inappropriate
Cefditoren (Spectracef)	PO	200–400 mg twice daily[b,d]	Inappropriate
Cefixime (Suprax)	PO	8 mg ÷ into 1 or 2 doses	Inappropriate
Cefotaxime (Claforan)	IV, IM	Inappropriate	100–180 mg ÷ into 4 to 6 doses
Cefpodoxime proxetil (Vantin)	PO	10 mg ÷ into 2 doses	Inappropriate
Ceftazidime (Fortaz, Tazicef)	IV, IM	Inappropriate	100–150 mg ÷ into 3 doses
Ceftriaxone (Rocephin)	IV, IM	Inappropriate	50–100 mg ÷ into 1 or 2 doses
Cefepime (Maxipime)	IV, IM	Inappropriate	100–150 mg ÷ into 2 or 3 doses
Carbapenems			
Ertapenem (Invanz)	IV, IM	Inappropriate	30 mg ÷ into 2 doses
Imipenem-cilastatin (Primaxin)	IV, IM	Inappropriate	60–100 mg ÷ into 4 doses
Meropenem (Merrem)	IV	Inappropriate	60–120 mg ÷ into 3 doses
Macrolides			
Azithromycin (Zithromax)	PO	10 mg on day 1, then 5 mg thereafter; 12 mg for pharyngitis	Inappropriate
Clarithromycin (Biaxin)	PO	15 mg ÷ into 2 doses	Inappropriate
Erythromycin base (numerous)	PO	30–50 mg ÷ into 4 doses	Inappropriate
Erythromycin ethylsuccinate (E.E.S., EryPed, Erythro)	PO	30–50 mg ÷ into 4 doses	Inappropriate
Erythromycin lactobionate (Erythrocin)	IV	Inappropriate	20–50 mg ÷ into 4 doses
Erythromycin stearate (numerous)	PO	30–50 mg ÷ into 4 doses	Inappropriate

Continued

TABLE 236.4 **Daily Dosage Schedules for Antimicrobial Agents in Pediatric Patients Beyond Newborn Period—cont'd**

Agent, Generic (Trade Name)	Route	Mild-to-Moderate Infections[a]	Severe Infections[a]
Lincosamides			
Clindamycin (Cleocin)	IV, IM	Inappropriate	20–40 mg ÷ into 3 or 4 doses
	PO	8–20 mg ÷ into 3 or 4 doses	Inappropriate
Vancomycin (Vancocin)	IV	Inappropriate	40–60 mg ÷ into 4 doses
Aminoglycosides			
Amikacin (Amikin)	IV, IM	Inappropriate	15–22.5 mg ÷ into 3 doses
Gentamicin (Garamycin)	IV, IM	Inappropriate	5–7.5 mg ÷ into 3 doses[e]
Kanamycin	IV, IM	Inappropriate	15–30 mg ÷ into 3 doses
Paromomycin	PO	25–35 mg ÷ into 3 doses	Inappropriate
Streptomycin	IM	Inappropriate	20–40 mg ÷ into 1 or 2 doses
Tobramycin (Nebcin)	IV, IM	Inappropriate	6–7.5 mg ÷ into 3 to 4 doses
Tetracyclines			
Doxycycline (numerous)	PO	2.2–4.4 mg ÷ into 1 or 2 doses	Inappropriate
Tetracycline	PO	25–50 mg ÷ into 4 doses	Inappropriate
Chloramphenicol	IV	Inappropriate	50–100 mg ÷ into 4 doses
Sulfonamides			
Erythromycin ethylsuccinate, sulfisoxazole (Pediazole, Eryzole)	PO	50 mg erythromycin/150 mg sulfa ÷ into four doses	Inappropriate
Sulfadiazine	PO	100–150 mg ÷ into 4 doses	Inappropriate
Trimethoprim-sulfamethoxazole (Bactrim, Septra, Sulfatrim, Cotrim)	PO	8–12 mg trimethoprim/40-60 mg sulfamethoxazole ÷ into 2 doses	Inappropriate
	IV	Inappropriate	10–20 mg trimethoprim/50–100 mg sulfamethoxazole ÷ into 4 doses
Fluoroquinolones			
Ciprofloxacin (Cipro)	PO	20–30 mg ÷ into 2 doses	Inappropriate
	IV	Inappropriate	20–30 mg ÷ into 2 doses
Rifampin (Rifadin)	PO	10–20 mg ÷ into 1 or 2 doses	20 mg ÷ into 2 doses
	IV	Inappropriate	20 mg ÷ into 2 doses
Metronidazole (Flagyl)	PO	15–50 mg ÷ into 3 or 4 doses	Inappropriate
	IV	Inappropriate	30 mg ÷ into 4 doses
Linezolid (Zyvox)	PO	Inappropriate	20–30 mg ÷ into 2 or 3 doses
	IV	Inappropriate	20–30 mg ÷ into 2 or 3 doses
Quinupristin-dalfopristin (Synercid)	IV	Inappropriate	22.5 mg ÷ 3 doses
Colistimethate sodium (Colistin, ColyMycin M)	IV, IM	Inappropriate	2.5–5 mg ÷ into 2 to 4 doses

IM, Intramuscularly; *IV,* intravenously; *PO,* orally.
[a]Total daily dosage (per kilogram). For larger children, maximal dosages may apply.
[b]Total dose.
[c]No longer available in the United States.
[d]Not approved for children younger than 12 years of age.
[e]A dose of 4 mg/kg once daily is used commonly in neonates. A dose of 67.5 mg/kg once daily in older children is investigational.

advisable to have the hospital laboratory determine serum antimicrobial concentrations. When this is not possible, careful follow-up is mandatory, and measurements of inflammatory indices, such as the erythrocyte sedimentation rate and C-reactive protein, are very useful in determining resolution of the infection.

Oral therapy can be considered for patients with osteomyelitis and suppurative arthritis only after an initial period of parenteral therapy, after results are available from cultures and susceptibility tests, and after the patient shows definite signs of resolution of inflammation. Oral therapy should be initiated before discharge from the hospital to ascertain compliance, determine serum antimicrobial concentrations when available, and observe for significant side effects that would preclude use of the oral antibiotic.

Food Interference With the Absorption of Some Oral Antibiotics

The absorption of some oral antimicrobial agents is decreased significantly when the drug is taken with food or near mealtime. These drugs include unbuffered penicillin G, penicillinase-resistant penicillins (i.e., nafcillin, oxacillin, cloxacillin, and dicloxacillin), ampicillin, and lincomycin. Dairy products and other foods or medications containing calcium or magnesium salts interfere with the absorption of tetracyclines. Absorption of penicillin V, buffered penicillin G, amoxicillin, cephalexin, cefaclor, chloramphenicol, erythromycin, and clindamycin is affected only slightly by food. When absorption is affected by the concurrent ingestion of food, antibiotics should be taken 1 or more hours before or 2 or more hours after meals. A dosage schedule of four times daily, rarely used for common infections, can be arranged for the drug to be given on arising, 1 hour before lunch and supper, and at bedtime. Most orally administered antibiotics can be administered twice or three times daily, a schedule that is accommodated easily by most parents.

Intravenous Versus Intramuscular Administration

Although a brief period occurs when the serum antimicrobial concentration is higher after intravenous administration of an antimicrobial agent than after intramuscular administration, no therapeutic advantage of intravenous as opposed to intramuscular administration has been demonstrated. Intravenous administration should be used if the patient is in shock or is suffering from a bleeding diathesis. When prolonged parenteral therapy is anticipated, the pain of injection and the small muscle mass of infants and young children preclude the intramuscular route and render intravenous therapy preferable. The physician must

TABLE 236.5 **Dosage Schedules for Antimicrobial Agents Used in Neonates**

		DOSAGE (mg/kg) AND INTERVAL OF ADMINISTRATION				
		WEIGHT <1200 g	WEIGHT 1200–2000 g		WEIGHT >2000 g	
Antibiotic	**Route**	**Age 0–4 wk**	**Age 0–7 Days**	**Age >7 Days**	**Age 0–7 Days**	**Age >7 Days**
Penicillin G, crystalline (U)	IV	25,000–50,000 q12h	25,000–50,000 q12h	25,000–50,000 q8h	25,000–50,000 q8h	25,000–50,000 q6h
Penicillin G, procaine (U)	IM		50,000 q24h	50,000 q24h	50,000 q24h	50,000 q24h
Penicillin G, benzathine (U)	IM		50,000 once	50,000 once	50,000 once	50,000 once
Penicillinase-Resistant Penicillins						
Oxacillin	IV, IM	25 q12h	25–50 q12h	25–50 q8h	25–50 q8h	25–50 q6h
Nafcillin	IV, IM	25 q12h	25–50 q12h	25–50 q8h	25–50 q8h	25–50 q6h
Broad-Spectrum Penicillins						
Ampicillin IV, IM						
Meningitis		50 q12h	50 q12h	50 q8h	50 q8h	50 q6h
Other infections		25 q12h	25 q12h	25 q8h	25 q8h	25 q6h
Meropenem	IV	20 q12h	20 q12h	20 q12h	20 q12h	20 q12h or q8h
Cephalosporins						
Cefazolin	IV, IM	20 q12h	20 q12h	20 q12h	20 q12h	20 q8h
Cefotaxime	IV, IM	50 q12h	50 q12h	50 q8h	50 q12h	50 q6h or q8h
Ceftriaxone	IV, IM	50 q24h	50 q24h	50 q24h	50 q24h	75 q24h
Ceftazidime	IV, IM	30 q12h	30 q12h	30 q12h	30 q12h	30 q12h
Cefepime	IV, IM	30 q12h	30 q12h	30 q12h	30 q12h	30 q12h to 50 q8h
Clindamycin	IV, IM	5 q12h	5 q12h	5 q8h	5 q8h	5 q6h
Erythromycin	PO	10 q12h	10 q12h	10 q8h	10 q12h	10 q6h or q8h

IM, Intramuscularly; *IV,* intravenously; *PO,* orally.
Modified from Sáez-Llorens X, McCracken GH, Jr. Clinical pharmacology of antibacterial agents. In: Remington JS, Klein JO, editors. *Infectious Diseases of the Fetus and Newborn Infant.* 4th ed. Philadelphia: WB Saunders; 1995:1325.

TABLE 236.6 **Dosage Schedule for Antibiotics Based on Postconceptional Age**[a]

		DOSAGE (mg/kg) AND INTERVAL OF ADMINISTRATION: GESTATIONAL AGE PLUS WEEKS OF LIFE			
Antibiotic	**Route**	**≤26**	**27–34**	**35–41**	**≥42**
Amikacin	IV, IM	7.5 q24h	7.5 q18h	7.5 q12h	7.5 q8h
Gentamicin	IV, IM	2.5 q24h	2.5 q18h	2.5 q12h[b]	2.5 q8h[b]
Tobramycin	IV, IM	2.5 q24h	2.5 q18h	2.5 q12h	2.5 q8h
Vancomycin	IV	10–15 q24h	10–15 q18h[c]	10–15 q12h[c]	10–15 q8h[c] or q6h

IM, Intramuscularly; *IV,* intravenously.
[a]Dosages should be adjusted according to serum drug concentrations.
[b]Single daily dosing is used commonly in neonates: 3–3.5 mg/kg (<35 wk) or 4 mg/kg (≥35 wk).
[c]At 28 days of life, vancomycin is administered at 20 mg/kg per dose; the interval remains the same.

be alert for thrombophlebitis, which can result from prolonged intravenous administration, and for sterile abscesses, which can develop after intramuscular administration.

Chloramphenicol, erythromycin, linezolid, tetracyclines, and vancomycin should be administered intravenously rather than intramuscularly. Chloramphenicol was thought to be absorbed poorly from intramuscular sites, although additional data suggested that such is not the case. Intramuscular injection of parenteral tetracyclines and erythromycin causes local irritation and pain, and intramuscular injection of vancomycin causes tissue necrosis. Care should be given to the administration of intramuscular injections.[31,221] Sites that minimize the risk for local neural, vascular, or tissue injury should be selected. The preferred site varies with the age of the child: the upper anterolateral aspect of the thigh in infants, the ventrogluteal area in children older than 2 years of age, and the deltoid area for older children. Inadvertent intra-arterial injection of benzathine penicillin G can cause tissue damage.

"Push" Versus "Steady" or "Continuous Drip" Intravenous Administration

Antimicrobial agents can be administered intravenously by the "push" method, in which case the drug is infused in 5 to 15 minutes; by "steady drip" in 1 to 2 hours; or by "continuous drip," whereby the drug is given throughout the period of administration. The push method results in high antibacterial activity in serum for short periods, whereas the steady and continuous drip methods produce lower but more sustained activity. The risk for development of adverse effects influences whether an antimicrobial agent should be administered by push or by steady drip. Pharmacodynamic studies suggest optimization of bactericidal activity when aminoglycosides are given by push once daily because the activity of these agents is concentration dependent. By contrast, β-lactams are given preferably in several doses or by a continuous drip to maintain concentrations of drug at the infection site that exceed the MIC of the pathogen for 50% or longer of the dosing interval (time-dependent pharmacodynamic principle). Rapid administration (<5 minutes) of large intravenous doses of penicillin should be avoided because of possible adverse CNS effects. Aminoglycosides given by the intravenous route should be infused in 20 to 60 minutes to obtain optimal peak concentrations. Antimicrobial activity, especially for penicillins, can deteriorate if drugs are kept in solution at room temperature for prolonged periods, as may occur with use of the continuous drip method. Fresh solutions of penicillins should be administered every 6 to 8 hours when the continuous drip method is used.

Diffusion of Antimicrobial Agents Across Biologic Membranes

Diffusion of any drug across a biologic membrane depends on the molecular size of the drug, the degree of protein binding (only the unbound portion of the drug crosses), the degree of ionization at physiologic pH (only the unionized portion is available for equilibration), and solubility in lipids. Thus, the lipid solubility of the unionized and unbound fraction of an antimicrobial agent determines the capability of the drug to diffuse to the site of infection. Antibiotics usually are not distributed evenly throughout the body.[263,264]

Diffusion of antimicrobial agents from blood into a joint space, pleural and pericardial fluid, and middle ear fluid is relatively unimpeded, and high concentrations of many drugs are achieved in these sites after systemic administration. More than 60% of the peak serum concentration of various penicillins and cephalosporins is present in the inflamed joint space.[260] Loculations of fluid in the presence of fibrous adhesions may limit the passage of antimicrobial agents into infected areas.

Diffusion of antibiotics from blood into CSF or into the aqueous humor of the eye is limited. Drugs that are highly soluble in lipids, un-ionized, and minimally bound to proteins (e.g., chloramphenicol, isoniazid, rifampin, and sulfonamides) pass into CSF in high concentrations, even in the absence of inflammation, whereas drugs such as the macrolides diffuse into CSF little, if at all. Fluoroquinolones pass readily into the CSF space but do not have an indication for use for meningitis in children. Penicillins, cephalosporins, and aminoglycosides pass more effectively into CSF when the membrane is inflamed; variable, but often low, concentrations of drug in CSF can be present even in the early stages of meningitis. The β-lactams are pumped actively out of the CSF space by the choroid plexus, a process that is inhibited partially by inflammation.

Duration of Therapy

Physicians must rely on empirically derived schedules of therapy for rapid and complete resolution of disease and minimal risk in terms of clinical or microbiologic failure or drug toxicity. Numerous studies evaluating the duration of therapy have been performed for streptococcal pharyngitis. The results are consistent in suggesting that the following are appropriate: 10 days of oral therapy with penicillins, cephalosporins, or macrolides; 5 days of azithromycin; or a single intramuscular dose of benzathine penicillin G. Opinions vary and data are conflicting regarding the duration of treatment for diseases such as osteomyelitis, suppurative arthritis, and infections of the urinary tract. Radetsky[286] wrote an enlightening history of the recommendations for the duration of treatment in bacterial meningitis and pointed out: "Even in the absence of specific data certain numbers have an unaccountable power to satisfy and reassure. 7, 10, 14 and 21 days have consistently appeared. Even in the trials performed at the dawn of the antimicrobial era, these numbers were chosen."

Dosage Schedules in Children With Renal or Hepatic Insufficiency

The kidneys are the major organs of excretion for most antimicrobial agents, including penicillins, cephalosporins, aminoglycosides, and tetracyclines (with the exception of doxycycline). Because impaired excretion can result in high and possibly toxic serum and tissue antimicrobial concentrations, alterations in dosage schedules should be considered in children with diminished renal function. Antibiotics that require careful dosage adjustment for renal impairment include aminoglycosides, ciprofloxacin, imipenem-cilastatin, meropenem, piperacillin/tazobactam, tetracyclines, TMP-SMX, and vancomycin. Agents requiring dosage adjustments only when renal failure is severe include most penicillins, cephalosporins, and clindamycin. Drugs that are eliminated by nonrenal mechanisms and therefore do not require adjustment of the dosage schedule for renal impairment include chloramphenicol, cloxacillin, dicloxacillin, doxycycline, erythromycin (including the newer macrolides), metronidazole, linezolid, nafcillin, oxacillin, and rifampin.[362]

Dosage schedules for patients with renal insufficiency can be altered by administering the usual dosage for the initial dose and increasing the interval between doses or decreasing individual doses (or both, in the case of renal shutdown). Although numerous guidelines have been developed to assist the physician, these formulas have been generated from studies of adults with renal impairment, and pediatricians must be cautious in adapting the formulas for use in infants and young children.[362] Serum antimicrobial concentrations should be monitored when aminoglycosides, vancomycin, and other drugs with potential toxicity are administered to children with renal insufficiency. Hepatic disorders can alter plasma protein binding, tissue binding, hepatic metabolism, and the distribution of antimicrobials that are metabolized or excreted by the liver.[356] Few data exist regarding adjustment of dosage schedules for antibiotics that are metabolized by the liver in patients with hepatic insufficiency.[205] It would be prudent to avoid the use of tetracyclines and to exercise caution when prescribing chloramphenicol, clindamycin, metronidazole, macrolides, rifampin, and penicillinase-resistant penicillins to patients with underlying hepatic disease.

Topical Use of Antimicrobial Agents

Topical antimicrobial agents are used for a variety of indications: bacitracin or polymyxin ointments are available (in many cases without prescription) for first aid of minor cuts, abrasions, and burns; tetracycline, erythromycin, and clindamycin have been used for the treatment of pustular acne; and metronidazole is approved for the topical treatment of inflammatory lesions and erythema associated with rosacea. Erythromycin, chloramphenicol, sulfonamide, gentamicin, tobramycin, tetracycline, and a combination of TMP and polymyxin B ointment or drops are used for the treatment of conjunctivitis, styes, and other minor infections of the eye. Silver nitrate drops or erythromycin or tetracycline ointment is used for the prevention of gonococcal ophthalmia in newborn infants. A controlled trial involving newborn infants in Africa demonstrated equivalent or superior efficacy of a 2.5% ophthalmic solution of povidone-iodine in contrast to topical silver nitrate or erythromycin for prophylaxis against ophthalmia neonatorum caused by *C. trachomatis, N. gonorrhoeae,* staphylococci, or gram-negative bacteria.[164] Ofloxacin drops (Floxin Otic) are approved for the treatment of otitis externa, chronic suppurative otitis media, and acute otitis media in children with tympanostomy tubes.[38] Ciprofloxacin and dexamethasone otic solution (Ciprodex) is approved for children 6 months of age and older who have tympanostomy tubes, to treat acute otitis media caused by *S. aureus, S. pneumoniae, H. influenzae, M. catarrhalis,* and *P. aeruginosa,* as well as acute otitis externa caused by *S. aureus* and *P. aeruginosa.* Mupirocin is effective in vitro against most *S. aureus* (including methicillin-resistant strains) and group A streptococci and is approved for the treatment of impetigo. At present, approximately 10% of CAMRSA strains are resistant to mupirocin; in some areas, the rate is as high as 30%. Mupirocin applied to the anterior nares may be of value in eradicating nasal carriage of methicillin-resistant staphylococci. However, the few well-designed controlled studies that exist do not support the routine use of mupirocin, except possibly for patients undergoing dialysis, because prolonged use of mupirocin has been associated with resistance to this agent, and recolonization is a common occurrence.[77] Most antibiotics used topically, such as bacitracin, neomycin, and polymyxin B, are of limited use as systemic agents. Retapamulin ointment (Altabax), a pleuromutilin antibacterial, was approved by the FDA in 2007 for topical treatment of impetigo caused by *S. aureus* (methicillin-susceptible isolates only) or *S. pyogenes* in patients aged 9 months or older. The dosage is twice-daily applications for 5 days.

Absorption after application to the conjunctivae or large areas of denuded skin can be significant, but application to normal skin does not result in detectable concentrations of antimicrobial activity in blood or urine. Sensitization does not appear to be an important problem with most topical antibiotics, although some patients with chronic dermatoses may react to certain agents such as neomycin. Antimicrobial agents of value for systemic use should not be applied extensively to the surface of the body or used routinely in closed units (e.g., burn units) because of the risk for inducing resistance.

The Committee on Drugs of the American Academy of Pediatrics concluded that topical antimicrobial agents may prevent infection after minor cuts, abrasions, and burns, but in most instances, gentle cleansing of minor wounds and burns is sufficient antisepsis.[8] Systemic antibiotics, rather than topical drugs, are recommended for chronic pyoderma, including impetigo, especially when more than several lesions are present.

Intermittent administration of inhaled tobramycin (twice daily for 4 weeks followed by 4 drug-free weeks) is indicated for the management of children and adults with cystic fibrosis and *P. aeruginosa* infection. Clinical data from a large, randomized, placebo-controlled trial indicate that tobramycin treatment improves pulmonary function, decreases the density of *P. aeruginosa* in sputum, reduces the risk for hospitalization, and is well tolerated. The diminished microbial reduction during the third cycle of treatment was not explained by the development of resistance to tobramycin.[290]

The use of antimicrobial-coated central venous catheters is not accepted practice in pediatrics, but limited evidence supports its potential usefulness, particularly if rates of catheter-related bloodstream infections exceed 3.3/1000 catheter days and if standard protective procedures already have been implemented.[269] Rates of bacterial colonization and bloodstream infections associated with the use of central venous catheters in high-risk adult patients were found to be lower in patients whose catheters were impregnated with minocycline and rifampin than in those impregnated with chlorhexidine and silver sulfadiazine.[95]

Current Use of Antimicrobial Agents for Prophylaxis

Chemoprophylaxis refers to the use of drugs to prevent infection. Antimicrobial treatment refers to the use of drugs after infection has taken place or when early signs of infectious disease are present or infection is suspected. The use of antimicrobial agents for prophylaxis has proved to be of value in many circumstances (Table 236.7) and currently is considered to be of probable value or is investigational for the prevention of infections in many other situations. Prophylaxis is of greatest value when the following criteria are met: use of a single drug with a narrow spectrum of activity, use of a drug with limited side effects or toxicity, and prevention of colonization by an organism of known susceptibility and one that is unlikely to become resistant during the period of drug use. Current recommendations from the American Academy of Pediatrics include the following circumstances: (1) site-related infections: otitis media, urinary tract infection, and endocarditis; (2) exposed host: *B. pertussis* exposure, *N. meningitidis* exposure, traveler's diarrhea, perinatal group B streptococci exposure, bite wound (i.e., human, animal, or reptile), infants born to HIV-infected mothers, close exposure to influenza in unimmunized hosts, susceptible contacts of index cases of invasive *H. influenzae* type b disease, and exposure to aerosolized spores of *B. anthracis;* (3) vulnerable host (pathogen): oncology or immunosuppressed patients (with *P. jirovecii* or fungi), organ transplant patients (with cytomegalovirus, *P. jirovecii,* or fungi), HIV-infected children (with *P. jirovecii* or polysaccharide encapsulated bacteria), preterm neonates (with *Candida* sp.), patients with anatomic or functional asplenia (with polysaccharide-encapsulated bacteria), chronic granulomatous disease (with *S. aureus* and certain other catalase-positive bacteria and fungi), congenital immunodeficiencies (with various pathogens), rheumatic fever (with group A streptococci), and neonatal herpes simplex virus disease.[12]

Use of Antimicrobial Agents for Children in School or Group Daycare

Infants and children usually return to their school or daycare during a course of antimicrobial therapy. Because of problems with the administration of drugs outside the home, physicians should prescribe medications that are given infrequently, are relatively stable at ambient temperatures, and need only simple directions. Drugs that are administered in once- or twice-daily schedules are preferred. Chewable tablets, when available, may be of value in reducing the need for the school or daycare provider to measure specific amounts of liquid suspension and to refrigerate suspensions. Single-dose regimens, such as intramuscular benzathine penicillin G for group A streptococcal infections, may be advantageous. Guidelines for administration of medications in schools have been published by the Council on School Health of the American Academy of Pediatrics and should be useful to the physician for prescribing drugs to children who attend school.[10]

Restriction on Use of Antimicrobial Agents for Infants and Children

Many antimicrobial agents are approved for use in adults but have not been approved by the FDA for use in infants and children. The reasons for lack of approval are drugs with insufficient experience in children, such as tigecycline (Tygacil); agents with real or suspected toxicity in children (e.g., damage to articular cartilage in juvenile animals associated with administration of the fluoroquinolones) that should be used only when necessary; and antibiotics for which the manufacturers have chosen not to submit data on use in children to the FDA, such as metronidazole (Flagyl) and cefotetan (Cefotan). These agents appear to be safe and effective in infants and children as a result of use by pediatricians, but no well-controlled studies of their efficacy or safety in this age group

TABLE 236.7 Antimicrobial Prophylaxis in Children

Prevention of Infection in Certain Patients	Antimicrobial Agent
Group A streptococcal infection in patients with a history of rheumatic fever	Benzathine penicillin G IM, penicillin V PO
Bacterial endocarditis in patients at risk during surgical procedures:	
• Dental procedures, surgery on the upper respiratory tract	Amoxicillin PO; clindamycin, cephalexin, cefadroxil, azithromycin, or clarithromycin in penicillin-allergic patients
• Gastrointestinal tract surgery or instrumentation	Cefazolin
• Esophageal, gastroduodenal (high-risk)	Cefazolin
• Biliary tract	Cefoxitin or metronidazole plus gentamicin *or* Cefazolin plus metronidazole *or* Clindamycin plus gentamicin or ciprofloxacin
• Colorectal, appendectomy (uncomplicated)	
• Genitourinary tract surgery or instrumentation	Amoxicillin PO, ampicillin IV, ampicillin plus gentamicin, cefazolin, or vancomycin plus gentamicin (for penicillin-allergic patients)
Neonatal sepsis caused by group B streptococcus	Penicillin (preferred) or ampicillin IM or IV (intrapartum)
Gonococcal ophthalmia in newborn infants	Silver nitrate or erythromycin ophthalmic ointment
Meningococcal disease in contacts	Rifampin, ceftriaxone
Haemophilus influenzae type b disease in contacts	Rifampin
Recurrent episodes of acute otitis media	Amoxicillin, sulfisoxazole
Postoperative infections	Penicillinase-resistant penicillins or first- or second-generation cephalosporins
Tuberculosis infections in close contacts	Isoniazid
Recurrent urinary tract infections	Trimethoprim-sulfamethoxazole, nitrofurantoin
Sepsis in patients with functional asplenia	Penicillin, amoxicillin, trimethoprim-sulfamethoxazole

IM, Intramuscularly; *IV,* intravenously; *PO,* orally.

have been performed. Although a drug that has been approved for adults may be used in children at the discretion of the physician, the prudent physician chooses to use such a drug only when it is uniquely appropriate for the infectious illness and records the basis for choice of the unapproved drug.

Home Intravenous Antibiotic Therapy

Home intravenous antibiotic therapy is now available in most communities and permits discharge from the hospital earlier than in the past. The safety, effectiveness, and cost-efficiency of such a program have been proved, and these factors are of particular value for children who require 3 to 6 weeks of therapy for severe osteomyelitis or suppurative arthritis or who have chronic disease that can be managed in the home, such as cystic fibrosis or malignant disease. In many cases, home care enables the patient to resume normal activities, including return to school. The following are factors that are necessary before consideration of home care:

1. Availability of a team that includes the physician, the pharmacist, a vendor who will supply the drug and supplies, and an intravenous specialty nurse
2. A disease that is stable and requires only continued antimicrobial therapy
3. Unavailability of a suitable oral antibacterial agent (see the earlier discussion on use of oral preparations for serious infections) and availability of a stable parenteral antibiotic with low toxicity that the patient can tolerate (as demonstrated in the hospital) and preferably with a long half-life to allow infrequent dosing
4. A member of the household who is able to administer the antibiotic and provide aseptic care of the venous access device
5. Appropriate follow-up that can be maintained for monitoring safety and effectiveness

If problems with venous access arise and ceftriaxone is appropriate therapy, the drug can be administered successfully in the outpatient setting by the intramuscular route once daily by a nurse.[129,302]

Drug-Drug Interactions

Drug-drug interactions can lead to therapeutic failure because of lack of effective activity of one or both drugs or serious adverse events resulting from toxic serum concentrations of one or both drugs.[130] Most children do not require daily medications for chronic diseases; thus, drug-drug interactions occur less commonly in pediatric than in geriatric patients, but the potential for interactions exists and must be considered when prescribing antibiotics. Because drug-drug interactions are not limited to prescription medications, inquiry into the use of over-the-counter medications should be made. Mechanisms for drug-drug interactions are classified as follows: physiochemical, in which one drug is physically incompatible in solution with another; pharmacokinetic, whereby one drug interferes with the absorption, distribution, metabolism, or excretion of the other; and pharmacodynamic, whereby one drug affects the activity of a second drug. Examples of each mechanism include inactivation of aminoglycosides by extended-spectrum penicillins, decreased absorption of tetracyclines with coadministration of antacids, antagonism of sulfonamide activity by procaine as a result of competition for PABA binding sites, and interference with the CYP450 oxidase enzyme system as observed with rifampin and macrolide drugs or with the azole antifungal agents and cyclosporine.

SUMMARY AND CONCLUSIONS

A summary of the information contained in this chapter is presented in the following questions that the physician must consider for appropriate use of antimicrobial agents in children:

1. Before the drug is administered:
   a. Have appropriate cultures been obtained for a specific microbiologic diagnosis?
   b. Has the patient received this drug or related compounds previously? If so, did the patient tolerate the drug? Were there any signs of toxicity or sensitization?
   c. Does the patient have a condition that requires exclusion of some drugs? For example, children with glucose-6-phosphate dehydrogenase deficiency may have induced hemolysis when a sulfonamide, nitrofurantoin, or primaquine is administered.
2. Factors to be considered when writing orders for the administration of antimicrobial agents in a hospital:
   a. If the drug is given by mouth, will coadministration with food interfere with absorption, or is diarrhea a risk?
   b. If a parenteral route is used, should the drug be administered by the intravenous or the intramuscular route?
   c. If the drug is administered by the intravenous route, is push, steady drip, or continuous drip preferred?
   d. Should the drug be instilled directly at the site of infection?
   e. Will the drug diffuse to the site of infection?
   f. Should incision and drainage of the infected area be performed before or after beginning therapy? Incision and drainage should be considered whenever a significant collection of pus is present. If a drainage procedure is performed, material should be obtained for culture and susceptibility testing.
   g. Does the patient have renal or hepatic insufficiency that requires alteration of the dosage schedule?
   h. Are any special precautions required for household contacts? Prophylaxis may be warranted in special circumstances of infection occurring in the household, daycare center, or nursery school.
3. Use of antimicrobial agents in children who are treated as outpatients:
   a. Have the names and functions of the drugs been communicated to the patient and the parent? Do any of the drugs prescribed interact with each other?
   b. Is the dosage schedule simple and satisfactory for the family circumstances (e.g., the child's school schedule or the schedule of the working parents)?
   c. Does the child have an adequate supply of the drug until it can be purchased? If not, the use of starter packages is of value. Administration of the first dose in the clinic is advantageous because it provides knowledge of acceptance and tolerability of the drug by the child.
   d. Are parents given instructions for reporting the clinical course by telephone? Is an appointment made for the next visit?
   e. Does the patient or parent know how to assess adequacy of response to the drug? Does the parent know how to take the child's temperature?
   f. Is the total amount of drug prescribed adequate for the course? Will refills of the prescription be needed?
   g. Is the drug provided in a convenient dosage form? Will the package be provided with an adequate means of measuring the drug? Does the agent require refrigeration?
   h. Has the patient or parent been informed of signs of side effects or toxicity?
   i. Are generic equivalents of the drug adequate?
   j. Will the patient be able to pay for the drug if it is purchased elsewhere (away from the clinic)? If applicable, will a third party pay for this prescription? (In some states, prescriptions by brand name may not be filled because reimbursement by the third-party payer, such as Medicaid, is insufficient.)
4. After the patient's course:
   a. How long should the patient take the drug?
   b. When should the initial choice of antimicrobial agents be reconsidered? When the results of cultures and appropriate susceptibility tests are available, should the initial choice be reevaluated and altered, if necessary?
   c. What studies should be performed to monitor the safety and adequacy of the regimen? Hematologic indices must be measured during the administration of certain antibiotics to detect any adverse reaction. Vigilance is important to detect symptoms or signs attributable to adverse reactions.
   d. Are repeat cultures necessary? In certain cases, the most appropriate criterion of efficacy is evaluation of the results of cultures.
   e. What clinical and laboratory signs of efficacy should be monitored? Signs may differ for different diseases and various drugs but should be considered by the physician when the course of therapy is designed.

BOX 236.2 Factors Contributing to Antimicrobial Failure

Host Related
Foreign body present
Anatomic defect
Defect in immune response to infection
Poor absorption of enteral antibiotic

Disease Related
Antibiotic inappropriate for the disease
Ancillary therapy not instituted (e.g., surgical drainage)
Sequestered focus of infection (undetected or inaccessible)

Organism Related
Acquired resistance to an antimicrobial agent
Superinfection with resistant bacteria

Drug Related
Inadequate adherence
Improper dosage schedule: route, dose, or duration
Inadequate diffusion to the site of infection
Drug-drug interactions: antibiotic inactivation or antagonism
Deterioration of drug during storage

5. What factors should be considered if the patient fails to respond to the antimicrobial agent? If the patient does not respond appropriately to the course of therapy, various factors must be considered, including those related to the disease, host, drug, or organism (Box 236.2).
6. What steps can be taken to prevent reinfection? For example, in certain circumstances prophylactic antibiotics, immunizations, or surgical procedures may be warranted.

Acknowledgements

We thank George H. McCracken Jr and colleagues for their contributions to this chapter in previous editions.

NEW REFERENCES SINCE THE SEVENTH EDITION

6. Alm RA, McLaughlin RE, Kos VN, et al. Analysis of *Staphylococcus aureus* clinical isolates with reduced susceptibility to ceftaroline: an epidemiological and structural perspective. *J Antimicrob Chemother*. 2014;69:2065-2075.
10. American Academy of Pediatrics Council on School Health. Policy statement—Guidance for the administration of medication in school. *Pediatrics*. 2009;124:1244-1251.
11. American Academy of Pediatrics Subcommittee on Management of Acute Otitis Media. The diagnosis and management of acute otitis media. *Pediatrics*. 2013;131:e964-e999.
12. American Academy of Pediatrics. Antimicrobial prophylaxis. In: Kimberlin DW, Brady MT, Jackson MA, Long SS, eds. *Red Book: 2015 Report of the Committee on Infectious Diseases*. 30th ed. Elk Grove Village, IL: American Academy of Pediatrics; 2015:959-974.
13. Andes D, Craig WA. In vivo pharmacodynamic activity of the glycopeptide dalbavancin. *Antimicrob Agents Chemother*. 2007;51:1633-1642.
22. Baddour LM, Wilson WR, Bayer AS, et al. Infective endocarditis in adults: diagnosis, antimicrobial therapy, and management of complications: a scientific statement for healthcare professionals from the American Heart Association. *Circulation*. 2015;132:1435-1486.
26. Barriere SL, Stryjewski ME, Corey GR, et al. Effect of vancomycin serum trough levels on outcomes in patients with nosocomial pneumonia due to *Staphylococcus aureus*: a retrospective, post hoc, subgroup analysis of the Phase 3 ATTAIN studies. *BMC Infect Dis*. 2014;14:183.
41. Blumer JL, Ghonghadze T, Cannavino C, et al. A multicenter, randomized, observer-blinded, active-controlled study evaluating the safety and effectiveness of ceftaroline compared with ceftriaxone plus vancomycin in pediatric patients with complicated community-acquired bacterial pneumonia. *Pediatr Infect Dis J*. 2016;35:750-756.
48. Boucher HW, Wilcox M, Talbot GH, et al. Once-weekly dalbavancin versus daily conventional therapy for skin infection. *N Engl J Med*. 2014;370:2169-2179.
53. Bradley JS, Puttagunta S, Rubino CM, et al. Pharmacokinetics, safety and tolerability of single dose dalbavancin in children 12-17 years of age. *Pediatr Infect Dis J*. 2015;34:748-752.
55. Brandon M, Dowzicky MJ. Antimicrobial susceptibility among Gram-positive organisms collected from pediatric patients globally between 2004 and 2011: results from the Tigecycline Evaluation and Surveillance Trial. *J Clin Microbiol*. 2013;51:2371-2378.
56. Bratzler DW, Dellinger EP, Olsen KM, et al. Clinical practice guidelines for antimicrobial prophylaxis in surgery. *Am J Health Sys Pharm*. 2013;70:195-283.
65. Cannavino CR, Nemeth A, Korczowski B, et al. A randomized, prospective study of pediatric patients with community-acquired pneumonia treated with ceftaroline versus ceftriaxone. *Pediatr Infect Dis J*. 2016;35:752-759.
69. Castanheira M, Mills JC, Costello SE, et al. Ceftazidime-avibactam activity tested against Enterobacteriaceae isolates from U.S. hospitals (2011 to 2013) and characterization of β-lactamase-producing strains. *Antimicrob Agents Chemother*. 2015;59:3509-3517.
73. Centers for Disease Control and Prevention. Guidelines for prevention and treatment of opportunistic infections among HIV-exposed and HIV-infected children. Available at: www.aidsinfo.nih.gov/contentfiles/lvguidelines/oi_guidelines_pediatrics.pdf.
74. Cerexa I, a subsidiary of Actavis plc. Ceftazidime-avibactam for injection anti-infective drugs advisory committee. Available at: www.fda.gov/downloads/advisorycommittees/committeesmeetingmaterials/drugs/anti-infectivedrugsadvisorycommittee/UCM425459.pdf2014.
79. Cho JC, Fiorenza MA, Estrada SJ. Ceftolozane/tazobactam: a novel cephalosporin/β-lactamase inhibitor combination. *Pharmacotherapy*. 2015;35:701-715.
83. Cohen-Wolkowiez M, Poindexter B, Bidegain M, et al. Safety and effectiveness of meropenem in infants with suspected or complicated intra-abdominal infections. *Clin Infect Dis*. 2012;55:1495-1502.
84. Cohen-Wolkowiez M, Watt KM, Hornik CP, et al. Pharmacokinetics and tolerability of single-dose daptomycin in young infants. *Pediatr Infect Dis J*. 2012;31:935-957.
106. Durata Therapeutics, Inc. Dalvance. Package insert 2014. Available at: http://content.stockpr.com/duratatherapeutics/files/docs/Dalvance+APPROVED+USPI.PDF.
107. Eberly MD, Eide MB, Thompson JL, Nylund CM. Azithromycin in early infancy and pyloric stenosis. *Pediatrics*. 2015;135:483-488.
110. Farrell DJ, Flamm RK, Sader HS, et al. Antimicrobial activity of ceftolozane-tazobactam tested against Enterobacteriaceae and *Pseudomonas aeruginosa* with various resistance patterns isolated in U.S. hospitals (2011-2012). *Antimicrob Agents Chemother*. 2013;57:6405-6410.
111. Farrell DJ, Sader HS, Flamm RK, et al. Ceftolozane/tazobactam activity tested against Gram-negative bacterial isolates from hospitalised patients with pneumonia in US and European medical centres (2012). *Int J Antimicrob Agents*. 2014;43:533-539.
118. Forest Laboratories, Inc. Teflaro. Package insert. 2010. Available at: www.allergan.com/assets/pdf/teflaro_pi.
127. Garazzino S, Castagnola E, Di Gangi M, et al. Daptomycin for children in clinical practice experience. *Pediatr Infect Dis J*. 2016;35:539-541.
134. Gonzalez-Ruiz A, Seaton RA, Hamed K. Daptomycin: an evidence-based review of its role in the treatment of Gram-positive infections. *Infect Drug Resist*. 2016;15:47-58.
145. Guzman Prieto AM, van Schaik W, Rogers MRC. Global emergence and dissemination of enterococci as nosocomial pathogens: attack of the clones? *Front Microbiol*. 2016;7:788.
148. Harrison CJ, Woods C, Stout G, Martin B, Selvarangan R. Susceptibilities of *Haemophilus influenzae*, *Streptococcus pneumoniae*, including serotype 19A, and *Moraxella catarrhalis* paediatric isolates from 2005 to 2007 to commonly used antibiotics. *J Antimicrob Chemother*. 2009;63:511-519.
163. Hyun DY, Mason EO, Forbes A, Kaplan SL. Trimethoprim-sulfamethoxazole or clindamycin for treatment of community-acquired methicillin-resistant *Staphylococcus aureus* skin and soft tissue infections. *Pediatr Infect Dis J*. 2009;28:57-59.
170. Jauregui LE, Babazadeh S, Seltzer E, et al. Randomized, double-blind comparison of once-weekly dalbavancin versus twice-daily linezolid therapy for the treatment of complicated skin and skin structure infections. *Clin Infect Dis*. 2005;41:1407-1415.
177. Jones RN, Sader HS, Flamm RK. Update of dalbavancin spectrum and potency in the USA: report from the SENTRY Antimicrobial Surveillance Program (2011). *Diagn Microbiol Infect Dis*. 2013;75:304-307.
181. Juul JJ, Mullins CF, Peppard WJ, et al. New developments in the treatment of acute bacterial skin and skin structure infectious: consideration for the effective use of dalbavancin. *Ther Clin Risk Manag*. 2016;12:225-232.
188. Kehl SC, Dowzicky MJ. Global assessment of antimicrobial susceptibility among Gram-negative organisms collected from pediatric patients between 2004 and 2012: results from the Tigecycline Evaluation and Surveillance Trial. *J Clin Microbiol*. 2015;53:1286-1293.
191. Kisgen JJ, Mansour H, Unger NR, et al. Tedizolid: a new oxazolidinone antimicrobial. *Am J Health Syst Pharm*. 2014;71:621-633.
198. Korczowski B, Antadze T, Giorgobiani M, et al. A multicenter, randomized, observer-blinded, active-controlled study to evaluate the safety and efficacy of

ceftaroline versus comparator in pediatric patients with acute bacterial skin and skin structure infection. *Pediatr Infect Dis J.* 2016;35(8):e239-e247.

203. Lagace-Wiens P, Walkty A, Karlowsky JA. Ceftazidime-avibactam: an evidence-based review of its pharmacology and potential use in the treatment of Gram-negative bacterial infections. *Core Evid.* 2014;9:13-25.
208. Leighton A, Gottlieb AB, Dorr MB, et al. Tolerability, pharmacokinetics, and serum bactericidal activity of intravenous dalbavancin in healthy volunteers. *Antimicrob Agents Chemother.* 2004;48:940-945.
213. Lieberman P, Nicklas RA, Oppenheimer J, et al. The diagnosis and management of anaphylaxis practice parameter: 2010 update. *J Allergy Clin Immunol.* 2010;126:477-4780.
215. Liscio JL, Mahoney MV, Hirsch EB. Ceftolozane/tazobactam and ceftazidime/avibactam: two novel β-lactamase inhibitor combination agents for the treatment of resistant Gram-negative bacterial infections. *Int J Antimicrob Agents.* 2015;46:266-271.
216. Liu C, Bayer A, Cosgrove SE, et al. Clinical practice guidelines by the Infectious Diseases Society of America for the treatment of methicillin-resistant *Staphylococcus aureus* infections in adults and children. *Clin Infect Dis.* 2011;52:e18-e55.
218. Locke JB, Zurenko GE, Shaw KJ, et al. Tedizolid for the management of human infections: in vitro characteristics. *Clin Infect Dis.* 2014;58:S35-S42.
224. Lucasti C, Popescu I, Ramesh MK, et al. Comparative study of the efficacy and safety of ceftazidime/avibactam plus metronidazole versus meropenem in the treatment of complicated intra-abdominal infections in hospitalized adults: results of a randomized, double-blind, phase II trial. *J Antimicrob Chemother.* 2013;68:1183-1192.
227. Lutsar I, Trafojer UM, Heath PT, et al. Meropenem vs standard of care for treatment of late onset sepsis in children of less than 90 days of age: study protocol for a randomised controlled trial. *Trials.* 2011;12:215.
230. Marbury T, Dowell JA, Seltzer E, et al. Pharmacokinetics of dalbavancin in patients with renal or hepatic impairment. *J Clin Pharmacol.* 2009;49:465-476.
238. McNeil JC, Kok EY, Forbes AR, et al. Healthcare-associated *Staphylococcus aureus* bacteremia in children: evidence for reverse vancomycin creep and impact of vancomycin trough values on outcome. *Pediatr Infect Dis J.* 2016;35:263-268.
245. Molina-Torres CA, Barba-Marines A, Valles-Guerra O, et al. Intracellular activity of tedizolid phosphate and ACH-702 versus *Mycobacterium tuberculosis* infected macrophages. *Ann Clin Microbiol Antimicrob.* 2014;13:13.
247. Moran GJ, Fang E, Corey GR, et al. Tedizolid for 6 days versus linezolid for 10 days for acute bacterial skin and skin-structure infections (ESTABLISH-2): a randomised, double-blind, phase 3, non-inferiority trial. *Lancet Infect Dis.* 2014;14:696-705.
250. Moya B, Zamorano L, Juan C, et al. Affinity of the new cephalosporin CXA-101 to penicillin-binding proteins of *Pseudomonas aeruginosa. Antimicrob Agents Chemother.* 2010;54:3933-3937.
255. Mushtaq S, Warner M, Ge Y, et al. In vitro activity of ceftaroline (PPI-0903M, T-91825) against bacteria with defined resistance mechanisms and phenotypes. *J Antimicrob Chemother.* 2007;60:300-311.
269. O'Grady NP, Alexander M, Burns LA, et al. Guidelines for the prevention of intravascular catheter-related infections. *Clin Infect Dis.* 2011;52:e162-e193.
283. Prokocimer P, Bien P, Deanda C, et al. In vitro activity and microbiological efficacy of tedizolid (TR-700) against Gram-positive clinical isolates from a phase 2 study of oral tedizolid phosphate (TR-701) in patients with complicated skin and skin structure infections. *Antimicrob Agents Chemother.* 2012;56:4608-4613.
284. Prokocimer P, Bien P, Surber J, et al. Phase 2, randomized, double-blind, dose-ranging study evaluating the safety, tolerability, population pharmacokinetics, and efficacy of oral torezolid phosphate in patients with complicated skin and skin structure infections. *Antimicrob Agents Chemother.* 2011;55:583-592.
285. Prokocimer P, De Anda C, Fang E, et al. Tedizolid phosphate versus linezolid for treatment of acute bacterial skin and skin structure infections: the ESTABLISH-1 randomized trial. *JAMA.* 2013;309:559-569.
287. Ragab AR, Al-Mazroua MK, Al-Harony MA. Incidence and predisposing factors of vancomycin-induced nephrotoxicity in children. *Infect Dis Ther.* 2013;2:37-46.
304. Rybak JM, Marx K, Martin CA. Early experience with tedizolid: clinical efficacy, pharmacodynamics, and resistance. *Pharmacotherapy.* 2014;34:1198-1208.
305. Sader HS, Castanheira M, Flamm RK, et al. Ceftazidime/avibactam tested against Gram-negative bacteria from intensive care unit (ICU) and non-ICU patients, including those with ventilator-associated pneumonia. *Int J Antimicrob Agents.* 2015;46:53-59.
306. Sader HS, Farrell DJ, Castanheira M, et al. Antimicrobial activity of ceftolozane/tazobactam tested against *Pseudomonas aeruginosa* and Enterobacteriaceae with various resistance patterns isolated in European hospitals (2011-12). *J Antimicrob Chemother.* 2014;69:2713-2722.
309. Sahm DF, Deane J, Bien PA, et al. Results of the surveillance of tedizolid activity and resistance program: in vitro susceptibility of gram-positive pathogens collected in 2011 and 2012 from the United States and Europe. *Diagn Microbiol Infect Dis.* 2015;81:112-118.
322. Shirley DT, Froh DK. Agranulocytosis in a pediatric patient treated with ceftaroline. *J Pediatric Infect Dis Soc.* 2016;5:e5-e8.
323. Shorr AF, Lodise TP, Corey GR, et al. Analysis of the phase 3 ESTABLISH trials of tedizolid versus linezolid in acute bacterial skin and skin structure infections. *Antimicrob Agents Chemother.* 2015;59:864-871.
325. Smith JR, Roberts KD, Rybak MJ. Dalbavancin: a novel lipoglycopeptide antibiotic with extended activity against gram-positive infections. *Infect Dis Ther.* 2015;4:245-258.
327. Snydman DR, McDermott LA, Jacobus NV. Activity of ceftolozane-tazobactam against a broad spectrum of recent clinical anaerobic isolates. *Antimicrob Agents Chemother.* 2014;58:1218-1223.
328. Solomkin J, Hershberger E, Miller B, et al. Ceftolozane/tazobactam plus metronidazole for complicated intra-abdominal infections in an era of multidrug resistance: results from a randomized, double-blind phase 3 trial (ASPECT-cIAI). *Clin Infect Dis.* 2015;60:1462-1471.
333. Sucher AJ, Chahine EB, Cogan P, et al. Cetolozane/tazobactam: a new cephalosporin and β-lactamase inhibitor combination. *Ann Pharmacother.* 2015;49:1046-1056.
334. Sutherland CA, Nicolau DP. Susceptibility profile of ceftolozane/tazobactam and other parenteral antimicrobials against *Escherichia coli, Klebsiella pneumoniae,* and *Pseudomonas aeruginosa* from US hospitals. *Clin Ther.* 2015;37:1564-1571.
335. Takeda S, Nakai T, Wakai Y, et al. In vitro and in vivo activities of a new cephalosporin, FR264205, against *Pseudomonas aeruginosa. Antimicrob Agents Chemother.* 2007;51:826-830.
340. Tato M, Garcia-Castillo M, Bofarull AM, et al. In vitro activity of ceftolozane/tazobactam against clinical isolates of *Pseudomonas aeruginosa* and Enterobacteriaceae recovered in Spanish medical centres: results of the CENIT study. *Int J Antimicrob Agents.* 2015;46:502-510.
352. Tomczyk S, Lynfield R, Schaffner W, et al. Prevention of antibiotic-nonsusceptible invasive pneumococcal disease with the 13-valent pneumococcal conjugate vaccine. *Clin Infect Dis.* 2016;62:1119-1125.
360. Varada NL, Sakoulas B, Lei LR, et al. Agranulocytosis with ceftaroline high-dose monotherapy or combination therapy with clindamycin. *Pharmacotherapy.* 2015;35:608-612.
361. Vazquez JA, Gonzalez LD, Stricklin D, et al. Efficacy and safety of ceftazidime-avibactam versus imipenem-cilastatin in the treatment of complicated urinary tract infections, including acute pyelonephritis, in hospitalized adults: results of a prospective investigator-blinded, randomized study. *Curr Med Res Opin.* 2012;28:1921-1931.
363. Vergidis P, Razonable RR, Wheat LJ, et al. Reduction in false-positive *Aspergillus* serum galactomannan enzyme immunoassay results associated with use of piperacillin-tazobactam in the United States. *J Clin Microbiol.* 2014;52:2199-2201.
364. Villarino ME, Scott NA, Weis SE, et al. Treatment for preventing tuberculosis in children and adolescents: a randomized clinical trial of a 3-month, 12-dose regimen of a combination of rifapentine and isoniazid. *JAMA Pediatr.* 2015;169:247-255.
365. Wagenlehner FM, Sobel JD, Newell P, et al. Ceftazidime-avibactam versus doripenem for the treatment of complicated urinary tract infections, including acute pyelonephritis: RECAPTURE, a Phase 3 randomized trial program. *Clin Infect Dis.* 2016;63(6):754-762.
366. Wagenlehner FM, Umeh O, Steenbergen J, et al. Ceftolozane-tazobactam compared with levofloxacin in the treatment of complicated urinary-tract infections, including pyelonephritis: a randomised, double-blind, phase 3 trials (ASPECT-cUTI). *Lancet.* 2015;385:1949-1956.
369. Wilson W, Taubert KA, Gewitz M. Prevention of infective endocarditis: guidelines from the American Heart Association: a guideline from the American Heart Association Rheumatic Fever, Endocarditis, and Kawasaki Disease Committee, Council on Cardiovascular Disease in the Young, and the Council on Clinical Cardiology, Council on Cardiovascular Surgery and Anesthesia, and the Quality of Care and Outcomes Research Interdisciplinary Working Group. *Circulation.* 2007;116:1736-1754.
370. Workowski KA, Bolan GA. Sexually transmitted diseases treatment guidelines, 2015. *MMWR Recomm Rep.* 2015;64:1-137.
373. Zasowski EJ, Rybak JM, Rybak MJ. The β-lactams strike back: ceftazidime-avibactam. *Pharmacotherapy.* 2015;35:755-7570.
375. Zerbaxa. Drugs@FDA. Food and Drug Administration Web site. Available at www.accessdata.fda.gov/drugsatfda_docs/nda/2014/206829Orig1s000SumR.pdf.
376. Zhanel GG, Calic D, Schweizer F, et al. New lipoglycopeptides: a comparative review of dalbavancin, oritavancin and telavancin. *Drugs.* 2010;70:859-886.
377. Zhanel GG, Chung P, Adam H, et al. Ceftolozane/tazobactam: a novel cephalosporin/β-lactamase inhibitor combination with activity against multidrug-resistant gram-negative bacilli. *Drugs.* 2014;74:31-51.
379. Zhanel GG, Lawson CD, Adam H, et al. Ceftazidime-avibactam: a novel cephalosporin/β-lactamase inhibitor combination. *Drugs.* 2013;73:159-177.
380. Zhanel GG, Love R, Adam H, et al. Tedizolid: a novel oxazolidinone with potent activity against multidrug-resistant gram-positive pathogens. *Drugs.* 2015;75:253-270.
381. Zhanel GG, Sniezek G, Schweizer F, et al. Ceftaroline: a novel broad-spectrum cephalosporin with activity against methicillin-resistant *Staphylococcus aureus. Drugs.* 2009;69:809-831.

The full reference list for this chapter is available at ExpertConsult.com.

Antimicrobial Prophylaxis

237

Walter N. Dehority • Gary D. Overturf

Antimicrobial prophylaxis is the limited administration of an antimicrobial agent or agents before or immediately after exposure to an infectious agent, with the intent of preventing an infection. Prevention is always preferred, provided the means are available and the risk-benefit and cost-benefit ratios are acceptable. The focus of this chapter is on prevention of morbidity and mortality from bacterial infections through prophylactic, and often empirical, use of antimicrobial agents. For many prophylactic regimens, employment is justified by severity of the disease; and in many instances, an evidence base supporting their use is meager or nonexistent. For other regimens, such as those employed in surgery, substantial evidence of efficacy exists for many recommended regimens. Prophylaxis against viral infections such as human immunodeficiency virus and varicella will not be discussed but rather only prophylaxis against bacterial infections and some fungal (yeast) infections. For discussions of available prophylaxis against viral infections, consult chapters addressing specific viral agents.

GENERAL PRINCIPLES OF PROPHYLAXIS

Factors influencing efficacy of prophylactic regimens are related to the potential pathogen, the prophylactic agent, the host, and the disease to be prevented (Box 237.1). In addition, the pharmacology, pharmacodynamics, and pharmacokinetics of antimicrobial agents will affect the efficacy of prophylaxis and dictate dosage and timing of administrations of antibiotics and duration of use. Failure to consider these factors will often lead to ineffective prophylaxis, overuse of antimicrobial agents, promotion of resistant microorganisms, economic waste, and risk for development of toxicity or other significant side effects.

Bacterial Pathogen

Prophylaxis is likely more effective when a single pathogen is targeted. In general, the greater the number of targeted pathogens, the less effective, more toxic, and more expensive the regimen becomes. Ideally, prophylaxis should be administered at the time of exposure to the potential pathogen. If exposure is prolonged or continuous, prophylaxis becomes less effective and less desirable. Bacteria that are not endogenous to the host (i.e., not part of the host's normal flora) generally are targeted more effectively if the exposure is known and identified.

Disease

The severity of the disease to be prevented is a major consideration. Potentially fatal infections such as meningococcemia, infections that result in high morbidity such as endocarditis, and infections of surgically implanted devices are justifiably targeted. Prophylaxis usually is not required for minor illnesses (e.g., cuts, abrasions). The site of infection also is important. Adequate concentrations of antimicrobial agents are achieved readily in organs that are highly vascular and have no anatomic barriers, whereas infections in restricted anatomic compartments (e.g., middle ear) or those that involve prosthetic materials may require special consideration.

Antimicrobial Agent

The most desirable prophylactic regimen is one in which a single, inexpensive antimicrobial drug is used with a narrow spectrum, which is easily administered and well tolerated with minimal side effects. The less frequently an agent is given, the more reliable the compliance of the patient to the prophylactic regimen.[80] When prophylaxis can be achieved effectively with a single administration of an antimicrobial agent, prophylaxis is likely to approach the ideal.

PROPHYLAXIS IN NEONATES

Ophthalmia Neonatorum

Prophylaxis recommendations target *Neisseria gonorrhoeae* and *Chlamydia trachomatis.* Ideally, prophylaxis should be directed at infants who are exposed to these two pathogens, but routine mass identification of such groups with certainty is problematic. Although routine prophylaxis has been discontinued in some countries (United Kingdom, Sweden),[40] topical antibiotic prophylaxis for ophthalmia neonatorum for these two agents continues to be recommended in the United States.[160]

In the past, topical 1% silver nitrate solutions, available in single-dose ampules, were the standard prophylaxis, and tetracycline ophthalmic preparations were considered the alternative. Neither tetracycline nor silver nitrate is produced in the United States; instead single-dose tubes of an ophthalmic ointment containing 0.5% erythromycin are provided. All three agents are effective prophylaxis for gonococcal ophthalmia neonatorum.[72] However, because silver nitrate frequently causes chemical conjunctivitis, its use has been largely discontinued in most countries. Gentamicin ophthalmic ointment is associated with severe ocular reactions in neonates and should not be used for prophylaxis.[112] Erythromycin and tetracycline ophthalmic ointments appear to be as effective as silver nitrate solution for routine prophylaxis of gonococcal ophthalmia,[93,162] but silver nitrate probably is the most reliably effective agent against penicillinase-producing *N. gonorrhea.* If erythromycin ointment is not available because of antimicrobial shortages, ceftriaxone (25–50 mg/kg intravenously [IV] or intramuscularly [IM], not to exceed 125 mg in a single dose) may be used.[160]

The effectiveness of erythromycin or tetracycline in the prevention of ophthalmia caused by penicillinase-producing *N. gonorrhoeae* has not been established. No topical regimen has proven efficacy against *Chlamydia* conjunctivitis or prevention of invasive *Chlamydia* infections of the neonate, such as lower respiratory tract infection.[26,41,73] Furthermore, topical regimens do not eliminate *C. trachomatis* from the nasopharynx and do not prevent pneumonia. Therefore mothers identified with chlamydial colonization or infection are provided with effective treatment, as noted later.

Prophylaxis should be administered as soon as possible after birth. Each eyelid should be wiped gently with sterile cotton before local prophylaxis is administered. Care must be exercised to ensure that the solution or ointment is in the conjunctival sac and that it is not flushed from the eye after instillation. Administration of ophthalmic prophylaxis is law in most states. Most important, maternal treatment against *Chlamydia trachomatis* or gonorrhea infection should be provided if these infections are identified in pregnant women before delivery during routine screening. Infants born to mothers with active gonococcal infections at birth should receive a single dose of ceftriaxone (25–50 mg/kg IM, not to exceed 125 mg). Antimicrobial regimens for treatment of sexually transmitted infections of both infants and mothers are reviewed in the periodic updates of the Centers for Disease Control and Prevention (CDC) sexually transmitted infection treatment guidelines.[160]

Group B Streptococcal Infections

Prophylaxis is recommended for the prevention of early-onset (onset within the first week of life) neonatal group B streptococcal infections.[7,13,27,115,128,133] No recommendations for prophylaxis against late-onset infections exist. The current indications for treatment of neonates and maternal carriers or those mothers at risk for transmission of group B streptococcal infections to their infants is reviewed in Chapter 83 and available from the CDC[39] and the American Academy of Pediatrics (AAP).[7]

BOX 237.1 Factors Influencing Effective Prophylaxis

- Single versus multiple potential pathogens
- Time of exposure to the pathogen
- Source of pathogens
- Severity of the disease to be prevented
- Targeted organs that could become infected
- Spectrum of activity of the antimicrobial agent
- Pharmacokinetics and the pharmacodynamics of the selected agent
- Duration of chemoprophylaxis
- Cost, toxicity, side effects, and acceptability of the agent
- Likelihood and consequences of emerging resistance

Multiple regimens have been evaluated to reduce vertical transmission of group B streptococcus.[2] The antepartum use of oral antimicrobial agents to eradicate group B streptococcus colonization of mothers (antepartum chemoprophylaxis) has not been successful, even when sexual partners were treated concurrently.[115] Prophylaxis of neonates with penicillin G or ampicillin soon after birth (postnatal chemoprophylaxis) is ineffective in preventing early-onset group B streptococcal disease, primarily because in most patients infection occurs in utero and the infants do not have symptoms at or within a few hours after birth.

Therefore current recommendations focus on treatment of all colonized women identified by recommended universal testing.[7,39] The AAP and CDC recommend that lower vaginal and anorectal (single-swab) specimens for culture be obtained at 35 to 37 weeks' gestation, placed into selective broth medium, transported, and subcultured onto solid media.[13,39] Both hybridization assays and DNA amplification techniques for detection of group B streptococci also are available and serve as the only acceptable alternatives to culture.[23,79] Rapid nucleic amplification methods are available for testing women at the time of entry into labor and thus provide opportunities for treatment of women who may not have been tested at 35 to 37 weeks' gestation. Maternal group B streptococcus carriers identified antepartum or those without culture or identification at the time of delivery with rapid testing but with one or more risk factors (see Chapter 83) should be given intrapartum intravenous ampicillin (2 g initially, then 1 g every 4 hours) or penicillin G (5 million U initially, then 2.5–3 million U every 4 hours until delivery).[39] Penicillin-allergic women may be given clindamycin or erythromycin intravenously. Previous delivery of an infant with invasive group B streptococcal disease warrants intrapartum maternal chemoprophylaxis for each subsequent pregnancy, regardless of maternal colonization.

Intrapartum antibiotic prophylaxis prevents substantial numbers of cases of early-onset neonatal group B streptococcal infection[81] and decreases the incidence of maternal group B streptococcal postpartum complications, including endometritis.[96,107] Since the institution of intrapartum antimicrobial prophylaxis, the rate of invasive group B streptococcal disease has declined by greater than 65% in prescreened mothers, and administration of intravenous ampicillin reduces the risk for development of early-onset group B streptococcal infection by 36% in infants born to women with premature rupture of membranes.[22] However, the decrease in the rate of group B streptococcal disease may be associated with an increased rate of disease caused by gram-negative pathogens.

Necrotizing Enterocolitis

Neonatal necrotizing enterocolitis (NEC) is a multifactorial disease, with bowel wall necrosis of variable length and depth being the characteristic common feature. Factors including ischemic stress, disruption of the bowel mucosal barrier, and resultant bacterial proliferation and invasion of the intestinal wall are part of the pathogenesis of NEC. Therefore suppression of gastrointestinal flora with nonabsorbable oral antimicrobial agents has been used in an effort to prevent the development of NEC in premature infants. Administration of oral kanamycin or gentamicin prophylactically in the first few hours of life has resulted in contradictory data. Furthermore, selective overgrowth of resistant organisms in the bowel and significant systemic absorption of aminoglycosides from injured mucosa are potential risk factors. Therefore, currently, oral aminoglycosides are not recommended for the routine prophylaxis or treatment of NEC. One report[113] suggests that oral vancomycin given for 48 hours before introduction of oral feeding may be beneficial in preventing NEC. These observations on use of antibiotics for prevention of NEC have not been confirmed, and such prophylaxis is not recommended. Lastly, orally administered probiotics have been suggested to alter the bowel flora and to reduce the incidence or severity of NEC. A 2014 Cochrane review on the use of probiotics to prevent the development of NEC included 24 randomized controlled trials with just more than 5000 infants.[1] These studies were marked by extreme variability in inclusion criteria and the dosing and content of the probiotic supplements. In neonates younger than 37 weeks estimated gestational age (EGA) or with birth weight of less than 2500 g, NEC incidence was reduced by 57%, with a 35% reduction in mortality with the use of enteral probiotics. No cases of probiotic-associated bacteremia were reported. A 2015 Cochrane review assessing lactoferrin alone for the prevention of NEC included two randomized controlled trials with just more than 500 premature infants.[120] A 70% reduction in the incidence of NEC and mortality was documented (5% risk difference; number needed to treat of 20). Bacteremia in two premature neonates (26 2/7 weeks and 28 6/7 weeks EGA) receiving enteral probiotics has been reported with the use of *Bifidobacterium longum*, with DNA sequencing documenting identical strains to those contained in the probiotic capsules used.[25]

Intravascular Catheter Insertion

Infection with coagulase-negative staphylococci, primarily *Staphylococcus epidermidis*, is likely to occur in premature infants or infants who have indwelling vascular catheters. Low-grade sepsis is the most common clinical manifestation; however, meningitis, endocarditis, omphalitis, cellulitis, and other focal infections may occur. Two randomized trials of low-dose vancomycin added to total parenteral nutrition (TPN) fluids (25 μg of vancomycin per milliliter of fluid) suggested that such a prophylactic regimen significantly reduces coagulase-negative staphylococcal infections in small premature infants in neonatal intensive care units (NICUs).[85,144] Despite the possible effectiveness of vancomycin prophylaxis,[20] the AAP has not made a routine recommendation for low-dose vancomycin because of the potential promotion of emerging resistance in gram-positive pathogens.

Continuous administration of fluconazole has been studied in high-risk, low-birth-weight infants who are at risk for development of systemic infections caused by *Candida* spp. Currently, the AAP Committee on Infectious Diseases recommends fluconazole prophylaxis for extremely low-birth-weight infants in NICUs with moderate (5–10%) or high (>10%) rates of invasive candidiasis.[5] The recommended regimen for extremely low-birth-weight infants is to initiate fluconazole treatment intravenously during the first 48 to 72 hours after birth at a dose of 3 mg/kg and administer it twice a week for 4 to 6 weeks, or until intravenous access is no longer required for care. Oral absorption of fluconazole is very good in neonates who are feeding. This regimen has been recommended because it has not been associated with emergence of resistance.

Recent interest in antiinfective agents such as ethanol as a lock solution for treatment or elimination of colonization of chronic indwelling lines has been proposed as an acceptable alternative to antibiotics[118,129,138]; however, although these agents have been effective for treatment or elimination of potential pathogens in biofilms infecting lines, they remain only recommended for treatment of lines infected with organisms not responsive to recommended treatment.[116] A Cochrane review of antimicrobial lock prophylaxis in adults and children did demonstrate a moderate benefit in the prevention of gram-positive catheter-related sepsis, although with an unforeseeable impact on the development of resistance.[153] Several small studies (<30 patients each) have demonstrated a reduction in the rate of central line–associated bloodstream infections (CLABSIs) with the use of ethanol lock prophylaxis in children with TPN-dependent intestinal failure.[16,117,124,155] A randomized controlled trial of 307 pediatric oncology patients younger than 18 years demonstrated a significant reduction in CLABSIs with the use of ethanol locks, with a number needed to treat of 13. No serious adverse events were reported.[132]

DISEASE-TARGETED PROPHYLAXIS

Rheumatic Fever

Group A streptococcal infection of the pharynx is the precipitating cause of rheumatic fever. Appropriate antibiotic treatment of streptococcal pharyngitis prevents development of acute rheumatic fever in most cases.[51] Because at least one-third of episodes of acute rheumatic fever result from inapparent streptococcal infections[44] and some patients with symptoms do not seek medical care, not all instances of rheumatic fever are preventable. Prevention of first attack (primary prevention) is accomplished by proper identification, adequate antibiotic treatment, and eradication of streptococcal infection. An individual who has suffered an attack of rheumatic fever is at very high risk for recurrence after subsequent group A streptococcal pharyngitis and needs continuous chemoprophylaxis to prevent such recurrence (secondary prevention).[46] The prophylaxis of rheumatic fever also is discussed in Chapter 29.

Primary Prevention

Primary treatment of episodic recurrent group A streptococcal infections is important in the prevention of rheumatic fever and recurrent episodes. The diagnosis and treatment of group A streptococcal infections are discussed in Chapter 82, and the prevention of rheumatic fever and its prophylaxis are discussed in Chapter 29. Acceptable regimens for treatment of acute group A streptococcal infections are provided in Table 237.1.[6,17,67,157] In addition, once-daily dosing of amoxicillin (50 mg/kg per day to a maximum of 1 g per day) is now recommended as a means of primary prevention of acute rheumatic fever in addition to twice-daily dosed penicillin.[6,14,140]

Even when treatment is started as long as 9 days after the onset of acute illness, penicillin may effectively prevent primary attacks of rheumatic fever.[37] Therefore a brief delay (24–48 hours) for processing of the throat culture before initiation of antibiotic therapy does not increase the risk for development of rheumatic fever. However, therapy also shortens the duration of clinical symptoms, so initiation of therapy at the earliest possible time is favored.[21] Intramuscular benzathine penicillin G is preferred to oral penicillin, particularly for patients who are unlikely to complete a 10-day course of oral therapy and for patients with a personal or family history of rheumatic fever, rheumatic heart disease, or other factors that place them at substantial risk for development of rheumatic fever.[46]

Secondary Prevention

Continuous antibiotic administration is indicated in patients at risk for developing recurrent disease after having infection with group A streptococcus or for those children with congenital or acquired cardiac disease who are at risk for development of endocarditis. Both the AAP and the American College of Cardiology provide recommendations for prophylaxis.

An individual in whom streptococcal pharyngitis develops after a previous attack of rheumatic fever is at high risk for having a recurrent attack of rheumatic fever, even after asymptomatic infections or symptomatic infections that are treated optimally. Therefore prevention of recurrent rheumatic fever requires continuous antimicrobial prophylaxis rather than recognition and treatment of acute episodes of streptococcal pharyngitis.[46] Continuous prophylaxis is recommended for patients with a well-documented history of rheumatic fever (including cases manifested solely by Sydenham chorea) and for those with definite evidence of rheumatic heart disease. Such prophylaxis should be initiated as soon as acute rheumatic fever or rheumatic heart disease is diagnosed. A full therapeutic course of penicillin or other effective regimen should be given first to patients with acute rheumatic fever to eradicate residual group A streptococcus, even if a throat culture is negative at that time. Streptococcal infections occurring in family members of patients with rheumatic fever should be treated promptly.

An injection of 1.2 million units of benzathine penicillin G for patients weighing more than 27 kg (600,000 units for those weighing <27 kg) every 4 weeks is the recommended regimen for secondary prevention in most circumstances in the United States (see Table 237.1). In countries where the incidence of rheumatic fever is particularly high, in special circumstances, or in certain high-risk individuals, such as patients with residual rheumatic carditis, administration of benzathine penicillin G every 3 weeks is justified and recommended.[99,100] Long-acting penicillin is of particular value in patients with a high risk for having a recurrence of rheumatic fever, especially those with rheumatic heart disease, in whom recurrence is very serious. The advantages of giving benzathine penicillin G must be weighed against the inconvenience to the patient and the pain of injection, which causes some individuals to discontinue prophylaxis.

Successful oral prophylaxis (penicillin V or sulfadiazine; see Table 237.1) depends primarily on the patient's adherence to prescribed

TABLE 237.1 Prevention of Rheumatic Fever

Agent	Dose	Mode	Duration
Primary Prevention			
Benzathine penicillin G	600,000 units for patients ≤27 kg (60 lb) 1.2 million units for patients >27 kg (60 lb)	Intramuscularly	Once
Penicillin V	Children: 250 mg 2–3 times daily (<27 kg [60 lb]) Children ≥27 kg (60 lb) or adults: 500 mg 2–3 times daily	Orally	10 days
Amoxicillin	50 mg/kg/day once daily (maximum dose: 1 g)	Orally	10 days
For Individuals Allergic to Penicillin			
Erythromycin (azithromycin for 5 days may be substituted; see package insert for dosage)[a]	40 mg/kg/day divided 2–4 times daily (1 g maximum/day	Orally	10 days
Secondary Prevention			
Benzathine penicillin G	1.2 million units (>27 kg) or 600,000 units (<27 kg) every 3–4 wk *or*	Intramuscularly	See text
Penicillin V	250 mg twice daily *or*	Orally	See text
Sulfadiazine	0.5 g once daily for patients ≤27 kg (60 lb) 1 g once daily for patients >27 kg (60 lb)	Orally	See text
For Individuals Allergic to Penicillin and Sulfadiazine			
Erythromycin	250 mg twice daily	Orally	See text

[a]Clarithromycin for 10 days or azithromycin for 5 days in recommended doses is also effective.

Modified from Dajani A, Taubert K, Ferrieri P, et al. Treatment of acute streptococcal pharyngitis and prevention of rheumatic fever: A statement for health professionals. *Pediatrics.* 1995;96:758-764.

regimens.[45] Patients need to be given careful and repeated instructions about the importance of prophylaxis. Most failures of prophylaxis occur in nonadherent patients. Even with optimal adherence of the patient, the risk for having a recurrence is higher in individuals receiving oral prophylaxis than in those receiving intramuscular benzathine penicillin G.[60] Oral agents are more appropriate for patients at lower risk for having rheumatic recurrence. Accordingly, some physicians elect to switch therapy to oral prophylaxis when patients have reached late adolescence or young adulthood and have remained free of rheumatic attacks for at least 5 years.

Duration of appropriate prophylaxis has been defined for those with rheumatic fever without carditis for 5 years after the last episode or until 21 years of age, whichever is longer, whereas for those with carditis, prophylaxis should be at least 10 years or until age 21 years, whichever is longer.[6,24] For those with residual heart disease (e.g., persistent valvular disease), prophylaxis should be given at least 10 years after the last episode or until age 40 years, whichever is longer.[6,67]

Although sulfonamides are not effective in the eradication of group A streptococcus, they do prevent development of infection. Sulfonamide prophylaxis is contraindicated in late pregnancy because of transplacental passage of such drugs and potential competition with bilirubin for albumin-binding sites.

For patients who are allergic to penicillin and sulfisoxazole, erythromycin or another macrolide (e.g., azithromycin or clarithromycin) is recommended. No data have been published about the use of other penicillins, macrolides, or cephalosporins for the secondary prevention of rheumatic fever, but the AAP has stated that clarithromycin for 10 days or azithromycin for 5 days is adequate for treatment.[6]

Bacterial Endocarditis

In 2007,[157] and again in 2008,[158] recommendations for antimicrobial prophylaxis were changed significantly from 1997 guidelines.[47] The rationale for these changes included three central concepts. First, endocarditis is much more likely to result from frequent exposure to random bacteremias associated with daily activities than from bacteremia caused by a dental, gastrointestinal tract, or genitourinary procedure. Second, prophylaxis may prevent an exceedingly small number of cases of endocarditis (if any) in individuals who undergo any procedure, and the risk for adverse reactions to antibiotics probably exceeds the benefit in any form of prophylactic treatment. Third, maintenance of optimal oral health and hygiene may reduce the incidence of bacteremia from daily activities and is more important than prophylactic antibiotics for a dental procedure to reduce the risk for endocarditis.

Therefore recommendations for the use of antibiotic prophylaxis after 2007 were limited to the highest risk cardiac conditions. Cardiac conditions associated with the highest risk are listed in Box 237.2. Prophylaxis is no longer provided to all subjects who have the highest lifetime risk for endocarditis. For patients with high-risk conditions listed in Box 237.2, all dental procedures that involve manipulation of gingival tissues or the periapical region of teeth or perforation of the oral mucosa are reasonable for administration of dental prophylaxis. Events and procedures such as routine anesthetic injections through noninfected tissues, taking dental radiographs, placement or removal of prosthodontic or orthodontic appliances, adjustment of orthodontic appliances, placement of orthodontic brackets, shedding of deciduous teeth, and bleeding from trauma to the lips or oral mucosa do not require prophylaxis. The recommendations for regimens for oral and parenteral antibiotics listed in Table 237.2 are for all dental procedures for which dental prophylaxis is reasonable for persons with high-risk conditions.

Recommendations for antimicrobial prophylaxis for respiratory procedures are only for procedures that involve the incision or incisional biopsy of the respiratory mucosa, such as tonsillectomy and adenoidectomy. Therefore prophylaxis is not recommended for bronchoscopy unless an incision of the respiratory tract will be made. An antimicrobial regimen that includes coverage of viridans group streptococci[32] can be selected from Table 237.2.

When using prophylaxis for high-risk procedures of the gastrointestinal or genitourinary tract, possible involvement of enterococcal organisms must be considered, as well as the inclusion of mixed infections with aerobic and anaerobic gram-negative and gram-positive organisms.[22,56] However, only enterococci are frequent causes of endocarditis. In the revised recommendations of 2007, the administration of prophylactic

BOX 237.2 Cardiac Conditions Associated With the Highest Risk for Adverse Outcomes From Endocarditis for Which Prophylaxis With Dental Procedures Is Reasonable

- Prosthetic cardiac valve or prosthetic material used for cardiac valve repair
- A history of previous infectious endocarditis
- Congenital heart disease (CHD)
  - Unrepaired cyanotic CHD, including palliative shunts and conduits
  - Completely repaired congenital heart defect with prosthetic material or device inserted by surgery or catheter intervention during the first 6 months after the procedure
  - Repaired CHD with residual defects at the site or adjacent to the site of a prosthetic patch or prosthetic device (which inhibit endothelialization)
- Cardiac transplantation recipients who develop valvulopathy

TABLE 237.2 Prophylactic Antimicrobial Regimens for Dental Procedures

Situation	Agent	REGIMEN, SINGLE DOSE 30–60 MINUTES BEFORE PROCEDURE	
		Adults	***Children***
Oral	Amoxicillin	2 g	50 mg/kg
Unable to take oral medications	Ampicillin	2 g IV or IM	50 mg/kg IV or IM
	or		
	Cefazolin or ceftriaxone	1 g IV or IM	50 mg/kg IV or IM
Allergic to penicillins or ampicillin—oral	Cephalexin	2 g	50 mg/kg
	or		
	Clindamycin	600 mg	20 mg/kg
	or		
	Azithromycin or clarithromycin	500 mg	15 mg/kg
Allergic to penicillins or ampicillin and unable to take oral medications	Cefazolin or ceftriaxone	1 g IV or IM	50 mg/kg IV or IM
	or		
	Clindamycin	600 mg IV or IM	20 mg/kg IV or IM

IM, Intramuscularly; *IV,* intravenously.

Modified from Wilson W, Taubert K, Gewitz M, et al. Prevention of infective endocarditis. Guidelines from the American Heart Association. *Circulation.* 2007;116(15):1736-1754.

antibiotics solely to prevent endocarditis is not recommended for patients who undergo esophagogastroduodenoscopy or colonoscopy, which is in contrast to previous recommendations made in 1997. For patients with infections of the gastrointestinal or genitourinary tract who may have intermittent or sustained enterococcal bacteremia or for those who receive antibiotic therapy to prevent wound infection or sepsis associated with a gastrointestinal or genitourinary tract procedure, it is reasonable to include an agent active against enterococci, such as penicillin, ampicillin, piperacillin, or vancomycin. Similarly, for patients with high-risk conditions listed in Box 237.2, antibiotic therapy to eradicate the infection from the urine before surgery is reasonable for those who are scheduled for an elective cystoscopy or other urinary tract manipulation or those who have an enterococcal urinary tract infection or colonization. Amoxicillin or ampicillin is the preferred agent for enterococci, but vancomycin may be used in those intolerant of β-lactam antibiotics.

Incision of surgically scrubbed skin without an underlying or adjacent infection is not likely to cause bacteremia, and prophylaxis is not recommended. In contrast, procedures on infected skin, skin structure, or musculoskeletal tissues are likely to cause endocarditis. Therefore, for children with high-risk cardiac conditions, a therapeutic regimen administered for treatment of the infection should contain an agent active against staphylococci and β-hemolytic streptococci, such as an antistaphylococcal penicillin or cephalosporin. Vancomycin or clindamycin may be administered to children unable to tolerate β-lactam antibiotics or those who are known or suspected to be infected with a methicillin-resistant strain of *Staphylococcus aureus* (MRSA).

The 2007 changes in recommendations for prophylaxis for endocarditis represent substantial changes to all the recommendations before 1997. Therefore a summary of those recommendations is listed in Box 237.3. In addition, the recommendations to withhold prophylaxis to subjects with a number of conditions have not changed, and those conditions or situations are listed in Box 237.4. A retrospective analysis of cases of infective endocarditis in children younger than 18 years at 37 medical centers 4 years before and 3 years after the 2007 release of the new endocarditis guidelines for antimicrobial prophylaxis failed to document any increase in infective endocarditis (1157 cases identified; 1.6% difference in cases before and after guideline release, $P = .7$).[122]

Recurrent Otitis Media

Acute otitis media is one of the most common infections in infants and children and has a tendency to recur, particularly during the first few years of life. In addition to tympanostomy tube placement and adenoidectomy, antimicrobial prophylaxis is one of the options that may be considered for the management of recurrent otitis media.[36,55,127] Chemoprophylaxis of otitis media is discussed also in Chapter 16.

Updated guidelines from 2013 on the management of acute otitis media in children published by the AAP, however, do not recommend antibiotics for prophylaxis in children with a history of recurrent acute otitis media.[98]

Patients most likely to benefit from prophylaxis include those younger than 2 years, those in out-of-home child care, and Native American children.[89,121] Prophylaxis is directed against the most common potential pathogens that cause otitis media: *Streptococcus pneumoniae*, *Moraxella catarrhalis*, and nontypeable *Haemophilus influenzae*. Amoxicillin, at a

BOX 237.3 Summary of Changes and New Recommendations for Antibiotic Prophylaxis for Bacterial Endocarditis[a]

- Bacteremia resulting from daily activities is much more likely to cause endocarditis than bacteremia associated with a dental procedure.
- Only an extremely small number of cases of endocarditis might be prevented by antibiotic prophylaxis even if prophylaxis were 100% effective.
- Prophylaxis is now recommended only for high-risk procedures, and prophylaxis is no longer recommended for any other form of congenital heart disease except for those listed in Box 237.2.
- Prophylaxis is reasonable only for dental procedures that involve the manipulation of the gingival tissues or periapical region of the teeth or perforation of the oral mucosa, and only for those with very high-risk conditions.
- Antibiotic prophylaxis is reasonable for procedures on the respiratory tract, infected skin or skin structures, or musculoskeletal tissues only for patients with underlying cardiac conditions with the highest risk for adverse outcomes from endocarditis.
- Antibiotic prophylaxis solely to prevent endocarditis is no longer recommended for genitourinary or gastrointestinal tract procedures.
- Conditions previously listed as not requiring prophylaxis (1997) continue to not require prophylaxis and now include vaginal delivery, hysterectomy, and tattooing, although body piercing for patients with high-risk conditions for endocarditis should not be performed.

[a]Data from Wilson W, Taubert KA, Gewitz PB, et al. Prevention of infective endocarditis: Guidelines from the American Heart Association. A guideline from the American Heart Association Rheumatic Fever, Endocarditis, and Kawasaki Disease Committee, Council on Cardiovascular Disease in the Young, and the Council on Clinical Cardiology, Council on Cardiovascular Surgery and Anesthesia, and the Quality of Care and Outcomes Research Interdisciplinary Working Group. *Circulation*. 2007;116:1736-1754.

BOX 237.4 Conditions for Which Antibiotics Should Not Be Used Solely for Endocarditis Prophylaxis

Cardiac Conditions

- Isolated secundum atrial septal defects
- Surgical repair of atrial septal defect, ventricular septal defect, or patent ductus arteriosus (without residual and beyond 6 months of age)
- Previous coronary artery bypass graft surgery
- Mitral valve prolapse without valvular regurgitation
- Physiologic, functional, or innocent heart murmurs
- Previous Kawasaki disease without valvular dysfunction
- Previous rheumatic fever with valvular dysfunction
- Cardiac pacemakers (intravascular and epicardial and implanted defibrillators)

Respiratory Tract

- Endotracheal intubation
- Bronchoscopy with a flexible bronchoscope, with or without biopsy
- Tympanostomy tube insertion

Gastrointestinal Tract

- Endoscopy with or without gastrointestinal biopsy

Genitourinary Tract

- Vaginal hysterectomy
- Vaginal delivery
- Cesarean section
- In uninfected tissue:
  - Urethral catheterization
  - Uterine dilation and curettage
  - Therapeutic abortion
  - Sterilization procedures
  - Insertion or removal of intrauterine devices

Other

- Cardiac catheterization, including balloon angioplasty
- Implanted cardiac pacemakers, implanted defibrillators, and coronary stents
- Incision or biopsy of surgically scrubbed skin
- Circumcision

dose of 20 mg/kg, or sulfisoxazole, at a dose of 50 mg/kg, may be given orally each evening for a period of 3 to 6 months or during the winter months. Although many other antimicrobial agents are used for the treatment of otitis media, only amoxicillin and sulfisoxazole currently are considered as prophylactic agents because only these two agents have undergone critical analysis in prospective trials. Antimicrobial prophylaxis must be used with great caution and balanced against the potential for increasing the emergence of resistant organisms, particularly *S. pneumoniae,* and the possible occurrence of drug-associated toxicity (e.g., neutropenia, rash, or other). Other measures that may decrease the incidence of recurrent acute otitis media include eliminating smoking in the home, reducing group child care attendance, eliminating pacifiers, and administering influenza and the pneumococcal conjugate vaccines. If these measures do not prevent recurrent infections, referral to an otolaryngologist is recommended for evaluation and possible tympanostomy tube placement or adenoidectomy, or both procedures.

Recurrent Urinary Tract Infection

Urinary tract infection (UTI) occurs in approximately 5% of girls and 1% to 2% of boys.[165] Recurrent UTIs are noted in 30% to 50% of children with UTIs, with most recurrences taking place within 3 months after the initial episode. Eighty percent of recurrences are new infections caused by different colonic bacterial species that have become resistant to recently administered antibiotics. The recurrence rate is not altered by extending the duration of treatment.

Renal parenchymal infections and renal scarring are well-recognized complications of UTIs in children.[78,105,139] Parenchymal scarring is found in 10% to 15% of children with UTIs,[143,165] hypertension will develop in an estimated 10% of children with this complication, and renal insufficiency may develop in a smaller number.[83] Vesicoureteral reflux is noted in 30% to 50% of children with UTIs,[105] the frequency being related directly to the number of UTI episodes and inversely to age. Children with reflux have a much higher incidence (30–60%) of pyelonephritic scarring than do children without reflux. More than 90% of children with renal parenchymal scarring have had vesicoureteral reflux and a history of UTI.[143,165]

Children who have three or more UTIs in a 12-month period may benefit from suppressive antibiotic therapy for as long as 6 months to allow repair of intrinsic bladder defense mechanisms.[165] In children with anatomic defects or reflux, suppressive therapy may be needed for as long as the underlying defect exists.

Appropriate prophylactic agents should result in low serum but high urinary levels of the medication, have minimal effect on fecal flora, be well tolerated, and be inexpensive.[104] Methenamine mandelate (75 mg/kg divided every 12 hours, maximum dose 500 mg) is a suitable agent for prophylaxis because it releases formaldehyde in an acid medium. A pH of 5.5 or lower must be maintained in the urine to obtain optimal results. Ascorbic acid or other acidifying agents should be used to achieve the desired urine acidity. Other useful agents for prophylaxis in children with normal renal function are trimethoprim-sulfamethoxazole (TMP-SMX), nitrofurantoin, and nalidixic acid.[30,59,74,105,137] TMP-SMX can be given at 2 mg of TMP and 10 mg of SMX per kilogram in a single daily dose or at 5 mg of TMP and 25 mg of SMX per kilogram twice a week. TMP has the additional unique characteristic of diffusing into vaginal and urethral fluids, thereby decreasing bacterial colonization with members of the Enterobacteriaceae family and diminishing ascending reinfection.[74,145] Nitrofurantoin is recommended at 1 to 2 mg/kg (maximum dose, 100 mg/day), taken each night. It has been used effectively as prophylaxis for recurrent UTIs in infants and children. Pulmonary, neurologic, and hepatic adverse effects have been reported but are rare occurrences.[105] Nalidixic acid (not recommended for children younger than 3 months) is administered at 30 mg/kg divided every 12 hours. It is a bactericidal agent for most of the common gram-negative uropathogens. More recently, various cephalosporins and amoxicillin–clavulanic acid have been used as prophylactic agents with good results.[104] Prophylactic agents are best administered as a single dose at bedtime. Despite the previous studies suggesting efficacy of UTI antimicrobial prophylaxis, it remains controversial and largely unsupported by well-performed studies. In the largest randomized controlled trial conducted on antimicrobial prophylaxis for recurrent UTI in children, and the only study adequately powered to detect a reduction in recurrent UTI with antimicrobial prophylaxis, 607 children (mean age, 12 months) with vesicoureteral reflux were randomly assigned to receive either TMP-SMX or placebo, with a primary outcome of preventing recurrent UTIs.[150] Prophylaxis reduced the risk for recurrent UTI by 50% (risk difference of 12%) compared with placebo. However, the study was not powered to assess for a reduction in renal scarring, and no difference between groups was seen in this study for this variable. The risk for a recurrent UTI with an *E. coli* strain resistant to TMP-SMX was threefold higher in the prophylaxis group (63% vs. 19%).

No studies of prophylaxis in children without nocturnal continence have shown efficacy, and prophylactic regimens employing broad-spectrum antibiotics (e.g., amoxicillin, cephalexin) are associated with the emergence of recurrent infections caused by antibiotic-resistant organisms such as *Pseudomonas aeruginosa.*

POSTEXPOSURE PROPHYLAXIS

Prophylaxis targeted against specific organisms after an individual is exposed is discussed in this section.

Pertussis

Prompt administration of erythromycin or other approved macrolide drugs to those in close contact with a case of pertussis is effective in limiting secondary transmission. Close contacts are household members, attendees of group child care facilities, and other individuals who are in contact with the index infected individual for 4 hours or more a day. Chemoprophylaxis is recommended irrespective of age or vaccination status because immunity after receiving pertussis immunization is not absolute and may not prevent development of infection.[11] The recommended dose of erythromycin is 40 to 50 mg/kg per day (maximum, 2 g/day) to be given orally in four divided doses for 14 days. Both clarithromycin (15 mg/kg, up to a maximum of 1 g, divided twice daily for 7 days) and azithromycin at standard doses (10 mg/kg the first day, up to a maximum of 500 mg, followed by 5 mg/kg, up to a maximum of 250 mg, each of the days 2 through 5) have been shown to be as effective as erythromycin and are much better tolerated.[38] Infants younger than 5 months should receive 10 mg/kg per dose once daily for 5 days. Individuals who are allergic to erythromycin or macrolides or those who cannot tolerate their side effects may be given TMP-SMX, although the efficacy of this regimen has not been documented. The dose is 8 mg/kg per day (TMP) and 40 mg/kg per day (SMX) orally in two divided doses for 14 days.[38]

Persons who have been in contact with an infected individual should be monitored closely for respiratory symptoms for 2 weeks after the last contact. The risk for contracting pertussis in adults providing medical care to children should be recognized. Symptoms may be mild and not readily recognized as pertussis; however, such individuals can transmit the infection.

Meningococcal Infections

Close contacts of patients with invasive disease caused by *Neisseria meningitidis* (meningococcemia, meningitis, or both) are at higher risk for acquisition of infection than is the general population. Secondary cases and outbreaks may occur in households, group child care centers, nursery schools, colleges, and military camps.[10] The attack rate for household contacts is 0.3% to 1% (300 to >1000 times the rate in the general population). Spread from patients to medical care providers occurs infrequently unless intimate contact (e.g., mouth-to-mouth resuscitation, intubation, suctioning) occurs. Respiratory tract cultures are not recommended and are not of value in deciding who should receive prophylaxis.[10]

If chemoprophylaxis is to be used it should be administered as soon as possible, preferably within 24 hours of identification of the index case.[10] Treatment with penicillin G, ampicillin, or sulfonamides for meningococcal disease does not reliably eradicate nasopharyngeal carriage of *N. meningitidis,* whereas treatment with extended-spectrum cephalosporins (e.g., ceftriaxone and cefotaxime) does eliminate carriage. Therefore antimicrobial chemoprophylaxis should be administered to the index patient before discharge from the hospital if the patient has been treated with the first three antibiotics.

The antibiotic of choice in most instances is rifampin. The recommended regimen is 10 mg/kg (maximum, 600 mg) every 12 hours for a total of four doses in 2 days. A liquid preparation can be formulated, or the powder can be mixed with applesauce or a similar vehicle. The rifampin prophylaxis regimen recommended for *H. influenzae* type b disease (see later) also is effective for meningococcal prophylaxis. Rifampin prophylaxis has several shortcomings.[109,134] It fails to eradicate *N. meningitidis* in 10% to 20% of pharyngeal carriers.[101] It is not recommended for pregnant women. Side effects occur frequently and include headache, dizziness, gastrointestinal symptoms, discoloration of body secretions (saliva, tears, urine), staining of contact lenses, and hepatotoxicity. Finally, several studies have documented the emergence of resistant meningococcal strains after administration of rifampin prophylaxis.[134] Failure of rifampin prophylaxis in the contact of a case with rifampin-resistant invasive meningococcal disease has also been reported.[48]

If the meningococcal isolate is known to be susceptible to sulfonamides, sulfisoxazole may be recommended, but currently it is difficult to provide susceptibility data for most laboratories. The dose is 500 mg/day for infants, 500 mg every 12 hours for children 1 to 12 years of age, and 1 g every 12 hours for children older than 12 years and adults. The duration of prophylaxis is 2 days.

During an outbreak, a single intramuscular injection of ceftriaxone was significantly more effective than rifampin in eradicating meningococci at 1 week (97% vs. 75%) and at 2 weeks (97% vs. 81%) after prophylaxis.[134] Ceftriaxone administered as a single intramuscular dose (125 mg for children younger than 15 years and 250 mg for adults) now is recommended as an acceptable alternative for prophylaxis. Ceftriaxone has the advantages of ease of administration, possibly greater efficacy, and safety in pregnancy. For high-risk contacts 18 years or older, a single 500-mg oral dose of ciprofloxacin is a third option for meningococcal prophylaxis.

Haemophilus influenzae Type b Infections

The risk for development of secondary invasive disease with *H. influenzae* type b is age dependent.[19] The risk incidence of disease has declined dramatically with the routine use of *Haemophilus* conjugate vaccines. However, in the era when *H. influenzae* type b infections occurred frequently, household contacts younger than 1 year had the highest risk (6%) for acquisition of secondary illness; the risk in children 4 years or younger also was high (2.1%). Children older than 6 years and adults are at little or no risk. The risk for children attending group child care centers may be increased but appears to be less than that for household contacts.[32,61,103,110,119] Exposed hospital personnel do not require antimicrobial prophylaxis. Data on the risk for spread with invasive disease due to *Haemophilus* serotypes other than b, such as type a or type f, are unknown, and currently prophylaxis is not recommended for serotypes other than type b.

In addition to protecting vaccinated children against invasive disease, conjugate vaccines appear to decrease pharyngeal colonization, which further reduces *H. influenzae* type b transmission to unvaccinated children. Prophylaxis currently is recommended for all household contacts, regardless of age, if at least one of the contacts is younger than 4 years and not immunized completely.[8] Complete immunization is defined as having received a conjugate vaccine: (1) at least one dose at 15 months or older, (2) two doses between 12 and 14 months of age, or (3) two or more doses before 12 months of age with a booster at 12 months or older.

Prophylaxis for nursery and group child care center contacts is less well defined, and definitive recommendations are lacking. In general, prophylaxis is recommended for child care centers with the same regimen as that recommended for households if (1) the center is attended by unvaccinated or incompletely vaccinated children younger than 2 years where contact is 25 hours per week or more or (2) two or more cases of invasive *H. influenzae* type b disease occur among attendees within 60 days and unvaccinated, or incompletely vaccinated, children attend the facility.[151] In facilities where all contacts are older than 2 years, prophylaxis need not be given, regardless of vaccination status.

Rifampin in a single dose of 20 mg/kg per day (maximum, 600 mg) for 4 days effectively eliminates oropharyngeal carriage of *H. influenzae* type b in 95% of treated individuals.[8] This regimen has been shown to be effective in preventing secondary cases of invasive *H. influenzae* type b disease in household members, group child care settings, and classroom contacts.[19,32] Prophylaxis should be initiated as soon as possible because most secondary cases occur during the first week after identification of the index case.[19] The index patient also should receive rifampin prophylaxis, usually initiated during hospitalization and just before discharge.

If prophylaxis is given to limit secondary spread to a cohort (household or group child care), children vaccinated with any *H. influenzae* type b vaccine and unvaccinated susceptible children should receive prophylaxis.[8] Prophylaxis is not recommended for pregnant women.

Tuberculosis

The three goals of preventive therapy for tuberculosis are (1) to prevent asymptomatic (latent) infection from progressing to clinical (active) disease, (2) to prevent recurrence of past disease, and (3) to prevent initial infection after exposure to persons with active disease in individuals who have negative tuberculin skin test results. The first two goals are covered in detail elsewhere (see Chapter 96); prevention of initial infection after exposure is addressed here. Chemoprophylaxis is given in an attempt to prevent the establishment of infection, and the recipient is protected only as long as antituberculous therapy is continued.

In the United States, isoniazid administered for 9 months is the preferred drug for children for chemoprophylaxis against *Mycobacterium tuberculosis,* for susceptible children exposed to active tuberculosis, or for those with positive reactive skin tests or interferon-γ release assays (latent tuberculosis infection [LTBI]). The recommended daily dose of isoniazid is 10 to 15 mg/kg per day (maximum, 300 mg/day) to be given as a single dose. However, alternative regimens, including a 6-month regimen of daily or weekly isoniazid, may be considered for children who cannot comply with a 9-month regimen. For both the 9- and 6-month regimens, twice-weekly (each isoniazid dose 20–30 mg/kg, maximum 900 mg), directly observed therapy regimens are equal in efficacy to the daily regimens. On the basis of data from randomized controlled trials, the use of once-weekly rifapentene and isoniazid with directly observed therapy for 12 weeks is now an acceptable option for the treatment of LTBI in children 12 years and older.[12,82,146] Adherence has been shown to be superior with this regime, with equivalent efficacy when compared with 9 months of isoniazid. Dosing is as follows: rifapentene: 10 to 14 kg—300 mg, 14.1 to 25 kg—450 mg, 25.1 to 32 kg—600 mg, 32.1 to 49.9 kg—750 mg, and 50 kg and over—900 mg; for isoniazid: 15 mg/kg, rounded to the nearest 50 or 100 mg; maximum of 900 mg.

Approximately 9% of isolates in the United States are resistant to isoniazid. However, most experts still recommend isoniazid to treat children with LTBI, unless there is contact with a person with known isoniazid-resistant tuberculosis. If the source case is found to be have an isoniazid-resistant, rifampin-susceptible organism, isoniazid should be discontinued and rifampin (10–20 mg/kg, 600 mg maximum) should be given for a total of 4 months.[12] For those exposed to multidrug-resistant tuberculosis strains (defined as resistance to isoniazid and rifampin), neither the ideal regimen nor duration is known; however, drugs to consider include pyrazinamide, fluoroquinolones, and ethambutol, depending on the susceptibility of the isolate, and individual consultation with a specialist in the treatment of tuberculosis is advisable.

Persons exposed to an infectious case of tuberculosis should undergo tuberculin skin testing or testing with a blood interferon-γ release assay, have a chest radiograph, and receive isoniazid prophylaxis or another appropriate and approved regimen as recommended earlier. If the tuberculin test result is negative, the chest radiograph is normal, and the individual is not anergic, isoniazid or another appropriate regimen should be administered for 12 weeks and contact with the index patient should be broken. Isoniazid may be discontinued if the result of a repeated skin test or interferon-γ release assay after 12 weeks of prophylaxis remains negative. If the skin test result becomes positive, isoniazid is continued for a total of 9 months. Candidates for postexposure prophylaxis include persons with impaired immunity; household contacts, particularly children younger than 4 years; recent contacts, especially human immunodeficiency virus–positive contacts; and persons known to be anergic from populations with a high prevalence of tuberculosis.

Management of a neonate whose mother or other household contact has tuberculosis should be based on individual considerations. In the case of an infant born to a mother (or where a household contact is present) when the chest radiograph is negative but the mother or contact has a positive tuberculin skin test or interferon-γ release assay, the mother and contact are candidates for treatment of latent tuberculosis infection, but the infant needs no special evaluation or therapy and can breast-feed. If the mother or a household contact has suspected or active tuberculosis disease, this infection should be reported to the health department and appropriate therapy should be started immediately. If the mother has active disease, the infant should be evaluated for congenital infection and should be separated from the mother or contact, or both, or until the mother or household contact is wearing a mask and receiving treatment. When the infant is receiving isoniazid prophylaxis, separation is no longer necessary. When the mother has received effective therapy, for at least 2 weeks, she may breast-feed the infant.[12]

HOST-TARGETED PROPHYLAXIS

Human and Animal Bites

Human and animal bites are relatively common occurrences. According to the CDC, more than 4.7 million animal bites occur annually in the United States and account for approximately 1% of all pediatric emergency visits.[4,135,152] Dog bites account for 80% to 90% of animal bites that require medical care.[31] The organisms most frequently isolated in human bites are *S. aureus,* γ-hemolytic streptococci, *Bacteroides* spp., *Eikenella corrodens,* and *Fusobacterium* spp.[147] In animal bites, *Pasteurella multocida, S. aureus,* and anaerobic cocci are the main pathogens.[148]

Data on the use of prophylactic antimicrobial agents after bites are sparse, and the role of prophylaxis in patients who seek medical care early for bite wounds is uncertain.[18,53,89,135,142] However, because these wounds usually are contaminated with potential pathogens, the administration of prophylaxis (or early treatment) should be considered for patients who have the following risk factors: moderate or severe bite wounds, especially with edema or crush injury; puncture wounds (common in cat bites), especially if there is penetration of bone, tendon sheath, or joints; a facial, hand or foot, or genital area bite; wounds in immunocompromised and asplenic children; or wounds with delayed presentation with signs of infection (e.g., delay of 18 hours or more between the time of injury and the time of initial physician assessment).[18,31,52,102,135,166] For many of these indications, the use of antibiotics is in effect early treatment rather than prophylaxis because contamination of the wound occurs at the time of the bite. A Cochrane review identified eight randomized controlled trials of antimicrobial prophylaxis for the prevention of infection in animal bites. Significant benefit with the use of prophylaxis was demonstrated for human bites and in the three studies assessing hand bites (26% risk reduction for infection).[75,106]

Because most human and animal bites result in polymicrobial aerobic and anaerobic infections, prophylaxis should target these organisms. For initial prophylaxis, amoxicillin-clavulanic acid (30–50 mg/kg per day) probably is optimal therapy.[28,31,59,142] Prophylaxis is recommended for 3 to 5 days. For children with penicillin allergy, an extended-spectrum cephalosporin or TMP-SMX plus clindamycin has been recommended.[4] Although they are only moderately active against *P. multocida,* macrolides, including erythromycin 30 to 50 mg/kg per day and standard doses of clarithromycin or azithromycin, are accepted alternatives in penicillin-allergic children, specifically when these organisms are isolated. Other experts recommend clindamycin 30 mg/kg per day divided into three doses as an alternative in children allergic to penicillins or cephalosporins, as noted previously.

Asplenia

The spleen constitutes approximately 25% of the lymphoid mass. It filters blood at a rate of 150 mL/minute and plays an important role in the primary defense against bacteria that gain circulatory access.[149] The spleen has an active role in phagocytosis, is a major source of T lymphocytes, and produces immunoglobulin M antibodies, complement, opsonins, and tuftsin (a phagocytosis-promoting tetrapeptide).

Asplenia may be congenital or acquired. In the past, splenectomy was performed frequently and for a variety of indications; however, currently, a number of methods are available for splenic salvage after trauma. Overwhelming and often fatal septicemia and meningitis occur with increased frequency in asplenic individuals.[163] The frequency of sepsis is 60 times greater in children who undergo splenectomy or those with splenic dysfunction (e.g., sickle cell disease) than in normal children. The risk for sepsis or severe outcome from sepsis is greater in children who lose splenic function by disease or trauma before 2 years of age or in those who have congenital absence of the spleen. Numerous congenital cardiac conditions carry high risk for development of congenital asplenia. Fatality from sepsis in splenectomized individuals is 200 times more common than that in the normal population.[149] The risk for development of sepsis is greatest in patients who have undergone splenectomies for underlying immunologic or reticuloendothelial disorders, and the risk is lowest in children after splenectomy for trauma.[90] In all categories, risk is highest in young infants and children, but it extends to teenagers and adults as well. The period of heightened susceptibility to infection is the initial 1 to 2 years after splenectomy; however, fulminant infection has been reported as long as 25 years after splenectomy.

S. pneumoniae is the most common cause of septicemia in splenectomized individuals. Despite prompt diagnosis and treatment, pneumococcal septicemia is associated with a fatality rate as high as 50%. Overall, 80% of postsplenectomy infections are caused by bacteria with capsular polysaccharides, particularly *S. pneumoniae* and *H. influenzae.*[141,149] Although *N. meningitidis* also has a polysaccharide capsule, lack of terminal components of complement constitute the greatest risk for development of infection, and whether the incidence of sepsis is higher in persons with asplenia is unclear. However, because overwhelming meningococcal sepsis has been reported in patients with asplenia, it is reasonable to include these patients as an at-risk population for this pathogen.

To reduce the likelihood of serious infections after splenectomy, several measures are advisable. Splenectomy should be performed only when it is absolutely indicated. If possible, the best approach is to delay the surgical intervention until the child is 5 or 6 years of age. For children with congenital high-risk conditions, the 13-valent pneumococcal polysaccharide protein conjugate vaccine should be provided in the recommended schedules. Although multivalent pneumococcal polysaccharide vaccine (PPS23) provides incomplete protection for patients undergoing splenectomy, especially infants and young children, it should be administered to all patients who are older than 2 years, ideally 2 weeks before splenectomy is performed and 8 weeks after any conjugate pneumococcal immunization.[114] A booster dose of PPS23 is indicated 5 years after immunization, with no more than two total doses of PPS23 before the age of 65 years.[114] Vaccination against *H. influenzae* type b and *N. meningitidis* types A, C, Y, and W-135 with the appropriate polysaccharide or polysaccharide-protein conjugate vaccine recommended for use in children should be provided. The 2015 CDC recommendations advise immunization of individuals with functional or anatomic asplenia with one of the two meningococcal B vaccines (a two-dose series of the MenB-4C or a three-dose series of the MenB-FHbp vaccines) (Table 237.3).[62] The 2013 CDC recommendations advise immunization with a quadrivalent meningococcal vaccine in children with asplenia down to 2 months of age (MenACWY-CRM at 2, 4, 6, and 12 months of age or MenACWR-D at 9 and 12 months of age) (Table 237.4).[101]

In addition to pneumococcal and meningococcal immunization, asplenic children should be immunized with *H. influenzae* vaccines as recommended for normal children beginning at 2 months of age. Previously unimmunized asplenic children younger than 5 years of should be given *Haemophilus* conjugate vaccines according to the CDC catch-up schedule.

Antibiotic prophylaxis is recommended for many children with asplenia regardless of their immunization status. For children with sickle cell anemia or congenital asplenia, antibiotic prophylaxis should be initiated as soon as the diagnosis is established, preferably before 2 months of age. Although other children with asplenia or splenic dysfunction, such as those with thalassemia or with malignant neoplasms, may be candidates for antibiotic prophylaxis, there is less consensus for children with splenectomy following trauma. The AAP Committee on Infectious Diseases recommends that in addition to immunization,

TABLE 237.3 Recommendations for Meningococcal B Immunization for Children With Asplenia

Meningococcal Serogroup B	AGE AT SPLENECTOMY (ADMINISTER *ONE* VACCINE PRODUCT BELOW)			
	8 wk–6 mo	*7–23 mo*	*2–10 y*	*10–18 y*[a]
Bexsero[b]	Not indicated	Not indicated	Not indicated	Administer 2-dose series, 1 mo apart
Trumenbra[b]	Not indicated	Not indicated	Not indicated	Administer 3-dose series at 0, 1–2, and 6 mo apart

[a]If the patient has received one meningococcal vaccination (typically if >11 years), complete a 2-dose series if at least 8 weeks have passed after the first immunization. If patient has already received 2 doses, no further immunizations are necessary.
[b]Bexsero and Trumenbra are meningococcal serogroup B vaccines.

TABLE 237.4 Recommendations for Quadrivalent Meningococcal Immunization in Asplenic Children

Meningococcal MCV4	AGE AT ASPLENIA (ADMINISTER *ONE* VACCINE PRODUCT BELOW)			
	8 wk to 6 mo	*7–23 mo*	*2–10 y*	*10–18 y*[a]
Menveo[b]	Administer at 2, 4, 6, and 12 months of age	Administer 2-dose series 12 wk apart; give 2nd dose after 1 y of age	Administer 2-dose series ≥8 wk apart	Administer 2-dose series ≥8 wk apart
Menactra[b]	Not indicated	Not indicated	Administer 2-dose series ≥8 weeks apart	Administer 2-dose series ≥8 wk apart

[a]If the patient has received one meningococcal vaccination (typically if >11 years), complete a 2-dose series if at least 8 weeks have passed after the first immunization. If patient has already received 2 doses, no further immunizations are necessary.
[b]Menveo and Menactra are quadrivalent (MCV4) meningococcal vaccines (A,C,Y,W-135 serogroups). Avoid use of Menactra in children <2 years because of interference with serologic response to pneumococcal conjugate vaccine; do not use Menactra within 4 weeks of pneumococcal conjugate vaccination.
Notes: (1) If the first meningococcal conjugate quadrivalent vaccine is administered at ≥7 years, a booster dose should be given every 5 years after completing the primary series (listed in Table 237.4). (2) If the first meningococcal quadrivalent vaccine is administered at ≤7 years, the first booster should be given 3 years after completing the primary series (listed in Table 237.4), and then every 5 years thereafter. (3) If a child began a series of Menveo or Menactra, then it is preferred that the series be completed with the same vaccine, but either may be substituted if needed. (4) The meningococcal quadrivalent (MCV4) and serogroup B vaccines may be administered together, but should be given in different locations (e.g., opposite arms).

antimicrobial prophylaxis should be considered for all children with asplenia younger than 5 years and for those at least 1 year after splenectomy.[9] Penicillin is the agent of choice. Penicillin V given twice daily (125 mg twice daily for children younger than 3 years; 250 mg twice daily for children older than 5 years) significantly decreases the frequency of invasive pneumococcal infection. Erythromycin and TMP-SMX are alternative options in patients with documented hypersensitivity to penicillin. The duration of prophylactic coverage remains controversial; current practice is to provide penicillin prophylaxis indefinitely in immunocompromised patients, whereas the duration for other children is empirical.[9,141] Children with sickle cell disease may have prophylaxis safely discontinued after 5 years of age.

Hemoglobinopathies

Functional asplenia is the primary reason for susceptibility to pneumococcal infection in children with sickle cell anemia. Serum immunoglobulins are normal or increased in these children; however, they have a dysfunctional alternative complement pathway and decreased opsonic activity (which is mediated by both the alternative and the classic complement components) against *S. pneumoniae.* Leukocyte function also is defective in patients with sickle cell anemia; intracellular production of hydrogen peroxide, respiratory stimulation, and hexose monophosphate shunt activity are inadequate during phagocytosis. In contrast, leukocytes from splenectomized patients without sickle cell anemia exhibit normal phagocytic function accompanied by adequate metabolic stimulation. Immunologic dysfunction occurs less rapidly and less commonly in children with hemoglobin C sickle cell anemia and hemoglobin C β-thalassemia.[94,159]

Patients with sickle cell disease are at risk for development of overwhelming infection (septicemia and meningitis) by encapsulated bacteria, including *S. pneumoniae, H. influenzae* type b, and, rarely, *N. meningitidis. S. pneumoniae* is the most important and frequent cause of septicemia and meningitis in these patients.[159] The risk is particularly high in children younger than 3 years.[65] A trend toward increased frequency of invasive disease in the first 2 to 5 years after splenectomy also has been noted. Unlike very young children, school-aged children appear to be less vulnerable to pneumococcal invasive infection, even though they remain functionally asplenic.[66,159,164]

The efficacy of penicillin prophylaxis in preventing pneumococcal infection in infants and young children with sickle cell disease has been well documented in several reports.[9,57,65,66,123,164] A Cochrane review of prophylactic penicillin use in children with sickle cell anemia demonstrated a 63% reduction in pneumococcal infection, although the risk for infection was low overall, particularly after the age of 5 years.[77] Adverse effects were rare and minor.

The recommended dose of penicillin V is 125 mg twice daily in children younger than 3 years and 250 mg twice daily in children 3 years or older. Some physicians recommend use of amoxicillin (20 mg/kg per day) or TMP-SMX (4 mg TMP plus 20 mg SMX per kilogram daily) in children younger than 5 years to include coverage against *Haemophilus* organisms, which are less likely to be a concern in children who are immunized adequately. A systematic review assessing medication adherence in children with sickle cell anemia found increased adherence to prophylactic antimicrobials prescribed via the intramuscular compared with the oral route (90% vs. 44%). Overwhelming sepsis, infections overall, and emergency department visits were associated with antimicrobial nonadherence.[156]

Because overwhelming infection can occur in infants as young as 3 months, detection of sickle cell anemia should be accomplished in the neonatal period. Infants in whom sickle cell anemia is diagnosed should start a prophylactic antibiotic regimen no later than 3 to 4 months of age.[66] The optimal duration of prophylaxis is not defined clearly, and the age at which prophylactic penicillin can be discontinued safely is determined arbitrarily.[9] A concern is that penicillin prophylaxis may decrease the development of natural immunity against pneumococcal infection in children receiving prophylaxis, thereby rendering them more susceptible to development of infection after prophylaxis is discontinued.[33] Another concern is the accelerated development of penicillin-resistant strains of *S. pneumoniae.*[58,159] A multicenter study by the Prophylactic Penicillin Study II group suggests that in children with sickle cell anemia who have not had a previous severe pneumococcal infection or surgical splenectomy and are receiving comprehensive care, prophylaxis may be stopped safely at 5 years of age.[58] Continuous prophylaxis has limitations, and serious overwhelming infection can occur while patients are receiving prophylaxis. Patients or parents (or both) should be aware that any febrile illness is potentially serious, and immediate medical attention should be sought.[43,123]

Cerebrospinal Fluid Leakage

The value of antibiotic prophylaxis in patients with cerebrospinal fluid leakage has not been proved.[63,108] In the absence of meningeal inflammation, many antibiotics do not penetrate the blood-brain barrier and do not attain adequate levels in cerebrospinal fluid. Antibiotic prophylaxis often fails and frequently alters the normal flora of the respiratory tract, thereby resulting in colonization with resistant bacteria. Prophylaxis may be considered for a short duration while surgical repair is being planned.[108]

SURGICAL PROPHYLAXIS

The goal of prophylactic administration of antibiotics before or during surgery is to reduce or eliminate postoperative morbidity, shorten hospitalization, and reduce the overall costs attributable to infection. Wounds can be classified as clean, clean-contaminated, contaminated, and dirty. Table 237.5 provides the conditions for these wound categories. Dirty wounds are those with purulence, abscess, or preoperative perforation of the gastrointestinal, oropharyngeal, biliary, or tracheobronchial tracts or penetrating trauma with environmental flora. The appropriate doses for children (by weight) are provided in Table 237.6.[3]

An effective prophylactic regimen should be directed against the most likely infecting organisms but need not eradicate every potential pathogen. Therefore, for most procedures, the first-generation cephalosporin cefazolin, which is active against many streptococci and staphylococci, remains effective. When operations involve the bowel with exposure to aerobic and anaerobic bowl flora, then several agents, including second-generation cephalosporins (cefoxitin, cefotetan) or ampicillin/sulbactam, may suffice alone, or combinations such as cefazolin with metronidazole may be substituted; vancomycin can be used for prophylaxis when frequent infections with MSRA are prominent, but it may not be more effective than cefazolin, and persistent use may lead to the emergence of vancomycin-resistant organisms. It is common practice to give antibiotics at the time of anesthesia induction, which should result in adequate tissue and serum levels at the time of incision and intraoperative tissue manipulation. For most procedures lasting less than 4 hours, a single dose is recommended. Published studies often use one or two additional doses after the completion of surgery, but most experts do not believe that these are necessary, and no data support the use of antibiotics beyond 48 hours.

General Surgical Procedures

Skin incision, organ manipulation, and surgical trauma increase the likelihood for development of local infection. Surgical procedures traditionally are classified as clean, clean-contaminated, and contaminated (see Table 237.5). A fourth category of dirty wounds includes those known to be contaminated, when before surgery the skin or visceral space was compromised, introducing normal bowel or skin flora, or by contamination with a large number of environmental bacteria. Prophylactic antibiotics are effective in reducing postoperative infections after contaminated and clean-contaminated surgical procedures, whereas their efficacy is more controversial for clean surgical procedures. Clean surgical procedures generally carry a risk for development of postoperative wound infection that is less than 5% and, in many hospitals, less than 1%.

The critical period for development of infection is short, and optimal prophylaxis should be restricted to the perioperative period. Antibiotic prophylaxis of less than 24 hours' duration is effective both clinically and experimentally. Administration of antibiotics should be started at the time of induction of anesthesia or immediately before the surgical incision is made and discontinued within 24 hours. A 5-year retrospective review of nearly 250,000 pediatric surgical procedures demonstrated that only 82% of children in whom prophylaxis was warranted received prophylaxis and 40% of patients received prophylaxis when none was indicated. Risk of *Clostridium difficile* was fourfold higher in those children receiving antimicrobial prophylaxis.[130]

Addressing all situations of surgical prophylaxis is beyond the scope of this chapter, and the reader is referred to several publications and reviews on the subject.[49,76,84,86,125,151,154] Nationwide standards and goals for surgical prophylaxis have been established.[29] The consensus of these statements is that effective surgical prophylaxis must include the first dose of antimicrobial agents within 60 minutes before the surgical procedure and that dosing should be discontinued within 24 hours after the end of surgery. These documents and others provide the routine basis and evidence base for all current guidelines on surgical prophylaxis, including the recommended regimens and dosing for cardiothoracic, vascular, and abdominal or colonic surgery, as well as hip or knee arthroplasty, vaginal or abdominal hysterectomy, and neurosurgical procedures.[15]

Neurosurgical Procedures

The use of prophylactic antibiotics for clean neurosurgical procedures remains controversial.[64,70,108,127] However, because of the perceived benefits of prophylactic antibiotics in uncontrolled trials involving a large number of patients, of whom adults were the majority, and in view of the scarcity of definitive studies, current recommendations support the use of a short-course prophylactic regimen.[34,54,68,126,161] Prophylaxis for clean neurosurgical procedures is particularly valuable for high-risk groups (e.g., patients undergoing operative procedures in excess of 4 hours, operations in which craniotomies are performed, or patients with major underlying disease).[35,50,136]

Placement of cerebrospinal fluid shunts is one of the most common neurosurgical procedures in pediatric patients. An estimated 10,000 new shunt insertions and 6000 revisions are performed annually in the United States. The frequency of shunt infection varies from 1.5% to 39% (average, 10–15%).[91,131] The major route of infection is colonization of the device or the operative wounds during placement.[68] Retrograde spread from the distal end of the catheter or hematogenous seeding accounts for some instances of infection.

Most infections are noted within 15 days to 2 months of shunt placement.[95,131] Commensal skin flora are the predominant pathogens. Coagulase-negative staphylococci are the most common pathogens and account for approximately 70% of shunt infections. *S. aureus* is less common. Gram-negative bacilli are the least common and often are the result of retrograde infection from the peritoneum.[91,131]

The role of prophylactic antibiotics for placement of cerebrospinal fluid shunts has been controversial.[69] A meta-analysis of 1359 patients in 12 randomized, controlled trials indicated that short-term perioperative antimicrobial prophylaxis at the time of placement of a cerebrospinal fluid shunt significantly decreases the risk for subsequent development of device-related infection.[95] Various antimicrobial regimens, including antistaphylococcal penicillins, cephalosporins, TMP-SMX, vancomycin, gentamicin, and combinations, were used in these trials. The choice of an appropriate prophylactic regimen in a particular setting should be based on the local epidemiology of suspected pathogens, local patterns of antimicrobial susceptibility, cost, and expected toxicity. The duration of perioperative prophylaxis should not exceed 48 hours.[88,95] A longer

TABLE 237.5 Surgical Procedures and Probable Pathogens

Surgical Category	Most Likely Pathogens
Clean	
Neurosurgical	CNS, *Staphylococcus aureus*
Cardiovascular	CNS, *S. aureus*
Orthopedic	CNS, *S. aureus*
Clean-Contaminated	
Burn	Group A streptococci, *S. aureus*, GNB
Gastrointestinal	GNB, anaerobes, enterococci
Urogenital	GNB, enterococci
Respiratory	α-Hemolytic streptococci, anaerobes
Contaminated	
Ruptured viscera	GNB, anaerobes, enterococci
Traumatic wounds	*S. aureus*, group A streptococci, clostridia

CNS, Coagulase-negative staphylococci; *GNB*, gram-negative bacilli.

TABLE 237.6 **Preoperative Antimicrobial Prophylaxis**

Type of Surgery	Antimicrobial Agents	Dose
Neonatal (≤72 h old)	Ampicillin	50 mg/kg
	Gentamicin	2.5 mg/kg
Cardiac	Cefazolin	30 mg/kg
	Vancomycin[a]	15 mg/kg
Gastrointestinal		
Gastric/esophageal	Cefazolin[b]	30 mg/kg
Biliary	Cefazolin	30 mg/kg
Colorectal/appendix[c]	Cefoxitin	40 mg/kg
	or	
	Metronidazole	15 mg/kg
	plus	
	Gentamicin	2.5 mg/kg
	or	
	Cefazolin	30 mg/kg
	plus	
	Metronidazole	15 mg/kg
	or	
	Clindamycin	10 mg/kg
	plus	
	Gentamicin	2.5 mg/kg
	or	
	Ciprofloxacin	10 mg/kg
Ruptured viscus[d]	Cefoxitin	40 mg/kg
	with or without	
	Gentamicin	2 mg/kg
	or	
	Gentamicin	2.5 mg/kg
	plus	
	Metronidazole	10 mg/kg
	plus	
	Ampicillin	50 mg/kg
	or	
	Meropenem	20 mg/kg
Genitourinary	Ampicillin	50 mg/kg
	plus	
	Gentamicin	2 mg/kg
	or	
	Cefazolin	30 mg/kg
Head and neck[e]	Clindamycin	10 mg/kg
	with or without	
	Gentamicin	2.5 mg/kg
	or	
	Cefazolin	30 mg/kg
	plus	
	Metronidazole	15 mg/kg
Neurosurgery	Cefazolin	30 mg/kg
	or	
	Vancomycin[a]	15 mg/kg
Ophthalmic	Gentamicin, ciprofloxacin, Ofloxacin, moxifloxacin, Tobramycin	Multiple drops topically 2–4 hours prior to surgery
	or	
	Neomycin-gramicidin-polymyxin B	Multiple drops topically 2–24 h before surgery
	or	
	Cefazolin	100 mg subconjunctivally
Orthopedic[f]	Cefazolin	30 mg/kg
	or	
	Vancomycin[a]	15 mg/kg
Thoracic	Cefazolin	30 mg/kg
	or	
	Vancomycin[a]	15 mg/kg

[a]If MRSA is a consideration.
[b]For certain high-risk conditions (e.g., decreased gastric acidity, poor intestinal motility, esophageal obstruction).
[c]Uncomplicated/no perforation.
[d]Treatment required as well; may use the same agents.
[e]Incision through oral or pharyngeal mucosa.
[f]Internal fixation of fractures, spinal procedures with and without instrumentation, implantation of prosthetic materials.
Note: Selection of appropriate antimicrobial agents for surgical prophylaxis must take into account patient-specific and institutional-specific resistance patterns as well as the likelihood of colonization with specific organisms.
Modified from Antimicrobial prophylaxis. In: Kimberlin DW, Brady MT, Jackson MA, Long SS, eds. *Red Book: 2015 Report of the Committee on Infectious Diseases.* 30th ed. Elk Grove Village, IL: American Academy of Pediatrics; 2015:959–974.

duration of prophylaxis increases cost and the risk for development of adverse reactions and promotes alteration of the normal flora and the emergence of resistant bacteria.

Cardiovascular Surgery

Infectious complications of cardiovascular surgery can be very serious and life-threatening, and antimicrobial prophylaxis is used commonly in most medical centers.[87,92] Most available data are based on reports from adult patients,[42,71] with little specific information available on prophylactic antibiotic use in pediatric patients. The goal of prophylactic therapy is prevention of wound infection, mediastinitis, and endocarditis. A survey of 43 North American academic centers with pediatric cardiovascular surgery programs indicated that all centers use prophylactic antibiotics for all operative procedures.[97] Monotherapy prophylaxis was used by 91% of respondents and consisted almost exclusively of a first- or second-generation cephalosporin. In 95% of centers, prophylaxis was started just before surgery or intraoperatively. Prophylaxis was continued for 48 hours or less in most (68%) instances. Prophylactic antibiotics often were continued while thoracostomy tubes, mediastinal tubes, or transthoracic vascular catheters were in place but usually not for endotracheal tubes, arterial or percutaneous central venous catheters, or temporary pacing wires. A prospective analysis using historical controls of 283 neonates undergoing cardiac surgery (mean age, <2 weeks) demonstrated no increased risk for surgical site infections when perioperative antimicrobial prophylaxis was limited to 48 hours in infants with a closed sternum[111].

Table 237.6 provides the current antibiotics and dosages recommended for surgical prophylaxis by type of surgery. It is recommended that a single dose be used for prophylaxis and that it be given 1 to 2 hours before surgery to ensure that adequate levels are present in tissue at the time of the initiation of the procedure. For those agents that require longer administration times such as vancomycin, administration of the dose should be at least 2 hours before the procedure. Recommendations are generally for only a single dose, but adequate levels should be maintained throughout the procedure; therefore repeated doses during a long procedure should be given if the procedure extends beyond 2 times the half-life of a drug, such as cefazolin, which would require repeating the dose in 3 to 4 hours. Duration of the antimicrobial agents is never to extend more than 24 hours after the initiation of the procedure.

NEW REFERENCES SINCE THE SEVENTH EDITION

1. Alfaleh K, Anabrees J. Probiotics for prevention of necrotizing enterocolitis in preterm infants. *Cochrane Database Syst Rev*. 2014;(4):CD005496, 1-88.
3. American Academy of Pediatrics. Antimicrobial Prophylaxis in Pediatric Surgical Patients. In: Kimberlin D, Brady M, Jackson M, Long S, eds. *Red Book: 2015 Report of the Committee on Infectious Diseases*. 30th ed. Elk Grove Village, IL: American Academy of Pediatrics; 2015:961-969.
4. American Academy of Pediatrics. Bite Wounds. In: Kimberlin D, Brady M, Jackson M, Long S, eds. *Red Book: 2015 Report of the Committee on Infectious Diseases*. 30th ed. Elk Grove Village, IL: American Academy of Pediatrics; 2015:205-210.
5. American Academy of Pediatrics. Candidiasis. In: Kimberlin D, Brady M, Jackson M, Long S, eds. *Red Book: 2015 Report of the Committee on Infectious Diseases*. 30the ed. Elk Grove Village, IL: American Academy of Pediatrics; 2015:275-280.
6. American Academy of Pediatrics. Group A Streptococcal Infections. In: Kimberlin D, Brady M, Jackson M, Long S, eds. *Red Book: 2015 Report of the Committee on Infectious Diseases*. 30th ed. Elk Grove Village, IL: American Academy of Pediatrics; 2015:732-744.
7. American Academy of Pediatrics. Group B Streptococcal Infections. In: Kimberlin D, Brady M, Jackson M, Long S, eds. *Red Book: 2015 Report of the Committee on Infectious Diseases*. 30th ed. Elk Grove Village, IL: American Academy of Pediatrics; 2015:745-750.
8. American Academy of Pediatrics. *Haemophilus influenzae* Infections. In: *Red Book: 2015 Report of the Committee on Infectious Diseases*. 30th ed. Elk Grove Village, IL: American Academy of Pediatrics; 2015:368-376.
9. American Academy of Pediatrics. Immunization in Special Clinical Circumstances. In: Kimberlin D, Brady M, Jackson M, Long S, eds. *Red Book: 2015 Report of the Committee on Infectious Diseases*. 30th ed. Elk Grove Village, IL: American Academy of Pediatrics; 2015:86-88.
10. American Academy of Pediatrics. Meningococcal Infections. In: Kimberlin D, Brady M, Jackson M, Long S, eds. *Red Book: 2015 Report of the Committee on Infectious Diseases*. 30th ed. Elk Grove Village, IL: American Academy of Pediatrics; 2015:547-558.
11. American Academy of Pediatrics. Pertussis (Whooping Cough). In: Kimberlin D, Brady M, Jackson M, Long S, eds. *Red Book: 2015 Report of the Committee on Infectious Diseases*. 30th ed. Elk Grove Village, IL: American Academy of Pediatrics; 2015:608-621.
12. American Academy of Pediatrics. Tuberculosis. In: Kimberlin D, Brady M, Jackson M, Long S, eds. *Red Book: 2015 Report of the Committee on Infectious Diseases*. 30th ed. Elk Grove Village, IL: American Academy of Pediatrics; 2015:805-831.
16. Ardura M, Lewis J, Tansmore J, et al. Central catheter-associated bloodstream infection reduction with ethanol lock prophylaxis in pediatric intestinal failure. *JAMA Pediatr*. 2015;169:324-331.
25. Berteli C, Pillonel T, Torregrossa A, et al. *Bifidobacterium longum* bacteremia in preterm infants receiving probiotics. *Clin Infect Dis*. 2014;60:924-927.
48. Delaune D, Andriamanantena D, Merens A, et al. Management of a rifampicin-resistant meningococcal infection in a teenager. *Infection*. 2013;41:705-708.
62. Folaranmi T, Rubin L, Martin S, et al. Use of serogroup B meningococcal vaccines in persons aged >10 years at increased risk for serogroup B meningococcal disease: recommendations of the advisory committee on immunization practices, 2015. *MMWR Morb Mortal Wkly Rep*. 2015;64:608-612.
75. Henton J, Jain A. Cochrane corner: antibiotic prophylaxis for mammalian bites (intervention review). *J Hand Surg Eur Vol*. 2012;37:804-806.
77. Hirst C, Owusu-Ofori S. Prophylactic antibiotics for preventing pneumococcal infection in children with sickle cell disease. *Cochrane Database Syst Rev*. 2014;(11):CD003427, 1-24.
82. Jereb JA, Goldberg S, Powell K, et al. Recommendations for use of an isoniazid-rifapentene regimen with direct observation to treat latent *Mycobacterium tuberculosis* infection. *MMWR Morb Mortal Wkly Rep*. 2011;60:1650-1653.
98. Lieberthal A, Carroll A, Chonmaitree T, et al. The diagnosis and management of otitis media. *Pediatrics*. 2013;131:e964-e999.
101. MacNeil J, Rubin L, McNamara L, et al. Use of MenACWY-CRM vaccine in children aged 2 through 23 months at increased risk for meningococcal disease: recommendations of the advisory committee on immunization practices, 2013. *MMWR Morb Mortal Wkly Rep*. 2013;63:527-530.
106. Medeiros I, Saconato H. Antibiotic prophylaxis for mammalian bites. *Cochrane Database Syst Rev*. 2001;(2):CD001738, 1-20.
111. Murray M, Corda R, Turcotte R, et al. Implementing a standardized perioperative antibiotic prophylaxis protocol for neonates undergoing cardiac surgery. *Ann Thorac Surg*. 2014;98:927-933.
112. Nathawad R, Mendez H, Ahmad A, et al. Severe ocular reactions after neonatal ocular prophylaxis with gentamicin ophthalmic ointment. *Pediatr Infect Dis J*. 2011;30:175-176.
114. Nourti J, Whitney C. Prevention of pneumococcal disease among infants and children: use of 13-valent pneumococcal conjugate vaccine and 23 valent pneumococcal polysaccharide vaccine. *MMWR Morb Mortal Wkly Rep*. 2010;59:1-24.
117. Oliveira C, Nasr A, Brindle M, et al. Ethanol locks to prevent catheter-related bloodstream infections in parenteral nutrition: a meta-analysis. *Pediatrics*. 2012;129:318-329.
120. Pammi M, Abrams S. Oral lactoferrin for the prevention of sepsis and necrotizing enterocolitis in preterm infants. *Cochrane Database Syst Rev*. 2015;(2):CD007137, 1-3.
122. Pasquali S, He X, Mohamad Z, et al. Trends in endocarditis hospitalizations at US children's hospitals: impact of the 2007 American Heart Association antibiotic prophylaxis guidelines. *Am Heart J*. 2012;163:894-899.
124. Pieroni K, Nespor C, Ng M, et al. Evaluation of ethanol lock therapy in pediatric patients on long-term parenteral nutrition. *Nutr Clin Pract*. 2013;28:226-231.
130. Rangel S, Fung M, Graham D, et al. Recent trends in the use of antibiotic prophylaxis in pediatric surgery. *J Pediatr Surg*. 2011;46:366-371.
132. Schoot R, van Ommen C, Stijnen T, et al. Prevention of central venous catheter-associated bloodstream infections in paediatric oncology patients using 70% ethanol locks: a randomized controlled multi-centre trial. *Eur J Cancer*. 2015;51:2031-2038.
146. Sterling T, Villarino E, Borisov A, et al. Three months of rifapentene and isoniazid for latent tuberculosis infection. *NEJM*. 2011;365:2155-2166.
150. The RIVUR Trial Investigators. Antimicrobial prophylaxis for children with vesicoureteral reflux. *NEJM*. 2014;370:2367-2376.
153. van de Wetering M, van Woensel B, Lawrie T. Prophylactic antibiotics for preventing gram positive infections associated with long-term central venous catheters in oncology patients. *Cochrane Database Syst Rev*. 2013;(11):CD003295, 1-30.
155. Wales P, Kosar C, Carricato M, et al. Ethanol lock therapy to reduce the incidence of catheter-related bloodstream infections in home parenteral nutrition patients with intestinal failure: preliminary experience. *J Pediatr Surg*. 2011;46:951-956.
156. Walsh K, Cutrona S, Kavanaugh P. Medication adherence among pediatric patients with sickle cell disease: a systematic review. *Pediatrics*. 2014;134:1175-1183.
160. Workowski K, Bolan G. Sexually transmitted diseases treatment guidelines. *MMWR Morb Mortal Wkly Rep*. 2015;64:1-240.

The full reference list for this chapter is available at ExpertConsult.com.

238 Outpatient Intravenous Antimicrobial Therapy for Serious Infections

Alice L. Pong • John S. Bradley

Outpatient parenteral antimicrobial therapy (OPAT) is the means by which children can receive the benefits of parenteral (intravenous or intramuscular) therapy in an outpatient setting, usually the home, avoiding hospitalization with the associated exposure to nosocomial pathogens, inpatient costs, and psychological stress for child and family. The widespread acceptance of OPAT by physicians, families, and insurers has led to a tremendous increase in the outpatient treatment of serious infectious diseases.* Madigan and colleagues reported 2.5% of hospital discharges in a 17-month period involved OPAT.[39] However, this increased prevalence of OPAT has not necessarily been associated with increased

*References 5, 19, 20, 24, 27, 30, 38, 41, 43, 44, 48, 49, 51, 52, 55, 59.

support for formal OPAT programs. Surveys among adult and pediatric infectious disease providers report significant inconsistency in the level of resources, oversight, and expectations associated with OPAT at different institutions.[4,42] The standard of care provided to children through OPAT should equal or surpass that provided to hospitalized children. National guidelines for OPAT in adults and children have been published by the Infectious Diseases Society of America and define both benefits and risks.[60] This chapter explains the basic concepts behind OPAT for children in order to achieve the same outcomes of parenteral therapy provided in an inpatient setting. It should be considered unethical to limit resources and place the child at increased risk for complications of the infection or therapy, particularly in an effort to save money by insurers or institutions. The OPAT team, which includes the physician, OPAT coordinator, nurse, pharmacist, parent or caregiver, and third-party payer, needs to work closely to ensure a successful outcome for the child.

EVALUATING A CHILD AND PARENTS FOR OUTPATIENT PARENTERAL ANTIMICROBIAL THERAPY

Broad criteria are used to determine the medical feasibility of using OPAT (Box 238.1). The most important aspect in the assessment of a newborn, infant, or child for OPAT is a determination that ongoing parenteral therapy is required to treat the infection appropriately and continuous skilled nursing observation and care are not required for management. Development of complications of the infection in the child should be considered highly unlikely by the time OPAT is undertaken; unskilled clinical observations by the parents or caregivers should be considered adequate for care. Additional significant risk should not be placed on the child's recovery by enrollment in an OPAT program. Whenever possible, oral antibiotic therapy should be used instead of parenteral therapy. Kovacich and colleagues[35] reported that 32% of pediatric patients with complications related to a peripherally inserted central catheter (PICC) treated with OPAT, on review, could have had intravenous antibiotics discontinued before discharge from the hospital. Options for oral therapy include agents such as the fluoroquinolones ciprofloxacin and levofloxacin, and an oxazolidinone, linezolid, that have excellent absorption and tissue exposure characteristics but may have some potential toxicities that may not be present with older generic parenteral antibiotics. The use of oral fluoroquinolones over parenteral therapy if no other class of oral agent is available is supported by the American Academy of Pediatrics Committee on Infectious Diseases. Pediatric safety data exist for both levofloxacin[9] and moxifloxacin.[11]

BOX 238.1 Medical and Social Criteria for Outpatient Parenteral Antimicrobial Therapy (OPAT)

Medical Criteria for OPAT

- Medical diagnosis of infection with a suspected or documented pathogen
- Clinical response to antiinfective therapy (if therapy is started in the hospital)
- No assessed need for urgent medical, surgical, or laboratory interventions to achieve a clinical response to antiinfective therapy
- No significant risk for complications of the infection
- No requirement for continuous skilled nursing care

Social Criteria for OPAT

- Parents interested and motivated
- Parents capable of assessing the child for complications of infection and therapy
- 24-hour telephone access to the OPAT team
- Transportation for timely return to the clinic or hospital, if needed
- Home environment acceptable and resources available
- Parents documented to be capable of administering parenteral antiinfective agents, if required, before OPAT begins

A child usually is prescribed an OPAT regimen from either a hospital setting after inpatient intravenous therapy or an outpatient setting such as a clinic or emergency department. For a child being discharged from the hospital, an unequivocal response to parenteral antiinfective therapy should be demonstrated. Most often, appropriate cultures will have directed the use of antiinfective therapy active against the isolated pathogens. For children with no positive cultures, the signs and symptoms of the infection should be resolving with empirical therapy, as demonstrated by decreasing fever, improving function, and improvement in inflammatory markers. The child's infection should be judged by the clinician to be unlikely to progress or to result in complications. No further surgical or medical interventions should be anticipated during the remainder of the parenteral antimicrobial therapy course.

The child's clinical course during receipt of OPAT needs to be monitored to be certain that the anticipated response continues to occur. An outpatient visit usually is scheduled for a few days after discharge.

Before a child is enrolled in OPAT, an assessment of the parents or caregivers also is required (see Box 238.1). Because the parents are responsible for the nursing care of their child in the home, they must be willing and capable participants. Although most parents are very interested and highly motivated to return home with their child, not all are willing to perform or are capable of performing the required nursing functions. Work and school schedules may conflict with timely administration of antibiotics. Most parents are capable of providing limited medical assessment of their children, but, unfortunately, some are not. In addition, the home environment should have the resources required for the proposed medical care. For example, intravenous therapy administered to a child through a tunneled, central catheter requires specified conditions for antiinfective drug infusions and dressing changes, including the availability of a clean room with running water, and a refrigerator if storage of antimicrobials and diluents is necessary. Less stringent criteria clearly would apply for a child visiting the outpatient clinic daily to receive intramuscular antibiotic injections. Communication between the parents and medical personnel is essential. For parents or caregivers, telephone access to nurses and clinicians is critical. In addition, the parents should be able to bring their child back to the hospital or clinic for reevaluation if complications arise either from the infection or from therapy. Hence, access to adequate transportation within a medically appropriate time frame is required. Families with no available transportation, families who live in rural areas located several hours' travel from a medical facility, and OPAT during the winter season in which weather conditions may severely limit travel all should be considered before OPAT is started. In addition to observing their child and communicating information to medical providers, many parents may be asked to infuse antiinfective agents intravenously into their children. Doing so requires an additional level of skill in the parent or caregiver and assessment of parental competence for this function by the OPAT nursing and medical personnel.

OUTPATIENT PARENTERAL ANTIMICROBIAL THERAPY PROGRAM

The roles of physicians, OPAT coordinators, nurses, pharmacists, and parents or patients have been defined previously (Table 238.1).[60] When the clinician considers that the child's condition is sufficiently stable to pursue intravenous outpatient therapy from a hospital ward, a clinic, or an emergency department setting, the coordinator of the outpatient treatment program is notified. In facilities where there is no formal OPAT program, different aspects of this role may be filled by multiple people, including a hospital case manager, homecare coordinator, and/or clinic nurse. This person is capable of assessing the feasibility of implementing OPAT for that particular child and family and assessing reimbursement by third-party payers and obtaining authorizations, if needed. Insurance companies may require a much greater financial contribution by families for the cost of care after a child is discharged, in contrast to their obligation for ongoing inpatient hospital charges. The OPAT coordinator interviews parents and medical staff to determine the parents' willingness and their abilities to administer medications and to assess the home environment. After the clinician prescribes the

TABLE 238.1 Roles of Physician, Outpatient Parenteral Antimicrobial Therapy (OPAT) Coordinator, Nurse, Pharmacist, and Parent

Role	Physician[a]	OPAT Coordinator[a]	Pediatric Nurse[a]	Pediatric Pharmacist[a]	Parent or Patient
Assess medical stability for home therapy	+	+	–	–	–
Assess family for capability for OPAT	+	+	+	–	–
Create and implement OPAT treatment plan	+	+	+	+	–
Order nursing visits	+				
Order clinic visits, laboratory tests, imaging examinations	+				
Educate parents about infection and complications	+	+	+	–	–
Educate parents about therapy and complications	+	+	+	+	–
Manage treatment	+	+	+	–	+
Monitor intravenous catheter status	+	–	+	–	+
Monitor clinical status	+	–	+	–	+
Monitor antimicrobial therapy	+	–	+	+	+
Prepare antimicrobial therapy	–	–	+	+	+
Availability for complications	+	+	+	+	+
Outcome assessment	+	+	+	+	+

[a]Certification or experience in pediatrics.

antiinfective agents, required nursing visits, ongoing laboratory and imaging tests, and follow-up clinic visits, the OPAT coordinator puts together the resources required for successful therapy. With knowledge of the parents' abilities and resources, the medication and equipment requirements, and the home nursing visits required, the coordinator makes the final determination about the feasibility of the program. An example of an OPAT physician's order form that includes catheter management and medication orders, laboratory and imaging test orders, and clinic visits is shown in Fig. 238.1. These orders usually are included in hospital discharge orders and are often incorporated into the electronic medical record. The coordinator of the OPAT program, whether it is clinic or hospital based, should ensure that open lines of communication exist among the clinician, the home visiting nurse, the pharmacist, and the parents. All members of the OPAT team should be aware of their responsibilities. A defined, written plan for medical and nursing care should be established, a physician should be identified who is responsible for managing the infection and any potential complications related to OPAT. It is critical that both parents and members of the OPAT team have access to this physician or the physician's designee for questions about the infection and therapy, and that this physician is clearly identified (and is aware of the responsibility) before discharge, to allow questions to be answered and decisions to be made on the need for urgent evaluation at a medical institution (clinic or emergency department). In many centers, the physician discharging the patient from the hospital may not be the physician responsible for outpatient management. Communication between providers is critical. Although infectious disease consultation is reported to improve appropriate selection of antimicrobial agents,[1] most institutions do not require infectious disease consultation for OPAT to be prescribed. The physician assuming care of the patient should understand any potential complications of OPAT that might arise.

OPAT may be provided by periodic visits to the clinic, emergency department, or day infusion center[24] or be provided in the home by visiting nurses and parents. For children receiving therapy at home, the frequency of the required home pediatric nursing visits needs to be individualized for each child and depends on many factors—the clinical course while the child is receiving therapy, the seriousness of the infection, the ability of the parents to effectively examine the child, and the risk for development of complications that can be related to either the infection or therapy. For most children, home nursing visits are performed weekly and are accompanied by catheter dressing changes. For some patients, more frequent visits may be required, especially at the beginning of OPAT. After treatment at home has been delivered as anticipated and recovery from infection is proceeding as expected, visits may be decreased to once each week, particularly if the parents have demonstrated competency in providing nursing care, including managing an intravenous catheter, changing wound dressings, and providing clinical assessment. The home visiting nurse also may have the opportunity to establish ongoing assessment of the parents' ability to administer antiinfective agents in the home.

Physical assessment of neonates receiving OPAT may be particularly difficult for parents, and daily visits throughout the entire course of therapy by skilled pediatric home visiting nurses may be required. Daily visits also are important for children with less stable infections, such as central nervous system infections, because subtleties in the neurologic examination findings may not be appreciated by parents or caregivers and may provide clues to impending problems. Nursing aspects of pediatric OPAT have been outlined by successful programs.[30,38,56]

Pediatric competency in nursing is not standardized. Each state government in the United States licenses nurses on the basis of criteria specific for that state. However, just as for inpatient pediatric care, pediatric experience is an important qualification for the home visiting nurse caring for children. Unfortunately, home nursing agencies providing care to children are not required to have expertise in pediatric nursing. Therefore considerable discrepancy exists in pediatric competency among nursing agencies. Given the importance of pediatric expertise in evaluation and management of infected children in the home, the home nursing agency contracted to provide care is expected to have personnel with training and experience equivalent to that of nurses providing care in a pediatric inpatient setting. The home nursing agency should be able to document proficiency in delivering care to newborns, infants, and children to the clinician and the OPAT coordinator.

In many states, only licensed nurses (registered nurses and licensed vocational nurses) may infuse antiinfective agents. However, most states have no rules prohibiting parents from administering drugs. Accordingly, parents may be expected to infuse medications to their children if licensed nurses are not deemed by the home care agency and the physician to be necessary to provide this function. The physician should be aware

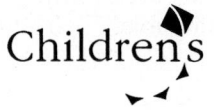

Children's Hospital - San Diego
3020 Children's Way
San Diego, California 92123-4282

Home Care Order Sheet for Infectious Diseases

Patient: ______________________

MR# ______________________

Account # ______________________

1. DISCHARGE DIAGNOSIS

2. NURSING REQUIREMENTS

a. Frequency of visits:

b. Complications to watch for (include with assessment at each visit):

c. Other nursing requirements

3. MEDICATIONS/ANTIBIOTICS (type, dose, dosing interval, duration):

a.

b.

c.

d. NS FLUSH ______ cc q ______ hrs e. Heparin flush ______ u/cc ______ cc ____ q hrs

4. LABORATORY TESTING:

☐ Via Venipuncture or ☐ Venous Access Device ☐ Other

a. Antibiotic levels

b. CBC

c. ESR, CRP

d. Chem 20

e. Cultures

5. OUTPATIENT VISITS (frequency while on therapy):

a. Infectious Disease Clinic (specify attending physician)

b. Other specialists

c. Primary care physician

6. OTHER TESTS TO BE SCHEDULED (imaging, etc.):

7. DC IV AND DC FROM HOMECARE WHEN THERAPY COMPLETE:

☐ YES ☐ RE-EVAL

8. ATTENDING PHYSICIAN

Dr. NOTIFIED OF PLAN BY

Signature ______________________ Date ______________

NON STOCK / RBF 1898 (06/96) ORIGINAL - Chart CANARY - Home Care Agency PINK - Infectious Diseases GOLD - Primary Care Physician

FIG. 238.1 An example of a physician's order sheet for outpatient intravenous antimicrobial therapy (OPAT) for serious infections at Rady Children's Hospital San Diego, California.

of the qualifications of the personnel responsible for the intravenous infusion of antiinfective agents.

The home visiting nurse should communicate with the physician about the medical status (e.g., the medical stability) of the child and plans for follow-up, before OPAT is started. Analogous to inpatient care, the nurses and physicians are expected to be on-call 24 hours each day.

Similarly, the pharmacist providing antiinfective therapy for OPAT should be familiar with the dosages and side effects of therapy provided to all pediatric age groups, from newborns to adolescents. Dosing errors in infants and children are not uncommon occurrences in health care facilities, given the broad range of doses administered.[33]

The parents should have written instructions for the tasks they are required to perform in the home, including information on sterile technique, administration of antimicrobials through sterile tubing and valves, flushing of catheters, and dressing changes. Their proficiency in management of the catheter and infusion of antiinfective agents should be demonstrated before the child is discharged from the hospital, emergency department, or clinic because some parents or caregivers may not be capable of performing these tasks adequately. Telephone numbers should be provided for the 24-hour on-call nursing and physician personnel. A list of complications of the medications and information on how the parent should perform a clinical assessment of the child's infection should be provided, along with a set of parameters requiring immediate notification of medical personnel. Plans for disposal of needles, dressings, and other medical waste also should be made before the child is sent home.

Visits to clinicians (i.e., primary care providers, surgeons, subspecialists) are scheduled as necessary according to the clinical status of the child and the degree of expertise required by the examiner. If the child is stable in an outpatient setting, the treating physician should determine the frequency of routine follow-up clinic visits unless the home visiting nurse or parent observes problems requiring more immediate attention. For any high-risk, relatively unstable child, daily physician visits may be important, particularly if skilled pediatric home nursing is not available; however, if daily physician visits become necessary, the value of OPAT versus inpatient hospitalization should be reassessed.

Although abuse of intravenous access seldom occurs, for an adolescent who may have a history of alcohol or drug dependence, the clinician should be particularly cautious in approving OPAT. For younger children with indwelling catheters, Münchausen syndrome by proxy may be a concern for infants and children who do not recover clinically as anticipated or have repeated unanticipated complications.

TABLE 238.2 Infections Treated With Outpatient Parenteral Antimicrobial Therapy Coordinator

Infection Treated	References	Design[a]
Collections of various infections	5, 8, 12, 22, 37, 56, 61	III
Appendicitis	6, 18, 54, 64	II
Catheter infection	34	III
Chronic suppurative otitis media	15	II
Cystic fibrosis	68	I
	13	II
	21, 28, 32, 38, 54, 58	III
Fever in immunocompromised children	44, 49, 66	I
	14, 49, 53	II
	30, 65	III
Meningitis	2, 3, 17	III
Mastoiditis	46	II
Neonatal infections	62	II
	7, 17	III
Osteoarticular infections	16, 40	III
Skin	10, 24	II
Urinary tract infection	20	II
	45	III
Peritonitis, peritoneal catheter related	36	III

[a]*I*, Randomized, prospective, comparative trial; *II*, prospective evaluation; *III*, retrospectively reviewed clinical experience.

INFECTIONS SUITABLE FOR OUTPATIENT PARENTERAL ANTIMICROBIAL THERAPY

Virtually any infection can be treated by OPAT at some point in the course of therapy by following the criteria listed in Box 238.1. For each child, a thorough assessment of the risks for development of complications of the infection must be made before outpatient therapy is considered. A partial list of infections treated with OPAT is given in Table 238.2; most of the studies are not prospective, randomized investigations comparing children receiving therapy in the hospital with those receiving therapy outside the hospital. Studies show the most common infections in pediatrics treated with OPAT are bone and joint, bloodstream, pulmonary, and gastrointestinal infections.[1,23,39] Other infections that have been treated with OPAT at some point include endocarditis; central nervous system infections, including meningitis, epidural abscess, subdural empyema, and brain abscess; urinary tract infections; upper respiratory tract infections, including severe acute otitis media, chronic suppurative otitis, and mastoiditis; fever with or without neutropenia in low-risk immunocompromised children; neonatal bacterial sepsis; and postoperative wound infections.

DELIVERY OF ANTIMICROBIAL THERAPY

Selection of an Antimicrobial Agent

Selection of antimicrobial therapy for OPAT is similar to selection of therapy for any child in that the primary goal is to achieve clinical and microbiologic cure with the most efficacious, least toxic, and most cost-effective agents. Selection of an agent that is more convenient to administer but that may not be as effective is not appropriate. However, of the agents that demonstrate equivalent activity against the child's pathogen, the preferred agent is the one that is given least frequently, is nontoxic, and requires the least frequent monitoring for adverse events. Preferred agents for the most common community-acquired pathogens are given in Table 238.3. Almost any pathogen, community acquired or nosocomial, bacterial, fungal, or viral, can be treated in the home if the medical and social criteria for OPAT can be met.

In general, β-lactam agents (i.e., penicillins, cephalosporins, and carbapenems) require less frequent monitoring than do aminoglycosides (i.e., gentamicin, tobramycin, and amikacin), glycopeptides (i.e., vancomycin, dalbavancin, oritavancin or telavancin), or oxazolidinones (e.g., linezolid or tedizolid). Agents that can be given intravenously during the course of a short period (5–15 minutes), such as β-lactam agents, are preferred to those that require up to an hour with each infusion (e.g., aminoglycosides and glycopeptides). Agents that can be given intramuscularly if intravenous access is temporarily lost are preferred to those that may be given only intravenously. Not only are these parameters designed to provide the optimal clinical outcome with minimal toxicity, they also are designed to facilitate therapy in the home. Dosing more frequently than every 8 hours poses a formidable challenge to many families, particularly those without extensive family support. Administration of two or three antibiotics that each require dosing three or four times each day is virtually impossible for most families to accomplish. These parameters are designed to maximize the potential for parents to be able to provide care at home with minimal risk. Although more frequent nursing visits may provide relief to parents, this is not always economically or logistically feasible. The charge for multiple nursing visits each day approaches the cost of a day in the hospital for a stable child, and most agencies do not have sufficient staff to provide more than one visit each week to a family.

Depending on the agent used, monitoring for antimicrobial toxicity in the outpatient setting should occur with the same frequency as that in the inpatient setting. Monitoring of renal function and serum antibiotic

TABLE 238.3 **Selection of Antimicrobial Agents for Common Pathogens in Community-Acquired Infections**

Pathogen	Antimicrobial Agent	Dosing Frequency (h)	Toxicity
Gram-Positive Bacteria			
Streptococcus pneumoniae	Penicillin G[a]	6	
	Ampicillin[a]	6–8	
	Cefuroxime[a]	8	
	Cefotaxime[a]	6–8	
	Ceftriaxone[a,b]	24	
	Linezolid[a]	8–12	Neutropenia, thrombocytopenia
	Vancomycin (for penicillin and cephalosporin nonsusceptible strains)[c]	8–12	Renal toxicity, ototoxicity
Staphylococcus aureus	Oxacillin[a]	6–8	
	Cefazolin[b]	8	
	Clindamycin[a]	8	Colitis
	Linezolid[a]	8–12	Neutropenia, thrombocytopenia
	Vancomycin[c]	8–12	Renal toxicity, ototoxicity
Streptococcus pyogenes	See *S. pneumoniae*		
Enterococcus	Ampicillin plus gentamicin[a,b]	Ampicillin: 6–8 Gentamicin: 8	Renal toxicity, ototoxicity (gentamicin)
	Vancomycin plus gentamicin[a,b]	Vancomycin: 8–12 Gentamicin: 8	Renal toxicity, ototoxicity (both gentamicin and vancomycin)
Gram-Negative Bacteria			
Haemophilus influenzae	Ampicillin[a]	6–8	
	Cefuroxime	8	
	Cefotaxime	8	
	Ceftriaxone[b]	24	
Escherichia coli	Ceftriaxone[b]	24	
	Ampicillin[a]	6–8	
	Cefotaxime[c]	6–8	
	Gentamicin[c] or tobramycin	8–24	Renal toxicity, ototoxicity
	Amikacin[c]	12-24	Renal toxicity, ototoxicity
Enterobacter, Serratia, Citrobacter (pathogens with inducible AmpC β-lactamases)	Cefepime[b]	8–12	
	Ertapenem[b]	12–24	
	Meropenem	8	
	Cefotaxime[a] or ceftriaxone plus an aminoglycoside[c] (gentamicin, tobramycin, amikacin)	Cefotaxime: 6–8 Ceftriaxone: 24 Gentamicin and tobramycin: 8–24 Amikacin: 24	Renal toxicity, ototoxicity (aminoglycoside)
	Ciprofloxacin[d]	12–24	Possible arthropathy
Pseudomonas aeruginosa	Meropenem[b]	8	
	Cefepime	8	
	Ceftazidime[a] plus an aminoglycoside[c]	Ceftazidime: 8 Aminoglycoside: see above	Renal toxicity, ototoxicity (aminoglycoside)
	Imipenem-cilastatin	6–8	Central nervous system irritability in children with underlying central nervous system inflammation
	Piperacillin-tazobactam[a] plus an aminoglycoside[c]	Piperacillin-tazobactam: 6 Aminoglycoside: see above	Renal toxicity, ototoxicity (aminoglycoside)
	Ciprofloxacin[d]	8–12	Possible arthropathy
Neisseria meningitidis	Ceftriaxone[b]	24	
	Penicillin G	6	
Fungal Pathogens			
Candida	Fluconazole IV[b]	24	
	Amphotericin B (lipid preparations are better tolerated)	24, or every other day; may return to infusion center for each injection to manage side effects	Fever, chills, anemia, hypokalemia, decreased glomerular function
	Caspofungin or micafungin	24	
Viral Pathogens			
Herpes simplex virus	Acyclovir	8	Neutropenia, renal toxicity
Cytomegalovirus	Ganciclovir	12–24	Neutropenia

[a]If organisms are documented to be susceptible.
[b]Preferred agents based on dosing frequency and side effects.
[c]Requires monitoring of renal function and serum concentrations.
[d]Not indicated for therapy unless no other therapy options exist.

concentrations is important for children being treated with aminoglycosides or vancomycin. For children receiving long-term β-lactam therapy, periodic monitoring of the peripheral white blood cell count and renal and hepatic function every 2 to 4 weeks may detect the uncommon but well-described antibiotic-mediated toxicities of this class of antibiotics before any clinical manifestations occur.

Delivery of Antimicrobial Agents

OPAT can be delivered by intramuscular or intravenous injection. In general, the need for more than two or three injections per day necessitates intravenous therapy. However, once-daily intramuscular therapy lasting 1 week or longer has not been associated with short-term complications in anecdotal reports.[7,8] Short polyethylene catheters normally used for inpatient intravenous therapy may be used for short-term therapy lasting less than 5 to 7 days.[24] On occasion, intravenous access will be lost, and the child will need to be reevaluated for ongoing parenteral therapy; if clinical improvement exceeds expectations, an early switch to oral convalescent therapy may be possible. If not, intravenous access may need to be reestablished. It may be performed in the home but more often will require the child and parent to return to the clinic or hospital. An intramuscular injection or injections may be given temporarily in the home, clinic, or emergency department until the intravenous catheter can be replaced.

For therapy lasting longer than 5 to 7 days, central catheters are preferred. PICC lines are widely available, practical, and cost-effective and have become the intravenous access of choice for extended therapy.[28,41,59,61] These catheters may be inserted through many different peripheral sites (usually the antecubital vein) by physicians or nurses with training in the placement of central catheters. Sedation usually is required for younger infants and children. Alternatively, more traditional subcutaneously tunneled central catheters with one or more ports (e.g., Hickman or Groshong) may be placed by a surgeon in the operating room with the child under general anesthesia. These tunneled catheters, which also may be used for blood sampling, are preferred for children requiring parenteral nutrition or other parenteral medications in addition to antimicrobials. Each type of central catheter requires sterile techniques for accessing the catheter and close monitoring of the catheter exit site during administration of therapy. The home visiting nurse agency should have written protocols for the care and use of central catheters that are consistent with standards set by The Joint Commission, which provides a program for Home Care Accreditation.[58] Complications associated with PICC lines include infection, occlusion, dislodgement, breakage, phlebitis, infiltration, leakage, and thrombosis.[35] Risk factors for complications include younger age, noncentral PICC tip location, discharge to a long-term care facility, and public insurance.[35]

Antiinfective agents may be infused directly into the catheter by the caregiver by way of an antibiotic-containing syringe simply attached to the catheter hub ("IV push"), followed by flushing of the catheter with saline or a heparin-containing solution. This method is often used for β-lactam agents. Alternatively, particularly for agents that cannot be infused quickly, an intravenous drip system must be used, or the agent must be infused by a pump. Pumps come in three basic designs: those with no electronic or moving parts; syringe pumps, in which the syringe containing the antiinfective agent is placed in a motorized pump designed to administer the dose during the course of a certain period; and electronic programmable pumps, which may have a variety of pump mechanisms and are programmed to control infusions of one or more agents administered during the course of different periods.

The least expensive pumps are those with no moving parts. One type of pump requires injection of the antibiotic solution, under some pressure, into a thick elastomeric "balloon." The pressure used to inject the antibiotic into the balloon then pushes the antibiotic through an infusion rate–limiting valve into the intravenous line and subsequently into the child. Other types of pumps are designed to place the antibiotic solution into a bag that then is placed into a device in which spring-loaded plates press on the solution contained in the bag, again pushing the antibiotic into the child through an infusion rate–limiting valve. These pumps generally use disposable infusion containers and are adequate for treatment with a single antibiotic administered up to a few times each day.

New tools for OPAT are becoming available each year. Resource guides to the equipment used for OPAT are available.[47] Unfortunately, for children, most of the equipment and resources available are designed for adults.

OUTCOME ANALYSIS

The anticipated outcome in the treatment of an infection is clinical and microbiologic cure with no complications of therapy. OPAT program outcomes should be evaluated at regular intervals by the entire OPAT team to determine whether local criteria for the OPAT program have provided the same standard of care as that in the hospital and offer opportunities for improved quality of care. Although the psychosocial benefits of OPAT for children from a secure home environment were the original impetus for the establishment of pediatric programs, the economic benefits of outpatient therapy have been easier to document for both adults and children, although current published data in children are sparse.[5,10,25,26,29,32,43,63,67,69] The cost of treatment is substantially less for outpatient therapy when neither hospital facilities nor 24-hour skilled nursing care is necessary. With shorter periods of hospitalization associated with OPAT, the risk for acquiring a nosocomial viral or bacterial infection should diminish and further decrease the overall cost of care.

However, complications may occur in children receiving OPAT, just as they occur in inpatients.[16,23,24,31,37,50] The infection being treated may not be under control or may relapse while the child is being monitored by parents or home nursing personnel. Errors in antibiotic dosing and administration may occur,[33] particularly if parents are given the responsibility of preparing and administering antibiotics in the home. Complications of antiinfective therapy, including adverse drug reactions, may increase when the number of antiinfective agents and doses administered to a child increases. Gomez and colleagues[23] reported catheter complications in 29% and adverse drug reactions in 29% of children receiving OPAT. Madigan and Banerjee also reported 29% of pediatric OPAT patients with catheter or drug related complications.[39]

In another pediatric study of children receiving long-term therapy for osteomyelitis, 51% of courses in 54 children were associated with adverse drug events.[16] Catheter- and pump-related complications often arise during therapy, with 26% of 98 children in one study having catheter complications, most commonly occlusion or clotting and dislodgement, also related to longer duration of therapy.[28,31,50] Parents may not be compliant with clinic visits and may not be in the home when the home nursing agency has scheduled a visit. Family members or neighbors other than those trained to care for the child may provide care without the knowledge of the home nursing agency or physician. The clinician may need to rehospitalize the child if doing so is required to complete parenteral therapy safely.

TJC publishes standards and reviews home care outcomes by evaluating specified parameters, including unscheduled inpatient admissions, early discontinuation of parenteral therapy, interruptions in parenteral therapy, catheter-related infections, and adverse drug reactions.[57]

Until recently, data on outcomes from various home nursing agencies were not made available to contracting physicians, hospitals, or payers. Outcome data now are required to be collected by home health organizations, which eventually will help standardize the assessment of OPAT programs. The physician or OPAT coordinator should request outcomes data from any home nursing agency proposing to care for a child by OPAT.

SUMMARY

Successful use of OPAT requires integrated delivery of care for children who are assessed to be at low risk for development of complications from their infections and therapy and do not require skilled nursing care. Parents fulfill the role of a pediatric nurse in the hospital and should be capable of providing a focused, limited assessment of their child and communicating any concerning changes in the child's medical condition or concerns regarding adverse drug reactions or catheter or pump malfunction to the appropriate medical personnel. The antiinfective agents, infusion equipment, and medical follow-up all should be designed for the outpatient setting compatible with the training and resources available to parents or caregivers in the home. Outcomes of pediatric OPAT should be equivalent to or better than those achieved in an inpatient setting.

NEW REFERENCES SINCE THE SEVENTH EDITION

1. Akar A, Singh N, Hyun DY. Appropriateness and safety of outpatient parenteral antimicrobial therapy in children: Opportunities for pediatric antimicrobial stewardship. *Clin Pediatrics.* 2014;53:1000-1003.
4. Bannerjee R, Beekmann SE, Doby EH, et al. Outpatient parenteral antimicrobial therapy practices among pediatric infectious diseases consultants: results of an emerging infections network survey. *J Pediatr Infect Dis Soc.* 2014;3:85-88.
35. Kovacich A, Tamma PD, Advani S, et al. Peripherally inserted central venous catheter complications in children receiving outpatient parenteral antibiotic therapy (OPAT). *Infect Control Hosp Epidemiol.* 2016;37:420-424.
39. Madigan T, Banerjee R. Characteristics and outcomes of outpatient parenteral antimicrobial therapy at an academic children's hospital. *Pediatr Infect Dis J.* 2013;4:346-349.
42. Muldoon EG, Switkowski K, Tice A, et al. A national survey of infectious disease practitioners on their use of outpatient parenteral antimicrobial therapy (OPAT). *Infect Dis.* 2015;47:39-45.

The full reference list for this chapter is available at ExpertConsult.com.

Antiviral Agents 239

Gail J. Harrison

The age of modern antiviral therapy began in the early 1950s, when methisazone, a derivative of the thiosemicarbazones (early antituberculosis compounds), was found also to have activity against vaccinia and variola viruses.[39,40,239,487,584,619] In 1959, the first antiherpes compound, idoxuridine, was synthesized; in 1962, it was approved for the topical treatment of herpetic keratitis.[140,323,474] Shortly thereafter, in 1964, trifluridine also was used to treat herpetic keratitis.[324,325,611] Also in 1964, the first description of vidarabine as an antiviral agent active against herpes simplex virus (HSV) was published, and amantadine was shown to have activity against influenza virus.[136,512] Two years later, amantadine was approved first for the prophylaxis and subsequently for the treatment of influenza A virus infection.[515] Shortly thereafter, in 1972, vidarabine was approved for the treatment of herpes encephalitis.[607] The year 1972 also marked the first description of ribavirin as a broad-spectrum antiviral agent, with activity against both DNA and RNA viruses, and in 1985, the aerosolized form of the drug was approved for the treatment of respiratory syncytial virus (RSV) bronchiolitis.[139,565] In 1977, acyclovir was reported to be a potent and selective inhibitor of the replication of both HSV and varicella-zoster virus (VZV) and boasted the added advantage of a favorable safety profile.[138,165,550] Subsequently, several structural analogues of acyclovir led to the development of antiviral agents with expanded antiviral spectra, such as ganciclovir, and agents with more favorable bioavailability, such as with the prodrugs valacyclovir and valganciclovir.[128,391] In the 1990s, the introduction of cidofovir, a broad-spectrum, long-lasting antiviral agent, and the neuraminidase inhibitors zanamivir and oseltamivir, which treat both influenza A and influenza B viruses, added new dimensions to antiviral therapy.[84,125,261,358,540] In 2007, the oral antiviral agent maribavir, and in 2011, the oral antiviral agent letermavir, both with unique anti–cytomegalovirus (CMV)-specific activity, were granted US Food and Drug Administration (FDA) orphan drug fast track status, and the antivirals are now in phase III clinical trials in immunocompromised patients with or at risk for resistant CMV infections.[611] Peramivir was the first intravenous antiviral for treatment of influenza A and B infection and was licensed by the FDA in 2014. The research now being conducted no doubt will expand our antiviral armamentarium to combat viruses that may be used as biologic weapons as well as to prevent the emergence of resistant viruses and spawn creative strategies such as multidrug therapy and targeted delivery systems.[209,251]

Even though diseases caused by viruses (Box 239.1) now may be treated with a variety of antiviral agents, the close relationship between the viral replicative cycle and its host cell metabolism unfortunately has caused the development of safe and effective antiviral agents to lag behind the development of other antimicrobials, such as antibiotics and antifungals. Clinically successful antiviral agents target and inhibit virus-specific functions while keeping cellular toxicity to a minimum. In addition, as a further testament to the codependency between viruses and host cells, some antiviral agents actually require cellular metabolism for antiviral activity, such as the terminal phosphorylation of acyclovir monophosphate to the active triphosphate form.

Antiviral agents can be categorized as virucidals, antiviral chemotherapeutic agents or drugs, and immunomodulators. Virucidal agents inactivate the virus on contact and include detergents, solvents, and ultraviolet light. These agents are not useful for treatment of human viral disease because healthy tissue also is destroyed. They may, however, be used to inactivate viruses on the surface of the skin or inanimate objects. Antiviral treatments that physically destroy both virus and the tissues infected or transformed by them include cryotherapy, laser therapy, and podophyllin and are used primarily to treat recalcitrant or life-threatening warts on mucocutaneous or laryngotracheal tissue. The host immune response also is important and in many cases essential for recovery from viral disease or even maintenance of a latent or inactivated state of the virus. Therefore successful antiviral treatment may necessitate relief from immunosuppression when it is feasible, such as for patients with Epstein-Barr virus (EBV)–induced lymphoproliferative disease who are undergoing cancer chemotherapy or organ transplantation. It also may include the use of biologic response modifiers, or immunomodulators, that manipulate the immune system to enhance its ability to contain viral infection. Examples of immunomodulators include immune globulin and monoclonal antibody preparations, cytokines such as interferons, and even novel approaches such as virus-specific cytotoxic T-cell lines designed to reconstitute host immunity.[22,36] In addition, supportive treatments, including fluid resuscitation, blood product transfusions, mechanical ventilation, and extracorporeal membrane oxygenation, are important for serious viral disease.[24,121] Finally, updated knowledge about specific antiviral therapy licensed for hepatitis viruses is reviewed in Chapters 47, 157, and 177, and antiretroviral therapy is reviewed in Chapter 192.

Antiviral chemotherapeutic agents usually inhibit virus-specific events (Fig. 239.1), such as adsorption or attachment to the host cell (pleconaril), penetration and uncoating of the viral genome (amantadine), viral gene expression and nucleic acid synthesis (acyclovir, ganciclovir), and even viral assembly of intact, infectious viral particles (interferons). Therefore antiviral agents exhibit their "antiviral effect" primarily while viral replication is active at the host cell level. If the antiviral compound is withdrawn or discontinued, viral replication resumes. Furthermore, the currently available antiviral agents do not appear to eliminate viruses that are latent or in other dormant or nonreplicative states. The goal

BOX 239.1 Virus-Associated Diseases That May Be Treated With Antiviral Agents That Are Currently Available or Under Clinical Development

DNA Viruses

- Herpes simplex virus
  - Gingivostomatitis
  - Keratoconjunctivitis
  - Eczema herpeticum
  - Whitlow
  - Genital ulcers
  - Esophagitis
  - Hepatitis
  - Encephalitis
  - Aseptic meningitis
  - Neonatal disease
- Varicella-zoster virus
  - Chickenpox
  - Zoster
  - Acute retinal necrosis
  - Pneumonitis
  - Hepatitis
  - Cerebral vasculitis and stroke
- Cytomegalovirus
  - Retinitis
  - Pneumonitis
  - Esophagitis and colitis
  - Fever and leukopenia syndrome
  - Congenital disease
- Epstein-Barr virus
  - Mononucleosis syndrome
  - Posttransplantation lymphoproliferative disease
- Herpes B virus
  - Encephalitis
- Adenoviruses
  - Disseminated disease
  - Hemorrhagic cystitis
  - Pneumonitis
  - Colitis
  - Conjunctivitis
- Hepatitis B virus
  - Acute and chronic hepatitis
- Variola virus
  - Smallpox
- Vaccinia virus
  - Vaccine-associated complications
- Papillomaviruses
  - Cutaneous and genital warts
  - Laryngeal papillomatosis
- Polyomaviruses (BK, JC, SV40)
  - Hemorrhagic cystitis
  - Progressive multifocal encephalopathy

RNA Viruses

- Influenza viruses
  - Influenza syndrome and complications
- Parainfluenza viruses
  - Laryngotracheobronchitis
  - Pneumonitis
- Respiratory syncytial virus
  - Bronchiolitis
  - Pneumonitis
- Measles virus
  - Measles syndrome
  - Encephalitis
  - Pneumonitis
- Enteroviruses
  - Aseptic meningitis and meningoencephalitis
  - Myocarditis
  - Neonatal disease
- Arenavirus
  - Lassa fever
- Hepatitis C virus
  - Acute and chronic hepatitis
- Ebola virus
  - Ebola virus hemorrhagic fever

of antiviral therapy, for the most part, is to inhibit active viral replication to such a degree that the host immune response is able to contain or in some instances even to eliminate the infection.

Antiviral agents usually have a narrow range of activity that can be predicted by their molecular mechanism of action. For example, rimantadine and amantadine have high activity against the RNA-containing influenza A virus, limited activity against influenza B virus, and virtually no activity against the DNA herpesviruses,[125,136] whereas acyclovir, a deoxyguanosine analogue that requires monophosphorylation by the viral enzyme thymidine kinase (TK) for activation, has significant activity against DNA viruses (HSV), which carry TK, but no activity against RNA viruses such as influenza virus. Viruses infecting a host also may become resistant to a specific agent to which they originally were susceptible, usually by induced or selected mutations. Resistance is therefore most likely to occur in viruses that infect the host with a high viral load and that have a high intrinsic viral mutation rate as well as in viruses that infect hosts who are exposed to selective drug pressure during chronic, low-dose, or repeated treatment with an antiviral agent.[274] Both resistant and sensitive viruses are capable of causing serious disease, especially in an immunocompromised host. Currently, most antiviral agents are administered as single therapeutic agents. However, double and triple combination antiviral drug therapy, now a routine therapy in modern antiretroviral regimens, is also important in selected circumstances for treatment of other viral diseases in immunocompromised hosts or where presence or emergence of drug-resistant viruses is likely.[25,245,251,443,445] Combination strategy increases antiviral effectiveness, prevents the emergence of drug resistance, and allows the administration of lower, less toxic dosages.[34,45,263,504,505]

ANTIVIRAL AGENTS ACTIVE AGAINST RNA VIRUSES

Table 239.1 provides a list of antiviral agents active against RNA viruses, including their clinical indications and usual dosages.

Amantadine and Rimantadine

Spectrum of Activity

Amantadine (1-adamantanamine hydrochloride) and rimantadine (α-methyl-1-adamantane methylamine hydrochloride) are tricyclic amines with specific activity against influenza A viruses (Fig. 239.2). Mean inhibitory concentrations of 0.1 to 0.4 μg/mL for amantadine have been reported, and rimantadine is 4 to 10 times more active than amantadine against susceptible subtypes of influenza A virus.[77,249,467] Amantadine also has in vitro activity against rubella virus, but efficacy was not confirmed in animal models.[453,454,513,555] Much higher concentrations (10–50 μg/mL) appear to inhibit influenza B virus and parainfluenza viruses, but these high concentrations cannot be achieved safely in humans.[513] Research and development continue with designs of more

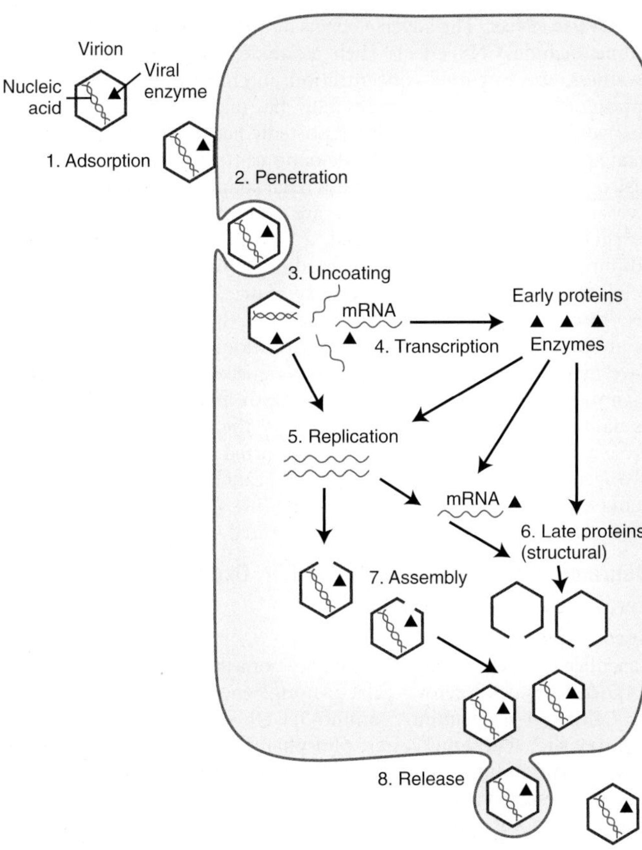

FIG. 239.1 Basic steps in intracellular (DNA) replication. *1,* Adsorption of virion to the cell membrane. *2,* Penetration. *3,* Uncoating, removal of the protein coat. *4,* Early gene expression, transcription of viral proteins. *5,* Replication, synthesis of DNA strands. *6,* Late gene expression, transcription of messenger RNA, and translation of late protein synthesis. *7,* Maturation and assembly of virions. *8,* Release.

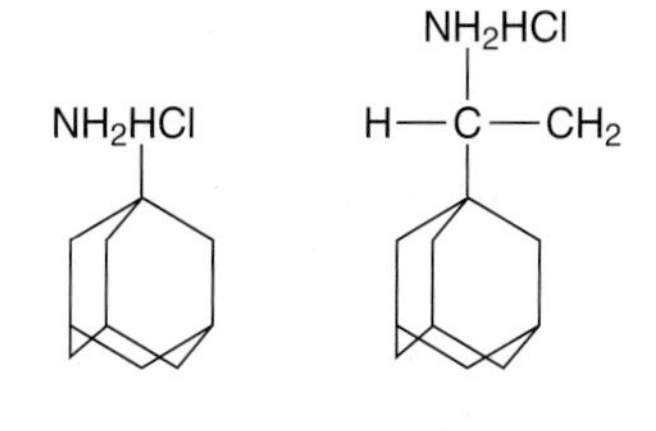

TABLE 239.1 Clinical Indications and Usual Treatment Dosages for Licensed Antiviral Agents Active Against RNA Viruses

Agent	Indication	Dosage
Amantadine	Influenza A	2.2–4.4 mg/kg/dose PO bid (max, 100–200 mg daily)
Rimantadine	Influenza A	2.5 mg/kg/dose PO bid (max 150 mg daily)
Oseltamivir	Influenza A and B	2 mg/kg/dose PO bid (max 150 mg daily)
Zanamivir	Influenza A and B	5 mg/dose inhaled bid
Ribavirin	Respiratory syncytial virus	6 g/300 mL inhaled daily in an 18-h period *or* 2–6 g/100 mL inhaled in a 2-h period tid
	Hepatitis C	600 mg PO bid (with interferon alfa)

adamantane-like inhibitors of the M2 proton channel against influenza A virus.[157,467] The adamantanes also have significant activity against hepatitis C virus (HCV) and rhabdoviruses (vesicular stomatitis virus and rabies virus).[527,534,612]

Mechanism of Action and Resistance

The mechanism of action of both amantadine and rimantadine against influenza A virus appears to be primarily inhibition of the ion channel function of the M2 protein in the membrane of the virus, possibly affecting two stages of viral replication: uncoating and, to a lesser extent, assembly.[23,125,244,467] Amantadine and rimantadine resistance occurs when mutations cause an amino acid change in one of four critical sites (amino acids 26, 27, 30, and 31) in the transmembrane channel or domain of the M2 viral protein.[343] Such mutations occur frequently and rapidly during therapy because approximately 30% of adults and children who receive amantadine or rimantadine therapy for at least 5 days shed resistant influenza virus.[247,250] These resistant strains are genetically stable, may be transmitted to close contacts, and can produce disease.[46,247,632] Immunocompromised patients may shed drug-resistant influenza viruses for prolonged periods, and resistant strains can persist even after drug administration has been discontinued.[343] However, debate has begun among experts concerning whether patients in whom a resistant strain is identified should be isolated until viral shedding has ceased.[234] Adamantane-resistant strains of influenza A subtype H3N2 and subtype H1N12009 have produced community outbreaks and epidemics.[46,246,247,632] Some strains of highly pathogenic A(H5N1) avian influenza are susceptible to adamantanes, but most strains of A(H5N1) should be considered resistant.[298] Strains of influenza A virus resistant to amantadine also are resistant to rimantadine, and vice versa, but they are usually susceptible to ribavirin and neuraminidase inhibitors. The mechanism of action against rabies virus appears to be by inhibition of later steps in replication, probably at the level of uncoating, when the virus is released into the intracytoplasmic compartment of infected cells.[567]

NH_2HCl NH_2HCl, H—C—CH_2

Amantadine   Rimantadine

FIG. 239.2 Structure of amantadine and rimantadine.

Pharmacokinetics

Amantadine is absorbed rapidly and nearly completely after oral administration, with peak plasma concentrations of 0.5 to 0.8 μg/mL attained within 2 hours of administration.[56,255] It is excreted almost unchanged in urine. Nasal and salivary secretions also contain high levels of amantadine, and the drug is present in cerebrospinal fluid (CSF) as well at approximately half the plasma level. Dose reductions, adjusted according to creatinine clearance, are required in patients with renal insufficiency and renal failure.[285,504,621] Rimantadine, on the other hand, is more slowly absorbed than amantadine, with peak plasma levels of 0.4 to 0.6 μg/mL achieved within 2 to 4 hours of administration.[15,16,255,433] Rimantadine is also present in high concentration in nasal secretions. It is excreted in urine, but only after extensive metabolism by the liver. Dose reduction is therefore recommended in patients with renal or hepatic disease.[86,613] Hemodialysis does not appear to clear either drug, so supplemental doses usually are not recommended after dialysis.[546] When they are administered to chronically ill, institutionalized older adult patients, dosages also may need to be adjusted.[424,461] In addition, aerosolized forms of amantadine and rimantadine have been evaluated in human volunteers.[253,259]

Clinical Indications, Dosage, and Adverse Effects

Clinical indications. Amantadine and rimantadine are equally effective for the treatment of disease caused by susceptible subtypes of influenza A virus.[125,343,613] If they are administered within the first 48 hours of symptoms, both agents significantly reduce the signs and symptoms of influenza in both adults and children by significantly shortening the duration of fever and respiratory and systemic symptoms by 1 day.[125,142,375,585,614,625] The duration and amount of viral shedding from the nasopharyngeal tract also are decreased, and otologic complications may be reduced.[152] Both agents are effective for prophylaxis against influenza A virus infection and disease, with approximately 50% overall effectiveness in preventing infection with the virus and approximately 60% to 70% overall effectiveness (up to 90% in some studies) in preventing clinical disease and, in individuals with breakthrough clinical disease, in reducing the severity of the disease.* The spontaneous emergence of resistant strains during rimantadine or amantadine therapy and subsequent transmission of these resistant strains may lessen the effectiveness of prophylaxis in some families and nursing homes.[247,398] Amantadine and rimantadine are both available as tablets (100 mg) and syrup (50 mg/5 mL) for oral administration.

Emergence of resistance to adamantanes has limited the use of amantadine and rimantadine as single agents for influenza treatment. Since 2005, all circulating H3N2 subtypes of influenza A virus have been resistant to amantadine and rimantadine. Also resistant to adamantanes is the 2009 pandemic subtype influenza A(H1N1)pdm2009, which replaced the previously susceptible seasonal H1N1 subtype when it emerged. Influenza B is intrinsically resistant to the adamantanes. Amantadine has also been included in treatment protocols for patients with rabies encephalitis.[612]

Dosage.

The usual dose of amantadine for children is 4.4 to 8.8 mg/kg per day divided twice daily (many experts recommend 5 mg/kg per day), with a maximal recommended daily dose of 200 mg. The usual dose of rimantadine for children is 5 mg/kg per day divided twice daily, with a maximal recommended daily dose of 150 mg.[15,234,433,613] Older children and adolescents may take the usual adult dose for each drug, which is 200 mg/day given once daily or, for better tolerance, divided into two 100-mg doses daily.[15] Older adult patients should receive 100 mg daily or less if renal insufficiency is present. To be effective, these agents should be given as soon as possible after the onset of symptoms.[126,125] The duration of treatment of established influenza should be 3 to 7 days, or at least 2 days after the cessation of systemic signs and symptoms.[125] Prevention of influenza is accomplished best through annual vaccination; however, rimantadine and amantadine may be used to prevent or to lessen influenza symptoms in both adults and children.[112,125,127] Prophylaxis should be administered during the period of risk, whether exposure is in the family, community, or nosocomial setting.[202] In general, prophylaxis should continue for at least 10 days after a known exposure occurs in an unprotected individual.[202] For patients who receive the combination of inactivated vaccine and oral prophylaxis, rimantadine or amantadine should be continued for at least 2 to 4 weeks after vaccination, when maximal antibody response from the vaccine is expected to occur. For patients who are at high risk but did not receive the vaccine, oral prophylaxis should be continued for as long as the period of risk is anticipated and may be extended to the end of the community's influenza season. Doses of both drugs should be adjusted for patients with renal disease, and doses of rimantadine should be adjusted for patients with hepatic disease.[86,285,504,613] Prolonged treatment may be associated with side effects, especially in older adults.[461] If side effects occur, the daily dose may be reduced to 100 mg and still be effective in most cases. The emergence of resistant strains during the period of drug administration may lessen the effectiveness of prophylaxis in some patients.[247,398] Combination with aerosolized ribavirin or the neuraminidase inhibitors may enhance the antiviral effect of amantadine or rimantadine against influenza A virus.[34,245,284,444,526]

An amantadine dose of 200 mg daily, combined with therapeutic coma, ketamine infusion, and management of cerebral vasospasms, known as the Milwaukee Protocol for Rabies, has been used to treat rabies encephalitis.[612] However, recent critical appraisal of this protocol has not substantiated its efficacy for treatment of rabies encephalitis.[630]

Amantadine also has applications for noninfectious conditions. For example, high-dose amantadine has been used to treat dyskinesia in Parkinson disease.[347] A recent case report showed that amantadine may be useful in the treatment of unresponsive wakefulness syndromes, such as persistent vegetative state, due to central nervous system (CNS) disease.[368]

*References 125, 143, 150, 202, 305, 306, 425, 449, 496, 602, 633.

Adverse effects. The adverse effects of both amantadine and rimantadine include CNS effects such as anxiety, depression, insomnia, dizziness, and impaired concentration; in children, these side effects appear to be rare, but they may be manifested as behavioral changes.[112,125,150,542] Rimantadine reportedly has fewer CNS side effects than amantadine.[125,150,254,418] Hallucinations, tremors, and seizures also may occur, especially in patients with renal failure who have high plasma levels of amantadine. In addition, rare cases of coma and fatal cardiac dysrhythmia have been reported.[468,504] A prudent procedure is to administer amantadine and rimantadine with caution to individuals being treated for seizures or neuropsychiatric disorders or to patients also receiving other medications that affect the nervous system, such as antihistamines.[418] Furthermore, institutionalized older adults may have increased plasma levels and experience side effects more often than younger patients.[461] On occasion, gastrointestinal symptoms such as nausea and vomiting may accompany the oral administration of these agents in all age groups. Most reported adverse effects of these two agents have been reversible, with significant long-term complications being exceedingly rare. Of note, amantadine also is used to treat parkinsonism and drug-induced extrapyramidal reactions.[515]

Neuraminidase Inhibitors (Zanamivir, Oseltamivir, Peramivir, and Laninamivir)

Spectrum of Activity

Zanamivir (5-[acetylamino]-4-[(aminoiminomethyl)-amino]-2,6-anhydro-3,4,5-trideoxy-D-glycero-D-galacto-non-2-enoic acid) and oseltamivir ([3*R*,4*R*,5*S*]-4-acetylamino-5-amino-3[1-ethylpropoxy]-1-cyclohexene-1-carboxylic acid ethyl ester phosphate [1:1]) are analogues of *N*-acetylneuraminic acid, the cell surface receptor for influenza viruses, and were designed to inhibit the viral neuraminidase of influenza viruses (Fig. 239.3). Oral oseltamivir and inhaled zanamivir are licensed in the United States. The cyclopentane peramivir ([1*S*,2*S*,3*S*,4*R*]-3-[(1*S*)-1-acetamido-2-ethyl-butyl]-4-(diaminomethylideneamino)-2-hydroxy-cyclopentane-1-carboxylic acid) and laninamivir ([4*S*,5*R*,6*R*]-acetamido-4-carbamimidamido-6-[(1*R*,2*R*)-3-hydroxy-2-methoxypropyl]-5-6-dihydro-4*H*-pyran-2-carboxylic acid) are newer neuraminidase inhibitors currently in clinical trials in the United States.

These four agents are potent and specific inhibitors of the neuraminidases of influenza A (seasonal H3N2, seasonal H1N1, H1N1pdm2009, and avian influenza viruses, including highly pathogenic H5N1 and H9N2) and influenza B viruses. Up to 90% of tested strains are inhibited at concentrations of 0.05 to 100 μmol/L.[221,334,589]

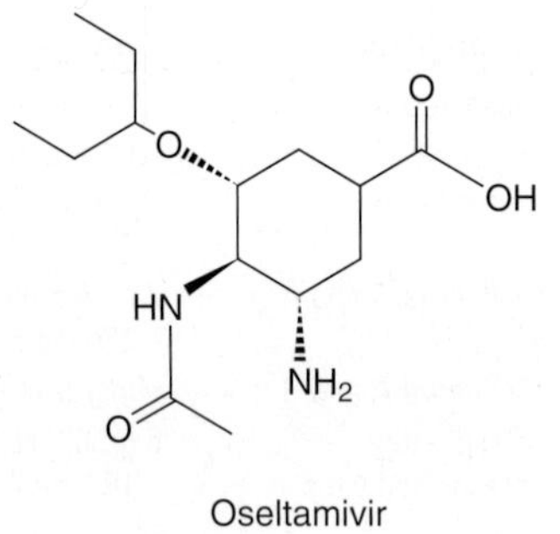

Oseltamivir

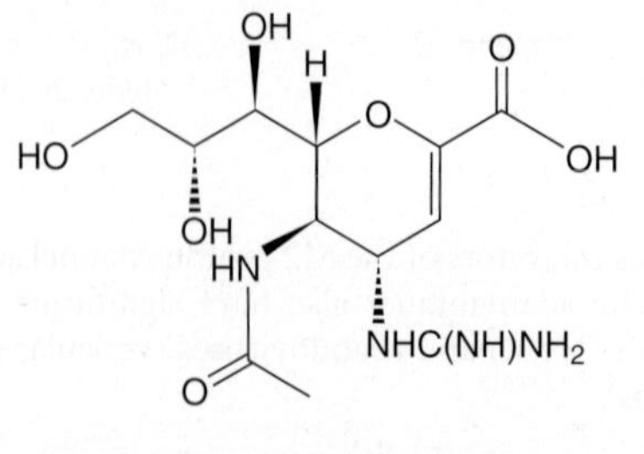

Zanamivir

FIG. 239.3 Structure of the neuraminidase inhibitors oseltamivir and zanamivir.

Peramivir has also shown efficacy for the treatment of influenza A and B, especially H1N1pdm2009, in at least four efficacy trials.[53] Peramivir, intravenous form, was first licensed in Japan and Korea in 2010, and in 2014 was approved by the FDA. Peramivir was first authorized for emergency use in the United States and other countries for treatment of adults and children with severe influenza during the 2009 H1N1 pandemic. It also was administered through emergency investigational new drug regulations[263,280] and appeared to be well tolerated and associated with recovery.[263] However, because peramivir under emergency use authorization was limited to critically ill patients for whom other therapy had failed or in whom oral drug absorption was unreliable or inhalation drug not feasible, the efficacy and safety of peramivir could not be adequately assessed. Peramivir intravenous preparation is now approved by the FDA for treatment of adults with symptomatic but uncomplicated influenza, who have had symptoms for less than 2 days, and shows similar efficacy and safety profiles compared with oral oseltamivir.[434,604]

Long-acting inhaled laninamivir octanoate is a new neuraminidase inhibitor, with activity against highly pathogenic avian influenza virus H5N1 in addition to influenza A (seasonal H3N2, seasonal H1N1, and H1N1pdm2009) and influenza B.[177,268,515,523] Laninamivir is licensed and available in Japan and in phase III clinical trials in the United States.[299,535,625] Influenza A (AH5N1, AH1N1) and B virus strains with reduced susceptibility to neuraminidase inhibitors (oseltamivir, zanamivir, and peramivir) have also been detected in hospitalized patients and community-acquired cases of influenza.[35,177,268,281,294-297,299,556,568]

Because influenza virus changes seasonally and antiviral resistance may evolve or emerge suddenly, any statements on presumed spectrum of antiviral activity of any neuraminidase inhibitor should be taken in the context of ongoing viral surveillance.[177,294,303,515,528]

These compounds also are capable of inhibiting neuraminidases from other pathogens and mammalian cells, but only at extremely high concentrations.

Mechanism of Action and Resistance

Neuraminidase permits influenza virus to penetrate through the mucoproteins present in respiratory secretions to the surfaces of cells, and inhibition of this enzyme prevents viral access and infection of cells. Neuraminidase also destroys receptors recognized by viral hemagglutinin and is therefore necessary for optimal release of influenza virus particles from infected cells. Inhibition prevents cell-to-cell spread of virus within the respiratory tract and lessens the intensity of the initial infection.[116,125,334,437,589] Mutations that induce amino acid changes in viral neuraminidase alter enzyme stability or activity, mutations in hemagglutinin produce a reduced affinity for cell receptors, and mutations in both produce resistant influenza viruses.[125,225–228] Cross-resistance to both zanamivir and oseltamivir, as well as to oseltamivir and peramivir, also can occur, especially if the mutation is in the hemagglutinin portion.[413] Resistance occurs either by spontaneous mutation or by selection during antiviral treatment and has been documented by in vitro passage of the virus in increasing concentrations of the agents, in patients receiving these antiviral agents, and in newly emerged strains that acquire a change in neuraminidase through mutation or reassortment. In 2007, influenza A(H1N1) seasonal acquired a change in neuraminidase, designated H275Y, that resulted in oseltamivir resistance, but zanamivir susceptibility was retained. In 2009, oseltamivir-susceptible influenza A(H1N1)pdm2009 emerged, replacing the oseltamivir-resistant seasonal H1N1. Beginning in 2009, individual cases of oseltamivir resistance, usually in immunocompromised patients receiving treatment, as well as community clusters of oseltamivir-resistant influenza A(H1N1) pdm2009, began to be detected.[92,158] Sporadic oseltamivir resistance has also been detected in avian influenza A(H5N1). Clinical trials of oral oseltamivir for the treatment of naturally occurring influenza detected resistance in 1% to 2% of posttreatment isolates from adults and adolescents and in 5% to 8% of isolates from younger children.[125,227,285,628] Currently, most seasonal H1N1 strains circulating in 2008–2009 were resistant to oseltamivir, and the overall occurrence of influenza A H1N1 subtypes resistant to oseltamivir is estimated at a rate of 2.6%, with an association between oseltamivir resistance and pneumonia in four clinical studies.[35,246,296,299,576]

Peramivir resistance has also been documented in both influenza A, including pandemic A(H1N1)pdm2009, and influenza B.[458] A point mutation at H273Y in one influenza B isolate from a human patient conferred double resistance to both oseltamivir and peramivir.[268] Most peramivir- and oseltamivir-resistant influenza strains remain susceptible to zanamivir at this time.

Zanamivir resistance appears rare, documented in case reports of either influenza A or B virus infection in patients who were usually immunocompromised hosts receiving antiviral medications for prolonged periods.[224,225,252,256,260,420,576] Large randomized trials of healthy individuals have not documented zanamivir resistance, but individualized case reports and small case series have shown that zanamivir resistance has emerged.[225,252,256,260,420] In one study from Australia, analysis of 391 influenza A(H1N1) seasonal isolates documented zanamivir resistance in 9 (2.3%) isolates.[297] Influenza B viruses with mutations in the neuraminidase active site conferring resistance to oseltamivir, peramivir, and zanamivir have been reported from several geographic sites.[177,268,515,528] Overall, there are currently at least 50 different documented amino acid substitutions that have produced mutations conferring reduced antiviral susceptibility to oseltamivir, zanamivir, peramivir, or laninamivir in influenza A and B viruses.[442,446] Preliminary evidence suggested that some mutant resistant strains may have reduced infectivity or virulence compared with susceptible strains,[571] but resistant strains have caused outbreaks and epidemics.[246] Therefore difference in influenza virulence cannot be predicted by the antiviral susceptibility pattern of the strain.

Pharmacokinetics

Zanamivir is administered as an inhaled dry powder and is deposited in the oropharynx and, to a lesser extent, in the tracheobronchial tree and lungs.[125] Approximately 4% to 17% of inhaled drug is absorbed systemically, and levels of 17 to 142 ng/mL can be detected in serum 1 to 2 hours after administration of a typical inhaled dose of 10 mg in adults.[88] Serum levels in pediatric patients who received an inhaled dose were extremely low (<10 ng/mL) or undetectable, which may be related to the ability of the patient to cooperate with the inhaled drug delivery system. The oral bioavailability of zanamivir is extremely low, with less than 5% of the administered dose absorbed, and therefore it is not administered in this form. Intravenous and intramuscular preparations of zanamivir also have been tested in clinical trials, but these forms are not available clinically at this time.[85,88,199,246] Intravenous zanamivir provides a sustained antiviral effect.[194] It also penetrates lung tissue. Zanamivir administered intravenously at doses of 100 mg, 200 mg, and 600 mg provides concentrations in epithelial lung fluid 12 hours after dosing of 74, 146, and 419 ng/mL, respectively.[523] In contrast, inhaled zanamivir concentrations provide much higher levels of 396 to 891 ng/mL to the respiratory tract. Zanamivir is not metabolized, and approximately 90% of zanamivir is excreted unchanged in urine.[88]

Oseltamivir, in contrast, has good oral bioavailability. The prodrug compound oseltamivir phosphate is metabolized by hepatic esterases to the parent active compound oseltamivir carboxylate.[125] Approximately 75% to 80% of the administered dose is absorbed, and peak plasma concentrations are reached within 3 to 4 hours but may be delayed, but not reduced, if the drug is given with food. A typical 75-mg dose will provide plasma concentrations of 0.3 to 0.5 μg/mL. Both the prodrug and the active form are eliminated unchanged through the kidneys, and dosages should be adjusted for patients with renal insufficiency or renal failure. Whether the drug dosage should be adjusted for patients with hepatic disease or liver failure is unclear from the available evidence. Information from a small number of pediatric patients suggests that the drug may be eliminated faster in younger children. Geriatric patients, however, appear to metabolize the drug similarly to young adults. Oseltamivir phosphate and oseltamivir carboxylate both may be found in breast milk, but often in concentrations lower than considered therapeutic for infants.[222]

Peramivir administered orally in doses ranging from 100 to 800 mg daily is not well absorbed and produces only modest antiviral effect.[38] Peramivir has been administered intravenously in doses of 200, 400, and 600 mg daily, or approximately 4 to 10 mg/kg once daily.[301] Plasma concentration of approximately 20 ng/mL within 24 hours of infusion has been documented, which is far in excess of the reported half maximal inhibitory concentration (IC_{50}) of peramivir against susceptible influenza strains. Pediatric dosing for peramivir suggests that 10 mg/kg daily produces adequate plasma levels and good antiviral effect with few adverse effects.[524] Pregnant or postpartum women may require higher doses on the basis of limited pharmacokinetic studies that have demonstrated increased plasma volume, increased volume of distribution of peramivir, and shorter half-life.[111] The half-life of peramivir varies between 7 and 20 hours in patients with normal renal function. Peramivir is excreted in the urine as the unchanged form, and dosage adjustments are needed in renal impairment. Patients with proven influenza infection show antiviral effects, with decreased viral shedding between days 2 and 6 of treatment (7–20%) and with clinical improvement and recovery.[524]

Laninamivir octanoate is the prodrug of the active compound laninamivir. It is administered as a single inhalation of either 20 mg or 40 mg to treat influenza infection. It is retained in the tissues and eliminated from the body very slowly, with a plasma half-life of 2 hours and lasting at least 3 days. Urinary excretion appears to occur. Clinical trials show that one inhalation of laninamivir is an effective and well-tolerated treatment for children and adults with seasonal influenza, including oseltamivir-sensitive and oseltamivir-resistant influenza A(H1N1) virus infection.[523,599]

Clinical Indications, Dosage, and Adverse Effects

Clinical indications. Zanamivir and oseltamivir have been shown to be effective in treating both influenza A and influenza B infection.[84,261,316,399,598,599] However, susceptibility of type B and H5NI and H1N1 subtypes of type A influenza may be reduced for oseltamivir.[567] When they are administered within the first 2 days of illness, they provide relief from symptoms up to 1.5 days earlier than placebo does and reduce the quantity and duration of viral shedding.* In some studies, the frequency of secondary complications, such as sinusitis, bronchitis, and otitis media with effusion (but not pneumonia), also was reduced.[125,594] Both antiviral agents are effective for the prophylaxis of influenza A and influenza B infection in both adults and children in family, community, transplant recipient, and nursing home situations.[303] They appear to be 30% to 50% effective in preventing viral infection and 64% to 84% effective in preventing disease.[125,252,258,402,426,594] However, up to 89% efficacy in preventing disease in families has been reported, and in older adult patients in nursing homes, 92% of cases of influenza may be prevented if the agents are administered to those who also have received influenza vaccine.[125,252,402] Oseltamivir may be administered to a patient of any age to treat influenza.

Peramivir may be administered intravenously, under investigational or emergency investigational new drug or clinical trials, to patients unable to tolerate oral oseltamivir or inhaled zanamivir.[380,496] The temporary emergency use authorization for peramivir for treatment of 2009 H1N1 influenza, granted by the FDA and managed through the Centers for Disease Control and Prevention (CDC), terminated in June 2010.[53,263] On the basis of results of clinical trials and experience with the emergency use authorization, 300- to 600-mg doses of peramivir appear to be effective for treatment of high-risk patients infected with susceptible influenza A or B virus strains.[53,263,346] Peramivir probably should not be used to treat patients with oseltamivir-resistant influenza infection (H275Y mutation), patients with mutations of neuraminidase E119D or R292K (which confer peramivir resistance), or patients suspected of having influenza caused by zanamivir resistance because it is likely not to be effective.

Laninamivir may be administered in some countries as a single inhalation to treat influenza A H1N1 and H5N1 infections in adults and children. A dose of laninamivir, 20 to 40 mg, administered in a single inhalation, is retained in the respiratory tissues for a prolonged time, providing very high levels, in excess of the IC_{50} of susceptible influenza strains. This high level may reduce the risk for emergence of resistant strains. Inhaled or intranasal laninamivir also enters the plasma, and renal excretion correlates with creatinine clearance. Pharmacokinetic studies suggest that dose adjustment may be necessary only in severe renal insufficiency.[301,599]

*References 84, 125, 256, 343, 402, 420, 427, 471, 581, 603.

Intravenous zanamivir, which remains investigational at this time, appears effective in treating high-risk, critically ill patients, including immunocompromised patients, with oseltamivir- or peramivir-resistant influenza A infection.[158,194,208,303,458]

Dosage. Zanamivir is administered by oral inhalation with an inhalation device provided with the product. Each inhalation dose is 5 mg, and two inhalations twice daily for 5 days is the usual recommended dosage for all age groups. Use of this drug and device is dependent on the understanding and cooperation of the patient; therefore it is not indicated for use in children younger than 7 years and may be of limited use in older children and adults who are unable to cooperate with the delivery system. No reduction in dosage is needed for patients with impaired renal function because very little of the inhaled drug is absorbed systemically.

Zanamivir has also been administered by nebulizer at a dosage of 16 to 32 mg (usually 24 mg) in 1 to 2 mL of sterile water every 6 hours for 5 to 10 days.[224]

Zanamivir has been administered intravenously in doses of 600 mg at a constant rate during 30 minutes, every 12 hours for 5 days, under investigational, compassionate use to individual patients and currently is being evaluated in clinical trials (https://clinicaltrials.gov).[149,158,243] Pediatric dosing in the clinical trials is weight based and age adjusted. A dose of 4 to 10 mg/kg per dose every 12 hours has been evaluated.[157] Younger children appear to require higher doses; children who weigh less than 11 kg may be given up to 24 mg per dose if renal function is normal. Some institutions have administered up to 16 to 24 mg/kg per dose every 12 hours. All trials agree that a maximum of 600 mg/dose should be given twice daily, and this maximum dose should be used for children who are older than 13 years or weigh more than 37 kg and have normal renal function. Doses should be adjusted in renal impairment according to creatinine clearance.

Oseltamivir is administered orally and is available in 75-mg capsules and a 12-mg/mL suspension. The usual adult dosage is 75 mg twice daily for treatment and once or twice daily for as long as 6 weeks for prophylaxis. The pediatric dose is 2 mg/kg per dose given twice daily (4 mg/kg per day divided twice daily).[125] Double dosing of oral oseltamivir (up to 150 mg twice daily for adults and older children) was recommended for some patients during the 2009 H1N1 influenza A pandemic and may be used for treatment of severe seasonal or pandemic influenza or influenza caused by a strain thought to have reduced susceptibility to oseltamvir.[111]

Peramivir has been administered intravenously to adults in doses between 300 and 600 mg once daily, during a 60-minute infusion.[544,626] Weight-based dosing suggests a once-daily dose of approximately 4 to 10 mg/kg. Duration of treatment is recommended for 5 to 10 days.[301,302] Pediatric dosing, for ages 3 months to 15 years, has been studied. A once-daily dose of 10 mg/kg, with a maximum daily dose of 600 mg, appears to be clinically and virologically effective and safe in infants and children with influenza.[524,564] Neonates should be dosed at 6 mg/kg daily and infants at 8 to 10 mg/kg daily, according to FDA guidance (https://www.fda.gov). Dosage adjustments are needed in renal impairment. Patients with severe or end-stage renal disease should probably receive 100 mg daily and after each dialysis because peramivir is cleared by dialysis (https://www.fda.gov).

The dose of laninamivir is 20 to 40 mg, administered in a single inhalation to treat the entire illness. Dosage adjustments are necessary only in severe renal impairment.[301,563,599]

Adverse effects. Both neuraminidase inhibitors are generally well tolerated, with few if any serious adverse effects observed in clinical trials. Zanamivir inhalation, however, may produce local irritation or bronchospasm in some patients. Oseltamivir has been associated with nausea and vomiting, which may be lessened by administration of the drug with food, and, rarely, psychosis and other psychiatric disorders, and renal, metabolic and cardiac reactions such as bradycardia and QT prolongation.[125,238] The most commonly observed side effect of inhaled laninamivir is gastrointestinal. The most common side effects of intravenous peramivir are nausea, vomiting, diarrhea, and neutropenia. Rarely, skin reactions and anaphylaxis have occurred with peramivir administration. Intravenous zanamivir appears well tolerated on the basis of limited clinical experience at this time.

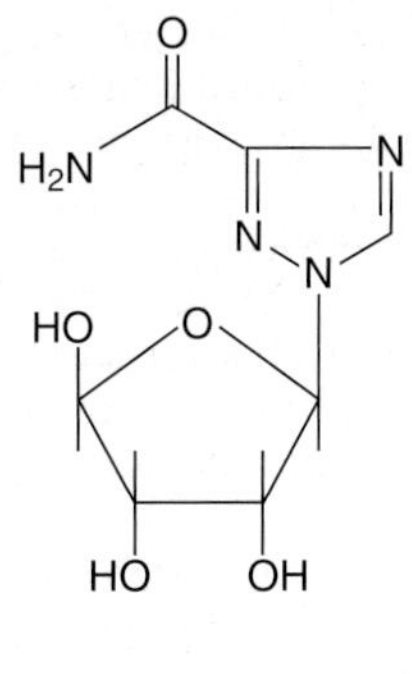

Ribavirin

FIG. 239.4 Structure of ribavirin.

Ribavirin

Spectrum of Activity

Ribavirin (1-β-D-ribofuranosyl-1,2,4-triazole-3-carboxamide) is a synthetic guanosine analogue with broad-spectrum antiviral activity (Fig. 239.4).[536] It inhibits the in vitro replication of a wide variety of RNA viruses, including orthomyxoviruses, such as influenza A and B viruses; paramyxoviruses, such as RSV, parainfluenza viruses, and measles virus; arenaviruses, such as Lassa fever virus; bunyaviruses, which cause viral encephalitis; togaviruses, such as HCV; enteroviruses, such as enterovirus 71, polioviruses, and coxsackie B virus; rabies virus; and retroviruses, including human immunodeficiency virus (HIV) type 1.[175,289,332,359,361,372,455,525,612] Also inhibited by ribavirin are many DNA viruses, such as adenoviruses, hepatitis A virus, CMV, and poxviruses (e.g., vaccinia virus).[151] It inhibits most orthomyxoviruses and paramyxoviruses at concentrations of 3 to 10 μg/mL and Lassa fever virus at 4 to 40 μmol/L.[292] Because most of its clinical use has been for the treatment of RNA viruses, ribavirin is included in this section of the chapter.

Mechanism of Action and Resistance

Ribavirin most likely exerts its antiviral effects by altering the cellular nucleotide pools and by interfering with viral mRNA formation.[76,175,558] The compound is phosphorylated by host cell enzymes to monophosphate, diphosphate, and triphosphate active forms, each with specific antiviral actions.[572] For example, ribavirin monophosphate competitively interferes with the synthesis of guanosine triphosphate and, subsequently, with viral nucleic acid synthesis. Ribavirin triphosphate inhibits the RNA polymerase of influenza virus and also interferes with the capping of its viral mRNA.[175,332,455,609,620] In addition, the diphosphate and triphosphate forms of ribavirin appear to inhibit the reverse transcriptase activity of HIV-1.[182] The mechanism of action of ribavirin against HCV and other viruses, however, is not well understood. Ribavirin also exerts an effect on the host immune system by inhibiting mast cell secretory responses and diminishing immunoglobulin E (IgE) responses.[488] Antiviral resistance is not well characterized and appears to be a rare occurrence. No ribavirin-resistant RSV isolates have been identified during clinical trials, and information is scant regarding the resistance of other viruses to ribavirin.[236,383,509]

Pharmacokinetics

Ribavirin can be administered by aerosol, orally, and intravenously. Aerosol administration of ribavirin with a small-particle aerosol generator delivers very high concentrations (>1000 μg/mL) of the drug to the respiratory tract.[345] Aerosolized drug also is absorbed systemically, and peak plasma levels after 8 hours of continuous aerosol administration range from 0.5 to 2.2 μg/mL; after 20 hours, they reach 0.8 to 3.3 μg/mL. After oral administration, bioavailability is 33% to 45%, and peak plasma levels of 1.3 to 3.2 μg/mL have been observed 1 to 2 hours after administration. Intravenous administration of ribavirin produces 10-fold higher plasma levels in less than 1 hour than after the administration of equivalent doses by different routes.[459] Higher doses used to treat Lassa fever produce plasma levels of up to 24 μg/mL. Ribavirin also crosses the blood-brain barrier and is present in CSF at approximately 70% of the plasma level.[122,287] The drug is metabolized by the liver, and approximately 40% of the dose is excreted by the kidneys.[459] The triphosphate form also concentrates in erythrocytes at an erythrocyte-to-plasma ratio of 40:1 and is slowly eliminated with a half-life of 40 days or longer. Hemodialysis and hemofiltration do not remove significant amounts of ribavirin from the body.[350]

Clinical Indications, Dosage, and Adverse Effects

Clinical indications. Ribavirin aerosol is licensed for the treatment of RSV bronchiolitis and pneumonia in children.[233] Treatment shortens the duration of viral shedding and improves the fever, respiratory rate, arterial oxygen saturation, and lower respiratory tract signs on physical examination in severely ill patients who receive the antiviral agent early in the course of their illness.*

No clear benefit has been observed in otherwise healthy, low-risk patients with mild disease or in those who receive treatment late in the course of the disease. Studies of infants receiving mechanical ventilation have reported conflicting results in clinical benefit.[410,422,537] However, despite numerous clinical studies, indications for treatment remain controversial because efficacy has not been documented convincingly in all studies and the benefits observed generally have been mild and difficult to quantitate objectively.[233] Nonetheless, because antiviral treatment clearly appeared to provide benefit to some children, in 1996, the American Academy of Pediatrics recommended that ribavirin be considered for the treatment of hospitalized infants and children with severe lower respiratory tract infection caused by RSV. Currently, the American Academy of Pediatrics recommends that inhaled ribavirin may be considered for use in selected, high-risk patients with documented, potentially life-threatening RSV infection.[12] From 1996 to 2015, prescription of inhaled ribavirin for bronchiolitis in otherwise healthy infants hospitalized with bronchiolitis has declined, and most pediatric infectious diseases specialists are reserving the antiviral for use in seriously or critically ill and high-risk infants and children.[41,87] Use of inhaled, oral, and intravenous ribavirin in allogeneic hematopoietic stem cell transplant recipients with RSV and other respiratory viruses has continued, with case series supporting clinical benefit in these high-risk patients, with few serious side effects.[96,219,229,390,520]

Patients thought to potentially benefit the most from inhaled ribavirin treatment are those younger than 6 weeks; those with chronic illnesses, such as congenital heart disease and chronic lung disease; premature infants; immunosuppressed children with primary immune disorders or those undergoing allogeneic hematopoietic stem cell marrow or solid-organ transplantation; and those with neurologic or neuromuscular disorders.[520,521] Treatment with ribavirin also appears to decrease nasopharyngeal secretion of RSV-specific IgE and IgA responses.[494] Long-term follow-up of treated patients suggests no adverse effects but possible improvement in pulmonary function.[265,313,379] Treatment may benefit immunocompromised children who have serious or prolonged RSV infection, such as those with congenital severe combined immunodeficiency.[405] Aerosolized, oral, or intravenous ribavirin, especially combined with intravenous immune globulin or RSV hyperimmune globulin, also may be of benefit to bone marrow transplant recipients and solid-organ transplant recipients with RSV lower tract disease.[135,213,379,382,423,606] Intravenous or oral administration appears less costly than aerosolized treatments.[135,213,423] Anecdotal reports and case series suggest that early administration of inhaled or oral ribavirin, with our without palivizumab, to immunocompromised patients with cancer or transplant recipients, during early upper respiratory tract disease, may be more efficacious than supportive care alone in preventing progression to lower tract disease or pneumonia.[96,170,405,520] Some centers have used oral ribavirin therapy for RSV infection, instead of inhaled or intravenous administration. Small studies and case series have shown similar therapeutic outcomes between oral and inhaled ribavirin therapy for RSV infection and lower respiratory tract disease after hematopoietic stem cell and solid-organ transplantation.[219,229,371,390,462] Laboratory confirmation of RSV infection by viral culture or rapid diagnostic tests that detect viral antigen in respiratory secretions is recommended for all patients before treatment with ribavirin is initiated or continued beyond 12 to 24 hours.

*References 223, 235, 265, 313, 410, 422, 475, 532, 535, 605.

Ribavirin also is licensed in capsule form for the treatment of chronic hepatitis caused by HCV, and in combination with interferon alfa, it produces a sustained decrease in HCV RNA levels, improvement in systemic symptoms such as fatigue, reduction in transaminases, and improvement in liver histologic features. These clinical benefits have been observed during initial treatment in previously untreated patients, in individuals initially unresponsive to interferon alone, and in patients treated for relapse.[55,58,137,147,198,286,404,481]

Treatment with high doses of orally or intravenously administered ribavirin significantly reduces mortality rates in patients with Lassa fever.[71,311,403] Ribavirin also appears to benefit patients suffering from other hemorrhagic fever syndromes, including Argentine, Sabiá, Bolivian, and Crimean-Congo hemorrhagic fevers, as well as those who have hemorrhagic fever with renal failure syndrome.[172,185,290,291,333] Ribavirin has also been used to treat La Crosse encephalitis, but clinical trials have not shown a clear therapeutic benefit.[406] In addition, ribavirin may benefit patients with other causes of viral encephalitis, including rabies, but clinical trials have not been performed, and proven benefit is lacking.[89] Oral ribavirin also may be of benefit prophylactically in individuals who are exposed to hemorrhagic fever syndromes, including Lassa fever.[282] Treatment of hantavirus pulmonary syndrome with intravenously administered ribavirin is being evaluated in clinical trials.

Ribavirin may benefit individuals with influenza A or B virus infection. In one randomized study of young adults suffering from influenza, aerosol treatment significantly reduced fever, systemic signs and symptoms, and virus titer in respiratory secretions.[536] Another study showed clinical benefit with high-dose oral ribavirin, but other studies have not confirmed a measurable clinical benefit or virologic response consistently with aerosolized or oral ribavirin.[50,344,512,536,554] Intravenous ribavirin also has been used anecdotally to treat serious, life-threatening influenza.[257,477] Early treatment with aerosolized or intravenous ribavirin in bone marrow and stem cell transplant recipients infected with parainfluenza virus may help prevent progression to lower tract disease and pneumonia or treat viremia and myocarditis, but controlled trials documenting efficacy and effect on overall mortality rates have not been published.[166,257,320,603] Ribavirin also has been used to treat measles pneumonia in immunocompetent and immunocompromised patients, with clinical benefit reported in some.[191,230,321] Ribavirin has also been included in treatment protocols for patients with rabies encephalitis, with unproven benefit.[387,612]

Clinical benefit, but not cure, also has been documented in case reports of children with subacute sclerosing panencephalitis caused by measles virus.[286,287,432,532] In these reports, repeated courses of large doses of ribavirin administered intravenously, combined with interferon alfa, provided serum and CSF levels that exceeded the minimal inhibitory concentrations needed to inhibit the virus in vitro and improved or stabilized seizures and neurologic status in treated patients.[287] Case reports and small series using ribavirin to treat serious adenoviral disease, including pneumonia and disseminated adenoviral disease, have been published, but no controlled trials documenting clinical benefit have been published.[32,64,94,206,397,430] Despite documented antiretroviral activity, treatment of HIV-infected patients with oral ribavirin has not shown clinical, virologic, or immunologic benefits consistently.[122,182,314] Recently in 2017, there have been published reports of use of intravenous and oral ribavirin to treat severe fever with thrombocytopenia syndrome (SFTS), an emerging, summertime, severe and often fatal tick-borne disease in China, Japan, and Korea.[300]

Dosage. A number of different dosages and routes of administration have been used to administer ribavirin to a variety of patients experiencing various infections. In normal and immunocompromised patients of all ages, the usual dosage of ribavirin, when it is administered topically by aerosol to the respiratory tract for treatment of influenza and lower respiratory tract disease caused by RSV, parainfluenza virus, and measles virus, is 6 g of drug reconstituted in a final volume of 300 mL of sterile water (final concentration, 20 mg/mL); a small-particle aerosol generator (SPAG-2 unit) is used to administer the drug continuously during a period of 12 to 18 hours for 3 to 7 days.* The drug may be delivered to an infant oxygen hood or tent, by facemask, or through pressure- or volume-cycled ventilators, provided ventilatory pressure is monitored and the device is checked for precipitation, which may cause ventilator dysfunction.[197,452]

Intermittent high-dose inhaled therapy, with drug administered at 60 mg/mL for 2 hours three times daily for 5 days, also appears to be effective and may be better tolerated in some older patients.[169] Longer courses of aerosolized therapy for up to 14 days have been used in severely immunocompromised patients with prolonged viral shedding and severe disease.[370]

Oral doses of up to 600 mg twice daily for 24 to 48 weeks, usually combined with interferon alfa, are used to treat hepatitis C in adults.[55,58,137,147,283,404,481] High doses of oral ribavirin also appear to be effective in treating influenza in normal hosts and RSV infection in immunocompromised hosts.[372,462,520] Even higher doses of oral ribavirin (2-g loading dose, followed by 2 g/day divided every 8 hours for 10 days) have been used for the treatment of Lassa fever and other hemorrhagic fever syndromes in adults.[172,185,282,291,311,333,403] Oral doses of ribavirin at 20 mg/kg per day for up to 14 days have been administered to transplant recipients with RSV infection.[83]

The intravenous dose of ribavirin used to treat Lassa fever is a 2-g loading dose (25–33 mg/kg estimated pediatric dose), followed by 1-g doses (15–16 mg/kg estimated pediatric dose) every 6 hours for 4 days and then 500-mg doses (8 mg/kg estimated pediatric dose) every 8 hours for 3 days to complete a 7- to 10-day course of treatment.[311,403] This intravenous dosage regimen also has been used to treat measles pneumonia, severe influenza with complications, pneumonia caused by RSV and parainfluenza virus in immunocompromised patients, and disseminated adenovirus disease.[191,230,382,477] Continuous intravenous infusions of ribavirin have been used in patients with severe disease caused by influenza and parainfluenza viruses.[257] Doses used to treat subacute sclerosing panencephalitis in children have been considerably higher and administered for longer periods.[287,432] In one report, pediatric patients received interferon alfa combined with 10 mg/kg of ribavirin administered intravenously every 8 hours daily for 7 days. Escalating doses of 20 mg/kg and then 30 mg/kg given every 8 hours daily for 7 days at 7-day intervals then were administered.[287] The highest dose tolerated was given for 7 days, repeated in 7-day intervals, and administered for a period of 6 months.

Adverse effects. Adverse effects of aerosolized ribavirin are unusual but include local irritation causing facial rash and conjunctivitis. Abnormalities in pulmonary function, including worsening of respiratory distress and bronchospasm, also have been reported.[212,236,530] In addition, one case of water intoxication associated with aerosolized ribavirin administration has been reported.[577] Older children, adolescents, and adults may be noncompliant with treatment or may even have anxiety attacks or experience other forms of psychological stress as they are being confined for continuous treatment for a 12- to 18-hour period. In these cases, intermittent, high-dose regimens may be better tolerated and might enhance compliance of the patient.[169] Precipitation of the drug in ventilator tubing systems and on filtering devices may cause ventilator dysfunction and respiratory distress or failure in mechanically ventilated patients, especially those receiving high-dose intermittent administration, but such events may be minimized by frequent monitoring of ventilator pressure, frequent cleaning of the tubing, and frequent changing of the filters.[197,410,422,452] Adverse hematologic effects, such as anemia, have not been documented consistently in patients who received aerosolized ribavirin. The environmental exposure to aerosolized ribavirin by health care workers providing direct care to a virus-infected patient may, in some instances, cause headache, conjunctivitis, contact lens damage, watery eyes, and bronchospasm in those with underlying reactive airway disease.[68,212,488,524]

These potential adverse effects are probably more likely to be seen in instances in which ribavirin is administered by hood, tent, or facemask than when it is administered to mechanically ventilated patients.[69] Environmental exposure of health care workers and family members may be reduced by providing routine patient care during periods when the aerosol generator has been turned off, by turning off the aerosol generator during periods of more urgent care, and by using protective equipment such as masks and goggles. Dose-related, reversible, usually

*References 50, 166, 223, 235, 236, 321, 344, 370, 397, 410, 422, 430, 536, 537, 570, 606.

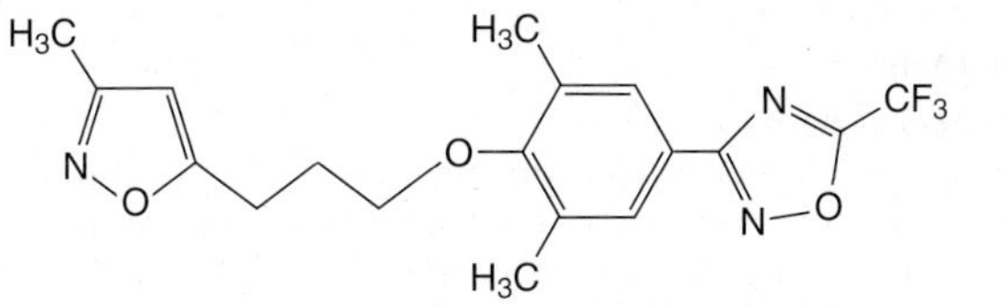

Pleconaril

FIG. 239.5 Structure of pleconaril.

mild anemia occurs frequently during and after long-term oral therapy and intravenous administration of ribavirin.[283,314,405] Rarely, severe anemia may occur and necessitate dose reduction or cessation of therapy.[406] Reversible increases in serum bilirubin, serum iron, and uric acid concentrations also have been documented during oral therapy. On rare occasion, intravenous administration of ribavirin has produced chills and rigors.[184,212]

Ribavirin has shown teratogenic, mutagenic, and embryotoxic effects in preclinical animal models.[272] Therefore investigators recommend that exposure of pregnant women to ribavirin, either therapeutically or through environmental exposure, be minimized or prevented whenever possible or practical.

Pleconaril and Pocapavir

Spectrum of Activity

Pleconaril and pocapavir are investigational viral capsid inhibitors with activity again various human wild-type and vaccine strain of polio and nonpolio enteroviruses and human rhinoviruses.

Pleconaril (3-[3,5-dimethyl-4[[3-(3-methyl-5-isoxazolyl)propyl]oly] phenyl]-5-(trifluoromethyl)-1,2,4-oxadiazole) is an antiviral agent and capsid inhibitor, with significant and specific activity against picornaviruses, both enteroviruses and rhinoviruses (Fig. 239.5). It was developed in the 1990s as a capsid-binding antiviral agent. In vitro, pleconaril inhibits the replication of most serotypes of enteroviruses at concentrations between 0.01 and 0.1 μg/mL. Echovirus 11, a commonly isolated enterovirus in the United States, appears to be the most sensitive enterovirus tested to date (inhibited at a mean concentration of 0.006 μg/mL), although resistant strains have been reported. Most rhinovirus serotypes are inhibited at slightly higher concentrations of 0.21 to 0.78 mg/mL but still within ranges safely achievable in patients.

Pocapavir [1,3-dichloro-2-(oxy)benzene] (V-073 or SCH-48973) is capsid inhibitor, investigational candidate, developed in the 1990s; it currently is being evaluated in clinical trials for treatment of wild-type and vaccine strain poliovirus infections and has variable antiviral activity against nonpolio enteroviruses.[119,407,579] In vitro, pocapavir inhibits human enteroviruses at an IC_{50} of 0.02 to 0.11 μg/L, with 80% of isolates inhibited at an IC_{50} of 0.9 μg/mL, or from 0.001 to 0.15 μmol/L, with 90% of enterovirus isolates inhibited at half maximal effective concentration (EC_{50}) values of less than 0.56 μmol/L.[82]

Mechanism of Action and Resistance

Pleconaril binds efficiently to a specific hydrophobic pocket within the viral capsid of picornaviruses and exhibits an antiviral effect by interfering with uncoating, attachment, and cell-to-cell transmission of infectious viral particles.[495] The drug induces a more rigid structure within the viral capsid, which then interferes with viral uncoating and release of viral RNA.[193,408,465,466,489,495] Pleconaril also appears to change the conformation of the canyon floor of the virus capsid when it integrates with the underlying pocket, thereby interfering with attachment of the virus to host cell receptors.[465,466] Resistance of picornaviruses to pleconaril both has been reported in vitro and has developed in vivo during treatment of enterovirus infections, especially in immune compromised patients.[47]

Pocapavir resistance in vitro involves a single amino acid change in one of either of two virus capsid proteins: VP1 or VP3 of enteroviruses. The isoleucine residue at position 194 in capsid protein VP1 is replaced with phenylalanine or methionine, or the alanine at position 24 in VP3 is replaced with valine in resistant strains.[119] Resistance occurs in vitro and may emerge in vivo during antiviral treatment.

Pharmacokinetics

The pharmacokinetics of pleconaril vary with the age of the group tested. After oral administration of single doses of 200 to 400 mg to adults, peak plasma concentrations of 1.1 to 2.4 μg/mL are achieved in 1.5 to 5 hours, with an average elimination half-life of 25 hours.[2] Repeated dosing for a 7-day period increases plasma concentrations to 1.33 to 3.4 μg/mL. When pleconaril is taken with food, especially a meal high in fat, absorption is enhanced significantly.[1,328] Single oral doses of 5 mg/kg in children provide plasma concentrations of approximately 1.3 μg/mL, with a more rapid elimination half-life of approximately 6 hours.[327] Neonates also absorb pleconaril well, but they do not exhibit dose-proportionate pharmacokinetics as adults do.[328] The drug also has a large volume of distribution and concentrates in tissues such as the liver, brain, and nasal epithelium, where viral replication and virus-induced disease are likely to occur.[328] Pleconaril appears to be excreted in feces and urine.

Pocapavir is well absorbed orally, but there are limited pharmacokinetic data available at this time.[119] Mean concentration of drug levels after oral administration have been measured in clinical trials well above the needed antiviral inhibitory concentrations.[119]

Clinical Indications, Dosage, and Adverse Effects

Clinical indications. Pleconaril, after clinical trial data were reviewed, was disapproved for licensure by the FDA in 2002 because of its modest effectiveness and possible side effects. Pleconaril currently is not licensed for therapeutic use, and it is not available at this time for compassionate use.[421,610] However, clinical trials continue to evaluate pleconaril for treatment of serious enteroviral disease as well as rhinovirus infection in neonates and children (https://clinicaltrials.gov). Pleconaril has shown efficacy in clinical trials against picornavirus infections in adults, children, and neonates.[3,4] In pretreated adults experimentally infected with coxsackie A21 virus, pleconaril significantly reduced viral titers as well as the clinical parameters of fever, nasal mucus production, and systemic symptoms compared with placebo.[248,495,510] In another trial, pleconaril resolved the symptoms of illness 2 days earlier than placebo, and patients who received pleconaril did not require as much concomitant medication for symptomatic relief as did those who received placebo.[495] In two placebo-controlled trials in adults with aseptic meningitis caused by enterovirus, pleconaril treatment reduced the duration of headache and other symptoms of meningitis by 2 to 3 days and allowed treated patients to return to work and routine daily activities 2 days earlier than patients who received placebo.[495,510] In a placebo-controlled trial in pediatric patients with aseptic meningitis caused by enterovirus, pleconaril significantly improved illness scores and reduced the duration of headache in older children, but clinical efficacy was difficult to assess in infants and younger children.[4] Viral shedding from the throat also was reduced in the treatment group.[505]

In addition to treatment of the "common cold" and "viral meningitis," another potential use of pleconaril is for the treatment of serious, persistent, or life-threatening illness caused by enteroviruses. More than 90 patients with unusual or life-threatening infections with enterovirus have received pleconaril on a compassionate-use basis.[193,610] These patients included immunocompromised patients with chronic meningitis, neonates with disseminated disease, patients with myocarditis,[495,610] and individuals with poliomyelitis associated with vaccine or wild-type poliovirus.[490] In all groups, most of the patients showed clinical and virologic responses. In a randomized clinical trial in neonates with virologically proven enterovirus sepsis, pleconaril showed shorter times to viral culture and polymerase chain reaction (PCR) test negativity and greater survival among pleconaril recipients compared with placebo recipients.[421]

Pocapavir has been developed as a poliovirus antiviral drug to control poliomyelitis outbreaks in the posteradication era. Efforts spearheaded by the Poliovirus Antivirals Initiative, began in 2007, continue to support clinical development of this and other antivirals active against poliovirus.[407] Prolonged excretion of vaccine-derived polioviruses by immune-deficient persons, especially those persons with primary B-cell immunodeficiency syndromes who inadvertently receive live, attenuated oral poliovirus vaccine and may continue to excrete vaccine-derived virulent virus into the environment, are a potential risk to polio eradication.[119] Immunized adults challenged with monovalent poliovirus type 1 vaccine and subsequently treated with pocapavir had reduced time to virus negativity in the stool compared with placebo recipients.[119] This indication, to reduce vaccine strain virus shedding in stool, is the primary proposed role for pocapavir. In addition pocapavir may be used to treat inadvertent exposure to vaccine poliovirus during manufacturing or research facilities, as well as outbreak control.[579]

Dosage. Pleconaril is manufactured as a hard gelatin capsule and an oral solution. A nasal spray formulation has also been developed and tested in clinical trials against rhinovirus infection. The capsule contains 200 mg of drug, and doses used in adults and older children have been 200 to 400 mg every 8 hours for 7 days (21 doses). An oral solution also has been prepared for pediatric and neonatal use. It contains 40 mg/mL of pleconaril, medium-chain triglycerides, two surfactants (Tween 80 and Arlacel), 1.5% saccharin, and cherry-peppermint flavoring. Doses of 5 mg/kg, 7.5 mg/kg, and 8 mg/kg of the oral solution administered every 8 to 12 hours for 7 days (14–21 doses) have been used in clinical trials of young children, infants, and neonates.[495,421]

Adult dosage of pocapavir 1600 mg per day is being evaluated in current clinical trials. No pediatric or neonatal dosing regimens are available at this time.[119]

Adverse effects. Oral pleconaril is generally well tolerated by all age groups. Adverse effects associated with pleconaril treatment include nausea, diarrhea, stomach upset or discomfort, and headache. Serious toxicities have not been documented to date, and preclinical studies did not show teratogenicity or fetal toxicity. Prolongation of menstrual cycle bleeding in young women taking pleconaril for 6 weeks for upper respiratory virus infections was observed in one clinical trial. Pocapavir is generally well tolerated, with reports of headaches in adults, and possibly mild liver enzyme elevations noted in clinical trials.[119]

ANTIVIRAL AGENTS ACTIVE AGAINST DNA VIRUSES

Table 239.2 provides a list of antiviral agents active against DNA viruses, including their clinical indications and usual dosages.

Acyclovir

Spectrum of Activity

Acyclovir, 9-[(2-hydroxyethoxy)methyl]-9*H*-guanine (also known as acycloguanosine), is an analogue of the nucleoside deoxyguanosine that has selective activity against the herpes family of viruses (Fig. 239.6).[130,165] It has the most potent antiviral activity against HSV type 1 and inhibits the virus at concentrations of 0.02 to 0.9 μg/mL.[592,608] Inhibitory concentrations of HSV type 2 and VZV are also high, at 0.3 to 2.2 μg/mL and 0.8 to 4.0 μg/mL, respectively.[54,550,592,608] In addition, EBV replication is inhibited by acyclovir at a mean concentration of 1.6 μg/mL, but the drug has no effect on cells latently infected with EBV.[114,266,373,566] CMV also is inhibited by very high concentrations of acyclovir (2–57 μg/mL).[54] Acyclovir has in vitro activity against simian herpesvirus B and hepatitis B virus (HBV).[49,285,592]

Mechanism of Action and Resistance

Acyclovir is phosphorylated to acyclovir monophosphate by viral TK. Cellular enzymes then convert the monophosphate form to acyclovir triphosphate, the active form of the drug.[608] Acyclovir triphosphate is

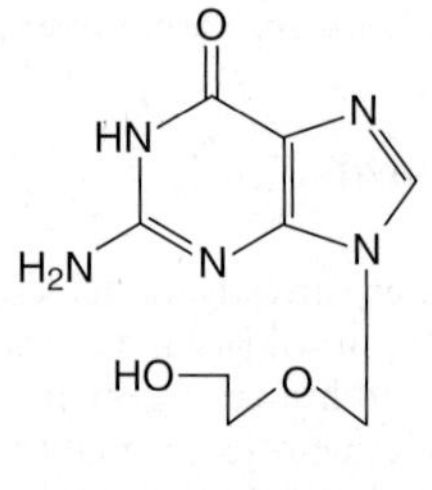

Acyclovir

FIG. 239.6 Structure of acyclovir.

TABLE 239.2 Clinical Indications and Usual Treatment Dosages for Licensed Antiviral Agents Active Against DNA Viruses

Agent	Indication	Dosage
Acyclovir	HSV, mucocutaneous	5% ointment 6 × daily
		15 mg/kg/dose PO 5 × daily (max 200 mg/dose)
		5–10 mg/kg/dose IV q8h
	HSV, encephalitis	10–15 mg/kg/dose IV q8h
	HSV, neonatal	20 mg/kg/dose IV q8h
	VZV, chickenpox and zoster	20 mg/kg/dose (max 800 mg) PO q6h
		10–20 mg/kg/dose (500 mg/m²/dose) IV q8h
Valacyclovir	HSV	500–1000 mg/dose PO bid
	VZV, zoster	1000 mg/dose PO bid
Penciclovir	HSV, mucocutaneous	1% cream q2h
Famciclovir	HSV, mucocutaneous	125–500 mg PO bid
	VZV, zoster	500 mg PO tid
Ganciclovir	CMV	5–6 mg/kg/dose IV q12h—induction
		5 mg/kg/dose qd 5 days/wk
		or
		1000 mg PO tid
		or
		500 mg PO 6 × daily—maintenance
Valganciclovir	CMV	900 mg PO bid—induction
		900 mg PO qd—maintenance
		15–18 mg/kg/dose every 12 h or bid
Foscarnet	CMV	60 mg/kg/dose IV q8h—induction
		90–120 mg/kg/dose daily—maintenance
Cidofovir	CMV	5 mg/kg/dose IV weekly
		Or
		1 mg/kg/dose IV 3 ×/wk—induction
		5 mg/kg q2wk—maintenance

CMV, Cytomegalovirus; *HSV*, herpes simplex virus; *VZV*, varicella-zoster virus.

present in HSV-infected cells at 40 to 100 times the concentration found in uninfected cells, and it competitively inhibits viral DNA polymerase in infected cells. Acyclovir triphosphate also is incorporated into viral DNA and, because it lacks the 3′-hydroxyl group, acts as a chain terminator during viral DNA synthesis. The DNA polymerase enzymes of the various herpesviruses differ in their degree of inhibition by acyclovir triphosphate, and for EBV and CMV, which do not contain viral TK, this inhibition accounts for most of the antiviral effect of the drug.[144,200] Host cellular growth also can be inhibited by acyclovir, but only at levels thousands of times higher than those that inhibit viral replication. This relatively selective mechanism of antiviral action provides a uniquely high therapeutic index.

Three basic mechanisms of resistance have been identified for herpesviruses to become resistant to acyclovir: deficient TK activity caused by absent or low production of viral TK, altered TK activity caused by abnormal substrate specificity so that the enzyme is present and able to phosphorylate but just does not phosphorylate acyclovir, and altered DNA polymerase.[95] Most clinical isolates of HSV that are resistant to acyclovir have deficient TK activity, and most resistant VZV isolates have altered TK activity or altered DNA polymerase.[460,573] The prevalence of acyclovir-resistant HSV isolates in normal hosts is less than 1%, but it can be as high as 10% to 20% in immunocompromised hosts receiving acyclovir therapy for 2 weeks or longer.[107,129,171,205,269] Emergence of acyclovir-resistant HSV type 1 through both viral thymidine kinase and DNA polymerase mutations in hematopoietic stem cell transplantation patients has been observed in 28% of patients shedding HSV type 1 and also has been associated with relapsed malignancies and higher mortality rates.[318] Resistant strains of VZV, on the other hand, are unusual.[115] Resistant HSV and VZV isolates retain virulence and can cause disease, especially extensive mucocutaneous lesions in immunocompromised hosts, but invasive diseases such as keratitis, uveitis, meningoencephalitis, and pneumonia also have occurred with resistant strains of HSV.[107,171,205,269,308,580] Immunocompromised hosts may shed resistant strains of HSV for prolonged periods and may experience recurrent disease with either sensitive or resistant strains. Such mutants are also cross-resistant to other antiviral agents that require viral TK for phosphorylation and activation (e.g., penciclovir and ganciclovir), but they are inhibited by antiviral agents that have different mechanisms of action (e.g., foscarnet, cidofovir, and trifluridine).

Pharmacokinetics

Acyclovir is available for topical, oral, and intravenous administration. Systemic absorption of acyclovir after topical application to intact skin is minimal (<0.01 μg/mL), and in one study in which acyclovir ointment was applied to zoster lesions in immunocompromised patients, plasma concentrations of less than 0.1 to 0.78 μg/mL were observed, thus suggesting some degree of percutaneous absorption.[124,592] The bioavailability of oral acyclovir is low (15–21%), with peak plasma concentrations of 0.4 to 0.8 μg/mL observed after the intake of one 200-mg capsule and concentrations of up to 1.6 μg/mL observed after an 800-mg dose.[57] When an equivalent dose in liquid suspension is administered to children, slightly lower peak plasma levels of 1.0 μg/mL are observed.[565] Intravenous infusion of 5 mg/kg for 1 hour provides peak plasma levels of 9.8 μg/mL, whereas plasma levels of 20.7 μg/mL are produced after a 10-mg/kg infusion.[63] Most of the administered dose of acyclovir is excreted unchanged in urine.[592] The elimination half-life of acyclovir is 2.5 to 3 hours in adult patients with normal renal function, slightly longer (3.8 hours) in neonates, and up to 20 hours in anuric patients.[57,196,273] Therefore dose adjustment, according to creatinine clearance, is needed in patients with renal insufficiency or renal failure.[362] Probenecid administration decreases renal clearance and prolongs the half-life of acyclovir. Acyclovir is distributed widely into a variety of body fluids, including saliva (13% of plasma levels), vaginal secretions (15–170% of plasma levels), zoster vesicular fluid (90–100% of plasma levels), aqueous humor (37% of plasma levels), breast milk (>300% of plasma levels), amniotic fluid and placenta (>200% of plasma levels), and CSF (50% of plasma levels).[196,293,294,340,363,416] More than half the drug is removed by hemodialysis, but very little is removed after peritoneal dialysis.[351,362]

Clinical Indications, Dosage, and Adverse Effects

Clinical indications. Topical acyclovir may decrease healing time and viral shedding slightly in mucocutaneous lesions of patients experiencing primary infection with HSV.[124] Little if any clinical benefit has been documented in patients with recurrent herpes simplex lesions; however, some patients report a soothing sensation after application of ointment to the lesions. Topical therapy also may produce a mild clinical benefit in immunocompromised patients with zoster lesions.[592] Oral acyclovir significantly reduces viral shedding, clinical symptoms, and time until lesion healing in normal and immunocompromised patients with a variety of mucocutaneous lesions (e.g., orolabial, pharyngeal, genital, rectal, gingivostomatitis, whitlow, skin) associated with primary HSV infection.[13,491,608] It also has been used to treat eye disease, including dendritic corneal ulcers.[120,264]

Oral acyclovir provides benefit to normal and immunocompromised children, adolescents, and adults with primary infection with VZV (varicella or chickenpox). Treatment reduces the duration of fever by 24 hours, the mean number of skin lesions, and the time to total crusting of lesions by 2 days. Postexposure prophylaxis with oral acyclovir also may reduce the risk for acquiring varicella by close and household contacts of patients with varicella. Administration of oral acyclovir during pregnancy is likely to clinically benefit a mother with varicella, but whether it reduces the risk for congenital or neonatal disease is not clear at this time. Recurrent HSV disease also is improved with oral acyclovir therapy. When it is administered during the prodrome or at the very first sign of lesions, treatment reduces viral shedding and time to lesion healing by 1.5 to 2 days.[482,593] Long-term, continuous suppressive therapy with oral acyclovir may be of benefit in some patients with frequent episodes of recurrent mucocutaneous disease, but asymptomatic shedding and person-to-person transmission still may occur.[214,492] Patients with recurrent skin disease, whitlow, or erythema multiforme may benefit from long-term suppressive therapy with oral acyclovir. Oral acyclovir suppression also reduces recurrences of genital herpes simplex during the last trimester of pregnancy and decreases the need for cesarean delivery.[74,513,516-518] Short-term prophylaxis administered during a period of risk for recurrence (e.g., sunlight exposure) may reduce the clinical recurrence of mucocutaneous disease. Oral acyclovir reduces virus shedding, time to skin lesion healing, and the duration of zoster-associated pain.[43,113] Treatment combined with steroids also appears to decrease the frequency and severity of postherpetic neuralgia in older adult patients, but specific trials conducted in children have not been performed because children seldom experience postherpetic neuralgia. Oral acyclovir also may reduce recurrence of HSV and VZV infections in bone marrow and solid-organ transplant recipients. Its effect on CMV and EBV disease in these patients, however, is minimal, if any.[566] Continuous suppressive therapy with oral acyclovir reduces cutaneous recurrences after neonatal infection when it is administered after a 14- to 21-day course of intravenous therapy has been completed.[339] Whether long-term oral suppressive therapy in neonates also prevents CNS recurrence is unclear at this time. Bell palsy associated with HSV infection may be treated with a combination of acyclovir and prednisone.[6] EBV-associated diseases have been treated with acyclovir, with variable clinical benefit.[513,526] Oral hairy leukoplakia, however, appears to respond to oral acyclovir treatment.[484,582] Treatment of patients with infectious mononucleosis reduces viral shedding but does not alter the disease course.[541] No clinical benefit has been documented when acyclovir was used to treat chronic hepatitis B.[49]

Intravenous acyclovir is used to treat all severe or life-threatening diseases caused by HSV and VZV, including encephalitis, hepatitis, neonatal disease, acute retinal necrosis syndrome, mucocutaneous disease, and zoster, with or without visceral dissemination, in both normal and immunocompromised patients.[63,231,336,342,353,457,591,624] Pediatric patients suffering from severe herpetic gingivostomatitis may benefit as well.[13] Early clinical trials also showed efficacy in the treatment of primary genital HSV infection.[123] In addition, normal patients with complications of varicella, including pneumonitis, encephalitis, and hepatitis, should receive intravenous acyclovir.[231] Other diseases associated with VZV in which acyclovir treatment is beneficial include zoster ophthalmicus with complications such as keratitis, anterior uveitis, and contralateral hemiplegia, as well as acute retinal necrosis syndrome.[457,539] Intravenous acyclovir is also highly effective in reducing the incidence of disease associated with HSV and VZV in marrow and solid-organ transplant recipients. Moreover, it may help reduce serious CMV disease in selected marrow and solid-organ transplant recipients, although it clearly is not as effective as ganciclovir or other antiviral agents with specific activity against CMV.[28,29,60,417,587] Treatment of human herpes infection with simian virus B requires high doses of intravenous acyclovir administered for a prolonged period, followed by suppressive therapy.[281] Despite in vitro activity, clinical benefit has not been documented in patients with hepatitis B.[49]

As of November 2012, a shortage of intravenous acyclovir related to manufacturing delays was announced. If the shortage is still in effect, or if another shortage occurs, ganciclovir, or foscarnet secondarily, is recommended for most patients who would ordinarily have received intravenous acyclovir (https://redbook.solutions.aap.org/ss/acyclovir-shortage.aspx). Cidofovir also has activity against HSV and VZV and may also be considered in selected patients.

Dosage. Topical acyclovir as a 5% ointment can be applied to local lesions every 3 to 4 hours five to six times daily for 7 days.[124] If the disease is unresponsive or severe, systemic therapy with oral or intravenous acyclovir should be initiated.

Oral acyclovir is formulated as 200-mg capsules, 800-mg tablets, and a 200-mg/5 mL banana-flavored suspension. The usual dose used to treat mucocutaneous lesions caused by primary infection with HSV in adults and adolescents is 200 mg administered five times daily for 10 days. The usual pediatric oral dose is 15 mg/kg per dose (maximum, 200 mg per dose) administered five times daily for 10 days. Recurrent HSV disease in adults and adolescents may be treated with a variety of different regimens: 800 mg three times daily for 2 days, 400 mg three times daily for 5 days, or 200 mg five times daily for 5 days.[323,324,593] Suppressive doses of 400 mg administered twice daily, often for many years, seem to be safe and effective.[214] This dose, administered to pregnant women with recent primary or recurrent genital herpes, also appears to decrease recurrences at or near delivery and to diminish the need for cesarean delivery.[74,340,559] After intravenous therapy has been completed, neonatal suppressive therapy is recommended at a dose of 300 mg/m^2 per dose administered three times daily for 6 months.[339] Because neonatal prophylaxis decreases but does not eliminate the risk for CNS recurrence and because the emergence of resistant strains has been documented, all early cutaneous lesions that recur despite compliance with oral prophylaxis, as well as other signs and symptoms suggestive of recurrent visceral or CNS disease, should be evaluated carefully in young infants, and the need for systemic therapy should be considered.[339] Oral acyclovir must be administered in higher doses to treat varicella and other VZV-associated diseases.[608] Adults and adolescents require 800-mg doses administered five times daily for 7 to 10 days or until lesions have crusted over.[33,595] The pediatric dose of acyclovir to treat varicella or chickenpox is 20 mg/kg (up to 800 mg maximum) per dose (80 mg/kg/day) administered four times daily for 5 days or until lesions have crusted.[9,160]

The usual dose for intravenous administration of acyclovir to treat serious disease associated with HSV beyond the neonatal period is 5 to 10 mg/kg per dose administered as a 1-hour infusion every 8 hours.[473,592,608] Treatment for a duration of 7 days is usually sufficient for mucocutaneous disease, but it should be continued until all lesions are healed and followed by long-term suppression if the patient remains immunocompromised. Herpes encephalitis should be treated for at least 14 days or longer, depending on clinical response and clearance of HSV DNA from the CSF.[337,336,355,607]

The recommended dose to treat all forms of neonatal HSV disease (skin, eye, and mouth disease; disseminated with visceral involvement; or encephalitis) is a high-dose regimen of 20 mg/kg per dose administered every 8 hours (60 mg/kg per day).[10] This high dose of intravenous acyclovir, although not currently formally approved by the FDA, has been shown to be safe and effective in neonates.[174,336] Duration of intravenous treatment is at least 14 days for skin, eye, and mouth disease and at least 21 days or until HSV DNA has cleared from the CSF, whichever is longer, for encephalitis and disseminated disease.[337,336] Persistence of HSV DNA in the CSF of neonates treated for 21 days with high-dose acyclovir is seen, and these patients usually have a more severe clinical course and poor neurodevelopmental outcome.[451] Intravenous acyclovir treatment for neonatal HSV disease should be followed by suppression treatment with oral acyclovir at 300 mg/m^2 per dose every 8 hours until at least 6 months of age to reduce risk for recurrences and to improve neurodevelopmental outcome.[10] Clinical studies have documented that these higher doses are safe in neonates but may cause renal insufficiency in older children and adults. Treatment of VZV-associated disease requires higher doses of acyclovir: 500 mg/m^2 per dose (10–20 mg/kg per dose) administered every 8 hours (total, 1500 mg/m^2 per day) for at least 5 to 7 days or until all lesions have been crusted over for 24 to 48 hours.[592,608] In all clinical indications, the dosage of intravenously administered acyclovir should be adjusted according to creatinine clearance in patients with renal insufficiency and renal failure.

Adverse effects. Adverse effects of acyclovir are unusual.[330] Topical application of the ointment may produce pain or local irritation, usually caused by the polyethylene glycol base.[124,592] Hand washing must be performed after each local application to lesions to avoid autoinoculation or person-to-person transmission. Oral acyclovir may cause nausea and diarrhea, rash, or headache.[592] Long-term oral administration of acyclovir appears to be safe in adults but may be associated with neutropenia in 46% of infants who receive suppression after treatment of neonatal HSV infection.[339,419] Intravenously administered acyclovir is generally well tolerated. However, extravasation of the drug (pH 9–11) can cause inflammation, ulceration, and necrosis of surrounding tissue.[330,438,529,569] Phlebitis also can develop. Neurotoxicity occurs rarely, usually in patients with renal insufficiency who have high serum concentrations.[42,181,232,590] Neurotoxicity associated with acyclovir is characterized by lethargy, confusion, tremor, and rarely seizures and coma. Renal tubular damage, crystalline nephropathy, or interstitial nephritis may occur in approximately 5% of patients.[476,506] These renal complications are more likely to develop in patients who are not adequately hydrated or in whom the drug has been infused at a rate faster than the recommended infusion time of 1 hour. Keeping urine-specific gravity below 1.010 is a reasonable guideline to ensure adequate hydration. No excess frequency of adverse events has been reported to date in pregnant women who receive acyclovir or in their fetuses or newborns.[74,91,340,513,518,624] Therefore, on the basis of available information, acyclovir seems to be safe when it is administered during pregnancy, especially during the last trimester, and does not appear to have any significant adverse effects.

Valacyclovir

Spectrum of Activity

Valacyclovir (L-valine, 2-[(2-amino-1,6-dihydro-6-oxo-9*H*-purin-9-yl) methoxy]ethyl ester monohydrochloride, also known as valacyclovir hydrochloride) is the hydrochloride salt of the L-valine ester of acyclovir.[44] It has essentially the same selective spectrum of antiviral activity against the herpesviruses as acyclovir does.[51]

Mechanism of Action and Resistance

Valacyclovir is converted rapidly to acyclovir and therefore has the same mechanisms of action and resistance as acyclovir.[51] Viral isolates that are resistant to acyclovir will be resistant to valacyclovir.

Pharmacokinetics

The pharmacokinetics of valacyclovir has not been studied in the pediatric population, but information gained from adults can be applied, in many ways, to pediatric patients. After oral administration, valacyclovir is absorbed rapidly from the gastrointestinal tract. It is metabolized by first pass through the intestinal tract and also by the liver into acyclovir and L-valine.[51] It has the advantage over acyclovir of having 54% bioavailability (vs. 20% for acyclovir), which is not altered by food.[545] A single dose of 1 g of valacyclovir administered to an adult produces plasma levels of 0.4 to 0.8 μg/mL. The half-life is 2.5 to 3 hours, similar to that of acyclovir, and is prolonged in patients with renal insufficiency or renal failure.[597,601] The drug is removed by hemodialysis. The rate but not the extent of conversion of valacyclovir to acyclovir is prolonged in patients with liver disease.

Clinical Indications, Dosage, and Adverse Effects

Clinical indications. Valacyclovir has been reported to be effective in treatment of primary and recurrent mucocutaneous disease caused by HSV-1, HSV-2, and VZV.[51,51,59,369,483,465] Randomized clinical trials conducted in adult patients showed valacyclovir to be superior to placebo and comparable to acyclovir in reducing the number and duration of lesions, pain, and time to healing in patients with primary and recurrent genital herpes and zoster.[59,483,552,617] It is also comparable to acyclovir for suppression of genital herpes recurrences. Furthermore, in a study of 27 CMV-seropositive heart transplant recipients, valacyclovir appeared to be equal or superior to oral acyclovir in preventing both laboratory and clinical parameters of CMV reactivation.[162] Because valacyclovir is converted to acyclovir, it is likely to be effective for all the clinical indications for which acyclovir has been shown to be effective.

Dosage. Valacyclovir is available only in 500-mg caplets; therefore a pediatric liquid formulation is not available at this time. The usual dose is 1 g twice daily for 10 days for primary genital herpes and 500 mg twice daily for 3 to 5 days for recurrent disease.[51,59,369,510] A daily dose of 500 mg has been used safely for longer than a year to suppress recurrences of HSV disease.[392] The dose to treat VZV-associated disease is higher than that for HSV-associated disease. A dose of 1 g three times a day for at least 7 days is usually necessary to treat zoster, and therapy should be continued until the lesions have dried.[52] The dose of valacyclovir should be adjusted according to creatinine clearance in patients with renal insufficiency or renal failure.

Adverse effects. The adverse effects of oral valacyclovir are similar to those of oral acyclovir and include gastrointestinal disturbances such as nausea, vomiting, and diarrhea.[51] Headache and behavioral changes also have been observed. Overdosage may produce precipitation of acyclovir in the renal tubules as well as CNS toxicity.

Penciclovir

Spectrum of Activity

Penciclovir (9-[4-hydroxy-3-hydroxymethylbut-1-yl] guanine) is an acyclic guanosine analogue with a selective spectrum of activity against the herpesviruses similar to that of acyclovir[67] (Fig. 239.7). This compound inhibits HSV-1 at very low concentrations (0.2–0.6 μg/mL) and HSV-2 at slightly higher concentrations (0.3–2.4 μg/mL).[26,67,216,600] At even higher concentrations (0.9–4.0 μg/mL), it inhibits VZV.[26,27] The compound has very little activity against CMV, and concentrations greater than 50 μg/mL are required to inhibit CMV. However, penciclovir does have activity against HBV.[118,349,522]

Mechanism of Action and Resistance

Like acyclovir, penciclovir is preferentially phosphorylated by viral TK in virus-infected cells to penciclovir monophosphate and by cellular enzymes to penciclovir triphosphate, which is the active form of the drug.[161] Penciclovir triphosphate competitively inhibits viral DNA polymerase. It is approximately 100 times less potent than acyclovir triphosphate in inhibiting viral DNA polymerase, but an antiviral effect is achieved because it is present in high concentrations for a prolonged period (7–20 hours) in virus-infected cells. However, unlike acyclovir, penciclovir is not a chain terminator during DNA synthesis. Penciclovir triphosphate also inhibits the DNA polymerase of HBV. Emergence of HSV strains resistant to penciclovir has been minimal.[366] Similar to HSV isolates resistant to acyclovir, isolates resistant to penciclovir may have viral TK gene mutations that produce mutants with deficient or altered TK activity, or they may have mutations in DNA polymerase genes.[101] Strains of acyclovir-resistant HSV that are TK-deficient mutants also will be resistant to penciclovir, but strains of acyclovir-resistant HSV that are TK altered may be susceptible to penciclovir.[68,463]

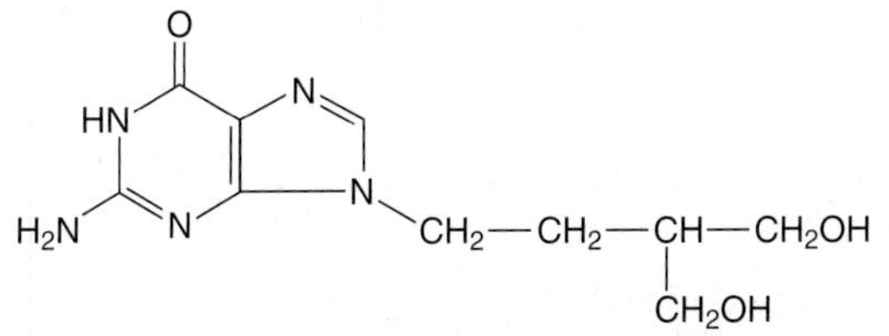

Penciclovir

FIG. 239.7 Structure of penciclovir.

Pharmacokinetics

Penciclovir is poorly absorbed after oral administration.[192] Adults who received a 10-mg/kg intravenous infusion of penciclovir had plasma levels of 12 μg/mL, but no pediatric information is available. Penciclovir 1% cream is not absorbed systemically. The systemic pharmacokinetics of penciclovir is discussed under famciclovir.

Clinical Indications, Dosage, and Adverse Effects

Penciclovir is available in the United States as a 1% cream in a propylene glycol base and is licensed for the treatment of herpes labialis lesions on the lips and face. Maximal clinical benefit occurs when the cream is applied to the lesions early, at the first clinical sign of disease, every 2 hours while awake for 3 to 5 days.[509,551] Application of penciclovir cream may be associated with local skin reactions, most likely caused by the propylene glycol base. An intravenous form of penciclovir has been tested in Europe, but it is not available in the United States. Penciclovir is not absorbed orally, but it is available as the oral prodrug famciclovir, which is converted rapidly to penciclovir. Dosages and systemic adverse effects of penciclovir are discussed under famciclovir.

Famciclovir

Spectrum of Activity

Famciclovir, 2-[(2-amino-9*H*-purin-9-yl)]-1,3-propanedial diacetate, is the prodrug of the antiviral agent penciclovir, which has selective activity against HSV-1, HSV-2, VZV, and HBV.

Mechanism of Action and Resistance

Famciclovir undergoes rapid transformation to penciclovir, which is monophosphorylated by viral TK to penciclovir monophosphate; the monophosphate, in turn, is converted by cellular enzymes to penciclovir triphosphate, the active form of the antiviral compound. Penciclovir then competitively inhibits viral DNA polymerase and, thereby, viral replication. The prolonged intracellular half-life observed with penciclovir also is observed with famciclovir. Penciclovir-resistant strains of HSV and VZV occur when mutations produce deficient or altered TK or altered DNA polymerase. Most TK-deficient acyclovir-resistant strains of HSV are also resistant to penciclovir.

Pharmacokinetics

Famciclovir is the diacetyl-6-deoxy analogue of the antiviral compound penciclovir. After oral administration, famciclovir is absorbed rapidly from the gastrointestinal tract with excellent (77%) bioavailability, and then it is metabolized in the liver by deacetylation and oxidation to form penciclovir. Single oral doses of 250 and 500 mg of famciclovir administered to adults produce peak plasma penciclovir levels of 1.6 to 1.9 μg/mL and 2.7 to 4.0 μg/mL, respectively. Administration of famciclovir with food reduces peak plasma concentrations by slowing the absorption time but does not alter the overall bioavailability of the drug. The half-life for penciclovir is 2 to 3 hours, after which it is excreted by filtration and active tubular secretion by the kidneys. Nonrenal clearance by fecal excretion also occurs for as much as one-third of the oral dose. Excretion of penciclovir is decreased in patients with renal insufficiency and renal failure, and in patients with liver disease, peak plasma levels may be reduced.[61] Penciclovir is removed from the body by hemodialysis. After oral administration of famciclovir to rats, penciclovir is concentrated in breast milk; however, no studies have been performed in lactating mothers to confirm such concentration in humans.

Clinical Indications, Dosage, and Adverse Effects

Clinical indications. In adult clinical trials, oral famciclovir was as effective as oral acyclovir and superior to placebo in treatment of recurrent mucocutaneous infections with HSV and VZV in both normal and immunocompromised patients.[110,393,497,583] When famciclovir was given early in the course of illness, time to lesion crusting and healing, duration of viral shedding, and length of acute pain all were shortened. In some studies, the duration of postherpetic neuralgia in older adult patients with zoster also was shortened.[583] Although to date it has not been studied specifically in clinical trials of patients with primary HSV and VZV infection, famciclovir probably also will provide clinical benefit in these conditions.[381] In addition, famciclovir is effective as suppressive therapy to reduce HSV recurrences and viral shedding.[146,415] Famciclovir also has been used to treat chronic HBV infection and for prophylaxis against recurrent HBV infection in liver transplant recipients.[237,393] No clinical trials in pediatric patients have been conducted.

Dosage. Famciclovir is available in 125-, 250-, and 500-mg tablets. An oral suspension for pediatric use is not available. The usual recommended oral dose of famciclovir to treat primary and recurrent mucocutaneous HSV disease is 125 mg twice daily for 5 days.[497] Dosages of suppressive therapy are slightly higher, 250 mg twice daily for as long as 1 year. Of note, clinical trials showed that single daily doses of 250 mg were not as effective as the twice-daily regimen in suppressing recurrences. For immunocompromised patients, especially those infected with HIV, even higher doses (500 mg twice daily for 7 days) may be necessary.[507] Treatment of VZV-associated disease, such as zoster, also requires higher doses (500 mg twice or three times daily for 10 days).[583] All dosage regimens should be reduced, according to creatinine clearance, in patients with renal insufficiency or renal failure.

Adverse effects. Adverse effects of treatment with oral famciclovir are unusual and include gastrointestinal disturbances, such as nausea and diarrhea; rash; CNS complaints, such as confusion, hallucinations, and disorientation; neutropenia; and elevated liver transaminases.[110,134,502]

Ganciclovir

Spectrum of Activity

Ganciclovir, 9-(1,3-dihydroxy-2-propoxymethyl)guanine (also known as DHPG), is an analogue of deoxyguanosine, similar to acyclovir, yet different in that it has an additional hydroxymethyl group on the acyclic side chain[179,183,470,531] (Fig. 239.8). This antiviral compound has selective activity against the herpesviruses, with uniquely potent antiviral activity against CMV. Ganciclovir inhibits HSV-1 and HSV-2 at 0.05 to 0.6 μg/mL, VZV at 0.4 to 10 μg/mL, CMV at 0.02 to 3.4 μg/mL, and EBV at 1.5 μg/mL. Human herpesvirus types 6 (HHV-6), 7 (HHV-7), and 8 (HHV-8) also may be inhibited by ganciclovir.[329] It has in vitro activity against adenoviruses and HBV as well.[179,211,430,537] High concentrations (30 to >700 μg/mL) of ganciclovir will inhibit the growth of most uninfected mammalian cells; bone marrow–derived cells, however, appear to be uniquely sensitive and can be inhibited at much lower concentrations (<0.7 μg/mL).

Ganciclovir

FIG. 239.8 Structure of ganciclovir.

Mechanism of Action and Resistance

Ganciclovir is monophosphorylated in infected cells by virus-induced enzymes: TK in HSV-infected cells and protein kinases that are encoded by the UL97 phosphotransferase gene in CMV-infected cells.[54,179,376,531] Cellular enzymes complete the phosphorylation to ganciclovir triphosphate, the active form of the compound, which is concentrated in infected cells. Ganciclovir triphosphate competitively inhibits the incorporation of deoxyguanosine triphosphate into viral DNA, where it slows and stops viral DNA chain elongation and produces short, noninfectious viral DNA fragments.[240] Ganciclovir also preferentially inhibits viral DNA polymerase.[384] Ganciclovir resistance has been detected in 8% to 38% of immunocompromised adult and pediatric patients who have received prolonged administration of ganciclovir, and such resistance is an important clinical problem.[104,155,210,511,543,578]

Patients may be infected with single or multiple strains of CMV, with both drug-sensitive and drug-resistant strains mixed in the population or in different body compartments.[173] Resistant strains may be induced or infect a patient primarily, emerge quickly after only weeks of therapy, or evolve more slowly and emerge sequentially after several months of antiviral prophylaxis or therapy.[105,173,304,493,608,618] These resistant mutants also retain virulence and are capable of producing serious and progressive disease.[62,173,304,500,538] Ganciclovir resistance in CMV strains occurs by at least two mechanisms: (1) point mutations or deletions in the UL97 gene that reduce intracellular phosphorylation of ganciclovir and (2) point mutations in the viral DNA polymerase UL54 (pol) gene that alter the function of the polymerase.[104,384,535,553] Most strains of CMV that are resistant to ganciclovir have UL97 mutations (most commonly at codons 460, 520, 594, and 595) and reduced phosphorylation, but they remain susceptible to foscarnet and cidofovir.[103,104,553] The most common specific UL97 mutations associated with ganciclovir resistance include A594V, L595S, M4601I/V, C592G, H520Q, and C603W (Fig. 239.9A). Each of these specific mutations increases the EC_{50} of ganciclovir against CMV by 5- to 10-fold, whereas C592G causes only a 3-fold increase in EC_{50}. Other, less known mutations may also be detected and confer functional resistance. However, CMV strains that are resistant to ganciclovir because of a mutation in the UL54 DNA polymerase gene also may be resistant to foscarnet or cidofovir, or to both.[384,503] Moreover, multiple highly resistant strains of CMV may occur if both UL97 phosphotransferase and UL54 DNA polymerase gene

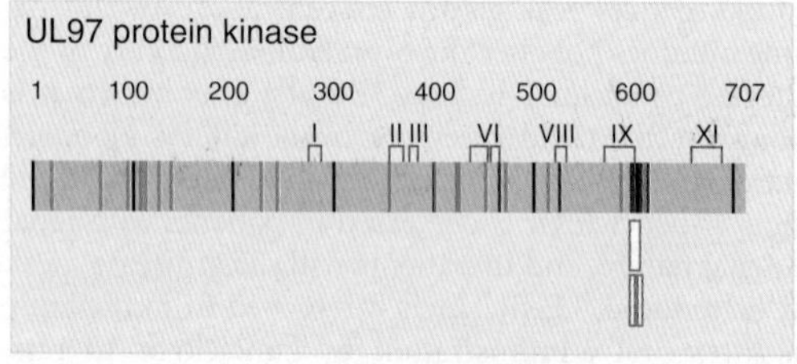

A

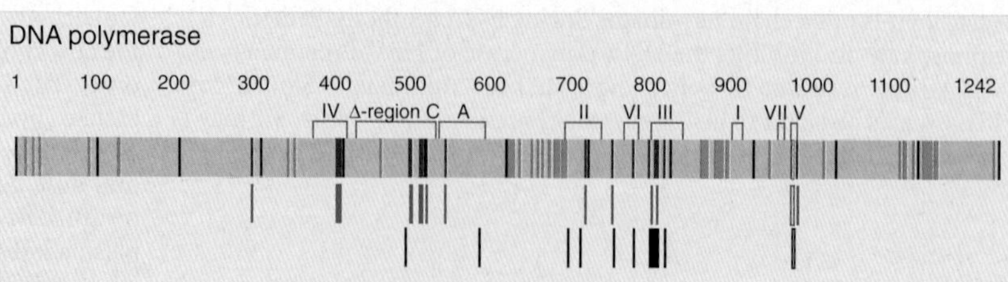

B

FIG. 239.9 Mutations associated with resistance to antiviral drugs. (A) The representation of the amino acid sequence of the UL97 kinase is shown with mutations associated with ganciclovir and maribavir resistance shown in *red* and *blue,* respectively. Polymorphisms observed in clinical specimens are shown in *green.* Conserved regions are designated by *blue brackets.* (B) The DNA polymerase amino acid sequence is depicted with mutations associated with ganciclovir, cidofovir, and foscarnet resistance shown in *red, blue,* and *black,* respectively. Conserved motifs are designated with *blue brackets.* (From James S, Prichard M. The genetic basis of human cytomegalovirus resistance and current trends in antiviral resistance analysis. Infect Disord Drug Targets 2011;11[5]:504-513.)

mutations are present.[105,535] Resistance conferred by UL54 mutations usually emerges after UL97 mutations have occurred.[210,535] Ganciclovir resistance in HSV occurs in TK-deficient, acyclovir-resistant strains of the virus.

Pharmacokinetics

Intravenous administration of a 5-mg/kg dose of ganciclovir in adults produces peak plasma levels of 8 to 11 μg/mL.[179,187] Similar pharmacokinetics in 10 pediatric patients aged 9 months to 12 years has been observed.[201] A study of the pharmacokinetics of ganciclovir in 27 neonates aged 2 to 49 days who were administered intravenous ganciclovir for treatment of congenital CMV disease showed a dose of 6 mg/kg to be the most appropriate dose for that age group, down to 32 weeks of gestation.[580,631] After intravenous administration, ganciclovir is distributed in CSF at 24% to 70% of plasma levels, and 38% of plasma levels enter brain tissue.[108,110] Drug levels in aqueous, vitreous, and subretinal fluid in the eye are comparable to serum levels, and even higher levels can be achieved with intravitreal implants.[20,187,352,396,431] Ganciclovir also accumulates in breast milk in animal models.[7] The plasma half-life is 2 to 4 hours in adults with normal renal function and longer than 24 hours in patients with renal insufficiency and renal failure.[541] The drug is eliminated by renal excretion, and dose reduction is required for patients with impaired creatinine clearance. Hydration will enhance elimination of the drug, and hemodialysis removes 60% of ganciclovir in plasma.[541] Ganciclovir also can be administered orally.[547] Its oral bioavailability is rather poor: 5% under fasting conditions and 6% to 9% if it is administered with food.[15,364] Oral doses of 1000 mg administered to adults every 8 hours produce plasma levels of 0.9 to 1.2 μg/mL.[15,505] The valine ester prodrug of ganciclovir, valganciclovir, has high oral bioavailability and efficacy equal to that of intravenous ganciclovir for prevention and treatment of mild to moderate CMV disease in transplant recipients and treatment of congenitally infected newborns.[163,319,394]

Clinical Indications, Dosage, and Adverse Effects

Clinical indications. Ganciclovir is used for the treatment of established CMV disease; for early or preemptive therapy in immunocompromised patients with virologic markers of active infection that are predictive of CMV disease; and for prophylaxis of high-risk patients, such as those who are CMV seropositive or who have received transplants from CMV-seropositive donors.[81] Ganciclovir is licensed for treatment and chronic suppression of sight-threatening CMV retinitis in immunocompromised patients and for prevention of CMV disease in transplant recipients. Clinical trials have demonstrated efficacy in these conditions.* Treatment with ganciclovir also is beneficial in immunocompromised individuals with other forms of invasive CMV disease, including pneumonia, colitis, esophagitis, myocarditis, encephalitis, persistent fever and leukopenia syndrome, and viral sepsis syndrome.† Treatment of established CMV pneumonia in bone marrow and stem cell transplant recipients is difficult, and the disease may not respond to ganciclovir treatment, with or without immune modulators or globulins.[167] Most clinical trials have been performed in adults, but children and infants with CMV disease benefit from treatment as well.

Ganciclovir treatment also has been evaluated in newborns congenitally infected with CMV with CNS involvement.[336,539,631] In addition, ganciclovir is used for preemptive therapy for patients (primarily recipients of solid-organ, marrow, and stem cell transplants) with virologic markers that are predictive of serious CMV disease.[73,218,266,549] Prophylaxis with ganciclovir to prevent CMV infection and disease in immunocompromised patients, including solid-organ and bone marrow transplant recipients and patients with acquired immunodeficiency syndrome (AIDS), also has been beneficial in most groups studied.[73,153,159,217,549,615,616] Prophylaxis reduces the risk for the acquisition of serious CMV disease or, in some groups, prolongs the incubation period, but it does not eliminate the risk.[159,217,553,615] Ganciclovir prophylaxis is also effective in preventing HSV infection in immunocompromised patients.[217] Ganciclovir appears to decrease HBV DNA levels and to improve hepatic enzymes in patients with posttransplantation infection or reactivation with HBV.[211] In addition, ganciclovir has been used to treat patients with serious disease associated with adenovirus infection, but clinical trials proving efficacy have not been performed.[575]

Dosage. Ganciclovir is supplied as a solution for intravenous infusion. The intravenous infusions are delivered best in a concentration of 10 mg/mL or less and administered during a 1-hour period. Intravitreal implants are also available and are designed to slowly release relatively large doses of ganciclovir locally into the eye during a period of many months.

Ganciclovir therapy for serious CMV disease outside the newborn period usually is administered in two phases, induction and maintenance. The recommended dose for induction therapy for serious CMV disease in adults and children with normal renal function is 5 mg/kg per dose administered intravenously every 12 hours for 2 to 3 weeks. Successful induction therapy is accompanied by clinical and virologic response. Maintenance therapy at doses of 5 mg/kg per dose administered intravenously every 12 to 24 hours should be continued in severely immunocompromised patients who are at risk for relapse.

Selected patients may receive oral ganciclovir for maintenance therapy, when available. Historically, ganciclovir 250- and 500-mg capsules and oral solution for oral administration were used for maintenance. These oral formulations of ganciclovir are rarely used now, since the introduction of valganciclovir oral capsules and solution, which provide superior bioavailability over oral ganciclovir.

The usual recommended dose for oral ganciclovir in adults was 1000 mg three times daily or, alternatively, 500 mg administered six times daily. The pediatric dose for maintenance oral therapy is not established. The duration of maintenance therapy should be individualized for each patient, but such therapy usually lasts through the period of greatest risk, such as rejection or immune suppression, or may be lifelong, as in patients with AIDS. Some patients who experience CMV disease, such as solid-organ transplant recipients with minimal immune suppression and minimal or no rejection, will respond dramatically to induction therapy and will not require long-term maintenance therapy.

A dose of 6 mg/kg administered every 12 hours for 6 weeks is recommended to treat newborns with moderate to severe congenital CMV disease.[336,338,360,631] This dose appears to be adequate for term newborns and premature newborns as young as 32 weeks' gestation, provided renal function seems to be normal for age. The dose for extremely premature newborns is not known and should be individualized according to the clinical judgment of the infectious diseases specialist. Oral valganciclovir is also recommended in newborns who are able to take and absorb oral medications for 6 months for treatment of congenital CMV disease.

Preemptive therapy, 5 mg/kg per dose administered every 12 hours, is initiated when virologic markers for active, invasive infection, such as positive cultures for CMV from bronchoalveolar lavage samples or the presence of CMV DNAemia or antigenemia, are identified by routine virologic surveillance.[548,553] After an induction period of 7 to 14 days, maintenance therapy usually is continued for 100 to 120 days after transplantation or longer if the patient remains at high risk for relapse of CMV disease. Prophylaxis with ganciclovir is administered immediately before transplantation and for a defined period after transplantation in patients who are at high risk, such as those who are CMV seropositive before transplantation and those who receive marrow or solid-organ transplants from a CMV-seropositive donor.[72,159,203,217,507,511,615,616]

Patients who do not respond to induction therapy, who relapse or progress during maintenance therapy with ganciclovir, or who have rising plasma levels of CMV DNA may have a resistant strain of CMV. Antiviral resistance has been documented in immunocompromised patients and newborns.[186] The addition of another antiviral with different mechanisms of action, such as foscarnet or cidofovir, may be beneficial. Maribavir may also be available by compassionate use in selected patients. If clinical or virologic responses still are not maintained, the possibility of a multiply resistant CMV strain should be considered. Patients with disseminated adenovirus disease have received doses of 5 mg/kg every 12 hours for 14 or more days, but clinical benefit has not been proved.[430]

Adverse effects. Adverse effects of ganciclovir can be both local and systemic. Local reactions, such as phlebitis, irritation, blistering, and ulceration at or around the infusion site, can occur and usually are attributed to the alkaline pH (pH 11) of the intravenous solution. Local

*References 73, 131, 159, 217, 218, 266, 279, 414, 511, 615.
†References 81, 108, 117, 148, 153, 167, 479, 480, 505, 507, 508.

reactions can be minimized by paying careful attention to the infusion site or by administering the antiviral agent through a central venous catheter. The most common systemic toxicity associated with ganciclovir administration is dose-dependent, reversible neutropenia, which occurs in one-third to one-half of patients (adults, children, and newborns) who receive this antiviral for longer than 2 weeks.[131,179] Thrombocytopenia also can occur, most often in patients with AIDS who are receiving other antiviral agents, including antiretrovirals.[277] If the neutropenia is severe (absolute neutrophil count <500/mm^3), ganciclovir administration should be halted temporarily until the neutrophil count recovers. Ganciclovir then may be readministered, if it is still clinically indicated, at the same or half the original dose while the patient is carefully monitored for recurrence of the neutropenia. Some experts have used recombinant granulocyte-macrophage colony-stimulating factor successfully to treat ganciclovir-induced neutropenia.[242] Anemia associated with ganciclovir administration is an unusual occurrence. Other adverse effects associated with ganciclovir include CNS disturbances, such as headache, behavioral changes, psychosis, seizures, and coma; mild nephrotoxicity with azotemia; liver dysfunction with elevated transaminases; and rash. Ganciclovir also is mutagenic, carcinogenic, and immunosuppressive. In addition, preclinical animal studies showed reproductive toxicity, with teratogenicity, embryotoxicity, and testicular atrophy.[179] Long-term studies in children who received ganciclovir as newborns are being conducted to determine the long-term effects of ganciclovir administration, if any. To date, none has been reported in case reports or case series. Also, caretakers who prepare and administer ganciclovir to patients should take precautions to minimize direct exposure to the antiviral agent.

Valganciclovir

Spectrum of Activity

Valganciclovir (L-valine, 2-[(2-amino-1,6-dihydro-6-oxy-9*H*-purin-9-yl)methoxy]-3-hydroxypropyl ester) is a prodrug of ganciclovir and therefore has the same selective spectrum of activity as ganciclovir against herpesviruses, especially CMV, as well as limited activity against adenoviruses and HBV.

Mechanism of Action and Resistance

Valganciclovir is the L-valyl ester (prodrug) of ganciclovir.[394] It is metabolized rapidly in the body to ganciclovir. Ganciclovir then is monophosphorylated by viral protein kinase (coded for by UL97 genes) in CMV-infected cells and further phosphorylated to the active form ganciclovir triphosphate by cellular kinases. Viral DNA synthesis is inhibited by ganciclovir triphosphate (see ganciclovir for details). Isolates of CMV become resistant to valganciclovir by mutations in UL97, the viral kinase gene, or in UL54, the viral DNA polymerase gene. Mutations in UL97 confer resistance to ganciclovir and therefore to valganciclovir, whereas mutations in UL54 confer double or triple resistance to ganciclovir, foscarnet, and cidofovir. Mutations in both genes can produce highly resistant strains of CMV.

Pharmacokinetics

Valganciclovir is well absorbed after oral administration and is rapidly hydrolyzed in the intestine and liver to ganciclovir.[464] The bioavailability of valganciclovir is high, approximately 60% (vs. 6–9% for ganciclovir), and an oral dose of 900 mg administered to adults produces ganciclovir blood levels equivalent to a 5-mg/kg dose administered intravenously.[75,317,394] Absorption is enhanced significantly with the ingestion of food, so physicians recommend that valganciclovir be taken with food or meals. The drug is excreted by the kidneys, and renal insufficiency produces prolonged excretion and a longer half-life (see ganciclovir). Oral valganciclovir solution has been administered to neonates and infants up to 6 months of age, at a dosage of 16 mg/kg per dose (range of 15–18 mg/kg per dose) every 12 hours, adjusted for renal function, if necessary. A dosing algorithm for pediatric patients, including infants younger than 4 months, based on body surface area and renal function, instead of weight, may also be used.[70] Valganciclovir is 41% bioavailable and provides stable and constant plasma concentrations and antiviral effects comparable to intravenously administered ganciclovir.[340,518] Pharmacokinetic studies have shown stable and effective antiviral plasma concentrations (mean trough, 0.51 μg/mL; and mean 2-hour peak, 3.81 μg/mL) and penetration into the CSF of infants.[378,435] Valganciclovir oral solution should be adjusted monthly for weight gain and also may be mixed with small amounts of formula or breast milk in a measured syringe to facilitate newborns and infants to take the antiviral.

Clinical Indications, Dosage, and Adverse Effects

Valganciclovir is available in 450-mg tablets, and the usual adult dose is 900 mg (two 450-mg tablets) twice daily for 14 days (induction therapy), followed by a maintenance dose of 900 mg administered once daily.[394] An oral solution (50 mg/mL concentration) is also licensed and available.[335] Valganciclovir is licensed for induction and maintenance treatment of CMV retinitis in immunocompromised patients, but clinical trials have shown that valganciclovir is beneficial to a variety of patients with a number of different CMV infections.[394] Antiviral prophylaxis or preemptive treatment for CMV DNAemia with valganciclovir for 100 to 200 days after transplantation in high-risk transplant recipients significantly reduces the incidence of CMV disease and improves graft survival.[617] Oral valganciclovir suppression in pediatric kidney transplant recipients for up to 200 days has been shown to be effective and to have a favorable safety profile.[586]

Treatment of newborns with symptomatic congenital CMV infection with oral valganciclovir (15–18 mg/kg per dose every 12 hours) appears beneficial, similar to intravenous ganciclovir benefits, providing improved head circumference, improved developmental milestones, and reduced risk for hearing loss and progression. A randomized clinical trial comparing 6 weeks versus 6 months of treatment in congenitally infected newborns has recently shown the longer 6-month duration of treatment to be more beneficial.[11] In some centers, treatment up to 12 months of age has shown benefit for prevention of hearing loss progression.[14] There are case reports of the use of valganciclovir or ganciclovir to treat newborns with asymptomatic congenital CMV with hearing loss, and some experts have advocated treatment of selected newborns with congenital hearing loss, especially if they have high or prolonged viral DNA levels in plasma.[326] However, conclusions about the efficacy of such treatment cannot be made from these reports at this time and await results of randomized clinical trials.[354,622] Currently, antiviral treatment of symptom-free newborns with congenital CMV and normal hearing is not recommended.

As with ganciclovir, if a patient treated with valganciclovir experiences progression of disease or recurrence during maintenance therapy, a resistant strain of CMV should be considered a possibility and antiviral treatment adjusted accordingly.[312] Adverse effects associated with the oral administration of valganciclovir include diarrhea and dose-dependent, reversible neutropenia.[394]

Neonates with congenital CMV disease treated with oral valganciclovir experience neutropenia approximately 19% of the time. Also reported has been a mild elevation of liver enzymes, as well as possible changes in patterns of sleeping or gastrointestinal upset in some infants.

Foscarnet

Spectrum of Activity

Foscarnet (phosphonoformic acid or trisodium phosphonoformate hexahydrate) is a pyrophosphate analogue that selectively inhibits herpesviruses[448] (Fig. 239.10). It also has activity against HIV and HBV.[30,176] At concentrations of 100 to 300 μmol/L, CMV is inhibited; whereas slightly lower concentrations (80–200 μmol/L) inhibit HSV types 1 and 2, VZV, EBV, and HHV-8.[448] Concentrations between 20 and 200 μmol/L appear to inhibit HBV. Foscarnet also inhibits most acyclovir-resistant HSV and VZV strains and most ganciclovir-resistant CMV strains.[195,389,498] Combinations of ganciclovir and foscarnet are

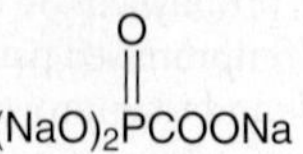

FIG. 239.10 Structure of foscarnet.

synergistic against CMV, and combinations of zidovudine and foscarnet appear to be synergistic against HIV.[176,389] At high concentrations (500–1000 µmol/L), foscarnet inhibits cellular DNA synthesis in uninfected cells.[106]

Mechanism of Action and Resistance

Foscarnet is not a nucleoside analogue, and it does not require phosphorylation or any other form of intracellular metabolism to be activated. Rather, it is a pyrophosphate analogue that directly inhibits viral and cellular DNA polymerase.[132,145] Selective viral inhibition is accomplished by noncompetitive and reversible blocking of the pyrophosphate binding site of the viral polymerase, in much lower concentrations than it inhibits cellular DNA polymerases. Because foscarnet does not require phosphorylation by viral TK or other kinases, it inhibits TK-deficient and altered strains of HSV and VZV that are resistant to acyclovir as well as UL97 phosphotransferase mutants of CMV that are resistant to ganciclovir. However, strains of herpesviruses of all types that are resistant to acyclovir or ganciclovir by mutation of the viral DNA polymerase gene are also resistant to foscarnet.[31,500]

Pharmacokinetics

Intravenous administration of 60 mg of foscarnet every 8 hours to adults produces plasma levels of 450 to 575 µmol/L; 90 mg administered every 12 hours produces plasma levels of 420 to 746 µmol/L.[145,498] CSF levels are usually approximately 60% of plasma levels, and vitreous concentrations in the eye are the same as or slightly higher than plasma levels.[262] Most (80%) of the dose of foscarnet is eliminated unmetabolized from the body through the kidneys, and plasma clearance decreases if renal function is impaired. The remaining 20% appears to be deposited in teeth and bone, where it accumulates and remains for months. The drug is removed by hemodialysis, but not appreciably by peritoneal dialysis.[8,386] Oral foscarnet has poor bioavailability (<10%) and causes diarrhea, and it is unlikely to be available for patient use.[447] Pharmacokinetic data in infants and children have not been published. However, preclinical studies showed that deposition of foscarnet in teeth and bones is greater in younger than in older animals.

Clinical Indications, Dosage, and Adverse Effects

Clinical indications. Foscarnet is licensed for both induction and maintenance treatment of CMV retinitis in immunocompromised patients and for treatment of mucocutaneous disease caused by acyclovir-resistant HSV.* Foscarnet also may be of benefit in patients with varicella or zoster caused by acyclovir-resistant VZV.[498] Because the combination of foscarnet and ganciclovir appears to be synergistic in vitro, immunocompromised patients who experience progression or relapse of CMV disease while receiving therapy with one or the other antiviral agent may benefit from combination therapy in some instances.[25,156,195,309] Foscarnet also may be used for the treatment or prophylaxis of serious or life-threatening CMV disease when ganciclovir is contraindicated or otherwise deemed clinically undesirable because of its myelosuppressive effects.[25,485,623] The antiretroviral properties of foscarnet, when it is combined with other antiviral agents, also may be beneficial in patients with HIV infection or AIDS.[48,310,456,560,561]

Dosage. Treatment with foscarnet usually is divided into two phases, induction and maintenance. The usual dosage of foscarnet for induction therapy is 60 mg/kg per dose administered intravenously every 8 hours for 3 weeks; maintenance therapy is 90 to 120 mg/kg per day administered indefinitely or through the period of risk.[322] The dose of foscarnet should be given slowly, during the course of 2 hours (or no faster than 1 mg/kg per minute), to reduce renal toxicity. Creatinine clearance should be used to adjust dosage regimens in patients with renal insufficiency or renal failure. Published experience on the use of foscarnet in pediatric patients is limited, but undoubtedly, certain pediatric patients benefit from receiving foscarnet therapy.[596] In these cases, the same per-kilogram dosage regimens can be used for most patients. Prehydration with saline and the use of probenecid with each dose are recommended in some patients to reduce renal toxicity.

*References 145, 156, 309, 365, 386, 456, 500, 519, 520, 596.

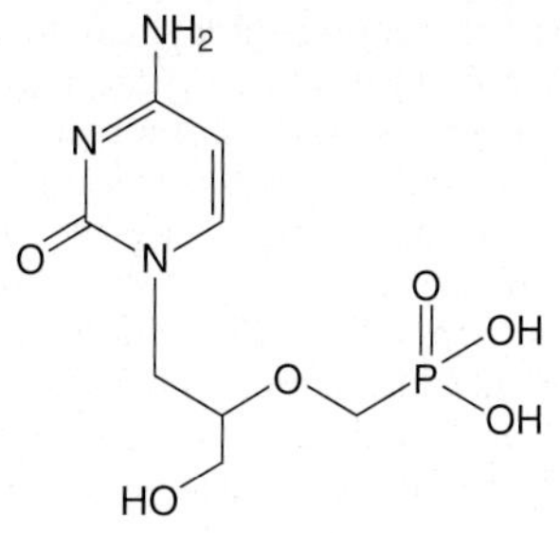

Cidofovir

FIG. 239.11 Structure of cidofovir.

Adverse effects. Foscarnet is associated with serious adverse effects and should be used only after thorough consideration of the risks and benefits involved.[106,145] Renal toxicity with azotemia, proteinuria, crystalluria, renal tubular acidosis or necrosis, and interstitial nephritis can occur in as many as a third of patients who receive foscarnet.[143,315] Renal toxicity generally occurs after the first week of therapy and usually is reversible. The risk for the development of renal toxicity is increased if the drug is given by rapid infusion or administered in high doses, if the patient is dehydrated, or if other nephrotoxic drugs are administered concomitantly with foscarnet.[439] Hydration, including saline loading, and administration of each dose during the course of at least 2 hours appear to reduce the risk for development of renal toxicity. Foscarnet binds divalent metal ions such as calcium in the body, and metabolic abnormalities, including hypocalcemia and hypercalcemia (total or ionized), hypophosphatemia and hyperphosphatemia, hypomagnesemia, and hypokalemia, may occur in approximately one-third of patients who receive foscarnet.[307] Symptoms of these acute metabolic abnormalities include perioral tingling, numbness or paresthesias of the limbs, and, if severe, seizures, tetany, and cardiac dysrhythmias. Administration of the dose during the course of at least 2 hours also reduces the risk for development of metabolic abnormalities. Foscarnet also can be deposited and concentrate in bone, with as yet unclear long-term consequences.[145] CNS side effects also occur in approximately one-fourth of patients and include headache, tremor, seizures, and behavioral changes. Abnormal liver function test results have been noted, and high urinary concentrations of foscarnet may produce painful genital ulcerations and rash in some patients.[267,539] Preclinical studies showed foscarnet to be mutagenic and associated with anomalies of skeletal development in young animals.[142]

Cidofovir and Brincidofovir

Spectrum of Activity

Cidofovir, (*S*-1-3-hydroxy-2-[phosphonomethoxypropyl])cytosine dihydrate (also known as HPMPC), is an acyclic phosphonate nucleotide analogue of deoxycytidine monophosphate with broad-spectrum in vitro antiviral activity against all DNA viruses, including herpesviruses (HSV types 1 and 2; CMV, EBV, and VZV; and HHV types 6, 7, and 8), adenoviruses, polyomaviruses (JC and BK viruses), papillomaviruses, and poxviruses (vaccinia, variola or smallpox, cowpox, monkeypox, camelpox, and molluscum contagiosum and orf viruses) (Fig. 239.11).* Cidofovir exhibits its most specific and potent antiviral activity against CMV (minimal inhibitory concentration, 0.25 µmol/L).[99,98,154,168] The compound also is very active against VZV (0.79 µmol/L), HSV-1 (12.7 µmol/L), and acyclovir-resistant, TK-deficient HSV-1 strains (6.24 µmol/L).[275,412,540] Cidofovir inhibits HSV-2 at concentrations of 31.7 µmol/L, adenoviruses at 10.8 µmol/L, and vaccinia virus at 12.7 µmol/L.[141,220,533] Strains of CMV UL97 mutants that are resistant to ganciclovir are inhibited by cidofovir, and cidofovir in combination with ganciclovir or foscarnet shows synergistic inhibition of CMV in vitro.[499]

*References 18, 98, 99,141, 154, 168, 207, 220, 275, 412, 439, 440, 499, 529, 530, 533, 540, 584.

Brincidofovir (3-hexadecyloxy-propyl-cidofovir [HDP-CDV or CMX001]) is the lipid conjugate of the acyclic nucleoside phosphonate antiviral cidofovir. It is a broad-spectrum antiviral agent active in vitro against double-stranded DNA viruses; these include all the herpesviruses, including acyclovir-resistant herpes simplex virus; adenoviruses; polyomaviruses, including BK viruses; and poxviruses, including variola small pox and vaccinia virus.[429,450,588] Brincidofovir also may be used to treat ganciclovir-resistant CMV infection, unless the resistance is acquired through UL54 mutation. In addition, it may have in vitro activity against RNA viruses, such as Ebola virus, in its lipid moiety form.[189,409]

Mechanisms of Action and Resistance

Cidofovir inhibits the replication of CMV and other viruses by selective inhibition of viral DNA polymerase.[99,275,412] The compound is phosphorylated by cellular enzymes to the active form cidofovir diphosphate. Cidofovir diphosphate inhibits both viral and cellular DNA polymerase; however, because the concentration necessary to inhibit cellular DNA synthesis is hundreds of times higher than that needed to inhibit viral DNA synthesis, cidofovir appears to selectively inhibit viral DNA synthesis at concentrations safely administered to humans. Cidofovir diphosphate has a long intracellular half-life that provides prolonged and persistent antiviral activity and allows infrequent dosing regimens in humans.[188,276,540] Because the compound does not require TK for initial phosphorylation, it is active against TK-deficient and TK-altered acyclovir-resistant HSV strains.[412] Resistance to cidofovir is unusual but can occur by mutations in viral DNA polymerase genes (codons 375 to 540 and possibly 978 to 988), most likely in patients who have received prolonged or repeated periods of treatment with ganciclovir or foscarnet. Strains of CMV that are resistant to cidofovir are also usually resistant to ganciclovir, and occasionally, triple mutants resistant to ganciclovir, foscarnet, and cidofovir occur.[154,574]

Brincidofovir is cleaved of its lipid moiety to be cidofovir, which is then converted through phosphorylation intracellularly into the active antiviral cidofovir diphosphate, which inhibits viral DNA polymerase by serving as an alternate substrate and results in inhibition of DNAsynthesis, for action against DNA viruses. However, for action against the RNA virus Ebola virus, intracellular phosphorylation may not be necessary for antiviral inhibition.

Pharmacokinetics

After an intravenous infusion of 5 mg/kg of cidofovir, peak plasma levels range from 11.6 to 26.1 μg/mL, with the latter occurring after administration of probenicid.[133,499,574] The plasma half-life is 2 to 3 hours, but the intracellular half-life is prolonged (between 17 and 65 hours).[540] CSF penetration by cidofovir is not well studied, but in at least one patient, the drug did not appear to cross the blood-brain barrier in detectable amounts. After topical administration to the eye or intact skin, systemic absorption is low, with peak plasma levels usually less than 0.5 μg/mL.[357,358] However, patients with abraded or denuded skin may have significant absorption.[52] The systemic absorption that occurs after intralesional or subcutaneous administration is not well characterized at this time. Intravitreal administration produces sustained antiviral effects in animal models.[188] Cidofovir is not well absorbed orally, with less than 5% bioavailability. However, bioavailable alkoxyalkyl esters of cidofovir are in development and may lead to an oral compound in the near future.[331] Aerosolized cidofovir also is being studied in animal models and appears to deliver high concentrations of antiviral to the lungs.[72] Cidofovir is eliminated through the kidney by glomerular filtration and active tubular secretion, and more than 90% of the original dose can be recovered unchanged in urine.

Brincidofovir, because of its lipid conjugation, has high oral bioavailability, higher intracellular concentrations of active drug, lower plasma concentrations of cidofovir, and increased antiviral potency against double-stranded DNA viruses.[190] Oral dosing of 4 mg/kg per dose administered every week or 2 mg/kg per dose twice weekly, or adult dosing of 100 to 200 mg per week, exceed inhibitory concentrations of most double-stranded DNA viruses of medical importance in humans. After 100 mg and 200 mg oral doses, mean trough levels of brincidofovir were between 10 to 17 ng/mL and 10 to 30 ng/mL, respectively, under fasting conditions. An intravenous formulation of brincidofovir is also under early clinical development.

Clinical Indications, Dosage, and Adverse Effects

Clinical indications. Cidofovir is licensed for induction and maintenance treatment of CMV retinitis in immunocompromised adults with AIDS.[499,562] Clinical trials have shown that cidofovir significantly delays progression of CMV retinitis in previously untreated patients as well as in those who previously failed to respond to or were intolerant of foscarnet or ganciclovir therapy.[357,358,377,469,472,522] Cidofovir also has been shown to be effective for the treatment of CMV infection and disease in marrow and stem cell transplant recipients. In addition, it has been used, in selected patients, for preemptive treatment of CMV infection after marrow and stem cell transplantation.[93,377,469] One study also showed that cidofovir helped prevent posttransplantation CMV-associated atherosclerosis in rats.[78] Patients infected with CMV strains resistant to ganciclovir or foscarnet, or both, may benefit from receiving cidofovir treatment.[154] Cidofovir is used by clinicians to treat immunocompromised children with serious CMV disease despite the lack of published experience in children.[80,90]

Cidofovir has broad-spectrum antiviral activity, and published case reports show that it has been used to treat patients with serious infections caused by a wide variety of DNA viruses. For example, patients with acyclovir- and foscarnet-resistant HSV infection have been treated successfully with topical and systemic cidofovir.[79,348,356,358] It also may be effective in treatment of selected patients with acyclovir-resistant VZV infections.[533] Moreover, one report showed that treatment with cidofovir and anti-CD20 monoclonal antibody was associated with remission and regression of posttransplantation EBV-associated lymphoproliferative disease.[241] The use of cidofovir to treat patients with AIDS and HHV-8 viremia and disease also has been reported.[65,401] Human papillomavirus–induced epithelial cell proliferation may be responsive to treatment with topical and intralesional administration of cidofovir.[557] Several small, uncontrolled case series have described the successful use of cidofovir to treat juvenile laryngeal papillomatosis, hypopharyngeal and esophageal papillomatous lesions, anogenital condylomas, and cervical intraepithelial neoplasia.[21,100,454,516,538,627] Furthermore, intravenous and intralesional therapy with cidofovir has been used to treat individual patients, including children, with refractory disseminated respiratory papillomatosis of the lung.[21,378,388] Human BK polyomavirus–associated acute hemorrhagic cystitis in immunocompromised patients has been treated with cidofovir, with varying results.[37,178] Case reports and small clinical trials evaluating cidofovir treatment in patients with progressive multifocal leukoencephalopathy who have AIDS or other immunocompromising conditions have not shown consistent benefit in survival or sustained improvement in neurologic status.[19,109,204,292,428,478,501,519] Successful cidofovir treatment of adenovirus disease in marrow and stem cell transplant recipients has been published in reports of case series, with the best results noted in patients in whom the disease was localized and treatment was initiated early.[64,206,278,367,400,486] Controlled clinical trials evaluating eye drops containing an investigational topical solution of cidofovir to treat patients with acute keratoconjunctivitis caused by adenovirus have not shown consistent benefit in the doses used.[270,271] Poxviruses are inhibited by cidofovir in concentrations safely achievable in humans, and at least one case report of successful treatment of orf (ecthyma contagiosum) has been published.[17,207] In addition, in vitro and animal model data suggest that cidofovir may be effective as short-term, postexposure prophylaxis of smallpox and other related poxvirus infections in humans as well as in the treatment of complications that may occur after inoculation with smallpox (vaccinia-like) vaccine.[18,98,99,141,154,499,486] However, no clinical trials in humans to evaluate the efficacy of cidofovir for the treatment of poxvirus infections have been published.[441]

Brincidofovir remains investigational at this time, and phase II and phase III clinical trials in adults and pediatric patients are underway (https://clinicaltrials.gov). In addition, more than a thousand patients have been administered brincidofovir under clinical trial or compassionate use, and case reports have shown safety and efficacy for a variety of viral infections in immunocompromised hosts. The clinical efficacy of brincidofovir for prophylaxis of CMV has shown significant benefit[395]; however, for treatment of CMV and adenovirus infections, in particular, it has not shown overwhelmingly positive results in clinical trials to date.

Dosage. The usually recommended dose for induction therapy with cidofovir is 5 mg/kg given as an intravenous infusion during the course of 1 hour administered once weekly for 2 consecutive weeks. Some clinicians suggest a reduced dosage regimen of 1 mg/kg administered three times weekly to reduce the risk for renal toxicity.[278] Maintenance therapy usually is administered as 1-hour infusions of 5 mg/kg once every 2 weeks to complete a total of at least five doses. These doses should be decreased to 1 to 3 mg/kg if renal insufficiency is present and discontinued if significant elevation of serum creatinine concentration or proteinuria occurs. Probenecid should be administered orally with each dose of cidofovir, 3 hours before and then 2 and 8 hours after completion of the intravenous infusion. Prehydration with normal saline before each infusion also is recommended. Topical preparations of eye drops containing 0.2% to 1% cidofovir and creams containing 1% cidofovir are being investigated.[271,270] The usual concentration used for intralesional injection is 2.5 mg/mL.[340,388]

Brincidofovir oral dosing in phase II and III clinical trials has been 2 mg/kg per dose twice weekly or 4 mg/kg per dose once weekly for adults and children. For individuals weighing more than 50 kg, 100 mg twice weekly or 200 mg once weekly has been used. The usual maximum dose per week has been 4 mg/kg per dose or 200 mg/dose weekly. Some clinical trials have used 40 mg/kg once-weekly dosing, with escalations to 100 mg and 200 mg doses weekly. Brincidofovir appears to be well absorbed under fasting conditions with a time to maximum plasma drug concentration proportional to the dose administered and ranging from 2 to 3 hours in adults. Half-life of the drug increases as the dose increases, with ranges from 6 to 24 hours. Brincidofovir is not detected in urine, but its elimination product cidofovir is detected after brincidofovir administration. No pharmacokinetics is available yet for neonates and infants; however, dose escalation pharmacokinetic studies evaluating 0.25, 0.5, 1, and 2 mg/kg per dose may be conducted in the future. Dosing in renal impairment usually does not require adjustment, based on current information. Dosing after dialysis is 1 mg/kg one to two times per week given after dialysis. There are no recommendations for adjustment in hepatic impairment. At this time, no information on use of brincidofovir in pregnancy or excretion in breast milk of breast-feeding women is available.

Adverse effects. Cidofovir is nephrotoxic and produces clinically apparent proximal tubular dysfunction, including Fanconi syndrome and acute renal failure, in as many as half the patients who receive the drug.[411,499] Early laboratory signs of renal toxicity include proteinuria, glycosuria, azotemia, and metabolic acidosis. Therefore patients receiving cidofovir should have a urinalysis and serum tests for renal function performed before taking each dose. The risk for development of renal toxicity can be reduced but not eliminated by probenecid and saline prehydration. Moreover, renal toxicity is more likely to occur if other nephrotoxic agents, such as aminoglycosides, amphotericin B, or foscarnet, are administered concurrently with cidofovir.[629] In clinical trials of patients with AIDS, administration of cidofovir also was associated with neutropenia. Ocular toxicity, including ocular hypotony (decreased intraocular pressure) and anterior uveitis and iritis, also has been reported in patients receiving cidofovir therapy.[5] Therefore frequent monitoring by an ophthalmologist, including measurement of intraocular pressure, is recommended for patients receiving cidofovir therapy. Intravitreal administration of cidofovir has produced uveitis, vitreitis, reduced intraocular pressure, and loss of vision.[341,436] Local or topical treatment with cidofovir may produce local reactions in the skin.

Brincidofovir has significant gastrointestinal side effects, including nausea and diarrhea. Diarrhea is especially common, reported in up to 70% of recipients in the higher range dosing, and is potentially serious in nature. Compared with cidofovir, brincidofovir has little or no nephrotoxicity, although isolated case reports of reversible nephrotoxicity have emerged.[180]

Information on drug interactions of brincidofovir is lacking at this time.

Maribavir and Letermovir

Spectrum of Activity and Mechanisms of Resistance

Maribavir (1263W94, VP-41263) and letermovir (AIC246, MK 8228) are oral investigational antivirals with potent activity solely against CMV.[66]

Maribavir is a benzimidazole riboside compound (benzimidavir) with potent activity primarily against CMV documented. It competes with adenosine triphosphate (ATP) for binding to pUL97, does not require intracellular phosphorylation, and is independent of pUL54. Maribavir directly inhibits UL97 kinase, an early viral gene product involved in viral DNA elongation, packaging, and egress or shedding of viral capsids from viral nuclei. It is active against ganciclovir-resistant CMV.

Resistance to maribavir may develop on therapy, especially if the patient has documented high viral load at the start of treatment with maribavir.[288,514] Various mutations have been shown to confer maribavir resistance by modifying the UL97 ATP binding site. The UL97 mutations elicited by ganciclovir and maribavir are different, but cross-resistance can occur if a single p-loop mutation occurs. CMV isolates that are resistant to maribavir usually remain susceptible to ganciclovir (and vice versa). Because maribavir inhibits UL97, it will impair phosphorylation of ganciclovir; therefore these two antivirals should not be coadministered at the same time in serious CMV infections. Maribavir and foscarnet, however, have been combined successfully in selected situations.

Letermovir is a viral terminase complex inhibitor with a potent, yet narrow, spectrum of antiviral activity only against human CMV. It has no activity against any other viruses. It has a novel mechanism of action by inhibiting CMV DNA synthesis at a late step by targeting the UL56 subunit of the terminase enzyme complex. It may have activity against CMV strains resistant to ganciclovir, foscarnet, and cidofovir and does not exhibit cross-resistance with other antiviral drugs. It is the protocol viral terminase complex inhibitor and the most advanced one in clinical development at this time.

High-grade resistance mutations in the UL56 terminase gene are readily selected in vitro under letermovir. In addition, in phase II prophylaxis trials, emergence of UL56 mutation V236M in the amino acid region 230–270 was associated with clinical resistance.[102,215,374]

Pharmacokinetics

Maribavir demonstrates rapid absorption after oral administration, linear pharmacokinetics, and in vivo anti-CMV activity in humans. Mean oral availability in humans ranges 25% to 40%, and it can be recovered in the urine. Peak plasma levels occur approximately 1 to 3 hours after oral administration. There is minimal accumulation of the drug at steady state.[385]

Letermovir demonstrates rapid absorption after oral administration. Doses may need to be adjusted in patients with renal and hepatic impairment.

Clinical Indications, Dosage, and Adverse Effects

Clinical indications. Maribavir remains investigational, and clinical trials are evaluating how it may be used to treat ganciclovir-resistant CMV infections in immunocompromised patients.[164] However, because it does not penetrate the CSF reliably, if there is a suspicion of or risk for CMV CNS disease, maribavir should not be used for treatment of CMV meningoencephalitis.

Letermovir has been investigated in clinical trials for prevention and treatment of CMV in immunocompromised hosts. Its lack of significant cross-resistance with other anti-CMV antivirals and its lack of myelosuppression make it a favorable option for clinical trials. Its clinical indication has not yet been determined, but it may be used as an antiviral for CMV-specific primary prophylaxis in allogeneic hematopoietic stem cell transplant recipients.[97]

Dosage. Maribavir is an oral antiviral agent. It has been administered in clinical trials in doses ranging from 300 to 600 mg/day up to 1200 to 2400 mg/day. Most trials have used 400 mg twice daily for 10 days in clinical trials of adults.

Letermovir is also an oral antiviral agent. It has been administered in clinical trials in doses ranging from 40 mg twice per day to 80 mg daily to as high as 320 mg daily in adults. Based on early pharmacokinetic trials, daily doses of 120 mg or 240 mg appear to achieve desirable levels without side effects.[97] No pediatric, neonate, or infant pharmacokinetic data are available at this time.

Adverse effects. Maribavir commonly causes disturbances in taste, but has not demonstrated any other significant side effects to date in clinical trials.

Letermovir appears safe in clinical trials based on information to date, with the only significant side effect noted being gastrointestinal symptoms.

NEW REFERENCES SINCE THE SEVENTH EDITION

3. Abzug M, Michaels M, Wald E, et al. A randomized, double-blind, placebo-controlled trial of pleconaril for the treatment of neonates with enterovirus sepsis. *J Pediatric Infect Dis Soc.* 2016;5(1):53-62.
10. American Academy of Pediatrics, Committee on Infectious Diseases. Respiratory syncytial virus. In: Kimberlin D, Brady M, Jackson MA, Long S, eds. *Red Book: 2015 Report of the Committee on Infectious Diseases.* 30th ed. Elk Grove Village, IL: American Academy of Pediatrics; 2015:667.
41. Beaird O, Frelfield A, Ison M, et al. Current practices for treatment of respiratory syncytial virus and other non-influenza respiratory viruses in high-risk patient populations: a survey of Institutions in the Midwestern Respiratory Virus Collaborative. *Transpl Infect Dis.* 2016;18(2):210-215.
47. Benschop K, Wildenbeest J, Koen G, et al. Genetic and antigenic structural characterization for resistance of echovirus 11 to pleconaril in an immunocompromised patient. *J Gen Virol.* 2015;96(Pt 3):571-579.
66. Bowman L, Melaragno J, Brennan D. Letermovir for the management of cytomegalovirus infection. *Expert Opin Investig Drugs.* 2017;26(2):235-241.
69. Bradley D, Moreira S, Subramoney V, et al. Pharmacokinetics and safety of valganciclovir in pediatric heart transplant recipients 4 months of age and younger. *Pediatr Infect Dis J.* 2016;35(12):1324-1328.
82. Buontempo P, Cox S, Wright-Minogue J, et al. SCH 48973: a potent, broad-spectrum, anti enterovirus compound. *Antimicrob Agents Chemother.* 1997;41(6):1220-1225.
83. Burrows F, Carlos L, Benzimra M, et al. Oral ribavirin for respiratory syncytial virus infection after lung transplantation: efficacy and cost-efficiency. *J Heart Lung Transplant.* 2015;34(7):958-962.
87. Carande E, Pollard A, Drysdale S. Management of respiratory syncytial virus bronchiolitis: 2015 survey of members of the European Society for Paediatric Infectious Diseases. *Can J Infect Dis Med Microbiol.* 2016;2016:9139537.
96. Chemaly R, Ghantoji S, Shah D, et al. Respiratory syncytial virus infections in children with cancer. *J Pediatr Hematol Oncol.* 2014;36(6):e376-e381.
97. Chemaly R, Ullman A, Stoelben S, et al. Letermovir for cytomegalovirus prophylaxis in hematopoietic cell transplantation. *N Engl J Med.* 2014;370(19):1781-1789.
105. Chou S. Approach to drug-resistant cytomegalovirus in transplant recipients. *Curr Opin Infect Dis.* 2015;28(4):293-299.
119. Collett M, Hincks J, Benschop K, et al. Antiviral activity of pocapavir in a randomized, blinded, placebo-controlled human oral poliovirus vaccine challenge model. *J Infect Dis.* 2017;215(3):335-343.
138. De Clercq E, Guangdi L. Approved antiviral drugs over the past 50 years. *Clin Microbiol Rev.* 2016;29(3):695-747.
164. El Chaer F, Shah D, Chemaly R. How I treat resistant cytomegalovirus infection in hematopoietic cell transplantation recipients. *Blood.* 2016;128(23):2624-2636.
174. Ericson J, Gostelow M, Autmizgine J, et al. Safety of high-dose acyclovir in infants with suspected and confirmed neonatal herpes simplex virus infections. *Pediatr Infect Dis J.* 2017;36(4):369-373.
180. Faure E, Galperine T, Cannesson O, et al. Case report: brincidofovir – induced reversible severe acute kidney injury in 2 solid-organ transplant for treatment of cytomegalovirus infection. *Medicine (Baltimore).* 2016;95(44):e5226.
186. Fisher C, Knudsen J, Lease E, et al. Risk factors and outcomes of ganciclovir resistant cytomegalovirus infection in solid organ transplant recipients. *Clin Infect Dis.* 2017;65(1):57-63.
189. Florescu D, Kalil A, Hewlett A, et al. Administration of brincidofovir and convalescent plasma in a patient with Ebola virus disease. *Clin Infect Dis.* 2015;61(6):969-973.
190. Florescu D, Keck M. Development of CMX001 (Brincidofovir) for the treatment of serious diseases or conditions caused by ds DNA viruses. *Expert Rev Anti Infect Ther.* 2014;12(10):1171-1178.
215. Goldner T, Hempel C, Ruebsamen-Schaeff H, et al. Geno- and phenotypic characterization of human cytomegalovirus mutants selected in vitro after letermovir (AIC246) exposure. *Antimicrob Agents Chemother.* 2014;58(1):610-613.
219. Gorcea C, Tholouli E, Turner A, et al. Effective use of oral ribavirin for respiratory syncytial viral infections in allogeneic haematopoietic stem cell transplant recipients. *J Hosp Infect.* 2017;95(2):214-217.
222. Greer LG, Leff RD, Rogers VL, et al. Pharmacokinetics of oseltamivir in breast milk and maternal plasma. *Am J Obstet Gynecol.* 2011;204(6):524e1-524e4.
229. Gueller S, Duenzinger U, Wolf T, et al. Successful systemic high-dose treatment of respiratory syncytial virus-induced infections occurring pre-engraftment in allogeneic hematopoietic stem cell transplant recipients. *Transpl Infect Dis.* 2013;15(4):435-440.
238. Hama R. The mechanisms of delayed onset type adverse reactions to oseltamivir. *Infect Dis (Lond).* 2016;48(9):651-666.
261. Heneghan CJ, Onakpoya I, Thompson M, et al. Zanamivir for influenza in adults and children: systematic review of clinical study reports and summary of regulatory comments. *BMJ.* 2014;348:g2547.
288. Houldcroft C, Bryant J, Depledge D, et al. Detection of low frequency multi-drug resistance and novel putative maribavir resistance in immunocompromised pediatric patients with cytomegalovirus. *Front Microbiol.* 2016;7:1317-1320.
300. In P, Kim HI, Kwon KT. Two treatment cases of severe fever and thrombocytopenia syndrome with oral ribavirin and plasma exchange. *Infect Chemother.* 2017;49(1):72-77.
312. James S, Prichard M. The genetic basis of human cytomegalovirus resistance and current trends in antiviral resistance analysis. *Infect Disord Drug Targets.* 2011;11(5):504-513.
318. Kakiuchi S, Tsuji M, Nishimura H, et al. Association of the emergence of acyclovir-resistant herpes simplex virus type 1 with prognosis in hematopoietic stem cell transplantation patients. *J Infect Dis.* 2017;215(6):865-873.
326. Kawada J, Torli Y, Kawano Y, et al. Viral load in children with congenital cytomegalovirus infection identified on newborn hearing screening. *J Clin Virol.* 2015;65:41-45.
347. Kong M, Ba M, Ren C, et al. An updated meta-analysis of amantadine for treating dyskinesia in Parkinson's disease. *Oncotarget.* 2017;8(34):57316-57326.
368. Lehnerer SM, Scheibe F, Buchert R, Kliesch S, Meisel A. Awakening with amantadine from a persistent vegetative state after subarachnoid hemorrhage. *BMJ Case Rep.* 2017;Jul 24.
385. Ma J, Nafziger A, Villano S, et al. Maribavir pharmacokinetics and the effects of multiple dose maribavir on cytochrome P450 (CYP) 1A2, CYP 2C9, CYP 2C19, CYP 2D6, CYP 3A, N-acetyltransferase-s, and xanthine oxidase activities in healthy adults. *Antimicrob Agents Chemother.* 2006;50(4):1130-1135.
390. Marcelin J, Wilson J, Razonable R, Mayo Clinic Hematology/Oncology and Transplant Infectious Diseases Service. Oral ribavirin therapy for respiratory syncytial virus infections in moderately to severely immunocompromised patients. *Transpl Infect Dis.* 2014;16(2):242-250.
395. Marty F, Winston D, Rowley S, et al. CMX001 to prevent cytomegalovirus disease in hematopoietic-cell transplantation. *N Engl J Med.* 2013;369(13):1227.
407. McKinlay M, Collett M, Hincks J, et al. Progress in the development of poliovirus antiviral agents and their essential role in reducing risks that threaten eradication. *J Infect Dis.* 2014;210(suppl 1):S447-S453.
409. McMullan L, Flint M, Dyall J, et al. The lipid moiety of brincidofovir is required for in vitro antiviral activity against Ebola virus. *Antiviral Res.* 2016;125:71-78.
421. Modlin J. Treatment of neonatal enterovirus infections. *J Pediatric Infect Dis Soc.* 2016;5(1):6304.
429. Mullane K, Nuss C, Ridgeway J, et al. Brincidofovir treatment of acyclovir-resistant disseminated varicella zoster virus infection in an immunocompromised host. *Transpl Infect Dis.* 2016;18(5):785-790.
434. Nakamura S, Miyazaki T, Izumikawa K, et al. Efficacy and safety of intravenous peramivir compared with oseltamivir in high risk patients infected with influenza A and B viruses: a multicenter randomized controlled study. *Open Forum Infect Dis.* 2017;4(3):ofx129.
435. Natale F, Bizzari B, Cardi V, et al. Ganciclovir (valganciclovir) penetrates into the cerebrospinal fluid of an infant with congenital cytomegalovirus infection. *Ital J Pediatr.* 2015;41:26.
438. Neocleous C, Andonopoulou E, Adramerina A, et al. Tissue necrosis following extravasation of acyclovir in an adolescent: a case report. *Acta Med Acad.* 2017;46(1):55-58.
450. Olson V, Smith S, Foster S, et al. In vitro efficacy of brincidofovir against variola virus. *Antimicrob Agents Chemother.* 2014;58(9):5570-5571.
451. Otto W, Myers A, LaRussa B, et al. Clinical markers and outcomes of neonates with herpes simplex virus deoxyribonucleic acid persistence in cerebrospinal fluid in disseminated and central nervous system infection. *J Pediatric Infect Dis Soc.* 2017;[Epub ahead of print].
374. Lischka P, Michel D, Zimmermann H. Characterization of cytomegalovirus breakthrough events in a phase 2 prophylaxis trial of Letermovir (AIC246, MK 8228). *J Infect Dis.* 2016;213(1):23-30.
514. Schubert A, Ehlert K, Schuler-Luettmann S, et al. Fast selection of maribavir resistant cytomegalovirus in a bone marrow transplant recipient. *BMC Infect Dis.* 2013;13:330.
520. Shah D, Ghantoji S, Shah J, et al. Impact of aerosolized ribavirin on mortality in 280 allogeneic haematopoietic stem cell transplant recipients with respiratory syncytial virus infections. *J Antimicrob Chemother.* 2013;68(8):1872-1880.
579. Torres-Torres S, Myers A, Klatte J, et al. First use of investigational antiviral drug pocapavir (v-073) for treating neonatal enteroviral sepsis. *Pediatr Infect Dis J.* 2015;34(1):52-54.
586. Varela-Fascinetto G, Benchimol C, Reyes-Acevedo R, et al. Tolerability of up to 200 days of prophylaxis with valganciclovir oral solution and/or film-coated tablets in pediatric kidney transplant recipients at risk of cytomegalovirus disease. *Pediatr Transplant.* 2017;21(1).
604. Wester A, Shetty AK. Peramivir injection in the treatment of acute influenza: a review of the literature. *Infect Drug Resist.* 2016;9:201-214.
588. Voigt S, Hofman J, Edelmann A, et al. Brincidofovir clearance of acyclovir-resistant herpes simplex virus – 1 and adenovirus infection after stem cell transplantation. *Transpl Infect Dis.* 2016;18(5):791-794.
611. Wilhelmus K. Antiviral treatment and other therapeutic interventions for herpes simplex epithelial keratitis. *Cochrane Database Syst Rev.* 2015;(1):CD002898.
630. Zeller FA, Jackson AC. Critical appraisal of the Milwaukee protocol for rabies: this failed approach should be abandoned. *Can J Neurol Sci.* 2016;43(1):44-51.

The full reference list for this chapter is available at ExpertConsult.com.

Antifungal Agents

240

Andreas H. Groll • Thomas J. Walsh

Invasive fungal infections are important causes of morbidity and mortality in children with severe underlying illnesses. These infections remain difficult to diagnose and can be rapidly fatal. As a consequence, early and appropriate antifungal chemotherapy is pivotal for successful management and survival. For decades, options for antifungal chemotherapy were limited to amphotericin B deoxycholate (D-AmB) with or without the addition of flucytosine. The 1990s, however, witnessed major progress through the introduction of the antifungal triazoles fluconazole and itraconazole and the development of less toxic formulations of amphotericin B. More recent advances include the advent of novel, potent, and broad-spectrum antifungal triazoles and the clinical development of echinocandins, a distinct class of antifungal agents that target the fungal cell wall (Fig. 240.1). This chapter is devoted to the clinical pharmacology of systemic antifungal agents; emphasis is placed on pharmacokinetics, dosing, and safety in pediatric age groups.

AGENTS FOR TREATMENT OF INVASIVE MYCOSES

Polyene Antibiotics

Amphotericin B Deoxycholate

First isolated in the 1950s as a natural product of a soil actinomycete,[228] amphotericin B belongs to a family of approximately 200 polyene macrolide antibiotics and consists of seven conjugated double bonds, an internal ester, a free carboxyl group, and a glycoside side chain with a primary amino group (Fig. 240.2). The compound is amphoteric (capable of reacting as either an acid or a base), is not orally or intramuscularly absorbed, and is virtually insoluble in water. For parenteral use, amphotericin B has been solubilized with deoxycholate as a micellar suspension, and this formulation has been produced for more than 50 years and is available in several generic forms.[52] Current data indicate that these formulations are comparable in activity to the original deoxycholate formulation.[511]

Mechanism of action. Amphotericin B, similar to other polyenes, acts primarily by binding to ergosterol, the principal sterol in the cell membrane of most fungi. This interaction with ergosterol results in the formation of ion channels, loss of protons and monovalent cations, depolarization, and concentration-dependent cell death. Although with less avidity, the compound also binds to cholesterol, the main sterol of mammalian cell membranes; this action accounts for most of the toxicities associated with this drug. A second mechanism of action of amphotericin B may involve oxidative damage of the cell through a cascade of oxidative reactions linked to its own oxidation, with formation of free radicals or an increase in membrane permeability. In addition to its antifungal activity, amphotericin B and its lipid formulations differentially augment innate host defense mechanisms against fungal pathogens.[86,167,252,601,602]

Antifungal activity. Amphotericin B has a broad spectrum of antifungal activity that includes most fungi pathogenic in humans. True microbiologic resistance to antifungal polyenes has been associated with qualitative or quantitative differences in the sterol composition of the cell membrane, but this resistance also may be related to increased catalase activity with decreased susceptibility to oxidative damage.[252] Resistance to amphotericin B remains uncommon in *Candida* spp. other than *Candida lusitaniae, Candida guilliermondii,* and *Candida lipolytica.* Some isolates of *Candida glabrata, Candida parapsilosis,* and *Candida tropicalis* also may be resistant to amphotericin B.[662,685,720] *Aspergillus terreus*[313,623] and some of the emerging pathogens such as *Trichosporon asahii*[15,691,692] *Fusarium* spp.,[84,543] *Scedosporium apiospermum,*[639,694] *Lomentospora (Scedosporium) prolificans,*[63,405] and certain dematiaceous fungi[259] may be completely resistant to safely achievable serum concentrations of amphotericin B. Acquisition of secondary resistance is an uncommon occurrence and has not been a clinical problem.[251]

Pharmacodynamics. In time-kill studies, amphotericin B displays concentration-dependent fungicidal activity against susceptible *Candida albicans, Cryptococcus neoformans,* and *Aspergillus fumigatus.*[341,342,538] In addition to its concentration-dependent fungicidal dynamics, a prolonged postantifungal effect (PAFE) of amphotericin B of up to 12 hours' duration has been demonstrated in *C. albicans* and *C. neoformans.*[188,648] Studies in laboratory animals support the concentration-dependent kill kinetics of amphotericin B in vitro. In neutropenic pharmacokinetic and pharmacodynamic mouse models of disseminated candidiasis and pulmonary aspergillosis, peak plasma concentration (C_{max})/minimal inhibitory concentration (MIC) was the parameter that provided the best correlation with outcome as measured by the residual organismal burden in tissue.[27,718] These laboratory findings indicate that single daily doses rather than continuous infusion will be most effective. Therefore, the dosage of amphotericin B should not be uncritically reduced, and infusion for durations longer than that recommended by the manufacturer should be avoided.

Pharmacokinetics. After intravenous administration, amphotericin B rapidly dissociates from its carrier deoxycholate and becomes highly protein bound before distributing into tissues.[118] The disposition of the compound follows a three-compartment model, with rapid initial clearance from plasma followed by a biphasic pattern of elimination with a β half-life of 24 to 48 hours and a prolonged terminal (γ) half-life of 15 days or more.[40] Tissue levels of amphotericin B in laboratory animals are highest in liver, spleen, bone marrow, kidney, and lung; concentrations in body fluids other than plasma are generally low.[314,376] However, despite mostly undetectable concentrations in the cerebrospinal fluid (CSF) and comparatively low concentrations in brain tissue across all species, amphotericin B is effective in the treatment of fungal infections of the central nervous system (CNS). After administration of a single dose of 0.6 mg/kg to adult human volunteers, two-thirds of the parent was excreted unchanged in the urine (20.6%) and feces (42.5%) with more than 90% accounted for in mass balance calculations at 1 week, and no metabolites were observed by HPLC or mass spectrometry.[53,54,140,548] Accordingly, adjustment of dose is not necessary in patients with unrelated renal or hepatic dysfunction.

Reported pharmacokinetic data in pediatric age groups are characterized by a high interindividual variability, which may be related to differences in underlying diseases and modes of administration (Table 240.1).[44,61,351,470,615] However, infants and children appear to clear the drug from plasma more rapidly than do adults, as indicated by a negative correlation between age and clearance.[61,351,469] Because distribution into tissues appears to be the main route of clearance from plasma, the faster clearance in individuals of younger age may be explained by the larger relative volume of parenchymatous organs in contrast to that in adults.[459] Currently, dosage recommendations for all pediatric age groups do not differ from those in adult patients.

Adverse effects. Infusion-related reactions and dose-limiting nephrotoxicity are major problems associated with the use of D-AmB and often limit successful therapy.[83] Infusion-related reactions (i.e., fever, rigors, chills, myalgia, arthralgia, nausea, vomiting, and headaches) are thought to be mediated by the release of cytokines, particularly tumor necrosis factor-alpha (TNFα) from monocytes in response to the drug.[32] These reactions can be noted in as many as 73% of patients prospectively monitored at the bedside.[684] In a prospective interventional study of pediatric patients with cancer, investigators observed fever, rigors, or both associated with the infusion of D-AmB in 19 of 78 treatment courses (24%).[470] However, these characteristic adverse effects of

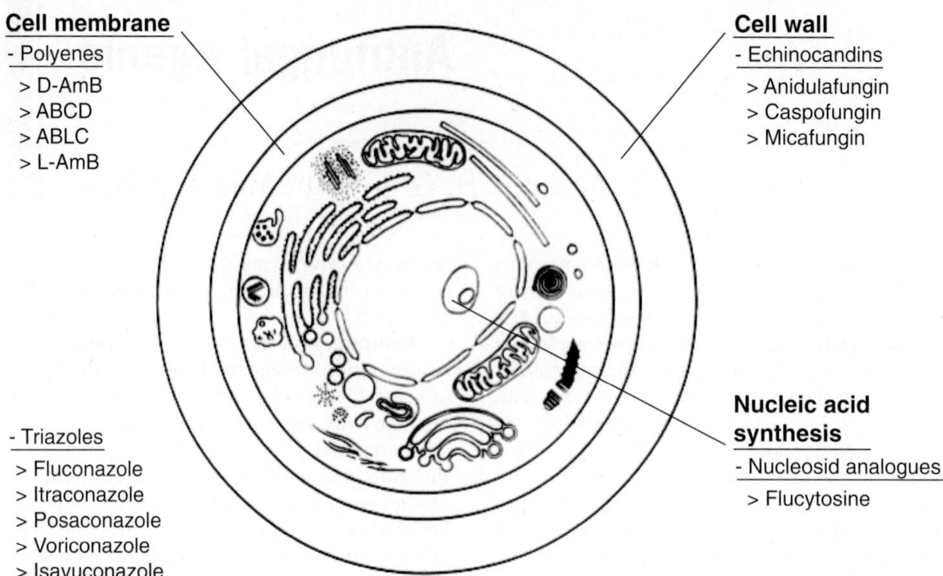

FIG. 240.1 Cellular targets of approved antifungal agents for treatment of invasive mycoses. (Modified from Groll AH, Piscitelli SC, Walsh TJ. Antifungal pharmacodynamics: concentration-effect relationships in vitro and in vivo. *Pharmacotherapy.* 2001;21[suppl 8]:133-148.)

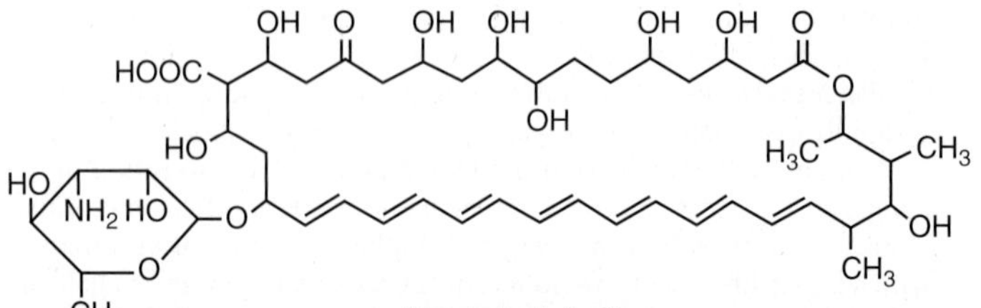

Amphotericin B

FIG. 240.2 Structural formula of amphotericin B.

TABLE 240.1 Pharmacokinetic Parameters of Amphotericin B Deoxycholate in Pediatric Patients[a]

Population/Reference	Dosage (mg/kg)	C_{max} (μg/mL)	$AUC_{0-\infty}$ (μg/mL/h)	Vd_{ss} (L/kg)	Cl (L/h/kg)	$t_{1/2}$ (h)
Preterm neonates[615] (*n* = 5, 0.5–7.5 mo)	1/md	0.96	NA	4.1	0.122	39
Preterm neonates[44] (*n* = 13, 0.06–1.8 mo)	0.5/md	0.96	NA	1.5	0.036	14.8
Infants/children[351] (*n* = 13, 0.08–18 y)	0.5/sd	1.5	NA	0.37	0.026	9.9
Infants/children[61] (*n* = 12, 0.3–14 y)	0.68/md	2.9	NA	0.76	0.027	18.1
Infants/children[470] (*n* = 20, 2.2–14.3 y)	0.98/sd	2.43	22.0	0.92	0.039	15.1
Children/adults[13] (*n* = 20, 4–66 y)	1/md	2.9	36	1.1	0.028	39

[a]All values are given as means.
$AUC_{0-\infty}$, Area under the concentration versus time curve from time zero to infinity; *Cl*, plasma clearance; *C_{max}*, peak plasma concentration; *md*, multiple-dose data; *NA*, not assessed; *sd*, single-dose data; *$t_{1/2}$*, elimination half-life; *Vd_{ss}*, apparent volume of distribution at steady state.

amphotericin B are observed only rarely in the neonatal setting.[338] In clinical practice, infusion-related reactions associated with amphotericin B therapy may be blunted by slowing the infusion rate but often require premedication with acetaminophen 10 to 15 mg/kg, hydrocortisone 0.5 to 1 mg/kg, or meperidine 0.2 to 0.5 mg/kg.[685] Less common acute adverse effects are hypotension, hypertension, flushing, and vestibular disturbances; bronchospasm and true anaphylaxis are rare occurrences.[251] Cardiac arrhythmias and cardiac arrest resulting from acute potassium release may occur with rapid infusion (<60 minutes), especially if the patient has preexisting hyperkalemia or renal impairment.[95,233,448]

The hallmarks of amphotericin B–associated dose-limiting nephrotoxicity are azotemia, wasting of potassium, and wasting of magnesium. The mechanisms of amphotericin B-induced nephrotoxicity have been recently reviewed.[396] Renal tubular acidosis and impaired urinary concentration ability rarely are of clinical significance.[230,575] Relevant electrolyte wasting occurs in approximately 12% of prospectively monitored patients.[684] Hypokalemia can be quite refractory to replacement until hypomagnesemia is corrected.[575] Azotemia is a common occurrence. In a large prospective clinical trial, the baseline serum creatinine rose by more than 100% in 34% of 344 unstratified pediatric and adult patients receiving D-AmB for empirical therapy of fever and neutropenia.[684] Azotemia can be exacerbated by concomitant nephrotoxic agents, in particular by cyclosporine and tacrolimus.[716] In series reporting safety data of D-AmB 0.5 to 1 mg/kg in premature neonates, the frequency of azotemia ranged from zero to 15%,[96,226,338,378,383] a finding indicating that the compound is much better tolerated in this setting than was reported early during its use.[43]

Nephrotoxicity associated with the use of amphotericin B has the potential to lead to renal failure and dialysis[722]; however, azotemia usually is reversible after discontinuation of the drug.[179,378,685] Avoiding concomitant nephrotoxic agents, appropriate hydration and normal saline loading (3 mEq Na^+/kg per day)[32,33,281] may greatly lessen the likelihood and severity of azotemia associated with amphotericin B therapy.

Other potentially relevant adverse effects of amphotericin B include a demyelinating encephalopathy[462] and normocytic, normochromic anemia associated with low erythropoietin levels after long-term administration.[141] Because D-AmB is topically irritating, a central line should be used for infusion, and local instillation of amphotericin B should be considered only in conjunction with expert consultation.

Therapeutic monitoring. Historically, 1-hour postinfusion plasma concentrations of twice the MIC of the fungal isolate have been proposed as targets for treatment of yeast infections.[176] However, monitoring of amphotericin B concentrations in plasma or CSF appears to be of little value because relationships between plasma and tissue concentrations and clinical efficacy or toxicity have not been adequately characterized.[251]

The toxicity of amphotericin B and the practice of normal saline loading warrant close monitoring of serum electrolytes, urea, and creatinine. D-AmB must not be infused in less than 60 minutes and only under particularly careful cardiac monitoring in newborns, as well as in patients with hyperkalemia and renal impairment, where arrhythmias resulting from acute potassium release may develop.[95,246]

Drug interactions. Drug-drug interactions caused by shared metabolic pathways are unknown for amphotericin B. Hypokalemia may be aggravated by diuretics and corticosteroids, cause rhabdomyolysis, and enhance the effects of nonpolarizing muscle relaxants. Similarly, hypomagnesemia may become especially profound in patients with cancer and chemotherapy-associated nephropathy. Impairment of glomerular filtration by amphotericin B may enhance plasma levels and, thereby, toxicity of many renally cleared drugs, including aminoglycosides, vancomycin, flucytosine, and cyclosporine.[251] Finally, the simultaneous infusion of granulocytes has been associated with acute pulmonary reactions,[730] and the two interventions should be chronologically separated as much as possible.

Indications. With the exception of resource-limited settings, few indications are left for antifungal treatment of opportunistic mycoses with D-AmB. These indications include candidemia and acute tissue-invasive candidiasis, particularly in neonates, and induction therapy for cryptococcal meningitis; however, in the absence of adequate clinical trials, D-AmB is still a valid option for treatment of severe forms of the endemic mycoses (Tables 240.2 to 240.4). Depending on both the type of infection and the host, the recommended daily dosage ranges from 0.7 to 1 mg/kg per day administered over 2 to 4 hours as tolerated.[251] Continuous infusion has no pharmacodynamic rationale,[27,718] no significant impact on renal toxicity,[197] and should not be used.

For empirical antifungal therapy in the persistently febrile neutropenic host, the historical standard dosage has been 0.5 to 0.6 mg/kg per day.[196,528] Efficacy of prophylactic intravenous amphotericin B in the setting of anticancer therapy has not been documented,[253] and a large, randomized, multicenter study failed to show any preventive benefit of aerosolized amphotericin B in neutropenic patients at high risk for developing invasive mold infections.[585] However, aerosolized amphotericin B may have a preventive role in patients who have undergone lung transplantation.[169]

On principle, treatment should be started at the full target dose, with careful bedside monitoring during the first hour of infusion to allow for prompt intervention for infusion-related reactions.[685] With the exception of uncomplicated candidemia and induction therapy of cryptococcal meningoencephalitis, the duration of treatment is ill defined for most infections.

Amphotericin B Lipid Formulations

During the late 1990s, three novel formulations of amphotericin B were approved in the United States and most of Europe: AmB colloidal dispersion (ABCD, Amphocil, or Amphotec), AmB lipid complex (ABLC or Abelcet), and a small unilamellar liposomal formulation (L-AmB, AmBisome). Because of their reduced nephrotoxicity in contrast to D-AmB, these compounds allow for the safer delivery of higher dosages of the parent molecule (amphotericin B). However, data from animal models also suggest that higher dosages are required for equivalent antifungal efficacy.[290,729]

Physicochemical properties and pharmacokinetics. The carriers of the lipid formulations are composed of biodegradable, amphiphilic bilayered membranes in which the hydrophilic heads of the lipid molecules face

TABLE 240.2 **Principal Options for Medical Management of Invasive Infections by Opportunistic Yeast**[a]

Fungal Disease	Management
Esophageal candidiasis	Fluconazole, itraconazole, voriconazole Caspofungin, micafungin Amphotericin B deoxycholate
Candidemia or invasive candidiasis	Fluconazole, voriconazole Caspofungin, micafungin Amphotericin B deoxycholate, liposomal amphotericin B *Second-line options:* One of the above with change in class Amphotericin B lipid complex Amphotericin B deoxycholate plus flucytosine
Cerebral cryptococcosis	Amphotericin B deoxycholate plus flucytosine, followed by fluconazole *Second-line options:* Amphotericin B deoxycholate plus fluconazole; fluconazole plus flucytosine; liposomal amphotericin B
Extracerebral manifestations	Fluconazole Amphotericin B deoxycholate ± flucytosine Liposomal amphotericin B

[a]In alphabetical order according to class (azoles/echinocandins/polyenes); for details, approval status, and age-specific dosages, see the text.

TABLE 240.3 **Principal Options for Medical Management of Invasive Infections by Opportunistic Molds**

Fungal Disease	Management[a]
Invasive aspergillosis	Voriconazole (isavuconazole)[b]
	Liposomal amphotericin B
	Second-line options:
	One of the above with change in class
	Posaconazole
	Caspofungin
	Amphotericin B lipid complex, amphotericin B deoxycholate
	Liposomal amphotericin B plus caspofungin
	Voriconazole plus caspofungin
	Consolidation therapy: Itraconazole, posaconazole, voriconazole
Non-*Aspergillus* hyalohyphomycetes	Voriconazole, posaconazole
	Liposomal amphotericin B, amphotericin B lipid complex, amphotericin B deoxycholate
Mucormycosis	Liposomal amphotericin B, amphotericin B lipid complex
	Second-line or consolidation:
	(Isavuconazole),[b] posaconazole
Dematiaceous molds	Voriconazole, posaconazole
	Liposomal amphotericin B, amphotericin B lipid complex, amphotericin B deoxycholate

[a]In alphabetical order according to class (azoles/echinocandins/polyenes); for details, approval status and age-specific dosages, see the text.
[b]Option for postpubertal adolescents; no pediatric dosage exists.

TABLE 240.4 **Principal Options for Medical Management of Invasive Infections by Endemic Molds**

Fungal Disease	Management[a]
Histoplasmosis	Liposomal amphotericin B followed by itraconazole
	Itraconazole[b]
	Secondary alternative options:
	Amphotericin B deoxycholate, amphotericin B lipid complex
	Fluconazole, posaconazole, voriconazole
Coccidioidomycosis	Amphotericin B deoxycholate, amphotericin B lipid complex, liposomal amphotericin B, followed by azoles
	Fluconazole[c]
	Itraconazole[b]
	Secondary alternative options:
	Posaconazole, voriconazole
Blastomycosis	Amphotericin B deoxycholate, followed by itraconazole
	Liposomal amphotericin B or amphotericin B lipid complex, followed by itraconazole
	Itraconazole[b]
	Secondary alternative options:
	Voriconazole
Paracoccidioidomycosis	Amphotericin B deoxycholate, amphotericin B lipid complex, liposomal amphotericin B
	Itraconazole,[b] voriconazole
Penicilliosis	Amphotericin B deoxycholate
	Itraconazole,[b] voriconazole
Sporotrichosis	Amphotericin B deoxycholate, followed by itraconazole
	Liposomal amphotericin B or amphotericin B lipid complex, followed by itraconazole
	Itraconazole[b]
	Terbinafine (lymphocutaneous disease only)

[a]In alphabetical order according to class (polyenes/azoles); for details and age-specific dosages, see the text.
[b]Clinically stable patients with mild to moderate disease and no central nervous system involvement, or as consolidation or maintenance therapy.
[c]Agent of first choice in (1) consolidation therapy of meningeal coccidioidomycosis, (2) *Coccidioides* meningitis, or (3) coccidioidomycosis in stable patients with mild-to-moderate disease or as consolidation or maintenance therapy.

outward to shield the hydrophobic tails. The membranes may form either spherical vesicles termed liposomes or bilayered complexes or dispersions with no specific vesicular structure. Incorporated into these water-soluble carriers, amphotericin B becomes soluble in plasma and available for distribution. Each of the lipid formulations of amphotericin B possesses distinct physicochemical and pharmacokinetic properties. All three, however, preferentially distribute to organs of the mononuclear phagocytic system (MPS) and functionally spare the kidney. Whereas the micellar dispersion of ABCD behaves kinetically very similarly to D-AmB, the small unilamellar liposomal preparation has a prolonged circulation time in plasma, achieves strikingly high C_{max} and area under the plasma concentration-time curve (AUC) values, and is taken up only slowly by the MPS. In contrast, the large, ribbon-like aggregates of ABLC are efficiently opsonized by plasma proteins and rapidly taken up by the MPS, thus resulting in lower peak plasma and AUC values (Table 240.5).[249,290] Whether and how the distinct physicochemical and pharmacokinetic features of each formulation translate into different pharmacodynamic properties in vivo is largely unknown. However, experimental head-to-head comparisons of all four formulations of amphotericin B against defined invasive mycoses suggest that important differences exist in antifungal efficacy depending on the agent, dose, type, and site of infection.[121,243,487]

TABLE 240.5 Physicochemical Properties and Multiple-Dose Pharmacokinetic Parameters of the Four Amphotericin B Formulations[a]

Properties and Parameters	D-AmB	ABCD	ABLC	L-AmB
Lipids (molar ratio)	Deoxycholate	Cholesteryl sulfate	DMPC/DMPG (7:3)	HPC/CHOL/DSPG (2:1:0.8)
Mol% AmB	34%	50%	50%	10%
Lipid configuration	Micelles	Micelles	Membrane-like	SUVs
Diameter (μm)	0.05	0.12-0.14	1.6-11	0.08
Dosage (mg AmB/kg)	1	5	5	5
C_{max} (μg/mL)	2.9	3.1	1.7	58
$AUC_{0-\infty}$ (μg/mL/h)	36	43	14	713
Vd_{ss} (L/kg)	1.1	4.3	131	0.22
Cl (L/h/kg)	0.028	0.117	0.476	0.017

[a]Data represent mean values, stem from adult patients, and were obtained after different rates of infusion.

$AUC_{0-\infty}$, Area under the concentration versus time curve from time zero to infinity; *CHOL*, cholesterol; *Cl*, plasma clearance; *C_{max}*, peak plasma concentration; *DMPC*, dimyristoyl phosphatidylcholine; *DMPG*, dimyristoyl phosphatidylglycerol; *DSPG*, distearoyl phosphatidylglycerol; *HPC*, hydrogenated phosphatidylcholine; *SUV*, small unilamellar vesicles; *Vd_{ss}*, apparent volume of distribution at steady state.

Modified from Groll AH, Muller FM, Piscitelli SC, et al. Lipid formulations of amphotericin B: clinical perspectives for the management of invasive fungal infections in children with cancer. *Klin Pädiatr.* 1998;210:264-273.

Safety and antifungal efficacy. Safety and antifungal efficacy of ABCD, ABLC, and L-AmB were demonstrated in an array of phase II and III clinical trials in immunocompromised, mostly adult patients with a wide spectrum of underlying disorders.[131,283,371,549,557,688,716,725] The overall response rates in these trials ranged from 53% to 84% in patients with invasive candidiasis and 34% to 59%, respectively, in patients with presumed or documented invasive aspergillosis.[249,290] A few randomized controlled trials were completed in which one of the newer formulations was compared with D-AmB. These studies consistently showed at least equivalent therapeutic efficacy and reduced nephrotoxicity of the investigated lipid formulation. Infusion-related side effects of fever, chills, and rigor were less frequent with L-AmB only.[19,83,684,715,714] Substernal chest discomfort, respiratory distress, and sharp flank pain may occur during infusion of L-AmB[322,552]; in comparative studies, hypoxic episodes associated with fever and chills occurred more frequently in ABCD recipients than in recipients of D-AmB.[85,715] Mild increases in serum bilirubin and alkaline phosphatase have been observed with all three formulations, as well as mild increases in serum transaminases with L-AmB. Nevertheless, no case of fatal liver disease has occurred.[249,290,729] An increased rate of hyperphosphatemia has been reported for L-AmB[343]; however, true hyperphosphatemia has to be carefully differentiated from pseudohyperphosphatemia that is due to interferences of L-AmB with assay systems for determination of serum phosphorus.[318,446]

Experience in pediatric patients. Considerable numbers of pediatric patients have been treated with ABCD, ABLC, or L-AmB on protocols in the clinical trials cited earlier.[617] Separately published pediatric data are discussed in the following subsections.

ABCD. ABCD is a complex of amphotericin B and sodium cholesteryl sulfate in an approximate 1:1 molar ratio that forms disklike colloidal structures on dissolution.[249] Estimated pharmacokinetic parameters in children are not significantly different from those in adult patients under conditions of steady state: mean AUC from 0 to 24 hours (AUC_{0-24}) is 7.10 mg/L/h (normalized to a 1-mg/kg per day dose); mean volume of distribution (V_d) is 4.57 L/kg, and mean total clearance (Cl) is 0.144 L/h/kg.[13]

A double-blind, randomized trial comparing ABCD (4 mg/kg per day) with D-AmB (0.8 mg/kg per day) for empirical antifungal therapy of febrile neutropenic patients that also included a larger number of pediatric patients found that ABCD was as effective but significantly less nephrotoxic than D-AmB.[715] Among children (0–15 years; mean, 8.8 years) with presumed or proved invasive fungal infections refractory to or intolerant of amphotericin B who were treated on five different open-label studies of ABCD with dosages that ranged from 0.8 to 7.5 mg/kg (mean, 4.5 mg/kg), 67% of patients reported infusion-related reactions, but nephrotoxicity, defined as an increase in serum creatinine to 2 times or more of the baseline value, was reported in only 12%.[570]

The published experience in the neonatal setting is limited to 16 infants with very low birth weight (779 ± 170 g; 25 ± 2 weeks) with invasive candidiasis and a serum creatinine concentration of 1.2 mg/dL or greater.[393] Infants received 3 mg/kg ABCD on day 1, followed by 5 mg/kg per day thereafter; a second agent was permitted for candidemia that persisted for 7 or more days. Of 14 evaluable patients, 13 cleared the organism after therapy with ABCD alone ($n = 8$) or in combination with another agent ($n = 5$), and overall survival was 75%.

These data overall indicate no fundamental differences in disposition, safety, and antifungal efficacy of ABCD in contrast to adult populations. The US Food and Drug Administration (FDA)-approved indication has been treatment of probable or proven invasive aspergillosis refractory to or intolerant of D-AmB, and the approved dosage was 3 to 4 mg/kg per day, administered over the course of 2 hours. Marketing of ABCD has been discontinued in the United States and most of Europe due to a higher rate of infusion-related reactions relative to D-AmB in controlled clinical trials[85,716] and the existence of better tolerated alternatives.

ABLC. ABLC is composed of dimyristoyl phosphatidylcholine/dimyristoyl phosphatidylglycerol (DMPC/DMPG) in a 1:1 molar ratio of lipid to amphotericin B and forms large, ribbon-like structures. The pharmacokinetic properties of ABLC were studied in whole blood in three pediatric patients with cancer who received the compound at 2.5 mg/kg over the course of 6 weeks for hepatosplenic candidiasis.[698] Steady state was achieved by day 7 of therapy; after the final dose, the mean AUC_{0-24} was 11.9 ± 2.6 mg/L/h, the mean C_{max} was 1.69 ± 0.75 mg/L, and clearance was 0.218 L/kg/h. In the six patients evaluable for safety assessment, mean serum creatinine levels were stable at the end of therapy and at 1-month follow-up and no increase in hepatic transaminases occurred. Five of the patients had infusion-related reactions to the first dose, which were prospectively monitored without prior premedication; however, infusion-related adverse reactions were well controlled thereafter by conventional premedications. All evaluable patients responded to therapy.

Safety and antifungal efficacy of ABLC were studied in 111 treatment episodes in pediatric patients (21 days to 16 years of age) refractory to or intolerant of conventional antifungal agents through an open-label, emergency-use protocol in the United States.[696] ABLC was administered at a mean daily dosage of 4.85 mg/kg (range, 1.1–9.5 mg/kg per day) for a mean duration of 38.9 days (range, 1–198 days). The mean serum creatinine for the entire study population did not significantly change between baseline (1.23 ± 0.11 mg/dL) and cessation of ABLC therapy (1.32 ± 0.12 mg/dL) over 6 weeks. No significant differences were observed between baseline and end-of-therapy levels of serum potassium, magnesium, hepatic transaminases, alkaline phosphatase, and hemoglobin. Among 54 cases fulfilling criteria for evaluation of antifungal efficacy, a complete or partial therapeutic response was obtained in 38 patients (70%).

The safety and efficacy of ABLC also were assessed in 548 children and adolescents who were enrolled in the Collaborative Exchange of Antifungal Research registry. Most patients were either intolerant of or refractory to conventional antifungal therapy. Response data were evaluable for 255 of the 285 patients with documented single or multiple pathogens. A complete (cured) or partial (improved) response was achieved in 54.9% of patients. No significant difference was noted between the rates of new hemodialysis versus baseline hemodialysis. Elevations in serum creatinine of greater than 1.5 times baseline and greater than 2.5 times baseline values were seen in 24.8% and 8.8% of all patients, respectively. The overall response rate and safety profile in pediatric patients were consistent with earlier reported findings of smaller trials.[719]

Eleven infants age 6 months and younger with candidemia were enrolled in the US open-label, emergency-use protocol.[696] Of the 11 patients, 7 maintained a stable mean serum creatinine; in 4 patients, a rise in serum creatinine was observed, but in each case, the increase was less than 40% of the baseline value. No differences were observed between baseline and end-of-therapy mean bilirubin levels. Among the 8 evaluable infants, a complete response was observed in 6 (75%). A population pharmacokinetic study in 28 mostly premature neonates with invasive *Candida* infections demonstrated that the disposition of ABLC in neonates is similar to that observed in other age groups; weight was the only factor that influenced clearance.[731] The safety of ABLC in neonates is further supported by a retrospective case-control study in 35 infants with very low birth weight who received the compound for at least 2 weeks; treatment with ABLC was well tolerated and did not increase serum creatinine or decrease potassium.[41]

The current data suggest no fundamental differences in disposition, safety, and antifungal efficacy of ABLC in contrast to adults. The FDA-approved indication is treatment of invasive fungal infections refractory to or intolerant of D-AmB, and the approved dosage is 5 mg/kg per day administered over the course of 2 hours.

L-AmB. L-AmB (AmBisome) consists of small, unilamellar spherical vesicles (true liposomes) composed of hydrogenated soy phosphatidylcholine and distearoyl phosphatidylglycerol stabilized by cholesterol and combined with amphotericin B in a 2 : 0.8 : 1 : 0.4 molar ratio.[249] Of note, a number of generic liposomal formulations of amphotericin B of various compositions exist in low- and middle-income countries.[7] However, these agents are pharmacologically not interchangeable with L-AmB in the form of AmBisome. The pharmacokinetic properties of L-AmB in pediatric patients beyond the neonatal period were investigated in a formal phase II, dose-escalation trial investigating dosages of 2.5, 5, and 7.5 mg/kg in immunocompromised patients, as well as by using a population-based approach. The results of these studies indicate that the disposition of L-AmB in pediatric patients is not substantially different from that in adults and that weight is a covariate that determines clearance and volume of distribution.[294,590] A pharmacokinetic pilot study was conducted in 12 children at risk for developing invasive fungal infections who received once-weekly, high-dose L-AmB (10 mg/kg over 2 hours) as prophylaxis. L-AmB was well tolerated and showed measurable amphotericin B plasma concentrations 7 days after the dose.[433] Similarly, among a cohort of 46 high-risk patients who received L-AmB as prophylaxis at a dosage of 2.5 mg/kg twice weekly, measurable plasma concentrations were observed at the end of the dosing interval.[77] These findings suggest that once weekly[272,433] as well as twice weekly[77] administration may provide useful protection against fungal infections.

Many pediatric patients have been enrolled in clinical trials with L-AmB but have not been reported separately.[438,684] Two hundred four children (mean age, 7 years) with neutropenia and fever of unknown origin were randomized in an open-label, multicenter trial to receive conventional D-AmB at 1 mg/kg per day ($n = 63$), L-AmB at 1 mg/kg per day ($n = 70$), or L-AmB at 3 mg/kg per day ($n = 71$) for empirical antifungal therapy.[531] Twenty-nine percent of patients treated with L-AmB 1, 39% of patients treated with L-AmB 3, and 54% of patients treated with D-AmB experienced adverse effects ($P = .01$); nephrotoxicity, defined as 100% or more increase in serum creatinine from baseline, was noted in 8%, 11%, and 21%, respectively (not significant [NS]). Hypokalemia (<2.5 mmol/L) occurred in 10%, 11%, and 26% of patients, respectively ($P = .02$); increases in serum transaminase levels (≥110 U/L) occurred in 17%, 23%, and 17%, respectively (NS); and increases in serum bilirubin (≥35 μmol/L) occurred in 11%, 12%, and 10% of patients, respectively. L-AmB at either 1 or 3 mg/kg per day was significantly safer and at least equivalent to D-AmB with regard to resolution of fever of unknown origin. L-AmB was well tolerated and effective in cohorts of immunocompromised children requiring antifungal therapy for proved or suspected infections, including patients with bone marrow transplants for primary immunodeficiencies[503] patients with cancer[100,550] and critically ill patients.[599] A phase IV analysis of 141 courses of L-AmB administered for a mean of 17 days' duration at a mean maximum dosage of 2.5 mg/kg for various indications to pediatric patients with cancer and hematopoietic stem cell transplantation (HSCT) revealed a low rate of adverse events (4%), necessitating discontinuation. Whereas mean aspartate transaminase, alanine transaminase, alkaline phosphatase, and bilirubin values were slightly higher at the end of treatment ($P = .01$), bilirubin and creatinine values were not different from baseline.[348]

L-AmB 2.5 to 7 mg/kg per day was evaluated prospectively in 24 infants with very low birth weight (mean birth weight, 847 ± 244 g; mean gestational age, 26 weeks) with systemic candidiasis. The mean duration of therapy was 21 days; the cumulative L-AmB dose was 94 mg/kg. Fungal eradication was achieved in 92% of the episodes; 20 (83%) infants were considered clinically cured at the end of treatment. No major adverse effects were recorded. One infant developed increased bilirubin and hepatic transaminase levels during therapy. Four (17%) infants died; in 2 of them (8%), the cause of death was attributed directly to systemic candidiasis.[326] In a second study undertaken by the same investigators, high-dose (5–7 mg/kg per day) L-AmB was evaluated prospectively in 41 episodes of systemic candidiasis occurring in 37 neonates (36 of 37 were premature infants with very low birth weights). Twenty-eight, five, and eight infants received 7, 6 to 6.5, and 5 mg/kg per day, respectively. Median duration of therapy was 18 days; median cumulative dose was 94 mg/kg. Fungal eradication was achieved in 39 of 41 (95%) episodes. Fungal eradication was achieved more rapidly in patients treated early with high doses and in patients who received high-dose L-AmB as first-line therapy.[325] Further prospective[37] and retrospective[416] cohort studies attest to the safety of L-AmB in infants with very low birth weight. Of note, the higher mortality reported in a single center analysis for infants with invasive candidiasis treated with lipid formulations relative to conventional D-AmB or fluconazole[39] is likely due to differences in acuity of illnesses and comorbidities rather than pharmacokinetic considerations.

Current data indicate no substantial differences in pharmacokinetics and pharmacodynamics of L-AmB between pediatric and adult patients. The FDA-approved dosages are 3 mg/kg per day (empirical antifungal therapy in febrile neutropenic patients), 3 to 5 mg/kg per day (therapy of invasive infections intolerant or refractory to D-AmB), 6 mg/kg per day for cryptococcal meningitis, and 3 mg/kg on days 1 through 5, 14, and 21 for immunocompetent and 4 mg/kg on days 1 through 5, 10, 17, 24, 31, and 38 for immunocompromised patients with visceral leishmaniasis, administered over the course of 2 hours. In Europe, L-AmB is approved for first-line treatment of invasive mycoses, empirical antifungal therapy, and treatment of leishmaniasis.

Indications. The lipid formulations of AmB have been a major advance in the management of invasive opportunistic fungal infections in immunocompromised patients. All three compounds have less renal toxicity than conventional amphotericin B, as defined by development of azotemia; distal tubular toxicity also may be somewhat reduced. Infusion-related reactions of fever, chills, and rigor occur substantially less frequently only with L-AmB, and no new toxicities have been noted. The available pharmacokinetic and safety data from children so far indicate no fundamental differences from data obtained in the adult population.

Therapeutically, the lipid formulations are at least as effective as is conventional amphotericin B deoxycholate for treatment of most opportunistic human mycoses, and these formulations can be effective if conventional amphotericin B has failed. The specific clinical indications of the lipid formulations are discussed in the respective fungal disease chapters and are summarized in Tables 240.2 to 240.4.

Flucytosine

Flucytosine (5-fluorocytosine [5-FC]; Ancobon; Ancotil; and generic) is a low-molecular-weight, water-soluble, synthetic fluorinated pyrimidine analogue (Fig. 240.3). It is taken up into the fungal cell by the fungus-specific enzyme cytosine permease and is converted in the cytoplasm by cytosine deaminase to 5-fluorouracil, a potent antimetabolite that causes RNA miscoding and inhibits DNA synthesis at the level of thymidylate synthase (Fig. 240.4).[170] Flucytosine is relatively nontoxic to mammalian cells because of the absence or very low level of activity of cytosine deaminase. In the United States, flucytosine is available only as an oral formulation; an intravenous formulation is available outside the United States in select countries.

Antifungal activity. The antifungal activity of flucytosine in vitro is essentially limited to *Candida* spp., *C. neoformans, Cryptococcus gattii, Saccharomyces cerevisiae, Rhodotorula* spp., and some dematiaceous molds.[159,205,219,292,518,520,642] Flucytosine generally is thought to have no or weak activity against *Aspergillus* spp. and other hyaline molds,[217,419] although this lack of activity in vitro may be pH dependent[626] and does not correlate with the documented efficacy in animal models.[628] Notably, whereas *Candida krusei* appears to be less susceptible to flucytosine, the compound is highly active against *C. glabrata.*[170,205,518] Synergistic or additive effects in combination with amphotericin B have been observed against *Candida*[431,450] and *Aspergillus* spp.[627] and in combination with amphotericin B, fluconazole, voriconazole, and posaconazole against *C. neoformans.*[47,271,432,477,586] Combination with echinocandins was additive or indifferent in vitro against *Candida* spp.[328]

Two mechanisms of resistance have been reported: (1) mutations in enzymes necessary for cellular uptake and transport of flucytosine or its metabolism and (2) increased synthesis of pyrimidine that competes with the fluorinated antimetabolites of the compound.[162,671] In pretreatment isolates, intrinsically resistant strains have been found in 3% to 8% of *C. albicans,* in 0% to 8% of non-*albicans Candida* spp., and in 2% or fewer of *C. neoformans* isolates.[432,518] In an analysis of 8803 clinical isolates comprising 18 *Candida* spp. obtained from more than 200 medical centers worldwide, primary resistance to flucytosine was an uncommon occurrence among *Candida* spp. (95% sensitive, 2% intermediate, and 3% resistant), with the exception of *C. krusei* (5% sensitive, 67% intermediate, and 28% resistant).[518] Development of resistance to flucytosine can be observed during treatment,[205] and it is thought to be caused predominantly by selection of resistant clones.[671]

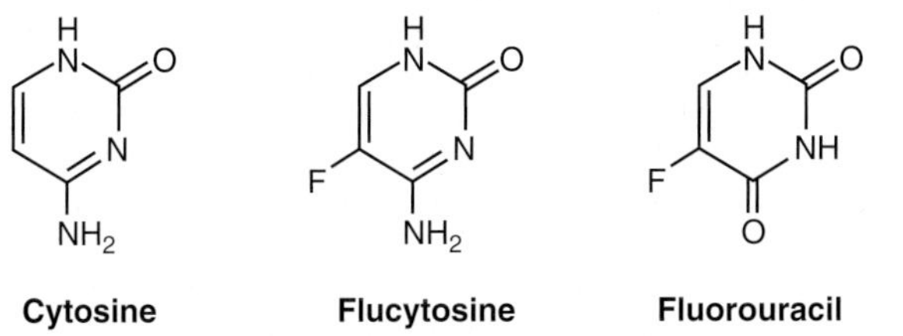

Cytosine **Flucytosine** **Fluorouracil**

FIG. 240.3 Structural formulas of cytosine, flucytosine, and fluorouracil.

As a consequence, flucytosine is rarely given alone but instead is given in combination with amphotericin B or fluconazole.

Pharmacodynamics. Time-kill assays against *Candida* spp. and *C. neoformans* demonstrated a predominantly concentration-independent fungistatic (99% reduction in colony-forming units) activity of flucytosine at concentrations exceeding the MIC of the investigated isolates.[389,655] A prolonged PAFE against these organisms was noted consistently that was dependent on concentration and duration of exposure and ranged from 0.8 to 10 hours.[441,577,578,740] Investigation of pharmacokinetic and pharmacodynamic relationships in a neutropenic mouse model of disseminated candidiasis that used the residual fungal burden in kidney tissue as the endpoint of antifungal efficacy revealed that both the time above the MIC and the AUC/MIC ratio were important in predicting efficacy; maximal efficacy was observed when levels exceeded the MIC for only 20% to 25% of the 24-hour dosing interval.[29] In experiments that used a pharmacodynamic model of disseminated candidiasis and bridging to humans by population pharmacokinetics and Monte Carlo simulation, an in vivo drug exposure breakpoint for flucytosine was apparent when serum levels were greater than the MIC for 45% of the dosing interval. The Monte Carlo simulations suggested that, using a human dose of 100 mg/kg per day in four divided doses, flucytosine resistance was defined at an MIC of 32 mg/L. Target attainment rates after administration of 25, 50, and 100 mg/kg per day were similar.[301] These data collectively suggest that lower dosages or less frequent dosing may yield identical antifungal efficacy while further reducing potential toxicities of flucytosine that are thought to be concentration dependent.[205]

Pharmacokinetics. Flucytosine is absorbed readily from the gastrointestinal tract, and oral bioavailability exceeds 80% (Table 240.6). C_{max} occurs 1 to 2 hours after administration. As a water-soluble compound, flucytosine has negligible protein binding (4%) and is widely distributed in the body, with a volume of distribution that approximates that of total body water. Mean CSF concentrations usually are 65% to 90% of simultaneous plasma concentrations. The drug penetrates well into peritoneal fluid, inflamed joints, and other fluid compartments, including the eye.[72,141,251]

In humans, less than 1% of a given dose of flucytosine is thought to undergo hepatic metabolism.[410] Some evidence suggests that bacteria of the gastrointestinal flora deaminate flucytosine to resorbable 5-fluorouracil,[274,411] a finding that may account for some of the toxicities observed after oral administration of the drug. Approximately 95% of a given dose of flucytosine is excreted into the urine in unchanged, active form by simple glomerular filtration.[251] Because the compound's elimination parallels the glomerular filtration rate, adjustment of the dosage is necessary in patients with impaired renal function.[144] In patients undergoing hemodialysis, a dose of 37.5 mg/kg is recommended after dialysis; in those undergoing hemofiltration, the dosage needs to be adjusted to the individual filtration rate.[312,374] In peritoneal dialysis, the compound can be administered systemically or intraperitoneally.[440]

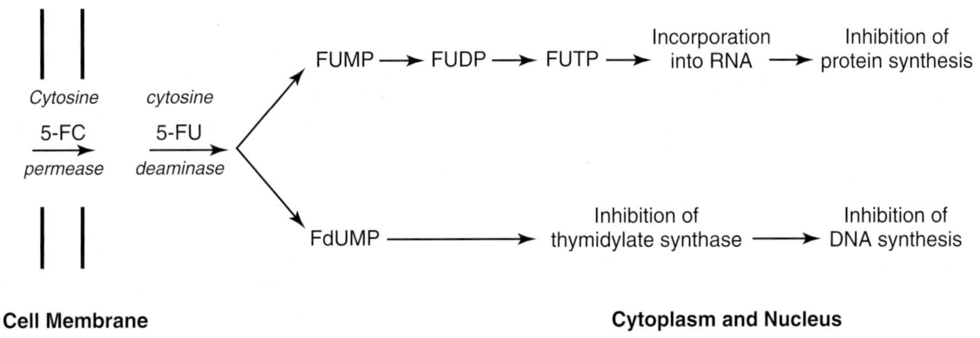

Cytosine permease: 5-FC → ; cytosine deaminase: 5-FU →

FUMP → FUDP → FUTP → Incorporation into RNA → Inhibition of protein synthesis

FdUMP → Inhibition of thymidylate synthase → Inhibition of DNA synthesis

Cell Membrane **Cytoplasm and Nucleus**

FIG. 240.4 Schematic of intracellular pathways and mechanism of action of flucytosine. *5-FC,* Flucytosine; *FdUMP,* 5-fluorodeoxyuridine monophosphate; *5-FU,* 5-fluorouracil; *FUDP,* 5-fluoridine diphosphate; *FUMP,* 5-fluoridine monophosphate; *FUTP,* 5-fluoridine triphosphate. (Modified from Groll AH, Piscitelli SC, Walsh TJ. Antifungal pharmacodynamics: concentration-effect relationships in vitro and in vivo. *Pharmacotherapy.* 2001;21[suppl. 8]:133-148; and Vermes A, Guchelaar HJ, Dankert, J. Flucytosine: a review of its pharmacology, clinical indications, pharmacokinetics, toxicity and drug interactions. *J Antimicrob Chemother.* 2000;46:171-179.)

TABLE 240.6 Pharmacokinetics of Flucytosine in Adults

Parameter or Characteristic	Value
Oral bioavailability	≥80%
C_{max}	50–120 µg/mL[a]
T_{max}	1-2 h
Protein binding	4%
Vd_{ss}	0.6–0.7 L/kg
$t_{1/2}\beta$	3–6 h
Clearance	≥95% renal
Unchanged drug in urine	≥95%
Relative cerebrospinal fluid levels	65–90%

[a]At steady state in patients with cryptococcal meningitis receiving 4 × 2 g/day orally.
Modified from Groll AH, Piscitelli SC, Walsh TJ. Antifungal pharmacodynamics: concentration-effect relationships in vitro and in vivo. *Pharmacotherapy*. 2001;21(suppl 8):133-148.
C_{max}, Peak plasma concentration; T_{max}, time until occurrence of peak plasma concentration; Vd_{ss}, volume of distribution at steady state.

Although the data are limited, impaired liver function does not appear to alter the disposition of flucytosine.[141]

In infants and children, the pharmacokinetic properties of flucytosine have not been systematically characterized. However, because of very similar physicochemical and pharmacokinetic properties, developmental changes in disposition similar to those found with fluconazole can be anticipated. Indeed, a similarly marked interindividual variability in clearance and volume of distribution has been reported in neonates[44] that renders uniform dosing recommendations in this population impossible.

A starting dosage for both adults and children of 100 mg/kg daily divided into three or four doses is recommended currently. Monitoring of plasma concentrations is essential to adjust dosage to changing renal function and avoid toxicity. After oral administration, near peak levels 2 hours after dosing overlap with trough levels as patients reach steady state, and thus these levels are sufficient for therapeutic monitoring.[205] In practice, plasma levels between 40 (trough) and less than 100 mg/L (peak) correlate with antifungal efficacy and seldom are associated with hematologic adverse effects.[205,672] However, retrospective evaluations in the United Kingdom revealed that only a fraction of plasma levels ordered for therapeutic monitoring were in this concentration range.[504,613]

Adverse effects. Common adverse effects associated with flucytosine that occur in 5% to 6% of patients include gastrointestinal intolerance and reversible elevations of hepatic transaminases and alkaline phosphatase. Rarer side effects are skin rashes, blood eosinophilia, and crystalluria.[251] Hematologic adverse effects have been reported in overall 6% of patients receiving oral flucytosine and may include neutropenia, thrombocytopenia, or pancytopenia. Notably, hematologic adverse effects occur less frequently if plasma levels of flucytosine do not exceed 100 mg/L.[205,251]

Drug interactions. Orally administered, nonresorbable antibiotics and administration of aluminum-based or magnesium hydroxide–based antacids may delay but do not impair absorption of the compound from the gastrointestinal tract.[251] 5-FC undergoes only minor hepatic metabolism, and it is not known to interfere with the cytochrome P (CYP)450 enzyme system. However, any drug that can cause a reduction in the glomerular filtration rate may lead to increased flucytosine serum levels and thereby has the potential to enhance 5-FC–associated toxicity. This phenomenon almost invariably is encountered with concomitant administration of amphotericin B, but it can occur similarly with numerous antimicrobial agents, anticancer drugs, and cyclosporine, to name only the most common examples.[141] The anticancer drug cytosine arabinoside (Ara-C) competitively inhibits the action of 5-FC, and these drugs should not be given concomitantly.[99]

Clinical indications. Because of the propensity of susceptible organisms to develop resistance in vitro,[529] 5-FC traditionally is not administered as a single agent. Ample laboratory and clinical experience exists regarding the combination of D-AmB and 5-FC (see Table 240.2).[170,251,671] Randomized clinical trials established the use of D-AmB in combination with 5-FC as standard for induction therapy of cryptococcal meningitis in non–human immunodeficiency virus (HIV)-infected and HIV-infected patients.[59,657] In a recent large randomized three-arm clinical trial in HIV-infected patients with cryptococcal meningitis, D-AmB 1 mg/kg per day plus 5-FC 100 mg/kg per day, as compared with D-AmB alone, was associated with improved survival.[142] Treatment with D-AmB plus 5-FC in this[142] and a previous small but well-designed trial[89] was associated with significantly increased rates of yeast clearance from cerebrospinal fluid, indicating that the combination of D-AmB and 5-FC is the most rapidly fungicidal regimen.[89] While controlled data for standard doses of ABLC are limited,[595] L-AmB has been shown to be equally effective to D-AmB at doses of 3 and 6 mg/kg and day,[269] and pharmacokinetic/pharmacodynamic bridging from a murine model of cryptococcal meningoencephalitis suggests near maximum efficacy with a dosage of 6 mg/kg per day of L-AMB or the combination of L-AmB 3 mg/kg per day plus 5-FC.[483]

Although no comparative trials have been performed, the cumulative clinical experience supports the combination of amphotericin B with 5-FC for the treatment of *Candida* infections involving deep tissues, particularly in critically ill patients and when non-*albicans Candida* spp. are involved.[205,303,420,631] This includes *Candida* meningitis, endophthalmitis, endocarditis, vasculitis, and peritonitis, as well as osteoarticular, renal, and disseminated candidiasis.[251,685]

The combination of 5-FC with fluconazole is an option for cryptococcal meningitis, when treatment with conventional or liposomal amphotericin B is not feasible.[373,442,444,481] Options for situations when 5-FC is not available include monotherapy with amphotericin B or the combination of amphotericin B and fluconazole.[142,400] The combination of 5-FC and fluconazole also may be useful as second-line therapy for individual patients with invasive *Candida* infections involving aqueous body compartments.

Antifungal Triazoles

The antifungal azoles are a class of synthetic compounds that have one or more azole rings and—attached to one of the nitrogen atoms—a more or less complex side chain. Whereas the imidazoles have two nitrogen atoms, the triazoles have three in the five-member ring. The triazole ring confers improved resistance to metabolic degradation, greater target specificity, and an expanded spectrum of activity.[236,235] The imidazoles miconazole and ketoconazole were the first azole compounds developed for systemic treatment of human mycoses. Severe toxicities associated with the drug carrier (miconazole) and erratic absorption and significant interference with the human CYP450 system (ketoconazole), however, limited their clinical usefulness.[251] The triazoles fluconazole and itraconazole (Fig. 240.5), in contrast, have become extremely useful components of the antifungal armamentarium. Overall, they are well tolerated and possess a broad spectrum of activity. Whereas fluconazole and itraconazole have been available since the 1990s, a next generation of antifungal triazoles entered clinical practice a decade ago; these so-called second-generation triazoles include voriconazole, posaconazole, and isavuconazole (Fig. 240.6).[293]

Mechanism of action. The antifungal azoles, as a class, target ergosterol biosynthesis by inhibiting the fungal CYP450-dependent enzyme lanosterol 14-α-demethylase. This inhibition interrupts the conversion of lanosterol to ergosterol and thus leads to accumulation of aberrant 14-α-methylsterols and depletion of ergosterol in the fungal cell membrane (Fig. 240.7). These effects alter cell membrane properties and function and, depending on organism and compound, may lead to cell death or inhibition of cell growth and replication. In addition, the azoles also inhibit CYP450-dependent enzymes of the fungal respiration chain, but the contribution of this action to their overall activity is unclear. Interaction with structurally similar mammalian CYP450-dependent enzyme systems is responsible for most toxicities and drug interactions of this class of compounds.[251,663]

Antifungal activity. Fluconazole and itraconazole are active principally against dermatophytes, *Candida* spp., *C. neoformans, C. gattii, T. asahii*, and other uncommon yeast organisms, as well as against dimorphic fungi such as *Histoplasma capsulatum, Coccidioides* spp., *Blastomyces*

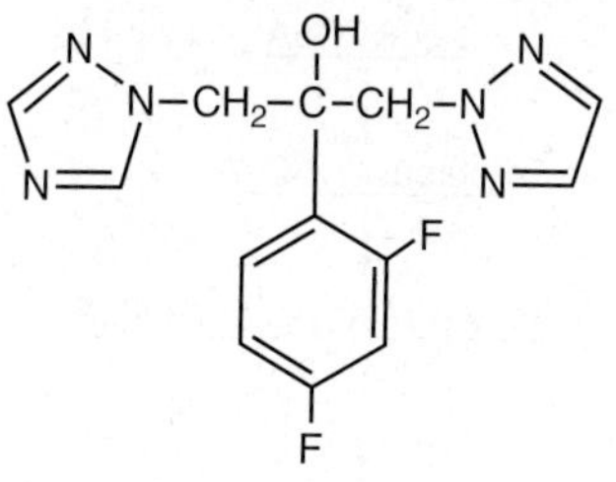

Fluconazole

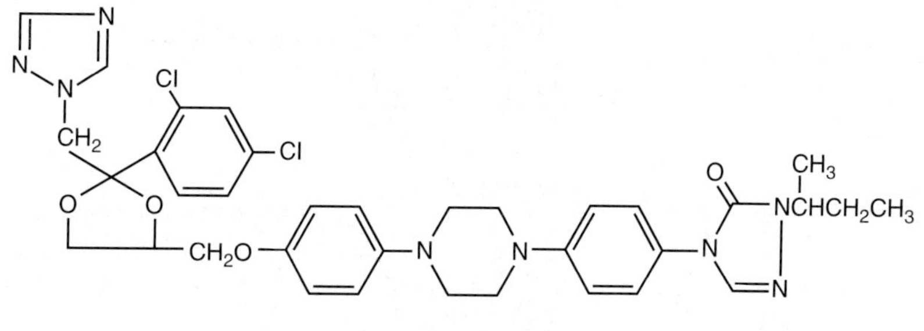

Itraconazole

FIG. 240.5 Structural formulas of the first-generation systemic antifungal triazoles fluconazole and itraconazole.

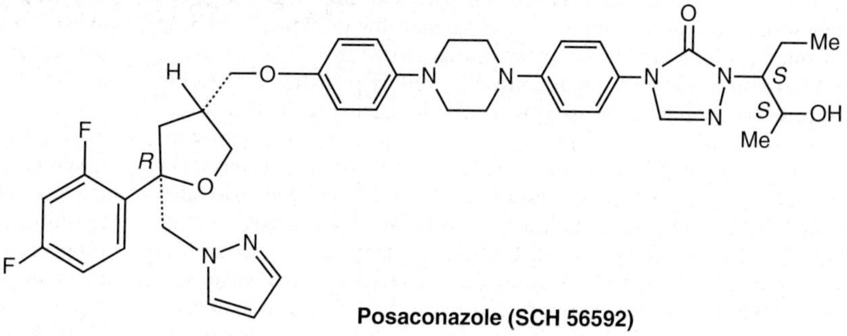

Posaconazole (SCH 56592)

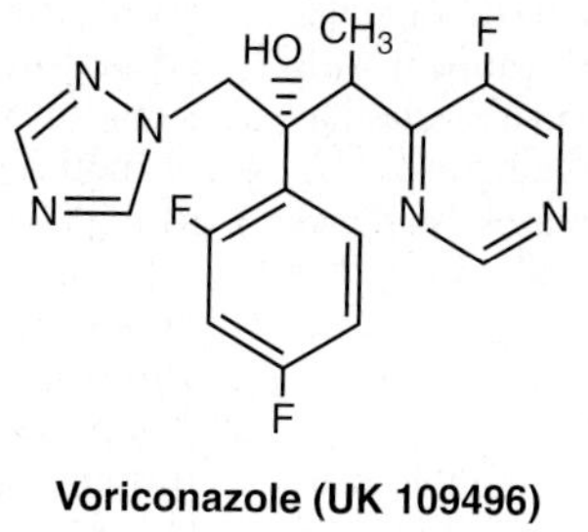

Voriconazole (UK 109496)

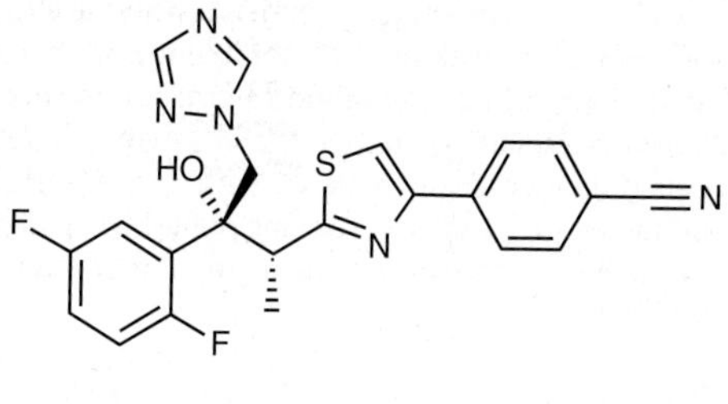

Isavuconazole (BAL4815)

FIG. 240.6 Structural formulas of the second-generation systemic antifungal triazoles posaconazole, voriconazole, and isavuconazole.

dermatitidis, Paracoccidioides brasiliensis, and *Sporothrix schenkii.*[236,235,642] These drugs have less activity against *C. glabrata* and none against *C. krusei.*[251,546] Clinically useful activity against *Aspergillus* spp. and dematiaceous molds is restricted to itraconazole, and both itraconazole and fluconazole are considered inactive against *Fusarium* spp. and the Mucorales.[251] The second-generation triazoles voriconazole, posaconazole, and isavuconazole have enhanced target activity and are active against a wide spectrum of clinically important fungi, including *Candida* spp., *T. asahii, C. neoformans, Aspergillus* spp., *Fusarium* spp., and other hyaline molds, as well as dematiaceous and dimorphic molds.[8,111,116,119,251,293] In contrast to fluconazole and itraconazole, all are active against *C. glabrata* and *C. krusei;* posaconazole and isavuconazole also are active against Mucorales, a feature that distinguishes it from all other azole compounds.[260]

Resistance. Several mechanisms of azole resistance in *Candida* spp. have been identified and include, but are not limited to, molecular alterations at the target binding site, increased target expression, and induction of cellular efflux pumps.[49,521,571,714] In contrast to pathogenic bacteria, genetic exchange mechanisms are largely unknown in fungi. Exposure-induced cumulative molecular events that lead to stable azole resistance have been reported; however, in the clinical setting, resistance is encountered most commonly in the form of a primarily resistant species or through selection of resistant subclones during exposure to azoles.[546,714]

Acquisition of microbiologic and clinical azole resistance was reported first in patients with chronic mucocutaneous candidiasis who were receiving long-term therapy with ketoconazole.[304] In the 1990s, before the advent of highly active antiretroviral therapy, azole-resistant oropharyngeal and esophageal candidiasis became a major clinical conundrum in patients with advanced HIV infection.[540,556] Emergence of *C. glabrata* and *C. krusei* infections in association with fluconazole prophylaxis has been observed in several bone marrow transplant

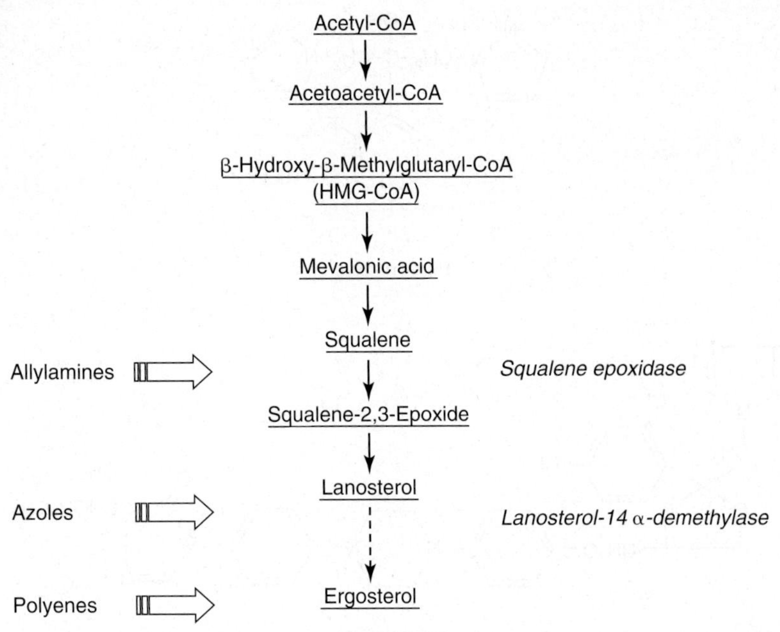

FIG. 240.7 Ergosterol biosynthesis and targets of current antifungal agents. *CoA,* Coenzyme A. (Modified from Groll AH, Walsh TJ. Uncommon opportunistic fungi: new nosocomial threats. *Clin Microbiol Infect* 2001;7[suppl 2]:8-24.)

centers[316,427,724,723] and in large cancer centers.[350] However, a large prospective series from Seattle showed an altogether low incidence of breakthrough candidemia (4.6%; in two-thirds caused by *C. glabrata* or *C. krusei*) and a low attributable mortality (20%) in patients receiving fluconazole prophylaxis despite frequent colonization with fluconazole-resistant *Candida* spp.[427] More recently, emergence of azole-resistant *C. parapsilosis* bloodstream infections has been reported in a laboratory based sentinel surveillance in South Africa: Of 531 *C. parapsilosis* isolates, only 199 (37%) were susceptible to fluconazole and voriconazole, limiting the choice of antifungal agents for management of candidemia in a resource-limited region.[234] Although cross-resistance of *Candida* spp. to antifungal azoles is a common occurrence,[50,229,463,507] it is not obligate; for example, patients with microbiologic and clinical fluconazole-resistant mucosal candidiasis may respond to itraconazole or second-generation triazoles.[280,563] Nonetheless, patients who have been exposed to azoles and who have breakthrough candidemia or an azole-resistant *Candida* isolate have a high likelihood of cross-resistance, and treatment with alternative agents is advised.[234,409,495] Acquired resistance to azoles has been documented in patients with *C. neoformans* meningitis,[70,604,605] and increasingly, reports are being published of secondary azole resistance and azole cross-resistance in filamentous fungi, especially *Aspergillus* spp.[110,152,454,521,609,618,659,660,673]

Fluconazole

Fluconazole (Diflucan; generic forms) is a synthetic, low-molecular-weight, water-soluble bis-triazole (see Fig. 240.5). Relative to ketoconazole, the compound has similar potency but is much more specific and therefore better tolerated. Fluconazole is active against *Candida* spp., *C. neoformans, C. gattii, T. asahii,* and endemic dimorphic fungi, but not against *Aspergillus* spp. and other hyaline or dematiaceous molds. Fluconazole has intermediate activity against *C. glabrata* and is inactive against *C. krusei.*[227,236,519,642]

Pharmacodynamics. Fluconazole generally is considered to be a fungistatic agent.[252] Time-kill assays performed over incubation periods of 24 to 48 hours in susceptible *Candida* spp. and *C. neoformans* showed fungistatic activity of fluconazole with variable concentration-related growth effects.[94,93,157,341,342] However, time-kill studies that used extended periods of incubation up to 14 days and nonproliferating growth conditions demonstrated direct fungicidal activity of fluconazole against *C. albicans.*[612] These observations raise the possibility that fluconazole may ultimately be able to eliminate *Candida* spp. without help from host defenses. Whether fungicidal activity in vitro portends a therapeutic advantage, however, continues to be a matter of debate.[670] In serum-free growth media, fluconazole displays no measurable PAFE against *C. albicans* and *C. neoformans*, but concentration-dependent PAFEs of 1 to 3.6 hours were observed in the presence of fresh serum. Finally, pretreatment of *C. albicans* with fluconazole increased its vulnerability to killing by polymorphonuclear leukocytes.[188,444]

In vivo pharmacodynamic studies of fluconazole in murine models of disseminated *C. albicans* candidiasis using the fungal burden in kidney tissue as an endpoint for antifungal efficacy collectively suggested that the AUC/MIC ratio is the pharmacodynamic parameter that best predicts antifungal efficacy of fluconazole[28,399,614] and that dosing regimens that produce prolonged sub-MIC concentrations are associated with development of resistance.[24] The linear pharmacokinetics and the available experimental and clinical data are in support of once-daily dosing regimens. Pharmacodynamic models and several animal studies demonstrate a correlation between the MIC of fluconazole and antifungal efficacy.[17,46,494,545,553,686] A postmarketing analysis of 1295 patient-episode-isolate events from 12 published clinical studies demonstrates success rates of 85% for those episodes in which the fluconazole MIC was 8 mg/L or less, 67% for those episodes in which the MIC was 16 to 32 mg/L, and 42% for those episodes with isolates that had an MIC of 64 mg/L or higher.[517] Of note, the additional consideration of wild-type MIC distributions and epidemiologic cutoff values has led to the proposition of species-specific clinical breakpoints that may be more sensitive to detect emerging resistance to common *Candida* species.[514] The pharmacokinetics and pharmacodynamics of antifungal agents in treating resistance fungi in children has been recently reviewed in detail elsewhere.[619]

Pharmacokinetics. Fluconazole is formulated for oral and parenteral use, and its disposition is independent of route and formulation. Fluconazole exhibits linear plasma pharmacokinetics that fit best into a two-compartment open model.[88]

Independent of food or intragastric pH, the oral bioavailability of fluconazole is greater than 90%. C_{max} occurs 1 to 2 hours after ingestion. Multiple dosing increases C_{max} approximately 2.5-fold. Steady state generally is reached within 4 to 7 days after once-daily dosing, but it can be achieved rapidly by doubling the dose on the first day.[227,236] Because of the free solubility in water, protein binding is low. Fluconazole distributes well into virtually all tissue sites and body fluids. The ratio of CSF and serum concentrations ranges from 0.5 to 0.9 during the dosing interval, and penetration into brain tissue and the different compartments of the eye is excellent. Fluconazole is relatively stable to metabolic conversion; more than 90% of a dose is excreted by the kidney, with approximately 80% recovered as unchanged, active drug and 11% recovered as inactive metabolites.[88,227,236] Because excretion of fluconazole parallels the glomerular filtration rate, the dosage must be adjusted in patients with renal impairment. A 50% reduction is required in patients with a creatinine clearance of 50 mL/min or less, and a 75% reduction is required in patients with a creatinine clearance of less than 21 mL/min; the initial loading dose need not be adjusted.[65,236] Fluconazole is dialyzable; in patients undergoing hemodialysis, 100% of the target dose is given after each dialysis session. In continuous venovenous hemofiltration and hemodiafiltration, dosing at the higher end of the dosing range (i.e., 800 mg/day in adults) is suggested.[64,584] A dose of 150 mg in a single 2-L dialysate bag has been used for continuous ambulatory peritoneal dialysis.[212,227,464,478,580,639] Hepatic insufficiency per se does not require adjustments of dosing, but careful monitoring of additional hepatic toxicity is required.[558] Finally, infants and children requiring extracorporeal membrane oxygenation (ECMO) were shown to have a higher volume of distribution but similar clearance relative to controls not on ECMO and may require higher loading doses for treatment.[704,705]

The plasma pharmacokinetic properties of fluconazole in pediatric age groups reflect developmental changes in the volume of distribution and clearance that are characteristic for a highly water-soluble drug with minor metabolism and predominantly renal elimination (Table 240.7). Except for premature neonates, in whom clearance initially is decreased, pediatric patients tend to have an increased weight-normalized clearance rate from plasma that leads to a shorter half-life in contrast to that in adults.[87,366,380,465,576,589,635] Whereas population-based pharmacokinetic studies do not exist for children, gestational age at birth, postnatal age, and creatinine level were identified as parameters of impact on clearance of fluconazole in premature infants.[679,680] Because exposure over the course of time appears to be the most predictive pharmacodynamic parameter,[28,399] fractionating the dose is not required in infants and children, despite the shorter half-life in these age groups. From a practical standpoint, a dosage of 12 mg/kg per day in children approximates the plasma exposure achieved in adults receiving the licensed therapeutic dose of 400 mg/day.[380] This pediatric dosage, which does not include neonates, also is consistent with that recommended in the FDA package labeling.

Adverse effects. In adults, fluconazole has been administered safely over prolonged periods at dosages of up to 1200 mg/day; dose-escalation to 1600 mg/day resulted mainly in increased hepatotoxicity, and dose-limiting neurotoxicity was observed at 2000 mg/day.[18] Compiled data from adult patients who received the drug at dosages of 100 to 400 mg/day over the course of at least 7 days indicate an overall incidence of at least possibly related adverse effects of 16%; significant adverse effects or laboratory abnormalities leading to the discontinuation of the drug were noted in overall 2.8%.[236] Nausea, vomiting, and other gastrointestinal symptoms are seen in fewer than 5% and skin rashes and headaches in fewer than 2% and are usually reversible; asymptomatic hepatic transaminase elevations were reported in as many as 7% of adult patients.[125,236]

In pediatric patients of all age groups, at dosages up to 12 mg/kg per day, fluconazole generally is well tolerated. The most common reported side effects in pediatric patients include gastrointestinal disturbances (8%), increases in hepatic transaminases (5%), and skin reactions (1%); toxicity-related discontinuation of therapy with fluconazole occurs in approximately 3% of patients.[480] In a systematic review of the compound's safety in pediatric patients including 90 articles and 4209 patients, the rate of toxicity induced discontinuations was 1%; hepatic toxicity and gastrointestinal disturbances were the most frequent adverse effects.[181] Severe side effects, including severe hepatotoxicity and exfoliative skin reactions, have been rarely reported in association with fluconazole therapy.[125,245]

Drug interactions. Fluconazole undergoes minimal CYP450-mediated metabolism; it inhibits CYP2C9, CYP3A4 and CYP2C19 in vitro and interacts with enzymes involved in glucuronidation, thus leading to certain significant drug-drug interactions.[125,240,261,526] Most important, concurrent therapy with cisapride, pimozide, quinidine, erythromycin, and newer antihistamines results in inhibition of the metabolic pathways of these drugs and potentially serious ventricular arrhythmias associated with QTc prolongation and is therefore strictly contraindicated.[251] By similar mechanisms, fluconazole can precipitate phenytoin toxicity,[445] may lead to increased plasma concentrations of cyclosporine, tacrolimus, and sirolimus,[377,491] and may potentiate the effects of short-acting benzodiazepines, carbamazepine, warfarin, sulfonylurea drugs, rifabutin, and nifedipine.[349,377,486,568] Fluconazole also may interfere with the plasma clearance of cyclophosphamide, a widely used anticancer agent that must be metabolized by CYP450 enzymes to produce alkylating species. This interaction may potentially result in a relevant reduction in the therapeutic efficacy of cyclophosphamide.[735] Further potential interactions with anticancer drugs have been observed with vincristine,[630] busulfan,[92] and all-*trans*-retinoic acid.[587] This adverse interaction with vincristine is a serious concern in pediatric oncology that includes all of the currently licensed triazoles.[456] The interaction may results in vasomotor collapse, seizures, and paralytic ileus. As vincristine is widely used in pediatric lymphoid malignancies, awareness of this potentially serious interaction with systemic antifungal triazoles is important.

Clinical indications. The clinical indications for fluconazole are summarized in Tables 240.2, 240.4, 240.8, and 240.9. Fluconazole is highly effective against superficial infections caused by dermatophytes and *Pityrosporum* spp.,[115,210,267] and it has excellent activity in the treatment of mucosal candidiasis, including vaginal, oropharyngeal, esophageal, and chronic mucocutaneous candidiasis.[201,250,287,418]

Several controlled studies including both neutropenic and non-neutropenic adult patients indicated that intravenous fluconazole 400

TABLE 240.7 Pharmacokinetic Parameters of Fluconazole in Pediatric Patients[a]

Age Group	Vd_{ss} (L/kg)	Cl (L/h/kg)	$t_{1/2}\beta$ (h)
Preterm <1500 g			
Day 1	1.18	0.010	88
Day 6	1.84	0.019	67
Day 12	2.25	0.031	55
Term neonates	1.43	0.036	28
Infants >1–6 mo	1.02	0.037	19
Children, 5–15 y	0.84	0.031	18
Adult volunteers	0.65	0.015	30

[a]Data represent mean values.

Cl, Total plasma clearance; $t_{1/2}\beta$, elimination half-life; Vd_{ss}, apparent volume of distribution at steady state.

Data from references 87, 366, 380, 465, 576, and 589.

TABLE 240.8 Options for Medical Management of Superficial Infections by Dermatophytes

Fungal Disease	Management[a]
Tinea capitis	Griseofulvin for a total of 6–8 wk Fluconazole, itraconazole for 4 wk Terbinafine for 4 wk
Tinea unguium	Itraconazole for 3–4 mo Terbinafine for 6 wk (fingernail) or 12 wk (toenail)
Tinea corporis, facialis, pedis	Topical antifungal azoles: Miconazole, clotrimazole, econazole, ketoconazole, sulconazole, oxiconazole bid for 2–4 wk Topical allyl/benzylamines, thiocarbamates: Terbinafine, naftifine, butenafine, tolnaftate daily to twice daily for 2–4 wk Other topical agents: Ciclopirox olamine bid for 2–4 wk *Refractory infections/immunocompromised patients:* Griseofulvin for 2–4 wk Fluconazole for 2–4 wk Itraconazole for 2–4 wk Terbinafine for 2–4 wk

[a]In alphabetical order according to class; for details and age-specific dosages, see the text.

Data from Friedlander SF, Suarez S. Pediatric antifungal therapy. *Dermatol Clin.* 1998;16:527-537; and Howard RM, Frieden IJ. Dermatophyte infections in children. *Adv Pediatr Infect Dis.* 1999;14:73-107.

TABLE 240.9 Options for Medical Management of Superficial Infections by Yeasts

Fungal Disease	Management[a]
Candida dermatitis Tinea versicolor	*Topical antifungal azoles:* Miconazole, sulconazole, econazole, oxiconazole, clotrimazole bid for 2–4 wk *Topical polyenes:* Amphotericin B or nystatin bid/qid for 2–4 wk *Other topical agents:* Ciclopirox olamine bid for 2–4 wk *Refractory infections/immunocompromised patients:* Fluconazole for 2–4 wk Itraconazole for 2–4 wk
Oropharyngeal candidiasis	*Topical polyenes:* Nystatin or amphotericin B four times daily for ≥2 wk *Topical antifungal azoles:* Clotrimazole lozenges five times daily for ≥2 wk *Refractory infections/immunocompromised patients:* Fluconazole for ≥2 wk Itraconazole for ≥2 wk Voriconazole Posaconazole Amphotericin B deoxycholate Echinocandin lipopeptides
Vulvovaginal candidiasis	*Topical antifungal azoles:* Miconazole, clotrimazole, butoconazole, terconazole, tioconazole qhs for ≥7 days *Topical polyenes:* Nystatin qhs for 14 days *Systemic antifungal azoles:* Fluconazole 150 mg PO × 1 day/50 mg PO × 3 days *Refractory infections/immunocompromised patients:* Fluconazole for ≥2 wk Itraconazole for ≥2 wk Amphotericin B deoxycholate

[a]In alphabetical order according to class; for details and age-specific dosages, see the text.
bid, Twice daily; *PO,* orally; *qhs,* at bedtime; *qid,* 4 times daily.
Data from Bennett JE. Antifungal agents. In: Mandell GL, Bennett JE, Dolin R, editors. *Principles and Practice of Infectious Diseases.* 4th ed. New York: Churchill Livingstone; 1995:401–410; and Walsh TJ, Gonzalez C, Lyman CA, et al. Invasive fungal infections in children: recent advances in diagnosis and treatment. *Adv Pediatr Infect Dis.* 1996;11:187-290.

to 800 mg/day is as effective as D-AmB 0.5 to 1 mg/kg per day against candidemia and other forms of invasive candidiasis, but it is better tolerated.[15,20,498,522,544,546] Fluconazole thus can be used for invasive *Candida* infections caused by susceptible organisms in patients who are in stable condition.[498,546,670] In patients who have received antifungal azoles for prophylaxis, however, breakthrough infections are likely to be caused by fluconazole-resistant *Candida* spp.,[366,427] and alternative agents are recommended. The recommended pediatric dosage range of fluconazole beyond the neonatal period is 6 to 12 mg/kg per day; in view of the faster clearance rate and the absence of population pharmacokinetics, however, 12 mg/kg per day may be the most appropriate dosage.[117,123,257,656]

Although controlled data are lacking in this special population,[122] fluconazole is a useful agent for treatment of invasive *Candida* infections in the neonatal setting. In six published series including 10 or more patients with proved invasive *Candida* infections, treatment with fluconazole at a daily dosage of usually 5 to 6 mg/kg was successful in 83% to 97%, and crude mortality ranged from 10% to 33%. In none of the 125 patients was fluconazole discontinued because of toxicity.[71,82,171,172,198,311,681] For infants, population-based pharmacokinetics and Monte Carlo simulation showed that for the treatment of invasive candidiasis, a dose of at least 12 mg/kg per day in the first 90 days after birth is needed to achieve an AUC/MIC index greater than 50 for *Candida* spp. with MIC less than 8 µg/mL in 90% or more of infants at less than 30 weeks' gestation and 80% of infants at 30 to 40 weeks' gestation, respectively; according to the model, infants with serum creatinine of 1.3 mg/dL or greater have a slower clearance rate, and dose adjustment is indicated if creatinine does not improve within 96 hours.[679,680] A loading dose of 25 mg/kg has been advocated for rapid attainment of target therapeutic drug concentrations.[525]

Fluconazole has been useful in the treatment of focal *Candida* urinary tract infections and uncomplicated funguria, and it has been used successfully in *Candida* peritonitis, endocarditis, osteomyelitis, meningitis, and endophthalmitis.[251,384] Further potential indications for fluconazole beyond the treatment of acute invasive *Candida* infections include consolidation therapy for chronic disseminated candidiasis[14,330] and cryptococcal meningitis.[562,657] High-dose fluconazole is an option for systemic infections caused by the yeast *T. asahii.*[16,259] Fluconazole is the current drug of choice for treatment of coccidioidal meningitis,[214,569] and it has proven effectiveness in nonmeningeal coccidioidal infections.[102,245] Fluconazole appears comparatively less active than itraconazole in the treatment of paracoccidioidomycosis, blastomycosis, histoplasmosis, and sporotrichosis.[158,213,270,331,332,496,497,712]

Fluconazole can prevent mucosal candidiasis in patients with HIV infection or cancer,[244,479,530] and it has proved efficacy in preventing invasive *Candida* infections in high-risk patients with acute leukemia or with bone marrow or liver transplants.[232,554,727] Fluconazole, given at 400 mg once daily to adults from the start of the conditioning regimen until day 75, can reduce the frequency of invasive *Candida* infections and lower mortality at day 110 after allogeneic bone marrow transplantation,[607] and it also may provide persistent protection against invasive candidiasis and *Candida*-related death. Fluconazole can decrease the frequency of severe, gut-related graft-versus-host disease (GVHD), and it has an independent overall survival benefit of 17% at 8 years after the end of treatment.[426] Fluconazole also has been shown to reduce the incidence of *Candida* infections in very-low-birth-weight infants, although without impact on overall mortality.* Thus, in the absence of safety concerns, fluconazole prophylaxis is a valid option for centers with a high frequency (>10%) of invasive *Candida* infections in low-birth-weight infants of less than 1000 g or in the setting of a nosocomial outbreak by a fluconazole-susceptible *Candida* spp. A prospective controlled observational study is still needed to address the neurodevelopmental safety concerns in infants exposed at this young age. Population pharmacokinetics and Monte Carlo simulation support a dose of 3 or 6 mg/kg twice weekly during the first 42 days of life for early prevention of candidiasis in infants born at 23 to 29 weeks of gestation, and a 6-mg/kg dose every 72 hours or 3 mg/kg daily for late prevention.[57,679,680] In the United States, fluconazole has no pediatric label below 6 months of age, and it is not formally approved for prophylaxis in the neonatal setting[106]; in countries of the European Union, the compound is approved for all pediatric age groups with the exception of premature neonates.

Itraconazole

Itraconazole (Sporanox, Sempera; generic forms)is a high-molecular-weight, highly lipophilic triazole (see Fig. 240.5). Structurally related to ketoconazole, it has a broader spectrum of antifungal activity that includes dermatophytes, *Candida* spp. (*C. krusei* excluded), *C. neoformans* and *C. gattii, Aspergillus* spp., some non-*Aspergillus* hyalohyphomycetes, various dematiaceous molds, and the dimorphic fungi. Itraconazole binds more avidly to its fungal target than does ketoconazole, but more weakly to human CYP450, thus leading to comparatively fewer mechanism-associated adverse effects.[235]

Pharmacodynamics. In vitro, itraconazole exerts species- and strain-dependent fungistatic or fungicidal pharmacodynamics. Time-kill experiments in serum-free and serum-containing media demonstrated the concentration-independent, fungistatic activity of itraconazole against *Candida* spp. and *C. neoformans.*[94,93,212,740] However, against *Aspergillus* spp., itraconazole displayed time- and concentration-dependent fungicidal activity with 87% to greater than 97% killing within 24 hours of exposure to the drug.[411] Potentially relevant persistent effects have not been reported thus far.

*References 57, 67, 75, 114, 120, 186, 277, 333-336, 415, 576, 649.

The principal feasibility of a correlation between in vitro susceptibility and outcome was demonstrated in mice with experimental disseminated aspergillosis.[153] Relationships between drug concentrations and antifungal efficacy of itraconazole were assessed in a model of invasive pulmonary aspergillosis in methylprednisolone/cyclosporine-immunosuppressed rabbits. In this model, an inhibitory sigmoid maximum effect model predicted a significant pharmacodynamic relationship (r = .87, P < .001) between itraconazole concentrations in plasma and antifungal efficacy as a function of the burden of *A. fumigatus* in lung tissue.[62]

In patients, however, the main rationale for monitoring plasma levels has been the erratic oral bioavailability of itraconazole, particularly in neutropenic patients. Historically, the target plasma level for itraconazole has been estimated at 0.25 mg/L (high-performance liquid chromatography [HPLC]) at trough, based on the concentration that inhibits 90% of a large set of clinical isolates.[81,144] Later, the predictive value of threshold concentrations of prophylactic itraconazole in a large cohort in patients undergoing intensive chemotherapy for acute leukemia was found to be 0.5 mg/L at trough (HPLC) by means of multivariate logistic regression analysis.[224]

In a phase 1 and II clinical trial of oral cyclodextrin-itraconazole in HIV-infected children with oropharyngeal candidiasis, the relationships between pharmacodynamic parameters and therapeutic response as assessed by standardized scoring of mucosal disease after 14 days of therapy fitted to inhibitory maximum effect pharmacodynamic models. Best fits were observed: AUC, AUC/MIC, C_{max}, and C_{max}/MIC (r = 0.483 to 0.595; P < .01).[246]

Pharmacokinetics. Itraconazole is available as capsules, as oral solution in hydroxypropyl-β-cyclodextrin (HP-β-CD), and as parenteral solution in HP-β-CD[3] that has been discontinued in the United States but is available in various other countries. Absorption of itraconazole from the capsule form depends on a low intragastric pH and is compromised in the fasting state, and it becomes erratic in patients with cancer and granulocytopenia or hypochlorhydria.[125,245,251] Absorption can be somewhat improved when the capsules are taken with food or an acidic beverage.[143,245] The oral solution of itraconazole in HP-β-CD has improved oral bioavailability that is further enhanced in the fasting state; however, this formulation may cause carrier-associated gastrointestinal intolerance.[50,547]

After oral administration of the capsule, C_{max} is measured within 1 to 4 hours; following once-daily dosing, steady state is achieved after 7 to 14 days.[235,245,273] In adult patients with cancer who were receiving the standard regimen of 2.5 mg/kg of HP-β-CD itraconazole twice daily, mean trough levels were 0.8 mg/L under conditions of steady state[532]; systemic absorption of the carrier was negligible.[144] After administration of the parenteral solution, drug and carrier rapidly dissociated and followed their own disposition; after the recommended regimen of 200 mg twice daily for 2 days followed by 200 mg daily for 5 days, mean trough levels were 0.53 µg/mL. The carrier HP-?-CD was not significantly metabolized, and virtually 100% was eliminated from plasma within 24 hours in unchanged form through glomerular filtration.[245]

Itraconazole exhibits dose-dependent pharmacokinetics with nonlinear increases in the AUC with increasing and split dosages.[235,246,532] Itraconazole is highly (95%) protein bound; only 0.2% circulates as free drug.[288] Although concentrations in nonproteinaceous body fluids are negligible, tissue concentrations in many organs, including the brain, may exceed corresponding plasma levels by 2 to 10 times.[143,288]

Itraconazole is metabolized extensively in the liver by numerous pathways to more than 30 metabolites and is excreted in metabolized form into bile and urine. The major metabolite, hydroxyitraconazole, possesses antifungal activity similar to that of itraconazole. It is eliminated more rapidly, but its plasma concentrations at steady state are 1.5 to 2 times higher than those of the parent compound.[144,245,591] The elimination half-life of itraconazole is 20 to 24 hours after single dosing and 35 to 40 hours under terms of steady state, a finding reflecting saturable excretion mechanisms.[394] The dosage of oral itraconazole does not need to be adjusted in patients with renal insufficiency or dialysis.[447] In patients with severe hepatic insufficiency, the elimination half-life of itraconazole can be prolonged, and additional hepatic toxicity or possible drug interactions should be monitored carefully.

Several studies have investigated the pharmacokinetics of the oral HP-?-CD solution of itraconazole in pediatric patients (Table 240.10).[146,175,246,282,581] In 26 infants and children ages 6 months to 12 years with cancer (n = 20) or liver transplantation who received the compound at 5 mg/kg once daily, plasma concentrations were substantially lower than those reported in adult patients with cancer, particularly in children younger than 2 years of age.[146,532] In 16 neutropenic children (1.7–14.3 years of age) who received HP-β-CD itraconazole for antifungal prophylaxis in a split dosing regimen of 2.5 mg/kg twice daily, peak and trough levels of itraconazole were substantially higher; nonetheless, a similar trend toward lower plasma concentrations occurred in the group of children 5 years of age and younger.[581] In a cohort of 26 HIV-infected children and adolescents (1.25–18 years), HP-β-CD itraconazole was safe and effective for treatment of oropharyngeal candidiasis at dosages of 2.5 mg once per day or 2.5 mg twice daily given for at least 14 days.[246] Many (77%) of the patients were receiving concomitant therapy with protease inhibitors or clarithromycin, drugs that are strong inhibitors of the CYP3A4-dependent metabolism of itraconazole.[526] Peak and trough levels measured after administration of the split-dosage regimen were similar to those observed in patients with cancer who were receiving the same dosage regimen.[581] Of note, population-based pharmacokinetics in pediatric cystic fibrosis and allogeneic bone marrow transplant patients receiving the oral solution

TABLE 240.10 Pharmacokinetics of Itraconazole After Administration of Hydroxypropyl-β-Cyclodextrin Oral Solution to Immunocompromised Infants and Children[a]

	Children With Cancer/ Liver Transplant[b] (n = 8, 0.5–2 y) 5 mg/kg daily × 14 days	Children With Cancer[b] (n = 7, 2–5 y) 5 mg/kg daily × 14 days	Children With Cancer[b] (n = 11, 6–12 y) 5 mg/kg daily × 14 days	Children With Cancer[c] (n = 9, 2–5 y) 2.5 mg/kg bid × 14 days	Children With Cancer[c] (n = 6, 6–12 y) 2.5 mg/kg bid × 14 days
C_{max} (µg/mL)	0.571 ± 0.416	0.534 ± 0.431	0.631 ± 0.358	1.024 ± 0.351	1.524 ± 0.770
T_{max} (h)	1.9 ± 0.1	2.9 ± 2.5	3.1 ±2.1	n/a	n/a
C_{min} (µg/mL)	0.159 ± 0.218	0.179 ± 0.100	0.233 ± 0.14	0.711 ± 0.251	1.072 ± 0.408
$AUC_{0-\infty}$ (µg/mL/h)	6.930 ± 5.83	7.33 ± 5.42	8.77 ± 5.05	NA	NA
$t_{1/2}\beta$ (h)	47.4 ± 55.0	30.6 ±25.3	28.3 ± 9.6	NA	NA
Accumulation factor	6.2 ± 5.0	3.3±3.0	8.6 ± 7.4	NA	NA

[a]Pharmacokinetic parameters were obtained after daily dosing over 14 days. All values represent mean values ± SD.

[b]Data from de Repentigny L, Ratelle J, Leclerc JM, et al. Repeated-dose pharmacokinetics of an oral solution of itraconazole in infants and children. *Antimicrob Agents Chemother.* 1998;42:404-8.

[c]Data from Schmitt C, Perel Y, Harousseau J, et al. Pharmacokinetics of itraconazole oral solution in neutropenic children during long-term prophylaxis. *Antimicrob Agents Chemother.*2001;45:1561-4.

Accumulation factor, AUC_{0-24} day 14/$AUC_{0-\infty}$ day 1.

$AUC_{0-\infty}$, Area under the concentration versus time curve from zero to infinity; *C_{max}*, peak plasma levels; *C_{min}*, minimum plasma levels; *n/a*, not assessed; *$t_{1/2}\beta$*, elimination half-life; *T_{max}*, time until occurrence of peak plasma concentration.

or the capsule formulation as antifungal prophylaxis suggests a starting dose of 5 mg/kg twice daily.[282]

Despite considerable interpatient variability that results from both variable absorption and hepatic metabolism, the pharmacokinetic properties of itraconazole in pediatric patients appear not to be fundamentally different from those of adults. A starting dosage of 2.5 mg/kg twice daily can be advocated, based on the available pharmacokinetic data.[146,175,246,581] Trough levels should be monitored, and dosing should be adjusted to maintain plasma concentrations of the parent itraconazole of greater than 0.5 mg/L by HPLC.[702] Of note, itraconazole is not formally approved for pediatric age groups in either the United States or the European Union.

Adverse effects. Itraconazole usually is well tolerated, with a pattern similar to that of fluconazole and a frequency of adverse effects approximately identical to that seen with fluconazole.[125] In 189 patients treated for systemic fungal infections at dosages of 50 to 400 mg/day for a median of 5 months, the rate of possibly or definitely related adverse effects was 39%.[647] Most of the observed reactions were transient and included nausea and vomiting (<10%), hypertriglyceridemia (9%), hypokalemia (6%), elevated hepatic transaminases (5%), rash or pruritus (2%), headaches or dizziness (<2%), and pedal edema (1%). Four percent of patients discontinued itraconazole treatment because of adverse effects. Gastrointestinal intolerance is the dose-limiting toxicity of the oral HP-β-CD formulation. In a comparative study in adult patients with acute leukemia, 46% of patients receiving a daily dose of 800 mg stopped treatment early because of severe nausea and vomiting. Crossover to the identical dose of the capsule formulation was well tolerated by all patients; patients receiving 400 mg/day of the solution had no gastrointestinal adverse effects.[223] Only a few cases of more severe hepatic injury or hepatitis have been described.[375] Itraconazole can have negative inotropic effects; because of a low but possible risk for cardiac toxicity, itraconazole should not be administered to patients with ventricular dysfunction.[9,379]

Cyclodextrin-itraconazole solution was safe and well tolerated for at least 14 days in reported phase I and II pharmacokinetic studies in immunocompromised pediatric patients.[146,246,581] Vomiting (12%), abnormal liver function tests (5%), and abdominal pain (3%) were the most common adverse effects considered definitely or possibly related to HP-β-CD itraconazole solution in an open study in 103 neutropenic pediatric patients with cancer who received the drug at 5 mg/kg daily or 2.5 mg/kg twice daily for antifungal prophylaxis for a median duration of 37 days; 18% of patients withdrew from the study because of adverse events.[203] In another report on pediatric patients with cancer who were receiving prophylactic oral itraconazole, adverse effects that led to the cessation of the itraconazole prophylaxis occurred in 11% of all 44 courses.[603]

Drug interactions. In contrast to fluconazole, both the propensity for and the extent of drug-drug interactions are greater.[242,245] Itraconazole is a substrate of CYP3A4, but it also interacts with the heme moiety of CYP3A, thus resulting in noncompetitive inhibition of oxidative metabolism of many CYP3A substrates. An interaction also can result from inhibition of P-glycoprotein-mediated efflux; P-glycoprotein is extensively co-localized and exhibits overlapping substrate specificity with CYP3A.[240,261] Inhibition of hepatic CYP450 enzyme systems may lead to increased and potentially toxic concentrations of coadministered drugs. Most important, the coadministration of cisapride, pimozide, bepridil, mizolastine, terfenadine, astemizole, oral midazolam, quinidine, dofetilide, triazolam, sertindole, eletriptan, nisoldipine, and levacetylmethadol with itraconazole can lead to serious cardiac arrhythmias and is thus strictly contraindicated.[240,295,526] Similarly contraindicated is the coadministration of 3-hydroxy-3-methylglutaryl coenzyme A (HMG CoA)-inhibitor cholesterol-lowering agents such as atorvastatin, lovastatin, and simvastatin, which are associated with rhabdomyolysis,[240,476] and ergot alkaloids metabolized by CYP3A4, which may result in ergotism. Potentially toxic levels of the coadministered drug also can be reached when itraconazole is given along with phenytoin, carbamazepine, benzodiazepines, cyclosporine, tacrolimus, sirolimus, methylprednisolone, budesonide, digoxin, warfarin, sulfonylurea compounds, ritonavir, indinavir, haloperidol, clarithromycin, verapamil, felodipine, busulfan, and vinca alcaloids.[78,240,357,456,486,527,566,665] The interaction between vincristine and itraconazole, which has led to fatalities in some cases, occurs most frequently in the setting of antifungal prophylaxis. Increased metabolism of itraconazole resulting in decreased plasma levels can be induced by rifampin, rifabutin, isoniazid, carbamazepine, phenobarbital, and phenytoin.[240,526,646] As a consequence, patients who receive itraconazole along with one of the drugs listed here or in the summary of product characteristics should be followed closely, and plasma concentrations of ideally both compounds, as well as hepatic function, should be monitored carefully.

Clinical indications. The clinical indications for itraconazole are summarized in Tables 240.2 to 240.4, 240.8, and 240.9. Itraconazole is a useful agent for dermatophytic infections, [115,265] pityriasis versicolor,[6,208,235,264] vaginal candidiasis,[616] and oropharyngeal and esophageal candidiasis.[1,146,246,563] While the experience with itraconazole in the primary treatment of cryptococcal meningitis is scant, itraconazole has been used with success for long-term treatment of cryptococcal meningitis in patients with HIV infection.[562,657]

Itraconazole may be a second-line option for treatment of invasive *Aspergillus* infections, in particular as maintenance or consolidation therapy in non-neutropenic patients.[155,620] Beyond invasive aspergillosis, itraconazole may be useful in the management of infections by certain dematiaceous molds.[260,596] Itraconazole is a current treatment of choice for lymphocutaneous sporotrichosis[145,331,542] and non–life-threatening, nonmeningeal paracoccidioidomycosis, blastomycosis, and histoplasmosis in non-immunocompromised patients,[112,160,466,474,634,713] as well as induction and maintenance therapy of mild to moderate, nonmeningeal histoplasmosis in HIV-infected patients.[710,711,713] Although earlier uncontrolled clinical trials suggested a somewhat inferior efficacy against nonmeningeal and meningeal coccidioidomycosis in comparison with fluconazole,[237,644,645] a randomized, double-blind comparative study in patients with progressive, nonmeningeal coccidioidomycosis showed a trend toward slightly greater efficacy when either of the drugs were given at a daily dosage of 400 mg.[215] Nonetheless, amphotericin B remains the treatment of choice for endemic mycoses in most immunocompromised patients and for those with life-threatening infections.[251]

Itraconazole was as effective as conventional amphotericin B but better tolerated when used for empirical antifungal therapy in persistently neutropenic patients with cancer.[80] Prophylactic itraconazole may reduce the incidence of proved or suspected invasive fungal infections in patients with hematologic malignancies[437] and those who have undergone HSCT.[423,726] Efficacy in the prevention of invasive aspergillosis is supported by a large meta-analysis,[225] but not by a randomized, comparative trial.

Posaconazole

Posaconazole (Noxafil) (see Fig. 240.6) is a novel lipophilic antifungal triazole with potent and broad-spectrum activity against opportunistic, endemic, and dermatophytic fungi in vitro. This activity extends to organisms that often are refractory to existing triazoles or amphotericin B or to echinocandins, such as *C. glabrata, C. krusei, A. terreus,* and *Fusarium* spp. Posaconazole also possesses clinically relevant activity against some members of the order Mucorales both in vitro and in vivo.[190,260,565,636]

Pharmacodynamics. Posaconazole is considered fungistatic against *Candida* and fungicidal against *Aspergillus* spp.[260] In time-kill assays, posaconazole showed concentration- and time-dependent fungicidal activity against *A. fumigatus*.[248,412,413] In vivo, in a neutropenic kidney target murine model of *C. albicans* infection and in an inhalational murine model of invasive pulmonary aspergillosis, the AUC/MIC ratio was the parameter predictive of antifungal efficacy.[25,307] In a phase II clinical trial in patients with invasive aspergillosis, higher average plasma concentrations of posaconazole were associated with higher response rates.[695] Mean plasma concentrations of posaconazole of 719 ng/mL and 1250 ng/mL resulted in overall response rates of 53% and 75% in salvage therapy of invasive aspergillosis.

While pharmacokinetic analysis of the two pivotal prophylaxis trials with the oral suspension did not report significant concentration-effect relationships[361,364] a pharmacodynamics assessment performed by the FDA has established an efficacy target for prophylaxis of 700 ng/mL for the purpose of dosing guidance for alternative formulations.[315]

Pharmacokinetics. Posaconazole is available as oral suspension, as solid oral tablet, and as intravenous solution in sulfobuthylether-beta-cyclodextrin. The oral suspension achieves optimal exposure when it is administered in two to four divided doses with food or a nutritional supplement; common gastrointestinal comorbidities in leukemia and hematopoietic stem-cell transplant patients may negatively affect absorption.[361,364,365] The oral suspension has dose-proportional pharmacokinetics in the 50- and 800-mg dose range, with saturation of absorption occurring at doses higher than 800 mg; after repeat dosing, steady state is achieved after 7 to 10 days with a sixfold to eightfold accumulation of plasma concentrations,[135] and marked accumulation within alveolar cells of the lung.[126] The solid oral tablet contains a pH-sensitive polymer matrix that inhibits the release of posaconazole prior to reaching the small intestine; it confers enhanced bioavailability and less variability in exposure, and gastric filling, pH and motility have no effect on absorption.[356,362,363] In a phase IB dose-ranging multicenter study in adults, a dose of 300 mg once daily (day 1: 300 mg twice daily) attained the prespecified exposure target of a $C_{average}$ of between 500 and 2500 ng/mL in 97% of the 51 subjects[177]; in a subsequent phase III study in adult patients at high risk for invasive fungal disease, the tablet formulation demonstrated a safety profile similar to that reported for posaconazole oral suspension, and most of the 210 patients (99%) achieved steady-state $C_{average}$ exposures in plasma of greater than 500 ng/mL.[129] Likewise, in a phase IB dose-ranging multicenter study in adults, 300 mg once daily (day 1: 300 mg twice daily) of the intravenous solution attained the prespecified exposure target in 95% of patients.[403] However, when administered peripherally at the same infusion site, multiple dosing of intravenous posaconazole led to unacceptably high rates of infusion-site reactions.[337] Independent of the formulation, posaconazole has a large volume of distribution in the order of 5 L/kg and displays a prolonged elimination half-life of approximately 20 hours. Posaconazole is metabolized to a small extent by uridine diphosphate (UDP) glucuronidation; it is not significantly metabolized through the CYP450 enzyme system but is primarily excreted in unchanged form in the feces (Table 240.11).[260,360,709] Posaconazole is a substrate and inhibitor of P-glycoprotein. However, investigation of the relationship between human multidrug resistance gene *(MDR1)* mRNA expression and posaconazole exposure showed no correlation. Thus, the moderate variability in the compound's pharmacokinetics is unlikely to be caused by interindividual differences in P-glycoprotein expression.[136]

Adverse effects. The overall safety of posaconazole was assessed in two open-label clinical trials of more than 400 patients with invasive fungal infections who received posaconazole suspension 800 mg/day in divided doses. Treatment-related adverse events occurred in 38% of patients (164 of 428); the most common were nausea (8%), vomiting (6%), headache (5%), abdominal pain (4%), and diarrhea (4%). Treatment-related abnormal liver function test results were observed in 3% of patients. No clinically significant differences occurred in mean QTc interval change from baseline. Serious adverse events considered possibly or probably related to posaconazole occurred in 35 (8%) patients. The most common severe adverse events were altered drug level, increased hepatic enzymes, nausea, rash, and vomiting (1% each). No significant trends related to age, sex, or race were observed, and no unique treatment-related adverse events were identified in patients during long-term exposure (>6 months) in contrast to those identified during shorter-duration therapy.[505,536] In two large, prospective, randomized comparative clinical trials investigating posaconazole for prevention of invasive fungal infections in high-risk patients with leukemia or HSCT, posaconazole was well tolerated, and the rate of study drug discontinuations in posaconazole-treated patients was not different from that in subjects in the control cohort receiving fluconazole or itraconazole.[132,650]

Drug interactions. Posaconazole is not significantly metabolized through the CYP450 enzyme system; therefore, CYP450-mediated drug-drug interactions have limited potential to affect posaconazole pharmacokinetics.[360] Posaconazole is a potent inhibitor of cytochrome P3A4, but it has no effect on 1A2, 2C8, 2C9, 2D6, or 2E1 isoenzymes.[709] Concomitant administration of posaconazole with terfenadine, astemizole, cisapride, pimozide, halofantrine, and quinidine can lead to serious cardiac arrhythmias and is thus strictly contraindicated.[572,573] Similarly contraindicated is the coadministration of HMG CoA-inhibitor cholesterol-lowering agents such as atorvastatin, lovastatin, and simvastatin, which are associated with rhabdomyolysis, and ergot alkaloids metabolized by CYP3A4, which may result in ergotism. Potentially toxic levels of the coadministered drug can be reached when posaconazole is given along with phenytoin, carbamazepine, benzodiazepines, cyclosporine, tacrolimus, sirolimus, methylprednisolone, digoxin, warfarin, sulfonylurea compounds, ritonavir, indinavir, atazanavir, haloperidol, clarithromycin, verapamil, nifedipine, diltiazem, nisoldipine, rifabutin, and vinca alkaloids. Because of a relevant decrease in posaconazole concentrations, concomitant use with rifabutin, phenytoin, efavirenz, fosamprenavir, cimetidine, or esomeprazole should be avoided.[91,572,573]

Clinical efficacy. Posaconazole has been targeted for prevention and treatment of serious infections caused by opportunistic and endemic fungal organisms. Posaconazole has demonstrated strong antifungal efficacy in phase II clinical trials in immunocompromised patients with primary or refractory oropharyngeal and esophageal candidiasis.[606,666] In a randomized, comparative phase III trial, posaconazole 100 mg daily (with day 1 dose 200 mg) was as effective as was fluconazole 100 mg daily (with day 1 dose 200 mg), in the primary treatment of HIV-associated oropharyngeal candidiasis: 155 of 169 (91.7%) patients receiving posaconazole in contrast to 148 of 160 (92.5%) of patients receiving fluconazole achieved a complete clinical response (cure).[667] Posaconazole 800 mg in divided doses also was investigated as salvage therapy in a large phase II study including 330 patients with invasive fungal infections intolerant to or refractory to standard therapies and a contemporaneous external control of 279 patients.[535] Most patients (86%) were refractory to previous therapy. Successful outcomes at the end of treatment in the posaconazole cohort and in the contemporaneous external control cohort were 42% versus 26% in aspergillosis (107 and 86 patients; separately published[695]), 39% versus 50% in fusariosis (18 vs. 4 patients), 56% versus 50% in zygomycoses (11 vs. 8 patients), 69% versus 43% in coccidioidomycosis (16 vs. 7 patients), 52% versus 53% in candidiasis (23 vs. 30 patients), 48% versus 58% in cryptococcosis (31 vs. 64 patients), 81% versus 0% in chromoblastomycosis (11 vs. 2 patients), and 64% versus 60% in other invasive fungal infections (30

TABLE 240.11 Principal Pharmacokinetic Properties of Posaconazole, Voriconazole, and Isavuconazole

	Posaconazole	Voriconazole	Isavuconazole
Formulation	PO	PO, IV	PO, IV
Dose linearity	Yes	No	Yes
Oral bioavailability (%)	>50	>90	>90
Protein binding (%)	>95	58	>99
Volume of distribution (L/kg)	>5	2	>5
Elimination half-life (h)	25	6	>80
Substrate/inhibitor of CYP450	—/3A4	3A4, 2C9, 2C19 / 3A4, 2C9, 2C19	3A4, 3A5/CYP3A4, CYP2C8, CYP2C9, CYP2C19,CYP2D6.
Elimination through			
Feces (%/% metabolites)	77/—	<20/?	46/100
Urine (%/% metabolites)	14/100	80/100	45/98

Data from references 134, 135, 243, 360, 533, 582, 583, 709.
UDP-GT, UDP glucuronosyltransferase.

vs. 20 patients). In a subset analysis of 39 patients with mostly refractory proved or probable CNS infections, posaconazole demonstrated clinical efficacy against cryptococcal meningitis (success rate in 29 patients [48%]) and against infections caused by opportunistic or endemic molds (5 of 10 patients [50%]).[527,535] These data are in agreement with the compound's extended spectrum of activity in vitro and demonstrate efficacy for treatment of refractory invasive opportunistic and endemic mycoses. A retrospective analysis of the manufacturer's compassionate-use program including 91 patients with proved or probable mucormycosis refractory or intolerant to prior antifungal therapy revealed a 60% success rate (complete and partial responses) at 12 weeks after initiation of therapy, thus providing first evidence for the clinical utility of posaconazole as second-line or consolidation therapy of mucormycosis.[653] Posaconazole has also been shown in a randomized, placebo- and active-controlled multicenter trial to be effective against toenail onychomycosis.[183]

The use of posaconazole for antifungal prophylaxis has had an important impact on reducing mortality of invasive fungal infections in patients with acute leukemia.[268] Two pivotal preventive randomized phase III studies in high-risk patients with HSCT and GVHD[650] and acute leukemias[132] have been conducted. In the first study, patients received either posaconazole 200 mg three times daily or fluconazole 400 mg daily, respectively, with the start of immunosuppression for a total of 16 weeks. Treatment with posaconazole led to a decreased incidence of invasive fungal infections at 16 weeks (5% vs. 9%; P = .07), with a statistically significant decrease in invasive *Aspergillus* infections (2% vs. 7%; P = .006). Seven days after end of treatment, fewer patients had invasive fungal disease (2% vs. 8%; P = .004) and fewer patients had invasive aspergillosis (1% vs. 6%; P = .001). No differences in overall mortality rates occurred at 12 weeks.[650] In the second study, patients received posaconazole 200 mg three times daily and either fluconazole 400 mg daily or itraconazole 200 mg twice daily, respectively. Treatment was started with each cycle after a drop of the absolute neutrophil count (ANC) to 500/μL or less for up to 12 weeks. Significantly fewer patients enrolled in the posaconazole arm of the trial developed an invasive fungal infection at day 7 after the end of treatment in contrast to the comparator arm (2% vs. 8%; P = .01); most important, treatment with posaconazole resulted in a significant decrease in the rate of invasive aspergillosis (1% vs. 7%; P = .001). At day +100 after randomization, the rate of invasive fungal infections was 5% and 11% (P = .01), respectively, and patients treated with posaconazole had a significantly improved survival probability (P = .035).[132] These two important studies demonstrate the preventive efficacy of posaconazole, in particular against invasive *Aspergillus* infections in high-risk patients, and a statistically significant survival benefit in patients with acute myeloblastic leukemia/myelodysplastic syndrome who are undergoing remission induction chemotherapy.

Approval status and dosing. In the United States, posaconazole is approved for treatment of oropharyngeal candidiasis, including disease refractory to itraconazole or fluconazole (oral suspension), and for prophylaxis of invasive *Candida* and *Aspergillus* infections in high-risk patients 13 years of age and older with HSCT and GVHD or those with hematologic malignancies and prolonged neutropenia (oral suspension and delayed-release tablets; intravenous solution for subjects ≥18 years). In the European Union, the compound is similarly approved for prophylaxis in high-risk adult patients, but also for treatment of aspergillosis, fusariosis, chromoblastomycosis, and coccidioidomycosis refractory to or intolerant of standard therapies in patients 18 years of age and older (see Tables 240.3, 240.4, and 240.9).

The recommended doses in patients 18 years of age and older for primary treatment of oropharyngeal candidiasis with the oral suspension is 100 mg/day (with day 1 dose 100 mg twice daily) and 400 mg twice daily for refractory disease; for prophylaxis of invasive *Candida* and *Aspergillus* infections, the recommended dose is 200 mg of the suspension three times daily or 300 mg once daily of the delayed-release tablets and the intravenous solution, respectively, with a loading dose of 300 mg twice daily on day 1 for each formulation. The dose of the oral suspension for salvage treatment is 400 mg twice daily given with food; for patients not tolerating solid food, the delayed-release tablets or the intravenous solution may be given at the identical doses as used for antifungal prophylaxis. Because of the improved target attainment, the delayed-release tablets should preferentially be administered when posaconazole is given by the oral route.[694]

Current data indicate no need for adjustments to dosage based on differences in age, gender, race,[574] or renal or hepatic function.[137,134] The pharmacokinetic properties of posaconazole in pediatric patients (<18 years of age) have not been conclusively studied. Early data obtained in 12 pediatric patients 8 years of age and older receiving the oral suspension indicated no fundamental differences in trough plasma concentrations in contrast to that of adults.[365] A twice-daily dosing algorithm based on allometric scaling for posaconazole resulted in adequate exposure in children with chronic granulomatous disease.[707] However, similar to published clinical experiences,[66,429,664] a pediatric phase IB dose finding trial was discontinued for failure to achieve the pharmacokinetic target due to absorption issues.[36] The intravenous solution and a new oral suspension formulation are currently under clinical investigation in order to provide pharmacokinetic and safety data on which to base safe and effective dosing of this important compound to pediatric patients.

Despite the described problems with absorption, successful salvage treatment with posaconazole has been reported in small numbers of pediatric patients with invasive fungal infections.[74,381] In these and other reports, posaconazole oral suspension was well tolerated and safe without signals for increased or unexpected toxicities relative to the adult population.*

Voriconazole

Voriconazole (Vfend; generic forms) (see Fig. 240.6) is a synthetic antifungal triazole with activity against a wide spectrum of clinically important yeasts and molds, including *Candida* spp., *C. neoformans*, *Aspergillus*, and other hyaline molds, dematiaceous molds, and dimorphic molds, both in vitro and in animal models. A notable exemption is the Mucorales, against which voriconazole is intrinsically inactive.[242,323,321,460]

Pharmacodynamics. Against *Candida* spp. and *C. neoformans*, voriconazole exhibited non–concentration-dependent fungistatic activity; against *A. fumigatus*, voriconazole displayed time-dependent fungicidal activity.[340,411] A concentration-dependent PAFE of 0.2 to 4.1 hours has been observed in the presence of serum against *C. albicans*.[216] In a murine kidney target model of disseminated candidiasis, the AUC/MIC ratio was the pharmacodynamic parameter that correlated best with efficacy. Using 10 *C. albicans* isolates of different voriconazole susceptibilities, the free drug AUC/MIC ratios were similar to all the organisms studied and similar to those observed for other azoles.[26] The AUC/MIC ratio also correlates with antifungal activity in vitro against *A. fumigatus*.[317] Concentration-response relationships of voriconazole in patients were analyzed in a total of 825 subjects from nine previously published clinical trials using logistic regression and Monte Carlo simulation. Whereas logistic regression analysis showed a nonlinear concentration-response relationship with the probability lower at the extremes, Monte Carlo simulation revealed that a trough/MIC ratio of 2:5 was associated with a near-maximal probability of response and that this parameter can be used as the exposure target, on the basis of either an observed MIC or reported MIC_{90} values of the suspected fungal pathogen(s).[643]

Pharmacokinetics. Voriconazole is available in oral and intravenous formulations. Oral bioavailability exceeds 90% in adults in the fasted state, but it is considerably lower (65%) in children,[683] which may be due to intestinal first-pass metabolism.[737] In adults, the compound has nonlinear pharmacokinetics between the dosages of 3 mg/kg and 4 mg/kg, while being linear in this dosage range in children.[683,690] Plasma protein binding is 58%, and the mean volume of distribution accounts for 2 L/kg. Tissue and CSF levels may exceed trough plasma levels severalfold. The plasma half-life is 6 hours, with elimination occurring primarily by oxidative hepatic metabolism to at least eight metabolites that are eliminated through the urine; less than 2% of a dose of voriconazole is excreted unchanged in urine. The major isoenzyme involved in voriconazole metabolism is CYP2C19, but CYP2C9 and CYP3A4 also contribute (see Table 240.11). In addition to considerable intrasubject variability, wide between-subject variability exists in the disposition of

*References 36, 66, 74, 135, 164, 165, 365, 381, 429, 664, 707, 736.

voriconazole that is at least in part related to a genetic CYP2C19 polymorphism.[242,289,455,523,533] The latter may be particularly relevant in Japanese patients, who have a higher incidence of poor and intermediate metabolizer phenotypes.[467] Recent guidelines from the Clinical Pharmacogenetics Implementation Consortium (CPIC) provide evidence-based recommendations for therapeutic drug monitoring or use of an alternative antifungal agent depending upon the CYP2C19 genotype.[457] Based on this variability, the significant correlations between exposure and effect,[643] and significant effects of therapeutic drug monitoring on treatment responses and adverse effects,[401,501] therapeutic drug monitoring is advocated in patients with life-threatening invasive fungal infections with a target trough concentration of between 1 and 5 mg/L of voriconazole, depending on safety and tolerability.[388,401,638,643]

Adverse effects. Voriconazole has an acceptable safety profile. The accrued clinical data indicate that side effects include four distinct clinical categories: transient liver enzyme abnormalities (10–20%), skin reactions (<10%), visual hallucinations or confusion (<10%), and transient, dose-related visual disturbances (photopsia with altered or enhanced perception of light, blurred vision; 25% to 45%).[242] With regard to the visual disturbances, no morphologic correlation was noted in animal models, and the underlying mechanism remains to be elucidated.[321] Drug-related adverse effects requiring the discontinuation of voriconazole were infrequent in comparative clinical trials and ranged from 2% to 13%.[12,284,693]

Serious hepatic reactions, including hepatic failure, have been observed during treatment with voriconazole; therefore, evaluation of liver function tests before and during treatment with voriconazole is advised. Azole therapy has been associated with QTc prolongation; for this reason, voriconazole should be administered with caution to patients with proarrhythmic conditions.[242] Phototoxicity is relatively common in children and has been reported to occur in close to 50% of children treated for 6 months or longer.[597] A possible link between long-term use of voriconazole, immunosuppression, and chronic phototoxicity with aggressive squamous cell carcinoma and melanoma has been reported in adult and pediatric patients.[138,443,597,728] As a consequence, the indication for further and prolonged voriconazole treatment in immunocompromised patients who develop phototoxicity needs to be evaluated extremely carefully.[597] Caution is also warranted with the concurrent use of methotrexate, as severe skin toxicity has been observed.[661] Moreover, fluorosis and periostitis also have been reported during long-term voriconazole use because of its elevated fluoride content.[625,708] Voriconazole is teratogenic in animals and may cause fetal harm when it is administered to a pregnant woman.[242]

Drug interactions. Voriconazole is both substrate and inhibitor of CYP2C19, CYP2C9, and CYP3A4, and, therefore, numerous clinically relevant and potentially hazardous drug-drug interactions must be considered and the drug product label consulted.[240,242] Voriconazole significantly increases exposure to cyclosporine, tacrolimus, benzodiazepines, methadone, fentanyl, alfentanil, oxycodone, vinca alkaloids, statins, omeprazole, warfarin, sulfonylurea drugs, phenytoin, protease inhibitors other than indinavir, and non-nucleoside reverse transcriptase inhibitors, thus requiring dosage adjustment or monitoring. Voriconazole exposure is significantly decreased by St. John's wort, phenytoin, ritonavir, efavirenz, rifabutin, carbamazepine, rifampin, and phenobarbital. Concurrent use of the last three enzyme inducers with voriconazole is contraindicated (risk for subtherapeutic levels of voriconazole), as is the concurrent use of terfenadine, astemizole, cisapride, quinidine, pimozide (risk of QTc prolongation resulting from increased exposure to these agents), ergotamine (risk for ergotism resulting from increased exposure), and sirolimus (increased exposure). Although voriconazole and sirolimus are relatively contraindicated due to the precipitous and approximately 10-fold rise of sirolimus, the combination may be used with 90% initial dosage reduction of the m-TOR inhibitor and with careful therapeutic drug monitoring of both agents. Dosage adjustments of voriconazole are also necessary when the drug must be used concurrently with phenytoin or rifabutin.[91,240,242,321,346]

Clinical efficacy. Voriconazole has demonstrated excellent clinical efficacy in phase II and III clinical trials in patients with oropharyngeal candidiasis and esophageal candidiasis.[12,280] In salvage studies in patients with fungal infections refractory or intolerant to treatment, complete and partial responses were seen in 43% to 48% of patients with invasive aspergillosis,[154,508,690] in 45% to 52% of patients with invasive candidiasis,[508] in 30% to 63% of patients with scedosporiosis,[508,690] in 45% of patients with fusariosis,[508] and in 38% of patients with cryptococcosis.[508]

A large, multinational, randomized phase III clinical trial of voriconazole and amphotericin B deoxycholate followed by other licensed antifungal agents for primary therapy of invasive aspergillosis revealed superior outcomes in voriconazole-treated patients.[284] At week 12, successful outcomes were noted in 52.8% of the patients in the voriconazole group and in 31.6% of those in the amphotericin B group (absolute difference, 21.2 percentage points; 95% confidence interval [CI], 10.4 to 32.9). The survival rate at 12 weeks was 70.8% in the voriconazole group and 57.9% in the amphotericin B group (hazard ratio, 0.59; 95% CI, 0.40–0.88). Voriconazole-treated patients had significantly fewer severe drug-related adverse events. A randomized double-blind clinical trial comparing open-label voriconazole plus blinded anidulafungin or blinded placebo for treatment of proved or probable invasive aspergillosis in patients with hematologic malignancies or allogeneic HSCT showed a statistical trend ($P = .07$) favoring the combination therapy with respect to the overall survival at 6 weeks, the primary endpoint of the study.[425] In a post-hoc analysis of patients diagnosed on the basis of positive galactomannan, which accounted for 78% of the study population, overall survival at 6 weeks was significantly higher in the combination arm. Although the clinical implications of this study are still debated, regulatory approval of the combination for invasive aspergillosis has failed. A randomized comparative study of voriconazole versus amphotericin B deoxycholate followed by fluconazole for treatment of candidemia in non-neutropenic patients showed similar response rates at end of treatment and similar survival rates at 3 months.[367] Twelve weeks after the end of treatment, successful outcomes were observed in 41% of patients in both treatment groups. Voriconazole cleared blood cultures as quickly as amphotericin B/fluconazole, and significantly fewer serious adverse events and cases of renal toxicity occurred. In a large, international collaborative study of voriconazole versus liposomal amphotericin B for empirical therapy, voriconazole did not meet the prespecified statistical endpoint for non-inferiority in a composite endpoint but was associated with significantly fewer breakthrough invasive fungal infections, particularly those caused by invasive aspergillosis.[693] Finally, several reports also suggested the potential usefulness of voriconazole for treatment of infections by unusual hyaline and dematiaceous fungi,[508] as well as for treatment of cerebral mold infections.[588]

Voriconazole also has been investigated as primary antifungal prophylaxis.[421,721] A multicenter, randomized, double-blind trial compared voriconazole 200 mg twice daily to fluconazole 400 mg once daily in 600 adult allogeneic HSCT patients. There was no difference in the cumulative rates of proved, probable, and presumptive invasive fungal infections at 6 months (7.3% vs. 11.2% [$P = .12$]); however, a trend was noted toward fewer infections by *Aspergillus* (9% vs. 17%, $P = .09$). Fungus-free survival rates (78% and 75%, respectively) were similar, as were overall survival rates and rates of premature study drug withdrawal.[721] A second study compared voriconazole 200 mg twice daily to itraconazole 200 mg twice daily in 489 allogeneic HSCT recipients. Efficacy was assessed by a composite endpoint, including survival at 180 days after transplantation and no breakthrough infections and no discontinuation of the study drug for more than 14 days during the first scheduled 100 days. Using this endpoint, voriconazole was superior to itraconazole, with a 49.1% versus 34.5% success rate ($P = .0004$). However, the rate of proved and probable invasive fungal infections was low (3% vs. 6%).[421]

Approval status and dosing. Voriconazole is approved in the United States and the European Union for treatment of invasive aspergillosis, fusariosis, and scedosporiosis; treatment of esophageal candidiasis; and primary treatment of candidemia and certain forms of invasive candidiasis in non-neutropenic patients (see Tables 240.2 and 240.3).[109,194] The recommended intravenous dosages for adults and adolescents (12 to 14 years and ≥50 kg; 15 to 17 years regardless of body weight) are 6 mg/kg twice daily on day 1, followed by 4 mg/kg twice daily. Oral doses in adults are 400 mg twice daily on day 1 (≥40 kg, 200 mg twice daily), followed by 200 mg twice daily (<40 kg, 100 mg twice daily).[194]

TABLE 240.12 Simulated Plasma Concentrations of Voriconazole After Multiple Doses of 3 and 4 mg/kg in Pediatric Versus Adult Patients

	VALUE[a]			
	Pediatric Patients (2–11 y)		Adult Patients	
Parameter	3 mg/kg	4 mg/kg	3 mg/kg	4 mg/kg
AUC_{tau} (ng/h/mL)	10,670	14,227	13,855	38,605
$C_{average}$ (ng/mL)	889	1,186	1,155	3,217

[a]Data are reported as medians following 6 mg/kg every 12 hours on day 1 and maintenance dose 3.

Whereas in pediatric patients, an increase in dosage by a factor of 1.3 leads to proportional increase in the mean average plasma concentration ($C_{average}$) and in the mean area under the concentration versus time curve (AUC_{tau}), adult patients display a 2.8-fold, hyperproportional increase in exposure, indicating nonlinear disposition. As a consequence, pediatric patients given 4 mg/kg do not achieve the same exposure as adults given 4 mg/kg, the dosage that has led to the approval of voriconazole for first-line treatment of invasive aspergillosis.

Modified from Walsh TJ, Karlsson MO, Driscoll T, et al. Pharmacokinetics and safety of intravenous voriconazole in children after single- or multiple-dose administration. *Antimicrob Agents Chemother.* 2004;48:2166–2172.

In patients with renal insufficiency, no adjustment of dosage is needed for the oral formulation; because of the renal clearance of the intravenous carrier, patients with a creatinine clearance of less than 50 mL/min should receive voriconazole by the oral route. In patients with mild-to-moderate hepatic function abnormalities, half of the daily maintenance dosage is recommended after the initial loading dose. Recommendations for severe liver failure are lacking.[242,321]

Whereas the disposition of voriconazole in infants younger than 2 years of age has not been systematically investigated,[161] initial pharmacokinetic studies in children 2 to 11 years of age revealed a faster weight-normalized clearance rate than in adults and lower exposure at similar dosages (Table 240.12).[689] This and several subsequent formal pharmacokinetic studies revealed that children need higher exposures relative to adults and that young adolescents 12 to 14 years of age with low body weight (<50 kg) appear to metabolize voriconazole similarly to children.[173,174,207,329,683] As a consequence, an intravenous dosage of 8 mg/kg twice daily (with day 1 dose 9 mg/kg twice daily) and an oral dose of the suspension of 9 mg/kg twice daily has been adopted by the European Medicines Agency (EMA) for children 2 years of age to younger than 12 years and 12 to 14 years weighing less than 50 kg.[194,207] Of note, the pediatric dosing regimens outlined here have also been explored in Japanese patients and found to be appropriate for this special population.[453] Considering the significant relationships between exposure and outcome described earlier, therapeutic drug monitoring should be performed in pediatric patients with life-threatening invasive fungal infections.[239,388,401,473]

Voriconazole has been administered safely and successfully to children younger than 12 years of age who had no therapeutic alternative. Of 58 immunocompromised children with proven or probable invasive fungal infection refractory to or intolerant of conventional antifungal therapy, 26 patients (45%) had a complete or partial response and 4 patients (7%) discontinued therapy because of intolerance. A total of 23 patients had voriconazole-related adverse events, most commonly elevations in hepatic transaminases or bilirubin ($n = 8$), skin rash ($n = 8$), abnormal vision ($n = 3$), and photosensitivity reactions ($n = 3$).[690] A large retrospective post-approval cohort study in 107 immunocompromised pediatric patients who received 252 courses of voriconazole for a median of 65 days (range, 1–1001) reported further safety data. Irrespective of causal relationships, increases in hepatic transaminases (53.5%), serum bilirubin (23.6%), and alkaline phosphatase (10.9%), skin eruptions (5.6%), and neurologic adverse events (4.8%) were mostly mild to moderate. Adverse events necessitating discontinuation of voriconazole occurred in 18 courses (7.1%). Treatment success was observed in 16 of 37 patients with proved, probable, or possible infections, and in 203 of 215 courses of empirical therapy or prophylaxis.[524] In other pediatric studies providing sufficient information, the rate of drug discontinuations because of adverse events was between 5% and 19%. Increases in hepatic transaminases were the most commonly observed adverse advents, followed by skin eruptions, and no consistent correlation between dose or exposure and adverse events have been established.[163] Voriconazole also has been used with success and acceptable tolerance in many patients with cystic fibrosis and allergic bronchopulmonary aspergillosis[291] and as antifungal prophylaxis in patients with hematologic malignancies or allogeneic HSCT.[164,414,422,449,736]

Isavuconazole

Isavuconazonium sulfate (Cresemba) is the water-soluble prodrug of isavuconazole, a broad-spectrum antifungal triazoles with activity against yeasts, molds, and dimorphic fungi. Isavuconazole is available as intravenous solution and as capsules for oral administration and approved for treatment of invasive aspergillosis and mucormycosis.[105,193,439]

Pharmacodynamics. Similar to other members of its class, isavuconazole is considered fungistatic against yeasts and mostly fungicidal against opportunistic moulds.[439] In vitro, prolonged antifungal effects of up to 5 hours duration have been demonstrated against *C. albicans.*[701] In a neutropenic murine model of disseminated candidiasis, the AUC/MIC ratio was the pharmacodynamic index that correlated best with efficacy. Pharmacodynamic targets for *C. albicans* were similar to those observed with other triazoles; however, targets for non-*albicans Candida* species were more than 10-fold lower than those for *C. albicans.*[385] In a persistently neutropenic rabbit model of invasive pulmonary aspergillosis, isavuconazole demonstrated dosage- and concentration-dependent response in reducing mortality, organism-mediated pulmonary injury, residual fungal burden, serum galactomannan index (GMI), and serum (1→3)-β-D-glucan levels.[512] Within the same model system, the AUC/MIC ratio correlated with suppression of the galactomannan index (GMI), and bridging of this experimental pharmacodynamic target to human population PK data showed the applicability of this efficacy endpoint for patients with invasive aspergillosis.[352] Similarly, using population pharmacokinetic data, Monte Carlo simulations, and the non-neutropenic murine efficacy index corresponding to 90% survival, isavuconazole exposures were achieved in >90% of simulated patients to treat MICs up to and including 1 mg/L according to EUCAST methodology, and >90% up to and including 0.5 mg/L according to CLSI methodology, respectively.[156] These investigations confirm the current dosing regimen and are helpful in setting interpretive breakpoints for in vitro resistance testing.

Pharmacokinetics. After systemic administration, the prodrug isavuconazonium sulfate is converted by plasma esterases to isavuconazole and the inactive cleavage product. The conversion is rapid and complete, with greater than 98% of a dose being converted to isavuconazole. The cleavage product is eliminated by metabolism and subsequent renal excretion of the metabolites.[105,193,439] In pharmacokinetic studies in healthy volunteers, maximum plasma concentrations (C_{max}) of isavuconazole were observed at 1.5 to 3 hours after oral administration or at the end of the 1-hour infusion. C_{max} and AUC values increased proportionally to the administered dose; there was a four- to fivefold accumulation during once-daily dosing, which is in line with the long terminal elimination half-life of isavuconazole of 84.5 to 117 hours, and the oral bioavailability was calculated at 98%. At steady state, after daily doses of 50 and 100 mg, the volume of distribution amounted to 308 to 542 L and systemic clearance was 2.4 to 4.1 L/h.[582,583] In a population-based pharmacokinetic model including data from nine phase I and one phase III clinical trial, a 2-compartment model with Weibull absorption function and first-order elimination process adequately described plasma isavuconazole concentrations; the mean estimate for isavuconazole clearance was 2.36 L/h, and those for the volumes of the central and peripheral compartments 49.1 and 417 L, respectively.[156] Isavuconazole is metabolized by the liver and excreted in metabolized form into urine and feces; in vitro studies indicate that CYP3A4, CYP3A5, and subsequently uridine diphosphate-glucuronosyltransferases (UGT) are involved.[109,193]

Adverse effects. Among 403 patients enrolled in two registration-relevant clinical trials, the most frequently reported adverse reactions of isavuconazole were gastrointestinal disturbances (13–26%), headache (17%), elevated liver chemistry tests (16%), hypokalemia (14%), dyspnea (12%), cough (12%), peripheral edema (11%), and back pain (10%). Serious adverse reactions occurred in 223 of 403 (55%) of patients, and 56 of 403 (14%) of patients permanently discontinued treatment due to an adverse reaction.[105] In trial 1, a randomized, double-blind comparison of isavuconazole (200 mg intravenously three times a day on days 1 and 2, then either intravenously or orally once daily) versus voriconazole (6 mg/kg intravenously twice daily on day 1, 4 mg/kg intravenously twice daily on day 2, then intravenously 4 mg/kg twice daily or orally 200 mg twice daily from day 3 onwards), most patients (247 [96%] receiving isavuconazole and 255 [98%] receiving voriconazole) had treatment-emergent adverse events (P = .122). Proportions of patients with treatment-emergent adverse events by system organ class were similar overall. However, isavuconazole-treated patients had a lower frequency of hepatobiliary disorders (23 [9%] vs. 42 [16%]; P = .016), eye disorders (39 [15%] vs. 69 [27%]; P = .002), and skin or subcutaneous tissue disorders (86 [33%] vs. 110 [42%]; P = .037). Drug-related adverse events were reported in 109 (42%) patients receiving isavuconazole and 155 (60%) receiving voriconazole (P < .001). In this pivotal trial, isavuconazole was well tolerated, with fewer study-drug–related adverse events relative to voriconazole.[408]

Drug interactions. Isavuconazole is a substrate of CYP3A4 and CYP3A5. In vitro, isavuconazole is an inhibitor of CYP3A4, CYP2C8, CYP2C9, CYP2C19, and CYP2D6. Isavuconazole is also an inhibitor of P-gp-, BCRP-and OCT2-mediated drug transporters. In vitro, isavuconazole is also an inducer of CYP3A4, CYP2B6, CYP2C8, and CYP2C9.[105,193,241] Because of the lack of a pediatric label, a detailed description of drug-drug interactions of isavuconazole is beyond the scope of this chapter, and the respective drug product label with the full prescribing information should be consulted.

Clinical efficacy. The clinical efficacy of isavuconazole has been investigated in phase II and III clinical trials in patients with uncomplicated esophageal candidiasis, candidemia or invasive candidiasis, and invasive mold disease caused by *Aspergillus* and other filamentous fungi, as well as those causing mucormycosis.[736,689,699,702]

In a dose-ranging phase II trial of isavuconazole in 160 patients with uncomplicated esophageal candidiasis evaluating different dosing regimens of isavuconazole and fluconazole 100 mg once daily (day 1: 200 mg), endoscopically confirmed clinical success rates after a minimum of 14 days of treatment were similar to those of fluconazole for each arm; there were no differences in the percentages of relapse at day 28 post end of treatment.[675] The efficacy and safety of isavuconazole in patients with candidemia and other forms of invasive candidiasis were investigated in a phase III randomized, double-blind trial comparing isavuconazole 200 mg IV three times daily for 2 days, followed by 200 mg IV daily versus caspofungin (70 mg IV daily on day 1, followed by 50 mg IV daily) with the option for a switch to oral isavuconazole (isavuconazole arm) or voriconazole (caspofungin arm) after day 10. The primary efficacy endpoint was successful overall response (based on successful clinical and mycological responses, and no use of alternative systemic antifungal therapy post end of treatment) at the end of IV therapy (EOIV). Among 400 evaluable patients, the primary endpoint of successful overall response at EOIV (isavuconazole, n/N = 120/199 [60.3%]; caspofungin, n/N = 143/201 [71.1%]; adjusted difference [95%CI]: −10.8 [−19.9, −1.8]) did not meet the prespecified non-inferiority margin. However, key secondary endpoints, all-cause mortality, and other outcomes including safety were similar in both arms.[368]

The efficacy of isavuconazole against invasive aspergillosis was studied in a phase III, double-blind, randomized trial. Adult patients with suspected invasive mold disease were randomized to receive 200 mg isavuconazole intravenously three times a day on days 1 and 2, then either intravenously or orally once daily or voriconazole 6 mg/kg intravenously twice daily on day 1, 4 mg/kg intravenously twice daily on day 2, then intravenously 4 mg/kg twice daily or orally 200 mg twice daily from day 3 onward. A total of 527 adult patients were randomly assigned (258 received study medication per group); all-cause mortality from first dose of study drug to day 42 was 19% with isavuconazole and 20% with voriconazole with an adjusted treatment difference of −1.0% (95% CI −7.8 to 5.7), meeting criteria for non-inferiority. In the cohort of 231 patients who had proven or probable invasive aspergillosis, all-cause mortality was 18.7% in the isavuconazole arm and 22.2% in the voriconazole arm, respectively, with an adjusted treatment difference of −2.7% (95% CI −13.6 to 8.2). Overall treatment success for proven/probable invasive aspergillosis at end of therapy was 35.0% (43/123) versus 38.9% (42/108) (95% CI, −16.3 to −8.4], not significant).

Isavuconazole was as effective as voriconazole and well tolerated with fewer study-drug–related adverse events relative to voriconazole.[408] The efficacy of isavuconazole for treatment of mucormycosis was assessed in a single-arm open-label phase III trial (VITAL study) using the identical dosing regimen as before and compared with amphotericin B in a matched case-control analysis. In this study, 37 patients with mucormycosis received isavuconazole for a median of 84 days (range, 2–882). By day 42, four patients (11%) had a partial response, 16 (43%) had stable disease, one (3%) had disease progression, three (8%) had missing assessments, and 13 (35%) had died. Day 42 crude all-cause mortality in seven (33%) of 21 primary-treatment isavuconazole cases was similar to 13 (39%) of 33 amphotericin B-treated matched controls (weighted all-cause mortality: 33% vs. 41%; P = 0.595).[428] Efficacy of isavuconazole has also been demonstrated in a limited number of patients with cryptococcosis and infections caused by dimorphic fungi who were enrolled in the VITAL open-label nonrandomized phase III clinical trial,[633] attesting to the potentially broader clinical usefulness of this agent.

Approval status and dosing. Isavuconazole is approved in both the United States and the European Union for patients 18 years of age and older for treatment of invasive aspergillosis and for treatment of mucormycosis.[105,193] In the European Union, the indication for treatment of mucormycosis is limited to patients for whom amphotericin B is inappropriate.[193] The approved dosage for both the intravenous and the oral capsule formulations is a loading dose of 200 mg isavuconazole (corresponding to 372 mg isavuconazonium sulfate) every 8 hours for six doses (48 hours), followed by a maintenance dose of 200 mg of isavuconazole once daily starting 12 to 24 hours after the last loading dose. No dose adjustment is required based on age, gender, or race. In patients with mild, moderate, or severe renal impairment, and in patients with mild or moderate hepatic impairment, no dose adjustment is necessary; for patients with severe hepatic impairment, no data exist and caution is warranted.[105,193] The pharmacokinetics and safety of isavuconazole in pediatric patients (<18 years) have not been studied yet; formal investigation plans for pediatric development of the compound exist for both the United States and the European Union but remain to be executed.

Echinocandin Lipopeptides

The echinocandins are a distinct class of semisynthetic amphiphilic lipopeptides that are composed of a cyclic hexapeptide core linked to a variably configured lipid side chain. The first compound of this class was cilofungin (LY 121019), an echinocandin B derivative with activity limited to *Candida* spp. However, clinical development was abandoned because of concerns regarding toxicity associated with the intravenous polyethylene glycol formulation vehicle.[221,251,561] Since the 1990s, a second generation of semisynthetic echinocandins with extended antifungal spectrum against *Candida* and *Aspergillus* spp., excellent safety profiles, and favorable pharmacokinetic characteristics has been developed: anidulafungin (Eraxis and Ecalta), caspofungin (Cancidas and generic forms), and micafungin (Mycamine) (Fig. 240.8). With few exceptions, current data indicate that these agents are not fundamentally different with respect to spectrum, pharmacodynamics, pharmacokinetics, safety, and antifungal efficacy.

Mechanism of action. The echinocandins act by noncompetitive inhibition of the synthesis of (1→3)-β-D-glucan, a polysaccharide in the cell wall of many pathogenic fungi (Fig. 240.9). Together with chitin, the ropelike glucan fibrils are responsible for the cell wall's strength and shape. They are important in maintaining the osmotic integrity of the fungal cell and play a key role in cell division and cell growth.[149,150,279] The proposed molecular target of the echinocandins, glucan synthase, is a heteromeric enzyme complex composed of at least one large integral

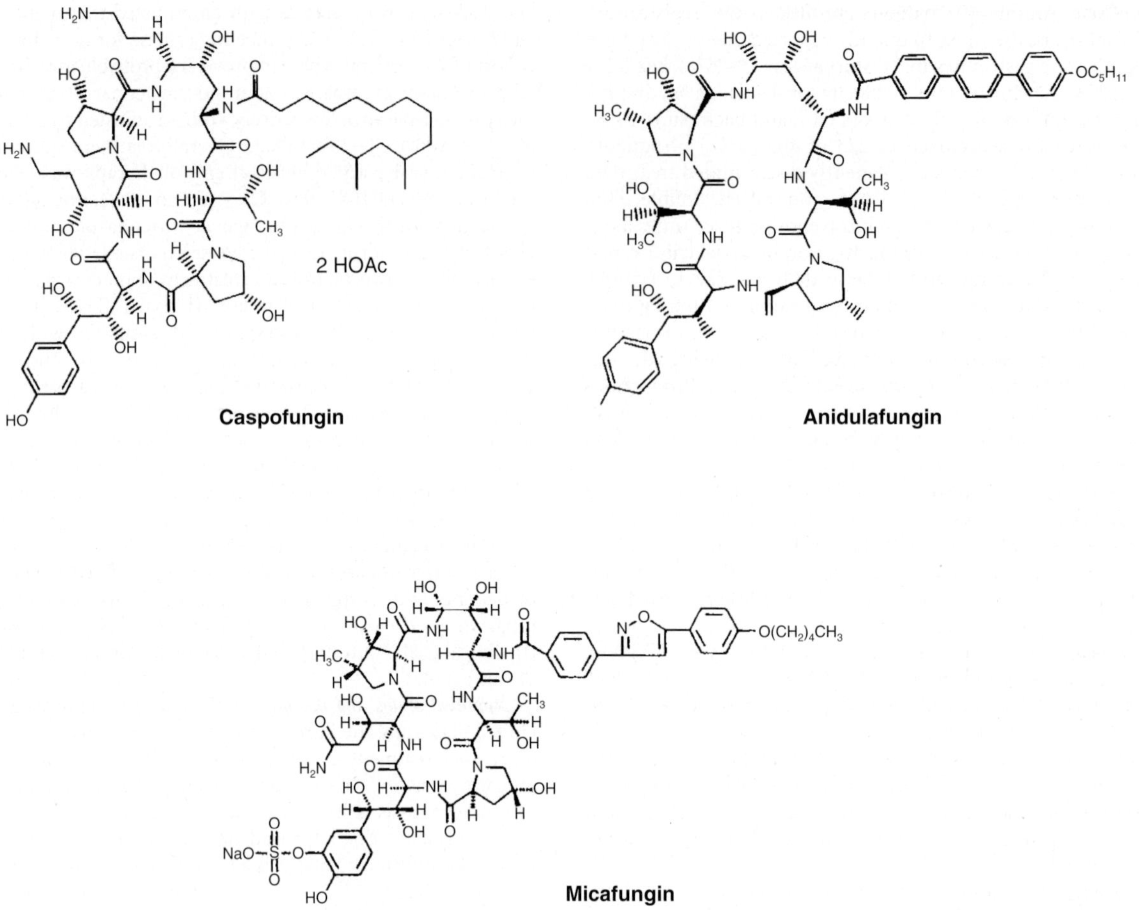

Caspofungin

Anidulafungin

Micafungin

FIG. 240.8 Structural formulas of echinocandin lipopeptides: anidulafungin, caspofungin, and micafungin.

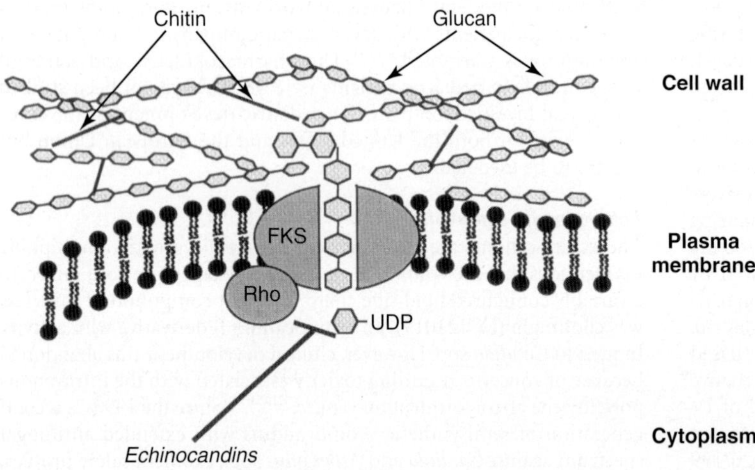

FIG. 240.9 Schematic of the proposed mechanism of action of echinocandin lipopeptides. Echinocandins inhibit the synthesis of cell wall 1,3-β-glucan at the level of the cell membrane. *FKS* is the proposed catalytic subunit, and *Rho* the proposed regulatory subunit of the glucan synthase complex. (Modified from Kurtz MB, Douglas CM. Lipopeptide inhibitors of fungal glucan synthase. *J Med Vet Mycol.* 1997;35:79-86.)

membrane protein encoded by the *FKS* gene that binds the substrate (UDP-glucose), and one small regulatory subunit, Rho1p, a guanosine diphosphate (GTP)-binding protein; other, as-yet unidentified, components also may be involved.[369,632] Additional immunomodulatory effects through unmasking of (1→3)-β-D-glucan with proinflammatory host cytokine release have been described and may contribute to in vivo efficacy of the echinocandins.[387]

Antifungal activity. The echinocandins have potent and broad-spectrum fungicidal in vitro activity against most *Candida* spp., including azole-resistant strains and biofilms, and potent inhibitory activity against *Aspergillus* spp. Their antifungal efficacy against these organisms in vivo has been demonstrated in various animal models. The current echinocandins have variable activity against dematiaceous and endemic mold and are considered inactive against most Hyalohyphomycetes, Mucorales, *C. neoformans,* and *T. asahii.* All echinocandins have demonstrated preventive and therapeutic activity in animal models of *Pneumocystis jirovecii* (formerly *Pneumocystis carinii*) pneumonitis. Preclinical in vitro and in vivo studies consistently have shown no antagonism between echinocandins and other antifungal agents but have shown indifference, additivity, or synergy when tested against *Aspergillus* spp., *C. albicans,* and non-*albicans Candida* spp.[190,244,248,251,509,667]

Resistance. Whereas the echinocandins show no cross-resistance to amphotericin B, co-resistance to both azoles and echinocandins in clinical isolates of *C. glabrata* may occur[515,741] and is of concern[509,598] as it may be associated with increased all-cause mortality in patients.[700] Very recently, a mutator phenotype caused by a mismatch repair defect has been described that is prevalent in *C. glabrata* clinical isolates and confers a higher propensity to breakthrough in preclinical experiments, and that may at least partially explain the elevated rates of triazole and multidrug resistance associated with *C. glabrata*.[276] Nevertheless, the frequency of resistance to echinocandins in otherwise susceptible fungal yeast species remains overall low.[509,598] Resistance to echinocandins during the course of therapy also has been reported for *C. krusei*.[506] Reduced echinocandin susceptibility may occur by three mechanisms: adaptive stress responses, which result in elevated cell wall chitin content and paradoxical growth in vitro at supraminimum inhibitory concentrations that greatly exceed those achieved in plasma (paradoxical effect); acquired *FKS* mutations, which confer reduced glucan synthase sensitivity, elevated MICs and clinical failure; and intrinsic *FKS* mutations. Intrinsic *FKS* mutations are naturally occurring mutations in the *C. parapsilosis* group and *C. guilliermondii* that confer elevated MIC levels but a lower level of reduced glucan synthase sensitivity in contrast to acquired *FKS* mutations. Of note, some *FKS* mutants have been shown to have significantly reduced fitness and virulence, which may contribute to the low incidence of echinocandin resistance reported in large surveillance studies.[69,369,500,509,598] New, species-specific clinical breakpoints that consider wild-type MICs, epidemiologic cutoff values, and pharmacokinetic and pharmacodynamic relationships have been proposed that are more sensitive to detect emerging resistance associated with FKS mutations and better able to predict risk for clinical failure.[31,509,516]

Relative to *Candida* spp., much less is currently known about echinocandin resistance among *Aspergillus* spp.; however, clinical breakthrough cases have been reported, and resistance has been confirmed in vivo.[218,305,521]

Pharmacodynamics. The echinocandins demonstrate a species-dependent mode of antifungal activity. Whole-cell in vitro assays reveal fungicidal activity against most *Candida* spp. but not against *Aspergillus* spp.[51,624] Microscopic examination of drug-exposed *A. fumigatus* shows a dose-dependent formation of microcolonies with progressively truncated, swollen hyphal elements that appear to be cell wall deficient but are able to regain their cell walls on subculture in the absence of drug.[168,370,482,541] These observations demonstrate differences in functional target sensitivity that are not fully understood. Time-kill studies in *Candida* spp. demonstrated predominantly concentration- and time-dependent fungicidal activity and rate-of-kill at concentrations greater than the MIC for all three compounds.[187,189,510] In addition, PAFEs between 5 and 12 hours at concentrations above the MIC have been demonstrated.[188,413]

In persistently neutropenic rabbit models, anidulafungin showed highly predictable concentration-effect relationships in experimental disseminated candidiasis; however, no concentration-effect relationships were observed in experimental pulmonary aspergillosis, despite full exploration of the dosage range.[247] Pharmacodynamic studies in murine kidney target models of disseminated candidiasis showed that the AUC/MIC ratio is the pharmacodynamic parameter that predicts efficacy of the echinocandins.[21,22,23,398] In a murine model of invasive pulmonary aspergillosis, the C_{max}/MEC ratio appeared to be the parameter most closely associated with efficacy.[717] Pharmacokinetic and pharmacodynamic correlations of all echinocandins have been explored in patients with esophageal and oropharyngeal candidiasis.[254] Using large datasets from two phase III clinical trials of micafungin for invasive candidiasis, a significant relationship between the AUC/MIC ratio of micafungin and mycological response was found by population pharmacokinetics and regression analysis; Monte Carlo simulation revealed lower AUC/MIC target for *C. parapsilosis* relative to other *Candida* spp., supporting the concept of species-specific echinocandin susceptibility breakpoints.[21]

Pharmacokinetics. The three currently available echinocandins are available only for intravenous administration. They exhibit dose-proportional plasma pharmacokinetics with a triexponential elimination pattern. Their β half-life is between 10 and 15 hours, thus allowing for once-daily dosing without major accumulation after multiple dosing. All echinocandins are highly (≥95%) protein-bound and distribute into all major organ sites, including the brain; however, concentrations in uninfected CSF are low. Within the lung, anidulafungin and micafungin have been shown to predominantly concentrate in alveolar macrophages. The echinocandins are chemically degraded or metabolized by the liver and slowly excreted into urine and feces; only small fractions (≤2%) of a dose are excreted into urine in unchanged form (Table 240.13).[125,137,139,254,668,687] The current echinocandins are not dialyzable, and no adjustment in dose is required for patients with renal insufficiency or renal failure. Similarly, no adjustment in dose is necessary for patients with mild-to-moderate (all) or severe (anidulafungin, micafungin) hepatic failure. Whether the minor differences in individual pharmacokinetic parameters such as AUC, peak plasma levels, volume of distribution, and clearance of the echinocandins are of clinical significance remains to be elucidated.

Adverse effects. At current dosages, anidulafungin, caspofungin, and micafungin generally are well tolerated. Fewer than 10% of patients enrolled in the various randomized comparative clinical trials discontinued echinocandin therapy because of drug-related adverse events.[148,359,451,539,654,697] Increased liver transaminases, gastrointestinal symptoms, skin rash, and headache probably or definitely associated with echinocandin treatment have been reported to occur at a frequency of less than 5% each. Like other basic polypeptides, the echinocandins have the theoretical potential to cause release of histamine.[148,359,451,539,654,697] Symptoms such as rash, facial swelling, pruritus, sensation of warmth, and anaphylactic reactions have been reported in isolated cases. Because of transient elevations of hepatic transaminases in interaction studies in healthy volunteers,[258] the concomitant use of caspofungin and cyclosporine currently is not recommended; clinical experience, however, indicates that both drugs can be given safely under careful monitoring.[238,424,640]

Drug interactions. In vitro studies showed that anidulafungin does not significantly inhibit the activities of clinically important human CYP450 isoforms at clinically relevant concentrations and that it is not an inhibitor of P-glycoprotein. Interaction studies demonstrated that no adjustment of dosage of either drug is warranted when anidulafungin

TABLE 240.13 Principal Pharmacokinetic Properties of the Echinocandin Lipopeptides Caspofungin, Anidulafungin, and Micafungin

Properties	Caspofungin	Anidulafungin	Micafungin
Formulation	IV	IV	IV
Dose linearity	Yes	Yes	Yes
Oral bioavailability (%)	n/a	n/a	n/a
Protein binding (%)	97	84	99
Volume of distribution (L/kg)	N/A	0.7-0.9	0.24
Elimination half-life (h)	8-10	24	15
Substrate/inhibitor of CYP450	NA	NA	NA
Routes of elimination	Degradation/metabolization, urine > feces	Degradation only, feces	Metabolization, feces > urine

CYP450, Cytochrome P450; *NA,* not applicable.
Data from references 243, 256, 258, and 668.

is coadministered with cyclosporine, tacrolimus, voriconazole, liposomal amphotericin B, or rifampin.[107]

Caspofungin is not a substrate of P-glycoprotein and is a poor substrate and a weak inhibitor of CYP450 enzymes.[42,732] Clinical studies demonstrated that the pharmacokinetic properties of caspofungin are not altered by itraconazole, amphotericin B, mycophenolate, nelfinavir, or tacrolimus. Caspofungin has no effect on the pharmacokinetics of itraconazole, amphotericin B, or the active metabolite of mycophenolate. Caspofungin can reduce the AUC of tacrolimus by approximately 20%, but it has no effect on cyclosporine levels. Inducers of drug clearance or mixed inducer and inhibitors, namely efavirenz, nelfinavir, nevirapine, phenytoin, rifampin, dexamethasone, and carbamazepine, may reduce caspofungin concentrations, and dose adjustment to a daily dose of 70 mg of caspofungin should be considered.[104,258,621]

Micafungin is a weak inhibitor of CYP3A in vitro, but it is neither a P-glycoprotein substrate nor inhibitor in vitro. In clinical studies, micafungin had no effect on mycophenolate mofetil, cyclosporine, tacrolimus, prednisolone, fluconazole, and voriconazole pharmacokinetics, but it increased the AUC of sirolimus, nifedipine, and itraconazole by approximately 20%. Patients receiving sirolimus, nifedipine, or itraconazole in combination with micafungin should be monitored for toxicity of these drugs, and sirolimus, nifedipine, and itraconazole dosage should be reduced if necessary. Amphotericin B, mycophenolate mofetil, cyclosporine, tacrolimus, prednisolone, sirolimus, nifedipine, fluconazole, itraconazole, voriconazole, ritonavir, and rifampin were shown to have no effects on the pharmacokinetics of micafungin.[108,256]

Caspofungin

Clinical efficacy. The clinical efficacy of caspofungin against *Candida* spp. was demonstrated first in phase II and 3 studies in immunocompromised patients with esophageal candidiasis.[30,676,677] A multicenter, randomized, double-blind phase III clinical trial investigated the efficacy of caspofungin for primary treatment of invasive *Candida* infections in 224 mostly nonneutropenic patients with D-AmB (0.6–1 mg/kg) as comparator agent. Among patients receiving at least one dose of the study drug, 73% of patients in the caspofungin cohort and 61.7% of patients in the D-AmB cohort had therapeutic success at the end of intravenous therapy. Among patients who received five or more doses, the response rates were 80.7% and 64.9%, respectively. No difference occurred in relapse or survival, but caspofungin was better tolerated.[451] Further large randomized clinical trials in patients with candidemia and other forms of invasive candidiasis showed similar outcomes of the standard dose of caspofungin relative to 100 and 150 mg daily of micafungin[499] and no general advantage of a high-dose (150 mg/day) caspofungin treatment regimen.[68] In deep-seated invasive candidiasis, including peritonitis, abdominal abscesses, chronic disseminated candidiasis, and arthritis, caspofungin was effective and safe at regular doses and up to 100 mg daily.[130]

A multicenter phase II salvage trial of caspofungin in 83 patients with definite or probable invasive aspergillosis revealed a complete or partial response in 45% of patients receiving at least one dose of caspofungin; in patients receiving the drug for more than 7 days, the response rate was 56%.[406] Rates of complete or partial responses in subsequent exploratory phase II clinical trials for primary treatment of proved or probable invasive aspergillosis appear to correlate with patients' comorbidities and range from 33%[678] and 42%[285] to 54%.[133] Caspofungin in combination with a triazole or polyene has been shown to be safe and effective in phase II trials and is an option for salvage therapy of invasive aspergillosis.[98,255,404]

In a large, randomized, double-blind clinical trial including 1095 patients, caspofungin was as effective as liposomal amphotericin B for empirical antifungal therapy in persistently febrile granulocytopenic patients, but it was better tolerated. The proportion of patients who survived at least 7 days after therapy was greater in the caspofungin group (92.6% vs. 89.2%).[697] Finally, randomized prospective comparisons suggest that caspofungin may be useful for prophylaxis in high-risk patients with hematologic malignancies.[103,430]

Approval status and dosing. Caspofungin is licensed in both the United States and Europe in patients 3 months of age or older with candidemia and certain forms of invasive *Candida* infections, as second-line therapy for invasive aspergillosis, and for empirical antifungal therapy in granulocytopenic patients [104,191]. In the United States, caspofungin also is approved for treatment of esophageal candidiasis (see Tables 240.2, 240.3, and 240.9).[104] The adult dosage regimen is 50 mg daily, with a single 70-mg loading dose on day 1, administered over 1 hour. No dosage adjustment is required in patients with renal insufficiency and mild hepatic insufficiency. In patients with moderate hepatic insufficiency (Child-Pugh category B), a maintenance dose of 35 mg/day is recommended after the loading dose of 70 mg. No recommendations exist for patients with severe hepatic insufficiency (Child-Pugh category C).[104,192,258]

In children and adolescents 2 to 17 years of age, the pharmacokinetics and safety of caspofungin were investigated using both a weight-based and a body surface-area regimen. Whereas a maintenance dosage of 1 mg/kg per day achieved suboptimal exposure, dosing with 50 mg/m^5 per day provided similar or slightly higher exposure relative to adults (Table 240.14).[682] In conjunction with pharmacokinetic data obtained in small children,[472] the dosage of 50 mg/m^5 per day (with day 1 dose 70 mg/m^5 per day and maximum daily dose of 70 mg) has been selected for pediatric patients between 3 months and 17 years of age.[104,195] This dosing regimen has been confirmed by a population pharmacokinetic study including 124 pediatric patients ages 3 months to 17 years enrolled in four clinical trials.[390] In neonates up to 3 months of postnatal age, limited pharmacokinetic data obtained in a small cohort of patients suggest that a dosage of 25 mg/m^5 per day results in similar bloodstream exposures as 50 mg/m^5 per day in older patients.[195,485,567] The experience with anidulafungin and micafungin, however, suggests that higher doses are likely needed to treat CNS infection.

Caspofungin appears to be well tolerated in pediatric patients. In the previously mentioned phase I and II dose-finding studies, none of

TABLE 240.14 Single-Dose Caspofungin Pharmacokinetics in Pediatric vs. Adult Patients[a]

	CHILDREN (2–11 Y)			
Dosage	**1 mg/kg**	**50 mg/m^5**	**Adolescents (12–17 y) 50 mg/m^5**	**Adults 50 mg**
$AUC_{0\text{-}24\,h}$ (µg/h/mL)	41.5	96.4	77.6	70.6
C1 (µg/mL)	6.59	13.9	7.67	7.67
C24 (µg/mL)	0.45	1.09	1.35	1.35
$t_{1/2}\beta$ (h)	7.2	7.6	11.7	11.7
Cl (mL/min/m^5)	8.57	7.78	6.07	6.07

[a]Least square means are reported for AUC, C1 (peak plasma concentration [C_{max}]), and C24 (minimum plasma concentration [C_{min}]), and harmonic means for $t_{1/2}\beta$. Data were obtained in groups of 6 to 10. Data in pediatric patients were compared with those obtained in 32 adult patients with mucosal candidiasis. In comparison with adult values, a 1-mg/kg dosage does not achieve the target trough concentration of caspofungin of 1 µg/mL and leads to a lower exposure as measured by the $AUC_{0\text{-}24\,h}$; the dosage regimen of 50 mg/m^5 leads to similar or slightly higher trough concentrations and similar or slightly higher exposure ($AUC_{0\text{-}24\,h}$).

Modified from Walsh TJ, Adamson PC, Seibel NL, et al. Pharmacokinetics, safety, and tolerability of caspofungin in children and adolescents. *Antimicrob Agents Chemother.* 2005;49:4536-4545.

AUC, Area under the concentration versus time curve from 0 to 24 hours; *Cl,* clearance; $t_{1/2}\beta$, elimination half-life.

the patients developed a serious drug-related adverse event or discontinued because of toxicity.[472,567,682] In a phase III estimation trial with safety as the primary objective, 82 patients between the ages of 2 and 17 years with persistent fever and neutropenia were randomly assigned to receive caspofungin or liposomal amphotericin B 3 mg/kg daily in a 2:1 ratio. Rates of drug-related adverse events were similar (clinical 48.2% vs. 46.2%; laboratory 10.7% vs. 19.2%); serious drug-related adverse events occurred in 1.8% of caspofungin-treated patients and in 11.5% of amphotericin B–treated patients. Overall success rates were not different.[407] A prospective phase II trial in 49 patients with invasive *Candida* or *Aspergillus* infections revealed no serious drug-related adverse events and an overall response rate of 73%.[738] In the combined analysis of caspofungin safety in all five clinical registration trials involving 171 pediatric patients 1 week to 17 years of age, the most common drug-related adverse events were fever (11.7%), increased alanine transaminase level (6.5%), and rash (4.7%); few events were serious (0.6%) or required treatment discontinuation (1.2%).[739] Favorable safety experiences also have been reported in immunocompromised pediatric patients who received the compound for various indications, mostly in combination with other antifungal agents,[100,166,206,238,452] and in neonates with refractory invasive candidiasis.[468,484,485] Breakthrough infections with rare fungal pathogens not inherently susceptible to echinocandins have been reported in individual patients and may need to be considered in cases of treatment failure.[458,734]

Anidulafungin

Clinical efficacy. The clinical efficacy of anidulafungin against *Candida* spp. was demonstrated in phase II or III studies in immunocompromised patients with esophageal candidiasis and candidemia. Anidulafungin had efficacy equivalent to that of fluconazole in esophageal candidiasis in a randomized, double-blind, international multicenter study; success was documented in 242 of 249 evaluable anidulafungin-treated patients (97.2%) and in 252 of 255 fluconazole-treated patients (98.8%). Adverse events leading to discontinuation were reported in 29 anidulafungin-treated patients (10%) versus 23 fluconazole-treated patients (8%).[358] In a dose-ranging study in 123 patients with invasive candidiasis randomized to anidulafungin 50, 75, or 100 mg once daily, success rates at end of therapy were 84%, 90%, and 89%, respectively.[359] A subsequent randomized, double-blind phase III noninferiority trial compared anidulafungin 100 mg once daily with fluconazole 400 mg once daily in a total of 245 mostly nonneutropenic patients with invasive candidiasis.[539] More patients receiving anidulafungin had clinical and microbiologic success at the end of intravenous therapy (75.6% vs. 60.2%); similar superiority was found at the 2- and 6-week follow-up after the end of all therapy (64.6% vs. 49.2% and 55.9% vs. 44.1%, respectively). The rate of death from all causes was 31% in the fluconazole group and 23% in the anidulafungin group ($P = .13$). A randomized double-blind clinical trial comparing open-label voriconazole plus blinded anidulafungin or blinded placebo for treatment of proved or probable invasive aspergillosis in patients with hematologic malignancies or allogeneic HSCT showed a statistical trend ($P = .07$) favoring the combination therapy with respect to the overall survival at 6 weeks, the primary endpoint of the study.[425] In an unscheduled post-hoc analysis of patients diagnosed on the basis of positive galactomannan, which accounted for 78% of the study population, overall survival at 6 weeks was significantly higher in the combination arm. Although the clinical implications of this study are still debated, regulatory approval of this combination has failed.

Approval status and dosing. Anidulafungin is licensed in both the United States and Europe for patients 18 years of age or older for candidemia and certain forms of invasive *Candida* infections in non-neutropenic patients.[107,192] In the United States, the compound is also licensed for esophageal candidiasis (see Table 240.2).[107] The recommended dose regimen consists of 100 mg (day 1: 200 mg) for invasive candidiasis and 50 mg daily (day 1:100 mg), for esophageal candidiasis, administered at a rate of 1.1 mg/min or higher. No dosage adjustment is needed in patients with renal impairment, patients undergoing hemodialysis, and patients with hepatic impairment (Child-Pugh classes A, B, and C).[107,192,549]

A pediatric phase I and II multicenter study of the pharmacokinetics and safety of anidulafungin has been completed in 19 granulocytopenic children with cancer. Patients were divided into two age cohorts (2 to 11 and 12 to 17 years) and were enrolled into sequential groups to receive 0.75 or 1.5 mg/kg per day[56] (Table 240.15). No drug-related serious adverse events were recorded. Pharmacokinetic parameters were similar across age groups and dosage cohorts and similar relative to adult patients. Following single and multiple daily doses of 0.75 mg/kg and 1.5 mg/kg, plasma concentration data corresponded to those in adults following a daily 50 and 100 mg dose, respectively.[56] In infants and neonates at risk for invasive candidiasis receiving 1.5 mg/kg per day anidulafungin after a single loading dose of 3 mg/kg, drug exposure levels after multiple doses were similar between neonates and infants and similar to those in children receiving similar weight-based dosing and in adult patients receiving 100 mg/day. No drug-related serious adverse events were observed.[124] Bridging studies from laboratory animals, however, indicate that a regimen of 3 mg/kg, followed by 1.5 mg/kg per day, is suboptimal for treatment of *Candida* meningoencephalitis and that higher dosages will be required to treat this condition.[701] No further data are available at this point, and the pediatric development program of the compound has not been formally completed.

Micafungin

Clinical efficacy. Micafungin was studied in open-label dose-ranging trials of endoscopically proved esophageal candidiasis in patients with HIV infection.[513,622] A double-blind comparative study investigating 50, 100, and 150 mg/day versus fluconazole 200 mg/day for HIV-associated esophageal candidiasis showed similar endoscopic cure rates and safety

TABLE 240.15 Single-Dose Anidulafungin Pharmacokinetics in Pediatric vs. Adult Patients[a]

	PEDIATRIC PATIENTS (2–17 Y)		ADULTS	
Dosage	**0.75 mg/kg**	**1.5 mg/kg**	**50 mg**	**100 mg**
C_{max} (μg/mL)	4.02	6.09	2.51	3.82
$AUC_{0\text{-}24\,h}$ (μg/h/mL)	48.0	9.7	53.3	104.8
$t_{1/2}\beta$ (h)	20.8	19.5	39.3[b]	42.3[b]
Cl (L/h/kg)	0.0175	0.0191	NA	NA
Vd_{ss} (L/kg)	0.45	0.49	0.72	0.78

[a]Pharmacokinetic parameters are expressed as mean values. Data were obtained in groups of six pediatric patients with compromised immunity and neutropenia per age group and dosage level, and were compared with those obtained in 26 adult healthy volunteers.

[b]$t_{1/2}\gamma$.

AUC, Area under the concentration versus time curve from 0 to 24 hours; *Cl,* clearance; C_{max}, peak plasma concentration; *NA,* not available; $t_{1/2}\beta$, elimination half-life; Vd_{ss}, volume of distribution at steady state.

Data from Benjamin DK Jr, Driscoll T, Seibel NL, et al. Safety and pharmacokinetics of intravenous anidulafungin in children with neutropenia at high risk for invasive fungal infections. *Antimicrob Agents Chemother.* 2006;50:632–638; and Vasquez JA, Sobel JD: Anidulafungin: a novel echinocandin. *Clin Infect Dis.* 2006;43:215–222.

profiles for micafungin at doses of 100 and 150 mg/day and fluconazole.[148] A further randomized, double-blind comparative trial in 523 patients 16 years of age and older with esophageal candidiasis investigated micafungin 150 mg/day versus fluconazole 200 mg/day.[147] For the primary endpoint of endoscopic cure, treatment difference was 0.3% (micafungin, 87.7%; fluconazole, 88.0%). A large randomized, double-blind noninferiority trial compared micafungin 100 mg once daily and liposomal amphotericin B 3 mg/kg once daily for first-line therapy of candidemia and other forms of invasive candidiasis in a total of 531 adult patients. The overall success rate in both treatment arms was similar (89.6% vs. 89.5%). No differences in survival were noted. Fewer severe treatment-related adverse events and adverse events that led to treatment discontinuation were observed in the micafungin arm.[371,557] In a second large, phase III, randomized clinical trial of a total of 595 patients with candidemia and other forms of invasive candidiasis, micafungin at 100 mg/day, micafungin at 150 mg/day, and caspofungin at 50 mg/day (with day 1 dose 70 mg) were equivalent in terms of efficacy, adverse events, and mortality.[178,499] A multinational, noncomparative open-label trial investigated micafungin for proved and probable invasive aspergillosis alone or in combination with another antifungal agent. A favorable response rate at the end of therapy was seen in 35.6% (80 of 225) of patients. Of those treated with only micafungin, favorable responses were seen in 6 of 12 (50%) of the primary and 9 of 22 (40.9%) of the salvage therapy group, with corresponding numbers in the combination treatment groups of 5 of 17 (29.4%) and 60 of 174 (34.5%) of the primary and salvage treatment groups, respectively.[151] Finally, micafungin 50 mg/day (<50 kg, 1 mg/kg) versus fluconazole 400 mg/day (<50 kg, 8 mg/kg) was investigated for prevention of invasive fungal infections in 882 patients undergoing HSCT. Prophylaxis was given from the start of the conditioning regimen until 5 days after engraftment. The overall success rate was significantly higher for patients randomized to receive micafungin (80.0% vs. 73.5%; $P = .03$). Drug-related adverse events were comparable.[654]

Approval status and dosing. In the United States, micafungin is licensed in adults and pediatric patients at least 4 months of age for prevention of *Candida* infections in patients undergoing HSCT, for treatment of candidemia and defined forms of invasive candidiasis, and for treatment of esophageal candidiasis (see Table 240.2).[108] In Europe, the compound is licensed for use in neonates, children, and adults for treatment of invasive candidiasis and as prophylaxis of *Candida* infections in patients with allogeneic HSCT and those with prolonged neutropenia; it is also licensed for treatment of esophageal candidiasis in individuals 16 years of age and older.[191] The recommended dosage is 100 mg/day for invasive candidiasis (US: ≤30 kg, 2 mg/kg; EU: ≤40 kg, 2 mg/kg), 150 mg/day for esophageal candidiasis (US: ≤340 kg, 3 mg/kg, >30 kg 2.5 mg/kg [maximum 150 mg]; EU: ≤40 kg, 3 mg/kg), and 50 mg/day (≤40 kg, 1 mg/kg) for the preventive indication. According to the European label, for invasive candidiasis, the dose may be increased to 200 mg/day in patients weighing more than 40 kg or 4 mg/kg per day in patients weighing 40 kg or less if the patient's response is inadequate.[194] The approved doses for children and neonates less than 4 months of age is 2 mg/kg and per day for prophylaxis of invasive candidiasis and 4 to 10 mg/kg and per day for treatment of invasive candidiasis. The SPC states that in this population, 4 mg/kg approximates drug exposures achieved in adults receiving 100 mg/day and that, if infection of the CNS is suspected, a higher dosage (e.g., 10 mg/kg) should be used. It also states that the safety and efficacy of doses of 4 and 10 mg/kg for the treatment of invasive candidiasis with CNS involvement has not been adequately established in controlled clinical studies.[195] Renal dysfunction, dialysis, or hepatic dysfunction does not alter the pharmacokinetics of micafungin and accordingly, no dose adjustments are required.[108,278]

The pharmacokinetics and safety of micafungin have been studied in 70 febrile granulocytopenic children 2 to 17 years of age. Micafungin was well tolerated at dosages of 0.5 to 3 mg/kg per day; pharmacokinetics were linear and similar to those observed in adults (Table 240.16).[590] Further pharmacokinetic studies in different populations of children of the same age range dosed between 1 and 4.5 mg/kg per day resulted in similar observations.[11,55,651] Population-based pharmacokinetic modeling of the data of the first dose-ranging study[299] and of pharmacokinetic data of 229 patients ages between 4 months and less than 17 years from four phase I and two phase III clinical trials[297] that used AUC_{24} target ranges of adults confirmed that dose regimens of 1, 2, and 3 mg/kg per day micafungin are appropriate for the prevention of invasive candidiasis, the treatment of invasive candidiasis, and the treatment of esophageal candidiasis, and that cutoffs of 40 or 50 kg for weight-based dosing resulted in heavier children being appropriately dosed. Of note, in the setting of prophylaxis, alternate dosing of micafungin (3 mg/kg) every other day provides drug exposure similar to standard dosing of 1 mg/kg given daily,[434] and alternate dosing may provide an alternative for antifungal prophylaxis in high-risk patients.[76,434]

The pharmacokinetics in neonates were explored in a phase I single-dose, multicenter, open-label, sequential-dose trial of micafungin 0.75 mg/kg, 1.5 mg/kg, and 3 mg/kg in 18 premature infants weighing more than 1000 g. On average, half-life was shorter and clearance more rapid in contrast to older children and adults.[286] Population pharmacokinetics modeling of the neonatal pharmacokinetics data and Monte Carlo simulation suggest that a larger neonatal dose is required to produce drug exposure comparable to those predicted on the basis of weight in children and adults; additional population pharmacokinetics based on open-label pharmacokinetics studies in which doses up to 15 mg/kg per day were safely administered support a target dose of

TABLE 240.16 Single-Dose Micafungin Pharmacokinetics in Pediatric Versus Adult Patients[a]

	PEDIATRIC PATIENTS (2–17 Y)			ADULTS	
Dosage	**1 mg/kg**	**2 mg/kg**	**4 mg**	**50 mg**	**100 mg**
C_{max} (μg/mL)	10.8	15.3	30.3	3.6	7.1
$AUC_{0\text{-}24\,h}$ (μg/h/mL)	40.3	83.0	191.4	33.9	59.9
$t_{1/2}\beta$ (h)	12.5	13.2	11.6	12.5	13.0
Cl (L/h/kg)	0.021	0.020	0.017	0.017[b]	0.018[b]
Vd_{ss} (L/kg)	0.33	0.31	0.28	0.31[b]	0.32[b]

[a]Pharmacokinetic parameters are expressed as mean values. Data were obtained in groups of seven to 15 pediatric patients with compromised immunity and neutropenia per age group and dosage level and were compared with those obtained in cohorts of eight to nine adult patients with hematopoietic stem cell transplantation.

[b]Weight normalization calculated by assuming an average body weight of 70 kg.

AUC, Area under the concentration versus time curve from 0 to 24 hours; *Cl,* clearance; C_{max}, peak plasma concentration; $t_{1/2}\beta$, elimination half-life; Vd_{ss}, volume of distribution at steady state.

Modified from Seibel NL, Schwartz C, Arrieta A, et al. Safety, tolerability, and pharmacokinetics of micafungin (FK463) in febrile neutropenic pediatric patients. *Antimicrob Agents Chemother.* 2005;49:3317–3324; and Groll AH, Stergiopoulou T, Roilides E, et al. Micafungin: pharmacology, experimental therapeutics and clinical applications. *Expert Opin Investig Drugs.* 2005;14:489–509.

10 mg/kg for neonates, particularly in view of the substantial risk for secondary brain involvement.[58,298,300,608] Although the treatment results in the pivotal candidemia study showed no signal for decreased efficacy at dosages between 2 and 4 mg/kg in this population,[534] a dose of at least 4 mg/kg in neonates with invasive candidiasis and a dose of 10 mg/kg in the case of CNS involvement is advocated.

A noncomparative phase II study investigated the activity of micafungin in combination with other agents (primarily liposomal amphotericin B) in 58 pediatric patients with mostly refractory invasive aspergillosis. The mean daily dose was 2.0 ± 1.2 mg/kg per day, and the mean duration of dosing was 67 ± 85 days. Overall response was 26 of 58 (45%). Thirteen patients (22%) discontinued micafungin, primarily because of a progression of underlying disease or invasive aspergillosis.[202] The comparative safety of micafungin was investigated in the pediatric subpopulation of a double-blind, phase III trial in patients with invasive candidiasis or candidemia. Patients were randomized to receive intravenous micafungin 2 mg/kg per day or liposomal amphotericin B 3 mg/kg per day for a minimum of 14 days. There was no difference in the success rates (69.2% vs. 74.1%). The incidence of serious adverse events (3.8% vs. 9.3%) and the rate of patients discontinuing therapy because of an adverse event (3.8% vs. 16.7%) were lower in patients treated with micafungin.[534] In a pooled analysis of adverse events data from six clinical trials that included close to 300 patients, 26.7% of patients had a treatment-related adverse event and 2.4% had a treatment-related adverse event that led to treatment discontinuation. No trends were seen with respect to dose or duration of treatment, and the types and rates of events were similar to those observed in adults.[34,35] Data from a large uncontrolled study of micafungin 1 mg/kg per day as prophylaxis during the neutropenic phase post allogeneic HSCT conducted in Korea[502] and of two large postapproval studies conducted by the manufacturer in Japan in the prophylactic and therapeutic setting[344,345] that enrolled a total of close to 600 pediatric patients of all age groups further attest to the safety of the compound. Last, in a systematic review of safety data of nine clinical trials involving 116 premature and nonpremature infants less than 2 years of age, treatment-related adverse events were recorded in 23% of patients; relative to low-birth-weight infants, more extremely low-birth-weight (15%) and very-low-birth-weight (40%) infants experienced treatment-related adverse events, but there was no relation to micafungin dose or duration.[417]

In Europe, the Summary of Product Characteristics for micafungin recommends careful monitoring of liver function and early discontinuation in the presence of significant and persistent elevation of alanine transaminase and aspartate transaminase values. It also recommends that micafungin treatment be conducted on a careful risk-benefit assessment, particularly in patients with liver diseases or concomitant hepatotoxic-genotoxic therapies.[191] This recommendation is based on preclinical data from a high-dose, long-term exposure model in rats treated with micafungin for either 3 or 6 months (equivalent to 12.5% or 25% of the total life span of the rat, respectively). The observed development of foci of altered hepatocytes and liver tumors in this species was dependent on both dose and duration of micafungin treatment. The human relevance of this finding is presently not known.

Agents for Systemic Treatment of Mycoses of the Skin and Its Appendages

Griseofulvin

Griseofulvin (Fig. 240.10) was isolated originally in 1939 as a natural product of *Penicillium griseofulvum*.[493] However, only in the late 1950s was it reported to be effective as an antifungal agent.[220] Griseofulvin has been used since extensively for the systemic treatment of superficial dermatophyte infections in both adults and children.

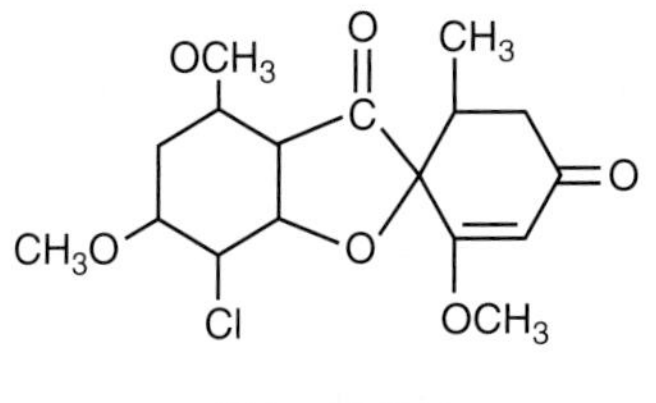

Griseofulvin

FIG. 240.10 Structural formula of griseofulvin.

Mechanism of action. Griseofulvin interferes with fungal microtubule formation. It disrupts the cell's mitotic spindle formation and thus arrests the metaphase of cell division.[262] Several additional mechanisms of action have been proposed, including inhibition of nucleic acid synthesis, interference with the synthesis of cell wall chitin, and anti-inflammatory properties.[267] Griseofulvin is deposited in keratin precursor cells and produces an unfavorable environment for fungal invasion; infected skin, hair, and nails are replaced with tissue not infected by the dermatophyte.

Antifungal activity. As evident from its mechanism of action, griseofulvin is a fungistatic compound. It is active against *Trichophyton, Microsporon*, and *Epidermophyton* spp. The drug has no activity against yeastlike organisms such as *Candida* spp., *Pityrosporum* spp., and *C. neoformans*. It also is inactive against opportunistic hyaline and dematiaceous molds and the dimorphic (endemic) molds.[199,208]

Pharmacokinetics. Griseofulvin is commercially available for oral administration only as generic griseofulvin microsize and griseofulvin ultramicrosize in suspension and tablet forms. Griseofulvin is weakly water soluble and poorly absorbed from the gastrointestinal tract. In contrast to nonmicrocrystalline drug preparations, microsize and ultramicrosize formulations display enhanced absorption, particularly when polyethylene glycol is used as dispersion carrier in the ultramicrosize formulations. Oral bioavailability of the microsize formulation is variable and ranges from 25% to 70%; ultramicrosize griseofulvin, in contrast, is almost completely absorbed.[73,267]

After oral administration, C_{max} occurs approximately 4 hours after dosing. Griseofulvin distributes to keratin precursor cells and is concentrated in skin, hair, nails, liver, adipose tissue, and skeletal muscles. In skin, over time, a concentration gradient is established, with the highest concentrations found in the outermost stratum corneum.[185,594] Non–protein-bound drug is carried in the extracellular fluid, in sweat, and through transepidermal fluid loss; in addition, reversible protein binding and high lipid solubility cause griseofulvin to partition into the stratum corneum, where its concentrations exceed that of serum. Within 48 to 72 hours after discontinuation of the drug, plasma concentrations of griseofulvin are markedly reduced, and the compound no longer is detectable in the stratum corneum.[73,267]

Griseofulvin is oxidatively demethylated and conjugated with glucuronic acid primarily in the liver; its major metabolite, 6-desmethylgriseofulvin, is microbiologically inactive.[392] The elimination of the compound from plasma is bi-exponential, with a terminal elimination half-life of 9 to 21 hours.[555] Approximately one third of a single dose of microsize griseofulvin is excreted in feces, and 50% is excreted in urine within 5 days. In urine, the drug is excreted mainly as free and glucuronized 6-desmethylgriseofulvin. Unchanged drug in the urine accounts for less than 1% of the dose.[391,392]

Separate pharmacokinetic data for pediatric patients have not been published; however, the compound is approved for children older than 2 years of age. The recommended pediatric dosage of microsize griseofulvin is 10 to 20 mg/kg per day, with a maximum of 1 g, administered in two divided doses; the recommended pediatric dosage of ultramicrosize griseofulvin is 5 to 10 mg/kg per day (maximum, 750 mg), also given in two divided doses.[182,210]

Adverse effects. Griseofulvin has an acceptable safety profile. More common adverse effects include headaches and a variety of gastrointestinal symptoms. Griseofulvin can cause photosensitivity and exacerbate lupus and porphyria. Cases of erythema multiforme–like reactions, toxic epidermal necrolysis, and a reaction resembling serum sickness have been reported. Proteinuria, nephrosis, hepatotoxicity, leukopenia, menstrual irregularities, and mental confusion have been reported rarely in association with griseofulvin therapy. Griseofulvin has been noted to produce estrogen-like effects in children and reversible diminution of hearing.[73,208,267] Griseofulvin is contraindicated in patients with porphyria or hepatocellular failure. The compound has been shown to be teratogenic in animals and should not be administered to pregnant women. Griseofulvin also has mutagenic and carcinogenic potential; the significance of these observations for humans, however, is unclear.[210,208]

Drug interactions. Griseofulvin has been noted to enhance the clearance of oral contraceptives, cyclosporine, theophylline, aspirin, and warfarin. Concurrent use of phenobarbital may lead to decreased levels of griseofulvin. Finally, concurrent ingestion of alcohol may lead to a disulfiram-like reaction.[210,208]

Indications. Griseofulvin remains an option for the treatment of tinea capitis, particularly when caused by *Microsporon*,[115,184,200] and for refractory tinea corporis (see Table 240.8).[275,592] For tinea capitis, 6 to 8 weeks of treatment usually are required.[182,306] The usual duration of therapy for refractory tinea corporis is 4 weeks.[182,210] Nail infections, which are increasingly observed in the pediatric population,[222] usually fail to respond to therapy with griseofulvin and are better treated with itraconazole or terbinafine.[265] Because griseofulvin is not effective against other fungal infections (see Table 240.9), the infecting organism always should be identified as a dermatophyte before therapy is initiated. In vitro resistance of dermatophytes to griseofulvin has been reported and may be the cause of therapeutic failure.[38]

Terbinafine

The allylamine terbinafine (Fig. 240.11) (Lamisil; and generic forms) is a synthetic antifungal agent that is useful for topical and systemic (oral tablets and suspension) treatment of superficial infections of the skin and its appendages by dermatophytes and yeasts, as well as possibly for treatment of cutaneous sporotrichosis. Terbinafine acts by inhibiting the biosynthesis of fungal ergosterol at the level of squalene epoxidase (see Fig. 240.8), thus leading to depletion of ergosterol and accumulation of toxic squalenes in the fungal cell membrane.[45]

Antifungal activity. Terbinafine has exceptionally potent and fungicidal in vitro activity against dermatophytes.[200] It also is highly active against *Aspergillus* spp., certain Hyalohyphomycetes, dematiaceous and dimorphic fungi, and *P. jiroveci*. Its in vitro activity against yeasts appears more variable.[217,251,319,560] Comparative in vitro studies have indicated that terbinafine may be more active against *Aspergillus* spp. than itraconazole[593] or amphotericin B,[579] more active than itraconazole against *S. schenkii*,[347] and less active or comparably active relative to the azoles against yeasts.[593]

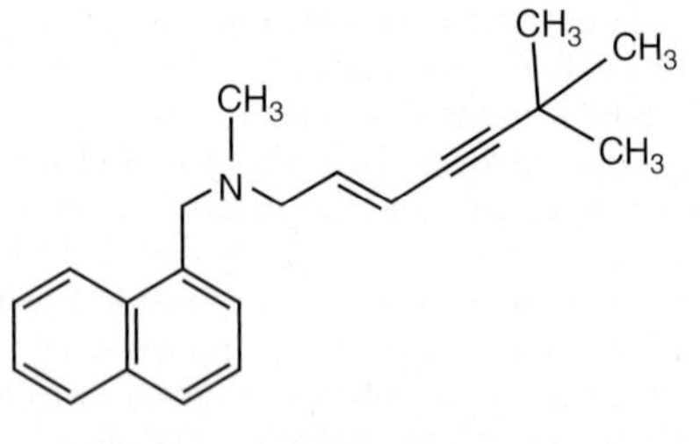

Terbinafine

FIG. 240.11 Structural formula of terbinafine.

Synergy with triazoles against *C. albicans*,[204,706] *C. glabrata*,[48] *C. neoformans*,[204] *A. fumigatus*,[82,461] non-*Aspergillus* hyalohyphomycetes,[435,436,489,560] and Mucorales[231] has been reported. Although more variable, synergy with amphotericin B also has been demonstrated for filamentous and yeast like fungi.[560] Unfortunately, because of the limited systemic distribution of terbinafine, this in vitro activity and synergy has limited in vivo efficacy in treatment of deeply invasive fungal infections. Terbinafine resistance in clinical dermatophyte isolates is a rare occurrence[320]; only two cases have been documented, in which the resistance mechanism was identified as a single amino acid substitution in squalene epoxidase.[490]

Pharmacokinetics. The pharmacokinetic properties of terbinafine in adults are well characterized.[45] Independent of food, oral bioavailability is 70% to 80%. Over the adult dosage range of 125 to 750 mg once daily, terbinafine displays linear plasma pharmacokinetics. C_{max} of 0.5 to 2.7 g/L is measured within 2 hours,[316,353,354] and steady state is reached after 10 to 14 days after only twofold accumulation.[45] As a lipophilic drug, terbinafine is strongly bound to plasma proteins. The compound is distributed extensively to tissues and accumulates throughout adipose tissues, dermis, epidermis, and nail. It exhibits a triphasic distribution pattern in plasma, with a terminal half-life up to 3 weeks; microbiologically active concentrations can be measured in plasma for weeks to months after the last dose, a finding consistent with a slow redistribution from peripheral tissue and adipose tissue sites.[45,354,471] Terbinafine undergoes extensive and complex hepatic biotransformation that involves at least seven CYP450 enzymes[674]; 15 mycologically inactive metabolites have been identified, mainly in urine.[354] Studies employing radiolabeled drug demonstrated that urinary excretion accounts for more than 70% and fecal elimination for 10% of radioactivity; the extent of enterohepatic recycling is unknown.[308,310] As a consequence of the compound's extensive hepatic metabolism and urinary excretion, caution is warranted in treating patients with severe hepatic and renal impairment (creatinine clearance ≤50 mL/min).[45]

The pharmacokinetic properties of terbinafine and five known major metabolites in plasma and urine were investigated after single and repeated oral administration of 125 mg/day to 12 pediatric patients for up to 56 days (mean age, 8 years; age range, 5 to 11 years; weight range, 17–34 kg) (Table 240.17).[310] No differences were found regarding the metabolism of terbinafine relative to healthy adults.[309] Steady state was reached at least on day 21, and no further accumulation occurred between days 21 and 56.[308,475] Comparison of the kinetic parameters of terbinafine after single administration of 125 mg showed comparable C_{max} and T_{max} (time until occurrence of C_{max}) values and a 40% higher AUC; when dose was calculated as milligrams per kilogram or milligrams per square meter, children showed a lower AUC (range, 29–45%) in contrast to that in adults, a finding indicating a higher, weight-normalized volume of distribution into lipophilic tissue. Children had shorter β-phase elimination half-lives, but the γ-phase terminal half-life determined after multiple dosing during washout was similar to that in adults. Thus, in children weighing 17 to 34 kg, a dose of 125 mg terbinafine

TABLE 240.17 Pharmacokinetic Parameters of Terbinafine in Children After a Single Dose of 125 mg Compared With Similar Parameters in Healthy Adults[a]

Parameters	Children With Tinea Capitis (n = 12)	Healthy Adults (n = 16)	Statistical Comparison
Age (y)	8 ± 2	26 ± 4	—
Weight (kg)	26 ± 5	64 ± 6	—
C_{max} (μg/mL)	0.706 ± 0.277	0.565 ± 0.329	NS
T_{max} (h)	2.1 ± 1.1	5 ± 0.7	NS
$AUC_{0-\infty}$ (μg/mL/h)	2.967 ± 0.965	2.135 ± 1.131	$P < .05$
$t_{1/2}\beta$ (h)	14.7 ± 4.3	27 ± 12	$P < .001$

[a]Mean values ± SD.

$AUC_{0-\infty}$, Area under the concentration versus time curve from zero to infinity; *C_{max}*, peak plasma concentration; *NS*, not significant; $t_{1/2}\beta$, elimination half-life; *T_{max}*, time until occurrence of peak plasma concentration.

Modified from Jones TC. Overview of the use of terbinafine (Lamisil) in children. *Br J Dermatol.* 1995;132:683–689.

yields pharmacokinetic properties similar to those in adults without drug accumulation, and dose calculation of milligrams per kilogram or milligrams per square meter would lead to lower drug levels than those recorded in adults.[2,308,324,475] Exploration of lower doses (62.5 mg/day) in eight children weighing 19 to 35 kg revealed an approximate reduction in trough level of 50%, indicating linearity of plasma pharmacokinetics in children.[324] Based on the experience with dosages of 10 mg/kg and less in adults and the described pharmacokinetic profile in children, a dose of 250 mg/day has been proposed for children weighing more than 40 kg, a dose of 125 mg/day for children weighing 20 to 40 kg, and 62.5 mg/day for children weighing less than 20 kg.[324]

Adverse effects. In adults, terbinafine usually is well tolerated at doses of up to 500 mg/day, and it has a relatively low incidence of adverse effects. Primary adverse effects include gastrointestinal upsets, headache, and skin reactions in 2% to 7% of patients. Terbinafine can cause hepatitis and liver failure. Potentially severe hepatotoxicity is estimated to occur in one in 120,000 patients, and asymptomatic rises in liver enzyme activities are likely to occur at a frequency of one in 200. As a consequence, the drug should not be administered in patients with an underlying liver problem, and liver function tests results should be obtained before terbinafine is prescribed. Less common but relevant adverse effects include mostly reversible loss of taste and/or smell; severe skin eruptions, including generalized erythematous pustulosis and drug-induced lupus erythematosus; Stevens-Johnson syndrome; blood dyscrasias; visual disturbances; and depressive symptoms.[5] No evidence indicates that these idiosyncratic effects are increasing in incidence with the increasing use of terbinafine.[492] Terbinafine has not been shown to be carcinogenic or mutagenic; its use is not recommended during pregnancy or in nursing mothers.

Several clinical studies have documented the safety of terbinafine in pediatric patients.[90,97,209,211,263,324,355,394,475,600] Terbinafine, administered for a median duration of 4 weeks (range, 1 to 28 weeks) was safe in children between 2 and 17 years of age who received the drug for various dermatophyte and yeast infections of the skin: of a total of 196 patients enrolled in six studies, 22 adverse events were observed in 15 patients. Adverse events probably associated with the use of terbinafine occurred in six of these patients (3%), but in none of these patients did terbinafine therapy have to be discontinued.[326] Terbinafine was similarly well tolerated in two double-blind, randomized trials in children with tinea capitis.[184,209,394]

Drug interactions. Multiple CYP450 enzymes are involved in the metabolism of terbinafine. However, with the possible exception of CYP2D6 substrates, in vitro studies revealed little or no effect on the metabolism of many characteristic CYP substrates.[674] Inhibition of CYP2D6-mediated metabolism may be relevant with the concomitant use of tricyclic antidepressants, β blockers, selective serotonin reuptake inhibitors, and type B monoamine oxidase inhibitors.

In clinical interaction studies, no pharmacokinetic or pharmacodynamic interactions were observed with the concomitant administration of terfenadine,[551] midazolam,[10] and alfentanil.[564] Terbinafine can (1) reduce the clearance of theophylline[641]; (2) increase levels of nortryptiline,[658] amitryptiline,[101] desipramine,[402] imipramine,[629] paroxetine[733] and dextromethorphan[4]; (3) increase or reduce warfarin exposure[266,703]; and (4) reduce the trough cyclosporine concentration in patients with transplants.[395] Clearance of terbinafine may be decreased by cimetidine and increased by rifampin.[251]

Clinical indications. Terbinafine is approved by the FDA in patients older than 18 years of age for the treatment of onychomycosis of toenails and fingernails caused by dermatophytes. It may be indicated for treatment of other superficial infections of the skin and its appendages caused by dermatophytes,[5,45,210] for cutaneous and lymphocutaneous sporotrichosis,[113,308] for subcutaneous phaeohyphomycosis[79,537] (see Tables 240.4 and 240.8), and for seborrheic dermatitis.[669] Recommended durations of treatment for tinea capitis, tinea corporis, and tinea pedis, fingernail onychomycosis, and toenail onychomycosis in adults are 4, 2, 6, and 12 weeks, respectively.[324,592]

Several studies have explored the clinical efficacy of terbinafine in children and adolescents.[90,97,211,324,355,394,475,600] The overall mycological and clinical efficacy for 152 children ages 2 to 17 years with various dermatophyte and yeast infections of the skin exceeded 95%.[324] In a prospective, randomized clinical trial in 210 children comparing treatment with 4 weeks of terbinafine versus 8 weeks of griseofulvin for *Trichophyton* tinea capitis, both regimens showed overall similar efficacy.[211] In a subsequent study of the duration of treatment in 176 patients, both 2 and 4 weeks of treatment were clinically superior to a 1-week regimen and had similar treatment efficacy, a finding suggesting that a 2-week course may be sufficient for patients with *Trichophyton* tinea capitis.[209] A similar study performed in 134 patients with *Microsporon* tinea capitis investigating 6, 8, 10, or 12 weeks of therapy demonstrated that 6 weeks of therapy were equivalent to griseofulvin.[394] Meta-analyses of terbinafine for the treatment of tinea capitis showed safety and efficacy similar to that of griseofulvin and itraconazole for infections caused by *Trichophyton* spp.,[115,200] superior efficacy to griseofulvin in children with *T. tonsurans* infection, but less clinical efficacy than griseofulvin in children with *Microsporon* infections.[115] A systematic review of 26 studies published between 1976 and 2011 on systemic treatment of onychomycosis in children found efficacy and safety profiles of terbinafine, itraconazole, griseofulvin, and fluconazole similar to those previously reported for adults.[265]

The broad-spectrum fungicidal in vitro activity, systemic availability, and lack of significant side effects suggested potential usefulness of terbinafine against deep-seated fungal infections. However, terbinafine was ineffective in animal models of pulmonary and disseminated aspergillosis,[339,580] systemic sporotrichosis,[327] cerebral phaeohyphomycosis, disseminated candidiasis, and pulmonary cryptococcosis,[559] findings explained by nonsaturable protein-binding kinetics.[580] Against experimental pulmonary pneumocystosis, terbinafine was active in some,[127,128] but not all,[699] models.

TOPICAL ANTIFUNGAL AGENTS

Apart from fungal keratitis, the use of topical antifungal agents is confined to superficial infections of the skin and mucosal surfaces. The decision to treat superficial infections of the skin and mucosal surfaces with a topical or systemic agent depends mainly on the site and extent of the infection. Immunocompromised children, however, usually require systemic therapies, as do patients with tinea capitis and onychomycosis (see Tables 240.8 and 240.9).[182,275]

Topical Therapeutics for Superficial Skin Infections

Dermatophytosis is caused by the filamentous fungi *Microsporon* spp., *Trichophyton* spp., and *Epidermophyton floccosum*. Many different agents and formulations are available for topical treatment of dermatophytic skin infections (i.e., tinea corporis, facialis, or pedis), including allylamines and azoles. Agents for treatment of *Candida* dermatitis and tinea (pityriasis) versicolor (caused by *Malassezia furfur* or *Malassezia pachydermatis*) include various topical azoles and topical polyenes. Most topical agents are applied twice daily well beyond the clinical resolution of the infection. A detailed review of the pharmacologic properties of these topical drugs and of the treatment of cutaneous mycoses is beyond the scope of this chapter and can be found elsewhere.[182,210,275,306]

Topical Therapeutics for Mucosal Candidiasis

Agents for the topical treatment of vulvovaginal candidiasis include a large variety of antifungal azoles and the polyene nystatin.[60,611,610] Azole agents may be absorbed to a minor extent and potentially can interfere with the metabolism of concomitant drugs. For example, potentiation of the anticoagulatory effects of acenocoumarol was noted after vaginal administration of miconazole capsules to two postmenopausal patients[372] and after oral administration of miconazole gel in three elderly patients with oral candidiasis.[488]

Antifungal azoles such as clotrimazole and miconazole and antifungal polyenes such as amphotericin B and nystatin are effective in the treatment of oropharyngeal candidiasis. Many clinical trials evaluated the usefulness of these agents for prevention of fungal infections in immunocompromised patients with cancer or HSCT. Although most agents have documented efficacy in the prevention of oropharyngeal candidiasis, they are not effective in preventing invasive mycoses and in improving infection-related and overall mortality in this setting.[180,253,302,397,637,652]

FUTURE DIRECTIONS

Pediatric age groups display important differences in host biology, predisposing conditions, epidemiology, and presentation of fungal infections relative to the adult population. Since the late 1990s, major advances have been made in the field of medical mycology. Most importantly, an array of new antifungal agents has entered the clinical arena. Although the final pediatric approval of some of these agents remains to be established, the development of pediatric therapies has moved forward in an exemplary manner. Invasive fungal infections will remain important causes of morbidity and mortality in immunocompromised pediatric patients. The availability of alternative therapeutic options is an important advance; at the same time, however, antifungal therapy has become increasingly complex, and clinical surveys indicate a substantial need for improvement in antifungal prescribing.[382,386] In addition to information on prior antifungal therapies, microbiologic data, existing comorbidities, and concurrent medications, guidance through the available antifungal armamentarium and pivotal clinical trials through pediatric specific recommendations[239,296] is needed more than ever in the management of the individual patient.

NEW REFERENCES SINCE THE SEVENTH EDITION

4. Abdel-Rahman SM, Marcucci K, Boge T, et al. Potent inhibition of cytochrome P-450 2D6-mediated dextromethorphan O-demethylation by terbinafine. *Drug Metab Dispos.* 1999;27:770-775.
7. Adler-Moore JP, Gangneux JP, Pappas PG. Comparison between liposomal formulations of amphotericin B. *Med Mycol.* 2016;54:223-231.
11. Albano E, Azie N, Roy M, et al. Pharmacokinetic and safety profiles of repeated-dose prophylactic micafungin in children and adolescents undergoing hematopoietic stem cell transplantation. *J Pediatr Hematol Oncol.* 2015;37:e45-e50.
31. Arendrup MC, Cuenca-Estrella M, Lass-Flörl C, Hope WW. Breakpoints for antifungal agents: an update from EUCAST focussing on echinocandins against *Candida* spp. and triazoles against *Aspergillus* spp. *Drug Resist Updat.* 2013; 16:81-95.
36. Arrieta A, Sung L, Berthold F, et al. Safety, tolerability, and pharmacokinetics of posaconazole oral Suspension in neutropenic children. In: Abstracts of the 53th Interscience Conference on Antimicrobial Agents and Chemotherapy. Washington, DC: American Society for Microbiology; 2013.
55. Benjamin DK Jr, Deville JG, Azie N, et al. Safety and pharmacokinetic profiles of repeated-dose micafungin in children and adolescents treated for invasive candidiasis. *Pediatr Infect Dis J.* 2013;32:e419-e425.
57. Benjamin DK Jr, Hudak ML, Duara S, et al. Effect of fluconazole prophylaxis on candidiasis and mortality in premature infants: a randomized clinical trial. *JAMA.* 2014;311:1742-1749.
66. Bernardo VA, Cross SJ, Crews KR, et al. Posaconazole therapeutic drug monitoring in pediatric patients and young adults with cancer. *Ann Pharmacother.* 2013;47:976-983.
75. Blyth CC, Barzi F, Hale K, Isaacs D. Chemoprophylaxis of neonatal fungal infections in very low birthweight infants: efficacy and safety of fluconazole and nystatin. *J Paediatr Child Health.* 2012;48:846-851.
76. Bochennek K, Balan A, Müller-Scholden L, et al. Micafungin twice weekly as antifungal prophylaxis in paediatric patients at high risk for invasive fungal disease. *J Antimicrob Chemother.* 2015;70:1527-1530.
77. Bochennek K, Tramsen L, Schedler N, et al. Liposomal amphotericin B twice weekly as antifungal prophylaxis in paediatric haematological malignancy patients. *Clin Microbiol Infect.* 2011;17(12):1868-1874.
83. Botero Aguirre JP, Restrepo Hamid AM. Amphotericin B deoxycholate versus liposomal amphotericin B: effects on kidney function. *Cochrane Database Syst Rev.* 2015;(11):CD010481.
100. Caselli D, Cesaro S, Ziino O, et al. A prospective, randomized study of empirical antifungal therapy for the treatment of chemotherapy-induced febrile neutropenia in children. *Br J Haematol.* 2012;158(2):249-255.
105. CDER—Center for Drug Evaluation and Research. Cresemba Label Information *(April 2015).* Washington, DC: US Food and Drug Administration, Center for Drug Evaluation and Research. www.accessdata.fda.gov/drugsatfda_docs/label/2015/207500s001,207501s001lbl.pdf.
106. CDER—Center for Drug Evaluation and Research. Diflucan Label Information *(March 2014).* Washington, DC: US Food and Drug Administration, Center for Drug Evaluation and Research. www.accessdata.fda.gov/drugsatfda_docs/label/2014/019949s058,019950s062,020090s042lbl.pdf.
109. CDER—Center for Drug Evaluation and Research. Vfend Label Information *(February 2015).* Washington, DC: US Food and Drug Administration, Center for Drug Evaluation and Research. www.accessdata.fda.gov/drugsatfda_docs/label/2015/021266s038,021267s047,021630s028lbl.pdf.
114. Che D, Zhou H, Li T, Wu B. Duration and intensity of fluconazole for prophylaxis in preterm neonates: a meta-analysis of randomized controlled trials. *BMC Infect Dis.* 2016;16:312.
115. Chen X, Jiang X, Yang M, et al. Systemic antifungal therapy for tinea capitis in children. *Cochrane Database Syst Rev.* 2016;(5):CD004685.
120. Cleminson J, Austin N, McGuire W. Prophylactic systemic antifungal agents to prevent mortality and morbidity in very low birth weight infants. *Cochrane Database Syst Rev.* 2015;(10):CD003850.
122. Clerihew L, McGuire W. Antifungal therapy for newborn infants with invasive fungal infection. *Cochrane Database Syst Rev.* 2012;(6):CD003953.
123. Cohen-Wolkowiez M, Benjamin DK Jr. Editorial commentary: fluconazole therapeutic drug monitoring in children with cancer: not today. *Clin Infect Dis.* 2014;59:1534-1536.
129. Cornely OA, Duarte RF, Haider S, et al. Phase 3 pharmacokinetics and safety study of a posaconazole tablet formulation in patients at risk for invasive fungal disease. *J Antimicrob Chemother.* 2016;71:718-726.
142. Day JN, Chau TT, Wolbers M, et al. Combination antifungal therapy for cryptococcal meningitis. *N Engl J Med.* 2013;368(14):1291-1302.
156. Desai A, Kovanda L, Kowalski D, et al. Population pharmacokinetics of isavuconazole from Phase 1 and Phase 3 (SECURE) trial in adults and target attainment in patients with invasive aspergillosis and other filamentous fungi. *Antimicrob Agents Chemother.* 2016;60(9):5483-5491.
164. Döring M, Blume O, Haufe S, et al. Comparison of itraconazole, voriconazole, and posaconazole as oral antifungal prophylaxis in pediatric patients following allogeneic hematopoietic stem cell transplantation. *Eur J Clin Microbiol Infect Dis.* 2014;33:629-638.
165. Döring M, Eikemeier M, Cabanillas Stanchi KM, et al. Antifungal prophylaxis with posaconazole vs. fluconazole or itraconazole in pediatric patients with neutropenia. *Eur J Clin Microbiol Infect Dis.* 2015;34:1189-1200.
175. Drogouti E, Pana ZD, Tragiannidis A, et al. Clinical pharmacology of itraconazole in children and adolescents. *Curr Fungal Infect Rep.* 2015;9:65-73.
177. Duarte RF, López-Jiménez J, Cornely OA, et al. Phase 1b study of new posaconazole tablet for prevention of invasive fungal infections in high-risk patients with neutropenia. *Antimicrob Agents Chemother.* 2014;58:5758-5765.
181. Egunsola O, Adefurin A, Fakis A, et al. Safety of fluconazole in paediatrics: a systematic review. *Eur J Clin Pharmacol.* 2013;69:1211-1221.
186. Ericson JE, Kaufman DA, Kicklighter SD, et al. Fluconazole prophylaxis for the prevention of candidiasis in premature infants: a meta-analysis using patient-level data. *Clin Infect Dis.* 2016;63(5):804-810.
191. European Medicines Agency. Cancidas Summary of Product Characteristics. www.ema.europa.eu/docs/en_GB/document_library/EPAR_-_Product_Information/human/000379/WC500021033.pdf.
192. European Medicines Agency. Ecalta Summary of Product Characteristics. www.ema.europa.eu/docs/en_GB/document_library/EPAR_-_Product_Information/human/000788/WC500020673.pdf.
193. European Medicines Agency. Isavuconazole Summary of Product Characteristics. www.ema.europa.eu/docs/en_GB/document_library/EPAR_-_Product_Information/human/002734/WC500196128.pdf.
194. European Medicines Agency. Mycamine Summary of Product Characteristics. www.ema.europa.eu/docs/en_GB/document_library/EPAR_-_Product_Information/human/000734/WC500031075.pdf.
195. European Medicines Agency. Vfend Summary of Product Characteristics. www.ema.europa.eu/docs/en_GB/document_library/EPAR_-_Product_Information/human/000387/WC500049756.pdf.
197. Falagas ME, Karageorgopoulos DE, Tansarli GS. Continuous versus conventional infusion of amphotericin B deoxycholate: a meta-analysis. *PLoS ONE.* 2013;8(10):e77075.
207. Friberg LE, Ravva P, Karlsson MO, Liu P. Integrated population pharmacokinetic analysis of voriconazole in children, adolescents, and adults. *Antimicrob Agents Chemother.* 2012;56:3032-3042.
234. Govender NP, Patel J, Magobo RE, et al. Emergence of azole-resistant Candida parapsilosis causing bloodstream infection: results from laboratory-based sentinel surveillance in South Africa. *J Antimicrob Chemother.* 2016;71:1994-2004.
239. Groll AH, Castagnola E, Cesaro S, et al. Fourth European Conference on Infections in Leukaemia (ECIL-4): guidelines for diagnosis, prevention, and treatment of invasive fungal diseases in paediatric patients with cancer or allogeneic haemopoietic stem-cell transplantation. *Lancet Oncol.* 2014;15:e327-e340.
241. Groll AH, Desai A, Han D, et al. Pharmacokinetic assessment of drug-drug interactions of isavuconazole with the immunosuppressants cyclosporine, mycophenolic acid, prednisolone, sirolimus, and tacrolimus in healthy adults. *Clin Pharmacol Drug Dev.* 2017;6(1):76-85.
265. Gupta AK, Paquet M. Systemic antifungals to treat onychomycosis in children: a systematic review. *Pediatr Dermatol.* 2013;30(3):294-302.
268. Halpern AB, Lyman GH, Walsh TJ, et al. Evidence-based review of primary antifungal prophylaxis during curative-intent therapy for acute myeloid leukemia. *Blood.* 2015;126:2790-2797.
269. Hamill RJ, Sobel JD, El-Sadr W, et al. Comparison of 2 doses of liposomal amphotericin B and conventional amphotericin B deoxycholate for treatment

of AIDS-associated acute cryptococcal meningitis: a randomized, double-blind clinical trial of efficacy and safety. *Clin Infect Dis.* 2010;51:225-232.

272. Hand EO, Ramanathan MR. Safety and tolerability of high-dose weekly liposomal amphotericin B antifungal prophylaxis. *Pediatr Infect Dis J.* 2014;33:835-836.
275. Hawkins DM, Smidt AC. Superficial fungal infections in children. *Pediatr Clin North Am.* 2014;61:443-455.
276. Healey KR, Zhao Y, Perez WB, et al. Prevalent mutator genotype identified in fungal pathogen *Candida glabrata* promotes multi-drug resistance. *Nat Commun.* 2016;7:11.
289. Hicks JK, Crews KR, Flynn P, et al. Voriconazole plasma concentrations in immunocompromised pediatric patients vary by CYP2C19 diplotypes. *Pharmacogenomics.* 2014;15:1065-1078.
296. Hope WW, Castagnola E, Groll AH, et al. ESCMID guideline for the diagnosis and management of *Candida* diseases 2012: prevention and management of invasive infections in neonates and children caused by *Candida* spp. *Clin Microbiol Infect.* 2012;18 Suppl 7:38-52.
297. Hope WW, Kaibara A, Roy M, et al. Population pharmacokinetics of micafungin and its metabolites M1 and M5 in children and adolescents. *Antimicrob Agents Chemother.* 2015;59:905-913.
315. Jang SH, Colangelo PM, Gobburu JV. Exposure-response of posaconazole used for prophylaxis against invasive fungal infections: evaluating the need to adjust doses based on drug concentrations in plasma. *Clin Pharmacol Ther.* 2010;88:115-119.
320. Jo Siu WJ, Tatsumi Y, Senda H, et al. Comparison of in vitro antifungal activities of efinaconazole and currently available antifungal agents against a variety of pathogenic fungi associated with onychomycosis. *Antimicrob Agents Chemother.* 2013;57:1610-1616.
336. Kaufman DA, Morris A, Gurka MJ, et al. Fluconazole prophylaxis in preterm infants: a multicenter case-controlled analysis of efficacy and safety. *Early Hum Dev.* 2014;90(suppl 1):S87-S90.
337. Kersemaekers WM, van Iersel T, Nassander U, et al. Pharmacokinetics and safety study of posaconazole intravenous solution administered peripherally to healthy subjects. *Antimicrob Agents Chemother.* 2015;59:1246-1251. Erratum in: Antimicrob Agents Chemother. 2016;60:4426.
344. Kobayashi C, Hanadate T, Niwa T, et al. Safety and effectiveness of micafungin in Japanese pediatric patients: results of a postmarketing surveillance study. *J Pediatr Hematol Oncol.* 2015;37:e285-e291.
345. Kobayashi C, Hanadate T, Niwa T, et al. Safety and efficacy of micafungin for prophylaxis against invasive fungal infections in Japanese patients undergoing hematopoietic stem cell transplantation: results of a post-marketing surveillance study. *J Infect Chemother.* 2015;21:438-443.
352. Kovanda LL, Petraitiene R, Petraitis V, et al. Pharmacodynamics of isavuconazole in experimental invasive pulmonary aspergillosis: implications for clinical breakpoints. *J Antimicrob Chemother.* 2016;71:1885-1891.
356. Kraft WK, Chang PS, van Iersel ML, et al. Posaconazole tablet pharmacokinetics: lack of effect of concomitant medications altering gastric pH and gastric motility in healthy subjects. *Antimicrob Agents Chemother.* 2014;58:4020-4025.
362. Krishna G, Ma L, Martinho M, O'Mara E. Single-dose phase I study to evaluate the pharmacokinetics of posaconazole in new tablet and capsule formulations relative to oral suspension. *Antimicrob Agents Chemother.* 2012;56:4196-4201.
363. Krishna G, Ma L, Martinho M, Preston RA, O'Mara E. A new solid oral tablet formulation of posaconazole: a randomized clinical trial to investigate rising single- and multiple-dose pharmacokinetics and safety in healthy volunteers. *J Antimicrob Chemother.* 2012;67:2725-2730.
368. Kullberg BJ, Thompson G, Pappas P, et al. Isavuconazole versus caspofungin in the treatment of candidaemia and other invasive *Candida* infections: the ACTIVE trial. In: Electronic abstracts of the 27th European Conference on Clinical Microbiology and Infectious Diseases (ECCMID). European Society of Clinical Microbiology and Infectious Diseases (ESCMID): Oral presentation 227 (2016).
379. Lee HJ, Lee B, Park JD, et al. Association of systolic blood pressure drop with intravenous administration of itraconazole in children with hemato-oncologic disease. *Drug Des Devel Ther.* 2015;9:6489-6495.
382. Lehrnbecher T, Kaiser J, Varwig D, et al. Antifungal usage in children undergoing intensive treatment for acute myeloid leukemia: analysis of the multicenter clinical trial AML-BFM 93. *Eur J Clin Microbiol Infect Dis.* 2007;26:735-738.
385. Lepak AJ, Marchillo K, VanHecker J, et al. Isavuconazole pharmacodynamic target determination for *Candida* species in an in vivo murine disseminated candidiasis model. *Antimicrob Agents Chemother.* 2013;57:5642-5648.
386. Lestner JM, Versporten A, Doerholt K, et al. Systemic antifungal prescribing in neonates and children: outcomes from the Antibiotic Resistance and Prescribing in European Children (ARPEC) Study. *Antimicrob Agents Chemother.* 2015;59:782-789.
388. Lewis R, Brüggemann R, Padoin C, et al. Triazole antifungal therapeutic drug monitoring. 6th European Conference on Infections in Leukemia (ECIL-6). www.kobe.fr/ecil/telechargements2015/ECIL6-Triazole-TDM-07-12-2015-Lewis-R-et-al.pdf.
396. Loo AS, Muhsin SA, Walsh TJ. Toxicokinetic and mechanistic basis for the safety and tolerability of liposomal amphotericin B. *Expert Opin Drug Saf.* 2013;12:881-895.
400. Loyse A, Wilson D, Meintjes G, et al. Comparison of the early fungicidal activity of high-dose fluconazole, voriconazole, and flucytosine as second-line drugs given in combination with amphotericin B for the treatment of HIV-associated cryptococcal meningitis. *Clin Infect Dis.* 2012;54:121-128.
401. Luong ML, Al-Dabbagh M, Groll AH, et al. Utility of voriconazole therapeutic drug monitoring: a meta-analysis. *J Antimicrob Chemother.* 2016;71:1786-1799.
403. Maertens J, Cornely OA, Ullmann AJ, et al. Phase 1B study of the pharmacokinetics and safety of posaconazole intravenous solution in patients at risk for invasive fungal disease. *Antimicrob Agents Chemother.* 2014;58:3610-3617.
408. Maertens JA, Raad II, Marr KA, et al. Isavuconazole versus voriconazole for primary treatment of invasive mould disease caused by *Aspergillus* and other filamentous fungi (SECURE): a phase 3, randomised-controlled, non-inferiority trial. *Lancet.* 2016;387(10020):760-769.
417. Manzoni P, Wu C, Tweddle L, Roilides E. Micafungin in premature and non-premature infants: a systematic review of 9 clinical trials. *Pediatr Infect Dis J.* 2014;33:e291-e298.
422. Maron GM, Hayden RT, Rodriguez A, et al. Voriconazole prophylaxis in children with cancer: changing outcomes and epidemiology of fungal infections. *Pediatr Infect Dis J.* 2013;32:e451-e455.
428. Marty FM, Ostrosky-Zeichner L, Cornely OA, et al. Isavuconazole treatment for mucormycosis: a single-arm open-label trial and case-control analysis. *Lancet Infect Dis.* 2016;16:828-837.
429. Matthias KR, Nix DE, Peloquin CA, Graham ML. Poor absorption of high-dose posaconazole in pediatric bone marrow transplant patients. *Ann Pharmacother.* 2012;46:e22.
439. Miceli MH, Kauffman CA. Isavuconazole: a new broad-spectrum triazole antifungal agent. *Clin Infect Dis.* 2015;61:1558-1565.
446. Miller MM, Johnson PN, Hagemann TM, et al. Pseudohyperphosphatemia in children treated with liposomal amphotericin B. *Am J Health Syst Pharm.* 2014;71:1462-1468.
452. Mori M, Imaizumi M, Ishiwada N, et al. Pharmacokinetics, efficacy, and safety of caspofungin in Japanese pediatric patients with invasive candidiasis and invasive aspergillosis. *J Infect Chemother.* 2015;21:421-426.
453. Mori M, Kobayashi R, Kato K, et al. Pharmacokinetics and safety of voriconazole intravenous-to-oral switch regimens in immunocompromised Japanese pediatric patients. *Antimicrob Agents Chemother.* 2015;59:1004-1013.
456. Moriyama B, Henning SA, Leung J, et al. Adverse interactions between antifungal azoles and vincristine: review and analysis of cases. *Mycoses.* 2011;54:e877-e879.
457. Moriyama B, Obeng AO, Barbarino J, et al. Clinical Pharmacogenetics Implementation Consortium (CPIC) Guidelines for CYP2C19 and voriconazole therapy. *Clin Pharmacol Ther.* 2016, Epub ahead of print.
458. Morris SK, Allen UD, Gupta S, Richardson SE. Breakthrough filamentous fungal infections in pediatric hematopoetic stem cell transplant and oncology patients receiving caspofungin. *Can J Infect Dis Med Microbiol.* 2012;23:179-182.
467. Narita A, Muramatsu H, Sakaguchi H, et al. Correlation of CYP2C19 phenotype with voriconazole plasma concentration in children. *J Pediatr Hematol Oncol.* 2013;35:e219-e223.
473. Neely M, Margol A, Fu X, et al. Achieving target voriconazole concentrations more accurately in children and adolescents. *Antimicrob Agents Chemother.* 2015;59:3090-3097.
483. O'Connor L, Livermore J, Sharp AD, et al. Pharmacodynamics of liposomal amphotericin B and flucytosine for cryptococcal meningoencephalitis: safe and effective regimens for immunocompromised patients. *J Infect Dis.* 2013;208:351-361.
502. Park HJ, Park M, Han M, et al. Efficacy and safety of micafungin for the prophylaxis of invasive fungal infection during neutropenia in children and adolescents undergoing allogeneic hematopoietic SCT. *Bone Marrow Transplant.* 2014;49:1212-1216.
506. Pelletier R, Alarie I, Walsh TJ. Emergence of disseminated candidiasis due to *Candida krusei* during treatment with caspofungin. *Med Mycol.* 2005;43:559-564.
511. Petraitis V, Petraitiene R, Lin P, et al. Efficacy and safety of generic amphotericin B in experimental pulmonary aspergillosis. *Antimicrob Agents Chemother.* 2005;49:1642-1645.
512. Petraitis V, Petraitiene R, Moradi PW, et al. Pharmacokinetics and concentration-dependent efficacy of isavuconazole for treatment of experimental invasive pulmonary aspergillosis. *Antimicrob Agents Chemother.* 2016;60:2718-2726.
582. Schmitt-Hoffmann A, Roos B, Heep M, et al. Single-ascending-dose pharmacokinetics and safety of the novel broad-spectrum antifungal triazole BAL4815 after intravenous infusions (50, 100, and 200 milligrams) and oral administrations (100, 200, and 400 milligrams) of its prodrug, BAL8557, in healthy volunteers. *Antimicrob Agents Chemother.* 2006;50:279-285.
583. Schmitt-Hoffmann A, Roos B, Maares J, et al. Multiple-dose pharmacokinetics and safety of the new antifungal triazole BAL4815 after intravenous infusion and oral administration of its prodrug, BAL8557, in healthy volunteers. *Antimicrob Agents Chemother.* 2006;50:286-293.
595. Sharkey PK, Graybill JR, Johnson ES, et al. Amphotericin B lipid complex compared with amphotericin B in the treatment of cryptococcal meningitis in patients with AIDS. *Clin Infect Dis.* 1996;22:315-321.

597. Sheu J, Hawryluk EB, Guo D, et al. Voriconazole phototoxicity in children: a retrospective review. *J Am Acad Dermatol.* 2015;72:314-320.
598. Shields RK, Nguyen MH, Clancy CJ. Clinical perspectives on echinocandin resistance among *Candida* species. *Curr Opin Infect Dis.* 2015;28:514-522.
599. Sideri G, Falagas ME, Grigoriou M, et al. Liposomal amphotericin B in critically ill paediatric patients. *J Clin Pharm Ther.* 2012;37:291-295.
610. Sobel JD. Recurrent vulvovaginal candidiasis. *Am J Obstet Gynecol.* 2016;214:15-21.
618. Steinmann J, Hamprecht A, Vehreschild MJ, et al. Emergence of azole-resistant invasive aspergillosis in HSCT recipients in Germany. *J Antimicrob Chemother.* 2015;70:1522-1526.
619. Stergiopoulou T, Walsh TJ. Clinical pharmacology of antifungal agents to overcome drug resistance in pediatric patients. *Expert Opin Pharmacother.* 2015;16:213-226.
625. Tarlock K, Johnson D, Cornell C, et al. Elevated fluoride levels and periostitis in pediatric hematopoietic stem cell transplant recipients receiving long-term voriconazole. *Pediatr Blood Cancer.* 2015;62:918-920.
630. Teusink AC, Ragucci D, Shatat IF, Kalpatthi R. Potentiation of vincristine toxicity with concomitant fluconazole prophylaxis in children with acute lymphoblastic leukemia. *Pediatr Hematol Oncol.* 2012;29:62-67.
633. Thompson GR 3rd, Rendon A, Ribeiro Dos Santos R, et al. Isavuconazole treatment of cryptococcosis and dimorphic mycoses. *Clin Infect Dis.* 2016;63:356-362.
651. Undre NA, Stevenson P, Freire A, Arrieta A. Pharmacokinetics of micafungin in pediatric patients with invasive candidiasis and candidemia. *Pediatr Infect Dis J.* 2012;31:630-632.
656. Van der Elst KC, Pereboom M, van den Heuvel ER, et al. Insufficient fluconazole exposure in pediatric cancer patients and the need for therapeutic drug monitoring in critically ill children. *Clin Infect Dis.* 2014;59:1527-1533.
659. van der Linden JW, Arendrup MC, Warris A, et al. Prospective multicenter international surveillance of azole resistance in *Aspergillus fumigatus. Emerg Infect Dis.* 2015;21:1041-1044.
661. van Hasselt JG, van Eijkelenburg NK, Huitema AD, et al. Severe skin toxicity in pediatric oncology patients treated with voriconazole and concomitant methotrexate. *Antimicrob Agents Chemother.* 2013;57:2878-2881.
664. Vanstraelen K, Colita A, Bica AM, et al. Pharmacokinetics of posaconazole oral suspension in children dosed according to body surface area. *Pediatr Infect Dis J.* 2016;35:183-188.
670. Vendetti N, Bryan M, Zaoutis TE, et al. Comparative effectiveness of fungicidal vs. fungistatic therapies for the treatment of paediatric candidaemia. *Mycoses.* 2016;59:173-178.
673. Verweij PE, Ananda-Rajah M, Andes D, et al. International expert opinion on the management of infection caused by azole-resistant *Aspergillus fumigatus. Drug Resist Updat.* 2015;21-22:30-40.
675. Viljoen J, Azie N, Schmitt-Hoffmann AH, Ghannoum M. A phase 2, randomized, double-blind, multicenter trial to evaluate the safety and efficacy of three dosing regimens of isavuconazole compared with fluconazole in patients with uncomplicated esophageal candidiasis. *Antimicrob Agents Chemother.* 2015;59:1671-1679.
700. Wang E, Farmakiotis D, Yang D, et al. The ever-evolving landscape of candidaemia in patients with acute leukaemia: non-susceptibility to caspofungin and multidrug resistance are associated with increased mortality. *J Antimicrob Chemother.* 2015;70:2362-2368.
705. Watt KM, Gonzalez D, Benjamin DK Jr, et al. Fluconazole population pharmacokinetics and dosing for prevention and treatment of invasive candidiasis in children supported with extracorporeal membrane oxygenation. *Antimicrob Agents Chemother.* 2015;59:3935-3943.
728. Wong JY, Kuzel P, Mullen J, et al. Cutaneous squamous cell carcinoma in two pediatric lung transplant patients on prolonged voriconazole treatment. *Pediatr Transplant.* 2014;18:E200-E207.
734. Yilmaz Karapinar D, Karadaş N, Önder Siviş Z, et al. Rare severe mycotic infections in children receiving empirical caspofungin treatment for febrile neutropenia. *Braz J Infect Dis.* 2015;19:549-552.
736. Yunus S, Pieper S, Kolve H, et al. Azole-based chemoprophylaxis of invasive fungal infections in paediatric patients with acute leukaemia: an internal audit. *J Antimicrob Chemother.* 2014;69:815-820.
737. Zane NR, Thakker DR. A physiologically based pharmacokinetic model for voriconazole disposition predicts intestinal first-pass metabolism in children. *Clin Pharmacokinet.* 2014;53:1171-1182.

The full reference list for this chapter is available at ExpertConsult.com.

241 Drugs for Parasitic Infections*

With increasing travel, immigration, use of immunosuppressive drugs, and the spread of HIV, physicians anywhere may see infections caused by parasites. The tables that follow list first-choice and alternative drugs for most parasitic infections. Box 241.1 provides the principal adverse effects of these drugs. Table 241.1 summarizes the known prenatal risks of antiparasitic drugs, and Table 241.2 lists brand names and manufacturers of the drugs.

PRINCIPAL ADVERSE EFFECTS OF ANTIPARASITIC DRUGS

Adverse effects of antiparasitic drugs vary with dosage, duration of administration, concomitant therapy, renal and hepatic function, immune competence, and the age of the patient. The principal adverse effects of antiparasitic agents are listed Box 241.1. The designation of adverse effects as frequent, occasional, or rare is based on published reports and on the experience of *Medical Letter* consultants.

*This chapter is reproduced from: Drugs for parasitic infections. *Med Lett.* 2013;11(suppl):e1–e31. *The Medical Letter* publications are protected by US and international copyright laws. Forwarding, copying or any other distribution of this material is strictly prohibited. For further information call: 800-211-2769.

BOX 241.1 Principal Adverse Effects of Antiparasitic Agents

Albendazole (Albenza)
Frequent: Abdominal pain; increased serum transaminases
Occasional: Reversible alopecia; leukopenia
Rare: Rash; hepatic toxicity; renal toxicity

Amphotericin B Deoxycholate (Fungizone)
Frequent: Renal damage; hypokalemia; thrombophlebitis at site of peripheral vein infusion; anorexia; headache; nausea; weight loss; bone marrow suppression with reversible decline in hematocrit; chills, fever,

BOX 241.1 Principal Adverse Effects of Antiparasitic Agents—cont'd

vomiting during infusion, possibly with delirium, hypotension or hypertension, wheezing, and hypoxemia, especially in cardiac or pulmonary disease
Occasional: Hypomagnesemia; normocytic, normochromic anemia
Rare: Hemorrhagic gastroenteritis, blood dyscrasias, rash, blurred vision, peripheral neuropathy, convulsions, anaphylaxis, arrhythmias, acute liver failure, reversible nephrogenic diabetes insipidus, hearing loss, acute pulmonary edema, spinal cord damage with intrathecal use

Amphotericin B Lipid Formulations (AmBisone, Abelcet, Amphotec)
Similar to amphotericin B but generally better tolerated. Nephrotoxicity is less common and less severe with the lipid-based formulations. Acute infusion reactions are worse with Amphotec, less with Abelcet and least with AmBisome. Liver toxicity has been reported.

Artemether (Artenam)
Occasional: Neurologic toxicity, possible increase in length of coma, increased convulsions, prolongation of QTc interval

Artemether/Lumefantrine (Coatem, Riamet)
Frequent: Abdominal pain, anorexia, headache, dizziness, diarrhea, vomiting, nausea, palpitations, arthralgia, myalgia, asthenia, fatigue, pruritus, rash, sleep disorder, cough
Occasional: Somnolence, involuntary muscle contractions, paresthesia, hypoesthesia, abnormal gait, ataxia
Rare: Hypersensitivity

Artesunate
Occasional: Ataxia, slurred speech, neurological toxicity, possible increase in length of coma, increased convulsions, prolongation of QTc interval

Atovaquone (Mepron, Malarone [With Proguanil])
Frequent: Rash, nausea
Occasional: Diarrhea, increased aminotransferases, cholestasis

Azithromycin (Zithromax)
Occasional: Nausea, diarrhea, abdominal pain, headache, dizziness, vaginitis
Rare: Angioedema, cholestatic jaundice, photosensitivity, reversible dose-related hearing loss, QT prolongation

Benznidazole (Rochagan)
Frequent: Allergic rash, dose-dependent polyneuropathy, GI disturbance, psychic disturbances

Benzyl Alcohol (Ulesfia Lotion)
Frequent: Eye irritation, contact dermatitis

Bithionol (Bitin)
Frequent: Photosensitivity reactions, vomiting, diarrhea, abdominal pain, urticaria
Rare: Leukopenia, toxic hepatitis

Chloroquine HCL and Chloroquine Phosphate (Aralen)
Occasional: Pruritus; vomiting; headache; confusion; depigmentation of hair; skin eruptions; corneal opacity; weight loss; partial alopecia; extraocular muscle palsies; exacerbation of psoriasis, eczema, and other exfoliative dermatoses; myalgias; photophobia
Rare: Irreversible retinal injury (especially when total dosage exceeds 100 g), discoloration of nails and mucous membranes, nerve-type deafness, peripheral neuropathy and myopathy, heart block, blood dyscrasias, hematemesis

Clarithromycin (Biaxin)
Occasional: Nausea, diarrhea, abdominal pain, abnormal taste, headache, dizziness
Rare: Reversible dose-related hearing loss, pseudomembranous colitis, pancreatitis, torsades de pointes

Clindamycin (Cleocin)
Frequent: Diarrhea, allergic reactions
Occasional: Pseudomembranous colitis, sometimes severe, can occur even with topical use
Rare: Blood dyscrasias, esophageal ulceration, hepatotoxicity, arrhythmia due to QTc prolongation

Crotamiton (Eurax)
Occasional: Rash

Dapsone
Frequent: Rash, transient headache, GI irritation, anorexia, infectious mononucleosis-like syndrome
Occasional: Cyanosis due to methemoglobinemia and sulfhemoglobinemia; other blood dyscrasias, including hemolytic anemia; nephrotic syndrome; liver damage; peripheral neuropathy; hypersensitivity reactions; increased risk of lepra reactions; insomnia; irritability; uncoordinated speech; agitation; acute psychosis
Rare: Renal papillary necrosis, severe hypoalbuminemia, epidermal necrolysis, optic atrophy, agranulocytosis, neonatal hyperbilirubinemia after use in pregnancy

Diethylcarbamazine Citrate (Hetrazan)
Frequent: Allergic or febrile reactions, which may be severe, in patients with microfilaria in the blood or the skin; GI disturbance
Rare: Encephalopathy

Diloxanide Furoate (Furamide)
Frequent: Flatulence
Occasional: Nausea, vomiting, diarrhea
Rare: Diplopia, dizziness, urticaria, pruritus

Eflornithine (Difluoromethylornithine, DFMO, Ornidyl)
Frequent: Anemia, leukopenia
Occasional: Diarrhea, thrombocytopenia, seizures
Rare: Hearing loss

Fluconazole (Diflucan)
Occasional: Nausea, vomiting, diarrhea, abdominal pain, headache, rash, increased aminotransferases
Rare: Severe hepatic toxicity, exfoliative dermatitis, anaphylaxis, Stevens-Johnson syndrome, toxic epidermal necrolysis, hair loss

Flucytosine (Ancobon)
Frequent: Blood dyscrasias, including pancytopenia and fatal agranulocytosis; GI disturbance, including severe diarrhea and ulcerative colitis; rash; hepatic dysfunction
Occasional: Confusion, hallucinations
Rare: Anaphylaxis

Furazolidone (Furoxone)
Frequent: Nausea, vomiting
Occasional: Allergic reactions, including pulmonary infiltration, hypotension, urticaria, fever, vesicular rash, hypoglycemia, headache
Rare: Hemolytic anemia in G6PD deficiency and neonates, disulfiram-like reaction with alcohol, MAO-inhibitor interactions, polyneuritis

Continued

BOX 241.1 Principal Adverse Effects of Antiparasitic Agents—cont'd

Iodoquinol (Yodoxin, and generics)
Occasional: Rash, acne, slight enlargement of the thyroid gland, nausea, diarrhea, cramps, anal pruritus
Rare: Optic neuritis, atrophy and loss of vision, peripheral neuropathy after prolonged use in high dosage (for months), iodine sensitivity

itraconazole (Sporanox, and generics)
Occasional: Nausea, epigastric pain, headache, dizziness, edema, hypokalemia, rash, hepatic toxicity
Rare: Congestive heart failure

Ivermectin, Oral (Stromectol)
Occasional: Mazzotti-type reaction seen in onchocerciasis, including fever; pruritus; tender lymph nodes; headache; and joint and bone pain
Rare: Hypotension

Ivermectin, Lotion (Sklice)
Occasional: Conjunctivitis, ocular hyperemia, eye irritation, dandruff, burning sensation of the skin

Ketoconazole (Nizoral)
Frequent: Nausea, vomiting
Occasional: Decreased testosterone synthesis, gynecomastia, oligospermia and impotence in men, abdominal pain, rash, hepatitis, pruritus, dizziness, constipation, diarrhea, fever and chills, photophobia, headache
Rare: Fatal hepatic necrosis, liver injury with jaundice, transient elevated transaminase, severe epigastric burning and pain, interference with adrenal function, anaphylaxis

Malathion (Ovide)
Occasional: Local irritation

Mebendazole (Vermox)
Occasional: Diarrhea, abdominal pain
Rare: Leukopenia, agranulocytosis, hypospermia

Mefloquine (Lariam)
Frequent: Vertigo, lightheadedness, nausea, other GI disturbances, nightmares, visual disturbances, headache, insomnia
Occasional: Confusion
Rare: Psychosis, hypotension, convulsions, coma, paresthesias

Meglumine Antimoniate (Glucantime)
Similar to sodium stibogluconate

Melarsoprol (Mel B)
Frequent: Myocardial damage, albuminuria, hypertension, colic, Herxheimer-type reaction, encephalopathy, vomiting, peripheral neuropathy
Rare: Shock

Metronidazole (Flagyl)
Frequent: Nausea, headache, anorexia, metallic taste
Occasional: Vomiting, diarrhea, insomnia, weakness, dry mouth, stomatitis, vertigo, tinnitus, paresthesias, rash, dark urine, urethral burning, disulfiram-like reaction with alcohol, candidiasis
Rare: Pseudomembranous colitis; leukopenia; pancreatitis; seizures; peripheral neuropathy; encephalopathy; cerebellar syndrome with ataxia, dysarthria, and MRI abnormalities

Miconazole (Monistat)
Occasional: Phlebitis, thrombocytosis, chills, intense, persistent pruritus, rash, vomiting, hyperlipidemia, dizziness, blurred vision, local burning and irritation with topical use
Rare: Anemia, thrombocytopenia, hyponatremia, renal insufficiency, anaphylaxis, cardiac and respiratory arrest with initial dose

Miltefosine (Impavido)
Frequent: Nausea, vomiting, diarrhea, motion sickness, increased creatinine

Niclosamide (Niclocide)
Occasional: Nausea, abdominal pain

Nifurtimox (Lampit)
Frequent: Anorexia, nausea, vomiting, gastric pain, insomnia, headache, vertigo, excitability, myalgia, arthralgia, peripheral polyneuritis
Rare: Convulsions, fever, pulmonary infiltrates, pleural effusion

Nitazoxanide (Alinia)
Occasional: GI disturbance, headache
Rare: Yellow discoloration of sclera, allergic reactions, increased creatinine, dizziness, flatulence, malaise, salivary gland enlargement, discolored urine, anemia, leukocytosis

Ornidazole (Tiberal)
Occasional: Dizziness, headache, GI disturbance
Rare: Reversible peripheral neuropathy

Oxamniquine (Vansil)
Occasional: Headache, fever, dizziness, somnolence and insomnia, nausea, diarrhea, rash, increased aminotransferases, ECG changes, EEG changes, orange-red discoloration of urine
Rare: Seizures, neuropsychiatric disturbances

Paromomycin (Aminosidine, Humatin)
Frequent: GI disturbance with oral use
Rare: Eighth cranial nerve damage (mainly auditory) and renal damage when aminosidine is given IV, vertigo, pancreatitis

Pentamidine Isethionate (Pentam 300, NebuPent)
Frequent: Hypotension, hypoglycemia often followed by diabetes mellitus, vomiting, blood dyscrasias, renal damage, pain at injection site, GI disturbance
Occasional: May aggravate diabetes, shock, hypocalcemia, liver damage, cardiotoxicity, delirium, rash
Rare: Herxheimer-type reaction, anaphylaxis, acute pancreatitis, hyperkalemia

Permethrin (Nix)
Occasional: Burning, stinging, numbness, increased pruritus, pain, edema, erythema, rash

Praziquantel (Biltricide)
Frequent: Abdominal pain, diarrhea, malaise, headache, dizziness
Occasional: Sedation, fever, sweating, nausea, eosinophilia
Rare: Pruritus, rash, edema, hiccups

Primaquine Phosphate
Frequent: Hemolytic anemia in G6PD deficiency
Occasional: Neutropenia, GI disturbance, methemoglobinemia
Rare: CNS symptoms, hypertension, arrhythmias

Proguanil (Paludrine, Malarone [With Atovaquone])
Occasional: Oral ulceration, hair loss, scaling of palms and soles, urticaria
Rare: Hematuria (with large doses), vomiting, abdominal pain, diarrhea (with large doses), thrombocytopenia

BOX 241.1 Principal Adverse Effects of Antiparasitic Agents—cont'd

Pyrantel Pamoate (Antiminth)

Occasional: GI disturbance, headache, dizziness, rash, fever

Pyrethrins With Piperonyl Butoxide (A-200)

Occasional: Allergic reactions

Pyrimethamine (Daraprim)

Occasional: Blood dyscrasias, folic acid deficiency

Rare: Rash, vomiting, convulsions, shock, possibly pulmonary eosinophilia, fatal cutaneous reactions with pyrimethamine-sulfadoxine (Fansidar)

Quinacrine

Frequent: Disulfiram-like reaction with alcohol, nausea and vomiting, colors skin and urine yellow

Occasional: Headache, dizziness

Rare: Rash, fever, psychosis, extensive exfoliative dermatitis in patients with psoriasis

Quinine Dihydrochloride and Quinine Sulfate

Frequent: Cinchonism (tinnitus, headache, nausea, abdominal pain, visual disturbance)

Occasional: Deafness, hemolytic anemia, other blood dyscrasias, photosensitivity reactions, hypoglycemia, arrhythmias, hypotension, fever

Rare: Blindness, sudden death if injected too rapidly, hypersensitivity reaction with TTP-HUS

Sodium Stibogluconate (Pentostam)

Frequent: Myalgia and arthralgia (typically, large joint, may or may not be symmetric); malaise, fatigue, and weakness; headache; anorexia; nausea; increased aminotransferases; increased amylase and lipase; T-wave flattening or inversion

Occasional: Abdominal pain, liver damage, bradycardia, leukopenia, thrombocytopenia, rash, vomiting

Rare: Diarrhea, pruritus, myocardial damage, hemolytic anemia, renal damage, shock, sudden death

Spiramycin (Rovamycine)

Occasional: GI disturbance

Rare: Allergic reactions

Sulfonamides

Frequent: Allergic reactions (rash, photosensitivity, drug fever)

Occasional: Kernicterus in newborn, renal damage, liver damage, Stevens-Johnson syndrome (particularly with long-acting sulfonamides), hemolytic anemia, other blood dyscrasias, vasculitis

Rare: Transient acute myopia, pseudomembranous colitis, reversible infertility in men with sulfasalazine, CNS toxicity with trimethoprimsulfamethoxazole in patients with AIDS

Suramin Sodium

Frequent: Vomiting, pruritus, urticaria, paresthesias, hyperesthesia of hands and feet, peripheral neuropathy, photophobia

Occasional: Kidney damage, blood dyscrasias, shock, optic atrophy

Tetracyclines (Doxycycline [Vibramycin], Tetracycline Hydrochloride [Sumycin])

Frequent: GI disturbance, bone lesions and staining and deformity of teeth in children age ≤8 years and in the newborn when given to pregnant women after the fourth month of pregnancy

Occasional: Malabsorption; enterocolitis; photosensitivity reactions; increased azotemia with renal insufficiency (except doxycycline, but exacerbation of renal failure with doxycycline has been reported); hepatic injury; parenteral doses may cause serious liver damage, especially in pregnant women and patients with renal disease receiving ≥1 g daily; esophageal ulcerations; cutaneous and mucosal hyperpigmentation

Rare: Allergic reactions, including serum sickness and anaphylaxis; pseudomembranous colitis; blood dyscrasias; drug-induced lupus; autoimmune hepatitis; increased intracranial pressure; fixed-drug eruptions; transient acute myopia; blurred vision; diplopia; papilledema; photoonycholysis and onycholysis; aggravation of myasthenic symptoms with IV injection, reversed with calcium; possibly transient neuropathy; hemolytic anemia

Tinidazole (Tindamax)

Occasional: Metallic taste, GI symptoms, rash

Rare: Weakness

Trimethoprim (Proloprim)

Frequent: Nausea and vomiting with high doses

Occasional: Megaloblastic anemia, thrombocytopenia, neutropenia, rash, fixed drug eruption

Rare: Pancytopenia, hyperkalemia

Trimethoprim/Sulfamethoxazole (Bactrim, Septra)

Frequent: Rash, fever, nausea and vomiting

Occasional: Hemolysis in G6PD deficiency, acute megaloblastic anemia, granulocytopenia, thrombocytopenia, pseudomembranous colitis, kernicterus in newborn, hyperkalemia

Rare: Agranulocytosis, aplastic anemia, hepatotoxicity, Stevens-Johnson syndrome, aseptic meningitis, fever, confusion, depression, hallucinations, deterioration in renal disease, intrahepatic cholestasis, methemoglobinemia, pancreatitis, ataxia, CNS toxicity in patients with AIDS, renal tubular acidosis, hyperkalemia

AIDS, Acquired immunodeficiency syndrome; *CNS,* central nervous system; *ECG,* electrocardiogram; *EEG,* electroencephalogram; *G6PD,* glucose-6 phosphate dehydrogenase; *GI,* gastrointestinal; *IV,* intravenous; *MAO,* monoamine oxidase; *MRI,* magnetic resonance imaging; *TTP-HUS,* thrombotic thrombocytopenic purpura/hemolytic-uremic syndrome.

TABLE 241.1 Safety of Antiparasitic Drugs in Pregnancy

Drug	Toxicity in Pregnancy	Recommendations	FDA
Albendazole (Albenza)	Teratogenic and embryotoxic in animals	Caution*; contraindicated for long-term use	C
Amphotericin B (Fungizone)	None known	Caution*	B
Amphotericin B liposomal (AmBisome)	None known	Caution*	B
Artemether/lumefantrine (Coartem, Riamet)[1]	Embryo-fetal loss in rats and and rabbits	Contraindicated during 1st trimester; caution 2nd and 3rd trimesters*	C
Artesunate[1]	Embryocidal and teratogenic in rats	Contraindicated during 1st trimester; caution 2nd and 3rd trimesters*	NA

Continued

TABLE 241.1 Safety of Antiparasitic Drugs in Pregnancy—cont'd

Drug	Toxicity in Pregnancy	Recommendations	FDA
Atovaquone (Mepron)	Maternal and fetal toxicity in animals	Caution*	C
Atovaquone/proguanil (Malarone)[2]	Maternal and fetal toxicity in animals	Caution*	C
Azithromycin (Zithromax)	None known	Probably safe	B
Benznidazole (Rochagan)	Unknown	Contraindicated	NA
Benzyl alcohol lotion (Ulesfia Lotion)	Unknown	Probably safe	B
Chloroquine (Aralen)	None known with doses recommended for malaria prophylaxis	Probably safe in low doses	C
Clarithromycin (Biaxin)	Teratogenic in animals	Contraindicated	C
Clindamycin (Cleocin)	None known	Caution*	B
Crotamiton (Eurax)	Unknown	Caution*	C
Dapsone	None known; carcinogenic in rats and mice; hemolytic reactions in neonates	Caution,* especially at term	C
Diethylcarbamazine (DEC; Hetrazan)	Not known; abortifacient in one study in rabbits	Contraindicated	NA
Diloxanide (Furamide)	Safety not established	Caution*	NA
Doxycycline (Vibramycin)	Tooth discoloration and dysplasia inhibition of bone growth in fetus; hepatic toxicity and azotemia with IV use in pregnant patients with decreased renal function or with overdosage	Contraindicated	D
Eflornithine (Ornidyl)	Embryocidal in animals	Contraindicated	C
Fluconazole (Diflucan)	Teratogenic	Contraindicated for high dose; caution* for single dose	C
Flucytosine (Ancoban)	Teratogenic in rats	Contraindicated	C
Furazolidone (Furoxone)	None known; carcinogenic in rodents; hemolysis with G6PD deficiency in newborn	Caution*; contraindicated at term	NA
Hydroxychloroquine (Plaquenil)	None known with doses recommended for malaria prophylaxis	Probably safe in low doses	C
Itraconazole (Sporanox)	Teratogenic and embryotoxic in rats	Caution*	C
Iodoquinol (Yodoxin)	Unknown	Caution*	C
Ivermectin (Sklice, Stromectol)[3]	Teratogenic in animals	Contraindicated	C
Ketoconazole (Nizoral)	Teratogenic and embryotoxic in rats	Contraindicated; topical probably safe	C
Lindane	Absorbed from the skin; potential CNS toxicity in fetus	Contraindicated	C
Malathion, topical (Ovide)	None known	Probably safe	B
Mebendazole (Vermox)	Teratogenic and embryotoxic in rats	Caution*	C
Mefloquine (Lariam)[4]	Teratogenic in animals	Caution*	B
Meglumine (Glucantine)	Not known	Caution*	NA
Metronidazole (Flagyl)	None known; carcinogenic in rats and mice	Caution*	B
Miconazole (Monistat)	None known	Caution*	C
Miltefosine (Impavido)	Teratogenic in rats and induces abortions in animals	Contraindicated; effective contraception must be used for 2 months after the last dose	NA
Niclosamide (Niclocide)	Not absorbed; no known toxicity in fetus	Probably safe	B
Nifurtimox (Lampit)	Retarded growth in rats and mice	Caution*; contraindicated during 1st trimester	NA
Nitazoxanide (Alinia)	None known	Probably safe	B
Oxamniquine (Vansil)	Embryocidal in animals	Contraindicated	NA
Paromomycin	Poorly absorbed; toxicity in fetus unknown	Oral capsules probably safe	C
Pentamidine (Pentam 300, NebuPent)	Safety not established	Caution*	C
Permethrin (Nix)	Poorly absorbed; no known toxicity in fetus	Probably safe	B
Praziquantel (Biltricide)	None known	Caution	B
Primaquine	Hemolysis in G6PD deficiency	Contraindicated	C
Pyrantel pamoate (Antiminth)	Absorbed in small amounts; no known toxicity in fetus	Probably safe	C
Pyrethrins and piperonyl butoxide (A-200)	Poorly absorbed; no known toxicity in fetus	Probably safe	C
Pyrimethamine (Daraprim)[5]	Teratogenic in animals	Caution*; contraindicated during 1st trimester	C
Quinacrine (Atabrine)	Safety not established	Caution*	NA
Quinidine	Large doses can cause abortion	Probably safe	C
Quinine (Qualaquin)	Large doses can cause abortion; auditory nerve hypoplasia, deafness in fetus; visual changes, limb anomalies, visceral defects also reported	Caution*	C
Sodium stibogluconate (Pentostam)	Not known	Caution*	NA
Spiramycin (Rovamycine)[5]	None known	Probably safe	NA
Sulfonamides	Teratogenic in some animal studies; hemolysis in newborn with G6PD deficiency; increased risk of kernicterus in newborn	Caution*; contraindicated at term	C
Suramin sodium (Germanin)	Teratogenic in mice	Caution*	NA

TABLE 241.1 Safety of Antiparasitic Drugs in Pregnancy—cont'd

Drug	Toxicity in Pregnancy	Recommendations	FDA
Tetracycline (Sumycin)	Tooth discoloration and dysplasia, inhibition of bone growth in fetus; hepatic toxicity and azotemia with IV use in pregnant patients with decreased renal function or with overdosage	Contraindicated	D
Tinidazole (Tindamax)	Increased fetal mortality in rats	Caution*	C
Trimethoprim	Folate antagonism; teratogenic in rats	Caution*	C
Trimethoprim/sulfamethoxazole (Bactrim)	Same as sulfonamides and trimethoprim	Caution*; contraindicated at term	C

CNS, Central nervous system; FDA, US Food and Drug Administration; *G6PD*, glucose-g phosphate dehydrogenase; *IV*, intravenous; *NA*, FDA pregnancy category not available.

*Use only for strong clinical indication in absence of suitable alternative.

1. Based on the few studies available, artemesinins have been relatively safe during pregnancy (Adam I, et al. *Am Trop Med Parisitol.* 2009;103:205), but some experts would not prescribe them in the 1st trimester (Clark RL. *Reprod Toxicol.* 2009;28:285; Manyando C, et al. *Malaria J.* 2012;11:141).
2. Safety in pregnancy is unknown; in a few small studies; outcomes were normal in women treated with the combination in the 2nd and 3rd trimester (Boggild AK, et al. *Am J Trop Med Hyg.* 2007;76:208).
3. Ivermectin has been inadvertently given to pregnant women during mass treatment programs; the rates of congenital abnormalities were similar in treated and untreated women. Because of the high risk of blindness from onchocerciasis, the use of ivermectin after the first trimester is considered acceptable according to the World Health Organization.
4. Mefloquine can be used for prophylaxis or treatment of malaria in pregnant women based on a review of published data (Schlagenhauf P, et al. *Clin Infect Dis.* 2012;54:e124).
5. Women who develop toxoplasmosis during the first trimester of pregnancy should be treated with spiramycin (3–4 g/d). After the first trimester, if there is no documented transmission to the fetus, spiramycin can be continued until term. If transmission has occurred in utero, therapy with pyrimethamine and sulfadiazine should be started. Pyrimethamine is a potential teratogen and should be used only after the first trimester (Montoya JG, Remington JS. *Clin Infect Dis.* 2008;47:554).

TABLE 241.2 Manufacturers of Drugs Used to Treat Parasitic Infections

Generic Name	Brand Name	Manufacturer
albendazole	Albenza	Amedra
amphotericin B	Fungizone, generics	X-Gen
amphotericin B, liposomal	AmBisome	Gilead
artemether[1]	Artenam	Arenco, Belgium
artemether/lumefantrine	Coartem, Riamet	Novartis
artesunate[2]		Guilin, Shanghai
atovaquone	Mepron	GlaxoSmithKline
atovaquone/proguanil	Malarone	GlaxoSmithKline
azithromycin	Zithromax	Pfizer
benznidazole[2]	Rochagan	
bithionol[1]	Bitin	
chloroquine	Aralen	Sanofi
clarithromycin	Biaxin	Abbvie
clindamycin	Cleocin	Pfizer
crotamiton	Eurax	Ranbaxy
dapsone		Jacobus
diethylcarbamazine citrate (DEC)[2]	Hetrazan	
dihydroartemisin/piperaquine	Euratesim	Sigma-Tau, Italy
diloxanide furoate[1]	Furamide, Entamide	
doxycycline	Vibramycin	Pfizer
eflornithine (difluoromethylornithine, DFMO)[2]	Ornidyl	Sanofi
fluconazole	Diflucan	Pfizer
flucytosine	Ancobon	Valeant
fumagillin[1]	Flisint	Sanofi, France
furazolidone[1]	Furoxone	
iodoquinol	Yodoxin	Glenwood
itraconazole	Sporanox	Janssen
ivermectin	Stromectol	Merck
	Sklice	Sanofi
ketoconazole	Nizoral	Janssen
lumefantrine/artemether	Coartem, Riamet	Novartis
malathion	Ovide	Taro
mebendazole		
mefloquine		
meglumine antimonate[1]	Glucantime	Sanofi, France
melarsoprol[2]	Mel-B	
metronidazole	Flagyl	Pfizer
miconazole[1]	Monistat	
Miltefosine[2,3]	Impavido, Miltex	Paladin, Canada
niclosamide[1]	Yomesan	
nifurtimox[2]	Lampit	Bayer HealthCare
nitazoxanide	Alinia	Romark
ornidazole[1]	Tiberal	
oxamniquine[1]	Vansil, Mansil	Pfizer, UK
paromomycin[1]	Leshcutan (topical)	Sun Pharma
pentamidine isethionate	Pentam 300, NebuPent	APP Pharmaceuticals
permethrin	Nix	Insight, Bayer
	Elimite	Renaissance Pharma
piperaquine/dihydroartemisin	Euratesim	Sigma Tau, Italy
praziquantel	Biltricide	Bayer
primaquine phosphate USP		Sanofi
proguanil[1]	Paludrine	
proguanil/atovaquone	Malarone	GlaxoSmithKline
propamidine isethionate[1]	Brolene	Aventis
pyrantel pamoate	Pin-X, Reese's Pinworm	Penn Labs, Reese
pyrethrins and piperonyl butoxide	Rid	Bayer
pyrimethamine USP	Daraprim	Amedra
quinidine gluconate		
quinine dihydrochloride[1]		
quinine sulfate	Qualaquin	AR Scientific
rifampin	Rifadin	Sanofi
sodium stibogluconate[2]	Pentostam	GlaxoSmithKline, UK
spiramycin[1]	Rovamycine	Sanofi, France
sulfadiazine		
suramin sodium[2]	Germanin	Bayer, Germany
tinidazole	Tindamax	Mission
trimethoprim-sulfamethoxazole	Bactrim	Sun Pharma
triclabendazole[1]	Egaten	Novartis
trimetrexate[1]	Neutrexin	

1. Not available in the United States; may be available through a compounding pharmacy such as Expert Compounding Pharmacy, 6744 Balboa Blvd, Lake Balboa, CA (800-247-9767) or Medical Center Pharmacy, New Haven, CT (203-688-7064). Other compounding pharmacies may be found through the National Association of Compounding Pharmacies (800-687-7850) or the Professional Compounding Centers of America (800-331-2498, www.pccarx.com).
2. Available from the CDC Drug Service, Centers for Disease Control and Prevention, Atlanta, GA 30333; 404-639-3670 (evenings, weekends, or holidays: 770-488-7100; fax: 404-639-3717).
3. Available from the CDC for treatment of infections with free-living amebae; available from the manufacturer through an IND application from the FDA for treatment of other infections.

Acanthamoeba Keratitis

Drug of choice	Keratitis is typically associated with contact lens use.[1] A topical biguanide, 0.02% chlorhexidine or polyhexamethylene biguanide (PHMB, 0.02%), either alone or combined with a diamidine, propamidine isethionate (Brolene) or hexamidine (Desomodine), have been used successfully.[2] They are administered hourly (or alternating every half hour) day and night for the first 48 hours and then continued on a reduced schedule for days to months.[3] None of these drugs is commercially available or approved for use in the United States, but they can be obtained from compounding pharmacies. Leiter's Park Avenue Pharmacy, San Jose, CA (800-292-6773; www.leiterrx.com) is a compounding pharmacy that specializes in ophthalmic drugs. Expert Compounding Pharmacy, 6744 Balboa Blvd., Lake Balboa, CA 91406 (800-247-9767) and Medical Center Pharmacy, New Haven, CT (203-688-7064) are also compounding pharmacies. Other compounding pharmacies may be found through the National Association of Compounding Pharmacies (800-687-7850) or the Professional Compounding Centers of America (800-331-2498, www.pccarx.com). Propamidine is available over the counter in the United Kingdom and Australia. Hexamidine is available in France. Debridement is most useful during the stage of corneal epithelial infection; keratoplasty in medically unresponsive keratitis was successful in 31 eyes in 30 patients.[4] Most cysts are resistant to neomycin; its use is no longer recommended. Azole antifungal drugs (ketoconazole, itraconazole) have been used as oral or topical adjuncts. Successful treatment with topical or oral voriconazole has been reported in a small number of patients who had not responded to PHMB, chlorhexidine, and hexamidine.[5,6] Use of corticosteroids is controversial. Prolonged therapy (≥6 months) may be necessary.[2]

1. Carvalho FR, et al. *Cornea.* 2009; 28:516.
2. Dart JK, et al. *Am J Ophthalmol.* 2009;148:487.
3. Visvesvara GS. *Curr Opin Infect Dis.* 2010;23:590.
4. Kitzmann AS, et al. *Ophthalmology.* 2009;116:864.
5. Bang BS, et al. *Am J Ophthalmol.* 2010;149:66.
6. Tu EY,et al. *Cornea.* 2010;29:1066.

Amebiasis *(Entamoeba histolytica)*

	Drug	Adult Dosage	Pediatric Dosage
Asymptomatic			
Drug of choice:	Iodoquinol[1]	650 mg PO tid × 20 d	30–40 mg/kg/d (max 2 g) PO in 3 doses × 20 d
Or	Paromomycin[2]	25–35 mg/kg/d PO in 3 doses × 7 d	25–35 mg/kg/d PO in 3 doses × 7 d
Or	Diloxanide furoate[3]*	500 mg PO tid × 10 d	20 mg/kg/d PO in 3 doses × 10 d
Mild to Moderate Intestinal Disease			
Drug of choice[4]:	Metronidazole	500–750 mg PO tid × 7–10 d	35–50 mg/kg/d PO in 3 doses × 7–10 d
Or	Tinidazole[5]	2 g once PO daily × 3 d	>3 y: 50 mg/kg/d (max 2 g) PO in 1 dose × 3 d
Followed by	Iodoquinol[1]	650 mg PO tid × 20 d	30–40 mg/kg/d (max 2 g) PO in 3 doses × 20 d
Or	Paromomycin[2]	25–35 mg/kg/d PO in 3 doses × 7 d	25–35 mg/kg/d PO in 3 doses × 7 d
Severe Intestinal and Extraintestinal Disease			
Drug of choice:	Metronidazole	750 mg PO (or IV) tid × 7–10 d	35–50 mg/kg/d PO (or IV) in 3 doses × 7–10 d
Or	Tinidazole[5]	2 g once PO daily × 5 d	>3 y: 50 mg/kg/d (max 2 g) PO in 1 dose × 5 d
Followed by	Iodoquinol[1]	650 mg PO tid × 20 d	30–40 mg/kg/d (max 2 g) PO in 3 doses × 20 d
Or	Paromomycin[2]	25–35 mg/kg/d PO in 3 doses × 7 d	25–35 mg/kg/d PO in 3 doses × 7 d

*Availability problems. See Table 241.1.
1. Iodoquinol should be taken after meals.
2. Paromomycin should be taken with a meal.
3. Not available commercially. It may be obtained through compounding pharmacies such as Expert Compounding Pharmacy, 6744 Balboa Blvd, Lake Balboa, CA 91406 (800-247-9767) or Medical Center Pharmacy, New Haven, CT (203-688-7064). Other compounding pharmacies may be found through the National Association of Compounding Pharmacies (800-687-7850) or the Professional Compounding Centers of America (800-331-2498, www.pccarx.com).
4. Nitazoxanide may be effective against a variety of protozoan and helminth infections (Bobak DA. *Curr Infect Dis Rep.* 2006;8:91; Diaz E, et al. *Am J Trop Med Hyg.* 2003;68:384). It is effective against mild to moderate amebiasis, 500 mg PO bid × 3 d (Rossignol JF, et al. *Trans R Soc Trop Med Hyg.* 2007;101:1025; Escobedo AE, et al. *Arch Dis Child.* 2009;94:478), but perhaps less so than metronidazole (Becker S, et al. *Am J Trop Hyg.* 2011;84:581). Nitazoxanide is FDA approved only for treatment of diarrhea caused by *Giardia* or *Cryptosporidium* (*Med Lett Drugs Ther.* 2003;45:29). It is available in 500-mg tablets and an oral suspension and should be taken with food.
5. Tinidazole, a nitroimidazole similar to metronidazole, appears to be as effective as metronidazole and better tolerated (*Med Lett Drugs Ther.* 2004;46:70). It should be taken with food to minimize adverse GI effects. For children and patients unable to take tablets, a pharmacist can crush the tablets and mix them with cherry syrup (Humco, and others). The syrup suspension is good for 7 days at room temperature and must be shaken before use (Fung HB, Doan TL. *Clin Ther.* 2005;27:1859). Ornidazole, a similar drug, is also used outside the United States.

Amebic Meningoencephalitis, Primary and Granulomatous[1]

	Drug	Adult Dosage	Pediatric Dosage
Primary Amebic Meningoencephalitis (PAM): *Naegleria fowleri*[2,3]			
Drug of choice:	Amphotericin B (conventional formulation)[4]	0.25 mg/kg IV over 4–6 h. If tolerated, 0.5 mg/kg IV the following day, increasing to 1.5 mg/kg IV once/d as tolerated (max 1.5 mg/kg/d)	0.25 mg/kg IV over 4–6 h. If tolerated, 0.5 mg/kg IV the following day, increasing to 1.5 mg/kg IV once/d as tolerated (max 1.5 mg/kg/d)
Or		1 mg/kg IV once/d plus 0.5 mg/d intraventricularly (can start with 0.025–0.050 mg/d and increase to 0.5 mg/d)[5] (max 1.5 mg/kg once/d total dosage by both IV and intraventricular routes)	1 mg/kg IV once/d plus 0.5 mg/d intraventricularly (can start with 0.025–0.050 mg/d and increase to 0.5 mg/d)[5] (max 1.5 mg/kg once/d total dosage by both IV and intraventricular routes)
	Rifampin	10 mg/kg IV once/d (max 600 mg/d)	10 mg/kg IV once/d (max 600 mg/d)
	Fluconazole	12 mg/kg IV once/d	12 mg/kg IV once/d
	Azithromycin	500 mg IV once/d	20 mg/kg IV once/d (max 500 mg/d)
Granulomatous Amebic Encephalitis (GAE): *Acanthamoeba* spp.[6–8]			
	Pentamidine[9]	4 mg/kg IV once/d	4 mg/kg IV once/d
	Sulfadiazine	1.5 g q6h PO	200 mg/kg/d PO in 4–6 doses (max 6 g/d)
	Flucytosine	37.5 mg/kg PO q6h (max 150 mg/kg/d)	37.5 mg/kg PO q6h (max 150 mg/kg/d)
	Fluconazole	12 mg/kg IV once/d	12 mg/kg IV once/d
	Miltefosine[10]	<45 kg: 100 mg/d PO in 2 doses ≥45 kg: 150 mg/d PO in 3 doses	2.5 mg/kg/d PO in 2 doses (max 100 mg/d)
Granulomatous Amebic Encephalitis (GAE): *Balamuthia mandrillaris*[11–16]			
	Azithromycin	500 mg IV once/d	20 mg/kg IV once/d (max 500 mg/d)
	Clarithromycin	14 mg/kg/d PO in 2 doses (max 2 g/d)	14 mg/kg/d PO in 2 doses (max 2 g/d)
	Pentamidine[9]	4 mg/kg IV once/d	4 mg/kg IV once/d
	Sulfadiazine	1.5 g PO q6h	200 mg/kg/d PO in 4–6 doses (max 6 g/d)
	Flucytosine	37.5 mg/kg PO q6h (max 150 mg/kg/d)	37.5 mg/kg PO q6h (max 150 mg/kg/d)
	Fluconazole	12 mg/kg IV once/d	12 mg/kg IV once/d
	Miltefosine[10]	<45 kg: 100 mg/d PO in 2 doses ≥45 kg: 150 mg/d PO in 3 doses	2.5 mg/kg/d PO in 2 doses (max 100 mg/d)

1. Meningoencephalitis caused by the free-living amebae *Naegleria fowleri, Acanthamoeba* spp., and *Balamuthia mandrillaris* has a mortality rate of >90%; effective treatment has not been established. Treatment recommendations are based on case reports of survivors, animal studies, and in vitro drug testing. Treatment decisions must be tailored to the clinical situation of each patient. Diagnostic assistance, specimen collection guidance, shipping instructions, and treatment recommendations are available through the CDC Emergency Operations Center at 770-488-7100.
2. Seidel JS, et al. *N Engl J Med.* 1982;306:346.
3 Vargas-Zepeda J, et al. *Arch Med Res.* 2005;36:83.
4. Although liposomal amphotericin B crosses the blood-brain barrier better than conventional amphotericin, it has been found to be less effective against PAM caused by *Naegleria fowleri* in mice. Amphotericin B methyl ester was also found to be less effective in the mouse model (Schuster FL, Visvesvara GS. *Int J Parasitol.* 2004;34:1001). Because of the extremely poor prognosis of PAM due to *Naegleria fowleri,* aggressive treatment, including the use of intraventricular amphotericin, should be considered.
5. Chapman SW, et al. In: Kauffman C, ed. *Essentials of Clinical Mycology.* 2nd ed. New York: Springer; 2011:41–55.
6. Immunocompromised patients with cutaneous acanthamoebiasis have been successfully treated with (1) pentamidine, flucytosine, and azithromycin in combination with topical chlorhexidine and 2% ketoconazole cream (Oliva S, et al. *South Med J.* 1999;92:55); (2) pentamidine in combination with topical chlorhexidine and 2% ketoconazole cream followed by oral itraconazole (Slater CA, et al. *N Engl J Med.* 1994;331:85); and (3) amphotericin B lipid complex and voriconazole (Walia R, et al. *Transplant Soc.* 2007;9:51). Miltefosine, both oral and topical, has also shown success in treating cutaneous disease (Aichelburg AC, et al. *Emerg Infect Dis.* 2008;14:1743; Walochnik J, et al. *J Antimicrob Chemother.* 2009;64:539).
7. Aichelburg AC, et al. *Emerg Infect Dis.* 2008;14:1743.
8. Seijo Martinez M, et al. *J Clinical Microbiol.* 2000;38:3892.
9. Addition of pentamidine is based on clinical judgement. Although it has good amebacidal activity in vitro and has been used successfully in the past to treat GAE in combination with the drugs listed, pentamidine is associated with adverse effects, including nephrotoxicity, leukopenia, elevated liver enzymes, and hypoglycemia. Additionally, pentamidine does not cross the normal, intact blood-brain barrier well.
10. Miltefosine is not approved for any indication in the United States. Case reports and in vitro data suggest it may have some antiamebic activity (Aichelburg AC, et al. *Emerg Infect Dis.* 2008;14:1743; Martinez DY, et al. *Infect Dis Soc Am.* 2010;51:e7; Schuster FL, et al. *J Eukaryot Microbiol.* 2006;53:121). Miltefosine (Impavido) is manufactured in 10- or 50-mg capsules by Paladin (Canada) and is available in the United States from the CDC for treatment of infections with free-living amebae. The drug is contraindicated in breastfeeding and pregnant women; a negative pregnancy test before drug initiation and effective contraception during and for 4 months after treatment is recommended (Murray HW, et al. *Lancet.* 2005;366:1561).
11. Cary LC, et al. *Pediatrics.* 2010;125:e699.
12. Deetz TR, et al. *Clin Infect Dis.* 2003;37:1304.
13. Martinez DY, et al. *Clin Infect Dis.* 2010;51:e7.
14. Orozco LD, et al. *J Clin Neurosci.* 2011;18:1118.
15. Bravo FG, et al. *Curr Opin Infect Dis.* 2011;24:112.
16. Doyle JS, et al. *J Neurosurgery.* 2011;114:458.

Ancylostoma caninum (Eosinophilic Enterocolitis)

Drug of choice:	Albendazole[1,2]	400 mg PO once	400 mg PO once
Or	Mebendazole	100 mg PO bid × 3 d	100 mg PO bid × 3 d
Or	Endoscopic removal		

1. Not FDA approved for this indication.
2. Albendazole must be taken with food; a fatty meal increases oral bioavailability.

Ancyclostoma Duodenale

See Hookworm

Angiostrongyliasis (*Angiostrongylus cantonensis, Angiostrongylus costaricensis*)

Drug of choice: *A. cantonensis* causes predominantly neurotropic disease.[1] *A. costaricensis* causes gastrointestinal disease. Most patients infected with either species have a self-limited course and recover completely. Analgesics, corticosteroids, and periodic removal of cerebrospinal fluid can relieve symptoms from increased intracranial pressure.[2] Treatment of *A. cantonensis* is controversial and varies across endemic areas.[3] No antihelminthic drug is proven to be effective, and some patients have worsened with therapy. Mebendazole or albendazole each with or without a corticosteroid appear to shorten the course of infection.[4] Ocular angiostrongyliasis is managed by early and complete surgical removal of larva.[5]

1. Wang QP, et al. *Lancet Infect Dis.* 2008;8:621.
2. Ramirez-Avila L, et al. *Clin Infect Dis.* 2009;48:322.
3. Diao Z, et al. *Emerg Infect Dis.* 2011;17:e1.
4. Sawanyawisuth K, Sawanyawisuth K. *Trans R Soc Trop Med Hyg.* 2008;102:990; Chotmongkol V, et al. *Am J Trop Med Hyg.* 2009;81:443.
5. Diao Z, et al. *Trop Doctor.* 2011;41:76.

Anisakiasis (*Anisakis* spp.)

Drug	Adult Dosage	Pediatric Dosage
Treatment of choice[1]:	Surgical or endoscopic removal	

1. Gastric anisakiasis can usually be diagnosed and treated by endoscopic removal of the worm (Hochberg NS, Hamer DH. *Clin Infect Dis.* 2010;51:806). Enteric anisakiasis is more difficult to diagnose; capsule or double-balloon endoscopy has been used (Yasunaga H, et al. *Am J Trop Med Hyg.* 2010;83:104; Nakaji K. *Intern Med.* 2009;48:573). Disease can be managed without worm removal as the worms eventually die. Surgery may be needed in the event of intestinal obstruction or peritonitis (Repiso Ortega A, et al. *Gastroenterol Hepatol.* 2003;26:341). Successful treatment of anisakiasis with albendazole 400 mg PO bid × 3–5 d has been reported, but diagnosis was presumptive (Moore DA, et al. *Lancet.* 2002;360:54; Pacios E, et al. *Clin Infect Dis.* 2005;41:1825).

Ascariasis (*Ascaris lumbricoides,* Roundworm)

	Drug	Adult Dosage	Pediatric Dosage
Drug of choice[1]:	Albendazole[2,3]	400 mg PO once	400 mg PO once
Or	Mebendazole	100 mg bid PO × 3 d or 500 mg once	100 mg PO bid × 3 d or 500 mg once
Or	Ivermectin[2,4]	150–200 μg/kg PO once	150–200 μg/kg PO once

1.Nitazoxanide may be effective against a variety of protozoan and helminth infections (Bobak DA, *Curr Infect Dis Rep.* 2006;8:91; Diaz E, et al. *Am J Trop Med Hyg.* 2003;68:384). It is effective against mild to moderate amebiasis, 500 mg bid × 3 d (Rossignol JF, et al. *Trans R Soc Trop Med Hyg.* 2007;101:1025; Escobedo AE, et al. *Arch Dis Child.* 2009;94:478). It is FDA approved only for treatment of diarrhea caused by *Giardia* or *Cryptosporidium* (*Med Lett Drugs Ther.* 2003;45:29). Nitazoxanide is available in 500-mg tablets and an oral suspension; it should be taken with food.
2. Not FDA approved for this indication.
3. Albendazole must be taken with food; a fatty meal increases oral bioavailability.
4. Gonzalez P, et al. *Curr Pharm Biotechnol.* 2012;13:1103. Safety of ivermectin in young children (<15 kg) and pregnant women remains to be established; animal studies have shown adverse effects on the fetus (el-Ashmawy IM, et al. *Res Vet Sci.* 2011;90:116). Taking ivermectin with a meal increases its bioavailability (Guzzo CA, et al. *J Clin Pharmacol.* 2002;42:1122).

Babesiosis

	Drug	Adult Dosage	Pediatric Dosage
Drug of choice[1]:	Atovaquone[2,3]	750 mg PO bid × 7–10 d	40 mg/kg/d PO in 2 doses × 7–10 d
Plus	Azithromycin[2]	500–1000 mg PO on day 1, then 250–500 mg PO on day 2–10	10 mg/kg (max 500 mg/dose) PO on day 1, then 5 mg/kg/d (max 250 mg dose) PO on day 2–10
Or	Clindamycin[2,4]	300–600 mg IV qid or 600 mg PO tid × 7–10 d	20–40 mg/kg/d (max 600 mg/dose) IV or PO in 3 or 4 doses × 7–10 d
Plus	Quinine[2,5]	650 mg PO tid or qid × 7–10 d	24 mg/kg/d (max 600 mg/dose) PO in 3 doses × 7–10 d

1. *Babesia microti* is the most common cause of human babesiosis in the United States (Vannier E, Krause PJ. *N Engl J Med.* 2012;366:2397), but disease caused by *B. duncani* or *B. divergens*-like organisms also has been documented (Persing DH, et al. *N Engl J Med.* 1995;332:298; Herwaldt B, et al. *Ann Intern Med.* 1996;124:643). In Europe, most cases have been attributed to *B. divergens* whereas a few have been caused by *B. venatorum* or *B. microti* (Herwaldt BL, et al. *Emerg Infect Dis.* 2003;9:942; Hunfeld KP, et al. *Int J Parasitol.* 2008;38:1219). *B. microti-like* organisms have been identified as etiologic agents in cases reported from Japan and Taiwan. Concurrent babesiosis, Lyme disease, and/or human granulocytic anaplasmosis may occur (Thompson C, et al. *Clin Infect Dis.* 2001;33:676). Symptoms of *B. microti* infection typically are mild to moderate and are treated with atovaquone plus azithromycin (Krause PJ, et al. *N Engl J Med.* 2000;343:1454). Clindamycin plus quinine is recommended for severe symptoms with *B. microti* infection and for all *B. divergens* infections (Wormser GP, et al. *Clin Infect Dis.* 2006;43:1089; Vannier E, Krause PJ. *N Engl J Med.* 2012;366:2397). Clindamycin plus quinine is also the treatment of choice for infections caused by *B. duncani, B. divergens*-like organisms, or *B. venatorum.* Exchange tranfusion should be considered for severely ill patients and those with high (>10%) parasitemia or pulmonary, renal, or hepatic compromise when infection is caused by *B. microti* and is recommended for cases of *B. divergens* infection. Highly immunosuppressed patients should be treated for a minimum of 6 weeks and at least 2 weeks past the last positive smear (Krause PJ, et al. *Clin Infect Dis.* 2008;46:370). High doses of azithromycin (600–1000 mg) have been used in combination with atovaquone for the treatment of immunocompromised patients (Weiss LM, et al. *N Engl J Med.* 2001;344:773). Resistance to atovaquone plus azithromycin has been reported in immunocompromised patients treated with a single subcurative course of this regimen (Wormser GP, et al. *Clin Infect Dis.* 2010; 50:381).
2. Not FDA approved for this indication.
3. Atovaquone is available in an oral suspension that should be taken with a meal to increase absorption.
4. Oral clindamycin should be taken with a full glass of water to minimize esophageal ulceration.
5. Quinine should be taken with or after a meal to decrease gastrointestinal adverse effects.

Balamuthia mandrillaris

See Amebic Meningoencephalitis, Primary

Balantidiasis *(Balantidium coli)*

	Drug	Adult Dosage	Pediatric Dosage
Drug of choice:	Tetracycline[1,2]	500 mg PO qid × 10 d	40 mg/kg/d (max. 2 g) PO in 4 doses × 10 d
Alternative:	Metronidazole[1]	500–750 mg PO tid × 5 d	35–50 mg/kg/d PO in 3 doses × 5 d
Or	Iodoquinol[1,3]	650 mg PO tid × 20 d	30–40 mg/kg/d (max 2 g) PO in 3 doses × 20 d

1. Not FDA approved for this indication.
2. Use of tetracyclines is contraindicated in pregnancy and in children <8 years. Tetracycline should be taken 1 hour before or 2 hours after meals and/or dairy products.
3. Iodoquinol should be taken after meals.

Baylisascariasis *(Baylisascaris procyonis)*

	Drug	Adult Dosage	Pediatric Dosage
Drug of choice:	The combination of albendazole 37 mg/kg/d PO and high-dose steroids has been used successfully.[1,2] Albendazole 25 mg/kg/d PO × 20 d started as soon as possible (up to 3 d after possible infection) might prevent clinical disease and is recommended for children with known exposure (ingestion of raccoon stool or contaminated soil).[3] Mebendazole, levamisole or ivermectin could be tried if albendazole is not available. Ocular baylisascariasis has been treated successfully using laser photocoagulation therapy to destroy the intraretinal larvae.[4]		

1. Peters JM, et al. *Pediatrics.* 2012;129:e806.
2. Haider S, *Emerg Infect Dis.* 2012;18:347.
3. Murray WJ, Kazacos KR. *Clin Infect Dis.* 2004;39:1484.
4. Garcia CA, et al. *Eye (Lond).* 2004;18:624.

Blastocystis spp.

	Drug	Adult Dosage	Pediatric Dosage
Drug of choice:	Clinical significance of these organisms is controversial.[1] Treatment options include metronidazole 750 mg PO tid × 10 d, trimethoprim/sulfamethoxazole 1 DS tab PO bid × 7 d or iodoquinol 650 mg PO tid × 20 d.[2] Metronidazole resistance may be common in some areas.[3] Nitazoxanide has been effective in clearing organisms and improving symptoms.[4]		

1. Poirier P, et al. *PLoS Pathogens.* 2012;8:e1002545.
2. Tan KS, *Clin Microbiol Rev.* 2008;21:639.
3. Yakoob J, et al. *Br J Biomed Sci.* 2004;61:75.
4. Diaz E, et al. *Am J Trop Med Hyg.* 2003;68:384; Rossignol JF. *Clin Gastroenterol Hepatol.* 2005;3:987.

Capillariasis *(Capillaria philippinensis)*

	Drug	Adult Dosage	Pediatric Dosage
Drug of choice:	Mebendazole[1]	200 mg PO bid × 20 d	200 mg PO bid × 20 d
Alternative:	Albendazole[1,2]	400 mg PO daily × 10 d	400 mg PO daily × 10 d

1. Not FDA approved for this indication.
2. Albendazole must be taken with food; a fatty meal increases oral bioavailability.

Chagas' Disease

See Trypanosomiasis

Clonorchis sinensis

See Fluke

Cryptosporidiosis (*Cryptosporidium*)

	Drug	Adult Dosage	Pediatric Dosage
Immunocompetent			
Drug of choice:	Nitazoxanide[1]	500 mg PO bid × 3 d	1–3 y: 100 mg PO bid × 3 d 4–11 y: 200 mg PO bid × 3 d >12 y: 500 mg PO bid × 3 d
Immunocompromised			
Drug of choice:	No drug has proven efficacy in cryptosporidiosis in immunosuppressed patients.[2] For HIV-infected patients, potent antiretroviral therapy is the mainstay of treatment. Nitazoxanide (treatment duration of 5–21 d),[3] paromomycin, or a combination of paromomycin and azithromycin may be tried to decrease diarrhea and recalcitrant malabsorption of antimicrobial drugs, which can occur with chronic cryptosporidiosis.[4]		

1. Nitazoxanide may be effective against a variety of protozoan and helminth infections (Bobak DA. *Curr Infect Dis Rep.* 2006;8:91; Diaz E, et al. *Am J Trop Med Hyg.* 2003;68:384). It is effective against mild to moderate amebiasis, 500 mg bid × 3 d (Rossignol JF, et al. *Trans R Soc Trop Med Hyg.* 2007;101:1025; Escobedo AA, et al. *Arch Dis Child.* 2009;94:478), but perhaps less so than metronidazole (Becker S, t al. *Am J Trop Med Hyg.* 2011;84:581). Nitazoxanide is FDA approved only for treatment of diarrhea caused by *Giardia* or *Cryptosporidium* (*Med Lett Drugs Ther.* 2003;45:29). It is available in 500-mg tablets and an oral suspension and should be taken with food.
2. Leitch GJ, He Q. *J Biomed Res.* 2012;25:1.
3. Krause I, et al. *Pediatr Infect Dis J.* 2012;31:1135.
4. Pantenburg B, et al. *Expert Rev Anti Infect Ther.* 2009;7:385.

Cutaneous Larva Migrans (Creeping Eruption, Dog and Cat Hookworm)

	Drug	Adult Dosage	Pediatric Dosage
Drug of choice[1]:	Albendazole[2,3]	400 mg PO daily × 3 d	400 mg PO daily × 3 d
Or	Ivermectin[2,4]	200 μg/kg PO daily × 1–2 d	200 μg/kg PO daily × 1–2 d

1. Heukelbach J, Feldmeier H. *Lancet Infect Dis.* 2008;8:302; Bowman DD, et al. *Trends Parasitol.* 2012;26:162.
2. Not FDA approved for this indication.
3. Albendazole must be taken with food; a fatty meal increases oral bioavailability.
4. Gonzalez P, et al. *Curr Pharm Biotechnol.* 2012;13:1103. Safety of ivermectin in young children (<15 kg) and pregnant women remains to be established; animal studies have shown adverse effects on the fetus (el-Ashmawy IM, et al. *Res Vet Sci.* 2011;90:116). Taking ivermectin with a meal increases its bioavailability (Guzzo CA, et al. *J Clin Pharmacol.* 2002;42:1122).

Cyclosporiasis (*Cyclospora cayetanensis*)

	Drug	Adult Dosage	Pediatric Dosage
Drug of choice[1]:	Trimethoprim/sulfamethoxazole[2]	TMP 160 mg/SMX 800 mg (1 double-strength tab) PO bid × 7–10 d	TMP 10 mg/kg/SMX 50 mg/kg/d PO in 2 doses × 7–10 d
Alternative:	Ciprofloxacin[2]	500 mg PO bid × 7 d	—

1. Ortega YR, Sanchez S. *Clin Microbiol Rev.* 2010;23:218. In one study of HIV-infected patients with *Cyclospora* infection, ciprofloxacin treatment led to resolution in 87% of patients compared to 100% with TMP/SMX (Verdier RI, et al. *Ann Intern Med.* 2000;132:885). HIV-infected patients may need higher dosage and long-term maintenance. Nitazoxanide (see also footnote 3) has also been used in a few patients, some of whom were sulfa allergic (Zimmer SM, et al. *Clin Infect Dis.* 2007; 44:466; Diaz E, et al. *Am J Trop Med Hyg.* 2003;68:384).
2. Not FDA approved for this indication.
3. Nitazoxanide may be effective against a variety of protozoan and helminth infections (Bobak DA, *Curr Infect Dis Rep.* 2006;8:91; Diaz E, et al. *Am J Trop Med Hyg.* 2003;68:384). It is effective against mild to moderate amebiasis, 500 mg bid × 3 d (Rossignol JF, et al. *Trans R Soc Trop Med Hyg.* 2007;101:1025; Escobedo AA, et al. *Arch Dis Child.* 2009;94:478), but perhaps less so than metronidazole (Becker S, et al. *Am J Trop Hyg.* 2011;84:581). Nitazoxanide is FDA approved only for treatment of diarrhea caused by *Giardia* or *Cryptosporidium* (*Med Lett Drugs Ther.* 2003;45:29). It is available in 500-mg tablets and an oral suspension and should be taken with food.

Cysticercosis

See Tapeworm

Diphyllobothrium Latum

See Tapeworm

Cystoisosporiasis (*Cystoisospora belli,* Formerly Known as *Isospora)*

	Drug	Adult Dosage	Pediatric Dosage
Drug of choice[1]:	Trimethoprim-sulfamethoxazole (TMP-SMX)[2]	TMP 160 mg/SMX 800 mg (1 double-strength tab) PO bid × 10 d	TMP 10 mg/kg/d/SMX 50 mg/kg/d PO in 2 doses × 10 d

1. *Isospora belli* has been renamed and included in the *Cystoisospora* genus. Usually a self-limited illness in immunocompetent patients. Immunosuppressed patients may need higher doses and longer duration (TMP-SMX qid for up to 3 to 4 wk (*Morbid Mortal Wkly Rep.* 2009;58 RR4:1). They may also require secondary prophylaxis (TMP-SMX DS 3 times/wk). In sulfa-allergic patients, pyrimethamine 50–75 mg daily in divided doses (plus leucovorin 10–25 mg/d) has been effective (Weiss LM, et al. *Ann Intern Med.* 1988;109:474).
2. Not FDA approved for this indication.

Dientamoeba fragilis[1]

	Drug	Adult Dosage	Pediatric Dosage
Drug of choice[2]:	Paromomycin[4,5]	25–35 mg/kg/d PO in 3 doses × 7 d	25–35 mg/kg/d PO in 3 doses × 7 d
Or	Iodoquinol[3,4]	650 mg PO tid × 20 d	30–40 mg/kg/d (max. 2 g) PO in 3 doses × 20 d
Or	Metronidazole[4]	500–750 mg PO tid × 10 d	35–50 mg/kg/d PO in 3 doses × 10 d

1. Stark D, et al. *Am J Trop Med Hyg.* 2010;82:614; Vandenberg O, et al. *Pediatr Infect Dis J.* 2007;26:88; Barratt JL, et al. *Parasitology.* 2011;138:557.
2. In one study, single-dose ornidazole, a nitroimidazole similar to metronidazole that is available in Europe, was effective and better tolerated than 5 days of metronidazole (Kurt O. *Clin Microbiol Infect.* 2008;14:601).
3. Iodoquinol should be taken after meals.
4. Not FDA approved for this indication.
5. Paromomycin should be taken with a meal.

Dracunculus medinensis (Guinea Worm)

	Drug	Adult Dosage	Pediatric Dosage
Drug of choice:	No drug is curative against *Dracunculus*. A program for monitoring local sources of drinking water to eliminate transmission has dramatically decreased the number of cases worldwide. The treatment of choice is slow extraction of worm combined with wound care and pain management.[1]		

1. *MMWR Morbid Mortal Wkly Rep.* 2011;60:1450.

Echinococcus

See Tapeworm

Entamoeba histolytica

See Amebiasis

Enterobius vermicularis (Pinworm)

	Drug	Adult Dosage	Pediatric Dosage
Drug of choice[1]:	Albendazole[2,3]	400 mg PO once; repeat in 2 wk	400 mg PO once; repeat in 2 wk
Or	Mebendazole	100 mg PO once; repeat in 2 wk	100 mg PO once; repeat in 2 wk
Or	Pyrantel pamoate[4]	11 mg/kg base PO once (max 1 g); repeat in 2 wk	11 mg/kg base PO once (max 1 g); repeat in 2 wk

1. Since family members are usually infected, treatment of the entire household is recommended; retreatment after 14–21 d may be needed.
2. Not FDA approved for this indication.
3. Albendazole must be taken with food; a fatty meal increases oral bioavailability.
4. Available without a prescription. Pyrantel pamoate suspension can be mixed with milk or fruit juice.

Fasciola hepatica

See Fluke

Filariasis[1,2]

	Drug	Adult Dosage	Pediatric Dosage
Wuchereria bancrofti, Brugia malayi, Brugia timori			
Drug of choice[3]:	Diethylcarbamazine[4,5]	6 mg/kg/d PO in 3 doses × 1 or 12 d[6]	6 mg/kg/d PO in 3 doses × 1 or 12 d[6]
Loa loa			
Drug of choice[7]:	Diethylcarbamazine[4,5]	9 mg/kg/d PO in 3 doses × 21 d[6]	9 mg/kg/d PO in 3 doses × 21 d[6]
Mansonella ozzardi			
Drug of choice:	See footnote 8		
Mansonella perstans			
Drug of choice:	See footnote 9		
Mansonella streptocerca			
Drug of choice[10]:	Diethylcarbamazine[4,5]	6 mg/kg/d PO in 3 doses × 12 d[6]	6 mg/kg/d PO in 3 doses × 12 d[6]
Or	Ivermectin[5,11]	150 µg/kg PO once	150 µg/kg PO once
Tropical Pulmonary Eosinophilia[12]			
Drug of choice:	Diethylcarbamazine[4,5]	6 mg/kg/d in 3 doses × 12–21 d[6]	6 mg/kg/d in 3 doses × 12–21 d[6]
***Onchocerca volvulus* (River Blindness)**			
Drug of choice:	Ivermectin[11,13]	150 µg/kg PO once, repeated every 6–12 mo until asymptomatic	150 µg/kg PO once, repeated every 6–12 mo until asymptomatic

1. Antihistamines or corticosteroids may be required to decrease allergic reactions to components of disintegrating microfilariae that result from treatment, especially in infection caused by *Loa loa.*

2. Endosymbiotic *Wolbachia* bacteria, which are present in most human filariae except *Loa loa,* are essential to filarial growth, development, embryogenesis and survival and represent an additional target for therapy. Doxycycline 100 or 200 mg/d PO × 6–8 wk in lymphatic filariasis, onchocerciasis, and *Mansonella perstans* has resulted in substantial loss of *Wolbachia* and decrease in both micro- and macrofilariae (Bockarie MJ, et al. *Expert Rev Anti Infect Ther.* 2009;7:595; Hoerauf A. *Curr Opin Infect Dis.* 2008;21:673; Coulibaly YI, et al. *N Engl J Med.* 2009;361:1448). Use of tetracyclines is contraindicated in pregnancy and in children <8 y.

3. Most symptoms are caused by the adult worm. A single-dose combination of albendazole (400 mg PO) with either ivermectin (200 µg/kg PO) or diethylcarbamazine (6 mg/kg PO) is effective for reduction or suppression of *W. bancrofti* microfilaria; none of these drug combinations kills all the adult worms (Taylor MJ, et al. *Lancet.* 2010;376:1175).

4. Diethylcarbamazine is available from the CDC [(407) 718-4745; email: parasites@cdc.gov].

5. Not FDA approved for this indication.

6. Multidose regimens have been shown to provide more rapid reduction in microfilaria than single-dose diethylcarbamazine, but microfilaria levels are similar 6–12 months after treatment (Andrade LD, et al. *Trans R Soc Trop Med Hyg.* 1995;89:319; Simonsen PE, et al. *Am J Trop Med Hyg.* 1995;53:267). A single dose of 6 mg/kg is used in endemic areas for mass treatment, but there are no studies directly comparing the efficacy of the single-dose regimen to a 12-day course. One review concluded that the 12-day regimen did not have a higher macrofilaricidal effect than single dose (Hoerauf A. *Curr Opin Infect Dis.* 2008;21:673; Figueredo-Silva J, et al. *Trans R Soc Trop Med Hyg.* 1996;90:192; Noroes J, et al. *Trans R Soc Trop Med Hyg.* 1997;91:78). For patients with microfilaria in the blood, some *Medical Letter* consultants recommend starting with a lower dosage and scaling up: day 1: 50 mg; day 2: 50 mg tid; day 3: 100 mg tid; day 4–14: 6 mg/kg/d in 3 doses (for *Loa loa* day 4–14: 9 mg/kg/d in 3 doses). Diethylcarbamazine should not be used for treatment of *Onchocerca volvulus* due to the risk of increased ocular side effects (including blindness) associated with rapid killing of the worms. It should be used cautiously in geographic regions where *O. volvulus* coexists with other filariae. See also footnote 13.

7. Bossinesq M. *J Travel Med.* 2012;19:140. In heavy infections with *Loa loa,* rapid killing of microfilariae can provoke encephalopathy. Apheresis has been reported to be effective in lowering microfilarial counts in patients heavily infected with *Loa loa* (Ottesen EA. *Infect Dis Clin North Am.* 1993;7:619). Albendazole may be useful for treatment of loiasis when diethylcarbamazine is ineffective or cannot be used, but repeated courses may be necessary (Klion AD, et al. *Clin Infect Dis.* 1999;29:680; Tabi TE, et al. *Am J Trop Med Hyg.* 2004;71:211). Ivermectin has also been used to reduce microfilaremia, but albendazole is preferred because of its slower onset of action and lower risk of precipitating encephalopathy (Klion AD, et al. *J Infect Dis.* 1993;168:202; Kombila M, et al. *Am J Trop Med Hyg.* 1998;58:458). Diethylcarbamazine, 300 mg PO once/wk, has been recommended for prevention of loiasis (Nutman TB, et al. *N Engl J Med.* 1988; 319:752).

8. Diethylcarbamazine has no effect. A single dose of ivermectin 200 µg/kg PO reduces microfilaria densities and provides both short- and long-term reductions in *M. ozzardi* microfilaremia (Gonzalez AA, et al. *W Indian Med J.* 1999;48:231). These parasites have been shown to contain *Wolbachia* which suggests doxycycline might be effective. See also footnote 2.

9. Diethylcarbamazine, melbendazole and ivermectin have not been found to be effective against *M. perstans.* Doxycycline is the drug of choice for disease acquired in West Africa (Coulibaly YI, et al. *N Engl J Med.* 2009;361:1448). Strains from Uganda appear not to have *Wolbachia* (Grobusch MP, et al. *Parasitol Res.* 2003;90:405). There is no effective therapy for patients with these strains or those who cannot take doxycycline (pregnant women, young children). See also footnote 2.

10. Diethylcarbamazine is potentially curative due to activity against both adult worms and microfilariae. Geographic overlap with *Onchocerca volvulus* and inability of most labs to distinguish between the species limits its use. Ivermectin is active only against microfilariae and can lead to long-term suppression (Fischer P, et al. *J Infect Dis.* 1999;180:1403). These parasites have been shown to contain *Wolbachia* which suggests doxycycline might be effective. See also footnote 2.

11. Gonzalez P, et al. *Curr Pharm Biotechnol.* 2012;13:1103. Safety of ivermectin in young children (<15 kg) and pregnant women remains to be established; animal studies have shown adverse effects on the fetus (el-Ashmawy IM, et al. *Res Vet Sci.* 2011;90:116). Taking ivermectin with a meal increases its bioavailability (Guzzo CA, et al. *J Clin Pharmacol.* 2002;42:1122).

12. Vijayan VK. *Curr Opin Pulm Med.* 2007;13:428. Relapses occur and can be treated with a repeated course of diethylcarbamazine.

13. Diethylcarbamazine should not be used for treatment of this disease because rapid killing of the worms can lead to blindness. Periodic treatment with ivermectin (every 3–12 mo), 150 µg/kg PO, can prevent blindness due to ocular onchocerciasis (Udall DN, *Clin Infect Dis.* 2007;44:53). Skin reactions after ivermectin treatment are often reported in persons with high microfilarial skin densities. Ivermectin has been inadvertently given to pregnant women during mass treatment programs; the rates of congenital abnormalities were similar in treated and untreated women. Because of the high risk of blindness from onchocerciasis, the use of ivermectin after the first trimester is considered acceptable according to the WHO. Addition of 6–8 weeks of doxycycline to ivermectin is increasingly common. Doxycycline (100 mg/day PO for 6 weeks), alone or followed by a single 150 µg/kg PO dose of ivermectin, resulted in long-term amicrofilaridermia and elimination of *Wolbachia* species (Hoerauf A, et al. *Lancet.* 2001;357:1415; Hoerauf A, et al. *Parasitol Res.* 2009;104:437).

Fluke, Hermaphroditic

	Drug	Adult Dosage	Pediatric Dosage
***Clonorchis sinensis* (Chinese Liver Fluke)[1]**			
Drug of choice:	Praziquantel[2]	75 mg/kg/d PO in 3 doses × 1–2 d	75 mg/kg/d PO in 3 doses × 1–2 d
Or	Albendazole[3,4]	10 mg/kg/d PO × 7 d	10 mg/kg/d PO × 7 d
***Fasciola hepatica* (Sheep Liver Fluke)[1]**			
Drug of choice[5]:	Triclabendazole[7]*	10 mg/kg PO once or twice	10 mg/kg PO once or twice
Alternative:	Bithionol*	30–50 mg/kg on alternate days × 10–15 doses	30–50 mg/kg on alternate days × 10–15 doses
Or	Nitazoxanide[3,6]	500 mg PO bid × 7 d	1–3 y: 100 mg PO bid × 7 d 4–11 y: 200 mg PO bid × 7 d >12 y: 500 mg PO bid × 7 d
***Fasciolopsis buski, Heterophyes heterophyes, Metagonimus yokogawai* (Intestinal Flukes)**			
Drug of choice:	Praziquantel[2,3]	75 mg/kg/d PO in 3 doses × 1 d	75 mg/kg/d PO in 3 doses × 1 d
***Metorchis conjunctus* (North American Liver Fluke)**			
Drug of choice:	Praziquantel[2,3]	75 mg/kg/d PO in 3 doses × 1 d	75 mg/kg/d PO in 3 doses × 1 d
Nanophyetus salmincola			
Drug of choice:	Praziquantel[2,3]	60 mg/kg/d PO in 3 doses × 1 d	60 mg/kg/d PO in 3 doses × 1 d
***Opisthorchis viverrini* (Southeast Asian Liver Fluke)[1]**			
Drug of choice:	Praziquantel[2]	75 mg/kg/d PO in 3 doses × 2 d	75 mg/kg/d PO in 3 doses × 2 d
Or	Albendazole[3,4]	10 mg/kg/d PO × 7 d	10 mg/kg/d PO × 7 d
Paragonimiasis *(P. westermani, P. miyazaki, P. skrjabini, P. hueitungensis, P. heterotrema, P. utcerobilaterus, P. africanus, P. mexicanus, P. kellicotti)* (Lung Fluke)[1]			
Drug of choice:	Praziquantel[2,3]	75 mg/kg/d PO in 3 doses × 2 d	75 mg/kg/d PO in 3 doses × 2 d
Alternative:	Triclabendazole[7]*	10 mg/kg PO once or twice	10 mg/kg PO once or twice
	Bithionol*	30–50 mg/kg on alternate days × 10–15 doses	30–50 mg/kg on alternate days × 10–15 doses

*Availability problems. See Table 241.2.

1. Marcos LA. *Curr Opin Infect Dis.* 2008;21:523; Hong ST, Fang Y, *Parasitol Int.* 2012;61:17; Keiser J, et al. *Curr Opin Infect Dis.* 2010;25:513.
2. Praziquantel should be taken with liquids during a meal.
3. Not FDA approved for this indication.
4. Albendazole must be taken with food; a fatty meal increases oral bioavailability.
5. Unlike infections with other flukes, *Fasciola hepatica* infections may not respond to praziquantel. Triclabendazole (Egaten) appears to be safe and effective, but data are limited (Keiser J, et al. *Expert Opin Investig Drugs.* 2005;14:1513). It is available from Victoria Pharmacy, Zurich, Switzerland (www.pharmaworld.com; 011-4143-344-60-60) and should be given with food for better absorption. Nitazoxanide also appears to have efficacy in treating fascioliasis in adults and in children (Favennec L, et al. *Aliment Pharmacol Ther.* 2003;17:265; Rossignol JF, et al. *Trans R Soc Trop Med Hyg.* 1998;92:103; Kabil SM, et al. *Curr Ther Res.* 2000;61:339).
6. Nitazoxanide may be effective against a variety of protozoan and helminth infections (Bobak DA. *Curr Infect Dis Rep.* 2006;8:91; Diaz E, et al. *Am J Trop Med Hyg.* 2003;68:384). It is effective against mild to moderate amebiasis, 500 mg bid × 3 d (Rossignol JF, et al. *Trans R Soc Trop Med Hyg.* 2007;101:1025; Escobedo AE, et al. *Arch Dis Child.* 2009;94:478), but perhaps less so than metronidazole (Becker S, et al. *Am J Trop Med Hyg.* 2011;84:581). Nitazoxanide is FDA approved only for treatment of diarrhea caused by *Giardia* or *Cryptosporidium* (*Med Lett Drugs Ther.* 2003;45:29). Nitazoxanide is available in 500-mg tablets and an oral suspension and should be taken with food.
7. Keiser J, et al. *Expert Opin Investig Drugs.* 2005;14:1513. See footnote 5 for availability.

Giardiasis *(Giardia duodenalis)*

	Drug	Adult Dosage	Pediatric Dosage
Drug of choice:	Tinidazole[1]	2 g PO once	≥3 y: 50 mg/kg PO once (max 2 g)
Or	Metronidazole[2]	250 mg PO tid × 5–7 d	15 mg/kg/d PO in 3 doses × 5–7 d
Or	Nitazoxanide[3]	500 mg PO bid × 3 d	1–3 y: 100 mg PO bid × 3 d 4–11 y: 200 mg PO bid × × 3 d >12 y: 500 mg PO bid × 3 d
Alternative[4]:	Paromomycin[2,5,6]	25–35 mg/kg/d PO in 3 doses × 5–10 d	25–35 mg/kg/d PO in 3 doses × 5–10 d
Or	Furazolidone*	100 mg PO qid × 7–10 d	6 mg/kg/d PO in 4 doses × 7–10 d
Or	Quinacrine[7,8]*	100 mg PO tid × 5 d	6 mg/kg/d PO in 3 doses × 5 d (max 300 mg/d)

*Availability problems. See Table 241.2.

1. A nitroimidazole similar to metronidazole, tinidazole appears to be as effective as metronidazole and better tolerated (*Med Lett Drugs Ther.* 2004;46:70). It should be taken with food to minimize adverse GI effects. For children and patients unable to take tablets, a pharmacist can crush the tablets and mix them with cherry syrup (Humco, and others). The syrup suspension is good for 7 days at room temperature and must be shaken before use (Fung HB, Doan TL. *Clin Ther.* 2005; 27:1859). Ornidazole, a similar drug, is also used outside the United States.
2. Not FDA approved for this indication.
3. Nitazoxanide may be effective against a variety of protozoan and helminth infections (Bobak DA. *Curr Infect Dis Rep.* 2006;8:91; Diaz E, et al. *Am J Trop Med Hyg.* 2003;68:384). It is effective against mild to moderate amebiasis, 500 mg bid × 3 d (Rossignol JF, et al. *Trans R Soc Trop Med Hyg.* 2007;101:1025; Escobedo AA, et al. *Arch Dis Child.* 2009;94:478), but perhaps less so than metronidazole (Becker S, et al. *Am J Trop Med Hyg.* 2011;84:581. Nitazoxinide is FDA approved only for treatment of diarrhea caused by *Giardia* or *Cryptosporidium* (*Med Lett Drugs Ther.* 2003;45:29). It is available in 500-mg tablets and an oral suspension and should be taken with food.
4. Additional option: albendazole (400 mg/d PO × 5 d in adults and 10 mg/kg/d PO × 5 d in children) (Yereli K, et al. *Clin Microbiol Infect.* 2004;10:527; Karabay O, et al. *World J Gastroenterol.* 2004;10:1215). Refractory disease: combination therapy with tinidazole or metronidazole plus paromomycin, furazolidone, or quinacrine has been successful (Nash TE, et al. *Clin Infect Dis.* 2001;33:22; Lopez-Velez R, et al. *Am J Trop Med Hyg.* 2010;83:171). In one study, nitazoxanide was used successfully in high doses (1.5 g PO bid × 30 d) to treat a case of *Giardia* resistant to metronidazole and albendazole (Abboud P,et al. *Clin Infect Dis.* 2001;32:1792).
5. Paromomycin should be taken with a meal.
6. Poorly absorbed; may be useful for treatment of giardiasis in pregnancy.
7. Not available commercially. It may be obtained through compounding pharmacies such as Expert Compounding Pharmacy, 6744 Balboa Blvd, Lake Balboa, CA 91406 (800-247-9767) or Medical Center Pharmacy, New Haven, CT (203-688-7064). Other compounding pharmacies may be found through the National Association of Compounding Pharmacies (800-687-7850) or the Professional Compounding Centers of America (800-331-2498, www.pccarx.com).
8. Quinacrine should be taken with liquids after a meal.

Gnathostomiasis *(Gnathostoma spinigerum)*[1]

	Drug	Adult Dosage	Pediatric Dosage
Treatment of choice:	Albendazole[2,3]	400 mg PO bid × 21 d	400 mg PO bid × 21 d
Or	Ivermectin[2,4]	200 μg/kg/d PO × 2 d	200 μg/kg/d PO × 2 d
Either ±	Surgical removal		

1. All patients should be treated with medication whether surgery is attempted or not. Herman JS, Chiodini PL. *Clin Microbiol Rev.* 2009;22:484; Ramirez-Avila L, et al. *Clin Infect Dis.* 2009;48:322.
2. Not FDA approved for this indication.
3. Albendazole must be taken with food; a fatty meal increases oral bioavailability.
4. Gonzalez P, et al. *Curr Pharm Biotechnol.* 2012;13:1103. Safety of ivermectin in young children (<15 kg) and pregnant women remains to be established; animal studies have shown adverse effects on the fetus (el-Ashmawy IM, et al. *Res Vet Sci.* 2011;90:116). Taking ivermectin with a meal increases its bioavailability (Guzzo CA, et al. *J Clin Pharmacol.* 2002;42:1122).

Gongylonemiasis (*Gongylonema* spp.)[1]

	Drug	Adult Dosage	Pediatric Dosage
Treatment of choice:	Surgical removal		
Or	Albendazole[2,3]	400 mg/d PO × 3 d	400 mg/d PO × 3 d

1. Pasuralertsakul S, et al. *Am Trop Med Parasitol.* 2008;102:455; Molavi G, et al. *J Helminth* 2006;80:425.
2. Not FDA approved for this indication.
3. Albendazole must be taken with food; a fatty meal increases oral bioavailability.

Hookworm *(Ancylostoma duodenale, Necator americanus)*

	Drug	Adult Dosage	Pediatric Dosage
Drug of choice:	Albendazole[1,2]	400 mg PO once	400 mg PO once
Or	Mebendazole	100 mg PO bid × 3 d or 500 mg once	100 mg PO bid × 3 d or 500 mg once
Or	Pyrantel pamoate[1,3]	11 mg/kg base (max 1 g) PO daily × 3 d	11 mg/kg base (max 1 g) PO daily × 3 d

1. Not FDA approved for this indication.
2. Albendazole must be taken with food; a fatty meal increases oral bioavailability.
3. Available without a prescription. Pyrantel pamoate suspension can be mixed with milk or fruit juice.

Hydatid Cyst

See Tapeworm

Hymenolepis nana

See Tapeworm

Isospora belli

See Cystoisosporiasis

Leishmaniasis[1]

	Drug	Adult Dosage	Pediatric Dosage
Visceral[2,3]			
Drug of choice:	Liposomal amphotericin B	See footnote 4	See footnote 4
Alternative:	Sodium stibo-gluconate*	20 mg antimony kg/d IV or IM × 28 d	20 mg antimony kg/d IV or IM × 28 d
Or	Meglumine antimonate*	20 mg antimony kg/d IV or IM × 28 d	20 mg antimony kg/d IV or IM × 28 d
Or	Miltefosine[5,6]*	2.5 mg/kg/d PO (max 150 mg/d) × 28 d	2.5 mg/kg/d PO (max 150 mg/d) × 28 d
OR	Amphotericin B[7]	1 mg/kg IV daily × 15–20 d or every second day for 4–8 wk (total usually 15–20 mg/kg)	1 mg/kg IV daily × 15–20 d or every second day for 4–8 wk (total usually 15–20 mg/kg)
Or	Paromomycin[7,8]* sulfate	15 mg/kg/d IM × 21 d	15 mg/kg/d IM × 21 d
Cutaneous[1,2,9]			
Drugs of choice:	Sodium stibo-gluconate*	20 mg antimony kg/d IV or IM × 20 d	20 mg antimony kg/d IV or IM × 20 d
OR	Meglumine antimonate*	20 mg antimony kg/d IV or IM × 20 d	20 mg antimony kg/d IV or IM × 20 d
Or	Miltefosine[5,10]*	2.5 mg/kg/d PO (max 150 mg/d) × 28 d	2.5 mg/kg/d PO (max 150 mg/d) × 28 d
Alternative[11]:	Paromomycin[7,12]*	Topically 2 ×/d × 10–20 d	Topically 2 ×/d × 10–20 d
Or	Pentamidine[7]	2–3 mg/kg IV or IM daily or every second day × 4–7 doses	2–3 mg/kg IV or IM daily or every second day × 4–7 doses
Mucosal[1,2,13]			
Drug of choice:	Sodium stibogluconate*	20 mg antimony kg/d IV or IM × 28 d	20 mg antimony kg/d IV or IM × 28 d
Or	Meglumine antimonate*	20 mg antimony kg/d IV or IM × 28 d	20 mg antimony kg/d IV or IM × 28 d
Or	Amphotericin B[7,14]	0.5–1 mg/kg IV daily or every second day for 4–8 wk	0.5–1 mg/kg IV daily or every second day for 4–8 wk
Or	Miltefosine[5,15]*	2.5 mg/kg/d PO (max 150 mg/d) × 28 d	2.5 mg/kg/d PO (max 150 mg/d) × 28 d

*Availability problems. See Table 241.2.

1. Murray HW. *Am J Trop Med Hyg.* 2012;86:434.
2. *Medical Letter* reviewers recommend consultation with physicians experienced in management of this disease. To maximize effectiveness and minimize toxicity, the choice of drug, dosage, and duration of therapy should be individualized based on the region of disease acquisition, likely infecting species, number, significance and location of lesions, and host factors such as immune status (Murray HW. *Lancet.* 2005;366:1561). Some of the listed drugs and regimens are effective only against certain *Leishmania* species/strains and only in certain areas of the world (Sundar S, Chakravarty J. *Expert Opin Pharmacother.* 2013;14:53).
3. Visceral infection is most commonly due to the Old World species *L. donovani* (kala-azar) and *L. infantum* (referred to as *L. chagasi* in the New World) (van Griensven J, Diro E. *Infect Clin Dis Clin North Am.* 2012;26:309).
4. Liposomal amphotericin B is the only lipid formulation of amphotericin B FDA approved for treatment of visceral leishmania, largely based on trials in patients infected with *L. infantum* (Balasegaram M, et al. *Expert Opin Emerg Drugs.* 2012;17:493). It is the treatment of choice for visceral leishmaniasis in the United States and Southern Europe and the treatment of choice for visceral disease in pregnancy. The total dose administered seems to be more important than the number of infusions or duration of therapy. The target dose for a nonimmunocompromised host is 18–21 mg/kg over 5 d.Two doses of 10 mg/kg have been used successfully in children with disease acquired in the Mediterranean (Syriopoulou V, et al. *Clin Infect Dis.* 2003;36:560). For visceral leishmaniasis acquired in the Indian subcontinent 10 mg/kg/d as a single dose or 5-d treatment with 3 mg/kg (total 15 mg/kg) has been effective (Murray HW, et al. *Lancet.* 2005;366:1561; Bern C, et al. *Clin Infect Dis.* 2006;43:917; Sundar S, et al. *N Engl J Med.* 2010;362:504). The FDA-approved dosage regminen is 3 mg/kg/d IV on days 1–5, 14, and 21 and for immunocompromised patients is 4 mg/kg on days 1–5, 10, 17, 24, 31, and 38. The relapse rate in immunocompromised patients is high; maintenance therapy (secondary prevention) is generally given indicated, but there is no consensus on dosage and duration.
5. Dorlo TP, et al. *J Antimicrob Chemother.* 2012;67:2576. Miltefosine (Impavido) is manufactured in 10- or 50-mg capsules by Paladin (Canada) and is available in the United States from the manufacturer through an IND application from the FDA. The drug is contraindicated in breastfeeding and pregnant women; a negative pregnancy test before drug initiation and effective contraception during and for 4 months after treatment is recommended (Murray HW, et al. *Lancet.* 2005;366:1561).
6. Miltefosine is effective for both antimony-sensitive and -resistant *L. donovani* (Indian).
7. Not FDA approved for this indication.
8. Paromomycin IM has been effective against *Leishmania* in India and against visceral leishmaniasis in East Africa, although higher doses (20 mg/kg) or longer duration of therapy may be needed (Musa AH, et al. *PLoS Negl Trop Dis.* 2010;4:e855; Hailu A, et al. *PLoS Negl Trop Dis.* 2010;4:e709. There are insufficient data to support its use in pregnancy (Sundar S, et al. *N Engl J Med.* 2007;356:2571; Sundar S, Chakravarty J. *Expert Opin Investig Drugs.* 2008;17:787). There is limited experience in paromomycin in South America or the Mediterranean, where it has been tried as second-line combination therapy with sodium stibogluconate.
9. Cutaneous infection is most commonly due to the Old World species *L. major* and *L. tropica* and the New World species *L. mexicana, L. (Vianna) braziliensis, L. (V.) panamensis* and others.
10. Machado PR, Penna G. *Curr Opin Infect Dis.* 2012;25:141. Miltefosine has been effective in trials for treatment of cutaneous leishmaniasis due to *L.(V.) panamensis* in Bolivia and Colombia, and for *L.(V.) braziliensis* in Brazil but not for treatment of *L.(V.) braziliensis* or *L. mexicana* in Guatemala, suggesting geography as well as species affects efficacy (Soto J, et al. *Am J Trop Med Hyg.* 2008;78:210, Machado PR, et al. *PLoS Negl Trop Dis.* 2010;4:e912; Soto J, et al. *Clin Infect Dis.* 2004;38:1266; Rubiano LC. et al. *J Infect Dis.* 2012;205:684). It has also has been effective for treatment of *L. major* acquired in Afghanistan and Iran (Mohebali, et al. *Acta Trop.* 2007;103:33; van Thiel PP, et al. *Clin Infect Dis.* 50:80). For forms of disease that require long periods of treatment, such as diffuse cutaneous leishmaniasis and post kala-azar dermal leishmaniasis, miltefosine might be a useful treatment (Berman JJ. *Expert Opin Drug Metab Toxicol.* 2008;4:1209).
11. Azole drugs (fluconazole, ketoconazole, itraconazole) have been used to treat cutaneous disease, with plausible efficacy (Blum JA, Hatz CS. *J Travel Med.* 2009;16:123). For treatment of *L. major* cutaneous lesions, a study in Saudi Arabia found that oral fluconazole, 200 mg once/d × 6 wk appeared to modestly accelerate the healing process (Alrajhi AA, et al. *N Engl J Med.* 2002;346:891). Fluconazole 8 mg/kg/d PO × 4–6 wk may have efficacy against *L. braziliensis* (Sousa AQ, et al. *Clin Infect Dis.* 2011;53:693). Intralesional injections of sodium stibogluconate or topical paromomycinare also used for uncomplicated lesions when subsequent mucosal leshmaniasis is unlikely (Soto J, et al. *Clin Infect Dis.* 2013;56:1255). Ketoconazole 600 mg/day PO × 28–30 d has been effective against *L. major, L. panamensis,* and *L. mexicana.* Studies with liposomal amphotericin are limited; the FDA total approved dose of 21 mg/kg may be effective (Wortmann G, et al. *Am J Trop Hyg.* 2010;83:1028). Thermotherapy may be an option for some cases of cutaneous *L. tropica* infection (Reithinger R, et al. *Clin Infect Dis.* 2005;40:1148). A device that generates focused and controlled heating of the skin is being marketed (ThermoMed; ThermoSurgery Technologies Inc., Phoenix, AZ, 602-264-7300; www.thermosurgery.com). In a few studies, localized thermal heat was as effective as multiple doses of sodium stibogluconate or meglumine antimoniate for up to 18 months with less toxicity (Safi N, et al. *Mil Med.* 2012;177:345; Lopez L, et al. *Trials.* 2012;13:58; Bumb RA, et al. *Br J Dermatol.* 2013;Jan 8).
12. Topical paromomycin should be used only in geographic regions where cutaneous leishmaniasis species have low potential for mucosal spread. A formulation of 15% paromomycin/12% methylbenzethonium chloride (Leshcutan) in soft white paraffin for topical use has been reported to be partially effective against cutaneous leishmaniasis due to *L. major* in Israel and Tunesia and *L. mexicana* and *L. (V.) braziliensis* in Guatemala, where mucosal spread is very rare (Arana BA, et al. *Am J Trop Med Hyg.* 2001;65:466; Kim DH, et al. *PLoS Negl Trop Dis.* 2009;3:e381; Ben Salah A, et al. *N Engl J Med.* 2013;368:524). The methylbenzethonium is irritating to the skin; lesions may worsen before they improve.
13. Mucosal infection (espundia) is most commonly due to New World species *L. (V.) braziliensis, L. (V.) panamensis,* or *L. (V.) guyanensis.*
14. Liposomal amphotericin 20–35 mg/kg divided in 3–5 doses may be active for mucosal disease (Amato VS, et al. *Am J Trop Med Hyg.* 2011;85:818).
15. Miltefosine has been effective for mucosal leishmania due to *L.(V.) braziliensis* in Bolivia (Soto J, et al. *Clin Infect Dis.* 2007;44:350; Soto J, et al. *Am J Trop Med Hyg.* 2009;81:387).

Lice *(Pediculus humanus, P. capitis, Phthirus pubis)*[1]

	Drug	Adult Dosage	Pediatric Dosage
Drug of choice:	Pyrethrins with piperonyl butoxide[2]	Topically, 2 × at least 7 d apart	Topically, 2 × at least 7 d apart
Or	0.5% ivermectin lotion[3]	Topically, once	Topically, once
Or	0.9% spinosad susp[4]	Topically, 2 × at least 7 d apart	Topically, 2 × at least 7 d apart
Or	1% permethrin[2]	Topically, 2 × at least 7 d apart	Topically, 2 × at least 7 d apart
Or	5% benzyl alcohol lotion[5]	Topically, 2 × at least 7 d apart	Topically, 2 × at least 7 d apart
Or	0.5% malathion[6]	Topically, 2 × at least 7 d apart	Topically, 2 × at least 7 d apart
Alternative:	Ivermectin[7,8,9]	200 or 400 μg/kg PO	>15 kg: 200 or 400 μg/kg PO

1. Pediculocides should not be used for infestations of the eyelashes. Such infestations are treated with petrolatum ointment applied 2–4 ×/d × 8–10 d. For pubic lice, treat with 1% permethrin, pyrethrins with piperonyl butoxide, or ivermectin.
2. Permethrin and pyrethrin are pediculocidal; retreatment in 7–10 d is needed to eradicate the infestation. Some lice are resistant to pyrethrins and permethrin (Meinking TL, et al. *Arch Dermatol.* 2002;138:220). *Medical Letter* consultants prefer pyrethrin products with a benzyl alcohol vehicle. Pyrethrins with piperonyl butoxide are recommended for use in children ≥2 y; permethrin for children ≥2 mo.
3. Not ovicidal, but lice that hatch from treated eggs die within 48 hours after hatching. Recommended for use in children ≥6 mo (*Med Lett Drugs Ther.* 2012;54:61; Pariser DM, et al. *N Engl J Med.* 2012;367:1687).
4. Not ovicidal, but causes neuronal excitation in insects leading to paralysis and death. The formulation also includes benzyl alcohol, which is pediculocidal. Two applications 7 days apart are needed. Recommended for children ≥4 y (*Med Lett Drugs Ther.* 2011;53:50).
5. Benzyl alcohol prevents lice from closing their respiratory spiracles and the lotion vehicle then obstructs their airway, causing them to asphyxiate. It is not ovicidal. Two applications at least 7 d apart are needed. Recommended for use in children ≥6 mo. Resistance, which is a problem with other drugs, is unlikely to develop (*Med Lett Drugs Ther.* 2009;51:57).
6. Malathion is both ovicidal and pediculocidal; 2 applications at least 7 d apart are generally necessary to kill all lice and nits. Recommended for children ≥6 y.
7. Not FDA approved for this indication.
8. Gonzalez P, et al. *Curr Pharm Biotechnol.* 2012;13:1103. Safety of ivermectin in young children (<15 kg) and pregnant women remains to be established; animal studies have shown adverse effects on the fetus (el-Ashmawy Im, et al. *Res Vet Sci.* 2011;90:116). Taking ivermectin with a meal increases its bioavailability (Guzzo CA, et al. *J Clin Pharmacol.* 2002;42:1122).
9. Ivermectin is pediculocidal, but not ovicidal; more than one dose is generally necessary to eradicate the infestation (Jones KN, English JC 3d. *Clin Infect Dis.* 2003;36:1355). The number of doses and interval between doses has not been established; animal studies have shown adverse effects on the fetus (el-Ashmawy IM, et al. *Res Vet Sci.* 2011;90:116). In one study of treatment of head lice, 2 doses of ivermectin (400 μg/kg) 7 days apart were more effective than treatment with topical malathion (Chosidow O, et al. *N Engl J Med.* 2010;362:896). In one study of treatment of body lice, a regimen of 3 doses of ivermectin (12 mg each) administered at 7-d intervals was effective (Fouault C, et al. *J Infect Dis.* 2006;193:474).

Loa loa

See Filariasis

Malaria, Treatment *(Plasmodium falciparum,[1] P. vivax,[2] P. ovale, P. malariae,[3] and P. knowlesi[4])*

	Drug	Adult Dosage	Pediatric Dosage
Oral (Uncomplicated or Mild Infection)[5]			
P. falciparum *or Unidentified Species*[6] *Acquired in Areas of Chloroquine-Resistant* P. falciparum[7]			
Drug of choice:	Atovaquone/proguanil[7]	4 adult tabs PO once/d or 2 adult tabs PO bid × 3 d[8]	<5 kg: not indicated 5–8 kg: 2 peds tabs PO once/d × 3 d 9–10 kg: 3 peds tabs PO once/d × 3 d 11–20 kg: 1 adult tab PO once/d × 3 d 21–30 kg: 2 adult tabs PO once/d × 3 d 31–40 kg: 3 adult tabs PO once/d × 3 d >40 kg: 4 adult tabs PO once/d × 3 d[8]

*Availability problems. See table 241.2.

1. Chloroquine-resistant *P. falciparum* occurs in all malarious areas except Central America (including Panama north and west of the Canal Zone), Mexico, Haiti, the Dominican Republic, Paraguay, northern Argentina, North and South Korea, Georgia, Armenia, most of rural China, and some countries in the Middle East (chloroquine resistance has been reported in Yemen, Saudi Arabia, and Iran). For treatment of multiple-drug-resistant *P. falciparum* in Southeast Asia, especially the greater Mekong region that includes Myanmar, Thailand, Cambodia, and Vietnam, where mefloquine resistance is frequent, atovaquone/proguanil, quinine plus either doxycycline or clindamycin, or artemether/lumefantrine may be used.
2. Chloroquine-resistant *P. vivax* is a significant problem in Papua-New Guinea and Indonesia. There are also reports of resistance from Myanmar, Vietnam, Korea, India, the Solomon Islands, Vanuatu, Indonesia, Guyana, Brazil, Colombia, and Peru (Baird JK. *Clin Microbiol Rev.* 2009;22:508).
3. Chloroquine-resistant *P. malariae* has been reported from Sumatra (Maguire JD, et al. *Lancet.* 2002;360:58).
4. Human infection with the simian species, *P. knowlesi*, has been reported in Malaysia where it was initially misdiagnosed as *P. malariae*. Additional cases have been reported from Thailand, Myanmar, Singapore, the Thai-Burma border, and the Philippines (Cox-Singh J, et al. *Clin Infect Dis.* 2008;46:165; *MMWR* 2009;58:229). Treatment with the usual antimalarials, such as chloroquine and atovaquone/proguanil, appears to be effective. In cases of severe infection, IV artesunate combined with oral artemether/lumefantrine or artesunate/mefloquine has been used successfully (Barber BE, et al. *Clin Infect Dis.* 2013;56:383).
5. Uncomplicated or mild malaria may be treated with oral drugs. Severe malaria (e.g., impaired consciousness, parasitemia >5%, shock) should be treated with parenteral drugs (Griffin KS, et al. *JAMA.* 2007;297:2264). Malaria breakthrough infection in a patient on prophylaxis should be treated with a different drug than the drug taken for prophylaxis.
6. Primaquine is given as part of primary treatment to prevent relapse after infection with *P. vivax* or *P. ovale.* Vivax malaria is a potentially more dangerous infection than previously thought (Baird JK, et al. *Microbiol Rev.* 2013; 26:36). See also footnote 20.
7. Atovaquone/proguanil is available as a fixed-dose combination tablet: adult tablets (Malarone; atovaquone 250 mg/proguanil 100 mg) and pediatric tablets (Malarone pediatric; atovaquone 62.5 mg/proguanil 25 mg). To enhance absorption and reduce nausea and vomiting, it should be taken with food or a milky drink. Safety in pregnancy is unknown and use is generally not recommended, In a few small studies outcomes were normal in women treated with the combination in the 2nd and 3rd trimester (Pasternak B, et al. *Arch Intern Med.* 2011;171:259; Boggild AK, et al. *Am J Trop Med Hyg.* 2007;76:208). The drug should not be given to patients with severe renal impairment (creatinine clearance <30 mL/min). There have been isolated case reports of resistance in *P. falciparum* in Africa, but *Medical Letter* consultants do not believe there is a high risk for acquisition of *Malarone*-resistant disease (Schwartz E, et al. *Clin Infect Dis.* 2003;37:450; Farnert A, et al. *BMJ.* 2003;326:628; Kuhn S, et al. *Am J Trop Med Hyg.* 2005;72:407; Happi CT, et al. *Malaria J.* 2006;5:82).
8. Although approved for once-daily dosing, *Medical Letter* consultants usually divide the dose in two to decrease nausea and vomiting.

Malaria, Treatment *(Plasmodium falciparum,*[1] *P. vivax,*[2] *P. ovale, P. malariae,*[3] and *P. knowlesi*[4])—cont'd			
	Drug	**Adult Dosage**	**Pediatric Dosage**
Or	Artemether/ lumefantrine[9,10]	6 doses over 3 d (4 tabs/dose at 0, 8, 24, 36, 48 and 60 h)	6 doses over 3 d at same intervals as adults: 5–15 kg: 1 tab/dose ≥15–25 kg: 2 tabs/dose ≥25–35 kg: 3 tabs/dose ≥35 kg: 4 tabs/dose
Or	Quinine sulfate	650 mg PO q8h × 3 or 7 d[11]	30 mg/kg/d PO in 3 doses × 3 or 7 d[11]
Plus	Doxycycline[12,13,14]	100 mg PO bid × 7 d	4 mg/kg/d PO in 2 doses × 7 d
Or plus	Tetracycline[12,13]	250 mg PO qid × 7 d	25 mg/kg/d PO in 4 doses × 7 d
Or plus	Clindamycin[12,15,16]	20 mg/kg/d PO in 3 doses × 7 d[17]	20 mg/kg/d PO in 3 doses × 7 d[17]
Alternative:	Mefloquine[18,19]	750 mg PO followed 12 h later by 500 mg	15 mg/kg PO followed 12 h later by 10 mg/kg
P. vivax *Acquired in Areas of Chloroquine-Resistant* P. vivax[2]			
Drug of choice:	Quinine sulfate	650 mg PO q8h × 3 or 7 d[11]	30 mg/kg/d PO in 3 doses × 3–7 d[11]
Plus	Doxycycline[12,13,14]	100 mg PO bid × 7 d	4 mg/kg/d PO in 2 doses × 7 d
Plus	Primaquine phosphate[6,20]	30 mg base/d PO × 14 d	0.5 mg/kg/d PO × 14 d
Alternative[21]:	Atovaquone/proguanil[7,22]	4 adult tabs PO once/d or 2 adult tabs bid[8] × 3 d	<5 kg: not indicated 5–8 kg: 2 peds tabs PO once/d × 3 d 9–10 kg: 3 peds tabs PO once/d × 3 d 11–20 kg: 1 adult tab PO once/d × 3 d 21–30 kg: 2 adult tabs PO once/d × 3 d 31–40 kg: 3 adult tabs PO once/d × 3 d >40 kg: 4 adult tabs PO once/d × 3 d[8]
	Mefloquine[18]	750 mg PO followed 12 h later by 500 mg	15 mg/kg PO followed 12 h later by 10 mg/kg
Either plus	Primaquine phosphate[6,20]	30 mg base/d PO × 14 d	0.5 mg/kg/d PO × 14 d
Plasmodium *spp. in Areas Without Chloroquine Resistance*[1–4]			
Drug of choice:	Chloroquine phosphate[6,23]	1 g (600 mg base) PO, then 500 mg (300 mg base) 6 h later, then 500 mg (300 mg base) at 24 and 48 h	10 mg base/kg (max 600 mg base) PO, then 5 mg base/kg 6 h later, then 5 mg base/kg at 24 and 48 h
Or	Regimen used for chloroquine-resistant species listed above		

9. The artemisinin-derivatives, artemether and artesunate, are both frequently used globally in combination regimens to treat malaria. Both are available in oral, parenteral and rectal formulations, but manufacturing standards are not consistent (Karunajeewa HA, et al. *JAMA.* 2007;297:2381; Ashley EA, White NJ. *Curr Opin Infect Dis.* 2005;18:531). Based on the few studies available, artemesinins have been relatively safe during pregnancy (Adam I, et al. *Am Trop Med Parisitol.* 2009;103;205), but some experts would not prescribe them in the 1st trimester (Clark RL. *Reprod Toxicol.* 2009;28:285; Manyando C, et al. *Malaria J.* 2012;11:141).

10. Artemether/lumefantrine is available as a fixed-dose combination tablet (Coartem in the United States and in countries with endemic malaria, Riamet in Europe and countries without endemic malaria); each tablet contains artemether 20 mg and lumefantrine 120 mg. It is FDA approved for treatment of uncomplicated malaria and should not be used for severe infection or for prophylaxis. The tablets should be taken with fatty food (tablets may be crushed, mixed with 1–2 tsp water, and taken with milk). Artemether/lumefantrine should not be used in patients with cardiac arrhythmias, bradycardia, severe cardiac disease, or QT prolongation. Concomitant use of drugs that prolong the QT interval or are metabolized by CYP2D6 is contraindicated (*Med Lett Drugs Ther.* 2009;51:75).

11. Available in the United States in a 324-mg capsule; 2 capsules suffice for adult dosage. In Southeast Asia, relative resistance to quinine has increased and treatment should be continued for 7 days. For infections acquired elsewhere treatment can be given for 3 d. Quinine should be taken with or after meals to decrease gastrointestinal adverse effects. It is generally considered safe in pregnancy.

12. Not FDA approved for this indication.

13. Use of tetracyclines is contraindicated in pregnancy and in children <8 yd. Tetracycline should be taken 1 hour before or 2 hours after meals and/or dairy products.

14. Doxycycline should be taken with adequate water to avoid esophageal irritation. It can be taken with food to minimize gastrointestinal adverse effects.

15. Oral clindamycin should be taken with a full glass of water to minimize esophageal ulceration.

16. For use in pregnancy and in children <8 y.

17. Lell B, Kremsner PG. *Antimicrob Agents Chemother.* 2002;46:2315; Ramharter M, et al. *Clin Infect Dis.* 2005;40:1777.

18. At this dosage, adverse effects include nausea, vomiting, diarrhea, and dizziness. Disturbed sense of balance, ringing of the ears, toxic psychosis (and other psychiatric effects) and seizures can also occur. Mefloquine can be used for treatment of malaria in pregnant women. The FDA reclassified mefloquine to pregnancy category B based on a review of published data (Schlagenhauf P, et al. *Clin Infect Dis.* 2012;54:e124). It should be avoided for treatment of malaria in persons with active depression or with a history of psychosis or seizures and should be used with caution in persons with any psychiatric illness. Mefloquine should not be used in patients with conduction abnormalities; it can be given to patients taking β-blockers if they do not have an underlying arrhythmia. Mefloquine should not be given together with quinine or quinidine, and caution is required in using quinine or quinidine to treat patients with malaria who have taken mefloquine for prophylaxis. Mefloquine should not be taken on an empty stomach; it should be taken with at least 8 oz of water.

19. *P. falciparum* with resistance to mefloquine is a significant problem in the malarious areas of Thailand and in areas of Myanmar and Cambodia that border on Thailand. It has also been reported on the borders between Myanmar and China, Laos and Myanmar, and in Southern Vietnam. In the United States, a 250-mg tablet of mefloquine contains 228 mg mefloquine base. Outside the United States, each 275-mg tablet contains 250 mg base.

20. Primaquine phosphate can cause hemolytic anemia, especially in patients whose red cells are deficient in G6PD. This deficiency is most common in African, Asian, and Mediterranean peoples. Patients should be screened for G6PD deficiency before treatment. Limited evidence suggests G6PD-deficient patients may be safely treated with a single weekly dose of primaquine 0.75 mg/kg for 8 wk. Resistance is not known to occur at a dose of 0.5 mg/kg daily for 14 d: suspected resistant strains may be treated with this daily dose for 28 d. Relapse despite adherence to a full primaquine dose may be due to a poor metabolizer phenotype. Primaquine should not be used during pregnancy. It should be taken with food to minimize nausea and abdominal pain.

21. Combination therapy with dihydroartemisinin/piperaquine (Euartesim) plus primaquine has demonstrated safety, efficacy, and tolerability for treatment of *P. vivax* (Sutanto I, et al. *Antimicrob Agents Chemother.* 2013;57:1128).

22. *Medical Letter* consultants recommend this combination. Published data on safety or efficacy for cure of *P. vivax* is lacking (Baird JK, et al. *Antimicrob Agent Chemother.* 2011;55:1827).

23. Chloroquine should be taken with food to decrease gastrointestinal adverse effects. If chloroquine phosphate is not available, hydroxychloroquine sulfate is as effective; 400 mg of hydroxychloroquine sulfate is equivalent to 500 mg of chloroquine phosphate.

Continued

Malaria, Treatment (*Plasmodium falciparum*,[1] *P. vivax*,[2] *P. ovale*, *P. malariae*,[3] and *P. knowlesi*[4])—cont'd

	Drug	Adult Dosage	Pediatric Dosage
Parenteral (Severe Infection)[5]			
All* Plasmodium *spp. (Chloroquine Sensitive and Resistant)			
Drug of choice[6,24]:	Quinidine gluconate[25]	10 mg/kg IV loading dose (max 600 mg) in normal saline over 1–2 h, followed by continuous infusion of 0.02 mg/kg/min until PO therapy can be started	10 mg/kg IV loading dose (max 600 mg) in normal saline over 1–2 h, followed by continuous infusion of 0.02 mg/kg/min until PO therapy can be started
Or	Quinine dihydrochloride[25]*	20 mg/kg IV loading dose in 5% dextrose over 4 h, followed by 10 mg/kg over 2–4 h q8h (max 1800 mg/d) until PO therapy can be started	20 mg/kg IV loading dose in 5% dextrose over 4 h, followed by 10 mg/kg over 2–4 h q8h (max 1800 mg/d) until PO therapy can be started
Or	Artesunate[9,26]* *Plus* a second oral drug[26]	2.4 mg/kg/dose IV × 3 d at 0, 12, 24, 48 and 72 h	2.4 mg/kg/dose IV × 3 d at 0, 12, 24, 48 and 72 h

24. Exchange transfusion is controversial but has been helpful for some patients with high-density (>10%) parasitemia, altered mental status, pulmonary edema, or renal complications (Van Genderen PJ, et al. *Transfusion.* 2009;Nov 20).
25. Continuous electrocardiographic, blood pressure, and glucose monitoring are recommended. Quinine IV is not available in the United States. Quinidine may have greater antimalarial activity than quinine. The loading dose should be decreased or omitted in patients who have received quinine or mefloquine. If more than 48 h of parenteral treatment are required, the quinine or quinidine dose should be reduced by 30–50%. Intrarectal quinine has been tried for the treatment of cerebral malaria in children (Achan J, et al. *Clin Infect Dis.* 2007;45:1446).
26. Oral artesunate is not available in the United States; the IV formulation is available through the CDC Malaria branch (M-F 9 am-5 pm ET, 770-488-7788 or 855-856-4713, or after hours, 770-488-7100) under an IND for patients with severe disease who do not have timely access, cannot tolerate, or fail to respond to IV quinidine (*Med Lett Drugs Ther.* 2008;50:37). To avoid development of resistance, adults treated with artesunate must also receive oral treatment doses of either atovaquone/proguanil, doxycycline, clindamycin or mefloquine; children should take either atovaquone/proguanil, clindamycin, or mefloquine (Nosten F, et al. *Lancet.* 2000;356:297; van Vugt M. *Clin Infect Dis.* 2002;35:1498; Smithuis F, et al. *Trans R Soc Trop Med Hyg.* 2004;98:182). If artesunate is given IV, oral medication should be started when the patient is able to tolerate it (SEAQUAMAT group, *Lancet.* 2005;366:717; Duffy PE, Sibley CH, *Lancet.* 2005;366:1908). Reduced susceptibility to artesunate characterized by slow parasitic clearance has been reported in Cambodia (Rogers WO, et al. *Malaria J.* 2009;8:10; Dundorp AM, et al. *N Engl J Med.* 2009;361:455).

Malaria, Self-Presumptive Treatment[1]

	Drug	Adult Dosage	Pediatric Dosage
Drug of Choice:	Atovaquone/proguanil[2,3]	4 adult tabs once/d or 2 adult tabs bid × 3 d[4]	<5 kg: not indicated 5–8 kg: 2 peds tabs once/d × 3 d 9–10 kg: 3 peds tabs once/d × 3 d 11–20 kg: 1 adult tab once/d × 3 d 21–30 kg: 2 adult tabs once/d × 3 d 31–40 kg: 3 adult tabs once/d × 3 d >40 kg: 4 adult tabs once/d × 3 d[4]
Or	Artemether/lumefantrine[2,5,6]	6 doses over 3 d (4 tabs/dose at 0, 8, 24, 36, 48, and 60 hours)	6 doses over 3 d at same intervals as adults 5–15 kg: 1 tab/dose 15–25 kg: 2 tabs/dose 25–35 kg: 3 tabs/dose >35 kg: 4 tabs/dose
Or	Quinine sulfate	650 mg PO q8h × 3 or 7 d[7,8]	30 mg/kg/d PO in 3 doses × 3 or 7 d[7]
Plus	Doxycycline[2,9,10]	100 mg PO bid × 7 d	4 mg/kg/d PO in 2 doses × 7 d

1. A traveler can be given a course of medication for presumptive self-treatment of febrile illness. The drug given for self-treatment should be different from that used for prophylaxis. This approach should be used only in very rare circumstances when a traveler would not be able to get medical care promptly.
2. Not FDA approved for this indication.
3. Atovaquone/proguanil is available as a fixed-dose combination tablet: adult tablets (Malarone; atovaquone 250 mg/proguanil 100 mg) and pediatric tablets (Malarone pediatric; atovaquone 62.5 mg/proguanil 25 mg). To enhance absorption and reduce nausea and vomiting, it should be taken with food or a milky drink. Safety in pregnancy is unknown and use is generally not recommended. In a few small studies outcomes were normal in women treated with the combination in the 2nd and 3rd trimester (Pasternak B, et al. *Arch Intern Med.* 2011;171:259; AK Boggild et al. *Am J Trop Med Hyg.* 2007;76:208). The drug should not be given to patients with severe renal impairment (creatinine clearance <30 mL/min). There have been isolated case reports of resistance in *P. falciparum* in Africa, but *Medical Letter* consultants do not believe there is a high risk for acquisition of Malarone-resistant disease (Schwartz E, et al. *Clin Infect Dis.* 2003;37:450; Farnert A, et al. *BMJ.* 2003;326:628; Kuhn S, et al. *Am J Trop Med Hyg.* 2005;72:407; Happi CT, et al. *Malaria J.* 2006;5:82).
4. Although approved for once-daily dosing, *Medical Letter* consultants usually divide the dose in two to decrease nausea and vomiting.
5. Artemether is frequently used globally in combination regimens to treat malaria. It is available in oral, parenteral, and rectal formulations, but manufacturing standards are not consistent (Karunajeewa HA, et al. *JAMA.* 2007;297:2381; Ashley EA, White NJ. *Curr Opin Infect Dis.* 2005;18:531). Based on the few studies available, artemesin derivatives have been relatively safe during pregnancy (Adam I, et al. *Am Trop Med Parisitol.* 2009;103;205; Manyando C, et al. *Malaria J.* 2012;11:141), but some experts would not prescribe them in the 1st trimester (Clark RL. *Reprod Toxicol.* 2009;28:285).
6. Artemether/lumefantrine is available as a fixed-dose combination tablet (Coartem in the United States and in countries with endemic malaria, Riamet in Europe and countries without endemic malaria); each tablet contains artemether 20 mg and lumefantrine 120 mg. It is FDA approved for treatment of uncomplicated malaria and should not be used for severe infection or for prophylaxis. The tablets should be taken with fatty food (tablets may be crushed and mixed with 1–2 tsp water, then taken with milk). Artemether/lumefantrine should not be used in patients with cardiac arrhythmias, bradycardia, severe cardiac disease, or QT prolongation. Concomitant use of drugs that prolong the QT interval or are metabolized by CYP2D6 is contraindicated (*Med Lett Drugs Ther.* 2009;51:75).
7. For treatment of multiple-drug-resistant *P. falciparum* in Southeast Asia, especially Thailand, where mefloquine resistance is frequent, atovaquone/proguanil, quinine plus either doxycycline or clindamycin, or artemether/lumefantrine may be used. For infections acquired elsewhere treatment can be given for 3 d.
8. Available in the United States in a 324-mg capsule; 2 capsules suffice for adult dosage. In Southeast Asia, relative resistance to quinine has increased and treatment should be continued for 7 d. Quinine should be taken with or after meals to decrease gastrointestinal adverse effects. It is generally considered safe in pregnancy.
9. Use of tetracyclines is contraindicated in pregnancy and in children <8 y. Tetracycline should be taken 1 hour before or 2 hours after meals and/or dairy products.
10. Doxycycline should be taken with adequate water to avoid esophageal irritation. It can be taken with food to minimize gastrointestinal adverse effects.

Malaria, Prevention[1]

	Drug	Adult Dosage	Pediatric Dosage
All *Plasmodium* spp. in Chloroquine-Resistant Areas[2–5]			
Drug of choice:	Atovaquone/proguanil[6,7]	1 adult tab/d[8]	5–8 kg: ½ peds tab/d[7,8] 9–10 kg: ¾ peds tab/d[7,8] 11–20 kg: 1 peds tab/d[7,8] 21–30 kg: 2 peds tabs/d[7,8] 31–40 kg: 3 peds tabs/d[7,8] >40 kg: 1 adult tab/d[7,8]
Or	Doxycycline[6,9,10]	100 mg PO daily[11]	2 mg/kg/d PO, up to 100 mg/d[11]
Or	Mefloquine[6,12,13]	250 mg PO once/wk[14]	≤ 9 kg: 5 mg/kg salt once/wk[14] 9–19 kg: ¼ tab once/wk[14] >19–30 kg: ½ tab once/wk[14] >31–45 kg: ¾ tab once/wk[14] >45 kg: 1 tab once/wk[14]
Alternative[15]:	Primaquine[16,17] phosphate	30 mg base PO daily	0.5 mg/kg base PO daily
All *Plasmodium* spp. in Chloroquine-Sensitive Areas[2–5]			
Drug of choice[6,18]:	Chloroquine phosphate[6,19,20]	500 mg (300 mg base) PO once/wk[21]	5 mg/kg base PO once/wk, up to adult dose of 300 mg base[21]

1. No drug guarantees protection against malaria. Travelers should be advised to seek medical attention if fever develops after they return. Insect repellents, insecticide-impregnated bed nets and proper clothing are important adjuncts for malaria prophylaxis (*Treat Guidel Med Lett.* 2009;7:83). Malaria in pregnancy is particularly serious for both mother and fetus; prophylaxis is indicated if exposure cannot be avoided.

2. Chloroquine-resistant *P. falciparum* occurs in all malarious areas except Central America (including Panama north and west of the Canal Zone), Mexico, Haiti, the Dominican Republic, Paraguay, northern Argentina, North and South Korea, Georgia, Armenia, most of rural China and some countries in the Middle East (chloroquine resistance has been reported in Yemen, Saudi Arabia, and Iran).

3. Chloroquine-resistant *P. vivax* is a significant problem in Papua-New Guinea and Indonesia. There are also reports of resistance from Myanmar, Vietnam, Korea, India, the Solomon Islands, Vanuatu, Indonesia, Guyana, Brazil, Colombia, and Peru (Baird JK, *Clin Microbiol Rev.* 2009;22:508).

4. Chloroquine-resistant *P. malariae* has been reported from Sumatra (Maguire JD, et al. *Lancet.* 2002;360:58).

5. Human infection with the simian species, *P. knowlesi,* has been reported in Malaysia, where it was initially misdiagnosed as *P. malariae.* Additional cases have been reported from Thailand, Myanmar, Singapore, the Thai-Burma border, and the Philippines (Cox-Singh J, et al. *Clin Infect Dis.* 2008;46:165; *MMWR.* 2009;58:229).

6. Vivax malaria is a potentially more dangerous infection that previously thought (Baird JK, et al. *Microbiol Rev.* 2013;26:36). Some *Medical Letter* consultants recommend primaquine as first choice for primary prophylaxis in areas where *P. vivax* is endemic. Atovaquone/proguanil, doxycycline, mefloquine, and chloroquine have no activity against latent liver stages of *P. vivax* or *P. ovale.* In one randomized study travelers taking mefloquine (52%) or doxycycline (53%) developed acute *P. vivax* malaria more than 1 mo after travel, while travelers taking daily primaquine had a 6% attack rate (Schwartz I, Regev-Yochay G. *Clin Infect Dis.* 1999;29:1502). Other *Medical Letter* consultants prescribe primaquine phosphate 30 mg base/d (0.6 mg base/kg/d for children) in addition to another drug taken during travel for 14 d after departure from areas where *P. vivax* or *P. ovale* are endemic (presumptive anti-relapse therapy). Since this is not always effective for prevention (Schwartz E, et al. *N Engl J Med.* 2003;349:1510), still others prefer to rely on surveillance to detect cases when they occur, particularly when exposure was limited or doubtful. See also footnote 17.

7. Atovaquone/proguanil is available as a fixed-dose combination tablet: adult tablets (Malarone; atovaquone 250 mg/proguanil 100 mg) and pediatric tablets (Malarone pediatric; atovaquone 62.5 mg/proguanil 25 mg). To enhance absorption and reduce nausea and vomiting, it should be taken with food or a milky drink. Safety in pregnancy is unknown and use is generally not recommended. In a few small studies outcomes were normal in women treated with the combination in the 2nd and 3rd trimester (Paternak B, et al. *Arch Intern Med.* 2011;171:259; Boggild AK, et al. *Am J Trop Med Hyg.* 2007;76:208). The drug should not be given to patients with severe renal impairment (creatinine clearance <30 mL/min). There have been isolated case reports of resistance in *P. falciparum* in Africa, but *Medical Letter* consultants do not believe there is a high risk for acquisition of *Malarone*-resistant disease (Schwartz E, et al. *Clin Infect Dis.* 2003;37:450; Aarnert A, et al. *BMJ.* 2003;326:628; Kuhn S, et al. *Am J Trop Med Hyg.* 2005;72:407; Happi CT, et al. *Malaria J.* 2006;5:82).

8. Beginning 1–2 d before travel and continuing for the duration of stay and for 1 wk after leaving malarious zone. In one study of malaria prophylaxis, atovaquone/proguanil was better tolerated than mefloquine in nonimmune travelers (Overbosch D, et al. *Clin Infect Dis.* 2001;33:1015). The protective efficacy of *Malarone against P. vivax* is variable ranging from 84% in Indonesian New Guinea (Ling J, et al. *Clin Infect Dis.* 2002; 35:825) to 100% in Colombia (Soto J, et al. *Am J Trop Med Hyg.* 2006;75:430). Some *Medical Letter* consultants prefer alternate drugs if traveling to areas where *P. vivax* predominates.

9. Use of tetracyclines is contraindicated in pregnancy and in children <8 y. Tetracycline should be taken 1 h before or 2 h after meals and/or dairy products.

10. Doxycycline should be taken with adequate water to avoid esophageal irritation. It can be taken with food to minimize gastrointestinal adverse effects.

11. Beginning 1–2 d before travel and continuing for the duration of stay and for 4 wk after leaving malarious zone. Doxycycline can cause gastrointestinal disturbances, vaginal moniliasis, and photosensitivity reactions.

12. *P. falciparum* with resistance to mefloquine is a significant problem in the malarious areas of Thailand and in areas of Myanmar and Cambodia that border on Thailand. It has also been reported on the borders between Myanmar and China, Laos and Myanmar, and in Southern Vietnam. In the United States, a 250-mg tablet of mefloquine contains 228 mg mefloquine base. Outside the United States, each 275-mg tablet contains 250 mg base.

13. Mefloquine can be used during pregnancy. The FDA reclassified mefloquine to pregnancy category B based on a review of published data (Schlagenhauf P, et al. *Clin Infect Dis.* 2012;54:e124). It is not recommended for use in travelers with active depression or with a history of psychosis or seizures and should be used with caution in persons with psychiatric illness. Mefloquine should not be used in patients with conduction abnormalities; it can be given to patients taking β-blockers if they do not have an underlying arrhythmia.

14. Beginning 1–2 wk before travel and continuing weekly for the duration of stay and for 4 wk after leaving malarious zone. Most adverse events occur within 3 doses. Some *Medical Letter* consultants favor starting mefloquine 3 weeks prior to travel and monitoring the patient for adverse events; this allows time to change to an alternative regimen if mefloquine is not tolerated. Mefloquine should not be taken on an empty stomach; it should be taken with at least 8 oz of water. For pediatric doses < ½ tablet, it is advisable to have a pharmacist crush the tablet, estimate doses by weighing, and package them in gelatin capsules. There is no data for use in children <5 kg, but based on dosages in other weight groups, a dose of 5 mg/kg can be used.

15. The combination of weekly chloroquine (300 mg base) and daily proguanil (200 mg) is recommended by the World Health Organization for use in selected areas; this combination is no longer recommended by the CDC. Proguanil (Paludrine; AstraZeneca, United Kingdom) is not available alone in the United States but is widely available in Canada and Europe. Prophylaxis is recommended during exposure and for 4 weeks afterwards. Proguanil has been used in pregnancy without evidence of toxicity (Phillips-Howard PA, Wood D. *Drug Saf.* 1996;14:131).

16. Not FDA approved for this indication.

17. Primaquine used as primary prophylaxis has proven good safety, tolerability, and efficacy when used in nonpregnant, G6PD-normal travelers (Hill DR, et al. *Am J Trop Med Hyg.* 2006;75:402–15). Beginning the day of travel and for 5 days following travel, this regimen prevents primary attacks of *P. falciparum* and *P. vivax,* and of secondary attacks (relapses) by *P. vivax* in the months following travel. Primaquine can cause hemolytic anemia, especially in patients whose red cells are deficient in G6PD. This deficiency is most common in African, Asian, and Mediterranean peoples. Patients should be screened for G6PD deficiency before treatment. Limited evidence suggests G6PD-deficient patients may be safely treated with a single weekly dose of primaquine 0.75 mg/kg for 8 weeks. Resistance is not known to occur at a dose of 0.5 mg/kg daily for 14 days: suspected resistant strains may be treated with this daily dose for 28 days. Relapse despite adherence to a full primaquine dose may be due to a poor metabolizer phenotype. Primaquine should not be used during pregnancy. It should be taken with food to minimize nausea and abdominal pain.

18. Alternatives for patients who are unable to take chloroquine include atovaquone/proguanil, mefloquine, doxycycline, or primaquine dosed as for chloroquine-resistant areas.

19. Chloroquine should be taken with food to decrease gastrointestinal adverse effects. If chloroquine phosphate is not available, hydroxychloroquine sulfate is as effective; 400 mg of hydroxychloroquine sulfate is equivalent to 500 mg of chloroquine phosphate.

20. Has been used extensively and safely for prophylaxis in pregnancy.

21. Beginning 1–2 wk before travel and continuing weekly for the duration of stay and for 4 wk after leaving malarious zone.

Microsporidiosis

	Drug	Adult Dosage	Pediatric Dosage
Ocular *(Encephalitozoon hellem, E. cuniculi, Vittaforma [Nosema] corneae)*			
Drug of choice:	Fumagillin[1]*		
	Plus		
	albendazole[2,3]	400 mg PO bid	15 mg/kg/d in 2 doses (max 400 mg/dose)
Intestinal *(E. bieneusi, E. [Septata] intestinalis)*			
E. bieneusi			
Drug of choice:	Fumagillin[4]*	20 mg PO tid × 14 d	
E. intestinalis			
Drug of choice:	Albendazole[2,3]	400 mg PO bid × 21 d	15 mg/kg/d in 2 doses (max 400 mg/dose)
Disseminated (*E. hellem, E. cuniculi, E. intestinalis, Pleistophora sp., Trachipleistophora* spp. and *Anncaliia [Brachiola] vesicularum*)			
Drug of choice[5]:	Albendazole[2,3]	400 mg PO bid	15 mg/kg/d in 2 doses (max 400 mg/dose)

*Availability problems. See Table 241.2.

1. Chan CM, et al. *Ophthalmology.* 2003;110:1420. Ocular lesions due to *E. hellem* in HIV-infected patients have responded to fumagillin eyedrops prepared from Fumidil-B (bicyclohexyl ammonium fumagillin) used to control a microsporidial disease of honey bees (Garvey MJ, et al. *Ann Pharmacother.* 1995;29:872), available from Leiter's Park Avenue Pharmacy, San Jose, CA (800-292-6773; www.leiterrx.com), a compounding pharmacy that specializes in ophthalmic drugs. For lesions due to *V. corneae,* topical therapy is generally not effective and keratoplasty may be required (Davis RM, et al. *Ophthalmology.* 1990;97:953).
2. Not FDA approved for this indication.
3. Albendazole must be taken with food; a fatty meal increases oral bioavailability.
4. Oral fumagillin (Flisint; Sanofi-Aventis, France) has been effective in treating *E. bieneusi* in patients with HIV or solid organ transplants (Molina J-M, et al. *N Engl J Med.* 2002;346:1963; Lanternier F, et al. *Transpl Infect Dis.* 2009;11:83) but has been associated with thrombocytopenia and neutropenia. Potent antiretroviral therapy may lead to microbiologic and clinical response in HIV-infected patients with microsporidial diarrhea. Octreotide (Sandostatin) has provided symptomatic relief in some patients with large-volume diarrhea.
5. Molina J-M, et al. *J Infect Dis.* 1995;171:245. There is no established treatment for *Pleistophora.* For disseminated disease due to *Trachipleistophora* or *Anncaliia,* itraconazole 400 mg PO once/d plus albendazole may also be tried (Coyle Cm, et al. *N Engl J Med.* 2004;351:42).

Mites

See Scabies

Moniliformis moniliformis[1]

	Drug	Adult Dosage	Pediatric Dosage
Drug of choice:	Pyrante pamoate[2,3]	11 mg/kg base PO once, repeat twice, 2 wk apart	11 mg/kg base PO once, repeat twice, 2 wk apart

1. Messina AF, et al. *Pediatr Infect Dis.* 2011;30:728.
2. Not FDA approved for this indication.
3. Available without a prescription. Pyrantel pamoate suspension can be mixed with milk or fruit juice.

Naegleria spp.

See Amebic Meningoencephalitis, Primary

Necator americanus

See Hookworm

Oesophagostomum bifurcum[1]

	Drug	Adult Dosage	Pediatric Dosage
Drug of choice:	Albendazole	400 mg PO once	15 mg/kg PO once (max 400 mg)
Or	Pyrantel pamoate[2,3]	11 mg/kg base (max 1 g) PO once/d × 3 d	11 mg/kg base (max 1 g) PO once/d × 3 d

1. Ziem JB, et al. *Ann Trop Med Parasitol.* 2004;98:385.
2. Available without a prescription. Pyrantel pamoate suspension can be mixed with milk or fruit juice.
3. Not FDA approved for this indication.

Onchocerca volvulus

See Filariasis

Opisthorchis viverrini

See Fluke

Paragonimus westermani

See Fluke

Pediculus captis, humanus, Phthirus pubis

See Lice

Pinworm

See Enterobius

Pneumocystis jirovecii (formerly *carinii*) Pneumonia[1]

	Drug	Adult Dosage	Pediatric Dosage
Moderate to Severe Disease[2]			
Drug of choice:	TMP-SMX	TMP 15–20 mg/kg/d, SMX 75–100 mg/kg/d PO or IV in 3 or 4 doses (change to PO after clinical improvement) × 21 d	TMP 15–20 mg/kg/d, SMX 75–100 mg/kg/d PO or IV in 3 or 4 doses (change to PO after clinical improvement) × 21 d
Alternative:	Pentamidine	3–4 mg/kg IV daily × 21 d	3–4 mg/kg IV daily × 21 d
Or	Primaquine[3,4]	30 mg base PO daily × 21 d	0.3 mg/kg base PO (max 30 mg) daily × 21 d
Plus	Clindamycin[3,5]	600–900 mg IV tid or qid × 21 d, or 300–450 mg PO tid or qid × 21 d (change to PO after clinical improvement)	15–25 mg/kg IV tid or qid (max 600 mg/dose) × 21 d, or 10 mg/kg PO tid or qid (max 300–450 mg/dose) × 21 d (change to PO after clinical improvement)
Mild to Moderate Disease			
Drug of choice:	TMP-SMX	2 double-strength tablets (160 mg/800 mg each) PO tid × 21 d	TMP 15–20 mg/kg/d, SMX 75–100 mg/kg/d PO in 3 or 4 doses × 21 d
Alternative:	Dapsone[3]	100 mg PO daily × 21 d	2 mg/kg/d (max 100 mg) PO × 21 d
Plus	Trimethoprim[3]	15 mg/kg/d PO in 3 doses	15 mg/kg/d PO in 3 doses
Or	Primaquine[3,4]	30 mg base PO daily × 21 d	0.3 mg/kg base PO daily (max 30 mg) × 21 d
Plus	Clindamycin[3,5]	300–450 mg PO tid or qid × 21 d	10 mg/kg PO tid or qid (max 300–450 mg/dose) × 21 d
Or	Atovaquone[6]	750 mg PO bid × 21 d	1–3 mo: 30 mg/kg/d PO in 2 doses × 21 d 4–24 mo: 45 mg/kg/d PO in 2 doses × 21 d >24 mo: 30 mg/kg/d PO in 2 doses × 21 d
Primary and Secondary Prophylaxis[7]			
Drug of choice:	TMP-SMX	1 tab (single or double strength) daily or 1 double-strength tab PO 3 d/wk	TMP 150 mg/SMX 750 mg/m²/d PO in 2 doses 3 d/wk
Alternative:	Dapsone[3]	50 mg PO bid or 100 mg PO daily	≥1 mo: 2 mg/kg/d (max 100 mg) PO or 4 mg/kg (max 200 mg) PO once/wk
Or	Dapsone[3]	50 mg PO daily or 200 mg PO each wk	
Plus	pyrimethamine[8]	50 mg PO daily or 75 mg PO each wk	
Or	Atovaquone[3,6]	1500 mg/d PO in 1 or 2 doses	1–3 mo: 30 mg/kg/d PO 4–24 mo: 45 mg/kg/d PO >24 mo: 30 mg/kg/d PO
Or	Pentamidine	300 mg aerosol inhaled monthly via *Respirgard II* nebulizer	≥5 y: 300 mg inhaled monthly via Respirgard II nebulizer

SMX, Sulfamethoxazole; *TMP,* trimethoprim.

1. Pneumocystis has been reclassified as a fungus (Gilroy SA, Bennett NJ. *Semin Respir Crit Care Med.* 2011;32:775).
2. In severe disease with room air PO_2 ≤70 mm Hg or Aa gradient ≥35 mm Hg, prednisone or its IV equivalent should also be used. For adults: days 1–5: 40 mg PO bid; days 6–10: 40 mg PO daily; days 11–21: 20 mg PO daily. For children: days 1–5: 2 mg/kg/d PO in 2 doses; days 6–10: 1 mg/kg/d PO in 2 doses; days 11–21: 0.5 mg/kg/d PO daily (Kaplan JE, et al. *Morbid Mortal Wkly Rep.* 2009;58[RR04]:1; *Morbid Mortal Wkly Rep.* 2009;58[RR11]:1).
3. Not FDA approved for this indication.
4. Primaquine phosphate can cause hemolytic anemia, especially in patients deficient in G6PD. This deficiency is most common in African, Asian, and Mediterranean peoples. Patients should be screened for G6PD deficiency before treatment. Primaquine should not be used during pregnancy. It should be taken with food to minimize nausea and abdominal pain.
5. Oral clindamycin should be taken with a full glass of water to minimize esophageal ulceration.
6. Atovaquone is available in an oral suspension that should be taken with a meal to increase absorption.
7. Primary/secondary prophylaxis in patients with HIV can be discontinued after CD4 count increases to >200 × 10^6/L for >3 mo.
8. Plus leucovorin 25 mg with each dose of pyrimethamine. Pyrimethamine should be taken with food to minimize gastrointestinal adverse effects.

River Blindness

See Filariasis

Roundworm

See Ascariasis

Sarcocystis spp. (Intestinal and Muscular)

	Drug	Adult Dosage	Pediatric Dosage
Drug of choice:	Sarcocystis in humans is acquired by ingesting sporocysts in infected meat. Infection is characterized by nausea, abdominal pain and diarrhea. Most muscle infections are mild or subclinical, although severe and prolonged muscle pain has been reported.[1] Albendazole was reported to be efficacious.[2]		

1. Fayer R. *Clin Microbiol Rev.* 2004;17:894; *MMWR Morb Mortal Wkly Rep.* 2012;61:37.
2. Arness MK, et al. *Am J Trop Med Hyg.* 1999;61:548.

Scabies *(Sarcoptes scabiei)*[1]

	Drug	Adult Dosage	Pediatric Dosage
Drug of choice:	5% Permethrin	Topically, 2 × at least 7 d apart	Topically, 2 × at least 7 d apart
Alternative:	Ivermectin[2,3]	200 μg/kg PO 2 × at least 7 d apart[4]	200 μg/kg PO, 2 × at least 7 d apart[4]
	10% crotamiton	Topically overnight on days 1, 2, 3, 8	Topically overnight on days 1, 2, 3, 8

1. Meinking TL, et al. Infestations. In: Schachner LA, Hansen RC, eds. *Pediatric Dermatology.* 4th ed. St Louis: Mosby; 2011:1535; Hay RJ, et al. *Clin Microbiol Infect.* 2012;18:313.
2. Not FDA approved for this indication.
3. Gonzalez P, et al. *Curr Pharm Biotechnol.* 2012;13:1103. Safety of ivermectin in young children (<15 kg) and pregnant women remains to be established; animal studies have shown adverse effects on the fetus (el-Ashmawy IM, et al. *Res Vet Sci.* 2011;90:116). Taking ivermectin with a meal increases its bioavailability (Guzzo CA, et al. *J Clin Pharmacol.* 2002;42:1122).
4. Currie Bj, McCarthy JS. *N Engl J Med.* 2010;362:717. A second ivermectin dose taken 2 weeks later increased the cure rate to 95%, which is equivalent to that of 5% permethrin (Usha V, et al. *J Am Acad Dermatol.* 2000;42:236). Ivermectin, either alone or in combination with a topical scabicide, is the drug of choice for crusted scabies in immunocompromised patients (del Giudice P. *Curr Opin Infect Dis.* 2004;15:123).

Schistosomiasis *(Bilharziasis)*[1]

	Drug	Adult Dosage	Pediatric Dosage
S. haematobium			
Drug of choice:	Praziquantel[2,3]	40 mg/kg/d PO in 1 or 2 doses × 1 d	40 mg/kg/d PO in 2 doses × 1 d
S. intercalatum[4]			
Drug of choice:	Praziquantel[2,3]	40 mg/kg/d PO in 1 or 2 doses × 1 d	40 mg/kg/d PO in 2 doses × 1 d
S. japonicum			
Drug of choice:	Praziquantel[2,3]	60 mg/kg/d PO in 2 or 3 doses × 1 d	60 mg/kg/d PO in 3 doses × 1 d
S. mansoni			
Drug of choice:	Praziquantel[2,3]	40 mg/kg/d PO in 1 or 2 doses × 1 d	40 mg/kg/d PO in 2 doses × 1 d
Alternative:	Oxamniquine[5]*	15 mg/kg PO once[6]	20 mg/kg/d PO in 2 doses × 1 d[6]
S. mekongi			
Drug of choice:	Praziquantel[2,3]	60 mg/kg/d PO in 2 or 3 doses × 1 d	60 mg/kg/d PO in 3 doses × 1 d

*Availability problems. See Table 241.2.

1. Praziquantel is the choice worldwide for treatment and prevention of schistomiasis (Liu R, et al. *Parasit Vectors.* 2011;4:201). Artemisinin treatment early after exposure may decrease the risk of acute disease (Ross AG, et al. *Lancet Infect Dis.* 2007;7:218; Liu R, et al. *Parasitol Res.* 2012;110:2071). It was less effective than praziquantel in an open-label trial of 212 children in Kenya (Obonyo CO, et al. *Lancet Infect Dis.* 2010;10:603).
2. Praziquantel should be taken with liquids during a meal.
3. Retreatment in 2–6 weeks increases cure (Doenhoff MJ, et al. *Curr Opin Infect Dis.* 2008;21:659; Gray DJ, et al. *BMJ.* 2011;342:d2651).
4. Geographically restricted to Central Western Africa and the island of São Tomé. Usually a disease of the lower GI tract; there are also case reports of complications including central nervous system, liver, and cardiopulmonary involvement (Murinello A, et al. *J Port Gastrenterol.* 2006;13:97).
5. Oxamniquine, which is not available in the United States, is generally not as effective as praziquantel. It has been useful, however, in some areas in which praziquantel is less effective (Ferrari ML, et al. *Bull World Health Organ.* 2003;81:190; Harder A, *Parasitol Res.* 2002;88:395). Oxamniquine is contraindicated in pregnancy. It should be taken after food.
6. In East Africa, the dose should be increased to 30 mg/kg PO, and in Egypt and South Africa to 30 mg/kg/d PO × 2 d. Some experts recommend 40–60 mg/kg PO over 2–3 d in all of Africa (Shekhar KC. *Drugs.* 1991;42:379).

Sleeping Sickness

See Trypanosomiasis

Strongyloidiasis *(Strongyloides stercoralis)*

	Drug	Adult Dosage	Pediatric Dosage
Drug of choice[1]:	Ivermectin[2]	200 µg/kg/d PO × 2 d	200 µg/kg/d PO × 2 d
Alternative:	Albendazole[3,4]	400 mg PO bid × 7 d	400 mg PO bid × 7 d

1. In immunocompromised patients or disseminated disease (strongyloides hyperinfection syndrome) additional doses or use of other drugs may be necessary. Veterinary subcutaneous and enema formulations of ivermectin have been used in severely ill patients with hyperinfection who were unable to take or reliably absorb oral medications (Marty fm, et al. *Clin Infect Dis.* 2005;41:e5; Lichtenberger p, et al. *Transpl Infect Dis.* 2009;11:137).
2. Gonzalez p, et al. *Curr Pharm Biotechnol.* 2012;13:1103. Safety of ivermectin in young children (<15 kg) and pregnant women remains to be established; animal studies have shown adverse effects on the fetus (el-Ashmawy im, et al. *Res Vet Sci.* 2011;90:116). Taking ivermectin with a meal increases its bioavailability (Guzzo ca, et al. *J Clin Pharmacol.* 2002; 42:1122).
3. Not FDA approved for this indication.
4. Albendazole must be taken with food; a fatty meal increases oral bioavailability.

Tapeworm Infection

	Drug	Adult Dosage	Pediatric Dosage
Adult (Intestinal Stage)			
Diphyllobothrium latum *(Fish)*, Taenia saginata *(Beef)*, Taenia solium *(Pork)*, Dipylidium caninum *(Dog)*			
Drug of choice:	Praziquantel[1,2]	5–10 mg/kg PO once	5–10 mg/kg PO once
Alternative:	Niclosamide[3]*	2 g PO once	50 mg/kg PO once
Hymenolepis Nana (Dwarf Tapeworm)			
Drug of choice:	Praziquantel[1,2]	25 mg/kg PO once	25 mg/kg PO once
Alternative:[4]	Niclosamide[3]*	2 g PO daily × 7 d	11–34 kg: 1 g PO on day 1 then 500 mg/d PO × 6 days > 34 kg: 1.5 g PO on day 1 then 1 g/d PO × 6 days
Larval (Tissue Stage)			
Echinococcus granulosus *(Cystic Echinococcosis)*			
Treatment of choice:		See footnote 5	
Drug of choice:	Albendazole[6]	15 mg/kg/d (max 800 mg) PO in 2 doses × 1–6 mo	15 mg/kg/d (max 800 mg) PO in 2 doses × 1–6 mo
Echinococcus multilocularis *(Alveolar Echinococcosis)*			
Treatment of choice:		See footnote 7	
Drug of choice:	Albendazole[6]	15 mg/kg/d (max 800 mg) PO in 2 doses × >2 y	
Taenia solium *(Cysticercosis)*			
Treatment of choice:		See footnote 8	
Alternative:	Albendazole[6]	15 mg/kg/d (max 800 mg) PO in 2 doses × 8–30 d; can be repeated as necessary	15 mg/kg/d (max 800 mg) PO in 2 doses × 8–30 d; can be repeated as necessary
Or	Praziquantel[1,2]	50 mg/kg/d PO × 15 d	50 mg/kg/d PO × 15 d

*Availability problems. See Table 241.2.
1. Not FDA approved for this indication.
2. Praziquantel should be taken with liquids during a meal.
3. Niclosamide must be thoroughly chewed or crushed and swallowed with a small amount of water.
4. Nitazoxanide may be an alternative (Ortiz JJ, et al. *Trans R Soc Trop Med Hyg.* 2002;96:193; Chero JC, et al. *Trans R Soc Trop Med Hyg* 2007;101:203; Diaz E, et al. *Am J Trop Med Hyg.* 2003;68:384).
5. Treatment of uncomplicated hepatic or abdominal cysts is stage-dependent and ranges from surgical resection to watch and wait (Brunetti E, et al. *Acta Trop.* 2010;114:1). Patients may benefit from surgical resection (for larger cysts) or percutaneous drainage of cysts. Percutaneous aspiration-injection-reaspiration with ultrasound guidance plus albendazole therapy (1 wk before and for 30 d after) has been effective for management of hepatic hydatid cyst disease (Golemanov B, et al. *Am J Trop Med Hyg.* 2011;84:48; Gupta N, et al. *J Gastrointest Surg.* 2011;15:1829). Praziquantel may also be useful preoperatively or in case of spillage of cyst contents during surgery.
6. Albendazole must be taken with food; a fatty meal increases oral bioavailability.
7. Surgical excision is the only reliable means of cure (but is rarely possible) and should be followed by prolonged albendazole therapy (Kern P. *Curr Opin Infect Dis.* 2010;23:505). Reports have suggested that in nonresectable cases, long-term (months to years) use of albendazole (400 mg bid) can stabilize and rarely cure infection (Moro P, Schantz PM. *Int J Infect Dis.* 2009;13:125; Chappius F. *Rev Med Suisse.* 2012;8:989).
8. Advances in neuroimaging using CT and MRI have facilitated the ability to make an accurate diagnosis (Del Brutto OH. *ScientificWorld J.* 2012;2012:159821; Nash TE, Garcia HH. *Nat Rev Neurol.* 2011;7:584). Initial therapy for patients with inflamed parenchymal cysticercosis should focus on symptomatic treatment with antiseizure medication (Sinha S, Sharma BS. *J Clin Neurosci.* 2009;16:867). Patients with live parenchymal cysts who have seizures should be treated with albendazole together with steroids and an antiseizure medication (Garcia HH, et al. *Curr Opin Infect Dis.* 2011;24:423). Patients with subarachnoid cysts or giant cysts in the fissures should be treated for at least 30 days (Proaño JV, et al. *N Engl J Med.* 2001;345:879). Surgical intervention (especially neuroendoscopic removal) or cerebrospinal fluid diversion followed by albendazole and steroids is indicated for obstructive hydocephalus. Arachnoiditis, vasculitis or cerebral edema is treated with albendazole or praziquantel plus prednisone (60 mg/d) or dexamethasone (4–6 mg/d). Any cysticidal drug may cause irreparable damage when used to treat ocular or spinal cysts, even when corticosteroids are used. An ophthalmic exam should always precede treatment to rule out intraocular cysts.

Toxocariasis

See Visceral Larva Migrans

Toxoplasmosis *(Toxoplasma gondii)*

	Drug	Adult Dosage	Pediatric Dosage
CNS Disease[1]			
Drug of choice:	Pyrimethamine[2]	200 mg PO × 1 then 50–75 mg/d PO × 3–6 wk	2 mg/kg/d PO × 2 d, then 1 mg/kg/d (max 25 mg/d) × 3–6 wk
Plus	Sulfadiazine[3]	1–1.5 g PO qid × 3–6 wk	100–200 mg/kg/d divided q6h PO × 3–6 wk
Or	Clindamycin[4,5,6]	1.8–2.4 g/d IV or PO in 3 or 4 doses	5–7.5 mg/kg/d IV or PO in 3 or 4 doses (max 600 mg/dose)
Or	Atovaquone[4,5,7]	1500 mg PO bid	1500 mg PO bid
Alternative:	TMP-SMX[4]	TMP 15–20 mg/kg/d, SMX 75–100 mg/kg/d PO or IV in 3 or 4 doses	TMP 15–20 mg/kg/d, SMX 75–100 mg/kg/d PO or IV in 3 or 4 doses
Primary Infection in Pregnancy			
Treatment of choice: See footnote 8			

SMX, Sulfamethoxazole; *TMP*, trimethoprim.

1. Treatment is followed by chronic suppression with lower dosage regimens of the same drugs. In the United States, for primary prophylaxis of HIV patients with CD4 <100 × 10^6 cells/L (outside the United States, CD4 <200 × 10^6 cells/L), either TMP-SMX, pyrimethamine with dapsone, or atovaquone with or without pyrimethamine can be used (TMP-SMX is generally preferred due to once-daily dosing). Primary or secondary prophylaxis may be discontinued when the CD4 count increases to >200 × 10^6 cells/L for >3 mo (*MMWR Morb Mortal Wkly Rep.* 2009;58[RR4]:1). In ocular toxoplasmosis with macular involvement, corticosteroids are recommended in addition to antiparasitic therapy (Montoya JG, Liesenfeld O. *Lancet.* 2004;363:1965).
2. Plus leucovorin 10–25 mg with each dose of pyrimethamine. Pyrimethamine should be taken with food to minimize gastrointestinal adverse effects.
3. Sulfadiazine should be taken on an empty stomach with adequate water.
4. Not FDA approved for this indication.
5. Clindamycin has been used in combination with pyrimethamine to treat CNS toxoplasmosis in HIV-infected patients who developed sulfonamide sensitivity while on sulfadiazine. Atovaquone has also been used to treat sulfonamide-intolerant patients (Chirgwin K, et al. *Clin Infect Dis.* 2002;34:1243).
6. Oral clindamycin should be taken with a full glass of water to minimize esophageal ulceration.
7. Atovaquone is available in an oral suspension that should be taken with a meal to increase absorption.
8. Women who develop toxoplasmosis during the first trimester of pregnancy should be treated with spiramycin (3–4 g/d). After the first trimester, if there is no documented transmission to the fetus, spiramycin can be continued until term. Spiramycin is not currently available in the United States but can be obtained at no cost from Aventis through an IND from the FDA (301-796-1600) following confirmation of the diagnosis by a recognized laboratory (e.g., Palo Alto Medical Foundation, Toxoplasmosis Laboratory 650-853-4828). If transmission has occurred in utero, therapy with pyrimethamine and sulfadiazine should be started. Pyrimethamine is a potential teratogen and should be used only after the first trimester (Montoya JG, Remington JS. *Clin Infect Dis.* 2008;47:554). Congenitally infected newborns should be treated with pyrimethamine every 2 or 3 days and a sulfonamide daily for about 1 y (Remington JS. *Infectious Disease of the Fetus and Newborn Infant,* 7th ed. Philadelphia: Saunders; 2011:918).

Trichinellosis *(Trichinella spiralis* and Other *Trichinella* spp.)

	Drug	Adult Dosage	Pediatric Dosage
Drug of choice[1]:	Steroids for severe symptoms	prednisone 30–60 mg PO daily ×10–15 d	
Plus	Albendazole[2,3]	400 mg PO bid × 8–14 d	400 mg PO bid × 8–14 d
Alternative:	Mebendazole[2]	200–400 mg PO tid × 3 d, then 400–500 mg tid × 10 d	200–400 mg PO tid × 3 d, then 400–500 mg tid × 10 d

1. Gottstein B, et al. *Clin Microbiol Rev.* 2009;22:127.
2. Not FDA approved for this indication.
3. Albendazole must be taken with food; a fatty meal increases oral bioavailability.

Trichomoniasis *(Trichomonas vaginalis)*

	Drug	Adult Dosage	Pediatric Dosage
Drug of choice[1]:	Tinidazole[2]	2 g PO once	50 mg/kg once (max 2 g)
Or	Metronidazole[3]	2 g PO once	15 mg/kg/d PO in 3 doses × 7 d

1. Sexual partners should be treated simultaneously with same dosage. If treatment failure occurs with metronidazole 2 g single dose and reinfection is excluded, treat with metronidazole 500 mg PO bid × 7 d. For patients taking 7 d of metronidazole, metronidazole or tinidazole 2 g PO daily × 5 d should be considered. Consultation and susceptibility testing is available from the CDC 404-718-4141 (*MMWR Morbid Mortal Wkly Rep.* 2010;59[RR-12]:1).
2. A nitroimidazole similar to metronidazole, tinidazole appears to be at least as effective as metronidazole and better tolerated. It should be taken with food to minimize adverse GI effects. For children and patients unable to take tablets, a pharmacist can crush the tablets and mix them with cherry syrup (Humco, and others). The syrup suspension is good for 7 days at room temperature and must be shaken before use (Fung HB, Doan TL. *Clin Ther.* 2005;27:1859). Ornidazole, a similar drug, is also used outside the United States.
3. Metronidazole has been associated with higher rates of parasitologic and clinical failure compared to tinidazole (Bachmann LH, et al. *Clin Infect Dis.* 2011; 53[Suppl 3]:S160).

Trichostrongylus Infection

	Drug	Adult Dosage	Pediatric Dosage
Drug of choice:	Pyrantel pamoate[1,2]	11 mg/kg base PO once (max 1 g)	11 mg/kg base PO once (max 1 g)
Alternative:	Mebendazole[1]	100 mg PO bid × 3 d	100 mg PO bid × 3 d
Or	Albendazole[1,3]	400 mg PO once	400 mg PO once

1. Not FDA approved for this indication.
2. Available without a prescription. Pyrantel pamoate suspension can be mixed with milk or fruit juice.
3. Albendazole must be taken with food; a fatty meal increases oral bioavailability.

Trichuriasis (*Trichuris trichiura*, Whipworm)

	Drug	Adult Dosage	Pediatric Dosage
Drug of choice:	Albendazole[1,2]	400 mg PO × 3 d	400 mg PO × 3 d
Alternative:	Mebendazole	100 mg PO bid × 3 d	100 mg PO bid × 3 d
Or	Ivermectin[1,3,4]	200 mcg/kg/d PO × 3 d	200 mcg/kg/d PO × 3 d

1. Not FDA approved for this indication.
2. Albendazole must be taken with food; a fatty meal increases oral bioavailability.
3. Gonzalez P, et al. *Curr Pharm Biotechnol.* 2012;13:1103. Safety of ivermectin in young children (<15 kg) and pregnant women remains to be established; animal studies have shown adverse effects on the fetus (el-Ashmawy IM, et al. *Res Vet Sci.* 2011;90:116). Taking ivermectin with a meal increases its bioavailability (Guzzo CA, et al. *J Clin Pharmacol.* 2002;42:1122).
4. Ivermectin alone is less effective than albendazole or mebendazole. Addition of ivermectin to albendazole or mebendazole improved cure rates in one study (Knopp S, et al. *Clin Infect Dis.* 2010;51:1420).

Trypanosomiasis

	Drug	Adult Dosage	Pediatric Dosage
***T. cruzi* (American Trypanosomiasis, Chagas' Disease)[1]**			
Drug of choice:	Benznidazole[2]*	5–7 mg/kg/d PO in 2 doses × 60 d	<12 y: 10 mg/kg/d PO in 2 doses × 60 d >12 y: 5–7 mg/kg/d PO in 2 doses × 60 d
Or	Nifurtimox*	8–10 mg/kg/d PO in 3–4 doses × 90 d	1–10 y: 15–20 mg/kg/d PO in 4 doses × 90 d 11–16 y: 12.5–15 mg/kg/d PO in 4 doses × 90 d
***T. brucei gambiense* (West African Trypanosomiasis, Sleeping Sickness)[3]**			
Hemolymphatic Stage			
Drug of choice[4]:	Pentamidine[5]	4 mg/kg/d IM or IV × 7 d	4 mg/kg/d IM or IV × 7 d
Alternative:	Suramin*	100 mg (test dose) IV, then 1 g IV on days 1,3,5,14, 21	2 mg/kg (test dose) IV, then 20 mg/kg IV on days 1,3,5,14, 21
Late Disease With Central Nervous System Involvement			
Drug of choice:[6]	Eflornithine[7]*	400 mg/kg/d IV in 4 doses × 14 d	400 mg/kg/d IV in 4 doses × 14 d
Or	Eflornithine[7]*	400 mg/kg IV in 2 doses × 7 d	
Plus	nifurtimox	15 mg/kg/d PO in 3 doses × 10 d	
Alternative:	Melarsoprol[8]	2.2 mg/kg/d IV × 10 d	2.2 mg/kg/d IV × 10 d
***T. b. rhodesiense* (East African Trypanosomiasis, Sleeping Sickness)[3]**			
Hemolymphatic Stage			
Drug of choice:	Suramin*	100 mg (test dose) IV, then 1 g IV on days 1,3,5,14, 21	2 mg/kg (test dose) IV, then 20 mg/kg IV on days 1,3,5,14, 21
Late Disease With CNS Involvement			
Drug of choice:	Melarsoprol[8]	2.2 mg/kg/d IV × 10 d	2.2 mg/kg/d IV × 10 d

*Availability problems. See Table 241.2.

1. Treatment of chronic or indeterminate Chagas' disease with benznidazole has been associated with negative seroconversion in children and reduced progression of cardiac disease in adults (Viotti R, et al. *Ann Intern Med.* 2006;144:724; de Andrade AL. *Lancet.* 1996;348:1407; Bern C, et al. *Clin Microbiol Rev.* 2011;24:655; LeLoup G, et al. *Curr Opin Infect Dis.* 2011; 24:428). Congenital transmission of Chagas disease occurs in 1–10% of children born to infected mothers.The safety of antitrypanasomal drugs in pregnancy is unknown. The treatment of mothers after delivery and cessation of breastfeeding is recommended (*MMWR Morb Mortal Wkly Rep.* 2012;61:477; Carlier Y, et al. *PLoS Negl Trop Dis.* 2011;5:e1250).
2. Benznidazole should be taken with meals to minimize gastrointestinal adverse effects. It is contraindicated during pregnancy.
3. Blum JA, et al. *Eur J Clin Microbiol Infect Dis.* 2012; Malvy D, Chappuis F. *Clin Microbiol Infect.* 2011;17:986.
4. Pentamidine and suramin have equal efficacy, but pentamidine is better tolerated.
5. Not FDA approved for this indication.
6. In one study, eflornithine for 7 d combined with nifurtimox × 10 d was more effective and less toxic than eflornithine × 14 d (Priotto F, et al. *Lancet.* 2009;374:56).
7. Eflornithine is highly effective in *T.b. gambiense,* but not in *T.b. rhodesiense* infections. In two studies of treatment of central nervous system disease due to *T.b. gambiense*, there were fewer serious complications with eflornithine than with melarsoprol (Kennedy PG. *Ann Neurol.* 2008;64:116; Chappuis F, et al. *Clin Infect Dis.* 2005;41:748). Eflornithine is available in limited supply only from the World Health Organization.
8. Kuepfer I, et al. *PLoS Negl Trop Dis.* 2012;6:e1695. Corticosteroids have been used to prevent arsenical encephalopathy (Pepin J, et al. *Trans R Soc Trop Med Hyg.* 1995;89:92).

Visceral Larva Migrans[1] *(Toxocariasis)*

	Drug	Adult Dosage	Pediatric Dosage
Drug of choice:	Albendazole[2,3]	400 mg PO bid × 5 d	400 mg PO bid × 5 d
Or	Mebendazole[2]	100–200 mg PO bid × 5 d	100–200 mg PO bid × 5 d

1. Optimum duration of therapy is not known; some *Medical Letter* consultants would treat × 20 d. For severe symptoms or eye involvement, treatment is extended 2–4 weeks and corticosteroids can be used in addition (Rubinsky-Elefant G, et al. *Ann Trop Parasitol.* 2010;104:3; Turrientes MC, et al. *Emerg Infect Dis.* 2011;17:1263).
2. Not FDA approved for this indication.
3. Albendazole must be taken with food; a fatty meal increases oral bioavailability.

Whipworm

See Trichuriasis

Wuchereria bancrofti

See Filariasis

242 Immunomodulating Agents

Justin E. Caron • Harry R. Hill • Timothy R. La Pine

There has been considerable clinical interest and basic science research into the functional mechanisms of the immune response and the identification of the specific biologic factors that modulate this response. This research has established that a critical and delicate balance in the regulation of both cellular and humoral function is essential for complete immunologic response to invasive pathogens and that alteration of this regulation may have potential clinical significance. Attempts to augment immune function in the challenged host or during specific immunodeficiency states have focused on numerous modifiers of immune biologic response. There are thousands of citations in the peer-reviewed medical literature on this topic. These efforts, in combination with advances made in hybridoma, recombinant DNA technology, nanotechnology, and proteomics, have resulted in numerous clinical trials conducted to explore the therapeutic utility of immunomodulating agents in the treatment of specific human disease states.[67] Select biologic agents used to manipulate immune regulation for the prevention and management of infectious diseases in infants and children are discussed.

MONOCLONAL ANTIBODIES

The use of serum antibody therapy, in the late 1800s, was among the first clinical attempts to modulate the immune response in the treatment of human sepsis. By the middle 1930s, serum-based therapy was the standard of care for many infectious illnesses, particularly pneumonia. Controlled trials during that time demonstrated that the administration of type-specific pneumococcal serum reduced the mortality rate by 50% in patients with pneumococcal pneumonia.[62, 61,103] With the introduction of antimicrobial pharmacologic agents in the 1940s, the use of serum antibody therapy for sepsis became less popular. The development of hybridoma technology by Kohler and Milstein[180] in 1975, however, provided the means to generate virtually unlimited amounts of monoclonal antibodies for potential clinical use. This technology, in combination with the advances in recombinant DNA technology, has allowed researchers to generate highly specific human monoclonal antibodies and to humanize murine monoclonal antibodies.[41,345] Monoclonal antibodies now are considered attractive molecules to be used potentially as antimicrobial and antiviral agents and immunomodulators, to deliver pharmacologic substances to sites of inflammation, or even to target certain cancerous tissues. This advance has led to the development of monoclonal antibody–based therapies to treat sepsis, septic shock, hemolytic uremic syndrome (HUS), viral diseases, and a number of inflammatory diseases in infants, children, and adults.

Monoclonal Antibody Preparations in Sepsis and Bacterial Infections

A monoclonal antibody could, in theory, be generated that would alter the clinical course of any infectious or inflammatory disease state. This hypothesis has fostered numerous studies evaluating the use of monoclonal antibodies in a variety of clinical diseases, particularly those related to alloimmune and autoimmune phenomena.[75,93,133,211,272] The use of monoclonal antibodies to alter the pathogenesis of sepsis and septic shock also has received considerable experimental and clinical attention. These efforts have focused on two phases in the development of the septic shock syndrome: (1) to block bacteria and their components that induce shock and (2) to modify the release and action of the proinflammatory mediators that lead to septic shock. Other efforts to alter the pathogenesis of bacterial infections have focused on targeting specific bacterial virulence factors, by using passive immunization strategies for potential use in alternative treatment regimens.[11,87,137,290] Here, we discuss the use of monoclonal antibody therapy in neonatal sepsis, followed by passive immune strategies in *Pseudomonas* infections.

Monoclonal antibody preparations to block bacteria or their components in the development of septic shock were initially used in early studies using type-specific antisera against *Streptococcus pneumoniae, Neisseria meningitidis,* and *Haemophilus influenzae.*[62] Attempts using monoclonal antibody therapy to alter the pathogenesis of bacterial sepsis leading to septic shock have focused on group B streptococcus (GBS) and *Escherichia coli.* These two bacteria are significant causes of neonatal morbidity and mortality. Infants usually acquire these bacterial infections from exposure in the birth canal; however, only a few of the exposed infants actually develop bacterial sepsis. Factors predisposing infants to acquisition of infection with these organisms include prematurity, prolonged rupture of membranes, and maternal sepsis. Neonatal infections occur more commonly with bacteria that possess specific capsular polysaccharides (i.e., the type III polysaccharide of GBS or the K-1 capsule of *E. coli*). Bacteria bearing these capsules are able to avoid opsonization and subsequent phagocytic killing by polymorphonuclear leukocytes (PMNs). Neonates with deficiencies of type-specific antibodies to these bacterial capsular antigens as a result of prematurity, which contributes to decreased maternal transplacental antibody transport, or inadequate maternal stores are predisposed to acquisition of GBS and *E. coli* infections.[147] These observations led investigators to hypothesize that passive antibody administration may be beneficial in preventing or reducing neonatal morbidity and mortality observed with these bacterial infections.

Rebecca Lancefield in 1933 originally demonstrated a protective efficacy for GBS antibody therapy using rabbit antisera. She established that this protective efficacy is type specific and classified three types of GBS strains. Antisera raised against type II or type III GBS did not protect against infection with type I bacteria. These experiments also suggested that antibodies to group B non–type-specific determinants (i.e., expressed on all GBS bacteria) are not protective.[113,197,195,196] Further experiments by Lancefield and coworkers with type I GBS demonstrated that antibodies to both carbohydrate and protein capsular components can be protective.[197,195] The first human studies to suggest that the administration of antibody to the infecting strain of bacteria could improve survival rates from early-onset GBS in infants occurred in the middle 1970s.[300,302,303,305] In these studies, fresh whole blood either containing or lacking opsonic antibody was administered to infants with early-onset GBS disease. All nine infants who demonstrated a rise in opsonic antibody after transfusion survived. In contrast, three of the six infants (50%) who received blood lacking antibody to their infection strain died.[300] Subsequent studies suggested that intravenous immune globulin (IVIG) could offer some protection against GBS infections in experimental animal models.[106,152] Because of their lack of specificity and decreased opsonic activity, however, polyclonal-type IVIG antibody preparations have had only variable and limited ability to alter the course and outcome of GBS or other bacterial infections in clinical trials.[143]

More recently, the International Neonatal Immunotherapy Study Collaborative Group conducted a randomized controlled trial of neonates with proven or suspected infection, which included 3493 infants receiving antibiotics, assigned to either polyvalent immunoglobulin G (IgG) immune globulin or placebo.[42] There was no significant difference in primary outcome, which was death or major disability at 2 years.[42] A Cochrane database meta-analysis of 9 studies (including the International Neonatal Immunotherapy Study) with 3973 infants with suspected or proven infection found no reduction in mortality rates during hospital stay, or death or major disability at 2 years.[257] In subgroup analysis, no decrease in mortality during hospital stay was found following

IgM-enriched IVIG administration in 4 studies of 266 neonates.[257] Routine use of IVIG or IgM-enriched IVIG is currently not recommended to prevent sepsis-related mortality in neonates.

The development of monoclonal antibodies to GBS type III occurred in the early 1980s.[301–303,305] The GBS type III–specific antibodies, which were of the IgM class, protected rats against intraperitoneal infection with homologous type GBS. Survival rates were 95% to 100% for rats protected by monoclonal antibody compared with 17% for unprotected rats. Protection was afforded even when therapy was delayed up to 24 hours after inoculation. Antibody administration resulted in the rapid accumulation of PMNs at the site of infection and prevented the depletion of bone marrow granulocyte stores commonly seen in animal models and human neonates with GBS infection.[302] Monoclonal IgG and IgA antibody preparations also have been generated to type III GBS.[30,243,301] A protective effect in animal models of GBS infection for all three immunoglobulin isotypes has been established.[303] In GBS infections, the ability of an antibody isotype preparation to activate the complement system is related directly to its protective and opsonic activity.[305] IgM is much more active in triggering complement than are monoclonal IgG and IgA preparations,[199,305] a finding that may explain why monoclonal IgM is quantitatively more effective against GBS infections.[146,149,305] Although human monoclonal IgM antibodies to GBS are available and have demonstrated effectiveness in reducing mortality in animal models of GBS sepsis, they have yet to be tried clinically to prevent or to attenuate GBS sepsis and septic shock in human neonates.[275,305]

Concomitant with the studies of monoclonal antibody preparations for use in experimental models of GBS infections were similar studies using monoclonal preparations in *E. coli* sepsis. *E. coli* is an antigenically complex, gram-negative bacterium having more than 150 somatic (O) and 100 capsular (K) antigens. Several factors associated with *E. coli* have been implicated as contributing to the virulence of these organisms. Among these, the K-1 capsular polysaccharide and lipopolysaccharide (LPS) have received the most attention.[35] The K-1 capsular polysaccharide on *E. coli* as a contributing factor to the virulence of this organism was suggested first by Robbins and colleagues in 1974.[282] Subsequent studies established that *E. coli* strains that possess the K-1 capsular polysaccharide are resistant to opsonization through the alternative complement pathway.[37,312] Several investigators have shown that antibody preparations to the K-1 capsular polysaccharide are opsonic and protective against lethal *E. coli* bacteremia in animals.[36] Although protection has been demonstrated primarily with IgM antibody, polyclonal hyperimmune IgG has shown some protection in animal models of lethal *E. coli* sepsis.[274] Because the serum from neonates is deficient in opsonic activity for *E. coli*, some investigators suggested that the administration of antibody against *E. coli* K-1 would enhance neonatal resistance to infections with this organism.[38,73] Investigators since have developed murine and human monoclonal IgM antibodies to *E. coli* K-1 and demonstrated that these antibodies are opsonic and protective against lethal *E. coli* infections in animal models.[274]

Other efforts have targeted Shiga-like toxin (Stx) producing *E. coli* (STEC), which is commonly produced by *E. coli* strain O157:H7. STEC is associated with HUS, which causes microangiopathic hemolytic anemia and is a leading cause of renal failure in children. There are two main Shiga-like toxins, Stx1 and Stx2, which pass across the inflamed colonic mucosa in infection and bind to target glycoprotein receptors in the kidney, thereby damaging the endothelium and resulting in platelet aggregation and microthrombosis.[270] HUS usually results from infection with Stx2-producing *E. coli*. Neutralizing antibodies to Stx2 are currently under investigation. A phase I clinical trial showed urtoxazumab, a humanized IgG1 monoclonal antibody targeting Stx2, to be well-tolerated in adults and STEC-infected pediatric patients.[213] An earlier study of STEC-infected mice showed 100% survival when urtoxazumab was administered within 24 hours, but the agent was ineffective when administered at 48 hours, at which point Stx production had already reached its peak.[347] Single-domain antibodies, such as those produced by the camelid family, comprise a novel type of monoclonal antibody preparation engineered to be just as specific as conventional antibodies, but offering several advantages lending to ease of manufacture, including increased permeability and a much smaller size (12–16 kDa) because they are composed of only a single domain. Mejias and colleagues[234] demonstrated that camelid single-agent antibodies, composed of a single heavy-chain variable domain (VHH), were capable of neutralizing Stx2 at nanomolar concentrations in STEC-infected mice in vivo, with 0.05 pmol required to protect 80% of naïve weaned mice challenged with 4×10^{11} CFU/kg of Stx2-producing *E. coli* O157:H7.[234] Because antibiotic treatment is not recommended in STEC infection, these alternative treatment modalities warrant further study and may show some promise in the treatment or prevention of HUS.

Staphylococci are major causes of acquired infections in prematurely born infants. Antibiotic resistance among staphylococcal species in these immunocompromised patients is of significant concern. Numerous monoclonal antibody–based preparations targeting staphylococcal virulence factors have been proposed. Pagibaximab, a humanized mouse chimeric monoclonal antibody targeting lipoteichoic acid (LTA) in gram-positive bacteria, has been evaluated in multiple clinical trials for the prevention of staphylococcal sepsis in very-low-birth-weight (VLBW) neonates.[334,333] Phase I/II trials showed pagibaximab to be safe and efficacious, but a phase IIb/III trial failed to show a reduction in sepsis in VLBW neonates.[8,265] A Cochrane data base review of 2 randomized controlled trials, assessing INH A-21 (a high-titer antistaphylococcal antibody IVIG preparation) in 512 and 1983 neonates, respectively, found no significant reduction in the risk of staphylococcal infection between INH A-21 and placebo.[299] This same review found no significant difference in the risk of infection for Altastaph (a polyclonal, pooled immune globulin to type 5 and 8 capsular polysaccharide) as compared with placebo in 206 VLBW neonates.[299]

During the past several decades, the importance of pneumococcal vaccination for individuals at risk for acquiring infection has been underscored by the emergence of antibiotic resistance among pneumococcal strains and the increased prevalence of invasive pneumococcal disease in immunocompromised patients. Unfortunately, pure pneumococcal capsular polysaccharide vaccines are poorly immunogenic in many immunodeficient patients who are at risk for acquiring infection. This concern has led to the development of monoclonal antibodies against type-specific pneumococcal infections. A human monoclonal IgM antibody has been generated and shown to provide type-specific protection against lethal pneumococcal infections in mice, even in the presence of complement deficiency.[351] Thus, type-specific monoclonal antibody preparations likely could provide protection against pneumococcal infection in high-risk immunocompromised humans, if such preparations can be safely administered intravenously in humans.

Gram-negative bacteria comprise an important cause of multidrug-resistant infections in pediatric intensive care units.[346] Alternative treatment regimens are needed to help combat drug-resistant bacterial strains, particularly *Pseudomonas* infections. *Pseudomonas aeruginosa* is an important cause of opportunistic and nosocomial infections, particularly in critically ill and immunocompromised patients, and it carries both a high mortality rate and a high likelihood for multidrug resistance. *P. aeruginosa* is a gram-negative bacillus that is distinguished from the Enterobacteriaceae by the production of oxidase. *P. aeruginosa* contains LPS in the outer membrane, along with relatively impermeable porins that, combined with multidrug efflux pumps, confer considerable resistance to many antimicrobial agents. Flagella, pili, and a mucoid exopolysaccharide slime layer facilitate binding of *P. aeruginosa* to host epithelial cells. Other virulence factors produced by *P. aeruginosa* include exotoxin A and exoenzyme S, which are injected into host cells by using a type III injection secretion system.

Studies have evaluated the use of monoclonal antibody therapy to treat *P. aeruginosa* infections in critically ill patients. A multicenter, phase II randomized, double-blind, placebo-controlled trial assessed the use of KB001, an anti-PcrV PEGylated (polyethylene glycol–linked) monoclonal antibody fragment, in mechanically ventilated patients with pulmonary *Pseudomonas* colonization.[112] KB001 is an engineered, human Fab fragment that binds to PcrV, which is a component of the type III secretory (TTS) apparatus (also known as the injectisome), that gram-negative bacteria including *Pseudomonas* use to inject TTS toxins directly into adjacent host eukaryotic cells.[290] This results in cytotoxic injury and is proposed to contribute to acute lung injury. In this multicenter phase II study, Francois and colleagues[112] demonstrated that intravenous infusion of KB001 was well tolerated at 3 and 10 mg/kg compared with placebo, and it was readily detected up to the 28-day end point. Although the study did not achieve clinical significance, KB001-treated patients had fewer episodes of *Pseudomonas* pneumonia and more 28-day *Pseudomonas*-free survivors.[112] KB001 was also evaluated in patients with chronic cystic fibrosis who received a single intravenous dose at 3 or 10 mg/kg. At 28 days, there was no significant decrease in symptoms, pulmonary function test results, or sputum culture *Pseudomonas* density; however, there was a dose-dependent decrease in sputum markers of inflammation, including myeloperoxidase, interkeukin-1 (IL-1), and IL-8, with significant reduction in neutrophil elastase and sputum neutrophil counts.[237] Monoclonal antibodies targeting the LPS-O polysaccharide moiety of *P. aeruginosa* and Psl, an exopolysaccharide involved in biofilm formation, have also been investigated.[87,137] Moreover, a monoclonal biphasic antibody targeting both PcrV and Psl, BiS4αPa, has been described.[137] Another passive immune approach to *Pseudomonas* infections is the use of IVIG, which has was shown to improve bacteremia and acute lung injury significantly in mice, either prophylactically or 3 hours after bacterial inoculation, in concordance with measurable anti-PcrV titers in the IVIG.[304] This study showed that although IVIG had no bactericidal activity in vitro, the addition of ceftazidime did, thus resulting in release of higher levels of TNF-α and increased mortality in the mice.

Monoclonal Antibody Therapy for Viral Infections

Monoclonal antibodies directed against viral glycoprotein complexes or that immunomodulate through other mechanisms are also being developed and evaluated for human use for a variety of viral diseases. Palivizumab, a humanized F protein monoclonal antibody, is routinely administered to preterm infants and other high-risk infants for immunoprophylaxis against respiratory syncytial virus (RSV) infection and disease.[10,39] It also is used for prophylaxis against RSV infection in older high-risk subjects, such as transplant recipients and children with cystic fibrosis.[10,39] In addition, palivizumab is administered in some patients to treat established RSV infections in immunocompromised patients awaiting immune reconstitution. A recombinant human antirabies monoclonal antibody has been tested in India. It appears to be safe and as efficacious as conventional serum-derived rabies immune globulin (RIG) and may soon replace the use of RIG for postexposure prophylaxis.[122,245,246] Monoclonal antibodies directed against vaccinia virus have been developed and tested in preclinical animal models as potential therapeutic antibodies for treatment of smallpox,[72] especially in viral glycoprotein complexes. The antiangiogenic monoclonal antibody bevacizumab (Avastin) is also been used to treat recurrent respiratory papillomatosis.[26]

Cytomegalovirus (CMV) is a ubiquitous virus that is often asymptomatic in the immunocompetent host, but it may cause significant morbidity and mortality in immunocompromised persons and life-threatening congenital infections or long-term disability including hearing loss and intellectual disability when acquired by the fetus in utero from mothers with primary CMV infection. CMV glycoproteins (gB, gH/gL/gO, and gM/gN) mediate viral entry into fibroblasts, whereas a pentameric complex (gH/gL/UL128-131) is required for viral entry into epithelial cells, endothelial cells, and macrophages.[111] These glycoprotein complexes are important potential targets for therapeutic neutralizing antibodies. The mechanism by which CMV crosses the placenta and infects the fetus is incompletely understood, but the process likely occurs when CMV bound by low affinity, IgG anti-CMV gB antibodies binds the neonatal Fc receptor expressed by syncytiotrophoblasts (normally used for transcytosis of maternal IgG for passive immunity), resulting in transcytosis of IgG-virion complexes, followed by focal infection of cytotrophoblasts, and spread of infection to stromal fibroblasts, villous capillary endothelial cells, and leukocytes in the fetal compartment.[221] This process is in contrast to high-affinity binding of CMV by IgG anti-CMV gB antibodies that is known to be required to prevent fetal transmission, presumably because the high-affinity antibody remains bound to the virus following transcytosis into syncytiotrophoblasts, thereby preventing infection of the cytotrophoblasts and stromal fibroblasts.[171,221]

Passive immunization with monoclonal antibodies and hyperimmune globulin (HIG) is currently being investigated for the prevention of CMV transmission in pregnant women. A phase II trial, evaluating therapy with HIG in women with primary CMV infection, showed a small (but not statistically significant) decrease in the risk of fetal transmission of CMV in 61 women who received HIG (30% transmission; 18 fetuses or infants), compared with 62 women with primary CMV infection who received placebo (44% transmission; 18 fetuses or infants; $P = .13$).[278] Fouts and associates[111] demonstrated, through serial depletions on CMV antigen expressing cells, that the major neutralizing component in HIG preventing epithelial cell entry is antibody directed against a pentameric complex gH/gL/UL128/UL130/UL131, and the dominant component preventing fibroblast entry is antibody against gH/gL. Lilleri and colleagues[210] investigated the presence of neutralizing antibodies in pregnant women with primary CMV infection and found that titers of IgG antibodies to the pentameric complex gH/gL/UL128-131 and gH/gL appeared earlier and were significantly higher in women who did not transmit the CMV virus to the fetus (nontransmitters) compared with women who did (transmitters).[210] Serum absorption of antipentameric antibodies with a soluble pentameric complex abolished the ability of the sera of CMV-infected women to neutralize viral infection of epithelial cells. This finding indicates that maternal antibodies to the pentameric complex play an important protective role against maternal-fetal transmission of CMV and are thus attractive targets for the development of passive immunization strategies. RG7667, a combination of two neutralizing monoclonal antibodies (MCMV5322A: anti-gH/gL; and MCMV3068A: anti-gH/gL/UL128-131), was evaluated in a phase I trial; this combination was shown to block CMV cell entry in fibroblasts, epithelial cells, endothelial cells, and macrophages and was safe and well tolerated in healthy adults.[162]

Researchers have examined the possible blockade of the proinflammatory cascade that accompanies severe infections.[1,20,117,194] The experimental attempts using monoclonal antibodies to modify the release and action of the proinflammatory mediators that lead to septic shock have focused on the proinflammatory effects of the cytokine family, endotoxin, and the functions of neutrophils and complement. Eculizumab (Soliris), a humanized monoclonal anti-C5 complement antibody that prevents the activation of terminal complement pathway, was approved by the US Food and Drug Administration (FDA) for treatment of atypical HUS and paroxysmal nocturnal hemoglobinuria.[261,320] The safety profile of eculizumab remains unclear, however, with rare reports of *Aspergillus niger* peritonitis[325] and meningococcal disease[101] in adults. Meningococcal bacteremia and elevated liver function test results have been reported in the pediatric population.[261] Nonetheless, case reports have shown eculizumab to be an effective treatment in atypical HUS.[261] Eculizumab is not indicated in the treatment of STEC-related HUS.

Treatment with monoclonal antibodies, such as rituximab, an antiCD20 therapeutic monoclonal antibody, and infliximab, an anti–tumor necrosis factor-α (TNF-α) monoclonal antibody, in patients with immune disorders increases the risk for certain infections, such as nontuberculous mycobacteria, as well as increased risk of malignancy including lymphoma.[45,138,277] Rituximab also profoundly depresses B-lymphocyte number and may lead to profound, persisting hypogammaglobulinemia.

CYTOKINES

Lymphokines and Monokines

The cytokines are a family of small, soluble protein molecules responsible for cell-to-cell communication. They are produced by several cell types and play crucial roles in many biologic processes, including growth, inflammation, immunity, and hematopoiesis. During infection, genes for nearly all the cytokines are expressed. The biologic activity of the prototype cytokines, the lymphokines and monokines, include interleukins and TNF-α; these molecules, along with the granulocyte colony-stimulating factors (G-CSFs), have received considerable attention as potential immunomodulatory agents. In response to pathogen invasion, these cytokines perform a complex series of interactions to initiate a cascade of biologic events resulting in the propagation and subsequent regulation of the inflammatory response, thereby leading to pathogen alienation while maintaining host preservation. Thus, the cytokine family, through a complex web of interactions, functions to initiate and then both to upregulate and downregulate the inflammatory response. On the basis of their roles of either upregulating or downregulating immune responsiveness, the cytokines generally and historically have been classified as either proinflammatory or antiinflammatory molecules. Although many cytokines have the potential to perform dual functions, either directly or indirectly, their proinflammatory or antiinflammatory properties are of considerable basic science and clinical therapeutic interest.[34,63,88,109,194,200,209,259]

Some prominent proinflammatory cytokines and their cellular sources are listed in Table 242.1. TNF-α and IL-1 generally are considered to be prominent early proinflammatory mediators. They induce gene expression of other proinflammatory cytokines, including IL-6 and IL-8, thereby leading to neutrophil activation, recruitment, and degranulation. TNF-α and IL-1 also activate a secondary cascade of inflammatory mediators, including arachidonic acid–derived prostaglandin I_2, thromboxane A_2, prostaglandin E_2, platelet-activating factor (PAF), and the complement system. The CSFs and IL-3 also are proinflammatory cytokines that induce bone marrow stem cell production of granulocytes and monocytes, in addition to activating neutrophils and inducing production of IL-1 and TNF-α.[34,63,88,109,194,200,209,259]

Prominent among the antiinflammatory cytokines (Table 242.2) are IL-4, IL-10, IL-13, and transforming growth factor-β. These cytokines may block endotoxin induction of IL-1 and TNF-α and suppress lymphocyte and monocyte function. In addition, the IL-1 receptor antagonist blocks the proinflammatory action of IL-1 by binding its receptor.[34,63,88,109,194,200,209]

Considerable experimental and clinical interest has focused on the proinflammatory cytokines TNF-α and IL-1 as important early mediators in the pathogenesis of sepsis and septic shock syndrome. The basis for the potential therapeutic utility of these two cytokines in human disease states involves two clinically distinct hypotheses: (1) excessive cytokine production results in host immune injury, leading to severe shock; and (2) deficient cytokine production renders a host susceptible to infection by invasive pathogens.[194]

The hypothesis that cytokine overproduction can lead to severe lethal shock is demonstrated in several animal models and is suggested in patients with overwhelming sepsis. The outer membranes of gram-negative bacteria contain LPSs or endotoxin, which induce the early proinflammatory cytokines TNF-α, IL-6, and IL-1. Although these cytokines may protect the host from infection, if they are expressed in excessive amounts, their effects can result in multiple organ failure and death. During severe sepsis, the levels of both TNF-α and IL-1 increase proportionately with the degree of hypotension and organ failure. The combination of these two cytokines can result in synergism over their individual effects by severalfold and can lead to lethal septic shock syndrome.[50,51] In animal models of shock and gram-negative sepsis, TNF-α levels rise rapidly after injection of bacteria or endotoxin and

TABLE 242.1 Proinflammatory Cytokines

Cytokine	Function	Predominant Cell Source
Tumor necrosis factor-α	Stimulates interleukin-6 and colony-stimulating factors Depresses erythropoiesis, stimulates interleukin-8 and interleukin-9 Promotes tumor necrosis and endotoxic shock	Monocytes and macrophages
Interleukin-1	Stimulates proliferation and differentiation of T and B lymphocytes Stimulates T lymphocytes to produce interleukin-2 Promotes colony-stimulating factor, interleukin-8 and interleukin-9 production, and endotoxic shock	Macrophages, astrocytes, monocytes, fibroblasts, keratinocytes, B lymphocytes, corneal epithelium, and other cell types
Interleukin-2	Stimulates growth of T lymphocytes Stimulates B-lymphocyte and monocyte differentiation Increases cytotoxicity of T lymphocytes and natural killer cells	Activated T lymphocytes
Interleukin-3	Multipotential hematopoietic cell growth factor Stimulates early B and T lymphocytes Mast cell growth factor	Activated T lymphocytes, natural killer cells
Interleukin-5	Stimulates eosinophil formation and differentiation Augments T lymphocyte cytotoxicity and proliferation of B lymphocytes	T lymphocytes, mast cells
Interleukin-7	Supports growth of pre-B lymphocytes Stimulates T lymphocytes	B lymphocytes, bone marrow fibroblasts, monocytes
Interleukin-8	Stimulates neutrophil, monocyte, and lymphocyte activation chemotaxis	Monocytes
Interleukin-9	Stimulates neutrophil, monocyte, and lymphocyte activation chemotaxis Stimulates erythroid progenitors, helper T-lymphocyte growth factor	T lymphocytes
Interleukin-11	T-lymphocyte–dependent stimulator of B lymphocytes	Bone marrow fibroblasts
Interleukin-12	Stimulates helper T-lymphocyte differentiation and interleukin-2 production Stimulates interferon-γ production Increases cytotoxicity of natural killer cells	T and B lymphocytes, lymphoblastoid cells
Interleukin-14	Stimulates proliferation of activated B lymphocytes Inhibits immunoglobulin secretion from B lymphocytes	T lymphocytes
Interleukin-15	Stimulates T-lymphocyte function and proliferation Enhances natural killer cell function	Monocytes and macrophages
Interleukin-16	Promotes migration of T lymphocytes	T lymphocytes
Interleukin-17	Stimulates interleukin-6 and interleukin-8 production	T lymphocytes
Interleukin-18	Stimulates interferon-γ and tumor necrosis factor-α production	Macrophages, mononuclear cells, and dendritic cells
Granulocyte colony-stimulating factor	Stimulates neutrophil colony formation	Monocytes and fibroblasts
Granulocyte-macrophage colony-stimulating factor	Stimulates granulocyte and monocyte formation Induces tumor necrosis factor	T lymphocytes, natural killer cells, endothelial cells, fibroblasts, and keratinocytes
Macrophage colony-stimulating factor	Activates monocytes and granulocytes Stimulates macrophage colony formation Induces interleukin-1 and tumor necrosis factor	Fibroblasts, monocytes, and endothelial cells

TABLE 242.2 **Antiinflammatory Cytokines**

Cytokine	Function	Predominant Cell Source
Interleukin-4	Stimulates proliferation of T and B lymphocytes and megakaryocytes A growth factor for mast cells and erythroid precursors	T lymphocytes
Interleukin-6	Blocks endotoxin induction of interleukin-1 and tumor necrosis factor B- and T-lymphocyte–stimulating activity	Monocytes, T and B lymphocytes, fibroblasts, epithelial and endothelial cells
Interleukin-10	Blocks production of interleukin-1 and tumor necrosis factor Inhibits primary allogeneic T-lymphocyte responses Inhibits interleukin-2, interleukin-8, and granulocyte-macrophage colony-stimulating factor	T and B lymphocytes, macrophages and monocytes
Interleukin-13	Blocks production of interleukin-1, tumor necrosis factor, and interleukin-8 Suppresses nitric oxide formation	T lymphocytes
Interleukin-1 receptor antagonist	Binds interleukin-1 receptors, blocking interleukin-1 effects	Monocytes and macrophages
Transforming growth factor-β	Reduces endotoxin-induced interleukin-1 and tumor necrosis factor production	Monocytes and macrophages

reach peak concentrations at 60 to 90 minutes, whereas IL-1 levels rise more slowly, peaking at 180 minutes. A similar time course response has been observed in human subjects injected with endotoxin.[51,236] Children with septicemia and purpura fulminans and children with meningococcal disease demonstrated an association between morbidity and mortality and high serum levels of TNF-α and IL-1.[119,245] These studies and others implicate TNF-α and IL-1 as prominent modulators in the development of the septic shock syndrome and suggest that a potential therapeutic benefit may be obtained by inhibiting the production of these cytokines and reducing their proinflammatory effects.

Experimental attempts to attenuate the excessive proinflammatory cytokine activity of TNF-α and IL-1 have focused on (1) inhibiting release of endotoxin. (2) blocking endotoxin–target cell binding and preventing the transmembrane signaling mechanisms leading to production of TNF-α and IL-1, (3) controlling the synthesis of TNF-α and IL-1 by inhibiting or suppressing specific cytokine gene transcription and translation, (4) inhibiting release of TNF-α and IL-1, (5) administering TNF-α and IL-1 neutralizing antibodies and soluble receptors, (6) producing and administering TNF-α and IL-1 receptor antagonists that block specific cytokine binding to target cell receptors, and (7) blocking TNF-α or IL-1 intracellular transmembrane signaling mechanisms and preventing their action on target cells.[200]

The use of monoclonal antiendotoxin antibodies to inhibit the binding of endotoxin to its target cells has received considerable attention. Numerous in vitro and in vivo animal experiments have suggested that blocking of endotoxin leads to improved survival by inhibiting proinflammatory cytokine production and expression.[247] The initial clinical studies in patients with gram-negative bacteremia who were treated with immunoglobulin preparations directed against endotoxin demonstrated a significant reduction in mortality rates.[21,293] Further studies suggested a reduction of septic shock in similarly treated high-risk surgical patients.[21] These observations led to the development of several clinical trials using human monoclonal antiendotoxin antibodies. HA-1A is a human monoclonal antibody against the lipid A moiety of bacterial endotoxin. The mechanism of HA-1A action is to block endotoxin triggering of the intracellular events leading to proinflammatory cytokine synthesis. In placebo-controlled clinical trials of HA-1A, either HA-1A or placebo was infused during the course of 20 minutes to patients with severe sepsis. These patients also received cardiopulmonary support and antibacterial therapy. The etiologic agents of sepsis included *E. coli, Pseudomonas,* and *Klebsiella* and *Enterobacter* spp. The investigators reported that HA-1A significantly reduced the incidence of mortality in adults with septic shock and gram-negative bacteremia. The mortality rate for those patients who were in severe shock before receiving HA-1A was reduced by 42%.[352] Although these early clinical studies using HA-1A were encouraging, a protective role for antiendotoxin antibodies was not established in subsequent clinical trials.[161,216] Antiendotoxin therapy may be more effective if it is given earlier during the sepsis syndrome before the development of shock. Because bacterial lysis caused by antibiotics is an ongoing process and results in further release of endotoxin, multiple doses of antiendotoxin antibodies also may prove beneficial in treating sepsis. The future clinical use of antiendotoxin antibodies may be in combination with other immunomodulation therapies, directed at simultaneously blocking several steps in both the propagation and action of proinflammatory cytokines.

Studies of cytokine inhibition have focused on controlling TNF-α and IL-1 with anti–TNF-α antibodies directed at these specific cytokines and their receptors. Control of proinflammatory cytokine synthesis is specific for each individual cytokine and requires an understanding of the unique temporal relationships among molecules during the propagation of inflammatory responses. A critical aspect of TNF-α and IL-1 gene expression in a variety of cell types has been the reported exquisite sensitivity of these cytokines to bacterial endotoxin.[63,88,194,200] Human blood monocytes synthesize TNF-α and IL-1 in the presence of endotoxin. In the absence of endotoxin, however, gene expression occurs, but protein translation does not take place.[294] Thus, these cells may be viewed as being primed for bacterial endotoxin exposure. TNF-α and IL-1 transcription is suppressed by the antiinflammatory cytokines IL-10, IL-13, and transforming growth factor-β, but the clinical therapeutic benefits these cytokines have in treating septic shock remain to be defined.[65,139,239,295] Agents blocking the lipoxygenase pathway of arachidonate metabolism also have been implicated in the reduction of TNF-α and IL-1 synthesis, and corticosteroids have been shown to suppress both TNF-α and IL-1 transcription and synthesis, but only when they have been administered before transcription has been initiated.[107,291]

The use of corticosteroids in infants and children with bacterial meningitis demonstrated that treatment with a combination of dexamethasone and antibiotics results in lower cerebrospinal fluid levels of TNF-α than occurs with treatment with placebo and antibiotics.[245] In addition, patients treated with corticosteroids had fewer neurologic symptoms.[174] Subsequent multicenter trials, however, failed to establish a protective effect of corticosteroid use in the treatment of children with meningitis.[327] One possible explanation for this discrepancy may be that corticosteroids almost exclusively suppress endotoxin-induced, proinflammatory cytokine gene transcription but have little or no effect on proinflammatory cytokine translation.[88,307] Thus, some investigators have suggested that the early administration of corticosteroids, before transcription has been initiated, would block cytokine synthesis. Timing of corticosteroid administration therefore may account for some of the clinical variability seen with its use in children with meningitis. Clinical trials are focusing on TNF-α and IL-1 synthesis with the administration of corticosteroids either before or while antibiotics are administered. Similarly, the temporal use of antibiotics, corticosteroids, and antiendotoxin therapy may result in an additive therapeutic benefit.

Neutralizing monoclonal antibodies against murine or human TNF-α have been shown to decrease mortality rates in several experimental animal models of sepsis.[27,225,319] Studies with soluble TNF-α receptors or their immunoadhesin constructs also have demonstrated an immunoprotective effect of TNF-α blockade in animal models of endotoxemia or bacteremia.[25] Although anti–TNF-α antibodies are being used with caution in humans, anti–TNF-α treatment in a limited number of patients with established septic shock resulted in increased vascular hemodynamics and left ventricular stroke volume.[131] The in vitro use of free soluble TNF-α receptors to bind TNF-α results in a 10- to 50-fold increase in binding affinity over that observed with anti–TNF-α monoclonal antibodies.[132] Results from phase II clinical trials using soluble TNF-α receptors, however, have not shown improvement in survival rates; moreover, administration of high doses actually increased the incidence of mortality.[132,288]

Certain naturally occurring substances inhibit IL-1 synthesis and action, but they also have effects on many of the other cytokines. Specific inhibitors of IL-1, however, have been identified. Most prominent of these is the IL-1 receptor inhibitor that competes with the binding of IL-1 to its cell surface receptor. Recombinant IL-1 receptor antagonist (IL-1ra) that blocks IL-1 effects has been studied in various animal models.[4,256] For instance, IL-1ra prevents death from endotoxic shock in rabbits.[256] The therapeutic use of IL-1ra in treating septic shock in early phase II human clinical trials showed improved survival rates at 28 days.[108] The subsequent randomized phase III trials, however, failed to show improvement in patients with severe shock.[107] Further clinical studies are ongoing. IL-1ra also has been used in treatment trials of patients with acute myelogenous leukemia. The uncontrolled production of IL-1 by leukemic blasts has been proposed to result in the continued proliferation of these cells and the development of acute myelogenous leukemia. Studies have shown that IL-1ra blocks the spontaneous proliferation and production of granulocyte-macrophage CSF (GM-CSF), IL-1, and IL-6 in the peripheral blood and bone marrow cells of these patients.[276] The potential clinical use of IL-1ra is being investigated in patients with psoriasis, rheumatoid arthritis, and myelogenous leukemia.[134] Similarly, combination therapy with the simultaneous blockade of both TNF-α and IL-1 is being investigated in endotoxin models of shock and a number of clinical disease states.[286]

Another approach to attenuate excessive proinflammatory cytokine responses is the use of pharmacologic agents. Salyer and colleagues[289] demonstrated that pentoxifylline, a methylxanthine derivative that blocks TNF-α transcription and production, could override some of the effects of TNF-α on PMNs. In this study, the profound decrease in human PMN chemotactic ability caused by excessive TNF-α was restored to normal by treatment with pentoxifylline. The specific mechanisms of this effect of pentoxifylline effect are not known, but the drug has been shown to restore PMN membrane fluidity inhibited by TNF-α that is critical for cell movement.[252,254] Furthermore, pentoxifylline can block PMN adhesion to endothelium and result in decreased PMN respiratory burst activity, which is thought to be responsible for the improved survival rates seen in pentoxifylline-treated animal models of endotoxin-induced septic shock.[258] Some of the clinical trials using pentoxifylline in surgical patients with early evidence of systemic inflammation have suggested a cardioprotective effect, although other studies have been less convincing.[100,310] Pentoxifylline also has been evaluated in preterm infants with sepsis. A meta-analysis of 6 randomized controlled trials with 416 infants found that pentoxifylline used as adjuncts to antibiotics in neonates with sepsis decreased all-cause mortality (typical relative risk, 0.57; 95% confidence interval [CI], 0.35–0.93; typical risk difference, −0.08; 95% CI, −0.14 to −0.01; number needed to treat to benefit = 13; 95% CI, 7–100).[262] No adverse effects attributable to pentoxifylline were noted. Pentoxifylline did not change the risk of necrotizing enterocolitis (NEC) in neonates with sepsis. Amrinone, a phosphodiesterase inhibitor, also has been shown to reduce TNF-α levels in LPS-challenged mice.[120] Thus, these and other pharmacologic agents may be useful in preventing or reducing some of the adverse and even fatal effects that are mediated by proinflammatory cytokines.

IVIG may have a potential inhibitory effect on proinflammatory cytokine activity. Patients in the active phase of Kawasaki disease have increased levels of TNF-α and IL-1. These cytokines have been postulated to stimulate local inflammatory responses by regulating leukocyte adherence and activation, thereby leading to the vascular damage that is a critical clinical aspect of this disease. Another suggestion is that the effects of IVIG therapy in Kawasaki disease, and perhaps in other diseases, may result from the attenuating production of the proinflammatory cytokines TNF-α and IL-1.[6,16,146] Animal models of LPS-induced TNF-α and IL-1 synthesis demonstrate a suppression of mononuclear cell synthesis of these proinflammatory cytokines when they are treated with IVIG.[18] The peripheral blood mononuclear cell production of TNF-α and IL-1, however, in patients with Kawasaki disease who were receiving IVIG therapy showed decreased synthesis of IL-1 but not of TNF-α.[203,202] The role of IVIG as an immunomodulator has been suggested in an ever-growing number of clinical disease states because of its broad immunoregulatory potential.[16,142] IVIG is indicated for the treatment of Kawasaki disease,[251] and it has also used in the treatment of severe autoimmune neutropenia of infancy[49] and in cases of fetal and neonatal alloimmune thrombocytopenia.[118]

The hypothesis that diminished levels of cytokines may render a host susceptible to development of infection was introduced by Weatherstone and Rich.[331] They suggested that the increased susceptibility to infection observed in premature neonates may be secondary to deficient proinflammatory cytokine production. In their study, these investigators measured cord blood monocyte secretion of TNF-α and IL-1 with and without stimulation of LPS. IL-1 activity by LPS-stimulated preterm monocytes did not differ from that observed by LPS-stimulated adult monocytes. TNF-α activity, however, in the LPS-stimulated monocytes from preterm neonates was significantly lower than that in both stimulated and unstimulated adult monocytes. Thus, these investigators concluded that diminished production of TNF-α may predispose the preterm infant to acquisition of infection. This finding has not been supported by the studies of infected animals, which show markedly elevated TNF-α levels, and subsequent studies in preterm infants have not established a deficiency in TNF-α.[339] Williams and colleagues[339] and Peat and coworkers[266] have, in contrast, shown that mononuclear cells from term neonates produced enhanced levels of TNF-α in response to GBS or endotoxin. Ongoing studies are defining the role of cytokine production in neonatal and other infections.

The proinflammatory cytokine IL-2 acts on activated T lymphocytes and to some extent on B lymphocytes and natural killer (NK) cells and causes them to proliferate or differentiate. IL-2 is synthesized by both T cells and NK cells.[238,329] Decreased IL-2 production or IL-2 receptor expression has been noted in a number of clinical disease states, most notably in cases of severe combined immunodeficiency disease. Lesser degrees of abnormalities may occur in acquired immunodeficiency syndrome (AIDS), type 1 diabetes mellitus, systemic lupus erythematosus, and hypogammaglobulinemia.[194,200,209] The most intriguing potential for IL-2 in the treatment of disease involves its use in tumor therapy.[284] IL-2 currently is approved for the treatment of metastatic renal carcinoma. Use of IL-2–activated NK cells results in a decrease in tumor burden in approximately 20% of patients, although serious side effects occur. In addition to its potential role as an antitumor agent, IL-2 shares many of the same effects as interferon-γ (IFN-γ) and may someday function as a therapeutic agent in infection, autoimmunity, and immunodeficiency.[200,284]

Both IL-8 and IL-9 have been investigated in various human disease states, primarily because of their powerful role in stimulating neutrophil function, including activation, adhesion, and chemotaxis. Patients with cystic fibrosis, bronchiectasis, and chronic bronchitis have demonstrated elevated levels of IL-8 in their sputum.[279] The sputum from these patients is highly chemotactic to neutrophils, but with treatment with monoclonal antibodies to IL-8, this chemotactic effect was inhibited. Aerosolized IL-8 inhibitors have been used in patients with cystic fibrosis and have resulted in decreased inflammation in these patients.[227,279] IL-8 inhibitors are being evaluated in infants with bronchopulmonary dysplasia. Researchers have speculated that the persistently elevated levels of IL-8 in the tracheal fluid of ventilated preterm infants lead to neutrophil accumulation and the development of pulmonary fibrosis, which may be reduced by IL-8 inhibitors.[169,181] Similar studies are being conducted with IL-9 inhibitors. Thus, these cytokines may play an important role in the acute inflammatory response leading to chronic disease states, and blocking of this response may be of therapeutic benefit. The proinflammatory IL-5 has not been implicated in a specific human disease state, but its strong B-cell proliferative effects suggest that it has a possible role in the pathogenesis of immunodeficiency, and its potent effects on eosinophil production, activation, and migration implicate its action in allergic responses.[44]

The proinflammatory activities of IL-12 and IL-18 are also of current immunologic interest. IL-12 is an integral immune regulator that is produced primarily by macrophages and dendritic cells.[254] IL-12 has been shown to induce the production of IFN-γ by T cells and natural NK cells.[219,220,254] IL-18 is another cytokine with many proinflammatory functions.[229] IL-18 was defined initially as IFN-γ–inducing factor.[52,89,201] IL-12 and IL-18, both alone and in synergy, regulate IFN-γ production in response to infection with intracellular parasites and bacteria and in certain autoimmune diseases.* The regulation of these cytokines may be therapeutically beneficial in certain disease states.[95,127,224] The other proinflammatory cytokines also are in various developmental stages of experimental investigation. As we learn more about their specific actions, we will better be able to determine their use as potential immunomodulating agents.

The antiinflammatory cytokines have limited clinical use. IL-4 can block both IL-1 and TNF-α transcription.[139,295] IL-4 has been shown to inhibit human neutrophil adhesion to human endothelial cells while enhancing the adhesion of eosinophils.[242] These effects have not been implicated in specific human diseases, but an IL-4 action is suggested in allergic responses. Although IL-6 has both antiinflammatory and proinflammatory effects, the levels of this cytokine were found to correlate with mortality rates in children with gram-negative and gram-positive sepsis, thereby suggesting that monitoring of IL-6 levels may be of prognostic value.[323] Similarly, IL-10 has been shown to block production of IL-1, IL-6, IL-8, IL-12, and TNF-α, as well as GM-CSF, in animal models.[78,222] IL-10 also has effects on mast cells, T cells, and NK cells, and it inhibits primary allogeneic T-cell responses. Thus, IL-10 may have a potential role in treating acute and chronic inflammation and may be effective in suppressing transplant rejection.[22,78] Studies examining the safety and immunomodulatory effects of the intravenous injection of IL-10 in humans demonstrate that it is well tolerated and results in decreased production of both TNF-α and IL-1.[34] Additional clinical studies have been conducted on the potential immunoregulatory effects of the antiinflammatory cytokines and may indicate the therapeutic use of these agents in human disease states.

IL-17 is a proinflammatory cytokine implicated in the regulation of many inflammatory states. IL-17 is produced by several cell types, including activated T-cell subsets, NK cells, and neutrophils.[91,212,314] IL-17 is involved in the regulation of inflammatory bowel disease and systemic lupus erythematosus.[183] IL-17 production is markedly deficient in patients with autosomal dominant hyper-IgE (Job syndrome) who have neutrophil chemotactic defects and recurrent bacterial and candidal infections.[193] More recently, decreased intracellular and extracellular production of IL-17 by cord blood mononuclear cells suggested that IL-17 may contribute to the human neonates' increased susceptibility to microbial infections.[59,60] Furthermore, the addition of IL-17 to cord blood mixed mononuclear cells significantly enhances production of the proinflammatory cytokines IL-6, TNF-α, IL-1β, and IL-8 in response to GBS.[59,60] IL-23 promotes the development and survival of IL-17–producing cells. The IL-17/IL-23 axis has been implicated in mediating initial neutrophil responses during infection. Dysregulation of this pathway is suggested in autoimmune diseases (i.e., multiple sclerosis, Crohn disease, and rheumatoid arthritis).[91,92,313] IL-17/IL-23 levels are elevated in patients with systemic lupus erythematosus and correlate with symptoms.[207,344,348] Current efforts are under investigation to modulate the IL-17/IL-23 axis to regulate autoimmunity and inflammation.[175] In a phase III randomized controlled trial of treatment with the anti–IL-17A monoclonal antibody, secukinumab (Cosentyx), in 397 patients with psoriatic arthritis,[15] patients were assigned to 300 mg, 150 mg, or 75 mg subcutaneous secukinumab or placebo.[15] Subcutaneous secukinumab at 300- and 150-mg doses significantly improved the signs and symptoms of psoriasis, defined as at least 20% improvement in the American College of Rheumatology response criteria (ACR20). Common adverse outcomes included respiratory infections and nasopharyngitis. Secukinumab is now approved by the FDA for use in the treatment of moderate to severe plaque psoriasis in adults. Ustekinumab (Stelara), a monoclonal antibody to the shared p40 subunit of IL-12 and IL-23, is also FDA approved for the treatment of treatment of moderate to severe plaque psoriasis in adults, after the agent was shown to be effective in achieving at least ACR20 at 24 weeks, with continued benefit at 52 weeks.[281] Brodalumab, a monoclonal antibody to the IL-17A receptor, has also been shown to be effective for the treatment of psoriasis in clinical trials, and was approved by the FDA in February 2017, despite termination of the Study of Efficacy and Safety of Brodalumab Compared With Placebo and Ustekinumab in Moderate to Severe Plaque Psoriasis Subjects (AMAGINE) phase III trials after two suicides were reported, with lingering uncertainty regarding reports of suicidal ideation.[79,233]

The removal of cytokines from blood of septic patients has received attention. The continuous removal of cytokines in the systemic inflammatory response syndrome by hemofiltration and hemodialysis is currently being used.[348] Cytokine adsorption has also received attention. CytoSorb, a hemoadsorption system, has been reported to decrease proinflammatory marker concentrations and significantly reduce supportive vasopressor requirements in patients with septic shock[153] and cardiogenic shock.[46] A randomized controlled trial in 43 patients with septic shock and acute lung injury showed that CytoSorb was safe and significantly reduced IL-6 concentrations compared with controls.[292] A randomized controlled trial in patients undergoing cardiopulmonary bypass (CPB), however, did not show a significant reduction in proinflammatory cytokine concentrations following hemoadsorption.[23] CPB has been shown to trigger proinflammatory cytokine production in an unpredictable manner because of contact activation of blood and white blood cells by artificial surfaces in the extracorporeal circuit.[82] The lack of significant IL-6 production found by Bernardi and colleagues[23] may be attributable to the much shorter duration of CPB (191 ± 56 minutes) than in patients in prior case reports (4 hours to 4 days), as the investigators point out in their study. An additional clinical trial evaluating the use of CytoSorb during CPB is currently under way.[19] The use of synthetic polymer resins,[173] immobilized antibody systems,[253] and activated carbon[13] is also under investigation. The polymyxin B filtration system has been shown to protect mice from the endotoxin-induced shock,[47] and it is under investigation in adult patients with gram-negative sepsis in intensive care units.[74] These efforts to reduce the proinflammatory cytokine load may have a role in the treatment of septic shock.

Colony-Stimulating Factors

CSFs are involved principally in the production of neutrophils and monocytes. They were discovered because of their ability to stimulate the formation of colonies of granulocytes and monocyte-macrophages in cultured bone marrow cells and were named according to the primary cell colony type that they elicited. GM-CSF induces peripheral blood macrophages and granulocytes. It also has other pleiotropic effects, including stimulation of precursors of megakaryocytes, mast cells, and eosinophils. In addition, GM-CSF has effects on neutrophil migration and phagocytosis. G-CSF induces peripheral blood granulocytes. Its actions are on both the production and the function of neutrophils, including migration, phagocytosis, and superoxide generation. Macrophage CSF (M-CSF) induces peripheral mononuclear phagocytes. IL-3 increases mast cell populations, as well as the induction of granulocytes, macrophages, eosinophils, and megakaryocytes.[90,91,130,191,201,208,235]

Clinical studies with GM-CSF and G-CSF as adjuvant therapy have been performed in individuals with distinct lymphopoietic disorders (i.e., congenital agranulocytosis, cyclic neutropenia, Shwachman-Diamond syndrome) or those disorders that are the consequences of cytotoxic chemotherapy, AIDS, and aplastic anemia. The CSFs can stimulate granulocyte and monocyte populations in these individuals, but the response is restricted to the number of available stem cells. CSF treatment can partially or completely reverse congenital neutropenia and has shown great promise in regeneration of lymphopoietic cells after administration of cytotoxic chemotherapy and high-dose chemotherapy followed by autologous bone marrow transplantation. Recombinant human GM-CSF (rhGM-CSF) also has been shown to be beneficial in patients with aplastic anemia.[12,13,321] Hammond and colleagues[135] demonstrated a dramatic increase in neutrophil counts in children with cyclic neutropenia who were treated with recombinant human G-CSF (rhG-CSF). Cyclic neutropenia is a rare disorder characterized by regular, 21-day cyclic fluctuations in the number of blood neutrophils, monocytes, eosinophils, lymphocytes, platelets, and reticulocytes. Although the exact

*References 89, 95, 127, 150, 157, 172, 224, 255, 308, 313, 314, 324, 332, 349.

mechanism of this disorder is not known, it is attributed to a regulatory abnormality affecting proliferation of stem cells. These infants have recurrent aphthous stomatitis, pharyngitis, lymphadenopathy, fever, and numerous infections during the periods of neutropenia. The length of cycling in treated infants decreased from 21 days to 1 day, and the neutrophil turnover rate increased nearly fourfold, thus significantly reducing the frequency of infection. The use of rhG-CSF also has shown promise for infants and children with neutrophil production disorders. Infants with congenital agranulocytosis, Kostmann syndrome, and Shwachman-Diamond syndrome, disorders characterized by severe, persistent absolute neutropenia, show a dramatic increase in neutrophil count after treatment with rhG-CSF.[33] In addition, rhG-CSF and rhGM-CSF have been used in neutropenic patients with AIDS. Despite the concern that the effects of GM-CSF to activate macrophages may in turn promote replication of human immunodeficiency virus (HIV), current studies are defining the role of rhGM-CSF and rhG-CSF in patients with AIDS.[129,208]

Thus, CSFs have emerged as significant modulators of human immune function and lymphopoiesis. Because the CSFs can functionally activate mature granulocytes and monocytes, considerable attention has focused on their future role in treating individuals at risk for acquiring infection. English and colleagues[94] reported decreased GM-CSF production by neonatal T cells. Because a major factor contributing to the increased susceptibility of human neonates to severe infections is their inability to produce adequate numbers of neutrophils in response to bacterial infections, these neonates may benefit from CSF treatment during severe infection.[29] Similar treatment in immunologically stressed patients with burns and trauma also may prove beneficial.[77,250]

INTERFERONS

Interferon-α and Interferon-β

The IFNs are glycoproteins that were discovered because of their antiviral properties. They are known to possess antitumor and immunomodulatory activities in addition to their antiviral effects.[17] The IFNs have been classified into three major groups: α, β, and γ. IFN-α and IFN-β were previously known as type I IFNs and have similar protein structures and bind the same receptor. IFN-γ, formerly type II IFN, has a much different structure and its own receptor.[9] IFN-α is produced by leukocytes. The earliest demonstration of its clinical usefulness was in the treatment of AIDS-related Kaposi sarcoma. In these initial studies, a Kaposi sarcoma tumor response occurred in 30% to 50% of the patients treated with recombinant IFN-α.[128,188,240,244] Researchers have speculated that IFN-α exerts its antitumor effect by activating cytotoxic T cells. Since then, placebo-controlled clinical trials have shown that IFN-α also may have significant antiretroviral effect in HIV-infected patients.[186,198] Clinical trials have been conducted to determine the effect of early treatment with IFN-α in reducing progression of HIV disease and to determine the therapeutic effect of IFN-α in combination with other drugs in the treatment of HIV infection and HIV-related diseases.[185,187]

IFN-α also has been used in various parts of the world for the treatment of chronic myeloid leukemia, hairy cell leukemia, basal cell carcinoma, multiple myeloma, hepatitis B and C, and condylomata acuminata (genital warts). In chronic myeloid leukemia, early treatment with IFN-α was reported to elicit complete hematologic remission in more than 70% of the patients treated. Many of these patients had total elimination of the Philadelphia chromosome, which is a hallmark of the disease.[315–317] Complete to 80% remissions also have been reported in the treatment of hairy cell leukemia.[273] Intralesional injection of IFN-α into basal cell carcinoma of the skin resulted in 81% tumor remission, as determined by biopsy.[70,164] Despite the variability of the outcomes among reports on the use of IFN-α in the treatment of multiple myeloma, it has been approved as therapy for these patients in a number of European countries.[223]

IFN-α also is used for the treatment of hepatitis B and C.[201] Clinical responses have been reported to be of long duration, often with complete loss of both hepatitis B surface antigen and evidence of viral replication. In chronic hepatitis C, complete responses to therapy, determined by the decline of serum aspartate aminotransferase to normal levels, have been observed in 50% to 70% of the patients treated. Although serum aspartate aminotransferase levels in one-half of the patients who had improved returned to pretreatment levels within 6 to 12 months after discontinuation of therapy, nearly 20% achieved sustained remission.[80,86,156,182,267] Studies also have shown that IFN-α is useful in treating condylomata acuminata caused by papillomaviruses.[43] Intralesional injections of IFN-α completely eliminated warts in more than 50% of the patients treated. IFN-α therapy also is suggested to reduce the number of lesions in juvenile laryngeal papillomatosis after systemic use.[217] Thus, IFN-α has therapeutic potential as both an antitumor agent and an antiviral agent.

IFN-β also has received attention as an antiviral and antitumor agent. Its clinical usefulness as a single-agent therapy is suggested in relapsing multiple sclerosis. The mechanism of IFN-β therapeutic action in multiple sclerosis is unknown.[165] Ongoing studies are investigating IFN-β therapy in combination with IFN-α in the treatment of various malignant neoplasms.

Interferon-γ

IFN-γ is produced by $CD4^+$ and $CD8^+$ cells as well as by NK cells.[144] Investigators have reported that circulating mononuclear cells and T cells from neonates are markedly deficient in their ability to produce IFN-γ in response to a variety of stimuli, compared with adult cells.[207,297,298,340] Studies using recombinant IFN-γ have shown that preincubation of neonatal neutrophils, which are deficient in their chemotactic ability, with recombinant IFN-γ enhances their chemotactic response to a level equal to that of adult neutrophils.[128] Other studies have shown that neonatal mixed mononuclear cells are deficient in the production of the IFN-γ–stimulating cytokines IL-12 and IL-18 in response to GBS.[148,150,170] In vitro treatment with recombinant IL-12 and IL-18 can correct this defect in IFN-γ production in response to GBS. These findings suggest that a potential role exists for the regulation of IFN-γ in neonatal host defense.

Job syndrome was first described by Davis, Schaller, and Wedgwood[81] in 1965 in two patients with recurrent staphylococcal abscesses. Patients with this syndrome often develop chronic sinopulmonary infections and mucocutaneous *Candida* infections. Hill and coworkers[151] observed that the patients with Job syndrome also have a profound defect in neutrophil chemotactic responsiveness along with extreme hyper-IgE. This defect in neutrophil chemotaxis is intermittent and occurs predominantly when the patient is symptomatic.[76,145,151] Because production of IFN-γ by mononuclear leukocytes in patients with hyper-IgE is markedly deficient or absent, in vitro studies were conducted to determine the effect of recombinant IFN-γ on the chemotactic responsiveness of neutrophils from patients with this syndrome. After pretreatment with IFN-γ, the chemotactic response of the neutrophils from patients with Job syndrome increased significantly, with an average enhancement of 300% above baseline to levels not significantly different from those of matched healthy controls.[168,349] In four patients with Job syndrome, preliminary trials of IFN-γ therapy with hyper-IgE suggested clinical benefit in three of these patients, with a significant decrease in eczema as well as in pulmonary symptoms and secretions.

Patients with chronic granulomatous disease (CGD) have an inherited deficiency in the proteins required for nicotinamide adenine dinucleotide phosphate oxidase activity. Phagocytes with this enzymatic defect are able to engulf bacteria but cannot generate the respiratory burst necessary to kill the organisms. Consequently, patients with CGD suffer severe, chronic, recurrent, life-threatening infections. The usefulness of treating patients with CGD with IFN-γ was suggested by studies showing that this lymphokine can stimulate the respiratory burst of normal phagocytes. Results of studies by Ezekowitz and colleagues[98] and Sechler and coworkers[296] showed that when macrophages from patients with CGD were treated with IFN-γ in vitro, a respiratory burst occurred, and superoxide anion was generated. Sechler and colleagues[296] further demonstrated a partial correction in neutrophils and monocytes from patients with CGD after subcutaneous treatment with recombinant IFN-γ. These initial results suggested that when administered in vivo to patients with CGD, recombinant IFN-γ could partially correct the defective ability of phagocytes to kill bacteria. Ezekowitz and coworkers[99,144] extended these findings in a double-blind, placebo-controlled trial. They showed that recombinant IFN-γ significantly decreased the relative risk for development of serious infection in patients with CGD, but these studies failed to demonstrate an effect of IFN-γ on respiratory burst activity. This cytokine most likely affects the arginine–nitric oxide pathway in neutrophils and macrophages. Patients who received IFN-γ had a 70% reduction in the risk for development of serious infection compared with control subjects. Overall, IFN-γ decreases the risk for development of infection and the duration of hospitalization in patients with CGD. When IFN-γ is administered with prophylactic antibiotics, an additive effect occurs, resulting in a nearly 20% increase in the infection-free rate of patients with CGD compared with IFN-γ alone.[99] IFN-γ was licensed by the FDA in December 1990 for the treatment of patients with CGD. The authors of the collaborative studies recommended its use with the addition of prophylactic antibiotics for treatment of patients diagnosed with CGD.[115]

Clinical interest in the use of IFN-γ has focused on adjunctive immunotherapy in fungal infections. A randomized controlled trial evaluated the use of IFN-γ in 90 patients with HIV-associated cryptococcal meningitis, in which patients were assigned to one of three arms: (1) intravenous amphotericin B and oral flucytosine (standard therapy); (2) standard therapy plus two doses of IFN-γ; or (3) standard therapy plus six doses of IFN-γ.[167] The rate of fungal clearance, defined as the mean rate of decrease in CSF cryptococcal CFU (early fungicidal activity [EFA]), was significantly more rapid in the IFN-γ treatment arms than in the standard therapy arm (difference in EFA was −0.15 logCFU/mL per day [$P = .02$] standard treatment vs. IFN-γ two doses; and −0.15 logCFU/mL per day [$P = .006$] standard treatment vs. IFN-γ six doses), although there was no significant difference in mortality between the groups at 2 weeks.

More recently, a randomized prospective phase IIIb case series evaluated the use of recombinant IFN-γ in combination with anidulafungin (Eraxis) in 11 patients with invasive *Candida* and/or *Aspergillus* infections.[83] Eight patients were treated, and three were assigned to the control group and received placebo rather than IFN-γ. Two patients with invasive aspergillosis died, and one patient with *Candida* endocarditis developed intracerebral mycotic aneurysm. Peripheral blood mononuclear cells (PBMCs) were isolated before, during, and after treatment to assess the effect of IFN-γ on cytokine production. IFN-γ enhanced PBMC production of IL-17 and IL-22, cytokines that play a crucial role in fungal host defense, in response to *Candida* blastoconidia and hyphae in six of eight patients.[83] IFN-γ also increased the expression of human leukocyte antigen (HLA)-DR–positive monocytes in patients with a baseline starting at less than 50% (and thus considered immunosuppressed), suggesting partial restoration of immune function.[83]

TOLL-LIKE RECEPTORS

Toll-like receptors (TLRs) are pathogen pattern-recognition receptors central to innate immune responses.[166] TLRs are a family of type 1 integral membrane glycoproteins that detect pathogens and initiate cytokine production by activation of nuclear factor κB (NF-κB). The ligands recognized by TLRs consist of a wide range of evolutionarily conserved motifs, such as LPS, single- and double-stranded RNA, and zymosan. Collectively, these motifs are called pathogen-associated molecular patterns (PAMPs). TLR recognition of PAMPs contributes to the immediate response and broad specificity of innate immune recognition toward bacterial, viral, fungal, and parasitic pathogens. Twelve TLRs have been described in mammals, with at least 10 known in humans.[2,3,6]

The role of TLRs as immunomodulating agents is of contemporary interest. Amlie-Lefond and colleagues[5] described the potential use of TLR agonists as protective agents against biothreat pathogens. TLR-1 to TLR-10 in humans act to augment the immune response. TLR agonists can bolster this response and potentially offer protection against specific infections or diseases. Stimulation of TLR-7 and TLR-8 has shown antiviral and antineoplastic properties in humans. A drug known to do this, imiquimod (Aldara), has been shown to be beneficial against human papillomavirus, molluscum contagiosum, genital warts, and basal cell carcinoma.[5,71,318] Imiquimod has also been used to treat cutaneous squamous cell carcinoma in situ,[264] although it is not FDA approved for this indication, and there is a case report of invasive squamous cell carcinoma that developed following topical imiquimod treatment of carcinoma in situ.[123] Stimulation of TLR-2 by using pretreatment with PAM3CSK4, a TLR-2 agonist, has been studied in mice and was shown to increase bacterial clearance and decrease mortality in a mouse model of methicillin-resistant *Staphylococcus aureus* pneumonia.[66] TLR9 stimulation with CpG-oligodeoxynucleotide (CpG-ODN), which is found in bacterial and viral DNA, following introduction of a burn injury in a mouse model, with subsequent establishment of a secondary lung infection with *S. pneumoniae*, was shown to improve mouse survival significantly at 1 and 3 days when CpG-ODN was administered at 2 hours after traumatic injury.[328] Lung washout samples analyzed at 1 day by time-of-flight mass cytometry showed increased expression of IL-17 in TCRγδ T cells in the CpG-ODN–treated group (compared with the control group, which received saline). TCRγδ-negative CpG-ODN–treated mice showed decreased pathogen clearance, a finding suggesting that TLR-9–stimulated IL-17–producing TCRγδ T cells play a role in host defense against *S. pneumoniae* lung infection.

Immunomodulatory oligonucleotides stimulate TLRs and induce cytokine production. Immunomodulatory oligonucleotides offer potential clinical use for treatment of a number of inflammatory diseases, including severe acute respiratory syndrome, for which clinical trials are under way.[5] Similar use of immunomodulatory oligonucleotides in patients with renal carcinomas and HIV infection also is under investigation. Evidence suggests that TLR-3 activation can enhance innate immune response and enhances production of IFN-α.[189] These features render TLR-3 agonists attractive agents in the treatment of HIV-related infections and infections in certain immunocompromised patients.

TLR expression in human neonates is currently being defined.[287] TLR-2, TLR-4, and TLR-8 functions have been described in neonates. Researchers have speculated that deficiency of TLR activation may contribute to the neonate's increased susceptibility to infection.[326] The results of TLR expression in neonates have varied. In general, similar expression of TLR-1 to TLR-4 occurs in neonates and adults. Low-birth-weight or premature infants, however, demonstrate significantly decreased expression of TLR-4.[110,318] Most studies describe decreased cytokine production to TLR agonists in neonates compared with adults. In particular, TNF-α production is significantly lower in response to LPS stimulation of TLR-4 in neonates compared with adults, and it is speculated that this decreased stimulation may contribute to the neonate's increased susceptibility to *E. coli* and other gram-negative infections.[58,192] Similarly, Levy and colleagues[206] demonstrated that TLR-8 agonists are beneficial in activating costimulatory responses in neonatal antigen-presenting cells and suggested that this type of agent may be used adjuvantly to enhance the neonatal immune response.

NEUTROPHILS AND COMPLEMENT

Recruitment of neutrophils from the bloodstream to extravascular sites of inflammation is a critical event in host defense against bacterial infection and in the repair of tissue damage. Under certain circumstances, accumulation of neutrophils may contribute to vascular and tissue injury. Thus, the regulatory mechanisms involved in neutrophil activation, recruitment, and subsequent degranulation are of potential clinical significance. Neutrophil adherence to and migration through capillary endothelium are critical early events in the acute inflammatory response. The adhesive interactions between leukocytes and endothelial cell surfaces are regulated by two novel families of glycoproteins: the integrins and the selectins. The β_2 integrins are membrane-bound glycoprotein receptors found on the surface of PMNs. The β_2 integrins CD11 and CD18 are required for adherence of PMNs to endothelial cell surfaces. The selectins also are membrane-bound glycoproteins that mediate neutrophil adhesion to endothelial cells. They include L-selectin, which is found on the surface of PMNs, and P-selectin and E-selectin, which are expressed on the surface of activated endothelial cells.[28,57,309,335,354]

The interaction between the β_2 integrins and the selectins serves to regulate PMN responses during inflammation. In general, the selectins P and E on the activated endothelial cell surface and L-selectin on the PMN cell surface function to facilitate PMN rolling and tethering to activated capillary endothelium. Once this tethering has occurred and the PMN itself is activated, the β_2 integrin CD11/CD18 receptors on the PMN form a tight adhesion with the endothelial cell surface that facilitates PMN attachment and polarization and leads to migration.[28,57,309,354] Congenital β_2 integrin CD11/CD18 deficiency states have been described (leukocyte adhesion deficiency type I). These patients have profound PMN adhesion and motility defects and recurrent life-threatening infections, along with delayed separation of the umbilical cord and juvenile periodontitis.[97,114] A second type, leukocyte adhesion deficiency type II, has been described as being caused by a deficiency of sialyl Lewis^X, the PMN ligand for E-selectin on endothelial cells.[258,269] Researchers also have shown that the tethering of PMNs to P-selectin on activated endothelial cells is critical for PMN priming by PAF and that monoclonal antibodies to P-selectin can block this response.[214] Monoclonal antibodies to P-selectin have been used in animal models of ischemia and reperfusion injury and have been shown to reduce significantly the severe edema and endothelial cell injury observed after reperfusion.[341] Similarly, monoclonal antibodies to P-selectin have resulted in significant endothelial cell preservation in animal models of lung injury and cardiac ischemia.[243,336] Monoclonal antibodies to E-selectin and L-selectin also are being tested in animal models.[228] With the rapid advances occurring in identification of new molecules that influence endothelial cell–leukocyte interactions, we will gain greater understanding of the complexity of cellular communication during inflammation.

BACTERICIDAL/PERMEABILITY-INCREASING FACTOR AND DEFENSINS

In addition to their respiratory burst activity in antimicrobial defense, human neutrophils have been shown to contain a variety of granule-associated antibacterial proteins and peptides.[280] These include bactericidal/permeability-increasing protein (BPI) and the defensin family of peptides. BPI is a 55-kDa receptor present in neutrophil granules, which contain two domains. One of the domains binds with LPS to increase membrane permeability and the lysis of gram-negative bacteria, whereas the other promotes the opsonization of gram-negative bacteria.[154] Neutrophil BPI functions best in inflamed tissues, where it acts in concert with defensins and the membrane attack complex of complement to cause cell lysis.

Meningococcemia is a severe gram-negative infection that occurs predominantly in infants and young adults. Mortality rates of meningococcemia range from 10% to 20%.[9,40,141,337,343,353] Endotoxin levels may be profoundly elevated and correlate with the severity of the illness.[37] Recombinant BPI (rBPI) has been used as an adjunct to antimicrobial therapy in children with severe meningococcal sepsis[204]; 14 of 193 patients with severe meningococcal disease who received rBPI (2 mg/kg during 30 minutes) died, compared with 20 of 203 control infants, an insignificant difference. Among the surviving treated patients, however, a modest improvement was noted in long-term functional outcome, a finding suggesting a possible beneficial effect in decreasing complications associated with septic shock.[121,204] Neonates have been shown to have reduced release and activity of BPI that may contribute to their enhanced susceptibility to gram-negative bacterial infections.[205]

The defensins are strongly cationic, single-chain peptides contained in neutrophil primary, or azurophilic, granules with molecular weights between 3 and 4.5 kDa. Defensins comprise 50% of the protein content of the neutrophil primary granules.[116,350] These peptides possess broad antimicrobial activity against gram-positive and gram-negative bacteria, fungi, mycobacteria, and some viruses. The defensins create voltage-sensitive pores in microbial membranes, with resulting cell lysis. They are divided into α and β defensins. Humans have six human α defensins (HAD-1 to HAD-6) and two human β defensins (HBD-1 and HBD-2).

The α defensins, HAD-1 to HAD-6, are made by neutrophils and compose 30% to 50% of the primary granule content.[140] Defensins appear at the site of inflammation. They are present after neutrophil degranulation induced by LPS, IL-8, C5a, and other stimuli. They also are found on the epithelial surfaces of the bronchi and in bronchial lavage fluid of patients with various types of inflammatory lung disease. The antimicrobial activity of the defensins is inhibited by high salt content, which may be clinically important in the immune response of patients with cystic fibrosis.[125]

The β defensins are produced by epithelial cells of the respiratory and gastrointestinal tracts.[31,298] HBD-1 is expressed constitutively by epithelial cells in the bronchi and the intestine, whereas HBD-2 synthesis is upregulated by inflammatory stimuli, including LPS, TNF-α, bacterial infection, and injury. Thus, HBD-1 acts to kill organisms in the absence of inflammation, whereas HBD-2 acts primarily as part of the inflammatory process.

In inflammatory lung disease, such as chronic bronchitis and chronic obstructive lung disease, both α defensins HAD-1 to HAD-6 and β defensin HBD-2 may be increased significantly, perhaps contributing to airway inflammation.[350] There are no reported clinical disorders of defensin production. Potential roles for the defensins as immunoregulatory-antimicrobial agents are being investigated.

Endotoxin and other proinflammatory mediators activate the complement system and the chemotactic properties of C5a, which recruits neutrophils to sites of infection. Interruption of this process at various levels may be possible with use of monoclonal antibody strategies that counteract the effects of the complement leading to septic shock. Although monoclonal antibodies directed at the specific components of the complement cascade have not been tested in human clinical trials, the use of monoclonal antibodies to inhibit C5a in primates challenged with *E. coli* improved the survival rate and reduced the incidence of adult respiratory distress syndrome.[7,32]

PLATELET-ACTIVATING FACTOR

PAF is a potent phospholipid inflammatory mediator with many biologic effects. Its synthesis is regulated by phospholipase A_2, an enzyme associated with the arachidonic acid pathway. PAF has a very short half-life in vivo because of its rapid degradation by PAF acetylhydrolase. PAF is synthesized by many cell types, including macrophages, neutrophils, platelets, eosinophils, endothelial cells, and hepatocytes.[338] Intravenous infusion of PAF into animals results in pulmonary hypertension, bronchoconstriction, neutropenia, thrombocytopenia, and ischemic bowel necrosis.[24,64,136] Production of PAF is stimulated in numerous clinical disease states, including hypoxia and ischemia, and after administration of biologic agents such as LPS, GM-CSF, TNF-α, IL-1, bradykinin, and thrombin.[102,190,231,232,271,284,342] Corticosteroids decrease levels of PAF by the induction of its natural inhibitor, PAF acetylhydrolase.[126] PAF has been shown to stimulate the production of many other mediators of inflammation, including TNF-α, complement breakdown products, oxygen radicals, catecholamines, prostaglandins, thromboxane, and the leukotrienes.[104,160,190,283,322,353] It also activates endothelial cells and neutrophils and monocytes, thereby leading to their adherence and migration.[230] Thus, PAF is a ubiquitous phospholipid mediator with many biologic effects and interactions within the inflammatory cascade.

The regulation of PAF has been studied in numerous potential clinical disease states, including sepsis and septic shock.[158] In clinical phase III trials in septic patients and patients in septic shock who received a PAF antagonist, a significant reduction in the mortality rate was noted.[85] The role of PAF, however, in the pathogenesis of NEC has received considerable attention.[54,55] NEC is an often-fatal gastrointestinal disease that predominantly affects premature infants. Exogenous administration of PAF into rat mesenteric circulation causes ischemic bowel necrosis and disease similar to that seen in neonatal NEC.[159] Endotoxin-induced intestinal injury is associated with increased PAF levels, and the infusion of high doses of endotoxin into animals produces a similar pathologic model of NEC, which can be prevented by administration of dexamethasone, PAF acetylhydrolase, or PAF receptor antagonists.[53,163] These animal studies suggest a link between PAF and its regulation and the development of NEC and implicate PAF as a potential endogenous inflammatory mediator in the pathogenesis of neonatal NEC.

Evidence in humans supports an association between PAF and human neonatal NEC. PAF levels are higher in infants with NEC compared with control subjects, and PAF acetylhydrolase activity is lower in infants with NEC.[56] PAF acetylhydrolase is suppressed with prematurity.[52] Because enteral feedings are necessary for the development of NEC, PAF levels were measured in feeding premature infants. In these studies, feedings alone increased circulating PAF levels but not PAF acetylhydrolase, and infants fed human breast milk had lower PAF levels and a lower incidence of NEC, a finding suggesting a protective effect of human milk through PAF regulation.[218] Human milk is known to have a number of factors protective against infectious disease, including PAF acetylhydrolase.[48,124] Because PAF acetylhydrolase activity is present in human milk and absent in formulas, the suggestion has been made that the protective activity observed in human milk against the development of NEC may result from blocking of PAF-related inflammatory responses.[48] The modulation of the many interactions of PAF within the inflammatory cascade may have future clinical potential in regulating neonatal NEC and other inflammatory disease states.

NITRIC OXIDE

Nitric oxide is a membrane-permeable gas that functions in the regulation of vascular tone and in the inhibition of platelet aggregation and leukocyte adhesion. In addition, nitric oxide has been shown to have antitumor and antimicrobial activity. Under normal conditions, nitric oxide synthase induces endothelial cell production of nitric oxide. The signal transduction pathway for nitric oxide is linked to pathways involving vasodilation. Some evidence indicates that the L-arginine–nitric oxide pathway is activated in sepsis, in which the effects of nitric oxide on the vasculature are associated with the severe vascular failure observed during septic shock.[68,69,179,241,248,249] Thus, inhibition of production of nitric oxide has been proposed as a novel approach for the treatment of the severe hypotension associated with septic shock.[330]

The increased production of nitric oxide observed during septic shock may have several harmful effects. Nitric oxide may be largely responsible for sepsis-induced hypotension. In vitro studies implicate nitric oxide in sepsis-induced myocardial depression, although nitric oxide synthase inhibitors have not been shown to prevent endotoxin-induced myocardial depression in vivo. Nitric oxide also has direct cytotoxic effects, and its overproduction in septic shock can lead to tissue injury and organ failure.[68,105,177] In addition, in vitro experiments suggest that nitric oxide may enhance the release of proinflammatory cytokines during septic shock.[96,248] Production of nitric oxide may, however, have some beneficial effects during septic shock. It is implicated in maintaining visceral and other microvasculature blood flow, both as a counterregulatory mechanism to the vasoconstrictive mediators released during sepsis and by its ability to block platelet adhesion, reducing potential microvasculature stasis and thrombosis.[178,226] In addition, high levels of nitric oxide have antimicrobial activity and enhance LPS-induced production of cytokine,[191] although whether these levels of nitric oxide reflect actual physiologic states has yet to be determined.

Because hypotension during sepsis is an important predictor of organ injury and death, use of nitric oxide synthase inhibitors may improve survival in severe septic shock by increasing mean arterial pressure. Nitric oxide synthase inhibitors have been shown to restore vascular responsiveness to catecholamines in animal models of endotoxin-induced septic shock.[155] In addition, nitric oxide synthase inhibition has been shown to normalize mean arterial pressure in anesthetized animals challenged with endotoxin or TNF-α without causing hypertension.[177] These considerations have led to the use of nitric oxide synthase inhibitors to treat hypotension in patients with sepsis and in patients receiving cytokine therapy for cancer.[176,215] Although these agents can alter mean arterial pressure, beneficial effects on clinical outcomes, including survival, are only suggested in human clinical trials.[248] Studies of endotoxin-challenged rats showed that partial nitric oxide synthase inhibition improved survival, whereas complete inhibition of nitric oxide production clearly was harmful, suggesting a beneficial effect with selective partial nitric oxide inhibition. Studies of nitric oxide inhibition that is more selective are being explored, and in the future such therapy may have clinical utility in the treatment of infectious disease states.

NANOTECHONOLOGY AND OTHER NOVEL TECHNIQUES

Nanomedicine is the application of nanoscale materials to medical treatment, diagnosis, and monitoring. There has been considerable interest in the biomedical application of nanotechnology, particularly by the pharmaceutical industry for the development and improvement of drug delivery systems. The use of nanotechnology in the modification and improvement of the immune response to infectious diseases has also been an active area of investigation. Nanoparticle carrier platforms include biodegradable polymers, viruses and viral-like particles, liposomes, nanoemulsions, and gold microparticles, among others.[184] Nanoparticles can be loaded with immunomodulating compounds such as cytokines, immune-stimulating ligands, vaccine adjuvants, and DNA or RNA. For example, biodegradable nanoparticles with CpG-ODN (TLR-9 ligand) attached to the nanoparticle surface by biotinylation can be loaded with envelope protein antigen from the West Nile Virus, as an adjuvant to immunization, thus targeting intracellular TLR-9 activation and eliciting a robust Th1 polarized response in mice.[84] Poly(lactic-co-glycolic acid) (PGLA) polymer nanoparticles, an FDA-approved delivery platform, can be densely packed with small interfering RNA (siRNA) and delivered to the murine genital tract of mice infected with a lethal dose of intravaginal herpes simplex virus type 2, thereby improving survival dramatically from 9 days in untreated mice to >28 days in treated mice.[311]

Another advantage of nanoparticle delivery platforms is the ability specifically to target ligands to macrophages, for uptake of immunomodulatory agents and antibiotics. For example, tumor-associate macrophages (TAMs) that have adopted a protumor phenotype express high levels of mannose receptors, which can be targeted by ligand binding with mannosylated endosomal escape nanoparticles loaded with siRNA, thus allowing for manipulation of the NF-κB pathway to induce antitumor characteristics in macrophages.[260] Macrophage mannose receptors are also upregulated in parasitic infections, and mannose ligand-grafted chitosan nanoparticles have been used to deliver amphotericin B directly to macrophages infected with *Leishmania*, an obligate intracellular protozoan parasite that infects macrophages.[14] This could potentially improve treatment and decrease the considerable toxic side effects associated with amphotericin treatment. Macrophage-specific nanodelivery platforms are also being investigated for use in the treatment of *Mycobacterium tuberculosis* infection, with the hope of developing alternative regimens for multidrug-resistant tuberculosis.[306]

Finally, adoptive cell transfer (ACT) technologies may also provide potential alternative treatment strategies for existing and emerging infectious diseases. ACT is already a promising therapy for cancer, in which tumor-infiltrating lymphocytes (TILs) from a sample of the patient's tumor are developed into multiple cell cultures with IL-2, assayed for tumor specific recognition, expanded to up to 10^{10} lymphocytes, and then reinfused into the patient following lymphodepletion (to remove T-regulatory cells and lymphocytes that compete with the transferred cells).[285] Adoptive T-cell immunotherapy has shown great promise in the treatment of metastatic melanoma, with cancer regression as high as 50% in patients with melanoma.[285] Adoptive T-cell transfer has also been proposed for the treatment of invasive fungal infections in immunocompromised patients, particularly patients undergoing hematopoietic stem cell transplantation (HSCT) for hematologic malignancies.[263] Invasive *Aspergillus* infections have a very high rate of mortality in HSCT recipients. A clinical trial evaluated the adoptive transfer of donor PBMC-derived *Aspergillus*-specific T cells in 10 haploidentical HSCT recipients with *Aspergillus* pneumonia and galactomannan antigenemia.[268] The negative control group consisted of 13 patients with invasive *Aspergillus* and/or galactomannan antigenemia who did not receive adoptive immunotherapy. Galactomannan antigenemia fell to normal levels within 6 weeks in the immunotherapy group but remained elevated in the control group for the duration of monitoring (15 weeks; $P < .002$ vs. control subjects). Nine of 10 patients in the treatment group cleared invasive *Aspergillus* in 7.8 ± 3.4 weeks, and 1 patient died ($P = .062$ vs. control subjects); six of 13 patients in the control group died. None of the patients who received immunotherapy developed graft versus host disease.

CONCLUSION

The initial attempts to augment immune function in the treatment of sepsis consisted of serum antibody therapy. The development of and refinements in hybridoma and recombinant technologies have provided the means to generate highly specific monoclonal antibodies. Although monoclonal antibodies directed toward bacteria and their components currently are not used during a course of sepsis, the future of these antibodies may lie in their combination with antimicrobial pharmacologic agents to treat infections with certain pathogens. The advances in basic science and clinical research also have demonstrated that the cytokine family plays many crucial roles in the pathogenesis of septic shock. The interactions among the proinflammatory cytokines initiate the cascade of biologic events leading to the propagation and regulation of inflammation. Although the proinflammatory cytokines are effective in augmenting immune responses, their overexpression can lead to severe septic shock. The use of neutralizing monoclonal antibodies to endotoxin, anti–TNF-α antibodies, and soluble TNF-α and IL-1 receptors, as well as IL-1 receptor antagonists, in human clinical trials of septic shock, however, has shown limited therapeutic potential. The future clinical use of cytokine inhibition may include a combination of a number of both recombinant and pharmacologic agents temporally administered to regulate multiple proinflammatory cytokine–mediated steps in the development of septic shock. The hematopoietic growth factors have demonstrated considerable clinical effect, especially in individuals with distinct lymphopoietic disorders and in patients receiving immunosuppressive chemotherapy. IFN-α, IFN-β, and IFN-γ have received considerable attention as potential immunomodulators. IFN-α has shown broad clinical application as an antitumor agent, as well as an antiviral agent; IFN-β is being used with some success in patients with relapsing multiple sclerosis. The stimulatory effect of IFN-γ on human neutrophils is demonstrated in infants and children with specific neutrophil disorders and in neonatal sepsis. TLR agonists are emerging as attractive therapeutic agents in a number of infectious diseases. Investigations defining the actions of the integrins and the selectins, bactericidal/permeability-increasing factor and defensins, and PAF and nitric oxide may provide novel future clinical therapeutic approaches to attenuate acute inflammatory responses. Nanotechnology and adoptive cell transfer are technologies that will also provide novel therapeutic approaches and improve existing treatments for infectious diseases. As we learn more about the complexity of intracellular and extracellular interactions and the delicate balance of these molecules in regulating immune responses, we will be better able to implement their clinical use in regulating infectious disease states in infants and children.

NEW REFERENCES SINCE THE SEVENTH EDITIONS

8. Anonymous. Safety and Efficacy of Pagibaximab Injection in Very Low Birth Weight Neonates for Prevention of Staphylococcal Sepsis. https://clinicaltrials.gov/show/NCT00646399.
10. Anonymous. Updated guidance for palivizumab prophylaxis among infants and young children at increased risk of hospitalization for respiratory syncytial virus infection. *Pediatrics.* 2014;134(2):415-420.
11. Antachopoulos C, Walsh TJ. Immunotherapy of *Cryptococcus* infections. *Clin Microbiol Infect.* 2012;18(2):126-133.
14. Asthana S, Gupta PK, Jaiswal AK, et al. Overexpressed macrophage mannose receptor targeted nanocapsules-mediated cargo delivery approach for eradication of resident parasite: in vitro and in vivo studies. *Pharm Res.* 2015;32(8):2663-2677.
15. Baeten D, Sieper J, Braun J, et al. Secukinumab, an interleukin-17A inhibitor, in ankylosing spondylitis. *N Engl J Med.* 2015;373(26):2534-2548.
19. Baumann A, Buchwald D, Annecke T, et al. RECCAS - REmoval of Cytokines during CArdiac Surgery: study protocol for a randomised controlled trial. *Trials.* 2016;17(1):137.
23. Bernardi MH, Rinoesl H, Dragosits K, et al. Effect of hemoadsorption during cardiopulmonary bypass surgery: a blinded, randomized, controlled pilot study using a novel adsorbent. *Crit Care.* 2016;20(1):96.
39. Brady MT, Byington CL, Davies HD, et al. Updated guidance for palivizumab prophylaxis among infants and young children at increased risk of hospitalization for respiratory syncytial virus infection. *Pediatrics.* 2014;134(2):415-420.
42. Brocklehurst P, Farrell B, King A, et al. Treatment of neonatal sepsis with intravenous immune globulin. *N Engl J Med.* 2011;365(13):1201-1211.
45. Browne SK, Zaman R, Sampaio EP, et al. Anti-CD20 (rituximab) therapy for anti-IFN-gamma autoantibody-associated nontuberculous mycobacterial infection. *Blood.* 2012;119(17):3933-3939.
46. Bruenger F, Kizner L, Weile J, et al. First successful combination of ECMO with cytokine removal therapy in cardiogenic septic shock: a case report. *Int J Artif Organs.* 2015;38(2):113-116.
49. Bux J, Behrens G, Jaeger G, et al. Diagnosis and clinical course of autoimmune neutropenia in infancy: analysis of 240 cases. *Blood.* 1998;91(1):181-186.
59. Caron JE, La Pine TR, Augustine NH, et al. Multiplex analysis of toll-like receptor-stimulated neonatal cytokine response. *Neonatology.* 2010;97(3):266-273.
66. Chen YG, Zhang Y, Deng LQ, et al. Control of methicillin-resistant *Staphylococcus aureus* pneumonia utilizing TLR2 agonist Pam3CSK4. *PLoS ONE.* 2016;11(3):e0149233.
79. Danesh MJ, Kimball AB. Brodalumab and suicidal ideation in the context of a recent economic crisis in the United States. *J Am Acad Dermatol.* 2016;74(1):190-192.
82. Day JR, Taylor KM. The systemic inflammatory response syndrome and cardiopulmonary bypass. *Int J Surg.* 2005;3(2):129-140.
83. Delsing CE, Gresnigt MS, Leentjens J, et al. Interferon-gamma as adjunctive immunotherapy for invasive fungal infections: a case series. *BMC Infect Dis.* 2014;14:166.
84. Demento SL, Bonafe N, Cui W, et al. TLR9-targeted biodegradable nanoparticles as immunization vectors protect against West Nile encephalitis. *J Immunol.* 2010;185(5):2989-2997.
87. DiGiandomenico A, Warrener P, Hamilton M, et al. Identification of broadly protective human antibodies to *Pseudomonas aeruginosa* exopolysaccharide Psl by phenotypic screening. *J Exp Med.* 2012;209(7):1273-1287.
101. Fakhouri F, Hourmant M, Campistol JM, et al. Terminal complement inhibitor eculizumab in adult patients with atypical hemolytic uremic syndrome: a single-arm, open-label trial. *Am J Kidney Dis.* 2016;68:84-93.
111. Fouts AE, Chan P, Stephan J-P, et al. Antibodies against the gH/gL/UL128/UL130/UL131 complex comprise the majority of the anti-cytomegalovirus (anti-CMV) neutralizing antibody response in CMV hyperimmune globulin. *J Virol.* 2012;86(13):7444-7447.
112. Francois B, Luyt CE, Dugard A, et al. Safety and pharmacokinetics of an anti-PcrV PEGylated monoclonal antibody fragment in mechanically ventilated patients colonized with Pseudomonas aeruginosa: a randomized,double-blind, placebo-controlled trial. *Crit Care Med.* 2012;40(8):2320-2326.
117. Gaur S, Kesarwala H, Gavai M, et al. Clinical immunology and infectious diseases. *Pediatr Clin North Am.* 1994;41(4):745-782.
118. Gilardin L, Bayry J, Kaveri SV. Intravenous immunoglobulin as clinical immune-modulating therapy. *CMAJ.* 2015;187(4):257-264.
123. Goh MS. Invasive squamous cell carcinoma after treatment of carcinoma in situ with 5% imiquimod cream. *Australas J Dermatol.* 2006;47(3):186-188.
137. Haq IJ, Gardner A, Brodlie M. A multifunctional bispecific antibody against Pseudomonas aeruginosa as a potential therapeutic strategy. *Ann Transl Med.* 2016;4(1):12.
138. Harigai M, Nanki T, Koike R, et al. Risk for malignancy in rheumatoid arthritis patients treated with biological disease-modifying antirheumatic drugs compared to the general population: A nationwide cohort study in Japan. *Mod Rheumatol.* 2016;26:1-9.
153. Hinz B, Jauch O, Noky T, et al. CytoSorb, a novel therapeutic approach for patients with septic shock: a case report. *Int J Artif Organs.* 2015;38(8):461-464.
162. Ishida JH, Burgess T, Derby MA, et al. Phase 1 randomized, double-blind, placebo-controlled study of RG7667, an anticytomegalovirus combination monoclonal antibody therapy, in healthy adults. *Antimicrob Agents Chemother.* 2015;59(8):4919-4929.
167. Jarvis JN, Meintjes G, Rebe K, et al. Adjunctive interferon-gamma immunotherapy for the treatment of HIV-associated cryptococcal meningitis: a randomized controlled trial. *AIDS.* 2012;26(9):1105-1113.
171. Kauvar LM, Liu K, Park M, et al. A high-affinity native human antibody neutralizes human cytomegalovirus infection of diverse cell types. *Antimicrob Agents Chemother.* 2015;59(3):1558-1568.
184. Krishnamachari Y, Geary SM, Lemke CD, et al. Nanoparticle delivery systems in cancer vaccines. *Pharm Res.* 2011;28(2):215-236.
192. La Pine T, Augustine N, Caron J. Toll-like receptors and tumor necrosis factor α production in neonatal host defense. *J Invest Med.* 2007;55:S143.
210. Lilleri D, Kabanova A, Revello MG, et al. Fetal human cytomegalovirus transmission correlates with delayed maternal antibodies to gH/gL/pUL128-130-131 complex during primary infection. *PLoS ONE.* 2013;8(3):e59863.
213. Lopez EL, Contrini MM, Glatstein E, et al. Safety and pharmacokinetics of urtoxazumab, a humanized monoclonal antibody, against Shiga-like toxin 2 in healthy adults and in pediatric patients infected with Shiga-like toxin-producing *Escherichia coli. Antimicrob Agents Chemother.* 2010;54(1):239-243.
221. Maidji E, McDonagh S, Genbacev O, et al. Maternal antibodies enhance or prevent cytomegalovirus infection in the placenta by neonatal Fc receptor-mediated transcytosis. *Am J Pathol.* 2006;168(4):1210-1226.
233. Mease PJ, Genovese MC, Greenwald MW, et al. Brodalumab, an anti-IL17RA monoclonal antibody, in psoriatic arthritis. *N Engl J Med.* 2014;370(24):2295-2306.
234. Mejias MP, Hiriart Y, Lauche C, et al. Development of camelid single chain antibodies against Shiga toxin type 2 (Stx2) with therapeutic potential against hemolytic uremic syndrome (HUS). *Sci Rep.* 2016;6:24913.
237. Milla CE, Chmiel JF, Accurso FJ, et al. Anti-PcrV antibody in cystic fibrosis: a novel approach targeting Pseudomonas aeruginosa airway infection. *Pediatr Pulmonol.* 2014;49(7):650-658.

251. Newburger JW, Takahashi M, Gerber MA, et al. Diagnosis, treatment, and long-term management of Kawasaki disease: a statement for health professionals from the Committee on Rheumatic Fever, Endocarditis and Kawasaki Disease, Council on Cardiovascular Disease in the Young, American Heart Association. *Circulation.* 2004;110(17):2747-2771.
256. Ohlsson A, Lacy JB. Intravenous immunoglobulin for suspected or proven infection in neonates. *Cochrane Database Syst Rev.* 2015;(3):CD001239.
260. Ortega RA, Barham W, Sharman K, et al. Manipulating the NF-kappaB pathway in macrophages using mannosylated, siRNA-delivering nanoparticles can induce immunostimulatory and tumor cytotoxic functions. *Int J Nanomedicine.* 2016;11:2163-2177.
261. Palma LM, Langman CB. Critical appraisal of eculizumab for atypical hemolytic uremic syndrome. *J Blood Med.* 2016;7:39-72.
262. Pammi M, Haque KN. Pentoxifylline for treatment of sepsis and necrotizing enterocolitis in neonates. *Cochrane Database Syst Rev.* 2015;(3):CD004205.
263. Papadopoulou A, Kaloyannidis P, Yannaki E, et al. Adoptive transfer of *Aspergillus*-specific T cells as a novel anti-fungal therapy for hematopoietic stem cell transplant recipients: Progress and challenges. *Crit Rev Oncol Hematol.* 2016;98:62-72.
264. Patel GK, Goodwin R, Chawla M, et al. Imiquimod 5% cream monotherapy for cutaneous squamous cell carcinoma in situ (Bowen's disease): a randomized, double-blind, placebo-controlled trial. *J Am Acad Dermatol.* 2006;54(6):1025-1032.
265. Patel M, Kaufman DA. Anti-lipoteichoic acid monoclonal antibody (pagibaximab) studies for the prevention of staphylococcal bloodstream infections in preterm infants. *Expert Opin Biol Ther.* 2015;15(4):595-600.
268. Perruccio K, Tosti A, Burchielli E, et al. Transferring functional immune responses to pathogens after haploidentical hematopoietic transplantation. *Blood.* 2005;106(13):4397-4406.
270. Picard C, Burtey S, Bornet C, et al. Pathophysiology and treatment of typical and atypical hemolytic uremic syndrome. *Path Biol (Paris).* 2015;63(3):136-143.
277. Ramos JM, Garcia-Sepulcre MF, Rodriguez JC, et al. Mycobacterium marinum infection complicated by anti-tumour necrosis factor therapy. *J Med Microbiol.* 2010;59(Pt 5):617-621.
278. Revello MG, Lazzarotto T, Guerra B, et al. A randomized trial of hyperimmune globulin to prevent congenital cytomegalovirus. *N Engl J Med.* 2014;370(14):1316-1326.
281. Ritchlin C, Rahman P, Kavanaugh A, et al. Efficacy and safety of the anti-IL-12/23 p40 monoclonal antibody, ustekinumab, in patients with active psoriatic arthritis despite conventional non-biological and biological anti-tumour necrosis factor therapy: 6-month and 1-year results of the phase 3, multicentre, double-blind, placebo-controlled, randomised PSUMMIT 2 trial. *Ann Rheum Dis.* 2014;73(6):990-999.
285. Rosenberg SA, Restifo NP, Yang JC, et al. Adoptive cell transfer: a clinical path to effective cancer immunotherapy. *Nat Rev Cancer.* 2008;8(4):299-308.
290. Sawa T, Ito E, Nguyen VH, et al. Anti-PcrV antibody strategies against virulent *Pseudomonas aeruginosa. Hum Vaccin Immunother.* 2014;10(10):2843-2852.
292. Schädler D, Porzelius C, Jörres A, et al. A multicenter randomized controlled study of an extracorporeal cytokine hemoadsorption device in septic patients. *Crit Care.* 2013;17(suppl 2):P62.
299. Shah PS, Kaufman DA. Antistaphylococcal immunoglobulins to prevent staphylococcal infection in very low birth weight infants. *Cochrane Database Syst Rev.* 2009;(2):CD006449.
304. Shimizu M, Katoh H, Hamaoka S, et al. Protective effects of intravenous immunoglobulin and antimicrobial agents on acute pneumonia in leukopenic mice. *J Infect Chemother.* 2016;22(4):240-247.
306. Singh R, Nawale L, Arkile M, et al. Phytogenic silver, gold, and bimetallic nanoparticles as novel antitubercular agents. *Int J Nanomedicine.* 2016;11:1889-1897.
311. Steinbach JM, Weller CE, Booth CJ, et al. Polymer nanoparticles encapsulating siRNA for treatment of HSV-2 genital infection. *J Control Release.* 2012;162(1):102-110.
320. Tschumi S, Gugger M, Bucher BS, et al. Eculizumab in atypical hemolytic uremic syndrome: long-term clinical course and histological findings. *Pediatr Nephrol.* 2011;26(11):2085-2088.
325. Vellanki VS, Bargman JM. *Aspergillus niger* peritonitis in a peritoneal dialysis patient treated with eculizumab. *Ren Fail.* 2014;36(4):631-633.
328. Wanke-Jellinek L, Keegan JW, Dolan JW, et al. Beneficial effects of CpG-oligodeoxynucleotide treatment on trauma and secondary lung infection. *J Immunol.* 2016;196(2):767-777.
333. Weisman LE. Antibody for the prevention of neonatal nosocomial staphylococcal infection: a review of the literature. *Arch Pediatr.* 2007;14(suppl 1):S31-S34.
334. Weisman LE, Thackray HM, Steinhorn RH, et al. A randomized study of a monoclonal antibody (pagibaximab) to prevent staphylococcal sepsis. *Pediatrics.* 2011;128(2):271-279.
346. Xu W, He L, Liu C, et al. The effect of infection control nurses on the occurrence of *Pseudomonas aeruginosa* healthcare-acquired infection and multidrug-resistant strains in critically-ill children. *PLoS ONE.* 2015;10(12):e0143692.
347. Yamagami S, Motoki M, Kimura T, et al. Efficacy of postinfection treatment with anti-Shiga toxin (Stx) 2 humanized monoclonal antibody TMA-15 in mice lethally challenged with Stx-producing *Escherichia coli. J Infect Dis.* 2001;184(6):738-742.

The full reference list for this chapter is available at ExpertConsult.com.

243 Probiotics

Jonathan D. Crews

The resident microbes of the human microbiota contribute to the overall health of infants and children. Changes in the composition and diversity of intestinal microbial communities have been observed in various clinical conditions. Probiotics and prebiotics have been advanced as safe and effective methods to manipulate intestinal microbiota to prevent or treat disease in humans.

The study of the beneficial health effects of microorganisms began in 1908, when Elie Metchnikoff linked the longevity of Bulgarian peasants with the lactobacilli in the yogurt they consumed. In the early 1900s, Henry Tissier isolated *Bifidobacterium* from the stool of a healthy infant and claimed it could displace pathogenic bacteria in the gut.[95] In the 21st century, an enormous amount of basic and translational research has focused on the characterization and manipulation of the intestinal microbiota. In 2007, a major advance occurred with the formation of the Human Microbiome Project, sponsored by the National Institutes of Health, which aimed to determine the composition of the human microbiome, identify factors that affect its composition, and investigate the mechanisms by which the microbiome affects human health.[73]

This chapter surveys probiotics and their application to the prevention and treatment of disease in newborns, infants, and children. Infectious diseases related to probiotic use also are reviewed.

DEFINITIONS

Probiotic Microorganisms

Probiotics is a general term for different species and strains of bacteria or yeast, usually commensal microorganisms of mammalian microbiota, which can promote health. The term is derived from Greek, meaning "for life." The Food and Agriculture Organization of the United Nations and the World Health Organization define probiotics as "live microorganisms that, when administered in adequate amounts, confer a health benefit on the host."[67,103] Probiotic preparations may be administered as a single strain or mixture of multiple strains. They are available as stand-alone products—tablets, capsules, wafers, powder sachets, and liquid—and as ingredients in food and beverages. More than 100 probiotic products are available globally.[95]

BOX 243.1 Microbial Species Used as Probiotics for Prevention and Treatment of Human Disease

Bacteria

Lactobacillus
- *L. acidophilus*
- *L. bulgaricus*
- *L. casei*
- *L. delbrueckii*
- *L. fermentum*
- *L. helveticus*
- *L. johnsonii*
- *L. paracasei*
- *L. plantarum*
- *L. reuteri*
- *L. rhamnosus*

Bifidobacterium
- *B. bifidum*
- *B. breve*
- *B. infantis*
- *B. lactis*
- *B. longum*

Streptococcus
- *S. salivarius*
- *S. thermophilus*

Enterococcus faecium (SF68 strain)

Escherichia coli (Nissle 1917 strain)

Clostridium butyricum

Bacillus
- *B. clausii*
- *B. coagulans*
- *B. subtilis*

Yeast

Saccharomyces boulardii

The most common probiotic bacteria are strains of *Lactobacillus* and *Bifidobacterium* species. They are gram-positive commensals found in the human gastrointestinal tract. Additional probiotic bacteria include *Bacillus clausii*, *Clostridium butyricum*, *Escherichia coli* Nissle 1917, and *Streptococcus thermophilus*. *Saccharomyces boulardii*, a yeast organism, is a popular and well-studied probiotic (Box 243.1).

Lactobacillus species are gram-positive, nonmotile, non–spore forming bacilli. They produce lactic acid as an end product of carbohydrate fermentation and have been referred to as lactic acid bacteria. They grow best under microaerophilic conditions and form small to medium gray colonies that demonstrate α-hemolysis on blood agar. They are resident microorganisms in the human mouth, gastrointestinal tract, and vagina. The *Lactobacillus* genus has more than 170 species.[57] Although not all lactobacilli are acid tolerant and bile resistant, the strains used as probiotics have these features. Several *Lactobacillus* species are found in probiotic products: *L. acidophilus*, *L. bulgaricus*, *L. casei*, *L. paracasei*, *L. reuteri*, and *L. rhamnosus*.[57,59]

Bifidobacterium species are gram-positive, nonmotile, non–spore forming, anaerobic organisms that are widely distributed among the gastrointestinal tracts of mammals, birds, and some insects. Bifidobacteria are one of the dominant bacterial members of the intestinal microbiota of infants.[149] *Bifidobacterium bifidum* was initially isolated from the stool of a healthy infant in 1906.[95] *Bifidobacterium longum* is one of the most abundant species in the human intestinal tract, and it is widely available as a probiotic.[151] Other *Bifidobacterium* species used in probiotic products include *B. breve*, *B. infantis*, and *B. lactis*.[59]

Saccharomyces boulardii was first identified from the surface of lychee and mangosteen fruit in 1920 by Henri Boulard.[95] It is considered a strain of *Saccharomyces cerevisiae*, a yeast used in baking and brewing. *S. boulardii* (i.e., *S. cerevisiae* var *boulardii*) has distinct metabolic and physiologic properties that make it better suited as a probiotic than *S. cerevisiae*.[34] *S. boulardii* grows optimally at 37°C, and is resistant to gastric acid and bile acids. Compared with bacterial probiotics, it has the benefit of being naturally resistant to antibiotics.[34]

Prebiotics and Synbiotics

Prebiotics are nondigestible food ingredients that benefit the host by selectively stimulating the growth or activity of indigenous bacteria.[53,54] The most common prebiotics are carbohydrates, which can be selectively fermented by species of resident intestinal microbiota. Examples include fructo-oligosaccharides (FOSs), inulin (i.e., FOS group), galacto-oligosaccharides, and lactulose.

Prebiotics increase stool colony counts of bifidobacteria and lactobacilli. They exert health effects through various mechanisms, including influencing the composition of the intestinal microbiota, improving intestinal barrier function, and direct modulation of the immune system.[118,131] For example, short-chain fatty acids (SCFAs) are important fermentation byproducts of prebiotics. They can interact with enterocytes and immune cells to strengthen the intestinal epithelium and modulate inflammation.

Human breast milk contains many oligosaccharides, which serve as natural prebiotics.[41] Human milk oligosaccharides promote and stimulate the growth of beneficial, indigenous strains of bacteria, especially *Bifidobacterium* and *Bacteroides* species. Prebiotics are added to several commercial infant formulas.

A synbiotic product contains prebiotics and probiotics.[146] The combination of prebiotic dietary carbohydrates with probiotic bacteria can improve the survival and promote the activity of the probiotic strain, thereby enhancing the overall effect.

MECHANISM OF ACTION

The means through which probiotics influence health outcomes remains incompletely understood. Numerous mechanisms of action have been proposed based on basic and translational research. The current framework is that certain mechanisms are widespread and common to various probiotic genera, whereas others are species or strain specific. Although a single probiotic strain may produce health benefits through multiple mechanisms, no individual probiotic should be expected to employ all the proposed mechanisms.[67] Research articles have reviewed the evidence describing the mechanisms of action specific to *Lactobacillus* species, *Bifidobacterium* species, and *S. boulardii*.[86,102,127]

Many clinical studies have demonstrated that probiotics can influence the composition of the intestinal microbiota.[94] The studies show that during intestinal dysbiosis (i.e., disruption or imbalance of microbiota), probiotics can promote the partial or complete restoration of intestinal microbiota. Reestablishment of a healthy intestinal microbiota is thought to be important for probiotics to exert their beneficial health effects. Swidsinski and colleagues studied 60 women receiving ciprofloxacin and metronidazole for bacterial vaginosis. Using fluorescence in situ hybridization, they found that *S. boulardii* CNCM I-1745, when administered concurrently or after the antibiotic regimen, reduced the antibiotic-associated changes of the fecal microbiota and improved the rate of microbial recovery.[136] In a clinical trial of 49 healthy adult patients, there was a lower rate of antibiotic-associated diarrhea and less pronounced shift in microbial communities when *S. boulardii* CNCM I-1745 was given with amoxicillin-clavulanate.[76]

Probiotics appear to influence microbial composition through three mechanisms: direct and indirect antimicrobial effects, the ability to enhance the integrity and function of the intestinal mucosal barrier, and immune modulation.[113] Several types of antimicrobial effects have been described for probiotics. They can exert colonization resistance, by which the colonization of enteric pathogens is hindered as the probiotic strain adheres to the intestinal epithelium or competes for necessary metabolites.[13] Several probiotic strains produce antimicrobial products, including bacteriocins, hydrogen peroxide, and organic acids. Bifidobacteria can produce bacteriocins that possess antibacterial activity against *Clostridium difficile* and *E. coli*.[91] Some probiotic strains can neutralize the bacterial toxins produced by enteropathogens. For example, *S. boulardii* can cleave *C. difficile* toxins and inactivate cholera toxin.[102]

The intestinal barrier function is disrupted in several illnesses, including infectious diarrhea, irritable bowel syndrome, and inflammatory bowel disease. Maintenance of the integrity of the epithelial and mucosal layers of the colon is important in intestinal function. SCFAs are a metabolic byproduct of several probiotic strains and a major energy source for intestinal epithelial cells. They are instrumental in cell proliferation, cell differentiation, and mucus secretion.[61] Probiotics can promote intestinal barrier integrity by enhancing the mucous layer and strengthening the tight junctions of the intestinal epithelial mucosa.[127]

Animal models and observations in human studies support an association between intestinal microbial colonization and the development of the immune system. Probiotics appear to influence both local and systemic immune function through effects on the intestinal epithelium, gut-associated lymphoid tissue, and host immune cells.[116] Local intestinal inflammation can be lessened through stabilization of intestinal barrier integrity, induction of antiinflammatory cytokines, and release of secretory immunoglobulin A (IgA).[127,133] Probiotics can enhance the production of protective cytokines, such as interleukin-10 and transforming growth factor-β, which inhibit epithelial cell apoptosis and enhance epithelial regeneration.[113] Prebiotic oligosaccharides after fermentation into SCFAs have antiinflammatory effects on intestinal mucosa.[61] Several strains of lactobacilli and bifidobacteria appear to influence the systemic immune system through effects on intestinal dendritic cells, regulatory T cells, IgA-producing B cells, and effector T and B cells.[116]

PROBIOTICS AND PREBIOTICS FOR PREVENTION AND TREATMENT OF CLINICAL CONDITIONS

Probiotic use is increasing. The National Health Interview Study found that 3.9 million adults in the United States consumed probiotic products in 2012, a fourfold increase from 2007.[28] Moreover, 294,000 US children 4 to 17 years of age used probiotics in the 30 days before the 2012 survey.[18] Probiotic use is also increasing among inpatients. In a sample of 60 US hospitals, the number of hospitalizations during which probiotics were prescribed increased 2.9-fold between 2006 and 2012.[168]

The rise in probiotic consumption has paralleled a surge in clinical research investigating their therapeutic and preventive potential. Numerous randomized, controlled trials (RCTs), albeit many with small sample sizes, have examined the effects of probiotics in various childhood disorders. Multiple meta-analyses have been derived pooled effect estimates from these trials. The meta-analyses have tended to evaluate probiotics as a therapeutic class, aggregating trials that employed different probiotic strains. This approach has been criticized due to growing evidence that probiotic strains have different mechanisms of action and health effects. In response, several investigators have performed meta-analyses of specific strains for various indications.[26,48,140,152] In addition to differences in the probiotic strains, clinical trials vary in probiotic dose, timing, and duration; study populations; and methods of administration. These differences are certain to modify the outcome of probiotic trials.

The regulatory status of commercial probiotic products varies throughout the world.[77] In the United States, probiotic products are marketed as dietary supplements with generally recognized as safe (GRAS) status and do not require premarketing review by the Food and Drug Administration.[68,159] In Europe, the European Food Safety Authority regulates probiotic products and their health claims. In most countries, there is limited regulatory oversight of the manufacturing process of probiotic products. Several issues related to the quality of probiotic products have been documented in many countries, including misidentification and mislabeling of probiotic strains, inaccurate labeling of viable organisms per dose, and contamination of products with potential pathogens.[77,104]

Acute Infectious Diarrhea

Acute infectious diarrhea is a major cause of morbidity and mortality among children worldwide, particularly among children younger than 5 years. Multiple randomized trials have investigated whether probiotics can reduce diarrheal symptoms in children with infectious diarrhea. Most studies focus on young children with acute viral gastroenteritis, although some include children with bacterial or parasitic intestinal infections. *Lactobacillus rhamnosus* GG (LGG) and *S. boulardii* are the most frequently used strains in probiotic trials for infectious diarrhea. Other probiotic strains have been studied in randomized trials, including *L. reuteri* DSM 17938, *L. acidophilus* LB, *E. coli* Nissle 1917, *L. paracasei* strain ST11, and various multistrain combinations.[43,65,66,128,141,152]

Several meta-analyses demonstrate that probiotics can shorten the duration of acute diarrhea in children.[6,39,48,138,142] The 2010 Cochrane review, which included 63 RCTs, found that probiotics shortened diarrheal symptoms. The mean duration of diarrhea decreased by 24.8 hours (95% confidence interval [CI], 15.9–33.6 hours) and the risk of diarrhea lasting 4 or more days decreased by 59% (risk ratio [RR], 0.41; 95% CI, 0.32–0.53) in people receiving a probiotic.[6]

Lactobacillus rhamnosus GG significantly reduced the duration of diarrhea by 1 day (mean difference, 1.1 days; 95% CI, −1.7 to −0.4) when data from 11 clinical trials (N = 2444 participants) were examined. LGG performed more effectively at a higher daily dose (≥10^{10} colony-forming units [CFUs]) than a lower daily dose (<10^{10} CFUs).[142] *Saccharomyces boulardii* also appears to alleviate symptoms of acute infectious diarrhea. A 2014 systematic review of 22 clinical trials found that *S. boulardii* reduced stool frequency on days 2 and 3 of illness and reduced the overall duration of diarrhea by 19.7 hours (95% CI, 13.3–26.1 hours).[48]

Several organizations recommend probiotics for children with acute infectious diarrhea. The American Academy of Pediatrics (AAP) supports "the use of probiotics, specifically LGG, early in the course of acute infectious diarrhea."[146] The European Society for Pediatric Gastroenterology, Hepatology, and Nutrition (ESPGHAN) endorses the use of LGG (daily dose of ≥10^{10} CFUs) or *S. boulardii* (daily dose of 250–750 mg) as an adjunct to rehydration therapy for acute gastroenteritis.[58,138]

Probiotics also have the potential to prevent acute diarrhea, particularly in children attending group childcare centers. RCTs performed in Mexico, Indonesia, Israel, and India found a modest benefit in the prevention of diarrheal illnesses in children attending childcare centers.[3,60,135,163] Several probiotic organisms were studied, including *L. reuteri*, *L. casei*, and *B. lactis*. However, because rotavirus was an important cause of diarrheal disease in several of the trials, the results might not be generalizable to regions with widespread use of rotavirus vaccine.

Antibiotic-Associated Diarrhea

Approximately 10% to 20% of children receiving antibiotics experience diarrhea.[74,80,147] Factors that increase the risk of antibiotic-associated diarrhea (AAD) in children include young age (<2 years) and broad-spectrum antibiotics, including aminopenicillins (especially when administered with clavulanate), cephalosporins, and clindamycin.[80,93] AAD can result from disruption of intestinal microbiota, overgrowth by enteric pathogens (especially *Clostridium difficile*), and metabolic alterations resulting in altered colonic digestion and absorption.[93]

Probiotics can minimize the disruption of the intestinal microbiota caused by systemic antibiotics.[76,94] Multiple RCTs found a modest benefit when probiotics were given concurrent with antibiotic therapy.[8,52,79,122,157] *Saccharomyces boulardii* and LGG are the strains most extensively studied in AAD.[139,140] Clinical trials evaluating multistrain products have had mixed results.[30,52,144] Yogurt consumption has not been shown to prevent AAD in children or adults.[114]

Meta-analyses support the use of probiotics in the prevention of AAD.[55,64,74] In a 2015 Cochrane review that included 22 RCTs (N = 3898 participants), the incidence of AAD among children in the probiotic group was lower than the control group (8% vs. 19%; RR, 0.46; 95% CI, 0.35–0.61). The number needed to prevent one case of diarrhea was 10.[55] The AAP and ESPGHAN endorse the use of LGG or *S. boulardii* to prevent AAD in children.[137,146]

Clostridium difficile colonizes the intestinal tract after alteration of normal intestinal flora, most commonly after antibiotic therapy. Individuals with recurrent *C. difficile*–associated diarrhea (CDAD) have markedly diminished microbial diversity compared with healthy controls.[27] Meta-analyses indicate that probiotics may reduce the risk of CDAD by 65%.[56,75] These studies, however, may not be generalizable to children because the included trials primarily studied adult patients. Nonetheless, preliminary studies of probiotics to prevent CDAD in children have yielded promising results.[79,137,140]

Nosocomial Diarrhea

A 1994 clinical trial suggested that probiotics could prevent hospital-acquired diarrhea. In this randomized, placebo-controlled trial, hospitalized children 5 to 24 months of age who were given formula supplemented with *B. bifidum* and *S. thermophilus* had a lower rate of hospital-onset diarrhea than controls (7% vs. 31%; P = .04). Children receiving the supplemented formula also shed rotavirus at a lower rate.[123] A 2011 meta-analysis (N = 3 RCTs) found that administration of LGG for the duration of hospitalization deceased the incidence of symptomatic rotavirus gastroenteritis.[143] However, the included trials had methodologic limitations, and the results may not be generalizable to settings with a low incidence of health care–acquired rotavirus. In subsequent trials, neither *L. reuteri* DSM 17938 nor *B. lactis* BB-12 was effective in preventing hospital-onset diarrhea.[69,153,161] Strict adherence to hand hygiene, standard precautions, and appropriate isolation are the most important interventions to prevent hospital-acquired diarrhea. There is insufficient evidence to support the routine use of probiotics to prevent health care–associated diarrhea in children.

Persistent Diarrhea

Persistent diarrhea is a common condition in resource-limited countries among children 5 years of age or younger. A 2013 Cochrane review concluded that probiotics can reduce stool frequency and shorten the duration of persistent diarrhea, although the evidence remains limited.[14] A randomized trial enrolling 235 children hospitalized in India with persistent diarrhea reported a shorter duration of diarrhea and shorter hospital stays for children taking LGG.[12]

Functional Gastrointestinal Disorders

Multiple clinical trials have evaluated the effect of probiotics on functional gastrointestinal disorders, including infantile colic, irritable bowel syndrome (IBS), functional abdominal pain disorders, and chronic constipation. Studies suggest probiotics are beneficial for infantile colic, IBS, and abdominal pain disorders, but they appear to have no effect on functional constipation.

Although the cause of infantile colic is unknown, it is considered a gastrointestinal disturbance. Infants with colic have decreased fecal microbial diversity compared with age-matched controls.[38] When *L. reuteri* DSM 17938 is administered to infants with colic, particularly breastfed infants, a positive therapeutic effect has been observed. A meta-analysis ($N = 6$ RCTs) found that infants in the *L. reuteri* group ($n = 213$), when compared with the placebo group ($n = 210$), had decreased crying time at 2 weeks and 3 weeks but not at 4 weeks.[167] The effect may be limited to breastfed infants because the only unsuccessful trial in the meta-analysis included formula-fed infants.[134] *Lactobacillus reuteri* DSM 17938 may also decrease the incidence of other functional gastrointestinal disorders in young infants.[71]

Probiotics can reduce abdominal pain and discomfort in children with IBS and functional abdominal pain disorders.[78,108] In 2017, a Cochrane review ($N = 13$ RCTs) reported that children with recurrent abdominal pain or IBS experienced a reduction in pain when treated with a probiotic.[108] However, the studies were of low to moderate quality due to heterogeneity, incomplete outcome data, and small sample size. The probiotic strains evaluated in the included studies were LGG, *L. reuteri*, or multistrain products. *S, cerevisiae* CNCM I-3856 and *Bifidobacterium* species have also been studied in adults with IBS.[26,169] Further research is needed to characterize the optimal probiotic regimen (i.e., strain, dose, and timing) for children with IBS or functional abdominal pain.

Probiotics do not improve functional constipation.[78] Current recommendations from the North American Society for Pediatric Gastroenterology, Hepatology, and Nutrition (NAPSGHAN) and ESPGHAN do not support their use for the treatment of childhood constipation.[145]

Helicobacter Pylori Infection

RCTs demonstrate that probiotics, when administered with triple therapy to children with *Helicobacter pylori*, can improve the eradication rate and decrease therapy-related side effects, particularly diarrhea.[85] An increase in adherence to treatment may explain the increased cure rate.[17] These trials are encouraging, but the optimal probiotic strain has not been identified. Further evidence is needed in children before probiotics are routinely used with standard *H. pylori* treatment.[146]

Inflammatory Bowel Disease

Pediatric patients often receive probiotics as adjunctive treatment for inflammatory bowel disease (IBD).[165] However, there are few large, well-designed clinical trials on their use with ulcerative colitis (UC) or Crohn disease (CD). A small study of 29 children with UC found that those receiving a commercial probiotic product containing eight strains achieved and maintained remission at a higher rate than those receiving placebo.[97] However, systematic reviews have not found a consistent benefit for probiotics in UC in induction or maintenance of disease remission.[89,107] There has been less clinical research on the use of probiotics in CD. Cochrane reviews have concluded there is no evidence to support their use in CD.[22,120]

Liver Disease

Given evidence of the interplay between the intestinal microbiota and the liver (i.e., gut-liver axis), early efforts are underway to investigate whether probiotics are effective in the prevention and treatment of pediatric liver disease.[101] Increased intestinal permeability and alterations in intestinal microbiota have been observed among children with nonalcoholic fatty liver disease (NAFLD), the most common chronic liver disease in children living in industrialized countries.[109] Three small clinical trials suggest that probiotics, when administered to obese children with NAFLD, modestly improve levels of alanine aminotransferase and decrease hepatic steatosis regardless of body mass index.[5,47,154]

Individuals with hepatic encephalopathy may benefit from probiotics. Clinical trials enrolling adult patients suggest that probiotics can hasten recovery and decrease plasma ammonia concentrations but do not affect overall mortality rates.[35]

Allergic and Atopic Diseases

Disturbances in the composition of the gut microbiota may play a role in the pathophysiology of allergic diseases by modifying local intestinal immunity and altering systemic immune programming. The hygiene hypothesis suggests that reduction in general microbial exposure during early childhood may increase susceptibility to allergic disease by reshaping the development of the immune system. Probiotics have been advanced as a method to prevent inappropriate immune development through maintenance of healthy intestinal microbiota.

Several clinical trials examined whether probiotic use during pregnancy or infancy, or both, influence the risk of developing allergic diseases. Overall, the research suggests that probiotics have a modest effect on the prevention of atopic dermatitis in at-risk infants (i.e., those with an immediate family member with allergic disease).[32,50,51,115,171] There is very limited evidence that probiotics have an impact on the development of allergic rhinitis, food allergies, or asthma/wheezing.[32,44,171]

In a 2007 study, pregnant women carrying children at high risk for atopic disease were randomized to receive a multistrain probiotic preparation (i.e., *L. rhamnosus* GG, *L. rhamnosus* DSM 7061, *B. breve* Bb99, and *Propionibacterium freudenreichii*) or placebo for 2 to 4 weeks before pregnancy, with their children receiving the same product for 6 months. By 2 years of age, children receiving probiotic therapy had a lower rate of atopic dermatitis (odds ratio [OR], 0.74; 95% CI, 0.55–0.98) and immunoglobulin E (IgE) –associated atopic dermatitis (OR = 0.66; 95% CI, 0.46–0.95).[81] A 2012 meta-analysis ($N = 13$ RCTs) reported a 25% reduction in the incidence of atopic dermatitis and IgE-associated atopic dermatitis. This effect, however, was documented only in the first 2 years of life and appeared to disappear by 5 years of age. There was significant heterogeneity among the included trials.[115]

Prebiotics may reduce the risk of developing allergic disease. Although there are fewer trials, the results are promising and suggest that giving prebiotics to infants may reduce the incidence of atopic dermatitis.[111]

The AAP and the European Academy of Allergy and Clinical Immunology do not endorse probiotics or prebiotics to prevent allergic disease due to limited scientific evidence.[106,146] In contrast, the World Allergy Organization (WAO) recommends prebiotics and probiotics to prevent atopic dermatitis. For infants who are not exclusively breastfed, the WAO recommends prebiotic supplementation.[33] They also support probiotics for pregnant women at high risk for having an allergic child, women breastfeeding infants at high risk for allergic disease, and infants at high risk for allergic disease. They acknowledge that the recommendations are based on low-quality evidence, but the WAO concludes that the potential benefits outweigh any safety concerns. The WAO does not specify a particular prebiotic product or a probiotic strain, dose, or duration.[49]

There is less research on the role of probiotics in the treatment of allergic diseases. A few preliminary studies found that probiotics may reduce symptoms of allergic rhinitis or atopic dermatitis. However, further studies are needed before definitive conclusions can be reached.[20,170]

Human Immunodeficiency Virus Infection

Individuals with human immunodeficiency virus (HIV) infection have a fecal microbiota profile distinct from healthy controls.[164] Preliminary studies suggest probiotics may improve the well-being of HIV-infected patients. Several studies have documented a modest increase in CD4 counts during probiotic use.[24,100] However, the effect of probiotics on HIV-associated diarrhea, including antiretroviral-associated diarrhea, has been mixed.[24] Overall, the evidence remains inconclusive on whether probiotics should be routinely administered to HIV-infected people.

Upper and Lower Respiratory Tract Infections

Growing evidence supports the notion that alterations in the intestinal microbiota can modulate the function of the innate immune system.[148] This finding has prompted investigation of the impact of probiotics on the prevention of respiratory infections.[46] In an RCT enrolling 638 childcare attendees 3 to 6 years of age, use of a fermented dairy drink containing *L. casei* mildly decreased the incidence of upper respiratory infections (URIs) compared with placebo (incidence rate ratio = 0.82; 95% CI, 0.68–0.99).[96] A 2015 Cochrane review (N = 12 RCTs) involving infants, children, and adults (N = 3720) found that probiotics appeared to prevent acute URIs, as measured by the number of people experiencing one or more episodes (OR = 0.53; 95% CI, 0.37–0.76) or three or more episodes (OR = 0.53; 95% CI, 0.36–0.80). There was also a lower rate of antibiotic prescriptions and a lower incidence of URI-related school absences in the probiotic group. However, when the URI rate (i.e., URI events per person-year) was measured, there was no difference between the probiotic and placebo groups. Several trials included in the analysis were determined to be of low or very low quality.[62]

Necrotizing Enterocolitis and Neonatal Sepsis

Meta-analyses have consistently found probiotics to reduce the incidence of necrotizing enterocolitis (NEC) among preterm neonates.[4,16,110] For example, a 2014 meta-analysis (N= 24 RCTs), which included 5529 preterm (<37 weeks' gestational age) or low-birth-weight (<2500 g) infants, found that probiotics decreased the incidence of NEC stage 2 or higher (RR, 0.43; 95% CI, 0.33–0.56) and mortality (RR, 0.65; 95% CI, 0.52–0.81).[4] Similar results were observed for very-low–birth-weight infants (<1500 g); however, the number of extremely-low-birth-weight (ELBW) infants (<1000 g) was too small to perform a meaningful analysis.

Several publications suggest that probiotics may decrease the incidence of late-onset sepsis, improve feeding tolerance, and shorten hospitalization.[2,117] Many different probiotic strains have been studied in neonates, including *L. acidophilus*, *L. reuteri*, *L. rhamnosus*, *B. bifidum*, *B. breve*, *B. infantis*, *S. boulardii*, and multistrain products.[9,63,72,87,150] Although many of these probiotic strains proved useful, there is evidence that not all probiotic strains are beneficial for preterm infants.[1] For example, a large and rigorous clinical trial (N= 1310) found that *Bifidobacterium breve* BBG-001 had no impact on the incidence of NEC, late-onset sepsis, or mortality for preterm infants.[31]

Neonatal centers throughout the United States and Europe routinely administer probiotics to preterm infants.[160] Some experts, however, have concerns about the increasing use of probiotics in preterm neonates. They cite issues with the quality of trials included in meta-analyses, the heterogeneity among published studies, the lack of an established probiotic regimen (i.e., strain, dose, and timing), and the absence of quality control regulations to ensure consistency and safety of probiotic products.[98,99] The AAP does not endorse the routine use of probiotics in preterm infants, but it does acknowledge there is "some evidence" to support their use to prevent NEC in infants weighing more than 1000 g.[146]

SAFETY OF PROBIOTICS AND PREBIOTICS IN INFANTS AND CHILDREN

Probiotics and prebiotics appear to be safe for infants and children. An analysis of 74 clinical trials, containing 7798 children who received a probiotic, did not identify any major safety concerns. No serious adverse events attributable to probiotics were reported, nor were there any infections from the administered probiotics. However, the documentation and reporting of adverse events was poor among many of the included studies.[156] Nonetheless, probiotics, although not without risk, appear to be safe for healthy infants and children. For high-risk or special patient groups, the safety of administering products containing live microorganisms requires careful consideration. The risks of probiotic use must be carefully balanced with the potential benefits.

Severe infections, including sepsis and meningitis, caused by probiotic microorganisms can occur in infants and children. Although uncommon, these events can be serious or fatal. Populations at risk include immunocompromised patients, preterm and low-birth-weight neonates, children with intestinal disorders, and patients with indwelling venous catheters.[42]

There is concern that probiotics may transfer antibiotic-resistance genes to pathogenic bacteria. Although there is no evidence that this has occurred, there is evidence to support the principle. Many probiotic strains possess genes that confer resistance to one or more antibacterial agents.[70,158] Xiao and colleagues, during a study evaluating the antibiotic susceptibility of *Bifidobacterium* species in commercial probiotic products in Japan, found *B. lactis* strains that harbored a plasmid-mediated *tet*(W) gene that conferred tetracycline resistance.[166] Mater and associates described the in vivo transfer of vancomycin resistance (i.e., *vanA* cluster) from a clinical *Enterococcus faecium* strain to a commercial strain of *L. acidophilus* during digestive passage in mice.[92] Lund and Edlund demonstrated the potential for a probiotic *E. faecium* strain (i.e., SF68) to receive the *vanA* gene cluster.[88] Collectively, these studies highlight the possibility of gene transfer between probiotic organisms and other microbes.

The purity of probiotic supplements, given the lack of regulatory oversight of the manufacturing process, is an important concern. Commercial probiotic products contaminated with cow's milk allergens have caused severe allergic reactions in children.[83, 90] In October 2014, a preterm neonate developed gastrointestinal mucormycosis related to contamination of a probiotic product with *Rhizopus oryzae*.[155]

INFECTIOUS DISEASES RELATED TO PROBIOTIC USE

As living microorganisms, probiotics have the potential to cause infectious diseases. Bloodstream infections are the most commonly reported infection. Serious, invasive infections have included meningitis, pneumonia, intraabdominal abscesses, and orthopedic hardware infections.

Bacteremia from *Lactobacillus* and *Bifidobacterium* species and fungemia from *Saccharomyces* species have been documented in infants and children.[10,36,45,129] However, the risk of bloodstream infections during probiotic use is very low. From 1995 to 2000, lactobacilli represented 0.2% of all positive blood cultures in Finland. There was no temporal change in the incidence of *Lactobacillus* bacteremia despite a substantial increase in the use of LGG during the study period.[126]

Bloodstream infections from probiotic organisms seem to be rare in immunocompromised patients. A large cancer center reported a low incidence of bloodstream infections due to *Lactobacillus* and *Saccharomyces* among hematopoietic stem cell transplant recipients.[29]

Invasive infections from *Lactobacillus* species have been described in neonates, children, and adults.[23,36,37,82] Bacteremia from *Lactobacillus* is the most commonly reported infection related to probiotic use. Not every infection from *Lactobacillus*, however, is attributable to probiotic use. Studies have demonstrated that lactobacilli isolated from human infections can be unrelated to the lactobacilli organisms in probiotic products.[7,112] Studies demonstrate that lactobacilli, as resident intestinal microbes, can originate from the host's microbiota. Infections from *Lactobacillus* have included neonatal sepsis, endocarditis, pneumonia, meningitis, liver abscess, intraabdominal abscess, and prosthetic joint infection.[19,21,23,40,119,124,130,132] Risk factors include immunocompromised status, indwelling central venous catheters, probiotic use, and recent surgical intervention.

Lactobacillus infections in children have been successfully treated with penicillin, ampicillin, clindamycin, or combination therapy (i.e.,β-lactam antibiotic plus aminoglycoside).[36,82] Lactobacilli tend to be resistant to vancomycin and fluoroquinolones; have variable susceptibility to penicillin, cephalosporins, and aminoglycosides; and have low minimum inhibitory concentrations (MICs) for piperacillin-tazobactam, clindamycin, and carbapenems.[84,125]

Bacteremia from *Bifidobacterium* has been documented among premature neonates receiving probiotics to prevent NEC. These rare cases have occurred in patients with abdominal pathology, including omphalocele, intestinal necrosis, and NEC.[15,45,162] A case of *Bifidobacterium breve* bacteremia was also reported in a child with acute lymphoblastic leukemia.[11]

Infections from *S. cerevisiae* and *S. boulardii* have been described in children and adults.[10,105,121] Fungemia is the most common clinical syndrome described, although endocarditis, pneumonia, liver abscess, peritonitis, and urinary tract infections have occurred.[105] Most fungemia cases have occurred in critically ill patients in intensive care units (ICUs). Risk factors include receipt of *S. boulardii* probiotic products, presence of indwelling central venous catheter, and receipt of broad-spectrum antibiotics.[10,105] *Saccharomyces* species can enter the bloodstream by intestinal translocation or external contamination of venous catheters. For example, an outbreak of *S. boulardii* fungemia included ICU patients who were not consuming probiotic supplements but were roommates of patients receiving lyophilized probiotic products.[25]

The management of *Saccharomyces* fungemia includes removal of indwelling vascular lines and antifungal therapy. Amphotericin B is the most frequently used agent, and clinical isolates of *Saccharomyces* are consistently susceptible to it. Fluconazole has also been used successfully to treat fungemia, although resistance has occasionally been reported.[105]

NEW REFERENCES SINCE THE SEVENTH EDITION

1. Abrahamsson TR. Not all probiotic strains prevent necrotising enterocolitis in premature infants. *Lancet*. 2016;387:624-625.
2. Aceti A, Gori D, Barone G, et al. Probiotics and time to achieve full enteral feeding in human milk-fed and formula-fed preterm infants: systematic review and meta-analysis. *Nutrients*. 2016;8:E471.
3. Agustina R, Kok FJ, van de Rest O, et al. Randomized trial of probiotics and calcium on diarrhea and respiratory tract infections in Indonesian children. *Pediatrics*. 2012;129:e1155-e1164.
4. AlFaleh K, Anabrees J. Probiotics for prevention of necrotizing enterocolitis in preterm infants. *Cochrane Database Syst Rev*. 2014;(4):CD005496.
5. Alisi A, Bedogni G, Baviera G, et al. Randomised clinical trial: the beneficial effects of VSL#3 in obese children with non-alcoholic steatohepatitis. *Aliment Pharmacol Ther*. 2014;39:1276-1285.
6. Allen SJ, Martinez EG, Gregorio GV, et al. Probiotics for treating acute infectious diarrhoea. *Cochrane Database Syst Rev*. 2010;(11):CD003048.
7. Aroutcheva A, Auclair J, Frappier M, et al. Importance of molecular methods to determine whether a probiotic is the source of *Lactobacillus* bacteremia. *Probiotics Antimicrob Proteins*. 2016;8:31-40.
8. Arvola T, Laiho K, Torkkeli S, et al. Prophylactic *Lactobacillus* GG reduces antibiotic-associated diarrhea in children with respiratory infections: a randomized study. *Pediatrics*. 1999;104:e64.
9. Athalye-Jape G, Rao S, Patole S. *Lactobacillus reuteri* DSM 17938 as a probiotic for preterm neonates: a strain-specific systematic review. *JPEN J Parenter Enteral Nutr*. 2016;40:783-794.
10. Atici S, Soysal A, Karadeniz Cerit K, et al. Catheter-related *Saccharomyces cerevisiae* fungemia following *Saccharomyces boulardii* probiotic treatment in a child in intensive care unit and review of the literature. *Med Mycol Case Rep*. 2017;15:33-35.
11. Avcin SL, Pokorn M, Kitanovski L, et al. *Bifidobacterium breve* sepsis in child with high-risk acute lymphoblastic leukemia. *Emerg Infect Dis*. 2015;21:1674-1675.
12. Basu S, Chatterjee M, Ganguly S, et al. Effect of *Lactobacillus rhamnosus* GG in persistent diarrhea in Indian children: a randomized controlled trial. *J Clin Gastroenterol*. 2007;41:756-760.
13. Baumler AJ, Sperandio V. Interactions between the microbiota and pathogenic bacteria in the gut. *Nature*. 2016;535:85-93.
14. Bernaola Aponte G, Bada Mancilla CA, Carreazo NY, et al. Probiotics for treating persistent diarrhoea in children. *Cochrane Database Syst Rev*. 2013;CD007401.
15. Bertelli C, Pillonel T, Torregrossa A, et al. *Bifidobacterium longum* bacteremia in preterm infants receiving probiotics. *Clin Infect Dis*. 2015;60:924-927.
16. Billimoria ZC, Pandya S, Bhatt P, et al. Probiotics—to use, or not to use? An updated meta-analysis. *Clin Pediatr (Phila)*. 2016;55:1242-1244.
17. Bin Z, Ya-Zheng X, Zhao-Hui D, et al. The efficacy of *Saccharomyces boulardii* CNCM I-745 in addition to standard *Helicobacter pylori* eradication treatment in children. *Pediatr Gastroenterol Hepatol Nutr*. 2015;18:17-22.
18. Black LI, Clarke TC, Barnes PM, et al. Use of complementary health approaches among children aged 4-17 years in the United States: National Health Interview Survey, 2007-2012. *Natl Health Stat Reports*. 2015;78:1-19.
19. Botros M, Mukundan D. *Lactobacillus* endocarditis with prosthetic material: a case report on non-surgical management with corresponding literature review. *Infect Dis Rep*. 2014;6:5497.
20. Boyle RJ, Bath-Hextall FJ, Leonardi-Bee J, et al. Probiotics for treating eczema. *Cochrane Database Syst Rev*. 2008;(4):CD006135.
21. Broughton RA, Gruber WC, Haffar AA, et al. Neonatal meningitis due to *Lactobacillus*. *Pediatr Infect Dis*. 1983;2:382-384.
22. Butterworth AD, Thomas AG, Akobeng AK. Probiotics for induction of remission in Crohn's disease. *Cochrane Database Syst Rev*. 2008;(3):CD006634.
23. Cannon JP, Lee TA, Bolanos JT, et al. Pathogenic relevance of *Lactobacillus*: a retrospective review of over 200 cases. *Eur J Clin Microbiol Infect Dis*. 2005;24:31-40.
24. Carter GM, Esmaeili A, Shah H, et al. Probiotics in human immunodeficiency virus infection: a systematic review and evidence synthesis of benefits and risks. *Open Forum Infect Dis*. 2016;3:ofw164.
25. Cassone M, Serra P, Mondello F, et al. Outbreak of *Saccharomyces cerevisiae* subtype *boulardii* fungemia in patients neighboring those treated with a probiotic preparation of the organism. *J Clin Microbiol*. 2003;41:5340-5343.
26. Cayzeele-Decherf A, Pelerin F, Leuillet S, et al. *Saccharomyces cerevisiae* CNCM I-3856 in irritable bowel syndrome: an individual subject meta-analysis. *World J Gastroenterol*. 2017;23:336-344.
27. Chang JY, Antonopoulos DA, Kalra A, et al. Decreased diversity of the fecal microbiome in recurrent *Clostridium difficile*-associated diarrhea. *J Infect Dis*. 2008;197:435-438.
28. Clarke TC, Black LI, Stussman BJ, et al. Trends in the use of complementary health approaches among adults: United States, 2002-2012. *Natl Health Stat Reports*. 2015;79:1-16.
29. Cohen SA, Woodfield MC, Boyle N, et al. Incidence and outcomes of bloodstream infections among hematopoietic cell transplant recipients from species commonly reported to be in over-the-counter probiotic formulations. *Transpl Infect Dis*. 2016;18:699-705.
30. Correa NB, Peret Filho LA, Penna FJ, et al. A randomized formula controlled trial of *Bifidobacterium lactis* and *Streptococcus thermophilus* for prevention of antibiotic-associated diarrhea in infants. *J Clin Gastroenterol*. 2005;39:385-389.
31. Costeloe K, Hardy P, Juszczak E, et al. *Bifidobacterium breve* BBG-001 in very preterm infants: a randomised controlled phase 3 trial. *Lancet*. 2016;387:649-660.
32. Cuello-Garcia CA, Brozek JL, Fiocchi A, et al. Probiotics for the prevention of allergy: a systematic review and meta-analysis of randomized controlled trials. *J Allergy Clin Immunol*. 2015;136:952-961.
33. Cuello-Garcia CA, Fiocchi A, Pawankar R, et al. World Allergy Organization–McMaster University guidelines for allergic disease prevention (GLAD-P): prebiotics. *World Allergy Organ J*. 2016;9:10.
34. Czerucka D, Piche T, Rampal P. Review article: yeast as probiotics—*Saccharomyces boulardii*. *Aliment Pharmacol Ther*. 2007;26:767-778.
35. Dalal R, McGee RG, Riordan SM, et al. Probiotics for people with hepatic encephalopathy. *Cochrane Database Syst Rev*. 2017;(2):CD008716.
36. Dani C, Coviello CC, Corsini II, et al. *Lactobacillus* sepsis and probiotic therapy in newborns: two new cases and literature review. *AJP Rep*. 2016;6:e25-e29.
37. De Groote MA, Frank DN, Dowell E, et al. Lactobacillus rhamnosus GG bacteremia associated with probiotic use in a child with short gut syndrome. *Pediatr Infect Dis J*. 2005;24:278-280.
38. de Weerth C, Fuentes S, Puylaert P, et al. Intestinal microbiota of infants with colic: development and specific signatures. *Pediatrics*. 2013;131:e550-e558.
40. Doern CD, Nguyen ST, Afolabi F, et al. Probiotic-associated aspiration pneumonia due to *Lactobacillus rhamnosus*. *J Clin Microbiol*. 2014;52:3124-3126.
41. Donovan SM, Comstock SS. Human milk oligosaccharides influence neonatal mucosal and systemic immunity. *Ann Nutr Metab*. 2016;69(suppl 2):42-51.
42. Doron S, Snydman DR. Risk and safety of probiotics. *Clin Infect Dis*. 2015;60(suppl 2):S129-S134.
43. Dubey AP, Rajeshwari K, Chakravarty A, et al. Use of VSL[sharp]3 in the treatment of rotavirus diarrhea in children: preliminary results. *J Clin Gastroenterol*. 2008;42(suppl 3):S126-S129.
44. Elazab N, Mendy A, Gasana J, et al. Probiotic administration in early life, atopy, and asthma: a meta-analysis of clinical trials. *Pediatrics*. 2013;132:e666-e676.
45. Esaiassen E, Cavanagh P, Hjerde E, et al. *Bifidobacterium longum* subspecies *infantis* Bacteremia in 3 extremely preterm infants receiving probiotics. *Emerg Infect Dis*. 2016;22:1664-1666.
46. Esposito S, Rigante D, Principi N. Do children's upper respiratory tract infections benefit from probiotics? *BMC Infect Dis*. 2014;14:194.
47. Famouri F, Shariat Z, Hashemipour M, et al. Effects of probiotics on nonalcoholic fatty liver disease in obese children and adolescents. *J Pediatr Gastroenterol Nutr*. 2017;64:413-417.
48. Feizizadeh S, Salehi-Abargouei A, Akbari V. Efficacy and safety of *Saccharomyces boulardii* for acute diarrhea. *Pediatrics*. 2014;134:e176-e191.
49. Fiocchi A, Pawankar R, Cuello-Garcia C, et al. World Allergy Organization–McMaster University guidelines for allergic disease prevention (GLAD-P): Probiotics. *World Allergy Organ J*. 2015;8:4.
52. Fox MJ, Ahuja KD, Robertson IK, et al. Can probiotic yogurt prevent diarrhoea in children on antibiotics? A double-blind, randomised, placebo-controlled study. *BMJ Open*. 2015;5:e006474.
53. Gibson GR, Probert HM, Loo JV, et al. Dietary modulation of the human colonic microbiota: updating the concept of prebiotics. *Nutr Res Rev*. 2004;17:259-275.

54. Gibson GR, Roberfroid MB. Dietary modulation of the human colonic microbiota: introducing the concept of prebiotics. *J Nutr.* 1995;125:1401-1412.
55. Goldenberg JZ, Lytvyn L, Steurich J, et al. Probiotics for the prevention of pediatric antibiotic-associated diarrhea. *Cochrane Database Syst Rev.* 2015;(12):CD004827.
56. Goldenberg JZ, Ma SS, Saxton JD, et al. Probiotics for the prevention of *Clostridium difficile*-associated diarrhea in adults and children. *Cochrane Database Syst Rev.* 2013;(5):CD006095.
57. Goldstein EJ, Tyrrell KL, Citron DM. *Lactobacillus* species: taxonomic complexity and controversial susceptibilities. *Clin Infect Dis.* 2015;60(suppl 2):S98-S107.
58. Guarino A, Ashkenazi S, Gendrel D, et al. European Society for Pediatric Gastroenterology, Hepatology, and Nutrition/European Society for Pediatric Infectious Diseases evidence-based guidelines for the management of acute gastroenteritis in children in Europe: update 2014. *J Pediatr Gastroenterol Nutr.* 2014;59:132-152.
59. Guarner F, Khan AG, Garisch J, et al. World Gastroenterology Organisation Global Guidelines: probiotics and prebiotics, October 2011. *J Clin Gastroenterol.* 2012;46:468-481.
60. Gutierrez-Castrellon P, Lopez-Velazquez G, Diaz-Garcia L, et al. Diarrhea in preschool children and *Lactobacillus reuteri*: a randomized controlled trial. *Pediatrics.* 2014;133:e904-e909.
61. Hamer HM, Jonkers D, Venema K, et al. Review article: the role of butyrate on colonic function. *Aliment Pharmacol Ther.* 2008;27:104-119.
62. Hao Q, Dong BR, Wu T. Probiotics for preventing acute upper respiratory tract infections. *Cochrane Database Syst Rev.* 2015;(2):CD006895.
63. Hartel C, Pagel J, Rupp J, et al. Prophylactic use of *Lactobacillus acidophilus/Bifidobacterium infantis* probiotics and outcome in very low birth weight infants. *J Pediatr.* 2014;165:285-289, e281.
65. Henker J, Laass M, Blokhin BM, et al. The probiotic *Escherichia coli* strain Nissle 1917 (EcN) stops acute diarrhoea in infants and toddlers. *Eur J Pediatr.* 2007;166:311-318.
66. Henker J, Laass MW, Blokhin BM, et al. Probiotic *Escherichia coli* Nissle 1917 versus placebo for treating diarrhea of greater than 4 days duration in infants and toddlers. *Pediatr Infect Dis J.* 2008;27:494-499.
67. Hill C, Guarner F, Reid G, et al. Expert consensus document. The International Scientific Association for Probiotics and Prebiotics consensus statement on the scope and appropriate use of the term probiotic. *Nat Rev Gastroenterol Hepatol.* 2014;11:506-514.
68. Hoffmann DE, Fraser CM, Palumbo FB, et al. Science and regulation. Probiotics: finding the right regulatory balance. *Science.* 2013;342:314-315.
69. Hojsak I, Tokic Pivac V, Mocic Pavic A, et al. *Bifidobacterium animalis* subsp. *lactis* fails to prevent common infections in hospitalized children: a randomized, double-blind, placebo-controlled study. *Am J Clin Nutr.* 2015;101:680-684.
70. Imperial IC, Ibana JA. Addressing the antibiotic resistance problem with probiotics: reducing the risk of its double-edged sword effect. *Front Microbiol.* 2016;7:1983.
71. Indrio F, Di Mauro A, Riezzo G, et al. Prophylactic use of a probiotic in the prevention of colic, regurgitation, and functional constipation: a randomized clinical trial. *JAMA Pediatr.* 2014;168:228-233.
72. Jacobs SE, Tobin JM, Opie GF, et al. Probiotic effects on late-onset sepsis in very preterm infants: a randomized controlled trial. *Pediatrics.* 2013;132:1055-1062.
73. Johnson CL, Versalovic J. The human microbiome and its potential importance to pediatrics. *Pediatrics.* 2012;129:950-960.
74. Johnston BC, Goldenberg JZ, Parkin PC. Probiotics and the prevention of antibiotic-associated diarrhea in infants and children. *JAMA.* 2016;316:1484-1485.
76. Kabbani TA, Pallav K, Dowd SE, et al. Prospective randomized controlled study on the effects of *Saccharomyces boulardii* CNCM I-745 and amoxicillin-clavulanate or the combination on the gut microbiota of healthy volunteers. *Gut Microbes.* 2017;8:17-32.
77. Kolacek S, Hojsak I, Canani RB, et al. Commercial probiotic products: a call for improved quality control. A position paper by the ESPGHAN Working Group for Probiotics and Prebiotics. *J Pediatr Gastroenterol Nutr.* 2017;Apr 11.
78. Korterink JJ, Ockeloen L, Benninga MA, et al. Probiotics for childhood functional gastrointestinal disorders: a systematic review and meta-analysis. *Acta Paediatr.* 2014;103:365-372.
79. Kotowska M, Albrecht P, Szajewska H. *Saccharomyces boulardii* in the prevention of antibiotic-associated diarrhoea in children: a randomized double-blind placebo-controlled trial. *Aliment Pharmacol Ther.* 2005;21:583-590.
80. Kuehn J, Ismael Z, Long PF, et al. Reported rates of diarrhea following oral penicillin therapy in pediatric clinical trials. *J Pediatr Pharmacol Ther.* 2015;20:90-104.
81. Kukkonen K, Savilahti E, Haahtela T, et al. Probiotics and prebiotic galacto-oligosaccharides in the prevention of allergic diseases: a randomized, double-blind, placebo-controlled trial. *J Allergy Clin Immunol.* 2007;119:192-198.
82. Land MH, Rouster-Stevens K, Woods CR, et al. *Lactobacillus* sepsis associated with probiotic therapy. *Pediatrics.* 2005;115:178-181.
83. Lee TT, Morisset M, Astier C, et al. Contamination of probiotic preparations with milk allergens can cause anaphylaxis in children with cow's milk allergy. *J Allergy Clin Immunol.* 2007;119:746-747.
84. Lee MR, Tsai CJ, Liang SK, et al. Clinical characteristics of bacteraemia caused by *Lactobacillus* spp. and antimicrobial susceptibilities of the isolates at a medical centre in Taiwan, 2000-2014. *Int J Antimicrob Agents.* 2015;46:439-445.
85. Li S, Huang XL, Sui JZ, et al. Meta-analysis of randomized controlled trials on the efficacy of probiotics in *Helicobacter pylori* eradication therapy in children. *Eur J Pediatr.* 2014;173:153-161.
86. Lievin-Le Moal V, Servin AL. Anti-infective activities of *Lactobacillus* strains in the human intestinal microbiota: from probiotics to gastrointestinal anti-infectious biotherapeutic agents. *Clin Microbiol Rev.* 2014;27:167-199.
88. Lund B, Edlund C. Probiotic *Enterococcus faecium* strain is a possible recipient of the vanA gene cluster. *Clin Infect Dis.* 2001;32:1384-1385.
89. Mallon P, McKay D, Kirk S, et al. Probiotics for induction of remission in ulcerative colitis. *Cochrane Database Syst Rev.* 2007;(4):CD005573.
90. Martin-Munoz MF, Fortuni M, Caminoa M, et al. Anaphylactic reaction to probiotics. Cow's milk and hen's egg allergens in probiotic compounds. *Pediatr Allergy Immunol.* 2012;23:778-784.
91. Martinez FA, Balciunas EM, Converti A, et al. Bacteriocin production by *Bifidobacterium* spp. A review. *Biotechnol Adv.* 2013;31:482-488.
92. Mater DD, Langella P, Corthier G, et al. A probiotic *Lactobacillus* strain can acquire vancomycin resistance during digestive transit in mice. *J Mol Microbiol Biotechnol.* 2008;14:123-127.
93. McFarland LV. Antibiotic-associated diarrhea: epidemiology, trends and treatment. *Future Microbiol.* 2008;3:563-578.
94. McFarland LV. Use of probiotics to correct dysbiosis of normal microbiota following disease or disruptive events: a systematic review. *BMJ Open.* 2014;4:e005047.
95. McFarland LV. From yaks to yogurt: the history, development, and current use of probiotics. *Clin Infect Dis.* 2015;60(suppl 2):S85-S90.
96. Merenstein D, Murphy M, Fokar A, et al. Use of a fermented dairy probiotic drink containing *Lactobacillus casei* (DN-114 001) to decrease the rate of illness in kids: the DRINK study. A patient-oriented, double-blind, cluster-randomized, placebo-controlled, clinical trial. *Eur J Clin Nutr.* 2010;64:669-677.
97. Miele E, Pascarella F, Giannetti E, et al. Effect of a probiotic preparation (VSL#3) on induction and maintenance of remission in children with ulcerative colitis. *Am J Gastroenterol.* 2009;104:437-443.
98. Mihatsch WA, Braegger CP, Decsi T, et al. Critical systematic review of the level of evidence for routine use of probiotics for reduction of mortality and prevention of necrotizing enterocolitis and sepsis in preterm infants. *Clin Nutr.* 2012; 31:6-15.
100. Miller H, Ferris R, Phelps BR. The effect of probiotics on CD4 counts among people living with HIV: a systematic review. *Benef Microbes.* 2016;7:345-351.
101. Miloh T. Probiotics in pediatric liver disease. *J Clin Gastroenterol.* 2015;49(suppl 1):S33-S36.
102. More MI, Swidsinski A. *Saccharomyces boulardii* CNCM I-745 supports regeneration of the intestinal microbiota after diarrheic dysbiosis—a review. *Clin Exp Gastroenterol.* 2015;8:237-255.
103. Morelli L, Capurso L. FAO/WHO guidelines on probiotics: 10 years later. *J Clin Gastroenterol.* 2012;46(suppl):S1-S2.
104. Morovic W, Hibberd AA, Zabel B, et al. Genotyping by PCR and high-throughput sequencing of commercial probiotic products reveals composition biases. *Front Microbiol.* 2016;7:1747.
105. Munoz P, Bouza E, Cuenca-Estrella M, et al. *Saccharomyces cerevisiae* fungemia: an emerging infectious disease. *Clin Infect Dis.* 2005;40:1625-1634.
106. Muraro A, Halken S, Arshad SH, et al. EAACI food allergy and anaphylaxis guidelines. Primary prevention of food allergy. *Allergy.* 2014;69:590-601.
108. Newlove-Delgado TV, Martin AE, Abbott RA, et al. Dietary interventions for recurrent abdominal pain in childhood. *Cochrane Database Syst Rev.* 2017;(3):CD010972.
109. Nobili V, Alkhouri N, Alisi A, et al. Nonalcoholic fatty liver disease: a challenge for pediatricians. *JAMA Pediatr.* 2015;169:170-176.
110. Olsen R, Greisen G, Schroder M, et al. Prophylactic probiotics for preterm infants: a systematic review and meta-analysis of observational studies. *Neonatology.* 2016;109:105-112.
111. Osborn DA, Sinn JK. Prebiotics in infants for prevention of allergy. *Cochrane Database Syst Rev.* 2013;(3):CD006474.
112. Ouwehand AC, Saxelin M, Salminen S. Phenotypic differences between commercial *Lactobacillus rhamnosus* GG and *L. rhamnosus* strains recovered from blood. *Clin Infect Dis.* 2004;39:1858-1860.
113. Patel R, DuPont HL. New approaches for bacteriotherapy: prebiotics, new-generation probiotics, and synbiotics. *Clin Infect Dis.* 2015;60(suppl 2):S108-S121.
114. Patro-Golab B, Shamir R, Szajewska H. Yogurt for treating antibiotic-associated diarrhea: systematic review and meta-analysis. *Nutrition.* 2015;31:796-800.
116. Prescott SL, Bjorksten B. Probiotics for the prevention or treatment of allergic diseases. *J Allergy Clin Immunol.* 2007;120:255-262.
117. Rao SC, Athalye-Jape GK, Deshpande GC, et al. Probiotic supplementation and late-onset sepsis in preterm infants: A meta-analysis. *Pediatrics.* 2016;137:e20153684.
118. Roberfroid M, Gibson GR, Hoyles L, et al. Prebiotic effects: metabolic and health benefits. *Br J Nutr.* 2010;104(suppl 2):S1-S63.
119. Robin F, Paillard C, Marchandin H, et al. *Lactobacillus rhamnosus* meningitis following recurrent episodes of bacteremia in a child undergoing allogeneic hematopoietic stem cell transplantation. *J Clin Microbiol.* 2010;48:4317-4319.
120. Rolfe VE, Fortun PJ, Hawkey CJ, et al. Probiotics for maintenance of remission in Crohn's disease. *Cochrane Database Syst Rev.* 2006;(4):CD004826.

121. Roy U, Jessani LG, Rudramurthy SM, et al. Seven cases of *Saccharomyces* fungaemia related to use of probiotics. *Mycoses*. 2017;60:375-380.
122. Ruszczynski M, Radzikowski A, Szajewska H. Clinical trial: effectiveness of *Lactobacillus rhamnosus* (strains E/N, Oxy and Pen) in the prevention of antibiotic-associated diarrhoea in children. *Aliment Pharmacol Ther*. 2008;28:154-161.
123. Saavedra JM, Bauman NA, Oung I, et al. Feeding of *Bifidobacterium bifidum* and *Streptococcus thermophilus* to infants in hospital for prevention of diarrhoea and shedding of rotavirus. *Lancet*. 1994;344:1046-1049.
124. Sadowska-Krawczenko I, Paprzycka M, Korbal P, et al. *Lactobacillus rhamnosus* GG suspected infection in a newborn with intrauterine growth restriction. *Benef Microbes*. 2014;5:397-402.
125. Salminen MK, Rautelin H, Tynkkynen S, et al. *Lactobacillus* bacteremia, species identification, and antimicrobial susceptibility of 85 blood isolates. *Clin Infect Dis*. 2006;42:e35-e44.
126. Salminen MK, Tynkkynen S, Rautelin H, et al. *Lactobacillus* bacteremia during a rapid increase in probiotic use of *Lactobacillus rhamnosus* GG in Finland. *Clin Infect Dis*. 2002;35:1155-1160.
127. Sarkar A, Mandal S. Bifidobacteria—insight into clinical outcomes and mechanisms of its probiotic action. *Microbiol Res*. 2016;192:159-171.
128. Sarker SA, Sultana S, Fuchs GJ, et al. *Lactobacillus paracasei* strain ST11 has no effect on rotavirus but ameliorates the outcome of nonrotavirus diarrhea in children from Bangladesh. *Pediatrics*. 2005;116:e221-e228.
129. Sato S, Uchida T, Kuwana S, et al. Bacteremia induced by *Bifidobacterium breve* in a newborn with cloacal exstrophy. *Pediatr Int*. 2016;58:1226-1228.
130. Sherid M, Samo S, Sulaiman S, et al. Liver abscess and bacteremia caused by *Lactobacillus*: role of probiotics? Case report and review of the literature. *BMC Gastroenterol*. 2016;16:138.
131. Shokryazdan P, Faseleh Jahromi M, Navidshad B, et al. Effects of prebiotics on immune system and cytokine expression. *Med Microbiol Immunol*. 2017; 206:1-9.
132. Somayaji R, Lynch T, Powell JN, et al. Remote transient *Lactobacillus animalis* bacteremia causing prosthetic hip joint infection: a case report. *BMC Infect Dis*. 2016;16:634.
133. Stier H, Bischoff SC. Influence of *Saccharomyces boulardii* CNCM I-745 on the gut-associated immune system. *Clin Exp Gastroenterol*. 2016;9:269-279.
134. Sung V, Hiscock H, Tang ML, et al. Treating infant colic with the probiotic *Lactobacillus reuteri*: double blind, placebo controlled randomised trial. *BMJ*. 2014;348:g2107.
135. Sur D, Manna B, Niyogi SK, et al. Role of probiotic in preventing acute diarrhoea in children: a community-based, randomized, double-blind placebo-controlled field trial in an urban slum. *Epidemiol Infect*. 2011;139:919-926.
136. Swidsinski A, Loening-Baucke V, Schulz S, et al. Functional anatomy of the colonic bioreactor: impact of antibiotics and *Saccharomyces boulardii* on bacterial composition in human fecal cylinders. *Syst Appl Microbiol*. 2016;39:67-75.
137. Szajewska H, Canani RB, Guarino A, et al. Probiotics for the prevention of antibiotic-associated diarrhea in children. *J Pediatr Gastroenterol Nutr*. 2016;62:495-506.
138. Szajewska H, Guarino A, Hojsak I, et al. Use of probiotics for management of acute gastroenteritis: a position paper by the ESPGHAN Working Group for Probiotics and Prebiotics. *J Pediatr Gastroenterol Nutr*. 2014;58:531-539.
139. Szajewska H, Kolodziej M. Systematic review with meta-analysis: *Lactobacillus rhamnosus* GG in the prevention of antibiotic-associated diarrhoea in children and adults. *Aliment Pharmacol Ther*. 2015;42:1149-1157.
140. Szajewska H, Kolodziej M. Systematic review with meta-analysis: *Saccharomyces boulardii* in the prevention of antibiotic-associated diarrhoea. *Aliment Pharmacol Ther*. 2015;42:793-801.
141. Szajewska H, Ruszczynski M, Kolacek S. Meta-analysis shows limited evidence for using *Lactobacillus acidophilus* LB to treat acute gastroenteritis in children. *Acta Paediatr*. 2014;103:249-255.
142. Szajewska H, Skorka A, Ruszczynski M, et al. Meta-analysis: *Lactobacillus* GG for treating acute gastroenteritis in children—updated analysis of randomised controlled trials. *Aliment Pharmacol Ther*. 2013;38:467-476.
143. Szajewska H, Wanke M, Patro B. Meta-analysis: the effects of *Lactobacillus rhamnosus* GG supplementation for the prevention of healthcare-associated diarrhoea in children. *Aliment Pharmacol Ther*. 2011;34:1079-1087.
144. Szymanski H, Armanska M, Kowalska-Duplaga K, et al. *Bifidobacterium longum* PL03, *Lactobacillus rhamnosus* KL53A, and *Lactobacillus plantarum* PL02 in the prevention of antibiotic-associated diarrhea in children: a randomized controlled pilot trial. *Digestion*. 2008;78:13-17.
145. Tabbers MM, DiLorenzo C, Berger MY, et al. Evaluation and treatment of functional constipation in infants and children: evidence-based recommendations from ESPGHAN and NASPGHAN. *J Pediatr Gastroenterol Nutr*. 2014;58:258-274.
147. Turck D, Bernet JP, Marx J, et al. Incidence and risk factors of oral antibiotic-associated diarrhea in an outpatient pediatric population. *J Pediatr Gastroenterol Nutr*. 2003;37:22-26.
148. Turner RB, Woodfolk JA, Borish L, et al. Effect of probiotic on innate inflammatory response and viral shedding in experimental rhinovirus infection—a randomised controlled trial. *Benef Microbes*. 2017;8:207-215.
149. Turroni F, Duranti S, Bottacini F, et al. *Bifidobacterium bifidum* as an example of a specialized human gut commensal. *Front Microbiol*. 2014;5:437.
150. Underwood MA. Impact of probiotics on necrotizing enterocolitis. *Semin Perinatol*. 2017;41:41-51.
151. Underwood MA, German JB, Lebrilla CB, et al. *Bifidobacterium longum* subspecies *infantis*: champion colonizer of the infant gut. *Pediatr Res*. 2015;77:229-235.
152. Urbanska M, Gieruszczak-Bialek D, Szajewska H. Systematic review with meta-analysis: *Lactobacillus reuteri* DSM 17938 for diarrhoeal diseases in children. *Aliment Pharmacol Ther*. 2016;43:1025-1034.
153. Urbanska M, Gieruszczak-Bialek D, Szymanski H, et al. Effectiveness of *Lactobacillus reuteri* DSM 17938 for the prevention of nosocomial diarrhea in children: a randomized, double-blind, placebo-controlled trial. *Pediatr Infect Dis J*. 2016;35:142-145.
154. Vajro P, Mandato C, Licenziati MR, et al. Effects of *Lactobacillus rhamnosus* strain GG in pediatric obesity-related liver disease. *J Pediatr Gastroenterol Nutr*. 2011;52:740-743.
155. Vallabhaneni S, Walker TA, Lockhart SR, et al. Notes from the field: fatal gastrointestinal mucormycosis in a premature infant associated with a contaminated dietary supplement—Connecticut, 2014. *MMWR Morb Mortal Wkly Rep*. 2015;64:155-156.
156. van den Nieuwboer M, Brummer RJ, Guarner F, et al. Safety of probiotics and synbiotics in children under 18 years of age. *Benef Microbes*. 2015;6:615-630.
157. Vanderhoof JA, Whitney DB, Antonson DL, et al. *Lactobacillus* GG in the prevention of antibiotic-associated diarrhea in children. *J Pediatr*. 1999;135:564-568.
158. Varankovich NV, Nickerson MT, Korber DR. Probiotic-based strategies for therapeutic and prophylactic use against multiple gastrointestinal diseases. *Front Microbiol*. 2015;6:685.
159. Venugopalan V, Shriner KA, Wong-Beringer A. Regulatory oversight and safety of probiotic use. *Emerg Infect Dis*. 2010;16:1661-1665.
160. Viswanathan S, Lau C, Akbari H, et al. Survey and evidence based review of probiotics used in very low birth weight preterm infants within the United States. *J Perinatol*. 2016;36:1106-1111.
161. Wanke M, Szajewska H. Lack of an effect of *Lactobacillus reuteri* DSM 17938 in preventing nosocomial diarrhea in children: a randomized, double-blind, placebo-controlled trial. *J Pediatr*. 2012;161:40-43, e41.
162. Weber E, Reynaud Q, Suy F, et al. *Bifidobacterium* species bacteremia: risk factors in adults and infants. *Clin Infect Dis*. 2015;61:482-484.
163. Weizman Z, Asli G, Alsheikh A. Effect of a probiotic infant formula on infections in child care centers: comparison of two probiotic agents. *Pediatrics*. 2005;115:5-9.
164. Williams B, Landay A, Presti RM. Microbiome alterations in HIV infection a review. *Cell Microbiol*. 2016;18:645-651.
165. Wong AP, Clark AL, Garnett EA, et al. Use of complementary medicine in pediatric patients with inflammatory bowel disease: results from a multicenter survey. *J Pediatr Gastroenterol Nutr*. 2009;48:55-60.
166. Xiao JZ, Takahashi S, Odamaki T, et al. Antibiotic susceptibility of bifidobacterial strains distributed in the Japanese market. *Biosci Biotechnol Biochem*. 2010;74:336-342.
167. Xu M, Wang J, Wang N, et al. The efficacy and safety of the probiotic bacterium *Lactobacillus reuteri* DSM 17938 for infantile colic: a meta-analysis of randomized controlled trials. *PLoS ONE*. 2015;10:e0141445.
168. Yi SH, Jernigan JA, McDonald LC. Prevalence of probiotic use among inpatients: a descriptive study of 145 U.S. hospitals. *Am J Infect Control*. 2016;44:548-553.
169. Yuan F, Ni H, Asche CV, et al. Efficacy of *Bifidobacterium infantis* 35624 in patients with irritable bowel syndrome: a meta-analysis. *Curr Med Res Opin*. 2017;1-7.
170. Zajac AE, Adams AS, Turner JH. A systematic review and meta-analysis of probiotics for the treatment of allergic rhinitis. *Int Forum Allergy Rhinol*. 2015;5:524-532.
171. Zuccotti G, Meneghin F, Aceti A, et al. Probiotics for prevention of atopic diseases in infants: systematic review and meta-analysis. *Allergy*. 2015;70:1356-1371.

The full reference list for this chapter is available at ExpertConsult.com.

PART

V

Prevention of Infectious Diseases

244 Health Care–Associated Infections

W. Charles Huskins • Julia Shaklee Sammons • Susan E. Coffin

Health care–associated (nosocomial) infections (HCAIs) are infections that occur as a consequence of health care. Many are associated with the use of modern invasive devices and procedures that breach normal host defenses and allow microbial invasion. Other infections result from exposure to pathogens in the health care environment that are transmitted from colonized or infected people or from contaminated objects and surfaces, water, or air; they may occur in those who have compromised immune systems or are particularly susceptible to infection, such as preterm infants. HCAIs also may occur in people delivering health care (i.e., occupationally acquired infections in health care providers).

HISTORICAL BACKGROUND

The history of HCAIs and their control is tightly linked to developments in institutional medical care.[652] Although not broadly recognized, efforts to study and prevent infection among hospitalized children have contributed significantly to the development of infection control and prevention efforts in general.

Semmelweis' classic studies of puerperal fever in the Vienna Lying-In Hospital in the mid-1800s provided insights into the cause and prevention of perinatal infections in neonates, not just their afflicted mothers.[653] Children also suffered greatly from the epidemics of contagious diseases that spread through hospitals during the 18th and 19th centuries.[234] This problem led to the opening of wards and entire hospitals designated for the treatment of patients with infectious diseases in the early 20th century.[652] By the mid-20th century, a number of interventions had been developed to minimize the spread of contagious diseases in hospitals, including the use of quarantine areas for new admissions, confinement of each child in an individual cubicle, creation of cohorts for patients admitted during community epidemics, use of masks by people caring for patients, exclusion of visitors, strict control of the health of nurses and physicians caring for the patients, and implementation of exhaust fans to prevent airborne transmission of measles and varicella.[67,86,293,417,437]

Outbreaks of *Staphylococcus aureus* infection in hospitalized infants had been documented in the late 1800s and early 1900s,[101,357] but the pandemic of *S. aureus* infections that plagued hospitals in the 1950s and 1960s drew special attention to the impact of infections caused by this organism. Outbreaks of staphylococcal disease were particularly devastating in neonatal nurseries, where epidemics caused by specific phage types caused substantial morbidity and mortality.[640] The seriousness of the hospital-acquired staphylococcal infection problem spawned more comprehensive efforts to document the impact and consequences of hospital-acquired infections[609–611] and served as the impetus to develop organized infection control programs, particularly in Great Britain (with its tradition of infection control sisters) and North America.

In 1970, a hospital-acquired infection surveillance and control program was established at Children's Hospital in Boston, and data were reported to the nascent National Nosocomial Infections Study at the Centers for Disease Control and Prevention (CDC).[240] The study emphasized the association of hospital-acquired infections with exposure to invasive devices and procedures. Additional epidemiologic studies of infections in pediatric patients cared for in intensive care units (ICUs) during the 1970s and early 1980s strengthened the association between the use of invasive devices and procedures and hospital-acquired infections.[263,299,310,454]

Advances in viral diagnostics in the 1970s led to greater appreciation of the importance of viruses as a significant cause of hospital-acquired infections, particularly in pediatric patients.[737,765] Spread of respiratory and gastrointestinal viruses, especially respiratory syncytial virus (RSV) and rotavirus, was documented as a severe problem on pediatric wards.[189,283,486,616,765]

In the past 40 years, problematic pathogens continue to emerge and reemerge as causes of HCAIs. Gram-positive bacteria, including coagulase-negative staphylococci, *S. aureus,* enterococci, and streptococci, have remained significant pathogens in hospitalized patients.[224,271,335,688] Antimicrobial-resistant bacteria, such as methicillin-resistant *S. aureus* (MRSA), vancomycin-resistant enterococci (VRE), and gram-negative bacilli resistant to third-generation cephalosporins, aminoglycosides, carbapenems, and quinolones are especially problematic.[305,330,363,441,442,585] Although MRSA has received the most attention in the media, gram-negative pathogens, such as carbapenemase-producing Enterobacteriaceae, *Burkholderia, Stenotrophomonas,* and *Acinetobacter* are even more problematic because they are resistant to most (or all) available antibiotics, and the pipeline of new active agents is very limited.[75]

Overuse of antibiotics is in part responsible for the continued increase in *Clostridium difficile* infections,[120] but the clonal spread of more virulent strains of *C. difficile* (e.g., NAP-1) has been a major problem for adults and children.[411,435,476,731] Many studies have documented an increase in *C. difficile* infection among hospitalized children over the past decade.[169,360,528,631,632,786]

As increasing numbers of severely ill and immunosuppressed children are cared for in hospitals, the incidence of fungal infection has increased dramatically, especially infection caused by *Candida* and *Aspergillus.*[1,224,229,475] Health care–associated acquisition of respiratory viruses, such as RSV, parainfluenza virus, and adenovirus, can cause severe and sometimes lethal pneumonia in these patients. HCAIs also can be caused by bloodborne pathogens, such as the human immunodeficiency virus (HIV), hepatitis B, hepatitis C, and parvovirus B19 among patients and health care workers.[113,119,109,277,547,691,727]

International outbreaks of infection, including severe acute respiratory syndrome (SARS), Middle East respiratory syndrome (MERS), pandemic influenza, and Ebola virus disease,[45,529,598,721] have been fueled by transmission in health care facilities. Health care workers have borne a substantial burden of disease from these infections.

For the past 2 decades, HCAIs have been viewed through the lens of efforts to improve the quality and safety of health care.[329,370] Most states require public reporting of institutional rates of HCAIs, and the Center for Medicare and Medicaid Services (CMS) requires facilities providing care for Medicare and Medicaid patients to report rates of HCAIs, with comparative data available for public viewing on the CMS's Hospital Compare website (www.hospitalcompare.hhs.gov). These infections are broadly recognized as important contributors to the preventable harms that affect patients as a consequence of health care, and a consortium of leading professional societies and governmental groups has issued a call to action for their elimination.[104] Initiatives to reduce HCAIs have been among the most prominent of the patient safety success stories,[117,577,576] and many multicenter collaborative networks are actively working on prevention of HCAIs in children.[64,314,444,490,647]

The U.S. Department of Health and Human Services is engaged in these efforts through its National Action Plan to Prevent Health Care–Associated Infections: Roadmap to Elimination (https://health.gov/hcq/prevent-hai-action-plan.asp) and the Partnership for Patients (https://partnershipforpatients.cms.gov/), a program that focuses on reducing preventable harms, including HCAIs, and readmissions. President Obama also took a leadership role in addressing the worldwide crisis in antimicrobial resistance through the President's Council of Advisors on Science and Technology Report to the President on Combating Antimicrobial Resistance (https://obamawhitehouse.archives.gov/sites/default/files/microsites/ostp/PCAST/pcast_carb_report_sept2014.pdf) and the White House's subsequent National Action Plan for Combating Antibiotic-Resistant Bacteria (https://obamawhitehouse.archives.gov/sites/default/files/docs/national_action_plan_for_combating_antibotic-resistant_bacteria.pdf).

The remaining sections of this chapter expand on these themes by describing HCAIs due to spread of communicable infections in health care facilities, infections related to invasive devices and procedures, infections caused by special pathogens, infections occurring in special populations, the components of programs to prevent these infections, and programs to optimize antimicrobial stewardship.

SPREAD OF COMMUNICABLE INFECTIONS IN HEALTH CARE FACILITIES

General Principles

HCAIs that occur as a result of spread of communicable infections common in the community are a major concern for all facilities providing health care to children. Several principles regarding the epidemiology of these infections, modified from those initially published by Hall,[280] are summarized here. First, their appearance and spread on the wards parallels closely the disease activity in the community. Second, exposure to these pathogens usually results in infection in any host who lacks specific immunity; consequently, a susceptible child is at risk regardless of the nature or severity of his or her underlying disease or medical treatment. Third, these infections are often more severe in patients who have underlying diseases (e.g., prematurity, pulmonary or cardiac disease) or who are immunocompromised. Fourth, children hospitalized as a result of the community-acquired infections comprise the most important reservoir for microorganisms causing these infections, but mildly symptomatic or asymptomatically colonized adult caregivers and visitors may be important reservoirs for some agents (e.g., RSV, pertussis). Fifth, prevention depends primarily on the timely implementation of and adherence to isolation precautions designed to interrupt the modes of transmission of the microorganisms involved. In some situations, other interventions are indicated, such as chemoprophylaxis for infants exposed to pertussis and immune globulin for high-risk individuals exposed to measles. Sixth, unless postdischarge surveillance is performed, the frequency of these infections can be underestimated because of short hospital stays and some infections (e.g., *C. difficile* infection) may be incubating at the time of discharge and manifest only after the child returns home.

Modes of Transmission

Airborne transmission involves spread of microorganisms by droplet nuclei, which are small particles (<5 μm) generated by the desiccation of larger respiratory droplets, especially those expelled by coughing. Because they are extremely light, droplet nuclei can travel very long distances on air currents. The small droplet nuclei can remain suspended in inhaled air, evading the mechanical host defenses of the upper respiratory tract, to reach the distal airways and alveoli.[502] Diseases spread by airborne transmission of respiratory droplet nuclei include measles, tuberculosis, smallpox, and under certain circumstances, influenza and varicella.[159,404,504,592,736]

Droplet transmission involves transfer of microorganisms by large respiratory droplets, such as those generated by coughing or sneezing, which typically travel short distances in the air before settling. Important pathogens spread by this route include *Bordetella pertussis, Neisseria meningitidis,* and group A streptococci.

Contact transmission is the principal mode of transmission for most HCAIs. Direct contact transmission involves physical contact between a person harboring the microorganism and a susceptible host, such as a caregiver with a herpetic whitlow who transmits the virus to a neonate. Indirect contact transmission involves transfer of microorganisms by an intermediary person, object, or surface. The hands of caregivers are a common source of indirect contact transmission,[76] but fomites and contaminated environmental surfaces are also important for certain pathogens (e.g., RSV, *C. difficile,* MRSA, *Acinetobacter baumannii, Pseudomonas aeruginosa,* norovirus).[544,755]

Endogenous infection or autoinfection is caused by a patient's own colonizing flora, usually as a consequence of host defenses that are compromised by severe underlying disease, immunosuppressive therapy, or invasive devices and procedures. Endogenous infections may be caused by microorganisms that are a part of the normal microbiome (e.g., coagulase-negative *Staphylococcus*) or that are acquired from exposure to the health care environment, usually by indirect contact transmission, and become persistent colonizers (e.g., VRE). These infections can be considered as a special case of contact transmission.

Common vehicle (i.e., common source) transmission involves the widespread dissemination of a microorganism to many people by a contaminated item or substance. Examples include recent outbreaks of hepatitis B and C due to blood contamination of reused items[113,277] and outbreaks caused by nonenteric gram-negative bacilli, such as *P. aeruginosa,* that thrive in medications, solutions, or wet equipment and are relatively resistant to preservatives, antiseptics, and disinfectants.

Vector transmission of microorganisms on (i.e., extrinsic) or within (i.e., intrinsic) insects is possible, but it is rare in hospitals.[46,123,225]

Some infections may be spread by more than one mode of transmission. For example, varicella zoster virus may be spread by airborne and contact transmission.

Standard and Transmission-Based Precautions

The CDC's Healthcare Infection Control Practices Advisory Committee's (HICPAC) guideline for isolation precautions describes strategies to prevent spread of communicable infections in health care facilities.[668] These strategies involve the use of *standard precautions,* which should be used for all hospitalized patients at all times, and *transmission-based precautions,* which are used for patients with suspected or confirmed infections that may be transmissible to other patients or health care workers. Transmission-based precautions include *airborne precautions, droplet precautions,* and *contact precautions,* each of which is designed to interrupt one of the described modes of transmission. The key components of standard precautions and transmission-based precautions are outlined in Boxes 244.1 and 244.2 and are described in more detail later in this chapter (see Infection Prevention and Control Programs in Health Care Facilities).

Respiratory Viruses

RSV is the most common health care–associated respiratory virus infection, especially among children younger than 2 years of age, because RSV infection accounts for a substantial number of hospital admissions of young children during epidemic periods.[77,282,332,396,660,743] In the absence of effective infection prevention and control programs, attack rates can be high because immunity after infection is short lived, inoculation of virus into the nose or eyes reliably leads to infection, infected children excrete high titers of virus in their copious secretions, and RSV survives for long periods in the environment.[284,286,281,282] Risk factors for health care–associated RSV infection are prematurity, heart and lung disease, immunocompromising conditions, and duration of hospitalization.[287–289,396,448,675,743]

The transmission of RSV can be markedly reduced by scrupulous attention to hand hygiene and the use of gloves and gowns when touching patients or their immediate inanimate environment.[272,402,740] Goggles and masks can be effective in further reducing the RSV attack rate among personnel.[9,238] However, it is unclear whether masks and eye protection are effective because they prevent direct deposition of respiratory droplets on the eyes or nose or merely because they reduce the likelihood that staff will rub their eyes or noses with contaminated hands. Covering only the nose and mouth with a mask is probably not very effective.[285] The HICPAC isolation guideline recommends use of contact precautions for care of hospitalized patients with RSV and does not require use of a mask.[668]

Some investigators have demonstrated that cohorting infected patients combined with the use of barriers can reduce spread of RSV.[193,375,452] However, it is not clear whether cohorting by clinical symptoms alone is effective or all admitted patients must be screened for RSV infection to identify children with minimal symptoms who may be excreting the virus. The added value of strict cohorting instead of rigorous use of barrier precautions has not been demonstrated. Universal gloving for all patient contacts during RSV infection has also been advocated; one study found that this policy was also associated with reduced rates of

BOX 244.1 Standard Precautions[a]

A. Handwashing

- Wash hands after touching blood, body fluids, secretions, excretions, and contaminated items, whether gloves are worn or not.
- Wash hands immediately after gloves are removed, between patient contacts, and when otherwise indicated to avoid transfer of microorganisms to other patients or environments.
- It may be necessary to wash hands between tasks and procedures on the same patient to prevent cross-contamination of different body sites.
- Use a plain (nonantimicrobial) soap for handwashing.
- Use an antimicrobial agent or a waterless antiseptic agent for specific circumstances (e.g., control of outbreaks or hyperendemic infections), as defined by the infection control program.

B. Gloves

- Wear gloves (clean, nonsterile gloves are adequate) when touching blood, body fluids, secretions, excretions, and contaminated items.
- Put on clean gloves just before touching mucous membranes and nonintact skin.
- Change gloves between tasks and procedures on the same patient after contact with material that may contain a high concentration of microorganisms.
- Remove gloves promptly after use, before touching noncontaminated items and environmental surfaces, and before going to another patient, and wash hands immediately to avoid transfer of microorganisms to other patients or environments.

C. Mask, Eye Protection, and Face Shield

- Wear a mask and eye protection or a face shield to protect mucous membranes of the eyes, nose, and mouth during procedures and patient care activities that are likely to generate splashes or sprays of blood, body fluids, secretions, and excretions.

D. Gown

- Wear a gown (a clean, nonsterile gown is adequate) to protect skin and prevent soiling of clothing during procedures and patient care activities that are likely to generate splashes or sprays of blood, body fluids, secretions, or excretions.
- Select a gown that is appropriate for the activity and amount of fluid likely to be encountered.
- Remove a soiled gown as promptly as possible, and wash hands to avoid transfer of microorganisms to other patients or environments.

E. Patient Care Equipment

- Handle used patient care equipment soiled with blood, body fluids, secretions, and excretions in a manner that prevents skin and mucous membrane exposures, contamination of clothing, and transfer of microorganisms to other patients and environments.
- Ensure that reusable equipment is not used for the care of another patient until it has been cleaned and reprocessed appropriately.
- Ensure that single-use items are discarded properly.

F. Environmental Control

- Ensure that the hospital has adequate procedures for the routine care, cleaning, and disinfection of environmental surfaces, beds, bedrails, bedside equipment, and other frequently touched surfaces, and ensure that these procedures are followed.

G. Linen

- Handle, transport, and process used linen soiled with blood, body fluids, secretions, and excretions in a manner that prevents skin and mucous membrane exposure and contamination of clothing and that avoids transfer of microorganisms to other patients and environments.

H. Occupational Health and Bloodborne Pathogens

- Take care to prevent injuries when using needles, scalpels, and other sharp instruments or devices; when handling sharp instruments after procedures; when cleaning used instruments; and when disposing of used needles.
- Never recap used needles or otherwise manipulate them using both hands or any other technique that involves directing the point of a needle toward any part of the body; rather, use a one-handed scoop technique or a mechanical device designed for holding the needle sheath.
- Do not remove used needles from disposable syringes by hand, and do not bend, break, or otherwise manipulate used needles by hand.
- Place used disposable needles and syringes, scalpel blades, and other sharp items in appropriate puncture-resistant containers, which are located as close as practical to the area in which the items were used, and place reusable syringes and needles in a puncture-resistant container for transport to the reprocessing area.
- Use mouthpieces, resuscitation bags, or other ventilation devices as an alternative to mouth-to-mouth resuscitation methods in areas where the need for resuscitation is predictable.

I. Patient Placement

- Place a patient who contaminates the environment or who does not (or cannot be expected to) assist in maintaining appropriate hygiene or environmental control in a private room.
- If a private room is not available, consult with infection control professionals regarding patient placement or other alternatives.

[a]Standard precautions apply to all patients, regardless of their diagnosis or presumed infection status. Standard precautions apply to any planned or potential contact with blood; all body fluids, secretions, and excretions except sweat, regardless of whether they contain visible blood; nonintact skin; and mucous membranes.

From Siegel JD, Rhinehart E, Jackson M, et al. *Guideline for Isolation Precautions: Preventing Transmission of Infectious Agents in Healthcare Settings 2007*. Centers for Disease Control and Prevention, Healthcare Infection Control Practices Advisory Committee, 2007. Available at: http://www.cdc.gov/hicpac/2007IP/2007isolationPrecautions.html.

central line–associated bloodstream infection (CLABSI).[781] The role of palivizumab as routine seasonal prophylaxis or as postexposure prophylaxis for high-risk patients has been examined in uncontrolled studies with generally positive but not conclusive results.[191,272,350,384,531]

Multidisciplinary programs to promote awareness of the potential for transmission of RSV and optimize the use of prevention measures using all or various combinations of these strategies. They have demonstrated effectiveness in reducing the incidence of health care–associated RSV infection.[15,272,348,400,402,446]

HCAIs due to parainfluenza virus and human metapneumovirus are similar to RSV in their epidemiology and prevention.[282,332,498,517] Health care–associated influenza is a common cause of intercurrent fever in hospitalized children during epidemic periods,[283,743] and outbreaks in neonatal ICUs have been described.[157,506,748] Asthma was identified as a risk factor for health care–associated seasonal influenza.[401] Although the 2009–10 pandemic of H1N1 influenza raised concerns about the potential for increased spread of influenza in health care facilities, the risk for transmission among hospitalized children appeared to be no different from that for seasonal influenza,[218,541] perhaps because of heightened awareness and more rigorous use of barrier precautions.

The modes of transmission of influenza have not been precisely defined. Although direct, indirect, and droplet contact are likely to be important, the potential for airborne transmission and the relative contributions of these various modes of transmission in health care

BOX 244.2 Transmission-Based Precautions[a]

Airborne Precautions

A. Patient Placement

- Place the patient in a private room that has monitored negative air pressure in relation to the surrounding areas; 6–12 air changes per hour; and appropriate discharge of air outdoors or monitored high-efficiency filtration of room air before the air is circulated to other areas in the hospital.
- Keep the room door closed and the patient in the room.
- When a private room is not available, place the patient in a room with a patient who has active infection with the same microorganism, unless otherwise recommended, but with no other infection.
- When a private room is not available and cohorting is not desirable, consultation with infection control professionals is advised before patient placement.

B. Respiratory Protection

- Wear respiratory protection when entering the room of a patient with known or suspected infectious pulmonary tuberculosis.
- A susceptible person should not enter the room of patients known or suspected to have measles (rubeola) or varicella (chickenpox) if other immune caregivers are available.
- If susceptible people must enter the room of a patient known or suspected to have measles or varicella, they should wear respiratory protection.
- People immune to measles or varicella need not wear respiratory protection.

C. Patient Transport

- Limit the movement and transport of the patient from the room to essential purposes only.
- If transport or movement is necessary, minimize patient's dispersal of droplet nuclei by placing a surgical mask on the patient if possible.

D. Additional Precautions for Preventing Transmission of Tuberculosis

- Consult the CDC Guidelines for Preventing the Transmission of Tuberculosis in Health-Care Facilities for additional prevention strategies.

Droplet Precautions

A. Patient Placement

- Place the patient in a private room.
- When a private room is not available, place the patient in a room with a patient who has active infection with the same microorganism but no other infection.
- When a private room is not available and cohorting is not achievable, maintain spatial separation of at least 3 feet between the infected patient and other patients and visitors.
- Special air handling and ventilation are not necessary, and the door may remain open.

B. Mask

- Wear a mask when working within 3 feet of the patient. (Logistically, some hospitals may want to implement wearing of a mask to enter the room.)

C. Patient Transport

- Limit the movement and transport of the patient from the room to essential purposes only.
- If transport or movement is necessary, minimize patient dispersal of droplets by placing a surgical mask on the patient, if possible.

Contact Precautions

A. Patient Placement

- Place the patient in a private room.
- When a private room is not available, place the patient in a room with a patient who has active infection with the same microorganism but no other infection.
- When a private room is not available and cohorting is not achievable, consider the epidemiology of the microorganism and the patient population when determining patient placement. Consultation with infection control professionals is advised before patient placement.

B. Gloves

- Wear gloves (clean, nonsterile gloves are adequate) when entering the room.
- During the course of providing care for a patient, change gloves after having contact with infective material that may contain high concentrations of microorganisms (i.e., fecal material and wound drainage).
- Remove gloves before leaving the patient's environment, and wash hands immediately with an antimicrobial agent or a waterless antiseptic agent.
- After glove removal and handwashing, ensure that hands do not touch potentially contaminated environmental surfaces or items in the patient's room to avoid transfer of microorganisms to other patients or environments.

C. Gown

- Wear a gown (a clean, nonsterile gown is adequate) when entering the room if you anticipate that your clothing will have substantial contact with the patient, environmental surfaces, or items in the patient's room or if the patient is incontinent or has diarrhea, an ileostomy, a colostomy, or wound drainage not contained by a dressing.
- Remove the gown before leaving the patient's environment.
- After gown removal, ensure that clothing does not contact potentially contaminated environmental surfaces to avoid transfer of microorganisms to other patients or environments.

D. Patient Transport

- Limit the movement and transport of the patient from the room to essential purposes only.
- If the patient is transported out of the room, ensure that precautions are maintained to minimize the risk for transmission of microorganisms to other patients and contamination of environmental surfaces or equipment.

E. Patient Care Equipment

- When possible, dedicate the use of noncritical patient care equipment to a single patient (or a cohort of patients infected or colonized with the pathogen requiring precautions) to avoid sharing between patients.
- If use of common equipment or items is unavoidable, adequately clean and disinfect them before use for another patient.

F. Additional Precautions for Preventing the Spread of Vancomycin Resistance

- Consult the Healthcare Infection Control Practices Advisory Committee (HICPAC) report on preventing the spread of vancomycin resistance for additional prevention strategies.

[a]Transmission-based precautions are followed when indicated in addition to standard precautions.

From Siegel JD, Rhinehart E, Jackson M, et al. *Guideline for Isolation Precautions: Preventing Transmission of Infectious Agents in Healthcare Settings 2007.* Centers for Disease Control and Prevention, Healthcare Infection Control Practices Advisory Committee, 2007. Available at: http://www.cdc.gov/hicpac/2007IP/2007isolationPrecautions.html.

facilities and the potential differences in transmission of seasonal versus pandemic influenza remain unclear.[106] For seasonal influenza, the CDC recommends use of droplet precautions, with the use of respiratory protection equivalent to a fitted N95 filtering facepiece respirator or equivalent N95 respirator during aerosol-generating procedures (http://www.cdc.gov/flu/professionals/infectioncontrol/healthcaresettings.htm).

Annual influenza vaccination of high-risk individuals and health care workers is important to limit the impact of transmission in health care facilities.[116] Issues related to vaccination of health care workers against influenza are discussed later in this chapter (see Infection Prevention and Control Programs in Health Care Facilities). Antiviral medications are an adjunct to vaccination for treatment to reduce viral shedding and chemoprophylaxis to prevent infection after exposure.[219]

Health care–associated adenovirus infections occur sporadically throughout the year, and outbreaks of respiratory tract infection and pharyngoconjunctival fever among hospitalized children have been described. Outbreaks in ICUs and units caring for immunocompromised patients have been associated with severe disease and substantial mortality rates.[473,678,766] In addition to direct and indirect contact, adenovirus may be spread by droplet contact, necessitating the use of droplet and contact precautions.

Health care–associated coronavirus infections may be more common than recognized.[236,332] Although standard precautions are sufficient for most serotypes of coronavirus, the CDC recommends contact and airborne precautions for MERS and SARS (http://www.cdc.gov/coronavirus/mers/infection-prevention-control.html).

Rhinovirus infections are generally mild, although serious lower tract disease has been documented in children with underlying disorders.[133] Standard Precautions are sufficient as a control measure in most situations.

Pertussis

Outbreaks of pertussis in hospitals and chronic care institutions are well documented.[114,220,382,423,661,697,717,738] In many situations, health care workers were responsible for spreading pertussis to hospitalized children.[114,132,382,423,738] The beneficial impact but high cost of controlling the intrahospital spread of pertussis was illustrated during a large, community-wide epidemic of pertussis in Cincinnati in 1993.[135]

Prevention of health care–associated pertussis depends on the appropriate isolation of children with suspected infection, use of droplet precautions, antimicrobial treatment of confirmed cases to minimize the potential for transmission, prompt identification and management of exposed patients and health care workers, and chemoprophylaxis for exposed individuals.[143,381,668] Hospital staff who have symptoms suggesting pertussis must be evaluated and treated promptly, and infected individuals should be excluded from work for at least the first 5 days of the recommended course of treatment. Health care workers should receive booster doses of pertussis vaccine (i.e., tetanus toxoid, reduced diphtheria toxoid, and acellular pertussis [Tdap]) to help prevent transmission in health care facilities.[116]

Gastrointestinal Viruses

Rotavirus is a common cause of endemic and epidemic health care–associated gastrointestinal virus infection.[88,156,258,588,602,680,745] The risk of HCAIs is closely associated with hospitalization during seasonal outbreaks, young age, and the length of hospitalization.[88,145,178,745] The risk for transmission from infected children is enhanced because infected children may shed the virus in their stool for many days after symptoms resolve, asymptomatically infected patients also may shed virus, and the virus can survive for extended periods on environmental surfaces.[26,145,239,636,770]

The primary mode of transmission is indirect contact with the contaminated hands of caregivers, and scrupulous adherence to contact precautions and appropriate disinfection of environmental surfaces are critically important.[678,749] The use of rotavirus vaccine appears to have decreased the risk of health care–associated rotavirus concomitant with reductions in the numbers of children hospitalized due to community-acquired infection.[24,789]

Health care–associated norovirus infection—most often due to genogroup II.4 that can cause more severe disease—is a major problem, although wards with elderly populations have been affected more significantly than pediatric wards.[181,472] Contamination of environmental surfaces is particularly common and contributes to transmission.[503,544] A HICPAC isolation guideline recommends use of contact precautions and appropriate disinfection of environmental surfaces, with additional recommendations to be considered in outbreak situations.[447]

Other intestinal viruses have been documented to cause endemic and epidemic nosocomial gastrointestinal infection, including enteric adenoviruses,[156,373] caliciviruses,[694] astroviruses,[177,383] and toroviruses.[333] Contact precautions should be used to prevent transmission of these enteric pathogens.[668]

Clostridium Difficile

Toxin-producing *C. difficile* acquired in the community may be spread in health care settings, although this is difficult to distinguish from spread of *C. difficile* from reservoirs in the health care facility such as infected patients or the health care environment. *C. difficile* infection is discussed later (see Health Care–Associated Infections Related to Special Pathogens).

Other Gastrointestinal Bacteria

Gastrointestinal bacterial pathogens, such as *Salmonella, Shigella, Campylobacter, Yersinia, Escherichia coli,* and *Vibrio cholerae,* may cause outbreaks of health care–associated diarrhea in areas where gastrointestinal infections caused by these organisms are endemic.* However, they are so uncommon in modern health care facilities that in the absence of an outbreak, the yield of routine stool cultures in the evaluation of health care–associated diarrhea is extremely low.[81,149,784]

Varicella Zoster Virus

Outbreaks of health care–associated varicella in hospitals have been documented in numerous reports.[233,276,404,642] The reports demonstrate conclusively that varicella can be transmitted by the airborne route, although spread by direct and droplet contact may well be more efficient. A study that used a polymerase chain reaction (PCR) assay detected airborne virus in the hospital rooms of patients with active infection and in air samples obtained in the hallway just outside the patients' negative-pressure isolation rooms.[637]

Transmission of varicella can be minimized if infected patients are cared for using airborne precautions in single rooms with separate exhaust systems and negative air pressure relative to the hallway.[21,668] Contact precautions to prevent direct and indirect contact transmission (i.e., gloves and gowns) are also important. Because infected people are infectious for 24 to 48 hours before distinctive symptoms and signs appear, prompt recognition and isolation of patients and visitors who may be in the contagious phase of varicella is critical. Caregivers who are not immune to varicella should not care for these patients.

Options for postexposure prophylaxis, including passive immunization and use of varicella vaccine and acyclovir, are discussed in the American Academy of Pediatrics' *Red Book.*[187] Hospitalized exposed children should remain in isolation from day 8 to day 21 after exposure. If passive immunization is administered, isolation should be continued until day 28 after exposure.[16]

The use of varicella vaccine has diminished the risk for health care–associated varicella by decreasing the number of children hospitalized with varicella, reducing the size of the pool of susceptible children in hospital wards, and providing protective immunity to health care workers who did not have a history of prior infection.[116] However, incompletely vaccinated children and health care workers and people who develop breakthrough infection pose a risk for transmission.

Cytomegalovirus

Two studies using molecular typing techniques have documented probable patient-to-patient spread of cytomegalovirus (CMV) in a neonatal ICU and a chronic care unit.[176,693] In both situations, the infected children had been in close proximity and were cared for by common caregivers for extended periods.

The risk of CMV transmission from infected patients to health care workers is very low. A meta-analysis of studies that examined the risk

*References 48, 98, 103, 203, 252, 302, 349, 485, 587, 617, 654, 702, 741.

of CMV among pediatric nurses indicates that CMV infection in this population occurs at a rate that is comparable to that for control populations (i.e., women of comparable age who are not nurses).[7] A subanalysis of these data suggests that nursery nurses may have a slightly higher rate of infection than control populations.[7] However, studies of CMV infection in nursery nurses that involved molecular typing of CMV isolates showed that the infected nurses did not acquire CMV from the infants in their care[7] and presumably contracted their infections from children in their own households, through sexual contact, or from other community sources.

Given the frequency of asymptomatic CMV excretion from children (e.g., approximately 1% of newborns excrete the virus), health care workers should assume that any child may be excreting virus and should practice hand hygiene and use of standard precautions as a part of routine patient care.[668] Additional interventions are not indicated, and pregnant staff members do not need to be given special assignments.

Herpes Simplex Virus

Health care–associated transmission of herpes simplex virus (HSV) type 1 to neonates has been confirmed through studies using molecular typing.[290,422,629,742] Direct contact transmission from a hospital worker with herpes labialis and indirect contact transmission from one infected neonate to another were the most likely routes, although transmission from an asymptomatic parent or caregiver was possible.

Health care–associated HSV infections among health care workers, patients, and family members have been described in ICUs.[6,559] Herpetic whitlow has been observed among nurses, presumably as a result of direct transmission during suctioning of oral and respiratory secretions from infected patients.[6] The use of standard precautions, particularly the use of gloves during contact with oral and respiratory sections, and hand hygiene is adequate to prevent transmission of HSV.[547]

Measles, Mumps, and Rubella Viruses

Transmission of measles in health care facilities remains a threat, and hospitals can serve as nidi for community-wide infection.[74,118,115,129] Measles is transmitted by airborne droplet nuclei, as demonstrated by an outbreak in a pediatrician's office.[592]

Prevention of health care–associated measles hinges on the prompt recognition of infected or potentially infected patients and placement of these patients in isolation rooms with negative air pressure relative to that of the hallway.[118,668] Despite prompt recognition, the identification and management of exposed patients, their family members, and health care workers is time consuming and expensive.[762] Prophylactic vaccination of exposed susceptible individuals within 3 days of the exposure reliably prevents measles, whereas administration of immune globulin within 3 days attenuates disease but does not guarantee that the exposed individual will not develop contagious infection.[186] To avoid outbreaks of measles among health care workers, health care facilities should require new employees involved in patient care to provide evidence of immunity or appropriate vaccination or to receive vaccination with measles vaccine or measles-mumps-rubella (MMR) vaccine.[116,376]

Outbreaks of health care–associated mumps and rubella have been reported less commonly than measles.[303,565,703,767] The primary concern about the spread of both infections is the potential for complications in health care workers—mumps orchitis in men and rubella in pregnant staff.

Information regarding the transmission of both viruses is limited, but it probably occurs primarily by droplet contact. Droplet precautions should be observed during close contact with infected patients.[668] Because transmission of mumps occurs before and within 5 days of parotitis onset, isolation should be imposed during this period.[387] Patients with congenital rubella syndrome may excrete large amounts of virus in their urine and respiratory secretions for extended periods. Gowns and gloves should be worn for contact with these patients for the first year of life unless nasopharyngeal and urine cultures are negative by 3 months of age.[668] There is no known effective postexposure prophylaxis for mumps- or rubella-exposed individuals.

As with prevention of measles, new employees involved in patient care should provide evidence of immunity or appropriate vaccination or receive vaccination with MMR vaccine as a condition of employment.[116]

Parvovirus B19

The wide spectrum of disease caused by parvovirus B19 coupled with well-documented health care–associated outbreaks of infection has fueled efforts to understand the transmission and control of this virus in hospitals. An experimental study of acute parvovirus B19 infection in normal adults detected virus in respiratory secretions during a period of viremia and systemic symptoms 6 to 13 days after inoculation.[22] Detectable virus in respiratory secretions disappeared as viremia and systemic symptoms diminished, and virus was not demonstrable in respiratory secretions when rash, arthralgias, and arthritis occurred several days later.[22] From studies of parvovirus B19 infection in health care facilities, it is apparent that the virus can be transmitted by acutely infected patients, probably due to high levels of virus in their blood and respiratory secretions.[49,216,374,440,560,590] The risk of transmission from chronically infected, immunocompromised patients is less clear; however, from one report, it appears that these patients can transmit infection.[440]

The mode of transmission is not clear but probably involves direct or indirect contact with respiratory secretions or droplet transmission. Droplet precautions should be maintained during contact with infected patients, and gloves should be worn when handling fomites contaminated with respiratory secretions.[668]

Parvovirus B19 has also been transmitted by plasma-derived factor replacement products used to treat hemophilia because the virus is resistant to the viral inactivation processes currently used in the manufacture of these products.[36,635,691] Screening blood donations for parvovirus B19 using nucleic acid tests has decreased but not eliminated the potential for transmission of the virus through transfusion of plasma-derived factor replacement products.[691]

Hepatitis A Virus

In the prevaccination era, hepatitis A virus caused rare but large epidemics in health care facilities.[34,198,362,522,754] Mildly symptomatic children who excrete virus in their stool can cause widespread transmission, and many secondary cases can occur before the infection is detected and contained.

Controlling a health care–associated hepatitis A outbreak is difficult and may require the assistance of the local health department. To limit the potential for indirect contact transmission, hospitalized infected children should be grouped together. Hand hygiene and use of barrier precautions should be emphasized to prevent direct and indirect contact transmission.[668] Postexposure prophylaxis, which may involve immune globulin or hepatitis A vaccination depending on age and underlying conditions, should be administered to all exposed, susceptible individuals.[188] Symptomatic health care providers should be furloughed until 1 week after the onset of symptomatic infection or until all susceptible people have received immune globulin.[70]

Enteroviruses

Outbreaks of health care–associated enterovirus have been reported, with most occurring in neonatal nurseries.[40,65,126,298,317,342,361,386,583,710] As for hepatitis A, hand hygiene and barrier precautions are of paramount importance to prevent transmission, and cohorting of infected infants is prudent.[668] One report describes the value of early diagnosis using a PCR assay.[31] The upper respiratory tract may be involved in acute enteroviral infection, but the use of masks by caregivers is not recommended.[668]

Tuberculosis

Health care–associated tuberculosis in pediatric patients occurs almost exclusively as a result of transmission of *Mycobacterium tuberculosis* from infected adults—parents, visitors, and health care workers—to children and other adults.[35,251,491,521,700,760] Probable transmission from infected children in health care settings has been described.[471,582] However, the risk of transmission from a child is very small because children infrequently have cavitary disease and consequently have fewer tubercle bacilli in their endobronchial secretions and because young children do not tend to generate aerosols of airborne droplet nuclei.[696] Nonetheless, transmission from children can occur as evidenced by extensive transmission from a 9-year-old child with bilateral cavitary disease.[159]

The risk of health care–associated tuberculosis in adult hospitals has been minimized by prompt recognition and treatment of pulmonary tuberculosis, adequate isolation of infectious patients in rooms with negative air pressure relative to that of the hallway, and proper use of personal protective equipment.[339] If rooms with appropriate ventilation are unavailable, alternative engineering solutions, such as well-placed and maintained ultraviolet lights, may be useful.[339] Personnel entering the rooms of infected patients should wear respiratory protection devices. Particulate respirators with a National Institute for Occupational Safety and Health (NIOSH) certification of N95 or better satisfy the CDC specifications for these devices.[339] These devices must be fit tested on the individuals using them according to the standards of the Occupational Health and Safety Administration (OSHA).[339]

Prompt identification of tuberculosis in parents, visitors, and health care workers in hospitals caring for pediatric patients is essential for reducing the risk for health care–associated tuberculosis in children and is cost saving compared with conducting postexposure follow-up investigations.[154] Health care workers should be screened yearly for evidence of tuberculosis.[339]

Invasive Bacterial Infections

Health care–associated transmission of *Neisseria meningitidis* is rare.[142,208,604] Nonetheless, *N. meningitidis* is spread by droplet transmission, and health care workers should use droplet precautions during the care of patients with suspected invasive meningococcal disease until the patient has completed 24 hours of parenteral antimicrobial therapy.[668]

Microbiology laboratory workers have developed fatal disease after working with cultures of this microorganism.[122,121] Clinical and research microbiologists who may be exposed routinely to isolates of *N. meningitidis* should receive meningococcal conjugate vaccine and booster doses every 5 years if they remain at increased risk.[116]

Health care–associated transmission of *Haemophilus influenzae* and *Streptococcus pneumoniae* has been a rare phenomenon.* The risk has likely been diminished substantially with vaccination.

Invasive bacterial infections in neonates, including infections caused by *S. aureus,* group B streptococci, *Citrobacter* spp., and *Enterobacter sakazakii,* are discussed later (see Health Care–Associated Infections in Special Populations).

Ectoparasites

Many outbreaks of scabies have been reported from a variety of health care institutions. The presence of crusted scabies, which is associated with defects in cellular immunity, increases the risk for transmission dramatically because of the large number of mites in these lesions.[413] Although health care–associated transmission of pediculosis is possible, the direct or indirect contact necessary to spread this infection (i.e., head-to-head contact or sharing of combs) is less likely in medical settings than at home.

Intestinal Helminths

Person-to-person transmission of *Enterobius vermicularis* (i.e., pinworm), *Strongyloides stercoralis, Hymenolepis nana,* and *Taenia solium* is possible because these microorganisms do not require an intermediate host and because the eggs or larvae excreted in the stool are infectious.[414] However, evidence for health care–associated transmission of these microorganisms is limited.[414]

HEALTH CARE–ASSOCIATED INFECTIONS DUE TO INVASIVE DEVICES AND PROCEDURES

HCAIs can occur from contact with intravascular catheters and infusions, respiratory therapy, instrumentation of the urinary tract, and surgical procedures. Children are at risk for other HCAIs related to medical treatments, including infections associated with the receipt of blood products. More is written about these infections in the chapters on common bloodborne pathogens.

*References 25, 37, 44, 136, 163, 171, 231, 315, 461, 477, 488, 527, 556, 684, 761.

Infections Related to Intravascular Catheters and Infusions

Infections related to intravascular catheters may be local or systemic. Local infections may involve the catheter exit site, subcutaneous track of tunneled catheters, or subcutaneous pocket of an implanted catheter.[483,533] Phlebitis is a common local complication but is usually caused by chemical or mechanical irritation and is less common in children than adults.[244] Suppurative thrombophlebitis is rare in children.[355] Bloodstream infections related to intravascular catheters can have serious complications, including development of endocarditis, septic thrombophlebitis, and infection at distal sites due to hematogenous seeding, and they independently increase mortality rates, length of stay, and hospital cost.[211,266,483,533]

Clinical and surveillance definitions for bloodstream infections related to central venous catheters differ, although they are often used interchangeably.[312,483] Catheter-related bloodstream infections are clinical events that require investigation to establish the catheter as the definitive source of infection (i.e., through quantitative blood cultures, differential time to positivity, or culture of the catheter itself, if removed).[484]

For surveillance purposes, central line–associated bloodstream infection (CLABSI) is the term used by the CDC's National Healthcare Safety Network (NHSN) to capture primary bloodstream infections in patients with central lines.[201] This definition is simpler for surveillance purposes. There is concern that NHSN definitions may overestimate catheter-related infections among some patients with impaired mucosal integrity in whom bacterial translocation may affect the pathogenesis of bloodstream infections.[227] This led to the development of modified definitions for infections in this subgroup of patients, identified as mucosal barrier injury CLABSI (MBI-CLABSI).[184,214,650] The CDC's NHSM website (http://www.cdc.gov/nhsn) provides updates on NHSN definitions and methods. Although the focus in this chapter is primarily on clinical events related to catheters, most epidemiologic data on bloodstream infections come from the use of surveillance definitions.

Most endemic catheter-associated bloodstream infections in children are associated with central venous catheters.[455] Peripheral venous catheters, especially catheters made with modern, nonthrombogenic materials, are rarely associated with bloodstream infections,[244,245,455,665] although few data are systematically collected, and the risk may be underestimated.[243,734] Peripheral arterial catheters were historically associated with lower infection rates compared with central venous catheters[200,235]; however, evidence suggests that rates of colonization and infection of these catheters may be similar to those observed for central lines.[369,439,537,620] The risk for bloodstream infection associated with peripheral arterial catheters appears to be highest among patients with femorally inserted catheters.[215,436]

The remainder of this section focuses on infections in central venous catheters. With prevention efforts, rates of catheter-associated bloodstream infections in the United States have decreased dramatically; the CDC's NHSN reported a 46% decline in CLABSIs between 2008 and 2013.[201] However, device-associated infections comprise approximately 25% of all HCAIs reported to NHSN,[453] and CLABSIs represent the most common device-associated infection in hospitalized children.[201] A NHSN report included data from 4567 hospitals from 53 states, territories, and the District of Columbia, of which 82 (1.8%) were dedicated children's or women and children's hospitals.[201]

Rates of bloodstream infection associated with central venous catheters in pediatric ICUs and inpatient wards and with neonatal ICUs are shown in Table 244.1 and Fig. 244.1. Rates of infection are highest among children in hematology/oncology and bone marrow transplantation units.[201] Catheter-associated infections are also common among children with intestinal failure (i.e., short-gut syndrome) who depend on parenteral nutrition. Among premature infants, infection rates are inversely proportional to birth weight. These data do not distinguish rates of infection associated with specific catheter types nor whether a specific catheter is the source of infection in patients who have multiple catheters in place concurrently.

Gram-positive organisms, including coagulase-negative staphylococci, *S. aureus,* and enterococci are most commonly identified in catheter-associated infections.[97,465,670,775] Although rates of CLABSI have decreased overall in recent years, the incidence density rate of *S. aureus* CLABSIs

TABLE 244.1 Pooled Means of Central Line–Associated Bloodstream Infection Rates by Pediatric Unit Reported to National Healthcare Safety Network[a]

Type of Unit	Number of Units Reporting	Bloodstream Infection Rates (%)[b]
Pediatric Intensive Care		
Medical	31	0.8
Medical/surgical	315	1.2
Cardiothoracic	43	1.3
Step-down	17	1.4
Pediatric Inpatient Wards		
Medical	70	1.1
Medical/surgical	320	0.9
Orthopedic	11	0.5
Rehabilitation	7	0.8
Surgical	12	1.1
Bone Marrow Transplantation		
Temporary line	16	2.2
Permanent line	17	2.4
Hematology/Oncology		
Temporary line	49	2.1
Permanent line	55	2.1

[a]Data from January to December 2013.
[b]Central line–associated bloodstream infections/1000 central line days.
Modified from Dudeck MA, Edwards JR, Allen-Bridson K, et al. National Healthcare Safety Network (NHSN) Report, data summary for 2013, device-associated module. *Am J Infect Control.* 2015;43:206–221.

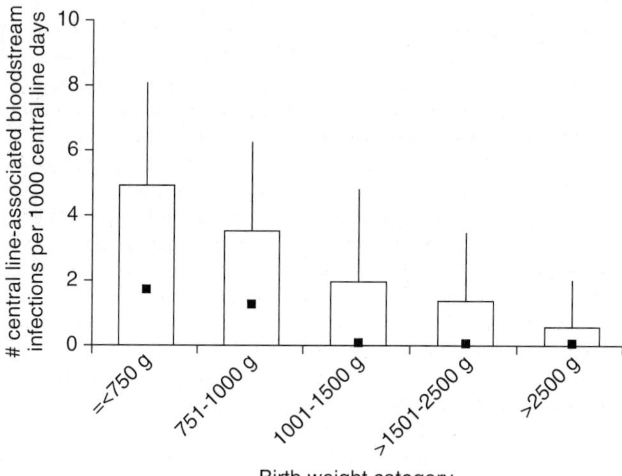

FIG. 244.1 Distribution of central line–associated bloodstream infection rates in level III neonatal intensive care units (ICUs) reported to the National Healthcare Safety Network (NHSN). Box plots of the distribution of central line–associated bloodstream infection rates in neonatal ICUs show the 50th percentile or median *(solid squares),* 75th percentile *(upper bound of each rectangle),* and 90th percentile *(upper bound of the line extending above each rectangle).* The number of participating neonatal ICUs in each of the birthweight classes ranged from 389 to 433. (Modified from Dudeck MA, Edwards JR, Allen-Bridson K, et al. National Healthcare Safety Network [NHSN] report, data summary for 2013, device-associated module. *Am J Infect Control.* 2015;43:206–221.)

among pediatric ICUs in the United States has remained the same.[217] Identification of gram-negative bacilli, including *Enterobacter* spp., *P. aeruginosa, Klebsiella pneumoniae,* and *Escherichia coli,* has increased to approximately one third of reported infections.[670] *Candida* spp. have also become increasingly prevalent[670,776] and comprised 15% of reported catheter-associated infections among a collaborative of pediatric ICUs.[520]

Antimicrobial resistance is a concern for all common pathogens isolated from bloodstream infections, including *S. aureus* and gram-negative bacilli.[96,670] Fifty percent of *S. aureus* infections were caused by MRSA in a collaborative of pediatric ICUs.[520] Bloodstream infections due to VRE may be more prevalent among high-risk groups such as pediatric oncology patients and should be considered when selecting empiric therapy based on local epidemiology.[353] Nontuberculous mycobacteria and *Nocardia* spp. also can cause bloodstream infections.[11]

The four major mechanisms for contamination of intravascular catheters are migration of microorganisms colonizing the skin at the insertion site along the external catheter surface and into the blood vessel (i.e., extraluminal contamination), contamination of the catheter or catheter hub through contact with hands of health care workers (i.e., intraluminal contamination), hematogenous seeding from another focus of infection, and contamination of the infusate.[151,152,533,534] The first two mechanisms are most important and vary in their contributions to infection depending on the duration of catheterization.[579] Extraluminal contamination predominates in the first 10 days (likely related to contamination during insertion), whereas the potential for intraluminal contamination increases with duration of catheterization and is most common after 30 days, most likely due to contamination during routine catheter maintenance and use.[579] Contamination of infusates is relatively uncommon; however, several epidemics have been associated with contaminated intravenous infusions,[424,425,457,662] medications,[51,270,457,543] and blood products.[108]

Additional pathogenic determinants of bloodstream infection include catheter material, host factors leading to the formation of a fibrin sheath,[482] and intrinsic virulence of the microorganism. Adherence properties of microorganisms are critical. Production of an extracellular polymeric substance by organisms such as coagulase-negative staphylococci, *S. aureus,* and *P. aeruginosa* leads to formation of a microbial biofilm in which microorganisms can become embedded and proliferate relatively protected from host defenses and antimicrobial agents.[5,196,321,478] *Candida* spp. also routinely produce biofilms, particularly in the presence of glucose-containing fluids.[82]

Risk factors for catheter-related bloodstream infection include heavy colonization of the skin at the catheter exit site[151,152,534,580] or catheter hub,[170,420] longer duration of insertion (>3 days),[153,244,245] prolonged hospitalization before catheterization,[469] presence of multiple concurrent central venous catheters,[144] substandard catheter care,[469] and host factors (e.g., neutropenia, prematurity),[469] including an extant mural or atrial thrombus.[151,152,534] The level and composition of nurse staffing have also been associated with bloodstream infections in adult surgical ICUs. Low ratios of nurses to patients and regular nurses (as opposed to pool nurses to patients have been associated with higher risks of bloodstream infections.[230,600]

Dedicated pediatric studies are limited, but age younger than 2 years, duration of catheterization (>7 days), and receipt of parenteral nutrition or blood transfusions have been independently associated with catheter-associated bloodstream infections in pediatric ICU patients.[175,210,268,469,520,779] A study of children at a tertiary care center found that catheter breakage was associated with significantly increased risk of bloodstream infection within 30 days of repair.[443] Additional novel risk factors identified in single studies include presence of a gastrostomy tube, nonoperative cardiovascular disease, ICU catheter placement,[779] and catheter placement at an external facility before hospital transfer.[377] Among pediatric oncology patients, placement of the catheter within 1 month, previous bacteremia in any central line, frequent platelet transfusions, and host factors, including recent neutropenia, relapsed malignancy, and bone marrow transplantation within the prior 100 days, have been associated with an increased risk of bloodstream infection.[19,353,354,599] Infusion of parenteral nutrition with lipids increases the risk of infection with coagulase-negative staphylococci and *Candida* in neonates.[32,87,228,623]

Among central venous catheters, nontunneled (percutaneously inserted) catheters account for most catheter-associated bloodstream infections, whereas totally implantable catheters carry the lowest risk,[316,398,495,657,698,769,778] although these comparisons may be confounded by several factors, including age and underlying severity of illness.[32,87,327,769,778] Tunneled catheters carry a lower infection risk compared with nontunneled catheters because a cuff prevents migration of microorganisms into the catheter tract. However, in a study of children with acute lymphoblastic leukemia undergoing induction chemotherapy, the catheter type (i.e., tunneled vs. nontunneled) used at the time of diagnosis had no impact on subsequent risk of bloodstream infection in this high-risk group.[53]

Peripherally inserted central (venous) catheters (PICCs) are used commonly in children, but data suggest the risk of PICC-associated infections in ICUs approaches that of centrally inserted venous catheters.[134,469] Duration of catheter dwell increases the risk of PICC-associated infection among neonates, although this finding has been inconsistent between studies.[268,494,655] Rates of infection are similar for catheters placed in the umbilical vein or artery.[392]

Catheter insertion site influences infection risk for adults, likely due to the density of local skin microorganisms. A meta-analysis showed that catheters inserted into the internal jugular vein carry a higher risk of colonization and infection compared with subclavian catheters, whereas femorally inserted catheters carry the highest risk, although the investigators suggested that interpretation might be limited by study heterogeneity and limitations in study design.[549] A Cochrane Review concluded that subclavian catheters were associated with less colonization and fewer thrombotic complications than femoral catheters in short-term catheterization, but no difference was found between subclavian and internal jugular venous catheters.[55] Femoral catheters have not been associated with higher rates of colonization and infection among children.[469,520,594]

Several methods have been used to identify the catheter as the source of infection, although no microbiologic gold standard for diagnosis of catheter-related bloodstream infection exists.[42] Proposed methods include collection of paired blood cultures from the catheter and a peripheral vein before starting therapy.[483] If a peripheral sample cannot be obtained, at least two samples should be drawn through different catheter lumens. If the catheter is removed because of suspected infection, catheter tip culture can be performed to determine whether it is colonized. Semiquantitative (roll-plate) or quantitative catheter culture techniques (i.e., luminal flushing or sonication) are the most reliable modalities and are preferred over qualitative broth cultures.[460,580,619,662,669]

Clinical criteria for definitive diagnosis of catheter-related bloodstream infections have been published[483] and require positive percutaneous culture results with concordant microbial growth from the catheter tip or catheter-drawn cultures that meet criteria for quantitative culture or differential time to positivity.[483] Quantitative blood cultures are the most accurate, but the differential time-to-positivity technique can be almost as sensitive (provided the same volume of blood is used to inoculate both blood culture bottles) and is less labor intensive.[619] Because peripheral blood cultures are drawn less frequently in children due to difficulty in obtaining peripheral specimens or concerns about drawing large blood volumes, the catheter is often implicated presumptively if no other source of infection is identified. This assumption has implications for management (including catheter removal) and is discussed further later.[483]

Empiric antimicrobial therapy for children with suspected bloodstream infection is similar to that for adults. Choice of therapy should be based on severity of illness, the nature and severity of underlying conditions, and epidemiology and susceptibility patterns of local pathogens. The clinical practice guideline cited previously contains detailed management recommendations.[483] In most cases, empiric therapy should include coverage of gram-positive and gram-negative bacteria. Because of the increased prevalence of MRSA across institutions, vancomycin is often included. Empiric combination therapy for multidrug-resistant, gram-negative bacilli such as *P. aeruginosa* should be added for patients who are severely ill, neutropenic, or known to be colonized with these organisms. Empiric antifungal therapy may be considered for septic patients with risk factors for candidemia, including receipt of parenteral nutrition, prolonged use of broad-spectrum antibiotics, hematologic malignancy, receipt of bone marrow or a solid organ transplant, or known colonization with *Candida* spp. After culture information is available, treatment can be tailored or discontinued as appropriate.

There is substantial evidence that most uncomplicated bloodstream infections in children can be treated effectively without catheter removal.[221,483,769] However, catheter removal should be strongly considered for difficult-to-treat bacteria, such as *S. aureus*, *P. aeruginosa*, and mycobacteria.[483] Treatment of catheter-associated fungemia without catheter removal has a relatively low success rate and may be associated with higher mortality rates.[165,246,484] Although a retrospective study of adults with catheter-associated candidemia found no difference in outcomes between early and late catheter removal, it did not address long-term outcomes such as recurrence.[526] This finding will require further consideration in future practice guidelines. Catheters should be removed immediately in patients with severe sepsis, embolic phenomena, septic thrombophlebitis, or endocarditis or if infection continues despite more than 72 hours of targeted therapy.

Clinical practice guidelines review the use of antibiotic lock therapy in the treatment of catheter-related bacteremia when catheter salvage is the goal.[483] The concept behind lock therapy is that organisms embedded in biofilms on intraluminal surfaces of long-term catheters may be killed more effectively by antibiotic concentrations 100 to 1000 times higher than standard concentrations of therapeutic parenteral antibiotics.[483] Antibiotic lock solutions are typically mixed with heparin in sufficient volumes to fill the lumen, allowed to dwell, and then removed. This approach is recommended in conjunction with systemic therapy for selected organisms. Lock therapy is not recommended for infections due to *S. aureus* and *Candida* spp. unless unusual extenuating circumstances are identified.[483] Use of adjunctive urokinase or other thrombolytic agents is not recommended.[30,397,483]

Duration of therapy varies by pathogen type but is typically 7 to 14 days.[483] With catheter removal, shorter courses (5–7 days) may be appropriate for uncomplicated infections with less virulent organisms such as coagulase-negative staphylococci. Persistently positive blood cultures despite targeted therapy or recrudescence of infection shortly thereafter should prompt catheter removal. Catheter removal from patients with persistent fever but no positive culture results and no evidence of infection elsewhere is controversial and should be approached on a case-by-case basis.

Some success has been reported in treating uncomplicated exit site infections without catheter removal. A trial of combined local and systemic antimicrobial treatment is warranted before a decision to remove the catheter is made. In contrast, treatment outcomes of tunnel or pocket infections usually are poor if the catheter is retained.[483,769]

A guideline for the prevention of catheter-related infections was updated,[469] and several reviews have summarized novel technologies for prevention of these infections.[151,304,580] Significant improvement in infection rates has been achieved within the context of organized initiatives and the use of care bundles for catheter insertion and maintenance. Key preventive measures are emphasized in this discussion.

Use of intravascular catheters should be limited to only when necessary. Reducing exposure to central venous catheters is one of the simplest ways to reduce bloodstream infection risk. Adherence to preventive measures during catheter insertion has significantly reduced bloodstream infections in adults, and these practices are often applied using insertion bundles.[52,577,752] Use of an insertion checklist and a fully stocked catheter cart or kit is recommended to ensure optimal practices are followed.[469] Key preventive measures during insertion include performance of hand hygiene and use of maximal sterile barrier precautions (e.g., sterile gowns, gloves, drapes).[469,581] Use of an alcoholic chlorhexidine antiseptic is preferred over povidone-iodine.[125,151,243,458,469] The catheter site should be covered with sterile gauze or a sterile, transparent, semipermeable dressing.[469] Routine application of topical antimicrobial agents is not recommended,[151,533,534] except for hemodialysis catheters.[469]

Ongoing preventive measures during catheter maintenance are critical. A pediatric quality improvement collaborative showed that maximizing compliance with insertion bundles was insufficient to reduce bloodstream infection rates in pediatric ICUs, underscoring the importance of scrupulous practices related to routine catheter use and maintenance.[338,347,490,648,774] Many improvement initiatives over the past decade have advocated maintenance care bundles—simultaneous implementation of multiple preventive practices to achieve maximal reductions in infections.[207] These bundles include daily assessment of catheter necessity and adherence to aseptic technique during catheter hub and catheter site care. Catheter hubs are common sites of catheter colonization; hubs should be cleansed using mechanical friction during each access with 70% ethanol, alcoholic chlorhexidine, or povidone-iodine.[469] Numerous studies have demonstrated the benefit of daily chlorhexidine bathing in reducing CLABSI in adult settings[190,499,509,572] and in pediatric and neonatal ICUs.[492,578] This practice is now recommended for all ICU patients with central venous catheters.[469] The US Food and Drug Administration recommends care in the use of chlorhexidine for skin antisepsis for premature infants or infants younger than 2 months of age because products with this chemical can cause irritation or chemical burns.[8]

Prevention guidelines also highlight the importance of minimizing catheter manipulation and provide detailed guidance for maintaining closed systems and when to change infusion sets.[469,534] Minimizing the frequency of catheter access is a common preventive strategy at many hospitals, although there are few data to support the practice.

Special approaches to prevention are recommended when infection rates remain unacceptably high despite adherence to basic preventive practices. These interventions include use of chlorhexidine-containing dressings[102,242,291,415,456,728] for central venous catheters in patients older than 2 months[469] and the use of antiseptic- or antibiotic-impregnated catheters.[151,533,534,580] Although most studies of impregnated catheters have considered adults, pediatric data are mounting,[60,128] including a randomized, controlled trial enrolling pediatric ICU patients that found the use of antibiotic-impregnated catheters significantly reduced rates of bloodstream infection compared with standard central venous catheters.[260] However, the antiinfective effect of these catheters is not permanent and may be limited to a relatively short period after insertion. Their long-term impact on antimicrobial resistance has not been evaluated, although prospective studies suggest that this risk is likely low.[533,633]

Multiple controlled studies have evaluated the use of antibiotic or antiseptic locks for the prevention of catheter-related bloodstream infections.[494] Numerous studies of antimicrobial lock therapy have demonstrated significant reductions in bloodstream infection risk,[241,534,539,780] including a meta-analysis of randomized clinical trials that showed a 69% reduction in CLABSIs among a variety of patient populations, including hemodialysis patients, adult and pediatric oncology patients, critically ill neonates, and patients receiving parenteral nutrition.[783] Multiple antibiotic and antiseptic lock solutions have been evaluated. Due to concerns regarding emergence of antimicrobial resistance in exposed organisms, antimicrobial lock therapy is recommended for patients at highest risk, including those with long-term hemodialysis catheters, patients with limited venous access and history of recurrent infection, and those at risk for severe sequelae from infection.[469]

Infections Related to Respiratory Therapy

Most infections related to respiratory therapy are associated with mechanical ventilation. Infections related to the use of other respiratory equipment, such as small-volume medication nebulizers, have also been described, although usually in the setting of epidemics related to the use of contaminated equipment.[68,150,470,497] This discussion focuses primarily on ventilator-associated events or complications.

Major infections include tracheitis, tracheobronchitis, and pneumonia. Mechanical ventilation may also increase the risk of sinusitis and otitis media among nasally intubated patients because nasotracheal tubes interfere with normal drainage of the sinus ostia and eustachian tubes.[54,273] Most of the clinical and surveillance data exist for ventilator-associated pneumonia (VAP).

VAP has been reported in 9% to 27% of intubated patients and is associated with prolonged ventilation, increased length of stay, higher mortality rates, and increased hospital costs.[274,346,534] Estimated rates of pneumonia for ventilated adults have been lower in recent years, ranging from 5% to 15%.[365] VAP rates for children in pediatric and neonatal ICUs are available from the CDC's 2013 NHSN report.[201] Similar to catheter-associated bloodstream infections, infection rates among neonates are inversely proportional to birth weight.[201] Comparisons between adult and pediatric rates of infection are limited due to recent changes in surveillance definitions. The VAP surveillance definition no longer applies to adult patients and was replaced by ventilator-associated events (VAEs) in 2013.[201] VAE definitions include criteria for ventilator-associated conditions (VACs), infection-related ventilator-associated conditions (IVACs), possible pneumonia, and probable pneumonia.[365]

The CDC convened a Neonatal and Pediatric VAE working group to modify the VAE definition for use in children.[139] Until new definitions are finalized and available for use, VAP surveillance continues for pediatric critical care locations,[201] and the term *VAP* continues to be used to describe clinical events involving pneumonia in ventilated patients. Aside from NHSN reports of infection rates, dedicated studies of VAP in infants and children are limited, although several reviews have summarized the existing pediatric literature.[223,575,744,777] Most of the information discussed is from adult studies.

Most cases of VAP are bacterial in origin and polymicrobial. The duration of mechanical ventilation before symptom onset is an important determinant of the most likely pathogens. Early pneumonia (<4 days) is more likely caused by antibiotic-sensitive community pathogens, such as *S. pneumoniae* and *Haemophilus* spp., whereas late infections (>4 days) are more often related to antibiotic-resistant organisms.[18,323,346,533] This difference reflects the frequency of exposure to prior antimicrobial therapy and the epidemiology of local ICU pathogens. The distinction may be less meaningful for patients who are frequently admitted to health care settings.

Major pathogens include gram-positive and gram-negative bacteria; *S. aureus* (including MRSA) and *P. aeruginosa* are isolated most frequently.[14,271,323] Other pathogens include *Streptococcus* spp., Enterobacteriaceae, and *Acinetobacter* spp.[250,323,596] Risk factors for infection with multidrug-resistant pathogens include prior intravenous antibiotics within 90 days, hospitalization for 5 or more days before diagnosis, septic shock, preceding acute respiratory distress syndrome (ARDS), and acute renal replacement therapy before infection onset.[346] Anaerobic bacteria are uncommonly implicated[323] but may play a role in polymicrobial infections, particularly when pneumonia results from aspiration. Nosocomial viruses and fungi rarely cause pneumonia in immunocompetent hosts. Although *Candida* spp. are sometimes isolated from lower respiratory tract samples, they are rarely the primary cause of pneumonia.[18]

VAP occurs when bacteria invade the pulmonary parenchyma of a patient receiving mechanical ventilation.[141] This process is directly linked to aspiration of oropharyngeal or gastric secretions that harbor potentially pathogenic organisms.[18,323] Colonization with pathogenic bacteria is facilitated by several factors, including enhanced bacterial adherence to mucosal surfaces in severely ill or debilitated patients, bacterial overgrowth of the stomach when acid-suppressing medications are used, and reductions in microbial diversity and pathogen selection due to antibiotic exposure.[535,707]

Endotracheal tubes interfere with normal protective airway reflexes and prevent effective coughing. Contaminated secretions pool and leak around the endotracheal tube. This process is exacerbated during changes in position or deflation of the subglottic cuff of the endotracheal tube cuff. Bacterial biofilms also form on the inner surface of the tube, providing a direct route for microbial invasion into the lower airway.[535]

Regurgitation of bacteria from the stomach into the pharynx can provide another route for bacteria into the airway. Normal gastric pH prevents heavy contamination of stomach contents, but bacteria proliferate when stomach acid is neutralized by antacids or histamine-2 (H_2) blockers. However, the degree to which gastric colonization contributes to risk for pneumonia is unclear.[707] Other potential pathways for infection include use of contaminated equipment or medications, often in outbreak settings,[438] and bacteremia with hematogenous spread.[18]

After pathogens enter the lower airway, host defenses are important in determining whether infection results. Diseases that compromise mucociliary clearance or the ability of the immune system to contain and inactivate pathogens dramatically increase infection risk.

Risk factors for VAP in adults include host factors that increase susceptibility to pneumonia, such as advanced age, underlying chronic lung disease, and immunosuppression; treatment factors that enhance colonization of the oropharynx or stomach with pathogenic bacteria; factors that promote reflux of gastric contents and aspiration into the lower airway, such as depressed mental status, supine positioning, nasogastric tubes, and enteral feeding; conditions that increase the duration of ventilation; and factors that hinder adequate pulmonary toilet, such as thoracic or abdominal surgery and immobilization.[707]

Although dedicated pediatric studies are limited, it is likely that many of the adult risk factors are also important for children. Prospective studies of critically ill children found that a genetic syndrome, postsurgical admission diagnosis, duration of stay in a pediatric ICU, prior antibiotic therapy, use of narcotic medications, enteral feeds, reintubation, and transport out of the ICU were independently associated with VAP.[14,212,249,274,385,554,695] Trauma,[709] female gender,[695] tracheostomy,[554] and gastroesophageal reflux disease[2] have also been associated with VAP in children in single studies.

The diagnosis of VAP can be challenging. Clinical diagnosis requires evaluation of a combination of clinical, radiographic, and microbiologic data. Relevant clinical findings include fever, leukocytosis or leukopenia, purulent secretions, and worsening gas exchange. Auscultation is often hindered by sounds of the ventilation system itself (particularly with high-frequency ventilation), and a variety of underlying pulmonary diseases and conditions (e.g., fluid overload) may produce sounds indistinguishable from those present in pneumonia. Radiographic findings include new or progressive pulmonary infiltrates, cavitation, air bronchograms, and pneumatoceles. Air bronchograms are the most sensitive for detecting pneumonia,[744] but chest radiograph findings have only limited specificity, because significant overlap exists between pneumonia and other pulmonary conditions.

Microbiologic data are important in the diagnosis and in guiding subsequent treatment. Samples of lower respiratory tract secretions and blood cultures should be obtained for all patients with suspected VAP. Tracheal aspirates can be misleading in an asymptomatic patient because endotracheal tubes are often colonized with potential pathogens.[261] Several invasive and noninvasive methods for obtaining respiratory specimens have been evaluated.[90,666,724] Current clinical practice guidelines recommend noninvasive sampling (i.e., endotracheal aspiration) with semiquantitative cultures for diagnosis[346] because current evidence does not show a difference in outcomes between sampling methods.[346] Gram stains are helpful in ruling out pneumonia when results are negative, but they have very poor positive predictive value[538] because localized irritation or superficial infection of the trachea can produce purulent secretions.

Empiric therapy for VAP should be based on the duration of intubation and hospitalization, prior or current antibiotic therapy, severity of clinical disease, nature and severity of underlying conditions, and epidemiology and resistance patterns of local pathogens. Several adult studies have shown that delayed initiation or inappropriate antibiotic therapy is associated with poor outcomes.[18] Initial broad-spectrum therapy with adequate coverage of *S. aureus* (and possibly MRSA), *P. aeruginosa*, and other gram-negative bacilli, as guided by local epidemiology, usually is appropriate and can be narrowed based on subsequent culture data and clinical and radiographic findings.[18,346]

Prolonged treatment of patients for whom the diagnosis is questionable should be avoided because this practice may lead to endotracheal colonization with antimicrobial-resistant bacteria. Treatment duration for VAP has not been evaluated for children. As for adults, uncomplicated cases should be treated for 7 days. For complicated cases or those with necrotizing pneumonia, at least 14 days of therapy should be administered. Shorter courses (<7 days) may be appropriate for children with ventilator-associated tracheitis without evidence of pneumonia.[716]

Comprehensive guidelines for prevention of health care–associated pneumonia[707] and VAP[141] are available and were updated in 2014.[365] Key strategies include three major themes: reducing aspiration of secretions, reducing colonization of the aerodigestive tract, and preventing use of contaminated equipment.[141] Many strategies are implemented as practice bundles that are aimed at producing more robust results when combined.[33,63,158,535,711,718]

Strategies for prevention include limiting the duration of ventilation and using noninvasive approaches when possible. Daily assessment of readiness to wean or extubate and spontaneous breathing trials are recommended.[141,366,729] Although a randomized clinical trial enrolling ventilated children failed to demonstrate a reduction in time to extubation with the use of a weaning protocol, most children included in the study were weaned from ventilator support in less than 2 days.[586] Minimizing sedation decreases the duration of ventilation.[365]

Aspiration can be minimized by maintaining patients in a semirecumbent position by elevating the head of the bed by 30 to 45 degrees.[365] Head-of-bed elevation has also been associated with reductions in clinically suspected pneumonia[750] and shorter ventilator stays.[367] Keeping the endotracheal tube free of secretions is also important in preventing aspiration. Use of a cuffed endotracheal tube is recommended[365]; cuffed tubes have been proved safe in pediatric patients and are routinely used in infants and children.[365] Suctioning should be performed by gently using a sterile, single-use catheter, and sterile fluids should be used to loosen secretions and clear the suction catheter. Other measures to reduce aspiration include avoiding unplanned extubation and reintubation and avoiding gastric overdistention.

To minimize contamination of respiratory equipment, sterile water should be used to rinse reusable devices. Tubing should be maintained in a dependent position relative to the endotracheal tube, and condensate should be routinely discarded. Circuits should remain closed during condensate removal. The ventilatory circuit should be changed only when visibly soiled or malfunctioning.[365] All respiratory equipment should be stored and disinfected properly.[141] Items with direct or indirect contact with mucous membranes or respiratory secretions should be cleaned thoroughly and sterilized or disinfected in a manner consistent with high-level disinfection. Hand hygiene and use of gloves during contact with objects or surfaces contaminated with respiratory secretions are also important.

Strategies to reduce colonization of the aerodigestive tract include regular oral care (e.g., toothbrushing).[365] Oral care with antiseptics such as chlorhexidine appears to be most beneficial for cardiac surgery patients.[365] Study results from metaanalyses of noncardiac surgery patients have shown reductions in rates of VAP for adults, but the impact on duration of ventilation, ICU length of stay, and mortality rates has not been demonstrated.[365,389,664] One study of adults showed that daily oral care with chlorhexidine might be harmful for some patients, but this finding will require further consideration in future prevention guidelines.[367]

Prophylactic antibiotic regimens have been used to modulate oropharyngeal colonization.[141,707] Selective decontamination of the digestive tract uses a combination of topical, nonabsorbable oral, and systemic antimicrobial agents to prevent secondary bacterial colonization and preemptively treat possible respiratory tract infection with commensal organisms.[182] Selective oropharyngeal decontamination is similar but includes application of topical oropharyngeal antimicrobial agents only. Selective decontamination of the digestive tract[173,182,379,671] has reduced mortality rates for adult ICU patients in randomized clinical trials, including a systematic review, but it is not recommended routinely because of increased selective pressure on antibiotic-resistant organisms and risk of *C. difficile* infection.[141,366,707]

Infections Related to Instrumentation of the Urinary Tract

Catheter-associated urinary tract infections (CAUTIs) are the most common HCAIs in hospitalized adults worldwide.[311] In contrast, CAUTIs comprise a much smaller proportion of device-related HCAIs in pediatric patients, likely due to differences in urinary tract catheterization between adults and children. However, data from the CDC's NHSN show that pooled mean rates of CAUTIs are similar for adult and pediatric ICUs.[201]

Although diagnostic criteria for CAUTIs vary and are often reported differently for various studies, surveillance definitions have been established and are updated annually.[312,573] Urinary tract infections (UTIs) are considered catheter associated if the patient had an indwelling catheter in place for more than 2 calendar days on the date of the event. Symptomatic UTIs are defined by signs or symptoms of infection (e.g., fever, urgency, frequency, dysuria, suprapubic tenderness) and a quantitative urine culture with 10^4 or more colony-forming units (CFUs) per milliliter of urine containing no more than two species.[573]

The most common organisms causing CAUTIs are those colonizing the perineum.[670] Infections in patients with short-term indwelling catheters (<30 days) are usually caused by single organisms, whereas infections in patients with long-term catheters (>30 days) are more often polymicrobial.[311] *E. coli* is the most commonly identified organism.[2,311,540] Other gram-negative bacteria (e.g., Enterobacteriaceae, *P. aeruginosa*), *Enterococcus* spp., and *Candida* spp. are also isolated.[2,165,311,431,432,540] Receipt of antimicrobial agents increases the risk of infection with resistant bacteria or fungi. In a single-center pediatric study, antibiotic exposure within the prior 2 months was more common for children with infections with *P. aeruginosa* as compared with children with infection due to *E. coli*.[66]

Microbial colonization of the urine is the first step in the pathogenesis of UTI; the urinary catheter facilitates this by perturbing host defenses and providing uropathogens easier access into the bladder. However, infection is not an inevitable result of bladder colonization, and many chronically catheterized patients have evidence of urine colonization for long periods without clinical evidence of infection. Pathogens may be introduced at catheter insertion, by ascension along the external catheter surface, or intraluminally through contamination of the collecting tube or drainage bag. A detailed culturing study of catheterized patients suggested that roughly two thirds of infections are caused by extraluminal spread of microorganisms along the external catheter surface, whereas the other one third are intraluminally acquired.[712] This finding is supported by numerous studies of catheterized adults that correlated microorganisms colonizing the urethral meatus with those most frequently causing infection.[95]

After catheter insertion, adherence of microbes along the internal and external surfaces of the catheter leads to colonization, facilitating the rapid formation of biofilms that migrate to the bladder within 1 to 3 days.[311,331,626] Movement of microorganisms into the bladder is facilitated by obstruction of urine flow and reflux of urine into the bladder (i.e., raising the collection system above the level of the bladder), but many bacteria can migrate upstream even in properly maintained systems. In the bladder, microorganisms multiply in the small but persistent reservoir of urine that is incompletely drained by the catheter.[95]

The reported incidence of catheter-associated bacteriuria is 3% to 8% per day; duration of catheterization is the most important risk factor.[311] Other risk factors for catheter-associated bacteriuria in adults include female sex, catheter insertion outside the operating room, catheter care violations, older age, and rapidly fatal underlying illness.[311]

The epidemiology of bacteriuria and UTIs has been evaluated for children, although most studies are outdated.[61,66,165,394,431,432,540] Duration of catheterization is also an important risk factor for infection in children.[408] In a large, prospective study of 525 hospitalized children with urinary catheters, median duration of catheterization was 7 days (range, 2–77 days).[432] A retrospective analysis of CAUTIs in a tertiary care children's hospital found that more than 80% of CAUTIs were identified in critically ill children and that 75% occurred in girls. Most patients had at least one chronic underlying condition, and approximately one third had an anatomic or functional abnormality of their genitourinary tract.[166]

The diagnosis of symptomatic CAUTIs is often challenging because many catheterized patients do not have symptoms such as urgency, frequency, or dysuria, and fever is often the most commonly identified sign. Pyuria is a reasonably good predictor of significant concentrations of gram-negative rods in the urine of catheterized patients, but it is a poor predictor of significant concentrations of enterococci or *Candida*[713] However, pyuria alone is not diagnostic of infection in catheterized patients, particularly those with long-term indwelling catheters.[311] Conversely, the absence of pyuria in a symptomatic, catheterized patient suggests an alternative diagnosis.

Definitive diagnosis of catheter-associated UTIs depends heavily on quantitative urine culture. For patients with short-term catheters, specimens should be collected from the aspiration port using aseptic technique. With long-term catheters, removing the catheter and collecting a specimen from a freshly placed catheter before initiating therapy is preferred.[311] Specimens should not be collected from the drainage bag.

Empiric antimicrobial therapy for UTI should be based on the severity of clinical disease, the nature and severity of underlying conditions, and knowledge of local epidemiology. Parenteral therapy is typically used until secondary bacteremia is excluded. Therapy with a broad-spectrum agent targeting gram-negative bacilli, potentially including *P. aeruginosa*, and enterococci usually is appropriate. Antifungal therapy can usually be withheld, unless yeast elements are identified on urinalysis or urine Gram stain. Based on the patient's clinical status and culture results, the treatment regimen can be tailored accordingly or discontinued.

Seven days of antimicrobial therapy is recommended for the treatment of most CAUTIs; longer courses (10–14 days) are used for patients with a delayed response or with evidence of pyelonephritis.[311] If the infection is uncomplicated and the child has responded clinically, oral therapy can be used to complete the course. If possible, indwelling urinary catheters should be removed. Infections involving nephrostomy or suprapubic catheters often recur if the catheters must remain in place. When nephrostomy tubes must be used for extended periods, suppressive antimicrobial therapy may be considered after treatment is completed, although there is a risk for secondary infection with resistant bacteria or yeast with this approach.

Detailed guidelines for the prevention of CAUTIs have been published[267,311] and updated in 2014.[426] Many of these strategies have been incorporated into prevention bundles that include standardized training and catheter insertion and maintenance practices; use of a prevention bundle was associated with a significant reduction in CAUTI rates in a tertiary care children's hospital.[166] Additional interventions, including nurse-based or electronic physician reminder systems to reduce inappropriate catheterization, have significantly reduced the rates of CAUTI among children and adults.[89,165,481]

Reducing unnecessary use of urinary catheters is the most important and effective preventive measure. Key prevention strategies include catheter insertion by trained personnel; attention to hand hygiene and aseptic technique during insertion; proper securement of indwelling catheters; maintenance of a sterile, continuously closed drainage system with unobstructed urine flow (i.e., keeping the collection tubing free of kinks or dependent loops); maintaining the drainage bag below the level of the bladder; and removal of the catheter as soon as possible.[427]

Although systemic antibiotics have reduced or delay the onset of catheter-associated bacteriuria or infection in adult studies,[95] their use at the time of catheter insertion, removal, or replacement is not routinely recommended owing to the potential for adverse effects and the development of antimicrobial resistance.[311] Other types of interventions have been studied, primarily in adults, and most have had limited or inconsistent benefits.[95,311,459] At Routine use of methenamine salts or cranberry products is not recommended for prevention of CAUTIs.

Infections Related to Surgical Procedures

Patients undergoing surgical procedures are at risk for a variety of HCAIs, including bacteremia, pneumonia, and UTIs (often related to indwelling medical devices), but surgical site infections (SSIs) are the most common.[59,566] Voluntary reporting of postoperative complications to the American College of Surgeons' National Surgical Quality Improvement Project (NSQIP) has generated specialty-specific data on the incidence of SSIs among children (Table 244.2).[91] SSIs have a significant impact on patient outcomes, including increased duration of hospitalization, health care costs, and increased risk of death.[20]

Consensus criteria for SSIs are available from the CDC's NHSN.[10] SSIs are further categorized as incisional infections (superficial or deep) or as organ or space infections (http://www.cdc.gov/nhsn/PDFs/pscManual/9pscSSIcurrent.pdf?agree=yes&next=Accept). Surveillance definitions require that infections arise within 30 days of surgery, unless an implant or homograft is left in place, in which case the infection surveillance period should be extended to 90 days. Surveillance definitions require reporting of an SSI that develops after a procedure in which infection was identified (e.g., drainage of an intraabdominal infection), although these cases should be flagged as having infection at the time of surgery. Stitch abscesses are not considered SSIs.

Traditionally, the NHSN has provided simple risk adjustment measures to account for differences in case mix and allow for meaningful comparisons between surgeons or hospitals. Three equally weighted factors were previously included: composite measure of severity of illness (i.e., American Society of Anesthesiology [ASA] score); wound classification of I to IV (i.e., clean, clean-contaminated, contaminated, and dirty-infected); and procedure duration.[155] The NHSN developed

TABLE 244.2 Rates of Surgical Site Infections for Pediatric Surgical Specialties, American College of Surgeons National Surgical Quality Improvement Program, 2010

	SURGICAL SITE INFECTION RATES (%)[a]	
Specialty	**All Cases**	**Neonates**
Neurosurgery	6.3	12.6
General surgery	3.8	6.2
Plastic surgery	3.1	0
Orthopedics	2.5	2.7
Otolaryngology	1.1	0
Urology	1.5	2.4

[a]Rates have been risk adjusted using NSQIP hierarchical model.
Modified from Bruny JL, Hall BL, Barnhart DC, et al. American College of Surgeons National Surgical Quality Improvement Program Pediatric: A beta phase report. *J Pediatr Surg.* 2013;48:74–80.

procedure-specific risk models for each procedure category reported to the NHSN that incorporate existing patient- and hospital-specific data elements. These models have improved predictive performance compared with traditional risk stratification and are intended to facilitate improved external benchmarking.[505]

In pediatric studies, independent risk factors for infection include those related to procedures, such as longer surgery duration,[59,164,167,194] prolonged preoperative hospitalization,[164,167,194] emergency surgery,[58,194,730] longer length of incision,[164,194] and procedures performed by trainees.[730] Patient-related factors that are associated with an increased risk of SSIs include younger age or prematurity,[92,451,659] nonwhite race,[92] obesity, and underlying diseases, including genetic conditions.[58,345,450,493] Potentially modifiable risk factors identified in a 2011 study included postoperative ICU admission, urinary catheter placement, and use of an implantable device.[92]

Additional data exist for specific surgery types. Children undergoing cardiovascular surgery are at high risk for infection due to the complexity of congenital heart disease and the aggressive medical management required for support preoperatively and postoperatively. A prospective study of more than 300 children undergoing cardiovascular surgery found an infection rate of 7.1%; infection rates were higher among patients with delayed sternal closure[206,434] and those with increased severity of illness (i.e., higher pediatric risk of mortality [PRISM] score).[566] Subsequent studies identified prolonged duration of surgery,[13,344,513] younger age[13,50,344,513] (<30 days[689]), cyanotic heart disease,[50] undergoing more than one cardiothoracic procedure,[309] having a preoperative medical device,[689] and parenteral nutrition as independent risk factors.[41,689] Gram-positive organisms are the most common cause of infection after cardiac surgical procedures;[507] however, one case series reported that gram-negative pathogens were isolated from approximately one third of children with postoperative mediastinitis.[434]

Reported rates of infection after cerebrospinal fluid shunting procedures vary widely.[393,532] Approximately 10% of newly placed shunts become infected within 1 year of placement.[673] Risk factors for initial shunt infections include prior neurosurgical procedure, age between 6 and 12 months, and presence of a gastrostomy tube. Additional risk factors include prematurity, perioperative cerebrospinal fluid leak, surgical revisions and replacement of cerebrospinal fluid shunts, and myelomeningocele.[337,380,532,601,673,674,676,692] Skin organisms, including *S. epidermidis* and *S. aureus*, are the most common causes of shunt infections. Adolescents have an increased incidence of shunt infections due to *Propionibacterium* spp., which can be difficult to diagnose.[4]

SSIs are common in orthopedic patients, particularly after spinal fusion. The risk of SSI is markedly elevated for children with underlying neurologic or neuromuscular conditions. The rate of infection after spinal fusion for idiopathic scoliosis is 0.5% to 1.6%, but the rate of infection for children with underlying conditions can exceed 20%.[450] Factors such as bowel incontinence, malnutrition, and instrumentation that extends to the pelvis are thought to contribute to this marked difference in risk of infection. Other risk factors for infection include an ASA score greater than 2, obesity, and antibiotic prophylaxis with clindamycin were independent risk factors for infection.[419] Gram-positive organisms are the predominant cause of postoperative infections in children with idiopathic scoliosis, whereas gram-negative organisms are more common in children who have undergone repair of nonidiopathic scoliosis.[450,630]

The pathogenesis of SSIs involves complex relationships of microbial characteristics, host factors, and the nature of the surgical procedure. Intraoperative contamination of the wound is presumed to be the most common mechanism of SSI. Even with careful skin preparation and expert technique, microbial contamination is virtually universal. Although skin organisms are a common cause of infection, a significant number of these organisms reside in skin appendages, such as sebaceous glands and hair follicles, which may not be eradicated by topical antiseptics.[462] Careful surgical technique is required to minimize contamination and avoid conditions that favor microbial growth postoperatively. Conditions include damaged or devascularized tissue resulting from rough handling or overuse of electrocautery and hematomas and seromas, which provide optimal bacterial growth conditions. Postoperative factors also contribute to the risk of SSI, although their relative importance remains unclear.[463]

SSIs rarely occur within 48 hours of surgery, except in cases of infection with *S. pyogenes* or *Clostridium* spp.; fever within 48 hours of surgery is unlikely to be related to the surgical site.[699] Management of SSIs may require a combination of surgical debridement and antimicrobial therapy, depending on the location and extent of infection. Superficial incisional infections may be treated topically or with oral antibiotics alone, whereas deep incisional and organ or space infections typically require debridement and drainage in addition to antimicrobial therapy. If fluid collections are inaccessible or attempts at drainage may compromise the patient's condition, antibiotics may be tried alone, although the clinical response must be closely monitored.

The presence of prosthetic or foreign material increases risk of infection and complicates infection management. In particular, shunt infections are unlikely to resolve without shunt removal.[782] In some special cases, antimicrobial therapy can successfully suppress infection with foreign material while postoperative healing takes place (e.g., plates and screws to stabilize bones after orthopedic procedures). However, device removal is typically recommended to achieve cure. The likelihood of salvage of an infected prosthesis improves if the infection is detected within 3 weeks of implantation, the implant remains stable and the surrounding tissue is healthy, and the patient receives appropriate systemic antimicrobial therapy.[788] With prosthetic joint infections, most patients require a minimum of 6 to 8 weeks of antimicrobial therapy.[788]

Evidence-based and best-practice guidelines for the prevention of SSIs are largely based on adult studies but have been generally applied to the prevention of pediatric surgical infections.[12,84,462] Multicenter learning collaboratives and use of bundles of prevention practices have been associated with reductions in rates of surgical sites infections.[615,732] Preoperative measures are designed to reduce the nature and degree of microbial contamination and include appropriate hair removal, hand antisepsis by surgical staff, and preoperative skin disinfection. The impact of preoperative antiseptic baths or showers on infection rates remains controversial, although this practice has been adopted by many institutions,[12,462,758] and the practice has reduced the number of bacteria colonizing the skin.[12,462] More substantial reduction of bacteria is seen with multiple showers or with showers immediately preceding surgery, suggesting that timing may be important.[12] Similarly, preoperative use of chlorhexidine shampoo was found to be superior to iodophor products in reducing the number of scalp microorganisms before neurosurgical procedures in children.[403]

Many adult studies have demonstrated that the preoperative use of topical antimicrobials in patients known to be colonized with *S. aureus* was associated with a reduced risk of SSIs.[69,130,558] A meta-analysis evaluated the effect of intranasal mupirocin used alone or as a component of a prevention bundle and found it was associated with reduced rates of *S. aureus* infections in surgical patients (i.e., patients with or without documented nasal carriage of *S. aureus*).[649] Mupirocin resistance was infrequently reported in the studies included in the meta-analysis, but it has been reported after widespread use of nasal mupirocin in other studies.[489]

Screening of all surgical patients for colonization is costly and not recommended as a routine practice,[23] but targeted or universal decolonization may be considered for high-risk groups, such as those undergoing placement of prosthetic devices, if the rate of SSIs remains elevated despite full implementation of routine prevention bundles.

Although removing hair appears to provide a cleaner operative site, current evidence suggests that shaving is associated with higher rates of infection, presumably due to microscopic skin trauma and liberation of resident skin flora from deep skin structures.[12] If hair removal is necessary, evidence suggests that clippers should be used instead of razors.[719] If required, most recommend hair removal is done immediately before surgery, but a meta-analysis found no difference in infection rates between hair removal 1 day before or the day of surgery.[719] However, the studies were small, and authors of the meta-analysis suggested that more research is needed.

Appropriate perioperative use of antimicrobial prophylaxis is an important measure to prevent infection.[83] The American College of Surgeons recommends prophylactic antimicrobial agents be used if an implant is placed, there is a high risk of infection (e.g., after clean-contaminated or contaminated procedures), or the consequences of a postoperative infection are likely to be severe.

A comprehensive meta-analysis of metaanalyses included 250 clinical trials with more than 4800 patients to determine whether antibiotic prophylaxis could be effective in preventing SSIs across a variety of procedures and found that perioperative antibiotics significantly reduced infection risk across the 23 types of surgery evaluated.[76] The protective effect was sustained across different levels of surgical cleanliness.[76] A 2014 study of children undergoing general, cardiac, and spinal surgery found that risk of SSI was 70% greater for patients who did not receive appropriate perioperative antimicrobial prophylaxis.[658]

Guidelines for procedure-specific antimicrobial agents were updated in 2013 by The American Academy of Pediatrics' Committee on Infectious Diseases and the American Society of Health System Pharmacists.[83] The most effective time for antibiotic administration is within 60 minutes of skin incision, except for agents such as vancomycin that require longer infusion times and therefore should be administered 1 to 2 hours before surgery. If surgery is prolonged, repeat dosing should be performed after two half-lives of the administered agent have elapsed. Because prolonged postoperative use does not reduce the risk of infection but does increase the risk of infections due to resistant organisms, antimicrobial agents should be stopped within 24 hours after the procedure.[160,463]

A variety of intraoperative practices and procedures are used to prevent contamination of the surgical site. Appropriate surgical hand antisepsis by surgical personnel reduces the number of bacteria on the hands and the potential for contamination through visible or microscopic breaks in surgical gloves. A systematic review found that use of an alcohol rub was as effective as aqueous scrubbing.[719] Skin antisepsis also reduces the number of viable bacteria at the surgical site. Evidence from randomized clinical trials and metaanalyses suggests that use of chlorhexidine is superior to that of iodophors in preventing SSIs and results in cost savings.[162,405] Operating room traffic should be minimized because activity increases bacterial counts in the air, but the effect on infection risk is likely small. Bacterial counts can also be minimized by regularly servicing operating room ventilation systems and maintaining adequate ventilation parameters.[17]

Proper surgical technique is critical in preventing infection.[12] Closed-suction drainage systems are frequently used in orthopedic operations to drain fluids from the surgical wound and reduce occurrence of hematoma, although recent systematic reviews and metaanalyses have been unable to demonstrate that this practice is associated with a reduced risk of postoperative infection.[550,753,785] Several studies have demonstrated that confidential feedback of surgeon-specific rates of infection to individual surgeons allows them to adjust their practices accordingly and reduces overall infection rates.[23,725]

Other infection-prevention interventions recommended for adult surgical patients include maintaining glycemic control and normothermia and use of supplemental oxygen to prevent tissue hypoxia.[23] Few data are available to determine the impact of these measures in pediatric surgical patients. Tight glycemic control may have untoward consequences in special populations of children, particularly infants. A multicenter trial of tight glycemic control in pediatric cardiac surgery patients is in progress.[237]

HEALTH CARE–ASSOCIATED INFECTIONS CAUSED BY SPECIAL PATHOGENS

Methicillin-Resistant *Staphylococcus Aureus*

MRSA has long been recognized as a nosocomial pathogen and accounted for more than 50% of *S. aureus* HCAIs in adult patients reported to the CDC in the 1990s.[514] In contrast, point prevalence surveys performed in the late 1990s by the Pediatric Prevention Network documented that only 2% of pediatric HCAIs were caused by MRSA.[271,689]

The epidemiology of health care–associated MRSA has changed dramatically over the past decade. Recent data suggest that approximately one third of all *S. aureus* device-related infections in neonatal ICUs are caused by methicillin-resistant strains.[306] Similarly, a nationwide study estimated that approximately one-third of nonneonatal hospital–onset *S. aureus* bacteremia resulted from methicillin-resistant strains.[364]

The molecular epidemiology of health care–associated MRSA infections has also changed over the past decade. In many institutions, community-associated MRSA strains, which are defined by the presence of the SCC*mec*IV cassette, a unique mobile genetic element, have become endemic.[343,466] Studies of the transmission dynamics of MRSA in the health care setting suggest that colonization pressure higher than 10% is associated with a marked increase in the risk of MRSA transmission to critically ill children. The risks of in-hospital transmission are similar for health care–associated and community-associated strains of MRSA.[570]

The changing epidemiology of health care–associated MRSA infections has had an unfortunate impact on patients. Compared with patients with HCAIs due to methicillin-sensitive strains of *S. aureus,* patients with similar infections due to MRSA often have worse outcomes with increased rates of death, longer durations of hospitalization, and higher total hospital costs.[146,147,213,364] Risk factors for MRSA HCAIs include exposure to broad-spectrum antibiotics, prolonged hospital stay, and use of indwelling medical devices.

Prevention of health care–associated MRSA infections has been the topic of several guidelines from experts in the fields of infectious diseases and hospital epidemiology.[23,328,511,667] Recommended practices for all acute care facilities include strict adherence to hand hygiene, use of contact precautions for patients with MRSA infection or colonization, rigorous decontamination of the patient care environment and medical equipment. antimicrobial stewardship, and active surveillance for health care–associated MRSA infections.[99]

For settings in which MRSA transmission persists despite full implementation of the described interventions, experts recommend active surveillance for MRSA colonization among patients who are recognized to be at high-risk or newly admitted.[99] When coupled with the use of contact precautions for MRSA-positive patients, this strategy enhances recognition and control of previously silent reservoirs. Data from a study performed in a tertiary care neonatal ICU suggested that active surveillance and cohorting might not be sufficient to prevent MRSA infections in hospitalized neonates, who may have MRSA infection before colonization can be recognized.[569]

Decolonization has been demonstrated in multiple studies to reduce MRSA transmission in settings where there is a high level of endemic transmission or an outbreak, including when a colonized health care worker was epidemiologically linked to MRSA transmission. A large, cluster-randomized, multicenter trial compared the impact of various control strategies on rates of MRSA infections in adult ICU patients. Investigators found that universal decolonization with intranasal mupirocin and daily chlorhexidine baths reduced the risk of MRSA infection and bloodstream infections compared with MRSA screening and isolation or MRSA screening, isolation, and targeted decolonization of patients found to be colonized with MRSA.[320] However, cost-effectiveness analyses of these strategies have yielded conflicting results.[259,319,479] In many neonatal ICUs, MRSA and methicillin-sensitive

S. aureus infections are common causes of health care–associated infections. A published observational study suggested that active surveillance for *S. aureus* and decolonization prevented *S. aureus* infections. In this study, decolonization was attempted by twice-daily application of intranasal mupirocin and two baths with 2% chlorhexidine for infants older than 36 weeks' gestational age or more than 4 weeks or daily bathing for 5 days for infants older than 2 months of age.[571]

Although decolonization therapy can reduce the transmission of MRSA in the health care setting, multiple studies have demonstrated that a large proportion of patients and health care workers who undergo decolonization become recolonized.[192] Factors that have been associated with failure to eradicate MRSA carriage include wounds, eczema, indwelling medical devices, and mupirocin-resistant MRSA.[292,677]

Universal use of contact precautions (i.e., use of gown and gloves for all patient contacts regardless of whether a patient is known to be colonized or infected with a resistant organism) can reduce the frequency of ICU health care worker clothing contamination.[772] However, the economic costs and burdens of this approach argue against its use except in response to an outbreak.

Vancomycin-Resistant Enterococci

In contrast to methicillin-resistant strains of *S. aureus,* people with VRE colonization or infection typically have an identifiable exposure to a high-risk health care setting, a medical device, or procedure. Vancomycin resistance in *Enterococcus faecium* or *Enterococcus faecalis* arises most frequently from acquisition of a mobile genetic element that carries with it the *vanA* or *vanB* resistance gene. Although exposure to vancomycin provides selection pressure that facilitates the expansion of VRE in a colonized host, it does not induce a vancomycin-sensitive strain of *Enterococcus* to become resistant. However, antibiotic exposure has been repeatedly associated with an increased risk of colonization and infection with VRE. In a previously uncolonized patient, antibiotic use reduces populations of commensal flora, thereby lessening colonization resistance and enhancing the capacity of VRE to establish colonization in a patient who is exposed to VRE. In a patient who is already colonized with VRE, antibiotic exposure reduces the density of colonization of other flora and allows expansion of the organism.[511] In hospitalized children, vancomycin exposure and mechanical ventilation immunosuppression, and older age were independently associated with bacteremia due to VRE, compared with vancomycin-sensitive *Enterococcus.*[279]

Three major sources are important in the transmission of VRE to patients: health care workers' hands, shared patient equipment, and the health care environment. Several observations support the importance of contaminated health care workers' hands in the transmission of VRE. First, VRE can easily be recovered from the hands and gloves of caregivers of VRE-positive patients.[524] Second, VRE has been recovered from computer keyboards used exclusively by health care workers, indicating that hand carriage of VRE can spread the organism beyond the environment of a colonized patient.[307] Third, having a health care worker who is simultaneously providing care to a VRE-positive and a VRE-negative patient has been demonstrated to be a risk factor for VRE acquisition.[79]

Many studies have demonstrated that VRE can persist on inanimate objects and the patient care environment for long periods.[515] Transmission can occur when a patient comes into contact with inadequately decontaminated shared patient equipment (e.g., pulse oximeters, rectal thermometers) or is admitted to an inadequately cleaned hospital room that previously housed a VRE-positive patient.[78,197]

Prevention of transmission of VRE relies on many of the same principles used to prevent transmission of other multidrug-resistant organisms in the health care setting. Similar to preventing MRSA transmission, strategies for interrupting patient-to-patient transmission of VRE rely on interrupting indirect transmission of the organism by health care workers' hands, shared patient equipment, or the health care environment.

As described in HICPAC's "Management of Multidrug-Resistant Organisms in Healthcare Settings, 2006,"[667] a comprehensive approach to the control of epidemiologically important organisms, including VRE, should include active surveillance for infection, application of standard and transmission-based isolation precautions, disinfection of the patient care environment, and judicious use of antibiotics.[667] Several studies have demonstrated that health care workers' hands or gloves are frequently contaminated after providing care for a VRE-colonized patient.[71,723] VRE can contaminate health care workers' hands even if gloves have been worn (presumably by unrecognized inoculation of the hand during the process of glove removal)[723] or if the environment or equipment of a VRE-colonized patient was touched.[71] Transmission-based precautions to prevent patient-to-patient spread of VRE also can reduce the prevalence of VRE among hospitalized patients.[542,704]

Antibiotic exposure does not induce resistance to vancomycin but has been associated with an increased risk for colonization or infection with VRE. It remains unclear whether alterations in the agents or duration of antibiotic therapy can reduce the prevalence of VRE. However, most experts agree that limiting the spectrum and duration of antibiotic therapy to that which is required based on the known or suspected pathogens can have a beneficial impact on the spread of many multidrug-resistant organisms by lessening of selection pressure.[667]

Multidrug-Resistant Gram-Negative Bacilli

Multidrug-resistant gram-negative bacilli (MDR-GNB) have emerged as an important and increasingly frequent cause of HCAIs. Data reported to the NHSN in 2014 revealed that 18% of HCAIs due to *Enterobacteriaceae* spp. were caused by extended-spectrum β-lactamase strains and that 16% of *Pseudomonas aeruginosa* isolates were multidrug resistant.[759] Although most isolates included in this report came from adult institutions, pediatric HCAIs due to extended-spectrum β-lactamase (ESBL)–producing *E. coli* and *Klebsiella* spp., multidrug-resistant *Acinetobacter baumanii* and *P. aeruginosa,* and carbapenemase-producing Enterobacteriaceae are rapidly emerging.[441]

In the United States, outbreaks of MDR-GNB have been reported in neonatal ICUs,[715] pediatric long-term care facilities,[747] and cystic fibrosis centers.[131] In a study of a nationwide sample of more than 368,000 pediatric samples collected from 1999 to 2012, demonstrated increases in the prevalence of *Klebsiella* spp. and *E. coli* with extended-spectrum β-lactamases in virtually all pediatric populations, including young children and outpatients, with an overall prevalence approaching 4%.[428]

Carbapenem-resistant *Enterobacteriaceae* have also emerged as a threat to children. Longitudinal analysis of pediatric isolates submitted from 1999 to 2012 to a national databank revealed that the overall prevalence of these organisms remained low at 0.08% of studied isolates. However, carbapenem resistance was most common in *Enterobacter* spp. isolates from blood cultures and patients who were 1 to 5 years of age or critically ill.[430]

Similar to other epidemiologically important drug-resistant pathogens (e.g., MRSA, VRE), MDR-GNB have frequently been isolated from the environment and equipment surrounding a colonized or infected patient. Although fewer studies have examined risk factors for endemic transmission or infection with MDR-GNB than for MRSA and VRE, outbreak investigations have frequently implicated contaminated respiratory therapy equipment (including mechanical ventilators), inappropriate use of multiuse vials of medications or diluents and urinary catheters, and inadequately cleaned patient environments as reservoirs of these organisms.[557] Additional studies have implicated exposure to broad-spectrum antibiotics and underlying gastrointestinal, neurologic, or renal disease, with an increased risk of ESBL-producing GNB in pediatric populations.[429,441,589,735,763]

The same prevention and control measures used to limit transmission of resistant gram-positive organisms in health care settings are presumed to be effective in preventing HCAIs due to MDR-GNB.[667] Studies have demonstrated that these organisms are often disseminated by health care workers' gloves, gowns, and hands after glove removal.[501] Hand hygiene remains the cornerstone of practices to prevent the transmission of MDR-GNB from patient to patient. Additional measures include identifying and controlling the reservoir of these organisms, typically through the use of standard and contact precautions, effective cleaning and disinfection of the shared patient equipment and the health care environment, and antimicrobial stewardship. Because relatively few pediatric hospitals routinely perform surveillance cultures for MDR-GNB, most infection prevention programs continue to rely on clinical cultures to identify patients who carry a resistant gram-negative organism. The duration of carriage of these organisms is not known but is presumed to be prolonged, and contact precautions are typically continued for patients with MDR-GNB at least until the time of hospital discharge.[464]

Clostridium Difficile

Although toxin-producing *C. difficile* is a well-recognized cause of antimicrobial-associated diarrhea in adults, the pediatric burden has been previously underappreciated. A prospective study of health care–associated diarrhea in hospitalized children and adolescents found that as a group, viral causes were most common; however, *C. difficile*–associated diarrhea was the most common single cause and was more common in older children.[395] Population-based and multicenter studies document a marked increase in pediatric hospitalizations associated with *C. difficile* infection.[356,360,528,787] Data from 2011 estimate that the national burden of health care–associated *C. difficile* infection among children 1 to17 years of age is approximately 6.3 cases per 100,000 people. The prevalence of asymptomatic carriage of toxigenic strains of *C. difficile* is very high among infants, particularly those who are hospitalized, and colonization rates can exceed 40%.[138,412]

Because *C. difficile* is seldom found in the stool of healthy women and clusters of colonized infants can often be detected in nurseries,[138] health care–associated transmission instead of vertical transmission is the presumed mode by which neonates acquire this microorganism. Rates of colonization fall during the first 24 months of life. By 3 years of age, approximately 1% to 3% of young children are colonized with toxigenic *C. difficile*, a rate similar to that observed among asymptomatic adult populations.[334,607,663]

An epidemic strain of *C. difficile* (i.e., NAP-1) emerged and disseminated in Canada and the United States during the mid-2000s and involved patients in the community and health care facilities.[435,476] This strain caused severe disease in populations thought to be at low risk, including peripartum women and children.[111] Several studies suggest that the prevalence of NAP-1 strains among children with *C. difficile* infection is 20% to 30%.[595,731] However, a single-center study of *C. difficile* isolates from children in 2013 found the prevalence of NAP-1 strains to be less than 1%.[368] These disparate findings suggest there may be substantial geographic variation in the prevalence of this hypervirulent strain.

Risk factors for health care-associated *C. difficile* infection in children are similar to those identified for adults. Disease usually is associated with recent antimicrobial therapy. Virtually every class of antibiotics has been implicated, although at least one study implicated fluoroquinolones in particular.[634] Another study found that exposure to three or more classes of antibiotics was the only independent risk factor for severe disease in a cohort of hospitalized children.[359] Patients with comorbid conditions such as malignancy, solid organ transplantation, and inflammatory bowel disease have an increased risk of disease.[360,528,548,634,708,726] An indwelling gastrostomy or jejunostomy feeding tube also is an independent risk factor for disease in children.[634] Two adult studies have explored the relationship of humoral immunity and *C. difficile*–associated diarrhea and found that patients who had serum antibodies against *C. difficile* toxin A were less like to develop disease when colonized or to develop recurrent disease.[388] The implications of these findings on the epidemiology of this disease for children remain unknown.

C. difficile can be found on the hands of personnel and in the patient's immediate environment.[256] Direct or indirect contact is responsible for the spread of this microorganism from patient to patient. Barriers (i.e., gowns and gloves) and hand hygiene reduce transmission. Vigorous environmental cleaning is important because *C. difficile* spores can heavily contaminate the environment and survive for long periods. Conventional cleaning agents may not be sporicidal, and some authorities recommend use of dilute bleach to disinfect rooms of patients with *C. difficile* infection, particularly while they have diarrhea.[256]

Emerging and Reemerging Pathogens

A variety of unusual, potentially fatal infections may be transmitted in health care settings. International air travel has increased the mobility of the world's population, making it possible for people to travel long distances during the incubation period of infections acquired in remote settings.[651] A high index of suspicion for these infections and prompt institution of appropriate isolation precautions are necessary to reduce the risk for health care–associated transmission.

The West African Ebola epidemic of 2014 and 2015 is a sobering example of the dramatic risks that a community-based outbreak can pose to a health care system. Ebola is a hemorrhagic fever caused by a flavivirus, and it can be transmitted person to person through blood and body fluid exposures. The characteristic clinical course, which culminates in marked diarrhea and bleeding from mucous membranes, puts health care workers at high risk of exposure. This risk is compounded by the small inoculum required to establish infection. As was evident in the West African outbreak, shortages of trained personnel and protective equipment can lead to extensive transmission in health care settings, with many patients and health care workers becoming infected.[72,722]

Due to international travel, countries throughout the globe had to use strict screening protocols to identify individuals who might have had early or subclinical Ebola infection. To respond to this risk, the CDC issued a national plan of preparedness that relied on a tiered approach with Frontline Healthcare Facilities that were capable and responsible for screening and isolating people who might have been exposed to Ebola and who were under investigation; Ebola Assessment Hospitals that could hospitalize and care for a person with suspected or confirmed Ebola for up to 5 days, during which time laboratory evaluation could be performed to confirm Ebola infection or establish an alternate diagnosis; and Ebola Treatment Centers that provided extended care for critically ill patients with confirmed Ebola for the duration of their illness.[483] Key to all protocols used to provide care to patients with suspected or confirmed Ebola infection is to isolate the patient, limit unnecessary visitors and staff contact with the patient, and protect health care workers from exposure through the use of specialized personal protective equipment and heightened monitoring when donning and doffing this equipment.[168]

Middle Eastern respiratory syndrome (MERS) is a viral respiratory infection caused by a novel coronavirus that emerged in Saudi Arabia in 2012.[172] The origins of this virus are not fully understood, but camels appear to be a common reservoir of this virus and the presumed source in many cases of community-onset infection. Most people infected with MERS develop fever, cough, and progressive respiratory distress. The case-fatality rate of MERS infections exceeds 50%. Like other coronaviruses, MERS coronavirus is spread through contact and respiratory droplets. Analysis of hospital-based outbreaks suggests that the virus also spreads by droplet nuclei (i.e., particles <5 μm in diameter that can travel long distances on air currents).[29]

Health care workers are at high risk for infection if they provide care to a MERS patient without using appropriate respiratory protection. An outbreak that occurred in South Korea in 20015 highlights the risk of travel-associated MERS. Delayed recognition of MERS infection in a traveler who was hospitalized with respiratory failure 9 days after he returned to South Korea from Saudi Arabia initiated a multihospital outbreak that lasted more than 2 months and infected 186 patients, 36 of whom died. The CDC recommends that all individuals with acute onset of febrile respiratory illnesses be screened for recent international travel.[492]

Plague is endemic in portions of the western United States and in other countries. Although rare, a recently reported case from Colorado demonstrates the potential for animal-to-human and human-to-human transmission of plague.[613] When caring for patients with known or suspected infection due to *Yersinia. pestis,* health care workers should wear masks if the patient has signs or symptoms of pulmonary involvement.[326] Tetracycline, doxycycline, sulfonamides, chloramphenicol, and perhaps fluoroquinolones can be used for prophylaxis of contacts.[326]

Some of the potential agents of bioterrorism are highly transmissible and can result in secondary health care–associated cases if a primary bioterrorism attack were to occur.[28,73,179,300,326,500] Smallpox is the most feared of the potential agents of biological warfare because it can be transmitted by droplet nuclei over large distances, the case-fatality ratio is approximately 30%, there is no effective treatment, and much of the world's population is nonimmune or was immunized in the distant past.[300] Even a very limited number of cases of smallpox would be a global public health emergency, and detailed plans for containment would be needed. Hospitalized patients with smallpox would require airborne and contact isolation precautions, and health care workers caring for these patients must be vaccinated.[300,705]

HEALTH CARE–ASSOCIATED INFECTIONS IN SPECIAL POPULATIONS

Neonates

Most healthy term neonates are born sterile but quickly become colonized with microorganisms derived from their mothers and the immediate environment. Predominant colonizers are coagulase-negative staphylococci on the skin and umbilicus and in the nose and α-hemolytic streptococci in the mouth. Acquisition of intestinal flora is more complex. Lactobacilli predominate in breastfed babies, whereas more adult flora composed of *Bacteroides* spp., other anaerobes, and *E. coli* colonize formula-fed babies.[263] These commensals help inhibit colonization with pathogenic microorganisms. Because pathogens can spread quickly in crowded nurseries, rooming-in and early discharge reduce the risk for colonization of normal neonates.[296,449]

The timing and nature of colonization of premature and full-term infants requiring care in neonatal ICUs is substantially different from that for healthy term infants. Colonization of these infants is substantially delayed, perhaps due to limited contact with their mothers, delayed enteral feeding, and administration of parenteral antimicrobial agents.[257,263,542] As colonization develops, the density and diversity of strains is also different from those found in healthy term infants. During the initial weeks of life, the compositions of skin, respiratory, and gastrointestinal microbiomes from a premature infant are similar.[574] Although coagulase-negative staphylococci colonize the skin, umbilicus, and nose of term and preterm infants,[263] molecular typing studies have demonstrated that particular strains of coagulase-negative staphylococci can persist in neonatal ICUs over extended periods, are transmitted on the hands of caregivers, and cause bloodstream infections in some infants.[322,445,555,687] Compared with healthy term infants, hospitalized neonates often have a larger proportion of intestinal flora composed of aerobic gram-negative bacilli, including *E. coli*, *Klebsiella* spp., *Enterobacter* spp., *P. aeruginosa*, *S. marcescens*, and *Citrobacter* spp.[257,263]

Several investigators have prospectively collected stool samples from neonatal ICU patients and compared isolates recovered from stool with those subsequently recovered from blood during episodes of late-onset sepsis. Molecular analysis suggests that colonization of the gut with pathogenic organisms often precedes bacteremia.[105,683]

S. aureus remains a significant pathogen in neonates; it may colonize a variety of sites, particularly the umbilicus and nose.[263] In term neonates, staphylococcal skin and soft tissue infections, including superficial skin infections, mastitis, and omphalitis, are the most common types of neonatal *S. aureus* infection. Risk factors for neonatal colonization with *S. aureus* include maternal colonization, anogenital carriage, prematurity, low birth weight, and exposure to medical devices.[340,358] Direct contact with colonized caregivers is presumed to be the predominant mode of transmission, although colonized mothers and visitors may also play an important role. Environmental contamination, with transmission of fomites by the hands of caregivers, has also been identified as a risk factor for MRSA acquisition.[57] Molecular analysis of strains isolated during clusters of MRSA infections or colonization have often demonstrated diversity in the isolated strains, suggesting multiple reservoirs leading to transmission.[569,591]

Colonization of the skin, nose, umbilicus, or rectum precedes infection,[318] but there is poor correlation between rates of colonization and infection. When active surveillance is performed, the number of colonized infants typically far exceeds the number of infected infants; conversely, outbreaks of staphylococcal infection can occur in nurseries with low colonization rates. For this reason and because of cost considerations, surveillance cultures to detect colonized infants are not routinely recommended except under outbreak conditions.

MRSA has been a sporadic but recurrent problem in many neonatal ICUs for many years. However, infants in neonatal ICUs and otherwise healthy neonates are being affected by broader trends in the incidence of MRSA infection (see Health Care–Associated Infections Caused by Special Pathogens). Data from the CDC demonstrated that approximately one-fourth of all *S. aureus* infections in hospitalized neonates were attributable to MRSA.[410] Risk factors for these infections include cesarean delivery (likely due to the longer postnatal hospital stay), male sex, surgical procedures, improper infection control practices associated with circumcision, and contact with an infected health care worker.[56,519,591] Control of MRSA outbreaks includes emphasis on standard infection control practices, such as hand hygiene, use of isolation precautions, environmental disinfection, and proper disinfection/sterilization of patient care equipment.

A report demonstrated the capacity of whole-genome sequencing to aid in the identification and management of an outbreak of MRSA in a neonatal ICU.[372] Screening for colonization during the course of an outbreak can identify asymptomatically colonized individuals, but the role of routine screening of infants and of health care workers is less clear.[253,569]

Decolonization of colonized or infected infants may be effective in reducing the risk of invasive infection with methicillin-sensitive *S. aureus* or MRSA.[571] The most common decolonization regimens include chlorhexidine gluconate baths and intranasal mupirocin. Although chlorhexidine is not formally approved for use in infants less than 2 months of age, it has been adopted by many neonatal ICUs. A 2014 survey revealed that 86% of responding academic neonatal ICUs used chlorhexidine.[341] The most common indications for use included skin antisepsis at the time of dressing change and catheter insertion. One report described a reduction in neonatal CLABSI associated with adoption of regular bathing of neonates with central lines with 2% chlorhexidine gluconate.[578,714] Several studies have examined the safety of chlorhexidine in neonates and found negligible absorption after bathing or cord care and no recognized toxicity.[127] Nonetheless, the paucity of high-quality, large studies demonstrating long-term safety of this agent have limited universal adoption.

Safety concerns are associated with other antiseptic agents that have been used on neonates. Iodophors may cause adsorption of iodine, and alcohols may cause chemical burns. These agents are not appropriate to use for bathing. A variety of antiseptic agents have been used for cord care, including triple dye (i.e., aqueous mixture of brilliant green, proflavine hemisulfate, and crystal violet), alcohol, bacitracin, chlorhexidine, and mupirocin, although extensive efficacy and safety data are not available for any of these compounds.[265]

Between 50% and 75% of women with group B streptococcal vaginal colonization transmit this microorganism to their neonates in the absence of chemoprophylaxis, although only 1% to 2% of colonized infants become infected. Although somewhat controversial, the CDC defines these and other infections transmitted from the birth canal as nosocomial infections.[247,250] However, the impact of conventional infection control interventions on early-onset (i.e., within the first 7 days of life) invasive group B streptococcal infection is limited. Intrapartum prophylaxis of women is a far more effective intervention to reduce infection rates in neonates.[107,646] Group B streptococci can be associated with late-onset infections (i.e., after 7 days of life) that are considered HCAIs in hospitalized neonates. Outbreaks of group B streptococcal infection due to indirect contact transmission in nurseries have been well documented.[204,264,525]

Preterm infants are particularly susceptible to infection caused by a variety of yeasts and, to a lesser extent, filamentous fungi; *Candida* spp. are the most common fungal pathogens that infect hospitalized neonates.[27] Infants likely become colonized on their skin and gastrointestinal tracts due to carriage of *Candida*, which can then predispose to invasive infection.[546,551,608] Risk factors for colonization or infection with *Candida* include treatment with H_2-blockers, broad-spectrum antibiotics, age older than 7 days, vaginal birth, and delayed enteral feeding.[622] Risk factors for bloodstream infection and the use of prophylactic fluconazole have been discussed previously (see Infections Related to Intravascular Catheters and Infusions). Risk factors for *Malassezia furfur* infection are similar to those for *Candida*, but the association with lipid emulsion is particularly strong because this organism is obligatorily lipophilic.[161,433,597] Infections caused by filamentous fungi are rare and are usually associated with contaminated devices or practices that facilitate cutaneous invasion.[496,608]

Citrobacter koseri (previously classified as *C. diversus*) has been responsible for a number of outbreaks of HCAIs among neonates.[418,552,771] Although most infants colonized with this microorganism do not develop clinical disease, infection typically results in meningitis due to the particular neurotropism of this bacterium. Neonatal *Citrobacter* meningitis is usually accompanied by formation of one or more brain abscesses and is associated with serious long-term neurologic sequelae. Sporadic outbreaks of *Citrobacter* infection have been reported,[418,552,771] and several published outbreak investigations have implicated transmission of this bacterium from the hands of caregivers to neonatal patients.[552,771] Molecular techniques have demonstrated that *C. koseri* also can be acquired perinatally by vertical transmission.[295]

Enterobacter sakazakii is a rare cause of HCAI in neonates.[701] Similar to infections caused by *C. koseri,* infections caused by this bacterium are usually severe, often involving meningitis and brain abscess.[62,110,137,391,672,739] Outbreaks of *E. sakazakii* infection have implicated a variety of products,[110,391] including intrinsically contaminated powdered milk formulas.[62,110,512,672,739] Because powdered formulas are not marketed as sterile products, feeding practices in neonatal ICUs need to balance the relative nutritional benefits of particular products against the small but real risk of infection with *E. sakazakii* and other potential pathogens.

Newer obstetric practices, such as fetal surgery, may pose unique infectious threats to the fetus and newborn, although few cases of prenatal infection have been reported.[195] Water births have also been associated with infectious complications, as demonstrated by the report of a case of *Legionella* pneumonia in an infant after a prolonged delivery in a pool with contaminated water.[226]

Hand hygiene is the most effective intervention to prevent spread of pathogenic microorganisms.[80] However, the hands of some staff may remain colonized with these microorganisms for prolonged periods despite scrupulous hand cleansing.[263] Use of artificial nails or nail wraps has been associated with carriage of *P. aeruginosa* on the hands of health care workers in a neonatal ICU.[222] Health care workers should not be allowed to wear artificial nails or nail wraps when providing hands-on patient care.[621] Alcohol-based hand rubs are the most effective agents in reducing hand colonization with pathogenic bacteria and are the preferred method for hand hygiene when hands are not visibly soiled.[80]

Preceding sections contain specific recommendations for the prevention of HCAIs caused by community pathogens and infections related to the use of invasive devices. Other general references regarding the prevention of infections in normal nurseries and neonatal ICUs have been published, including recommendations regarding the design of facilities, appropriate staffing, and general infection prevention procedures.[19,139,603] Several interventions designed specifically to prevent HCAIs in high-risk infants deserve additional comment.

The Vermont Oxford Network, which conducts the evidence-based quality improvement collaborative for neonatology, is a large, multicenter network of neonatal units organized for the purpose of implementing evidenced-based interventions to improve the quality of care of neonates[313,520] Data from a group of 669 neonatal ICUs spanning the years 2000 through 2009 describe a significant reduction in late bacterial infections. In 2000, 21.1% of surviving infants weighing 501 to 1500 g experienced a late bacterial or fungal infection, whereas the rate of late infections was 15.0% for similar infants in 2009.[313]

Many investigators have attempted to manipulate the flora that colonize hospitalized infants in neonatal ICUs to interfere with colonization by potential pathogens.[254,448,551] Some of the studies using viridans streptococci demonstrated favorable results, but this approach has not been pursued, in part due to concern about the potential for adverse events.[265,351,487,593] One study examined the impact of universal glove use before all patient care and venous catheter manipulations. In a single-center study, investigators observed a reduction in the frequency of bloodstream infections due to gram-positive organisms.[348,351] Caution has been sounded, however, to the adoption of this practice until additional data are available due to the well-recognized unintended consequences associated with glove use (e.g., lower compliance with hand hygiene, reduced episodes of hands-on patient care).[140]

Infants of extremely low birth weight have immature, fragile skin that is predisposed to drying and cracking and may not be an adequate barrier to prevent invasion by bacteria colonizing the skin. Products containing emollients that include fatty acids have been developed to reduce transepidermal fluid loss and improve skin barrier function in very-low-birth-weight infants. A randomized, controlled trial of the effect of an emollient ointment (Aquaphor) in infants with a birth weight of 501 to 1000 g and a gestational age of 30 weeks or less was conducted in 53 neonatal ICUs participating in the Vermont Oxford Network.[198] Although this intervention was associated with improved skin condition, the treatment group had a higher rate of late-onset bacterial sepsis (although there was no effect on mortality rates). In contrast, two randomized, controlled trials conducted in Bangladesh found that sunflower seed oil reduced the rate of late-onset infection and mortality rates for preterm infants with a gestational age of 33 weeks or less.[159,161,160] The increased risk of infection that is observed among premature infants in neonatal ICUs in limited resource settings compared with the United States likely contributes to the differential impact of these interventions.

Because premature infants lack sufficient levels of opsonizing antibodies, many trials have examined the efficacy of intravenous immunoglobulin in preventing infection in premature infants,[41,206,345,415,702] only one of which demonstrated any benefit in reducing overall infection rates.[41] In contrast, a large trial that randomized almost 3500 infants with suspected or proven infection found therapy with intravenous immunoglobulin had no impact on death or major disability.[83] A published Cochrane review analyzed all published studies and concluded that "routine administration of intravenous immunoglobulin (IVIG) or IgM-enriched IVIG to prevent mortality in infants with suspected or proven neonatal infection is not recommended. No further research is recommended."[536]

Because preterm infants have limited neutrophil pools and limited neutrophil function, several randomized, controlled studies have examined the prophylactic and therapeutic effect of granulocyte-macrophage colony-stimulating factor (GM-CSF) and granulocyte colony-stimulating factor (G-CSF) on infections in preterm infants. In all of these studies, infants receiving these agents had higher peripheral blood neutrophil counts than infants receiving placebo. However, the evidence of the beneficial effects of treatment with these agents is limited.[94,101,457,467]

Leukocytes in stored blood products may have adverse effects on immune function, especially in preterm infants. However, a study examining the effect of a universal prestorage red blood cell leukoreduction program found no effect on bloodstream infection and mortality rates but was associated with improvements in other clinical outcomes.[210] Use of postnatal corticosteroids to prevent or treat chronic lung disease in preterm infants has been associated with higher rates of HCAIs[640] and other short-term and long-term adverse outcomes.[141]

Immunocompromised Children

Children with congenital or acquired immunocompromising conditions are at high risk for HCAIs. The risk for these infections is related to host factors, such as the nature and severity of immunocompromise, use of indwelling medical devices, and frequency and nature of exposure to the health care environment.

The epidemiology of and risk factors associated with HCAIs in immunocompromised children have been best characterized for children with oncologic conditions. Investigators from St. Jude Children's Research Hospital have described the epidemiology of HCAIs for their patients and reported that CLABSIs comprised approximately one third of all identified HCAIs.[435] A large, multicenter collaborative engaged 32 multidisciplinary teams from pediatric hematology-oncology units and demonstrated a significant reduction in CLABSIs associated with implementation of a catheter care bundle; the mean infection rate fell from 2.85 to 2.02 cases per 1000 catheter days over the 32-month program.[94] A single-center, well-controlled study determined the attributable outcomes of CLABSI in pediatric oncology patients. These investigators found that a single CLABSI was associated with a 21-day increased length of stay and almost $70,000 increase in health care costs.[773]

Risk factors associated with CLABSIs in pediatric oncology patients include neutropenia, platelet transfusion, and recent catheter placement.[353,475] Injury of the mucosal barriers of the oropharynx and gastrointestinal tract pose a unique threat of bloodstream infection. A new CLABSI surveillance definition was introduced in 2013 to identify the events that may arise due to translocation of bacteria across a disrupted epithelium rather than breeches in technique during the placement or use of a catheter.[537]

The risk for HCAIs in children undergoing bone marrow or solid organ transplantation can be influenced by factors related to the patient's underlying health status, microbiologic characteristics of the donor and recipient of the graft, the duration and nature of immunosuppression required for successful engraftment of the transplanted organ, and the duration and nature of exposure to medical devices and the health care setting.[353] Solid organ transplant recipients are at risk for SSIs and for bacterial and fungal infections associated with the use of medical devices. Severe manifestations of common childhood viruses, particularly respiratory viruses, can also pose a threat to a child who has recently undergone organ transplantation. Visitor screening, annual influenza vaccination of health care providers and family members, and appropriate use of sick leave are thought to reduce the risk of health care–associated viral infections.[278,706]

Immunocompromised children require the same strategies described earlier to prevent HCAIs when they undergo an invasive procedure, surgery, or have a medical device. For children with nonpermanent immunocompromising conditions (e.g., those receiving chemotherapy or initiating antiretroviral therapy), all elective surgeries and invasive procedures should be deferred until their immunocompromised state has resolved.

The increased susceptibility to opportunistic pathogens necessitates heightened infection prevention measures for some children with the most profound degree of immunosuppression. Numerous outbreaks due to low-virulence organisms commonly found in the environment, such as mold infections related to construction in or near a health care facility, have been reported.[564] Because airborne fungal spores can enter the health care environment, the CDC recommends that the most severely immunocompromised patients, such as neutropenic patients undergoing allogeneic stem cell transplantation, remain in a protective environment that includes added engineering measures such as a positive-pressure patient care environment, high-efficiency particulate air filtering, selective air-handling units, and high numbers of air exchanges per hour (>12/hour).[651]

Despite the broad adoption of these recommendations by many centers that care for high-risk oncology patients in the United States, relatively few studies have demonstrated their effectiveness. A meta-analysis was unable to demonstrate that measures to control the air quality reduced the risk of invasive mold infections,[645] and a systematic review described an association between high-efficiency particulate air filtration and a reduction in fungal infections only when the analysis was limited to nonrandomized studies.[205]

Children With Burns

Relatively few reports describe the epidemiology of HCAIs in pediatric burn patients, and most are likely outdated.[148,248,644,733,756] Using modified CDC definitions, investigators found infection of the burn wound occurred in 10% of patients, or an incidence density of 5.6 burn infections per 1000 patient-days.[756] Data from 2013 that was submitted to the NHSN from adult and pediatric critical care burn units found the median rate of CLABSI was 2.2 cases per 1000 catheter-days.[201] Although pediatric-specific data are not available for dedicated pediatric burn units, it is reasonable to presume that the rates of rates of HCAIs are similar in adult and dedicated pediatric burn centers. New definitions for burn infection were developed and endorsed by a consensus conference convened by the American Burn Association[269] and have been incorporated into NHSN definitions.[312]

The risk and microbiology of burn infections are related to the size of the burn wound and the time of onset of the infection. Infections in burn patients can arise from endogenous organisms (often organisms colonizing the wound) or exogenous organisms. Colonization of a burn typically proceeds from gram-positive organisms, antibiotic-susceptible gram-negative organisms, and fungal and antibiotic-resistant gram-negative organisms.[584] Gram-positive cocci, including methicillin-susceptible *S. aureus* and MRSA, were the most common cause of burn infection in patients with relatively small burns (<30% of body surface area), whereas gram-negative bacteria (especially *P. aeruginosa*) were more common causes of infection in patients with extensive burns (>30% of body surface area).

Interventions to reduce the incidence of HCAIs in burn patients include the use of barrier techniques to reduce cross-colonization of patients, measures to prevent cross colonization of patients during hydrotherapy treatments, topical antibiotics to retard growth of microorganisms in the burn wound, appropriate use of systemic antibiotics, and early excision and closure of the burn wound. The Shriners Burns Hospital in Boston has been successful in controlling infections in severely burned children using these methods and bacteria-controlled nursing units (i.e., laminar airflow units providing controlled temperature and humidity combined with barrier precautions).[757] A randomized, controlled trial of selective decontamination of the digestive tract using polymyxin E, tobramycin, and amphotericin B in severely burned children found no evidence of benefit.[43]

Children With Cystic Fibrosis

In 2003, Saiman and Siegel reviewed the epidemiology of important pathogens in people with cystic fibrosis and convened an international consensus conference to develop evidence-based guidelines for standardized microbiologic and infection control practices for those with cystic fibrosis.[624] Key elements of this guideline included the need to interrupt the transmission of *Burkholderia cepacia* complex, *P. aeruginosa,* and MRSA among individuals with cystic fibrosis in health care settings. The 2014 guideline emphasized standard infection control practices, such as appropriate hand hygiene, proper use of isolation precautions, and effective procedures for cleaning and disinfecting or sterilizing reused equipment contaminated with respiratory secretions.[625] These updated guidelines include several novel recommendations intended to limit person-to-person transmission of pathogens that threaten the health of patients with cystic fibrosis based on the observation that they can harbor critical microorganisms (e.g., *P. aeruginosa, B. cepacia*) for months before detection on respiratory tract cultures. Contact precautions are recommended for use in inpatient and ambulatory settings for all patients with cystic fibrosis. Patients should be advised to avoid close contact with each other, with at least 6 feet separating them in all clinical settings. They also are advised to wear a mask at all times while they are within a facility that provides health care.

In inpatient settings, the guideline recommends contact isolation and a single-patient room for patients with cystic fibrosis, regardless of colonization status. However, patients who are not colonized with MRSA, *B. cepacia* complex, and multidrug-resistant *P. aeruginosa* may share a room with a patient who does not have cystic fibrosis and who is at low risk for infection with these bacteria if a single-patient room is not available. All patients, whether colonized with these bacteria or not, should avoid contact with other patients with cystic fibrosis. All patients should receive annual influenza vaccination and age-appropriate pneumococcal vaccination.

Children Undergoing Dialysis

Children with chronic renal failure who are undergoing hemodialysis or peritoneal dialysis have multiple risk factors for HCAIs. Renal failure is associated with impaired immune function, including phagocyte dysfunction due to uremia. Children with renal failure often require frequent contacts with the health care system, including hospitalization, further increasing the risk of acquiring multidrug-resistant organisms. The indwelling medical devices required for dialysis pose additional risks. Studies of adult patients with end-stage renal disease have demonstrated an increased risk of infection associated with an immunocompromised condition related to an underlying disease process or use of immunosuppressing therapies, anemia, or iron overload.[38]

Infection of dialysis access devices for hemodialysis or peritoneal dialysis remains the most common type of HCAI among patients with end-stage renal disease.[38] For hemodialysis patients, the risk for bacteremia is influenced by the type of vascular access device in use. Arteriovenous fistulas are associated with the lowest risk of bacteremia, in contrast to nontunneled dialysis catheters, for which the risk for bacteremia can approach 22.5 infections per 1000 dialysis procedures, which is 7-fold to 10-fold higher than the rate of infections reported for patients undergoing dialysis through an arteriovenous fistula during the same period.[308,720] Adult studies have demonstrated that comorbid conditions (particularly diabetes mellitus and hypertension) are independently associated with an increased risk of bacteremia for patients undergoing hemodialysis.[409] Gram-positive organisms are the most common cause of bacteremia in patients undergoing hemodialysis; *S. aureus* and coagulase-negative staphylococci are the most frequently isolated pathogens.

Many of the same practices used to prevent catheter-associated bloodstream infections in patients with conventional central venous catheters are considered standard of care for patients with hemodialysis catheters, although there are several important differences. In contrast to exit sites for conventional venous catheters, current guidelines recommend that antiseptic or antibacterial ointment (i.e., povidone-iodine or bacitracin/gramicidin/polymyxin B) be placed at the exit site of hemodialysis catheters after insertion and after each dialysis session provided the catheter material is compatible with the substance.[533]

Efforts to increase the use of arteriovenous fistulas and improve the access techniques have resulted in substantial reductions in the rate of bacteremia among adult dialysis patients. For hemodialysis patients with a history of multiple episodes of bacteremia, several metaanalyses[390,780] and a randomized trial have demonstrated that use of antibiotic or antiseptic locks between dialysis sessions were associated with a reduced risk of subsequent bacteremia.[690] Although few data are available from studies of pediatric patients, application of these same strategies to pediatric patients undergoing hemodialysis is likely to reduce the risk for bacteremia in this patient population.

Peritonitis is the most common HCAI in patients undergoing intermittent or continuous peritoneal dialysis. In addition to raising the risk of infection-related death, peritonitis poses long-term risks for patients who require chronic dialysis. Repeated or protracted episodes of inflammation of the peritoneum can result in permanent fibrosis of the peritoneal membrane and render peritoneal dialysis ineffective. Pediatric data suggest gram-positive organisms account for 44% of cases of culture-positive peritonitis. Approximately half of the gram-positive isolates were *S. aureus,* and the remaining isolates were coagulase-negative staphylococci. Approximately 50% of pediatric peritonitis cases in this population are caused by gram-negative organisms, whereas less than 5% of episodes are caused by fungi.[124]

Using data from the International Pediatric Peritoneal Dialysis Registry, the International Society for Peritoneal Dialysis has published guidelines for the treatment and prevention of peritonitis in pediatric patients.[751] They recommend that antibiotics be administered by the intraperitoneal route for the treatment of peritonitis. Empiric antibiotics should be selected based on available data on local resistance patterns of likely infecting organisms. Vancomycin is not routinely recommended for empiric therapy unless the institution's rate of MRSA exceeds 10% or the patient has a history of MRSA colonization or infection.[751] Definitive therapy should be tailored after the organism has been isolated and susceptibility data are available. The recommended duration of therapy is based on the infecting organism but ranges from 2 to 3 weeks for most bacterial pathogens. Replacement of the peritoneal catheter is recommended for cases of refractory or relapsing bacterial peritonitis, in the setting of a tunnel infection, and for fungal peritonitis.

Prevention of HCAIs in children undergoing peritoneal dialysis rests on the same principles used to prevent intravascular infections: scrupulous adherence to aseptic technique during catheter insertion and access and close attention to the care of the catheter exit site. A multicenter collaborative defined the most important strategies (i.e., best-care bundles) to prevent infections in pediatric patients with end-stage renal disease receiving peritoneal dialysis.[516] The collaborative observed an overall rate of peritonitis of 0.46 episodes per patient-year and found that the site-specific rate of peritonitis was inversely related to the degree of compliance with the peritoneal dialysis care catheter bundle.[656] Consensus guidelines for the prevention and treatment of catheter-related infections and peritonitis in pediatric patients receiving peritoneal dialysis were updated in 2012.[751]

Children in Long-Term Care Facilities

Several reports have described the burden and spectrum of HCAIs among children in long-term care facilities. A prospective, longitudinal study of four pediatric facilities described the spectrum of endemic nosocomial infections over a 2-year period in the 1990s.[746] The cumulative incidence of infection was 40%. Upper respiratory tract infections and UTIs were the most common types of infection and accounted for 37% and 31% of infections, respectively. Most UTIs occurred in a small group of patients with functional or anatomic genitourinary abnormalities related to neural tube defects or neuromuscular disorders, although the investigators did not differentiate between symptomatic infections and asymptomatic bacteriuria. A later report described the burden of device-related infections in this population.[294] The incidence of CAUTI was more than twice as common among pediatric ICUs reporting data to the National Nosocomial Infections Surveillance System, whereas the incidences of VAP and central venous catheter–associated bloodstream infections were equivalent or slightly lower than that reported from pediatric ICUs. A single-center retrospective study performed at a 109-bed pediatric long-term care facility in 2009 reported the incidence of HCAIs to be 6.21 infections per 1000 resident-days.[3] In this study, streptococcal and staphylococcal skin infections were the most commonly identified infections.

Due to limited active surveillance in many pediatric long-term care facilities, there is likely underrecognition of endemic HCAIs that occur in these settings. The residential setting and the behavioral activities of children, however, likely contribute to a significant risk of clusters or outbreaks of HCAIs due to respiratory and gastrointestinal pathogens. In a 4-year retrospective study of three pediatric long-term care facilities, investigators identified a total of 62 outbreaks that involved 700 patients.[510] Outbreaks due to respiratory viruses were most common and were associated with the largest numbers of confirmed cases in residents and staff. Gastroenteritis, particularly that due to norovirus, was relatively common and associated with large numbers of suspected cases. Because of the heterogeneity in the populations of patients served and the ongoing improvement efforts underway at virtually all sites where health care is provided, caution must be exercised when selecting a benchmark with which to compare a facility's rates of HCAIs.

Guidelines for the infrastructure and essential activities of infection control programs and key prevention practices in long-term care facilities have been published, although they do not specifically address issues unique to children in long-term care facilities.[232,679,682] Key prevention measures are effective hand hygiene, appropriate use of barriers and isolation precautions, proper care of patients with indwelling devices (e.g., tracheostomies) or who require invasive procedures (e.g., bladder catheterization), prevention of decubitus ulcers, age-appropriate immunization (including yearly influenza vaccine), and early detection and control of outbreaks of infection.

Similar to reports from adult facilities, adherence to hand hygiene practices can be suboptimal. In a multicenter study, investigators observed an overall rate of hand hygiene compliance that was approximately 40% and found that compliance was much lower for nonclinical than clinical staff (14% vs. 61%).[93]

INFECTION PREVENTION AND CONTROL PROGRAMS IN HEALTH CARE FACILITIES

This section highlights key elements of a comprehensive program to prevent and control HCAIs in health care facilities that provide inpatient care for pediatric patients. A detailed description of the development, implementation, and maintenance of an effective program is beyond the scope of this chapter, but several excellent and authoritative references on this topic are available.[183,336,399,474,764]

Many external groups and organizations have significant influence on infection prevention and control programs in health care facilities. Their activities are outlined in Table 244.3.

Organization and Activities of Health Care Infection Control Programs

In 1998, a consensus panel of national experts published a report on the requirements for infrastructure and activities of HCAI prevention and control programs.[641] The specific recommendations of the panel are listed in Table 244.4, accompanied by an indication of the strength of the recommendation, and they are described in more detail in the

TABLE 244.3 **External Groups and Organizations Influencing Health Care–Associated Infection Prevention and Control Programs**

Group or Organization	Activities
Division of Healthcare Quality Promotion (DHQP), National Center for Emerging and Zoonotic Infectious Diseases (NCEZID), Centers for Disease Control and Prevention (CDC)	Provides data and guidance on prevention of health care–associated infections (HCAIs); antimicrobial resistance; adverse drug events; blood, organ and tissue safety; immunization safety; and other related adverse events or medical errors in health care affecting patients and health care personnel Investigates and responds to emerging infections and related adverse events among patients and health care personnel Conducts epidemiologic and basic and applied laboratory research to identify new strategies to prevent HCAIs, antimicrobial resistance, and related adverse events or medical errors Serves as the national reference laboratory for the identification and antimicrobial susceptibility testing of pathogens that cause HCAIs
National Healthcare Safety Network (NHSN)	Collects and reports data on the incidence of HCAIs, antimicrobial use and resistance, and process measures tightly linked with prevention of HCAIs
Healthcare Infection Control Practices Advisory Committee (HICPAC)	Provides guidance to DHQP regarding surveillance, prevention, and control of HCAIs; publishes evidence-based guidelines for HCAI prevention
US Department of Health and Human Services (HHS)	Develops the National Action Plan to Prevent Health Care—Associated Infections: Roadmap to Elimination, which includes components for acute care hospitals, ambulatory surgical centers, end-stage renal disease facilities, and long-term care facilities
Center for Medicare and Medicaid Services (CMS)	Requires reporting of some HCAIs by facilities providing care to Medicare and Medicaid beneficiaries Comparative data available for public viewing on the CMS Hospital Compare website Leads the Partnership for Patients, which aims to reduce preventable harms, including HCAIs
State health departments	Require public reporting of institutional rates of HCAIs, with specifics varying by state
Professional societies:	Advocate for public policy related to prevention of HCAIs
Society of Healthcare Epidemiology of America (SHEA)	Develop and collaborate on publication of evidence-based guidelines for HCAI prevention
Association for Professionals in Infection Control and Epidemiology (APIC)	Provide training for health care epidemiologists and infection preventionists Sponsor scientific meetings on HCAI prevention
Infectious Diseases Society of America (IDSA)	Publish journals, including articles on HCAI prevention
The Joint Commission	Provides accreditation standards for infection prevention and control programs; promulgates National Patient Safety Goals, which includes goals related to prevention of HCAIs
National Quality Forum	Selects measures of health care quality
Occupational Safety and Health Administration (OSHA) of the US Department of Labor	Issues regulations to minimize occupational hazards to health care workers, including exposure to bloodborne pathogens and tuberculosis
Institute of Medicine (IOM)	Publishes scientific reports related to improving patient safety and reducing HCAIs
Institute for Healthcare Improvement (IHI)	Provides guidance documents on performance improvement regarding patient safety, including preventing HCAIs Conducts campaigns to improve patient safety Provides training for patient safety officers
Children's Hospital Association	Coordinates performance improvement collaboratives to reduce HCAIs
Vermont Oxford Network	Collects and reports outcomes of neonatal care, including late-onset sepsis Coordinates improvement collaboratives to improve outcomes, including reducing late-onset sepsis
National Surgical Quality Improvement Project	Coordinates an outcomes-based program to measure and improve the quality of surgical care, including prevention of surgical site infections
Consumers Union	Publishes reports and ranking of hospitals with respect to HCAI prevention Advocates for patient safety

report.[641] A similar document outlining the elements of infection prevention and control in long-term care facilities has been published.[679] Another guideline describes the skills and competencies of people who lead these programs.[352] These publications do not deal specifically with pediatric issues, although the recommendations are generally applicable to facilities providing care to children.

Surveillance Strategies

Surveillance of HCAIs is necessary to understand the specific infection problems of individual facilities, to provide a means of evaluating the effectiveness of interventions to reduce the frequency of these infections, and to facilitate detection of outbreaks of infection. Infection prevention and control programs should have a surveillance plan for the health care facility that is based on the prioritized risks associated with care provided to patients in the facility and sound epidemiologic principles.[406]

The CDC NHSN surveillance methodology has become the de facto standard for surveillance. Although not without limitations, the methodology is well defined and time tested and allows institutions to benchmark themselves in relation to other institutions through periodic data summaries from the NHSN.[202] NHSN methodology is used extensively by states and by the CMS for public reporting of rates of HCAIs (see Table 244.3). The CDC's NHSN has posted definitions for HCAIs with detailed instructions on the application of its methods on its website (http://www.cdc.gov/nhsn/enrolled-facilities/index.html).

Surveillance should examine adherence to processes that are tightly linked to outcomes. For example, facilities should monitor adherence with hand hygiene, transmission-based isolation precautions,[85,639] and intervention bundles to prevent CLABSI, CAUTI, and SSI.[63,490,523,577] These process measures can be used to guide and monitor improvement efforts.

Surveillance and reporting of communicable infections to state departments of health is a duty of infection prevention and control programs. It is often done in collaboration with the facility's microbiology laboratory.

Outbreak Investigation

Because outbreaks of HCAIs are often associated with significant patient morbidity and mortality, clusters of infection should be investigated

TABLE 244.4 **Consensus Panel Recommendations for the Requirements for Infrastructure and Essential Activities of Infection Control and Epidemiology in Hospitals**

Recommendation	Category[a]
Critical Data and Information	
Surveillance of nosocomial infections must be performed.	I
Surveillance data must be analyzed appropriately and used to monitor and improve infection control and health care outcomes.	I
Clinical performance and assessment indicators used to support external comparative measurements should meet the criteria delineated by the Society for Healthcare Epidemiology of America (SHEA) and Association of Professionals in Infection Control and Epidemiology (APIC).	II
Policies and Procedures	
Written infection prevention and control policies and procedures must be established, implemented, and updated periodically.	II and III
Policies and procedures should be monitored periodically for performance.	II and III
Regulations, Guidelines, and Accreditation Requirements	
Health care facilities should use infection control personnel to assist in maintaining compliance with relevant regulatory and accreditation requirements.	II
Infection control personnel should have appropriate access to medical or other relevant records and to staff members who can provide information on the adequacy of the institution's compliance with regard to regulations, standards, and guidelines.	II
The infection control program should collaborate with and provide liaison to appropriate local and state health departments for reporting of communicable diseases and related conditions and to assist with the control of infectious diseases.	II and III
Employee Health	
The infection control program personnel should work collaboratively with the facility's employee health program personnel.	II
At the time of employment, all facility personnel should be evaluated by the employee health program for conditions related to communicable diseases.	II and III
Appropriate employees or other health care workers should have periodic medical evaluations to assess for new conditions related to infectious diseases that may have an impact on patient care, the employee, or other health care workers, including review of immunization and tuberculosis skin test status if appropriate.	II and III
Employees must be offered appropriate immunizations for communicable diseases.	I and III
The employee health program should develop policies and procedures for the evaluation of ill employees, including assessment of disease communicability, indications for work restrictions, and management of employees who have been exposed to infectious diseases, including postexposure prophylaxis and work restrictions.	I
Prevention of Transmission of Infectious Diseases	
All health care facilities must have the capacity to identify the occurrence of outbreaks or clusters of infectious diseases.	I
All health care facilities must have access to the services of personnel trained and experienced in conducting outbreak investigations.	II
When an outbreak occurs, the infection control team must have adequate resources and the authority to ensure a comprehensive and timely investigation and the implementation of appropriate control measures.	II
Education and Training of Health Care Workers	
Health care facilities must provide ongoing educational programs in infection prevention and control to health care workers.	II and III
Educational programs should be evaluated periodically for effectiveness, and attendance should be monitored.	II and III
Personnel	
The personnel and supporting resources, including secretarial services, available to the hospital epidemiology and infection control program should be proportional to the size, complexity, and estimated risk for the population served by the institution.	II
All hospitals should have the continuing services of trained hospital epidemiologists and infection control professionals.	I
Infection control professionals should be encouraged to obtain certification in infection control.	II
Health care facilities should provide or make available in a timely fashion sufficient office space, equipment, statistical and computer support, and clinical microbiology and pathology laboratory services to support the surveillance, prevention, and control program of the institution.	II

[a]Categories: I, strongly recommended for implementation based on evidence from at least one properly randomized, controlled trial or evidence from at least one well-designed clinical trial without randomization or evidence from cohort or case-control analytic studies (preferably from more than one center) or evidence from multiple time-series studies. II, recommended for implementation based on published clinical experience or descriptive studies or reports of expert committees or opinions of respected authorities. III, recommended when required by government rules or regulations.

From Scheckler WE, Brimhall D, Buck AS, et al. Requirements for infrastructure and essential activities of infection control and epidemiology in hospitals: a consensus panel report. *Infect Control Hosp Epidemiol.* 1998;19:114–124.

promptly. A single, highly unusual infection (e.g., postoperative group A streptococcal infection) is sufficient cause for an investigation. Clusters of HCAIs caused by an uncommon microorganism, a common microorganism with an unusual antimicrobial susceptibility pattern, or a series of infections at the same anatomic site (e.g., outbreak of diarrhea) also are indications for an investigation. However, some outbreaks are more difficult to recognize because they occur intermittently, involve multiple microorganisms, involve infection at various anatomic sites, or have long incubation periods.

Box 244.3 provides an outline of the steps involved in investigating a cluster of HCAIs. Detailed discussions of the methods used for outbreak investigation can be found elsewhere.[47,183,336,399,474,764] Published outbreak investigations are an invaluable resource because they provide insight into potential causes. However, it is hazardous to jump to conclusions regarding the cause of a particular cluster of infections based on the results of a prior investigation. Careful investigation is necessary to establish or refute epidemiologic links between cases and potential causes.

Molecular genotyping techniques are an important adjunct to traditional epidemiologic methods and can serve as a powerful tool to confirm or refute a particular source or mode of transmission of a particular microorganism. Several reports have described the use of whole-genome sequencing in outbreak investigations and the insight this method provided in understanding the spread of health care–acquired pathogens.[372,685]

BOX 244.3 Approach to the Investigation of Clusters of Health Care–Associated Infections

1. Confirm the diagnosis.
2. Make a case definition.[a]
3. Search for additional cases.
4. Plot the epidemic curve.
5. Compare rates before the epidemic with current rates using statistical tests to prove that an epidemic exists.
6. Perform a literature review.
7. Open lines of communication with leaders of relevant departments, the microbiology laboratory, and the hospital administration.
8. Keep detailed records of events and conversations.
9. Review charts of all cases, and compile a line listing of relevant information.
10. Formulate a hypothesis about a likely reservoir and mode of transmission.[a]
11. Institute temporary control measures.
12. Perform a case-control study to develop epidemiologic evidence to support or refute the hypotheses.
13. Update control measures.
14. Document the reservoir and mode of transmission microbiologically. Confirm the relatedness of isolates using molecular genotyping techniques if necessary.[a]
15. Document the efficacy of control measures.
16. Write a report and distribute it to appropriate individuals.
17. Change policies and procedures if necessary.

[a]Molecular genotyping techniques may be employed early in the course of the investigation to evaluate the relatedness of pathogens associated with the cluster, reservoirs, and modes of transmission.

Policies and Procedures

Policies and procedures are necessary to optimize and standardize hospital routines and patient care practices. Certain generic policies and procedures apply to all departments, such as those for hand hygiene, isolation precautions, prevention of transmission of infectious diseases from and to visitors and health care workers, reprocessing of reusable patient care items, and disposal of medical waste. Other policies and procedures should be tailored to the potential infection risks relevant to specific departmental activities. Individual guidelines on various topics published by the CDC's HICPAC (http://www.cdc.gov/hicpac/pubs.html), a compendium of guidelines on the prevention of HCAIs in acute care hospitals published by the Society for Healthcare Epidemiology of America (SHEA),[100,199,209,366,426,468,618] and guidelines published by other professional societies serve as useful references for these efforts.

However, merely developing policies, procedures, and standardized practices is insufficient. Achievements in the prevention of HCAIs primarily have resulted from reliably incorporating evidence-based practices into routine patient care. Effective leadership and application of principles and practices of implementation and improvement science are critical to the success of this effort.[324,627,628]

Hand Hygiene

Proper hand hygiene, which includes handwashing using soap and water and hand antisepsis using a waterless, alcohol-based agent, reduces carriage of potential pathogens on the hands of health care workers.[80,561] Hand hygiene is widely regarded as the quintessential infection prevention measure.

Indications and procedures for hand hygiene are reviewed in detail in the SHEA and HICPAC guidelines and a guidance document produced under the auspices of the World Health Organization (WHO).[80,209,639] The WHO approach was developed as a user-centric model and has five moments for hand hygiene: before patient contact; before performing an aseptic task, after actual or potential contact with body fluids, after contact with the patient or his or her immediate surroundings, and after contact with the patient care environment outside the immediate surroundings.[639] The WHO has also provided a strategy for measurement of adherence with the five moments and behavior change strategies to improve adherence.[638,768]

Handwashing with soap and water must be performed when hands are visibly soiled to remove organic material and associated microorganisms. When hands are not visibly soiled, hand antisepsis using an alcohol-based, waterless product is preferred because it reduces the number of pathogenic bacteria that transiently colonize the hands more effectively than handwashing.[80,562] Hand hygiene is also necessary after removing gloves—an indication that many health care professionals fail to fully appreciate—because gloves can have macroscopic and microscopic holes that lead to hand contamination and because hands can be contaminated in the process of removing soiled gloves.[371]

Individuals wearing artificial nails are more likely to harbor pathogenic gram-negative bacilli and yeast on their fingertips, and these organisms are less effectively cleared from artificial nails by use of an alcohol-based agent than from natural nails.[297,480] Use of artificial nails or nail wraps was associated with carriage of *P. aeruginosa* on the hands of health care workers and infection among high-risk infants in a neonatal ICU.[222,275] For these reasons, the HICPAC hand hygiene guideline recommends that health care workers not wear artificial fingernails or extenders when providing patient care and that natural nails should be kept less than 0.25 inches long.[80,21]

Isolation Precautions

Proper use of isolation precautions is important for all health care facilities but especially critical in facilities caring for pediatric patients. Children hospitalized as the result of infections acquired in the community represent a substantial proportion of pediatric admissions, and transmission of these infections to other susceptible patients is a significant problem (see Spread of Communicable Infections in Health Care Facilities). Effective use of appropriate isolation precautions markedly reduces transmission of these agents.

HICPAC isolation guideline recommends the use of two tiers of precautions: standard precautions and transmission-based precautions.[668,667]

Standard Precautions

Standard precautions synthesize the goals of protecting health care workers from bloodborne pathogens and protecting health care workers and patients from transmission of microorganisms from moist body substances.[668] Standard precautions apply to any planned or potential contact with blood; all body fluids, secretions, and excretions except sweat, regardless of whether they contain visible blood; nonintact skin; mucous membranes; and supplies, equipment, or surfaces contaminated with these substances (see Box 244.1). Standard precautions should be used in the care of all patients at all times, regardless of their diagnosis or presumed infection status.[668]

Transmission-Based Precautions

Other precautions are needed to prevent transmission of contagious diseases (e.g., varicella, measles, tuberculosis, pertussis) and other epidemiologically important microorganisms (e.g., multidrug-resistant microorganisms, *C. difficile*) from infected or colonized patients. Transmission-based precautions are designed to provide the necessary measures in addition to those already specified by standard precautions to interrupt known modes of transmission of these microorganisms.[668] The three types of transmission-based precautions are airborne, droplet, and contact precautions (see Box 244.2).

1. Airborne precautions are designed to prevent transmission of microorganisms spread by droplet nuclei (e.g., measles, varicella, tuberculosis), which can be carried on air currents over substantial distances.[668] Special air handling and ventilation are required.[668]
2. Droplet precautions are designed to prevent transmission of microorganisms spread by large respiratory droplets that travel only short distances before settling.[668] Special air handling and ventilation are not required.
3. Contact precautions are designed to prevent transmission of microorganisms spread by direct and indirect contact.[668]

Because some infections are spread by more than one mode of transmission, types of precautions may need to be combined (e.g., varicella requires airborne precautions and contact precautions). Patients infected or colonized with more than one microorganism also may require a combination of systems.

The HICPAC guideline lists clinical syndromes and conditions warranting empiric use of transmission-based precautions in addition to standard precautions to prevent transmission of epidemiologically important pathogens until infection with these microorganisms is excluded.[609] To ensure that appropriate empiric precautions are implemented promptly, hospitals must have systems in place to evaluate patients for these infections as a part of their routine preadmission and admission care.

Visitors

Visitors with communicable diseases can inadvertently expose hospitalized patients and health care workers unless procedures to identify and exclude them are in place. Varicella, measles, and tuberculosis are the most problematic infections because they are spread by airborne transmission, enabling infected visitors to expose a large number of individuals in a short period. Visitors with pertussis, viral respiratory and gastrointestinal infections, parvovirus B19 infection, rubella, and mumps can pose a significant hazard to patients and health care workers with whom they have close contact.

Procedures to identify potentially infected visitors should include visiting children because they are the most likely people to be infected with these agents. Adult visitors and parents or guardians of visiting children should be asked a set of screening questions about fever, rash, respiratory and gastrointestinal symptoms, and recent exposure to other children with chickenpox, measles, or whooping cough. People without significant symptoms or exposures should be allowed to visit with no restrictions. Those who are otherwise well but have a recent history of a minor illness may be allowed to visit but potentially with restrictions, such as no visits by child visitors to the activity room and no sharing of food, drinks, or toys. People with fever, symptoms consistent with active respiratory or gastrointestinal infections, or rash consistent with a viral exanthem should not be allowed to visit. Individuals with significant exposures to chickenpox or measles who are susceptible to these infections and those with exposure to pertussis who may be in the incubation period of the disease should not be allowed to visit. This screening process should be repeated each day that the person visits the hospital. This procedure does not guarantee that people are not in the incubation phase of a contagious disease at the time of their visit (e.g., varicella) but can be useful in limiting exposures.

Many pediatric facilities implemented blanket restrictions on visitation by children during the influenza A H1N1 pandemic of 2009.[612] Some facilities impose annual restrictions on visitation by young children during winter to prevent transmission of respiratory virus infections, but the nature, frequency and effect of these restriction policies have not been described.

SHEA published an expert guidance document providing recommendations for hand hygiene and use of barrier precautions by visitors.[508] It recommends use of contact precautions by visitors to patients colonized or infected with extensively drug-resistant, gram-negative organisms and possibly by visitors of patients infected with enteric pathogens (e.g., *C. difficile*, norovirus). Use of contact precautions is not recommended for visitors to patients with MRSA or VRE. The guideline acknowledges that requirements for the use of barriers should be balanced by the potential negative psychosocial impact on children and interference with bonding, breastfeeding, and delivery of family-centered care and by practical concerns regarding enforcement.

Occupational Health

Health care workers require protection from the significant infectious risks inherent in patient care, and patients and other health care workers need to be protected from exposure to health care workers with communicable diseases. Integrating management and prevention strategies to accomplish these two goals requires close collaboration between hospital infection prevention and control programs and employee health departments. A HICPAC guideline for infection control in health care workers contains comprehensive recommendations for evaluation of illnesses, postexposure evaluation and management, and prevention of occupationally acquired infections in health care workers.[70]

Evaluation of Ill Health Care Workers

Hospital staff and volunteers with symptoms such as persistent fever, conjunctivitis, skin lesions or rashes, diarrhea, and persistent cough should be evaluated for a communicable disease. Possible cases of varicella, herpes zoster on an exposed area of the body, herpetic whitlow, adenoviral conjunctivitis, measles, mumps, rubella, pertussis, staphylococcal skin infection, enteric infection in a food service worker, and active pulmonary tuberculosis should be investigated promptly and confirmed with laboratory tests if necessary.

Many health care workers choose to have these problems evaluated by their primary care providers. However, employee health departments have an interest in completing or collaborating in these assessments, especially if there is a question about whether the condition was acquired in the workplace, requires a furlough from work, or might have exposed patients or other health care workers.

Postexposure Evaluation and Management of Health Care Workers

A structured approach to the assessment and management of exposures of health care workers to patients with infectious diseases is critical for promptly providing postexposure prophylaxis, if indicated, and to allay anxiety while avoiding unnecessary interventions and loss of workdays. The first step is to develop criteria for assessing the nature of the exposure because many reported encounters do not pose a significant risk of infection. Some exposures (e.g., varicella, hepatitis B) may require an assessment of the susceptibility of the health care worker to infection, and procedures should describe the indications for laboratory tests and the interpretation of results.

Postexposure prophylaxis regimens for various exposures are discussed in a HICPAC guideline,[70] and those for bloodborne infections are available in various other guidelines[643] (https://stacks.cdc.gov/view/cdc/20711) Additional information for postexposure prophylaxis can be obtained by searching the Centers for Disease Control and Prevention website (http://www.cdc.gov). Counseling regarding the risks and consequences of the exposure is an important component of this service.

Prevention of Occupationally Acquired Infections by Health Care Workers

Because vaccination against infectious diseases is a highly cost-effective prevention strategy, hospitals should offer vaccinations free of charge. Vaccination against measles (or demonstration of immunity) has been regarded as a quality of care indicator for occupational health programs since 1994.[376] In 2013, the CMS required acute care hospitals in the United States to report influenza vaccination of health care workers as part of the Hospital Inpatient Quality Reporting Program.

Yearly influenza vaccination of health care workers is recommended by the Advisory Committee on Immunization Practices.[116] Although vaccination rates of health care workers have improved substantially, they remain suboptimal.[421] Interventions to improve vaccination rates are provision of vaccine free of charge, enhanced access to vaccination, reminders or incentives, active management of the vaccination program requiring active declination, and mandatory immunization policies. Mandatory immunization policies are most effective[421,563]; however, despite endorsement by the American Academy of Pediatrics,[185] the Pediatric Infectious Diseases Society (PIDS), SHEA, and the Infectious Diseases Society of America (IDSA) (http://www.idsociety.org/uploadedFiles/IDSA/Policy_and_Advocacy/Current_Topics_and_Issues/Immunizations_and_Vaccines/Health_Care_Worker_Immunization/Statements/IDSA_SHEA_PIDS%20Policy%20on%20Mandatory%20Immunization%20of%20HCP.pdf), mandatory vaccination has not been adopted universally.

Given the significant occupational risk for hepatitis B infection in hospitals, hepatitis B vaccination should be offered routinely to health care workers.[643] The OSHA bloodborne pathogens standard requires hospitals to offer free hepatitis B vaccination, and workers who do not wish to be vaccinated must sign a specific informed refusal. Other vaccines, such as the varicella vaccine and acellular pertussis vaccine, can help to eliminate or at least drastically reduce occupational acquisition of these diseases.

In addition to hepatitis B vaccination, the OSHA bloodborne pathogens standard mandates other prevention measures, including the development of an exposure control plan that identifies employees with occupational risk for exposure to bloodborne pathogens; annual training for these individuals regarding the risk for bloodborne infection and prevention measures; provision of personal protective clothing and equipment; work practice controls, including equipment and procedures for the safe handling and disposal of needles and sharp instruments; and procedures for identification, transportation, storage, and disposal of contaminated items and waste.[530]

In 2005, The CDC published detailed guidelines to prevent and control transmission of *M. tuberculosis* to health care workers.[339]

Reprocessing of Reusable Patient Care Items

Many HCAI outbreaks have been related to use of contaminated equipment. Consequently, hospital infection prevention and control programs must work closely with all hospital departments reprocessing reusable patient care items to ensure proper selection, implementation, and quality monitoring of reprocessing methods.[614]

Education and Training of Heath Care Workers

Providing education and training in general principles and specific aspects of hospital infection prevention and control is one of the primary responsibilities of program staff. Staff members should be familiar with principles of adult learning, assessing the educational needs of the audience, defining learning objectives, determining optimal instructional formats, using effective teaching and communication skills, and weighing the merits of various educational tools.

Product Evaluation

Many new medical products are introduced to the health care market every year. Although some products have the potential to reduce infectious risks, data to substantiate the safety and efficacy claims of manufacturers often are limited. Many devices marketed to hospitals caring for children have never been tested in children. Because these products often are substantially more expensive than existing products, there must be a compelling rationale for their use. Infection prevention and control staff members can provide valuable assistance to hospital committees in assessing the potential benefits of new products and, when appropriate, can design and conduct appropriate product evaluations trials.

ANTIMICROBIAL STEWARDSHIP PROGRAMS IN HEALTH CARE FACILITIES

The rapid emergence of pathogens resistant to multiple antimicrobial agents (e.g., VRE, ESBL- and carbapenemase-producing gram-negative bacteria) and the widespread dissemination of these resistant microorganisms constitute an unprecedented worldwide crisis[75] (see http://www.cdc.gov/drugresistance/threat-report-2013/ and http://www.who.int/antimicrobial-resistance/events/UNGA-meeting-amr-sept2016/en/). The mechanisms involved in the emergence and spread of antimicrobial resistance are complex but are no doubt facilitated by intense selective pressure caused by overuse and misuse in hospitals of antimicrobial agents, particularly newer, broad-spectrum agents.

Studies demonstrate that most hospitalized children, particularly in settings such as ICUs and transplantation units, receive empiric, targeted, or prophylactic treatment with antimicrobial agents.[39,255,545] Hospitals that used higher volumes of antimicrobial agents are also more likely to use broad-spectrum agents.[255] Inappropriate use of antimicrobial agents is common,[416,553] although the definition of the term *appropriateness* is not standardized and is subject to interpretation.[180,606]

In 2007, IDSA and SHEA published a guideline for institutional antimicrobial stewardship programs (ASPs).[174] In 2012, the IDSA, SHEA, and PIDS published a policy statement on antimicrobial stewardship.[686] Children's hospitals responded by developing ASPs.[518] A 2014 NHSN survey of acute care hospitals in the United States reported that 50% of the 76 responding children's hospitals had an ASP that contained all seven of the CDC's Core Elements of Hospital Antibiotic Stewardship Programs.[567] A comparative analysis of children's hospitals with or without a formal ASP demonstrated lower use of all antimicrobial agents in hospitals that had a formal ASP.[301]

The Core Elements of Hospital Antibiotic Stewardship Programs[568] are summarized in Box 244.4 and described in more detail on the CDC website (http://www.cdc.gov/getsmart/healthcare/implementation/core-elements.html). The CDC has collaborated with the National Quality Forum to develop a playbook for ASPs based on these core elements (http://www.qualityforum.org/Publications/2016/05/Antibiotic_Stewardship_Playbook.aspx). All acute care hospitals receiving reimbursement by CMS and accreditation by The Joint Commission are required to have an ASP based on these core elements.

In 2016, SHEA and IDSA published comprehensive evidence-based guidelines for implementation and measurement of antibiotic stewardship interventions for inpatient populations. The guideline provides detailed recommendations that expand particularly on strategies and interventions that address the Action component of the CDC's Core Elements. Augmenting this guidance is a growing literature on addressing antimicrobial stewardship for hospitalized children, including patient populations, conditions, and antimicrobials that represent appropriate targets and effective interventions to improve antimicrobial use for these targets.[254,262,301,378,606,605,681]

BOX 244.4 Centers for Disease Control and Prevention Core Elements of Hospital Antibiotic Stewardship Programs[a]

1. Leadership commitment: Dedicate necessary human, financial, and information technology resources.
2. Accountability: Appoint a physician leader responsible for program outcomes.
3. Drug expertise: Appoint a pharmacist leader responsible for working to improve antibiotic use.
4. Action: Implement recommended actions.
5. Tracking: Monitor antibiotic prescribing and resistance patterns.
6. Reporting: Report information on antibiotic use and resistance regularly to doctors, nurses, and relevant staff.
7. Education: Educate clinicians about resistance and optimal prescribing.

[a]Described in more detail at http://www.cdc.gov/getsmart/healthcare/implementation/core-elements.html.

Modified from Pollack LA, Srinivasan A. Core elements of hospital antibiotic stewardship programs from the Centers for Disease Control and Prevention. *Clin Infect Dis.* 2014;59(suppl 3):S97–S100.

NEW REFERENCES SINCE THE SEVENTH EDITION

4. Achermann Y, Goldstein EJ, Coenye T, et al. *Propionibacterium acnes*: from commensal to opportunistic biofilm-associated implant pathogen. *Clin Microbiol Rev.* 2014;27:419-440.
8. Food and Drug Administration. Drug safety labeling changes; 2012. http://www.fda.gov/Safety/MedWatch/SafetyInformation/Safety-RelatedDrugLabelingChanges/ucm307387.htm.
19. Ammann RA, Laws HJ, Schrey D, et al. Bloodstream infection in paediatric cancer centres—leukaemia and relapsed malignancies are independent risk factors. *Eur J Pediatr.* 2015;174:675-686.
23. Anderson DJ, Podgorny K, Berrios-Torres SI, et al. Strategies to prevent surgical site infections in acute care hospitals: 2014 update. *Infect Control Hosp Epidemiol.* 2014;35(suppl 2):S66-S88.
29. Assiri A, McGeer A, Perl TM, et al. Hospital outbreak of Middle East respiratory syndrome coronavirus. *N Engl J Med.* 2013;369:407-416.
33. Azab SF, Sherbiny HS, Saleh SH, et al. Reducing ventilator-associated pneumonia in neonatal intensive care unit using "VAP prevention bundle": a cohort study. *BMC Infect Dis.* 2015;15:314.
36. Azzi A, Morfini M, Mannucci PM. The transfusion-associated transmission of parvovirus B19. *Transfus Med Rev.* 1999;13:194-204.
39. Baggs J, Fridkin SK, Pollack LA, et al. Estimating national trends in inpatient antibiotic use among US hospitals from 2006 to 2012. *JAMA Intern Med.* 2016;176:1639-1648.

41. Barker GM, O'Brien SM, Welke KF, et al. Major infection after pediatric cardiac surgery: a risk estimation model. *Ann Thorac Surg*. 2010;89:843-850.
42. Baron EJ, Miller JM, Weinstein MP, et al. A guide to utilization of the microbiology laboratory for diagnosis of infectious diseases: 2013 recommendations by the Infectious Diseases Society of America (IDSA) and the American Society for Microbiology (ASM)(a). *Clin Infect Dis*. 2013;57:e22-e121.
45. Bautista E, Chotpitayasunondh T, Gao Z, et al. Clinical aspects of pandemic 2009 influenza A (H1N1) virus infection. *N Engl J Med*. 2010;362:1708-1719.
53. Bergmann K, Hasle H, Asdahl P, et al. Central venous catheters and bloodstream infection during induction therapy in children with acute lymphoblastic leukemia. *J Pediatr Hematol Oncol*. 2016;38:e82-e87.
64. Billett AL, Colletti RB, Mandel KE, et al. Exemplar pediatric collaborative improvement networks: achieving results. *Pediatrics*. 2013;131(suppl 4):S196-S203.
68. Block C, Ergaz-Shaltiel Z, Valinsky L, et al. Deja vu: *Ralstonia mannitolilytica* infection associated with a humidifying respiratory therapy device, Israel, June to July 2011. *Euro Surveill*. 2013;18:20471.
69. Bode LG, Kluytmans JA, Wertheim HF, et al. Preventing surgical-site infections in nasal carriers of *Staphylococcus aureus*. *N Engl J Med*. 2010;362:9-17.
72. Boozary AS, Farmer PE, Jha AK. The Ebola outbreak, fragile health systems, and quality as a cure. *JAMA*. 2014;312:1859-1860.
83. Bratzler DW, Dellinger EP, Olsen KM, et al. Clinical practice guidelines for antimicrobial prophylaxis in surgery. *Am J Health Syst Pharm*. 2013;70:195-283.
88. Bruijning-Verhagen P, Quach C, Bonten M. Nosocomial rotavirus infections: a meta-analysis. *Pediatrics*. 2012;129:e1011-e1019.
91. Bruny JL, Hall BL, Barnhart DC, et al. American College of Surgeons National Surgical Quality Improvement Program Pediatric: a beta phase report. *J Pediatr Surg*. 2013;48:74-80.
93. Buet A, Cohen B, Marine M, et al. Hand hygiene opportunities in pediatric extended care facilities. *J Pediatr Nurs*. 2013;28:72-76.
94. Bundy DG, Gaur AH, Billett AL, et al. Preventing CLABSIs among pediatric hematology/oncology inpatients: national collaborative results. *Pediatrics*. 2014;134:e1678-e1685.
99. Calfee DP, Salgado CD, Milstone AM, et al. Strategies to prevent methicillin-resistant *Staphylococcus aureus* transmission and infection in acute care hospitals: 2014 update. *Infect Control Hosp Epidemiol*. 2014;35(suppl 2):S108-S132.
100. Calfee DP, Salgado CD, Milstone AM, et al. Strategies to prevent methicillin-resistant *Staphylococcus aureus* transmission and infection in acute care hospitals: 2014 update. *Infect Control Hosp Epidemiol*. 2014;35:772-796.
105. Carl MA, Ndao IM, Springman AC, et al. Sepsis from the gut: the enteric habitat of bacteria that cause late-onset neonatal bloodstream infections. *Clin Infect Dis*. 2014;58:1211-1218.
107. Centers for Disease Control and Prevention. Hospital-associated measles outbreak—Pennsylvania, March-April 2009. *MMWR Morb Mortal Wkly Rep*. 2012;61:30-32.
127. Chapman AK, Aucott SW, Gilmore MM, et al. Absorption and tolerability of aqueous chlorhexidine gluconate used for skin antisepsis prior to catheter insertion in preterm neonates. *J Perinatol*. 2013;33:768-771.
130. Chen AF, Wessel CB, Rao N. *Staphylococcus aureus* screening and decolonization in orthopaedic surgery and reduction of surgical site infections. *Clin Orthop Relat Res*. 2013;471:2383-2399.
134. Chopra V, Anand S, Krein SL, et al. Bloodstream infection, venous thrombosis, and peripherally inserted central catheters: reappraising the evidence. *Am J Med*. 2012;125:733-741.
139. Cocoros NM, Kleinman K, Priebe GP, et al. Ventilator-associated events in neonates and children—a new paradigm. *Crit Care Med*. 2016;44:14-22.
141. Coffin SE, Klompas M, Classen D, et al. Strategies to prevent ventilator-associated pneumonia in acute care hospitals. *Infect Control Hosp Epidemiol*. 2008;29 (Suppl 1):S31-S34.
143. Committee on Infectious Diseases, American Academy of Pediatrics. Pertussis (whooping cough). In: Kimberlin DW, Brady MT, Jackson MA, Long SS, eds. *Red Book: 2015 Report of the Committee on Infectious Diseases*. 30th ed. Elk Grove, IL: American Academy of Pediatrics; 2015:608-621.
144. Concannon C, van Wijngaarden E, Stevens V, et al. The effect of multiple concurrent central venous catheters on central line-associated bloodstream infections. *Infect Control Hosp Epidemiol*. 2014;35:1140-1146.
160. Dagan O, Cox PN, Ford-Jones L, et al. Nosocomial infection following cardiovascular surgery: comparison of two periods, 1987 vs. 1992. *Crit Care Med*. 1999;27:104-108.
166. Davis KF, Colebaugh AM, Eithun BL, et al. Reducing catheter-associated urinary tract infections: a quality-improvement initiative. *Pediatrics*. 2014;134:e857-e864.
169. de Blank P, Zaoutis T, Fisher B, et al. Trends in *Clostridium difficile* infection and risk factors for hospital acquisition of *Clostridium difficile* among children with cancer. *J Pediatr*. 2013;163:699-705, e1.
172. de Groot RJ, Baker SC, Baric RS, et al. Middle East respiratory syndrome coronavirus (MERS-CoV): announcement of the Coronavirus Study Group. *J Virol*. 2013;87:7790-7792.
175. DeBiasi RL, Song X, Cato K, et al. Preparedness, evaluation, and care of pediatric patients under investigation for Ebola virus disease: experience from a pediatric designated care facility. *J Pediatric Infect Dis Soc*. 2016;5:68-75.
180. DePestel DD, Eiland EH 3rd, Lusardi K, et al. Assessing appropriateness of antimicrobial therapy: in the eye of the interpreter. *Clin Infect Dis*. 2014;59(suppl 3):S154-S161.
183. Dhar S, Cook E, Oden M, et al. Building a successful infection prevention program: key components, processes, and economics. *Infect Dis Clin North Am*. 2016;30:567-589.
185. Committee on Infectious Diseases, American Academy of Pediatrics. Hepatitis A. In: Kimberlin DW, Brady MT, Jackson MA, Long SS, eds. *Red Book: 2015 Report of the Committee on Infectious Diseases*. 30th ed. Elk Grove, IL: American Academy of Pediatrics; 2015:391-399.
186. Committee on Infectious Diseases, American Academy of Pediatrics. Influenza immunization for all health care personnel: keep it mandatory. *Pediatrics*. 2015;136:809-818.
187. Committee on Infectious Diseases, American Academy of Pediatrics. Measles. In: Kimberlin DW, Brady MT, Jackson MA, Long SS, eds. *Red Book: 2015 Report of the Committee on Infectious Diseases*. 30th ed. Elk Grove, IL: American Academy of Pediatrics; 2015:535-547.
188. Committee on Infectious Diseases, American Academy of Pediatrics. Varicella zoster infections. In: Kimberlin DW, Brady MT, Jackson MA, Long SS, eds. *Red Book: 2015 Report of the Committee on Infectious Diseases*. 30th ed. Elk Grove, IL: American Academy of Pediatrics; 2015:846-860.
195. Done E, Gratacos E, Nicolaides KH, et al. Predictors of neonatal morbidity in fetuses with severe isolated congenital diaphragmatic hernia undergoing fetoscopic tracheal occlusion. *Ultrasound Obstet Gynecol*. 2013;42:77-83.
197. Drees M, Snydman DR, Schmid CH, et al. Prior environmental contamination increases the risk of acquisition of vancomycin-resistant enterococci. *Clin Infect Dis*. 2008;46:678-685.
199. Dubberke ER, Carling P, Carrico R, et al. Strategies to prevent *Clostridium difficile* infections in acute care hospitals: 2014 update. *Infect Control Hosp Epidemiol*. 2014;35(suppl 2):S48-S65.
201. Dudeck MA, Edwards JR, Allen-Bridson K, et al. National Healthcare Safety Network report, data summary for 2013, device-associated module. *Am J Infect Control*. 2015;43:206-221.
206. Edwards MS, Baker CJ. Median sternotomy wound infections in children. *Pediatr Infect Dis*. 1983;2:105-109.
207. Edwards JD, Herzig CT, Liu H, et al. Central line-associated blood stream infections in pediatric intensive care units: longitudinal trends and compliance with bundle strategies. *Am J Infect Control*. 2015;43:489-493.
209. Ellingson K, Haas JP, Aiello AE, et al. Strategies to prevent healthcare-associated infections through hand hygiene. *Infect Control Hosp Epidemiol*. 2014;35:937-960.
214. Epstein L, See I, Edwards JR, et al. Mucosal barrier injury laboratory-confirmed bloodstream infections (MBI-LCBI): descriptive analysis of data reported to National Healthcare Safety Network (NHSN), 2013. *Infect Control Hosp Epidemiol*. 2016;37:2-7.
217. Fagan RP, Edwards JR, Park BJ, et al. Incidence trends in pathogen-specific central line-associated bloodstream infections in US intensive care units, 1990-2010. *Infect Control Hosp Epidemiol*. 2013;34:893-899.
237. Gaies MG, Langer M, Alexander J, et al. Design and rationale of safe pediatric euglycemia after cardiac surgery: a randomized controlled trial of tight glycemic control after pediatric cardiac surgery. *Pediatr Crit Care Med*. 2013;14:148-156.
246. Garnacho-Montero J, Diaz-Martin A, Garcia-Cabrera E, et al. Impact on hospital mortality of catheter removal and adequate antifungal therapy in *Candida* spp. bloodstream infections. *J Antimicrob Chemother*. 2013;68:206-213.
249. Gautam A, Ganu SS, Tegg OJ, et al. Ventilator-associated pneumonia in a tertiary paediatric intensive care unit: a 1-year prospective observational study. *Crit Care Resusc*. 2012;14:283-289.
254. Gerber JS, Kronman MP, Ross RK, et al. Identifying targets for antimicrobial stewardship in children's hospitals. *Infect Control Hosp Epidemiol*. 2013;34:1252-1258.
259. Gidengil CA, Gay C, Huang SS, et al. Cost-effectiveness of strategies to prevent methicillin-resistant *Staphylococcus aureus* transmission and infection in an intensive care unit. *Infect Control Hosp Epidemiol*. 2015;36:17-27.
260. Gilbert RE, Mok Q, Dwan K, et al. Impregnated central venous catheters for prevention of bloodstream infection in children (the CATCH trial): a randomised controlled trial. *Lancet*. 2016;387:1732-1742.
262. Goldman JL, Lee BR, Hersh AL, et al. Clinical diagnoses and antimicrobials predictive of pediatric antimicrobial stewardship recommendations: a program evaluation. *Infect Control Hosp Epidemiol*. 2015;36:673-680.
266. Goudie A, Dynan L, Brady PW, et al. Attributable cost and length of stay for central line-associated bloodstream infections. *Pediatrics*. 2014;133:e1525-e1532.
268. Greenberg RG, Cochran KM, Smith PB, et al. Effect of catheter dwell time on risk of central line-associated bloodstream infection in infants. *Pediatrics*. 2015;136:1080-1086.
274. Gupta S, Boville BM, Blanton R, et al. A multicentered prospective analysis of diagnosis, risk factors, and outcomes associated with pediatric ventilator-associated pneumonia. *Pediatr Crit Care Med*. 2015;16:e65-e73.
278. Guzman-Cottrill JA, Phillipi CA, Dolan SA, et al. Free vaccine programs to cocoon high-risk infants and children against influenza and pertussis. *Am J Infect Control*. 2012;40:872-876.

301. Hersh AL, De Lurgio SA, Thurm C, et al. Antimicrobial stewardship programs in freestanding children's hospitals. *Pediatrics.* 2015;135:33-39.
306. Hocevar SN, Edwards JR, Horan TC, et al. Device-associated infections among neonatal intensive care unit patients: incidence and associated pathogens reported to the National Healthcare Safety Network, 2006-2008. *Infect Control Hosp Epidemiol.* 2012;33:1200-1206.
319. Huang SS, Septimus E, Avery TR, et al. Cost savings of universal decolonization to prevent intensive care unit infection: implications of the REDUCE MRSA trial. *Infect Control Hosp Epidemiol.* 2014;35(suppl 3):S23-S31.
320. Huang SS, Septimus E, Kleinman K, et al. Targeted versus universal decolonization to prevent ICU infection. *N Engl J Med.* 2013;368:2255-2265.
330. Iwamoto M, Mu Y, Lynfield R, et al. Trends in invasive methicillin-resistant *Staphylococcus aureus* infections. *Pediatrics.* 2013;132:e817-e824.
332. Jain S, Self WH, Wunderink RG, et al. Community-acquired pneumonia requiring hospitalization among U.S. adults. *N Engl J Med.* 2015;373:415-427.
334. Jangi S, Lamont JT. Asymptomatic colonization by *Clostridium difficile* in infants: implications for disease in later life. *J Pediatr Gastroenterol Nutr.* 2010;51:2-7.
336. Jarvis WR, ed. *Bennett and Brachman's Hospital Infections.* 6th ed. Philadelphia: Lippincott Williams & Wilkins; 2014.
341. Johnson J, Bracken R, Tamma PD, et al. Trends in chlorhexidine use in US neonatal intensive care units: results from a follow-up national survey. *Infect Control Hosp Epidemiol.* 2016;37:1116-1118.
345. Kagen J, Lautenbach E, Bilker WB, et al. Risk factors for mediastinitis following median sternotomy in children. *Pediatr Infect Dis J.* 2007;26:613-618.
346. Kalil AC, Metersky ML, Klompas M, et al. Management of adults with hospital-acquired and ventilator-associated pneumonia: 2016 clinical practice guidelines by the Infectious Diseases Society of America and the American Thoracic Society. *Clin Infect Dis.* 2016;63:e61-e111.
351. Kaufman DA, Blackman A, Conaway MR, et al. Nonsterile glove use in addition to hand hygiene to prevent late-onset infection in preterm infants: randomized clinical trial. *JAMA Pediatr.* 2014;168:909-916.
352. Kaye KS, Anderson DJ, Cook E, et al. Guidance for infection prevention and healthcare epidemiology programs: healthcare epidemiologist skills and competencies. *Infect Control Hosp Epidemiol.* 2015;36:369-380.
354. Kelly MS, Conway M, Wirth KE, et al. Microbiology and risk factors for central line-associated bloodstream infections among pediatric oncology outpatients: a single institution experience of 41 cases. *J Pediatr Hematol Oncol.* 2013;35:e71-e76.
356. Khanna S, Baddour LM, Huskins WC, et al. The epidemiology of *Clostridium difficile* infection in children: a population-based study. *Clin Infect Dis.* 2013;56:1401-1406.
360. Kim J, Smathers SA, Prasad P, et al. Epidemiological features of *Clostridium difficile*-associated disease among inpatients at children's hospitals in the United States, 2001-2006. *Pediatrics.* 2008;122:1266-1270.
364. Klieger SB, Vendetti ND, Fisher BT, et al. *Staphylococcus aureus* bacteremia in hospitalized children: incidence and outcomes. *Infect Control Hosp Epidemiol.* 2015;36:603-605.
365. Klompas M, Branson R, Eichenwald EC, et al. Strategies to prevent ventilator-associated pneumonia in acute care hospitals: 2014 update. *Infect Control Hosp Epidemiol.* 2014;35(suppl 2):S133-S154.
366. Klompas M, Branson R, Eichenwald EC, et al. Strategies to prevent ventilator-associated pneumonia in acute care hospitals: 2014 update. *Infect Control Hosp Epidemiol.* 2014;35:915-936.
367. Klompas M, Li L, Kleinman K, et al. Associations between ventilator bundle components and outcomes. *JAMA Intern Med.* 2016;176:1277-1283.
368. Kociolek LK, Patel SJ, Shulman ST, et al. Molecular epidemiology of *Clostridium difficile* infections in children: a retrospective cohort study. *Infect Control Hosp Epidemiol.* 2015;36:445-451.
377. Krishnaiah A, Soothill J, Wade A, et al. Central venous catheter-associated bloodstream infections in a pediatric intensive care unit: effect of the location of catheter insertion. *Pediatr Crit Care Med.* 2012;13:e176-e180.
378. Kronman MP, Hersh AL, Gerber JS, et al. Identifying antimicrobial stewardship targets for pediatric surgical patients. *J Pediatric Infect Dis Soc.* 2015;4:e100-e108.
380. Kulkarni AV, Drake JM, Lamberti-Pasculli M. Cerebrospinal fluid shunt infection: a prospective study of risk factors. *J Neurosurg.* 2001;94:195-201.
381. Kuncio DE, Middleton M, Cooney MG, et al. Health care worker exposures to pertussis: missed opportunities for prevention. *Pediatrics.* 2014;133:15-21.
385. Kusahara DM, Enz Cda C, Avelar AF, et al. Risk factors for ventilator-associated pneumonia in infants and children: a cross-sectional cohort study. *Am J Crit Care.* 2014;23:469-476.
406. Lee JH, Hornik CP, Benjamin DK Jr, et al. Risk factors for invasive candidiasis in infants >1500 g birth weight. *Pediatr Infect Dis J.* 2013;32:222-226.
407. Benjamin DK, Stoll BJ, Fanaroff AA, et al. Neonatal candidiasis among extremely low birth weight infants: risk factors, mortality rates, and neurodevelopmental outcomes at 18 to 22 months. *Pediatrics.* 2006;117:84-92.
411. Lessa FC, Mu Y, Bamberg WM, et al. Burden of *Clostridium difficile* infection in the United States. *N Engl J Med.* 2015;372:825-834.
421. Lindley MC, Bridges CB, Strikas RA, et al. Influenza vaccination performance measurement among acute care hospital-based health care personnel—United States, 2013–14 influenza season. *MMWR Morb Mortal Wkly Rep.* 2014;63:812-815.
425. Liu Y, Liu K, Yu X, et al. Identification and control of a *Pseudomonas* spp (*P. fulva* and *P. putida*) bloodstream infection outbreak in a teaching hospital in Beijing, China. *Int J Infect Dis.* 2014;23:105-108.
426. Lo E, Nicolle LE, Coffin SE, et al. Strategies to prevent catheter-associated urinary tract infections in acute care hospitals: 2014 update. *Infect Control Hosp Epidemiol.* 2014;35(suppl 2):S32-S47.
429. Logan LK, Meltzer LA, McAuley JB, et al. Extended-spectrum β-lactamase-producing Enterobacteriaceae infections in children: a two-center case-case-control study of risk factors and outcomes in Chicago, Illinois. *J Pediatric Infect Dis Soc.* 2014;3:312-319.
430. Logan LK, Renschler JP, Gandra S, et al. Carbapenem-resistant Enterobacteriaceae in children, United States, 1999–2012. *Emerg Infect Dis.* 2015;21:2014-2021.
434. Long CB, Shah SS, Lautenbach E, et al. Postoperative mediastinitis in children: epidemiology, microbiology and risk factors for gram-negative pathogens. *Pediatr Infect Dis J.* 2005;24:315-319.
444. Lyren A, Brilli R, Bird M, et al. Ohio Children's Hospitals'' solutions for patient safety: a framework for pediatric patient safety improvement. *J Healthc Qual.* 2016;38:213-222.
450. Mackenzie WG, Matsumoto H, Williams BA, et al. Surgical site infection following spinal instrumentation for scoliosis: a multicenter analysis of rates, risk factors, and pathogens. *J Bone Joint Surg Am.* 2013;95:800-806, S801–2.
453. Magill SS, Edwards JR, Bamberg W, et al. Multistate point-prevalence survey of health care-associated infections. *N Engl J Med.* 2014;370:1198-1208.
463. Manian FA. The role of postoperative factors in surgical site infections: time to take notice. *Clin Infect Dis.* 2014;59:1272-1276.
467. Marlow N, Morris T, Brocklehurst P, et al. A randomised trial of granulocyte-macrophage colony-stimulating factor for neonatal sepsis: childhood outcomes at 5 years. *Arch Dis Child Fetal Neonatal Ed.* 2015;100:F320-F326.
468. Marschall J, Mermel LA, Fakih M, et al. Strategies to prevent central line-associated bloodstream infections in acute care hospitals: 2014 update. *Infect Control Hosp Epidemiol.* 2014;35:753-771.
469. Marschall J, Mermel LA, Fakih M, et al. Strategies to prevent central line-associated bloodstream infections in acute care hospitals: 2014 update. *Infect Control Hosp Epidemiol.* 2014;35(suppl 2):S89-S107.
479. McKinnell JA, Bartsch SM, Lee BY, et al. Cost-benefit analysis from the hospital perspective of universal active screening followed by contact precautions for methicillin-resistant *Staphylococcus aureus* carriers. *Infect Control Hosp Epidemiol.* 2015;36:2-13.
483. Mermel LA, Allon M, Bouza E, et al. Clinical practice guidelines for the diagnosis and management of intravascular catheter-related infection: 2009 Update by the Infectious Diseases Society of America. *Clin Infect Dis.* 2009;49:1-45.
492. Milstone AM, Elward A, Song X, et al. Daily chlorhexidine bathing to reduce bacteraemia in critically ill children: a multicentre, cluster-randomised, crossover trial. *Lancet.* 2013;381:1099-1106.
493. Milstone AM, Maragakis LL, Townsend T, et al. Timing of preoperative antibiotic prophylaxis: a modifiable risk factor for deep surgical site infections after pediatric spinal fusion. *Pediatr Infect Dis J.* 2008;27:704-708.
506. Munoz-Price LS, Banach DB, Bearman G, et al. Isolation precautions for visitors. *Infect Control Hosp Epidemiol.* 2015;36:747-758.
509. Munoz P, Menasalvas A, Bernaldo de Quiros JC, et al. Postsurgical mediastinitis: a case-control study. *Clin Infect Dis.* 1997;25:1060-1064.
510. Murray MT, Pavia M, Jackson O, et al. Health care-associated infection outbreaks in pediatric long-term care facilities. *Am J Infect Control.* 2015;43:756-758.
516. Neu AM, Miller MR, Stuart J, et al. Design of the standardizing care to improve outcomes in pediatric end stage renal disease collaborative. *Pediatr Nephrol.* 2014;29:1477-1484.
518. Newland JG, Gerber JS, Weissman SJ, et al. Prevalence and characteristics of antimicrobial stewardship programs at freestanding children's hospitals in the United States. *Infect Control Hosp Epidemiol.* 2014;35:265-271.
520. Niedner MF, Huskins WC, Colantuoni E, et al. Epidemiology of central line-associated bloodstream infections in the pediatric intensive care unit. *Infect Control Hosp Epidemiol.* 2011;32:1200-1208.
528. Nylund CM, Goudie A, Garza JM, et al. *Clostridium difficile* infection in hospitalized children in the United States. *Arch Pediatr Adolesc Med.* 2011;165:451-457.
533. O'Horo JC, Maki DG, Krupp AE, et al. Arterial catheters as a source of bloodstream infection: a systematic review and meta-analysis. *Crit Care Med.* 2014;42:1334-1339.
535. Oboho IK, Tomczyk SM, Al-Asmari AM, et al. 2014 MERS-CoV outbreak in Jeddah—a link to health care facilities. *N Engl J Med.* 2015;372:846-854.
536. Ohlsson A, Lacy JB. Intravenous immunoglobulin for suspected or proven infection in neonates. *Cochrane Database Syst Rev.* 2015;(3):CD001239.
546. Pammi M, Holland L, Butler G, et al. *Candida parapsilosis* is a significant neonatal pathogen: a systematic review and meta-analysis. *Pediatr Infect Dis J.* 2013;32:e206-e216.

548. Pant C, Deshpande A, Altaf MA, et al. *Clostridium difficile* infection in children: a comprehensive review. *Curr Med Res Opin.* 2013;29:967-984.
551. Parm U, Metsvaht T, Sepp E, et al. Risk factors associated with gut and nasopharyngeal colonization by common gram-negative species and yeasts in neonatal intensive care units patients. *Early Hum Dev.* 2011;87:391-399.
554. Patria MF, Chidini G, Ughi L, et al. Ventilator-associated pneumonia in an Italian pediatric intensive care unit: a prospective study. *World J Pediatr.* 2013;9:365-368.
563. Pitts SI, Maruthur NM, Millar KR, et al. A systematic review of mandatory influenza vaccination in healthcare personnel. *Am J Prev Med.* 2014;47:330-340.
564. Pokala HR, Leonard D, Cox J, et al. Association of hospital construction with the development of healthcare associated environmental mold infections (HAEMI) in pediatric patients with leukemia. *Pediatr Blood Cancer.* 2014;61:276-280.
567. Pollack LA, Plachouras D, Sinkowitz-Cochran R, et al. A concise set of structure and process indicators to assess and compare antimicrobial stewardship programs among EU and US hospitals: results from a multinational expert panel. *Infect Control Hosp Epidemiol.* 2016;37:1201-1211.
568. Pollack LA, Srinivasan A. Core elements of hospital antibiotic stewardship programs from the Centers for Disease Control and Prevention. *Clin Infect Dis.* 2014;59(suppl 3):S97-S100.
569. Popoola VO, Budd A, Wittig SM, et al. Methicillin-resistant *Staphylococcus aureus* transmission and infections in a neonatal intensive care unit despite active surveillance cultures and decolonization: challenges for infection prevention. *Infect Control Hosp Epidemiol.* 2014;35:412-418.
570. Popoola VO, Carroll KC, Ross T, et al. Impact of colonization pressure and strain type on methicillin-resistant *Staphylococcus aureus* transmission in children. *Clin Infect Dis.* 2013;57:1458-1460.
571. Popoola VO, Colantuoni E, Suwantarat N, et al. Active surveillance cultures and decolonization to reduce *Staphylococcus aureus* infections in the neonatal intensive care unit. *Infect Control Hosp Epidemiol.* 2016;37:381-387.
573. Centers for Discase Control and Prevention. CDC/NHSN surveillance definitions for specific types of infections; 2017. https://www.cdc.gov/nhsn/pdfs/pscmanual/17pscnosinfdef_current.pdf.
574. Prince AL, Antony KM, Chu DM, et al. The microbiome, parturition, and timing of birth: more questions than answers. *J Reprod Immunol.* 2014;104–105:12-19.
578. Quach C, Milstone AM, Perpete C, et al. Chlorhexidine bathing in a tertiary care neonatal intensive care unit: impact on central line-associated bloodstream infections. *Infect Control Hosp Epidemiol.* 2014;35:158-163.
591. Reich PJ, Boyle MG, Hogan PG, et al. Emergence of community-associated methicillin-resistant *Staphylococcus aureus* strains in the neonatal intensive care unit: an infection prevention and patient safety challenge. *Clin Microbiol Infect.* 2016;22(645):e641-e648.
595. Rhee SM, Tsay R, Nelson DS, et al. *Clostridium difficile* in the pediatric population of Monroe County, New York. *J Pediatric Infect Dis Soc.* 2014;3:183-188.
598. Riley S, Fraser C, Donnelly CA, et al. Transmission dynamics of the etiological agent of SARS in Hong Kong: impact of public health interventions. *Science.* 2003;300:1961-1966.
599. Rinke ML, Milstone AM, Chen AR, et al. Ambulatory pediatric oncology CLABSIs: epidemiology and risk factors. *Pediatr Blood Cancer.* 2013;60:1882-1889.
601. Rogers EA, Kimia A, Madsen JR, et al. Predictors of ventricular shunt infection among children presenting to a pediatric emergency department. *Pediatr Emerg Care.* 2012;28:405-409.
603. Rogowski JA, Staiger D, Patrick T, et al. Nurse staffing and NICU infection rates. *JAMA Pediatr.* 2013;167:444-450.
605. Ross RK, Hersh AL, Kronman MP, et al. Cost of antimicrobial therapy across US children's hospitals. *Infect Control Hosp Epidemiol.* 2015;36:1242-1244.
606. Ross RK, Hersh AL, Kronman MP, et al. Impact of Infectious Diseases Society of America/Pediatric Infectious Diseases Society guidelines on treatment of community-acquired pneumonia in hospitalized children. *Clin Infect Dis.* 2014;58:834-838.
607. Rousseau C, Lemee L, Le Monnier A, et al. Prevalence and diversity of *Clostridium difficile* strains in infants. *J Med Microbiol.* 2011;60:1112-1118.
612. Ruch-Ross HS, Zapata LB, Williams JL, et al. General influenza infection control policies and practices during the 2009 H1N1 influenza pandemic: a survey of women's health, obstetric, and neonatal nurses. *Am J Infect Control.* 2014;42:e65-e70.
613. Runfola JK, House J, Miller L, et al. Outbreak of human [neumonic plague with dog-to-human and possible human-to-human transmission—Colorado, June-July 2014. *MMWR Morb Mortal Wkly Rep.* 2015;64:429-434.
620. Safdar N, O'Horo JC, Maki DG. Arterial catheter-related bloodstream infection: incidence, pathogenesis, risk factors and prevention. *J Hosp Infect.* 2013;85:189-195.
625. Saiman L, Siegel JD, LiPuma JJ, et al. Infection prevention and control guideline for cystic fibrosis: 2013 update. *Infect Control Hosp Epidemiol.* 2014;35(suppl 1):S1-S67.
630. Salsgiver E, Crotty J, LaRussa SJ, et al. Surgical site infections following spine surgery for non-idiopathic scoliosis. *J Pediatr Orthop.* 2016;http://journals.lww.com/pedorthopaedics/Abstract/publishahead/Surgical_Site_Infections_following_Spine_Surgery.99312.aspx?trendmd-shared=0.
631. Sammons JS, Localio R, Xiao R, et al. *Clostridium difficile* infection is associated with increased risk of death and prolonged hospitalization in children. *Clin Infect Dis.* 2013;57:1-8.
632. Sammons JS, Toltzis P, Zaoutis TE. Clostridium difficile infection in children. *JAMA Pediatr.* 2013;167:567-573.
634. Sandora TJ, Fung M, Flaherty K, et al. Epidemiology and risk factors for *Clostridium difficile* infection in children. *Pediatr Infect Dis J.* 2011;30:580-584.
635. Santagostino E, Mannucci PM, Gringeri A, et al. Transmission of parvovirus B19 by coagulation factor concentrates exposed to 100 degrees C heat after lyophilization. *Transfusion.* 1997;37:517-522.
643. Schillie S, Murphy TV, Sawyer M, et al. CDC guidance for evaluating health-care personnel for hepatitis B virus protection and for administering postexposure management. *MMWR Recomm Rep.* 2013;62(RR-10):1-19.
649. Schweizer M, Perencevich E, McDanel J, et al. Effectiveness of a bundled intervention of decolonization and prophylaxis to decrease gram positive surgical site infections after cardiac or orthopedic surgery: systematic review and meta-analysis. *BMJ.* 2013;346:f2743.
650. See I, Iwamoto M, Allen-Bridson K, et al. Mucosal barrier injury laboratory-confirmed bloodstream infection: results from a field test of a new National Healthcare Safety Network definition. *Infect Control Hosp Epidemiol.* 2013;34:769-776.
656. Sethna CB, Bryant K, Munshi R, et al. Risk factors for and putcomes of catheter-associated peritonitis in children: The SCOPE Collaborative. *Clin J Am Soc Nephrol.* 2016;11:1590-1596.
658. Shah GS, Christensen RE, Wagner DS, et al. Retrospective evaluation of antimicrobial prophylaxis in prevention of surgical site infection in the pediatric population. *Paediatr Anaesth.* 2014;24:994-998.
663. Sherertz RJ, Sarubbi FA. The prevalence of *Clostridium difficile* and toxin in a nursery population: a comparison between patients with necrotizing enterocolitis and an asymptomatic group. *J Pediatr.* 1982;100:435-439.
664. Shi Z, Xie H, Wang P, et al. Oral hygiene care for critically ill patients to prevent ventilator-associated pneumonia. *Cochrane Database Syst Rev.* 2013;(8):CD008367.
670. Sievert DM, Ricks P, Edwards JR, et al. Antimicrobial-resistant pathogens associated with healthcare-associated infections: summary of data reported to the National Healthcare Safety Network at the Centers for Disease Control and Prevention, 2009–2010. *Infect Control Hosp Epidemiol.* 2013;34:1-14.
673. Simon TD, Butler J, Whitlock KB, et al. Risk factors for first cerebrospinal fluid shunt infection: findings from a multi-center prospective cohort study. *J Pediatr.* 2014;164:1462-1468, e1462.
676. Simon TD, Whitlock KB, Riva-Cambrin J, et al. Revision surgeries are associated with significant increased risk of subsequent cerebrospinal fluid shunt infection. *Pediatr Infect Dis J.* 2012;31:551-556.
679. Smith A, Saiman L, Zhou J, et al. Concordance of gastrointestinal tract colonization and subsequent bloodstream infections with gram-negative bacilli in very low birth weight infants in the neonatal intensive care unit. *Pediatr Infect Dis J.* 2010;29:831-835.
681. Smith MJ, Gerber JS, Hersh AL. Inpatient antimicrobial stewardship in pediatrics: a systematic review. *J Pediatric Infect Dis Soc.* 2015;4:e127-e135.
687. Soeorg H, Huik K, Parm U, et al. Genetic relatedness of coagulase-negative staphylococci from gastrointestinal tract and blood of preterm neonates with late-onset sepsis. *Pediatr Infect Dis J.* 2013;32:389-393.
691. Soucie JM, Monahan PE, Kulkarni R, et al. Evidence for the continued transmission of parvovirus B19 in patients with bleeding disorders treated with plasma-derived factor concentrates. *Transfusion.* 2013;53:1143-1144.
692. Spader HS, Hertzler DA, Kestle JR, et al. Risk factors for infection and the effect of an institutional shunt protocol on the incidence of ventricular access device infections in preterm infants. *J Neurosurg Pediatr.* 2015;15:156-160.
706. Szymczak JE, Smathers S, Hoegg C, et al. Reasons why physicians and advanced practice clinicians work while sick: a mixed-methods analysis. *JAMA Pediatr.* 2015;169:815-821.
708. Tai E, Richardson LC, Townsend J, et al. *Clostridium difficile* infection among children with cancer. *Pediatr Infect Dis J.* 2011;30:610-612.
711. Talbot TR, Carr D, Parmley CL, et al. Sustained reduction of ventilator-associated pneumonia rates using real-time course correction with a ventilator bundle compliance dashboard. *Infect Control Hosp Epidemiol.* 2015;36:1261-1267.
718. Tang HJ, Chao CM, Leung PO, et al. Achieving "zero" CLABSI and VAP after sequential implementation of central line bundle and ventilator bundle. *Infect Control Hosp Epidemiol.* 2015;36:365-366.
721. WHO Ebola Response Team. Ebola virus disease in West Africa—the first 9 months of the epidemic and forward projections. *N Engl J Med.* 2014;371:1481-1495.
722. WHO Ebola Response Team, Agua-Agum J, Ariyarajah A, et al. West African Ebola epidemic after one year—slowing but not yet under control. *N Engl J Med.* 2015;372:584-587.
726. Thompson CM Jr, Gilligan PH, Fisher MC, et al. *Clostridium difficile* cytotoxin in a pediatric population. *Am J Dis Child.* 1983;137:271-274.
732. Toltzis P, O'Riordan M, Cunningham DJ, et al. A statewide collaborative to reduce pediatric surgical site infections. *Pediatrics.* 2014;134:e1174-e1180.
733. Tran S, Chin AC. Burn Sepsis in Children. *Clin Pediatr Emerg Med.* 2014;15:149-157.

735. Tsai MH, Chu SM, Hsu JF, et al. Risk factors and outcomes for multidrug-resistant gram-negative bacteremia in the NICU. *Pediatrics*. 2014;133:e322-e329.
750. Wang L, Li X, Yang Z, et al. Semi-recumbent position versus supine position for the prevention of ventilator-associated pneumonia in adults requiring mechanical ventilation. *Cochrane Database Syst Rev*. 2016;(1):CD009946.
753. Watanabe T, Muneta T, Yagishita K, et al. Closed suction drainage is not necessary for total knee arthroplasty: a prospective study on simultaneous bilateral surgeries of a mean follow-up of 5.5 years. *J Arthroplasty*. 2016;31:641-645.
758. Webster J, Osborne S. Preoperative bathing or showering with skin antiseptics to prevent surgical site infection. *Cochrane Database Syst Rev*. 2015;(2):CD004985.
759. Weiner LM, Fridkin SK, Aponte-Torres Z, et al. Vital signs: preventing antibiotic-resistant infections in hospitals—United States, 2014. *MMWR Morb Mortal Wkly Rep*. 2016;65:235-241.
762. Wendorf KA, Kay M, Ortega-Sanchez IR, et al. Cost of measles containment in an ambulatory pediatric clinic. *Pediatr Infect Dis J*. 2015;34:589-593.
771. Williams C, McGraw P, Schneck EE, et al. Impact of universal gowning and gloving on health care worker clothing contamination. *Infect Control Hosp Epidemiol*. 2015;36:431-437.
773. Wilson MZ, Rafferty C, Deeter D, et al. Attributable costs of central line-associated bloodstream infections in a pediatric hematology/oncology population. *Am J Infect Control*. 2014;42:1157-1160.
776. Wisplinghoff H, Ebbers J, Geurtz L, et al. Nosocomial bloodstream infections due to *Candida* spp. in the USA: species distribution, clinical features and antifungal susceptibilities. *Int J Antimicrob Agents*. 2014;43:78-81.
781. Yin J, Schweizer ML, Herwaldt LA, et al. Benefits of universal gloving on hospital-acquired infections in acute care pediatric units. *Pediatrics*. 2013;131:e1515-e1520.
783. Zacharioudakis IM, Zervou FN, Arvanitis M, et al. Antimicrobial lock solutions as a method to prevent central line-associated bloodstream infections: a meta-analysis of randomized controlled trials. *Clin Infect Dis*. 2014;59:1741-1749.
785. Zhou XD, Li J, Xiong Y, et al. Do we really need closed-suction drainage in total hip arthroplasty? A meta-analysis. *Int Orthop*. 2013;37:2109-2118.
787. Zilberberg MD, Tillotson GS, McDonald C. *Clostridium difficile* infections among hospitalized children, United States, 1997–2006. *Emerg Infect Dis*. 2010;16:604-609.
789. Zlamy M, Kofler S, Orth D, et al. The impact of rotavirus mass vaccination on hospitalization rates, nosocomial rotavirus gastroenteritis and secondary blood stream infections. *BMC Infect Dis*. 2013;13:112.

The full reference list for this chapter is available at ExpertConsult.com.

245 Active Immunizing Agents

Penelope H. Dennehy • Ian C. Michelow • Michael P. Koster • Michael A. Smit • Jerome Larkin

Prevention of infectious diseases in children by immunization is one of the outstanding accomplishments of medical science. Children enjoy better health today because of effective immunization programs, which in many countries have markedly diminished the morbidity and mortality of previously common contagious diseases. The striking decline in the United States in vaccine-preventable childhood diseases is demonstrated in Table 245.1.[4] Immunization programs have led to the global eradication of smallpox, elimination of measles and poliomyelitis in some regions of the world, and substantial reductions in the morbidity and mortality attributed to diphtheria, tetanus, and pertussis. The World Health Organization (WHO) estimates that 2 to 3 million child deaths are prevented by vaccinations annually (http://www.who.int/mediacentre/factsheets/fs378/en/).

To achieve this progress in child health, scientific technology and medical practice have combined efforts to (1) understand the biology of causal infectious agents, (2) purify these agents and some of their components, (3) develop and test safe and effective vaccines, (4) manufacture and administer the vaccines to appropriate segments of the population, (5) develop appropriate indications and implement schedules for immunizations, and (6) identify necessary contraindications.

Infectious diseases can be prevented through immunization by stimulating an active immunologic defense (e.g., from humoral antibody) through the administration of antigens, usually before natural exposure to an infectious agent (i.e., active immunization) or by temporarily supplying preformed human or animal antibody to persons before or soon after exposure to certain infectious agents (i.e., passive immunization). Active immunizations, including the currently available vaccines, are discussed in this chapter. The composition of major vaccines and their routes of administration are listed in Table 245.2.

ACTIVE IMMUNOPROPHYLAXIS: CONSIDERATIONS AND RECOMMENDATIONS

Vaccines

An ideal immunizing agent should include several characteristics. The agent should be easy to produce in well-standardized preparations that are readily quantifiable and stable in immunobiologic potency. It should be easy to administer and not produce disease in the recipient or susceptible contacts. It should induce long-lasting (ideally permanent) immunity that is measurable by available and inexpensive techniques. It should be free of contaminating and potentially toxic substances, and adverse reactions should be minimal and have minor consequences. All of these objectives rarely, if ever, are met with the currently available vaccines because they are neither completely safe nor completely effective. Partial immunity or undesirable side effects or reactions, or both, including rare severe reactions, can occur. Nonetheless, vaccines in current use are highly effective and very safe.

All active immunizing agents (i.e., vaccines) contain one or more antigens that stimulate a protective immunologic response. Some are live attenuated viruses or bacteria; other vaccines consist of killed microorganisms or contain inactivated components such as exotoxins (i.e., toxoids). In some vaccines, the antigen is a highly defined, single constituent, such as *Haemophilus influenzae* type b (Hib) polysaccharide, whereas in others, the antigen component is less well defined, such as live viruses or whole-cell pertussis vaccines composed of killed *Bordetella pertussis* organisms.

Immunizing agents are administered in suspending fluids such as sterile water, saline solution, or complex tissue culture fluid that can contain proteins or other constituents from the medium from which the vaccine was produced (e.g., serum proteins, egg antigens, other tissue culture–derived antigens). Certain preservatives, stabilizers, or antibiotics are added to some vaccines, and in some cases, the additives can result in hypersensitivity reactions. To enhance immunogenicity, particularly for vaccines containing inactivated microorganisms or their extracted components, adjuvants such as aluminum compounds are added.

Immunization Schedules

The vacinee's age and timing of immunization are critical for the success of vaccination. The vaccine schedule is based on many factors, including the epidemiology of naturally occurring disease, age-specific risk of complications caused by the natural disease, anticipated immunologic

TABLE 245.1 Reduction in Morbidity of Some Vaccine-Preventable Diseases in the United States

Disease	Maximum No. of Cases (y)	Cases in 2015	% Decrease
Diphtheria	206,939 (1921)	0	100
Pertussis	265,269 (1934)	20,762	92
Tetanus	1314 (1922–1926)	29	98
Poliomyelitis, paralytic	21,269 (1952)	0	100
Measles	894,134 (1941)	188	>99
Mumps	152,209 (1968)	1329	>99
Rubella	57,686 (1969)	5	>99
Congenital rubella syndrome	20,000 (1964–1965)	1	>99
Haemophilus influenzae type b	20,000 (before 1987)	29	>99
Invasive pneumococcal disease (>5 y)	15,933 (2000)	1177	93
Hepatitis B	21,102 (1990)	3370	84
Varicella	158,364 (1992)	9789	94

Modified from Centers for Disease Control and Prevention. Notice to readers: final 2015 reports of nationally notifiable infectious diseases and conditions. *MMWR Morb Mortal Wkly Rep.* 2016;651306–21.

TABLE 245.2 Vaccines Available in the United States for Pediatric Use and Routes of Administration[a]

Vaccine	Type	Recommended Route
BCG	Live bacteria	ID (preferred) or SC
Diphtheria-tetanus (DT, Td)	Toxoids	IM
DTaP	Toxoids and inactivated bacterial components	IM
DTaP–hepatitis B–IPV (combination)	Toxoids and inactivated bacterial components, recombinant viral antigen, inactivated virus	IM
DtaP-IPV/Hib (combination)	Toxoids and inactivated bacterial components, polysaccharide-protein conjugate, inactivated virus	IM
DtaP-IPV (combination)	Toxoids and inactivated bacterial components, inactivated virus	IM
Hepatitis A	Inactivated virus	IM
Hepatitis B	Recombinant viral antigen	IM
Hepatitis A–hepatitis B (combination)	Inactivated virus and recombinant viral antigen	IM
Hib conjugate	Bacterial polysaccharide-protein conjugate	IM
Hib–hepatitis B (combination)	Bacterial polysaccharide-protein conjugate and recombinant viral antigen	IM
Hib conjugate–meningococcal conjugate CY (combination)	Bacterial polysaccharide-protein conjugate combined with bacterial polysaccharide	
Human papilloma virus (HPV2, HPV4, and HPV9)	Recombinant viral antigens	IM
Influenza (IIV)	Inactivated viral components	IM
Influenza (LAIV)	Live attenuated viruses	Intranasal spray
Japanese encephalitis	Inactivated virus	SC
Meningococcal polysaccharide (MPSV4)	Bacterial polysaccharide	SC
Meningococcal conjugate (MCV4)	Bacterial polysaccharide-protein conjugate	IM
Meningococcal serogroup B (MenB)	Bacterial lipoprotein	IM
MMR	Live attenuated viruses	SC
MMRV	Live attenuated viruses	SC
Pneumococcal polysaccharide (PPSV23)	Bacterial polysaccharide	IM or SC
Pneumococcal conjugate (PCV13)	Bacterial polysaccharide-protein conjugate	IM
Poliovirus (IPV)	Inactivated viruses	IM or SC
Rabies	Inactivated virus	IM
Rotavirus (RV1 and RV5)	Live attenuated viruses	oral
Tdap	Toxoids and inactivated bacterial components	IM
Tetanus	Toxoid	IM
Typhoid	Bacterial capsular polysaccharide	IM
Typhoid	Live attenuated bacteria	Oral
Varicella	Live attenuated virus	SC
Yellow fever	Live attenuated virus	SC

[a]Only major childhood vaccines and selected others are included.

BCG, Bacille Calmette-Guérin (tuberculosis); *DT*, diphtheria-tetanus toxoids (for children <7 y); *DTaP*, diphtheria-tetanus toxoids–acellular pertussis vaccine (for children <7 y); *Hib*, *Haemophilus influenzae* type b conjugate vaccine; *ID*, intradermal; *IM*, intramuscular; *IPV*, inactivated poliovirus vaccine; *MMR*, live measles-mumps-rubella viruses vaccine; *MMRV*, live measles-mumps-rubella-varicella viruses vaccine; *SC*, subcutaneous; *Td*, tetanus-diphtheria toxoid (for children ≥7 y and adults); *Tdap*, diphtheria–reduced tetanus toxoids–acellular pertussis vaccine (for children ≥10 y and adults).

response of the host to the antigens, duration of immunity that can be induced, and recommended ages for routine health care visits. Vaccines are recommended at the youngest age at which significant risk for the natural disease and its complications exist and at which a protective immunologic response to the vaccine can occur.

An example is measles vaccine, which in the United States is recommended routinely at 12 to 15 months of age because in the first year of life many children have residual, transplacentally acquired maternal measles serum antibody that interferes with the antibody response. However, during measles outbreaks or for travel of infants to measles-endemic areas, measles vaccination is recommended for infants as young as 6 months because the risk of complications with measles is high among children younger than 1 year.[38,471] These infants should be vaccinated again at 12 to 15 months of age. Similarly, in countries where measles causes significant morbidity and mortality for infants younger than 9 months, the Global Advisory Group of the WHO's Expanded Programme on Immunization (EPI) has recommended giving measles vaccine to infants as young as 6 months of age.[697]

The recommended doses of vaccine are determined by the number necessary to achieve a uniform and predictable immunologic response and to sustain protection. Some immunizing agents require the administration of more than one dose for development of an adequate antibody response and require a booster dose to maintain protection. Examples are pertussis, diphtheria, and tetanus vaccines. Intervals between doses are based on the kinetics of primary and secondary antibody responses.

Route of Administration

An example of the effect of the route of administration on immunologic response is provided by poliomyelitis vaccines. Inactivated poliovirus vaccines given intramuscularly induce systemic immunity through serum antibody production, but they do not consistently evoke local secretory immunoglobulin A (IgA) antibodies in the intestinal tract and thereby effectively prevent subsequent transmission of wild-type virus. Because live attenuated oral polio vaccine (OPV) induces optimal intestinal and systemic antibody, it was the preferred vaccine for routine immunization of children in the United States against poliomyelitis for 3 decades and remains the recommended vaccine by the WHO for global eradication.[701] Vaccines containing adjuvants must be injected deep into the muscle mass because if they are administered subcutaneously or intradermally, they can cause local irritation, inflammation, granuloma formation, or necrosis.[29,408]

Injectable vaccines should be administered in areas unlikely to cause local neural, vascular, or tissue injury (Table 245.3).[29,408] Although the upper, outer quadrant of the buttocks has been used as a frequent site of immunization, this area ordinarily should not be used because the gluteal region consists mostly of fat in young children and because of potential injury to the sciatic nerve. Ideally, intramuscular injections should be given in the anterolateral aspect of the upper part of the thigh or the deltoid muscle of the upper part of the arm. The anterolateral aspect of the thigh is preferred for infants because of its muscle mass relative to other sites. For older children, the deltoid muscle usually is sufficiently large for intramuscular injection. The incidence of significant pain in 18-month-old children injected intramuscularly in the thigh is greater than that after deltoid injections and can result in transient limping.[363] The deltoid is the preferred site for intramuscular administration of vaccines in children 18 months of age or older, although some physicians prefer the anterolateral aspect of the thigh for toddlers.[29,408]

Subcutaneous inoculations usually should be given in the thigh of infants and the deltoid area of older children. Intradermal vaccines should be administered on the volar aspect of the forearm.

Recommended routes for administration of vaccines are provided in their package inserts and are summarized in recommendations for immunizations by the Committee on Infectious Diseases of the American Academy of Pediatrics (AAP)[29] and the Advisory Committee on Immunization Practices (ACIP) of the Centers for Disease Control and Prevention (CDC).[408]

Vaccine Dose

The recommended dose of each immunizing agent is derived from theoretical considerations and vaccine trials. Because inactivated immunizing agents cannot replicate in the host, these vaccines must contain an adequate antigenic mass to stimulate the desired immunologic response. Long-lasting immunity with these vaccines requires repeated doses. Exceeding the recommended dose can be hazardous because of excessive local or systemic concentrations of immunizing agents, whereas administration of doses smaller than those recommended may result in inadequate response and protection.[29,408]

TABLE 245.3 Site and Needle Length by Age for Intramuscular Immunization

Age Group	Needle Length, inches (mm)	Suggested Injection Site
Neonate (preterm and term) and infants age <1 mo	⅝ (16)	Anterolateral thigh muscle
Term infant, age 1–12 mo	1 (25)	Anterolateral thigh muscle
Toddlers and children	⅝ –1 (16–25)	Deltoid muscle of the arm
	1–1¼ (25–32)	Anterolateral thigh muscle
Adolescents and young adults		
Female and male, <60 kg	1 (25)	Deltoid muscle of the arm
Female, 60–70 kg	1 (25)	Deltoid muscle of the arm
Female, 70–90 kg	1 (25) – 1½ (38)	Deltoid muscle of the arm
Female, >90 kg	1½ (38)	Deltoid muscle of the arm
Male, 70–118 kg	1 (25) – 1½ (38)	Deltoid muscle of the arm
Male, >118 kg	1½ (38)	Deltoid muscle of the arm

Modified from American Academy of Pediatrics. Active immunization. In: Kimberlin DW, Brady MT, Jackson MA, Long SS, eds. *Red Book: 2015 Report of the Committee on Infectious Diseases.* 30th ed. Elk Grove Village, IL: American Academy of Pediatrics; 2015:1–56.

Lapsed Immunizations

Intervals between multiple doses of an antigen longer than those recommended do not affect the antibody responses achieved, provided the immunization series is completed. Restarting the series after interruption of the vaccine schedule or giving additional doses is not necessary.

Simultaneous Administration of Multiple Vaccines

Because most vaccines can be given simultaneously without impairing effectiveness or safety, multiple vaccines are given to children concurrently.[392] Simultaneous administration of vaccines is particularly important for inadequately immunized children whose return for further immunization is doubtful or for patients with imminent travel plans.

An inactivated vaccine and a live virus vaccine can be administered simultaneously at different sites without interference with the immune response. Exceptions are yellow fever and cholera vaccines because antibody responses are diminished if they are administered simultaneously. If possible, administration of these vaccines should be separated by at least an interval of 3 weeks.[408] In the case of live virus vaccines, the immune response to one live virus vaccine can be impaired if it is given within 4 weeks of another.[408] Parenteral live virus vaccines not administered on the same day should be given at least 4 weeks apart. This consideration is the basis of the recommended minimal interval of 1 month (i.e., 4 weeks) between doses of measles vaccine, such as for a previously unimmunized person who is entering college. Guidelines for spacing live and killed antigen vaccines are given in Table 245.4.

TABLE 245.4 Guidelines for Spacing the Administration of Live and Inactivated Antigens

Antigen Combination	Recommended Minimum Interval Between Doses
Two or more inactivated[a]	None; can be administered simultaneously or at any interval between doses
Inactivated plus live	None, can be administered simultaneously or at any interval between doses
Two or more live injectible[b]	28-day minimum interval, if not administered simultaneously

[a]In people with functional or anatomic asplenia, quadrivalent meningococcal conjugate vaccine (MCV4-D; Menactra) should not be given until at least 4 weeks after all doses of 13-valent pneumococcal conjugate vaccine (PCV13) have been administered because of interference with the immune response to the PCV13 series because both vaccines are conjugated to diphtheria toxin carrier protein. PCV13 and 23-valent pneumococcal polysaccharide vaccine (PPSV23) should not be administered simultaneously and should be spaced at least 8 weeks apart; when both vaccines are indicated, PCV13 should be administered first, if possible.

[b]An exception is made for some live oral vaccines (e.g., Ty21a typhoid vaccine, oral poliovirus vaccine, oral rotavirus vaccine) that can be administered simultaneously or at any interval before or after inactivated or live parenteral vaccines.

Modified from American Academy of Pediatrics. Active immunization. In: Kimberlin DW, Brady MT, Jackson MA, Long SS, eds. *Red Book: 2015 Report of the Committee on Infectious Diseases*. 30th ed. Elk Grove Village, IL: American Academy of Pediatrics; 2015:1–56.

Record Keeping, Patient Information, Informed Consent, and Reporting

Accurate record keeping by physicians is required, and parents (or patients) should keep up-to-date immunization records for their children. The 1986 National Childhood Vaccine Injury Act (NCVIA) requires that for routinely recommended childhood vaccines, health care providers record in the child's permanent medical record the date of administration of the vaccine, manufacturer, lot number, and name of the health care provider administering the vaccines.[29]

All children and their parents or caregivers should be informed about the benefits and risks of the vaccines to be administered. For vaccines currently specified in the NCVIA, Vaccine Information Statements (VISs) have been prepared by the CDC and must be used by vaccine administrators.

Informed consent should be obtained before the administration of vaccines. Some physicians and other health care providers may choose to obtain the parent's signature, but current law does not require written consent. An appropriate alternative to written consent is to note in the patient's record that the VISs have been provided and discussed with the parent, patient, or legal guardian.[29]

To increase knowledge about adverse reactions, all temporally associated events severe enough to require the patient to seek medical attention should be reported to the Vaccine Adverse Events Reporting System (VAERS); VAERS forms can be obtained by calling 800-822-7967 or by accessing the website (http://vaers.hhs.gov). Health care providers who administer vaccines are required in the United States to report to the VAERS specific adverse events in recipients of the vaccines covered by the NCVIA (Health Resources and Services Administration: http://www.hrsa.gov/vaccinecompensation/vaccinetable.html.). This system for reporting adverse events associated with vaccination was established by the US Department of Health and Human Services to foster recognition of vaccine-related reactions and further study to establish possible causation.

Decreased occurrence of vaccine-preventable infectious diseases has resulted in a greater number of adverse events temporally related to immunization than cases of disease. Although in some cases, such as vaccine-associated paralytic poliomyelitis, vaccine has been established as the cause, in other circumstances, such as brain damage alleged to be attributed to whole-cell pertussis vaccine, causation by vaccine has not been proved.[14]

Increased public visibility of vaccine reactions contributed to a marked increase in vaccine litigation in the 1980s as compensation was sought through the judicial system by those alleged to have suffered serious vaccine-related sequelae. A marked increase in manufacturers' actual and anticipated liability costs and subsequent escalating increases in the price of vaccines occurred concomitantly. These and other developments, such as threats to the vaccine supply, concerns by parents about vaccine safety, and recognition of the benefits derived from improved coordination and planning of vaccine programs, led to passage of the 1986 NCVIA and the National Vaccine Injury Compensation Program (https://www.hrsa.gov/vaccinecompensation/index.html), a no-fault system to compensate victims of certain presumed vaccine-related events.

The Department of Health and Human Services administers the compensation program. Decisions on compensation are made by the US Court of Federal Claims and are based on the Vaccine Injury Table, which was revised since passage of the original legislation in response to new findings and analysis by several Institute of Medicine (IOM) committees. Compensation for injuries occurring after the program's effective date of October 1, 1988, is provided by excise taxes on each vaccine. The program has been successful in reducing vaccine-related litigation, stabilizing vaccine prices, and creating a favorable environment for the introduction of new vaccines.[262]

Vaccine Recommendations and Schedules

In developing recommendations for immunization, many factors are considered, including the vaccine's characteristics, scientific knowledge about the principles of immunization, assessment of the benefits of the vaccine, the risk of the disease and its complications, vaccine costs, and risk of adverse reactions. Changes in relative benefits and risks necessitate continued review of recommendations.

In the United States, recommendations for immunization of infants and children are made by the ACIP of the CDC and the AAP's Committee on Infectious Diseases. These committees work closely together, and in most circumstances, their recommendations are similar. The two committees and the American Academy of Family Practice (AAFP) issue a single vaccine schedule each year. The 2016 schedule for routine administration of childhood vaccines is given in Fig. 245.1 and Table 245.5.

A major change in 1996 was the establishment of a routine preadolescent immunization visit at 11 to 12 years of age.[125] The dose of adult tetanus-diphtheria–acellular pertussis (Tdap) vaccine should be given at that time, as should a dose of the meningococcal conjugate vaccine and the first dose of human papillomavirus (HPV) vaccine. At this preadolescent visit, children not previously vaccinated with hepatitis B, varicella, or the second dose of measles-containing vaccine (or any combination of these vaccines) should be given the necessary immunizations and scheduled for future visits to receive any vaccines not administered during this visit.

Other countries have similar national mechanisms for formulating immunization schedules and recommendations that are based on the local epidemiology of diseases and available vaccines. In low-resource countries, practices are guided by the WHO's EPI. Current recommendations are listed at the website (http://www.who.int/immunization/policy/Immunization_routine_table2.pdf?ua=1).

As new vaccines and scientific knowledge become available, vaccine recommendations and schedules are modified and changed. Examples of changes in the past 2 decades include the use of pneumococcal conjugate vaccine beginning at 2 months of age, universal toddler hepatitis A immunization, and recommendations for administration of a second dose of varicella vaccine, and the introduction of acellular pertussis vaccines for adolescents and adults.

Implementation of Vaccine Programs

In addition to the availability of safe and effective vaccines and appropriate schedules for their use, effective means of implementation and delivery are necessary for the success of vaccine programs. In the United States, high rates of immunization among school-aged children have been achieved, in part because of public health programs for vaccine administration, government support for vaccine purchase, and state laws requiring immunization for school entry. In contrast to rates of approximately 95% or higher among school-aged children, immunization

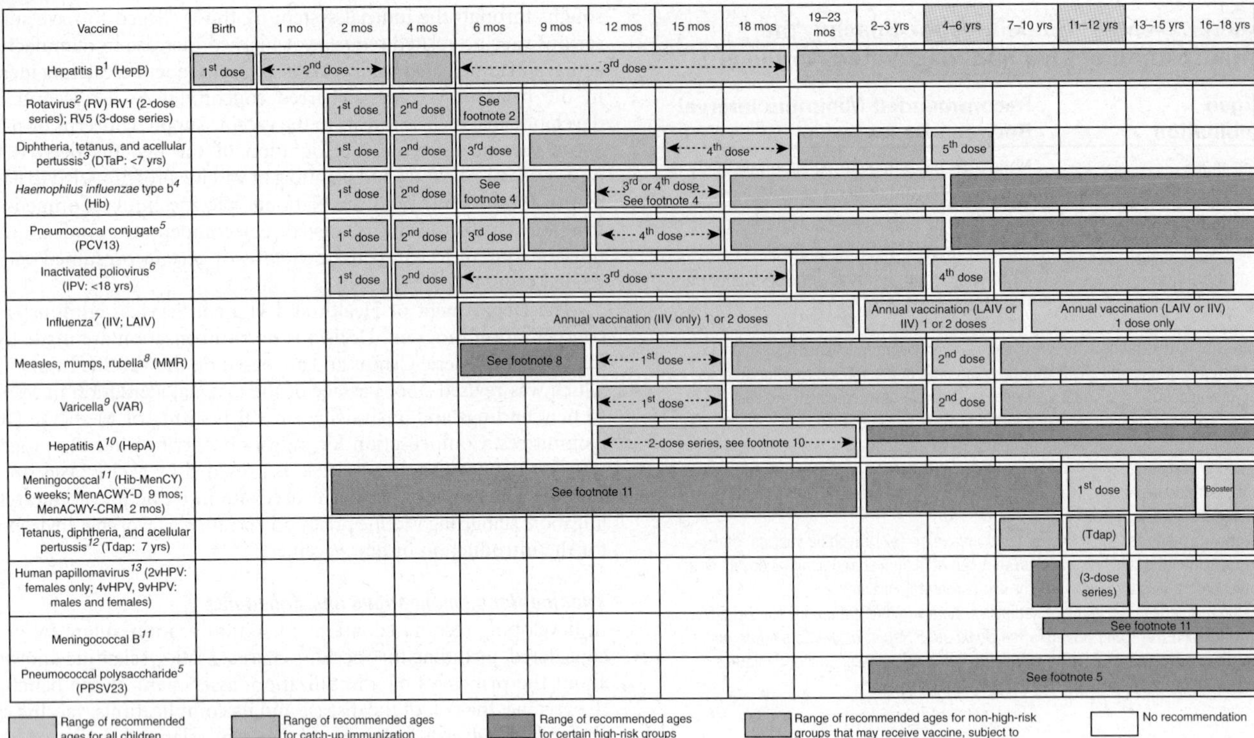

Vaccine
Birth
1 mo
2 mos
4 mos
6 mos
9 mos
12 mos
15 mos
18 mos
19–23 mos
2–3 yrs
4–6 yrs
7–10 yrs
11–12 yrs
13–15 yrs
16–18 yrs
Hepatitis B¹ (HepB)
1st dose
2nd dose
3rd dose
Rotavirus² (RV) RV1 (2-dose series); RV5 (3-dose series)
1st dose
2nd dose
See footnote 2
Diphtheria, tetanus, and acellular pertussis³ (DTaP: <7 yrs)
1st dose
2nd dose
3rd dose
4th dose
5th dose
Haemophilus influenzae type b⁴ (Hib)
1st dose
2nd dose
See footnote 4
3rd or 4th dose, See footnote 4
Pneumococcal conjugate⁵ (PCV13)
1st dose
2nd dose
3rd dose
4th dose
Inactivated poliovirus⁶ (IPV: <18 yrs)
1st dose
2nd dose
3rd dose
4th dose
Influenza⁷ (IIV; LAIV)
Annual vaccination (IIV only) 1 or 2 doses
Annual vaccination (LAIV or IIV) 1 or 2 doses
Annual vaccination (LAIV or IIV) 1 dose only
Measles, mumps, rubella⁸ (MMR)
See footnote 8
1st dose
2nd dose
Varicella⁹ (VAR)
1st dose
2nd dose
Hepatitis A¹⁰ (HepA)
2-dose series, see footnote 10
Meningococcal¹¹ (Hib-MenCY) 6 weeks; MenACWY-D 9 mos; MenACWY-CRM 2 mos)
See footnote 11
1st dose
Booster
Tetanus, diphtheria, and acellular pertussis¹² (Tdap: 7 yrs)
(Tdap)
Human papillomavirus¹³ (2vHPV: females only; 4vHPV, 9vHPV: males and females)
(3-dose series)
Meningococcal B¹¹
See footnote 11
Pneumococcal polysaccharide⁵ (PPSV23)
See footnote 5
Range of recommended ages for all children
Range of recommended ages for catch-up immunization
Range of recommended ages for certain high-risk groups
Range of recommended ages for non-high-risk groups that may receive vaccine, subject to individual clinical decision making
No recommendation

This schedule includes recommendations in effect as of january 1, 2016. Any dose not administered at the recommended age should be administered at a subsequent visit, when indicated and feasible.The use of a combination vaccine generally is preferred over separate injections of its equivalent component vaccines. Vaccination providers should consult the relevant advisory committee on immunization practices (ACIP) statement for detailed recommendations, available online at http://www.cdc.gov/vaccines/hcp/acip-recs/index.html. Clinically significant adverse events that follow vaccination should be reported to the vaccine adverse event reporting system (VAERS) online (http://www.vaers.hhs.gov) or by telephone (800-822-7967). Suspected cases of vaccine-preventable diseases should be reported to the state or local health department. Additional information, including precautions and contraindications for vaccination, is available from CDC online (http://www.cdc.gov/vaccines/recs/vac-admin/contraindocations.htm) or by telephone (800-CDC-INFO [800-232-4636]).

This schedule is approved by the advisory committee on immunization practices (http//www.cdc.gov/vaccines/acip), the american academy of pediatrics (http://www.aap.org), the american academy of family physicians (http://www.aafp.org), and the american college of obstetricians and gynecologists (http://www.acog.org).

NOTE: The above recommendations must be read along with the footnotes of this schedule.

FIG. 245.1 Recommended immunization schedule for people from birth to 18 years of age in the United States in 2016. An expanded version of the table and its 13 footnotes can be found at https://www.cdc.gov/vaccines/schedules/hcp/imz/child-adolescent.html. (From Centers for Disease Control and Prevention. Immunization schedules. http://www.cdc.gov/vaccines/schedules/hcp/child-adolescent.html.)

rates for infants and young children in the 1980s were significantly lower.[713] In a survey of 21 primarily urban areas throughout the United States, 11% to 58% (median, 44%) of children who entered school in 1991 and 1992 were fully vaccinated by their second birthday. Failure to immunize young children was a major factor in the outbreaks of measles in major urban areas in the United States in 1989 through 1991.[634]

The measles epidemic and the recognition of low immunization rates prompted a national campaign to achieve the US Public Health Service's goal of a 90% vaccine coverage rate for children by the time they were 2 years of age. Initiatives have included improved access to vaccines, education of health care providers in the community, and the development of standards for pediatric immunization practice.[498] The standards have been endorsed by the AAP, AAFP, and other major professional organizations and serve as guidelines to be followed for improving the delivery of vaccines. They include evaluation of the patient's immunization status at all medical visits, use of valid contraindications, simultaneous administration of all indicated vaccines, and routine audits of the immunization status of patients by providers. These and other initiatives resulted in increasing immunization rates among young children.

According to the National Immunization Survey, coverage rates for children 19 to 35 months of age in 2015 were 72.2% for completion of the combined vaccine series, which includes four or more doses of diphtheria, tetanus toxoids, and acellular pertussis vaccine (DTaP); three or more doses of poliovirus vaccine; one or more doses of measles-containing vaccine; full series of Hib vaccine (i.e., three or four doses, depending on product type); three or more doses of hepatitis B vaccine (HepB); one or more doses of varicella vaccine; and four or more doses of pneumococcal conjugate vaccine (PCV).[344] Vaccination coverage rates in the United States for preschool-aged children consistently have been greater than 70% since 2013.

Vaccine Contraindications, Precautions, and Use in Special Circumstances

Recommendations for the use of specific vaccines include contraindications and use in special circumstances, such as immunocompromised patients (from underlying disease or therapy such as high-dose corticosteroids) and pregnancy.[29,408] Established, generic contraindications are moderate or severe illness, a previous anaphylactic reaction to the specific vaccine, and a severe hypersensitivity reaction (e.g., anaphylaxis) to a vaccine constituent.

The decision to defer immunization in a febrile child should be based on the physician's assessment of the severity of the illness rather than the degree of fever. Children with minor illness and low-grade fever usually should be vaccinated, especially if a child is unlikely to return promptly for the deferred immunization.

Administration of live virus vaccines such as varicella and measles-mumps-rubella (MMR) vaccines usually is contraindicated in patients with altered immunity. However, the morbidity and mortality rates of measles and the lack of complications from vaccination of children infected with human immunodeficiency virus (HIV) prompted recommendations that these children, unless significantly immunocompromised, receive the MMR vaccine.[17,126,471]

Because of a theoretical risk to the developing fetus, administration of live virus vaccines in most cases is not recommended for pregnant women.[36,408] However, inadvertent administration of vaccine is not necessarily a reason for termination of the pregnancy, and some live

TABLE 245.5 Catch-Up Immunization Schedule for People Age 4 Months Through 18 Years Who Start Late or Are >1 Month Behind—United States, 2017[a]

Vaccine	Minimum Age for Dose 1	MINIMUM INTERVAL BETWEEN DOSES			
		Dose 1 to 2	Dose 2 to 3	Dose 3 to 4	Dose 4 to 5
Children 4 Months–6 Years of Age					
Hepatitis B[1]	Birth	4 wk	8 wk *and* at least 16 wk after first dose Minimum age for the final dose is 24 wk	—	—
Rotavirus[2]	6 wk	4 wk	4 wk[2]	—	—
Diphtheria, tetanus, and acellular pertussis[3]	6 wk	4 wk	4 wk	6 mo	6 mo[3]
Haemophilus influenzae type b[4]	6 wk	4 wk if first dose was administered before first birthday 8 wk (as final dose) if first dose was administered at age 12–14 mo No further doses needed if first dose was administered at age ≥15 mo —	4 wk[4] if current age is younger than 12 mo and first dose was administered before age 7 mo and at least 1 previous dose was PRP-T (ActHib, Pentacel, Hiberix) or unknown 8 wk and age 12–59 mo (as final dose)[4] If current age is younger than 12 mo *and* first dose was administered at age 7–11 mo *or* If current age is 12–59 mo *and* first dose was administered before first birthday *and* second dose administered <15 mo *or* If both doses were PRP-OMP (PedvaxHIB; Comvax) *and* were administered before first birthday No further doses needed if previous dose was administered at age ≥15 mo	8 wk (as final dose); dose necessary only for children 12–59 mo who received 3 doses before first birthday	—
Pneumococcal[5]	6 wk	4 wk if first dose administered before first birthday 8 wk (as final dose for healthy children) if first dose was administered at or after first birthday No further doses needed for healthy children if first dose administered at age ≥24 mo	4 wk if current age is <12 mo and previous dose given at <7 mo of age 8 wk (as final dose for healthy children) if previous dose given between 7–11 mo (wait until at least 12 mo old); *or* if current age is ≥12 mo and at least 1 dose was given before age 12 mo No further doses needed for healthy children if previous dose administered at age ≥24 mo	8 wk (as final dose); dose necessary only for children 12–59 mo of age who received 3 doses before age 12 mo or for children at high risk who received 3 doses at any age	— —

Continued

TABLE 245.5 Catch-Up Immunization Schedule for People Age 4 Months Through 18 Years Who Start Late or Are >1 Month Behind—United States, 2017[a]—cont'd

Vaccine	Minimum Age for Dose 1	MINIMUM INTERVAL BETWEEN DOSES			
		Dose 1 to 2	Dose 2 to 3	Dose 3 to 4	Dose 4 to 5
Inactivated poliovirus[6]	6 wk	4 wk[6]	4 wk[6]	6 mo[6] (minimum age of 4 y for final dose).	—
Measles, mumps, rubella[8]	12 mo	4 wk	—	—	—
Varicella[9]	12 mo	3 mo	—	—	—
Hepatitis A[10]	12 mo	6 mo	—	—	—
Meningococcal[11] (Hib-MenCY ≥6 wk; (MenACWY-D ≥9 mo; MenACWY-CRM ≥2 mo)	6 wk	8 wk[11]	See footnote 11	See footnote 11	—

Vaccine	Minimum Age for Dose 1	MINIMUM INTERVAL BETWEEN DOSES		
		Dose 1 to Dose 2	Dose 2 to Dose 3	Dose 3 to Dose 4
Children and Adolescents 7–18 Years of Age				
Meningococcal[11] (MenACWY-D ≥9 mo; MenACWY-CRM ≥2 mo)	N/A	8 wk11	—	—
Tetanus, diphtheria; tetanus, diphtheria, and acellular pertussis[12]	7 y[12]	4 wk	4 wk if first dose of DTaP/DT was administered before first birthday 6 mo (as final dose) if first dose of DTaP/DT or Tdap/Td was administered at or after first birthday	6 mo if first dose of DTaP/DT was administered before first birthday
Human papillomavirus[13]	9 y	Routine dosing intervals are recommended[13]		
Hepatitis A[10]	N/A	6 mo	—	—
Hepatitis B[1]	N/A	4 wk	8 wk *and* at least 16 wk after first dose	—
Inactivated poliovirus[6]	N/A	4 wk	4 wk[6]	6 mo[6]
Measles, mumps, rubella[8]	N/A	4 wk	—	—
Varicella[9]	N/A	3 mo if age <13 y 4 wk if age ≥13 y	—	—

[a]The recommendations must be read with the numeric footnotes of this schedule (https://www.cdc.gov/vaccines/schedules/hcp/imz/catchup.html/).
N/A, Not applicable.
From Centers for Disease Control and Prevention. Immunization schedules. http://www.cdc.gov/vaccines/schedules/hcp/child-adolescent.html.

virus vaccines, such as those for yellow fever and poliomyelitis, can be given safely to pregnant women. Inactivated bacterial and viral vaccines such as tetanus toxoids, hepatitis B, and influenza vaccine, which are composed of antigenic components or killed organisms, can and should be given during pregnancy if indicated.

In some recipients, vaccines can cause severe reactions, which may be a contraindication or precaution to subsequent administration of the specific vaccine. An example is a child in whom a fever of 40.5°C (105°F) or higher develops after receiving DTaP vaccine and for whom administration of further doses of pertussis-containing vaccine is not indicated in most cases. This recommendation is based on the unproven but reasonable presumption that children who experience adverse reactions after receiving pertussis immunization are at risk for similar reactions of equal or greater magnitude on subsequent immunization.[188]

Anaphylactic reactions caused by allergenic components of a vaccine (e.g., gelatin or egg protein in vaccine prepared in embryonated chicken eggs) have occurred rarely. Vaccines posing a potential risk for egg-sensitive people include those against measles, mumps, inactivated influenza, and yellow fever. Before administering vaccines to people with possible hypersensitivity to vaccine constituents, physicians should review current recommendations for these vaccines. In other circumstances, specific immunizations may be contraindicated because of previous reactions and the child's medical history, such as with DTaP (e.g., evolving neurologic disorders) and MMR (e.g., immune thrombocytopenia associated temporally with vaccination).[408]

Misconceptions

Appropriate and safe use of vaccines requires knowledge of the patient's relevant medical history, adverse reactions associated with previous receipt of vaccines, and specific indications and contraindications. Without this information, vaccines may be administered inadvertently or not given in circumstances in which immunization is indicated, thereby resulting in missed opportunities for receiving the recommended immunization and susceptibility of the child to a preventable disease. Examples of common misconceptions concerning contraindication to vaccines are given in Box 245.1.

International Travel

Foreign travel often is an indication for giving vaccines not routinely administered to children. The risk of exposure to certain vaccine-preventable diseases may be greater than in the United States, and travelers may be exposed to infections that are uncommon or do not occur in the United States. Examples include vaccines against hepatitis A, typhoid fever, yellow fever, and Japanese encephalitis (JE) (Table 245.6), depending on the location and circumstances of the person's visit. Some countries may require yellow fever vaccination for entry. The second dose of measles vaccine should be given to children and adolescents who have received only one dose (provided 4 weeks or more have elapsed since administration of the first dose), irrespective of age because the risk of exposure to measles cases may be substantial in some foreign countries. Children and adolescents should have received all vaccines routinely recommended for their age.

Information on vaccine requirements for international travel is provided in a semiannually revised publication by the CDC, *Health Information for International Travel*[678] (https://wwwnc.cdc.gov/travel/page/yellowbook-home). Information also is available from the CDC International Travelers Hotline (800-232-4636) or the CDC Traveler's Health website (http://wwwnc.cdc.gov/travel/).

Vaccine Safety

Immunizations are among the most cost-effective and widely used public health interventions. Public health recommendations for vaccine programs and practices represent a dynamic balancing of risks and benefits. Vaccine safety or risk monitoring is necessary to weigh these factors accurately and adjust vaccination policies accordingly.

No vaccine is perfectly safe or effective. As the incidence of vaccine-preventable diseases is reduced, public concern refocuses from the risk of contracting disease to the health risks associated with vaccines. A higher standard of safety typically is expected for vaccines compared with other medical interventions because in contrast to most pharmaceutical products that are administered to ill people for curative purposes, vaccines usually are given to healthy people to prevent disease acquisition. Public tolerance of adverse reactions due to products given to healthy people, especially healthy infants, is substantially lower than that to products administered to people who are already ill.

The lower tolerance of risk for vaccines necessitates investigating possible causes of rare adverse events after administration of vaccinations more aggressively than would be acceptable for other pharmaceutical products. Because vaccination is such a common event, any health problem that occurs after immunization can be attributed to the vaccine. Health effects reported as being associated with vaccines may be true adverse reactions or may be associated with vaccination only by coincidence. Because a temporal relationship alone does not prove causation, cause-and-effect relationships often are impossible to establish. Epidemiologic and related studies must be performed to ascertain the incidence and nature of adverse reactions to vaccines. The studies are important in ensuring a scientific rationale for recommendations for vaccine use and optimal public and professional acceptance of vaccines.

The topic of vaccine safety became prominent during the mid-1970s with increases in the number of lawsuits filed on behalf of patients

BOX 245.1 Misconceptions About Vaccine Contraindications

- Mild acute illness with low-grade fever or mild diarrheal illness in an otherwise well child.
- Current antimicrobial therapy or the convalescent phase of illness.
- Reaction to previous vaccine dose that involved only soreness, redness, or swelling in the immediate vicinity of the vaccination site or temperature of less than 40.5°C (105°F).
- Prematurity. The appropriate age for initiating most immunization in the prematurely born infant is the usual recommended chronologic age. Vaccine doses should not be reduced for preterm infants.
- Pregnancy of mother or other household contact. Vaccine viruses in MMR vaccine are not transmitted by vaccine recipients. Although varicella vaccine and influenza vaccine viruses have been transmitted by a healthy vaccine recipient to contacts, the frequency is rare, only mild or asymptomatic infection has been reported, and use of vaccine is not contraindicated by pregnancy of the child's mother or other household contacts.
- Recent exposure to an infectious disease.
- Breastfeeding. The only vaccine virus that has been isolated from breast milk is rubella vaccine virus. No evidence indicates that breast milk from women immunized against rubella is harmful to infants.
- A history of nonspecific allergies or relatives with allergies.
- Allergies to penicillin or any other antibiotic, except anaphylactic reactions to neomycin or streptomycin. These reactions occur rarely, and none of the vaccines licensed in the United States contains penicillin.
- Allergies to duck meat or duck feathers. No vaccine available in the United States is produced in substrates containing duck antigens.
- Family history of convulsions in persons considered for pertussis or measles vaccination.
- Family history of sudden infant death syndrome in children considered for DTaP vaccination.
- Family history of an adverse event, unrelated to immunosuppression after vaccination.
- Malnutrition.

DTaP, Diphtheria-tetanus–acellular pertussis; *MMR*, measles-mumps-rubella.
Modified from American Academy of Pediatrics. Active immunization. In: Kimberlin DW, Brady MT, Jackson MA, Long SS, eds. *Red Book: 2015 Report of the Committee on Infectious Diseases*. 30th ed. Elk Grove Village, IL: American Academy of Pediatrics; 2015:1–56.

TABLE 245.6 Recommended Immunizations for Travelers to Developing Countries

Immunizations	LENGTH OF TRAVEL		
	Brief (<2 wk)	**Intermediate (2 wk–3 mo)**	**Long-Term Residential (>3 mo)**
Review and complete age-appropriate childhood schedule	+	+	+
DTaP, poliovirus, pneumococcal, and *Haemophilus influenzae* type b vaccines may be given at 4-week intervals if necessary to complete the recommended schedule before departure. Rotavirus vaccine has maximum ages for the first and last doses; consideration should be given to the timing of an infant's travel so that the infant will be able to receive the vaccine series.			
Measles: Infants 6–11 mo of age should receive 1 dose of MMR vaccine before departure. Two additional doses are given if younger than 12 mo of age at first dose.			
Varicella			
Hepatitis A[a]			
Hepatitis B[b]			
Vaccines against the following diseases should be considered depending on the geographic area and circumstances of the visit:			
Japanese encephalitis[c]	±	±	+
Meningococcal disease[d]	±	±	±
Rabies[e]	±	+	+
Typhoid fever[f]	±	+	+
Yellow fever[g]	+	+	+

[a]Indicated for travelers to areas with intermediate or high endemic rates of hepatitis A virus infection.
[b]If insufficient time to complete 6-month primary series, an accelerated series can be given.
[c]For regions with endemic infection. For high-risk activities in areas experiencing outbreaks, vaccine is recommended, even for brief travel.
[d]Recommended for regions of Africa with endemic infection and during local epidemics and required for travel to Saudi Arabia for the Hajj.
[e]Indicated for persons at high risk for animal exposure (especially dogs) and for travelers to countries with endemic infection.
[f]Indicated for travelers who will consume food and liquids in areas of poor sanitation.
[g]For regions with endemic infection.
DTaP, Diphtheria-tetanus–acellular pertussis.
Modified from American Academy of Pediatrics. Immunizations in special clinical circumstances. In: Kimberlin DW, Brady MT, Jackson MA, Long SS, eds.. *Red Book: 2015 Report of the Committee on Infectious Diseases.* 30th ed. Elk Grove Village, IL: American Academy of Pediatrics; 2015:101–107; Centers for Disease Control and Prevention. Health information for international travel, 2016: international travel with infants and young children. http://wwwnc.cdc.gov/travel/yellowbook/2016/international-travel-with-infants-children/vaccine-recommendations-for-infants-children

presumably injured by the diphtheria-tetanus-pertussis (DTP) vaccine.[280] Legal decisions were made and damages awarded despite the lack of scientific evidence to support claims of vaccine injury.[280] As a result of the liability, prices soared, and several manufacturers halted production. A shortage of vaccines resulted, and public health officials became concerned about the return of epidemic diseases. To reduce liability and respond to public health concerns, Congress passed the NCVIA in 1986.

The NCVIA mandates that all health care providers report certain adverse events that occur after the administration of vaccination with routinely recommended childhood vaccines. As a result, the VAERS was established by the US Food and Drug Administration (FDA) and the CDC in 1990. VAERS provides a mechanism for the collection and analysis of adverse events associated with vaccines currently licensed in the United States. Adverse events are defined as health effects occurring after immunization that may or may not be related to the vaccine. VAERS data are monitored continually to detect previously unknown adverse events or increases in known adverse events.[187]

The gaps that exist in the scientific knowledge of rare vaccine adverse events prompted the CDC to develop the Vaccine Safety Datalink (VSD) project.[185] It involved forming partnerships with four large health maintenance organizations to monitor vaccine safety continually. VSD is an example of a large, linked database and includes information on more than 6 million people. The VSD project enables planned vaccine safety studies and timely investigations of hypotheses. The CDC has established an Immunization Safety Office (http://www.cdc.gov/vaccinesafety/iso.html) that identifies possible vaccine side effects and conducts studies to determine whether health problems are caused by vaccines.

Reference Sources

Several comprehensive sources of information about pediatric vaccines are available. The AAP publishes *The Red Book: Report of the Committee on Infectious Diseases* every 3 years. The next edition will be published in 2018. In the interval between editions, the AAP publishes recommendations in its newsletter *AAP News* and subsequently in *Pediatrics.* The ACIP issues vaccine recommendations and relevant information in *Morbidity and Mortality Weekly Report.* Manufacturers provide product information for each vaccine in the FDA-approved package inserts.

VACCINES RECOMMENDED FOR ROUTINE ADMINISTRATION

Diphtheria Toxoid

The introduction of diphtheria toxoid–containing vaccine in the 1940s led to a dramatic reduction in the incidence of diphtheria in the United States. From 1980 through 2004, 57 cases of diphtheria were reported in the United States, an average of 2 to 3 per year,[405] and only five cases have been reported since 2000. A confirmed case has not been reported in the United States since 2003.[31] However, diphtheria remains a potentially significant public health problem. Serologic surveys in the United States and England have suggested that many adults are not immune.[219,405,449]

Although a study published in 1996 demonstrated that most adults in the United States do have protective concentrations of serum antitoxin,[321] data obtained from a national population-based serosurvey published in 2002 revealed that the prevalence of immunity to diphtheria, as determined by the level of diphtheria antitoxin, progressively decreased from 91% among children 6 to 11 years of age to approximately 30% among those 60 to 69 years of age.[472] Of the reported cases with known patient age since 1980, 58% were among people 20 years of age or older and 44% were among people 40 years of age or older. Most cases have occurred in unimmunized or inadequately immunized people.

The current age distribution of cases corroborates the finding of inadequate levels of circulating antitoxin in many adults. Adequate immunization has not eliminated the potential for transmission of *Corynebacterium diphtheriae* completely because immunization does not prevent carriage of *C. diphtheriae* in the nasopharynx or on the skin.[90,405]

C. diphtheriae requires infection with a virus to acquire the genetic information for toxin production, which is the primary mediator of disease. When isolated, strains of *C. diphtheriae* should be tested for toxin production to establish causality in clinical disease. Non–toxin-producing strains can cause an undifferentiated pharyngitis that is usually self-limited. Because the organism requires tellurite for growth, the microbiology laboratory must be alerted to the fact that diphtheria is suspected when specimens are submitted. Polymerase chain reaction (PCR) methods can help in making the diagnosis if antibiotics have been given before obtaining cultures.

C. diphtheriae is further subdivided in to four biotypes: *gravis*, *intermedius*, *mitis*, and *belfanti*. All four biotypes have the potential to produce toxin. Humans are the reservoir for *C. diphtheriae* and may be asymptomatic. Transmission occurs by respiratory droplets or contaminated fomites. Asymptomatic carriers and those with disease can shed the organism for weeks after infection. Shedding is terminated within 48 hours of initiating appropriate antimicrobial therapy.

As a result of inadequate immunity in adults, infants, and children, an epidemic of diphtheria occurred in the 1990s throughout the former Soviet Union, including Russia, Ukraine, and the central Asian republics. Case-fatality rates ranged from 3% to 23%.[285,334] Diphtheria continues to be a significant cause of morbidity and mortality in developing countries,[285] and it therefore remains a source of possible exposure during travel to endemic countries. Because humans are the only known reservoir for *C. diphtheriae,* universal immunization with a diphtheria toxoid–containing vaccine is the only effective control measure.

Preparations

Diphtheria toxoid is produced by growing toxigenic *C. diphtheriae* in liquid medium. The filtrate is incubated with formaldehyde to convert toxin to toxoid and then is adsorbed onto an aluminum salt adjuvant.

Diphtheria toxoid is available in combination with DTaP for routine immunization of infants and children younger than 7 years and for adolescents and adults 11 to 64 years of age as a single booster (Tdap). Two brands of Tdap are available: Boostrix (approved for people ≥10 years of age) and Adacel (approved for people 11 to 64 years of age). DTaP and Tdap vaccines do not contain thimerosal as a preservative. Diphtheria toxoid also is available as a DTaP–inactivated poliovirus (IPV)–hepatitis B combination, a DTaP–inactivated poliovirus (IPV)–Hib conjugate combination, and in combination with tetanus toxoid (i.e., DT and Td) for use when pertussis vaccination is contraindicated. No diphtheria-only vaccine is available. Hib, pneumococcal, and meningococcal conjugate vaccines containing diphtheria toxoid or CRM197 protein, a nontoxic variant of diphtheria toxin used as an adjuvant, are not substitutes for diphtheria toxoid immunization.[31]

Pediatric formulations (i.e., DT and DTaP) contain an amount of tetanus toxoid similar to adult Td, but they contain three to four times as much diphtheria toxoid. The concentration of diphtheria toxoid (D) for children younger than 7 years per 0.5-mL intramuscular dose of DTaP or DT vaccine is 6.7 to 25 limit of flocculation (Lf) units, depending on the vaccine manufacturer. Vaccines approved for children 7 years or older and adults (i.e., Tdap and Td) contain only a fraction of the diphtheria toxoid (d = 2–2.5 Lf) because of adverse reactions related to dose and age.[31,90,405]

Immunogenicity

After a primary series of three properly spaced diphtheria toxoid doses in adults or four doses in infants, a protective level of antitoxin (≥0.1 IU of antitoxin/mL) is reached in more than 95% of vaccinees. Diphtheria toxoid has been estimated to have a clinical efficacy rate of 97%. Immune response to diphtheria toxoid was measured after administration of each adult Tdap vaccine and compared with that elaborated after Td vaccine. Seroprotective antidiphtheria levels, defined as a titer of 0.1 IU/mL or more, and booster response rates to diphtheria were determined to be noninferior after administration of Tdap compared with Td vaccination.[405]

Adverse Events

Other than local reactions of pain and swelling at the site of vaccine injection, immunization does not cause significant adverse events. These local reactions have been attributed to hypersensitivity reactions in response to the pertussis component and are not a contraindication for administration of further vaccination if otherwise indicated.

Regarding adverse reactions reported after administration of Tdap, vaccination with Boostrix was associated with a statistically higher rate of moderate to severe headache compared with Td, and vaccination with Adacel was associated with higher rates of mild injection site pain and low-grade fever compared with the Td vaccine. No serious adverse events have been reported for Boostrix. There have been two reports of serious adverse events, both characterized as neuropathic reactions, in adults, possibly related to having received Adacel (none reported in adolescents), and in both cases, symptoms resolved completely within several days.[90]

When administered in the third trimester of pregnancy as recommended by the ACIP, there has been no association with increases in poor birth outcomes or maternal adverse events.[90,243,488,625]

Indications

Primary immunization consists of five doses of diphtheria toxoid, provided as DTaP or as DT if pertussis is contraindicated.[31,90,405] The first three doses are administered routinely to children who are 2, 4, and 6 months of age. A fourth dose is administered 6 to 12 months after the third dose, between 12 to 18 months of age, to maintain adequate antibody concentrations for the ensuing preschool years. For those not immunized in infancy, the initial dose is followed by two doses given 2 and 8 to 14 months later. A single booster dose given when the child is 4 to 6 years of age (before school entry) is indicated unless the preceding dose was given after the fourth birthday. Interruption of the recommended schedule or delay in administering subsequent doses during primary immunization does not reduce immunity or necessitate restarting the series.

In 2005, the FDA licensed two vaccines containing tetanus toxoid, reduced diphtheria toxoid, and acellular pertussis antigens (i.e., Tdap) for routine use in adolescents and adults. Tdap is recommended only for a single dose across all age groups, including as a one-time-only substitute for the next scheduled or recommended Td booster in individuals who previously completed their primary vaccination series with DTP or DTaP. The preferred age for Tdap vaccination is 11 to 12 years. Adolescents 11 to 18 years of age who completed their primary series with DTP or DTaP are encouraged to receive Tdap. Tdap may be given without regard to prior immunization history (e.g., those who received Td less than 10 years earlier) to a patient for whom pertussis immunization is indicated.

Although longer intervals between Td and Tdap could decrease the occurrence of local reactions, the benefits of protection against pertussis outweigh the potential risk for adverse events.[170] Every 10 years thereafter, a tetanus booster should be provided by Td vaccine. Adolescents between the ages of 11 and 18 years who have never been vaccinated against tetanus, diphtheria, or pertussis initially should receive Tdap followed by Td for the subsequent two doses at 4 weeks or more and 6 to 12 months after that.

No pertussis-containing vaccine has been FDA approved for children between the ages of 7 and 10 years. If pertussis vaccine is not contraindicated, children 7 through 10 years of age who are not fully vaccinated (i.e., have not received five doses of DTaP or four doses of DTaP if the fourth dose was administered on or after the fourth birthday) should receive a single dose of Tdap to provide protection against pertussis. If additional doses of tetanus and diphtheria toxoid–containing vaccines are needed for children 7 through 10 years of age after Tdap vaccine is substituted as the first dose, Td vaccine should be provided for the subsequent two doses at 4 weeks or more and 6 to 12 months after that if indicated for the catch-up series.[31,171] Tdap is recommended in this age group because of its reduced antigen content compared with DTaP, resulting in reduced reactogenicity.[171] Pregnant woman should receive Tdap early in the third trimester of each pregnancy.[171]

After exposure to a case of strongly suspected or proven diphtheria, asymptomatic, previously immunized people should receive a booster of an age-appropriate diphtheria toxoid–containing vaccine if they have not received a booster dose of a diphtheria toxoid–containing vaccine within 5 years. For people 10 years or older, Tdap is preferred over Td if a pertussis booster vaccine was not previously received.[31] If not previously immunized, carriers should receive age-appropriate diphtheria toxoid–containing vaccine (i.e., DTaP [or DT], Tdap, or Td) as soon as identified and should complete the entire series. Patients recovering from diphtheria infection should be immunized because infection does not confer immunity.

Precautions and Contraindications

The only contraindication to diphtheria toxoid is a history of severe hypersensitivity developing after receipt of a previous vaccine dose. Vaccination with diphtheria or tetanus toxoid is not associated with an increased risk of convulsions. Local reactions alone do not preclude continued use.

Haemophilus influenzae Type b Vaccine

Before the introduction of routine infant and childhood vaccination against Hib in 1985, this pathogen was the major cause of invasive bacterial infections in young children in the United States. It was the most common cause of bacterial meningitis and epiglottitis and a significant cause of septic arthritis, osteomyelitis, septicemia, occult febrile bacteremia, pneumonia, pericarditis, and cellulitis in children younger than 5 years, in whom it caused an estimated 12,000 cases of meningitis and 8000 additional cases of invasive Hib disease annually.[198] The cumulative risk for Hib disease was approximately one among every 200 US children in the first 5 years of life, with the peak incidence of Hib meningitis occurring among infants between 6 and 12 months of age. In high-risk populations, such as American Indians and Alaska Natives, rates of disease in the absence of immunizations were higher, and a greater proportion of cases of meningitis occurred early in the first year of life than in low-risk populations.[198,343,680] Although rates of Hib disease among these vulnerable populations have decreased in the postvaccine era, they remain 8 to 10 times higher compared with white and black children younger than 5 years.[89]

In 2000, before the widespread introduction of Hib vaccines in resource-poor countries, the WHO estimated that at least 8 million cases of serious disease in children and approximately 371,000 deaths were attributable to Hib annually.[699] As of 2014, 192 of the 193 WHO member states (99.5%) had adopted conjugated Hib vaccines in their routine immunization programs. As a consequence, invasive Hib disease has been virtually eliminated in many industrialized countries, and its incidence has declined by more than 90% in resource-poor countries with effective national immunization programs. However, the WHO estimates that only 56% of the eligible population globally receives three doses of Hib vaccine, and coverage rates are as low as 21% in the western Pacific.

Hib remains the most common cause of nonepidemic bacterial meningitis among unvaccinated children younger than 1 year. The mortality rate for Hib meningitis treated with appropriate antibiotics is approximately 4%, and 15% to 30% of survivors have hearing impairment or severe permanent neurologic sequelae.[89]

Because most cases of Hib disease occur in infancy, vaccines that induce protection before the age of 6 months are necessary for effective control of Hib disease. The Hib polysaccharide capsule is the major virulence factor, and bactericidal antibodies directed against the polysaccharide antigens are protective. Capsular type b is responsible for more than 90% of systemic *H. influenzae* infections. However, purified polysaccharide vaccines are poor immunogens and children's T-lymphocyte–independent immunoglobulin M (IgM) response is largely ineffective, particularly in children younger than 18 months who lack immunologic memory. Covalent linkage of the purified capsular polysaccharide, polyribosylribitol phosphate (PRP), to a protein carrier creates a conjugate glycoprotein that is T-lymphocyte dependent and elicits protective antibody in infants and young children and significantly greater concentrations of circulating anti-PRP at all ages than does the unconjugated polysaccharide. T-cell–dependent antigens involve helper T-lymphocyte activation of a B-cell humoral antibody response. T-cell–dependent antigens also are able to prime a booster response and induce immunologic memory (i.e., anamnestic response).

The introduction of Hib conjugate vaccines in the United States, first in children at least 18 months of age in 1987 and for routine infant immunization in 1990, dramatically decreased the incidence of meningitis and bacteremia caused by Hib. As of 2000, the incidence of invasive Hib disease in the United States had decreased by 99% since the prevaccine era, with an incidence rate of less than one case per 100,000.[143] During 2000 through 2012, the average annual incidence of invasive disease in young children was lower than the Healthy People 2020 goal of 0.27 case per 100,000 children.[89] The remarkably rapid reduction in incidence of disease was partly the result of the ability of the vaccine to reduce asymptomatic oropharyngeal colonization in vaccinated children that also had the indirect effect of reducing exposure and infection in those not immunized (i.e., community or herd immunity).[63,338] Colonization rates have declined from up to 7% in the prevaccine era to less than 1% in the vaccine era.

Preparations

Three single-antigen Hib conjugate vaccine products and two combination vaccine products that contain Hib conjugate are available in the United States. All Hib vaccines contain polyribosylribitol phosphate (PRP), the organism's polysaccharide capsular antigen. Three licensed single-antigen Hib conjugate vaccines—PRP-OMP (PedvaxHIB, Merck), PRP-T (ActHIB, Sanofi Pasteur), and PRP-T (Hiberix, GlaxoSmithKline)—are approved for use in early infancy (Table 245.7).

Each conjugate vaccine is chemically and immunologically unique. PRP preparations are composed of the type b PRP antigen conjugated to a protein, but they have different protein carriers, sizes of the saccharide component, and chemical linkages. The carrier proteins for PRP-OMP and PRP-T are an outer membrane protein from *Neisseria meningitidis* and tetanus toxoid, respectively. Since July 2000, the entire Hib vaccine supply for the United States has been thimerosal free. The dose of each Hib conjugate vaccine is 0.5 mL and given intramuscularly.

Two licensed combination vaccines containing Hib are available in the United States: DTaP/IPV/PRP-T (Pentacel, Sanofi Pasteur), which is approved for immunization at 2, 4, 6, and 15 to 18 months of age, and MenCY/PRP-T (MenHibRix, GlaxoSmithKline), a combination conjugate vaccine approved in 2012 for children 6 weeks to 18 months of age to prevent meningococcal serogroups C and Y and Hib. Use of DTaP/PRP-T (TriHIBit, Sanofi Pasteur) was discontinued in 2011, and PRP-OMP/Hep B (Comvax, Merck) was discontinued in 2014.

TABLE 245.7 *Haemophilus influenzae* Type b Vaccine Schedules

VACCINE		AGE AT VACCINATION			
Type	**Trade Name**	**2 mo**	**4 mo**	**6 mo**	**12–15 mo**
PRP-T	ActHIB	X (1st)	X (2nd)	X (3rd)	X
	Pentacel[a]	X (1st)	X (2nd)	X (3rd)	X
	Hiberix	X (1st)	X (2nd)	X (3rd)	X
	MenHibrix[b]	X (1st)	X (2nd)	X (3rd)	X
PRP-OMP	PedvaxHIB	X (1st)	X (2nd)	—	X

[a]Combination vaccine with DTaP/IPV + PRP-T.
[b]Combination vaccine with MenCY + PRP-T.
PRP-OMP, Polyribosylribotol phosphate conjugated to the outer membrane protein complex from *Neisseria meningitides*; *PRP-T*, polyribosylribotol phosphate conjugated to tetanus toxoid.

Immunogenicity and Efficacy

Placebo-controlled field trials of Hib conjugate vaccines in infants in the United States demonstrated almost 100% protection and provided the basis for the initial approval of these vaccines for use in this country. In a Navajo population of infants at high risk for Hib disease who were vaccinated at 2 and 4 months of age with PRP-OMP or placebo, vaccine efficacy was 100% at 1 year of age and 93% in total.[577] Licensure of PRP-T was based on immunogenicity in a three-dose schedule that was comparable to that of the other two products. A clinical trial in Great Britain found the efficacy of PRP-T comparable to that of PRP-OMP.[84,649]

Although the data are limited, some evidence suggests that administration of the first dose of the Hib vaccine before the child reaches the age of 6 weeks may result in immunologic tolerance to the Hib antigen and reduce the immune response to subsequent doses.[473] Therefore, Hib vaccines, including combination vaccines that contain Hib conjugate, should not be given to an infant younger than 6 weeks.

Long-term protection induced by invasive Hib disease in unvaccinated children is associated with an anti-PRP antibody concentration of greater than 0.15 µg/mL, whereas concentrations greater than 1.0 µg/mL are considered to be markers of long-term protective immunity in vaccinated children.[89] Children who have invasive Hib infection before 24 months of age may remain at risk for another Hib infection, and they should be immunized according to the age-appropriate schedule for unimmunized children.[32] Children who develop invasive disease despite two to three Hib vaccines and those with recurrent invasive Hib warrant an immunologic evaluation. Nontypeable *H. influenzae* lacks a polysaccharide capsule that renders the Hib vaccine ineffective against this cause of acute otitis media (AOM), acute sinusitis, bronchitis, and community-acquired pneumonia.

Adverse Events

Hib vaccines are well tolerated. Local reactions occur in approximately 25% of recipients but typically are mild and last less than 24 hours.[232,680] Systemic reactions such as fever and irritability are infrequent occurrences. When conjugate vaccines are administered concurrently with DTaP vaccine, the incidence of systemic reactions is similar to that observed when only DTaP is given.[232]

Indications

Routine vaccination against Hib disease is recommended for all children beginning at approximately 2 months of age.[32,89] Two or three doses, depending on the product, given at 2-month intervals (optimal) are indicated by the time that the child is 6 months of age. PedvaxHIB is given as a two-dose primary series at 2 and 4 months, whereas ActHIB, Hiberix, Pentacel, and MenHibRix are approved for immunization at 2, 4, 6, and 15 to 18 months of age (see Table 245.7). The recommended age to initiate the primary series is 2 months, with a minimum age of 6 weeks. The minimum interval between doses is 4 weeks, with at least 8 weeks separating the last dose in the primary series and the booster.

Excellent immune responses have been achieved when vaccines from different manufacturers have been interchanged in the primary series.[53,77,312] PRP-T and PRP-OMP are considered interchangeable for primary and booster vaccinations. If more than a single brand of vaccine is used, the child should receive a three-dose primary series. A final dose of any product, irrespective of the previous vaccines received, is acceptable when the child is 12 to 15 months of age for completion of the Hib vaccine immunization schedule. When feasible, the conjugate vaccine product used for the first dose should be used for subsequent doses in children younger than 12 months.

For American Indian and Alaska Natives, PRP-OMP is the preferred vaccine for the primary series doses. Hib meningitis incidence peaks at a younger age among American Indian and Alaska Native infants.[218,608] PRP-OMP vaccine produces a protective antibody response after the first dose and provides early protection that American Indian and Alaska Native infants particularly need.[20,232,230]

For children in whom immunization for Hib infection has not been initiated by the time that they reach 7 months of age, the recommended schedules depend on the child's age and the choice of conjugate vaccine.[32,89] Previously unimmunized children between 15 and 59 months should be immunized with at least a single dose of any licensed conjugate Hib vaccine. For previously unimmunized children 5 years or older, immunization is indicated only if they have an underlying condition predisposing to Hib disease, such as anatomic or functional asplenia, sickle cell disease, immunoglobulin deficiency and immunoglobulin G2 subclass deficiency, early component complement deficiencies, and HIV infection or if they are recipients of hematopoietic stem cell transplants or are immunosuppressed because of chemotherapy or radiation therapy. More than one dose may be recommended for this population.[32,89]

Precautions and Contraindications

Adverse reactions to Hib-containing monovalent vaccines are uncommon, usually mild, and usually resolve within 12 to 24 hours.[232,230,282,352] Rates of adverse reactions to Hib combination vaccines are similar to those observed with separately administered vaccines.[79,319,493] More complete information about adverse reactions to a specific vaccine is available in the package insert for each vaccine.

Vaccination with a Hib-containing vaccine is contraindicated in infants younger than 6 weeks. Vaccination with a Hib-containing vaccine is contraindicated for people known to have a severe allergic reaction to any component of the vaccine. The tip caps of the Hiberix prefilled syringes can contain natural rubber latex, and the vial stoppers for Comvax, ActHib, and PedvaxHIB contain natural rubber latex, which can cause allergic reactions in people who are latex sensitive. Vaccination with these vaccines is therefore contraindicated for those known to have a severe allergic reaction to dry natural rubber latex. The vial stoppers for Pentacel and MenHibRix do not contain latex.

As with all pertussis-containing vaccines, benefits and risk should be considered before administering Pentacel to those with a history of fever higher than 40.5°C, hypotonic-hyporesponsive episode, persistent inconsolable crying lasting 3 or more hours within 48 hours after receipt of a pertussis-containing vaccine, or seizures within 3 days of receiving a pertussis-containing vaccine.

Hib monovalent and combination conjugate vaccines are inactivated vaccines and can be administered to people with immunocompromising conditions. However, immunologic response to the vaccine may be suboptimal.[408]

Hepatitis A Vaccine

The occurrence of hepatitis A is highest in developing countries and reflects the primary route of transmission: fecal-oral, person-to-person spread. In the United States, before vaccine became available, hepatitis A was a common infection that caused substantial morbidity with significant associated costs.[151,400] In 1995, the hepatitis A vaccine was licensed by the FDA, and during the decades that followed, acute hepatitis A infection in the United States dramatically declined, from 31,032 reported infections in 1995 to an all-time low of 1398 in 2011.[270,494] In 2012 and 2013, however, the first increases in cases occurred since 1995, with 1562 and 1781 reported cases, respectively.[494]

In the prevaccine era, the incidence of hepatitis A varied considerably among different populations.[270,619] A shift occurred in the epidemiology of hepatitis A in the United States after the introduction of hepatitis A vaccine. Disease in the United States most commonly occurred in children 5 to 14 years of age.[270] After vaccines were licensed, rates of infection among children declined more rapidly than did rates among adults, resulting in similar rates among all age groups. Historically, rates of infection were highest among Alaska Natives and American Indians, and most cases occurred in a small number of states and counties in the western and southwestern regions of the country. During the decades after vaccine licensure, we have seen near-elimination of age-specific, racial, and geographic disparities.[270,494]

Individuals at risk for hepatitis A infections include close contacts of people infected with hepatitis A virus (HAV), travelers to developing countries, those who engage in homosexual and bisexual activity, and injecting drug users. However, in approximately 50% of reported cases, no risk factor is identified.[33] These infections likely are attributable to fecal-oral spread from asymptomatic contacts. Because children frequently have asymptomatic infections and can shed virus for prolonged periods, they play an important role in transmission of HAV. Children and infants shed virus for longer periods than adults do, up to several months after the onset of clinical illness. In one study involving adults without an identified source of infection, 52% of their households included a child younger than 6 years.[270]

It has long been recognized that the control and ultimate elimination of hepatitis A by active immunization could best be achieved through universal childhood immunization.[651] However, it was not until 2005 that hepatitis A vaccine was licensed for use in children from 12 to 23 months of age. Before then, it had been restricted to children older than 2 years and consequently could not be incorporated readily into routine infant vaccinations. In May 2006, the ACIP recommended including hepatitis A vaccine in the routine infant immunization schedule.[270]

Before vaccine was available, community-wide outbreaks, recurring every 3 to 10 years in high-risk communities, accounted for much of the occurrence of hepatitis A infection and disease. Outbreaks among children attending childcare and the staff are common occurrences and have been associated with community outbreaks.[326] However, the prevalence of hepatitis A infection among childcare center staff and the children and adolescents who previously attended is not increased, a finding suggesting that infections within childcare settings most commonly reflect transmission within the community that extends to these settings.[326] Transmission of HAV also can occur in institutions for the developmentally disabled and in neonatal intensive care units. Transmissions from hospitalized patients to health care professionals have been reported.[33]

In addition to direct person-to-person transmission, infection can be acquired by the ingestion of contaminated water or food, especially that imported from endemic countries. An outbreak in 2013 from contaminated pomegranate seeds, which were imported to the United States from Turkey, infected 165 people across 10 states; 42% were hospitalized, three developed fulminate hepatitis, and one required liver transplantation.[494]

Preparations

Inactivated and attenuated HAV vaccines have been developed.[239] However, only inactivated vaccines are licensed in the United States. Inactivated HAV vaccine is prepared by methods similar to those used for inactivated poliomyelitis vaccine. Virus is propagated in human diploid fibroblast cell cultures, formalin inactivated, and adsorbed to aluminum hydroxide adjuvant. Two inactivated HAV vaccines are licensed in the United States: Havrix (SmithKline Beecham Biologicals) and Vaqta (Merck & Co.). Vaqta and Havrix have two formulations, an adult and a pediatric product with different antigen content (Table 245.8). The pediatric formulation is indicated for people 12 months to 18 years of age. The vaccines can be used interchangeably.[95]

Limited data indicate that hepatitis A vaccine may be administered simultaneously with other vaccinations.[33] A combination HAV and hepatitis B vaccine (Twinrix) is licensed in the United States for people 18 years and older. All HAV-containing vaccines are administered intramuscularly.

Immunogenicity and Efficacy

Inactivated hepatitis A vaccine is highly immunogenic. After receiving a single dose, 95% of children and most adults seroconvert within 1 month.[33,270] After receipt of a second dose in children, seroconversion approximates 100%. Hepatitis A vaccine is immunogenic in children younger than 2 years old who do not have passively acquired maternal antibody.[536,643] In two large clinical trials of inactivated hepatitis A vaccine in children older than 2 years, the protective efficacy rate was greater than 90%.[358,682] In a double-blind, placebo-controlled, randomized study in Thailand involving approximately 34,000 vaccinees, the protective efficacy rate against clinical hepatitis A was 94% after administration of two doses given 1 month apart; it was 100% after subsequent administration of a 12-month booster dose.[358]

Vaccination has been effective in controlling outbreaks in communities with high rates of disease.[270] For example, in a New York State community in which HAV was highly endemic among children, a single dose of vaccine was 100% effective beginning 3 weeks after immunization in preventing symptomatic disease.[682] Moreover, observations from countries where routine hepatitis A vaccination of infants or children has been implemented suggest a strong herd immunity effect.[221,240] The duration of protection after vaccination is likely to be prolonged. Protective antibody levels of anti-HAV were observed in 99% of children evaluated 5 to 6 years after receiving Vaqta.[681] Kinetic models of antibody decline indicate that protective levels of antibody could exist for more than 25 years in adults and up to 20 years in children.[650,652] No data are available to determine whether and when children will need a hepatitis A booster vaccine. In an ongoing study designed to address the need for a booster dose, no cases of hepatitis A among children 9 years after initial vaccination have been reported.[683]

Reduced vaccine immunogenicity has been observed in infants with passively acquired anti–hepatitis A antibody who are administered hepatitis A vaccines.[221,428,433] Studies demonstrated that despite lower antibody levels in infants born to anti–hepatitis A–positive mothers, most infants with passively acquired antibody had an anamnestic response to a booster dose 1 to 6 years later.[221,269,380] In most infants, maternally acquired anti–hepatitis A antibody declines to undetectable levels by the time the child reaches 12 months of age.[432] Hepatitis A vaccine is highly immunogenic for all infants when administered when they are older than 1 year, irrespective of maternal antibody status.[72,221]

Concurrent administration of immune globulin and vaccine inhibits the peak serum antibody concentration achieved but not the rate of seroconversion.[666] Because antibody concentrations reach much higher than protective levels, this inhibition is not considered clinically significant and supports passive-active immunoprophylaxis when indicated.

TABLE 245.8 Recommended Doses and Schedules for Inactivated Hepatitis A Vaccines

Age (y)	Vaccine Trade Name	Hepatitis A Antigen Dose	Volume per Dose (mL)	No. of Doses	Schedule
1–18	Havrix	720 ELU	0.5	2	Initial and 6≥12 mo later
1–18	Vaqta	25 U[a]	0.5	2	Initial and 6≥18 mo later
≥19	Havrix	1440 ELU	1.0	2	Initial and 6≥12 mo later
≥19	Vaqta	50 U[b]	1.0	2	Initial and 6≥18 mo later
≥18	Twinrix[c]	720 ELU	1.0	3 or 4	Initial, 1 and 6 mo later *or* Initial, 7 days and 21–30 d, followed by a dose at 12 mo

[a]Antigen units; each unit is equivalent to 1 μg of viral protein.
[b]A combination of hepatitis B (Engerix-B, 20 μg) and hepatitis A (Havrix, 720 ELU) vaccine.
[c]Twinrix is licensed for use in people ≥18 years in 3-dose and 4-dose schedules.
ELU, Enzyme-linked immunosorbent assay units.
Modified from American Academy of Pediatrics. Hepatitis A. In: Kimberlin DW, Brady MT, Jackson MA, Long SS, eds. *Red Book: 2015 Report of the Committee on Infectious Diseases*. 30th ed. Elk Grove Village, IL: American Academy of Pediatrics; 2015:391–9.

Adverse Events

Except for rare reports of anaphylaxis and anaphylactoid reaction in adults in Europe and Asia, serious reactions to inactivated HAV vaccine have not been reported.[269,380] Pain, tenderness, and infection at the injection site can occur.[358]

Indications

HAV immunization is recommended routinely for children 12 through 23 months of age, for people who are at increased risk for infection, for those who are at increased risk for severe manifestations of hepatitis A if infected, and for anyone who wants to obtain immunity.[22,33,151,156,270]

All children in the United States should receive hepatitis A vaccine routinely according to the licensed two-dose schedule, with the initial dose administered at 1 year of age (i.e., 12 to 23 months) and the second dose 6 to 12 months later. Children who are not immunized by 2 years of age can be immunized at subsequent visits.

Hepatitis A vaccination is recommended routinely for the following people who are at increased risk for infection[22,33,270]:

- All susceptible people traveling to or working in countries that have a high or intermediate hepatitis A endemicity should be vaccinated or receive immune globulin before departure.[151] HAV vaccine at the age-appropriate dose is preferred to immune globulin. The first dose of HAV vaccine should be administered as soon as travel is considered. One dose of single-antigen vaccine administered at any time before departure can provide adequate protection for most healthy people. Travelers who are younger than 12 months should receive a single dose of immune globulin (0.02 mL/kg), which provides effective protection for up to 3 months; 0.06 mL/kg for travel provides protection up to 6 months.
- Susceptible household members and other close personal contacts of international adoptees newly arriving from countries with high or intermediate hepatitis A endemicity should be vaccinated.[27,156] Data from a study conducted at three adoption clinics in the United States indicate that 1% to 6% of newly arrived international adoptees have acute HAV infection. The risk of HAV infection among close personal contacts of international adoptees is estimated at 106 (range, 90–819) per 100,000 household contacts of international adoptees within the first 60 days after their arrival in the United States. HAV vaccine should be administered to all previously unvaccinated people who anticipate close personal contact (e.g., household contact, regular babysitters) with an international adoptee from a country with high or intermediate endemicity during the first 60 days after arrival of the adoptee in the United States. The first dose of the two-dose HAV vaccine series should be administered as soon as adoption is planned, ideally two or more weeks before the arrival of the adoptee.
- Male adolescents and adults who have sex with men should be immunized. Outbreaks of hepatitis A among men who have sex with men have been reported often, including in urban areas in the United States, Canada, and Australia.
- Adolescent and adult users of injection and noninjection drugs should be vaccinated. Periodic outbreaks among injection and noninjection drug users have been reported in many parts of the United States and in Europe.
- Susceptible patients with chronic clotting disorders who receive clotting factor concentrates should be immunized. Reported outbreaks of hepatitis A in patients with hemophilia receiving solvent-detergent–treated factor VIII and factor IX concentrates were identified during the 1990s, primarily in Europe, although one case was reported in the United States.
- People at risk for occupational exposure (e.g., handlers of HAV-infected primates, people working with HAV in a research laboratory setting) should be immunized. Outbreaks of hepatitis A have been reported among people working with nonhuman primates that were born in the wild rather than those born and raised in captivity.
- People with chronic liver disease are at increased risk for fulminant hepatitis A. Susceptible patients who are awaiting or have received liver transplants should be immunized.

Although the ACIP guidelines do not recommend routine vaccination of food handlers, vaccination of these workers should be considered in areas where state and local health authorities or private employers determine that vaccination is cost-effective.

Postexposure Prophylaxis

People who have been exposed to HAV but have not received HAV vaccine should have one dose of single-antigen HAV vaccine or immune globulin as soon as possible.[151] Table 245.9 provides prophylaxis guidance and dosages. The efficacy of immune globulin or vaccine for postexposure prophylaxis when administered more than 2 weeks after exposure has not been established. Information about the relative efficacy of vaccine compared with immune globulin after exposure is limited, and no data are available for people older than 40 years or those with underlying medical conditions.

All previously unimmunized people with close personal contact with a person with serologically confirmed HAV infection, such as household and sexual contacts, should receive vaccine or immune globulin within 2 weeks after the most recent exposure. Serologic testing of contacts is not recommended because testing adds unnecessary cost and may delay administration of postexposure prophylaxis.

Outbreaks of HAV infection at childcare centers have been recognized since the 1970s, but their frequency has decreased as HAV immunization rates for children have increased and as hepatitis A incidence among children has declined. HAV vaccine or immune globulin should be administered to all previously unimmunized staff members and attendees of childcare centers or homes if one or more cases of hepatitis A are recognized in children or staff members or cases are recognized in two or more households of center attendees. In centers that provide care only to children who do not wear diapers, vaccine or immune globulin need be given only to classroom contacts of an index-case patient.

TABLE 245.9 Recommendations for Postexposure Immunoprophylaxis of Hepatitis A Virus

Time Since Exposure	Age of Patient	Recommended Prophylaxis[a]
≤2 wk	<12 mo	IGIM, 0.02 mL/kg
	12 mo–40 y	HAV vaccine
	≥41 y	IGIM, 0.02 mL/kg but HAV vaccine can be used if IGIM is unavailable
	People of any age who are immunocompromised, have chronic liver disease, or a contraindication to vaccination	IGIM, 0.02 mL/kg
≥2 wk	<12 mo	No prophylaxis
	≥12 mo	No prophylaxis, but HAV vaccine may be indicated for ongoing exposure

[a]Dosage and schedule of HAV vaccine as recommended according to age in Table 245.8.

HAV, Hepatitis A virus; *IGIM*, immune globulin intramuscular.

Modified from American Academy of Pediatrics. Hepatitis A. In: Kimberlin DW, Brady MT, Jackson MA, Long SS, eds. *Red Book: 2015 Report of the Committee on Infectious Diseases*. 30th ed. Elk Grove Village, IL: American Academy of Pediatrics; 2015: 391–399.

When an outbreak occurs (i.e., hepatitis A cases identified in two or more families), vaccine or immune globulin also should be considered for members of households that have children (i.e., center attendees) in diapers. Children and adults with hepatitis A should be excluded from the center until 1 week after onset of illness, until the postexposure prophylaxis program has been completed in the center, or until directed by the health department. Although precise data concerning the onset of protection after postexposure prophylaxis are not available, allowing prophylaxis recipients to return to the childcare center setting immediately after receipt of the vaccine or immune globulin dose seems reasonable.

Schoolroom exposure usually does not pose an appreciable risk for infection, and postexposure prophylaxis is not indicated when a single case occurs and the source of infection is outside the school. However, HAV vaccine or immune globulin can be used for unimmunized people who have close contact with the index patient if transmission within the school setting is documented.

Usually, health care–associated HAV in hospital personnel has occurred through spread from patients with acute HAV infection for whom the diagnosis was not recognized. Careful hygienic practices should be emphasized when a patient with jaundice or known or suspected hepatitis A is admitted to the hospital. When outbreaks occur, HAV vaccine or immune globulin is recommended for people in close contact with infected patients. There is no recommendation for routine preexposure use of HAV vaccine for hospital personnel.

If a food handler is diagnosed with hepatitis A, HAV vaccine or immune globulin should be provided to other food handlers at the same establishment. Food handlers with acute HAV infection should be excluded for 1 week after the onset of illness. Because common-source transmission to patrons is unlikely, postexposure prophylaxis with HAV vaccine or immune globulin typically is not indicated but may be considered if the food handler directly handled food during the time when he or she likely was infectious and had diarrhea or poor hygiene practices and if prophylaxis can be provided within 2 weeks of exposure. Routine HAV immunization of food handlers is not recommended.

Precautions and Contraindications

Hepatitis A vaccine should not be administered to people with a hypersensitivity reaction to any of the vaccine components, such as alum or, in the case of Havrix, phenoxyethanol.[15] Safety data for pregnant women are not available, but the risk is considered to be low or nonexistent because the vaccine contains inactivated, purified viral proteins.

Hepatitis B Vaccine

Hepatitis B virus (HBV) infection is a leading cause of acute hepatitis and a major public health problem of global importance. Its incidence is especially high in many Asian and African countries. Individuals with chronic infection are at risk for chronic hepatitis, cirrhosis, and primary hepatocellular carcinoma. Rates of new infection are highest among adults, but chronic infection is more likely to occur in individuals infected as infants or children. They are at increased risk for chronic and malignant liver disease, and as chronic carriers, they serve as the reservoir for transmission of HBV.

The initial strategies for prevention of hepatitis B through vaccination reflect the various epidemiologic patterns of HBV infection in different areas of the world.[116] In the United States, for example, infection is of comparatively low endemicity and occurs primarily in adolescents and adults. The risk of infection, however, is much greater in certain populations. Examples include those born and living in areas or among groups in which HBV is highly endemic and those with lifestyles predisposing to the acquisition of HBV, such as male homosexual activity, intravenous drug abuse, and promiscuous heterosexual activity.[11] In geographic areas in which HBV infection is highly endemic, infection usually is acquired at birth or during childhood, a pattern prompting the recommendation for universal vaccination of infants. Many countries have adopted hepatitis B vaccine into their national campaigns, and children recently immigrated to the United States from endemic areas confirm this trend, with higher levels of neutralizing antibodies found in newer immigrants.[709]

In 1991, the CDC initiated a comprehensive hepatitis B vaccination strategy to eliminate transmission of HBV in the United States.[116] Critical elements of this strategy included preventing perinatal transmission of HBV by identifying and providing immunoprophylaxis to infants of hepatitis B virus surface antigen (HbsAg)–positive mothers and universal hepatitis B vaccination of infants to interrupt transmission and prevent future infection. This approach provided effective programs for routine childhood immunization, protection without any need to identify specific risk factors, and protection before significant exposure occurred. The positive effects of universal infant immunization had been observed in Taiwan, where the strategy of universal infant immunization already was being used. In Taiwan, the overall prevalence rate of HBV for children 1 to 10 years of age decreased from 9.8% in 1984 to 1.3% in 1994.[182]

In 1994, the ACIP expanded the recommendations to include previously unvaccinated children 11 to 12 years old.[124] In October 1997, these recommendations were expanded to include all unvaccinated children from birth to 18 years old and made hepatitis B vaccine available through the Vaccines for Children (VFC) program for those from birth to 18 years of age who were eligible for the program.[135] The goal of the 1997 recommendations was to increase access to hepatitis B vaccine by encouraging the vaccination of previously unvaccinated children and adolescents when they were seen for routine medical visits.[15] Expansion of the recommended age group for receiving vaccination and for VFC eligibility simplified previous recommendations and eligibility criteria for receiving HBV vaccine. The other ACIP priorities for giving hepatitis B vaccination to children remained unchanged and included the following groups: all infants; children in populations at high risk for HBV infection, such as Alaska Natives, Pacific Islanders, and children who reside in households of first-generation immigrants from countries where HBV infection is moderately or highly endemic; previously unvaccinated children 11 to 12 years of age; and older adolescents and adults in defined at-risk groups.[124,116]

Between 1990 and 2004, the incidence of HBV infection in the United States declined by 75%. The decline was greatest among children and adolescents. Coincident with the decline in HBV incidence, vaccine coverage for children 19 to 35 months of age increased from 16% to 92% from 1991 to 2004.[147] Among adolescents 13 to 15 years old, vaccine coverage increased from 0% to 74% between 1993 and 2004 according to CDC data. Since its inception in 1991, many aspects of the national immunization strategy to eliminate HBV transmission have been implemented with great success, especially the routine vaccination of all infants. Nonetheless, many challenges remain.

Despite the overall decline in hepatitis B incidence and the recommendations for routine vaccination of infants and children, increasing proportions of new HBV infections in the United States occur among adolescents and adults who have defined risk factors, including those with multiple sex partners (i.e., more than one partner during the preceding 6 months), men who have sex with men, and injecting drug users.[441] The primary means of preventing these infections is to identify settings such as correctional facilities, sexually transmitted disease clinics, and drug treatment centers where adolescents and adults with high-risk drug and sexual practices can be routinely accessed and vaccinated. In correctional facilities where previously unvaccinated inmates are offered HBV vaccination, 60% to 80% of inmates accepted offered vaccination.[677]

Although universal screening of all pregnant women has been widely adopted across the United States, fewer than half of all HBsAg-positive pregnant women are identified through prenatal screening.[261] These women with unknown HBsAg status are not screened consistently, even when they are hospitalized during labor and delivery; consequently, their infants do not receive appropriate postexposure prophylaxis.[635] The birth dose of HBV vaccine, which can serve as a safety net for infants born to mothers for whom testing was not performed or not performed correctly, was administered to only 45% of infants born in the United States in 2004, less than the rate of 54% seen before July of 1999, when recommendations were made to suspend the birth dose of hepatitis B vaccine temporarily until a thimerosal-free vaccine became available.[440]

To enhance existing strategies aimed at prevention of perinatal HBV transmission, the ACIP recommended in December of 2005 that all delivery hospitals institute specific policies and procedures to improve identification of infants born to HBsAg-positive mothers and mothers with unknown HBsAg status.[464] These recommendations were made to ensure administration of appropriate postexposure prophylaxis and a birth dose of HBV vaccine to all medically stable infants. A study of prospectively collected data from 5 of 64 US-funded Perinatal Hepatitis B Prevention Programs from 2007 through 2013 found that perinatal hepatitis B virus infection occurred among 1.1% of infants, despite 94.9% of infants receiving hepatitis B vaccine and hepatitis B immune globulin within 12 hours of birth.[583] Infants born to mothers who were younger, hepatitis B e antigen (HbeAg) positive, or who had a high viral load or received fewer than three hepatitis B vaccine doses were at greatest risk for infection.

The 2005 ACIP statement also updated recommendations to improve vaccination coverage of adolescents and children by implementing immunization record reviews for all children 11 to 12 years old and children younger than 19 years who were born in countries with high or intermediate HBV endemicity and by vaccinating all unvaccinated adolescents in settings that provide health care services to this age group.[464]

Preparations

Hepatitis B vaccines consisting of inactivated, purified HBsAg derived from chronic hepatitis B plasma were introduced in the early 1980s. In the late 1980s, two recombinant vaccines (Recombivax HB, Merck & Co.; Engerix-B, SmithKline Beecham Biologicals) were licensed in the United States and are available in single-antigen and combined formulations. Only the recombinant vaccines are available in the United States, but plasma-derived vaccines are widely used in other areas of the world. The recombinant vaccines contain 5 to 40 μg/mL of HBsAg protein. Pediatric formulations contain no thimerosal or only trace amounts.

Vaccine is administered intramuscularly in the anterolateral thigh or deltoid area, depending on the age and size of the recipient. Administration in the buttocks or intradermally has been associated with decreased immunogenicity and is not recommended at any age.

Immunogenicity and Efficacy

The recommended series of three doses of vaccine induces a protective antibody response in more than 95% of infants, children, adolescents, and adults younger than 40 years.[34,464] In field trials, the efficacy rates have been 80% to 95% and usually correlate with immunogenicity. Protection against disease is virtually 100% for people who develop adequate serum antibody concentrations (anti-HBs ≥10 mIU/mL) after receiving vaccination. Adults older than 40 years and immunosuppressed people are less likely to develop protective anti-HBs concentrations.

Hepatitis B vaccine is highly immunogenic. Postvaccination serologic testing is not indicated except for infants born to HBsAg-positive women, people with ongoing occupational exposure to blood, and people with immunosuppressive conditions. Active immunization in combination with passive immunoprophylaxis with hepatitis B immune globulin (HBIG) administered within 12 to 24 hours after birth to infants born to chronically infected mothers is more than 90% effective in preventing transmission of HBV to the infant. Active postexposure vaccination without HBIG administered soon after birth has been effective in preventing perinatal transmission and is used in areas where the use of HBIG is impractical.[310]

Vaccine-induced protection against symptomatic infection in a normal host is prolonged and correlates with immunologic memory, which has been demonstrated in immunized children and adults for at least 12 years after vaccination. Children immunized at birth are protected for at least 10 years. The need for routine booster doses has not been demonstrated.

Vaccine failures related to HBV variants with mutations in the *S* gene leading to conformational changes in the HBsAg protein, the major target for neutralizing anti-HBs antibody, have occurred in fully vaccinated children and perinatally exposed infants who received appropriate active and passive postexposure prophylaxis and in many cases had protective anti-HBs antibody levels.[356] Although no evidence establishes that these escape mutations pose a threat to the effectiveness of current hepatitis B vaccine programs, surveillance to detect emergence of HBV variants in immunized populations is warranted.[464,717]

Adverse Events

Other than soreness at the injection site, reactions to hepatitis B vaccine rarely occur. Postvaccination surveillance performed after licensure of the plasma-derived vaccine indicated a possible association between Guillain-Barré syndrome and receipt of the first vaccine dose, but no evidence indicates an association of Guillain-Barré syndrome with recombinant vaccine.[464,465] Anaphylaxis has been estimated to occur in one of 600,000 doses distributed.[464,465] Several nonfatal pediatric cases have been reported.

Indications

Routine immunization with hepatitis B vaccine is recommended for all infants in the United States and should be completed by 6 to 18 months of age for all infants born to HBsAg-negative mothers.[34,464] Delivery hospitals should develop policies that ensure administration of a birth dose for all infants weighing 2000 g or more at birth unless a physician's order to defer immunization is in place and the serologic status of the mother is in the infant's medical record. Administering the first dose of hepatitis B vaccine soon after birth should minimize the risk of infection because of errors in maternal HBsAg testing or reporting or from exposure to people with chronic HBV infection in the household and can increase the likelihood of completing the vaccine series. For infants weighing less than 2 kg who are born to HBsAg-negative mothers, initiation of vaccine should begin at 1 month of chronologic age. Administration of the second dose of vaccine is recommended 1 to 2 months after administration of the first dose, followed by a third dose when the infant is 6 to 18 months of age.

Only single-antigen hepatitis B vaccine can be used for doses given to infants between birth and 6 weeks of age. Single-antigen or combination vaccine may be used to complete the series; four doses of vaccine can be administered if a birth dose is given and a combination vaccine containing a hepatitis B component is used to complete the series.

Routine screening of all pregnant women for HBsAg is recommended because of the necessity for administering a birth dose of vaccine and HBIG.[34,464] Infants born to HBsAg-positive mothers, including preterm and low-birth-weight infants, should be given HBIG (0.5 mL) within 12 hours after birth at a separate injection site, as well as the birth dose of HBV vaccine.[34,464] If a preterm infant weighing less than 2000 g is born to an HBsAg-positive mother, the birth dose of hepatitis B vaccine should not be counted toward completion of the vaccine series, and three additional doses of hepatitis B vaccine should be administered beginning when the child is 1 month of age. In addition to receiving HBIG and the hepatitis B vaccine series within 12 hours of birth, infants of HBsAg-positive mothers should be tested for HBsAg and antibody to HBsAg (i.e., anti-HBs) at 9 to 12 months of age (or 1–2 months after the final dose of the vaccine series, if the series is delayed) to identify those with chronic HBV infection and those who may require revaccination.[464,582]

A woman whose HBsAg status is unknown at delivery should undergo blood testing as soon as possible to determine it. The infant should receive the first dose of hepatitis B vaccine within 12 hours. If the woman is found to be HBsAg positive, her infant should receive HBIG as soon as possible within 7 days. In populations for which HBsAg testing of pregnant women is not feasible, all infants should receive hepatitis B vaccine at birth and 2 months and complete the series by the time they reach 6 months of age.

Hepatitis B vaccination is recommended for all children and adolescents younger than 19 years in the United States. Children who have not been immunized previously may begin the vaccine series during any visit. All children 11 to 12 years of age should have a review of their immunization records and receive the complete hepatitis B vaccine series if they have not been vaccinated previously. All children and adolescents younger than 19 years who were born in Asia, the Pacific Islands, Africa, or other intermediate- or high-endemic countries or have at least one parent who was born in one of these areas should have a review of their immunization records and complete the hepatitis B vaccine series if they were not vaccinated previously.[464]

TABLE 245.10 **Recommended Doses and Schedules of Hepatitis B Virus Vaccines in the United States**

Group	VACCINE Recombivax HB Dose μg (mL)	 Engerix-B Dose μg (mL)
Infants of HBsAg-negative mothers and children and adolescents <20 y	5 (0.5)	10 (0.5)
Infants of HBsAg-positive mothers (HBIG also recommended)	5 (0.5)	10 (0.5)
Children 1–10 y	5 (0.5)[a]	10 (0.5)[a,b]
Adolescents 11–15 y	10 (0.5)[c]	N/A
Adolescents 11–19 y	5 (0.5)[a]	10 (0.5)[a,b]
Adults (≥20 y)	10 (1.0)	20 (1.0)[b]
Patients undergoing dialysis and other immunocompromised persons		
<20 y[d]	5 (0.5)	10 (0.5)
≥20 y	40 (1.0)[e]	40 (2.0)[f]
Unvaccinated adults with diabetes mellitus 19–59 y[g]	10 (1.0)	20 (1.0)

[a]Pediatric formulation licensed for use in a 3-dose schedule at 0, 12, and 24 months for children 5 to 16 y and at 0, 1, and 6 mo for adolescents 11 to 16 y.
[b]Also licensed as a 4-dose schedule at 0, 1, 2, and 12 mo for all age groups.
[c]Adult formulation administered on a 2-dose schedule at 0 mo and then 4 to 6 mo later, licensed for adolescents 11 to 15 y.[136]
[d]Higher doses may be more immunogenic, but no specific recommendations have been made.
[e]Special formulation for patients undergoing dialysis given at 0, 1, and 6 mo.
[f]Two 1.0-mL doses administered as one or two injections in a 4-dose schedule at 0, 1, 2, and 6 mo.
[g]Three doses administered at 0, 1, and 6 months.[172]
HBIG, Hepatitis B immune globulin; *HBsAg*, hepatitis B surface antigen.
Modified from American Academy of Pediatrics. Hepatitis B. In: Kimberlin DW, Brady MT, Jackson MA, Long SS, eds. *Red Book: 2015 Report of the Committee on Infectious Diseases.* 30th ed. Elk Grove Village, IL: American Academy of Pediatrics; 2015:400–23; Centers for Disease Control and Prevention. A comprehensive immunization strategy to eliminate transmission of hepatitis B virus infection in the United States: recommendations of the Advisory Committee on Immunization Practices (ACIP). Part 1: immunization of Infants, children, and adolescents. *MMWR Recomm Rep.* 2005;54RR-16):1–32.

Vaccination also is recommended for those with one or more of the following risk factors for acquiring HBV infection[34]:

- Sexually active adolescents and adults who have a recently acquired sexually transmitted disease, are seeking evaluation or treatment for a sexually transmitted infection, are identified as sex workers, or have had one or more sex partners in the previous 6 months
- Sexually active men who have sex with men
- Household contacts or sexual partners of HBsAg-positive people
- Injecting drug users
- People at occupational risk for infection through exposure to blood or blood-contaminated body fluids, such as health care workers and public safety workers
- Residents and staff of institutions for the developmentally disabled
- Patients undergoing hemodialysis (vaccination of those with early renal failure is encouraged before they require hemodialysis)
- Patients with human immunodeficiency virus (HIV) infection, chronic liver disease, or diabetes mellitus
- Members of households with international adoptees who are HBsAg positive
- Travelers, especially children, to areas with high and intermediate rates of infection with HBV who have close contact with the local population or are likely to have contact with blood, such as in a medical setting or by sexual contact with residents
- Inmates in long-term correctional facilities

In addition to active and passive immunoprophylaxis of infants born to HBsAg-positive mothers, postexposure prophylaxis is recommended in the following circumstances:

- Sexual partner of an HBsAg-positive person. A single dose of HBIG within 14 days of the last sexual contact and initiation of the three-dose hepatitis B vaccination is recommended for susceptible people.
- Household exposure or close contact of an unvaccinated infant younger than 12 months old to a primary caregiver who has acute or chronic hepatitis B infection. Infants in this circumstance should receive HBIG and be vaccinated against hepatitis B. If at the time of exposure only one dose of vaccine has been administered, the second dose should be administered if the interval is appropriate, or HBIG should be administered if immunization is not yet due. If the infant has been immunized fully or has received at least two doses of vaccine, the infant should be presumed protected, and HBIG is not required.
- Accidental percutaneous or per mucosal exposure of a susceptible person to HBsAg-positive blood, such as a needlestick or other accident involving blood in a hospital or an injury to a susceptible person caused by the bite of an HBsAg-positive child. For this indication, HBIG and vaccine are given. Recommendations in these circumstances are complex and based on the availability of the blood source for HBsAg testing and the hepatitis B vaccination status of the exposed person.

Booster doses are not recommended except for patients undergoing hemodialysis and possibly other immunocompromised patients, who should undergo annual antibody testing to assess the need. An additional dose is indicated for those whose serum anti-HBsAg concentration is less than 10 mIU/mL.

The current recommended doses and schedule for the use of hepatitis B vaccines licensed in the United States in infants and other age groups are shown in Table 245.10, and more information can be found elsewhere.[34,464,465] For completing the hepatitis B vaccine series and achieving complete vaccination for hepatitis B, the two licensed hepatitis B vaccines are interchangeable when administered in doses recommended by the manufacturers.[34,464] In September 1999, the FDA approved an optional two-dose schedule of Recombivax HB for vaccination of adolescents 11 to 15 years of age. The ACIP recommended that this schedule be included in the VFC program in February 2000.[136] With the two-dose schedule, the adult dose of Recombivax HB is administered to adolescents 11 to 15 years old, with the second dose given 4 to 6 months after the first dose. In immunogenicity studies enrolling adolescents 11 to 15 years of age, antibody concentrations and seroprotection rates were similar with the two-dose schedule and the currently licensed three-dose schedule. Follow-up data collected during the course of 2 years indicated that the rate of decline in concentration of antibody for the two-dose schedule was similar to that for the three-dose schedule.

No data are available to assess long-term protection or immune memory after vaccination with the two-dose schedule, and whether booster doses of vaccine will be required is not known. Children and adolescents who have begun vaccination with a dose of the pediatric formulation should complete the three-dose series with this dose. Similarly, if the formulation administered to an adolescent at the start of a series is not known, the series should be completed with the three-dose schedule.

A combination of hepatitis B (Engerix-B, 20 μg) and hepatitis A (Havrix, 720 enzyme-linked immunosorbent assay units [ELU]) vaccine (i.e., Twinrix) is licensed for use in people 18 years or older in a three-dose schedule administered at birth, 1 month, and 6 or more months later. An alternative four-dose schedule was approved in 2007; vaccinations are given at birth, day 7, and between days 21 and 30 and followed by a booster dose at 12 months.[34]

In December of 2006, the ACIP approved recommendations for hepatitis vaccine use in adults.[465] In settings in which high proportions of adults are at risk for HBV infection, the ACIP recommends universal hepatitis B vaccination for all unvaccinated adults. Settings include sexually transmitted infection treatment facilities, HIV testing and treatment facilities, facilities providing drug abuse treatment and prevention services, health care settings targeting services to injection drug users, correctional facilities, health care settings serving men who have sex with men, chronic hemodialysis facilities and end-stage renal disease programs, and institutions and nonresidential care facilities for people with developmental disabilities.

For other primary care and specialty medical settings in which adults at risk for HBV infection receive care, the ACIP recommends that health care providers inform all patients about the health benefits of vaccination, including the risk of acquiring HBV infection, and other people for whom vaccination is recommended. They should vaccinate adults who report a risk of developing HBV infection and any adults requesting protection from HBV infection. To promote vaccination in all settings, health care providers should implement standing orders to identify adults recommended for hepatitis B vaccination and administer vaccination as part of routine clinical services, not require acknowledgment of an HBV infection risk factor for adults to receive vaccine, and use available reimbursement mechanisms to remove financial barriers to receiving hepatitis B vaccination.

In 2011, the ACIP recommended that all previously unvaccinated adults 19 through 59 years of age with type 1 or type 2 diabetes mellitus be vaccinated against hepatitis B as soon as possible after a diagnosis of diabetes is made. Unimmunized adults with diabetes mellitus who are 60 years or older may be vaccinated at the discretion of the treating clinician after assessing their risk.[172]

Contraindications

The only contraindication to receiving HBV vaccination is a history of anaphylaxis to a previous dose of vaccine. Data on the safety of HBV vaccines are not available for pregnant women, but because the vaccines contain only HBsAg and not live virus, they should not harm the developing fetus. Because HBV infection during pregnancy can result in transmission to the neonate, susceptible women at increased risk for infection should be vaccinated during pregnancy. Inadvertent vaccination of HBsAg-positive people has no deleterious effects.

Human Papillomavirus Vaccine

Genital HPV infection is thought to be the most common sexually transmitted viral infection, accounting for more than 14 million new cases annually in the United States.[579] The estimated prevalence of HPV infection among 15- to 19-year-olds is 32.9%, and among 20-to 24-year-old, sexually active women, it is 53.8%.[579] Prevalence is thought to be similar among males.[249] HPV typically infects girls and women soon after sexual exposure.[208,690] Median time from first intercourse to first detection of HPV is only 3 months.[208] The estimated lifetime risk of acquiring HPV infection by those with at least one sexual partner is more than 84% for women and more than 91% for men.[189] More than 80% of women and men acquire HPV infection by 45 years of age.[189]

More than 40 HPV types can infect the genital tract and are classified on the basis of their association with cervical cancer.[492] The low-risk, nononcogenic HPV types (i.e., types 6 and 11) are associated with anogenital warts, mild cervical dysplasia, and recurrent respiratory papillomatosis. The high-risk, oncogenic HPV types are causally linked to several human cancers in women and men, including cancers of the cervix, vulva, vagina, anus, and penis and a subset of head and neck cancers.[439] Infection with HPV causes almost all cases of cervical cancer, and before vaccine development, it was the second most common cause of death from cancer among women globally, surpassed only by breast cancer.[439] Cervical cancer remains a significant cause of cancer death worldwide.[265] The development of cervical cancer often occurs decades after initial infection. HPV types 16 and 18 account for 70% of cervical cancers.[196] A variety of other types account for the remaining 30% of cervical cancers, and these types vary in their distribution globally.

Although the incidence of HPV is high, most infections clear without intervention. Seventy percent of new infections clear within 1 year, and 91% clear within 2 years.[196] Persistent infection with high-risk HPV types, defined as detection of the same viral type at two or more visits 6 months apart, is the most important risk factor for developing cervical cancer precursor lesions. Studies have demonstrated that persistent infection with a high-risk HPV type is associated with a greater than 10-fold risk of high-grade cervical cancer precursors.[350,483]

Three prophylactic HPV subunit vaccines are licensed and recommended for use in the United States.[457,533] Use of these vaccines has significantly decreased the prevalence of vaccine-type HPV infection. In one study, vaccine-type HPV prevalence in the study population decreased by 75% among women and more than 90% among vaccinated women.[379] Areas with high HPV vaccine coverage have seen decreases in anogenital warts.[244,245,547] The impact on the incidence of HPV-related cervical and other anogenital cancers will take years to assess because the cancers can occur decades after infection. Incidence of recurrent respiratory papillomatosis and associated cancers also is likely to decrease as a result of widespread vaccination.

Preparations

In 2006, the FDA licensed the first HPV vaccine for use in girls and women 9 through 26 years of age in the United States, and this was done for use in boys and men 9 through 26 years of age in 2009.[35,167,456] The quadrivalent vaccine (Gardasil, Merck & Co.) contains HPV types 6, 11, 16, and 18 virus-like particles (VLPs) and protects against four HPV types, which together cause 70% of cervical cancers (i.e., HPV types 18 and 16) and 90% of genital warts (i.e., HPV types 6 and 11).

The quadrivalent HPV vaccine (HPV4) is prepared from the highly purified VLPs of the major capsid (L1) protein of HPV types 6, 11, 16, and 18. The L1 proteins are produced by *Saccharomyces cerevisiae* and self-assemble into VLPs. The VLPs mimic the HPV virus, but they contain no viral DNA. Each 0.5-mL dose contains 20 µg of HPV 6 L1 protein, 40 µg of HPV 11 L1 protein, 40 µg of HPV 16 L1 protein, and 20 µg of HPV 18 L1 protein.

A bivalent vaccine (HPV2) (Cervarix, GlaxoSmithKline), which is directed against two oncogenic HPV types (i.e., 16 and 18), was licensed for use in girls and women 10 through 25 years of age in 2009 and not licensed for males.[35,159]

A 9-valent vaccine (9vHPV) (Gardasil 9, Merck), which protects against the same four HPV types as the quadrivalent HPV vaccine plus HPV 31, 33, 45, 52, and 58 VPs, was approved by the FDA in 2014 and recommended by the ACIP in 2015.[277,533] It was licensed for use in men and women 9 to 26 years of age.[277]

The HPV vaccines use alum as an adjuvant and do not contain thimerosal or antibiotics. The vaccines should be stored at 2°C to 8°C (36°F–46°F) and not frozen.[159]

Primary vaccination dosing schedules with HPV vaccines are the same and consist of three 0.5-mL doses administered intramuscularly. The second and third doses should be administered 2 and 6 months after administration of the first dose. In 2016, the ACIP recommended that 9- to 14-year-old children receive two HPV vaccine doses instead of the previously recommended three doses because studies showed good immune responses compared with earlier groups receiving three doses.[474] The recommendation for three doses remained the same for ages 15 to 26 years. The FDA also announced approval of the two-dose schedule for the 9vHPV vaccine.[278] Due to licensing and manufacturing issues, 9vHPV will be the primary HPV vaccine going forward.

Immunogenicity and Efficacy

Data from randomized, controlled trials (RCTs) have shown consistently that prophylactic HPV VLP vaccines are immunogenic and efficacious in preventing infection and lesions caused by the targeted HPV types.[336,402,439,476,616] Vaccine efficacy seems to be mediated by a type-specific humoral immune response.

Evaluations of the quadrivalent HPV4 vaccine have demonstrated that vaccinated individuals develop high antibody titers to the respective HPV types that exceed the antibody titers seen with natural HPV infection.[616] However, the level of antibody that confers a protective response is unknown.[616] For the HPV4 VLP vaccine, an antibody response significantly greater than placebo was sustained for at least 3 years without booster doses.[336,663] Although vaccine efficacy studies have been done only enrolling adolescents 13 years or older, immunogenicity bridging studies have been performed with children as young as 9 years of age. Antibody titers to HPV types 6, 11, 16, and 18 were found to be higher in younger adolescents than in young adults. From these data, investigators inferred that protection exists against cervical cancer, cancer precursor lesions, and genital warts, even for young adolescent girls who receive the HPV4 vaccine.

The results from four RCTs demonstrate that a regimen of three intramuscular injections of HPV VLP vaccine provides high-level protection from infection and lesions caused by targeted HPV types.[402,439] A combined analysis of HPV4 vaccine efficacy in phase II and phase III clinical trials showed 100% protection against precancerous lesions (i.e., carcinoma in situ II/III or adenoma in situ) caused by HPV type 16 or 18 and 99% protection against genital wart development.[476]

A randomized, multicenter, double-blind study found the 9vHPV vaccine antibody response to HPV types 6, 11, 16, and 18 to be noninferior to the response with the HPV4 vaccine.[378] From this result, the 9vHPV vaccine can be inferred to have the same protective efficacy as the HPV4 vaccine. The 9vHPV vaccine prevented infection and disease related to HPV types 31, 33, 45, 52, and 58; for high-grade cervical, vulvar, or vaginal disease related to these HPV types, the vaccine had a 96.7% efficacy rate.[378]

It is not known whether HPV vaccines provide long-term protection or booster doses will be necessary. The quadrivalent HPV4 vaccine does not have efficacy against existing disease or infection caused by HPV.

HPV2 vaccine efficacy was evaluated in two randomized, double-blind, controlled clinical trials in females 15 through 25 years of age. In the analysis, 99% or more of participants developed an HPV 16 and 18 antibody response 1 month after completing the three-dose series. After concomitant administration of HPV2 with tetanus toxoid, diphtheria toxoid, and acellular pertussis vaccine and/or with meningococcal conjugate vaccine in females 11 through 18 years of age compared with those after administration at separate visits, the antibody responses for bivalent vaccine antigens were noninferior.[159]

In summary, HPV vaccines are highly effective in preventing HPV-16 and HPV-18–related cervical precancerous lesions in females. The HPV4 vaccine is highly effective in preventing HPV-6 and HPV-11–related genital warts in females and males, and HPV4 vaccine also is effective in preventing anal precancerous lesions in males. Vaccines offer no protection against progression of infection to disease from HPV acquired before immunization.[35]

Adverse Events

HPV vaccines appear to be generally safe and well tolerated.[620] The HPV4 and 9vHPV vaccines have similar safety profiles.[533] The most common adverse events are local injection site reactions such as mild to moderate pain, redness, pruritus, or swelling.[533] For females 9 to 26 years of age, 9vHPV compared with HPV4 vaccine recipients had more injection site adverse events, including swelling (40.3% vs. 29.1%) and redness (34.0% vs. 25.8%).[533]

In analyses of local and general adverse events after bivalent HPV2 vaccine administration versus control vaccines, 92% reported injection site pain, 48%, had redness, and 44% had swelling in the HPV2 group. These findings compared with 64% to 87%, 24% to 28%, and 17% to 21% in the control groups for the same findings. Fatigue, headache, and myalgia were the most common general symptoms reported.[159]

Additional data on vaccine safety, including data on pregnancy and fetal and infant outcomes, are being collected. Data will continue to be collected in postlicensure studies.

Indications

The ACIP issued recommendations for the use of the HPV4 vaccine in March 2007, the bivalent HPV2 vaccine in May 2010, and the 9vHPV in March 2015.[159,160,167,457,456,533] Routine vaccination with three doses of vaccine is recommended for girls 11 to 12 years of age. The vaccination series can be started in girls as young as 9 years of age at the discretion of physicians and parents. Catch-up vaccination is recommended for girls and women 13 to 26 years of age who have not been vaccinated previously or who have not completed the full vaccination series.

Only HPV4 and 9vHPV vaccines are recommended for routine immunization of boys at 11 or 12 years of age (the series can be started at 9 years of age), and it is recommended for boys and men 13 through 21 years of age not previously immunized.[209] Men 22 through 26 years of age may be immunized on request. Vaccine is recommended for men who have sex with men and males who are immunocompromised (including those with HIV infection) through 26 years of age.

Ideally, vaccination should be administered before potential exposure to HPV through sexual contact occurs. HPV vaccines are not licensed for use in people older than 26 years.[35]

Vaccine is administered in a three-dose schedule, and the second and third doses should be administered 2 and 6 months after the first dose. Immunogenicity data allow for some degree of flexibility in the dosing schedule, which is often an important consideration in providing multidose vaccines to adolescents for whom contact with health providers can be sporadic. For both vaccines, the minimum interval from dose 1 to dose 2 is 4 weeks. The minimum interval from dose 2 to dose 3 should not be less than 12 weeks. For ages 9 to 14 years, vaccine can be administered in a two-dose schedule, with the second dose administered at least 6 months after the first dose. The three-dose schedule should be used for ages 15 to 26 years.[474]

HPV vaccine can be administered at the same visit when other age-appropriate vaccines, such as Tdap, Td, and MCV4 (meningococcal), are provided.[508] Women who have received an HPV vaccine must continue to have regular Papanicolaou test screening. HPV vaccines do not provide protection against all HPV types associated with development of cancer, and vaccines do not alter the progression of HPV infection acquired before immunization.

People through 26 years of age with evidence of current HPV infection, such as cervical dysplasia, a positive HPV DNA test result, or anogenital warts or a history of anogenital warts, should receive HPV immunization because infection with all vaccine HPV types is unlikely and the vaccine can provide protection against HPV infection with types not already acquired.[35] Vaccine recipients should be advised that data from clinical trials do not indicate the vaccine will have any therapeutic effect on existing abnormalities found by Papanicolaou testing, on HPV infection, or on genital warts. However, HPV vaccination can provide protection against infection with HPV types not already acquired.

Lactating women can receive HPV4 or 9vHPV vaccine, but the bivalent vaccine has not been studied in lactating women. Patients of the appropriate age who are immunocompromised due to disease or medication can receive HPV vaccine. However, the immune response to vaccination and vaccine effectiveness may be less than in those who are immunocompetent.

Contraindications and Precautions

HPV4 and 9vHPV vaccines are contraindicated for people with a history of immediate hypersensitivity to yeast or to any vaccine component.[533] Bivalent HPV2 vaccine is contraindicated for people with a history of immediate hypersensitivity to any vaccine component. HPV2 vaccine in the prefilled syringe formulation should not be administered to latex-sensitive individuals because the rubber stopper contains latex.[35]

HPV vaccine is listed under pregnancy category B and is not recommended for use in pregnancy.[159,457] If an adolescent becomes pregnant during the vaccination period, subsequent doses should be deferred until after parturition. The vaccine has not been associated causally with adverse outcomes of pregnancy or adverse effects on the developing fetus. However, data on vaccination during pregnancy are limited.

Influenza Vaccine

Influenza virus infection continues to cause significant morbidity and mortality despite the availability of effective vaccines and antiviral therapy for prevention and treatment of influenza. In the United States, epidemics of influenza typically occur during the winter months and have been associated with an average of approximately 36,000 deaths per year, and between 1976 and 2007, estimated cases ranged from 3000 to 49,000 each year.[158,638]

Influenza viruses cause disease among all age groups.[300,301,486] Rates of infection are highest among children, but rates of serious illness and death are highest among those 65 years or older, children 2 years or younger, and people of any age who have medical conditions that increase the risk of complications from influenza.[65,64,299,486] The impact of influenza on normal children and those with underlying high-risk conditions is appreciable, and the burden of disease in young children attributed to influenza is underrecognized.[542] Attack rates among normal children have been estimated at 10% to 40% each year, and approximately 1% of influenza infections result in hospitalization.[302,542] Influenza also causes a significant burden in outpatient settings, especially for those 2 to 17 years of age.[279]

A major difficulty in the development and provision of satisfactory immunizing agents for the prevention of influenza is the antigenic variation of the viruses. Periodic minor antigenic changes in influenza A or B virus are the major factors in the continuing occurrence of yearly influenza. Although outbreaks usually are limited in magnitude, the resulting morbidity and mortality remain discouragingly high. Major antigenic changes in influenza A virus, as occurred in 1957 to 1958 (Asian strain), in 1968 to 1969 (Hong Kong strain), and again in 2009 (pH1N1) account for the pandemic spread of disease associated with greater overall morbidity and mortality. The CDC estimates that in the 2009 pandemic the H1N1 influenza virus caused more than 60 million Americans to become ill and led to more than 270,000 hospitalizations and 12,500 deaths.[371] People younger than 65 years accounted for 90% of hospitalizations and deaths. With typical seasonal influenza, approximately 90% of the people who die are older than 65 years.

Preparations

An assortment of influenza vaccines are licensed for use in the United States: inactivated trivalent influenza vaccine (IIV3), adjuvanted inactivated trivalent influenza vaccine (aIIV3), recombinant trivalent influenza vaccine (RIV3), inactivated quadrivalent influenza vaccine (IIV4), inactivated quadrivalent cell culture-based influenza vaccine (ccIIV4), and live attenuated quadrivalent influenza vaccine (LAIV).[101,315]

The trivalent vaccines contain three virus strains (usually two type A and one type B), and the composition is changed periodically in anticipation of the prevalent influenza strains expected to circulate in the United States in the following winter. The quadrivalent vaccines include an additional type B strain.[315] Most vaccines are prepared from virus grown in the allantoic sac of the chick embryo. Exceptions include one IIV4 preparation with virus propagated through canine kidney cells and the RIV3 preparation, which is manufactured without the use of influenza viruses.[315]

IIV3, aIIV3, IIV4, and ccIIV4 are inactivated influenza vaccines (IIVs) that contain no live virus. IIVs distributed in the United States consist of subvirion vaccine, prepared by disrupting the lipid-containing membrane of the virus, or purified surface-antigen vaccine. All IIV formulations are available for intramuscular use, except ccIIV4, which is intradermal.

IIV4 is licensed and recommended for children 6 months or older and for adults, including those with or without chronic medical conditions. Vaccine is available in pediatric (0.25-mL dose) and adult (0.5-mL dose) formulations. IIV3 and ccIIV4 (using the 0.5-mL dose) are licensed and recommended for children 4 years or older and for adults. RIV3, also in the 0.5-mL dose, is licensed and recommended for those18 years or older.

IIV is administered intramuscularly into the anterolateral thigh of infants and young children and into the deltoid muscle of older children and adults. RIV3 is administered intramuscularly into the deltoid muscle. The volume of vaccine depends on age. Infants and toddlers 6 months through 35 months of age should receive a dose of 0.25 mL, and all individuals 36 months or older should receive 0.5 mL per dose. Children younger than 9 years who are being immunized against influenza for the first time should receive two doses of TIV given 4 weeks apart before the start of the influenza season. IIV is shipped and stored at 2°C to 8°C (35°F–46°F).

The intradermal formulation of IIV4 is licensed for the 2016–2017 influenza season for use in individuals 18 through 64 years of age.[315] It is administered preferably over the deltoid muscle and only by using the device included in the vaccine package. Vaccine is supplied in a single-dose, prefilled microinjection system (0.1 mL). The intradermal formulation of IIV4 is shipped and stored at 2°C to 8°C (35°F–46°F).

Many manufacturers produce inactivated influenza vaccine each year for the US market. Vaccines are available in single-dose syringes and vials or multidose vials and in preservative-free formulations. Approved age indications vary by manufacturer and product. Clinicians should obtain inactivated influenza vaccine appropriate for the age groups they plan to vaccinate. The ACIP does not recommend use of influenza vaccine outside the vaccine's FDA-approved age indication. Tables listing each year's influenza vaccines are available in the annual ACIP and AAP influenza statements and on the CDC influenza website (https://www.cdc.gov/flu/professionals/vaccination/vaccine_safety.htm). Package inserts should be consulted for recommended age groups and possible contraindications for each vaccine in addition to information regarding additional components of various vaccine formulations.

LAIV is cold adapted, developed by passaging the viruses at successively lower temperatures in tissue culture so that replication occurs only in the upper respiratory tract.[74] LAIV is licensed by the FDA for healthy individuals 2 through 49 years of age. It has not been recommended for those with a history of asthma or other high-risk medical conditions associated with an increased risk of complications from influenza.

LAIV is administered intranasally in a prefilled, single-use sprayer containing 0.2 mL of vaccine. A removable dose-divider clip is attached to the sprayer to administer 0.1 mL separately into each nostril. Children younger than 9 years being immunized against influenza for the first time should receive two doses of LAIV given 4 weeks apart before the start of the influenza season. The LAIV formulation licensed in the United States must be shipped and stored at 2°C to 8°C (35°F–46°F). After the vaccine is warmed to room temperature for intended use, it must be used within 30 minutes.

Trivalent influenza vaccines contain A (H1N1), A (H3N2), and B viral antigens. The quadrivalent influenza vaccines include an additional B viral antigen because of the difficulty of predicting which B virus lineage will predominate during a given season.

Immunogenicity and Efficacy

Children 6 months or older typically have protective levels of anti-influenza antibody against specific influenza virus strains after receiving the recommended number of doses of seasonal inactivated influenza vaccine.[226,305,417,499,702,704] Immunogenicity studies using the influenza A (H1N1) 2009 monovalent vaccine indicated that more than 90% of children 9 years or older responded to a single dose with anti-influenza antibody levels considered to be protective. Young children had inconsistent responses to a single dose of the influenza A (H1N1) 2009 monovalent vaccine across studies, with 20% of children 6 to 35 months of age responding to a single dose with protective anti-influenza antibody levels. However, in all studies, 80% to 95% of vaccinated infants, children, and adolescents developed protective anti-influenza antibody levels to the 2009 H1N1 influenza virus after two doses.[56,506,538]

In most seasons, one or more seasonal vaccine antigens are changed compared with the previous season. In consecutive years when vaccine antigens change, children younger than 9 years who received only one dose of vaccine in their first year of vaccination are less likely to have protective antibody responses when administered only a single dose during their second year of vaccination compared with children who received two doses in their first year of vaccination.[258,502,668]

When the vaccine antigens do not change from one season to the next, priming children 6 to 23 months of age with a single dose of vaccine in the spring followed by a dose in the fall results in similar antibody responses compared with a regimen of two doses in the fall.[257] However, one study conducted during a season when the vaccine antigens did not change compared with the previous season estimated 62% effectiveness against influenza-like illness for healthy children who had received only one dose in the previous influenza season and only one dose in the study season compared with 82% for those who received two doses separated by 4 weeks or more during the study season.[10]

The antibody response for children at higher risk for influenza-related complications (e.g., children with chronic medical conditions) may be lower than those reported typically for healthy children.[71,316] However, antibody responses among children with asthma are similar to those of healthy children and are not substantially altered during asthma exacerbations requiring short-term prednisone treatment.[522]

Vaccine effectiveness studies also have indicated that two doses are needed to provide adequate protection during the first season that young children are vaccinated. Among children younger than 5 years who have never received influenza vaccine previously or who received only one dose of influenza vaccine in their first year of vaccination, vaccine effectiveness is lower compared with children who received two doses in their first year of being vaccinated. Two large, retrospective studies of young children who had received only one dose of IIV in their first year of being vaccinated found no decrease in influenza-like illness–related office visits compared with unvaccinated children.[10,558] Similar results were reported in a case-control study of children 6 to 59 months of age in which laboratory-confirmed influenza was the outcome measured.[602] These results, along with the immunogenicity data indicating that antibody responses are substantially higher when young children are given two doses, are the basis for the recommendation that all children 6 months to 8 years of age who are being vaccinated for the first time should receive two vaccine doses separated by 4 weeks or more.

Estimates of vaccine efficacy or effectiveness among children 6 months or older have varied by season and study design. In a randomized trial conducted during five influenza seasons (1985–90) in the United States for children 1 to 15 years of age, annual vaccination reduced laboratory-confirmed influenza A substantially (77–91%).[501] A 1-year, placebo-controlled study reported vaccine efficacy rates against laboratory-confirmed influenza illness of 56% for healthy children 3 to 9 years of age and 100% for healthy children and adolescents 10 to 18 years old.[197]

A randomized, double-blind, placebo-controlled trial conducted during two influenza seasons among children 6 to 24 months of age indicated that the efficacy rate was 66% against culture-confirmed influenza illness during the 1999–2000 influenza season but did not reduce culture-confirmed influenza illness substantially during the 2000–01 influenza season.[351] A case-control study conducted during the 2003–04 season indicated vaccine effectiveness of 49% against laboratory-confirmed influenza.[602] An observational study of children 6 to 59 months of age with laboratory-confirmed influenza compared with children who tested negative for influenza reported vaccine effectiveness of 44% in the 2003–04 influenza season and 57% during the 2004–05 season.[255] Partial vaccination (i.e., only one dose for children being vaccinated for the first time) was not effective in either study.

During an influenza season (2003–04) with a suboptimal vaccine match, a retrospective cohort study conducted among approximately 30,000 children 6 months to 8 years of age indicated vaccine effectiveness of 51% against medically attended, clinically diagnosed pneumonia or influenza (i.e., no laboratory confirmation of influenza) among fully vaccinated children and 49% among approximately 5000 children 6 to 23 months old.[558]

Another retrospective cohort study of similar size conducted during the same influenza season in Denver but limited to healthy children 6 to 21 months of age estimated clinical effectiveness of 2 IIV doses to be 87% against pneumonia or influenza-related office visits.[10]

Among children, TIV effectiveness may increase with age.[501,711] A systematic review of published studies estimated vaccine effectiveness at 59% for children 2 years or older but concluded that additional evidence was needed to demonstrate effectiveness among children 6 months to 2 years old.[370]

Because of the recognized influenza-related disease burden among children with other chronic diseases or immunosuppression and the long-standing recommendation for vaccination of these children, randomized, placebo-controlled studies to determine efficacy in high-risk children are needed but are currently unavailable. Although data about influenza vaccine in specific immunocompromised states are limited, the Infectious Diseases Society of America (IDSA) publishes guidelines for specific immune-compromising diagnoses.[568] In a nonrandomized, controlled trial enrolling children 2 to 6 years old and 7 to 14 years old who had asthma, vaccine efficacy was 54% and 78% against laboratory-confirmed influenza type A infection and 22% and 60% against laboratory-confirmed influenza type B infection, respectively. Vaccinated children 2 to 6 years of age with asthma did not have substantially fewer type B influenza virus infections compared with the control group in this study.[623]

The association between vaccination and prevention of asthma exacerbations is unclear. Vaccination provided protection against asthma exacerbations in some studies.[403,511]

IIV has reduced AOM in some studies. Two studies reported that IIV decreased the risk of influenza-related otitis media by approximately 30% among children with mean ages of 20 and 27 months, respectively.[194,339] However, a large study conducted among children with a mean age of 14 months indicated that IIV was not effective against AOM.[351] Influenza vaccine effectiveness against a nonspecific clinical outcome such as AOM, which is caused by a variety of pathogens and is not typically diagnosed using influenza virus culture, is expected to be relatively low.

The relative effectiveness of LAIV and IIV for medically attended, laboratory-confirmed influenza was evaluated using US Influenza Vaccine Effectiveness Network data.[192] For the 2013–14 season, children 2 to 8 years of age who received LAIV had significantly higher odds of influenza (odds ratio, 5.36) than those who received IIV[192] The greater odds of illness with influenza A/H1N1pdm09 included the 2010–11 and 2013–14 seasons. Another study of the 2013–14 season found the effectiveness of LAIV against influenza A/(H1N1)pdm09 to be 17%, compared with 60% for IIV, for children 2 to 17 years of age.[284]

After the ACIP recommendation for preferential use of LAIV during the 2014–15 season for children 2 to 8 years of age, another study examined vaccine effectiveness by type.[716] In this study with 9311 participants at 5 US sites, the preference for use of LAIV in young children was not supported. Based on these and several other studies, LAIV was not recommended for use for any age for the 2016–17 season.[101,315]

Adverse Events

All inactivated influenza vaccines contain killed viruses and therefore cannot produce signs or symptoms of influenza caused by active virus infection. The most common symptoms associated with IIV administration are soreness at the injection site and fever. Fever, usually occurring 6 to 24 hours after immunization, affects 10% to 35% of children younger than 2 years. Mild systemic symptoms, such as nausea, lethargy, headache, muscle aches, and chills also can occur after receipt of IIV.

Before the 2010–11 influenza season, an increased risk of febrile seizures after IIV3 administration had not been observed in the United States.[313,329] The CDC and the FDA conducted enhanced monitoring for febrile seizures after influenza vaccination because of reports of an increased risk of fever and febrile seizures in young children in Australia that were associated with a 2010 Southern Hemisphere vaccine produced by CSL Biotherapies. The risk was up to nine febrile seizures per 1000 doses during the 2010–11 influenza season. Due to the increased risk, the ACIP does not recommend the US licensed Afluria (CSL Biotherapies' IIV3) for children younger than 9 years.[164]

For the 2010–11 season, surveillance for US licensed influenza vaccines detected safety signals for febrile seizures in younger children after IIV administration.[426,645] On further review, the increased risk was found for children 6 months through 4 years of age, ranging from the day of vaccination to the day after vaccination (i.e., 0–1-day risk window). The risk was found to be higher when children received concomitant PCV13, and the risk peaked at about 16 months of age.[645] No increased risk was observed for children 5 years or older after IIV or for children of any age after LAIV. The magnitude of the increased risk of febrile seizures in young children in the United States (<1 case/1000 children vaccinated) was substantially lower than the risk observed in Australia in 2010.

After evaluating the data on febrile seizures from the 2010–11 influenza season and taking into consideration benefits and risks of vaccination, no policy change was recommended for use of IIV or PCV13. According to the CDC, surveillance data on febrile seizures in young children after administration of influenza vaccine for the 2011–12 influenza season (i.e., same vaccine formulation as for the 2010–11 season) were consistent with those from the 2010–11 influenza season. No changes in the use of IIV or PCV13 are recommended, although surveillance is ongoing.[315]

LAIV usually is well tolerated and may produce mild signs or symptoms related to influenza virus infection that include headache and runny nose or nasal congestion in vaccinees. Transmission of LAIV strains to unimmunized contacts has been documented only once in prelicensure studies. The proposed explanation for the uncommon occurrence of transmission is that the vaccine virus is shed for a shorter duration and in a much smaller quantity than are wild-type strains.

Indications

Routine annual influenza vaccination is recommended for all people 6 months or older.[37,101,315] To permit time for production of protective antibody levels,[91,317] vaccination optimally should occur before the onset of influenza activity in the community. Vaccination providers should offer vaccination as soon as the vaccine is available. Vaccination should be offered throughout the influenza season (i.e., as long as influenza viruses are circulating in the community).[101,315] Due to the previously described issues with vaccine effectiveness, LAIV was not recommended by the ACIP for any age group for the 2016–17 influenza season.[315]

Particular focus should be on the administration of IIV for all children and adolescents who have underlying medical conditions associated with an increased risk of complications from influenza, including the following:

- Asthma or other chronic pulmonary diseases, including cystic fibrosis
- Hemodynamically significant cardiac disease
- Immunosuppressive disorders or therapy
- HIV infection
- Sickle cell anemia and other hemoglobinopathies
- Diseases that require long-term aspirin therapy, including juvenile idiopathic arthritis or Kawasaki disease
- Chronic renal dysfunction
- Chronic metabolic disease, including diabetes mellitus
- Any condition that can compromise respiratory function or handling of secretions or can increase the risk of aspiration, such as neurodevelopmental disorders, spinal cord injuries, seizure disorders, or neuromuscular abnormalities

Although universal immunization for all individuals 6 months or older is recommended, particular immunization efforts should be made for the following groups to prevent transmission of influenza to those at risk, unless contraindicated:

- Household contacts and out-of-home care providers of children younger than 5 years and at-risk children of all ages should be immunized.
- Any female who is pregnant, is considering pregnancy, has just delivered, or is breastfeeding during the influenza season should be immunized.. Studies have shown that infants born to immunized women have better influenza-related health outcomes. However, the estimated median seasonal vaccination coverage among women with a live birth was only 47% during the 2009–10 influenza season, even though pregnant women and their infants are at higher risk for complications. Data from some studies suggest that influenza vaccination during pregnancy may decrease the risk of preterm birth.
- Health care personnel or health care volunteers should be immunized.. Despite the recent AAP recommendation for mandatory influenza immunization for all health care personnel,[76,101] many remain unvaccinated. The CDC estimated that only 77% of health care personnel received the seasonal influenza vaccine for the 2014–15 season.[81] The AAP recommends mandatory vaccination of health care personnel because they frequently come into contact in their clinical settings with patients at high risk for influenza illness.
- Close contacts of immunosuppressed individuals should be immunized.

Previously unimmunized children between 6 months to 9 years of age should receive two doses of influenza vaccine before the onset of influenza season. Available data suggest that children younger than 9 years who did not receive the second dose of influenza vaccine in the initial year that influenza vaccine was given may not be adequately protected the next influenza season with only one dose. In this group, levels of protection can be suboptimal, especially if the antigenic specificity of the predominant strains has changed from the previous year. The AAP recommends that two doses be given to these children the following influenza season.[101] This recommendation applies only to the influenza season that follows the first year that a child younger than 9 years old receives influenza vaccine (Fig. 245.2).

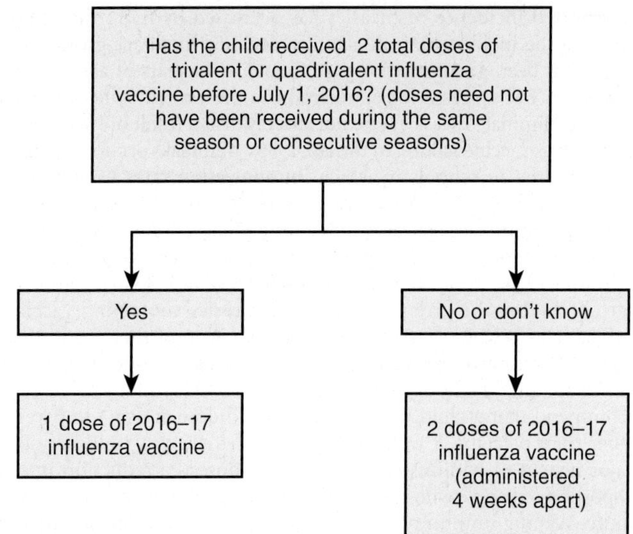

FIG. 245.2 Influenza vaccine dosing algorithm for children age 6 months through 8 years for the US 2016–17 influenza season. (From Centers for Disease Control and Prevention. Prevention and control of seasonal influenza with vaccines recommendations of the Advisory Committee on Immunization Practices—United States, 2016–17 influenza season. https://www.cdc.gov/mmwr/volumes/65/rr/rr6505a1.htm.)

Precautions and Contraindications

IIVs are contraindicated for infants younger than 6 months and children who have a moderate to severe febrile illness on the basis of clinical judgment of the pediatrician.[179] People with acute febrile illness usually should not be vaccinated until their symptoms have abated. However, minor illnesses with or without fever do not contraindicate the use of influenza vaccine, particularly in children with mild upper respiratory tract infection or allergic rhinitis.[101,315]

Pregnancy is not a contraindication to influenza vaccine administration. Vaccination with IIVs are advised for pregnant girls and women who have an underlying high-risk condition.

IIVs can be used to prevent influenza in those who are in close contact with most immunosuppressed individuals, such as those receiving care in a protective environment after undergoing hematopoietic stem cell transplantation.

Severe allergic and anaphylactic reactions can occur in response to several influenza vaccine components, but such reactions are rare. Currently available influenza vaccines are prepared by means of inoculation of virus into chicken eggs, with the exception of the RIV3 and ccIIV4 preparations.[315] The use of influenza vaccines for people with a history of egg allergy was reviewed by the ACIP.[315] For the 2016–17 influenza season, the ACIP recommended that people with egg allergy who report only hives after egg exposure should receive IIVs, with several additional safety measures. For the 2016–17 influenza season, the ACIP recommended the following:

- People with a history of egg allergy who have experienced only hives after exposure to egg should receive influenza vaccine.[315]
- People who report having had reactions to egg involving symptoms such as angioedema, respiratory distress, lightheadedness, or recurrent emesis or who required epinephrine or another emergency medical intervention, particularly those that occurred immediately or within minutes to hours after egg exposure, should receive influenza vaccine.[315]

Measles Vaccine

Since the introduction of an inactivated and a live virus, attenuated measles vaccine (i.e., Edmonston B strain) in the United States in 1963, the reported incidence of measles has decreased by more than 99%. Although the incidence of measles has declined in all age groups, the decline has been greatest among children 5 to 14 years of age.

Measles was targeted for elimination in the United States by 1982. Efforts to eliminate measles were not successful as a result of two factors. The first was vaccine failure. In the late 1980s, outbreaks occurred among older children in schools in which immunization rates usually were greater than 95%.[459,505] Attack rates were 1% to 5% because of the accumulation of measles-susceptible individuals from vaccine failure. The recurrent measles outbreaks among vaccinated school-aged children in the mid-1980s prompted the ACIP and the AAP in 1989 to recommend that all children be given two doses of measles-containing vaccine, preferably as MMR.[13,109] Although administration of the second dose originally was recommended at entry to primary school (ACIP) or middle/secondary school (AAP), the ACIP, the AAP, and the AAFP now recommend that a child be given the second dose at age 4 to 6 years rather than delaying it until the child is 11 to 12 years old.[38,471] The major benefit of administering the second dose is a reduction in the proportion of people who remain susceptible because of primary vaccine failure. Waning immunity is not a major cause of vaccine failure and has little influence on transmission of measles, and revaccination of children who have low concentrations of measles antibody produces only a transient rise in antibody concentration.[454,458,505,518,669]

The second factor leading to outbreaks of measles was the failure to implement current immunization strategies, especially in the inner cities, where a high proportion of preschool-aged children had not been vaccinated. From 1989 through 1991, the proportion of unvaccinated people with measles increased, as reflected by outbreaks among unvaccinated inner-city preschool-aged children. Many barriers to providing timely immunization to these children were identified during investigation of the measles resurgence that occurred between 1989 and 1991. Reported cases of measles declined rapidly after the 1989–91 resurgence because of intensive efforts to vaccinate preschool-aged children. Measles vaccination levels among 2-year-old children increased from 70% in 1990 to 91% in 1997. From 2001 to 2008, a median of 56 measles cases were reported to the CDC annually.[523]

In 2000, the United States achieved measles elimination, defined as interruption of year-round endemic measles transmission.[382] However, importations of measles into the United States continue to occur, posing risks for measles outbreaks and sustained measles transmission. Since 2000, the annual number of cases has ranged from a low of 37 in 2004 to a high of 667 in 2014.[267,287] Most cases have been among people who are not vaccinated against measles. Most cases are imported from other countries or linked to imported cases. Most imported cases originate in Asia, Africa, and Europe and occur among US citizens traveling abroad and people visiting the United States from other countries.[614] Since 1993, the largest outbreaks of measles in the United States have occurred in populations that refuse vaccination for religious or personal belief reasons.[534,610] Most outbreaks have involved limited spread from measles imported from outside the United States. The increased numbers of outbreaks and measles importations into the United States underscore the ongoing risk of measles among unvaccinated people and the importance of vaccination against measles.

The recommended age for receiving routine vaccination with measles vaccine has been lowered in the past decade from 15 months to 12 to 15 months of age.[141] The decision to lower the age for receiving routine primary vaccination was based on the observation that most children are susceptible to measles by the time that they reach 12 months of age because of waning transplacental immunity.[447,455] Most mothers have vaccine-induced immunity rather than immunity conferred by infection with wild virus. Because antibody concentrations induced by measles vaccination typically are lower than those induced by natural measles, measles-specific antibodies acquired transplacentally are lower in infants of vaccinated mothers, and these infants are susceptible at an earlier age.

Preparations

The live measles virus vaccine (Moraten strain) available in the United States is prepared in chick fibroblast cell culture. Each dose of vaccine contains neomycin, sorbitol, and hydrolyzed gelatin as a stabilizer. Preparations include MMR and measles-mumps-rubella-varicella (MMRV) vaccines. MMRV vaccine was licensed in the United States in September 2005 and may be used instead of MMR and varicella vaccine to implement the recommended two-dose vaccine schedule for prevention of measles, mumps, rubella, and varicella among children 12 months to 12 years of age. Single-component measles vaccine is not available in the United States.

Inadequate protection against measles can result from the administration of improperly stored vaccine. Before reconstitution, measles vaccine must be stored at a temperature between 2°C and 8°C (35.6°F–46.4°F) or colder and must be protected from light, which may inactivate the virus. Reconstituted vaccine should be stored in a refrigerator and discarded if not used within 8 hours.

Immunogenicity and Efficacy

Immunization produces a mild or unapparent, noncommunicable infection. Measles antibodies develop in approximately 95% of children vaccinated at 12 months of age and in 98% of children vaccinated at 15 months of age.[455] Studies indicate that serologic evidence of measles immunity develops in more than 99% of people who receive two doses of measles vaccine, separated by at least 1 month, on or after their first birthday.[191,206] Although vaccine-induced antibody titers are lower than those after natural disease, persistence of protective titers for as long as 16 years after administration of vaccine has been demonstrated.[410,458] Most vaccinated people who appear to lose antibody have an anamnestic response after revaccination, indicating that they most likely are still immune.[514] A small percentage of vaccinated individuals may lose protection after several years as a result of secondary vaccine failure.[466]

Adverse Events

Vaccine-associated symptoms, consisting of fever higher than 39.4°C (102.9°F) or rash occurring 5 to 10 days after immunization, develop in 5% to 18% of recipients.[421,530] Serious complications related to vaccine use occur far less frequently than after natural measles.[525]

Thrombocytopenia occurs at a rate of one case for every 30,000 to 40,000 doses distributed. Based on data from Sweden and Finland, the IOM concluded that a causal association exists between MMR and thrombocytopenia.[362] The decrease in platelet count presumably is caused by the measles component and usually is not clinically apparent. However, thrombocytopenic purpura occurring after vaccination has been reported.

Central nervous system disease, specifically encephalitis or encephalopathy, is reported at a rate of less than one case per 1 million doses of vaccine administered. Because the incidence of encephalitis or encephalopathy after the administration of measles vaccination to healthy children is lower than the observed incidence of encephalitis of unknown origin, some or most of the reported severe neurologic disorders may be only temporally, rather than causally, related to measles immunization. The risk of subacute sclerosing panencephalitis (SSPE) developing in vaccinated children is extremely low and is estimated to be approximately one twelfth of the risk for SSPE developing after a case of natural measles (0.7 SSPE cases/1 million vaccine doses vs. 8.5 cases/1 million natural measles infections).[82,106,362] Vaccine-strain measles virus never has been confirmed in a case of SSPE.[38]

Reactions to measles vaccine are not age related and occur only in susceptible vaccinees. After revaccination, reactions should be expected only in those who failed to respond to the first immunization.

No convincing evidence establishes that any vaccine causes autism or autistic spectrum disorder. Concern has been raised about a possible relation between MMR vaccine and autism by some parents of children with autism. Symptoms of autism often are noticed by parents during the second year of life and may manifest after administration of MMR by weeks or months. Two independent nongovernmental groups, the IOM and the AAP, reviewed the evidence regarding a potential link between autism and MMR vaccine.[328,360,361] Both groups independently concluded that available evidence does not support an association and that the United States should continue its current MMR vaccination policy.

Indications

Unless otherwise contraindicated, measles vaccine is indicated for people susceptible to measles.[38,471] The recommended age for receiving the first dose of measles vaccine is 12 to 15 months. In high-risk areas, such as those with recurrent measles transmission, the initial dose should be administered when the child reaches 12 months of age. The second dose is given routinely at 4 to 6 years and no later than 11 to 12 years of age. The minimal interval between the two doses is 4 weeks.

Adults born before 1957 usually can be considered immune to measles because of previous natural infection. Those born after 1956 and for whom immunoprophylaxis is indicated should receive two doses of vaccine.

During outbreaks, when the likelihood of exposure to measles is high, measles vaccine should be given to infants as young as 6 months. Seroconversion rates are significantly less for children vaccinated before reaching 1 year of age than those for older children. Children immunized before their first birthday then should be revaccinated with MMR at 12 to 15 months of age, with a third dose given according to local policy.

Measles remains endemic in many areas of the world. Although vaccination against measles is not a requirement for entry into any country, susceptible children, adolescents, and adults born after 1956 should be offered measles vaccination (usually as MMR) before embarking on international travel. Infants 6 months or older who are traveling to areas where measles is endemic or epidemic should be vaccinated before departure and revaccinated at 12 to 15 months. Vaccination of infants younger than 6 months is not necessary because most young infants are protected by maternally derived antibodies.

Exposure of susceptible individuals to measles is not a contraindication to administering vaccination; MMR vaccine given within 72 hours of exposure may provide protection. For vaccine-eligible people 12 months or older who are exposed to measles, administration of MMR vaccine is preferable to using immune globulin if administered within 72 hours of initial exposure. If exposure does not result in infection, immunization will protect against future infection.

MMRV vaccine may be used instead of MMR and varicella vaccine to implement the recommended two-dose vaccine schedule for children 12 months to 12 years of age. At the time of its licensure, use of MMRV vaccine was preferred for the first and second doses over separate injections of equivalent component vaccines (i.e., MMR vaccine and varicella vaccine), which was consistent with the ACIP's 2006 general recommendations on the use of combination vaccines.[407]

In February 2008, on the basis of preliminary data from two studies conducted after licensure that suggested an increased risk of febrile seizures 5 to 12 days after vaccination among children 12 to 23 months of age who had received the first dose of MMRV vaccine compared with children the same age who had received the first dose of MMR vaccine and varicella vaccine administered as separate injections at the same visit, the ACIP issued updated recommendations regarding MMRV vaccine use.[155] The updated recommendations expressed no preference for use of MMRV vaccine over separate injections of equivalent component vaccines for the first and second doses.

The final results of the two postlicensure studies indicated that among children 12 to 23 months of age, one additional febrile seizure occurred 5 to 12 days after vaccination per 2300 to 2600 children who had received the first dose of MMRV vaccine compared with children who had received the first dose of MMR vaccine and varicella vaccine administered as separate injections at the same visit.[394] Data from postlicensure studies do not suggest that children 4 to 6 years of age who received the second dose of MMRV vaccine had an increased risk of febrile seizures after vaccination compared with children the same age who received MMR vaccine and varicella vaccine administered as separate injections at the same visit.[395]

In June 2009, after consideration of the postlicensure data and other evidence, the ACIP adopted new recommendations regarding use of MMRV vaccine for the first and second doses and identified a personal or family (i.e., sibling or parent) history of seizure as a precaution for the use of MMRV vaccine.[450] For the first dose of measles, mumps, rubella, and varicella vaccines at 12 to 47 months of age, the MMR vaccine and varicella vaccine or MMRV vaccine may be used. Providers who are considering administering MMRV vaccine should discuss the benefits and risks of vaccination options with the parents or caregivers. Unless the parent or caregiver expresses a preference for MMRV vaccine, the CDC recommends that MMR vaccine and varicella vaccine should be administered for the first dose in this age group. For the second dose of measles, mumps, rubella, and varicella vaccines at any age (i.e., 15 months to 12 years) and for the first dose at an age older than 48 months, use of MMRV vaccine usually is preferred over separate injections of its equivalent component vaccines (i.e., MMR vaccine and varicella vaccine). This recommendation is consistent with the ACIP's 2011 general recommendations regarding use of combination vaccines, which state that use of a combination vaccine usually is preferred over its equivalent component vaccines.[408]

Precautions and Contraindications

Immunocompromised patients with conditions such as lymphoreticular or other generalized malignant disease and primary or secondary immunodeficiency states should not be given live virus, attenuated measles vaccine.[38,471] After cessation of their chemotherapy, these individuals usually should not receive measles vaccine for at least 3 months. However, because the intensity and type of immunosuppressive therapy, radiation therapy, underlying disease, and other factors determine when immunologic responsiveness will be restored, arriving at a definitive recommendation for an interval after cessation of immunosuppressive therapy when measles vaccine can be safely and effectively administered often is not possible.

An exception to the contraindication of administering measles vaccine to immunocompromised patients is asymptomatic HIV-infected patients, for whom measles vaccination given as MMR at 12 to 15 months of age is recommended. The need to protect HIV-infected people who are at increased risk for severe complications if infected with measles has been balanced against the risk of adverse reactions. Measles vaccine is not recommended for HIV-infected people with evidence of severe immunosuppression. A case of progressive measles pneumonitis occurred in a person with acquired immunodeficiency syndrome (AIDS) and severe immunosuppression to whom MMR vaccine was administered,[126] and morbidity related to measles vaccination has been reported for people with severe immunosuppression unrelated to HIV infection. The antibody response to measles vaccine in severely immunocompromised HIV-infected people is diminished.[58]

In the United States, the incidence of measles currently is very low. Among HIV-infected people who do not have evidence of severe immunosuppression, no serious or unusual adverse events have been reported after receiving measles vaccination.[470,512,519,615] MMR vaccination is recommended for all asymptomatic HIV-infected people who do not have evidence of severe immunosuppression and for whom measles vaccination would otherwise be indicated. MMR vaccination also should be considered for all symptomatic HIV-infected people who do not have evidence of severe immunosuppression.[568] Testing asymptomatic people for HIV is not necessary before administering MMR.[17]

Systemically absorbed corticosteroids can suppress the immune system of an otherwise healthy person. However, neither the minimal dose nor the duration of therapy sufficient to cause immune suppression is well defined. Although the immunosuppressive effects of corticosteroid treatment vary, many clinicians consider that a corticosteroid dose equivalent to or greater than a prednisone dose of 2 mg/kg per day or a total of 20 mg/day is sufficiently immunosuppressive to raise concern about the safety of administering live virus vaccines. People who have received systemic corticosteroids in doses of 2 mg/kg per day or 20 mg daily or on alternate days for an interval of 14 days or longer should avoid receiving vaccination with MMR for at least 1 month after cessation of corticosteroid therapy.[471,568] People who have received prolonged or extensive topical, aerosolized, or other local corticosteroid therapy that causes clinical or laboratory evidence of systemic immunosuppression also should avoid receiving vaccination with MMR for at least 1 month after cessation of therapy.[471]

The live attenuated measles virus vaccine used for immunization is not communicable. Contacts of immunocompromised patients should be vaccinated to prevent the spread of natural measles to these patients.

Although no direct evidence has demonstrated that measles vaccine is harmful to a pregnant woman or her fetus, the vaccine should not be administered to women known to be pregnant or who are considering becoming pregnant because of the theoretical risk of fetal infection

TABLE 245.11 Suggested Intervals Between Immune Globulin Administration and Measles or Varicella Vaccination

Product and Indication	Route	DOSE U or mL	DOSE mg/kg	Interval (mo)[a]
RSV monoclonal antibody (Synagis)	IM	—	15 (monoclonal)	None
Tetanus (as TIG)	IM	250 U	10	3
Hepatitis A prophylaxis (as IG)				
Contact prophylaxis	IM	0.02 mL/kg	3.3	3
International travel	IM	0.06 mL/kg	10	3
Hepatitis B prophylaxis (as HBIG)	IM	0.06 mL/kg	10	3
Rabies prophylaxis (as RIG)	IM	20 IU/kg	22	4
Varicella prophylaxis (as VariZIG)	IM	125 U/10 kg (maximum, 625 U)	20–40	5
Measles prophylaxis (as IG)				
Standard	IM	0.25 mL/kg	40	5
Immunocompromised contact	IM	0.50 mL/kg	80	6
Botulinum immune globulin Intravenous (human, as BabyBIG)	IV	1.5 mL/kg	75	6
Blood transfusion				
Washed RBCs	IV	10 mL/kg	Negligible	None
RBCs, adenine-saline added	IV	10 mL/kg	10	3
Packed RBCs	IV	10 mL/kg	20–60	5
Whole blood	IV	10 mL/kg	80–100	6
Plasma/platelet products	IV	10 mL/kg	160	7
CMV immune globulin	IV	3 mL/kg	150	6
IGIV				
Replacement therapy for immune deficiencies	IV	—	330–400	8
Therapy for ITP	IV	—	400	8
Varicella prophylaxis		—	400	8
Therapy for ITP	IV	—	1000	10
Therapy for ITP or Kawasaki disease	IV	—	1600–2000	11

[a]These intervals should provide sufficient time for decreases in passive antibodies in all children to allow an adequate response to measles or varicella vaccine. Physicians should not assume that children are fully protected against measles during these intervals. Additional doses of immune globulin or measles vaccine may be indicated after exposure to measles.
BabyBIG, Botulinum immune globulin; *CMV*, cytomegalovirus; *HBIG*, hepatitis B immune globulin; *IG*, immune globulin; *IM*, intramuscular; *ITP*, immune thrombocytopenic purpura; *IV*, intravenous; *IGIV* intravenous immune globulin; *RIG*, rabies immune globulin; *RBCs*, red blood cells; *RSV*, respiratory syncytial virus; *TIG*, tetanus immune globulin; *VariZIG*, varicella-zoster immune globulin.
Modified from American Academy of Pediatrics. Active Immunization in People Who Recently Received Immune Globulin and Other Blood Products. In: Kimberlin DW, Brady MT, Jackson MA, Long SS, editors. *Red Book: 2015 Report of the Committee on Infectious Diseases*. 30th ed. pp. 38-40, Elk Grove Village, IL: American Academy of Pediatrics; 2015 and Kroger A, Sumaya C, Pickering L, et al. General recommendations on immunization—recommendations of the Advisory Committee on Immunization Practices (ACIP). *MMWR Recomm Rep*. 2011;60:1-64.

associated with a live virus vaccine. Women vaccinated with MMR should avoid conception for 28 days after being vaccinated.[139]

Because measles vaccination may diminish cutaneous manifestations of cell-mediated immunity temporarily, a tuberculin test performed several days to 6 weeks after receiving immunization can yield a false-negative result. Although natural measles infection can exacerbate tuberculosis, no evidence indicates that measles vaccination is associated with such an effect. Tuberculin skin testing is not a prerequisite for administering measles immunization. If a tuberculin test is indicated, it should be performed on the day of immunization or postponed for 4 to 6 weeks because measles vaccination may suppress tuberculin reactivity temporarily.

For people who are allergic to eggs, the risk of having serious allergic reactions such as anaphylaxis after receiving MMR vaccine is extremely low, and skin testing with vaccine cannot predict an allergic reaction to vaccination.[38,369,386] Obtaining a skin test is not required before administering MMR to people who are allergic to eggs. Similarly, the administration of gradually increasing doses of vaccine is not required.[471] Data indicate that most anaphylactic reactions to measles- and mumps-containing vaccines are not associated with hypersensitivity to egg antigens but rather to other components of the vaccines, such as the gelatin stabilizer.[311,340,385,419]

Children with a history of thrombocytopenic purpura or thrombocytopenia may be at risk for clinically significant thrombocytopenia after receiving immunization with MMR.[70,362] The decision to vaccinate should be based on the benefits of immunity to measles, mumps, and rubella and the risk of recurrence or exacerbation of the thrombocytopenia after receiving vaccination or from natural infection with measles or rubella. For children in whom thrombocytopenia develops in the month after receiving a dose of measles-containing vaccine, withholding the second dose of measles vaccine is prudent if the incidence of measles remains low.

Receipt of antibody-containing blood products (i.e., whole blood, plasma, or parenteral immune globulin) may interfere with seroconversion in response to the measles vaccine. High doses of immune globulin preparations can inhibit the immune response to measles vaccine for 3 or more months, depending on the dosage.[603] The length of time that passively acquired antibody persists depends on the concentration and quantity of the blood product received (Table 245.11).[38,471]

As with any condition that induces fever during the second year of life, children predisposed to having febrile seizures may experience seizures after receiving measles vaccination. Most convulsions that develop after receiving measles immunization are simple febrile seizures and occur in children without known risk factors. Febrile seizures that occur after the administration of vaccinations do not increase the risk of epilepsy or other neurologic disorders.[66] The risk of seizures after receiving measles vaccination may be increased for children with a history of convulsions or those with a history of convulsions in first-degree family members.[662] Although the exact risk cannot be determined, it appears to be low. The recommendation to immunize children with a personal history of seizures or those with a history of seizures in first-degree family members is based on factors indicating that the benefits greatly outweigh the risks. Prophylactic use of anticonvulsants usually is not feasible because therapeutic concentrations of many currently prescribed anticonvulsants are not achieved for some time after the initiation of therapy.

Meningococcal Vaccine

N. meningitidis causes a spectrum of infections, including meningitis, bacteremia, and rarely bacteremic pneumonia. Meningococcal disease develops rapidly and is fatal in 10% to 15% of cases. Of patients who recover, 11% to 19% have permanent hearing loss, neurologic disability, loss of limbs, or other serious sequelae.

In the United States since the introduction of Hib and pneumococcal polysaccharide-protein conjugate vaccines for infants, *N meningitidis* has become the leading cause of bacterial meningitis in children and remains an important cause of bacteremia and sepsis.[586,686] Disease most often occurs in previously healthy children 2 years or younger; the peak incidence occurs among children younger than 1 year.[442] Another peak occurs among adolescents and young adults 16 through 21 years of age. Historically, college freshman who lived in dormitories and military recruits in boot camp had a higher rate of disease compared with people who are the same age and who are not living in such accommodations.

Close contacts of patients with meningococcal disease are at increased risk for infection. The attack rate for household contacts is 500 to 800 times the rate in the general population. Patients with persistent complement component deficiencies (i.e., C5 to C9, properdin, or factor H or factor D deficiencies) or anatomic or functional asplenia are at increased risk for invasive and recurrent meningococcal disease. Although surveillance data for cases of meningococcal disease among HIV-infected persons are limited in the United States, a growing body of evidence demonstrates an increased risk of meningococcal disease among HIV-infected people.[445]

There are 12 known serogroups of *N. meningitidis*. Six serogroups (i.e., A, B, C, W, X, and Y) are responsible for invasive human disease. Serogroups A and X are rare in the United States. Distribution of the other serogroups in the United States has shifted in the past 2 decades.[205] Serogroups B, C, and Y each account for approximately 30% of reported cases. Approximately three fourths of cases among adolescents and young adults are caused by serogroups C, Y, or W135. Among infants, 50% to 60% of cases are caused by serogroup B.

For unknown reasons, the incidence of meningococcal disease has declined since the peak of disease in the late 1990s.[205] Approximately 800 to 1200 cases are reported annually in the United States. The decline began before the implementation of routine adolescent conjugate polysaccharide meningococcal immunization and has occurred in all serogroups, including those not included in the available vaccines.

In the United States, the incidences of serogroups C and Y, which represent most cases of meningococcal disease, are at historic lows. However, a peak in disease incidence among adolescents and young adults 16 to 21 years of age has persisted, even after routine vaccination of adolescents was recommended in 2005. From 2006 through 2010, the first 5 years after routine use of meningococcal vaccine was recommended, the CDC received reports of approximately 30 cases of serogroup C and Y meningococcal disease among people who had received the vaccine. The case-fatality ratio was similar among people who had received vaccine compared with those who were unvaccinated. Of the 13 reports of breakthrough disease for which data on underlying conditions were available, four people had underlying conditions or behaviors associated with an increased risk of bacterial infections, including type 1 diabetes mellitus, current smoking, history of bacterial meningitis and recurrent infections, and aplastic anemia, paroxysmal nocturnal hemoglobinuria, and receipt of eculizumab, an immune modulator that blocks complement protein C5.[443]

Serogroup B disease incidence has declined despite the fact that serogroup B is not contained in any of the existing conjugate polysaccharide meningococcal vaccines. Approximately 50 to 60 cases of serogroup B meningococcal disease occur annually among adolescents and young adults 11 through 24 years of age in the United States.[205]

Outbreaks occur in communities and institutions, including childcare centers, schools, colleges, and military recruit camps. In the United States, approximately 98% of cases of meningococcal disease are sporadic; however, outbreaks of meningococcal disease continue to occur.[93] From 2009 through 2015, there were seven outbreaks of serogroup B meningitis at US universities that resulted in 43 cases and 3 deaths.

In other parts of the world, the number of cases is much higher.[368] In the sub-Saharan African meningitis belt, which extends from Ethiopia to Senegal, peaks of serogroup A meningococcal disease occur regularly during the dry season. Major epidemics occur every 8 to 12 years. In each epidemic, tens of thousands of cases and thousands of deaths can occur. Approximately 350 million people are at risk. The phased introduction of MenAfriVac, a novel serogroup A meningococcal conjugate vaccine that is being implemented through preventive national campaigns in meningitis belt countries for all individuals 1 to 29 years of age, holds great promise to end epidemic meningitis.[406]

Meningococcal disease continues to cause epidemics outside the meningitis belt.[368] Serogroup W135 has emerged as an epidemic strain causing disease in Saudi Arabia in association with the Hajj pilgrimage. Since 2002, serogroup W meningococcal disease has also been reported in sub-Saharan African countries during epidemic seasons. More recently, serogroup W outbreaks have occurred in South America. Serogroup X, previously a rare cause of sporadic meningitis, has been responsible for outbreaks between 2006 and 2010 in Kenya, Niger, Togo, Uganda, and Burkina Faso.[705] Prolonged outbreaks of serogroup B meningococcal disease have occurred in New Zealand, France, and Oregon. Serogroup Y emerged in Colombia and Venezuela, where it became the common disease-causing serogroup in 2006.[571]

Preparations

MenACWY vaccines. Four meningococcal vaccines that contain purified capsular polysaccharide alone or that are conjugated to a carrier protein are licensed and available in the United States for the prevention of invasive disease caused by *N. meningitidis* serogroups A, C, W135, and Y (Table 245.12).

Quadrivalent meningococcal polysaccharide vaccine (MPSV4; Menomune, Sanofi Pasteur) was licensed in 1981 for use in children 2 years or older. Each vaccine dose contains 50 mg of each of the four purified bacterial capsular polysaccharides from serogroups A, C, Y, and W135. MPSV4 is available as a single dose or multidose (10-dose) vial of lyophilized vaccine, with a corresponding single-dose or multidose vial of diluent. After reconstitution of the lyophilized vaccine with the diluent, each dose consists of a 0.5-mL solution for injection. Vaccine supplied in single-dose vials should be used immediately after reconstitution. Vaccine supplied in multidose vials may be used for up to 35 days after reconstitution if stored at 2°C to 28°C (35°F–46°F). MPSV4 is administered subcutaneously and can be given concurrently with other vaccines but at different anatomic sites.

Two meningococcal conjugate vaccines (i.e., MenACWY-D [Menactra, Sanofi Pasteur] and MenACWY-CRM [Menveo, Novartis Vaccines]) are licensed for use in people 2 through 55 years of age. MenACWY-D is a liquid solution supplied in 0.5-mL single-dose vials. Each dose contains 4 µg each of the four capsular polysaccharides from serogroups A, C, Y, and W135 conjugated to 48 µg of diphtheria toxoid. MenACWY-CRM consists of two components: 10 µg of lyophilized meningococcal serogroup A capsular polysaccharide conjugated to CRM197 (MenA) and 5 µg each of capsular polysaccharide of serogroup C, Y, and W135 conjugated to CRM197 in 0.5 mL of phosphate buffered saline, which is used to reconstitute the lyophilized MenA component before injection. The reconstituted vaccine should be used immediately but may be held at or below 25°C (77°F) for up to 8 hours. Meningococcal conjugate vaccines are administered intramuscularly as a single 0.5-mL dose and can be given concurrently with other recommended vaccines. Limited data suggest that different conjugate vaccine products can be used interchangeably.[204]

MenACWY-D and MenACWY-CRM are also licensed for infants but with different administration schedules. MenACWY-D is licensed as a two-dose primary series, 3 months apart, for children 9 through 23 months of age. MenACWY-CRM is licensed for use in children 2 through 23 months of age. For children initiating vaccination at 2 months of age, MenACWY-CRM is administered as a four-dose series at 2, 4, 6, and 12 months of age. For children initiating vaccination at 7 months through 23 months of age, MenACWY-CRM is administered as a two-dose series with the second dose administered in the second year of life and at least 3 months after the first dose.

TABLE 245.12 **Licensed Meningococcal Vaccines—United States, 1981–2015**

Formulation	Type	Trade Name	Manufacturer	Licensed (y)	Age Group	Doses	Serogroups
MPSV4[a]	Polysaccharide	Menomune	Sanofi Pasteur	1981	≥2 y	Single dose	A, C, W, and Y
MenACWY-D[b]	Conjugate	Menactra	Sanofi Pasteur	2005	11–55 y	Single dose	A, C, W, and Y
MenACWY-D[b]	Conjugate	Menactra	Sanofi Pasteur	2007	2–10 y	Single dose	A, C, W, and Y
MenACWY-D[b]	Conjugate	Menactra	Sanofi Pasteur	2011	9–23 mo	2-dose series	A, C, W, and Y
MenACWY-CRM[c]	Conjugate	Menveo	Novartis	2010	11–55 y	Single dose	A, C, W, and Y
MenACWY-CRM[c]	Conjugate	Menveo	Novartis	2011	2–10 y	Single dose	A, C, W, and Y
MenACWY-CRM[c]	Conjugate	Menveo	Novartis	2011	2–23 mo	4-dose series	A, C, W, and Y
Hib-MenCY-TT[d]	Conjugate	MenHibrix	GlaxoSmithKline	2012	6 wk–18 mo	4-dose series	C and Y
MenB-FHbp[e]	Recombinant	Trumenba	Wyeth	2014	10–25 y	3-dose series	B
MenB-FHbp[e]	Recombinant	Trumenba	Wyeth	2014	10–25 y	2-dose series	B
MenB-4C[f]	Recombinant	Bexsero	Novartis	2015	10–25 y	2-dose series	B

[a]Package insert available at http://www.fda.gov/downloads/BiologicsBloodVaccines/Vaccines/ApprovedProducts/UCM308370.pdf.
[b]Package insert available at http://www.fda.gov/downloads/BiologicBloodVaccines/Vaccines/ApprovedProducts/UCM131170.pdf.
[c]Package insert available at http://www.fda.gov/downloads/BiologicsBloodVaccines/Vaccines/ApprovedProducts/UCM201349.pdf.
[d]Package insert available at http://www.fda.gov/downloads/BiologicsBloodVaccines/Vaccines/ApprovedProducts/UCM308577.pdf.
[e]Package insert available at http://www.fda.gov/downloads/BiologicsBloodVaccines/Vaccines/ApprovedProducts/UCM421139.pdf.
[f]Package insert available at http://www.fda.gov/downloads/BiologicsBloodVaccines/Vaccines/ApprovedProducts/UCM431447.pdf.

In June 2012, a combination conjugate vaccine against Hib (i.e., PRP-T) and *N. meningitidis* serogroups C and Y (i.e., Hib-MenCY-TT [MenHibrix, GlaxoSmithKline]) was licensed. Hib-MenCY-TT contains 5 µg of *N. meningitidis* serogroup C capsular polysaccharide, 5 µg of *N. meningitidis* serogroup Y capsular polysaccharide, and 2.5 µg of *Haemophilus influenzae* serogroup B capsular polysaccharide, with each conjugated to tetanus toxoid. The vaccine is lyophilized and should be reconstituted with a 0.9% saline diluent . After reconstitution of the lyophilized vaccine with the diluent, each dose consists of a 0.5-mL solution for injection. Hib-MenCY-TT is administered intramuscularly and is approved as a four-dose series for children at 2, 4, 6, and 12 through 18 months.

MenB vaccines. In October 2014, the first serogroup B meningococcal vaccine, MenB-FHbp (Trumenba, Wyeth Pharmaceuticals) was licensed. A second serogroup B vaccine, MenB-4C (Bexero, Novartis Vaccines), was licensed in January 2015 (see Table 245.12). Both vaccines are licensed for use in people 10 through 25 years of age.

MenB-FHbp is a bivalent vaccine consisting of two recombinant lipidated factor H binding protein (FHbp) antigens, one from FHbp subfamily A and one from subfamily B. FHbp is one of many proteins found on the surface of meningococci and contributes to the ability of the bacterium to avoid host defenses. The FHbp proteins are individually produced in *Escherichia coli.* Each 0.5-mL dose contains 60 µg of each FHbp variant, 0.018 mg of polysorbate 80, and 0.25 mg of Al^{3+} as $AlPO_4$ in 10 mM histidine buffered saline at pH 6.0. The vaccine is administered as a 0.5-mL dose intramuscularly. MenB-FHbp is licensed as for a three-dose series and a two-dose series. In April 2016, the FDA approved a label change giving MenB-FHbp a flexible three-dose schedule of 0, 1 to 2 months, and 6 months and a two-dose schedule of 0 and 6 months.

MenB-4C is a multicomponent vaccine consisting of three recombinant proteins (i.e., neisserial adhesion A [NadA], factor H binding protein [FHbp] fusion protein, and neisserial heparin binding antigen [NHBA] fusion protein) and outer membrane vesicles (OMVs) containing outer membrane protein PorA serosubtype P1.4 (i.e., New Zealand epidemic strain N298/254). The three recombinant proteins are individually produced in *E. coli.* The OMV antigenic component is produced by fermentation of *N. meningitidis* strain NZ98/254 (expressing outer membrane protein PorA serosubtype P1.4), followed by inactivation of the bacteria by deoxycholate, which also mediates vesicle formation. The antigens are adsorbed onto aluminum hydroxide. Each 0.5-mL dose of MenB-4C contains 50 µg each of recombinant proteins NadA, NHBA, and FHbp; 25 µg of OMV; 1.5 mg of aluminum hydroxide (0.519 mg of Al^{3+});, 3.125 mg of sodium chloride; 0.776 mg of histidine; and 10 mg of sucrose at pH 6.4 to 6.7. The vaccine is administered as a 0.5-mL dose intramuscularly. MenB-4C is licensed as a two-dose series, with doses administered at least 1 month apart.

Immunogenicity and Efficacy

MenACWY vaccines. The polysaccharide capsule of *N meningitidis* is an important determinant of virulence. Serum antibody to capsular polysaccharide protects against disease by activating complement-mediated bacteriolysis or opsonization, or both. Complement-dependent bactericidal activity induced by immunization with meningococcal vaccine is measured by use of a serum bactericidal antibody assay with a human (hSBA) complement source. A defined bactericidal antibody titer that indicates protection against invasive meningococcal disease is assay dependent. When sera are tested using a human complement source, SBA titers of 1:4 or higher are considered protective. Studies have demonstrated that almost all people who developed invasive serogroup C meningococcal disease had sera that lacked bactericidal activity to the pathogenic meningococcal strain.[304,307] In contrast, people with detectable SBA against a specific strain rarely developed disease.

The characteristics of MPSV4 are similar to other polysaccharide vaccines (e.g., pneumococcal polysaccharide). The vaccine is usually not effective in children younger than 18 months. The response to the vaccine is typical of a T-cell independent antigen, with an age-dependent response and poor immunogenicity in children younger than 2 years. Little boost in antibody titer occurs with repeated doses; the antibody that is produced is relatively low-affinity IgM, and switching from IgM to IgG production is poor.

Protective antibody concentrations are achieved within 10 to 14 days of administration of MPSV4. The vaccine elicits protective levels of bactericidal antibody to all four serogroups in more than 97% of recipients as measured at 28 days after vaccination. The antibody responses to each of the four polysaccharides in the polysaccharide vaccine are serogroup specific and independent. Group A polysaccharide induces antibody in some children as young as 3 months, although a response comparable to that in adults is not achieved until the child is 4 to 5 years of age.[531] The serum antibody response to serogroup C is age dependent, with a poor response in children younger than 2 years.[303] Serum concentrations of antibodies against group A and C polysaccharides decrease markedly during the first 3 years after receipt of a single dose of vaccine. The decrease in antibody occurs more rapidly in infants and young children than in adults.[384,712]

Field trials of A and C meningococcal vaccines in Europe and Africa have demonstrated efficacy rates against serogroup A of 85% to 95% 1 year after vaccination.[531,667] After 3 years, efficacy rates were 67% for older children but only 10% for children younger than 4 years at the time of immunization with serogroup A vaccine.[553] In an epidemic, serogroup C vaccine demonstrated clinical efficacy rates similar to those for the serogroup A vaccine.[633]

Serogroup Y and W135 antigens are immunogenic and safe in children older than 2 years. However, clinical efficacy has not been demonstrated for these preparations.[12,57,664]

People with deficiencies of the terminal components of serum complement and those with anatomic or functional asplenia have antibody responses to quadrivalent meningococcal vaccines consistent with protection.[565,567] However, the clinical efficacy of vaccination has not been evaluated in these people.

Meningococcal conjugate vaccines prime the immune system, and immunologic memory persists even in the absence of detectible bactericidal antibodies. Although vaccine-induced immunologic memory often protects against infection with other encapsulated bacteria such as Hib, detectable circulating antibody appears to be important for protection against *N. meningitidis*.[304] Effectiveness of the three meningococcal conjugate vaccines, which were licensed after MPSV4, was inferred by comparing SBA responses induced by the new vaccines compared with SBA responses induced by MPSV4 in people 2 through 55 years of age or by achieving a seroresponse at or above a predefined bactericidal antibody titer among children 2 through 23 months of age.

Protective antibody concentrations are achieved within 8 days after administration of MenACWY-D.[78] In studies conducted among people 11 to 55 years of age comparing the immunogenicity of conjugate vaccine with that of the polysaccharide vaccine at 28 days after vaccination, the percentage of those achieving at least a fourfold increase in bactericidal titer for each serogroup was higher in the MPSV4 group than in the MenACWY-D group for people older than 18 years. Nonetheless, the criteria for demonstrating immunologic noninferiority to MPSV4 were still achieved. The percentage of those with at least a fourfold rise was highest for serogroup W135 and lowest for serogroup Y. The percentage of people achieving a protective level of bactericidal antibody was greater than 97% for all serogroups in the MenACWY-D and MPSV4 groups.

Response to revaccination with MenACWY-D was assessed by administering MenACWY-D to people previously vaccinated with MPSV4 or MenACWY-D and to vaccine- naïve control subjects. All people in all three groups achieved protective bactericidal antibody titers at 8 and 28 days after receiving MenACWY-D. Those initially primed with MenACWY-D achieved higher bactericidal antibody concentrations than those of the naïve controls for all serogroups except A. In contrast, bactericidal antibody titers of those primed with MPSV4 were lower than those of vaccine-naïve controls on days 8 and 28 for all serogroups.

In study participants 11 to 18 years of age, noninferiority of MenACWY-CRM to MenACWY-D was demonstrated for all four serogroups.[166] The proportions of people with seroresponses were statistically higher for serogroups A, W, and Y in the MenACWY-CRM group, compared with the MenACWY-D group. The clinical relevance of higher postvaccination immune responses is not known.

The immunogenicity of MenACWY-CRM in children 2 through 10 years of age was evaluated in a multicenter, randomized, controlled trial.[327] After a single MenACWY-CRM dose, seroresponses to group C, Y, and W135 in children 2 through 5 years and 6 through 10 years of age were noninferior to responses after a single MenACWY-D dose.

MPSV4 is administered subcutaneously, whereas MCV4 is administered intramuscularly. More than 100 people have inadvertently received the MCV4 vaccine by the subcutaneous route. For a subset of these individuals, the CDC determined that although the serologic responses were lower after MCV4 was administered subcutaneously compared with intramuscularly, the proportions of individuals who achieved antibody levels thought to be protective were similar. The CDC therefore did not recommend that those who had received MCV4 needed to be reimmunized.[149]

In clinical trials Hib-MenCY-TT was coadministered with DTaP-HepB-IPV and 7-valent pneumococcal conjugate vaccine (PCV7) at ages 2, 4, and 6 months and with MMR, varicella, and PCV7 vaccines at 12 to 15 months of age. No decreased immunogenicity of coadministered vaccines was observed.[96,460] A randomized, controlled, multicenter study evaluated the percentage of subjects with hSBA titers of 1:8 or higher at 2 months after the second dose was administered at 4 months of age. In the group vaccinated with Hib-MenCY-TT, 94% and 83% of children achieved hSBA antibody titers of 1:8 or higher for meningococcal serogroups C and Y, respectively, after the second dose.[507]

When the MenACWY-D vaccine was licensed in 2005, some experts predicted that the vaccine would be effective for up to 10 years, providing protection through the period of highest risk in late adolescence and early adulthood. Since the 2005 ACIP recommendations, additional data have improved our understanding of meningococcal conjugate vaccines, including the duration of vaccine-induced immunity. Antibody persistence studies indicate that circulating antibody declines 3 to 5 years after a single dose of MenACWY-D or MenACWY-CRM.[296,388,665] Results from a vaccine effectiveness study demonstrate waning effectiveness, and many adolescents are not protected 5 years after vaccination.[203] ACIP concluded that a single dose of meningococcal conjugate vaccine administered at age 11 or 12 years is unlikely to protect most adolescents through the period of increased risk at ages 16 through 21 years. On the basis of this information, in 2011, ACIP recommended adding a booster dose at 16 years of age.[169]

MenB vaccine. The immunogenicity of both serogroup B meningococcal vaccines (i.e., MenB-4C and MenBFHbp) has been evaluated in numerous published clinical trials.[391,461,546,556,576,575,591,640] Both vaccines appear to provide short-term immunogenicity in healthy populations. Studies on vaccine efficacy are not available. Licensure was based on the ability of the vaccines to elicit detection of bactericidal antibody that is presumed to indicate protection. Studies regarding antibody persistence are limited. Immunogenicity studies in populations at increased risk for invasive meningococcal disease have not been completed.

MenB-FHbp has been administered concomitantly with the following: quadrivalent human papillomavirus (HPV) vaccine[591] but not 9-valent HPV vaccine, with MenACWY (unpublished data), and with Tdap vaccine (Adacel, Sanofi Pasteur [unpublished data]).

Adverse Events

MenACWY vaccines. MPSV4 has been used extensively in mass-immunization programs and in the military and among international travelers. Adverse reactions to MPSV4 usually are mild; the most frequent reactions are pain and redness at the injection site that last for 1 or 2 days.[62] Estimates of the incidence of local reactions range from 4% to 56%. Transient fever occurs in as many as 5% of vaccine recipients in some studies but is less common in older children and adults.

The most frequently adverse events reported to VAERS for MenACWY-D include fever (16.8%), headache (16.0%) injection-site erythema (14.6%), and dizziness (13.4%). Syncope has been identified as an adverse event after any vaccination, with a higher proportion of syncope events reported to VAERS occurring in adolescents than other age groups.[154] Syncope was listed in 10% of reports involving MenACWY-D. Twenty-four deaths (0.3%) were reported.

The most frequently reported adverse events for MenACWY-CRM were injection-site erythema (19.7%) and injection site swelling (13.7%). Syncope was listed in 8.8% of reports involving MenACWY-CRM. One death (0.4%) was reported.

Rates of local and systemic adverse events observed after administration of Hib-MenCY-TT were comparable to rates observed after administration of Hib-TT. Hib-MenCY-TT was found to be safe and immunogenic for Hib and meningococcal serogroups C and Y.

MenB vaccine. The safety of both serogroup B meningococcal vaccines (i.e., MenB-4C and MenBFHbp) have been evaluated in numerous published clinical trials.[391,461,556,575,591,597] There were no deaths considered to be related to either vaccine. The most frequently reported severe local and systemic adverse events for MenB-4C include injection site pain (20–29%), fever of 38°C or higher (1–5%), headache (4–6%), fatigue (4–6%), myalgias (12–13%), and joint pain (2%). For MenBFHbp, the most frequently reported severe local and systemic adverse events include injection site pain (5–8%), fever of 38°C (2–8%), headache (1%), fatigue (1–4%), myalgias (1–3%), and joint pain (1%).

Indications

Meningococcal polysaccharide vaccine. Routine vaccination of civilians with MPSV4 is not recommended.[204] Use of MPSV4 should be limited to people older than 55 years or when MenACWY is not available.

TABLE 245.13 Recommended Meningococcal Vaccines for Immunocompetent Children

Age	Vaccine	Status
2 mo–10 y	MenACWY-D[a] MenACWY-CRM[b] HibMenCY-TT[c]	Not routinely recommended
10–25 y	MenB-FHbp *or* MenB-4C	Not routinely recommended
11–21 y	MenACWY-D *or* MenACWY-CRM	Primary: Age 11–12 y: 1 dose Age 13–18 y: 1 dose if not previously immunized Age 19–21 y: not routinely recommended but may be given as catch-up immunization for those who have not received a dose after their 16th birthday Booster: 1 dose recommended for adolescents if first dose administered before 16th birthday

[a]Licensed only for people 9 mo to 55 y.
[b]Licensed only for people 2 mo to 55 y.
[c]Licensed only for children 6 wk to 18 mo.
Modified from American Academy of Pediatrics. Meningococcal infections. In: Kimberlin DW, Brady MT, Jackson MA, Long SS, eds. *Red Book: 2015 Report of the Committee on Infectious Diseases.* 30th ed. Elk Grove Village, IL: American Academy of Pediatrics; 2015:547–58.

TABLE 245.14 Meningococcal Vaccine Recommendations by Risk Group

MenACWY Vaccines	MenB Vaccines
Complement deficiency[a]	Complement deficiency[a]
Anatomic or functional asplenia[b]	Anatomic/functional asplenia[b]
Outbreak[c]	Outbreak[c]
Microbiologists[d]	Microbiologists[d]
HIV infection	
Travelers[e]	
First-year college students[f]	
Military recruits	

[a]Inherited or chronic deficiencies of C3, C5–C9, properdin, factor D, or factor H or those receiving eculizumab.
[b]Includes sickle cell disease.
[c]The CDC defines outbreaks and those at risk.
[d]Only microbiologists who routinely work with *N meningitidis.*
[e]To areas with hyperendemic or epidemic meningococcal disease.
[f]Unvaccinated or inadequately vaccinated first-year college students who live in residence halls.
Modified from Committee on Infectious Diseases, American Academy of Pediatrics. Recommendations for serogroup B meningococcal vaccine for persons 10 years and older. *Pediatrics.* 2016;138:e20161890.

Meningococcal conjugate vaccines. Routine childhood immunization with meningococcal conjugate vaccine (i.e., MenACWY) is recommended for adolescents 11 through 18 years of age, but it is not recommended for children 2 months through 10 years of age because the infection rate is low for this age group; the immune response is less robust than in older children, adolescents, and adults; and duration of immunity is unknown.[28,39,204] Recommendations for routine use of MenACWY in adolescents are shown in Table 245.13 and are as follows:[28,39,204]

- Adolescents should be immunized routinely at the 11- to 12-year of age health care visit, when immunization status and other preventive health services can be addressed. A booster dose at 16 years of age is recommended for adolescents immunized at 11 through 12 years of age.
- Adolescents 13 through 18 years of age should be immunized routinely with a meningococcal conjugate vaccine if not previously immunized. Adolescents who receive the first dose at 13 through 15 years of age should receive a one-time booster dose at 16 through 18 years of age.
- Adolescents who receive their first dose of meningococcal conjugate vaccine at or after 16 years of age do not need a booster dose unless they have risk factors.
- People 19 to 21 years of age are not routinely recommended to receive meningococcal conjugate vaccine, but vaccine may be administered as a catch-up dose for those who have not received a dose after their 16th birthday.

The ACIP and the AAP recommend routine use of meningococcal conjugate vaccines (e.g., MenACWY) for people 2 months or older who have certain medical conditions that increase the risk of meningococcal disease, including those who have persistent (e.g., genetic) deficiencies in the complement pathway (e.g., C3, properdin, factor D, factor H, C5-C9), people receiving eculizumab (because the drug binds C5 and inhibits the terminal complement pathway), and people with functional or anatomic asplenia, including people with sickle cell disease (Table 245.14).[28,39,204] In 2016, the ACIP recommended that people 2 months or older with HIV infection also be given meningococcal conjugate vaccines based on data indicating an increased risk of disease.[445] Specific recommendations for immunization of high-risk children with meningococcal conjugate vaccines are shown in Table 245.15.[28,39,204,445]

MenB vaccines. Routine vaccination with meningococcal serogroup B vaccine is recommended for those 10 years or older who are at increased risk for serogroup B disease (see Tables 245.14 and 245.15), including the following groups: (1) people with persistent complement component diseases, including inherited or chronic deficiencies in C3, C5-C9, properdin, factor D, or factor H, and people receiving eculizumab; (2) people with anatomic or functional asplenia, including sickle cell disease; and (3) healthy people who are at increased risk because of a serogroup B meningococcal disease outbreak.[211,276,444] The AAP and the CDC do not express a preference for the two licensed vaccines, but the same product must be used for the entire series.

A three-dose schedule for MenB-FHbp is recommended for people at increased risk for meningococcal serogroup B disease. For healthy people 16 to 23 years of age who are not at increased risk for meningococcal serogroup B disease, the ACIP has a permissive recommendation that allows use of one of the meningococcal serogroup B vaccines if the patient desires to be immunized.[211,444] If an adolescent so chooses and MenB-FHbp is selected, the ACIP recommends a two-dose schedule. If a patient receives a second dose of MenB-FHbp less than 6 months after the first dose, a third dose should be given at least 6 months after the first.

Postexposure Immunoprophylaxis

Because secondary cases can occur several weeks or more after onset of disease in the index case, meningococcal vaccine is an adjunct to chemoprophylaxis when an outbreak is caused by a serogroup prevented by a meningococcal vaccine. For control of meningococcal outbreaks caused by vaccine-preventable serogroups (i.e., A, C, Y, and W135), the preferred vaccine for adults and children 2 years and older is a meningococcal conjugate vaccine (i.e., MenACWY).[204] For outbreaks caused by serogroup B meningococcal disease, vaccination with a serogroup B meningococcal vaccine is recommended for those 10 years or older identified as being at increased risk because of the outbreak.[178]

Precautions and Contraindications

Vaccination with MenACWY, MPSV4, or Hib-MenCY-TT is contraindicated for people known to have a severe allergic reaction to any component of the vaccine, including diphtheria or tetanus toxoid. The ACIP does not consider a history of Guillain-Barré syndrome to be a contraindication or precaution for meningococcal vaccination.[204] Because MenACWY, MPSV4, and Hib-MenCY-TT are inactivated vaccines, they can be administered to people who are immunosuppressed as a result

TABLE 245.15 Recommended Immunization Schedule and Intervals for Children at Risk for Invasive Meningococcal Disease[a]

Age	Subgroup	Primary Immunization	Booster Dose[b]
2–18 mo[c]	Children who have persistent complement deficiencies, have functional or anatomic asplenia are at risk during a community outbreak attributable to a vaccine serogroup	4 doses of HibMenCY-TT at 2, 4, 6, and 12–15 mo[c]	Person remains at increased risk and first dose received at following age: For 2 mo–6 y of age: should receive additional dose of MenACWY 3 y after primary immunization; boosters should be repeated every 5 y thereafter For ≥7 y of age: should receive additional dose of MenACWY 5 y after primary immunization; boosters should be repeated every 5 y thereafter
2–23 mo with high-risk conditions	Children who have persistent complement deficiencies, have functional or anatomic asplenia, have HIV, travel to or are residents of countries where meningococcal disease is hyperendemic or epidemic are at risk during a community outbreak attributable to a vaccine serogroup	4 doses of MenACWY-CRM (Menveo) at 2, 4, 6, and 12 mo	
9–23 mo with high-risk conditions	Children who have persistent complement deficiencies, travel to or are residents of countries where meningococcal disease is hyperendemic or epidemic are at risk during a community outbreak attributable to a vaccine serogroup	2 doses of MenACWY (Menactra), 12 wk apart[d]	
2–55 y with high-risk conditions and not immunized previously[e,f]	People who have persistent complement deficiencies, have functional or anatomic asplenia, have HIV People who travel to or are residents of countries where meningococcal disease is hyperendemic or epidemic are at risk during a community outbreak attributable to a vaccine serogroup	2 doses of MenACWY, 8–12 wk apart 1 dose of MenACWY[e]	
≥10 y with high-risk conditions	People who have persistent complement deficiencies, have functional or anatomic asplenia are at risk during a community outbreak attributable to a vaccine serogroup	2 doses of MenB-4C 4 wk apart *or* 3 doses of MenB-FHbp administered at 0, 2 and 6 mo	—

[a]Includes children who have persistent complement deficiencies (e.g., C5–C9, properdin, factor H or factor D) and anatomic or functional asplenia; travelers to or residents of countries in which meningococcal disease is hyperendemic or epidemic; and children who are part of a community outbreak of a vaccine-preventable serogroup.
[b]If child remains at increased risk of meningococcal disease.
[c]Infants and children who received Hib-MenCY-TT and are traveling to areas with highly endemic rates of meningococcal disease, such as the African "meningitis belt," are not protected against serogroups A and W and should receive a quadrivalent meningococcal vaccine licensed for children age ≥2 mo before travel.
[d]Because of high risk of invasive pneumococcal disease, children with functional or anatomic asplenia should not be immunized with MenACWY-D (Menactra) before age 2 y to avoid interference with the immune response to the pneumococcal conjugate vaccine (PCV) series.
[e]If MenACWY-D is used, administer at least 4 weeks after completion of all PCV doses.
[f]If an infant is receiving the vaccine before travel, two doses can be administered as early as 2 months apart.
Modified from American Academy of Pediatrics. Meningococcal Infections. In: Kimberlin DW, Brady MT, Jackson MA, Long SS, eds. *Red Book: 2015 Report of the Committee on Infectious Diseases.* 30th ed. Elk Grove Village, IL: American Academy of Pediatrics; 2015:547–58.

of disease or medications; however, response to the vaccine may be less than optimal.

No RCTs have been conducted primarily to evaluate use of MPSV4 or MenACWY vaccines in pregnant or lactating women. VAERS reports of exposure to MPSV4 during pregnancy have not identified adverse effects among pregnant women or newborns of women vaccinated during pregnancy. From the VAERS reports available for women found to be pregnant at the time of MenACWY-D vaccination, no major safety concerns associated with vaccination have been identified in the mother or fetus. Pregnancy should not preclude vaccination with MenACWY or MPSV4, if indicated.[204] Women of childbearing age who become aware that they were pregnant at the time of MenACWY vaccination should contact their health care provider or the vaccine manufacturer so that their experience can be captured in the manufacturer's registry of vaccination during pregnancy.

Before administering MenB vaccines, treating clinicians should consult the package insert for a full list of precautions, warnings, and contraindications.[211,444] Pregnancy and breastfeeding are precautions because neither vaccine has been evaluated in these situations. A severe allergic reaction to a previous dose of MenB vaccine or any of its components is a contradiction.

Mumps Vaccine

Live virus mumps vaccine became available in the United States in 1967 and was recommended for routine use in 1977. The incidence of reported mumps cases decreased rapidly after vaccine licensure until 1986 through 1987, when a resurgence of mumps occurred resulting in 20,638 reported cases.[111,199] The resurgence was attributed to a susceptible cohort of adolescents and young adults entering high school and college who were not targeted for vaccination and spared from natural infection by declining disease rates. In 1989, the ACIP and AAP implemented a two-dose combined MMR schedule given at 4 to 6 or at 11 to 12 years of age.[110] By the early 2000s, on average, fewer than 270 cases were reported annually, and seasonal peaks were no longer seen.[67]

Before vaccine licensure in 1967 and during the early years of vaccine use, most reported cases occurred in the 5- to 9-year age group, with 90% of cases occurring among children 15 years of age and younger. In the late 1980s, a shift toward older children occurred. Since 1990, people 15 years or older have accounted for 30% to 40% of cases per year.

In 2006, an outbreak of 6584 cases occurred and was centered on highly two-dose vaccinated college students in the American Midwest.[229] The 2006 outbreak underscored limitations in the 1998 recommendations about prevention of mumps transmission in health care and other settings with a high risk of mumps transmission. After reviewing data from this outbreak and previous evidence of mumps vaccine effectiveness and transmission, the ACIP issued updated recommendations, specifying that all children and adults in certain high-risk groups, including students at post–high school educational institutions, health care personnel, and international travelers, should receive two doses of mumps-containing vaccine.[110] In the next 2 years, the number of reported cases returned to usual levels, and outbreaks involved fewer than 20 cases.

Outbreaks have continued to occur, particularly in high-density, close-contact settings, despite high two-dose coverage. Because two doses of mumps-containing vaccine are not 100% effective, most mumps cases in settings of high immunization coverage such as the United States most often occur among people who have received two doses. In the 2009–10 season, a large outbreak occurred in the northeastern United States, affecting more than 3500 people, primarily members of traditional observant communities in New York and New Jersey.[163] There was also an outbreak in the US territory of Guam, with 505 cases reported.[500] Most patients had received two doses of MMR vaccine and were exposed in communal settings. In 2011 through 2013, there were several smaller mumps outbreaks reported on college campuses in California,[173] Virginia, and Maryland. However, they had limited spread, and national case counts for these years were at several hundred cases per year.

In 2014, several outbreaks affiliated with universities were reported from multiple states, including one community outbreak in Ohio linked to a university that involved over 400 people and an outbreak affecting the National Hockey League. Outbreaks have been reported from several university campuses in 2015 through 2016, including a number of smaller outbreaks with limited spread. The two largest outbreaks were from Iowa and Illinois, each involving several hundred university students; both held wide-scale vaccination campaigns that included providing a third dose of MMR as a control measure.[7]

In 2016, the greatest number of mumps cases since the outbreaks of 2006 was reported. These outbreaks involved 45 states and more than 2800 individuals. Six states (i.e., Arkansas, Illinois, Indiana, Iowa, Massachusetts, and Oklahoma) reported more than 100 cases in 2016.

Preparations

The live attenuated mumps virus vaccine (i.e., Jeryl Lynn strain) used in the United States is prepared in chick embryo cell culture and is available in combination as MMR and MMRV. The AAP and ACIP recommend that combined MMR vaccine be used when any of the individual components is indicated, and MMRV is recommended if the vaccinee is 12 months through 12 years of age.

Each dose of vaccine contains neomycin, sorbitol, and hydrolyzed gelatin as stabilizers. Before reconstitution, MMR vaccine must be stored at 2°C to 8°C (35.6°F–46.4°F) or colder and protected from light to avoid inactivation. After reconstitution, the vaccine should be used within 8 hours or discarded.

Immunogenicity and Efficacy

The vaccine induces an asymptomatic, noncommunicable infection. After vaccination with MMR vaccine, approximately 94% of infants and children develop detectable mumps antibodies with (range, 89–97%).[85,254,264,396,425,544,548,588,589,647,648] Vaccination induces relatively low levels of antibodies compared with natural infection.[347,675] After a second dose of MMR vaccine, most people mounted a secondary immune response, approximately 50% had a fourfold increase in antibody titers, and the proportion with low or undetectable titers was significantly reduced from 20% before vaccination with a second dose to 4% at 6 months after vaccination.[92,306,422]

Although antibody measurements are often used as a surrogate measure of immunity, no serologic tests are available for mumps that consistently and reliably predict immunity. The immune response to mumps vaccination probably involves the humoral and cellular immune response, but no definitive correlates of protection have been identified.

Clinical studies conducted before vaccine licensure involving approximately 7000 children found a single dose of mumps vaccine to be approximately 95% effective in preventing mumps disease.[348,624,675] However, vaccine effectiveness estimates have been lower in postlicensure studies. The median vaccine effectiveness against mumps has been estimated at 78% for one dose and 88% for two doses.[471] In the United States, estimated vaccine effectiveness for one dose of mumps-containing vaccine is between 81% and 91% in junior high and high school settings[180,183,341,389,626,684] and between 64% and 76% among household or close contacts.[452,626] Population and school-based studies conducted in Europe and Canada report comparable estimates of 49% to 92% for vaccine effectiveness.[104,181,202,233,241,335,431,555,584,612,641]

Fewer studies have been conducted to assess the effectiveness of two doses of mumps-containing vaccine. In the United States, outbreaks among populations with high two-dose coverage found two doses of mumps-containing vaccine to be 80% to 92% effective in preventing clinical disease.[452,581] In the 1988 through 1989 outbreak among junior high school students, the risk of mumps was five times higher for students who received one dose compared with students who received two doses.[341] Population and school-based studies in Europe and Canada estimate two doses of mumps-containing vaccine to be 66% to 95% effective.[104,202,233,241,335,578,612] Despite relatively high two-dose vaccine effectiveness, high two-dose vaccine coverage may not be sufficient to prevent all outbreaks.[5,216,229]

Studies indicate that one dose of MMR vaccine can provide persistent antibodies to mumps. Most people (70–99%) examined approximately 10 years after initial vaccination had detectable mumps antibodies.[92,306,422] T-lymphocyte immunity to mumps was found in 70% of adults vaccinated in childhood compared with 80% of adults who acquired a natural infection during childhood.[213,332] In two-dose recipients, mumps antibodies were detectable in 74% to 95% of people followed over 12 years after receipt of a second dose of MMR vaccine, but antibody levels declined with time.[227,422] Mumps antigen–specific lymphoproliferative responses have been detected in vaccine recipients without detectable mumps antibodies, but the role of these responses in protection against mumps disease is not clear.[377,653]

Adverse Events

The use of mumps vaccine is associated with very few side effects. Parotitis and fever have been reported rarely. Hypersensitivity reactions, including rash, pruritus, and purpura, have been associated temporally with vaccination, but they are transient and usually mild. Administration of MMR is not harmful if it is given to an individual already immune to one or more of the viruses.[40,471]

The frequency of reported central nervous system dysfunction after vaccination is not greater than the observed background rate for unimmunized people.[471] The IOM concluded that evidence is inadequate to establish a causal relationship between the Jeryl Lynn strain of mumps vaccine used in the United States and aseptic meningitis, encephalitis, or sensorineural deafness.[362]

Indications

Routine active immunization as MMR of children 12 to 15 months of age is recommended.[40,471] Most children receive a second dose of mumps vaccine in childhood as a result of the recommendation for routine measles revaccination with MMR. Susceptible older children, adolescents, and adults also should be vaccinated against mumps.

Evidence of immunity through documentation of vaccination is defined as one dose of live mumps vaccine for preschool-aged children and adults not at high risk for exposure and infection and two doses of live mumps vaccine for school-aged children (i.e., kindergarten to grade 12) and adults at high risk for exposure and development of infection (i.e., health care workers, international travelers, and students at post–high school education institutions). Additional recommendations for outbreak control include administering a second dose of MMR for preschool-aged children and adults not at high risk for exposure and acquisition of infection if these people are part of a group that is experiencing an outbreak.[150]

To ensure high levels of immunity, especially among groups at high risk for exposure and development of infection, every opportunity should be used to provide the first or second dose of MMR vaccine to those without adequate evidence of immunity (e.g., documentation of vaccination). No formal recommendation for a third MMR dose exists, but the CDC has provided guidelines for public health agencies considering its use as a control measure during mumps outbreaks.[266] Factors that can trigger a recommendation include outbreaks in populations with two-dose MMR vaccination coverage of greater than 90%, intense exposure settings such as universities, evidence of sustained transmission for greater than 2 weeks, and high attack rates (>5 cases/1000 people).

Mumps remains endemic throughout most of the world. Although vaccination against mumps is not a requirement for entry into any country, susceptible children, adolescents, and adults born after 1956 should be offered mumps vaccination, usually as MMR, before engaging in international travel.

Mumps vaccine has no proven value in the prevention of disease in susceptible individuals after exposure to mumps, probably because the time required to develop protective antibody titers after immunization exceeds the incubation period of clinical mumps. However, if the exposure does not result in infection, the vaccine confers subsequent immunity.

Precautions and Contraindications

For people who are allergic to eggs, the risk of serious allergic reactions such as anaphylaxis after receiving MMR is extremely low, and skin testing with vaccine cannot predict an allergic reaction to vaccination.[40,369,386] Performing skin testing is not required before administering MMR to people who are allergic to eggs. Similarly, the administration of gradually increasing doses of vaccine is not required.[471] Data indicate that most anaphylactic reactions to measles- and mumps-containing vaccines are not associated with hypersensitivity to egg antigens but rather with hypersensitivity to other components of the vaccines, such as the gelatin stabilizer.[311,340,385,419]

Because of the theoretical risk of fetal damage, mumps vaccine should not be administered to women known to be pregnant or who are considering becoming pregnant. Women vaccinated with MMR should avoid conception for 28 days after vaccination.[471]

Lymphoreticular or other generalized malignancy and primary or secondary immunodeficiency states represent contraindications to the use of mumps vaccine. Exceptions are children with HIV infection who are immunized against measles with MMR (see Measles Vaccine). Because infection after vaccination is noncommunicable, susceptible close contacts of immunosuppressed patients should be vaccinated to avoid exposure to mumps in these patients.

After cessation of immunosuppressive therapy, mumps vaccine usually is withheld for at least 3 months. Because the intensity and type of immunosuppressive therapy, radiation therapy, underlying disease, and other factors determine when immunologic responsiveness will be restored, making a definitive recommendation for an interval after cessation of immunosuppressive therapy when mumps vaccine can be safely and effectively administered often is not possible.

The effect of immune globulin preparations on the response to mumps vaccine is unknown. High doses of immune globulin preparations can inhibit the immune response to measles vaccine for 3 or more months, depending on the dosage.[29] If mumps vaccine is given as the MMR vaccine, the recommendations for measles vaccine should be followed (see Table 245.11).

Administration of mumps vaccine should be avoided if the individual is receiving immunosuppressive dosages of systemic corticosteroids. The effects of corticosteroids vary, but many clinicians consider that a dose equivalent to 2 mg/kg per day or 20 mg/day of prednisone is sufficiently immunosuppressive to raise concern about the safety of vaccination with live virus vaccines.

Pertussis Vaccine

Pertussis (i.e., whooping cough), which is caused by the fastidious, gram-negative, pleomorphic bacillus *B. pertussis,* continues to produce significant morbidity and mortality worldwide among young children.[491] In the absence of vaccination, the WHO estimated that approximately 1 million deaths would have occurred from the disease and its complications. In the United States, the number of cases has been reduced by approximately 95% during the vaccine era.

Despite an effective vaccine, pertussis continues to occur in the United States in all age groups. Since the historic low point achieved in the 1980s, the incidence of pertussis has increased steadily. Outbreaks have occurred recently in California, Washington, and Minnesota. In the California outbreak, there was a degree of clustering within populations for whom vaccination rates, largely due to nonmedical exemptions, were low.[60] Nonmedical exemption laws appear to increase the rates of pertussis in local areas of undervaccination in the unvaccinated and vaccinated population.[60,706]

Surveillance data collected by the CDC's National Immunization Program for the periods from 1994 through 1996 and 1997 through 2000 demonstrated that the incidence of pertussis increased 60% among adolescents and adults and 11% among infants younger than 6 months.[142] Data from the National Notifiable Disease Surveillance System reveal an escalation in the increase in all age groups between 2001 and 2004.[90] Incidence rates for the pediatric population peak for infants younger than 6 months and again during adolescence between 11 and 18 years of age.[21] The increase in the number of cases among young infants suggests that a true increase in pertussis circulation has occurred. The number of cases among children old enough to receive vaccine has remained stable. The likely reason that pertussis remains endemic in the United States despite high vaccination rates is that neither infection nor immunization provides life-long immunity.

Humans are the only known reservoir for pertussis. Vaccine effectiveness falls off rapidly after immunization, with rates of 68% after the first year dropping to 8.9% after 4 years.[393] Pregnant woman who have received Tdap in the third trimester of pregnancy had significant declines in immunity 9 to 15 months after delivery.[1]

The experiences of countries where rates of pertussis vaccination have markedly declined provide strong support for continuing routine immunization of infants and young children.[188] In the United Kingdom, as a result of adverse publicity about pertussis vaccination, a decrease in immunization rates for 2-year-old children from 77% in 1974 to 30% in 1978 was followed by an epidemic of 102,500 cases of pertussis. A similar experience occurred in Japan, which reported 13,105 cases and 41 deaths in 1979 after routine immunization had been suspended temporarily in 1975.

In the United States during the 1980s, publicity about alleged serious reactions to pertussis vaccine generated public controversy about the risk of receiving pertussis vaccine. This resulted in costly litigation and escalating vaccine costs and jeopardized vaccine supply and development.[490,532] The experience in countries such as England and Japan, the severity of pertussis in young infants, and the usually benign or self-limited sequelae of pertussis vaccination clearly justify continuing routine childhood immunization. Several risk-benefit analyses provided additional evidence in support of vaccination.[188,349]

Effective primary preventive programs necessitate immunizing young infants, usually beginning at 2 months of age, because the morbidity and mortality of pertussis are greatest for infants, especially those younger than 6 months.[123,188] Approximately 26% of reported cases in the United States occur in infants younger than 6 months. During the period from 1997 through 2000, the case-fatality rate for infants younger than 6 months was 0.8%; 63% of these infants were hospitalized with frequent complications, including pneumonia (11.8%), seizures (1.4%), and encephalopathy (0.2%).[142] From 2000 through 2004, 100 pertussis-related deaths were reported; 90% were among infants younger than 4 months, and 76% occurred in infants younger than 2 months.[90]

In 2014, 23,971 cases of pertussis were reported to the CDC; 9935 cases occurred during an outbreak in California to produce a rate of 26 cases per 100,000 people, with a rate of 1746 cases per 100,000 infants younger than 12 months. Three deaths were attributed to this outbreak, all were infants with an onset of illness at less than 5 weeks of age.[691]

Maintaining high rates of immunization in children beyond infancy, with booster immunization for adolescents and adults, may reduce the risk of infection in infants by decreasing the incidence of infection in older family members and the resultant transmission of *B. pertussis* within the household. Vaccination, including boosters, is essential because the disease is highly infectious, and transmission often occurs before adults seek medical care.

Preparations

Whole-cell pertussis vaccine was introduced in the United States in the 1920s. Not until the 1940s to 1950s, however, did pediatric whole-cell pertussis vaccine become routinely recommended for children. This vaccine, unavailable in the United States since 2002, consisted of a suspension of inactivated *B. pertussis* combined with diphtheria and tetanus toxoids (DTP).[90]

To reduce the incidence of local and systemic reactions caused by whole-cell vaccines, less reactogenic pediatric acellular vaccines composed of one or more purified components of *B. pertussis* combined with diphtheria and tetanus toxoids (DTaP) were developed. Initially licensed in 1991 for use as the fourth or fifth dose in the series, DTaP was licensed in 1997 for all five doses in the series.

TABLE 245.16 **Acellular Pertussis Vaccines Licensed for Use in the United States**

Vaccine	Trade Name	Vaccine Manufacturer	No. of Pertussis Antigens	Antigenic Content	Dose Series Approved
DTaP Vaccines for Children Age <7 Years					
DTaP	Daptacel	Sanofi Pasteur	5	PT, FHA, PE, 2 types of FIM	All 5 doses
DTaP	Infanrix	GlaxoSmithKline Biologicals	3	PT, FHA, PE	All 5 doses
DTaP-IPV	Kinrix	GlaxoSmithKline Biologicals	3	PT, FHA, PE	Booster dose for 5th dose of DTaP and 4th dose of IPV, children 4 through 6 years of age
DTaP-hepatitis B-IPV	Pediarix	GlaxoSmithKline Biologicals	3	PT, FHA, PE	First 3 doses, children 6 wk–6 y of age
DTaP-IPV/Hib	Pentacel	Sanofi Pasteur	5	PT, FHA, PE, 2 types of FIM	First 4 doses, children 6 wk–4 y of age
DTaP-IPV	Quadracel	Sanofi Pasteur	5	PT, FHA, PE, 2 types of FIM	Booster dose for 5th dose of DTaP and 4th dose of IPV, children 4–6 y of age
Tdap Vaccines for Adolescents					
Tdap	Adacel	Sanofi Pasteur	5	PT, FHA, PE, 2 types of FIM	Single dose at 11–12 y of age instead of Td
Tdap	Boostrix	GlaxoSmithKline Biologicals	3	PT, FHA, PE	Single dose at 11–12 y of age instead of Td

DTaP, Diphtheria–tetanus–acellular pertussis; *FHA*, filamentous hemagglutinin; *FIM*, fimbriae; *Hib*, *Haemophilus influenzae* type b vaccine; *IPV*, inactivated poliovirus vaccine; *PE*, pertactin; *PT*, pertussis toxin; *Td*, tetanus and reduced diphtheria toxoids; *Tdap*, tetanus–diphtheria–acellular pertussis.
Modified from American Academy of Pediatrics. Pertussis (whooping cough). In: Kimberlin DW, Brady MT, Jackson MA, Long SS, eds. *Red Book: 2015 Report of the Committee on Infectious Diseases.* 30th ed. Elk Grove Village, IL: American Academy of Pediatrics; 2015:608–21.

Numerous acellular vaccines formulated from the different components have been tested in children. All currently US licensed vaccines contain detoxified or inactivated pertussis toxin (i.e., pertussis toxoid) and filamentous hemagglutinin.[231] Most vaccines include one or both of the following *B. pertussis* antigens: pertactin (PRN, a 69-kd outer membrane protein) and fimbriae proteins (FIM, agglutinogens). Various vaccines have different amounts of each component. No pertussis-only vaccine is available.

From 2001 until 2008, numerous changes were made to the list of licensed acellular pertussis–containing vaccines available in the United States. Several acellular vaccines are available for use in the primary vaccination series for children younger than 7 years (Table 245.16).

For enhanced control of pertussis, routine revaccination of adolescents and adults with an acellular pertussis vaccine is recommended to minimize the morbidity associated with infection in these age groups and to reduce the reservoir of infection. Tdap vaccines contain the same pertussis antigen components as are in the pediatric vaccines (some in reduced quantities). The tetanus and diphtheria components are the same as for the current adult formations of Td, with reduced diphtheria content as recommended for use in people 7 years of age or older.

The ACIP recommends that whenever feasible, the same DTaP vaccine product should be used for all doses of the vaccination series. If the vaccine provider does not know or does not have available the type of DTaP previously administered, any of the available licensed DTaP vaccines can be used to complete the vaccination series.[138]

Immunogenicity

The Multicenter Acellular Pertussis Trial evaluated the immunogenicity and safety of 13 acellular pertussis–containing vaccines compared with whole-cell DTP administered to infants at 2, 4, and 6 months of age in the United States.[231] Serologic correlates of immunity to diphtheria and tetanus toxoids, defined as antibody levels 0.1 IU/mL or greater, were achieved after vaccination with acellular vaccines and were comparable with those achieved with DTP vaccination. Pertussis immunity, determined by at least a fourfold rise in antibody titer to pertussis toxin and filamentous hemagglutinin, was equal to or greater than results with DTP after immunization with either of the two DTaP vaccines.[253]

Efficacy

For whole-cell and acellular vaccines, serologic correlates of immunogenicity have not been established for assessing efficacy. Field and other epidemiologic studies must be performed to demonstrate efficacy. Studies in the United States of household contacts exposed to pertussis indicate that the efficacy of whole-cell vaccine was 80% or greater.[123,188,513] Studies reporting lower rates of vaccine efficacy often reflect the use of different criteria for the diagnosis of pertussis and lesser effectiveness of the vaccine in protecting against mild infection than against severe disease.[268] Vaccine-induced immunity persists for at least 3 years and subsequently diminishes with time.

Pertussis in individuals previously vaccinated is less severe and is associated with fewer complications than in unvaccinated people. In a case-control study of pertussis, immunization of both parents decreased the incidence of disease by 51% among infants younger than 4 months.[691] Vaccine effectiveness in pregnant women is 91%.[50]

In studies of the efficacy of eight acellular pertussis vaccines in infants, rates of prevention of pertussis ranged from 58% to 93%.[541] Comparing efficacy of the different products, however, often is not possible because of differences in study design, vaccine schedule (i.e., number of doses and age of administration), case definitions of pertussis, and other confounding variables. The acellular vaccines appear to be similar in efficacy to most whole-cell vaccines. Whereas in two large trials in Sweden and Italy, several acellular vaccines demonstrated substantially greater efficacy than seen in the one US whole-cell vaccine previously approved, other whole-cell vaccines studied appeared to be slightly more effective than acellular vaccines in other trials.[252] The vaccines in the Swedish and Italian trials were given in a three-dose schedule, in contrast to the four-dose primary schedule for vaccination of young children in the United States.

Adverse Events

Local and febrile reactions to whole-cell vaccines occur in more than one half of DTP recipients.[200] These manifestations usually develop within the first 24 hours and are brief in duration. More serious reactions to whole-cell vaccines are uncommon. The reactions include prolonged crying for 3 hours or longer occurring within the first 48 hours of receiving vaccination (1% to 3% of DTP recipients) and a temperature of 40.5°C or greater (≥104.9°F) within 48 hours (0.3%); a hypotonic-hyporesponsive episode described as collapse or shock-like state within 48 hours and seizure within 3 days of vaccination was estimated to occur once per 1750 doses.[200] Episodes of inconsolable crying, high fever, and hypotonic-hyporesponsive episodes after receipt of DTP vaccine resolved without sequelae.

Most post-DTP seizures occurring within 48 hours of receipt of vaccine are brief, self-limited, and generalized and occur in association with fever. These seizures have not been demonstrated to result in the subsequent development of epilepsy or other neurologic sequelae. Predisposing factors include an underlying convulsive disorder, a personal history of previous convulsion, and a family history of convulsions.[128] A small increase in the risk of febrile seizure but no increased risk in the development of epilepsy after immunization has been reported.[627]

The incidence of local and febrile reactions after the administration of acellular vaccines is significantly lower.[231,541] Comparison of rates of adverse events with different acellular vaccines versus whole-cell vaccines demonstrated similar safety profiles for each of the vaccines.[193,585] The most common adverse events include injection site reactions (e.g., erythema, induration, tenderness) and mild system symptoms, including slight to moderate fever, drowsiness, irritability, and loss of appetite.

Rates of local reactions increase with each subsequent dose of DTaP vaccine.[537,642] Booster doses of acellular pertussis vaccine may be associated with extensive local swelling (i.e., limb swelling), especially with vaccines having a high diphtheria content.[554] The pathogenesis of this reaction is not understood, but it spontaneously resolves without sequelae and is not associated with an increased risk of similar adverse events occurring after receipt of the fifth dose.[41] Severe reactions to acellular vaccines such as prolonged crying of 3 hours or more, temperature greater than or equal to 40.5°C (104.9°F), hypotonic-hyporesponsive episodes, and seizures are rare.[193,231,309,323,541,585,644] As with local and febrile reactions, their occurrence with acellular pertussis vaccination is significantly less frequent than that after whole-cell vaccination.

Syncope can occur after immunization with Tdap, is more common among adolescents and young adults, and can result in serious injury if a vaccine recipient falls. Vaccinees should be seated and observed for 15 minutes after immunization. If syncope occurs, patients should be observed until symptoms resolve.[41]

When administered in the third trimester of pregnancy as recommended by the ACIP, there has been no association with an increased risk of maternal or neonatal death, preeclampsia, hemorrhage, uterine rupture, caesarean section, renal failure, premature delivery, decreased birth weight, or prolonged stay in a neonatal intensive care unit with administration of Tdap. Increases in poor birth outcomes or maternal adverse events have not been observed among women receiving multiple Tdap vaccines during pregnancies spaced less than 5 years apart.[243,488,625] This finding was confirmed in a review of reported adverse events following the recommendation that pregnant women received Tdap during the third trimester of each pregnancy regardless of prior vaccine history.[489]

Serious Neurologic Illness

The National Childhood Encephalopathy Study (NCES), a large case-control study from Great Britain that was published in 1985, estimated that the occurrence of acute neurologic illness resulting in hospitalization was 1 case per 140,000 DTP vaccinations.[481] In a 10-year follow-up study published in 1993, neurologic sequelae were found to be common occurrences, but no more so than in children with unrelated, acute neurologic illness in infancy,[480] and reviews of the data have disputed the conclusion that pertussis vaccine can cause neurologic sequelae.[14,128,622] Later data from Canada evaluating more than 12,000 pediatric hospitalizations for serious neurologic illness between 1993 and 2002 found no association after administration of more than 6.5 million doses between development of encephalopathy and receipt of DTaP vaccination.[41] Taken together, the data do not support a role for whole-cell pertussis vaccine in causing brain damage.[115]

Indications

Vaccination against pertussis with DTaP is recommended routinely for children at 2, 4, and 6 months of age, followed by a fourth dose at 12 to 18 months of age and a fifth dose at 4 to 6 years of age.[21,41,90] Immunization can be started when the child is as young as 6 weeks of age if pertussis is prevalent in the community. The interval between administrations of the three doses of the initial series can be as short as 4 weeks. The AAP and ACIP recommend exclusive use of acellular pertussis vaccines for all doses of the pertussis vaccine series.[21,41,90] DTP is no longer available in the United States. However, in many countries, including several in Europe and developing countries, whole-cell vaccine remains the recommended product.

A single dose of Tdap is recommended universally for people 11 years or older, including adults, in place of the initial Td booster vaccine. The preferred schedule is to administer Tdap at the preventive visit for the 11- or 12- year-old children who have completed their primary DTP/DTaP series.[21,41,90] Adolescents and adults 11 years or older who received Td but not Tdap should receive a single dose of Tdap to provide protection against pertussis. Tdap can be administered regardless of the time since receipt of the last tetanus- or diphtheria-containing vaccine.[41] Adolescents between the ages of 11 and 18 years who have never been vaccinated against tetanus, diphtheria, or pertussis should initially receive a single dose of Tdap followed by Td for the subsequent two doses at 4 weeks or more and 6 to 12 months later.

No pertussis-containing vaccine is FDA approved for children between the ages of 7 and 10 years. If pertussis vaccine is not contraindicated, children 7 through 10 years of age who are not fully vaccinated (i.e., have not received five doses of DTaP or four doses of DTaP if the fourth dose was administered on or after the fourth birthday) should receive a single dose of Tdap to provide protection against pertussis. If additional doses of tetanus and diphtheria toxoid–containing vaccines are needed for children 7 through 10 years of age, Tdap vaccine is substituted as the first dose. The subsequent two doses should be Td vaccine at 4 weeks or more and 6 to 12 months after the previous dose if indicated for the catch-up series.[29,90]

Women should receive Tdap before becoming pregnant. Women who have not been immunized previously with Tdap should receive Tdap during pregnancy, preferably during the early third trimester (i.e., after 20 weeks' gestation). If it is not administered during pregnancy, Tdap should be administered in the immediate postpartum period.[171,175] Additional immunization with Tdap should be administered in the early third trimester of each additional pregnancy. Every 10 years thereafter, booster vaccination should be provided by Td.

As further protection against transmission of pertussis to infants who are at greatest risk for pertussis-related morbidity or mortality compared with other age groups, the cocoon strategy is recommended to immunize mothers, families, and close contacts against pertussis to decrease their likelihood of acquisition and subsequent transmission of *B. pertussis* to infants. Adolescents and adults (i.e., parents, siblings, grandparents, child care providers, and health care personnel) who have or anticipate having close contact with an infant younger than 12 months should receive a single dose of Tdap to protect against pertussis if they have not previously received Tdap. Ideally, these people should receive Tdap at least 2 weeks before beginning close contact with the infant.[41,171]

Contraindications and Precautions

The contraindications and precautions for administering pertussis vaccine are based on adverse reactions associated with whole-cell vaccine. Although reactions occurring after the administration of DTaP are much less common than are those associated with DTP, the contraindications and precautions for DTaP are the same.[21,41,90] Adverse events temporally related to pertussis immunization that contraindicate further administration of DTaP are as follows:

- An immediate anaphylactic reaction. Subsequent immunization with any of the three components of the vaccine should be avoided.
- Encephalopathy occurring within 7 days. Children who experienced encephalopathy within 7 days after administration of a previous dose of diphtheria and tetanus toxoids and pertussis vaccine (i.e., DTP, DTaP, or Tdap) not attributable to another identifiable cause should not receive additional doses of a vaccine that contains pertussis. Encephalopathy in this context is defined as a severe, acute, central nervous system disorder (e.g., coma, prolonged seizures) unexplained by another cause and may manifest as major alterations in consciousness or generalized or focal seizures that persist for more than a few hours without recovery within 24 hours. Additional doses of DT (or Td) vaccine should be substituted for any pertussis-containing vaccine.

Postvaccination reactions constituting precautions are as follows:

- Moderate or severe acute illness with or without a fever
- Guillain-Barré syndrome within 6 weeks after a previous dose of tetanus toxoid–containing vaccine

- A convulsion, with or without fever, occurring within 3 days of receiving DTP or DTaP vaccination
- Persistent, severe, inconsolable screaming or crying for 3 hours or more within 48 hours of DTP or DTaP vaccination
- Hypotonic-hyporesponsive episode occurring within 48 hours of DTP or DTaP vaccination
- Temperature of 40.5°C (104.9°F) or greater that is unexplained by another cause and occurs within 48 hours of DTP or DTaP vaccination

With these adverse events occurring in temporal association with DTaP vaccination, the decision to administer additional doses of pertussis vaccine should be considered carefully. Children for whom vaccination is deferred because of moderate or severe acute illness should be vaccinated when their condition improves. In circumstances such as a pertussis outbreak in which the potential benefits of pertussis immunization outweigh the possible risks, vaccination is indicated, particularly because these events have not been proved to cause permanent sequelae. The risk of these reactions occurring after receipt of DTaP is substantially lower than after receipt of DTP.

For children with an evolving neurologic disorder in the first year of life, pertussis immunization should be deferred until the nature and cause of the disorder have been established. A personal history of having a stable neurologic condition (i.e., previous convulsion unrelated to DTaP vaccination, a history of seizure disorder, well-controlled seizures, or cerebral palsy) or a family history of convulsions is not a contraindication, and pertussis immunization should be administered on schedule.

Certain conditions after DTaP vaccine, such as temperature of 40.5°C (104.9°F) or higher, collapse or shock-like state, persistent crying, or convulsions with or without fever, are a precaution to subsequent doses of DTaP. However, occurrence of one of these adverse reactions after DTaP vaccine in childhood is not a contraindication or precaution to administration of Tdap to an adolescent or adult. A history of severe Arthus hypersensitivity reaction after a previous dose of a tetanus or diphtheria toxoid–containing vaccine administered less than 10 years earlier should lead to deferral of Tdap or Td immunization for 10 years after administration of the tetanus or diphtheria toxoid–containing vaccine.[21,41,90]

Pneumococcal Vaccine

S. pneumoniae is a leading bacterial pathogen, especially among young children, elderly people, and people with predisposing conditions. In children, it is the most common cause of otitis media, occult bacteremia, and bacterial pneumonia requiring hospitalization. After the widespread introduction of conjugate Hib vaccination and subsequent marked decline in occurrence of Hib meningitis, *S. pneumoniae* became a leading cause of bacterial meningitis in children in the United States.

In some populations, such as Alaska Natives, the incidence of bacteremia is markedly higher than that reported in other geographic areas of the United States.[228] Groups considered at high risk for invasive pneumococcal disease (IPD) include children with sickle cell disease, asplenia, Hodgkin disease, congenital humoral immunodeficiency, HIV infection, and nephrotic syndrome and recipients of organ transplants. Children who have received cochlear implants are at particular risk for developing meningitis.[144,552] Other chronic diseases associated with an increased risk of development of severe pneumococcal disease include chronic cardiovascular and pulmonary diseases, diabetes mellitus, and renal failure. The role of these chronic diseases in predisposing individuals to pneumococcal infection has been demonstrated primarily in adults. Mortality rates are highest among those who have bacteremia or meningitis, elderly people, and patients with impaired humoral immunity or certain chronic diseases.

The purified polysaccharide vaccine has been effective in reducing severe disease in the adult population,[99] but it has little impact in young children because the vaccine is not immunogenic in children younger than 2 years.[42] The polysaccharide vaccine has not been effective in preventing otitis media caused by *S. pneumoniae*.[42] Several factors made the development of new preventive strategies for pneumococcal disease a high priority.[212,214] Morbidity and mortality rates of pneumococcal infection appear to be particularly high in developing countries. The increasing incidence of antimicrobial-resistant pneumococci further underscores the need for developing effective pneumococcal vaccines for young children.[88] Resistance of *S. pneumoniae* to multiple antibiotics increased rapidly in the United States and even more rapidly in other parts of the world.[381] Children younger than 2 years have the highest rate of IPD but do not develop an effective antibody response to polysaccharide vaccine. Children 2 to 5 years of age may have relatively poor responses to serotypes 6B, 14, 19F, and 23F, which are common causes of pediatric infections and the most prevalent penicillin-resistant serotypes.

These factors prompted the development of conjugated polysaccharide–protein vaccines, two of which have been licensed in the United States. These vaccines are similar in design to the licensed Hib conjugate vaccines. Because of the large number of serotypes of *S. pneumoniae* that cause disease, development of these conjugate pneumococcal vaccines was more difficult than the development of similar vaccines for Hib. Each pneumococcal antigen must be coupled to a protein carrier, and the vaccine must be prepared to ensure that antigen is sufficient to induce an immune response but insufficient to elicit an adverse reaction.

One potential problem with conjugate pneumococcal vaccines is the need to immunize against many different serotypes of pneumococci. Because of local reactions to the protein component, conjugate vaccines that contain all implicated serotypes have proved difficult to produce. Initial decisions for serotype inclusion need to be carefully planned for specific groups. For instance, vaccine containing types 4, 6B, 9V, 14, 18C, 19F, and 23F (i.e., PCV7) is necessary for prevention of otitis media in the United States, whereas types 1, 2, and 5 need to be added to prevent pneumonia in developing countries.

The use of conjugate vaccines against limited serotypes has led to emergence of pneumococcal serotypes (e.g., 19A) that were previously less common but have proved equally concerning for IPD and emerging resistance.[102,161,364] Emergence of replacement serotypes led to the expansion of the previous vaccine to the 13-valent pneumococcal conjugate vaccine (PCV13) in the United States.[162] Routine infant immunization using these conjugate vaccines led to significant reductions in the instances of *S. pneumoniae* disease.[263] Since the widespread introduction of PCV7 in infants in 2000, rates of IPD have decreased markedly in the United States.[263] The incidence of all IPDs has decreased by 80% for children younger than 2 years and by up to 90% for infections caused by vaccine and vaccine-related serotypes.[42,161,686] An increase in nonvaccine serotype disease has occurred, but it is small compared with the overall reductions in vaccine-type disease.[52,102,145,161]

A decline in the incidence of vaccine-type disease among unvaccinated children and adults has occurred since the introduction of routine vaccination for infants in the United States.[145] Rates of IPD among infants younger than 2 months have decreased significantly, providing evidence that vaccinating children 2 to 23 months of age has led to changes in pneumococcal carriage in infants who were too young to receive PCV7.[543] In surveillance of children with sickle cell disease from 1998 to 2009, rates of IPD fell by 53%.[528] As of 2012, PCVs are included in national immunization programs in 86 of 194 WHO member states, with similar expectations of IPD decrease.[174]

Herd immunity is estimated to prevent twice as many cases as do the direct effects of vaccination alone.[145,161] Although the exact mechanism of herd immunity is uncertain, one hypothesis is that vaccinated children are less likely to have nasal carriage of pneumococcus and therefore less pneumococcal transmission to their contacts.[222] Use of conjugate vaccines has reduced nasopharyngeal carriage of vaccine serotypes with PCV7 and PCV13.[201,223,224] Pneumococcal conjugate vaccination also has led to increased nasopharyngeal colonization of children with nonvaccine serotypes.[293,479] In surveillance of IPD cases among children younger than 5 years, the introduction of PCV7 decreased penicillin-nonsusceptible cases by 64%, with serotypes not in PCV7 causing 78% to 97% of penicillin-nonsusceptible IPD.[331] This underscores the need for ongoing surveillance of emerging nonvaccine serotypes with respect to nasopharyngeal colonization, antibiotic nonsusceptibility and of rates of IPD.[613]

Preparations

Two pneumococcal vaccines are available for use in children in the United States. The first is a 13-valent vaccine (PCV13) licensed in 2010

(Prevnar, Wyeth Vaccines), which contains the capsular polysaccharides from serotypes contained in the previous PCV7 (i.e., 4, 6B, 9V, 14, 18C, 19F, and 23F) and six additional serotypes (i.e., 1, 3, 5, 6A, 7F, and 19A) conjugated to mutant diphtheria toxin (CRM197).[42] Serotypes included in PCV7 and potentially cross-reactive serotypes (i.e., 6A, 9A, 9L, 18B, and 18F) accounted for 86% of cases of bacteremia, 83% of cases of meningitis, and 65% of AOM cases occurring in children younger than 6 years in the United States during 1978 to 1994.[509] In 2007, the Active Bacterial Core surveillance estimated 4600 cases of IPD among children younger than 5 years in the United States, with 2900 attributable to serotypes covered by PCV13 versus 60 cases covered by PCV7.[161] The incidence of IPD from PCV13 or nonPCV7 serotypes was reduced by 64% and 93%, respectively, among children younger than 5 years by 2013, driven mostly by reductions of serotypes 19A and 7F.[487]

The second vaccine (i.e., PPV23 [Pneumovax]) is composed of purified, capsular polysaccharide antigens of 23 pneumococcal serotypes. Although 90 different serotypes have been identified, vaccine serotypes in the 23-valent vaccine are historically responsible for 85% to 90% of adult infections and almost 100% of invasive disease and 85% of otitis media cases in children.[112,294] Each vaccine is recommended in a dose of 0.5 mL that is given intramuscularly.

Immunogenicity and Efficacy

The immunogenicity of the conjugate polysaccharide vaccine appears to be determined by the pneumococcal polysaccharide serotype, rather than by the carrier protein. Some serotypes (i.e., 14, 18C, and 19F) are excellent immunogens because they elicit antibody protection after a single dose, whereas others (i.e., 6B and 23F) require three doses of vaccine.[259] Conjugate vaccine elicits immunologic memory.[259] The antibody concentrations achieved after the initial series of three doses usually are sustained for only a few months and then decline to almost preimmunization levels. A dose of pneumococcal vaccine (i.e., polysaccharide or conjugate) given in the second year of life elicits an amnestic-type response.

Prelicensure clinical efficacy of PCV7 was studied in a large, prospective, placebo-controlled efficacy trial in northern California involving 38,000 children. The vaccine was 89% effective in preventing invasive disease caused by any pneumococcal serotype and 97% effective against disease caused by the seven vaccine serotypes.[80] For noninvasive disease, a decrease of 7% in the number of cases of otitis media and 23% in doctor visits for recurrent otitis (i.e., six or more visits per year) occurred for vaccinated children. The study also demonstrated an 11% decrease in the number of clinical cases of pneumonia and efficacy of 26% against a first episode of radiograph-confirmed pneumonia in vaccinees.[333,600]

Prelicensure immunogenicity of PCV13 was studied in a randomized, double-blind, active-controlled trial in which 663 US infants received at least one dose of PCV7 or PCV13. The study was powered for noninferiority of immunoglobulin antibody response measured by enzyme immunoassay and included subset analysis of functional antibody responses measured by opsonophagocytosis assay (OPA).[25,707] The noninferiority criterion (i.e., immunoglobulin geometric mean concentrations) was met for all shared serotypes; although slightly lower in the PCV13 group, the functional OPA response was similar, suggesting PCV13 has similar efficacy as PCV7 against shared serotypes. After a fourth dose of PCV13, the additional six serotypes also produced a functional OPA response in 97% to 100%.

The ability of PCV7 to protect children against AOM was evaluated in an efficacy trial conducted in Finland.[260] For prevention of AOM caused by pneumococci of any serotype, efficacy was estimated to be 34%, whereas efficacy against AOM irrespective of cause was 6%. Efficacy against AOM caused by vaccine-related serotypes was 57%, but an increase of 33% in the rate of AOM episodes caused by nonvaccine serotypes occurred in the group receiving the heptavalent vaccine compared with controls. Despite of the increase in disease caused by nonvaccine serotypes, the net effect on pneumococcal AOM was a reduction of 34%.

RCTs enrolling African children and using a nine-valent pneumococcal conjugate vaccine demonstrated efficacy in the prevention of radiologically confirmed pneumonia and vaccine-type IPD.[220,398] The vaccine was efficacious in preventing vaccine-type invasive disease in HIV-infected children.[398] One of the trials demonstrated a reduction in the all-cause mortality rate for vaccine recipients.[220] These data make a compelling case for extending the benefits of pneumococcal conjugate vaccination to developing countries.

Vaccination with purified polysaccharide vaccine results in serologic type-specific antibody in most healthy adults and older children. Immunocompromised patients may respond less well. In children younger than 2 years, the antibody response is poor to most serotypes, including those most likely to cause infection, such as types 6A and 14.[130,112,294] Patients with AIDS have impaired antibody responses to vaccination, but asymptomatic HIV-infected adults do respond.[130,112]

Vaccine efficacy in preventing serious pneumococcal infection has been demonstrated for the purified polysaccharide vaccine primarily in immunocompetent adults, including elderly people and those with chronic diseases such as chronic pulmonary and cardiac disorders and diabetes mellitus, which predispose these patients to development of pneumococcal infections. Efficacy against vaccine serotypes ranges from 61% to 75% in adults.[99,594] Investigations in adults in whom vaccine protection against pneumococcal infection has been substantially less have been criticized for methodologic problems.[130,112] Efficacy in the limited studies of children has been consistent with that for adults. In children with sickle cell disease or anatomic asplenia, an octavalent vaccine was highly effective in preventing bacteremic infection.[51]

Adverse Events

Pneumococcal conjugate vaccines appear to be safe, and in 13 clinical trials, the safety profile of PCV13 was comparable to that of PCV7.[25,42,509] The reactions most commonly reported have been local reactions at the injection site, but they occur at a lower frequency than do local reactions with other childhood vaccines such as DTP.[80]

Local reactions at the injection site, such as erythema and pain, are reported for approximately 50% of recipients of the purified polysaccharide vaccine.[42] However, more severe local and systemic reactions, such as fever and myalgia, are rare events that occur in less than 1% of vaccine recipients. Severe systemic reactions such as anaphylaxis rarely have been reported.[692] Preterm infants show safety results comparable with those for term infants.[463] In adults who were revaccinated within 1 to 2 years in early studies, local reactions occurred more commonly than did those after initial immunization.[130,112] However, subsequent investigations, including studies of children, indicated no increase in the incidence or severity of local or systemic reactions on revaccination after longer intervals.[401,557]

Indications

Recommendations for the use of PCV13 have been issued by the AAP and the ACIP.[25,509] The AAP and ACIP recommend universal use of PCV13 in children 59 months or younger. For children to whom no prior PCV7 or PCV13 has been administered before they reach 7 months of age, four doses of PCV13 are recommended. Doses should be administered routinely at 2, 4, 6, and 12 to 15 months of age. For children younger than 24 months who have not received their recommended four doses of PCV7, a dose of PCV13 should be administered at the next scheduled vaccination; the total number of doses is based on the child's age and described elsewhere.[25,42,509]

A single supplemental dose of PCV13 is recommended for all children 14 months to 59 months who have previously received all four doses of PCV7. A single dose of PCV13 is recommended for children 60 months to 18 years of age who are fully immunized with PCV7 and have underlying medical conditions that increase their risk of IPD. For children 6 through 18 years of age, PCV13 should be given regardless of previous PCV7 or PPSV23 administration.[87] If not previously administered, children 24 months to 18 years of age should receive the PPV23 to expand serotype coverage.

The AAP recommends PPV23 for children 24 months or older and PCV13 for all children 59 months of age or older who belong to one or more of the following risk groups:

- Immunocompetent children with chronic heart disease, chronic lung disease, diabetes mellitus, cerebrospinal fluid leaks, or cochlear implants

- Children with functional or anatomic asplenia, including sickle cell disease or other hemoglobinopathies, congenital or acquired asplenia, or splenic dysfunction
- Children with immunocompromising conditions, including HIV infection; chronic renal failure and nephrotic syndrome; diseases associated with treatment with immunosuppressive drugs or radiation therapy, including malignant neoplasms, leukemias, lymphomas, and Hodgkin disease; or solid organ transplantation and congenital immunodeficiency

For previously vaccinated children 18 years or younger who are at high risk for severe pneumococcal infection, revaccination with PPV23 after 5 years is recommended.[25,87,509] For children between the ages of 6 and 18 years who have not received PCV13 but have received at least one PPSV23 dose, a single PCV13 dose should be given at least 8 weeks after the last PPSV23 dose, regardless of previously given PCV7.[176] This includes children who have functional (e.g., sickle cell disease) or anatomic asplenia, children and adolescents with HIV infection, and those who have a rapid antibody decline (i.e., nephrotic syndrome, renal failure, or organ transplantation).[295] Revaccination with PPV23 should be considered for high-risk older children and adults who were vaccinated 6 years or more earlier, but no more than two total PPV23 doses are necessary. The interval between polysaccharide and conjugate vaccines should be at least 8 weeks, regardless of the order given.[399]

Contraindications

No contraindications to initial vaccination exist.[25,509] The safety of pneumococcal vaccine in pregnant women has not been evaluated, but adverse consequences for the fetus have not been observed in neonates whose mothers were vaccinated inadvertently during pregnancy. Ideally, women at high risk for pneumococcal disease should be vaccinated before pregnancy. For people who have had a severe reaction, such as anaphylaxis or a localized, severe hypersensitivity response, revaccination should be avoided.

Poliovirus Vaccine

The widespread implementation of poliovirus vaccine programs resulted in a dramatic reduction in the incidence of paralytic poliomyelitis throughout the world. In contrast to the prevaccine era, when more than 18,000 cases of paralytic disease occurred in the United States annually, the last known case in this country caused by indigenous wild-type virus occurred in 1979.[178] Other than rare imported cases, the only cases of paralytic poliomyelitis in the United States since then have been vaccine related.

The effectiveness of polio vaccination led the WHO to launch the Global Polio Eradication Initiative in 1988, when approximately 350,000 people succumbed to polio each year. The initiative initially made rapid gains; the number of new wild poliovirus cases decreased by 99% between 1988 and 2005. However, ongoing transmission threatened the success of the polio eradication program, and the Polio Eradication and Endgame Strategic Plan 2013–18 was developed under the auspices of the WHO to eradicate wild poliovirus, vaccine-associated paralytic polio (VAPP), and circulating vaccine-derived poliovirus (VDPV).[701] The phased plan was implemented in places where OPV was used routinely. At least one dose of inactivated polio vaccine (IPV) was introduced in 2015, and bivalent OPV (bOPV, types 1 and 3) replaced trivalent OPV (tOPV) starting in 2016. The type 2 component of tOPV is being removed because it causes more than 90% of all cVDPV cases and approximately 40% of vaccine-associated paralytic polio cases, it interferes with the immune response to the other two types, and wild poliovirus type 2 has been eradicated since 1999.

As of 2016, four of the six regions of the WHO have been certified polio-free: the Americas (1994), Western Pacific (2000), Europe (2002), and South East Asia, including India (2014). Eighty percent of the world's population currently lives in polio-free areas. However, Afghanistan, Nigeria, and Pakistan are the three remaining reservoirs of endemic disease, largely because regional conflicts and poor health care infrastructures hinder widespread immunization campaigns. Countries with ongoing outbreaks of cVDPV include Guinea, Lao People's Democratic Republic, Madagascar, Myanmar, Nigeria, and Ukraine.[516,539,701]

The elimination of poliovirus infection has been achieved primarily through the use of OPV (i.e., Sabin strain). This product had been the vaccine of choice for children in the United States since the early 1960s because it induced optimal intestinal immunity, was painless to administer, and secondarily immunized some contacts by fecal-oral spread of the vaccine virus and contributed to the immunity of the population.[105] Because 8 to 10 cases of vaccine-associated paralytic polio occurred annually and the risk of exposure to wild poliovirus had been markedly reduced or eliminated in the United States, expanded use of IPV (i.e., Salk strain) was recommended by the CDC and the AAP beginning in 1997.[16,129]

In 1999, as a result of progress in the global eradication of poliomyelitis, the need for further reduction in the risk of acquiring vaccine-associated paralytic polio, and the acceptance of IPV by parents and physicians,[131] IPV was recommended for the first two doses of poliovirus vaccine for routine childhood vaccination.[18,134] To eliminate the risk of vaccine-associated paralytic polio completely, an all-IPV schedule was recommended in January of 2000 for routine childhood vaccination in the United States.[19,137,134] IPV is the only vaccine used in developed countries.

Since 2000, there have been ongoing outbreaks of paralytic poliomyelitis caused by circulating VDPVs that are neurovirulent polioviruses derived from the Sabin OPV vaccine strain. The epidemics have occurred among underimmunized children living in certain economically deprived regions. The low immunization rates in these areas have permitted these viruses to circulate for long periods and, by continuous mutation, to acquire biologic properties that are indistinguishable from naturally occurring wild polioviruses. Interruptions in OPV administration and the previous eradication of the corresponding serotype of indigenous wild poliovirus were the critical risk factors for all VDPV outbreaks.[387] Circulation of VDPVs underscores the critical importance of eliminating the last pockets of wild poliovirus, maintaining universally high levels of polio vaccine coverage (>90% of young children), withdrawing all OPVs as soon as wild poliovirus has been eradicated globally, and continuing poliovirus surveillance into the foreseeable future.

Preparations

Trivalent IPV is the only vaccine available for routine infant and childhood immunization in the United States. IPV is prepared by inactivation of naturally occurring polioviruses by treatment with formaldehyde. Five trivalent IPV vaccines are available in the United States: IPOL (single-component vaccine [Sanofi Pasteur]), Pediarix (in combination with DTaP vaccine and HBV vaccine [GlaxoSmithKline]), Pentacel (in combination with DTaP and Hib vaccines [Sanofi Pasteur]), Quadracel (in combination with DTaP vaccine [Sanofi Pasteur]), and Kinrix (in combination with DTaP vaccine [GlaxoSmithKline]). These vaccines are produced in monkey kidney (Vero) cells except for Pentacel, which is grown in human diploid cells, and each contains 40, 8, and 32 D-antigen units of poliovirus types 1, 2, and 3, respectively. The single-component vaccine is the only IPV preparation that contains preservative.

The trivalent OPV formulations contain approximately $10^{6.5}$ 50% tissue culture infectious doses ($TCID_{50}$), $10^{5.5}$ $TCID_{50}$, and $10^{6.2}$ $TCID_{50}$ of poliovirus types 1, 2, and 3, respectively, in a 10:1:3 ratio. The unequal contribution of each type to the trivalent preparation represents a balanced formulation designed to account for the more efficient replication of type 2 OPV virus in the gastrointestinal tract and to avoid interference with the replication of the two latter types. The live oral OPV strains are grown in Vero cells and do not contain a preservative. OPV is no longer available in the United States.

Monovalent OPV (mOPV) vaccines (types 1 and 3) are recommended for use in supplementary immunization campaigns where only wild poliovirus type 1 or type 3 alone is circulating, with the purpose of controlling outbreaks. Two doses of mOPV administered within 2 weeks is used as part of the short-interval additional dose approach, which is intended to rapidly boost population immunity in certain settings.[670]

Immunogenicity and Efficacy

Neutralizing antibodies are detectable to all three poliovirus types in 99% of recipients of IPV after two doses and in 100% after the third dose.[468,606] Detectable antibody persists at protective levels for at least 5 years, although geometric mean titers decline considerably.[630] A meta-analysis revealed that vaccine efficacy of the currently licensed enhanced-potency IPV formulations ranges from 33% to 47% after one dose and 79% to 90% after two doses in infants older than 10 weeks.[308]

An optimal immune response to trivalent OPV requires multiple doses. In developed countries, three doses given at least 2 months apart are sufficient, with antibody prevalence to all three types being approximately 96% after the third dose.[468] Detectable serum antibody to all three types persists in 84% to 98% of vaccinees 5 years after receiving primary immunization.[411]

OPV efficacy was directly evaluated during a type 1 poliovirus outbreak in Taiwan in the early 1980s. During this outbreak, vaccine efficacy was estimated to be 82%, 96%, and 98% for one, two, and three or more doses, respectively.[390] In tropical countries, the series of OPV at 6, 10, and 14 weeks of age recommended by the WHO EPI fails to produce active immunity in a significant proportion of infants. Low seroconversion rates have been documented in many locations, averaging 73%, 90%, and 70% for types 1, 2, and 3, respectively.[526] Diarrheal disease at the time of immunization is a major factor.[496] The impact of diarrhea on seroconversion persists despite the administration of three or four OPV doses.

The monovalent OPV vaccines have higher type-specific seroconversion rates than does the trivalent vaccine and are considered more effective when used in response to an outbreak caused by one poliovirus type.[103]

Adverse Events

No serious adverse events have been associated with use of the currently available IPV vaccine.[19,43,134] Because IPV vaccine contains trace amounts of streptomycin, neomycin, and polymyxin B, allergic reactions are possible in recipients with hypersensitivity to one or more of these antibiotics.

The OPV vaccine can cause vaccine-associated paralytic polio, the overall risk for which is approximately one case per 2.4 million doses distributed. The rate after the first dose is approximately one case per 750,000 doses, including vaccine recipient and contact cases. Immunodeficiency-related VDPV excretion by people with primary immunodeficiencies is a rare complication of OPV use and is associated with chronic excretion and fatal disease.[98]

Indications

The polio vaccination series in the United States consists of four doses of IPV administered subcutaneously or intramuscularly.[19,43,134] The first and second doses are administered at 2 and 4 months of age, respectively. The third dose is usually given at 6 to 18 months of age, and a fourth dose is given routinely at 4 to 6 years of age, before school entry. Administration of a fourth dose is not necessary if the third dose was given on or after the child's fourth birthday. IPV is a component of Pediarix, Pentacel, Quadracel, and Kinrix. Pediarix may be given from 6 weeks through 6 years of age. Pentacel may be used 6 weeks through 4 years of age, and Quadracel and Kinrix may be used for children 4 to 6 years of age.

The WHO continues to recommend OPV as the vaccine of choice for global eradication of wild poliovirus in endemic areas and during epidemics. Since 2015, at least one additional dose of IPV is recommended from 14 weeks of age, with or without a concurrent OPV dose, in preparation for withdrawing all OPV after global eradication has been certified. Since 2016, trivalent OPV has been switched to bivalent OPV (i.e., types 1 and 3). In the immunization schedule of the WHO EPI, doses of OPV are recommended at birth and when the child is 6, 10, and 14 weeks of age.[29] In geographic areas with endemic polio, a dose may be given when the neonate is discharged from the hospital (i.e., the zero dose). Supplementary doses often are given during mass community programs in these areas. Breastfeeding does not interfere with successful immunization with OPV.

Routine poliovirus vaccination is not necessary in adults residing in the United States. These individuals are at minimal risk for exposure, and most are adequately protected because of vaccination during childhood. However, vaccination is recommended for individuals who have an increased risk of exposure, including people traveling to countries where poliomyelitis is epidemic or endemic, members of communities of specific population groups experiencing wild poliovirus disease, health care workers in close contact with patients who may be excreting wild poliovirus, and laboratory workers in contact with specimens that may contain wild-type poliovirus. Previously immunized adults who are at increased risk for exposure to poliomyelitis, such as those traveling to countries where poliomyelitis is still endemic, should receive a single dose of IPV. Available data do not indicate the need for more than a single lifetime booster dose of IPV. Adults who are unvaccinated or whose vaccination status is not documented should receive a primary vaccination series with IPV. This consists of two doses of IPV at 4- to 8-week intervals and a third dose 6 to 12 months after the second dose.

Precautions and Contraindications

IPV is contraindicated in people who have ha an anaphylactic reaction after receiving a previous dose of IPV or an anaphylactic reaction to one of the antibiotics in the vaccine preparation (i.e., streptomycin, polymyxin B, or neomycin).[19,43,134] Poliomyelitis vaccination usually is contraindicated in pregnant women because of the theoretical risk of harm to the fetus. However, no deleterious effects from IPV administered during pregnancy have been demonstrated; and if immediate protection against poliomyelitis is needed, IPV may be given.

Rotavirus Vaccine

Rotavirus infection is the most common cause of severe diarrhea disease in infants and young children worldwide and continues to have a major global impact on childhood morbidity and mortality, causing an estimated 527,000 deaths of children younger than 5 years each year or approximately 5% of all childhood deaths worldwide.[521] In the United States before the introduction of vaccine in 2006, an estimated 3 million rotavirus infections occurred every year, and 95% of children had at least one rotavirus infection by 5 years of age. Rotavirus infection was responsible for more than 400,000 physician visits, more than 200,000 emergency department (ED) visits, 55,000 to 70,000 hospitalizations, and 20 to 60 deaths each year of children younger than 5 years.[298,688] In the prevaccine era, rotavirus accounted for 30% to 50% of all hospitalizations for gastroenteritis among US children younger than 5 years.[217]

Rotavirus gastroenteritis is preventable with live oral rotavirus vaccines. In 1998, the only approved rotavirus vaccine, a tetravalent rhesus-based rotavirus vaccine (RRV-TV) (Rotashield, Wyeth Laboratories), was withdrawn from the market in the United States because of an association with intussusception among vaccinated infants.[495] In 2006, a bovine-based pentavalent rotavirus vaccine (RotaTeq, Merck & Co.) was licensed by the FDA for use in infants in the United States. The ACIP of the CDC and the AAP have recommended universal vaccination of US infants against rotavirus.[24,217] In 2008, a live attenuated human rotavirus vaccine (Rotarix, GlaxoSmithKline) was licensed in the United States.

The epidemiology of rotavirus disease in the United States has changed dramatically since rotavirus vaccines became available in 2006. National declines in rotavirus detection have been reported, ranging from 58% to 90% in each of the seven postvaccine years compared with all seven prevaccine years combined. A biennial pattern of rotavirus activity emerged in the postvaccine era, with years of low activity and highly erratic seasonality alternating with years of moderately increased activity and seasonality similar to that seen in the prevaccine era.[9] Other US studies show the large public health impact of routine rotavirus vaccination in reducing the circulation of rotavirus among US children. Declines in laboratory-confirmed rotavirus hospitalization[632] and reductions in outpatient visits, emergency room visits, acute gastroenteritis, and rotavirus-coded hospitalizations have been reported.[215] From 2007 through 2011, more than 176,000 hospitalizations, 242,000 emergency department visits, and 1.1 million outpatients visits due to diarrhea were averted, resulting in costs savings of $924 million over the 4-year period.[427]

Preparations

Two rotavirus vaccines are licensed for use in the United States. The pentavalent rotavirus vaccine (RV5) is an oral vaccine that contains five live reassortant rotaviruses. The rotavirus parent strains of the reassortants were isolated from human and bovine hosts. Four reassortant rotaviruses express one of the outer capsid proteins (i.e., G1, G2, G3, or G4) from the human rotavirus parent strain and the attachment protein (i.e., P7[5]) from the bovine rotavirus parent strain. The fifth reassortant virus expresses the attachment protein (i.e., P1A[8]) from the human rotavirus parent strain and the outer capsid protein (i.e., G6) from the bovine rotavirus parent strain. The reassortants are propagated in Vero cells using standard tissue culture techniques.

RV5 vaccine is provided in a squeezable plastic dosing tube with a twist-off cap designed to allow for the vaccine to be administered directly to infants by mouth. Each tube contains a single 2-mL dose of the vaccine as a buffered-stabilized liquid solution.

The human rotavirus vaccine (RV1) is a G1 P1A[8] virus attenuated by passage in cell culture. RV1 is provided as a lyophilized powder that is reconstituted with a supplied diluent before administration.

Both rotavirus vaccines must be stored at refrigerator temperatures (2°C–8°C [35°F–46°F]) and protected from light. RV1 diluent may be stored at room temperature. The vaccines must not be frozen. The shelf life of properly stored vaccine is 24 months. RV5 should be administered as soon as possible after being removed from refrigeration. RV1 should be administered within 24 hours of reconstitution. Reconstituted RV1 may be stored at refrigerator or room temperature.

No studies have addressed the interchangeability of the rotavirus vaccines.

Immunogenicity and Efficacy

The immune correlates of protection from rotavirus infection and disease are not fully understood. In a large phase III clinical trial of RV5, an increase in titer of rotavirus group-specific serum IgA antibodies was used as one of the measures of the immunogenicity. Serum samples were obtained from a subset of study participants before they were immunized and approximately 2 weeks after they received the third dose. Seroconversion was defined as a threefold or greater increase in antibody titer from baseline. Seroconversion rates for IgA antibody to rotavirus were 95% among vaccine recipients and 14% among recipients of the placebo.[660]

The efficacy of RV5 was evaluated in two phase III trials.[83,660] In these trials, the efficacy of RV5 after completion of a three-dose regimen against rotavirus gastroenteritis of any severity was 74%, and against severe rotavirus gastroenteritis, it was 98 percent. Efficacy was observed against all G1 to G4 and G9 serotypes, but relatively few non-G1 rotavirus cases were reported. RV5 reduced the incidence of office visits by 86%, emergency department visits by 94%, and hospitalizations for rotavirus gastroenteritis by 96%. The efficacy of RV5 in the second rotavirus season after immunization was 63% against rotavirus gastroenteritis of any severity and 88% against severe rotavirus gastroenteritis.

Neither breastfeeding nor concurrent administration of other childhood vaccines appears to diminish the efficacy of a three-dose series of RV5. The efficacy of RV5 between doses of a three-dose series and with less than three doses (i.e., incomplete regimen) was explored in post hoc analyses of the large efficacy study of RV5. The vaccine reduced the rates of combined hospitalizations and ED visits for G1 through G4 rotavirus gastroenteritis by 100% between doses 1 and 2 and 91% between doses 2 and 3. RV5 reduced the rates of rotavirus gastroenteritis regardless of serotype by 82% between doses 1 and 2 and 84% between doses 2 and 3.[237]

Phase III clinical trials of RV1 efficacy have involved more than 21,000 infants 6 through 12 weeks of age, primarily in two studies in Latin America and Europe.[569,658] After completion of a two-dose RV1 regimen, the efficacy of rotavirus vaccine against severe rotavirus gastroenteritis (i.e., Latin American study) was 85%, and against any rotavirus gastroenteritis (i.e., European study), it was 87%. RV1 reduced hospitalization for rotavirus gastroenteritis by 85% to 100%, depending on the study. The efficacy of fewer than two doses is not known.

Adverse Events

Safety with respect to intussusception was evaluated for 71,725 subjects enrolled in phase III efficacy trials of RV5.[83,660] For the prespecified 42-day postimmunization end point, six cases of intussusception were observed in the RV5 group versus five cases of intussusception in the placebo group (multiplicity-adjusted relative risk, 1.6). The data did not suggest an increased risk of intussusception relative to placebo. Among vaccine recipients, no confirmed cases of intussusception occurred within the 42-day period after administration of the first dose, which was the period of highest risk for the previously licensed RRV-TV vaccine. No evidence of clustering of cases of intussusception was observed within a 7- or 14-day window after immunization for any dose. For the 1-year follow-up period after administration of the first dose, 13 cases of intussusception were observed in the RV5 group versus 15 cases of intussusception in the placebo group (multiplicity-adjusted relative risk = 0.9).

Some studies performed outside the United States detected a low level of increased risk of intussusception after rotavirus immunization shortly after the first dose. The level of risk observed in these postmarketing studies is substantially lower than the risk of intussusception after immunization with RotaShield, the previous rotavirus vaccine.[100,524,655] US postmarketing studies have also identified a small increased risk of intussusception with RV5 and RV1, usually within a week after the first or second vaccine dose. This additional risk is estimated to range from about one case per 20,000 to 100,000 US infants who receive rotavirus vaccine.[73,325,601,679,708]

Both vaccines are well tolerated and have a low reactogenicity profile when given alone. They do not cause clinically significant increases in reactogenicity when coadministered with other routine childhood vaccines.[234,563] For both vaccines, the incidence of fever, vomiting, diarrhea, and irritability were measured in the clinical trials. For RV5, no significant difference versus placebo was observed in the incidence of fever or severe fever and irritability or severe irritability. A 3% increase in the incidence of diarrhea and vomiting was observed with RV5, but these symptoms were mild and did not require treatment.[83,236,660] For RV1, no difference versus placebo was observed in the incidence of diarrhea, fever or severe fever, vomiting or severe vomiting, and irritability or severe irritability within 14 days of immunization with any dose.[235,535,657,659] There was no statistically significant increased risk of death or other serious adverse events with either vaccine compared with placebo.

Vaccine virus shedding in stool has been documented for both rotavirus vaccines. Rotavirus shedding occurs in approximately 9% of RV5 recipients after the first dose but rarely after subsequent doses.[236] For RV1, live rotavirus shedding in stool occurs in approximately 25% of recipients, with peak excretion occurring about day 7 after the first dose. With the use of more sensitive real-time PCR tests for rotavirus shedding, detection rates for viral shedding were demonstrated in 20% to 30% in recipients of RV5 and in 80% to 90% of those receiving RV1.[355,611] Both vaccines have been transmitted from vaccine recipients to unvaccinated siblings, but no significant gastrointestinal symptoms were seen in the unvaccinated sibling after transmission.[527,559] Shedding and transmission are not considered significant safety concerns because of the attenuated nature of the rotavirus vaccine strains and the lack of severe gastrointestinal symptoms after transmission.

In 2010, porcine circovirus or porcine circovirus DNA was detected in both rotavirus vaccines.[68,297,413,469] There is no evidence that this virus is a safety risk or causes illness in humans.[412]

Indications

Infants should receive three doses of RV5 administered orally at 2, 4, and 6 months of age or two doses of the RV1 at 2 and 4 months of age.[24,217] The first dose should be administered when the child is between 6 and 14 weeks of age (i.e., on or before 14 weeks, 0 days of age). Subsequent doses should be administered at a minimum of 4-week intervals, and all doses of vaccine should be administered by the time the child is 32 weeks of age (i.e., on or before 32 weeks, 0 days).

Immunization should not be initiated for infants older than 14 weeks because of insufficient data on the safety of the first dose of rotavirus vaccine in older infants. Vaccine should not be administered after 8 months of age because of insufficient data on the safety and efficacy of rotavirus vaccine in infants after this age. For infants for whom the first dose of rotavirus vaccine is inadvertently administered off-label at 15 weeks or older, the rest of the rotavirus immunization series should be completed according to the schedule defined earlier because timing of the first dose should not affect the safety and efficacy of the second and third doses.

The rotavirus vaccine series should be completed with the same product whenever possible. However, vaccination should not be deferred if the product used for a prior dose or doses is not available or is not known. In this situation, the provider should continue or complete the series with the product that is available. If any dose in the series was RV5 (RotaTeq) or the vaccine brand used for any prior dose in the series is not known, a total of three doses of rotavirus vaccine should be administered. Infants documented to have had rotavirus gastroenteritis before receiving the full course of rotavirus immunizations should still start or complete the three-dose schedule because the initial infection frequently provides only partial immunity.

Infants who are being breastfed can receive rotavirus vaccine. Like other childhood vaccines, rotavirus vaccine can be administered to infants with transient, mild illnesses, with or without low-grade fever.[408] Rotavirus vaccine can be administered together with DTaP, Hib, IPV, hepatitis B, and pneumococcal conjugate vaccines.

The AAP and ACIP support immunization of preterm infants under the following conditions. The infant is at least 6 weeks of age, the infant is clinically stable, and the first dose of vaccine is given at the time of discharge or after the infant has been discharged from the hospital nursery.

Infants living in households with people who have or are suspected of having an immunodeficiency disorder or impaired immune status or with a pregnant woman can be immunized. To minimize potential virus transmission, all members of the household should employ measures such as good handwashing after contact with the feces of the immunized infant (e.g., after changing a diaper) for at least 1 week after the first dose of rotavirus vaccine has been given.

An infant who regurgitates, spits out, or vomits during or after receiving a dose of rotavirus vaccine should not have that dose re-administered. The infant can receive the remaining recommended doses of rotavirus vaccine at appropriate intervals. If a recently immunized child is hospitalized for any reason, no precautions other than standard precautions need be taken to prevent the spread of vaccine virus in the hospital setting.

Contraindications and Precautions

Rotavirus vaccine should not be administered to infants who have severe hypersensitivity to any component of the vaccine or individuals who have experienced a serious allergic reaction to a previous dose of rotavirus vaccine.[24,217] The RV1 oral applicator contains latex rubber. RV5 may be preferred for children at high risk for latex sensitization.

Practitioners should consider the potential risks and benefits of administering rotavirus vaccine to infants with known or suspected altered immunocompetence. Children and adults who are immunocompromised because of congenital immunodeficiency, bone marrow transplantation, or solid organ transplantation sometimes experience severe, prolonged, and even fatal rotavirus gastroenteritis. However, no safety or efficacy data are available for the administration of rotavirus vaccine to infants who are potentially immunocompromised with the exception of infants with severe combined immune deficiency (SCID). SCID is a contraindication for the use of both rotavirus vaccines.[157] Gastroenteritis, including severe diarrhea and prolonged shedding of vaccine virus, has been reported in infants who were administered live oral rotavirus vaccines and later identified as having SCID.[61]

Rotavirus vaccine should not be administered to infants with acute, moderate to severe gastroenteritis until the condition improves. Rotavirus vaccine has not been studied among infants with concurrent acute gastroenteritis, in whom its immunogenicity and efficacy theoretically can be compromised. Infants with moderate to severe illness should be immunized as soon as they have recovered from the acute phase of the illness.

Infants with preexisting chronic gastrointestinal conditions and who are not undergoing immunosuppressive therapy should benefit from rotavirus vaccine immunization, and the benefits outweigh the theoretical risks. However, the safety and efficacy of rotavirus vaccine have not been established for infants with these preexisting conditions (e.g., congenital malabsorption syndromes, Hirschsprung disease, short-gut syndrome, persistent vomiting of unknown cause).

A history of intussusception is a contraindication for the use of both rotavirus vaccines.[165] Some data suggest that infants with a history of intussusception may be at higher risk for a repeat episode than other infants.

Rubella Vaccine

Rubella is a viral disease that usually manifests as a mild febrile rash illness in adults and children; however, 20% to 50% of infected people are asymptomatic. Rubella can have severe adverse effects on the fetuses of pregnant women who contract the disease during the first trimester of pregnancy. It causes a wide range of congenital defects known as congenital rubella syndrome (CRS). The primary objective of the rubella vaccination program is to prevent intrauterine rubella infection. The primary strategies for rubella control in the United States are universal childhood vaccination, prenatal screening of pregnant women for rubella immunity, and vaccination of rubella-susceptible women after delivery.

In the prevaccine era, epidemics of rubella occurred every 6 to 9 years, with the last major epidemic in the United States taking place in 1964 through 1965.[694] The incidence of reported cases of rubella fell sharply after routine rubella immunization of young children was initiated in the United States in 1969. From the estimated 2 million cases per year in the prevaccine era, fewer than 1000 cases were reported in 1983.

During 1989 through 1991, a resurgence of rubella occurred, primarily because of outbreaks among unvaccinated adolescents and young adults who initially were not recommended for vaccination and in religious communities with low rubella vaccination coverage.[107] As a result of the rubella outbreaks, two clusters of approximately 20 CRS cases occurred.[424,475] Outbreaks during the mid-1990s occurred in settings where young adults congregated and involved unvaccinated people who belonged to specific racial or ethnic groups.[121] Further declines occurred as rubella vaccination efforts increased in other countries in the WHO Region of the Americas. From 2001 through 2004, reported rubella and CRS cases were at an all-time low, with an average of 14 reported rubella cases a year, four CRS cases, and one rubella outbreak (defined as three or more cases linked in time or place).[550]

In October 2004, 35 years after initiation of the rubella immunization program, an independent panel of international experts was convened by the CDC to assess progress toward elimination of rubella and CRS. Based on data showing fewer than 25 cases of rubella reported each year since 2001, at least 95% vaccination coverage among school-aged children, an estimated 91% population immunity, adequate surveillance to detect rubella outbreaks, and a pattern of virus genotypes consistent with virus originating in other parts of the world, panel members concluded unanimously that rubella was no longer is endemic in the United States.[549]

Rubella continues to be endemic in many parts of the world. Internationally imported rubella cases may give rise to indigenous transmission. From 2005 through 2011, a median of 11 rubella cases was reported each year in the United States (range, 4–18). Two rubella outbreaks involving three cases and four total CRS cases were reported. Among the 67 rubella cases reported from 2005 through 2011, a total of 28 cases (42%) were known importations.[551] In 2011, an expert panel reviewed available data and unanimously agreed that rubella elimination had been maintained in the United States.[520]

From 2012 through 2015 a total of 29 rubella cases (range, 5–9 cases/year) and 6 CRS cases (range, 1–3 cases/year) have been reported in the United States. The United States needs to continue its vigilance against rubella and CRS by maintaining high vaccination rates among children; ensuring vaccination among women of childbearing age, especially women born outside the United States; continuing surveillance of rubella and CRS; and responding rapidly to any outbreak.[146]

Preparations

Since 1979, RA 27/3 (*Rubella abortus*, 27th specimen, third extract) vaccine, prepared in human diploid tissue culture, has been the only vaccine available in the United States; it replaced the earlier HPV-77 and Cendehill vaccines. RA 27/3 induces higher antibody titers and more closely parallels the immune response after natural infection than did previous vaccines.[314,420,425,515,676] Two rubella-containing vaccines, MMR and MMRV, are available. Both vaccines should be kept at 2°C to 8°C (35.6°F–46.4°F) or colder during storage and should be protected from light to avoid inactivation of the virus. After reconstitution, the vaccine should be used within 8 hours.

Immunogenicity and Efficacy

Immunization with rubella vaccine induces humoral and cell-mediated immunity. At least 95% of susceptible vaccinees 12 months or older develop antibody titers that are protective after a single dose of vaccine.[275,281,288,607,639,676] After a second dose of rubella vaccine, approximately 99% had detectable rubella antibody and approximately 60% had a fourfold increase in titer.[372,404,423]

Follow-up studies indicate that one dose of rubella vaccine can provide long-lasting immunity. Vaccine-induced rubella antibodies have persisted in more than 90% of vaccinees 16 years after receiving a single dose of vaccine, but antibody levels decreased over time.[190,345,353,421,540] Although levels of vaccine-induced rubella antibodies can decrease over time, data from surveillance of rubella and CRS suggest that waning immunity with increased susceptibility to rubella disease does not occur. Among people receiving two doses, approximately 91% to 100% had detectable antibodies 12 to 15 years after receiving the second dose.[227,423]

Outbreaks of rubella in vaccinated populations are rare. Studies demonstrate rubella vaccine is approximately 97% effective in preventing clinical disease after a single dose (range, 94–100%).[69,225,283]

Lifelong protection against clinical reinfection or asymptomatic viremia, or both, usually results from a single dose of vaccine given early in childhood. In some cases, vaccinees exposed to natural rubella developed a rise in antibody titer unassociated with clinical symptoms. Reinfection is associated only rarely with viremia. Significant pharyngeal shedding also is observed infrequently. Person-to-person transmission, however, has not been reported. Reinfection caused by wild-type rubella virus also may be observed in individuals with previous natural rubella infection. The risk of CRS developing from rubella reinfection during pregnancy is extremely low.[561]

Adverse Events

Rubella vaccines usually are well tolerated. The most frequent complaints after vaccination are fever, lymphadenopathy, or rash, which occur in 5% to 15% of children 5 to 12 days after receiving vaccination.[44] Transient peripheral neuritis (i.e., paresthesia and pain in the arms and legs) has been observed uncommonly, primarily in older age groups.[580]

Approximately 3% of children have transient joint manifestations, including arthralgia and, less commonly, arthritis 1 to 3 weeks after being immunized. Although 25% of women report having joint pain after being vaccinated, arthritis with objective clinical findings lasting less than 10 days occurs in 13% to 15%. Cases of persistent or recurrent joint symptoms have been reported but are rare events. In 1992, the IOM reviewed the existing data on rubella and adverse joint events and concluded that the evidence available was consistent with a causal relationship between rubella vaccination and chronic arthritis in women, although data on current vaccine strains are limited.[354] The incidence of joint manifestations after immunization is lower than that after natural infection at the corresponding age.

Rubella revaccination is well tolerated, even among college-aged and older vaccinees, and it is associated with a much lower incidence of adverse reactions than primary rubella immunization of young adult populations. Reported rates of joint-related complaints of 4% to 18% after revaccination are lower than those reported after primary vaccination.[186,590]

Indications

Live virus rubella vaccine usually is recommended for all children 12 months or older. It is given as MMR or MMRV when children are 12 to 15 months of age.[44,471] A second dose of rubella vaccine administered as MMR or MMRV is given at the time they enter school, usually 4 to 6 years of age, according to recommendations for routine measles immunization. The vaccine should be provided to previously unimmunized preschool-aged children or older schoolchildren despite a history of having clinical rubella, unless serologic tests confirm immunity.

Emphasis should be placed on the immunization of the postpubertal male and female population, especially college students and those in the military. Rubella vaccine also should be administered to adolescent girls and women of childbearing age who lack a history of previous vaccination. Other opportunities for immunization include premarital screening, routine gynecologic examinations, visits for neonatal and well-child care, or other medical visits. The immediate postpartum period is an excellent time for giving immunizations. Rubella vaccine can be given after administration of anti-Rho(D) immune globulin, but serologic testing to determine whether seroconversion has occurred should be performed at least 8 weeks after vaccination. When practical, potential vaccinees may be screened for susceptibility. However, vaccination of girls and women of childbearing age is justifiable and may be preferable, without previous serologic testing of women not known to be pregnant.

Adults in the United States who were born in countries where rubella vaccination was not offered are at higher risk for contracting rubella and having infants with CRS. Health care practitioners who treat foreign-born adults should document the rubella immunity of these patients with a written record of rubella-containing vaccine or by serologic testing. Susceptible adults, especially women of childbearing age, should be vaccinated. During rubella outbreaks, all susceptible people who have no contraindications to rubella vaccine should be identified and vaccinated.

Precautions and Contraindications

Specific contraindications to the administration of live rubella vaccine include pregnancy; severe febrile illness; known history of anaphylactic reaction to rubella vaccine, gelatin, or neomycin, which are contained in the vaccine; and immunodeficiency conditions (i.e., malignancy, primary immunodeficiency disease, immunosuppressive or corticosteroid therapy, and radiation therapy).[44,471] People with mild immunosuppression, such as those with asymptomatic HIV infection or those taking short-term or low-dose corticosteroids, may be vaccinated.

Postpubertal women of childbearing age who are known to be pregnant or who are attempting to become pregnant should not be vaccinated. Vaccinated women should be counseled about the need to avoid pregnancy for 28 days after receiving vaccination.[471] Although pregnancy is a contraindication to administering rubella vaccination, the maximal theoretical risk to the fetus is estimated to be 2.6%.[545] From 1979 until 1989, the CDC registered 321 susceptible women who inadvertently had received RA 27/3 rubella vaccine within 3 months before or after conception and carried their pregnancies to term. None of their infants had defects compatible with CRS, although 2% had serologic evidence of intrauterine infection.[113] Because rubella virus has been isolated from the products of conception of women vaccinated during pregnancy, continued caution with respect to vaccination during pregnancy is advised. However, the evidence available indicates that rubella vaccination inadvertently given during pregnancy ordinarily does not represent a reason to consider interruption of pregnancy.

Although vaccine virus may be isolated from the pharynx, vaccinees do not transmit rubella to others, except in the case of a vaccinated breastfeeding mother. In this situation, the infant may be infected through breast milk, and a mild rash illness may develop, but serious adverse effects have not been noted. Infants infected through breastfeeding respond normally to rubella vaccination at 15 months of age. Breastfeeding is not a contraindication to receiving rubella vaccination.

Concern about potential transmission of disease from immunized children to susceptible contacts, including pregnant women, has not been supported by studies of susceptible household contacts. Susceptible children whose household contacts are pregnant may be vaccinated.

People with a history of thrombocytopenia may experience thrombocytopenia after receipt of MMR vaccine. The decision to vaccinate should depend on the benefits of immunity compared with the risk of recurrence or exacerbation of thrombocytopenia after vaccination or during natural infection with measles or rubella.

Rubella vaccine should not be given during an interval beginning 2 weeks before and extending 3 months after the administration of immune globulin or blood transfusion. Because rubella vaccine usually is given as MMR or MMRV, and evidence suggests that high doses of immune globulin preparations can inhibit the immune response to measles vaccine for 3 or more months, depending on the dosage, rubella vaccination with MMR or MMRV necessitates deferral for longer periods (see Measles Vaccine).[44,471,603]

Tetanus Toxoid

The efficacy of active immunization against tetanus was demonstrated most dramatically in military personnel during World War II, when tetanus toxoid virtually eliminated tetanus in injured servicemen. Since the 1940s, routine immunization of civilians in the United States with tetanus toxoid has been successful in almost eliminating tetanus. In most cases, disease has been reported in unimmunized or inadequately immunized individuals.[114] The primary three-dose series of a tetanus toxoid–containing vaccine confers protective immunity for 10 years or longer.[90,405]

Without a tetanus booster, immunity wanes over time. The potential for occurrence of tetanus is indicated by the significant number of adults in the United States who lack protective concentrations of serum antibody.[289] Between 2001 and 2008, 233 cases of tetanus were reported in the United States with a case-fatality rate of 13%. In 22 of these cases, the children were between the ages of 5 and 19 years, and 16 had received one or no tetanus immunizations. There were no deaths in this age group.[168]

Neonatal tetanus also has been almost eliminated in the United States. However, it is a leading cause of morbidity in neonates in developing countries. As a result, global elimination of neonatal tetanus remains a goal of the WHO. Because the spores of tetanus are distributed widely in the environment, the risk of infection among the unimmunized is constant. This is a fact not necessarily appreciated by parents who refuse immunization in the belief that widespread immunization in the general population will confer some protection on the unimmunized, as was demonstrated by two cases of tetanus in children in Oklahoma in 2012.[246,375]

Preparations

Tetanus toxoid is prepared by formaldehyde treatment of *Clostridium tetani* toxin.[90,405] It has been prepared in fluid and aluminum salt-adsorbed preparations, but in the United States, only the latter is available. Fluid toxoid preparations result in a significantly shorter duration of immunity than that induced by aluminum-adsorbed antigens; therefore, adsorbed antigens are recommended.

Tetanus toxoid is available in combination with diphtheria toxoid and acellular pertussis vaccine (DTaP) for routine administration to infants and children younger than 7 years and for adolescents and adults 11 years or older as a single booster (Tdap). For all people for whom pertussis vaccine is contraindicated, tetanus toxoid is combined with diphtheria toxoid as DT or Td (see Diphtheria Toxoid).

The first two Tdap vaccines approved for use in adolescents and adults in the United States—Boostrix (GlaxoSmithKline Biologicals) and Adacel (Sanofi Pasteur)—were licensed in 2005. Preparations of DT, Td, and Tdap are identical in the amounts of tetanus toxoid they contain, but they differ in the quantity of diphtheria toxoid. The dose of Tdap is the same as that of DT or Td (0.5 mL) and is administered intramuscularly.

Immunogenicity and Efficacy

Adequate primary immunization provides sufficient protective titers of antitoxin for at least 10 years and ensures prompt, anamnestic responses to subsequent booster injections. Immune response to tetanus toxoid was measured after administration of each adult Tdap vaccine and compared with that elaborated after Td vaccine. Seroprotective anti-tetanus antibody concentrations, defined as a titer 0.1 IU/mL or greater, and booster response rates to tetanus were determined to be noninferior after vaccination with Tdap compared with Td vaccination.[90,405]

Adverse Events

Local reactions of pain, swelling, and induration can occur, but these reactions in children usually are attributable to the pertussis component contained in the vaccine rather than to response to tetanus toxoid.[47] Hypersensitivity reactions can occur in adolescents and adults but rarely are severe. Neurologic reactions occurring after the administration of tetanus toxoid are rare events. Reactions include brachial neuritis and Guillain-Barré syndrome.

Regarding adverse reactions reported after Tdap, vaccination with Boostrix was associated with a statistically higher rate of moderate to severe headache compared with Td, and that with Adacel was associated with higher rates of mild injection site pain and low-grade fever compared with the Td vaccine. No serious adverse events have been reported for Boostrix. Two cases of serious adverse advents (both characterized as neuropathic reactions) in adults possibly related to having received Adacel (none reported in adolescents) have been reported, and in both cases, symptoms resolved completely within several days.[90,405]

Indications

Preexposure indications. For primary immunization, doses of tetanus toxoid provided as DTaP should be administered when the child is 2, 4, and 6 months of age.[21,47,90] A fourth dose is given 6 to 12 months after the third dose (i.e., at 12 to 18 months of age) to maintain adequate serum antibody concentrations for the ensuing preschool years. For children younger than 7 years not immunized in infancy, an initial dose of DTaP is given with subsequent doses 2, 4, and 10 to 16 months later, followed by a single booster dose at age 4 to 6 years, just before school entry.

In 2005, the FDA licensed two Tdap vaccines for routine use in adolescents and adults. Adacel (Sanofi Pasteur) is approved for people 11 to 64 years of age, and Boostrix (GlaxoSmithKline Biologicals) is approved for children and adolescents 10 years or older. These vaccines are approved for one-time use only in individuals who have previously completed their primary vaccination series with DTP or DTaP as a substitute for their next Td booster.[171] The preferred age for Tdap vaccination is 11 to 12 years. Catch-up vaccination with Tdap is encouraged for adolescents 13 to 18 years old who completed their primary series with DTP or DTaP and have not received a Td or Tdap booster.

Adolescents 11 through 18 years of age who received Td but not Tdap are encouraged to receive a single dose of Tdap to provide protection against pertussis if they have completed the recommended childhood DTP/DTaP immunization series. Tdap should be administered regardless of the interval since the last tetanus or diphtheria toxoid–containing vaccine. Although longer intervals between Td and Tdap may decrease the occurrence of local reactions, the benefits of protection against pertussis outweigh the potential risk of adverse events.[47,171] Every 10 years thereafter, tetanus booster should be provided by Td.

Adolescents between the ages of 11 and 18 years who have never been vaccinated against tetanus, diphtheria, or pertussis should receive Tdap initially, followed by Td for the subsequent two doses 4 or more weeks and then 6 to 12 months later. For children between the ages of 7 and 10 years who have not been vaccinated previously, Tdap vaccine should substitute an initial dose of Td in the catch-up series, followed by two subsequent doses of Td vaccine at 4 or more weeks, and 6 to 12 months after the previous dose.[47,171] Interruption of the recommended schedule or delay in administering subsequent doses during primary immunization does not reduce immunity.

Antepartum indications. In areas of the world where the risk of acquiring neonatal tetanus is significant, previously unimmunized, pregnant women should receive two antepartum doses of a tetanus toxoid–containing vaccine spaced at least 4 weeks apart. The second dose should be given at least 2 weeks before delivery. The woman should complete the three-dose series in 6 to 12 months.[318,405] Tdap should be substituted for the first Td dose if Tdap has not been administered previously. In the United States, immunization with Tdap is recommended during each pregnancy, preferably in the early third trimester.[171,175] If vaccination is not provided before delivery or during pregnancy, women who have not received Tdap vaccine previously should receive a single dose of Tdap in the immediate postpartum period, preferably before being discharged from their hospital or birthing center.

Postexposure wound management. The potential need for immunoprophylaxis is an integral aspect of wound management at the time of trauma or injury. The recommended use of tetanus toxoid in

TABLE 245.17 Recommended Tetanus Prophylaxis in Wound Management

	CLEAN, MINOR WOUNDS		ALL OTHER WOUNDS[a]	
History of Tetanus Toxoid	**Td or Tdap[b]**	**TIG**	**Td or Tdap[b]**	**TIG**
<3 doses or unknown	Yes	No	Yes	Yes
≥3 doses	No[c]	No	No[d]	No

[a]Including wounds contaminated with dirt, feces, soil, and saliva; puncture wounds; avulsions; and wounds resulting from missiles, crushing, burns, and frostbite.
[b]For children <7 y; diphtheria–tetanus–acellular pertussis (DTaP) or diphtheria-tetanus (DT) (depending on vaccine status of patient) is preferred to tetanus toxoid (TT) alone. Tdap is preferred over Td for underimmunized children ≥7 y who have not received Tdap previously.[47] Td is preferred to TT for adolescents who received Tdap previously or when Tdap is not available.
[c]Yes if ≥10 y since last tetanus-containing vaccine dose.
[d]Yes if ≥5 y since last tetanus-containing vaccine dose. More frequent boosters are not needed and can accentuate side effects.
Td, Tetanus-diphtheria; *Tdap,* tetanus–diphtheria–acellular pertussis; *TIG,* tetanus immune globulin.

addition to tetanus immune globulin at the time of injury is given in Table 245.17. To ensure adequate immunity, children and adults receiving tetanus toxoid for wound management should be given age-appropriate preparations of vaccines containing diphtheria and pertussis, unless contraindicated, and tetanus toxoid. Tdap is preferred over Td if the person has not received Tdap previously.[47,171] Specific recommendations depend on the individual's immunization status, the nature of the wound, and the duration of time between when the injury occurred and evaluation and treatment were undertaken.

After prophylaxis is provided, primary immunization should be completed subsequently in those lacking the recommended number of doses. This conservative approach to the frequent administration of booster doses of tetanus toxoid in wound management for previously immunized people is supported by the prolonged immunity from tetanus vaccination and the increased incidence of hypersensitivity reactions associated with receipt of frequent booster injections.[529] Patients convalescing from tetanus infection should complete active immunization because infection often does not confer immunity.

Precautions and Contraindications

A history of having an immediate, severe hypersensitivity reaction to tetanus toxoid–containing preparations that is severe or anaphylactic in type is a contraindication to receiving further vaccination.[21,47,90,405] People who experience Arthus-type hypersensitivity reactions after receiving tetanus toxoid or temperature greater than 39.4°C (103°F) after a previous dose of a tetanus toxoid–containing preparation usually have high serum tetanus antitoxin concentrations and should not be given doses of Td more frequently than every 10 years, even if they have a tetanus-prone wound.[47] If an anaphylactic reaction to a previous dose of tetanus toxoid is suspected, intradermal skin testing may be helpful in determining whether to discontinue tetanus toxoid vaccination.[367]

Because tetanus toxoid administration has been associated with recurrence of Guillain-Barré syndrome in rare cases,[359] the decision to give additional doses in people with a history of this syndrome within 6 weeks after receipt of tetanus toxoid should be based on consideration of the benefit of revaccination and the comparative risk of recurrence of Guillain-Barré syndrome.[128] No physician-diagnosed cases of anaphylaxis, Arthus reactions, or Guillain-Barré syndrome in any adolescent or adult after either Tdap vaccine have been reported.

Varicella Vaccine

In the prevaccine era, varicella was endemic in the United States and virtually all people acquired varicella by the time they reached adulthood. Varicella infection was responsible for an estimated 4 million cases, 11,000 hospitalizations, and 100 deaths each year in the United States.[133] Approximately 90% of cases were children, with the highest incidence for children 1 to 6 years old.

After introduction and routine use of varicella vaccine in 1995, the incidence of varicella fell by 90%, deaths from varicella declined by 66%, and rates of hospitalization for varicella decreased by 80%.[322,504,715] However, a high frequency of breakthrough varicella (i.e., chickenpox occurring in a previously vaccinated person) in immunized children and continuing outbreaks of varicella in schools and in childcare centers occurred, despite high rates of vaccination.[292] Studies showed that over time the vaccine's effectiveness was less than 90%,[592] and in one study of healthy children, the rate of seroconversion after one dose of the vaccine was only 76%.[477] In June 2006, the CDC and AAP recommended a routine two-dose varicella vaccination policy for children (i.e., first dose at 12 to 15 months and second dose at 4 to 6 years) and catch-up vaccinations for children, adolescents, and adults who previously had received only one dose.[23,451]

Since recommendation of a routine second dose of vaccine in 2006, the incidence of varicella has declined further among children. Data show that administration of two doses of varicella vaccine is associated with higher antibody titers, presumably offering better protection from varicella.[415] Results from a controlled study of the effectiveness of two doses of varicella vaccine indicated that administration of two doses was highly effective in preventing varicella in the first 2.5 years after implementation of the two-dose schedule to prevent disease.[595] Odds of developing varicella were 95% lower for children who received two doses compared with one dose of varicella vaccine.

Preparations

Three varicella-containing vaccines are approved for use in the United States: varicella vaccine (Varivax), combination MMRV vaccine (ProQuad), and herpes zoster vaccine (Zostavax). Varicella vaccine was licensed in the United States in 1995. It is a preparation of the Oka strain of varicella-zoster virus (VZV) obtained from the vesicle fluid of a healthy child with varicella that has been attenuated by serial propagation in human embryo lung fibroblasts, guinea pig embryonic cells, and human diploid cell cultures. The vaccine contains trace amounts of neomycin, fetal bovine serum, sucrose, residual components of human diploid (MRC-5) cells, and gelatin. The vaccine does not contain preservatives.

Varicella vaccine is lyophilized and stored frozen at −15°C or colder until reconstituted. Any freezer that reliably maintains an average temperature of −15°C and has a separate sealed freezer door is acceptable for storing vaccine. The vaccine also may be stored at refrigerator temperature (2°C–8°C) for as long as 72 hours before reconstitution. Vaccine stored at 2°C to 8°C that is not used within 72 hours should be discarded. Reconstituted vaccine should be stored at room temperature and discarded if it is not used within 30 minutes.

In September 2005, a combined live attenuated MMRV vaccine was licensed for use in children 12 months through 12 years of age.[148] The attenuated measles, mumps, and rubella vaccine viruses in MMRV are identical and of equal titer to those in the MMR vaccine. The titer of Oka/Merck VZV is higher in MMRV vaccine than in single-antigen varicella vaccine. Each 0.5-mL dose contains a small quantity of hydrolyzed gelatin, human albumin, residual components of MRC-5 cells, neomycin, bovine calf serum, and other buffer and media ingredients. Unlike single-antigen varicella vaccine, MMRV vaccine cannot be stored at refrigerator temperature. MMRV vaccine must be stored frozen at an average temperature of −15°C or lower for up to 18 months. After reconstitution, the vaccine should be used immediately to minimize loss of potency and should be discarded if it is not used within 30 minutes. The diluent should be stored separately at room temperature or in the refrigerator. MMRV vaccine contains no preservative.

In May 2006, the FDA approved herpes zoster vaccine for use in people 60 years or older. No indications for use of this vaccine in children exist.

Immunogenicity and Efficacy

Varicella vaccine is highly immunogenic in susceptible children. Seroconversion has occurred in more than 96% of children 12 months to 12 years of age after one dose of vaccine.[685] Preexisting antibody, if present at 12 months of age, does not appear to interfere with antibody response. As with other viral vaccines, the antibody response after immunization is lower than that from natural disease. Adolescents and adults have age-related decreases in the ability to develop a primary response to varicella virus.[291] Seroconversion rates of 78% to 82% after one dose and 99% after two doses have been reported in those older than 12 years.[291,685]

In studies in the United States and Japan, serum antibodies to varicella have been detected for as long as 10 to 20 years after immunization in more than 95% of immunized children.[59,376] Antibody concentrations have persisted for at least 1 year in 97% of adults and adolescents who were administered two doses of vaccine 4 to 8 weeks apart.[291] Cell-mediated immunity to VZV has been detected in 87% of children and 94% of adults 5 years after vaccination.[714]

MMRV vaccine was licensed on the basis of equivalence of immunogenicity of the antigenic components, rather than clinical efficacy. Clinical studies involving healthy children 12 to 23 months of age indicated that those who received a single dose of MMRV vaccine developed levels of antibody to measles, mumps, rubella, and varicella similar to those of children who received MMR and varicella vaccines concomitantly at separate injection sites.[414]

Varicella vaccine has been demonstrated to be highly effective in preventing varicella in children and in reducing the severity of infection if they do become infected. In prelicensure clinical trials, vaccine was 70% to 90% effective in preventing varicella and more than 95% effective in preventing severe disease.[416,674] Several postlicensure studies have shown similar results, with vaccine effectiveness ranging from 83% to 100% in preventing varicella and 87% to 100% in preventing severe disease.[195,365,654] In follow-up studies, chickenpox developed in 0.2% to 2.3% of vaccinated children per year after exposure to wild-type varicella virus, a rate that does not seem to increase with length of time after immunization.[661] These vaccine failure cases are mild, with fewer skin lesions, lower rates of fever, and faster recovery, and they are less contagious than are moderate to severe cases of varicella.[75,593,661,671] These infections have been called *breakthrough varicella*.

Although findings of some studies have suggested otherwise, most investigations have not identified time since vaccination as a risk factor for breakthrough varicella. Some investigations have identified asthma, use of corticosteroids, and vaccination at younger than 15 months as risk factors for breakthrough varicella.[251,286,365,646,656] Breakthrough varicella infection can result from several factors, including interference of vaccine virus replication by circulating antibody, impotent vaccine resulting from storage or handling errors, or inaccurate record keeping. Interference from live viral vaccine administered before varicella vaccine can reduce vaccine effectiveness.

A study of 115,000 children in two health maintenance organizations from 1995 to 1999 found that children who received varicella vaccine less than 30 days after MMR vaccination had a 2.5-fold increased risk of breakthrough varicella compared with those who received varicella vaccine before, simultaneously with, or more than 30 days after receiving MMR.[656] Inactivated vaccines (i.e., DTaP, Hib, IPV, and hepatitis B) and OPV did not increase the risk of breakthrough varicella if they were administered less than 30 days before administration of varicella vaccine.

For adults and adolescents who have seroconverted, varicella vaccine provides protective efficacy rates of approximately 70% after household exposure. In the remaining 30%, attenuated disease with fewer skin lesions and little or no systemic toxicity develops, as in children.[291]

Adverse Events

Varicella vaccine produces relatively few adverse reactions.[596,693] The most common adverse reactions that occur after receipt of varicella vaccine are local reactions, such as pain, soreness, erythema, and swelling. Based on information from the manufacturer's clinical trials of varicella vaccine, local reactions after receiving the first dose are reported by 19% of children and by 24% of adolescents and adults.[596,693] These local adverse reactions usually are mild and self-limited.

A varicella-like rash at the site of injection is reported by 3% of children and by 1% of adolescents and adults after receipt of the second dose. In both circumstances, a median of two lesions has occurred. These lesions usually occur within 2 weeks and usually are maculopapular rather than vesicular.[596,693]

In postlicensure studies, the adverse event most frequently reported is a mild vesicular rash that occurs in approximately 5% of vaccinees.[133,290] Most of these generalized rashes occur within 3 weeks, and most are maculopapular. In one study, vesicular rashes that occurred within 2 weeks of vaccination were more likely to be caused by wild-type varicella, whereas rashes that occurred more than 2 weeks after vaccination were more likely to be caused by the Oka vaccine strain.[596]

Systemic reactions can occur. Fever within 42 days of vaccination is reported by 15% of children and 10% of adolescents and adults. Most of these episodes of fever have been attributed to concurrent illness rather than to the vaccine.

Clinical trials of MMRV that compared events that occurred within 42 days of receiving MMRV or MMR and varicella vaccine separately in different anatomic sites found the frequencies of local reactions and generalized varicella-like rash similar to those described for varicella vaccine.[414] A temperature of 38.9°C (102°F) or higher within 42 days of vaccination was more common in the MMRV group (22%) than in the group that received MMR and varicella vaccine at different sites (15%). A measles-like rash also occurred more frequently in MMRV recipients (3%) than in those receiving separate injections (2%). Fever and measles-like rash usually occurred 5 to 12 days after receipt of vaccination. In a postlicensure study, an increased risk of seizure was seen among children 12 to 23 months of age receiving MMRV vaccine compared with those who received MMR and varicella vaccines given separately in the 7- to 10-day postvaccination period.[394]

Varicella vaccine is a live virus vaccine and may result in a latent infection, similar to that caused by wild-type varicella virus. Consequently, zoster caused by the vaccine virus has been reported, mostly among vaccinated children. Based on reports to VAERS, the rate of herpes zoster after varicella vaccination is 2.6 cases per 100,000 vaccine doses distributed.[133] The incidence of herpes zoster after natural varicella infection in healthy people younger than 20 years is 68 cases per 100,000 person-years,[320] and for all ages, it is 215 cases per 100,000 person-years.[242] However, the latter rates should be compared cautiously because they are based on populations monitored for longer periods than the vaccinees were monitored.

Cases of herpes zoster have been confirmed by PCR to be caused by vaccine virus and wild-type virus, a finding suggesting that some herpes zoster disease in vaccinees may result from antecedent natural varicella infection.[133,330] Most cases of herpes zoster that occur after administration of vaccine have been mild and have not been associated with complications such as postherpetic neuralgia.

Transmission of the vaccine virus occurs rarely and most often from immunocompromised vaccinees. Of the 15 million doses of varicella vaccine distributed, on only three occasions has transmission from immunocompetent people been documented by PCR analysis.[418,574] All three cases resulted in mild disease without complications. In one case, a child 12 months old transmitted the vaccine virus to his pregnant mother.[437,574] The mother elected to terminate the pregnancy, but fetal tissue tested by PCR was negative for varicella vaccine virus. The other two documented cases involved transmission from healthy children 1 year of age to a healthy sibling 4.5 months of age and to a healthy father.[133] Transmission also has occurred from a person with herpes zoster caused by vaccine strain virus.[94] Transmission has not been documented in the absence of a vesicular rash after vaccination. No evidence indicates reversion to virulence of the vaccine strain during transmission; siblings of leukemic vaccine recipients who acquired vaccine virus had mild rash in 75% of cases and symptomless seroconversion in 25%.[55]

Indications

Monovalent varicella vaccine and MMRV have been licensed for use for healthy children 12 months through 12 years of age.[26,23,49,155,450,451] Children in this age group should receive two 0.5-mL doses of varicella vaccine administered subcutaneously, separated by at least 3 months. The recommendation for at least a 3-month interval between doses is based on the design of the studies evaluating two doses in this age group; if the second dose inadvertently is administered between 28 days and 3 months after the first dose, the second dose does not need to be repeated.

All healthy children routinely should receive the first dose of varicella-containing vaccine at 12 through 15 months of age. The second dose of vaccine is recommended routinely when children are 4 through 6 years of age (i.e., before a child enters kindergarten or first grade) but can be administered at an earlier age. Because of the minimal potential for increased febrile seizures after the first dose of MMRV vaccine in children 12 through 15 months of age, the AAP and ACIP recommend a choice of MMR plus monovalent varicella vaccine or MMRV for toddlers receiving their first immunization of this kind.[26,450] Parents should be counseled about the rare possibility of their child developing a febrile seizure 1 to 2 weeks after immunization with MMRV for the first immunizing dose. For the second dose at 4 through 6 years of age, MMRV usually is preferred over MMR plus monovalent varicella to minimize the number of injections. Varicella vaccine should be administered to all children in this age range unless there is evidence of immunity to varicella or a contraindication to administration of the vaccine.

A catch-up second dose of varicella vaccine should be offered to all children 7 years and older who have received only one dose. A routine health maintenance visit at 11 through 12 years of age is recommended for all adolescents to evaluate immunization status and administer necessary vaccines, including the varicella vaccine.

Individuals 13 years or older without evidence of immunity should receive two 0.5-mL doses of varicella vaccine separated by at least 28 days. The recommendation for at least a 28-day interval between doses is based on the design of the studies evaluating two doses in this age group. For people who previously received only one dose of varicella vaccine, a second dose is necessary. Only monovalent varicella vaccine is licensed for use in this age group.

Women should be assessed prenatally for evidence of varicella immunity. On completion or termination of their pregnancies, women who do not have evidence of varicella immunity should receive the first dose of varicella vaccine before discharge from the health care facility. The second dose should be administered 4 to 8 weeks later at the postpartum or other health care visit. To ensure administration of varicella vaccine, standing orders are recommended for health care settings where completion or termination of pregnancy occurs.

Postexposure prophylaxis. Data from the United States and Japan in a variety of settings indicate that varicella vaccine is 70% to 100% effective in preventing illness or modifying the severity of illness if it is used within 3 days and possibly up to 5 days after exposure.[573,672] The ACIP recommends administration of varicella vaccine to people without evidence of immunity 12 months or older, including adults, as soon as possible within 72 hours and possibly up to 120 hours after varicella exposure.[451] Varicella vaccine may prevent or modify disease and should be considered in these circumstances if there are no contraindications to its use. A second dose should be given at the age-appropriate interval after the first dose. Physicians should advise parents and their children that the vaccine may not protect against disease in all cases because some children might have been exposed at the same time as the index case. However, if exposure to varicella does not cause infection, postexposure immunization with varicella vaccine will result in protection against subsequent exposure. There is no evidence that administration of varicella vaccine during the presymptomatic or prodromal stage of illness increases the risk of vaccine-associated adverse events or more severe natural disease.

In 2006, the ACIP approved a revised definition for evidence of immunity to varicella.[451] Revised criteria for evidence of immunity to varicella include any of the following:

- Documentation of age-appropriate vaccination
- Preschool-aged children 12 months or older: one dose
- School-age children, adolescents, and adults: two doses
- Laboratory evidence of immunity or laboratory confirmation of disease
- Birth in the United States before 1980
- Diagnosis of varicella or verification of history of varicella disease by a health care provider
- History of herpes zoster based on health care provider diagnosis

Precautions and Contraindications

Varicella-containing vaccines are contraindicated for pregnancy, severe febrile illness, known history of anaphylactic reaction to vaccine components, and immunodeficiency states (i.e., malignancy, primary immunodeficiency disease, immunosuppressive or corticosteroid therapy, and radiation therapy).[26,23,49,155,450,451]

Varicella vaccine should not be administered to people who have had an anaphylactic-type reaction to any component of the vaccine, including gelatin and neomycin. Most people with allergy to neomycin have resulting contact dermatitis, a reaction that is not a contraindication to immunization. Monovalent varicella vaccine does not contain preservatives or egg protein, and although the measles and mumps vaccines included in MMRV vaccine are produced in chick embryo culture, the amounts of egg cross-reacting proteins are not significant. Children with egg allergy routinely can be given MMRV without previous skin testing.

Varicella vaccine should not be administered routinely to children who have congenital or acquired T-lymphocyte immunodeficiency, including those with leukemia, lymphoma, and other malignant neoplasms affecting the bone marrow or lymphatic systems, and children receiving long-term immunosuppressive therapy. An exception includes certain children infected with HIV (discussed later). Children with impaired humoral immunity can be immunized.

Immunodeficiency should be excluded before immunization of children with a family history of hereditary immunodeficiency. An immunodeficient or HIV-seropositive household family member does not contraindicate vaccine use in other family members.

In people with possible altered immunity, immunization against chickenpox should use only monovalent varicella vaccine. The Oka vaccine strain remains susceptible to acyclovir. If a high-risk patient develops vaccine-related varicella, acyclovir should be used as treatment.

Before routine immunization of healthy children against varicella was instituted in the United States in 1995, many young children with leukemia were susceptible to chickenpox. Considering the variation in intensity of chemotherapy regimens and the decreasing incidence of varicella in the United States, these high-risk children should not be immunized routinely. Immunization of susceptible leukemic children without evidence of immunity in remission should be undertaken only with expert guidance and with availability of antiviral therapy in case complications occur.

Live virus vaccines usually are withheld for an interval of at least 3 months after immunosuppressive cancer chemotherapy has been discontinued. However, the interval until immune reconstruction varies with the intensity and type of immunosuppressive therapy, radiation therapy, underlying disease, and other factors. It often is not possible to make a definitive recommendation for an interval after cessation of immunosuppressive therapy when live virus vaccines can be administered safely and effectively.

Screening for HIV infection is not indicated before routine VZV immunization. Varicella vaccine should be considered for nonimmune HIV-infected children with a $CD4^+$ T-lymphocyte percentage of 15% or greater, especially if they are receiving antiretroviral therapy.[482] Eligible children should receive two doses of monovalent varicella vaccine with a 3-month interval between doses and return for evaluation if they experience a postimmunization varicella-like rash. Hundreds of HIV-infected children have been safely immunized in the United States, and the vaccine is tolerated much as it is in healthy immunized children. Varicella vaccine has protected these children against varicella and herpes zoster by preventing infection with wild-type VZV.

Varicella vaccine should not be administered to people who are receiving high doses of systemic corticosteroids (i.e., 2 mg/kg per day or more of prednisone or its equivalent or 20 mg/day of prednisone or its equivalent) for 14 days or more. The recommended interval between discontinuation of corticosteroid therapy and immunization with varicella vaccine is at least 1 month. Varicella vaccine may be administered to people receiving inhaled, nasal, and topical corticosteroids. The results of one small study indicate that two doses of the varicella vaccine in 29 children with nephrotic syndrome between 12 months and 18 years of age usually were well tolerated and immunogenic, including children receiving low-dose, alternate-day prednisone.

Household contacts of immunocompromised people should be immunized if they have no evidence of immunity to decrease the likelihood that wild-type VZV will be introduced in the household. Transmission of vaccine-strain VZV from healthy people has been documented in seven instances, resulting in eight secondary cases. Even in families with immunocompromised people, including people with HIV infection, no precautions are needed after immunization of healthy children in whom a rash does not develop. Immunized people in whom a rash develops should avoid direct contact with immunocompromised hosts without evidence of immunity for the duration of the rash.

Receipt of antibody-containing blood products (i.e., whole blood, plasma, or parenteral immune globulin) may interfere with seroconversion to varicella vaccine. The length of time that such passively acquired antibody persists depends on the concentration and quantity of the blood product received[408] (see Table 245.11).

Although no direct evidence demonstrates that varicella vaccine is harmful to a pregnant woman or her fetus, the vaccine should not be administered to women known to be pregnant or considering becoming pregnant within the month because of the theoretical risk of fetal infection associated with a live virus vaccine. Vaccinated women should avoid conception for 1 month after receiving vaccination.

The manufacturer established a Varicella Vaccination in Pregnancy Registry to monitor the maternal-fetal outcomes of pregnant women inadvertently given varicella vaccine. The registry was closed in October 2013 because the low rate of exposure of varicella-susceptible women of childbearing age to VZV-containing vaccines, in addition to the rarity of the outcome, contributed to the low feasibility of the registry providing more robust data on the risk of congenital varicella syndrome within a reasonable timeframe.[453] A summary of 18 years of registry data found no cases of congenital varicella syndrome and no increased prevalence for other birth defects after exposure to VZV-containing vaccines during pregnancy. However, the number of exposures was insufficient to exclude a very low risk of congenital varicella syndrome in varicella-susceptible women exposed during the high-risk period.[689]

A study of nursing mothers and their infants showed no evidence of excretion of vaccine strain in human milk or of transmission to infants who are breastfeeding. Varicella vaccine should be administered to nursing mothers who lack evidence of immunity.

Reye syndrome has occurred in children infected with varicella who receive salicylates. Whether varicella vaccine may induce Reye syndrome is not known, but the vaccine manufacturer recommends that salicylates not be given within at least 6 weeks after administration of varicella vaccine.

Diseases for Which Combination Vaccines Are Available

Many new and improved vaccines have been introduced over the past 20 years. Incorporation of these vaccines into already complex childhood immunization schedules has posed a challenge. In the 2016 Recommended Immunization Schedule in the United States, a minimum of 22 separate injections are needed to immunize a child from birth to 2 years of age.[210,560] At some visits, the administration of three to five separate injections can be indicated.

Combination vaccines represent one solution to the problem of increased numbers of injections. These vaccines incorporate into a single product antigens that prevent several diseases. Combinations licensed in recent years in the United States are shown in Table 245.18.

Licensed combination vaccines can be used when any components of the combination are indicated and its other components are not contraindicated and if licensed by the FDA for that dose in the series.[408] Use of combination vaccines can reduce the number of injections patients receive and alleviate parental concerns about the number of injections. Potential advantages of combination vaccines include improved vaccine coverage rates, timely vaccination coverage for children who need catch-up vaccination, reduced shipping and stocking costs, reduced costs for extra health care visits necessitated by deferral of vaccination, and facilitation of adding new vaccines into vaccination programs.

Potential disadvantages of combination vaccines include adverse events that may occur more frequently after administration of a combination vaccine compared with administration of separate antigens at the same visit, such as those that occur with the MMRV vaccine and combination DTaP-hepatitis B-IPV vaccine[450,637]; confusion and uncertainty about selection of vaccine combinations and schedules for subsequent doses, especially when vaccinations are given by multiple providers who might be using different products; reduced immunogenicity of one or more components[238]; extra doses of certain antigens in the fixed product (e.g., a provider who uses DTaP-hepatitis B-IPV vaccine will give an extra dose of hepatitis B component); and a shorter shelf-life than the individual component vaccines. The economic impact of the use of combination vaccines is unclear because combination products have the potential for increased or decreased costs compared with single-antigen component vaccines.

The minimum age for administration of a combination vaccine is the oldest minimum age for any of the individual components; the minimum interval between doses is equal to the greatest minimum interval of any of the individual components. When patients have received the recommended immunizations for some of the components in a combination vaccine, administering the extra antigens in the combination vaccine is permissible if they are not contraindicated and doing so will reduce the number of injections required. However, excessive doses of toxoid vaccines (i.e., diphtheria and tetanus) can result in extensive local reactions.

Only combination vaccines licensed by the FDA should be used. Separate vaccines should not be combined into the same syringe for administration together unless mixing is indicated for the patient's age and is explicitly specified on the FDA-approved product label inserts. Only one combination vaccine (i.e., DTaP-IPV/Hib vaccine [Pentacel])

TABLE 245.18 Combination Vaccines Licensed in the United States[a]

Vaccine[b]	Trade Name (year licensed)	Age Range	Routinely Recommended Ages
DTaP-HepB-IPV	Pediarix (2002)	6 wk–6 y	Three-dose series at 2, 4 and 6 mo
DTaP-IPV/Hib	Pentacel (2008)	6 wk–4 y	Four-dose series at 2, 4, 6, and 15–18 mo
DTaP-IPV	Kinrix (2008)	4–6 y	Fifth dose of DTaP and fourth dose of IPV
DTaP-IPV	Quadracel (2015)	4–6 y	Fifth dose of DTaP and fourth or fifth dose of IPV
HepA-HepB	Twinrix (2001)	≥18 y	Three doses on a schedule of 0, 1, and 6 mo
Hib-MenCY	MenHibrix (2012)	2 –23 mo	Four-dose series at 2, 4, 6, and 15–18 mo
MMRV	ProQuad (2005)	12 mo–12 y	Two doses, the first at 12–15 mo, the second at 4–6 y

[a]Excludes measles-mumps-rubella (MMR), DTaP, Tdap, Td, and IPV vaccines, for which individual components are not available. DTaP/Hib (TriHIBit) and Hib/HepB (Comvax) are no longer manufactured.

[b]A hyphen (-) between vaccine products indicates that products are supplied in their final form by the manufacturer and do not require mixing or reconstitution by the user. A slash (/) indicates that the products must be mixed or reconstituted by the user.

DTaP, Diphtheria–tetanus–acellular pertussis; *HepA*, hepatitis A; *HepB*, hepatitis B; *Hib*, *Haemophilus influenzae* type b; *IPV*, inactivated poliovirus; *MenCY*, meningococcal group CY; *MMRV*, measles-mumps-rubella-varicella.

Modified from American Academy of Pediatrics. Combination vaccines. In: Kimberlin DW, Brady MT, Jackson MA, Long SS, eds. *Red Book: 2015 Report of the Committee on Infectious Diseases*. 30th ed. Elk Grove Village, IL: American Academy of Pediatrics; 2015:36–7.

contains separate antigen components for which FDA approves mixing by the user. The safety, immunogenicity, and efficacy of unlicensed combinations are unknown.

Licensure of a combination vaccine by the FDA is based on studies demonstrating that the product's immunogenicity (or efficacy) and safety are comparable or equivalent to monovalent or combination products licensed previously. FDA licensure also indicates that a combination vaccine may be used interchangeably with monovalent formulations and other combination products with similar component antigens produced by the same manufacturer to continue the vaccination series. For example, DTaP, DTaP/Hib, and future DTaP vaccines that contain similar acellular pertussis antigens from the same manufacturer may be used interchangeably if licensed and indicated for the patient's age.[152]

Licensure of a vaccine by the FDA does not necessarily indicate that the vaccine is interchangeable with products from other manufacturers. Data are readily available for diseases with known serologic correlates of protective immunity. For diseases without surrogate laboratory markers, prelicensure field vaccine efficacy (phase III) trials or postlicensure surveillance usually are required to determine protection.[478] The ACIP prefers that doses of vaccine in a series come from the same manufacturer; however, if this is not possible or if the manufacturer of doses of vaccine given previously is unknown, providers should administer the vaccine that they have available.

VACCINES WITH SELECTIVE INDICATIONS FOR CHILDREN AND ADOLESCENTS

Bacille Calmette-Guérin Vaccine

Effective control of tuberculosis in the United States has been achieved by the early identification and treatment of cases, followed by surveillance of household and other close contacts and institution of appropriate preventive measures for those at high risk for disease development. In the United States, the mainstay of preventive therapy is isoniazid chemoprophylaxis, which is used in asymptomatically infected people to prevent the progression of infection to disease. In selected instances, however, the potential for acquiring disease, poor compliance by contacts instructed to take chemoprophylaxis, or failure of chemoprophylaxis may justify the use of immunoprophylaxis.[127]

Bacille Calmette-Guérin (BCG) is not usually recommended for immunoprophylaxis in the United States because of the low risk of infection with *Mycobacterium tuberculosis*, the unpredictable effectiveness of the vaccine against adult pulmonary tuberculosis, and the vaccine's potential interference with tuberculin skin test reactivity. Elsewhere in the world, BCG vaccine is used in more than 100 countries and is recommended routinely at birth by the WHO[696] (http://www.who.int/immunization/policy/Immunization_routine_table2.pdf?ua=1). Of primary concern to pediatricians is the risk to an infant born to a mother with tuberculosis or living within a household with other identified individuals with tuberculosis.[48]

Preparations

BCG is the only approved vaccine against tuberculosis. BCG is a live attenuated strain derived from *Mycobacterium bovis.* All currently available BCG vaccines are derived from the original strain at the Pasteur Institute in Paris, but they have been propagated by different methods in many laboratories and therefore vary in their immunogenic and reactogenic properties. BCG (Merck) is the only vaccine licensed in the United States. Comparative evaluations of this preparation and other BCG vaccines have not been performed.

BCG is administered only percutaneously using a sterile multiple-puncture device. The standard dose of BCG vaccine is 0.2 to 0.3 mL of reconstituted lyophilized BCG. At least 10 new potential vaccines to prevent tuberculosis are in clinical development.[274] Nevertheless, BCG will remain in use in the foreseeable future and may continue to be used as a prime vaccine in a prime-boost immunization schedule in conjunction with new tuberculosis vaccines.[383] BCG preparations instilled in the treatment of bladder cancer are not intended to be used as vaccines.[127]

Immunogenicity and Efficacy

BCG is used primarily in young infants in an attempt to prevent disseminated and other life-threatening manifestations of *M. tuberculosis* disease. However, BCG does not prevent infection with *M. tuberculosis.* The efficacy of different BCG vaccines seems to vary broadly. Two meta-analyses of published clinical trials and case-control studies concerning the efficacy of BCG vaccines concluded that BCG has relatively high protective efficacy (approximately 80%) against meningeal and miliary tuberculosis in children.[207,562] The protective efficacy against pulmonary tuberculosis, however, differed significantly among the studies, precluding a specific conclusion. Protection afforded by BCG in one meta-analysis was estimated to be 50%.[207]

Adverse Events

Four billion doses of BCG have been administered with a proven safety record.[383] BCG vaccination usually results in scarring at the site of injection. However, the vaccine has been associated uncommonly (1–2% of vaccinations) with local adverse reactions such as subcutaneous abscess and lymphadenopathy, which are not usually serious. Osteitis affecting the epiphyses of long bones is a rare complication that develops in 1 of 1 million vaccinees and may occur as long as several years after receiving BCG immunization. The rate may be higher among neonates. Disseminated fatal disease occurs rarely (0.1–1 case/1 million vaccinees), primarily in people with severely impaired immune systems.[127,409,438,621]

Antituberculosis therapy, except for pyrazinamide, is recommended to treat osteitis and disseminated disease caused by BCG. Some experts also recommend treatment of chronic suppurative lymphadenitis caused by BCG. People with complications caused by BCG should be referred to a tuberculosis expert for management.

Indications

In the United States, administration of BCG should be considered only in limited and select circumstances, such as unavoidable risk of exposure to *M. tuberculosis* and failure or unfeasibility of other methods of control of tuberculosis. The ACIP and AAP have published recommendations for the use of BCG to control tuberculosis in children.[33,169] Healthy infants from birth to 2 months of age may be given BCG without tuberculin skin testing; thereafter, BCG is given only to children with a negative tuberculin skin test result. BCG immunization should be considered for infants and children who are not infected with HIV in the following circumstances:

- The child is exposed continually to a person or people with contagious pulmonary tuberculosis resistant to isoniazid and rifampin, and the child cannot be removed from this exposure.
- The child is exposed continually to a person or people with untreated or ineffectively treated contagious pulmonary tuberculosis, and the child cannot be removed from the exposure or given antituberculosis therapy.

Careful assessment of the potential risks and benefits of BCG vaccine and consultation with personnel in local area control programs for tuberculosis are strongly recommended before the use of BCG. When BCG vaccine is given, care should be taken to observe the precautions and directions for administration on the product label. Other childhood vaccines can be administered concurrently with BCG.

Skin Test Reactivity

Recipients of BCG should have repeat tuberculin skin tests 2 to 3 months after immunization to establish that tuberculin cellular reactivity has developed. Failure to react dictates the need for repeat BCG vaccination followed by repeat tuberculin testing.[127] The tuberculin reaction to the BCG vaccine available in the United States usually results in 7 to 15 mm of induration after vaccination and diminishes gradually during subsequent years. Without revaccination or repeated exposure to *M. tuberculosis,* reactivity usually disappears within 10 years.[127] The size of the area of induration may be correlated with the number of doses of BCG.[357] However, tuberculin skin test sensitivity does not correlate with BCG efficacy.[337] In BCG recipients, differentiating between a tuberculin reaction representing acquired tuberculous infection and persistent postvaccination reactivity is difficult.

Because the degree and duration of protection against tuberculous disease afforded by BCG are uncertain, a positive tuberculin reaction may be indicative of disease. BCG recipients with a positive tuberculin skin test result should be carefully evaluated with risk assessment, radiography, and other diagnostic tests, including an interferon-γ release assay (IGRA), which does not produce cross-reactions after sensitization by BCG.[467]

Precautions and Contraindications

BCG vaccine should not be administered to individuals with burns, skin infections, and certain primary or secondary immunodeficiencies, including HIV infection, because of the risk of disseminated BCG disease. The use of BCG vaccine also is contraindicated in people receiving immunosuppressive medications, including high-dose corticosteroids.

In the United States, where the risk of acquiring tuberculosis is low, BCG vaccine should not be administered to children with known or suspected asymptomatic HIV infection.[127,510] However, in countries where the risk of contracting tuberculosis is high and HIV surveillance of pregnant women and infants is limited, the WHO has recommended that asymptomatic HIV-infected children receive BCG vaccine at birth or shortly thereafter.[696,695] However, the WHO recommends that BCG should not be administered to infants known to be infected with HIV even in resource-poor regions because the risk of disseminated BCG in these infants is significantly high, approaching 1%.[698,699] Although no harmful effects of BCG vaccine on the fetus have been documented, women should avoid receiving vaccination during pregnancy.

Cholera Vaccine

The global burden of cholera is difficult to estimate due to underreporting, but experts place the annual number of cases at 2.9 million with 95,000 deaths.[8] In 2009, 45 countries reported 221,226 cholera cases with 4946 deaths to the WHO, with 98% of cases and 99% of deaths reported from Africa.[566] In, 2010, an outbreak of cholera occurred in Haiti with more than one-half million cases and more than 7000 confirmed deaths. It was the first epidemic in the Western Hemisphere since the 1991 epidemic in Peru.[6] After it emerged in Haiti, cholera spread to other countries, including the Dominican Republic and Cuba.

From 2001 through 2013, 123 confirmed cases of cholera in the United States were acquired abroad; of these, 63 were associated with the epidemic in Hispaniola.[436] Most cases of disease have occurred in travelers to cholera-affected areas or people who have eaten contaminated food brought or imported from these areas.[122] Although cholera remains a significant public health concern in African, Asian, and South American countries, even in these countries the risk to US travelers is low. People following the usual tourist itinerary that use standard accommodations in countries reporting cholera are at very low risk for infection.[566]

Preparations

There are two major types of oral vaccines against cholera: killed whole cell-based and genetically attenuated live vaccines.[345] A single cholera vaccine CVD 103-HgR (Vaxchora; PaxVax, Redwood City, CA) is available in the United States. This vaccine is an attenuated live oral genetically modified *V. cholerae* O1 strain (CVD 103-HgR) and was licensed by FDA in 2016 for United States travelers 18 to 64 years of age visiting endemic countries.

Two other vaccines are prequalified by WHO and are available in many countries outside the United States: WC/rBS (Dukoral; Crucell, the Netherlands) and Modified WC-only (Shanchol; Shantha Biotechnics, Medchal, Hyderabad, India). The WC/rBS vaccine is a whole, killed cell–based vaccine that contains *Vibrio cholerae* O1 with purified recombinant B subunit of cholera toxoid. The modified WC-only vaccine is also a whole, killed cell-based vaccine but lacks the B subunit. The WC-only vaccine was originally manufactured by the government of Vietnam. Although inexpensive to produce, it did not elicit antitoxic immunity. In 2007, the WC-only vaccine was modified with international efforts to create a low-cost vaccine that is produced in India[572,599]

Immunogenicity and Efficacy

In a randomized, placebo-controlled, double-blind trial of the CVD 103-HgR vaccine with an oral cholera challenge in 197 health human volunteers, vaccine efficacy was found to be 90% at 10 days and 80% 3 months after a single vaccine dose.[184] Although the CVD 103-HrG vaccine provides protective vibriocidal antibodies in 90% of vaccinees, it is specific to *V. cholerae* serogroup 01 and does not confer protection to O139 or other non-O1 serogroups.[184] CVD 103-HrG vaccines have the benefit of being efficacious with a onetime dose instead of the two spaced doses required of the killed, whole cell vaccines.

WC/rBS vaccine confers protection specific to *V. cholerae* serogroup O1.[345] Immunization does not protect against *V. cholerae* serogroup O139 or other species of *Vibrio.* Field trials in Bangladesh, Peru, and Sweden have shown that the WC/rBS vaccine confers 85% to 90% protection for 6 months in all age groups after administration of two doses 1 week apart. In Bangladesh, protection declined rapidly after 6 months in young children, but it was still approximately 60% effective in older children and adults after 2 years. Because of the limited duration of protection, the WC/rBS vaccine is not recommended to be used in children younger than 2 years.

The modified killed, whole cell–only vaccine had been studied in several trials and found to be safe and highly effective, with seroconversion rates of vibriocidal antibodies ranging from 53% to 91%.[54,572,599,628] Limited data on the safety and immunogenicity of the modified whole-cell–based vaccine in children at least 1 year of age appear promising.[572]

Adverse Events

In clinical trials of the newly licensed CVD 103-HgR vaccine, there was no difference between placebo and vaccine recipients with respect to diarrhea, asthenia, headache, abdominal pain, anorexia, nausea and vomiting, or fever.[184]

Millions of doses of WC/rBS vaccine have been supplied worldwide.[345] According to manufacturer information from clinical trials and postmarketing surveillance, mild gastrointestinal symptoms (e.g., abdominal pain, cramping, diarrhea, nausea) are most commonly reported, occurring at a frequency of 0.1% to 1%. Serious adverse events, including a flulike syndrome, rash, arthralgia, and paresthesias, are rare, occurring in less than one of 10,000 doses distributed. In several RCTs, the modified, killed, whole cell–only vaccine also demonstrated a low frequency of mild symptoms and no major adverse events.[54,572,628]

Indications

In June 2016, the ACIP voted to recommend cholera vaccine (CVD 103-HgR, Vaxchora) for adult (18–64 years old) travelers to an area of active toxigenic V. cholerae O1 transmission. Special consideration should be given for those at higher than average risk, such as health care professionals in endemic areas, aid workers in refugee camps, and those traveling to remote areas where cholera epidemics are occurring and access to medical care is limited. No country requires proof of cholera immunization as a condition for entry, and the WHO recommends against such a requirement. Some local authorities, however, may require immunization; to determine local requirements, travelers should consult the embassies of the countries to which they will be traveling.

Precautions and Contraindications

Oral cholera vaccine should not be administered to people with a hypersensitivity reaction to any of the vaccine components. Administration of oral cholera vaccine should be postponed for people with acute gastrointestinal illness or acute febrile illness.

Japanese Encephalitis Virus Vaccine

Japanese encephalitis (JE) virus, the most important cause of epidemic mosquito-borne arboviral encephalitis in Asia, has a wide clinical spectrum, ranging from asymptomatic infection to permanent neurologic sequelae associated with a high rate of disability (i.e., 709,000 disability-adjusted life-years), and a high case-fatality rate of 20% to 30% or even higher among children younger than 10 years. The annual incidence of JE among 3 billion people at risk in 24 countries in Southeast Asia and the Western Pacific is 1.8 case per 100,000 people despite the availability of effective vaccines in many regions.[700]

The JE virus is a zoonotic flavivirus that cannot be eliminated because its animal reservoirs are widespread. However, human infection could be controlled by universal human immunization in endemic areas. The envelope glycoprotein of the JE virus contains the major epitopes that are targeted by neutralizing antibodies.

Historically, an inactivated mouse brain–derived vaccine (JE-VAX) controlled JE virus infection successfully among human populations in Japan, Korea, and Taiwan since 1968.[517] This vaccine is no longer available in the United States and is being phased out elsewhere because of greater reactogenicity, higher cost, and larger number of doses compared with the newer-generation vaccines.

Preparations

The 15 JE vaccines in use in Asia are classified in four categories: inactivated mouse brain–derived vaccines, inactivated Vero cell–derived vaccines, live attenuated vaccines, and live recombinant (chimeric) vaccines. In the United States, the inactivated Vero cell–derived, alum-adjuvanted vaccine, JE-VC (Ixiaro, Intercell Biomedical, United Kingdom, distributed by Novartis Vaccines and Diagnostics in the United States) is indicated for use in individuals 2 months and older.[177] It is derived from the attenuated SA 14-14-2 JEV strain.

The primary vaccination series for JE-VC is two intramuscular doses administered 28 days apart. The dose for children younger than 3 years is 0.25 mL, and 0.5 mL is given to children 3 years or older.[177] The vaccine does not contain stabilizers, antibiotics, or thimerosal and should be stored at 2°C to 8°C (35°F–46°F) and protected from light.

A primary hamster kidney cell—derived, live attenuated vaccine (CD.JEVAX) has been used widely in China since 1988 and is used widely in Asia now. It is based on the SA 14-14-2 JEV strain. Primary immunization consists of a single 0.5- mL subcutaneous dose in children 8 months or older. It contains gelatin, human serum albumin, and other stabilizers.

A live attenuated, recombinant (chimeric) JE virus vaccine (IMOJEV, JE-CV, ChimeriVax-JE) was licensed in Australia in 2010 and is used widely in Asia. The premembrane and envelope coding sequences derived from the SA 14-14-2 JEV strain were engineered to replace the homologous sequences of the live attenuated yellow fever vaccine virus, which is used as a vector. This vaccine is propagated in Vero cells. Primary immunization is a single dose of 0.5 mL given subcutaneously at 9 months or older, and a booster dose is indicated for children.

Immunogenicity and Efficacy

The JE-VC vaccine was licensed in the United States on the basis of its ability to induce JE virus–neutralizing antibodies as a surrogate for protection and safety evaluations in approximately 5000 adults.[587] The accepted immunologic surrogate of protection is a serum neutralizing antibody titer of at least 1 : 10 as determined by a 50% plaque reduction neutralization assay ($PRNT_{50}$) result.[700]

Vaccine effectiveness for the inactivated JE-VC vaccine is at least 93%, 80% to 99% for the live attenuated JE vaccines, and at least 90% for the live recombinant vaccines. Long-term immunogenicity data are limited. A booster vaccine is recommended 2 years after the primary series to induce a robust anamnestic response.[700]

Mass immunization campaigns with live attenuated and inactivated mouse brain–derived JE vaccines significantly reduce JE disease in a community. No data are available for the inactivated Vero cell–derived and live recombinant vaccines.

Adverse Reactions

The inactivated Vero cell–derived vaccines, live attenuated vaccines, and live recombinant vaccines all have acceptable safety profiles. The most common local reactions to JE-VC are rash, fever, headache, myalgia, and fatigue, but severe reactions occur in 1.6 of 100,000 administered doses,[177,700] as described on the CDC website (http://www.cdc.gov/vaccines/acip/recs/grade/je-child.html). Severe adverse events include febrile convulsions, thrombocytopenic purpura, and encephalitis.[247] The other vaccine preparations are associated with similar reactogenicity and tolerability as that of JE-VC.

Indications

The risk of JE for most travelers to Asia is low but varies on the basis of destination, duration, season, and activities. All travelers to countries with endemic JE should be informed of the risks of JE and use personal protective measures (i.e., bed nets and mosquito repellants) to reduce the risk of mosquito bites. For some travelers who will be in high-risk settings, JE vaccine can further reduce the risk of infection. The CDC recommends JE vaccine for travelers who plan to spend a month or longer in areas with endemic infection during the JE virus transmission season.[30,271] JE vaccine should be considered for shorter-term travelers if they plan to travel away from an urban area and have an itinerary or activities that increase the risk of JE virus exposure. Information on the location of JE virus transmission and detailed information on vaccine recommendations and adverse events can be obtained from the CDC website (https://wwwnc.cdc.gov/travel).

Primary immunization with JE-VC should be completed at least 1 week before potential exposure to JE virus. If the primary series was administered more than 1 year earlier, a booster dose is recommended for individuals older than 16 years before potential reexposure.[248] Data on the response to a booster dose administered more than 2 years after the primary series and the need for and timing of additional booster doses are not available. There is no information about the utility of booster doses for children. The sparse available data suggest that the different JE vaccines are interchangeable without causing adverse reactions or compromising immunogenicity.

Precautions and Contraindications

A severe allergic reaction after a previous dose of JE-VC is a contraindication to administration of subsequent doses.[271] JE-VC contains protamine sulfate, a compound known to cause hypersensitivity reactions in some people.

Practitioners should use caution when considering the use of JE vaccine in pregnant women. Vaccination with JE vaccines usually should be deferred because of a theoretical risk to the developing fetus. However, pregnant women who must travel to an area in which the risk of JE exposure is high should be vaccinated with an inactivated JE vaccine if the benefits outweigh the risks of vaccination for the mother and developing fetus.

Breastfeeding is not a contraindication to vaccination with inactivated JE vaccine. However, whether JE-VC is excreted in human milk is not known. Because many drugs are excreted in human milk, practitioners should use caution when considering the use of inactivated JE vaccine in breastfeeding women.

No data exist on the use of JE-VC in immunocompromised people or patients receiving immunosuppressive therapies.

Rabies Vaccine

Rabies is a viral zoonosis transmitted in saliva and other tissue of infected mammals. The virus enters the central nervous system of the host and causes an acute, progressive encephalomyelitis that is almost universally fatal. Postexposure prophylaxis is possible because of the long incubation period, usually weeks to months, of this infection. The time of incubation correlates with the length of the axon along which the virus migrates to eventually infect the central nervous system. Children are at particular risk of exposure to rabies from an infected dog, cat, or other animal because they are less likely to take aversive measures if attacked and are more likely to sustain an injury to the head or neck. Accordingly, children are likely to have shorter incubation periods especially with an exposure injury on the head or neck.

In this century, the number of human deaths in the United States attributed to rabies has declined from 100 or more each year to an average of 2 or 3 each year. Two programs have been responsible for this decline. First, animal control and vaccination programs begun in the 1940s and oral rabies vaccination programs in the 2000s have eliminated domestic dogs as reservoirs of rabies in the United States. Second, effective human rabies vaccines and immunoglobulins have been developed.

Wild animals are the most important source of infection for humans and domestic animals. Insectivorous bats carrying variants of the rabies virus have been responsible for most human cases of rabies in the continental United States in recent years. Transmission has occurred from minor and unrecognized bites from infected bats. Wild carnivores, especially raccoons, skunks, and foxes, are the terrestrial animals most often infected with rabies. Wildlife rabies occurs throughout the continental United States; only Hawaii remains consistently free of rabies. Domestic animals, including dogs, cats, and ferrets, can be infected, with three times as many reports of rabies annually in cats compared with dogs.

Human exposure to rabies from a domestic animal in the United States is a rare occurrence. In most other countries (e.g., Asia, Africa, and Latin America), dogs remain the most important potential source of infection. International travelers in areas where canine rabies is endemic are at increased risk for exposure to rabies.

Rabies was diagnosed in a total of 37 people in the United States since 2003.[485] Seventy percent of them acquired the disease in the United States or Puerto Rico. Organ or tissue transplantation was identified as the source of infection for 19% of individuals. Bats were implicated as the source of infection in 65%, with a bat bite reported in seven cases bat contact without a reported bite in six cases and a rabies virus associated with bats without a known exposure identified in four cases. Thirty percent of human rabies deaths reported to the CDC since 2003 appear to have been related to rabid animals outside the United States.

Preparations

Two rabies vaccines are available for preexposure and postexposure prophylaxis in the United States: human diploid cell vaccine (HDCV) and purified chicken embryo cell (PCEC). Both vaccines are licensed for intramuscular administration. HDCV (Imovax Rabies, Sanofi Pasteur) is derived from the Pitman-Moore strain grown in human diploid cell culture. PCEC (RabAvert, Chiron Corporation-Novartis) is prepared from the fixed rabies virus strain Flury LEP grown in primary culture of chicken fibroblasts. The HDCV and PCEC vaccines each contain the WHO-recommended standard of at least 2.5 IU of rabies virus antigen per 1.0-mL intramuscular dose. Although not licensed for use in the United States, two intradermal rabies vaccines are recommended by the WHO and used in countries where the two tissue culture vaccines (i.e., HDCV and PCEC) are prohibitively expensive.[132]

Immunogenicity and Efficacy

Viral neutralizing antibodies are produced within 7 to 10 days, and protective immunity usually persists for 2 years or longer. Although a definitive protective titer has not been identified, the WHO and CDC adhere to working guidelines for an acceptable response to immunization.[118] The CDC specifies complete viral neutralization at a 1:5 or greater titer by the rapid fluorescent-focus inhibition test as acceptable; the WHO specifies 0.5 IU/mL or more as acceptable.

Given the essentially universal fatal prognosis of infection after symptoms develop, no randomized, placebo-controlled human trials have documented the efficacy of vaccine for preexposure or postexposure prophylaxis. However, substantial field experience and direct evidence from controlled animal studies demonstrate a protective effect. The paucity of human cases attests to the efficacy of postexposure prophylaxis with the currently recommended vaccine and immune globulin preparations.

Rabies has not been reported in the United States in any patient who received the recommended postexposure measures. Cases of human rabies occurring after postexposure prophylaxis have resulted from failure to adhere to established guidelines, such as those of the CDC or the WHO.[117,250,272,598,673]

Adverse Events

Reactions occurring after administration of HDCV or PCEC vaccine are less serious and less common than those associated with the previously available vaccines.[132] Local reactions at the injection site occur in 30% to 74% of injections, and mild systemic reactions such as fever, headache, nausea, abdominal pain, muscle aches, and dizziness occur in 5%to 40% of vaccine recipients. In one report, approximately 6% of people had an immune complex–like reaction 2 to 21 days after receipt of the booster dose of HDCV.[108] This systemic hypersensitivity reaction occurred less frequently in people receiving primary vaccination. The reactions have been associated with the presence of β-propiolactone–altered human albumin in HDCV and the development of IgE antibodies to this allergen.[273]

Indications and Precautions

When used as indicated, both types of rabies vaccine are considered equally safe and effective for preexposure and postexposure prophylaxis as described in the ACIP recommendations.[448,570] Usually, an immunization series is initiated and completed with one vaccine product. No clinical studies have been conducted that documented a change in efficacy or the frequency of adverse reactions when the series is completed with a second vaccine product. Ideally, an immunization series should be completed with the same product unless serious allergic reactions occur. Corticosteroids, immunosuppressive conditions, and concurrent administration of antimalarial agents can interfere with the adequate development of an active immune response. Postvaccination titers should be checked in these circumstances or if a significant interruption in vaccine schedule has occurred, especially in the context of a more significant exposure, and in consultation with local public health authorities.

For adults, rabies vaccination always should be administered in the deltoid area. For children, the anterolateral aspect of the thigh also is acceptable. The gluteal area never should be used for HDCV or PCEC injections because administration of HDCV in this area results in lower neutralizing antibody titers and decreased immunogenicity.[272]

Postexposure prophylaxis. The essential components of rabies postexposure prophylaxis are wound treatment and, for previously unvaccinated people, concurrent administration of human rabies immune globulin (HRIG) and vaccine (Table 245.19).[448,570] The combination of active and passive immunization is indicated for the treatment of all bite and all non-bite exposures inflicted by animals suspected or proven to be rabid. Recommendations for the management of people with possible exposure to rabies include giving meticulous attention to thorough cleansing of the wound with soap and water. The decision to give rabies immunoprophylaxis depends on the circumstances precipitating the exposure, the species and condition of the animal inflicting the wound, and the prevalence of rabies in local animal populations. Bite and nonbite exposures, including scratches, abrasions, open wounds, and mucous membranes contaminated with saliva, are considered significant. Because the need for preventive measures is based on these specific circumstances, the local department of health should be consulted promptly concerning the necessity for initiating postexposure prophylaxis.

When possible, the brains of wild animals (i.e., skunks, foxes, coyotes, raccoons, and bats), stray dogs or cats, or symptomatic animals implicated in an exposure should be examined in certified laboratories for evidence of rabies. Immunization always should be initiated promptly and discontinued only if laboratory results are negative. Individuals exposed to healthy dogs or cats that are available for observation do not require immediate prophylactic treatment. Implicated healthy domestic dogs or cats should be quarantined and observed for at least 10 days. If symptoms develop that suggest rabies, the exposed individual should begin postexposure prophylaxis, and the brain of the animal should be examined. An unknown or unavailable animal must be regarded as potentially rabid.

Studies conducted in the United States by the CDC have documented that a regimen of one dose of HRIG and five doses of rabies vaccine (1.0 mL for each dose) given on days 0, 3, 7, 14 and 28 was safe and induced an excellent antibody response in all recipients.[448] In March 2010, the ACIP changed recommendations to one dose of HRIG with four doses of rabies vaccine (1.0 mL for each dose) given on days 0, 3, 7, and 14. The number of doses recommended for people with altered immunocompetence has not changed; they should be administered a five-dose vaccination regimen (days 0, 3, 7, 14, and 28) along with one dose of HRIG.[570] If anatomically feasible, the full dose of HRIG (20 IU/kg) should be infiltrated thoroughly in the area around and into the wounds. Any remaining volume should be injected intramuscularly at a site distant from that of vaccine administration. The dose of HRIG should not exceed that recommended and should not be given beyond the seventh day because HRIG can partially suppress active antibody production.

People previously fully vaccinated do not require HRIG and should receive only vaccine (two doses 3 days apart) because an amnestic response will occur after the administration of a booster regardless of

TABLE 245.19 **Rabies Postexposure Prophylaxis for Individuals Not Previously Immunized**

Animal Type	Evaluation and Disposition of the Animal	Postexposure Prophylaxis Recommendations
Wild		
Skunks, raccoons, foxes, and most other carnivores; bats	Regard as rabid unless animal proven negative by laboratory tests[a]	Consider immediate vaccination and if not previously vaccinated, use rabies immune globulin
Domestic		
Dogs, cats, and ferrets	Healthy and available for 10 days observation	Persons should not begin prophylaxis unless animal develops clinical signs of rabies[b]
	Rabid or suspected rabid	Immediately vaccinate
	Escaped (unknown)	Consult public health officials
Other		
Livestock, small rodents, large rodents (woodchucks and beavers), lagomorphs (rabbits and hares), and other mammals	Consider individually	Consult public health officials Bites of squirrels, hamsters, guinea pigs, gerbils, chipmunks, rats, mice, other small rodents, rabbits, and hares rarely require antirabies prophylaxis

[a]The animal should be euthanized and tested as soon as possible. Holding for observation is not recommended. Discontinue vaccine if immunofluorescence test results of the animal are negative.

[b]During the 10-day observation period, begin postexposure prophylaxis at the first sign of rabies in a dog, cat, or ferret that has bitten someone. If the animal exhibits clinical signs of rabies, it should be euthanized immediately and tested.

Modified from Manning SE, Rupprecht CE, Fishbein D, et al. Human rabies prevention—United States, 2008: recommendations of the Advisory Committee on Immunization Practices. *MMWR Recomm Rep*. 2008;57(RR-3):1–28.

the antibody titer.[448] Serum for antibody testing should be obtained from people whose prophylaxis history or immune status is uncertain, and the course of postexposure active and passive immunoprophylaxis as described for nonimmune individuals should be initiated immediately. If serologic testing demonstrates adequate anti-rabies antibody, postexposure prophylaxis can be discontinued.

Once initiated, rabies prophylaxis should not be interrupted or discontinued because of local or mild systemic adverse reactions to rabies vaccine. Usually, the reactions can be successfully managed with antiinflammatory and antipyretic agents such as ibuprofen or acetaminophen. When a person with a history of serious hypersensitivity to rabies vaccine must be revaccinated, antihistamines can be administered. Epinephrine should be readily available to counteract any anaphylactic reactions, and the person should be observed carefully immediately after receiving vaccination.

Preexposure prophylaxis. Active immunization should be considered for high-risk groups (i.e., veterinarians, animal handlers and control officers, selected laboratory workers, people visiting countries where rabies is hyperendemic, and people whose pursuits may involve frequent contact with rabid animals, such as spelunkers). People whose risk of exposure is less but whose access to immediate competent medical care is restricted also should be considered for preexposure prophylaxis.

The primary series consists of three doses (1.0 mL/dose) administered on days 0, 7, and 21 or 28, given intramuscularly in the deltoid area. The three-dose series provides long-term protective immunity, and routine serologic testing for rabies antibody after primary immunization is not necessary. For individuals who may be immunosuppressed, measurement of anti-rabies antibodies should be performed. In the case of continued or frequent exposure, serum samples should be tested every 2 years and a booster dose of rabies vaccine provided when the antibody titer falls below the minimum accepted level.[448]

Precautions and Contraindications

Because of the potential consequences of inadequately treated rabies exposure and because no indication exists that fetal abnormalities have been associated with rabies vaccination, pregnancy is not considered a contraindication to postexposure prophylaxis.[448] If the risk of exposure to rabies is substantial, preexposure prophylaxis also can be indicated during pregnancy.

People who have a history of serious hypersensitivity to rabies vaccine should be revaccinated with caution. Although serious systemic, anaphylactic, or neuroparalytic reactions are rare events during and after the administration of rabies vaccines, the reactions pose a serious dilemma for the patient and the attending physician. A patient's risk of acquiring rabies must be carefully considered before deciding to discontinue vaccination. Advice and assistance on the management of serious adverse reactions for people receiving rabies vaccines may be sought from the state health department or the CDC.

Typhoid Vaccine

Typhoid fever, an acute, life-threatening febrile illness caused by the bacterium *Salmonella enterica* serovar *typhi (S. typhi),* remains a serious public health problem throughout the developing world. Although disease prevalence varies greatly depending on the specific population studied, current global estimates suggest that 27 million cases of typhoid and 270,000 deaths occur annually.[97] In the United States and much of the developed world, typhoid fever has virtually disappeared.[97] Approximately 400 cases of typhoid fever, mostly among travelers, are reported to the CDC each year. Most reported cases in the United States are acquired during travel to developing countries.[374] The primary indication for typhoid vaccination in the United States is international travel to an endemic area.[373] In developing countries without safe water and sanitation, mass immunization is a potentially effective strategy to limit the severity and impact of typhoid fever.[3]

The changing epidemiology of typhoid fever underscores the importance of vaccination of international travelers and high-risk populations in endemic regions. Studies report that the highest incidence rate is found among children younger than 5 years and results in more severe disease than in earlier periods.[604,609] *S. typhi* is increasingly resistant to ampicillin, chloramphenicol, and cotrimoxazole; even quinolone resistance is reported in many parts of the world.[97,366] Case-fatality rates, which had decreased from 10% to 1% with appropriate antibiotic therapy, could rise again without safe, effective, and affordable vaccination strategies, especially as rates of resistance increase across the globe.

Preparations

The three types of typhoid vaccines are inactivated, whole-cell vaccines; live attenuated bacterial vaccines; and subunit vaccines.[503] The parenteral, heat-phenol–inactivated, whole-cell vaccine widely used for many years was highly immunogenic but also was highly reactogenic and no longer is available in the United States. It is the only vaccine approved for use in children as young as 6 months and is still available in several developing countries because of its affordability, although the manufacture of this vaccine may not be up to international standards.

Two vaccines are licensed for use in the United States: an oral live, attenuated vaccine (TY21a, Vivotif Berna) and a purified Vi (virulence) capsular polysaccharide of *S. typhi* vaccine (ViCPS) (Typhim Vi, Aventis Pasteur) for intramuscular use. Table 245.20 provides information on

TABLE 245.20 Dosage and Schedule for Typhoid Fever Vaccination

Vaccination	Age (y)	Dose/Route of Administration	No. of Doses	Dosing Schedule	Boosting Interval
Oral Live Attenuated TY21a Vaccine					
Primary series	≥6	1 capsule[a]/oral	4	Days 0, 2, 4, 6	NA
Booster	≥6	1 capsule[a]/oral	4	Days 0, 2, 4, 6	Every 5 y
Vi Capsular Polysaccharide Vaccine					
Primary series	≥2	0.50 mL/IM	1	NA	NA
Booster	≥2	0.50 mL/IM	1	NA	Every 2 y

[a]Administer with cool liquid no warmer than 37°C (98.6°F).
NA, Not applicable.
Modified from Jackson BR, Iqbal S, Mahon B, et al. Updated recommendations for the use of typhoid vaccine—Advisory Committee on Immunization Practices, United States, 2015. *MMWR Morb Mortal Wkly Rep.* 2015;64:305–8.

vaccine dosage and administration. The time required for primary vaccination is different for the two vaccines, as are the lower age limits for use in children.

Ty21a is an oral, live attenuated vaccine consisting of a stable mutant, Ty21a, developed by chemical mutagenesis of a pathogenic *S. typhi* strain. This vaccine was licensed in the United States in 1989 for use in adults and children 6 years or older and is available as an enteric-coated capsule (i.e., must be swallowed whole). The four-dose primary vaccine series in the United States and Canada (three-dose series in other parts of the world) is administered as one capsule every other day, taken 1 hour before a meal, for a total of four capsules. The capsules should be kept refrigerated (not frozen), and all four doses must be taken to achieve maximum efficacy. Each capsule should be taken with cool liquid no warmer than 37°C (98.6°F) approximately 1 hour before a meal. This regimen should be completed 1 week before potential exposure. The vaccine manufacturer recommends that Ty21a not be administered to infants or children younger than 6 years.

A parenteral subunit vaccine, ViCPS, was licensed in 1994 for use in adults and children as young as 2 years of age. Primary vaccination with ViCPS consists of one 0.5-mL (25-µg) dose administered intramuscularly and should be given at least 2 weeks before potential exposure. The manufacturer does not recommend the vaccine for children younger than 2 years.

Various protein conjugated Vi polysaccharide vaccines have been developed and are used in countries other than the United States, Two were recently licensed in India for use in children 3 months or older.[366,631]

In circumstances of continued or repeated exposure to *S. typhi,* booster doses are recommended to maintain immunity after primary immunization. The optimal booster schedule for either vaccine has not been determined. Current recommendations for revaccination with either vaccine are provided in Table 245.20. No data have been reported comparing the use of one vaccine as a booster after primary immunization with the other.

Efficacy

Although field trials have demonstrated approximately 80% efficacy of typhoid vaccines in US travelers,[446] no comparative studies have been performed.[366] For the heat-phenol–inactivated, whole-cell vaccine, efficacy ranged from 51% to 88% and lasted for as long as 7 years. The oral, live attenuated Ty21a vaccine stimulates humoral (i.e., serum IgG and mucosal IgA antibodies) and cell-mediated immune responses. In trials of the Ty21a vaccine, efficacy ranged from 42% to 96% after administration of the initial series of three doses, with the lower efficacies seen in trials from areas with highly endemic disease.[429,605] The optimal schedule for booster immunizations has not been determined for this vaccine. Protective immunity persisted for at least 7 years in field trials in endemic countries where herd immunity may have an effect.[324] Revaccination is recommended with the same four-capsule regimen every 5 years for as long as continued exposure is likely to occur.

Immunization with ViCPS results in seroconversion, defined as a fourfold rise in serum anti-Vi antibody, in 80% of vaccinees within 2 weeks in endemic and nonendemic areas.[324,342,397] Because the vaccine is administered parenterally, mucosal immunity does not develop. The efficacy of ViCPS vaccine in clinical trials was 72% at 17 months[2] and 64% at 21 months[397] after administration of a single dose. A cluster-randomized trial in India enrolling 37,673 children 2 years or older demonstrated 61% effectiveness.[629] Polysaccharide vaccines do not stimulate T cells and cannot establish immunologic memory. Additional doses of ViCPS therefore do not elicit a booster effect. Revaccination with a single dose is recommended every 2 years for people who remain at risk.

Conjugate Vi vaccines trials have used various carrier proteins, and one study of more than 12,000 children 2 to 5 years old demonstrated 90% efficacy over a trial period of 4 years using recombinant exoprotein A of *Pseudomonas aeruginosa* (Vi-rEPA).[434] Anti-Vi IgG titers were higher and longer lasting with conjugate Vi vaccines compared with Vi alone in adults and children from endemic areas.[631]

None of the typhoid vaccines approaches 100% efficacy, and a large inoculum of *S. typhi* can overcome vaccine-induced immunity. Vaccines do not substitute for proper hygiene and appropriate food handling practices.

Adverse Events

Reactions to the oral Ty21a vaccine usually are mild and consist of transient gastrointestinal upset, fever, headache, and an occasionally rash. These reactions occur in less than 5% of recipients.[366] Adverse systemic effects are reported in less than 1% of vaccinees, and neither the development of bacteremia nor person-to-person transmission has been reported.[324]

Reactions to the ViCPS vaccine also occur infrequently and are reported in approximately 7% of recipients[366] These reactions include tenderness at the injection site, erythema and induration, fever, and rarely, rashes. Systemic complaints occur in less than 2%.[324] In contrast, reactions to the inactivated, whole-cell vaccine occur more commonly and are more severe; they include fever in as many as 24% of recipients, headache, and severe local pain or swelling in as many as 35% of vaccinees. Between 13% and 24% of vaccinees have missed school or work because of adverse reactions.[430]

Reactions to the conjugate Vi vaccines were mild and limited to fever and mild erythema. There were no serious adverse events.[434,631]

Indications

Typhoid vaccination in the United States is recommended only for the following groups[366,503]:

- Travelers in areas where typhoid fever is endemic and for whom the risk of exposure is recognized; risk of exposure is greatest with travel to the Indian subcontinent, Latin America, Asia, the Middle East, and Africa
- People with intimate exposure to a documented *S. typhi* carrier, as occurs with continuing household contact
- Laboratory workers who have frequent contact with *S. typhi* and people living in areas outside the United States with endemic typhoid infection

Vaccination is not recommended for people attending summer camp or for those in areas of natural disaster or for control of common-source outbreaks. Doses and schedules for the different typhoid vaccines are given in the recommendations of the CDC.[366,503]

Contraindications

Ty21a is a live attenuated vaccine and should not be given to immunocompromised patients, including those receiving high doses of corticosteroids and people with HIV infection.[366,503] Ty21a vaccine also should not be administered during a gastrointestinal illness or concurrent with certain antibiotics. The *2015 Red Book* recommends avoiding antimicrobial therapy for at least 24 hours before the first dose of oral typhoid vaccine through 7 days after the last dose.[45] Reports are conflicting regarding the use of the antimalarial agents atovaquone and proguanil; however, chloroquine and mefloquine do not appear to interfere with the immune response to oral Ty21a. Neither of the available typhoid vaccines should be given to anyone with a history of severe local or systemic reactions after receiving a previous dose of vaccine.

Ty21a is not approved for children younger than 6 years, and ViCPS is not approved for children younger than 2 years. The whole-cell, inactivated vaccine available outside of the United States is approved for use in children between 6 months and 2 years of age.

Information is not available on the safety of these vaccines when they are used during pregnancy. It is prudent on theoretical grounds to avoid vaccinating pregnant women.

Yellow Fever Vaccine

Yellow fever occurs only in sub-Saharan Africa and tropical South America, where it causes an estimated 200,000 cases and 30,000 deaths annually.[564] During the past 2 decades, 90% of all yellow fever cases were reported from countries in West Africa, where travelers are thought to be at the highest risk of travel-associated yellow fever.[617] Clinical disease ranges from a mild, nonspecific febrile illness to severe disease with jaundice and hemorrhage.

Yellow fever is an important vaccine-preventable disease among travelers to areas where yellow fever occurs. The yellow fever epidemic zones include Bolivia, Brazil, Colombia, Ecuador, French Guiana, Guyana, Paraguay, Peru, Suriname, Venezuela, and much of sub-Saharan Africa. From 1970 to 2013, 10 cases of yellow fever were reported in unvaccinated travelers from the United States and Europe who traveled to West Africa (five cases) or South America (five cases). The unvaccinated traveler's risk of acquiring yellow fever probably is increasing because potential zones of transmission of yellow fever are expanding to include urban areas with large populations of susceptible humans and abundant competent mosquito vectors. Vaccination is the most effective preventive measure against yellow fever, a disease that has no specific treatment and may cause the death of 20% to 50% of patients.[484]

Preparations

Yellow fever vaccines are derived from the original 17D yellow fever vaccine strain. The live attenuated 17D-204 and 17DD yellow fever strains are the yellow fever vaccines most commonly used.[484] The only yellow fever vaccine licensed in the United States is the 17D-204 vaccine, which is prepared in chick embryos (YF-Vax, Sanofi Pasteur).[618]

Primary immunization consists of a single, subcutaneous injection of 0.5 mL of reconstituted, freeze-dried vaccine for adults and children. The vaccine should be stored at 2°C to 8°C. Because the vaccine does not contain a preservative, reconstituted vaccine that remains unused after 1 hour must be properly disposed.

Immunogenicity and Efficacy

Seroconversion rates of 93% have been documented for young children receiving yellow fever vaccine.[710] Thirteen observational studies showed a seropositivity rate of 92% at least 10 years after receiving the vaccine and 80% at least 20 years after vaccination.[617] Immunity develops by the tenth day after primary vaccination. The titer of virus-neutralizing antibodies in the sera of vaccinees is used as a surrogate for vaccine effectiveness.

No human efficacy studies have been performed with yellow fever vaccine. However, the number of yellow fever cases was substantially reduced after the introduction of the vaccine, supporting its protective role in humans. Worldwide, only 18 cases of yellow fever have been reported in vaccine recipients after the administration of more than 540 million doses; 16 (89%) had received a vaccine dose within the previous 10 years.[617]

Adverse Events

The 17D-204 and 17DD yellow fever vaccines are among the safest and most effective viral vaccines.[484] Since 1965, approximately 8 million doses of 17D-derived yellow fever vaccine have been administered to US travelers, and approximately 300 million doses have been administered to people in areas where yellow fever is endemic. Although 10% to 30% of people who receive vaccine report headaches, myalgia, and low-grade fever that begin within a few days after vaccination and last 5 to 10 days, less than 1% report temporarily curtailing their usual activities.

Historically, yellow fever vaccine–associated adverse events were seen primarily among infants and manifested as encephalitis. However, with the current yellow fever vaccine, serious adverse events associated with vaccine rarely occur. A systematic review found that no serious adverse events were reported in four RCTs of infants and children ($n = 1866$).[636]

Three well-characterized serious adverse events may occur after yellow fever vaccine administration: immediate hypersensitivity or anaphylactic reactions, yellow fever vaccine–associated neurologic disease (YEL-AND), and yellow fever vaccine–associated viscerotropic disease (YEL-AVD). Immediate hypersensitivity reactions, characterized by rash, urticaria, or bronchospasm, or a combination of these features is uncommon (1.8 cases/100,000 doses). Unrecognized allergy to eggs or chicken or to the hydrolyzed gelatin used to stabilize the vaccine may be responsible for hypersensitivity reactions.

YEL-AND is a serious but rarely fatal adverse event that occurs among people of all ages. YEL-AND manifests as several distinct clinical syndromes, including meningoencephalitis (i.e., neurotropic disease), Guillain-Barré syndrome, acute disseminated encephalomyelitis (ADEM), and bulbar palsy, starting 3 to 28 days after vaccination, usually in first-time recipients.[140] Meningoencephalitis occurs as a result of direct yellow fever vaccine viral invasion of the central nervous system (CNS) with infection of the meninges or the brain, or both. The other neurologic syndromes (e.g., Guillain-Barré syndrome, ADEM) represent autoimmune manifestations in which antibodies or T cells produced in response to the vaccine cross-react with neuronal epitopes and lead to central or peripheral nerve damage. The incidence of YEL-AND in the United States is 0.8 case per 100,000 doses.

In 2001, a previously unrecognized, potentially fatal adverse reaction among recipients of YF vaccine was first described. This syndrome previously was reported as febrile multiple organ dysfunction or failure and now is called yellow fever vaccine–associated viscerotropic disease. YEL-AVD mimics naturally acquired wild-type yellow fever disease, with the vaccine virus proliferating and disseminating throughout the host's tissues. Since it was initially described, more than 65 confirmed or suspected cases have been reported globally. On the basis of an analysis of cases for which information is available, YEL-AVD has occurred only after a recipient's first yellow fever vaccination; no cases of YEL-AVD occurring in people receiving booster doses of the vaccine have been reported. The median time from vaccination to disease onset is approximately 4 days. The case-fatality ratio for reported cases is approximately 60%. The incidence of YEL-AVD in the United States is 0.4 case per 100,000 doses.

Several risk estimates for YEL-AVD have been published. On the basis of VAERS data, the reporting rate of YEL-AVD is 3 to 4 cases per 1 million doses distributed.[435,462]

The recognition of these adverse events may be challenging because the neurologic syndromes (e.g., encephalitis, myelitis) can be difficult to distinguish from bacterial meningitis, encephalitis, or malaria, and the viscerotropic syndrome can be difficult to distinguish from hemorrhagic fevers, viral hepatitis, and many other causes of multisystem failure.

Indications

Yellow fever vaccine is recommended for people 9 months or older traveling to or residing in areas where yellow fever is endemic.[618] Because of the increased risk of neurologic complications, infants 6 to 8 months of age should be considered for vaccination only when travel to high-risk areas is unavoidable and high-level protection against mosquito exposure is not feasible. Infants younger than 6 months have a substantially increased risk of neurologic disease, and vaccination should not be given to this age group. Vaccination for international travel to certain destinations is required.

Yellow fever vaccination requirements for specific countries are available on the CDC Traveler's Health website (http://wwwnc.cdc.gov/travel/yellowbook/2016/infectious-diseases-related-to-travel/yellow-fever). To obtain an international certificate of vaccination, a yellow fever vaccine approved by the WHO and administered at a designated yellow fever vaccine center is required. Yellow fever vaccine centers in the United States can be identified by contacting state or local health departments or visiting the CDC website (http://wwwnc.cdc.gov/travel/yellow-fever-vaccination-clinics/search). If the risks of potential serious adverse events caused by the yellow fever vaccine are considered greater than the potential benefits for exposed individuals, a medical waiver letter can be provided, and guidance is provided on the CDC website (http://wwwnc.cdc.gov/travel/yellowbook/2016/infectious-diseases-related-to-travel/yellow-fever#4731).

Historically, the WHO international health regulations required revaccination at 10-year intervals. However, evidence from several studies indicated that yellow fever immunity persists for many decades. In 2015, the CDC's ACIP issued a recommendation that only a single dose of yellow fever vaccine is required to provide long-lasting protection for most travelers except for pregnant women, hematopoietic stem cell transplant recipients and HIV-infected people. The WHO has removed the booster requirement from the international health regulations as of 2016.[617]

Yellow fever vaccines can be administered at the same time as inactivated vaccines and other live attenuated viral vaccines, except for the MMR vaccine, because the immune responses against yellow fever, mumps, and rubella are inhibited.[408] These vaccines should be given 30 days apart.

Precautions and Contraindications

The risk of having adverse reactions appears to be age related.[618] Infants younger than 9 months should not receive yellow fever vaccine because of the increased risk of vaccine-associated neurotropic disease developing in this age group.[30] Immunization should be delayed until an infant is at least 9 months of age. In unusual circumstances, physicians considering vaccinating infants 6 to 8 months of age should contact the applicable division of the CDC for advice (i.e., CDC Division of Vector-Borne Infectious Diseases or the CDC Division of Global Migration and Quarantine: 800-232-4636).

No major adverse effects of yellow fever vaccine on the developing fetus have been demonstrated. A slight increased risk was observed for minor, mostly skin, malformations in infants. A higher rate of spontaneous abortions in pregnant women receiving the vaccine was reported but not substantiated. Vaccine administration to pregnant women usually is not indicated because the vaccine is a live virus. Pregnant women should be considered for vaccination only when travel to high-risk areas is required and protection against mosquito exposure is not feasible. Considering that immune responses to vaccination during pregnancy may vary, serologic testing can be considered to document a protective immune response to the vaccine.

Three YEL-AND cases have been reported in exclusively breastfed infants whose mothers were vaccinated with yellow fever vaccine. All three infants were younger than 1 month and diagnosed with encephalitis. Until more data are available, yellow fever vaccine should be avoided in breastfeeding women. However, when travel of breastfeeding mothers to a yellow fever–endemic area cannot be avoided, these women should be vaccinated.

Yellow fever vaccine, which is a live attenuated virus vaccine, poses a risk of developing encephalitis or other serious adverse events for patients with conditions that commonly result in immunosuppression (i.e. AIDS or symptomatic HIV infection, primary immunodeficiencies, thymic disease with abnormal immune function such as thymoma or myasthenia gravis, malignancy, transplantation, and radiation therapy). The vaccine should be avoided by these people. Although not specifically tested, the vaccine is presumed to pose risks for patients receiving immunosuppressive or immunomodulatory therapies (e.g., high-dose systemic corticosteroids, alkylating drugs, antimetabolites, tumor necrosis factor-α inhibitors, interleukin-1 and interleukin-6 blocking agents, other monoclonal antibodies such as rituximab and alemtuzumab) and should be avoided in most cases according to the drug manufacturers. A history of thymectomy or indirect radiation therapy is not considered a contraindication.

Family members of immunosuppressed people, who themselves have no contraindications, may receive yellow fever vaccine. If travel to an epidemic or endemic area is necessary, the patient should be instructed in ways to avoid mosquitoes and given a vaccine waiver letter.

People with a history of systemic anaphylaxis to eggs or chicken should not be vaccinated because the vaccines contain egg proteins and on rare occasion may induce immediate allergic reactions. People may also develop allergies to the vaccine because it contains gelatin and latex from the vial stopper. Less severe or local manifestations of allergy to eggs or to feathers are not contraindications to yellow fever vaccine administration and do not warrant performing vaccine skin testing.[36] If international quarantine regulations are the only reason to immunize a patient known to be hypersensitive to eggs, a medical waiver letter should be provided. If immunization of an individual with a questionable history of egg hypersensitivity is considered essential because of the high risk of exposure, an intradermal skin test can be given as directed in the vaccine package insert.[618]

Vaccines Related to Bioterrorism

Anthrax and smallpox vaccines are potentially available to protect children against bioterrorist attacks with *Bacillus anthracis* and variola. Anthrax vaccine is not approved by the FDA for use in children. The AAP updated its recommendations on exposure to anthrax through bioterrorism in 2014.[86] Until there are sufficient data to support FDA approval, anthrax vaccine will be made available for children at the time of an event as an investigational vaccine through an expedited process that requires institutional review board approval, including the use of appropriate consent documents. Information on the process required for use of anthrax vaccine in children will be available on the CDC website at the time of an event (https://www.cdc.gov/anthrax/).[703]

The only smallpox vaccine licensed in the United States is ACAM2000, a live virus vaccine.[153] In the absence of a smallpox outbreak, preexposure smallpox immunization is not recommended for children.[46] Anthrax and smallpox vaccines are reviewed in the relevant disease-specific chapters of this textbook.

Investigational Vaccines

Routine immunizations for children have virtually eliminated many infectious diseases from the United States. These successes have encouraged research to develop vaccines to prevent other serious viral and bacterial diseases affecting children. A 1985 report by the IOM of the National Academy of Sciences reviewed the benefits that would be associated with the development and use of new and improved vaccines in the United States.[212] The report listed 14 diseases for which vaccines were desirable. A 1999 study by the IOM observed that considerable progress had been made since the 1985 study.[213] Seven of 14 vaccines listed in the 1985 study as domestic priorities for development are now licensed. They include acellular pertussis vaccine, LAIV, and vaccines against hepatitis A and B, Hib, varicella, and rotavirus.

The 1999 IOM report used a new quantitative model to compare the cost and health benefits of developing candidate vaccines.[213] This model can be used to evaluate the potential impact of a new vaccine on public health. In the 1999 report, the model was used to evaluate diseases for which candidate vaccines were being developed. The report divided 26 candidate vaccines into four groups, arranged from most to least favorable for development. The four vaccines in the top tier include a cytomegalovirus vaccine given to adolescents, a universal influenza vaccine, a group B *Streptococcus* vaccine for high-risk adults and pregnant women, and an *S. pneumoniae* vaccine for infants and seniors. Other diseases for which vaccines would be desirable included *Chlamydia trachomatis,* enterotoxigenic *E. coli,* Epstein-Barr virus, *Helicobacter pylori,* hepatitis C virus, herpes simplex virus, human papilloma virus (HPV), *M. tuberculosis, Neisseria gonorrhoeae,* respiratory

BOX 245.2 Pathogens With Important Public Health Implications That Have No Licensed Vaccines

Campylobacter jejuni
Chikungunya virus
Dengue virus
Enterotoxigenic *Escherichia coli*
Enterovirus 71 (EV71)
Group B *Streptococcus* (GBS)
Herpes simplex virus
Human immunodeficiency virus type 1 (HIV-1)
Influenza virus (i.e., no universal vaccine)
Leishmania spp. (i.e., leishmaniasis)
Mycobacterium tuberculosis (i.e., tuberculosis)
Necator americanus and *Ancylostoma duodenale* (i.e., human hookworm disease)
Nipah virus
Nontyphoidal *Salmonella* spp. (i.e., salmonellosis)
Norovirus
Plasmodium spp. (i.e., malaria)
Respiratory syncytial virus (RSV)
Salmonella enterica subspecies (i.e., paratyphoid fever)
Schistosoma mansoni, S. haematobium, and *S. japonicum* (i.e., schistosomiasis)
Shigella spp. (i.e., shigellosis)
Staphylococcus aureus
Streptococcus pneumoniae
Streptococcus pyogenes
Trypanosoma cruzi (i.e., Chagas disease)
Zika virus

syncytial virus, parainfluenza virus, *Shigella*, and groups A and B streptococci. Two vaccines listed in the 1999 study are now licensed: pneumococcal conjugate vaccine for infants and seniors and HPV vaccine.

Progress in vaccine development is periodically reviewed and published by National Institute of Allergy and Infectious Diseases (NIAID) scientists in The Jordan Report.[497] The 2012 report discusses progress in vaccine development and states that we now have licensed vaccines against Hib and pneumococcal types that cause high childhood morbidity and mortality rates, against hepatitis A and B, against rotaviruses, and against varicella. We also have improved vaccines against such diseases as influenza and pertussis.

Advances in biotechnology, increased understanding of the virulence factors of infectious agents, and knowledge of the host immune response have led to new approaches for vaccine development.[256] Technological advances in making vaccines, including protein conjugation of bacterial polysaccharides, DNA vaccines, viral chimeras, viral vectors, and other novel platforms have been developed. Vaccines are being developed by the application of these newer technologies to numerous infectious agents for which effective vaccines are not currently available. The development of vaccines for these pathogens requires solution of several immunologic problems, including pathogen variability, short effector memory, evoking functional responses, and identification of antigens that generate protective responses.[539]

The 2012 Jordan Report states that many challenges remain. Progress on vaccines to prevent some high-burden diseases has been frustratingly slow, although there is a growing pipeline of novel vaccines against dengue, malaria, tuberculosis, and others. The Report lists approximately 600 vaccine candidates in development against an estimated 110 pathogens. Considering the resource constraints in vaccine development, approaches that are most likely to produce high-priority vaccines need to be identified.

A special issue of *Vaccine* published in June 2016 focuses on the research and development pipeline of vaccines against 25 pathogens for which no licensed vaccines currently exist but for which there is high public health importance, as identified by the WHO Product Development for Vaccines Advisory Committee (PDVAC).[687] PDVAC is a body of independent experts that was established in 2014 to guide the WHO and the vaccine development community along the pathway toward the goal of licensure and deployment in countries with the highest disease burden. These vaccines are listed in Box 245.2.

NEW REFERENCES SINCE THE SEVENTH EDITION

1. Abu Raya B, Srugo I, Kessel A, et al. The decline of pertussis-specific antibodies after tetanus, diphtheria, and acellular pertussis immunization in late pregnancy. *J Infect Dis*. 2015;212:1869-1873.
4. Adams DA, Thomas KR, Jajosky RA, et al. Summary of notifiable infectious diseases and conditions—United States, 2014. *MMWR Morb Mortal Wkly Rep*. 2016;63:1-152.
5. Advisory Committee on Immunization Practices, Centers for Disease Control and Prevention. Immunization of health-care personnel: recommendations of the Advisory Committee on Immunization Practices (ACIP). *MMWR Recomm Rep*. 2011;60(RR-7):1-45.
7. Albertson JP, Clegg WJ, Reid HD, et al. Mumps outbreak at a university and recommendation for a third dose of measles-mumps-rubella vaccine—Illinois, 2015-2016. *MMWR Morb Mortal Wkly Rep*. 2016;65:731-734.
8. Ali M, Nelson AR, Lopez AL, et al. Updated global burden of cholera in endemic countries. *PLoS Negl Trop Dis*. 2015;9:e0003832.
9. Aliabadi N, Tate JE, Haynes AK, et al. Sustained decrease in laboratory detection of rotavirus after implementation of routine vaccination—United States, 2000-2014. *MMWR Morb Mortal Wkly Rep*. 2015;64:337-342.
13. American Academy of Pediatrics Committee on Infectious Diseases. Updated recommendations on the use of meningococcal vaccines. *Pediatrics*. 2014;134:400-403.
16. American Academy of Pediatrics Committee on Infectious Diseases. Immunization of adolescents: recommendations of the Advisory Committee on Immunization Practices, the American Academy of Pediatrics, the American Academy of Family Physicians, and the American Medical Association. American Academy of Pediatrics Committee on Infectious Diseases. *Pediatrics*. 1997;99:479-488.
28. American Academy of Pediatrics. Active immunization. In: Kimberlin DW, Brady MT, Jackson MA, Long SS, eds. *Red Book: 2015 Report of the Committee on Infectious Diseases*. 30th ed. Elk Grove Village, IL: American Academy of Pediatrics; 2015:13-43.
29. American Academy of Pediatrics. Arboviruses. In: Kimberlin DW, Brady MT, Jackson MA, Long SS, eds. *Red Book: 2015 Report of the Committee on Infectious Diseases*. 30th ed. Elk Grove Village, IL: American Academy of Pediatrics; 2015:240-246.
30. American Academy of Pediatrics. Committee on Native American Child Health and Committee on Infectious Diseases. Immunizations for Native American children. American Academy of Pediatrics. *Pediatrics*. 1999;104:564-567.
31. American Academy of Pediatrics. Diphtheria. In: Kimberlin DW, Brady MT, Jackson MA, Long SS, eds. *Red Book: 2015 Report of the Committee on Infectious Diseases*. 30th ed. Elk Grove Village, IL: American Academy of Pediatrics; 2015:325-329.
32. American Academy of Pediatrics. infections. In: Kimberlin DW, Brady MT, Jackson MA, Long SS, eds. *Red Book: 2015 Report of the Committee on Infectious Diseases*. 30th ed. Elk Grove Village, IL: American Academy of Pediatrics; 2015:368-376.
33. American Academy of Pediatrics. Hepatitis A. In: Kimberlin DW, Brady MT, Jackson MA, Long SS, eds. *Red Book: 2015 Report of the Committee on Infectious Diseases*. 30th ed. Elk Grove Village, IL: American Academy of Pediatrics; 2015:391-399.
34. American Academy of Pediatrics. Hepatitis B. In: Kimberlin DW, Brady MT, Jackson MA, Long SS, eds. *Red Book: 2015 Report of the Committee on Infectious Diseases*. 30th ed. Elk Grove Village, IL: American Academy of Pediatrics; 2015:400-423.
35. American Academy of Pediatrics. Human papilloma viruses. In: Kimberlin DW, Brady MT, Jackson MA, Long SS, eds. *Red Book: 2015 Report of the Committee on Infectious Diseases*. 30th ed. Elk Grove Village, IL: American Academy of Pediatrics; 2015:576-583.
36. American Academy of Pediatrics. Immunization in special clinical circumstances. In: Kimberlin DW, Brady MT, Jackson MA, Long SS, eds. *Red Book: 2015 Report of the Committee on Infectious Diseases*. 30th ed. Elk Grove Village, IL: American Academy of Pediatrics; 2015:68-107.
37. American Academy of Pediatrics. Influenza. In: Kimberlin DW, Brady MT, Jackson MA, Long SS, eds. *Red Book: 2015 Report of the Committee on Infectious Diseases*. 30th ed. Elk Grove Village, IL: American Academy of Pediatrics; 2015: 476-493.
38. American Academy of Pediatrics. Measles. In: Kimberlin DW, Brady MT, Jackson MA, Long SS, eds. *Red Book: 2015 Report of the Committee on Infectious Diseases*. 30th ed. Elk Grove Village, IL: American Academy of Pediatrics; 2015: 535-547.
39. American Academy of Pediatrics. Meningococcal Infections. In: Kimberlin DW, Brady MT, Jackson MA, Long SS, eds. *Red Book: 2015 Report of the Committee on Infectious Diseases*. 30th ed. Elk Grove Village, IL: American Academy of Pediatrics; 2015:547-558.

40. American Academy of Pediatrics. Mumps. In: Kimberlin DW, Brady MT, Jackson MA, Long SS, eds. *Red Book: 2015 Report of the Committee on Infectious Diseases.* 30th ed. Elk Grove Village, IL: American Academy of Pediatrics; 2015:564-568.
41. American Academy of Pediatrics. Pertussis (whooping cough). In: Kimberlin DW, Brady MT, Jackson MA, Long SS, eds. *Red Book: 2015 Report of the Committee on Infectious Diseases.* 30th ed. Elk Grove Village, IL: American Academy of Pediatrics; 2015:608-621.
42. American Academy of Pediatrics. Pneumococcal infections. In: Kimberlin DW, Brady MT, Jackson MA, Long SS, eds. *Red Book: 2015 Report of the Committee on Infectious Diseases.* 30th ed. Elk Grove Village, IL: American Academy of Pediatrics; 2015:626-638.
43. American Academy of Pediatrics. Poliovirus Infections. In: Kimberlin DW, Brady MT, Jackson MA, Long SS, eds. *Red Book: 2015 Report of the Committee on Infectious Diseases.* 30th ed. Elk Grove Village, IL: American Academy of Pediatrics; 2015:644-650.
44. American Academy of Pediatrics. Rubella. In: Kimberlin DW, Brady MT, Jackson MA, Long SS, eds. *Red Book: 2015 Report of the Committee on Infectious Diseases.* 30th ed. Elk Grove Village, IL: American Academy of Pediatrics; 2015:688-695.
45. American Academy of Pediatrics. Salmonella Infections. In: Kimberlin DW, Brady MT, Jackson MA, Long SS, eds. *Red Book: 2015 Report of the Committee on Infectious Diseases.* 30th ed. Elk Grove Village, IL: American Academy of Pediatrics; 2015:695-702.
46. American Academy of Pediatrics. Smallpox (variola). In: Kimberlin DW, Brady MT, Jackson MA, Long SS, eds. *Red Book: 2015 Report of the Committee on Infectious Diseases.* 30th ed. Elk Grove Village, IL: American Academy of Pediatrics; 2015:709-712.
47. American Academy of Pediatrics. Tetanus (Lockjaw). In: Kimberlin DW, Brady MT, Jackson MA, Long SS, eds. *Red Book: 2015 Report of the Committee on Infectious Diseases.* 30th ed. Elk Grove Village, IL: American Academy of Pediatrics; 2015:773-778.
48. American Academy of Pediatrics. Tuberculosis. In: Kimberlin DW, Brady MT, Jackson MA, Long SS, eds. *Red Book: 2015 Report of the Committee on Infectious Diseases.* 30th ed. Elk Grove Village, IL: American Academy of Pediatrics; 2015:805-831.
49. American Academy of Pediatrics. Varicella-zoster. In: Kimberlin DW, Brady MT, Jackson MA, Long SS, eds. *Red Book: 2012 Report of the Committee on Infectious Diseases.* 30th ed. Elk Grove Village, IL: American Academy of Pediatrics; 2015:846-860.
50. Amirthalingam G, Andrews N, Campbell H, et al. Effectiveness of maternal pertussis vaccination in England: an observational study. *Lancet.* 2014;384(9953): 1521-1528.
60. Atwell JE, Van Otterloo J, Zipprich J, et al. Nonmedical vaccine exemptions and pertussis in California, 2010. *Pediatrics.* 2013;132:624-630.
67. Barskey AE, Glasser JW, LeBaron CW. Mumps resurgences in the United States: a historical perspective on unexpected elements. *Vaccine.* 2009;27: 6186-6195.
68. Baylis SA, Finsterbusch T, Bannert N, et al. Analysis of porcine circovirus type 1 detected in Rotarix vaccine. *Vaccine.* 2011;29:690-697.
69. Beasley RP, Detels R, Kim KS, et al. Prevention of rubella during an epidemic on Taiwan. HPV-77 and RA 27-3 rubella vaccines administered subcutaneously and intranasally HPV-77 vaccine mixed with mumps and/or measles vaccines. *Am J Dis Child.* 1969;118:301-306.
73. Belongia EA, Irving SA, Shui IM, et al. Real-time surveillance to assess risk of intussusception and other adverse events after pentavalent, bovine-derived rotavirus vaccine. *Pediatr Infect Dis J.* 2010;29:1-5.
79. Black CL, Yue X, Ball SW, et al. Influenza vaccination coverage among health care personnel—United States, 2014-15 influenza season. *MMWR Morb Mortal Wkly Rep.* 2015;64:993-999.
80. Black S, Greenberg DP. A combined diphtheria, tetanus, five-component acellular pertussis, poliovirus and *Haemophilus influenzae* type b vaccine. *Expert Rev Vaccines.* 2005;4:793-805.
85. Borgono JM, Greiber R, Solari G, et al. A field trial of combined measles-mumps-rubella vaccine. Satisfactory immunization with 188 children in Chile. *Clin Pediatr (Phila).* 1973;12:170-172.
86. Bradley JS, Peacock G, Krug SE, et al. Pediatric anthrax clinical management. *Pediatrics.* 2014;133:e1411-e1436.
87. Brady MT, Byington CL, Davies HD, et al. Immunization for *Streptococcus pneumoniae* infections in high-risk children. *Pediatrics.* 2014;134:1230-1233.
89. Briere EC, Rubin L, Moro PL, et al. Prevention and control of *Haemophilus influenzae* type b disease: recommendations of the advisory committee on immunization practices (ACIP). *MMWR Recomm Rep.* 2014;63(RR-01):1-14.
92. Broliden K, Abreu ER, Arneborn M, et al. Immunity to mumps before and after MMR vaccination at 12 years of age in the first generation offered the two-dose immunization programme. *Vaccine.* 1998;16:323-327.
93. Brooks R, Woods CW, Benjamin DK Jr, et al. Increased case-fatality rate associated with outbreaks of *Neisseria meningitidis* infection, compared with sporadic meningococcal disease, in the United States, 1994-2002. *Clin Infect Dis.* 2006;43:49-54.
96. Bryant KA, Marshall GS, Marchant CD, et al. Immunogenicity and safety of *H influenzae* type b–*N meningitidis* C/Y conjugate vaccine in infants. *Pediatrics.* 2011;127:e1375-e1385.
97. Buckle GC, Walker CL, Black RE. Typhoid fever and paratyphoid fever: systematic review to estimate global morbidity and mortality for 2010. *J Glob Health.* 2012;2:010401.
98. Burns CC, Diop OM, Sutter RW, et al. Vaccine-derived polioviruses. *J Infect Dis.* 2014;210(suppl 1):S283-S293.
101. Byington CL, Maldonado YA, Barnett ED, et al. Recommendations for prevention and control of influenza in children, 2016–2017. *Pediatrics.* 2016;138:pii: e20162527.
104. Castilla J, Garcia Cenoz M, Arriazu M, et al. Effectiveness of Jeryl Lynn-containing vaccine in Spanish children. *Vaccine.* 2009;27:2089-2093.
105. Centers for Disease Control and Prevention. Addition of history of intussusception as a contraindication for rotavirus vaccination. *MMWR Morb Mortal Wkly Rep.* 2011;60:1427.
111. Centers for Disease Control and Prevention. Estimates of deaths associated with seasonal influenza—United States, 1976-2007. *MMWR Morb Mortal Wkly Rep.* 2010;59:1057-1062.
121. Centers for Disease Control and Prevention. Licensure of a 13-valent pneumococcal conjugate vaccine (PCV13) and recommendations for use among children—Advisory Committee on Immunization Practices (ACIP), 2010. *MMWR Morb Mortal Wkly Rep.* 2010;59:258-261.
125. Centers for Disease Control and Prevention. Mumps outbreak on a university campus—California, 2011. *MMWR Morb Mortal Wkly Rep.* 2012;61: 986-989.
129. Centers for Disease Control and Prevention. Notice to readers: newly licensed smallpox vaccine to replace old smallpox vaccine. *MMWR Morb Mortal Wkly Rep.* 2008;57:207-208.
132. Centers for Disease Control and Prevention. Pertussis—United States, 1997-2000. *MMWR.* 2002;51:73-76.
135. Centers for Disease Control and Prevention. Poliomyelitis prevention in the United States: introduction of a sequential vaccination schedule of inactivated poliovirus vaccine followed by oral poliovirus vaccine. Recommendations of the Advisory Committee on Immunization Practices (ACIP). *MMWR Recomm Rep.* 1997;46(RR-3):1-25.
138. Centers for Disease Control and Prevention. Progress in introduction of pneumococcal conjugate vaccine—worldwide, 2000-2012. *MMWR Morb Mortal Wkly Rep.* 2013;62:308-311.
145. Centers for Disease Control and Prevention. Rubella and congenital rubella syndrome—United States, January 1, 1991-May 7, 1994. *MMWR Morb Mortal Wkly Rep.* 1994;43:391, 397-401.
146. Centers for Disease Control and Prevention. Seasonal influenza vaccine safety: a summary for clinicians, 2016. https://www.cdc.gov/flu/professionals/vaccination/vaccine_safety.htm.
147. Centers for Disease Control and Prevention. Syncope after vaccination—United States, January 2005-July 2007. *MMWR Morb Mortal Wkly Rep.* 2008;57: 457-460.
148. Centers for Disease Control and Prevention. Tetanus surveillance—United States, 2001-2008. *MMWR Morb Mortal Wkly Rep.* 2011;60:365-369.
161. Centers for Disease Control and Prevention. Updated recommendations for use of tetanus toxoid, reduced diphtheria toxoid, and acellular pertussis vaccine (Tdap) in pregnant women—Advisory Committee on Immunization Practices (ACIP), 2012. *MMWR Morb Mortal Wkly Rep.* 2013;62:131-135.
163. Centers for Disease Control and Prevention. Use of 13-valent pneumococcal conjugate vaccine and 23-valent pneumococcal polysaccharide vaccine among children aged 6-18 years with immunocompromising conditions: recommendations of the Advisory Committee on Immunization Practices (ACIP). *MMWR Morb Mortal Wkly Rep.* 2013;62:521-524.
166. Centers for Disease Control and Prevention. Use of Japanese encephalitis vaccine in children: recommendations of the advisory committee on immunization practices, 2013. *MMWR Morb Mortal Wkly Rep.* 2013;62:898-900.
170. Centers for Disease Control. Mumps prevention. *MMWR Morb Mortal Wkly Rep.* 1989;38:388-392, 397-400.
171. Centers for Disease Control. Mumps—United States, 1985-1988. *MMWR Morb Mortal Wkly Rep.* 1989;38:101-105.
172. Centers for Disease Control. Pneumococcal polysaccharide vaccine: Recommendations of the Advisory Committee on Immunization Practices (ACIP). *MMWR.* 1989;38:64-68, 73-76.
175. Centers for Disease Control. Rubella and congenital rubella—United States, 1983. *MMWR Morb Mortal Wkly Rep.* 1984;33:237-242, 247.
178. Centers for Disease Control. Surveillance of tetanus, 1987 and 1988. *Wkly Epidemiol Rec.* 1990;65:261-263.
180. Chaiken BP, Williams NM, Preblud SR, et al. The effect of a school entry law on mumps activity in a school district. *JAMA.* 1987;257:2455-2458.
181. Chamot E, Toscani L, Egger P, et al. Estimation of the efficacy of three strains of mumps vaccines during an epidemic of mumps in the Geneva canton (Switzerland). *Rev Epidemiol Sante Publique.* 1998;46:100-107.

183. Cheek JE, Baron R, Atlas H, et al. Mumps outbreak in a highly vaccinated school population. Evidence for large-scale vaccination failure. *Arch Pediatr Adolesc Med.* 1995;149:774-778.
187. Chen WH, Cohen MB, Kirkpatrick BD, et al. Single-dose live oral cholera vaccine CVD 103-HgR protects against human experimental infection with *Vibrio cholerae* O1 El Tor. *Clin Infect Dis.* 2016;62:1329-1335.
188. Cherry JD, Brunell PA, Golden GS, et al. Report of the task force on pertussis and pertussis immunization—1988. *Pediatrics.* 1988;81:933-984.
189. Chesson HW, Dunne EF, Hariri S, et al. The estimated lifetime probability of acquiring human papillomavirus in the United States. *Sex Transm Dis.* 2014;41:660-664.
190. Christenson B, Bottiger M. Long-term follow-up study of rubella antibodies in naturally immune and vaccinated young adults. *Vaccine.* 1994;12:41-45.
192. Chung JR, Flannery B, Thompson MG, et al. Seasonal effectiveness of live attenuated and inactivated influenza vaccine. *Pediatrics.* 2016;137:e20153279.
198. Cochi SL, Broome CV, Hightower AW. Immunization of US children with *Hemophilus influenzae* type b polysaccharide vaccine. A cost-effectiveness model of strategy assessment. *JAMA.* 1985;253:521-529.
199. Cochi SL, Preblud SR, Orenstein WA. Prospectives on the relative resurgence of mumps in the United States. *Am J Dis Child.* 1988;142:499-507.
203. Cohn A Proceedings of the Advisory Committee on Immunization Practices (ACIP) meeting. Paper presented at the Advisory Committee on Immunization Practices (ACIP) meeting; 2010; Atlanta, GA.
204. Cohn AC, MacNeil JR, Clark TA, et al. Prevention and control of meningococcal disease: recommendations of the Advisory Committee on Immunization Practices (ACIP). *MMWR Recomm Rep.* 2013;62(RR-2):1-28.
205. Cohn AC, MacNeil JR, Harrison LH, et al. Changes in *Neisseria meningitidis* disease epidemiology in the United States, 1998-2007: implications for prevention of meningococcal disease. *Clin Infect Dis.* 2010;50:184-191.
209. Committee on Infectious Diseases, American Academy of Pediatrics. Recommended childhood and adolescent immunization schedule—United States, 2016. *Pediatrics.* 2016;137:e20154531.
210. Committee on Infectious Diseases, American Academy of Pediatrics. HPV vaccine recommendations. *Pediatrics.* 2012;129:602-605.
211. Committee on Infectious Diseases, American Academy of Pediatrics. Recommendations for serogroup B meningococcal vaccine for persons 10 years and older. *Pediatrics.* 2016;138:pii: e20161890.
214. Committee to Study Priorities for Vaccine Development, Institute of Medicine. *Vaccines for the 21st Century: A Tool for Decision Making.* Washington. DC: National Academies Press; 2000.
215. Cortes JE, Curns AT, Tate JE, et al. Rotavirus vaccine and health care utilization for diarrhea in U.S. Children. *N Engl J Med.* 2011;365:1108-1117.
216. Cortese MM, Jordan HT, Curns AT, et al. Mumps vaccine performance among university students during a mumps outbreak. *Clin Infect Dis.* 2008;46:1172-1180.
218. Coulehan JL, Michaels RH, Hallowell C, et al. Epidemiology of *Haemophilus influenzae* type B disease among Navajo Indians. *Public Health Rep.* 1984;99: 404-409.
225. D'Amelio R, Biselli R, Fascia G, et al. Measles-mumps-rubella vaccine in the Italian armed forces. *JAMA.* 2000;284:2059.
229. Dayan GH, Quinlisk MP, Parker AA, et al. Recent resurgence of mumps in the United States. *N Engl J Med.* 2008;358:1580-1589.
231. Decker MD, Edwards KM. *Haemophilus influenzae* type b vaccines: history, choice and comparisons. *Pediatr Infect Dis J.* 1998;17(suppl):S113-S116.
233. Deeks SL, Lim GH, Simpson MA, et al. An assessment of mumps vaccine effectiveness by dose during an outbreak in Canada. *CMAJ.* 2011;183:1014-1020.
237. Dennehy PH, Vesikari T, Matson DO, et al. Efficacy of the pentavalent rotavirus vaccine, RotaTeq(R) (RV5), between doses of a 3-dose series and with less than 3 doses (incomplete regimen). *Hum Vaccin.* 2011;7:563-568.
239. D'Hondt E. Possible approaches to develop vaccines against hepatitis A. *Vaccine.* 1992;10:S48-S52.
241. Dominguez A, Torner N, Castilla J, et al. Mumps vaccine effectiveness in highly immunized populations. *Vaccine.* 2010;28:3567-3570.
243. Donegan K, King B, Bryan P. Safety of pertussis vaccination in pregnant women in UK: observational study. *BMJ.* 2014;349:g4219.
244. Donovan B, Franklin N, Guy R, et al. Quadrivalent human papillomavirus vaccination and trends in genital warts in Australia: analysis of national sentinel surveillance data. *Lancet Infect Dis.* 2011;11:39-44.
245. Donovan B, Grulich AE. The quadrivalent HPV vaccine is effective prophylaxis against HPV-related external genital lesions in young men. *Evid Based Med.* 2011;16:157-158.
246. Douvoyiannis M, Belamarich PF, Goldman DL. Tetanus after vaccine refusal and an opportunity for the pediatric infectious diseases specialist. *Clin Pediatr (Phila).* 2015;54:513-516.
249. Dunne EF, Nielson CM, Stone KM, et al. Prevalence of HPV infection among men: a systematic review of the literature. *J Infect Dis.* 2006;194:1044-1057.
254. Ehrenkranz NJ, Ventura AK, Medler EM, et al. Clinical evaluation of a new measles-mumps-rubella combined live virus vaccine in the Dominican Republic. *Bull World Health Organ.* 1975;52:81-85.
256. Ellis RW, Rappuoli R, Ahmed S. New technologies for making vaccines. In: Plotkin S, Orenstein W, Offit P, eds. *Vaccines.* 6th ed. Philadelphia, PA: Saunders-Elsevier; 2013:1182-1199.
263. Feikin DR, Kagucia EW, Loo JD, et al. Serotype-specific changes in invasive pneumococcal disease after pneumococcal conjugate vaccine introduction: a pooled analysis of multiple surveillance sites. *PLoS Med.* 2013;10:e1001517.
264. Feiterna-Sperling C, Bronnimann R, Tischer A, et al. Open randomized trial comparing the immunogenicity and safety of a new measles-mumps-rubella vaccine and a licensed vaccine in 12- to 24-month-old children. *Pediatr Infect Dis J.* 2005;24:1083-1088.
265. Ferlay J, Soerjomataram I, Dikshit R, et al. Cancer incidence and mortality worldwide: sources, methods and major patterns in GLOBOCAN 2012. *Int J Cancer.* 2015;136:E359-E386.
266. Fiebelkorn A, Barskey A, Hickman C, et al. Mumps. In: Prevention CfDCa, ed. *Manual for the Surveillance of Vaccine-Preventable Diseases.* 5th ed. Atlanta, GA: US Department of Health and Human Services, Centers for Disease Control and Prevention; 2012.
267. Fiebelkorn AP, Redd SB, Gastanaduy PA, et al. A comparison of postelimination measles epidemiology in the United States, 2009-2014 versus 2001-2008. *J Pediatric Infect Dis Soc.* 2017;6:40-48.
274. Fletcher HA, Schrager L. TB vaccine development and the End TB Strategy: importance and current status. *Trans R Soc Trop Med Hyg.* 2016;110:212-218.
275. Fogel A, Moshkowitz A, Rannon L, et al. Comparative trials of RA 27-3 and Cendehill rubella vaccines in adult and adolescent females. *Am J Epidemiol.* 1971;93:392-398.
276. Folaranmi T, Rubin L, Martin SW, et al. Use of serogroup B meningococcal vaccines in persons aged ≥10 years at increased risk for serogroup B meningococcal disease: recommendations of the Advisory Committee on Immunization Practices, 2015. *MMWR Morb Mortal Wkly Rep.* 2015;64:608-612.
277. Food and Drug Administration. *December 10, 2014 approval letter—Gardasil 9.* Silver Spring, MD: US Department of Health and Human Services; 2014.
278. Food and Drug Administration. *October 7, 2016 approval letter for human papillomavirus 9-valent vaccine, recombinant to include a 2-dose regimen for individuals 9 through 14 years of age.* Silver Spring, MD: US Department of Health and Human Services; 2016.
279. Fowlkes A, Steffens A, Temte J, et al. Incidence of medically attended influenza during pandemic and post-pandemic seasons through the Influenza Incidence Surveillance Project, 2009-13. *Lancet Respir Med.* 2015;3:709-718.
281. Freestone DS, Reynolds GM, McKinnon JA, et al. Vaccination of schoolgirls against rubella. Assessment of serological status and a comparative trial of Wistar RA 27/3 and Cendehill strain live attenuated rubella vaccines in 13-year-old schoolgirls in Dudley. *Br J Prev Soc Med.* 1975;29:258-261.
282. Fritzell B, Plotkin S. Efficacy and safety of a *Haemophilus influenzae* type b capsular polysaccharide-tetanus protein conjugate vaccine. *J Pediatr.* 1992;121: 355-362.
283. Furukawa T, Miyata T, Kondo K, et al. Rubella vaccination during an epidemic. *JAMA.* 1970;213:987-990.
284. Gaglani M, Pruszynski J, Murthy K, et al. Influenza vaccine effectiveness against 2009 pandemic influenza A(H1N1) virus differed by vaccine type during 2013-2014 in the United States. *J Infect Dis.* 2016;213:1546-1556.
287. Gastanaduy PA, Redd SB, Fiebelkorn AP, et al. Measles—United States, January 1-May 23, 2014. *MMWR Morb Mortal Wkly Rep.* 2014;63:496-499.
288. Gatchalian S, Cordero-Yap L, Lu-Fong M, et al. A randomized comparative trial in order to assess the reactogenicity and immunogenicity of a new measles mumps rubella (MMR) vaccine when given as a first dose at 12-24 months of age. *Southeast Asian J Trop Med Public Health.* 1999;30:511-517.
295. Giebink GS. Preventing pneumococcal disease in children: recommendations for using pneumococcal vaccine. *Pediatr Infect Dis.* 1985;4:343-348.
296. Gill CJ, Baxter R, Anemona A, et al. Persistence of immune responses after a single dose of Novartis meningococcal serogroup A, C, W-135 and Y CRM-197 conjugate vaccine (Menveo® or Menactra®) among healthy adolescents. *Hum Vaccin.* 2010;6:881-887.
304. Goldschneider I, Gotschlich EC, Artenstein MS. Human immunity to the meningococcus. I. The role of humoral antibodies. *J Exp Med.* 1969;129: 1307-1326.
306. Gothefors L, Bergstrom E, Backman M. Immunogenicity and reactogenicity of a new measles, mumps and rubella vaccine when administered as a second dose at 12 y of age. *Scand J Infect Dis.* 2001;33:545-549.
307. Gotschlich EC, Goldschneider I, Artenstein MS. Human immunity to the meningococcus. IV. Immunogenicity of group A and group C meningococcal polysaccharides in human volunteers. *J Exp Med.* 1969;129:1367-1384.
308. Grassly NC. Immunogenicity and effectiveness of routine immunization with 1 or 2 doses of inactivated poliovirus vaccine: systematic review and meta-analysis. *J Infect Dis.* 2014;210(suppl 1):S439-S446.
314. Grillner L. Neutralizing antibodies after rubella vaccination of newly delivered women: a comparison between three vaccines. *Scand J Infect Dis.* 1975;7:169-172.
315. Grohskopf LA, Sokolow LZ, Broder KR, et al. Prevention and control of seasonal influenza with vaccines. *MMWR Recomm Rep.* 2016;65:1-54.

318. Group GA. Expanded programme on immunization. Global Advisory Group—Part II. Achieving the major disease control goals. *Wkly Epidemiol Rec.* 1994;69:29-31, 34-35.
319. Guerra FA, Blatter MM, Greenberg DP, et al. Safety and immunogenicity of a pentavalent vaccine compared with separate administration of licensed equivalent vaccines in US infants and toddlers and persistence of antibodies before a preschool booster dose: a randomized, clinical trial. *Pediatrics.* 2009;123:301-312.
325. Haber P, Patel M, Izurieta HS, et al. Postlicensure monitoring of intussusception after RotaTeq vaccination in the United States, February 1, 2006, to September 25, 2007. *Pediatrics.* 2008;121:1206-1212.
331. Hampton LM, Farley MM, Schaffner W, et al. Prevention of antibiotic-nonsusceptible *Streptococcus pneumoniae* with conjugate vaccines. *J Infect Dis.* 2012;205:401-411.
332. Hanna-Wakim R, Yasukawa LL, Sung P, et al. Immune responses to mumps vaccine in adults who were vaccinated in childhood. *J Infect Dis.* 2008;197:1669-1675.
341. Hersh BS, Fine PE, Kent WK, et al. Mumps outbreak in a highly vaccinated population. *J Pediatr.* 1991;119:187-193.
345. Hill HA, Elam-Evans LD, Yankey D, et al. Vaccination coverage among children aged 19-35 months—United States, 2015. *MMWR Morb Mortal Wkly Rep.* 2016;65:1065-1071.
346. Hillary IB, Griffith AH. Persistence of rubella antibodies 15 years after subcutaneous administration of Wistar 27/3 strain live attenuated rubella virus vaccine. *Vaccine.* 1984;2:274-276.
347. Hilleman MR, Buynak EB, Weibel RE, et al. Live, attenuated mumps-virus vaccine. *N Engl J Med.* 1968;278:227-232.
348. Hilleman MR, Weibel RE, Buynak EB, et al. Live attenuated mumps-virus vaccine. IV. Protective efficacy as measured in a field evaluation. *N Engl J Med.* 1967;276:252-258.
352. Holmes SJ, Fritzell B, Guito KP, et al. Immunogenicity of *Haemophilus influenzae* type b polysaccharide-tetanus toxoid conjugate vaccine in infants. *Am J Dis Child.* 1993;147:832-836.
353. Horstmann DM, Schluederberg A, Emmons JE, et al. Persistence of vaccine-induced immune responses to rubella: comparison with natural infection. *Rev Infect Dis.* 1985;7(suppl 1):S80-S85.
354. Howson CP, Katz M, Johnston RB Jr, et al. Chronic arthritis after rubella vaccination. *Clin Infect Dis.* 1992;15:307-312.
355. Hsieh YC, Wu FT, Hsiung CA, et al. Comparison of virus shedding after lived attenuated and pentavalent reassortant rotavirus vaccine. *Vaccine.* 2014;32:1199-1204.
366. Jackson BR, Iqbal S, Mahon B, et al. Updated recommendations for the use of typhoid vaccine—Advisory Committee on Immunization Practices, United States, 2015. *MMWR Morb Mortal Wkly Rep.* 2015;64:305-308.
368. Jafri RZ, Ali A, Messonnier NE, et al. Global epidemiology of invasive meningococcal disease. *Popul Health Metr.* 2013;11:17.
372. Johnson CE, Kumar ML, Whitwell JK, et al. Antibody persistence after primary measles-mumps-rubella vaccine and response to a second dose given at four to six vs. eleven to thirteen years. *Pediatr Infect Dis J.* 1996;15:687-692.
376. Johnson MG, Bradley KK, Mendus S, et al. Vaccine-preventable disease among homeschooled children: two cases of tetanus in Oklahoma. *Pediatrics.* 2013;132:e1686-e1689.
377. Jokinen S, Osterlund P, Julkunen I, et al. Cellular immunity to mumps virus in young adults 21 years after measles-mumps-rubella vaccination. *J Infect Dis.* 2007;196:861-867.
378. Joura EA, Giuliano AR, Iversen OE, et al. A 9-valent HPV vaccine against infection and intraepithelial neoplasia in women. *N Engl J Med.* 2015;372:711-723.
379. Kahn JA, Widdice LE, Ding L, et al. Substantial decline in vaccine-type human papillomavirus (HPV) among vaccinated young women during the first 8 years after HPV vaccine introduction in a community. *Clin Infect Dis.* 2016;63:1281-1287.
388. Keyserling H, Papa T, Koranyi K, et al. Safety, immunogenicity, and immune memory of a novel meningococcal (groups A, C, Y, and W-135) polysaccharide diphtheria toxoid conjugate vaccine (MCV-4) in healthy adolescents. *Arch Pediatr Adolesc Med.* 2005;159:907-913.
389. Kim-Farley R, Bart S, Stetler H, et al. Clinical mumps vaccine efficacy. *Am J Epidemiol.* 1985;121:593-597.
391. Kimura A, Toneatto D, Kleinschmidt A, et al. Immunogenicity and safety of a multicomponent meningococcal serogroup B vaccine and a quadrivalent meningococcal CRM197 conjugate vaccine against serogroups A, C, W-135, and Y in adults who are at increased risk for occupational exposure to meningococcal isolates. *Clin Vaccine Immunol.* 2011;18:483-486.
393. Klein NP, Bartlett J, Fireman B, et al. Waning Tdap effectiveness in adolescents. *Pediatrics.* 2016;137:e20153326.
396. Klinge J, Lugauer S, Korn K, et al. Comparison of immunogenicity and reactogenicity of a measles, mumps and rubella (MMR) vaccine in German children vaccinated at 9-11, 12-14 or 15-17 months of age. *Vaccine.* 2000;18:3134-3140.
399. Kobayashi M, Bennett NM, Gierke R, et al. Intervals Between PCV13 and PPSV23 Vaccines: recommendations of the Advisory Committee on Immunization Practices (ACIP). *MMWR Morb Mortal Wkly Rep.* 2015;64:944-947.
404. Kremer JR, Schneider F, Muller CP. Waning antibodies in measles and rubella vaccinees—a longitudinal study. *Vaccine.* 2006;24:2594-2601.
406. Kristiansen PA, Jorgensen HJ, Caugant DA. Serogroup A meningococcal conjugate vaccines in Africa. *Expert Rev Vaccines.* 2015;14:1441-1458.
412. Kuehn BM. FDA: Benefits of rotavirus vaccination outweigh potential contamination risk. *JAMA.* 2010;304:30-31.
420. Le Bouvier GL, Plotkin SA. Precipitin responses to rubella vaccine RA 27-3. *J Infect Dis.* 1971;123:220-223.
422. LeBaron CW, Forghani B, Beck C, et al. Persistence of mumps antibodies after 2 doses of measles-mumps-rubella vaccine. *J Infect Dis.* 2009;199:552-560.
423. LeBaron CW, Forghani B, Matter L, et al. Persistence of rubella antibodies after 2 doses of measles-mumps-rubella vaccine. *J Infect Dis.* 2009;200:888-899.
424. Lee SH, Ewert DP, Frederick PD, et al. Resurgence of congenital rubella syndrome in the 1990s. Report on missed opportunities and failed prevention policies among women of childbearing age. *JAMA.* 1992;267:2616-2620.
427. Leshem E, Moritz RE, Curns AT, et al. Rotavirus vaccines and health care utilization for diarrhea in the United States (2007-2011. *Pediatrics.* 2014;134:15-23.
431. Lewis JE, Chernesky MA, Rawls ML, et al. Epidemic of mumps in a partially immune population. *Can Med Assoc J.* 1979;121:751-754.
434. Lin FY, Ho VA, Khiem HB, et al. The efficacy of a Salmonella typhi Vi conjugate vaccine in two-to-five-year-old children. *N Engl J Med.* 2001;344:1263-1269.
436. Loharikar A, Newton AE, Stroika S, et al. Cholera in the United States, 2001-2011: a reflection of patterns of global epidemiology and travel. *Epidemiol Infect.* 2015;143:695-703.
442. MacNeil JR, Bennett N, Farley MM, et al. Epidemiology of infant meningococcal disease in the United States, 2006-2012. *Pediatrics.* 2015;135:e305-e311.
443. Macneil JR, Cohn AC, Zell ER, et al. Early estimate of the effectiveness of quadrivalent meningococcal conjugate vaccine. *Pediatr Infect Dis J.* 2011;30:451-455.
444. MacNeil JR, Rubin L, Folaranmi T, et al. Use of serogroup B meningococcal vaccines in adolescents and young adults: recommendations of the Advisory Committee on Immunization Practices, 2015. *MMWR Morb Mortal Wkly Rep.* 2015;64:1171-1176.
445. MacNeil JR, Rubin LG, Patton M, et al. Recommendations for use of meningococcal conjugate vaccines in HIV-infected persons—Advisory Committee on Immunization Practices, 2016. *MMWR Morb Mortal Wkly Rep.* 2016;65:1189-1194.
446. Mahon BE, Newton AE, Mintz ED. Effectiveness of typhoid vaccination in US travelers. *Vaccine.* 2014;32:3577-3579.
452. Marin M, Quinlisk P, Shimabukuro T, et al. Mumps vaccination coverage and vaccine effectiveness in a large outbreak among college students—Iowa, 2006. *Vaccine.* 2008;26:3601-3607.
453. Marin M, Willis ED, Marko A, et al. Closure of varicella-zoster virus-containing vaccines pregnancy registry—United States, 2013. *MMWR Morb Mortal Wkly Rep.* 2014;63:732-733.
456. Markowitz LE, Dunne EF, Saraiya M, et al. Human papillomavirus vaccination: recommendations of the Advisory Committee on Immunization Practices (ACIP). *MMWR Recomm Rep.* 2014;63(RR-05):1-30.
458. Markowitz LE, Preblud SR, Fine PE, et al. Duration of live measles vaccine-induced immunity. *Pediatr Infect Dis J.* 1990;9:101-110.
460. Marshall GS, Marchant CD, Blatter M, et al. Co-administration of a novel Haemophilus influenzae type b and *Neisseria meningitidis* serogroups C and Y-tetanus toxoid conjugate vaccine does not interfere with the immune response to antigens contained in infant vaccines routinely used in the United States. *Hum Vaccin.* 2011;7:258-264.
461. Marshall HS, Richmond PC, Nissen MD, et al. A phase 2 open-label safety and immunogenicity study of a meningococcal B bivalent rLP2086 vaccine in healthy adults. *Vaccine.* 2013;31:1569-1575.
463. Martinon-Torres F, Czajka H, Center KJ, et al. 13-valent pneumococcal conjugate vaccine (PCV13) in preterm versus term infants. *Pediatrics.* 2015;135:e876-e886.
467. Mazurek GH, Jereb J, Vernon A, et al. Updated guidelines for using interferon gamma release assays to detect *Mycobacterium tuberculosis* infection—United States, 2010. *MMWR Recomm Rep.* 2010;59(RR-5):1-25.
469. McClenahan SD, Krause PR, Uhlenhaut C. Molecular and infectivity studies of porcine circovirus in vaccines. *Vaccine.* 2011;29:4745-4753.
471. McLean HQ, Fiebelkorn AP, Temte JL, et al. Prevention of measles, rubella, congenital rubella syndrome, and mumps, 2013: summary recommendations of the Advisory Committee on Immunization Practices (ACIP). *MMWR Recomm Rep.* 2013;62(RR-04):1-34.
474. Meites E, Kempe A, Markowitz LE. Use of a 2-dose schedule for human papillomavirus vaccination—updated recommendations of the Advisory Committee on Immunization Practices. *MMWR Morb Mortal Wkly Rep.* 2016;65:1405-1408.
475. Mellinger AK, Cragan JD, Atkinson WL, et al. High incidence of congenital rubella syndrome after a rubella outbreak. *Pediatr Infect Dis J.* 1995;14:573-578.
485. Monroe BP, Yager P, Blanton J, et al. Rabies surveillance in the United States during 2014. *J Am Vet Med Assoc.* 2016;248:777-788.

487. Moore MR, Link-Gelles R, Schaffner W, et al. Effect of use of 13-valent pneumococcal conjugate vaccine in children on invasive pneumococcal disease in children and adults in the USA: analysis of multisite, population-based surveillance. *Lancet Infect Dis.* 2015;15:301-309.
488. Morgan JL, Baggari SR, McIntire DD, et al. Pregnancy outcomes after antepartum tetanus, diphtheria, and acellular pertussis vaccination. *Obstet Gynecol.* 2015;125:1433-1438.
489. Moro PL, Cragan J, Tepper N, et al. Enhanced surveillance of tetanus toxoid, reduced diphtheria toxoid, and acellular pertussis (Tdap) vaccines in pregnancy in the Vaccine Adverse Event Reporting System (VAERS), 2011-2015. *Vaccine.* 2016;34:2349-2353.
490. Mortimer EA Jr. Pertussis and pertussis vaccine. In: Aronoff SC, ed. *Advances in Pediatric Infectious Diseases.* Vol. 5. Chicago: Year Book Medical Publisher; 1990:1-27.
493. Murphy TV, Denniston MM, Hill HA, et al. Progress toward eliminating hepatitis A disease in the United States. *MMWR Suppl.* 2016;65:29-41.
495. Murphy TV. *Haemophilus influenzae* vaccines: 1997. *Adv Pediatr Infect Dis.* 1997;13:279-304.
497. National Institute of Allergy and Infectious Diseases. *The Jordan Report—Accelerated Development of Vaccines, 2012.* Washington, DC: National Institutes of Health; 2012.
500. Nelson GE, Aguon A, Valencia E, et al. Epidemiology of a mumps outbreak in a highly vaccinated island population and use of a third dose of measles-mumps-rubella vaccine for outbreak control—Guam 2009 to 2010. *Pediatr Infect Dis J.* 2013;32:374-380.
503. Newton A, Routh J, Barbara E, Mahon B. Typhoid and paratyphoid fever. In: Brunette G, ed. *CDC Health Information for International Travel, 2016.* New York: Oxford University Press; 2016.
507. Nolan T, Richmond P, Marshall H, et al. Immunogenicity and safety of an investigational combined *Haemophilus influenzae* type B-*Neisseria meningitidis* serogroups C and Y-tetanus toxoid conjugate vaccine. *Pediatr Infect Dis J.* 2011;30:190-196.
508. Noronha AS, Markowitz LE, Dunne EF. Systematic review of human papillomavirus vaccine coadministration. *Vaccine.* 2014;32:2670-2674.
512. Onorato I, Markowitz L, Oxtoby M. Childhood immunization, vaccine-preventable diseases and infection with human immunodeficiency virus. *Pediatr Infect Dis J.* 1988;6:588-595.
516. Organization WH Global Polio Eradication Initiative. http://polioeradication.org/.
520. Papania MJ, Wallace GS, Rota PA, et al. Elimination of endemic measles, rubella, and congenital rubella syndrome from the Western hemisphere: the US experience. *JAMA Pediatr.* 2014;168:148-155.
521. Parashar UD, Gibson CJ, Bresse JS, et al. Rotavirus and severe childhood diarrhea. *Emerg Infect Dis.* 2006;12:304-306.
527. Payne AB, Link-Gelles R, Azonobi I, et al. Invasive pneumococcal disease among children with and without sickle cell disease in the United States, 1998 to 2009. *Pediatr Infect Dis J.* 2013;32:1308-1312.
528. Payne DC, Edwards KM, Bowen MD, et al. Sibling transmission of vaccine-derived rotavirus (RotaTeq) associated with rotavirus gastroenteritis. *Pediatrics.* 2010;125:e438-e441.
532. Peter G. Vaccine crisis: an emerging societal problem. *J Infect Dis.* 1985;151:981-983.
533. Petrosky E, Bocchini JA Jr, Hariri S, et al. Use of 9-valent human papillomavirus (HPV) vaccine: updated HPV vaccination recommendations of the advisory committee on immunization practices. *MMWR Morb Mortal Wkly Rep.* 2015;64:300-304.
534. Phadke VK, Bednarczyk RA, Salmon DA, et al. Association between vaccine refusal and vaccine-preventable diseases in the United States: a review of measles and pertussis. *JAMA.* 2016;315:1149-1158.
540. Plotkin SA, Buser F. History of RA27/3 rubella vaccine. *Rev Infect Dis.* 1985;7(suppl 1):S77-S78.
541. Plotkin SA. Increasing Complexity of Vaccine Development. *J Infect Dis.* 2015;212(suppl 1):S12-S16.
544. Popow-Kraupp T, Kundi M, Ambrosch F, et al. A controlled trial for evaluating two live attenuated mumps-measles vaccines (Urabe Am 9-Schwarz and Jeryl Lynn-Moraten) in young children. *J Med Virol.* 1986;18:69-79.
545. Preblud SR. Some current issues relating to rubella vaccine. *JAMA.* 1985;254:253-256.
546. Read RC, Baxter D, Chadwick DR, et al. Effect of a quadrivalent meningococcal ACWY glycoconjugate or a serogroup B meningococcal vaccine on meningococcal carriage: an observer-blind, phase 3 randomised clinical trial. *Lancet.* 2014;384:2123-2131.
547. Read TR, Hocking JS, Chen MY, et al. The near disappearance of genital warts in young women 4 years after commencing a national human papillomavirus (HPV) vaccination programme. *Sex Transm Infect.* 2011;87:544-547.
548. Redd SC, King GE, Heath JL, et al. Comparison of vaccination with measles-mumps-rubella vaccine at 9, 12, and 15 months of age. *J Infect Dis.* 2004;189(suppl 1):S116-S122.
549. Reef SE, Cochi SL. The evidence for the elimination of rubella and congenital rubella syndrome in the United States: a public health achievement. *Clin Infect Dis.* 2006;43(suppl 3):S123-S125.
550. Reef SE, Redd SB, Abernathy E, et al. Evidence used to support the achievement and maintenance of elimination of rubella and congenital rubella syndrome in the United States. *J Infect Dis.* 2011;204(suppl 2):S593-S597.
556. Richmond PC, Marshall HS, Nissen MD, et al. Safety, immunogenicity, and tolerability of meningococcal serogroup B bivalent recombinant lipoprotein 2086 vaccine in healthy adolescents: a randomised, single-blind, placebo-controlled, phase 2 trial. *Lancet Infect Dis.* 2012;12:597-607.
559. Rivera L, Pena LM, Stainier I, et al. Horizontal transmission of a human rotavirus vaccine strain—a randomized, placebo-controlled study in twins. *Vaccine.* 2011;29:9508-9513.
560. Robinson CL, Advisory Committee on Immunization Practices ACAIWG. Advisory Committee on Immunization Practices recommended immunization schedules for persons aged 0 through 18 years—United States, 2016. *MMWR Morb Mortal Wkly Rep.* 2016;65:86-87.
566. Routh J, Newton A, Mintz E. Cholera. In: Brunette G, ed. *CDC Health Information for International Travel, 2016.* New York: Oxford University Press; 2016.
568. Rubin LG, Levin MJ, Ljungman P, et al. 2013 IDSA clinical practice guideline for vaccination of the immunocompromised host. *Clin Infect Dis.* 2014;58:309-318.
571. Safadi MA, Cintra OA. Epidemiology of meningococcal disease in Latin America: current situation and opportunities for prevention. *Neurol Res.* 2010;32:263-271.
575. Santolaya ME, O'Ryan M, Valenzuela MT, et al. Persistence of antibodies in adolescents 18-24 months after immunization with one, two, or three doses of 4CMenB meningococcal serogroup B vaccine. *Hum Vaccin Immunother.* 2013;9:2304-2310.
576. Santolaya ME, O'Ryan ML, Valenzuela MT, et al. Immunogenicity and tolerability of a multicomponent meningococcal serogroup B (4CMenB) vaccine in healthy adolescents in Chile: a phase 2b/3 randomised, observer-blind, placebo-controlled study. *Lancet.* 2012;379:617-624.
578. Sartorius B, Penttinen P, Nilsson J, et al. An outbreak of mumps in Sweden, February-April 2004. *Euro Surveill.* 2005;10:191-193.
579. Satterwhite CL, Torrone E, Meites E, et al. Sexually transmitted infections among US women and men: prevalence and incidence estimates, 2008. *Sex Transm Dis.* 2013;40:187-193.
581. Schaffzin JK, Pollock L, Schulte C, et al. Effectiveness of previous mumps vaccination during a summer camp outbreak. *Pediatrics.* 2007;120:e862-e868.
582. Schillie S, Murphy TV, Fenlon N, et al. Update: shortened interval for postvaccination serologic testing of infants born to hepatitis B-infected mothers. *MMWR Morb Mortal Wkly Rep.* 2015;64:1118-1120.
583. Schillie S, Walker T, Veselsky S, et al. Outcomes of infants born to women infected with hepatitis B. *Pediatrics.* 2015;135:e1141-e1147.
584. Schlegel M, Osterwalder JJ, Galeazzi RL, et al. Comparative efficacy of three mumps vaccines during disease outbreak in Eastern Switzerland: cohort study. *BMJ.* 1999;319:352.
588. Schwarz AJ, Jackson JE, Ehrenkranz NJ, et al. Clinical evaluation of a new measles-mumps-rubella trivalent vaccine. *Am J Dis Child.* 1975;129:1408-1412.
591. Senders S, Bhuyan P, Jiang Q, et al. Immunogenicity, tolerability and safety in adolescents of bivalent rLP2086, a meningococcal serogroup B vaccine, coadministered with quadrivalent human papilloma virus vaccine. *Pediatr Infect Dis J.* 2016;35:548-554.
597. Sheldon EA, Schwartz H, Jiang Q, et al. A phase 1, randomized, open-label, active-controlled trial to assess the safety of a meningococcal serogroup B bivalent rLP2086 vaccine in healthy adults. *Hum Vaccin Immunother.* 2012;8:888-895.
601. Shui IM, Baggs J, Patel M, et al. Risk of intussusception following administration of a pentavalent rotavirus vaccine in US infants. *JAMA.* 2012;307:598-604.
607. Singh R, John TJ, Cherian T, et al. Immune response to measles, mumps & rubella vaccine at 9, 12 & 15 months of age. *Indian J Med Res.* 1994;100:155-159.
608. Singleton R, Hammitt L, Hennessy T, et al. The Alaska *Haemophilus influenzae* type b experience: lessons in controlling a vaccine-preventable disease. *Pediatrics.* 2006;118:e421-e429.
610. Smith CK, McNeal MM, Meyer NR, et al. Rotavirus shedding in premature infants following first immunization. *Vaccine.* 2011;29:8141-8146.
611. Smith PJ, Marcuse EK, Seward JF, et al. Children and adolescents unvaccinated against measles: geographic clustering, parents' beliefs, and missed opportunities. *Public Health Rep.* 2015;130:485-504.
612. Snijders BE, van Lier A, van de Kassteele J, et al. Mumps vaccine effectiveness in primary schools and households, the Netherlands, 2008. *Vaccine.* 2012;30:2999-3002.
614. Sotir MJ, Esposito DH, Barnett ED, et al. Measles in the 21st century, a continuing preventable risk to travelers: data from the GeoSentinel Global Network. *Clin Infect Dis.* 2016;62:210-212.
617. Staples JE, Bocchini JA Jr, Rubin L, et al. Yellow fever vaccine booster doses: recommendations of the Advisory Committee on Immunization Practices, 2015. *MMWR Morb Mortal Wkly Rep.* 2015;64:647-650.
620. Stokley S, Jeyarajah J, Yankey D, et al. Human papillomavirus vaccination coverage among adolescents, 2007-2013, and postlicensure vaccine safety monitoring, 2006-2014—United States. *MMWR Morb Mortal Wkly Rep.* 2014;63:620-624.
622. Stratton KR, Howe CJ, Johnston RB Jr. Adverse events associated with childhood vaccines other than pertussis and rubella. Summary of a report from the Institute of Medicine. *JAMA.* 1994;271:1602-1605.

624. Sugg WC, Finger JA, Levine RH, et al. Field evaluation of live virus mumps vaccine. *J Pediatr*. 1968;72:461-466.
625. Sukumaran L, McCarthy NL, Kharbanda EO, et al. Association of Tdap vaccination with acute events and adverse birth outcomes among pregnant women with prior tetanus-containing immunizations. *JAMA*. 2015;314:1581-1587.
627. Sun Y, Christensen J, Hviid A, et al. Risk of febrile seizures and epilepsy after vaccination with diphtheria, tetanus, acellular pertussis, inactivated poliovirus, and *Haemophilus influenzae* type B. *JAMA*. 2012;307:823-831.
632. Tate JE, Mutuc JD, Panozzo CA, et al. Sustained decline in rotavirus detections in the United States following the introduction of rotavirus vaccine in 2006. *Pediatr Infect Dis J*. 2011;30(suppl):S30-S34.
639. Tischer A, Gerike E. Immune response after primary and re-vaccination with different combined vaccines against measles, mumps, rubella. *Vaccine*. 2000;18:1382-1392.
640. Toneatto D, Ismaili S, Ypma E, et al. The first use of an investigational multi-component meningococcal serogroup B vaccine (4CMenB) in humans. *Hum Vaccin*. 2011;7:646-653.
641. Toscani L, Batou M, Bouvier P, et al. Comparison of the efficacy of various strains of mumps vaccine: a school survey. *Soz Praventivmed*. 1996;41:341-347.
647. Usonis V, Bakasenas V, Chitour K, et al. Comparative study of reactogenicity and immunogenicity of new and established measles, mumps and rubella vaccines in healthy children. *Infection*. 1998;26:222-226.
648. Usonis V, Bakasenas V, Kaufhold A, et al. Reactogenicity and immunogenicity of a new live attenuated combined measles, mumps and rubella vaccine in healthy children. *Pediatr Infect Dis J*. 1999;18:42-48.
653. Vandermeulen C, Clement F, Roelants M, et al. Evaluation of cellular immunity to mumps in vaccinated individuals with or without circulating antibodies up to 16 years after their last vaccination. *J Infect Dis*. 2009;199:1457-1460.
665. Vu DM, Welsch JA, Zuno-Mitchell P, et al. Antibody persistence 3 years after immunization of adolescents with quadrivalent meningococcal conjugate vaccine. *J Infect Dis*. 2006;193:821-828.
668. Walter EB, Neuzil KM, Zhu Y, et al. Influenza vaccine immunogenicity in 6- to 23-month-old children: are identical antigens necessary for priming? *Pediatrics*. 2006;118:e570-e578.
669. Ward B, Boulinanne N, Ratnam S, et al. Cellular immunity in measles vaccine failure: demonstration of measles antigen-specific lymphoproliferative responses despite limited serum antibody production after revaccination. *J Infect Dis*. 1995;172:1591-1595.
670. Wassilak SG, Oberste MS, Tangermann RH, et al. Progress toward global interruption of wild poliovirus transmission, 2010-2013, and tackling the challenges to complete eradication. *J Infect Dis*. 2014;210(suppl 1):S5-S15.
676. Weibel RE, Villarejos VM, Klein EB, et al. Clinical and laboratory studies of live attenuated RA 27/3 and HPV 77-DE rubella virus vaccines. *Proc Soc Exp Biol Med*. 1980;165:44-49.
678. Weinberg MS. Vaccine recommendations for infants and children. In: Brunette G, ed. *CDC Health Information for International Travel, 2016*. New York: Oxford University Press; 2016:490-521.
679. Weintraub ES, Baggs J, Duffy J, et al. Risk of Intussusception after monovalent rotavirus vaccination. *N Engl J Med*. 2014;370:513-519.
684. Wharton M, Cochi SL, Hutcheson RH, et al. A large outbreak of mumps in the postvaccine era. *J Infect Dis*. 1988;158:1253-1260.
687. Giersing BK, Modjarrad K, Kaslow DC, Moorthy VS. Report from the World Health Organization's Product Development for Vaccines Advisory Committee (PDVAC) meeting, Geneva, September 7-9, 2015. WHO Product Development for Vaccines Advisory Committee; WHO Product Development for Vaccines Product Development Advisory Committee. *Vaccine*. 2016;34:2865-2869.
688. Widdowson MA, Meltzer MI, Zhang X, et al. Cost-effectiveness and potential impact of rotavirus vaccination in the United States. *Pediatrics*. 2007;119:684-697.
689. Willis E, Marko A, Marin M, et al. 1048Pregnancy registry for varicella-zoster virus-containing vaccines: 18-year summary of pregnancy outcomes. *Open Forum Infect Dis*. 2014;1(suppl 1):S307.
691. Winter K, Glaser C, Watt J, et al. Pertussis epidemic—California, 2014. *MMWR Morb Mortal Wkly Rep*. 2014;63:1129-1132.
694. Witte JJ, Karchmer AW, Case G, et al. Epidemiology of rubella. *Am J Dis Child*. 1969;118:107-111.
696. World Health Organization. Global Advisory Committee on Vaccine Safety, report of meeting held 3-4 December 2009. *Wkly Epidemiol Rec*. 2010;85:29-33.
697. World Health Organization. *Haemophilus influenzae* type b (Hib) vaccination position paper—July 2013. *Wkly Epidemiol Rec*. 2013;88:413-426.
698. World Health Organization. Japanese encephalitis vaccines: WHO position paper—February 2015. *Wkly Epidemiol Rec*. 2015;90:69-87.
699. World Health Organization. Polio vaccines: WHO position paper—March, 2016. *Wkly Epidemiol Rec*. 2016;91:145-168.
701. World Health Organization. WHO position on measles vaccines. *Vaccine*. 2009;27:7219-7221.
702. Wright JG, Quinn CP, Shadomy S, et al. Use of anthrax vaccine in the United States: recommendations of the Advisory Committee on Immunization Practices (ACIP), 2009. *MMWR Recomm Rep*. 2010;59(RR-6):1-30.
705. Xie O, Pollard AJ, Mueller JE, et al. Emergence of serogroup X meningococcal disease in Africa: need for a vaccine. *Vaccine*. 2013;31:2852-2861.
706. Yang YT, Debold V. A longitudinal analysis of the effect of nonmedical exemption law and vaccine uptake on vaccine-targeted disease rates. *Am J Public Health*. 2014;104:371-377.
708. Yih WK, Lieu TA, Kulldorff M, et al. Intussusception risk after rotavirus vaccination in U.S. Infants. *N Engl J Med*. 2014;370:503-512.
709. Yun K, Urban K, Mamo B, et al. Increasing hepatitis B vaccine prevalence among refugee children arriving in the United States, 2006-2012. *Am J Public Health*. 2016;106:1460-1462.
716. Zimmerman RK, Nowalk MP, Chung J, et al. 2014-2015 Influenza vaccine effectiveness in the United States by vaccine type. *Clin Infect Dis*. 2016;63:1564-1573.

The full reference list for this chapter is available at ExpertConsult.com.

Passive Immunization 246

Danica J. Schulte

PRINCIPLES OF PASSIVE IMMUNITY

Definition

Passive immunization is the administration of antibodies to provide immediate protection against a microbial agent, or toxin. Passive immunization is used to provide temporary immunity in an unimmunized person exposed to an infectious disease when active immunization is unavailable (e.g., respiratory syncytial virus [RSV] infection), is contraindicated (e.g., varicella in an immunocompromised child), or has not been given before exposure (e.g., tetanus, rabies).

Passive immunization also is used in the management of certain disorders associated with toxins (e.g., diphtheria), for certain bites (e.g., snake, spider), in drug overdose (e.g., digoxin), as a specific (e.g., Rh0[D] immunoglobulin) or nonspecific (e.g., antithymocyte globulin) immunosuppressant, and in the treatment of certain infectious diseases.

The following four types of preparations are used in passive immunization (Table 246.1):

1. Standard human immune serum globulin (HISG) for general use, which is available as immunoglobulin for intramuscular use (IGIM), intravenous use (IGIV), and subcutaneous use (IGSC)
2. Special high-titer immunoglobulins with a known antibody content for specific illnesses
3. Animal sera and antitoxins
4. Monoclonal antibodies (Table 246.2)

Most of the licensed special immunoglobulins are for intramuscular use only. Plasma, serum, and breast milk also can be used in passive immunization.

Passive immunization is not always effective. The duration is short, varying between 1 and 6 weeks. Undesirable reactions can occur, especially if the antibody is of nonhuman origin. High-titer special

TABLE 246.1 **Antibody Preparations Available for Passive Immunity in the United States**

Product	Abbreviations and Brand Names	Principal Use
Standard Human Immune Serum Globulins for Intramuscular or Subcutaneous Use		
Immunoglobulin, intravenous	IGIV, IVIG	Treatment of antibody deficiency, immune thrombocytopenic purpura, Kawasaki disease, other immunoregulatory and inflammatory diseases
Immunoglobulin, intramuscular	IGIM, IG, ISG	Treatment of antibody deficiency; prevention of measles, hepatitis A
Immunoglobulin, subcutaneous	IGSC	Treatment of antibody deficiency
Special Human Immune Globulins for Intramuscular or Subcutaneous Use		
Hepatitis B immunoglobulin	HBIG, HyperHEP B, Nabi-HB, HepaGamB	Prevention of hepatitis B
Varicella-zoster immunoglobulin	VariZIG	Prevention or modification of chickenpox
Rabies immunoglobulin	RIG	Prevention of rabies
Tetanus immunoglobulin	TIG	Prevention or treatment of tetanus
Vaccinia immunoglobulin	VIG, VIGIM	Prevention or treatment of vaccinia, prevention of smallpox
Rh0(D) immunoglobulin	RhoGAM, MICRhoGAM, HyperRHO S/D, BayRho-D	Prevention of Rh hemolytic disease
Special Human Immunoglobulins for Intravenous Use		
Cytomegalovirus immunoglobulin	CMV-IGIV, CMVIG, CytoGam	Prevention or treatment of cytomegalovirus infection
Hepatitis B immunoglobulin, intravenous	HBIGIV, HepaGam B, Nabi-HB NovaPlus	Prevention of hepatitis B (including liver transplantation)
Vaccinia immunoglobulin, intravenous	VIGIV	Prevention or treatment of vaccinia, prevention of smallpox
Rh0(D) immunoglobulin, intravenous	WinRho SDF, Rhophylac	Treatment of immune thrombocytopenic purpura
Botulinum immunoglobulin	BIG, BabyBIG	Treatment of newborn botulism
Animal Sera and Globulins		
Tetanus antitoxin (equine)	TAT	Prevention or treatment of tetanus (when TIG is unavailable)
Diphtheria antitoxin (equine)	DAT	Treatment of diphtheria
Botulinum antitoxins (equine)	BAT	Treatment of botulism
Latrodectus mactans antivenin (equine)	Antivenin	Treatment of black widow spider bites
Crotalidae polyvalent antivenin (equine)	—	Treatment of most snake bites
Crotalidae polyvalent immune Fab (ovine)	—	Treatment of most snake bites
Micrurus fulvius antivenin (equine)	—	Treatment of coral snake bites

immunoglobulins and IGIVs are identical to regular immunoglobulins and IGIVs, except that they are derived from patients hyperimmunized or convalescing from a specific infection or selected from donors with high titers in response to a specific antigen. They are useful in several disorders in which regular immunoglobulin and IGIV are of little or no value.

Animal Sera and Antitoxins

Animal sera and antitoxins are derived from the serum of immunized animals, usually horses (i.e., equine formulations). Because these sera are foreign proteins, they carry a significant risk for sensitization. They should be administered only when specifically indicated, after sensitivity tests, and by a physician prepared to deal with a hypersensitivity reaction.

A careful medical history must be obtained before an animal serum is injected. Patients must be asked about asthma, hay fever, urticaria, and previous injections of animal serum. Patients with a history of asthma, allergic rhinitis, or other allergic symptoms on exposure to horses may be dangerously sensitive to the corresponding serum, and the serum should be given only with the utmost caution.

Sensitivity Tests for Animal Serum

A skin prick test, followed by an intradermal skin test, always should be performed before injection of an animal serum, regardless of whether the patient has had the serum previously.[23] A skin prick test is performed by applying a drop of a 1:100 dilution of the serum in saline to the site of a superficial scratch, prick, or puncture on the volar aspect of the forearm and observing it for 20 minutes. A positive control (i.e., 0.1% histamine phosphate) and negative control (i.e., saline) should also be applied. A positive reaction consists of erythema with wheal formation 3 mm greater than the negative control. However, previous use of antihistamines may render results of these tests negative.

If the skin prick test result is negative, an intradermal test is performed by injecting 0.02 mL of a 1:1000 saline dilution; positive (i.e., 0.1% histamine phosphate) and negative control tests should be performed. The reaction is read 10 to 30 minutes after the injection and is positive if a wheal appears that is 3 mm greater than the negative control. If the test result is negative, it should be repeated with 0.02 mL of a 1:100 dilution. For people with a negative history of animal allergy and no previous exposure to animal sera, the 1:100 dilution may be used initially if the skin prick test result is negative.

Although intradermal skin tests have resulted in fatalities, skin prick tests have not, but they can still be associated with immediate reactions. A skin test never should be performed or serum injected unless a syringe containing 1 mL of 1:1000 epinephrine is within immediate reach and supportive care is available.

Skin tests can indicate the probability of sensitivity. However, a negative skin test result does not guarantee the absence of sensitivity. A specific history of allergy or a positive skin test reaction with horse serum is sufficient reason for special caution. A positive history of sensitivity to horse dander is an indication of the need for extreme caution.

Administration of Animal Serum

If the history and sensitivity test reactions are negative, the indicated dose of serum may be given intramuscularly, with epinephrine at hand.[23] The patient should be watched closely for an hour for adverse reactions.

Intravenous injection may be indicated if a high concentration of circulating antibody is required rapidly, as in botulism or diphtheria. The manufacturer's instructions should be consulted.

If the skin test reaction is positive or there is a history of allergy to animal serum but the need for the serum is unquestioned (and epinephrine is at hand), a procedure commonly referred to as desensitization can be undertaken, although any significant desensitization is unlikely to occur. This procedure establishes temporary tolerance to the serum. Desensitization should be performed by trained personnel with the necessary emergency equipment and drugs immediately available.

TABLE 246.2 US-Adopted Nomenclature for Monoclonal Antibodies

The suffix *–mab* or *–nab* is used for all monoclonal antibodies and fragments. Letters preceding the suffix identify the product source.[a]

Letter	Source
u	Human
e	Hamster
o	Mouse
i	Primate
a	Rat
xi	Chimeric
zu	Humanized

The disease state targeted by the monoclonal antibody is specified by a syllable preceding one of the letters above.[b]

Syllable	Target Disease or System
–vir	Viral disease
–bac	Bacterial disease
–lim	Immune system
–les	Infectious lesions
–circ	Cardiovascular system
Syllable	**Tumors**
–col	Colon
–mel	Melanoma
–mar	Mammary
–got	Testis
–gov	Ovary
–pr(o)	Prostate
–tum	Miscellaneous

[a]Examples are *o* for mouse, as in muromonab, and *u* for human, as in adalimumab.
[b]Combinations of target and source designations result in endings such as *–limumab* (i.e., immune system, human) and *–ciximab* (i.e., circulatory system, chimeric, with the consonant *r* dropped).

Desensitization consists of periodic (i.e., 15-minute intervals) injections or infusions of progressively larger doses of the serum, starting at a very low dose, until tolerance is achieved. Schedules for intravenous and intradermal, subcutaneous, or intramuscular desensitization are given in the *2015 Red Book.*[23] Administration of sera after desensitization has been achieved must be continuous or protection from desensitization is lost rapidly.

Hypersensitivity Reactions to Animal Serum

Hypersensitivity reactions to animal serum are of four general types:

1. Anaphylactic reactions consisting of urticaria or other rashes; respiratory distress with wheezing, dyspnea, cough, hoarseness, or stridor; cardiovascular reactions, including tachycardia, hypotension, arrhythmia, cyanosis, shock, and unconsciousness; and gastrointestinal reactions, such as cramps, diarrhea, and vomiting, all occurring seconds to minutes after an injection has been administered
2. Acute febrile reactions consisting of moderate or severe hyperpyrexia within 2 hours after an injection has been given
3. Serum sickness reactions consisting of urticaria, arthritis, adenopathy, and fever occurring hours to days after an injection has been administered, depending on the dose and the presence or degree of previous sensitization (i.e., serum sickness occurs within hours or a few days after the second injection and within 7 to 12 days after the first injection)
4. Various delayed reactions, including peripheral neuritis, nephritis, Guillain-Barré syndrome, and myocarditis

Treatment of Hypersensitivity Reactions to Animal Serum

For anaphylactic reactions, 1 : 1000 epinephrine at a dose of 0.01 mL/kg (maximum dose, 0.5 mL) is given subcutaneously or intramuscularly immediately. If improvement is not achieved immediately, 1 : 10,000 epinephrine at a dose of 0.01 mL/kg is given intravenously. This dose can be repeated every 10 minutes for up to three doses. The 1-mL 1 : 1000 epinephrine vials must be diluted 1 : 10 in physiologic saline (i.e., 1 : 10,000) and injected slowly at a dose of 0.01 mL/kg; a 1 : 10,000 dilution in a 10-mL vial also is available.

Administration of epinephrine may be repeated in 5 to 15 minutes if the response is not satisfactory. Vasopressors and positive-pressure oxygen are helpful. For severe urticaria or edema, particularly edema of the larynx, intramuscular injection of antihistamines and corticosteroids is indicated. Administration of serum therapy (if necessary) should be resumed 6 to 8 hours later or after all visible signs of reaction have subsided.

Mild febrile reactions (temperatures <39°C [<102.8°F]) are treated with ibuprofen or acetaminophen. Severe febrile reactions can cause seizures and death and should be treated rigorously with sponge baths or other cooling means to reduce the temperature promptly. Serum sickness and serum neuritis usually are treated with corticosteroids.

Human Immune Serum Globulin

HISG, or gamma globulin, is available in three forms for general use: IGIM, IGIV, and IGSC. IGIM is used primarily for the prevention of certain infectious disorders and less commonly for the treatment of antibody immunodeficiencies. IGIV is used in the treatment of primary and secondary antibody deficiencies, many immunoregulatory disorders (e.g., immune thrombocytopenic purpura, Kawasaki disease), and neurologic disorders (e.g., Guillain-Barré syndrome, peripheral neuritis). IGSC is used exclusively for the treatment of antibody deficiency.

Intramuscular Immunoglobulin

Pharmacology. IGIM is prepared from pooled human serum by the Cohn alcohol fractionation procedure, thereby deriving its alternative name of Cohn fraction II. This procedure and viral inactivation steps remove most other serum proteins, hepatitis viruses, and human immunodeficiency viruses (i.e., HIV-1 and HIV-2), thereby providing a safe product for intramuscular injection. It is reconstituted as a sterile, approximately 16% solution (160 mg/mL) with or without preservative. It contains a wide spectrum of antibodies to viral and bacterial antigens.

IGIM is greater than 95% immunoglobulin G (IgG), but trace quantities of IgM and IgA and other serum proteins are present. IgM and IgA are therapeutically insignificant because of their rapid half-lives (about 7 days) and low immunoglobulin concentrations. Immunoglobulin contains all IgG allotypes (i.e., GM and KM allotypes, which are antigenic determinants on γ and κ light chains, respectively).

IGIM is approved only for intramuscular or subcutaneous use, and intravenous injection of IGIM usually is contraindicated. IGIM aggregates in vitro to high-molecular-weight complexes (i.e., 9.5S to 40S) that are strongly anticomplementary. These aggregates probably are responsible for the occasional systemic reactions to IGIM. The incidence of these reactions is increased if the patient has received IGIM previously or if it is inadvertently given intravenously. Agammaglobulinemic boys with affected male relatives (suggesting X-linked inheritance) may have a lower incidence of reactions.[471] Small intradermal injections of IGIM are not of value except as a placebo, and they are contraindicated.

Intramuscular immunoglobulin in antibody immunodeficiency. IGIM is used infrequently for IgG replacement therapy in immunodeficiency. The usual dosage is 100 mg/kg per month, about equivalent to 0.7 mL/kg per month of the 16% (160 mg/mL) product. Two or three such injections are given at the onset of therapy as a loading dose, often over a 3- to 5-day period. The maximal maintenance dosage should not exceed 20 or 30 mL/wk.

Few studies on optimal dosage are available. However, the Medical Research Council Working Party[471] found that 25 mg/kg per week (100 mg/kg per month) was therapeutically equivalent to 50 mg/kg per week but that 10 mg/kg per week was inadequate. Use of IGIM by this route has been supplanted largely by IGIV administration.

IGIM should be given at multiple sites to avoid giving more than 5 mL at any one site (i.e., 10 mL in a large adult). The buttocks are the preferred site, but the anterior of the thighs also can be used. Tenderness, sterile abscesses, fibrosis, and sciatic nerve injury may result from these injections. The danger of sciatic nerve injury is especially great in a small malnourished infant with inadequate muscle and fat in the gluteal regions. Large doses of IGIM should not be given to patients with severe thrombocytopenia because of the risk for development of hematoma and infection.

The injections are given initially at monthly intervals. If the patient continues to have infection or if a characteristic symptom (e.g., cough, conjunctivitis, diarrhea, arthralgia, purulent nasal discharge) recurs at the end of the injection period, the interval between doses is decreased to 3 or 2 weeks. Because IgG catabolism increases during acute infections, extra injections of IGIM often are given.

Because high serum levels of IgG cannot be maintained, serial immunoglobulin assays are unnecessary in assessing the effectiveness of treatment. The maximal increase in serum IgG level after a standard IGIM injection varies from patient to patient and from dose to dose because of different rates of absorption, local proteolysis at the injection site, and distribution within tissues.

An intramuscular injection of 100 mg/kg of IGIM usually raises the IgG serum level by 100 mg/dL after 2 to 4 days.[669] A recent IGIM injection usually does not obscure the diagnosis of hypogammaglobulinemia.

Intramuscular immunoglobulin and special intramuscular immunoglobulins for prevention of infectious diseases. IGIM is recommended for prophylaxis of hepatitis A and measles. The recommended doses are found in the sections on these disorders. Special high-titer IGIMs are available for several disorders, such as hepatitis B and varicella. These products are identical to IGIM except for the high titers of specific antibodies. These products also are discussed in the sections on these disorders.

Adverse effects of intramuscular immunoglobulin. Rare anaphylactic reactions to intramuscular injections of immunoglobulin have been reported, particularly in patients requiring repeated injections.[208] The Medical Research Council Working Party[471] observed these reactions in 33 (19%) of 175 patients treated during a 10-year period. After approximately 40,000 injections, 85 reactions occurred; in eight patients, the injections were stopped as a result of these adverse effects, and one death was recorded. The reactions occurred at any stage of treatment and were unrelated to any particular lot number of IGIM or its anticomplementary activity. Symptoms include anxiety, nausea, vomiting, malaise, flushing, facial swelling, cyanosis, and loss of consciousness. Immediate treatment with epinephrine and antihistamines is indicated.

People who experience these reactions should be evaluated before receiving a repeat injection. Skin testing should be performed with several lots of IGIM.[208] A skin test result that is positive for an old but not a new lot of immunoglobulin may indicate a particular idiosyncratic reaction to a particular lot. Under these circumstances, incremental doses of immunoglobulin from a new lot are recommended. In other patients, IgE antibodies to IgG develop and result in positive, immediate skin test reactions to all IGIM lots. In many other patients, no cause of the reactions can be found. Some of these patients can tolerate gradually increasing doses of immunoglobulin, particularly if they are premedicated with a nonsteroidal antiinflammatory agent, diphenhydramine, or corticosteroids. In a few patients, antibodies have developed to the IgA present in minute quantities in immunoglobulin, and these IgA antibodies can be detected by serology.[743] This topic is discussed further in the Adverse Effects of Intramuscular Immunoglobulin section.

Administration of exogenous gamma globulin may inhibit the endogenous synthesis of gamma globulin. In a few patients given IGIM or IGIV from early infancy, depressed IgG levels returned to normal when the injections were stopped. Amer and colleagues[20] reported decreased IgG levels in premature infants given monthly IGIM injections since birth.

IGIM injections or infusions can inhibit antibody responses to live virus vaccines such as measles or varicella. Siber and associates[640] recommend an interval of 3 months between IVIG or IGIM therapy and administration of live virus vaccines after immunoglobulin doses of less than 40 mg/kg, an interval of 6 months after doses of 40 to 80 mg/kg, an interval of 8 months after doses of 80 to 400 mg/kg, and an interval of 12 months after large doses (1–2 g/kg).[23]

Late side effects after IGIM injections are uncommon occurrences, but fibrosis of the buttocks or localized subcutaneous atrophy may develop at the site of repeated injections in some patients. Repeated injections of IGIM may result in high levels of mercury from the thimerosal preservative. Although symptoms of acrodynia (i.e., mercury toxicity) developed in one patient as a result of such therapy,[457] most remained asymptomatic.

Intravenous Immunoglobulin

IGIV is further-treated Cohn fractionated human immunoglobulin that has been rendered free of complexes and is safe for intravenous infusion. These products can be given in large quantities for antibody deficiencies[124]; for several autoimmune, inflammatory, and neurologic disorders[64,201]; and for prevention of transplant rejection.[350,351]

Pharmacology. The first IGIV produced in the United States in 1981 was Gamimune, a reduced and alkylated 5% solution containing 10% maltose.[41] The second IVIG produced was prepared by acidification and treatment with pepsin; the lyophilized powder could be reconstituted as a 3%, 6%, or 12% solution (Sandoglobulin). Since then, several IGIVs have been introduced by different manufacturers.[528]

Several methods of treating Cohn fraction II, including treatment with proteolytic enzymes, ultracentrifugation, chromatography, reduction of sulfhydryl bonds by alkylation, and incubation at low pH, have been used to eliminate high-molecular-weight complexes. Solvent and detergent treatment, pasteurization, and addition of the fatty acid caprylate are used to ensure that viral inactivation occurs,[309] and various stabilizers, such as maltose, albumin, or sucrose, are then added. Variations in manufacturing techniques result in unique characteristics in the different immunoglobulin products.[528]

Although these products vary somewhat across brands and batches,[650,668] they are for the most part therapeutically equivalent and usually are selected on the basis of cost and convenience. IgG subclass differences exist.[46,650] Antibody titers to specific pathogens also may vary across lots and among different IGIVs.[234] Products have different IgA contents, which can be a consideration for patients with anti-IgA antibodies.[46] Premixed liquids have the advantage of convenience because the reconstitution step is not required; however, most solutions must be kept refrigerated.

The IGIV products currently available have all IgG subclasses, adequate serum half-lives (i.e., 15 to 25 days), a wide spectrum of antibody activity, and minimal anticomplementary activity, and they are free of bacterial and viral contamination.[329] Individual donors are checked for viral pathogens, and the final product is checked for sterility. The ability of the fractionation process to remove viral and prion particles is validated by spiking test pools with model pathogens and subjecting them to the same fractionation process used by the plasma pools for human use. Some of them are 5% to 10% solutions, and others are lyophilized powders that are reconstituted as 3% to 12% solutions.[528,670]

IGIV has several advantages over IGIM. Larger quantities of IgG can be given, high levels of serum IgG can be achieved rapidly, painful intramuscular injections are avoided, tissue pooling and local proteolysis are avoided, and home administration and self-administration are easier to perform.

Administration of intravenous immunoglobulin. Administration of IGIV requires venous access, which is sometimes a problem in small children or obese patients. It also requires close monitoring during the infusion, which usually takes 2 to 5 hours.[667] The initial rate is 0.01 mL/kg per minute, and if no side effects occur, it can be doubled at 15- to 30-minute intervals to a maximal rate of 0.08 mL/kg per minute. Rates above 5 mL/kg per hour (0.08 mL/kg per minute) are not recommended. Vital signs should be monitored frequently, and trained personnel should be available to treat adverse reactions. Adverse effects tend to be associated with rapid rates of infusion, patients with concurrent acute infections, previously untreated patients, or significant time elapse between infusions (>6-week intervals).

IGIV is contraindicated in patients who have had an anaphylactic reaction to IGIV or other blood products. It should be administered with great caution to patients who have IgG subclass deficiencies along with IgA deficiency or anti-IgA antibodies, or both.[183]

In responsible, older patients receiving infusions without adverse effects, infusion by home self-administration can be accomplished with considerable cost savings.[52,390,659] However, in most cases, IGIV infusions are performed in the clinic setting or by a home infusion service.

A few investigators have given high concentrations (i.e., 9–12% solutions) infused rapidly during a period of 20 to 40 minutes, which may be tolerated by some patients.[615] However, it should not be done except by experienced personnel equipped to manage adverse reactions.

The brand, lot number, dose, premedication, and adverse reactions should be recorded. Cold solutions should be warmed to room temperature before administration.

Premedication, such as acetaminophen or diphenhydramine, is often given 30 minutes before infusions are started, particularly for the first infusion or for patients who have had prior reactions. Intravenous hydrocortisone (i.e., 5 to 6 mg/kg in children and 100 to 150 mg/kg in adults) or oral prednisone can be used for prevention of anticipated severe reactions.

Side effects of intravenous immunoglobulins. Certain brands of IVIG may cause more adverse reactions. In one study involving patients with Kawasaki disease, the two IGIVs used were equivalent therapeutically, but one had a 12-fold (2% vs. 25%) increase in side effects.[590]

Immediate reactions, such as headaches, shaking chills, nausea and vomiting, myalgias, or arthralgias that occur during or shortly after the infusions, are common occurrences.[198,667,669] They may occur in as many as 10% of recipients, especially with a first infusion or in individuals with prior reactions.[668] They can be treated by slowing or stopping the infusions and giving nonsteroidal antiinflammatory drugs, diphenhydramine, hydrocortisone, or other steroids. Occasionally, switching to a different product (usually one available as a solution) may alleviate the reactions.

Severe immediate reactions. Anaphylaxis, shortness of breath, hypotension, hypertension, and other immediate reactions are uncommon events. Because they rarely involve IgE antibodies, they are called anaphylactoid reactions, and they may be associated with cytokine release, complement activation, or vasoactive substance in the preparations.

Immediate reactions in immunoglobulin A–deficient patients. An occasional IgA-deficient patient exposed to blood, plasma, or any form of immunoglobulin may develop IgE anti-IgA antibodies, which can cause a reaction to the small amount of IgA in imunoglobulin.[125] IgG anti-IgA in high titers may cause a complement-mediated anaphylactic reaction.[743] These reactions are rare, and testing patients for IgA deficiency before administration of IGIV is unnecessary. Patients with profound antibody deficiency do not develop anti-IgA antibodies. For the sensitized patient, the use of a low-IgA-content product or premedication is indicated. Although IgA deficiency is rare, patients with this condition should not be given IGIV unless it is absolutely indicated.

Aseptic meningitis. Headache is a common occurrence during or after IGIV infusions, but some patients develop severe headaches 6 to 24 hours after the infusion, sometimes associated with photophobia, stiff neck, and nausea.[365,732] Several of these patients have had spinal taps that show cerebrospinal fluid (CSF) pleocytosis but negative viral and bacterial cultures. The symptoms usually resolve within 96 hours. This complication may recur despite changing brands of IGIV. Most occur when IGIV is used in large doses (e.g., 2 g/kg) for neurologic diseases. Individuals with a history of migraine may be more susceptible to aseptic meningitis.[621] These patients may tolerate slow infusions of subcutaneous immunogobulin.[572,671] Headaches and aseptic meningitis often can be avoided by premedication with steroids or with antimigraine medications.

Renal complications. Renal failure, usually temporary, has been reported with IGIV, particularly among patients with a history of renal disease.[572,668] When such a problem is anticipated, IGIV should be given slowly at no more than 0.5 g/kg per day.[668]

Thrombotic complications. Several thrombotic events, including stroke, myocardial infarction, transient ischemic events, and central vein thrombosis, have occurred after IGIV infusions.[668] These events may be associated with high doses and rapid infusion, particularly among patients with preexisting cardiovascular illness, obesity, immobility, or hematologic malignancy.[42,668,779] However, further research is needed to establish the risk of thrombotic events in patients without these risk factors.[43]

Rare side effects. Transient neutropenia, hemolytic anemia, acidosis, and symptoms of hyperviscosity occur rarely.[117,668]

Transmission of pathogens, including hepatitis C, by intravenous immunoglobulin. Because IGIV is derived from human donors, a remote chance of transmission of viral or other pathogens exists. Tests of donors and the final products are performed, and newer testing for prions is in place but is not of proven reliability. No instance of HIV infection or Jakob-Creutzfeldt or new-variant Jakob-Creutzfeldt disease have been linked to the use of IGIV. Nonetheless, some patients with immunodeficiency receiving long-term IGIV therapy have developed progressive central nervous system problems.[797]

In the early 1990s, hepatitis C was transmitted by experimental IGIV lots,[423,514] some European preparations,[86,87,421,768] and some commercially available US lots.[143,612] Until the report of an outbreak of hepatitis C in 1994,[143] no US cases of hepatitis associated with a commercially available IVIG had been reported. Transmission occurred shortly after hepatitis C–seropositive donors were excluded from the donor pools used in the manufacture of IGIV.

A plausible explanation for the lack of transmission before this US Food and Drug Administration (FDA) policy was instituted is that the hepatitis C antibodies neutralized trace amounts of hepatitis C virus not eliminated during the fractionation. As of October 1994, 137 suspected cases were reported, 88 of which were confirmed.[143,614] Of the 88 patients, 51 (58%) had primary immunodeficiencies, and 63% eventually became symptomatic.

Bjoro and associates[87] reported that immunocompromised patients had a severe and rapidly progressive course of hepatitis C infection and that responses to interferon (IFN) were poor. Razvi and colleagues[573] did not confirm this finding in US patients. Newer manufacturing processes and more rigorous testing seemingly have eliminated the risk of hepatitis C transmission.

Intravenous immunoglobulin and intramuscular immunoglobulin inhibition of vaccine antibody responses. Live virus vaccines can have diminished immunogenicity when given shortly before or during the several months after receipt of immunoglobulin. Immunoglobulin administration inhibits the response to measles vaccine for a prolonged period, and inhibition of rubella vaccine also has been demonstrated. The interval between measles vaccine and immunoglobulin depends on the dose of immunoglobulin. The period of inhibition of response to varicella vaccine is not known, and the recommendation is to follow that for measles vaccine administration. Immunoglobulin does not impair responses to oral polio vaccine, oral rotavirus vaccine, or yellow fever vaccine.

In contrast to live virus vaccines, administration of immunoglobulin has not been demonstrated to cause significant inhibition of immune responses to inactivated vaccines and toxoids. Vaccines should be administered at sites different from those of IGIM. IGIV recipients should be immunized according to the recommended schedule for routine childhood immunization. The 2015 pediatric *Red Book* gives detailed recommendations.[23]

Intravenous immunoglobulin in primary immunodeficiencies. Administration of IGIV is indicated for patients with profound primary antibody deficiency (i.e., quantitative and qualitative), for patients with combined immunodeficiencies, and for those with secondary immunodeficiency along with significant antibody deficiency (Box 246.1). Regular infusions of IGIV can keep patients with primary antibody immunodeficiencies free of infections for long periods or lessen the severity and frequency of chronic infections.[581]

Patients with hereditary agammaglobulinemias, common variable immunodeficiency, and immunodeficiencies with hyper-IgM clearly benefit from replacement therapy. In combined antibody and cellular defects and in secondary antibody immunodeficiencies, administration of IVIG serves as an important ancillary treatment, but it does not correct the associated T-cell defect or underlying cause of the secondary immunodeficiency.

The recommended dose of IGIV is 400 to 600 mg/kg, usually given every 3 to 4 weeks.[528,667] It should be given every 3 weeks if symptoms develop late in the period between monthly infusions. In general, the trough IgG level should be maintained at approximately 400 mg/dL higher than the pretreatment level, which normalizes the IgG level in most patients (e.g., 600–1000 mg/dL).

BOX 246.1 Immunodeficiencies for Which Human Immune Globulin May Be Beneficial

Antibody Deficiencies

Congenital agammaglobulinemias
Common variable immunodeficiency
Immunodeficiencies with hyper-IgM
Transient hypogammaglobulinemia of infancy (sometimes)
IgG subclass deficiency with or without IgA deficiency (sometimes)
Antibody deficiency with normal immunoglobulins

Combined Deficiencies

Severe combined immunodeficiencies (all types)
Wiskott-Aldrich syndrome
Ataxia-telangiectasia
Short-limbed dwarfism
X-linked lymphoproliferative syndrome

Secondary Immunodeficiencies

Malignant neoplasms with antibody deficiencies: multiple myeloma, chronic lymphocytic leukemia, and other cancers
Protein-losing enteropathy with hypogammaglobulinemia
Nephrotic syndrome with hypogammaglobulinemia
Pediatric acquired immunodeficiency syndrome
Intensive care patients: trauma, surgery, or shock
After transplantation
Burns
Prematurity

Certain patients who experience continued infections may receive even higher doses (i.e., 600–800 mg/kg every 3 to 4 weeks).[207,358] Patients receiving these larger doses may have less frequent sinopulmonary infections, improved pulmonary function, and decreased number of days of illness and hospitalization compared with patients receiving lower doses.[667] Some investigators recommend giving even higher doses (i.e., keeping trough levels >800 mg/dL) in an effort to prevent pulmonary complications.[207,358] Some patients with severe disease do not respond to higher doses or more frequent infusions because of permanent tissue damage or deep-seated chronic infection.

IGIV also is used in patients with antibody deficiency but with normal or almost normal immunoglobulin levels. These patients often need higher or more frequent doses of IGIV because their IgG catabolism is increased as a result of their high serum IgG levels. On rare occasions, IGIV is indicated for infants with transient hypogammaglobulinemia and persistent infection. IGIV also has been used in patients with IgG subclass deficiencies, but controlled studies demonstrating efficacy are lacking.[85,390,643]

Special uses of intravenous immunoglobulin in antibody deficiencies. A syndrome of polymyositis or chronic encephalitis, or both, caused by persistent enteroviral infection in patients with agammaglobulinemia has been treated successfully with very high doses of IGIV containing specific antibody to the virus.[470,565] However, some patients do not respond.[181]

A very high dose of IGIV (up to 2 g/kg per day) is used occasionally in patients with primary immunodeficiency who develop parvovirus B19 infection, autoimmune disease such as immune thrombocytopenic purpura, or persistent respiratory viral infection.[667]

Subcutaneous Human Immunoglobulin

An alternative to injection of IGIM or infusion of IGIV is slow subcutaneous infusion of immunoglobulin.[4,81,80,244] This route is used extensively in Europe with a 16% preservative-free immunoglobulin. A preservative-free 16% product (Vivaglobin) was licensed in 2006 in the United States for subcutaneous use.[513] However, 10% to 12% solutions for IGIV also can be used safely.[671]

These products usually are infused into the abdominal wall or thigh with a battery-operated portable infusion pump.[80,244] The usual dose is 100 to 150 mg/kg per week, the same monthly dose as recommended for IGIV, given at a rate of 0.05 to 0.20 mL/kg per hour. Larger doses and more rapid infusions can be accomplished by using multiple injection sites. If a patient is beginning IGSC therapy and an immediate therapeutic level is sought, loading doses of IGIV at double the monthly maintenance dose can be given 1 week before the start of IGSC. Peak serum IgG levels after IGSC occur 48 to 96 hours after the infusion.

IGSC infusions, which can be self-administered, are well tolerated, safe, and preferred by some patients because the adverse reactions are considerably less.[80,244,293] Premedication is rarely needed. They are more suitable than IGIV for home self-administration.[243,244]

Stiehm and coworkers[671] used this route successfully in patients with poor intravenous access, aseptic meningitis after IGIV infusion, anaphylactic reactions after receiving IGIV infusion, or rapid gastrointestinal protein loss. IGSC has been used safely in IgA-deficient adults with frequent respiratory infections,[293] during pregnancy,[82] and in children.[4]

Rapid administration of IGSC has been achieved by using two pumps at four infusion sites and increasing the rate to 20 mL/h per pump, allowing the entire infusion to be completed in little more than an hour.[244]

Immunoglobulin Administration by Oral, Intrathecal, Aerosol, and Local Routes

Many types of antibody have been given by unusual routes with various degrees of success. None except intravitreous injection of monoclonal antibody is standard care.

Oral immunoglobulin. Breast milk is the ultimate oral passive immune agent with preventive benefit for newborns. Oral immunoglobulin administered to provide antimicrobial activity to the gastrointestinal tract mimics the action of antibody-rich colostrum and breast milk. In humans, little or no ingested immunoglobulin is absorbed intact into the systemic circulation.[44] Some oral immunoglobulin traverses the entire gastrointestinal tract undigested, particularly in premature infants.[75] Oral immunoglobulin may neutralize microorganisms, inhibit colonization, and prevent microbial attachment to the gastrointestinal mucosa.

Rotavirus infection. Barnes and colleagues[70] fed human immunoglobulin or placebo for 7 days to premature infants in a nursery in which rotavirus was endemic. Rotavirus-associated diarrhea developed in 6 of 11 babies given placebo and in 1 of 14 given oral immunoglobulin. Oral administration of immunoglobulin in low-birth-weight infants may be a useful strategy in treating rotavirus infections, but further clinical trials are needed to assess efficacy.[535]

Losonsky and coworkers[434] administered oral human immunoglobulin to two children with severe combined immunodeficiency and chronic rotavirus infection and demonstrated a decrease in the amount of free rotavirus excretion and survival of the immunoglobulin through the gastrointestinal tract. Kanfer and associates[361] used oral human immunoglobulin to treat rotavirus infection that occurred after bone marrow transplantation. In 2015, Williams reported the use of enteral immunoglobulin in four pediatric stem cell transplant recipients with good results.[767]

Bovine hyperimmune colostral immunoglobulin enriched in rotavirus antibodies (from immunized cows) also has been used in the prevention of rotavirus infection. Davidson and colleagues[186] prevented rotavirus infection in 55 children admitted to an Australian hospital by administering a 10-day course of bovine colostrum; nine of 65 control children became infected.

Turner and Kelsey[716] added at least 360 mL of cow colostrum to the formula of 31 term infants 3 to 7 months of age for an average of 101 days (range, 16–202 days). Rotavirus infections occurred in 11 (35%) of the colostrum-fed group and 14 (42%) of the control group, an insignificant difference, but symptomatic infection occurred in 1 (3%) of the infants receiving colostrum and 6 (18%) of the controls.

This product also has been used in two studies of the treatment of rotavirus diarrhea in Bangladesh.[481,609] In both studies, less diarrhea, fewer days of illness, less stool output, and more rapid clearance of rotavirus from the stool occurred. Guarino and coworkers[286] used oral human immunoglobulin (300 mg/kg) as a single dose and observed more rapid recovery from rotavirus diarrhea. Oral immunoglobulin is a promising but unproved agent for the prevention and treatment of rotavirus infection.

Necrotizing enterocolitis. Eibl and colleagues[206] were able to prevent necrotizing enterocolitis in all 90 infants given oral immunoglobulin rich in serum IgA. Six cases occurred among 91 control infants. Rubaltelli and colleagues[592] in Italy achieved similar results with oral monomeric IgG.

Cryptosporidial infection. Bovine colostrum was used successfully to treat cryptosporidial diarrhea in HIV infection.[634] Borowitz and Saulsbury[102] used oral immunoglobulin successfully to treat cryptosporidial infection in a child with acute leukemia.

Other diarrheas. Oral human immunoglobulin has been used after bone marrow transplantation and lung transplantation to prevent the development of viral gastroenteritis[239,361] and to treat nonspecific diarrhea in immunodeficient patients.[473] Commercial products from bovine colostrum are available in Sweden and India.[235,548] Considerable experimental study findings in veterinarian medicine are available for other oral immunoglobulins.

Aerosolized and intratracheal immunoglobulin. Aerosolized and intratracheal immunoglobulin has been used with encouraging results in experimental models of pneumonia caused by RSV, pneumococci, staphylococci, *Yersinia pestis,* and parainfluenza and influenza viruses.[270,314,531,569,570,586] Aerosolized monoclonal antibodies also are being studied for specific infections, bioterrorist toxins (e.g., anthrax, ricin), and lung immunomodulation.[218,415,559,738]

Rimensberger and colleagues[582] conducted a placebo-controlled trial of aerosolized human immunoglobulin (not RSV-IVIG) in the treatment of RSV infection. No significant benefit was found, but the treatment was well tolerated.

Heikkinen and coworkers[306] used an IgA-enriched human immunoglobulin as a nasal spray twice daily for 8 weeks to reduce respiratory infections in children between 1 and 4 years of age attending childcare. A 42% reduction was achieved among the 19 children receiving the immunoglobulin compared with the 20 children in the placebo group. The study authors suggested that this treatment also could decrease the incidence of otitis media.

Intrathecal immunoglobulin. Human immunoglobulin has been used intrathecally for the treatment of viral encephalomyelitis in patients with antibody deficiency.[215] Monoclonal antibodies occasionally are given intrathecally in cancer therapy.[665] The use of antitoxin intrathecally in tetanus is discussed in the section on tetanus.

Other administration routes. Local application of antibody has been used in the prevention and treatment of surgical and traumatic wounds.[373,558] Injections of the monoclonal antibody bevacizumab (Lucentis) into the vitrea to treat macular degeneration are being tested.[176] Inner ear injection of infliximab, a tumor necrosis factor (TNF) monoclonal antibody, has been used in autoimmune neurosensory hearing loss.[730] Intraarticular immunoglobulin had no clinical benefit for patients with rheumatoid arthritis.[57]

Immunoglobulin in Secondary Immunodeficiencies

Many chronically ill patients have a primary illness that results in immunosuppression and increased susceptibility to infection. These secondary immunodeficiencies are considerably more common than primary immunodeficiency and are particularly common developments in hospitalized patients. Although most patients have cellular (T-cell) deficiencies, some have antibody deficiencies that are isolated or combined with other immune defects. These patients may have low immunoglobulin levels, poor antibody responses to antigenic challenge, low levels of natural antibodies that may result from loss of immunoglobulin, loss of immune cells, or the toxic effect of therapy or infection on the immune system. Box 246.1 lists diseases and conditions in which secondary antibody immunodeficiency can occur.

Laboratory criteria that support the use of IGIV include significant hypogammaglobulinemia (serum IgG <200 mg/dL or total immunoglobulin [IgG + IgM + IgA] <400 mg/dL), absent or unexpectedly low titers of natural antibodies, absent or poor response to antigenic challenge (i.e., tetanus or pneumococcal vaccines), and lack of an antibody response to the infecting organism.[669] Some of the more common secondary immunodeficiencies with antibody defects are discussed in the following sections.

Hematologic and Oncologic Diseases

Antibody deficiencies can occur with multiple myeloma, chronic lymphocytic leukemia, lymphoma, and advanced cancer, aggravated by the immunosuppressive agents used in their therapy. A double-blind multicenter study concluded that the prophylactic infusion of 400 mg/kg of IGIV every 3 weeks reduced the incidence of bacterial infections in patients with chronic lymphocytic leukemia.[172] The treatment group had fewer infections with *Streptococcus pneumoniae* and *Haemophilus influenzae,* but no difference was observed in infections caused by other gram-negative bacteria, fungi, or viruses.

This beneficial effect has been confirmed in subsequent studies,[177,240,289] and although concern has been raised about its cost-effectiveness,[753] IGIV has been shown to reduce the incidence of infections in patients with multiple myeloma[157] and in those receiving chemotherapy for lung cancer.[617] However, Blombery and colleagues[90] found no benefit in the routine use of peritransplantation IVIG to reduce infectious complications in patients with multiple myeloma undergoing autologous hematopoietic stem cell transplantation.

Protein-Losing States: Enteropathy, Nephrotic Syndrome, and Plastic Bronchitis

In some pediatric patients, antibody deficiency results from massive proteinuria (i.e., nephrosis), diarrhea (i.e., protein-losing enteropathy), or loss into the lung (i.e., plastic bronchitis) associated with accelerated IgG loss. Most of these patients have minimal trouble with recurrent infection, probably because antibody synthesis is intact and most likely accelerated. However, if the loss of IgG greatly exceeds synthetic capacity, symptomatic severe hypogammaglobulinemia may result. IGIV infusions can be used diagnostically in such cases. A large intravenous infusion, followed by serial measurements of serum IgG levels, can document an accelerated IgG half-life (i.e., <10 days).

These patients are candidates for IGIV therapy if they have recurrent infections or very low IgG levels (e.g., <200 mg/dL). Administration of large and repeated doses of IGIV is necessary. Occasionally, antibody infusions help to control the severe diarrhea of protein-losing enteropathy.[133] IGSC has been used in this situation because its delayed release into the circulation can generate higher long-term IgG levels than can be achieved with an equivalent IGIV monthly dose.[671]

Intensive Care Patients: Trauma, Surgery, and Septic Shock

Patients undergoing severe stress associated with trauma or extensive surgery have profound exposure and susceptibility to infection and a spectrum of immune deficiencies, including cutaneous anergy, leukocyte dysfunction, hypogammaglobulinemia, and transiently impaired antibody synthesis.[265,492,771] Bowel stasis and hypotension may promote gram-negative sepsis or endotoxemia, or both, along with the development of severe and often irreversible shock.

Early studies by Ziegler and associates[796] and Baumgartner and colleagues[74] suggested that when antisera to a mutant J5 *Escherichia coli* endotoxin with anti–lipid A activity is used in bacteremic or surgical intensive care unit (ICU) patients, the incidence and severity of severe shock could be reduced. However, Calandra and colleagues,[130] used a human IGIV to J5 *E. coli* in 71 patients with gram-negative infections and shock and could not confirm their results. No differences were found in mortality rates, onset of time to shock, and complications.

Just and coworkers[355] administered IGIV and antibiotics to 50 patients in the ICU thought to have infection and compared their outcomes with 54 control patients who received antibiotics alone. Although no difference in survival occurred, they found a trend indicating that the IGIV-antibiotic group had a shortened stay in the ICU, a shorter period in which respiratory therapy was required, improved renal function, and a favorable effect on infection. Ferrara and colleagues[227] reported that IGIV was a viable adjunct treatment option for certain cases of drug-resistant bacterial infections, and there was a clear survival advantage with the use of IGIV in adult sepsis syndromes by suppressing inflammation.

Rodriquez and colleagues[588] gave an IgM-enriched IGIV or albumin to 56 patients with sepsis undergoing abdominal surgery and found a reduction of sepsis from 55% to 25%. Another multicenter study of 352 postsurgical patients confirmed the observation that standard IGIV (400 mg/kg at weekly intervals) reduced the incidence of infections and shortened the stay in the ICU in contrast to patients treated with placebo or hyperimmune core-lipopolysaccharide immunoglobulin.[332]

Werdan[759] reviewed the use of IGIV in sepsis and suggested certain specific subgroups could benefit (e.g., postoperative sepsis, septic shock with endotoxinemia, sepsis with neutropenia). Although certain subgroups may benefit from the use of IGIV for sepsis, there is a need for further clinical trials to make a recommendation for use.[15,629,656] Tagami and colleagues reviewed the role of IGIV as an adjunctive treatment in 1324 patients with pneumonia and septic shock from July 2010 through March 2013, and found no reduction in mortality rates.[695] A single-institution study from Egypt suggested that IGIV was beneficial in children younger than 2 years of age in the ICU who had sepsis.[209] Studies of IGIV in trauma patients requiring surgery[188,197,263,694] and in patients with head trauma[771] have shown questionable efficacy.

Monoclonal antibodies to endotoxin have been tested in clinical trials of patients in septic shock, but none had proven efficacy.[499,760,795] Monoclonal antibody to TNF-α also has shown no efficacy in the treatment of adults with septic shock.[3,169] Monoclonal antibodies to interleukin-6 (IL-6) or IL-1 receptor likewise have not been effective in the treatment of shock.[246]

Prematurity

All premature infants have low levels of maternally derived IgG at birth, and levels approaching 100 mg/dL develop in the first months of life in most.[65] The IgG levels may be further depressed by pulmonary disease (with transudation into the lungs), fever and stress (with increased IgG catabolism), and multiple blood sampling.[519] Their sluggish antibody responses, concurrent IgM and IgA deficiencies, and immature complement, phagocytic, and T-cell systems render low-birth-weight infants extraordinarily susceptible to development of infection.[426]

Attempts to decrease the incidence of infections in premature infants by using periodic immunoglobulin injections began in the 1960s. Four controlled studies enrolling a total of 363 infants used immunoglobulin doses of 80 to 240 mg/kg per month during their stay in the nursery (two studies), for 4 months, and for 1 year.[20,171,194,663] In two studies, a slight decrease in the number and severity of infections was observed, but there was no difference in survival. These mixed results suggest that immunoglobulin at the doses used had no prophylactic value for these patients.

In the past few decades, the increasing rate of survival of premature infants and the availability of IGIV have reawakened interest in the use of antibody to prevent infections in premature infants. An initial double-blind clinical trial by Baker and colleagues[58] suggested that IGIV at a dose of 0.5 g/kg at frequent intervals in the first weeks of life significantly reduced the frequency of sepsis, particularly that caused by *Staphylococcus epidermidis*. Subsequent studies, however, did not show a clear benefit.

Meta-analyses of prospective, randomized, placebo-controlled prevention studies (representing 5000 infants) were performed by Jenson and Pollock[343,344] and Ohlsson and Lacy.[520,522,523] These studies had different entry criteria, doses, and brands of IGIV, but most infants weighed less than 2000 g, were given IGIV therapy within the first week of life, and received doses of at least 400 mg/kg per month; culture-proven sepsis was used as an end point. Overall, a slight reduction (3%) was seen in the incidence of sepsis, but there were no differences in mortality rates, length of stay, or other complications of prematurity, such as necrotizing enterocolitis, bronchopulmonary dysplasia, and intraventricular hemorrhage. The International Neonatal Immunotherapy Study Collaborative Group concluded that IGIV had no effect on outcomes of suspected or proven neonatal sepsis.[284]

Shamin and coworkers[627] gave sufficient IGIV for 6 months to 15 of 30 matched premature infants with severe bronchopulmonary dysplasia to maintain their IgG levels above 400 mg/dL, whereas the untreated infants had levels below 200 mg/dL. The number of infections, notably pneumonia, was significantly reduced in the IGIV group (i.e., 5 episodes of pneumonia and 4 other infections) in contrast to the control group (i.e., 15 episodes of pneumonia and 12 other infections). In 2011, a large collaborative study of 113 hospitals in nine countries evaluated the use of IGIV in neonatal sepsis and found no effect on the outcome of suspected or proven neonatal sepsis.[284]

The evidence still supports the 1990 National Institutes of Health (NIH) consensus statement that IGIV should not be given routinely to infants of low birth weight[501] but that it may be of value in selected premature infants at high risk for infection. IGIV is sometimes beneficial for premature infants with a history of serious infections and underlying lung disease; most have hypogammaglobulinemia and should be regarded as having transient hypogammaglobulinemia of infancy.

Hyperimmune IGIV, or monoclonal antibodies enriched in antibodies against specific microbial antigens (e.g., *Staphylococcus aureus*), may be beneficial for certain high-risk newborn and premature infants. Two large, multicenter, double-blind clinical trials of *S. aureus* hyperimmune human immunoglobulins enrolled infants with very low birth weights. One (Altastaph) used immunoglobulin from donors immunized with a staphylococcal vaccine against serotypes 5 and 8.[78,450] The other (Veronate) used immunoglobulin from donors with a high titer to ClfA, a staphylococcal fibrinogen-binding protein.[91,135,189,367] Neither trial showed a significantly decreased severity or incidence of staphylococcal infections. The anti–lipoteichoic acid monoclonal antibody, pagibaximab, demonstrated safety and tolerability, but it did not reduce overall rates of neonatal sepsis.[546]

Transplantation

Conditioning regimens to eliminate or reduce the host's hematopoietic and immune systems before transplantation (i.e., bone marrow and solid organ) render these patients extremely susceptible to infection, particularly cytomegalovirus (CMV) infections.[717] IGIV and CMV intravenous immunoglobulin (CMV-IGIV) have been used to prevent infection and to modify graft-versus-host disease and prevent solid organ transplant rejection.

Early studies of IGIV therapy after allogeneic bone marrow transplantation were modestly successful in preventing infections, decreasing graft-versus-host reaction, and increasing survival rates.[6,73,173,271,687,685,686] This effect was less dramatic when CMV infection was controlled by ganciclovir and screening of blood products.[288] Two more multicenter studies showed only a modest or no effect on modifying acute graft-versus-host reactions or mortality rates.[175,773] In single-center studies, CMV-IGIV was of no benefit in CMV-positive lung transplant recipients[399] or liver transplant recipients.[276]

IGIV is beneficial for adult kidney transplant recipients with high titers of human leukocyte antigen (HLA) antibodies, resulting in a shorter time to transplantation, reduced HLA antibody titers, and improved allograft survival rates.[350,351] The use of IGIV together with other immunomodulatory therapies, such as anti-CD 20, are being studied to reduce infectious complications in renal transplant recipients.[741]

Burns

Bacterial sepsis, particularly *Pseudomonas* spp. and *E. coli* sepsis, is the leading cause of death of the 300,000 patients hospitalized annually in the United States for burns.[491,492] The protein loss in these patients induces hypogammaglobulinemia in proportion to the severity of the burn. High-dose IGIV prolongs survival in experimentally burned mice infected with *Pseudomonas* spp., and preliminary studies of hyperimmune immunoglobulin and plasma administered to human burn patients were encouraging, but proof of efficacy is lacking[372,560,681] (discussed later).

Human Immunodeficiency Virus Infection

Chapter 192B discusses HIV infection.

Intravenous Immune Globulin in Immunoregulatory and Neurologic Disorders

High-dose IGIV has immunosuppressive and antiinflammatory effects that render it a valuable agent in the treatment of several autoimmune,

treatment was delayed until the fourth or fifth day. Other investigators have reported similar findings.[701,702]

Tasman and associates[701,702] emphasized the importance of intravenous administration of antitoxin because rapid achievement of high blood levels results in rapid neutralization of antitoxin and the appearance within 30 minutes of antitoxin in saliva. They showed that the mortality rate and the severity of the myocarditis and neuritis in experimental diphtheria in guinea pigs could be reduced by giving antitoxin intravenously rather than intramuscularly.

McCloskey and Smilack[462] determined the antitoxin content of standard human immunoglobulin. None of the lots tested contained diphtheria antitoxin in a sufficient titer to allow its use for antitoxin therapy. They suggested that an IGIV with higher-titer antitoxin be developed to eliminate the risk of giving horse serum intravenously. Such a product is produced and used in the Ukraine.[222]

Recommendations

Diphtheria antitoxin of equine origin is indicated for all suspected or proven cases of diphtheria.[26] It is available in vials containing 20,000 U from the CDC. Before administration, skin tests must be performed to determine sensitivity. If the patient has a previous history of serum reactions or the test results are positive, a schedule of desensitization as outlined earlier must be followed.

The amount of antitoxin given depends on the location and the extensiveness of the membrane, the degree of systemic toxicity, and the duration of illness. The preferred route is intravenous, although intramuscular administration has been used historically in milder cases. In all cases, diphtheria antitoxin should be given promptly rather than be delayed while awaiting bacterial confirmation of the diagnosis.[26]

In cutaneous diphtheria, antitoxin is of uncertain value. When used, the dose is 20,000 to 40,000 U to prevent toxic sequelae. For pharyngeal or laryngeal disease, the dose is 20,000 to 40,000 U; for nasopharyngeal disease, the dose is 40,000 to 60,000 U; and for extensive disease with neck edema or disease of more than 3 days' duration, the dose is 80,000 to 120,000 U.[26] Although antimicrobial therapy is a valuable aid in the treatment of diphtheria, it is not a substitute for antitoxin therapy.

Routine use of antitoxin in an asymptomatic, exposed, susceptible patient is not recommended. With heavy exposure or for an extremely susceptible host, 5000 to 10,000 U of antitoxin given intramuscularly can be used in addition to antibiotics and diphtheria immunization. Proof of efficacy is lacking, however.

In 1936, Wade Hampton Frost demonstrated that diphtheria toxoid given to school children was effective in preventing disease and resultant death.[236] Diphtheria antitoxin is used to prevent diphtheria and is contained in the currently used diphtheria-pertussis-tetanus (DTaP) and tetanus-diphtheria (Tdap) vaccines.

Because human IGIV has various amounts of diphtheria antitoxin, it cannot be used as a replacement for animal antitoxin.[26]

Pertussis

Pertussis antiserum was used in the 1930s for the treatment of pertussis.[104] Human pertussis immunoglobulin was developed in the 1960s but was shown to have no additive benefit to antibiotics in the treatment of pertussis,[61,488] and it is no longer available commercially.

Granström and coworkers[272] used an experimental human hyperimmune serum from subjects immunized with a two-component acellular vaccine to treat 33 children, and an equal number received an albumin placebo. Both groups received the same antibiotic and supportive treatment. The treated children had decreased coughing and whooping, particularly if treatment was started early in the course of disease. There was no significant difference in the duration of hospitalization. Ichimaru and colleagues[328] successfully used a high-titer human IGIV preparation to treat a severely ill 1-year-old child.

Bruss and associates[120] studied a 4% high-titer human pertussis immunoglobulin in 26 children with pertussis and found that the product was safe at three dose levels (250, 750, and 1500 mg/kg). It provided good serum pertussis IgG levels with a half-life of 38 days. High titers of anti-pertussis antibodies were produced, and other studies have correlated the titers with protection against disease in animal models after an aerosolized challenge.[121,611] Little antibody appeared in nasal secretions. Efficacy was not evaluated in this study, but the suggestion was made that treated infants had a shorter duration of paroxysms and that the product was effective in the treatment of aerosol-induced pertussis in mice.[121]

A subsequent randomized, double-blind, placebo-controlled phase III trial that enrolled 25 infants was terminated because of unavailability of study product and poor recruitment. Preliminary analysis did not suggest a clinical benefit in symptoms such as cough, apnea, and oxygen desaturation in contrast to placebo.[296]

Recommendations

Because of the lack of well-designed, placebo-controlled, double-blind trials of immunomodulating agents, no recommendation exists for the role of passive immunity for pertussis.

Respiratory and Other Bacterial Infections

Respiratory tract infections caused by group A streptococci, *S. pneumoniae, H. influenzae* type b, and to a lesser extent, *Neisseria meningitidis, Chlamydia pneumoniae,* and *Mycoplasma pneumoniae* occur more frequently in patients with primary antibody deficiencies, and these infections can be reduced markedly by the regular administration of IGIV or IGIM.[227,419,514] IGIV represents a viable adjunct treatment option for certain cases of drug-resistant bacterial infections, and there is a clear survival advantage with the use of IGIV in adult sepsis syndromes by suppressing inflammation.[227] Specific animal antisera to some of these organisms were used in the early 1930s for the treatment of severe infections (e.g., meningitis), even after the introduction of sulfonamides.[16] Efficacy varied but was clearly better than no treatment at all, and a combination of sulfonamides and antibody seemed to be synergistic.[16]

Small doses of IGIM (100 mg/kg per month) did not prevent or improve the course of respiratory infections in normal children.[71,231] However, Nydahl-Persson and colleagues[511] gave 24 children with repeated bacterial respiratory infection (i.e., pneumonia or otitis media) trimethoprim-sulfamethoxazole or IGIV (400 mg/kg per month). Both agents were effective in reducing the number of infections compared with a control group.

Santoshan and associates[608] administered a human IGIM prepared from the sera of donors immunized with pneumococcal, meningococcal, and *H. influenzae* type b polysaccharide vaccines (i.e., bacterial polysaccharide immunoglobulin [BPIG]) to Apache Indian infants living on reservations in Arizona. Of the 703 infants studied, 222 infants in the study group received three doses of BPIG (0.5 mL/kg) at 2, 6, and 10 months of age, and the 218 infants in the control group received saline injections at the same ages. During the study period, seven cases of invasive *H. influenzae* type b disease and four cases of invasive pneumococcal disease occurred in the control group in contrast to one and two cases, respectively, in the BPIG-treated group, which was a significant difference ($P < .05$).

Otitis Media

Immunologically normal, otitis media–prone children seem to derive little preventive or therapeutic benefit from low-dose immunoglobulin given intramuscularly (100 mg/kg per month)[352] or intravenously (200 mg/kg per month).[360]

In patients with primary immunodeficiency, the frequency and severity of episodes of otitis media are diminished dramatically by the use of immunoglobulin in large doses. In children with secondary antibody deficiency associated with HIV infection, IGIV in large doses (400 mg/kg per month) reduced the frequency of otitis media by 60%.[484,485] Patients with subtle immunologic abnormalities such as IgG subclass deficiencies, IgA deficiency, and polysaccharide antibody deficiencies may have recurrent episodes of otitis media that can be reduced with a large dose of IGIV (e.g., 400 mg/kg per month).[360,389,511,638,643]

BPIG reduced the number of episodes of pneumococcal otitis media in high-risk Native American infants,[638] but it did not decrease the total number of episodes of otitis media. Large doses of RSV-IVIG (750 mg/kg per month) reduced the frequency of non-RSV otitis among young infants.[646] This product may have high antibody titers to bacteria and other viruses.[213] Ishizaka and coworkers[335] successfully treated seven children with recurrent pneumococcal otitis media with IGIV.

The studies previously discussed indicate that low-dose IGIM is ineffective in the prevention or treatment of otitis media, but high doses of IGIV (e.g., >400 mg/kg per month) may reduce the frequency and severity of otitis media in immunodeficient and otitis-prone normal children, probably by reducing virus- and bacteria-mediated disease.[301] Englund and Glezen[211] suggested that passive immunization transplacentally from a recently immunized pregnant mother with *H. influenzae* or pneumococcal vaccine also should be considered.

IGIV should not be used routinely for otitis media–prone normal children. However, in extreme cases, it can be considered after failure of prophylactic antibiotics and pneumococcal immunization.

Sinusitis

Sinusitis is a common occurrence in immunodeficient patients and is difficult to prevent or eradicate, even with optimal treatment. Mofenson and colleagues[484] found that neither IGIV (400 mg/kg per month) nor thrice-weekly sulfonamide prophylaxis prevented sinusitis from developing in children with HIV infection. Prospective data demonstrated that IGIV replacement treatment does not reduce or resolve chronic sinusitis,[227] but Desrosiers and Kilty[192] suggest IGIV may be an option for very refractory patients after endoscopic sinus surgery. In patients with no or subtle immune defects (e.g., IgG subclass deficiencies, polysaccharide antibody deficiencies), high-dose IGIV sometimes can decrease the frequency and severity of sinusitis.[109,161,567,643]

Lower Respiratory Tract Infections

Although high-dose IGIV had proven benefit in preventing pneumonia in immunodeficient patients,[128] there is no evidence that it can prevent pneumonia in normal patients. Anecdotal cases of IGIV used as adjunctive therapy for refractory viral pneumonia have been reported.[600,679]

Cystic Fibrosis

Winnie and associates[772] suggested that IGIV might improve pulmonary function in pulmonary exacerbations of cystic fibrosis. All patients received antibiotics, were older than 12 years, and had no long-term benefit from IGIV. Van Wye and coworkers[731] had similar results with the use of hyperimmune *Pseudomonas* IGIV in patients with cystic fibrosis.

A controlled trial of *Pseudomonas* hyperimmune IGIV in 116 patients with cystic fibrosis was discontinued because a 6-month interim analysis showed no reduction in acute pulmonary exacerbations.[562]

Balfour-Lynn and colleagues[63] suggested that high-dose IGIV had short-term benefit for improving pulmonary function and decreasing the need for steroids in selected patients with cystic fibrosis and respiratory obstruction receiving inhaled and oral steroids. In one study of 186 infants with cystic fibrosis, 92 receiving palivizumab and 94 receiving placebo over a single RSV season, the outcomes were similar for the two groups, and more research is required to recommend palivizumab prophylaxis in children with cystic fibrosis.[583,584]

Burn Infections

Kefalides and associates[372] reduced the mortality rate for severely burned children by administering plasma (1 mL/kg for each 1% of surface area burned) or IGIM (1 mL/kg on days 1, 3, and 5) from 40% to 20%. They concluded that solutions containing antibodies (i.e., plasma or immunoglobulin) were more effective in reducing the complications of infections than were other colloids. However, Stone and colleagues[681] could not achieve any clinical benefit from IGIM therapy (0.4 mL/kg every third day until skin coverage) in 60 burned subjects compared with 40 controls.

Convalescent plasma, special immunoglobulin with high antibody titer to *Pseudomonas,* and *Pseudomonas* vaccines also have been used in burn patients in an attempt to reduce infections, but without proof of efficacy.[180,196,349,498,637] An observational study suggested that the combined use of IGIV and polymyxin B reduced the number of septic episodes and shortened the length of hospital stay for severely burned children.[444]

Firoz and colleagues[233] summarized 5 years of experience with 82 patients with toxic epidermal necrolysis in a burn unit in San Antonio. They found no mortality benefit for the use of IGIV compared with supportive care.

Gram-Negative Infections

The most extensive use of immunoglobulin for infections in adults involved trauma, shock, and postoperative patients thought to have gram-negative infections (reviewed earlier with secondary immunodeficiency).[74,130,188,227,260,355,795,796] In 2002, a meta-analysis involving 492 patients receiving polyclonal IGIV for sepsis and septic shock suggested a benefit, particularly among adults,[14] but results of later clinical trials of the use of IGIV as an adjunctive therapy for sepsis have been mixed.[15]

Newborn Sepsis

Newborns and premature infants in particular are highly susceptible to bacterial sepsis and its sequelae. In addition to antibiotics, leukocytes, granulocyte colony-stimulating factor, and IGIV have been used as adjunctive therapy. Numerous studies on the prevention and treatment of newborn sepsis are available, and some suggest only slight benefit in preventing sepsis. Ohlsson and Lacy[521–523] reviewed the literature on the use of IGIV for suspected or proven infection in neonates and found insufficient evidence exists to support the routine administration of IGIV for neonatal sepsis. In 2011, the International Neonatal Immunotherapy Study Collaborative Group, a large collaborative study of 113 hospitals in nine countries, supported this conclusion. They evaluated the use of IGIV in neonatal sepsis and found no effect on the outcome of suspected or proven neonatal sepsis.[284]

IGIV may be considered for septic premature infants not responding well to conventional therapy, but the evidence does not support its use. It may be particularly valuable for neutropenic septic infants because it can help to mobilize leukocytes from the storage pool.

Staphylococcal Infections

Staphylococcal infections with various degrees of severity are ubiquitous. They include superficial skin infections, acute infections such as abscesses and wound infections, deep-seated indolent cellulitis, and three toxin-mediated diseases: scalded skin syndrome, toxic shock, and acute food poisoning. Antibiotics usually are effective in controlling the infections, but in some instances, the organism is antibiotic resistant or the disease is rapidly progressive. IGIV can have adjunctive benefit in some of these situations.[373,744]

In addition to the use of IGIV, novel antistaphylococcal antibodies are being developed and tested in clinical trials. Antibody products are directed against a variety of targets on the staphylococcal organism (i.e., capsule, lipoteichoic acid, and toxins). These products are in phase I and II trials. Antibodies are being developed for prevention and treatment of staphylococcal disease.[519]

Altastaph is a hyperimmune polyclonal immunoglobulin preparation that targets CP5 and CP8 capsular polysaccharides. It was shown to prevent *S. aureus* bacteremia in mice, but two phase II clinical trials failed to demonstrate efficacy.[78,242,596]

Staphylococcal Toxic Shock Syndrome

Patients with staphylococcal TSS have a rapid onset of fever, shock, macular desquamating rash, and multisystem organ failure.[21,474,628] The pathogenesis of the disorder results from infection with a strain that releases toxic shock syndrome toxin-1 (TSST-1).[21] Approximately 20% of all staphylococcal isolates carry the gene for this toxin.[435] TSST-1 is a potent superantigen that directly activates the 5% of T cells that have a Vβ2 T-cell receptor[435]; activation results in the rapid release of multiple cytokines and a clinical picture of rapidly progressive illness. Studies have implicated methicillin-resistant *S. aureus* (MRSA) in severe TSS.[341]

IGIV contains antitoxins that neutralize the staphylococcal (and streptococcal) superantigens.[700] It has been used successfully in animal models of TSS [21] and several patients.[516,541,616] Although no controlled clinical trials have been performed for staphylococcal TSS, most authorities recommend large IGIV doses (at least 400 mg/kg) in addition to antibiotic treatment and circulatory support.[21] IGIV also downregulates cytokine synthesis and action and inhibits immune activation, thereby providing additional benefits.[21]

Higuchi and coauthors[313] reported a large family that had recurrent episodes of staphylococcal TSS associated with normal immunoglobulin levels but low serum antibody titers to staphylococcal superantigens. Two boys in the family achieved successful prophylaxis with regular IGIV infusions.

Neonatal Staphylococcal Infections

Administration of passive immunity may have value for neonatal staphylococcal infections. Infection with *S. epidermidis*, is the most common cause of sepsis in premature infants, and it is aggravated in part by the use of catheters and parenteral lipid infusions.[58,234] Infections with *S. aureus* are also problems in neonatal ICUs. Use of passive immunity directed at reducing *S. aureus* infections has been tested.

One controlled study showed that IGIV decreased the incidence of infections but did not eliminate them.[58] This benefit has not been found in all trials of IGIV in newborns. Although the administration of IGIV increased IgG levels in newborns, the overall morbidity and death rates for nosocomially acquired sepsis were unchanged.

This variation can be explained by different amounts of staphylococcal antibodies in different IGIV brands and lots, particularly opsonic antibodies, which have been shown in animal models to be the most important correlate of clinical protection.[234] Because antibody variation exists in lots of IGIV made from pools of thousands of donors, it is not surprising that Krediet and colleagues[398] could not reliably increase the opsonic titers of premature infants by administering single-donor, fresh frozen plasma.

Because pooled IGIV has not decreased mortality rates for this high-risk population, the development of organism-specific immunoglobulin has been explored. INH-A21 (Veronate) is a plasma-derived, donor-selected, polyclonal antistaphylococcal human immunoglobulin. A phase II, multicenter, double-blind clinical trial of this antibody was conducted for 512 low-birth-weight infants (50 to 1250 g), but no clinically significant differences were seen in the incidence of *S. aureus* or coagulase-negative *Staphylococcus*.[91]

In a phase III trial with a larger enrollment, 1983 infants received placebo or the study drug (i.e., INH-A21). The investigators were unable to demonstrate benefit in protection against late-onset sepsis resulting from *S. aureus* or coagulase-negative *Staphylococcus*. The incidence of sepsis in the placebo group was 5% and 6% in the treatment group.[189]

Pagibaximab is a humanized mouse chimeric monoclonal antibody directed against lipoteichoic acid, a cell wall component of gram-positive bacteria. Phase I, II, and III studies demonstrated safety and tolerability but no observed reduction in sepsis.[546,757,758]

In the past decade, highly virulent and antibiotic-resistant strains of *S. aureus* have emerged. They are responsible for aggressive infections, including necrotizing fasciitis, and pulmonary necrosis. The virulence factors are being elucidated, and Panton-Valentine leukocidin (PVL), a product of the *pvl* gene, correlates with higher morbidity and mortality rates for patients with MRSA infections.[93] The precise role that PVL plays in the pathogenesis of severe *S. aureus* infections is unclear, but it may provide a target for antibody neutralization in a severe toxin-mediated disease process.[113] Children with PVL-positive MRSA infections mount a robust antibody response to PVL, but the antibody does not seem to protect against future infections with the same organism.[311]

Neutralization of *S. aureus* PVL by IGIV in vitro has been demonstrated, and it neutralizes pore formation and the cytopathic effect of *S. aureus*.[245] Because of this in vitro data and its use in other diseases with toxin production such as TSS, the use of IGIV in aggressive infections caused by PVL-producing *S. aureus* can be considered as adjuvant therapy along with early debridment and active antimicrobial therapy.[300,783]

Refractory Staphylococcal Infections

Another use of immunoglobulin is for the treatment of antibiotic-resistant chronic staphylococcal infection along with intravenous antibiotics. Waisbren[744] treated 16 of these patients with an antibiotic and gamma globulin combination, with recovery observed in 13 of them. Hyperimmune plasma and immunoglobulin from patients immunized with staphylococcal toxoids are widely used in Russia with apparent success.[373]

Recommendations

Large doses of IGIV are indicated for the treatment of staphylococcal TSS.[38] The recommended regimen is a single dose of 1 to 2 g/kg or 400 mg/kg daily for 5 days. A repeated dose may be necessary because of rapid clearance of IGIV in this illness.[38] The value of IGIV in refractory chronic staphylococcal infections has not been proved, although anecdotal reports of efficacy exist.[744]

IGIV is not recommended routinely for the prevention of infection in premature newborn infants. IGIV can have adjunctive benefit in the treatment of neonates with sepsis, particularly those with neutropenia.[344] Development of specific antistaphylococcal immunoglobulins to prevent staphylococcal infection in infants with very low birth weights continues to be an active area of investigation.[626]

Streptococcal Infections

Circulating antibody may play a role in the prevention and treatment of group A streptococcal infection.[362] Newborns rarely develop invasive streptococcal illness, in part because of protective transplacental antibodies.[362] Equine antitoxin was used with some success in the treatment of erysipelas and scarlet fever in the 1920s and 1930s.[438,690]

Invasive Group A Streptococcal Infections

Invasive group A streptococcal infections, including septicemia, necrotizing fasciitis or myositis, and TSS, are increasing in severity and frequency.[27] Streptococcal pyrogenic exotoxins, including types A, B, and C, and mitogenic factor elaborated by certain strains of streptococci may be responsible for these serious complications of infection. Streptococcal pyrogenic exotoxins are potent superantigens that activate certain T lymphocytes directly and lead to the massive production of multiple cytokines, with resultant shock, fever, and organ failure. IGIV contains neutralizing antibodies that respond to these antigens,[508,509] but the titers vary across batches.[618]

Patients with invasive soft tissue infections with group A *Streptococcus* may benefit from high-dose IGIV.[182,258,508] In contrast to these reports, Mehta and colleagues[472] could not document a benefit for IGIV in patients admitted to the ICU with invasive group A infections from any cause.

Streptococcal Toxic Shock Syndrome

Many case reports have attested to the value of IGIV in streptococcal TSS since the report by Barry and coauthors in 1992.[17,72,185,417,431,553] Kaul and colleagues[368] reported a study of 21 consecutive patients at several Canadian medical centers in 1994 and 1995 who were treated with IGIV and compared them with 32 similar patients not given IGIV at the same centers for the 3 preceding years. Both groups received appropriate antibiotics and were similar with regard to demographics, severity score, and timing of intervention. The median IGIV dose was 2 g/kg. The survival rate for the IGIV-treated group was significantly greater at 7 and 30 days (90% and 67%, respectively) than that for the untreated controls (50% and 34%, respectively; $P = .02$), and the days of hospitalization were insignificantly shortened (29 vs. 39). Serum from the IGIV-treated patients caused a marked inhibition of lymphocyte mitogenic activity to their own bacterial isolates after a single IGIV dose. This study excluded children from the analysis because of ethical considerations and the overall lower mortality rate for the younger age groups.

In a large, multicenter, retrospective trial of children with streptococcal TSS,[625] IGIV was administered to 84 of 192 children with streptococcal TSS, and the overall mortality rate and overall hospital and drug costs were evaluated. The investigators found no added benefit of IGIV infusion and reported the increased costs for IGIV administration. However, in a study by Linner and colleagues that was reported in 2014, both IGIV and clindamycin therapy contributed to significantly improved survival of patients with streptococcal TSS.[431]

PANDAS Syndrome and Sydenham Chorea

Murphy and colleagues[493] and Swedo and coauthors[689] reported a syndrome of tics or obsessive-compulsive behavior, or both, occurring in prepubertal children soon after the onset of a streptococcal infection. They called the syndrome pediatric autoimmune neuropsychiatric disorders associated with streptococcal disease (PANDAS). They suggested a benefit for treatment of PANDAS with IGIV.[554] The National Institute of Mental Health is conducting a trial examining the benefits of IGIV for patients with PANDAS (http://clinicaltrials.gov/ct2/show/NCT01281969).

Sydenham chorea is a movement disorder that follows streptococcal infection. Successful treatment of Sydenham chorea with IGIV has been anecdotally reported.[729,746]

Recommendations

The use of IGIV can be considered as adjunctive therapy for TSS or necrotizing fasciitis in severely ill patients. Various regimens of IGIV, including 150 to 400 mg/kg per day for 5 days or a single dose of 1 to 2 g/kg, have been used, but the optimal regimen is unknown.[27] Repeated administration of IGIV may be necessary after a few days because of rapid IGIV catabolism.

IGIV may be beneficial for severe streptococcal soft tissue infections such as necrotizing fasciitis. IGIV has no proven benefit in PANDAS syndrome,[528] but studies are ongoing.

Tetanus, Tetanus Antitoxin, and Tetanus Immunoglobulin

Antitoxin for the treatment of tetanus was introduced into medicine by Behring and Kitasato in 1890; large doses (50 to 100 mL) of serum from horses immunized with tetanus toxin were used. The dose was increased gradually to 300 to 500 mL, which is equivalent to 300 to 500 U of antitoxin. As the means to increase the production and concentration of antitoxin developed and a high mortality rate persisted, the dosage of antitoxin was increased until doses as high as 200,000 U, repeated at weekly intervals, were recommended.[549] Despite such heroic therapy, no solid proof of efficacy was obtained.

In 1960, Brown and colleagues,[115] using sequential analysis, found that the mortality rate was 49% for 41 patients with tetanus who received 200,000 U of antitoxin, a statistically significant difference that established therapeutic efficacy. Extensive controlled studies established that mortality rates did not improve when larger doses (100,000–500,000 U) were used.[437,722–724]

Similarly, Patel and associates[547] could find no difference in the mortality rates of patients with tetanus treated with antitoxin doses of 5000 to 60,000 U. Adequate blood levels of antitoxin were observed in all cases, even in fatal cases, with a dose of 10,000 U. In mild cases, no antitoxin was necessary. They and others have reported considerable differences in mortality rates, ranging from 0% to 98%; the rate depends primarily on the severity of illness rather than on the dose of antitoxin.

Athavale and colleagues[54] established that antitoxin had benefit in tetanus neonatorum and in tetanus in children up to 12 years of age. Antitoxin affected the mortality rate in mild and moderate cases but not in severe ones. A dose of 10,000 U was as effective as one of 30,000 U.

The mechanism of action of antitoxin is to neutralize the toxin before it is transported to the nervous system through the circulation. Antitoxin also can neutralize toxin locally and prevent its systemic absorption. Antitoxin can be given locally at the site of production of toxin (e.g., site of a wound), intravenously in severe cases, or intramuscularly in less severe cases.

In 1962, an estimated 750,000 annual doses of equine tetanus antitoxin were needed in the United Kingdom, which is equivalent to more than a million doses in the United States.[594] Serum sickness occurs in 6% to 14% and fatal anaphylaxis in 1 of 100,000 injections of equine-derived antitoxin. Hyperimmune human tetanus immunoglobulin (TIG), first available in the early 1960s, gradually has replaced equine tetanus antitoxin.

Rubbo and Suri[593] and Rubinstein[594] showed that TIG given intramuscularly (5–10 U/kg) provides adequate circulating antitoxin levels. It is maintained in the circulation for considerably longer than is equine tetanus antitoxin.

The efficacy of TIG is equivalent to that of equine tetanus antitoxin. McCracken and associates[464] compared the results of 550 U of TIG with 10,000 U of tetanus antitoxin in the treatment of tetanus neonatorum. Among the 65 infants in each treatment group, no difference was observed in severity, length of hospitalization, need for sedation or gavage feeding, or mortality rate. Blake and colleagues[88] analyzed 545 tetanus cases reported to the CDC from 1965 to 1971 and found no difference in the outcome of patients treated with equine tetanus antitoxin or TIG.

The first use of intrathecal antitoxin was recorded in 1898 by Charles Church and Rambord from the Pasteur Institute and by Cushing in 1899.[549] In 1902, a French surgeon reviewed 27 cases of tetanus treated with intrathecal antitoxin and concluded that there was no additional benefit.[769]

Gupta and associates[291] gave TIG intrathecally to alternate patients with early tetanus. Among 49 patients given intrathecal TIG (250 U), three deteriorated, and one died; among 48 patients given intramuscular TIG (1000 U), 15 deteriorated, and 10 died. No side effects occurred. Herrero and coworkers[312] could not prove a benefit for administering intrathecal antitoxin for tetanus neonatorum. Although an early meta-analysis of intrathecal therapy cast doubt on its efficacy,[5] studies from India[247] and Brazil[478] and a larger meta-analysis[356] suggested a beneficial effect for intrathecal antibody.

TIG can be given along with tetanus toxoid for passive-active immunization. A dose of 250 U of TIG given intramuscularly at a site different from that of the toxoid does not interfere with the active antibody response.[463]

Lee and Lederman[420] measured the tetanus antitoxin titers in 29 lots of IGIV and found considerable variation, although all lots had titers greater than 4 U/mL (mean, 21 U/mL). All lots would provide sufficient anti–tetanus toxin antibody if used at doses of 100 mg/kg as an alternative to TIG or tetanus antitoxin.

Recommendations

Prophylaxis. If a nonimmunized person sustains a serious injury or a bite, 250 to 500 U of TIG should be given intramuscularly as soon as possible.[38] A larger dose is used in the event of an extensive wound or delay in treatment. TIG is available for intramuscular administration in individual vials containing 250 U. Alum-precipitated toxoid to initiate active immunity is given at a different site with a separate syringe.

Human IGIV also can be used if TIG is not available and should be administered at a dose of 200 to 400 mg/kg.[38] The use of IGIV is not FDA approved and the anti-tetanus antibody levels in IGIV are not routinely assessed.

If TIG or IGIV is unavailable, tetanus antitoxin (equine) can be administered after screening and testing for serum sensitivity have been performed.[38] Equine antitoxin for human use is available in several countries, but not in the United States, where TIG is available.

Treatment. In addition to administration of antibiotics and management of the wound, TIG should be given, but the optimal dose has not been established. At least 500 U is recommended, but doses as high as 3000 to 6000 U have been used. Some of the TIG is infiltrated near the wound, and the remainder is administered intramuscularly.[38] If the wound is extensive, TIG can be diluted with saline to infiltrate the entire area. TIG also is indicated for the treatment of tetanus neonatorum. Recent meta-analyses suggest that intrathecal use is beneficial for adults and infants.[356] A study of infants with neonatal tetanus showed mild improvement in outcome in infants who received intrathecal TIG.[11]

Equine tetanus antitoxin has been used when TIG is unavailable, but this product is not available in the United States. It should be given in a single dose of 100,000 U, with 50,000 U given intramuscularly and 50,000 given intravenously after appropriate testing for sensitivity. On recovery, the patient should undergo primary immunization.

McCracken and associates[464] found that 500 U of TIG given intramuscularly and 10,000 U of equine antitoxin were equally efficacious for tetanus neonatorum,. Intrathecal TIG has been recommended in certain clinical situations,[291,356,469] but it is not always beneficial.[77,312] TIG is not licensed for intrathecal use.

PASSIVE IMMUNITY IN VIRAL INFECTIONS

Enteroviruses

Poliovirus

Before the development of poliomyelitis vaccines in the mid-1950s, IGIM was used extensively for the prevention of poliomyelitis. Bodian[94,95] showed that Red Cross IGIM had neutralizing antibody to all three strains of poliovirus in approximately equal titers and that rhesus monkeys given intramuscular poliovirus could be protected against disease by the subcutaneous administration of IGIM.

Bloxsom,[92] in an uncontrolled study performed during a 1948 Texas epidemic, gave 841 contacts an average dose of 2 mL of IGIM and observed only four cases at 1, 2, 3, and 42 days after administration of the IGIM injection. His interpretation was that IGIM had been given too late to prevent the first three cases and that protection had worn off in the fourth case.

A committee on immunization of the National Foundation for Infantile Paralysis recommended in March 1951 that a controlled study be conducted on the efficacy of IGIM for the prevention of poliomyelitis during epidemics. Hammon and associates[299] subsequently undertook a massive field study in communities in three states during poliomyelitis epidemics.

Fifty-five thousand children between the ages of 1 and 11 years received IGIM (average dose, 0.14 mL/lb) or gelatin in a double-blind fashion. During the first week after injection was administered, 12 cases occurred among the IGIM recipients and 16 cases among the gelatin recipients. In the two groups, 3 and 23 cases occurred in the second week and 6 and 38 cases occurred in the third to fifth weeks, respectively. When protection was incomplete, decreased severity was observed. Protection waned by 6 weeks and disappeared by 8 weeks. These clinical results were confirmed by isolation of the virus or a rise in antibody titer in affected patients.

IGIM was an inefficient method of poliomyelitis prophylaxis in that it prevented only one case for every 500 to 2000 injections and only for a brief time. Its chief value was for close family contacts of affected children and for aborting severe local epidemics. IGIV failed to improve outcomes of patients with postpolio syndrome.[84,395]

Recommendations. The use of IGIM rarely is indicated for the prevention of poliomyelitis. An exposed unimmunized subject can be given 0.31 mg/kg of IGIM. An unimmunized patient who is traveling to an endemic or epidemic area and who cannot have vaccine can be given this dose of IGIM for temporary protection.

An immunodeficient patient inadvertently exposed to live attenuated polio vaccine who is excreting poliovirus in stool may be a candidate for receiving IGIV and oral immunoglobulin in an effort to rid the gastrointestinal tract of the virus.

Other Enteroviruses

Enteroviruses, particularly echoviruses and coxsackieviruses, can cause severe disease in neonates[334,429] and in immunodeficient patients, particularly those with X-linked agammaglobulinemia or common variable immunodeficiency.[577] IGIM and IGIV have been used in both groups for the prevention and treatment of these infections.[577]

Meningoencephalitis. Chronic enteroviral meningoencephalitis with severe neurologic findings may develop in agammaglobulinemic patients; however, the incidence has decreased since routine treatment with IGIV has been instituted for these patients. IGIV does not prevent all cases, likely as a result of different titers of antibodies to different enteroviral serotypes. McKinney and coworkers[467] summarized the results of treatment of 42 patients with chronic enterovirus meningoencephalitis: 10 received IGIM or plasma (one survived), 10 received IGIV (seven survived), and 12 received both intraventricular IGIV and systemic IGIV (10 survived).

Misbah and colleagues[480] reviewed 15 patients with chronic enteroviral meningoencephalitis not included in the McKinney report, some of whom had been described by others.[202,394] Of the five patients treated with IGIV, three survived, and of 10 treated with IGIV and intraventricular or intrathecal IGIV, five survived. Mellouli and colleagues[475] successfully treated an agammaglobulinemic boy who developed echovirus meningoencephalitis while receiving IGIV with intraventricular immunoglobulin through an Ommaya reservoir in addition to aggressive intravenous therapy.

Quartier and associates[565] reported complete clinical and virologic remission in two patients with X-linked agammaglobulinemia, as determined by culture and polymerase chain reaction (PCR) assay. The first patient was treated with IGIV and a brief course of pleconaril. The second patient was treated with IGIV and pleconaril, but intraventricular immunoglobulin was added when CSF pleocytosis persisted after 11 months of therapy. Complete clinical and virologic remission persisted at the 20-month follow-up. This study indicated that CSF PCR assay can be used in addition to viral culture as a guide to successful therapy.

Neonatal enteroviral infection. Severe and sometimes fatal disseminated enterovirus infection can develop in neonates.[566] Case reports have suggested a benefit with the use of IGIV.[334,348,726] Kimura and coworkers[384] treated coxsackievirus B3 infection in four term infants with IGIV. The three who were treated early survived, but the infant treated 6 days after the onset of infection died. Abzug and associates[6] treated nine infants with echovirus and coxsackievirus B infection with IGIV but without apparent benefit; however, three of five infants who received high-titer IGIV had a shortened period of viremia. Rentz and colleagues[578] suggested that the maternal plasma might be used in lieu of IGIV as a source of high-titer antibody for newborns with a severe enteroviral infection. Yen and colleagues evaluated the benefit of IGIV therapy for severe neonatal enteroviral infections and found that serum aspartate aminotransferase (AST) levels correlated with disease severity and that early IGIV therapy could improve survival.[785]

Nagington and colleagues[494] used IGIM successfully in an echovirus 11 outbreak in a special care nursery, but Kinney and coworkers[385] could not demonstrate a benefit for using IGIM in a similar nursery with the same virus. Pasic and associates[545] administered IGIV at 400 mg/kg prophylactically during a nursery echovirus 6 outbreak and thought that the severity of illness was decreased, although viral transmission continued.

Recommendations. IGIV may be used for critically ill neonates with disseminated enterovirus infection, although its benefit has not been proved. In an outbreak situation with a known serotype and the availability of IGIV with significant titer to this serotype, IGIV should be considered.[704] Multiple doses of 500 mg/kg and single doses of 750 to 1000 mg/kg have been used.[6,348,384,726]

For chronic enteroviral meningoencephalitis, McKinney and colleagues[467] recommend that sufficient IGIV be administered to maintain an IgG serum trough level of 900 to 1000 mg/dL. Higher doses may be needed if the IGIV titer for the infecting virus is low. Quartier and coworkers[565] used 500 mg/kg of IGIV every 24 to 48 hours for 2 weeks, followed by 500 mg/kg two to three times per week for 6 weeks and then gradual reductions, but with maintenance of the trough IgG level at greater than 800 mg/dL.

Administration of IGIV by intraventricular catheter should be considered for patients who do not improve despite receiving aggressive therapy with IGIV. IGIV for intraventricular administration should have a neutral pH, be given slowly, and be at room temperature.[467] Dwyer and Erlendsson[202] used 6% IGIV intraventricularly, starting at doses of 120 mg/day and increasing to 600 mg/day during the first week of treatment, followed by doses of 300 mg/day for 1 to 4 weeks. Quartier and colleagues[565] administered 300 mg of IGIV daily for 15 days and then 300 mg three times per week to a patient whose intravenous IGIV therapy had failed. The duration and frequency of intraventricular immunoglobulin and IGIV must be individualized and determined by clinical and virologic response and normalization of CSF and ventricular fluid. IGIV with a high titer to the infecting serotype should be used for systemic and intraventricular therapy.

Hepatitis A

The widest use for human IGIM has been for the prevention of hepatitis A, but this indication has been decreased by the widespread use of hepatitis A vaccine.[28] The efficacy of IGIM was demonstrated in 1945 by Stokes and Neefe[680] in aborting an epidemic in a children's summer camp, by Havens and Paul[304] in controlling an institutional epidemic, and by Gellis and associates[248] in preventing hepatitis A in the Mediterranean theater of operations at the close of World War II. The administration of combined IGIM and hepatitis A vaccine and scrupulous cleanliness can be used to interrupt the intestinal-oral circuit of transmission to abort an incipient epidemic.

IGIM is efficacious in preventing hepatitis A if it is given within 2 weeks of the last exposure.[9,28] Protection typically persists for 6 to 8 weeks. Stokes and associates[677] found that a single dose of IGIM (0.02 mL/

kg) provided a degree of protection for up to 9 months in individuals residing at an institution in which hepatitis A was endemic.

The effectiveness of IGIM in hepatitis A varies from 80% to 95%, depending on how soon it is administered after exposure and the severity of the exposure.[750] IGIM suppresses clinical manifestations of the disease, but anicteric hepatitis is not prevented, and the ratio of anicteric to icteric hepatitis may be as high as 12:1.[404] The period of protection exceeds the expected duration of the IGIM, supporting the concept of passive-active immunity. The hypothesis is that as a result of continuous exposure, a mild illness ensues, which confers long-lasting immunity.[404,676,749]

In initial studies, Stokes and Neefe[679] used an IGIM dose of 0.15 mL/lb, whereas others used doses of 0.06 to 0.12 mL/lb.[250,304] In 1951, Stokes and associates[677] showed that doses as low as 0.01 mL/lb were effective in limiting spread but did not completely prevent hepatitis. Hsia and colleagues[322] in 1954 also found that a dose of 0.01 mL/lb was effective in preventing hepatitis among family contacts. However, in 1958, Ward and associates[751] were able to reduce the case incidence of hepatitis among institutionalized patients from 19.5 to 7.4 cases per 1000 patients with 0.01 mL/lb and 1.7 cases per 1000 patients with 0.06 mL/lb. The larger dose may be particularly important for adults because they are subject to more severe disease.

The use of serologic tests for hepatitis A provides a way to determine the immunity of a subject, the presence of inapparent infection, the titer of hepatitis A virus (HAV) in lots of IGIM, and the validity of the passive-active immunity concept.[677,680] In other earlier studies, Krugman[400] showed that an IGIM preparation with a titer of 1:3200 was effective in neutralizing the infectivity of MS-1 serum, a substance that contains HAV. Farcet and colleagues evaluated the HAV antibody titer in plasma pools from March 2003 through September 2008 and determined the HAV titers adequate for HAV protection for those receiving antibody replacement for primary immune deficiency.[219]

Most current lots of IGIM have anti-HAV antibodies when they are assayed by a competitive-inhibition radioimmunoassay. Titers greater than 1:100 are protective.[651]

Recommendations

Household and sexual contacts. All previously unimmunized people with close contact with a person with HAV should be given a single IGIM dose of 0.02 mL/kg or single-antigen hepatitis A vaccine as soon as possible after being exposed.[9,28,735] For healthy people between the ages of 12 months and 40 years, single-antigen hepatitis A vaccine at the age-appropriate dose is preferred. For those older than 40 years, those younger than 12 months, immunocompromised individuals, people who have had chronic liver disease, and those for whom vaccine is contraindicated, IGIM is preferred.[504] Serologic testing for hepatitis A is unnecessary and may delay the administration of IGIM. The use of IGIM longer than 2 weeks after exposure has occurred but is not indicated.[28,232]

School exposure. IGIM usually is not necessary for children and their teachers exposed to a single case of hepatitis A in the classroom of a day school. However, if several children are infected or if transmission in the school is documented, IGIM (0.02 mL/kg) or vaccination is indicated for unimmunized students and teachers who have close contact with the index case. IGIM prophylaxis is recommended for children and staff exposed at a boarding school or in a school for developmentally disabled children, where opportunities for transmission by the fecal-oral route are increased.

Institutional outbreaks. Hepatitis A outbreaks in institutions such as boarding schools, childcare centers, custodial care centers, and prisons require aggressive action; however, the frequency of these outbreaks have decreased with increasing vaccination rates. Vaccine or IGIM should be administered to all previously unimmunized staff members and attendees if one or more cases of hepatitis A are recognized among children or staff or two or more cases among households with attendees at the centers. Vaccine or IGIM should be given to all household members with those in diapers at the centers if two or more families are affected.[9,28] If an outbreak of hepatitis A is traced to a food handler, IGIM or vaccine should be given to close contacts and other restaurant employees.[136]

Hospital and clinic exposure. When an outbreak occurs, vaccine or IGIM is recommended for people in close contact with the infected patient.[9]

Common source exposure. Common source exposure cases usually are identified too long after the exposure occurs for IGIM to be effective. If a person has been exposed within the previous 2 weeks, IGIM or vaccine can be given (0.02 mL/kg).[9]

Community outbreaks. Unless a source of the infection is identified, mass use of IGIM is ineffective and not recommended because it will not interfere with transmission.[53] Immunization is recommended.

Foreign travel. Individuals going to developing countries should receive vaccine 1 month before departure. Travelers who are administered vaccine can be assumed to be protected within 4 weeks after receiving the first vaccine dose.[148,232] If the departure date is less than 2 weeks away, 0.02 mL/kg of IGIM and vaccine can be used.[28] IGIM provides immediate protection and does not interfere with efficacy of the vaccine. If exposure to hepatitis A will continue beyond 3 months, the IGIM dose should be 0.06 mL/kg and repeated every 5 months if exposure to hepatitis A continues and the patient cannot be immunized.[9]

Primate exposure. Certain subhuman primates such as chimpanzees can carry HAV. Animal handlers should observe scrupulous hygiene and be given hepatitis A vaccine. If bitten and unimmunized, they should receive 0.02 mL/kg of IGIM and vaccine.[148]

Needle exposure. IGIM is indicated for susceptible people accidentally inoculated with blood or serum from a patient with hepatitis A. The recommended dose is 0.02 mL/kg; pregnancy is not a contraindication to the administration of IGIM.

Newborn infants of infected mothers. Perinatal transmission of HAV is rare. If the mother becomes symptomatic with acute hepatitis A between 2 weeks before and 1 week after delivery, the infant can be given 0.02 mL/kg of IGIM. Efficacy has not been established.[148]

Hepatitis B and Hepatitis B Immunoglobulin

Hepatitis B virus causes a wide spectrum of illness, ranging from asymptomatic seroconversion to fulminant hepatitis. Although most healthy patients recover completely, the carrier state occurs commonly in exposed immunocompromised patients, such as newborns, patients taking immunosuppressive medications, and patients with primary or secondary immunodeficiencies.

Transmission occurs after exposure to blood or other body fluids, through inoculation or sexual contact, and by close personal contact such as may occur in childcare centers. The main route of transmission used to be by blood transfusion, but with donor testing, this route is no longer common in developed countries. An important route of perinatal transmission is from the mother to the newborn infant, who is likely to remain chronically infected for a lifetime. This route usually can be prevented by active and passive immunization.

Immune Globulin Use in Hepatitis B

The initial study of IGIM in hepatitis B was conducted in 1945 by Grossman and associates,[283] who treated alternate battle casualties given whole blood or plasma with two 10-mL injections of IGIM 1 month apart. The incidence of icteric hepatitis was 1.3% among 384 IGIM-treated patients and 9.9% among 384 control patients. The highly significant difference suggested a beneficial effect of IGIM.

In 1947, Duncan and associates[200] reported the results from a similar study, although they gave only one 10-mL injection. Hepatitis occurred in 1.2% of 2406 patients in the IGIM-treated group and in 0.9% of patients in the control group, which was an insignificant difference. However, the mean incubation period was significantly prolonged for the IGIM-treated group (to 103 days) compared with the control group (87 days).

Holland and associates[317] could not alter the incidence or severity of posttransfusion hepatitis for 84 open-heart surgery patients by giving two 10-mL doses of IGIM 1 month apart compared with 83 non–IGIM-treated controls. These findings were confirmed in a large cooperative study of 5189 transfused cardiovascular patients given 10 mL of IGIM during the first, fourth, and seventh postoperative weeks.[268] Redeker and associates[574] could not demonstrate that IGIM protected spouses of individuals with type B hepatitis. Similarly, Kuhns and colleagues[407] could not reduce the incidence of posttransfusion hepatitis B with 20 mL of IGIM. Both latter studies used IGIM with low titers of antibody to hepatitis B surface antigen (anti-HBs).

Several factors probably are responsible for the variation in effectiveness of IGIM in hepatitis B. One is the degree of exposure to hepatitis B virus, which can be massive (e.g., blood transfusion) or minimal (e.g., household contact). A second factor is the different levels of antibody to hepatitis B surface antigen (anti-HBs) in different lots of IGIM. Because IGIM does not always contain high titers of anti-HBs, it is not recommended for hepatitis B prophylaxis. Standard immunoglobulin is not effective for postexposure prophylaxis against HBV infection because the concentration of anti-HBs is too low.[29]

Hepatitis B Immunoglobulin

Soon after hepatitis B surface antigen (HBsAg) and its antibody (anti-HBs) were identified, researchers could measure and select lots (or donors) with titers of anti-HBs of at least 1 : 100,000 by radioimmunoassay. This product, hepatitis B immunoglobulin (HBIG), has been licensed since 1978 for the prevention of hepatitis B.[28,140,142]

In 1971, Krugman and associates[401,404,405] evaluated high-titer HBIG in institutionalized children injected with the infective serum MS-2. Hepatitis developed in all 11 children exposed to MS-2 serum, and five remained HBsAg carriers after 320 days. Among five children given MS-2 serum and standard immunoglobulin, hepatitis developed in three, but none became a carrier. Of 10 children exposed to MS-2 serum and HBIG, six were completely protected, one had a transient infection, and three developed classic hepatitis. They concluded that HBIG was 70% effective under these circumstances. Their later studies confirmed that HBIG could reduce the incidence, severity, and carrier rate of HBsAg significantly after prenatal exposure to hepatitis B virus.[402]

Szmuness and associates[691] tested the efficacy of HBIG versus IGIM by giving standard IGIM or HBIG to institutionalized children at admission and at 4-month intervals for 1.5 to 2 years and compared the incidence of hepatitis with that among untreated patients. Both globulin-treated groups had a lower attack rate (11% [treated] vs. 25% [untreated]) and a lower incidence of persistent hepatitis B antigen (0% [treated] vs. 13.5% [untreated). IGIM and HBIG were effective in preventing or modifying nonparenterally transmitted hepatitis B in an endemic setting. Anti-HBs developed in 55% of the patients treated with standard IGIM, whereas antibody developed in only 23% of the patients treated with HBIG, suggesting that passive-active immunity occurred more frequently in the group that received standard IGIM than in the group that received HBIG.

Seeff and associates[620] gave HBIG or standard IGIM to 302 individuals definitively exposed orally or parenterally to material that was infectious for hepatitis B. The incidence of clinical and subclinical hepatitis during the first 6 months was 0.7% for the HBIG-treated group and 6.1% for the IGIM-treated group. At 6 months, 32% of the IGIM recipients and 6% of the HBIG recipients had antibody, a finding indicative of minimal passive-active immunity in the HBIG-treated group.

Grady[269] reported similar results with HBIG after accidental exposure. The incidence of hepatitis at 6 months was 7% (of 251 patients) with standard IGIM, 5% (of 208 patients) with intermediate-titer HBIG, and 2% (of 253 patients) with high-titer HBIG. This protection waned after 6 months, and differences in the groups became less apparent after 9 months, possibly because of reexposure, delayed onset of infection, or failure of passive-active immunity

Prevention of Vertical Transmission

Beasley and associates[75,76] studied the efficacy of HBIG in preventing perinatal transmission of the hepatitis B virus carrier state from a mother to her newborn infant. HBIG or placebo was given at birth to the infants of hepatitis B early antigen (HBeAg)–positive, HBsAg-positive carrier mothers, and the infants were monitored for at least 15 months. Of 61 placebo recipients, 92% became carriers; of 67 infants who received 1 mL of HBIG at birth, 54% became carriers; and of 57 infants who received 0.5 mL of HBIG at birth and at 3 and 6 months, 26% became carriers. Passive-active immunization, indicated by the presence of anti-HBs, occurred in 27% of the single-dose group and in 61% in the three-dose group.

On the basis of these and other studies[346,577] suggesting that multiple HBIG doses were more effective in interrupting vertical transmission of the HBsAg carrier state than a single HBIG dose, advisory committees in the early 1980s recommended that all infants of HBsAg-positive mothers be given HBIG (0.5 mL) immediately after birth and again at 3 and 6 months.[140,142] However, many of these infants became infected sometime after their last HBIG dose (i.e., in the second or third year of life), indicating a need for more durable active immunity. Shi and colleagues[633] systematically reviewed the effect of HBIG given in pregnancy to interrupt mother-to-child transmission of hepatitis B. They evaluated 37 randomized, controlled trials between January 1990 and December 2008 and concluded that there may be some benefit in HBIG use in pregnancy to prevent intrauterine transmission.

Wong and associates[778] studied the efficacy of hepatitis B vaccine given in conjunction with HBIG in the prevention of vertical transmission of the carrier state from mother to infant. They gave hepatitis B vaccine (36 infants), hepatitis B vaccine plus one dose of HBIG (35 infants), hepatitis B vaccine plus seven monthly HBIG doses (35 infants), or placebo (35 infants) to infants of HBsAg-positive mothers. In all vaccine groups, development of a persistent carrier state was reduced significantly compared with the placebo group (21% with hepatitis B vaccine alone, 2.9% with hepatitis B vaccine plus one dose of HBIG, and 6.8% with hepatitis B vaccine plus seven doses of HBIG vs. 73.2% for placebo groups). Anti-HBs developed in all infants of the treatment groups, indicating that HBIG did not interfere with active immunization.

This and other studies[693] indicate that HBIG given at the same time as hepatitis B vaccine provides optimal passive-active immunity for long-lasting prevention of the carrier state, and this dose of 0.5 mL is the current recommendation. Studies of adults confirm that HBIG given before or simultaneously with the first dose of hepatitis B vaccine does not interfere with the antibody response to hepatitis B vaccine.[789] This approach can protect 85% to 95% of infants from perinatally acquired HBV infection.[151]

HBIG is not of value in the treatment of acute[7] or chronic[576] hepatitis B infection.

Hepatitis B Immunoglobulin in Liver Transplantation

Liver transplantation in a patient infected with hepatitis B is associated with a high rate of its recurrence in the new liver and subsequent death (50% in 2 years). Intravenous HBIG has proven efficacy and a dose-dependent response in the prevention of HBV recurrence after liver transplantation.[170] It has been the mainstay of posttransplantation prophylaxis for recurrent HBV since the early 1990s.[123] The HBIG doses needed to prevent reinfection are very high, and HBIG primarily is given intravenously.[706]

HBIG given intravenously or by the usual intramuscular route can reduce the rate of recurrence of hepatitis B.[603] In a retrospective analysis of 359 transplantations, the rate of hepatitis B recurrence was 74% ± 6% among 67 patients given no HBIG, 74% ± 5% among 83 patients given HBIG for 2 months, and 36% ± 4% among the 209 patients given HBIG for 6 months or longer.

Grazi and coworkers[274] reduced significantly the recurrence rate in HBsAg-positive, hepatitis B virus DNA–negative cirrhotic individuals undergoing liver transplantation with the use of HBIG for 1 year after transplantation. Recurrence was seen in 8 (80%) of 10 controls and four (16%) of 25 HBIG-treated patients. Other reports are available.[703,705]

In addition to HBIG therapy, pretransplantation and posttransplantation antiviral drugs such as lamivudine or entecavir are used. When administered in the immediate pretransplantation period to patients with a high viral burden, these drugs enhance the effectiveness of HBIG because less virus must be neutralized.[13,323,366,585,703] Long-term maintenance of antivirals with discontinuation of HBIG after several months may be feasible.[164,719,777]

Preliminary studies of monoclonal antibodies to hepatitis B antigens are being conucted.[155,264,794]

Recommendations.

Prophylaxis. HBIG is recommended after a person's parenteral or mucous membrane (e.g., oral, sexual, ophthalmic) has contact with blood or body fluids from individuals with hepatitis B or with

TABLE 246.4 Postexposure Recommendations for Hepatitis B Immunoglobulin and Hepatitis B Vaccine

	HEPATITIS B IMMUNOGLOBULIN		HEPATITIS B VACCINE	
Type of Exposure to Hepatitis B	**Dose**	**Recommended Timing**	**Dose**	**Recommended Timing**
Perinatal				
Infant of HBsAg-positive mother	0.5 mL IM	Within 12 h of birth	0.5 mL	First dose within 12 h, repeat 2 times
Infant of mother whose HBsAg status is unknown	0.5 mL IM	Within 7 days of birth if mother is found to be HBsAg positive	0.5 mL	First dose within 12 h, repeat 2 times
Premature infant (<2000 g) whose mother's HBsAg status is unknown	0.5 mL IM	Within 12 h of birth (unless maternal HBsAg test result is negative by this time)	0.5 mL	First dose within 12 h, repeat 3 times
Mucous Membrane or Percutaneous With Known Nonoccupational Exposure				
Nonvaccinated	0.06 mL/kg IM	Immediately	0.5 mL[a]	First dose immediately, repeat 2 times
Previously vaccinated, known responder	None	None	None	—
Previously vaccinated, unknown response	0.06 mL/kg IM	Test patient for anti-HBs; omit HBIG[b] if anti-HBs is >10 mIU/mL	0.5	Give booster[b]
Previously vaccinated, known nonresponder	0.06 mL/kg IM	Immediately, may repeat in 1 mo if <10 mIU/mL[c]	0.5 mL[a]	Give booster immediately, repeat 2 times if necessary
Sexual, Known Exposure				
Nonvaccinated	0.06 mL/kg IM	Immediately, but no later than 14 days	0.5 mL[a]	First dose immediately, repeat 2 times
Vaccinated[b]	None	None	0.5 mL	Give booster if unknown response

[a]Dose is for individuals younger than 20 years. The adult vaccine dose is 1 mL. The dose for immunosuppressed patients and patients undergoing dialysis varies with the vaccine used. Vaccine doses given in the table are for Recombivax HB or Engerix-B.

[b]Recent CDC recommendations for exposure (sexual, sexual assault, percutaneous, or mucosal) from a source with unknown hepatitis B status are to forgo vaccine and HBIG if the exposed patient is already immunized and has written documentation of complete vaccine series and did not receive serologic testing for response. Individual assessments of potential risk must be made.

[c]People who have not responded to two vaccine series are discussed in the text.

HBIG, Hepatitis B immunoglobulin; *anti-HBs*, antibody to hepatitis B surface antigen; *HBsAg*, hepatitis B surface antigen.

HBsAg-positive materials (e.g., blood, plasma) and for neonates born to HBsAg-positive mothers (see Table 246.3).[29]

Exposure to blood that contains or may contain hepatitis B surface antigen. No prospective studies have tested the efficacy of a combination of HBIG and hepatitis B vaccine in preventing hepatitis B after accidental exposure, including exposure by the percutaneous, ocular, and mucous membrane routes or by human bites that penetrate the skin. Health care workers at risk for accidents should receive hepatitis B vaccine because preexposure immunization is the most effective means to prevent HBV transmission.[29] For unimmunized people, the combination of HBIG and hepatitis B vaccine is recommended after significant accidental exposure (Table 246.4).

If the exposed patient is unimmunized and the blood or secretions come from an individual known to be HBsAg positive or the infection status of the source is unknown but the source is at high risk, immediate prophylaxis is indicated. A single dose of HBIG (0.06 mL/kg or 5 mL for adults) should be given intramuscularly as soon as possible, preferably within 24 hours of exposure.[29] Hepatitis B vaccine should be given simultaneously at a different site and repeated after 1 and 6 months (see Table 246.4). After massive exposure (i.e., by blood transfusion), much larger doses of HBIG may be indicated.

If the exposed patient has been immunized but the serologic response is not known, anti-HBs titers should be determined and the individual treated according to the results; if nonresponsive (i.e., anti-HBs <10 mIU/mL by radioimmunoassay), HBIG and a full series of vaccine should be given. For patients with a contraindication to vaccine, two doses of HBIG (0.06 mL/kg) should be used, the second administered 1 month after the first. Two doses of HBIG also should be given to an exposed health care worker who is known to have no response to two series of hepatitis B vaccine.[29]

The CDC recommendation[148] for nonoccupational exposures is to administer vaccine alone to previously immunized individuals as a booster dose without the need to document serologic response if the exposed person has written documentation of a completed hepatitis B vaccine series. The *Red Book*[29] agrees with this booster vaccine approach. I recommend a more individualized approach for assessing risks of the addition of HBIG.

Perinatal exposure. Among mothers who are HBsAg positive and HBeAg positive, 85% of their untreated infants will become infected and be chronic carriers, and chronic hepatitis, cirrhosis, or hepatic cancer will develop in some of them. If the mother is HBsAg positive only, the risk for her offspring of becoming a carrier is less but still significant. More than 90% of infants infected perinatally develop chronic HBV infection.[29] These infants should receive HBIG prophylaxis and hepatitis B vaccine.

Infants born to mothers who are HbsAg positive. For optimal passive-active immunity, HBIG (0.5 mL) is given to the newborn at birth (preferably in the delivery room but within 12 hours at the latest). Hepatitis B vaccine (at a dose that is one half of the adult dose) is begun simultaneously and repeated at 1 and 6 months (see Table 246.3). This combination is only about 90% effective in preventing the carrier state because intrauterine infection is not prevented.

Term infants born to mothers not tested for HBsAg. If the HBsAg status of the mother is unknown, hepatitis B vaccine should be given to the term infant within 12 hours, and HBIG should be administered as soon as the mother is shown to be a carrier. Its effectiveness is diminished markedly if administration is delayed beyond 48 hours after birth but is recommended to be given up to 7 days after birth.[29]

The mother should be tested immediately. If she is HBsAg negative, the vaccine series is continued as recommended for other infants. If the mother is found to be HBsAg positive, HBIG and hepatitis B vaccine should be given to her infant, even if a significant delay has occurred. After the final dose of the vaccine series, the infant can be tested for HBsAg and anti-HBs at 9 to 18 months to determine the success of the HBIG and vaccine regimen. Testing should not be performed before 9 months of age to avoid detection of anti-HBs from HBIG administered during infancy and to maximize the likelihood of detecting late HBV infections.[29] If HBsAg is found, the infant is a carrier. If anti-HBs is detected, the child was successfully immunized. Administration of HBIG at birth should not interfere with polio or DTaP vaccines starting at 2 months of age.

Premature infants. Premature infants with birth weights less than 2000 g who are born to women not tested for HBsAg should be given HBIG (0.5 mL) within 12 hours of birth unless the mother's HBsAg test result can be available within 12 hours and is negative. Immunization should be started immediately and repeated for a total of four doses (rather than the usual three doses) because of the poorer response of preterm infants to the vaccine.[29]

Sexual exposure to hepatitis B or a carrier of hepatitis B. Sexual exposure (including rape) to an individual who has hepatitis B or is a carrier is an indication for administration of HBIG (0.06 mL/kg intramuscularly; maximum, 5 mL) and initiation of hepatitis B vaccination. HBIG should be given as soon as possible but not after 14 days after exposure. If only HBIG is given, a second dose of HBIG is recommended after 30 days. The CDC[148] also recommends booster vaccine alone in this situation if written documentation is available for a completed hepatitis B vaccine series.

Possible exposure. After possible exposure (e.g., percutaneous, ingestion, sexual) to an unidentified person or body fluid for which the HBsAg status is unknown, the decision to treat with HBIG must be made individually on the basis of the likelihood that the source is HBsAg positive and the seriousness of the exposure. Hepatitis B vaccine should be initiated immediately if the exposed person is not immunized. Current *Red Book* and CDC recommendations[29] suggest that in cases of an unknown source, vaccine alone is acceptable for an unvaccinated exposed patient and that no treatment is required if the exposed person has written documentation of previous immunization. I recommend a more individual approach to assess risks.

Ideally, the source subject should be tested for HBsAg positivity; if the results are available within 7 days for a percutaneous exposure and 14 days for a sexual exposure,[29] HBIG (0.06 mL/kg; maximum, 5 mL) can be given immediately and again at 1 month if the source is HBsAg positive and the patient did not or could not receive vaccine. When the source subject cannot be tested or the source is likely to be HBsAg positive, HBIG is administered immediately.

If the exposed individual is a high-risk patient (e.g., immunodeficient, immunosuppressed, institutionalized, undergoing hemodialysis) or is in an environment or health care unit for which past environmental control measures have been ineffective, HBIG should be given in addition to hepatitis B vaccine.

HBIG is not indicated on a routine basis after administration of blood transfusions. School or hospital exposure or usual household exposure is not an indication for HBIG, but household exposure is an indication for vaccine for unimmunized exposed individuals.[29]

Liver transplantation. For patients who are HBsAg positive at the time they undergo liver transplantation or in the rare situation in which the donor of the liver is HBsAg positive, administration of HBIG is recommended in the preoperative period and after transplantation to prevent recurrence in the transplanted liver.[274,490,603,604,701,703,708]

The typical regimen is to use very high HBIG doses (i.e., 2000 IU [10 mL]/wk) before transplantation and immediately after transplantation along with antiviral medications.[703] The HBIG is continued for several months to years, and the dose is determined by monitoring of the hepatitis B viral burden by PCR. After several months, the HBIG dose may be reduced or discontinued, but the antivirals are continued, as discussed earlier.[777]

Hepatitis C

Early studies suggested that lots of polyvalent IGIM or HBIG not screened for hepatitis C antibodies provided some protection against the acquisition of non-A, non-B hepatitis (presumably hepatitis C) after heart surgery or hemodialysis.[387,607,648]

Two studies provide some evidence for a prophylactic effect of IGIM. Piazza and colleagues[556] gave polyvalent IGIM (from pools containing antibodies to hepatitis C virus [HCV]) or placebo monthly for 4 to 20 months to the seronegative sexual partners of 884 patients who were seropositive for HCV. One of the 450 (representing 560 subject-years) in the IGIM group became infected, compared with 6 of 449 (500 subject-years) in the placebo group (P = .03; relative risk, 10.7). The study authors concluded that sexual transmission of hepatitis C occurs and that immunoglobulin has a protective effect.

Féray and associates[225] reviewed the records of 218 patients with hepatitis C coinfection undergoing liver transplantation who received an HBIG product that contained antibody to HCV. The incidence of HCV viremia 1 year after transplantation was significantly lower (25 [54%] of 46) among patients receiving HBIG than those not receiving it (162 [94%] of 172; P < .001). They also reviewed 210 transplanted HCV-seronegative patients and found that hepatitis C developed within 1 year in 18 (26%) of 68 patients who received the HBIG product containing anti-HCV antibody, in contrast to 40 (47%) of 86 patients who did not receive HBIG, a significant difference (P < .001) suggesting a preventive effect of hepatitis C antibodies.

Also supporting this concept was the observation that HCV was transmitted by pooled human immunoglobulin in the early 1990s, shortly after HCV antibody–positive donors were excluded from the donor pool.[146,614] These antibodies presumably neutralized the small amounts of HCV in the unscreened lots. Yu and colleagues[788] demonstrated that HCV antibodies in unscreened immunoglobulin lots containing HCV antibodies prevented low-dose infection in chimpanzees. Screened IGIM lots after 1991 lacking HCV antibodies did not prevent infection.

Because HBIG can prevent recurrence of hepatitis B among patients with hepatitis B undergoing liver transplantation,[274,604] researchers have postulated that hepatitis C antibodies might prevent recurrence in hepatitis C–positive liver transplant recipients. Studies are ongoing to develop monoclonal antibodies, immunomodulators, and vaccines to effectively neutralize HCV.[12,100,253,369,370,532,748] Bavituximab is a monoclonal antibody that targets phosphatidylserine, a specific phospholipid component of cell membranes that become exposed on the outer membrane of cells infected with HCV. A phase I study demonstrated mild adverse events for six patients.[12]

Experimental Hepatitis C Immunoglobulin

Experimental HCV-IGIV is derived from human plasma units rejected for HBIG or IGIV manufacture because of the presence of hepatitis C antibodies. It does not contain hepatitis C, as tested by PCR. Krawczynski and colleagues[397] showed that HCV-IGIV delayed but did not prevent experimental hepatitis C infection in chimpanzees, in contrast to regular IGIV without hepatitis C antibodies.

Willems and colleagues[766] gave HCV-IGIV to 26 hepatitis C–positive liver transplant recipients during the ahepatic and postoperative periods without decreasing the rate of recurrence of hepatitis C. Davis and colleagues[187] reported a multicenter, double-blind study of HCV-IGIV (Civacir, Nabi) in hepatitis C–positive liver-transplant recipients. No effect occurred on HCV RNA levels, but some decrease in liver enzyme activities compared with control patients was observed. The use of antibody to prevent the development of hepatitis C after liver transplantation has not been successful, which was attributed to limitations of dosing and the inability of HCV-IGIV to neutralize the HCV RNA in phase II trials.[187]

Recommendations. No passive immune product is available for hepatitis C prophylaxis.

Herpesviruses

The common herpesviruses that cause human infection are CMV, Epstein-Barr virus (EBV), herpes simplex virus types 1 and 2, varicella-zoster virus, and human herpesviruses 6, 7, and 8. Although these DNA viruses produce latent infection that can reactivate, particularly in immunodeficient patients, the major uses of immunoglobulins have been in the prevention of primary varicella-zoster virus infection and prevention and treatment of CMV infection in transplant recipients and in pregnant women and their fetuses with primary infection.

Cytomegalovirus

Use of cytomegalovirus intravenous immunoglobulin or intravenous immunoglobulin in transplantation. CMV infection remains a major complication after hematopoietic cell transplantation and solid organ transplantation. Seronegative individuals who receive an allograft from a seropositive donor are at the highest risk for acquiring CMV infection. Polyvalent IGIV and hyperimmune CMV intravenous immunoglobulin (CMV-IGIV [CMVIG]) have been used since the 1980s to prevent development of CMV infection in bone marrow and solid organ transplant recipients.[774] Clinical trials in the 1990s demonstrated the efficacy of prophylaxis with IGIV in preventing CMV infection and pneumonia. CMVIG is prepared from the plasma of donors with high anti-CMV titers, but polyvalent IGIV also contains anti-CMV antibodies at a lower titer. Early studies used CMVIG or IGIV alone, but later studies have combined immunoglobulin with antiviral agents.

Early studies of renal and liver transplant recipients showed the efficacy of CMVIG or IGIV.[654] Two meta-analyses demonstrated decreased CMV mortality rates with the use of CMVIG or IGIV in bone marrow and solid organ transplant recipients.[776] Others have shown a similar prophylactic benefit for IGIV or CMVIG.[476,639] Ruutu and coworkers[599] showed no prophylactic benefit for CMVIG in CMV-seronegative bone marrow transplant recipients. A multicenter retrospective review[571] of CMVIG prophylaxis in addition to intravenous ganciclovir in pediatric lung transplant recipients did not demonstrate a decrease in post-transplant CMV infection or morbidity rates.

Several factors that have reduced the need for CMVIG or IGIV in transplant recipients include the realization of a markedly reduced risk for development of CMV if the donor and recipient are CMV antibody negative (D^-/R^-), use of CMV-seronegative or filtered blood products, early detection of CMV by PCR, and use of ganciclovir-valganciclovir prophylaxis or early treatment.[297]

Snydman and colleagues,[653] in an open-label, multicenter study of liver transplantation, found that the combination of CMVIG and ganciclovir was superior to different immunosuppressive regimens in historical controls. Campbell and colleagues[132] recommended universal prophylaxis for the patients at highest risk, children receiving liver transplants (D^+/R^-), but the role of immunoglobulin was uncertain.

For heart and lung transplant recipients, the use of CMVIG for CMV infection prophylaxis has been recommended by some groups if the donor or the recipient is CMV seropositive. Weill and associates[754] showed that combined ganciclovir and CMVIG reduced the incidence of CMV infection in high-risk lung transplant recipients compared with historical controls. In a retrospective study, Ruttmann and colleagues[598] showed decreased morbidity resulting from CMV infection in lung transplant recipients given CMVIG and ganciclovir compared with the use of ganciclovir alone. A meta-analysis examining the use of CMV hyperimmune globulin (CMVIG) for the prevention of CMV infection and disease in solid organ transplant recipients demonstrated that prophylactic administration of CMVIG was associated with improved total survival and a reduced frequency of CMV-related disease and deaths.[99]

Zamora and associates[792] recommended intravenous ganciclovir and CMVIG for all lung transplant recipients when the donor or recipient is CMV seropositive; and in the situation of D^+/R^-. They gave seven infusions of CMVIG in the first 90 days after transplantation. Other investigators[99,184,725] and consensus statements[45,561] permit the use of combined therapy with CMVIG for high-risk heart and lung transplant recipients and other solid organ recipients, despite the absence of definitive controlled studies. The use of IGIV for the treatment of hemophagocytic lymphohistiocytosis associated with CMV infection also has been reported.[320]

Use of cytomegalovirus intravenous immunoglobulin in perinatal cytomegalovirus infection. Another use of CMVIG may be the treatment of in utero CMV infection.[503] Two infusions of CMVIG were given intraperitoneally at 28 and 29 weeks' gestation to a CMV-infected fetus. The therapeutic benefit was unclear because the infant had intracranial calcifications at 2 weeks of age but was free of neurologic symptoms at 1 year of age. Matusuda and colleagues[458] and Sato and associates[610] used serial anti-CMV immunoglobulin injections into the fetal abdominal cavity to treat acute CMV infection in a fetus with a good fetal outcome.

Nigro and associates[507] treated a pregnant woman with primary CMV infection and in utero infection of one twin fetus with intravenous CMVIG at 30 weeks' gestation. CMVIG also was injected into the amniotic sac. The affected twin had better growth, decreased placental thickening, and lessened cord edema. Although born with CMV infection and hepatosplenomegaly, the child was normal at the age of 2 years.

Nigro and colleagues[505] gave 31 pregnant women with primary CMV infection at least one dose of CMVIG (200 U/kg) during pregnancy. Ultrasonic evidence of CMV infection was seen in 15 fetuses. Nine women received additional CMVIG into their amniotic sac or umbilical cord. Only one woman gave birth to an infant with CMV infection, compared with seven of 14 women who did not receive CMVIG during pregnancy. All of these women had in utero infection confirmed by CMV-positive (culture or PCR) amniotic fluid. The infants of mothers who received CMVIG during the first half of the pregnancy were followed in a case-control study evaluating their outcomes compared with those of 32 congenitally infected infants whose mothers did not receive CMVIG during pregnancy.[506] The risk for having a CMV-affected child with psychomotor retardation and hearing deficit was significantly higher in the untreated group, leading the study authors to conclude that immunoglobulin administered during the first half of pregnancy to women with primary CMV infection decreases neurologic sequelae associated with in utero CMV infection.

Another group[737] compared infected infants born to women with primary CMV infection before 17 weeks' gestation who were treated with 200 U/kg of Cytotect (CMVIG product available in Europe) with those who were untreated and participants in a natural history study. At 1 year of age, four of 31 infants of Cytotect-treated mothers had poor outcome compared with the 16 infants from 37 untreated mothers. Results from a double-blind, randomized, placebo-controlled trial of Cytotect prophylaxis in 124 patients suggested protection against in utero fetal infection (44% in the placebo group vs. 30% in the treated group).[446] However, treatment with CMVIG did not significantly modify the course of primary CMV infection, and the clinical outcomes were similar for the two groups.[579]

Recommendations. Patients undergoing allogeneic human stem cell transplantation who are at risk for CMV disease (e.g., a CMV-seropositive recipient or a CMV-seronegative recipient and a CMV-seropositive donor) should receive prophylactic antiviral therapy or preemptive antiviral therapy after early detection of infection by CMV PCR. Routine use of CMVIG is not recommended for prevention of CMV disease.[96]

Similarly, for solid organ recipients, the highest risk is a CMV-seropositive donor and a CMV-seronegative recipient, in which case antiviral prophylaxis is used. Antiviral prophylaxis rather than CMVIG or IGIV is used in kidney and liver transplantation.[342,623] In high-risk situations such as heart and lung transplantation with a CMV-seropositive donor or recipient, some centers use CMVIG in addition to antiviral therapy, despite lack of proof by multicenter, randomized studies.[99,561,725]

CMVIG or IGIV in combination with antiviral agents is used to treat severe CMV disease, such as pneumonia, in transplant recipients.[241,533,550,575,790] For CMVIG, 400 mg/kg on days 1, 2, and 7 and 200 mg/kg on days 14 and 21 have been used in addition to antiviral therapy,[575] although others have used a lower dose (100 mg/kg every other day for 2 weeks).[249] IGIV administered as 500 mg/kg every other day for 10 to 59 days, followed by 500 mg/kg once or twice weekly for an extended period, also has been reported.[531] Garcia-Gallo and colleagues[243] reported the use of CMVIG as an adjunct to antiviral therapy to prevent development of pneumonitis in lung transplant recipients with invasive CMV disease and as preemptive therapy (with ganciclovir) in posttransplant recipients with a persistent CMV viral load.

CMVIG for in utero CMV infection is not recommended routinely, but several studies have demonstrated its safety and efficacy. Its use may be of value in selected situations of confirmed primary maternal infection or fetal infection.

Epstein-Barr Virus

EBV, the etiologic agent of infectious mononucleosis, causes severe infection in immunocompromised patients and males with X-linked lymphoproliferative syndrome. IGIV has been given to EBV-seronegative males with X-linked lymphoproliferative syndrome in an attempt to prevent EBV infection, but EBV infection developed in some of them despite IGIV adminstration.[230]

Transplant recipients with EBV-induced posttransplantation lymphoproliferative syndrome or hepatitis have been treated successfully with a combination of IGIV or CMVIG, antiviral therapy, and IFN-α.[190,515,696] Ramirez-Arila and associates[568] studied the concentrations of antibody to EBV in four lots of CMV-IVIG and found that standard EVIG contained higher concentrations of anti EBV antibody than the CMV-IVIG. They also observed that the CMV-IVIG was 1.8 times more expensive than standard IVIG.

A similar approach was unsuccessful in X-linked lymphoproliferative syndrome.[525] CMVIG was used in one case because it contains higher titers of anti-EBV antibody than IGIV.[190] One case of fulminant EBV hepatitis was treated successfully with liver transplantation, antiviral therapy, and CMVIG.[224]

A multicenter trial indicated that CMVIG given to liver transplant recipients did not prevent posttransplantation lymphoproliferative disease or other EBV disease.[276] However, the EBV serology was unavailable for 50 of the 82 donors, hampering interpretation of the results.

Ohta and colleagues[524] reported marked improvement of a patient with chronic EBV hepatitis after kidney transplantation by treatment with the anti-CD20 monoclonal antibody rituximab after failure to reduce immunosuppression. Rituximab has been used successfully in the treatment of EBV-induced posttransplantation lymphoproliferative disease in stem cell transplantation[221,636,683] and solid organ transplantion.[165,303,310,699,784]

Rituximab also has been used in preemptive therapy in stem cell transplantation based on EBV viral load.[167,728] Boesch and colleagues[97] reported the successful use of rituximab to treat an adolescent without immunodeficiency who developed EBV-associated lymphoproliferative disease that involved massive submucosal infiltration of B cells in the lingual tonsils, trachea, and bronchi and resultant near-complete airway obstruction that was unresponsive to steroids. A 28-year-old recipient of an orthotopic liver transplant was successfully treated with antiviral therapy and IGIV for EBV-related posttransplantation lymphoproliferative disease refractory to rituximab.[712] Some centers use IGIV or CMVIG in addition to antiviral therapy as prophylaxis in high-risk transplant recipients.[277]

Recommendations. Current approaches to EBV-induced posttransplantation lymphoproliferative disease include reduction of immunosuppression and consideration of preemptive therapy or treatment with rituximab,[657] although antiviral medication, anticytokine therapy, chemotherapy, and immunotherapy all have been used. In a literature review, Giulino and colleagues[257] found evidence of a better response to rituximab in children compared with adults and suggested that rituximab might be appropriate as first-line therapy for posttransplantation lymphoproliferative disease in children. The role of IGIV or CMVIG in addition to the use of anti-CD20 monoclonal antibodies has not been clearly defined.

Herpes Simplex Infections

Neutralizing antibody has a protective effect in herpes simplex virus (HSV) infection in the newborn period. Mothers with a reactivated herpes infection during delivery are 10-fold less likely to transmit HSV to their newborn infants during vaginal delivery than are mothers with primary HSV infection at delivery, presumably because of the transplacental transfer of antiherpes antibody.[30,564] IGIV-containing HSV antibodies have not been used in the prevention of neonatal herpes infection, although Whitley[761] proposed that HSV monoclonal antibody or hyperimmune IGIV should be evaluated for treatment of disseminated neonatal disease.

Masci and colleagues[456] compared monthly IGIV (400 mg/kg) with intermittent acyclovir treatment (800 mg twice daily for 1 week each month) in patients with recurrent genital HSV infection for 6 months and found fewer recurrences in the IGIV-treated group.

Recommendations. IGIV is not recommended for the prevention or treatment of HSV infections.

Varicella-Zoster Virus and Varicella-Zoster Immunoglobulin

Immunoglobulin for varicella. After success was achieved with IGIM in the prevention of measles and hepatitis, IGIM was evaluated for the prevention of varicella. Although Funkhouser[238] in 1948 showed some beneficial effects for the use of standard IGIM in the prevention of varicella in an uncontrolled study, Greenberg and colleagues[278] and Schaeffer and Toomey[612] were unable to prevent chickenpox in exposed children with IGIM doses of 2.5 to 20 mL.

Others have reported anecdotal evidence for the efficacy of IGIM in large doses during the early stages of chickenpox and herpes zoster. These claims included prompt relief of pain in zoster[756] and rapid resolution of skin lesions.[418,586] However, even high-titer zoster immunoglobulin does not prevent dissemination of herpes zoster.[667]

In 1962, Ross[591] gave 242 children IGIM in doses of 0.1 to 0.6 mL/lb within 3 days of exposure to chickenpox; 209 similarly exposed, uninjected children were used as controls. The attack rate was the same (97%) in both groups, indicating that IGIM does not prevent varicella under these conditions. However, with doses of IGIM above 0.2 mL/lb, the severity of the disease was reduced, as indicated by a decreased number of pox and reduced temperature. Children receiving the largest dose of IGIM (0.6 mL/lb) had maximal temperatures of 38.9°C (102°F) compared with 41.1°C (106°F) for controls and had 40 pox compared with 207 for controls. Other investigators have reported similar but uncontrolled observations that immunoglobulin modifies the severity of chickenpox.[333,713]

Varicella-zoster immunoglobulin for varicella. The prophylactic value of large immunoglobulin doses in decreasing the incidence and severity of varicella led to a trial of high-titer plasma or immunoglobulin preparations to prevent varicella.[62] They include zoster immunoglobulin (ZIG) and plasma (ZIP) from convalescing zoster patients and varicella-zoster immunoglobulin (VZIG) prepared from high-titer plasma from normal adults.

In 1969, Brunell and associates[119] selected convalescing patients with zoster whose complement-fixing antibody titers were 1:256 or greater and prepared ZIG from their plasma; this material had titers considerably higher than did standard immunoglobulin. Exposed children from six families in which chickenpox was occurring were given ZIG or immunoglobulin at doses of 2 mL. In none of six children receiving ZIG did chickenpox develop, whereas it developed in all six children given standard immunoglobulin. No antibody developed in the ZIG-treated group, indicating that the disease was prevented.

Because this dose did not prevent varicella in leukemic children or other high-risk patients, a larger dose (5 mL) was used in a later study to successfully modify or to prevent varicella in eight of nine high-risk children.[118,116] Severe varicella developed in one child given a less potent preparation of ZIG. These observations were confirmed in two later studies. Judelsohn and associates[354] gave ZIG to 56 exposed high-risk children; mild varicella occurred in seven patients and was prevented in the others, most of whom were susceptible as determined by absence of serum antibody. Gershon and colleagues[251] gave ZIG to 15 seronegative, high-risk exposed children; varicella was severe in one, mild in nine, and subclinical in five. Subclinical infection was determined by the acquisition of membrane antibody as detected by fluorescent microscopy.

Orenstein and associates[530] studied 553 exposed, high-risk patients who received ZIG of two different titers (≥1:1280 vs. 1:2560). They found that the clinical attack rate after receipt of ZIG correlated with the type of exposure (i.e., varicella developed in 36% with household exposure, 7.7% with hospital exposure, and 0% with school exposure), the rise in antibody titer (i.e., 45% of patients without a fourfold titer increase became ill in contrast to 22% of patients with a fourfold or greater rise in titer), and the titer of the administered ZIG (i.e., significantly more complications and deaths occurred in recipients of the lower titer ZIG).

Because of the limited supply of ZIG and ZIP, VZIG from normal adults became the commercially available product in the United States. Zaia and associates[791] compared the efficacy of ZIG and VZIG in immunocompromised children exposed to varicella. Varicella attack rates and the clinical severity in recipients of VZIG and ZIG were not significantly different. A higher incidence of subclinical infection was indicated by the rise in antibody titer in ZIG recipients (31.3%) compared with that in VZIG recipients (16%). A larger dose of VZIG (2.5 mL/10 kg vs. 1.25 mL/10 kg) reduced the frequency of subclinical infection from 20% to 4.3%. Varicella developed in several high-risk patients with demonstrable serum antibody at exposure, indicating that history-negative, seropositive patients are at risk for clinical varicella-zoster infection and should be given VZIG regardless of antibody titer.

In 2006, VZIG became unavailable and was replaced by VariZIG (available through FFF Enterprises: 800-843-7477, http://www.fffenterprises.com), which is similar to VZIG. It is an immunoglobulin product made from human plasma and contains high levels of anti-varicella immunoglobulin and is approved for administration to high-risk individuals after exposure.[152,150] IGIV and acyclovir prophylaxis are reasonable alternatives for postexposure prophylaxis if VariZIG is not available.

Intravenous immunoglobulin for varicella prophylaxis. In 1984, Paryani and colleagues[542,543] observed that IGIV at doses of 4 mL/kg to 6 mL/kg resulted in serum varicella-zoster virus antibody titers comparable to those in patients receiving VZIG at standard doses. Subsequently, Chen and Liang[159] demonstrated that varicella was prevented by a single dose of IGIV at 200 mg/kg in five children with leukemia.

Immunocompromised patients who are receiving IGIV at 400 mg/kg are thought to be protected for 3 weeks after infusion and do not require additional VZIG on exposure.[40] However, Ferdman and Church[226] reported that varicella occurred in two patients (one was a 21-year-old woman) receiving 500 mg/kg of IGIV after exposure to varicella 7 and 11 days after infusion. Another child receiving 400 mg/kg IGIV developed varicella 9 days after infusion. Both had mild disease and responded well to acyclovir. The investigators suggest that for patients with profound immunodeficiency, VZIG can be given in addition to IGIV.

Kavaliotis and associates[369] found that an IGIV dose of 1 g/kg given within 6 to 24 hours of exposure was 90% effective in preventing varicella in an oncology unit, with no additional advantage observed with administration of VZIG. All of the children who contracted VZV received prophylactic treatment consisting of a single infusion of varicella-zoster immunoglobulin (VZIG) at a dose of 1 mL/kg (group A) or intravenous immunoglobulin (IVIG) at a dose of 1 g/kg (group B) or VZIG plus IVIG at the previously described doses (group C).

Tokat and colleagues[709] described a 32-year-old man with severe varicella pneumonia that progressed to acute respiratory distress syndrome. IGIV (400 mg/kg for 5 days) was given with a successful outcome.

Recommendations. The decision to administer VariZIG or IGIV or acyclovir to prevent chickenpox is based on the patient's susceptibility, the type of exposure, and the patient's immune competence.

Determination of susceptibility. With the exception of bone marrow transplant recipients, most immunocompromised individuals with previous varicella infection are considered immune; however, their immune status should be confirmed with varicella antibody titers. Healthy adults reared in the United States are considered immune if they have a history of varicella, zoster, or vaccination. Immunocompromised children and adults without a history of varicella are considered susceptible because of their higher risk of severe infection. Bone marrow transplant recipients are considered susceptible regardless of the varicella history of the donor or recipient. If varicella or herpes zoster[453] develops after transplantation, the patient then is considered to be immune.[145,721]

An immunocompromised, unimmunized child without a history of chickenpox is considered susceptible even if antibody titers are present because receipt of blood products containing immunoglobulin may result in transient seropositivity. Alternatively, patients who received VariZIG may have had asymptomatic varicella with the subsequent development of varicella antibodies, but they may not be protected on reexposure.[21] The value of antibody titer to determine susceptibility in these patients is controversial. However, oncology patients who have been vaccinated for varicella before illness and have been seropositive for varicella antibodies before receipt of blood products are considered immune and do not routinely need VariZIG. The severity of immune compromise is also a factor, and bone marrow transplant recipients are considered susceptible despite prior history of immunization or disease.

VariZIG is not recommended for immunodeficient patients who have been vaccinated in the past, provided they previously were shown to have varicella antibody, even if they are seronegative at the time of exposure. These individuals are expected to have mild disease.[721] Verifying varicella immunity with antibody before forgoing VariZIG administration in this situation is a reasonable approach because administration of VariZIG can be delayed up to 10 days and remain efficacious.

Type of exposure. Individuals residing in the same household as a patient with varicella, people who have had face-to-face contact with a patient considered infectious, and patients sharing the same hospital room are considered to have significant exposure. Because the duration of exposure that results in transmission is not known, each exposure must be evaluated individually. Contact with a varicella vaccine recipient with a varicella rash must be considered a significant exposure for an immunodeficient patient because the vaccinee may have wild-type virus infection; vaccine strain virus rarely has been transmitted.[145]

BOX 246.3 Candidates for Varicella-Zoster Immune Globulin (VariZIG) After Significant Exposure

- Immunocompromised children without a history of varicella and without documented response to immunization[a]
- Susceptible, pregnant women
- Newborn infants whose mothers had an onset of varicella within 5 days of delivery or within 48 hours after delivery
- All hospitalized premature infants born at <28 weeks' gestation or <1000 g at birth, regardless of maternal history
- Hospitalized premature infants of >28 weeks' gestation whose mothers have no history of chickenpox or who are seronegative; may consider its use for other premature infants

[a]Severity of immune compromise is a factor in the decision to give VariZIG despite immunization and disease history.

Candidates for varicella-zoster immunoglobulin or intravenous immunoglobulin.

Normal adults, children, and adolescents. Normal children, adolescents, and adults exposed to chickenpox or zoster usually are not candidates for receiving VariZIG or IGIV (Box 246.3). Because of the prolonged incubation period for varicella, the chickenpox vaccine can be given if the exposed individual is older than 12 months.

Immunocompromised children and adults. The principal use of VariZIG is to prevent chickenpox in susceptible immunocompromised children exposed to zoster or chickenpox (see Box 246.3). This group includes those with primary immunodeficiency and those with secondary immunodeficiency, including HIV infection and neoplastic disease, and those receiving immunosuppressive therapy (e.g., systemic steroids, chemotherapy).[51,517,530] Susceptible pregnant women are also candidates for VariZIG because of their increased risk of severe varicella pneumonia.[68,416,652]

Term and premature newborns. Newborns who acquire varicella after birth are not at high risk for severe disease and are not candidates for receiving VZIG, with the possible exception of those whose mothers have severe skin disease.[416] Newborn infants born to mothers in whom varicella developed within 5 days before or 2 days after delivery are at high risk for severe varicella because they have not received transplacental protective antibodies.[721] Others, questioning the validity of these limits, have treated a small number of infants born to mothers in a window ranging from 7 days before delivery to 5 days after delivery with IGIV (500 mg/kg) and a prophylactic acyclovir regimen.[325]

Exposed hospitalized premature infants born at less than 28 weeks' gestation or less than 1000 g should receive VariZIG. These infants are susceptible, regardless of the maternal history of varicella, because of incomplete transplacental transfer of maternal antibody. Hospitalized premature infants with significant exposure who were born at more than 28 weeks' gestation and whose mothers do not have a history of varicella or are seronegative also are considered candidates for receiving VariZIG because transplacental antibody would not be present.[416,453,721]

Gold and colleagues[262] showed that gestational age of more than 28 weeks and birth weight above 1000 g do not always accurately predict the presence of maternal varicella antibody. Ogilvie[517] suggested that infants born before 30 weeks' gestation be given VariZIG and that some infants born after 28 weeks will lose their maternal antibody by 60 days of age. She recommends antibody testing on exposure if it can be performed quickly to assess the need for passive immune prophylaxis. Linder and colleagues[430] also found that only 24% of premature neonates born at 29 to 35 weeks had positive fluorescent antibody to membrane antigen (FAMA) titers at 2 months of age.

Gold and associates[262] recommended the routine use of VariZIG in the neonatal ICU if the FAMA assay is not available to determine susceptibility. Previous administration of blood products in the neonatal ICU may render these results uninterpretable.

Dosage. The VariZIG brand of VZIG is supplied in lyophilized vials of 125 U (reconstituted to a 5% solution for intramuscular use). The dose of VariZIG is 125 U/10 kg given intramuscularly. The minimal dose for infants is 125 U (one vial), and the maximal dose is 625 U for adults (five vials).[38,151]

Although VariZIG should be given to susceptible candidates as soon as possible after exposure for maximal protection, it can be given up to 10 days after exposure.[138,150] A second dose is not needed for subsequent exposure unless it occurs beyond 3 weeks after administration of the VariZIG dose.[21] IGIV (400 mg/kg) is an acceptable alternative if the child has a bleeding diathesis and cannot receive intramuscular injections or VariZIG is not available.[721]

VariZIG is not recommended for the treatment of chickenpox, zoster, disseminated varicella, or postherpetic neuralgia. Zoster immunoglobulin did not prevent dissemination of zoster in immunocompromised patients.[667]

Human Immunodeficiency Virus Infection

The rationale for use of IGIV in patients with advanced HIV disease is their increased susceptibility to common bacterial and viral infections, poor primary antibody responses to vaccine antigens despite hypergammaglobulinemia, and in young children, a limited antibody spectrum to common bacterial pathogens. Although the central immune defect in acquired immunodeficiency syndrome (AIDS) is a loss of helper T-cell (CD4+) number and function, the polyclonal B-cell activation and defective helper T-cell function result in a significant B-cell deficiency.[83,512]

In children with AIDS, bacterial infections occur more commonly than opportunistic infections. Immune-mediated thrombocytopenic purpura and viral diseases (i.e., RSV, parvovirus, and other disorders amenable to IGIV prophylaxis or therapy) also can develop in patients with AIDS.

After preliminary uncontrolled studies suggested a benefit for IGIV in children with advanced HIV infection,[131,641] two large, multicenter, controlled studies undertaken by the National Institutes of Health–supported Pediatric AIDS Clinical Trial Group determined the efficacy of IGIV in decreasing infections and improving survival in AIDS patients.[500,661]

In the first study, 372 children received 400 mg/kg of IGIV every 4 weeks or an albumin control for 2 years.[500] Thirty percent of all children in the IGIV-treated group had serious infections in contrast to 42% in the placebo group. Children who were less ill (i.e., those with CD4+ lymphocyte counts >200 cells/mL) benefited in particular from IGIV. Children in this category had fewer serious infections and were hospitalized less frequently than those in the placebo group, and their CD4+ counts dropped less rapidly than those of the placebo group.[483] The mortality rate for both groups was identical. Children with CD4+ counts less than 200 cells/mL (i.e., those with severely impaired immunity) who were given IGIV had no significant decrease in infections, days of hospitalization, or deaths compared with their counterparts in the placebo group.

The study authors concluded that IGIV significantly reduced the risk of serious infection for some children with symptomatic HIV infection, primarily those with CD4+ counts between 200 and 500 cells/mL. In a follow-up study, the placebo group was allowed to cross over to receive IGIV, with a drop in the rate of serious infections and hospitalizations.[486]

In a second trial of IGIV in which all the children received zidovudine, a significant decrease in serious bacterial infections was found, but this benefit was limited to children who did not receive trimethoprim-sulfamethoxazole prophylaxis for *Pneumocystis jiroveci* pneumonia.[661] The consensus of an HIV Working Group[780] was that HIV-infected children with significant hypogammaglobulinemia or documented poor antibody formation might be candidates for receiving IGIV therapy. IGIV also may be beneficial for HIV-infected children who have recurrent infections not controlled by antibiotics or chronic nonspecific diarrhea with failure to thrive. IGIV also was shown to prevent serious infections in adults with advanced HIV infection.[382]

In addition to preventing serious bacterial infections, IGIV given to children with HIV infection reduced the number of nonserious bacterial infections (by 60% for ear infections, 13% for skin infections, and 10% for other upper respiratory tract infections) and viral infections by approximately one third in both trials.[480,484,482,661] In an additional study, 135 children with symptomatic and asymptomatic perinatally acquired HIV infection in addition to uninfected infants were given monthly IVIG infusions over 12 months. The study authors found significant reductions in the frequency of common bacterial infections in the HIV-symptomatic group compared with the asymptomatic and the control groups.[526] Another study showed that monthly IGIV could be safely discontinued in children who are clinically stable and receiving highly active antiretroviral therapy (HAART).[280]

Regular IGIV infusion improved left ventricular function in HIV-infected children with dilated cardiomyopathy.[432] It is also effective in treating certain other complications of HIV infection, including thrombocytopenia,[129,410] red cell aplasia associated with parvovirus B19 infection,[391] Guillain-Barré syndrome,[256] and certain drug reactions.[229]

IGIV, even in high doses, provides no antiviral activity in HIV infection.[528] Attempts to use HIV-specific antibody to prevent HIV infection or to provide an antiviral effect have met with very limited success.

These studies have used human immune plasma or hyperimmune HIV immunoglobulin (HIVIG) from asymptomatic HIV-seropositive patients, porcine antisera, or monoclonal antibodies.[674] In two of three controlled clinical trials of immune plasma in adult patients with AIDS, a modest clinical benefit was achieved, as judged by decreased opportunistic infections, a slight increase in CD4+ cell counts, and improved survival. However, no striking decreases in viral burden were seen.[337,424,740]

In a double-blind, placebo-controlled, multicenter study, HIV-seropositive pregnant women receiving zidovudine were given HIVIG monthly during the last trimester of pregnancy, and their newborns were given one HIVIG dose at birth. No effect on the rate of maternal-fetal HIV transmission compared with that in a similar group given regular IGIV was found.[673] The rate of transmission in both groups was unexpectedly low (<5%), and the study was discontinued after 800 patients had been enrolled because the study was not statistically powered to detect a slight reduction in transmission rates.

Another study examined the antiviral effect of large doses of HIVIG in 30 children with moderately advanced HIV infection who were receiving stable antiviral treatment and showed a measurable viral burden.[672] No striking beneficial effect was observed as indicated by plasma HIV RNA levels, cellular viral culture titers, or immunologic assays.

Despite these failures, efforts to develop antibody preparations that can neutralize the virus continue. These preparations would be particularly valuable after needlestick, perinatal, or sexual exposure.[672] Under study are monoclonal antibodies to neutralizing regions of the virus, antibodies to coreceptors that may interfere with HIV attachment, and combinations of antibodies with different specificities, including combinations of HIVIG with monoclonal antibodies.[47,126,409,427,428,538] An effective neutralizing antibody also would provide valuable information toward an effective vaccine.

Recommendations. IGIV may be beneficial in symptomatic children with HIV infection to prevent bacterial and viral infections and treat certain complications (e.g., thrombocytopenia, anemia of parvovirus infection, and autoimmune hemolytic anemia [Duncan syndrome]), but it has no direct antiviral activity. Because the administration of HAART plays a critical role in the reconstitution of the immune system, specifically the cellular immune system and resultant increase in humoral immunity, additional passive immunity administered with IGIV has not had a substantial benefit for children with well-controlled HIV infection. HIVIG or plasma derived from infected patients has little or no antiviral activity or clinical benefit for HIV-infected adults or children, and the administration of HIVIG during pregnancy did not provide added reduction in maternal-fetal transmission of HIV.

Measles

The first successful prophylaxis of measles with convalescent serum was reported by Cenci in 1907.[118] Convalescent serum was used in the United States first in 1916 by Park and Freeman[539] and Zingher,[798] who gave 4 or 8 mL of serum to 41 recently exposed children at New York Metropolitan Hospital. Measles did not develop in any of the 20 children who received the 8-mL dose and developed in only 3 of the 20 children who received the 4-mL dose. In 1926, Park and Freeman[539] found that 6 to 10 mL of convalescent serum was 92% efficacious in preventing measles in recently exposed individuals, a finding confirmed and extended by Stillerman and associates.[675] Placental extracts containing serum antibodies also were used in the prevention and modification of measles.[466]

Stokes and colleagues[679] and Ordman and associates[529] confirmed in 1944 that immunoglobulin given immediately after exposure could prevent or modify measles, and given in the early stages of clinical illness, it could lessen its severity. In 1955, Greenberg and coworkers[279] observed that a lower incidence of measles encephalitis in IGIM-modified measles.

A major use of IGIM in the 1960s was to diminish the side effects of the Edmonston strain of measles vaccine. In 1962, Krugman and associates[403] observed that the simultaneous administration of 0.02 mL/lb of immunoglobulin at the time of Edmonston measles vaccination reduced the incidence of high fever from 40% to 14% and the incidence of rash from 10% to 2%. The mean titer of measles antibody achieved was somewhat reduced by the IGIM, and a slight decrease in the rate of seroconversion occurred; nonetheless, the vaccine and IGIM combination was 95% effective.[678] The current measles vaccine is less reactogenic and does not require concomitant IGIM injections.

Audet and colleagues[55] report that the measles neutralizing antibody titer in recent IGIV lots is decreasing because of the lower titer of vaccine-induced antibodies compared with natural infection among donors. Although not tested, IGIM probably has lower titers of measles antibodies, and the recommended prophylactic doses may be inadequate.

Recommendations. IGIM or IGIV can be given to susceptible contacts within 6 days of exposure to prevent or to modify measles.[31] Infants younger than 1 year, immunocompromised patients, and pregnant women are at risk for severe disease and should receive immunoprophylaxis. Because HIV-infected patients with significant immunodeficiency may contract measles after exposure despite receiving immunization, they should also receive passive immunoprophylaxis.[250] IGIM is not recommended for healthy household or other close contacts if they have received at least one measles-containing vaccine, unless they are immunocompromised. Measles vaccine has some efficacy if it is given within 72 hours of exposure and is preferred for the management of outbreaks among healthy individuals older than 1 year of age.[31]

The standard dose of IGIM is 0.25 mL/kg for healthy patients and 0.5 mL/kg for immunocompromised patients. The maximal dose is 15 mL. IGIV at comparable doses also can be used, but titers may be diminished in recent years.[55]

Immunodeficient children receiving regular IGIV treatments at doses of at least 400 mg/kg should be protected for up to 3 weeks after administration.[31] Administration of IGIM to a healthy infant precludes the use of measles vaccine for 5 months if the dose was 0.25 mL/kg and 6 months if the dose was 0.5 mL/kg. For larger doses, longer intervals are needed (e.g., 8–11 months).[31]

IGIV in addition to other immunomodulators has been used for the treatment of acute measles infection[495] and subacute sclerosing panencephalitis (SSPE), a delayed, rare, degenerative neurologic disease complicating wild-type measles infection.[266]

Mumps

Mumps immunoglobulin has limited efficacy as postexposure prophylaxis, and this product no longer is manufactured in the United States.[32,174]

Parvovirus

Human parvovirus B19, also called erythrovirus, is the cause of the benign childhood exanthem called fifth disease. It may also cause polyarthropathy, transient aplastic crises in patients with hemolytic anemia, chronic red cell aplasia in immunocompromised patients, and hemophagocytic syndrome.[112,331,786] Patients susceptible to chronic parvovirus infection include those with congenital[700] or acquired immunodeficiencies,[166,391] those receiving immunosuppressive therapy,[220,786] and organ transplant recipients.[363,451] In utero parvovirus infection can result in hydrops fetalis.[711] The use of parvovirus DNA PCR has facilitated establishment of the diagnosis in immunodeficient patients unable to make antibodies or in patients who have passively acquired parvovirus antibodies.

Parvovirus B19 has tropism for marrow erythroid progenitor cells because the cells express the blood group P antigen, the cellular receptor for the virus. Because most adults have encountered and made antibodies to parvovirus, IGIV is an excellent source of anti–parvovirus B19 antibodies.[619] IGIV has been used successfully to treat parvovirus-induced red cell aplasia.[179,411] Successfully treated patients have decreased viremia, reticulocytosis, and resolution of the anemia within 2 weeks. Sometimes, relapse or persistent infection occurs, requiring maintenance IGIV therapy, particularly in patients with HIV infection and low $CD4^+$ cell counts.[390]

For treatment of chronic infection in immunodeficient patients, IGIV therapy often is effective and should be considered.[33,227] IGIV has been used successfully to treat parvovirus B19 anemia resulting from chemotherapy[468] or rituximab therapy,[631] or both.[336,658] However, IGIV was not of value in four children with persistent parvovirus infection undergoing chemotherapy for acute lymphocytic leukemia.[227] IGIV also has been used successfully for treatment of parvovirus B19 anemia in renal transplant recipients.[163,452,534,655]

Viguier and coauthors[736] administered 1 g/kg of IGIV for 2 days to treat successfully a 33-year-old woman with parvovirus B19–associated polyarteritis nodosa and fever, palpable purpura, intense myalgia, paresthesias, and polyarthritis of the hand joints. IGIV has been used with success in parvovirus B19–associated chronic fatigue syndrome in three adults[379] and one teenage boy.[465]

IGIV has been used as a supplement to transfusions in severe in utero parvovirus infection with hydrops fetalis. Selbing and coworkers[622] described a 24-week pregnant woman with severe preeclampsia whose fetus had ascites and pericardial effusion. She was given 25 g of IGIV, with resolution of the ascites, effusion, and anemia. Matsuda and colleagues[459] treated a parvovirus B19–infected hydropic fetus with two injections of immunoglobulin into the fetal peritoneum, with resolution of the anemia and the hydrops.

Rugolotto and colleagues[595] treated an anemic newborn due to intrauterine parvovirus infection with IGIV (1 g/kg every 3 weeks for 8 months). Heegaard and coauthors[305] reported similar success with IGIV in addition to in utero transfusions. Earlier attempts to treat older infants with persistent parvovirus-induced congenital anemia with IGIV were unsuccessful.[114]

Dennert and colleagues[191] performed a pilot study on the use of IGIV for 17 patients with chronic dilated cardiomyopathy and a significant parvovirus B19 viral load. Endomyocardial biopsies demonstrated a significant reduction in viral load and improvement in cardiac function. IGIV has also been used to successfully treat fulminant hepatitis resulting from parvovirus B19 in a 2-year-old Chinese boy.[134]

Human neutralizing monoclonal antibodies have been generated from infected individuals[254] for possible future therapeutic use.

Recommendations. Red cell aplasia caused by parvovirus infection in immunodeficient patients, including those with HIV infection, should be treated with IGIV (400 mg/kg per day for 5 days or 1 g/kg per day for 2 days).[112,391,489] If relapse is likely to occur because of the patient's severe immunocompromised status, IGIV (400 mg/kg) can be given every 4 weeks.

Neonates with persistent congenital anemia caused by parvovirus B19 should receive IGIV (400 mg/kg) for 5 days, with additional doses given if the anemia does not resolve. Pregnant women carrying fetuses with in utero hydrops fetalis caused by parvovirus B19 infection also may be candidates for IGIV therapy, as discussed in the Parvovirus section.

Rabies and Rabies Immunoglobulin

Rabies is the ideal disease for passive immunization because the exact moment, the exact source, and the exact location of exposure usually are known. The long incubation period and the fact that the virus remains localized to the wound for several days enhance the effectiveness of passive immunization. Although a rabies serum was prepared initially in 1889 by Babes and Lepp,[56] experiments of Habel[294] in mice, guinea pigs, and monkeys involving the use of rabbit hyperimmune serum demonstrated that antibody worked by two mechanisms: neutralizing the virus while it is still in tissues and retarding the spread of virus within the nervous system, thereby prolonging the incubation period and permitting active immunity by vaccine to become established.

On the basis of these studies, a World Health Organization (WHO) Expert Committee in 1950 recommended that a field trial of the efficacy of hyperimmune rabies serum in conjunction with vaccine be conducted.[216] It was undertaken in Iran because multiple bites by a single rabid wolf coming into isolated villages occurred, and this severe exposure had an associated 40% to 50% mortality rate. In 1954, a single rabid wolf bit 27 individuals, 17 of whom were bitten on the head. These 17 were divided into three groups: five received vaccine alone, seven received vaccine and one dose of antirabies serum, and five received vaccine and two doses of antirabies serum.[66] Of the five people treated with vaccine alone, three died of rabies; one in seven in the one-dose antiserum group died, and none of the five in the two-dose antiserum group died.

Antibody studies conducted on these patients indicated that a single or double dose of antiserum, followed by 14 to 21 daily doses of vaccine, resulted in significant levels of circulating antibody for as long as 50 days.[295] The antibody found early is supplied passively; after the tenth day, the antibody present is a result of the vaccine. Optimal treatment requires passive and active immunization.

Before 1971, the only available antiserum was of equine origin. It is still the only product available in some countries. Since 1971, human rabies immunoglobulin (RIG) has been available in the United States and many other countries and is preferred because of the lessened risk of serum reactions.[642] Human antibody has a half-life in the circulation twice that of equine antibody, and higher levels of passive antibody are maintained. However, the antibody response to the vaccine given concomitantly is suppressed more effectively.[433]

A case of fatal rabies was reported in a 19-year-old man bitten on the finger by a rabid mongoose despite the recommended postexposure prophylaxis (i.e., RIG and five doses of human diploid cell rabies vaccine).[635] Possible reasons for failure included inadequacy of the recommended dose of RIG; vaccine injection into the gluteal region, where more fat is found than in the recommended deltoid region; and decreased antibody response to the vaccine as a result of a possible immunodeficiency state.

Prevention of rabies consists of three essential components: thorough washing of the wound with a 20% soap solution followed by irrigation with povidone-iodine,[89,597] passive immunization with rabies antibody, and active immunization. Although most cases of failure are caused by lack of adherence to these three strategies,[557] isolated cases of rabies occurring despite appropriate management have been reported.

Wilde and associates[765] reported failure of prophylaxis in five Thai children who received multiple bites on the face and head. They suggested that failure to infiltrate all wounds with RIG and surgical closure before the wound was infiltrated might have been factors. Hemachudha and coauthors[307] reported failure of prophylaxis in a child with minor scratches on the nose and in a woman with a deep wound on the cheek. They suggested that direct inoculation of virus into nerve endings might have occurred.

Goudsmit and associates[267] found that a human monoclonal antibody combination was equivalent to RIG when it was used with vaccine in a hamster model of rabies. Bakker and colleagues[59,60] reported clinical data from two phase I studies evaluating the monoclonal antibody cocktail CL184 against rabies for use in resource-limited areas where there is no access to human or equine rabies immunoglobulin.

Two phase II trials have been completed in the United States and the Philippines. A third is being conducted in India.[103,261]

Recommendations. Human RIG is recommended for nonimmunized individuals for all bites by animals in which rabies cannot be ruled out and for nonbite exposure to animals proved to be or suspected of being rabid.[31,141] Treatment should be given as early as possible after exposure and followed by vaccine administration. The decision to administer postexposure prophylaxis should be based on guidelines.[34]

Two human RIG products are available in the United States: BayRab and Imogam Rabies-HT. Both are prepared from the plasma of hyperimmunized donors. The recommended dose of 20 IU/kg of RIG must not be exceeded because higher doses can suppress immunologic response of the simultaneously administered vaccine. The entire dose of RIG should be infiltrated around the wounds as soon as possible after the bite.[498] If this is not anatomically feasible, any remaining RIG should be given intramuscularly.[34]

Wilde and colleagues,[765] recognizing the difficulty in infiltrating multiple wounds with a small volume of RIG, suggested dilution of the RIG. The WHO[781] recommends dilution of the RIG twofold to threefold in saline to ensure an adequate volume for infiltration. RIG should not be frozen, and if it is frozen, it should not be used. In addition to passive immunization with RIG on the first day of treatment, exposed patients should receive active immunization with rabies vaccine in four doses over 2 weeks.

Purified equine RIG–containing rabies antibodies may be available outside the United States and is associated with a low rate of serum sickness (<1%). Equine RIG is administered at a dose of 40 IU/kg, and desensitization before administration may be required.

Administration of one of the three vaccines licensed in the United States should be started at the same time as RIG; however, the vaccine and RIG should not be administered in the same syringe or with the same syringe or needle. Only two of the licensed vaccines are produced and available in the United States: human diploid cell rabies vaccine and purified chicken embryo cell vaccine. The vaccines are equally effective and administered in multiple separate doses. Vaccine should be given in the deltoid muscle or, for an infant, in the anterolateral aspect of the thigh and at an anatomic site removed from the injury or injection sites of RIG. The vaccine should be administered on days 0, 3, 7, and 14 after exposure, with day 0 designated as the day of initial presentation. This new schedule replaces the previously recommended schedule that included a fifth dose administered on day 28.[31]

If RIG is not available immediately, immunization should be started and RIG given if it is available within 7 days.[34,141,498] If vaccine is not available immediately, RIG should be administered and the vaccine given as soon as possible. If both RIG and vaccine are delayed, both should be given whenever available, regardless of the interval between exposure and treatment.[34,141,498]

The administration of passive antibody can inhibit the response to rabies vaccines; therefore, the recommended dose should not be exceeded. Vaccine never should be administered in the same parts of the body or with the same syringe used to give RIG. Hypersensitivity reactions to RIG are rare.

RIG is not recommended for patients who previously received a full postexposure vaccine course of human diploid cell rabies vaccine, rabies virus adsorbed, or purified chicken embryo cell vaccine; those who have received a three-dose preexposure intramuscular series of these vaccines; those who have received a three-dose preexposure intradermal human diploid cell rabies vaccine used in the United States; or those who have been immunized with any vaccine and have a documented rabies titer.[34,141,498]

Postexposure prophylaxis of immunodeficient patients is problematic. Jaijaroensup and coauthors[340] reported poor or nondetectable neutralizing antibody in five HIV-infected patients who received intradermal vaccine and proposed that higher doses of vaccine or additional boosters be considered. Serologic failure of preexposure and postexposure rabies immunizations in children with HIV infection has been reported.[536,707] The number of doses of rabies vaccine recommended for people with altered immunocompetence has not changed; for these people, postexposure prophylaxis should be continued and comprises a five-dose vaccination regimen with one dose of RIG.

RIG is not indicated for the treatment of rabies. Hemachudha and colleagues[308] described a patient with rabies who developed total limb and facial paralysis after receiving RIG.

Respiratory Syncytial Virus

Acute RSV infection of the respiratory tract is the most common cause of hospitalization of infants and young children and a significant public health expense. For high-risk patients such as premature infants and infants with chronic lung disease, RSV infection can be severe and life-threatening. The observation that passively transferred maternal antibody provided some protection from RSV infection[518] led to the development of passive immunity products to prevent and to modify the severity of infection. No effective vaccine exists.

Respiratory Syncytial Virus Intravenous Immunoglobulin

The first immune modulator used for the prevention of RSV infection was RSV-IGIV (RespiGam), a 5% polyclonal human IGIV prepared from healthy donors with high RSV-neutralizing antibody titers. RSV-IGIV was licensed in 1996 after studies in high-risk infants demonstrated its efficacy. Groothuis and colleagues[281] conducted a prospective, blinded, randomized trial at five centers and showed that 58 premature infants who received RSV-IGIV at 750 mg/kg per month during the winter months had a significantly lower incidence of RSV lower respiratory tract disease than that observed in 58 premature control infants who did not receive RSV-IGIV (6.9% vs. 24.1%; $P = .01$). The RSV-IGIV–treated patients also had a lower incidence of moderate-to-severe RSV lower respiratory tract disease ($P = .006$), fewer days of hospitalization ($P = .020$), and fewer days in the ICU ($P = .05$).

Another large, multicenter, double-blind, placebo-controlled RSV-IGIV study[563] of 510 infants with prematurity or bronchopulmonary dysplasia demonstrated a decreased number of hospitalizations (13.5% vs. 8.0%; $P = .047$), decreased total number of RSV-related hospital days ($P = .045$), and decreased days with oxygen use ($P = .007$). Use of RSV-IGIV also decreased days of hospitalization for any respiratory illness by 38% and total respiratory illness hospital days by 46%, presumably because of antibodies to other respiratory pathogens. An added benefit of RSV-IGIV prophylaxis was a decreased incidence of otitis media (number of episodes: 0.15 per patient vs. 0.78 per control; $P = .003$).[301,644]

In 1997, the American Academy of Pediatrics recommended RSV-IGIV for high-risk children with prematurity or bronchopulmonary dysplasia[22] but not for infants with cyanotic congenital heart disease[282,647] because of the risk of serious side effects. RSV-IGIV is no longer available.

Palivizumab

In 1996, palivizumab (Synagis), a humanized IgG1 monoclonal antibody against the fusion (F) glycoprotein of RSV,[259,682] entered clinical trials. Palivizumab neutralizes type A and type B RSV and is 50 to 100 times more potent than RSV-IGIV.[606] A multicenter, randomized, double-blind, placebo-controlled study of 1502 high-risk infants (i.e., premature infants and infants younger than 2 years with bronchopulmonary dysplasia) demonstrated the efficacy of 15 mg/kg of palivizumab given intramuscularly every 30 days.[330] It resulted in significantly decreased number of RSV hospitalizations (55%; $P < .001$), RSV hospital days ($P < .001$), and days of oxygen therapy ($P < .001$).

Palivizumab was licensed in 1998. It was the first monoclonal antibody approved for the prevention of an infectious disease. Postlicensure studies have supported its effectiveness.[551,589,649] Although debate continues about the cost-effectiveness of palivizumab in some countries,[371,527,688] palivizumab prophylaxis for high-risk infants has become the standard of practice in the United States.[24]

In 2003, Feltes and colleagues[223] reported the results of an international, randomized, double-blind, placebo-controlled trial of palivizumab prophylaxis in 1287 children with congenital heart disease. With the use of palivizumab, the study showed a 45% reduction in RSV hospitalizations, a 56% reduction in the total number of hospital days, and a 73% reduction in the total number of hospital days with oxygen. European cardiologists and the American Academy of Pediatrics recommend use of palivizumab for infants with hemodynamically significant heart disease (i.e., uncorrected, partially corrected, or with residual disease), pulmonary hypertension or chronic lung disease, and hemodynamically significant dilated or hypertrophic cardiomyopathy causing cyanosis or requiring cardiac medication.[38,710]

The use of palivizumab for more than one season has been a concern because of the theoretical risk for side effects resulting from the development of an antibody to the murine component.[414,510] Null and colleagues[510] found that only one child of 55 receiving palivizumab for a second season developed an anti-palivizumab titer of greater than 1:40. This child had a titer of 1:160 on day 30 that fell to 1:10 on day 120 (i.e., 30 days after the fourth injection), suggesting a nonspecific reactivity. No associated adverse events occurred, and the palivizumab trough concentrations were as expected.

Palivizumab or other RSV antibodies are not indicated for the treatment of RSV infection, although some have used palivizumab for treatment of adult and pediatric patients in high-risk settings.[158,381,624] In a small pharmacokinetic study, Saez-Llorens and colleagues[601] found that although palivizumab was safe, it had no clinical benefit for previously healthy children with acute RSV infection. Banna and colleagues[67] successfully used palivizumab and steroid therapy to treat an adult woman with RSV-related pneumonia after stem cell transplantation. An experimental RSV monoclonal antibody (Medi-493), given intravenously, showed no benefit for intubated patients with RSV infection and respiratory failure.[449] Studies of high-titer monoclonal antibodies may yield different results.[237,613,624]

Passive Immunity in Respiratory Syncytial Virus Treatment

Although a single dose of 1500 mg/kg of RSV-IGIV was of no benefit in normal and high-risk children with RSV infection,[587,589] DeVincenzo and associates[193] gave a single dose of RSV-IGIV (1500 mg/kg) to 11 bone marrow transplant recipients after the onset of RSV infection. All but one patient also received ribavirin. Only one patient died in this group, which compares favorably with historical controls given ribavirin therapy alone.

Ghosh and coworkers[252] gave IGIV (500 mg/kg) every other day and aerosolized ribavirin to 14 adult bone marrow transplant recipients with RSV upper respiratory tract infection to prevent pneumonia and death. Infection resolved in 10 patients, pneumonia developed in 4, and 2 died. Aerosolized human IGIV was of no clinical benefit in the treatment of patients with RSV infection.[582]

Recommendations. Palivizumab is indicated for prevention of RSV infection during the RSV infection season for high-risk premature infants or infants with chronic lung disease.[35] The period of prophylaxis should be individualized, depending on the duration of the local RSV infection season.

Candidates for prophylaxis. Certain patient groups are candidates for prophylaxis[35]:

1. Infants younger than 24 months with chronic lung disease requiring medical treatment in the 6 months before the start of the RSV infection season may benefit from prophylaxis. Two seasons of treatment may be required for some infants who require ongoing medical treatment.
2. Premature infants without chronic lung disease who were born before 32 weeks' gestation may benefit from prophylaxis. For these infants, the major risk factors to consider are gestational age and the chronologic age at the start of RSV season.
3. Infants born at 28 weeks, 6 days; gestation or earlier may benefit from prophylaxis during RSV season when that occurs in the first 12 months of life, whereas infants born at 29 to 32 weeks' gestation may benefit most from prophylaxis up to 6 months of age,[35] although decisions should be individualized. After an infant qualifies for initiation of prophylaxis at the start of RSV season, administration of prophylaxis should continue throughout the season and not stop on the basis of the chronologic age.[35]
4. Premature infants of 32 to 35 weeks' gestation who are 3 months or younger at the start of RSV season, including those born during the RSV season, and have one of two risk factors may benefit from prophylaxis: attends child care in a setting with multiple infants or young toddlers or has one or more older siblings (or other child) younger than 5 years living in the household. Prophylaxis should continue until the infant is 3 months of age.[35]
5. Infants younger than 12 months during RSV season with congenital abnormalities of the airway or neuromuscular disease may be considered for immunoprophylaxis if their condition compromises handling of respiratory secretions.[35]
6. Children younger than 24 months with hemodynamically significant cyanotic or acyanotic heart disease may benefit from prophylaxis. Criteria include children requiring medication for congestive heart failure and children with moderate to severe pulmonary hypertension. Children with hemodynamically insignificant heart disease are not candidates for palivizumab. This category includes atrial septal defect, small ventricular septal defect, pulmonic stenosis, mild coarctation of the aorta, and patent ductus arteriosus. Children who have had

surgical correction and do not require medications for congestive heart failure also are not candidates for prophylaxis. After cardiopulmonary bypass, a postoperative dose of palivizumab can be given to maintain protection because decreased levels of antibody have resulted from cardiopulmonary bypass.[224]

7. Infants who are severely immunocompromised can be considered for prophylaxis, although there are no studies on which to base a recommendation.

Possible indications. Possible indications for use include the following:

1. Nosocomial outbreaks can be an indication. No data exist to support palivizumab use in controlling an RSV outbreak in a hospital setting. However, palivizumab in addition to implementation of strict isolation practices has been used in this setting and may be of value in aborting a nosocomial outbreak of RSV infection.[1,178,364,412,644] Current dosing recommendations for outpatients may not be adequate for some hospitalized premature infants.[782]
2. Patients with cystic fibrosis who are younger than 2 years of age may be candidates for RSV prophylaxis, but no data exist on which to base a recommendation.
3. Older, high-risk infants who received palivizumab the previous season but remain unwell, are immunocompromised, or have recently undergone a procedure such as transplantation or operation may benefit from a second season of palivizumab. This includes immunodeficient infants receiving IGIV because IGIV has only low titers of RSV antibodies.

Dosage and administration. Prophylaxis is given monthly from just before the start of the local RSV infection season until the end of the season. Usually, five injections are given from November to March, but starting earlier or extending into April may be required. It is important to be aware of local outbreak data. If an infant develops RSV infection while receiving prophylaxis, palivizumab should be continued because more than one RSV strain could infect the patient in a single season.[35]

The dose of palivizumab for prophylaxis is 15 mg/kg per month given intramuscularly. It is supplied in 50- and 100-mg vials. Palivizumab is not indicated for the treatment of RSV infections.

Rotavirus

Several reviews have summarized the role of oral immunoglobulin in the prevention and treatment of rotavirus infection.[98,186,298,535,755] Its effectiveness varies, in part because of differences in antibody titer in the various products.[70,204,286,287,315,481,609] Human immunoglobulin has been used to prevent rotavirus infection; Barnes and colleagues[70] and Pammi and colleagues[535] gave human gamma globulin orally to low-birth-weight infants in a nursery in which rotavirus was endemic. Patients given human immunoglobulin had a more attenuated disease than the placebo controls.

Human immunoglobulin has been infused into the duodenum to treat two children with prolonged rotavirus infection.[286] One patient responded rapidly, but the other had a prolonged course. Losonsky and coworkers[434] gave human immunoglobulin to three immunodeficient patients and demonstrated that it survived passage of the gastrointestinal tract in an immunologically active form.

Pooled colostrum concentrate from hyperimmunized pregnant cows with high titers to several rotavirus serotypes has been used in several studies.[122] In a controlled study, bovine immune colostrum did not prevent development of symptomatic rotavirus infection in infants, but treated patients had a decrease in the duration of diarrhea.[718] Immune bovine colostrum also was used prophylactically for 2 weeks in 10 infants in a childcare center, with evidence of a protective effect.[204]

A double-blind, placebo-controlled trial of oral lyophilized rotavirus bovine colostrum in Bangladesh showed that a 4-day course decreased diarrhea, the need for oral rehydration, and viral shedding.[609] Mitra and associates[481] also showed that cow colostrum[716] significantly shortened the duration of diarrhea and decreased stool output. Hilpert and colleagues[315] demonstrated that rotavirus colostrum decreased virus excretion in infants with rotavirus diarrhea.

A lactobacillus engineered to express a neutralizing antibody fragment of a llama immunoglobulin (i.e., lactobodies) was given orally to experimental animals with rotavirus diarrhea. It markedly shortened disease duration, severity, and viral load.[537,727] A recently licensed vaccine for rotavirus seems safe and effective.[36]

Recommendations. Because rotavirus infection usually is self-limited, no commercial passive antibody product has been developed, although it would be useful in developing countries. The neutralizing titer of human immunoglobulin probably is not high enough to be consistently beneficial. Oral vaccines may decrease the need for antibody-based therapies.

Rubella

Immunoglobulin rarely is used for prevention of rubella because of its uneven efficacy. Early studies suggested some prophylactic benefit. In 1952, Korns[396] showed that one lot of IGIM at a dose of 0.1 mL/lb provided partial protection against the development of epidemic rubella. However, the titers of rubella antibodies varied significantly between lots and did not provided consistent protection.

Studies in epidemic situations have shown that 5 mL of IGIM can prevent development of clinical rubella,[273] but Brody and coworkers[110] showed that an IGIM dose of 0.55 mg/kg resulted in a decreased clinical attack rate but also a high incidence of subclinical infection. Military recruits were protected by a 15-mL dose of IGIM administered before exposure.[321]

Extensive studies on IGIM prophylaxis for rubella conducted by Green[275] and Krugman and Ward[405] did not demonstrate a protective effect of IGIM (0.12 to 0.2 mL/lb). Lundström and coworkers[442] gave 251 exposed pregnant women 4 mL of convalescent rubella IGIM and 28 exposed pregnant women 24 mL of standard IGIM. Rubella developed in 6 (2.4%) of the 251; three of these six women aborted, and one had an infant with probable congenital rubella. None of the 28 women given 24 mL of standard IGIM contracted rubella. Their subsequent study demonstrated that convalescent rubella IGIM given to pregnant women with clinically manifested rubella did not protect against congenital rubella or lessen the probability of fetal damage.[443]

Recommendations. IGIM prophylaxis is not indicated for children and nonpregnant adults exposed to an infected contact because of the mildness of the infection. IGIM is not recommended for most exposed pregnant women because the clinical syndrome may be masked and congenital rubella not prevented.

For exposed pregnant women who will not consider abortion if rubella develops, IGIM may have some value in reducing the chance for fetal infection. A dose of 0.55 mL/kg of IGIM given intramuscularly is the recommended dose. However, mothers who have received prophylaxis after exposure have delivered infants with congenital rubella.[37] Administration of immunoglobulin eliminates the value of IgG antibody testing to detect maternal infection.

Vaccinia, Variola, and Vaccinia Immunoglobulin

Vaccinia virus is closely related antigenically to smallpox (variola) virus, and immunity to vaccinia virus through vaccination prevents smallpox.[502] Although smallpox has been eradicated from the world since 1977, the virus exists in a few research laboratories and is a potential weapon in biologic warfare.

Vaccination is still given to members of the military, to some health care workers, and to laboratory workers who handle cultures or animals contaminated with vaccinia virus, some recombinant vaccinia viruses, and other orthopoxviruses (e.g., monkeypox, cowpox). Passive immunization occasionally is necessary after laboratory accidents, inadvertent vaccination of high-risk individuals, and exposure of high-risk individuals to a recently vaccinated individual.

Passive immunization against variola was known as early as 1895, when Hlava and Honl[316] showed that schoolchildren could be protected from variola by the injection of 3 to 10 mL of serum from a cowpox-immune calf. At the same time, protective human antibodies developed after vaccination, and passive transmission of these antibodies from mothers to infants was demonstrated.[664] Thereafter, effective prevention of smallpox by well-organized mass vaccination campaigns diminished interest in passive immunization.

Janeway, quoted by Enders,[210] found neutralizing vaccinia antibody in immunoglobulin in 1944, and Verlinde and Spaander[733] in 1949 found high titers of the antibodies in convalescent immunoglobulin from recently vaccinated individuals. In 1956, Gispen and associates[255] developed a human vaccinia immunoglobulin (VIG) that did not interfere with active immunity, and they proposed its use with vaccine as prophylaxis against vaccinia encephalitis. Human VIG is derived from the plasma of vaccinated donors.[144]

The value of human VIG in treating smallpox or disseminated vaccinia is based on the presence of viremia, which leads to secondary dissemination. Administration of neutralizing antibody can prevent or limit the spread of infection and modify clinical expression of the disease.

Studies on the efficacy of VIG in treating smallpox and vaccinia complications were initiated by Kempe and colleagues in 1955.[62,377] They used a VIG that was prepared from recently vaccinated donors with a neutralizing titer of 1:256 to 1:512, in contrast to titers of 1:16 or 1:32 in standard IGIM. The households of new admissions to the Madras (India) Smallpox Hospital were visited, and alternate family contacts received VIG 0.2 mL/lb for adults and 0.05 to 0.2 mL/lb for children.[377] After 25 days, eight cases of smallpox developed in 75 contacts not given VIG, and two cases developed in 56 contacts given VIG, a significant difference. A similar, more extensive study disclosed 21 cases of smallpox (four severe) among 379 contacts serving as controls and five cases of smallpox (none severe) among 326 contacts given VIG.[378]

Kempe[376] reported the results of 300 cases of smallpox vaccination (vaccinia) complications treated with VIGIM, including 62 cases of generalized vaccinia, 132 cases of eczema vaccinatum, 23 cases of vaccinia necrosum, 12 cases of vaccinia encephalitis, and 28 cases of autoinoculation. VIGIM was given prophylactically to 44 eczematoid children requiring smallpox vaccine (0.6 to 1.2 mL/kg). VIGIM did not affect the course of vaccinia encephalitis. Of 28 patients with autoinoculation who received VIGIM, 27 did well. Among the 132 patients with eczema vaccinatum given VIGIM, nine deaths occurred; this 7% mortality rate compares favorably with the usual mortality rate of 30% to 40% associated with supportive care only. All 62 patients with generalized vaccinia who were given VIGIM did well, although four children required a second course.

Of the 23 patients with vaccinia necrosum who received VIGIM, seven died (30%); however, this disease usually is fatal, and immune defects were present in most of the patients.[69] These results strongly supported the efficacy of VIGIM and subsequently were confirmed by studies in Sweden[441] and the United Kingdom.[632]

In 1997, Kesson and coauthors[380] reported a severely immunocompromised patient with progressive vaccinia who had inadvertently received a vaccinia melanoma oncolysate vaccination but was successfully treated with VIGIM and ribavirin. Nanning[496] studied the effect of VIGIM on postvaccinia encephalitis. He gave a placebo or 2 mL of VIG to Dutch military recruits at the time of primary vaccination; three cases of encephalitis occurred among 43,630 vaccinated recruits given VIG, compare with 13 cases among 53,044 recruits in the control group. This 77% reduction is statistically significant.

Intramuscular Vaccinia Immunoglobulin and Intravenous Vaccinia Immunoglobulin

Two types of VIG are now available, VIGIM (for intramuscular use) and IV-VIG (for intravenous use). IV-VIG was approved in the United States in 2005 for specific indications—treatment of infections that involve accidental implantation in the eye (except for isolated keratitis), mouth, or other hazardous areas; eczema vaccinatum; progressive vaccinia; severe generalized vaccinia; and vaccinia in patients with burns, impetigo, varicella-zoster, poison ivy, or severe eczema. Both VIG preparations are prepared from the plasma of vaccinated donors.

IV-VIG used at a dose of 100 mg/kg results in a more rapid and higher antibody peak than does an injection of VIGIM.[319] The first civilian treated with VIGIV was a woman with vaccinia blepharoconjunctivitis; she also received topical antiviral medication.[324] Another laboratory worker with ocular vaccinia was treated with a single dose of VIGIV.[425]

IV-VIG is available from CDC under an IND protocol that has guidelines for dosage and administration. The CDC Clinical Consultation Team can be contacted through the Clinicians Information Hotline for VIG requests to treat vaccine-related adverse events (877-554-4625, http://www.bt.cdc.gov/agent/smallpox/index.asp).

Recommendations. Complications of vaccination are the usual indications for VIG. They include accidental or intentional vaccination of a patient with a contraindication to the vaccine, autoinoculation of the eye, eczema vaccinatum, severe generalized vaccinia, and vaccinia necrosum.

The initial dose of VIGIM is 0.6 mL/kg. In adults, the dose must be divided and administered over 24 to 36 hours. Repeated doses can be given at 2- to 3-day intervals for vaccine complications until recovery begins, as evidenced by no new lesions. VIG should be given as soon as possible after diagnosis is established.[8,146]

For unimmunized patients exposed to smallpox, VIGIM in combination with vaccine can be given. A dose of 0.6 mL/kg should be given as soon as possible, preferably within 1 to 3 days.[8,461,718] Current recommendations from the US Army Medical Research Institute of Infectious Diseases suggest that VIGIM may be of value in postexposure prophylaxis of smallpox when it is given within the first week after exposure and concurrently with vaccination. Vaccination alone is recommended for those without contraindications. Both vaccine and VIGIM should be given if more than 1 week has elapsed since exposure occurred.

The current supplies of VIGIM do not permit its routine use in combination with vaccine for bioterrorism exposure.[146] However, if additional supplies become available, a VIGIM dose of 0.3 mL/kg in combination with vaccine can be used.

Cidofovir also has been used.[106,107] VIGIM is not indicated for established smallpox, postvaccinial encephalitis, or hypersensitivity and toxic rashes that occur after vaccination. However, the lack of efficacy of VIGIM in the past does not exclude a potential beneficial effect for IV-VIG. The pathogenesis of vaccinial encephalitis is poorly understood and may involve both infection and immune response,[318] and VIGIV may be beneficial.

Inadvertent vaccination of a pregnant woman occasionally results in fetal complications, with an estimated fetal vaccinia case rate of one case per 10,000 to 100,000 vaccinated pregnant women. Although IV-VIG has not been licensed for this purpose, but it can be offered for use as an investigational product. Some investigators suggest use of IV-VIG if it is given within 10 days of vaccination of a pregnant woman.[141,497,721]

In ocular vaccinia, VIGIM is contraindicated for isolated vaccinial keratitis because it may increase corneal scarring[425] as suggested by animal studies. If additional indications for VIGIM exist, such as conjunctivitis, blepharitis, and eczema vaccinatum, keratitis is not a contraindication for use of VIGIM. Scarring can occur from vaccinial keratitis in the absence of VIGIM treatment. IV-VIG has been used in an experimental rabbit model of vaccinia virus keratitis.[18] In this study, the use of IV-VIG neither exacerbated nor ameliorated the keratitis but did not cause the corneal scarring seen with the use of VIGIM. Topical medications such as trifluridine also are recommended.[552]

In summary, VIG products appear to be generally safe, with few instances of allergic or adverse reactions. The intramuscular and intravenous products are well tolerated, and because intravenous administration results in a more favorable pharmacokinetic profile than the intramuscular preparation, this may be the preferred product for significant vaccinia exposures. The recommended dosage of VIGIV (Cangene) for the management of severe complications of smallpox (vaccinia) vaccination (indications previously listed) is 6000 U/kg, to be given as soon as symptoms appear.[44] The intravenous product has clinical advantages over the intramuscular product that include absence of mercury, rapid absorption, and more favorable pharmacokinetics.[775]

IV-VIG at a very high dose was used in the treatment of a smallpox vaccinee with undiagnosed acute myelogenous leukemia who developed progressive vaccinia. The total dose given to this patient was 16,740,000 U over 4 days, with good resolution.[149] The CDC has developed clinical evaluation tools for smallpox vaccine adverse reactions, which are available on their website (http://emergency.cdc.gov/agent/smallpox/vaccination/clineval).

Regional Viruses

Argentine Hemorrhagic Fever

Junin virus, the etiologic agent of Argentine hemorrhagic fever (AHF), causes a febrile illness with high mortality rates from vascular or neurologic complications.[555] Patients may improve or have severe hemorrhagic or neurologic manifestations (or both) within the first 2 weeks of illness.[447] Maiztegui and colleagues[447] found that immune plasma given before the ninth day of illness to 91 patients reduced the mortality rate to 1.1%, compared with a mortality rate of 16.5% for the 97 patients given normal plasma ($P < .01$). Ten of the patients who received immune plasma relapsed with fever and cerebellar signs after several weeks, as did eight others who were not part of the study. The neurologic relapse was self-limited in all but one patient, who died.

With a case-fatality rate of the illness without treatment between 15% and 30%, the use of a live attenuated vaccine has markedly reduced the incidence of AHF.[212] Present specific therapy involves the transfusion of immune plasma with defined doses of neutralizing antibodies during the prodromal phase of illness.[19] However, alternative forms of treatment are called for because of the current difficulties in early detection of AHF, related to its decrease in incidence, troubles in maintaining adequate stocks of immune plasma, and the absence of effective therapies for severely ill patients that progress to a neurologic-hemorrhagic phase.[212]

Difficulty in obtaining immune plasma, possible neurologic complications of plasma treatment, and lack of efficacy late in the course of the disease have led to the use of ribavirin, despite its limitation late in the disease.[213] An effective, live attenuated viral vaccine is in use, with a protective efficacy of 95% against AHF.[19,448]

Ebola Infection

Ebola virus, a filovirus, causes severe and often fatal hemorrhagic fever. In March 2014, the largest Ebola outbreak in history occurred in West Africa. This outbreak has spurred research therapies, including monoclonal antibodies[101,479,580] and vaccines,[327] to treat the disease.[383]

Kudoyarova-Zubavichene and coworkers[406] reviewed the use of hyperimmune goat or equine serum in the prevention and treatment of Ebola infection. Goat hyperimmune serum protects guinea pigs from experimental infection if it is given less than 24 hours before exposure and provides some benefit if it is given within 72 hours after exposure. This product was used for emergency prophylaxis in four patients exposed by laboratory accidents. Mild infection developed in one definitely exposed patient, but Ebola disease did not develop in the other three patients with questionable exposure. All four patients also received recombinant human INF-α_2. Equine serum has protected baboons from low-dose virus challenge but not cynomolgus monkeys from a high-dose virus challenge.[339] Equine serum given to monkeys on the day of infection and 5 days later did not prevent death.[338]

Gupta and coauthors[292] reported that a murine polyclonal immune serum protected 100% of normal mice and mice with severe combined immunodeficiency after a lethal challenge. Wilson and colleagues[770] were able to protect mice with monoclonal antibodies to Ebola glycoprotein for up to 2 days after infection. Parren and associates[540] were able to protect guinea pigs by giving a human neutralizing antibody up to 1 hour after infection with Ebola virus. Protection of mice by neutralizing monoclonal antibody before and up to 2 days after virus was also shown.[697] Antibody may be a useful agent in the prevention of Ebola disease. Other human monoclonal antibodies are being developed.[203,454,455,793]

Recommendations. The use of antibody in the prevention and treatment of Ebola infection has not been proved, but monoclonal antibodies and vaccines are being developed.

Tickborne Encephalitis

Tickborne encephalitis is caused by a flavivirus that is endemic in Russia and eastern and central Europe. Several neurologic syndromes are associated with this infection: febrile headache, aseptic meningitis, meningoencephalitis, meningomyeloencephalitis, and postencephalitic syndrome.[199] Meningoencephalitis is the most severe form, and it can result in death or permanent paresis. Effective vaccines are available[199,290] and have been successful in dramatically lowering the incidence of this disease.[408]

Passive immunization with a hyperimmune human globulin has been used for postexposure prophylaxis in endemic countries, but it may result in antibody-dependent enhancement of infection.[386,745] Arras and colleagues[50] question these case reports in contrast to the large number of doses of passive antibody given. Günther and Hagland[290] contend that hyperimmunoglobulin is not indicated for children younger than 14 years because of concerns that antibody may worsen the disease. The lack of efficacy trials also led to questioning of the use of this product.[10]

In 1995, von Hedenstrüm and colleagues[742] recommended hyperimmunoglobulin for postexposure prophylaxis in addition to immunization. In a review of 656 patients with tickborne encephalitis in southern Germany, Kaiser[359] concluded that postexposure prophylaxis with hyperimmunoglobulin was less effective than with vaccine and should be used only when necessary. It is thought that vaccine is the best method for disease prevention.

Acknowledgments

I am grateful to Drs. E. Richard Stiehm and Margaret A. Keller, authors of this chapter in the sixth edition of this book, and Dr. Deborah Lehman, author of this chapter in the seventh edition.

NEW REFERENCES SINCE THE SEVENTH EDITION

13. Akcam AT, Ulku A, Rencuzogullari A, et al. Antiviral combination therapy with low-dose hepatitis B immunoglobulin for the prevention of hepatitis B virus recurrence in liver transplant recipients: a single-center experience. *Transplant Proc.* 2015;47:1445-1449.
14. Alejandria MM, Lansang MA, Dans LF, et al. Intravenous immunoglobulin for treating sepsis, severe sepsis and septic shock. *Cochrane Database Syst Rev.* 2013;(9):CD001090.
42. Ammann EM, Haskins CB, Fillman KM, et al. Intravenous immune globulin and thromboembolic adverse events: a systematic review and meta-analysis of RCTs. *Am J Hematol.* 2016;91:594-605.
43. Ammann EM, Jones MP, Link BK, et al. Intravenous immune globulin and thromboembolic adverse events in patients with hematologic malignancy. *Blood.* 2016;127:200-207.
68. Bapat P, Koren G. The role of VariZIG in pregnancy. *Expert Rev Vaccines.* 2013;12:1243-1248.
84. Bertolasi L, Frasson E, Turri M, et al. A randomized controlled trial of IV immunoglobulin in patients with postpolio syndrome. *J Neurol Sci.* 2013;330:94-99.
101. Bornholdt ZA, Turner HL, Murin CD, et al. Isolation of potent neutralizing antibodies from a survivor of the 2014 Ebola virus outbreak. *Science.* 2016;351:1078-1083.
105. Bradley JS, Peacock G, Krug SE, et al. Pediatric anthrax clinical management: executive summary. *Pediatrics.* 2014;133:940-942.
152. Centers for Disease Control and Prevention. Updated recommendations for use of VariZIG—United States, 2013. *MMWR Morb Mortal Wkly Rep.* 2013;62:574-576.
155. Cerino A, Bremer CM, Glebe D, et al. A human monoclonal antibody against hepatitis B surface antigen with potent neutralizing activity. *PLoS ONE.* 2015;10:e0125704.
156. Chalk CH, Benstead TJ, Keezer M. Medical treatment for botulism. *Cochrane Database Syst Rev.* 2014;(2):CD008123.
177. Cowan J, Cameron DW, Knoll G, et al. Protocol for updating a systematic review of randomised controlled trials on the prophylactic use of intravenous immunoglobulin for patients undergoing haematopoietic stem cell transplantation. *BMJ Open.* 2015;5:e008316.
179. Crabol Y, Terrier B, Rozenberg F, et al. Intravenous immunoglobulin therapy for pure red cell aplasia related to human parvovirus b19 infection: a retrospective study of 10 patients and review of the literature. *Clin Infect Dis.* 2013;56:968-977.
264. Golsaz Shirazi F, Mohammadi H, Amiri MM, et al. Monoclonal antibodies to various epitopes of hepatitis B surface antigen inhibit hepatitis B virus infection. *J Gastroenterol Hepatol.* 2014;29:1083-1091.
284. INIS Collaborative Group, Brocklehurst P, Farrell B, et al. Treatment of neonatal sepsis with intravenous immune globulin. *N Engl J Med.* 2011;365:1201-1211.
289. Gunther G, Dreger B. Post-marketing observational study on 5% intravenous immunoglobulin therapy in patients with secondary immunodeficiency and recurrent serious bacterial infections. *Microbiol Immunol.* 2013;57:527-535.
327. Huttner A, Dayer JA, Yerly S, et al. The effect of dose on the safety and immunogenicity of the VSV Ebola candidate vaccine: a randomised double-blind, placebo-controlled phase 1/2 trial. *Lancet Infect Dis.* 2015;15:1156-1166.
239. Gairard-Dory AC, Degot T, Hirschi S, et al. Clinical usefulness of oral immunoglobulins in lung transplant recipients with norovirus gastroenteritis: a case series. *Transplant Proc.* 2014;46:3603-3605.
323. Hu TH, Chen CL, Lin CC, et al. Section 14. Combination of entecavir plus low-dose on-demand hepatitis B immunoglobulin is effective with very low hepatitis B recurrence after liver transplantation. *Transplantation.* 2014;97(suppl 8):S53-S59.
383. Kilgore PE, Grabenstein JD, Salim AM, et al. Treatment of Ebola virus disease. *Pharmacotherapy.* 2015;35:43-53.

395. Koopman FS, Beelen A, Gilhus NE, et al. Treatment for postpolio syndrome. *Cochrane Database Syst Rev*. 2015;(5):CD007818.
431. Linner A, Darenberg J, Sjolin J, et al. Clinical efficacy of polyspecific intravenous immunoglobulin therapy in patients with streptococcal toxic shock syndrome: a comparative observational study. *Clin Infect Dis*. 2014;59:851-857.
479. Misasi J, Gilman MS, Kanekiyo M, et al. Structural and molecular basis for Ebola virus neutralization by protective human antibodies. *Science*. 2016;351:1343-1346.
522. Ohlsson A, Lacy JB. Intravenous immunoglobulin for preventing infection in preterm and/or low birth weight infants. *Cochrane Database Syst Rev*. 2013;(7):CD000361.
523. Ohlsson A, Lacy JB. Intravenous immunoglobulin for suspected or proven infection in neonates. *Cochrane Database Syst Rev*. 2013;(7):CD001239.
546. Patel M, Kaufman DA. Anti-lipoteichoic acid monoclonal antibody (pagibaximab) studies for the prevention of staphylococcal bloodstream infections in preterm infants. *Expert Opin Biol Ther*. 2015;15:595-600.
568. Ramirez-Avila L, Garner OB, Cherry JD. Relative EBV antibody concentrations and cost of standard IVIG and CMV-IVIG for PTLD prophylaxis in solid organ transplant patients. *Pediatr Transplant*. 2014;18:599-601.
579. Revello MG, Lazzarotto T, Guerra B, et al. A randomized trial of hyperimmune globulin to prevent congenital cytomegalovirus. *N Engl J Med*. 2014;370:1316-1326.
580. Reynard O, Volchkov VE. Characterization of a novel neutralizing monoclonal antibody against Ebola virus GP. *J Infect Dis*. 2015;212(suppl 2):S372-S378.
584. Robinson KA, Odelola OA, Saldanha IJ. Palivizumab for prophylaxis against respiratory syncytial virus infection in children with cystic fibrosis. *Cochrane Database Syst Rev*. 2014;(5):CD007743.
585. Roche B, Roque-Afonso AM, Nevens F, et al. Rational basis for optimizing short and long-term hepatitis B virus prophylaxis post liver transplantation: role of hepatitis B immune globulin. *Transplantation*. 2015;99:1321-1334.
629. Shankar-Hari M, Spencer J, Sewell WA, et al. Bench-to-bedside review: immunoglobulin therapy for sepsis—biological plausibility from a critical care perspective. *Crit Care*. 2012;16:206.
656. Soares MO, Welton NJ, Harrison DA, et al. Intravenous immunoglobulin for severe sepsis and septic shock: clinical effectiveness, cost-effectiveness and value of a further randomised controlled trial. *Crit Care*. 2014;18:649.
683. Styczynski J, Gil L, Tridello G, et al. Response to rituximab-based therapy and risk factor analysis in Epstein Barr virus-related lymphoproliferative disorder after hematopoietic stem cell transplant in children and adults: a study from the Infectious Diseases Working Party of the European Group for Blood and Marrow Transplantation. *Clin Infect Dis*. 2013;57:794-802.
694. Tagami T, Matsui H, Fushimi K, et al. Intravenous immunoglobulin use in septic shock patients after emergency laparotomy. *J Infect*. 2015;71:158-166.
695. Tagami T, Matsui H, Fushimi K, et al. Intravenous immunoglobulin and mortality in pneumonia patients with septic shock: an observational nationwide study. *Clin Infect Dis*. 2015;61:385-392.
741. Vo AA, Jordan SC. Benefits, efficacy, cost-effectiveness and infectious complications in transplant patients desensitized with intravenous immunoglobulin and anti-CD20 therapy. *Clin Exp Immunol*. 2014;178(suppl 1):48-51.
746. Walker K, Brink A, Lawrenson J, et al. Treatment of sydenham chorea with intravenous immunoglobulin. *J Child Neurol*. 2012;27:147-155.
767. Williams D. Treatment of rotavirus-associated diarrhea using enteral immunoglobulins for pediatric stem cell transplant patients. *J Oncol Pharm Pract*. 2015;21:238-240.
785. Yen MH, Huang YC, Chen MC, et al. Effect of intravenous immunoglobulin for neonates with severe enteroviral infections with emphasis on the timing of administration. *J Clin Virol*. 2015;64:92-96.

The full reference list for this chapter is available at ExpertConsult.com.

Public Health Aspects of Infectious Disease Control

247

Kathleen H. Harriman • Laurene Mascola

PUBLIC HEALTH AND INFECTIOUS DISEASE CLINICIANS

Infectious disease physicians and other clinicians who provide care for patients with known or suspected infectious diseases play an essential role in infectious disease surveillance and are important public health partners. Systematic infectious disease surveillance is critical in informing disease prevention and control efforts, and public health practitioners rely on clinicians to report cases of infectious disease.

In addition to the routine reporting of reportable infectious diseases, which is essential for public health surveillance, often the first notification to public health authorities of an unusual case or cluster of disease cases is made by an astute clinician. Only after public health authorities are alerted to an unusual case or cluster of disease cases through reporting by a clinician or analysis of surveillance data may an investigation take place and any necessary control measures be implemented.

Frontline clinicians play a crucial role in recognizing patients with an unusual constellation of symptoms, symptoms of a disease of public health importance that is rarely seen in the United States, a severe presentation of what is typically a less severe infectious disease, or a severe illness with the hallmarks of infectious disease for which a diagnosis cannot be found. Such cases take on even more importance when the patient has a history of international travel, exposure to exotic animals, or other unusual exposures. When such cases are reported to public health, often they can be evaluated with diagnostic methods that may not be available commercially.

This chapter describes the mutually beneficial collaboration between public health and infectious disease clinicians.

PUBLIC HEALTH

"The success or failure of any government in the final analysis must be measured by the well-being of its citizens. Nothing can be more important to a state than its public health; the state's paramount concern should be the health of its people."

—Franklin Delano Roosevelt, 1932

The US Centers for Disease Control and Prevention (CDC) defines public health as the science of protecting and improving the health of families and communities through promotion of healthy lifestyles, research on disease and injury prevention, and detection and control of infectious diseases.[26] This chapter focuses on the prevention and control of infectious diseases, although the same principles can be applied to many other health problems.

INFECTIOUS DISEASE SURVEILLANCE

One of the essential services of public health is monitoring the health of the population. Public health surveillance is one method used to monitor the incidence of infectious diseases. The CDC Working Group on Public Health Surveillance Systems defines public health surveillance as "the ongoing, systematic collection, analysis, interpretation, and dissemination of data about a health-related event for use in public health action to reduce morbidity and mortality and to improve health" and notes that outbreak identification requires "an increase in frequency of disease above the background occurrence of the disease."[10]

The Institute of Medicine's 1988 report on the future of public health highlighted the role and goals of surveillance by recognizing that one of the three core functions of public health—assessment—relies on public health surveillance to identify and describe problems, guide decisions about appropriate actions, and monitor progress.[68]

In 2011, the US Council of State and Territorial Epidemiologists stated that the overarching goal of surveillance is "[t]o provide actionable health information to public health staff, government leaders, and the public to guide public health policy and programs."[92]

Uses of infectious disease surveillance data include identifying outbreaks, informing and evaluating disease prevention and control efforts, determining vaccination strategies and assessing vaccine safety and effectiveness, monitoring antimicrobial resistance, monitoring health care–associated infections, and guiding allocation of resources for disease prevention, control, and treatment programs.

In the United States, the CDC and state, local, and territorial health departments carry out public health functions, including infectious disease surveillance. Public health authorities at the CDC, state, and territorial health departments collaborate in determining which diseases should be nationally notifiable to the CDC. Additionally, reporting of specified infectious diseases is required by law in each state. Although health care providers and laboratories are typically designated reporters, state laws vary with regard to the persons who are responsible for reporting, the diseases or conditions that are reportable, and the circumstances under which reporting is to occur.[6] Specific information is generally available online or on request from state or local public health agencies.

Although public health is responsible for evaluating and taking action on infectious diseases identified through disease surveillance, unless a report of disease is initiated by a health care provider, infection preventionist, or laboratory, no information is generated. Without baseline data on the incidence of infectious diseases, an increase or decrease in cases might not be recognized. Timely and accurate public health surveillance data can lead to earlier outbreak detection and more rapid implementation of prevention and control measures. In addition, the impact of intervention activities and other public health activities can be evaluated more accurately, leading to a more rational establishment of priorities and resource allocation.

However, the collection of data without analysis, interpretation, and dissemination of the data is of no value. Public health surveillance data obtained by both traditional and nontraditional means, such as syndromic surveillance, can be used for immediate public health action, program planning and evaluation, and formulating research hypotheses.[13,12] When used properly, surveillance data help in directing disease prevention and control activities and evaluating their impact.

Incentives to primary reporting sources to maintain good reporting, such as ongoing feedback, are essential for maintaining a useful surveillance system. After surveillance data are analyzed, the results are relayed to the primary reporting source and to others interested in the data. Such feedback serves to sustain interest in the reporting system and thereby maintains the quality of data obtained and continuously updates persons at each level of the surveillance system about the changing patterns of disease occurrence and new strategies for disease prevention and control.

One vehicle for the feedback of national surveillance information is the *Morbidity and Mortality Weekly Report,* which is published by the CDC.[37] The CDC also publishes periodic summaries of surveillance activities relating to specific diseases. In addition, regular summaries of surveillance activities are published by many state and local health departments as well as the World Health Organization (WHO).[100] Today, most public health agencies have publically accessible websites, and most of these summaries are easily available online.

Increased use of automated reporting systems using electronic health records and laboratory results has streamlined the reporting process and improved the completeness and timeliness of surveillance data.[20] In addition, social media is increasingly playing a role in infectious disease surveillance. Public health practitioners use social media to monitor trends, collect data, and provide information; the public uses social media to monitor and report diseases and obtain information. The use of social media and online resources will continue to enhance public health surveillance.

HOW PUBLIC HEALTH CAN ASSIST CLINICIANS

Clinicians can contact public health agencies for consultation when they encounter patients who may have infectious diseases with known, unknown, or unclear etiologies, or when an outbreak is suspected. When a clinician encounters a patient who has an unusual or severe presentation of what appears to be an infectious disease or becomes aware of a cluster of patients with similar symptoms, public health may be able to assist with determining a diagnosis. Public health also investigates suspected outbreaks of infectious disease and implements outbreak control measures.

Point-of-care bidirectional communication between public health practitioners and clinicians can facilitate clinical decision making based on the most current public health information. For example, public health practitioners can inform clinicians about infectious diseases known to be circulating in the area of the patient's residence and about infectious diseases patients may have been exposed to during travel. Public health practitioners can also provide recommendations for treatment and isolation of infected patients and postexposure prophylaxis for their contacts, including first responders such as emergency medical services personnel.

In addition, public health laboratories can be extremely helpful to clinicians. Although clinical laboratories provide excellent service for routine testing, they may not be able to test for more obscure pathogens. If an unusual disease is suspected, public health laboratories can perform testing for an array of possible agents, including biologic threats. Public health practitioners and laboratories also may be able to assist clinicians in establishing a diagnosis when the differential diagnosis contains several possible infectious disease entities with similar clinical presentations. New infectious disease diagnostic technologies will continue to be developed and are likely to be initially available only at public health laboratories.

Public health laboratories can often also detect more common pathogens such as *Neisseria meningitidis* or *Streptococcus pneumoniae* in clinical specimens that have not grown in culture in clinical laboratories by using nucleic acid–based assays such as polymerase chain reaction (PCR) because the sensitivity of the PCR test is not affected by prior antibiotic treatment.[83] Public health laboratories may also perform PCR testing for other diseases such as measles, which can be diagnostically challenging in an era of low incidence.

In addition to identifying disease-causing pathogens, public health laboratories are able to use molecular methods to perform strain typing that further characterizes pathogens and may identify novel strain types. Such testing may also detect new agents and identify outbreaks. A public health laboratory first identified 2009 pandemic H1N1 influenza A, which at the time was a novel influenza strain.

Advancement in laboratory methods has also enhanced the usefulness of surveillance data in outbreak detection by linking bacterial isolates obtained from geographically scattered cases. CDC coordinates PulseNet,[39] a national network of public health and food regulatory agency laboratories that connects foodborne illness cases to detect outbreaks. PulseNet uses a variety of methods to subtype *Escherichia coli* (O157 and other Shiga toxin–producing *E. coli*), *Campylobacter, Listeria monocytogenes, Salmonella, Shigella, Vibrio cholerae, Vibrio parahaemolyticus,* and *Cronobacter* isolates. Pulsed-field gel electrophoresis (PFGE), multiple-locus variable-number tandem repeat analysis (MLVA), and whole-genome sequencing (WGS) are PulseNet's main subtyping (or "fingerprinting") tools. These molecular fingerprints, or patterns, are submitted electronically to a dynamic database at CDC. This database is available on demand to participants, which allows for rapid comparison of the patterns and identification of clusters of cases, which can lead to identification and removal of contaminated food products from the homes of consumers thereby preventing further disease. In addition to foodborne outbreaks, PulseNet has also identified outbreaks caused by bacteria from animal and water sources.

The use of culture-independent diagnostic tests (CIDTs) is rapidly changing the way that clinical laboratories diagnose patients with infectious diseases. Antigen-based tests and nucleic acid–based assays that do not depend on culture and produce no isolate have become increasingly common. Almost all *Clostridium difficile, Legionella* spp., *Bordetella pertussis* and influenza cases are now diagnosed by CIDTs.[73] The use of CIDTs for enteric infections such as *Campylobacter* and Shiga toxin–producing *E. coli* is also very common.[66] The use of CIDTs has implications for public health surveillance because bacterial isolates are needed for molecular characterization, which may be used in addition to other data to attribute illness to specific sources. In addition, isolates are necessary for antimicrobial resistance testing. Although PCR testing is available for many of the known genes that cause antimicrobial resistance, new resistance genes would not be detected. Therefore, public health laboratories will continue to request some CIDT-positive specimens from clinical laboratories for culture and isolate-based monitoring until new testing methods, such as metagenomics and next-generation sequencing technology that work directly on clinical specimens, become established.[39,47]

Another CDC online tool is MicrobeNet, which can be used by clinicians, hospitals, and public health to rapidly identify rare and emerging infections. Traditionally, clinicians or laboratorians who needed to identify rare bacteria or fungi or to confirm an infectious disease diagnosis due to an uncommon organism needed to send a sample to the CDC and await test results. MicrobeNet provides access to the CDC's virtual microbe library of more than 2400 rare and emerging infectious bacteria and fungi and helps public health laboratories and hospitals quickly identify some of the most difficult pathogens to grow and detect.[36]

OUTBREAK INVESTIGATION

When faced with an unusual case or cluster of cases that may be of public health concern, public health authorities conduct an investigation in an attempt to determine or confirm a diagnosis, describe the scope of the problem, and, if unknown, identify a cause. Front-line clinicians may be called on to assist in such investigations.

When investigating a possible outbreak, a useful approach is for investigators to address the inquiry systematically using the CDC's 10-step method[41]:

Prepare for Fieldwork

The following are the steps in preparing for fieldwork:

1. Establish the existence of an outbreak
2. Verify the diagnosis
3. Define and identify cases
4. Describe and orient the data in terms of time, place, and person
5. Develop hypotheses
6. Evaluate hypotheses
7. Refine hypotheses and carry out additional studies
8. Implement control and prevention measures
9. Communicate findings

Several exercises illustrating these principles, including communicable and noncommunicable disease outbreaks, can be found at the CDC's training site for epidemic intelligence service officers.[28]

PUBLIC HEALTH PREVENTION AND CONTROL MEASURES

After an unusual case or cluster of cases is recognized and an investigation has occurred, many tools are available for public health intervention, if it is indicated. Two important interventions, immunization and the treatment of individual patients, are not considered in this chapter because they are addressed at length elsewhere in this book.

Other public health tools that are not discussed here but are also relevant to the prevention and control of infectious diseases include modifications to human behaviors that affect exposure to infectious diseases such as sexual behavior and injection drug use, water and food sanitation, food preparation methods, burial practices, and so on.

Additionally, various prevention and control measures can be applied to animals, such as vaccination and treatment or prophylaxis, that decrease their risk for spreading diseases to humans.[71] Finally, prevention and control measures can be applied to the environment, such as proper disposal of waste, vector control, and appropriate design and proper maintenance of buildings and other equipment that can reduce opportunities for disease transmission. An example of such a control measure would include proper maintenance of spas or cooling towers to prevent *Legionella* transmission.[24]

Isolation

Isolation is the separation of persons who have a specific infectious illness from those who are healthy, and the restriction of their movement to stop the spread of that illness during the period of communicability.[40] Indications for isolation of patients with infectious diseases have changed greatly in the twentieth century with increasing knowledge about modes of transmission and with antimicrobial therapy, which rapidly renders patients with many diseases noninfectious. The American Academy of Pediatrics (AAP) *Red Book: Report of the Committee on Infectious Diseases* is an excellent resource for information about isolation recommendations.[2]

Quarantine

In addition to containing the spread of communicable illnesses through isolation, another less commonly used control measure is quarantine. Quarantine is the separation and restriction of movement of susceptible persons who, although not yet ill, have been exposed to an infectious agent and therefore may become infectious.[30] When quarantine is used it is imposed for a period equal to the longest usual incubation period of the disease.

The history and practice of quarantine began as early as the 14th century in Italy to control plague by requiring ships arriving in Venice from infected ports to anchor for 40 days before landing.[33] The Italian word, *quaranta,* meaning 40, evolved into the commonly used word *quarantine.*

In recent years, health departments in the United States have rarely implemented quarantine. However, it was used during the 2003 severe acute respiratory syndrome (SARS) outbreak, and it may also be used for susceptible persons who have been exposed to measles and did not receive timely postexposure prophylaxis.

Preexposure and Postexposure Prophylaxis

The word prophylaxis is used in this section to describe the use of antimicrobial or immunologic agents to prevent infection before or after exposure to an infectious disease. The decision to initiate preexposure or postexposure prophylaxis and the choice and dosage of agents require careful consideration of both the child's clinical status and the epidemiologic factors that may place the child at risk for acquiring the disease. Public health authorities should be notified of cases and exposures of reportable infectious diseases. A public health investigation may be conducted to ensure that all exposed persons have been identified and, when necessary, treated or placed under observation or even quarantine. In addition, public health practitioners can often provide useful additional information on recommended prophylaxis regimens. For detailed information on the use of prophylaxis to prevent specific infectious diseases, the regularly updated AAP *Red Book: Report of the Committee on Infectious Diseases* should be consulted.[2] In addition, the US Advisory Committee for Immunization Practices recommendations also contain information about prophylaxis for vaccine-preventable diseases.[25]

COMMON PATTERNS OF DISEASE SPREAD

Animal-to-Person Spread

Many infectious diseases are transmitted from animals to humans (zoonoses). Of all emerging diseases in the 20th and 21st centuries, more than 75% are zoonotic in origin.[56] Clinicians who routinely inquire about animal contacts as part of the clinical and epidemiologic history of an ill patient frequently find valuable clues to an obscure diagnosis.

Details of the clinical manifestations, differential diagnosis, and treatment of zoonoses are found in the appropriate chapters elsewhere in this book. For a complete description of the circumstances under which each agent is spread from animal to person, consult a textbook of zoonoses. Often, emerging and reemerging infectious diseases in humans, such as SARS, Middle East respiratory syndrome (MERS), and Ebola virus, are found to have an animal reservoir.[1,59]

Person-to-Person Spread

As members of groups—including their families, schools, camps, child care centers, and religious organizations—children are at risk for acquiring or spreading infectious agents that are transmitted from person to person. Knowledge of the typical patterns of spread can be useful in planning surveillance or in designing prevention and control measures. For example, recognition that diarrheal illnesses can result from person-to-person spread in child care centers and that it can indicate inadequate hygienic practices may justify specific surveillance for diarrhea in that setting.

In this section, disease transmission in the household, child care centers, and schools is briefly discussed. The important areas of disease transmission in child care centers and hospitals are discussed in separate chapters in more depth. Maternal transmission of specific infections to the fetus or neonate is also reviewed elsewhere in this book.

EXAMPLES OF EXPOSURE SOURCES

Contaminated Food

Many foods have been shown to be the vehicle of transmission in outbreaks caused by a wide range of bacteria, viruses, and parasites, in addition to many naturally occurring toxins and human-made chemicals. Inherent contamination of meat, poultry, and eggs with *Salmonella,* Shiga toxin–producing *E. coli, Listeria,* and other pathogens, as well as deficiencies in food storage and preparation and ingestion of raw or improperly cooked animal products in both eating establishments and the home, still contribute to outbreaks and sporadic cases of gastrointestinal infectious diseases.[48,60,61,64] In addition, practices with known risks such as drinking unpasteurized milk can result in infection.[31]

Outbreaks of infection and secondary hemolytic uremic syndrome resulting from infection with Shiga toxin–producing *E. coli* strains such as O157:H7 and O104:H4 have been related to juice,[97] ground beef,[87] spinach,[14] sprouts,[9] unpasteurized milk,[51,57] and other food items. In addition, new problems can result from changes in the food industry and in patterns of food consumption.[50] In recent years, several large outbreaks of salmonellosis have been associated with the widespread distribution of fresh produce, a previously rare vehicle of *Salmonella* transmission.[5]

The CDC publishes the Foodborne Outbreak Online Database,[32] and although the number of outbreaks reported to public health authorities represents only a small fraction of those that occur, these reports can provide important insight into the epidemiology of foodborne disease.

Clinicians must work in conjunction with public health authorities by confirming diagnoses through appropriate diagnostic methods and promptly reporting findings or suspicions of foodborne illness so that foodborne outbreaks can be recognized in a timely fashion to control and prevent these illnesses most effectively.

Recreational Water

Water can be a source of infectious disease, and outbreaks of waterborne disease associated with recreational water use, such as swimming or wading[46,63,86]; use of hot tubs, spas, and water parks[16,67,72]; and exposure to decorative fountains[93] have been reported. Diseases transmitted in this manner include shigellosis, cryptosporidiosis, norovirus gastroenteritis, viral conjunctivitis, giardiasis, legionellosis, enterohemorrhagic *E. coli* O157:H7, and *Pseudomonas* dermatitis ("hot tub folliculitis").[90]

Deaths may occur, especially with cases of primary amebic meningoencephalitis caused by any of several free-living amebae in persons who had recently been swimming, typically in warm, stagnant water.[7,78] In the United States, these infections have traditionally been reported in southern-tier states, with more than half of infections occurring in Texas and Florida.[38] However, in 2010 and 2012, *Naegleria fowleri* infections were documented in Minnesota, an area at much higher latitude than previous US cases.[69]

Unpasteurized Milk

Unpasteurized or "raw" milk has been demonstrated as the vehicle of transmission in outbreaks of brucellosis, tuberculosis, and diphtheria, as well as outbreaks of diseases caused by group A streptococci, *Salmonella, Shigella, Campylobacter, Listeria, Yersinia enterocolitica,* and staphylococcal toxin.[49,75] Exposure to unpasteurized milk should be rare in the United States. Unfortunately, the use of raw milk as a "health food" continues to account for outbreaks of disease, particularly outbreaks caused by *E. coli* O157:H7, *Salmonella,* and *Campylobacter*.[31,57,75,84] In addition, children sometimes drink raw milk while visiting dairy farms on school field trips, during other youth activities, or during travel to other countries, which puts them at risk for infectious diarrhea and Shiga toxin–producing *E. coli*–related renal failure.

VECTORBORNE DISEASE

Vectors such as mosquitoes and ticks can transmit infectious diseases. Examples of tick-borne diseases in the United States include anaplasmosis, babesiosis, ehrlichiosis, Lyme disease, Rocky Mountain spotted fever, tick-borne relapsing fever, tick paralysis, and tularemia.[23,52] Mosquito-borne diseases that have been found in the United States include West Nile virus infection, eastern equine encephalitis, La Crosse encephalitis, St. Louis encephalitis, and western equine encephalitis.[42] Outbreaks of locally transmitted cases of malaria in the United States have been small and relatively isolated,[35] but several dengue outbreaks have been detected in the United States since 1980, including seven outbreaks in southern Texas along the United States–Mexico border, one outbreak in Hawaii in 2001, and two outbreaks in southern Florida in 2009 and 2010.[94] Other vectorborne infections that can be carried back from foreign travel include Zika virus, chikungunya, dengue, Rift Valley fever, yellow fever, and many others. In addition, fleas can spread endemic or murine typhus, plague, and cat-scratch fever, and body lice can spread epidemic typhus, relapsing fever, and trench fever.

The CDC has excellent online resources for vectorborne diseases,[27] and local and state public health practitioners can provide clinicians with information on vectorborne diseases in the geographic regions they serve and other regions where patients may have traveled. In addition, public health laboratories may be able to assist in establishing a diagnosis.

Personal protection against vectors such as mosquitoes and ticks includes avoiding vector-infested areas and having an awareness of peak exposure times and places, wearing protective clothing, using insect repellents applied to skin or clothing and spatial repellents, using bed nets, and frequently inspecting for and promptly removing attached ticks.[82] These individual preventive measures can be practiced in any circumstance where exposure to infected mosquitoes or ticks may occur.

Bioterrorism and Natural Disasters

Unfortunately, an important responsibility of public health authorities is to help prepare the nation and clinicians for the possibility of biologic, radiologic, or chemical terrorism and natural disasters. Children have special vulnerabilities to biologic terrorism and chemical agents because of their unique physiology and the limited availability of age-appropriate and weight-appropriate antidotes and treatments.[58,81] Also, clinicians' unfamiliarity with presenting clinical syndromes from either biologic or chemical exposures could delay appropriate diagnosis and treatment.[45,58,89]

Another issue is that the Strategic National Stockpile, a national repository of antimicrobial agents, chemical antidotes, antitoxins, and other life-support medications and equipment, can only stockpile US Food and Drug Administration (FDA)-licensed items and only for their FDA-approved indications.[95] Often FDA indications for antimicrobial and other therapeutic agents for children after a biologic agent release are lacking, causing the stockpile to be deficient in certain therapeutic agents for children.

Terrorism preparedness is a unique and hopefully rare component of general emergency and disaster preparedness. However, natural disasters are more common, and infections that are typically rare in the United States can result from compromised personal hygiene, wounds and injuries, contaminated food and water, and exposure to insect vectors. Prompt recognition and appropriate management by clinicians of unusual diseases are critical during and after disaster situations.

COMMON DISEASE TRANSMISSION SETTINGS

Households

Spread of disease in households is common, and transmission can be considered in two stages: introduction of the agent into the family, usually by a single member, and spread to other family members.[8] Spread to other members can be described in terms of rapidity and intensity, the latter commonly measured by the secondary infection rate (or secondary attack rate), which is defined as the proportion of the contacts of the index carrier or index case who become infected (or ill) in a given interval after exposure. The secondary infection rate varies from agent to agent and may be affected by the age, sex, and infectivity of the introducer; the size of the family; crowding; the age of household contacts; previous immunity; and interventions attempted, including vaccination, isolation, treatment, and prophylaxis. The ratio of the secondary attack rate to the incidence of disease in the community is a measure of the importance of the family as a focus of disease.[55,77]

Child Care Centers

It is well known that infectious disease agents are easily transmitted among children in child care centers and that outbreaks occur in these settings[22,74,101] (see Chapter 248). Interventions that have proved valuable for reducing infections within child care centers include formal written policies for infection prevention and control within the child care center, formal education of child care center staff concerning infection prevention practices, good hand hygiene by both staff and children, appropriate cleaning of contaminated surfaces and items, separation of food preparation and diaper changing areas, exclusion of certain ill children, cohorting ill children when exclusion is not possible, and ensuring adequate age-appropriate immunization of child care attendees and staff and optimal ratios of children to staff.[62,98]

Schools

Typically, infectious disease spread in schools is less than that in families and child care centers. However, schools may serve to spread infection from family to family. Settings that result in a greater level of person-to-person contact than is found in typical classroom settings, such as participation in school sports[17] or attendance at boarding schools, summer camps, and college dormitories, also can result in more efficient transmission of disease.[3,65,88,91] In recent years, measles, mumps, influenza, meningococcal disease, norovirus, and methicillin-resistant *Staphylococcus aureus* outbreaks have occurred in these settings.[17,19,15,18,76,96]

HEALTH INFORMATION FOR INTERNATIONAL TRAVEL

International travel, whether by child or adult, necessitates preparation beforehand to obtain the proper immunizations and contingency plans for the possibility of encountering unsanitary food or water during the travel.[43,53,70,80] Illnesses acquired abroad may not be manifested until after returning home, with consequent diagnostic difficulty. Clinicians should query parents regarding travel when children have unusual symptoms or acute febrile rash illnesses.

Active and passive immunization are covered elsewhere in this book, and updated travel-related immunization information is available at the CDC's traveler's health website.[42,43,80] Disease-specific information for travelers and clinicians is available in the CDC's "Yellow Book" at that website,[42] including information on international travel with infants and children.[99] In addition, travel notices are available that can alert travelers and clinicians to infectious disease outbreaks occurring throughout the world. It should also be noted that measles remains endemic in much of the world outside of the Western Hemisphere, including some European countries. Infants traveling to parts of the world where measles is circulating should be vaccinated as young as 6 months of age.[21]

Safe water may be found in many hotels in large cities throughout the world, but only water from adequately chlorinated sources can be considered truly safe. Where chlorinated water is not available, canned or bottled carbonated beverages and beverages made from boiled water or that contain alcohol may be safe; however, an outbreak caused by commercially bottled water contaminated by non-O1 *Vibrio cholerae* has been described.[11] Ice made from untreated water may contaminate an otherwise safe beverage, either directly or by leaving contaminated water on the outside of the container. The CDC has prepared guidance on preparation and storage of safe water that can be found online.[29]

Food should also be selected carefully. In areas of the world where hygiene and sanitation are poor, travelers should avoid salads, uncooked vegetables, unpasteurized milk, and milk products such as cheese and should eat only fruits and vegetables that can be peeled by the traveler or have been cooked and are still hot. In addition to the recommendation that all children receive hepatitis A vaccine, persons who are traveling to countries with high or intermediate levels of endemic hepatitis A infection are recommended to receive hepatitis A vaccine before departure.[54]

Children younger than 2 years of age have a high risk for acquiring traveler's diarrhea.[4,79,85] Traveler's diarrhea is caused by several bacterial pathogens, including *E. coli, Shigella, Campylobacter, Salmonella, Aeromonas, Plesiomonas,* and noncholera vibrios. Noroviruses are also an important cause of morbidity among travelers, and outbreaks on cruise ships are frequently reported.[34] Some travelers may be at increased risk because genetic risk factors associated with susceptibility to specific pathogens have been identified.[4]

Immediate medical attention should be sought for an infant or child with blood or mucus in the stool, fever with rigors, or persistent vomiting or diarrhea with dehydration. Because infants and small children are particularly at risk for becoming dehydrated, parents need to be aware of the signs of dehydration and be prepared to use oral rehydration solutions containing appropriate concentrations or electrolytes as a preventive measure while medical attention is being obtained. WHO oral rehydration solutions are widely available at stores and pharmacies in most developing countries.

For more information on traveler's diarrhea, including antimicrobial treatment and oral rehydration therapy, please see the CDC Yellow Book.[42]

For travel to areas where vectorborne diseases circulate, guidance on general protective measures for mosquitoes, ticks, and other arthropods, including the use of insect repellents for children, can be found in the CDC Yellow Book.[82]

SUMMARY

By working together to leverage the strengths and resources of both, clinicians and public health practitioners are partners in protecting and improving the health of the community.

NEW REFERENCES SINCE THE SEVENTH EDITION

1. Adney DR, van Doremalen N, Brown VR, et al. Replication and Shedding of MERS-CoV in Upper Respiratory Tract of Inoculated Dromedary Camels. *Emerg Infect Dis*. 2014;20(12):1999-2005.
2. American Academy of Pediatrics. In: Kimberlin DW, Brady MT, Jackson MA, Long SS, eds. *Red Book: 2015 Report of the Committee on Infectious Diseases*. 30th ed. Elk Grove Village, IL: American Academy of Pediatrics; 2015.
3. Anderson BJ, McGuire DP, Reed M, et al. Prophylactic valacyclovir to prevent outbreaks of herpes gladiatorum at a 28-day wrestling camp: a 10-year review. *Clin J Sport Med*. 2016;26(4):272-278.
7. Booth PJ, Bodager D, Slade TA, et al. Notes from the Field: Primary Amebic Meningoencephalitis Associated with Hot Spring Exposure during International Travel: Seminole County, Florida, July 2014. *MMWR Morb Mortal Wkly Rep*. 2015;64(43):1226.
19. Centers for Disease Control and Prevention. Mumps outbreak on a university campus: California, 2011. *Morb Mortal Wkly Rep*. 2012;31(48):986-989.
21. Centers for Disease Control and Prevention. Prevention of measles, rubella, congenital rubella syndrome, and mumps, 2013: summary recommendations of the Advisory Committee on Immunization Practices (ACIP). *MMWR Recomm Rep*. 2013;62(RR-04):1-34.
22. Centers for Disease Control and Prevention. West Nile Virus and other nationally notifiable arboviral diseases—United States, 2014. *MMWR Morb Mortal Wkly Rep*. 2015;64(34):929-934.
23. Centers for Disease Control and Prevention. Diagnosis and management of tickborne rickettsial diseases: Rocky Mountain Spotted Fever and Other Spotted Fever Group Rickettsioses, Ehrlichioses, and Anaplasmosis—United States. *MMWR Recomm Rep*. 2016;65(2):1-44.
24. Centers for Disease Control and Prevention. Centers for Disease Control and Prevention. *Legionella* water system maintenance. Available at: http://www.cdc.gov/legionella/water-system-maintenance.html.
43. Christenson JC. Preparing families with children traveling to developing countries. *Pediatr Ann*. 2008;37(12):806-813.
44. Cleg WJ, Linchangco PC, Arwady MA, et al. Measles outbreak in a child care center, Cook County, Illinois, 2015. *J Pediatric Infect Dis Soc*. 2016;Epub ahead of print.
46. Cope JR, Prosser A, Nowicki S, et al. Preventing community-wide transmission of *Cryptosporidium:* a proactive public health response to a swimming pool-associated outbreak—Auglaize County, Ohio, USA. *Epidemiol Infect*. 2015;143(16):3459-3467.
48. Crowe SJ, Mahon BE, Viera AR, et al. Vital signs: multistate foodborne outbreaks—United States, 2010–2014. *MMWR Morb Mortal Wkly Rep*. 2015;64(43):1221-1225.
49. Davis KR, Dunn AC, Burnett C, et al. *Campylobacter jejuni* Infections Associated with Raw Milk Consumption—Utah, 2014. *MMWR Morb Mortal Wkly Rep*. 2016;65(12):301-305.
50. Doyle MP, Erickson MC, Alali W, et al. Food Industry's Current and Future Role in Preventing Microbial Foodborne Illness within the United States. *Clin Infect Dis*. 2015;61(2):252-259.
58. Hamele M, Poss WB, Sweney J. Disaster preparedness, pediatric considerations in primary blast injury, chemical, and biological terrorism. *World J Crit Care Med*. 2014;3(1):15-23.
59. Han HJ, Wen HL, Zhou CM, et al. Bats as reservoirs of severe emerging infectious diseases. *Virus Res*. 2015;205:1-6.
60. Heiman KE, Garalde VB, Gronostaj M, et al. Multistate outbreak of listeriosis caused by imported cheese and evidence of cross-contamination of other cheeses, USA, 2012. *Epidemiol Infect*. 2015;30:1-11.
61. Heiman KE, Mody RK, Johnson SD, et al. *Escherichia coli* O157 Outbreaks in the United States, 2003–2012. *Emerg Infect Dis*. 2015;21(8):1293-1301.
63. Hlavsa MC, Roberts VA, Kahler AM, et al. Outbreaks of Illness Associated with Recreational Water—United States, 2011–2012. *MMWR Morbid Mortal Wkly Rep*. 2015;64(24):668-672.
64. Hoffman N, Luo Y, Monday SR, et al. Tracing origins of the *Salmonella* Bareilly strain causing a food-borne outbreak in the United States. *J Infect Dis*. 2016;213(4):502-508.
77. Levri KM, Reynolds L, Liko J, et al. Risk Factors for Pertussis Among Hispanic Infants: Metropolitan Portland, Oregon, 2010–2012. *Pediatr Infect Dis J*. 2016;35(5):488-493.
87. Rangel JM, Sparling PH, Crowe C, et al. Epidemiology of *Escherichia coli* O157:H7 outbreaks, United States, 1982–2002. *Emerg Infect Dis*. 2005;11(4):603-609.
90. Segna KG, Koch LH, Williams JV. "Hot tub" folliculitis from a nonchlorinated children's pool. *Pediatr Dermatol*. 2011;28(5):590-591.
93. Smith SS, Ritger K, Samala U, et al. Legionellosis Outbreak Associated With a Hotel Fountain. *Open Forum Infect Dis*. 2015;2(4):1-7.
95. U.S. Government Accountability Office. Efforts to address the medical needs of children in a chemical, biological, radiological, or nuclear incident. April 2013. Available at: http://www.gao.gov/assets/660/654264.pdf.
96. Venuto M, Garcia K. Analyses of the contributing factors associated with foodborne outbreaks in school settings (2000–2010). *J Environ Health*. 2015;77(7):16-20.
98. Wagner J, Clodfelter S. Preventing diseases and outbreaks at child care centers using an education, evaluation, and inspection method. *J Environ Health*. 2014;76(7):18-23.
101. Yagupsky P. Outbreaks of *Kingella kingae* infections in daycare facilities. *Emerg Infect Dis*. 2014;20(5):746-753.

The full reference list for this chapter is available at ExpertConsult.com.

248 Infections in Out-of-Home Child Care

Sheryl L. Henderson • Ellen R. Wald

When parents are employed outside of the home or are otherwise unable to care for their preschool children during all or part of the day, they make arrangements for child care during their time away. The term child care encompasses a large variety of options in the absence of a parent or legal guardian. These include (1) small family child care homes that provide care for six or fewer children, usually in the home of the care provider; (2) large family child care homes that provide care for seven to 12 children, usually in the home of the care provider; (3) large child care centers housed in nonresidential settings that provide care for at least seven children in one location; and (4) facilities that care for ill children who are temporarily unable to attend their regular child care setting for health reasons.[15]

Of the estimated 20 million children younger than 5 years identified in the 2010 US Census, approximately 12 million (60%) attended some type of regular child care arrangement at least once a week. Approximately half of these received care provided by parents or relatives. Nearly 4.5 million (23%) preschool-aged children were cared for in an out-of-home organized child care facility (such as a child care center, nursery, or preschool), and 2.4 million (12%) had care provided by a nonrelative either in their own home or a family child care setting.[183] Federal statistics on the health and well-being of children indicate that in 2012, approximately 61% of children in the United States, aged 3 to 6 years, who were not yet attending kindergarten were enrolled in center-based child care—that is, child care centers, prekindergarten, nursery school, Head Start programs, and other early childhood education programs.[105]

The child care center for preschool-aged children is an optimal setting for infectious agents to be readily transmitted among children and staff. Therefore policies and practices that attend to the control and prevention of infectious disease are a major component of child care licensing procedures.[15,16] All states in the United States have licensing regulations for out-of-home child care. However, they are primarily directed toward child care centers, thus missing the majority of children attending child care homes.

FACTORS AFFECTING TRANSMISSION OF INFECTIOUS AGENTS

Numerous studies have demonstrated increased numbers of infections in children attending out-of-home group child care compared with those cared for at home.[27,76,87,99,100,153,208-210,284] The first year of child care attendance has been identified as a period of increased incidence of infectious illness among child care attendees in several studies. However, after this time period, incidence decreases, and results suggest that earlier child care attendance is protective of respiratory[27,87,154] or gastrointestinal[99,100,153] illness before school entry.

Multiple factors can contribute to the transmission of infectious agents in the group child care setting (Box 248.1), the most important of which are host factors relating to the immunologic susceptibility of young children. Children younger than 5 years do not naturally have fully developed immunity against the polysaccharide antigens of respiratory pathogens such as *Streptococcus pneumoniae, Haemophilus influenzae, Neisseria meningitidis,* and *Kingella kingae.*[287] The natural tendency for intimacy in an age group that has not established acceptable toileting practices and is not knowledgeable or fully capable of basic hygienic practices increases the chances of transmission from an infected child to another or to staff. In larger child care centers, children are usually placed in age cohorts, and thus the immunologically less mature are more contagious to each other and have greater tendency to develop illness. Respiratory and gastrointestinal pathogens frequently contaminate toys and environmental surfaces. Infants and toddlers are indiscriminate in mouthing objects and fingers, thus contributing to the potential organisms that naturally populate the saliva and the respiratory tract to be transmitted readily from child to child.

Unique risk factors identified as particularly important in the spread of gastrointestinal organisms are large numbers of diaper-aged children in centers where staff members who diaper children are also responsible for food preparation.[30,131] Separating diaper-aged children from those who are older is important to limit spread of enteric illness. If meals are prepared in the child care setting, separating this activity from toilet areas is essential. Current national guidelines recommend separate staff for handling food and diapering children in facilities large enough to have adequate staffing.[14,19] In addition, overcrowding, understaffing, and poorly designed physical environments can foster transmission of infectious agents in child care facilities. A lack of or inadequate number of hand-washing facilities or hand-sanitizing solutions for children and providers creates an almost insurmountable barrier to infection control. Other risk factors are related to the age of the participants, the number of children, and the ratio of staff to children. The last is determined in part by the age of the children; younger children require higher staff-to-child ratios. In overcrowded situations with inadequate staff, infection can be spread easily because of inappropriate hand hygiene or inattention to other facets of infection control. Parental situations may also factor into increased risk because parents may choose not to withdraw ill children from attendance at child care because of the expense and inconvenience of creating alternate child care arrangements, thus further exposing other children and staff to infectious agents. Availability and accessibility of resources for care of ill children in these situations would also reduce the risk for further spread of illness.

MODES OF TRANSMISSION OF INFECTIOUS DISEASES IN OUT-OF-HOME CHILD CARE

The major modes of transmission of infectious agents in out-of-home child care are respiratory, gastrointestinal (primarily fecal-oral), direct person-to-person contact, indirect contact with contaminated fomites, and contact with infected body fluids—blood, urine, or saliva. Some infections may be transmitted in more than one way (e.g., herpes simplex virus [HSV] can be spread through direct contact with broken skin or mucosal exposure to infected body fluids). The most important pathogens and their modes of transmission of infection in out-of-home child care are shown in Table 248.1. Respiratory and gastrointestinal infections are the most common causes of illness in infants, toddlers, and preschoolers, regardless of whether these children attend out-of-home child care.[155]

Respiratory

For some microbiologic species causing infection, the mode of transmission is the airborne route. Direct contact with the infected individual is not necessary for the spread of the infection. When an infected person coughs, sneezes, or sings, the organism is aerosolized into small droplets (<5 μm) and can remain suspended in the air for several hours. These aerosol nuclei are capable of traveling distances on air currents. Agents known to be transmitted by this means include the measles and varicella viruses and *Mycobacterium tuberculosis.*

Most commonly, respiratory organisms are spread by the production of droplets laden with infective particles. When an infected person talks, sneezes, or coughs, droplets containing these microorganisms are formed, expelled, and may land on the mucosa of another individual. These droplets may also be transmitted directly from mucosa to mucosa when close physical contact occurs. More often, droplets land on nonporous surfaces (e.g., cribs, tables, toys, chairs) or on clothes and paper (fomites) and remain infective for minutes to hours. Hand contact with contaminated surfaces and fomites can result in infection if the hands touch the nasal or conjunctival mucosa.[134,155] Agents that can be transmitted by droplet spread from mucosa to mucosa, from finger to mucosa, or by fomites include most respiratory viruses (respiratory syncytial virus [RSV], rhinovirus, human metapneumovirus, coronavirus, human herpesvirus type 6 [HHV-6], influenza virus, parainfluenza virus, adenovirus, parvovirus B19, measles virus, mumps virus, rubella virus, and varicella zoster virus), *Bordetella pertussis, Haemophilus influenzae* type b (HIB), *S. pneumoniae, N. meningitidis,* and *Streptococcus pyogenes.*[101,114,115,130,133,134] Finger-to-mucosa spread of respiratory pathogens is the most important and common mechanism for transmission of viral and bacterial infections and is a mechanism of self-inoculation.[143] Consequently, hand hygiene that includes hand washing and the use of alcohol-based sanitizers is an essential element of preventing spread of infection.[155,237]

BOX 248.1 Risk Factors for Infectious Disease in Child Care Facilities

Children

Immunologic susceptibility to infectious agents
Lack of or poor hygiene around toileting
Natural tendency to intimacy
Frequent oral contact with objects in the environment
Lack of awareness and practice of good hygiene

Caregivers

Insufficient training in infection control
Lack of policy regarding immunization
Inadequate screening for infectious diseases

Environmental Issues

Inappropriate staff-to-child ratios
Overcrowding
Failure to separate age groups
Poorly designed physical layout

- Inadequate or poorly placed sinks
- Toilet areas and food preparation areas and personnel are not separate

Parents

Pressure to admit sick children to out-of-home child care

Gastrointestinal

Gastrointestinal pathogens are most commonly spread by the fecal-oral route. The number of organisms required to produce infection will determine whether infection occurs by person-to-person spread or whether a food or fluid intermediary is required. Organisms such as rotavirus, *Giardia lamblia,* and *Shigella* spp. require very low inoculum to transmit infection and can be carried on the hands (without obvious gross contamination) after person-to-person contact or by the touching of infected surfaces. In contrast, *Salmonella,* rarely a cause of diarrheal outbreaks in the child care setting, requires large numbers of organisms to produce infection. For these pathogens, an intermediary step of food or beverage contamination is required to allow organisms to replicate up to the necessary inocula.

Numerous studies have demonstrated fecal organisms on child care center environmental surfaces with which infants and toddlers have had contact, as well as on the hands of care providers.[98,168,280,289] Contamination of the environment is highest when the child care attendees are younger than 3 years. This age predilection correlates with the number of children still wearing diapers.[266,281] Several important pathogens, including fecal bacteria, rotavirus, hepatitis A virus (HAV), and *G. lamblia* cysts, are able to survive on environmental surfaces for periods ranging from hours to weeks,[71,179] therefore increasing opportunities for transmission in the absence of effective environmental cleaning standards.

TABLE 248.1 Pathogens and Modes of Transmission of Infection in Day Care

Mode of Transmission	Bacteria	Viruses	Parasites
Respiratory	*Haemophilus influenzae* type b *Streptococcus pneumoniae* *Neisseria meningitidis* Group A *Streptococcus* *Bordetella pertussis* *Mycobacterium tuberculosis* *Kingella kingae*	Adenovirus Coronavirus Human metapneumovirus Influenza A and B Measles Mumps Parainfluenza Parvovirus B19 Respiratory syncytial Rhinovirus Rubella Varicella zoster	
Fecal-oral	*Campylobacter* spp. *Clostridium difficile* Shiga toxin–producing *Escherichia coli* (e.g., O157:H7) *Salmonella* spp. *Shigella* spp.	Enteroviruses Hepatitis A Enteric adenovirus Astrovirus Calicivirus (norovirus and sapovirus) Enterovirus Rotavirus Astrovirus	*Cryptosporidium parvum* *Enterobius vermicularis* *Giardia lamblia*
Person-to-person by skin contact	Group A *Streptococcus* *Staphylococcus aureus*	Herpes simplex Varicella zoster (shingles)	*Pediculus capitis* *Sarcoptes scabiei* *Trichophyton* spp. *Microsporum* spp.
Contact with urine or saliva		Cytomegalovirus Herpes simplex virus	
Contact with blood		Hepatitis B virus Hepatitis C virus Cytomegalovirus Human immunodeficiency virus	

Skin to Skin

Bacterial, viral, and parasitic infections of the skin can be transmitted person to person by direct contact. Bacterial pathogens such as *S. pyogenes* and *Staphylococcus aureus* usually are not invasive unless a break in the integument occurs, such as after minor trauma (e.g., insect bites). HSV may be transmitted from skin or mucosa to skin by direct contact, again only if the skin is broken. Infestations such as scabies and lice are transmitted person to person by mobile parasites. The superficial dermatophytes responsible for tinea infections (*Trichophyton, Microsporum,* and *Epidermophyton*) are transmitted by person-to-person spread or by contact with infected fomites such as combs, hairbrushes, and hats.

Blood, Urine, and Saliva

Hepatitis B virus (HBV), hepatitis C virus (HCV), and human immunodeficiency virus (HIV) are blood-borne pathogens with rare potential to be transmitted in the child care setting. Although both hepatitis B and HIV can be demonstrated at very low levels in urine and saliva, exchange of these body fluids is very unlikely to transmit infection. Enzymes present in saliva can inactivate the HIV virus. Risk for transmission of HIV through saliva increases if there is visible blood present in saliva (which may occur if the biter has bleeding gums or periodontal disease).

Bites in child care are always of concern because this is a behavioral manifestation primarily exhibited by preschoolers. The highest risk for transmission of a blood-borne pathogen by a bite would be to the biter if blood is drawn or already present (e.g., severe dermatitis) or to the person bitten if infected blood is present in saliva.[29] Reports of HBV transmission through biting are rare and occurred before the vaccine era[201] To date, there have been no reports of transmission of HIV through biting in a child-care setting.[43]

At child care centers, transmission of cytomegalovirus (CMV) or HSV most commonly occurs among attendees by contamination of toys with saliva. CMV is primarily shed in urine and saliva, although it is present in blood and seminal fluid. Asymptomatic infants and toddlers can shed virus in urine and saliva for months[5,45,93] Early studies demonstrated contaminated fomites and environmental surfaces as potential sources of transmission[102,216] Care providers and family members can become infected with CMV by the finger-to-mucosa route after contamination of hands by urine or saliva.[46] This is of concern because the greatest consequence of CMV infection is primary infection of a pregnant care provider leading to symptomatic congenital infection with CMV.

PREVENTION AND CONTROL OF INFECTIONS IN OUT-OF-HOME CHILD CARE

The American Academy of Pediatrics (AAP), the American Public Health Association, and the National Resource Center for Health and Safety in Child Care and Early Education have developed consensus guidelines on planning and practices in child care that promote the health and safety of children in out-of-home child care, including practices that prevent and control the spread of infection. This includes information on collecting, reviewing, and maintaining health records of children and staff, planning the physical space of the facility, methods of cleaning and disinfecting spaces, educating staff and families on recognizing potentially infectious illnesses, and establishing exclusion policies for specific infections.[14,16,19]

Written Policies

Each child care facility should have written policies for preventing and managing child and staff illness due to transmissible agents. Policies should define roles and responsibilities of child care staff in preventing infectious illnesses. Written documentation should include policies for hand hygiene and personal hygiene procedures, environmental cleaning procedures; collecting, filing, and updating health and immunization records on all children and staff; education of child care personnel about health issues; communicating with parents; determining when a child or staff member should be excluded from the facility because of infection and when they can return; and working with public health officials in reporting and managing any outbreaks. Policies should also define the use of Standard Precautions and procedures to minimize risk to potentially infectious blood and body fluids. Large child care centers benefit from having a health professional consultant for their health and safety procedures.[14]

Hand Hygiene

The key factor in prevention of disease in the child care setting is maintenance of optimal hygienic standards based on recognized mechanisms of transmission of infection. Hand hygiene is considered the single most important preventive measure.[38,125,176,223,237] Hands are in constant motion and readily spread respiratory and enteric pathogens around the environment. Adequate hand hygiene includes hand washing with soap and water for 20 seconds and the use of alcohol-based sanitizers.

Two randomized intervention studies showed a modest benefit of increased attention to hand washing in preventing respiratory infections in children younger than 2 years and in preventing episodes of diarrhea in children older than 2 years.[229,230] Two other studies have evaluated the role of alcohol-based sanitizers in the homes of children in out-of-home child care in reducing the secondary spread of illness. One demonstrated a reduction in gastrointestinal illness among family members[237] and the other a reduction in respiratory illnesses.[184] Applicability to the child care environment also has been evaluated as part of several multipronged interventional programs.[155] A meta-analysis of studies evaluating the effect of hand hygiene interventions on reducing respiratory and gastrointestinal illness in community settings showed interventions that involved hand hygiene education plus the use of ordinary soaps had the greatest decrease in gastrointestinal and respiratory illnesses. The majority of studies evaluated were performed in child care centers and involved children younger than 5 years. No significant differences in benefits were noted with the use of alcohol-based sanitizers or antibacterial soaps compared with hand washing with nonantibacterial soap.[8]

Environment and Physical Plant Standards

In the planning of child care facilities, space and equipment needs that minimize the risk for transmission of infectious agents must be considered. Because fecal contamination is related strongly and inversely to age, having physical premises large enough to separate diapered children from older children is important. Food handling and storage areas should be separated from the toileting and diapering space. When tables in the play area are used for food, they must be sanitized before food service. Because contamination of hands is the most critical factor in transmission of infection, hand-washing facilities must be easily available to staff and children. Such facilities are especially important in the diaper-changing, toileting, and food preparation areas, and separate sinks should be used in each of these areas. The hand-washing sinks should be made of nonporous materials and preferably be hands-free and in easy reach of soap and towel dispensers.

Because feces-contaminated surfaces are major vehicles for the spread of enteric infections, particular care must be taken in planning the space and selecting equipment for diaper changing and toileting activities. The choice of equipment should be based on durability and ease of cleaning and disinfecting. Sinks, supplies, and waste containers should be placed within easy reach of the diapering table. The toddler area should be equipped with training toilets and junior-sized toilets with appropriate steps. The use of potty chairs is strongly discouraged.[15]

Kotch and colleagues performed a randomized intervention trial comparing frequency of diarrheal illnesses and related absences in 23 matched child care centers in North Carolina.[175] All received education on hygienic practices, but the intervention centers also had equipment installed for diapering, food handling, and hand washing that was designed to reduce transmission of pathogens (e.g., hands-free operations, nonporous surfaces). The intervention group showed a decrease in frequency of diarrheal illness (0.9 vs. 1.58 illnesses per 100 child-days). Caregivers in the intervention group had a significantly lower proportion of days absent due to illness compared with the control group (0.77% vs. 1.73%).

Food Preparation

Given the high transmissibility of enteric agents in a child care setting, much attention must be given to procedures involving food preparation. Areas for food preparation and storage should be separate from diapering and toileting areas. Food should not be brought into diapering and toileting areas. Ideally, there should be separate personnel for food handling and caregiving. This may not be possible in smaller child care or family home settings. If this is the case, then food preparation should occur before handling any diapers, and hand hygiene should be practiced diligently. Hands should be washed with soap before handling food. If any personnel has illness concerning for an enteric pathogen (vomiting, diarrhea, jaundice), infectious skin lesions that cannot be covered, or difficult-to-control respiratory secretions, they should not be preparing food.[14]

Immunization and Screening of Children and Staff

Primary immunizations in infants and toddlers have greatly reduced many of the infectious illnesses that were easily transmitted among children in closed settings decades ago. The vaccine-preventable diseases for a preschool child are diphtheria, tetanus, pertussis, polio, influenza, measles, mumps, rubella, varicella, rotavirus, *H. influenzae* infection, *S. pneumoniae*, hepatitis A, and hepatitis B infections. Studies have shown that children who attend registered child care facilities are more likely to be up to date in their immunizations than are children cared for at home.[148] Laws requiring age-appropriate vaccination of children attending licensed child care programs exist in almost all states. Children should be immunized appropriately for age before entering child care, unless there is a medical contraindication or exemption for religious or philosophical reasons.

Employees and volunteers should have a health assessment before initiating work with children. This includes documenting and updating records of immunizations or immunity to HAV and HBV, measles, mumps, rubella, varicella, diphtheria, tetanus, polio, pertussis (to include one dose of acellular pertussis), and influenza. Recommendations for vaccination of children and adults are updated regularly by the Advisory Committee on Immunization Practices.[7] Staff should receive annual influenza vaccinations, especially because young infants are a most vulnerable population for significant morbidity with influenza illness.

Before initiating work in a child care setting, adult and adolescent staff should be screened for tuberculosis (TB) by skin testing or a blood interferon-γ release assay. If the initial screening is negative, those at risk should have annual TB testing. If positive, a chest radiograph should be performed and the staff member evaluated and cleared by a health care provider or public health official before beginning child care activities.[14,16]

Exclusion Policy

The use of exclusion policies for specific infectious illnesses reflects not only risk for transmission to others but also the recognition that when children have moderate to severe illnesses, they may require more individualized care. When stool is not easily contained in a diaper, or toilet-trained children have accidental stooling because of diarrhea, transmissibility of enteric pathogens increases significantly. Similarly, respiratory agents shed in secretions are readily transmissible through coughing, sneezing, or contamination of hands or environmental surfaces. Even more increased attention to personal, hand, and environmental hygiene is necessary.[14]

The indications for exclusion of children from child care and their subsequent return to care vary based on the infection. In some cases children known to have highly infectious illnesses should not be allowed to attend child care until treatment is initiated (e.g., group A *Streptococcus* [GAS] infections), the symptoms have resolved (e.g., diarrhea caused by *Shigella*, rotavirus, or *Giardia*), or transmissibility has waned, as in pertussis, varicella, measles, and mumps. In addition, there are certain symptom complexes for which children should be excluded if the specific pathogen or the contagiousness of their illness is unknown (e.g., if a child has a high fever and a rash or diarrhea of unknown etiology). A list of recommendations for exclusion is presented in Table 248.2. There are some children attending group child care who remain unimmunized or underimmunized because of either contraindications for health reasons (e.g., immunocompromised state) or exemptions for a family's philosophical, religious, or personal beliefs. In the event of an outbreak of a vaccine-preventable disease (such as measles), these children should be excluded from child care until return is indicated by disease-specific guidelines and decisions made in conjunction with public health officials.[14,15] There are conditions that do not necessarily require exclusion from child care. These include (1) asymptomatic excretion of some

TABLE 248.2 Recommendations for Temporary Exclusion From Child Care for Infections

Symptom Complexes	Infectious Etiology	Temporarily Exclude?	If Excluded, Readmit When
Illness that prevents child from participating comfortably in activities		Yes	Exclusion criteria are resolved and child is able to participate without compromising staff's ability to care for other children
Illness that results in a greater need for care than the program staff can provide without compromising their ability to care for other children		Yes	
Other health conditions that may indicate severe illness (e.g., severely ill appearance, fever, lethargy, lack of responsiveness, persistent crying, difficulty breathing or quickly spreading rash)		Yes	
Abdominal Pain	*Viral* *Bacterial* Group A *Streptococcus* pharyngitis	No, unless: Severe pain causing child to double over or scream Bloody/black stools No urine output for 8 h Diarrhea Vomiting Jaundice Fever with behavior change Looks or acts very ill	Pain resolves Able to participate Exclusion criteria are met

Continued

TABLE 248.2 Recommendations for Temporary Exclusion From Child Care for Infections—cont'd

Symptom Complexes	Infectious Etiology	Temporarily Exclude?	If Excluded, Readmit When
Cold symptoms: e.g., runny nose, scratchy throat, coughing, sneezing, watery eyes, fever	*Viral* Adenovirus Coxsackie virus Enterovirus Parainfluenza virus Respiratory syncytial virus Rhinovirus Coronavirus Influenza *Bacterial* Mycoplasma *Bordetella pertussis*	No, unless: Fever accompanied by behavior change Looks or acts very ill Difficulty breathing Blood-red or purple rash not associated with injury Meets other exclusion criteria	
Conjunctivitis	Bacterial Viral	No, unless child meets other exclusion criteria	For bacterial conjunctivitis: after parent has discussed with health professional Antibiotics may or may not be prescribed Exclusion criteria are resolved
Cough	Upper respiratory infection, usually viral Sinus infection, usually viral but may be bacterial Lower respiratory infection, usually viral but may be bacterial Croup, viral Pertussis	No, unless severe cough, rapid or difficult breathing, wheezing if not already evaluated and treated, cyanosis	Exclusion criteria are resolved
Fever	Viral Bacterial Parasitic	No, unless: Behavior change Unable to participate Care would compromise staff's ability to care for other children	Able to participate Exclusion criteria are resolved
Diarrhea	Usually viral Bacterial Parasitic	Yes, if: Stool is not contained in the diaper Diarrhea is causing "accidents" for toilet-trained children Stool frequency exceeds two or more stools above normal for that child Blood or mucus in stool Black stool Dry mouth No urine output in 8 h Jaundice Fever with behavior change Looks or acts very ill	Diapered children have their stool contained by the diaper Toilet-trained children do not have toileting accidents Stool frequency is fewer than two above normal for that child Able to participate without compromising staff's ability to care for them Cleared to return by health professional for all cases of bloody diarrhea and diarrhea caused by Shiga toxin–producing *E. coli, Shigella, Salmonella, Cryptosporidium*, or *Giardia*
Mouth sores	Oral thrush (candida) Herpes simplex virus Enterovirus (e.g., Coxsackie virus)	No, unless: Drooling steadily because of mouth sores Unable to participate Care would compromise staff's ability to care for other children	Able to participate Exclusion criteria are resolved
Rash	Viral Skin infections and infestations (i.e., scabies, ringworm) Severe bacterial infections: *N. meningitides, S. pneumoniae, S. aureus*	No, unless: Rash with behavior change or fever Has oozing or open wound Bruising not associated with injury Joint pain with rash Unable to participate Tender, red area of skin, particularly if increased in size or tenderness	Able to participate in activities On antibiotic (see indications for specific etiologies) Exclusion criteria are resolved
Sore throat	Viral Group A *Streptococcus*	No, unless: Unable to swallow Excessive drooling with breathing difficulty Fever with behavior change Child meets other exclusion criteria	Able to swallow Able to participate On medication at least 24 h for strep throat Exclusion criteria are resolved
Vomiting	Usually viral	Yes, if: Vomited more than two times in 24 h Vomiting and fever Green or bloody emesis No urine output in 8 h Looks or acts very ill	Vomiting ends Able to participate Exclusion criteria are resolved

Modified from American Academy of Pediatrics. *Managing Infectious Diseases in Child Care and Schools: a Quick Reference Guide.* 3rd ed. Elk Grove Village, Ill: American Academy of Pediatrics; 2013.

enteropathogens, (2) purulent or nonpurulent conjunctivitis, (3) a rash without a fever or behavioral change, (4) CMV infection, (5) the carrier state of HBV infection, (6) HIV infection, and (7) parvovirus B19 infection in an immunocompetent host. For many infections, the highest risk for transmission of disease occurs before the appearance of recognizable symptoms. After illness occurs, other children already have been exposed, and exclusion is a less effective strategy. For this reason, exclusion has not been shown to be successful in reducing the frequency of viral upper respiratory tract infections.

Prophylaxis of Close Contacts

Prophylaxis is a strategy that may be useful in the management of some infections that occur in child care centers. For example, if a child has had invasive disease caused by *N. meningitidis,* rifampin prophylaxis for all child care contacts may prevent secondary or associated cases. If a child has pertussis, exposed children may be protected by a booster immunization, if appropriate, and administration of a macrolide for prophylaxis. During community epidemics, vaccination can be used as a strategy to prevent secondary infections. For example, immunization with MMR vaccine can be successful in terminating epidemics of measles in elementary or high schools. Varicella vaccine also can be used throughout a community and up to 3 days after exposure to curtail the spread of disease.

Education

An integral part of the control of infection within a child care center is education of families and staff (including caregivers and custodians). The staff must understand the general principles of transmission and control of infections. Education before job placement and frequent in-service trainings reinforce the importance of some basic techniques, especially hand hygiene. Supervision is essential to ensure compliance with policies.[176]

Parents should be educated regarding recognition of illness, especially illnesses for which the child would receive the best care and attention at home or at a facility for ill children. The rationale and importance of compliance with child care center rules should be emphasized. The child care program should inform parents of the need to share information about communicable illnesses in the child or a family member.

INFECTIOUS AGENTS IN CHILD CARE

Infections Spread by the Respiratory Route

Upper Respiratory Infections

Respiratory viruses (rhinovirus, coronavirus, respiratory syncytial virus, human metapneumovirus, parainfluenza viruses 1 to 4, influenza viruses A and B, and adenoviruses) are the most common causes of infection in preschool-aged children.[33,101,115,292] The range of clinical manifestations includes asymptomatic infection, simple upper respiratory infection (rhinitis), acute otitis media, pharyngitis, croup, tracheitis, bronchiolitis, and pneumonitis. Disease may be mild or severe and involve a single level or more than one level of the respiratory tree. Human bocavirus, first characterized by molecular analysis in 2005, has been identified in the respiratory tract of children with respiratory illness. However, more than 80% are identified in the setting of viral coinfection using molecular techniques.[300] Bocavirus is also present in asymptomatic shedders. Its role as a pathogen has yet to be fully elucidated.[42,163,196,300] Children may experience multiple infections with the same agent because of antigenic diversity within virus subtypes (e.g., influenza A virus), existence of multiple subtypes (e.g., rhinoviruses, coronaviruses), and failure of immunity to develop after a single exposure (e.g., respiratory syncytial virus). Viruses are shed from the site of infection (conjunctiva, nose, throat), even before clinical symptoms develop, thereby rendering control of the spread of these infections in child care difficult. Documentation that children in out-of-home child care (large family or other child care centers) experience more respiratory infections than those noted in children in home care is ample.[94,111,154,189,190,208,209,259,263,284]

The availability of molecular techniques for viral identification has improved the ability and sensitivity of detecting viruses in respiratory secretions that may be pathogens or colonizers. In a 2-year longitudinal study of 225 children from three child care centers, Martin and colleagues identified more than one virus in 47% of specimens (455 total) that were obtained at the time of mild or moderate illness. Only one virus was detected in 32% and none in 18%.[197]

Bacterial coinfection causing complications can occur with viral upper respiratory infection. The most common complication is acute otitis media. Sinusitis, pneumonia, and meningitis are more invasive complicating infections. The overall incidence of these complications has dramatically decreased with the implementation of universal vaccination with conjugated HIB in 1987[248] and conjugated pneumococcal vaccines in 2000 and 2010.

The peak age incidence of acute otitis media is between 6 and 18 months, similar to that of viral upper respiratory tract infections. Most children have had at least one episode of acute otitis media by the time they reach their second birthday, and approximately one-third will have had at least three episodes by that time.[271] Not surprisingly, because the frequency of episodes of viral respiratory infections is increased in children attending out-of-home child care, these children experience a notable increase in the frequency of episodes of otitis media.[228,259,262,263,284] Two reviews strongly supported the notion that attendance at child care is a major risk factor for acquiring acute otitis media.[233,279] Wald and colleagues[284] provided data indicating that the risk for hospitalization for performance of myringotomy with tube placement was highest for children in large child care environments. Similarly, the risk for contracting recurrent acute otitis media and persistent middle-ear effusion also is higher for children in child care than for those who receive care at home.[83,108,260,275] Researchers do not recommend that children with mild respiratory infections or otitis media be excluded from child care or be separated from the group of well children unless they act systemically ill or have fever with behavior change, difficulty breathing, purpuric or petechial rash, severe cough, or cyanosis.[14] Furthermore, the strategy of exclusion from child care for mild respiratory illnesses has not been shown to achieve an overall reduction in infections for children in child care facilities.

Systemic Viral Infections

Parvovirus B19. Parvovirus B19, the etiologic agent of erythema infectiosum, or fifth disease, is spread by the respiratory route. Typically, the virus infects and destroys red blood cell precursors until the virus is neutralized by the development of antibody. Viral replication, viremia, and nasopharyngeal shedding occur approximately 1 week before the development of clinical symptoms. This benign disease of childhood (in a normal host) may occur in preschool- and school-aged children. The classical clinical illness is characterized by an erythematous rash on the face that gives a "slapped-cheek" appearance. This rash may follow 1 to 3 weeks after a mild, nonspecific illness with fever, myalgias, and headache. This maculopapular rash begins on the proximal ends of the extremities extending to the distal portions and trunk. After several days, these lesions may develop into a lacy reticular pattern and then fade. Infection can be asymptomatic in as many as 50% of children.

Less typical presentations include the papulopurpuric gloves-and-socks syndrome and rubelliform or petechial rashes. A community outbreak of parvovirus with petechial rash among children in Wisconsin has been described.[97] Children who are immunosuppressed may develop a more chronic infection resulting in a severe anemia because of the delayed clearance of the virus. Similarly, children with hemolytic disorders such as sickle cell disease can develop profound anemia during the period of aplasia.

The clinical importance of parvovirus B19 in the context of child care infections is transmission from an infected preschool-aged child to a pregnant mother or child care provider.[121] Infection of the fetus may lead to nonimmune hydrops secondary to infection of erythrocyte progenitor cells. Estimates of fetal loss when a pregnant woman of unknown antibody status is exposed to parvovirus are 2.5% after household exposure and 1.5% after occupational exposure in a school or child care facility.[23]

Children are not excluded from group child care when rash is present as they are no longer contagious. Children need not be excluded from child care unless other exclusion criteria are met (i.e., fever with behavior change). However, an infected child who has a blood disorder or is immunocompromised can shed large amounts of virus and should be excluded.[14,274] Routine exclusion of pregnant women from a child care center where erythema infectiosum is identified is not recommended.[15,138]

Hand-Foot-and-Mouth Disease. Hand-foot-and-mouth disease (HFMD) is a clinical syndrome characterized by a vesicular exanthema on the distal parts of the extremities and mild stomatitis. Infections are often asymptomatic or mild, but they can be associated with fever and significant pain with the vesicles. Severe stomatitis can lead to dehydration. HFMD is most commonly caused by the enteroviruses Coxsackie A16 and enterovirus 71, although other enteroviruses have been identified. Transmission is person to person through contact with infected saliva, vesicles, respiratory secretions, or stool. Outbreaks usually occur during summer or autumn months in the United States. Two outbreaks of Coxsackie virus A16 HFMD have been reported in children attending child care.[106,107] In recent years, outbreaks of HFMD associated with Coxsackie virus A6 have been described worldwide; one outbreak in four geographically distinct states in the United States related to Coxsackie A6 occurred during winter months. Of the 63 cases, 34 were in children younger than 2 years. The symptoms were more severe than those usually associated with Coxsackie virus A16.[59] The most significant clinical concern is the acquisition of Coxsackie virus infection during pregnancy, which may lead to spontaneous abortion.[107,214] Exclusion from group child care is not routinely recommended because symptomatic and asymptomatic children may shed virus in stool for several weeks.[14]

Local Bacterial Infections

Streptococcus pyogenes *or Group A* Streptococcus. GAS is a frequent cause of respiratory and skin infections. The most common expression of infection with GAS is the development of pharyngitis and fever in a school-aged child. Usually, the throat infection is accompanied by tender anterior cervical nodes. In classical infection, none of the usual signs of viral upper respiratory disease—coryza, cough, and conjunctivitis—are present. This classical presentation, however, is rare in children younger than 3 years. Streptococcal infection of a preschool-aged child more often takes the form of a protracted upper respiratory infection. More typically, these patients have low-grade fever, persistent nasal discharge, anorexia, and cervical adenopathy. Given the rarity of rheumatic fever in young children, it is recommended to not test these young children unless they have contact with an older sibling with GAS infection or an outbreak is present.[252]

Although exposure of child care attendees to an index case of streptococcal pharyngitis can be assumed to result in secondary cases, relatively few epidemics of GAS infection have been reported in child care facilities.[103,152,254] An outbreak occurred in a child care center in which preschool children shared facilities with kindergarten children in an after-school program. During a 3-month period, 47% of the child care population had positive pharyngeal cultures for GAS or positive results on a rapid antigen-detection test.[254]

GAS can also be transmitted person to person by skin-to-skin contact and colonize healthy skin. Superficial infection (impetigo) may then occur at sites of traumatized skin (e.g., insect bites or scratches). Often GAS and *S. aureus* are both isolated from sites of impetigo. Erysipelas and cellulitis due to GAS can result in an abrupt onset of fever and dramatic cutaneous erythema and tenderness often accompanied by regional adenopathy. Outbreaks of perianal cellulitis have been reported from child care centers.[206,239] A cluster of 12 cases of perianal cellulitis, characterized by a well-demarcated rash around the anus with itching, rectal pain, blood-streaked stools, and occasionally a purulent discharge, was reported from a kindergarten setting in Denmark.[220]

The diagnosis of streptococcal skin infection can be made by careful performance of wound or surface cultures (obtained after carefully cleansing the area around the lesions) or examination of tissue aspirates. Spread of typical impetigo occurs commonly within families and presumably also would occur within child care centers. Children with GAS infections of the throat or skin should be excluded from group child care for 24 hours after the initiation of appropriate antibiotic treatment.[14,15]

Invasive Bacterial Disease

Kingella kingae. *K. kingae* is a fastidious gram-negative coccobacillus that colonizes the oropharynx and is becoming increasingly recognized as an important cause of osteoarticular infections in young children (<4 years).[37,96,296] It has also been identified in cases of bacteremia and endocarditis[96,295] Colonization rates are highest in children younger than 2 years. Similar to other bacterial pathogens, the organism colonizes the upper respiratory tract of young children. The presence of different strains changes over time. The tonsils are identified as the primary site for colonization. Preceding stomatitis and upper respiratory viral infections have been recognized as risk factors for invasive disease.[21,96] Disrupted mucosa may provide entry into the bloodstream, increasing the risk for disease at distant sites. Children with osteoarticular disease may often present subacutely, with symptoms related to the affected limb, but with low-grade or no fever and elevated inflammatory markers.

Methods of diagnostic detection have improved over the past several years, including the ability to identify *K. kingae* by molecular techniques. This has contributed to the increase in identification of this pathogen in clusters of infection. In-depth studies from Israel have identified *K. kingae* as the most common microbe causing osteoarticular infections in children aged 6 months to 3 years.[299,96]

K. kingae can persist in the upper respiratory tract of asymptomatic children over long periods of time. Studies have demonstrated that the absence or presence of colonizing bacteria is variable and strains may replace one another over time.[22] *Kingella* carriage rates in the general population are estimated to be 3% to 17%.[64,96,297] Outbreaks of osteomyelitis and septic arthritis associated with *K. kingae* have been reported in child care settings in Minnesota,[171] France,[37] and Israel.[296,298] In 2007, a cluster of cases in a child care center in North Carolina was reported associated with a case of endocarditis. Genetically similar *Kingella* isolates were obtained from symptom-free children in the same child care.[244] Colonization rates in these child care centers ranged from 7% to 42%. Bidet and colleagues described the first European cluster of *Kingella* osteoarticular infections. There were five child care attendees out of 24 who presented with arthritis or osteomyelitis in a 1-month period in France. The colonization rate among children who were not receiving antibiotics was 46% to 53%.[32,37]

Neisseria meningitidis. *N. meningitidis* is a gram-negative, polysaccharide-encapsulated diplococcus that colonizes the nasopharynx. With the reduction of invasive HIB and *S. pneumoniae* disease because of effective immunization strategies, *N. meningitidis* is a leading cause of bacterial meningitis in the United States. Type B is the predominant subtype in the United States.[193] Meningococcemia is a major manifestation of invasive meningococcal disease with significant morbidity. Less commonly, pericarditis, pneumonia, arthritis, otitis media, or epiglottitis can occur. Active surveillance (2006–12) in the United States observed the highest rates of invasive meningococcal disease among infants younger than 1 year, although the case-fatality rate was the lowest in this age group. Hematogenous dissemination from the colonized nasopharynx may result in invasive disease. Transmission is person to person through infected respiratory droplets. Household contacts exposed to patients with meningococcal disease have a significantly higher risk for acquiring infection than does the general population.[203,205]

Most cases of meningococcal disease are sporadic; however, there are several reports of outbreaks in closely grouped communities, including military barracks and college dormitories. In addition, the risk for acquiring secondary disease caused by *N. meningitidis* is increased in the child care setting.[160,185,212,234] In a Belgian report,[88] exposure in a child care nursery during a prolonged meningococcal epidemic conferred a risk for infection that was 76 times greater than that in children of similar age who received care at home.

Prompt institution of chemoprophylaxis with rifampin is the recommended strategy for management of all intimate child contacts of a person with invasive *N. meningitidis* disease to prevent development of secondary or associated illness. A single oral dose of ciprofloxacin or azithromycin or an intramuscular dose of ceftriaxone is an alternative for adult contacts. Pregnant women should not receive rifampin or ciprofloxacin. Throat culture to identify those who would require prophylaxis is not recommended. In addition to household and other high-risk contacts, all child care contacts (children and adults) of an index case with meningococcal disease within 7 days of onset should receive chemoprophylaxis.[15] In an outbreak, meningococcal conjugate vaccine may also be used for prevention of secondary cases if the outbreak serotype is one that is contained in the vaccine and the contacts are in an appropriate age group for immunization.[15] Management of exposures and outbreaks should be performed in conjunction with public health officials.

As of this writing, six vaccines are licensed in the United States for *N. meningitidis*. Four contain components against the serogroups A, C, Y, and W135, three of which are conjugate vaccines licensed to begin a primary series during infancy. In 2014 and 2015, two recombinant serogroup type B vaccines were approved for use in children and youth aged 10 to 25 years.[194]

Children with meningococcal disease should be excluded from child care until they have received antimicrobial treatment for at least 24 hours.

Mycobacterium tuberculosis. Infection caused by *M. tuberculosis* in a preschool-aged child is a sentinel event. It represents the exposure of that child to an adolescent or adult with active tuberculosis disease. Children this young are much less likely to have cavitary lesions in their lungs and thus are less likely to be contagious. The identification of an infected child should prompt a public health investigation to identify the index case. Cases of tuberculosis in children have been traced to attendance at child care.[122,186,211] Children identified as having active tuberculosis may attend group child care if public health officials have approved and determined that (1) they have started and are adherent to therapy, (2) they are noninfectious, (3) their symptoms have decreased, and (4) they are able to participate in the activities of the child care center. Children with latent TB disease are not contagious and do not need to be excluded from group child care.[15] Screening of personnel who work in child care settings, including both staff and volunteers at high risk for exposure to TB, is essential to prevent tuberculosis in childhood. Child care staff members diagnosed with active TB disease are excluded from caring for children until they are determined to be noncontagious.[15]

Infections of the Gastrointestinal Tract

Parasitic Infections

Giardia lamblia. *G. lamblia* is the most common intestinal parasite of humans and a major cause of diarrhea in child care centers.[39,227,243] Infection can be caused by the ingestion of as few as 10 cysts. Transmission is fecal-oral and most commonly results from person-to-person spread, although waterborne outbreaks have been documented.[169] Parents of child care attendees are at risk for acquiring infection.[223] Asymptomatic excretion does occur and is most common in children younger than 3 years.[30,224,227] Demonstration of *G. lamblia* cysts on environmental surfaces indicates additional potential for transmission.[71] Cysts can remain infective on cool, moist environmental surfaces or in cool waters for months, increasing the chance of ingestion. Infection with this parasite causes infestation of the duodenum and proximal jejunum and results in asymptomatic carriage more often than clinical disease.[158]

After an incubation period of approximately 2 weeks, symptomatic patients experience diarrhea, intermittent abdominal pain, anorexia, and flatulence. The most notable feature of the infection is its tendency to become protracted, thereby leading to weight loss, failure to thrive, and anemia. Diagnosis is made by identifying organisms using sensitive and specific enzyme immunoassays or direct fluorescent antibody assays of stool samples. Occasionally, trophozoites or cysts are identified by microscopic examination of stool or duodenal aspirates. Treatment is not recommended for asymptomatic individuals shedding *G. lamblia* cysts. For symptomatic individuals, treatment may be undertaken. Relapses occur in approximately 15% of patients, often requiring a second course of treatment. After resolution of symptoms, either by virtue of treatment or by spontaneous cure, patients may continue to shed cysts for a very long time.[158,224]

Children are excluded from group child care if there is diarrhea present that is not contained in the diaper or causes accidents in older children or if the child cannot participate in center activities. Follow-up testing is not required if the child or staff member does not have diarrhea.

Cryptosporidium. *Cryptosporidium* parasites (primarily *C. parvum and C. hominum)* have been mainly identified as an opportunistic infection causing diarrhea in immunocompromised hosts. Infection usually results in self-limited illness in immunocompetent children and adults.[73] The usual clinical symptoms are frequent watery diarrhea that may be associated with low-grade fever, abdominal pain, and weight loss. Vomiting occurs in approximately 30% of patients. The illness is usually self-limited in healthy individuals, although the diarrhea can last as long as 2 or 3 weeks. Oocysts can be shed in stool of immunocompetent individuals up to 60 days after gastrointestinal symptoms resolve.[164]

Cryptosporidium oocysts can be found in the soil, water, or food or on surfaces contaminated by feces. Transmission is fecal-oral. The most common source of transmission and outbreaks has been the ingestion of contaminated water (either drinking or recreational exposure).[192] Increased incidence of cryptosporidiosis occurs during summer and early fall months corresponding to months with increased recreational water activities.[58] The oocysts can survive chlorine in water treated at recommended levels for recreation.[250] In 2011–12 more than half (52%) of the reported 69 outbreaks of diarrhea associated with treated recreational water in the United States were due to *Cryptosporidium.*[150] Like *G. lamblia, Cryptosporidium* has a very low infectious dose for humans. Infection can occur with as few as 10 to 30 oocysts.[67] Spread of infection is facilitated in child care centers because oocysts shed in the feces of infected persons are highly resistant to common disinfectants. Many outbreaks of diarrhea caused by *Cryptosporidium* have been reported from child care centers.[11,12,72,77,142,270] Asymptomatic children and adults shed oocysts for weeks after infection.

The diagnosis is made by examination of stool for oocysts by direct immunofluorescent antibody method. Direct microscopy can be performed with special stains such as the modified Kinyoun acid-fast stain. Alternative methods include enzyme immunoassays specific for *Cryptosporidium* antigen. Routine stool examinations for ova and parasites can miss the cryptosporidium oocysts. Generally, treatment is not required for immunocompetent individuals. The recommended treatment is a 3-day course of nitazoxanide for anyone aged 1 year and older. Treatment can reduce the duration of diarrhea and shedding of oocysts in stool.[13]

Exclusion from child care is recommended if stool cannot be contained in the diaper, older children are having accidents, stool frequency is 2 times or more above normal for that child, blood or mucus is found in the stool, or child is not able to participate in usual activities of the child care center. This latter situation causes excess work for staff and may compromise care of other children.

Bacterial Pathogens

Shigella. Infection with *Shigella* organisms causes illness of variable severity but easy transmissibility. Accordingly, *Shigella* is one of the most common causes of diarrhea outbreaks in the child care population.[48,25,120] Infection can be caused by as few as 10 organisms. Fecal-oral transmission is the primary mode of transmission. *Shigella* organisms can survive in water for up to 6 months as well as on food, and have been implicated in both water-borne and food-borne illnesses. There are four species (*S. sonnei* [the predominant species in the United States], *S. flexneri, S. dysenteriae,* and *S. boydii*) responsible for human shigellosis.

Shigellosis is primarily a disease of young children. In the US reporting of laboratory-confirmed infection, the highest incidence rates are among children age 4 years and younger. Younger children have the highest attack rate during outbreaks and are the most effective transmitters of infection.[273] Child care personnel and family contacts also experience high attack rates.[151,269] Surveillance data from the National Outbreak Reporting System (NORS) identified *Shigella* as the most common bacterial etiology of outbreaks of acute gastroenteritis spread person to person in 2009–10.[135,290] Of the 2259 outbreaks reported, 4% were caused by *Shigella,* and of those with reported settings ($n = 30$), nearly all (97%) were in child care centers.[290]

After an incubation period of 1 to 3 days, fever and watery diarrhea, followed by crampy abdominal pain, tenesmus, and mucoid bloody stools, occurs in patients with classical disease. In many cases, the illness is mild and self-limited, is indistinguishable from other causes of gastroenteritis, and often does not require treatment.

Stool culture for *Shigella* is diagnostic. Detection of *Shigella* by multiplex nucleic acid techniques is also becoming more available. Treatment of shigellosis with an appropriate antimicrobial effectively terminates the illness. Antimicrobial treatment decreases the duration of symptoms and fecal shedding. Untreated persons continue to excrete organisms for several weeks. Susceptibility varies both within and outside the United States, and therefore testing of stool isolates is indicated. Isolates with increasing resistance to ampicillin and trimethoprim-sulfamethoxazole are being reported. Therefore it is important to isolate the organism and determine susceptibility in order to provide optimal treatment.[25,161]

It is essential that child care centers and health professionals work with public health agencies in evaluating and managing outbreaks. Symptomatic staff and attendees should have stool cultured if a case of *Shigella* is identified. Children or staff with confirmed *Shigella* infection should be excluded. They can return to child care when diarrhea has stopped for at least 24 hours. Some states may require a negative stool culture obtained after 24 hours of diarrheal cessation before a child care staff or attendee may return.[14,15]

Salmonella. *Salmonella* is the most common cause of bacterial diarrhea in many parts of the United States and is the cause of numerous outbreaks a year. The most common serotypes are *Salmonella* serovars *typhimurium, enteritidis* and *newport.* Infection usually occurs after the ingestion of contaminated food or beverages and has also been reported after contact with colonized reptiles such as turtles.[139,285] These modes of transmission underscore the importance of hand hygiene, proper food handling and cooking, and avoiding exposure of preschool children to reptiles and amphibians. Person-to-person spread seldom occurs, except in infancy, when the infective dose is low.[293]

The most common expression of infection with *Salmonella* is uncomplicated gastroenteritis. The illness begins approximately 12 to 36 hours after exposure and often is characterized by initial vomiting followed by diarrhea. Abdominal pain and fever are frequent accompaniments; occasionally, stools contain mucus and blood. Although most cases are self-limited, *Salmonella* infection can be distinguished from other causes of gastroenteritis by its occasionally protracted course. Nearly half of children younger than 5 years may excrete *Salmonella* organisms up to 3 months after infection. Infants younger than 1 year have the highest incidence of invasive *Salmonella* disease in the United States. Children younger than 4 years have the highest age-specific incidence of nontyphoidal *Salmonella* infection in the United States.[15]

The diagnosis is made by stool culture. In general, antimicrobials are not recommended for those with asymptomatic nontyphoidal *Salmonella* infection or uncomplicated gastroenteritis. Antimicrobial therapy can prolong the duration of fecal shedding of organisms. Management of certain hosts, such as neonates and immunocompromised patients, is controversial. Although some experts recommend antimicrobial therapy for these groups, few data support this recommendation.

Exclusion from child care is recommended if diarrhea cannot be contained in the diaper of a diapered child or if an older child has accidents. When stools are normal, little reason exists to restrict attendance. Obtaining stool cultures from asymptomatic contacts is not necessary for nontyphoidal *Salmonella.* If *Salmonella typhi* or *paratyphi* is identified in the stool of a child or staff member, they should be treated and excluded until three stools obtained 48 hours or more after antibiotics end, are negative.[14,15]

Clostridium difficile. *Clostridium difficile* is the classical cause of pseudomembranous colitis in patients who have received or are receiving antimicrobial agents, and it rarely causes disease unassociated with antimicrobial use. The organism, a gram-positive, spore-forming rod, is distributed widely in soil and in the gastrointestinal tract of humans. Infection is acquired by ingestion of spores from the environment or an infected person. Disease is a consequence of the elaboration of one or more toxins by vegetative organisms. Clinical symptoms include fever, diarrhea, and abdominal cramps. Stools may contain blood and mucus. The illness varies in severity from mild to life-threatening. Early studies demonstrated an increased association of *C. difficile* toxin with diarrheal disease during an evaluation of five outbreaks in three child care centers.[172,173] During outbreaks of *C. difficile* diarrhea in child care centers, environmental contamination was increased, as was recovery of *C. difficile* from the hands of children and staff.[173]

The epidemiology of *C. difficile* infection in the general population has changed dramatically since the early 2000s, with an increase in incidence and severity in adults. Epidemiologic studies of *C. difficile* in hospitalized children show similar trends.[36,174,236] Population-based studies indicate that in children, 50% to 71% of cases are community-acquired infections.[170,288]

The ability to identify the true incidence of *C. difficile* disease in children younger than 3 years is complicated by the fact that as many as 30% to 70% of infants younger than 1 year are colonized by toxigenic and nontoxigenic strains without signs of disease.[26,162,181,235,278] This colonization rate decreases over the next 2 years of life. Children aged 3 years and older have the same rates of *C. difficile* infection as the general adult population (<3%).[162]

Hand hygiene with the use of soap and water is important in the setting of an outbreak. The *C. difficile* spores are not inactivated by alcohol-based sanitizers. Children and personnel should be excluded from group child care until they are asymptomatic.

***Shiga toxin–producing strains of* Escherichia coli.** Infection with Shiga toxin–producing strains of *E. coli* (STEC) is characterized by bouts of often bloody diarrhea and abdominal pain. The bacteria have the potential to cause significant morbidity in children. Approximately 5% to 10% of infected children develop hemolytic uremic syndrome (HUS). Hemorrhagic colitis is also a complication of this infection.

Ruminants such as cattle are the main reservoir for STEC. Transmission is fecal-oral. Infection occurs through ingestion of contaminated food or water or through direct contact with an infected person, carrier animal (such as in petting zoos), or contaminated fomites. Numerous outbreaks have occurred associated with raw meat, unpasteurized milk, contaminated foods, and recreational water.

The most common *E. coli* serotype causing illness is O157:H7. However, several other types have been associated with bloody diarrhea and with HUS.

Numerous STEC outbreaks have been reported in child care settings.[10,35,226,257] In 1986, an outbreak of diarrhea caused by *E. coli* O157:H7 was reported from a child care center attended by 107 children.[257] Thirty-four percent of attendees became ill, with a significant increase in risk for younger children. Approximately one-third of the children with diarrhea had bloody stools, and HUS developed in three children. Although infection with *E. coli* O157:H7 usually occurs after the ingestion of contaminated foods, person-to-person spread of infection most likely occurred in this epidemic. The diarrheal illness also was documented in family members of ill children.

Subsequent epidemiologic studies in Minnesota confirmed the mode of transmission for *E. coli* O157:H7 to be person to person in the child care setting.[35] Outbreaks of another strain with severe sequelae (*E. coli* O104:H4) have been reported in adults in Europe.[113]

A systematic analysis of 90 outbreaks occurring worldwide (1982–2006) identified about 20% of cases arising from secondary spread. The highest proportion of secondary cases was among children younger than 6 years.[255]

Antibiotic treatment has not been recommended for persons with diarrhea caused by *E. coli* O157:H7.[294]

Infected children should be excluded from group child care until diarrhea resolves and two stool cultures are negative (obtained 48 hours after any antibiotic treatment if used).[15] Unfortunately, fecal shedding of *E. coli* O157:H7 may be quite prolonged in young children.[267] Any symptomatic contact of a person with STEC should have stools cultured. In an outbreak situation, child care centers should be closed to new admissions. Control and management of outbreaks should be performed in conjunction with public health officials.

Viral Gastrointestinal Pathogens

Viral enteric pathogens are common causes of acute gastroenteritis in group child care settings. Norovirus has become the leading cause of acute gastroenteritis (AGE) since the widespread introduction of the rotavirus vaccine in 2006. It has been responsible for multiple outbreaks of AGE each year in the United States. The caliciviruses, norovirus and Sapovirus, are nonenveloped RNA viruses that have a worldwide distribution. Sapovirus is much less frequently an agent of gastroenteritis than is norovirus but has been implicated in child care outbreaks.[140]

Transmission is by person-to-person spread through the fecal-oral route or through contaminated food or water. Noroviral particles found in vomitus are potentially infectious through the airborne route during forceful vomiting. Norovirus is antigenically diverse, therefore repeated bouts of diarrhea may occur with exposure to different viral variants. Norovirus is highly contagious; a very small inoculum is required to establish infection. Outbreaks frequently are observed in closed populations, including child care centers and on cruise ships. The attack rate usually is high. Several reports highlight the transmissibility of the Caliciviridae in the child care setting.[126,157]

A cross-sectional survey in the Netherlands of the presence of stool pathogens in preschool child-parent pairs (907 households) was recently published. Monthly stool sampling for 16 enteric organisms with multiplex polymerase chain reaction (PCR) was performed along with symptom questionnaires and the collection of demographic data. The most commonly isolated viruses associated with child care attendance (52% of respondents) were the Caliciviridae (norovirus and Sapovirus). Clinical symptoms of AGE were significantly associated with norovirus II, astrovirus, and adenovirus 41.[145]

Astroviruses are also common causes of diarrheal illness in child care. Outbreaks have been reported in child care settings[9,253] and other closed populations. Children younger than 4 years are infected most commonly, and the illness has a winter predominance. Transmission is usually person to person by the fecal-oral route. This illness is indistinguishable from the other viral causes of gastroenteritis, presenting with watery diarrhea that may be accompanied by vomiting, fever, or abdominal pain. Healthy, symptom-free individuals can shed virus for several weeks.

Infections Spread by Skin Contact

Staphylococcus aureus

S. aureus is part of the endogenous flora of humans; the nose is the primary site of carriage in adults and children. At any one time, approximately 30% of people carry *S. aureus* in their anterior nares.[195] Transmission is primarily through person-to-person skin contact but also occurs through direct contact with contaminated environmental surfaces.

During the 1990s there was an increasing prevalence of disease caused by methicillin-resistant *S. aureus* (MRSA) in children without predisposing risk factors such as contact with the health care system.[51,144] Studies of colonization in child care centers demonstrated likely transmission within the child care setting.[1,146,245]

This community-acquired MRSA (CA-MRSA) has a genetic predisposition for causing skin and soft tissue infections (e.g., abscesses, carbuncles, and furuncles). More rarely, CA-MRSA causes severe invasive infections such as bacteremia, endocarditis, osteomyelitis, pyomyositis, or necrotizing pneumonia. Methicillin-susceptible strains of *S. aureus* (MSSA) cause similar clinical findings. Surveys of the incidence of CA-MRSA disease in hospital and community settings (including child care) have demonstrated the most rapid increase of infections among young children.[78,116,204]

A survey of MRSA isolates derived from national databases of hospital discharges over a 10-year period from 1998 to 2007 demonstrated a 16-fold increase in hospitalization rates for CA-MRSA infections in children. The proportion of *S. aureus* abscesses caused by the CA-MRSA phenotype increased from 8.7% to 60.3% over this same time period.[204] An epidemiologic survey (2001–02) using data from the Active Bacterial Core Surveillance program demonstrated the incidence of disease related to CA-MRSA was highest among individuals younger than 2 years. Of the 1647 patients with CA-MRSA isolates, 77% had skin and soft tissue infection.[116]

Children with documented MRSA should not be excluded from child care for colonization or for skin or soft tissue infections. Any open and draining wounds should be covered.

Scabies

Scabies is an infection of the skin caused by infestation with the female mite *Sarcoptes scabiei.* It is an obligate parasite that undergoes its complete life cycle in humans. Transmitted by person-to-person spread from an infested individual, the mite buries itself beneath the stratum corneum and burrows along for its 30-day life span while laying two to three eggs per day. The larval and nymphal mites scatter after hatching to embed themselves in skin at distant sites. Some 3 to 6 weeks later, a pruritic eruption (worse at night) develops and leads to excoriation, bleeding, and crusting. The distribution of lesions varies with age. In adults and older children, the eruption, which consists of papules, vesicles, and nodules, occurs commonly in the interdigital spaces of the hands, on the extensor surface of the elbows, and around the umbilicus, waist, axillary lines, and genital area. In infants and young children, vesicular and eczematous lesions can be found on the hands and feet, as well as on the face and head.

Although scabies is spread primarily by close personal contact, skin-to-skin transmission can result from prolonged casual contact; this is observed in child care centers.[238] Mites can survive on inanimate surfaces for 2 to 3 days, a period that permits transmission by fomites such as clothes, bed linen, and furniture. An outbreak of scabies was reported in a hospital-affiliated child care facility. Elimination of the problem required a coordinated effort with simultaneous treatment of all potentially infected individuals.[238]

The diagnosis is made by scraping the lesions and demonstrating the mite, ova, or mite feces. Treatment of the index case should be undertaken with a scabicide, preferably 5% permethrin in children older than 2 months. Lindane should not be used because of safety concerns. Asymptomatic contacts should be treated simultaneously because they may be infected unknowingly and may be capable of transmitting the mite during this asymptomatic period. Clothing and bed linens that had contact with the skin of infected persons during the 3 days before treatment should be laundered in hot water. Alternatively, items can be stored in plastic for at least 4 days.[15]

An infected child should be excluded from child care until treatment has occurred which is usually overnight.

Head Lice

Head lice (*Pediculus capitis)* infestation occurs commonly in children attending child care, preschool, and elementary school. It affects children of every socioeconomic status. The insect, a hemophagocytic ectoparasite, obtains nourishment by sucking capillary blood from the scalp. Female lice attach egg cases (nits) to the hair shafts at or very near the scalp. The eggs hatch 8 to 11 days later, and the louse nymphs are released.

The diagnosis is often made by close inspection of the scalp. Nits are observed readily, although live lice may be difficult to see, especially in light infestations.

Treatment is with topical pediculicides, used as directed with care. These include permethrin lotions and pyrethrin-based products. Resistance has been identified with these products. Additionally products such as malathion, benzyl alcohol lotion, spinosad suspension, or ivermectin lotion may be used. Lindane shampoo should not be used because of safety concerns.[15] Nits can be removed mechanically with spiral combs.

Head lice is transferred by direct head-to-head contact and rarely by fomites such as hats, combs, clothing, or bedding. However, such items used by the infected person within 2 days can be washed in high temperatures (130°F [54.4°C]) and dried on a hot air cycle.[15] If lice infestation is diagnosed in a child in child care, he or she should not be sent home early, but families of other children and the child's household should be notified so that they can be evaluated. Children with lice can return to child care after treatment has occurred.

Infections Spread by Contact With Blood, Urine, or Saliva

Cytomegalovirus

CMV is a common cause of infection in preschool-aged children. Most often, the infection is completely asymptomatic.[94] Rarely, the child may experience a febrile illness with lymphadenopathy and hepatosplenomegaly. In the United States, approximately 0.7% of newborns are infected with CMV in utero and shed virus at birth.[167] Of these, approximately 90% are symptom free.[261,44] CMV is the leading known cause of sensorineural hearing loss in infants. Sources of CMV in the child care setting are infants and children who have been infected by their mothers by vertical transmission in utero, perinatally, or postpartum through breast-feeding (~6%). Infection in preschool-aged children leads to viral shedding into saliva and urine. Transmission likely occurs by direct contact with infected saliva or through fomites (toys and blankets) contaminated with saliva, rather than by respiratory droplets.[258] Shedding of CMV is as chronic among infected toddlers in child care centers as it is in children with perinatal or congenital infection.[5,217,218]

Strangert and colleagues[264] reported the isolation of CMV from 7 of 10 children between 21 and 30 months of age in one child care center. Strom[265] found that 13 of 18 (72%) children between 24 and 36 months of age in a single nursery excreted CMV. Children younger than 3 years who acquire CMV after birth excrete CMV in urine and saliva for 6 to 42 months (mean, 18 months).[5] Other investigators demonstrated that peak rates of infection occur in children between 1 and 3 years of age, when viral excretion may be documented in as many as 70% of children in child care.[2,156,165,207,216,218]

Household contact is a common source of CMV in young children. A population-based study evaluating risk factors for CMV among 4 to 10 year olds in the United States participating in the NHANES III identified CMV status of household members (mother and siblings) to be a strong predictor of CMV seroprevalence in the child. In this study, previous child care attendance was not shown to be a significant predictor.[261]

The greatest risk for morbidity is the acquisition of CMV during early pregnancy in child care providers or mothers of children attending child care.[4,2,3,6] Such acquisition may lead to clinically evident congenital CMV infection (microcephaly, hepatosplenomegaly, chorioretinitis, psychomotor retardation, and deafness) in approximately 5% to 10% of infected children. Another 10% to 15% of infants experience occult, but potentially damaging, infection that results in milder degrees of hearing loss and learning disabilities.[258] Because of the high rates of asymptomatic excretion by children, it is important for child care personnel to be aware of the risks of transmission and routinely practice appropriate hand hygiene.[15]

Herpes Simplex Virus

HSV is a DNA virus that commonly infects mucosal epithelial cells. Inoculation and replication at the site of infection are followed by the establishment of latency in sensory ganglia. Primary infection with HSV type 1 most often occurs in the oral mucosa. Approximately 15% of young children younger than 3 years will have gingivostomatitis as the manifestation of primary HSV-1 infection.[20,65,240] Symptoms of primary infection range from asymptomatic to severe, painful ulcerations of the oral mucosa and perioral regions that can lead to dehydration in a child who is unable to swallow. Stomatitis may be accompanied by signs of upper respiratory infection, fever, pharyngitis, and regional lymphadenopathy. Reactivation of virus most often manifests as asymptomatic shedding of virus in the saliva or as the presence of labial ulcerations (i.e., cold sores). Other sites of recurrent lesions may be seen, such as herpetic whitlow resulting from a child autoinoculating his or her fingers through sucking. Children who have perinatally acquired HSV may have recurrent infections at sites related to the original infection.

Transmission in a group child care setting is through direct contact with herpetic lesions, or fomites contaminated with infected saliva. Studies have demonstrated high attack rates of HSV infection and stomatitis in orphanages[65,132] and child care settings.[240,177] One study of 90 children in a child care center (aged 0–37 months) in Japan identified four clusters of infection over the 4 years of observation. Horizontal transmission was confirmed by genetic analysis of the isolated viruses.[177]

Children with herpetic gingivostomatitis do not need to be excluded from group care unless there is difficulty controlling drooling. Children and staff with recurrent infection do not need to be excluded. Covering recurrent lesions with clothing or bandages during child care is sufficient.[15]

Human Immunodeficiency Virus

The potential transmission of HIV by blood or body fluid exposure can cause great concern for families and staff. However, the risk for nonsexual, nonpercutaneous transmission is extremely low. Studies of risk to health care workers with percutaneous exposure to known HIV-infected blood by needlestick has been estimated to be less than three in 1000 exposures.[34] To date, HIV infection has not been reported to be transmitted in a child care center.

There are rare case reports of transmission of HIV within households with an infected member.[49,110,119,283] In most cases, transmission occurred in a setting with ongoing exposure of nonintact skin (e.g., eczema) or mucosal surfaces to infected blood or body fluids. Three children have been identified who were likely infected through the practice of premastication of food by an HIV-infected caregiver. In two cases, the premastication occurred at a time the caregiver was known to have had bleeding gums or mouth sores.[119] In light of its rare horizontal transmission to nonsexual contacts within households with an infected member, HIV would not be expected to spread in child care settings.[117,166]

One potential high-risk situation may involve HIV-positive children who are persistent biters or who have extensive weeping skin lesions. However, several reports indicate a lack of transmission to individuals bitten or scratched by a person infected with HIV.[95,232,251,276] An incident was reported from London in which 21 elementary school–aged children repeatedly stuck themselves and their classmates with diabetic needles on the playground. When it was determined that one of the children was HIV positive with high viral load, 19 children received antiretroviral medication for postexposure prophylaxis. There were no HIV seroconversions.[272]

Since the institution of guidelines to identify HIV-positive women during pregnancy and intervene with peripartum antiretroviral medication,[50] the incidence of perinatal HIV infection in the United States has declined dramatically.[53] Recent estimates are that fewer than 200 infants are born in the United States with HIV infection. Children who are born in countries with high rates of HIV infection and immigrate or are adopted into the United States should be screened for HIV infection. Personnel should be trained in the use of standard precautions and use gloves for potential exposures to blood or body fluids. Blood and bodily fluid from everyone should be treated as if it potentially carries a blood-borne pathogen. Children who have weeping skin lesions that cannot be covered or bleeding problems should be excluded from child care until the problem is resolved.[14]

Vaccine-Preventable Diseases

Since the beginning of the vaccine era in the early 20th century, many of the infectious illnesses that were easily spread among children and household contacts are now significantly decreased in number. A comparison of annual morbidity of 10 infectious diseases for which universal vaccination is recommended for US children showed an approximately 95% to 100% decrease in morbidity for all infections (2007 vs. baseline 20th-century annual morbidity data).[221] Currently 14 vaccines are recommended for children in the United States before entry into elementary school. These provide protection to young infants and children through the development of individual and herd immunity. Because of the success of vaccine programs, fewer practitioners in countries with robust vaccine programs have seen the clinical manifestations of these infections. However, there continues to be a need for awareness of the clinical presentations of these diseases because unimmunized or underimmunized children (by family choice or because of immunocompromised status) may carry these organisms into or be exposed to them in group child care settings. States have differing regulations for vaccination exemptions by families for religious or philosophical reasons. Accordingly, rates of unimmunized children vary by geographic location. When outbreaks of vaccine-preventable illnesses do occur, public health officials should be notified and involved in management. Exclusion of unvaccinated children from child care may be recommended for their health and that of those who are unable to be immunized because of age or health status. Many infections are still present in high rates in other countries, and children born in these countries who immigrate may be asymptomatic carriers of infectious organisms (e.g., hepatitis A).

Diphtheria

Diphtheria is caused by production of toxin by the bacteria *Corynebacterium diphtheria*. Clinical presentation may include nasal symptoms, membranous pharyngitis, obstructive laryngotracheitis, or skin manifestations. The prominent symptoms are usually a severe sore throat and croup accompanied by toxemia.

A probable case of diphtheria was reported in the United States in 2012.[62] The case before that was reported in 2003. Diphtheria is still present and endemic in countries with low rates of vaccination and predominantly in tropical areas of the world. In 2014, more than 7000 cases were reported worldwide by the World Health Organization.

C. diphtheriae is spread by respiratory droplets after intimate contact with someone who is infected or is a carrier. Individuals are susceptible if they have not been immunized or have been immunized only partially. Treatment is with antitoxin and antibiotics (erythromycin or penicillin). Prophylaxis can be accomplished with erythromycin or penicillin if an individual is found to be a carrier. Immunization with a diphtheria toxoid–containing vaccine is effective in preventing disease and spread of infection.

Haemophilus influenzae *Type B*

Historically, HIB was the major bacterial pathogen of childhood and was responsible for many cases of meningitis, epiglottitis, pneumonia, facial cellulitis, and septic arthritis. These infections primarily occurred in children between 2 months and 5 years of age, with a peak occurring in those between 6 and 18 months of age. The organism colonizes the nasopharynx before becoming blood-borne; hematogenous dissemination results in a distant focus of infection. The bacteria are transmitted on respiratory droplets.

The availability and universal use of effective vaccines for the prevention of HIB infection have dramatically changed the epidemiology of infections caused by this pathogen.[248] Conjugate vaccines were introduced in 1987. Although there has been a marked decline in invasive disease since then, cases of invasive HIB disease are still reported sporadically. The Active Bacterial Core Surveillance Report identified 11 cases of HIB invasive disease in in the United States in 2013 and 12 cases in 2014, three were younger than 1 year.[63]

Schulte and coworkers[241] reviewed the pattern of invasive HIB infection in New York State after the introduction of the conjugate vaccine. These investigators demonstrated a dramatic decline in the incidence of HIB disease in children younger than 5 years, among both those in child care and those in home care. In 2007, a voluntary recall of HIB vaccine by one supplier led to underimmunizaton of children younger than 15 months because immunization schedules required adjustment. The following year an increase in cases of HIV invasive disease (five children ≤3 years of age) was reported from the state of Minnesota (higher than in the previous 16 years). Of these cases, the majority of children were underimmunized because of parental refusal. Although cases were present, a simultaneous survey of nasopharyngeal carriage of HIB showed low rates of carriage in this age group.[191]

Rifampin is the medication of choice for prophylaxis of at-risk individuals exposed to a case of HIB disease. In the rare instance of invasive HIB disease in a child care center, public health officials should be involved in management. All personnel and child care attendees should receive rifampin prophylaxis if two or more cases of invasive HIB disease have occurred in the center within 60 days and unimmunized or underimmunized children attend. If only one case has occurred in the child care center, all attendees who are unimmunized or not completely immunized should be monitored carefully and be medically evaluated if ill or febrile.[15] Children with HIB disease should be excluded until cleared by a health care provider.

Streptococcus pneumoniae

Pneumococci are a common cause of bacterial infections of the upper and lower respiratory tracts, including otitis media, sinusitis, and pneumonia.[242] As respiratory pathogens, they can also cause other upper respiratory tract infections, such as conjunctivitis, and important systemic illnesses, including occult bacteremia, bacteremic periorbital cellulitis, and meningitis.

S. pneumoniae is spread easily in the child care setting related to the high rates of nasal carriage in young children. It is transmitted on respiratory droplets. Numerous studies have demonstrated the horizontal transmission of *S. pneumoniae* and its relationship to nasal carriage among children in child care centers.

In 2000, a pneumococcal conjugate vaccine containing seven common serotypes of *S. pneumoniae* (PCV7) was licensed in the United States. Subsequently, a reduction in nasopharyngeal colonization rates with the serotypes of *S. pneumoniae* contained in the vaccine was documented among young children.[81,80,136] A secondary effect of the conjugate vaccines was the decrease of both colonization and disease among the contacts of vaccinees.[124]

The implementation of PCV7 also had an impact on the rates of carriage and disease caused by penicillin-nonsusceptible strains.[178,249] Active surveillance data from 1996 to 2004 demonstrated an 81% decrease in invasive disease caused by penicillin-nonsusceptible pneumococci in children younger than 2 years.[178] However, soon after the introduction of PCV7, replacement, non-PCV7 pneumococcal strains were identified in the nasopharynx of healthy, symptom-free children, and were also the cause of invasive disease (e.g., meningitis or bacteremia).[79,147,219]

In 2010, a 13-valent pneumococcal conjugate vaccine was licensed that incorporated antigens of the more invasive pneumococcal serotypes including serotype 19A, which had emerged as a predominant non-PCV7 serotype often causing severe disease. PCV13 replaced PCV7 in recommendations for universal vaccination of infants.[57] Since then, several studies have documented a decrease in nasopharyngeal carriage in preschool children of PCV13 strains of pneumococcus,[91,127] including nonsusceptible strains.[82] Declining rates of acute otitis media,[112,182,268] hospitalizations for pneumonia,[128,129] and other invasive pneumococcal diseases such as meningitis[137] were demonstrated in multiple studies.

Children with pneumococcal disease (local or invasive) do not need to be excluded from child care unless they are unable to fully participate or require additional care by staff. There is no recommendation for chemoprophylaxis of contacts of an individual with pneumococcal disease.

Influenza

Influenza is a common cause of upper respiratory infection in preschool-aged children. The severity of infection is variable, from mild nasal congestion to a severe sepsis syndrome. Influenza can cause significant morbidity in people of all ages; children younger than 5 years carry a large burden of disease. Secondary lower respiratory tract infections with *S. aureus* or *S. pneumoniae,* among other pathogens, contribute to much of the morbidity in severe cases.

Influenza is transmitted person to person through infected droplets with a cough or sneeze, or indirectly from contaminated objects. Secondary transmission to household and child care contacts is a common occurrence.

Epidemics occur seasonally during the colder months of the year. However, in 2009 to 2012 a pandemic of influenza A (H1N1) strain was seen globally that began in the spring. During this pandemic there was an observed fourfold increase in mortality among children compared with previous years.[61]

Because of variation in influenza A antigens, components of influenza vaccines are adjusted annually. The antigens for H1N1 have subsequently been included in the seasonal vaccine. A trivalent inactivated influenza vaccine is recommended for seasonal immunization of persons older than 6 months.

Children with influenza should not be excluded from child care unless they are unable to participate, or if caring for the child would compromise the ability of staff to care for other children.[14]

Varicella

Varicella, or chickenpox, is a highly contagious infection that is spread easily by the airborne route and by respiratory droplets. It is characterized by a pruritic, generalized vesicular rash that occurs in one to six crops, each crop separated by 24 to 36 hours. Fever usually is mild. The most common complication is secondary bacterial pyoderma, and although uncommon, pneumonia and secondary invasive infection caused by *S. pyogenes* can cause significant morbidity. Varicella zoster virus remains latent in sensory ganglia after primary infection but can be reactivated as herpes zoster or "shingles," in which case it is manifested as a vesicular eruption involving one to three sensory dermatomes. If infection is acquired in early pregnancy, varicella embryopathy (limb bands or amputation) has been noted in a small fraction of children.

Live, attenuated varicella vaccine became available for universal use in the United States in children between 12 and 18 months of age in

1995. The availability of this vaccine altered the epidemiology of varicella in the United States dramatically. The vaccine has been demonstrated to be highly effective during most outbreaks of varicella in child care[70,159] and in clinical practice.[282] The general effectiveness of the vaccine is 83% to 86% against all forms of the disease and 97% to 100% against moderate to severe disease. However, through active surveillance, breakthrough disease in children who had received one dose of varicella disease was reported. Outbreaks were reported in elementary schools with high rates of vaccine coverage[52,277] and in a Connecticut child care center in which 25 children contracted varicella (68% of whom were vaccinated). Disease was milder among vaccinated children.[118] These observations led to the recommendation by the Advisory Committee on Immunization Practices in 2006 for a universal two-dose varicella vaccine schedule. The first dose is given when the child is 12 to 15 months of age and a second dose at 4 to 6 years of age.[55] A retrospective cohort analysis of claims data evaluating trends in hospitalizations related to varicella disease demonstrated an 84% decline of hospitalizations in 2012 compared with 1994 (before licensure of the varicella vaccine), and a 38% decline comparing the one- and two-dose vaccine periods.[188]

About 10% to 15% of children may develop a popular or vesicular rash at the site of vaccination 5 to 26 days after receiving the immunization. If this does occur without further spread of rash or systemic symptoms, the child may attend child care with the lesions covered. A child with active chickenpox should be excluded from the child care setting until all lesions are scabbed over and the child is able to participate in activities. A child or staff member with varicella zoster need only be excluded if the rash cannot be covered.[14]

Measles

Measles (rubeola) is a highly contagious respiratory infection with a household attack rate of 90%. Infants and children less than 5 years of age are at the highest risk for complications. Measles virus is spread by droplets, hand transmission, and the airborne route. The illness usually is moderate to severe; high fever and prominent respiratory symptoms (cough and coryza) and conjunctivitis are present for several days before onset of the rash. Diarrhea occasionally may be a prominent feature. After the rash erupts, the fever and respiratory symptoms persist for several more days. Pneumonia and encephalitis are complications of measles virus infection; each occurs at an incidence of 1 per 1000 cases.

In the year 2000, endemic measles was determined to be eliminated in the United States.[215] However, outbreaks continue to be reported each year. In 2014, there were 23 measles outbreaks, totaling 667 cases; the largest involved 383 cases among unvaccinated members of a closed community. In early 2015, a notable outbreak of 136 cases occurred at an amusement park during the holiday season. It is thought that the virus was introduced by a foreign traveler, and molecular testing confirmed it was the same strain as was responsible for an outbreak in the Philippines the previous year.[301]

In 2015, an outbreak was reported in a child care center in Illinois, primarily affecting the most vulnerable: infants who were too young to be immunized.[69] Twelve of the 15 cases were in infants, aged 3 to 11 months, who attended the same group child care. There were 14 infants in the child care room that were exposed, indicating a high attack rate. One of the early cases was initially diagnosed with Kawasaki disease and was not diagnosed with measles until another infected infant was identified.

Measles is effectively prevented by immunization. Current recommendations are to immunize twice: once when the child is between 12 and 15 months of age, and again at 4 to 6 years of age. For exposed, susceptible children, vaccination is recommended with the mumps, measles, and rubella (MMR) vaccine within 72 hours of exposure. During an outbreak, vaccine may be given to children 6 to 11 months of age. However, a child who receives measles vaccine before 1 year of age must still receive the vaccine at 12 to 15 months of age; the first is not counted toward the two required for full protection. Immune globulin can be given within 6 days to an exposed, susceptible individual for whom the live viral vaccine is contraindicated or in whom exposure was more than 72 hours before medical evaluation. This includes infants younger than 12 months and immunocompromised individuals.[15] Children with measles and any exposed unimmunized children should be excluded from the group care setting until at least 2 weeks after the onset of rash in the last case of measles.

Rubella

Rubella, another exanthematous disease of childhood, is much milder than rubeola but attacks a similar age group. Incidence of rubella in the United States dramatically decreased with universal immunization. Endemic rubella was determined to be eliminated from the Americas in 2009.[24,180]

Rubella is a highly contagious RNA virus that is transmitted by the respiratory route. Clinically it is characterized by mild fever, lymphadenopathy (postauricular and occipital), and rash. The illness is difficult to distinguish from other viral exanthems. Up to 50% of infections may be asymptomatic.

If rubella is contracted during the first or early second trimester of pregnancy, a severe fetal infection resulting in microcephaly, deafness, congenital heart defects, eye disorders, and psychomotor retardation may result. Acquisition of infection during pregnancy may be a potential hazard for child care personnel or mothers of children who attend child care if an outbreak of rubella occurs in the child care setting. In a large outbreak of rubella in Nebraska in 1999, 14 children (nine of whom were <12 months old) and 2 parents acquired their infection in a child care center.[84]

The incidence of congenital rubella syndrome can be minimized by appropriate immunization of preschoolers and personnel. Any child or personnel with noncongenital rubella infection should be excluded from the group child care setting until 7 days after the onset of rash. In outbreak situations, any exposed, unimmunized, or underimmunized children should be excluded from a group setting until they are immunized, or excluded for 21 days after rash onset of the last outbreak case. Children with congenital rubella syndrome may shed virus in urine or nasopharyngeal secretions and be considered contagious until at least 1 year of age. They can be declared noncontagious if two cultures of clinical specimens obtained 1 month apart are negative for rubella virus after 3 months.[15]

Pertussis

Pertussis, or whooping cough, is a highly communicable respiratory disease caused by *Bordetella pertussis.* The attack rate and severity of disease are highest in the first year of life. The illness classically is divided into three phases: catarrhal, paroxysmal, and convalescent. In the first stage, the child has no fever but has symptoms, primarily rhinorrhea, and a cough. When the nasal symptoms resolve, however, the cough becomes and remains very prominent for many weeks. The cough is characterized by paroxysms that are followed by an inspiratory effort (whoop) or leave the child exhausted and occasionally apneic. Individuals are most infectious during the catarrhal phase and the first 2 weeks of cough. The convalescent stage is the many weeks necessary for complete recovery. Infected children younger than 1 month are at greatest risk for significant morbidity and mortality. Treatment with a macrolide is effective in decreasing the shedding of organisms, and prompt treatment will shorten the course of the disease.

Complete immunization with a five-dose series of acellular pertussis vaccine is effective in preventing most cases of pertussis, although illness does occur in partially and occasionally in fully immunized children.[68] Pertussis continues to cause disease in vaccinated and unvaccinated persons, with peaks in incidence occurring every few years. In 2012, a pertussis epidemic occurred in the State of Washington, with highest incidence among infants younger than 1 year and children 10 to 14 years of age.[60] Similar age trends were seen nationwide in the many geographic areas affected by the epidemic. There were 48,277 cases of pertussis reported that year, the highest number since 1955. After a person has been exposed to a case, macrolides provide effective prophylaxis and are the first-line drugs. Trimethoprim-sulfamethoxazole is an alternate in a person who is older than 2 months and unable to tolerate a macrolide, or who has documented macrolide-resistant pertussis.

Prophylaxis is recommended for exposure in child care. If appropriate, booster doses of acellular diphtheria-tetanus-pertussis vaccine should be given to exposed children in a child care or household setting. A child who has pertussis or has been exposed to a case of pertussis and has symptoms should be excluded from group child care until receipt of 5 days of an appropriate course of a macrolide (azithromycin or erythromycin).[14] If no treatment is received, then exclusion is for 21 days after onset of cough. Immunization status should be updated if a person is underimmunized. Adolescents who have received their primary series of tetanus-diphtheria-pertussis should receive a single dose of the tetanus-diphtheria (Tdap) vaccine at age 11 or 12 years. It is recommended that individuals who are in contact with children younger than 12 months also receive a pertussis booster with the Tdap vaccine. Women should receive Tdap vaccine with each pregnancy regardless of previous vaccination status.[15]

Poliomyelitis

Through the Global Polio Eradication Initiative, polio is on the verge of being eradicated worldwide with major vaccination efforts of multiple organizations. Only 73 cases from two countries were reported in 2015.[104,199] Poliovirus is an enterovirus. Although most infections with this virus are subclinical, in the preimmunization era, polio was the major cause of acquired paralytic disease, especially in older children and young adults. In some developing countries, it was a major health problem until very recently.

Poliomyelitis is prevented effectively by use of either the live oral poliovirus vaccine or the inactivated, enhanced-potency parenteral vaccine (IPV).[225] The Advisory Committee on Immunization Practices of the Centers for Disease Control and Prevention (CDC) and the AAP recommend a four-dose all-IPV vaccine schedule for routine immunization of all infants and children in the United States.

Mumps

Mumps is a relatively benign infection of childhood that often is asymptomatic. The most prominent clinical feature is parotitis. Occasionally, a clinically significant central nervous system infection causes unilateral sensorineural deafness. This infection had been dramatically reduced by widespread use of the MMR vaccine. However, large outbreaks continue to occur in the United States. In 2006, there was an outbreak primarily among vaccinated young adults in the Midwest,[86] and in 2009, an outbreak occurred primarily among vaccinated school-aged children in a religious community in New York and New Jersey.[28,56]

There was a dramatic increase in numbers of cases in 2012–2014, with the CDC reporting 1057 cases in 2015 and 1661 cases in the first half of 2016. Since the early 2000s the age of highest incidence of mumps has shifted from the preschool child to adolescents and young adults. This is possibly a result of waning immunity. Children with mumps should be excluded from the group child care setting until 5 days after the onset of parotid swelling.

Rotavirus

Before the introduction of rotavirus vaccine for the immunization of infants in 2006, rotavirus was the most common identifiable infectious cause of gastroenteritis leading to hospitalization in young children, and accounting for more than 25% of diarrheal cases in the United States.[40,89,149,198,286] It is currently a significant cause of diarrhea in developing countries, contributing substantially to the worldwide mortality figures for gastroenteritis.

A very low inoculum of rotavirus is needed to cause infection. The virus can be recovered from asymptomatic hosts, especially neonates and infants.[66] It is shed in large numbers in the stool of patients with symptoms, thereby contributing to the high prevalence of the virus on environmental surfaces during outbreaks.[291] Viral shedding occurs both before and after symptoms have appeared.[222] Most illnesses caused by rotavirus occur in the cooler months in temperate climates but occur year-round in tropical areas. The peak attack rate is in the 6- to 24-month-old age group. Before the introduction of vaccine, many outbreaks were reported in group child care settings.[31,213,222,231] In prospective studies of diarrheal illness in children attending child care, rotavirus was implicated in 6% to 24% of cases of gastroenteritis,[31,30,149,266] as well as in 20% to 40% of outbreaks.[31]

In early 2006, a bovine rotavirus-based pentavalent vaccine was licensed for use in US infants. Three doses of the vaccine are given orally at 2, 4, and 6 months of age.[17] In 2008, a monovalent attenuated human rotavirus was licensed for a two-dose schedule given orally at 2 and 4 months.

Both have been shown to be effective against rotavirus of any severity.[41,47,75,90,187,256] A review of a claims database for one health care system (2008–11) demonstrated much lower rates of hospitalizations and emergency department visits coded for unspecified gastroenteritis and rotavirus among households in which an infant had been vaccinated against rotavirus, thus demonstrating indirect protection among household members.[74]

Treatment of children with rotavirus diarrhea is supportive. Exclusion criteria from child care are the same as those for any diarrheal illness. Children should be excluded if the stool cannot be contained in the diaper or accidents occur in toilet-trained children. Return to child care is appropriate when the stool is controlled and the child's illness does not put extra burden on child care staff.

Hepatitis A Virus

Before the institution of universal immunization of young children, HAV, an enterovirus, was a common cause of acute hepatitis in children. As with other enteric pathogens, this organism is transmitted by the fecal-oral route. Manifestations of infection vary remarkably according to age. In young children (<6 years), infection with HAV may be entirely asymptomatic or associated with relatively mild and nonspecific symptoms such as low-grade fever, anorexia, nausea, vomiting, and diarrhea in 30% of patients. Jaundice, a more specific marker of liver disease, occurs in fewer than 10% of children younger than 6 years.[123] In contrast, adults with hepatitis A often are icteric in conjunction with other gastrointestinal symptoms. Infection, when symptomatic, usually lasts several weeks but occasionally can become protracted.

Transmission is primarily by person-to-person spread, but fomites may play an important role because the organism can persist and remain infective in the dried state for months.[200] HAV is shed in high density in the stool of infected persons from 2 weeks before until 1 week after the onset of clinical symptoms.

Intramuscular immunoglobulin given within 2 weeks of exposure to susceptible individuals (infants <12 months of age) is very effective in preventing symptomatic disease. Unimmunized children older than 12 months can be vaccinated as postexposure prophylaxis.[15] Since the recommendation for universal vaccination of children 12 to 23 months of age, there has been a significant reduction in the incidence of acute HAV disease.[54] Clusters of infection have been reported among close contacts of asymptomatic, newly arrived international adoptees from countries with high rates of HAV.[109] The AAP, Advisory Committee on Immunization Practices (ACIP), and CDC recommend vaccination of close contacts of internationally adopted children at risk for HAV, including parents and babysitters.[18]

HAV vaccine is recommended for children beginning at age 12 months. If a person in the child care setting does contract HAV, or there are two or more households affected by HAV, unimmunized child care contacts should receive HAV vaccine or intravenous immune globulin. Children and adults (especially food handlers) with HAV disease should be excluded from the group child care setting until 1 week after the onset of illness or after they are cleared by public health officials.[15]

Hepatitis B Virus

HBV is a DNA-containing virus that causes infections with a wide range of clinical manifestations from asymptomatic seroconversion to fatal hepatitis. Infection is more likely to be asymptomatic in children than in adults.[202] Common symptoms include fever, fatigue, anorexia, malaise, and jaundice. Other gastrointestinal symptoms, such as nausea, vomiting, and diarrhea, may be prominent. Joint symptoms (arthritis and arthralgias) and cutaneous lesions (papular acrodermatitis) may be noted early in the course of the illness.

The most common modes of transmission of HBV in adults are contact with blood and sexual activity. Young children usually acquire infection with HBV by vertical transmission from their mother at delivery. The maternal infection may be acute or chronic. Infection acquired vertically by an infant usually is asymptomatic, but it leads to chronic carriage of hepatitis B surface antigen in most cases. With increasing immigration and adoption of infants from HBV-endemic areas, more HBV-carrier children will be identified.[141] It is important to screen children from areas where the prevalence of hepatitis B is more than 2% as they arrive to the United States.

Transmission of HBV within the child care setting is rare but has been reported.[85,92,247] In one US case, the probable source was a bite by a child who was a carrier of HBV.[247] In the other, a child care worker with chapped hands was exposed to the blood of a child who was an HBV carrier.[92] The third involved an aggressive 21-month-old child with weeping dermatitis and a history of biting other children. Other investigations failed to demonstrate transmission in child care facilities despite long-term contact, including one situation with a high potential for blood exposure.[246]

Implementation of the current recommendation to screen all pregnant women for HBV and to undertake universal immunization against hepatitis B in infancy is the most effective way to prevent the spread of this infection. Infants born to mothers positive for hepatitis B surface antigen are recommended to receive hepatitis B immune globulin in addition to the vaccine.

Because of the low risk for transmission within the group child care setting, the AAP, American Public Health Association, and CDC do not recommend exclusion of HBV-infected children from child care or HBV screening of children as a criterion for entry. A child known to have active HBV should be excluded from child care if they have weeping sores that cannot be covered, generalized dermatitis, a bleeding problem, or aggressive behavior (e.g., biting or scratching) that may draw blood of the person with HBV. Child care personnel should use Standard Precautions and gloves, handling all blood and body fluids as if they are potentially infected.[15]

NEW REFERENCES SINCE SEVENTH EDITION

10. Al-Jader LN, Walker AM, Williams HM, Willshaw GA, Cheasty T. Outbreak of *Escherichia coli* O157 in a nursery: lessons for prevention. *Arch Dis Child.* 1999;81(1):60-63.
14. American Academy of Pediatrics. *Managing Infectious Diseases in Child Care and Schools: A Quick Reference Guide.* 3rd ed. Elk Grove Village, IL: American Academy of Pediatrics; 2013.
15. American Academy of Pediatrics. *Red Book: The Report of the Committee on Infectious Diseases.* 30th ed. Elk Grove Village, IL: American Academy of Pediatrics; 2015.
19. American Academy of Pediatrics Pennsylvania Chapter. *Model Child Care Health Policies.* In: Aronson SS, ed. 5th ed. Elk Grove Village, IL: American Academy of Pediatrics; 2014. www.ecels-healthychildcarepa.org.
22. Amit U, Flaishmakher S, Dagan R, et al. Age-Dependent Carriage of *Kingella kingae* in Young Children and Turnover of Colonizing Strains. *J Pediatric Infect Dis Soc.* 2014;3(2):160-162.
24. Andrus JK, de Quadros CA, Solorzano CC, et al. Measles and rubella eradication in the Americas. *Vaccine.* 2011;29(suppl 4):D91-D96.
26. Bacon AE, Fekety R, Schaberg DR, et al. Epidemiology of *Clostridium difficile* colonization in newborns: results using a bacteriophage and bacteriocin typing system. *J Infect Dis.* 1988;158(2):349-354.
27. Ball TM, Holdberg CJ, Aldous MB, et al. Influence of attendance at day care on the common cold from birth through 13 years of age. *Arch Pediatr Adolesc Med.* 2002;156(2):121-126.
28. Barskey AE, Schulte C, Rosen JB, et al. Mumps outbreak in Orthodox Jewish communities in the United States. *N Engl J Med.* 2012;367(18):1704-1713.
29. Bartholomew CF, Jones AM. Human bites: a rare risk factor for HIV transmission. *AIDS.* 2006;20(4):631-632.
32. Basmaci R, Ilharreborde B, Bidet P, et al. Isolation of *Kingella kingae* in the oropharynx during K. kingae arthritis in children. *Clin Microbiol Infect.* 2012;18(5):134-136.
36. Benson L, Song X, Campos J, et al. Changing epidemiology of *Clostridium difficile*-associated disease in children. *Infect Control Hosp Epidemiol.* 2007;28(11):1233-1235.
37. Bidet P, Collin E, Basmaci R, et al. Investigation of an outbreak of osteoarticular infections caused by *Kingella kingae* in a childcare center using molecular techniques. *Pediatr Infect Dis J.* 2013;32(5):558-560.
42. Broccolo F, Falcone V, Esposito S, et al. Human bocaviruses: Possible etiologic role in respiratory infection. *J Clin Virol.* 2015;72:75-81.
43. Canadian Pediatric Society. A bite in the playroom: Managing human bites in child care settings. *Paediatr Child Health.* 2008;13(6):515-526.
44. Cannon M, Stowell J, Clark R, et al. Repeated measures study of weekly and daily cytomegalovirus shedding patterns in saliva and urine of healthy cytomegalovirus-seropositive children. *BMC Infect Dis.* 2014;14(569).
46. Cannon MJ, Westbrook K, Levis D, et al. Awareness of and behaviors related to child-to-mother transmission of cytomegalovirus. *Prev Med.* 2012;54(5):351-357.
50. Centers for Disease Control and Prevention. Active Bacterial Core Surveillance (ABC's); 2016. http://www.cdc.gov/abcs/reports-findings/survreports/hib14.html.
53. Centers for Disease Control and Prevention. Licensure of a 13-Valent Pneumococcal Conjugate Vaccine (PCV13) and Recommendations for Use Among Children—Advisory Committee on Immunization Practices (ACIP), 2010. *MMWR Morb Mortal Wkly Rep.* 2010;59(9):258-261.
55. Centers for Disease Control and Prevention. Multiply resistant shigellosis in a day-care center—Texas. *MMWR Morb Mortal Wkly Rep.* 1986;35(48):753-755.
62. Centers for Disease Control and Prevention. Summary of Notifiable Diseases—2012. *MMWR Morb Mortal Wkly Rep.* 2014;61(53).
64. Ceroni D, Dubois-Ferriere V, Anderson R, et al. Small risk of osteoarticular infections in children with asymptomatic oropharyngeal carriage of *Kingella kingae. Pediatr Infect Dis J.* 2012;31(9):983-985.
69. Clegg WJ, Linchangco PC, Arwady MA, et al. Measles Outbreak in a Child Care Center, Cook County, Illinois, 2015. *J Pediatric Infect Dis Soc.* 2016.
74. Cortese MM, Dahl RM, Curns AT, et al. Protection against gastroenteritis in US households with children who received rotavirus vaccine. *J Infect Dis.* 2015;211(4):558-562.
75. Cortese MM, Tate JE, Simonsen L, et al. Reduction in gastroenteritis in United States children and correlation with early rotavirus vaccine uptake from national medical claims databases. *Pediatr Infect Dis J.* 2010;29(6):489-494.
79. Dagan R. Serotype replacement in perspective. *Vaccine.* 2009;27(suppl 3):C22-C24.
82. Dagan R, Juergens C, Trammel J, et al. Efficacy of 13-valent pneumococcal conjugate vaccine (PCV13) versus that of 7-valent PCV (PCV7) against nasopharyngeal colonization of antibiotic-nonsusceptible *Streptococcus pneumoniae. J Infect Dis.* 2015;211(7):1144-1153.
87. de Hoog M, Venekamp R, van der Ent C, et al. Impact of early daycare on healthcare resource use related to upper respiratory tract infections during childhood: prospective WHISTLER cohort study. *BMC Med.* 2014;12:107.
90. Desai AP, Sharma D, Crispell EK, et al. Decline in Pneumococcal Nasopharyngeal Carriage of Vaccine Serotypes After the Introduction of the 13-Valent Pneumococcal Conjugate Vaccine in Children in Atlanta, Georgia. *Pediatr Infect Dis J.* 2015;34(11):1168-1174.
93. Dollard SC, Keyserling H, Radford K, et al. Cytomegalovirus viral and antibody correlates in young children. *BMC Res Notes.* 2014;7:776.
99. Enserink R, Simonsen J, Mughini-Gras L, et al. Transient and sustained effects of child-care attendance on hospital admission for gastroenteritis. *Int J Epidemiol.* 2015;44(3):988-997.
100. Enserink R, Ypma R, Donker GA, et al. Infectious disease burden related to child day care in the Netherlands. *Pediatr Infect Dis J.* 2013;32(8):e334-e340.
102. Faix R. Survival of cytomegalovirus on environmental surfaces. *J Pediatr.* 1985;106(4):649-652.
104. Farag NH, Wadood MZ, Safdar RM, et al. Progress Toward Poliomyelitis Eradication—Pakistan, January 2014–September 2015. *MMWR Morb Mortal Wkly Rep.* 2015;64(45):1271-1275.
105. Federal Interagency Forum on Child and Family Statistics. America's Children: Key National Indicators of Well-Being; 2015. http://www.childstats.gov.
112. Fortunato F, Martinelli D, Cappelli MG, et al. Impact of Pneumococcal Conjugate Universal Routine Vaccination on Pneumococcal Disease in Italian Children. *J Immunol Res.* 2015;2015:206757.
113. Frank C, Werber D, Cramer JP, et al. Epidemic profile of Shiga-toxin-producing *Escherichia coli* O104:H4 outbreak in Germany. *N Engl J Med.* 2011;365(19):1771-1780.
127. Gounder PP, Bruce MG, Bruden DJ, et al. Effect of the 13-valent pneumococcal conjugate vaccine on nasopharyngeal colonization by *Streptococcus pneumoniae*—Alaska, 2008–2012. *J Infect Dis.* 2014;209(8):1251-1258.
128. Greenberg D, Givon-Lavi N, Ben-Shimol S, et al. Impact of PCV7/PCV13 introduction on community-acquired alveolar pneumonia in children <5 years. *Vaccine.* 2015;33(36):4623-4629.
129. Griffin MR, Mitchel E, Moore MR, et al; Centers for Disease Control and Prevention (CDC). Declines in pneumonia hospitalizations of children aged <2 years associated with the use of pneumococcal conjugate vaccines—Tennessee, 1998–2012. *MMWR Morb Mortal Wkly Rep.* 2014;63(44):995-998.
133. Hall AJ, Wikswo ME, Manikonda K, et al. Acute gastroenteritis surveillance through the National Outbreak Reporting System, United States. *Emerg Infect Dis.* 2013;19(8):1305-1309.
137. Harboe ZB, Dalby T, Weinberger DM, et al. Impact of 13-valent pneumococcal conjugate vaccination in invasive pneumococcal disease incidence and mortality. *Clin Infect Dis.* 2014;59(8):1066-1073.
140. Hassan-Rios E, Torres P, Munoz E, et al. Sapovirus gastroenteritis in preschool center, Puerto Rico, 2011. *Emerg Infect Dis.* 2013;19(1):174-175.
145. Heusinkveld M, Mughini-Gras L, Pijnacker R, et al. Potential causative agents of acute gastroenteritis in households with preschool children: prevalence, risk factors, clinical relevance and household transmission. *Eur J Clin Microbiol Infect Dis.* 2016;35(10):1691-1700.

150. Hlavsa MC, Roberts VA, Kahler AM, et al. Outbreaks of Illness Associated with Recreational Water–United States, 2011–2012. *MMWR Morb Mortal Wkly Rep.* 2015;64(24):668-672.
153. Hullegie S, Bruijning-Verhagen P, Uiterwaal CS, et al. First-year Daycare and Incidence of Acute Gastroenteritis. *Pediatrics.* 2016;137(5).
162. Jangi S, Lamont JT. Asymptomatic colonization by *Clostridium difficile* in infants: implications for disease in later life. *J Pediatr Gastroenterol Nutr.* 2010;51(1):2-7.
163. Jartti T, Hedman K, Jartti L, et al. Human bocavirus—the first 5 years. *Rev Med Virol.* 2012;22(1):46-64.
164. Jokipii L, Jokipii AMM. Timing of symptoms and oocyst excretion in human cryptosporidiosis. *N Engl J Med.* 1986;315(26):1643-1647.
170. Khanna S, Baddour LM, Huskins WC, et al. The epidemiology of *Clostridium difficile* infection in children: a population-based study. *Clin Infect Dis.* 2013;56(10):1401-1406.
172. Kim J, Smathers SA, Prasad P, et al. Epidemiological features of *Clostridium difficile*-associated disease among inpatients at children's hospitals in the United States, 2001–2006. *Pediatrics.* 2008;122(6):1266-1270.
175. Kotch JB, Isbell P, Weber DJ, et al. Hand-washing and diapering equipment reduces disease among children in out-of-home child care centers. *Pediatrics.* 2007;120(1):e29-e36.
180. Lambert N, Strebel P, Orenstein W, et al. Rubella. *Lancet.* 2015;385(9984):2297-2307.
181. Larson HE, Barclay FE, Honour P, et al. Epidemiology of *Clostridium difficile* in infants. *J Infect Dis.* 1982;146(6):727-733.
182. Lau WC, Murray M, El-Turki A, et al. Impact of pneumococcal conjugate vaccines on childhood otitis media in the United Kingdom. *Vaccine.* 2015;33(39):5072-5079.
183. Laughlin L. Who's Minding the Kids? Child Care Arrangements: Spring 2011. Current Population Reports P70-135. Washington, DC: US Census Bureau; 2013.
187. Leshem E, Tate JE, Steiner CA, et al. Acute gastroenteritis hospitalizations among US children following implementation of the rotavirus vaccine. *JAMA.* 2015;313(22):2282-2284.
188. Leung J, Lopez AS, Blostein J, et al. Impact of the US Two-dose Varicella Vaccination Program on the Epidemiology of Varicella Outbreaks: Data from Nine States, 2005–2012. *Pediatr Infect Dis J.* 2015;34(10):1105-1109.
193. MacNeil JR, Bennett N, Farley MM, et al. Epidemiology of infant meningococcal disease in the United States, 2006-2012. *Pediatrics.* 2015;135(2):e305-e311.
194. MacNeil JR, Rubin L, Folaranmi T, et al. Use of Serogroup B Meningococcal Vaccines in Adolescents and Young Adults: Recommendations of the Advisory Committee on Immunization Practices, 2015. *MMWR Morb Mortal Wkly Rep.* 2015;64(41):1171-1176.
196. Martin ET, Fairchok MP, Kuypers J, et al. Frequent and prolonged shedding of bocavirus in young children attending daycare. *J Infect Dis.* 2010;201(11):1625-1632.
197. Martin ET, Fairchok MP, Stednick ZJ, et al. Epidemiology of multiple respiratory viruses in childcare attendees. *J Infect Dis.* 2013;207(6):982-989.
199. Mbaeyi C, Saatcioglu A, Tangermann RH, et al. Progress Toward Poliomyelitis Eradication—Afghanistan, January 2014August 2015. *MMWR Morb Mortal Wkly Rep.* 2015;64(41):1166-1170.
201. McIntosh ED, Bek MD, Cardona M, et al. Horizontal transmission of hepatitis B in a children's day-care centre: a preventable event. *Aust N Z J Public Health.* 1997;21(7):791-792.
215. Papania MJ, Wallace GS, Rota PA, et al. Elimination of endemic measles, rubella, and congenital rubella syndrome from the Western hemisphere: the US experience. *JAMA Pediatr.* 2014;168(2):148-155.
224. Pickering LK, Woodward WE, Dupont HL, et al. Occurrence of *Giardia-lamblia* in Children in Day-Care-Centers. *J Pediatr.* 1984;104(4):522-526.
226. Raffaelli RM, Paladini M, Hanson H, et al. Child care-associated outbreak of *Escherichia coli* O157:H7 and hemolytic uremic syndrome. *Pediatr Infect Dis J.* 2007;26(10):951-953.
235. Sammons JS, Toltzis P, Zaoutis TE. *Clostridium difficile* Infection in children. *JAMA Pediatr.* 2013;167(6):567-573.
236. Sandora TJ, Fung M, Flaherty K, et al. Epidemiology and risk factors for *Clostridium difficile* infection in children. *Pediatr Infect Dis J.* 2011;30(7):580-584.
249. Sharma D, Baughman W, Holst A, et al. Pneumococcal carriage and invasive disease in children before introduction of the 13-valent conjugate vaccine: comparison with the era before 7-valent conjugate vaccine. *Pediatr Infect Dis J.* 2013;32(2):e45-e53.
250. Shields JM, Hill VR, Arrowood MJ, et al. Inactivation of *Cryptosporidium parvum* under chlorinated recreational water conditions. *J Water Health.* 2008;6(4): 513-520.
252. Shulman ST, Bisno AL, Clegg HW, et al. Clinical practice guideline for the diagnosis and management of group A streptococcal pharyngitis: 2012 update by the Infectious Diseases Society of America. *Clin Infect Dis.* 2012;55(10): e86-e102.
268. Tamir SO, Roth Y, Dalal I, et al. Changing Trends of Acute Otitis Media Bacteriology in Central Israel in the Pneumococcal Conjugate Vaccines Era. *Pediatr Infect Dis J.* 2015;34(2):195-199.
272. Thomas HL, Liebeschuetz S, Shingadia D, et al. Multiple needle-stick injuries with risk of human immunodeficiency virus exposure in a primary school. *Pediatr Infect Dis J.* 2006;25(10):933-936.
274. Thurn J. Human parvovirus B19: historical and clinical review. *Rev Infect Dis.* 1988;10(5):1005-1011.
278. Tullus K, Aronsson B, Marcus S, et al. Intestinal colonization with *Clostridium difficile* in infants up to 18 months of age. *Eur J Clin Microbiol Infect Dis.* 1989;8(5): 390-393.
285. Walters MS, Simmons L, Anderson TC, et al. Outbreaks of salmonellosis from small turtles. *Pediatrics.* 2016;137(1).
287. Weintraub A. Immunology of bacterial polysaccharide antigens. *Carbohydr Res.* 2003;338(23):2539-2547.
288. Wendt JM, Cohen JA, Mu Y, et al. *Clostridium difficile* infection among children across diverse US geographic locations. *Pediatrics.* 2014;133(4):651-658.
290. Wikswo ME, Hall AJ. Outbreaks of acute gastroenteritis transmitted by person-to-person contact—United States, 2009–2010. *MMWR Surveill Summ.* 2012;61(9):1-12.
296. Yagupsky P. Outbreaks of *Kingella kingae* infections in daycare facilities. *Emerg Infect Dis.* 2014;20(5):746-753.
297. Yagupsky P, Bar-Ziv Y, Howard CB, et al. Epidemiology, etiology, and clinical features of septic arthritis in children younger than 24 months. *Arch Pediatr Adolesc Med.* 1995;149(5):537-540.
299. Yagupsky P, Porsch E, St Geme JW 3rd. *Kingella kingae:* an emerging pathogen in young children. *Pediatrics.* 2011;127(3):557-565.
301. Zipprich J, Winter K, Hacker J, et al. Measles outbreak—California, December 2014–February 2015. *MMWR Morb Mortal Wkly Rep.* 2015;64(6):153-154.

The full reference list for this chapter is available at ExpertConsult.com.

Animal and Human Bites 249

Morven S. Edwards

Many children delight in teasing dogs, and without caution go too near them, by which they get miserably torn and mangled. … What these boys had been doing to enrage the dog we cannot tell, but suspect they had been tormenting him in some way, thinking that as he was chained he could not injure them. But they were mistaken in this, and one of them is likely to be bitten very severely.[7]

Anonymous, 1830

HISTORICAL ASPECTS

The consequences of bites resulting from provoking dogs were of concern in the 19th century just as they are today. In early reports, infected bite wounds were noted to contain fusiform bacilli and spirochetal organisms. We now know that the many aerobic and anaerobic organisms composing the normal flora of an animal's mouth are potential bite wound pathogens. Human bites, recorded since the biblical era, are the most frequent type of bite after dog and cat bites. Reports of infection occurring after human bites in children have been noted in the United States since at least 1910.[52]

The importance of debridement and drainage in treatment of infected bite wounds was understood in the preantibiotic era, but these infections carried a high morbidity rate. In a report from 1936, amputation was required in one-third of cases in which treatment was delayed for 24 hours or longer.[92] Adjuncts to cleansing, such as electrocauterization and even radiation therapy, were used in efforts to prevent or to treat infection, but not until the introduction of penicillin was the outcome of bite wound infections improved over that achieved by symptomatic therapy alone.

EPIDEMIOLOGY

More than 150 million cats and dogs are kept as pets in the United States.[72] The estimated annual incidence is 1 to 2 million dog bites, 400,000 cat bites, 250,000 human bites, and 45,000 snake bites.[37] Rabbits, skunks, squirrels, horses, rats, hogs, and monkeys cause at least 1% of bite injuries. Pet ferret attacks have caused severe facial injuries.[27] Taken together, bites from nondomestic animals, generally thought to pose a higher risk for transmission of rabies, constitute less than 1% of reported bite wounds. The right arm is bitten most frequently, presumably because of defensive attempts by victims using their dominant arm. At least three-fourths of bites are located on extremities. Facial bites represent only 10% of the total, but two-thirds of them are sustained by children younger than 10 years.

Children are the most common victims of animal bites. More than one-half of all dog bites occur in persons younger than 20 years of age with a peak incidence in children 5 to 9 years of age.[78] Costs attributable to dog bites exceed $1 billion per year in the United States.[73] Many bites do not require medical intervention and are not reported. Up to 1% of all pediatric emergency department visits during the summer months are for treatment of animal bites.[22] Five percent of children seeking care for a dog bite require hospital admission.[20] Most bites occur in late afternoon and early evening hours. Boys sustain dog bites twice as often as girls, but girls are bitten more frequently by cats.

Large dogs account for most animal bites and are implicated in most bites with a fatal outcome. Ten to 20 fatal human attacks occur yearly in the United States. At least 25 breeds of dogs were cited in 238 fatalities from dog bites during the past 25 years.[82] The most common breed is the pit bull, which accounted for 39% of wounds in one series of 650 pediatric dog bite injuries.[35] The severity of wounds inflicted by pit bull breeds is due to their biting force and their tendency to inflict multiple bites and to bite and grind their molars into tissue. In most instances (53%), the dog inflicting a bite belongs to the child's immediate or extended family. Stray dogs account for only 10% of bites inflicted. When the circumstances are known, most mammalian bites are provoked, although the victim may not have agitated an animal intentionally.

Infection is a common complication of animal bites. Between 10% and 20% of dog bites and as many as 50% of cat bites for which medical care is sought become infected.[55] With the exception of monkey bites, which have a high infection rate, infection seldom develops after bites by other mammals. Factors influencing the risk for development of infection include the patient's age, type and location of the wound, and length of time that transpires between the bite and initiation of treatment. Wounds of the hand are more likely to become infected than are those of the arm, leg, or face. Puncture wounds become infected more often than lacerations, superficial wounds, or wounds with skin and soft tissue defects. Infection is likely to develop when wounds are repaired surgically or when care is delayed more than 24 hours after injury.

The incidence of infection after human bites is approximately 10% to 30%. In children, human bites are typically superficial, and the infection rate is low (~10%). Human bites have a peak incidence in the spring and early summer and on Saturdays, especially for the adolescent age group. Alcohol and drug use may play a role. Bites occur more commonly in males than in females, except for the 15- to 20-year-old age groups, in which females are bitten more frequently. Most bites in teenagers are associated with aggressive behavior. Among 322 children who suffered human bites, 21% were younger than 5 years, 21% were 5 to 10 years, and 58% were older than 10 years.[65]

Biting is a common occurrence in the out-of-home care setting. The incidence peaks in midmorning and during the early school year in September. Toddlers are bitten more often than infants and other preschoolers, and boys are bitten more often than girls.[86] Approximately 50% of all children enrolled in out-of-home care suffer bite wounds. Most of these bites are minor and do not break the skin. A higher proportion of bites in younger children (such as preschoolers) are to the face, whereas most bites in adolescents are on the upper extremities and hands.

Bites as a sign of child abuse are noted more commonly in the 0- to 4-year-old age group; the age of the abusing parents is usually younger than 20 years for mothers and younger than 22 years for fathers. An attempt should be made to identify the biter and measure distances between circular bite marks to ascertain the spread. In addition, biting children may have learned this behavior from abusive adults and may themselves be victims of human bites.

MICROBIOLOGY

The oral flora of the biting animal, rather than skin flora of the victim, is the source of most isolates from bite wounds, but both can be sources for infection.[1] Infections usually are polymicrobial and contain mixed aerobic-anaerobic isolates. Table 249.1 lists bacterial isolates from the wounds of 50 patients with dog bites and 57 with cat bites that were infected at presentation to an emergency department for care.[88] A median of five bacterial isolates were found per culture. Slightly more than one-half of the wounds yielded both aerobes and anaerobes, and

TABLE 249.1 Bacteria Isolated From 50 Infected Dog Bites and 57 Infected Cat Bites

	NO. OF PATIENTS (%)	
Bacteria	***Dog Bite***	***Cat Bite***
Aerobes		
Pasteurella	25 (50)	43 (75)
Streptococci	23 (46)	26 (46)
Staphylococcus aureus	10 (20)	2 (4)
Other staphylococci	13 (23)	18 (31)
Neisseria	8 (16)	11 (19)
Corynebacterium	6 (12)	16 (28)
EF-4b	5 (10)	9 (16)
Moraxella	5 (10)	20 (35)
Enterococcus	5 (10)	7 (12)
Bacillus	4 (8)	6 (11)
Pseudomonas	3 (6)	3 (5)
Actinomyces	3 (6)	2 (4)
Brevibacterium	3 (6)	2 (4)
Weeksella	2 (4)	4 (7)
Eikenella corrodens	1 (2)	1 (2)
Capnocytophaga	1 (2)	4 (7)
Acinetobacter	0	4 (7)
Other	19 (38)	19 (33)
Anaerobes		
Fusobacterium	16 (32)	19 (33)
Bacteroides	15 (30)	16 (28)
Porphyromonas	14 (28)	17 (30)
Prevotella	14 (28)	11 (19)
Propionibacterium	10 (20)	10 (18)
Peptostreptococcus	8 (16)	3 (5)
Eubacterium	2 (4)	1 (2)
Others	1 (2)	5 (9)

Modified from Talan DA, Citron DM, Abrahamia FM, et al. Bacteriologic analysis of infected dog and cat bites. *N Engl J Med.* 1999;340:85-92.

anaerobes alone were isolated from slightly more than one-third of the wounds. *Pasteurella* spp. were the most common pathogen in dog and cat bites (50% and 75%, respectively), with *Pasteurella canis* being isolated most often from dog bites and *Pasteurella multocida* subspecies *multocida* and *septica* isolated most often from cat bites. *Pasteurella* carrier rates are as high as 66% for dogs and 90% for cats, so it is not surprising that this organism is associated so commonly with infected bite wounds. Infection has occurred as a consequence of bites by large cats, including lions,[15] cougars,[56] and tigers,[17] as well as house cats. The type of wound commonly inflicted (i.e., puncture by cats versus laceration by dogs) might explain the species-specific disparity in infection rates.

Other aerobic agents commonly isolated from infected dog or cat bites include streptococci, staphylococci, *Moraxella, Neisseria,* and corynebacteria. Although streptococci often are β-hemolytic, *Streptococcus pyogenes* was isolated from only 12% of dog bites and from none of the infected cat bites in one large series.[88] *Staphylococcus aureus* was isolated frequently from infected dog bites but infrequently from cat bite wounds. Species such as *Capnocytophaga canimorsus* and *Neisseria weaveri* are notable because infections in association with these species have occurred in splenectomized persons and in those with immunocompromising conditions.[5,60] *Neisseria animaloris* and *Neisseria zoodegmatis* are newly recognized as causes of animal bite wound infections.[50] Animal bites are implicated as a vehicle for transmission of a number of systemic infectious diseases caused by viruses, fungi, and mycobacteria in addition to bacteria (Box 249.1).[77] Macaque monkeys kept as pets can transmit herpes B virus.[2] Transmission of such unusual pathogens as orf virus, *Pseudallescheria boydii,* or *Mycobacterium chelonae* by bites of a goat, dog, or ferret, respectively, has been described.[53,61,80] Cats can transmit such unusual infections as diphtheria, coccidioidomycosis, and tularemia.[11,33,91] Tularemia can also be transmitted by the bite of such diverse species as wild boar, coyote, hog, lamb, muskrat, opossum, raccoon, rat, skunk, squirrel, snapping turtle, and weasel.[16,66]

The bacteriology of human bite wounds also reflects the human oral flora of the biter. Human saliva and dental plaque can contain more than 42 different species of bacteria in concentrations of 10^9 colony-forming units per milliliter. Table 249.2 lists common human bite wound isolates and their relative frequency of isolation.[10,14,44,71,87] α-Hemolytic streptococci, especially *Streptococcus anginosus,* are the most frequent isolates. Other common bacterial isolates include *S. pyogenes, S. aureus, Haemophilus* spp., *Eikenella corrodens,* and oral anaerobes, especially *Fusobacterium, Prevotella, Veillonella,* and *Peptostreptococcus* spp. *E. corrodens* produces a small colony that "pits" or "corrodes" the agar surface and has a light yellow pigment and an odor like that of hypochlorite bleach.

BOX 249.1 Diseases Transmitted by Animal Bite Wounds

Blastomycosis	*Mycobacterium chelonae*
Brucellosis	*Mycobacterium marinum*
Cat-scratch disease	*Mycobacterium fortuitum*
Coccidioidomycosis	Orf
Diphtheria	Plague
Hemorrhagic fever	Rabies
Herpes B virus	Rat-bite fever[a]
Leptospirosis	Sporotrichosis
Monkeypox	Tularemia

[a]Both infections caused by *Streptobacillus moniliformis* and *Spirillum minus.*

TABLE 249.2 Approximate Prevalence and Bacteriology of Isolates From Human Bite Wound Infections[a]

		PRESENT IN:	
Isolate	**Prevalence (%)**	***OB***	***CFI***
Aerobes			
Streptococci			
α-Hemolytic	28–90	+	+
Streptococcus anginosus	52	+	+
β-Hemolytic			
Group A	14–26	+	+
Other	12	+	+
γ-Hemolytic	3–33	+	–
Enterococci	6–11	–	+
Staphylococcus aureus	13–55	+	+
Coagulase-negative staphylococci	6–53	+	+
Haemophilus influenzae	2–6	+	+
Haemophilus spp. (other)	11–20	+	+
Eikenella corrodens	10–30	+	+
Micrococcus spp.	3–5	–	+
Moraxella spp.	3	+	–
Neisseria spp.	11–15	+	+
Corynebacterium spp.	28–41	+	+
Acinetobacter calcoaceticus	2–6	–	+
Campylobacter spp.	16	+	+
Escherichia coli	6	+	–
Klebsiella pneumoniae	3–6	+	+
Enterobacter spp.	3–4	+	–
Nocardia spp.	3	–	+
Anaerobes			
Acidaminococcus spp.	2	+	+
Actinomyces spp.	4–8	+	+
Bacteroides ovatus	6	–	+
Bacteroides ureolyticus	3–11	+	–
Bacteroides spp. (unspeciated)	12–33	+	+
Bifidobacterium spp.	11	–	+
Clostridium perfringens	4	+	–
Prevotella melaninogenica	15–22	+	+
Prevotella intermedia	11–26	+	+
Prevotella oralis	6–17	+	+
Prevotella buccae	15	+	+
Prevotella disiens	4	–	+
Prevotella loescheii	3	+	+
Porphyromonas species	2	+	+
Eubacterium species	3–11	+	+
Fusobacterium nucleatum	12–33	+	+
Fusobacterium necrophorum	4–6	–	+
Fusobacterium species (other)	17	–	+
Peptostreptococcus anaerobius	3	+	–
Peptostreptococcus asaccharolyticus	22	+	+
Peptostreptococcus intermedius	3	+	–
Peptostreptococcus (Finegoldia) magnus	2–17	+	+
Peptostreptococcus micros	12–20	+	+
Gemella morbillorum	3	+	–
Peptostreptococcus prevotii	3	+	–
Peptostreptococcus species (other)	3–22	+	+
Veillonella parvula	9–11	+	+
Veillonella species (other)	6–18	+	+
Spirochetes	5–30	+	+

[a]Based on a compilation of data from references 10, 14, 44, 71, and 87.
CFI, Clenched-fist injury; *OB*, occlusional bite wound; +, present; –, absent.

BOX 249.2 Diseases Transmitted by Human Bite Wounds

Actinomycosis
Cytomegalovirus infection
Hepatitis B virus infection
Hepatitis C virus infection
Herpesvirus infection
HIV infection
Invasive group A streptococcal infection
Syphilis
Tetanus
Toxic shock syndrome
Tuberculosis
Whitlow

BOX 249.3 Potential Complications of Animal Bite Wounds

Arthritis
Brain abscess
Endocarditis
Endophthalmitis
Meningitis
Mycotic aneurysm
Orbital cellulitis
Osteomyelitis
Pneumonia
Sepsis
Synovitis
Tendinitis
Tenosynovitis

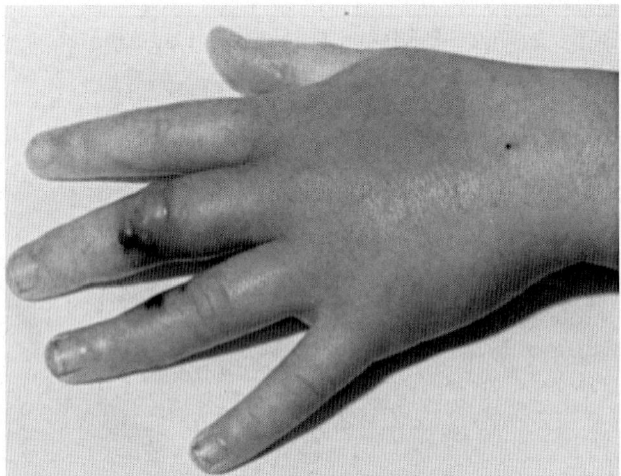

FIG. 249.1 Dog bite wound–associated tenosynovitis in a 4-year-old girl. *Enterococcus* was isolated from the wound culture.

Cultures of virtually all infected bite wounds grow bacterial pathogens; wound cultures of patients who initially are seen less than 8 hours after incurring an injury, before the development of clinical infection, yield potential pathogens in 85% of cases.[38] The bacteriology of early-treated, colonized wounds is remarkably similar to the bacteria isolated from wounds evaluated later with established infection. The average bite wound yields between 3.4 and 5.4 bacterial isolates, including 1.7 to 2.4 aerobes and 1.7 to 3 anaerobes. Anaerobes are isolated from more than 50% of human bite wounds, almost always in mixed culture with aerobes, and they are associated more often with more serious infections, amputation, and the presence of abscesses.[87] Many of the anaerobes isolated from human bite wounds, especially *Prevotella* and *Porphyromonas* spp., are β-lactamase producers.

In addition to oral bacterial infection, human bites have been associated with viral infections, such as those caused by herpes simplex virus,[68] cytomegalovirus,[68] hepatitis B virus,[51] hepatitis C virus,[26] and possibly human immunodeficiency virus (HIV),[6] as well as syphilis,[28] tuberculosis,[38] actinomycosis,[12] and tetanus[70] (Box 249.2).

CLINICAL MANIFESTATIONS

Signs of infection after animal bites develop within hours to several days after injury. Infection is the usual reason that patients seek medical attention more than 8 to 12 hours after injury, whereas those seen earlier are more concerned with prophylaxis or surgical repair. Findings suggestive of wound infection include localized swelling, erythema, and pain with or without serosanguineous or purulent drainage (Fig. 249.1). The clinical findings vary with the infecting organism, site of injury, and type of bite. The jaws and teeth of dogs are likely to produce multiple puncture wounds as well as jagged lacerations with devitalized tissue. These lesions can be associated with depressed skull fractures, sometimes in more than one cranial region. Puncture wounds, particularly those inflicted by cat bites, often are deceptively innocuous. Inoculation of organisms deep into poorly vascularized areas, such as tendon sheaths, fascia, joints, and bones, is likely to result in an infected wound.

The characteristic findings of *P. multocida* infection include a rapid onset of intense pain, swelling, and erythema, often within hours after injury. Cellulitis is usually evident within 24 to 36 hours after the bite. Despite these intense local symptoms, patients generally are afebrile, and less than 20% have lymphangitis and regional adenitis. Patients with wound infection caused by staphylococci or streptococci usually experience less intense pain, have a delay between injury and the onset of symptoms of days rather than hours, and may have a more diffuse, less fiery cellulitis. Gas in tissues of the forearm clinically suggestive of clostridial gas gangrene has occurred in infections caused by *S. anginosus* and *Streptococcus mutans* after horse bite lacerations.[67] Wound infection clinically resembling that caused by *P. multocida* from which the related but more unusual gram-negative rod *Actinobacillus lignieresii* was isolated has been reported in a child who sustained a facial bite by a horse.[21]

Some of the complications resulting from direct extension or generalized spread of infection caused by animal bites are summarized in Box 249.3. Tenosynovitis caused by *P. multocida* can be apparent within hours or can manifest days to weeks after injury, when persistence of swelling, tenderness, or pain and a mass overlying the involved tendon sheath suggest the diagnosis. *Pasteurella* osteomyelitis that develops after a cat bite is characterized by pain, swelling, and tenderness over the involved bone.[54] When the periosteum has been entered, osteomyelitis can develop despite early administration of local and antibiotic treatment. Bites to the cranium occur with relative frequency in small children because their heads are at the level of the mouth of medium- to large-sized dogs. Complications of perforating cranial bites in children include compound depressed skull fractures, brain abscess, dural lacerations, and extensive intracerebral injuries, which can prove fatal.[3,15] Brain abscess and meningitis can occur as complications of these injuries.

In patients with systemic infections transmitted by animal bites, the incubation periods and clinical manifestations vary with the causative agent. For example, streptobacillary rat-bite fever occurs after an incubation period of less than 1 week, whereas spirillary rat-bite fever, or sodoku, has a 2-week asymptomatic interval after the bite. For many of the infections listed in Box 249.1, the bite wound serves as the site of inoculation and has healed completely during the incubation period.[36,62,83] For example, fatal encephalitis has resulted from the bite or scratch of a monkey that is actively shedding herpes B virus. Post-exposure prophylaxis with an antiviral such as acyclovir can prevent life-threatening illness.[2] Isolation of *C. canimorsus* is common among patients with splenectomy, alcoholism, and chronic lung disease.[76] The symptoms heralding the onset of systemic infections caused by animal bites are discussed in their respective chapters.

A high index of suspicion can be required to trace the infection to the animal source. For example, most cases of human plague in the United States result from bites by infected fleas, but contact with a domestic cat infected with *Yersinia pestis* can be the source of infection.[32] With tularemia, an ulcerative or pustular lesion develops at the bite site 4 to 7 days after injury and is associated with fever, chills, and painful regional adenopathy. In a case of *Mycobacterium marinum* infection that developed after a dolphin bite, one of several discrete fluctuant masses containing the isolate developed in an area just proximal to the original wound.[30] *Mycoplasma* has been implicated in "seal finger" from

BOX 249.4 Potential Complications of Human Bite Wounds

Abscess	Scarlet fever
Cellulitis	Septic arthritis
Compartment syndrome	Sepsis
Fracture	Tendon severance or injury
Necrotizing fasciitis	Tenosynovitis
Nerve severance or injury	Toxic shock syndrome
Osteomyelitis	

a seal skin, tooth, or claw injury, an infection characterized by severe pain and massive swelling and erythema 4 to 8 days after injury.[9] With cat-scratch disease caused by *Bartonella henselae*, a papule or pustule may be present at the original bite site when systemic signs develop. An ulceration at the site of a rodent bite has been described with sporotrichosis.[49]

Human bites can be categorized as those resulting in paronychial infection, occlusional bites, and clenched-fist injuries. Potential complications of human bites are noted in Box 249.4. Paronychia is an infection of the structures of the distal phalanx, either those surrounding the nail or the bone itself. The area is red, tender, and swollen and may have associated purulence.

Most occlusional wounds are minor and require routine care with cleansing and bandaging. The infection rate after occlusional bite wounds is 10% to 30%, and 87% of these may require hospitalization.[8] Wounds to the hand and with any edema or crush injury and those that involve a bone or a joint have a greater potential to become infected. Infections usually present as cellulitis. With early treatment, these injuries rarely result in serious complications. The infection generally spreads proximally, and fewer than 5% of cases have associated fever, lymphangitis, or lymphadenopathy. A malodorous discharge or abscess can be present if anaerobes are involved. Complications may be limited to skin defects when skin avulsion has occurred, but septic arthritis and osteomyelitis may develop if the joint or bone is involved.[45] In immunocompromised hosts, such as those with hematologic malignant disease or neutropenia, sepsis may occur. Amputation can be necessary as a result of the initial bite or as a consequence of chronic infection.[63] Tendon injury, primary nerve injury and tenosynovitis, compartment syndrome, and resultant secondary nerve damage can occur.

Clenched-fist injuries, or "fight bites," are the most serious of human bite wounds and occur when the closed fist of one person strikes another in the teeth and a break in the skin occurs.[47] The most common cause is a fight, although the injury can occur during contact sports. The metacarpophalangeal joint of the middle finger of the dominant hand is most often involved. The break in the skin may be only 2 to 5 mm in length but often results in penetration into the joint or even into bone. Patients and physicians may underestimate the potentially serious nature of these wounds. Bacteria penetrate the knuckle area during the initial contact and, on relaxation of the hand, are carried by the tendons proximally into the potential spaces of the hand. Infection can spread laterally, between the collateral and accessory ligaments, or dorsally into the thin-walled bursa overlying the metacarpal head or into the palmar deep spaces of the hand. The swelling usually spreads proximally from the site of injury. Patients often avoid seeking attention initially because of the circumstances surrounding the injury and 6 to 8 hours later seek medical attention with a painful, throbbing, swollen, infected hand. Purulent exudate can be foul smelling if anaerobes are present.

The range of motion of the hand usually is limited by swelling and edema but also can be limited as a result of tendon or nerve injury or severance. Osteomyelitis of the small bones of the hand can present as continued pain, swelling, and erythema with or without drainage 10 days to 3 weeks after the injury has occurred. Osteomyelitis and septic arthritis caused by *E. corrodens*, often in association with α-hemolytic streptococci, frequently are insidious and persistent and may lead to amputation, especially if treated with the wrong antibiotics. Permanent limitation of range of motion and joint stiffness can occur.

DIAGNOSIS AND TREATMENT

The most important aid to establishing the diagnosis of infection after bite wounds is the proper use of wound cultures. A culture specimen need not be obtained from children evaluated in the immediate postinjury period (the first 12 hours) unless the bite is located on the face or hand or signs of infection are present. Isolates from an uninfected but contaminated wound do not predict the future development of infection. Routine determination of the microorganisms colonizing bites on the face or hands is useful because of the potentially devastating consequences of infection at these locations. After the wound has been cleansed, culture should be performed routinely when evaluation is at an interval exceeding 12 hours from the time of injury, except for wounds evaluated more than 24 hours after injury with no signs of infection.

When material is obtained for wound culture, the microbiology laboratory should be informed that the source of the specimen is a bite wound. This information should optimize accuracy because *P. multocida* can be mistaken morphologically for *Neisseria* or *Haemophilus influenzae*. Appropriate media must be used for the isolation of anaerobes, and gram-negative rods should be considered pathogens. A blood culture should be performed if fever or systemic toxicity is evident, although bacteremia occurs rarely. Diagnostic imaging is indicated when the periosteum has potentially been penetrated. Magnetic resonance imaging or computed tomographic imaging can detect periosteal defects, particularly in children with cranial bite wounds. For patients in whom wound infection has extended locally, sutures, if present, should be removed and material from the involved tissue obtained for study. Material should be aspirated from areas of cellulitis and drained from areas of frank abscess formation. If osteomyelitis is suspected, a bone biopsy should be submitted for Gram stain, culture, and histopathologic evaluation. If the course of the wound infection is indolent, acid-fast stains and mycobacterial cultures should be performed. Serum for serologic testing should be obtained from patients with symptoms suggesting a systemic infection. The details of the indicated diagnostic evaluation for systemic infections transmissible by animal and human bites are specified in the appropriate chapters.

The basic elements of management are outlined in Box 249.5. The wound should be cleansed with clean water or saline, and any foreign body or debris and necrotic tissue should be removed. Cautious debridement is indicated for some wounds, with care being taken to not create a potential skin defect. The wound should be irrigated, with a large syringe and needle or catheter tip used as a moderate-pressure jet to diminish the bacterial inoculum. Puncture wounds should be cleansed but not irrigated because irrigation may damage tissues further.

The value and risks associated with primary closure remain controversial. Data support surgical closure with interrupted sutures or adhesive strips for patients with wounds less than 12 hours old and without any signs of infection. Early primary closure has also been successful for wounds to the face and neck. The blood supply to the head and face area is superior to that of most other anatomic areas, and these areas are rarely dependent; therefore, edema and swelling resolve more rapidly or do not develop. In one prospective study, primary closure in patients presenting less than 8 hours after injury was associated with only slightly higher development of wound infection than that occurring after non–bite wound lacerations.[18] Most nonpuncture animal bite wounds except those involving the hands or feet can be treated by primary closure without substantially increasing the risk for development of infection.[34] Wounds to the hands should be observed and left open for either delayed primary or secondary closure. Infected wounds should not be closed initially, but approximation of margins and closure by either delayed primary or secondary intent is advisable for infected nonfacial wounds.

Some clinicians prefer to approximate wound edges with adhesive strips or tissue adhesive rather than to suture wounds. In cases of clenched-fist injury, a hand surgeon should examine the wound to determine whether the joint capsule or bone has been compromised. Surgical consultation with an appropriate specialist is appropriate for complicated wounds and for most hand wounds. Elevation of a swollen or inflamed part is crucial to healing. The elevation should be maintained above the level of the heart. Legs and hands also can be elevated with pillows.

Definitive data on which to base the use of antibiotic prophylaxis after animal bites are lacking. Prospective clinical trials that have addressed the issue find significantly lower infection rates for prophylaxis of wounds in patients presenting at 9 to 24 hours after injury but not for those presenting less than 9 hours after injury.[85] Prophylactic dicloxacillin, cephalexin, or erythromycin was not beneficial therapy for low-risk dog bite wounds in another prospective study because infection rates for wounds in both the antibiotic and control groups did not exceed 5%.[22] A meta-analysis of eight randomized trials totaling 783 patients with dog bite wounds found that prophylactic antibiotics did reduce the incidence of infection.[19] The estimated cumulative incidence of infection was 16% in controls, and the relative risk was 0.56 (95% confidence interval, 0.38–0.82) in patients given antibiotics. Treatment of approximately 14 patients was required to prevent one infection. Some consider antibiotic use therapeutic rather than prophylactic in this setting and suggest that antibiotic therapy be given in all cases of dog bites except those initially evaluated more than 24 hours after injury with no clinical signs of infection.[93]

BOX 249.5 Management Procedures for Bite Wounds

Obtain history from patient
- Situation leading to injury
- Place of occurrence
- Patient allergies
- Other medications (potential interactions)

Perform evaluation of patient
- Nerve function
- Tendon function
- Vascular integrity
- Range of motion
- Potential bone and joint involvement

Diagram or photograph wound
Mark leading edge of cellulitis
Culture wound (if infected)
Irrigate wound (do not irrigate puncture wounds)
Debride wound cautiously
Obtain diagnostic imaging for penetrating injuries overlying bones or joints, if fracture suspected or foreign body suspected
Drain abscesses
Operative debridement (for removal of devitalized tissue and for severe bites, as indicated)
Administer antimicrobial agents (prophylactic therapy, 3–5 days; longer duration for established infection)
Elevate injured area
Close the wound (see text)
Immobilize wound area (3 days for hands)
Have the patient exercise the injured area (if previously immobilized)
Administer tetanus toxoid
Submit health department report (if required)

Administration of a 3- to 5-day course of broad-spectrum antimicrobial therapy for children with fresh wounds and those with cat bite wounds may decrease the rate of infection.[4] Antimicrobial therapy should also be initiated in the following circumstances: wounds with signs of infection; all cat bite wounds; moderate to severe bites, especially if edema or crush injury is present; puncture wounds, particularly if bone, joint, or tendon sheath penetration may have occurred; facial wounds; all hand or foot bite wounds; wounds in the genital area; and wounds in asplenic or immunocompromised persons.[38,90]

Antimicrobial agents should be selected according to the most likely pathogens and their usual susceptibility patterns to antimicrobial agents.[39,44] If cultures are performed, therapy should be adjusted according to the organisms isolated and their susceptibility to antimicrobial agents. The activity of antibiotics commonly used against the usual bite wound pathogens is outlined in Table 249.3. Common pathogens to be considered in the selection of antimicrobial therapy include streptococci, *S. aureus, Haemophilus* spp., *E. corrodens, P. multocida,* and β-lactamase–producing oral anaerobes. Methicillin-resistant staphylococci are relatively common flora in healthy cats but isolation of methicillin-resistant *S. aureus* (MRSA) from infected bite wounds occurs uncommonly.[72,74]

The oral agent of choice for dog, cat, mammal, and human bites is amoxicillin–clavulanic acid. For penicillin-allergic children, the combination of either an extended-spectrum cephalosporin *or* trimethoprim-sulfamethoxazole in conjunction with clindamycin can be substituted.[4] The intravenous agent of choice is ampicillin-sulbactam; piperacillin-tazobactam can be used as an alternative.[4] For penicillin-allergic children, the combination of either an extended-spectrum cephalosporin *or* trimethoprim-sulfamethoxazole in conjunction with clindamycin *or* a carbapenem should be administered.[4] Consideration should be given, for children with severe bite wound infections, to providing coverage with vancomycin for MRSA while cultures are pending.

First-generation cephalosporins are of limited utility because of poor activity against *E. corrodens,* and some anaerobes and should not be used as empirical monotherapy. Erythromycin also has poor activity against *P. multocida, E. corrodens,* and *Fusobacterium nucleatum,* and

TABLE 249.3 Comparative in Vitro Antimicrobial Activity of Selected Oral Antimicrobial Agents Against Common Bite Wound Pathogens

	Staphylococcus aureus[a]	*Eikenella corrodens*	*Streptococcus*	*Haemophilus*	*Pasteurella*	Anaerobes
Amoxicillin	–	+	v	v	v	v
Amoxicillin–clavulanic acid	v	+	+	+	+	+
Cephalexin	v	–	v	–	v	–
Cefaclor	v	–	v	v	v	–
Cefuroxime	v	v	v	v	v	–
Meropenem	v	+	+	+	+	+
Dicloxacillin	v	–	v	–	–	–
Erythromycin	v	–	v	–	v	–
Azithromycin	v	v	v	–	v	v
Clarithromycin	v	v	v	–	v	–
Trimethoprim-sulfamethoxazole	+	+	v	+	+	–
Moxifloxacin	+	+	+	+	+	+
Clindamycin	+	–	+	–	–	+

[a]Methicillin-resistant *S. aureus* can be a pathogen in bite wounds.
+, Active; –, poorly active or inactive; *v*, variable.

its use as monotherapy can lead to therapeutic failure. Newer macrolides, including azithromycin, show improved activity compared with erythromycin against the spectrum of bite wound pathogens, but *Haemophilus* spp. and *F. nucleatum* remain relatively resistant.[44]

The quinolones exhibit broad activity against the pathogens implicated in bite wounds.[42,87] Linezolid has greater activity than the macrolides against the gram-positive organisms and fusobacteria isolated from human bite wounds, but some aerobic gram-negative organisms are at the susceptibility breakpoint.[41] Ceftaroline has excellent activity against *P. multocida* and other *Pasteurella* species and aerobic gram-positive organisms, including MRSA.[43] Antimicrobial therapy should be adjusted in accordance with the patient's individual isolates and susceptibility pattern.

If any question exists about the prompt filling of a prescription because of financial or other concerns, a dose of intramuscular or intravenous antibiotics should be administered and hospitalization considered. Patients' wounds should be reexamined within 48 hours. If outpatient therapy is initiated and the cellulitis advances, hospitalization is indicated. Indications for hospitalization also include patient noncompliance and virtually all clenched-fist injuries.

The duration of antimicrobial therapy is determined by the type and severity of infection. Prophylactic antimicrobial agents typically are given for 3 to 5 days. A suggested duration of therapy, assuming that proper drainage has been established for infected wounds, is 10 days for cellulitis or localized abscess, 2 to 3 weeks for tenosynovitis, and 3 to 6 weeks for osteomyelitis. When improvement is evident, treatment can be completed orally. At least 4 weeks of intravenous therapy should be administered to patients with endocarditis. Although the number of patients is too small for the required dosage to be established with certainty, ampicillin (400 mg/kg per day) has been used successfully for the treatment of *P. multocida* meningitis.[46]

In every child sustaining a bite wound, immunization status should be determined to assess the need for tetanus prophylaxis and whether rabies prophylaxis should be undertaken (see the appropriate chapters).

REPTILE BITES

Approximately 4700 people in the United States are bitten yearly by poisonous snakes.[84] Approximately one-half occur in people younger than 20 years. The curiosity of children can contribute to this exposure because many are bitten while handling poisonous snakes. Boys are more likely than girls to incur snake bites requiring antivenom therapy.[69] An average of five persons die of snake bites each year.[58]

Venomous snakes are divided into four families, two of which, the Crotalidae (rattlesnakes, copperheads, and water moccasins) and the Elapidae (coral snakes), are found in the United States. Snake venoms are among the most complex of proteins. The local effects of the venom of pit vipers (Crotalidae), which is rich in proteolytic activity, include swelling, pain, edema, ecchymosis, and tissue necrosis with the formation of bullae. Systemic effects result from increased blood vessel permeability and hemolysis and may include hematuria, hematemesis, and disseminated intravascular coagulopathy. The venom of the eastern coral snake causes minimal local tissue destruction. It is a neurotoxin that produces paresthesia of the involved extremity, followed by involvement of the cranial nerves and bulbar paralysis.

Goldstein and associates[40] isolated 58 aerobic and 28 anaerobic organisms after culturing the venom from 15 rattlesnakes. The aerobes most commonly isolated were *Pseudomonas aeruginosa, Proteus* spp., and *Staphylococcus epidermidis.* Among the anaerobes, *Clostridium* spp. were the isolates found most frequently; *Bacteroides fragilis* also was recovered. Defecation of prey during ingestion contributes to this preponderance of gastrointestinal flora. When the fangs are cleansed carefully before collection, the venom itself is sterile, thus indicating that bacterial isolates potentially contaminating snake bite wounds are a reflection of the oral flora.

Alligators are generally not aggressive toward humans.[59] In persons sustaining alligator bite wounds, infection is caused most commonly by *Aeromonas hydrophila.* A report of mixed infection with *A. hydrophila, Enterobacter agglomerans,* and *Citrobacter diversus* and the frequency with which *Proteus vulgaris* and *Pseudomonas* spp. are isolated from alligator mouths suggest that treatment of alligator bites should be directed at gram-negative species.[29] *Vibrio* infection should be suspected in victims of shark bites as well as in all wounds exposed to salt water.[75] *Aeromonas* spp. and other gram-negative bacilli, as well as *S. aureus* and anaerobes, can infect shark bites.[79] The exotic pet industry is growing in the United States, and the common green iguana is a popular pet. Few cases of infections from iguana bites have been reported, and most bites do not have serious effects because these creatures are generally nonaggressive, but *Serratia marcescens* cellulitis has been observed.[31,48] The mouths of Komodo dragons harbor many species of bacteria, including *Escherichia coli*, staphylococci, and streptococci, but Komodo dragon bites to humans are rare.[13]

The inflammatory changes of envenomation can be difficult to differentiate from those of infection. Some experts suggest use of a broad-spectrum antibiotic for injuries with severe tissue involvement but not for bites with minor or minimal envenomation.[81] Others suggest that prophylactic antibiotics are not required in snake bite victims.[64,89] Amoxicillin-clavulanate is an appropriate oral antimicrobial and ampicillin-sulbactam *plus* gentamicin is an appropriate parenteral regimen for empirical treatment of reptile bite wounds.[4] Piperacillin-tazobactam can be used as an alternative to ampicillin-sulbactam. The oral alternatives for penicillin-allergic children are the same as those given for other animal bite wounds. The suggested parenteral regimen for a penicillin-allergic child is clindamycin *plus* an extended spectrum cephalosporin or gentamicin or aztreonam or quinolone *or* a carbapenem. Treatment should be guided by the results of cultures and susceptibility testing.

PREVENTION

Bite wounds are, at least in part, preventable injuries. Prevention strategies include appropriate infection control measures in the sports setting and education of young athletes as well as their coaches and trainers. Bites can occur in the out-of-home care setting, even when caregivers are vigilant. A cross-sectional survey of 5- to 15-year-olds found that dog bite prevention knowledge was poor, particularly among younger children.[23] Video-based dog bite prevention interventions are effective in improving short-term knowledge in preschool- and school-aged children.[24,57] There is as yet no direct evidence that educational programs actually lead to a reduction in dog bite rates in children and adolescents. Educating young children could improve their attitude and behavior toward dogs, and data are needed to evaluate dog bite rates as outcomes of such interventions.[25]

NEW REFERENCES SINCE THE SEVENTH EDITION

2. Akhras N, Blackwood RA. Monkey bites: Case report and literature review. *Clin Pediatr (Phila).* 2012;52:574-576.
4. American Academy of Pediatrics. Bite wounds. In: Kimberlin DW, Brady MT, Jackson MA, Long SS, eds. *Red Book: 2015 Report of the Committee on Infectious Diseases.* 30th ed. Elk Grove Village: American Academy of Pediatrics; 2015:205-210.
13. Borek HA, Charlton NP. How not to train your dragon: a case of Komodo dragon bite. *Wild Environ Med.* 2015;26:196-199.
24. Dixon CA, Pomerantz WJ, Hart KW, et al. An evaluation of a dog bite prevention intervention in the pediatric emergency department. *J Trauma Acute Care Surg.* 2013;75:S308-S312.
35. Garvey EM, Twitchell DK, Ragar R, et al. Morbidity of pediatric dog bites: a case series at a level one pediatric trauma center. *J Pediatr Surg.* 2015;50:343-346.
43. Goldstein EJC, Citron DM, Merriam CV, et al. Ceftaroline versus isolates from animal bite wounds: Comparative *in vitro* activities against 243 isolates, including 156 *Pasteurella* species isolates. *Antimicrob Agents Chemother.* 2012;56:6319-6323.
50. Heydecke A, Andersson B, Holmdahl T, et al. Human wound infections caused by *Neisseria animaloris* and *Neisseria zoodegmatis*, former CDC group EF-4a and EF-4b. *Infect Ecol Epidemiol.* 2013;3:20312.
57. Lakestani N, Donaldson ML. Dog bite prevention: effect of a short educational intervention for preschool children. *PLoS ONE.* 2015;10:e0134319.
72. Muniz IM, Penna B, Lilenbaum W. Treating animal bites: susceptibility of staphylococci from oral mucosa of cats. *Zoonoses Public Health.* 2013;60:504-509.
74. Ogden RK Jr, Hedican EB, Stach LM, et al. Antibiotic management of animal bites in children during the methicillin-resistant *Staphylococcus aureus* era. *J Pediatric Infect Dis Soc.* 2013;2:379-381.
84. Seifert SA, Boyer LV, Benson BE, et al. AAPCC database characterization of native U.S. venomous snake exposures, 2001–2005. *Clin Toxicol (Phila).* 2009;47:327-335.

The full reference list for this chapter is available at ExpertConsult.com.

250 Bioterrorism

Robert J. Leggiadro

The intentional delivery of *Bacillus anthracis* spores through mailed letters or packages established the clinical reality of bioterrorism in the United States in the autumn of 2001.[12,52] An understanding of the epidemiology, clinical manifestations, and management of the more credible biologic agents is critical to limiting morbidity and mortality from a bioterrorism attack.[20,37,47,59]

Implementation of an effective response to deliberate release of biologic agents by terrorists requires detection and reporting of cases as soon as possible.[7,16] Prompt recognition of unusual clinical syndromes and increases above seasonal levels in the incidence of common syndromes or deaths from infectious agents is critical to an effective response.[7,27,47,57]

HISTORY

The concept of biologic warfare or terrorism is not a new one. In 1346, the Tatar force attacking Kaffa (also Caffa, now Feodossia, Ukraine) was struck by a plague epidemic.[17,82] To take advantage of this development, the Tatars catapulted the corpses of their plague victims into Kaffa. An outbreak of plague did occur in the city, representing one of the first biologic attacks recorded.[17,82]

Smallpox first was used as a biologic weapon during the French and Indian War of 1754 to 1767.[17] Apparently, British troops deliberately infected Native Americans with smallpox by giving them blankets from infected patients.

A secret branch of the Japanese army, Unit 731, reportedly caused outbreaks of plague by dropping plague-infected fleas over populated areas of China in World War II.[45] Bomb experiments of weaponized anthrax spores were conducted by the Allies on uninhabited Gruinard Island near the coast of Scotland and resulted in heavy contamination in 1942.[69] Viable anthrax spores persisted until the island was decontaminated with formaldehyde and seawater in 1986.

In response to a perceived German biologic warfare threat, the United States began research into the offensive use of biologic agents in 1943 at Camp Detrick (renamed Fort Detrick in 1956) in Frederick, Maryland.[17] President Nixon stopped all offensive biologic and toxin weapon research and production by executive order in 1969. Included among the agents destroyed as a result of this action were *B. anthracis,* botulinum toxin, *Francisella tularensis, Coxiella burnetii,* Venezuelan equine encephalitis virus, *Brucella suis,* and staphylococcal enterotoxin B. Begun in 1953, the US defensive program at Fort Detrick continues today as the US Army Medical Research Institute of Infectious Diseases (USAMRIID).[17]

The Biological and Toxin Weapons Convention was ratified in 1972 and went into effect in 1975.[81] It prohibits the development, production, stockpiling, or transfer of biologic weapons agents (microbial pathogens and toxins) for other than peaceful purposes and any devices used to deliver these agents. One hundred forty-three states are parties to the convention, with an additional 18 signatories. Unfortunately, the treaty was not accompanied by effective provisions for verification.

Although the Soviet Union signed the convention at its inception in 1972, it formed and funded an organization known most recently as Biopreparat (Chief Directorate for Biological Preparations) 2 years later.[23] This organization was designed to carry out offensive biologic weapons research, development, and production concealed behind legal and civil biotechnology research. Its capacity for production of biologic weapons included plague, tularemia, glanders, brucellosis, anthrax, smallpox, and Venezuelan equine encephalomyelitis.[2]

An incident at a military microbiology facility in Sverdlovsk (now Yekaterinburg) in the former Soviet Union in 1979 proved to be a grim warning of the dangers of biologic weapons science.[61] An accidental aerosolized release of anthrax spores resulted in at least 79 cases of anthrax, including 68 deaths. This largest reported outbreak of inhalational anthrax occurred in people living or working within a 4-km zone downwind of the facility.

Iraq's biologic warfare program commenced in earnest in 1985 after initial explorations in the late 1970s.[84] By the end of the Persian Gulf War in 1991, Iraqi scientists had investigated the biologic warfare potential of five bacterial strains, one fungal strain, five viruses, and four toxins. The United Nations Special Commission suspects that from 1991 to 1995, Iraq actively preserved biologic weapons capability, including botulinum toxin, anthrax, and *Clostridium perfringens* spores.[23]

The Japanese cult Aum Shinrikyo made several unsuccessful attempts at disseminating anthrax from rooftops and trucks in central Tokyo in the early 1990s before successfully releasing sarin nerve gas into Tokyo's subways and killing a dozen people in 1995.[83] A large community outbreak of salmonellosis was caused by the intentional contamination of restaurant salad bars for political reasons by members of a religious commune in The Dalles, Oregon, in 1984.[76]

EPIDEMIOLOGY

Potential biologic weapons share several characteristics. Ease of acquisition and production is a primary consideration. Other ideal properties include the potential to be aerosolized (particle size, 1–10 μm) and dispersed over a wide geographic area as well as resistance to sunlight, desiccation, and heat. The potential to cause lethal or debilitating disease and person-to-person transmission are important features, as is lack of effective therapy or prophylaxis.[30,37,45]

Any small or large outbreak of disease merits evaluation as a potential biologic event.[67] Unusually high rates of disease (e.g., a cluster of life-threatening pneumonia cases in previously healthy adults) as well as unusual clinical syndromes should signal a warning. After definitions of the cause and rate of attack have been determined, an epidemic curve based on the number of cases during a specific time can be calculated. The epidemic curve in a biologic event triggered by a point-source exposure most likely would be compressed, with a peak occurring in a matter of hours or days. The occurrence of a second curve peak would be possible with contagious agents as a result of person-to-person transmission. The steep epidemic curve expected in a bioterrorism attack is similar to what would be seen with other point-source exposures, such as food-borne outbreaks.

Several epidemiologic clues may be helpful in determining whether further investigation into an outbreak as a potential biologic attack is warranted. Major indicators are a large epidemic, especially in a discrete population; more severe disease than expected for a given pathogen; and a disease unusual for a given geographic area (e.g., pulmonic tularemia in an urban setting). Multiple simultaneous epidemics of different diseases, outbreaks with both human and zoonotic consequences, and unusual strains or susceptibility profiles are additional helpful parameters. Variable attack rates as a function of agent release relative to the interior or exterior of a building also would be useful.[67] Although most bioterrorism attacks will be covert,[7,16] intelligence revealing plans for an attack, terrorist claims of deliberate release, or direct physical evidence of an attack obviously would point to a biologic event.

The emergence of mosquito-borne West Nile virus encephalitis in New York City in the summer of 1999 is an example of a naturally occurring outbreak that had elements of a potential bioterrorist attack.[7,27,71] This outbreak represented a disease occurring in an unusual (previously nonendemic) area as well as one with zoonotic (birds) in

BOX 250.1 Critical Biologic Agents

Bacteria
Anthrax
Plague
Q fever
Tularemia
Brucellosis

Viruses
Smallpox
Viral encephalitis
Viral hemorrhagic fevers

Toxins
Botulinum toxin
Staphylococcal enterotoxin B

addition to human consequences. It marked the first documented appearance of West Nile virus in the Western Hemisphere and the first arboviral outbreak in New York City since the yellow fever epidemics of the 19th century.[27] A large avian die-off, affecting primarily crows, preceded the outbreak in humans by at least several weeks.

CRITICAL BIOLOGIC AGENTS

In addition to anthrax, critical biologic agents include brucellosis, plague, Q fever, and tularemia; smallpox, viral encephalitis, and viral hemorrhagic fever; and illnesses related to botulinum and staphylococcal enterotoxin B toxins (Box 250.1).[7,53,57] The five more credible biologic agents are discussed further.

Anthrax

Bacillus anthracis is a large sporulatory, gram-positive rod with three distinct life cycles featuring multiplication of spores in soil, animal (herbivore) infection, and human infection.[55] Anthrax continues to occur in developing countries where the organism is highly endemic and the use of animal anthrax vaccine is not comprehensive (e.g., Iran, Iraq, Turkey, Pakistan, and sub-Saharan Africa). Human cases may be classified as either agricultural or industrial. Herders, butchers, and slaughterhouse workers in direct contact with infected animals are susceptible to acquiring agricultural infection, and workers in mills that process animal hair and those handling bone meal may acquire industrial infection.[68]

The four forms of human anthrax are cutaneous, inhalational, gastrointestinal, and injectional.[35] The most common form is cutaneous, which is acquired through contact with an infected animal or animal products. The much less common inhalational form results from the deposition of spores in the lungs, and gastrointestinal anthrax occurs after the ingestion of infected meat. Because human-to-human transmission of anthrax has not been reported, standard precautions are recommended for hospitalized patients with all forms of anthrax infection.[46,74]

In the United States, 224 cases of cutaneous anthrax were reported between 1944 and 1994.[46] Most cases in recent decades were a result of exposure to wool or animal hair.[68] Cases of cutaneous, inhalational, and gastrointestinal anthrax have been reported in persons who made or handled imported animal-hide drums or participated in drumming events where imported animal-hide drums contaminated with *B. anthracis* spores were used.[22,33,49]

The clinical features and course of the first 10 confirmed cases of inhalational anthrax associated with bioterrorism in the United States in the fall of 2001 have been reported.[52] Epidemiologic investigation indicated that the outbreak was a result of intentional delivery of *B. anthracis* spores through mailed letters or packages. The median incubation period was 4 days and ranged from 4 to 6 days. Several clinical features of these patients were not emphasized in earlier reports of inhalational anthrax, a previously rare disease. Drenching sweating, nausea, and vomiting were common manifestations of the initial phase of illness in this outbreak. Pleural effusions were a remarkably consistent clinical feature. No predominant underlying diseases or conditions were noted.

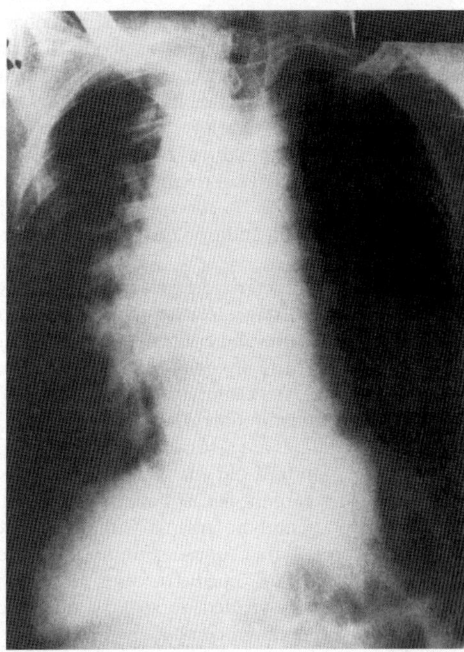

FIG. 250.1 Chest radiograph showing a widened mediastinum secondary to hemorrhagic mediastinitis in a patient with a fatal case of inhalational anthrax. (From LaForce FM, Bumford FH, Feeley JC, et al. Epidemiologic study of a fatal case of inhalation anthrax. *Arch Environ Health.* 1969;18:798-805.)

None of the 10 patients had an initially normal chest radiograph. In addition to characteristic mediastinal widening (Fig. 250.1), paratracheal or hilar fullness, pleural effusions, and parenchymal infiltrates were noted. Computed tomography of the chest was more sensitive than chest radiography in revealing mediastinal lymphadenopathy, and an elevation in the proportion of neutrophils or band forms represented an early diagnostic clue.

Inhalational anthrax previously was reported to be a biphasic illness with influenza-like symptoms such as fever, cough, malaise, fatigue, and chest discomfort in the first phase, followed briefly by 1 to 2 days of improvement before development of the acute phase 2 to 5 days later.[18] However, this brief period of improvement between the initial and fulminant phases of illness was not observed in the first intentional outbreak associated with mail.[48]

The 55% survival rate in these patients was higher than previously reported (<15%). Limited data on treatment of survivors suggest that early treatment with a fluoroquinolone and at least one other active drug (e.g., rifampin, clindamycin, or vancomycin) may improve survival.[12,74] A systematic review of 82 cases of inhalational anthrax from 1900 to 2005 revealed several findings.[41] Initiation of antibiotic or anthrax antiserum therapy during the prodromal phase of disease was associated with a substantial improvement in short-term survival. In addition, both multidrug antibiotic regimens and pleural fluid drainage were associated with decreased mortality.[5] Nasal congestion, rhinorrhea, and sore throat, infrequently seen in this series, might help distinguish influenza-like illness from inhalational anthrax.[21]

Newer diagnostic methods for *B. anthracis* infection include polymerase chain reaction assay, immunohistochemistry, and sensitive serologic tests. If meningitis has not been ruled out, the Centers for Disease Control and Prevention (CDC) recommend a regimen including a fluoroquinolone, such as ciprofloxacin; a drug that inhibits protein synthesis, such as linezolid; and a drug that penetrates the central nervous system, such as meropenem. If meningitis has been ruled out with the use of a lumbar puncture, a two-drug regimen that includes a fluoroquinolone plus linezolid or clindamycin is recommended.[1,10] Corticosteroids should be considered for meningitis or significant mediastinal edema.[5,48]

Passive immunization with a polyclonal or monoclonal antibody product may offer adjunctive value to antibiotic therapy, especially if the organisms are resistant to multiple antibiotics.[34] Raxibacumab is a human immunoglobulin G1 monoclonal antibody directed against protective antigen, a component of anthrax toxin. A single dose of raxibacumab improved survival in rabbits and monkeys with symptomatic inhalational anthrax.[62] In trigger-based intervention studies, human anthrax immunoglobulin induced up to 75% survival in rabbits depending on the dose and severity of toxemia at the time of treatment. In nonhuman primates, up to 33% survival was observed in treated animals.[63] The CDC recommends antitoxin treatments in cases of systemic anthrax.[40]

Cutaneous anthrax is characterized by a skin lesion evolving from a papule, through a vesicular stage, to a depressed black eschar, often surrounded by significant edema and erythema.[25,70,74] The lesion, which may mimic a spider bite, is usually painless and located on exposed parts of the body (i.e., face, neck, and arms). The incubation period ranges from 1 to 12 days but commonly is less than 7 days. With effective antimicrobial therapy, fatalities are rare occurrences (<1%). Cutaneous anthrax occurred in a 7-month-old infant who was exposed at his mother's workplace as a result of the fall 2001 attack. This infant displayed severe microangiopathic hemolytic anemia with renal involvement, coagulopathy, and hyponatremia, unusual findings with cutaneous anthrax.[31] A systematic review of 73 pediatric cases, most of which were cutaneous or gastrointestinal, yielded no striking differences in the presentation of anthrax in children compared with adults.[11]

Injectional anthrax is characterized by skin lesions similar to those seen in "skin-popping" drug users. Unlike cutaneous anthrax, injectional anthrax is not associated with eschar formation on the skin, and the mortality, even with treatment, is considerably higher, at 34%.[75]

The organism grows readily on sheep blood agar and forms rough, gray-white colonies 4 to 5 mm in size with characteristic comma-shaped or "comet tail" protrusions.[55] *B. anthracis* is differentiated from other *Bacillus* spp. by an absence of the following: hemolysis, motility, growth on phenylethyl alcohol blood agar, gelatin hydrolysis, and salicin fermentation. Biosafety level 2 conditions for safe specimen processing in the microbiology laboratory and prompt confirmation of suspected isolates at CDC or the USAMRIID in Fort Detrick are warranted.[46,68]

Postexposure vaccination with an inactivated, cell-free anthrax vaccine is indicated along with ciprofloxacin, doxycycline, or amoxicillin chemoprophylaxis after a proven biologic event has occurred.[74,79] Recommendations for postexposure prophylaxis (and prolonged therapy after initial therapy for inhalational or cutaneous anthrax) include a 60-day course of antibiotics followed by careful clinical observation. Preexposure vaccination may be indicated for the military and other select populations or for groups for which a calculable risk can be assessed.[79]

Smallpox

After a worldwide eradication program, the last known endemic case of smallpox occurred in Somalia in 1977, and the World Health Organization declared smallpox eradicated in 1980.[39] No animal reservoir exists. Current recognized stocks of variola virus are authorized only at the CDC in Atlanta and a Russian state laboratory in Koltsovo. However, additional variola isolates, either long held unreported or acquired through security breaches, also may exist. The World Health Assembly agreed to postpone setting a date for destruction of the world's remaining smallpox virus stocks in May 2014.[8] The decision on a time line for destruction has been postponed four other times so that crucial research may be completed. Routine vaccination against smallpox ceased in the United States in 1972 and for military personnel in 1990. In December 2002, in response to the possible threat of an intentional release of smallpox virus, the US government implemented a program to immunize select military and public health personnel against smallpox.[80] Release of an aerosol would be the most likely route of transmission during an act of bioterrorism.

Smallpox is transmitted by respiratory secretions and requires close person-to-person contact. The incubation period generally is 12 to 14 days, with a range of 7 to 17 days. The prodromal illness of classic variola major features an acute onset of malaise, fever, rigors, vomiting, headache, and backache. Two to 3 days later, a discrete rash appears on the face, hands, forearms, and mucous membranes; it spreads to the legs and then centrally to the trunk during the second week of illness.

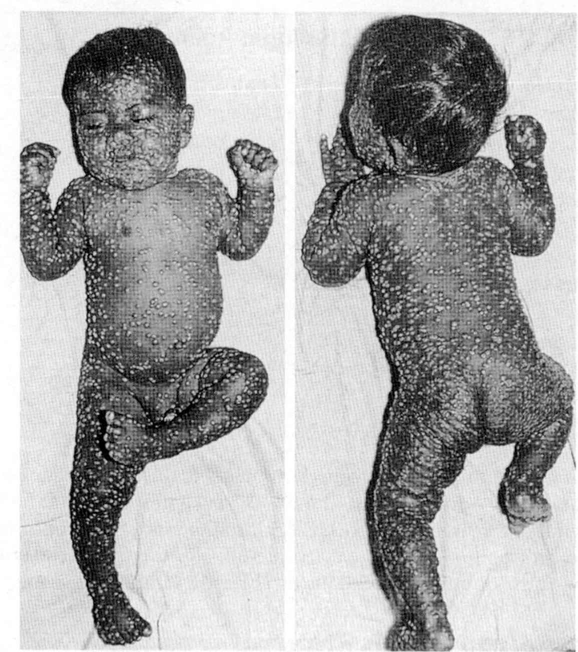

FIG. 250.2 The lesions of smallpox are at the same stage of development on each area of the body, are deeply embedded in the skin, and are more densely concentrated on the face and extremities. (From Henderson DA. Smallpox: clinical and epidemiologic features. *Emerg Infect Dis.* 1999;5:537-539.)

Lesions progress from macules to papules to pustular vesicles during the course of 1 to 2 days. Umbilicate scabs form 8 to 14 days after onset and leave depressions and depigmented scars.[38]

In contrast to varicella (chickenpox), the rash of smallpox is centrifugal, with a concentration of lesions on the face and extremities, including the palms and soles, versus the trunk in varicella (Fig. 250.2). Smallpox lesions also are synchronous in stage of development, whereas the lesions of chickenpox appear in crops every few days, which results in lesions at very different stages of maturation in different areas of the skin. Any confirmed case of smallpox represents an international emergency and must be reported to national authorities through local and state health departments.[39]

Historically, the mortality rate associated with smallpox was 30% for unvaccinated contacts, and currently no antiviral therapy of proven efficacy has been developed. Supplies of vaccinia vaccine and vaccinia immune globulin intravenous (VIGIV) are available only through the CDC.[39] Postexposure vaccination and strict quarantine are indicated for all household and other face-to-face contacts of suspected smallpox cases.[39]

In a limited outbreak with few cases, hospitalized patients should receive care in negative-pressure rooms with high-efficiency particulate air filtration. In addition, precautions using gloves, gowns, and masks are indicated. Home isolation and care are appropriate for most patients in larger outbreaks.[39]

Between January 24 and October 31, 2003, 37,901 volunteers in 55 jurisdictions received 38,885 smallpox vaccinations through the US Department of Health and Human Services program, with a take rate of 92%.[15] The Vaccine Adverse Event Reporting System (VAERS) received 822 adverse event reports related to these vaccines, an overall reporting rate of 217 per 10,000 vaccinees; 722 nonserious reports to VAERS included multiple signs and symptoms of mild systemic and self-limited local reactions, including fever, rash, pain, and headache.[15]

No cases of preventable life-threatening adverse reactions, such as eczema vaccinatum, progressive vaccinia, or fetal vaccinia, were reported. No cases of vaccinia contact transmission occurred. No vaccinee or contact of this program received VIGIV. Rigorous smallpox vaccine safety screening, educational programs, and older vaccinees may have contributed to low rates of preventable life-threatening adverse reactions.[15]

Of the adverse events, 100 were designated serious, resulting in 85 hospitalizations, two permanent disabilities, 10 life-threatening illnesses, and three deaths. Among the serious adverse events, 21 cases were classified as myocarditis or pericarditis and 10 as ischemic cardiac events that were not anticipated on historical data. Two cases of generalized vaccinia and one case of postvaccinial encephalitis also were detected.[15]

The first confirmed case of eczema vaccinatum in the United States related to smallpox vaccination since routine vaccination was discontinued in 1972 was reported in 2007.[80] A 28-month-old child with refractory atopic dermatitis developed eczema vaccinatum after exposure to his father, a member of the US military who had recently received smallpox vaccine. The child's mother also developed vaccinia infection.[80]

Treatment of the child included VIGIV, used for the first time in a pediatric patient; cidofovir, never previously used for human vaccinia infection; and ST-246, an investigational agent being studied for the treatment of orthopoxvirus infection.[80]

The child recovered without apparent sequelae or significant scarring. Although it is difficult to assess and differentiate the effects of specific therapeutic interventions, the child's immune system almost certainly played a role in the eventual control of the infection. This case illustrates the need for meticulous prevaccination screening and the potential hazards of widespread vaccination.[80]

ACAM2000, a second-generation smallpox vaccine produced in cell culture from a clonally purified master seed stock of vaccinia derived from the New York City Board of Health strain of vaccinia, has replaced the original Dryvax vaccine in the Strategic National Stockpile.[19,36] Replication-deficient smallpox vaccines, such as the modified vaccinia Ankara (MVA), and antivirals may offer a safer, more inclusive method of addressing smallpox vaccine–associated adverse reactions, including in individuals at risk for complications.[19,32,36,73]

Plague

Plague, a zoonotic illness caused by the gram-negative bacillus *Yersinia pestis,* is primarily a disease of rodents, with transmission occurring through infected fleas. Human disease is acquired through rodent flea vectors as well as respiratory droplets from animals to humans and humans to humans. Transmission of plague to humans in the United States primarily is by the bites of fleas from infected rodents. From 2001 to 2012, the annual number of plague cases reported in the United States ranged from one to 17 (median, three), most commonly in the southwestern United States.[43] Eleven cases were reported in the first 8 months of 2015 for unclear reasons.[43] Now an endemic zoonosis in the United States, plague is likely to continue causing rare but severe human illness in western states. Historically, plague was often linked to poor sanitation that resulted in rodent infestations.[54] However, plague in New Mexico has increasingly occurred in more affluent areas, a result of continued suburban and exurban development in enzootic plague foci.[72] Indications of a deliberate release of plague bacilli would include the occurrence of cases in locations not known to have enzootic infection, in persons without known risk factors, and in the absence of previous rodent deaths.[45] Travelers can acquire plague in one area and become ill in another area where plague is not endemic (i.e., peripatetic plague).[44]

The three clinical forms of human plague are bubonic, primary septicemic, and pneumonic. Bubonic plague, characterized by the development of an acute regional lymphadenopathy, is the most frequent clinical form and accounts for 76% of US cases.[43] Septicemic plague without obvious lymphadenopathy may be more difficult to diagnose than bubonic plague because of nonspecific manifestations (i.e., fever, chills, abdominal pain, nausea, vomiting, diarrhea, tachycardia, tachypnea, and hypotension).[45] Delay in establishing the diagnosis and initiating appropriate therapy may lead to death.[43,45,58]

However, the pneumonic form would be the most likely manifestation as a result of release of an aerosol during a biologic attack.[30,45] This clinical form is the least common, but it has the highest mortality rate; it is almost always fatal if antibiotics are not begun within 24 hours of the onset of symptoms. A 2014 outbreak in Colorado represents the largest outbreak of pneumonic plague in the United States since 1924. The source of the outbreak was a dog with pneumonic plague. Four persons developed plague after exposure to the ill dog; one of the patients also had close contact with the index patient after he developed plague pneumonia, supporting possible human-to human transmission.[29,65] The incubation period for primary pneumonic plague is 1 to 3 days. Fever, chills, headache, and rapidly progressive weakness are characteristic of all clinical forms of plague. Cough, dyspnea, and hemoptysis are distinctive of primary pneumonic plague. The sudden appearance of a large number of previously healthy patients with fever, cough, shortness of breath, chest pain, and a fulminant course leading to death should suggest the possibility of pneumonic plague or inhalational anthrax immediately. The presence of hemoptysis would strongly suggest plague.[4,45]

Y. pestis may be identified in clinical specimens by Gram, Wright-Giemsa, Wayson, and immunofluorescence staining methods in addition to standard bacterial culture. Appropriate clinical specimens include lymph node aspirates and blood as well as tracheal washes or sputum smears if pneumonic plague is suspected. Tests used to confirm a suspected diagnosis include antigen detection, immunoglobulin M enzyme immunoassay, and polymerase chain reaction assay.[13,45] When plague is suspected, both the state and public health laboratory and public health authorities should be notified promptly.[78]

Effective therapy is available in the form of streptomycin, gentamicin, chloramphenicol, doxycycline, and ciprofloxacin.[45] Parenteral aminoglycoside therapy is recommended in a contained casualty setting (modest number of patients requiring treatment); oral therapy is recommended in a mass casualty scenario.[45] The potential benefits of doxycycline and ciprofloxacin in the treatment of pneumonic plague infection in children substantially outweigh the risks.[16,45] An inactivated, whole-cell *Y. pestis* vaccine was discontinued by its manufacturers in 1999 and no longer is available.[45]

In addition to standard precautions, droplet precautions are indicated for all patients with suspected plague until pneumonia is excluded and appropriate therapy has been initiated. Droplet precautions should be continued in patients with confirmed pneumonic plague for 48 hours after the initiation of appropriate therapy.[45] Only standard precautions are recommended for bubonic plague.

Tularemia

The etiologic agent of this zoonotic illness is *F. tularensis*, a gram-negative coccobacillus. The disease may be acquired from ticks and deer flies, contact with animals such as rabbits and rodents, ingestion of contaminated water, or inhalation of aerosols.[77] In a bioterrorist event, inhalation of an aerosol would be the most likely route of infection.[4,24] Human-to-human transmission of tularemia has never been reported. Tularemia is not a common disease, but it continues to cause approximately 100 reported human cases annually in the United States. Although outbreaks do occur, the majority of reported tularemia cases in the United States are sporadic. Approximately 40% of all tularemia cases reported to the CDC each year occur in Arkansas, Oklahoma, and Missouri. Because the distribution of tularemia may be changing gradually, it should be considered even in areas where it has rarely been reported. All suspected or confirmed cases must be reported to health authorities.[77]

Clinical forms of the disease include ulceroglandular, glandular, oculoglandular, oropharyngeal, pneumonic, and typhoidal, the type reflecting the organism's portal of entry.[26,51] Either pneumonic alone or typhoidal, with or without a pneumonic component, would be the most likely clinical manifestation of tularemia as a result of aerosol release during a biologic attack.[4,24,77] A novel intraerythrocytic phase during *F. tularensis* infection was shown in a murine model of pulmonary tularemia.[42] The incubation period for tularemia is 3 to 6 days, with a range of 1 to 21 days. Typhoidal tularemia may be manifested as fever of unknown origin. Standard precautions are indicated for hospitalized patients with all forms of tularemia.[24]

The diagnosis is established most often by serologic testing, and isolation of *F. tularensis* from clinical specimens requires cysteine-enriched media or inoculation of laboratory mice. In addition to a need for special media, the laboratory should always be informed when tularemia is suspected because of the potential hazard to laboratory personnel. Suspected isolates should be confirmed by the CDC or USAMRIID through local or state health departments.[24]

Effective therapeutic agents include streptomycin, gentamicin, tetracycline, ciprofloxacin, and chloramphenicol; postexposure prophylaxis with doxycycline or ciprofloxacin may be considered.[24] The benefits of tetracycline or ciprofloxacin therapy outweigh the risks in children younger than 8 years in select clinical situations, including tularemia.[24,56] There is no vaccine available for tularemia.[1]

Botulism

Seven distinct but related neurotoxins, A through G, are produced by different strains of *Clostridium botulinum,* an anaerobic gram-positive rod. The most common types in US food-borne outbreaks are A, B, and E; outbreaks with unusual botulinum toxin types (i.e., C, D, F, and G or E not acquired from an aquatic food) would suggest deliberate release.[3] Classical neuroparalytic disease is acquired through the ingestion of preformed neurotoxin. Other forms include localized infection (wound botulism) and *C. botulinum* intestinal colonization in infants with in vivo toxin production (infant botulism). Botulism in the United States is seen most often in small clusters or single cases associated with home-canned foods. Although airborne transmission of botulinum neurotoxin does not occur naturally, aerosolization of preformed toxin would be the most likely route of transmission in a bioterrorism event.[3,30] Sabotage of food supplies is also possible. Botulism is not transmitted from human to human; standard precautions are recommended for hospitalized patients.

The incubation period for food-borne botulism generally is 12 to 36 hours (range, 6 hours to 8 days). The clinical manifestations of disease acquired by inhalation would be the same as those for food-borne botulism. Early manifestations include blurred vision, diplopia, and dry mouth. Patients are afebrile with a clear sensorium.

Later clinical features indicative of more severe disease include dysphonia, dysarthria, dysphagia, ptosis, and a symmetric, descending, progressive muscular weakness with respiratory failure.[3] Clinical suspicion is critical because a recognized source of exposure may be absent in a biologic attack. Botulism is a reportable disease.

A toxin neutralization bioassay in mice is used to identify botulinum toxin in serum, stool, or food. *C. botulinum* also may be cultured from stool and food. Electromyography can be helpful diagnostically. Heptavalent (A–G) botulinum antitoxin (HBAT) of equine origin, which has been approved by the US Food and Drug Administration and is available from the CDC, should be administered as soon as possible to patients symptomatic with botulism.[1,3,50] A pentavalent toxoid (PBT) of *C. botulinum* toxin types A, B, C, D, and E is no longer available for use as a vaccine.[64]

Viral Hemorrhagic Fever

The term viral hemorrhagic fever (VHF) refers to a clinical illness associated with fever and a bleeding diathesis caused by a virus belonging to one of four distinct families: Filoviridae (e.g., Ebola, Marburg), Arenaviridae (e.g., Lassa fever), Bunyaviridae (e.g., Rift Valley fever), and Flaviviridae (e.g., yellow fever). VHF agents are RNA viruses normally transmitted to humans from animal reservoirs or arthropod vectors. Geographic distribution of these agents is as follows: Ebola and Marburg, Africa; Lassa, West Africa; New World arenaviruses, the Americas; Rift Valley fever, Africa and the Middle East; and yellow fever, Africa and the Americas. Most of these agents are considered serious, potential biologic threats because of their potential to be aerosolized and their high morbidity and mortality rates. Clinical features vary with the specific virus, but all are capable of causing fever, myalgia, prostration, petechiae, hemorrhage, and shock.[9]

Treatment generally is supportive, although ribavirin has some in vitro and in vivo activity against arenaviruses and bunyaviruses but not against filoviruses or flaviviruses. VHF-specific barrier precautions, as well as airborne precautions, are recommended for any patient with suspected or documented VHF. Effective prophylaxis after exposure to a VHF agent is not available, although guidelines for the use of oral ribavirin as postexposure prophylaxis for Lassa fever have been proposed on the basis of an extensive review of the literature and experience in the field.[6,9] Clinical trials are needed to evaluate new therapies and vaccines against Ebola virus disease.[28]

PREPAREDNESS AND RESPONSE

Being prepared for a bioterrorist attack or any other large-scale infectious disease outbreak relies on similar critical elements.[27,47,60,66,71] Clinician awareness and education are paramount. Because practicing physicians most likely will be the first group to encounter diseases caused by biologic weapons, they must be familiar with the signs and symptoms of the more credible biologic agents (e.g., smallpox, anthrax).[47,60,66] Recognition of an unusual case or cluster of illnesses should prompt a report to the local public health authorities.[14,27] Improved communication between human and animal health authorities is warranted because many potential bioterrorist agents, such as anthrax, brucellosis, Q fever, plague, and tularemia, are zoonotic diseases.[27] Knowledge of the processes by which the hospital laboratory, the local or state health department, or the CDC performs diagnostic studies to implicate or to exclude biologic agents also is important.[7,27,47] Local, state, and federal public health agencies must coordinate plans for dealing with a large-scale outbreak caused by a biologic event.[7,14,27,71] They should address rapid investigation of the outbreak, public education, mass distribution of antibiotics and vaccines, the capacity to care for mass casualties, and proper, expeditious treatment of the dead.[7,27,47,71]

NEW REFERENCES SINCE THE SEVENTH EDITION

1. Adalija AA, Toner E, Inglesby TV. Clinical management of potential bioterrorism-related conditions. *N Engl J Med.* 2015;372:954-962.
8. Blogs.nature.com/news/2014/05. WHO postpones decision on destruction of smallpox stocks-again. May 28, 2014.
10. Bradley JS, Peacock G, Krug SE, et al. American Academy of Pediatrics clinical report: Pediatric anthrax clinical management executive summary. *Pediatrics.* 2014;133:940-942.
11. Bravata DM, Holty JE, Wang E, et al. Inhalational, gastrointestinal, and cutaneous anthrax in children: a systematic review of cases: 1900–2005. *Arch Pediatr Adolesc Med.* 2007;161:896-905.
19. Clinical guidance for smallpox vaccine use in a postevent vaccination program. *MMWR Recomm Rep.* 2015;64(RR-2):1-26.
28. Florescu DF, Kalil AC, Hewlett AL, et al. Administration of brincidofovir and convalescent plasma in a patient with Ebola virus disease. *Clin Infect Dis.* 2015;61:969-973.
29. Foster CL, Mould K, Reynolds P, et al. Sick as a dog. *N Engl J Med.* 2015;372:1845-1850.
32. Frey SE, Winokur PL, Salata RA, et al. Safety and immunogenicity of IMVAMUNE smallpox vaccine using different strategies for a post event scenario. *Vaccine.* 2013;31:3025-3033.
35. Hanczaruk M, Reischl U, Holzmann T, et al. Injectional anthrax in heroin users, Europe, 2000–2012. *Emerg Infect Dis.* 2014;20:322-323.
40. Hendricks KA, Wright ME, Shadomy SV, et al. Centers for Disease Control and Prevention expert panel on prevention and treatment of anthrax in adults. *Emerg Infect Dis.* 2014;20(2):e130687.
43. Human plague—United States, 2015. *MMWR Morb Mortal Wkly Rep.* 2015;64:918-919.
54. Kugeler KJ, Staples JE, Hinckley AF, et al. Epidemiology of human plague in the United States, 1900-2012. *Emerg Infect Dis.* 2015;21:16-22.
63. Mytle N, Hopkins RJ, Malkevich NV, et al. Evaluation of intravenous anthrax immune globulin for treatment of inhalation anthrax. *Antimicrob Agents Chemother.* 2013;57:5684-5692.
65. Outbreak of human pneumonic plague with dog-to-human and possible human-to-human transmission—Colorado, June–July 2014. *MMWR Morb Mortal Wkly Rep.* 2015;64:429-434.
72. Schotthoefer AM, Eisen RJ, Kugeler KJ, et al. Changing economic indicators of human plague, New Mexico, USA. *Emerg Infect Dis.* 2012;18:1151-1154.
73. Smee DF. Orthopoxvirus inhibitors that are active in animal models: an update from 2008 to 2012. *Future Virol.* 2013;8:891-901.
75. Sweeney DA, Hicks CW, Cui X, et al. Anthrax infection. *Am J Respir Crit Care Med.* 2011;184:1333-1341.
77. Tularemia—United States, 2001–2010. *MMWR Morb Mortal Wkly Rep.* 2013;62:963-966.

The full reference list for this chapter is available at ExpertConsult.com.

PART

VI

Approach to the Laboratory Diagnosis of Infectious Diseases

251 Bacterial Laboratory Diagnosis

Paula A. Revell • Lakshmi Chandramohan

Laboratory tests can lead to or confirm diagnoses as well as aid in choosing appropriate therapy. The challenge of the clinical diagnostic laboratory is to provide accurate, clinically relevant information in a timely manner. However, a recent report by the Institute of Medicine highlighted the fact that diagnostic errors are underappreciated and occur with unacceptable frequency.[46] Effective collaboration between physicians and laboratories is key to minimizing this type of error. To this point, laboratory diagnosis of bacterial infections begins at the bedside, not in the laboratory, with the appropriate collection and transport of specimens. This initial step is critical in making an accurate laboratory diagnosis, as no level of technical expertise or amount of specialized technology can correct for an improperly collected or transported specimen. Most bacteriology testing depends on the cultivation and identification of living organisms, and as such, more than any other area of the clinical laboratory, microbiology is affected by inappropriate specimen management practices. Examples of common problems include incorrect or insufficient specimen labeling, insufficient volume of specimen collected, incorrect transport media, and delays in transport of the specimen to the laboratory. Some common principles for quality specimen collection and transport are listed in Box 251.1.

CULTURE-BASED DETECTION

Whereas technologic advancements have been made in the area of direct pathogen identification by use of molecular methods and mass spectrometry, the isolation of live organisms is still critical, in particular because of the need to determine antimicrobial susceptibility results. Bacterial culture depends on the growth of organisms on various different types of culture media, including selective, differential, and enriched.

Each particular type of specimen has distinct requirements for optimal collection and transport as well as recommended media types to support growth of suspected organisms. The individual specimen-specific collection and cultivation requirements, as well as strategies for identification and diagnosis of various bacterial infections, are described in the following sections.

Specimen-Specific Collection and Cultivation Requirements

Bloodstream Infection

Sepsis has long been associated with significant morbidity and mortality; according to the Centers for Disease Control and Prevention (CDC) National Center for Health Statistics, sepsis was the 11th leading cause of death in the United States in 2013.[100] Given the significant impact of sepsis, the detection of microorganisms circulating in the bloodstream of a patient is among the most critical roles of the clinical microbiology laboratory. Detection of bacterial pathogens is typically accomplished through the incubation of a blood sample in a bottle that contains a specialized liquid medium on a continuously monitored blood culture system. A positive blood culture can confirm a cause of the septic event as well as allow appropriate antimicrobial susceptibility testing and thus optimal antibiotic therapy. The automated blood culture systems routinely used in microbiology laboratories are described as continuously monitored because the system takes periodic readings to evaluate possible growth of microorganisms. Several systems are currently available with differences in detection methods, but all perform comparably. This constant monitoring is accomplished without entering the bottle, and thus the contamination rate for these systems is lower than that of the lysis-centrifugation system (Isolator, Wampole Laboratories).

The single variable with the greatest impact on the sensitivity of detection of bacterial pathogens in blood is the volume of blood that is cultured.[22,56] Whereas this observation is based primarily on data from studies of adult patients, several studies show that increasing the volume of blood cultured increases the sensitivity of detection in a pediatric population as well.[23,30] In addition, multiple studies have demonstrated that low-level bacteremia in pediatric patients is common, and thus by increasing the volume of blood cultured, the likelihood of detecting low-level bacteremia increases.[49] Because pediatric patients have a wide range of blood volumes, there is not one recommended volume for optimal blood culture collection. The most common approach to guiding appropriate volume of blood cultured from pediatric patients is the implementation of a weight-based guideline.[38]

As is the case with any specimen, blood cultures should be transported to the laboratory in a timely manner. Several studies have shown that delays in entry of blood culture bottles to the blood culture system can result in falsely negative cultures (decreasing sensitivity of detection) and increases in time to detection (delaying the reporting of positive results).[82] Optimally, the blood culture bottle should be loaded onto the blood culture system within 4 hours of collection. If delay in entry to the blood culture system is required, during the delay time, the sample should not be incubated at 37°C (98.6°F) because preincubation may significantly compromise results.[95] Optimal temperature for transport of blood culture bottles is room temperature.

Before the introduction of automated, continuously monitored blood culture detection systems, the detection of certain fastidious organisms required incubation times up to 2 weeks. However, with use of the automated systems, both routine and fastidious organisms will be detected within a 5-day incubation time. This 5-day incubation time is adequate for detection of fastidious organisms such as *Brucella, Francisella, Haemophilus, Actinobacillus, Cardiobacterium, Eikenella, Kingella, Abiotrophia,* and *Granulicatella*.[21,96] Importantly, there are limitations to the routine blood culture; for example, *Streptobacillus moniliformis* is sensitive to even low levels of the anticoagulant SPS, which is added to some aerobic blood culture bottles. In cases with suspected rat-bite fever, the recommendation would be to include an anaerobic blood culture bottle because the anaerobic bottles contain a lower level of SPS.[85] Certain organisms are so slow growing that they will likely be missed with the routine 5-day incubation time of a standard blood culture; examples of these pathogens are filamentous fungi, *Nocardia* spp., and slow-growing mycobacterial species. Because these microorganisms do require longer incubation times and different media than the routine blood culture provides, it is best to send separate specimens for specialized fungal or mycobacterial testing if these organisms are suspected.

After the blood culture is flagged as positive, organism identification and susceptibility testing can be performed. Although traditional identification and antimicrobial susceptibility results can take up to 48 hours to obtain, the introduction of mass spectrometry and molecular technologies to the clinical microbiology laboratory has dramatically decreased the time to definitive organism identification.[31] Several rapid molecular tests are available that can identify organisms to species or genus level and for a limited number of drugs can provide information on antimicrobial resistance.[11] Two examples of gram-positive organisms with known resistance phenotypes that can be identified with rapid molecular tests are *Enterococcus faecium* resistant to vancomycin and *Staphylococcus aureus* resistant to methicillin. For gram-negative organisms, although information regarding species-level identification can be obtained, there are no molecular assays that can predict susceptibility. Importantly, the addition of rapid identification by molecular tests or mass spectrometry does not replace the need to grow the organism in order to perform traditional susceptibility testing.

BOX 251.1 Principles for Quality Specimen Collection and Transport

Use sterile technique to minimize contamination.
Collect as close to the site of infection as possible.
Collect at optimal times to recover the pathogens of interest.
Obtain a sufficient quantity of the specimen to perform the requested tests.
Use appropriate collection devices and specimen containers to ensure recovery of all organisms.
Collect all microbiology specimens before the institution of antibiotics.
Properly label and seal the specimen container before transport.
Minimize transport time or maximize transport media. There is always some loss of viability during transport.

Respiratory Tract Infections

Although most respiratory tract infections have viral causes, the focus of this chapter is on bacterial pathogens. The laboratory diagnosis of respiratory tract infections is complicated by the fact that the respiratory tract is normally colonized with a complex and robust microbiologic community. Importantly, many of the organisms that are normal colonizers of the respiratory tract can also be pathogenic when they are overgrown or out of balance with the normal ecology of the respiratory tract. Common components of normal respiratory flora that are also respiratory tract pathogens include but are not limited to *Streptococcus pneumoniae, Haemophilus influenzae, S. aureus, Neisseria meningitidis,* and *Moraxella catarrhalis.* It is important to note that the newly available, highly sensitive molecular panels for identification of respiratory pathogens may include bacterial organisms that can be components of normal flora. The significance of a positive molecular result in the setting of existing normal respiratory flora is complicated and must be interpreted with caution.

For the purposes of laboratory testing, the respiratory tract is divided in two on the basis of anatomy; the upper respiratory tract includes the areas from the anterior nasal passages to the larynx, and the lower respiratory tract includes the structures beyond the larynx. Typically, samples collected from the upper respiratory tract include swabs and washes and are not considered sterile, whereas samples collected from the lower respiratory tract typically require more invasive collection techniques, such as bronchoalveolar lavage or lung biopsy, and may be considered sterile. Because of the difficult and invasive nature of true lower respiratory specimen collection, laboratories often accept specimens that require less-invasive techniques, such as expectorated sputa or tracheal aspirates, in an effort to diagnose a lower respiratory tract infection. However, these less-invasive specimens are not sterile and must be considered in the context of normal respiratory flora.

Upper respiratory tract infections account for more physicians' office visits than any other type of infection,[18] and although most of these infections are the result of viral infections, bacterial etiologies are also important. Examples of infections that fall into the "upper respiratory" category include pharyngitis, otitis media, and otitis externa.

The etiology of pharyngitis can be made by culture and nucleic acid or antigen-based methods. Typically, the specimen is collected on a throat or oropharyngeal swab; swabs made of synthetic fibers are optimal, and there may be an advantage to use of a flocked swab for optimal sample collection.[41] In the pediatric patient population, agents other than *Streptococcus pyogenes* (group A streptococcus) can cause pharyngitis and must be considered. Not all laboratories routinely identify organisms other than group A streptococci (GAS), and thus special requests should be made to ensure appropriate testing. In addition to GAS, large colony-forming, β-hemolytic organisms from the Lancefield groups C and G, as well as *Arcanobacterium haemolyticum,* may cause pharyngitis with clinical symptoms similar to those of GAS pharyngitis.[94] Detection of GAS nucleic acid by various molecular methods has been shown to offer superior sensitivity to antigen-based detection. However, these tests are unable to distinguish whether the presence of GAS nucleic acid reflects organism carriage or the cause of pharyngitis. An argument against the routine use of molecular methods is the potential for high numbers of false-positive results due to GAS detection in asymptomatic carriers. Therefore it is important to highlight that the use of any GAS diagnostic test requires adherence to clinical guidelines detailing the indications for testing.[35]

Otitis externa and otitis media are usually diagnosed clinically and managed empirically; however, in cases of spontaneous perforation of the tympanic membrane or when myringotomy/tympanocentesis is performed, fluid can be sent for culture and microbiologic evaluation. Fluid is the optimal specimen for bacterial culture. Nasopharyngeal specimens are not representative of the etiologic agents of otitis media.[43]

Laboratory diagnosis of lower respiratory tract infections, primarily pneumonia, is complicated by the difficulty of collecting appropriate lower respiratory tract samples. In addition, delays in transport of specimens to the laboratory may result in overgrowth of significant pathogens by nonpathogenic colonizing flora or the loss of significant pathogens.[16,67] Whereas organisms isolated from specimens such as pleural fluid or tissue from lung biopsy must always be considered significant, these highly invasive procedures are relatively rarely performed. The most common specimens collected to aid in diagnosis of pneumonia include sputa and tracheal washes or aspirates. Results from cultures of these specimen sources in any scenario are complicated by the presence of normal upper airway flora, and the determination of significance for any given isolated organism is difficult.[16] To aid in the determination of the quality of either sputa or bronchial aspirate specimens, laboratories perform microscopy-based screening of specimens and reject samples that are not adequate. Specimen quality is evaluated on the basis of the presence and quantity of organisms, squamous epithelial cells, and polymorphonuclear leukocytes. A large number of squamous epithelial cells represents oropharyngeal contamination, and these specimens should be rejected with a recommendation for recollection (with the exception of cases in which *Legionella* or mycobacterial infections are suspected).[86] The presence of large numbers of polymorphonuclear leukocytes can indicate a quality specimen; however, there are exceptions to this observation. In the case of tracheal secretions or aspirates from ventilated, low-birth-weight infants, large numbers of polymorphonuclear leukocytes were associated with the length of intubation and not the development of respiratory symptoms.[86] Although bronchoalveolar lavage is not as commonly performed because of the more invasive nature of the procedure, bronchoalveolar lavage specimens provide quality lower respiratory tract samples. The procedure includes the wedging of the bronchoscope channel into an airway lumen followed by the injection of saline through the lumen. The injected saline is aspirated out in several aliquots. The initial aliquot removed will be contaminated with upper airway secretions and should be discarded before bacterial culture. In an effort to aid in establishing significance of various pathogens isolated from bronchoalveolar lavage cultures, some laboratories perform quantitative cultures and establish cutoffs for significance.[13]

Central Nervous System Infections

Because of the significant morbidity and mortality associated with bacterial meningitis, the rapid and timely identification of the causative agent is critical. Cerebrospinal fluid (CSF) specimens are collected by lumbar puncture and must be transported to the laboratory at room temperature and processed without delay. Owing to the rapid changes in the pH of the CSF on removal from the patient and the hypotonic nature of CSF, the viability of microorganisms is reduced as time passes, potentially increasing the likelihood of false-negative culture results[28]; in addition, host cells may lyse, resulting in an altered cell count. If sequential tubes of CSF are collected, the first tube is not ideal for microbiologic studies because of the possibility of contamination with skin flora or blood from the initial lumbar puncture, which can alter culture results. The second tube should be sent for microbiologic studies whenever possible. Although bacterial stain and culture can be performed on small amounts of fluid, it is recommended to send larger amounts of CSF because of the typically low number of microorganisms present in the specimen. For isolation of mycobacteria from CSF, a minimum of 5 mL of specimen is recommended.[3]

On receipt into the laboratory, CSF specimens should be routinely Gram stained and set up for bacterial culture. Sensitivity of the Gram stain can be improved by concentrating the specimen by cytocentrifugation before staining.[84] Positive Gram stain results can offer useful information about organism morphology and Gram stain phenotype; but large numbers of organisms are needed for visualization, and a negative Gram stain result does not indicate a lack of pathogenic organisms in the CSF.[53] Staining with acridine orange (a fluorescent stain) increases the sensitivity of detection of microorganisms, but this stain does not provide information about the Gram-stain phenotype (e.g., gram positive or gram negative).[52,55] CSF specimens should be inoculated onto both chocolate agar and sheep blood agar and incubated for 72 hours. Routine inoculation of broth-based media is not necessary and may result in isolation of contaminants.[65,90] Inoculation of broth media may add value in cases in which anaerobic or other unusual organisms are suspected or when hardware is in place. Direct bacterial antigen testing of CSF by latex agglutination is not recommended.[72]

Although CSF culture is the diagnostic reference standard for bacterial meningitis, the sensitivity is limited (ranging from 70% to 90%), particularly when antibiotics have been previously administered.[79] Nucleic acid amplification tests, such as polymerase chain reaction (PCR)-based multiplex panels, offer a high level of sensitivity and specificity and, as such, have significant utility in detecting pathogens from a single CSF sample. Additionally, the amplification of DNA from nonviable bacteria could potentially facilitate diagnosis in culture negative cases.[51,66,97,99] The Film Array Meningitis/Encephalitis (ME) Panel (BioFire Diagnostics) is the only US Food and Drug Administration (FDA)-cleared PCR-based panel for detecting pathogens including bacteria, viruses, and yeast from CSF specimens obtained from patients with signs and symptoms of meningitis or encephalitis. Importantly, because of the need to perform antimicrobial susceptibility testing, nucleic acid testing should only be considered as an adjunct to routine bacterial culture.[70]

Urinary Tract Infections

Pediatric urinary tract infections are most commonly caused by gram-negative enteric bacteria. *Escherichia coli* causes 80% of infections. Other common pathogens include but are not limited to *Klebsiella* spp., *Proteus* spp., *Enterobacter* spp., group B streptococcus and *Enterococcus* spp., and occasionally *Pseudomonas* spp.[6,102] As is the case for respiratory tract pathogens, urinary tract pathogens must be isolated and identified in and among a background of other normal bacterial flora. To distinguish organisms that colonize the distal urethra from true urinary tract pathogens, quantitative bacterial culture is performed on urine specimens. A recent meta-analysis evaluating the impact of preanalytic practices on diagnostic accuracy of urine cultures emphasized that midstream collection with cleansing is ideal[54]; however, these specimens are difficult to obtain in many pediatric age groups. Catheterized specimens are an acceptable choice for patients in whom the clean-catch method is not possible. Soiled diapers and urine collected by affixing a bag to the perineum are not acceptable specimens. To prevent misleading results, it is important that urine specimens be kept refrigerated if they are not inoculated in a timely manner (<2 hours); in cases of prolonged storage of urine at ambient temperature, false-positive culture results can be obtained. Regardless of the specimen, a known volume of urine, 0.001 mL for catheter samples or clean-catch samples, is inoculated onto plate media. This plating technique allows the number of colony-forming units (CFU) per milliliter of urine to be quantified. Current recommendations based on previous studies state that 50,000 CFU/mL of a single uropathogenic organism in a properly collected urine specimen in the presence of pyuria is indicative of a urinary tract infection.[91] Any quantity of bacterial growth from urine collected through a suprapubic aspiration is considered significant.

Gastrointestinal Infections

The most common manifestation of gastrointestinal (GI) infection in pediatrics is acute diarrhea, and as is the case with pharyngitis, the most common cause is not bacterial. Viral, parasitic, or immune-related issues most commonly cause diarrhea. However, the ability to rule out a bacterial cause is critical, and thus the clinical microbiology laboratory must have appropriate processes in place to isolate and to identify bacterial stool pathogens. Feces should be collected in a sterile container and transported to the laboratory in a timely fashion to avoid overgrowth with normal flora and the potential loss of pathogenic organisms. If rapid transport to the laboratory is not possible, transport media such as Cary-Blair can be used to stabilize the organisms during transport to the laboratory. Because of the presence of high quantities of commensal flora in feces, stool cultures require a combination of both selective and differential media to identify potential pathogens. Most standard stool cultures will include at least two selective and differential media types; commonly used media formulations for the isolation of pathogens such as *Salmonella* and *Shigella* include but are not limited to MacConkey agar, xylose-lysine-deoxycholate agar, and Hektoen enteric agar. Other examples of media formulated for the detection of specific stool pathogens are cefsulodin-irgasan-novobiocin (CIN) agar for isolation of *Yersinia* species, thiosulfate–citrate–bile salts–sucrose (TCBS) agar for the isolation of *Vibrio* species, and Campylobacter agar for the isolation of *Campylobacter jejuni* and *Campylobacter coli.* Another important pediatric enteric pathogen is Shiga toxin–producing *E. coli* (STEC); most reported STEC infections in the United States are caused by *E. coli* O157:H7, with an estimated 73,000 cases occurring each year.[63] Non-O157 STEC organisms can also cause diarrheal illness and have been associated with outbreaks and sporadic illness.[48] Direct plating methods for the detection of *E. coli* O157:H7 should be performed on a selective and differential agar, such as sorbitol-MacConkey agar (SMAC), cefixime-tellurite-sorbitol-MacConkey agar (CT-SMAC), or CHROMagar O157. The toxin genes can be detected by molecular methods, or toxin can be detected by enzyme immunoassay after broth enrichment.[42]

There is no single definition of what pathogens are routinely screened for in the stool culture. Owing to the variability in the stool culture process, the clinician must inquire as to what pathogens are routinely screened for and which pathogens may require a request for specialized culture methods in the testing laboratory.

Several recently developed PCR-based, multiplex GI panels offer a reduction in time to result and detect a broad range of organisms including bacterial, viral, and protozoal pathogens. The three FDA-cleared nucleic acid based syndromic GI panels—xTag GI Pathogens Panel (GPP) (Luminex), FilmArray GI Panel (BioFire Diagnostics), and Verigene Enteric Pathogens test (Nanosphere)—detect *Campylobacter* spp., *Salmonella* spp., *Vibrio* spp., *E. coli* O157, *Yersinia enterocolitica, Shigella,* and bacterial toxin (STEC), whereas *Plesiomonas shigelloides* and *Aeromonas* spp. are only included in the FilmArray panel.[101] Implementation of these panels has been shown to increase pathogen detection and has potential to reduce nosocomial transmission events and decrease inappropriate antibiotic therapy.[7,12,71,80,87] However, given that these are culture-independent methods, no antimicrobial susceptibility data are available with a positive result. The absence of susceptibility results may have a greater impact on pediatric patient populations because infants and children are more likely to need antimicrobial therapy than adults. Specifically for cases of salmonellosis or shigellosis, the resistance profile of these pathogens varies widely, and appropriate therapy requires susceptibility testing.[26] Clinical laboratories that offer these multiplex panels may perform reflex bacterial cultures as needed so that susceptibility testing can be completed, but this is not a standard practice, and as such the clinician should be aware of the laboratory practices before ordering these molecular tests.[26] Additionally, these panels may not be appropriate in certain situations such as hospital-onset diarrhea, for which *Clostridium difficile* testing might be all that is required. A final consideration is whether these panels should be restricted to certain patient populations (e.g., immunocompromised) or made available to all.[9,57]

NON–CULTURE-BASED DETECTION METHODS

Several non–culture-based approaches are used to detect bacterial infections, including microscopy, detection of bacterial antigens or antibodies against the organism, and detection of nucleic acids by molecular methods. A detailed overview of these detection methods for bacteria is provided in this section.

Microscopy

Direct microscopic observation of the specimen is a simple yet reliable technique for demonstrating the presence of microorganisms as well as inflammatory cells in the specimen. Differential (Gram, Kinyoun, Giemsa) and fluorescent (acridine orange, auramine-rhodamine) stains are most commonly used. The Gram stain is a rapid, inexpensive method for assessing the presence of an etiologic agent in the specimen. Preliminary assessments from a stained specimen can indicate the Gram phenotype (positive or negative), the morphology (cocci vs. bacilli), and the spatial arrangement (clusters, chains, or diploid formation). Other differential stains routinely used for bacterial identification are the Kinyoun stain for *Mycobacterium* spp., the modified Kinyoun stain for *Nocardia* spp. and *Streptomyces* spp., and the Wright-Giemsa stain for bacteria *(Borrelia)* or bacterial inclusions *(Anaplasma, Ehrlichia)* in clinical specimens. Fluorescent stains are generally more sensitive than differential stains; however, the Gram phenotype is not available by this type of stain. Although useful information may be collected through a positive direct stain, a negative stain result does not rule out the presence of microorganisms, and thus all direct bacterial stains should be followed by culture.

Mass Spectrometry

Matrix-assisted laser desorption/ionization time-of-flight mass spectrometry (MALDI-TOF-MS) is a technology that provides rapid identification of a variety of pathogens isolated from clinical specimens within hours.[15,27] This technology uses unique protein spectral profiles of the microorganisms to identify organisms based on known catalogued databases of these profiles.[24,29,40] In contrast to traditional biochemical-based methods of identification of microorganisms, MALDI-TOF-MS allows the identification of organism with minimal culture growth and as such shortens the time to identification significantly.[8,31,64] Two commercially available MALDI-TOF-MS platforms are cleared by the FDA for organism identification on culture isolates, but no system has yet been cleared for organism identification of direct specimens.[14,36,83,89]

Molecular Diagnostic Techniques

Nucleic acid amplification tests (NAATs) detect bacterial nucleic acid from either direct specimen or cultured bacterial isolates. NAATs have become increasingly important tools for the detection and identification of infectious diseases. The introduction of nucleic acid–based testing has provided increased sensitivity of detection and decreased time to detection for many bacterial pathogens. Molecular tests that are widely used in clinical microbiology include both highly complex tests that require specialized staff and are performed in batches as well as the more recently available "on demand" assays that can be performed in a more clinically relevant time period and by nonlaboratory personnel. Molecular techniques can be particularly useful for the detection and identification of fastidious organisms (those that have specialized growth conditions or are slow or noncultivable under laboratory conditions). There are numerous molecular tests to aid in the identification of poorly cultivable or atypical organisms, including *Chlamydia trachomatis, Neisseria gonorrhoeae, Mycobacterium tuberculosis, Bordetella pertussis, Bartonella henselae, Mycoplasma pneumoniae,* and many others. The number of pathogens that can be detected by NAATs is rapidly increasing, as are the specimen types from which molecular testing can be performed.

Molecular Methods for Atypical Organisms

Bordetella pertussis

Although infection with *B. pertussis* can occur at any age, babies younger than 6 months, infants, and young children are at highest risk.[69] *B. pertussis* infection mostly remains a clinical diagnosis; however, laboratory detection is often sought for confirmation. Isolation of the organism by culture has been the historical standard test for confirmation of diagnosis and is essential if evaluation of antimicrobial resistance is required. However, successful isolation of the organism declines significantly beyond the first 2 weeks of illness and with prior antibiotic therapy.[33,92] Furthermore, *B. pertussis* is fastidious and requires 3 to 6 days of incubation to form detectable colonies by culture. *B. pertussis* often will not grow if cultures are not initiated within 48 hours of sample collection.[59] As per CDC recommendation, PCR detection of *B. pertussis* DNA has become increasingly available for the timely diagnosis of pertussis.[5] Optimal specimens for PCR testing include nasopharyngeal swabs and aspirates. Throat swabs and anterior nasal swabs have low rates of DNA recovery and should be avoided for *B. pertussis* testing.[5] The increased specificity and rapidity of PCR testing allow the results to be available within 24 to 48 hours. There are currently no FDA-approved *B. pertussis* PCR assays, and there are no standardized protocols, reagents, or reporting formats for *B. pertussis* PCR testing. Consequently, PCR assays vary widely among laboratories. Most *B. pertussis* PCR assays use a single DNA target, the insertion sequence IS481 that is present in multiple copies in the *B. pertussis* chromosome and in fewer copies on the chromosomes of *Bordetella holmesii* and *Bordetella bronchiseptica.*[81] The presence of IS481 in the chromosomes of nonpertussis strains can lead to false positivity.[37] Therefore interpretation of PCR results should be done carefully in conjunction with evaluation of clinical symptoms.

Tuberculosis

The poor sensitivity of standard laboratory tests for the detection of *M. tuberculosis* is a major obstacle to diagnosis of tuberculosis in children. In addition, the nonspecific clinical presentation, paucibacillary nature of pediatric disease, and inability to expectorate sputum in children further complicate the laboratory diagnosis of tuberculosis.[50] Adequate clinical specimens are often difficult to obtain from children younger than 8 years because of lack of sputum production, and first-morning gastric aspirates are an important specimen for pediatric patients.[88] Even with best practice, *M. tuberculosis* is isolated in less than 50% of clinically suspected pediatric cases.[1] Therefore most cases are still diagnosed on the basis of clinical and radiographic findings. However, rapid laboratory confirmation of tuberculosis can lead to earlier treatment initiation, targeted antimicrobial therapy, and better clinical outcomes.[10] Tests based on nucleic acid amplification have become an important tool for the diagnosis of tuberculosis and, when results are positive, can detect *M. tuberculosis* directly from a specimen with a rapid turnaround time of hours or days in contrast to the weeks required with culture. Whereas the currently available molecular methods are rapid and have excellent specificities, their sensitivities do not equal those of culture-based methods, particularly in cases of smear-negative specimens.[58,73] Unfortunately, most pediatric tuberculosis cases are smear negative.

Several molecular methods for detection of tuberculosis are FDA cleared or approved. The enhanced amplified *M. tuberculosis* direct test (E-MTD, Gen-Probe) and the Amplicor *M. tuberculosis* test (Roche Diagnostic Systems) are FDA approved for detection of *M. tuberculosis* complex in smear-positive respiratory specimens.[58,73] The Gen-Probe test is also approved for use with smear-negative respiratory specimens from patients thought to have tuberculosis. The E-MTD test (isothermal transcription mediated) and the Amplicor test (PCR based) rely on amplification of a portion of the 16S rRNA followed by hybridization and detection of a probe specific for *M. tuberculosis* complex bacteria. None of these tests has been approved for direct detection from extrapulmonary specimens. There are no specific recommendations made on the use of molecular testing in the diagnosis of tuberculosis in children who cannot produce sputum and in the diagnosis of extrapulmonary tuberculosis.

Clostridium difficile

Laboratory methods for detection of *C. difficile* have undergone considerable evolution since the organism's etiologic association with antibiotic-associated infectious diarrhea and pseudomembranous colitis or *C. difficile*–associated disease in hospitalized patients was established. The diagnostic gold standards for *C. difficile* detection included anaerobic bacterial culture coupled with toxin detection or tissue culture cytotoxic assay, both of which are time-consuming, expensive, and technically challenging.[14] Although rapid detection kits (i.e., immunoassay) are commercially available, they lack sufficient sensitivity and specificity without serial testing.[17,25,32] The emergence of community-acquired *C. difficile* cases without antecedent antibiotic exposure in addition to the emergence of a quinolone-resistant "hypervirulent" strain of *C. difficile* (designated BI/NAP1/027) in adult and pediatric patients led to significant technical improvements in diagnostic laboratory testing.[62,74] One diagnostic approach to the identification of *C. difficile* is to use a rapid, real-time PCR–based molecular assay that targets the disease-producing *C. difficile* toxin genes. Factors that decrease the viability of organisms (e.g., treatment with antibiotics) lower the sensitivity of detection for culture and rapid immunoassays, but loss of viability does not affect molecular assays. There are currently at least 12 FDA-cleared assays available for detection of *C. difficile*.[2] Most methods are based on real-time PCR with the following exceptions: illumigene *C. difficile* assay (Meridian Bioscience), a loop amplification–based method; and Portrait Toxigenic assay (Great Basin Corp.), an isothermal amplification and chip-based method. All these tests yield results in fewer than 24 hours, with sensitivities reported at greater than 95% and negative predictive values of 99%.[4,93] However, positive *C. difficile* PCR assays on stool specimens in infants younger than 12 months usually represent colonization, and testing should be performed in infants only when other possible causes of diarrhea have been ruled out.[8]

Neisseria gonorrhoeae *and* Chlamydia trachomatis

Adolescents and young adults have higher rates of infection with *Chlamydia trachomatis* (CT) and *Neisseria gonorrhoeae* (GC) than any other age group does,[75] and nucleic acid amplification testing has greatly facilitated sensitive and specific screening in this population. These assays are extremely sensitive with a limit of detection as low as a single gene copy.[19,39] In addition, testing of urine specimens offers noninvasive sample collection. These tests provide the ability to test for both GC and CT in the same specimen. The most commonly used FDA-approved assays are for testing on cervical swabs from women and urethral swabs and urine from men and women. Importantly, none of these assays is approved for testing of specimens from children. The identification of sexually transmitted diseases like *C. trachomatis* and *N. gonorrhoeae* infections in children should raise suspicion for sexual assault, and there are both medical and legal implications to the diagnosis of sexually transmitted diseases in infants and children.[44] Thus testing requires the use of a highly specific method; the gold standard for detection of GC/CT in children and infants has been culture from appropriate specimens.[98]

Sequence-Based Technologies

Sequence-based technologies have been used to improve the speed and accuracy of identification of organisms that are difficult to identify by conventional methods or to detect and identify uncultivable organisms. New high-throughput sequencing technologies, also known as next-generation sequencing, have replaced the commonly used Sanger sequencing for clinical microbiology application.[45,61,76] For bacterial identification, 16S ribosomal genes are common targets of interest.[20] There are several open-access ribosomal sequence databases that can be used to produce alignments of the 16S ribosomal sequences and subsequent species assignment. By comparing the organism's 16S rRNA gene sequence with sequences found in databases of known organisms, the identity of etiologic agents from clinical specimens can be successfully determined.[20,34,47,68] Other technologies, such as pyrosequencing and single-cell and whole-genome sequencing methods, are also promising and powerful tools in clinical microbiology.[60,77,78] These methods are able to generate megabases of sequence information about the whole organism yet are currently in the research use–only phase and are not widely used in diagnostic microbiology laboratories.

NEW REFERENCES SINCE THE SEVENTH EDITION

2. Antonara S, Leber AL. Diagnosis of *Clostridium difficile* infections in children. *J Clin Microbiol.* 2016;54(6):1425-1433.
7. Binnicker MJ. Multiplex molecular panels for diagnosis of gastrointestinal infection: performance, result interpretation, and cost-effectiveness. *J Clin Microbiol.* 2015;53(12):3723-3728.
9. Bloomfield MG, Balm MN, Blackmore TK. Molecular testing for viral and bacterial enteric pathogens: gold standard for viruses, but don't let culture go just yet? *Pathology.* 2015;47(3):227-233.
11. Buehler SS, Madison B, Snyder SR, et al. Effectiveness of practices to increase timeliness of providing targeted therapy for inpatients with bloodstream infections: a laboratory medicine best practices systematic review and meta-analysis. *Clin Microbiol Rev.* 2016;29(1):59-103.
12. Buss SN, Leber A, Chapin K, et al. Multicenter evaluation of the BioFire FilmArray gastrointestinal panel for etiologic diagnosis of infectious gastroenteritis. *J Clin Microbiol.* 2015;53(3):915-925.
26. Cronquist AB, Mody RK, Atkinson R, et al. Impacts of culture-independent diagnostic practices on public health surveillance for bacterial enteric pathogens. *Clin Infect Dis.* 2012;54(suppl 5):S432-S439.
30. Dien Bard J, McElvania TeKippe E. Diagnosis of bloodstream infections in children. *J Clin Microbiol.* 2016;54(6):1418-1424.
31. Dixon P, Davies P, Hollingworth W, et al. A systematic review of matrix-assisted laser desorption/ionisation time-of-flight mass spectrometry compared to routine microbiological methods for the time taken to identify microbial organisms from positive blood cultures. *Eur J Clin Microbiol Infect Dis.* 2015;34(5):863-876.
35. Felsenstein S, Faddoul D, Sposto R, et al. Molecular and clinical diagnosis of group A streptococcal pharyngitis in children. *J Clin Microbiol.* 2014;52(11):3884-3889.
45. Hasman H, Saputra D, Sicheritz-Ponten T, et al. Rapid whole-genome sequencing for detection and characterization of microorganisms directly from clinical samples. *J Clin Microbiol.* 2014;52(1):139-146.
46. Balogh EP, Miller BT, Ball JR, eds. *Improving Diagnosis in Health Care.* Washington, DC: National Academies Press; 2015.
54. LaRocco MT, Franek J, Leibach EK, et al. Effectiveness of preanalytic practices on contamination and diagnostic accuracy of urine cultures: a laboratory medicine best practices systematic review and meta-analysis. *Clin Microbiol Rev.* 2016;29(1):105-147.
57. Liesman RM, Binnicker MJ. The role of multiplex molecular panels for the diagnosis of gastrointestinal infections in immunocompromised patients. *Curr Opin Infect Dis.* 2016;29(4):359-365.
61. Long SW, Williams D, Valson C, et al. A genomic day in the life of a clinical microbiology laboratory. *J Clin Microbiol.* 2013;51(4):1272-1277.
66. Meyer T, Franke G, Polywka SK, et al. Improved detection of bacterial central nervous system infections by use of a broad-range PCR assay. *J Clin Microbiol.* 2014;52(5):1751-1753.
70. Nesher L, Hadi CM, Salazar L, et al. Epidemiology of meningitis with a negative CSF Gram stain: under-utilization of available diagnostic tests. *Epidemiol Infect.* 2016;144(1):189-197.
71. Nicholson MR, Van Horn GT, Tang YW, et al. Using multiplex molecular testing to determine the etiology of acute gastroenteritis in children. *J Pediatr.* 2016;176:50-56.
76. Padmanabhan R, Mishra AK, Raoult D, et al. Genomics and metagenomics in medical microbiology. *J Microbiol Methods.* 2013;95(3):415-424.
79. Ramautar AE, Halse TA, Arakaki L, et al. Direct molecular testing to assess the incidence of meningococcal and other bacterial causes of meningitis among persons reported with unspecified bacterial meningitis. *Diagn Microbiol Infect Dis.* 2015;83(3):305-311.
80. Rand KH, Tremblay EE, Hoidal M, et al. Multiplex gastrointestinal pathogen panels: implications for infection control. *Diagn Microbiol Infect Dis.* 2015;82(2):154-157.
87. Spina A, Kerr KG, Cormican M, et al. Spectrum of enteropathogens detected by the FilmArray GI Panel in a multicentre study of community-acquired gastroenteritis. *Clin Microbiol Infect.* 2015;21(8):719-728.
97. Wootton SH, Aguilera E, Salazar L, et al. Enhancing pathogen identification in patients with meningitis and a negative Gram stain using the BioFire FilmArray(®) meningitis/encephalitis panel. *Ann Clin Microbiol Antimicrob.* 2016;15:26.
100. Xu J, Murphy SL, Kochanek KD, et al. Deaths: final data for 2013. *Natl Vital Stat Rep.* 2016;64(2):1-119.
101. Zhang H, Morrison S, Tang YW. Multiplex polymerase chain reaction tests for detection of pathogens associated with gastroenteritis. *Clin Lab Med.* 2015;35(2):461-486.

The full reference list for this chapter is available at ExpertConsult.com.

Fungal Laboratory Analysis

252

David A. Bruckner

Historically, fungi were regarded as insignificant causes of infection. The dramatic increase in invasive fungal infections has been directly related to organ transplant recipients, particularly during the post-transplantation period, and patients with malignant neoplasms and debilitating immunologic or metabolic disorders, such as systemic lupus erythematosus, diabetes mellitus, and alcohol or injection drug abuse.

Until recently, fungi were allowed to carry multiple scientific names based on the sexual (teleomorph) and asexual (anamorph) stages of their life cycle. In many cases, it was difficult to establish the relationship of these forms. As of 2013, the dual naming is no longer permitted, so there will only be one name for a fungus. The main criteria for classification are genetic rather than phenotypic.[3] This may affect species names of medically important fungi.

SPECIMEN COLLECTION

When an infectious process is suspected, the most appropriate tests directed toward the detection of the etiologic agent must be ordered. Knowledge of the pathophysiology of the disease process is important in determining the type of specimen and optimal time for specimen collection. These collections must include sufficient quantity of specimens for culture, direct microscopy and detection of the etiologic agent using antigen tests, molecular tests, special stains, and antibody methods. All specimens should be considered hazardous, and universal precautions must be used for all specimen collection procedures. Procedures used for specimen collection for direct detection or culture of bacteria can be used for fungi (Table 252.1).[2,4] Microbiologists and pathologists are available to guide physicians in selecting the most appropriate specimen for culture and other tests to achieve rapid detection and recovery of the microorganism causing the infection. Most clinical laboratories have established guidelines for specimen collection with minimal volumes of specimen to be collected. In addition, specimens should be collected in sterile containers before the initiation of therapy to ensure that optimal recovery of organisms is achieved. Specimens collected for 24 hours, such as urine and sputa, are unsuitable for fungal culture because of bacterial overgrowth. Swab specimens are considered inadequate for the recovery of fungi, particularly when multiple culture tests (bacteriology, mycology, mycobacteriology, and virology) from the same swab specimen are requested. In many instances, surgeons send tissue for a histologic diagnosis and neglect to submit a request for culture. If an infection caused by a dimorphic fungus such as *Coccidioides immitis* is suspected, the physician should notify the laboratory because of hazards associated with culture of this organism. A poorly collected specimen may result in the failure to recover the organism, or it may lead to therapy directed at a contaminating or commensal organism.

Specimens should be transported to the laboratory as soon as possible under optimal conditions, which usually are advised in the laboratory specimen collection manual that should be available to all physicians. Specimen transport and storage at room temperature is recommended. Ideally, specimens should be received in the laboratory within 2 hours of being collected. If a delay occurs in setting up cultures, the specimen should be held at room temperature or 4°C (39.2°F) to prevent bacterial overgrowth. Unacceptable specimens that should not be processed include specimens in containers that leak, specimens received many days after collection, and specimens held under inappropriate temperature conditions. Some fungal isolates, such as *Cryptococcus* spp. and *Histoplasma capsulatum,* do not survive well at refrigerated or freezing temperatures.

DIRECT DETECTION

In the laboratory, direct wet mounts or smears can be prepared, and a portion of the specimen can be used for culture (Table 252.2). Blood, cerebrospinal fluid (CSF), and urine also can be used for the detection of antigens and nucleic acids by enzyme immunoassay, lateral flow devices, latex agglutination, magnetic resonance, polymerase chain reaction, and radioimmunoassay.[1,2,4–9] These assays have proved useful for the detection of infections caused by *Aspergillus* spp., *Blastomyces dermatitidis, Cryptococcus neoformans,* and *H. capsulatum.* Although molecular methods may be used for the direct detection of fungal infections (Table 252.3), most have been validated in specific laboratories as a laboratory developed test (LDT) for clinical use but are not readily available in most clinical laboratories. Direct microscopic examination, including frozen sections of tissue to provide an immediate presumptive diagnosis, should be performed on most specimens. A definitive diagnosis may be made when specific fungal elements pathognomonic for fungal infections are detected in direct specimen stains. Examples include *Blastomyces dermatitidis, C. neoformans, Coccidioides posadasii, C. immitis,* and *Pneumocystis jiroveci.* Detection of wide and narrow, wavy, or ribbonlike nonseptate hyphae is consistent with a *Mucorales* spp. infection. Direct specimen examinations always must be followed with culture because the direct examination can never be used to rule out infection, and recovery of the organism may be necessary for speciation or susceptibility testing.

Fungemia can be directly detected from whole blood using the T2Candida magnetic resonance method.[7] Candida can be directly detected from blood culture broth in approximately 1 hour using the FilmArray Blood Culture Identification kit or Candida QuickFISH BC method.[6,8] Although the number of *Candida* species detected are limited, these methods are significant improvements in direct detection of etiologic agents causing serious infections and use of antifungal therapeutics.

Serology may be used to diagnose fungal infections because either other direct detection methods were negative or the organism failed to grow in culture. In general, serology is not as sensitive as are other direct methods, such as antigen detection, particularly in immunocompromised patients. Serology has been useful in the diagnosis of *C. immitis, C. posadasii,* and *H. capsulatum* infections and can be used to follow successful therapy in coccidioidomycosis.[9] Serologic methods include complement fixation, enzyme immunoassay, immunodiffusion, lateral flow devices, and latex agglutination.

During infections, fungal cell wall antigens are released into surrounding tissue and body fluids (blood, CSF, respiratory secretions, and urine).[9] The results from antigen-based tests are much more rapid than culture. Their detection can be useful in supporting a clinical diagnosis when culture and histopathology are negative. Detection of glucuronoxylomannan has been successfully used to diagnose and follow *C. neoformans* and *Cryptococcus gattii* infections. This test is highly sensitive, and circulating capsular polysaccharide can be quantitated to determine a patient's therapeutic response.

Invasive aspergillosis is a diagnostic challenge, and the development of a galactomannan test (polysaccharide cell wall component of *Aspergillus*) had been helpful in certain patient populations. Test results have better predictability among patients with hematologic malignancies than among those receiving a solid-organ transplant. False-positive test results are common in lung transplant recipients. Urine antigen tests for the diagnosis of blastomycosis, coccidiomycosis, and histoplasmosis are sensitive and more rapid than culture or serologic results. Other fluids can be used with these tests for detection of blastomycosis and histoplasmosis, but

TABLE 252.1 **Specimen Collection Guidelines**

Specimen	Recommendations	Transport Device/Comments
Abscess/wounds	Collect as per bacterial culture.	Collect in sterile container with as much material as possible. If swab is used, use exclusively for mycology. RT
Blood	Use fungal media for mold recovery and collect as per product insert. Yeast (*Candida*) can be readily recovered from bacterial blood culture systems.	BacT/Alert, BACTEC, VersaTREK, or Septi-Chek (biphasic) bottles. Isolator (lysis-centrifugation). RT, never refrigerate.
Bone marrow	Collect as per bacterial culture.	Collect in sterile container, Isolator, or heparin (green top) tube. If clotted, may have to homogenize or cut into pieces to place on mycology media. RT
CSF	Collect as per bacterial culture. Fluid volumes greater than 1 mL should be centrifuged or filtered.	Collect in sterile container. RT, never refrigerate. Always perform direct examination.
Eye	Corneal scrapings should be inoculated directly onto mycology media. Vitreous fluid should be collected by needle aspiration.	Direct inoculation onto mycology media without cycloheximide. Vitreous fluid can be placed in a sterile container, or the syringe with needle removed can be sent to the laboratory. RT.
Fluids other than CSF and urine	Collect as per bacterial culture. Fluid volumes greater than 1 mL should be centrifuged or filtered.	Collect in sterile container. RT. Always perform direct exam.
Hair	Use Wood lamp to help select infected hairs and obtain hair roots. Also scrape border of infected area if lesions are present.	Place 10–12 hair roots in sterile container. RT.
Nails	Swab surface with 70% alcohol. Clip nails or scrape with scalpel. Collect softened material from beneath nail bed.	Use sterile container or directly inoculate mycology media. RT.
Prostatic secretions	Empty bladder before giving prostate massage. For detection of *Blastomyces* and less commonly *Coccidioides, Cryptococcus,* and *Histoplasma.*	Place in sterile container or directly inoculate mycology plates. RT.
Respiratory	Collect as per bacterial culture using same rejection criteria for sputum. Early morning sputum is the preferred specimen.	Use sterile container. RT.
Skin	Disinfect surface area with 70% alcohol to remove bacterial contaminants. Scrape skin surface at the edge of the lesion or collect with soft-bristled toothbrush.	Use sterile container or directly inoculate mycology media. RT.
Tissue/biopsy	Collect specimen per surgical technique. Examine tissue for granules.	Use sterile container to which a small amount of sterile saline or water may be added to keep tissue moist. RT.
Urine	Collect as per bacterial culture. Early morning specimen is preferred. Use midstream collection technique.	Use sterile wide-mouthed container. RT.
Vaginal	Collect specimen as per bacterial culture. Primarily for *Candida* infections.	Swab transport device or sterile container. RT.

CSF, Cerebrospinal fluid; *RT,* room temperature.

the test may have to be validated by the laboratory before the results can be used clinically. β-D-Glucan is a major cell wall component of most fungi, with the exception of *Mucorales* and low amounts in *Cryptococcus* and *Blastomyces.* This serum antigen has been used as a diagnostic marker for invasive fungal infections. False-positive test results for β-D-glucan and galactomannan have occurred in patients exposed to specific bacteria and products containing these polysaccharides.

Molecular methods have found a successful rapid clinical diagnostic home for detecting fungemias (see Table 252.3). A number of laboratory-developed molecular tests for the detection of fungal pathogens using specimens other than blood are available in specialized centers, but none have been approved by the US Food and Drug Administration, although they may be approved for use in Europe.[9]

PRIMARY ISOLATION MEDIA

The most reliable and sensitive means for definitive diagnosis of a fungal infection is isolation of the organism on culture media.[2,4,5] A variety of media are commercially available for primary isolation of fungal organisms (Table 252.4). The medium chosen should support the growth of fungal isolates while inhibiting bacterial organisms from specimens collected from nonsterile sites. Traditional antibiotics used include chloramphenicol, gentamicin, penicillin, and streptomycin. Antibacterial agents can inhibit actinomycetes; therefore media without antibiotics should be chosen if this agent is suspected, or a combination of media with and without antibiotics could be used.

Media may use cycloheximide, a protein synthesis inhibitor, to suppress the growth of saprophytic fungi. It also inhibits *Aspergillus, Candida, Cryptococcus, Trichophyton,* and most *Mucorales* spp. Cycloheximide can be used in combination with various antibacterial agents listed earlier.

Chromogenic media are useful for the recovery and identification of *Candida* spp.[4] Dermatophyte test medium (DTM) was designed specifically for the culture and isolation of dermatophytes. Other media used can be those containing caffeic acid for the detection of *C. neoformans* and *C. gattii* by its phenol oxidase activity or media overlaid with olive oil (long-chain fatty acid source) for the recovery of *Malassezia furfur.*

When processing tissue, avoid the use of a mortar and pestle or tissue grinder. Hyphal elements, particularly aseptate hyphae, are easily destroyed in this process, rendering culture recovery of *Mucorales* impossible. Recommendations are to mince the tissue with a scissors or scalpel blade into 1-mm cubes and to place these fragments onto the agar surface.

Nonselective media will permit the recovery of rapidly growing yeast and fungi as well as of fastidious, slow-growing fungi. Selective media will enhance the recovery of slower-growing dimorphic fungi while inhibiting the faster-growing yeast and fungi that may contaminate the medium and render isolation of the slower-growing organisms impossible.

In general, a battery of media, including media containing sheep blood (BHI and Sabouraud brain-heart infusion agar [SABHI]), is used for the recovery of fungal isolates. Although sheep blood inhibits conidiation, it does improve the recovery of fungal isolates. Agar plates or screw-capped tubes can be used for isolating fungal isolates. Most mycologists prefer agar plates because of the ease of handling the cultures, and the larger surface area provides for better isolation of colonies. Plates usually are

TABLE 252.2 **Methods for Direct Microscopic Detection of Fungi in Human Specimens**

Stain/Method	Use	Comments
Calcofluor white	Fluorochrome binds to chitin and cellulose in fungal cell wall.	Rapid detection of fungi and *Pneumocystis*. Staining time is 1 min; requires fluorescent microscope. Organisms fluoresce blue-white. May be used with Evans blue to suppress background fluorescence. Can be used with KOH to digest specimens.
Candida QuickFISH	Identifies three *Candida* spp. from blood culture broth.	Need fluorescent microscope and slide station. Expensive but 20 min to identify isolates.
Fontana-Masson	Detects *Cryptococcus* and dematiaceous fungi.	Stains melanin black or dark brown. Many nondematiaceous fungi will also stain.
Giemsa	Stains most bacteria and fungi.	Used for the detection of *Histoplasma* and *Talaromyces marneffei* in blood and bone marrow. *Pneumocystis* trophozoites and intracystic sporozoites can be detected. Organisms stain blue-purple.
Gridley	Stains fungal cell wall.	Cell wall stains purple-red with yellow background.
Gomori methenamine silver	Stains most organisms in tissue.	Fungi including *Pneumocystis* cysts stain gray-black. Difficult-to-control staining reaction and may be difficult to interpret because of background staining.
Gram	Is used primarily for detection of bacteria	Yeast cells and pseudohyphae stain gram positive; *Cryptococcus* stains gram positive surrounded by a capsular halo; hyphae will stain gram negative.
Hematoxylin and eosin	Is used to demonstrate nucleus and cytoplasmic inclusions in cells.	Fungi nucleus stain violet to blue-purple; cytoplasm stains pink. Can see fungal pigments.
India ink (Nigrosin)	Helps detect capsule of *Cryptococcus*, which appears as a clear halo around the organism. Capsule may be difficult to detect in some infections.	To help detect capsule of *Cryptococcus* capsule, which appears as a clear halo around the organism may be difficult to detect.
Mucin (Mayer or Southgate mucicarmine)	Stains mucopolysaccharide or fungal capsule.	Cryptococcal capsule stains red. *Blastomyces* and *Rhinosporidium* may also stain.
Papanicolaou	Is used to detect the presence of malignant cells.	Fungal elements stain pink. Some fungi may not stain.
Periodic acid–Schiff (PAS)	Stains glycogen, mucin, mucoproteins, and glycoprotein.	A mucin stain used to stain the capsular mucopolysaccharide of fungi. Capsule will have a pink-magenta or purple color.
Potassium hydroxide	Detects yeast and hyphal elements in wet mounts.	Used as a clearing agent to make fungi more visible in tissue, hair, nails, and body fluids. Digests proteinaceous material of host cells, leaving fungi intact.
Toluidine blue	Detects *Pneumocystis* cysts.	Cell wall stains purple.
Wright	Stains most bacteria and fungi.	Used for the detection of *Histoplasma* and *Talaromyces marneffei* in blood and bone marrow. *Pneumocystis* trophozoites and intracystic sporozoites can be detected. Organisms stain blue-purple.

BAL, Bronchial alveolar lavage or wash; *CSF*, cerebrospinal fluid; *DFA*, direct fluorescent antibody; *EIA*, enzyme immunoassay.

TABLE 252.3 **Nonmicroscopic Direct Fungal Detection Methods**

Organism	Specimen	Test	Comments
Antibody			
Blastomyces	Blood	CF, ID	X-rx with other dimorphic fungi
Coccidioides	Blood	CF, EIA, ID	Ab develop 4–6 wk after exposure; used to follow therapy
Histoplasma	Blood, CSF	CF, EIA, ID	X-rx with other dimorphic fungi
Antigen			
Aspergillus	Blood, BAL, CSF	Galactomannan	False-positive results with other filamentous fungi and bacteria
Blastomyces	Blood, CSF, urine	EIA	X-rx with other dimorphic fungi
Coccidioides	Blood, BAL, CSF, urine	EIA	X-rx with other dimorphic fungi
Cryptococcus	Blood, CSF, urine	EIA, LA, LFD	Highly sensitive and specific
Histoplasma	Blood, urine	EIA	X-rx with other dimorphic fungi
Pneumocystis	Blood, BAL	1,3-β-D-glucan	Lacks sensitivity and specificity
Molecular			
Candida	Blood culture broth	BCID (FilmArray)	5 species, 1 h, rapid ID but expensive
	Whole blood	T2Candida	5 species, 4 h, rapid ID, sensitive but expensive
	Whole blood or blood culture broth	Europe, LDT	Tests not approved by FDA
Aspergillus	Blood, BAL, CSF	Europe, LDT	Tests not approved by FDA
Pneumocystis	BAL	LDT	Tests not approved by FDA

Ab, Antibody; *BAL*, bronchial alveolar lavage; *CF*, complement fixation; *CSF*, cerebral spinal fluid; *EIA*, enzyme immunoassay; *FDA*, US Food and Drug Administration; *ID*, immunodiffusion; *LDT*, laboratory-developed test; *LFD*, lateral flow device; *X-rx*, cross-reacts.

TABLE 252.4 **Primary Isolation Media**

Media	Supplements	Use
CHROMagar, Candida or Albicans ID agar	Chromogenic substrates and antibiotics	Medium used for isolation and differentiation for recovery of clinically important yeasts. Assimilation of chromogenic substrates and colony color development allow presumptive identification of common *Candida* species. *Candida* spp. detected is manufacturer dependent.
Dermatophyte test medium	Chloramphenicol, cycloheximide, gentamicin	Selective and differential medium for recovery of dermatophytes *(Epidermophyton, Microsporum, Trichophyton)*. Medium turns from yellow to red with growth of dermatophytes.
Inhibitory mold agar (IMA)	Chloramphenicol; gentamicin may be added	Selective and enriched medium used to isolate cycloheximide-sensitive fungi *(Candida, Cryptococcus, Histoplasma,* mucoraceous fungi, some *Aspergillus)* and inhibit bacterial growth.
Mycosel (Mycobioti)	Chloramphenicol and cycloheximide	Selective medium for isolation of dimorphic fungi and dermatophytes. Chloramphenicol inhibits bacterial growth, and cycloheximide inhibits rapidly growing molds and yeasts.
Potato flake agar	Can be made selective by addition of chloramphenicol and cycloheximide	Used to stimulate production of conidia and pigment.
Sabouraud brain-heart infusion agar (SABHI)	Used with (selective) or without antibiotics. Antibiotics include chloramphenicol, ciprofloxacin, cycloheximide, penicillin, and streptomycin. Could add sheep blood for recovery of *Histoplasma*	General-purpose medium for growth of most fungi, including yeast phase of dimorphic fungi.
Sabouraud dextrose agar (SDA)	None Addition of olive oil on surface	General-purpose medium supporting growth of aerobic actinomycetes and all fungi. Selective for cultivation of *Malassezia furfur.*
Yeast extract phosphate medium	Ammonium hydroxide and chloramphenicol	Selective medium promotes recovery of slow-growing dimorphic fungi. Chloramphenicol inhibits bacterial growth and ammonium hydroxide inhibits growth of other fungi.

sealed with air-permeable tape or shrink-wrap to prevent inadvertent opening of the plate and also to slow down or to retard dehydration of the media because many plates are held for 4 weeks in the laboratory before the specimen is signed out as negative. Examination of culture plates or agar tubes should be performed in a certified biologic safety cabinet. Most fungi will grow on routine bacteriology plates; however, the incubation time usually is short and may not allow sufficient time for the fungi to grow and be visually noticed on the plates.

NEW REFERENCES SINCE THE SEVENTH EDITION

1. Arvanitis M, Anagnostou T, Fuchs BB, Caliendo AM, Mylonakis E. Molecular and nonmolecular diagnostic methods for invasive fungal infections. *Clin Microbiol Rev*. 2014;27:490-526.
2. CLSI. Principles and procedures for detection of fungi in clinical specimens: Direct examination and culture. Approved guidelines. CLSI document M54-A. Wayne, PA 2012; Clinical and Laboratory Standard Institute.
3. De Hoog GS, Chaturvedi V, Denning DW, et al. Name changes in medically important fungi and their implications in clinical practice. *J Clin Microbiol*. 2015;53:1056-1061.
4. Jorgensen JH, Pfaller MA. *Ed-in-Chief. Manual of Clinical Microbiology*. 11th ed. Washington DC: ASM Press; 2015.
6. Pardo J, Klinker KP, Borgert SI, et al. Clinical and economic impact of antimicrobial stewardship interventions with the FilmArray blood culture identification panel. *Diag Microbiol Infect Dis*. 2016;84:159-164.
7. Pfaller MA, Wolk DM, Lowery TJ. T2MR & T2Candida: Novel technology for the rapid diagnosis of candidemia and invasive candidiasis. *Future Microbiol*. 2015;11:103-117.
8. Phoompoung P, Chayakulkeeeeree M. Recent progress in the diagnosis of pathogenic *Candida* species in blood culture. *Mycopathologia*. 2016;10:1007-1013.
9. Powers-Fletcher MV, Hanson KE. Nonculture diagnostics in fungal disease. *Infect Dis Clin North Am*. 2016;30:37-49.

The full reference list for this chapter is available at ExpertConsult.com.

253 Viral Laboratory Diagnosis

Romney M. Humphries • Marjorie J. Miller

In the past, diagnostic testing for viral agents consisted primarily of isolation of virus in tissue culture and serologic studies. These tests were often perceived as too impractical, nonproductive, and slow to warrant implementation in the hospital laboratory. Fortunately, technologic developments and an expanding commercial availability of reagents and test kits have enabled laboratories to provide effective virologic diagnostic services with turnaround time to results and charges similar to those for other areas of the microbiology laboratory. Although an increasing number of these reagents are being approved or licensed as in vitro diagnostic devices, a major hurdle to implementing these in the laboratory is the requirement for laboratory verification of manufacturer-established performance characteristics for each test before implementation. Such verification studies often are extensive and taxing to laboratory resources, although manufacturers may offer educational and technical support to assist the laboratory, if permitted by local regulations. Practical guidance for verification studies has been published elsewhere.[6,20,64]

Presently, virologic services offered by clinical laboratories may range from referral of specimens to a reference laboratory, to limited detection of viral antigens or nucleic acids or an extended menu of qualitative and quantitative molecular assays. This chapter presents the general aspects of diagnosis of viral infections, including specimen selection, collection, and transport; conventional and modified culture for virus isolation and identification; and rapid detection of viral antigens and nucleic acids directly in specimens. Specific aspects of diagnosis are presented in the respective chapters covering the viral agents.

SPECIMEN COLLECTION AND TRANSPORT

Laboratory diagnosis of viral infections depends primarily on the collection of appropriate specimens, in sufficient volume, at the correct time during the course of the illness using optimal transport and storage conditions. Improvements in the sensitivity and accuracy of laboratory assays will be rendered insignificant if preanalytic considerations are overlooked.

Specimen Collection Sites

The selection of appropriate specimens as early in the acute phase of the illness as possible is critical to the recovery of viruses. A guide to recommended collection sites for specific viral syndromes is presented in Table 253.1. In general, the extent of the diagnostic investigation should be dictated by the characteristics of the illness being studied. For example, in common respiratory illnesses such as pharyngitis or croup, collection of a single specimen from the throat usually is sufficient. In other situations in which an illness is severe or unique, collection of specimens from multiple sites is important. In addition, in unusual cases, serum should be obtained for frozen storage in case subsequent serologic studies are required.

In severe illnesses, invasive procedures (e.g., brain, cardiac, liver, lung biopsies, and needle aspiration of body fluids) frequently must be performed to obtain material for laboratory study. Many medical specialists argue against using these invasive procedures because little can be done to treat viral illnesses. However, in our experience, the knowledge gained from a positive viral identification justifies some risk incurred in collecting specimens. At present, antiviral drugs are similar to antibacterial and antifungal agents in that they generally can be used effectively only after definitive identification of the etiologic agent. Demonstration of a viral etiology in diseases such as encephalitis, pneumonia, or cardiac disease can prevent the unnecessary administration of antibiotics and steroids. In many cases, overuse of services, patient trauma, and overall cost can be reduced when a viral agent is confirmed. Finally, the prognosis of a particular illness is more accurate when the specific etiology is known.

Collection of Specimens

Specimens for virus culture or direct examination are generally obtained as they are for other microbiologic studies. The primary purpose of a transport medium is to provide a protective protein, neutral pH, and antibiotics for control of microbial contamination and, most important, prevention of desiccation. Many viral transport and storage media are available commercially. Saline or holding media that contain serum should be avoided. Useful liquid transport media (i.e., 2-mL aliquots in screw-capped vials) consist of tryptose phosphate broth with 0.5% bovine albumin; Hanks balanced salt solution with 5% gelatin or 10% bovine albumin; or buffered sucrose phosphate (0.2 mol/L, 2-SP), which has been used as a combined transport medium for viral, chlamydial, and mycoplasmal culture requests and is appropriate for long-term frozen storage of specimens and isolates. Many of these transport media also have been evaluated and found acceptable for use in rapid methods (e.g., enzyme-linked immunosorbent assay [ELISA] and nucleic acid amplification tests [NAATs]).[15]

Convenient and practical collection devices, such as UTM Kits (Copan), or Universal Viral Transport Kits (Becton Dickenson), consist of a swab, usually a nylon flocked swab on a plastic shaft, and a self-contained transport medium. Calcium alginate swabs, which are toxic to herpes simplex virus (HSV), and wooden shafts, which may be toxic to viruses and the cell culture system itself, should not be used. Nylon flocked swabs should be used over traditional swabs whenever possible, because these are associated with both enhanced absorbance to, and subsequent release of, specimen from the swab.[1,78]

Throat

Specimens from the throat should be obtained with a swab in a manner similar to that used for bacterial culture. The posterior pharyngeal wall and tonsillar surfaces, any inflamed or erythematous areas, and any visible lesions are swabbed firmly without contact with the tongue and anterior oral cavity.

Nose and Nasopharynx

Specimens should be collected with nasopharyngeal swabs that have thin, flexible shafts by inserting the swab into the nasopharynx and rotating it to obtain the maximal number of ciliated, columnar epithelial cells and then placing the swab in transport medium. Alternatively, nasopharyngeal secretions can be obtained from infants by nasal washing. In this method, a small amount of sterile phosphate-buffered saline (3–7 mL) is squeezed into the nose with a nasal bulb aspirator (1 oz, tapered) and then immediately withdrawn and placed in a sterile, screw-capped container. Nasopharyngeal aspirates also may be obtained with a mucus collection device. An appropriately sized catheter is inserted nasally into the posterior of the nasopharynx; intermittent suction is applied as the catheter is withdrawn. Aspirate is washed through the tubing with 5 to 8 mL of transport medium or sterile phosphate-buffered saline. Nasopharyngeal washes and aspirates should be placed into a viral-specific transport medium, which enhances sensitivity of both direct antigen tests and molecular methods. Although washes and aspirates were traditionally preferred for direct antigen detection, studies have shown equivalent collection of exfoliated virus-infected epithelia by flocked swabs. Nasopharyngeal specimens collected using flocked swabs yield sensitivity equivalent to that of aspirates for direct antigen detection and, in many cases, better sensitivity for NAATs.[48,78] Generally, oropharyngeal and especially nasal specimens[1,29] are thought to be of lower sensitivity than nasopharyngeal specimens, although some suggest collection of combined nasopharyngeal and oropharyngeal specimens for optimal sensitivity for respiratory virus detection by NAAT.[29,36]

Other Respiratory Specimens (Sputum, Tracheal Aspirates, Bronchial Washings, Bronchoalveolar Lavage)

Collection depends on the volume obtained. Volumes of 0.5 mL or larger should be placed in a sterile container and sealed tightly. If the volume is less than 0.5 mL, the specimen is placed in 2 mL of transport medium.

Eye

Exudate or pus should be removed first with a sterile swab. Conjunctival specimens may be obtained by pressing a swab premoistened with sterile saline firmly against the inflamed areas. The swab is returned to the self-contained transport device. Corneal scrapings should be obtained by an ophthalmologist or other trained person and placed in transport medium immediately.

Body Fluids Other Than Blood

Body fluids such as urine (clean voided, 5–10 mL), cerebrospinal fluid (CSF) (2–5 mL), pleural effusion, and peritoneal, pericardial, or joint fluid should be collected under sterile conditions and placed in securely sealed, sterile containers. For small volumes (≤0.5 mL), the specimen may be placed in transport medium.

Lesions

For lesions, fresh vesicles should be selected because detection of virus decreases significantly as lesions age. They should be gently swabbed with sterile saline. The vesicle is ruptured and both fluid and cells collected from the base of the lesion. Material obtained from several lesions may be pooled. Desiccation must not be allowed to occur; swabs should be submitted moistened with their self-contained transport medium or, if that is unavailable, placed in 2 mL of transport medium. Specimens may be collected with a swab or aspirated with a 26-gauge needle attached to a tuberculin syringe. Aspirated fluid should be rinsed

TABLE 253.1 **Specimen Collection Guide for the Diagnosis of Viral Infections Based on the Viral Syndrome and Etiologic Agent Suspected**

Main Location or Category of Illness	Clinical Diagnosis	SPECIMEN COLLECTION SOURCE: *Most Practical*	*Most Definitive*	*Other Sources*	Etiologic Agent Suspected[a]
Upper respiratory tract	Common cold, nasopharyngitis	Nasopharynx	Nasopharynx	Nasopharyngeal/nasal, oropharyngeal swab, nasal swab, stool, blood	Rhinoviruses, coronaviruses, parainfluenza viruses, RSV, enteroviruses, adenoviruses
	Pharyngitis	Throat	Throat	Stool, blood	Adenoviruses, enteroviruses, Epstein-Barr virus, influenza viruses, parainfluenza viruses
	Herpangina, other enanthems	Throat	Lesions	Stool, blood	Enteroviruses, HSV
	Laryngitis, laryngotracheitis	Throat	Larynx or trachea	Nasopharyngeal/nasal wash	Parainfluenza viruses, influenza viruses
	Parotitis, other salivary gland enlargement	Throat	Stensen duct	Urine, blood, cerebrospinal fluid	Mumps virus, enteroviruses
Lower respiratory tract	Bronchitis, bronchiolitis, pneumonia	Nasopharynx	Bronchoalveolar lavage, bronchial washing biopsy	Blood, sputum, nasopharyngeal/ nasal wash, stool	RSV, human metapneumovirus, parainfluenza viruses, adenoviruses, influenza viruses, cytomegalovirus
	Pleurodynia	Throat	Throat	Stool	Enteroviruses
	Pleural effusion	Pleural fluid	Pleural fluid	Throat, stool, blood	Enteroviruses, adenoviruses
Heart	Myocarditis, pericarditis, conduction defects	Throat	Pericardial fluid, biopsy	Stool, blood, urine	Enteroviruses, influenza viruses, adenoviruses
Central nervous system	Meningitis	Throat	Cerebrospinal fluid	Stool, blood, urine	Enteroviruses, mumps virus, arboviruses, HSV-2, lymphocytic choriomeningitis virus
	Encephalitis	Throat	Brain biopsy	Cerebrospinal fluid, stool, blood, urine	Arboviruses, mumps virus, enteroviruses, HSV-1, influenza viruses
	Guillain-Barré syndrome, cerebellar ataxia, transverse myelitis, poliomyelitis	Throat	Throat	Stool, blood, cerebrospinal fluid	Influenza viruses, arboviruses, enteroviruses, Epstein-Barr virus
Genital tract	Orchitis, epididymitis	Throat	Testicular biopsy	Stool, blood, urine	Mumps, enteroviruses, lymphocytic choriomeningitis virus
	Herpes genitalis	Lesions	Lesions	Vagina, cervix, urethra	HSV
Urinary tract	Cytomegalovirus infection	Urine	Urine	Throat, blood	Cytomegalovirus
	Hematuria and/or pyuria	Throat, urine	Urine	Blood, stool	Arboviruses, enteroviruses, mumps virus, adenoviruses, BK virus if immune compromised
Gastrointestinal tract	Nausea and/or vomiting	Throat	Throat	Stool, blood	Enteroviruses, influenza viruses, noroviruses
	Diarrhea	Stool	Stool	Throat	Rotaviruses, enteroviruses, adenoviruses, noroviruses
	Abdominal pain	Throat	Throat	Stool, blood	Enteroviruses, adenoviruses
	Acute abdomen mesenteric adenitis	Throat	Mesenteric lymph node biopsy, peritoneal fluid	Stool, blood	Enteroviruses, adenoviruses
	Hepatitis	Throat	Liver biopsy	Stool, blood	Hepatitis A, B, C, E, and G viruses, Epstein-Barr virus, adenoviruses, enteroviruses, cytomegalovirus
	Pancreatitis	Throat	Duodenal fluid	Stool, blood	Enteroviruses
	Reye syndrome	Throat	Liver biopsy	Blood	Influenza viruses, varicella virus
	Hepatosplenomegaly	Throat	Blood, liver biopsy	Stool, urine	Adenoviruses, enteroviruses, Epstein-Barr virus, cytomegalovirus

Reticuloendothelial system	Generalized lymphadenopathy	Throat	Blood, lymph node biopsy	Stool, urine	Adenoviruses, enteroviruses, Epstein-Barr virus, cytomegalovirus
	Immunodeficiency	Blood	Blood	Lymph nodes	HIV
Bone or joints	Osteomyelitis	Bone	Bone	Throat, blood, urine, skin lesion	Rubella virus, vaccinia virus
	Arthritis	Joint fluid	Joint fluid	Throat, blood, urine	Rubella virus, arboviruses
Muscle	Myositis	Throat	Muscle biopsy	Stool, blood	Influenza virus, enteroviruses
Skin	Exanthematous disease	Throat	Vesicular fluid, skin biopsy	Stool, blood, urine, eye	Measles virus, rubella virus, varicella virus, enteroviruses, HSV
Eye	Conjunctivitis, including pharyngoconjunctival fever	Conjunctiva	Conjunctiva	Throat, stool	Adenoviruses, enteroviruses
Eye	Keratoconjunctivitis	Conjunctiva, cornea	Conjunctiva, cornea	Throat, stool	Adenoviruses, herpes simplex virus, varicella virus
	Retinitis	Vitreous, aqueous fluid	Vitreous, aqueous fluid		Cytomegalovirus, herpes simplex virus, varicella virus
Fever	Nonspecific febrile illness (human-to-human transmission)	Throat	Blood	Stool, urine, cerebrospinal fluid	Enteroviruses, influenza viruses, adenoviruses, cytomegalovirus
	Nonspecific febrile illness (arthropod vector)	Blood	Blood	Throat, urine, cerebrospinal fluid	Arboviruses
	Fever of unknown origin	Blood	Blood	Urine, stool, throat	Hepatitis A, B, C, E, and G viruses, cytomegalovirus, herpes simplex virus, Epstein-Barr virus, adenoviruses
Congenital infection	Rubella virus	Throat	Blood	Nasopharynx, biopsy material, cerebrospinal fluid, lens of eye	Rubella virus, cytomegalovirus, Zika virus
	Cytomegalovirus infections	Urine, saliva	Urine (first 21 days life)		
	Zika virus	Urine, blood	Urine, blood (first 48 hours life)		
	HIV infection	Blood	Blood	Lymph node	HIV
Perinatal and neonatal infections	Herpes simplex virus, cytomegalovirus, enterovirus infections	Throat, urine	Blood	Urine, nasopharynx, stool, skin lesions, cerebrospinal fluid	Enteroviruses, RSV, influenza viruses, herpes simplex virus, cytomegalovirus

[a]This list includes only the more commonly associated agents. It is likely that with more general use of viral diagnostic services, new virus and disease associations will be made.
HIV, Human immunodeficiency virus; *HSV,* herpes simplex virus; *RSV,* respiratory syncytial virus.

into 1 to 2 mL of transport medium. Syringes should not be submitted to the laboratory with the needle attached.

For direct antigen detection by immunofluorescence (direct fluorescent antibody [DFA]), the vesicle is ruptured as previously described and epithelial cells are collected by firmly swabbing the base of the lesion. Cells are transferred to a clean glass slide by firmly rolling the swab back and forth over a 5- to 10-mm area (dime size) or, if a ringed slide is used, into the center of the ring. For differentiation of HSV types 1 and 2 (HSV-1 and HSV-2) and varicella-zoster virus (VZV) by DFA, three slides should be prepared.

Stool and Rectal Specimens

Fecal specimens should be collected only when the specific primary diagnosis is diarrhea or when concomitant serologic study with paired sera can be performed. Both enteroviruses and adenoviruses can be detected and recovered readily from stool, but because these agents are carried in the lower gastrointestinal tract for considerable periods of time after acute infection, use of this source for establishing the diagnosis of specific illnesses is limited.

For recovery of enteroviruses, fresh stool specimens are better than rectal swabs; 2 to 5 g (2–3 tsp) of formed or liquid specimen should be transferred to a sterile, leak-proof container. However, from a practical point of view, a rectal swab is the simplest method of specimen collection. A rectal swab can be obtained immediately, whereas collection of a stool specimen usually entails considerable delay. Of importance is that the swab contain visible stool; the swab should be inserted 3 to 5 cm into the rectum, rolled against the mucosa, and then transported in transport medium.

Blood

Some viruses can be recovered from serum or red blood cells (RBCs), but in general, leukocytes are a better source of virus. Fresh blood (optimally 5 mL) is collected in a suitable anticoagulant (i.e., heparin, ethylenediaminetetraacetic acid [EDTA], or acid citrate dextrose) and transported to the laboratory for processing to enrich for leukocytes. EDTA is the anticoagulant of choice because it is an acceptable transport for culture, as well as for molecular methods such as hybridization and PCR.

Bone Marrow

Approximately 2 mL should be aspirated into a tube or syringe containing heparin anticoagulant, mixed thoroughly to prevent clotting, and transported without further additives or diluents.

Biopsy Specimens

For biopsy specimens, fresh tissue obtained from the affected site should be placed in 2 mL of transport medium to prevent desiccation.

Autopsy Specimens

Most postmortem specimens are almost useless for viral cultivation because of the manner in which autopsies usually are performed. If labile agents are to be recovered, the autopsy should be performed within 4 hours of death. All tissues (as 1- to 2.5-cm cubes) for study should be obtained aseptically, and individual tissue should be collected with sterile instruments and placed in separate sterile containers. Because the usual autopsy routine entails fixation of specimens, of vital importance is that specimens for viral isolation not be placed in containers with fixatives such as formalin or other preservatives.

Transport to the Laboratory

The method of handling specimens from the time of collection to laboratory processing is critical not only for preservation of virus infectivity for recovery in culture but also for optimal preservation of nucleic acid integrity before molecular detection methods. In general, the less time that transpires between collection and processing by the laboratory, the greater is the chance of detecting the virus. Specimens should not be frozen or exposed to temperatures higher than 22°C (71.6°F). For short-term storage (<5 days) of most viruses, the specimen should be held at 4°C (39.2°F) until it can be processed in the laboratory. For transport to the laboratory, this temperature can be achieved with the use of cold packs or ice. Transport of specimens at 4°C is less critical for testing by molecular-based assays, provided an appropriate transport medium is used and the delay is not greater than 1 day.[15]

When considerable delay between collection and culture will elapse (e.g., transport to other laboratories, holiday schedules, and so on), special preparation is necessary. Such preparation needs to be individualized and based on the most likely viral cause of a particular illness. For example, when an enteroviral etiologic agent is suspected, freezing the specimen (−70°C [−94°F]) and shipping it with dry ice are satisfactory. In contrast, a urine specimen from a patient with possible cytomegalovirus (CMV) infection should not be frozen. It should be shipped under wet ice at 4°C (39.2°F) because CMV in urine is stable for several days at this temperature. For specific characteristics of individual viruses, see the respective chapters in this book.

LABORATORY DIAGNOSIS OF VIRAL INFECTIONS

In recent years, technologic advances have provided powerful and achievable methods for the detection of viruses in clinical specimens. Widespread availability of commercial reagents and kits for molecular detection and quantitation of viral nucleic acids in specimens has made these methods accessible for many hospitals. In some instances, qualitative NAATs can be performed in the clinic, at the point of care. Laboratories may combine both culture and nonculture approaches to optimize viral disease diagnosis, although most have eliminated culture in deference to the superior sensitivity, specificity, and turnaround times achievable by molecular methods. Table 253.2 summarizes optimal methods for the laboratory identification of specific viruses, and more in depth information is presented in the individual chapters of this book.

Virus Isolation

Isolation of viruses in culture is no longer routinely performed by many clinical laboratories but remains available in many reference and public health laboratories. Unlike rapid methods, which are limited to the detection of specific viral antigens or nucleic acids, culture is open-ended and permits detection of unexpected or new viruses. In addition, a broad range of specimens can be evaluated by culture, whereas more rapid methods are licensed for use with a defined and limited number of specimens. Viruses that can be isolated in culture and readily identified include adenoviruses, HSV, VZV, CMV, enteroviruses, rhinoviruses, influenza and parainfluenza viruses, respiratory syncytial virus (RSV), rubella virus, mumps virus, and measles virus. For optimal laboratory diagnosis, indicating the name of the suspected virus on the requisition is important because some viruses require specific cell lines, procedures for identification, or both. Cultures are maintained for different time frames before finalizing a report of negative results, depending on the virus being sought. For example, HSV cultures usually are observed for 5 to 7 days, CMV for 1 month, and all others for 2 to 4 weeks.

Traditional Culture

For traditional culture, clinical samples are inoculated onto one or more cell lines, selected based on the submitted specimen and suspected virus. Cultures are observed at regular intervals for evidence of viral infection characterized by the appearance of cytopathic effect, the ability to hemadsorb or hemagglutinate RBCs, or immunofluorescence with monoclonal antibodies. Adenoviruses, CMV, HSV, VZV, rhinoviruses, and enteroviruses can be identified and reported by their characteristic cytopathic effect. Parainfluenza and influenza viruses, in contrast, may or may not produce cytopathic effect but can be detected with the traditional hemadsorption method, in which a suspension of guinea pig RBCs is added to the cell culture. The RBCs adhere to tissue culture cells infected with these viruses. RSV is identified presumptively by its typical cytopathic effect (syncytium formation) and definitively by immunofluorescence with monoclonal antibodies. The traditional method for isolation and identification of rubella virus is by evaluating for interference of the cytopathic effect of a second virus, usually echovirus 11. Finally, although rarely performed, definitive identification of viral serotypes (e.g., adenovirus and enterovirus) by the neutralization test can be done for epidemiologic purposes. For the most part, the

TABLE 253.2 **Common Laboratory Methods for Diagnosis of Specific Viral Illnesses**[a]

Virus	Culture	Antigen Detection	Serology	Nucleic Acid Amplification Test	Most Useful Method for Diagnosis
Adenoviruses	Not routine	DFA ELISA	Reference or public health laboratory	Detected by some multiplexed respiratory virus NAATs Single-analyte commercial NAAT available	NAAT
Arboviruses of North and South America, including Zika	Reference or public health laboratory	Not routine	Reference or public health laboratory	Reference or public health laboratory	Serology or NAAT
Coronaviruses	Not practical by routine methods (except SARS-CoV, which should not be cultured outside public health laboratories)	Not routine	Not routine	Detected by some multiplexed respiratory virus NAATs	NAAT
Rhinoviruses	Not routine, must be differentiated from enteroviruses by acid lability	Not routine	Not routine	Detected by some multiplexed respiratory virus NAATs	NAAT
Enteroviruses	Not routine, some coxsackieviruses are difficult to culture by routine methods	Not routine	Not routine	NAAT from CSF Detected by some multiplexed respiratory virus NAATs	NAAT
Cytomegalovirus	Not routine	Not routine	Routine	Both qualitative and quantitative NAATs routine	NAAT
Epstein-Barr virus (EBV)	Not practical by routine methods	Not routinely performed	Routine	Quantitative NAATs routine	NAAT
Herpes simplex virus	Routine	DFA	Routine	Commercial NAAT	NAAT (especially from CSF) culture
HIV	Not routine	p24 antigen assay	Routine	Quantitative NAATs routine	Serology NAAT
Human metapneumovirus (hMPV)	Not routine	DFA	Not routine	Detected by some multiplexed respiratory virus NAATs Single-analyte commercial NAAT available	NAAT
Influenza viruses	Not routine	DFA RICT	Not routine	Multiple NAATs available, including those that subtype virus Detected by some multiplexed respiratory virus NAATs	NAAT

Continued

TABLE 253.2 Common Laboratory Methods for Diagnosis of Specific Viral Illnesses[a]—cont'd

Virus	Culture	Antigen Detection	Serology	Nucleic Acid Amplification Test	Most Useful Method for Diagnosis
Measles virus	Not routine	Not routine	Routine	Reference or public health laboratory	Serology NAAT
Mumps virus	Not routine	Not routine	Routine	Reference or public health laboratory	Serology NAAT
Parainfluenza viruses	Not routine	DFA	Not routine	Detected by some multiplexed respiratory virus NAATs	NAAT
Respiratory syncytial virus	Not routine	DFA RICT	Not routine	Detected by some multiplexed respiratory virus NAATs	DFA RICT NAAT
Rabies virus (animal infections)	Not routinely performed	DFA at public health laboratory	Public health laboratory	Public health laboratory	Submit to public health laboratory
Rubella virus	Not routine	Not routine	Routine	Not routine	Serology NAAT
Poxviruses	Not routine	Not routine	Not useful for diagnosis	Vaccinia virus PCR at public health laboratory	Clinical diagnosis (molluscum) or submit to public health laboratory
Varicella-zoster virus	Not routine	DFA	Not routine	Routine, as laboratory developed tests	DFA NAAT
Hepatitis A virus	Not routine	Not routine	Routine	Not routine	Serology
Hepatitis B virus	Not practical by routine methods	Not routine	Routine	Routine	Serology (diagnosis) NAAT (to monitor treatment)
Hepatitis C virus	Not practical by routine methods	Not routine	Routine	Both qualitative and quantitative NAATs routine	Serology (diagnosis) NAAT (diagnosis and to monitor treatment)
Norovirus	Not practical by routine methods	ELISA	Not routine	Routine	NAAT
Rotavirus	Not routine	ELISA	Not routine	Routine on some commercial multiplex NAATs	ELISA
Adenovirus 40 and 41	Not practical by routine methods	ELISA	Not routine	Routine on some commercial multiplex NAATs	ELISA NAAT

[a]For details, see chapters for the specific viral agents in this textbook.

CSF, Cerebrospinal fluid; *DFA*, direct fluorescent antibody; *ELISA*, enzyme-linked immunosorbent assay; *NAAT*, nucleic acid amplification test; *PCR*, polymerase chain reaction; *RICT*, rapid immunochromatographic test; *SARS-CoV*, severe acute respiratory syndrome–corona virus.

neutralization test has been replaced by nucleic acid sequencing approaches to serotyping, which have equivalent specificities.[43,51]

NAATs, serologic tests, or a combination of the two are recommended for viruses that are difficult or impossible to isolate in commonly employed cell lines or that require special techniques for detection of their presence. For instance, although mumps virus can be isolated in the same cell lines used for other paramyxoviruses and detected by hemadsorption or hemagglutination, NAAT and serology are preferred methods for establishing diagnosis. Buccal or oral swabs collected early in disease are tested by reverse transcriptase polymerase chain reaction (RT-PCR) assay for mumps virus. If negative, acute and convalescent serum specimens may reveal diagnosis in patients with signs and symptoms of mumps. Similarly, when measles is suspected, diagnosis is confirmed most easily by serologic studies or NAAT. Paired sera collected 1 week apart usually reveal a fourfold antibody titer rise. Alternatively, demonstration of a single measles-specific immunoglobulin M antibody or detection of measles RNA by RT-PCR performed on oropharyngeal or nasopharyngeal swabs or urine establishes diagnosis. It should be noted that specimens for NAAT should be collected no more than 3 days after onset of rash, although RNA may be detected as late as 14 days after rash onset.

Modified Culture

Several physical and chemical methods enhance the detection of virus in culture. One common technique, termed the shell vial assay (SVA), entails centrifugation of the specimen onto a cell monolayer and detection of early antigen. This method is used by most laboratories that continue to perform viral cultures because it significantly decreases the time to result (i.e., 1–3 days) compared with traditional culture (5–30 days). Antigen is detected by immunofluorescence or occasionally by immunoperoxidase staining with monoclonal antibodies directed against a specific virus, before the appearance of cytopathic effect. SVAs are used extensively for detection of HSV, CMV, VZV, adenovirus, RSV, influenza virus, parainfluenza virus, measles virus, and human metapneumovirus.

Pooled antibodies directed against seven commonly isolated respiratory viruses (i.e., adenovirus; influenza viruses A and B; parainfluenza virus types 1, 2, and 3; and RSV) are commercially available.[46,55,63] To be adequately sensitive for each of these respiratory viruses, either two or more single cell lines in shell vial are used or mixed cell lines are applied to shell vial cultures. The commercially available R-Mix (Diagnostic Hybrids) mixed cell line, for example, consists of one cell line to support replication of RSV, adenovirus, and parainfluenza (i.e., A549) and another to support replication of influenza (i.e., Mv1Lu). R-Mix Too was developed after recognition that severe acute respiratory syndrome–coronavirus (SARS-CoV) readily infected Mv1Lu cell lines[23]; R-Mix Too mitigates the risk for inadvertent amplification of SARS-CoV in the routine clinical laboratory by replacing Mv1Lu with MDCK cell lines.

A second modification of cell culture is for the rapid detection of HSV using an enzyme-linked virus-inducible system (ELVIS).[71] This system consists of a mixture of modified baby hamster kidney cells and MRC-5 cells. The modified baby hamster kidney cells contain an HSV-inducible promoter and an *Escherichia coli* LacZ reporter gene that produces β-galactosidase only when cells are infected with HSV. After the addition of a substrate for the β-galactosidase, infected cells stain blue, whereas uninfected cells remain colorless. ELVIS appears to be comparable to culture for the detection of HSV-positive specimens (95% and 100% sensitivity) in a similar time frame, 1.4 to 1.7 days.[45]

Direct Detection

Cytology

Historically, rapid detection of viral infection relied on light microscopy and evaluation of tissues and exfoliated cells for viral inclusions or other cytopathic effects. Cytologic identification of virus is most useful in illnesses with vesicular exanthems such as HSV or VZV infection. A scraping of the base of an HSV or VZV lesion (Tzanck smear) reveals multinucleated giant and balloon cells when stained with hematoxylin and eosin, Wright, or Giemsa stain. In contrast, vesicular lesions caused by enteroviral infections do not contain giant or balloon cells, and allergy-related lesions contain eosinophils. Cytologic study of urine in congenital CMV infection reveals cells with the characteristic "owl's eye" intranuclear inclusions in 25% to 50% of cases, and nasal or pharyngeal smears in measles may reveal typical giant cells. These types of stains are no longer routinely performed in most diagnostic virology laboratories because they have been replaced by immunofluorescence or NAATs, which are more sensitive and specific. Whereas the Tzanck smear cannot differentiate HSV from VZV and the presence of multinucleated giant cells is necessary to make the diagnosis, immunofluorescence can identify the causative agent specifically, and the presence of viral antigen in balloon or giant cells is diagnostic.

Antigen Detection

Antigen-detection methods are available for most commonly isolated viruses. Advantages of these methods include speed, standardized reagents and kits, the ability to detect nonviable, nonculturable, or difficult-to-grow viruses, and the ability to detect antigen when culture may be negative late in the course of infection. Generally, these methods are not as sensitive as NAAT or an optimized culture; thus NAAT or culture backup is recommended. DFA, indirect immunofluorescent assay (IFA), and ELISA, as well as lateral flow immunoassay platforms, are used most commonly for antigen detection in the clinical laboratory.

Immunofluorescence

Antigen detection by immunofluorescence requires collection of the appropriate cell types (i.e., those in which the virus propagates) in adequate numbers for evaluation. In some cases, the specimen is placed on the slide directly (e.g., HSV or VZV detection), but usually the sample is transported to the laboratory for processing and slide preparation (e.g., for respiratory virus detection). As is the case for all methods discussed in this chapter, the importance of adequate specimen collection cannot be overemphasized. When stringent specimen quality criteria are applied (e.g., ≥60 columnar epithelial cells per sample for influenza testing), DFA sensitivity approaches that of NAATs.[61] However, such adequate specimens are infrequently collected, even when staff are trained in proper collection techniques.[42]

DFA methods use virus-specific monoclonal antibody labeled with fluorescein dye to detect antigen and usually require approximately 30 to 45 minutes to complete. If processing of the specimen is required and slides are prepared in the laboratory, additional time is necessary. For IFA, unlabeled monoclonal antibody is added to the sample and incubated, followed by a wash and the addition of fluorescein-labeled antimouse immunoglobulin. After an additional incubation and wash, the slide can be examined for typical fluorescence. IFA can be completed in 2 to 3 hours. The advantage of using DFA or IFA is the ability to determine specimen adequacy and to perform small-batch and demand testing. A high-quality microscope and skilled, experienced personnel are required for optimal preparation and evaluation of the specimen.

The first DFA reagent available for use in the diagnostic laboratory was for the detection of HSV in genital, dermal, oral, and anal lesions. The test should not be used for detection of HSV in CSF, asymptomatic genital specimens, tracheal aspirates, or bronchoalveolar lavage (BAL) specimens. Sensitivity of the DFA (and culture) for HSV detection varies by the stage of the lesion. DFA or culture detected HSV in 96.7% of vesicles, 79.2% of pustules, 44.7% of ulcers, and 16.7% of crusts.[39] In contrast, detection of HSV by NAAT is less influenced by lesion stage[19] and may increase yield of a positive result by 13% of vesicles, 28% of ulcers, and 20% of crusts.[68] Nonetheless, lesion duration and morphology remain strongly associated with the likelihood of HSV detection by NAAT, and negative results were obtained in 41.4% of vesicles, 48.4% of ulcers, and 76.9% of crusts.

DFA was also used historically for detection of VZV and remains a reliable test for primary disease in unvaccinated individuals. However, the utility of DFA for detecting VZV in the post–varicella vaccine era is diminished by the fact that breakthrough disease in previously vaccinated patients presents as a macular or papular rash, from which virus-infected cells for DFA testing cannot be readily collected. In such instances, NAAT should be performed on a swab or scraping of the rash, which is associated with 95% to 100% sensitivity.[42,79]

Detection of CMV antigen in lung tissue or BAL specimens and in liver tissue has been used for diagnosis of CMV pneumonia or hepatitis.

However, the sensitivity of DFA is less than that of CMV culture, SVA, or NAAT. The preferred specimen for diagnosis of CMV pneumonia by DFA is a lung biopsy, although BAL specimens are collected far more commonly. A comparison of the cellular portion, supernate, and whole BAL for isolation of CMV in culture suggested that CMV is associated with the cell-free rather than the cellular component.[10] The pp65 antigenemia assay consists of separation of leukocytes from whole blood, spotting or cytocentrifuging cells onto microscope slides, fixation and permeabilization, staining with anti-pp65 monoclonal antibodies, and detection by fluorescein-labeled or peroxidase-labeled secondary antibodies. pp65-Positive leukocytes are quantitated. This assay has widely been replaced in clinical practice by CMV DNA qualitative and quantitative PCR. The main limitation of the pp65 antigenemia assay is that it can only be performed on blood, whereas NAATs have been validated on several specimen types.

Finally, DFA and IFA are useful for the rapid detection of common respiratory virus in nasopharyngeal washes, aspirates, and suctions. DFA for RSV has been evaluated extensively. As is the case for VZV, RSV is relatively labile, and antigen detection actually may be more sensitive than culture. However, the DFA is less sensitive than NAAT, detecting only 73.9% of NAAT-positive cases in one study.[40] In addition, because up to 30% of specimens submitted for establishing the diagnosis of RSV contain other viruses,[5,9] multiplex NAATs or DFAs that evaluate for other respiratory viruses may be advisable when evaluating the patient with respiratory tract infection. The sensitivity of DFA and IFA for detection of influenza virus A and B, parainfluenza virus 1, 2, and 3, and adenovirus antigens varies, so NAATs must be performed if these are negative, for optimal diagnosis.

Enzyme-Linked Immunosorbent Assays

Standardized, well-characterized commercial kits for the detection of viral antigen by ELISA are available for HSV, RSV, influenza virus A and B, rotavirus, norovirus, adenovirus, HIV (p24), human T-lymphotropic virus (HTLV) 1 and 2, and hepatitis B virus (HBV). Intracellular and extracellular antigen can be detected; the methods are generally simple technically and are less affected by suboptimal specimen handling than are viral cultures. ELISAs come in two basic formats, either a classical microtiter or self-contained rapid immunochromatographic tests (RICT). The microtiter format uses antibodies lining the surface of the solid phase to capture viral antigen, which in turn is reacted with an enzyme-labeled secondary antibody, followed by detection with the addition of substrate and color development. Results are read spectrophotometrically and thus are objective, thereby eliminating some of the difficulties inherent in microscopic techniques, which require technical skill and expertise for evaluation of specimens. A major limitation of these approaches compared with DFA is that the adequacy of the specimen cannot be ascertained.

RICTs use a membrane as the solid support to retain viral antigen, to which enzyme-labeled antibodies are added to react with trapped antigen. Antigen-antibody complexes are detected using a chromogenic substrate, which is read visually. Although they are rapid (15–20 minutes) and simple to perform, RICTs tests are more expensive, require more hands-on time, and do not result in objective end points. False-positive results and interpretation can be a problem. Some membrane-based methods use analyzer reader devices to standardize result interpretation, which have been shown to improve sensitivity and specificity of these assays.[16] Detection of influenza and RSV antigens in nasopharyngeal aspirates, washes, suctions, and swabs has been evaluated extensively in standard and membrane ELISA formats.

Many of the RICTs are Clinical Laboratory Improvement Amendments (CLIA) waived, meaning they may be performed in emergency departments, outpatient clinics, and physician offices for point-of-care diagnosis of influenza A and B and RSV in patients with compatible respiratory symptoms. The clinical performance of these RICTs may vary significantly from the specifications listed in the package insert and year to year based on circulating virus type and subtype. Similarly, these tests have limited sensitivity compared with NAATs, and negative results should be interpreted with caution, in particular during peak influenza season, and should be backed up by NAAT. For instance, the sensitivity of the BinaxNOW Influenza A & B was 75% for influenza A virus and 72% for influenza B during one influenza season, but only 48.9% and 36%, respectively, for a subsequent season, because of antigenic drift in the seasonal influenza virus.[24] Similarly, the reported sensitivity of various RICTs to detect novel influenza viruses, such as the 2009 (H1N1) pandemic and the H3N2v 2012 influenza strains, was 0% to 70%,[17,18] depending on test manufacturer. The performance of RICTs also depends on the prevalence of the virus among patients with febrile respiratory tract infections. When the prevalence of influenza in children with compatible symptoms was 5%, the predictive value of a positive RICT was found to be 50% in contrast to RT-PCR and the predictive value of a negative test to be 98%.[25] Conversely, when the prevalence of influenza was 21%, the positive predictive value was 85% and the negative predictive value was 91%.[25] Finally, performance of the RICTs decreases as time from onset of symptoms increases. Thus, for optimal diagnosis, these should be used when disease prevalence is high and in patients with 4 days or less of symptoms. The Centers for Disease Control and Prevention in the United States also reports annually on the availability of these tests; these data are available at http://www.cdc.gov/flu/professionals/diagnosis/clinician_guidance_ridt.htm.

Children shed high titers of RSV; therefore RICTs for RSV performs significantly better in the pediatric population than do influenza tests. However, optimal performance is based on patient age and timing of specimen collection relative to onset of symptoms. The BinaxNOW RSV was positive in 79% to 91% of children younger than 1 year of age in contrast to NAAT-confirmed or culture-confirmed RSV infection, but in only 52% of those 1 year of age and older[47] to 25% of adults.[54] The assay was positive in 92% of patients with 0 to 1 day of symptoms, 78% with 2 to 4 days, and 65% with 5 or more days of symptoms.[47] Similar to influenza, performance of RSV RICTs varies significantly year to year and with virus prevalence.[12]

Rotavirus antigen detection by standard ELISA has been studied thoroughly. Many of the assays have excellent sensitivity (93–100%) and specificity (98–100%) in contrast to that of electron microscopy. Detection of rotavirus by ELISA may be preferred over more sensitive methods, such as RT-PCR. In one study of 648 children with acute gastroenteritis and 500 healthy controls, ELISA was found to have higher clinically specificity for rotavirus than was RT-PCR. Although more rotavirus was detected in both cases and controls by the RT-PCR, these were at low viral loads and in children who had been vaccinated against rotavirus, suggesting rotavirus was not the cause of gastroenteritis in the symptomatic children.[74] RICTs also are available for rotavirus antigen detection and, as is typical of this format, are somewhat less sensitive than standard ELISA, with approximately 10^7 virions/mL required for detection of a positive specimen. An excellent ELISA for detection of adenovirus 40 and 41 in stool specimens is available and yields a reported sensitivity and specificity of 96%.[33,80]

Nucleic Acid Detection

Molecular methods for the detection, identification, and characterization of microorganisms are being adapted increasingly for use in the clinical laboratory. These assays provide a timely and specific diagnosis, although the cost of reagents can range from $30 to more than $200 per test. NAATs were first developed in-house primarily for the identification of viruses that are not readily cultured (e.g., HSV from CSF) and for those in which time to detection by traditional means is too long to affect patient care (e.g., CMV). The past several years have witnessed an explosion in the number of NAATs for the rapid detection of all viruses commonly encountered in clinical practice, including many that are cleared by the US Food and Drug Administration (FDA) as in vitro diagnostic devices. When all costs are accounted for, including length of stay, frequency of diagnostic testing, and antibiotic use, diagnosis of respiratory viruses in children by a multiplex molecular method has been shown to be associated with cost savings equaling the cost of the assay or higher.[44]

Increased use of molecular testing for the diagnosis of viral infections has stimulated several recent developments, including automation of nucleic acid extraction, amplification, detection, and reporting and interpretation of results. Several "sample to answer" platforms are now commercially available, allowing use of these technologies in smaller laboratories situated in community hospitals or emergency departments that do not have expertise in sophisticated molecular diagnostics, although careful application of techniques to avoid nucleic acid cross-contamination is required. Recently, several commercial, CLIA-waived cartridge-based NAATs have come to the market, enabling rapid, point-of-care testing in the clinic.

In most cases, NAATs offer enhanced sensitivity and specificity over the other assays described in this chapter. However, clinical specimens sometimes contain inhibiting substances that interfere with the performance of NAATs. Internal control nucleic acids, generally in the form of bacteriophages or murine viruses, may be spiked into clinical specimens to monitor for inhibition. Additional limitations of NAATs are the potential for sample to sample or amplicon cross-contamination, leading to false-positive results and the inability to distinguish between actively replicating virus and residual viral nucleic acids. Similarly, because NAATs are significantly more sensitive than traditional methods, it is becoming apparent that some populations may be colonized with low levels of virus that are undetectable by culture or antigen based testing.[74]

NAATs approved or cleared by the FDA at the time of writing are discussed in the following sections with respect to their application for the diagnosis and monitoring of certain viral infections. The analytical and clinical performance characteristics of these tests are well defined, and these assays undergo routine quality assurance monitoring. Because the list of FDA-approved/cleared molecular assays is ever expanding, readers are directed to the FDA website (http://www.fda.gov/MedicalDevices/ProductsandMedicalProcedures/InVitroDiagnostics/ucm330711.htm) for a comprehensive up-to-date list of FDA-approved/cleared tests. In addition, laboratories may develop NAATs through use of analyte-specific reagents that are widely available for a variety of viral targets. These laboratory-developed tests can then be validated for clinical use in accordance with CLIA requirements, which must include assessment of accuracy or bias, precision, linearity, limit of detection, interfering substances, and stability. The sensitivity and specificities of these laboratory-developed assays will vary across laboratories, and thus results from different laboratories cannot be used for comparison.

CLIA-Waived Nucleic Acid Amplification Tests

Recently, two CLIA-waived NAATs were cleared by the FDA for the detection of influenza (Table 253.3). The Alere i Influenza A & B assay is performed on nasopharyngeal swabs and uses a nicking endonuclease amplification reaction for ultrarapid amplification of DNA or RNA, which is detected by fluorescently labeled molecular beacons. The assay yields results within 15 minutes, with all steps performed onboard the Alere platform.[50] The Cobas Liat system similarly detects influenza A and B nucleic acids within 20 minutes, by Taqman probe–based RT-PCR.[9] Both systems are rapid to perform in the clinic, requiring less than 3 minutes hands-on time to prepare testing. Early data suggest the Alere i Influenza A & B assay may be less sensitive than conventional PCR performed in the laboratory, with sensitivity ranging from 77.8% for influenza A to 75% for influenza B.[32] Nonetheless, sensitivity was significantly improved over rapid ELISA tests performed in the clinic,

TABLE 253.3 Comparison of Select Single-Analyte and Multiplexed Nucleic Acid Amplification Tests for the Qualitative Detection of Viral Targets

Assay (Manufacturer)	Targets	Extraction	Method[a]	Approved Specimens	Time to Results
CLIA-Waived (Point of Care) NAATs					
Alere i Influenza A & B (Alere)	Influenza A Influenza B	N/A	Helicase dependent amplification	Nasopharyngeal swab	15 min
cobas Liat Influenza A/B (Roche)	Influenza A Influenza B	N/A	Taqman RT-PCR	Nasopharyngeal swab	20 min
Single-Analyte NAATs					
Adenovirus R-gene (bioMerieux)	Adenovirus	Offline	Taqman RT-PCR	Nasopharyngeal swab Nasopharyngeal wash/aspirate	1 h
Lyra Adenovirus Assay (Quidel)	Adenovirus	Offline	Taqman RT-PCR	Nasal swab Nasopharyngeal swab	2 h
ProAdenoTM+ Assay (Hologic)	Adenovirus	Offline	Taqman RT-PCR	Nasopharyngeal swab	4 h
Xpert EV (Cepheid)	Enterovirus	Online	Taqman RT-PCR	Cerebrospinal fluid	2.5 h
COBAS AmpliPrep/COBAS TaqMan HCV Qualitative test	HCV	Online	Taqman RT-PCR	Plasma Serum	6 h
AmpliVue HSV 1+2 (Quidel)	HSV-1 HSV-2	N/A	Helicase-dependent amplification with detection by DNA test strip hybridization and visual output	Cutaneous lesion swab Mucocutaneous lesion swab	1 h
ARIES HSV 1 & 2 Assay (Luminex)	HSV-1 HSV-2	Online	RT-PCR	Cutaneous lesion swab Mucocutaneous lesions swab	2 h
BD ProbeTec Herpes Simplex Viruses Q[x] Amplified DNA Assay	HSV-1 HSV-2	Online	Strand displacement amplification (SDA)	Anogenital lesion swab	3 h
MultiCode-RTx Herpes Simplex 1 & 2 (Luminex)	HSV-1 HSV-2	Offline	RT-PCR and multicode chemistry	Vaginal lesion swab	4 h
Simplexa HSV 1 & 2 Direct (DiaSorin)	HSV-1 HSV-2	N/A	RT-PCR with Scorpion Probes	Genital swab CSF	1.5 h
Xpert Norovirus (Cepheid)	Norovirus GI Norovirus GII	Online	RT-PCR with Molecular Beacons	Stool	1.5 h
Aptima Zika Virus Assay	Zika virus	Online (Panther system)	Transcription-mediated amplification (TMA)	Plasma Serum	3.5 h

Continued

TABLE 253.3 Comparison of Select Single-Analyte and Multiplexed Nucleic Acid Amplification Tests for the Qualitative Detection of Viral Targets—cont'd

Assay (Manufacturer)	Targets	Extraction	Method[a]	Approved Specimens	Time to Results
Multiplexed NAATs					
Lyra Direct HSV 1+2/VZV Assay (Quidel)	HSV-1 HSV-2 VZV	N/A	Taqman RT-PCR	Cutaneous lesion swab Mucocutaneous lesion swab	1 h
ProFlu+ Assay (Hologic)	Influenza A Influenza B RSV	Offline	Taqman RT-PCR	Nasopharyngeal swab	4 h
ProFAST+ (Hologic)	Influenza A H1 Influenza A/H3 Influenza A H1N1 (2009)	Offline	Taqman RT-PCR	Nasopharyngeal swab	4 h
Quidel Molecular Influenza A+B (Quidel)	Influenza A Influenza B	Offline	Taqman RT-PCR	Nasopharyngeal swab Nasal swab	3 h
Simplexa FluA/B & RSV (Diasorin)	Influenza A Influenza B RSV	Offline	RT-PCR and Scorpion Probes	Nasopharyngeal swab	3 h
Simplexa FluA/B & RSV Direct (Diasorin)	Influenza A Influenza B RSV	N/A	RT-PCR and Scorpion Probes	Nasopharyngeal swab	1.5 h
Simplexa Flu A/B & RSV Kit (Diasorin)	Influenza A Influenza B RSV	Offline	RT-PCR and Scorpion Probes	Nasopharyngeal swab	3 h
Simplexa Influenza A H1N1 (2009) (Diasorin)	Influenza A Influenza A/H1N1 (2009)	Offline	RT-PCR and Scorpion Probes	Nasopharyngeal swab	3 h
Xpert Flu (Cepheid)	Influenza A Influenza A 2009 H1N1 Influenza B	Online	RT-PCR with Molecular Beacons	Nasal aspirate/ wash Nasopharyngeal swab	1.5 h
Xpert Flu/RSV XC (Cepheid)	Influenza A Influenza B RSV	Online	RT-PCR with Molecular Beacons	Nasal aspirate/wash Nasopharyngeal swab	1.5 h
Lyra Parainfluenza Virus Assay (Quidel)	Parainfluenza 1 Parainfluenza 2 Parainfluenza 3	Offline	Taqman RT-PCR	Nasal swab Nasopharyngeal swab	2 h
Prodesse ProParaflu+ Assay (Hologic)	Parainfluenza 1 Parainfluenza 2 Parainfluenza 3	Offline	Taqman RT-PCR	Nasopharyngeal swab	4 h
Lyra RSV + hMPV Assay (Quidel)	RSV hMPV	Offline	Taqman RT-PCR	Throat swab	2 h

[a]For details on test method, refer to the text.

CLIA, Clinical Laboratory Improvement Amendments; *CSF,* cerebrospinal fluid; *HCV,* hepatitis C; *hMPV,* human metapneumovirus; *HSV,* herpes simplex virus; *NAAT,* nucleic acid amplification test; *RSV,* respiratory syncytial virus; *RT-PCR,* reverse transcriptase polymerase chain reaction; *VZV,* varicella-zoster virus.

which were only 25% to 71.4% sensitive for influenza A and B. In contrast, the Liat system was shown to have sensitivity of 99.2% for influenza A and 100% for influenza B in one early study.[4]

Single-Analyte Nucleic Acid Amplification Tests

Many single-analyte NAATs are available for detection of viruses in clinical specimens (see Table 253.3). NAATs have become the gold standard test for many viral infections. For example, NAATs on CSF are the procedure of choice for diagnosis of HSV encephalitis, although at the present, only one singleplex assay, the Simplexa HSV 1 & 2 Direct, has been cleared by the FDA for this indication (see Table 253.3). Several commercial HSV NAATs (see Table 253.3) are cleared for testing of cutaneous and mucocutaneous lesions. These assays detect and differentiate HSV-1 and HSV-2 and are associated with enhanced sensitivity in contrast to culture. NAATs are able to identify asymptomatic HSV, detect the presence of HSV for a longer period (in older lesions and even fixed tissue), and have greater diagnostic value than culture and clinical observations for assessing genital HSV and treatment efficacy in patients with recurrent genital HSV.[31,49]

Similar to HSV, detection of enterovirus in CSF by NAAT is the standard, because of slow growth or failure of certain serotypes to grow in culture. The sensitivity of the commercial enterovirus NAATs is 83% to 100%, whereas culture of CSF yields an isolate in only 36% of patients with enteroviral meningitis.[52] Such assays are particularly helpful because CSF evaluation for pleocytosis is not always reliable for diagnosis of enteroviral meningitis.[67] The Xpert EV is the only FDA-cleared assay for this indication. It is a cartridge-based assay designed to be run on demand, in emergency departments, yielding results in a time frame suitable for making medical management decisions.

Single-analyte, commercial NAATs are also available for the qualitative detection of adenovirus, hepatitis C virus (HCV), norovirus, and Zika virus from a variety of specimens (see Table 253.3). Many laboratory-developed tests are commonly available at both reference and hospital laboratories for other viral agents.

Multiplexed Assays

Multiplexed assays for the detection of influenza A and influenza B are listed in Table 253.3. These assays replace DFA and rapid antigen tests as a sensitive and specific means by which to rapidly detect these viruses. Several of these assays have the added benefits of also detecting RSV and providing a differentiation between the influenza A virus subtypes. All of the assays described in this section have excellent performance, with published sensitivities and specificities of more than 95% for their specific targets, when performed per manufacturer instructions.

The Prodesse ProFAST+ (Hologic) assays are multiplex real-time RT-PCR for the qualitative detection and discrimination of seasonal influenza A/H1, A/H3, and 2009 H1N1 viral nucleic acids. The assay targets the hemagglutinin gene and does not detect influenza B or C. In contrast, the Prodesse ProFlu+ (Hologic) assay targets the matrix gene for influenza A, the nonstructural genes NS-1 and NS-2 from influenza B, and the polymerase gene of RSV A and RSV B. In both assays, specimen is processed on an off-line nucleic acid extractor, and NAAT is performed on a Cepheid SmartCycler II instrument. The assay is based on Taqman chemistry, in which a target-specific probe with a 5′ fluorophore and a 3′ fluorescence resonance energy transfer (FRET) quencher anneals to the viral cDNA. While the probe is intact, fluorescence is quenched by FRET by the quencher molecule. However, during DNA amplification, the 5′ to 3′ exonuclease activity of Taq DNA polymerase cleaves the fluorophore from the probe, displacing it from the quencher, and allowing fluorescence. Assays for the detection of adenovirus (ProAdeno+), and parainfluenza (ProParaflu+) are also available from the Hologic Prodesse line of assays. Like the Prodesse assays, the Quidel Lyra Influenza A + B assay uses Taqman chemistry for the detection of influenza A and B. The Lyra assays also multiplexed assays for HSV-1, HSV-2, and VZV from lesions, human metapneumovirus and RSV from throat swabs, and parainfluenza 1, parainfluenza 2, and parainfluenza 3 from nasopharyngeal swabs.

The Simplexa assays (DiaSorin) are performed on the 3M integrated cycler instrument. These assays are either performed direct from specimen (e.g., FluA/B & RSV Direct) or following off-line nucleic acid extraction (e.g., FluA/B & RSV). In these assays, RT-PCR is detected through use of bifunctional scorpion primer/probe molecules in which the 5′ end of the primer is covalently linked to the probe. The probe is a self-complementary stem sequence with a fluorophore at one end a quencher at the other. When the probe anneals to the amplicon, the fluorophore and quencher separate, leading to an increase in fluorescence. Sensitivity of the Simplexa Flu A/B & RSV Direct assay was reported for influenza A as 82% to 96%, for influenza B as 76% to 99%, and for RSV as 95% to 98%.[40] Specificity is greater than 99% for all three targets. Finally, the Cepheid Xpert Flu is a cartridge-based assay that uses real-time PCR with molecular beacon detection and is performed on the GeneXpert instrument. Molecular beacon probes that have self-complimentary ends that form a stem-loop structure in their native state, keeping a 5′ fluorophore and a 3′ quencher in close proximity. On hybridization to the target cDNA, fluorophore and quencher are separated, yielding signal. The GeneXpert assays are moderate complexity, with less than 15 minutes hands-on time required to pipette the sample into the cartridge and start the assay; results are available in less than 1 hour.

Highly Multiplexed Assays

Until recently, NAATs for infectious diseases testing were relatively simple, detecting at most eight targets because of limitations in sensitivity and specificity when attempting to detect multiple analytes. However, in recent years, highly multiplexed NAATs have been developed for the detection of a wide variety of viruses that might be present in a single clinical sample, providing the key advantage of traditional culture. Such so-called syndromic panels are best suited to sample types and situations in which a wide range of viruses (or other pathogens) may cause similar symptoms, such as with respiratory tract infections, meningitis/encephalitis, or gastroenteritis. Four main companies have developed panels to date, including Luminex, BioFire, GenMark, and Nanosphere, although several others have methods in development. The currently available diagnostic panels approved for use by the FDA are listed in Table 253.4. Some of these include detection of bacterial pathogens, yeast, or parasites. The primary value of these syndromic panels is improved sensitivity coupled with the detection of etiological agents that are not routinely tested for by other means (e.g., viral causes of diarrhea, coronaviruses in respiratory specimens, and parechovirus in CSF).[57]

In the original Luminex xTag assays, viral nucleic acids are coextracted from specimens spiked with an internal control (MS2 phage), using an off-line automated extractor. Multiplex RT-PCR is then performed using primers specific to the viral targets and the control; these primers contain a tag sequence for target-specific primer extension (TSPE). The target-specific primers are then extended through addition of biotinylated deoxycytidine triphosphate to the reaction mixture, which is incorporated into the TSPE products. Following TSPE, products are mixed with color-coded microspheres with antitags. The antitag binds the tags present on the TSPE products, hybridizing the amplicons to the beads. The beads are read through solution-based microarray on the Luminex 100/200 or MAGPIX systems by two lasers—the first identifies the virus-specific color-coded bead, and the second determines whether amplicon is hybridized to the bead. The clinical performance of the xTAG Respiratory Virus Panel is well established, but the assay has several limitations. Sensitivity for certain adenoviruses (species C, serotypes 7a and 41) is poor, and primers for detection of rhinovirus cross-react with enterovirus.[22,56,65] Similar to the Respiratory Virus Panel, the Gastrointestinal Pathogen Panel sensitivity is only 17.9% to 80% for adenovirus detection as compared to single-analyte PCRs.[26,35] A key limitation of both the Respiratory Virus Panel and Gastrointestinal Pathogen Panel tests is the risk for false-positive findings as a result of cross-contamination by amplified nucleic acids, which are pipetted manually between stages of the assay. Additional limitations include time-to-results, which is 8 to 10 hours, and technical hands-on time. Luminex recently released the NxTAG Respiratory Pathogen Panel, which addresses many of these concerns. This method streamlines the process to include a single integrated multiplex PCR and bead hybridization step, which is followed by detection on the MAGPIX system. These modifications also reduce the risk for cross-contamination because the system is closed following addition of extracted nucleic acids to the test wells. Two studies have evaluated the NxTAG to date compared with singleplex RT-PCRs. Sensitivity for all targets was excellent, with the exception of the coronaviruses HKU1 and OC43, wherein only two of three specimens tested were detected,[8] although a second study found 94% sensitivity for HKU1 and 100% for OC43.[73]

Like the Luminex assays, the eSensor XT-8 (GenMark) is performed by extracting viral nucleic acids with addition of a bacteriophage internal control. End-point PCR is performed, after which exoculease is used to create single-stranded DNA. This is hybridized to ferrocene-labeled signal probes specific to the different viral targets and application to a single-file microarray of preassembled gold-plated electrodes coated with single-stranded oligonucleotide capture probes. If present, target DNA-probe complexes hybridize the capture probes, binding the ferrocene label in proximity to the gold electrode; an electrical current is applied, and captured target DNA is analyzed by electrochemical detection using voltammetry. The eSensor XT-8 has excellent sensitivity and specificity for viral targets detected by the assay.[60,62] The Verigene assays are performed on the Verigene processor, on which automated nucleic acid extraction, multiplexed RT-PCR, and hybridization to a slide array are performed. Detection occurs through Nanosphere's proprietary gold nanoparticle hybridization technology. Amplicons from RT-PCR are hybridized to a microarray followed by silver-coated gold nanoparticle probe hybridization. Product is detected by light scattering off the nanoprobes. Overall, the time to results is 2 hours, with very little hands-on time (pipetting of specimens to the test cartridge at the start of the assay and removal to the reader at the end of the assay). However, throughput is low, with only one sample per processer. The Verigene Flex Test includes detection of up to 16 viral and bacterial targets (see Table 253.4); however, users define which combination of targets are selected and reported at the time of test ordering. The laboratory is only charged for those analytes reported. Additional results initially not reported can be revealed, at an additional cost. Such a model has the advantage of allowing scalable respiratory virus testing for different patient populations, or during different respiratory seasons. From the laboratory perspective, testing is streamlined and economical.

Finally, the FilmArray panels (BioFire) are fully closed systems with a specimen-in, result-out format. These sealed systems minimize the contamination concerns associated with Luminex and GenMark assays. Nucleic acids are detected by a nested multiplex PCR; product is detected using end-point melting curve data on the FilmArray instrument. The assay requires little hands-on time, and results are available in just over 1 hour. A significant drawback of the system is the throughput because only one sample can be processed on the instrument at a time. Thus larger laboratories may need multiple instruments to meet test volume. The FilmArray Respiratory Panel is cleared for the detection of 15 viruses and subtypes. Similar to the xTAG RVP assays, detection of adenovirus is problematic,[18,59] particularly species C; serotypes 2 and 6 are poorly detected. The FilmArray Meningitis/Encephalitis panel includes several viral targets (see Table 253.4), with excellent sensitivity and specificity compared with PCR, with the exception of human herpesvirus-6 (HHV-6), of which only 85.7% of cases were detected.[41]

Viral Nucleic Acid Quantitation Assays

Quantitative NAATs (qNAATs) play an important role in the diagnosis and management of viral disease.[27] Viral load assays are used to predict disease progression, distinguish symptomatic from asymptomatic infection, monitor the development of antiviral resistance, and assess the efficacy of antiviral therapy. Table 253.5 lists the FDA-approved quantitative molecular assays currently available.

TABLE 253.4 Comparison of the Highly Multiplexed Assays for the Detection of Respiratory Viruses

Test	Method	Specimen	Time to Result	Targets
Respiratory Panels				
xTAG RVP (Luminex)	End-point RT-PCR with microsphere-based detection	Nasopharyngeal swab	8–10 h	Adenovirus hMPV Influenza A Influenza A H1 Influenza A H3 Influenza B Parainfluenza-1 Parainfluenza-2 Parainfluenza-3 Rhinovirus RSV A RSV B
NxTAG Respiratory Pathogen Panel (Luminex)	End-point RT-PCR with microsphere-based detection on the MagPix system	Nasopharyngeal swab	5 h	Adenovirus Coronavirus HKU1 Coronavirus NL63 Coronavirus 229E Coronavirus OC42 Human bocavirus hMPV Influenza A Influenza A H1 Influenza A H3 Influenza B RSV A RSV B Parainfluenza 1 Parainfluenza 2 Parainfluenza 3 Parainfluenza 4 Rhinovirus/enterovirus *Chlamydophila pneumoniae* *Mycoplasma pneumoniae*
FilmArray Respiratory Panel (BioFire)	Onboard nucleic acid extraction followed by RT-PCR and microarray detection	Nasopharyngeal swab	1 h	Adenovirus Coronavirus NL63 Coronavirus 229E Coronavirus OC43 Coronavirus HKU1 hMPV Influenza A Influenza A/H1 Influenza A/H3 Influenza A/H1-2009 Influenza B Parainfluenza 1 Parainfluenza 2 Parainfluenza 3 Parainfluenza 4 RSV Rhinovirus/enterovirus *Bordetella pertussis* *Chlamydophila pneumoniae* *Mycoplasma pneumoniae*

TABLE 253.4 Comparison of the Highly Multiplexed Assays for the Detection of Respiratory Viruses—cont'd

Test	Method	Specimen	Time to Result	Targets
Respiratory Pathogens Flex test (Nanosphere/ Luminex)			2 h	Adenovirus hMPV Influenza A H1 Influenza A H3 Influenza A Influenza B Parainfluenza 1 Parainfluenza 2 Parainfluenza 3 Parainfluenza 4 Rhinovirus RSV A RSV B *Bordetella pertussis* *Bordetella parapertussis/B. bronchiseptica* *Bordetella holmesii*
eSensor Respiratory Virus Panel (GenMark)	Multiplex PCR with DNA hybridization and electrochemical detection	Nasopharyngeal swab	6 h	Adenovirus B/E Adenovirus C hMPV Influenza A H1 Influenza A H3 Influenza A H1N1 (2009) Influenza B Parainfluenza virus 1 Parainfluenza virus 2 Parainfluenza virus 3 RSV A RSV B Rhinovirus
Gastrointestinal (GI) Panels				
FilmArray GI Panel (BioFire)	Onboard nucleic acid extraction followed by RT-PCR and microarray detection	Stool in Carey Blair Transport media	1 h	Adenovirus F 40/41 Astrovirus Norovirus GI/GII Rotavirus A Sapovirus (I, II, IV, and V) *Campylobacter* spp. *Clostridium difficile* *Plesiomonas shigelloides* *Salmonella* *Yersinia enterocolitica* *Vibrio* spp. *E. coli* O157 Enteroaggregative *E. coli* Enteropathogenic *E. coli* Enterotoxigenic *E. coli lt/st* Shiga-like toxin–producing *E. coli stx1/stx2* Shigella/enteroinvasive *E. coli* *Cryptosporidium* *Cyclospora cayetanensis* *Entamoeba histolytica* *Giardia lamblia*
Nanosphere		Stool	2 h	Norovirus Rotavirus *Campylobacter* spp. *Salmonella* spp. Shiga toxin 1 Shiga toxin 2 *Shigella* spp. *Vibrio* group *Yersinia enterocolitica*

Continued

TABLE 253.4 Comparison of the Highly Multiplexed Assays for the Detection of Respiratory Viruses—cont'd

Test	Method	Specimen	Time to Result	Targets
xTAG Gastrointestinal Pathogen Panel		Stool	5 h	Adenovirus 40/41 Norovirus GI/GII Rotavirus A *Campylobacter* *C. difficile* *Escherichia coli* O157 Enterotoxigenic *E. coli* LT/ST *Salmonella* *Shigella* *Vibrio cholera* *Cryptosporidium* *Entamoeba histolytica* *Giardia*
Meningitis Panels				
FilmArray Meningitis/Encephalitis Panel (BioFire)	Onboard nucleic acid extraction followed by RT-PCR and microarray detection	CSF	1 h	CMV Enterovirus HSV-1 HSV-2 Human herpesvirus 6 Human parechovirus VZV *Escherichia coli K1* *Haemophilus influenzae* *Listeria monocytogenes* *Neisseria meningitidis* *Streptococcus agalactiae* *Streptococcus pneumoniae* *Cryptococcus neoformans/gattii*

CMV, Cytomegalovirus; *CSF,* cerebrospinal fluid; *hMPV,* human metapneumovirus; *HSV,* herpes simplex virus; *RSV,* respiratory syncytial virus; *RT-PCR,* reverse transcriptase polymerase chain reaction; *VZV,* varicella-zoster virus.

TABLE 253.5 US Food and Drug Administration–Approved Quantitative Molecular Assays

Target	Specimen	Linear Range	Method	Test Name	Manufacturer
HBV	Plasma, serum	$10–10^9$ IU/mL	Real-time PCR	Abbott Real-time HBV	Abbott Molecular, Inc., Des Plaines, IL
	Plasma, serum	$20–1.7 \times 10^8$ IU/mL	Real-time PCR	COBAS AmpliPrep/COBAS TaqMan HBV Test v2.0	Roche Molecular Diagnostics Pleasanton, CA
HCV	Plasma, serum	$12–1.0 \times 10^8$ IU/mL	Real-time RT-PCR	Abbott real-time HCV	Abbott Molecular, Inc., Des Plaines, IL
	Serum	$615–7.7 \times 10^6$ IU/mL	bDNA	VERSANT HCV RNA 3.0 Assay	Siemens Healthcare Diagnostics, Deerfield, IL
	Plasma, serum	$15–1.0 \times 10^8$ IU/mL	Real-time RT-PCR	COBAS AmpliPrep/ COBAS TaqMan HCV Test v2.0	Roche Molecular Diagnostics Pleasanton, CA
HIV	Plasma	$40–1.0 \times 10^7$ cp/mL	Real-time RT-PCR	Abbott Real-time HIV-1	Abbott Molecular, Inc., Des Plaines, Ill
	Plasma	$176–3.47 \times 10^6$ cp/mL	NASBA	NucliSens HIV-1 QT	bioMerieux, Inc., Durham, NC
	Plasma	$20–1.0 \times 10^7$ cp/mL	Real-time RT-PCR	COBAS AmpliPrep/ COBAS TaqMan HIV-1 Test v2.0	Roche Molecular Diagnostics, Pleasanton, CA
	Plasma	$75–5.0 \times 10^5$ cp/mL	bDNA	VERSANT HIV-1 RNA 3.0 Assay	Siemens Healthcare Diagnostics, Deerfield, IL
CMV	Plasma	$137–9.1 \times 10^7$ IU/mL	Real-time PCR	COBAS AmpliPrep/ COBAS TaqMan CMV Test	Roche Molecular Diagnostics, Pleasanton, CA
	Plasma	$119–7.9 \times 10^7$ IU/mL	Real-time PCR	*artus* CMV RGQ MDx Kit	Qiagen, Inc., Gaithersburg, MD

CMV, Cytomegalovirus; *HBV,* hepatitis B virus; *HCV,* hepatitis C virus; *HIV,* human immunodeficiency virus; *PCR,* polymerase chain reaction; *RT-PCR,* reverse-transcriptase polymerase chain reaction.

qNAAT assays for the management of HIV were the first to be used routinely for the early detection of infection, resolution of indeterminate Western blot results, evaluation of suspected prenatal and intrapartum infection, and monitoring of the viral load for prognosis and evaluation of therapeutic efficacy. The goal of antiretroviral therapy is a reduction of HIV-1 RNA below the limits of detection of the more sensitive assays (<20 to 75 cp/mL).[27,70,76] Detection and quantitation of serum HBV DNA can assist in diagnosis of early acute infection, distinguish active from inactive infection, and monitor response to antiviral therapy. In early acute infection in which HBsAg is not detectable or yields equivocal results, detection of HBV DNA may be used to make the diagnosis. Viral load can predict the course of chronic HBV infection as well. Viral loads are high in chronic active, replicative infection and are low or undetectable in chronic inactive infection. The aim of antiviral therapy is long-term suppression of viral replication; increasing HBV DNA levels may signal emergence of drug-resistant strains.[30,75] Detection and quantitation of HCV RNA is useful for establishing the diagnosis of acute hepatitis before seroconversion, for detection of chronic HCV in seronegative patients, for resolution of indeterminate serologic results, and to monitor patients for disease progression and response to therapy.[3,7,11,38] qNAATs are essential for management of chronic HCV. Viral load and genotype determine the likelihood of sustained viral response (SVR) and potential duration of treatment. Response to treatment is measured by achievement of SVR, defined as the absence of demonstrable viral replication 12 to 24 weeks after completion of a full course of treatment.

As is typical of other herpes group viruses, CMV possesses a high prevalence rate, establishes latency, and although usually asymptomatic in the normal host, causes disease in immunologically compromised hosts. Transplant recipients, patients with HIV or acquired immunodeficiency syndrome (AIDS), patients with cancer, and newborns are usually at highest risk for severe disease. Optimal patient management relies on laboratory testing. Quantitative assays are useful for early detection of CMV infection, differentiating latent infection from active disease, predicting disease progression, and monitoring response to antiviral therapy.[14,37,72,77] In general, higher viral loads correlate with risk for disease development, and lower levels are associated with asymptomatic infection. Recommendations for serial monitoring using qNAATs have been published.[14,37,72] Generally, threefold to fivefold changes in viral load may represent a biologically significant change in viral replication. Viral load thresholds that can guide therapeutic decisions in patient management across transplant groups are not yet well established because of variability in qNAAT assay design among laboratories and previous lack of a reference standard. The availability of FDA-approved assays calibrated against the World Health Organization (WHO) international standard should clarify interpretation of results and aid in the establishment of significant viral load thresholds within different immunosuppressed populations.[14,72]

FDA-approved qNAAT assays do not exist for Epstein-Barr virus (EBV), BK virus (BKV), and adenoviruses; however, quantitation of these viruses is routinely performed.[27] As mentioned earlier, laboratory-developed tests vary in assay design and thus yield results that cannot be compared across laboratories. No standardized threshold values have been determined for the purpose of clinical management. Differences include specimen type (whole blood, plasma, peripheral blood mononuclear cells [PBMCs]) and volume, nucleic acid extraction method, PCR primers and probes, amplification chemistry, calibrators used to create standard curves, and result reporting (copies or IU per milliliter, copies per PCR, and copies per DNA concentration).

Conventional diagnostic methods generally are not useful in the evaluation of EBV-related disorders in immunosuppressed patients. Culture is not practical or useful, and serology is difficult to interpret in the setting of immunosuppression. PCR offers the possibility of rapid detection of EBV in a variety of clinical specimens and allows a semiquantitative or quantitative estimate of viral load. PCR has been used for establishing the diagnosis of AIDS-related central nervous system lymphoma, EBV-related lymphoproliferative disorders, and other EBV-associated diseases (e.g., infectious mononucleosis, fatal infectious mononucleosis, chronic active EBV infection, and EBV-associated hemophagocytic syndromes) in which increased DNA concentrations are associated with more severe clinical categories.[34,53] PCR is particularly useful for the early identification and diagnosis of lymphoproliferative disorders (e.g., posttransplantation lymphoproliferative disorder [PTLD]) in pediatric patients after they have undergone liver transplantation, for monitoring EBV levels so that immunosuppression can be adjusted, and as a prognostic marker.[28,53] Viral load measurement of EBV is routinely used to diagnose or predict impending PTLD. High levels are nearly always associated with PTLD, and increasing DNAemia predicts impending PTLD before appearance of signs and symptoms. Standardization of blood compartment used and calibration of qNAAT assays to the WHO EBV standard should clarify significant quantitative thresholds for the management of PTLD.[34,69] Primary infection with BKV typically occurs in childhood and usually results in chronic, asymptomatic infection in immunocompetent individuals. Whereas clinical disease is rare in immunocompetent adults, BKV infections are a significant cause of morbidity and mortality in immunosuppressed patients, particularly in renal transplant recipients and those with hematologic malignancies. Disease manifestations in renal transplants include BKV nephropathy (BKVN), which may result in renal dysfunction and graft loss. Asymptomatic hematuria, hemorrhagic cystitis, and renal impairment may occur in bone marrow transplant recipients and patients with hematologic malignancy. BKVN affects 1% to 10% of renal transplant recipients with frequencies of graft loss between 10% and 80% within 5 years. BKV quantitative PCR can facilitate early diagnosis of BKVN, guide management of immunosuppressive therapy, and monitor response to intervention. Prospective studies have shown that high-level BKV viruria (1–3 months after transplantation) precedes sustained viremia (1–12 weeks before polyomavirus-associated nephropathy [PVAN]), which in turn precedes allograft dysfunction. Reduction of immunosuppression or treatment with cidofovir when the viral load reaches a specific level has been associated with improved clinical outcomes. BKV quantitative cutoffs that indicated the need for renal biopsy were DNA loads greater than 10^7 copies/mL in urine or plasma loads greater than 10^4 that persist for longer than 3 weeks.[58,66]

Human adenoviruses are associated with a variety of diseases affecting all organ systems. Most disease in immunocompetent individuals is self-limited; however, severe or fatal disseminated disease may occur in bone marrow, stem cell, or solid organ transplant recipients. Treatment includes administration of cidofovir and reduction of immunosuppression. Viral load testing is increasingly being used to predict disease dissemination (>10^4 copies/mL) and monitor antiviral therapy, although viral load thresholds are still to be determined.[21]

SUMMARY

Methods for the laboratory diagnosis of viral infections, including culture, SVA, antigen detection, and molecular diagnostic methods, have been reviewed. The use of these tests in some combination is most practical because a single test may not yield a diagnosis. For many viruses, culture has been the gold standard or reference method for evaluation of the new, rapid tests. However, culture is neither 100% sensitive nor always diagnostic of symptomatic infection. With the newer methods, particularly molecular diagnostic methods, the gold standard is changing, and evaluation of new techniques must be compared against a spectrum of laboratory and clinical data. Standards for performance and guidelines for the use and interpretation of molecular techniques are becoming available. Quantitative (vs. qualitative) viral results may be useful for interpreting tests, particularly with regard to viruses causing latent infection or for monitoring therapy or disease progression. Finally, interpretation of any result requires integration of the clinical history, laboratory data, treatment records, and observation of trends over time.

NEW REFERENCES SINCE THE SEVENTH EDITION

3. Belousova V, Abd-Rabou AA, Mousa SA. Recent advances and future directions in the management of hepatitis C infections. *Pharmacol Ther.* 2015;145:92-102.
4. Binnicker MJ, Espy MJ, Irish CL, et al. Direct detection of influenza A and B Viruses in less than 20 minutes using a commercially available rapid PCR assay. *J Clin Microbiol.* 2015;53(7):2353-2354.
7. Caliendo AM, Valsamakis A, Zhou Y, et al. Multilaboratory comparison of hepatitis C virus viral load assays. *J Clin Microbiol.* 2006;44(5):1726-1732.
8. Chen JH, Lam HY, Yip CC, et al. Clinical evaluation of the new high-throughput Luminex NxTAG respiratory pathogen panel assay for multiplex respiratory pathogen detection. *J Clin Microbiol.* 2016;54(7):1820-1825.
9. Chen L, Tian Y, Chen S, et al. Performance of the Cobas® Influenza A/B assay for rapid PCR-based detection of influenza compared to Prodesse ProFlu+ and viral culture. *Eur J Microbiol Immunol (Bp).* 2015;5(4):236-245.
14. Dioverti MV, Razonable RR. Clinical utility of cytomegalovirus viral load in solid organ transplant recipients. *Curr Opin Infect Dis.* 2015;28(4):317-322.
16. Dunn J, Obuekwe J, Baun T, et al. Prompt detection of influenza A and B viruses using the BD Veritor System Flu A+B, Quidel® Sofia® Influenza A+B FIA, and Alere BinaxNOW® Influenza A&B compared to real-time reverse

transcription-polymerase chain reaction (RT-PCR). *Diagn Microbiol Infect Dis.* 2014;79(1):10-13.
26. Gu Z, Zhu H, Rodriguez A, et al. Comparative evaluation of broad-panel PCR assays for the detection of gastrointestinal pathogens in pediatric oncology patients. *J Mol Diagn.* 2015;17(6):715-721.
27. Gullett JC, Nolte FS. Quantitative nucleic acid amplification methods for viral infections. *Clin Chem.* 2015;61(1):72-78.
29. Hammitt LL, Kazungu S, Welch S, et al. Added value of an oropharyngeal swab in detection of viruses in children hospitalized with lower respiratory tract infection. *J Clin Microbiol.* 2011;49(6):2318-2320.
30. Han SH, Tran TT. Management of chronic hepatitis B: an overview of practice guidelines for primary care providers. *J Am Board Fam Med.* 2015;28(6):822-837.
32. Hazelton B, Gray T, Ho J, et al. Detection of influenza A and B with the Alere i Influenza A & B: a novel isothermal nucleic acid amplification assay. *Influenza Other Respir Viruses.* 2015;9(3):151-154.
34. Kanakry JA, Hegde AM, Durand CM, et al. The clinical significance of EBV DNA in the plasma and peripheral blood mononuclear cells of patients with or without EBV diseases. *Blood.* 2016;127(16):2007-2017.
36. Kim C, Ahmed JA, Eidex RB, et al. Comparison of nasopharyngeal and oropharyngeal swabs for the diagnosis of eight respiratory viruses by real-time reverse transcription-PCR assays. *PLoS ONE.* 2011;6(6):e21610.
37. Kotton CN, Kumar D, Caliendo AM, et al. Updated international consensus guidelines on the management of cytomegalovirus in solid-organ transplantation. *Transplantation.* 2013;96(4):333-360.
38. Kumar S, Jacobson I. Optimal management of the hepatitis C patient: review of the AASLD/IDSA guidelines. *Curr Hepatology Rep.* 2014;13:314-320.
40. Landry ML, Ferguson D. Comparison of Simplexa Flu A/B & RSV PCR with cytospin-immunofluorescence and laboratory-developed TaqMan PCR in predominantly adult hospitalized patients. *J Clin Microbiol.* 2014;52(8):3057-3059.
41. Leber AL, Everhart K, Balada-Llasat JM, et al. Multicenter evaluation of the BioFire FilmArray meningitis encephalitis panel for the detection of bacteria, viruses and yeast in cerebrospinal fluid specimens. *J Clin Microbiol.* 2016;54(9):2251-2261.
50. Nie S, Roth RB, Stiles J, et al. Evaluation of Alere i Influenza A&B for rapid detection of influenza viruses A and B. *J Clin Microbiol.* 2014;52(9):3339-3344.
53. Nowalk A, Green M. Epstein-Barr Virus. *Microbiol Spectr.* 2016;4(3).
57. Petterson J, York V, Ward P, et al. The value of a multiplexed gastrointestinal pathogen panel in 2 distinct patient populations. *Diagn Microbiol Infect Dis.* 2016;85(1):105-108.
58. Pham PT, Schaenman J, Pham PC. BK virus infection following kidney transplantation: an overview of risk factors, screening strategies, and therapeutic interventions. *Curr Opin Organ Transplant.* 2014;19(4):401-412.
60. Pierce VM, Hodinka RL. Comparison of the GenMark Diagnostics eSensor respiratory viral panel to real-time PCR for detection of respiratory viruses in children. *J Clin Microbiol.* 2012;50(11):3458-3465.
66. Sawinski D, Goral S. BK virus infection: an update on diagnosis and treatment. *Nephrol Dial Transplant.* 2015;30(2):209-217.
69. Semenova T, Lupo J, Alain S, et al. Multicenter evaluation of whole-blood Epstein-Barr viral load standardization using the WHO international standard. *J Clin Microbiol.* 2016;54(7):1746-1750.
70. Sollis KA, Smit PW, Fiscus S, et al. Systematic review of the performance of HIV viral load technologies on plasma samples. *PLoS ONE.* 2014;9(2):e85869.
72. Tan SK, Waggoner JJ, Pinsky BA. Cytomegalovirus load at treatment initiation is predictive of time to resolution of viremia and duration of therapy in hematopoietic cell transplant recipients. *J Clin Virol.* 2015;69:179-183.
73. Tang YW, Gonsalves S, Sun JY, et al. Clinical Evaluation of the Luminex NxTAG Respiratory Pathogen Panel. *J Clin Microbiol.* 2016;54(7):1912-1914.
74. Tate JE, Mijatovic-Rustempasic S, Tam KI, et al. Comparison of 2 assays for diagnosing rotavirus and evaluating vaccine effectiveness in children with gastroenteritis. *Emerg Infect Dis.* 2013;19(8):1245-1252.
75. Terrault NA, Bzowej NH, Chang KM, et al. AASLD guidelines for treatment of chronic hepatitis B. *Hepatology.* 2016;63(1):261-283.
76. US Department of Health and Human Services, Office of AIDS Research Advisory Council. Guidelines for the use of antiretroviral agents in HIV-1 infected adults and adolescents. 2016; http://aidsinfo.nih.gov/contentfiles/adultandadolescentGL.pdf.
77. Vora SB, Englund JA. Cytomegalovirus in immunocompromised children. *Curr Opin Infect Dis.* 2015;28(4):323-329.

The full reference list for this chapter is available at ExpertConsult.com.

254 Parasitic Laboratory Diagnosis

David A. Bruckner • Robyn Shimizu-Cohen

Parasitic infections usually are associated with tropical areas; however, many infections (*Dientamoeba fragilis, Entamoeba histolytica, Enterobius vermicularis, Giardia duodenalis,* and *Toxoplasma gondii*) have worldwide distribution. With the ability of travelers to move freely throughout the world, clinical laboratories must be able to recommend specimen collection and detection and identification methods for all types of parasitic infections. It is helpful if the physician informs the laboratory of the parasitic infection that is suspected or the travel history of the patient because some organisms are detected more easily using specific methods (e.g., *Giardia* and *Cryptosporidium*—direct fluorescent antibody [DFA], enzyme immunoassay [EIA], or lateral flow assay [LFA] techniques) or alternative methods (e.g., microfilaria—Nuclepore filtration or Knott concentration procedure). The methods used, as with the rest of microbiology, are undergoing significant change, with a number of US Food and Drug Administration (FDA)- approved very sensitive nucleic acid amplification tests that can be used to detect a limited number of parasitic infections.[6,7,12] These methods are slowly being adopted for use, so the older classical methods to detect infections still prevail.[3,5,10]

The life cycle of the parasite and the time of infection are important factors in determining the type of specimens to be collected and the techniques used to detect the infection (Table 254.1). Multiple specimens might have to be examined before the etiologic agent can be detected (e.g., colon aspirates or biopsy tissue for *E. histolytica,* blood for malaria or acute Chagas disease). Detection of antibodies to *Taenia solium, Strongyloides stercoralis, T. gondii, Trypanosoma cruzi,* and *E. histolytica* may be helpful in determining a diagnosis. All specimens must be considered infectious and must be handled with universal safety precautions using personal protective equipment (PPE).

The diagnosis of most parasitic infections is dependent on macroscopic or microscopic examination and antigen detection methods (DFA, EIA, LFA) of blood, feces, respiratory, tissue, and genitourinary specimens. Specimens must be collected using methods that allow for the preservation of parasites when they are transported to the laboratory. Most stool specimens are collected at home or in a physician's office that may be a considerable distance from the laboratory performing the stool examination. Trophozoites disintegrate rapidly and do not form cysts after passage; therefore stool specimens should be collected in containers from stool collection kits that have preservatives. The preservatives fix the specimens so that the trophozoites can be recognized easily on permanent stained slides and prevent the continued development of larvae and eggs. Exceptions to the use of preservatives involve new polymerase chain reaction (PCR) methods that use fresh stool or stool collected in Cary-Blair transport medium. In laboratories that have personnel with limited or no experience in detecting common or unusual parasitic infections, it is recommended that specimens be sent to referral laboratories with experienced personnel if there is reticence in performing routine examinations.

If questions of when and how to collect specimens to maximize the recovery of parasites occur, the specific laboratory to be used should be consulted about the collection methods of choice.

TABLE 254.1 Diagnostic Stages and Anatomic Sites of Parasites

	Blood	CNS	Eye	GI	GU	Li/Sp	Lung	Lymph Node	Muscle	Skin	Other
Protozoa											
Acanthamoeba spp.		t	**C/T**							C/T	
Babesia spp.	**RBC**										Serology
Balantidium coli				**C/T**							
Cryptosporidium spp.				**Oocyst**							
Cyclospora cayetanensis				**Oocyst**							
Cystoisospora belli				**Oocyst**							
Dientamoeba fragilis				**t**							
Entamoeba histolytica		t		**C/T**		t	t				Serology
Giardia duodenalis				**C/T**							
Leishmania donovani	A (**WBC**)					**A**					Serology
Leishmania spp.										**A**	Serology
Microsporidia			**S**	**S**	**S**		**S**	**S**	**S**		
Naegleria spp.		**t**								C/T	
Plasmodium spp.	**RBC**										Serology
Toxoplasma gondii	t (WBC)	C	C			C/T	C/T	C/T	C		Serology
Trichomonas vaginalis					t						
Trypanosoma cruzi	T (plasma)								**A**		Serology
Trypanosoma gambiense	**T (plasma)**	**T**									
Trypanosoma rhodesiense	**T (plasma)**	**T**									
Helminths											
Ancylostoma duodenale				**a/E**							
Ascaris lumbricoides				**a/E**			L				
Brugia malayi	**MF**							a			
Clonorchis sinensis				**E**		a					
Diphyllobothrium latum				**a/E**							
Dipylidium caninum				**a/E**							
Echinococcus spp.		L				L	L				Serology
Enterobius vermicularis				**a/E**							
Fasciola hepatica				**E**		a					
Fasciolopsis buski				**a/E**							
Heterophyes spp.				**a/E**							
Hymenolepis spp.				**a/E**							
Loa loa	**MF**		MF								
Metagonimus spp.				**a/E**							
Necator americanus				**a/E**							
Onchocerca volvulus			MF							**a/MF**	
Opisthorchis spp.				**E**		a					
Paragonimus spp.				E			**a/E**				
Schistosoma spp.	a			**E**	**E**						Serology
Strongyloides stercoralis				**a/L**							Serology
Taenia spp.		L	L	**a/E**						L	
Trichinella spiralis				a/L					**a/L**		Serology
Trichuris trichiura				**a/E**							
Wuchereria bancrofti	**MF**							a			

Bold type indicates parasites most frequently detected at that source.
a, Adult; *A*, amastigote; *CNS*, central nervous system; *C*, cyst; *E*, eggs; *GI*, gastrointestinal tract; *GU*, genitourinary tract; *L*, larvae; *Li/Sp*, liver/spleen; *MF*, microfilaria; *RBC*, red blood cell; *S*, spores; *t*, trophozoite; *T*, trypomastigote; *WBC*, white blood cell.

STOOL SPECIMENS FOR DETECTION OF INTESTINAL PARASITES

Liquid or semisolid fresh stool specimens should be examined within 30 to 60 minutes, respectively, from the time of collection for protozoan trophozoites. Because most clinical laboratories cannot perform the examination in this time frame, stool specimens should be placed in preservative immediately after passage (Table 254.2). Most stool collection kits contain a combination of vials such as sodium acetate–acetic acid–formalin (SAF) and polyvinyl alcohol (PVA); however, one-vial kits are becoming the system of choice. Mercury-, PVA-, and formalin-free preservatives are commonly available. Specimens should be collected before radiologic examination with barium is performed, which may prevent the detection of intestinal parasites for up to 10 days after administration. Other substances or medications that also can interfere with the detection of intestinal parasites for a prolonged period of time include antibiotics (aminoglycosides, metronidazole, and tetracycline), antimalarial agents, bismuth, mineral oil, and nonabsorbent antidiarrheal agents. The specimen should be collected in a clean, wide-mouthed container and must not be contaminated with toilet water or urine. When collected, the specimen should be immediately transferred to a container with preservative. After being mixed with the preservative,

TABLE 254.2 Common Intestinal Tract Specimen Preservatives[a]

Stool Preservative	Concentrate	Permanent Stain	Immunoassay	Advantages	Disadvantages
Formalin	Yes	No	Yes	Easy to prepare and has a long shelf life; preserves helminth eggs and larvae and protozoan cysts well; can be used with modified acid-fast and trichome stains; can be used with most immunoassays	Does not preserve trophozoite morphology adequately; not suitable for permanent stains; specimen does not adhere to slide
MIF	Yes	No	No	Has a long shelf life; fixes and stains parasite forms simultaneously	Two solutions must be mixed immediately before use; trophozoite morphology is poorly preserved; not suitable for modified acid-fast or trichrome stains; iodine interferes with immunoassays
PVA	Yes	Yes	No	Excellent preservation of trophozoite morphology; suitable for PCR assays	Contains Hg, making disposal quite costly; morphology of larvae and eggs makes identification difficult; unsuitable for modified stains; PVA interferes with immunoassays
PVA, modified	Yes	Yes	No	Does not contain mercury; disposal is less expensive	Copper or zinc (substitute for mercury) does not preserve trophozoite and cyst morphology as well as mercury, making identification difficult; PVA interferes with immunoassays
SAF	Yes	Yes	Yes	Does not contain mercury; disposal is less expensive; has a long shelf life; permanent stain of choice is iron hematoxylin; preserves helminth eggs and larvae and protozoan cysts well; can be used with most immunoassays and special stains	Must use albumin-coated slides for permanent stains; contains formalin
Schaudinn	No	Yes	No	Excellent preservation of trophozoite morphology	Contains Hg, making disposal quite costly; not recommended for concentrates and has poor adhesive properties for liquid and mucoid specimens
Schaudinn, modified	Yes	Yes	Yes	Does not contain Hg, PVA, or formalin	Uses Zn as substitute for Hg May need to coat slide with albumin for better specimen adhesion.
Universal fixative (Total-Fix)	Yes	Yes	Yes	No formalin, Hg or PVA	

[a]Consult product inserts to determine whether specimens in these preservatives can be used with special stains, immunoassays, or molecular testing.
MIF, Merthiolate-iodine-formalin; *PCR,* polymerase chain reaction; *PVA,* polyvinyl alcohol; *SAF,* sodium acetate–acetic acid–formalin.

the specimen can be stored at room temperature until it is transported to the laboratory.

FDA-approved nucleic acid–based PCR testing is used to detect a limited number of intestinal protozoan infections and may include bacterial and viral causes of diarrhea in the same test. Specimens used in these assays are either fresh stool, stool placed in Cary-Blair transport medium, or preservative-fixed stool. Tests are of moderate complexity, and results are available in 1 to 5 hours. These tests are first-generation qualitative tests with a result of presence or absence of parasites. Multiplex assays may be less sensitive than single-plex assays. Quantitative assays may eventually prove to be useful to follow therapy, but these have not been applied to routine patient care in parasitology.[2,4]

Physicians should recommend that three specimens are collected on alternate days within 10 days to rule out most intestinal infections. The probability of detecting stool parasites with a single stool specimen is as low as 50%. Multiple specimens collected from the same patient on the same day should not be accepted. Many intestinal protozoa, such as *Giardia,* have a cyclical population cycle, and the concentration of trophozoites and cysts in the stool can vary considerably from day to day. Whether more than one specimen is necessary for PCR testing has not been evaluated.

OTHER SPECIMENS FOR DETECTION OF INTESTINAL PARASITES

Sigmoidoscopy samples may be submitted for the detection of *E. histolytica.* No fewer than six (mucosal) specimens should be submitted to the laboratory. Aspirates or scrapings can be collected and sent to the laboratory for direct wet mount observations, immunoassay, or PCR (not commercially available). Preservatives such as Schaudinn fluid or PVA can be used to fix the samples to microscopic slides. Biopsy specimens should be submitted to the pathology laboratory for histologic preparation.

Duodenal aspirates and biopsy specimens can be collected for the detection of *Cryptosporidium, Giardia,* and *Strongyloides.* Collection techniques similar to those mentioned for the detection of *E. histolytica* can be used. In addition, duodenal contents may be sampled using the Entero-Test. The nylon string can be sent directly to the laboratory for processing and microscopic examination for parasitic organisms.

Strongyloides larvae might be detected in respiratory or other tissue and fluid specimens during autoinfection or hyperinfection cycles. Serologic testing can be used to detect *Strongyloides* infections with low worm burdens.

E. vermicularis infections are detected best using the cellulose tape method. Specimens should be collected in the early morning before bathing or having a bowel movement. The adhesive side of the cellulose tape is pressed against the anal folds; and after completion of sampling, the tape is placed with the adhesive side down onto a microscope slide. *Enterobius* eggs and adults may be trapped on the tape (commercial collection kits are available). Multiple specimens (four to six) may be collected on consecutive days to rule out the presence of infection. Eggs from infections with *Taenia* adult worms also may be detected using this method.

STOOL PROCESSING AND EXAMINATION FOR PARASITES

Stool specimens can be examined by light microscopically as wet mounts, concentrates, and stained slides; by DFA, EIA, LFA, and immunoblot for specific antigens; and by nucleic acid methods. Most of these techniques detect only a limited number of pathogenic parasites. To detect the majority of the stool pathogens, all specimens should be examined by microscopy using a concentration technique and a permanently stained slide (Fig. 254.1).

If fresh, unpreserved specimens are received, a direct wet mount should be performed for the detection of motile protozoan trophozoites and protozoan cysts. Helminth eggs and larvae also may be seen. If necessary, a few drops of saline may be used to emulsify the stool, and a drop is placed on a microscopic slide and covered with a 22 × 22 mm coverslip. The wet mount should be examined using ×100 and ×400 magnifications. A drop of iodine solution may be added to highlight parasite internal structures; however, parasite motility will be lost. A concentrate and a permanent stained slide also should be prepared from this fresh specimen.

Common concentration techniques include the flotation method using zinc sulfate ($ZnSO_4$) and formalin-ethylacetate sedimentation method. Specimens fixed in formalin, merthiolate-iodine-formalin (MIF), PVA, SAF, or Schaudinn can be used. The flotation method gives a cleaner preparation to observe cysts and eggs, but the high specific gravity of $ZnSO_4$ tends to distort cysts and eggs, rendering identification difficult. Heavier eggs (e.g., *Ascaris* or operculated eggs) will not float and will be found in the sediment; therefore one should examine the surface film and sediment for a complete examination. The sedimentation method is used most widely in laboratories. Parasites and fecal debris are pelleted to the bottom of the tube by centrifugation. After the supernatant is discarded, the sediment is examined for parasites at ×100 and ×400 magnifications.

Permanent stained slides should be prepared on every stool specimen that is examined for ova and parasites. The stained slide is used primarily to detect and identify protozoa, trophozoites, and cysts. Gomori trichrome (Wheatley modification) and iron hematoxylin stains frequently are used in laboratories. Both stains have advantages and disadvantages that should be weighed, as should the expertise of laboratory personnel, before selecting the stain of choice for the laboratory.

Certain parasites are not detected easily by wet mount or routine permanent stained slides stained with Gomori trichrome (Wheatley modification) and iron hematoxylin. They include *Cryptosporidium* spp., *Cyclospora cayetanensis, Cystoisospora belli,* and microsporidia. The oocysts of *Cryptosporidium, Cyclospora,* and *Cystoisospora* can be detected by the modified acid-fast stain; however, some oocysts are refractory to stain. Similarly, the spores of microsporidia can be stained with a variety of stains, but not all spores stain evenly with the same stain.

Cultures of fresh stool or contents of the large intestine have been used to detect *E. histolytica;* however, this methodology is not practical for most clinical laboratories.

EIA, LFA, and immunoblot kits are commercially available for the detection of *E. histolytica/Entamoeba dispar* group, *G. duodenalis,* and *Cryptosporidium* spp. For the *E. histolytica/E. dispar* group, only fresh or frozen stool can be used in the assay. Formalin interferes with reagents to detect *E. histolytica* and cannot be used. EIA kits are available that will discriminate between these organisms using fresh or frozen stool. EIA kits for the detection of *Giardia* and *Cryptosporidium* can be used with fresh, frozen, or formalin-fixed stool. DFA tests have been developed to detect *Giardia* and *Cryptosporidium.* Depending on the manufacturer, either fresh or formalin-fixed specimens can be used.

PCR analysis also has been used to detect *E. histolytica, G. duodenalis, Cryptosporidium* spp., and *C. cayetanensis,* along with bacterial and viral pathogens. Specimens include fresh stool, stool placed in Cary-Blair transport medium, or preservative-fixed stool. Results can be available in 1 to 5 hours, depending on the manufacturer. These tests are expensive, but having a same-day result and increased patient satisfaction may outweigh the expense. If one PCR stool test can detect the same parasites

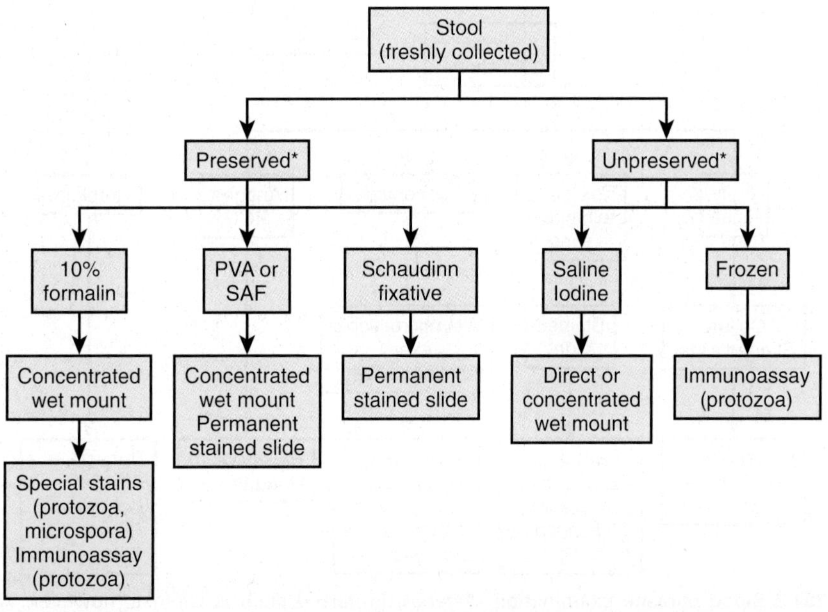

FIG. 254.1 Parasite stool examination. *Asterisk,* Worms (cestodes, nematodes, trematodes)—fix in 70% ethanol. *PVA,* Polyvinyl alcohol; *SAF,* sodium acetate–acetic acid–formalin.

that may require three stool specimens using routine methods, the cost will be nearly equivalent.

DFA, EIA, LFA, and immunoblot kits are readily available. DFA, EIA, LFA, and immunoblot kits have excellent sensitivity and specificity compared with microscopy. The disadvantage of using DFA, EIA, LFA, or immunoblot kits is that they detect only one or two pathogens at one time, so other pathogens might be missed. Additional parasite examinations would have to be performed to detect other parasitic pathogens.

Detection of *S. stercoralis* is enhanced by culturing a small amount of fresh stool on an agar plate and looking for larval tracks across the plate, as evidenced by lines of bacterial growth. Other methods include the Baermann concentrate, Harada-Mori, or Petri dish filter paper slant. It is possible that hookworm eggs could hatch, and the larvae would have to be differentiated from *Strongyloides* larvae.

BLOOD PARASITES

Although most laboratories will see blood parasites only during proficiency testing (Fig. 254.2), *Babesia* spp., *Leishmania donovani*, microfilaria, *Plasmodium* spp., and *Trypanosoma* spp. may be found.[8] Depending on the parasite and infectious numbers, they may also be seen in cerebrospinal fluid, macrophages, plasma, tissue, or red blood cells. Maintaining proficiency to correctly identify *Plasmodium* to species or to recognize the amastigote stages of *Leishmania* is difficult for many laboratorians because these infections are seen so infrequently in the United States. Physicians should inform laboratory personnel about specific diagnoses or infections they are considering and the travel and medication history of the patient. If the patient took partial prophylaxis for malaria, a longer time should be spent examining the blood film owing to low parasitemia. Similarly, differences in periodicity of microfilaria in the blood exist, and the timing of collection of specimens becomes more important. Alternative concentration techniques not normally used in most laboratories, such as Nuclepore filtration or the Knott concentration procedure, can be used to detect microfilaria in low numbers. Without the knowledge of what infection the physician may be considering, these concentration procedures are not routinely performed on blood or other specimens, and the diagnosis of infections could be delayed or missed. Requests for the diagnosis of malaria must be considered to be STAT requests owing to the morbidity and mortality mostly associated with *Plasmodium falciparum* infections.

Although some parasites (trypanosomes and microfilaria) can be detected by their motility in whole blood, identification is dependent on morphology as seen with a permanent stain. The blood film stain of choice is Giemsa, although Wright stain can also be used, or Delafield hematoxylin stain can be used for the microfilarial sheath. Because Giemsa stains may not differentiate the microfilaria nuclei adequately, Delafield hematoxylin stain may be necessary to speciate the microfilaria.

Blood films can be prepared in clinics or at the bedside (finger or earlobe sticks); however, the recommendation is that blood be collected in ethylenediaminetetraacetic acid (EDTA, lavender-topped tube) so that multiple slides (thick and thin blood films) can be prepared in the laboratory and antigen detection methods can be used. EDTA-collected blood provides the best overall morphology of parasites, and the tubes should be filled to the proper level to reduce distortion of the blood cells and organisms by the anticoagulant. Heparin tubes (green-topped tubes) also can be used; however, these blood-filled tubes cannot be used for PCR testing. The blood should be examined for parasites within 4 to 6 hours of being collected.

Blood should be drawn immediately when parasitemia is suspected. For malaria, blood should be drawn every 6 to 8 hours for 36 hours to rule out infection. Pediatric patients may have blood samples drawn at 10-hour intervals. One set of negative blood films does not rule out the presence of malaria. When the parasitemia level is low, procedures other than thick films, such as antigen detection, serology, or PCR analysis, may be the more sensitive method to detect *Babesia*, Chagas disease, malaria, or microfilaria. Serology has not been shown to be an effective method to detect active infections of African trypanosomiasis in nonendemic areas.

Blood Processing and Examination for Parasites

If the physician does not indicate the specific blood parasite suspected, fresh blood should be used as a wet mount to look for the presence of microfilaria or trypanosomes by their characteristic shape and motility. If these parasites are detected, a permanent stained slide will have to be performed to identify the organisms to species. When thick and thin blood films are examined for the presence of parasites, no fewer than 300 microscopic oil fields (×1000) should be examined before finalizing a result for the presence of *Babesia* or malaria. One may use lower magnification when looking for the presence of trypanosomes (×400) or microfilaria (×100), but the entire film should be observed before finalizing a result. Thin films are used for the detection of blood parasites, for enumeration of infected cells, and also to determine the species of parasite. When the films are air dried, the film can be fixed with 100% methanol and stained with Giemsa stain or Wright stain without the methanol

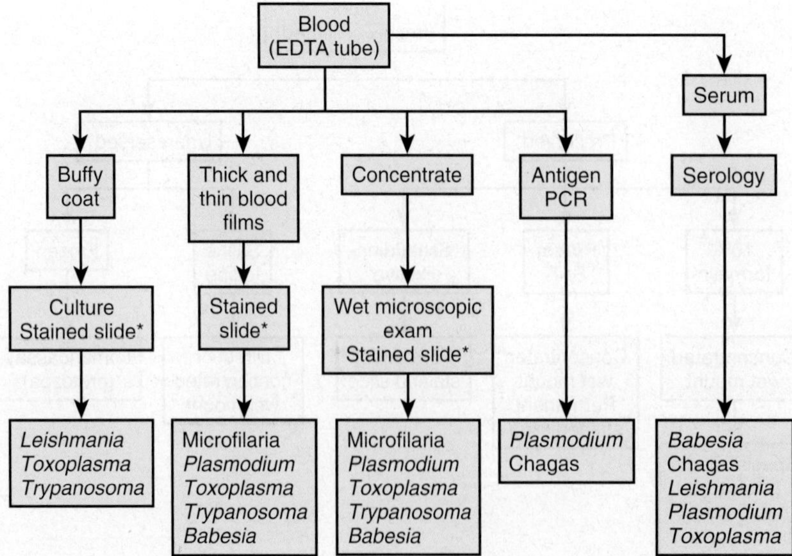

FIG. 254.2 Blood parasite examination. *Asterisk,* Preferred stain is Giemsa; however, Wright stain is also acceptable. *EDTA,* Ethylenediamine tetraacetic acid; *PCR,* polymerase chain reaction.

fixation process. If *Babesia* or malarial parasites (*P. falciparum, Plasmodium knowlesi,* and *Plasmodium vivax*) are present, one should quantitate the number of infected red blood cells. This quantification can be expressed as the number of infected cells per 100 red blood cells observed in the blood film. Serial specimens collected at various times during therapy can be used to monitor the success or failure of therapy. Continued presence of parasites in blood films without a marked decrease in parasitemia within the first 24 hours is an indication of therapeutic failure.

Thick films are prepared with one or two drops of blood that should be stirred in a small circle for 10 to 20 seconds at various intervals as it dries on the slide to prevent the blood from sloughing from the slide during the staining process. The thicker the film, the more likely the blood will slough. Detecting and identifying the presence of parasites on thick films is extremely difficult, particularly with inexperienced laboratory personnel. When the thick film has dried, the blood film is laked with water or buffer before staining if Wright stain is used, or the films can be placed directly into Giemsa stain without prior laking. Laking disrupts the red cell membrane, allowing the hemoglobin to be removed and leaving parasites, white blood cells, and platelets intact. The search for microfilaria can be performed at a lower magnification, whereas the search for *Babesia,* malaria, and trypanosomes must be done with oil magnification looking at 200 to 300 oil microscopic fields.

Concentration techniques also can be used to detect *Babesia, Leishmania,* malaria, microfilaria, and trypanosomes. Microhematocrit capillary tubes can be centrifuged, and the parasitized red blood cells and trypanosomes can be detected near the buffy coat interface. The tube can be scored and snapped, and the buffy coat can be used to prepare films. Alternatively, the tube can be observed under a microscope at the buffy coat interface for the presence of motile trypanosomes.

Microfilaria can be concentrated using the Knott procedure or Nuclepore membrane filtration technique. Normally, a 5-µm filter is used, but if *Mansonella perstans* microfilaria is suspected, a 3-µm filter is recommended. Most laboratories would not be familiar with or normally use concentration techniques unless specifically asked to do so.

Antigen tests for malaria have been developed and approved by the FDA for clinical use. These tests are extremely useful for laboratories that have limited expertise and exposure to specimens containing malaria or *Babesia.* It is difficult to differentiate malaria from babesiosis with infections when only very young trophozoites are microscopically observed. In this situation, the malarial antigen test can be very helpful. Antigens detected in these tests include histidine-rich protein-2, lactate dehydrogenase, and aldolase. False-negative antigen test results are known to occur owing to mutations of histidine-rich protein-2 in *P. falciparum* infection.[1] The sensitivity of the antigen tests to detect infections caused by *P. vivax, Plasmodium malariae,* or *Plasmodium ovale* is considerably reduced compared with *P. falciparum.*[9] The histidine-rich protein-2 remains in the blood for a considerable period of time after therapy, so it cannot be used to follow therapy. False-positive antigen test results are known to occur in patients with hepatitis, leishmaniasis, rheumatoid arthritis, and schistosomiasis.

PCR testing for malaria is available from most referral laboratories, but it should not be used as the first test for the detection and identification of malaria. Blood films and antigen detection tests should be the first tests ordered.

The Centers for Disease Control and Prevention (CDC) have an excellent website (www.cdc.gov/malaria) on the detection and treatment of malaria.

UROGENITAL SPECIMENS

Trichomonas vaginalis is the most common parasitic pathogen; however, schistosome eggs, microfilaria, and microsporidia also may be recovered from urogenital specimens. Many *T. vaginalis* infections are diagnosed on clinical signs and symptoms without a specimen being collected. The detection of *T. vaginalis* usually is based on direct observation in wet mounts prepared from vaginal and urethral discharges, prostatic secretions, and urine sediment. Urine specimens should be obtained from first-voided urine in the morning. Specimens collected for the detection of *T. vaginalis* should not be refrigerated because *T. vaginalis* is susceptible to cold temperatures. Specimens can be diluted with a drop of saline and observed under low power in reduced illumination for the presence of motile flagellates. Stained slides, such as Giemsa or Papanicolaou smears, also can be used, but the most infections with *T. vaginalis* are identified by the direct wet mount. This method is rapid and inexpensive; however, it lacks sensitivity, so there can be a significant number of false-negative specimens.

Culture (InPouch TV) can be used and is recommended by the CDC for patients suspected of harboring *T. vaginalis* infections when no organisms were detected by the direct wet mount method. Specimens can be collected with a brush, swab, or sponge. Specimens should be inoculated as soon as possible into the media. Cultures showing no organisms after incubation for 4 days can be reported as negative. When specimen transport is an issue, commercially available DFA, EIA, and nucleic acid detection kits are an excellent alternative. Nucleic acid amplification tests use the same transport as used for the detection of *Neisseria gonorrhoeae* and *Chlamydia trachomatis,* including ThinPrep and SurePath transport. Use of this transport for the patient allows for only one specimen to be collected. Some nucleic amplification tests have results available in approximately 1 hour, making them comparable to the direct wet mount but with greater sensitivity.[11] The alternative detection methods can be quite expensive.

The Knott concentration procedure and the Nuclepore membrane filtration technique have been used for the detection of microfilaria in the urine. Microfilaria most frequently detected using these methods are *Wuchereria bancrofti* and *Onchocerca volvulus* (after therapy).

Schistosoma haematobium eggs found in the urine can be concentrated by sedimentation, centrifugation, or the Nuclepore membrane filtration procedure. The preferred specimen is urine collected at midday, when the patient is most active and most likely to have eggs in the urine.

Serology

A serologic diagnosis may be required when the parasites reside in tissues or other body sites and it is difficult to acquire a diagnostic specimen (e.g., in a patient with chronic Chagas disease or neural cysticercosis). Serology testing may also be useful when parasites, eggs, or larvae are in very low numbers in specimens and are difficult to detect (e.g., in a patient with babesiosis, fascioliasis, malaria, paragonimiasis, or strongyloidiasis).

A positive serologic test in an individual who resides in an endemic area must be interpreted with caution because the result may reflect past exposure and be unrelated to current clinical condition. A positive test in an individual without any past exposure may indicate a recent infection; however, this result must be correlated with the patient's clinical picture.

The detection of immunoglobulin A (IgA), IgE, IgG, and IgM antibodies to specific parasite antigens may or may not be helpful in establishing a diagnosis. With the exception of serology tests for the diagnosis of toxoplasmosis and the screening of the blood supply for antibodies to *Trypanosoma cruzi,* most of the other parasitic serology tests have limited laboratory availability. Although some of the tests have been validated as laboratory developed tests (LDTs), except for *T. gondii* and *T. cruzi,* there are no established external proficiency testing programs such as those offered through the College of American Pathologists. Even though the test methodology may be the same between different laboratories, reagents used in the tests may not have been standardized if they do not use the same kit manufacturer. This can lead to variable results.

In the United States, most serologic tests for the diagnosis of a parasitic infection are limited to the most commonly acquired extraintestinal infections. These are available at a few referral laboratories, specialized testing centers, and the CDC. Information on availability of parasite serology tests can be acquired from referral laboratories or from the CDC (DPDX@CDC.gov or 404-718-4100). The CDC offers the most comprehensive services for tests available and will also provide some information on unusual serologic testing not available in the United States.

OTHER SPECIMENS

Other important pathogenic parasites, such as ocular infections with *Acanthamoeba* and *Toxoplasma gondii,* can be detected in other anatomic sites and are addressed in specific chapters.

NEW REFERENCES SINCE THE SEVENTH EDITION

1. Baker J, Gatton ML, Peters J, et al. Transcription and expression of *Plasmodium falciparum* histidine-rich proteins in different stages and strains: implications for rapid diagnostic tests. *PLoS ONE*. 2016;6:e22593.
2. Cimino RO, Jeun R, Juarez M, et al. Identification of human intestinal parasites affecting an asymptomatic peri-urban Argentinian population using multi-parallel quantitative real-time polymerase chain reaction. *Parasit Vectors*. 2015;8:380.
3. Garcia LS. *Diagnostic Medical Parasitology*. 6th ed. Washington D.C.: ASM Press; 2016.
4. Gotfred-Rasmussen H, Lund M, Enemark HL, et al. Comparison of sensitivity and specificity of 4 methods for detection of *Giardia duodenalis* in feces: Immunofluorescence & PCR are superior to microscopy of concentrated iodine-stained samples. *Diagn Microbiol Infect Dis*. 2016;84:187-190.
5. Jorgensen JH, Pfaller MA. ed-in-chief. *Manual of Clinical Microbiology*. 11th ed. Washington D.C.: ASM Press; 2015.
6. Khare R, Espy MJ, Cebelinski E, et al. Comparative evaluation of two commercial multiplex panels for detection of gastrointestinal pathogens by use of clinical stool specimens. *J Clin Microbiol*. 2016;52:3667-3673.
7. Molling P, Nilsson P, Ennefors T, et al. Evaluation of the BD Max Enteric Parasite panel for clinical diagnostics. *J Clin Microbiol*. 2016;54:443-444.
9. Nkrumah B, Acquah SE, Ibrahim L, et al. Comparative evaluation of two rapid field tests for malaria diagnosis: Partec rapid malaria test and Binax Now malaria rapid diagnostic test. *BMC Infect Dis*. 2011;11:143-150.
10. Procop GW, Koneman EW. *Koneman's Color Atlas and Textbook of Diagnostic Microbiology*. Philadelphia: Lippincott, Williams & Wilkins; 2016.
11. Van der Pol B. Clinical laboratory testing for *Trichomonas vaginalis* infection. *J Clin Microbiol*. 2016;54:7-12.
12. Verweij JJ, Stensvold CR. Molecular testing for clinical diagnosis and epidemiological investigations of intestinal parasitic infections. *Clin Microbiol Rev*. 2014;27:371-418.

The full reference list for this chapter is available at ExpertConsult.com.

Index

Page numbers followed by "*f*" indicate figures, "*t*" indicate tables, "*b*" indicate boxes, and "*e*" indicate online content.

A

B

G

H

J

K

L

M

N

P

Q

S

V

W